Applied Therapeutics

The Clinical Use of Drugs

TENTH EDITION

Edited By

Brian K. Alldredge, PharmD
Professor of Clinical Pharmacy and Associate Dean, Academic Affairs
Department of Clinical Pharmacy
School of Pharmacy
University of California, San Francisco
San Francisco, California

Robin L. Corelli, PharmD
Professor of Clinical Pharmacy
Department of Clinical Pharmacy
School of Pharmacy
University of California, San Francisco
San Francisco, California

Michael E. Ernst, PharmD, BCPS, FCCP
Professor (Clinical)
Department of Pharmacy Practice and Science
College of Pharmacy
Department of Family Medicine
Carver College of Medicine
The University of Iowa
Iowa City, Iowa

B. Joseph Guglielmo, PharmD
Professor and Chair
TA Oliver Chair in Clinical Pharmacy
Department of Clinical Pharmacy
School of Pharmacy
University of California, San Francisco
San Francisco, California

Pamala A. Jacobson, PharmD
Associate Professor
Department of Experimental and Clinical Pharmacology
College of Pharmacy
University of Minnesota
Minneapolis, Minnesota

Wayne A. Kradjan, PharmD, BCPS
Dean Emeritus and Professor Emeritus
College of Pharmacy
Oregon State University
Oregon Health & Science University
Corvallis, Oregon

Bradley R. Williams, PharmD, FASCP, CGP
Professor of Clinical Pharmacy and Clinical Gerontology
Titus Family Department of Clinical Pharmacy and Pharmaceutical Economics and Policy
Schools of Pharmacy and Gerontology
University of Southern California
Los Angeles, California

Wolters Kluwer Health | Lippincott Williams & Wilkins
Philadelphia • Baltimore • New York • London
Buenos Aires • Hong Kong • Sydney • Tokyo

Acquisitions Editor: David B. Troy
Project Manager: Meredith L. Brittain
Marketing Manager: Joy Fisher-Williams
Designer: Doug Smock
Compositor: Aptara, Inc.

Two Commerce Square
2001 Market Street
Philadelphia, PA 19103 USA
LWW.com

Tenth Edition

Printed in China

Library of Congress Cataloging-in-Publication Data

Koda-Kimble and Young's applied therapeutics : the clinical use of drugs.
– 10th ed. / edited by Brian K. Alldredge . . . [et al.].
p. ; cm.
Applied therapeutics
Rev. ed. of: Applied therapeutics : the clinical use of drugs / edited
by Mary Anne Koda-Kimble ... [et al.]. 9th ed. c2009.
Includes bibliographical references and index.
ISBN 978-1-60913-713-7
I. Koda-Kimble, Mary Anne. II. Alldredge, Brian K. III. Applied therapeutics.
IV. Title: Applied therapeutics.
[DNLM: 1. Drug Therapy–methods. WB 330]
615.5′8–dc23

2011047631

Care has been taken to confirm the accuracy of the information presented and to describe generally accepted practices. However, the authors, editors, and publisher are not responsible for errors or omissions or for any consequences from application of the information in this book and make no warranty, expressed or implied, with respect to the currency, completeness, or accuracy of the contents of the publication. Application of the information in a particular situation remains the professional responsibility of the practitioner.

The authors, editors, and publisher have exerted every effort to ensure that drug selection and dosage set forth in this text are in accordance with current recommendations and practice at the time of publication. However, in view of ongoing research, changes in government regulations, and the constant flow of information relating to drug therapy and drug reactions, the reader is urged to check the package insert for each drug for any change in indications and dosage and for added warnings and precautions. This is particularly important when the recommended agent is a new or infrequently employed drug.

Some drugs and medical devices presented in the publication have Food and Drug Administration (FDA) clearance for limited use in restricted research settings. It is the responsibility of the health care provider to ascertain the FDA status of each drug or device planned for use in their clinical practice.

9 8 7 6 5 4 3 2 1

CCS0112

Dedication

The Editors wish to express their sincere thanks and longstanding admiration to the creators of Applied Therapeutics, Drs. Mary Anne Koda-Kimble and Lloyd Young. They are truly educational visionaries whom we deeply respect as the innovators and pioneers in the teaching of patient-centered drug therapeutics. Their passion has touched the lives of countless health care professional students, clinicians, and patients throughout the world. As their colleagues and friends, we are forever indebted for their contributions and we consider it a privilege to carry forward their legacy—renamed as Koda-Kimble and Young's Applied Therapeutics*—into future editions.*

Preface

It has been nearly 40 years since the first edition of *Applied Therapeutics: The Clinical Use of Drugs* was published. The landscape of health care has evolved radically during this time, much of it spurred by remarkable advancements in drug discovery and clinical therapeutics. Despite these changes, the founding principle for this innovative text—a patient-centric, case-based approach to learning—remains integral to the current edition. Our authors present more than 860 patient cases that stimulate the reader to integrate and apply therapeutic principles in the context of specific clinical situations. Students and practitioners are provided with a glimpse into the minds of clinicians as they assess and solve therapeutic problems toward the development of their own critical-thinking and problem-solving skills. Every chapter in this edition has been revised and updated to reflect our ever-changing knowledge of drugs and the application of this knowledge to the individualized therapy of patients. Additionally, content within several sections has been extensively reorganized, with new chapters introduced to expand important topics. Among these are new chapters in the Arthritic Disorders, Women's Health, Neurologic Disorders, Neoplastic Disorders, and Pediatrics sections.

Readers familiar with past editions of the text will notice some welcome changes in the tenth edition. The overall design has been updated for visual appeal and to allow the reader to more quickly distinguish cases from surrounding text. In lieu of the traditional chapter outline, all chapters now contain a Core Principles section at the beginning, which provides the most important "take home" information from the chapter. Each Core Principle is mapped to specific cases within the chapter where the principle is discussed in detail. Key references and websites are listed at the end of each chapter, whereas the full reference lists for each chapter have been moved online.

A particularly significant change to the tenth edition is the incorporation of online multimedia content, much of it author-created, for many of the chapters. These include images, videos, narrated presentations, animations, and podcasts, which can be found on the textbook's website (see the "Additional Resources" section, which follows this preface, for more information). The incorporation of supplemental multimedia into the tenth edition marks a commitment on the part of the editorial team to ensure that *Koda-Kimble and Young's Applied Therapeutics* increases its role as a viable and dynamic resource that can appeal to multiple learning styles and future generations. We welcome your feedback as we undertake planning for the next edition.

The authors have drawn on information from the literature, current standards, and their own clinical experiences to share the process involved in making sound and thoughtful therapeutic decisions. *However, it remains the responsibility of every practitioner to evaluate the appropriateness of a particular opinion in the context of the actual clinical situation, bearing in mind any recent developments in the field. We strongly urge students and practitioners to consult several appropriate information sources when working with new and unfamiliar drugs.*

ACKNOWLEDGMENTS

We are deeply indebted to the many dedicated people who have given of themselves to complete the tenth edition of *Koda-Kimble and Young's Applied Therapeutics.* As always, we are most grateful to our contributing authors who have been attentive to meeting our stringent time deadlines and unique writing format. We especially thank those authors who graciously provided multimedia to accompany their chapter, and we gratefully recognize the additional time and effort this entailed. We hold their creativity in the highest regard. The exceptional work of our section editors, Judith Beizer, Marcia Buck, Shareen El-Ibiary, Marcus Ferrone, Patrick Finley, Timothy Ives, Mark Kirstein, Lisa Kroon, Kelly Lee, Myrna Munar, Jean Nappi, Tricia Russell, and Joseph Saseen, cannot be overstated. These content experts gave us critical feedback necessary in both the organizational structure of the textbook and in the individual editing of chapters; without their dedication and assistance, this edition would not be possible. We would also like to thank Facts and Comparisons for allowing us to use their data for the construction of some of our tables.

Two individuals from Lippincott Williams and Wilkins, Meredith Brittain and Loftin (Paul) Montgomery, Jr., deserve special recognition for their efforts. Their exceptional patience, attention to detail, and firm guidance helped us all stay on task. This edition would not have come to completion without their partnership. Mary Tod (copyediting), Ed Schultes, Jr. (multimedia production), and Jeri Litteral (typesetting) all played key roles in the production of the tenth edition, and we sincerely thank them for their assistance in completing this edition. Most importantly, we would be remiss not to acknowledge the love, understanding, and support of our spouses, children, and in some cases, grandchildren. They selflessly gave to us the many early mornings, late nights, and weekends we spent writing and editing.

As in past editions, we continue to dedicate our work to our students who inspire us and to the many patients we have been privileged to care for. Our patients have repeatedly taught us how critical it is to tailor our knowledge to their specific circumstances, to listen well, and to welcome them as true partners in their care.

Brian K. Alldredge
Robin L. Corelli
Michael E. Ernst
B. Joseph Guglielmo
Pamala A. Jacobson
Wayne A. Kradjan
Bradley R. Williams

Additional Resources

The Tenth Edition of *Koda-Kimble and Young's Applied Therapeutics: The Clinical Use of Drugs* includes additional resources for both instructors and students, available on the book's companion website at http://thepoint.lww.com/AT10e.

STUDENT RESOURCES

Students who have purchased *Koda-Kimble and Young's Applied Therapeutics: The Clinical Use of Drugs*, Tenth Edition have access to the following additional resources for each chapter:

- An audio recording of that chapter's core principles
- A full online reference list for that chapter

In addition, at least one of the following supplements each chapter to enhance the chapter content:

- Audio files (most recorded by author)
- PowerPoints (most created by author)
- PowerPoints with audio (most created/recorded by author)
- Animations
- Videos (some created by author)
- Additional content (created by author)
- Interactive versions of the algorithms found in the book
- Full-color images

INSTRUCTOR RESOURCES

Approved adopting instructors will be given access to the following additional resources:

- PowerPoint slides
- Image bank (includes all images and tables in the book)
- Pathophysiology image collection

In addition, purchasers of the text can access the searchable Full Text On-line by going to the *Koda-Kimble and Young's Applied Therapeutics: The Clinical Use of Drugs*, Tenth Edition website at http://thepoint.lww.com/AT10e. See the inside front cover for more details, including the passcode you will need to gain access to the website.

Section Editors

Judith L. Beizer, PharmD, CGP, FASCP
Clinical Professor
Department of Clinical Pharmacy Practice
College of Pharmacy & Allied Health Professions
St. John's University
Jamaica, New York

Marcia L. Buck, PharmD, FCCP, FPPAG
Associate Professor, Pediatrics
School of Medicine
Clinical Coordinator, Pediatrics
Department of Pharmacy
University of Virginia
Charlottesville, Virginia

Shareen Y. El-Ibiary, PharmD, BCPS
Associate Professor of Pharmacy Practice
Department of Pharmacy Practice
Midwestern University, College of Pharmacy—Glendale
Glendale, Arizona

Marcus Ferrone, PharmD, BCNSP
Associate Professor of Clinical Pharmacy
Director, Drug Products Services Laboratory
Department of Clinical Pharmacy
School of Pharmacy
University of California, San Francisco
San Francisco, California

Patrick R. Finley, PharmD, BCPP
Professor of Clinical Pharmacy
Department of Clinical Pharmacy
School of Pharmacy
University of California, San Francisco
San Francisco, California

Timothy J. Ives, PharmD, MPH, FCCP, BCPS
Professor
Eshelman School of Pharmacy
The University of North Carolina at Chapel Hill
Chapel Hill, North Carolina

Mark N. Kirstein, PharmD
Associate Professor
Department of Experimental and Clinical Pharmacology
College of Pharmacy
University of Minnesota
Minneapolis, Minnesota

Lisa A. Kroon, PharmD, CDE
Professor of Clinical Pharmacy
Department of Clinical Pharmacy
School of Pharmacy
University of California, San Francisco
Clinical Pharmacist, General Internal Medicine and Diabetes Clinics
University of California, San Francisco Medical Center
San Francisco, California

Kelly C. Lee, PharmD, BCPP
Assistant Professor of Clinical Pharmacy
Skaggs School of Pharmacy and Pharmaceutical Sciences
University of California, San Diego
La Jolla, California

Myrna Y. Munar, PharmD
Associate Professor
Department of Pharmacy Practice
College of Pharmacy
Oregon State University
Oregon Health and Science University
Portland, Oregon

Jean M. Nappi, PharmD, FCCP, BCPS
Professor
Clinical Pharmacy and Outcome Sciences
South Carolina College of Pharmacy
Clinical Pharmacy Specialist in Cardiology
Medical University of South Carolina
Charleston, South Carolina

Tricia M. Russell, PharmD, BCPS, CDE
Assistant Professor
Department of Pharmacy Practice
Wilkes University, Nesbitt College of Pharmacy & Nursing
Wilkes-Barre, Pennsylvania

Joseph J. Saseen, PharmD, FCCP, FASHP, BCPS
Professor
University of Colorado Anschutz Medical Campus
Schools of Pharmacy and Medicine
Director, PGY2 Ambulatory Care/Family Medicine Residency
Clinical Pharmacy Specialist
Department of Family Medicine
Aurora, Colorado

Contributors

Steven R. Abel, PharmD, FASHP
Associate Dean for Clinical Programs
Bucke Professor and Head
Department of Pharmacy Practice
Purdue University College of Pharmacy
West Lafayette, Indiana

Jessica L. Adams, PharmD
Human Immunodeficiency Virus Pharmacology Fellow
Eshelman School of Pharmacy
University of North Carolina Chapel Hill
Chapel Hill, North Carolina

Brian K. Alldredge, PharmD
Professor and Associate Dean
Department of Clinical Pharmacy
School of Pharmacy
University of California, San Francisco
San Francisco, California

Judith A. Alsop, PharmD
Health Sciences Clinical Professor
Department of Clinical Pharmacy
School of Pharmacy
University of California, San Francisco
Director, Sacramento Division, California Poison Control System
University of California, Davis Health System
San Francisco and Sacramento, California

J.V. Anandan, PharmD
Adjunct Associate Professor
Eugene Applebaum College of Pharmacy and Health Sciences
Wayne State University
Pharmacy Specialist
Department of Pharmacy Services
Henry Ford Hospital
Detroit, Michigan

Heather M. Arnold, PharmD, BCPS
Critical Care Clinical Pharmacist
Department of Pharmacy
Barnes-Jewish Hospital
St. Louis, Missouri

Magdalene M. Assimon, PharmD
Nephrology Pharmacotherapy Research Fellow
Department of Pharmacy Practice
Albany College of Pharmacy and Health Sciences
Albany, New York

Francesca T. Aweeka, PharmD
Professor
Department of Clinical Pharmacy
School of Pharmacy
University of California, San Francisco
San Francisco, California

Jennifer H. Baggs, PharmD, BCPS
Clinical Staff Pharmacist
Department of Pharmacy
University Medical Center
Tucson, Arizona

Maria Ballod, PharmD
Nutrition Support Pharmacist
Department of Pharmacy
Instructor of Pharmacy
College of Medicine
Mayo Clinic
Jacksonville, Florida

Andrew D. Barnes, PharmD
Clinical Professor
School of Pharmacy
University of Washington
Director, Critical Care Residency, Pharmacy Services
University of Washington Medicine
Seattle, Washington

David T. Bearden, PharmD
Clinical Associate Professor
Department of Pharmacy Practice
College of Pharmacy
Oregon State University
Portland, Oregon

Sandra Benavides, PharmD
Assistant Professor
Pharmacy Practice
College of Pharmacy
Nova Southeastern University
Clinical Pharmacist
Department of Pharmacy
Joe DiMaggio Children's Hospital
Fort Lauderdale and Hollywood, Florida

Rosemary R. Berardi, PharmD, FCCP, FASHP, FAPhA
Professor of Pharmacy
College of Pharmacy
University of Michigan
Ann Arbor, Michigan

Paul M. Beringer, PharmD, FASHP, FCCP
Associate Professor
Department of Clinical Pharmacy
University of Southern California
Los Angeles, California

Jeff F. Binkley, PharmD, BCNSP, FASHP
Assistant Professor
Department of Clinical Pharmacy
University of Tennessee College of Pharmacy
Director of Pharmacy
Maury Regional Medical Center
Memphis and Columbia, Tennessee

KarenBeth H. Bohan, PharmD, BCPS
Associate Professor
Department of Pharmacy Practice
Wilkes University
Clinical Pharmacist
Department of Pharmacy
Wilkes-Barre General Hospital
Wilkes-Barre, Pennsylvania

Laura M. Borgelt, PharmD, BCPS, FCCP
Associate Professor
Departments of Clinical Pharmacy and Family Medicine
University of Colorado Anschutz Medical Campus
Aurora, Colorado

Jolene R. Bostwick, PharmD, BCPS, BCPP
Clinical Assistant Professor
Department of Clinical, Social, and Administrative Sciences
University of Michigan College of Pharmacy
Clinical Pharmacist in Psychiatry
Department of Pharmacy Services
University of Michigan Health System
Ann Arbor, Michigan

Nicole J. Brandt, PharmD, CGP, BCPP, FASCP
Associate Professor
Department of Pharmacy Practice and Science
University of Maryland, Baltimore
Clinical Pharmacist, Geriatrics
Veterans Affairs
Baltimore, Maryland

Tina Penick Brock, MSPharm, EdD
Professor and Associate Dean
Department of Clinical Pharmacy
School of Pharmacy
University of California, San Francisco
San Francisco, California

Michael R. Brodeur, PharmD, CGP, FASCP
Associate Professor
Department of Pharmacy Practice
Albany College of Pharmacy and Health Sciences
Albany, New York

Glen R. Brown, PharmD
Clinical Professor
Faculty of Pharmaceutical Sciences
University of British Columbia
Clinical Pharmacy Specialist, Critical Care
Department of Pharmacy
St. Paul's Hospital
Vancouver, British Columbia, Canada

Marcia L. Buck, PharmD, FCCP, FPPAG
Associate Professor, Pediatrics
School of Medicine
University of Virginia
Clinical Coordinator, Pediatrics
Department of Pharmacy
University of Virginia
Charlottesville, Virginia

Jamie J. Cavanaugh, PharmD
Clinical Instructor
Division of Pharmacy Practice and Experiential Education
Eshelman School of Pharmacy
University of North Carolina at Chapel Hill
Chapel Hill, North Carolina

Stanley W. Chapman, PharmD, MD
Professor Emeritus
Department of Medicine
University of Mississippi Medical Center
Jackson, Mississippi

Steven W. Chen, PharmD, FASHP
Associate Professor
Department of Clinical Pharmacy and Pharmaceutical Economics and Policy
Hygeia Centennial Chair in Clinical Pharmacy
University of Southern California School of Pharmacy
Los Angeles, California

Michael F. Chicella, PharmD
Clinical Coordinator
Department of Pharmacy
Children's Hospital of The King's Daughters
Norfolk, Virginia

Jennifer W. Chow, PharmD
Pediatric Clinical Specialist
Department of Pharmacy
Children's Hospital of The King's Daughters
Norfolk, Virginia

Cary R. Chrisman, PharmD
Assistant Professor
Department of Clinical Pharmacy
University of Tennessee College of Pharmacy
Clinical Pharmacist, Department of Pharmacy
Methodist Medical Center
Memphis and Oak Ridge, Tennessee

Thomas E. Christian, BSPharm, BCPS
Pharmacy Therapeutics Manager, Infectious Disease Coordinator
Department of Pharmacy
PeaceHealth Southwest
Vancouver, Washington

John D. Cleary, PharmD
Professor and Vice Chair of Research
Department of Pharmacy Practice
Assistant Professor, Medicine
Department of Infectious Diseases
University of Mississippi Schools of Pharmacy and Medicine
Jackson, Mississippi

Michelle Condren, PharmD, AE-C, CDE
Associate Professor and Vice Chair
Department of Clinical and Administrative Sciences—Tulsa
College of Pharmacy
Associate Professor, Pediatrics
School of Community Medicine
University of Oklahoma
Tulsa, Oklahoma

Amanda H. Corbett, PharmD, BCPS, FCCP, AAHIVE
Clinical Assistant Professor
Eshelman School of Pharmacy
University of North Carolina
Chapel Hill, North Carolina

Robin L. Corelli, PharmD
Professor of Clinical Pharmacy
Department of Clinical Pharmacy
School of Pharmacy
University of California, San Francisco
San Francisco, California

Timothy W. Cutler, PharmD, CGP
Associate Professor of Clinical Pharmacy
Department of Clinical Pharmacy
School of Pharmacy
University of California, San Francisco
San Francisco, California

Larry H. Danziger, PharmD
Professor of Pharmacy Practice
Department of Pharmacy Practice
University of Illinois at Chicago
Chicago, Illinois

Eli N. Deal, PharmD, BCPS
Clinical Pharmacist, Internal Medicine
Department of Pharmacy
Barnes-Jewish Hospital
St. Louis, Missouri

Ellen R. DeGrasse, PharmD, BCPS
Clinical Assistant Professor
Department of Pharmacy
University of Washington School of Pharmacy
Seattle, Washington

Philip T. Diaz, MD
Professor
Department of Internal Medicine
The Ohio State University
Columbus, Ohio

Betty J. Dong, PharmD, FASHP, FCCP
Professor of Clinical Pharmacy
Department of Clinical Pharmacy
School of Pharmacy
Clinical Pharmacist, Thyroid Clinic
University of California, San Francisco
San Francisco, California

Andrew J. Donnelly, PharmD, MBA, FASHP
Clinical Professor
Department of Pharmacy Practice
University of Illinois at Chicago College of Pharmacy
Director of Pharmacy Services
Department of Pharmacy
University of Illinois Medical Center at Chicago
Chicago, Illinois

Julie A. Dopheide, PharmD, BCPP
Associate Professor of Clinical Pharmacy, Psychiatry and the Behavioral Sciences
University of Southern California Schools of Pharmacy and Medicine
Los Angeles County and University of Southern California Medical Center
Los Angeles, California

Richard H. Drew, PharmD, MS, BCPS, FCCP
Professor
Campbell University College of Pharmacy and Health Sciences
Associate Professor of Medicine (Infectious Diseases)
Duke University School of Medicine
Duke Medical Center
Durham, North Carolina

Arkadiusz Z. Dudek, MD, PhD
Associate Professor
Department of Medicine
Division of Hematology-Oncology Transplantation
University of Minnesota
Minneapolis, Minnesota

Julie B. Dumond, PharmD, BCPS, AAHIVE
Research Assistant Professor
Division of Pharmacotherapy and Experimental Therapeutics
Eshelman School of Pharmacy
University of North Carolina at Chapel Hill
Chapel Hill, North Carolina

Robert E. Dupuis, PharmD
Clinical Associate Professor
Eshelman School of Pharmacy
University of North Carolina at Chapel Hill
Chapel Hill, North Carolina

Shareen Y. El-Ibiary, PharmD, BCPS
Associate Professor of Pharmacy Practice
Department of Pharmacy Practice
Midwestern University, College of Pharmacy—Glendale
Glendale, Arizona

Rene A. Endow-Eyer, PharmD, BCPP
Psychiatric Clinical Pharmacy Specialist
Department of Pharmacy Service
Veterans Affairs San Diego Healthcare System
San Diego, California

Michael E. Ernst, PharmD, BCPS, FCCP
Professor (Clinical)
Department of Pharmacy Practice and Science
College of Pharmacy
Department of Family Medicine
Carver College of Medicine
The University of Iowa
Iowa City, Iowa

Gregory A. Eschenauer, PharmD, BCPS
Clinical Pharmacist
Infectious Diseases
Department of Pharmacy
University of Pittsburgh Medical Center
Pittsburgh, Pennsylvania

Sanaz Farhadian, PharmD
Academic Detailing Pharmacist
Department of Pharmacy
Veterans Affairs San Diego Healthcare System
San Diego, California

Elizabeth Farrington, PharmD, FCCP, FCCM, FPPAG, BCPS
Clinical Assistant Professor
Department of Pharmacotherapy and Experimental Education
Eshelman School of Pharmacy
University of North Carolina
Chapel Hill, North Carolina
Pharmacist III
Pediatrics
New Hanover Regional Medical Center
Betty H. Cameron Women's and Children's Hospital
Wilmington, North Carolina

Jonathan D. Ference, PharmD, BCPS
Associate Professor
Department of Pharmacy Practice
Wilkes University Nesbitt College of Pharmacy and Nursing
Director of Pharmacotherapy Education
Wyoming Valley Family Medical Residency Program
Wilkes-Barre, Pennsylvania

Victoria F. Ferraresi, PharmD, FASHP, FCSHP
Associate Professor of Clinical Pharmacy
Department of Clinical Pharmacy
School of Pharmacy
University of California, San Francisco
Director of Pharmacy Services
Pathways Home Health and Hospice
San Francisco and Sunnyvale, California

Christopher K. Finch, PharmD, BCPS
Associate Professor
Department of Clinical Pharmacy
University of Tennessee
Assistant Director
Clinical Pharmacy Services
Department of Pharmacy
Methodist University Hospital
Memphis, Tennessee

Patrick R. Finley, PharmD, BCPP
Professor of Clinical Pharmacy
Department of Clinical Pharmacy
School of Pharmacy
University of California, San Francisco
San Francisco, California

Douglas N. Fish, PharmD
Professor and Chair
Department of Clinical Pharmacy
University of Colorado School of Pharmacy
Clinical Specialist in Critical Care/Infectious Diseases
Department of Pharmacy
University of Colorado Hospital
Aurora, Colorado

Randolph V. Fugit, PharmD, BCPS
Clinical Assistant Professor
Department of Clinical Pharmacy Practice
University of Colorado at Denver Health Sciences Center
Internal Medicine Clinical Specialist
Department of Pharmacy
Denver Veterans Affairs Medical Center
Denver, Colorado

Mark W. Garrison, PharmD, FCCP
Assistant Dean and Associate Professor
Department of Pharmacotherapy
College of Pharmacy
Washington State University
Deaconess Medical Center
Spokane, Washington

James J. Gasper, PharmD
Assistant Clinical Professor
Department of Clinical Pharmacy
School of Pharmacy
University of California, San Francisco
Psychiatric Clinical Pharmacist
Community Behavioral Health Services
San Francisco Department of Public Health
San Francisco, California

Katherine R. Gerrald, PharmD, BCPS
Assistant Professor of Pharmacy Practice
Department of Pharmacy Practice
Presbyterian College School of Pharmacy
Clinton, South Carolina

Jane M. Gervasio, PharmD, BCNSP, FCCP
Vice Chair and Associate Professor
Department of Pharmacy Practice
Butler University
Indianapolis, Indiana

Virginia L. Ghafoor, PharmD
Clinical Pharmacy Specialist
Pain Management
University of Minnesota Medical Center
Division of Fairview Health Services
Minneapolis, Minnesota

Jeffery A. Goad, PharmD, MPH
Associate Professor of Clinical Pharmacy
Department of Clinical Pharmacy and Pharmaceutical Economics and Policy
School of Pharmacy
University of Southern California
Los Angeles, California

Julie A. Golembiewski, PharmD
Clinical Associate Professor
Pharmacy Practice and Anesthesiology
University of Illinois at Chicago
Clinical Pharmacist
Hospital Pharmacy and Anesthesiology
University of Illinois Medical Center
Chicago, Illinois

Luis S. Gonzalez, III, PharmD, BCPS
Associate Clinical Preceptor of Pharmacy and Therapeutics
University of Pittsburgh School of Pharmacy
Manager, Clinical Pharmacy Services
Pharmaceutical Care Services
Conemaugh Memorial Medical Center
Pittsburgh and Johnstown, Pennsylvania

Mildred D. Gottwald, PharmD
Director
Clinical Research
Gilead Sciences
Foster City, California

Kathleen G.E. Green, MS, PharmD
Clinical Assistant Professor
Experimental and Clinical Pharmacology
University of Minnesota College of Pharmacy
Pharmacy Clinical Leader, Oncology/Bone Marrow Transplantation
Department of Pharmacy
University of Minnesota Medical Center, Fairview
Minneapolis, Minnesota

B. Joseph Guglielmo, PharmD
Professor and Chair
TA Oliver Chair in Clinical Pharmacy
Department of Clinical Pharmacy
School of Pharmacy
University of California, San Francisco
San Francisco, California

Karen M. Gunning, PharmD, BCPS, FCCP
Associate Professor (Clinical)
Departments of Pharmacotherapy and Family and Preventive Medicine
University of Utah College of Pharmacy & School of Medicine
Clinical Pharmacist
University of Utah Sugarhouse Family Health Center
University of Utah Healthcare
Salt Lake City, Utah

Sally K. Guthrie, PharmD
Associate Professor
Department of Clinical and Social Administrative Sciences
College of Pharmacy
University of Michigan
Ann Arbor, Michigan

Mark R. Haase, PharmD, FCCP, BCPS
Associate Professor
Department of Pharmacy Practice
Health Sciences Center School of Pharmacy
Texas Tech University
Amarillo, Texas

Mary F. Hebert, PharmD, FCCP
Professor
Department of Pharmacy
University of Washington
Seattle, Washington

Emily L. Heil, PharmD, BCPS
Infectious Diseases Clinical Pharmacy Specialist
Department of Pharmacy
University of Maryland Medical Center
Baltimore, Maryland

David W. Henry, PharmD, MS, BCOP, FASHP
Associate Professor and Chair
Department of Pharmacy Practice
University of Kansas School of Pharmacy
Pediatric Hematology/Oncology Pharmacy Specialist
University of Kansas Hospital
Lawrence and Kansas City, Kansas

Richard N. Herrier, PharmD
Clinical Professor
Department of Pharmacy Practice and Science
College of Pharmacy
University of Arizona
Tucson, Arizona

Karl M. Hess, PharmD, FCPhA
Assistant Professor of Pharmacy Practice and Administration
Western University of Health Sciences
College of Pharmacy
Pomona, California

Mark T. Holdsworth, PharmD
Associate Professor of Pharmacy and Pediatrics and Pharmacy Practice Head
College of Pharmacy
Executive Chair, Human Research Review Committee
University of New Mexico Health Sciences Center
Albuquerque, New Mexico

Curtis D. Holt, PharmD
Clinical Professor
Department of Surgery
University of California, Los Angeles
Los Angeles, California

Priscilla P. How, PharmD, BCPS
Assistant Professor
Department of Pharmacy, Faculty of Science
National University of Singapore
Principal Clinical Pharmacist
Department of Medicine, Division of Nephrology
National University Hospital
Singapore, Singapore

Karen Suchanek Hudmon, DrPH, MS, RPh
Associate Professor
Department of Pharmacy Practice
Purdue University
West Lafayette, Indiana

Matthew K. Ito, PharmD, FCCP, FNLA, CLS
Professor
Department of Pharmacy Practice
Oregon State University/Oregon Health Sciences University
College of Pharmacy
Portland, Oregon

Gail S. Itokazu, PharmD
Clinical Associate Professor
Department of Pharmacy Practice
University of Illinois, Chicago
Clinical Pharmacist
Department of Pharmacy
John H. Stroger Jr. Hospital of Cook County
Chicago, Illinois

Timothy J. Ives, PharmD, MPH, FCCP, BCPS
Professor
Eshelman School of Pharmacy
University of North Carolina at Chapel Hill
Chapel Hill, North Carolina

Kellie L. Jones, PharmD, BCOP
Clinical Associate Professor
Department of Pharmacy Practice
Purdue University
Indianapolis, Indiana

Nicole A. Kaiser, RPh, BCOP
Clinical Assistant Professor
School of Pharmacy, The University of Colorado
Oncology Clinical Pharmacy Specialist
Department of Pharmacy
The Children's Hospital
Denver, Colorado

James S. Kalus, PharmD, BCPS
Senior Pharmacy Manager
Department of Pharmacy Services
Henry Ford Hospital
Detroit, Michigan

Angela D.M. Kashuba, BScPharm, PharmD, DABCP
Associate Professor
Eshelman School of Pharmacy
University of North Carolina at Chapel Hill
Chapel Hill, North Carolina

Michael B. Kays, PharmD, FCCP
Associate Professor
Department of Pharmacy Practice
Purdue University College of Pharmacy
Indianapolis, Indiana

George A. Kenna, PhD, RPh
Assistant Professor of Psychiatry
Warren Alpert Medical School
Center for Alcohol Addiction Studies
Brown University
Clinical Pharmacist
Department of Pharmacy
Westerly Hospital
Providence and Westerly, Rhode Island

Jiwon Kim, PharmD, BCPS
Assistant Professor
Department of Clinical Pharmacy and Pharmaceutical Economics and Policy
University of Southern California School of Pharmacy
Clinical Pharmacist
Department of Pharmacy
University of Southern California University Hospital
Los Angeles, California

Mark N. Kirstein, PharmD
Associate Professor
Department of Experimental and Clinical Pharmacology
College of Pharmacy
University of Minnesota
Minneapolis, Minnesota

Katie L. Kiser, PharmD, BCPS
Assistant Professor
Department of Pharmacy Practice and Science
University of Maryland School of Pharmacy
Baltimore, Maryland

Daren L. Knoell, PharmD, FCCP
Professor
Departments of Pharmacy and Internal Medicine
Davis Heart and Lung Research Institute
The Ohio State University
Columbus, Ohio

Lee A. Kral, PharmD, BCPS
Adjunct Assistant Professor
Department of Anesthesia
The University of Iowa Carver College of Medicine
Clinical Pharmacy Specialist, Pain Management
Department of Pharmaceutical Care
The University of Iowa Hospitals and Clinics
Iowa City, Iowa

Bridgette L. Kram, PharmD
Surgical/Trauma Intensive Care Unit Clinical Pharmacist
Department of Pharmacy
Wesley Medical Center
Wichita, Kansas

Robert A. Kratzke, MD
Associate Professor
Department of Medicine
Division of Hematology-Oncology Transplantation
University of Minnesota
Minneapolis, Minnesota

Donna M. Kraus, PharmD, FAPhA, FPPAG
Pediatric Clinical Pharmacist
Associate Professor of Pharmacy Practice
Departments of Pharmacy Practice and Pediatrics
Colleges of Pharmacy and Medicine
University of Illinois at Chicago
Chicago, Illinois

Lisa A. Kroon, PharmD, CDE
Professor of Clinical Pharmacy
Department of Clinical Pharmacy
School of Pharmacy
University of California, San Francisco
Clinical Pharmacist, General Internal Medicine and Diabetes Clinics
University of California, San Francisco Medical Center
San Francisco, California

Jonathan P. Lacro, PharmD, BCPS, BCPP
Associate Clinical Professor
Departments of Pharmacy & Pharmaceutical Science and Psychiatry
University of California, San Diego
Director, Pharmacy Education and Training
Department of Pharmacy
Veterans Affairs San Diego Healthcare System
San Diego, California

Alan H. Lau, PharmD
Professor
Director, International Clinical Pharmacy Education
College of Pharmacy
University of Illinois at Chicago
Chicago, Illinois

Kelly C. Lee, PharmD, BCPP
Assistant Professor of Clinical Pharmacy
Skaggs School of Pharmacy and Pharmaceutical Sciences
University of California, San Diego
La Jolla, California

Michelle Lee, PharmD
Infectious Disease Pharmacist
Department of Pharmacy
Methodist Hospital of Southern California
Arcadia, California

Susan H. Lee, PharmD
Surgery/Critical Care Clinical Pharmacist
Department of Pharmacy
Veterans Affairs Puget Sound Medical Center
Seattle, Washington

Lisa K. Lohr, PharmD, BCPS, BCOP
Clinical Assistant Professor
College of Pharmacy
University of Minnesota
Oncology Pharmacy Specialist/Oncology Medication Therapy Management Provider
Masonic Cancer Center (University of Minnesota/Fairview)
Minneapolis, Minnesota

Rex S. Lott, PharmD, BCPP
Professor
Department of Pharmacy Practice & Administrative Sciences
Idaho State University College of Pharmacy
Mental Health Clinical Pharmacist
Department of Pharmacy and Mental Health
Boise Veterans Affairs Medical Center, Boise, Idaho
Clinical Associate Professor
University of Washington School of Medicine
Department of Psychiatry and Behavioral Sciences
Seattle, Washington

Sherry Luedtke, PharmD, FPPAG
Associate Professor
Department of Pharmacy Practice
Texas Tech Health Sciences Center School of Pharmacy
Amarillo, Texas

May Mak, PharmD
Assistant Professor
Department of Clinical Pharmacy and Pharmaceutical Economics and Policy
University of Southern California
Los Angeles, California

Joel C. Marrs, PharmD, BCPS (AQ Cardiology), CLS
Assistant Professor
University of Colorado Anschutz Medical Campus
School of Pharmacy
Clinical Pharmacy Specialist
Department of Pharmacy
Denver Health
Aurora, Colorado

Darius L. Mason, PharmD, BCPS
Assistant Professor
Department of Pharmacy Practice
Albany College of Pharmacy and Health Science
Albany, New York

James W. McAuley, PhD, FAPhA
Associate Professor
Departments of Pharmacy Practice and Neurology
The Ohio State University College of Pharmacy
Columbus, Ohio

James P. McCormack, BSc(Pharm), PharmD
Professor
Faculty of Pharmaceutical Sciences
University of British Columbia
Vancouver, British Columbia, Canada

Jennifer McNulty, MD
Associate Clinical Professor
Department of Obstetrics and Gynecology
Division of Maternal Fetal Medicine
University of California, Irvine
Staff Perinatologist
Long Beach Memorial Medical Center
Long Beach, California

Scott T. Micek, PharmD, BCPS, FCCP
Clinical Pharmacist, Critical Care
Department of Pharmacy
Barnes-Jewish Hospital
St. Louis, Missouri

Robert K. Middleton, PharmD
Director of Pharmacy
Department of Pharmacy
Ministry Saint Clare's Hospital
Weston, Wisconsin

Molly G. Minze, PharmD
Assistant Professor
Department of Pharmacy Practice
Texas Tech Health Sciences Center
School of Pharmacy
Abilene, Texas

Myrna Y. Munar, PharmD
Associate Professor
Department of Pharmacy Practice
College of Pharmacy
Oregon State University
Oregon Health and Science University
Portland, Oregon

Milap C. Nahata, PharmD, MS
Professor and Division Chair
Director, Institute of Therapeutic Innovations and Outcomes
College of Pharmacy
Professor of Internal Medicine and Pediatrics
College of Medicine
Associate Director, Pharmacy
Ohio State University Medical Center
The Ohio State University
Columbus, Ohio

Jean M. Nappi, PharmD, FCCP, BCPS
Professor
Clinical Pharmacy and Outcome Sciences
South Carolina College of Pharmacy
Clinical Pharmacy Specialist in Cardiology
Medical University of South Carolina
Charleston, South Carolina

Paul E. Nolan, Jr., PharmD
Professor
Department of Pharmacy Practice & Science
College of Pharmacy
University of Arizona
Cardiovascular Clinical Pharmacist
University Medical Center
Tucson, Arizona

Edith A. Nutescu, PharmD, FCCP
Clinical Professor
Pharmacy Practice and Center for Pharmacoeconomic Research
University of Illinois at Chicago College of Pharmacy
Director, Antithrombosis Center
University of Illinois at Chicago Medical Center
Chicago, Illinois

Cindy L. O'Bryant, PharmD, BCOP
Associate Professor
Department of Clinical Pharmacy
University of Colorado
Oncology Clinical Specialist
Department of Pharmacy
University of Colorado Cancer Center
Aurora, Colorado

Rory E. O'Callaghan, PharmD
Clinical Pharmacist
Adjunct Assistant Professor of Pharmacy Practice
University of Southern California School of Pharmacy
Los Angeles, California

Julie L. Olenak, PharmD
Associate Professor
Department of Pharmacy Practice
Wilkes University
Nesbitt College of Pharmacy and Nursing
Wilkes-Barre, Pennsylvania

Neeta Bahal O'Mara, PharmD, BCPS, CCP
Clinical Pharmacist
Dialysis Clinic, Inc.
North Brunswick, New Jersey

Makala B. Pace, PharmD, BCOP
Clinical Pharmacy Specialist
Division of Pharmacy
Thoracic/Head & Neck Medical Oncology
The University of Texas
MD Anderson Cancer Center
Houston, Texas

Robert Lee Page, II, PharmD, MSPH, FCCP, FASHP, FAHA, FASCP, BCPS, CGP
Associate Professor
Departments of Clinical Pharmacy & Physical Medicine
University of Colorado Schools of Pharmacy and Medicine
Clinical Specialist
Division of Cardiology
University of Colorado Hospital
Aurora, Colorado

Louise Parent-Stevens, PharmD, BCPS
Clinical Assistant Professor
Department of Pharmacy Practice
College of Pharmacy
University of Illinois at Chicago
Clinical Pharmacist
Department of Family Medicine
University of Illinois Medical Center
Chicago, Illinois

Patricia L. Parker, PharmD, BCPS
Health Sciences Associate Clinical Professor
Department of Clinical Pharmacy
School of Pharmacy
University of California, San Francisco
Clinical Coordinator
Department of Pharmacy
University of California, Davis Medical Center
Sacramento, California

Katherine Tipton Patel, PharmD, BCOP
Clinical Pharmacy Specialist
Division of Pharmacy
Thoracic/Head and Neck Medical Oncology
The University of Texas
MD Anderson Cancer Center
Houston, Texas

Margaret M. Pearson, PharmD, MS
Director, Department of Pharmacy
Mississippi State Department of Health
Jackson, Mississippi

Jennifer Tran Pham, PharmD, BCPS
Clinical Assistant Professor
Departments of Pharmacy Practice and Pediatrics
University of Illinois at Chicago College of Pharmacy
Neonatal Clinical Pharmacist
Department of Pharmacy
University of Illinois at Chicago Medical Center at Chicago
Chicago, Illinois

Brian A. Potoski, PharmD
Assistant Professor
Departments of Pharmacy and Therapeutics
University of Pittsburgh School of Pharmacy
Associate Director, Antibiotic Management Program
University of Pittsburgh Medical Center
Presbyterian University Hospital
Pittsburgh, Pennsylvania

David J. Quan, PharmD
Clinical Professor of Pharmacy
Department of Clinical Pharmacy
School of Pharmacy
University of California, San Francisco
Clinical Pharmacist
Department of Pharmaceutical Services
University of California, San Francisco Medical Center
San Francisco, California

Ralph H. Raasch, PharmD, FCCP, BCPS
Associate Professor
Department of Pharmacy Practice and Experiential Education
Eshelman School of Pharmacy
University of North Carolina at Chapel Hill
Chapel Hill, North Carolina

Andrei M. Rakic, MD
Assistant Professor of Clinical Anesthesiology
Department of Anesthesiology
University of Illinois at Chicago
Anesthesiologist and Pain Physician
Department of Anesthesiology
University of Illinois Medical Center
Chicago, Illinois

Erin C. Raney, PharmD, BCPS
Associate Professor
Department of Pharmacy Practice
Midwestern University College of Pharmacy—Glendale Campus
Clinical Pharmacist
Midwestern University Multispecialty Clinic
Glendale, Arizona

Alison M. Reta, PharmD
Clinical Pharmacist
Adjunct Assistant Professor of Pharmacy Practice
University of Southern California School of Pharmacy
Los Angeles, California

John R. Rogosheske, PharmD
Clinical Assistant Professor
College of Pharmacy
University of Minnesota
Clinical Pharmacist
Department of Pharmacy Services
University of Minnesota Medical Center, Fairview
Minneapolis, Minnesota

Carol J. Rollins, PharmD, MS, RD, BCNSP
Clinical Associate Professor
Department of Pharmacy Practice and Science
The University of Arizona
Interim Assistant Director, Clinical Pharmacy
Department of Pharmacy, University Medical Center
Tucson, Arizona

Rebecca A. Rottman-Sagebiel, PharmD, BCPS, CGP
Clinical Assistant Professor
Pharmacy Education and Research Center
University of Texas at Austin
Geriatric Clinical Pharmacy Specialist
Department of Pharmacy
South Texas Veterans Health Care System
San Antonio, Texas

Melody Ryan, PharmD, MPH
Associate Professor
Department of Pharmacy Practice and Science
College of Pharmacy
Department of Neurology
College of Medicine
University of Kentucky
Clinical Pharmacy Specialist
Department of Pharmacy
Veterans Affairs Medical Center
Lexington, Kentucky

Joseph J. Saseen, PharmD, FCCP, FASHP, BCPS
Professor
University of Colorado Anschutz Medical Campus
Schools of Pharmacy and Medicine
Director, PGY2 Ambulatory Care/Family Medicine Residency
Clinical Pharmacy Specialist
Department of Family Medicine
Aurora, Colorado

Eric F. Schneider, PharmD, BCPS
Associate Dean, Northwest Campus
Associate Professor of Pharmacy Practice
Associate Professor of Family and Preventive Medicine
University of Arkansas for Medical Sciences
Fayetteville, Arkansas

Patricia M. Schuler, PharmD
Associate Professor
Depart of Clinical Pharmacy and Outcome Sciences
South Carolina College of Pharmacy
Clinical Specialist—Cardiology
Department of Pharmacy
The Medical University of South Carolina
Charleston, South Carolina

Catrina R. Schwartz, PharmD
Clinical Assistant Professor
Department of Pharmacotherapy
Washington State University College of Pharmacy
Spokane, Washington

Timothy H. Self, PharmD
Professor of Clinical Pharmacy
College of Pharmacy
University of Tennessee Health Science Center
Director, PGY2 Internal Medicine Pharmacy Residency
Department of Pharmacy
Methodist University Hospital
Memphis, Tennessee

Amy Hatfield Seung, PharmD, BCOP
Clinical Specialist, Hematologic Malignancies
Department of Pharmacy
Johns Hopkins Hospital
Baltimore, Maryland

Sachin R. Shah, PharmD, BCOP, FCCP
Associate Professor
Department of Pharmacy Practice
Texas Tech University Health Science Center—School of Pharmacy
Advanced Clinical Pharmacist
Department of Pharmacy
Veterans Administration North Texas Health Care System
Dallas, Texas

Carrie A. Sincak, PharmD, BCPS
Vice Chair of Acute Care and Associate Professor
Department of Pharmacy Practice
Midwestern University Chicago College of Pharmacy
Downer's Grove, Illinois
Clinical Pharmacist
Department of Internal Medicine
Loyola University Medical Center
Maywood, Illinois

Harleen Singh, PharmD
Clinical Associate Professor
Department of Pharmacy Practice
Oregon State University
Clinical Specialist Pharmacist
Department of Pharmacy
Veterans Affairs Medical Center
Portland, Oregon

Julian Hoyt Slade, III, PharmD, BCOP
Clinical Pharmacy Specialist
Gastrointestinal Medical Oncology
Division of Pharmacy
University of Texas
MD Anderson Cancer Center
Houston, Texas

Jessica C. Song, MA, PharmD
Clinical Pharmacy Supervisor
PGY1 Pharmacy Residency Coordinator
Department of Pharmacy Services
Santa Clara Valley Medical Center
San Jose, California

Suellyn J. Sorensen, PharmD, BCPS
Clinical Pharmacist Specialist
Infectious Diseases, Pulmonary, and Neurology
Director, Midwest AIDS Education and Training Center Indiana
Department of Pharmacy
University Hospital of Indiana University Health
Indianapolis, Indiana

Marilyn R. Stebbins, PharmD
Health Sciences Clinical Professor
Department of Clinical Pharmacy
School of Pharmacy
University of California, San Francisco
Pharmacy Utilization Director
CHW Medical Foundation Mercury Medical Group
Department of Pharmacy
Catholic Healthcare West Medical Foundation
San Francisco and Sacramento, California

Glen L. Stimmel, PharmD, BCPP
Professor of Clinical Pharmacy, Psychiatry and the Behavioral Sciences
University of Southern California School of Pharmacy
Keck School of Medicine
Los Angeles, California

Steve Stricker, PharmD, MS, BCOP
Assistant Professor
Department of Pharmacy Practice
Samford University McWhorter School of Pharmacy
Birmingham, Alabama

David J. Taber, PharmD, BCPS
Clinical Assistant Professor
Department of Clinical Pharmacy and Outcomes Sciences
South Carolina College of Pharmacy
Clinical Pharmacy Specialist
Department of Pharmacy Services
Medical University of South Carolina
Charleston, South Carolina

Kimberly B. Tallian, PharmD, BCPP, FASHP, FCCP, FCSHP
Associate Clinical Professor, Pharmacy
University of California, San Francisco and University of California, San Diego
Pharmacy Clinical Manager
Department of Pharmacy
Scripps Memorial Hospital—La Jolla
La Jolla, California

Yasar O. Tasnif, PharmD
Clinical Assistant Professor
Cooperative Pharmacy Program
University of Texas—Pan American
Edinburg, Texas

Daniel J. G. Thirion, PharmD, FCSHP
Clinical Associate Professor
Faculte de Pharmacie
University of Montreal
Pharmacist
Department of Pharmacy
McGill University Health Center
Montreal, Quebec, Canada

Lisa A. Thompson, PharmD
Assistant Professor
Department of Clinical Pharmacy
University of Colorado School of Pharmacy
Oncology Clinical Specialist
Department of Pharmacy
University of Colorado Cancer Center
Aurora, Colorado

Dominick P. Trombetta, PharmD, BCPS, CGP, FASCP
Associate Professor
Department of Pharmacy Practice
Wilkes University
Wilkes-Barre, Pennsylvania

Toby C. Trujillo, PharmD, BCPS
Associate Professor
Department of Clinical Pharmacy
University of Colorado School of Pharmacy
Clinical Specialist, Cardiology/Anticoagulation
Department of Pharmacy
University of Colorado Hospital
Aurora, Colorado

Kimey D. Ung, PharmD, BCPS
Clinical Pharmacy Specialist
Center for Women Obstetrics Division
Long Beach Memorial Medical Center and Miller Children's Hospital
Assistant Clinical Professor
Department of Clinical Pharmacy
School of Pharmacy
University of California, San Francisco
Long Beach and San Francisco, California

Geoffrey C. Wall, PharmD, FCCP, BCPS, CGP
Professor of Clinical Sciences
Department of Clinical Sciences
Drake University College of Pharmacy
Clinical Pharmacist
Iowa Inflammatory Bowel Disease Center
Des Moines, Iowa

Sheila K. Wang, PharmD, BCPS (AQ –ID)
Assistant Professor
Department of Pharmacy Practice
Midwestern University Chicago College of Pharmacy
Clinical Pharmacist, Infectious Disease
Department of Pharmacy
Rush University Medical Center
Chicago, Illinois

Brian Watson, PharmD, BCPS
Clinical Pharmacy Specialist, Critical Care
Department of Pharmacy
Union Memorial Hospital
Clinical Assistant Professor
University of Maryland School of Pharmacy
Baltimore, Maryland

Kristin Watson, PharmD, BCPS
Assistant Professor
Department of Pharmacy Practice and Sciences
University of Maryland School of Pharmacy
Baltimore, Maryland

C. Wayne Weart, PharmD, BCPS, FASHP, FAPhA
Professor of Clinical Pharmacy and Outcome Sciences
South Carolina College of Pharmacy
Professor of Family Medicine
Medical University of South Carolina
Charleston, South Carolina

Lynn Weber, PharmD, BCOP
Clinical Pharmacist in Oncology/Hematology
Pharmacy Residency Coordinator and PGY-1 Residency Director
Department of Pharmacy
Hennepin County Medical Center
Minneapolis, Minnesota

Timothy E. Welty, PharmD, FCCP
Professor
Department of Pharmacy Practice
University of Kansas School of Pharmacy
Lawrence, Kansas

C. Michael White, PharmD, FCP, FCCP
Professor and Head
Department of Pharmacy Practice
University of Connecticut
Director, Evidence-based Practice Center
University of Connecticut/Hartford Hospital
Storrs and Hartford, Connecticut

Bradley R. Williams, PharmD, FASCP, CGP
Professor of Clinical Pharmacy and Clinical Gerontology
Titus Family Department of Clinical Pharmacy and Pharmaceutical Economics and Policy
Schools of Pharmacy and Gerontology
University of Southern California
Los Angeles, California

Casey B. Williams, PharmD, BCOP
Adjunct Clinical Assistant Professor
Department of Pharmacy Practice
University of Kansas School of Pharmacy
Hematology/Oncology Clinical Coordinator and Residency Director
Department of Pharmacy
University of Kansas Hospital
Lawrence and Kansas City, Kansas

Craig Williams, PharmD
Associate Professor
Department of Pharmacy Practice
Oregon State University
Clinical Specialist
Department of Family Medicine
Oregon Health Sciences University Hospital
Portland, Oregon

Dennis M. Williams, PharmD
Associate Professor
Division of Pharmacotherapy and Experimental Therapeutics
Eshelman School of Pharmacy
University of North Carolina at Chapel Hill
Clinical Specialist
Department of Pharmacy
University of North Carolina Hospitals
Chapel Hill, North Carolina

Ann K. Wittkowsky, PharmD, CACP, FASHP, FCCP
Clinical Professor
Department of Pharmacy
University of Washington School of Pharmacy
Director, Anticoagulation Services
Department of Pharmacy
University of Washington Medical Center
Seattle, Washington

Katie A. Won, PharmD, BCOP
Clinical Associate
College of Pharmacy
University of Minnesota
Clinical Pharmacist, Oncology
Department of Pharmacy
Hennepin County Medical Center
Minneapolis, Minnesota

Annie Wong-Beringer, PharmD, FCCP, FIDSA
Associate Professor
Department of Clinical Pharmacy
University of Southern California
Infectious Diseases Pharmacist
Department of Pharmacy
Huntington Hospital
Los Angeles, California

Wendy O. Zizzo, PharmD
Associate Professor
Behavior Sciences/Alcohol and Other Drug Studies
San Diego City College
San Diego, California

Paolo V. Zizzo, DO
Assistant Clinical Professor
Department of Medicine
University of California, San Diego
Medical Staff, Department of Medicine
Tri City Medical Center
San Diego and Oceanside, California

Reviewers

Steven R. Abel, PharmD, FASHP
Associate Dean for Clinical Programs
College of Pharmacy
Head, Department of Pharmacy Practice
Bucke Professor of Pharmacy Practice
Purdue University
Indianapolis, Indiana

Saafan Al-Safi, BScPharm, RPh, PhD
Professor in Clinical Pharmacy & Therapeutics
International Advisor in Clinical Pharmacy
Ontario College of Pharmacists
Toronto, Canada

William L. Baker, PharmD, BCPS
Assistant Clinical Professor of Pharmacy Practice
University of Connecticut School of Pharmacy
Storrs, Connecticut

Veronica Bandy, PharmD, MS, FCPhA, FCSHP
Director of IPP Programs
Assistant Clinical Professor
Department of Pharmacy Practice
University of the Pacific
Stockton, California

John D. Bowman, MS
Associate Professor
Department of Pharmacy Practice
Texas A&M HSC Rangel College of Pharmacy
Kingsville, Texas

Elias B. Chahine, PharmD, BCPS
Assistant Professor of Pharmacy Practice
Clinical Pharmacists
Palm Beach Atlantic University Gregory School of Pharmacy
West Palm Beach, Florida

Eunice P. Chung, PharmD
Associate Professor of Pharmacy Practice and Administration
Director of Curriculum Development Pharmacy Practice
Western University of Health Sciences, College of Pharmacy
Pomona, California

Charles C. Collins, BS, PhD
Professor of Pharmaceutical Sciences
Bill Gatton College of Pharmacy
East Tennessee State University
Johnson City, Tennessee

Stephanie Counts, PharmD
Associate Professor
Pharmacy Practice
Midwestern University—Glendale
Glendale, Arizona

Monika N. Daftary, PharmD
Associate Professor
Clinical and Pharmacy Administrative Sciences
Howard University College of Pharmacy
Washington, District of Columbia

Sudip Das, PhD
Associate Professor
Pharmacy
Butler University
Indianapolis, Indiana

Crystal Deas, PharmD, BCPS
Assistant Professor of Pharmacy Practice
Pharmacy Practice Primary Care Residency
Harding University
Searcy, Arkansas

Lea S. Eiland, PharmD, BCPS
Associate Clinical Professor and Associate Department Head
Pharmacy Practice
Auburn University
Huntsville, Alabama

Glen E. Farr, PharmD
Professor and Associate Dean for Continuing Education
The University of Tennessee Health Science Center
Knoxville, Tennessee

Rebecca S. Finley, PharmD
Founding Dean
Pharmacy
Thomas Jefferson University Jefferson School of Pharmacy
Philadelphia, Pennsylvania

Jill Fitzgerald, PhD
Professor of Literacy
University of North Carolina at Chapel Hill
Chapel Hill, North Carolina

Gina Garrison, BS, PharmD
Associate Professor
Pharmacy Practice
Albany College of Pharmacy and Health Sciences
Albany, New York

Nicole Harder, RN, BN, MPA
Coordinator, Simulation Learning Centers
University of Manitoba Faculty of Nursing
Winnipeg, Canada

Arthur F. Harralson, PharmD, BCPS
Professor and Chairman
Pharmacogenomics
Associate Dean for Academic Affairs Administration
Shenandoah University
Winchester, Virginia

Angela Kim-Sing, PharmD, ACPR, FCSHP
Director, Office of Experiential Education
Faculty of Pharmaceutical Sciences
The University of British Columbia
Vancouver, Canada

Chris King-Talley, PhD
Interdisciplinary Graduate Studies
University of Calgary
Calgary, Alberta, Canada

Harold Kirschenbaum, MS, PharmD
Associate Dean for Professional Affairs
Professor of Pharmacy Practice
Arnold & Marie Schwartz College of Pharmacy and Health Sciences
Long Island University
Long Island, New York

Brian M. Matayoshi, PhD
Professor of Physiology
Philadelphia College of Osteopathic Medicine - Georgia Campus
Suwanee, Georgia

Laurie Mauro, PharmD
Professor of Clinical Pharmacy
Director of Educational Assessment
Department of Pharmacy Practice
College of Pharmacy and Pharmaceutical Sciences
The University of Toledo
Toledo, Ohio

Beverly C. Mims, PharmD
Associate Professor
Pharmacy Practice
Howard University School of Pharmacy
Washington, District of Columbia

Stefanie Nigro, PharmD
Assistant Professor of Pharmacy Practice
University of Connecticut School of Pharmacy
Storrs, Connecticut

Kathleen Pace Murphy, MBA
Professor
University of Texas Health Science Center
Health Careers
Houston, Texas

Nathan Painter, PharmD, CDE
Assistant Clinical Professor
UCSD Skaggs School of Pharmacy and Pharmaceutical Sciences
La Jolla, California

Michael J. Peeters, PharmD, MEd, BCPS
Clinical Associate Professor
Department of Pharmacy Practice
University of Toledo College of Pharmacy & Pharmaceutical Sciences
Toledo, Ohio

Helen Pervanas, PharmD, RPh
Assistant Professor of Pharmacy Practice
Department of Pharmacy Practice-Worcester/Manchester
Massachusetts College of Pharmacy and Health Sciences
Worcester, Massachusetts

Christine M. Petraglia, RPh, MSEd
Holyoke Medical Center
Clinical Pharmacist
Holyoke, Massachusetts

John Poon, PharmD
Inpatient Pharmacist
Clinical Pharmacist
Kaiser Permanente Antioch Medical Center
Antioch, California

Keith Rodvold, PharmD
Professor
Pharmacy Practice
University of Illinois at Chicago College of Pharmacy
Chicago, Illinois

Jessica Rogers
Academic Coordinator
Education
Trillium College
Oshwa, Ontario, Canada

Martha Zervopoulos Siomos, DNP, MSN, ADM-BC, FNP-BC
Assistant Professor
Family Nurse Practitioner
Rush University College of Nursing
Chicago, Illinois

Candace Smith, PharmD
Associate Clinical Professor and Chair
Clinical Pharmacy Practice Department
Clinical Pharmacy Practice
St. John's University and Allied Health Professions
Queens, New York

Linda Spooner, PharmD, BCPS
Associate Professor of Pharmacy Practice
Department of Pharmacy Practice
Massachusetts College of Pharmacy and Health Sciences
Worcester, Massachusetts

Michael Steinberg, PharmD, BCOP
Associate Professor of Pharmacy Practice
Department of Pharmacy Practice Worcester/Manchester School of Pharmacy
Massachusetts College of Pharmacy and Health Sciences
Worcester, Massachusetts

Michael C. Thomas, PharmD, BCPS
Assistant Professor
Pharmacy Practice (Emergency Medicine)
South University–Savannah
Savannah, Georgia

Andrea Traina, PharmD
Assistant Professor
St. John Fisher College Wegmans School of Pharmacy
Rochester, New York

April Vallerand, BSN, MSN, PhD Nursing
Associate Professor
Wayne State University College of Nursing
Detroit, Michigan

Arun Verma, PhD, MSc
Instructor
Division of Pharmacy Practice
The University of British Columbia
Vancouver, British Columbia, Canada

Kristina Ward, PharmD, BCPS
Clinical Associate Professor
Department of Pharmacy Practice
University of Rhode Island College of Pharmacy
Kingston, Rhode Island

Kathy Zaiken, PharmD
Assistant Professor
Pharmacy Practice
Massachusetts College of Pharmacy and Health Sciences
Boston, Massachusetts

Brief Table of Contents

SECTION 15: PSYCHIATRIC DISORDERS 1863

Section Editors: Patrick R. Finley and Kelly C. Lee

SECTION 16: SUBSTANCE ABUSE 2011

SECTION 17: NEOPLASTIC DISORDERS 2080

Section Editor: Mark N. Kirstein

SECTION 18: PEDIATRICS 2265

Section Editor: Marcia L. Buck

SECTION 19: GERIATRIC THERAPY 2359

Section Editor: Judith L. Beizer

Detailed Table of Contents

SECTION 8: DERMATOLOGIC DISORDERS 925

Section Editor: Timothy J. Ives

SECTION 9: ARTHRITIC DISORDERS 989

Section Editor: Tricia M. Russell

1

Assessment of Therapy and Medication Therapy Management

Marilyn R. Stebbins, Timothy W. Cutler, and Patricia L. Parker

CORE PRINCIPLES

		CHAPTER CASES
1	Medication Therapy Management Services (MTMS) are provided to patients in all care settings but were first described in the Medicare Modernization Act of 2003.	**Case 1-5 (Questions 1, 5)**
2	MTMS includes comprehensive medication therapy review, developing a personalized medication record, a medication action plan, and documentation of the encounter.	**Case 1-5 (Questions 1–4)**
3	Medication reconciliation and taking an accurate and complete medication history are crucial to a successful MTMS encounter.	**Case 1-1 (Questions 1–3)**
4	Data necessary to perform MTMS can be obtained from many sources, including the patient, the paper chart, the pharmacy information system, and the electronic health record.	**Case 1-5 (Questions 1, 5)**
5	A careful and complete patient interview should include a medical, medication, and social history and must be provided in a culturally sensitive manner.	**Case 1-1 (Questions 1–3), Table 1-1, Online Content**
6	A successful MTMS encounter must be well documented following the Problem Oriented Medical Record.	**Case 1-5 (Question 1), Table 1-2**
7	The first step in documenting an MTMS encounter involves subjective and objective data collection to identify the primary problem.	**Case 1-2 (Question 1), Case 1-3 (Question 1), Case 1-4 (Question 1)**
8	Once the subjective and objective information is obtained, the clinician must assess the drug therapy or disease-specific problem. The assessment is the clinician's clinical justification for the plan.	**Case 1-5 (Questions 1, 2)**
9	The final step in documenting the MTMS encounter is developing the medication action plan and processing any billing requirements.	**Case 1-5 (Questions 1, 2, 4)**
10	To ensure the needs of the patient are met, communication of the plan with the patient and patient's other providers is required.	**Case 1-5 (Question 3)**

With the passage of the Patient Protection and Affordable Care Act and the Health Care and Education Reconciliation Act of 2010, pharmacists and other providers have tremendous opportunities in the implementation of health care reform.[1,2] One of the hallmarks of this law is delivery system reform. As health care delivery systems change, pharmacists have an opportunity to improve overall quality of care, to become involved in coordinated health care approaches such as medical home teams and accountable care organizations, and to collaborate to improve care for high-risk patients and those with chronic conditions in primary-care settings. Pharmacists practicing in acute care settings will have additional opportunities as hospitals will have financial incentives to improve quality, reduce costs, and decrease hospital-acquired conditions.[1,2] With the pharmacists' expertise in medication therapy management, their leadership and involvement are crucial as these collaborative practices are being developed and implemented.

This chapter presents several approaches to assessing drug therapy and provides the framework for medication therapy management services (MTMS) across the continuum of care. The illustrations in this chapter primarily focus on the pharmacist; however, the principles used to assess patient response to drug therapy are of value to all health care providers.

MTMS was first described in the Medicare Modernization Act of 2003 (MMA 2003), which also established the first outpatient prescription drug benefit (also known as Medicare Part D) for those eligible for Medicare.[3] MTMS was defined in MMA 2003 as *a program of drug therapy management that may be furnished by a pharmacist and that is designed to assure . . . that covered Part D drugs under the prescription drug plan are appropriately used to optimize therapeutic outcomes through improved medication use, and to reduce the risk of adverse events, including adverse drug interactions.*

In 2003, the MMA defined eligibility criteria for MTMS, which were updated in 2010 to ensure that more Medicare beneficiaries would qualify for MTMS. MTMS-eligible beneficiaries must:

1. Take multiple Medicare Part D–covered drugs
2. Have multiple chronic diseases
3. Are likely to incur annual costs of at least $3,000 for all covered Part D drugs

Although MTMS is the term used in MMA 2003 to describe medication management for those eligible under the Medicare Part D benefit, the same approach is appropriate for any patient taking medications for chronic conditions. To respond to the need for further clarification of the term MTMS, 11 professional pharmacy associations more formally defined MTMS in a consensus document published in 2004.[4] According to this definition, MTMS can be applied to any patient in a variety of settings. Furthermore, this definition clarifies the type of activities involved in a medication therapy management (MTM) program.

MTMS has a direct relationship to pharmaceutical care. Pharmaceutical care has been described as *the responsible provision of drug therapy to achieve definite outcomes that are intended to improve a patient's quality of life.*[5,6] In fact, MTMS has been described as a service provided in the practice of pharmaceutical care.[7] However, unlike pharmaceutical care, MTMS is recognized by payers, has current procedural terminology (CPT) codes specifically for pharmacists, and has several clearly defined interventions. Therefore, MTMS will be the term used to describe the activity of MTM in various patient populations.

Both patient self-care and medication reconciliation are critical aspects of any MTMS encounter regardless of the setting (i.e., inpatient, community, ambulatory, or institutional). Patient self-care is defined by the World Health Organization as those *activities [that] individuals, families, and communities undertake with the intention of enhancing health, preventing disease, limiting illness, and restoring health. These activities are derived from knowledge and skills from the pool of both professional and lay experience. They are undertaken by lay people on their own behalf, either separately or in participative collaboration with professionals.*[8] Patient self-care requires the patient to take responsibility for the illness; however, the help of a professional to structure healthy self-care is important. For example, patients with diabetes who monitor their blood glucose levels regularly and adjust their diet according to the guidelines published from the American Diabetes Association (ADA) would be practicing self-care. Self-care is often the work that the patient performs between visits with the provider. The patient should be involved in his or her own care to ensure the best outcomes.

Medication reconciliation is the comprehensive evaluation of a patient's medication regimen any time there is a change in therapy in an effort to avoid medication errors such as omissions, duplications, dosing errors, or drug interactions, as well as to observe compliance and adherence patterns. This process should include a comparison of the existing and previous medication regimens and should occur at every transition of care in which new medications are ordered, existing orders are rewritten or adjusted, or when the patient has added nonprescription medications to his or her self-care.[9] Although not a new concept to the profession of pharmacy, there has been heightened awareness and intensified effort in this area of practice as a result of the Joint Commission. The Joint Commission is the national accrediting body for hospitals and other health care delivery organizations that has committed to improving patient care through an inspection and evaluation process. In 2005, the Joint Commission announced its National Patient Safety Goal (NPSG) 8A and 8B to *accurately and completely reconcile medications across the continuum of care.* This goal requires institutions to develop and test processes for medication reconciliation in ambulatory and acute care settings.[10] Currently, the Joint Commission is re-evaluating and refining the standards surrounding NPSG 8 so that they can be more readily and successfully implemented by institutions. The release of the new standards is anticipated in January 2011.

The general approach to an MTMS patient encounter in various clinical settings will be discussed in the next sections. Figure 1-1 provides an overview of a patient encounter that includes information gathering from various data sources; interviewing the patient while using effective communication skills; assessing the medical illness(es); developing a plan to manage the illness(es); documenting the service (including billing); and monitoring, follow-up, or referral for any additional issues that cannot be resolved during the encounter.

SOURCES OF PATIENT INFORMATION

Successful patient assessment and monitoring requires the gathering and organization of all relevant information.[6,11] The patient (or family member or other representative) is always the primary source of information. The provider asks the patient a series of questions to obtain subjective information that is helpful in making a diagnosis or evaluating ongoing therapy. Likewise, pharmacists, home care nurses, and other providers without direct access to patient data also must obtain subjective data or measure objective physical data to guide recommendations for therapy and to monitor previously prescribed therapy.

Data-Rich Environment

In a "data-rich environment," such as a hospital, long-term care facility, or outpatient medical clinic, a wealth of information is available to practitioners from the medical record, pharmacy profile, and medication administration record (MAR). In these settings, physicians, nurses, and patients are readily available. This facilitates timely, effective communication among providers involved in the drug therapy decision-making process. Objective data (e.g., diagnosis, physical examination, laboratory and other test results, vital signs, weight, medications, medication allergies, intravenous flow rates, and fluid balance) are readily available. Likewise, the cases presented throughout this text usually provide considerable data on which to make more thorough assessments and therapeutic decisions. The patient record provides

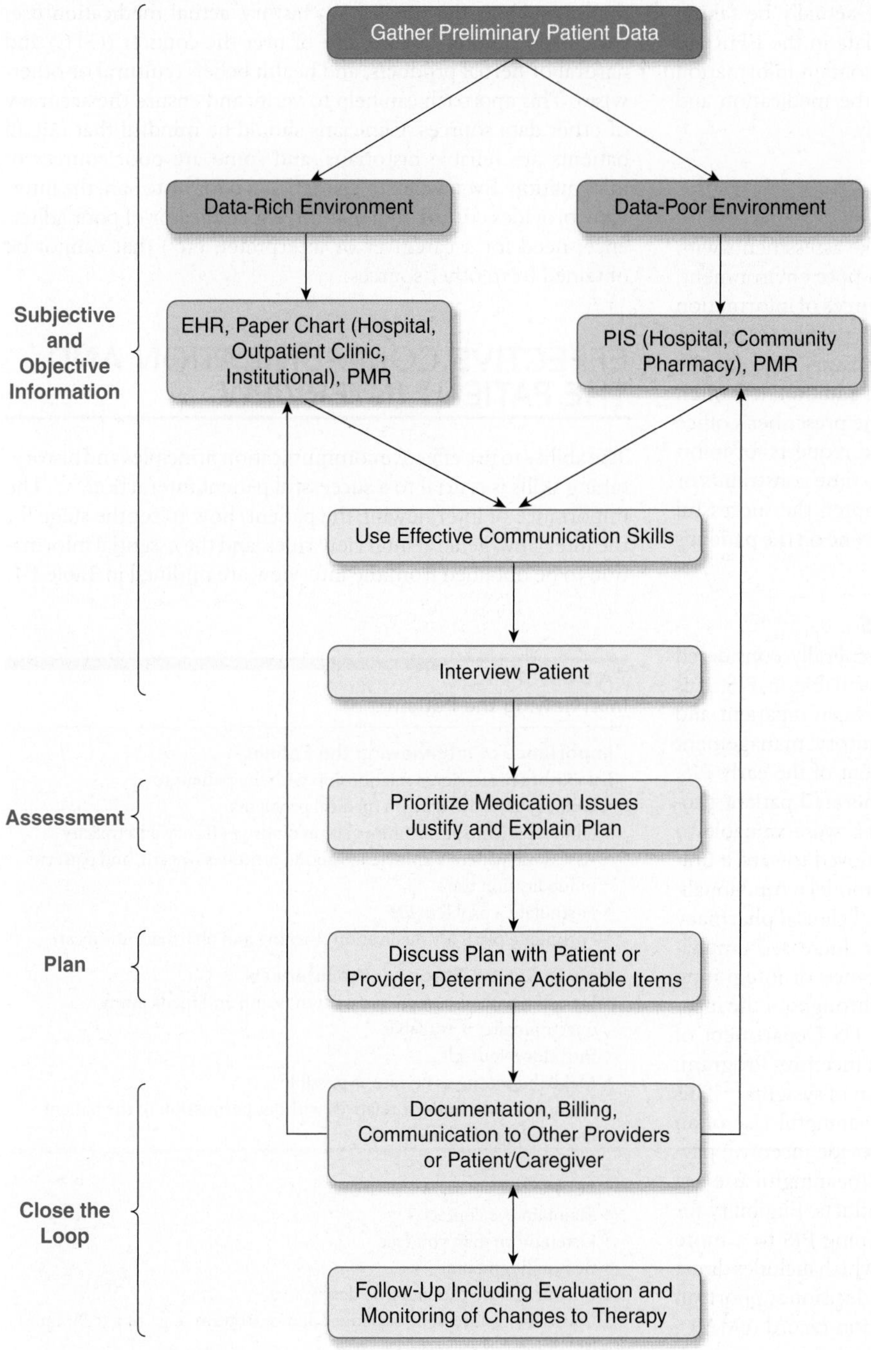

FIGURE 1-1 General approach to a patient encounter. EHR, electronic health record; PIS, pharmacy information system; PMR, personal medication record.

readily available information that is needed to identify and assess medical problems, which is necessary to design patient-specific care plans and document MTMS. In some settings, patient insurance information is important to help understand the formulary choices and access to medications.

PAPER CHARTS

A paper chart may be a source of valuable patient information. Paper charts may exist in a variety of settings, including the hospital, outpatient clinic, or institutional setting. This source of information is considered data rich but does have limitations. Paper charts are organized differently by site and by setting. The information contained in a hospital chart will be different from that contained in an outpatient clinic. Furthermore, it may be difficult to obtain a paper chart, or access may be delayed if another professional is using the chart. Significant data delays may occur in paper charts, as information such as laboratory results, test results, and chart notes may not be placed in the chart for several days after the test or documentation is complete. As a result, it is important to realize the limitations of this data-rich environment and that the information obtained during the patient interview is still extremely important.

ELECTRONIC HEALTH RECORD

An electronic health record (EHR) is an electronic version of the paper chart. These records are available in hospitals, clinics, and institutional settings, but the type of EHR and the organization of information will vary among the different settings and software applications. The EHR provides a wealth of information and is one of the most complete sources of reliable information. Unlike a paper chart, the EHR may be interfaced with the laboratory, pharmacy, and radiology systems so that data are available in real time with minimal delays. Unfortunately, clinicians may rely on the EHR too much for the patient information, and unless medication and problem lists are updated at every visit, this could lead to assumptions. For example, a patient who has metformin

500 mg twice daily listed in the EHR may actually be taking the medication once daily. Therefore, the data in the EHR are extremely useful, but it is still important to obtain information directly from the patient and to reconcile the medication and problem list and update the EHR accordingly.

Data-Poor Environment

In reality, clinicians are often required to make assessments with limited information. Even in a relatively data-poor environment, such as a community pharmacy, valuable sources of information are still available, including (a) the medication profile, (b) patient demographic data, (c) medication allergy history, and (d) the patient's insurance coverage information. In addition, it is often possible to consult with the prescriber (or the prescriber's office staff); however, contact may be delayed, and requests for information may be met with resistance owing to time constraints or other factors. As illustrated later in this chapter, the successful practitioner can make assessments and intervene on the patient's behalf even with limited information.

PHARMACY INFORMATION SYSTEMS

Pharmacy information systems (PIS) are generally considered data poor. When evaluating information available in PIS, it is important to the appreciate differences between inpatient and outpatient PIS. Pharmacy billing and inventory management were the motivation behind the establishment of the early PIS. These initial systems provided fill lists, generated patient profiles, and produced medication labels, which were valuable to institutional pharmacies as the profession moved toward a unit dose medication distribution system. More modern functionalities allow for some limited documentation of clinical pharmacy activities, but still, this system is data poor. Increased emphasis on patient safety highlights the importance of integrating PIS with other computerized systems used throughout the inpatient setting. An initiative set forth by the US Department of Health and Human Services, called the EHR Incentive Program, exemplifies the importance of the integration of systems.[12] This initiative, commonly referred to as the "Meaningful Use of an EHR," allows Medicare and Medicaid to provide incentive payments to providers and hospitals for the "meaningful use" of certified health information technology products. Eligibility for these incentive payments involves transitioning PIS to a more data-rich clinical information system (CIS), which includes direct computerized physician order entry, clinical decision support, an EHR, an electronic medication administration record (eMAR), and integration of various ancillary information systems such as pharmacy and laboratory services. Additional functionality incorporates the use of bar code technology, which allows the ability to track and promote quality assurance during the medication administration process. Information generated by the CIS is electronically transmitted to the pharmacy in real time, eliminating lost, illegible, or incomplete medication orders. Improved communication among various health care providers, decreased medication turnaround time, enhanced compliance with medication use policies and formularies, and reductions in medication errors are potential benefits of the EHR Incentive Program. Although increasing numbers of institutions are incorporating this technology into their practice settings, implementation of CIS in hospitals has not occurred for numerous reasons, including expense and system complexity.

Especially in a data-poor environment, it is important that the clinician be a proactive interviewer; in many instances, the interviewer becomes an investigator. The investigative approach is direct and requires strong problem-solving abilities and active listening skills. Questions should be formulated to obtain information such as the medication history, actual medication use, patient perception of care, use of over-the-counter (OTC) and natural or herbal products, and health beliefs (cultural or otherwise). This approach can help to verify and ensure the accuracy of other data sources. Clinicians should be mindful that not all patients are reliable historians, and some are poor sources of information. Even when the patient is a poor historian, the interview provides critical information (e.g., indicator of poor adherence, need for a caregiver or interpreter, etc.) that cannot be obtained from other sources.

EFFECTIVE COMMUNICATION AND THE PATIENT INTERVIEW

The ability to use effective communication principles and history-taking skills is crucial to a successful patient interaction.[6,11] The importance of interviewing the patient, how to set the stage for the interview, general interview rules, and the essential information to be obtained from the interview are outlined in Table 1-1.

TABLE 1-1
Interviewing the Patient

Importance of Interviewing the Patient

Establishes professional relationship with the patient to:
- Obtain subjective data on medical problems
- Obtain patient-specific information on drug efficacy and toxicity
- Assess the patient's knowledge about, attitudes toward, and pattern of medication use
- Formulate a problem list
- Formulate plans for medication teaching and pharmaceutical care

How to Set the Stage for the Interview
- Have the patient complete a written health and medication questionnaire, if available
- Introduce yourself
- Make the setting as private as possible
- Do not allow friends or relatives without permission of the patient
- Do not appear rushed
- Be polite
- Be attentive
- Maintain eye contact
- Listen more than you talk
- Be nonjudgmental
- Encourage the patient to be descriptive
- Clarify by restatement or patient demonstration (e.g., of a technique)

General Interview Rules
- Read the chart or patient profile first
- Ask for the patient's permission to conduct an interview or make an appointment to do so
- Begin with open-ended questions
- Move to close-ended questions
- Document interaction

Information to Be Obtained
- History of allergies
- History of adverse drug reactions
- Weight and height
- Drugs: dose, route, frequency, and reason for use
- Perceived efficacy of each drug
- Perceived side effects
- Adherence to prescribed drug regimen
- Nonprescription medication use (including complementary and alternative medications)
- Possibility of pregnancy in women of childbearing age
- Family or other support systems

Source: Teresa O'Sullivan, PharmD, University of Washington.

Information obtained from the patient is critical for assessment and planning in medication therapy management.

ONLINE CONTENT

For an example of a patient interview and medication history taking tips, please go to http://thepoint.lww.com/AT10e.

OBTAINING A PATIENT HISTORY

Those who provide MTMS should develop standardized forms to record patient information obtained from the patient interview. Standardization facilitates quick retrieval of information, minimizes the inadvertent omission of data, and enhances the ability of other practitioners to use shared records.[6,11]

For convenience, the patient interview and record can be divided into sections with subjective and objective data as well as an assessment and plan (including expected outcomes). Components of subjective and objective data are the medical history, medication history, and social history. In some situations, these histories can be supplemented by the generation of flowchart diagrams to monitor changes in specific variables (e.g., blood glucose concentration, blood pressure, weight) with time. These charts and documentation systems may be incorporated into the EHR, PIS, or a similar electronic platform.

Medical History

The medical history is essential to the provision of MTMS. It can be as extensive as the medical records that are maintained in an institution or physician's office, or it can be a simple patient profile that is maintained in a community pharmacy. The purpose of the medical history is to identify significant past medical conditions or procedures; identify, characterize, and assess current acute and chronic medical conditions and symptoms; and gather all relevant health information that could influence drug selection or dosing (e.g., function of major organs such as the gastrointestinal tract, liver, and kidney, which are involved in the absorption and elimination of drugs; height and weight, including recent changes in either; age and sex; pregnancy and lactation status; and special nutritional needs). Not all interviews require the interviewer to ask for this much general information; however, in a data-poor environment, more information is required directly from the patient. A more focused interview may be appropriate in settings in which the information required is available electronically or is specific to a single disease state. For example, in an anticoagulation clinic, the information that is elicited from the patient is often specific to the patient's anticoagulation therapy (e.g., bleeding incidents, newly started medications, dietary changes, missed warfarin doses, etc.).

CASE 1-1

QUESTION 1: P.J., a 45-year-old woman of normal height and weight, states that she has diabetes. What questions might the practitioner ask of P.J. to determine whether type 1 or type 2 disease should be documented in her medical history?

Patients usually can enumerate their medical problems in a general way, but the practitioner often will have to probe more specifically to refine the diagnosis and assess the severity of the condition. Diabetes mellitus is used to illustrate the types of questions that can be used to gather important health information and assess drug therapy. The following questions should generate information that will help to determine whether P.J. has type 1 or type 2 diabetes mellitus.

- **How old were you when you were told you had diabetes?**
- **Do any of your relatives have diabetes mellitus? What do you know of their diabetes?**
- **Do you remember your symptoms? Please describe them to me.**
- **What medications have you used to treat your diabetes?**

When questions such as these are combined with knowledge of the pathophysiology of diabetes, appreciation of the typical presenting signs and symptoms of the disease, and understanding of the drugs generally used to treat both forms of diabetes, meaningful MTM can be provided. Even simple assessments such as the observation of a patient's body size can provide information useful for therapeutic interventions. For example, a person with type 2 diabetes is more likely to be an overweight adult (see Chapter 53, Diabetes Mellitus).

Medication History

In the community pharmacy setting, patients generally present themselves in one of four ways: (a) with a self-diagnosed condition for which nonprescription drug therapy is sought, (b) with a newly diagnosed condition for which a drug has been prescribed, (c) with a chronic condition that requires refill of a previously prescribed drug or the initiation of a new drug, or (d) on referral from their health plan or provider, or self-referral for focused medication therapy review (MTR). In the first and second situations, the practitioner must confirm the diagnosis by using disease-specific questions as illustrated in Question 1. In the third situation, the practitioner uses the same type of questioning as in the first two situations; however, this time the practitioner needs to evaluate whether the desired therapeutic outcomes have been achieved. The practitioner must evaluate the information gleaned during follow-up visits in the context of the history and incorporate it into his or her assessment and medication action plan (MAP). In the fourth situation, in which patients require a focused MTR, the medication and medical history information are equally important. Without the medical history, it is not possible to evaluate whether the drug therapy is appropriate, and without an accurate medication history, it is not possible to determine whether the patient has reached the desired goals of therapy for her condition. The goal of the medication history is to obtain and assess the following information: the specific prescription and nonprescription drugs that the patient is taking (the latter includes OTC medications, botanicals, dietary supplements, recreational drugs, alcohol, tobacco, and home remedies); the intended purpose or indications for each of these medications; how taken (e.g., route, ingestion in relation to meals), how much, and how often these medications are used; how long these agents have been taken or used (start and stop dates); whether the patient believes that any of these agents are providing therapeutic benefit; whether the patient is experiencing or has experienced any adverse effects that could be caused by each of these agents (idiosyncratic reactions, toxic effects, adverse effects); whether the patient has stopped taking any of the medications for any reason; and allergic reactions and any history of hypersensitivity or other severe reactions to drugs. This information should be as specific as possible, including a description of the reaction, the treatment, and the date of its occurrence.

The approach and process by which the medication history is obtained does not necessarily change based on the setting of the encounter. A successful medication reconciliation process consists of a standardized systematic approach, with the initial step in this process involving the collection of the best medication history possible from every patient that enters any point in the health care system. The appropriate health care professional to obtain this information varies widely from one institution to the next, and may involve an array of individuals. Although pharmacists are uniquely qualified and have demonstrated increased accuracy in acquiring the medication history,[13] ultimately, medication reconciliation requires a multidisciplinary effort in which all available resources are integrated into each step of the process when appropriate.[14] Shared accountability by using key members of the health care team such as nurses, pharmacy technicians, pharmacists, and prescribers is essential in this process. Once an accurate medication history is obtained, this information is used to ensure that as the patient moves through the health care system, any deviation from prescribed regimen is deliberate and based on acute changes in the patient's condition. If an observed discrepancy is the result of an intended therapeutic decision by the prescribing clinician, appropriate documentation with either the reason for or intention to change, hold, or discontinue the medication should be completed in a manner that is clear to all members of the health care team. Unintentional variances in the medication lists should be considered as potential medication errors pending clarification from the prescribing clinician.

Because medication errors most commonly occur during transitions of care, the essential times to conduct medication reconciliation are when a patient is admitted to or discharged from a health care facility.[15,16] A crucial final step in the reconciliation process, and a vital piece of MTMS, occurs at discharge to avoid therapeutic duplication, drug interactions, and omissions of medications that may have been discontinued or placed on hold during hospitalization. On departure from a health care facility, a complete list of the patient's medications must be communicated to the patient and the next provider of service regardless of the setting. It is important to realize that efforts to implement a medication reconciliation process should not focus simply on fulfilling a Joint Commission standard but that this process allows for informed prescribing decisions and creates a safer environment for patients by improving the accuracy of medication administration throughout the continuum of care.

Perhaps the most important aspect of the medication history is to ensure that no assumptions related to medication use go unverified with the patient. The provider should ask questions related to how the current medication therapy is actually taken by the patient. The interviewer should then compare the use of medications as defined by the patient to the prescription information on the bottle or in the PIS/EHR. This information may identify discrepancies or misunderstandings between the prescriber and patient. As discussed previously, the patient may not have adequate health literacy, and the interpretation of the medication instructions printed on the bottle or described by a health professional may not be understandable to a patient. The review of the medication history is an opportune time to identify and clarify such misunderstandings.

CASE 1-1, QUESTION 2: P.J. has indicated that she is injecting insulin to treat her diabetes. What questions might be asked to evaluate P.J.'s use of and response to insulin?

The following types of questions, when asked of P.J., should provide the practitioner with information on P.J.'s understanding about the use of and response to insulin.

DRUG IDENTIFICATION AND USE

- **What type of insulin do you use?**
- **How many units of insulin do you use?**
- **When do you inject your insulin?**
- **Where do you inject your insulin? (Rather than the more judgmental question, "Do you rotate your injection sites?")**
- **Please show me how you usually prepare your insulin for injection. (This request of the patient requires the patient to demonstrate a skill.)**
- **What, if anything, keeps you from taking your insulin as prescribed?**

ASSESSMENT OF THERAPEUTIC RESPONSE

- **How do you know if your insulin is working?**
- **What blood glucose levels are you aiming for?**
- **What foods or meals do you find affect your blood sugars most?**
- **How often and when during the day do you test your blood glucose concentration?**
- **Do you have any blood glucose records that you could share with me?**
- **Please show me how you test your blood glucose concentration.**
- **What is your understanding of the hemoglobin A_{1c} blood test?**
- **When was the last time you had this test done?**
- **What were the results of the last hemoglobin A_{1c} test?**

ASSESSMENT OF ADVERSE EFFECTS

- **Do you ever experience reactions from low blood glucose?**
- **What symptoms warn you of such a reaction?**
- **When do these typically occur during the day?**
- **How often do they occur?**
- **What circumstances seem to make them occur more frequently?**
- **What do you do when you have a low blood glucose?**

The patient's responses to these questions on drug use, therapeutic response, and adverse effects will allow a quick assessment of the patient's knowledge of insulin and whether she is using it in a way that is likely to result in blood glucose concentrations that are neither too high nor too low. The responses to these questions also should provide the practitioner with insight about the extent to which the patient has been involved in establishing and monitoring therapeutic outcomes. Based on this information, the practitioner can begin to formulate the patient's therapeutic plan.

Social History

The social history is used to determine the patient's occupation and lifestyle; important family relationships or other support systems; any particular circumstances (e.g., a disability) or stresses in her life that could influence the MAP; and attitudes, values, and feelings about health, illness, and treatments.

CASE 1-1, QUESTION 3: A patient's occupation, lifestyle, insurance status, ability to pay, and attitudes often can determine the success or failure of drug therapy. Therefore, P.J.'s prescription drug coverage, nutritional history, her level of activity or exercise in a typical day or week, the family dynamics, and any particular stresses that may affect glucose control need to be documented and assessed. What questions might be asked of P.J. to gain this information?

WORK

- **Describe a typical workday and a typical weekend day.**

INSURANCE/COST

- **What type of prescription drug coverage do you have? How much do you pay for your insulin and diabetic supplies? How often do you go without your insulin or supplies because of their cost?**

EXERCISE

- **Describe your exercise habits. How often, how long, and when during the day do you exercise? Describe how you change your meals or insulin when you exercise.**

DIET

- **How many times per day do you usually eat? Describe your usual meal times.**
- **What do you usually eat for each of your main meals and snacks?**
- **Are you able to eat at the same time each day?**
- **What do you do if a meal is delayed or missed?**
- **Who cooks the meals at home? Does this person understand foods to prepare for someone with diabetes?**
- **How often do you eat meals in a restaurant?**
- **How do you order meals in a restaurant to maintain a proper diet for your diabetes? (*Note:* This is asked of patients who frequently dine in restaurants.)**

SUPPORT SYSTEMS

- **Who else lives with you? What do they know about diabetes? How do they respond to the fact that you have diabetes? How do they help you with your diabetes management? Does it ever strain your relationship? What are the issues that seem to be most troublesome? (*Note:* These questions apply equally to the workplace or school setting. Often, the biggest barrier to multiple daily injections is refusal of the patient to inject insulin while at work or school.)**

ATTITUDE

- **How do you feel about having diabetes?**
- **What worries or bothers you most about having diabetes? (*Note:* Participate in the patient's care. This approach is likely to enhance the patient–provider relationship, which should translate into improved care.)**

APPROACH TO AND ASSESSMENT OF PATIENT THERAPY

The provider–patient encounter will vary based on the location and type of services provided and access to necessary information. However, the general approach to the patient encounter should follow the problem-oriented medical record (POMR). Organizing information according to medical problems (e.g., diseases) helps to break down a complex situation (e.g., a patient with multiple medical problems requiring multiple drugs) into its individual parts.[4,5] The medical community has long used a *POMR* or *SOAP note* to record information in the medical record or chart by using a standardized format (Table 1-2). Each medical problem is identified, listed sequentially, and assigned a number. *Subjective* data and *objective* data in support of each problem are delineated, an *assessment* is made, and a *plan* of action identified. The first letter of the four key words (subjective, objective, assessment, and plan) serve as the basis for the SOAP acronym.

TABLE 1-2
Elements of the Problem-Oriented Medical Record[a]

Problem name: Each "problem" is listed separately and given an identifying number. Problems may be a patient complaint (e.g., headache), a laboratory abnormality (e.g., hypokalemia), or a specific disease name if prior diagnosis is known. When monitoring previously described drug therapy, more than one drug-related problem may be considered (e.g., nonadherence, a suspected adverse drug reaction or drug interaction, or an inappropriate dose). Under each problem name, the following information is identified:	
Subjective	Information that explains or delineates the reason for the encounter. Information that the patient reports concerning symptoms, previous treatments, medications used, and adverse effects encountered. These are considered nonreproducible data because the information is based on the patient's interpretation and recall of past events.
Objective	Information from physical examination, laboratory test results, diagnostic tests, pill counts, and pharmacy patient profile information. Objective data are measurable and reproducible.
Assessment	A brief but complete description of the problem, including a conclusion or diagnosis that is supported logically by the above subjective and objective data. The assessment should not include a problem or diagnosis that is not defined above.
Plan	A detailed description of recommended or intended further workup (laboratory tests, radiology, consultation), treatment (e.g., continued observation, physiotherapy, diet, medications, surgery), patient education (self-care, goals of therapy, medication use and monitoring), monitoring, and follow-up relative to the above assessment.

[a] Sometimes referred to as the *SOAP* (subjective, objective, assessment, plan) note.

The POMR is a general approach and helps to focus the encounter, which provides a structure for the documentation of the services provided. The following section will describe the POMR and SOAP note in more detail.

Problem List

Problems are listed in order of importance and are supported by the subjective and objective evidence gathered during the patient encounter. Each problem in the list can then be given an identifying number. All subsequent references to a specific problem can be identified or referenced by that number (e.g., "problem 1" or simply "1"). These generally are thought of in terms of a diagnosed disease, but they also may be a symptom complex that is being evaluated, a preventive measure (e.g., immunization, contraception), or a cognitive problem (e.g., nonadherence). Any condition that requires a unique management plan should be identified as a problem to serve as a reminder to the practitioner that treatment is needed for that problem. Different settings and activities or clinical services will determine the priority of the problems identified.

Medical problems can be *drug related*, including prescribing errors, dosing errors, adverse drug effects, adherence issues, and the need for medication counseling. Drug-related problems may be definite (i.e., there is no question that the problem exists) or possible (i.e., further investigation is required to establish whether the problem really exists). The most commonly encountered types of drug-related problems are listed in Table 1-3.[6,11]

TABLE 1-3
Drug-Related Problems

Drug Needed
Drug indicated but not prescribed; a medical problem has been diagnosed, but there is no indication that treatment has been initiated (maybe it is not needed)
Correct drug prescribed but not taken (nonadherence)
Wrong or Inappropriate Drug
No apparent medical problem justifying the use of the drug
Drug not indicated for the medical problem for which it has been prescribed
Medical problem no longer exists
Duplication of other therapy
Less expensive alternative available
Drug not covered by formulary
Failure to account for pregnancy status, age of patient, or other contraindications
Incorrect nonprescription medication self-prescribed by the patient
Recreational drug use
Wrong Dose
Prescribed dose too high (includes adjustments for renal and hepatic function, age, body size)
Correct prescribed dose but overuse by patient (overadherence)
Prescribed dose too low (includes adjustments for age, body size)
Correct prescribed dose but underuse by patient (underadherence)
Incorrect, inconvenient, or less-than-optimal dosing interval (consider use of sustained-release dosage forms)
Adverse Drug Reaction
Hypersensitivity reaction
Idiosyncratic reaction
Drug-induced disease
Drug-induced laboratory change
Drug Interaction
Drug–drug interaction
Drug–food interaction
Drug–laboratory test interaction
Drug–disease interaction

The distinction between medical problems and drug-related problems sometimes is unclear, and considerable overlap exists. For example, a medical problem (i.e., a disease, syndrome, symptom, or health condition) can be prevented, cured, alleviated, or exacerbated by medications. When assessing drug therapy, several situations could exist: treatment is appropriate and therapeutic outcomes have been achieved; drugs that have been selected are ineffective or therapeutic outcomes are partially achieved; dosages are subtherapeutic or medication is taken improperly; an inappropriate drug for the medical condition being treated has been prescribed or is being used; or the condition is not being treated.

Likewise, a drug-related problem can cause or aggravate a medical problem. Such drug-related problems could include hypersensitivity reactions; idiosyncratic reactions; toxic reactions secondary to excessive doses; adverse reactions (e.g., insulin-induced hypoglycemia or weight gain); drug–drug, drug–disease, drug–laboratory test, and drug–lifestyle interactions; or polypharmacy (using multiple medications), which may increase the risk of adverse drug events.[17]

Subjective and Objective Data

Subjective and objective data in support of a problem are important because assessment of patients and therapies requires the gathering of specific information to verify that a problem continues to exist or that therapeutic objectives are being achieved. Subjective data refer to information provided by the patient or another person that cannot be confirmed independently. This is the data most commonly obtained during a patient interview. Objective data refer to information observed or measured by the practitioner (e.g., laboratory tests, blood pressure [BP] measurements). The objective data are most commonly obtained from the EMR or paper chart (data-rich environment). However, some objective data can be obtained in data-poor environments. In the absence of a medical record, weight, height, pulse, BP, blood glucose readings, and other objective information can be gathered during the provider–patient encounter.

CASE 1-2

QUESTION 1: P.N., a 28-year-old man, has a BP of 140/100 mm Hg. What is the primary problem? What subjective and objective data support the problem, and what additional subjective and objective data are not provided but usually are needed to define this particular problem?

The primary problem is hypertension. No subjective data are given. The objective data are the patient's age, sex, and BP of 140/100 mm Hg. Each of these is important in designing a patient-specific therapy plan. Because hypertension often is an asymptomatic disease (see Chapter 14, Essential Hypertension), subjective complaints such as headache, tiredness or anxiety, shortness of breath (SOB), chest pain, and visual changes usually are absent. If long-term complications such as rupturing of blood vessels in the eye, glomerular damage, or encephalopathy were present, subjective complaints might be blurring or loss of vision, fatigue, or confusion. Objective data would include a report by the physician on the findings of the chest examination (abnormal heart or lung sounds if secondary heart failure [HF] has developed), an ocular examination (e.g., presence of retinal hemorrhages), and laboratory data on renal function (blood urea nitrogen, creatinine, or creatinine clearance). To place these complications in better perspective, the rate of change should be stated. For example, the serum creatinine has increased from a level of 1 mg/dL 6 months ago to a value of 3 mg/dL today. Vague descriptions such as "eye changes" or "kidney damage" are of little value, because progressive damage to these end organs results from uncontrolled high BP, and disease progression needs to be monitored more precisely.

CASE 1-3

QUESTION 1: D.L., a 36-year-old construction worker, tripped on a board at the construction site 2 days ago, sustaining an abrasion of his left shin. He presents to the emergency department with pain, redness, and swelling in the area of the injury. He is diagnosed as having cellulitis. What is the primary problem? What subjective and objective data support the problem? What additional subjective and objective data are not provided but usually are needed to define this particular problem?

The primary problem is cellulitis of the left leg. Useful pieces of subjective information are D.L.'s description of how he injured his shin at a construction site and his current complaints of pain, redness, and swelling. The fact that he was at a construction site is indirect evidence of a possible dirty wound. Further information must be obtained about how he cleaned the wound after the injury and whether he has received a booster dose of tetanus toxoid within the past 10 years. Objectively, the wound is on the left shin. No other objective data are given. Additional data to obtain would be to document the intensity of the redness on a one-to-four-plus scale, the size of the inflamed area as described by an area of demarcation, the circumference of his left shin compared with his right shin, the presence or absence of pus and any lymphatic involvement, his temperature, and a white blood cell count with differential.

CASE 1-4

QUESTION 1: C.S., a 58-year-old woman, has had complaints of fatigue, ankle swelling, and SOB, especially when lying down, for the past week. Physical examination shows distended neck veins, bilateral rales, an S_3 gallop rhythm, and lower extremity edema. A chest radiograph shows an enlarged heart. She is diagnosed as having HF and is being treated with furosemide and digoxin. What is/are the primary problem(s)? What subjective and objective data support the problem(s)? What additional subjective and objective data are not provided but usually are needed to define this (these) particular problem(s)?

The primary problem is systolic HF. Subjectively, C.S. claims to be experiencing fatigue, ankle swelling, and SOB, especially when lying down. She claims to have been taking furosemide and digoxin. An expanded description of these symptoms and her medication use would be helpful. The findings on physical examination and the enlarged heart on chest radiograph are objective data in support of the primary problem of HF. In addition, other objective findings that would help in her assessment would be the pulse rate, BP, serum creatinine, serum potassium concentration, digoxin blood level, a more thorough description of the rales on lung examination, extent of neck vein distension, and degree of leg edema. Pharmacy records could be screened to determine current dosages and refill patterns of the medications.

In this case, a second primary problem may be present. Current recommendations for the management of HF include use of an angiotensin-converting enzyme (ACE) inhibitor before or concurrent with digoxin therapy. Thus, a possible drug-related problem is the inappropriate choice of drug therapy ("wrong drug"). The patient or prescriber should be consulted to ascertain whether an ACE inhibitor has been used previously, any contraindications exist, or possible adverse effects were encountered.

Assessment

After the subjective and objective data have been gathered in support of specific listed problems, the practitioner should assess the acuity, severity, and importance of these problems. He or she should then identify all factors that could be causing or contributing to the problem. The assessment of the severity and acuity is important because the patient expects relief from the symptoms that are of particular concern at this time. During the initial encounter with a patient, it might be discovered that the medical problem is only a symptom complex and that a diagnosis is needed to more accurately identify the problem and further define its severity.

The assessment is usually performed during or immediately after the data gathering while the provider keeps in mind evidence-based practices. For example, if diabetes is assessed and pertinent subjective data (medication history, social history, diet, and exercise, etc.) and objective data exist (laboratory test results like hemoglobin A_{1c}, low-density lipoprotein cholesterol [LDL-C], BP, etc.), then the assessment of diabetes may be to determine whether the patient is meeting the goals for the disease as defined by the ADA. If the patient is not at goal, then the explanation of the reasons why would be described in the assessment, and the plan would then be centered on helping that patient get to goal. Sometimes, the distinction between subjective information provided by the patient and assessments made by the practitioner are confused in the POMR. What the patient reveals belongs in the subjective data, and how the provider interprets it belongs in the assessment. For example, a patient stating that she is having difficulty affording her medications belongs in the subjective information. However, a patient appearing to have cost-related nonadherence belongs in the assessment, as it is the provider's interpretation of what the patient has stated.

DRUG THERAPY ASSESSMENT

A responsibility of the practitioner is to monitor the response of patients to prescribed therapeutic regimens. The purpose of drug therapy monitoring is to identify and solve drug-related problems and to ensure that all therapeutic objectives are being achieved. Unless proven otherwise, the medical diagnosis should be assumed to be correct. On occasion, the diagnosis may not be readily apparent, or a drug-induced problem may have been diagnosed incorrectly as being a disease entity.

Nurses, pharmacists, physicians, physician assistants, and other health care practitioners share the responsibility to assess and monitor patient drug therapy. For the pharmacist, medication reconciliation and the drug therapy assessment may occur in many practice settings, including the community pharmacy while dispensing or refilling prescriptions or counseling patients, during MTMS encounters in the home or in the clinic, while assessing therapy for the hospitalized patient, or as part of routine monthly evaluations of patients residing in long-term care facilities. Many states have enacted legislation allowing pharmacists to develop collaborative drug therapy agreements with physicians for disease state management of common disorders such as asthma, diabetes, dyslipidemia, and hypertension. Additional services commonly provided by pharmacists through collaborative drug therapy agreements include anticoagulation monitoring, emergency contraception, and immunizations.[7] These services often involve more detailed drug therapy evaluation and assessment and may occur within or outside the traditional pharmacy setting. Regardless, the patient's need (this should be the primary consideration), time constraints, working environment (a determinant of the amount of patient information that is available), and practitioner's skill level govern the extent of monitoring. Similarly, the exact steps used to monitor therapy and the order in which they are executed need to be adapted to a practitioner's personal style. Thus, the examples given in this chapter should be used by the reader as a guide rather than as a recipe in a cookbook.

Plan

After the problem list is generated, subjective and objective data are reviewed, and the severity and acuity of the problems are assessed and prioritized, the next step in the problem-oriented (i.e., SOAP) approach is to create a plan, which at the minimum should consist of a diagnostic plan and an MAP that includes patient education. The plan is the action that was justified in the assessment. The plan is clear and direct and does not require explanation (this should be explained in the assessment). For example, if a patient is experiencing constipation while taking an opioid pain reliever, the plan would be to recommend a stool softener and stimulant laxative such as docusate sodium and bisacodyl. The plan should also include any follow-up that would be necessary as a result of to the action taken.

Patient Education

Educating patients to better understand their medical problem(s) and treatment is an implied goal of all treatment plans. This process is categorized as the development of a patient education plan. The level of teaching has to be tailored to the patient's needs, health literacy, willingness to learn, and general state of health and mind. The patient should be taught the knowledge and skills needed to achieve and evaluate his or her therapeutic outcome. An important component of the patient education plan emphasizes the need for patients to follow prescribed treatment regimens.

The POMR will allow the provider to focus the interview and encounter independent of the site or service offered. The POMR facilitates documentation of the provision of MTMS across multiple sites and services (across the continuum of care).

The next few sections will discuss how to approach MTMS in various clinical settings.

MEDICATION THERAPY MANAGEMENT SERVICES IN THE COMMUNITY PHARMACY OR AMBULATORY SETTING

The core elements of MTMS have been described by the American Pharmacists Association (APhA) and the National Association of Chain Drug Stores.[18] According to these organizations, the core elements of MTMS should include the following components:

1. Medication therapy review (MTR)
2. Personal medication record (PMR)
3. Medication action plan (MAP)
4. Intervention or referral
5. Documentation and follow-up

Medication Therapy Review (MTR)

The MTR may be a comprehensive review, including medication reconciliation, in which the provider reviews all of the medications the patient is currently taking, or it may be a focused review of one medication-related issue such as an adverse event. Examples of services provided during the MTR are described in Table 1-4. MTR is dependent on the information that is available from the patient or other data sources. Community pharmacies may be a data-poor environment, and access to necessary information may be limited. In some ambulatory clinics, the provider may have access to the EHR (data-rich environment).

TABLE 1-4
Examples of Services Provided During a Medication Therapy Review

- Assess the patient's health status
- Assess cultural issues, health literacy, language barriers, financial status, and insurance coverage or other patient characteristics that may affect the patient's ability to take medications appropriately
- Interview the patient or caregiver to assess, identify, and resolve actual or potential adverse medication events, therapeutic duplications, untreated conditions or diseases, medication adherence issues, and medication cost considerations
- Monitor medication therapy, including response to therapy, safety, and effectiveness
- Monitor, interpret, and assess patient laboratory values, especially as they relate to medication use/misuse
- Provide education and training on the appropriate use of medications
- Communicate appropriate information to other health professionals, including the use and selection of medication therapy

Source: American Pharmacists Association; National Association of Chain Drug Stores Foundation. Medication therapy management in pharmacy practice: core elements of an MTM service model (version 2.0). *J Am Pharm Assoc (2003)*. 2008;48(3):341–353.

Personalized Medication Record (PMR)

Regardless of the setting, a necessary tool to help with the gathering of the medication information is the PMR. This medication record should be updated after any change in medication therapy and should be shared with other health care providers. The patient is responsible for the upkeep of the PMR, but the PMR requires periodic review by the pharmacist or other provider. The goal of this record is to promote self-care and ownership of the medication regimen.[18] The PMR should be used at all levels of care, thereby facilitating the medication reconciliation process required across the continuum of care. An example of a PMR is shown in Figure 1-2.

Once the patient interview has occurred and the PMR has been updated, the provider may still require information to make an assessment. In such cases, the provider must do his or her best with the available information, or may obtain missing information such as the medical history or objective data from other providers. Lack of objective information is common in the community pharmacy setting, and the ability to address all problems effectively may be limited in this data-poor environment. In some encounters, obtaining the necessary information and medication reconciliation may take the entire visit, necessitating a follow-up encounter.

Medication Action Plan (MAP)

If adequate information is available to assess the current problem, an MAP should be developed. Because the MAP is patient centered and is prioritized according to the urgency of need, the provider and the patient should develop the plan together. An example of an MAP can be seen in Figure 1-3.

Intervention and Referral

The MAP often describes the intervention performed in an MTM encounter and may serve as documentation that can be shared with the patient and other health care providers (like the PMR). The primary purpose of the MAP is to make the action plan patient centered and to provide the patient with documentation of what they need to do next in the action plan. It also provides space for the patient to document what he or she did related to this action and when it was done. In some instances, the MAP may involve referral to another provider (a physician or pharmacist with additional qualifications) if the issue is beyond the scope of the intervening pharmacist. Some reasons for referral may include diabetes education by a certified diabetes educator, diagnosis of a new or suspected medical condition, or laboratory testing that may be beyond the scope of the pharmacist.

Coordination of care is a key element of MTMS and MTR.[4] This may include improving the communication between the patient and other health care providers, enhancing the patient's understanding of his or her health issues or concerns, maximizing health insurance coverage, advocating on behalf of the patient to get needed medications using available resources and programs, and various other functions that will improve the patient's understanding of his or her health care environment and promote self-care. Coordination of care may be the primary action taken on behalf of the patient and may be included in the MAP.

Patient: M.C. ALLERGIES: None Type of reaction: N/A	Primary Physician: Dr. Sara Smith (555-3971)	Pharmacist: Mary Doe (555-5551)	Date Prepared: 4/2/12	Date Updated: 5/2/12

Start Date	Medication (generic)	Dosage	Route	Times per Day	Scheduled Times	Purpose for Use	Remarks	Prescriber (Phone)	Stop Date
1/2/12	(lisinopril)	40 mg	By mouth	Once	9 a.m.	High blood pressure		Sara Smith, MD (555-3971)	
1/2/12	(metoprolol)	50 mg	By mouth	Twice	9 a.m. and 9 p.m.	High blood pressure		Sara Smith, MD (555-3971)	
1/2/12	(glipizide)	5 mg	By mouth	Once	9 a.m.	Diabetes	Take 30 minutes before breakfast	Sara Smith, MD (555-3971)	
1/2/12	(indomethacin)	50 mg	By mouth	Up to three times if needed	9 a.m., 4 p.m., 11 p.m.	Back pain	Take with food. Do not take this medicine with other anti-inflammatory medicines (e.g., ibuprofen, naproxen). Do not take this medication unless you have pain.	Sara Smith, MD (555-3971)	
4/2/12	Crestor® (rosuvastatin)	40 mg	By mouth	Once	9 a.m.	Cholesterol		Ted Hart, MD (555-1234)	

Bring this Personal Medication Record with you to all visits with health care providers and if you are admitted to a hospital. Contact your pharmacist regarding questions or updates.

FIGURE 1-2 Example of a Personal Medication Record (PMR).

Documentation and Follow-up

The development of a documentation process is a necessary component of MTMS.[18] Documentation should be standardized and based on the POMR format. All appropriate records, including the PMR and MAP, should be shared with other providers to promote communication and continuity of care. If the encounter requires follow-up, the documentation should reflect the timing of the follow-up care, and any expectations of the patient and providers should be included. Thorough documentation of the encounter allows all providers to quickly assess the progress of the patient and determine that the desired outcome has been achieved.

My Medication–Related Action Plan

Patient:	M.C.
Provider (Phone):	Dr. Sara Smith (555-3971)
Pharmacy/Pharmacist (Phone):	RiteMart/Mary Doe, PharmD (555-5551)
Date Prepared:	May 2, 2012

The list below has important Action Steps to help you get the most from your medications. Follow the checklist to help you work with your pharmacist and providers to manage your medications AND make notes of your actions next to each item on your list

Action Steps ⟶ What I need to do...	Notes ⟶ What I did when I did it...
☐ **For your muscle weakness and soreness** Stop Crestor® (rosuvastatin) 40 mg. We asked Dr. Hart to change to a lower dose or different agent such as simvastatin. Obtain blood test from Dr. Hart's office. Follow-up with Dr. Hart in 2 days.	
☐ **Medicine Cost** We have asked Dr. Hart to stop Crestor (rosuvastatin) as it is too expensive. A generic medicine such as simvastatin will cost you less and was recommended to Dr. Hart as an alternative. Continue to ask your pharmacist and doctor whether the medications you are taking are covered by your Medicare Part D plan and whether there are any alternatives that might be less expensive for you.	
☐ **For Pain** Talk to Dr. Sara Smith about other pain medicines because the indomethacin may not be the best choice for you because of side effects. Some choices might include other medicines such as Vicodin (hydrocodone and acetaminophen), over-the-counter acetaminophen, or medicines like naproxen or ibuprofen.	

My next appointment with my pharmacist is on: __________ (date) at ______ ☐AM ☐PM

This form is based on forms developed by the American Pharmacist Association and the National Association of Chain Drug Store Foundation. Reproduced with permission from APhA and NACDS Foundation.

FIGURE 1-3 Example of a Medication Action Plan (MAP).

An important aspect of documenting the encounter is to submit billing for the encounter when appropriate. Although billing for MTMS is not universally accepted by all payers, the introduction of the national provider identifier (NPI) and pharmacist-specific CPT codes may soon make this a reality.[7,19] The implementation of Medicare Part D in 2006 allowed pharmacists in pharmacies contracted with prescription drug plans to provide MTMS to plan-identified Medicare recipients. Pharmacists bill these plans through the contracted pharmacy by using an NPI and one of three CPT codes. The NPI number designates the provider to be paid, and the CPT determines the amount of payment based on the services rendered. The CPT codes specific to pharmacists providing MTMS include the following:

CPT 99605: Initial face-to-face assessment or intervention by a pharmacist with the patient for 1 to 15 minutes

CPT 99606: Subsequent face-to-face assessment or intervention by a pharmacist with the patient for 1 to 15 minutes

CPT 99607: Each additional 15 minutes spent face-to-face by a pharmacist with the patient; used in addition to 99605 or 99606

Although the NPI number and CPT codes allow pharmacists to bill for MTMS, the reimbursement varies by plan and negotiated contract and is beyond the scope of this text. Pharmacists have also developed patient self-pay reimbursement strategies as well as contracts with self-insured employers and state-run Medicaid programs to provide services.[20,21]

The Patient Protection and Affordable Care Act of 2010 and the Health Care and Education Reconciliation Act of 2010 describe the need for payment reform that promotes improved quality of care. Other providers also see these laws providing new opportunities for pharmacists to participate in care teams such as the patient-centered medical home and pay-for-performance programs to improve medication-related care coordination, quality scores, and patient outcomes.[22,23] The enhanced payment for improving quality in medication-related areas could be used to fund the pharmacist in this activity.

CASE 1-5

QUESTION 1: M.C. is a 76-year-old woman who comes to an appointment at the community pharmacy with her daughter for a focused MTR. She has a Medicare Part D prescription drug plan and is asking for help with her medication costs. She indicates that she has type 2 diabetes, hypertension, back pain, and hyperlipidemia. Her medications include lisinopril 40 mg once daily, metoprolol 50 mg twice daily, glipizide 5 mg once daily, indomethacin 50 mg up to three times daily as needed for pain, and rosuvastatin 40 mg once daily. M.C. tells you that she has trouble paying for her rosuvastatin (tier 3, $60 copayment) and would rather have something generic that costs less (tier 1, $5 copayment). Further, she complains of muscle soreness and weakness during the last 3 weeks. What objective information can be obtained in a community pharmacy setting? What is the primary problem? What additional information is necessary to determine the cause of her problem? How would a clinician assess and document her problem(s) in a SOAP format?

Although generally not considered a data-rich environment, increasing amounts of objective information can be gathered during the patient encounter at a community pharmacy. Specifically, information such as weight, BP, temperature, and finger-stick glucose and cholesterol levels can be measured if indicated for this patient. This information may be useful to the community pharmacist when performing the MTR to determine whether the medications are achieving the desired therapeutic outcomes. Although the patient presented for MTR, the primary complaint is the patient's self-reported muscle weakness and soreness during the last 3 weeks. Assuming that M.C. is a patient of this pharmacy, the practitioner could gather the necessary medication history from the PIS. Because the patient is present, this is a good opportunity to develop a PMR with M.C. While developing the PMR with the patient, the practitioner should gather additional information from M.C. about her medication use. For example, the name of one of M.C.'s medicines could be read with the practitioner continuing to ask open-ended questions such as, "How do you take this medication?" "What is your routine for taking your medication?" and "What types of problems, if any, have you had while using this medication?" This process will help to quickly identify any medication discrepancies between the pharmacy computer system and the patient's understanding of medication administration. If discrepancies are noted, the practitioner can clarify them with M.C. right away as part of the intervention. The PMR should also include a section to list medication allergies. The type of reaction should also be included on the PMR so that other providers will know the severity of the medication allergy (i.e., intolerance vs. anaphylactic reaction). Based on data gathered from the pharmacy computer and M.C., a PMR (depicted in Fig. 1-3) could be developed.

Reviewing the medications alone often does not provide enough information to determine whether M.C. is experiencing a medication-related event. Further questioning may be necessary. M.C. should be asked questions such as "What other medications have you tried in the past?" "How often do you experience muscle weakness and soreness?" "Which muscles are hurting?" "Show me where the problem is," "What do you think is causing the problem?" or "Describe the problem you are experiencing in more detail." Asking questions related to the onset of her symptoms of muscle soreness and weakness will help to determine whether this is a medication-related problem.

The practitioner can develop an assessment from this questioning and the PMR of the current problem that she is experiencing. As indicated on the PMR, M.C. started rosuvastatin most recently. The initiation of this medication corresponds to the onset of her recent soreness and weakness. β-Hydroxy-β-methylglutaryl-CoA (HMG-CoA) reductase inhibitors like rosuvastatin are known to cause myositis, or muscle breakdown, which may lead to weakness and muscle soreness. Furthermore, the prescribed dose is high for a woman of M.C.'s age. Based on this information, an assessment of the problem can be pursued. If rosuvastatin is the suspected agent, the plan would include actions necessary to solve the problem or to determine whether rosuvastatin is the cause of her muscle soreness and weakness. Unfortunately, not all of the necessary information is available (e.g., her baseline cholesterol, serum creatinine, liver function tests, or creatine kinase levels) to develop a formal plan of action to resolve the adverse medication event. However, part of the plan may be to obtain the laboratory test results necessary to identify or act on the adverse medication event. An example of the documentation of the SOAP note follows.

PRIMARY PROBLEM:
Muscle soreness and weakness (possible adverse medication event)

SUBJECTIVE:
M.C. reports weakness and soreness, predominantly in her legs during the past 3 weeks. She has difficulty rising from her chair after sitting for long periods and describes the pain as aching. The patient reports taking her medications as prescribed and rarely misses a dose.

OBJECTIVE:
Total Cholesterol: 137 mg/dL; LDL-C: 56 mg/dL; HDL: 54 mg/dL; Triglycerides: 136 mg/dL
Temperature: 98.5°F

ASSESSMENT:
M.C. has muscle weakness and soreness in her large muscle groups. She is currently at the recommended LDL-C goal level for a person with diabetes and hypertension per NCEP ATP III guidelines (very-high-risk LDL-C goal is <70 mg/dL).[24] Her current lipid therapy is rosuvastatin 40 mg once daily, which was started by her cardiologist 6 weeks ago. The initiation of rosuvastatin 40 mg correlates to the timing of her muscle soreness and weakness. HMG-CoA reductase inhibitors (i.e., rosuvastatin) are known to cause myositis or myalgias, and this patient is at particular risk given her age, sex, and starting dose. It is possible that the rosuvastatin could be causing her muscle soreness and weakness. Other lipid-lowering agents could be tried or the dose of rosuvastatin could be reduced, which might eliminate or reduce this adverse event. A creatine kinase level should be obtained to determine the severity of the myositis. A serum creatinine should also be measured, as myositis can lead to renal damage and rhabdomyolysis in severe cases; however, this is usually accompanied by fever and other symptoms that the patient is not currently experiencing.

PLAN:
1. **DRUG-RELATED ADVERSE EVENT:**
   - Discussed the possibility of an adverse medication event with the patient, which included the signs and symptoms of myalgias and myositis.
   - Contacted Dr. Hart (M.C.'s cardiologist) to discuss the current problem with rosuvastatin.
   - Per discussion with Dr. Hart, will obtain a creatine kinase level and serum creatinine.
   - Discontinue rosuvastatin per the pharmacist's recommendation. Dr. Hart agreed that M.C. should temporarily stop her rosuvastatin until her laboratory values are reviewed.
   - Alternative dosing of rosuvastatin 5 mg or another equivalent agent (atorvastatin 10 mg or simvastatin 20 mg) was discussed with Dr. Hart.
   - M.C. is to see Dr. Hart in the cardiology clinic in 2 days to discuss the laboratory values and alternative therapies.
   - Discussed the entire plan with M.C., and she verbalized understanding of steps that she is to take with respect to her current medication-induced problem.

CASE 1-5, QUESTION 2: From M.C.'s medication profile, what other problems can be identified with her medication therapy? What can be done to address these issues?

There are three remaining issues that may need to be addressed. The first issue relates to the pain medicine (indomethacin) that M.C. is taking. It is suggested that indomethacin may have a higher rate of central nervous system side effects in the elderly compared with other agents in the same class.[25] Furthermore, the American Geriatric Society guidelines on the management of mild to moderate persistent pain caution the use of nonsteroidal anti-inflammatory agents in older adults, preferring acetaminophen as a first-line agent.[26] Other prescription medications such as hydrocodone/acetaminophen or nonprescription medication such as acetaminophen alone could be used to help treat M.C.'s pain (see Chapter 7, Pain and Its Management, and Chapter 102, Geriatric Drug Use). Second, it is not clear from the current information whether the various providers are communicating. It is the responsibility of the pharmacist to help coordinate care among multiple prescribers as described by the APhA MTMS consensus document.[4] Therefore, it is important to be sure that both providers (Drs. Smith and Hart) receive a copy of the documentation of the issues addressed during the visit (SOAP note).

Finally, M.C. came into the pharmacy asking for help with her medication costs. To assess this problem, it is important to ask whether there are specific cost issues with a particular drug or whether it is her overall medication regimen that causes her concern. Another important question to ask is whether she has stopped taking any medications or changed the way that she takes her medications because of cost. Many patients will discuss cost and adherence issues with their pharmacist, because the point of sale for medications occurs at the pharmacy. However, they may not discuss this problem with the prescriber. Cost and nonadherence due to cost may be medication-related problems that the pharmacist must communicate to the prescriber on behalf of the patient. In assessing drug cost, there are several steps that can be taken. First, determine the patient's ability to pay for medications; implement low-cost, medically appropriate interventions targeted to patient needs; facilitate enrollment into relevant benefit programs; and confirm medication changes with the patient and prescribers (Table 1-5).

TABLE 1-5
Cost Containment Strategies

Patient With Prescription Drug Coverage
- Maximize generic drugs
- Maximize formulary coverage
- Switch to agents covered on the least expensive formulary tier
- If patient has Medicare Part D, determine eligibility for low-income subsidy through the Social Security Administration
- Consider mail-order prescription programs

Uninsured Patient
- Use low-cost generic programs (e.g., Rx Outreach, Costco, Wal-Mart, Target generic programs)
- Switch to therapeutically equivalent lower-cost brand name drugs when generics are unavailable
- Consider tablet splitting, if appropriate
- Consider pharmaceutical industry–sponsored patient assistance programs or foundation-sponsored copay-assistance programs
- Determine whether the patient is eligible for Medicaid, Medicare, Medicare Part D, or other assistance programs

For M.C., the rosuvastatin is her biggest concern, as it costs $60 per month and her Medicare Part D plan lists it as a nonpreferred (tier 3) agent on the formulary. With the possible discontinuation of her rosuvastatin, it is important for the pharmacist to anticipate her need for an alternative lipid-lowering agent and to determine whether there are cost-effective formulary alternatives that may be appropriate. This information can then be relayed to the prescriber. Furthermore, the alternative lipid-lowering formulary choice can be integrated into the plan developed for the primary issue of muscle soreness and weakness (see Case 1-5, Question 1). The integration of multiple problems is a complicated but important aspect of the MAP.

CASE 1-5, QUESTION 3: What additional information can be provided to M.C. at this time?

As discussed previously, an important part of MTMS involves the MAP. The MAP is a document that may empower the patient and promote self-care. The information on the MAP is important for both the patient and provider and facilitates communication among multiple providers. When a patient presents the PMR and MAP to all providers, complex medication information can be shared across the continuum of care. An example of M.C.'s MAP is included in Figure 1-3.

Because extensive information was communicated to the patient and other providers, follow-up (phone or face-to-face) would be appropriate and necessary to determine the resolution to the medication-related issues identified. Follow-up should occur in a timely manner, likely after M.C. has obtained the necessary laboratory test results and has been evaluated by her cardiologist as outlined in the plan. The follow-up should include questions related to the changes that were (or were not) made based on the practitioner recommendations and any new issues that have surfaced. Follow-up should be considered after any encounter in which an action plan is developed to determine whether the medication-related problem has been resolved. Additionally, problems may be identified and prioritized during the initial visit but, because of time constraints, may not be addressed. A follow-up visit allows for assessment of these problems.

CASE 1-5, QUESTION 4: Assuming that the pharmacy provider had an NPI number and a contract with M.C.'s Medicare Part D prescription drug plan, how could the 30 minutes spent with M.C. be billed to her insurance?

Provided that M.C. was identified by her Medicare prescription drug plan as eligible for MTMS, the practitioner could bill for the 30-minute encounter. Using the practitioner's NPI number and the appropriate CPT codes, the practitioner could bill for one CPT 99605 (for the first 15 minutes of initial face-to-face MTM encounter) and one CPT 99607 (for an additional 15 minutes spent with the patient in a face-to-face MTM encounter). M.C.'s Medicare Part D plan may require the practitioner to bill the prescription drug plan initially, and then the plan would pay the community pharmacy directly instead of reimbursing the individual pharmacist. Documentation of the visit would need to be stored at the site of the encounter in case any information was requested from M.C.'s prescription drug plan.

MEDICATION THERAPY MANAGEMENT IN THE ACUTE CARE SETTING

CASE 1-5, QUESTION 5: M.C. has just been hospitalized in a large medical center for renal failure and urosepsis. The pharmacist has access to the medical chart, nursing record, MAR, and a computer that directly links to the clinical laboratory. The pharmacists at this facility assess the patient's drug therapy and routinely provide clinical pharmacokinetic monitoring. How would the pharmacist approach M.C. differently in this inpatient setting compared with the pharmacist in Question 1 who worked in a community pharmacy?

Similar to the outpatient setting, the SOAP format is often used when documenting the encounter of the hospitalized patient; however, obtaining the information needed poses unique challenges. In this setting, subjective information may be more difficult to obtain at the time of assessment in those patients presenting with cognitive impairment resulting from their acute condition, such as the seriously ill or injured patient. Objective data, on the other hand, are more readily available and retrievable with access to pharmacy, laboratory, and other medical record information. On admission to the health care facility, the medication reconciliation process should be initiated to identify any variances in the admission orders when compared with the patient's home medication list. With acute medical problems superimposed on chronic conditions, it is not unusual to have new medications added and home medications held, changed, or discontinued.

Assessing the appropriateness of drug therapy requires a basic understanding of both pharmacokinetic (e.g., absorption, distribution, metabolism, and elimination of the drug) and pharmacodynamic (e.g., the relief of pain with an analgesic or reduction of BP with an antihypertensive agent) principles. This detailed assessment and monitoring is dependent on the availability of robust patient and laboratory data. The inpatient setting is a relatively data-rich environment in which access to needed information is generally readily available. Knowledge of the patient's height, body weight, and hepatic and renal function are essential for proper dosage considerations. The type of hospitalized patient will vary from the short-stay, otherwise healthy elective surgery patient to the critically ill, hemodynamically compromised patient. The pharmacist must be intimately aware of how pharmacokinetics and pharmacodynamics can be markedly altered throughout the hospitalization or disease-state process in each patient evaluated. This heightened awareness will allow for timely interventions and minimize medication errors resulting from improper or delayed dosage adjustments as the clinical status of the patient changes. Drug level monitoring may be suitable for certain medications and is of great clinical value; nevertheless, it is important to take into consideration clinical response to drug therapy along with the assessment of a specific laboratory value. Accurate interpretation of any drug level requires review of the nursing MAR (or eMAR), evaluating time of drug administration to that of serum sample acquisition. When serum drug levels are obtained, they must be reviewed for validity before alterations in medication regimens are made. If a serum drug concentration seems unusually high or low, the clinician must consider all of the various factors that might influence the serum concentration of the drug in that particular patient. When the reason for an unexpected abnormal serum drug concentration is not apparent, the test should be repeated before considering a dose change that may cause supratherapeutic or subtherapeutic concentrations resulting from erroneous data.

When M.C. was seen in the community pharmacy, the pharmacist assessed her chronic conditions (diabetes, hypertension, and hyperlipidemia, as well as her cost issues), and her drug therapy. Monitoring in the community pharmacy–based MTM program occurs at regular time intervals and is less sensitive to the day-to-day changes of the patient. However, in the inpatient setting, M.C. has acute conditions (renal failure and urosepsis) superimposed on her chronic conditions. Monitoring of medication therapy will occur frequently, resulting in a dynamic treatment plan for her acute and chronic conditions.

Although the inpatient setting is relatively data rich, the information gathered and the assessment and plan formulated in the facility must be communicated to other providers once the patient is discharged. At discharge, it is critical to ensure that the patient has follow-up with his or her primary care physician or coordinated care team in a timely fashion. At this point, it is again critical for the pharmacist to perform medication reconciliation to determine exactly what did happen once the patient returned home. This closes the loop at a critical time when the patient is prone to medication errors and readmission.

CONCLUSION

Interventions in any setting require interdisciplinary communication, assessment of patient-specific needs, and documentation of the visit. The health care system is complicated, and it is often difficult for the patient to effectively navigate. Consistency and follow-through are important to both patients and other providers regardless of MTMS setting. As illustrated in Figure 1-1, communication to the patient, documentation by using the SOAP note and the MAP, and follow-up are all closely correlated. To develop a successful and coordinated action plan, information must be gathered in an organized and concise fashion. This information, if properly documented and shared with other providers, will improve the coordination of care and lead to safe and effective medication use throughout the patient's experience with the health care system.

ACKNOWLEDGMENT

The authors acknowledge Mary Anne Koda-Kimble, Wayne Kradjan, Robin Corelli, Lloyd Young, B. Joseph Guglielmo, and Brian Alldredge for their contributions to the version of this chapter found in previous editions.

KEY REFERENCES AND WEBSITES

A full list of references for this chapter can be found at **http://thepoint.lww.com/AT10e**. Below are the key references and websites for this chapter, with the corresponding reference number in this chapter found in parentheses after the reference.

Key References

American Pharmacists Association; National Association of Chain Drug Stores Foundation. Medication therapy management in pharmacy practice: core elements of an MTM service model (version 2.0). *J Am Pharm Assoc (2003)*. 2008;48(3):341. (18)

Bluml BM. Definition of medication therapy management: development of professionwide consensus. *J Am Pharm Assoc (2003)*. 2005;45(5):566. (5)

Cipolle RJ et al., eds. *Pharmaceutical Care Practice: The Clinician's Guide*. 2nd ed. New York, NY: McGraw-Hill; 2004. (11)

Health Information Technology: Initial Set of Standards, Implementation Specifications, and Certification Criteria for Electronic Health Record Technology. *Fed Regist*. 2010;75(144):44589. (12)

Health Care and Education Reconciliation Act of 2010. Pub L No. 111-152, 124 Stat 1029. (2)

Hepler CD, Strand LM. Opportunities and responsibilities in pharmaceutical care. *Am J Hosp Pharm*. 1990;47(3):533. (6)

Medicare Prescription Drug, Improvement, and Modernization Act of 2003 (MMA). Cost and Utilization Management; Quality Assurance; Medication Therapy Management Program. Pub L No. 108-173, 117 Stat 2070. (4)

Patient Protection and Affordable Care Act (PPACA). Pub L No. 111-148, 124 Stat 119. (1)

Rovers JP, Currie JD, eds. *A Practical Guide to Pharmaceutical Care: A Clinical Skills Primer*. 3rd ed. Washington, DC: American Pharmacists Association; 2007. (7)

Key Websites

National Patient Safety Goals. Joint Commission on Accreditation of Healthcare Organizations. **http://www.jointcommission.org/PatientSafety/NationalPatientSafetyGoals/**. Accessed June 1, 2008. (10)

2 Interpretation of Clinical Laboratory Tests

Catrina R. Schwartz and Mark W. Garrison

CORE PRINCIPLES

	CHAPTER CASES
1 Laboratory findings should be used to compliment other subjective and objective findings and must not be evaluated in isolation. The values must be assessed in context of the clinical situation and incorporate understanding of human physiology.	**Case 2-1 (Questions 1–3), Case 2-4 (Question 1), Case 2-5 (Question 1), Case 2-7 (Question 1), Case 2-8 (Question 1)**
2 Lack of availability, expense, or inconvenience may limit the usefulness of some clinical laboratory tests. Estimations by means of equations or nomograms may be used in clinical practice to overcome these barriers.	**Case 2-2 (Questions 1, 2), Case 2-4 (Question 1)**
3 Test reliability is impacted by various factors including statistical and preanalytical variations, accuracy, and precision.	**Case 2-3 (Question 1), Table 2-1**
4 Laboratory findings can be helpful in assessing clinical disorders, establishing a diagnosis, assessing drug therapy, or evaluating disease progression.	**Case 2-6 (Question 1), Case 2-9 (Question 1), Case 2-10 (Question 1), Case 2-11 (Question 1)**

This chapter provides the reader with an overview of laboratory tests commonly used in clinical practice. Specialized laboratory tests, which are used to monitor specific disease states or specific drug therapies, are integrated into the case histories, questions, and answers in the disease-specific chapters of this textbook. Over-the-counter or patient-directed laboratory tests are briefly presented at the end of this chapter because of their increased availability and use. The most recent edition of a complete laboratory reference book should be reviewed when comprehensive understanding of clinical laboratory tests is required.[1,2]

GENERAL PRINCIPLES

Generally, laboratory tests should be ordered only if the results of the test will affect decisions about the care of the patient. Serum, urine, and other bodily fluids can be analyzed routinely; however, the economic cost and impact on the quality of life related to obtaining these data must always be balanced by benefit to patient-specific outcomes.

Reference Ranges

The term *reference range* is typically preferred in clinical practice rather than *normal range* as there are several factors that contribute to the "normal" value for each individual. Laboratory findings, within and outside the reference range, can be helpful in assessing clinical disorders, establishing a diagnosis, assessing drug therapy, or evaluating disease progression. In addition, baseline laboratory tests are often necessary to evaluate disease progression and response to therapy or to monitor the development of toxicities associated with therapy.

For a multimedia slide set describing general principles of laboratory testing, go to http://thepoint.lww.com/AT10e

When assessing laboratory findings it is important to be mindful that values outside the reference range may not require clinical intervention. Values must be assessed in context of the clinical situation and incorporate understanding of human physiology. Likewise, values that fall within the reference range may need further assessment secondary to limitations of the test or impact of biologic or physiologic considerations. Laboratory findings should also be used to compliment other subjective and objective findings and must not be evaluated in isolation.

Laboratory test results are specific to the clinical laboratory conducting the test and can vary based on the type of equipment and testing methods used. Consequently, clinicians should rely

TABLE 2-1
Preanalytical Variation: Factors Affecting the Test Result From the Time the Test Is Ordered Until It Arrives at the Laboratory

Variable	Example(s)
Incorrect test ordered	Albumin ordered to assess impact of recent dietary change (prealbumin better marker for acute changes)
Sample incorrectly labeled	Sample obtained from one patient and labeled with another name
Improper preparation for test	Fasting indicated but not followed: fasting glucose, complete lipid panel Pretest medications not administered in the appropriate manner Pretest diet restrictions not met: rare meat ingested before guaiac test
Medication	Medication interfered with testing procedure or by pharmacologic effect: β-agonist can reduce serum potassium concentrations, thiazides can increase serum uric acid levels
Improper timing of test	Vancomycin trough taken after first dose (rather than before the 4th dose) aPTT measured 2 hours after initial dose (rather than 6 hours after start) Fasting glucose test completed shortly after a meal, TSH measured 2 weeks after dose change (rather than 4–6 weeks after change)
Collection incomplete or improper	Abnormal 24-hour urine collection secondary to patient forgetting to void in provided container, blood specimen obtained from extremity with IV infusion site resulting in dilutional effect of glucose, BUN, and electrolytes, specimen collected in incorrect container.
Improper handling or storage	Hyperkalemia because of hydrolysis of blood specimen
Poor accuracy or precision	Faulty or outdated laboratory reagents in use
Technical	Result incorrectly read, computer keying error
Sex	Many laboratory findings are sex-dependent
Age	Neonatal, pediatric, adult, and geriatric populations have unique reference ranges for numerous laboratory tests
Pregnancy	Gestational status impacts numerous laboratory findings: alkaline phosphatase, cholesterol, iron, etc.
Posture	Being in upright position during laboratory sampling can increase albumin, calcium, iron, etc.
Exercise	Strenuous exercise before testing can impact lactate, creatine kinase, ALT, AST, uric acid, etc.
Normal physiologic fluctuations	Circadian rhythm can impact cortisol, serum iron, serum creatinine, WBC count, etc.
Medical procedures	Blood transfusion with red blood cells before hemoglobin A_{1c} measured result in normal A_{1c} for poorly controlled individual with diabetes, creatine kinase elevated secondary to recent cardioversion

A_{1c}, hemoglobin A_{1c} (also glycosylated hemoglobin); ALT, alanine aminotransferase; aPTT, activated partial thromboplastin time; AST, aspartate aminotransferase; BUN, blood urea nitrogen; IV, intravenous; TSH, thyroid-stimulating hormone; WBC, white blood cell.

on reference ranges listed by their own clinical laboratory when assessing laboratory tests.

Evaluating Laboratory Results

The reference ranges provided in this chapter are for general illustrative purposes. When applying this information to the clinical setting, appropriate clinical assessment and judgment should be applied. Patient-specific attributes such as the individual's age, sex, race, clinical presentation, lifestyle, and so forth are factors that may influence reported laboratory results and, therefore, must be taken into consideration. Statistical and preanalytical variations are common and must also be evaluated in context of the result obtained. Refer to Table 2-1 for examples of common preanalytical variables.

Test Reliability

As a result of probability, if the same test is completed multiple times on the same sample, typically 1 of 20 results or 5% will be reported outside of the provided reference range. Indicators of test reliability include accuracy, precision, sensitivity, and specificity. Precision refers to the repeatability of a laboratory test (i.e., test results fall within a similar value when repeated), whereas accuracy is the ability of a test to provide a result that is reflective of the "true" value (i.e., the test result matches the actual real value). Quality control and assurance practices at each laboratory are monitored regularly to ensure reliability of results. Typically, if a result is obtained that is significantly outside the reference range, the laboratory will repeat the test to confirm or refute the finding.

Research studies generally establish the sensitivity and specificity of laboratory tests. Clinically these are essential to distinguish the presence or absence of a disease or condition. Sensitivity is the ability of the test to correctly identify the disease or condition. If a test is 95% sensitive, then 95% of the individuals will be correctly identified as having the disease or condition, but 5% will have a negative test result even though they have the disease or condition (false negative). Specificity is the ability of the test to rule out individuals who do not have the disease or condition. If a test is 95% specific, then 95% of the individuals without disease will have a correct negative result, but 5% will be identified as having the disease or condition even though they are negative (false positive).

Units of Measure

The International System of Units (SI) reports clinical laboratory values using the metric system. The basic unit of mass for the SI system is the *mole*, which is not influenced by the added weight of salt or ester formulations. Therefore, the mole is technically and pharmacologically more meaningful than the gram because each physiological reaction occurs on a molecular level. Efforts to implement the SI system internationally for laboratory test reports have been resisted in the United States. Despite adopting SI transition policies in the late 1980s, major American medical journals have since reverted back to the traditional units for laboratory test reporting.[3,4] In this chapter, reference ranges for common laboratory tests are presented in both conventional and SI units, along with "conversion factors" to interchange traditional and SI units (Tables 2-2 and 2-3).

TABLE 2-2
Blood Chemistry Reference Values

Laboratory Test	Normal Reference Values: Conventional Units	Normal Reference Values: SI Units	Conversion Factor	Comments
Electrolytes				
Sodium	135–145 mEq/L	135–145 mmol/L	1	Low sodium is usually caused by excess water (e.g., ↑ serum antidiuretic hormone) and is treated with water restriction. ↑ in severe dehydration, diabetes insipidus, significant renal and GI losses.
Potassium	3.5–5 mEq/L	3.5–5 mmol/L	1	↑ with renal dysfunction, acidosis, K-sparing diuretics, hemolysis, burns, crush injuries. ↓ by diuretics, alkalosis, severe vomiting and diarrhea, heavy NG suctioning.
CO_2 content	22–28 mEq/L	22–28 mmol/L	1	Sum of HCO_3^- and dissolved CO_2. Reflects acid–base balance and compensatory pulmonary (CO_2) and renal (HCO_3^-) mechanisms. Primarily reflects HCO_3^-.
Chloride	95–105 mEq/L	95–105 mmol/L	1	Important for acid–base balance. ↓ by GI loss of chloride-rich fluid (vomiting, diarrhea, GI suction, intestinal fistulas, overdiuresis).
BUN	8–20 mg/dL	2.8–7.1 mmol/L	0.357	End product of protein metabolism, produced by liver, transported in blood, excreted renally. ↑ in renal dysfunction, high protein intake, upper GI bleeding, volume contraction.
Creatinine	0.6–1.2 mg/dL	53–106 μmol/L	88.4	Major constituent of muscle; rate of formation constant; affected by muscle mass (lower with aging); excreted renally. ↑ in renal dysfunction. Used as a primary marker for renal function (GFR).
CrCl	90–130 mL/min	1.5–2.16 mL/s	0.01667	Reflects GFR; ↓ in renal dysfunction. Used to adjust dosage of renally eliminated drugs.
Estimated GFR	90–120 mL/min per 1.73 m^2	n/a	n/a	Possibly a more accurate reflection of renal function than CrCl. Still influenced by muscle mass.
Cystatin C	<1.0 mg/dL	<0.749 μmol/L	0.749	Indicator of renal function—not influenced by patient muscle mass, age, or sex. May also help predict patients at risk for cardiovascular disease.
Glucose (fasting)	70–99 mg/dL	3.9–5.5 mmol/L	0.05551	↑ in diabetes or by adrenal corticosteroids.
Glycosylated hemoglobin	<4–5.6%	<4–5.6%	1	Used to assess average blood glucose during 1–3 months. Helpful for monitoring chronic blood glucose control in patients with diabetes. Values >8% seen in patients with poor glucose control.
Calcium—total	8.5–10.5 mg/dL	2.1–2.6 mmol/L	0.250	Regulated by body skeleton redistribution, parathyroid hormone, vitamin D, calcitonin. Affected by changes in albumin concentration. ↓ by hypothyroidism, loop diuretics, vitamin D deficiency; ↑ in malignancy and hyperthyroidism.
Calcium—unbound	4.5–5.6 mg/dL	1.13–1.4 mmol/L	0.250	Physiologically active form. Unbound "free" calcium remains unchanged as albumin fluctuates. Total calcium ↓ when albumin ↓.
Magnesium	1.5–2.4 mEq/L	0.75–1.2 mmol/L	0.51	↓ in malabsorption, severe diarrhea, alcoholism, pancreatitis, diuretics, hyperaldosteronism (symptoms of weakness, depression, agitation, seizures, hypokalemia, arrhythmias). ↑ in renal failure, hypothyroidism, magnesium-containing antacids.
Phosphate[a]	2.5–4.5 mg/dL	0.8–1.45 mmol/L	0.323	↑ with renal dysfunction, hypervitaminosis D, hypocalcemia, hypoparathyroidism. ↓ with excess aluminum antacids, malabsorption, renal losses, hypercalcemia, refeeding syndrome.
Uric acid	<7 mg/dL	<0.42 mmol/L	0.06	↑ in gout, neoplastic, or myeloproliferative disorders, and drugs (diuretics, niacin, low-dose salicylate, cyclosporine).
Proteins				
Prealbumin	15–36 mg/dL	150–360 mg/L	10	Indicates acute changes in nutritional status, useful for monitoring TPN.
Albumin	3.3–4.8 g/dL	33–48 g/L	10	Produced in liver; important for intravascular osmotic pressure. ↓ in liver disease, malnutrition, ascites, hemorrhage, protein-wasting nephropathy. May influence highly protein-bound drugs.
Globulin	2.3–3.5 g/dL	23–35 g/L	10	Active role in immunologic mechanisms. Immunoglobulins ↑ in chronic infection, rheumatoid arthritis, multiple myeloma.

(continued)

TABLE 2-2
Blood Chemistry Reference Values *(Continued)*

Laboratory Test	Normal Reference Values: Conventional Units	Normal Reference Values: SI Units	Conversion Factor	Comments
Cardiac Markers				
CK	<150 units/L	<2.5 μkat/L	0.01667	In tissues that use high energy (skeletal muscle, myocardium, brain). ↑ by IM injections, MI, acute psychotic episodes. Isoenzyme CK-MM in skeletal muscle; CK-MB in myocardium; CK-BB in brain. MB fraction >5%–6% suggests acute MI.
CK-MB	0–12 units/L	0–0.2 μkat/L	0.01667	
cTnI	<1.5 ng/mL	<1.5 mcg/L	1	More specific than CK-MB for myocardial damage, elevated sooner and remains elevated longer than CK-MB. cTnI >2.0 suggests acute myocardial injury.
Myoglobin	<90 mcg/L	<90 mcg/L	1	Early elevation (within 3 hours), but less specific for myocardial injury compared with CK-MB.
Homocysteine	4.6–11.9 μmol/L	4.6–11.9 μmol/L	1	Damages vessel endothelial, which may increase the risk for cardiac disease. Associated with deficiencies in folate, vitamin B_6, and vitamin B_{12}.
LDH	<200 units/L	<3.33 μkat/L	0.01667	High in heart, kidney, liver, and skeletal muscle. Five isoenzymes: LD1 and LD2 mostly in heart, LD5 mostly in liver and skeletal muscle, LD3 and LD4 are nonspecific. ↑ in malignancy, extensive burns, PE, renal disease.
BNP	<100 pg/mL	<100 ng/L	1	BNP >500 ng/L indicates left ventricular dysfunction. Released from heart with ↑ workload placed on heart (e.g., CHF).
NT-proBNP	<60 pg/mL males <150 pg/mL females	<60 ng/L males <150 ng/L females	1	Component of a precursor to BNP. NT-proBNP has similar clinical utility to BNP as a marker for cardiovascular disease.
CRP	0–1.6 mg/dL	0–16 mg/L	1	Nonspecific indicator of acute inflammation. Similar to ESR, but more rapid onset and greater elevation. CRP >3 mg/dL increases risk of cardiovascular disease.
hs-CRP	0–2.0 mg/L	0–2.0 mg/L	1	More sensitive measure of CRP; concentrations from 0.5–10 mg/L; hs-CRP <1.0 mg/L low risk for cardiovascular disease; 1.0–3.0 mg/L average risk; and >3.0 mg/L high risk for cardiovascular disease.
Liver Function				
AST	0–35 units/L	0–0.58 μkat/L	0.01667	Large amounts in heart and liver; moderate amounts in muscle, kidney, and pancreas. ↑ with MI and liver injury. Less liver specific than ALT.
ALT	0–35 units/L	0–0.58 μkat/L	0.01667	From heart, liver, muscle, kidney, pancreas. ↑ negligible unless parenchymal liver disease. More liver specific than AST.
ALP	30–120 units/L	0.5–2.0 μkat/L	0.01667	Large amounts in bile ducts, placenta, bone. ↑ in bile duct obstruction, obstructive liver disease, rapid bone growth (e.g., Paget disease), pregnancy.
GGT	0–70 units/L	0–1.17 μkat/L	0.01667	Sensitive test reflecting hepatocellular injury; not helpful in differentiating liver disorders. Usually high in chronic alcoholics.
Bilirubin—total	0.1–1 mg/dL	1.7–17.1 μmol/L	17.1	Breakdown product of hemoglobin, bound to albumin, conjugated in liver. Total bilirubin includes direct (conjugated) and indirect bilirubin. ↑ with hemolysis, cholestasis, liver injury.
Bilirubin—direct	0–0.2 mg/dL	0–3.4 μmol/L	17.1	
Miscellaneous				
Amylase	35–120 units/L	0.58–2.0 μkat/L	0.01667	Pancreatic enzyme; ↑ in pancreatitis or duct obstruction.
Lipase	0–160 units/L	0–2.67 μkat/L	0.01667	Pancreatic enzyme, ↑ acute pancreatitis, elevated for longer period than amylase.
PSA	0–4 ng/mL	0–4 mcg/L	1	↑ in benign prostatic hypertrophy (BPH) and also in prostate cancer. PSA levels of 4–10 ng/mL should be worked up. Risk of prostate cancer increased if free PSA/total PSA <0.25.
TSH	0.4–5 μunits/mL	0.4–5 munits/L	1	↑ TSH in primary hypothyroidism requires exogenous thyroid supplementation.
Procalcitonin	<0.5 ng/mL	<0.5 mcg/L	1	↑ Bacterial infections—low risk of sepsis if <0.5 ng/mL; high risk of severe sepsis if >2.0 ng/mL. May assist in when to start/stop antibiotic therapy.

(continued)

TABLE 2-2
Blood Chemistry Reference Values *(Continued)*

Laboratory Test	Normal Reference Values: Conventional Units	SI Units	Conversion Factor	Comments
Cholesterol				
Total	<200 mg/dL	<5.2 mmol/L	0.02586	Desirable = Total <200; LDL 70–160 (depends on risk factors); HDL >45 mg/dL; ↑ LDL or ↓ HDL are risk factors for cardiovascular disease. Consult NCEP and ATP guidelines for most current target goals and description of patient risk factors.
LDL	70–160 mg/dL	<4.13 mmol/L	0.02586	
HDL	40 mg/dL	1.03 mmol/L	0.02586	
Triglycerides (fasting)	<150 mg/dL	<1.70 mmol/L	0.0113	↑ by alcohol, saturated fats, drugs (propranolol, diuretics, oral contraceptives). Obtain fasting level.

[a] Phosphate as inorganic phosphorus.
ALP, alkaline phosphatase; ALT, alanine aminotransferase; AST, aspartate aminotransferase; ATP, Adult Treatment Panel; BNP, brain natriuretic peptide; BPH, benign prostatic hypertrophy; BUN, blood urea nitrogen; CHF, congestive heart failure; CK, creatine kinase (formerly known as creatine phosphokinase); CrCl, creatinine clearance; CRP, C-reactive protein; cTnI, cardiac troponin I; ESR, erythrocyte sedimentation rate; GFR, glomerular filtration rate; GGT, gamma-glutamyl transferase; GI, gastrointestinal; HDL, high-density lipoprotein; IM, intramuscularly; LDH, lactate dehydrogenase; LDL, low-density lipoprotein; MI, myocardial infarction; NCEP, National Cholesterol Education Program; NG, nasogastric; PE, pulmonary embolism; PSA, prostate-specific antigen; SI, International System of Units; TPN, total parenteral nutrition; TSH, thyroid-stimulating hormone.

FLUIDS AND ELECTROLYTES

Sodium

Reference Range: 135–145 mEq/L or mmol/L

Sodium is the predominant cation of extracellular fluid (ECF). Only a small amount of sodium (~5 mEq/L) is in intracellular fluid (ICF). Along with chloride, potassium, and water, sodium is important in establishing serum osmolarity and osmotic pressure relationships between ICF and ECF. Dietary intake of sodium is balanced by renal excretion of sodium, which is regulated by aldosterone (enhances sodium reabsorption), natriuretic hormone (increases excretion of sodium), and antidiuretic hormone (enhances reabsorption of free water). An increase in the serum sodium concentration could suggest either impaired sodium excretion or volume contraction. Conversely, a decrease in the serum sodium concentration to less-than-normal values could reflect hypervolemia, abnormal sodium losses, or sodium starvation. Although healthy individuals are able to maintain sodium homeostasis without difficulty, patients with kidney failure, heart failure, or pulmonary disease often encounter sodium and water imbalances. In adults, changes in serum sodium concentrations most often represent water imbalances rather than sodium imbalances. Hence, serum sodium concentrations are more reflective of a patient's fluid status rather than sodium balance.

HYPONATREMIA

Hyponatremia can result from dilution of the sodium concentration in serum or from a total body depletion of sodium. The finding of hyponatremia implies that sodium has been diluted throughout all body fluids because water moves freely across cell membranes in response to oncotic pressures. Dilutional hyponatremia occurs when the ECF compartment expands without an equivalent increase in sodium. Some clinical conditions (e.g., cirrhosis, congestive heart failure, renal impairment), as well as the administration of osmotically active solutes (e.g., albumin, mannitol), are commonly associated with dilutional hyponatremia. Hyponatremia that results from sodium depletion presents as a low serum sodium concentration in the absence of edema. Sodium-depletion hyponatremia can be caused by mineralocorticoid deficiencies, sodium-wasting renal disease, or replacement of sodium-containing fluid losses with nonsaline solutions.

HYPERNATREMIA

Hypernatremia represents a state of relative water deficiency and, therefore, excessive concentrations of sodium in all body fluids (hypertonicity). Hypernatremia can be caused by the loss of free water, loss of hypotonic fluid, or excessive sodium intake. Free water loss is uncommon, except in the presence of diabetes insipidus. Gastroenteritis is the most common cause of hypotonic fluid loss in infants and the elderly. Increased retention of sodium in patients with hyperaldosteronism can also increase serum sodium concentrations. Excessive salt intoxication is usually accidental or iatrogenic and most commonly results from inappropriate intravenous administration of hypertonic salt solutions. Some β-lactam antibiotics (e.g., ticarcillin) contain a modest sodium load and can cause fluid overload when high dosages are administered.

The primary defense against hypertonicity is thirst and subsequent fluid intake. Hypernatremic syndromes, therefore, usually occur in patients who are unable to drink sufficient fluids. For example, infants who cannot demand fluid are at greatest risk for the development of hypernatremia. Similarly, patients who are vomiting, comatose, or not allowed oral fluids are at risk for hypernatremia.

CASE 2-1

QUESTION 1: M.C., a 61-year-old woman with no known drug allergies (NKDA) is hospitalized with a chief complaint of increasing shortness of breath (SOB) and orthopnea during the past week. She has been treated previously for heart failure and has not taken any medication during the past 2 weeks. M.C. has severe (4+) pedal edema and is in respiratory distress. Laboratory tests were ordered and reported back as follows:

Sodium (Na), 123 mEq/L
Potassium (K), 4.1 mEq/L
Chloride (Cl), 90 mEq/L
Carbon dioxide (CO_2), 28 mEq/L

TABLE 2-3
Hematologic Laboratory Values

Laboratory Test	Normal Reference Values: Conventional Units	Normal Reference Values: SI Units	Comments
RBC count			
• Male	4.3–5.9 × $10^6/\mu L$	4.3–5.9 × $10^{12}/L$	
• Female	3.5–5.0 × $10^6/\mu L$	3.5–5.0 × $10^{12}/L$	↓ with anemias, bleeding, hemolysis. ↑ with polycythemia, chronic hypoxia.
Hct			
• Male	39%–49%	0.39–0.49	
• Female	33%–43%	0.33–0.43	Similar to Hct.
Hgb			
• Male	14–18 g/dL	140–180 g/L	
• Female	12–16 g/dL	120–160 g/L	
MCV	76–100 μm^3	76–100 fL[a]	Describes average RBC size; ↑ MCV = macrocytic, ↓ MCV = microcytic.
MCH	27–33 pg	27–33 pg	Measures average weight of Hgb in RBC.
MCHC	33–37 g/dL	330–370 g/L	More reliable index of RBC hemoglobin than MCH. Measures average concentration of Hgb in RBC. Concentration will not change with weight or size of RBC.
Reticulocyte count (adults)	0.1%–2.4%	0.001–0.024	Indicator of RBC production; ↑ suggests ↑ number of immature erythrocytes released in response to stimulus (e.g., iron in iron-deficiency anemia).
ESR			Nonspecific; ↑ with inflammation, infection, neoplasms, connective tissue disorders, pregnancy, nephritis. Useful monitor of temporal arteritis and polymyalgia rheumatica.
• Male	0–20 mm/h	0–20 mm/h	
• Female	0–30 mm/h	0–30 mm/h	
WBC count	4–11 × $10^3/\mu L$	4–11 × $10^9/L$	Consists of neutrophils, lymphocytes, monocytes, eosinophils, and basophils; ↑ in infection and stress.
ANC	2,000 cells/μL		ANC = WBC × (% neutrophils +% bands)/100; if <500 ↑ risk infection, if >1,000 ↓ risk infection.
Neutrophils	40%–70%	0.4–0.7	↑ in neutrophils suggests bacterial or fungal infection. ↑ in bands suggests bacterial infection.
Bands	3%–5%	0.03–0.05	
Lymphocytes	20%–40%	0.20–0.40	
Monocytes	0%–11%	0–0.11	
Eosinophils	0%–8%	0–0.08	Eosinophils ↑ with allergies and parasitic infections.
Basophils	0%–3%	<0.03	
Platelets	150–450 × $10^3/\mu L$	150–450 × $10^9/L$	<100 × $10^3/\mu L$ = thrombocytopenia; <20 × $10^3/\mu L$ = ↑ risk for severe bleeding.
Iron			
• Male	80–180 mcg/dL	14–32 $\mu mol/L$	Body stores two-thirds in Hgb; one-third in bone marrow, spleen, liver; only small amount present in plasma. Blood loss major cause of deficiency.
• Female	60–160 mcg/dL	11–29 $\mu mol/L$	↑ needs in pregnancy and lactation.
• TIBC	250–460 mcg/dL	45–82 $\mu mol/L$	↑ capacity to bind iron with iron deficiency.

[a] fL, femtoliter; femto, 10^{-15}; pico, 10^{-12}; nano, 10^{-9}; micro, 10^{-6}; milli, 10^{-3}.
ANC, absolute neutrophil count; ESR, erythrocyte sedimentation rate; Hct, hematocrit; Hgb, hemoglobin; MCH, mean corpuscular hemoglobin; MCHC, mean cell hemoglobin concentration; MCV, mean cell volume; RBC, red blood cell; SI, International System of Units; TIBC, total iron-binding capacity; WBC, white blood cell.

Blood urea nitrogen (BUN), 30 mg/dL
Serum creatinine (SCr), 1.3 mg/dL
Fasting glucose, 260 mg/dL

Should M.C. be given sodium chloride to return her serum sodium concentration to a normal value?

All body fluids are in osmotic equilibrium, and changes in serum sodium concentration are associated with shifts of water into and out of cells. M.C. has 4+ pedal edema and heart failure; her serum concentration of sodium is probably low because her plasma volume is increased relative to sodium. The serum sodium concentration in this case does not reflect total body sodium content. The usual treatment for this type of hyponatremia is salt and water restriction combined with diuresis in an attempt to remove the excess fluid associated with M.C.'s heart failure (see Chapters 10, Fluid and Electrolyte Disorders, and 19, Heart Failure). M.C. should not be given sodium chloride to return her serum concentration to normal. Her blood glucose level will be addressed later in this chapter.

Potassium

Reference Range: 3.5–5.0 mEq/L or mmol/L

Sodium is the major cation in the ECF, and potassium is the major intracellular cation in the body. The potassium ion in the ECF is filtered freely at the glomerulus of the kidney, reabsorbed in the proximal tubule, and secreted into the distal segments of the nephron. Because the majority of potassium is sequestered within cells, a serum potassium concentration is not a good measure of total body potassium. Intracellular potassium, however, cannot be measured easily. Fortunately, the clinical manifestations of potassium deficiency (e.g., fatigue, drowsiness, dizziness, confusion, electrocardiographic changes, muscle weakness, muscle pain) correlate well with serum concentrations. The serum potassium concentration is buffered and can be within normal limits despite abnormalities in total body potassium. During potassium depletion, potassium moves from the ICF into the ECF to maintain the serum concentration. When the serum concentration decreases by a mere 0.3 mEq/L, the total body potassium deficit is approximately 100 mEq. Serum potassium concentrations, therefore, can be misleading when interpreted in isolation from other considerations, and assumptions should not be made as to the status of total body potassium concentration based solely on a serum concentration measurement.

HYPOKALEMIA

The kidneys are responsible for about 90% of daily potassium loss (~40–90 mEq/day), and the remaining 10% of potassium excretion each day is managed by the gastrointestinal (GI) system and the dermatologic system (i.e., sweating). The kidneys, however, have only a limited ability to conserve potassium. Even when potassium intake has ceased, the urine will contain at least 5 to 20 mEq of potassium per 24 hours. Therefore, prolonged intravenous therapy with potassium-free solutions in a patient unable to obtain potassium in foods (e.g., nothing by mouth [NPO]) can result in hypokalemia. Hypokalemia can also be induced by osmotic diuresis (e.g., mannitol, glucosuria), thiazide or loop diuretics, excessive mineralocorticoid activity, or protracted vomiting. Although the fluid secreted along most of the upper GI tract contains only a modest amount of potassium (i.e., 5–20 mEq/L), vomiting can induce hypokalemia because of the combined effect from decreased food intake, loss of acid, alkalosis, and loss of sodium. The loss of large amounts of colonic fluid through severe diarrhea can cause potassium depletion because fluid in the colon is high in potassium content (i.e., 30–40 mEq/L). Insulin and stimulation of β_2-adrenergic receptors can also induce hypokalemia because both increase the movement of potassium into cells from the extracellular fluid. The magnitude of a potassium deficiency is difficult to establish because only 2% of the body's potassium is extracellular. Equation 2-1 can be used to estimate the potassium deficit with hypokalemia:

$$\text{Kdeficit (mmol)} = (K_{normal} - K_{measured}) \times \text{kg of body weight} \times 0.4 \quad \text{(Eq. 2-1)}$$

It is also important to note that hypomagnesemia often accompanies hypokalemia, as magnesium is necessary for the movement of sodium, potassium, and calcium in and out of cells. As a result, hypokalemic individuals not responding to potassium therapy may be refractory to treatment until hypomagnesemia is corrected. Often laboratories omit magnesium from the general electrolyte panel so this test may need to be specially ordered.

HYPERKALEMIA

Hyperkalemia most commonly results from decreased renal excretion of potassium, excessive exogenous potassium administration (especially when combined with a potassium-sparing diuretic), or excessive cellular breakdown (e.g., hemolysis, burns, crush injuries, surgery, infections). Metabolic acidosis also can induce hyperkalemia as hydrogen ions move into cells in exchange for potassium and sodium. Abnormal potassium concentrations in the serum primarily affect excitability of nerve and muscle tissue (e.g., myocardial tissue). As a result, arrhythmias can be induced by hyperkalemia or hypokalemia. Potassium also affects some enzyme systems and acid–base balance, as well as carbohydrate and protein metabolism.

CASE 2-1, QUESTION 2: M.C. also has type 1 diabetes mellitus, and is hospitalized a couple of months later for ketoacidosis. Her fasting blood glucose is 802 mg/dL, her urine output is 140 mL/hour, and her urine is positive (4+) for glucose and ketones. M.C.'s blood pH is 7.1, and her serum potassium concentration is 4.1 mEq/L. Although M.C.'s serum potassium concentration is normal, why is her serum potassium of concern?

When the pH of the blood is acidic, potassium shifts out of cells in response to increased concentrations of intracellular hydrogen ion. M.C.'s serum potassium concentration appears "normal" because acidosis has shifted potassium from intracellular storage sites into the circulating plasma volume. M.C's total-body potassium concentration is decreased as a result of both glycosuria and polyuria. As a result, treatment of M.C's diabetic ketoacidosis without supplemental potassium could result in significant hypokalemia. When her acidosis and hyperglycemia are treated, potassium ions will return intracellularly. If supplemental potassium is not provided, the serum potassium concentration will decrease dramatically. As a very general guideline, for every 0.1 decrease in pH from 7.4, the serum potassium concentration will be falsely elevated by about 0.6 mEq/L. With M.C's pH of 7.1, her reported serum potassium concentration of 4.1 mEq/L will actually be closer to 2.3 mEq/L when the acidosis is corrected (i.e., 0.6 mEq/L × three 0.1 pH units = falsely elevated by 1.8 mEq/L).

Carbon Dioxide Content

Reference Range: 22–28 mEq/L or mmol/L

The CO_2 content in the serum represents the sum of the bicarbonate concentration (HCO_3) and the concentration of dissolved CO_2 in the serum. The dissolved CO_2 represents a relatively small component of total CO_2 content, making CO_2 essentially a measure of the bicarbonate concentration in serum. Chloride and bicarbonate are the primary negatively charged anions that offset the positively charged cations (i.e., sodium, potassium).

Although several buffer systems (e.g., hemoglobin [Hgb], phosphate, protein) participate in regulating pH within physiological limits, the carbonic acid–bicarbonate system is the most important. From a clinical standpoint, most disturbances of acid–base balance result from imbalances of the carbonic acid–bicarbonate system. The importance of bicarbonate in maintaining physiological pH is presented in Chapter 9, Acid–Base Disorders.

Chloride

Reference Range: 95–105 mEq/L or mmol/L

Chloride is the principal inorganic anion of the ECF; changes in chloride concentration are usually related to sodium concentration in an effort to maintain a neutral charge. The serum chloride concentration per se has no real diagnostic significance. In fact, the only real reason for measuring the serum chloride is to validate the serum sodium concentration. The relationship between serum concentrations of sodium, bicarbonate, and chloride is described by Equation 2-2, where *R* represents the anion gap:

$$Cl^- + HCO_3^- + R = Na^+ \quad \text{(Eq. 2-2)}$$

As with bicarbonate, chloride contributes to maintaining acid–base balance. A decreased serum chloride concentration often accompanies metabolic alkalosis, whereas an increased serum chloride concentration may be indicative of a hyperchloremic metabolic acidosis. The serum chloride concentration, however, can also be slightly decreased in acidosis if organic acids or other acids are the primary cause of the acidosis. *Hyperchloremia*, in the absence of metabolic acidosis, is seldom encountered because chloride retention is usually accompanied by sodium and water retention. *Hypochloremia* can result from excessive GI loss of chloride-rich fluid (e.g., vomiting, diarrhea, gastric suctioning, intestinal fistulas). Because chloride ions are renally excreted with cations, hypochloremia may also result from significant diuresis.

Anion Gap

The *R* factor, or anion gap (AG), represents the contribution of unmeasured acids, such as lactate, phosphates, sulfates, and proteins. As displayed in Equation 2-2, a patient's anion gap is determined by subtracting the primary anions (Cl^- and HCO_3^-) from the primary cation (Na^+). Some clinicians include potassium in this determination and subtract the anions from both major cations (Na^+ and K^+). A normal anion gap is typically 5 to 12 mEq/mL if potassium is not incorporated in the calculation or less than 16 mEq/mL if potassium is considered.

An elevated anion gap may be indicative of a metabolic acidosis caused by an increase in lactic acids, ketoacids, salicylic acids, methanol, or ethylene glycol. A low anion gap may be the result of reduced concentrations of unmeasured anions (e.g., hypoalbuminemia) or from systematic underestimation of serum sodium (e.g., hyperviscosity of myeloma). Again, see Chapter 9, Acid–Base Disorders, for a more detailed discussion of the clinical use of the anion gap.

Blood Urea Nitrogen

Reference Range: 8–20 mg/dL or 2.8–7.1 mmol/L

Urea nitrogen is an end product of protein metabolism. It is produced solely by the liver, transported in the blood, and excreted by the kidneys. The serum concentration of urea nitrogen (i.e., BUN) is reflective of renal function because the urea nitrogen in blood is filtered completely at the glomerulus of the kidney, and then reabsorbed and tubularly secreted within nephrons. Acute or chronic renal failure is the most common cause of an elevated BUN. Although the BUN is an excellent screening test for renal dysfunction, it does not sufficiently quantify the extent of renal disease. In addition, several nonrenal factors such as unusually high protein intake and conditions that increase protein catabolism (or upper GI bleeding) can increase the BUN concentration. A patient's hydration status will also influence BUN; a water deficit tends to concentrate the urea nitrogen, and a water excess dilutes the urea nitrogen. The ratio of BUN to SCr can also be of clinical use. A normal ratio is roughly 15:1. Ratios greater than 20:1 are observed in patients with decreased blood flow to the kidney (e.g., prerenal disease such as dehydration or conditions involving reduced cardiac output) or conditions involving increased protein in the blood (e.g., dietary intake or an upper GI bleed). Situations in which the BUN:SCr ratio is less than 15:1 are seen in patients with renal failure, significant malnourishment (decreased intake of protein), or severe liver disease in which the liver is no longer able to form urea.

Creatinine

Reference Range: 0.6–1.2 mg/dL or 53–106 μmol/L

Creatinine is derived from creatine and phosphocreatine, major constituents of muscle. Its rate of formation for a given individual is remarkably constant and is determined primarily by an individual's muscle mass or lean body weight. Therefore, the SCr concentration is slightly higher in muscular subjects, but unlike the BUN, it is less directly affected by exogenous factors or liver impairment. Once creatinine is released from muscle into plasma, it is excreted renally almost exclusively by glomerular filtration. A decrease in the glomerular filtration rate (GFR) results in an increase in the SCr concentration. Thus, careful interpretation of the SCr concentration is used widely in the clinical evaluation of patients with suspected renal disease.

A doubling of the SCr level roughly corresponds to a 50% reduction in the GFR. This general rule of thumb only holds true for steady-state creatinine levels.[5]

CASE 2-1, QUESTION 3: M.C. was initiated on digoxin 0.125 mg orally once daily after IV loading doses. Serum creatinine was ordered to assess her renal function and need for potential dosage adjustment. The clinical laboratory determined her SCr was 1.2 mg/dL. Although this laboratory result is within normal limits, what would more accurately reflect her renal status?

An SCr of 1.2 mg/dL in M.C. does not necessarily reflect normal renal function. As patients become older, muscle mass represents a smaller proportion of total weight and creatinine production is decreased. Furthermore, the SCr concentration in female patients is generally 0.2 to 0.4 mg/dL (85%–90%) less than for males because females have less muscle mass. Because M.C. is a 61-year-old woman, a creatinine clearance (CrCl) determination would more accurately reflect her renal function status.

Creatinine Clearance

Reference Range: 90–130 mL/minute

Because creatinine is cleared almost exclusively through the glomerulus in the kidney, CrCl can be used as a clinically useful measure of a patient's GFR. CrCl serves as a valuable clinical parameter because many renally eliminated drugs are dose-adjusted based on the patient's renal function. To determine actual CrCl, the patient's urine is collected for a 24-hour period, and the concentration of urine creatinine (mg/dL), total volume of urine collected during the 24-hour period (mL/minute), and SCr (mg/dL) are determined. The patient-specific measured CrCl is determined using Equation 2-3:

$$\text{Measured 24 hr CrCl}_{(\text{mL/min})} = \frac{[\text{Urine conc}_{(\text{mg/dL})}] \times [\text{Total urine volume}_{(\text{mL/min})}]}{\text{SCr}_{(\text{mg/dL})}}$$

(Eq. 2-3)

Unfortunately, urine collections are time-consuming and expensive, and incomplete collections can substantially underestimate renal function. In lieu of measuring actual CrCl, simplistic equations are commonly used to estimate a patient's CrCl. The following Cockcroft-Gault formula incorporates age, body weight, and SCr.[6] Typically, clinicians use ideal body weight (IBW) in the calculation of estimated CrCl; however, actual body weight (ABW) may be used when ABW is less than IBW. Equation 2-4 has the highest correlation and the greatest accuracy in patients with SCr concentrations less than 1.5 mg/dL[7]:

$$\text{Estimated CrCl for males (mL/min)} = \frac{(140 - \text{Age})(\text{Body weight in kg})}{(72)(\text{SCr}_{(\text{mg/dL})})}$$

(Eq. 2-4)

The Cockcroft-Gault formula must be multiplied by 85% to calculate CrCl for females. Another commonly used approach to estimating CrCl is the Jelliffe method,[8] shown in Equation 2-5:

$$\text{Estimated CrCl for Males}(\text{mL/min/1.73m}^2) = \frac{98 - [(0.8)(\text{Age} - 20)]}{\text{SCr}_{(\text{mg/dL})}}$$

(Eq. 2-5)

This Jelliffe formula must be multiplied by 90% to calculate CrCl for females. The use of this method substantially underestimates CrCl for patients with SCr values less than 1.5 mg/dL,[9] whereas Cockcroft-Gault appears to have the highest correlation and greatest accuracy in patients with SCr values less than 1.5 mg/dL.[7] For patients with liver dysfunction, all methods of calculating CrCl from an SCr value are associated with significant overpredictions of CrCl.[9] Thus, methods for predicting CrCl should be used cautiously when attempting to adjust drug dosages in patients with liver disease.

CASE 2-2

QUESTION 1: A 24-hour CrCl determination was ordered for E.S., a 63-year-old, 60-kg white man. The following data were returned from the clinical laboratory (total collection time was 24 hours):

Total urine volume, 1,000 mL
Urine creatinine concentration, 42 mg/dL
SCr, 1.7 mg/dL

Determine both the measured and the estimated CrCl for E.S. based on the given data, and compare and contrast these results.

Using Equation 2-3, E.S. has a 24-hour measured CrCl of approximately 17 mL/minute. His estimated CrCl is 38 mL/minute using the Cockcroft-Gault method (Equation 2-4). Based on both methods, E.S.'s ability to clear renally eliminated drugs is impaired. An incomplete collection of urine during the 24-hour period or possible mishandling of the specimen can be explanations for the lower value seen with the measured CrCl. Because E.S. had an elevated SCr of 1.7 mg/dL, the accuracy of the Cockcroft-Gault estimation might also be compromised.

Estimated Glomerular Filtration Rate (GFR)

An alternative approach to the Cockcroft-Gault method of estimating an adult patient's clearance was developed as part of the Modification of Diet in Renal Disease (MDRD) study and has been referred to as the MDRD Equation.[10] The originally described equation has been modified into an abbreviated format (Eq. 2-6) as follows:

$$\text{Estimated GFR}_{(\text{mL/min per }1.73\text{m}^2)} = 186 \times (\text{SCr})^{-1.154} \times (\text{Age})^{-0.203} \times (0.742 \text{ if female}) \times (1.212 \text{ if African American}) \quad \textit{(Eq. 2-6)}$$

where SCr is the serum creatinine in mg/dL, age is in years, and the appropriate additional components are included for female or African American patients. The above equation is applicable to laboratories reporting SCr values that have not been standardized. Starting in 2005, laboratories began standardizing their SCr values using an isotope dilution mass spectrometry (IDMS) to minimize the variation observed in SCr results from different clinical laboratories. In settings in which the SCr results have been standardized, the initial parameter in the MDRD equation is adjusted downward and the following is used to estimate GFR:

$$\text{Estimated GFR}_{(\text{mL/min per }1.73\text{m}^2)} = 175 \times (\text{SCr})^{-1.154} \times (\text{Age})^{-0.203} \times (0.742 \text{ if female}) \times (1.212 \text{ if African American}) \quad \textit{(Eq. 2-7)}$$

When compared with the Cockcroft-Gault approach, MDRD estimations of GFR were more consistent with actual measurements of GFR. However, because both approaches rely on SCr, the influence of muscle mass and dietary intake still must be taken into consideration. A more detailed description of the MDRD equation to estimate GFR is addressed in Chapter 31, Chronic Kidney Diseases.

CASE 2-2, QUESTION 2: Based on previous information provided for E.S. in Question 1, determine his estimated GFR using the MDRD equation. Assume the SCr result of 1.7 mg/dL was obtained from a clinical laboratory that standardizes their SCr testing.

E.S. has an estimated GFR of 40.9 mL/minute and an average body surface area (BSA) of 1.73 m² when Equation 2-7 is used. This value is similar to the estimated value obtained using the Cockcroft-Gault method. Although estimated GFR is thought to be a more accurate indicator of renal function, the influence of muscle mass can still influence the result. If E.S. has reduced muscle mass, the results for both estimated GFR and estimated CrCl will be falsely elevated. In addition, in clinical practice when using the MDRD equation as a gauge for renal function, clinicians typically rely on a series of estimated GFR determinations during a period of 3 months to characterize an individual's renal function. This also assumes the patient is relatively stable with no significant fluctuations in renal function.

Cystatin C

Although SCr has long been the primary marker for renal function, cystatin C is a relatively new biomarker being investigated as a more precise measure of GFR. Cystatin C is cleared predominantly through the kidneys, and elevated levels are observed in patients with declining renal function. Reference ranges for cystatin C are similar to SCr (≤1.0 mg/L). In contrast to SCr, which is produced from muscle cells, cystatin C is produced by the blood cells and is not significantly influenced by factors such as muscle mass, diet, age, sex, and race. In addition, increases in serum cystatin C levels tend to occur earlier than increases in SCr, making it possible to detect renal insufficiency in patients at an earlier stage. This is particularly desirable in patients with diabetes, hypertension, or cardiovascular disease who may be at higher risk for the development of renal disease. Cystatin C is also being evaluated as a potential predictor of cardiovascular disease, and preliminary research has also been directed at the role of cystatin C in Alzheimer disease and demyelinating conditions like multiple sclerosis.

Glucose

Reference Range: 70–99 mg/dL or 3.9–5.5 mmol/L (fasting)

The fasting glucose concentration in the ECF is regulated closely by homeostatic mechanisms to provide body tissues with a ready source of energy. Insulin and glucagon play a critical role in this complex process. Because plasma glucose concentrations fluctuate in response to ingestion of meals, most glucose concentrations are measured in either the fasting state or the postprandial state, depending on the type of information desired. Generally, normal glucose values refer to the plasma glucose concentration in the fasting state. The specific laboratory assay of blood sugar determinations must also be considered because different assay methods vary in their specificity and sensitivity to glucose. Glucose testing using whole blood from capillary finger sticks is used in conjunction with blood glucose metering devices for patients with diabetes. Whole blood measurements using these devices are typically 15% lower than corresponding plasma glucose levels.

GLYCOSYLATED HEMOGLOBIN

Reference Range: 4%–5.6%

Hemoglobin (Hgb) is the oxygen-carrying component of the red blood cell (RBC). During the functional life span of RBCs (~4 months), glucose molecules irreversibly bind to Hgb, which results in glycosylated Hgb (A_{1c}). The concentration of Hgb A_{1c}, therefore, reflects a patient's average blood glucose concentration for the life span of circulating RBCs. In contrast, fasting glucose serum concentrations can fluctuate acutely based on either meals or insulin use. As a result, measurement of Hgb A_{1c} concentrations provides a much better tool for evaluating chronic diabetes therapy. In a patient without diabetes, about 5% of Hgb is glycosylated; however, poorly controlled patients with diabetes can have Hgb A_{1c} values greatly exceeding 8%. In one study of patients with elevated Hgb A_{1c} values, every 1% reduction in the elevated Hgb A_{1c} reduced the risk of microvascular complications by 37% and reduced the risk of acute myocardial infarction by 14%.[11] The interpretation of serum concentrations of plasma glucose, Hgb A_{1c}, and other related laboratory tests is presented in Chapter 53, Diabetes Mellitus.

HYPERGLYCEMIA AND HYPOGLYCEMIA

Hyperglycemia and hypoglycemia are nonspecific signs of abnormal glucose metabolism. Diabetes mellitus is the most common cause of hyperglycemia. Insufficient carbohydrate intake because of a missed meal is the most common cause of hypoglycemia in a patient receiving insulin or another hypoglycemic medication.

CASE 2-3

QUESTION 1: T.C., a 68-year-old man, visits his endocrinologist to assess control of his type 2 diabetes. His average blood sugar during the past 90 days recorded by his blood glucose monitor is 217 mg/dL. However, T.C.'s Hgb A_{1c} was 9%, which correlates with an average glucose concentration of roughly 240 mg/dL. T.C. is confused that these values are different because he routinely ensures his blood glucose machine is calibrated and coded properly. Why is the laboratory average different?

T.C. should not be alarmed with the difference in these values. His blood glucose monitor is likely working properly and adequately measuring fluctuations in his plasma glucose concentrations. However, the monitor may be reflecting a lower average glucose concentration because of the timing of his daily testing for glucose. For example, measuring blood glucose in a fasting state more frequently than after mealtime could contribute to lower average concentrations because fasting values are typically lower than postprandial concentrations. The Hgb A_{1c} is more indicative of his average blood sugar control during the past 90 days than the 90-day average recorded by his blood glucose monitor. A higher concentration of glucose in the blood positively correlates with a higher glycosylated Hgb. This value is typically reported as a percentage, with approximately 5% (100 mg/dL) considered as normal in a person without diabetes. As the Hgb A_{1c} percentage increases, each point raises the corresponding blood glucose value by about 35 mg/dL (e.g., 8% = 205 mg/dL, 9% = 240 mg/dL).

Osmolality

Reference Range: 280–300 mOsm/kg or mmol/kg

The osmolality of a solution is a measure of the number of osmotically active ions (i.e., particles present) per unit of solution. It is the total number of particles in the solution, not the weight of the particle or the nature of the particle, that determines osmolality. Because one mole of a substance contains 6×10^{23} molecules, equimolar concentrations of all substances in the undissociated state exert the same osmotic pressure. A mole of an ionized compound such as Na^+Cl^- contributes twice as many particles in solution as one mole of an undissociated compound such as glucose. In most situations, the primary determinants of serum osmolality in the ECF are sodium (and its accompanying anions), glucose, and BUN. If one corrects for the concentrations of glucose and BUN, the serum concentration of sodium closely mirrors the serum osmolality. A simplified formula (Eq. 2-8) useful for rule-of-thumb calculations is as follows:

$$\text{Osmolarity}_{(\text{mOsm/kg H}_2\text{O})} = 2[\text{Na}^+] + \frac{[\text{Glucose}]}{20} + \frac{[\text{BUN}]}{3} \quad \textbf{(Eq. 2-8)}$$

Serum osmolarity is useful when evaluating fluid and electrolyte disorders, particularly sodium imbalances. An increase in the measured serum osmolarity, relative to the calculated osmolarity, can be attributed to an increase in the number of solutes, a reduction in the amount of free water (e.g., patients with significant dehydration), or perhaps laboratory error. The difference between the measured serum osmolality and the calculated serum osmolality is commonly referred to as the "osmol gap" (see Chapter 10, Fluid and Electrolyte Disorders).

MULTICHEMISTRY PANELS

Frequently, multiple laboratory tests are needed for a given patient. Common clinical laboratory panels include a basic metabolic panel (BMP), comprehensive metabolic panel (CMP), electrolyte, hepatic function, and renal function panels (Table 2-4). Clinicians will often use the following abbreviated method to report a BMP in written medical records:

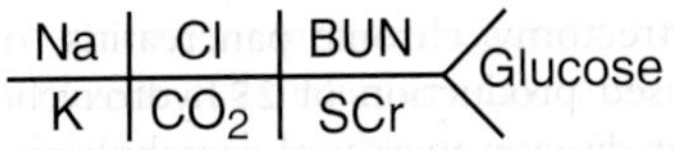

Multichemistry tests have become routinely used because they quickly provide basic information concerning organ function at relatively low cost. In addition, laboratory automation frequently makes it more cost effective to order a battery of tests within a panel versus a single test. A potential disadvantage of obtaining a battery of tests, however, is that clinicians may be inclined to pursue further laboratory testing when "abnormalities" are not clinically relevant. It is important to note that the individual laboratory tests included in a particular multichemistry panel may vary among clinical laboratories.

Calcium

Reference Range: 8.5–10.5 mg/dL or 2.1–2.6 mmol/L

The total calcium content resides primarily in the bone, with only about 1% freely exchangeable with that in the ECF. This reservoir of calcium in bones maintains the concentration of calcium in the plasma constant despite pronounced changes in the external balance of calcium. If the homeostatic factors (i.e., parathyroid hormone, vitamin D, calcitonin) that regulate the calcium content of body fluid are intact, a patient can lose 25% to 30% of total body calcium without a change in the concentration of calcium ion in the plasma.

About 40% of the calcium in the ECF is bound to plasma proteins (especially albumin), 5% to 15% is complexed with phosphate and citrate, and about 45% to 55% is in the unbound, ionized form. Most laboratories measure the total calcium

can be increased by strenuous exercise, intramuscular injections of drugs that are irritating to tissue (e.g., diazepam, phenytoin), acute psychotic episodes, crush injuries, or myocardial damage.

CK is composed of M and B subunits, which are further divided into three isoenzymes: MM, BB, and MB. The CK-MM isoenzyme is found predominantly in skeletal muscle, the CK-BB isoenzyme in the brain, and the CK-MB isoenzyme in the myocardium. Myocardial CK activity consists of 80% to 85% CK-MM and 15% to 20% CK-MB. Noncardiac tissues that contain large amounts of CK have either CK-MM or CK-BB. The MB fraction is rare in tissues other than the myocardium.

CK-MB typically begins to increase 3 to 6 hours after an acute myocardial infarction (MI), peaks at 12 to 24 hours, and accounts for about 5% or more of the total CK.[12] Myocardial damage appears to correlate with the amount of CK-MB released into the serum (i.e., the higher the amount of CK-MB, the more extensive the myocardial injury). Although CK-MB levels greater than 25 units/L are usually associated with an MI,[13] the absolute amount can vary, depending on the assay method. Generally, if the amount of CK-MB exceeds 6% of the total, myocardial injury has presumably occurred. Analysis of CK-MB provides a rapid, sensitive, specific, cost-effective, and definitive means of detecting MI.[14]

CASE 2-5

QUESTION 1: S.G., a 44-year-old woman, appears at the emergency department of a local hospital, with complaints of sudden-onset chest pain, diaphoresis, and nausea that began about 1 hour ago. S.G describes her pain as severe and not relieved by position change, antacids, or nitroglycerin. An electrocardiogram (ECG) reveals changes consistent with an acute MI. The total CK serum concentration is 118 units/L and the CK-MB is 5 units/L. S.G. was admitted to the coronary care unit to rule out an acute MI. Why are the total CK and CK-MB serum concentrations within the reference range in S.G., despite clear evidence supporting an acute MI?

The total CK and CK-MB are both within the reference range for S.G.; however, an MI cannot be excluded. CK serum concentrations usually do not rise above normal values until 4 to 8 hours after myocardial injury and usually peak in about 12 to 24 hours. About 10% of patients with suspected MIs fail to demonstrate an increase in the total CK, although serial CK-MB fractions will be increased. When CK-MB is greater than 6% of total CK, an MI has probably occurred even if the total CK is not elevated.[12]

Troponin

Reference Range: <1.5 ng/mL or <1.5 mcg/L

Troponins are proteins that regulate the calcium-mediated interaction of actin and myosin within muscles. There are two cardiac-specific troponins, cardiac troponin I (cTnI) and cardiac troponin T (cTnT). Whereas cTnT is present in cardiac and skeletal muscle cells, cTnI is present only in cardiac muscle.[15,16] Compared with the detection of CK-MB, the presence of troponin I is a more specific and sensitive indicator of myocardial damage.[17] Furthermore, the concentration of cTnI increases within 2 to 4 hours of an acute MI, enabling clinicians to quickly initiate appropriate therapy. Troponin also remains elevated for about 10 days compared with the 2- to 3-day elevation typically observed with CK-MB. cTnI levels greater than 2.0 ng/mL are suggestive of acute myocardial tissue injury. The use of troponin as a primary diagnostic test for acute MI has widely replaced CK-MB.[17] (See Chapter 18, Acute Coronary Syndromes.)

Myoglobin

Reference Range: 0–90 mcg/L

Myoglobin, a protein in heart and skeletal muscle cells, provides oxygen to working muscles. When muscle is damaged, myoglobin is released into the bloodstream. As a cardiac biomarker, myoglobin concentrations in serum rise within 3 hours after insult to the myocardial tissue, peak in about 8 to 12 hours, and return to normal in about a day. Because myoglobin serum concentrations rise more quickly than CK-MB after myocardial injury, they can be of value in helping rule out MI in the emergency department. Myoglobin serum concentrations, however, tend to be less specific for myocardial tissue compared with CK-MB. Trauma or ischemic injury to noncardiac tissue can increase serum myoglobin. Because troponin serum concentrations in serum also increase rapidly after myocardial damage, troponin is often preferred over myoglobin as a biomarker of cardiac damage.

Homocysteine

Reference Range: 4.6–11.9 μmol/L

Patients with deficiencies in folate, vitamin B_6, or vitamin B_{12} tend to have elevated serum levels of homocysteine. Homocysteine is believed to have a destructive effect on vascular epithelium. With time, patients with elevated homocysteine levels (>12 μmol/L) are believed to be at increased risk for cardiac disease.[18] Screening individuals with a positive family history for elevated homocysteine or those with atherosclerosis without typical risk factors or increased lipids has been advocated. Understanding the association between increased homocysteine levels and specific vitamin deficiencies, supplementation of folate, vitamin B_6, and vitamin B_{12} has been used clinically. However, data are too limited to suggest this approach reduces the incidence of acute MI or stroke.

Lactate Dehydrogenase

Reference Range: <200 units/L (adult)

The enzyme lactate dehydrogenase (LDH) is present in the heart, kidney, liver, and skeletal muscle. It is also abundantly present in erythrocytes and lung tissue. Because increased serum concentrations of LDH can be associated with diseases in many different organs and tissues, the diagnostic usefulness of an LDH determination is somewhat limited. There are, however, five isoenzymes of LDH. Although most tissues contain all five isoenzymes, some tissues have a predominance of one of the isoenzymes. LDH_1 and, to a lesser extent, LDH_2 predominate in the heart. Skeletal muscle and the liver have a predominance of LDH_5. LDH_3 and LDH_4 are found in a variety of tissues, including the lungs, RBCs, kidneys, brain, and pancreas. Consequently, identifying specific isoenzymes can increase the diagnostic usefulness of serum LDH determinations. For example, the elevated serum LDH associated with MI consists mostly of LDH_1 and LDH_2, whereas with acute liver disease there is a greater proportion of LDH_4 and LDH_5. Unfortunately, these isoenzyme patterns are not necessarily typical of all myocardial or liver diseases. With the availability of other myocardial enzymes, LDH as a diagnostic tool is used less frequently.

Brain Natriuretic Peptide

Reference Range: <100 pg/mL or <100 ng/L

Brain natriuretic peptide (BNP) is released from the heart when increased demands are placed on the myocardial tissue. Elevations in BNP are indicative of patients with congestive heart failure (CHF). In an effort to reduce workload on the heart, BNP counteracts the renin-angiotensin-aldosterone system and causes vasodilatory effects, along with natriuresis (increased excretion of sodium), all geared at reducing blood volume. Patients with some degree of CHF typically have BNP levels greater than 100 ng/L. BNP levels greater than 500 ng/L represent definite left ventricular dysfunction, and further evaluation is warranted to more fully characterize the extent of impaired cardiac function.[19] More recently, the *N*-terminal proBNP (NT-proBNP) is a component of BNP being used in the clinical setting to a greater extent. BNP has also been used as a tool for patients presenting to the emergency department with severe dyspnea; however, recent studies have not demonstrated additional benefits associated with using BNP to guide therapy or to use BNP as criteria for admission.

C-Reactive Protein

Reference Range: 0–1.6 mg/dL or 0–16 mg/L

C-reactive protein (CRP) is a nonspecific, acute-phase reactant helpful in the diagnosis and monitoring of inflammatory processes (e.g., rheumatoid arthritis) and infections. CRP is produced by the liver in response to an inflammatory process. Although an elevation in CRP indicates the presence of an acute inflammatory event, the nonspecific nature of the test does little to identify the cause or location of the inflammation. CRP is similar to an older test, the erythrocyte sedimentation rate (ESR), but it tends to be more sensitive than ESR and is also associated with a more rapid and greater response to acute inflammation. A potential use of CRP is in the diagnosis of acute MI and as a risk factor for cardiovascular disease.[20] A more sensitive test for CRP is now available and is referred to as hs-CRP or high-sensitivity CRP. The hs-CRP test measures the same acute-phase reactant, but it is able to detect much lower levels of CRP, making it useful for early detection of patients at risk of cardiovascular diseases. Risk assessment is stratified based on the following criteria: patients with hs-CRP values less than 1.0 mg/L have a low risk of cardiovascular disease; patients with an hs-CRP between 1.0 and 3.0 mg/L correspond with average risk; and patients with an hs-CRP greater than 3.0 mg/L are considered to be at high risk for cardiovascular diseases. It is important to realize that although hs-CRP is a new indicator for cardiovascular diseases, evaluation of other well-established patient risk factors still needs to be taken into consideration to determine the overall risk of cardiovascular disease. CRP has also been used to assess chronic inflammatory diseases such as rheumatoid arthritis and Crohn's disease. In addition, because viral infections do not typically increase CRP serum concentrations, the use of CRP as a diagnostic tool to differentiate viral versus bacterial infections might be clinically helpful.

LIVER FUNCTION TESTS

Aspartate Aminotransferase

Reference Range: 0–35 units/L or 0–0.58 μkat/L

The aspartate aminotransferase (AST) enzyme is abundant in heart and liver tissue and moderately present in skeletal muscle, the kidney, and the pancreas. In cases of acute cellular injury to the heart or liver, the enzyme is released into the blood from the damaged cells. In clinical practice, AST determinations have been used to evaluate myocardial injury and to diagnose and assess the prognosis of liver disease resulting from hepatocellular injury. The serum AST level is increased in more than 95% of patients after an MI. However, the increase in AST does not occur until 4 to 6 hours after the onset of myocardial injury. Peak AST concentrations are seen in the serum after 24 to 36 hours, returning to the normal range in about 4 to 5 days. The magnitude of the peak AST levels approximates the extent of myocardial damage (see Chapter 18, Acute Coronary Syndromes).

Serum AST values are elevated significantly in patients with acute hepatic necrosis, whether caused by viral hepatitis or a hepatotoxin (e.g., carbon tetrachloride). In these situations, the serum concentrations of both AST and alanine aminotransferase (ALT) will be increased, even before the appearance of clinical symptoms (e.g., jaundice). The AST and ALT serum concentrations can be increased by as much as 100 times the usual upper limits of normal in the presence of parenchymal liver disease. Patients with intrahepatic cholestasis, posthepatic jaundice, or cirrhosis usually experience more moderate elevations of AST, depending on the extent of cell necrosis. The AST serum concentration is usually higher than that of ALT in patients with cirrhosis, and the AST increase is usually about four to five times greater than the upper limit of normal.

Alanine Aminotransferase

Reference Range: 0–35 units/L or 0–0.58 μkat/L

The ALT enzyme is found in essentially the same tissues that have high concentrations of AST. However, elevations in serum ALT are more specific for liver-related injuries or diseases. Although ALT is relatively more abundant in hepatic tissue versus cardiac tissue than AST, the liver still contains 3.5 times more AST than ALT. Serum concentrations of both AST and ALT increase when disease processes affect liver cell structure, but ALT concentrations are not significantly increased as a result of an acute MI. Evaluating the ratio of ALT to AST can be potentially useful, particularly in the diagnosis of viral hepatitis. The ALT/AST ratio frequently exceeds 1.0 with alcoholic cirrhosis, chronic liver disease, or hepatic cancer. However, ratios less than 1.0 tend to be observed with viral hepatitis or acute hepatitis, which can be useful when diagnosing liver disease.

Alkaline Phosphatase

Reference Range: 30–120 units/L or 0.5–2.0 μkat/L

The alkaline phosphatases (ALPs) constitute a large group of isoenzymes that play important roles in the transport of sugar and phosphate. These isoenzymes of ALP have different physiochemical properties and originate from different tissues (e.g., liver, bone, placenta, intestine). In normal adults, ALP is derived primarily from liver and bone. Although only small amounts of ALP are present in the liver, this enzyme is secreted into the bile, and substantially elevated ALP serum concentrations can be seen with mild intrahepatic or extrahepatic biliary obstruction. Thus, the presence of early bile duct abnormalities can result in elevated ALP before increases in the serum bilirubin are observed. Drug-induced cholestatic jaundice (e.g., chlorpromazine or sulfonamides) can increase serum ALP concentrations. In mild cases of acute liver cell damage, ALP levels are seldom elevated. Even in cirrhosis, ALP concentrations are variable and depend on the degree of hepatic decompensation and obstruction.

The osteoblasts in bone produce large amounts of ALP, and marked serum elevations can be seen in Paget disease of the bone, hyperparathyroidism, osteogenic sarcoma, osteoblastic cancer metastatic to bone, and other conditions of pronounced osteoblastic activity. The serum ALP is increased during periods of rapid bone growth (e.g., infancy, early childhood, healing bone fractures) and during pregnancy because of the contributions of the placenta and fetal bones.

CASE 2-6

QUESTION 1: L.M., a 59-year-old woman currently taking atorvastatin 40 mg daily for hypercholesterolemia, complains of fatigue and myalgia during the past week since her last prescription refill. On assessment, her primary care provider determines she has been taking an incorrect dose. Instead of cutting an 80-mg tablet in half, she has been taking the entire tablet, thereby effectively doubling her dose. The physician orders liver function tests (LFTs), CK, and SCr to evaluate her myalgia. Laboratory results indicate the following:

AST, 51 units/L
ALT, 72 units/L
ALP, 82 units/L
CK, 216 units/L
SCr, 1.4 mg/dL

Why are these laboratory results of sufficient concern to warrant discontinuation or dose reduction of atorvastatin?

L.M.'s LFTs are elevated and are of concern, particularly in light of her other signs and symptoms. Statins have been implicated in causing elevations in LFTs on initiation of therapy and with dose increases. LFTs can be increased by up to three times the upper limit of normal. In the absence of jaundice or other clinical signs and symptoms, reduction of her atorvastatin dose will generally be sufficient in returning LFTs to normal values without adverse sequelae. L.M.'s values will likely return to baseline when her atorvastatin dose is reduced to 40 mg or discontinued. Additional monitoring after intervention would be indicated to confirm whether her LFTs stabilize or whether a trend of elevations is noted on multiple occasions. CK serum concentrations can also be increased in response to muscle injury or myalgia. When CK increases ten times the upper limit of normal, myopathy should be suspected. L.M.'s CK is mildly increased at this time, but not at an alarming value.

Gamma-Glutamyl Transferase

Reference Range: 0–70 units/L or 0–1.17 µkat/L

Although the enzyme gamma-glutamyl transferase (GGT) is found in the kidney, liver, and pancreas, its major clinical value is in the evaluation of hepatobiliary disease. An increase in the serum concentration of GGT parallels the increase of ALP in obstructive jaundice and infiltrative disease of the liver. However, increased ALP in the presence of a normal GGT is more suggestive of muscular or bone-related issues. GGT is one of the more sensitive liver enzymes for identifying biliary obstruction and cholecystitis. Because GGT is a hepatic microsomal enzyme, tissue concentrations increase in response to microsomal enzyme induction by alcohol and other drugs (e.g., carbamazepine, phenobarbital, phenytoin). As a result, GGT is a sensitive indicator of recent or chronic alcohol exposure.

Bilirubin

Total Bilirubin—Reference Range: 0.1–1.0 mg/dL or 1.7–17.1 µmol/L
Direct (Conjugated) Bilirubin—Reference Range: 0–0.2 mg/dL or 0–3.4 µmol/L

Bilirubin is primarily a breakdown product of Hgb and is formed in the reticuloendothelial system (Fig. 2-1, step 1). It is then transferred into the blood (step 2), where it is almost completely bound to serum albumin (step 3). When bilirubin arrives at the sinusoidal surface of the liver cells, the free fraction is

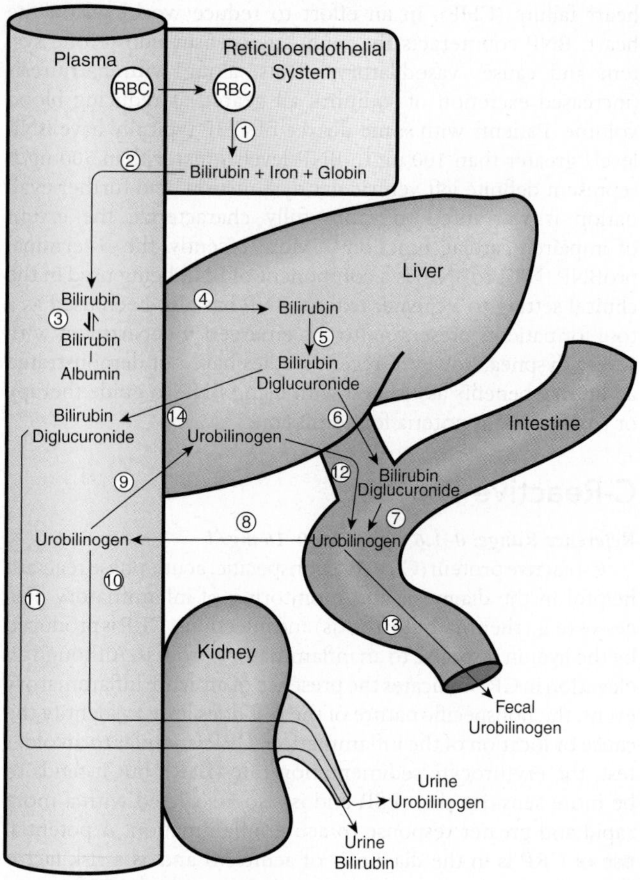

FIGURE 2-1 Bilirubin metabolism.

rapidly taken up into the cell (step 4) and converted primarily to bilirubin diglucuronide (step 5). A monoglucuronide is also formed that is metabolized predominantly to the diglucuronide. The conjugated bilirubin diglucuronide is then excreted into the bile (step 6) and appears in the intestine, where bacteria convert most of it to urobilinogen (step 7). The majority of urobilinogen is destroyed or excreted in the feces (step 13), but a small portion is reabsorbed into the blood (step 8) and either reabsorbed into the liver (step 9) and subsequently excreted into the bile (step 12) or excreted into the urine (step 10). Urobilinogen is responsible for the straw color of the urine and the yellowish-brown color of the feces. The mechanism by which conjugated bilirubin in the liver cell is transferred to the blood (step 14) is not well understood. However, in many types of liver disease, conjugated (direct) bilirubin is present in increased concentrations in the blood. When this concentration exceeds 0.2 to 0.4 mg/dL, bilirubin will begin to appear in the urine (step 11). Unconjugated (indirect) bilirubin is water insoluble and is highly bound to serum albumin; both factors account for its lack of excretion in the urine.[21]

HYPERBILIRUBINEMIA

CASE 2-7

QUESTION 1: A.R., a 42-year-old man with a 2-year history of hypertension controlled with hydrochlorothiazide and a 1-year history of Parkinson disease controlled by carbidopa/levodopa, is hospitalized after an episode of orthostatic hypotension. Admitting laboratory results show a hematocrit (Hct) of 27%. Because A.R. had a long history of alcoholism, additional laboratory tests were obtained. His results were as follows:

Total bilirubin, 3.5 mg/dL
Direct bilirubin, 0.5 mg/dL
ALP, 40 units/L
AST, 32 units/L
ALT, 27 units/L

Based on this information and Figure 2-1, what are three major causes of increased bilirubin in adults, and what might be the most logical cause of increased bilirubin in A.R.?

Increases in serum bilirubin can be categorized into three primary causes. First, hepatocellular injury interferes with the ability of the liver to conjugate bilirubin, leading to a disproportional increase of total bilirubin relative to the direct bilirubin (i.e., the indirect bilirubin will be increased). The normal AST and ALT values observed with A.R. indicate that hepatocellular damage is not likely the cause of the increased bilirubin. Therefore, a diagnosis of hepatocellular damage cannot be confirmed by the serum bilirubin concentrations alone. Second, hyperbilirubinemia can involve cholestatic or obstructive (posthepatic) causes. Blockage of the bile duct secondary to cholelithiasis (gallstone) or tumor will tend to increase conjugated (direct) bilirubin. In obstructive causes of hyperbilirubinemia, mild elevations in AST and ALT, as well as marked increases in ALP and GGT, are usually observed. Furthermore, increased excretion of excess conjugated bilirubin in the urine commonly results in dark brown–colored urine. Again, the clinical scenario illustrated with A.R. does not appear to support a cholestatic component as the cause of his increased bilirubin (ALP is within the reference range, and his direct bilirubin is only slightly elevated). The third primary cause of increased serum bilirubin involves hemolysis (prehepatic). In cases in which erythrocytes are rapidly hemolyzed (e.g., sickle cell disease, drug-induced hemolysis), serum concentrations of indirect bilirubin increase. If the liver is conjugating and eliminating bilirubin normally, total bilirubin will increase out of proportion to the direct bilirubin, and the other LFTs will appear within the reference range. This appears evident in A.R.'s case, making hemolysis the likely cause of his hyperbilirubinemia.

MISCELLANEOUS TESTS

Amylase and Lipase

Amylase (reference range: 35–120 units/L or 0.58–2.0 μkat/L) and lipase (reference range: 0–160 units/L or 0–2.67 μkat/L) are enzymes produced in the pancreas and secreted into the duodenum to assist in the digestive process. Amylase is responsible for breaking down complex carbohydrates into simple sugars and is also found in the saliva. Significant elevations in serum amylase are observed in patients with acute pancreatitis or pancreatic duct obstruction. Amylase levels tend to rise 6 to 48 hours after onset of the disease and usually return to normal 3 days after the acute event. In chronic pancreatitis or obstruction, amylase levels may remain elevated for longer periods. Other nonpancreatic conditions (e.g., bowel perforation, biliary disease, perforated peptic ulcer, ectopic pregnancy, mumps) can be associated with elevated serum amylase levels.

Lipase is responsible for breaking down triglycerides into fatty acids. Elevated serum lipase levels are also suggestive of pancreatic disease and tend to be more specific for pancreatic disease than amylase. The onset of lipase elevation is similar to amylase; however, lipase typically remains elevated for 5 to 7 days and can be useful in diagnosing patients in later stages of pancreatic disease. Narcotics (e.g., morphine) can constrict the sphincter of Oddi and increase serum concentrations of amylase and lipase.

Prostate-Specific Antigen

Reference Range: 0–4 ng/mL or 0–4 mcg/L

Prostate-specific antigen (PSA) is a protease glycoprotein produced almost exclusively by prostate epithelial cells. Serum concentrations of PSA are increased when the normal prostate glandular structure is disrupted by benign or malignant tumor or inflammation. More than half of men with benign prostatic hyperplasia have elevated serum PSA concentrations. PSA is also a valuable parameter for staging and monitoring the progression and response to therapy of prostate cancer.[22]

PSA serum concentrations increase after prostatic manipulation such as digital rectal examination (DRE), transrectal ultrasound, cystoscopy, or biopsy of the prostate. In addition, serum PSA will increase 24 to 48 hours after ejaculation. Although elevated serum concentrations of PSA can occur in men with benign prostatic hyperplasia, concentrations tend to be higher and encountered more often in men with cancer. As a result, the American Cancer Society[23] and the American Urological Association[24] currently recommend that health care providers offer a PSA blood test and DRE yearly to men older than 50 years. For men considered to be at high risk (family history or African American men), testing at age 45 years is suggested. Combination of both PSA and DRE was more effective in detecting prostate cancer than either test alone.

The serum half-life of PSA is 2 to 3 days, but serum PSA concentrations can remain high for several weeks after manipulation of the prostate. Men with PSA levels between 4 and 10 ng/mL should be evaluated further for potential prostate cancer. Circulating serum PSA is bound to plasma proteins, and the capability exists to measure both total and free (unbound) PSA concentrations. Increased risk of prostate cancer has been observed in men with a free PSA to total PSA ratio of less than 0.25.[25] An aggressive approach to localize prostate cancer for men with life expectancies more than 10 years is now favored.[22,26]

Thyroid-Stimulating Hormone

Reference Range: 0.4–5 μunits/mL or munits/L

Thyroid-stimulating hormone (TSH, also known as thyrotropin) is commonly used to monitor exogenous thyroid replacement therapy in individuals diagnosed with primary hypothyroidism. In addition, TSH may also be measured in conjunction with T_4 levels to diagnose this condition or secondary hypothyroidism. Causes of secondary hypothyroidism typically arise from damage, such as trauma or tumors, to the hypothalamus or pituitary gland. Secretion of thyrotropin-releasing hormone (TRH) (sometimes referred to as thyroid-releasing hormone) and TSH are substantially impaired or absent as a result of this damage. Conversely, primary hypothyroidism occurs in response to low levels of T_3 and T_4. Reduced levels stimulate TRH and TSH release in the absence of the negative feedback typically exerted by normal levels of T_3 and T_4; as a result, increased TSH is noted.

Exogenous thyroid hormone replacement therapy balances TSH secretion to achieve a euthyroid state. Individuals taking inappropriate replacement doses will exhibit alterations in TSH levels. In the absence of other clinical influences or interactions, a high TSH level indicates the need to supplement with additional thyroid medication, whereas a low TSH supports the reduction in exogenous supplementation. Causes of primary hypothyroidism include congenital defects, idiopathic hypothyroidism, thyroiditis (inflammation of the thyroid gland), or antithyroid medications. Chapter 52, Thyroid Disorders, provides a more detailed discussion of the clinical implications of altered thyroid laboratory findings.

Procalcitonin

Procalcitonin is a precursor for calcitonin and is typically undetectable in healthy individuals. Elevations in procalcitonin occur in patients with inflammation secondary to bacterial infections; however, a similar increase is not observed in patients with inflammation secondary to viral infections or noninfectious conditions. Interestingly, increases in calcitonin are not seen in patients with elevated procalcitonin. Because of the selective nature toward bacterial infections, procalcitonin has been used as an indicator for initiating and discontinuing antibiotic therapy. With concerns involving overuse or inappropriate use of antibiotics and the associated development of resistance, treatment algorithms have been established to minimize unwarranted antibiotic therapy or extended durations of therapy. In patients with sepsis or sepsis syndrome, procalcitonin levels less than 0.5 ng/mL are associated with a low risk of progression to severe sepsis and levels greater than 2.0 ng/mL represent a high risk for severe sepsis. Similarly, trials involving lower respiratory tract infections have suggested that antibiotic therapy should be discouraged in patients with procalcitonin levels less than 0.25 ng/mL, but encouraged for those with levels of 0.5 ng/mL or greater. These criteria have also been used as a guide for discontinuing therapy as infections resolve. The half-life of procalcitonin is roughly 1 day. The exact role procalcitonin plays as a marker for bacterial infection and as a guide for therapy has not been clearly characterized. Additional trials will help to accurately define the role of procalcitonin levels in this setting.

Cholesterol and Triglycerides

A detailed discussion of hypercholesterolemia and lipid disorders is provided in Chapter 13, Dyslipidemias, Atherosclerosis, and Coronary Heart Disease. For convenience, the current range of desired values for total cholesterol (TC), low-density lipoproteins (LDLs), high-density lipoproteins (HDLs), and fasting triglycerides (TGs) has been incorporated in Table 2-2. The reader is referred to Chapter 13, Dyslipidemias, Atherosclerosis, and Coronary Heart Disease, or to National Cholesterol Education Program and Adult Treatment Panel guidelines for a detailed description on the topic.[27]

HEMATOLOGY

There are several different hematologic cell types that originate from the hematopoietic stem cell. Each cell line has a defined role and unique contribution to the overall homeostatic process, and may be found in the bone marrow, lymph system, or blood. Typically, routine clinical laboratory testing involves measuring concentrations of mature myeloid cells found in the blood. Figure 2-2 illustrates the various lineages derived from the hematopoietic stem cell.[28] The cells derived from the myeloid linage are the focus of the following discussion. Readers are encouraged to refer to Section 17, Neoplastic Disorders, to gain further understanding of the clinical relevance of lymphoid and myeloid cells (Fig. 2-2).

Complete Blood Count

The complete blood count (CBC) is one of the most commonly ordered clinical laboratory tests. A CBC measures the red blood cells (RBCs), hemoglobin (Hgb), hematocrit (Hct), mean cell volume (MCV), mean cell Hgb concentration (MCHC), and total white blood cells (WBCs). Depending on the laboratory, an order for a CBC may also include platelets, reticulocytes, or leukocyte differential. An abbreviated method of noting hematologic parameters in clinical practice is noted in the following figure. In addition, a list of hematologic laboratory values are presented in Table 2-2.

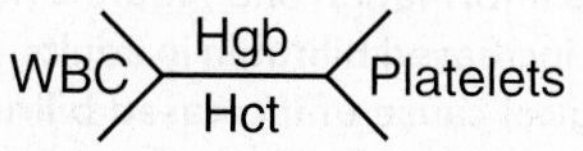

Red Blood Cells (Erythrocytes)

Males—Reference Range: 4.3–5.9 × $10^6/\mu L$ or 4.3–5.9 × $10^{12}/L$
Females—Reference Range: 3.5–5.0 × $10^6/\mu L$ or 3.5–5.0 × $10^{12}/L$

Erythrocytes or RBCs are produced in the bone marrow, released into the peripheral blood, circulated for approximately 120 days, and cleared by the reticuloendothelial system. The primary function of RBCs is to transport oxygen to tissues. The concentration of RBCs in the blood can be measured to detect anemia, calculate RBC indices, or calculate the Hct. Hct and Hgb concentrations are generally used to monitor quantitative changes in RBCs.

Hematocrit

Males—Reference Range: 39%–49% or 0.39–0.49
Females—Reference Range: 33%–43% or 0.33–0.43

Hct (packed cell volume) is determined by centrifuging a capillary tube of whole blood and comparing the height of the settled RBCs to the height of the column of whole blood. The percentage of RBCs to the blood volume is the Hct. A decrease in Hct may result from bleeding, the bone marrow suppressant effects of drugs, chronic diseases, genetic alterations in RBC morphology, or hemolysis. An increase in Hct may result from hemoconcentration, polycythemia vera, or polycythemia secondary to chronic hypoxia.

Hemoglobin

Males—Reference Range: 14–18 g/dL or 140–180 g/L
Females—Reference Range: 12–16 g/dL or 120–160 g/L

Hgb is the oxygen-carrying compound contained in RBCs. Therefore, total Hgb concentration primarily depends on the number of RBCs in the blood sample. As mentioned with Hct, medical conditions that impact the number of RBCs will also affect Hgb concentration. As discussed previously, glycosylated Hgb (A_{1c}) is a related test used to monitor diabetes mellitus.

Red Blood Cell Indices

RBC indices (also known as Wintrobe indices) are useful in the classification of anemias. These indices include the MCV, the mean cell hemoglobin (MCH), and the MCHC. These indices are calculated in Equations 2-9 to 2-11:

$$\text{MCV} = \frac{\text{Hct} \times 1{,}000}{\text{RBC (in millions}/\mu\text{L)}} = 76 - 100 \text{ (in } \mu\text{m}^3 \text{ or fL)} \quad \textit{(Eq. 2-9)}$$

$$\text{MCH} = \frac{\text{Hgb (in g/dL} \times 10)}{\text{RBC (in millions}/\mu\text{L)}} = 27 - 33 \text{ (in pg)} \quad \textit{(Eq. 2-10)}$$

$$\text{MCHC} = \frac{\text{Hgb (in g/dL)}}{\text{Hct}} = 33 - 37 \text{ (in g/dL)} \quad \textit{(Eq. 2-11)}$$

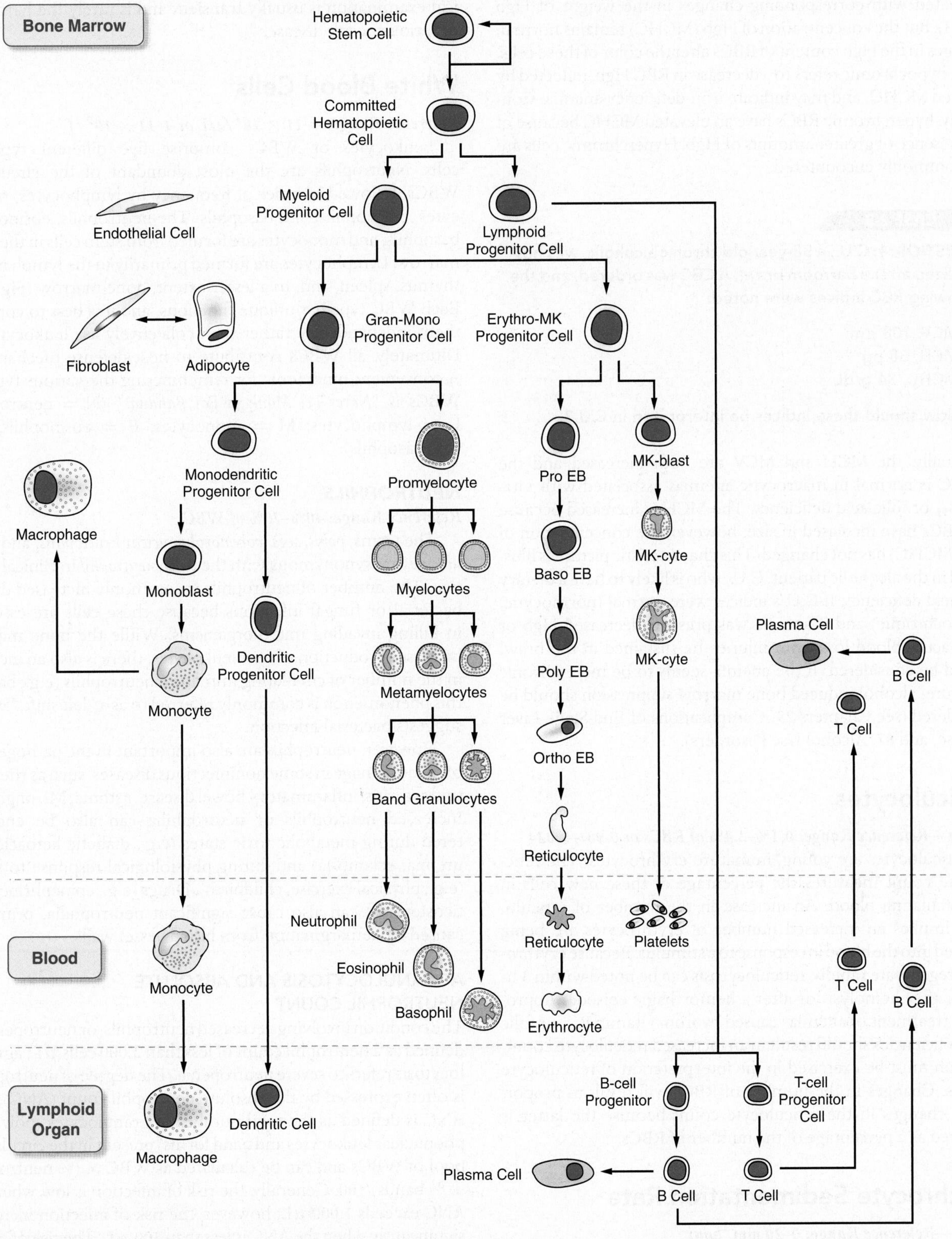

FIGURE 2-2 Hematopoietic stem cell lineage. (Adapted with permission from Greer JP, Foerster J, Rodgers GM et al., eds. *Wintrobe's Clinical Hematology*. 12th ed. Philadelphia, PA: Lippincott Williams & Wilkins; 2009:80.)

MEAN CELL VOLUME

The MCV detects changes in cell size. A decreased MCV indicates a microcytic cell, which can result from iron-deficiency anemia. A large MCV indicates a macrocytic cell, which can be caused by a vitamin B_{12} or folic acid deficiency. Underlying disease states (e.g., habitual alcohol ingestion, chronic liver disease, anorexia nervosa, hypothyroidism, reticulocytosis, hematologic disorders) may also present with an elevated MCV secondary to deficiencies in these vitamins.[29] The MCV can be normal in a patient with a "mixed" (microcytic and macrocytic) anemia. Note that a direct assessment of a blood smear by a microscopic examination is the gold standard for confirming RBC size.

MEAN CELL HEMOGLOBIN

The MCHC is a more reliable index of RBC Hgb than MCH. The former measures the concentration of Hgb, whereas the latter measures the weight of Hgb in the average RBC. In normochromic anemias, changes in the size of RBCs (MCV) are associated with corresponding changes in the weight of Hgb (MCH), but the concentration of Hgb (MCHC) remains normal. Changes in the Hgb content of RBCs alter the color of these cells. Thus, hypochromic refers to a decrease in RBC Hgb, reflected by reduced MCHC, and may indicate iron-deficiency anemia. Conversely, hyperchromic RBCs have an elevated MCHC because of the presence of greater amounts of Hgb. Hyperchromic cells are not commonly encountered.

CASE 2-8

QUESTION 1: C.U., a 58-year-old chronic alcoholic, was hospitalized after a barroom brawl. A CBC was ordered, and the following RBC indices were noted:

MCV, 108 μm^3
MCH, 38 pg
MCHC, 34 g/dL

How should these indices be interpreted in C.U.?

Usually, the MCH and MCV are both increased and the MCHC is normal in macrocytic anemias associated with vitamin B_{12} or folic acid deficiency. The MCH is increased because the RBCs have increased in size; however, the concentration of Hgb (MCHC) has not changed. This characteristic picture is illustrated in the alcoholic patient, C.U., who is likely to have a dietary folic acid deficiency. If C.U.'s indices were normal (normocytic, normochromic) and if anemia was present (decreased Hgb or Hct), acute blood loss from injuries he sustained in the brawl should be considered. If the anemia seems to be more chronic in nature, alcohol-induced bone marrow suppression should be considered (see Chapters 29, Complications of End-Stage Liver Disease, and 87, Alcohol Use Disorders).

Reticulocytes

Adults—Reference Range: 0.1%–2.4% of RBCs or 0.001–0.024

Reticulocytes are young, immature erythrocytes. The reticulocyte count measures the percentage of these new cells in the circulating blood. An increase in the number of reticulocytes implies an increased number of erythrocytes are being released into the blood in response to a stimulus. Because erythrocytes regenerate rapidly, reticulocytosis can be noted within 3 to 5 days after hemolysis or after a hemorrhagic episode. Appropriate treatment of anemias caused by iron, vitamin B_{12}, or folic acid deficiencies should result in an increased reticulocyte count. Caution must be exercised in the interpretation of reticulocyte counts. Changes in the number of RBCs will result in proportional changes in the reticulocyte count because the latter is reported as a percentage of the number of RBCs.

Erythrocyte Sedimentation Rate

Males—Reference Range: 0–20 mm/hour
Females—Reference Range: 0–30 mm/hour

The ESR is the rate at which erythrocytes settle to the bottom of a test tube through the forces of gravity and in response to fibrinogen levels in the blood. The ESR is a nonspecific value and may be increased abnormally in acute and chronic inflammatory processes, acute and chronic infections, neoplasms, infarction, tissue necrosis, rheumatoid-collagen disease, dysproteinemias, nephritis, and pregnancy. Laboratory technique can affect the sedimentation rate substantially. Because many factors can enhance the settling rate of RBCs, moderate to marked elevation of the ESR merely indicates an inflammatory component to a disease state. An increased ESR in the setting of a normal physical examination is usually transient and is rarely the harbinger of serious occult disease.[30]

White Blood Cells

Reference Range: 4–11 × $10^3/\mu L$ or 4–11 × $10^9/L$

Leukocytes or WBCs comprise five different types of cells. Neutrophils are the most abundant of the circulating WBCs, followed in order of frequency by lymphocytes, monocytes, eosinophils, and basophils. The neutrophils, eosinophils, basophils, and monocytes are formed from stem cells in the bone marrow. Lymphocytes are formed primarily in the lymph nodes, thymus, spleen, and, to a lesser extent, bone marrow (Fig. 2-2). Each WBC type has unique functions, and it is best to consider them independently rather than collectively as "leukocytes."[31] Ultimately, all WBCs contribute to host defense mechanisms. A convenient mnemonic for remembering the various types of WBCs is *"Never Let Monkeys Eat Bananas"* (N = neutrophils; L = lymphocytes; M = monocytes; E = eosinophils; and B = basophils).

NEUTROPHILS

Reference Range: 40%–70% of WBC

The terms, *polys, segs, polymorphonuclear neutrophils,* and *granulocytes* are synonymous with the term *neutrophil* in clinical practice. The number of neutrophils is commonly increased during bacterial or fungal infections because these cells are essential in killing invading micro-organisms. While the bone marrow increases production of new leukocytes, there is also an increase in the number of circulating immature neutrophils (e.g., bands); this phenomenon is commonly referred to as a "left shift," which suggests bacterial infection.

However, neutrophils are also important in the pathogenesis of tissue damage in some noninfectious diseases, such as rheumatoid arthritis, inflammatory bowel disease, asthma, MI, or gout.[32] Increased neutrophils or neutrophilia can also be encountered during metabolic toxic states (e.g., diabetic ketoacidosis, uremia, eclampsia) and during physiological response to stress (e.g., physical exercise, childbirth). Drugs (e.g., epinephrine, corticosteroids) can also cause significant neutrophilia, primarily caused by demargination from blood vessel walls.

AGRANULOCYTOSIS AND ABSOLUTE NEUTROPHIL COUNT

The condition involving decreased neutrophils, or neutropenia, is defined as a neutrophil count of less than 2,000 cells/μL; agranulocytosis refers to severe neutropenia. The degree of neutropenia is often expressed by the absolute neutrophil count (ANC). The ANC is defined as the total number of granulocytes (polymorphonuclear leukocytes and band forms) present in the circulating pool of WBCs and can be calculated as WBC × (% neutrophils + % bands)/100. Generally, the risk of infection is low when the ANC exceeds 1,000/μL; however, the risk of infection increases significantly when the ANC is less than 500/μL. The risk of developing bacteremia is increased further as the ANC decreases to less than 100/μL, a condition commonly referred to as "profound neutropenia" (see Chapter 72, Prevention and Treatment of Infections in Neutropenic Cancer Patients). The most common causes of neutropenia are metastatic carcinoma, lymphoma, and chemotherapeutic agents.

LYMPHOCYTES

Reference Range: 20%–40% of WBC

Lymphocytes constitute the second most common WBC in circulating blood. These leukocytes respond to foreign antigens by initiating the immune defense system. The vast majority of lymphocytes are located in the spleen, lymph nodes, and other organized lymphatic tissue. The lymphocytes circulating in blood represent less than 5% of the total amount in the body.

There are two major types of lymphocytes. T lymphocytes (thymic dependent) participate in cell-mediated immune responses, and B lymphocytes (bone marrow derived) are responsible for humoral antibody responses. Therefore, diseases affecting lymphocytes primarily manifest themselves as immune deficiency disorders that render the patient unable to defend against normal pathogens (see Chapter 73, Pharmacotherapy of Human Immunodeficiency Virus Infection) or as autoimmune diseases in which immune responses are directed against the body's own cells.[31]

Increased numbers of lymphocytes on a white count differential sometimes accompany lymphoma (see Chapter 92, Hematologic Malignancies) and viral infections such as infectious mononucleosis, mumps, and rubella. A relative lymphocytosis is sometimes encountered when the total lymphocytes have remained constant despite a decline in the total neutrophils.

MONOCYTES

Reference Range: 0%–11% of WBC

Monocytes are formed in the bone marrow and are the precursors to macrophages and antigen-presenting cells (dendritic cells), which are found in the body's tissues.[33] Macrophages and dendritic cells are phagocytic cells that engulf foreign antigens or dead or dying cells. Dendritic cells also present fragments of antigens to T and B lymphocytes. Monocytosis may be observed in mononucleosis, subacute bacterial endocarditis, malaria, and tuberculosis, as well as during the recovery phase of some infections.

EOSINOPHILS

Reference Range: 0%–8% of WBC

Because eosinophils have surface receptors that bind IgG and IgE, they can modify reactions associated with IgG- and IgE-mediated degranulation of mast cells. Primary lysosomal granules, small dense granules, and specific or secondary granules are the three types of granules found within eosinophils. The latter granules account for most of the biological activity of eosinophils and are toxic to parasites, tumor cells, and some epithelial cells.[34]

Eosinophils have phagocytic activity, catalyze the oxidation of many substances, facilitate killing of micro-organisms, initiate mast cell secretion, protect against various parasites, and play some role in host defense. Eosinophilia is probably most commonly associated with allergic reactions to drugs, allergic disorders (e.g., hay fever, asthma, eczema), invasive parasitic infections (e.g., hookworm, schistosomiasis, trichinosis), collagen vascular diseases (e.g., rheumatoid arthritis, eosinophilic fasciitis, eosinophilic-myalgia syndrome), and malignancies (e.g., Hodgkin disease).[35–37]

BASOPHILS

Reference Range: 0%–3% of WBC

During infection or inflammation, basophils leave the blood and mobilize as mast cells to the affected site and release granules. These granules contain histamine, serotonin, prostaglandins, and leukotrienes. Degranulation results in an increased blood flow to the site and may compound inflammatory processes. An increase in basophils commonly accompanies allergic and anaphylactic responses, chronic myeloid leukemia, myelofibrosis, and polycythemia vera. A decrease in the number of basophils is generally not readily apparent because of the small number of these cells in the blood.[31]

CASE 2-9

QUESTION 1: R.L., a 45-year-old man, is hospitalized with a sustained high fever of 39.4°C, SOB, and pleurisy. His cough is productive of rusty sputum, and he appears to be in acute distress. The results of the CBC and leukocyte differential are as follows:

Total WBC count, 18,000/μL
Neutrophils, 76%
Bands, 13%
Lymphocytes, 10%
Monocytes, 0
Eosinophils, 1%
Basophils, 0

On the basis of this laboratory report and other findings, a diagnosis of pneumococcal pneumonia is suspected. How is R.L.'s laboratory report consistent with bacterial infection?

WBCs are the host's chief defense system, and the neutrophil is the main component of that system. During bacterial infections, the leukocyte count and the neutrophils are generally increased, and a left shift (increase in bands) may be noticeable. The percentage of other types of WBCs is decreased proportionately because the number of neutrophils is increased.

As the infection progresses, the percentage of band cells may decrease as a result of an increase in the number of neutrophils that have a longer half-life. This decrease in bands does not necessarily indicate improvement. A decrease in the percentage of neutrophils with a decrease in the total WBC count is characteristic of effective antibiotic therapy.

CASE 2-10

QUESTION 1: S.Q., a 35-year-old woman, was treated for 7 days with dicloxacillin for cellulitis of the left leg. On the eighth day, an allergic urticarial rash developed. The CBC showed a total leukocyte count of 10,000/μL with 6% eosinophils. What is the significance of this eosinophil count?

In the clinical setting, absolute leukocyte counts may be used in conjunction with normal reference values. Absolute counts are calculated by multiplying the percentage of each individual cell by the total leukocyte count. Eosinophils are usually increased in allergic reactions; therefore, a drug-induced hypersensitivity reaction is a strong probability in S.Q., with an absolute count of 600 eosinophils/μL (i.e., 6% of 10,000 leukocytes). The clinician should be suspicious of an allergic drug reaction when absolute eosinophil counts exceed 300 cells/μL. Eosinophils may increase before, after, or concurrent with other evidence of allergy (e.g., rash). Eosinophilia without evidence of allergy is not sufficient cause to discontinue a suspected medication unless the eosinophilia is significant (i.e., >2,000 cells/μL). In addition, the absence of eosinophilia certainly does not rule out an allergic diagnosis in a patient exhibiting clear clinical manifestations of an apparent allergic reaction.

Thrombocytes

Reference Range: 150–450 × 10^3/μL or 150–450 × 10^9/L

Appropriate platelet (i.e., thrombocyte) function is essential to blood clotting. Decreased platelet counts or thrombocytopenia may lead to petechiae, ecchymosis, and spontaneous hemorrhage. Causes include decreased platelet production, accelerated destruction, loss from excessive bleeding or trauma, dilution of blood samples secondary to blood transfusion, sequestration secondary to hypersplenism, disseminated intravascular coagulation, infection, or systemic lupus erythematosus. Malignancy, rheumatoid arthritis, iron-deficiency anemia, polycythemia vera, and postsplenectomy syndromes are the most common causes of elevated platelet counts or thrombocytosis.

Coagulation Studies

The control of bleeding depends on the formation of a platelet plug and the formation of a stable fibrin clot. The formation of this clot, the complex interactions of plasma proteins and clotting factors, and the clinical application of laboratory tests of coagulation are described in Chapter 16, Thrombosis. The prothrombin time (PT), international normalized ratio (INR), and activated partial thromboplastin time (aPTT) are used to diagnose coagulation abnormalities or to monitor the effectiveness of patients receiving anticoagulation therapy. When used to assess drug therapy, achieving a value outside the reference range is in fact a therapeutically desirable outcome. These tests are described briefly in this chapter, with the understanding that the reader will refer to Chapter 16, Thrombosis, to gain the appropriate perspective on the clinical applicability of these tests.

ACTIVATED PARTIAL THROMBOPLASTIN TIME

Reference Range: 20–39 seconds

aPTT measures the intrinsic clotting system, which depends on factors VIII, IX, XI, and XII and the factors involved in the final common pathway of the clotting cascade (factors II, X, and V). aPTT is commonly used to monitor unfractionated heparin therapy.

PROTHROMBIN TIME

Reference Range: 10–14 seconds

Prothrombin is synthesized in the liver and is converted to thrombin during the blood clotting process. Thrombin formation is the critical event in the hemostatic process because thrombin creates fibrin monomers that ultimately assemble into a clot and stimulates platelet activation. The PT test directly measures the activity of clotting factors VII and X, prothrombin (factor II), and fibrinogen. Automated laboratory instruments measure PT by recording the time required for the blood to clot after tissue thromboplastin has been added to the patient's blood sample.

INTERNATIONAL NORMALIZED RATIO

Although INR is the recommended method to accurately monitor anticoagulant therapy, several potential problems have been identified with the INR system. Because of the variable sensitivity of thromboplastin reagents to decreases in specific clotting factors, there may be a lack of reliability of the INR system when it is used at the onset of warfarin therapy and for screening for a coagulopathy. Despite these potential problems with the INR system, the American College of Chest Physicians unanimously recommends using the INR system of reporting during initiation and maintenance of anticoagulant therapy.[38] However, attempts to standardize laboratory reporting have not completely eliminated the variability observed among different laboratories, so clinicians must be cautious when interpreting coagulation parameters obtained from more than one institution.

The INR is calculated using Equation 2-12, where the prothrombin ratio (PTR) is the ratio between the patient's PT and the laboratory's control PT, and the ISI is the international sensitivity index. Commercial manufacturers quantify the ISI for the specific thromboplastin reagent used in each lot and report this information in the product package insert. For a thorough review on the monitoring of anticoagulant therapy, see Chapter 16, Thrombosis.

$$\mathrm{INR} = \left\{\frac{\mathrm{PT\ (patient)}}{\mathrm{PT\ (control)}}\right\}^{\mathrm{ISI}} = \mathrm{PTR}^{\mathrm{ISI}} \quad \textit{(Eq. 2-12)}$$

URINALYSIS

A standard urinalysis begins with simple observation of the color and the gross general appearance of the urine specimen. The urine pH and specific gravity are then recorded. Formed elements in the urine are examined microscopically, and the urine is searched routinely for pathologically significant substances that are normally not present (e.g., glucose, blood, ketones, bile pigments).

Gross Appearance of the Specimen

The concentrated, first-morning urine specimen is usually analyzed to eliminate effects of undue dilution as a result of water intake. The color should be slightly yellow, depending on the degree of dilution, and the appearance should be clear. The appearance of the urine may reveal clouds of crystals, bilirubin, blood, porphyrins, proteins, food or drug colorings, or melanin. Discolored urine is abnormal. A red coloration of the urine may be imparted by blood, porphyria, or ingestion of phenolphthalein. A brown urine color may be caused by the acid hematin of blood or from melanin pigments. Excessive excretion of urobilinogen or the effects of drugs such as rifampin or phenazopyridine may cause a dark orange urine color. A blue to blue-green color of the urine may result from the systemic administration of methylene blue.

Specimen pH

When freshly produced, urine is normally mostly acidic (pH 4.5–8). Alkaline urine may indicate an aged specimen, systemic alkalosis, failure of renal acidifying mechanisms, or infection in the urinary tract.

Specific Gravity

A normal morning urine specimen should have a specific gravity of 1.002 to 1.030. The upper end of this range is close to the maximal concentrating ability of the kidney. A value of 1.010 supports relative hydration, whereas a value greater than 1.020 indicates relative dehydration.

Protein

Proteinuria is a classic sign of renal injury and a matter of concern. If proteinuria is found during the evaluation of a patient with a nonrenal illness, it suggests that the disease may also involve the kidneys (i.e., hypertension, diabetes).[39] A healthy adult generally excretes 30 to 130 mg/day of protein into the urine.

Protein in a urine sample is generally tested qualitatively on a random urine sample by a dipstick method and is usually reported on a scale of 0 (<30 mg/dL), 1+ (30–100 mg/dL), 2+ (100–300 mg/dL), 3+ (300–1,000 mg/dL), and 4+ (>1,000 mg/dL). A positive qualitative test for urine protein should be repeated after a few days because transient proteinuria can accompany various physiological and pathological states, even when kidney function is normal. Therefore, patients with congestive heart failure, seizures, or febrile illnesses and normal renal function need not undergo invasive renal function tests if the proteinuria is modest and likely to be transient. Another qualitative evaluation of proteinuria can be performed in about 2 weeks to confirm the diagnosis of transient proteinuria.[40] If subsequent qualitative test results are positive, a 24-hour urine sample should be collected to quantitatively test for protein and creatinine (see Creatinine Clearance section). In patients with a normal 24-hour urinary protein concentration, previous positive qualitative test results probably represent either false-positive results or a transient phenomenon.[39] A laboratory parameter being used with increased frequency to assess proteinuria is the urine albumin to urine creatinine ratio (UACR). This measurement tends to be less influenced by fluctuations in urine concentration and may offer a more reliable indication of proteinuria. UACR values are typically less than 30 mg/g; patients with values between 30 and 300 mg/g are considered to have microalbuminuria, and UACR values greater than 300 mg/g indicate macroalbuminemia. A more detailed discussion of the UACR will be addressed in Chapter 31, Chronic Kidney Diseases.

MICROSCOPIC EXAMINATION

The urine sediment is examined for RBCs, WBCs, casts, yeast, crystals, and epithelial cells.

RBCs should be absent in normal urine, although fewer than 4 to 6 RBCs per high-power field (HPF) would still be considered in the normal range. Bleeding or clotting disorders, some collagen diseases, and various bladder, urethral, and prostatic conditions may cause microscopic hematuria. In women, vaginal blood occasionally contaminates the urine specimen, but the presence of numerous squamous epithelial cells should be sufficient to alert clinicians to this artifact.

WBCs should be virtually absent in normal urine, although up to 5 WBCs/HPF would still be in the reference range. The presence of WBCs in the urine (pyuria) usually suggests an acute infection in the urinary tract (see Chapter 68, Urinary Tract Infections). Some noninfectious inflammatory diseases of the kidney, ureter, or bladder may also contribute WBCs to the urine sediment.

Casts are composed of proteinaceous or fatty material that outlines the shape of the renal tubules where they were deposited. The presence of casts in the urine must be interpreted in light of other factors related to the kidney and its function; however, fatty casts, RBC casts, and WBC casts are always significant. RBC casts usually suggest glomerular injury, and WBC casts suggest tubular or interstitial injury. Lipid casts with proteinuria are characteristic findings in patients with nephrotic syndrome or hypothyroidism.[41] The finding of hyaline casts alone in the presence of proteinuria suggests a renal origin for the protein. Hyaline or granular casts alone, however, only suggest some

TABLE 2-5
Therapeutic Drug Monitoring Reference Ranges

Drug	Peak Reference Range	SI Units	Trough Reference Range	SI Units	Notes
ANTIBIOTICS					
Peak and trough targets may vary with dosing interval, type or severity of infection, and patient-specific factors					
Amikacin	25–35 mcg/mL	43–60 μmol/L	<10 mcg/mL	<17 μmol/L	Traditional dosing
Gentamicin or Tobramycin	6–10 mcg/mL	13–21 μmol/L	<2 mcg/mL	<4.2 μmol/L	Traditional dosing
Gentamicin or Tobramycin	20 mcg/mL	42.5 μmol/L	Undetectable	Undetectable	Extended dosing
Vancomycin	Not recommended		10 mcg/mL	3 μmol/L	Recommended to keep >10 mcg/mL to avoid development of resistance
			15–20 mcg/mL	10–14 μmol/L	Complicated infections (bacteremia, endocarditis, osteomyelitis, meningitis, and hospital-acquired pneumonia caused by *S. aureus*

Drug	Therapeutic Reference Level	SI Units
ANTIEPILEPTIC DRUGS		
Therapeutic targets may vary with seizure control and patient-specific factors		
Carbamazepine	4–12 mcg/mL	17–51 μmol/L
Phenobarbital	10–40 mcg/mL	43–170 μmol/L
Phenytoin	10–20 mcg/mL	40–79 μmol/L
Primidone	4–12 mcg/mL	18–55 μmol/L
Valproic acid	50–125 mcg/mL	350–690 μmol/L
ANTIDEPRESSANTS AND RELATED AGENTS		
Therapeutic targets may vary with response and patient-specific factors		
Amitriptyline	120–250 ng/mL	433–903 nmol/L
Clozapine	200–350 ng/mL	0.6–1 μmol/L
Desipramine	100–300 ng/mL	281–1125 nmol/L
Doxepin	100–250 ng/mL	107–537 nmol/L
Imipramine	125–300 ng/mL	446–893 nmol/L
Lithium	0.6–1.2 mEq/L	0.6–1.2 nmol/L
Nortriptyline	50–170 ng/mL	190–646 nmol/L
ANTIARRHYTHMICS		
Clinically therapeutic targets may vary with response and patient-specific factors		
Amiodarone	0.5–2.5 mcg/mL	1.5–4 μmol/L
Digoxin	0.8–2 ng/mL	0.9–2.5 nmol/L
Flecainide	0.2–1 mcg/mL	0.5–2.4 μmol/L
Lidocaine	1.5–6 mcg/mL	6.4–26 μmol/L
Procainamide	4–10 mcg/mL	17–42 μmol/L
Quinidine	2–5 mcg/mL	6–15 μmol/L

TABLE 2-6
Laboratory Monitoring for Common Therapeutic Agents[a]

Drug or Drug Class	SCr, CrCl	BUN	Na	K	CO_2	Ca	Mg	Phos	Glu	CBC	WBC Indices	RBC Indices	LFT(s)	Lipids	TSH	Drug Level	Other	Notes
ACEI, ARB	✓			✓														
Acitretin									✓				✓	✓				
Aldosterone antagonists	✓	✓		✓														
Amiodarone				✓			✓								✓		Free T_4	Chest x-ray
Atypical antipsychotics									✓					✓				*Also see clozapine*
Calcipotriol/calcipotriene						✓												
Carbamazepine	✓	✓								✓			✓			✓	Calcium and Vit D levels	Genotyping, drug interactions possible
Clozapine									✓		✓						Absolute neutrophil count	
DMARDs	✓									✓			✓					
Digoxin	✓		✓	✓	✓	✓	✓									✓		
Diuretics	✓	✓	✓	✓	✓	✓	✓		✓								Uric acid	
Enoxaparin	✓																Platelets	Anti-Xa (obesity, renal dysfunction, pregnancy)
Ethosuximide													✓			✓		
Felbamate										✓								
Fenofibrate													✓					CK if muscle symptoms
Fexofenadine	✓																	Dose adjusted CrCl <80 mL/min
Flecainide				✓												✓		
Gemfibrozil										✓			✓					CK if muscle symptoms
Glitazones													✓					
Glyburide	✓								✓								A_{1c}	Not recommended CrCl <50 mL/min
HMG-CoA inhibitors													✓				Lipids, baseline CK	CK, TSH if muscle symptoms
Lithium	✓	✓	✓	✓	✓	✓				✓					✓	✓		Pregnancy test

Metformin	✓						✓					Hgb, Hct, Vit B_{12}, folic acid	
Niacin			✓	✓	✓			✓				Uric acid	CK if muscle symptoms
NSAIDs	✓					✓		✓					
Oxcarbazepine		✓								✓			
Phenytoin						✓					✓	Albumin, Calcium and Vit D levels	
PPIs												Vit B_{12}	
Ranitidine	✓											Vit B_{12}	Dose adjusted CrCl <50 mL/min
Retinoids (oral)					✓			✓	✓				Monthly pregnancy test
Theophylline											✓		Drug interactions possible
Thyroid replacement										✓		Free T_4	
Topiramate												Bicarbonate	Ammonia if symptomatic
Valproic acid						✓		✓			✓	Plt count, coagulation tests	Ammonia if symptomatic
Warfarin												INR, Hct	Genotyping, drug interactions possible

[a] Frequency and type of monitoring may vary based on clinical situation.

Adapted from Therapeutic Research Center. Recommended lab monitoring for common medications. *Pharm Lett*. 2010;26(260704).

A_{1c}, hemoglobin A_{1c}; ACEI, angiotensin-converting enzyme inhibitor; ARB, angiotensin receptor blocker; BUN, blood urea nitrogen; CBC, complete blood count; CK, creatine kinase; CrCl, creatinine clearance; DMARDs, disease-modifying antirheumatic drugs; Hct, hematocrit; Hgb, hemoglobin; HMG-CoA, 3-hydroxy-3-methylglutaryl-coenzyme A; INR, international normalized ratio; LFTs, liver function tests; NSAIDs, nonsteroidal anti-inflammatory drugs; Plt, platelet; PPIs, proton-pump inhibitors; RBC, red blood cell; SCr, serum creatinine; T_4, thyroxine; TSH, thyroid-stimulating hormone; Vit, vitamin; WBC, white blood cell.

defect in factors that affect cast formation, and are therefore difficult to interpret.

Crystals may originally appear as a cloud in the urine. Their formation is pH dependent, and they often appear only as the urine cools to room temperature or in concentrated urine. In acid urine, crystals may be uric acid or calcium oxalate; in alkaline urine, they may be phosphates. Crystals per se are not highly significant, although they may reflect a tendency toward the formation of renal calculi (see Chapter 30, Acute Kidney Injury).

CASE 2-11

QUESTION 1: R.C. is a 23-year-old man who was diagnosed with type 1 diabetes mellitus about 10 years ago; until now his diabetes has been well controlled with an aggressive insulin regimen. His sister brings him to the emergency department with a 3-day history of fever, chills, dysuria, malaise, and some confusion. He also complains of nausea and vomiting and a poor appetite. Because he has not been able to keep any food down for about 48 hours, he has not taken his insulin. A finger stick blood glucose is 545 mg/dL, and a stat midstream urinalysis and Gram stain indicate the following:

pH, 5.2
Appearance cloudy
Specific gravity, 1.033
Urine protein, 3+
Urine glucose, 4+
Urine ketones, positive
Urine bacteria, 4+
Urine WBC, too numerous to count (TNTC)
Squamous epithelial, few per HPF
Urine nitrite, positive
Gram stain, numerous gram-negative rods

What objective data from the urinalysis indicate that R.C. is critically ill?

The cloudy appearance of R.C.'s urine indicates the presence of bacteria, protein, and WBCs, which is substantiated by the data (4+ bacteria, 3+ protein, and TNTC WBCs). The lack of a significant amount of squamous epithelial cells, the presence of a significant amount of nitrite-producing bacteria, and the Gram stain indicate a clean-catch urine specimen and a urinary tract infection (UTI) involving gram-negative organisms. Because the renal threshold of glucose is typically 180 mg/dL, the presence of 4+ glucose in the urine indicates that the blood glucose concentration significantly exceeds this figure (substantiated by blood glucose of 545 mg/dL). Acidification of the urine and ketonuria occur after the release of ketone bodies into the bloodstream after the breakdown of fatty acids for energy utilization. It is likely that R.C. has a severe UTI and, most likely, diabetic ketoacidosis. (See Chapters 53, Diabetes Mellitus, and 68, Urinary Tract Infections, for thorough discussions of diabetes, diabetic ketoacidosis, and UTIs.)

THERAPEUTIC DRUG MONITORING

Many drugs have a wide dosing range that can achieve efficacy with low risk of toxicity. Drugs that have a narrow dosing range with high risk of toxicity or narrow therapeutic drugs have blood levels that are often evaluated by means of laboratory monitoring. Results from therapeutic drug monitoring assist clinicians with appropriate dosing adjustments to prevent toxicity and achieve appropriate clinical outcomes. Pharmacokinetic parameters as well as drug interactions may significantly impact the laboratory results and must be integrated into the clinical assessment of the data. Refer to Table 2-5 for a list of common therapeutic drug monitoring reference ranges. Similarly, for certain drugs and drug classes, there are recommended laboratory tests that should be performed to monitor their potential adverse effects on organ systems. Table 2-6[42] summarizes the laboratory monitoring for common therapeutic agents.

TABLE 2-7
FDA and Non–FDA-Approved Products Available for Patient-Directed Monitoring or Testing

Blood Chemistry

Blood glucose monitors
Glycosylated hemoglobin (A_{1c})
Lipids (TC, HDL, LDL, TG)
Prothrombin (PT, INR)

Screening for Disease or Infection

Middle ear monitor (otitis media)
Urinary tract infection
Urine dipsticks
Glucose, ketones, specific gravity, blood, pH, protein, nitrite, leukocytes
Anemia (Hgb)
Hepatitis C
HIV
Kidney disease (microalbuminuria)
Thyroid (TSH)
Fecal occult blood test

Fertility—Male

Fertility tests (sperm counts)
Paternity testing (DNA)
Hormone tests (testosterone, DHEA)

Fertility—Female

Ovulation tests (LH)
Pregnancy tests (hCG)
Menopause tests (FSH)
Maternity testing (DNA)
Hormone tests (estrogen, progesterone, testosterone)

Drugs of Abuse

Alcohol
Nicotine
THC (marijuana)
Cocaine
Opiates
Amphetamines
Methamphetamines
PCP
Barbiturates
Benzodiazepines
MDMA (ecstasy)

A_{1c}, glycosylated hemoglobin; DHEA, dehydroepiandrosterone; FDA, US Food and Drug Administration; FSH, follicle-stimulating hormone; hCG, human chorionic gonadotropin; HDL, high-density lipoprotein; Hgb, hemoglobin; HIV, human immunodeficiency virus; INR, international normalized ratio; LDL, low-density lipoprotein; LH, luteinizing hormone; MDMA, 3′4-methylelenedioxy-methamphetamine; PCP, phencyclidine; PT, prothrombin time; TC, total cholesterol; TG, triglyceride; THC, tetrahydrocannabinol; TSH, thyroid-stimulating hormone.

PATIENT-DIRECTED MONITORING AND TESTING

Often patient-directed self-monitoring is an essential component to successful management of certain disease states such as blood pressure monitoring for hypertension and blood glucose monitoring for diabetes mellitus. When used appropriately, data obtained from these monitoring devices can be used by health care providers and consumers to initiate or modify therapies accordingly.

Additional laboratory, self-monitoring tests or devices are also available for consumers to purchase for independent testing or screening purposes at home (Table 2-7). Some products provide an immediate result, whereas others require submitting a completed kit to a laboratory for analysis. Samples may be obtained from various sources, including urine, blood, saliva, stool, or hair samples. In 1992, sales of over-the-counter diagnostic tests in the United States were $750 million. By 2002, sales jumped to $2.8 billion annually.[43] The incidence of consumers using these products has significantly increased and likely will continue to climb due to increased access via the Internet as well as additional tests becoming available.

In the United States, some, but not all, patient-directed tests have been approved by the US Food and Drug Administration (FDA). A current listing of approved products is available though the FDA's Office of In Vitro Diagnostic Device Evaluation and Safety (OIVD) and can be accessed online at **http://www.fda.gov/MedicalDevices/ProductsandMedicalProcedures/InVitroDiagnostics/default.htm**. Consumers should be cautioned about the accuracy of tests that have not been approved and the validity of all test results, especially for diagnostic purposes, because many factors can impact or interfere with the sensitivity (probability of obtaining a positive result when sample is truly positive) and specificity (probability of obtaining a negative result when the sample is truly negative). Follow-up assessment with a health care provider should be encouraged to confirm or refute patient-directed test results. Table 2-7 provides examples of tests available.

KEY REFERENCES AND WEBSITES

A full list of references for this chapter can be found at **http://thepoint.lww.com/AT10e**. Below are the key references and websites for this chapter, with the corresponding reference number in this chapter found in parentheses after the reference.

Key References

Burtis CA, Ashwood ER, Bruns DE. *Tietz Textbook of Clinical Chemistry and Molecular Diagnostics*. 4th ed. Philadelphia, PA: WB Saunders Co; 2005. (1)

McPherson RA, Pincus MR. *Henry's Clinical Diagnosis and Management by Laboratory Methods*. 21st ed. Philadelphia, PA: WB Saunders Co; 2006. (2)

Key Websites

In vitro Diagnostics, US Food and Drug Administration. **http://www.fda.gov/MedicalDevices/ProductsandMedicalProcedures/InVitroDiagnostics/default.htm.**

Lab Tests Online. **http://labtestsonline.org.**

National Guideline Clearinghouse, US Department of Health and Human Services. **http://www.guidelines.gov.**

National Kidney Foundation. **http://www.kidney.org/professionals/.**

3 Anaphylaxis and Drug Allergies

Robert K. Middleton

CORE PRINCIPLES

	CHAPTER CASES
DRUG ALLERGIES	
1 Drug allergies are a subset of adverse drug reactions that are usually mediated by the immune system. Although typically unpredictable, there are several factors known to influence the frequency of allergic reactions including age, sex, genetics, prior drug exposure, and drug dose and route. A detailed drug history is key to assisting in the diagnosis of a drug allergy.	**Case 3-1 (Questions 1, 2)**
2 Skin testing for allergy to penicillin is an important diagnostic tool that assists in determining whether or not a patient is truly allergic to this class of drug. Patients presenting with a history of penicillin allergy but who have a negative penicillin scratch test and a negative intradermal test can be safely given β-lactam antibiotics.	**Case 3-1 (Question 3)**
3 There are varying degrees of cross-reactivity between various β-lactam antibiotics. Understanding the frequency of cross-reactivity is important in making treatment decisions if skin testing is not available. The frequency of cross-reaction between penicillins and cephalosporins has been reported to be 5% to 15%, but is likely much lower. The risk of a cephalosporin reaction in a patient with a penicillin allergy decreases with increasing cephalosporin generation, being lowest with the third- and fourth-generation drugs. The frequency of cross-reaction between penicillins and carbapenems or monobactams appears to be very low (approximately 1%).	**Case 3-1 (Question 4)**
ANAPHYLAXIS	
1 Anaphylaxis is a serious allergic reaction that has a rapid onset and might cause death. It is caused by the rapid release of immune mediators from tissue mast cells and peripheral blood basophils. Symptoms such as pruritus of the hands, feet, and groin; flushing; light-headedness; hypotension; tachycardia; and difficulty breathing can begin within minutes of exposure to the precipitating agent, which is most commonly foods, insect stings, and drugs. Prompt recognition and treatment are critical to ensure a favorable outcome.	**Case 3-2 (Questions 1, 2)**
2 Epinephrine is the drug of choice for treatment of anaphylaxis and should be given immediately upon suspicion of an anaphylactic reaction. Epinephrine should be given intramuscularly into the lateral thigh as often as every 5 minutes to treat symptoms. Intramuscular injection is preferred over the subcutaneous and intravenous (IV) routes due to rapid absorption and ease of administration. The patient should be placed in the Trendelenburg position and second-line treatments including oxygen, IV fluids, and a nebulized β-agonist initiated as needed. Antihistamines and corticosteroids are also commonly used to treat anaphylaxis although there are no data showing an impact on outcome from these therapies.	**Case 3-2 (Question 3)**

continued

GENERALIZED REACTIONS		
1	Generalized hypersensitivity reactions can manifest in a number of ways including drug fever, serum sickness, hemolytic anemia, vasculitis, and autoimmune disorders. Specific organ systems such as the lungs, liver, kidneys, and hematopoietic system can also be the target of allergic drug reactions.	**Case 3-3 (Question 1), Case 3-4 (Questions 1, 2), Case 3-5 (Questions 1, 2)**
PSEUDOALLERGIC REACTIONS		
1	Pseudoallergic reactions are drug reactions that exhibit clinical signs and symptoms of an allergic response, but are not immunologically mediated. Pseudoallergic reactions can be relatively benign (such as red man syndrome from vancomycin) or potentially life-threatening, clinically resembling immune-mediated anaphylaxis as from radiocontrast media. Several drugs are associated with pseudoallergic reactions including aspirin and nonsteroidal anti-inflammatory drugs, opiates, angiotensin-converting enzyme inhibitors, and injectable iron products.	**Case 3-6 (Questions 1, 2, 5), Case 3-7 (Question 1)**
2	The management of pseudoallergic reactions is the same as for true allergic reactions.	**Case 3-6 (Questions 3, 4), Case 3-7 (Question 2)**
PREVENTION AND MANAGEMENT OF ALLERGIC REACTIONS		
1	The keys to preventing an allergic reaction in a patient with history of allergy are a good description of the reaction and its causes, distinguishing between drug allergy and drug intolerance, and good documentation and communication of the reaction.	**Case 3-1 (Questions 1, 2), Case 3-8 (Question 1)**
2	In some cases, it is necessary to treat a patient with a drug to which they have a significant allergic reaction. To accomplish this, the process of tolerance induction (or desensitization) may be used. Tolerance induction starts with administration of a sub-allergenic dose of the drug to which a patient is allergic and the progressive administration of larger doses with the goal of modifying the patient's response. Once tolerance has been successfully induced, the patient must remain on the drug to maintain the state of tolerance. Tolerance induction should not be used in patients with a history of a severe non-IgE–mediated reaction such as hepatitis, hemolytic anemia, Stevens-Johnson syndrome, or toxic epidermal necrolysis.	**Case 3-9 (Questions 1, 2, 4)**
3	The oral route of tolerance induction is preferred over the IV route. Patients may experience a mild reaction during desensitization, although severe reactions are rare. Even after successful desensitization, patients may experience an allergic reaction during full dose therapy.	**Case 3-9 (Questions 2, 3)**
4	A graded drug challenge (also called test dosing) is a process of giving sub-therapeutic doses of a drug to a patient to determine if they are allergic. A graded drug challenge generally uses larger starting doses than tolerance induction and involves fewer steps. Graded drug challenge may be appropriate in patients with a distant or unclear history of drug allergy, when the reaction seems minor or when diagnostic testing is unavailable, or in cases where cross-reactivity is expected to be low. Graded challenge should not be used in patients with a history of a severe non-IgE–mediated reaction such as hepatitis, hemolytic anemia, Stevens-Johnson syndrome, or toxic epidermal necrolysis.	**Case 3-9 (Question 1)**

Adverse drug reactions occur in up to 20% of hospitalized patients and up to 25% of ambulatory patients. Studies have found that up to 6% of all hospitalizations are caused by an adverse drug event. Allergic or hypersensitivity reactions account for about one-third of all adverse drug reactions and may affect 10% to 15% of hospitalized patients.[1–4] In one study of more than 36,000 hospitalized patients, 731 adverse events were identified, with 1% being severe, life-threatening, allergic reactions.[5] The potential morbidity and mortality associated with allergic drug reactions can be significant.

Definition

Allergic reactions are a subset of adverse drug reactions. One classification divides adverse drug events into the following:

- Type A reactions are "predictable, usually dose dependent, and related to the pharmacologic actions of the drug."
- Type B reactions are "unpredictable, often dose independent, and are related to the individual's immunologic response or to genetic differences in susceptible patients."

- Type C reactions are chronic side effects related to the duration of therapy, for example, adrenal suppression from corticosteroids.
- Type D reactions are rare side effects, delayed in onset, and usually dose-related, such as carcinogenicity.[6]

Type B reactions can be further divided into drug intolerance (an undesired pharmacological effect that occurs at low or subtherapeutic doses and is not related to abnormalities in the metabolism, excretion, or bioavailability of the drug), drug idiosyncrasy (an unexpected effect often caused by underlying abnormalities of metabolism, excretion, or bioavailability), drug allergy (immune-mediated hypersensitivity), and pseudoallergic reactions, (non-immune mediated hypersensitivity reactions, also known as anaphylactoid reactions).[7,8] Under this classification, drug allergy or drug hypersensitivity is an unpredictable adverse drug reaction that is immunologically mediated.[9]

Predisposing Factors

Factors known to affect the incidence of allergic reactions can be categorized as being drug-related or patient-related.[10]

AGE AND SEX

Children are less likely to become sensitized than adults, presumably because younger age is likely to be associated with less cumulative drug exposure.[10–13] More female than male patients experience allergic reactions (up to 2.3:1), although this may vary by type of reaction, drug, patient age, and setting.[3,14]

GENETIC FACTORS

Patients with histories of allergic rhinitis, asthma, or atopic dermatitis who experience a systemic drug reaction tend to react more severely than others.[10,12,15] Familial occurrences of allergic reactions, although rare, have been reported. For example, erythema multiforme was described in three of five siblings treated with thiabendazole.[16] Ethnic predisposition to drug allergy is increasingly recognized. White patients are more likely to experience hypersensitivity reactions to abacavir than nonwhite patients, and black patients are more susceptible to angioedema from angiotensin-converting enzyme (ACE) inhibitors than are other ethnic groups.[17,18] A patient's ability to metabolize a drug is influenced by his or her genetic makeup and may affect the incidence of allergic reactions. Pharmacogenetics (i.e., the study of genetically determined variability to drug response) often centers on drug-metabolizing enzymes because many drugs are metabolized by enzymes that are encoded by variations in DNA sequences or genetic polymorphisms.[19]

Acetylator phenotype (e.g., fast acetylator or slow acetylator) is genetically determined, and several variations in the gene encoding for *N*-acetyltransferase (NAT) are recognized.[19] The slow acetylator phenotype is an autosomal recessive trait. Slow acetylators are at risk for sulfonamide hypersensitivity and also are more likely to develop antinuclear antibodies (ANA) and symptoms of systemic lupus erythematosus (SLE) when treated with procainamide or hydralazine.[20] Drug-induced lupus can be considered an allergic reaction because of its association with an immune response, as evidenced by an increase in ANA.

Anticonvulsant hypersensitivity syndrome, characterized by fever, generalized rash, lymphadenopathy, and internal organ involvement, is most associated with aromatic anticonvulsants (e.g., phenytoin, phenobarbital, and carbamazepine) and is more common in patients with a heritable deficiency in epoxide hydrolase.[21] This syndrome also is known as drug hypersensitivity syndrome and as DRESS (drug rash with eosinophilia and systemic symptoms) syndrome. A genetic defect also might be responsible for a serum sicknesslike reaction to cefaclor.[21]

Numerous polymorphisms are known for the cytochrome P-450 (CYP) isoenzyme family that catalyzes the oxidative metabolism of hundreds of drugs. The best studied of these are variations in genes that encode for CYP2D6, CYP2C9, CYP2C19, and CYP3A4. Examples of the phenotypic expression of these variations include poor metabolizers (who possess nonfunctional alleles and have reduced metabolic activity) and ultra rapid metabolizers (who have multiple copies of functional genes and have enhanced metabolic activity).[19] Genetic differences in CYP-metabolizing enzymes might explain the predisposition to drug allergy and hypersensitivity of some individuals, as well as other forms of drug toxicity and drug response.

Whereas genetic polymorphism in drug metabolizing enzymes is responsible for some allergic reactions, gene variations in the major histocompatibility complex (MHC) perhaps are more significant.[17] For example, dermatologic reactions and thrombocytopenia to gold and toxicity to penicillamine are linked to the presence of the HLA-DR3 allele in the MHC; severe cutaneous reactions to allopurinol are linked to presence of the HLA-B*5801 allele in the Han Chinese population, and the potentially life-threatening hypersensitivity syndrome seen with abacavir is strongly associated with the HLA-B*5701, HLA-DR7, and HLA-DQ3 haplotype.[17,20–24] In the latter case, presence of this haplotype in patients predicted abacavir hypersensitivity 100% of the time, and its absence had a 97% negative predictive value.[22] This haplotype appears more commonly in white patients than in other ethnic groups and explains the predisposition of white patients to this severe reaction. Genetic screening of patients for this haplotype before initiating abacavir therapy has significantly reduced the occurrence of hypersensitivity reactions.[25] In the future, it is hoped genes that are involved in life-threatening hypersensitivity reactions (e.g., anaphylaxis, hepatotoxicity, blood dyscrasias, Stevens-Johnson syndrome, toxic epidermal necrolysis) will be identified.

ASSOCIATED ILLNESS

Although genes clearly play a role in hypersensitivity reactions, environmental factors (e.g., concomitant illness) also are implicated. For example, the incidence of maculopapular rash with ampicillin therapy is significantly higher in patients with Epstein-Barr virus infections (e.g., infectious mononucleosis), lymphocytic leukemia, or gout.[10,26] Infection with herpes virus or Epstein-Barr virus also has been linked to DRESS syndrome[27,28]; and the occurrence of reactions to trimethoprim-sulfamethoxazole in patients who are HIV-positive is about 10-fold higher than in the HIV-negative population.[17] Liver or kidney disease may alter the metabolism or elimination of reactive drug metabolites, increasing the risk of an allergic response.

PREVIOUS DRUG ADMINISTRATION

A previous history of an allergic reaction to a drug being considered for treatment, or one that is immunochemically similar, is the most reliable risk factor for development of a subsequent allergic reaction.[10,11] A commonly encountered example is the patient with a history of a severe allergic reaction to penicillin, in whom all structurally related penicillin compounds should be avoided, and in whom the possibility of a hypersensitivity reaction should be considered when using other β-lactam antibiotics.[10]

DRUG-RELATED FACTORS

The dose, frequency of exposure, and route of administration can influence the incidence of drug allergy. For example, penicillin-induced hemolytic anemia requires high and sustained drug concentrations.[13] In β-lactam antibiotic IgE sensitivity, frequent intermittent courses, rather than continuous therapy, are more likely to result in drug sensitization.[19] The route of administration is important in terms of the risk of both sensitization and allergic reaction in a previously sensitized person. Topical administration carries the greatest risk of sensitization, followed by subcutaneous, intramuscular, and oral routes. The intravenous (IV) route is the least sensitizing route of administration.[8] However, in a patient who is already sensitized to a specific medication, the risk of an allergic reaction to that medication is greatest when it is given IV and least when given orally. This is thought to be a function of the rate of drug delivery.[10] Multiple drug therapy is associated with a greater risk of allergic reactions. This may be related to increased demands on metabolic pathways from multiple drugs, leading to the accumulation of reactive metabolites.[8]

Pathogenesis

Allergic drug reactions cannot be attributed to a single immunopathologic mechanism. Traditionally, an allergic drug reaction was thought to occur in two phases, initial sensitization and subsequent elicitation.[29] Most drugs are small molecules (<1000 Da) and are unable to stimulate an immune response. Sensitization occurs as a result of covalent binding of a drug or a metabolite to a carrier protein in a process referred to as haptenation.[7,30] This drug–protein (or drug metabolite–protein) complex is sufficiently large to induce the production of drug-specific T- or B-lymphocytes and IgM, IgG, and IgE. On re-exposure to the drug, the patient is likely to present with allergic symptoms.[19] Allergic reactions to β-lactam antibiotics occur by this mechanism. This theory, however, cannot explain several allergic phenomena. For instance, some chemically inert drugs (i.e., drugs that cannot form stable covalent bonds and do not have reactive metabolites) can still elicit an allergic response. Lidocaine and mepivacaine are examples. Furthermore, some patients have a strong allergic reaction to a drug on initial exposure, and some allergic reactions rapidly occur after drug exposure, a time period shorter than expected for the development of new antibodies. To account for some of these observations, other models for explaining allergic reactions have been proposed. The direct pharmacological interaction, or P-I, concept offers one explanation for these observations. This model suggests that some drugs are able to bind directly to T-cell receptors in a reversible, noncovalent manner. The drug–T-cell receptor complex interacts with MHC molecules, leading to activation and expansion of T cells that are directed against the drug.[31] On the other hand, the danger hypothesis proposes idiosyncratic drug reactions are the result of damaged or stressed cells that release "danger signals." Danger signals may be cytokines (e.g., interleukins, tumor necrosis factors) that act as co-stimulants to trigger an immune response once released. Similar to the P-I concept, neither covalent binding of drug to a carrier protein nor prior drug exposure is a prerequisite for an allergic response with the danger hypothesis. Rather, the drug itself, or a reactive metabolite, directly induces cell injury or stress, causing the release of danger signals. Once the drug is discontinued, generation of danger signals cease, and the clinical manifestations of the allergic reaction resolve.[32] Undoubtedly, the processes involved in allergic reactions are complex and might include some combination of each theory. Interested readers are referred to more in-depth reviews.[33,34]

DRUGS AS ALLERGENS AND IMMUNOLOGIC CLASSIFICATION

Although there are proposed changes to the nomenclature and classification of drug allergies,[35] the Gel and Coombs classification is the most common. In this system allergic drug reactions can be classified into one of four types (Table 3-1).[10,11]

TYPE I: IMMEDIATE HYPERSENSITIVITY REACTIONS

Type I reactions are typically mediated by the immune globulin IgE. Initial exposure to an antigen results in production of specific IgE antibodies that are expressed on the surface of mast cells in the tissue and basophils in the blood. On re-exposure, the antigen cross-links with two or more surface-bound IgE antibodies causing the release of several chemical mediators including histamine, tryptase, leukotrienes, prostaglandins, and cyotkines.[29]

ONLINE CONTENT **For a visual of reaction to allergen exposure, see http://thepoint.lww.com/AT10e.**

A period of several weeks is required after initial exposure and sensitization before a type I reaction can be elicited; once sensitized, however, a type I response can be elicited within minutes as a result of existing antibodies. In addition, a type I reaction can occur on re-exposure to small amounts of drug administered by any route.[29,36–38] Such reactions can be limited to single organs or may affect multiple organ systems. Reactions range in

TABLE 3-1
Immunological Classification of Allergic Drug Reactions

Immunologic Class	Antibody	Mechanism	Common Clinical Manifestations
Type I (immediate)	IgE	Drug–hapten reacts with IgE antibody on the surface of mast cells and basophils, resulting in the release of mediators	Urticaria, bronchospasm, anaphylaxis
Type II (cytotoxic)	IgG	Hapten–cell reaction: Drug interacts with cell surfaces, resulting in the formation of an immunogenic complex and the production of antibodies	Hemolytic anemia
–	IgM	Immune complex reaction: Drug reacts with antibody in circulation, forming a complex that with complement binds to the cell, resulting in injury (hematologic reactions only)	Granulocytopenia
–	–	Autoimmune reaction: Drug induces autoantibody production against platelets	Thrombocytopenia
Type III (immune complex)	IgG	Same as type II immune complex reactions (nonhematologic reactions)	Serum sickness, vasculitis
Type IVa-d (cell mediated)	–	Interaction of sensitized T lymphocytes with drug antigen	Contact dermatitis, chronic allergic rhinitis, maculopapular exanthema

Source: VanArsdel P. Drug Hypersensitivity. In: Bierman C, ed. *Allergic Diseases from Infancy to Adulthood*. Philadelphia, PA: WB Saunders; 1988:684; Pichler WJ et al. Drug hypersensitivity reactions: pathomechanism and clinical symptoms. *Med Clin North Am*. 2010;94:645.

severity from pruritus and urticaria to bronchospasm, respiratory distress, laryngeal edema, circulatory collapse, and death. Immune-mediated anaphylaxis is the classic example of a type I reaction. Reactions that clinically resemble anaphylaxis, but do not involve immunologic mediators (antibodies), are termed anaphylactoid reactions (see Case 3-6, Question 1).

TYPE II: CYTOTOXIC REACTIONS

Cytotoxic reactions involve the interaction of IgG or IgM and can occur by three different mechanisms (Table 3-1). Common clinical manifestations of cytotoxic reactions include hemolytic anemia, thrombocytopenia, and granulocytopenia. Penicillin-induced hemolytic anemia is the best-known example of a cytotoxic drug reaction. This reaction typically appears after 7 days of high-dose therapy.[13,39,40]

TYPE III: IMMUNE COMPLEX–MEDIATED REACTIONS

Immune complex–mediated reactions result from the formation of drug–antibody complexes in serum, which often deposit in blood vessel walls, resulting in activation of complement and endothelial cell injury.[36] Also referred to as serum sickness, these reactions typically manifest as fever, urticaria, arthralgia, and lymphadenopathy 7 to 21 days after exposure.[13,41]

TYPE IV: CELL-MEDIATED (DELAYED) REACTIONS

In cell-mediated (delayed) reactions, an antigen binds with sensitized T cells. Contact dermatitis is the most common manifestation of cell-mediated reactions, although systemic reactions can occur. The variety of clinical manifestations of delayed hypersensitivity has been attributed to distinct patterns of cytokine release and effector-cell recruitment, based on the type of T cells stimulated. For example, hypersensitivity reactions involving type 1 helper T cells are induced by interferon-γ and interleukin-2, whereas reactions involving type 2 helper T cells use interleukins 4 and 5. Each pattern of cytokine release recruits specific effector cells, such as macrophages, neutrophils, or other T cells, and is responsible for the unique clinical manifestations of the reaction. Based on this understanding, type IV reactions have been further subclassified as type IVa, type IVb, type IVc, and type IVd, corresponding to four unique patterns of T-cell and effector-cell involvement.[42]

An understanding of the immunologic mechanism can be helpful in the diagnosis and treatment of an allergic reaction; however, the exact immunologic mechanism is unknown for many allergic reactions to drugs. In addition, patients often present with several symptoms characteristic of more than one of the reactions described herein. The use of many drugs concurrently also makes it difficult to identify the drug responsible for the reaction. Therefore, a careful drug history and diagnostic tests (e.g., wheal and flare, in vitro detection of drug-specific IgE antibodies) often are necessary for an appropriate diagnosis and treatment of a patient.

Diagnosis

DISTINCTIVE FEATURES OF ALLERGIC REACTIONS

The first step in the diagnosis of an allergic drug reaction is to recognize and differentiate it from other adverse drug reactions. This can be accomplished by having a good understanding of the distinctive features of allergic drug reactions (Table 3-2).[9,11,26]

TABLE 3-2
Clinical Features of Allergic Drug Reactions

- Are unpredictable
- Occur only in susceptible individuals
- Have no correlation with known pharmacologic properties of the drug
- Require an induction period on primary exposure but not on readministration
- Can occur with doses far below therapeutic range
- Can affect most organs, but commonly involves the skin
- Most commonly manifests as an erythematous or maculopapular rash, but includes angioedema, serum sickness syndrome, anaphylaxis, and asthma
- Occur in a small proportion of the population (10%–15%)
- Disappear on cessation of therapy and reappear after readministration of a small dose of the suspected drug(s) of similar chemical structure
- Desensitization may be possible

Source: Assem E. Drug allergy and tests for its detection. In: Davies DM, ed. *Textbook of Adverse Drug Reactions*. New York: Oxford University Press; 1991:689; Schnyder B. Approach to the patient with drug allergy. *Immunol Allergy Clin North Am*. 2009;29:405.

CASE 3-1

QUESTION 1: J.A., a 73-year-old woman, is admitted from a nursing home with an infected decubitus ulcer. Cultures reveal *Staphylococcus aureus*, which is sensitive to oxacillin, cefazolin, and vancomycin. On questioning, J.A. reports having experienced a rash to penicillin in the past. Her current medications include oral docusate 100 mg twice daily (BID), oral enalapril 5 mg every morning, oral prednisone 20 mg daily, and oral ibuprofen 800 mg three times daily (TID). What information should be obtained to determine whether J.A.'s rash represents an allergic drug reaction?

The single most informative diagnostic procedure for allergic drug reactions is a detailed drug history (Table 3-3), which is helpful in obtaining the information necessary to determine whether a reaction represents a drug allergy and in identifying the culprit drug. In inquiring about prior allergic and medication encounters, it is important to document the drugs to which

TABLE 3-3
Detailed Drug History

- Name of the medication
- Route of administration
- Reason medication was prescribed
- Nature and severity of reaction
- Temporal relationships between drugs and reaction (dose, date initiated, duration, when during the course of treatment did the reaction occur)
- Prior allergy history
- When did the reaction occur (days to weeks vs. months to years)
- Similar reactions in family members
- Prior exposure to the same or structurally related medications
- Concurrent medications
- Management of the reaction (effect of drug discontinuation; therapies required to treat the reaction)
- Response to treatment
- Prior diagnostic testing or rechallenge
- Other medical problems (if any)

Source: Khan DA, Solensky R. Drug allergy. *J Allergy Clin Immunol*. 2010;125 (2 Suppl 2):S126; Celik G. Drug allergy. In: Adkinson NF, ed. *Middleton's Allergy: Principles and Practice*. 7th ed. St. Louis, MO: Mosby; 2008:1205; Marquardt DL et al. Anaphylaxis. In: Middleton E Jr et al, eds. *Allergy. Principles and Practices*. 4th ed. St. Louis, MO: Mosby; 1993:1365.

the patient has or has not previously reacted. This can sometimes alert the clinician about certain types of compounds to which the patient is likely to react. In addition, the acquired information allows the clinician to characterize the drug reaction and to appreciate how such a reaction might be manifested in the patient on exposure to the same, or an immunologically similar, compound in the future.

The temporal relationship between drugs and reactions often is the strongest piece of evidence implicating an allergic reaction to a particular agent. Drugs that the patient has received for long continuous periods before the onset of a reaction are less likely to be implicated than drugs that have been recently initiated or restarted.[43] Equally important is to determine when an adverse reaction has occurred. Many compounds have been reformulated over the years, resulting in removal of sensitizing impurities (e.g., penicillin, vancomycin). Therefore, it is possible that re-exposure to the agent will not result in an adverse event. Inquiring about whether the patient has received the drug since the first episode by asking the patient about other brands or names of other drugs in the same class (e.g., amoxicillin, ampicillin) will assist in determining whether the patient is likely to react to the drug on re-exposure. It usually is helpful to chart all the drugs the patient is currently taking, their dose, and start and stop dates of use. This can be compared with the onset and disappearance of the reaction.

CASE 3-1, QUESTION 2: On further questioning, J.A. reports having experienced an urticarial rash in the past when given ampicillin for a kidney infection approximately 2 years ago. The rash developed over her entire body less than a day after starting the antibiotic and disappeared 2 days after discontinuation. Her treatment course was completed with ciprofloxacin. She denies having had a viral infection at the time of the rash to ampicillin. She does not recall having experienced any adverse effects when she received penicillin before this reaction. No other recent changes in her treatment regimen were made before the occurrence of the rash. Why is it likely that J.A. is allergic to penicillin?

Several useful pieces of information gleaned from the drug history obtained from J.A. can be used to determine the likelihood of an allergic reaction to penicillin. J.A.'s rash appeared less than a day after initiation of ampicillin and other drugs had not been added; therefore, the rash probably was caused by ampicillin.

Another important method of identifying a potential drug-induced allergic reaction is to examine the patient's medication list to determine whether the patient is receiving an agent that commonly is implicated in causing the exhibited allergic manifestation. For example, amoxicillin and ampicillin are two of the top three drugs implicated in drug-induced rash.[14]

J.A. received penicillin previously without experiencing any adverse effects until an urticarial rash (a relatively common allergic manifestation) developed on subsequent exposure. This sequence of events follows the typical pattern of an allergic reaction. Allergic reactions commonly require an induction period to sensitize the person to the antigen; however, once sensitized, allergic symptoms typically occur immediately on re-exposure.[43] Therefore, a prior exposure to the same or structurally related compounds needs to be documented.

Finally, it is important to evaluate other medical problems that can elicit or mimic a reaction resembling drug allergy (see the previous section "Associated Illness"). Rashes to ampicillin commonly occur in patients with concurrent Epstein-Barr virus infection.[44] J.A. denies having a viral infection at the time of her rash, thereby strengthening the case that the rash was likely a manifestation of an allergic reaction.

SKIN TESTING

CASE 3-1, QUESTION 3: Why might skin testing for penicillin allergy be appropriate (or inappropriate) for J.A.?

Although J.A.'s elicited medication history strongly suggests that she is allergic to penicillin, a skin test and a drug rechallenge would more firmly establish her drug allergy. Penicillin degrades to major determinants (95%) and minor determinants (5%). Penicilloyl, the primary metabolite of penicillin, is referred to as the major determinant. The other derivatives are referred to as minor determinants. Of these, the parent compound (penicillin), penicilloate, and penilloate are the minor determinants most associated with allergic reactions. The terms major determinant and minor determinant refer to the frequency of antibody formation to these antigenic penicillin metabolite–protein complexes. These terms do not describe the severity of the allergic reaction. Indeed, the major determinant is thought to be responsible for accelerated reactions, but not anaphylaxis. The minor determinants are responsible for anaphylaxis and immediate systemic reactions.

Skin testing with these determinants is used to identify which patients have IgE antibodies to penicillin and which do not. The skin-testing antigen for the major determinant of penicillin is commercially available as penicilloyl polylysine (PPL; Pre-Pen), which was recently re-introduced into the United States after several years of absence.[45] Skin testing using Pre-Pen is a safe and effective procedure (Table 3-4), with less than 1% of positive responders developing systemic reactions.[40] In those in whom a false-negative response occurred, reactions were mild after penicillin administration and, in most cases, did not require drug discontinuation.[39,40] Skin testing with PPL identifies 80% of patients allergic to penicillin. When PPL is supplemented with skin tests for the minor determinants of penicillin, 99.5% of penicillin-allergic patients can be identified.[39] Of the minor determinants, only penicillin G is available in the United States, although a minor determinant mixture is marketed in Europe and Australia.[46] The negative predictive value of skin testing was demonstrated when 34 purportedly "penicillin-allergic patients" needed β-lactam antibiotics during hospitalization. Each subsequently tested negative to penicillin skin-testing and no allergic drug reactions occurred.[47]

Penicillin and its metabolites become antigenic when combined with proteins and can precipitate a hypersensitivity reaction in a patient on re-exposure. In patients with a history of penicillin hypersensitivity, skin test reactivity is affected by the length of time since the allergic reaction and by the nature of the past reaction. Skin test positivity is greatest 6 to 12 months after a reaction and decreases with time. Skin test positivity in one study was found to be only 40% of patients with a history of anaphylaxis, 17% with urticaria, and 7% for maculopapular rashes.[39] Skin testing should not be performed in patients receiving antihistamines because they block the response to the antigen and can result in misinterpretation. In patients receiving antihistamines (i.e., H_1- or H_2-receptor antagonists) or when skin testing is not possible because of severe skin disease, in vitro assays to detect drug-specific IgE antibodies have been developed for the major and minor determinants of penicillin.

To determine whether skin testing is appropriate for J.A., the risks and benefits must be weighed. Because the time of the last reaction was approximately 2 years ago, J.A. may still retain some skin-test positivity if the previous reaction was truly an allergic response to ampicillin. Testing with PPL (major determinant)

TABLE 3-4
Penicillin Skin Testing Procedure

Agent	Procedure	Interpretation
Penicilloyl polylysine (Pre-Pen) Major determinant	Puncture (scratch) test one drop of full-strength solution (6×10^{-5} mol/L)[a]	*No wheal or erythema or wheal <5 mm in diameter after 15 minutes:* proceed with intradermal test. *Wheal or erythema of 5 to 15 mm in diameter or more within 15 minutes:* choose alternative agent, consider desensitization if no other alternatives exist.
PPL	Intradermal test: inject sufficient volume PPL to raise an intradermal bleb of 3 mm in diameter[a] Saline: negative control Histamine: positive control (optional; useful if it is suspected that patient may be anergic)	Read at 20 minutes. Negative response: no increase in size of original bleb and no greater than reaction at control site. Positive response: itching and increase in size of original bleb to at least 5 mm and greater than saline control: choose alternative agent; consider desensitization if no other alternatives exist.
Penicillin G potassium (>1 week old) most important of the minor determinants	Scratch test one drop of 10,000 unit/mL solution	Same as scratch test with PPL (see above).
Penicillin G potassium	Intradermal test: 0.002 mL of 10,000 unit/mL solution	Same as intradermal test with PPL (see above).
—	Serial testing with 10, 100, or 1,000 unit/mL solutions can be performed in those with strong history or serious reactions	

[a] PPL is administered initially as a scratch test. If no wheal or erythema develops, then intradermal testing is performed.
PPL, penicilloyl polylysine.
Source: Pre-Pen benzylpenicilloyl polylysine injection solution [package insert]. Round Rock, TX: ALK-Abelló, Inc; 2010. http://www.prepen.com/package-insert. Accessed November 7, 2010.

and penicillin G (minor determinant) could be useful in determining whether J.A. is likely to experience an urticarial or anaphylactic reaction to penicillin or its derivatives. That J.A. is currently receiving prednisone should not alter the interpretation of the skin test results because the corticosteroids minimally affect the IgE-mediated immediate hypersensitivity reactions. The risks of developing serious systemic reactions to penicillin skin testing are minimal.

The benefit of penicillin skin testing for J.A., however, is questionable because she could be treated with an antibiotic other than a penicillin. The most practical approach to penicillin-allergic patients is simply to avoid the drug. Therefore, the patient's drug history should always be evaluated carefully. In the unlikely situation in which treatment with a penicillin is essential, penicillin skin testing would be useful.

CROSS-REACTIVITY

CASE 3-1, QUESTION 4: J.A. received a scratch test with PPL, which was negative; however, an intradermal test was positive. What treatment options are available to J.A. for her infection?

All penicillin derivatives should be avoided because J.A. had a positive skin-test reaction. Skin tests are not commercially available for cephalosporins and other β-lactam antibiotics. Although cephalosporin-skin testing (i.e., prick followed by intradermal instillation) has been proposed, no prospective studies have evaluated this approach and this practice is not without risk.[48,49] Therefore, clinicians must rely on cross-reactivity data to determine whether a nonpenicillin β-lactam antibiotic (e.g., a cephalosporin) can be used in a penicillin-allergic patient.

Cross-reactivity (i.e., cross-antigenicity) between penicillin and cephalosporins has been reported in 5% to 15% of patients[39,40]; however, the true incidence of cross-reactivity is considerably less because these initial percentages were based on the recollection of patients of an allergic history rather than by objective skin tests.

The risk of a cephalosporin reaction in a patient with a penicillin allergy decreases with increasing cephalosporin generation: 5% to 16.5% for first-generation, 4% for second-generation, and 1% to 3% for third-generation and fourth-generation cephalosporins.[50] The risk of a serious allergic reaction with the use of an advanced-generation cephalosporin in a penicillin-allergic patient might be no greater than the risk of any alternative antibiotic.[51] The cross-reactivity between penicillins and cephalosporins formerly was attributed primarily to their common β-lactam chemical-ring structure; however, side-chain–specific reactions are now recognized to be responsible for a significant portion of allergic reactions within and between the penicillin and cephalosporins families.[48,51,52] In a study of 30 patients with immediate allergic reactions to cephalosporins, less than 20% reacted to penicillin determinants (i.e., skin test positivity, radioallergosorbent testing positivity, or both).[52] (Radioallergosorbent testing is a radioimmune test to detect IgE antibodies responsible for hypersensitivity.) This cross-reactivity between penicillin and cephalosporins is significantly less than earlier reports (up to 50%); however, the results of this study could be attributable to the greater use of third-generation, rather than the first-generation cephalosporins, which share more chemical structure similarities with the penicillins. Additional support for the importance of side-chain–specific reactions of β-lactams comes from observational data noting that 30% of patients with immediate reactions to penicillins were selective for amoxicillin.[53] In patients with allergy to amoxicillin, studies have found 2% to 38% cross-reactivity with the cephalosporin cefadroxil; both drugs share the same side chain.[7] Patients allergic to ampicillin also may have a greater risk of allergic reaction to cephalosporins that share the same side chain, such as cephalexin, cefaclor, cephradine, and loracarbef.[7] Some patients also have multiple drug allergies and could manifest an allergic reaction to these drugs (and others that are not β-lactams) in a manner similar to their penicillin reaction.[39]

Cross-reactivity between penicillins and carbapenems (imipenem, meropenem, ertapenem, doripenem) and monobactams (e.g., aztreonam) has also been studied. In one report, about 50% of patients with a history of penicillin allergy exhibited hypersensitivity reactions to the carbapenem antibiotic imipenem-cilastatin.[39] More recent data, however, suggest that the rate of cross-reactivity is far lower, approximately 1%. One hundred twelve patients with a history of immediate reactions to a penicillin and a positive skin test to penicillin underwent skin testing with imipenem-cilastatin. One patient (0.9%) had a positive skin test. One hundred ten of the remaining 111 patients received gradually increasing intramuscular doses of imipenem-cilastatin with no reactions observed.[54] Similarly, 108 children with a history of an immediate hypersensitivity reaction to a penicillin and a positive skin test underwent intradermal skin testing to meropenem. One child (0.9%) had a positive skin test. The remaining 107 subjects received increasing doses of intramuscular meropenem with no reactions reported.[55] There also does not appear to be significant cross-reactivity between penicillins and the monobactam aztreonam.[56] Ceftazidime and aztreonam have an identical side-chain, however, and there is evidence of cross-reactivity between these two antibiotics.[57]

Although desensitization with an appropriate cephalosporin is a potential option for J.A. (see Case 3-9, Question 1), her infection is not life-threatening, and the organism is probably sensitive to a other antimicrobial agents. In this case, it would be prudent to treat J.A. with a non–β-lactam antibiotic. If J.A.'s skin tests to cephalosporin were undertaken, and had been negative, she could receive a cephalosporin despite her positive history beginning with a cautiously administered small (i.e., "test") initial dose.[39]

GENERALIZED REACTIONS

Drug allergies can be grouped into three categories: generalized reactions, organ-specific reactions, and pseudoallergic reactions. Generalized reactions involve multiple organ systems and variable clinical manifestations. Anaphylactic reactions, serum sickness reactions, drug-induced fever, hypersensitivity vasculitis, drug-induced vasculitis, and autoimmune drug reactions are the generalized drug reactions presented in this chapter.

Anaphylaxis

CASE 3-2

QUESTION 1: L.P., an 85-kg, 29-year-old man, presents to the emergency department with a chief complaint of a cat bite to the forearm two days prior. Physical examination reveals a man in moderate distress with multiple puncture wounds on the volar aspect of the right arm. The area surrounding the wounds is swollen, erythematous, and tender to the touch. L.P.'s history is notable for migraine headaches, which are managed with atenolol 25 mg once daily; exercise-induced asthma, controlled with an albuterol metered-dose inhaler as needed; diabetes managed through diet and weight control, and a history of a laparoscopic appendectomy 3 years prior. He has no known allergies. The wound is cleansed with a germicidal soap and 3 g ampicillin/sulbactam is started intravenously. Three minutes after starting the ampicillin/sulbactam, L.P. notes tingling and pruritus of both his hands and feet, and appears flushed. One minute later he complains of light-headedness, difficulty breathing, and a lump in his throat. His vital signs at this time are blood pressure (BP) 100/60 mm Hg (normal, 125/85); heart rate 70 beats/minute (normal, 60); and respiratory rate 27 breaths/minute (normal, 12). Chest auscultation reveals restricted airflow and stridor. Anaphylaxis is the diagnosis and emergency treatment is started. What subjective and objective evidence support the diagnosis of anaphylaxis in L.P.?

Anaphylaxis is a serious allergic reaction that has a rapid onset and can cause death.[58] The diagnosis is considered probable if one of three clinical criteria are met:[59]

1. an acute onset of a reaction (minutes to hours) with involvement of the skin, mucosal tissue, or both, and at least one of the following:
   a. respiratory compromise
   b. reduced blood pressure or symptoms of end-organ dysfunction
2. two or more of the following that occur rapidly after exposure to a likely allergen for that patient:
   a. involvement of the skin/mucosal tissue
   b. respiratory compromise
   c. reduced blood pressure or associated symptoms
   d. persistent gastrointestinal symptoms
3. reduced blood pressure, after exposure to a known allergen

Anaphylaxis results from the rapid release of immunologic mediators from tissue mast cells and peripheral blood basophils.

ONLINE CONTENT

For a visual of development of anaphylaxis, see http://thepoint.lww.com/AT10e.

The symptoms of anaphylaxis vary widely, depending on the route of exposure, rate of exposure, and dose of allergen.[36,38,60,61] Symptoms often begin within minutes of exposure, as in L.P., and most reactions occur within 1 hour. On rare occasions, anaphylaxis can appear several hours after exposure and late phase or biphasic attacks have occurred 1 to 72 hours after the initial attack (most commonly within 8 hours). In general, the severity of the anaphylaxis is directly proportional to the speed of onset. L.P. displays symptoms in many of the organs commonly involved in anaphylaxis. Although almost any organ system can be affected, the cutaneous, gastrointestinal (GI), respiratory, and cardiovascular systems are involved most frequently, either singly or in combination.[36,38,60,61] These "shock organs" contain the largest number of mast cells and are the most highly affected.

L.P. exhibits erythema (flushed appearance) and complains of pruritus of his hands and feet, both common initial symptoms of anaphylaxis; the groin also is commonly affected. These symptoms can progress to urticaria and angioedema, especially of the palms, soles, periorbital tissue, and mucous membranes. L.P. describes the early manifestations of angioedema (laryngeal edema) with complaints of a lump in his throat (this also may be described as throat tightness or constriction by some patients).

The upper and lower respiratory tracts also can be involved during an anaphylactic event. L.P. exhibits stridor, indicating upper airway involvement. Hoarseness is another sign of upper respiratory tract involvement. In addition, L.P. is tachypneic with poor airflow, suggesting his lower airway also is affected. L.P. does not display wheezing or acute emphysema, which are further clues of lower airway involvement. Respiratory symptoms can lead to suffocation and death.[60] In one autopsy series, laryngeal edema accounted for 25% of the fatalities and acute emphysema for another 25% of the deaths.[62] Cardiovascular symptoms also are ominous. Cardiovascular collapse and hypotensive shock (anaphylactic shock) are caused by peripheral vasodilation, enhanced vascular permeability, leakage of plasma, low cardiac output, and intravascular volume depletion. Thus, hypotension, as seen with L.P., is a common cardiac manifestation. Tachycardia also commonly occurs in patients with cardiac complications of anaphylaxis. L.P. does not show a significant increase in heart rate, however, he is taking the β-blocker atenolol. Other cardiac manifestations of anaphylaxis include a direct cardiodepressant effect and various electrocardiographic changes, including arrhythmias and ischemia.

Although not demonstrated by L.P., common GI manifestations such as abdominal cramping, diarrhea (which can be bloody), nausea, and vomiting also are manifested during an anaphylactic reaction.[36,38,60] In summary, L.P.'s rapid onset and progression of symptoms involving multiple organ systems (i.e., cutaneous, respiratory, and cardiovascular systems) are consistent with an anaphylactic reaction. L.P.'s anaphylaxis is a severe reaction given its speed of onset, the number of organ systems involved, and the degree of involvement. In particular, his respiratory and cardiovascular symptoms indicate a potentially life-threatening reaction.

CASE 3-2, QUESTION 2: What is the mechanism behind anaphylaxis and what is the likely cause of L.P.'s anaphylactic event?

Anaphylaxis occurs through one of three mechanisms.[36] In the first type of reaction, exposure to a foreign protein, either in its native state or as a hapten conjugated to a carrier protein, causes IgE-antibody formation. The IgE antibodies then bind to receptors on mast cells and basophils. On re-exposure, the antigen stimulates cellular degranulation through both antigen-IgE antibody formation and cross-linking, which result in massive release of preformed immunologic mediators from the mast cells and basophils. Histamine is the major mediator of anaphylaxis and the primary preformed cellular constituent. Histamine has multiple effects and is likely responsible for vasodilation, urticaria, angioedema, hypotension, vomiting, abdominal cramping, and changes in coronary flow.[38] Leukotrienes (e.g., leukotrienes C_4 and D, also known as slow-reacting substance of anaphylaxis), platelet activating factor, and prostaglandins are generated rapidly as a result of cellular degranulation, and other mediators of anaphylaxis (e.g., tryptase, chymase, carboxypeptidase A, tumor necrosis factor, and other cytokines and chemokines) are released as well.[36,60] Anaphylactic reactions to *Hymenoptera* venom (e.g., bee stings), insulin, streptokinase, penicillins, cephalosporins, local anesthetics, and sulfonamides occur through this IgE-mediated mechanism.

Anaphylaxis also can occur via the formation of immune complexes that activate the complement system and the subsequent formation of anaphylatoxins C3a, C4a, and C5a. Such anaphylatoxins can directly stimulate mast cell and basophil degranulation and mediator release. In 2008, cases resembling anaphylaxis in patients receiving heparin, particularly those also undergoing dialysis, were reported with almost 100 deaths occurring internationally. The culprit was found to be a contaminant (oversulfated chondroitin sulfate) that caused symptoms by this mechanism.[63,64]

The third mechanism by which substances, such as radiocontrast media and other hyperosmolar agents, can cause anaphylaxis is by the direct stimulation of mediator release (primarily histamine). The pathway by which this occurs is as yet unknown, but it is independent of IgE and complement.

Additionally, when no distinct mechanism can be associated with an anaphylactic event, the term idiopathic anaphylaxis is applied.[36,61]

Foods, insect stings, and drugs are the most common causes of anaphylaxis.[65] Antibiotics (particularly β-lactams and fluoroquinolones), nonsteroidal anti-inflammatory drugs (NSAIDs), neuromuscular blocking agents, radiocontrast media, chemotherapeutic agents, and monoclonal antibodies are the most common causes of drug-induced anaphylaxis. L.P.'s anaphylactic episode most likely is related to the first mechanism (i.e., IgE-antibody formation). L.P. is receiving a drug from a class of antibiotics well known to cause anaphylaxis. Specifically, L.P. may have received a prophylactic β-lactam antibiotic prior to his appendectomy, a standard of practice. Exposure to the antibiotic at that time stimulated IgE-antibody formation. After exposure to the β-lactam ampicillin/sulbactam in the emergency department, antibody–antigen complexes were formed, resulting in cellular degranulation and anaphylaxis. The temporal relationship of L.P.'s anaphylactic reaction to the administration of the antibiotic also strongly implicates ampicillin/sulbactam as the precipitating agent. Furthermore, L.P. was not exposed to agents known to cause anaphylaxis by one of the other known mechanisms. A review of L.P.'s surgical records is necessary to confirm his prior exposure to a sensitizing antibiotic.

CASE 3-2, QUESTION 3: Given L.P.'s signs and symptoms and the presumed cause of his anaphylactic reaction, how should he be treated?

Effective management of anaphylaxis requires quick recognition and aggressive therapeutic intervention because of the immediate life-threatening nature of the reaction, as illustrated by L.P. The severity of the anaphylactic reaction must be assessed quickly, the probable causative agent determined, the administration of the offending substance discontinued, and the absorption of the offending agent minimized if possible. Recent guidelines on the management of anaphylaxis list the following treatments in order of importance: epinephrine, patient position, oxygen, intravenous fluids, nebulized therapy, vasopressors, antihistamines, corticosteroids, and other agents.[59] All of these interventions must be undertaken promptly and the clinical status of the patient closely monitored. Vital signs, cardiac and pulmonary function, oxygenation, cardiac output, and tissue perfusion in particular must be immediately and continuously assessed.[36,60]

Although not definitively known to be the cause, the infusion of ampicillin/sulbactam should be stopped to prevent further exposure to the presumed precipitating agent. Additionally, the forearm wounds should be flushed with normal saline to remove any residual cleansing agent in the event that this is the cause of the reaction.

Pharmacological treatment of anaphylaxis has traditionally involved several drugs and drug classes such as epinephrine, antihistamines, and corticosteroids aimed at reversing the clinical manifestations of anaphylaxis and interrupting the biological pathways involved. Recent literature reviews, however, failed to find well-designed and well-conducted randomized controlled trials to support the use of these drugs.[66–69] Recommendations for use are based on tradition, case reports, case series, and expert opinion.

L.P. is showing early signs of anaphylactic shock that must be managed immediately. Studies have shown that failure to use epinephrine early in anaphylaxis is a risk factor for a poor outcome. Despite the lack of strong evidence to support its use, epinephrine is the drug of choice for the pharmacologic management of anaphylaxis and all national and international anaphylaxis guidelines recommend epinephrine as first-line treatment.[59,70] (For an EpiPen video demonstration, go to http://www.epipen.com/how-to-use-epipen.) The α-adrenergic effects of epinephrine increase systemic vascular resistance and increase blood pressure while decreasing mucosal edema and relieving upper airway obstruction, angioedema, and hives. These actions counter the vasodilating and hypotensive effects of histamine and the other mediators of anaphylaxis. In addition, the β-adrenergic effects of epinephrine promote bronchodilation and increase cardiac rate and contractility. Epinephrine also inhibits the release of mediators from basophils and mast cells.

The route of epinephrine administration is important. Most guidelines recommend intramuscular (IM) epinephrine, 0.01 mg/kg of a 1 mg/mL (1:1,000) solution to a maximum dose of 0.5 mg in an adult or 0.3 mg in a child injected into the lateral aspect of the thigh every 5 to 10 minutes as needed.[59,70] Epinephrine doses should be expressed in mass concentration (e.g., 1 mg in 1 mL) instead of ratios such as 1:1,000, which have been confused with epinephrine concentrations used in cardiac arrest (1:10,000) and caused dosing errors.[70] Epinephrine is vasodilatory in skeletal muscle and because skeletal muscle is highly vascular absorption is rapid. While some guidelines propose the subcutaneous route for epinephrine administration, subcutaneous tissue is less vascular than skeletal muscle, thus there is less rapid absorption of epinephrine. Additionally, epinephrine causes vasoconstriction in subcutaneous tissue, therefore slowing its own absorption. Studies have shown that IM epinephrine injections into the thigh achieve higher blood concentrations more rapidly than do subcutaneous or IM injections into the arm in healthy subjects.[71] The rate and extent of absorption from IM and subcutaneous routes of epinephrine administration, however, have not been studied in patients experiencing anaphylaxis and there is no evidence that epinephrine is ineffective when given IM or subcutaneously into the arm.[59] Epinephrine should be administered via the IV route in cases of anaphylaxis that have not responded to repeated doses of IM epinephrine and/or are progressing to shock, or in cases where cardiorespiratory arrest appears imminent. Low cardiac output and intravascular volume depletion from shock decrease tissue perfusion and possibly the absorption of subcutaneous or IM injections. In animal studies, the benefits of intermittent IV boluses of epinephrine are short lived and a continuous infusion of epinephrine provides optimal results.[72] In L.P.'s case, an initial dose of 0.5 mg of 1 mg/1 mL epinephrine solution should be injected IM into his lateral thigh. This should be repeated every 5 minutes until symptoms improve.

Some evidence suggests poor outcomes in patients who are in an upright position during anaphylactic shock. Pumphrey[73] studied 38 deaths from anaphylactic shock and in 10 cases where postural information was documented, patients died after being moved to an upright position. Four deaths occurred immediately after changing position. Movement of the patient from a supine to an upright position during shock possibly worsened already poor venous return, causing a sudden decrease in cardiac filling and subsequent circulatory collapse (referred to as empty ventricle syndrome).[73] Thus, placing L.P. in the Trendelenburg position (patient supine, inclined approximately 45 degrees with head at the lower end and legs at the upper end) might improve survival by enhancing perfusion to vital organs. After repositioning, oxygen should be started and normal saline infused at a rate sufficient to maintain perfusion to vital organs. Normal saline is the preferred crystalloid because it stays in the intravascular space longer than does dextrose and does not contain lactate (e.g., Lactated Ringer's solution), which could worsen metabolic acidosis. Circulating blood volume can decrease by as much as 35% in the first 10 minutes of anaphylactic shock because of vasodilation and fluid shifting from the intravascular to the extravascular space.[59] Therefore, vigorous fluid resuscitation might be necessary (e.g., 1 to 2 L of normal saline at a rate of 5 to 10 mL/kg in the first 5 minutes). Cerebral perfusion, as evidenced by adequate mentation, must always take precedence over BP readings when managing shock.

The effect of L.P.'s atenolol also must be considered. Patients taking a β-blocker, whether cardioselective or not cardioselective, could experience more severe episodes and more refractory episodes of anaphylaxis than patients not taking a β-blocker. This effect might be caused by a blunted response to epinephrine when given to treat anaphylaxis, resulting in refractory hypotension, bradycardia, and bronchospasm.[59] If L.P.'s BP and heart rate do not substantially improve shortly after initiating epinephrine, IV glucagon, which can stimulate heart rate and cardiac contractility independent of β-adrenergic blockade, should be given (Table 3-5). Airway protection is important because glucagon may cause emesis and there is a risk of aspiration, especially in drowsy or obtunded patients. Methylene blue, through its ability to reduce nitric oxide production (a known potent vasodilator) has been found to be effective in a small number of cases of anaphylaxis with refractory hypotension.[65,74] Other vasopressors such as dopamine (2–20 mcg/kg/minute) may be needed to maintain blood pressure if there is poor response to epinephrine and glucagon. Second-line treatment for anaphylaxis includes inhaled β-agonists, H_1 and H_2 antihistamines, and corticosteroids. In light of L.P.'s severe pulmonary reaction, he should receive a nebulized β-agonist (e.g., albuterol). If L.P.'s respiratory status fails to improve after pharmacologic intervention, intubation must be considered. Atenolol would not be expected to diminish the effect of albuterol because atenolol is a β_1 cardioselective β-blocker and the dose is low. Because histamine is the primary mediator of anaphylaxis, IV administration of an H_1 antihistamine such as diphenhydramine (50 mg every 6 hours until the reaction resolves) should be considered. Similarly, giving an H_2 antihistamine is a common practice. Both therapies present little acute risk to the patient, but as already noted, there are few data supporting their efficacy in treating anaphylaxis.[67] Because L.P. is not receiving any drugs known to interact with cimetidine and because he has no diseases that require dose adjustment, cimetidine may be given as outlined in Table 3-5.

Lastly, given the severity of his reaction and his pulmonary involvement, L.P. is a candidate for IV corticosteroids. Methylprednisolone, 125 mg every 6 hours for four doses, might be beneficial and is associated with minimal risk. Although commonly used, corticosteroids will not affect the acute course of the reaction due to their delayed onset of action (typically 4–6 hours after administration). Corticosteroids may impact a prolonged episode of anaphylaxis and could prevent or minimize the occurrence of a biphasic reaction, although this has not been proven in well-controlled trials. The effect of methylprednisolone on L.P.'s diabetes is not a factor because his condition is potentially life-threatening. Once stabilized, L.P. should be transferred to a critical care setting and monitored for a minimum of 24 hours because relapses of the anaphylactic reaction can occur.[36,38,60,61]

Serum Sickness

Serum sickness is a type III hypersensitivity reaction that results from the production of antibodies directed against heterologous protein or drug haptens with subsequent tissue deposition. The typical presentation of serum sickness (Table 3-6) includes fever, cutaneous eruptions (95%), lymphadenopathy, and joint symptoms (10%–50%).[75–78] Symptoms usually occur 1 to 2 weeks after exposure, but accelerated reactions can occur within 2 to 4 days in previously sensitized persons. Laboratory data are relatively nonspecific and are of little diagnostic value. For example, the erythrocyte sedimentation rate (ESR) and the serum

TABLE 3-5
Drug Therapy of Anaphylaxis

Drug	Indication	Adult Dosage	Complications
First-line Therapy			
Epinephrine	Hypotension, bronchospasm, laryngeal edema, urticaria, angioedema	0.3–0.5 mL of a 1 mg/1 mL solution IM every 5 minutes PRN; if progressing to cardiorespiratory arrest 1–3 mL of 1:10,000 (0.1–0.3 mg) IV for 3 minutes 1 mL of 1 mg/mL (1:1,000) in 250 mL of normal saline IV at a rate of 4–10 mcg/min (preferred over intermittent injections) 3–5 mL of 1:10,000 intratracheally every 10–20 minutes PRN	Arrhythmias, hypertension, nervousness, tremor
Oxygen	Hypoxemia	40%–100%	None
Albuterol		0.5 mL of 0.5% solution in 2.5 mL of saline via nebulizer (i.e., 2.5 mg)	Arrhythmias, hypertension, nervousness, tremor
IV fluids	Hypotension	1 L of normal saline every 20–30 minutes PRN (rates as high as 1–2 mL/kg/min may be necessary)	Pulmonary edema, CHF
Second-line Therapy			
Antihistamines	Hypotension, urticaria	—	—
H_1 receptor antagonists	—	Diphenhydramine 25–50 mg IV, IM, PO every 6–8 hours PRN Hydroxyzine 25–50 mg IM or PO every 6–8 hours PRN	Drowsiness, dry mouth, urinary retention; may obscure symptoms of continuing reaction
H_2 receptor antagonists		Cimetidine 300 mg IV for 3–5 minutes or PO every 6–8 hours PRN Ranitidine 50 mg IV for 3–5 minutes every 8 hours PRN or 150 mg PO BID PRN Famotidine 20 mg IV for 3–5 minutes every 12 hours PRN or 20 mg PO BID PRN	— —
Corticosteroids	Bronchospasm; patients undergoing prolonged resuscitation or severe reaction	Hydrocortisone sodium succinate 100 mg IM or IV every 3–6 hours for two to four doses or Methylprednisolone sodium succinate 40–125 mg IV every 6 hours for two to four doses	Hyperglycemia, fluid retention
Dopamine	Hypotension refractory to epinephrine	400 mg in 500 mL dextrose 5% at 2–20 mcg/kg/min	Hypertension, tachycardia, palpitations, arrhythmias
Norepinephrine	Hypotension refractory to epinephrine	4 mg in 1 L dextrose 5% IV at a rate of 2–12 mcg/min	Arrhythmias, hypertension, nervousness, tremor
Glucagon[b]	Refractory hypotension	1 mg IV for 5 minutes, followed by 5–15 mcg/min in fusion	Nausea, vomiting

[a]Although not effective during acute anaphylaxis, these agents may reduce or prevent recurrent or prolonged reactions.
[b]Glucagon may be particularly useful in patients taking β-adrenergic blockers, because it can increase both cardiac rate and contractility regardless of β-adrenergic blockade. Choice of agent and starting doses should be patient-specific, weighing safety and efficacy.
BID, twice a day; IM, intramuscularly; IV, intravenously; PO, orally; PRN, as needed.

concentration of circulating immune complexes usually are increased. Complements C3 and C4 are often low, whereas activation products C3a and C3a desarginine are elevated. Urinalysis might reveal proteinuria, hematuria, or an occasional cast.[75–78]

In most cases, serum sickness reactions are mild and self-limiting and resolve within a few days to weeks after withdrawal of the inciting agent. Antihistamines and aspirin can be used to relieve pruritus and arthralgias. In severe cases, corticosteroids might be used and can be tapered during 10 to 14 days.[75–78] At one time, heterologous serum (e.g., anti-thymocyte globulin made from rabbit or equine serum) was a leading cause of serum sickness. With the decline in use of these products, however, the most common causes of serum sickness today are penicillins and cephalosporins, although biological agents such as rituximab, infliximab, and natalizumab are increasingly associated with serum sickness.[79,80]

Drug Fever

CASE 3-3

QUESTION 1: M.M., a 57-year-old ill-appearing woman, is hospitalized with a 3-day history of difficulty breathing, left-sided chest pain on inspiration, fever, chills, and a productive cough. Her medical history is significant only for hypertension, well controlled on hydrochlorothiazide; she has no known drug allergies. M.M.'s physical findings on admission are temperature, 38°C; respirations, 20 breaths/minute; left-sided crackles heard on auscultation; oxygen saturation 85% on room air; and heart rate 85 beats/minute. A chest radiograph reveals an infiltrate in her left lower lobe. Her white blood cell (WBC) count is 17,500 cells/μL with the following differential:

TABLE 3-6
Hypersensitivity Reactions to Drugs: Serum Sickness

Clinical manifestations	Fever, cutaneous eruptions (95% of cases), lymphadenopathy, and joint systems (10%–50%). Onset 1–2 weeks after exposure, 2–4 days in sensitized individuals. Laboratory data relatively nonspecific: elevated ESR and circulating immune complexes. Complements C3 and C4 are often low, whereas activation products C3a and C3a desarginine are elevated. RF sometimes present. UA may reveal proteinuria, hematuria, or an occasional cast.
Prognosis	Usually mild and self-limiting. Most resolve within a few days to weeks after withdrawal of inciting agent.
Treatment	Aspirin and antihistamines can relieve arthralgias and pruritus. Corticosteroids may be required for severe cases and tapered for 10–14 days.

ESR, erythrocyte sedimentation rate; RF, rheumatoid factor; UA, urinalysis.
Source: Buhner D, Grant JA. Serum sickness. *Dermatol Clin.* 1985;3:107; Lawley TJ et al. A study of human serum sickness. *J Invest Dermatol.* 1985;85(1 Suppl): 129s; Erffmeyer JE. Serum sickness. *Ann Allergy.* 1986;56:105; Lin RY. Serum sickness syndrome. *Am Fam Physician.* 1986;33:157.

Polymorphonuclear neutrophil leukocytes (PMN), 83% (normal, 45%–79%)
Bands, 12% (normal, 0%–5%)
Lymphocytes, 10% (normal, 16%–47%)
Basophils, 0% (normal, 0%–1%)
Eosinophils, 1% (normal, 1%–2%)

Community-acquired pneumonia is the diagnosis, and M.M. is empirically started on ceftriaxone 1 g IV daily, azithromycin 500 mg IV daily, and oxygen at 2 L/minute. Other medications include oral acetaminophen 325 mg every 4 to 6 hours as needed for temperature greater than 38°C, oral famotidine 20 mg BID, and oral hydrochlorothiazide 12.5 mg daily. Seventy-two hours later, M.M. is breathing without pain at a respiratory rate of 12 breaths/minute, her lungs are clear to auscultation, and her oxygen saturation is 98% on room air. She appears much better and offers no new complaints. Her temperature during the previous 48 hours has ranged from 38.6°C to 40°C, her pulse has ranged from 90–100 beats/minute, and her WBC count is 22,000 with the following differential: PMN, 89%; bands, 5%; lymphocytes, 12%; basophils, 0%; and eosinophils, 7%. Drug-induced fever is considered. What evidence supports this diagnosis? What is the mechanism for drug fever?

Drug fever is described as a febrile reaction to a drug without cutaneous symptoms and is estimated to occur in 3% to 5% of inpatients.[81] Drug fever can be challenging to identify and can be misinterpreted as a new infectious process or failure of an existing infection to respond to treatment. Such failure to recognize a drug fever can lead to prolonged hospitalization and unnecessary tests or medications.[82] Table 3-7 lists the characteristics of hypersensitivity drug-induced fever. The most important finding in the case of M.M. is her clinical improvement with respect to her pulmonary status despite a high-grade fever and persistent leukocytosis; she also appears healthier than expected if she had an untreated infection. Whereas a drop in her WBC count would be anticipated given her improving respiratory function, her WBC count remains elevated, consistent with hypersensitivity drug fever. Notably, her eosinophil count is increased, a frequent sign of hypersensitivity reactions. Despite her high-grade fever, she has a relative bradycardia; that is, her heart rate is not as elevated as expected if an infectious process were ongoing. Further, the timing of the symptoms favors a drug-induced fever (i.e., within days of starting a new medication). A definitive diagnosis can be made only by stopping the suspected offending agent, however, because fever generally resolves within 48 to 72 hours if a rash is not present. When a rash is present, on the other hand, the fever may persist for several days after stopping the implicated drug.

Drug fever can be caused by various mechanisms, although it is ascribed most commonly to a hypersensitivity reaction. Other mechanisms include the pharmacologic action of the drug (e.g., cell destruction from antineoplastic agents releases endogenous pyrogens); altered thermoregulatory function (e.g., increased metabolic rate from thyroid hormone); decreased sweating from drugs with anticholinergic properties (e.g., atropine, tricyclic antidepressants, phenothiazines); drug-administration-related fever (e.g., amphotericin B, bleomycin); and idiosyncratic reactions (e.g., neuroleptic malignant syndrome from haloperidol, malignant hyperthermia from inhaled anesthetics).[81,83]

TABLE 3-7
Hypersensitivity Reactions to Drugs: Drug-Induced Fever

Frequency	True frequency is unknown because fever is a common manifestation and almost any drug can cause fever. Estimate is that 3%–5% of hospitalized patients experiencing adverse drug reaction suffer from drug fever alone or as part of multiple symptoms.
Clinical manifestations	Temperatures may be 38°C or higher and do not follow a consistent pattern. Although patients may have high fevers with shaking chills, patients generally have few symptoms or serious systemic illness. Skin rash (18%), eosinophilia (22%), chills (53%), headache (16%), myalgias (25%), and bradycardia (11%) can occur in patients with drug fever. Onset of fever after exposure to the offending agent is highly variable, ranging from an average of 6 days for antineoplastics to 45 days for cardiovascular agents. Occurrence of fever is independent of the dose of the offending agent.
Treatment	Although drug fever can be treated symptomatically (e.g., with antipyretics, cooling blankets), stopping the offending agent is the only therapy that will eliminate fevers. Patients generally defervesce within 48–72 hours of stopping the suspect drug.
Prognosis	Drug fever is usually benign, although one review[57] found a mean increased length of hospitalization of 9 days per episode of drug fever. Rechallenge with the offending drug usually results in rapid return of the fever. Although re-exposure to the suspect drug was previously thought to be potentially hazardous, there is little risk of serious sequelae.

Source: Patel RA, Gallagher JC. Drug fever. *Pharmacotherapy.* 2010;30:57; Tabor PA. Drug-induced fever. *Drug Intell Clin Pharm.* 1986;20:413; Mackowiak PA, LeMaistre CF. Drug fever: a critical appraisal of conventional concepts. An analysis of 51 episodes in two Dallas hospitals and 97 episodes reported in the English literature. *Ann Intern Med.* 1987;106:728; Cunha BA, Shea KW. Fever in the intensive care unit. *Infect Dis Clin North Am.* 1996;10:185.

CASE 3-3, QUESTION 2: What agent is the most likely cause of drug fever in M.M.?

Most of the information available on drug fever is based on case reports or small case series, and reviews of the literature.[82,84] Unfortunately, the literature is inconsistent with regard to the frequency of drug fever (e.g., very common, common, uncommon) and such descriptions are not supported by good clinical data. Nevertheless, some drugs are more commonly associated with drug fever than others. These include anti-infectives as a class (especially β-lactam antibiotics), antiepileptics, and antineoplastics. Drug fever has also been reported frequently with amphotericin B, azathioprine, hydroxyurea, methyldopa, procainamide, quinidine, and quinine.[81–85]

In M.M.'s case, ceftriaxone or azithromycin is the most likely cause of her ongoing fever, given the timing of the reaction relative to beginning the antibiotics and the frequency of febrile reactions attributed to them, especially to β-lactam antibiotics. Febrile reactions have not been associated with acetaminophen, and famotidine is rarely a cause of fever without other symptoms of an allergic reaction. Although diuretics such as hydrochlorothiazide can cause fever, M.M. was taking this medication before admission without any ill effects, making this drug an unlikely culprit.

CASE 3-3, QUESTION 3: How should M.M.'s drug fever be treated? Can M.M. receive cephalosporins in the future?

Because M.M. has responded clinically, her antibiotics should be discontinued and her fever curve, WBC count, heart rate, and respiratory status followed. An oral antibiotic from another drug class (e.g., a fluoroquinolone) should be started to complete a 7-day to 10-day antibiotic course of therapy. Acetaminophen and other antipyretics should be avoided unless M.M. becomes uncomfortable from the fever because they can mask the response to the discontinuation of her antibiotics.

As with any hypersensitivity reaction, rechallenge with the offending drug can cause a similar, or sometimes greater, response. In M.M.'s case, re-exposure to ceftriaxone (or another β-lactam antibiotic) or a macrolide might cause a febrile reaction. It is unclear, however, how large the risk of re-exposure truly is. Although drug fever sometimes precedes more serious hypersensitivity reactions, evidence suggests there may be little risk to re-exposure. Should M.M. require ceftriaxone (or another β-lactam or macrolide antibiotic) in the future, it would be prudent to administer the drug in a setting where M.M. can be monitored, at least initially, to ensure prompt treatment if an immediate hypersensitivity reaction develops.

Hypersensitivity Vasculitis

CASE 3-4

QUESTION 1: M.G., a 26-year-old woman with cystic fibrosis, is admitted for treatment of pneumonia. Sputum cultures obtained before admission reveal *Alcaligenes xylosoxidans* sensitive only to minocycline and chloramphenicol. M.G. is initiated on appropriate doses of these two antibiotics for a 2-week course. On day 8 of therapy, M.G. begins to complain of a rash on her legs. Physical examination reveals palpable purpura and a maculopapular rash on both lower extremities. Laboratory data reveal an elevated ESR and leukocytosis. What is the likely cause of M.G.'s rash and laboratory abnormalities?

TABLE 3-8
Criteria[a] for the Classification of Hypersensitivity Vasculitis

- Development of symptoms after age 16
- Medication at disease onset that may have been a precipitating factor
- Slightly elevated purpuric (hemorrhagic) rash over one or more areas of the skin that does not blanch with pressure and is not related to thrombocytopenia
- Maculopapular rash over one or more areas of the skin
- Biopsy showing granulocytes around an arteriole or venule

[a] The diagnosis of hypersensitivity vasculitis can be made if a patient exhibits at least three of these criteria.
Source: Calabrese LH et al. The American College of Rheumatology 1990 criteria for the classification of hypersensitivity vasculitis. *Arthritis Rheum.* 1990;33:1108.

M.G.'s presentation is suggestive of a diagnosis of hypersensitivity vasculitis. Hypersensitivity vasculitis, also called cutaneous leukocytoclastic angiitis, is characterized by inflammation of the small blood vessel walls. These reactions occur when immune complex deposition within the small veins and arterioles activates complement, causing the release of chemotactic factors. These factors attract polymorphonuclear cells that cause vessel damage.[86–88]

Drug-Induced Vasculitis

Approximately 10% of cases of cutaneous vasculitis are believed to be drug-related.[89] Approximately 100 drugs have been identified as causing vasculitis, including β-lactams, fluoroquinolones, NSAIDs, antiepileptics, and tumor necrosis factor blockers.[90–92] Interested readers are referred to more in-depth reviews.[91,93,94] The diagnosis of hypersensitivity vasculitis is based on five clinical criteria (Table 3-8), three of which must be present.[95] M.G. meets three of the five criteria, including age greater than 16 years, palpable purpura, and a maculopapular rash. In addition, minocycline, a medication that she was taking at the onset of the rash, has been associated with serum sickness and vasculitic-type reactions. Onset of symptoms typically occurs 7 to 10 days after initiation of drug therapy, but can occur sooner on re-exposure. Purpuric papules and macular eruptions, the most commonly observed findings, are usually symmetric and occur on the extremities (Table 3-9).[87] Hypersensitivity vasculitis can

TABLE 3-9
Hypersensitivity Reactions to Drugs: Clinical Manifestations of Drug-Induced Vasculitis

- Palpable purpura and maculopapular rash occurring symmetrically predominantly on the lower extremities
- Multiple organ systems may be involved:
  - *Renal:* microscopic hematuria to nephrotic syndrome and acute renal failure
  - *Liver:* enlarged liver, elevated enzymes
  - *Joints:* arthritis
  - *Gastrointestinal:* abdominal pain
- Laboratory data usually show nonspecific abnormalities of inflammation: elevated erythrocyte sedimentation rate and leukocytosis. Peripheral eosinophilia may be present and serum complement concentrations can be low. Histologic findings on biopsy reveal small blood vessels with leukocytoclastic or necrotizing vasculitis
- Onset typically 7–21 days after initiation of therapy

Source: Valeyrie-Allanore L et al. Drug-induced skin, nail and hair disorders. *Drug Saf.* 2007;30:1011; Martinez-Taboada VM et al. Clinical features and outcome of 95 patients with hypersensitivity vasculitis. *Am J Med.* 1997;102:186.

TABLE 3-10
Hypersensitivity Reactions to Drugs: Autoimmune Drug-Induced Lupus

Frequency	Less likely to affect women and black patients than idiopathic SLE. Drug-induced lupus is more common in individuals with slow acetylator phenotype.
Clinical manifestations	Milder disease than idiopathic SLE. Arthralgias, myalgias, fever, malaise, pleurisy, and slight weight loss. Mild splenomegaly and lymphadenopathy. *Onset:* Usually abrupt, occurring several months to years after continuous therapy with the offending drug. *Appearance*: Photosensitivity appears in about 25% of patients, but the classic butterfly malar rash, discoid lesions, oral mucosal ulcers, Raynaud phenomenon, and alopecia are unusual features with drug-induced lupus as opposed to idiopathic SLE. *Laboratory studies*: Positive ANA (predominantly single-stranded DNA and antihistone antibodies), anemia, and elevated erythrocyte sedimentation rate. Many patients demonstrate ANA without development of lupus disease. It is not necessary, therefore, to discontinue therapy in asymptomatic patients with positive ANA.
Treatment	Clinical features subside and disappear days to weeks after discontinuation of the offending drug. Serologic tests resolve more slowly. ANA may persist for a year or longer.
Prognosis	Drug-induced lupus does not predispose to development of idiopathic SLE. Lupus-inducing drugs do not appear to increase the risk of exacerbation of idiopathic SLE. Long-term treatment with interferon-λ may, however, worsen pre-existing SLE.

ANA, antinuclear antibody; SLE, systemic lupus erythematosus.
Source: Valeyrie-Allanore L et al. Drug-induced skin, nail and hair disorders. *Drug Saf.* 2007;30:1011; Antonov D et al. Drug-induced lupus erythematosus. *Clin Dermatol.* 2004;22:157.

involve multiple organ systems. Renal damage, ranging from microscopic hematuria to nephrotic syndrome and acute renal failure, is common in patients with disseminated disease.[87] An enlarged liver with elevated enzymes is indicative of hepatocellular involvement. Although the lungs and ears can be involved as well, clinical manifestations are usually mild.[87] Arthralgia also is commonly observed. Laboratory examinations usually show nonspecific abnormalities of inflammation such as an elevated ESR and leukocytosis. In patients with cystic fibrosis experiencing acute pneumonia, these laboratory abnormalities already could be present and, therefore, will not be helpful in establishing the diagnosis of hypersensitivity vasculitis in M.G.

CASE 3-4, QUESTION 2: What additional workup could be performed to confirm the diagnosis of drug-induced vasculitis in M.G.?

In addition to the previous workup, other laboratory and diagnostic procedures might demonstrate peripheral eosinophilia and low serum complement concentrations. A biopsy, which typically reveals granulocytes in the wall of a venule or arteriole and eosinophils at any location, would provide more definitive information.[94]

CASE 3-4, QUESTION 3: How should M.G.'s hypersensitivity vasculitis be treated?

The first step is to discontinue the minocycline therapy. Drug-induced vasculitic reactions typically resolve on their own without additional interventions. If the reaction is severe, corticosteroids can be used.

Autoimmune Drug Reactions

CASE 3-5

QUESTION 1: R.F., a 24-year-old white male medical student, has been treated for 5 months with isoniazid because of a positive skin test for tuberculosis. He now is in the clinic with complaints of new-onset myalgias and arthralgias. Laboratory values obtained the morning of the visit are within normal limits except for a positive ANA titer and an elevated ESR. What is the likely cause of R.F.'s symptoms and laboratory abnormalities?

Some drugs can induce an autoimmune process characterized by the presence of autoantibodies and, in some instances, clinical features of an autoimmune disorder. A drug-induced syndrome resembling systemic lupus erythematosus usually is characterized by myalgias, arthralgias, positive ANA titers, and an elevated ESR (Table 3-10). All of these characteristics are manifested by R.F.

The first case of drug-induced lupus erythematosus (DILE) was recognized more than 60 years ago and was associated with sulfadiazine.[96] Subsequently, more than 80 drugs have been associated with DILE including isoniazid, chlorpromazine, quinidine, methyldopa, and minocycline; however, hydralazine and procainamide are the drugs most frequently associated with this syndrome.[91,97–100] As with idiopathic SLE, DILE can be separated into systemic, subacute cutaneous, and chronic cutaneous lupus. An exact incidence of DILE is difficult to ascertain because of changing patterns of drug use; however, it is estimated that 10% of SLE cases are drug-induced with 15,000 to 30,000 cases in the United States annually.[89]

CASE 3-5, QUESTION 2: How can the diagnosis of drug-induced lupus be differentiated from SLE in R.F.?

In contrast to idiopathic SLE, DILE is less likely to affect women and black patients.[98] On average, patients with DILE are twice as old as those with idiopathic SLE at the time of diagnosis. Individuals with a slow acetylator phenotype have a greater tendency to exhibit DILE; ANA after exposure to lupus-inducing drugs also appear more rapidly.[101,102] In general, DILE is a milder disease than idiopathic SLE. Many patients with DILE, however, could fulfill the diagnostic criteria for SLE according to the American Rheumatism Association.[101] Arthralgias or myalgias accompanied by a positive ANA test can be the only clinical features for some patients with drug-induced lupus. Symptoms usually appear abruptly after several months to years of continuous therapy with the offending drug. Common complaints include fever, malaise, arthralgias, myalgias, pleurisy, and slight weight loss. Mild splenomegaly and lymphadenopathy have been reported occasionally. The skin is affected in about 25% of cases manifesting as photosensitivity on light exposed surfaces. The classic butterfly malar rash, discoid lesions, oral mucosal ulcers, Raynaud's phenomenon, and alopecia are unusual features in DILE in contrast to idiopathic SLE. In addition, the central nervous system and kidneys rarely are affected.[98] Laboratory abnormalities commonly include anemia and an elevated ESR. The evidence supporting a diagnosis of drug-induced lupus in R.F. includes white male predominance, abrupt onset and relatively mild symptomatology, and lack of the classic butterfly malar rash. More definitive tests include determining whether antibodies to single-stranded (indicative of drug-induced lupus) or double-stranded DNA (indicative of SLE) are present.

CASE 3-5, QUESTION 3: Should ANA have been monitored in an effort to detect drug-induced lupus at an earlier stage in this patient?

No. Although all patients with symptomatic drug-induced lupus test positive for ANA (which consist predominantly of single-stranded DNA and antihistone antibodies),[98] many patients taking lupus-inducing drugs become ANA positive without going on to experience lupus. In patients treated with procainamide, about 50% to 75% are positive for ANA after 12 months and 90% after 2 years or more of continuous therapy; only 10% to 20% of those patients actually experience lupus symptoms.[103–105] Similarly, up to 44% of patients are ANA positive after 3 years of hydralazine therapy, but DILE occurs in only 6.7% of patients after 3 years of treatment.[106] It is not necessary to discontinue therapy in asymptomatic patients with positive ANA because most of them will never exhibit clinical symptoms.[98]

CASE 3-5, QUESTION 4: How should R.F.'s drug-induced lupus be treated?

Musculoskeletal complaints can be treated with aspirin or an NSAID. More severe symptoms from pleuropulmonary or pericardial involvement may require the use of corticosteroids.[99] Clinical features of DILE usually subside and disappear in days to weeks with discontinuation of the offending drug. Occasionally, these symptoms linger or recur over a course of several months before eventually disappearing. Serologic tests tend to resolve more slowly: ANA may persist for a year or longer.[98,103] Drug-induced lupus does not predispose patients to the subsequent development of idiopathic SLE.[107] In most instances, lupus-inducing drugs do not increase the risk of exacerbation of idiopathic SLE[108]; however, long-term treatment with isoniazid may worsen pre-existing SLE.[109] R.F. has not yet completed his 6- to 9-month course of isoniazid therapy. An alternative agent should be prescribed for R.F. for at least an additional month and preferentially for up to 4 more months (see Chapter 65, Tuberculosis).

ORGAN-SPECIFIC REACTIONS

The drug allergies in this chapter have been grouped into categories of generalized reactions, organ-specific reactions, and pseudoallergic reactions. The generalized reactions have been described first, the organ-specific hypersensitivity drug reactions affecting the blood, liver, lung, kidney, and skin are described next, and pseudoallergic reactions follow.

Blood: Immune Cytopenias

Drug-induced immune cytopenias (e.g., granulocytopenia, thrombocytopenia, hemolytic anemia) result from type II–mediated allergic reactions (Table 3-1). A drug or drug metabolite binds to the surface of blood elements such as granulocytes, platelets, and red blood cells. IgG or IgM antibodies are formed and are directed against the drug or drug metabolite bound to the cell (i.e., hapten–cell reaction).[13] Typical symptoms associated with immune thrombocytopenia include chills, fever, petechiae, and mucous membrane bleeding. Granulocytopenia generally manifests with chills, fever, arthralgias, and a precipitous drop in the leukocyte count. Symptoms of hemolytic anemia can be subacute or acute and can be sufficiently severe to cause renal failure. The Coombs test is useful in identifying antibodies bound to red cells or circulating immune complexes directed against red cells. Antibiotics are the most commonly implicated class of drugs causing either neutropenia or hemolytic anemia.

Liver

Hypersensitivity reactions involving the liver can be classified as cholestatic or cytotoxic. Jaundice is usually the first sign of a cholestatic reaction, in addition to pruritus, pale stools, and dark urine. Cholestatic reactions usually are reversible on discontinuation of the offending agent. Cytotoxic reactions can involve hepatocellular necrosis or steatosis and can result in irreversible damage if not recognized early.

Lung

Pulmonary manifestations of drug hypersensitivity include asthma and infiltrative reactions. Asthma typically occurs as part of a generalized systemic reaction. Most reactions to drugs that involve asthma alone represent a pharmacologic side effect rather than a true allergic reaction.

Infiltrative reactions typically develop 2 to 10 days after exposure and manifest with cough, dyspnea, fever, chills, and malaise.[11] Infiltrative reactions vary in presentation from eosinophilic pneumonitis to acute pulmonary edema.

Kidney

The most common hypersensitivity reaction involving the kidney is interstitial nephritis. Typical findings include fever, rash, and eosinophilia. Methicillin is the drug most commonly associated with interstitial nephritis, although penicillins, sulfonamides, and cimetidine also have been implicated in renal hypersensitivity reactions.[11,13] (See Chapter 30, Acute Kidney Injury, for hypersensitivity reactions to specific drugs that adversely affect the kidney.)

Skin

Adverse reactions involving the skin are the most common clinical manifestation of drug allergy. Although several different types of cutaneous reactions are possible, most drug-induced skin eruptions can be classified as erythematous, morbilliform, or maculopapular in appearance.[13] In a surveillance study of drug-induced skin reactions, amoxicillin was the most common cause, followed by trimethoprim-sulfamethoxazole and ampicillin. Overall, allergic skin reactions were identified in 2% of hospitalized patients.[14]

Treatment of skin reactions includes discontinuation of the offending drug and general supportive care. (See Chapter 39, Dermatotherapy and Drug-Induced Skin Disorders.)

PSEUDOALLERGIC REACTIONS

CASE 3-6

QUESTION 1: C.C., a 37-year-old man with no known allergies, is hospitalized for treatment of methicillin-resistant *S. aureus* (MRSA) bacteremia associated with an infected central line. His medical history is significant for short-bowel syndrome requiring parenteral nutrition and one previous episode of MRSA line infection successfully treated with vancomycin. Similar to his last admission, vancomycin 750 mg IV for 60 minutes every 12 hours is begun. A trough level taken after the fifth dose, however, is 8 mg/L and the vancomycin dose is doubled to 1,500 mg IV every 12 hours, to be administered at the same rate. Fifteen minutes after the new dose of vancomycin is begun, C.C. experienced hypotension (100/70 mm Hg), tachycardia (85 beats/minute), generalized pruritus, and facial flushing. C.C. is diagnosed as having a pseudoallergic reaction to vancomycin. What subjective and objective data in C.C. are important in differentiating vancomycin pseudoallergic reaction from a true allergic reaction?

Pseudoallergic reactions (also called non-allergic hypersensitivity reactions) are drug reactions that exhibit clinical signs and symptoms of an allergic response, but are not immunologically mediated.[110] They can manifest as relatively benign symptoms or as severe, life-threatening events indistinguishable from anaphylaxis (Table 3-11).[110] The latter response is described as an anaphylactoid reaction because it resembles true anaphylaxis, but does not involve IgE-antibody formation.[13,110] The risk of such potentially severe reactions needs to be considered when prescribing agents known to be associated with anaphylactoid reactions. For example, the prophylactic use of antibiotics such as ciprofloxacin to prevent meningococcal infections during an outbreak was associated with a relatively high rate (1:1,000) of serious anaphylactoid reactions.[111] This would be of potentially greater importance in the setting of a mass prophylaxis program to combat exposure to anthrax. Unlike true allergic reactions, which require an induction period during which a patient becomes sensitized to an antigen, pseudoallergic reactions can occur on the first exposure to a drug. The development of pseudoallergic reactions can be dose related, manifesting when large doses of the drug are administered, when the dose is increased, or when the rate of IV administration is increased.[11]

C.C. has experienced a common pseudoallergic reaction to vancomycin, usually referred to as the "red man syndrome" or "red neck syndrome," which primarily occurs when large doses of vancomycin are administered rapidly. Differentiating between a true allergic response and a pseudoallergic response can be difficult because the signs and symptoms can be indistinguishable. For example, each of the symptoms experienced by C.C. (flushing, tachycardia, pruritus, and hypotension) is caused by histamine release and can occur during an anaphylactic episode (see Case 3-2, Question 2). To conclusively determine the cause of the reaction would require immunologic testing for antibodies to the suspect drug or agent, which is not always possible or practical. In this case, C.C. had uneventfully received vancomycin previously and has tolerated five doses during this hospitalization; therefore, it is unlikely that the reaction is immunologically mediated (i.e., a true allergic reaction). Furthermore, the reaction occurred after an increase in his vancomycin dose, which further supports the diagnosis of a pseudoallergic reaction.

CASE 3-6, QUESTION 2: Why did vancomycin cause a pseudoallergic reaction in C.C.?

Two general mechanisms have been proposed for pseudoallergic reactions: complement activation and direct histamine release.[36]

Complement activation is secondary to immune complex formation, leading to the production of C3a, C4a, and C5a. These anaphylatoxins directly stimulate tissue mast cell and basophil degranulation and the subsequent release of neurochemical mediators. Radiocontrast media, whole blood and blood products, and protamine cause pseudoallergic reactions via this mechanism of complement activation.[110]

Pseudoallergic reactions from direct drug-induced histamine release occur through an as yet unknown pathway. Direct drug-induced release of histamine does not involve complement activation or IgE-antibody formation. Several drugs (e.g., vancomycin, protamine, radiocontrast media, opiates, pentamidine, phytonadione, deferoxamine) are known to directly stimulate histamine release.[13,110]

TABLE 3-11
Hypersensitivity Reactions to Drugs: Pseudoallergic Reactions

Frequency	Highly variable, depending on the agent involved. For example, up to 30% of patients taking aspirin exhibit a cutaneous pseudoallergic response. On the other hand, pseudoallergic reactions to other agents, such as phytonadione and thiamine, are rare.
Clinical manifestations	Range from benign reactions (e.g., pruritus and flushing) to a life-threatening clinical syndrome indistinguishable from anaphylaxis. Commonly require a higher drug dose to elicit the response than a true IgE-mediated reaction. May arise less quickly (>15 minutes after exposure) than true allergic reaction.
Diagnostic workup	Skin tests and identification of specific antibodies are negative.
Treatment	Pseudoallergic reactions are treated the same as true allergic reactions (i.e., according to the clinical presentations of the patient). Thus, some reactions simply may require removal of the suspect agent, whereas some anaphylactoid reactions may require aggressive therapy (e.g., epinephrine, antihistamines, corticosteroids).
Prognosis	As with true allergic reactions, patients who have experienced a pseudoallergic drug reaction may have a similar reaction on re-exposure. The severity of response may lessen, however, with repeated administration. Furthermore, for some drugs, the frequency and severity of the reaction also may be influenced by the dose or rate of intravenous administration. Pretreatment regimens to reduce the frequency and the severity of responses have been developed for some drugs well known to cause pseudoallergic reactions (e.g., radiocontrast media).

Source: Pichler WJ et al. Drug hypersensitivity reactions: pathomechanism and clinical symptoms. *Med Clin North Am.* 2010;94:645; Schnyder B. Approach to the patient with drug allergy. *Immunol Allergy Clin North Am.* 2009;29:405; Sanchez-Borges M. NSAID hypersensitivity (respiratory, cutaneous, and generalized anaphylactic symptoms). *Med Clin North Am.* 2010;94:853.

Some drugs (e.g., radiocontrast media and protamine) cause pseudoallergic reactions via both complement activation and direct-histamine release mechanisms. Furthermore, some drugs (e.g., vancomycin, quaternary ammonium muscle relaxants, and ciprofloxacin) can cause both true allergic reactions and pseudoallergic reactions.[30]

CASE 3-6, QUESTION 3: How should C.C.'s pseudoallergic reaction be treated? Does treatment of pseudoallergic reactions differ from that of true allergic reactions?

The first step in treating C.C.'s reaction is to eliminate the underlying cause. Thus, his vancomycin infusion should be held until the reaction resolves. Because the reaction is histamine-mediated, administration of an antihistamine such as diphenhydramine 50 mg IV is warranted. Observation of his BP and heart rate is mandatory. Intravenous fluids should be administered if his BP continues to fall or fails to stabilize. Patients with allergic reactions should be treated based on their clinical signs and symptoms, regardless of the mechanism behind the reaction. Thus, for all intents and purposes, pseudoallergic reactions are treated in the same manner as true allergic reactions.

CASE 3-6, QUESTION 4: Can C.C. continue to receive vancomycin? How can future reactions be prevented?

It is not necessary to discontinue vancomycin therapy in C.C. This reaction can be prevented by administering smaller doses of the drug more frequently (e.g., 1,000 mg every 8 hours rather than 1,500 mg every 12 hours) or infusing the dose for a longer interval, typically 2 hours. Alternatively, pretreatment with an antihistamine 1 hour before vancomycin administration is effective. In addition, tachyphylaxis to vancomycin-induced red man syndrome is independent of pretreatment with antihistamine and is another characteristic that differentiates a pseudoallergic reaction from a true allergic reaction. Pretreatment regimens to prevent pseudoallergic reactions to various other drugs (e.g., radiocontrast media) also are well described and can be effective.

CASE 3-6, QUESTION 5: What other drugs are commonly associated with pseudoallergic reactions?

Many other agents have been associated with pseudoallergic reactions.[30] Some of the agents more commonly associated with pseudoallergic reactions are described next.

Aspirin/Nonsteroidal Anti-Inflammatory Drugs

After penicillins, aspirin is the drug most commonly reported as causing "allergic" reactions. Reactions to aspirin can be divided into three broad categories: respiratory reactions, cutaneous manifestations, and anaphylaxis. None of these reactions has been consistently associated with IgE.[112]

RESPIRATORY

The prevalence of bronchospasm with rhinoconjunctivitis is 0% to 28% in children with aspirin sensitivity. In adult asthmatics, the prevalence of aspirin sensitivity ranges from 5% to 20%. The prevalence of aspirin sensitivity during aspirin challenge in adult asthmatics with a history of aspirin-induced respiratory reaction ranges from 66% to 97%.[113] Symptoms usually occur within 30 minutes to 3 hours of ingestion. The triad seen in many sensitive patients is aspirin sensitivity, nasal polyps, and asthma. All potent inhibitors of cyclo-oxygenase can cause respiratory symptoms in aspirin-sensitive patients. Thus, patients who react to aspirin should be considered sensitive to NSAIDs, and vice versa. Weak cyclo-oxygenase inhibitors, such as acetaminophen, choline magnesium salicylate, salicylamide, salsalate, and sodium salicylate, are generally well tolerated in patients with aspirin sensitivity.[112]

CUTANEOUS

The prevalence of cutaneous reactions to aspirin depends on the type of reaction and the population studied. For example, urticaria-angioedema occurs in 0.5% of children, 3.8% of the general adult population, and in 21% to 30% of patients with a history of chronic urticaria. Disease activity at the time of aspirin challenge plays an important role in those with a history of chronic urticaria. In one study, 70% of patients whose urticaria was active at the time of challenge reacted to aspirin, compared with only 6.6% of patients whose urticaria was not active at the time of challenge. Furthermore, aspirin or NSAID may aggravate pre-existing urticaria.[112–114] Other dermatologic reactions to aspirin occur with less frequency; for example, eczema, purpura, and erythema multiforme occur in 2.4%, 1.5%, and 1% of the population, respectively.

ANAPHYLAXIS

The true prevalence of aspirin-induced or NSAID-induced anaphylaxis is unknown, but may range from 0.07% of the general population to 10% of patients with anaphylactic symptoms. Although IgE is not consistently associated with aspirin-related or NSAID-related reactions (including anaphylaxis), aspirin-induced or NSAID-induced anaphylaxis shares three characteristics with immune-mediated anaphylaxis that point to IgE as a cause. First, the reaction occurs after two or more exposures to the offending agent, suggesting that preformed IgE antibodies are responsible. Second, patients do not have underlying nasal polyposis, asthma, or urticaria. Third, the patient who reacts to aspirin or a single NSAID can tolerate a chemically unrelated NSAID, suggesting that a drug-specific IgE antibody has been formed.[112,115]

The NSAIDs that selectively inhibit cyclo-oxygenase-2 (COX-2) while sparing cyclo-oxygenase-1 (COX-1) include celecoxib, rofecoxib, and valdecoxib, among others. Celecoxib is the only COX-2 inhibitor currently marketed in the United States. Selective inhibition of COX-2 provides anti-inflammatory effects while minimizing the renal effects, GI toxicity, and antiplatelet effects seen with inhibition of COX-1. Aspirin and older NSAIDs are nonselective inhibitors of cyclo-oxygenase, inhibiting both COX-1 and COX-2. Anaphylactoid or hypersensitivity reactions have been reported with celecoxib and it appears that the rate of hypersensitivity is comparable to that of traditional NSAIDs.[115] Notably, celecoxib prescribing information states that, as with any NSAID, use is contraindicated in patients who have experienced asthma, urticaria, or allergic-type reactions after taking aspirin or other NSAIDs. Several reports, however, describe successful administration of celecoxib and other COX-2 selective agents to patients with aspirin-sensitive asthma or a history of hypersensitivity reactions to traditional NSAIDs, and evidence suggests that inhibition of COX-1 rather than COX-2 is key to initiating these events.[115–119] Nevertheless, COX-2 selective agents can still elicit allergic responses by other means (e.g., IgE-mediated hypersensitivity). Thus, appropriate precautions and monitoring should be followed when initiating therapy in any patient with a history of allergic reactions to aspirin or other NSAIDs.

and personnel trained to evaluate and address anaphylaxis is prudent.

LATEX ALLERGY

Natural latex is a milky fluid consisting of extremely small particles of rubber obtained from the rubber tree. Natural rubber includes all products made from, or containing, natural latex.[133] Many products commonly used in health care (e.g., gloves, BP cuffs, catheters, injection ports, rubber stoppers of medication vials) are made wholly or in part of latex. Over the past several years, the significance of latex allergy has become clear as cases of allergic reactions, some life-threatening, have been reported.[133] Health professionals must recognize the types of reactions latex can cause and must know how to minimize patient exposure to latex. Also, preparing parenteral drugs for latex-allergic patients can be difficult because of the number of materials involved that may contain latex.

Health professionals are at significant risk for developing latex allergy because of their frequent exposure to latex products. Other groups at risk for developing latex allergy are workers in businesses that manufacture latex products; patients with spina bifida; and people with allergies to avocado, potato, banana, tomato, chestnuts, kiwi fruit, and papaya.[133]

Three types of reactions to latex have been described: irritant contact dermatitis, allergic contact dermatitis (chemical sensitivity dermatitis), and immediate hypersensitivity.[133,134]

Irritant contact dermatitis is the most common reaction to latex and manifests as dry, itchy, irritated areas of the skin. This is not a true allergic reaction to latex.[133]

Allergic contact dermatitis is a delayed hypersensitivity reaction caused by exposure to chemicals added during the processing and manufacturing of latex. A rash, similar to that seen with poison ivy, usually begins 24 to 48 hours after exposure and may progress to oozing blisters.[133]

Immediate hypersensitivity to proteins in the latex is an IgE-mediated allergic response. The reaction can begin within minutes of exposure to latex or occur hours later. Symptoms vary from mild skin redness, hives, and itching to respiratory involvement (runny nose, sneezing, itchy eyes, trouble breathing, asthma). Rare cases of anaphylactic shock have been described.[133] Reports of the prevalence of latex allergy vary from 1% to 6% of the general population and 8% to 12% of health care workers. Latex allergy is diagnosed by obtaining an accurate description of the reaction and establishing a temporal relationship to latex exposure. Diagnostic kits are available to detect latex antibodies as well as to aid in the diagnosis of allergic contact dermatitis.[133,134]

Health care practitioners, particularly those in settings in which IV or intramuscular medications are administered, may be faced with preparing parenteral products for a latex-allergic patient. This often poses a challenge because latex is in many of the materials used to prepare parenteral products (e.g., rubber stoppers on medication vials, injection ports on IV bags, rubber plungers for syringes, IV transfer sets).[133,134] Many manufacturers are now preparing products in a latex-free form, which simplifies drug preparation. Furthermore, manufacturers of medical devices are now required to identify on their labels which products have natural latex and which have dry natural rubber.[134] Many institutions have instituted policies on the preparation of parenteral products for the "latex-sensitive" person. Readers are referred to these references for the details of these procedures.[135,136]

PREVENTION AND MANAGEMENT OF ALLERGIC REACTIONS

CASE 3-8

QUESTION 1: A.M., a 40-year-old woman, is hospitalized with a diagnosis of community-acquired pneumonia. Her medical history is noncontributory except for an uneventful course of ampicillin 6 months before admission for an ear infection. A.M. is empirically treated with cefuroxime 0.75 g IV every 8 hours. On day 2 of therapy, she develops a raised pruritic maculopapular rash on her back, abdomen, and upper extremities. Antacid, docusate sodium, albuterol by metered-dose inhaler, and multivitamins were initiated on the same day as the cefuroxime. How should A.M.'s allergic reaction be managed? How might her allergic reaction have been prevented?

When examining methods to prevent allergic reactions, three possibilities exist: (a) the patient has unknowingly been sensitized to a drug and experiences an allergic reaction on receiving the same or a similar drug again; (b) the patient has a history of an allergic reaction to a medication and mistakenly receives the same or a similar medication a second time and again develops an allergic reaction; and (c) the patient has a history of an allergic reaction to a medication and intentionally receives the same or similar medication again. As in the first situation, A.M.'s allergic reaction was unpredictable and, therefore, could not be prevented. To prevent future allergic reactions (i.e., the second situation), however, A.M.'s reaction should be well documented in the medical chart and pharmacy records. In addition, all patients should undergo a thorough drug history on hospitalization. Careful attention should be paid to differentiating drug intolerance (e.g., stomach upset) from true allergic reactions, and any allergic reactions elicited during an interview should be documented appropriately. Adequate communication of allergic reactions is the single most important method of preventing their occurrence.

As described earlier, the first step in managing an allergic reaction is to determine its cause. Given A.M.'s history of exposure to ampicillin, the timing of the reaction, and the low frequency of allergic reactions to her other medications, cefuroxime is the most likely candidate. Second, a decision regarding whether to stop the suspect drug should be made. This decision must be based on the severity of the reaction, the condition being treated, and the availability of suitable alternatives. When possible, an equally effective alternative drug should be substituted for the suspect agent, preferably one that is immunologically distinct to avoid cross-sensitivity (see Case 3-1, Question 4, for a discussion of cross-reactivity).[137] If a suitable alternative exists, the offending agent should be stopped and the reaction treated symptomatically if necessary. In the case of A.M., another antimicrobial (e.g., azithromycin, clarithromycin, trimethoprim-sulfamethoxazole) could be substituted for cefuroxime (Chapter 64, Respiratory Tract Infections) and her symptoms treated with an oral or parenteral antihistamine, as well as a low-potency topical corticosteroid if necessary.

Some cases are described by the third situation: a patient develops an allergic reaction (or has a well-documented history of drug allergy), and it is inappropriate or not possible to change to an alternative drug. If the sensitivity reaction is severe or life-threatening, desensitization should be considered (Case 3-9, Questions 1 and 2); premedication to prevent or minimize anaphylaxis is not effective.[30] If the reaction is minor (e.g., pruritus, rash, or GI symptoms), premedication or management of the reaction with antiallergy medications (e.g., antihistamines) might be sufficient to allow completion of therapy. It is rare in such cases for the reaction to progress to more serious allergic symptoms such as anaphylaxis[137]; however, suppression of allergic symptoms should be undertaken cautiously because many immunologic reactions are not IgE mediated and may progress to serious reactions, despite treatment. In general, allergy suppression should be reserved for prevention of mild reactions that are known or strongly suspected to be IgE mediated.[30,137]

Desensitization

β-LACTAMS

CASE 3-9

QUESTION 1: K.A. is a 24-year-old primigravida in her eighth week of pregnancy with a history of angioedema secondary to penicillin. Her initial pregnancy screening revealed a positive Venereal Disease Research Laboratory reaction and a fluorescent treponemal antibody absorption titer of 1:64. K.A. denies a history of genital lesions, currently does not exhibit clinical signs or symptoms of syphilis, and denies previous treatment for syphilis. Based on the serologic evidence and her history, a diagnosis of early latent syphilis is made. Current treatment guidelines indicate that penicillin is the drug of choice for K.A. How can a possible reaction to penicillin be prevented in K.A.? Is premedication an alternative to preventing a reaction?

There are situations where a drug is medically necessary in a patient with a known or suspected allergy to the drug, alternative therapy is not available, and diagnostic testing does not exist. In such cases there are two options: induction of tolerance (also called desensitization) or a graded challenge. Desensitization is the process of administering gradually increasing doses of a drug in an effort to modify a patient's response to the drug so that it can then be safely administered.[7] This process has been used successfully to manage both immune-mediated and non–immune-mediated reactions. A graded challenge (also called incremental test dosing) is the process of careful administration of sub-therapeutic doses of drug to determine if a patient is truly allergic. Although similar sounding, there are distinct differences between the two processes.[7] For example, unlike induction of tolerance, a graded challenge does not alter a patient's response to the drug. The initial drug doses used for inducing tolerance are sub-allergenic—as low as 1/10,000th of the final dose and the process can take several hours involving multiple doses, each slightly larger than the preceding dose. Starting doses for a graded challenge may be 1/100th of the final dose. The process generally involves fewer steps (as few as two) and can be typically accomplished more rapidly. If the graded challenge is completed and a therapeutic course of drug tolerated, a graded challenge is not required before future courses of the drug. Tolerance induction, on the other hand, is only maintained as long as the patient receives the suspect drug; any interruption of therapy will require the desensitization procedure to be repeated (see Case 3-9, Question 4).

The choice of drug desensitization or using a graded challenge depends on the likelihood of the patient having a true allergic reaction. A graded challenge may be appropriate in patients with a distant or unclear history of drug allergy; when the reaction seems minor or for which diagnostic testing is unavailable; or in cases where cross-reactivity is expected to be low. For example, a patient with a maculopapular rash to ceftriaxone may undergo a graded challenge to imipenem-cilastatin to assess tolerance. On the other hand, a patient with a well-described, severe IgE-mediated reaction to a drug may be better suited for tolerance induction. Importantly, graded challenge or tolerance induction should not be used in patients with a history of a severe non-IgE–mediated reaction such as hepatitis, hemolytic anemia, Stevens-Johnson syndrome, toxic epidermal necrolysis, or DRESS syndrome due to the risk of provoking a potentially life-threatening reaction.[7] Because K.A.'s reaction to penicillin may be potentially severe, premedication is not an option and desensitization to penicillin should be started. (See Chapter 69, Sexually Transmitted Diseases, for alternative therapy.)

CASE 3-9, QUESTION 2: How should K.A. be desensitized? Why should she be skin-tested before desensitization?

If possible before tolerance induction is begun, K.A. should be skin-tested (see Case 3-1, Questions 3 and 4) to confirm her penicillin allergy.[30,40,137] Patients who have a positive history of penicillin allergy, but whose skin tests are negative, can receive full therapeutic doses without desensitization with little risk of developing an allergic reaction. One author, for example, reported only one case of acute anaphylaxis in a skin test–negative patient given full therapeutic doses of penicillin in more than 1,500 skin tests; similar results have been reported by other investigators.[40,137] If skin testing cannot be performed or if K.A.'s skin test is positive, desensitization should be initiated. Acute oral desensitization to penicillin and other *β*-lactam antibiotics is well established; one such protocol is outlined in Table 3-12, although others have been used successfully.[138]

The oral route for *β*-lactam desensitization is preferred to the parenteral route because: (a) exposure by the oral route is less likely to cause a systemic allergic reaction than parenteral exposure; (b) fatal anaphylaxis from oral *β*-lactam drug therapy is rare; (c) preformed polymers and conjugates of penicillin major and minor determinants to *Penicillium* proteins are not well absorbed after oral administration; (d) blood levels rise gradually, favoring univalent haptenation; and (e) fatal or life-endangering

TABLE 3-12
***β*-Lactam Oral Desensitization Protocol**

Stock Drug Concentration (mg/mL)[a]	Dose No.	Amount (mL)	Drug Dose (mg)	Cumulative Drug (mg)
0.5	1[b]	0.05	0.025	0.025
0.5	2	0.10	0.05	0.075
0.5	3	0.20	0.10	0.175
0.5	4	0.40	0.20	0.375
0.5	5	0.80	0.40	0.775
5.0	6	0.15	0.75	1.525
5.0	7	0.30	1.50	3.025
5.0	8	0.60	3.00	6.025
5.0	9	1.20	6.00	12.025
5.0	10	2.40	12.00	24.025
50	11	0.50	25.00	49.025
50	12	1.20	60.00	109.025
50	13	2.50	125.00	234.025
50	14	5.00	250.00	484.025

[a]Dilutions using 250 mg/5 mL of pediatric suspension.
[b]Oral dose doubled approximately every 15 to 30 minutes.
Dosing for the oral protocol is arbitrary and should be adjusted for individual patients based on the clinical sensitivity and the desired drug dose end point.
Source: Sullivan TJ et al. Desensitization of patients allergic to penicillin using orally administered beta-lactam antibiotics. *J Allergy Clin Immunol.* 1982;69:275; Wendel GD Jr et al. Penicillin allergy and desensitization in serious infections during pregnancy. *N Engl J Med.* 1985;312:1229.

TABLE 3-13
β-Lactam Intravenous Desensitization Protocol

Stock Drug Concentration (mg/mL)[a]	Dose No.[b]	Amount per 50 mL (mg/mL)[c]	Cumulative Drug (mg)
0.005	1	0.0001	0.005
0.025	2	0.0005	0.030
0.125	3	0.0025	0.155
0.625	4	0.0125	0.780
3.125	5	0.0625	3.905
15.625	6	0.3125	19.530
31.25	7	0.625	50.780
62.50	8	1.25	113.280
125.00	9	2.5	238.280
250.00	10[d]	5.0	488.280

[a] Stock drug solutions are prepared using serial dilutions of the desired goal (e.g., 500 mg of β-lactam). Doses 1 through 5 represent fivefold dilutions; doses 6 through 10 represent twofold dilutions.
[b] Interval between doses is 1 to 30 minutes. If desensitization is interrupted for >2 half-lives of the β-lactam, desensitization should be repeated.
[c] Mix 1 mL of stock drug solution in 50 mL 5% dextrose/0.225 normal saline or other compatible solution. Infuse each dose for 20–45 minutes. Dilution volume may vary with patient age and weight.
[d] If all 10 doses are administered and tolerated, the remainder of a full therapeutic dose of the β-lactam should be administered.
Dosing for the IV protocol is arbitrary and should be adjusted for individual patients based on the clinical sensitivity and the desired drug dose end point.
Source: Borish L et al. Intravenous desensitization to beta-lactam antibiotics. *J Allergy Clin Immunol.* 1987;80(3 Pt 1):314.

reactions have not occurred using current methods. In addition, oral desensitization can be accomplished over several hours.[30] If oral desensitization is not possible (e.g., if oral absorption is questionable), parenteral desensitization can be instituted. Although the subcutaneous and intramuscular routes have been used, the IV route is quicker and allows better control over the rate and concentration of drug administered, and any untoward reaction can be detected promptly and treated rapidly.[30,139] Table 3-13 outlines an IV β-lactam desensitization protocol. Oral and parenteral desensitization methods have not been compared formally, however. Patients should not be premedicated before desensitization, because this may prevent detection of minor allergic responses that may precede more serious reactions. In addition, only experienced personnel should undertake desensitization in an appropriate setting where emergency resuscitative equipment is readily available because severe reactions can develop.[137] Thus, K.A. should undergo oral desensitization as outlined in Table 3-12 if her skin test is positive or if skin testing cannot be performed.

CASE 3-9, QUESTION 3: Is K.A. at risk for an allergic reaction during tolerance induction? If tolerance induction is successful, is she at risk for a reaction during full-dose penicillin therapy?

Acute β-lactam desensitization, regardless of the route or protocol chosen, is not without risk. Approximately 5% of patients experience mild cutaneous reactions during desensitization, although one study reported reactions in 20% of patients during oral desensitization.[30,140] If a reaction occurs during the desensitization procedure itself, the reaction may be treated and desensitization continued using lower doses, increased intervals between doses, or both, after the reaction has abated. Severe, fatal reactions during desensitization are rare.[139]

Uneventful β-lactam desensitization, however, does not guarantee patients will be without reaction during full-dose therapy. Approximately 25% to 30% of patients experience a mild reaction during therapy, and 5% experience more severe reactions, including drug-induced serum sickness, hemolytic anemia, or urticaria.[30] Reaction rates are no different in severely ill or pregnant patients compared with stable or nonpregnant patients, although those with cystic fibrosis may be more difficult to desensitize because of their high frequency of allergic reactions.[140,141] Despite the occurrence of reactions, full-dose therapy is possible for most tolerance-induction procedures, but suppression of the reaction (e.g., by diphenhydramine) may be required.[139] Tolerance induction is also dose-dependent as allergic symptoms can appear after a substantial increase in the dose after tolerance has been achieved.[30]

CASE 3-9, QUESTION 4: If K.A. requires penicillin at a later date, will she need to undergo desensitization again? What is chronic desensitization?

The desensitized state, once achieved, will persist for approximately 48 hours after the last full dose of antibiotic; after this time, drug sensitivity will return.[30,139] Thus, if K.A. requires future courses of penicillin, she will need to undergo desensitization once again. In some cases, those requiring long-term antibiotic therapy (e.g., for endocarditis), those who may require β-lactams at a future date (e.g., those with cystic fibrosis), or those who have occupational exposure to β-lactams, maintenance of the desensitized state can be considered. Chronic twice daily dosing of oral penicillin has safely resulted in "chronic desensitization." Similar to acute desensitization, once therapy is interrupted, the allergic state returns.[13,30]

OTHER DRUGS

CASE 3-9, QUESTION 5: Have patients allergic to drugs besides β-lactams been desensitized successfully?

Although most experience with desensitization is with penicillin and other β-lactams, desensitization also has been accomplished with numerous other drugs, including allopurinol, vancomycin, antineoplastic agents, aspirin, and monoclonal antibodies.[80,138,139] Interestingly, not all of these cases represent IgE-mediated hypersensitivity reactions. For example, reactions to trimethoprim-sulfamethoxazole commonly occur in patients infected with HIV and may not be IgE mediated. Yet, given its role in treating and preventing *Pneumocystis jiroveci* pneumonia, successful desensitization to trimethoprim-sulfamethoxazole is commonly used.[139]

KEY REFERENCES AND WEBSITES

A full list of references for this chapter can be found at **http://thepoint.lww.com/AT10e**. Below are the key references for this chapter, with the corresponding reference number in this chapter found in parentheses after the reference.

Key References

Antonov D, et al. Drug-induced lupus erythematosus. *Clin Dermatol.* 2004;22:157. (96)

Dedeoglu F. Drug-induced autoimmunity. *Curr Opin Rheumatol.* 2009;21:547. (89)

Frumin J, Gallagher JC. Allergic cross-sensitivity between penicillin, carbapenem, and monobactam antibiotics: what are the chances? *Ann Pharmacother.* 2009;43:304. (56)

Hoover T et al. Angiotensin converting enzyme inhibitor induced angio-oedema: a review of the pathophysiology and risk factors. *Clin Exp Allergy.* 2010;40:50. (120)

Kemp SF et al. Epinephrine: the drug of choice for anaphylaxis. A statement of the World Allergy Organization. *Allergy.* 2008;63:1061. (70)

Khan DA, Solensky R. Drug allergy. *J Allergy Clin Immunol.* 2010; 125(2 Suppl 2):S126. (7)

Lieberman P et al. The diagnosis and management of anaphylaxis practice parameter: 2010 update [published correction appears in *J Allergy Clin Immunol.* 2010;126:1104]. *J Allergy Clin Immunol.* 2010;126:477. (59)

Patel RA, Gallagher JC. Drug fever. *Pharmacotherapy.* 2010;30:57. (82)

Pichler WJ et al. Drug hypersensitivity reactions: pathomechanism and clinical symptoms. *Med Clin North Am.* 2010;94:645. (79)

Sanchez-Borges M. NSAID hypersensitivity (respiratory, cutaneous, and generalized anaphylactic symptoms). *Med Clin North Am.* 2010;94:853. (114)

Scherer K, Bircher AJ. Danger signs in drug hypersensitivity. *Med Clin North Am.* 2010;94:681. (8)

Schnyder B. Approach to the patient with drug allergy. *Immunol Allergy Clin North Am.* 2009;29:405. (80)

Solensky R. Drug desensitization. *Immunol Allergy Clin North Am.* 2004;24:425. (139)

ten Holder SM et al. Cutaneous and systemic manifestations of drug-induced vasculitis. *Ann Pharmacother.* 2002;36:130. (94)

Wedner HJ. Drug allergy prevention and treatment. *Immunol Allergy Clin North Am.* 1991;11:679. (137)

4

Managing Drug Overdoses and Poisonings

Judith A. Alsop

CORE PRINCIPLES

CHAPTER CASES

EPIDEMIOLOGY

1 In 2009, 2.48 million poisonings were reported to the American Association of Poison Control Centers. Half of these exposures occur in children younger than 6 years of age and usually involve a single substance that is found in the home such as personal care items, analgesics, and cleaning agents. The elderly have access to numerous and dangerous medications and have a higher rate of completed suicide attempts than other age groups.

Case 4-1 (Questions 2, 3)

GENERAL MANAGEMENT

1 The most important aspect of patient management is to support airway, breathing, and circulation (the "ABCs"). There is no "cookbook" method to treat all poisoned patients, so it is important to treat the patient, not the poison or the laboratory values. The assessment and treatment of the potentially poisoned patient can be separated into seven functions: (a) gather history of exposure, (b) evaluate clinical presentation (i.e., "toxidromes"), (c) evaluate clinical laboratory patient data, (d) remove the toxic source (e.g., irrigate eyes, decontaminate exposed skin), (e) consider antidotes and specific treatment, (f) enhance systemic clearance, and (g) monitor patient outcome.

Case 4-4 (Questions 1, 5, 6)

GASTROINTESTINAL DECONTAMINATION

1 The most appropriate method for gastrointestinal (GI) tract decontamination is unclear because sound comparative data for different methods of GI decontamination are not available. Lavage, emesis, and cathartics are rarely performed as there is no evidence they improve patient outcome. Activated charcoal is generally safe to use, but it should not be administered if the benefit is not greater than the risk. Whole bowel irrigation using a polyethylene glycol–balanced electrolyte solution can successfully remove substances (iron, lithium, sustained-release dosage forms) from the entire GI tract in a period of several hours.

Case 4-3 (Questions 6, 7), Case 4-4 (Questions 11, 12, 16), Case 4-5 (Question 3)

ANTIDOTES

1 An antidote is a drug that neutralizes or reverses the toxicity of another substance. Some antidotes displace drugs from receptor sites (e.g., naloxone for opioids, flumazenil for benzodiazepines), and some can inhibit the formation of toxic metabolites (e.g., *N*-acetylcysteine [NAC] for acetaminophen, fomepizole for methanol).

Case 4-4 (Questions 2, 4)

continued

TOXICOLOGY LABORATORY SCREENING

1 Urine drug screens can be useful in a patient with coma of unknown etiology, when the presented history is inconsistent with clinical findings, or when more than one drug might have been ingested. Qualitative screening is intended to identify unknown substances involved in the toxic exposure. A benzodiazepine screen can detect oxazepam, a common benzodiazepine metabolite, but will not detect alprazolam and lorazepam as they are not metabolized to oxazepam. Opioid screens may not detect synthetic opioids such as fentanyl and methadone. Quantitative testing determines how much of a known drug is present and can help determine the severity of toxicity and the need for aggressive interventions (e.g., hemodialysis).	**Case 4-4 (Questions 1, 7)**

TOXIDROMES

1 A toxidrome is a consistent constellation of signs and symptoms associated with some specific classes of drugs. The most common toxidromes are those associated with anticholinergic activity, increased sympathetic activity, and central nervous system (CNS) stimulation or depression. Anticholinergic drugs increase heart rate and body temperature, decrease GI motility, dilate pupils, and produce drowsiness or delirium. Sympathomimetic drugs increase CNS activity, heart rate, body temperature, and blood pressure. Opioids, sedatives, hypnotics, and antidepressants depress the CNS, but the specific class of CNS depressant often cannot be easily identified.	**Case 4-4 (Questions 1, 2, 5)**

SALICYLATES

1 Acute ingestion of 150 to 300 mg/kg aspirin causes mild to moderate intoxication, greater than 300 mg/kg indicates severe poisoning, and greater than 500 mg/kg is potentially lethal. Symptoms of intoxication include vomiting, tinnitus, delirium, tachypnea, metabolic acidosis, respiratory alkalosis, hypokalemia, irritability, hallucinations, stupor, coma, hyperthermia, coagulopathy, and seizures. Salicylate intoxication mimics other medical conditions and can be easily missed. Patients with a chronic salicylate exposure, acidosis, or CNS symptoms and those who are elderly are high-risk and should be considered for early dialysis.	**Case 4-1 (Question 3), Case 4-2 (Questions 1–6)**

IRON

1 Acute elemental iron ingestions of less than 20 mg/kg are usually nontoxic; doses of 20 to 60 mg/kg result in mild to moderate toxicity, and doses of greater than 60 mg/kg are potentially fatal. Symptoms of toxicity include nausea, vomiting, diarrhea, abdominal pain, hematemesis, bloody stools, CNS depression, hypotension, and shock. Patients with severe iron poisoning do not exhibit the second stage of so-called recovery but continue to deteriorate.	**Case 4-3 (Questions 2–14)**

TRICYCLIC ANTIDEPRESSANTS

1 Severe toxicity has been associated with doses of 15 to 25 mg/kg. Symptoms include tachycardia with prolongation of the PR, QTc, and QRS intervals, ST and T-wave changes, acidosis, seizures, coma, hypotension, and adult respiratory distress syndrome. A QRS segment greater than 100 milliseconds is commonly seen in severe tricyclic antidepressant overdoses.	**Case 4-4 (Questions 9–17)**

ACETAMINOPHEN

1 Toxicity is associated with acute ingestions greater than 150 mg/kg or more than 7.5 g total in adults. Symptoms in patients with toxicity include vomiting, anorexia, abdominal pain, malaise, and progression to characteristic centrilobular hepatic necrosis. Acetaminophen-induced hepatotoxicity is universal by 36 hours after ingestion, but patients who receive NAC within 8 to 10 hours after ingestion rarely exhibit hepatotoxicity. There is no consensus as to the best route of NAC administration, the optimal dosage regimen, or the optimal duration of therapy.	**Case 4-5 (Questions 1–15)**

This chapter reviews common strategies for the evaluation and management of drug overdoses and poisonings. Information for the management of specific drug overdoses is best obtained from a poison control center (reached by calling 1-800-222-1222 anywhere in the United States).

Epidemiologic Data

AMERICAN ASSOCIATION OF POISON CONTROL CENTERS AND DRUG ABUSE WARNING NETWORK

Toxicity secondary to drug and chemical exposure commonly occurs in children. The incidence of exposure to specific agents and the severity of outcomes varies based on the population studied (Table 4-1).[1–3] The number of reported toxic exposures in the United States in 2009 was approximately 2.48 million, according to the American Association of Poison Control Centers (AAPCC).[3] In most cases, little or no toxicity was associated with the exposure. Although 24.1% of patients received treatment at a health care facility, only 6.1% reported moderate or severe symptoms and 0.06% resulted in fatalities.

According to the Drug Abuse Warning Network (DAWN), almost 2 million US emergency department (ED) visits involved drug misuse or abuse in the year 2008. Of those cases, illicit drug use was mentioned more than 2.7 million times because many of the visits involved multiple drugs of abuse.[4] These disparate statistics from two national sources underscore the difficulty in determining the true incidence of poisoning and overdoses.[5]

AGE-SPECIFIC DATA

Stratifying patients by age can be useful in assessing the likelihood of severe toxicity from an exposure. Most unintentional ingestions by children 1 to 6 years of age occur because children are curious, becoming more mobile, and beginning to explore their surroundings, and they often put objects or substances into their mouths.[6] Of all reported poisonings, 38.9% occur in children younger than 3 years and 51.9% occur in children younger than 6 years of age.[3] According to AAPCC statistics, 11.26% of pediatric (younger than 6 years of age) poisoning cases were treated in a health care facility, and the remaining cases were managed at home.[3] Severe toxicity in young children is relatively uncommon as exposures usually involve the ingestion of relatively small amounts of a single substance.[6,7] Of pediatric cases reported to AAPCC, there were 769 (0.06%) life-threatening outcomes and 31 (0.00%) fatalities from a total of 1,290,784 pediatric cases.[3]

AAPCC epidemiologic data also report medication errors, which in the pediatric population commonly result from confusing units of measurement (e.g., teaspoons vs. milliliters or tablespoons vs. teaspoons), incorrect formulation or concentration administered, dispensing cup errors, and incorrect formulation or concentration dispensed from the pharmacy.[3]

In children older than 6 years of age, the reasons for toxic exposure to medications are less clear.[8] Adolescent children generally have poor knowledge of the toxicity of medications and can overdose themselves unintentionally.[6,9] The potential for suicide attempts or intentional substance abuse should not be ignored in older children. These intentional overdoses commonly involve mixed exposures to illicit drugs, prescribed medications, or ethanol, and are associated with more severe toxicity and death than unintentional toxic exposures.

For many teens, using prescription drugs is not considered dangerous as the drugs are not illegal like heroin or cocaine. In a 2007 survey, 9.5% of adolescents 12 to 17 years of age said they had used an illicit substance in the past month.[10] The lifetime use of opiates or opioids, other than heroin, in 12th graders has doubled from 6.6% in 1991 to 13.2% in 2008.[10]

In geriatric patients, overdoses tend to have a greater potential for severe adverse effects compared with overdoses in other age groups.[11] Although the elderly constitute 13% of the population, they account for 33% of the drug use and 16% of the suicides.[12] Patients age 65 or older take an average of 5.7 prescription medications along with 2 to 4 nonprescription drugs daily.[11,12] In 2007, the suicide rate for people 65 years and older was 14.3 per 100,000 population compared with the national average of 11.3 per 100,000.[13] The elderly are more likely to have underlying illnesses and often have access to a variety of potentially dangerous medications. This results in higher rates of completed suicides than in other age groups.[11,12]

TABLE 4-1
Substances Most Commonly Involved in Poisonings[a]

Children	Adults	Fatal Exposures (All Ages)
Personal care products	Analgesics	Sedatives/hypnotics/antipsychotics
Analgesics	Sedatives/hypnotics/antipsychotics	Cardiovascular agents
Cleaning substances	Antidepressants	Opioids
Topical products	Cleaning substances	Acetaminophen-containing products
Vitamins	Cardiovascular agents	Antidepressants
Antihistamines	Alcohols	Acetaminophen
Cough and cold products	Bites, envenomations	Alcohols
Pesticides	Pesticides	Stimulants and street drugs
Plants	Antiepileptic agents	Muscle relaxants
GI products	Personal care products	Cyclic antidepressants
Antimicrobials	Antihistamines	Antiepileptic agents
Arts and office supplies	Hormones and hormone antagonists	Fumes/gases/vapors
Alcohols	Antimicrobials	Aspirin
Hormones and hormone antagonists	Chemicals	Nonsteroidal anti-inflammatory drugs
Cardiovascular agents	Fumes/gases/vapors	Antihistamines
	Hydrocarbons	

[a]Poisoning exposures are listed in order of frequency encountered.
GI, gastrointestinal.
Source: Bronstein AC et al. 2009 Annual report of the American Association of Poison Control Centers' National Poison Data System (NPDS): 27th Annual Report. *Clin Toxicol (Phila)*. 2010;48:979.

Information Resources

COMPUTERIZED DATABASES

A vast number of substances can be involved in a poisoning or overdose. Reliable data about the contents of products, toxicities of substances, and treatment approaches need to be readily accessible. POISINDEX, a computerized database,[14] provides information on thousands of drugs by brand name, generic name, and street name, as well as foreign drugs, chemicals, pesticides, household products, personal care items, cleaning products, poisonous insects, poisonous snakes, and poisonous plants. Annual subscriptions to POISINDEX, updated quarterly, are expensive and are generally available only in large medical centers.[15]

PRINTED PUBLICATIONS

Textbooks and manuals also provide useful clinical information about the presentation, assessment, and treatment of toxicities. *Goldfrank's Toxicologic Emergencies*[16] and the pocket-size *Poisoning & Drug Overdose*[17] are valuable, less-expensive alternatives to computerized database programs. Books, however, are less useful than computerized databases because information must be condensed and cannot be updated as frequently. Some drug package inserts also refer to treatment of acute toxicities; however, the information can be inadequate or inappropriate.[18,19]

POISON CONTROL CENTERS

Poison control centers provide the most cost-effective and accurate information to health care providers and to the general public.[20,21] Poison centers are staffed by trained poison information specialists who have a pharmacy, nursing, or medical background. Physician backup is provided 24 hours a day by board-certified medical toxicologists. The nonphysician clinical toxicologists, pharmacists, and nurses who staff poison control centers are certified as specialists in poison information by the AAPCC or as clinical toxicologists by the American Board of Applied Toxicology.[22]

The poison information specialist must accurately and efficiently assess event-specific toxicity by telephone, without the benefit of direct observation of the patient. The specialist must communicate this assessment along with treatment information quickly, accurately, and professionally in a reassuring manner. Subsequent to telephone consultations, poison control center staff should initiate follow-up calls to determine the effectiveness of the recommended treatment and the need for additional evaluation or treatment.[23,24]

EFFECTIVE COMMUNICATION

Effective communication is essential to the assessment of potential poisonings. In most situations, the person seeking guidance on the management of a potentially toxic exposure is the parent of a small child who may have ingested a substance. The caller is usually anxious about the child and may feel guilty about the exposure. To calm the caller, the health care provider should quickly reassure the parent that telephoning for help was appropriate and that the best assistance possible will be provided.[24] If English is not the first language of the caller, or if there are other communication barriers (e.g., panic), solutions must be found to enhance outcomes. Most poison centers subscribe to translation services or have bilingual staff to communicate with non–English-speaking callers. Poison centers also have special equipment to serve the hearing- and speech-impaired populations.

Once calm, effective communication is established, the health care provider should first determine whether the patient is conscious and breathing and has a pulse. If life-threatening symptoms have occurred, the caller should call 9-1-1 for emergency services. If the health care provider does not have the knowledge or resources to provide poison information, he or she should refer the caller to the closest poison control center. Information on the location and phone number of the nearest poison control center can be found at **http://www.aapcc.org** or by calling 1-800-222-1222 in the United States.

GENERAL MANAGEMENT

Supportive Care and "ABCs"

Management of poisoned or overdosed patients is primarily based on symptomatic and supportive care. Specific antidotes exist only for a small percentage of the thousands of potential drugs and chemicals that can cause a poisoning.

The first aspect of patient management should always be basic support of airway, breathing, and circulation (the "ABCs"). The assessment and treatment of the potentially poisoned patient can be separated into seven primary functions: (a) gathering history of exposure, (b) evaluating clinical presentation (i.e., "toxidromes"), (c) evaluating clinical laboratory patient data, (d) removing the toxic source (e.g., irrigating eyes, decontaminating exposed skin), (e) considering antidotes and specific treatment, (f) enhancing systemic clearance, and (g) monitoring outcome.[25–27]

GATHERING HISTORY OF EXPOSURE

Comprehensive historical information about the toxic exposure should be gathered from as many different sources as possible (e.g., patient, family, friends, prehospital health care providers). This information should be compared for consistency and evaluated relative to clinical findings and laboratory results. The patient's history of the exposure is often inaccurate and should be confirmed with objective findings.[25,26,28] For example, a patient who presents to an ED with a supposed hydrocodone and carisoprodol overdose is expected to be lethargic or comatose. If the patient arrives wide awake with tachycardia and agitation, the caregiver should suspect exposure to other substances.

Specific information should be sought concerning the patient's state of consciousness, symptoms, probable intoxicant(s), and maximal amount and dosage form(s) of substance ingested, as well as when the exposure occurred. Medications, allergies, and prior medical problems also should be ascertained to facilitate development of treatment plans (e.g., a history of renal failure may indicate the need for hemodialysis to compensate for decreased renal drug clearance).[25,26]

EVALUATING CLINICAL PRESENTATION AND TOXIDROMES

A thorough physical examination is needed to characterize the signs and symptoms of overdose, and should be conducted serially to determine the evolution or resolution of the patient's intoxication. An evaluation of the presenting signs and symptoms can provide clues to the drug class causing the toxicity, confirm the historical data surrounding the toxic exposure, and suggest initial treatment.[25,29–31] The patient may be asymptomatic on presentation, even though a potentially severe exposure has occurred, if absorption of the drug or toxic substance is incomplete or if the substance has not yet been metabolized to a toxic substance.[32–34]

Characteristic toxidromes (i.e., a constellation of signs and symptoms consistent with a syndrome) can be associated with some specific classes of drugs.[26,30,31] The most common toxidromes are those associated with anticholinergic activity, increased sympathetic activity, and central nervous system (CNS) stimulation or depression. Anticholinergic drugs can increase heart rate and body temperature, decrease gastrointestinal (GI) motility, dilate pupils, and produce drowsiness or delirium. Sympathomimetic drugs can increase CNS activity, heart rate, body temperature, and blood pressure (BP). Opioids, sedatives, hypnotics, and antidepressants can depress the CNS, but the specific class of CNS depressant often cannot be easily identified.

Classic findings may not be present for all drugs within a therapeutic class. For example, opioids generally induce miosis, but meperidine can produce mydriasis. Furthermore, the association of symptoms with a particular class of toxic substances is difficult when more than one substance has been ingested. Practitioners should not focus only on the specific clinical findings associated with a toxidrome. Rather, they should consider all subjective and objective data gathered from the history of exposure, the patient's medical history, physical examination, and laboratory findings.[30]

INTERPRETATION OF LABORATORY DATA

DRUG SCREENS

A urine drug screen can be useful in identifying the presence of drugs and their metabolites in selected patients but is not indicated in all cases of drug overdose. Urine drug screens can be useful in a patient with coma of unknown etiology, when the presented history is inconsistent with clinical findings, or when more than one drug might have been ingested.[35,36]

PHARMACOKINETIC CONSIDERATIONS

The absorption, distribution, metabolism, and elimination of drugs in the overdosed patient can be quite different than when the drug is taken in usual therapeutic doses.[32–34] The expected pharmacodynamic and pharmacokinetic features of drugs can be substantially altered by large drug overdoses, especially with drugs that exhibit dose-dependent pharmacokinetics. The rate of drug absorption is generally slowed by large overdoses, and the time to reach peak serum drug concentrations can be delayed.[35,37] For example, peak serum concentrations of phenytoin can be delayed for 2 to 7 days after an orally ingested overdose.[38,39] The volume of distribution of an overdosed drug can be increased, and when usual metabolic pathways become saturated, secondary clearance pathways can be important. For example, large overdoses of acetaminophen saturate glutathione mechanisms of metabolism, resulting in hepatotoxicity.[40]

When the pharmacokinetic parameters of an overdosed drug are altered, serial plasma concentration measurements can better define the absorption, distribution, and clearance phases of the ingested substance. Pharmacokinetic parameters that have been derived from therapeutic doses should not be used to predict whether absorption is complete or to predict the expected duration of intoxication caused by large overdoses.[34,41,42]

DECONTAMINATION

After the airway and the cardiopulmonary system are supported, efforts should be directed toward removing the toxic substance from the patient (i.e., decontamination).[25,43] Decontamination presumes that both the dose and the duration of toxin exposure are important in determining the extent of toxicity and that prevention of continued exposure will decrease toxicity.[32–34,43] This intuitive concept is clearly relevant to ocular, dermal, and respiratory exposures, when local tissue damage is the primary problem. Respiratory decontamination involves removing the patient from the toxic environment and providing fresh air or oxygen to the patient. Decontamination of skin and eyes involves flushing the affected area with large volumes of water or saline to physically remove the toxic substance from the surface.[25,26]

GASTROINTESTINAL DECONTAMINATION

Because most poisonings and overdoses result from oral ingestions, measures to decrease or prevent continued GI absorption have commonly been used to limit the extent of exposure.[25,26,40] GI decontamination should be considered if the ingestion is large enough to produce potentially significant toxicity, or if the potential severity of the ingestion is unknown and the time since ingestion is less than1 hour. The following methods have historically been used: (a) evacuation of gastric contents by emesis or gastric lavage, (b) administration of activated charcoal as an adsorbent to bind the toxic substance remaining in the GI tract, (c) use of cathartics or whole bowel irrigation (WBI) to increase the rectal elimination of unabsorbed drug, or (d) a combination of any of these methods.[44–49]

ONLINE CONTENT

For a PowerPoint presentation about GI decontamination, go to http://thepoint.lww.com/AT10e.

The efficacy of GI decontamination varies, depending on when the process is initiated relative to the time of ingestion, dose ingested, and other factors. Furthermore, ipecac-induced emesis, gastric lavage, cathartics, and activated charcoal are not directly associated with improved patient outcomes.[44–49]

The most appropriate method for GI tract decontamination remains unclear because sound comparative data for different methods of GI decontamination are not available. Clinical research in healthy subjects, by necessity, must use nontoxic doses of drugs. Studies using nontoxic doses are not applicable to the overdose situation because alterations in GI absorption can occur with large doses. In addition, low-dose studies generally rely on pharmacokinetic end points such as peak plasma concentrations, area under the plasma concentration–time curve, or quantity of drug recovered from the urine.[44,45,47–49] In contrast, clinical studies of GI decontamination methods in patients who have ingested toxic doses of a substance use clinical outcomes or a directional change in serum drug concentrations.[44,45,48,49] These latter trials are not standardized with respect to the dose ingested or to the time interval between drug ingestion and GI decontamination.[44–49]

Ipecac-Induced Emesis and Gastric Lavage

Ipecac-induced emesis and gastric lavage primarily remove substances from the stomach. Their efficacy is affected significantly by the time the ingested substance remains in the stomach. Gastric lavage and ipecac-induced emesis are most effective when implemented before the substance moves past the stomach into the intestine (usually within 1 hour).[44,45]

The commonly used adult gastric lavage tube (36F) has an internal diameter too small to allow recovery of large tablet or capsule fragments. An even smaller diameter lavage tube is used for children.[45] Gastric lavage may be useful only if large amounts of a liquid substance were ingested and the patient arrived within 1 hour of the ingestion.[45] However, patients usually arrive in the ED more than an hour after ingestion, when absorption of the toxin has most likely already occurred. As a result, the efficacy of these procedures in overdose situations is minimal, and no studies have confirmed that use of gastric lavage or ipecac-induced emesis improves the outcome of the patient.[44,45,50] For these reasons, ipecac is no longer used, and gastric lavage is used only in rare, specific situations.

Activated Charcoal

In 1963, a review article concluded that activated charcoal was the most valuable agent available for the treatment of poisoning.[51]

This conclusion was based only on studies in fasting patients who had nontoxic exposures. Nevertheless, data from those studies were extrapolated to poisoned patients. Since then, activated charcoal has become the preferred method of GI decontamination for the treatment of toxic ingestions.[25,43,51–53]

The goal of therapy is to decrease the absorption of the substance and reduce or prevent systemic toxicity.[46] Unfortunately, there are no satisfactorily designed clinical studies assessing benefit from the use of activated charcoal to guide the use of this therapy. There is also no evidence that the administration of activated charcoal improves clinical outcomes.[46]

The use of activated charcoal at a dose of 1 g/kg should be considered when the patient has ingested a toxic substance that is known to be absorbed by activated charcoal within 1 hour of the ingestion. The potential for benefit is unknown if the activated charcoal is given more than 1 hour after ingestion.[46] It should be noted that iron and lithium are not absorbed by activated charcoal. Other forms of GI decontamination must be used to remove those substances from the GI tract.[46]

Generally the use of activated charcoal is safe. Although there are relatively few reports of adverse effects from the use of activated charcoal, there are numerous reports of complications, usually involving aspiration. It is essential that the patient has an intact or protected airway (intubation) before activated charcoal is administered, especially in drowsy patients or patients who may rapidly become obtunded.[46]

ONLINE CONTENT

To see activated charcoal in a lung x-ray, go to http://thepoint.lww.com/AT10e.

Vomiting with aspiration of activated charcoal occurs in about 5% of patients who receive activated charcoal.[46,53–55] The resulting pulmonary problems can be caused by aspiration of acidic stomach contents or the charcoal. Decreased oxygenation can occur immediately, or pulmonary effects can occur later.[55–59] Adult respiratory distress syndrome has resulted after the unintentional instillation of charcoal into the lung.[55] Aspiration of charcoal can result in chronic lung disease or fatalities, whereas the toxic exposure, for which the charcoal was administered, is often not lethal or even serious.[56,60]

Cathartics

Historically, sorbitol (a cathartic) was often administered with activated charcoal to enhance passage of the charcoal-substance complex through the GI tract. However, decreased transit time through the bowel has not been proven to decrease absorption as drug absorption does not take place in the large bowel.[47] Sorbitol is also associated with vomiting and aspiration.[47] Hypernatremia can also develop subsequent to the administration of repeat doses of activated charcoal with sorbitol.[61,62] Currently, most EDs use aqueous activated charcoal mixtures rather than charcoal–sorbitol combinations. Because cathartics are not effective in reducing drug absorption or increasing patient outcome, their use is no longer advised.[47]

Whole Bowel Irrigation

Whole bowel irrigation with a polyethylene glycol–balanced electrolyte solution (e.g., Colyte, GoLYTELY) can successfully remove substances from the entire GI tract in a period of several hours. WBI is effective with ingestions of sustained-release dosage forms, as well as substances that form bezoars (concretions of tablets or capsules), such as ferrous sulfate or phenytoin.[26,48,63] WBI is also indicated when the toxic agent is not adsorbed by activated charcoal (e.g., body-packer packets, lithium, iron, potassium).[25,26,48,63] This method of GI decontamination takes much longer to complete and is associated with poor patient compliance because large volumes of fluid (2 L/hour for adults until the effluent is clear) need to be ingested to be effective.[63] A nasogastric (NG) tube can be inserted, and the WBI fluid can be administered via NG tube so that lack of patient compliance is no longer a factor.[48]

ANTIDOTES AND SPECIFIC TREATMENTS

An antidote is a drug that neutralizes or reverses the toxicity of another substance. Some antidotes can displace a drug from receptor sites (e.g., naloxone for opioids, flumazenil for benzodiazepines), and some can inhibit the formation of toxic metabolites (e.g., *N*-acetylcysteine [NAC] for acetaminophen, fomepizole for methanol).[26,64,65] Some treatments are highly effective for the management of individual drug overdoses but do not meet the definition of an antidote. For example, sodium bicarbonate is used to treat the cardiotoxicity arising from tricyclic antidepressant (TCA) overdoses, and benzodiazepines are used to treat CNS toxicity associated with cocaine and amphetamine overdoses.[26,66–68] However, it is important to note that for antidotes to be effective, they must be readily available at the health care facility in adequate doses to treat the patient in a timely manner.[69]

ENHANCING SYSTEMIC CLEARANCE

Hemodialysis and manipulation of urine pH can enhance the clearance of substances. Hemodialysis can successfully treat some specific intoxications (e.g., methanol, ethylene glycol, aspirin, theophylline, lithium). Hemodialysis can also be used in patients with severe acid–base disturbances or renal dysfunction.[50] Alkalinization of the urine can enhance the elimination of drugs such as aspirin and phenobarbital.[70–72]

MONITORING OUTCOME

Selecting the appropriate parameters and length of time to monitor a patient who has been exposed to a toxic agent requires knowledge of toxic effects and the time course of the intoxication.[36,37] Most patients who are at risk for moderate or severe toxicity should be monitored in an intensive care unit (ICU) with careful assessments of cardiac, pulmonary, and CNS function.[73,74]

ASSESSMENT OF SALICYLATE INGESTION

Gathering a History

CASE 4-1

QUESTION 1: M.O., the mother of a 3-year-old child, states that her daughter, D.O., has ingested some aspirin tablets. What additional information should be obtained from or given to M.O. at this time?

Obtaining an initial assessment of the patient's status is essential. The caller's telephone number should be obtained in the event that the call is disconnected, initial recommendations need to be modified, or subsequent follow-up is needed. The health care provider should ask for patient-specific information with questions that are nonthreatening and nonjudgmental. The caller should be reassured that calling for help was the right thing to do.

Evaluating Clinical Presentation

CASE 4-1, QUESTION 2: On further questioning, M.O. states that D.O. is crying and complaining of a stomachache. Otherwise, the child appears to be acting normally. D.O. was found sitting on the bathroom floor with an aspirin bottle in her hand and some partially chewed tablets on the floor next to her. M.O. states that the child had the same look on her face that she has when she eats things that she does not like. M.O. reports that she can see white tablet material gummed on the child's teeth. The mother was gone no more than 5 minutes and had asked her 5- and 6-year-old sons to watch their sister. What additional information is needed to correctly assess the potential for toxicity in D.O.?

To determine the potential toxicity for an unintentional ingestion, it is important to assess the presence of symptoms and to identify the substance ingested. Inquiries should begin with open-ended questions to determine the facts that the caller is certain of versus what may have been assumed. The answers usually point to more specific information that is needed to accurately assess the exposure.[23]

D.O.'s symptoms presently are not life-threatening. Her behavior is consistent with being scared in response to the mother's anxiety. Once it has been established that the child does not need immediate life-saving treatment, the caller is generally more willing and able to answer additional questions.

M.O. already has provided information about the child's symptoms. More information is needed to determine the identity of the ingested substance, the time of ingestion, the brand of aspirin (to ensure that the product is not an aspirin-combination or even an aspirin-free formulation), the dosage form, the number of dosage units in a full container, and the number of remaining dosage units in the container. The parent should be careful to look for tablets under beds, rugs, or other locations out of sight (e.g., wastepaper baskets, toilets, pet food dishes, pockets). The dosage forms in the container should be identical in appearance, and the contents should be what are stated on the label. Information concerning the child's weight and health status, as well as whether the child is taking other medications, is also important. The child's weight is useful in determining the maximum milligram per kilogram dose of aspirin that was ingested.

When more than one child is present during an ingestion, the caller should be questioned as to whether other children also could have participated in the ingestion. In this situation, the children could have shared equally in the missing medication, all of the drug could have been fed to one child, or all of the drug could have been ingested by the oldest or most aggressive child. When it is unclear how much is missing among a group of children, each child should be evaluated and managed as if he or she may have ingested the total missing quantity.

Triage of Call

CASE 4-1, QUESTION 3: M.O. has now determined that a total of five tablets each containing 325 mg per tablet of aspirin are missing from the bottle. Because M.O. recalls having taken two aspirin tablets from this bottle, it is not likely that her daughter took more than three tablets. M.O. states that D.O. weighs 36 pounds. What treatment is needed for this child?

The maximal dose of aspirin ingested by this child is likely to be much less than the minimal dose required to cause significant symptoms based on her weight for her age (i.e., 36 pounds or approximately 16 kg). A dose of 150 mg/kg of aspirin is the smallest dose at which treatment or assessment at a health care facility is necessary.[72,75] D.O. is likely to have ingested a maximum of 975 mg of aspirin (i.e., three 325-mg tablets), which is about 60 mg/kg (975 mg divided by 16 kg). If this child is healthy, takes no medications, and is not allergic to aspirin, the child does not require any treatment. With this history of ingestion, the only adverse effect that might occur is some mild nausea. Providing information to the mother that her child had not ingested a toxic or dangerous amount will be reassuring.

For many years, aspirin was the most common cause of unintentional poisoning and poisoning deaths among children.[75–77] However, safety closure packaging and reduction of the total aspirin content in a full bottle of children's aspirin to approximately 3 g has steadily reduced the frequency of pediatric aspirin poisoning and deaths.[76–78] Although acute aspirin poisoning remains a problem, the largest percentage of life-threatening intoxications now results from therapeutic overdose.[72] Therapeutic overdoses occur when a dose is given too frequently, when both parents unknowingly dose the child with the drug, or when too large a dose is given. Therapeutic overdoses are especially problematic when excessive doses are given for a prolonged period and the drug is able to accumulate.[72]

Outcome for M.O.

Follow-up telephone consultation on toxic ingestions is important to identify children who unexpectedly develop symptoms that might need to be treated. A telephone call to M.O. 6 to 24 hours after her initial call would be appropriate to follow up on the child. On a call back to M.O., the parent stated that she gave D.O. lunch at the appropriate time. D.O. then watched cartoons, took her usual nap, and remained asymptomatic.

Acute and Chronic Salicylism

SIGNS AND SYMPTOMS

CASE 4-2

QUESTION 1: V.K., a 65-year-old, 55-kg woman with a history of chronic headaches, has taken 10 to 12 aspirin tablets daily for several months. On the evening of admission, she became lethargic, disoriented, and combative. Additional history revealed that she ingested up to 100 aspirin tablets on the morning of admission (about 10 hours earlier) in a suicide attempt. She complained of ringing in her ears, nausea, and three episodes of vomiting. Vital signs were BP 140/90 mm Hg, pulse 110 beats/minute, respirations 36 breaths/minute, and temperature 102.5°F. V.K.'s laboratory data obtained on admission were as follows:

Serum sodium (Na), 148 mEq/L
Potassium (K), 2.8 mEq/L
Chloride (Cl), 105 mEq/L
Bicarbonate, 10 mEq/L
Glucose, 60 mg/dL
Blood urea nitrogen (BUN), 35 mg/dL
Creatinine, 2.2 mg/dL

Arterial blood gas (ABG) values (room air) were as follows: pH, 7.25; P_{CO_2}, 20 mm Hg; and P_{O_2}, 95 mm Hg. A serum salicylate concentration measured approximately 12 hours after the acute ingestion was 88 mg/dL. Her hemoglobin was 9.6 g/dL with a hematocrit of 28.9% and a prothrombin time (PT) of 16.4 seconds. Is V.K. at high risk because of her ingestion?

The symptoms and severity of salicylate intoxication depend on the dose consumed; the patient's age; and whether the ingestion was acute, chronic, or a combination of the two.[77,79,80] This case illustrates an acute ingestion in someone who has also chronically ingested aspirin. Acute ingestion of 150 to 300 mg/kg of aspirin is likely to produce mild to moderate intoxication, greater than 300 mg/kg indicates severe poisoning, and greater than 500 mg/kg is potentially lethal.[72,75] V.K., who ingested approximately 600 mg/kg, has taken a potentially lethal dose. Chronic salicylate intoxication is usually associated with ingestion of greater than 100 mg/kg/day for more than 2 days.[72,75] V.K. has been taking 70 mg/kg/day for her headaches in addition to her acute ingestion. V.K. demonstrates many of the findings typical of severe acute salicylism (see Pathophysiology of Salicylate Intoxication and Assessment of Toxicity sections). V.K.'s prognosis is potentially poor because she is elderly and has taken a potentially lethal overdose of aspirin.

Pathophysiology of Salicylate Intoxication

CASE 4-2, QUESTION 2: Describe the pathophysiology and clinical features of acute and chronic salicylism.

Toxicity from salicylate exposure results in direct irritation of the GI tract, direct stimulation of the CNS respiratory center, stimulation of the metabolic rate, lipid and carbohydrate metabolism disturbances, and interference with hemostasis.[72,75,77,79,80] Toxic doses of salicylate directly stimulate the medullary respiratory center leading to nausea, vomiting, tinnitus, delirium, tachypnea, seizures, and coma, and influence several key metabolic pathways.[72,77–81] Direct stimulation of the respiratory drive increases the rate and depth of ventilation, which can result in primary respiratory alkalosis. The respiratory alkalosis causes increased renal excretion of bicarbonate, resulting in decreased buffering capacity. The patient usually presents with a partially compensated respiratory alkalosis.[72,78,79,81] Hypokalemia can result from increased GI and renal losses of potassium, as well as from systemic alkalosis.[72,79,80]

Although marked metabolic and neurologic abnormalities are most commonly observed in young children with advanced salicylate intoxication, adolescents or adults acutely poisoned with a large dose of salicylates can exhibit these symptoms as well.[72,78,79] Acute salicylism in a young child often takes a more severe course than that typically seen in adults. After acute ingestion, children quickly pass through the phase of pure respiratory alkalosis. Renal bicarbonate loss secondary to respiratory alkalosis reduces the buffering capacity more profoundly in a child and facilitates the development of metabolic acidosis.[72,77,79,81]

Salicylates have toxic effects on several biochemical pathways that contribute to metabolic acidosis and other symptoms.[72,79–81] Mitochondrial oxidative phosphorylation is uncoupled and results in an impaired ability to generate high-energy phosphates, increased oxygen use and carbon dioxide production, increased heat production and hyperpyrexia, increased tissue glycolysis, and increased peripheral demand for glucose. Salicylates also inhibit key dehydrogenase enzymes within the Krebs cycle, resulting in increased levels of pyruvate and lactate. The increased demand for peripheral glucose causes increased glycogenolysis, gluconeogenesis, lipolysis, and free fatty acid metabolism. The latter results in enhanced formation of keto acids and ketoacidosis.[77,81]

The patient may become severely volume depleted through several mechanisms.[72,79,81] Hyperthermia and hyperventilation produce increased insensible water loss, vomiting may promote GI fluid losses, and the solute load caused by altered glucose metabolism results in an osmotic diuresis. Depending on the patient's acid–base balance and net fluid and electrolyte intake and output, serum sodium and potassium concentrations may be normal, elevated, or decreased. Hypernatremia and hypokalemia are most common.[77,79]

Blood glucose concentration is usually normal or slightly elevated, although hypoglycemia may accompany chronic salicylism (e.g., as illustrated by V.K.) or occur late in acute intoxication. CNS glucose levels can be markedly reduced in the presence of normal blood glucose concentrations because increased CNS glucose utilization to generate high-energy phosphate exceeds the rate at which glucose can be supplied.[72,77,79,81]

Other manifestations of severe acute salicylism include a variety of neurologic signs and symptoms: disorientation, irritability, hallucinations, lethargy, stupor, coma, and seizures.[73,77] Hyperthermia may be marked and can result in the inappropriate administration of aspirin as an antipyretic. Coagulopathy can occur because of impaired platelet function, hypoprothrombinemia, reduced factor VII production, and increased capillary fragility, especially when aspirin is taken chronically.[79–81] Pulmonary edema and acute renal failure also can occur, but the former occurs more commonly after chronic intoxication.[79,81,82]

Chronic salicylism symptoms are similar to acute intoxications. However, patients with chronic exposures may have fewer GI symptoms but generally appear more ill and have more CNS symptoms.[75,83] In both adults and children, the principal signs of chronic salicylism are a partially compensated metabolic acidosis, increased anion gap, ketosis, dehydration, electrolyte loss, hyperventilation, tremors, agitation, confusion, stupor, memory deficits, renal failure, and seizures.[77,79,80,84] The severity of CNS manifestations is related to the cerebrospinal fluid (CSF) salicylate concentration.[78,79] CSF concentrations may increase in the presence of systemic acidosis because a greater fraction of salicylate is not ionized and can cross the blood–brain barrier. Therefore, metabolic acidosis is especially dangerous in a salicylate-intoxicated patient.[77,79]

Unless the history of salicylate intake is specifically sought, the problem may not be immediately apparent, especially in the elderly in whom such findings are likely to be attributed to other causes (e.g., encephalitis, meningitis, diabetic ketoacidosis, myocardial infarction).[27,79,83] Delay in diagnosis has been associated with increased mortality.[27,72,79,83] Unfortunately, plasma salicylate concentrations do not correlate well with the degree of poisoning in chronically intoxicated patients. It is more important to treat the patient according to the clinical status rather than his or her salicylate concentration.[72] Death in patients with salicylism, whether acute or chronic, results from CNS or cardiac dysfunction, or pulmonary edema.[77,79,83]

ASSESSMENT OF TOXICITY

CASE 4-2, QUESTION 3: What signs, symptoms, and laboratory values in V.K. are consistent with salicylate intoxication?

V.K. demonstrates many of the findings typical of severe acute salicylism. Hyperventilation has resulted from the direct respiratory stimulant effects of salicylate and as compensation for her metabolic acidosis (Pco_2, 20 mm Hg; pH, 7.25; serum bicarbonate, 10 mEq/L; respiratory rate, 36 breaths/minute). Hypokalemia (2.8 mEq/L) in the presence of metabolic acidosis represents severe potassium depletion because of increased renal and possibly GI losses. Hyperpyrexia caused by salicylate is present in V.K., although an infectious cause must also be considered. Her neurologic symptoms of lethargy, disorientation, and combativeness, as well as tinnitus, nausea, and vomiting, are commonly seen in severe salicylate intoxication. In addition, being elderly and taking a lethal amount of aspirin bodes ill for this patient's outcome.

LABORATORY EVALUATION

CASE 4-2, QUESTION 4: What objective evaluations should be assessed in a patient with presumed salicylate intoxication?

V.K.'s workup illustrates a thorough initial patient evaluation. Laboratory evaluation should include ABG values, serum electrolytes, BUN, serum creatinine, blood glucose, and a complete blood cell count.[77,79,80] Urine should be tested for specific gravity and pH.[77] In symptomatic patients, a PT or international normalized ratio (INR) and partial thromboplastin times are useful to assess the presence of salicylate-induced coagulopathy. Vitals signs should be monitored for an increased respiratory rate and hyperpyrexia.[78,79] Physical examination should include an evaluation of chest radiograph, cardiopulmonary and neurologic function, and measurement of urine output.[79]

A salicylate blood concentration should be obtained 6 hours after an acute ingestion at a known time, immediately and 6 hours after an acute ingestion at an unknown time, and immediately and every 2 to 6 hours in symptomatic patients.[27,68,77,79,85] Serum salicylate concentrations should be reassessed every 4 to 6 hours to verify that the original concentration represented a peak level and that the salicylate level is decreasing rather than increasing.[27,72,77,80,82] Obtaining the units of measurement on salicylate serum concentrations is essential because different laboratories report concentrations in different units (e.g., mg/dL, mcg/mL, mmol/L). An incorrect interpretation of the salicylate unit of measurement can result in overestimates or underestimates of the severity.[27]

Historically, the Done nomogram was used to determine the degree of toxicity from a known single acute salicylate ingestion by plotting the serum salicylate concentration by time since the ingestion.[86] However, clinical symptoms and laboratory findings are more useful in identifying the degree of acute intoxication, assessing patient prognosis, and guiding therapy.[85] In case of chronic ingestions, the nomogram is not useful, and other parameters such as acid–base and electrolyte balance should be used to determine severity of the case.[72,77]

The Done nomogram is also not useful in certain situations such as ingestion of enteric-coated or sustained-release salicylate products, when the time of ingestion is unknown, or when the patient is acidemic or has renal failure.[77,79,80,85–87] The nomogram is also less useful when salicylate serum concentrations are measured more than 12 hours after ingestion. Serum concentrations obtained less than 6 hours after ingestion in acute ingestion situations are also difficult to interpret because the drug level has not yet peaked and can result in an underestimation of the eventual degree of intoxication.[72,77,84,87] Salicylate concentrations can continue to rise for approximately 24 hours if a large amount has been taken or if enteric-coated tablets have been ingested. Enteric-coated tablets can clump together, forming a bezoar that slowly releases drug into the gut.[79,85] Because of these difficulties in interpreting salicylate concentrations, the Done nomogram is no longer used.[27]

MANAGEMENT

CASE 4-2, QUESTION 5: What would be a reasonable management plan for V.K.?

Management of salicylate intoxication depends on the degree of acid–base and electrolyte disturbances.[72,77,79] Activated charcoal is not indicated for V.K. because the ingestion occurred approximately 10 hours ago and she has a somewhat altered mental status.[46] The risk of aspiration is greater than the value of possibly adsorbing any remaining aspirin from the GI tract. In addition, V.K. already has symptoms of salicylate poisoning, indicating that the aspirin has already been absorbed. Others might argue that if she ingested 100 tablets, some of the drug may still be present in the GI tract and giving activated charcoal late may bind some of the drug still present.

V.K.'s hypokalemia, acidosis, and hypoglycemia must be corrected, and is probably best accomplished through the administration of intravenous (IV) hypotonic saline–dextrose solutions combined with potassium supplementation. This solution is administered at a rate that replaces the patient's deficits and keeps pace with continued losses.[72,77,79–81] Care should be taken to avoid overzealous fluid therapy, which can predispose the patient to cerebral or pulmonary edema.[79,81] Administration of an IV dextrose bolus is also indicated because V.K. is hypoglycemic (60 mg/dL).[77,79,81]

SODIUM BICARBONATE

It is important to correct V.K.'s acidosis because acidosis will increase CSF salicylate concentrations.[78,79] Correction of acidosis can be accomplished by adding sodium bicarbonate to her IV fluids.[72,77–80] V.K.'s serum sodium and potassium concentrations should be monitored closely as adding potassium to IV fluids will mostly likely be required.[86] Providing adequate ventilation to prevent respiratory alkalosis is essential. With a respiratory rate of 36 breaths/minute, placing the patient on a ventilator to assist with breathing might be considered. However, forced mechanical ventilation can interfere with the patient's need to compensate to maintain the serum pH. Patients on ventilators can become severely acidotic, which can result in death because of an inability to compensate adequately.[77,88]

SEIZURES

Seizures are not evident in V.K. but can be encountered in cases of severe salicylate poisoning. Seizures generally carry a poor prognosis and are indicative of severe salicylate intoxication that requires hemodialysis.[77] Other treatable causes of seizures (e.g., marked alkalosis, hypoglycemia, hyponatremia) can be present in individuals such as V.K. and should be ruled out. If seizures occur, benzodiazepines are the drugs of choice for treatment.[77]

COAGULOPATHY AND HYPERTHERMIA

Coagulopathy generally responds to vitamin K_1, which should be given if the PT or INR is prolonged.[77] GI bleeding or other hemorrhage can occur but is not common.[77,79,80] Mild hyperthermia usually does not require therapy, but cooling fans and mist may be required for extremely elevated temperatures.[77,81]

PULMONARY EDEMA

Noncardiogenic pulmonary edema commonly occurs in salicylate intoxications, especially when the overdose is attributable to chronic ingestions.[77,79,82] Pulmonary edema is associated with a high incidence of neurologic symptoms in patients and can occur even without fluid overload.[79,82] Increased alveolar capillary membrane permeability, prostaglandin effects, and a metabolic interaction with platelets releasing membrane permeability substances are the primary mechanisms for the cause of pulmonary edema associated with salicylate overdose. Treatment is aimed at reducing salicylate levels via alkalinization or hemodialysis.[82]

ALKALINIZATION

CASE 4-2, QUESTION 6: What measures will enhance salicylate elimination? Which of these may be indicated in V.K.?

Alkalinization of the urine and hemodialysis can enhance the excretion of salicylate in overdose situations.[72,78] Hemodialysis is preferred because it can also correct fluid and electrolyte imbalances.[79,82,83] Sodium bicarbonate is recommended for alkalinization to increase the arterial pH with the goal of minimizing salicylate transport into the CNS.[78,79,81]

Although large doses of sodium bicarbonate can enhance the renal elimination of the weak acid and shorten its half-life, this treatment does not favorably influence the morbidity or mortality of patients with salicylism. Alkalinization with forced fluid diuresis can also place the patient at risk for sodium and fluid retention, as well as pulmonary edema if too much fluid is given too quickly.[77,79,80,82] Whether the urine can be adequately alkalinized (pH >7) in severely intoxicated pediatric patients has been questioned because of the large acid load that is excreted.[72,77,78] Nevertheless, urine alkalinization with sodium bicarbonate should be attempted in severely salicylate-intoxicated adult patients such as V.K.

Potassium replacement in patients receiving alkalinization is essential.[77,79,81] These patients may require large amounts of potassium supplementation as a result of renal wasting of potassium. The risk for pulmonary edema can be minimized if this is done without forcing fluids.[77,79–81]

Hemodialysis should be considered in patients who show progression of severe salicylate intoxication and seizure activity, renal failure, or plasma salicylate concentrations in the potentially fatal range.[72,79,80,82,84] Patients with a chronic exposure, acidosis, or CNS symptoms and those who are elderly or ill are high-risk patients and should be considered for early dialysis.[79,84] Because V.K. has many of the risk factors, she is a candidate for emergent hemodialysis.

CLINICAL OUTCOME OF PATIENT V.K.

A repeat salicylate level 6 hours later (18 hours after ingestion) had increased to 93 mg/dL. Her chemistry panel revealed serum sodium, 144 mEq/L; potassium, 2.1 mEq/L; chloride, 100 mEq/L; bicarbonate, 9 mEq/L; glucose, 78 mg/dL; creatinine, 4.8 mg/dL; and BUN, 42 mg/dL. Her hemoglobin was now 8.5 g/dL with a hematocrit of 23% and a PT of 16.6 seconds. V.K.'s pH on blood gases remained in the 7.2 to 7.3 range. Urinary alkalinization was attempted with a high-dose IV sodium bicarbonate infusion in an attempt to reach a urine pH of 7.5. However, her urine pH never increased above pH 5.6. V.K. became fluid overloaded and exhibited dyspnea. She was placed on a ventilator with worsening of her symptoms. A chest radiograph showed pulmonary edema. V.K. became confused and agitated, pulling at her IV lines and trying to get out of bed. Nephrology was consulted to provide emergent hemodialysis to correct the acidosis, electrolyte abnormalities, and fluid overload. As the catheter was being placed, the patient had a tonic-clonic seizure. Lorazepam 2 mg IV was administered and the seizure stopped. At this time, the patient was unresponsive. The NG tube revealed the presence of copious amounts of bright red blood. She was rushed to surgery for an emergency laparotomy. On the way to the operating room, she had another seizure, went into respiratory arrest, coded, and could not be resuscitated.

ASSESSMENT OF IRON INGESTION

Gathering History and Communications

CASE 4-3

QUESTION 1: The grandmother of R.F., a 20-month-old boy, calls the ED because her grandson is vomiting and appears to have been playing with some green tablets. The child was left alone in his room for about 15 minutes to take a nap. Why might the consultation with this grandmother be expected to be more difficult than the consultation in Case 4-1, Question 1?

Phone calls to a health care provider, a health care facility, or a poison control center from individuals other than the parent are usually more difficult to manage as the caller may not be able to provide all patient-specific information needed (e.g., patient weight, chronic medications) to accurately assess the drug ingestion. Additional information is often needed from a parent. Furthermore, nonparent callers tend to be more upset about an unintentional ingestion and may have more difficulty than a parent in taking decisive action.

Triage of Call

CASE 4-3, QUESTION 2: Despite additional questioning, R.F.'s grandmother cannot identify the tablets and cannot find any labeling or empty medicine containers that could help in the tablet identification. R.F. is still vomiting, and some of the vomitus is green-colored like the tablets. There are three children in the household and two adults who take medications for various chronic illnesses. According to the grandmother, R.F. is healthy, and no one else in the household currently has the "flu" or other GI illness. The child's mother gave birth 3 weeks ago and is now at her obstetrician's office for a postnatal visit. What recommendations could be provided to R.F.'s grandmother at this time?

With this history, the practitioner should consider whether the information presented by R.F.'s grandmother is consistent with a drug ingestion and whether this incident is likely to be associated with a significant adverse outcome. Most 2-year-old children experience limited toxicity with unintentional drug ingestions because only a relatively small amount of substance is usually ingested.[6,7] Nevertheless, some substances (e.g., methanol, ethylene glycol, nicotine, caustic substances, camphor, chloroquine, clonidine, diphenoxylate-atropine, theophylline, oral hypoglycemic agents, calcium-channel blockers, TCAs) can produce significant toxicity when only small amounts are ingested.[7,89,90]

Although the history of drug ingestion in R.F. is somewhat vague, the description of a green tablet, the vomiting of green material, and the recent pregnancy of his mother suggest possible ingestion of prenatal iron tablets. Because this exposure would be categorized as an unknown toxicity with a realistic potential for severe toxicity if iron tablets were ingested, R.F. should be brought to the ED for evaluation. Depending on the distance to the hospital and the anxiety level of the grandmother, the practitioner might want to instruct the grandmother to call for emergency medical services transportation. She should be instructed to take the green tablets to the ED along with the child so the tablets can be identified. Other medications that are in the house should also be taken to the ED, and the mother should be contacted at the obstetrician's office.

Substance Identification

CASE 4-3, QUESTION 3: R.F.'s mother has been contacted and has confirmed that the only green tablets in the house are her prenatal iron supplements. She is close to the

hospital and will await the arrival of her son. R.F. arrived 20 minutes later along with one green tablet and an empty prescription container that was found by his older brother. R.F. is still vomiting but is awake and alert with a heart rate of 125 beats/minute, a respiratory rate of 28 breaths/minute, a temperature of 99.1°F, and pulse oximetry of 99%. How can the maximal potential severity of this ingestion be estimated at this time?

R.F.'s vital signs, when corrected for age, are normal. Attention should now focus on identifying the ingested substance and the maximal potential severity of the ingestion. Although this case involves an unknown ingestion, with a possibility of being a severe iron intoxication, the identity of the tablets still has not been verified. Therefore, R.F. must be carefully assessed, and the ingestion history reaffirmed.

All solid dosage prescription drugs are required by the US Food and Drug Administration (FDA) to have identification markings. Reference books (e.g., *Facts and Comparisons,*[91] *Physicians' Desk Reference*),[92] computerized databases (e.g., IDENTIDEX),[93] and the product manufacturers can assist in identifying solid dosage forms. Websites such as **http://www.pharmer.org**[94] and **http://www.drugs.com**[95] can also be useful in obtaining drug identification information.

The imprint code markings on the green tablet brought to the ED with R.F., the empty medication container, and the mother's assistance should be sufficient to correctly identify the tablet. The identification of this green tablet will most likely establish the toxicity potential because most childhood ingestions usually involve only one substance. Once the tablet has been identified, the maximal number of tablets ingested should be estimated.

The label on the empty medication container can provide information on the identity and number of tablets dispensed. The date the prescription was obtained, the number of estimated doses taken, and the number currently remaining in the medication container can be used to approximate the maximal number of tablets ingested.

R.F.'s vital signs and symptoms should be monitored at frequent intervals to evaluate whether his clinical status is consistent with expectations based on the suspected ingestion. Nausea, vomiting, diarrhea, and abdominal pain are commonly encountered early in the course of iron intoxication.[96–101] The absence of symptoms, however, should not be interpreted as an indication that a poisoning has not occurred, especially if the patient is being evaluated within a short time after the presumed ingestion.[96,98–101]

Evaluating Severity of Toxicity

CASE 4-3, QUESTION 4: R.F. weighs 22 pounds, appears to be in no apparent distress, and has stopped vomiting. About 30 mL of dark-colored vomitus was recovered, but no tablets are seen, and testing demonstrates that no blood is present in the vomitus. A maximum of 11 tablets was ingested based on the bottle label and the mother's recall. What degree of toxicity should be expected in R.F.?

The potential severity of ingestion can be estimated for commonly ingested drugs such as acetaminophen,[102] salicylates,[75] iron,[96] and TCAs[103] because of well-established dose–toxicity relationships. Acute elemental iron ingestions of less than 20 mg/kg are usually nontoxic, doses of 20 to 60 mg/kg result in mild to moderate toxicity, and doses of more than 60 mg/kg are severe and potentially fatal.[97,99,101]

The label on the prescription medication container, as well as independent verification of the tablet by R.F.'s mother and the tablet imprint, indicates that each tablet contained 300 mg of ferrous sulfate in an enteric-coated formulation. Because the dose–toxicity relationship of iron is based on the amount of elemental iron ingested, knowledge of the specific iron salt is important in calculating the ingested dose. Ferrous sulfate contains 20% elemental iron, ferrous gluconate contains 12%, and ferrous fumarate contains 33%.[96,97,99,100] Therefore, each 300-mg ferrous sulfate tablet contains 60 mg of elemental iron. R.F. ingested a maximum of 11 enteric-coated ferrous sulfate 300-mg tablets and he weighs 22 pounds (10 kg). His ingestion of approximately 66 mg/kg (60 mg per tablet × 11 tablets = 660 mg total divided by 10-kg patient weight) of iron places him at risk of severe toxicity. Although R.F.'s only symptom is vomiting at this time, absorption could be delayed because he ingested an enteric-coated formulation.

Abdominal Radiographs

CASE 4-3, QUESTION 5: R.F. is expected to experience potentially severe toxicity from his ingestion of iron. Why would an abdominal radiograph be useful to verify the number of iron tablets that were actually ingested?

Radio-opaque substances (e.g., iron, enteric-coated tablets, chloral hydrate, phenothiazines, heavy metals), theoretically, can be visualized in the GI tract by an abdominal radiograph.[104] The ability of a radiograph to demonstrate the presence of a radiodense substance depends on the dosage form, concentration, and molecular weight of the substance. The intact dosage form can often be detected if the tablet has not already disintegrated or dissolved.[104]

ONLINE CONTENT

To see X-rays of iron in the GI tract, go to http://thepoint.lww.com/AT10e.

Less than one-third of pediatric abdominal radiographs show positive evidence of tablets or granules after iron poisoning.[105] Children are more likely than adults to chew tablets rather than swallow them whole, and false-negative results can occur even when whole tablets have not already started to disintegrate. If the tablets were chewed, an abdominal radiograph to verify the number of ingested iron tablets is not likely to be useful. However, an abdominal radiograph after the completion of GI decontamination can help assess whether additional decontamination is needed.[104]

Gastrointestinal Decontamination

CASE 4-3, QUESTION 6: Why would gastric lavage or activated charcoal not be indicated for the management of R.F.'s iron ingestion?

When selecting a method of GI decontamination, consider the substance ingested, maximal potential toxicity expected from the drug dosage form, potential time course of toxicity, time elapsed between ingestion and the initiation of treatment, symptoms, and physical examination findings. Decontamination with activated charcoal is not indicated because R.F. has ingested iron tablets, which are not adsorbed by activated charcoal.[53,96,104] Gastric lavage would also not be effective because the removal of large undissolved iron tablets from the stomach is limited by the small internal diameter of the gastric lavage tube, especially in pediatric patients.[104,105]

Whole Bowel Irrigation

CASE 4-3, QUESTION 7: What other method of GI decontamination should be considered for R.F.?

Whole bowel irrigation with a polyethylene glycol electrolyte solution can be considered in this case. WBI fluid can be administered orally or infused by NG tube at a rate of 1.5 to 2 L/hour for adults and at a rate of 500 mL/hour for children.[63,106] Although the large volume of fluid to be ingested during a period of several hours and the frequent association of nausea and vomiting often result in poor patient compliance, R.F. is hospitalized and the fluid can be infused by NG tube. WBI should be continued until the rectal effluent is clear, which may take many hours.[63,106,107]

MONITORING EFFECTIVENESS OF TREATMENT

CASE 4-3, QUESTION 8: How should the effectiveness of GI decontamination be assessed in the ED?

The simplest method of assessing GI decontamination is to visually inspect the return fluid from the WBI for tablets or tablet fragments. Increasing serum iron concentrations, deteriorating clinical status, or evidence of radiodense tablets in the GI tract on abdominal radiograph would warrant more aggressive treatment.[97–99,105,107]

Serum Iron Concentrations

CASE 4-3, QUESTION 9: At this time, R.F. has no evidence of CNS or cardiovascular symptoms that can occur with toxic iron ingestions. He did have one large dark-colored diarrheal stool that tested negative for blood. A serum iron concentration, obtained about 3 hours after the ingestion, was 470 mcg/dL (normal, 60–160 mcg/dL). What conclusions as to severity or likely clinical outcome can be derived from this serum iron concentration?

The serum iron concentration provides an indication as to whether more aggressive therapy is needed.[101,105,108] The higher than normal serum iron concentration confirms the suspicion that R.F. has ingested iron tablets despite both his current lack of serious symptoms and the absence of tablet evidence in the rectal effluent or by abdominal radiograph.

The time course of absorption is probably the most difficult pharmacokinetic parameter to evaluate with toxic ingestions. For example, drug concentrations can continue to rise after an overdose despite GI decontamination.[98,100,101,108] This prolongation of absorption time is further complicated when sustained-release or enteric-coated dosage formulations have been ingested because the onset of symptoms is unpredictable.[99]

R.F.'s serum iron concentration of 470 mcg/dL suggests a serious ingestion because peak serum iron concentrations greater than 500 mcg/dL are usually predictive of significant toxicity.[98–101,105,108] This single serum iron concentration does not provide information as to whether the serum concentration is rising or declining or when the serum iron concentration will peak as a result of his iron ingestion.[109] Iron tablets may also clump together and form a bezoar. Bezoar formation can result in prolonged absorption and delay the onset of toxicity.[98,101] Samples for peak serum iron concentration should be obtained 4 to 6 hours after ingestion.[99–101,108] Although R.F.'s serum iron concentration was measured approximately 3 hours after ingestion, another serum iron measurement in 2 to 4 hours is needed because he ingested an enteric-coated formulation.

Blood Glucose, White Blood Cell Count, and Total Iron Binding Capacity

CASE 4-3, QUESTION 10: R.F. had WBI administered through the NG tube for 4 hours until the rectal effluent was clear. At this time, R.F. began to vomit numerous times and became drowsy and fussy. A second serum iron concentration was ordered (i.e., 6 hours after ingestion). What other laboratory tests could be helpful in assessing the potential toxicity of iron in R.F.?

Blood glucose concentrations and white blood cell counts usually are increased when serum iron concentrations are greater than 300 mcg/dL. A white blood cell count greater than 15,000/μL and a blood glucose concentration greater than 150 mg/dL within 6 hours of ingestion generally suggest a greater likelihood of severe iron intoxication.[98] These tests provide supplemental confirmation of iron intoxication and may be useful in medical facilities in which serum iron concentrations cannot be obtained. These laboratory tests are not routinely monitored in iron poisoning because of the poor sensitivity (about 50%).[99] Treatment should not be based on a white blood cell and glucose concentration alone.[98–100,105] If a patient with severe iron toxicity presents to a health care facility that cannot perform timely serum iron levels, either the blood iron sample must be sent to a laboratory that can do the testing quickly or the patient must be transferred to a health care facility that can do serum iron testing for patient monitoring.

It was once believed that if the serum iron concentration exceeded the total iron binding capacity concentration, it would indicate substantial iron toxicity. The correlation between the total iron binding capacity concentration and iron toxicity, however, has not held up, and the total iron binding capacity test is no longer used to monitor iron toxicity.[101]

Stages of Iron Toxicity

CASE 4-3, QUESTION 11: It is now 6 hours since R.F. ingested the iron tablets. His second serum iron concentration is not yet available. He continues to be fussy and drowsy but has missed his usual afternoon nap. He has several more episodes of vomiting. Why is R.F.'s relatively mild course at this time not particularly reassuring?

The time between the ingestion of an overdose of drugs and the development of severe toxicity can be delayed. It is unclear why there may be an asymptomatic period, but it may be secondary to delayed absorption of the ingested drug, the time required for the drug distribution, or the time needed to form a toxic metabolite. Consequently, R.F. may still exhibit further symptoms of severe toxicity. Four distinct stages of symptoms can be encountered with iron toxicity.[96–101]

STAGE I

Stage I symptoms usually occur within 6 hours of ingestion. During this time, nausea, vomiting, diarrhea, and abdominal pain are encountered and are probably secondary to the erosive effects of iron on the GI mucosa. The caustic effects of free iron can cause bleeding as evidenced by blood in the vomitus and stool.

In more severe intoxications, CNS and cardiovascular toxicity can be present during stage I.[98–101]

STAGE II

The second stage of iron toxicity has been suggested as a period of decreasing symptoms and an apparent improvement in the clinical condition. This stage can last for up to 12 to 24 hours after the ingestion and could be misinterpreted as resolving toxicity. This stage may represent the time needed for the absorbed iron to distribute throughout the body before systemic symptoms develop.[96] Alternatively, this stage might merely reflect patients who did not receive treatment early in the course of intoxication and appeared to be well before systemic effects developed. In most severe cases, stage II is not encountered and the patient's condition continues to progressively deteriorate.[98–101]

STAGE III

Stage III generally occurs 12 to 48 hours after iron ingestion and is characterized by CNS toxicity (e.g., lethargy, coma, seizures) and cardiovascular toxicity (e.g., hypotension, shock, pulmonary edema). Metabolic acidosis, hypoglycemia, hepatic necrosis, renal damage, and coagulopathy can be experienced at this stage.[98–101]

STAGE IV

The final stage is apparent 4 to 6 weeks after acute iron ingestion and consists of late-appearing GI tract sequelae that are secondary to the initial local toxicity. In this stage, prior tissue damage can progress to gastric scarring and strictures at the pylorus, resulting in permanent abnormalities of GI function.[98–101]

Patients can present to the health care facility in any stage of iron toxicity and can have a fatal outcome in any stage. Assigning a stage of toxicity should not be based on time since ingestion, but instead should be based on clinical symptoms.[100]

Deferoxamine Chelation

CASE 4-3, QUESTION 12: The clinical laboratory has reported that the second serum iron concentration that was obtained 6 hours after ingestion from R.F. has increased from 470 to 553 mcg/dL. The child has continued to vomit. R.F.'s mother states that the child looks "pale" to her. What criteria are most important in determining whether the antidote deferoxamine should be administered to R.F.?

Deferoxamine (Desferal) chelates iron by binding ferric ions in plasma to form the iron complex ferrioxamine.[99] Deferoxamine prevents iron toxicity at a cellular level by removing iron from mitochondria.[97] Unfortunately, deferoxamine is not a very effective antidote as a relatively small amount of iron is bound (approximately 9 mg of iron to 100 mg of deferoxamine).[109,110] The iron–deferoxamine complex primarily is excreted renally as ferrioxamine.[97,99,100] Renal elimination of the ferrioxamine usually results in a pinkish-orange urine, often described as "vin rose."[97,99,100] Deferoxamine therapy should be initiated when serum iron concentrations exceed 500 mcg/dL and when symptoms of iron toxicity (e.g., GI symptoms, hemorrhage, coma, shock, seizures) are present.[97–100] R.F. is experiencing symptoms, he presumably ingested up to 66 mg/kg of elemental iron, and iron absorption appears to be ongoing based on the increase in his serum iron concentration. Therefore, R.F. should be treated with deferoxamine.

DEFEROXAMINE DOSE

CASE 4-3, QUESTION 13: What dose of deferoxamine should be prescribed for R.F., and how should it be administered?

Deferoxamine is most effective when administered intravenously as a constant infusion owing to its short half-life (76 ± 10 minutes).[98,100,109] Clinically, a slow IV infusion is preferred instead of intramuscular administration because the IV dose can be better controlled, is less painful, and is better absorbed than an intramuscularly administered dose.[100–101] Deferoxamine at a dose of 15 mg/kg/hour is usually administered in a continuous IV infusion. However, doses up to 45 mg/kg/hour have been used in patients with severe iron poisoning.[98–101,109] Hypotension can result from administering IV boluses of deferoxamine too rapidly.[97,99,101,109,110] According to the manufacturer, the total deferoxamine dose should not exceed 6 g every 24 hours when administered to adults or children, but adverse effects have not been seen in patients who received more than 6 g every 24 hours.[100,110]

Deferoxamine should be initially administered to R.F. at a lower rate of about 8 mg/kg/hour, and his clinical status should be monitored closely. If the dose is tolerated, the rate can be increased every 5 minutes until the desired dose of 15 mg/kg/hour is achieved.[98]

MONITORING AND DISCONTINUATION

CASE 4-3, QUESTION 14: R.F. is admitted to the pediatric ICU 1 hour after the initiation of a deferoxamine infusion at 8 mg/kg/hour. How should deferoxamine therapy be monitored, and when should it be discontinued?

The rate of deferoxamine infusion should be increased if symptoms of severe iron toxicity develop, and the dosage should be decreased if adverse effects develop.[98,99,101,110] The infusion of deferoxamine should be continued until the serum iron concentration is less than 100 mcg/dL and symptoms of iron toxicity are no longer present.[110] Patients will require chelation therapy for about 1 to 2 days, depending on the severity of symptoms.[98–100] Chelation therapy that continues longer than necessary should be avoided because deferoxamine infusion for more than 24 hours has been associated with the development of acute respiratory distress syndrome.[98–100]

The urine color change to vin rose indicates ferrioxamine in the urine.[97,101] The disappearance of the vin rose color should not be used as a reliable marker of adequacy of deferoxamine therapy because not all patients experience vin rose urine.[97,101] There is also no correlation between amount of iron ingested, serum iron concentration, and the urine color change.[97]

Deferoxamine can interfere with some laboratory methods used to measure serum iron concentrations and cause falsely low values.[97,98,108,111] To monitor serum iron concentrations when deferoxamine has been started, using atomic absorptive spectroscopy is recommended.[110] When deferoxamine is initiated, the clinical laboratory should be contacted to clarify whether deferoxamine will interfere with their serum iron analysis.

Outcome of Patient R.F.

R.F. was admitted to the pediatric ICU overnight and treated with a constant infusion of deferoxamine at 15 mg/kg/hour for 13 hours. His GI symptoms were no longer apparent, he became more alert, and his vitals signs were stable. An analysis of a blood sample for free iron the next morning revealed a serum iron level of 67 mcg/dL. He was discharged home that afternoon.

ASSESSMENT OF CENTRAL NERVOUS SYSTEM DEPRESSANT VERSUS ANTIDEPRESSANT INGESTION

Validation of Ingestion

CASE 4-4

QUESTION 1: T.C., a 34-year-old unconscious woman, was found lying on the couch with a suicide note. The note stated that she had ingested 25 of her pills. On discovering T.C. unresponsive, T.C.'s 15-year-old daughter called paramedics. When the paramedics arrived, T.C.'s heart rate was 145 beats/minute, BP was 105/65 mm Hg, and respirations were 12 breaths/minute and shallow. T.C. was found in a pool of vomitus. T.C. responded only to painful stimuli. The paramedics immediately started an IV line after completing their assessment of her ABCs. Why should the drug overdose information from this suicidal patient be validated?

Assessing the accuracy of historical information in adult drug exposures is difficult, and many health care professionals question the validity of information, especially from suicidal patients.[25–28,30] The ingestion history could be inaccurate because the patient's altered mental status might prevent accurate recollection of what occurred. She may also try to intentionally mislead health care providers to minimize appropriate care. The supposition that the drug overdose history from a patient is unreliable is based on studies demonstrating poor correlation between stated drug ingestions and urine drug test results.[26–28,30,35,36,112] There are also numerous false-positive results that can be misleading because of drug interference.[113,114]

Urine drug screens generally detect all recent drug and substance use, rather than just an overdosed drug. Urine drug screen results, therefore, are not reliable indicators of acute exposures. Every effort should be made to validate the history with information from other sources. In suicidal patients, one should consider all drugs that may have been available to the patient, as well as the patient's presenting symptoms, laboratory tests, and information obtained from family members, police, paramedics, and other individuals who know the patient.[25–28,30]

Interventions by Protocol

CASE 4-4, QUESTION 2: In addition to managing the ABCs, what pharmacologic interventions should be authorized for the paramedics to administer to T.C. in addition to the initiation of an IV solution?

GLUCOSE AND THIAMINE

Emergency medical service personnel often have protocols directing them to treat patients who are unconscious from an unknown cause. These protocols generally include administration of glucose, thiamine, and naloxone.[26,30,64,115] If paramedics cannot measure a blood glucose concentration immediately, T.C. should be given 50 mL of 50% dextrose to treat possible hypoglycemia. The risks of hyperglycemia from this dose of glucose are negligible relative to the significant benefits if the patient is hypoglycemic. Thiamine should be administered concurrently with glucose because glucose can precipitate Wernicke-Korsakoff complex in thiamine-deficient patients[116] (see Chapter 87, Alcohol Use Disorders). Wernicke encephalopathy is a reversible neurologic disturbance consisting of generalized confusion, ataxia, and ophthalmoplegia. Korsakoff psychosis is believed to be irreversible and is associated with a more prolonged deficiency of thiamine.[116,117] This unconscious patient should also be evaluated for blood loss, sepsis, hypoxia, and evidence of head trauma.[25]

NALOXONE

The pure opioid antagonist, naloxone, is indicated for the treatment of respiratory depression induced by opioids,[115,118] but many emergency medical service protocols authorize paramedics to routinely administer naloxone to all patients with any decreased mental status.[118] Naloxone reportedly has reversed coma and acute respiratory depression in intoxicated patients who have no evidence of opioid use.[64,117] The response of these patients to naloxone might have been secondary to opioids that were not detected by the urine toxicology screens (e.g., oxycodone, methadone, fentanyl). Drug-induced CNS depression usually waxes and wanes, and reports of naloxone success in patients who have not used opioids could also have been the result of responses to needle sticks, movement, or other stimuli rather than a response to naloxone.

Administering naloxone to an opioid-addicted patient can precipitate withdrawal symptoms (e.g., agitation, combativeness, vomiting, diarrhea, lacrimation, rhinorrhea) that can further complicate the intoxication picture.[64] Small doses of naloxone should be administered initially to determine the patient's response to this medication. Violent and aggressive behavior can result when sudden increased consciousness is induced by naloxone.[30] This can complicate emergency care in an emergency transport vehicle and put caregivers and patients at risk for trauma.[64]

Initial Treatment

CASE 4-4, QUESTION 3: The paramedics arrive at the ED with T.C. 30 minutes after her daughter called them. T.C.'s heart rate in the ED is 148 beats/minute, BP is 90/55 mm Hg, and respirations have decreased from 12 breaths/minute, spontaneous and shallow, to 7 breaths/minute, with assisted ventilation from a bag-valve mask. T.C. remains unresponsive. The paramedics were unable to find any prescriptions or other medications in the house. The daughter believed that her mother was taking medication for depression, but she could not be more specific. The police will notify T.C.'s husband and try to obtain additional information about the ingested substance. What initial treatment should be provided for T.C. in the ED?

T.C. should be intubated and mechanically ventilated with 100% oxygen because of her shallow, slow respirations and the likelihood that vomitus could have been aspirated into her lungs. The BP taken by the paramedics was 105/65 mm Hg and now is 90/55 mm Hg. A bolus of IV fluid should be administered to T.C. to determine whether an increase in her intravascular fluid volume will increase her BP and improve her mental status.[25,43]

Antidotes

CASE 4-4, QUESTION 4: T.C.'s husband reports that T.C. is under the care of a psychiatrist for depression and two

prior suicide attempts. He does not know the identity of her medication, but attempts are underway to contact T.C.'s psychiatrist. What antidotes can be administered in the ED for diagnostic purposes? Should flumazenil (Romazicon) be administered?

Theoretically, antidotes such as naloxone, flumazenil, deferoxamine, and digoxin-specific antibody-FAB fragments could be administered in a hospitalized setting to identify an unknown toxin.[25,29,30,118–120] However, the cost and time required for administration, and increased risks from these antidotes, preclude their use for diagnostic purposes without some plausible suspicion of a specific drug ingestion. Although naloxone and flumazenil can reverse CNS depression caused by opioids and benzodiazepines, respectively, their use is not appropriate without historical, clinical, or toxicologic laboratory findings that suggest that one of these drugs is a cause of T.C.'s intoxication.[118,119]

Organ System Evaluations

CASE 4-4, QUESTION 5: How can the initial physical assessment, using an organ systems approach, help in identifying the drugs ingested by T.C.?

The patient's ABCs and CNS and cardiopulmonary functions should be assessed with special attention to clinical manifestations that suggest ingestion of a specific class of drugs.[30,43] T.C.'s history of depression suggests that antidepressants, antipsychotics, lithium, or benzodiazepines are candidates for ingestion in her case. An organ system evaluation will help determine whether these (or other) drugs might have been ingested. Nonprescription medications such as aspirin, acetaminophen, decongestants, and antihistamines, which are commonly available in most households, should also be considered because adult drug ingestions usually involve more than one drug.

CENTRAL NERVOUS SYSTEM FUNCTION

Changes in CNS function are probably the single most common finding associated with drug intoxication.[30] CNS depression or stimulation, seizures, delirium, hallucinations, coma, or any combination of these can be manifested in intoxicated patients. CNS changes can be the direct result of an ingested drug or may be additive to other underlying CNS processes or medical conditions.[120] Many drug overdoses can produce different clinical manifestations at various times during the intoxication, and different doses can produce different effects as well.[30,68]

Drugs with anticholinergic properties can produce disorientation, confusion, delirium, and visual hallucinations early in the course of the intoxication; coma can become apparent as toxicity progresses. Generally, overdoses with anticholinergic drugs do not produce true hallucinations, but rather pseudohallucinations. When a patient with an intact baseline mental status presents with psychosis, paranoia, or visual hallucinations, CNS stimulants such as cocaine or amphetamines should be considered.[30,66]

Drug intoxication–induced alterations in CNS function are initially difficult to distinguish from those caused by underlying psychiatric disorders, trauma, hypoxia, or metabolic disorders, such as hepatic encephalopathy or hypoglycemia. However, with the passage of time, decreased CNS function secondary to drug toxicity is more likely to wax and wane in severity in contrast to the more constant CNS depression that occurs with significant trauma or metabolic disorders. Drug toxicity also rarely produces focal neurologic findings. Changes in pupil size, reflexes, and vital signs can provide insights into the pharmacologic class of drug involved in the intoxication.[26,30,31]

CNS depression, seizures, disorientation, and other CNS changes that are commonly associated with drugs likely to be prescribed by psychiatrists should be evaluated carefully in T.C. For example, T.C.'s pupil size would most likely be dilated if she had ingested a TCA because of the anticholinergic effects of these drugs. TCA intoxications can also cause myoclonic spasms.[30] These spasms are often difficult to differentiate from seizure activity caused by TCA overdoses, although the spasms are often asymmetric and more persistent.[121]

CARDIOVASCULAR FUNCTION

Assessment of heart rate, rhythm, conduction, and measurements of hemodynamic function can also be used to help identify the type of drug ingested. Overdoses of sympathomimetic drugs usually increase heart rate. Overdoses of cardiac glycosides or β-blockers can slow the heart rate. Although drugs can increase or decrease heart rate directly, indirect cardiac effects (e.g., reflex tachycardia in response to hypotension) also need to be considered. Abnormal heart rates produced by drug overdoses are usually not treated unless hypotension or severe dysrhythmias are precipitated.[30,43]

PULMONARY FUNCTION

Evaluating the rate and depth of respiration and the effectiveness of gas exchange in an intoxicated patient can also help identify drugs that might have been ingested. A decrease in respiratory rate is commonly associated with the ingestion of CNS depressants. An increased respiratory rate and depth is generally associated with CNS stimulant toxicity. An increase in respiratory rate can also be secondary to respiratory compensation for a drug-induced metabolic acidosis.[30] Aspiration of gastric contents after vomiting is a common event in drug ingestions. Aspiration pneumonitis is the most common pulmonary abnormality associated with significant intoxications.[46] Noncardiogenic acute pulmonary edema has been associated with drug overdoses of salicylates[81–84] (especially with chronic intoxications) and the use of drugs of abuse (e.g., cocaine and heroin).[122–129]

TEMPERATURE REGULATION

Body temperature is an important and sometimes overlooked parameter when assessing potential intoxications.[30,43] Decreased mental status is often associated with a loss of thermoregulation, and this results in a body temperature that falls or increases toward the ambient temperature. Increased body temperature (hyperthermia) caused by overdoses of CNS stimulants (e.g., cocaine, amphetamines, ecstasy), salicylates, hallucinogens (e.g., phencyclidine), or anticholinergic drugs or plants (e.g., jimsonweed) can have serious consequences.[30,32,43] Body temperature should be measured rectally to obtain an accurate representation of core body temperature.[130]

Hyperthermia caused by drug overdoses is commonly encountered in hot, humid environments or when the intoxication is associated with physical exertion, increased muscle tone, or seizures. In these patients, it is important to obtain renal function tests (e.g., BUN, serum creatinine) and a serum creatine kinase measurement to determine whether rhabdomyolysis has occurred secondary to breakdown of muscle tissue.[30,43,130]

GASTROINTESTINAL FUNCTION

The GI tract should be assessed for decreased motility because drug absorption can be delayed or prolonged.[30,131,132] When this is the case, decontamination may be beneficial after an oral ingestion even if a long time has elapsed since the ingestion. The presence of blood in either emesis or stool may signal ingestion of a GI irritant or caustic substance.[133]

SKIN AND EXTREMITIES

The physical examination should include a thorough evaluation of the body surfaces. Look for causes of trauma that may also explain the patient's condition. Examination of the skin and extremities can provide evidence of drug intoxication, especially with IV or subcutaneous drug injection needle marks.[30] Drugs can be hidden in the rectum or vagina.[30] Look for drug patches (e.g., fentanyl) on hidden areas of the body such as the back of the neck or scrotum. Fluid-filled bullae at gravity-dependent sites that have been in contact with hard surfaces for a long time suggest prolonged coma.[30] Muscle tone also should be assessed.[30] Increased tone or myoclonic spasms can be caused by some drug overdoses (e.g., TCAs) and can produce rhabdomyolysis or hyperthermia.[30,130] Dry, hot, red skin may also be an indication of anticholinergic toxicity.[30,43]

In summary, an organ system assessment of T.C. can provide useful insights into the identity of drugs that might have been ingested, the viability of organ function that might have been adversely affected, and the treatment that should be instituted.

Laboratory Tests

CASE 4-4, QUESTION 6: What laboratory tests should be ordered for T.C.?

The laboratory assessment of an intoxicated patient should be guided by the history of the events surrounding the ingestion, clinical presentation, and past medical history.[25,134] The status of oxygenation, acid–base balance, and blood glucose concentration must be determined, especially in patients with altered mental status such as T.C.[43] Oxygenation can be assessed initially by pulse oximetry, and acid–base status by ABGs and serum electrolyte concentrations.[26,134,135] T.C. was given oxygen and a bolus of IV fluid on her arrival at the ED. Paramedics administered glucose during her transportation to the ED.

A medical history of organ dysfunction or medical disorders (e.g., diabetes, hypertension) that can damage organs of elimination (e.g., kidney, liver) will also guide the need for laboratory tests. A serum creatinine concentration and liver function tests (e.g., aspartate aminotransferase [AST], alanine aminotransferase [ALT]) should be ordered. Other more specific tests reflective of her past medical history can be ordered subsequent to dialogue with her psychiatrist. A complete blood cell count, complete chemistry panel, serum osmolality, and other baseline laboratory tests should be obtained.[30] Pregnancy tests should be considered in female patients of childbearing age because unwanted pregnancies are common causes of overdose.[136,137]

A baseline electrocardiogram (ECG) should be obtained when exposure to a cardiotoxic drug is suspected or whenever the cardiovascular or hemodynamic status is altered.[26,29,43,135] A 12-lead ECG should be ordered because T.C. is likely to have ingested a psychotropic agent. Continuous cardiac monitoring should be instituted because of the significant cardiotoxicity associated with overdoses of these agents. Patients with severe TCA overdoses frequently present with symptoms of coma, tachycardia with a prolonged QRS segment, seizures, hypotension, and respiratory depression.[138–141]

A chest radiograph is useful when the potential exists for either direct pulmonary toxicity or aspiration.[26,29] A chest radiograph is indicated because T.C. had vomitus in her mouth and TCAs are associated with the development of acute respiratory distress syndrome and pulmonary edema.[138,142,143]

Qualitative Screening

CASE 4-4, QUESTION 7: Why should (or should not) T.C.'s urine and blood be screened to assist in identifying the ingested substance?

Toxicology laboratory testing can be used to identify the substances involved in a toxic exposure, to exclude substances, or to measure the concentration of substances in serum or other biological fluids.[27,134,135] The identification and quantification of compounds should be considered as two distinct types of toxicologic testing.[27,144] *Qualitative* screening, intended to identify unknown substances, must be able to identify which substance or class of substances is involved in the toxic exposure. *Quantitative* testing is similar to therapeutic drug monitoring in that the presence of the substance usually is known, and the question being answered is how much is present.[27]

Screening various biological fluids suspected of having high concentrations of a parent drug and its metabolites can identify unknown substances. Urine is screened much more commonly than blood, whereas gastric fluid is rarely evaluated. A urine drug screen is preferred to a blood drug screen because urine generally contains a higher concentration of a drug and its metabolites than other body fluids.[145]

When reviewing the results of urine screening panels for drugs and other substances, one must remember that the presence of a substance in urine is not necessarily related to a concurrent toxicity. A positive result on a urine screening panel merely indicates that the patient has ingested or has been exposed to the substance, but it does not differentiate between toxic and nontoxic doses. If a drug and its metabolites are eliminated slowly into the urine for a prolonged time, and if the testing methodology detects small concentrations of the substance, urine drug screening could identify the presence of a substance days, weeks, or even months after the exposure (e.g., marijuana).[27,135]

It is important to know which drugs or substances are tested at a given laboratory. Many laboratories restrict the number of drugs for which they test because 15 drugs account for more than 90% of all drug overdoses.[35] Some urine toxicology screens only detect common drugs of abuse (e.g., amphetamines, barbiturates, benzodiazepines, cocaine, marijuana, opioids).[135] Some drugs of abuse are not detected on routine drug screening (e.g., gamma hydroxybutyrate, ketamine, flunitrazepam).[27] Some analyses detect only antibodies to drug metabolites. For example, a benzodiazepine screen detects oxazepam, a common benzodiazepine metabolite. However, alprazolam and lorazepam are not metabolized to oxazepam and will not be detected in a urine screen. Likewise, an opioid screen may not detect the synthetic opioids such as fentanyl and methadone.[135]

Results of qualitative toxicology screening tests are difficult to interpret. False negatives, false positives, cross-reactivity with related drugs, chronicity of exposure, and length of time since last exposure all complicate results.[113,114,135] Urine toxicology screen results rarely change clinical management of the patient. Monitoring mental, cardiovascular, and respiratory status and other laboratory parameters provide better clues than the results of a urine toxicology screen.[26,27,134,135,144]

Toxicology screening can be appropriate when the history of a suspected toxic exposure is unavailable, inaccurate, or inconsistent with the clinical findings.[27] However, it is important to know which drugs are detected on a given toxicology screen.[135] A comprehensive qualitative urine drug screen can be considered for T.C. because information about the substance(s) she ingested is not yet known.

Quantitative Testing

CASE 4-4, QUESTION 8: Why should a quantitative toxicology laboratory test be ordered (or not ordered) for T.C. as well?

After a qualitative urine analysis for drugs, a quantitative analysis of drug concentration in blood can help determine the severity of toxicity and the need for aggressive interventions (e.g., hemodialysis).[27,36,135,144] Quantitative tests are especially useful when assessing the potential toxicity of drugs with delayed clinical toxicity or when the toxicity primarily is caused by metabolites (e.g., ethylene glycol, methanol). The concentration of a drug in serum is sometimes much more predictive of end-organ damage than clinical findings (e.g., acetaminophen effect on the liver).

Quantifying the amount of drug in serum is useful when (a) the concentration of the substance correlates with toxic effects, (b) the turnaround time for results is rapid, and (c) treatment can be guided by the serum concentration.[35,134,144] To aid in the care of poisoned patients, stat quantitative serum concentrations of acetaminophen, carbamazepine, carboxyhemoglobin, digoxin, ethanol, ethylene glycol, iron, lithium, methanol, methemoglobin, phenobarbital, salicylates, and theophylline should be available at laboratories of large health care facilities.[26,27,36,134,144]

When blood samples are collected to quantitate potentially intoxicating substances, as much information as possible should be obtained about the time course of events to determine whether absorption and distribution of the substance is complete. Serial samples may be needed to determine whether significant absorption is still occurring.[32,33] In contrast to the interpretation of therapeutic serum concentrations of chronically administered drugs, the serum concentration of a substance ingested in an overdose is not likely to be at steady state.

Quantitative toxicologic testing will not benefit T.C. at this point in time because the identity of the ingested substance is unknown. Nevertheless, a serum ethanol concentration could be useful in this case because alcohol is often ingested concurrently in overdose situations.[134] Most poison centers also recommend obtaining a quantitative acetaminophen level on all intentional ingestions because serious hepatotoxicity can occur if acetaminophen ingestion is missed.[27,134,135]

Assessment

CASE 4-4, QUESTION 9: T.C.'s clinical status has not changed in the past 10 minutes. A urine toxicology screen, blood acetaminophen, blood alcohol, and ABGs have been ordered. The 12-lead ECG shows a prolonged QRS interval of 0.14 seconds (normal, <0.1 seconds). No antidotes have been administered. T.C.'s physical examination did not detect any evidence of trauma to her head. Her pupils were dilated and slowly responsive to light, and her bowel sounds were hypoactive. What conclusions can be made at this time with regard to the likely substance ingested by T.C.?

Although the ingested substance still has not been specifically identified, the available data provide some clues as to the likely pharmacologic class of drug that was ingested. The presence of CNS depression (T.C. is unresponsive), slowed ventricular conduction (prolonged QRS on ECG), tachycardia (heart rate, 148 beats/minute), hypotension (BP, 90/55 mm Hg), and decreased GI motility (hypoactive bowel sounds), and the history of a possible depressive illness (history from husband and daughter) are all consistent with a TCA drug overdose. The antidepressant could have been ingested alone or with other agents.

Antidepressant Toxicities

CASE 4-4, QUESTION 10: How would the different toxicities of the various available antidepressants affect the treatment of T.C.?

The major pharmacologic effects and toxicities of the antidepressants are similar for all drugs within the same class. When a specific drug within a therapeutic class has not yet been identified, the overdose should be managed as if the ingested drug can produce the most severe toxicity of any drug in the class. In this light, T.C.'s presumed antidepressant drug overdose should be evaluated and managed initially as TCA (e.g., amitriptyline) ingestion.[140,146] Antidepressants with different structures and actions (e.g., trazodone [Desyrel], fluoxetine [Prozac], sertraline [Zoloft]) generally do not produce toxicity as severe as that of the TCAs.[140,146,147]

Gastrointestinal Decontamination

CASE 4-4, QUESTION 11: If a TCA ingestion is presumed, why might GI decontamination be appropriate at this time?

The longer GI decontamination is delayed relative to the time of ingestion, the less effective it is likely to be because drug absorption will already have occurred. Because the time of ingestion is unknown and T.C. is unresponsive, she probably already has absorbed significant amounts of the drug, making her more vulnerable to aspiration. Additionally, T.C. might already have aspirated because she was found in a pool of vomitus. TCA overdoses can also cause seizures, which would be a relative contraindication to GI decontamination. In consideration of these concerns, many would not support GI decontamination for T.C.[44–47,55–58]

Others might support GI decontamination because TCAs have strong central and peripheral anticholinergic properties that slow GI emptying, which could result in erratic absorption and delayed toxicity, but T.C. would first need to be intubated to protect her airway. Furthermore, TCAs have a large volume of distribution (10–50 L/kg), and both the parent drug and its metabolite undergo enterohepatic recirculation. The half-life of TCAs in overdose situations is 37 to 60 hours. For those reasons, activated charcoal could be reasonably administered in an effort to adsorb any drug that may not yet be absorbed from the GI tract.[53]

Repeated doses of activated charcoal have been used to increase the elimination of TCAs because of the long half-life of TCAs and the enterohepatic recirculation. In clinical studies, multiple-dose activated charcoal has increased the elimination of amitriptyline, but the data are insufficient to support or exclude the use of this therapy.[50]

CASE 4-4, QUESTION 12: How should the effectiveness of GI decontamination be monitored in T.C.?

If activated charcoal is administered, T.C. must first be intubated to protect her airway, and the charcoal must be administered via NG tube because she is unconscious. The insertion of the NG tube could stimulate the gag reflex, causing vomiting and possible aspiration. T.C.'s lung sounds should be monitored closely to determine whether aspiration pneumonitis is developing, particularly because T.C. was found unconscious and had already vomited.

Activated charcoal, especially in multiple doses, can produce ileus, GI obstruction, or intestinal perforation, especially when administered to patients who have ingested drugs that slow GI motility.[50,53,106] Bowel sounds must be monitored frequently to determine that an ileus is not developing. Once the patient passes a charcoal-laden stool, the activated charcoal can be considered to have successfully passed through the GI tract.

Sodium Bicarbonate and Hyperventilation

CASE 4-4, QUESTION 13: According to T.C.'s psychiatrist, he prescribed amitriptyline 100 mg at bedtime for her severe depression. How does this new information alter T.C.'s treatment plan?

This information confirms the assumptions that a TCA was ingested. It also specifically identifies the drug ingested. In TCA ingestions, severe toxicity has been associated with doses of 15 to 25 mg/kg.[103] T.C. ingested a total of 2,500 mg based on her suicide note that said she took 25 tablets. If she weighs about 60 kg and was truthful about the amount taken, she ingested a significantly toxic dose (about 42 mg/kg).

On the ECG, TCA toxicity will manifest as tachycardia with prolongation of the PR, QTc, and QRS intervals, ST and T-wave changes, and abnormalities of the terminal 40-millisecond vector.[103,121,138,141,148–151] TCAs have anticholinergic, adrenergic, and quinidinelike membrane effects on the heart.[121,138,140,146,149] It is believed that the anticholinergic effect causes the tachycardia and the quinidinelike effect causes the ECG changes.

In addition, TCAs are sodium-channel blockers.[152] Sodium-channel blockade slows the maximum uptake stroke of phase 0 of the action potential and decreases automaticity. Blockade decreases conduction velocity in the Purkinje fibers, which increases the QRS interval.[149] Myocardial depression, ventricular tachycardia, and ventricular fibrillation are the most common causes of death from TCAs.[141] Therefore, admission to the ICU with continuous cardiac monitoring is essential for T.C.[148]

The primary therapy for reversing ventricular arrhythmias and conduction delays is alkalinization of the serum and sodium loading by administrating IV hypertonic sodium bicarbonate.[121,138,140,141,149,150,153] Indications for sodium bicarbonate include hypotension, prolonged QRS segment (longer than 100 milliseconds), right bundle branch block, and wide complex tachycardia.[140,150] Alkalinization increases serum protein binding of the TCAs and thereby reduces the amount of free active drug (probably a minor consideration).[121,138,141,150] Correction of the serum pH is beneficial because underlying acidosis increases TCA cardiotoxic effects.[150] Furthermore, sodium bicarbonate has been found useful even in patients with a normal pH because sodium bicarbonate purportedly overcomes the sodium-channel blockade and decreases cardiotoxicity.[150,152]

On the basis of T.C.'s tachycardia and a widened QRS segment on ECG, she should be treated with IV sodium bicarbonate with the goal of achieving an arterial pH of 7.5 to 7.55.[141,150] Sodium bicarbonate could have been administered earlier because the suspicion of an antidepressant overdose was strong initially, her ECG demonstrated QRS prolongation and worsening myocardial conduction, and her BP continued to decline from the time she was first seen by the paramedics. If not monitored closely, the use of IV sodium bicarbonate could introduce the risk of sodium overload and subsequent pulmonary edema.[103,151]

An alternative is to hyperventilate the patient to a pH of 7.5 by adjusting her ventilator setting, thereby decreasing the cardiotoxicity of the TCA.[138,141,151] The combination of IV bicarbonate and mechanical ventilation is more likely to produce severe alkalemia. Careful and frequent monitoring of the serum pH of patients on dual therapy is essential.[138,152]

MONITORING EFFICACY

CASE 4-4, QUESTION 14: How should the sodium bicarbonate therapy in T.C. be monitored?

Many patients intoxicated with TCAs present with severe acidosis. Large doses of sodium bicarbonate may be required to normalize the arterial pH. The efficacy of sodium bicarbonate administration can be evaluated by monitoring acid–base status using ABGs, especially if the patient is also being ventilated mechanically.[138,152,153]

Sodium bicarbonate should be administered IV as a bolus of 1 to 2 mEq/kg for a 1- to 2-minute period. Continuous ECG monitoring is needed to monitor results of the bolus on cardiac abnormalities. Repeat bolus doses are administered as needed until the QRS interval narrows and tachycardia slows. Blood pH should be tested after several boluses to determine whether a target pH of 7.5 to 7.55 has been obtained.[150] At a minimum, ABGs should be determined within an hour of starting sodium bicarbonate therapy to determine pH response to the bicarbonate.[153] Bolus bicarbonate can be followed by a constant sodium bicarbonate infusion of 150 mEq/L sodium bicarbonate to maintain an alkaline pH.[150] ABGs must be monitored frequently to ensure a response.[138,152,153] Serial ECGs to measure the QRS interval can evaluate the efficacy of sodium bicarbonate. A prolonged QRS interval will generally narrow to normal after the systemic pH has been increased to about 7.5.[153]

Seizures

CASE 4-4, QUESTION 15: T.C. gradually developed more severely altered mental status and became comatose, not responding even to painful stimuli. She suddenly experienced a tonic-clonic seizure, which lasted about 2 minutes and terminated spontaneously. Should anticonvulsant therapy be initiated for T.C. at this time?

CNS toxicity is common in TCA overdoses. Symptoms include agitation, hallucinations, coma, myoclonus, and seizures.[121,138–141] Seizures can cause significant increases in acidosis and increase cardiotoxicity. Seizures are often seen immediately before cardiopulmonary arrest. Because of the severe consequences of prolonged seizures, aggressive drug treatment with rapid onset of action is indicated, and benzodiazepines are the drugs of choice to treat these seizures.[138,141]

Drug overdose–induced grand mal seizures are most commonly single seizures that terminate before drug therapy can be administered.[140] Seizure activity is not expected to persist, so instituting long-term anticonvulsant therapy is not indicated. However, if her seizure did not stop within 1 to 2 minutes, a benzodiazepine would have been indicated.[121,138,140] The onset of action of phenobarbital is too delayed for managing acute seizures, and phenytoin is usually ineffective in treating drug toxicity–related seizures.[121] After a seizure, the patient may become more acidotic and hypotensive.[141] Blood gases, creatine kinase, and ECG changes should be monitored immediately after a seizure.

Interpretation of Urine Screens

CASE 4-4, QUESTION 16: T.C.'s BP fell to 88/42 mm Hg, and dopamine was started. Her pH on repeat ABGs was 7.26. T.C.'s ECG normalized after the administration of 150 mL of sodium bicarbonate by IV bolus. After dopamine, her BP increased to 102/68 mm Hg, and seizure activity ceased. The urine drug screen results were positive for amitriptyline and nortriptyline. Acetaminophen and alcohol were not detected in her blood. Does the presence of nortriptyline indicate that T.C. has ingested other drugs in addition to her amitriptyline?

Nortriptyline is a metabolite of amitriptyline and, therefore, was identified on the urine drug screen. Metabolites, as well as the parent compound, are often identified on comprehensive urine drug screens.[135]

Duration of Hospitalization

CASE 4-4, QUESTION 17: How long should T.C. be monitored?

T.C. should be admitted to the ICU and monitored until all evidence of CNS and cardiovascular toxicity has been reversed.[121] There is some controversy over how long symptomatic patients should be observed. Some believe symptomatic patients need cardiac monitoring for 24 hours after ingestion.[140] Others believe TCA overdose patients need to be monitored until they are symptomfree for 24 hours because of a few reports of late development of symptoms.[141] However, 98% of signs of cardiotoxicity and arrhythmias are seen within the first 24 hours after TCA ingestion.[121,139] Because the incidence of late-occurring symptoms is rare, most patients are discharged after they are fully awake.[138] After the toxicity has completely resolved, T.C. should be evaluated by a psychiatrist to determine whether she should be admitted for inpatient treatment of her suicidal ideation.[138–140]

Outcome of Patient T.C.

T.C. had no further seizure activity. She remained on a dopamine infusion for 8 hours and required several more boluses of IV sodium bicarbonate. The next afternoon, she started to awaken with her family at the bedside. She was tearful and expressed regret that her suicide attempt was not successful. She repeatedly told her family that they would be better off without her. Her psychiatrist saw her, and arrangements were made to transfer her to an in-patient psychiatric hospital once she was medically cleared.

ASSESSMENT OF ACETAMINOPHEN INGESTION

Mechanism of Hepatotoxicity

CASE 4-5

QUESTION 1: L.P., a 23-year-old woman who is about 32 weeks pregnant, presents to the ED 5 hours after ingesting 50 acetaminophen 500-mg tablets. She is depressed and hoped to end her pregnancy by ingesting acetaminophen. Her pregnancy was unplanned, and she has received no prenatal care. L.P. has vomited spontaneously four times since the ingestion and is complaining of abdominal pain; her heart rate is 100 beats/minute, BP is 100/70 mm Hg, and temperature is 97.5°F. L.P. does not have any chronic diseases, and the remainder of her medical history is unremarkable. How does an overdose of acetaminophen cause toxicity?

Acetaminophen is metabolized in the liver by glucuronidation and sulfation. The mixed-function oxidase system cytochrome P-450 (CYP) 2E1 metabolizes a portion of the acetaminophen to the highly reactive metabolite *N*-acetyl-*p*-benzoquinoneimine (NAPQI). In therapeutic doses, this metabolite is detoxified in the liver by glutathione. At toxic serum acetaminophen concentrations, the glucuronidation and sulfation metabolic pathways become saturated. Usually, NAPQI is detoxified by conjugation with glutathione, but increased amounts of the toxic metabolite deplete hepatic glutathione stores. When glutathione stores are decreased to about 30% of normal, the toxic metabolite binds to liver cells, resulting in the characteristic centrilobular hepatic necrosis seen in acetaminophen overdoses.[154–157]

ONLINE CONTENT

For a diagram that shows the mechanism of acetaminophen poisoning and treatment, go to http://thepoint.lww.com/AT10e.

Complication of Pregnancy

CASE 4-5, QUESTION 2: How does L.P.'s pregnancy change the management of her acetaminophen ingestion?

Pregnancy does not alter the initial approach to the assessment or treatment of potentially toxic ingestions, and assessment should focus initially on the mother.[158,159] Overdoses during pregnancy are often associated with attempted abortions, depression, prior loss of a child or children, potential loss of a lover, or economic reasons.[136,137,158,159] Intentional ingestions of analgesics, prenatal vitamins, iron, psychotropic agents, and antibiotics account for 74% of the overdoses during pregnancy.

The fetus is at risk when the mother overdoses on acetaminophen because acetaminophen crosses the placenta. The fetal liver can oxidize acetaminophen to its hepatotoxic metabolite by 14 weeks of gestation.[154] However, the fetal liver has only about 10% of the capability of the adult liver to metabolize acetaminophen. The fetal liver can conjugate acetaminophen with both glutathione and sulfate, but detoxification by glutathione conjugation appears to be decreased.[160,161]

In studies of maternal acetaminophen toxicity, most of the pregnant women survived without damage to themselves or their babies. However, there were also maternal and fetal deaths as a result of the overdoses.[160,162,163] Acetaminophen overdoses during pregnancy did not appear to increase the risk for birth defects or adverse pregnancy outcome unless the mother suffered severe toxicity, emphasizing the need to treat the mother promptly.[154,160,163]

Gastrointestinal Decontamination

CASE 4-5, QUESTION 3: What GI decontamination should be initiated for L.P.?

L.P.'s acetaminophen ingestion occurred 5 hours ago; therefore, the drug is likely to be totally absorbed, and no GI decontamination should be initiated.

Estimating Potential Toxicity

CASE 4-5, QUESTION 4: How should the potential toxicity of the acetaminophen ingestion be assessed in L.P.?

Acetaminophen toxicity results from ingestions greater than 150 mg/kg or more than 7.5 g total in adults. However, serum acetaminophen concentrations better predict acetaminophen-induced hepatotoxicity than the dose of acetaminophen acutely ingested.[164,165] The Matthew-Rumack nomogram (Fig. 4-1) is used in the United States to assess the potential for hepatotoxicity from acute overdoses of acetaminophen.[165] The treatment line is defined by a serum acetaminophen concentration of 200 mcg/mL at 4 hours after acetaminophen ingestion and 30 mcg/mL at 15 hours after ingestion on a semilogarithmic graph.[157] Others prefer to be more conservative and use the bottom line of 150 mcg/mL at 4 hours to begin treatment as histories of ingestion are often inaccurate. The serum acetaminophen concentration is plotted on a graph against the time of ingestion.[165] The nomogram predicts the probability that the AST or ALT will be greater than 1,000 international units/L and can be used to guide therapy by indicating whether a specific acetaminophen concentration is in the toxic range.[166] The nomogram is useful only for acute ingestions because it underestimates the potential for toxicity in chronic acetaminophen ingestions. It should be noted that although the nomogram is used to plot acetaminophen concentrations for all patients, it has been validated only in healthy nonalcoholic adult patients.[157]

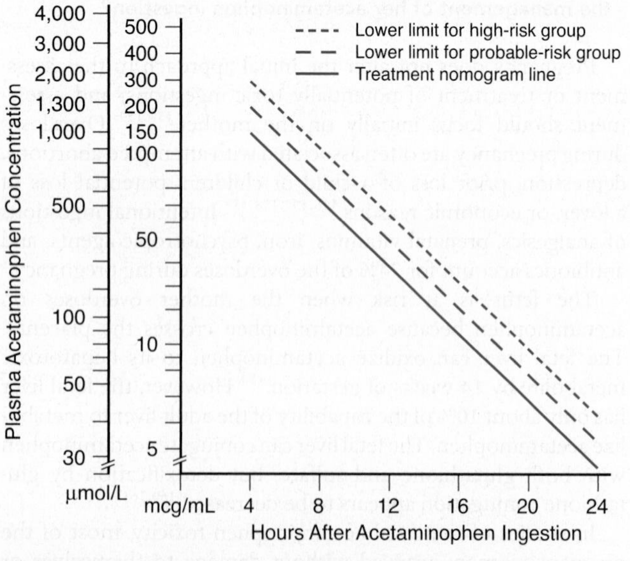

FIGURE 4-1 Nomogram for interpretation of severity of acetaminophen poisoning. Adapted with permission from Smilkstein MJ et al. Efficacy of oral *N*-acetylcysteine in the treatment of acetaminophen overdose: analysis of national multicenter study (1976–1985). *N Engl J Med.* 1988;319:1557.

Acetaminophen Treatment Nomogram

CASE 4-5, QUESTION 5: When is the preferred time to measure a serum acetaminophen concentration?

Acetaminophen absorption generally is complete within 1.5 to 2.5 hours after ingestion of solid or liquid dosage forms.[165] The Matthews-Rumack nomogram is not applicable before 4 hours after ingestion because it is based on complete drug absorption.[165] Most clinical laboratories can complete their assays and report acetaminophen serum concentration results within 2 hours.

Stages of Acetaminophen Toxicity

CASE 4-5, QUESTION 6: What are the clinical signs and symptoms of acetaminophen toxicity?

Early detection of an acetaminophen overdose is difficult because there are no characteristic early diagnostic findings. Toxicity appears in stages that may overlap and are not clear-cut. About 30 minutes to 24 hours after ingestion, the patient may exhibit anorexia, nausea, vomiting, malaise, and diaphoresis that can easily be attributed to other causes. The second stage of acetaminophen toxicity occurs about 24 to 48 hours after ingestion and is the stage in which hepatotoxicity develops. Hepatotoxicity is universal by 36 hours after ingestion. An AST measurement is the most sensitive measure of hepatotoxicity as AST abnormalities always precede evidence of actual liver impairment.[157,167,168]

In the third stage, 72 to 96 hours after ingestion, maximal liver dysfunction is evident with the return of anorexia, nausea, vomiting, and malaise. Symptoms can range from mild to fulminant liver failure with hepatic encephalopathy, coma, and hemorrhage. AST and ALT serum concentrations can be greater than 10,000 international units/L. There are also increases in bilirubin and INR measurements, as well as abnormalities in glucose and pH readings. Death, if it occurs, is usually a result of multiorgan failure or hemorrhage caused by hepatic failure. Most deaths occur 3 to 5 days after exposure. Patients who survive this stage go into recovery.[157,167,168]

Antidotes

CASE 4-5, QUESTION 7: What antidote for acetaminophen ingestion should be considered in L.P.? How does the antidote work, and when is it most effective?

Toxicity is determined by the results of a serum acetaminophen concentration measured at least 4 hours after ingestion.[165] NAC is the antidote for acetaminophen toxicity. NAC is a sulfhydryl donor that converts to cysteine, which is subsequently converted to glutathione.[154,166–168] NAC acts as a glutathione substitute and directly combines with the toxic acetaminophen metabolite, NAPQI, reducing it to a nontoxic cysteine conjugate.[167] NAC can also substitute for sulfation, which increases the nontoxic metabolism through that route as well. NAC increases intrahepatic microcirculation and is believed to possess hepatoprotective properties, showing some value even after liver damage has already occurred.[154,168]

Instituting therapy early with NAC is essential. When NAC is started within 8 to 10 hours of the ingestion, hepatotoxicity resulted in only 1.6% of cases. In patients who were started on NAC more than 10 hours after ingestion, 53% developed liver damage.[157,168]

Safety of *N*-Acetylcysteine in Pregnancy

CASE 4-5, QUESTION 8: Is NAC safe to use during pregnancy?

Acetaminophen overdose in pregnant women should be managed in the same manner as in nonpregnant patients.[160–163] If the life of the mother is not saved, the fetus will not survive (unless the child is near term and is emergently delivered); therefore, attention to the mother must be foremost. NAC therapy is not contraindicated in pregnant patients and might be helpful because it crosses the placenta and can protect the fetus from hepatotoxicity.[160,162,163]

NAC therapy appears to be protective for both mother and fetus.[154,157,160–163] When used as an antidote for acetaminophen overdose in pregnancy, NAC did not appear to result in toxic effects to the fetus.[154,157,160,162,163] The probability of fetal death was increased with the delay in NAC treatment after overdose and with acetaminophen overdose early in gestation.[157,160,168]

Route of Administration of *N*-Acetylcysteine

CASE 4-5, QUESTION 9: The 6-hour acetaminophen concentration in L.P. was 245 mcg/mL. By what route should NAC be administered?

This concentration of acetaminophen at 6 hours is above the treatment line on Figure 4-1. Because there was some delay from the time of ingestion to presentation at the ED and L.P. was already vomiting, it will be more difficult for L.P. to tolerate oral NAC. For this reason, IV NAC is recommended.

An FDA-approved sterile, pyrogen-free formulation of NAC is available as Acetadote.[169–171] The use of IV NAC is not completely risk-free because of a possible anaphylactoid reaction during the first dose of the IV NAC. The incidence of adverse reactions ranges from 14.3% to 23%. Asthmatic patients and patients with ectopy should receive the drug slowly and carefully, while being watched for symptoms of a reaction.[171]

A majority of the adverse reactions include nausea, vomiting, urticaria, flushing, and pruritus. Bronchospasm, angioedema, hypotension, and death have rarely occurred and must be carefully monitored when the IV route is being used.[169,172,173] Most reactions occur during or just after the first 15 minutes of the initial antidote infusion and appear to be dose related.[173] Because of the timing issue, the first dose of IV NAC is usually administered for 60 minutes instead of 15 minutes, even though a study comparing adverse reactions in the two infusion rates did not show clinically significant differences.[171,174]

Intravenous *N*-Acetylcysteine

CASE 4-5, QUESTION 10: How should IV NAC be administered to L.P.?

The FDA-approved IV NAC protocol is the same 20-hour dosing regimen used in Europe, known as the Prescott protocol.[169,170,171] A 150 mg/kg loading dose of NAC in 5% dextrose is infused IV slowly for 60 minutes while watching for symptoms of a possible anaphylactoid reaction. This is followed by a maintenance dose of 50 mg/kg infused for 4 hours, and then followed with a 100 mg/kg dose infused for 16 hours. This regimen provides a total of 300 mg/kg NAC during the 20 hours after the loading dose.[171] As soon as the patient is able to tolerate oral administration, the patient can be switched to oral NAC therapy.

Oral *N*-Acetylcysteine

CASE 4-5, QUESTION 11: Once she is able to tolerate oral NAC treatment, what dosing regimen would be appropriate for L.P.?

The standard oral NAC protocol is based on the original clinical studies.[166] The loading dose of NAC is 140 mg/kg orally using either the 10% or 20% mucolytic solutions that were formulated for inhalation therapy. Seventeen additional maintenance doses of 70 mg/kg of NAC are administered at 4-hour intervals after the initial dose, for a total of 72 hours of therapy. This provides a total of 1,330 mg/kg NAC during 72 hours.[169,175] Because oral NAC contains a sulfhydryl group, the substance has a very disagreeable taste and smell (like rotten eggs) that commonly results in nausea and vomiting for the patient. To mask the unpleasant taste and odor, NAC is diluted to a concentration of 5% using a carbonated beverage or fruit juice.[166] Because the entire dose of oral NAC passes through the liver, high concentrations are produced, which is seen as an advantage of oral therapy.[169]

Shorter oral NAC regimens are currently being used based on the efficacy of IV therapy.[176,177] Short-course oral NAC follows the same 20-hour time course as IV NAC. Patients receive the usual 140 mg/kg oral loading dose of NAC, followed by 70 mg/kg every 4 hours for five additional doses (20 hours of therapy). Serum acetaminophen, liver function tests, and INR are repeated at 20 hours after the loading dose, which is after the fifth maintenance dose. If 20-hour liver function tests and coagulation studies are normal and the acetaminophen level is less than the lower limits of detection, NAC can be stopped. A repeat set of liver function tests is recommended at 36 hours after ingestion. In other versions of the 20-hour NAC therapy, the dosage regimen is the same, but the laboratory studies are measured initially, and then at 16, 36, and 48 hours after ingestion.[177]

Efficacy of *N*-Acetylcysteine

CASE 4-5, QUESTION 12: Which route of NAC administration is more effective?

There is no proven evidence that one route of NAC administration is superior to the other.[168,169,178–180] Patient outcome after an acetaminophen overdose depends more on the time after the ingestion that treatment begins rather than on the route of administration of NAC. Patients who are started on NAC within 8 to 10 hours after ingestion, regardless of the route, rarely develop hepatotoxicity. Patients who present late or have a delay in the time of NAC treatment have higher rates of hepatoxicity.[154,168,169,175,179–181]

In one comparative study of IV NAC to oral NAC therapy, both were effective in reducing hepatotoxicity when therapy was initiated within 10 hours after ingestion. Vomiting delayed oral administration of the drug, but IV administration resulted in significantly longer delays in instituting therapy.[179] IV NAC avoids the problems of the vomiting patient, but oral NAC is safer. Oral

NAC is associated with nausea and vomiting, whereas IV NAC is associated with bronchospasm, urticaria, and angioedema during administration.[154,168] In addition, oral therapy is much less expensive.[181]

Although the time of initiation of therapy is one of the key factors in reducing hepatotoxicity from acetaminophen ingestions, length of therapy has become another factor.[180,182] Because the duration of therapy with the IV formulation is 21 hours, patients with severe toxicity may be undertreated. It is essential that the patient be re-evaluated at the end of the 21 hours to make sure that acetaminophen levels are not detectable and that liver enzymes are trending downward significantly. If there is still measurable acetaminophen and liver enzymes are still elevated, therapy with NAC must be continued.

Starting oral NAC may take less time to prepare than IV NAC therapy and is less expensive. If the patient presents early after an acetaminophen ingestion and does not have nausea and vomiting, oral therapy would be indicated. If the patient presents late (more than 10 hours after ingestion) with signs and symptoms of hepatotoxicity along with intractable nausea and vomiting, IV NAC should be instituted at once.[169,175]

Monitoring Efficacy of *N*-Acetylcysteine

CASE 4-5, QUESTION 13: How should the efficacy of NAC therapy be monitored in L.P.?

The effectiveness of NAC intervention in L.P. should be monitored by daily assessment of her acetaminophen concentration (as long as it is still measurable), AST, ALT, total bilirubin, glucose, and INR. The AST and ALT serum concentrations typically increase within 36 hours (range, 24–72 hours) after ingestion.[168,179] As the hepatic damage continues, the liver enzymes may peak at several tens of thousands units, even with NAC therapy. In most patients, AST and ALT begin to decline after 3 days and then return to baseline values.[168]

In a small number of patients, usually those who presented late after the ingestion, fulminant hepatic failure may develop. Symptoms of severe or persistent acidosis, coagulopathy, a significantly increased serum creatinine, and grade III to IV encephalopathy are consistent with fatal outcomes in patients with fulminant hepatic failure. Liver transplantation might be a consideration for these patients.[157,183–186]

Duration of *N*-Acetylcysteine Therapy

CASE 4-5, QUESTION 14: How long should NAC administration be continued?

The original NAC dosing protocol was based on an assumption that the half-life of acetaminophen was 4 hours. After five half-lives (20 hours), the acetaminophen should be metabolized and NAC could be discontinued. An NAC dose of 6 mg/kg/hour was determined to be necessary based on the rate of glutathione turnover relative to NAPQI production. To ensure that patients received an adequate NAC dose, the FDA recommended that this dose be changed to 18 mg/kg/hour for 72 hours.[187] This recommendation serves as the basis for the traditional 72-hour oral course of NAC therapy.

When using the traditional 72-hour oral course of NAC, therapy can be discontinued if the liver function tests are trending toward normal, other laboratory tests (i.e., coagulation studies, glucose, pH, bilirubin) are within normal ranges, and acetaminophen is no longer present in the serum. As long as acetaminophen is present, it can be metabolized to NAPQI and cause further toxicity.[168,176,187] Continued NAC will not be harmful to the patient and can be beneficial.

When using the shorter 20-hour course of oral NAC, if liver function tests and coagulation studies are normal and the 20-hour acetaminophen concentration can no longer be measured in the serum, NAC therapy can be stopped.[177] However, if 20-hour liver function tests or coagulation studies are abnormal, or if the 20-hour acetaminophen concentration measurement reveals acetaminophen still present in the serum, NAC therapy should be continued for at least another 24 hours.[178,179] Laboratory tests should be repeated every 24 hours, and the patient's progress must be monitored closely. If the patient is not improving, NAC should be continued until the patient recovers, receives a liver transplant, or dies.[157]

At this time, there is no consensus as to the best route of NAC administration, optimal dosage regimen, or optimal length of therapy.[168,169,187] There is consensus, however, that for optimal results, NAC therapy must be instituted within 10 hours after ingestion.[154,168,169,175,179,181] For patients who do not exhibit any signs of hepatotoxicity, shorter-course NAC therapy reduces the amount of NAC administered to the patient, decreases the quantity of laboratory tests, shortens hospital stay, and is less costly.[169,176,187]

N-Acetylcysteine Toxicity

CASE 4-5, QUESTION 15: How should the toxicity of NAC therapy be monitored in L.P.?

With the exception of vomiting, oral NAC is remarkably safe and has not been associated with toxicity.[154,168,169] Oral NAC must be retained for a minimum of 1 hour after ingestion to be successfully absorbed. If L.P. vomits within an hour after her oral NAC dose, the dose should be repeated. If she experiences protracted vomiting, administration of antiemetic drugs (e.g., ondansetron, metoclopramide) or placement of a duodenal feeding tube can improve GI tolerance.[169,188,189] If the patient cannot tolerate oral liquids, NAC therapy should continue via IV administration.

IV NAC therapy has been associated with anaphylactoid reactions in up to 14% of the patients. Although most reactions are not severe, bronchospasm, angioedema, and respiratory arrest have been reported.[154,168,169,187] Patients should be monitored for allergic and anaphylactoid reactions when NAC is administered IV. Most reactions can be avoided by infusing the NAC loading dose slowly for 60 minutes.[154,168,169]

Outcome of Patient L.P.

L.P. continued to have nausea and vomiting and had difficulty tolerating liquids. IV NAC was continued. An obstetrics consultation was requested to evaluate L.P.'s pregnancy. Fetal monitoring was instituted during her hospital admission. A sonogram was taken of the baby. Once L.P. saw her baby's image from the sonogram, her depressed mood seemed to lift. Approximately 36 hours after ingestion, her acetaminophen level was no longer detectable, and her liver function tests showed a mild elevation of her AST at 274 units/L and an ALT of 188 units/L. Her INR and total bilirubin values were normal at 0.7 seconds and 0.8 mg/dL, respectively.

L.P. was seen by a psychiatrist. She was scheduled for counseling and prenatal classes. L.P. seemed eager to attend the classes, and she talked enthusiastically about the baby when family members came to visit. Because of L.P.'s pregnancy, the decision was made to continue NAC for a full 72-hour course with the goal of protecting the fetal liver as much as possible. Six weeks later, she had a normal delivery of a healthy 6-pound, 1-ounce baby girl.

SUMMARY

Unfortunately, there is no cookbook method to treat all poisoned patients. Each exposure is unique: the patients, substances, symptoms, time of exposure, and circumstances differ in each case. Treatment of the poisoned patient often involves controversy because solid, evidence-based science to support a given decision is frequently lacking. When challenged with a poisoning exposure, consult with a poison control center. By calling 1-800-222-1222, the call will be connected to the poison center where consultation is available 24 hours a day nationwide.

KEY REFERENCES AND WEBSITES

A full list of references for this chapter can be found at **http://thepoint.lww.com/AT10e**. Below are the key references and websites for this chapter, with the corresponding reference number in this chapter found in parentheses after the reference.

Key References

Boyle JS et al. Management of the critically poisoned patient. *Scand J Trauma Resusc Emerg Med*. 2009;17:29. (29)

Bronstein AC et al. 2009 Annual report of the American Association of Poison Control Centers' National Poison Data System (NPDS): 27th Annual Report. *Clin Toxicol (Phila)*. 2010;48:979. (3)

Chyka PA et al. Position paper: single-dose activated charcoal. *Clin Toxicol (Phila)*. 2005;43:61. (46)

Committee on Poison Prevention and Control, Board on Health Promotion and Disease Prevention, Institute of Medicine of the National Academies. Poison control center activities, personnel, and quality assurance. *Forging a Poison Prevention and Control System*. Chapter 5. Washington, DC: The National Academies Press; 2004. (22)

Forsberg S et al. Coma and impaired consciousness in the emergency room: characteristics of poisoning versus other causes. *Emerg Med J*. 2009;26:100. (120)

Kociancic T, Reed MD. Acetaminophen intoxication and length of treatment: how long is long enough. *Pharmacotherapy*. 2003;23:1052. (187)

Manoguerra AS et al. Iron ingestion: an evidence-based consensus guideline for out-of-hospital management. *Clin Toxicol (Phila)*. 2005;43:553. (96)

[No authors listed]. Position paper: cathartics [published correction appears in *J Toxicol Clin Toxicol*. 2004;42:1000]. *J Toxicol Clin Toxicol*. 2004;42:243. (47)

[No authors listed]. Position paper: ipecac syrup [published correction appears in *J Toxicol Clin Toxicol*. 2004;42:1000]. *J Toxicol Clin Toxicol*. 2004;42:133. (44)

[No authors listed]. Position paper: whole bowel irrigation [published correction appears in *J Toxicol Clin Toxicol*. 2004;42:1000; dosage error in article text]. *J Toxicol Clin Toxicol*. 2004;42:843. (48)

Proudfoot AT et al. Position paper on urine alkalinization. *J Toxicol Clin Toxicol*. 2004;42:1. (70)

Rumack BH et al. Acetaminophen overdose: 662 cases with evaluation of oral acetylcysteine treatment. *Arch Intern Med*. 1981;141(3 Spec No):380. (166)

Liebelt EL. Targeted management strategies for cardiovascular toxicity from tricyclic antidepressant overdose: the pivotal role for alkalinization and sodium loading. *Pediatr Emerg Care*. 1998;14:293. (150)

Temple AR. Pathophysiology of aspirin overdosage toxicity, with implications for management. *Pediatrics*. 1978;62(5 Pt 2 Suppl):873. (81)

Vale JA et al. Position paper: gastric lavage. *J Toxicol Clin Toxicol*. 2004;42:933. (45)

Key Websites

CDC Injury Prevention and Control: Data and Statistics. **http://www.cdc.gov/injury/wisqars/index.html.**

Drug Abuse Warning Network. **https://dawninfo.samhsa.gov/data.**

5 End-of-Life Care

Victoria F. Ferraresi

CORE PRINCIPLES

		CHAPTER CASES
1	End-of-life care consists of palliative and hospice care. It is ideally introduced early in the disease progression to provide support to patients of all ages with a serious chronic or life-threatening illness. Medicare patients who enter a hospice program agree to relinquish their regular Medicare benefits as they relate to the terminal illness, and accept the palliative rather than curative approach that will be provided by hospice. The hospice provides all care related to the hospice diagnosis under a managed-care model at a fixed reimbursement.	Case 5-1 (Question 1)
2	In 2008, the Hospice Conditions of Participation were updated to include a review of the medication profile as part of the initial assessment of new patients. The medication regimens of hospice patients should be continually reviewed and updated, with unnecessary, ineffective, or duplicative medications discontinued.	Case 5-1 (Question 2)
3	Patients near end of life can experience a number of distressing symptoms. These should be anticipated and treated in a timely manner that is acceptable to the patients and their families.	Case 5-1 (Question 3)
4	Well-trained pharmacists can improve medication management for hospice patients, while helping the hospice manage their drug costs.	Case 5-1 (Question 2)
5	Many barriers exist regarding pain management and the use of opioids.	Case 5-1 (Question 4)
6	Effective pain management uses a variety of approaches.	Case 5-2 (Question 1)
7	Pain and symptom management may at times require an aggressive approach.	Case 5-3 (Questions 1–3)

HOSPICE AND PALLIATIVE CARE

Terminology

Hospice care and *palliative care* are similar, but distinct, terms sharing the common belief that the relief of suffering is a long-standing, central, and fully legitimate aim of medicine. *End-of-life care* refers to both hospice care and palliative care. The basic principle of end-of-life care is to optimize the quality of life for the patient and family in the last weeks and months of life, as well as to provide support for the family beyond the end of life into bereavement.

Palliative care, which includes hospice care, is ideally introduced early in the disease progression to provide support to patients of all ages with a serious chronic or life-threatening illness. It can be provided concurrently with other treatments to cure or reduce disease, or it can be provided independently. The word *palliation*, derived from the Latin word *pallium* (a cloak), has been defined as "treatment to reduce the violence of a disease." The World Health Organization and the National Consensus Project define palliative care as an approach that improves the quality of life of patients and their families who are facing a life-threatening illness, by preventing and relieving suffering through early identification and impeccable assessment and treatment of pain and other physical, psychosocial, and spiritual problems.[1–4] Palliative care:

- Affirms life and regards dying as a normal process
- Provides relief from pain and other distressing symptoms
- Intends neither to hasten nor postpone death
- Integrates the psychological and spiritual aspects of patient care
- Offers a support system to help patients live as actively as possible until death
- Uses a multidisciplinary team approach to address the needs of the patient and his or her family during the patient's illness and
- Provides bereavement counseling when indicated.[3]

In 2006, palliative medicine became a recognized subspecialty of internal medicine, awarded by the American Board of Medical Specialties.[5] Beginning in September 2011, the Joint Commission will offer an Advanced Certification Program for Palliative Care to recognize hospitals that provide high-quality palliative care services.[6]

Hospice, originally a place or way station for people making a pilgrimage, is considered both a philosophy of care and a place to deliver care. *Hospice care* focuses on the palliation of pain and other symptoms when active treatment to cure a terminal illness ends. Hospice care can be delivered in a building designated as a hospice, in the patient's home, or in a facility where the patient resides. As a programmatic model for delivering palliative care, hospice care provides an interdisciplinary team approach to the individualized symptom management (e.g., pain), as well as psychosocial, emotional, spiritual, and bereavement support for the patient and his or her family and caregivers during the last months of life.[7]

Hospice Care in the United States

According to estimates of the National Hospice and Palliative Care Organization, there were approximately 5,000 hospice programs in the United States in 2009. In that year, 41.6% of all deaths in the United States occurred under hospice care. Hospices provided care for patients with various terminal illnesses (e.g., cancer [40.1% of all admissions], heart disease [11.5%], debility unspecified [13.1%], dementia [11.2%], and lung disease [8.2%]).[7]

Younger adults and pediatric patients account for less than 1% of the hospice population. Although pediatric hospice programs are growing, fewer patients in this population received hospice care in 2006 compared with 2005.[8] Regulatory, financial, cultural, and educational barriers play a role in diminished access to hospice care for pediatric patients.[9] Some states now offer hospice care (under Medicaid and other state programs) to pediatric patients with expanded benefits to improve coordination of care.[10]

About 83% of hospice patients were 65 years of age or older, and one-third were 85 years or older. In 2009, 83.4% of hospice patients received this care as a benefit provided by Medicare. Almost all (93%) hospice programs are certified by the Centers for Medicare and Medicaid Services to provide care to beneficiaries under the Medicare Hospice Benefit.[7]

The Medicare Hospice Benefit

The Medicare Hospice Benefit is funded from Part A (the hospital portion) of Medicare.[11,12] Patients are eligible for this benefit if, in the opinion of two physicians (i.e., patient's primary-care physician and hospice medical director), the natural course of their disease will result in death within 6 months. Eligibility for hospice can continue beyond the initial certification if the hospice medical director recertifies eligibility at defined intervals, called certification periods. Other insurance payers generally follow this criterion. In electing this benefit, patients agree to relinquish their regular Medicare benefits as they relate to the terminal illness and accept the palliative rather than curative approach that will be provided by hospice. This benefit links all care related to the terminal illness to the selected Medicare-certified hospice program, which coordinates and provides all care. The regulatory framework for the provision of hospice care under Medicare is defined in 42 CFR Part 418, Medicare and Medicaid Programs: Hospice Conditions of Participation.[12]

Hospice care is provided (and reimbursed) under Medicare at four levels, all of which can be modified at any time based on a patient's condition or caregiving needs:

- Routine home care (day-to-day care in the home)
- Continuous home care (when more skilled care in the home is required owing to symptom management or a caregiving crisis)
- General inpatient care (reimbursement for an inpatient stay in a hospital or skilled nursing facility related to symptoms that cannot be managed in the home)
- Inpatient respite care (up to 5 days in a skilled nursing facility) to give the caregiver a break or respite

Most care, consisting of pain and symptom management and assistance with activities of daily living, as well as psychosocial support, is provided to hospice patients at the routine level of care.

Patients may freely visit their primary-care provider (i.e., physician or nurse practitioner) for any reason, including reasons unrelated to their terminal illness. The primary-care provider will be paid directly by Medicare. Patients may choose to use their regular Medicare benefits for other unrelated illnesses; visits to providers for care or treatments unrelated to the primary hospice diagnosis are not limited or restricted. Patients may revoke their election of the Medicare Hospice Benefit at any time (e.g., end hospice care to pursue curative treatment or seek treatment outside the hospice plan of care). Patients may, at a later date, choose to return to hospice care or change to a different hospice program, without restrictions or loss of benefits.[12]

Hospice programs receive a fixed daily payment to provide all care related to the terminal diagnosis (e.g., medications, supplies, durable medical equipment, procedures, home health aides, provider visits, spiritual care, bereavement services). The reimbursement rates for the four levels of hospice care under the Medicare Hospice Benefit are established each summer for the following fiscal year, effective October 1.[13] A baseline reimbursement rate is set, along with an adjustment for wage differentials (the wage index) based on the local cost of living.[14,15] As an example, Table 5-1 shows reimbursement rates for the provision of routine home care in San Francisco, California, and Jefferson City, Missouri, for fiscal year 2011. Historically, hospice reimbursement rates have been low and have not kept pace with rising costs. The total daily reimbursement for the two markets above have increased by 11% and 10.4%, respectively, from 2007 to 2011 (2.75% and 2.6% per year.) The Hospice wage index scale is being adjusted (and phased out) from 2009 to 2016, and, overall, this will decrease hospice reimbursement.[15–17]

TABLE 5-1

Example of Hospice Daily Payment Rates for Routine Level of Care, 2011 Fiscal Year (October 1, 2010–September 30, 2011)[13,14]

	A Unadjusted Payment Rate (B + C)	B Nonlabor Portion	C Labor Portion	D Wage Index	E Adjusted Labor Portion (C × D)	F Total Daily Payment (B + E)
San Francisco, CA	$146.63	$45.88	$100.75	1.6595	$167.19	**$213.07**
Jefferson City, MO	$146.63	$45.88	$100.75	0.9105	$91.73	**$137.61**

TABLE 5-2
Comparison of Hospice Reimbursement With Drug Price Escalation 2004–2009[13,14,21–26]

Year	Unadjusted Daily Reimbursement	% Annual Rate Increase	Prescription Drug Price Increases (%) Generic Products	Branded Products	Total
2011	$146.63	2.6%	NA	NA	NA
2010	$142.91	2.1%	NA	NA	NA
2009	$139.97	3.6%	0.3%	9.2%	5.5%
2008	$135.11	3.3%	0.3%	8.3%	5.3%
2007	$130.79	3.4%	0.5%	7.4%	4.9%
2006	$126.49	3.7%	0.2%	6.9%	4.9%
2005	$121.98	3.3%	0.4%	6.3%	4.7%
2004	$118.08	3.4%[a]	0.5%	6.7%	5.2%

[a] The unadjusted daily hospice rate for 2003 was $114.20.

Programs generally have high costs at the start of care because of personnel costs involved in the admission, assessment, and development of the initial plan of care, and obtaining medications, medical equipment, and medical supplies. High costs are also encountered nearer to the end of life, when new problems can appear and symptoms often intensify. The Centers for Medicare and Medicaid Services is considering hospice payment reform, consisting of higher payments at the start of care and near the end of life to account for greater care needs during these periods, differing payments based on where the beneficiary resides (home versus a facility), or on the type of care provided, and on quality outcomes.[15,16]

It is common for patients to be referred to hospice when death is imminent. Median lengths of stay have declined, from 71.8 days during the Medicare demonstration project (1980–1982) to 26 days in 2005 and to 21.1 days in 2009.[7,18–20] Approximately 34.4% of patients admitted to a hospice program in 2009 died or were discharged within 7 days.[7] Furthermore, drug costs continue to outpace increases in hospice reimbursement by at least a factor of two for brand name products based on data reported by Medco Health Solutions, a large pharmacy benefit manager (Table 5-2).[21–26] A Kaiser Family Foundation report cites a rise in retail prescription prices of 3.6% annually between 2000 and 2009, compared with the average inflation rate of 2.5%.[27] These variables (i.e., referrals to hospice later in the course of terminal illness, higher costs at the start of care, shortened lengths of stay, higher drug costs) have placed intense pressure on hospice programs to manage expenses. Because it is difficult to influence the time when patients are referred to hospice, the duration of time in hospice care, or the inherently higher costs when patients are first enrolled into hospice, the management of drug costs has taken a high priority in providing cost-effective hospice care.

Improving Patient Care and Managing Drug Costs

In 2008, the Hospice Conditions of Participation were updated to be more patient centered and outcome oriented, and the number of standards was increased from 48 to 96.[12] Coverage of medications continues to be mandated as follows, in §418.106 Drugs and biologicals, medical supplies, and durable medical equipment: "...drugs and biologicals related to the palliation and management of the terminal illness and related conditions, as identified in the hospice plan of care, must be provided by the hospice while the patient is under hospice care."

A new standard, §418.106, specifically addresses medication management and the review of the medication profile and specifies that "[t]he hospice must ensure that the interdisciplinary group confers with an individual with education and training in drug management as defined in hospice policies and procedures and State law... to ensure that drugs and biologicals meet each patient's needs."

The regulations specify that the initial and comprehensive assessment must "take into account" the drug profile (24 CFR §418.54). This is defined as "[a] review of all of the patient's prescription and over-the-counter drugs, herbal remedies and other alternative treatments that could affect drug therapy" and is to include the following:

- Effectiveness of drug therapy
- Drug side effects
- Actual or potential drug interactions
- Duplicate drug therapy
- Drug therapy currently associated with laboratory monitoring

Although the regulations do not specify who is to perform the medication assessment, pharmacists are uniquely qualified to fill this role.

Well-trained pharmacists can improve patient care and positively affect the fiscal margins of hospice programs by discouraging inappropriate use of medications, establishing evidence-based formularies, promulgating prior authorization policies for specific targeted drugs, establishing policies for adhering to the use of generic drugs, and managing the quantities of medications to be dispensed. In addition to managing drug expenditures, pharmacists provide drug information both to patients and providers, and work integrally with other members of the hospice health care team to improve the safe and effective use of medications.[28–42]

Referral to Hospice

ELIGIBILITY

CASE 5-1

QUESTION 1: M.P. is an 89-year-old woman referred to hospice for end-stage Alzheimer dementia. She lives in a residential care home for the elderly with a hired caregiver. Her husband has been unable to care for her at home for some time because she requires full assistance with all activities of daily living. She was recently hospitalized with aspiration pneumonia and a urinary tract infection, and completed a course of intravenous (IV) vancomycin and piperacillin/tazobactam. Her past medical history includes osteoporosis, coronary artery disease, chronic obstructive pulmonary disease (COPD), hypercholesterolemia, and hypothyroidism. She is not oriented to person, place, or date. Her speech is unintelligible or nonsensical. She cannot

feed herself, but will eat the thick pureed food that is fed to her. She is bed-bound and incontinent of urine and stool. She is restless and irritable at times, especially at night. Her Palliative Performance Scale (PPS) is 30%. Weight is 112 pounds, decreased from 135 pounds a year ago, and a recent serum albumin is 2.2 g/dL. What criteria does M.P. meet for eligibility for hospice services under the Medicare Hospice Benefit?

Patients with chronic diseases (e.g., Alzheimer disease, Parkinson disease, stroke, heart failure, lung disease) can be sufficiently ill and debilitated to need custodial care, but might not be sufficiently ill to meet the definition of a terminal illness. This differentiation between terminally ill versus chronically ill requiring custodial care is important because to qualify for hospice services under the Medicare Hospice Benefit, patients must be at a stage where death is expected within the next 6 months. For cancer diagnoses, the presence of widespread metastatic disease may make this prognosis more easily evident. However, for other chronic diseases, this is not as clear.

ONLINE CONTENT **For a graph that shows the factors to be taken into account when considering further anticancer therapy, benefit vs. cost, go to http://thepoint.lww.com/AT10e.**

The Medicare fiscal intermediaries have issued criteria to assist in the determination of eligibility for hospice care, as well as criteria to meet a 6-month terminal prognosis for a number of diseases. These criteria, or local coverage determinations (LCDs), provide guidelines for meeting an overall decline in clinical status, for meeting non–disease-specific data to establish a baseline, for establishing the effect of comorbidities (e.g., renal failure, liver disease), and for the submission of documentation for having met criteria. Criteria have been established for patients with cancer and noncancer diagnoses, and these criteria are used in the determination of eligibility for service and reimbursement.[43] Criteria for the noncancer diagnoses have been developed for amyotrophic lateral sclerosis, dementia as a result of Alzheimer disease and related disorders, heart disease, human immunodeficiency virus disease, liver disease, pulmonary disease, renal disease, stroke, and coma.

The determination of whether M.P. meets eligibility requirements for Medicare Hospice Benefits must be based on the established LCDs for dementia as a result of Alzheimer disease. These criteria include the following:

- Stage 7 or beyond, according to the Functional Assessment Staging Scale
  - Stage 7A: Can speak six or fewer intelligible words in a day or during an interview
  - Stage 7B: Speech ability limited to the use of a single intelligible word in a day or during an interview
  - Stage 7C: Cannot ambulate without assistance
  - Stage 7D: Cannot sit up without assistance
  - Stage 7E: Loss of ability to smile
  - Stage 7F: Loss of ability to hold head up independently
- Unable to ambulate without assistance
- Unable to dress without assistance
- Unable to bathe without assistance
- Urinary and fecal incontinence, intermittent or constant
- No consistently meaningful verbal communication; stereotypical phrases only or the ability to speak is limited to six or fewer intelligible words
- One of the following within the past 12 months: aspiration pneumonia, pyelonephritis or upper urinary tract infection,

TABLE 5-3
Palliative Performance Score (PPS) Version 2

PPS Level	Ambulation	Activity and Evidence of Disease	Self-Care	Intake	Conscious Level
100%	Full	Normal activity and work No evidence of disease	Full	Normal	Full
90%	Full	Normal activity and work Some evidence of disease	Full	Normal	Full
80%	Full	Normal activity with effort Some evidence of disease	Full	Normal or reduced	Full
70%	Reduced	Unable to do normal job/work Significant disease	Full	Normal or reduced	Full
60%	Reduced	Unable to do hobby/housework Significant disease	Occasional assistance necessary	Normal or reduced	Full or confusion
50%	Mainly sit/lie	Unable to do any work Extensive disease	Considerable assistance required	Normal or reduced	Full or confusion
40%	Mainly in bed	Unable to do most activity Extensive disease	Mainly assistance	Normal or reduced	Full or drowsy ± confusion
30%	Totally bed-bound	Unable to do any activity Extensive disease	Total care	Normal or reduced	Full or drowsy ± confusion
20%	Totally bed-bound	Unable to do any activity Extensive disease	Total care	Minimal to sips	Full or drowsy ± confusion
10%	Totally bed-bound	Unable to do any activity Extensive disease	Total care	Mouth care only	Drowsy or coma ± confusion
0%	Death				

Instructions: PPS level is determined by reading left to right to find a "best horizontal fit." Begin at left column reading downwards until current ambulation is determined, then, read across to next and downwards until each column is determined. Thus, "leftward" columns take precedence over "rightward" columns.

Reprinted with permission from Victoria Hospice Society. Palliative Performance Scale (PPSv2), version 2. Medical Care of the Dying. 4th ed. Victoria, British Columbia, Canada: Victoria Hospice Society; 2006:120. www.victoriahospice.org/sites/default/files/imce/PPS%20ENGLISH.pdf. Accessed April 17, 2011.Copyright © 2001 Victoria Hospice Society. The Palliative Performance Scale version 2 (PPSv2) tool is copyright to Victoria Hospice Society and replaces the first PPS published in 1996 [*J Pall Care* 9(4):26–32]. Victoria Hospice Society, 1952 Bay Street, Victoria, BC, V8R 1J8, Canada www.victoriahospice.org edu.hospice@viha.ca

septicemia, decubitus ulcers (multiple, stages 3 and 4), fever (recurrent after antibiotic treatment)
- Inability to maintain sufficient fluid and caloric intake with 10% weight loss during the previous 6 months or serum albumin less than 2.5 g/dL

The PPS score (Table 5-3) gradates the extent of disability and can be used to assist in the determination of hospice eligibility.[44] M.P. meets the previous criteria and is eligible for hospice because of her Alzheimer disease. She clearly is debilitated. She is unable to speak intelligently, cannot feed herself, is not oriented to time or place, is incontinent of urine and stool, has lost about 20% of her weight during the past year, has a serum albumin of 2.2 g/dL, and has a PPS rating of 30% (i.e., totally bed-bound, unable to do any activity, confused). In addition, she has a number of comorbidities, experienced a recent episode of aspiration pneumonia, and finished a course of antibiotic therapy.

MEDICATION MANAGEMENT

CASE 5-1, QUESTION 2: M.P. has no known allergies. Her current medications are memantine 10 mg twice daily, aspirin 81 mg once daily, alendronate 70 mg weekly, esomeprazole 20 mg daily, lovastatin 20 mg with dinner, megestrol 40 mg/mL 5 mL (200 mg) twice daily, levothyroxine 0.1 mg daily, multivitamin daily, beclomethasone metered-dose inhaler one puff daily, albuterol 2.5 mg/ipratropium 0.5 mg via nebulizer every 4 hours as needed for wheezing or shortness of breath, acetaminophen 325 to 650 mg every 6 hours as needed for mild pain or fever, olanzapine 5 mg at bedtime as needed for restlessness and aggressive behavior, milk of magnesia 30 mL daily for constipation, and a bisacodyl suppository 10 mg every 3 days as needed if no bowel movement. What is your assessment of M.P.'s medication regimen? Which medications are the hospice required to provide, and which might be discontinued?

Hospices are required to provide (pay for) medications related to the terminal diagnosis for the palliation of symptoms within the hospice plan of care (POC). The POC is the individualized plan of treatment developed for each patient formulated at the start of care and updated regularly by the interdisciplinary group (IDG). The Conditions of Participation mandate that the IDG be composed of a physician, registered nurse, social worker, and a pastoral or other counselor.[12] A registered nurse coordinates the implementation of the POC. Some hospice program IDGs have incorporated a pharmacist into the group to review medication issues.

The large array of medications being taken by M.P. is similar to the medication lists of many hospice patients. These patients are often elderly and have a long history of several chronic medical conditions for which they have been taking multiple medications. In most cases, the medication lists of patients who are admitted into a hospice program have seldom been reviewed, updated, or modified in light of the present medical situation. Admission to a hospice program represents a change in the level of care and is a most appropriate time for a review of all medications to ascertain the necessity of each, with the goal of optimizing efficacy and minimizing the potential for adverse effects, medication errors, and inappropriate costs.

Because M.P. is to be enrolled into a hospice program, her care should not be focused on curative treatments, but rather on the management of discomforting symptoms and on improving her quality of life in the time remaining. M.P.'s medications should be analyzed with the goal of simplification. Unnecessary medications should be discontinued and alternatives added to manage two or more symptoms concurrently. The following changes should be considered:

Acetaminophen. This analgesic is often helpful in relieving mild pain, particularly in immobile elderly patients. A trial of around-the-clock acetaminophen could be helpful.

Albuterol/ipratropium combination. The hospice program is not required to pay for medications related to M.P.'s COPD because it is not related to the Alzheimer disease. This combination inhalation formulation should be continued if she is able to participate in her nebulizer treatments and they improve her breathing as she is recovering from aspiration pneumonia. The hospice may decide to pay for it, however, if they determine that the pneumonia contributed to her overall decline (see Chapter 24, Chronic Obstructive Pulmonary Disease).

Alendronate. This bisphosphonate drug can be discontinued because the treatment of osteoporosis is not an important consideration at this terminal stage of her life nor is it in the hospice POC. Thus, hospice would not cover it. Furthermore, M.P. is bed-bound; alendronate should be ingested in the upright position, and patients should remain upright after taking the medication to decrease the risk of alendronate-induced esophageal irritation (see Chapter 105, Osteoporosis). Pain that she may experience from osteoporosis can be treated with analgesics.

Aspirin. The low-dose aspirin is intended to decrease the risk of cardiovascular clotting. The aspirin will not increase M.P.'s comfort or quality of life. Although the aspirin would not be covered by her Medicare Hospice Benefit, it can be continued unless her primary-care provider prefers its discontinuation.

Beclomethasone. This patient is not functioning well cognitively (i.e., not oriented to time, person, or place) and would be unable to effectively time the inhalation of a breath to the actuation of her metered-dose inhaler. A systemic corticosteroid (e.g., prednisone) might improve her COPD symptoms and also improve her appetite and sense of well-being. The potential for adverse effects is modest with short-term corticosteroid use.

Bisacodyl, Milk of Magnesia. Constipation in hospice patients is common because of decreased gastrointestinal motility with advanced age, decreased physical activity, lack of adequate fiber and fluid intake, and use of constipating medications (e.g., opioids, anticholinergics, psychotropic agents).[45,46] The milk of magnesia, with an occasional bisacodyl suppository, is a good laxative regimen for this patient. If an opioid is later prescribed for M.P., a mild stimulant laxative (e.g., senna) with a stool softener (e.g., docusate) would be indicated. If stool softeners, stimulants, and saline laxatives are ineffective in resolving opioid-induced constipation, oral sorbitol or lactulose (10 g/15 mL) in 30-mL dosages can be prescribed up to four doses a day if needed. (Sorbitol would be preferred because it is more cost-effective.) Mineral oil 30 mL daily is an option if the stool is hard; however, mineral oil would not be optimal for M.P. because of her risk of aspiration. In cases of refractory constipation, the use of methylnaltrexone bromide, an injectable opioid antagonist, can reverse opioid-induced constipation by antagonizing opioid effects within the gastrointestinal tract without affecting systemic analgesia.[47,48] This quaternary derivative of naltrexone does not cross the blood–brain barrier. Dosing is weight based; it is given subcutaneously as either 8 mg for patients weighing 38 to 62 kg (84 to 136 pounds) or 12 mg for patients weighing 62 to 114 kg (136 to 251 pounds) once a day. The most common adverse events are abdominal pain, flatulence, nausea, and dizziness.[49]

Esomeprazole. This proton-pump inhibitor would probably be unnecessary because alendronate-induced esophageal or gastrointestinal irritation would not be an issue subsequent to its discontinuation. However, if a proton-pump inhibitor is needed, nonprescription generic omeprazole or lansoprazole is preferred because they are more cost-effective.[50] Lansoprazole would be appropriate if the patient cannot swallow whole tablets.

Levothyroxine. This thyroid medication should be continued until M.P. is no longer able to swallow. This medication, however, would not be covered under her Medicare Hospice Benefit, which is based on her Alzheimer disease, rather than other thyroid end-of-life disease (e.g., cancer).

Lovastatin. Cholesterol-lowering agents are not necessary during the last 6 months of life and should be discontinued. Lovastatin would not improve the quality of life of M.P. at this stage of her terminal illness and would not be covered by her Medicare Hospice Benefit.

Megestrol. The progesterone derivative, megestrol, in doses of 400 to 800 mg daily, can substantially stimulate appetite.[51,52] If an undernourished hospice patient desires to eat more, the hospice may choose to provide an appetite stimulant. It is unclear whether stimulation of appetite in a cognitively impaired patient will result in weight gain or improved nutritional status. Because the benefits in this situation are unclear, the potential of adverse effects (e.g., venous thrombosis) of megestrol needs to be considered, especially in M.P., who is not ambulatory and had been taking low-dose aspirin for prevention of cardiovascular clotting.

Memantine. Because the *N*-methyl-D-aspartate antagonist, memantine, has been modestly effective in improving performance in patients with moderate to severe Alzheimer disease,[53,54] it is probably of limited utility for M.P. (see Chapter 103, Geriatric Dementias). It would be reasonable to discontinue M.P.'s memantine subsequent to discussion with appropriate hospice team members and M.P.'s family.

Multivitamins. Multivitamins and other nutritional supplements are unlikely to improve M.P.'s comfort or quality of life. The discontinuation of these drugs would simplify medication administration, decrease the potential for medication errors, and decrease costs.

Olanzapine. An antipsychotic (e.g., olanzapine, haloperidol, chlorpromazine) is often prescribed off-label to manage the agitation and confusion encountered by patients with dementia (see Chapter 103, Geriatric Dementias). At the time of admission to hospice, patients may be receiving atypical agents (e.g., olanzapine). Small doses of the first-generation antipsychotics, such as haloperidol and chlorpromazine, may be very useful in treating opioid-induced nausea and vomiting, although randomized clinical trials demonstrating efficacy are lacking.[55] They would be covered by M.P.'s Medicare Hospice Benefit. Chlorpromazine would be preferable when more sedation is desired.

ONLINE CONTENT

For a diagram that shows factors that influence nausea and vomiting in the central nervous system and the gastrointestinal tract, go to http://thepoint.lww.com/AT10e.

SYMPTOM MANAGEMENT

The American College of Physicians has developed clinical guidelines, based on a systematic review of evidence and on a report by the Agency for Healthcare Research and Quality, to improve palliative care at the end of life. These guidelines provide strong recommendations for the regular assessment of patients at the end of life for symptoms of pain, dyspnea, and depression, and for therapies of proven effectiveness for these symptoms. For patients with cancer, these include the use of opioids, nonsteroidal anti-inflammatory drugs, and bisphosphonates for pain; tricyclic antidepressants, selective serotonin reuptake inhibitors, and psychosocial interventions for depression; and opioids for unrelieved dyspnea and oxygen for short-term relief of hypoxemia. The guidelines do not address other variables of palliative care at the end of life or the management of other matters (e.g., nutritional support) because the quality of evidence is limited rather than because other issues or symptoms are unimportant.[56] The National Consensus Project for Quality Palliative Care recommends the measurement and documentation of pain and other symptoms using available scales with timely assessment and symptom management acceptable to both the patients and their families as a preferred practice.[4]

CASE 5-1, QUESTION 3: As soon as the hospice admission and assessment is completed, the nurse develops a plan for symptom management and orders a comfort kit for M.P. What are the components of this kit, and why is it useful?

Some hospices use a general comfort kit that contains specific medications to manage symptoms commonly encountered by most hospice patients, or they order medications to treat anticipated symptoms for a specific patient. These medications are placed in the home or facility where the patient resides. This facilitates the availability of medications to patients who encounter anticipated symptoms and is convenient when caregivers are instructed by the patient's primary-care provider to provide the medication to the patient. Patients living with cancer can encounter as many as 27 symptoms (median, 11), many of which occur together.[57] In one study, patients ($n = 176$) experienced an average of 6.6 to 6.8 distressing symptoms during the last week of life.[58] In general, the prevalence of each symptom is difficult to measure and demonstrates a high degree of variability. Pain (34%–96%), fatigue (32%–90%), and breathlessness (10%–95%) appear to be the most common in patients with a variety of terminal conditions, with the prevalence of pain in cancer patients reported as 35% to 96%.[59] Patients with terminal illnesses, including dementia as in M.P., also experience depression (3%–82%), anxiety (8%–79%), confusion (6%–93%), insomnia (9%–74%), nausea (6%–68%), constipation (23%–70%), diarrhea (3%–90%), and anorexia (21%–92%).[59] The disparity in symptom prevalence may be attributed to a host of variables (e.g., study design, patient population, underlying disease, inconsistent definitions, and where care was provided). The occurrence of symptoms, however, can vary significantly, even within the last week of life, and the need for frequent assessment of patients cannot be overemphasized. Morphine, lorazepam, haloperidol, prochlorperazine suppositories, and an anticholinergic agent are commonly ordered for hospice patients. Drugs that can palliate more than one symptom, such as morphine for pain or dyspnea, or haloperidol for agitation or nausea, are particularly suited to inclusion in a comfort kit.

Morphine. Every hospice cancer patient should have a short-acting opioid available for the palliation of unrelieved dyspnea and pain. Although morphine can cause respiratory depression, small doses are very effective in controlling dyspnea by multiple mechanisms: vasodilation, reduced peripheral vascular resistance, inhibition of baroreceptor responses, reduction of brainstem responsiveness to carbon dioxide (the primary mechanism of opioid-induced respiratory depression), and lessened reflex vasoconstriction caused by increased blood Pco_2 levels. Opioids can also reduce the anxiety associated with dyspnea and might also act directly on opioid receptors present in the airways (Table 5-4).[60–64]

Hospice patients generally do not have IV access (i.e., an IV catheter) into which medications can be easily administered. As a result, medications are primarily administered orally and, occasionally, by sublingual, buccal, transdermal, rectal, or subcutaneous (if an infusion is warranted) routes of administration. When patients lose the ability to swallow near the end of

TABLE 5-4
Treatment of Dyspnea at End of Life[60–64]

Nonpharmacologic methods	Pursed-lip breathing Upright position Relaxation Meditation Use of a fan or open window to circulate air over the face
Pharmacologic therapy	**Systemic opioids (short-acting)** in small doses given orally, sublingually, or via injection can be given every 1–2 hours as needed. **Long-acting agents** can be added to supplement the routine use of short-acting opioids. **Inhaled opioids** deliver medication via nebulization directly into the airway, avoiding first-pass metabolism, allowing use of smaller doses, theoretically minimizing side effects such as drowsiness. May cause local histamine release, leading to bronchospasm. Use nonpreservative sterile injectable products. More cumbersome and expensive owing to use of nebulizer and nonpreservative parenteral products; evidence does not show that nebulized opioids provide greater benefit than nebulized saline. Agents: morphine 2.5–10 mg in 2 mL of 0.9% saline; hydromorphone 0.25–1 mg in 2 mL of 0.9% saline; fentanyl 25 mcg in 2 mL of 0.9% saline Generally given every 2–4 hours as needed for breathlessness. **Benzodiazepines** are useful for the anxiety associated with breathlessness.

life (or have a condition that precludes swallowing), the sublingual or buccal routes of administration are the most useful, especially if drugs are lipophilic. Morphine is hydrophilic, and although some of it might be absorbed across the mucous membranes, the primary clinical effect probably results from gastrointestinal absorption after the drug has trickled down the back of the throat.

Oral morphine sulfate, in a concentration of 20 mg/mL, is commonly packaged in a 30-mL bottle at the beginning of hospice care. This bottle of morphine can provide sixty 10-mg doses, and at this concentration, only 0.5 mL of morphine needs to be administered. Oxycodone or hydromorphone, in comparable adjusted doses, can be substituted for morphine when needed.

Lorazepam. A short-acting benzodiazepine (e.g., lorazepam 0.5 mg every 4 hours as needed) is useful for the treatment of anxiety. Patients, especially those with respiratory symptoms, can experience episodes of extreme anxiety near the end of life. Caution should be used to not overuse these drugs in the elderly because they can increase the risk of falling or cause paradoxical reactions and worsen delirium or restlessness.

Haloperidol. Small doses of haloperidol (e.g., 0.5–1 mg) are useful for the treatment of restlessness, delirium, or nausea and vomiting.

Prochlorperazine. When patients cannot take oral medications to manage nausea and vomiting, rectal suppositories of prochlorperazine are often effective. Although it is necessary to consider the etiology of the nausea and vomiting, prochlorperazine is generally a good initial agent.

Anticholinergic agent. As death approaches, patients can have difficulty in clearing pharyngeal secretions, and as a result, generate a sound commonly known as a death rattle.[65] Although patients are often unconscious at this point, this sound can be very distressing to those nearby. An anticholinergic agent (e.g., glycopyrrolate, hyoscyamine, scopolamine, atropine) can be administered in an attempt to dry these pharyngeal secretions. This treatment modality is usually initiated after the patient has become obtunded; if begun too early, patients might develop problems with thickened bronchial or pulmonary secretions, tachycardia, delirium, dry mouth, or other adverse anticholinergic effects. Glycopyrrolate, available in a tablet or injectable formulation (and soon-to-be-available oral solution), is a good choice for an anticholinergic agent because it minimally crosses the blood–brain barrier. The 1-mg tablets could be crushed and placed under the tongue every 8 hours. Hyoscyamine is available as oral tablets, oral sustained-release tablets, sublingual tablets, oral liquid, oral solution, and injection. Either the sublingual tablets or oral solution of hyoscyamine can be given in a 0.125- to 0.25-mg dose sublingually every 4 hours as needed. Scopolamine transdermal patches have a slow onset of action (blood levels are detected 4 hours after application)[66] and are of limited utility in this situation. The oral or sublingual administration of atropine ophthalmic solution 1% is convenient to administer and is cost-effective. Assuming that 20 drops is approximately equivalent to 1 mL, patients can be given 0.5 to 1 mg (1–2 drops) of the atropine ophthalmic solution orally or sublingually every 4 hours as needed. Families and caregivers must be instructed not to use this in the eye.

CASE 5-1, QUESTION 4: The hospice nurse for M.P. has difficulty finding oral morphine sulfate available from a pharmacy and difficulty in finding a pharmacy willing to accept a faxed prescription. Why is morphine so difficult to obtain, and how should the nurse manage this problem?

Providing relief for pain or other symptoms with opioids is often difficult owing to numerous barriers. Patients and caregivers are often fearful of opioids, or mistakenly believe these medications will cause addiction or hasten death.[67] Pharmacists can create barriers by not having opioids in the pharmacy, sometimes because of the fear of robbery, fear of investigation by drug regulatory agencies, or insufficient appreciation of the usefulness of opioids in pain management and palliative care.[68] Pharmacists who are inexperienced in providing service to hospice patients might not be knowledgeable about federal regulations governing the provision of controlled substances to hospice patients. Federal statutes, as well as most state statutes, permit prescriptions for Schedule II controlled substances for hospice patients to be faxed. According to the Code of Federal Regulations (21CFR1306.11) paragraph (g): "A prescription prepared in accordance with 1306.05 written for a Schedule II narcotic substance for a patient enrolled in a hospice care program certified and/or paid for by Medicare under Title XVIII or a hospice program which is licensed by the state may be transmitted by the practitioner or the practitioner's agent to the dispensing pharmacy by facsimile. The practitioner or the practitioner's agent will note on the prescription that the patient is a hospice patient. The facsimile serves as the original written prescription for purposes of this paragraph (g) and it shall be maintained in accordance with 1304.04(h)."[69]

The process of ordering controlled substances for use by hospice patients at home can take many hours, and sometimes as much as an entire day. Hospice providers should anticipate possible difficulties when placing orders for Schedule II controlled substance medications. M.P.'s nurse should take the time to address any concerns M.P.'s caregivers and family may have about these medications (i.e., how they may affect her, any worries about addiction, side effects, etc.) and allow ample time to order them so that symptoms can be managed as they develop.

PAIN MANAGEMENT

For a diagram that shows a schema for the approach to pain management, go to http://thepoint.lww.com/AT10e.

ONLINE CONTENT

CASE 5-2

QUESTION 1: G.G., a 40-year-old woman, is admitted to hospice with stage IV ovarian cancer, metastatic to her pelvis, liver, and lungs. She was diagnosed after many months of nonspecific complaints of gastric distress and bloating. On laparotomy, she was evaluated as stage III and underwent a total abdominal hysterectomy and bilateral salpingo-oophorectomy and tumor debulking at that time. She has undergone subsequent chemotherapy and repeated tumor debulkings. In the past 6 months, her weight has decreased from 175 pounds to 153 pounds (she is 62 inches tall). Her primary complaints are constant nausea, constipation, and gripping abdominal pain, which she characterizes as burning and twisting. She quantifies the pain as 8 of 10 (on a 0- to 10-point scale) and describes the pain as one that moves into her groin and leg. Her family is unhappy about the drowsiness she experiences from her medications; they believe she is overmedicated. She has no known allergies. Her current medications include fentanyl transdermal system 75 mcg/hour every 72 hours, extended-release morphine sulfate capsules 50 mg three times daily (usually intended for once-daily administration), docusate sodium 250 mg daily, lansoprazole 30 mg daily, and lorazepam 0.5 mg every 4 hours as needed for nausea and anxiety. What is the most accurate assessment of her pain management regimen?

G.G. is currently using two long-acting opioids (i.e., fentanyl transdermal, sustained-release morphine), but is still unable to achieve relief of her pain, which is probably neuropathic pain (burning and twisting). The use of two long-acting agents is duplicative and should be replaced with one opioid. Methadone may be a better long-acting agent because it has activity against neuropathic pain (see Chapter 7, Pain and Its Management). When converting fentanyl and morphine to methadone, the following should be considered: (a) patient adherence and ability to follow prescription directions, (b) use of an appropriate conversion formula, (c) converting a transdermal formulation of fentanyl to an oral opioid formulation, and (d) a supplemental opioid for breakthrough pain.

Because of its long and variable elimination half-life, the dose of methadone should generally be adjusted only once every 4 to 6 days, and patients must be able and willing to precisely follow directions for its use. The methadone prescribing information should be used for the conversion, with a general rule of thumb being that the initial methadone dose should not exceed 30 mg (Table 5-5).[70,71]

Once the conversion is made, the calculated dose is adjusted and the dosing interval is set at every 12, 8, or 6 hours, based on patient age, previous use of opioids, and current clinical status. Clinical judgment is vital in individualizing a regimen for each patient based on his or her needs.

Before calculating the conversion to methadone for G.G., an important consideration in patients using transdermal fentanyl is an assessment of its absorption.[72] Fentanyl from the transdermal system is absorbed through several layers of the skin and deposited in the subcutaneous fat, from which it is

TABLE 5-5
Conversion of Oral Morphine Dose to Oral Methadone Requirement

Total Daily Baseline Oral Morphine Dose (i.e., Dose of Morphine Equivalents)	Estimated Daily Oral Methadone Requirement (as % of Total Daily Morphine Dose)
<100 mg	20%–30%
100–300 mg	10%–20%
300–600 mg	8%–12%
600–1,000 mg	5%–10%
>1,000 mg	<5%

absorbed into the systemic circulation. It is generally observed that transdermal fentanyl is not effective in very thin, cachectic patients. In those cases, the conversion would be made without including the fentanyl. The patch would be removed at initiation of the first methadone dose and supplemented with medication for breakthrough pain if needed. In patients using multiple patches, one patch can be removed every 3 days. Despite weight loss, G.G. (62 inches and 153 pounds) is not cachectic, and the fentanyl should be included when calculating the conversion of her current opioid dose to a comparable methadone dose. In this patient, her sustained-release morphine formulation (50 mg three times daily) is equivalent to 150 mg/day of oral morphine. Her fentanyl transdermal system 75 mcg/hour is equivalent to about 150 mg/day of oral morphine. Her total morphine equivalents per day are 150 mg plus 150 mg, or 300 mg. Using a 1 : 5 ratio for conversion of morphine equivalents to methadone, the calculated dose of oral methadone for this patient should be about 60 mg/day.

Although G.G. is relatively young, has been using opioids for some time, and has severe pain (quantified at 8 of 10), a methadone dose of 20 mg every 8 hours (i.e., 60 mg/day) might be excessive. She should be treated with 15 mg of methadone every 8 hours (45 mg/day), and the dose increased, if needed, based on her clinical response. This smaller initial dose would accommodate for some incomplete cross-tolerance from the morphine and fentanyl, and for any fentanyl that remains in her system for the next several days. Patients who have been on much higher doses of opioids, alternatively, can be converted during a period of several days (e.g., converting one-third of the previous daily dose of opioid every 3 days). This is an especially useful method for converting opioid doses for thin, cachectic patients who have been on multiple transdermal patches. A clinician should be in touch with G.G. frequently during the first several days after her conversion to methadone. A telephone call should be made 2 to 4 hours after the first dose to assess for efficacy and toxicity (primarily somnolence, confusion, or nausea). If pain relief does not last for the entire dosing interval, it can be adjusted, or G.G. can be instructed to take an extra dose of methadone.

An added benefit in changing to methadone for G.G. is a financial one for the hospice. Outpatient prescription prices for long-acting opioids are very steep and significantly add to hospice costs. The prudent use of methadone can improve overall pain management and keep costs in check. When methadone is not appropriate, generic extended-release morphine is a good second choice. Transdermal fentanyl should be reserved for patients who cannot take oral medication or for when there are significant compliance issues. Extended-release oxycodone should be used only when patients cannot tolerate morphine, have significant renal impairment, or have other contraindications to its use. By converting to methadone, G.G.'s daily cost for the opioid alone will decrease substantially, while still providing appropriate and effective pain management.

G.G. will also need a supplemental analgesic for breakthrough pain. Some practitioners use small doses of methadone, 2.5 mg or 5 mg, as often as every 3 hours. This is a good choice in a well-supervised (i.e., inpatient) setting with nurses familiar with the use of methadone. However, if caregivers treat methadone as if it were morphine, which is much more commonly used for breakthrough pain, the risk of overmedicating the patient is very real. This can have disastrous consequences, especially in frail, elderly patients. Because G.G. is not in an inpatient setting and has tolerated morphine well in the past, 30 mg or 1.5 mL of morphine 20 mg/mL can be prescribed to be taken every 2 hours as needed for breakthrough pain.

Aggressive Symptom Management and Palliative Sedation

CASE 5-3

QUESTION 1: D.V., a 35-year-old man with gastric cancer metastasized to the esophagus with periaortic involvement, is hospitalized. He was diagnosed 10 months ago, and his disease has progressed despite multiple courses of chemotherapy (most recently, irinotecan and cetuximab). A double-lumen, peripherally inserted central catheter line has been inserted. He has lost 65 pounds since diagnosis, weighs 150 pounds at 6 feet tall, and presents with abdominal pain, severe nausea, vomiting, obstipation (intractable constipation), and general malaise. D.V. describes his pain as a 7 of 10 in intensity and as "burning like a knife through my stomach." He uses 50 to 75 patient-controlled analgesia (PCA) bolus doses every 24 hours. He has no other medical problems. D.V. is referred to hospice care because he and his wife have agreed to stop chemotherapy and do not want to go back to the hospital. He states a history of allergic reactions to morphine, ondansetron, and diphenhydramine, although these reactions are not noted. He is presently receiving hydromorphone 2 mg/hour in an IV infusion with 1 mg PCA bolus dose every 5 minutes, hydromorphone 4 mg orally every 4 hours as needed for pain, fentanyl transdermal 275 mcg/hour every 3 days, ketamine 20 mg orally every 3 hours, senna two tablets twice daily, docusate sodium 250 mg twice, PEG 3350 17 g daily, lactulose 15 mL as needed for constipation, lorazepam 2 mg orally every 4 hours as needed for nausea or vomiting, metoclopramide 10 mg orally every 6 hours as needed for nausea or vomiting, promethazine 25 mg IV every 4 hours as needed for nausea or vomiting, baclofen 10 mg every 8 hours as needed for hiccups, and pantoprazole 40 mg once daily. What is your assessment of his medication regimen?

D.V.'s drug regimen is unnecessarily complicated for a patient at home. It may be possible to simplify it by looking at each problem anew. His pain is poorly managed as evidenced by his complaint of pain intensity at 7 of 10 (on a scale of 0–10), the use of multiple opioids, and the use of excessive PCA boluses. Once an infusion with PCA dosing is started, there is no need to continue other long-acting opioids (i.e., transdermal fentanyl) or oral agents for breakthrough pain. The PCA doses are serving as the rescue doses for breakthrough pain, and pain relief should be titrated using this method alone. Once pain is well controlled, an oral long-acting agent can be considered if the patient is able to swallow. To do otherwise creates a chaotic approach. Patients reporting allergic reactions to opioids should be carefully asked to describe the precise nature of the purported allergic reaction. True allergies to opioids are rare; patients often refer to an adverse reaction as an allergy, or have experienced an effect from the histamine release that is associated with opioids. Hydromorphone, especially injectable hydromorphone, is much more expensive and no more effective than morphine and is best reserved for use in patients who have a genuine allergy to morphine.

Although D.V. had been prescribed ketamine every 3 hours in the hospital, it is unrealistic to expect that this can be continued in the home setting. D.V. and his wife would probably be glad to discontinue it and replace it with an alternative because of his need to be dosed so often.

D.V.'s constipation is currently treated with multiple medications within the same therapeutic class. It would be more prudent to maximize the use of a single agent within a category, rather than using two products at less than the maximally recommended doses. D.V. can use a higher dose of senna (up to four tablets twice daily), and then, if necessary, add sorbitol (which is more cost effective than lactulose).

D.V. also takes multiple medications for his nausea and vomiting. The injectable promethazine can be converted to suppositories for use at home. He had also been directed to take lorazepam for his nausea and vomiting; however, benzodiazepines are not effective antiemetics. They are given to manage the anxiety associated with nausea and vomiting, and are particularly useful in managing the anticipatory nausea and vomiting that is commonly encountered during chemotherapy administration. Metoclopramide can be useful for D.V.'s nausea and vomiting if his physical examination reveals hypoactive bowel sounds. It is also useful for treating hiccups, and the need for baclofen can be reassessed.

CASE 5-3, QUESTION 2: A few days after arriving home, D.V. asks his hospice nurse, "Can't you just give me something to end it all?" He has not been sleeping well, is tired of taking so many medications, and wants to alleviate the burden he feels he is imposing on his wife.

In patients who are terminally ill, suffering may continue despite maximal palliative efforts. As a result, practitioners continually encounter patients' requests for the ending of their lives because of overwhelming suffering. Although controversial, most clinicians are significantly averse to this practice both ethically and legally.[73–80] Although substantial numbers of clinicians can imagine situations in which assisted suicide would be acceptable, few are willing to actively participate in the ending of a patient's life.[81,82]

In a small number of patients, it may be desirable to reduce suffering by the thoughtful use of medications to induce sedation.[83–86] It is not appropriate to increase opioid doses to achieve the desired sedated state. Medications used successfully to induce sedation for these patients include benzodiazepines, barbiturates, and propofol. No drug or drug class is superior to any other for this use.[87,88]

A trial of palliative sedation with intravenous lorazepam could be initiated and managed by the hospice nurse at a rate of 1 mg/hour and gradually increased if needed to the desired effect.[88] Although palliative sedation has a small potential to shorten life, the need to relieve terminal agitation could justify this risk. Palliative sedation should only be initiated as a last resort in severe cases not responsive to other palliative measures, and only after thorough discussion of the important clinical and ethical issues with the patient, family, and other clinical team members.

CASE 5-3, QUESTION 3: Repeated increases in the hydromorphone infusion basal rate (he is now at 25 mg/hour) had little effect on managing D.V.'s pain, and his consistent use

of up to 120 PCA attempts in 24 hours reflects his continued pain. He describes the intensity of his pain as 8 of 10. Before considering palliative sedation, what other therapeutic interventions can be implemented for D.V.?

Before considering palliative sedation, patients should be thoroughly assessed for insomnia and depression. Underlying reasons for insomnia should be explored and treated. Poor pain management is often the cause. In D.V., lidocaine 0.5 to 1 mg/kg/hour administered IV or subcutaneously might be useful to assist in the management of his severe neuropathic pain.[89–93] Lidocaine purportedly interrupts pain transmission by blocking sodium channels (see Chapter 7, Pain and Its Management).

D.V. was started on lidocaine 1 mg/kg/hour IV. A bolus dose was not given because of the short half-life of lidocaine. Overnight, his use of hydromorphone boluses dropped to one. He now reports his pain as 1 of 10 and that he slept through the night for the first time in months. During the next 2 days, the hydromorphone basal rate was tapered to 5 mg/hour. He did not experience any lidocaine toxicity, such as perioral numbness, metallic taste, or somnolence. D.V. continued on lidocaine, using no hydromorphone boluses for the next 2 weeks, until he died at home surrounded by his family.

KEY REFERENCES AND WEBSITES

A full list of references for this chapter can be found at http://thepoint.lww.com/AT10e. Below are the key references and website for this chapter, with the corresponding reference number in this chapter found in parentheses after the reference.

Key References

Bruera E et al, eds. *Textbook of Palliative Medicine*. New York, NY: Oxford University Press; 2006. (2)

National Consensus Project for Quality Palliative Care (2009). *Clinical Practice Guidelines for Quality Palliative Care, Second Edition*. http://www.nationalconsensusproject.org. Accessed March 11, 2011. (4)

Electronic Code of Federal Regulations. Title 42–Public Health, Chapter IV—Centers for Medicare and Medicaid Services, Department of Health and Human Services, Part 418—Hospice Care. http://ecfr.gpoaccess.gov/cgi/t/text/textidx?c=ecfr&sid=6265ddb45c786ea731b66312dcf31d44&rgn=div5&view=text&node=42:3.0.1.1.5&idno=42. Accessed July 18, 2011. (12)

American Society of Health-System Pharmacists. ASHP statement on the pharmacist's role in hospice and palliative care. *Am J Health Syst Pharm*. 2002;59:1770. (29)

Lycan J et al. Improving efficacy, efficiency and economics of hospice individualized drug therapy. *Am J Hosp Palliat Care*. 2002;19:135. (31)

Lee J, McPherson MF. Outcomes of recommendations by hospice pharmacists. *Am J Health Syst Pharm*. 2006;63:2235. (33)

Wilson S et al. Impact of pharmacist intervention on clinical outcomes in the palliative care setting. *Am J Hosp Palliat Care*. 2010 November 28. [Epub ahead of print] (41)

Victoria Hospice Society. Palliative Performance Scale (PPSv2), version 2. Medical Care of the Dying. 4th ed. Victoria, British Columbia, Canada: Victoria Hospice Society; 2006:120. http://www.victoriahospice.org/sites/default/files/imce/PPS ENGLISH.pdf. Accessed April 17, 2011. (44)

Qaseem A et al. Evidence-based interventions to improve the palliative care of pain, dyspnea, and depression at the end of life: a clinical practice guideline from the American College of Physicians. *Ann Intern Med*. 2008;148:141. (56)

U.S. Food and Drug Administration. Code of Federal Regulations Title 21. 21CFR1306.11(g). http://www.accessdata.fda.gov/scripts/cdrh/cfdocs/cfcfr/CFRSearch.cfm?fr=1306.11. Accessed April 24, 2011. (69)

Fass J, Fass A. Physician-assisted suicide: ongoing challenges for pharmacists. *Am J Health Syst Pharm*. 2011;68:846. (81)

Kirk TW et al. National Hospice and Palliative Care Organization (NHPCO) position statement and commentary on the use of palliative sedation in imminently dying terminally ill patients. *J Pain Symptom Manage*. 2010;39:914. (83)

Key Websites

American Academy of Hospice and Palliative Medicine (AAHPM). http://www.aahpm.org/

Center to Advance Palliative Care (CAPC). http://www.capc.org/

Children's Hospice and Palliative Care Coalition. http://www.childrenshospice.org

Centers for Medicare & Medicaid Services (CMS). http://www.cms.gov/center/hospice.asp

End of Life/Palliative Education Resource Center (EPERC). http://www.eperc.mcw.edu/eperc

Hospice Foundation of America (HFA). http://www.hospicefoundation.org/

Innovations in End-of-Life Care (an international journal of leaders in end-of-life care). http://www2.edc.org/lastacts/

International Association for Hospice & Palliative Care (IAHPC). http://www.hospicecare.com/

MedlinePlus. Hospice Care. http://www.nlm.nih.gov/medlineplus/hospicecare.html

National Hospice and Palliative Care Organization (NHPCO). http://www.nhpco.org/

The Population-based Palliative Care Research Network (PoPCRN). http://www.ucdenver.edu/academics/colleges/medicalschool/departments/medicine/GIM/Popcrn/Pages/PopcrnHome.aspx

End of Life Online Curriculum. http://endoflife.stanford.edu/M00_overview/intro_lrn_overv.html

NHPCO Pediatric Palliative Care and Hospice. http://www.nhpco.org/pediatrics

American Academy of Pediatrics. Section on Hospice and Palliative Medicine. http://www.aap.org/sections/palliative

The National Consensus Project for Quality Palliative Care. http://www.nationalconsensusproject.org

6 Nausea and Vomiting

Lisa K. Lohr

CORE PRINCIPLES

	CHAPTER CASES
MOTION SICKNESS	
1 Motion sickness is caused by discordant information about body position or motion received from visual, vestibular, or body proprioceptors. Acetylcholine is thought to be the primary neurotransmitter involved.	**Case 6-1 (Question 1)**
2 Transdermal scopolamine is recommended for prophylaxis of motion sickness for moderate to severe stimuli. Dimenhydrinate or promethazine are recommended for treatment of breakthrough symptoms. The most common adverse effects of these agents include drowsiness, confusion, and dry mouth.	**Case 6-1 (Question 2), Table 6-1**
CHEMOTHERAPY-INDUCED NAUSEA AND VOMITING	
1 Nausea and vomiting are initiated by several stimuli, and mediated by several neurotransmitters in the central nervous system, peripheral nervous system, and gastrointestinal tract. Because of the multiple neurotransmitter receptors involved, successful prophylaxis and treatment of chemotherapy-induced nausea and vomiting will almost always require medications with more than one mechanism of action.	**Case 6-2 (Question 1)**
2 The likelihood of nausea and vomiting depends on patient risk factors and most importantly on the emetogenicity of the chemotherapy agents prescribed. The antiemetic regimen should be appropriate for the chemotherapy agent with the highest emetogenicity level.	**Case 6-2 (Question 1), Table 6-2**
3 Patients receiving highly emetogenic chemotherapy should receive prophylaxis with a 5-serotonin receptor type 3 (5-HT_3) antagonist, dexamethasone, and fosaprepitant or aprepitant. Patients receiving moderately emetogenic chemotherapy should receive prophylaxis with a 5-HT_3 antagonist and dexamethasone (plus fosaprepitant or aprepitant for those chemotherapy agents posing a high risk of delayed nausea and vomiting).	**Case 6-2 (Question 2), Tables 6-3, 6-4, Figures 6-2, 6-3**
4 For breakthrough symptoms, patients should receive rescue antiemetics with a different mechanism of action than the prophylactic medications and receive more aggressive antiemetics before the next cycle of chemotherapy.	**Case 6-2 (Question 3), Tables 6-3, 6-4, Figures 6-2, 6-3**
RADIATION-INDUCED NAUSEA AND VOMITING	
1 Radiation can cause nausea and vomiting by the same pathways as chemotherapy. The risk depends on the area and size of the radiation field as well as the fractional dose of radiation and whether the patient has had chemotherapy in the past.	**Case 6-3 (Question 1), Table 6-5**
2 The recommended prophylaxis for radiation-induced nausea and vomiting includes a 5-HT_3 antagonist with dexamethasone for high-risk patients, and with or without dexamethasone for patients at moderate risk. Breakthrough symptoms may be treated with a 5-HT_3 antagonist or dopamine antagonist.	**Case 6-3 (Question 1), Table 6-5**

continued

POSTOPERATIVE NAUSEA AND VOMITING

1	The risk of postoperative nausea and vomiting depends on several patient, surgical and anesthetic factors. The antiemetic regimen should be proportional to the risk factors.	**Case 6-4 (Question 1), Table 6-6**
2	The most active agents in preventing postoperative nausea and vomiting are 5-HT_3 antagonists. For patients at moderate to high risk, a 5-HT_3 antagonist should be combined with dexamethasone or droperidol. Antiemetics used for rescue therapy should be of a different class than the prophylaxis agents used.	**Case 6-4 (Question 1), Table 6-6**

DEFINITION

Nausea and vomiting are unpleasant symptoms caused by self-limiting disorders or serious conditions such as cancer. These symptoms can range from mild, short-lived nausea to continuing severe emesis and retching. The emetic response can be described in three phases: nausea, vomiting, and retching. *Nausea* is the subjective feeling of the need to vomit. It includes an unpleasant sensation in the mouth and stomach and can be associated with salivation, sweating, dizziness, and tachycardia. *Vomiting* is the forceful expulsion of the stomach contents through the mouth, but is preceded by the relaxation of the esophageal sphincter, contraction of the abdominal muscles, and temporary suspension of breathing. *Retching* is the rhythmic contraction of the abdominal muscles without actual emesis. It can accompany nausea, or occur before or after emesis.

EPIDEMIOLOGY AND CLINICAL PRESENTATION

Nausea and vomiting are caused by many disorders. Central nervous system (CNS) causes include increased intracranial pressure, migraine headaches, brain metastases, vestibular dysfunction, alcohol intoxication, and anxiety. Infectious disease causes include viral gastroenteritis, food poisoning, peritonitis, meningitis, and urinary tract infections. Metabolic causes include hypercalcemia, uremia, hyperglycemia, and hyponatremia. Gastrointestinal disorders, such as gastroparesis, bowel obstruction, distension, and mechanical irritation, can cause nausea and vomiting. Among the many medications that can cause nausea and vomiting are cancer chemotherapy, antibiotics, antifungals, and opiate analgesics.

In addition to the suffering involved, uncontrolled vomiting can lead to dehydration, electrolyte imbalances, malnutrition, aspiration pneumonia, and esophageal tears. Nausea and vomiting often reduces food intake and can impair a person's ability to care for himself or herself. Significant reductions in quality-of-life scores have been demonstrated in cancer patients with chemotherapy-induced nausea and vomiting compared with patients who did not have those symptoms.[1]

PATHOPHYSIOLOGY

The CNS, the peripheral nervous system, and the gastrointestinal (GI) tract are all involved in initiating and coordinating the emetic response. In the CNS, the vomiting center (VC) receives incoming signals from other parts of the brain and the GI tract and then coordinates the emetic response by sending signals to the effector organs. The VC is located in the medulla oblongata of the brain, near the nucleus tractus solitarius (NTS). The VC is stimulated by neurotransmitters released from the chemoreceptor trigger zone (CTZ), the GI tract, the cerebral cortex, the limbic system, and the vestibular system (Fig. 6-1). The major neurotransmitter receptors associated with the emetic response include serotonin (the 5-hydroxytryptamine type 3, [5-HT_3]) receptors, neurokinin 1 (NK1) receptors, and dopamine receptors. Other receptors involved include corticosteroid, acetylcholine, histamine, cannabinoid, gabaminergic, and opiate receptors. Many of these receptors are targets for antiemetic therapy.

In the CNS, the CTZ is located in the area postrema on the floor of the fourth ventricle in the brainstem; it lies outside the blood–brain barrier. When the CTZ senses toxins and noxious substances in the blood or cerebrospinal fluid, it triggers the emetic response by releasing neurotransmitters that travel to the VC and the NTS. The major neurotransmitter receptors include serotonin, dopamine, and neurokinin 1.

The GI system also plays a large part in the initiation of the emetic response. The GI tract contains enterochromaffin cells in the GI mucosa. When these cells are damaged by chemotherapy, radiation, anesthetics, or mechanical irritation, serotonin is released, which can stimulate the vagal afferents as well as directly stimulate the VC and NTS. The vomiting center then initiates the emetic response.

The cerebral cortex and limbic system can stimulate the emetic center in response to emotional states such as anxiety, pain, and conditioned responses (anticipatory nausea and vomiting). The neurotransmitters involved in this pathway are less well understood. Disorders of the vestibular system, such as vertigo and motion sickness, stimulate the VC through acetylcholine and histamine release.

DIAGNOSIS

The initial evaluation of the patient with nausea and vomiting should include the onset of symptoms, the severity and duration of symptoms, hydration status, precipitating factors, current medical conditions and medications, and food and infectious contacts. The etiology of the nausea and vomiting should be determined, if possible, so that underlying conditions can be treated specifically. Supportive treatment should be initiated, if needed, including fluid and electrolyte replacement. If the nausea and vomiting is mild and self-limited, antiemetic therapy may not be required. For others, however, the appropriate antiemetic therapy will depend on the patient and the etiology of the nausea and vomiting.

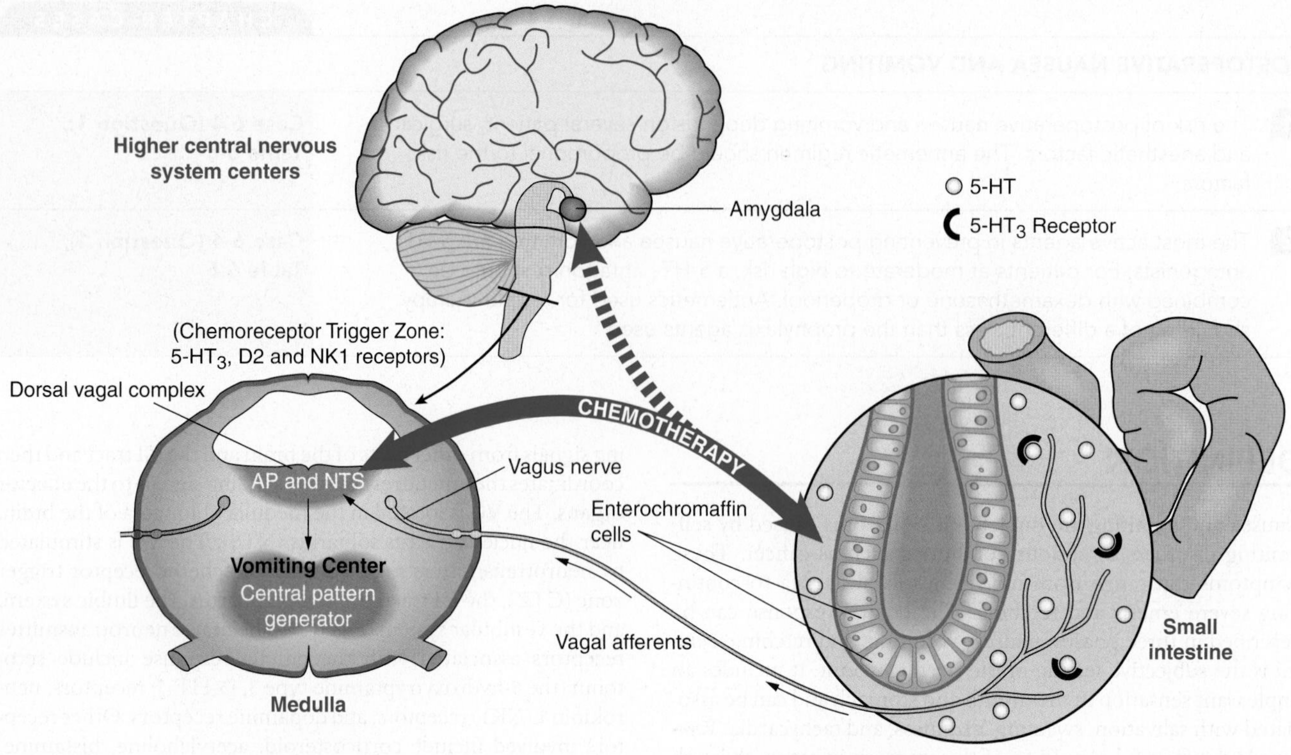

FIGURE 6-1 Pathways by which chemotherapeutic agents may produce an emetic response. AP, anterior pituitary; 5-HT, serotonin; 5-HT_3, serotonin type 3 receptor; NTS, nucleus tractus solitarius.

MOTION SICKNESS

Clinical Presentation and Risk Factors

CASE 6-1

QUESTION 1: P.C. is a 27-year-old woman who has no significant medical history, with the exception of moderate dysmenorrhea and motion sickness associated with travel by air. Previously, she has taken dimenhydrinate before airplane trips with moderate success. She is engaged to be married, and she and her fiancé have decided on a weeklong Caribbean cruise for their honeymoon. P.C. is concerned that she may also develop sea sickness and that dimenhydrinate may not control her symptoms, particularly in the event of rough weather at sea. Will P.C. be at higher risk for motion sickness?

The symptoms of motion sickness occur in response to an unusual perception of real or apparent motion. In these situations, there is sensory conflict about body position or motion through the visual, vestibular, or body proprioceptors. Acetylcholine is thought to be the primary neurotransmitter involved in signaling the VC, as is histamine, but to a lesser extent. Adrenergic stimulation can block this transmission. Symptoms begin with stomach discomfort and progress to salivation changes, sweating, dizziness, lethargy, retching, and emesis. The risk of motion sickness is low in children younger than 2 years of age. The risk is highest in children and adolescents compared with adults, and higher in women than men. In some individuals, sensitivity to motion sickness diminishes with time.[2] Travel by boat is most likely to cause symptoms; air, car, and train travel is less likely.[3,4] The severity of the motion sickness is highly dependent on the individual and also varies with the weather and position in the plane or boat. Because of P.C.'s history and her travel plans, she is at high risk for recurrence of her motion sickness symptoms.

Nonpharmacologic measures or natural remedies may be useful for reducing motion sickness.[2] These include riding in the middle of the boat or plane where the motion is less dramatic, lying in a semirecumbent position, fixing the vision on the horizon, avoiding reading, and closing the eyes if below deck or in the cabin. Many people recommend keeping active on a ship to "get their sea-legs" faster through habituation. The effectiveness of acupressure at the P6 point of the wrist (about three fingerbreadths above the wrist) is unclear. A controlled-stimulus trial compared two brands of wristbands with placebo; neither band was more effective than placebo in preventing symptoms of motion sickness.[5] Studies of ginger preparations also are equivocal. The action of ginger may be through enhanced gastric emptying and not on the vestibular system.[6,7]

Overview of Treatment

CASE 6-1, QUESTION 2: For P.C., what medications are available to prevent and treat motion sickness symptoms?

Anticholinergic agents and antihistamines that cross the blood–brain barrier effectively prevent and treat motion sickness.[3,4] In general, these medications are more effective in preventing than treating established symptoms. 5-HT_3 receptor antagonists and NK1 receptor antagonists have not been shown to be effective in preventing motion sickness.[2,6] Nonsedating antihistamines are not as effective as other antihistamines because they do not sufficiently cross the blood–brain barrier.[2,3] Scopolamine has been well studied for the prevention of motion sickness and is highly effective.[2,8] In a controlled trial, scopolamine was more effective than promethazine and both were more

TABLE 6-1
Medications for Prevention or Treatment of Motion Sickness in Adults

Medication (Trade Name)	Dosage	Recommended Use	Adverse Effects
Scopolamine (Transderm-Scop)	1.5 mg TOP behind the ear every 3 days. Apply at least 3 hours (preferably 6–8 hours) before exposure.	Long-term exposure (>6 hours) to moderate to intense stimulus. Alternative treatment for shorter or milder stimulus.	Dry mouth, drowsiness, blurred vision, confusion, fatigue, ataxia
Dimenhydrinate (Dramamine)	50–100 mg PO every 4–6 hours (max 400 mg/day). May be taken PRN or on scheduled basis if required.	Short- or long-term exposure to mild to moderate stimulus. Alternative for intense stimulus.	Drowsiness, dry mouth, thickening of secretions, dizziness
Promethazine (Phenergan)	25 mg PO every 4–6 hours. May be taken PRN or on scheduled basis if required. 25–50 mg IM every 4–6 hours for established severe symptoms. May be taken PRN or on scheduled basis if required.	In combination with dextroamphetamine for short exposure to intense stimulus. Alternative for longer or milder stimulus.	Drowsiness, orthostatic hypotension, dry mouth
Meclizine (Antivert, Bonine)	12.5–50 mg PO every 6–24 hours. May be taken PRN or on scheduled basis if required.	Alternative for mild stimulus or in combination for moderate to severe stimulus.	Drowsiness, dry mouth, thickening of secretions, dizziness
Dextroamphetamine (Dexedrine)	5–10 mg PO every 4–6 hours. May be taken PRN or on scheduled basis if required.	In combination with promethazine for short exposure of intense stimulus.	Restlessness, abuse potential, insomnia, overstimulation, tachycardia, palpitations, hypertension
Cyclizine (Marezine)	50 mg PO every 4–6 hours (max 200 mg/day). May be taken PRN or on scheduled basis if required.	Alternative for mild stimulus situations.	Drowsiness, dry mouth,

IM, intramuscular; PO, oral; PRN, as needed; TOP, topically.
Source: Priesol AJ. Motion sickness. Up To Date. http://www.uptodate.com/contents/motion-sickness?source=search_result&selectedTitle=1%7E51. Accessed September 27, 2010; Shupak A, Gordon CR. Motion sickness: advances in pathogenesis, prediction, prevention, and treatment. *Aviat Space Environ Med.* 2006;77:1213.

effective than placebo, meclizine, or lorazepam.[9] Scopolamine is available as a topical patch, which bypasses the problem of GI symptoms associated with motion sickness. Table 6-1 describes medications effective for motion sickness based on the intensity of the stimulus, adult doses, and potential adverse effects.

Because P.C. is a susceptible individual in a moderate-severe stimulus situation, prevention with a scopolamine patch applied behind the ear every 3 days, starting 6 to 8 hours before departure, should be recommended. If she experiences breakthrough symptoms, dimenhydrinate or promethazine may be useful. She should be advised about the potential adverse effects of these agents, which include drowsiness, confusion, and dry mouth.

CHEMOTHERAPY-INDUCED NAUSEA AND VOMITING

Clinical Presentation and Risk Factors

CASE 6-2

QUESTION 1: M.C., a 54-year-old woman with breast cancer, is in the clinic today to receive her first cycle of chemotherapy. Her chemotherapy will consist of intravenous (IV) docetaxel 75 mg/m^2, carboplatin dosed to achieve an area under the curve (AUC) of 6 mg/mL/minute. This will be repeated every 21 days. In addition, she will receive trastuzumab 4 mg/kg IV for one dose, then 2 mg/kg/week for 17 weeks. M.C. does not drink alcohol or smoke. Her only other medical condition is adult-onset diabetes, which is controlled with metformin and diet. She has had four children, now all grown, and had substantial morning sickness with each of her pregnancies. M.C.'s neighbor has told her that all chemotherapy causes severe nausea and vomiting. How likely is M.C. to experience nausea and vomiting?

Chemotherapy-induced nausea and vomiting (CINV) occurs in many patients receiving chemotherapy for cancer.[1] The mechanisms of the emetic response described at the beginning of this chapter apply to CINV as well. The major neurotransmitter receptors involved in these pathways include 5-HT$_3$, NK1, and dopamine receptors. CINV can occur in different phases. Acute-phase CINV symptoms occur within a few hours after the administration of the chemotherapy. These symptoms often peak several hours after administration and can last for the first 24 hours. Some antineoplastic agents can also cause nausea and vomiting symptoms for a longer time after chemotherapy administration. These delayed CINV symptoms peak in about 2 to 3 days and can last 6 to 7 days. Some patients experience acute symptoms without delayed symptoms. Some other patients experience delayed symptoms without acute symptoms, and many patients experience CINV in both the acute and delayed phases. Some patients who have received previous chemotherapy treatments may experience a conditioned response in which they have symptoms even before the chemotherapy starts. This is called *anticipatory nausea and vomiting,* and it is difficult to treat because it is primarily triggered by poor nausea and vomiting control in previous cycles. Breakthrough nausea and vomiting occur if the primary prophylactic antiemetics fail to work completely. Of course, regardless of the time course and cause, these are very distressing, unpleasant, and disruptive symptoms for the patient.

The likelihood of CINV depends on several factors.[1] Patient-related factors that increase the risk of acute-phase CINV include age younger than 50 years, female sex, poor control of symptoms in prior cycles, history of motion sickness or nausea with pregnancy, anxiety, or depression. A significant history of alcoholism actually protects against CINV. Delayed symptoms are more common in women, in those who have had poor emetic control in the acute phase, and in patients with anxiety or depression.

Chemotherapy-related factors also predict the likelihood of symptoms. Factors such as shorter infusion time, higher dose, and more chemotherapy cycles increase the risk of CINV. With multiday chemotherapy regimens, the symptoms usually peak on about the third to fourth day of chemotherapy, when the acute symptoms caused by the later days' doses are overlapping with the delayed symptoms from the first days' doses. The most predictive factor, however, is the chemotherapy agent's inherent ability to cause CINV, or its emetogenicity.[1,10,11] Antineoplastics that are most likely (>90% of patients) to cause symptoms are classified as highly emetogenic chemotherapy. Agents that cause nausea and vomiting in 30% to 90% of patients are classified as moderate-risk agents. Low emetogenicity agents cause symptoms in 10% to 30% of patients. Other chemotherapy agents have a minimal risk, causing CINV in less than 10% of patients. Table 6-2 lists selected chemotherapy agents in the various emetogenicity classes, noting that references differ in the estimation of emetic risk for some antineoplastic agents. The emetogenicity risk also depends on the dosage used and the route of administration.

Certain antineoplastic agents are more likely to cause delayed CINV symptoms. These include cisplatin, carboplatin, cyclophosphamide, doxorubicin, epirubicin, ifosfamide, and to a lesser degree, irinotecan and methotrexate. Patients receiving more than one of these agents are at high risk for delayed symptoms.

Most chemotherapy agents are given in combinations, rather than as single agents. Estimating the emetogenicity of chemotherapy combinations has always been difficult. The chemotherapy regimen that contains cyclophosphamide and either doxorubicin or epirubicin for breast cancer in females is highly emetogenic (symptoms in >90% of patients). The primary literature of the regimen should always be consulted to determine the emetic risk. Should that not be available, the antiemetic regimen should be geared toward the chemotherapy agent with the highest emetogenicity level given on that day.[1,12,13] For example, in a chemotherapy combination with one high-risk agent and one with a moderate risk, the antiemetic regimen should be appropriate for the high-risk chemotherapy agent.

Antiemetic efficacy, or complete emetic response, is usually defined as no emesis and no nausea or only mild nausea in the first 24 hours after chemotherapy administration. With currently recommended antiemetic regimens, most, but not all, patients will be protected from emesis in the acute phase (first 24 hours). Nausea, however, is more difficult to control. In addition, delayed CINV symptoms are more difficult to prevent.

Overview of Treatment

CASE 6-2, QUESTION 2: M.C. is at moderate risk for acute CINV. Her personal risk factors include female sex, history of morning sickness with pregnancy, and being a nondrinker. The docetaxel has a low risk of acute CINV, the carboplatin has a moderate risk of acute CINV with a high risk of delayed CINV, and the trastuzumab has a minimal risk of acute CINV. What antiemetics are available for M.C.?

Appropriate antiemetic therapy is based on the emetogenicity of the chemotherapy regimen and patient risk factors. Because the pathophysiologic response of nausea and vomiting involves many neurotransmitters, combinations of antiemetics from different therapeutic classes will be more effective in most situations than a single agent. The predominant classes of antiemetics used for CINV include 5-HT_3 antagonists, the NK1 antagonist, and corticosteroids.

5-HT_3 ANTAGONISTS

The 5-HT_3 antagonists inhibit the action of serotonin in the GI tract and the CNS and thereby block the transmission of emetic signals to the VC. 5-HT_3 antagonists are both highly effective and have minimal side effects. Several agents and dosage forms in this class are now available: ondansetron, granisetron, dolasetron, and palonosetron. Dosages of these agents are shown in Table 6-3. The route of administration should be matched to the clinical status of the patient. Oral tablets are appropriate for most patients, but intravenous, topical, or oral dissolving tablet formulations may be needed in patients who cannot take oral medications.

These agents have been widely studied, and some commonalities have emerged. All of the 5-HT_3 antagonists are considered to have equivalent efficacy.[14–19] All of these agents have a threshold effect and so a sufficiently large dose must be given to block the relevant receptors. In addition, the dose-response curve is relatively flat, such that escalating the dose beyond the threshold dose does not enhance efficacy. When given in appropriate doses, all of these agents have similar efficacy for acute CINV, with response rates of 60% to 80%, depending on study design.[1,12,14–19] The effectiveness of the 5-HT_3 receptor antagonists is enhanced by the addition of dexamethasone. The response rate increases by about 15% to 20% in regimens that include dexamethasone and a 5-HT_3 antagonist.[17,20] Oral and IV 5-HT_3 administration are equally effective assuming the patient can take oral medications. The side effects of all the 5-HT_3 antagonists are similar and fairly mild and include headache, constipation, diarrhea, and transient elevations of liver function tests. 5-HT_3 antagonists are one component of optimal antiemetic prophylaxis for acute CINV. They are not more effective than agents from other classes (notably dexamethasone, aprepitant, or prochlorperazine) for delayed CINV.[17,21–23] 5-HT_3 antagonists, therefore, are not generally recommended for delayed CINV. The 5-HT_3 antagonists are metabolized by different cytochrome P-450 enzymes, including CYP1A2, CYP2D6 and CYP3A4. Differences in the metabolic rate of 5-HT_3 antagonists attributable to CYP2D6 polymorphisms might account for differences in efficacy among individual patients.[17] However, these differences are not used clinically to choose initial antiemetic therapy at this time.

Ondansetron, granisetron, and dolasetron have similar pharmacokinetic parameters. Palonosetron, the newest member of the 5-HT_3 antagonist family, is distinguished by a longer elimination half-life than others in its class. Palonosetron was compared with single doses of 5-HT_3 antagonists with shorter half-lives in various studies. Palonosetron showed equivalent or somewhat superior efficacy, but questions have arisen regarding the lack of comparable treatment in the control arms.[18,24] One group of researchers described a three-drug combination of palonosetron, dexamethasone, and aprepitant in a noncomparative, phase II study with moderately emetogenic chemotherapy, and found that the three-drug combination was safe and effective.[25] Whether palonosetron is equivalent or superior to other 5-HT_3 antagonists should be determined by trials that compare palonosetron with another 5-HT_3 antagonist, with both treatment arms also containing dexamethasone and aprepitant in the acute and delayed phases. These trials have yet to be conducted. Currently, palonosetron is substantially more expensive than the generic forms of the other 5-HT_3 antagonists.

Palonosetron is normally administered as a single 0.25-mg IV or 0.5-mg oral (PO) dose before chemotherapy. With its long elimination half-life (about 40 hours), palonosetron should be

TABLE 6-2
Emetogenicity of Selected Antineoplastic Agents by Dose and Route of Administration

Chemotherapy Agent	Injectable Administration	Oral Administration
Aldesleukin (Proleukin)	>12–15 million units/m² = Moderate ≤12 million units/m² = Low	
Alemtuzumab (Campath)	Minimal	
Altretamine (Hexalen)		High
Arsenic trioxide (Trisenox)	Moderate	
Asparaginase (Elspar)	Minimal	
Azacitdine (Vidaza)	Moderate	
Bendamustine (Treanda)	Moderate	
Bevacizumab (Avastin)	Minimal	
Bexarotene (Targretin)		Low
Bleomycin (Blenoxane)	Minimal	
Bortezomib (Velcade)	Low	
Busulfan (Busulfex, Myleran)	Moderate	≥4 mg = Moderate <4 mg = Minimal
Cabazitaxel (Javtana)	Moderate	
Capecitabine (Xeloda)		Low
Carboplatin (Paraplatin)	Moderate with high risk of delayed CINV	
Carmustine (BiCNU)	>250 mg/m² = High ≤250 mg/m² = Moderate	
Chlorambucil (Leukeran)		Minimal
Cetuximab (Erbitux)	Minimal	
Cisplatin (Platinol)	≥50 mg/m² = High <50 mg/m² = Moderate High risk of delayed CINV	
Cladribine (Leustatin)	Minimal	
Clofarabine (Clolar)	Moderate	
Cyclophosphamide (Cytoxan)	>1,500 mg/m² = High ≤1,500 mg/m² = Moderate High risk of delayed CINV	≥100 mg/m²/d = Moderate <100 mg/m²/d = Low
Cytarabine (Ara-C, Cytosar-U)	>200 mg/m² = Moderate 100–200 mg/m² = Low <100 mg/m² = Minimal	
Dacarbazine (DTIC)	High	
Dactinomycin (Cosmegen)	Moderate	
Dasatinib (Sprycel)		Minimal
Daunorubicin (Cerubidine)	Moderate	
Decitabine (Dacogen)	Minimal	
Docetaxel (Taxotere)	Low	
Doxorubicin (Adriamycin)	Moderate High risk of delayed CINV	
Doxorubicin liposomal (Doxil)	Moderate	
Epirubicin (Ellence)	Moderate High risk of delayed CINV	
Erlotinib (Tarceva)		Minimal
Etoposide (VePeSid)	Low	Moderate
Everolimus (Afinitor)		Minimal
Fludarabine (Fludara)	Minimal	Low
Fluorouracil (Adrucil)	Low	
Gefitinib (Iressa)		Minimal
Gemcitabine (Gemzar)	Low	
Hydroxyurea (Hydrea)		Minimal
Idarubicin (Idamycin)	Moderate High risk of delayed CINV	
Ifosfamide (Ifex)	Moderate	
Imatinib (Gleevec)		Moderate
Interferon α2B (Intron A)	≥10 million units/m² = Moderate <10 million units/m² = Low	
Irinotecan (Camptosar)	Moderate Some risk of delayed CINV	
Ixabepilone (Ixempra)	Low	
Lapatinib (Tykerb)		Low
Lenalidomide (Revlimid)		Minimal
Lomustine (CeeNU)		Moderate
Mechlorethamine (Mustargen)	High	
Melphalan (Alkeran)	Moderate	Minimal
Mercaptopurine (Purinethol)		Minimal

(continued)

TABLE 6-2
Emetogenicity of Selected Antineoplastic Agents by Dose and Route of Administration (*Continued*)

Chemotherapy Agent	Injectable Administration	Oral Administration
Methotrexate (Trexall)	≥250 mg/m² = Moderate 50–249 mg/m² = Low <50 mg/m² = Minimal Some risk of delayed CINV	Minimal
Mitomycin (Mutamycin)	Low	
Mitoxantrone (Novantrone)	Low	
Nelarabine (Arranon)	Minimal	
Nilotinib (Tasigna)		Low
Oxaliplatin (Eloxatin)	Moderate	
Paclitaxel (Taxol)	Low	
Paclitaxel Protein Bound (Abraxane)	Low	
Panitumumab (Vectibix)	Minimal	
Pazopanib (Votrient)		Low
Pegasparaginase (Oncaspar)	Minimal	
Pemetrexed (Alimta)	Low	
Pentostatin (Nipent)	Low	
Pralatrexate (Folotyn)	Moderate	
Procarbazine (Matulane)		High
Rituximab (Rituxan)	Minimal	
Romidepsin (Istodax)	Low	
Sorafenib (Nexavar)		Minimal
Streptozocin (Zanosar)	High	
Sunitinib (Sutent)		Minimal
Temozolamide (Temodar)	Moderate	>75 mg/m²/d = Moderate ≤75 mg/m²/d = Low
Temsirolimus (Torisel)	Minimal	
Teniposide (Vumon)	Low	
Thalidomide (Thalomid)		Minimal
Thioguanine (Tabloid)		Minimal
Thiotepa (Thiotepa)	Low	
Topotecan (Hycamptin)	Moderate	Low
Trastuzumab (Herceptin)	Minimal	
Tretinoin (Vesanoid)		Low
Vinblastine (Velban)	Minimal	
Vincristine (Oncovin)	Minimal	
Vinorelbine (Navelbine)	Minimal	
Vorinostat (Zolinza)		Low

High = >90% (of patients would experience chemotherapy-induced nausea and vomiting [CINV] without antiemetic premedication); Moderate = 30%–90%; Low = 10%–30%; Minimal = <10%.
Source: Ettinger DS et al. Antiemesis: clinical practice guidelines in oncology. V2.2010. **http://www.nccn.org/professionals/physician_gls/pdf/antiemesis.pdf.** Accessed September 30, 2010; Grunberg SM et al. Evaluation of new antiemetic agents and definition of antineoplastic agent emetogenicity—an update. *Support Care Cancer.* 2005;13:80; American Society of Clinical Oncology et al. American Society of Clinical Oncology guideline for antiemetics in oncology: update 2006 [published correction appears in *J Clin Oncol.* 2006;24:5341]. *J Clin Oncol.* 2006;24:2932; Roila F et al. Guideline update for MASCC and ESMO in the prevention of chemotherapy- and radiotherapy-induced nausea and vomiting: results of the Perugia consensus conference. *Ann Oncol.* 2010;21(Suppl 5):v232.

effective for at least a few days, but little data are published using repeated doses in fewer than 7 days. Palonosetron has been studied in a three-dose regimen (administration on days 1, 3, 5) for multiday chemotherapy in an uncontrolled trial.[26] This regimen appeared to be safe and effective, but was not compared with any other regimen. It is not clear that palonosetron would have superior activity compared with repeated doses of the other 5-HT_3 antagonists.

It is difficult to identify the 5-HT_3 antagonist with the highest overall cost-effectiveness because drug acquisition costs vary between the inpatient and outpatient clinics and from institution to institution. Costs of the different agents should be compared at each practice site to determine the preferred agent.

CORTICOSTEROIDS

The mechanism of action of corticosteroids as antiemetics has not been fully determined. Some suggest that corticosteroids may decrease serotonin release, antagonize 5-HT_3, or activate corticosteroid receptors in the NTS of the medulla in the CNS.[20] Many studies validate the effectiveness of corticosteroids in the prophylaxis of CINV symptoms. Efficacy with both dexamethasone and methylprednisolone has been described, but dexamethasone is much more widely studied and almost exclusively used. Dexamethasone improves the antiemetic control of 5-HT_3 antagonists by about 15% to 20%.[20] In addition to its use in the acute phase of CINV, dexamethasone is one of the cornerstone agents used to prevent delayed CINV. It is inexpensive and available in both IV and oral formulations.

The optimal dose of dexamethasone with different emetic stimuli has been studied in controlled trials.[27] For moderately emetogenic chemotherapy in the acute phase, a single 8-mg dose was as effective as larger 24-mg doses or prolonged administration. In the setting of highly emetogenic cisplatin-based chemotherapy, higher doses of 12 or 20 mg were superior to doses of 4 and 8 mg. If dexamethasone is used with aprepitant in the acute phase, the lower 12-mg prechemotherapy dose is recommended because of inhibition of steroid metabolism by aprepitant (see the NK1 receptor antagonist section).[12] For prevention of delayed CINV symptoms, the most commonly used dose of dexamethasone is 8 mg twice daily on days 2 and 3 after chemotherapy without aprepitant. The dose for delayed CINV should be reduced to 8 mg daily when used with aprepitant.

Corticosteroids are sometimes underused because of the potential risk of side effects. The adverse effects of corticosteroids include insomnia, jitteriness, increased appetite, GI distress, and perineal irritation if the IV dexamethasone is infused too quickly.[18,27,28] For most patients, however, dexamethasone is well tolerated, especially because the therapy is typically short term at lower doses. Steroid-related hyperglycemia may occur, especially in patients with pre-existing diabetes.[20] These patients should be advised to monitor their glucose levels more frequently and contact their practitioner if the levels remain elevated. In the nondiabetic patient, hyperglycemia is uncommon. Tapering the corticosteroid dose after the end of treatment for CINV is usually unnecessary because the duration of therapy is short. Rare patients who have steroid withdrawal-like symptoms may, however, benefit from a short taper on repeated corticosteroid courses.

Corticosteroids also have antitumor properties and are a part of the antineoplastic regimen for some malignancies, such as lymphoma, lymphoid leukemia, and myeloma, and additional dexamethasone for the antiemetic protection is not necessary. In these cases, the corticosteroid should be administered just before the rest of the chemotherapy to provide antiemetic activity. If aprepitant is part of an antiemetic regimen in a situation where the corticosteroid is given for antitumor reasons, the dose of the corticosteroid should not be reduced.[12]

NEUROKININ 1 RECEPTOR ANTAGONISTS

The potential use of NK1 receptor antagonists as antiemetics became apparent when the role of substance P in the peripheral nervous system and CNS was recognized in the emetic stimulus pathway. Aprepitant, the first NK1 receptor antagonist available, is active in both the acute and delayed phases of CINV caused by moderately and highly emetogenic chemotherapy. Aprepitant is usually given as a 3-day oral regimen, 125 mg on day 1 and 80 mg on days 2 and 3. Early trials determined that aprepitant could not replace a 5-HT_3 antagonist, but that it would be used best in conjunction with corticosteroids and a 5-HT_3 antagonist.[29] Studies have shown that aprepitant-containing regimens were

TABLE 6-3
Antiemetic Agents for Chemotherapy-Induced Nausea and Vomiting (CINV)

Medication (Trade Name)	Class	Indication	Dose in Adults (Doses Should be Given 30–60 Minutes Before Chemotherapy)
Aprepitant (Emend)	NK1 antagonist	Acute and delayed	PO: 125 mg on day 1, 80 mg on days 2 and 3
Dexamethasone (Decadron)	Corticosteroid	Acute (high emetogenicity)	PO/IV: 12 mg (with aprepitant) or 20 mg (without aprepitant)
		Acute (moderate emetogenicity)	PO/IV: 8–12 mg
		Acute (low emetogenicity)	PO/IV: 4–8 mg
		Delayed	PO/IV: 8 mg daily days 2–4 or days 2 and 3 *or* PO: 4 mg BID days 2–4
Dolasetron (Anzemet)	5-HT_3 antagonist	Acute	PO: 100–200 mg
Dronabinol (Marinol)	Cannabinoid	Breakthrough	PO: 2.5–10 mg PO TID to QID
Droperidol (Inapsine)	Butyrophenone	Breakthrough	IV: 0.625–1.25 mg every 4–6 hours PRN
Fosaprepitant (Emend)	NK1 antagonist	Acute	IV: 150 mg ×1 dose *or* 115 mg initial dose (followed by aprepitant 80 mg PO on days 2 and 3
Granisetron (Kytril)	5-HT_3 antagonist	Acute	IV: 1 mg or 0.01 mg/kg PO: 2 mg TOP: 3.1 mg/24-h patch applied 24–48 hours before chemotherapy and kept on until 24 hours after chemotherapy or up to 7 days
Haloperidol (Haldol)	Butyrophenone	Breakthrough	PO/IV/IM: 0.5–1 mg every 6 hours PRN
Metoclopramide (Reglan)	Dopamine antagonist	Breakthrough	PO/IV: 10–40 mg every 6 hours PRN
Lorazepam (Ativan)	Benzodiazepine	Breakthrough	PO/IV/IM/SL: 0.5–2 mg every 6 hours PRN
Nabilone (Cesamet)	Cannabinoid	Refractory symptoms	PO: 1–2 mg BID (max 2 mg TID)
Olanzapine (Zyprexa)	Serotonin/dopamine antagonist	Acute/delayed/breakthrough	PO: 2.5–10 mg QHS or 2.5 mg BID *or* 2.5 mg TID plus 5 mg QHS
Ondansetron (Zofran)	5-HT_3 antagonist	Acute (moderate or high emetogenicity)	IV: 8–12 mg or 0.15 mg/kg PO: 16–24 mg
		Delayed	8 mg PO BID or 8 mg IV daily
Palonosetron (Aloxi)	5-HT_3 antagonist	Acute/delayed	IV: 0.25 mg PO: 0.5 mg
Prochlorperazine (Compazine)	Dopamine antagonist	Breakthrough Acute	PO/IV/IM: 5–10 mg (up to 20 mg) every 4–6 hours PRN *or* PR: 25 mg every 12 hours PRN PO/IV: 10 mg
Promethazine (Phenergan)	Dopamine antagonist	Breakthrough	PO/IV/IM/PR: 12.5–25 mg every 4–6 hours PRN

BID, twice daily; IM, intramuscular; IV, intravenous; NK1, neurokinin 1; PO, oral; PR, rectal; PRN, as needed; QHS, at bedtime; QID, four times daily; TID, three times daily. Source: Ettinger DS et al. Antiemesis: clinical practice guidelines in oncology. V2.2010. **http://www.nccn.org/professionals/physician_gls/pdf/antiemesis.pdf.** Accessed September 30, 2010; American Society of Clinical Oncology et al. American Society of Clinical Oncology guideline for antiemetics in oncology: update 2006 [published correction appears in *J Clin Oncol.* 2006;24:5341]. *J Clin Oncol.* 2006;24:2932; Roila F et al. Guideline update for MASCC and ESMO in the prevention of chemotherapy- and radiotherapy-induced nausea and vomiting: results of the Perugia consensus conference. *Ann Oncol.* 2010;21(Suppl 5):v232.

more effective in women than in men, which is fortunate because women have more acute and delayed symptoms than men.[29]

Aprepitant has been studied in the prevention of CINV with highly and moderately emetogenic chemotherapy.[17,29] These studies showed improved response rates when aprepitant was added to antiemetic regimens containing a 5-HT_3 antagonist plus dexamethasone.

Although CINV symptoms tend to worsen from cycle to cycle, the effects of aprepitant seem to be maintained during four cycles of chemotherapy in patients receiving moderately emetogenic chemotherapy.[30] The addition of aprepitant to the antiemetic regimen on cycle 2 (even when omitted from cycle 1) also seems to improve control of CINV symptoms.[31,32] For patients who have had inadequate response to an antiemetic regimen that did not include aprepitant, it may be useful to add it in later cycles.

The efficacy of aprepitant for the control of delayed CINV symptoms was confirmed in a trial of 489 patients comparing a standard aprepitant regimen (aprepitant, ondansetron, and dexamethasone on day 1, followed by aprepitant and dexamethasone on days 2 and 3, and dexamethasone on day 4) with a regimen without aprepitant (ondansetron and dexamethasone on days 1 through 4) in patients receiving highly emetogenic chemotherapy.[33] The aprepitant-containing regimen offered superior control of CINV in the acute, delayed, and overall periods. The study confirmed that aprepitant is superior to a 5-HT_3 antagonist during the delayed phase of CINV.

There is growing evidence that the prechemotherapy dose of aprepitant (or fosaprepitant) provides the majority of the benefit compared with the postchemotherapy doses.[17,34] This first dose of aprepitant blocks about 80% of the NK1 receptors in the CNS.[17,34] One study compared a single 150-mg IV dose of fosaprepitant to the standard three-day oral regimen (along with ondansetron and dexamethasone) in patients receiving highly emetogenic chemotherapy. There was no difference found in the antiemetic efficacy between the two groups.[35] Ongoing research is needed to further clarify the optimal dosing regimen.

Aprepitant is generally well tolerated with mild side effects, including fatigue, hiccups, headache, and diarrhea.[29,33] The overall adverse effects in standard aprepitant-containing regimens are not appreciably different from regimens without aprepitant. An intravenous prodrug, fosaprepitant, is now available, and an IV dose of 115 mg can replace the first prechemotherapy 125-mg PO dose of aprepitant.[34]

Aprepitant is metabolized by the CYP3A4 enzyme system. It is a moderate inhibitor and inducer of CYP3A4, and an inducer of CYP2C9.[1,29] Consequently, several drugs potentially interact with aprepitant. The most commonly encountered interaction is with the corticosteroids. Aprepitant increases the AUC of dexamethasone such that the dexamethasone dose (when used as an antiemetic) should be reduced by about one-half of the usual dose when these drugs are used together.[1,17,29] The interaction is greatest when the corticosteroid is administered orally. However, when the corticosteroid is also given as part of the antitumor regimen, the corticosteroid dose should not be reduced because of concern that the antineoplastic activity might be compromised.[12] Aprepitant may also enhance warfarin metabolism by inducing CYP2C9. International normalized ratio (INR) values in patients treated with warfarin and the standard aprepitant regimen are significantly reduced, especially on day 8 of the chemotherapy cycle.[17,29,36,37] The patient's coagulation status after aprepitant administration should be monitored, especially during the 7- to 10-day period after aprepitant. The dosage of warfarin should be adjusted if the INR is out of range. Several chemotherapy agents (paclitaxel, etoposide, ifosfamide, irinotecan, imatinib, vinca alkaloids, and others) are metabolized by the CYP3A4 enzyme system, and the metabolism of these agents may be altered by aprepitant. Aprepitant was used in clinical trials with some of these agents. Caution is warranted because the clinical relevance of this potential interaction is not known.[29,38] Other drugs that may interact with aprepitant include oral contraceptives, itraconazole, terfenadine, and phenytoin.[29]

OTHER ANTIEMETICS

Medications from other drug classes have also been used as antiemetics for CINV. These include dopamine antagonists (prochlorperazine, promethazine), benzodiazepines (lorazepam), butyrophenones (droperidol, haloperidol), benzamides (metoclopramide), and cannabinoids. Many of these agents were used widely until more effective antiemetic agents became available. These agents remain useful for breakthrough symptoms or for patients who are refractory to standard therapy. The dosages and indications for these agents are shown in Table 6-3. Many of these agents have more side effects than contemporary agents, especially sedation and extrapyramidal side effects, such as dystonia and akathisia. Lorazepam is commonly used as a rescue antiemetic. Its mechanism of action as an antiemetic is not completely understood, but it may involve disruption of the cortical impulses to the VC, as well as anxiolytic activity.

Olanzapine is an atypical antipsychotic agent that antagonizes several serotonin and dopamine receptors as well as other neurotransmitter receptors.[39] Its antiemetic action was first described in patients with refractory nausea or vomiting and advanced cancer. Olanzapine has activity both in the prevention of CINV in patients at high risk, as well as rescue treatment for patients with refractory nausea and vomiting. Studies have demonstrated its efficacy in preventing CINV in the setting of highly and moderately emetogenic chemotherapy. Newer, controlled trials show improved response rates when added to an antiemetic regimen of a 5-HT_3 antagonist plus dexamethasone, as well as comparable activity to aprepitant.[23,36,39,40] The usual dose of olanzapine used in these trials was 10 mg PO daily on days 1 through 5.

Olanzapine is also active as a rescue agent for patients with refractory CINV. In this setting, the usual dose of olanzapine is 2.5 to 10 mg daily in one to four divided doses. The common side effects of olanzapine include sleepiness, dry mouth, and dizziness, although these were not significant in the preliminary reports.[23,36,39,40] Olanzapine is a good choice for control of highly refractory CINV symptoms, but further study is warranted before it should be routinely recommended for prophylaxis of acute and delayed CINV.

Cannabinoids have long been used for refractory nausea and vomiting. This is based on the effect of the CNS cannabinoid receptors on the CTZ, the NTS, and the VC.[41] Small trials have shown conflicting effectiveness in the prevention of CINV.[42,43] A new oral cannabinoid, nabilone, was approved for the treatment of CINV in patients who do not respond adequately to other antiemetics.[41] Cannabinoids are associated with side effects, such as drowsiness, dry mouth, dysphoria, vertigo, and euphoria.[41,42] Although some patients have a clear preference for, and good response to, cannabinoids, side effects and a lack of pronounced efficacy limit their use in the general population of chemotherapy patients. These agents are usually reserved for patients who do not have adequate relief from other rescue medications, such as phenothiazines, benzodiazepines, or olanzapine.

CASE 6-2, QUESTION 3: M.C. is at moderate risk for acute nausea and vomiting and at high risk for delayed CINV symptoms, as a result of her chemotherapy regimen of docetaxel, carboplatin, and trastuzumab. What would be the most appropriate antiemetic regimen for M.C.?

The optimal prophylactic antiemetic regimens depend on the emetic risk of the chemotherapy regimen. Treatment guidelines have been developed by several groups, including the American

TABLE 6-4
Recommended Antiemetic Regimens for Chemotherapy-Induced Nausea and Vomiting (CINV) by Emetogenicity of Chemotherapy Regimen

Emetogenicity Potential	Acute-Phase CINV (Doses Should be Given 30–60 Minutes Before Chemotherapy)	Delayed-Phase CINV	Breakthrough CINV
High-risk IV chemotherapy regimens	Day 1: single dose $5\text{-}HT_3$ antagonist + dexamethasone + aprepitant/fosaprepitant	Dexamethasone days 2–4 + aprepitant days 2 and 3 (not needed if fosaprepitant 150-mg dose used)	Two agents for PRN use
Moderate-risk IV chemotherapy regimens with high risk of delayed CINV	Day 1: single dose $5\text{-}HT_3$ antagonist + dexamethasone + aprepitant/fosaprepitant	Dexamethasone days 2 and 3 + aprepitant days 2 and 3[a]	Two agents for PRN use
Other moderate-risk IV chemotherapy regimens	Day 1: single dose $5\text{-}HT_3$ antagonist + dexamethasone	None	One agent for PRN use
Low-risk IV chemotherapy regimens	Single dose dexamethasone or metoclopramide or prochlorperazine	None	Either none or one agent for PRN use
Minimal-risk IV chemotherapy regimens	None	None	Usually none
High-moderate risk PO chemotherapy regimens	$5\text{-}HT_3$ antagonist	None	One agent for PRN use
Low-risk PO chemotherapy regimens	None	None	One agent for PRN use

[a]NCCN guidelines also include as options dexamethasone alone days 2 and 3 or ondansetron/granisetron/dolasetron days 2 and 3 of chemotherapy.
$5\text{-}HT_3$, serotonin; CINV, chemotherapy-induced nausea and vomiting; PRN, as needed.
Source: Ettinger DS et al. Antiemesis: clinical practice guidelines in oncology. V2.2010. **http://www.nccn.org/professionals/physician_gls/pdf/antiemesis.pdf.** Accessed September 30, 2010; American Society of Clinical Oncology et al. American Society of Clinical Oncology guideline for antiemetics in oncology: update 2006 [published correction appears in *J Clin Oncol.* 2006;24:5341]. *J Clin Oncol.* 2006;24:2932; Roila F et al. Guideline update for MASCC and ESMO in the prevention of chemotherapy- and radiotherapy-induced nausea and vomiting: results of the Perugia consensus conference. *Ann Oncol.* 2010;21(Suppl 5):v232.

Society of Clinical Oncology (ASCO; **http://jco.ascopubs.org/content/24/18/2932.full.pdf+html**)[12]; the National Comprehensive Cancer Network (NCCN; **http://www.nccn.org/professionals/physician_gls/PDF/antiemesis.pdf**; guidelines can be accessed by creating a free login)[1]; and the Multinational Association of Supportive Care in Cancer (MASCC; **http://annonc.oxfordjournals.org.floyd.lib.umn.edu/content/21/suppl_5/v232.full.pdf+html**).[13] These evidence- and consensus-based guidelines, which are similar in regard to the roles of the various antiemetics, are summarized in Table 6-4 and Figure 6-2.

For M.C., the best regimen would include a single dose of a $5\text{-}HT_3$ antagonist plus dexamethasone 8 to 12 mg oral or IV plus oral aprepitant 125 mg on day 1, then oral dexamethasone 8 mg on days 2 through 4 and oral aprepitant 80 mg on days 2 and 3. She should be offered medications for breakthrough CINV symptoms, such as prochlorperazine and lorazepam. She should be warned of the potential adverse effects of dexamethasone, especially hyperglycemia, and counseled to check her blood sugars more frequently and contact her physician if they remain elevated. M.C. should be advised to maintain a record of her symptoms and contact her physician if the breakthrough medications are not working or if she cannot keep fluids down.

If M.C. had been prescribed a multiday chemotherapy regimen, prophylaxis with a $5\text{-}HT_3$ antagonist and dexamethasone should be offered for each day that moderately or highly emetogenic chemotherapy is administered.[1,12,13,44] Aprepitant might be useful with multiday chemotherapy regimens, although it has not been studied in this context. Preliminary studies indicated that aprepitant was safe to administer for a total of 5 days, but it is not clear whether the additional doses would increase the antiemetic effects. If multiday chemotherapy regimens have a high risk of delayed symptoms, then some therapy (e.g., dexamethasone plus prochlorperazine or metoclopramide, if aprepitant was already administered) for the delayed symptoms should be continued for at least 2 to 3 days after the last chemotherapy administration.

Modern antiemetic regimens achieve complete emetic control in about 70% to 90% of patients, but the response rate is lower for delayed CINV symptoms. If CINV symptoms are not adequately controlled, alterations in the prophylactic antiemetic regimen should be made for the next cycle (Fig. 6-3). Suggestions include upgrading to the next higher emetogenicity level recommendation, adding aprepitant if not already given, and scheduling antiemetic agents from other pharmacologic classes.

ONLINE CONTENT

For additional patient cases covering more CINV situations, go to http://thepoint.lww.com/AT10e.

Many patients may benefit from nondrug therapy for CINV symptoms, especially for anticipatory nausea and vomiting and anxiety. Techniques include guided imagery, hypnosis, relaxation techniques, systematic desensitization, and music therapy.[45] Acupuncture and acupressure techniques have been investigated for use in CINV, and some patients benefit from their use. The use of acupressure devices that stimulate the P6 point on the wrist have been proposed; however, in a controlled trial in patients with breast cancer, it was not found to be helpful.[46] If patients are troubled by CINV symptoms, it is recommended that they refrain from heavy meals for 8 to 12 hours before the chemotherapy. They should also avoid heavy, greasy foods and food with strong aromas. Chewing gum can mask the metallic taste that some patients perceive. Dry, salty foods can also help settle the stomach.

RADIATION-INDUCED NAUSEA AND VOMITING

Clinical Presentation and Risk Factors

CASE 6-3

QUESTION 1: E.G. is a 54-year-old man with newly diagnosed head and neck cancer who will receive radiation therapy concurrently with chemotherapy containing cisplatin and fluorouracil. His daily (Monday through Friday) radiation

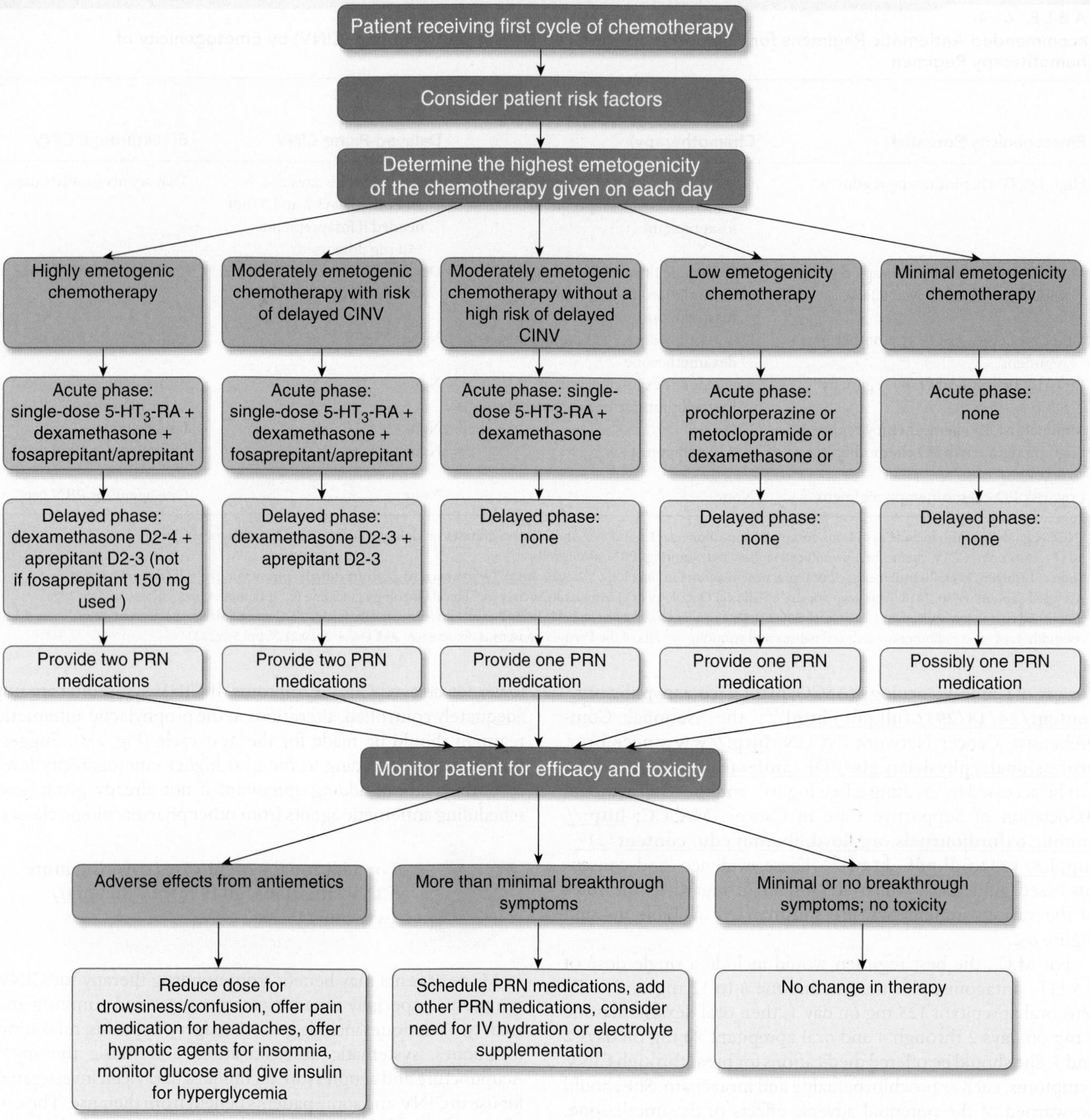

FIGURE 6-2 Algorithm for antiemetic selection for an initial chemotherapy cycle. CINV, chemotherapy-induced nausea and vomiting; D, days; 5-HT$_3$-RA, serotonin type 3 receptor antagonist; PRN, as needed.

treatments will last for 6 weeks. He has a heavy smoking history (35 pack-years) and "quit" last week, although it is not going well. After E.G.'s nausea and vomiting from the chemotherapy subsides, is he at risk for experiencing radiation-induced nausea and vomiting? What antiemetic prophylaxis is appropriate?

Radiation therapy can cause nausea and vomiting through the same basic pathways that chemotherapy does. Radiation-induced nausea and vomiting (RINV) affects 40% to 80% of patients receiving radiation therapy. The risk of RINV depends on several factors, namely the size and area to be irradiated, larger fractional doses of radiation, and whether the patient has had previous chemotherapy.[1,47,48] Patients with radiation areas larger than 400 cm^2 are more likely to have significant RINV symptoms. The radiation therapy oncologist will determine the size of the radiation field and fractional doses of radiation to maximize the efficacy of the radiation therapy. The high dose used in total body irradiation (associated with hematopoietic stem cell transplantation) causes RINV in greater than 90% of patients. Patients receiving radiation to the upper abdominal area experience nausea and vomiting about 50% to 80% of the time. Radiation to other areas of the body is less likely to cause nausea and vomiting. E.G. is at low risk for experiencing RINV because his radiation site will be in the head and neck region, his radiation site is not likely to be larger than 400 cm^2, and he will likely receive a smaller fractional dose, although he will be receiving concurrent chemotherapy.

Overview of Treatment

Just as with CINV, symptoms caused by radiation can be prevented with 5-HT$_3$ antagonists, corticosteroids, or both.

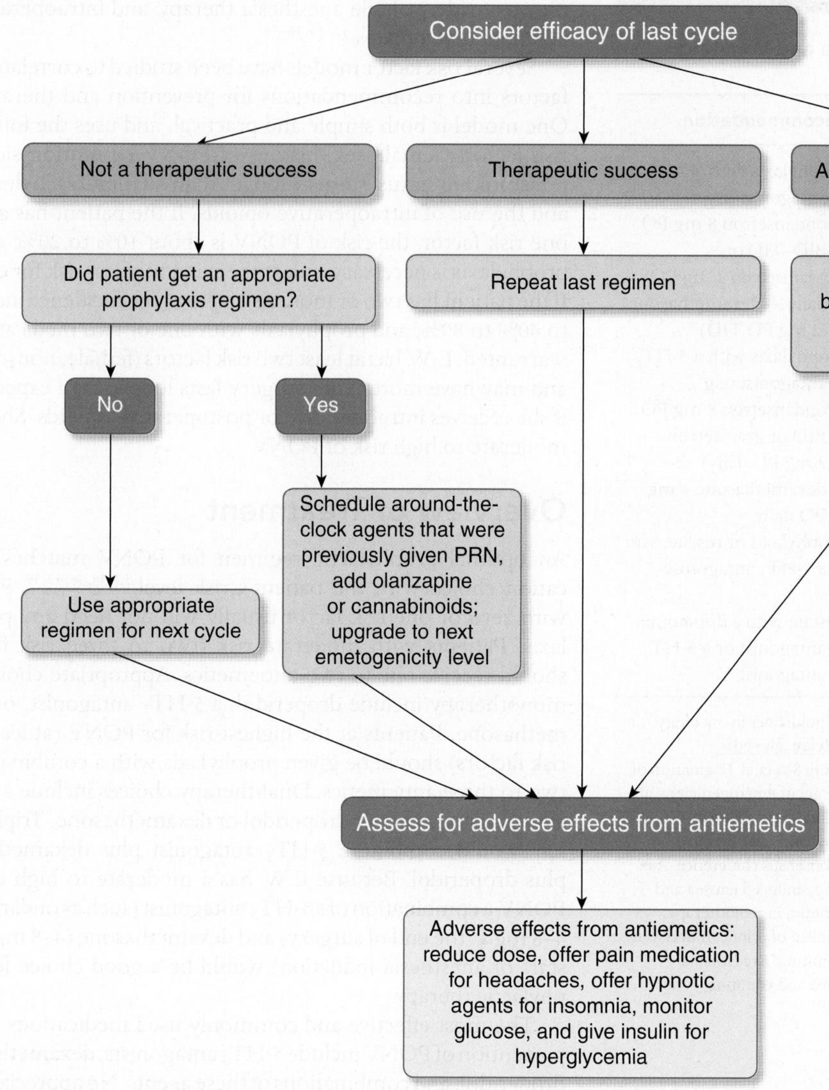

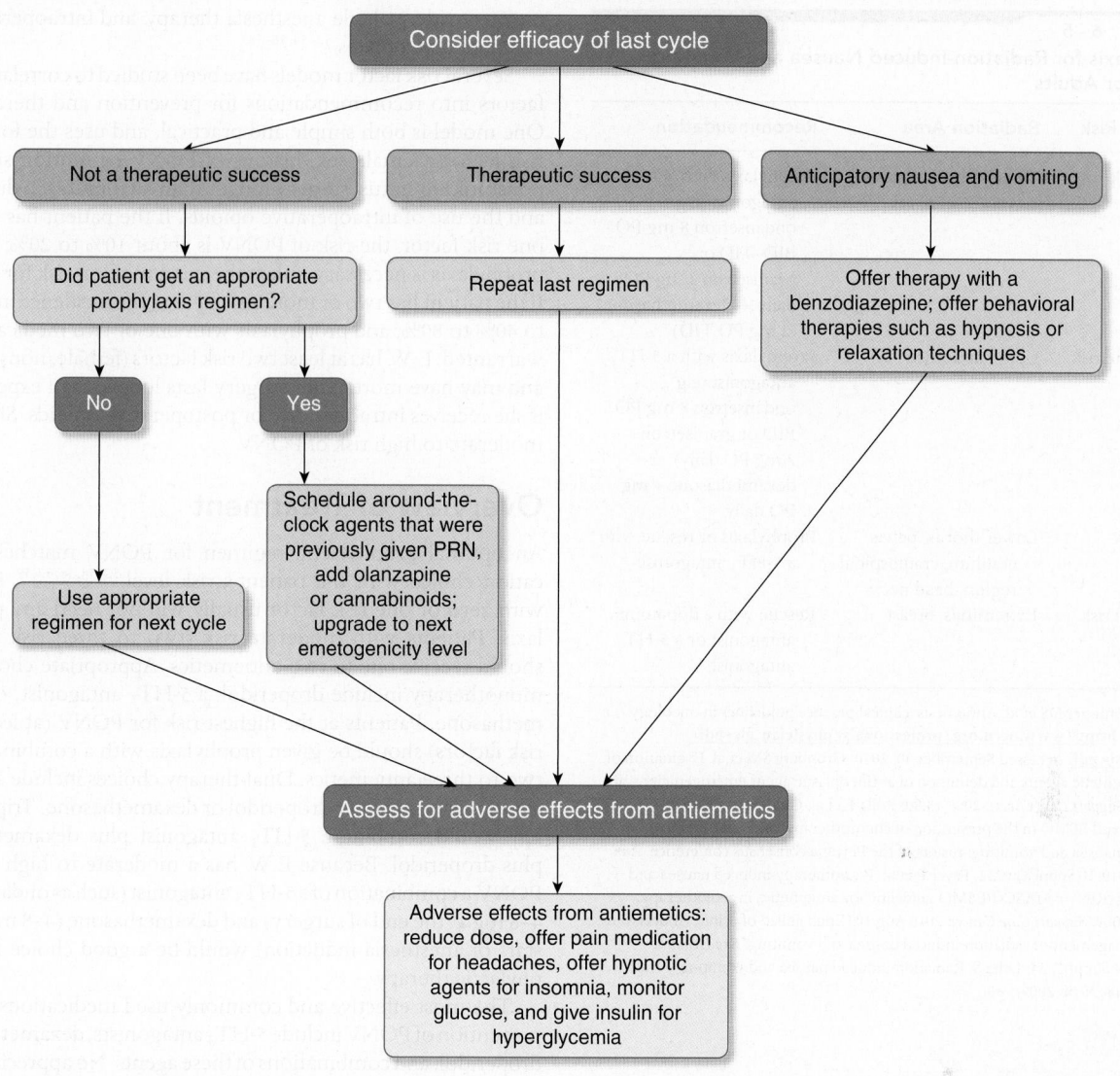

FIGURE 6-3 Algorithm for selection of antiemetic regimens for subsequent chemotherapy cycles. PRN, as needed.

Evidence- and consensus-based recommendations have been published by several multidisciplinary groups and are shown in Table 6-5. High-risk RINV is best treated with a combination of a 5-HT_3 antagonist and a corticosteroid.[1,47–51] Patients receiving concomitant chemotherapy and radiation should receive antiemetics appropriate for the chemotherapy regimen.[1] Patients receiving radiotherapy in the moderate RINV risk group can receive either prophylaxis or rescue therapy with a 5-HT_3 antagonist. Because E.G. is at low risk for having RINV symptoms, he does not need prophylaxis with a 5-HT_3 antagonist. If he experiences symptoms, rescue therapy with a dopamine antagonist or a serotonin antagonist should be offered.

POSTOPERATIVE NAUSEA AND VOMITING

Clinical Presentation and Risk Factors

CASE 6-4

QUESTION 1: E.W. is a 48-year-old woman who is scheduled for a laparoscopic cholecystectomy. The scheduled duration of her surgery is less than an hour. Her medical history includes hypertension. She does not have a history of motion sickness, and she is a nonsmoker. E.W. has never had surgery before. Her sister-in-law had severe nausea and vomiting after an outpatient surgical procedure last year, and E.W. is worried that it might happen to her. What is E.W.'s risk of having postoperative nausea and vomiting? What can be done to reduce her risk, and how can symptoms be treated if they occur?

Postoperative nausea and vomiting (PONV) is a common complication of surgery, affecting 25% to 30% of all patients, but up to 80% of patients in high-risk groups.[52] In surgical patients, PONV can lead to hospitalizations, stress on the surgical closure, hematomas, and aspiration pneumonitis. Patient-related, surgical, and anesthetic factors can increase the risk of PONV.[52–56] Patient risk factors include female sex, history of motion sickness, nonsmoking status, obesity, and a history of PONV. Some surgical risk factors for PONV include long duration of surgery and type of surgical procedure (e.g., laparoscopy, ear-nose-throat procedures, gynecologic surgeries, and strabismus repair). Anesthetic risk factors include the use of volatile anesthetics or nitrous oxide (as opposed to IV propofol) and the use of intraoperative or postoperative opioids. Children are twice as likely to have PONV as adults.[53,57] The risk increases with the child's age but declines after puberty.

TABLE 6-5
Prophylaxis for Radiation-Induced Nausea and Vomiting (RINV) for Adults

Emetic Risk	Radiation Area	Recommendation
High risk	Total body irradiation	Prophylaxis with a 5-HT_3 antagonist (e.g., ondansetron 8 mg PO BID–TID or granisetron 2 mg PO daily + dexamethasone (2 mg PO TID)
Moderate risk	Upper abdomen	Prophylaxis with a 5-HT_3 antagonist (e.g., ondansetron 8 mg PO BID or granisetron 2 mg PO daily) ± dexamethasone 4 mg PO daily
Low risk	Lower thorax, pelvis, cranium, craniospinal region, head/neck	Prophylaxis or rescue with a 5-HT_3 antagonist
Minimal risk	Extremities, breast	Rescue with a dopamine antagonist or a 5-HT_3 antagonist

Source: Ettinger DS et al. Antiemesis: clinical practice guidelines in oncology. V2.2010. http://www.nccn.org/professionals/physician_gls/pdf/antiemesis.pdf. Accessed September 30, 2010; Grunberg SM et al. Evaluation of new antiemetic agents and definition of antineoplastic agent emetogenicity—an update. *Support Care Cancer.* 2005;13:80; Roila F et al. Guideline update for MASCC and ESMO in the prevention of chemotherapy- and radiotherapy-induced nausea and vomiting: results of the Perugia consensus conference. *Ann Oncol.* 2010;21(Suppl 5):v232; Feyer P et al. Radiotherapy-induced nausea and vomiting (RINV): MASCC/ESMO guideline for antiemetics in radiotherapy: update 2009. *Support Care Cancer.* 2010 Aug 10 [Epub ahead of print]; Abdelsayed GG. Management of radiation-induced nausea and vomiting. *Exp Hematol.* 2007;35(4 Suppl 1):34; Urba S. Radiation-induced nausea and vomiting. *J Natl Compr Canc Netw.* 2007;5:60.

Certain anesthesia practices may reduce the risk of PONV. These include use of regional anesthesia (instead of general anesthesia), use of total IV anesthesia with propofol, use of intraoperative oxygen, adequate hydration, and avoidance of nitrous oxide, volatile anesthesia therapy, and intraoperative or postoperative opiates.[52–54,56–58]

Several risk factor models have been studied to correlate these factors into recommendations for prevention and therapy.[52,54] One model is both simple and practical, and uses the following risk factors: female sex, history of PONV or motion sickness, nonsmoking status, surgery longer than 60 minutes in duration, and the use of intraoperative opioids. If the patient has zero or one risk factor, the risk of PONV is about 10% to 20%, and no prophylaxis is necessary unless there is a medical risk for emesis. If the patient has two or more risk factors, the incidence increases to 40% to 80%, and prophylaxis with one or two medications is warranted. E.W. has at least two risk factors (female, nonsmoker) and may have more if her surgery lasts longer than expected or if she receives intraoperative or postoperative opioids. She has a moderate to high risk of PONV.

Overview of Treatment

An optimal prophylactic regimen for PONV matches medication choice with the patient's risk level.[52–54,56,57,59] Patients with zero or one risk factor usually will not need any prophylaxis. Patients with moderate risk (two to three risk factors) should receive one to two antiemetics. Appropriate choices for monotherapy include droperidol, a 5-HT_3 antagonist, or dexamethasone. Patients at the highest risk for PONV (at least four risk factors) should be given prophylaxis with a combination of two to three antiemetics. Dual-therapy choices include a 5-HT_3 antagonist plus either droperidol or dexamethasone. Triple therapy would combine a 5-HT_3 antagonist plus dexamethasone plus droperidol. Because E.W. has a moderate to high risk for PONV, a combination of a 5-HT_3 antagonist (such as ondansetron 4–8 mg at the end of surgery) and dexamethasone (4–8 mg at the start of anesthesia induction) would be a good choice for prophylactic therapy.

The most effective and commonly used medications for the prevention of PONV include 5-HT_3 antagonists, dexamethasone, droperidol, and combinations of these agents. No appreciable difference is found in efficacy or adverse effects between the 5-HT_3 antagonists; therefore, the costs of the different agents should be taken into consideration when selecting therapy.[52,60] Droperidol has long been used for PONV, but concerns have been raised

TABLE 6-6
Medications for Prevention and Treatment of Postoperative Nausea and Vomiting (PONV) in Adults

Medication	Prophylactic Dose	Treatment or Rescue Dose
Aprepitant	40 mg PO within 3 hours before induction of anesthesia	None
Dexamethasone	4–10 mg at the start of induction of anesthesia	2–4 mg IV
Dolasetron	12.5 mg IV at end of surgery	12.5 mg IV
Droperidol	0.625–1.25 mg IV at end of surgery	0.625–1.25 mg IV or IM every 4–6 hours
Metoclopramide	10–20 mg IV at end of surgery	10–20 mg IV or IM every 6 hours
Granisetron	0.35–1 mg IV at end of surgery	0.1 mg
Ondansetron	4–8 mg IV at end of surgery	1 mg IV every 8 hours
Palonosetron	0.075 mg IV immediately prior to induction of anesthesia	None
Prochlorperazine	5–10 mg IV at end of surgery	5–10 mg IV or IM every 4–6 hours
Promethazine	12.5–25 mg IV at induction or end of surgery	12.5–25 mg IV or IM every 4–6 hours
Scopolamine	1.5 mg TOP evening before surgery or at least 4 hours before end of surgery	

IM, intramuscular; IV, intravenous; PO, oral; TOP, topical patch.
Source: Gan TJ et al. Consensus guidelines for managing postoperative nausea and vomiting. *Anesth Analg.* 2003;97:62; Golembiewski J et al. Prevention and treatment of postoperative nausea and vomiting. *Am J Health Syst Pharm.* 2005;62:1247; Kloth D. New pharmacologic findings for the treatment of PONV and PDNV. *Am J Health Syst Pharm.* 2009;66(1 Suppl 1):S11; Ignoffo RJ. Current research on PONV/PDNV: practical implications for today's pharmacist. *Am J Health Syst Pharm.* 2009;66(1 Suppl 1):S19; Kovac AL. Prevention and treatment of postoperative nausea and vomiting. *Drugs.* 2000;59:213; Gan TJ et al. Society for Ambulatory Anesthesia guidelines for the management of postoperative nausea and vomiting. *Anesth Analg.* 2007;105:1615; Wilhelm SM et al. Prevention of postoperative nausea and vomiting. *Ann Pharmacother.* 2007;41:68; Golembiewski J, Tokumaru S. Pharmacological prophylaxis and management of adult postoperative/postdischarge nausea and vomiting. *J Perianesth Nurs.* 2006;21:385.

about the rare occurrence of QT prolongation and torsades de pointes.[59,61] Most clinicians believe droperidol to be safe, especially when doses are not excessive (up to 1.25 to 2.5 mg/dose for adults).[53,61,62] The mechanism by which dexamethasone protects against PONV is unclear, but its efficacy has been shown in many trials.[53,57,59] Combinations of medications with different mechanisms of action are more effective than monotherapy. Aprepitant has been studied in the prevention of PONV.[29,52,53] Studies have shown the activity of aprepitant and indicate similar activity compared with ondansetron.[29,52,53] Aprepitant, however, is significantly more expensive than generic ondansetron or dexamethasone, which is a consideration. The use of aprepitant is also limited by the potential for drug interactions.[56] Dexamethasone and 5-HT_3 antagonist combinations have been well studied and are highly effective.[52,53,57,59,62] Transdermal scopolamine is also effective but can have side effects.[52] Dosages for the prophylaxis and treatment of PONV are shown in Table 6-6. 5-HT_3 antagonists and droperidol seem to be more effective when given at the end of surgery. Corticosteroids are best given before the induction of anesthesia.[53,61]

Several methods for nonpharmacologic techniques for the prevention of PONV have been studied and have been shown to be effective, at least in some patient populations. These include acupuncture, transcutaneous nerve stimulation, acupressure at the P6 wrist point, hypnosis, and aromatherapy with isopropyl alcohol. Ginger remedies were not found to be more effective than placebo for PONV.[53]

Even with appropriate prophylaxis for PONV, some patients will experience breakthrough symptoms and require rescue therapy.[52] Patients who have not received prophylaxis with a 5-HT_3 antagonist can be offered a low dose of a 5-HT_3 antagonist for rescue. For rescue, only about one-quarter of the prophylaxis dose is needed.[53] For all patients who have breakthrough symptoms, it is important to choose an antiemetic from a different pharmacologic class than the agents used for prophylaxis.[52,54,59] Droperidol, promethazine, metoclopramide, and prochlorperazine are commonly used as rescue medications. If E.W. had breakthrough nausea, droperidol (0.625–1.25 mg IV or intramuscular every 4–6 hours as needed) would be a good choice for rescue therapy.

KEY REFERENCES AND WEBSITES

A full list of references for this chapter can be found at **http://thepoint.lww.com/AT10e.** Below are the key references and websites for this chapter, with the corresponding reference number in this chapter found in parentheses after the reference.

Key References

American Society of Clinical Oncology et al. American Society of Clinical Oncology guideline for antiemetics in oncology: update 2006 [published correction appears in *J Clin Oncol.* 2006;24:5341]. *J Clin Oncol.* 2006;24:2932. (12)

Feyer P et al. Radiotherapy-induced nausea and vomiting (RINV): MASCC/ESMO guideline for antiemetics in radiotherapy: update 2009. *Support Care Cancer.* 2010 Aug 10 [Epub ahead of print]. (47)

Gan TJ et al. Society for Ambulatory Anesthesia guidelines for the management of postoperative nausea and vomiting. *Anesth Analg.* 2007;105:1615. (57)

Golding JF, Gresty MA. Motion sickness. *Curr Opin Neurol.* 2005; 18:29. (6)

Ignoffo RJ. Current research on PONV/PDNV: practical implications for today's pharmacist. *Am J Health Syst Pharm.* 2009; 66(1 Suppl 1):S19. (55)

Roila F et al. Guideline update for MASCC and ESMO in the prevention of chemotherapy- and radiotherapy-induced nausea and vomiting: results of the Perugia consensus conference. *Ann Oncol.* 2010;21(Suppl 5):v232. (13)

Shupak A, Gordon CR. Motion sickness: advances in pathogenesis, prediction, prevention, and treatment. *Aviat Space Environ Med.* 2006;77:1213. (3)

Key Websites

Ettinger DS et al. Antiemesis: clinical practice guidelines in oncology. V2.2010. **http://www.nccn.org/professionals/physician_gls/pdf/antiemesis.pdf.** Accessed September 30, 2010. (1)

Priesol AJ. Motion sickness. Up To Date. **http://www.uptodate.com/contents/motion-sickness?source=search_result&selectedTitle=1%7E51.** Accessed September 27, 2010. (2)

7 Pain and Its Management

Lee A. Kral and Virginia L. Ghafoor

CORE PRINCIPLES

		CHAPTER CASES
1	Pain is an unpleasant sensory and emotional experience associated with actual or potential tissue damage. The perception of pain is individualized and affected by other comorbidities such as depression and anxiety. It is characterized as musculoskeletal, neuropathic, or visceral.	**Case 7-1 (Questions 1, 2)**
2	Pain management is complex and requires multimodal therapies, both pharmacologic and nonpharmacologic. Many factors affect analgesic selection, including comorbidities, available routes of administration, and cost. Multimodal therapy, especially with medications, requires monitoring for efficacy and adverse effects.	**Case 7-1 (Questions 3–6)**
3	Fibromyalgia and myofascial pain both present with musculoskeletal pain, but fibromyalgia is a syndrome of central neurotransmitter imbalance. Myofascial pain is a localized chronic pain at the neuromuscular junction. Muscle relaxants have shown minimal benefit for chronic pain.	**Case 7-2 (Questions 1–3)**
4	Anticonvulsants and antidepressants are the analgesics of choice for treating peripheral neuropathic pain either as monotherapy or combination therapy. Opioids and topical agents may also be used. Therapy is chosen depending on whether the pain is localized or more generalized in presentation.	**Case 7-3 (Questions 1, 2)**
5	Elderly patients and patients with multiple comorbidities are at high risk for adverse effects. Pharmacokinetic and pharmacodynamic drug interactions must be considered with use of antineuralgics and antidepressants.	**Case 7-3 (Questions 3, 4)**
6	Neuropathic pain may be caused by injury to peripheral nerves or to the central nervous system. Central neuropathic pain may present with peripheral symptoms that are localized or generalized. Pharmacotherapy has minimal effectiveness. Interventional therapies may serve an adjunctive role for pain relief to facilitate the primary goal of physical functional rehabilitation.	**Case 7-4 (Questions 1, 2)**
7	Pain is the most common symptom of osteoarthritis in older adults. There are several guidelines addressing osteoarthritis, and pain management is a balance between pain relief and prevention of side effects. Acetaminophen, nonsteroidal anti-inflammatory drugs, and opioids are beneficial in the treatment of pain but have unwanted side effects. Topical agents may be an alternative to systemic therapies in patients at risk for adverse gastrointestinal and renal effects.	**Case 7-5 (Questions 1–4)**
8	Abdominal pain is mediated by the enteric nervous system and does not always have a typical presentation. Pharmacologic therapy is often ineffective. Antidepressants in conjunction with cognitive behavioral pain management are recommended for management of functional abdominal pain syndrome.	**Case 7-6 (Questions 1, 2)**
9	Opioid therapy requires effective risk assessment to avoid medication abuse, misuse, and diversion. Monitoring recommendations should include use of written opioid agreements, urine drug testing, opioid risk screening tools, and electronic prescription monitoring program records.	**Case 7-6 (Questions 3–6)**

continued

10	Cancer pain may result from one or more causes related to direct tumor involvement, cancer therapy, and psychological factors. Pain management involves assessment of the patient to determine the etiology of pain and development of a care plan to address pain and symptom management.	**Case 7-7 (Question 1)**
11	Transdermal fentanyl and methadone are potent opioids commonly used in cancer pain management. Opioid conversion tables for fentanyl and methadone are different due to differences in pharmacokinetics in cancer patients. Treatment of incident, spontaneous, and end-of-dose pain should be part of the cancer pain management plan. Supplemental doses of short-acting opioids are recommended for breakthrough pain management.	**Case 7-7 (Questions 2–5)**
12	Medication adverse effects including sedation, constipation, nausea, vomiting, itching, and respiratory depression should be addressed in the pain management plan. Risk of QTc prolongation should be periodically evaluated with methadone. Complimentary and alternative medicine therapies are widely used by patients in the management of cancer pain, dyspnea, and nausea and vomiting. Neuraxial opioid administration may be appropriate for patients with intolerable pain who cannot tolerate systemic opioid therapy.	**Case 7-7 (Questions 6–9)**

Incidence, Prevalence, and Epidemiology

Pain is defined as "an unpleasant sensory and emotional experience associated with actual or potential tissue damage or described in terms of such damage."[1] The ability to experience pain is critical for survival because it informs the body of real or potential injury (e.g., touching a hot stove). The body is then able to respond to the threat and protect itself from further injury (e.g., refraining from touching or removing the hand from the hot stove). Pain is a hallmark of many chronic conditions, affecting more than 25% of Americans over the age of 20 years.[2] The most common types of pain include low back pain, headache, and joint pain.[2] Many people think that pain is a natural part of growing older, and up to 60% of people believe that pain is just something you have to live with.[3] Chronic pain is reported more often in women than men, and in non-Hispanic white patients compared with other races and ethnicities.[2] Chronic pain is also more common in those whose income is two times less than the level of poverty. Pain is more complex than just physiology. It is a subjective experience, and sometimes the amount of pain does not appear to equal the extent of tissue damage. A person's perception of pain is affected by environmental, emotional, cultural, spiritual, and cognitive factors. Unrelieved chronic pain affects not only physical well-being but also a person's psychological and social well-being, as well as relationships with loved ones. About one-third of people with chronic pain describe it as "disabling," with the Centers for Disease Control and Prevention reporting that chronic pain is the leading cause of disability in the United States and that the cost of chronic pain was estimated in 1998 to be $100 billion annually.[4] Pain is also the second leading cause of health-related work absenteeism, with at least 50 million workdays lost each year.[5]

Gureje et al. investigated an international population of chronic pain patients in the primary care setting.[6] They found a strong association between persistent pain disorders and psychological disorders. These were proportionally related, so the greater the pain disorder, the greater the psychological disorder. Factors that increase pain and suffering include sensory factors, cognitive factors, and emotional factors (Fig. 7-1). All are interrelated and illustrate the complex nature of chronic pain.

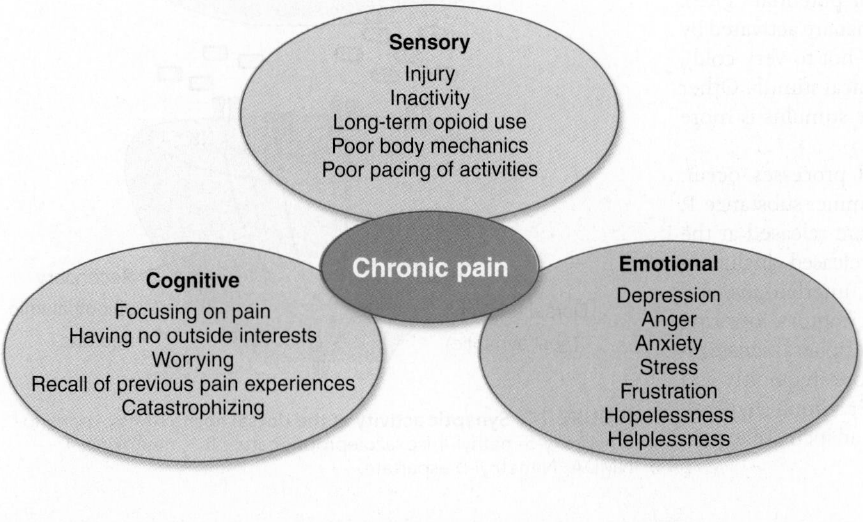

FIGURE 7-1 Factors affecting chronic pain.

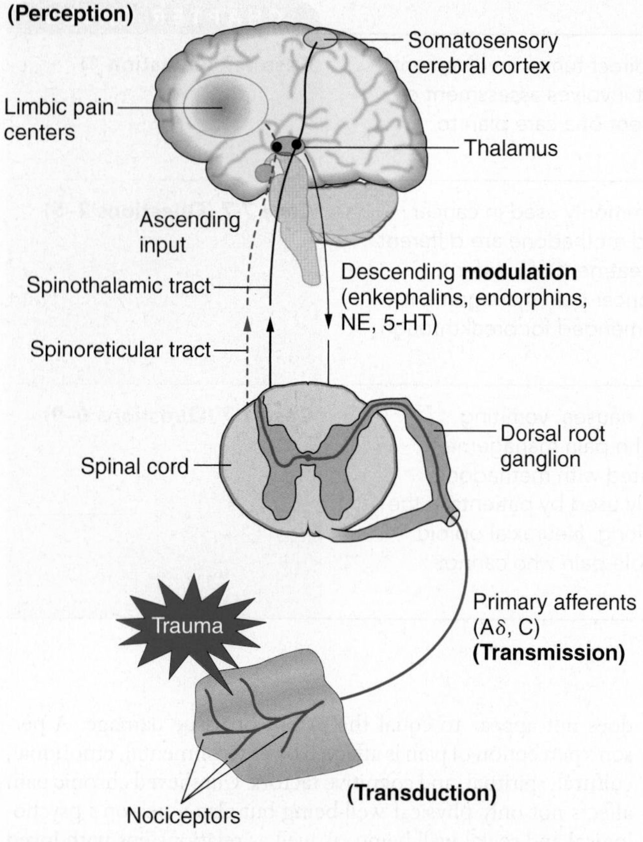

FIGURE 7-2 Pain pathways. 5-HT, serotonin; NE, norepinephrine.

Pathophysiology

ASCENDING PATHWAY

Nociception, or the sensation of pain, is composed of four basic processes: transduction, transmission, modulation, and perception (Fig. 7-2). *Transduction* is the process by which noxious stimuli are translated into electrical signals at peripheral receptor sites (free nerve endings located throughout the skin, muscle, joints, fascia, and viscera). Normal sensory stimuli do not activate the pain signal, but if the stimulus is powerful enough to surpass the threshold for innocuous activation, the receptors become *nociceptors* (pain receptors). These sensory receptors target mechanical (crushing or pressure), chemical (endogenous or exogenous), or thermal (hot or cold) stimuli. Some nociceptors are polymodal, transducing more than one type of stimuli. One of these types of nociceptors is called the transient receptor potential (TRP). This family has a large number of members that are activated by the whole spectrum of thermal stimuli (very hot to very cold), as well as some mechanical and various chemical stimuli. Other receptors are "silent," but are recruited if the stimulus is more intense or prolonged.

After stimulation of nociceptors, several processes occur. Proinflammatory mediators, including histamine, substance P, prostaglandins, bradykinins, and serotonin, are released at the site of injury. Immune mediators are also released, including tumor necrosis factor, nerve growth factors, interleukins, and interferons. These mediators sensitize the nociceptors, lowering the pain threshold in and around the injury (peripheral sensitization). The sensitized nociceptors may fire more frequently and erratically and are stimulated by much weaker stimuli (hyperalgesia). More frequent firing is correlated with an increase in pain intensity.

Transmission is the propagation of the electrical signal along primary afferent nerves, through the dorsal horn of the spinal cord to the central nervous system (CNS). Painful impulses are generated at the nociceptor, with voltage-gated sodium channels initiating the action potentials. Voltage-gated calcium channels are responsible for allowing calcium influx to the presynaptic terminal, causing neurotransmitter release. The message is then transmitted to the spinal cord via two primary afferent nerve types: myelinated A fibers and unmyelinated C fibers. The Aδ fibers are responsible for rapidly conducting impulses associated with thermal and mechanical stimuli. Transmission of signals along Aδ fibers results in sharp or stabbing sensations that alert the patient to an injury (also called "first pain"). This produces reflex signals, such as musculoskeletal withdrawal, to prevent further injury.

The smaller, unmyelinated C fibers respond to mechanical, thermal and chemical stimuli but conduct impulses at a much slower rate compared with Aδ fibers. Transmission of electrical impulses via C fibers results in pain that is dull, aching, burning, and diffuse (called "second pain"). Prolonged stimulation of C fibers causes an additive effect on the perceived intensity of second pain, called *wind-up.*

At the level of the dorsal horn of the spinal cord, the primary afferents cause calcium release into the presynaptic terminal. This leads to release of excitatory amino acids (EAAs) like glutamate into the synapse (Fig. 7-3). C fibers also release peptides such as substance P, neurokinins, and calcitonin gene-related peptide (CGRP). The EAAs then stimulate the postsynaptic receptors and the electrical signals stimulate second-order neurons in the CNS. The postsynaptic α-amino-3-hydroxy-5-methyl-4-isoxazoleproprionate (AMPA) receptors are sodium channel–mediated, and are responsible for the first pain mentioned previously. *N*-methyl-D-aspartate (NMDA) receptor channels allow both sodium and calcium passage. Usually a magnesium ion holds the channels closed; however, when there is sustained firing from the primary afferents, the magnesium ion is displaced

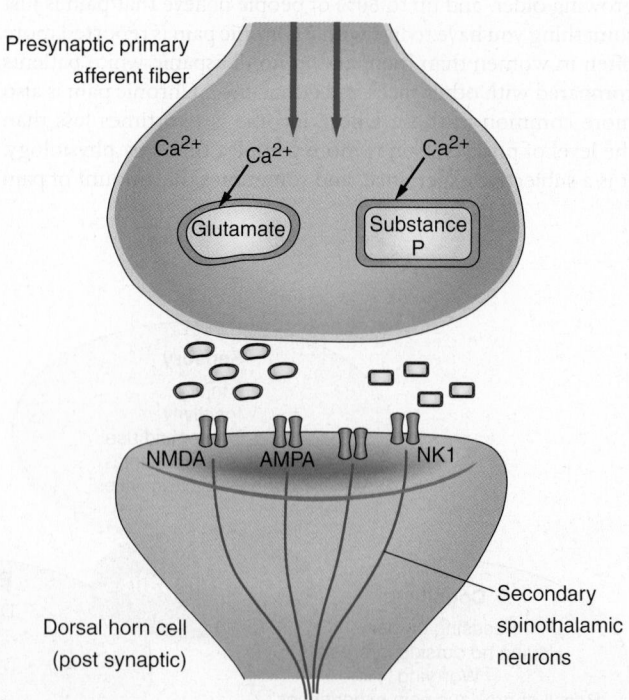

FIGURE 7-3 Synaptic activity at the dorsal horn. AMPA, α-amino-3-hydroxy-5-methyl-4-isoxazoleproprionate; NK1, neurokinin 1; NMDA, *N*-methyl-D-aspartate.

and the NMDA receptor is activated. This sensitizes the second-order neurons that will then discharge at a higher frequency. When sensitization occurs, the firing threshold is reduced, so even slightly painful stimuli (hyperalgesia) and nonpainful stimuli (allodynia) cause sustained activation of second-order neurons. NMDA receptor activation is linked to *wind-up* and *central sensitization* (decreased thresholds for response or increased vigor of responses after a sensitizing event) and may contribute to the maintenance of chronic pain conditions with processes occurring both at the dorsal horn level and in the supraspinal areas. Central sensitization may occur with all types of pain when prolonged primary afferent activation causes *plasticity* (adaptation) of the pain sensory thresholds in the CNS.

One of the most controversial effects of central sensitization is known as *opioid-induced hyperalgesia* (OIH). OIH may occur with intermittent or continuous administration of opioid therapy, often seen with higher doses in chronic pain patients. The use of opioids is associated with analgesic tolerance and activation of pronociceptive mechanisms leading to central sensitization and increased pain sensitivity.[7,8] Mechanisms associated with OIH include glutamate activation and upregulation of spinal dynorphin. Cholecystokinin, an excitatory neurotransmitter released from neurons in the rostral ventromedial medulla, activates pathways that upregulate spinal dynorphin.[9,10] Glutamate activation of NMDA receptors results in spinal neuron sensitization and increases pronociceptive mechanisms for pain transmission. Blockade of the NMDA receptor has been shown to reduce OIH and slow the development of opioid tolerance. Methadone, an opioid mu receptor agonist and NMDA receptor antagonist, can potentially prevent tolerance and OIH.[10,11]

Visceral nociception follows somatosensory pathways and also its own systems. Aδ and C fibers have been found in the heart, pleura, abdominal cavity, gallbladder, and testicles. Additionally the intestinal tract has its own neuronal system called the "brain-gut axis" that operates independently and in conjunction with the rest of the CNS. Like the somatosensory pathways, peripheral and central sensitization occurs with chronic visceral pain. Activation of the autonomic nervous system may also affect visceral sensitivity and the role of emotions in modulating visceral pain. Visceral pain may be referred to areas of the somatosensory system (e.g., a myocardial infarction causes left arm pain), leading to a complex presentation of an individual's pain.[12]

SUPRASPINAL MODULATION AND THE DESCENDING PATHWAY

Once nociceptive signals reach the CNS, they ascend to the thalamus, primarily via the spinothalamic tract. From the thalamus, tertiary neurons project to many structures in the brain, including the brainstem, diencephalon, primary and secondary somatosensory cortices, and fronto-limbic area. The somatosensory cortex is where the brain interprets the qualities of pain such as location, duration, and intensity. Tertiary neurons also project to the limbic system, which is involved in the affective or emotional component of pain. *Perception* is when the sensory (physical) and affective (psychological) components of the nociceptive message are integrated into the patient's overall experience. An individual does not experience pain until the brain has processed and interpreted the electrical nociceptive signal.

A second tract, called the spinoreticular tract, ascends to the thalamus, but also branches off at the brainstem to stimulate descending modulation. *Modulation* happens throughout the CNS and results in either an increase or a decrease in transmission. Neurons from the thalamus and brainstem release inhibitory neurotransmitters, such as norepinephrine (NE), serotonin (5-HT), γ-aminobutyric acid (GABA), glycine, endorphins, and enkephalins, which inhibit EAA activity in the ascending pathway. GABA is more active at supraspinal sites, and glycine is more active at spinal sites. The GABA-A receptor is a binding site for benzodiazepines and barbiturates, and the GABA-B receptor is a binding site for baclofen, causing muscle relaxation. Glycine has both pronociceptive and antinociceptive effects, depending on the receptor. Endogenous opioids are the most common group of inhibitory peptides, inhibiting EAA release from the presynaptic terminals and activation of second-order neurons in the postsynaptic terminals. Opioids also enhance the descending pathway via release of NE and 5-HT. In fact, activation of most of the supraspinal structures results in enhancement of NE and 5-HT effects.

Diagnosis and Clinical Presentation

Pain is a symptom and a reactionary response to real or potential bodily harm, but it is not currently defined as a specific disease state. It also cannot be measured objectively. It is a symptom that relies on a patient's subjective report and any physical findings indicative of underlying pathology. Health care teams take on the task of identifying the cause of the pain using everything from noninvasive imaging such as magnetic resonance imaging to invasive testing such as electromyelograms and spinal discography.

Pain can be classified in many ways. Some conditions are classified as syndromes because the patient presents with a constellation of symptoms that cannot be attributed to any definitive diagnosis or disease process (e.g., complex regional pain syndrome, fibromyalgia syndrome). Often clinicians simply state the location and type of pain (e.g., neuropathic pain in bilateral lower extremities). Cancer-related pain, whether from the disease process itself or the treatment of the disease (surgery, chemotherapy, or radiation), presents very much like noncancer pain, but is treated more aggressively. One of the most common ways to classify pain is to describe the time course. *Acute pain* is caused by an injury or illness. It alerts an individual to the injury and initiates withdrawal from the noxious stimulus. It typically has an easily identified cause and location. The course is predictable, and the pain is expected to diminish in hours, days, or weeks as the injury heals. It may be associated with an inflammatory response, producing redness and swelling. Inadequately treated acute pain can evoke physiologic hormonal responses that alter circulation and tissue metabolism; these can also produce tachypnea, tachycardia, widening of the pulse pressure, and increased sympathetic nervous system activity. It can also cause emotional distress. (See Chapter 8, Perioperative Care, for further discussion of acute pain management.)

Chronic pain serves no biologic purpose. It is characterized by persistent pain that lasts beyond the length of an illness or the healing of an injury. Sometimes there is no apparent cause. It may be either continuous or recurrent and of sufficient duration and intensity to adversely affect a patient's well-being, level of function, and quality of life. Risk factors for developing chronic pain include individual predisposition (e.g., female sex, increasing age, or a genetic predisposition), environmental factors (e.g., previous pain experiences or abuse), and psychological factors (e.g., anxiety, depression, or catastrophizing).[12]

Chronic pain can be further classified based on mechanism, symptoms, or location of injury. *Musculoskeletal* or *inflammatory pain* is described as constant, aching pain, often mediated by prostaglandins. It is usually caused by injury to the skeletal muscles or joints. Pain may be localized to the joints (as in rheumatoid arthritis and osteoarthritis) or more regional (as with myofascial pain or muscle strain). *Neuropathic pain* is described as tingling, sharp, shooting, stabbing, burning, or other uncomfortable feelings (*dysesthesias*) such as feeling like there are bugs crawling on

TABLE 7-1
Patient Evaluation

General history	Chief complaint History of present illness (HPI) Past medical history (PMH) Family history Social history Current medications, including allergies
Pain history	Onset Duration Quality Intensity Ameliorating factors Exacerbating factors Pain rating, if possible
Analgesic history	Current analgesics Dose/route Duration of use Effectiveness Adverse effects Past analgesics Dose/route Effectiveness Duration of use Adverse effects
Clinical examination	Clinician observations of patient behavior (grimacing, withdrawing, guarding) Physical examination Functional assessment

the skin. Neuropathic pain may be constant (as in diabetic peripheral neuropathy) or intermittent (as in trigeminal neuralgia). It is typically caused by injury within the nervous system or a nervous system response to persistent pain stimulus from outside the nervous system. *Visceral pain* can have a vague presentation, as the enteric and autonomic nervous systems are involved. Patients may report nausea or generalized abdominal discomfort (as in endometriosis, hepatitis, or pancreatitis). Some people report pain in the absence of physiologic tissue damage; however, their perception of the pain is very real. This is called *dysfunctional pain*. Conditions such as irritable bowel syndrome, fibromyalgia, interstitial cystitis, and some abdominal or pelvic pain fall into this category. In these conditions, pain appears to be generated by an imbalance in pronociceptive signals and antinociceptive signals in the CNS. Patients with dysfunctional pain syndromes are heavily influenced by factors that augment or diminish the CNS pathways (including stress, anxiety, depression, or illness).

Assessment

Pain is very subjective and difficult to measure in quantitative terms. It is essential to obtain a thorough history and examination, both physical and psychological. When obtaining a pain history, clinicians should gather details about the pattern, duration, location, and character of the pain. Find out what makes the pain worse and what makes it better, what medications and nonpharmacologic therapies have been tried in the past, and what was the result of that trial (positive or negative outcome) (Table 7-1).

Pain intensity should be measured using an appropriate pain scale according to the patient's ability to communicate (Table 7-2, Fig. 7-4).[13] Single-dimensional pain scales tend to be more accurate in the acute pain setting and not as helpful for chronic pain because they only capture a "snapshot" of what the patient is feeling. Chronic pain symptoms wax and wane during a long period, so more useful tools are multidimensional pain scales that evaluate function, including sleep, appetite, performance of activities of daily living, work, and social interactions. Examples of

TABLE 7-2
Pain Assessment Tools for Adults[13]

Tool	Method of Administration	Comments
Visual Analog Scale (VAS)	Verbal, visual	+ Reliable, sensitive to acute changes in pain −Requires paper/pencil, mechanical skills, decreased reliability with cognitive, visual or auditory impairment, not sensitive to long-term changes in pain
Numerical Rating Scales (NRS)	Verbal, visual	+ Reliable, good validity, detects treatment effects acutely −Decreased reliability with extremes of age −Requires abstract thought, difficult to use with cognitive, visual or auditory impairment −Not sensitive to long-term changes in pain
Verbal Description Scales (VDS)	Verbal, visual	4- or 5-point scales + Reliable, good validity, preferred by older adults, preferred by some over NRS or VAS −Dependent on literacy and language −Limited number of response categories, unequal intervals between anchors −Not very sensitive to changes in pain
Faces Pain Scale (FPS)	Visual	+ Reliable, good validity, good with poor literacy or language barrier + Possibly easier than NRS or VDS −Requires abstract thinking, not specific for pain
Brief Pain Inventory (BPI)	Verbal, written	+ Reliable + Intensity and interference components + Sensitive to change in condition over time −Doesn't assess quality of pain or affective component
McGill Pain Questionnaire (MPQ)	Verbal, written	Long form—30 minutes Short form—2–3 minutes + Reliable + Measures sensory and affective components + Valid in older patients −Not recommended for illiterate or cognitively impaired patients

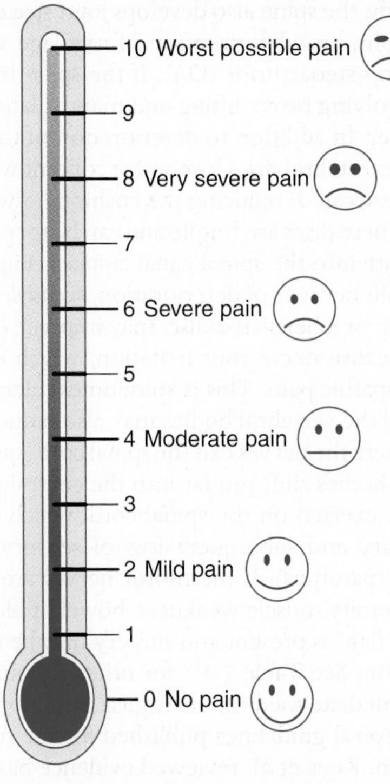

FIGURE 7-4 Pain assessment scale. (Adapted from Northeast Health Care Quality Foundation [NHCQF], the Medicare Quality Improvement Organization [QIO] for Maine, New Hampshire and Vermont, under contract with the Centers for Medicare & Medicaid Services [CMS], an agency of the U.S. Department of Health and Human Services.)

multidimensional tools include the McGill Pain Questionnaire and the Brief Pain Inventory.[14,15] Ultimately, the most useful assessment tools are the ones that each patient will provide, such as the number of hours they spend on their hobbies, or how well they can perform activities of daily living. Some of the most difficult patients to assess are children and patients with cognitive, visual, or hearing impairment. These patients may have difficulty describing and communicating their pain and discomfort. There are multiple assessment tools that are designed and tested in these special populations to increase the accuracy of pain assessment. In addition to physical and functional assessments, psychological evaluations help to identify those patients who may need more psychiatric or psychological therapy to help them cope with their chronic pain. Because controlled substances are commonly used to treat pain, some clinicians advocate for substance abuse screening (see Case 7-6, Question 4).

Overview of Treatment

Treatment of pain is based on guidelines whenever possible. However, the number of treatment guidelines for pain management is limited. More commonly clinicians choose a therapy based on the type of pain that patients present with (neuropathic, musculoskeletal, visceral, dysfunctional). For all types of pain, multimodal therapy including pharmacologic, physical rehabilitation, and cognitive behavioral therapy should be combined. Interventional therapies should be considered if possible.

A treatment plan must always include evaluation of the following factors: age, comorbidities (such as renal and liver disease), route of administration (the oral route may not be suitable), concurrent medications (for duplication or drug–drug interactions), laboratory abnormalities, and financial resources.

Acute pain is usually managed very effectively with nonsteroidal anti-inflammatory drugs (NSAIDs), acetaminophen, or opioids (see Chapter 8, Perioperative Care). Pharmacotherapy for chronic pain is more complex. First-line agents for the treatment of neuropathic pain consist of antidepressants, preferably serotonin and norepinephrine reuptake inhibitors (SNRIs) or tricyclic antidepressants (TCAs). These agents enhance the descending inhibitory pain pathway. Anticonvulsants (sodium-channel blockers, calcium-channel blockers, or GABA agonists) are also considered first-line therapy for many common types of neuropathic pain. They inhibit activation of sodium and calcium channels, block release of EAAs such as glutamate, or block the postsynaptic receptors. Some anticonvulsants also enhance the inhibitory effects of GABA. If the pain is localized, topical agents may be useful (e.g., capsaicin or local anesthetics). Addition of tramadol, tapentadol, or another opioid may be considered if the former agents fail to provide adequate analgesia. Combination therapy has been shown to be more effective in some cases (TCA-anticonvulsant or opioid-anticonvulsant combinations).[16] Nerve blocks and other interventional therapies may be helpful for short-term relief.

Chronic musculoskeletal pain usually responds to acetaminophen, salicylates, or NSAIDs, in addition to nonpharmacologic therapies such as heat and ice or physical rehabilitation modalities. Opioids are useful in the acute pain setting (immediately after injury or surgery) but are less helpful for chronic pain. Localized pain may be amenable to topical therapies (NSAIDs, capsaicin), and trigger points (taut muscle bands) may be amenable to injections. SNRIs may also be considered for this indication. Duloxetine is US Food and Drug Administration (FDA)-approved for treating musculoskeletal pain like low back pain or osteoarthritis pain.

Visceral pain is complex, and there are no clear treatment guidelines. Because it travels the somatosensory pathways, antidepressants or opioids that enhance inhibitory modulation are most commonly used. Additionally, anticonvulsants that reduce central sensitization and hyperalgesia may be helpful.

Trials of any pharmacologic therapy must be monitored for both efficacy and toxicity. Patients must have realistic expectations for any medication trial. Even the most effective analgesics are expected to achieve only about 30% to 50% improvement in chronic pain. This is why multimodal therapy is essential. NSAID therapy should be accompanied by monitoring for dyspepsia, peptic ulcers, and gastrointestinal (GI) bleeding, elevated blood pressure, and declining renal function, at a minimum. Antidepressants do not usually require laboratory monitoring but are known to cause dry mouth, constipation, urinary retention, and drowsiness. Some of the anticonvulsants require laboratory monitoring for liver toxicity, electrolyte imbalance, or bone marrow abnormalities. All anticonvulsants may cause drowsiness, dizziness, and cognitive dysfunction, with short-term memory loss and word-finding difficulty. Opioids require laboratory monitoring for long-term adverse effects such as osteoporosis, hypogonadism, and end-organ impairment, and patients must be asked about constipation, drowsiness, nausea, and vomiting. Drug interactions, both pharmacokinetic (e.g., hepatic enzyme interactions) and pharmacodynamic (e.g., additive sedation), are common with many of these agents, particularly when used in combination.

LOW BACK PAIN

Low back pain is the fifth most common reason for visits to primary-care providers.[17,18] Some have reported that low back pain episodes are self-limited and resolve within 30 days; however, Hestbaek et al. conducted a literature review in 2003 in which they concluded that low back pain is not a self-limiting condition and refuted the assumption that 80% to 90% of low back pain patients become pain free within 1 month.[19] Andersson et al. reported the rate of recurrence of back pain to be between 9% and 72%. The prevalence of back pain rises with increasing age up to 65 years, after which it drops off for unknown reasons.[20] There is an association between psychological factors and the occurrence of low back pain, including anxiety, depression, somatization symptoms, stress, and negative body image. Chronic low back pain patients have higher rates of emotional distress and depression (25%) relative to acute low back pain subjects (2.9%).[21] Socioeconomic risk factors include job dissatisfaction, physical work, psychologically stressful work, low educational achievement, and workers' compensation insurance.[22] Biomechanical and physical work factors such as heavy lifting, repetitive motion, nonneutral body postures, and vibration are established risks for back disorders.[23] Chronic low back pain also creates a large financial burden on the workplace. Low back pain accounts for almost $20 million in lost productivity annually, and patients who have been on disability for more than 1 year rarely return to work.[24]

Low back pain, by definition, affects the lumbosacral spine and associated muscles and nerves. In about 85% of cases, no pathophysiologic cause can be found.[25] The functional spinal unit is made up of two vertebral bodies, two zygapophyseal (facet) joints, the intervertebral disc, and the supporting ligamentous structures (Fig. 7-5). The facet joints of the spine form the junction where vertebral bodies meet. The joint space is maintained by cartilage and fluid in the joint. Like all weight-bearing joints of the body, the spine also develops joint space narrowing, bony hypertrophy, and deterioration of cartilage with normal use, resulting in osteoarthritis (OA). If the spine is used more, as with jobs involving heavy lifting and manual labor, the joints deteriorate faster. In addition to deterioration of the facet joint spaces, the intervertebral discs lose water content with time and may become desiccated, reducing the cushion between the vertebral bodies. These discs are fragile and can be torn or damaged and may herniate into the spinal canal *foramen* (Fig. 7-5). If vertebral bodies shift because of deterioration, *spondylolisthesis* may occur. This shift, or a herniated disc, may impinge on the spinal nerve root, or cause nerve root irritation, which can produce radicular neuropathic pain. This is sometimes referred to as *sciatica*. Shifting of the vertebral bodies may also reduce the size of the foramen where the nerves exit the spinal cord (*spinal stenosis*). If the vertebral bodies shift too far into the central spinal canal, pressure can be exerted on the spinal cord, which may lead to spinal cord injury and subsequent loss of sensory and motor nerve function (paralysis). If the motor nerves are affected (as with lower extremity muscle weakness, bowel or bladder incontinence), a "red flag" is present and surgery may be necessary to preserve function. See Table 7-3[26] for other serious conditions that call for immediate medical or surgical attention.

There are several guidelines published for the management of low back pain. Koes et al. reviewed evidence-based management guidelines from 13 different countries and 2 international committees that were published between 2000 and 2008.[27] The guidelines were based on scientific evidence, as well as group

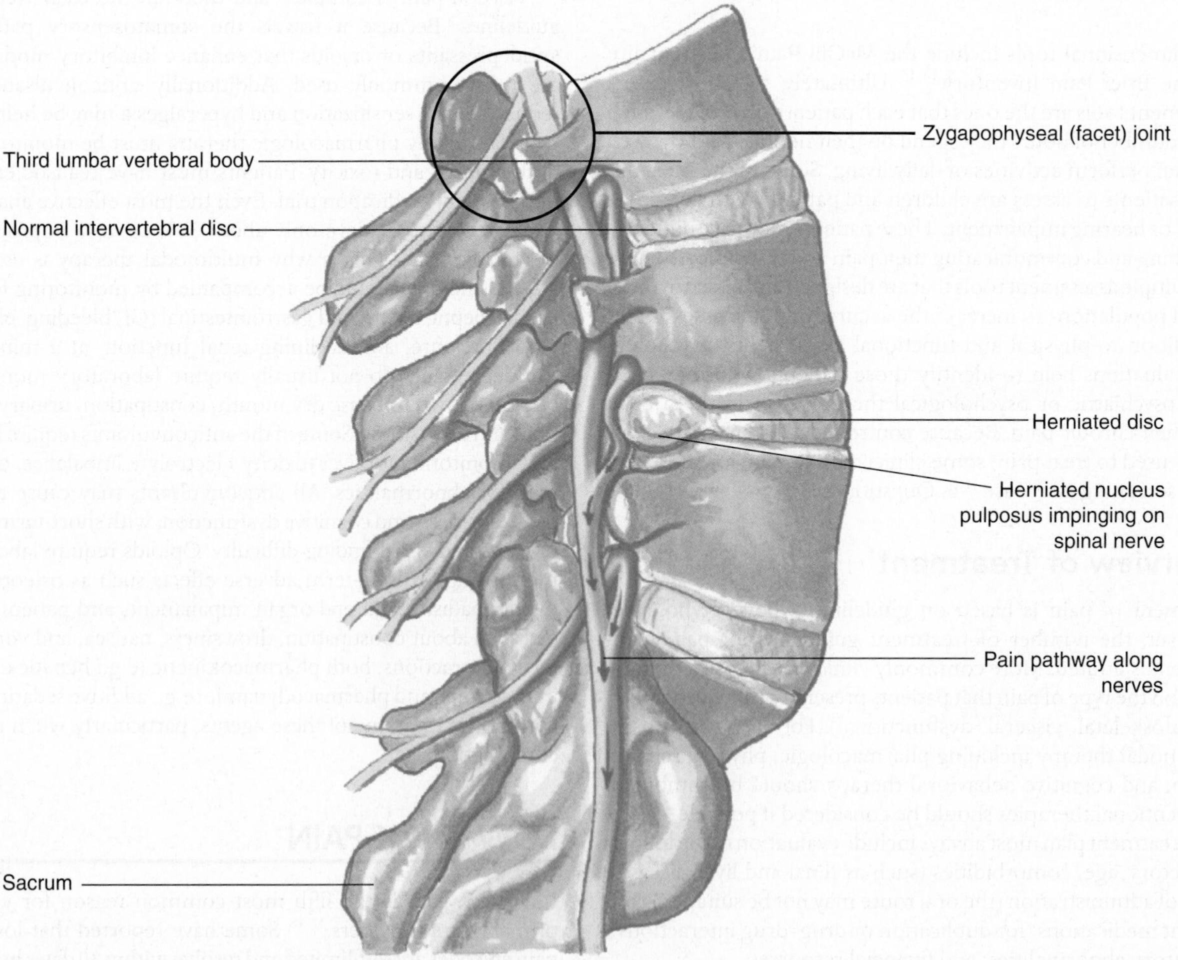

FIGURE 7-5 Spine anatomy and disc herniation.

TABLE 7-3
Red Flags for Potentially Serious Conditions That Cause Back Pain[26]

Possible Fracture	Possible Tumor or Infection	Possible Cauda Equina Syndrome
Major trauma, such as vehicle accident or fall from height	Age <20 or >50 years	Saddle anesthesia
Minor trauma or strenuous lifting in older or potentially osteoporotic patients	History of cancer	Recent onset of bladder dysfunction (urinary retention, increased frequency, overflow incontinence)
	Constitutional symptoms (recent fever, chills, unexplained weight loss)	Severe or progressive neurologic deficit in the lower extremities
	Risk factors for spinal infections:	Unexpected laxity of the anal sphincter
	Recent bacterial infection	
	IV drug abuse	
	Immune suppression	
	Pain that worsens when supine	Perianal/perineal sensory loss
	Severe nighttime pain	Major motor weakness:
		Quadriceps (knee extension weakness)
		Ankle plantar flexors, evertors, and dorsiflexors (foot drop)

IV, intravenous.

consensus and discussion. Table 7-4 presents a summary of common recommendations. All guidelines were in agreement on the use of simple analgesics such as over-the-counter acetaminophen and NSAIDs for first-line therapy for both acute and chronic low back pain. Both of these medication classes are considered effective for short-term use, although their effects are modest. Acetaminophen is considered the safest choice. Its mechanism of action is not well defined, but it has analgesic activity in the CNS. It has no peripheral clinical effect on prostaglandins, so lacks typical anti-inflammatory activity. Use of acetaminophen therefore avoids the GI, renal, and cardiovascular toxicities associated with NSAIDs. NSAIDs reduce pain and inflammation by inhibiting cyclo-oxygenases (COX-1 and COX-2) at the site of injury and along the ascending pain pathway. The NSAIDs are equally effective across the drug class, although some patients may respond to one agent better than another. They are better than placebo for back pain without sciatica, but not for back pain with sciatica.[28,29] COX-2 selective inhibitors are as effective as traditional NSAIDs for analgesia but are better tolerated.[30] Celecoxib is the only COX-2 selective inhibitor available in the United States. Acetaminophen may be used in combination with NSAIDs for additive analgesia. NSAID choices and doses may be found in Chapter 44, Rheumatoid Arthritis.

TABLE 7-4
Summary of Common Recommendations for Treatment of Low Back Pain[27]

Acute or Subacute Pain
Reassure patients that diagnosis is not serious
Advise to stay active
Prescribe medication if necessary
First-line: acetaminophen
Second-line: NSAIDs
Third-line: muscle relaxants, opioids, antidepressants, or anticonvulsants as coanalgesics
Discourage bed rest
Do not recommend supervised exercise program
Chronic Pain
Discourage use of alternative therapies (ultrasound, electrotherapy)
Short-term use of medication/manipulation
Supervised exercise therapy
Cognitive behavioral therapy
Multidisciplinary treatment

NSAIDs, nonsteroidal anti-inflammatory drugs.

Most guidelines recommend either muscle relaxants or weak opioids as third-line choices for short-term use in either acute or chronic low back pain. Despite the fact that muscle relaxants are used commonly, there is no evidence that they are effective for chronic low back pain. Agents such as cyclobenzaprine and tizanidine, as well as benzodiazepines like diazepam, show moderate efficacy in the short-term (<2 weeks) but are associated with a higher incidence of adverse effects than placebo.[31] Weak opioids have also shown modest relief with short-term use (<4 weeks).[32] There are several studies showing some efficacy for most long- and short-acting opioids, but they do not show any long-term functional improvement or return to work.[33,34] Tramadol and tapentadol also have a small number of trials supporting their use in chronic low back pain.[35,36] A Cochrane review updated in 2010 evaluated the use of long-term (>4 weeks) opioids for chronic low back pain. Tramadol was the only agent that was superior to placebo for pain relief and improved function.[37]

A few guidelines, including those from the American Pain Society (APS), recommend use of antidepressants or anticonvulsants for neuropathic pain symptoms.[32] Antidepressants, specifically the TCAs, have shown modest analgesia compared with placebo, but they have not been shown to be effective for acute low back pain, nor have they shown demonstrable improvement in function.[38,39] There have been a very small number of trials using the anticonvulsants, topiramate and gabapentin, for back pain. Anticonvulsants traditionally have been helpful for treating neuropathic pain (e.g., peripheral neuropathies) but produce only small improvements for back pain with radiculopathy.[40–43]

Clinical Presentation and Treatment of Low Back Pain

MULTIDIMENSIONAL PAIN ASSESSMENT

CASE 7-1

QUESTION 1: J.P. is a 48-year-old man who presents with low back and leg pain. He has had chronic back pain for several years, which has progressively gotten worse during the last several months. He reports an aching pain that is localized to his lumbosacral spine with some radiation into his buttocks and hips. He also describes burning pain into

his right leg. He rates his pain as 7 of 10 on the numeric pain scale. On good days his pain is 5 of 10. He recently did some yard work and had an acute exacerbation of his pain. He reports this felt like 10 of 10 on the numeric pain scale, and he was in bed for the following 2 days because of pain. He is usually able to do some chores around the house, but activity makes his pain worse. He sleeps poorly (only about 4–5 hours/night), and he does not go out or socialize very often because he is afraid this will exacerbate his pain. He used to golf and play softball but is not able to participate in these hobbies any more as a result of pain. He smokes two packs of cigarettes daily and drinks about a six-pack of beer each week. He was previously a plumber but had to quit his job earlier this year because of health problems. On physical examination he reports pain with forward flexion of his spine and spine rotation to the left. No pain is elicited with isolated manipulation of his hips and tailbone, and he has minimal discomfort with straight leg raise. His reflexes are intact, and he has full strength in his lower extremities. J.P. has pain with palpation along his lumbar paraspinal muscles and marked tenderness at the level of L4 to L5. He denies any lower extremity weakness and also denies loss of bowel or bladder control. He has not found anything that really helps his pain except rest and acetaminophen/codeine that his sister gave him. His past medical history includes hypertension, hyperlipidemia, depression, and morbid obesity. His current medications are lisinopril for hypertension, simvastatin for hyperlipidemia, a baby aspirin, and acetaminophen/codeine. He also takes three tablets of over-the-counter strength (200 mg/tablet) ibuprofen and three tablets of extra-strength (500 mg/tablet) acetaminophen about four times daily with minimal relief of his pain. His reflexes are intact, and he has full strength in his lower extremities. The remainder of his physical examination is unremarkable except that general deconditioning is noted. There are no laboratory tests or imaging studies available. He reports that his blood pressure is usually around 150/80 mm Hg with a pulse around 75 beats/minute. What are the clinically relevant findings (or absence of findings) for J.P.'s pain assessment, and how would you characterize his pain?

The presentation and assessment of back pain can be very complex given its multifactorial nature. Acute low back problems are defined by the Agency for Health Care Policy and Research as "activity intolerance attributable to lower back or back-related leg symptoms of less than 3 months' duration."[26] J.P.'s acute exacerbations would fit this definition. When J.P. has acute exacerbations of his back pain, the numeric pain scale is an accurate assessment tool (Table 7-2, Fig. 7-4). His rating of 10 of 10 indicates severe acute pain. Clinicians should also consider a patient's vital signs, which may be elevated with acute pain. If a patient is unable to communicate (e.g., on a respirator) changes in vital signs may be the only indicator of discomfort.

J.P.'s chronic back pain assessment must rely heavily on the history he provides, as there is minimal objective evidence to base the assessment on, other than his findings on physical examination or imaging studies. He indicated that his chronic pain is about 7 of 10 on the numeric pain scale. Even though the numeric pain scale has been validated for chronic pain, it is less useful in this setting because it only gives a snapshot of the whole pain picture. A multidimensional tool, like the Brief Pain Inventory (http://prc.coh.org/pdf/BPI%20Short%20Version.pdf) or the McGill Pain Questionnaire (http://www.chcr.brown.edu/pcoc/shortmcgillquest.pdf), are more useful tools to assess chronic pain (Table 7-2). Physical activities, sleep, diet, and social interactions may be affected by chronic pain. J.P. notes that his pain is worse with physical activity. He reports sleeping poorly and has limited physical activity and minimal social interaction. All of these factors contribute to a patient's pain experience and must be considered (Fig. 7-1).

Assessment of chronic pain is not only more complex, but is more extensive, as the perception and response to chronic pain is widely variable. Each patient experiences pain in his or her own way. A psychological assessment is essential to identify comorbidities such as depression or anxiety and any history of abuse (physical, verbal, sexual) or previous trauma, as well as to assess a patient's coping ability. J.P. has a diagnosis of depression that is currently not being treated pharmacologically. It may be helpful to ask J.P. about his spirituality and cultural values, as these may offer unique opportunities (or barriers) to any proposed treatment plan. Additionally, if opioids are being considered, many clinicians endorse the use of a substance abuse screening tool such as the Screener and Opioid Assessment of Patients with Pain (SOAPP), Opioid Risk Tool (ORT), or Diagnosis, Intractability, Risk, Efficacy (DIRE) score. J.P. drinks alcohol, smokes tobacco, and has used his sister's acetaminophen/codeine. These factors may warrant use of a screening tool to assess his risk for opioid abuse.

J.P.'s chronic pain has been present for several years and has gradually worsened. Based on his history and current physical examination, he appears to have mechanical musculoskeletal pain. He is a former plumber, which involves bending and lifting, which puts him at risk for facet joint arthritis. He describes the aching, localized pain that is typical of arthritis, either in his spine-hip junction (sacroiliac joint) or his zygapophyseal (facet) joints, which are the most common locations for lumbosacral pain. He demonstrated localized tenderness at the L4 to L5 level and had pain with spinal rotation to the left and with forward flexion of the spine. This is most consistent with facet joint disease. He also has muscle tenderness along the spine, which is very common, as the body attempts to accommodate structural spine abnormalities. Muscular pain may radiate into the mid back or into the buttocks, but does not travel below the knees. J.P. did not have pain that radiated below the knees. J.P. does not have any motor weakness, past experiences, or comorbidities that would indicate a red flag (Table 7-3).

J.P.'s physical examination reveals radicular pain in the L5 dermatome. Unlike muscular pain, radicular pain travels from the spine past the knee into the distal extremities. J.P. describes burning and shooting pain that radiates from his spine down his legs to his toes. These are hallmarks of neuropathic pain, although it appears to be multifactorial, which is very common with chronic low back pain. So J.P. appears to have both musculoskeletal and neuropathic pain. This mixed picture is very common with back pain and adds complexity to both diagnosis and treatment plans. For more information on musculoskeletal pain and neuropathic pain, see the Diagnosis and Clinical Presentation section.

IMPACT OF COMORBID MEDICAL ILLNESS ON PAIN ASSESSMENT

CASE 7-1, QUESTION 2: What comorbidities will affect J.P.'s presentation and pain assessment?

J.P. has a concurrent diagnosis of depression, which is quite common in patients with chronic pain. Between 30% and 54% of patients with chronic pain present with symptoms of depression.[44] This is two or three times higher than the general population.[45] Depression is often underrecognized in the face of pain as a presenting symptom. Many times primary care providers investigate for a functional cause of the pain, but overlook the psychosocial aspects of pain. Variables associated with depression in chronic pain are female sex, younger age, lower socioeconomic status, unmarried, Caucasian, and higher pain severity.[46] In fact, as pain severity worsens, depressive symptoms worsen, medical visits become more frequent, and health care costs increase.[47] The relative deficiency of NE and 5-HT that occur with depression makes the pain-blocking function of the descending pain pathway less effective. As a result, J.P. may feel more pain physiologically and also have a greater emotional response to his pain and other stressors. His depression may be contributing to his sleep disturbance and his diminished social interactions. Untreated depression may be detected with a multidimensional pain assessment tool. If identified and treated, his pain may improve concurrently with his depression. Other psychiatric comorbidities that commonly occur with chronic pain include anxiety, personality disorders, and substance abuse.

J.P. also has a diagnosis of hypertension. Although this will not directly contribute to his pain, any acute exacerbations may cause an increase in his pulse and blood pressure. Increases in blood pressure are associated with an increased incidence of stroke. The presence of hypertension is also a factor when developing a treatment plan. He is currently taking ibuprofen for pain, and NSAIDs are known to cause fluid retention, compromise renal function, and diminish the benefits of antihypertensives (like J.P.'s lisinopril). Corticosteroids, which may be used during an interventional pain procedure, may also increase blood pressure.

LOW BACK PAIN TREATMENT

CASE 7-1, QUESTION 3: How can current low back pain treatment guidelines be applied to J.P.'s pharmacologic regimen?

Acetaminophen is considered first-line therapy for low back pain. J.P. has been using acetaminophen up to 6,000 mg daily, which exceeds the recommended maximal daily dose of 4,000 mg. He has also been using some acetaminophen/codeine that he got from his sister. J.P. is at risk for liver toxicity from high doses of acetaminophen. Additionally, he has not found the acetaminophen to be helpful, so it should be stopped. J.P. is also taking ibuprofen, which is an NSAID and recommended as second-line therapy. He is taking 2,400 mg daily without benefit. His pain relief is unlikely to improve with a dose increase, but he may benefit from rotation to another NSAID with a different chemical structure. Naproxen is an inexpensive agent that is also available over-the-counter. He does not demonstrate any muscle spasm, so a muscle relaxant is not indicated, nor is it recommended for chronic back pain.[27] He has radicular pain, so a trial of gabapentin may be helpful. He has been using the codeine-containing product and notes that this has been helpful; however, opioids are not recommended for long-term management and have not shown substantial benefit with long-term use. He should be encouraged to reduce or discontinue use of the opioid.

Chang et al. recommends a trial of TCAs if NSAIDs and acetaminophen have failed.[48] This may also help his chronic insomnia, but the doses used for analgesia (typically less than 100 mg) may not be high enough to have true antidepressant effects. Selective serotonin reuptake inhibitors (SSRIs) may be used to treat depression, but have no independent analgesic effects. However, if his depression improves, we would expect to see a proportional improvement in his pain. Because SSRIs are better tolerated than TCAs, and TCAs have not demonstrated improvement in function in the long-term, J.P. should have a trial of a generic SSRI such as citalopram.

CHANGING ANALGESIC OR ROUTE OF ADMINISTRATION

CASE 7-1, QUESTION 4: J.P. returns after 3 months with a small improvement in his back pain. He is sleeping a bit better (6 hours per night). He is attending physical therapy sessions, although infrequently. He has been taking citalopram 20 mg daily for his depression and feels this is somewhat helpful for his mood. He has been taking naproxen 500 mg three times a day (TID) and gabapentin 300 mg TID for his pain. Neither of these has provided adequate relief. Another provider gave him a prescription for oxycodone 5 mg/acetaminophen 325 mg one to two tablets every 6 hours as needed. J.P. has been taking two tablets every 6 hours on a regular schedule. Although this helps his pain (30% improvement), the relief only lasts 3 to 4 hours, and then he is in pain for another 2 to 3 hours before he can take another dose. He also reports a lot of nausea with this regimen. He has heard about "pain patches" and wonders if these might be an option for him.

J.P. is getting about 30% improvement with oxycodone/acetaminophen, which is a good response for any analgesic, but the duration of relief is short and he is having nausea after each dose. He has asked about using a pain patch. What therapy might you suggest for J.P.? Is a pain patch a good choice?

There are several analgesic options available for patients who are unable to tolerate or ingest solid oral dosage forms (tablets and capsules). It is common for patients with feeding tubes and patients who have maxillofacial surgery to use alternative dosage forms such as oral liquids, topicals, or transdermal products (Table 7-5). J.P. has asked about a pain patch. It is likely that he is referring to a fentanyl transdermal system. Fentanyl patches are synthetic, extended-delivery options, but also are expensive, as are most of the long-acting agents, and his insurance company may not cover these. So a pain patch may not be the best choice for J.P. Because he is able to take oral medications, it would be most reasonable to simply rotate to an oral opioid that offers a longer duration of action.

When considering product rotation for J.P., it is important to consider drug formulation and availability, route of administration, drug interactions, adverse effects, and cost. The oxycodone/acetaminophen product that he is currently using is not providing an adequate duration of analgesia. He may need to use a long-acting opioid to achieve sustained analgesia. There are many long-acting opioid formulations available including long-acting morphine (tablets, capsules), oxycodone (tablets), hydromorphone (capsules), methadone (tablets), oxymorphone (tablets), and fentanyl (patch). Because he is getting good pain relief with oxycodone/acetaminophen, converting to a long-acting formulation of oxycodone seems the most logical choice. J.P. is currently taking eight 5-mg tablets of oxycodone daily (40 mg total per day). This may be directly converted to long-acting oxycodone 20 mg twice daily. (See more information about opioid conversions in Case 7-7, Question 5.) If he continues to have nausea after his doses of oxycodone/acetaminophen, he may need to rotate to another opioid or use a nonoral route of administration, an antiemetic, or a nonopioid analgesic.

J.P. has been using several different analgesics for his pain, including an NSAID, an anticonvulsant, an antidepressant, and an opioid. These agents will offer pharmacologic activity at several points in the pain pathway (Fig. 7-2) and offer additive analgesic effects.[49,50] However, multimodal therapy also carries the risk of additive adverse effects and possible drug interactions. For example, the anticonvulsant and the opioid may cause additive

TABLE 7-5
Analgesics for Patients Who Cannot Take Solid Oral Dosage Forms

Oral Liquids
Acetaminophen (elixir, liquid, solution, suspension, syrup)
Ibuprofen (suspension)
Naproxen (suspension)
Gabapentin (solution)
Carbamazepine (suspension)
Oxcarbazepine (suspension)
Nortriptyline (solution)
Oxycodone (solution)
Hydrocodone/acetaminophen (elixir, solution)
Morphine (solution)
Methadone (solution)
Other Oral Products
Lamotrigine (disintegrating tablet)
Fentanyl (mucous membrane lozenge, buccal tablet, buccal film)
Rectal Suppositories
Acetaminophen
Indomethacin
Hydromorphone
Morphine
Topicals
Diclofenac (gel)
Capsaicin (cream)
Local anesthetics (ointment, gel, cream)
Transdermal Patches
Diclofenac
Lidocaine
Capsaicin
Methyl salicylate
Fentanyl

sedation. The balance between adverse effects and analgesia must be considered with any changes in drug therapy. He is also taking lisinopril. Using an NSAID concurrently with an angiotensin-converting enzyme (ACE) inhibitor or an angiotensin receptor blocker may cause hyperkalemia or acute renal blood flow compromise. A nonacetylated salicylate such as salsalate may offer analgesia with a lower risk potential and fewer adverse effects and drug interactions. It has minimal effects on prostaglandin production.

MONITORING AND PREVENTION OF ANALGESIC SIDE EFFECTS

CASE 7-1, QUESTION 5: J.P. returns 6 months later, after seeing a pain specialist and a psychologist. He is now taking gabapentin 1,200 mg TID, meloxicam 7.5 mg daily, amitriptyline 25 mg every night at bedtime (QHS), and oxycodone CR 20 mg twice a day (BID). How would you monitor J.P.'s therapy?

Clinicians must assess each part of J.P.'s care plan, both the positive aspects and the negative aspects. Is J.P. meeting his goals on his personal care plan? Is he getting more sleep? Is he more physically active? Is he managing his stressors better? Is his pain improved? There are several monitoring tools that may be used in an ongoing fashion to record progress in the long-term. They assess what is called the "4 A's": analgesia, activities of daily living, adverse effects, and potential aberrant drug-related behavior (with opioids). (For an example, go to **http://www.painknowledge.org/physiciantools/Chart/Chart%20Note%20Tool%20Rev%201-17-08.pdf**.)

In addition to monitoring for efficacy, assessing for adverse effects of his medication is critical. Gabapentin may cause sedation, dizziness, edema, and cognitive impairment of short-term memory, concentration, and word-finding. His meloxicam, an NSAID, may cause GI upset or ulceration, so he should be advised to watch for black, tarry, sticky stools or any sign of internal bleeding. He may experience easy bruising and bleeding related to the platelet inhibitory effects of NSAIDs, and should have his serum creatinine and potassium checked regularly to monitor for NSAID-induced renal toxicity. His blood pressure should also be monitored regularly as this has been elevated in the past. His oxycodone may cause constipation, sedation, dry mouth, and urinary retention. If he is using the opioid regularly he should be advised to also use a bowel regimen with a stool softener or a motility agent. Additionally, if he is using the opioid long-term, he may need to have his testosterone levels checked and bone density testing done periodically to monitor for hypogonadism and osteoporosis, which are associated with chronic opioid therapy. J.P.'s amitriptyline may cause additive sedation, constipation, and urinary retention. He is unlikely to have problems with orthostatic hypotension, but this is common in older patients.

NONPHARMACOLOGIC THERAPIES FOR LOW BACK PAIN

CASE 7-1, QUESTION 6: What nonpharmacologic therapies may be beneficial for J.P.'s pain?

Koes et al. found that most guidelines recommend a supervised exercise program, cognitive behavioral therapy, and short-term pharmacologic therapy.[27] The APS recommends that epidural steroid injections and possibly surgery may be considered in patients with persistent radicular low back pain. Because J.P. has radicular pain into his legs and he has tried first-line therapies, he may be a candidate for an epidural steroid injection. This will only offer temporary relief, at best, but may provide him enough relief to participate more in physical rehabilitation. Studies show mixed results with both injections and surgery, so J.P. must be part of the decision-making process.[51]

In the past patients were advised to use bed rest for acute back pain; it is now recommended that patients remain physically active. This has been shown to improve pain and function at 3 to 4 weeks compared with bed rest.[52] Bed rest is not recommended for chronic back pain either. J.P. has very limited physical activity and was noted to be deconditioned. Inactivity can increase muscular pain. A referral for physical rehabilitation is a key component of management, specifically a supervised exercise regimen. There is no difference in benefit among different forms of exercise, so J.P. and his therapist may build a program that best fits his interests and needs. Physical rehabilitation also may include stretching and strengthening, but these are not effective unless used as part of a comprehensive exercise program. Other modalities such as cold packs to reduce inflammation in the acute phase of an injury and heat to relax muscles may be used, but there is no evidence supporting either of these therapies. Spine manipulation and low back corsets have shown some efficacy, but other physical modalities such as massage, ultrasound, traction, injections, acupuncture, or shoe lifts have not been shown to be effective.[32] J.P. may report that he has more pain after he starts an exercise regimen, as his muscles get reconditioned. J.P. should be encouraged and given assurances that physical activity that is at an appropriate level for his needs may cause him to hurt but will not harm him. He can also learn

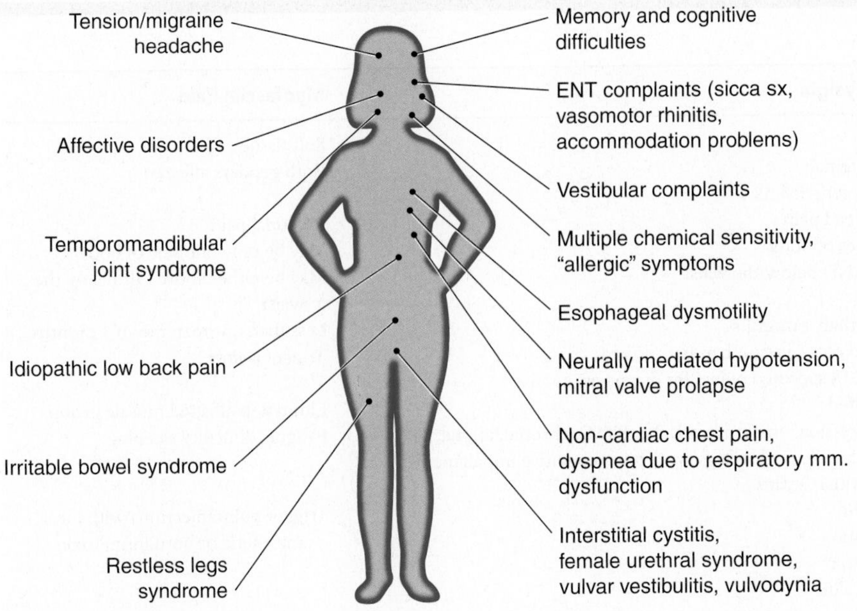

FIGURE 7-6 Systemic conditions that overlap with fibromyalgia. (Reprinted with permission from Clauw DJ. Fibromyalgia. In: Fishman SM et al, eds. *Bonica's Management of Pain*. 4th ed. Philadelphia, PA: Lippincott Williams & Wilkins; 2010:474.)

how to pace his activities so he does not overdo it with yard work as he has done in the past.

Cognitive behavioral therapy (CBT) is also an essential component of multidisciplinary management. CBT works on a patient's perception of pain and expectations, focusing on mood, catastrophizing, negative thinking, and poor coping skills. After J.P.'s depression is addressed, he can work with a therapist on coping skills and how to use self-regulation and manage stressors.

FIBROMYALGIA AND MYOFASCIAL PAIN

Fibromyalgia is a chronic debilitating condition with the primary symptoms of chronic widespread pain and fatigue. It affects between 3 and 6 million people in the United States, at a cost of $2,000 per patient per year. It is defined by the American College of Rheumatology (ACR) as pain that is both chronic (lasting longer than 3 months) and widespread (above and below the waist and on both sides of the body), with a finding of 11 of 18 specific tender points on physical examination. We have since learned that fibromyalgia tenderness is not limited to these tender points, prompting the ACR to re-evaluate its diagnostic criteria. They propose using a widespread pain index, in which patients indicate how many areas of their body have pain, and a symptom severity scale, in which patients rate the severity of fatigue, waking unrefreshed, and cognitive and somatic symptoms. Initial evaluation of these updated criteria correctly identified 88.1% of cases.[53] Fibromyalgia was previously thought to be a peripheral pain related to an inflammatory or muscular disorder, but in the past 10 years it has been shown that it may be the manifestation of CNS neurotransmitter dysfunction. Patients with fibromyalgia are more likely to have suffered a traumatic event previously, such as a motor vehicle accident or childhood sexual abuse.[54–57] Daily management of symptoms seems to be largely affected by an exaggerated response to personal stressors, noxious stimuli (hyperalgesia), and nonnoxious sensory stimuli (allodynia).[58–60] Studies have shown an imbalance in neurotransmitters in which excitatory neurotransmitters in the CNS of fibromyalgia patients are increased, including glutamate (a twofold increase) and substance P (a threefold increase), and inhibitory neurotransmitters, NE and 5-HT, are decreased.[61–65]

Fibromyalgia is associated with other comorbidities that need to be addressed for symptom management, even though treating these symptoms may not directly benefit the hallmark tenderness associated with the syndrome. Noncardiac chest pain, headache, memory problems, affective disorders, esophageal dysmotility, restless legs syndrome, interstitial cystitis, irritable bowel syndrome (IBS), vulvar pain in women, and chronic prostatitis in men are commonly present in individuals with fibromyalgia (Fig. 7-6).[66]

Myofascial pain is similar to fibromyalgia with its presentation of muscular pain, but involves pain arising from soft tissues and is more localized (Table 7-6). It affects all age groups and is associated with numerous other pain conditions. It is classically associated with muscle knots called "trigger points." A trigger point is described as a hyperirritable spot in skeletal muscle that is associated with a palpable "taut band" of muscle. Trigger points are hypothesized to evolve from excessive acetylcholine release from the motor endplate, leading to sustained muscle fiber contracture.

Development of trigger points is usually associated with mechanical overuse or overload of a muscle group (as with repetitive work). It is also associated with postural problems, prolonged static positions, emotional stress (causing muscles to tense), and nutritional deficiencies (such as vitamins B_1, B_6, B_{12}, and D, iron, magnesium, and zinc) or metabolic problems such as thyroid disease. It is thought that low-intensity exertions related to static posture cause small muscle fibers to be continuously activated, leading to the development of trigger points.[67] Nociceptors are abundant in muscle nerves, and there are a variety of nociceptors that can be stimulated by substances like prostaglandins, bradykinin, protons, ATP, 5-HT, and glutamate, which are released from damaged tissue. The neuropeptides, substance P and CGRP, are also found in the nociceptor terminals, which stimulate the inflammatory cascade, leading to peripheral sensitization and the clinical manifestation of muscle pain. Continuous activation of muscle nociceptors leads to release of substance P and glutamate from the presynaptic terminal at the dorsal root ganglion. These substances activate postsynaptic AMPA and NMDA receptors, respectively, and subsequently may lead to neuroplasticity (Fig. 7-3).

There have been three evidence-based guidelines published for the treatment of fibromyalgia: the APS in 2005, the European

TABLE 7-6
Comparing Fibromyalgia and Myofascial Pain

Criteria	Fibromyalgia	Myofascial Pain
Origin of pain	CNS	Soft tissues
Epidemiology	Usually female Possible genetic link	Both genders affected
Location/Spread	Widespread pain Both sides of body Above AND below the waist	Regional pain May be only one side of body May be either above OR below the waist
Duration	Greater than 3 months	Less than or greater than 3 months
Localized pain	Tender points (no taut bands) Need 11/18 specified points for diagnosis	Trigger points
Range of motion	Not limited	Limited in affected muscle group
Associated syndromes/symptoms	IBS, depression, anxiety, headache, PTSD, chronic fatigue, sleep disturbance, restless legs syndrome, cognitive impairment, interstitial cystitis	Fatigue, difficulty sleeping
Pharmacologic treatment	Pregabalin Duloxetine Milnacipran Amitriptyline Gabapentin Cyclobenzaprine Pramipexole Tizanidine	Trigger point injections with local anesthetic or botulinum toxin
Non-pharmacologic treatment	Physical rehabilitation, CBT	Physical rehabilitation, improving ergonomics and postural support

IBS = irritable bowel syndrome, PTSD = post-traumatic stress disorder, CBT = cognitive behavioral therapy

League Against Rheumatism (EULAR) in 2008, and the Association of the Scientific Medical Societies in Germany in 2008.[68–70] These guidelines recommended a multidisciplinary approach with pharmacologic and nonpharmacologic therapy. In the past, therapies have targeted skeletal muscles using NSAIDs and muscle relaxants, which were ineffective. Because newer evidence indicates a CNS neurotransmitter imbalance, the most effective pharmacologic approaches have targeted these imbalances. Antidepressants have been shown to reduce pain and improve function by increasing levels of 5-HT and NE in the CNS. Historically, the tertiary TCA, amitriptyline, and cyclobenzaprine (a muscle relaxant with a tricyclic structure) have been shown to improve pain, sleep, and sense of well-being, but their effect is modest and appears to be short-term.[71–73] Venlafaxine, as well as some older SSRIs (fluoxetine and paroxetine), have shown mixed results. The newer, more-selective SSRIs (such as citalopram) have had little benefit.[74–76] Duloxetine and milnacipran are both SNRIs that are FDA-approved for fibromyalgia. Milnacipran appears to have more NE activity than duloxetine. This difference does not appear to confer a therapeutic difference. Both of these agents improve average pain scores, Fibromyalgia Impact Questionnaire (**http://www.myalgia.com/FIQ/fiq.pdf**) scores, physical functioning, and overall sense of well-being.[77–81] See Table 7-7 for doses and precautions.

Pregabalin is an anticonvulsant that was approved by the FDA in 2007 for treating fibromyalgia. It targets the increased levels of glutamate in the CNS by binding to the $\alpha_2\delta$ subunit of voltage-gated calcium channels, preventing release of glutamate from presynaptic terminals (Fig. 7-3). This agent has been shown to improve average pain scores and patient perception of improvement, but failed to show improvement in Fibromyalgia Impact Questionnaire scores.[82,83] A long-term open-label study found that patients who did well in the short term maintained

TABLE 7-7
Pharmacologic Treatment of Fibromyalgia

Drug	Fibromyalgia Dosing	Adverse Effects	Comments
Amitriptyline	25–50 mg QHS	Dry mouth, constipation, urinary retention, orthostatic hypotension, somnolence	Caution in elderly patients
Cyclobenzaprine	10–30 mg QHS	Dry mouth, constipation, urinary retention, somnolence	Caution in elderly patients
Duloxetine[a]	30 mg daily × 1 week, then 60 mg daily	Nausea, dry mouth, constipation, fatigue, sweating, anorexia	Monitor liver transaminases
Milnacipran[a]	12.5 mg × 1 day, then 12.5 mg BID × 2 days, then 25 mg BID × 4 days, then 50 mg BID, may titrate to 100 mg BID	Nausea, headache, constipation, insomnia, hot flushes	Monitor blood pressure, heart rate
Pregabalin[a]	75 mg BID, titrate to 150 mg TID	Somnolence, dizziness, edema, cognitive effects	Reduce dose for renal impairment
Gabapentin	300 mg QHS, titrate to 600 mg TID	Somnolence, dizziness, edema, cognitive effects	Reduce dose for renal impairment

[a] Food and Drug Administration–approved to treat fibromyalgia.
BID, twice daily; QHS, every night at bedtime; TID, three times a day.

an improvement in pain for up to 6 months compared with placebo.[84] Gabapentin, a similar compound, has not been formally approved for fibromyalgia but has support for its use. Some insurance companies require a trial with gabapentin before allowing use of pregabalin because of its lower cost.[85] Hauser et al.[86] compared duloxetine, milnacipran, and pregabalin in fibromyalgia, and reported that duloxetine and pregabalin were better than milnacipran in improving pain and sleep. Duloxetine was better for symptoms of depression, and pregabalin and milnacipran were better for fatigue. Headache and nausea were more common with duloxetine and milnacipran, and diarrhea was more common with duloxetine.

Other drug therapies that have shown some benefit in treating fibromyalgia and its comorbidities include pramipexole, a dopamine agonist, which is beneficial in treating restless legs symptoms, as well as pain and fatigue.[87] Tizanidine, a central α_2 agonist, has also shown some improvement in sleep, pain, and other measures. The sedative sodium oxybate, a precursor of GABA, has also shown some efficacy, particularly with regard to restorative sleep and some pain measures.[88–90] However, it was denied approval by the FDA for fibromyalgia in 2010 because of its potential for abuse. NSAIDs, acetaminophen, and opioids are not recommended for treating fibromyalgia pain, although the weak opioid tramadol has shown some benefit.[69,91,92]

The mainstay of treatment for myofascial pain is trigger point injections. The goal is to reduce pain levels enough so that physical rehabilitation may commence to restore function. Some clinicians use a dry-needling technique. This involves placing a solid filament needle (like an acupuncture needle) into the trigger point to disrupt the muscle fibers, allowing relaxation of the taut band.

For a video that shows trigger point injection, go to http://thepoint.lww.com/AT10e.

Some clinicians inject medications into the trigger point. The current recommendation is to use 0.25% lidocaine or other local anesthetics.[93] Botulinum toxin has been used most recently, but the literature has offered mixed results with regard to its effectiveness.[94,95] None of the above techniques has been shown to be better than another. Several other pharmacologic therapies may be used, but none have more than anecdotal support. General approaches to pain management, including NSAIDs, antidepressants, anticonvulsants, and opioids, may be helpful for individual patients. Vitamin D deficiency has been linked to chronic musculoskeletal pain, although this is somewhat controversial.[96,97] Myofascial pain treatment is aimed at correcting precipitating behaviors including ergonomic factors. Physical rehabilitation is essential for teaching patients appropriate stretching and strengthening exercises, as well as postural support and stabilization.

Clinical Presentation and Treatment of Fibromyalgia

DISTINGUISHING FIBROMYALGIA FROM MYOFASCIAL PAIN

CASE 7-2

QUESTION 1: G.R. is a 38-year-old white woman who presents with chronic widespread muscle pain from her neck down past her buttocks. She also has headaches when her pain is severe. She has had this pain for several years and notes that her pain developed after a car accident in which she sustained a whiplash injury. She describes difficulty sleeping, poor concentration, and fatigue. Her pain rating is 8 of 10 on most days. She works part-time doing some home transcription. Nothing really helps her pain, and physical activity makes the pain worse, so she does not exercise. Her pain is also worse when she is stressed. She was previously told that she has fibromyalgia. Another provider told her she has myofascial pain, and several more have told her that "it's all in her head." Her past medical history includes depression and IBS. She has tried ibuprofen, cyclobenzaprine, SOMA (carisoprodol), and acetaminophen in the past without relief. She is currently taking tramadol 50 mg (1 tablet) four times daily (QID), which provides about 20% pain relief. She is also taking sertraline for depression. G.R. is married and has three children. She smokes one pack of cigarettes daily but denies drinking alcohol or using illicit drugs. She reports that her mother and sister have fibromyalgia and depression. She reports diffuse tenderness to palpation along her paraspinal muscles bilaterally, as well as her bilateral trapezius and levator scapulae muscles and her hips bilaterally. Several tender points are elicited. Her only remarkable laboratory result is vitamin D, 24 ng/mL (normal > 30 ng/mL).

Does G.R. have fibromyalgia or myofascial pain? What part(s) of her presentation supports this?

It is not unusual for clinicians to misdiagnose myofascial pain and fibromyalgia. Sometimes both patients and clinicians are looking for a diagnosis to explain this diverse and nonspecific collection of symptoms. G.R. likely has fibromyalgia, given her widespread pain that has been present for more than 3 months and was precipitated by a traumatic event (car accident). She reports sleeping poorly, fatigue, and the comorbidities of depression and IBS. On physical examination, she exhibits widespread musculoskeletal tenderness including, but not limited to, several of the identified fibromyalgia tender points, bilaterally, both above and below the waist. No "taut bands" are elicited, although her job as a transcriptionist leads to long periods where she may be in a static position, and this may contribute to a possible myofascial component. Her vitamin D level represents a mild deficiency.

FIBROMYALGIA TREATMENT

CASE 7-2, QUESTION 2: What pharmacologic and nonpharmacologic therapies could be recommended for G.R.?

An appropriate first step for G.R. is to develop a multidisciplinary approach, including physical rehabilitation, CBT, and pharmacologic therapy adjustments. She is currently taking an antidepressant (sertraline), which may be helpful for her depression but is likely not very helpful for her fibromyalgia. It may be possible to switch her to an SNRI like duloxetine or milnacipran, but not without checking with her other prescriber(s). She is currently using tramadol with some relief. She has not maximized her dose (maximum daily dose is 400 mg); however, she is also taking an SSRI, which may increase her CNS levels of 5-HT to a dangerous level. The risks and benefits of combining antidepressants with tramadol must be considered on a patient-by-patient basis. Because she is having trouble sleeping, she could be offered a trial of amitriptyline or pregabalin, both of which have sedating side effects. See Table 7-7 for dosing and precautions. Pregabalin is a recommended agent and has a different mechanism of action than the medications that she has previously tried. If her

TABLE 7-8
Oral Muscle Relaxants

Drug	Dose	Adverse Effects	Monitoring/Comments
Antispasmodic			
Cyclobenzaprine	5 mg TID, titrate to 10 mg TID	Dry mouth, constipation, urinary retention, somnolence, confusion, blurred vision	Also available in extended-release formulation
Metaxalone	300 mg TID–QID	GI upset, nausea, vomiting, dizziness, headache, somnolence, hemolytic anemia, leucopenia, jaundice	Contraindicated in anemia, liver impairment, renal impairment Monitor liver function, CBC
Methocarbamol	1,500 mg TID, or 1,000 mg QID	Itching, rash, indigestion, nausea, vomiting, dizziness, headache, nystagmus, somnolence, vertigo, blurred vision, arrhythmias, hypotension, leucopenia	Monitor heart rate, blood pressure
Orphenadrine citrate	100 mg BID	Syncope, nausea, vomiting, dry mouth, dizziness, blurred vision, palpitations	Monitor CBC, liver function
Chlorzoxazone	500–750 mg TID–QID	Lightheadedness, dizziness, somnolence, malaise, liver toxicity	Monitor liver function
Carisoprodol	250–350 mg TID and at bedtime	CNS depressant, dizziness, headache, somnolence	Monitor for weakness, dizziness, confusion
Antispastic			
Tizanidine	4 mg TID, titrate to max of 12 mg TID	Hypotension, somnolence, muscle weakness	Monitor blood pressure, liver function
Baclofen	10 mg TID, titrate to max of 20 mg QID	Somnolence, muscle weakness, ataxia	
Benzodiazepines (diazepam)	2 mg TID, titrate to max of 10 mg TID	CNS depressant, somnolence, weakness	Monitor sedation Risk of physical dependence
Dantrolene	25 mg daily × 7 days, 25 mg TID × 7 days, titrate to max of 100 mg QID	Hepatitis, tachycardia, confusion, nausea, vomiting, depression, fatigue, dizziness, somnolence, blood dyscrasias, rash, GI obstruction	Monitor liver function

BID, twice a day; CBC, complete blood cell count; GI, gastrointestinal; QID, four times a day; TID, three times a day.

insurance will not pay for this, she could try gabapentin instead. A vitamin D supplement should also be considered to correct her slightly low vitamin D levels. Although there is not strong evidence supporting vitamin D supplementation, there is little harm in correcting her slight deficiency.

Bernardy et al. conducted a systematic review of cognitive behavioral therapy for fibromyalgia, and found that this therapy improves coping with pain and reduces depressed mood and health care–seeking behavior.[98] Hauser et al. evaluated different regimens of aerobic activity with a meta-analysis and found that land- and water-based aerobic exercise, at a slight to moderate intensity, 2 to 3 times a week for at least 4 weeks resulted in improvement of depressed mood and increased Health-Related Quality of Life scores and physical fitness. This was maintained if the patient continued exercise at home.[99] Acupuncture has not been found to be beneficial.[100]

MUSCLE RELAXANT RECOMMENDATIONS

CASE 7-2, QUESTION 3: G.R. has used at least two different muscle relaxants. Is a muscle relaxant a good choice for G.R.?

Muscle relaxants are commonly used to treat chronic musculoskeletal pain. Because patients with fibromyalgia present with muscular pain, clinicians mistakenly believe that a skeletal muscle relaxant may be helpful. Cyclobenzaprine is considered a possible option for treating fibromyalgia pain. There is a small amount of evidence that it improves sleep in these patients (see above). There is also a study that shows improvement with tizanidine, but there are no data supporting continued use of carisoprodol. These agents belong to a chemically diverse family, but all work in the CNS, either in the brain or in the spinal cord. They are categorized as either antispasmodics or antispasticity agents. The antispasmodics are either benzodiazepines (e.g., diazepam) or nonbenzodiazepines (e.g., cyclobenzaprine) and are used for muscular pain and spasms associated with peripheral musculoskeletal conditions. The antispasticity agents reduce spasticity associated with upper motor neuron disorders like multiple sclerosis (e.g., dantrolene, baclofen) (Table 7-8). Chou et al. performed a systematic review of trials to compare efficacy and safety of skeletal muscle relaxants.[101] Although the evidence was considered to be of fair quality, they concluded that for the treatment of musculoskeletal pain, tizanidine, orphenadrine, carisoprodol, and cyclobenzaprine were more effective than placebo. There were not sufficient data of good quality to determine whether metaxalone, methocarbamol, chlorzoxazone, baclofen, or dantrolene were better than placebo for this indication.[101] At this time guidelines do not recommend chronic use of muscle relaxants for musculoskeletal pain. Because G.R. has not experienced any improvement in her pain with previous trials of muscle relaxants, switching to another is not likely to yield any improvement in her symptoms.

NEUROPATHIC PAIN AND POSTHERPETIC NEURALGIA

Pain may be centrally or peripherally mediated. Peripheral sensory neuropathy usually involves injury or insult to peripheral nerves, like postherpetic neuralgia (PHN), which affects spinal nerve dermatomes. The pain tends to be fairly localized, either regionally or along an associated dermatome. Central pain syndromes originate from injury to the CNS or alteration in central pain processing, as occurs with neuroplasticity. Central pain presents with a larger affected area, up to and including unilateral, head-to-toe pain that may be seen after a stroke.

Herpes zoster occurs in 500,000 Americans each year, and approximately 20% of these patients experience PHN.[102,103] Evidence-based guidelines for treating neuropathic pain have been sponsored by several international organizations in the last several years.[104,105] Most studies have been conducted in PHN and diabetic peripheral neuropathy (DPN), as these are the most common neuropathic pain conditions. Some types of neuropathic pain (e.g., spinal cord injury and human immunodeficiency virus–neuropathy) have been quite resistant to pharmacologic therapy. Studies to date have shown only partial relief of neuropathic pain regardless of pharmacologic treatment. Doses, adverse effects, and monitoring for these agents can be found in Table 7-9.

First-line treatments for neuropathic pain include SNRI antidepressants such as TCA's, venlafaxine, and duloxetine. These antidepressants demonstrate effective pain relief, even in patients without concurrent depression. The TCAs are inexpensive and easily administered once daily; however, they have significant anticholinergic adverse effects, such as dry mouth and constipation, that many patients do not tolerate. The secondary amine antidepressants, like nortriptyline, have fewer anticholinergic adverse effects than the parent compound amitriptyline and are similarly effective. TCAs are known to cause orthostatic hypotension and urinary retention in elderly patients and may cause cardiac arrhythmias with higher doses. Venlafaxine has been shown to be effective for certain types of peripheral neuropathic pain.[106] At lower doses it functions as an SSRI, so doses need to be titrated by 37.5-mg or 75-mg increments each week to reach a target dose of at least 200 mg daily. At this dose, venlafaxine offers SNRI activity. However, at higher doses (>225 mg/day), increases in blood pressure and heart rate caused by

TABLE 7-9
Pharmacologic Options for Treatment of Neuropathic Pain

Drug	Dose[a]	Adverse Effects	Monitoring/ Comments
Carbamazepine[b]	200 mg TID, titrate to max 400 mg TID	Diplopia, rash, hepatitis, neutropenia, aplastic anemia, dizziness, cognitive effects, hyponatremia	Check LFTs, CBC, sodium at baseline and every 3 months during therapy
Oxcarbazepine	75 mg BID, titrate to max 1,200 mg BID	Rash, cognitive effects, hyponatremia, sedation, blurred vision	Check sodium every 2 weeks for 3 months, then with dose increases
Lamotrigine	25 mg daily, titrate to max 200 mg BID	Desquamating rash, cognitive effects	Requires very slow titration to avoid rash
Topiramate[b]	25 mg BID, titrate to max 200 mg BID	Nausea, anorexia, paresthesias, metabolic acidosis, cognitive effects, nephrolithiasis	Check serum bicarbonate at baseline and every 3 months or with each dose increase
Lacosamide	50 mg BID, titrate to max 200 mg BID	Nausea, vomiting, dizziness, diplopia, ataxia, fatigue, rash, atrial fibrillation/flutter	ECG at baseline and with dose adjustments, especially in patients at risk for cardiac conduction abnormality Reduce dose for renal and liver impairment
Gabapentin[b]	300 mg daily, titrate to max 1,200 mg TID	Somnolence, dizziness, edema, cognitive effects	Reduce dose for renal impairment or elderly patients
Pregabalin[b]	75 mg BID, titrate to max 300 mg BID	Same as gabapentin	Same as gabapentin
Amitriptyline/nortriptyline	10 mg QHS, titrate to 100 mg QHS	Dry mouth, constipation, urinary retention, orthostatic hypotension, somnolence	Caution in elderly patients
Duloxetine[b]	30 mg daily, titrate to max 60 mg daily	Nausea, dry mouth, headache, diarrhea, fatigue, sweating, anorexia	Contraindicated with liver disease or concurrent alcohol consumption
Venlafaxine	37.5 mg daily, titrate to max 225 mg daily	Headache, nausea, sweating, sedation, hypertension, seizures, tachycardia	Serotonergic effects <150 mg and noradrenergic effects >150 mg Monitor blood pressure and heart rate
Opioids[b]	10–15 mg morphine every 4 hours or equianalgesic dose of other opioid	Somnolence, dry mouth, constipation, urinary retention	May cause confusion in elderly patients Use with a bowel regimen
Tramadol[b]	25 mg QID to max 100 mg QID	Somnolence, dry mouth, constipation	Caution with antidepressants
Capsaicin cream[b]	Apply QID	Rash, burning feeling on skin	Avoid contact with mucous membranes, eyes
Capsaicin patch[b]	Apply 1 patch for 1 hour, every 3 months	Skin irritation at application site, burning feeling on skin	Must be applied in medical office
Lidocaine patch[b]	Apply 1–3 patches daily for 12 hours	Skin reaction at site of application	

[a] All oral agents are titrated up to reduce adverse effects and titrated down when discontinuing therapy.
[b] Food and Drug Administration–approved for treating pain conditions.
BID, twice a day; CBC, complete blood cell count; ECG, electrocardiogram; LFTs, liver function tests; QHS, every night at bedtime; QID, four times a day; TID, three times a day.

increased NE activity may cause patients to stop therapy. Duloxetine has shown efficacy in treating diabetic peripheral sensory neuropathy with once-daily dosing.[107,108] Cardiac rhythm, blood pressure, and pulse rate do not seem to be affected by duloxetine. The most common adverse effect with duloxetine is nausea on initiation. The dose of duloxetine is titrated up over 2 weeks to minimize the nausea. Duloxetine is contraindicated in patients with liver disease or those who drink alcohol as there have been reports of liver failure with this medication

Anticonvulsants that bind to voltage-gated calcium channels are also considered first-line therapy for C fiber–related neuropathic pain (such as DPN and PHN), allodynia, and nonpainful dysesthesias (abnormal sensations). They have also been very helpful in reducing central sensitization by preventing the release of glutamate and blocking glutamate receptors. Gabapentin and pregabalin (gabapentinoids), both voltage-gated calcium-channel blockers, have shown efficacy and are FDA-approved for treating neuropathic pain, including PHN and DPN.[109,110] These agents must be taken two or three times daily and may cause dizziness, somnolence, peripheral edema, and cognitive problems. The somnolence is usually managed with a slow titration, but these combined effects may be significant in elderly patients. Although neither agent has many drug interactions, the doses must be reduced for renal insufficiency, as they are 100% renally eliminated.

Anticonvulsants that block sodium-channel, such as carbamazepine, oxcarbazepine, and lamotrigine, have been shown to be helpful for A∂ fiber–mediated pain such as trigeminal neuralgia that has sharp, shooting qualities. Carbamazepine is an older agent that requires routine monitoring of complete blood counts (CBCs) for blood dyscrasias, liver transaminases for possible hepatitis, and serum sodium for possible syndrome of inappropriate antidiuretic hormone (SIADH)–induced hyponatremia. It is also a strong cytochrome P-450 enzyme inducer, and there are numerous drug–drug interactions with carbamazepine. Oxcarbazepine has substantially fewer drug interactions and does not require monitoring of CBCs and liver transaminases because it does not form the 10,11-epoxide metabolite that carbamazepine does. It requires monitoring of serum sodium for the first 3 months of therapy and periodically thereafter, as it may cause SIADH and hyponatremia, especially within the first 3 months of therapy. Lamotrigine has few drug interactions except with valproic acid and does not require any laboratory monitoring. It may, however, cause a desquamating rash (Stevens-Johnson syndrome) if the dose is escalated too quickly. A newer agent, lacosamide, shows modest efficacy for treating DPN but is not FDA-approved for treating pain.

Topical agents such as local anesthetics and capsaicin are effective for treating localized areas of neuropathic pain, such as PHN. A 5% lidocaine patch is approved by the FDA for the treatment of PHN and is particularly helpful for treating allodynia. It is very well tolerated and easy to apply. It may be cut to the desired shape, and very minimal local anesthetic penetrates the skin, so there is no systemic toxicity. Various other topical lidocaine products are available (ointments and creams), but most do not penetrate the skin deep enough to reach the affected nerve endings. Capsaicin cream is available in several strengths, and there is now an FDA-approved 8% patch available for medical office use. Capsaicin depletes substance P in the periphery and down-regulates the TRPV1 receptors. Because it is derived from chili peppers, it causes a significant amount of burning until the substance P is depleted, and many patients do not tolerate the application of the cream several times daily to accomplish this. The patch is applied in the medical office for an hour, once every 3 months.

Opioid analgesics have shown the same efficacy as other agents in treating neuropathic pain, particularly PHN and DPN. However, they are not usually considered first-line therapy because of potential long-term effects such as hyperalgesia, tolerance, immunosuppression, and hypogonadism with osteoporosis. Constipation, sedation, nausea, and urinary retention occur commonly with opioids, and the constipation, in particular, must be treated concurrently with a bowel regimen such as a stool softener and a stimulant laxative. Tramadol, which has both weak opioid activity and SNRI activity, has been shown to be effective in several types of neuropathic pain. Its adverse effects are similar to those of both opioids and SNRIs, including constipation, sedation, and possibly seizures, which are a dose-limiting effect.

When analgesic classes were compared, the TCAs were equally effective and well tolerated compared with the gabapentinoids and substantially less expensive.[105]

There are some data that show that a combination of agents, such as an opioid and a gabapentinoid, or a TCA and a gabapentinoid, may offer more analgesia than either agent alone.[49,50] This analgesic polypharmacy may offer additive analgesia because different agents act on different parts of the pain-signaling pathways. If more than one agent is used, lower doses of each may reduce adverse effects. However, polypharmacy adds complexity to regimens, which may reduce compliance and cause confusion, particularly in elderly patients.

Clinical Presentation and Treatment of Postherpetic Neuralgia

NEUROPATHIC PAIN SYMPTOMS

CASE 7-3

QUESTION 1: K.J. is a 73-year-old man with a history of Hodgkin lymphoma. He is in remission after chemotherapy and radiation treatment. He is seen in consult for PHN attributable to a case of shingles during chemotherapy. The zoster episode was after his first chemotherapy cycle 2 years ago. The lesions covered an area around his right lower abdomen below the umbilicus in a 10- to 15-cm strip around the lower back and buttock. Sitting quietly, his pain is a 1 to 2 of 10. At its worst it is 7 to 8 of 10. Pain is aggravated by light touch or any jarring motion (such as riding in a car) or rubbing of clothes on the location of the zoster. He has two areas that have greater pain, one located in the lower right aspect of his back and the other in the right lower abdominal quadrant. He describes the pain as a burning sensation. He gets mild relief from topical aquaphilic ointment. If he stays busy, it sometimes takes his mind off the pain. He has not been sleeping well because of the pain. His past medical history includes Hodgkin lymphoma, in remission, low back pain, and benign prostatic hypertrophy (BPH). He currently takes acyclovir 400 mg daily, alprazolam 0.25 mg QHS as needed (PRN) for sleep, docusate 100 mg BID PRN for constipation, multivitamin one daily, tamsulosin 0.4 mg QHS, and zolpidem 5 mg QHS. K.J. is married, has never smoked, and denies alcohol and illicit drug use. His physical examination is unremarkable with the exception of scarring noted from the right lower abdomen to the back. Laboratory results and vital signs obtained at this visit are the following:

Serum creatinine, 1.2 mg/dL
Electrolytes, within normal limits
Blood pressure, 137/80 mm Hg
Heart rate, 77 beats/minute
Weight, 80 kg

Which of K.J.'s presenting symptoms are consistent with neuropathic pain and PHN?

K.J. is past the acute phase of his herpes zoster (shingles) pain, but now notices that the pain has a burning quality, localized over the region where his lesions have healed. This is quite typical for a PHN presentation. Another feature that indicates a neuropathic type of pain is his increase in pain with light touch or rubbing of his clothing (allodynia). It is a localized pain that does not radiate past the dermatomal distribution of his zoster infection. Opportunistic infections like herpes zoster are common in patients who are immunocompromised like K.J. when he was receiving chemotherapy.

POSTHERPETIC NEURALGIA TREATMENT

CASE 7-3, QUESTION 2: Which medication is the most appropriate option for treating K.J.'s PHN pain? What factors need to be considered when choosing a medication for K.J.?

The American Academy of Neurology (AAN) published PHN treatment guidelines in 2004. Since that time there have been many more studies published, but there has been very little change in the approach to treating neuropathic pain. The AAN guidelines state that TCA's (amitriptyline, nortriptyline, desipramine), gabapentin, pregabalin, opioids, and topical lidocaine patches are effective and should be used in the treatment of PHN. There is limited evidence to support nortriptyline versus amitriptyline, and the data are insufficient to recommend one opioid over another.[111]

Ideally, patients should be treated with the most effective therapy that has the lowest risk of adverse effects. K.J. has peripheral neuropathic pain in a localized area, which is typical of PHN, so a reasonable first-line choice would be a lidocaine patch; however, his pain is in a 10- to 12-cm strip that covers a fairly large surface area from his abdomen to his back. He would need to use at least two patches daily to cover this area, which is fewer than the maximal recommended dose of three patches daily, but it would be an effective barrier against the pain of clothing rubbing against this location. Another localized option would be capsaicin (either as a patch or a cream). Capsaicin cream is available over the counter and is substantially less expensive than lidocaine patches. Insurance plans may require a trial of capsaicin before approving the more-expensive lidocaine patch. Unfortunately, many patients cannot tolerate the burning associated with capsaicin.

Another first-line option would be a TCA, which may help him sleep. However, he has BPH, and the anticholinergic effects of a TCA may cause increased urinary retention. They also cause orthostatic hypotension and may be a risk for K.J. if he has to get up during the night to use the bathroom. If a TCA is used, an appropriate starting dose in an older patient is 10 mg of either amitriptyline or nortriptyline at bedtime, with gradual dose escalation as the patient tolerates. (See Table 7-9 for more complete information.) An SNRI such as duloxetine would have fewer anticholinergic adverse effects but is not FDA-approved for treating PHN.

A calcium-channel blocking anticonvulsant such as gabapentin is also a possibility. The sedating effects of gabapentin may help him sleep if his last dose is given at bedtime, and would not cause the urinary retention, constipation, and orthostatic hypotension that a TCA would. Given his age, a slow dose escalation starting at 100 mg TID would be appropriate. The most important aspect of monitoring for this agent would be for cognitive effects, such as short-term memory problems or difficulty with word-finding.

If the above options do not provide adequate analgesia, addition of an opioid such as morphine or oxycodone may be considered. As stated above, opioids offer additive relief when combined with other analgesics. Initially, a short-acting opioid should be used so that K.J. may be titrated to the optimal analgesic dose. Tramadol is another alternative with some TCA-like activity and mild opioid effects. However, if an opioid is added, it may increase the adverse effects of the above agents, including constipation, sedation, urinary retention, and cognitive effects. Whenever an opioid is added to a medication regimen, a bowel regimen must be implemented as well. A commonly used regimen includes a stool softener such as docusate sodium 100 mg BID and a mild stimulant laxative such as senna one to two tablets QHS. If this combination is not effective, an osmotic agent such as polyethylene glycol powder may be added.

MODIFYING THE NEUROPATHIC PAIN REGIMEN

CASE 7-3, QUESTION 3: K.J. returns after 2 months with complaints that he could not tolerate the burning of the capsaicin cream so discontinued this. He is currently using gabapentin 1,200 mg TID and tramadol 50 mg one tablet QID. He still has 5 of 10 burning pain over his right abdomen and back. He states that he has felt drowsy and has "unclear thoughts" with the gabapentin and does not feel that it has been very effective, despite titrating this to the maximal dose of 3,600 mg daily. His wife reports that he is withdrawing from friends and he does not feel as involved. He is sleeping better, however, and believes that the tramadol is somewhat helpful in "taking the edge off" his pain. Given this information, what would be an appropriate adjustment in his therapy?

Adverse cognitive effects like K.J. is having are common with anticonvulsants, especially in older patients. Problems with memory, concentration, and word-finding are common. No anticonvulsant is better than any other in this regard; however, some of the adverse effects are dose-related, and patients may exhibit tolerance to some of the effects (like sedation) with time. K.J. is at the maximal recommended daily dose of gabapentin and does not feel that this has been very helpful. At this time he may need to be tapered off the gabapentin. Sometimes patients do not notice analgesic effects of their medications until they are discontinued. It is a good practice to titrate oral analgesics upward when starting therapy and downward when discontinuing, to avoid a marked increase in pain and withdrawal syndromes that have been reported with both antidepressants and some anticonvulsants. He could reduce his dose by 300 mg every 3 to 5 days until his pain increases or he is off the gabapentin.

A different topical agent (although more expensive) would be the lidocaine patch. Because he and his wife are reporting some signs of depression, an antidepressant may be an option. An antidepressant was not chosen previously because of concerns about his BPH symptoms; however, a nontricyclic SNRI agent like duloxetine may be an effective alternative to treat his depression as well as his pain, although there are no studies reporting its effectiveness for this indication. Another option may be to switch to another anticonvulsant. Pregabalin has very similar pharmacologic activity to gabapentin, so it may not offer any additional analgesia over gabapentin. Possibly a sodium-channel blocking anticonvulsant like oxcarbazepine could be used for a trial. However, there are minimal data supporting the sodium-channel blockers for typical C fiber–mediated pain associated with PHN.

ANALGESIC DRUG–DRUG INTERACTIONS

CASE 7-3, QUESTION 4: K.J.'s doctor decides to order duloxetine and a lidocaine patch and taper off the gabapentin as tolerated. When she orders K.J.'s new regimen, she notes that there is a drug–drug interaction listed

with the duloxetine and tramadol. What would be your recommendations regarding potential drug–drug interactions with analgesics and, in particular, with K.J.'s regimen? What changes could be made?

Antidepressants either increase the concentrations of NE or 5-HT or both. Tramadol also has NE and 5-HT reuptake inhibitor activity, so it is possible to end up with a net excess of either of these neurotransmitters, or both. The consequence of an excess of NE is CNS excitation and possible seizures. The consequence of an excess of 5-HT is a possibly life-threatening syndrome called *serotonin syndrome.* Symptoms of serotonin syndrome include muscle rigidity, hyperpyrexia, mental status changes, and possible organ failure. None of these serious adverse effects are very predictable, although they are more likely with higher doses of either agent. However, any of the antidepressants may cause this interaction with tramadol and other serotonergic agents. Tramadol is commonly used with antidepressants, but the lowest effective doses should be used and patients should be counseled to watch for mental status changes.

Pharmacodynamic interactions are more likely to occur with analgesic polypharmacy. Because several analgesics may be used together to decrease the excitatory effects of the pain signal, there is always a risk of additive sedation, dizziness, or even respiratory depression. Several pharmacokinetic drug–drug interactions may occur with analgesics as well. In K.J.'s case, his duloxetine and tramadol are both substrates of cytochrome P-450 2D6 and may compete with each other for this enzyme. This may alter the blood levels and clinical effects of these agents. A table of agents commonly used in pain management, the relevant cytochrome P450 enzyme involved in its metabolism, and therefore potential drug interactions can be found in Table 7-10.

K.J. likely needs an antidepressant for his depression symptoms, so switching his tramadol to another opioid, such as oxycodone or morphine, should be considered to avoid the possibility of serotonin syndrome. He reported some relief with tramadol, and both oxycodone and morphine are effective in treating PHN.[50,112] He should be counseled on a possible increase in opioid-related adverse effects with the stronger opioid.

COMPLEX REGIONAL PAIN SYNDROME

Complex regional pain syndrome (CRPS) is defined by the International Association for the Study of Pain as a syndrome that usually develops after an initiating noxious event, is not limited to the distribution of a single peripheral nerve, and is apparently disproportional to the inciting event. It is associated at some point with evidence of edema, changes in skin blood flow, abnormal pseudomotor activity in the region of the pain, or allodynia or hyperalgesia.[113] It usually occurs after some type of injury, but may develop as a response to a CNS lesion like a stroke or spinal cord injury, or even without any known cause. It was previously known as reflex sympathetic dystrophy or causalgia, but has more recently been defined according to whether the cause is known or unknown. The overall incidence of CRPS is estimated to be anywhere from 5.46 to 26.2 per 100,000 person-years with women being three times more likely to be affected. The upper extremities are more likely to be affected than the lower extremities, and fractures are the most common inciting event.[114,115] Acutely, the inflammatory response causes peripheral sensitization and localized pain, vasodilation, release of inflammatory markers such as interleukin 6 and TNF-α, and accumulation of immunoglobulin in the affected area. This is coupled with an increase in CNS concentrations of proinflammatory cytokines, which may contribute to central sensitization. Clinical features tend to be disproportionately greater than expected with the

TABLE 7-10
Drug Interactions With Analgesics

CYP1A2	CYP2C9	CYP2C19	CYP2D6	CYP3A4
Substrates				
Amitriptyline	Amitriptyline	Amitriptyline	Amitriptyline, mexiletine	Alprazolam, methadone
Naproxen	Celecoxib	Citalopram	Nortriptyline, morphine	Amitriptyline, prednisone
R-warfarin	Diclofenac	Diazepam	Cyclobenzaprine, codeine	Buspirone, sertraline
Duloxetine	Fluoxetine	Indomethacin	Desipramine, oxycodone	Clonazepam, temazepam
Methadone	Ibuprofen	Topiramate	Doxepin, paroxetine	Codeine, zaleplon
Theophylline	Naproxen		Fluoxetine, sertraline	Cyclobenzaprine, zolpidem
Tizanidine	Piroxicam		Hydrocodone, tramadol	Diazepam, R-warfarin
	S-warfarin		Methadone, venlafaxine	Fentanyl, carbamazepine
	Phenytoin		Fentanyl, duloxetine	Lidocaine, erythromycin
Inducers				
Carbamazepine	Carbamazepine	Carbamazepine	Carbamazepine	Carbamazepine
Phenytoin	Fluoxetine	Phenytoin	Phenytoin	Oxcarbazepine
	Cimetidine			Phenytoin
	Metronidazole			
	Fluconazole			
Inhibitors				
Cimetidine	Carbamazepine	Fluoxetine	Celecoxib	Fluoxetine
Ciprofloxacin	Paroxetine	Indomethacin	Desipramine	Sertraline
	Sertraline	Paroxetine	Fluoxetine	Ketoconazole
	Valproic acid	Topiramate	Methadone	Cyclosporine
	Phenytoin		Paroxetine	
			Sertraline	
			Valproic acid	

CYP, cytochrome P-450.

inciting injury. They include sensory symptoms such as burning pain, allodynia, and hyperalgesia. There are also autonomic symptoms such as edema, sweating, and reduced skin blood flow. The affected extremity tends to be either warmer (earlier) or colder (later) than the unaffected extremity. These symptoms may be partly influenced by the sympathetic nervous system, called *sympathetically maintained pain*. Trophic changes such as abnormal nail growth, hair growth, fibrosis, thin glossy skin, or osteoporosis are also common. Motor symptoms include weakness of the affected extremity and a possible tremor.

Because the pathology of central pain syndromes is elusive, a specific treatment plan is also not possible. A global approach to management is necessary, targeting the physical symptoms of pain and vasomotor effects, and functional restoration. Tran et al. performed a systematic review of randomized, controlled trials for the treatment of CRPS, and Perez et al. published evidence-based guidelines for treating CRPS.[116,117] Pharmacologic therapies with literature support include corticosteroids (with or without cerebral infarction) and bisphosphonates, which inhibit bone resorption. Symptomatically they reduce pain and edema, and increase the range of motion of the affected limb. The free radical scavenger, dimethyl sulfoxide (DMSO), has shown a possible benefit in early (warm) CRPS, and *N*-acetyl cysteine shows some benefit for later (cold) CRPS. Gabapentin may offer relief early in the course of the syndrome, but does not show any long-term benefit. Other commonly used analgesics (NSAIDs, acetaminophen, opioids, antidepressants, other anticonvulsants, capsaicin) have shown only anecdotal efficacy in CRPS.

Interventional therapies such as intravenous (IV) regional blocks with local anesthetics and various other medications are commonly used to improve the vasomotor effects of CRPS, although they do not have strong literature support. They block the sympathetic nervous system, leading to vasodilation of the affected extremity. Stellate ganglion nerve blocks are used for upper extremity symptoms and lumbar sympathetic blocks are used for the lower extremities. These may provide short-term symptom improvement, allowing patients to undergo physical rehabilitation with less pain and more mobility. Subanesthetic infusions of ketamine have also shown some promise. The most invasive approach to managing peripheral CRPS symptoms is a spinal cord stimulator. This involves placing an electrode(s) in the epidural space at the level of the nerve root that innervates the affected extremity. A mild electrical current is sent via a small generator (about the size of a matchbook) that the patient can control with an external control. The stimulator provides patients with a sensation of "tingling" in the affected area(s) instead of pain. Studies have shown that spinal cord stimulation provides about 2 to 5 years of symptom relief and improvement in quality of life, but after 5 years there was no difference compared with patients who did not have the spinal cord stimulator, and these studies have not shown any improvement in function. This is accompanied by expenses greater than $10,000 and a high rate of complications (72% in the first 2 years). Physiotherapy (including physical and occupational therapy) has shown a beneficial effect on function and coping ability and is recommended as part of a standard therapeutic approach.[116,118]

Clinical Presentation and Treatment of Complex Regional Pain Syndrome

COMPLEX REGIONAL PAIN SYNDROME SYMPTOMS

CASE 7-4

QUESTION 1: B.E. is a 39-year-old woman who presents with right hand pain, especially in the thumb and index finger. Three months ago she fell from her bicycle, sustaining a fracture of the right thumb metacarpal and right index proximal phalanx. She underwent closed reduction with pinning of the right thumb metacarpal and was placed in a cast for 1 month. Initially her pain was localized at the base of her right thumb and was well controlled with hydromorphone or hydrocodone/acetaminophen. Three weeks ago the pin was removed, and physical therapy was initiated. Since then she has noticed that the pain has been progressively getting worse. The pain is more intense than it was, and it radiates down to the second and third digits and up to the radial aspect of her right forearm. She describes it as constant stabbing pain. She denies any numbness in her right forearm or fingers. A few days ago she noticed purplish color and progressive swelling in her right hand. Also, she has hypersensitivity to light touch in the right index and middle fingers and the radial aspect of her right forearm. She notes that her right hand has had progressive stiffness, and her range of motion is quite limited because of pain. Her physical therapist reports that the right hand looks much different in terms of color changes, swelling, and atrophic changes when compared with last week. Her past medical history includes systemic lupus erythematosus (with pleurisy, photosensitive rash, oral ulcers, Raynaud's, positive antinuclear antibody test, and positive double-stranded DNA), depression, and a left rotator cuff repair. She takes fluoxetine 40 mg daily, hydroxychloroquine sulfate 400 mg daily, and ibuprofen 400 mg as needed. She has previously experienced rashes with codeine and amitriptyline. B.E. is divorced with two children, earned a PhD, and works full time at a local college. She does not use any alcohol, tobacco, or recreational drugs. On physical examination her right hand has a purplish discoloration. Right upper extremity skin temperature 25.8°C. Left upper (unaffected) extremity skin temperature 29.6°C. Allodynia is noted on the dorsal aspect of the right index and middle fingers, as well as on the radial aspect of the right hand and forearm. Mild swelling in the right hand and hypotrophic changes of intrinsic hand muscles of the right hand are observed. There is limited range of motion of the right wrist in flexion (15 degrees) and extension (30 degrees), and she is not able to perform ulnar and radial deviation because of the pain. Muscle strength is 5 of 5 in the left upper extremity and 3 of 5 in the right wrist flexion/extension and hand grip. Sensation is intact in bilateral upper extremities. The rest of the physical examination was unremarkable. Her vital signs today are as follows:

Blood pressure, 126/75 mm Hg
Heart rate, 72 beats/minute
Respiratory rate, 16 breaths/minute
Weight, 82.3 kg
Body mass index, 30.22 kg/m^2

She has a pain rating of 6 of 10. The medical team believes that B.E. has CRPS and plans to perform a stellate ganglion block. What symptoms does B.E. have that are consistent with CRPS and central pain?

B.E. exhibits unilateral upper extremity pain after a known injury. She experienced increasing pain, discoloration, and swelling in the affected extremity with allodynia. Her physical therapist confirmed that the right hand looks much different in terms of color changes, swelling, and atrophic changes in the past week. Her physical examination reveals the classic symptoms of purplish discoloration and temperature difference between the affected and unaffected extremity, as well as allodynia on the dorsal aspect of the right index and middle fingers and the radial aspect of the right hand and forearm. Mild swelling in the right hand and hypotrophic changes of intrinsic hand muscles of the right hand were noted. Her skin temperature on the affected limb is lower than the unaffected limb by more than 2°C, indicating a significant difference. She has limited range of motion of the right wrist in flexion (15 degrees) and extension (30 degrees), and she was not able to perform ulnar and radial deviation because of pain. All of her symptoms are classically associated with CRPS.

COMPLEX REGIONAL PAIN SYNDROME TREATMENT

CASE 7-4, QUESTION 2: What should be recommended for treating CRPS in B.E.?

The team plans to perform an IV regional block on B.E., which may offer some short-term relief to allow her to continue participating in physical therapy, but this will not offer long-term relief. Her hand is already starting to exhibit vasoconstriction, so it may be too late to offer corticosteroids, but gabapentin may still have some benefit by reducing her allodynia. Also, a bisphosphonate such as alendronate may be helpful for her pain and to prevent bone resorption and osteoporosis.

PHARMACOTHERAPY OPTIONS FOR CHRONIC PAIN IN THE ELDERLY

Pain is common in older adults but often poorly assessed and managed, resulting in consequences that include sleep disturbances, malnutrition, decline in social and recreational activities, deterioration in physical functioning, falls, depression, anxiety, and impaired cognition. When assessing pain, it is important to select a tool that has been validated for age and cognitive function. The 0–10 Numeric Rating Scale (NRS) has been validated across all age groups and is useful in patients who do not have mental status deficits. Other scales tested in older adults who cannot comprehend the NRS include the Revised Faces Pain Scale (FPS-R) and Iowa Pain Thermometer.[119] The pain thermometer in Figure 7-4 demonstrates the NRS and FPS-R scales. Verbal pain assessment using the NRS can be easily done by simply asking the patient, "On a scale of 0 to 10, with 0 being no pain and 10 being the worst pain you can imagine, how much does it hurt right now? How much does it hurt at its worst? How much does it hurt at its least?" If the patient cannot understand the NRS, use the FPS-R and have the patient point to the face that shows how they feel about their pain.

OA-related pain is a frequent complaint in the elderly. There are six different professional organizations who have published recommendations on the treatment of OA (Table 7-11) in addition to guidelines by the American Geriatrics Society (AGS) for pain management.[120–122] The decision on which set of guidelines to use for OA is not clear. All of the guidelines are evidence-based but have different viewpoints on treatment, including pharmacotherapy, surgery, physical modalities, and complementary medicine. Case 7-5 will focus on selection of analgesics for older adults. A summary of the pathophysiology, diagnosis, and treatment of OA is found in Chapter 43, Osteoarthritis.

TABLE 7-11
Summary of Pharmacologic Therapy Recommendations[a] From Osteoarthritis Guidelines[120]

Medication	ACR	EULAR	OARSI	AAOS	NICE
Acetaminophen	1	1	1	1	1
Tramadol	2				
Opioids	2	2	2		2
NSAIDs	1	2	1	1	2
COX-2	2	2	1	2	2
Topical NSAID	2	1	1	2	1
Capsaicin	2	1	1		2
Topical salicylate	2	1			NR
Intraarticular steroids	1	2	2	Short-term	2
Intraarticular hyaluronic acid	2	2	2	NR	NR
Glucosamine and chondroitin		2	2	NR	NR

[a] Strength of recommendation: 1, first-line; 2, second-line; NR, not recommended.
AAOS, American Academy of Orthopedic Surgeons (2008); ACR, American College of Rheumatology (2000); COX-2, cyclo-oxygenase-2; EULAR, European League Against Rheumatism (2003, knee; 2005, hip); NICE, National Institute of Health and Clinical Excellence (2008); NSAID(s), nonsteroidal anti-inflammatory drug(s); ORSI, Osteoarthritis Research Society International (2008).

Clinical Presentation and Treatment of Osteoarthritis

OSTEOARTHRITIS SYMPTOMS

CASE 7-5

QUESTION 1: H.T. is a 72-year-old man seeking pharmacist consultation on over-the-counter (OTC) arthritis pain medications. He is a retired mechanic who likes to build vintage automobiles as a hobby. He has experienced bilateral knee pain for more than 10 years as a result of lifting heavy parts and squatting on the knees to make automobile repairs. During the past year, the pain has become worse on the inner part of the right knee. He complains of general stiffness in both knees early in the morning, but his right knee will continue to have a "grinding" sensation with movement. The pain can get so bad that his right knee "sometimes will give out." His primary-care physician started him on oxycodone 5 mg combined with acetaminophen 325 mg, which works for a while, but the relief does not last very long. He uses ibuprofen occasionally and Aspercreme to the knee joint when the pain gets bad. In addition to pain, he also has hypertension. H.T. states that other than knee pain he feels well and has no complaints. He denies social habits of smoking and frequent use of alcohol. His current pharmacy profile contains prescriptions for metoprolol ER 100 mg orally (PO) once daily for blood pressure and oxycodone 5 mg/acetaminophen 325 mg with one tablet PO BID for pain.

What symptoms of OA are experienced by H.T.?

Data from the National Health and Nutrition Examination Survey I indicate that symptomatic OA (e.g., pain, swelling, stiffness) of the knee affects 4.3 million (12.1%) adults older than 60 years of age with the prevalence higher in women.[123] Occupations that require regular knee bending, lifting, or carrying heavy loads can predispose the knee to OA. In men, such jobs may account as much as obesity for OA.[124]

H.T. reports symptoms of morning stiffness, pain with activity, occasional swelling, crepitus (grinding of the knee), and instability of the knee. Mechanical joint pain, typified by OA, generally causes only 5 to 10 minutes of morning stiffness, but affected joints become progressively more painful with activity. The pain can be localized to either the medial or lateral aspect of the joint depending on which compartment is involved. With more severe disease, contracture may be present, which increases the energy required to stand upright. Loss of ligament and muscle support can lead to instability of the joint, causing the knee to "give way" as a reaction to the pain. Swelling may or may not be present.[125,126]

ACETAMINOPHEN AND OPIOID COMBINATIONS

CASE 7-5, QUESTION 2: How should the current OA guidelines be applied in management of H.T.'s pain with oxycodone/acetaminophen?

Analgesic and anti-inflammatory medications are important in OA pain management but should be used concurrently with nutritional, physical, educational, and cognitive-behavioral interventions. Medication selection is based on the need to balance efficacy with adverse side effects, patient preference, and cost.[122] Acetaminophen is recommended as a first-line therapy in all guideline recommendations for OA (Table 7-11).[120] There is growing controversy about the maximal safe dose of acetaminophen, which has been widely accepted at 4,000 mg/day to minimize the risk of hepatocellular toxicity. A recent meta-analysis of recommendations for management of hip and knee OA found new evidence for increased risk of hospitalizations related to GI ulcers and bleeding with acetaminophen doses greater than 3,000 mg/day.[127] Acute renal insufficiency has been attributed to high acetaminophen levels associated with overdoses, which may lead to hepatotoxicity.[128] Dosage limits to 2,000 g to 3,000 mg/day have been suggested as a way to minimize the risk of renal or hepatic toxicity with prolonged use of acetaminophen.[129,130] However, lower doses of acetaminophen result in a reduction in the analgesic efficacy. Current AGS guidelines for treatment of persistent pain in older adults recommend acetaminophen 500 mg to 1,000 mg orally every 6 hours with a maximum of 4,000 mg daily.[121] The FDA published new acetaminophen OTC label requirements in 2009 to include a statement on the risk of consuming three or more alcoholic drinks every day while taking acetaminophen but did not change the maximal daily dose of 4,000 mg as a result of insufficient data on liver toxicity in healthy adults.[131]

Opioid use is most prevalent for management of OA in weight-bearing joints and low back pain. Current guidelines by the American Academy of Orthopedic Surgeons (AAOS), ACR, EULAR, Osteoarthritis Research Society International (OARSI), and the National Institute of Health and Clinical Excellence (NICE) (Table 7-11) recommend opioid therapy as a second-line option for patients who have an inadequate response or contraindications to other therapies.[120] An agreement between the clinician and patient should be established addressing treatment goals, use of opioid medication, management of side effects, and participation in other therapies to improve physical function before opioid therapy is started.[121] When initiating opioid therapy in older adults, a series of trials may be needed to determine the correct dose and frequency of use while minimizing side effects. Respiratory depression is less likely to occur if the opioid is initiated at a low dose and slowly titrated upward. Short-acting (i.e., immediate-release) opioids, such as hydromorphone or oxycodone, are recommended every 4 hours as needed for pain.[129,130] Patients taking a short-acting oral opioid as needed to reduce pain with movement should be instructed to take the medication 30 minutes before starting activity.

Use of long-acting (i.e., sustained-release) formulations should be reserved for patients who tolerate around-the-clock dosing of short-acting opioids. Tramadol and tapentadol are alternative analgesics with mild opioid activity that can be used for pain management if the patient cannot tolerate side effects with stronger opioids.[121] Table 7-12 provides analgesic recommendations in older adults. Constipation is almost unavoidable with chronic opioid therapy in older adults. To minimize constipation,

TABLE 7-12
Recommended Oral Analgesic Medications for Older Adults[120,121]

Drug	Recommended Starting Dose	Comments
Nonopioid Analgesics		
Acetaminophen (Tylenol)	500–1,000 mg every 6 hours	Maximum dose usually 4 g daily. Reduce maximum dose 50% to 75% in patients with hepatic insufficiency or history of alcohol abuse.
Celecoxib (Celebrex)	100 mg daily	Higher doses associated with higher incidence of gastrointestinal and cardiovascular side effects. Patients with indications for cardioprotection require aspirin supplement; therefore, older individuals will still require concurrent gastroprotection.
Naproxen sodium	220 mg twice daily	May have less cardiovascular toxicity.
Ibuprofen	200 mg three times a day	May have less cardiovascular toxicity.
Tramadol (Ultram)	25 mg every 4–6 hours	Maximum dose 300 mg/d. Risk of seizures if used in higher doses. May precipitate serotonin syndrome if used with selective serotonin reuptake inhibitors.
Tapentadol (Nucynta)	50 mg every 4–6 hours (equivalent to oxycodone 10 mg every 4–6 hours)	Clinical trials suggest lower incidence of gastrointestinal side effects compared with other opioids.
Opioid Analgesics		
Hydromorphone (Dilaudid)	1–2 mg every 3–4 hours	For breakthrough pain or around-the-clock dosing.
Morphine (immediate-release)	2.5–10 mg every 4 hours	Most commonly used for episodic or breakthrough pain. Toxic metabolites may limit usefulness in patients with renal insufficiency.
MS Contin or Oramorph SR (long-acting morphine)	15 mg every 12 hours	Usually started after initial dose determined by the effects of immediate-release opioid.
Oxycodone (immediate-release)	2.5–5 mg every 4–6 hours	Useful for acute recurrent, episodic or breakthrough pain.
OxyContin (long-acting oxycodone)	10 mg every 12 hours	Usually started after initial dose determined by effects of immediate-release opioid.

adequate hydration and use of a motility-inducing laxative containing senna or bisacodyl is recommended.[130]

Morphine and codeine should be avoided in older adults with chronic renal insufficiency owing to the potential for accumulation of active metabolites that may cause delirium, confusion, and excessive sedation. Meperidine, pentazocine, and propoxyphene are not recommended because of the accumulation of toxic metabolites that cause seizures or cardiac arrhythmias. In late 2010, the FDA voted to remove propoxyphene products from the US market because of the high risk of cardiac toxicity.

Transdermal buprenorphine was approved by the FDA in June 2010 for treatment of moderate to severe pain. Buprenorphine is a potent opioid with partial mu agonist and kappa antagonist activity. The pharmacokinetics of buprenorphine and ceiling limit for respiratory depressant effects make it a reasonable choice for older adults. Most of the published data on transdermal buprenorphine for musculoskeletal pain in older adults are currently from Europe.[132]

In H.T.'s case, the dose of acetaminophen is too low. However, he is taking a combination product, and an increase in acetaminophen increases the overall oxycodone intake. The pharmacist should talk to both H.T. and the clinician prescribing oxycodone/acetaminophen about the benefit of maximizing the acetaminophen dose. Oxycodone should be prescribed separately to avoid unintended opioid adverse effects. This will allow more individualized dosing of oxycodone and acetaminophen.[121] If the knee pain still persists after increasing the acetaminophen dose, the frequency of oxycodone use should be increased to 5 mg every 4 hours as needed depending on the recurrence of pain. Switching to a long-acting opioid, such as OxyContin, would be beneficial in H.T. if he continues to use the short-acting oxycodone frequently.

NONSTEROIDAL ANTI-INFLAMMATORY DRUGS

CASE 7-5, QUESTION 3: H.T. is currently on metoprolol for hypertension and uses OTC ibuprofen occasionally for knee pain. What is the potential risk of uncontrolled hypertension and cardiovascular events with NSAIDs?

Currently, the ACR, OARSI, and AAOS support nonselective NSAIDs as a first-line therapy for moderate to severe pain and inflammation associated with OA.[120] Toxicity remains the most troublesome aspect of prescribing NSAIDs for the treatment of OA. GI toxicity is highest among patients with a previous history of GI bleeding, age older than 60 years, concurrent use of corticosteroids, or concurrent anticoagulant therapy. Nephrotoxicity is also a significant problem and is more common in individuals with pre-existing renal disease or advanced age.[133] A summary of NSAID toxicity is found in Chapter 44, Rheumatoid Arthritis. Celecoxib, an NSAID selective for COX-2, is a second-line recommendation in the ACR, EULAR, AAOS, and NICE guidelines because of the risk of potential cardiovascular toxicity (Table 7-13).[120,133,134] The AGS guideline recommendations state that nonselective NSAIDs and COX-2 selective inhibitors may be considered rarely, and with extreme caution, in highly selected individuals.[121]

The effects of NSAIDs on blood pressure are attributable to multiple mechanisms. Inhibition of COX-2 is associated with reductions in both prostaglandin E_2 (PGE_2) and prostaglandin I_2 (PGI_2 or prostacyclin). Inhibition of PGE_2 synthesis may induce an acute relative reduction in daily urinary sodium excretion of 30% or more, which can lead to an increase in blood pressure.[135] Patients who have impaired renal function as a result of any comorbid medical condition may accumulate a considerable amount of salt and water within 1 to 3 weeks of initiating NSAID therapy. NSAIDs and COX-2 selective inhibitors may also impair the vasodilatory benefits of PGI_2, which may lead to an increase in the systemic vascular resistance, thus increasing the mean arterial blood pressure.[136]

The importance of background antihypertensive therapy in NSAID-induced blood pressure destabilization was evaluated by Wheaton et al. using the clinic systolic blood pressure as the primary end point.[136] Results indicated that rofecoxib (no longer available in the United States) induced significant increases in systolic blood pressure in patients taking angiotensin-converting enzyme inhibitors and β-blockers but not in those taking calcium-channel blockers. These results support the theory that calcium-channel blockers do not significantly depend on vascular prostacyclin as part of their mechanism of action.[135] Because NSAIDs have a destabilizing effect on blood pressure, they should be used with caution in patients with hypertension who are taking renin-angiotensin blocking agents or diuretics and in patients who have diabetes or early chronic kidney disease (glomerular filtration rate of 40–60 mL/minute). It is not recommended to prescribe NSAIDs on a chronic basis to patients with systolic heart failure.[135]

An observational study found an increased risk of cardiovascular events with rofecoxib, diclofenac, indomethacin, and meloxicam compared with nonusers of NSAIDs. NSAIDs that did not increase the risk of cardiovascular events included celecoxib, ibuprofen, naproxen, and piroxicam (Table 7-13).[134] The Nurses' Health Study compared the risk of cardiovascular events of acetaminophen and NSAIDs in women.[137] This study included a prospective cohort of approximately 71,000 women between 44 and 69 years of age who had 2,041 confirmed cardiovascular events during 12 years of observation. Compared with nonusers of NSAIDs or acetaminophen, women with regular consumption of acetaminophen ($\geq$22 days per month) had about the same risk of cardiovascular events (1.35 with a 95% confidence interval of 1.14–1.59),[135,137] which is similar to the risk of cardiovascular events with rofecoxib at 25 mg or less (Table 7-13).[134] The authors speculated that increases in blood pressure, inhibition of prostaglandin synthesis, and impaired endothelial function through depletion of glutathione induced by acetaminophen may contribute to the increased risk.[135,137]

H.T. should be cautioned about the potential for increased blood pressure, GI bleeding, and decreased kidney function with frequent use of ibuprofen. Currently, H.T.'s blood pressure is controlled on metoprolol with occasional use of ibuprofen. If he increases his use of ibuprofen, he should be advised on the use of a proton-pump inhibitor (available OTC) or misoprostol for GI protection and have his blood pressure checked.[121] The

TABLE 7-13
Risk of Cardiovascular Events With NSAID Use[134]

	Drug	Relative Risk for Cardiovascular Events (95% Confidence Interval)
Increased risk for cardiovascular events	Diclofenac	1.40 (1.19–1.65)
	Rofecoxib	1.36 (1.18–1.58)
	Indomethacin	1.36 (1.15–1.61)
	Meloxicam	1.24 (1.06–1.45)
No increase in risk for cardiovascular events	Piroxicam	1.16 (0.86–1.56)
	Ibuprofen	1.09 (0.99–1.20)
	Celecoxib	1.06 (0.92–1.22)
	Naproxen	0.99 (0.89–1.09)

NSAID, nonsteroidal anti-inflammatory drug.

TABLE 7-14

Comparison of Functional Abdominal Pain Syndrome and Pancreatitis[139]

Diagnosis	Location	Clinical Presentation	Aggravating Factors	Psychosocial Factors	Comorbid Diagnosis
Chronic pancreatitis (visceral)	Epigastric Localized Radiates to back and flank	Remits and relapses	Supine position Food	None	Diabetes Hypertriglyceridemia
Functional abdominal pain syndrome	Variable Diffuse	Persistent	Stress	Anxiety Depression Somatization	None

pharmacist should also provide recommendations on topical pain treatments as an alternative to ibuprofen.

TOPICAL MEDICATIONS

CASE 7-5, QUESTION 4: What topical agents are recommended for OA pain management?

The benefit of topical agents is the avoidance of adverse renal and GI effects. H.T. is currently using topical Aspercreme (trolamine 10%) for local relief of knee pain. Trolamine is a salicylate product that works as a rubefacient and presumably reduces pain by increasing local blood flow. Only the EULAR guidelines recommend topical salicylates as a first-line therapy owing to a lack of evidence on efficacy. NSAIDs (diclofenac gel) and capsaicin are recommended as first-line or second-line therapy in all guidelines (Table 7-11).[121] H.T. should be counseled that OTC capsaicin may be a better alternative to Aspercreme. H.T. should be instructed to talk to his primary-care physician about the use of diclofenac gel. Refer to the Chapter 44, Rheumatoid Arthritis, for topical products and Case 7-3, Question 2, in this chapter.

FUNCTIONAL ABDOMINAL PAIN SYNDROME

Functional abdominal pain syndrome (FAPS) is a chronic pain disorder localized to the abdomen that cannot be explained by a structural or metabolic disorder using currently available diagnostic methods. The reported prevalence of FAPS in North America ranges from 0.5% to 2% and does not differ from that of other countries. FAPS is more common in women (female to male ratio of 3:2) and peaks in the fourth decade of life. Patients with FAPS have high work absenteeism and health care utilization.[138]

Key features in the diagnosis of FAPS include abdominal pain that is present for at least 6 months and is not related to gut function. The patient will often have a decrease in daily activity with time. The principal criterion differentiating FAPS from other GI disorders, such as pancreatitis, is the lack of symptom relationship to food intake or defecation (Table 7-14).[139] Psychological disturbances are more likely when pain has persisted for a long period and manifests as symptom-related behaviors that dominate a patient's life (Table 7-15).[138]

Treatment of FAPS starts with the development of an effective clinician–patient relationship, and establishing reasonable limits for prescribing medication. Psychological counseling and CBTs are key components to successful management of the patient.

Clinical Presentation and Treatment of Chronic Abdominal Pain

FUNCTIONAL ABDOMINAL PAIN SYNDROME SYMPTOMS

CASE 7-6

QUESTION 1: M.T. is a 33-year-old woman with chronic abdominal pain. She first experienced recurrent episodes of abdominal pain at the age of 13 after menarche. At age 21, she was diagnosed with acute pancreatitis secondary to alcohol use. Her pain has persisted despite numerous trials of medications including gabapentin, sertraline, tramadol, and hydrocodone/acetaminophen. She has undergone multiple diagnostic evaluations for the abdominal pain, but all have resulted in negative findings. During the past year, M.T. has had eight visits to the emergency department for severe pain where she usually receives IV hydromorphone and then is discharged with a week's supply of oxycodone/acetaminophen. In addition to the emergency department visits, she has been hospitalized three times in the past year for abdominal pain.

Today, M.T. is being seen in the clinic by her primary-care physician for continued management of chronic abdominal pain, which she describes as "constantly aching." For 2 years M.T.'s primary-care physician has been prescribing oxycodone in conjunction with an opioid agreement focused on minimizing the use of emergency department visits for pain management. M.T. believes her current management with oxycodone 5 mg orally every 4 hours PRN for severe pain is insufficient and would like the 30-day supply limit increased from 180 tablets to 240 tablets.

TABLE 7-15

Symptom-Related Behaviors of Functional Abdominal Pain Syndrome

Expressing pain of varying intensity through verbal and nonverbal methods
Urgent reporting of intense symptoms disproportionate to available clinical and laboratory data
Minimizing or denying a role for psychosocial contributors, anxiety, depression; attributing symptoms of anxiety or depression to presence of pain
Requesting diagnostic studies or surgery to validate the condition as "organic"
Focusing attention on complete relief of symptoms
Seeking health care frequently
Taking limited personal responsibility for self-management
Making requests for narcotic analgesics when other treatment options have been implemented

The primary-care physician is concerned about M.T.'s functional status since starting opioid therapy. There has been no noticeable improvement in M.T.'s pain despite three increases in the 30-day oxycodone supply over the past 2 years. During the office visit, M.T. is emotionally labile at times and tearful when discussing her pain but is emphatic that she is not depressed. She states that she drinks one or two "highballs" (whisky and soda) about two times a week to help her relax when she is feeling "stressed out." M.T. denies smoking or illicit drug use. She is currently unemployed and seeking permanent disability because the pain interferes with her ability to work. Her physical examination is unremarkable except for diffuse abdominal tenderness. What is the clinical relevance of M.T.'s self-description of abdominal pain?

M.T.'s self-report of pain is consistent with FAPS. From the physiologic perspective, M.T.'s abdominal pain most likely originated from a combination of somatic and visceral components associated with menses and pancreatitis. When the pain symptoms occur frequently in conjunction with a stressor as in FAPS, the main mechanism for altered pain regulation relates to the failure to inhibit the amplification of normal regulatory afferent input through altered central mechanisms in the prefrontal, cingulated cortex, and limbic structures (e.g., cognitive and emotions centers of the brain). This impairment in homeostatic inhibition of pain may be related to reduced levels of 5-HT, NE, endorphin, and other neuropeptides that mediate descending pain transmission in the CNS. Recognition of the CNS as the primary modulator of pain in FAPS is essential to understanding its clinical presentation, diagnosis, and therapeutic strategies.[140]

FUNCTIONAL ABDOMINAL PAIN SYNDROME TREATMENT

CASE 7-6, QUESTION 2: What are the current recommendations for pharmacologic treatment of FAPS?

Treatment recommendations for patients with FAPS are empirical and not based on results from well-designed clinical trials. Clinical trials have not been targeted to this diagnostic entity, so treatments are typically designed on the basis of data from other chronic pain disorders. The cornerstone to management depends on an effective relationship between the clinician and patient. In this case, the primary-care physician needs to listen to M.T.'s concerns but set realistic and consistent limits when ordering tests, medical interventions, and medications. M.T. needs to be an active participant in the pain management plan and take responsibility of self-care.[138]

Antidepressants, such as TCAs in low daily dosages, may be useful in treating FAPS for both pain and depression owing to their combined noradrenergic and serotonergic effects. In other chronic pain conditions, TCAs generally have been more successful than using selective serotonin-reuptake inhibitors.[141] Newer agents with combined 5-HT and NE reuptake activity (e.g., SNRIs such as venlafaxine and duloxetine) have recognized pain-reducing effects with somatic pain conditions and may be useful in FAPS. To ensure treatment adherence, M.T. needs affirmation that antidepressant is not prescribed simply to treat depression. It is important that the clinician educate the patient on the role of antidepressant in the treatment of pain. Patient education resources such as diagrams help to show the physiologic basis for treatment of pain and describe descending inhibitory pathways.[142]

Anecdotal reports and observations on the use of medications for other chronic pain conditions are the basis for use in FAPS. Gabapentin and pregabalin clinical trials have established their effect for neuropathic pain, but benefit for visceral or central pain syndromes is not established. NSAIDs offer little benefit because their action is located in the peripheral nervous system. Long-term treatment with benzodiazepines is not recommended because of their abuse potential and tendency to interact with other medications. For patients who are refractory to usual doses of antidepressant medication, referral to psychiatry should be made for treatment with atypical antipsychotic agents such as quetiapine.[139,142]

RISK OF ADDICTION

CASE 7-6, QUESTION 3: There is concern about M.T.'s use of alcohol and escalating use of opioid medication. What is the risk that M.T. will become addicted to opioids?

Opioid use behaviors are stratified based on the risk of aberrant drug use. Aberrant drug use behaviors may occur along a spectrum from those less suggestive of addiction, such as an occasional, sanctioned increase in the opioid dose, to those that may be more suggestive of addiction, such as injecting oral formulations. Table 7-17 gives definitions of terms associated with opioid use.[143] M.T. has multiple behaviors that are less suggestive for addiction. M.T. has multiple behaviors in which some are more indicative of addiction while others can be explained given the etiology of FAPS. For example, high health care utilization for pain validation is not uncommon in patients with FAPS. Also, aggressive complaining about the need for more opioid medication may be driven by M.T.'s perception that the current dose prescribed by her primary-care physician no longer relieves her pain, implying tolerance has developed (Table 7-16).[143,144]

TABLE 7-16
Terms Related to Opioid Use[144]

Term	Definition
Abuse	Any use of an illegal drug, or the intentional self-administration of a medication for a nonmedical purpose such as altering one's state of consciousness (e.g., getting high).
Addiction	A primary, chronic, neurobiological disease with genetic, psychosocial, and environmental factors influencing its development and manifestations. It is characterized by behaviors that include one or more of the following: impaired control over drug use, compulsive use, continued use despite harm, and craving.
Physical dependence	A state of adaptation manifested by a drug class–specific withdrawal syndrome that can be produced by abrupt cessation, rapid dose reduction, decreasing blood level of the drug, or administration of an antagonist.
Pseudoaddiction	Condition characterized by behaviors that outwardly mimic addiction but are in fact driven by a desire for pain relief (e.g., constantly watching the clock to dose medication "on time" so pain does not become severe).[127]
Tolerance	A state of adaptation in which exposure to a drug induces changes that result in a diminution of one or more opioid effects with time.

TABLE 7-17
Opioid Use Risk Stratification[143]

More Suggestive of Addiction	Less Suggestive of Addiction
Concurrent abuse of alcohol or illicit drugs	Aggressive complaining about the need for more drugs
Evidence of a deterioration in the ability to function at work, in the family, or socially that appears to be related to drug use	Drug hoarding during periods of reduced symptoms
Injecting oral formulations	Openly acquiring similar drugs from other medical sources
Multiple dose escalations or other nonadherence with therapy despite warnings	Requesting specific drugs
Obtaining prescription drugs from nonmedical sources	Reporting psychic effects not intended by the physician
Prescription drug forgery	Resistance to a change in therapy associated with tolerable adverse effects accompanied by expression of anxiety related to the return of severe symptoms
Repeated resistance to changes in therapy despite clear evidence of physical or psychological effects	Unapproved use of the drug to treat another symptom
Repeatedly seeking prescriptions from other physicians or emergency departments	Unsanctioned dose escalation or other nonadherence with therapy on one or two occasions
Selling prescription drugs	
Stealing or borrowing drugs from others	

The factor that is most concerning for addiction is M.T.'s continued use of alcohol despite previous pancreatitis and misusing it to treat anxiety. There is also a risk of increased opioid side effects, especially sedation and respiratory depression, with concurrent use of alcohol. Multiple literature reports have confirmed there is a strong association between alcohol abuse and opioid addiction.[144–146] Guidelines for chronic opioid therapy strongly recommend clinicians conduct a risk assessment of substance abuse, misuse, or addiction before initiating opioid therapy.[144]

ASSESSMENT OF CHRONIC OPIOID THERAPY

CASE 7-6, QUESTION 4: M.T. really wants to continue with opioid therapy despite the concerns of her primary-care physician. Is M.T. a candidate for chronic opioid therapy?

There are multiple sources in the literature for information and guidelines on written agreements (i.e., contracts) between the clinician and patient for chronic opioid therapy (COT).

For an example of a written COT agreement, go to http://thepoint.lww.com/AT10e.

The written COT agreement should include goals of therapy, how opioids will be prescribed and taken, expectations for follow-up and monitoring, alternatives to COT, expectations regarding use of concomitant therapies, and potential for weaning and discontinuing. Indications for weaning or tapering the opioid include failure to make progress toward therapeutic goals, intolerable adverse effects, or repeated or serious aberrant drug-related behaviors. Patient compliance requirements within the written agreement should include pill counts to monitor overuse, random urine drug screens for illicit substances or opioids obtained from other sources, and limited prescribing to help the patient manage use if necessary (limit opioid supply or prescribe weekly or biweekly amounts).[144] In this case, M.T. has not made progress in meeting the goal of decreased emergency department utilization, and she has been resistant to trying other therapies despite the ineffectiveness of opioids in treating her pain. These behaviors would indicate M.T. is not a candidate for COT.

Screening tools that assess the potential risks for opioid misuse based on patient characteristics are helpful in determining eligibility for COT. Patient self-report questionnaires for assessing risk of aberrant drug-related behavior include the Screener and Opioid Assessment for Patients with Pain (SOAPP) version 1, the revised SOAPP (SOAPP-R), and the ORT.[144]

For copies of the revised SOAPP and the Current Opioid Misuse Measure (COMM), go to http://thepoint.lww.com/AT10e.

The DIRE instrument is clinician administered and designed to assess the potential efficacy of opioid therapy as well as harm.[144] In M.T.'s case, her DIRE score is 10, which would indicate she is not a suitable candidate for long-term opioid therapy. M.T.'s DIRE score and assessment are shown in Table 7-18.

For a blank DIRE form, see http://thepoint.lww.com/AT10e.

DISCONTINUING OPIOID THERAPY

CASE 7-6, QUESTION 5: M.T. is going to be discontinued from opioids as part of the pain management plan. How long should the opioid medication be weaned?

Guidelines from the APS strongly recommend that clinicians wean patients from chronic opioids if they have repeated aberrant drug-related behaviors, experience no progress toward meeting therapeutic goals, or experience intolerable adverse effects.[144] When weaning patients from long-term opioid therapy, the length of time the patient has been taking opioids needs to be considered. Approaches to weaning range from a slow 10% dose reduction per week to a more rapid 25% reduction every few days. Evidence to guide specific recommendations on the rate of reduction is lacking, although the slower rate may help reduce the unpleasant symptoms of opioid withdrawal.[144]

There is insufficient evidence to guide recommendations for the use of short-acting versus long-acting oral opioids, or as-needed versus around-the-clock dosing during taper.[144] In this case, M.T.'s oxycodone dose will be reduced slowly for 2 months in conjunction with starting psychological therapy for stress management and counseling for alcohol use. The quantity of

TABLE 7-18
M.T.'s DIRE Score

Score	Factor	Explanation
1	Diagnosis	1 = Benign chronic condition with minimal objective findings or no definite medical diagnosis (e.g., fibromyalgia, migraine headache, nonspecific back pain)
1	Intractability	1 = Few therapies have been tried and the patient takes a passive role in his or her pain management process
7	Risk	(psychological + chemical health + reliability + social support)
	Psychological	2 = Personality or mental health interferes moderately (e.g., depression or anxiety disorder)
	Chemical Health	1 = Active or very recent use of illicit drugs, excessive alcohol, or prescription drug abuse
	Reliability	2 = Occasional difficulties with compliance, but generally reliable
	Social Support	2 = Reduction in some relationships and life roles
1	Efficacy Score	1 = Poor function or minimal pain relief despite moderate to high opioid doses
10	**Total**	
	Score 7–13: not a suitable candidate for long-term opioid therapy	
	Score 14–21: good candidate for long-term opioid therapy	

DIRE, Diagnosis, Intractability, Risk, and Efficacy score.
Adapted with permission from Chou R et al. Clinical guidelines for the use of chronic opioid therapy in chronic noncancer pain. *J Pain.* 2009;10:113.

oxycodone 5-mg tablets will be reduced by 60 tablets per month until discontinued. M.T. will need to be monitored for signs of withdrawal, which include anxiety, tachycardia, sweating, and other autonomic symptoms. Should withdrawal symptoms occur, they may be lessened by clonidine 0.1 mg to 0.2 mg orally twice a day.[147]

COGNITIVE BEHAVIORAL THERAPIES

CASE 7-6, QUESTION 6: What nonpharmacologic therapies could be offered to M.T. to help with her pain management?

The psychological approach to CBT has been shown to be beneficial in the treatment of chronic pain including FAPS. CBT typically combines stress management, problem solving, goal setting, pacing of activities, and assertiveness into a strategy for self-management of pain. Biofeedback, meditation, guided imagery, and hypnosis can all be incorporated within a CBT plan (Table 7-19). The objective is to help patients acquire a sense of hopefulness and resourcefulness, and develop positive coping skills.[148]

Complementary and alternative therapies such as spinal manipulation, massage, and acupuncture are commonly used in patients with chronic pain, but data supporting their use in FAPS is limited. Transcutaneous electrical nerve stimulation has been tried in FAPS patients, but the results are inconclusive.[140,142]

TABLE 7-19
Cognitive Behavioral Therapy[148]

Meditation—intentional self-regulation of attention using a systematic focus on particular aspects of inner and outer body experience.
Biofeedback—self-regulatory technique that teaches a patient how to exert control over the physiological processes exacerbating pain. Biofeedback equipment conveys physiological responses as visual or auditory signals that the patient can observe on a computer monitor. With practice, the patient learns to control and change his or her physiological responses by manipulating the auditory or visual signals.
Guided imagery—useful method to help patients with pain to relax and achieve a sense of control and distraction. This modality involves the generation of different mental images, evoked either by oneself or with help from the practitioner.
Hypnosis—a state of heightened awareness and focused concentration that can be used to manipulate the perception of pain.

CANCER PAIN AND SYMPTOM MANAGEMENT

Pain is one of the most commonly experienced and feared symptoms of cancer. Cancer pain is defined as pain that results from treatment of the disease or the direct impact of tumor growth. During cancer treatment, 35% to 56% of patients will have pain with up to one-third of those patients having severe pain.[149] The type of cancer pain can be classified as somatic, neuropathic, or visceral. Approximately one-half of all cancer pain is somatic, arising from bone, muscle, ligament, subcutaneous tissue, or skin.

Somatic pain is frequent with breast cancer, genitourinary tumors, bone metastasis, and lymphatic malignancies. Neuropathic pain may be caused by surgery, cancer chemotherapy, radiation, herpes zoster (shingles), and tumor progression such as advanced head and neck cancer. Visceral pain often presents with GI cancers.[149–151]

Sixty-four percent of patients with advanced cancer report an increased frequency and intensity of pain compared with patients with early-stage cancer.[151] Factors influencing the degree of pain include the primary cancer, stage of disease, location of metastasis, and comorbid medical conditions.[150,152] Each pain complaint must be assessed for time of onset, body location, pattern of progression, impairment of physical function, psychosocial impact, and other associated symptoms such as nausea, fatigue, shortness of breath, constipation, and mental status changes. Table 7-20 gives a summary of common cancer pain causes and symptoms.[152]

The initial treatment of cancer pain is based on the severity as reported by the patient.[152] Factors to consider when starting an analgesic regimen include the pain etiology, patient tolerance (e.g., opioid doses), setting where the medication will be administered, and previous experience with analgesics that were efficacious or produced adverse effects. In general, mild pain (e.g., pain rated ≤4 of 10 in severity) can be managed with nonopioid or a combination of nonopioid and an opioid analgesic. Moderate to severe pain (e.g., pain rated >4 of 10 in severity) usually requires an opioid analgesic. The treatment of neuropathic pain may require the use of anticonvulsant or antidepressant medication. Nerve blocks and invasive surgical procedures are options for pain control that is refractory to conventional medication management.[152,153]

TABLE 7-20
Common Cancer Pain Presentation[152]

Syndrome	Associated Cancer or Treatment	Associated Signs and Symptoms
Bone metastasis	Breast cancer, lung cancer, multiple myeloma, prostate cancer	• Pain is usually described as dull or aching. • Pain is usually localized to the metastatic site. • Spine metastasis to the base of the skull may produce headache, pain associated with head movement, and pain in the face, neck, and shoulder.
Epidural spinal cord compression	Breast cancer, lung cancer, melanoma, multiple myeloma, prostate cancer, renal cancer	• Pain is usually midline. • Pain can be sharp and shooting in a radicular distribution if nerve roots are involved. • Cervical lesions: pain can radiate down one or both arms. • Thoracic lesions: pain is described as a "tight band" around the patient's chest. • Lumbosacral lesions: pain can radiate down one or both legs. • Other signs: bowel and bladder dysfunction.
Cervical plexopathy	Metastasis to the cervical lymph nodes; local extension of primary head and neck tumors	• Pain is characterized by aching discomfort that may radiate into the neck and shoulders.
Brachial plexopathy	Breast cancer, lung cancer, lymphoma	• Pain usually begins in the shoulder and is associated with shooting or electrical sensations in the thumb and index finger if the upper plexus is damaged by tumor. • Pain usually begins in the shoulder and radiates into the elbow, arm, and medial forearm and into the fourth and fifth digits if the lower plexus is damaged by tumor.
Lumbar plexopathy	Colorectal cancer, endometrial cancer, renal cancer, sarcoma, lymphoma	• Pain is usually felt in the lower abdomen, buttock and leg. • Perineal and perirectal pain may occur if tumor invades the sacral plexus. • Associated symptoms can include weakness, sensory loss, or urinary incontinence.
Peripheral neuropathies	Multiple myeloma Chemotherapy (vinca alkaloids, taxanes, platinum compounds, thalidomide) Postsurgical pain syndrome	• Sensory motor neuropathy is characterized by distal paresthesias, sensory loss, weakness, and muscle wasting. It may occasionally ascend upward in a manner similar to Guillain-Barre syndrome • Chemotherapy dose-related peripheral neuropathies are characterized by dysesthesias in the feet and hands, and hyporeflexia • Post-radical neck dissection: tight, burning sensation in the area of sensory loss; dysesthesias and shock-like pain may be present. • Postmastectomy pain: tight, constricting pain in the posterior wasll, axilla, and anterior chest wall that is exacerbated by movement • Postthoracotomy pain: aching sensation in the distribution of the incision with sensory loss with or without autonomic changes. • Postnephrectomy pain: numbness, fullness, or heaviness in the flank, anterior abdomen and groin associated with dysesthesias. • Post-limb amputation: pain occurs at the site of the surgical pain and is characterized by a burning, dysestic sensation that is exacerbated by movement

Presentation and Treatment of Cancer Pain

CANCER PAIN ETIOLOGY

CASE 7-7

QUESTION 1: L.V. is a 58-year-old man who was diagnosed with stage IV squamous cell carcinoma of the subglottis 2 months ago. The cancer is locally advanced with involvement of multiple cervical lymph nodes. He had a modified neck resection to remove the primary tumor and lymph nodes while sparing the larynx. Chemoradiation therapy began 3 weeks after surgery with cisplatin 100 mg/m^2 every 3 weeks (days 1, 22, and 43) and external beam radiation delivering 70 Gy fractionated over the course of 7 weeks. L.V. is now in his fourth week of radiation therapy and continues to have significant neck and shoulder pain described as "sudden shocklike sensations with movement" and rated 6 of 10 despite a recent increase in his long-acting oral morphine to 60 mg twice daily with immediate-release morphine 10 mg PO every 4 hours PRN for breakthrough pain. He also reports that his throat is getting so sore that he cannot bear to swallow and rates the pain 10 of 10. L.V. appears quite fatigued and lethargic during his appointment with the radiation oncologist. The physical examination is remarkable for dry oral mucous membranes, erythema and mild ulceration of the oropharynx, and allodynia with light palpitation of the trapezius and sternocleidomastoid with pain greater on the left side.

The radiation oncologist orders laboratory tests and the results are as follows:

General Chemistry:
Sodium, 132 mEq/L
Potassium, 4.2 mEq/L
Chloride, 101 mEq/L
CO_2, 26 mmol/L
Anion gap, 5 mEq/L
Glucose, random, 70 mg/dL
Urea nitrogen, 28 mg/dL
Creatinine, 1.5 mg/dL

Calcium, total, 9.0 mg/dL

CBC With Differential:

White blood cell count, 7.1 × $10^9/\mu L$
Red blood cell count, 3.25 × $10^6/\mu L$
Hemoglobin, 14 g/dL
Hematocrit, 43%
Mean cell volume, 91 × $10^6/\mu L$
Mean cell hemoglobin, 30 pg/cell
Mean cell hemoglobin concentration, 33 g/dL
Platelet, 369 × $10^3/\mu L$
Absolute neutrophils, 5 × 10^9/L
Absolute lymphocytes, 1.2 × 10^9/L
Absolute monocytes, 0.2 × 10^9/L
Absolute eosinophils, 0 × 10^9/L
Absolute basophils, 0 × 10^9/L

The radiation oncologist decides to admit L.V. to the hospital for dehydration and pain management. What are the possible etiologies of L.V.'s pain?

L.V. is presenting with a new complaint of a severe sore throat and persistent neck and shoulder pain. Laboratory data rule out infection and myelosuppression. His kidney function may be impaired by dehydration and cisplatin therapy. The most likely causes of L.V.'s pain are the recent surgical neck resection and mucositis from external beam radiation.

L.V. also has postoperative peripheral neuropathy characterized by shocklike sensation in the neck and shoulders after the resection of the tumor. The physical examination of L.V.'s neck and shoulders is remarkable for allodynia, which can be present with neuropathy. The cervical lymph node resection may have caused neuropathy due to nerve damage via crushing, pressure, incision, or inflammation. This results in ectopic firing and changes in the receptive field, causing nerve excitability and spontaneous activity (wind-up). Neuronal hyperexcitability may be related to overexpression of sodium channels and activation of the NMDA receptor.[154] Cervical plexopathy may also be contributing to the discomfort.

Mucositis occurs in up to 45% of individuals treated for head and neck cancer with the chemoradiation regimen L.V. is receiving.[154,155] Chemotherapy and radiation directly affect the proliferation of epithelial cells and connective tissue, causing damage to and loss of the mucosal barrier. On physical examination, the oropharynx is red and ulcerated, which is indicative of mucositis. Chapter 90, Adverse Effects of Chemotherapy and Targeted Agents, provides information on the signs and symptoms of mucositis. Pain associated with mucositis is dependent on the degree of tissue damage, sensitization of nociceptors, and activation of inflammatory and pain mediators. L.V.'s complaint of sore throat pain limiting his ability to swallow is a common presentation of mucositis. In head and neck cancer patients treated with radiation, pain intensity scores directly correspond to mucositis and increase at week 3, often peak at week 5, and persist for weeks after the end of treatment.[153]

In addition, L.V. may have cisplatin-related neurotoxicity. Approximately 30% to 40% of patients may experience sensory loss as a result of direct neuronal DNA damage and apoptotic cell death caused by cisplatin. Neurotoxicity is a dose-limiting side effect for all the platinum agents. Cisplatin peripheral toxicity can occur in patients who receive a cumulative dose of more than 400 to 500 mg/m^2.[156] All sensory modalities are involved, but loss of large fiber function is often prominent. Persistent dysesthetic pain (e.g., an unpleasant abnormal sensation, whether spontaneous or evoked) is a late phenomenon that may continue to progress for several months after cessation of cisplatin.

TRANSDERMAL FENTANYL DOSE CALCULATION

CASE 7-7, QUESTION 2: L.V. was started on IV hydromorphone using patient-controlled analgesia (PCA) with an average usage of 14 mg/day. He now rates his pain as 4 of 10. Owing to difficulty swallowing secondary to the mucositis and xerostomia, he had a gastric feeding tube placed for nutrition. The plan is to convert the IV hydromorphone to a transdermal fentanyl patch. What transdermal fentanyl patch dose should L.V. be started on, and what are the instructions for use?

For more than two decades, the World Health Organization's (WHO) analgesic ladder has been used to guide cancer pain management.[157] The ladder progresses in a stepwise manner starting with acetaminophen, NSAIDs, and adjuvant medications (e.g., coanalgesics such as anticonvulsants and antidepressants for neuropathic pain) as initial therapy. If the pain intensity is greater than 4 of 10 but not severe, weak opioid analgesics may be added to the pain regimen. For severe pain, strong opioids such as morphine, hydromorphone, fentanyl, and oxycodone are recommended in step 3 of the WHO analgesic ladder. The downside to using this algorithm is that cancer pain rarely progresses in the stepwise fashion that the WHO ladder implies. Therefore, several organizations including the APS, National Comprehensive Cancer Network, and American Cancer Society have proposed different strategies for managing cancer pain based on the assessment of the patient, development of an individualized care plan for pain, and symptom management.[152,158,159]

Before starting IV hydromorphone, L.V. has severe throat pain rated 10 of 10 and moderate-severe neck and shoulder pain rated 6 of 10. Because of the severity of pain and inability to swallow, IV opioid therapy using PCA is appropriate. Chapter 8, Perioperative Care, provides a discussion of PCA. Hydromorphone is a good choice for IV opioid therapy because it does not have active metabolites that could accumulate with renal insufficiency. The transdermal fentanyl patch is an excellent choice for L.V.'s eventual outpatient pain management because it will provide continuous release of opioid and is convenient to use.[160] Kadian, an extended-release morphine capsule, can be administered via the gastric feeding tube because the capsule is opened and contents flushed through the gastric feeding tube with water. Limitations to Kadian include patient manipulation of the gastric feeding tube with self-administration and potential for morphine side effects secondary to metabolite accumulation if renal insufficiency persists.

Transdermal fentanyl patches are intended for opioid-tolerant patients with stable chronic pain. Opioid-tolerant patients are those who have been taking daily, for a week or longer, at least 60 mg of oral morphine, 30 mg of oral oxycodone, or at least 8 mg of oral hydromorphone or an equianalgesic dose of another opioid. Respiratory depression associated with opioids is more likely to occur in opioid-naïve patients, patients with postoperative pain, and those with intermittent or mild pain that is managed with PRN opioid administration.[159,161] Before the current hospital admission, L.V. was taking 120 mg of long-acting oral morphine per day with additional oral morphine for breakthrough pain. L.V. is a good candidate for a transdermal fentanyl patch.

L.V.'s transdermal fentanyl regimen will need to be determined by converting IV hydromorphone using an equianalgesic dose approximation. Doses of two different opioids (or two different routes of administration of the same opioid) are considered to be equianalgesic if they provide the same degree of pain relief. Table 7-21[162] gives equianalgesic opioid doses. The calculations to convert L.V. from IV hydromorphone to transdermal

TABLE 7-21
Equianalgesic Opioid Dosing

Opioid	Equianalgesic Dose (mg) Oral	Parenteral	Comments
Morphine	30	10	Standard for comparison of opioid analgesics. Frequency for controlled release preparations: 8 or 12 hours for MS Contin or Oramorph. 12 or 24 hours for Kadian. 24 hours for Avinza. Embeda (morphine sulfate and naltrexone) is a diversion-deterrent formulation. Morphine not recommended in patients with severe renal impairment.
Hydromorphone (Dilaudid, Exalgo)	7.5	1.5	Exalgo (extended release) dosed every 24 hours. Can be used in patients with renal or liver impairment.
Fentanyl	—	0.1	Refer to Table 7-22 for transdermal fentanyl. Equianalgesic conversion ratios have not been established for transmucosal and transbuccal fentanyl formulations. Can be used in patients with renal or liver impairment.
Oxycodone	20	—	OxyContin (controlled release) is dosed every 8 or 12 hours. Can be used in patients with renal impairment.
Levorphanol (Levo-Dromoran)	4 acute 1 chronic	1 chronic	Long plasma half-life (12–16 hours but may be as long as 90–120 hours). Use with caution in older adults.
Buprenorphine (Buprenex, Butrans)[161,162]	0.3	0.4 (SL)	Available as sublingual tablets and injection. Analgesic ceiling of 32 mg/d SL. Butrans (transdermal buprenorphine) available. Suboxone (buprenorphine and naloxone) restricted to treatment of opioid dependence. Partial agonists not recommended for cancer pain management.
Meperidine (Demerol)[159,161]	100	300	Not recommended for routine clinical use. Normeperidine is a toxic metabolite that produces anxiety, tremors, myoclonus and generalized seizures.

SL, sublingual.

fentanyl (Duragesic) are shown in Figure 7-7. There are several published tables for converting morphine to transdermal fentanyl by researchers and manufacturers of transdermal fentanyl products. They provide slightly different dose conversion recommendations. Duragesic has wide morphine dose ranges, which may result in underdosing the transdermal fentanyl patch in cancer patients (Table 7-22).[161,163] Breitbart et al. recommend a 2:1 ratio of oral morphine to transdermal fentanyl (i.e., 2 mg oral morphine is equivalent to 1 mcg/hour transdermal fentanyl), resulting in higher transdermal fentanyl doses, which may be excessive for elderly patients.[164] A study by Donner et al. suggested a dose ratio of 60 mg/day oral morphine is equal to 25 mcg/hour transdermal fentanyl, which falls between the manufacturer's table and the study recommendations by Breitbart et al.[163–165] The Donner conversion ratio is used in most references because it is less likely to cause underdosing or overdosing.[165]

TABLE 7-22
Conversion from Oral Morphine to Duragesic[163]

Oral 24-Hour Morphine (mg/d)	Duragesic Dose (mcg/h)
60–134	25
135–224	50
225–314	75
315–404	100
405–494	125
495–584	150
585–674	175
675–764	200
765–854	225
855–944	250
945–1034	275
1035–1124	300

Reprinted with permission from Facts & Comparisons eAnswers. http://online.factsandcomparisons.com/MonoDisp.aspx?monoID=fandc-hcp12689&quick=332587%7c5&search=332587%7c5&isstemmed=True#firstMatch. Accessed March 30, 2011.

L.V.'s transdermal fentanyl patch dose is 116 mcg/hour (Fig. 7-7) using the dose ratio 60 mg/day oral morphine to 25 mcg/hour transdermal fentanyl. Because L.V.'s pain is well controlled based on the intensity rating of 4 of 10, the dose of transdermal fentanyl should be rounded down to the nearest available patch size, which is 100 mcg/hour. If L.V.'s pain was not controlled, the transdermal patch dose should be rounded up to the nearest available patch size.[161]

Patients who have been on opioid therapy for a prolonged time are likely to exhibit tolerance to the therapeutic effect. However, when switched to a different opioid, the level of tolerance may change (i.e., diminished tolerance to the new opioid) owing to the pharmacokinetic properties of the new opioid. This change in sensitivity to the new opioid is called incomplete cross tolerance.[161] Most opioid doses need to be reduced by 25% to 50% after the conversion calculation to account for the incomplete cross tolerance.[159] The exception to this is methadone and fentanyl. Conversion ratios for methadone and fentanyl have already accounted for incomplete cross tolerance, so no further reductions are generally needed. Therefore, L.V.'s transdermal fentanyl patch dose should not be reduced for incomplete cross tolerance.

After the initial transdermal patch is applied, it will take 12 hours to reach the minimal effective blood concentration and up

Step 1:
Determine the 24-hour total of the opioid that will be converted. For L.V., the 24-hour total of intravenous hydromorphone is 14 mg.

Step 2:
Select the equianalgesic dose ratio that corresponds to the opioid and route that will be converted from Table 7-21. Ratio calculations should be set up to correlate the actual dose with the equianalgesic equivalent as shown below:

$$\frac{\text{"X" mg total daily dose of new opioid}}{\text{mg total daily dose of current opioid}} = \frac{\text{equianalgesic factor of new opioid}}{\text{equianalgesic factor of current opioid}}$$

For conversion of L.V.'s hydromorphone dose, 1.5 mg intravenous hydromorphone is equianalgesic to 30 mg oral morphine:

$$\frac{\text{"X" mg total daily dose of new opioid}}{\text{14 mg intravenous hydromorphone}} = \frac{\text{30 mg oral morphine}}{\text{1.5 mg intravenous hydromorphone}}$$

Step 3:
Cross multiply the ratio to determine the total daily dose of oral morphine.

$(1.5)(X) = (14)(30)$
$1.5X = 420$
$X = 280$ mg of oral morphine

Step 4:
Determine L.V.'s transdermal fentanyl patch dose equivalent to 280 mg oral morphine.

Manufacturer's Conversion Ratio[163]
225–314 mg oral morphine/day = 75 mcg/hour transdermal fentanyl

Donner Study Ratio[165]
The conversion ratio of 60 mg/day oral morphine to 25 mcg/hour transdermal fentanyl will be used for the calculation.

$$\frac{\text{"X" mg total daily dose of new opioid}}{\text{280 mg oral morphine/day}} = \frac{\text{25 mcg/hour transdermal fentanyl}}{\text{60 mg oral morphine/day}}$$

$(60)(X) = (280)(25)$
$X = 116$ mcg/hour transdermal fentanyl

Breitbart Study Ratio[164]
The conversion ratio of 2 mg oral morphine to 1 mcg/hour transdermal fentanyl will be used for the calculation.

$$\frac{\text{"X" mg total daily dose of new opioid}}{\text{280 mg oral morphine/day}} = \frac{\text{1 mcg/hour transdermal fentanyl}}{\text{2 mg oral morphine}}$$

$(2)(X) = (280)(1)$
$X = 140$ mcg/hour transdermal fentanyl

FIGURE 7-7 Conversion of L.V. from intravenous hydromorphone to transdermal fentanyl.

to 36 hours to achieve the maximal concentration. The transdermal fentanyl patch must be changed every 72 hours to maintain the steady-state blood concentration. Elderly, cachectic, or debilitated patients may have altered pharmacokinetics (i.e., more rapid rate of release) as a result of poor subcutaneous fat stores, thus requiring the transdermal fentanyl patch be changed every 48 hours.[163]

L.V. should be instructed that the transdermal fentanyl patch should be applied to an intact, nonirritated and nonirradiated flat skin surface such as the chest, back, flank, or upper arm.[161] He should be warned about the risk of elevated body temperature (e.g., 40°C or 104°F) resulting in a faster release of fentanyl from the patch. The increased fentanyl level could cause serious respiratory depression. L.V. should be cautioned about avoiding external heating sources such as electric blankets, heating pads, tanning beds, sunbathing, hot baths, hot tubs, saunas, and heated water beds.[161] Fentanyl transdermal skin patches should not be used if damaged or cut as this may increase the absorption of the medication. L.V. should be told to wash his hands immediately if contact is made with the fentanyl gel that was inside the transdermal patch.

TRANSITION TO TRANSDERMAL FENTANYL

CASE 7-7, QUESTION 3: How should L.V. be transitioned from IV hydromorphone to the transdermal fentanyl patch?

Reducing the IV hydromorphone continuous infusion by 50% should occur 6 hours after the initial transdermal fentanyl patch is placed. Discontinuation of the IV hydromorphone continuous infusion and PCA dose should occur 12 hours after the initial transdermal fentanyl patch placement.[161] L.V. may need to use a short-acting (i.e., immediate-release) opioid until the maximal fentanyl blood concentration is achieved. Additional short-acting opioid may be needed for pain that occurs near the end of the 72-hour dose interval.

TABLE 7-23
Equianalgesic Doses for Actiq (Transmucosal Fentanyl) and Fentora (Buccal Fentanyl)[166]

Current Actiq Dose (mcg)	Initial Fentora Dose (mcg)
200	100
400	100
600	200
800	200
1,200	400
1,600	400

Reprinted with permission from Facts & Comparisons eAnswers. http://online.factsandcomparisons.com/MonoDisp.aspx?monoID=fandc-hcp12688&quick=366114%7c5&search=366114%7c5&isstemmed=True#firstMatch. Accessed March 30, 2011.

OPIOID THERAPY FOR BREAKTHROUGH PAIN MANAGEMENT

CASE 7-7, QUESTION 4: What are L.V.'s options for breakthrough pain management?

Breakthrough pain can be classified as spontaneous pain (frequently idiopathic, occurring with no known stimulus), incident pain (secondary to a stimulus that the patient may or may not be able to control), or end-of-dose failure (pain at the end of the dosing interval of the long-acting opioid).[161] Incident pain can be reduced by instructing the patient to take a dose of short-acting opioid 30 minutes before activity. Spontaneous breakthrough pain should be treated by administering a short-acting opioid as soon as the pain is experienced. For patients on long-acting opioid formulations experiencing end-of-dose failure, APS guidelines recommend supplementary doses of a short-acting opioid equivalent to 5% to 15% of the total daily dose to be taken every 2 hours as needed.[159] Short-acting opioid/acetaminophen products have a maximal dose to prevent liver toxicity with acetaminophen, thus creating a ceiling limit on the analgesic efficacy. Plain short-acting opioids (e.g., morphine, oxycodone, hydromorphone) should be used for patients requiring large doses for breakthrough pain.

In L.V.'s case, short-acting opioid solution (morphine, hydromorphone, or oxycodone) should be available for breakthrough pain before discontinuation of IV hydromorphone. The short-acting opioid can be administered in solution form through the gastric feeding tube or as oral tablets if L.V. can tolerate swallowing. L.V.'s oncologist would like to use oral morphine solution for breakthrough pain management. Because the transdermal fentanyl total daily dose is approximately equal to a total daily dose of 280 mg of oral morphine (Fig. 7-7), 10% of the total daily morphine dose would be 28 mg. The dose should be rounded to the nearest tablet size, which is 30 mg, if L.V. would eventually take morphine tablets.

If more than two supplemental doses of short-acting morphine 30 mg are required daily to keep L.V.'s pain under control, an increase in the transdermal fentanyl patch dose should be tried. For patients with pain rated 4 of 10 or less and not exceeding four supplemental doses per day, the long-acting opioid dose (e.g., transdermal fentanyl) should be increased by the amount equal to the daily total of supplemental short-acting opioid taken for pain. Moderate to severe pain may require an increase in the opioid total daily dose by 50% to 100%.[159]

Fentanyl administration by oral transmucosal (Actiq) or buccal (Fentora) routes is approved for breakthrough pain management in cancer patients. The dose of both formulations is determined by titration (i.e., starting with the lowest dose and increasing based on pain relief) rather than a percentage of the total daily dose.[166] Equianalgesic doses of Actiq and Fentora are given in Table 7-23. The oral transmucosal and buccal routes would not be preferred in L.V.'s case due to his dry oral mucous membranes secondary to radiation, which will impact absorption. Xerostomia is a common problem associated with radiation therapy of the head and neck and occurs in 80% of patients by week 7 of treatment. Problems related to xerostomia include difficulty speaking, chewing, swallowing, infections; mouth pain; and dental caries. Reports indicate up to 64% of patients may experience moderate-to-severe xerostomia 3 years after radiation treatment.[155,167] Chapter 90, Adverse Effects of Chemotherapy and Targeted Agents, provides information on topical treatment of mucositis and xerostomia.

METHADONE DOSE CALCULATION

CASE 7-7, QUESTION 5: L.V. has now completed chemoradiation therapy, and the mucositis pain has resolved. He continues to have persistent burning neuropathic pain rated 8 of 10 in the neck and shoulders and is using transdermal fentanyl 100 mcg/hour along with five doses of immediate-release oral morphine 30 mg per day. He is also taking gabapentin 900 mg orally three times a day and using a Lidoderm patch on each shoulder. L.V.'s oncologist wants to switch to oral methadone for neuropathic pain management. What is the oral methadone dose L.V. should be started on?

Methadone is an opioid agonist with analgesic activity at mu and delta receptors. Additional mechanisms of methadone that make it unique from other opioids and a good option for neuropathic pain include 5-HT and NE reuptake inhibition and antagonist effects at the NMDA receptor. Rotation to methadone is recommended when a patient has an inadequate response to other opioids or experiences intolerable side effects such as delirium, myoclonus, or nausea. A trial with methadone is warranted for L.V. because his neuropathic pain is not well controlled with transdermal fentanyl and other coanalgesics, including gabapentin and Lidoderm. Refer to Case 7-3 for treatment of neuropathic pain.

Unlike short-acting opioids, methadone has a long half-life that ranges from 15 to 60 hours with a duration of action of 6 to 12 hours.[159] The conversion to methadone is not proportional like other opioid equianalgesic dose calculations. Older opioid dosing tables list a single conversion factor as 20 mg of oral methadone (or 10 mg IV methadone) is equianalgesic to 30 mg of oral morphine. The single methadone conversion factor was intended for acute pain and does not account for chronic use. The conversion ratios vary with morphine dose. Contemporary tables contain three or more morphine to methadone ratios to adjust for the magnitude of the methadone dose potency with higher morphine daily dose requirements for chronic nonmalignant and cancer pain. The most commonly used morphine to methadone conversions are given in Table 7-24.[168]

L.V.'s total daily dose of morphine is between 340 mg and 390 mg after converting transdermal fentanyl and adding the immediate-release morphine. Figure 7-8 gives calculations to convert transdermal fentanyl to oral methadone in L.V. The dose of oral morphine falls within the dose range of 301 to 600 mg, which corresponds to a 10:1 oral morphine to oral methadone ratio (Table 7-24). L.V.'s total daily dose of methadone is approximately 34 mg or 39 mg, depending on the conversion ratio of transdermal fentanyl used (e.g., 34 mg will be used for this case based on the Donnor ratio). For most patients, the recommended methadone dose interval is every 8 hours. Older adults or frail

TABLE 7-24
Morphine to Methadone Equianalgesic Dose Ratio[168]

Oral Morphine Dose (mg/d)	<100	101–300	301–600	601–800	801–1000	≥1001
Oral morphine to oral methadone ratio	3:1	5:1	10:1	12:1	15:1	20:1

patients may need methadone dosed every 12 hours to reduce the occurrence of side effects such as sedation.[159,161]

L.V.'s total daily dose of methadone should be divided into three doses and administered on an 8-hour interval. However, methadone is available in tablets (5 mg and 10 mg) or oral solution. The problem with L.V.'s total daily methadone dose is that it does not divide evenly using tablets. Splitting methadone tablets is not recommended because of the inconsistency in the dose with unequal tablet portions. Methadone solution is not convenient to use, and the dose needs to be drawn accurately with an oral syringe to prevent overdosing. L.V. would need approximately 11 to 13 mg of oral methadone solution per dose, which may be difficult to calibrate with the oral syringe. Therefore, L.V.'s methadone dose should be rounded down to the nearest available tablet size (i.e., 10 mg). Using a rapid switch transition from transdermal fentanyl to methadone, L.V. should be instructed to remove the transdermal fentanyl patch and begin methadone 10 mg orally every 8 hours approximately 12 hours after the patch has been removed. L.V. can continue to use morphine sulfate immediate-release 30 mg every 2 hours as needed for breakthrough pain. The immediate-release morphine dose may need to be reduced if L.V. has a good response to methadone.

Because methadone has a long terminal half-life, it will take 4 or more days to achieve steady state. Unless L.V. is experiencing severe pain, the methadone dose should not be increased before 5 days. L.V. should be encouraged to use the immediate-release morphine during the transition period. The methadone dose can be adjusted based on the total daily dose of morphine used for pain control during the transition period.[161]

METHADONE TOXICITY SIGNS AND SYMPTOMS

CASE 7-7, QUESTION 6: What are the signs and symptoms of methadone toxicity that should be communicated to L.V.?

Step 1:
Determine the 24-hour total of the opioid that will be converted. For L.V., the transdermal fentanyl 100 mcg/hour patch will need to be converted to oral morphine. In addition, L.V. is using 150 mg/day of immediate-release oral morphine.

Donner Study Ratio[165]
The conversion ratio of 60 mg/day oral morphine to 25 mcg/hour transdermal fentanyl will be used for the calculation.

$$\frac{\text{"X" mg total daily dose of new opioid}}{\text{100 mcg/hour transdermal fentanyl}} = \frac{\text{60 mg/day oral morphine}}{\text{25 mcg/hour transdermal fentanyl}}$$

(25)(X) = (100)(60)
X = 240 mg oral morphine
Therefore, the total daily dose of oral morphine is 390 mg (240 mg + 150 mg)

Breitbart Study Ratio[164]
The conversion ratio of 2 mg oral morphine to 1 mcg/hour transdermal fentanyl will be used for the calculation.

$$\frac{\text{"X" mg total daily dose of new opioid}}{\text{100 mcg/hour transdermal fentanyl}} = \frac{\text{2 mg oral morphine}}{\text{1 mcg/hour transdermal fentanyl}}$$

(1)(X) = (2)(100)
X = 200 mg/day oral morphine
Therefore, the total daily dose of oral morphine is 340 mg (200 mg + 150 mg)

Step 2:
Select the equianalgesic dose ratio from the methadone table that corresponds to a total daily morphine use of 390 mg (using the Donner method in step 1).[161,169]

According to the methadone dose Table 7-24, morphine doses in the range of 301–600 mg correspond to a 10:1 ratio (oral morphine to oral methadone).

$$\frac{\text{"X" mg total daily dose oral methadone}}{\text{390 mg total daily dose oral morphine}} = \frac{\text{1 mg oral methadone}}{\text{10 mg oral morphine}}$$

(10)(X) = (390)(1)
10X = 390
X = 39 mg of oral methadone/day
If the total daily dose of 340 mg oral morphine is used for the calculation, the total daily dose of methadone would be 34 mg.

FIGURE 7-8 Conversion of L.V. from transdermal fentanyl to oral methadone.

In 2006, the FDA issued a public health advisory to alert prescribers and patients of the risk of fatal respiratory depression and QTc interval prolongation associated with methadone.[169] L.V. should be instructed to take methadone exactly as prescribed to prevent serious problems with breathing. He should be told about the signs and symptoms of methadone toxicity including shallow breathing, slowed respirations followed by periods of not breathing, slurred speech or difficulty talking, loud snoring, and inability to walk normally.[161] L.V. should be told to seek medical attention immediately if he experiences any of these signs and symptoms of methadone toxicity. He should also let family members living with him know about the risks of methadone so they can be aware of the signs and symptoms of methadone toxicity.

METHADONE TOXICITY MONITORING

CASE 7-7, QUESTION 7: What are the recommendations for monitoring cardiac toxicity associated with methadone?

Methadone can cause prolongation of the QTc interval and increase the risk for development of torsades de pointes (potentially fatal arrhythmia). Factors associated with QTc prolongation are methadone doses greater than 100 mg/day, hypokalemia, low prothrombin level (suggestive of reduced liver function), and drug interactions involving the cytochrome P-450 3A4 enzyme.[168,169]

Consensus guidelines have been published on cardiac monitoring for patients taking methadone. The guidelines recommend pretreatment screening, electrocardiogram evaluation, and risk stratification for QTc intervals exceeding 500 milliseconds. For a QTc interval exceeding 500 milliseconds, the consensus guidelines recommend reducing or discontinuing methadone (Table 7-25).[170]

OPIOID SIDE EFFECT MANAGEMENT

CASE 7-7, QUESTION 8: How should opioid side effects be managed?

Appropriate use of opioids requires minimizing the occurrence of side effects including sedation, nausea, vomiting, pruritus, myoclonus, and cognitive impairment.[171] Table 7-26 gives treatment for common opioid-related side effects. In cancer patients, multiple factors may contribute to the emergence of opioid side effects such as renal insufficiency, nausea and vomiting caused by changes in gut motility or chemotherapy, sedation owing to metabolic disturbances, and concomitant use of other sedatives or antiemetics. Tolerance to most of the opioid side effects develops in 3 to 7 days. If the side effects do not diminish with time, treatment may include switching to a different opioid or adding another medication to counteract the undesired effect.[159,171]

Respiratory depression is a serious adverse event and often is preceded by sedation. With methadone, the peak respiratory depressant effects typically occur later and persist longer than with other opioids. Naloxone is an opioid receptor antagonist that can be used to reverse respiratory depression caused by opioid medications. Opioid-tolerant patients are exquisitely sensitive to opioid antagonists. If naloxone is necessary, it should be titrated to effect (i.e., 0.02 mg IV push every 2 minutes) to prevent profound withdrawal, seizures, arrhythmias, and severe pain (e.g., the analgesic effect of opioids is reversed with naloxone).[159] Patients who are overdosed on methadone will require a continuous IV infusion of naloxone for 24 to 36 hours because of the long elimination half-life of methadone.

TABLE 7-25
Consensus Recommendations for Methadone QTc Prolongation[170]

Inform patients of arrhythmia risk before prescribing methadone.
Obtain patient history of structural heart disease, arrhythmia, and syncope.
Obtain a pretreatment ECG before starting methadone and follow up 30 days after starting methadone. Annual ECG is recommended. Additional ECG if the methadone dosage exceeds 100 mg/d or patient has unexplained syncope or seizures.
Reduce or discontinue methadone if the QTc interval exceeds 500 milliseconds.
Screen medication profile use of drugs that also may prolong or slow the elimination of methadone (i.e., SSRIs, antifungal agents, protease inhibitors, phenytoin, rifampin, phenobarbital, droperidol).

ECG, electrocardiogram; SSRIs, selective serotonin reuptake inhibitors.

TABLE 7-26
Pharmacological Treatments for Opioid-Related Side Effects[171]

Side Effect	Treatment
Constipation	Stool softener, laxative, methylnaltrexone, oral naloxone
Sedation	Methylphenidate, modafinil
Pruritus	Diphenhydramine, hydroxyzine
Nausea	Prochlorperazine, haloperidol, metoclopramide, ondansetron, antihistamine
Dysphoria	Haloperidol, opioid rotation
Cognitive impairment	Methylphenidate, modafinil, opioid rotation
Myoclonus	Clonazepam, dose reduction, opioid rotation

REFRACTORY CANCER PAIN MANAGEMENT

CASE 7-7, QUESTION 9: What are other options if pain is not controlled with conventional pharmacotherapy?

Neuraxial opioid administration (epidural or intrathecal) can be used to treat cancer pain that is refractory to conventional therapy with opioids and coanalgesic medications.[172] Cancer patients with a life expectancy less than 3 months typically have epidural medication administration through a catheter tunneled under the skin that is connected to an ambulatory infusion pump. Long-term neuraxial therapy must be administered through an implantable intrathecal pump to avoid infection complications. Indications for use of neuraxial therapy include neuropathic pain, mixed neuropathic-nociceptive pain, radicular pain from failed back syndrome, and CRPS (refer to Cases 7-1 and 7-4). Medication selection is based on the patient's allergy history and response to a screening trial. Opioids (morphine, hydromorphone, fentanyl), local anesthetics (bupivacaine, ropivacaine), clonidine, ziconotide, and baclofen are commonly used in neuraxial regimens.[172]

Complementary and alternative medicine therapies are widely used by patients in the management of cancer pain, dyspnea, and nausea and vomiting. Auricular acupuncture, therapeutic touch, and hypnosis may help with the management of cancer pain. Music therapy, massage, meditation, and hypnosis may help to reduce anxiety caused by dyspnea. Acupuncture and guided imagery may be beneficial in treating chemotherapy-induced nausea and vomiting.[171]

Oral cannabinoid formulations (dronabinol and nabilone) are approved by the FDA for chemotherapy-induced nausea and vomiting refractory to conventional antiemetic therapy. Several studies of the endogenous cannabinoid receptors (CB_1 and CB_2) have demonstrated efficacy in the management of pain. In the CNS, the CB_1 receptor is expressed in the areas involved in nociceptive processing, including the periaqueductal gray matter and dorsal horn of the spinal cord. The CB_2 receptor is expressed on cells of the immune system and is involved in modulation of inflammation and pain. CB_2 receptor activation has been shown to be analgesic in neuropathic pain models.[171,173] Medical use of cannabinoids has been debated in many states. In October 2009, the Department of Justice issued a memorandum to US Attorneys stating that federal resources should not be used to prosecute persons whose actions comply with their state's laws permitting medical use of marijuana. Currently, 14 states allow the use of medical marijuana via inhalation for various diseases and medical conditions including nonmalignant and cancer pain.[174]

KEY REFERENCES AND WEBSITES

A full list of references for this chapter can be found at **http://thepoint.lww.com/AT10e**. Below are the key references for this chapter, with the corresponding reference number in this chapter found in parentheses after the reference.

Key References

American Geriatrics Society Panel on Pharmacological Management of Persistent Pain in Older Persons. Pharmacological management of persistent pain in older persons. *J Am Geriatr Soc.* 2009;57:1331. (121)

Attal N et al. EFNS guidelines on the pharmacological treatment of neuropathic pain: 2010 revision. *Eur J Neurol.* 2010;17:1113. (16)

Carville SF et al. EULAR evidence-based recommendations for the management of fibromyalgia syndrome. *Ann Rheum Dis.* 2008;67:536. (69)

Chou R et al. Clinical guidelines for the use of chronic opioid therapy in chronic noncancer pain. *J Pain.* 2009;10:113. (144)

Chou R et al. Medications for acute and chronic low back pain: a review of the evidence for an American Pain Society/American College of Physicians clinical practice guideline [published correction appears in *Ann Intern Med.* 2008;148:247]. *Ann Intern Med.* 2007;147:505. (32)

Chou R et al. Comparative efficacy and safety of skeletal muscle relaxants for spasticity and musculoskeletal conditions: a systematic review. *J Pain Symptom Manage.* 2004;28:140. (101)

Drossman DA. Severe and refractory chronic abdominal pain: treatment strategies. *Clin Gastroenterol Hepatol.* 2008;6:978. (142)

Dubinsky RM et al. Practice parameter: treatment of postherpetic neuralgia: an evidence-based report of the Quality Standards Subcommittee of the American Academy of Neurology. *Neurology.* 2004;63:959. (111)

Dworkin RH et al. Recommendations for the pharmacological management of neuropathic pain: an overview and literature update. *Mayo Clin Proc.* 2010;85(3 Suppl):S3. (104)

Finnerup NB et al. The evidence for pharmacological treatment of neuropathic pain. *Pain.* 2010;150:573. (105)

Harvey WF, Hunter DJ. Pharmacologic intervention for osteoarthritis in older adults. *Clin Geriatr Med.* 2010;26:503. (120)

Koes BW et al. An updated overview of clinical guidelines for the management of non-specific low back pain in primary care. *Eur Spine J.* 2010;19:2075. (27)

Miaskowski C et al. *Guideline for the Management of Cancer Pain in Adults and Children, APS Clinical Practice Guideline Series, No. 3.* Glenview, IL: American Pain Society; 2005. (152)

Turk DC et al. Psychological approaches in the treatment of chronic pain patients—when pills, scalpels and needles are not enough. *Can J Psychiatry.* 2008;53:213. (148)

Key Websites

Partners against Pain. **www.partnersagainstpain.com.www.nhpoc.org**

8

Perioperative Care

Andrew J. Donnelly, Julie A. Golembiewski, and Andrei M. Rakic

CORE PRINCIPLES

	CHAPTER CASES
PREOPERATIVE MEDICATIONS	
1 Chronic medications that are necessary to maintain the patient's underlying physiological condition are generally administered up to, and including, the day of surgery. The decision to hold medications that cause bleeding (e.g., warfarin, clopidogrel), have hemodynamic (e.g., angiotensin-converting enzyme inhibitor) or hypoglycemic effects (e.g., insulin), or that can potentially interact with intraoperative and postoperative medications (e.g., buprenorphine) is made on an individual basis based on risk and benefit.	**Case 8-1 (Question 1)**
2 Premedication may be administered immediately before surgery to reduce the patient's anxiety about the upcoming surgery (e.g., midazolam) or to reduce the patient's risk for aspiration (e.g., sodium citrate).	**Case 8-2 (Question 1)**
INTRAVENOUS ANESTHETIC AGENTS	
1 General anesthesia, defined as a state of drug-induced unconsciousness, is most commonly achieved by the administration of an intravenous anesthetic agent. The choice of agent is based on patient characteristics.	**Case 8-3 (Question 1), Case 8-4 (Question 1), Case 8-5 (Question 1)**
VOLATILE INHALATION AGENTS	
1 Volatile inhalation agents are administered to maintain general anesthesia, although sevoflurane may also be used to induce general anesthesia (via a face mask). These agents vary in potency, pharmacokinetics, pharmacologic properties, and cost.	**Case 8-7 (Question 1), Case 8-8 (Question 1)**
NEUROMUSCULAR BLOCKING AGENTS	
1 Neuromuscular blocking agents (NMBAs) are administered to facilitate endotracheal intubation and to relax skeletal muscle during surgery. Succinylcholine, a depolarizing agent, has a fast onset, short duration of action, and a significant adverse effect profile. The nondepolarizing NMBAs (e.g., rocuronium, vecuronium, cisatracurium, pancuronium) differ in their routes of elimination and cardiovascular adverse effect profile.	**Case 8-9 (Questions 1, 2), Case 8-10 (Question 1)**
LOCAL ANESTHETICS	
1 Local anesthetics are routinely administered in the perioperative setting to provide local or regional anesthesia. Agents vary in their physiochemical properties, which account for differences in onset and duration of action. To minimize the risk for systemic local anesthetic toxicity (which can be life-threatening), attention must be paid to the total dose administered, the vascularity of the injection site, and patient characteristics (such as age and the presence of cardiac, renal, or hepatic dysfunction).	**Case 8-11 (Question 1), Case 8-12 (Question 1)**

continued

ANTIEMETIC AGENTS AND POSTOPERATIVE NAUSEA AND VOMITING	
1 Postoperative nausea and vomiting (PONV) is one of the most common complications after surgery. Identifying the number of risk factors is critical for assessing a patient's risk for experiencing PONV. Patients at moderate or high risk for experiencing PONV should receive one or more prophylactic antiemetics. If PONV develops despite antiemetic prophylaxis, administration of an antiemetic with a different mechanism of action is the most effective treatment.	**Case 8-13 (Questions 1–4)**
ANALGESIC AGENTS AND POSTOPERATIVE PAIN	
1 On-demand administration of an intravenous opioid (patient-controlled analgesia [PCA]) can provide excellent analgesia with the added benefit of allowing the patient control over his or her pain management. Appropriate patient selection, ordering, pump programming, therapy adjustments, monitoring, and patient education are critical for safe PCA use.	**Case 8-14 (Questions 1–7)**
2 Epidural analgesia can provide superior pain relief compared with an intravenous opioid for patients undergoing certain types of major surgery. An opioid and a local anesthetic are often administered in combination as a continuous infusion through the epidural catheter. Appropriate patient selection, ordering, pump programming, therapy adjustments, monitoring, and review of concurrent medications are critical for safe epidural analgesia.	**Case 8-15 (Questions 1–6)**
3 The pain management plan should be individualized, taking into consideration the invasiveness and type or location of the surgery, anticipated pain intensity after surgery, patient comorbidities, current medications, and previous response to analgesic medications. Maximizing the use of nonopioid analgesics (such as acetaminophen, nonsteroidal anti-inflammatory drugs, and local anesthetics) can improve analgesia and reduce the need for an opioid. Lower opioid use can mean fewer undesirable adverse effects, particularly nausea, vomiting, and excessive sedation.	**Case 8-16 (Question 1)**

The operating room (OR) is one of the most medication-intensive settings in a hospital. During the perioperative period (broadly defined as the preoperative, intraoperative, and postoperative periods), a patient may receive many medications. Most of them are used primarily in the OR setting and have limited application elsewhere in the institution. For other medications, their use in the OR may differ from that seen in other patient care areas. The OR is unique in that a significant number of the medications are administered as single doses by the anesthesia care provider (e.g., physician, nurse anesthetist, anesthesia assistant). To ensure continuity of care of the surgical patient, health care providers from all settings (e.g., acute care, home health care, extended care) should have a basic understanding of perioperative drug therapy.

This chapter reviews seven major classes of medications used during the perioperative period: preoperative medications, intravenous (IV) anesthetic agents, volatile inhalation agents, neuromuscular blocking agents, local anesthetics, antiemetic agents, and analgesic agents.

PREOPERATIVE MEDICATIONS

A preoperative evaluation ensures that the patient is medically prepared for surgery (e.g., pre-existing medical conditions such as diabetes, hypertension, or asthma are controlled or stable), allows the provider to discuss the most appropriate anesthetic and postoperative pain management options with the patient, and helps reassure and educate the patient. Once the plan is made, the anesthesia provider and the surgeon determine whether the patient should take his or her regularly scheduled medications up to and including the morning of surgery. These chronic medications are often necessary to maintain the patient's physiological condition. The decision to continue or withhold chronic medications before surgery depends on the patient's current medical condition and the potential for withdrawal symptoms, worsening of the patient's underlying physiological condition, drug interactions with anesthetic medications, perioperative hemodynamic instability, or postoperative complications such as bleeding.

Administration of preoperative medications (premedicants) to patients can be thought of as the start of their operative course. Many different medications are used preoperatively and can be grouped into the following classes: benzodiazepines, opioids, gastric motility stimulants, H_2-receptor antagonists, and antacids. A key point concerning preoperative medication is that not all patients will require premedicants. Patients should be assessed individually regarding their need for pharmacologic premedication. If required, premedicants should be selected based on patient-specific needs. Administration of a standard preoperative regimen to all patients should be avoided.

Goals of Premedication

Major goals of premedication are to decrease the patient's anxiety about the upcoming surgery and to produce sedation. In addition to relieving anxiety and producing sedation, premedication is occasionally used to provide analgesia, reduce anesthetic requirements, prevent autonomic responses that result in

TABLE 8-1
Indications, Routes of Administration, and Doses of Preoperative Agents[a] [1–4]

Agent	Indications	Routes of Administration	Doses[b]
Benzodiazepines			
Diazepam	Anxiolysis, amnesia, sedation	PO	*Adults:* 5–10 mg
Lorazepam	Anxiolysis, amnesia, sedation	PO	0.025–0.05 mg/kg (range, 1–4 mg for adults)
		IV	*Adults:* 0.025–0.04 mg/kg; *Pediatrics:* 0.01–0.03 mg/kg (titrate dose; max: 2 mg)
Midazolam	Anxiolysis, amnesia, sedation	PO	*Adults:* 20 mg; *Pediatrics:* 0.5–0.75 mg/kg (max: 20 mg)
		IM	*Adults:* 0.05–0.08 mg/kg (max: 10 mg); *Pediatrics:* 0.1–0.15 mg/kg (max: 10 mg)
		IV	*Adults:* 1–2.5 mg (titrate dose); *Pediatrics:* 0.025–0.05 mg/kg (titrate dose)
		IN	*Pediatrics:* 0.2 mg/kg (max: 15 mg)
Opioids			
Morphine	Analgesia, sedation	IM	*Adults:* 2–4 mg; *Pediatrics:* 0.02–0.05 mg/kg
		IV	Titrate dose
Fentanyl	Analgesia, sedation	IV	*Adults:* 25–100 mcg (titrate dose); *Pediatrics:* 0.05–2 mcg/kg
Anticholinergics			
Atropine (A)	Antisialagogue (S > G > A), sedation (S > A > G)	IM/IV	*Adults:* 0.3–0.6 mg; *Pediatrics:* 0.02 mg/kg IM, 0.01 mg/kg IV (max: 0.4 mg)
Scopolamine (S)	Sedation, amnesia, antisialagogue	IM/IV	*Adults:* 0.1–0.4 mg; *Pediatrics:* 0.02 mg/kg IM, 0.01 mg/kg IV (max: 0.4 mg)
Glycopyrrolate (G)	Antisialagogue	IM/IV	*Adults:* 0.1–0.3 mg; *Pediatrics:* 0.005–0.01 mg/kg (max: 0.3 mg)
Gastric Motility Stimulants			
Metoclopramide	Reduce gastric volume, antiemetic	PO	*Adults:* 10 mg; *Pediatrics:* 0.15 mg/kg
		IV	*Adults:* 0.1–0.2 mg/kg (5–10 mg); *Pediatrics:* 0.1–0.15 mg/kg
H_2-Receptor Antagonists			
Cimetidine	↑ Gastric pH	PO	*Adults:* 300 mg; *Pediatrics:* 7.5 mg/kg
		IV	*Adults:* 300 mg; *Pediatrics:* 7.5 mg/kg
Ranitidine	↑ Gastric pH	PO	*Adults:* 150 mg; *Pediatrics:* 2 mg/kg
		IV	*Adults:* 50 mg; *Pediatrics:* 0.5–1 mg/kg
Famotidine	↑ Gastric pH	PO	*Adults:* 40 mg; *Pediatrics:* 0.5 mg/kg
		IV	*Adults:* 20 mg; *Pediatrics:* 0.25 mg/kg
Nizatidine	↑ Gastric pH	PO	*Adults:* 150 mg–300 mg
Nonparticulate Antacids			
Citric acid and sodium citrate	↑ Gastric pH	PO	*Adults:* 30 mL

[a] General dosage guidelines; doses must be individualized based on patient-specific parameters.
[b] Doses listed are for agents when used as sole premedicant; doses may need to be reduced if premedicants are administered in combination (e.g., opioids, benzodiazepines).
IM, intramuscular; IN, intranasal; IV, intravenous; PO, oral.

intraoperative hemodynamic instability, decrease salivation and secretions, reduce gastric fluid volume, or increase gastric pH. Table 8-1 lists medications commonly used preoperatively and their major indications, routes of administration, and dosages.[1–4] Midazolam is by far the most commonly used premedicant.

Selection Criteria

Factors to consider when selecting a preoperative drug include the patient's American Society of Anesthesiologists (ASA) physical status class,[3] medical conditions, degree of anxiety, age, surgical procedure to be performed, length of procedure, postoperative admission status (e.g., inpatient vs. outpatient), drug allergies, previous experience with medications, and concurrent drug therapy. The ASA physical status classification system classifies patients as I through V. ASA-I patients are healthy with little medical risk, whereas ASA-V patients have little chance of survival. Severe systemic disorders (e.g., uncontrolled diabetes mellitus, coronary artery disease) are present in ASA-III through ASA-V patients. Selection of preoperative medications in this group of patients will be more difficult. These patients generally have limited physiological reserve; thus, administration of a cardiovascular depressant agent, for example, can be harmful. Furthermore, these patients will be taking a significant number of medications; hence, chances for drug interactions are increased. The patient's other medical conditions are important to consider to prevent the administration of contraindicated medications. For example, the benzodiazepines are contraindicated in pregnancy. A patient's age will play a role in the response seen with premedicant administration. The elderly are often more sensitive to preoperative opioids and benzodiazepines, as well as to the central nervous system (CNS) effects of anticholinergic agents.

Familiarity with the surgery to be performed will aid in selecting appropriate premedicants. In surgical cases in which painful procedures (e.g., vascular cannulation, peripheral nerve block) will be performed on the patient, an analgesic premedicant may be warranted. The length and type of the procedure is important to consider when selecting premedicants. For example, a patient undergoing emergency surgery who has not fasted is often administered a nonparticulate antacid because of the risk for aspiration of gastric contents. In outpatient surgery, agents with a long duration of action should be avoided because residual effects can prolong discharge time. Finally, it is important to review the patient's current drug therapy before selecting an agent to prevent potentially harmful drug interactions.

Timing and Routes of Administration

The timing and route of administration is almost as important as the choice of the agent. As a general rule, agents administered by the IV route produce the fastest onset of action and are often given after the patient arrives in the OR, whereas medications administered via the oral route are usually administered 30 to 60 minutes before the patient arrives in the OR. If possible, the intramuscular (IM) route should be avoided because it is painful and undesirable for the patient.

Administration of Chronic Medications Before Surgery

CASE 8-1

QUESTION 1: K.J., a 61-year-old man, is scheduled to undergo a carotid endarterectomy under general anesthesia. K.J.'s past medical history is significant for diabetes, hypertension, hyperlipidemia, and coronary artery disease. His current medications are enalapril 20 mg once daily, metoprolol XL 50 mg once daily, metformin XR 1,000 mg once daily, atorvastatin 40 mg once daily, aspirin EC 325 mg once daily, and clopidogrel 75 mg once daily. What medications should K.J. take the morning of surgery?

Consequences of stopping a chronic medication before, or failing to restart that medication after surgery, can be significant. For example, abrupt discontinuation of a β-blocker during the perioperative period in a patient who has been on chronic β-blocker therapy can increase the risk of death in the intraoperative and postoperative period. The American College of Cardiology/American Heart Association (ACC/AHA) recommends continuation of β-blocker therapy in patients undergoing surgery who are receiving a β-blocker for treatment of conditions with ACC/AHA Class I guideline indications for the drugs (e.g., angina, symptomatic arrhythmia, postmyocardial infarction).[5] Angiotensin-converting enzyme inhibitors (ACEIs) and angiotensin receptor blockers (ARBs) increase the risk of hypotension after induction of anesthesia when these agents are not withheld 24 hours before surgery.[6] In general, this hypotension is not responsive to conventional vasopressors (ephedrine, phenylephrine) but will respond to vasopressin.[7] Stopping the ACEI before surgery, however, can result in adverse postoperative effects such as rebound hypertension and atrial fibrillation. Therefore, the decision to continue or stop the ACEI or ARB before surgery is made on an individual basis, taking into consideration the indication for the ACEI or ARB and the type of surgery. Calcium-channel blockers, clonidine, amiodarone, digoxin, and statins should be continued. Preoperative withdrawal of a statin in a patient undergoing major vascular surgery, for example, increases the risk of myocardial infarction and cardiovascular death after surgery.[8] Diuretics are typically held the morning of surgery to minimize the risk of hypovolemia and electrolyte abnormalities.

Oral antidiabetic agents and noninsulin injectable agents are typically held the morning of surgery and not restarted until normal food intake resumes. In patients with renal dysfunction and those who may receive IV contrast media, metformin should be discontinued 24 to 48 hours before surgery to reduce the risk of perioperative lactic acidosis. For patients on insulin therapy, a portion of the morning dose of intermediate- or long-acting insulin is generally administered on the day of surgery after a check of the patient's blood glucose. Close blood glucose monitoring guides subsequent insulin doses to avoid hypoglycemia.[9]

Antiepileptics, antipsychotics, benzodiazepines, lithium, selective serotonin and norepinephrine reuptake inhibitors (SSRIs and SNRIs), tricyclic antidepressants (TCAs), and carbidopa/levodopa have a greater risk for withdrawal or disease decompensation than for perioperative complications. These medications should therefore be continued up to and including the morning of surgery.

Monoamine oxidase inhibitors (MAOIs) can interact with certain drugs used during anesthesia to produce cardiovascular instability. However, administration of an MAOI-safe anesthetic avoids the need to stop the MAOI before surgery (and relapse of the underlying disease) in a patient requiring an MAOI for refractory psychiatric illness.[10]

Nonselective nonsteroidal anti-inflammatory drugs (NSAIDs) reversibly inhibit platelet aggregation and are often stopped 1 to 3 days before surgery, depending on the duration of action of the drug. Celecoxib does not affect platelet aggregation and may be continued up to and including the day of surgery. Nonselective NSAIDs and celecoxib should be held if there is a concern for impaired renal function during or after surgery.

For patients on anticoagulant or antiplatelet therapy, the risks for thromboembolism must be balanced with the risk for bleeding during and after the surgical procedure. For patients on warfarin who are at high risk for perioperative thromboembolism, bridging anticoagulation therapy with IV heparin or low-molecular-weight heparin (LMWH) before surgery is recommended. Warfarin may not need to be discontinued if the patient is undergoing minor surgery (e.g., certain ophthalmic, dental, or dermatologic procedures). For patients who have had coronary stents recently placed, discontinuing antiplatelet therapy prematurely can significantly increase the risk of perioperative stent thrombosis and have catastrophic consequences.[11]

Traditionally, it was thought that patients who have been taking long-term corticosteroid therapy before surgery will experience adrenal insufficiency in the perioperative period and should receive a supplemental stress-dose of hydrocortisone or methylprednisolone during and up to 2 to 3 days after surgery.[12] A recent review of the literature, however, found that patients on long-term corticosteroid therapy only require continuation of their normal daily dose of corticosteroid in the perioperative period. These patients are generally able to increase their endogenous adrenal function above their baseline corticosteroid dose to meet the increased demand from surgery; a supplemental stress dose of corticosteroid is not necessary. These patients can be closely monitored, and if hypotension that is refractory to volume replacement does develop, a stress dose of a corticosteroid should be administered at that time. Patients who have a known dysfunctional hypothalamic-pituitary-adrenal axis deficiency (e.g., Addison disease), on the other hand, will require supplemental corticosteroid doses in the perioperative period as they cannot increase endogenous cortisol production to meet the increased demand from surgery.[13]

Opioid-dependent chronic pain patients who undergo surgery often experience more severe acute pain after surgery. These patients should receive either their chronic opioid medication or a comparable dose of an IV opioid the morning of surgery to meet their daily requirements to avoid uncontrolled pain and opioid-withdrawal symptoms. Opioid-dependent patients being treated with buprenorphine present a unique challenge for postoperative pain management. Buprenorphine is a partial mu-agonist and kappa antagonist that tightly binds to these receptors for a very long time. If buprenorphine is continued up to the morning of surgery, it prevents a pure mu-agonist such as morphine from providing effective analgesia. Although buprenorphine produces analgesia, it only partially stimulates the mu-receptor, resulting in a ceiling effect for analgesia. Increasing the dose of buprenorphine does not usually provide enough analgesia. In patients expected to have moderate to severe pain after surgery (requiring the use of an opioid), it is recommended that buprenorphine be discontinued 5 to 7 days before surgery. These patients may be transitioned to nonopioid pain medications and possibly methadone, which would then be continued up to and including the morning of surgery. The use of nonopioid analgesics or analgesic techniques (e.g., acetaminophen, peripheral nerve blockade, epidural analgesia) for perioperative analgesia should be maximized, regardless of whether or not buprenorphine is discontinued prior to surgery.[14]

For K.J., metformin should be discontinued 24 to 48 hours before surgery to minimize the risk for lactic acidosis during or after surgery. Metoprolol, on the other hand, should be taken up to and including the morning of surgery. K.J. has coronary artery disease and is undergoing a carotid endarterectomy, which is a vascular surgical procedure with a high risk of serious cardiovascular complications (such as stroke or myocardial infarction). Based on the ACC/AHA practice guidelines,[5] perioperative β-blocker therapy is recommended for K.J. The decision for K.J. to take enalapril and atorvastatin the morning of surgery is made by the anesthesia care provider. For K.T., it is likely that he will be asked to take his atorvastatin but hold his morning dose of enalapril to ensure hemodynamic stability during induction of general anesthesia. The decision for K.J. to take or hold aspirin and clopidogrel is made by the surgeon, based on risk of bleeding versus the benefit of cardiovascular protection. For K.T., it is likely that the surgeon will ask him to take the aspirin up to and including the morning of surgery but hold the clopidogrel for 7 days before surgery.

Aspiration Pneumonitis Prophylaxis

CASE 8-2

QUESTION 1: D.W., a 5-foot 4-inch, 95-kg, 38-year-old woman, ASA-II, is scheduled to undergo a laparoscopic cholecystectomy under general anesthesia. D.W. has type 2 diabetes. Physical examination is normal except for an abnormal airway, which is anticipated to complicate intubation. Her medications include glipizide and an antacid for dyspepsia. The procedure is scheduled as a same-day surgery. What factors predispose D.W. to aspiration, and what premedication, if any, should D.W. receive for aspiration prophylaxis?

DEFINITION

Aspiration pneumonitis, although uncommon, is a potentially fatal condition that occurs as a result of regurgitation and aspiration of gastric contents. Aspiration of undigested or semidigested gastric contents into the respiratory tract can cause obstruction and an inflammatory response. Acute chemical pneumonitis and subsequent acute lung injury (aspiration pneumonitis) can result from aspiration of acidic gastric secretions.[15] For adult patients, it is believed that aspiration of more than 25 mL of gastric fluid with a pH of less than 2.5 places them at greater risk for severe pneumonitis and pulmonary sequelae should aspiration occur.[1]

RISK FACTORS

Patients at greatest risk for regurgitation and aspiration include those with increased gastric acid, elevated intragastric pressure, gastric or intestinal hypomotility, digestive structural disorders, neuromuscular incoordination, and depressed sensorium. These can include pregnant women, obese patients, and patients with diabetes, as well as patients with a hiatal hernia, gastroesophageal reflux, esophageal motility disorders, or peptic ulcer disease.[1,16] Diabetic patients with reflux symptoms or poor glucose control may also benefit from pharmacologic prophylaxis. In addition to having delayed gastric emptying, obese patients will often present with increased abdominal pressure and an abnormal airway; both factors predispose these individuals to aspiration. Hormonal changes in pregnant women account for delayed gastric emptying and relaxation of the lower esophageal sphincter. An increase in intra-abdominal pressure is also seen during pregnancy. Labor can increase gastrin levels, increasing gastric volume and acidity as well as delaying gastric emptying. Patients undergoing emergency surgery frequently have full stomachs because they have not had time to fast appropriately.

Rapid sequence induction, effective application of cricoid pressure, maintaining a patent upper airway, avoiding inflation of the stomach with anesthetic gases, and inserting a large-bore gastric tube once the airway has been secured, as well as the use of regional anesthesia when possible, are probably the most important measures the anesthesia provider can take to reduce the patient's risk of aspiration.[17] Routine administration of pharmacologic aspiration prophylaxis is not cost-effective and does not reduce morbidity in healthy patients undergoing elective surgery.[18] Administration of pharmacologic aspiration prophylaxis should, however, be considered to prevent morbidity in patients at risk for aspiration.

D.W. has several factors that place her at risk for aspiration. She is obese with an abnormal airway. She also has diabetes and reports symptoms of dyspepsia that are relieved by antacids. These conditions will predispose D.W. to increased abdominal pressure, delayed gastric emptying, and increased risk of regurgitation. Her abnormal airway may delay intubation, increasing the amount of time D.W. is susceptible to aspiration. Therefore, aspiration prophylaxis with medications that buffer gastric acid and reduce gastric volume is prudent for D.W.

MEDICATIONS

Many medications (e.g., antacids, gastric motility stimulants, H_2-receptor antagonists) can reduce the risk of pneumonitis if aspiration occurs. These drugs, with the possible exception of metoclopramide, are relatively free of adverse effects and have a favorable risk-benefit profile.

ANTACIDS

Antacids, effective in raising gastric pH to greater than 2.5, should be given as a single dose (30 mL) approximately 15 to 30 minutes before induction of anesthesia. Nonparticulate antacids (e.g., citric acid and sodium citrate) are the agents of choice because the suspension particles in particulate antacids can act as foci for an inflammatory reaction if aspirated and increase the risk of pulmonary damage.[1] Antacids have two major advantages when used for aspiration pneumonitis prophylaxis; there is no "lag time" for onset of activity, and antacids are effective on the fluid already in the stomach. Their major disadvantages are (a) a short-acting buffering effect that is not likely to last as long as the surgical procedure (citric acid and sodium citrate must be administered no more than 1 hour before induction of anesthesia, with its duration possibly dependent on gastric emptying); (b) the potential for emesis (owing to their lack of palatability); (c) the possibility of incomplete mixing in the stomach; and (d) their administration adds fluid volume to the stomach.[1,18]

GASTRIC MOTILITY STIMULANTS

The gastric motility stimulant, metoclopramide, has no effect on gastric pH or acid secretion. This agent reduces gastric volume in predisposed patients (e.g., parturients, obese patients) by promoting gastric emptying. Preoperative metoclopramide increases lower esophageal sphincter pressure and reduces gastric volume.[1,18] Metoclopramide should be administered 60 minutes before induction of anesthesia when given orally. When given by the IV route, metoclopramide should be slowly (3–5 minutes) administered 15 to 30 minutes before induction of anesthesia. The effects of metoclopramide on gastric emptying have been variable, especially when used with other agents. For example, the concomitant administration of anticholinergics (e.g., glycopyrrolate, atropine) or prior administration of opioids can reduce lower esophageal sphincter pressure, which can offset the effects of metoclopramide on the upper gastrointestinal (GI) tract.[1,19]

H_2-RECEPTOR ANTAGONISTS

H_2-receptor antagonists reduce gastric acidity and volume by decreasing gastric acid secretion. Unlike antacids, the H_2-receptor antagonists do not produce immediate effects. Onset time for these agents when administered orally is 1 to 3 hours; good effects will be seen in 30 to 60 minutes when administered IV.[3] Duration of action of H_2-receptor antagonists is also important because the risk of aspiration pneumonitis extends through emergence from anesthesia. After IV administration, the cimetidine dose should be repeated in 6 hours if necessary, whereas therapeutic concentrations of ranitidine and famotidine persist for 8 and 12 hours, respectively.[3]

PROTON-PUMP INHIBITORS

Proton-pump inhibitors (PPIs; e.g., omeprazole) act at the final site of gastric acid secretion, making these agents very effective in suppressing acid secretion. When the effects of preoperative IV pantoprazole on gastric pH and volume were compared with IV ranitidine and placebo, both pantoprazole and ranitidine significantly reduced the volume and increased the pH of gastric contents when compared with placebo (saline). There was no difference, however, between the pantoprazole and ranitidine groups.[20] Therefore, there appears to be no need to use the more-expensive PPIs in patients at risk for pulmonary aspiration.

Because D.W.'s surgery is scheduled as a same-day surgery, D.W. will arrive at the hospital or surgical center approximately 90 minutes before the start of the procedure. A nonparticulate antacid such as citric acid and sodium citrate solution 30 mL orally can be administered to D.W. immediately before entering the OR. The anesthesia care provider may also administer an H_2-receptor antagonist instead of, or in addition to, the nonparticulate antacid.

INTRAVENOUS ANESTHETIC AGENTS

General Anesthesia

General anesthesia is a state of drug-induced unconsciousness. Other components of general anesthesia include amnesia, analgesia, immobility, and attenuation of autonomic responses to noxious stimuli.[21] Drugs used to induce general anesthesia should produce unconsciousness rapidly and smoothly while minimizing any cardiovascular changes. An IV induction agent is commonly administered for initiation of general anesthesia. The most common drug used for IV induction is propofol. Methohexital, etomidate, remifentanil, midazolam, and ketamine are less frequently used. Propofol can also be used to maintain general anesthesia, as drugs that do not accumulate during repeat or continuous dosing are ideal choices for maintenance therapy.

Mechanisms of Action

Most IV anesthetic agents produce CNS depression by action on the γ-aminobutyric acid (GABA) benzodiazepine chloride ion channel receptor. GABA is the principal inhibitory neurotransmitter in the CNS. The barbiturates (methohexital) bind to a receptor site on the GABA–receptor complex, reducing the rate of dissociation of GABA from its receptor. This results in increased chloride conductance through the ion channel, nerve cell hyperpolarization, and inhibition of nerve impulse transmission. Barbiturates can directly activate the chloride channels by mimicking the action of GABA. Benzodiazepines (midazolam) also bind to this GABA–receptor complex, and their subsequent potentiation of the inhibitory action of GABA is well described. At large doses, most of the benzodiazepine receptors will be occupied, and hypnosis (unconsciousness) will occur. The site of action of etomidate—and propofol—is also at the GABA receptor, with etomidate augmenting GABA-gated chloride currents and propofol enhancing the activity of the GABA-activated chloride channel. Ketamine acts at a different site than other induction agents. At anesthetic doses, ketamine produces dissociation between the cortex and the thalamus within the limbic system, resulting in a dissociative state; that is, the patient appears to be detached from his or her surroundings. Ketamine also produces analgesia and amnesia at these doses.[22]

Pharmacokinetics

The onset and duration of effect are the most important pharmacokinetic properties of IV anesthetic agents when used for induction of anesthesia. In general, the commonly used IV induction agents have a rapid onset of action and short clinical duration. The degree to which metabolism plays a role in the clinical duration of IV induction agents is variable; rapid metabolism can be a significant factor in the relatively shorter duration to full recovery of propofol.[22] Table 8-2 compares the pharmacokinetic properties of IV anesthetic agents.[22–24]

Adverse and Beneficial Effects

IV anesthetic agents can produce a variety of adverse and beneficial effects other than loss of consciousness (e.g., cardiovascular depression or stimulation, pain on injection, nausea and vomiting, respiratory depression or stimulation, CNS cerebroprotection or excitation, adrenocorticoid suppression, anxiolysis, amnesia, analgesia). Table 8-3 compares the relative significance of these effects among available agents.[22–24] The most

TABLE 8-2

Pharmacokinetic Comparison of Common Intravenous Anesthetic Agents[22–24]

Drug	Half-Life (hours)	Onset (seconds)	Clinical Duration (minutes)[a]	Hangover Effect[b]
Etomidate	2–5	≤30	3–12	+
Ketamine	1–3	30–60	10–20	++ – +++[c]
Methohexital	4	≤30	5–10	+
Midazolam	1–4	30–90	10–20	+++[d]
Propofol	0.5–7	≤45	5–10	0 – +

[a] Time from injection of agent to return to conscious state.
[b] Residual psychomotor impairment after awakening from induction dose.
[c] When ketamine is administered as the induction agent (e.g., 5–10 mg/kg IM).
[d] When midazolam is administered as the induction agent (e.g., 0.15 mg/kg IV).

TABLE 8-3
Effects of Intravenous Induction Agents[22–24]

Adverse Effect	Etomidate	Ketamine	Methohexital	Midazolam	Propofol	Remifentanil
Adrenocorticoid suppression	+	–	–	–	–	–
Cerebral protection	+	–	+	+	+	–
Cardiovascular depression	–	–	++	+	++	–/+[a]
Emergence delirium or euphoria	–	++	–	–	+	–
Myoclonus	+++	+	++	–	+	–/+[a]
Nausea/vomiting	+++	++	++	+	–[b]	++
Pain on injection	++	–	+	–	++	–
Respiratory depression	++	–	++	+/++	++	+/++[a]
Anxiolysis/amnesia	–	–/+[a]	–	++++	–/+[a]	–
Analgesia	–	+++	–	–	–	++++

[a] Dose-dependent effects.
[b] Has antiemetic effects
+ to ++++, likelihood of adverse effect relative to other agents; –, no effect.

troublesome are usually cardiovascular effects or CNS excitation reactions. Contribution to postoperative nausea and vomiting (PONV) and delirium, for example, can be significant and may delay full recovery and patient discharge from the postanesthesia care unit (PACU). This is of particular concern in the ambulatory surgery setting because the patient will be discharged home. CNS effects can include hiccups, myoclonus, seizure activity, euphoria, hallucinations, and emergence delirium. The cerebroprotective effect produced by methohexital, etomidate, and propofol results from a reduction in cerebral blood flow secondary to cerebral vasoconstriction. As a result, cerebral metabolic rate, cerebral blood flow, and intracranial pressure are reduced.[22–24] This effect is useful if these drugs are available in therapeutic concentrations at a time of potential cerebral ischemia.

Agent Selection

The selection of an IV anesthetic agent should be determined based on patient characteristics, which may include history of PONV, allergy profile, psychiatric history, or cardiovascular status.

Propofol: Antiemetic Effect and Full Recovery Characteristics

CASE 8-3

QUESTION 1: K.T., a 19-year-old woman, ASA-I, is admitted to the ambulatory surgery center for strabismus surgery to correct misalignment of her extraocular muscles. She is otherwise healthy, and all laboratory values obtained before surgery are within normal limits. The duration of K.T.'s surgery is anticipated to be approximately 90 minutes. Which IV induction agent should be used?

Propofol is a good choice here for several reasons. Strabismus surgery is considered highly emetogenic because operative manipulation of extraocular muscles can trigger the oculoemetic reflex. Therefore, precautions should be taken to reduce the possibility of nausea and vomiting postoperatively. Propofol produces the lowest incidence of PONV when compared with other IV induction agents and the volatile inhalation agents; it has even been associated with a direct antiemetic effect.[25] This effect does not preclude the need for prophylactic antiemetic therapy, but may contribute to the avoidance of emesis in K.T. immediately after surgery. Furthermore, ambulatory surgery demands rapid, full recovery from general anesthesia. Propofol, in particular, is associated with a more rapid recovery of psychomotor function and a patient-perceived superior quality of recovery.[24]

Etomidate Use in Cardiovascular Disease

CASE 8-4

QUESTION 1: L.M., a 73-year-old man, ASA-IV, is in need of repair of an abdominal aortic aneurysm. During a preoperative evaluation a few days before surgery, his blood pressure (BP) was 160/102 mm Hg, and his medical records revealed hypertension that was poorly controlled by hydrochlorothiazide 25 mg daily and metoprolol XL (Toprol) 100 mg daily. He also has angina that occasionally requires treatment with sublingual nitroglycerin. An exercise stress test showed electrocardiogram changes at a moderate exercise load. Two days before the elective aneurysm repair was scheduled, L.M. presented to the emergency department with a 4-hour history of severe back pain. His surgeon believes that there is a high likelihood that the aneurysm is leaking or expanding and schedules surgery immediately. What is the best plan for L.M.'s anesthetic induction and maintenance?

L.M. has significant cardiovascular disease, and care should be taken to minimize any cardiovascular depression, tachycardia, or hypertension during induction and maintenance of anesthesia. Of the currently available induction agents, etomidate has the most stable cardiovascular profile[24] and is associated with minimal cardiovascular depression. Opioids generally produce minimal cardiovascular effects and could potentially be used for induction. Propofol and ketamine can cause hemodynamic changes and are best avoided in L.M. Etomidate would be an excellent choice for induction, followed by an inhaled anesthetic agent such as sevoflurane or isoflurane to maintain anesthesia.

Methohexital for Electroconvulsive Therapy

CASE 8-5

QUESTION 1: T.B., a 33-year-old woman, ASA-I, will undergo an electroconvulsive therapy (ECT) procedure for treatment of her severe, medication-resistant depression. T.B. is scheduled to go home within 1 to 2 hours after the

procedure, which will be performed under general anesthesia. What IV induction agent should be used?

ECT procedures are an important method of treatment of severe and medication-resistant depression, mania, and other serious psychiatric conditions. During the ECT procedure, an electrical current is applied to the brain, resulting in an electroencephalographic spike and wave activity, a generalized motor seizure, and acute cardiovascular response. For an optimal therapeutic (antidepressant) response, T.B.'s seizure activity should last from 25 to 50 seconds. General anesthesia is administered to ensure amnesia, prevent bodily injury from the seizure, and control the hemodynamic changes. When selecting an IV induction agent, its effect on electroencephalographic seizure activity, its ability to blunt the hemodynamic response to ECT, and its recovery profile (e.g., short time to discharge, nonemetogenic) are important considerations. Because most IV induction agents have anticonvulsant properties, small doses must be used to allow adequate seizure duration. Methohexital is considered the gold standard.[26,27] Propofol, in smaller doses, can also be used. Combining a short-acting opioid such as remifentanil with propofol will allow a small dose of propofol to be used and the seizure duration to be prolonged. Although etomidate does not adversely affect the seizure duration, the hemodynamic response to ECT is accentuated because etomidate is cardiovascularly stable and cannot blunt the cardiovascular response to ECT. In addition, it can cause nausea and vomiting, resulting in delayed recovery. Midazolam reduces seizure activity, and ketamine increases the risk of delayed recovery by producing nausea and ataxia.[26,27] Therefore, methohexital, in a dose of 0.75 to 1 mg/kg IV, can be administered because it will not affect the seizure duration or prolong T.B.'s recovery time. Alternatively, a small dose of propofol (0.75 mg/kg) and remifentanil (up to 1 mcg/kg) are also appropriate.

Ketamine Use in Pediatrics

CASE 8-6

QUESTION 1: R.L., a 4-year-old boy, ASA-II, is scheduled for a painful debridement and dressing change that is anticipated to take approximately 15 minutes. He is brought to the procedure room near the OR along with his parents and is in distress over parting from them. He currently has no IV line in place and will not take any oral medication. How could sedation and analgesia be provided to R.L.?

Although ketamine can be given IM, administration by this route is painful and not optimal. However, it might be preferable to starting an IV in R.L. for a short, painful procedure. At a dose of 3 or 4 mg/kg IM, ketamine produces sedation with amnesia and analgesia. Intubation is unnecessary because ketamine causes little or no respiratory depression. However, this dose of ketamine produces a dissociative stare or trance (eyes are open but patient does not respond) and nystagmus generally lasting 30 to 60 minutes. R.L.'s parents should be informed about these potential effects. Ketamine may also be safely used in the emergency department to provide dissociative sedation for short, painful procedures in children (e.g., fracture reduction, laceration repair, abscess drainage). Appropriate guidelines for use of ketamine in this setting should be followed.[28]

VOLATILE INHALATION AGENTS

Currently, four volatile inhalation agents are available for use in the United States: desflurane, sevoflurane, isoflurane, and enflurane, with the latter being rarely used in clinical practice. The volatile inhalation agents are unique in that they can produce all components of the anesthetic state, to varying degrees (e.g., minimal, if any, analgesia). Immobility to surgical stimuli and amnesia are postulated to be the predominant effects produced by these agents. Unlike IV anesthetic agents, these drugs are administered into the lungs via an anesthesia machine, and as a result, it is easy to increase or decrease drug levels in the body. The anesthesia care provider can estimate, with the use of technology, the anesthetic partial pressure at the site of action (brain); this helps the anesthesia care provider maintain an optimal depth of anesthesia.[29]

Although the volatile inhalation agents could, theoretically, be used to produce general anesthesia by themselves, it is much more common to use a combination of drugs intended to take advantage of smaller doses of each drug while avoiding the disadvantages of high doses of individual agents. This practice is referred to as *balanced anesthesia*. For example, midazolam is used routinely to produce sedation, anxiolysis, and amnesia, whereas the administration of an IV anesthetic agent (e.g., propofol), followed by administration of a neuromuscular blocking agent (e.g., succinylcholine), can produce rapid loss of consciousness and muscle relaxation to facilitate endotracheal intubation. Volatile inhalation agents provide maintenance of general anesthesia, along with reflex suppression (e.g., lowering BP and heart rate) and some muscle relaxation. Opioids (e.g., fentanyl) also can induce reflex suppression, thereby lowering total anesthetic requirements. Subsequent doses of a nondepolarizing neuromuscular blocking drug might be necessary to provide adequate relaxation for the surgical procedure.

Uses

The volatile inhalation agents are primarily used in clinical practice to maintain general anesthesia. Sevoflurane also can be used to induce general anesthesia via a face mask because of its low pungency. Desflurane and sevoflurane, because of their low blood solubility, are ideally suited for maintenance of general anesthesia in ambulatory surgery patients and for inpatients when rapid wake-up is desired (e.g., neurosurgery procedures).

Site and Mechanism of Action

The goal of inhalation anesthesia is to develop and maintain a satisfactory (anesthetizing) partial pressure of anesthetic in the brain, which is the site of anesthetic action.[29] Although the mechanism of action of the volatile inhalation agents is not fully understood, these agents are believed to disrupt neuronal transmission in discrete areas throughout the CNS by either blocking excitatory, or enhancing inhibitory, transmission through synapses. Ion channels (especially GABA receptors) are likely targets of volatile inhalation anesthetic agent action.[21]

Anesthesia Machine and Circuit

A basic understanding of the anesthesia machine and circuit is helpful to understanding many of the concepts associated with the administration of volatile inhalation agents. Three parts of the anesthesia machine are critically important for the administration of volatile inhalation anesthetics. The *flowmeters* regulate the amount of nitrous oxide (an anesthetic gas), air, and oxygen delivered to the patient. The *vaporizers* regulate the concentration of volatile inhalation agent administered to the patient, and the *carbon dioxide absorber*, which contains either soda lime or barium hydroxide lime, removes carbon dioxide from exhaled air. The first step in the administration of a volatile inhalation agent to a patient is to begin the flow of background gases. Flow is measured in liters per minute. A mixture of nitrous oxide and oxygen is commonly used. This gas mixture flows to one of the vaporizers, where a portion of it enters the vaporizer and "picks up" the anesthetic vapor of the volatile inhalation agent. The concentration of volatile inhalation agent delivered by the vaporizer is proportional to the amount of gas mixture passing through it, which is regulated by adjusting the vaporizer's concentration dial. The gas and anesthetic vapor mixture exits the vaporizer and continues through the anesthetic circuit, where it is ultimately delivered to the patient via an endotracheal tube or face mask. The exhaled air from the patient, which contains the volatile inhalation agent and carbon dioxide, is returned to the circuit. If a semiclosed-circuit breathing system is being used, rebreathing of the exhaled volatile agent can occur if the fresh gas flow rate is low enough (e.g., ≤2 L/minute).[30]

Potency

Potency of the volatile inhalation agents is compared in terms of minimum alveolar concentration (MAC). MAC is the alveolar concentration of anesthetic at 1 atmosphere that prevents movement in 50% of subjects in response to a painful stimulus (e.g., surgical skin incision).[29] The lower an agent's MAC, the greater is the anesthetic potency. A value of 1.3 MAC is required to produce immobility in 95% of patients, whereas 1.5 MAC is required to block the adrenergic response to noxious stimuli.[29] Furthermore, the inhalation agents are additive in their effects on MAC; the addition of a second agent reduces the required concentration of the first agent. For example, when desflurane, isoflurane, and sevoflurane are administered with 60% to 70% nitrous oxide, their MAC values decrease from 6%, 1.15%, and 1.71% to 2.38%, 0.56%, and 0.66%, respectively.[29] Of the volatile inhalation agents routinely used, isoflurane has the lowest MAC and desflurane the highest (Table 8-4).[29]

Chemical Stability

Desflurane and isoflurane are very stable compounds and are not broken down by the moist soda lime or barium hydroxide lime contained in the carbon dioxide absorber of the anesthesia machine. Sevoflurane degrades in the presence of carbon dioxide absorbent to multiple by-products, with compound A being most important. In rats, compound A has caused nephrotoxicity,[31] but no clinically significant changes in serum creatinine and blood urea nitrogen have been demonstrated in human studies.[32–34] The administration of sevoflurane at low flow rates is one of the major factors that increases compound A concentration. The US Food and Drug Administration (FDA) requires that the sevoflurane package insert contain a warning that sevoflurane exposure should not exceed 2 MAC hours at flow rates of 1 to less than 2 L/minute, and flow rates less than 1 L/minute are not recommended. Nevertheless, even when low fresh gas flows are used for long periods and exposure to compound A is high, the levels of compound A are much less than what is believed to be a toxic level.[35]

If the carbon dioxide absorber (soda lime or barium hydroxide lime) is excessively dry, carbon monoxide can be produced when the volatile inhalation agents pass through the dry absorbent. This situation is most commonly encountered on a Monday morning in an anesthesia machine that has been idle during the weekend and has had a continuous flow of fresh gas through the absorbent. Carbon monoxide production can be prevented by ensuring that the vaporizer is turned off when not in use and at the end of the day.

AMSORB PLUS, an alkali hydroxidefree carbon dioxide absorbent containing calcium hydroxide (vs. sodium, barium, or potassium hydroxide), makes the chemical stability of volatile inhalation agents in the absorbent not a clinical concern. It does not generate compound A when used with sevoflurane or carbon monoxide under any clinical conditions.[36]

Pharmacokinetics

A series of anesthetic partial pressure gradients beginning at the anesthesia machine serve to drive the volatile inhalation agent across barriers to the brain. These gradients are as follows: anesthesia machine > delivered > inspired > alveolar > arterial > brain. The alveolar partial pressure provides an indirect measurement of the anesthetic partial pressure in the brain because the alveolar, arterial, and brain partial pressures rapidly equilibrate.[29]

Factors that influence the uptake and distribution of a volatile inhalation agent include the inspired concentration of the agent, alveolar ventilation, solubility of the agent in the blood (blood–gas partition coefficient), blood flow through the lungs, distribution of blood to individual organs (levels rise most rapidly in highly perfused organs—brain, kidney, heart, liver), solubility of the agent in tissue (tissue–blood partition coefficient), and mass of tissue.[29] If all other factors are equal, agents with low solubilities will equilibrate quickly and, as a result, have a faster wash-in (onset). Solubility is also a factor in the elimination of

TABLE 8-4
Pharmacologic and Pharmacokinetic Properties of the Volatile Inhalation Agents[29]

Property or Effect	Desflurane	Sevoflurane	Isoflurane	Enflurane
MAC in O_2 (adults)	6.0	1.71	1.15	1.7
Blood–gas partition coefficient[a]	0.42	0.69	1.46	1.91
Brain–blood partition coefficient[b]	1.29	1.7	1.6	1.4
Muscle–blood partition coefficient[c]	2.02	3.13	2.9	1.7
Fat–blood partition coefficient[d]	27.2	47.5	45	36
Metabolism	0.02%	3%	0.2%	2%
Molecular weight (g)	168	201	184.5	184.5
Liquid density[e]	1.45	1.505	1.496	1.517

[a] The greater the blood–gas partition coefficient, the greater the blood solubility.
[b] The greater the brain–blood partition coefficient, the greater the brain solubility.
[c] The greater the muscle–blood partition coefficient, the greater the muscle solubility.
[d] The greater the fat–blood partition coefficient, the greater the fat solubility.
[e] Density determined at 25°C for desflurane, isoflurane, and enflurane and at 20°C for sevoflurane.
MAC, minimum alveolar concentration to prevent movement in 50% of subjects.

volatile inhalation agents, in addition to metabolism and extent of tissue equilibration. Low-solubility agents are more rapidly washed out (eliminated) because more of the agent is removed from the blood in one passage through the lungs.[29] As can be seen in Table 8-4, desflurane has the lowest solubility of any of the volatile inhalation agents, with sevoflurane's solubility being lower than isoflurane's for blood. As a result of their low solubility, quicker responses to intraoperative concentration changes are seen with desflurane and sevoflurane as well as a faster emergence and awakening from anesthesia and a more rapid return to normal motor function and judgment when compared with isoflurane.[37–39]

As seen in Table 8-4, the metabolism of the volatile inhalation agents varies (e.g., desflurane is metabolized least). An important point is that metabolism does not alter the rate of induction or maintenance of anesthesia because the amount of anesthetic administered to the patient greatly exceeds its uptake.[29] Metabolism of sevoflurane has resulted in peak inorganic fluoride levels greater than 100 μM.[33] Historically, a fluoride level of 50 μM has been used as a cut-off for potential nephrotoxicity based on reports of methoxyflurane-associated nephrotoxicity at levels greater than 50 μM.[40] Despite this, sevoflurane has not been demonstrated to produce nephrotoxicity. Potential reasons for this include the fact that sevoflurane's low blood gas solubility may limit the degree of its metabolism once the anesthetic is discontinued and that sevoflurane, unlike methoxyflurane, undergoes minimal renal defluorination.[41]

Pharmacologic Properties

All volatile inhalation agents depress ventilation (with an elevation of $PaCO_2$) and dilate constricted bronchial musculature in a dose-dependent manner. As mentioned previously, sevoflurane can be used for mask induction of general anesthesia because it is not as pungent as desflurane, isoflurane, or enflurane. Administration of a pungent agent by mask for induction can cause coughing, breath-holding, laryngospasm, and salivation in the patient. All volatile inhalation agents depress myocardial contractility and decrease arterial BP in a dose-dependent manner. Isoflurane can increase heart rate, so cardiac output is usually maintained. Sevoflurane produces little increase in heart rate, so cardiac output may not be as well maintained as with isoflurane. Although enflurane can increase heart rate, cardiac output is usually decreased. Desflurane can produce sympathetic nervous system activation, resulting in a transient increase in BP and heart rate when concentrations are rapidly increased.[29,40] The sympathetic nervous system activation may be caused by stimulation of medullary centers via receptors in the upper airway and lungs.[42] Enflurane can sensitize the myocardium to the arrhythmogenic effects of epinephrine. The volatile inhalation agents decrease cerebral metabolic rate and produce cerebral vasodilation, resulting in increased cerebral blood flow and volume. Enflurane can cause epileptiform activity that can result in clinical tonic-clonic seizures. All volatile inhalation agents produce muscle relaxation and potentiate the actions of the neuromuscular blocking agents. The volatile inhalation agents relax uterine smooth muscle, which can contribute to perinatal blood loss. All volatile inhalation agents have been implicated as triggers of malignant hyperthermia (MH) and are contraindicated in MH-susceptible patients. Finally, all volatile inhalation agents are associated with postoperative nausea, vomiting, and shivering.[29,40]

Drug Interactions

Opioids, benzodiazepines, α_2-adrenergic agonists, and neuromuscular blocking agents potentiate the effects of the volatile inhalation agents. Thus, their administration permits use of lower dosages of the volatile inhalation agents, thereby reducing their potential for adverse effects.

Economic Considerations

The following items must be considered when examining the costs associated with the administration of volatile inhalation agents from an institutional perspective: cost of the volatile inhalation agent (including waste), cost of the equipment necessary to administer the volatile inhalation agent, cost of adjuvants used to treat adverse effects of the volatile agent, and time spent in the OR and PACU.

The cost of a volatile agent depends on (a) the cost per milliliter of the liquid anesthetic, (b) the amount of vapor generated per milliliter, (c) the amount of volatile agent that must be delivered from the anesthesia machine to sustain the desired alveolar concentration, and (d) the flow rate of the background gases.[43–45] The use of low flow rates can result in substantial reductions in the volatile anesthetic drug cost per case. An important point to keep in mind when comparing only the cost of the volatile inhalation agents themselves (e.g., excluding any benefits in terms of cost reduction that may be realized by a quicker discharge from the recovery room) is that the low-solubility volatile agents have to be administered at low flow rates to prevent their cost from being substantially higher than that of the more traditional agents (e.g., isoflurane) when administered at rates of 2 to 3 L/minute.

The cost of purchasing new vaporizers and upgrading or replacing agent analyzers that are used to administer and monitor volatile inhalation agents, respectively, can be significant. These costs become a concern when a new product is introduced onto the market.

Medications used to treat adverse effects associated with the volatile inhalation agents include β-blockers, opioids, benzodiazepines, vasopressors, and antiemetic agents. Antiemetic agents are routinely used to prevent or treat the PONV seen with the volatile inhalation agents. Intraoperative use of volatile inhalation agents is a leading cause of early (within the first 2 hours after surgery) postoperative vomiting.[46] Although the administration of an antiemetic agent adds to the cost, it is significantly less than the cost of an unanticipated admission to the hospital secondary to PONV.

Desflurane Use for Maintenance of General Anesthesia

SYMPATHETIC NERVOUS SYSTEM ACTIVATION

CASE 8-7

QUESTION 1: C.K., a 26-year-old man, ASA-I, is scheduled to undergo a laparoscopic hernia repair on an outpatient basis. During his preoperative evaluation on the morning of surgery, his BP was 115/75 mm Hg, and his heart rate was 70 beats/minute. The surgery is expected to last less than 2 hours, so a propofol induction is planned followed by maintenance of general anesthesia with desflurane without nitrous oxide. After induction of anesthesia, the desflurane concentration on the vaporizer was rapidly increased to 8%. Within 1 minute of the concentration increase, C.K.'s BP increased to 148/110 mm Hg, and his heart rate increased to 112 beats/minute. What could be causing C.K.'s increased BP and heart rate, and how could it have been prevented?

Desflurane can produce sympathetic nervous system activation with a resultant increase in BP and heart rate under certain circumstances. One of these is the rapid increase of desflurane concentration to 1.1 MAC as seen with C.K.[47] This hemodynamic response can be attenuated by the IV administration of fentanyl approximately 5 minutes before the increase in desflurane concentration.[48] Fentanyl is a good choice because it effectively blunts the increase in heart rate and BP, while having minimal cardiovascular depressant and postoperative sedative effects. Alternatively, nitrous oxide can be administered with desflurane, thereby allowing the desflurane concentration to be maintained at less than 1 MAC (6%).

Emergence Agitation in Children

CASE 8-8

QUESTION 1: P.F., a 3-year-old child, ASA-I, is undergoing a tonsillectomy. General anesthesia will be induced and maintained with sevoflurane and nitrous oxide. His surgery was uneventful, with a duration of 30 minutes. He was awakened from anesthesia and transferred to the PACU to recover. Shortly after he arrived, P.F. became extremely restless and began crying. The nurse and his mother were unable to console him. Could this reaction be attributed to sevoflurane, and if so, can it be prevented?

Emergence agitation after the administration of the short-acting inhaled anesthetics, desflurane and sevoflurane, is fairly common, with a reported incidence as high as 80%.[49] Emergence agitation is more common in young children, and its cause is not clear. Children become restless, cry, and exhibit involuntary physical activity that can result in self-injury. Caring for a child experiencing emergence agitation is difficult and very upsetting to the caregiver and the parents of the child. Premedication with oral midazolam[50] and administering analgesics to minimize postoperative pain[51] may reduce the incidence. A small dose of dexmedetomidine (0.3 mcg/kg IV), an α_2-agonist with sedative and analgesic properties, after induction of anesthesia reduces the incidence of emergence agitation without prolonging recovery in children undergoing sevoflurane anesthesia.[52] Although desflurane cannot be used to induce general anesthesia, switching to desflurane for maintenance of anesthesia after sevoflurane induction has been reported to reduce the severity of emergence agitation when it occurs.[53]

NEUROMUSCULAR BLOCKING AGENTS

Uses

Neuromuscular blocking agents are one of the most commonly used classes of drugs in the OR. They are used primarily as an adjunct to general anesthesia to facilitate endotracheal intubation and to relax skeletal muscle during surgery under general anesthesia.[54] Skeletal muscle relaxation optimizes the surgical field for the surgeon and prevents patient movement as a reflex response to surgical stimulation. Neuromuscular blocking agents are also used in the intensive care unit (ICU) to paralyze mechanically ventilated patients.[55] An important point to remember is that neuromuscular blocking agents have no known effect on consciousness or pain threshold. Consequently, adequate sedation (or anesthesia) and analgesia must be ensured when neuromuscular blocking agents are administered.

Mechanism of Action

When two molecules of acetylcholine (Ach) bind to the Ach subunits of the nicotinic cholinergic receptors located on the motor nerve endplate, the Ach receptor undergoes a conformational change that allows the influx of sodium and potassium into the muscle cell, the membrane depolarizes, and the muscle contracts. Neuromuscular blocking agents bind to these subunits and effectively block normal neuromuscular transmission. Two classes of neuromuscular blocking agents exist based on their mechanism of action: depolarizing and nondepolarizing. Succinylcholine, the only depolarizing neuromuscular blocking agent in clinical use today, acts like Ach to depolarize the membrane. Because succinylcholine is not metabolized as quickly as Ach at the neuromuscular junction, its action at the nicotinic receptor persists longer than Ach. Succinylcholine causes a persistent depolarization of the motor endplate because the sodium channels cannot reopen until the motor endplate repolarizes, producing a sustained skeletal muscle paralysis. The paralysis produced by depolarizing agents is preceded initially by fasciculations (transient twitching of skeletal muscle). The nondepolarizing neuromuscular blocking agents act as competitive antagonists to Ach at the Ach subunits of the nicotinic cholinergic receptors, thereby preventing Ach from binding and causing depolarization of the muscle membrane and muscle contraction.[54,56]

Monitoring Neuromuscular Blockade

In addition to clinical assessment (e.g., lack of movement) by the anesthesia provider and the surgeon, the degree of neuromuscular blockade produced by neuromuscular blocking agents is monitored by nerve stimulation with a peripheral nerve stimulator. Most commonly, the ulnar nerve is electrically stimulated, and the response of the innervated muscle, the adductor pollicis in the thumb, is visually assessed. Adequate neuromuscular blockade is present when the train-of-four (four electrical stimulations of 2 Hz delivered every 0.5 seconds) count is 1/4 or 2/4 (one or two visible muscle twitches of a possible four twitches).[55]

Classification

Neuromuscular blocking agents are commonly classified by the type of blockade produced (depolarizing vs. nondepolarizing), chemical structure (steroidal compound, Ach-like, benzylisoquinolinium compound), or duration of action (ultrashort, intermediate, long), as listed in Table 8-5.[57]

Adverse Effects

The underlying mechanisms for the cardiovascular adverse effects of neuromuscular blocking agents are listed in Table 8-6 and include blockade of autonomic ganglia (hypotension), blockade of muscarinic receptors (tachycardia), and release of histamine from circulating mast cells (hypotension).[56–58] In general, the steroidal compounds exhibit varying degrees of vagolytic effect, whereas the benzylisoquinolinium compounds are associated with varying degrees of histamine release. Although not reported as a problem when used short term in the OR, the use of neuromuscular blocking agents in ICU patients for extended periods can result in prolonged neuromuscular blockade or acute quadriplegic myopathy syndrome, albeit infrequently.[56] Of the currently available neuromuscular blocking agents, cisatracurium and vecuronium are devoid of clinically significant cardiovascular effects and are the agents of choice for patients with unstable cardiovascular profiles.[54,56,57] Succinylcholine is associated with a significant number of adverse effects, including

TABLE 8-5
Classification of Neuromuscular Blocking Agents[57]

Agent	Type of Block	Clinical Duration of Action[a]	Structure
Atracurium (Tracrium)	–	Intermediate	Benzylisoquinolinium
Cisatracurium (Nimbex)	–	Intermediate	Benzylisoquinolinium
Pancuronium (Pavulon)	–	Long	Steroidal
Rocuronium (Zemuron)	–	Intermediate	Steroidal
Succinylcholine (Anectine, Quelicin)	+	Ultrashort	Acetylcholine like
Vecuronium (Norcuron)	–	Intermediate	Steroidal

[a] Time from injection of agent to return to twitch height to 25% of control (time at which another dose of agent will need to be administered to maintain paralysis); in general, clinical duration of a standard intubating dose of ultrashort agents ranges from 3 to 5 minutes, intermediate agents from 30 to 40 minutes, and long agents from 60 to 120 minutes.
+, depolarizing; –, nondepolarizing.

hyperkalemia, arrhythmias, fasciculations, muscle pain, myoglobinuria, trismus, phase II block, and increased intraocular, intragastric, and intracranial pressures.[57,58] Succinylcholine, like inhalational anesthetics, can trigger MH.[56] Of these adverse effects, bradycardia, hyperkalemia (which can trigger arrhythmias and cardiac arrest in patients at risk), and MH crisis are severe and potentially life-threatening reactions. Nevertheless, succinylcholine is still used today because of its rapid onset and ultrashort duration of action as well as its ability to be administered IM in children in an emergent situation when IV access has not been established.

Drug Interactions

Several drugs interact with neuromuscular blocking agents. The volatile inhalation agents potentiate the neuromuscular blockade produced by nondepolarizing agents, thereby allowing a lower dose of the latter to be used when administered concomitantly. Other agents reported to potentiate the effects of neuromuscular blocking agents include the aminoglycosides, clindamycin, magnesium sulfate, quinidine, furosemide, lidocaine, amphotericin B, and dantrolene. Carbamazepine, phenytoin, corticosteroids (chronic administration), and theophylline antagonize the effects of neuromuscular blocking agents.[56,57] By appropriately monitoring the patient and dosing the neuromuscular blocking agent to effect, significant problems from drug interactions can be minimized.

Reversal of Neuromuscular Blockade

The action of neuromuscular blocking agents ceases spontaneously as plasma concentrations decline or when anticholinesterases (e.g., neostigmine, edrophonium, pyridostigmine) are administered. Anticholinesterases inhibit the enzyme acetylcholinesterase, which degrades Ach, and are used to reverse paralysis produced by nondepolarizing agents. Anticholinergic agents are coadministered (in the same syringe) with the anticholinesterases to minimize other cholinergic effects (e.g., bradycardia, bronchoconstriction, salivation, increased peristalsis, nausea, vomiting) caused by the increase in Ach concentration. Atropine is routinely administered with edrophonium, and glycopyrrolate with neostigmine or pyridostigmine, to take advantage of similar onset times and durations of action.[54,55,57] Reversal of neuromuscular blockade, as a general rule, is not attempted until spontaneous recovery is well established. Before extubation, adequacy of reversal is assessed with the use of a peripheral nerve stimulator and by clinical assessment of the patient (e.g., ability to sustain head lift for 5 seconds).[57,58]

Pharmacokinetics and Pharmacodynamics

RAPID SEQUENCE INDUCTION

CASE 8-9

QUESTION 1: R.D., a 36-year-old man, ASA-I, is admitted through the emergency department for an emergency appendectomy. R.D. is otherwise healthy, has no drug allergies, and is currently taking no medications. All laboratory values are normal. Admission notes reveal that R.D. ate dinner approximately 2 hours earlier. Because of this, the anesthesia provider plans to perform a rapid sequence induction using the Sellick maneuver. Which neuromuscular blocking agent would be most appropriate for R.D.?

Rapid sequence induction is indicated for patients at risk for aspiration of gastric contents should regurgitation occur. Patients who have recently eaten (with a full stomach), morbidly obese

TABLE 8-6
Causes of Cardiovascular Adverse Effects of Neuromuscular Blocking Agents[56–58]

Agent	Histamine Release[a]	Autonomic Ganglia	Vagolytic Activity	Sympathetic Stimulation
Atracurium[a]	++	–	–	–
Cisatracurium	–	–	–	–
Pancuronium	–	Weak block	++	++
Rocuronium[b]	–	–	+	–
Succinylcholine	+	Stimulates	–	–
Vecuronium	–	–	–	–

[a] Histamine release is dose and rate related; cardiovascular changes can be lessened by minimizing dose and injecting agent slowly.
[b] Produces an increase in heart rate of approximately 18% with intubating dose of 0.6 mg/kg; effect usually transient and resolves spontaneously.
+ – ++, likelihood of developing the cardiovascular adverse effect relative to the other agents; –, no effect.

TABLE 8-7

Pharmacokinetic and Pharmacodynamic Parameters of Action of Neuromuscular Blocking Agents[55–58]

Agent	Cl (mL/kg/min)	Vd_{ss} (L/kg)	Half-Life (minutes)	ED_{95} (mg/kg)	Intubating Dose (mg/kg)[a,b]	Onset (minutes)[c]	Clinical Duration of Action of Initial Dose (minutes)
Atracurium[d]	5–7	0.2	20	0.2–0.25	0.4–0.5	2–3	25–30
Cisatracurium	4.6	0.15	22	0.05	0.15–0.2	2–2.5	50–60
Pancuronium	1–2	0.3	80–120	0.07	0.04–0.1	3–5	80–100
Rocuronium[d]	4.0	0.3	60–70	0.3	0.6–1.2	1–1.5	30–60
Succinylcholine[d]	37	0.04	0.65	0.25	1.5	1	5–10
Vecuronium[d]	4.5	0.4	50–70	0.05–0.06	0.1	2–3	25–30

[a] Dose when nitrous oxide–opioid technique is used.
[b] Intermittent maintenance doses to maintain paralysis, as a general rule, will be approximately 20% to 25% of the initial dose.
[c] Time to intubation.
[d] Also can be administered as a continuous infusion to maintain paralysis. Suggested infusion ranges under balanced anesthesia are atracurium, 4–12 mcg/kg/min; cisatracurium, 1–2 mcg/kg/min; rocuronium, 6–14 mcg/kg/min; succinylcholine, 50–100 mcg/kg/min; vecuronium, 0.8–2 mcg/kg/min.
Cl, clearance; ED_{95}, effective dose causing 95% muscle paralysis; Vd_{ss}, steady-state volume of distribution.

patients, or patients with a history of gastroesophageal reflux are at risk for aspiration, as is the case for R.D. The goal of rapid sequence induction is to minimize the time during which the airway is unprotected by intubating the patient as fast as possible (e.g., within 60 seconds). In this technique, the patient is preoxygenated, after which an IV induction agent is administered, followed immediately by a neuromuscular blocking agent. Manual ventilation of the patient is not attempted after administration of these agents. Apnea occurs as the neuromuscular blocking agent takes effect; therefore, a neuromuscular blocking agent with as rapid an onset as possible is required to produce adequate intubating conditions as quickly as possible. The Sellick maneuver is often used during rapid sequence induction. It is performed by placing downward pressure on the cricoid cartilage, which compresses and occludes the esophagus and helps prevent passive regurgitation of gastric contents into the trachea. Intubation is then performed within 60 seconds.

Table 8-7 lists the onset times of normal intubating doses and other information pertaining to the use of neuromuscular blocking agents.[55–58] Succinylcholine has the fastest onset time, which makes it an appropriate agent to use in rapid sequence induction.[59]

Because R.D. is an otherwise healthy man with no contraindications to the use of succinylcholine, this agent should be used.

DEPOLARIZING AGENT CONTRAINDICATIONS

CASE 8-9, QUESTION 2: What would be the most appropriate choice of a neuromuscular blocking agent if R.D. presents with a history of susceptibility to MH, and why?

Succinylcholine is contraindicated in patients with skeletal muscle myopathies; after the acute phase of injury (i.e., 5–70 days after injury) after major burns, multiple trauma, extensive denervation of skeletal muscle, or upper motor neuron injury; in children and adolescents (except when used for emergency tracheal intubation or when the immediate securing of the airway is necessary); and in patients with a hypersensitivity to the drug.[54,57] Succinylcholine can also trigger MH and is absolutely contraindicated in MH-susceptible patients.[60]

The nondepolarizing neuromuscular blocking agents are safe to use in MH-susceptible patients.[61] Rocuronium has the fastest onset time of the nondepolarizing agents, although it is slightly slower than succinylcholine.[58] The onsets of the remaining intermediate- and long-duration agents can be shortened by increasing the dose, which not only results in a faster onset of action but also prolongs the duration of action. Rocuronium's time to maximal blockade, for example, can be reduced to 60 seconds with an initial dose of 1.2 mg/kg (vs. a normal initial dose of 0.6 mg/kg). Increasing the dose from 0.6 mg/kg to 1.2 mg/kg, however, will prolong the clinical duration from approximately 30 minutes to at least 60 minutes.[62] Rocuronium, with its rapid onset of action, would be a suitable alternative to succinylcholine in R.D.'s case. Its longer clinical duration of action could be a concern if the airway cannot be secured immediately or if the procedure is shorter than the duration of an intubating dose of rocuronium. Because this procedure will last longer than the duration of muscle relaxation provided by the intubating dose of rocuronium, this is not a concern.

Routes of Elimination

CASE 8-10

QUESTION 1: M.M., a 70-year-old woman, ASA-IV, is scheduled to undergo a 2-hour GI procedure. Pertinent laboratory findings are as follows:

Aspartate aminotransferase, 272 units/L
Alanine aminotransferase, 150 units/L
Blood urea nitrogen, 40 mg/dL
Serum creatinine, 1.8 mg/dL
Albumin, 2.6 g/dL

Which neuromuscular blocking agent would you recommend for M.M.?

When selecting a neuromuscular blocking agent, one of the factors that must be considered is the patient's renal and hepatic function. Neuromuscular blocking agents often depend on the kidneys and liver for varying amounts of their metabolism and excretion (Table 8-8).[54,55,58] Some agents, however, are primarily metabolized by plasma cholinesterase (pseudocholinesterase), Hofmann elimination (a nonbiological process that does not require renal, hepatic, or enzymatic function), or nonspecific esterases.

Hofmann elimination is a pH- and temperature-dependent process unique to atracurium and cisatracurium. One of the products produced by Hofmann elimination is laudanosine, a CNS stimulant in high concentrations. Laudanosine undergoes renal and hepatic elimination. Because of the short-term use of atracurium and cisatracurium in the OR, accumulation of laudanosine with resultant seizure activity is not a concern, even in patients with end-stage renal failure.[63] Because plasma cholinesterase levels may be decreased in patients with

TABLE 8-8
Elimination of Neuromuscular Blocking Agents[54,55,58]

Agent	Renal	Hepatic	Biliary	Plasma
Atracurium	10%		NS	Hofmann elimination, ester hydrolysis
Cisatracurium	NS		NS	Hofmann elimination
Pancuronium	80%	10%	5%–10%	
Rocuronium	10%–25%	10%–20%	50%–70%	
Succinylcholine				Plasma cholinesterase
Vecuronium	15%–25%	20%–30%	40%–75%	

NS, not significant.

renal or hepatic dysfunction, the duration of action of succinylcholine could be prolonged. The increased duration of action of succinylcholine in patients with low levels of normal plasma cholinesterase is generally not clinically significant. Patients with atypical plasma cholinesterase, however, cannot hydrolyze the ester bonds in succinylcholine. This results in a significantly increased duration of action in these patients.[64]

Unchanged neuromuscular blocking agents and their metabolites are excreted by the renal or biliary routes. The duration of action of the renally eliminated agent, pancuronium, will be increased in patients with renal failure. Vecuronium's duration of action can be increased in patients with liver disease, reflecting impaired metabolism or excretion rather than termination of effect by redistribution.[65] Although the main route of elimination of rocuronium is hepatobiliary, the duration of action of rocuronium can be significantly prolonged in chronic renal failure.[66]

Because M.M. has evidence of both significant renal and hepatic impairment, cisatracurium or atracurium would be appropriate choices for a neuromuscular blocking agent because their properties are not altered significantly by renal and hepatic failure. Furthermore, because these agents have an intermediate duration of action, they can easily be used in a 2-hour procedure. The availability of generic atracurium makes this agent a more economical choice; however, the greater propensity of atracurium to cause histamine release with resultant hypotension makes cisatracurium the most appropriate choice in this 70-year-old, ASA-IV patient.

LOCAL ANESTHETICS

Local and Regional Anesthesia

Some surgical procedures can be performed under regional anesthesia (anesthesia selective for part of the body, such as the area near the surgical site) rather than general anesthesia (total body anesthesia with the patient rendered unconscious). Epidural, spinal (intrathecal), peripheral nerve block, or local infiltration anesthesia can be chosen, depending on the location of the surgical site, extent of the surgery, patient health and physical characteristics, coagulation status, duration of surgery, and the desires and cooperativeness of the patient. For epidural anesthesia, the local anesthetic is administered into the epidural space, which is located between the dura and the ligament covering the spinal vertebral bodies and discs. To provide spinal anesthesia, the local anesthetic is injected into the cerebrospinal fluid within the subarachnoid (intrathecal) space. By injecting a local anesthetic in the tissue near a specific nerve or nerve plexus (peripheral nerve block), certain types of surgery can be performed under regional anesthesia rather than general anesthesia. Examples include carotid endarterectomy (cervical plexus), upper extremity surgery (brachial plexus), and hand surgery (ulnar, median, or radial nerve). Regional anesthesia can be selected to reduce or avoid the likelihood of complications such as postoperative pain, nausea, vomiting, laryngeal irritation, or dental complications, all of which are associated with general anesthesia. Potential advantages of spinal or epidural anesthesia include reduction of the stress response to surgery, improvement in cardiac function in patients with ischemic heart disease, fewer postoperative pulmonary complications, and the ability to continue epidural analgesia into the postoperative period.[67] Potential advantages of peripheral nerve block include continued analgesia into the postoperative period and fewer side effects or technical problems than epidural analgesia.[68] Disadvantages of spinal, epidural, or peripheral nerve block include the additional time and manipulations required to perform it, possible complications or pain from invasive catheter placements or injections, slow onset of effect, possible failure of technique, and potential toxicity from absorption of the drugs administered. Finally, local infiltration anesthesia can be used to provide localized anesthesia to allow a minor procedure (e.g., a deep laceration repair) to be performed or to provide postoperative analgesia at the site of surgical incision.

Uses of Local Anesthetic Agents

Local anesthetics are a mainstay of analgesia because they prevent the initiation or propagation of the electrical impulses required for peripheral and spinal nerve conduction. These agents can be administered by all routes previously discussed, depending on the drug chosen. Table 8-9 lists the common uses of currently available local anesthetics.[69,70] Local anesthetics are often given in combination with other agents, such as sodium bicarbonate (to increase the speed of onset and reduce pain on local infiltration), epinephrine (to prolong the duration of action and to delay vascular absorption of the local anesthetic, thereby minimizing plasma concentration and systemic toxicity), or opioids (to provide analgesia by a different mechanism of action).

TABLE 8-9
Clinical Uses of Local Anesthetic Agents[69,70]

Agent	Primary Clinical Use
Esters	
Chloroprocaine	Epidural
Cocaine	Topical
Tetracaine	Topical
Amides	
Bupivacaine	Local infiltration, nerve block, epidural, spinal
Lidocaine	Local infiltration, nerve block, spinal, epidural, topical, intravenous regional
Mepivacaine	Local infiltration, nerve block, epidural
Ropivacaine	Local infiltration, nerve block, epidural

Mechanism of Action

The two structural classes of local anesthetics are characterized by the linkage between the molecule's lipophilic aromatic group and hydrophilic amine group: amides and esters. Both amide and ester classes provide anesthesia and analgesia by reversibly binding to and blocking the sodium channels in nerve membranes, thereby decreasing the rate of rise of the action potential such that threshold potential is not reached. As a result, propagation of the electrical impulses required for nerve conduction is prevented. The axonal membrane blockade that results is selective depending on the drug, the concentration and volume administered, and the depth of nerve penetration. C fibers (pain transmission and autonomic activity) appear to be the most easily blocked, followed by fibers responsible for touch and pressure sensation (A-α, A-β, and A-δ), and finally, those responsible for motor function (A-α and A-β). At the most commonly used doses and concentrations, some non–pain-transmitting nerve fibers are also blocked. The blockade of sensory, motor, or autonomic (sympathetic, parasympathetic) fibers may result in adverse effects such as paresthesia, numbness and inability to move extremities, hypotension, and urinary retention. Systemic effects (e.g., seizures or cardiac arrhythmias) are related to the inherent cardiac and CNS safety margins of these drugs.[69,70]

Ropivacaine, like bupivacaine, has a long duration of action. Higher plasma concentrations of ropivacaine are required to produce mild CNS toxicity (lightheadedness, tinnitus, numbness of the tongue) in volunteers when compared with bupivacaine. In animal studies, ropivacaine was found to be less cardiotoxic than bupivacaine. As a result, some practitioners believe that ropivacaine is safer than bupivacaine. However, once plasma concentrations reach higher levels, all local anesthetics are capable of producing severe myocardial depression.[71] Prevention of local anesthetic systemic toxicity (LAST) is key, with attention paid to early detection of intravascular needle or catheter placement as well as predictors of local anesthetic plasma levels (e.g., dose, block site, patient factors, etc.) that will be discussed further in the Toxicity section.

Allergic Reaction

Localized skin hypersensitivity reactions (e.g., localized rash, itching, edema, burning) to local anesthetics are the most common types of allergic reactions. Ester-type local anesthetic agents (e.g., chloroprocaine) produce most of the allergic reactions, owing to their metabolite, para-aminobenzoic acid (PABA). True (systemic immunologic) allergy to amide-type local anesthetics is extremely rare. However, allergic reactions may occur to a preservative (methylparaben or other substances that are structurally similar to PABA) in the product. Because amide-type local anesthetics do not undergo metabolism to a PABA metabolite, a patient with a known allergy to an ester-type local anesthetic can safely receive an amide-type agent.[69,70,72] When selecting a product, it is best to administer a preservative free, epinephrine-free preparation to a patient with a known allergy to a local anesthetic.

Toxicity

Factors that influence the toxicity of local anesthetics include the total amount of drug administered, presence or absence of epinephrine, vascularity of the injection site, extremities of age (e.g., <4 months or >70 years of age), and presence of cardiac, renal, or hepatic dysfunction.[71] Systemic absorption of the local anesthetic is positively correlated with the vascularity of the injection site (IV > epidural > brachial plexus > subcutaneous). End-stage pregnancy, extremities of age, significant hepatic or renal dysfunction, and advanced heart failure can result in either higher peak levels or accumulation of local anesthetic with continued or repeated dosing. In general, local anesthetic doses should be reduced in patients with these conditions.[73]

Toxic levels of local anesthetics are most often achieved by unintentional intravascular injection, which results in excessive plasma concentrations. Systemic toxicity of local anesthetics involves the CNS and cardiovascular systems. Patients may initially complain of tinnitus, lightheadedness, metallic taste in the mouth, tingling, numbness, and dizziness. Hypotension may occur. These symptoms can quickly be followed by tremors, seizures, arrhythmias, unconsciousness, and cardiac or respiratory arrest as plasma levels rise.[69,74] If signs and symptoms of LAST occur, treatment includes airway management, benzodiazepines for seizure management, and if a cardiac arrest occurs, standard Advanced Cardiac Life Support should be initiated with minor modifications. Small (10–100 mcg) initial epinephrine doses are preferred, vasopressin is not recommended, calcium-channel blockers and β-blockers should be avoided, and ventricular arrhythmias should be treated with amiodarone. After airway management, 20% lipid emulsion therapy may be considered at the first signs of LAST (initial IV bolus dose of 1.5 mL/kg followed by 0.25 mL/kg/minute for at least 10 minutes after circulatory stability is achieved).[71]

Physicochemical Properties Affecting Action

The potency of a local anesthetic is primarily determined by the degree of lipid solubility. Local anesthetics such as bupivacaine are highly lipid soluble and can be given in concentrations of 0.25% to 0.5%. Less lipid-soluble agents, such as lidocaine, require concentrations of 1% to 2% for many anesthetic techniques.

Amide-type local anesthetics are metabolized primarily by microsomal enzymes in the liver. The cytochrome P-450 enzyme system is involved in the metabolism of lidocaine (CYP3A4) and ropivacaine (CYP3A2, CYP3A4, and CYP1A2). Agents that induce or inhibit these enzymes could affect the metabolism, and therefore the plasma concentration, of these drugs. Ester-type local anesthetics are hydrolyzed by plasma cholinesterase and, to a lesser extent, cholinesterase in the liver.[69,70]

Differences in the clinical activity of local anesthetics are explained by other physicochemical properties such as protein binding and pK_a (the pH at which 50% of the drug is present in the unionized form and 50% in the ionized form). Agents that are highly protein bound typically have a longer duration of action. Agents with a lower pK_a typically have a faster onset of action.[70]

Choice of local anesthetic is based on the duration of the surgical procedure (e.g., the duration of analgesia required). Usually, a local anesthetic that will, at least minimally, outlast the duration of surgery with a single injection is chosen; a continuous infusion can also be administered for titration of effect with shorter-acting agents. Important physicochemical and pharmacokinetic properties of local anesthetics are shown in Table 8-10.[69,70]

Regional Anesthesia in High-Risk Patients

CASE 8-11

QUESTION 1: M.S., a 52-year-old, 5-foot 9-inch, 105-kg black man, is undergoing an emergent minor hand repair procedure after a fall-related injury. His medical history is positive for type 1 diabetes mellitus for 41 years, angina,

TABLE 8-10
Physicochemical and Pharmacokinetic Properties of Local Anesthetic Agents[69,70]

Agent	pK_a	Potency	Toxicity	Onset	Duration[a]	Maximum Recommended Dose[b] Plain (mg)	With Epinephrine (mg)
Esters							
Cocaine[c]	–	–	–	–	–	1.5 mg/kg	–
Chloroprocaine	9.1	Low	Very low	Very fast	Short	800	1,000
Tetracaine	8.4	High	Moderate	Slow	Very long	100 (topical)	200
Amides							
Bupivacaine	8.1	High	High	Slow	Long	175	225
Lidocaine	7.8	Moderate	Moderate	Fast	Moderate	300	500
Mepivacaine	7.7	Moderate	Moderate	Moderate	Moderate	300	500
Ropivacaine	8.1	High	Moderate	Slow	Long	300	–

[a] Depends on factors such as injection site, dose, and addition of epinephrine. In general, a short duration is <1 hour, a moderate duration is 1–3 hours, and a long or very long duration of action is 3–12 hours when the local anesthetic is administered without epinephrine.
[b] Maximum recommended single dose for infiltration or peripheral nerve block in 70-kg adults.
[c] Topical use only; concentrations >4% are not recommended owing to increased risk for systemic adverse effects.

and hypertension. On OR admission, laboratory values of note are plasma glucose, 240 mg/dL, and BP, 145/92 mm Hg. His sister tells the anesthesia provider that he has been having increasing difficulty walking up stairs and, of late, is often short of breath. The anesthesia provider chooses to provide regional anesthesia via an axillary block; the anticipated duration of surgery is 2 hours. M.S. agrees with this plan. Why is this a good plan for M.S., and which local anesthetic should be chosen?

With his medical conditions of diabetes, angina, and hypertension, M.S. is at risk for complications from general anesthesia. General anesthesia is not absolutely necessary in this localized surgery. Regional anesthesia would be beneficial in M.S. because it does not disrupt autonomic function. In addition, his diabetes and obesity, and possibly full stomach (emergency surgery, diabetic gastroparesis), place him at significant risk for aspiration during both induction and emergence from general anesthesia. An axillary block with a local anesthetic could provide M.S. with adequate anesthesia and analgesia during and after his procedure.

The local anesthetic of choice is one with a duration at least that of the anticipated surgery and with a good safety profile should systemic absorption inadvertently occur. A local anesthetic containing epinephrine would increase the agent's duration of action and reduce the systemic absorption; however, such an agent is not indicated in M.S. because of his diabetes (peripheral vascular effects) and hypertension (added effect from catecholamine administration). Lidocaine as a single injection without epinephrine has a duration of action that may be too short for M.S.'s procedure. Mepivacaine, an intermediate-acting local anesthetic, or ropivacaine, a long-acting agent to provide longer-lasting postoperative analgesia, would be appropriate choices to use in M.S.

Alkalinization of Local Anesthetics

CASE 8-12

QUESTION 1: T.F., a 22-year-old man, is scheduled for a hernia repair. He has never undergone surgery and is very anxious. In the preoperative area, the nurse chooses to locally infiltrate 1% lidocaine to reduce the pain and discomfort from IV catheter placement. She injects a small amount of lidocaine under the skin. T.F. flinches and complains of pain from the injection. Can anything be done to reduce the pain from injection of lidocaine?

The onset of action of local anesthetics depends on their pK_a. Drugs with pK_as closest to body pH (7.4) will have the fastest onset because a high percentage of the local anesthetic molecules will be unionized and therefore will be able to cross the nerve membranes to their intracellular site of action. Local anesthetics are formulated in solutions with acidic pH to optimize their shelf-lives. When sodium bicarbonate is added to local anesthetic solutions, the pH is increased, the percentage of unionized drug is increased, and the onset of local anesthetic action can be shortened considerably. The amount of bicarbonate added to the solution depends on the pH of the local anesthetic agent. Because too much sodium bicarbonate will precipitate the local anesthetic, a dose of 0.1 mEq (0.1 mL of a 1-mEq/mL concentration) of sodium bicarbonate is added to 10 mL of bupivacaine, whereas 1 mEq (1 mL of a 1-mEq/mL concentration) is added to 10 mL of lidocaine. More importantly, alkalinized lidocaine can be significantly less painful for subcutaneous injection before IV catheter placement when compared with lidocaine at pH 5 (its pH in the commercially available vial).[75] However, if the lidocaine contains epinephrine, the addition of bicarbonate to the solution will destroy the activity of epinephrine (which is stable only in an acidic pH).

ANTIEMETIC AGENTS AND POSTOPERATIVE NAUSEA AND VOMITING

Impact of Postoperative Nausea and Vomiting

The two most common complications after surgery are postoperative pain and PONV. Patients who experience PONV are greatly dissatisfied with their surgical experience, and require additional resources such as nursing time, and medical and surgical supplies. Furthermore, vomiting can provoke the rupture of surgical sutures and cause wound pain and hematomas, and, if severe, more serious adverse events can occur (e.g., aspiration pneumonitis, increased intraocular pressure leading to loss of vision). PONV typically lasts less than 24 hours; however, symptom distress can continue at home, thereby preventing the patient from resuming normal activities or returning to work. It is important to remember that nausea is a separate subjective sensation and is not always followed by vomiting. Nausea can be more distressing to patients than vomiting.[76]

Mechanisms of and Factors Affecting Postoperative Nausea and Vomiting

The vomiting center is reflex activated through the chemoreceptor trigger zone (CTZ). Input from other sources can also stimulate the vomiting center. Afferent impulses from the periphery (e.g., manipulation of the oropharynx or GI tract), the cerebral cortex (e.g., unpleasant sights or smells, emotions, anxiety, hypotension, pain), and the endocrine environment (e.g., female sex) can also stimulate the vomiting center. In addition, disturbances in vestibular function (e.g., movement after surgery, middle ear surgery) can stimulate the vomiting center via direct central pathways and the CTZ. Neurotransmitter receptors that play an important role in impulse transmission to the vomiting center include dopamine type 2 (D_2), serotonin (5-HT_3), muscarinic cholinergic (M_1), histamine type 1 (H_1), and neurokinin type 1 (NK_1) (Fig. 8-1).[76–80] Opioid analgesics can activate the CTZ, as well as the vestibular apparatus, to produce nausea and vomiting.[76–80]

PONV is probably not caused by a single event, entity, or mechanism; instead, the cause is likely to be multifactorial. Factors that place adults at risk for developing PONV include female sex, history of PONV or motion sickness, nonsmoking status, use of postoperative opioids, duration of anesthesia, and general anesthesia with inhalation anesthetic agents.[81,82] A commonly used tool for determining an adult patient's risk of developing PONV has been developed; one point is assigned to each of the following risk factors: female sex, nonsmoker, history of PONV, and postoperative use of opioids.[83] The level of risk for developing PONV is low (<20%) for patients with zero or one risk factor and increases significantly with the presence of each additional risk factor (2 risk factors, 40%; 3 risk factors, 60%; and 4 risk factors, 80%).[83] For children, risk factors for postoperative vomiting include duration of surgery 30 minutes or longer, age 3 years or older, strabismus surgery, and a history of postoperative vomiting in the child or PONV in the mother, father, or siblings.[84] Similarly to adults, the level of risk for developing postoperative vomiting is low for children with zero or one risk factor and increases significantly with the presence of each additional risk factor (2 risk factors, 30%; 3 risk factors, 55%; and 4 risk factors, 70%).[83] In children, nausea is not easily measured and hence not routinely assessed.

CASE 8-13

QUESTION 1: J.E., a 34-year-old, 55-kg woman, is scheduled to undergo a gynecologic laparoscopy under general inhalation anesthesia on an outpatient basis. She has had one previous surgery, has no known medication allergies, and is a nonsmoker. On questioning, she reports that she experienced PONV after her first surgery. Her physical

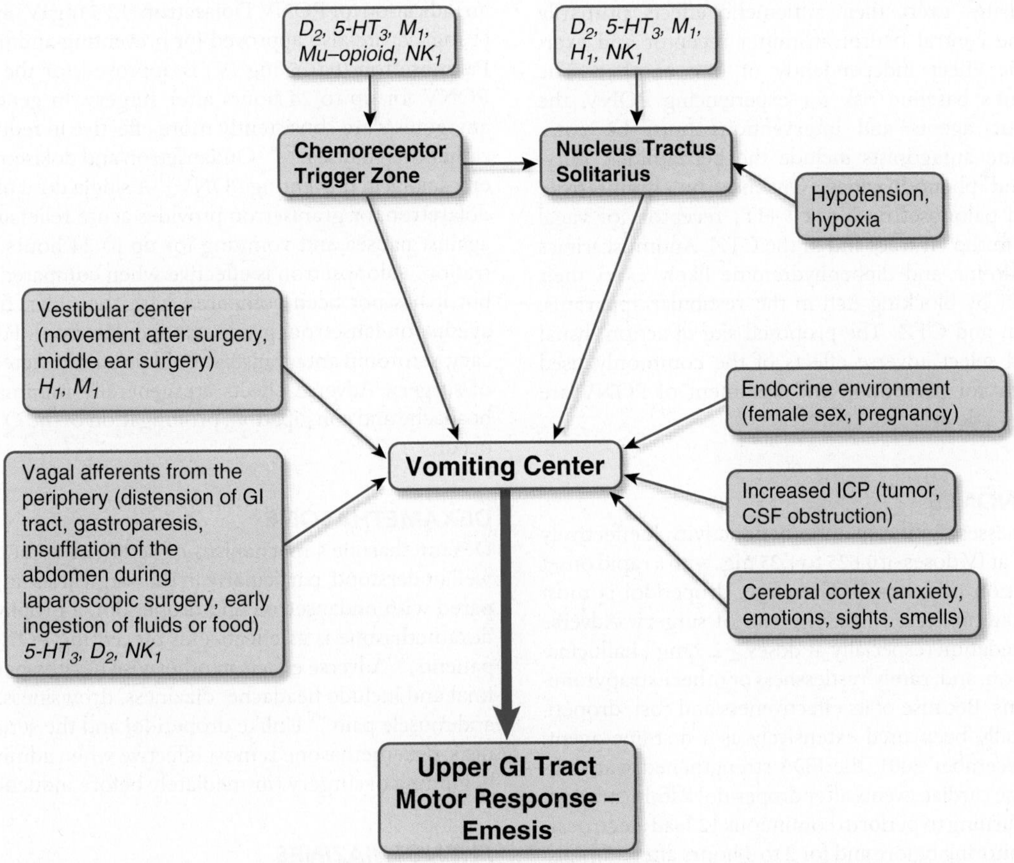

FIGURE 8-1 Mechanisms and neurotransmitters of postoperative nausea and vomiting. The chemoreceptor trigger zone (CTZ) is located in the area postrema of the midbrain. The vomiting center is also located in the midbrain, close to the nucleus tractus solitarius (NTS) and the area postrema. The CTZ, NTS, and area postrema are rich in 5-HT_3, H_1, M_1, D_2, and mu-opioid receptors. Antiemetic agents used to manage postoperative nausea and vomiting block one or more of these receptors. 5-HT_3, serotonin type 3 receptor; CSF, cerebral spinal fluid; D_2, dopamine type 2 receptor; GI, gastrointestinal; H_1, histamine type 1 receptor; ICP, intracranial pressure; M_1, muscarinic cholinergic type 1 receptor; NK_1, substance P neurokinin type 1 receptor.

examination is unremarkable. Is J.E. a candidate for prophylactic antiemetic therapy?

J.E. has several risk factors that make her susceptible to experiencing PONV. Adult women are two to three times more likely than adult men to develop PONV. Previous PONV also increases the likelihood of developing PONV threefold. In addition, a non-smoking status increases the risk of developing PONV. Using the simplified risk score for PONV, J.E. has four risk factors, anticipating that she will require postoperative opioids for pain management. In addition, the type of procedure J.E. is undergoing (gynecologic laparoscopy) may further increase her risk for developing PONV. Because of the presence of four risk factors, J.E. is at very high risk and should be administered at least two prophylactic antiemetic agents.

Prevention of Postoperative Nausea and Vomiting: Choice of Agent

CASE 8-13, QUESTION 2: Which antiemetic drugs would be most appropriate for J.E., and when should they be administered?

Antiemetic drugs can be classified as antimuscarinics (scopolamine, promethazine, diphenhydramine), serotonin antagonists (ondansetron, dolasetron, granisetron, palonosetron), benzamides (metoclopramide), butyrophenones (droperidol), phenothiazines (prochlorperazine), and NK_1 antagonists (aprepitant). These drugs exert their antiemetic effects primarily by blocking one central neurotransmitter receptor and exert their antiemetic effect independently of one another. The higher a patient's baseline risk for experiencing PONV, the more antiemetic agents and interventions must be combined. Dopamine antagonists include the benzamides, butyrophenones, and phenothiazines. Ondansetron, granisetron, dolasetron, and palonosetron block 5-HT_3 receptors of vagal afferent nerves in the GI tract and in the CTZ. Antimuscarinics such as scopolamine and diphenhydramine likely exert their antiemetic effect by blocking Ach in the vestibular apparatus, vomiting center, and CTZ. The proposed site of action, usual adult dose, and select adverse effects of the commonly used antiemetic drugs for prevention and treatment of PONV are summarized in Table 8-11.[3,76,78,81,82,85]

BUTYROPHENONES

Droperidol possesses significant antiemetic activity. It effectively prevents PONV at IV doses of 0.625 to 1.25 mg, with a rapid onset and short duration of action.[86] Therefore, droperidol is most effective when administered near the end of surgery. Adverse effects include sedation (especially at doses ≥2.5 mg), hallucinations, hypotension, and, rarely, restlessness or other extrapyramidal (EP) reactions· Because of its effectiveness and cost, droperidol has historically been used extensively as a first-line agent. However, in December 2001, the FDA strengthened warnings regarding adverse cardiac events after droperidol administration. With the new warning to perform continuous 12-lead electrocardiographic monitoring before and for 2 to 3 hours after administration of droperidol, it became an issue, from both expense and logistical viewpoints, to administer droperidol to an outpatient, a patient in the PACU (recovery room), or a patient in an unmonitored bed. Because low-dose droperidol has been used for more than 30 years to prevent PONV, several studies were undertaken to examine the effect of low-dose droperidol on the QT_C interval. When compared with placebo (saline), low-dose droperidol did not produce QT_C prolongation after surgery.[87] When compared with ondansetron, droperidol produced similar QT_C prolongation, and it was concluded that serotonin antagonists may not be safer than low-dose droperiol.[88] Finally, Nuttall et al.[89] retrospectively examined whether low-dose droperidol administration increased the incidence of torsades de pointes in patients undergoing general surgery. Of the 16,791 patients exposed to droperidol, no patient experienced torsades de pointes. These authors concluded that the FDA's black-box warning for low-dose droperidol is excessive and unnecessary.

BENZAMIDES

Metoclopramide, in doses of 10 to 20 mg, has been used in the prevention and treatment of PONV. However, variable results have been seen with this agent at these doses.[90] For maximal benefit, metoclopramide should be administered in a dose of 25 mg IV near the end of surgery (secondary to its rapid redistribution after IV administration); 10 mg IV administered at the beginning of surgery is not effective.[91] Adverse effects of metoclopramide include drowsiness and EP reactions, such as anxiety and restlessness. Metoclopramide should be administered by slow IV injection for at least 2 minutes to minimize the risk of EP reactions and cardiovascular effects such as hypotension, bradycardia, and supraventricular tachycardia.

SEROTONIN ANTAGONISTS

Ondansetron (4 mg IV) was the first 5-HT_3 antagonist to receive an indication for PONV. Dolasetron (12.5 mg IV) and granisetron (1 mg IV) are also approved for preventing and treating PONV. Palonosetron (0.075 mg IV) is approved for the prevention of PONV for up to 24 hours after surgery. In general, serotonin antagonists are consistently more effective in reducing vomiting rather than nausea.[82,92] Ondansetron and dolasetron are equally efficacious in preventing PONV.[93] A single dose of ondansetron, dolasetron, or granisetron provides acute relief and can protect against nausea and vomiting for up to 24 hours after administration. Palonosetron is effective when compared with placebo, but it has not been compared with the older, first-generation agents (ondansetron, granisetron, dolasetron). For optimal efficacy, serotonin antagonists should be administered near the end of surgery. Adverse effects are generally minimal and include headache and constipation; prolongation of the QT_C interval can occur.

DEXAMETHASONE

Dexamethasone's mechanism of action as an antiemetic is not well understood, particularly in the surgical setting. When compared with ondansetron and droperidol, a prophylactic dose of dexamethasone is as effective in preventing PONV in high-risk patients.[94] Adverse effects in otherwise healthy patients are minimal and include headache, dizziness, drowsiness, constipation, and muscle pain.[95] Unlike droperidol and the serotonin antagonists, dexamethasone is most effective when administered at the beginning of surgery (immediately before induction).[96]

PHENOTHIAZINES

Prochlorperazine has been used successfully to prevent PONV. Prochlorperazine (10 mg IM) was found to have superior efficacy (less nausea and vomiting, as well as less need for rescue antiemetics) when compared with ondansetron for preventing PONV.[97] Prochlorperazine may cause sedation, EP reactions, and

TABLE 8-11

Classification, Proposed Site(s) of Action, Usual Dose, and Adverse Effects of Select Antiemetic Drugs[3,76,78,81,82,85]

Antiemetic Drug	Proposed Receptor Site of Action	Usual Dose[a]	Duration of Action	Adverse Effects	Comments
Butyrophenones					
Droperidol	D_2	*Adult:* 0.625–1.25 mg IV *Pediatric:* 20–50 mcg/kg IV for prevention; 10–20 mcg/kg IV for treatment	≤12–24 hours	Sedation, restlessness or agitation, hallucinations, hypotension (especially in hypovolemic patients), EPS	Monitor ECG for QT prolongation, torsades de pointes
Phenothiazines					
Prochlorperazine	D_2	*Adult:* 5–10 mg IM or IV; 25 mg PR *Pediatric:*[b] 0.1–0.15 mg/kg IM, 0.1–0.13 mg/kg PO, 2.5 mg PR	4–6 hours (12 hours when given PR)	Sedation, hypotension (especially in hypovolemic patients), EPS	
Antimuscarinics					
Promethazine	D_2, H_1, M_1	*Adult:* 6.25–25 mg IM, IV, or PR[c]	4–6 hours	Sedation, hypotension (especially in hypovolemic patients), EPS, serious tissue injury from inadvertent arterial injection or IV extravasation	Limit concentration to 25 mg/mL; dilute in 10–20 mL of saline, inject through a running line, and advise patient to report IV site discomfort
Diphenhydramine	H_1, M_1	*Adult:* 12.5–25 mg IM or IV *Pediatric:* 1 mg/kg IV, PO (max: 25 mg for children younger than 12 years)	4–6 hours	Sedation, dry mouth, blurred vision, urinary retention	
Scopolamine	M_1	*Adult:* 1.5 mg transdermal patch	72 hours[d]	Sedation, dry mouth, visual disturbances, dysphoria, confusion, disorientation, hallucinations	Apply at least 4 hours before end of surgery; wash hands after handling patch; not appropriate for children, elderly, or patients with renal or hepatic impairment
Benzamides					
Metoclopramide	D_2	*Adult:* 25 mg IV *Pediatric:* 0.25 mg/kg IV	≤6 hours	Sedation, hypotension, EPS	Consider for rescue if N/V is believed to be caused by gastric stasis; reduce dose to 5 mg in renal impairment; give slow IV push
Serotonin Antagonists					
Ondansetron	5-HT_3	*Adult:* 4 mg IV *Pediatric:* 0.05–0.1 mg/kg IV	Up to 24 hours	Headache, lightheadedness, constipation, QT prolongation	
Dolasetron	5-HT_3	*Adult:* 12.5 mg IV *Pediatric:* 0.35 mg/kg IV	Up to 24 hours	Headache, lightheadedness, constipation, QT prolongation	
Granisetron	5-HT_3	*Adult:* 0.35 mg–1 mg IV *Pediatric:* Not known	Up to 24 hours	Headache, lightheadedness, constipation, QT prolongation	
Palonosetron		*Adult:* 0.075 mg IV	Up to 24 hours	Headache, constipation, QT prolongation	
NK_1 Antagonists					
Aprepitant	NK_1	*Adult:* 40 mg PO up to 3 hours before surgery	Up to 24 hours	Headache	
Other					
Dexamethasone	Unknown	*Adult:* 4 mg IV *Pediatric:* 0.15 mg/kg IV	Up to 24 hours	Genital itching, flushing	

[a]Unless otherwise indicated, pediatric doses should not exceed adult doses.

[b]Children >10 kg or older than 2 years only. Change from IM to PO as soon as possible. When administering PR, the dosing interval varies from 8 to 24 hours, depending on the child's weight.

[c]Maximum of 12.5 mg in children younger than 12 years.

[d]Remove after 24 hours. Instruct patient to thoroughly wash the patch site and their hands.

D_2, dopamine type 2 receptor; ECG, electrocardiogram; EPS, extrapyramidal symptoms (e.g., motor restlessness or acute dystonia); 5-HT_3, serotonin type 3 receptor; H_1, histamine type 1 receptor; IV, intravenous; IM, intramuscular; M_1, muscarinic cholinergic type 1; NK_1, neurokinin type 1 receptor; N/V, nausea or vomiting; PO, orally (by mouth); PR, per rectum.

cardiovascular effects. Because it has a short duration of action, multiple doses may be necessary.

ANTIMUSCARINICS

Scopolamine blocks afferent impulses at the vomiting center and blocks Ach in the vestibular apparatus and CTZ. Transdermal scopolamine is useful for prevention of nausea, vomiting, and motion sickness. Compared with placebo, transdermal scopolamine effectively reduces the incidence of emetic symptoms.[98] Common side effects include dry mouth and visual disturbances. Patients can also have trouble correctly applying the patch. It is important to apply the patch before surgery because its onset of effect is 4 hours. Patients should also be instructed to wash their hands after applying the patch and to dispose of the patch properly.

NEUROKININ-1 ANTAGONISTS

Aprepitant is the first NK_1 antagonist to be approved for prevention of PONV. Aprepitant has a long half-life and is administered orally before surgery. For prevention of PONV in patients undergoing abdominal surgery, aprepitant was similar in efficacy (defined as no vomiting and no use of rescue antiemetics in the first 24 hours after surgery) to ondansetron. Aprepitant, however, was significantly more effective than ondansetron in preventing vomiting at 24 and 48 hours after surgery. Aprepitant was well tolerated, with adverse effects similar to ondansetron.[99]

COMBINATION OF AGENTS

As discussed, droperidol, serotonin antagonists, dexamethasone, and transdermal scopolamine effectively prevent PONV. However, these agents fail to prevent PONV in approximately 20% to 30% of patients. Most of the agents effectively block one receptor believed to be involved in the activation of the vomiting center. However, because the cause of PONV is likely multifactorial, a combination of antiemetic agents (from different classes) is more efficacious for preventing PONV in a high-risk patient. In a factorial trial of six interventions for prevention of PONV in more than 5,000 high-risk patients undergoing surgery, patients were randomly assigned to 1 of 64 possible combinations of six different prophylactic interventions: 4 mg IV ondansetron or no ondansetron; 4 mg IV dexamethasone or no dexamethasone; 1.25 mg IV droperidol or no droperidol; propofol or a volatile inhalation anesthetic agent; nitrous oxide or nitrogen (i.e., no nitrous oxide); and remifentanil (an ultrashort-acting opioid) or fentanyl (a short-acting opioid).[94] Each antiemetic agent intervention (ondansetron, dexamethasone, droperidol) had similar efficacy and reduced the risk of PONV by about 26%. The risk was further reduced when a combination of any two antiemetics was administered, with no difference among the various combinations of agents. The risk was the lowest when all three antiemetic agents were administered.

For prophylaxis of PONV, J.E. should receive at least two antiemetic agents because she is at very high risk for experiencing PONV. Dexamethasone 4 mg IV can be administered at the beginning of surgery (just after induction of anesthesia) and 4 mg IV ondansetron (or 0.625 mg droperidol) should be administered approximately 30 minutes before the end of surgery. If an alternative agent (to ondansetron or droperidol plus dexamethasone) or third agent is warranted (because she is at such high risk), an antihistamine or antimuscarinic agent such as 25 mg IV diphenhydramine intraoperatively or a transdermal scopolamine patch, placed within 2 hours before the induction of general anesthesia, can be used.

Treatment of Postoperative Nausea and Vomiting

CASE 8-13, QUESTION 3: J.E. is taken to surgery. Anesthesia is induced with propofol and maintained with sevoflurane. Fentanyl is administered intraoperatively for analgesia. A prophylactic dose of dexamethasone is administered at the beginning of surgery, and ondansetron is administered near the end of surgery. Neuromuscular blockade produced by vecuronium is reversed with neostigmine and glycopyrrolate. In the recovery room, J.E. becomes nauseated and has several emetic episodes. What is the most appropriate treatment at this time?

Although dexamethasone and ondansetron are effective for both prevention and treatment of PONV, a rescue antiemetic is most efficacious if it works by a different mechanism of action than the prophylactically administered antiemetics.[100] Prophylactic dexamethasone or ondansetron can be effective for up to 24 hours. If nausea and emetic episodes occur in the recovery room, the prophylactic antiemetic agents were ineffective. Phenothiazines (prochlorperazine) and benzamides (metoclopramide) block dopaminergic stimulation of the CTZ, making these agents appropriate for J.E. Prochlorperazine may be preferred because metoclopramide's primary effect is in the GI tract rather than the CTZ. Diphenhydramine, which blocks Ach receptors in the vestibular apparatus as well as histamine receptors that activate the CTZ, would also be an appropriate choice for rescue for J.E. Because excessive sedation could delay J.E.'s discharge from the ambulatory surgery center, doses should not exceed 25 mg IV for diphenhydramine. In addition, it is important to assess J.E. for postoperative factors that could increase the likelihood of PONV. If postural hypotension is present, IV fluids and ephedrine would be appropriate therapy.

Anesthetic Agents With a Low Incidence of Postoperative Nausea and Vomiting

CASE 8-13, QUESTION 4: How could J.E.'s anesthetic regimen have been modified to reduce the likelihood of PONV?

Several changes could be made in the anesthetic regimen to reduce the likelihood of PONV. When propofol is used for both induction and maintenance of anesthesia, it reduces the risk of PONV similar to the administration of a single antiemetic.[94] Because perioperative administration of opioids is associated with PONV, the use of NSAIDs (oral agents preoperatively and postoperatively, parenteral acetaminophen or ketorolac intraoperatively and postoperatively), when appropriate, can reduce the need for postoperative opioids. In addition, surgical wound infiltration with a long-acting local anesthetic, such as bupivacaine, should also be used, as needed, to reduce postoperative incisional pain.

ANALGESIC AGENTS AND POSTOPERATIVE PAIN MANAGEMENT

Acute Pain

Surgery causes injury to the body, resulting in acute pain. Specifically, the tissue damage from surgery releases substances that directly stimulate or sensitize nociceptors (free nerve endings in the skin, muscle, bone, and connective tissue that detect damaging or unpleasant stimuli). These substances (e.g., bradykinin, serotonin, prostaglandins, and cytokines) mediate pain impulses, which then travel from the periphery (surgical incision) to the dorsal horn of the spinal cord. Glutamate and substance P are released in the dorsal horn to cause the pain impulses to ascend to higher centers in the brain. Nerves originating in the brainstem descend to the spinal cord and release substances (norepinephrine, serotonin, endogenous opioids) that modulate (inhibit) pain transmission. The final integration of all these processes is perception—this is when the patient "feels" the pain. Because cortical and limbic systems are involved, the same surgery can result in significant individual differences in pain perception.[101,102]

Most patients will have pain at rest after surgery, with the magnitude of the pain generally correlating to the invasiveness of the surgery. More intense pain would be expected after major abdominal surgery than after laparoscopic hernia repair, for example. In addition, certain types of movement after major surgery (e.g., coughing after major upper abdominal surgery or knee flexion after total knee replacement) can evoke pain that is more intense, less responsive to opioids, and longer lasting than pain at rest.[103] Nerve injury or peripheral or central nerve sensitization can occur, leading to pain hypersensitivity, pain in response to a stimulus that is not usually painful (allodynia), pain that is difficult to manage, or chronic pain after surgery. Immobility and body positioning after surgery, for example, can lead to musculoskeletal pain.[103–105] Patients vary in their response to pain (and interventions) and in their personal preferences toward pain management. Acute pain usually resolves when the injury heals (hours to days). Unrelieved acute postoperative pain has detrimental physiological and psychological effects, including impaired pulmonary function (leading to pulmonary complications); thromboembolism; tachycardia; hypertension and increased cardiac work; impairment of the immune system; nausea, vomiting, and ileus; chronic pain; and anxiety, fatigue, and fear.[105]

Adequate pain assessment and management are essential components of perioperative care. Education of patients and families about their roles, as well as the limitations and side effects of pain treatments, is critical to managing postoperative pain. Pain management must be planned for and integrated into the perioperative care of patients. Proactive planning includes obtaining a pain history based on the patient's own experiences with pain and a frank discussion of a realistic comfort–function goal for the patient (e.g., complete pain relief after major surgery is not a realistic goal). The intensity and quality of pain, as well as the patient's response to treatment and the degree to which pain interferes with normal activities, should be monitored. Ideally, pain should be prevented by treating it adequately because once established, severe pain can be difficult to control.

Management Options

Effective postoperative pain management should provide subjective pain relief while minimizing analgesic-related adverse effects, allow early return to normal daily activities, and minimize the detrimental effects from unrelieved pain. The following techniques can be used to manage postoperative pain: (a) systemic administration of opioids, NSAIDs, and acetaminophen; (b) on-demand administration of IV opioids, also known as *patient-controlled analgesia* (PCA); (c) epidural analgesia (continuous and on-demand, usually with an opioid–local anesthetic mixture); (d) local nerve blockade, such as local infiltration or peripheral nerve block; and (e) application of heat or cold, guided imagery, music, relaxation, or other nonpharmacologic intervention. Local anesthetics, opioids, acetaminophen, and NSAIDs can be used alone or in combination to create the optimal analgesic regimen for each patient based on factors such as efficacy of the agent to reduce pain to an acceptable level, type of surgery, underlying disease, adverse effects, and cost of therapy. For patients experiencing mild to moderate postoperative pain, local anesthetic wound infiltration, peripheral nerve blockade, or administration of a nonopioid analgesic such as an NSAID or acetaminophen are appropriate approaches to analgesia. For moderate or severe postoperative pain, an opioid is required. The choice of agent, dose, and route of administration depends on the clinical situation. For example, a patient who cannot take anything by mouth may receive an IV opioid in a dose appropriate for the severity of the pain and the presence or absence of risk factors for opioid-induced respiratory depression. A patient who is tolerating crackers and a soft drink before discharge from the surgery center should receive the first dose of the analgesic that will be prescribed for the patient at home. This will ensure that the analgesic (commonly, acetaminophen plus hydrocodone) will be effective and tolerated by the patient. For moderate to severe pain after more-invasive surgery, an IV opioid (e.g., morphine, hydromorphone), an epidural containing a local anesthetic and opioid, or a peripheral nerve block with local anesthetic is necessary. (For more information about general pain management, see Chapter 7, Pain and Its Management.) Analgesia for acute pain in the perioperative setting is best achieved by using a multimodal (balanced) approach with a combination of two or more analgesic medications or modalities that have different mechanisms of action to provide additive or synergistic analgesia with fewer adverse effects when compared with a single analgesic medication or modality.[105] Examples of multimodal analgesic regimens used in the perioperative setting include (a) local anesthetic wound infiltration, acetaminophen, NSAIDs, and if necessary, a weaker opioid analgesic (e.g., hydrocodone plus acetaminophen) after laparoscopic cholecystectomy, (b) continuous epidural analgesia (with opioid plus local anesthetic) with IV acetaminophen and, if necessary, a potent IV opioid for rescue analgesia in an area not covered by the epidural catheter, and (c) continuous peripheral nerve blockade, with acetaminophen, NSAIDs, and, if necessary, an opioid for rescue analgesia in an area not covered by the nerve block.[106]

PATIENT-CONTROLLED ANALGESIA

ADVANTAGES

CASE 8-14

QUESTION 1: J.A., a 50-year-old, 5-foot 4-inch, 50-kg woman, is immediately postoperative from a total abdominal hysterectomy for a neoplasm. Her laboratory values are remarkable for a serum creatinine of 1.3 mg/dL. She is allergic to penicillin. She will be admitted to the postsurgical floor for a planned stay of 2 to 3 days. What mode of pain management should be chosen for J.A.?

PCA is a popular method of administering analgesics and has been shown to provide an overall improvement in analgesia and greater patient satisfaction when compared with traditional intermittent IV opioid injections.[107] Patients treated with traditional intermittent IV dosing of opioids "as needed" can experience severe pain because the serum opioid concentration is allowed to fall to less than the minimum effective analgesic concentration (the concentration that provides approximately 90% pain relief). In addition, high peak plasma opioid concentrations can be seen with this administration method, often resulting in excessive nausea, vomiting, or sedation, as well as respiratory depression. Small, frequent opioid doses on demand, as seen in

PCA, minimize the peaks and valleys in serum concentrations seen with relatively larger intermittent IV doses and allow the patient control over his or her pain management. This is helpful in minimizing adverse effects associated with high peak serum concentrations and inadequate pain relief caused by subtherapeutic serum concentrations. Small, frequent, patient-controlled dosing of opioids is efficacious because opioids have a steep sigmoidal dose–response curve for analgesia, resulting in the ability of a small opioid dose to move the plasma concentration from being subtherapeutic to above the minimum effective plasma concentration that will provide effective pain relief. However, one must remember that these small, frequent on-demand doses are intended to *maintain* analgesia. The patient should be reasonably comfortable (e.g., from a loading dose) before the initiation of PCA.[108,109] In terms of safety, sedation generally precedes respiratory depression.[110] Therefore, if a patient becomes sedated, self-administration of additional patient-controlled bolus doses will stop, allowing the serum opioid concentration to fall to a safe level.

Therapy can be individualized by using small doses of opioids at preset intervals (e.g., 1 mg of morphine every 10 minutes), with the patient in control of his or her analgesic administration. An infusion pump with a programmed on-demand dose (the dose the patient can self-administer), number of minutes between allowable doses (lock-out interval), and maximum number of boluses per hour is equipped with a button that the patient presses to receive a dose. An IV bolus is the most common PCA route, with opioids being the drugs of choice to provide analgesia.

If the patient is educated to use PCA properly, it can be used to alleviate anticipated pain before movement or physical therapy in a pre-emptive fashion. J.A. has undergone a procedure for which moderate to severe pain is expected in the immediate postoperative period. J.A.'s pain requirement in the immediate postoperative period could be met with PCA opioid administration after first administering a loading dose of an IV opioid, which is titrated to achieve the appropriate level of analgesia. Analgesia can then be maintained with patient-controlled bolus doses. When her opioid requirements decline or when she can tolerate oral intake, she can then be switched to oral analgesics.

PATIENT SELECTION

CASE 8-14, QUESTION 2: J.A.'s surgeon decides to prescribe PCA for postoperative pain management. How should J.A. be evaluated for her ability to appropriately participate in her analgesic administration?

Patients receiving PCA therapy must be able to understand the concept behind PCA and to operate the drug administration button. J.A. must be alert, oriented, and willing to assume control of her own pain management. She must be able to comprehend the relationships between a stimulus (pain), a response (pushing the button), and a delayed result (pain relief). She must understand verbal or written instructions about the function and safety features of the infusion pump and how to titrate the drug as needed for satisfactory analgesia. The anticipated intensity of the patient's pain after surgery should be such that an IV opioid would be required for pain management. PCA has been used successfully in children, generally after ages 8 or 9 (adjusting doses appropriately), and in elderly patients. It is not indicated in patients who are expected to require parenteral opioids for analgesia for less than 24 hours because these patients will generally be able to tolerate oral analgesics shortly after surgery.

PATIENT INSTRUCTIONS

CASE 8-14, QUESTION 3: J.A. is nervous about giving herself an overdose while using PCA. What instructions should be provided to her?

Patients often worry about the safety of PCA, which can lead to reluctance to provide themselves with adequate pain relief. J.A. should be informed that she will be frequently assessed by the nurse (particularly during the first 24 hours of therapy). If she becomes sleepy from the opioid, she should not press the button. When this adverse effect of the opioid has worn off, she will wake up (plasma opioid level has fallen back into or below the therapeutic range) and she may then press the button to receive a dose of the opioid if she has pain. This is an important safety feature of PCA and is the reason family members must not push the button for the patient. However, J.A. should also know that she may have to press the button several times (after the lock-out interval has passed) before her pain is relieved. She must also be informed that she may require a larger PCA dose, so it is important for J.A. to assess her pain relief from her current ("usual") dose that most patients are initially started on after surgery. Accurate pain assessment after her prescribed dose is critical for ensuring that her dose is sufficient to provide the desired level of analgesia. She should also understand the possible adverse effects of her PCA medication and what can be done to prevent and treat these effects, as well as the advantages of providing herself with adequate analgesia (e.g., early ambulation). Finally, she should be told of the negligible risk of narcotic addiction from short-term PCA use and be given ample opportunity to ask questions.

CHOICE OF AGENT

CASE 8-14, QUESTION 4: Meperidine is ordered for J.A.'s PCA. Is this a reasonable drug choice for her?

Ideally, opioids for PCA administration have a rapid onset and intermediate duration of action (30–60 minutes), with no accumulation or adverse effects. The physicians, nurses, and pharmacists involved with the care of the patient should be familiar with the drug selected for PCA. Morphine is by far the most common choice for PCA, although other opioids such as fentanyl and hydromorphone can be used. Drug choice is based on past patient experiences, allergies, adverse effects, and special considerations, such as renal function. Meperidine has a metabolite, normeperidine, which is renally excreted, has a long half-life, and can cause cerebral irritation and excitation. Symptoms of CNS toxicity from normeperidine include agitation, shaky feelings, delirium, twitching, tremors, and myoclonus or tonic-clonic seizures. These symptoms can be seen when meperidine is administered in higher doses or for a prolonged period.[111] The presence of renal insufficiency increases the risk of accumulation of normeperidine.[111] Meperidine also inhibits serotonin reuptake and has a fairly high serotonergic potential. The risk of a patient developing the serotonin syndrome is greater when meperidine is coadministered with another drug that has moderate or high serotonergic potential (e.g., fluoxetine, fluvoxamine, paroxetine, venlafaxine).[112] For these reasons, meperidine is a poor choice for analgesia, particularly for J.A. who has diminished renal function. Morphine is conjugated with glucuronide in hepatic and extrahepatic sites (particularly the kidney) to its two major metabolites, morphine-3-glucuronide and morphine-6-glucuronide; both metabolites are excreted primarily in the urine. Morphine-6-glucuronide is an active metabolite that can accumulate in patients with renal failure, resulting in prolonged analgesia, sedation, and respiratory depression.[113] Because of

TABLE 8-12
Adult Analgesic Dosing Recommendations for Intravenous Patient-Controlled Analgesia[a,102,114,115]

Drug	Usual Concentration	Demand Dose (mg)		Lock-Out Interval (minutes)
		Usual	Range	
Fentanyl (as citrate)	10 mcg/mL	0.01–0.02	0.01–0.04	10
Hydromorphone hydrochloride	0.2 mg/mL	0.2–0.3	0.1–0.4	10
Morphine sulfate	1 mg/mL	1–2	0.5–2.5	10

[a] Analgesic doses are based on those required by a healthy 55- to 70-kg, opioid-naïve adult. Analgesic requirements vary widely among patients. Doses may need to be adjusted because of age, condition of the patient, and prior opioid use.

J.A.'s diminished renal function, morphine should probably be avoided because other options exist. Hydromorphone is not metabolized to an active 6-glucuronide metabolite, and fentanyl is metabolized to inactive metabolites. Either hydromorphone or fentanyl is an appropriate analgesic choice for J.A. Hydromorphone is chosen. Table 8-12 lists common doses and lock-out intervals for drugs administered by PCA.[102,114,115]

DOSING

CASE 8-14, QUESTION 5: J.A. was not receiving an opioid before surgery (e.g., she is opioid naïve). What dose of hydromorphone and what lock-out interval should be used for her initial PCA pump settings?

If J.A. is experiencing pain before PCA has been initiated, she should receive a loading dose of IV hydromorphone titrated to achieve baseline pain relief (may require up to 1 mg). Once adequate analgesia is achieved, demand doses of 0.2 mg with a lock-out interval of 10 minutes would be a good choice to maintain analgesia for this opioid-naïve patient. If J.A.'s pain is not relieved after two to three demand doses within 1 hour, the demand dose can be increased to 0.3 mg.

USE OF A BASAL INFUSION

CASE 8-14, QUESTION 6: After the first postoperative evening, J.A. tells you that she had a terrible time sleeping. She describes waking up in pain frequently, despite pressing her PCA button many times. She rates her pain as moderate to severe in intensity and fairly constant. A review of the history on her PCA device reveals successful delivery of 9 mg of hydromorphone (30 demand doses, 0.3 mg each) during the past 12 hours. J.A. is not sedated and reports no adverse effects from hydromorphone. How can J.A.'s pain management be improved?

Many PCA infusion pumps offer a continuous infusion setting for a basal infusion during intermittent dosing. Use of a basal (continuous) infusion has not been shown to improve analgesia and likely increases the risk of adverse effects (owing to the potential of an opioid overdose in some patients). Therefore, routine basal (continuous) infusion of opioids cannot be recommended for acute pain management. In an opioid-naïve patient such as J.A., however, continuing to increase the demand dose increases the risk of excessive sedation and respiratory depression (owing to high peak levels). Also, J.A. describes her pain as moderate to severe in intensity and fairly constant in nature when she does not regularly push the demand button. For J.A., a continuous infusion could be beneficial. As a rule of thumb, an opioid-naïve patient experiencing acute pain (that can change quickly) should receive no more than one-third of her average hourly usage as a continuous infusion or a maximum of 1 mg/hour of morphine (or its equivalent, which would be 0.2 mg/hour for hydromorphone). For J.A., a continuous infusion of 0.2 mg/hour hydromorphone should be initiated in addition to her demand dose of 0.3 mg every 8 minutes. Because the onset of action of hydromorphone is about 5 minutes and the peak effect occurs in 10 to 20 minutes, shortening the lock-out interval is not recommended because J.A. could access the next dose of hydromorphone before the effects of the initial dose can be appreciated. That could lead to dose-stacking and significant adverse effects, such as excessive sedation and respiratory depression.

ADVERSE EFFECTS

CASE 8-14, QUESTION 7: The next day, J.A. requested only a few demand doses and reports adequate pain relief with her PCA, but now complains of feeling slightly groggy and nauseated. Bowel sounds are noted on physical examination, and J.A. plans to try to take clear liquids later that morning. What are the adverse effects of PCA opioids, and how can J.A.'s complaints be addressed?

Opioids can produce sedation, confusion, euphoria, nausea and vomiting, constipation, urinary retention, and pruritus. These adverse effects can be managed by dose adjustments or pharmacologic intervention. Although rare, life-threatening respiratory depression is the most serious adverse effect of opioid administration.[110] Because sedation precedes respiratory depression, systematic assessment of sedation and respiratory parameters should be performed at frequent intervals (every 1 to 2 hours during the first 24 hours of therapy). The patient should be observed for how quickly he or she arouses when stimulated, and the rate, depth, and regularity of the patient's respirations should be assessed and compared with the patient's baseline status.[110,114] Particular attention must be paid to patients at high risk for respiratory depression from an opioid. These risk factors include age older than 65 years, obesity, pulmonary disease or other conditions that reduce ventilatory capacity, and known or suspected history of sleep apnea.[114] Technical problems must also be ruled out. The PCA pump should be checked to ensure that it is delivering the correct drug and dose, programming should be checked for accuracy (e.g., drug concentration, dosing interval), and the opioid reversal agent naloxone must be readily available. Monitoring for efficacy and adverse effects of PCA therapy should include pain intensity and quality, response to treatment, number of on-demand requests, analgesic consumption, BP, heart rate, respiratory rate and effort, and level of sedation, as well as the presence of other adverse effects of opioids such as nausea and itching.

J.A.'s PCA hydromorphone dose could be reduced to manage her sedation and nausea. However, her pain control must be carefully reassessed to ensure efficacy of the newly lowered dose. An order for a nonsedating antiemetic (such as ondansetron) could also be provided. NSAIDs (ketorolac IV or other NSAID orally) or acetaminophen (IV or oral) are not sedating; thus, they should be added to the analgesic regimen to provide analgesia and allow a reduction in her opioid dose. However, because of J.A.'s compromised renal function, acetaminophen is a better choice than an NSAID. If J.A. is able to take fluids orally, PCA should be discontinued and oral analgesics administered as needed. As healing occurs, her pain intensity should lessen, and oral opioid–acetaminophen products should manage her pain adequately.

EPIDURAL ANALGESIA

CASE 8-15

QUESTION 1: T.M., a 69-year-old man, enters the surgical ICU after surgery for colorectal cancer (lower anterior resection, urethral stents, ileorectal pull-through). His pain is managed through a lumbar epidural catheter. What are the benefits and risks of epidural analgesia, and why was this approach to postoperative analgesia chosen for T.M.?

ADVANTAGES AND DISADVANTAGES

Epidural analgesia can offer superior pain relief compared with traditional parenteral (IM, IV, and IV PCA) analgesia[116] as well as facilitate return of GI function, decrease pulmonary complications, and possibly decrease cardiovascular events.[117,118] Epidural PCA offers an advantage compared with parenteral opioids (including IV PCA) because it allows individualization of the analgesic requirements, lower total drug use, greater patient satisfaction,[119] and improved analgesia.[120] Epidural catheter placement is an invasive procedure that can result in unintentional dural puncture (causing postdural puncture headache), insertion site inflammation or infection, catheter migration, and, rarely, epidural hematoma.[115]

PATIENT SELECTION

Epidural analgesia should be chosen based on the need for good postoperative pain relief and reduced perioperative physiological responses. Postoperative pain should be localized at an appropriate level for catheter placement in the lumbar or thoracic location of the epidural space. Patients undergoing abdominal, gynecologic, obstetric, colorectal, urologic, lower limb (e.g., major vascular), or thoracic surgery are excellent candidates for epidural pain management. Absolute contraindications to epidural analgesia include severe systemic infection or infection in the area of catheter insertion, known coagulopathy, clinically significant abnormal platelet count or function, increased intracranial pressure, patient refusal, and anatomical abnormalities that make epidural catheter placement difficult or impossible.[121] T.M. is a good candidate for epidural analgesia based on the severity of pain associated with his surgery and the location and invasiveness of the surgical procedure.

CHOICE OF AGENT AND MECHANISMS OF ACTION

CASE 8-15, QUESTION 2: What drug or drug combination can be used for T.M.'s epidural infusion? What are the mechanisms of action of the analgesics commonly administered in the epidural space?

Most commonly, an opioid and a local anesthetic are administered in combination in the epidural analgesic infusion. Opioids in the epidural space are transported by passive diffusion and the vasculature to the spinal cord, where they act at opioid receptors in the dorsal horn. After epidural administration, opioids can reach brainstem sites by cephalad movement in the cerebrospinal fluid. In addition, lipophilic opioids (fentanyl, sufentanil) have substantial systemic absorption from the epidural space.[113,122] Opioids selectively block pain transmission and have no effect on nerve transmission responsible for motor, sensory, or autonomic function.[123] Local anesthetics, however, spread within the epidural space to anesthetize nerve roots as they exit the neural foramina (openings in the spinal column) and block nerve transmission. Depending on the drug, concentration, and depth of nerve penetration, local anesthetics produce sensory, motor, or autonomic blockade (see Local Anesthetics section). Table 8-13 describes the spinal actions, efficacy, and adverse effects of opioids and local anesthetics administered by the epidural route.[114,121,122,124]

As previously mentioned, opioids and local anesthetics are combined in the same solution because these two classes of drugs act synergistically at two different sites to produce analgesia, allowing the administration of lower doses of each drug to reduce the risk of adverse effects while providing effective analgesia. Table 8-14 lists the drugs, concentrations, and typical infusion rates for epidural administration.[115,122,123,125] Bupivacaine is commonly chosen as the local anesthetic agent. Because pain fibers are on the outer aspect of the nerve and are not heavily myelinated, a low concentration of bupivacaine ($\leq$0.125%) can be administered to block these fibers without significantly blocking motor fibers. The choice of opioid is based on pharmacokinetic differences among the available agents. Onset, duration, spread of agent in the spinal fluid (dermatomal spread), and systemic absorption are affected by the lipophilicity of the drug.[124] Highly lipophilic opioids such as fentanyl and sufentanil have a faster onset of action, a shorter duration of action (from a

TABLE 8-13

A Comparison of the Spinal Actions, Efficacy, and Adverse Effects of Opioids and Local Anesthetics[a,114,121,122,124]

	Opioids	Local Anesthetics
Actions		
Site of action	Substantia gelatinosa of dorsal horn of spinal cord[b]	Spinal nerve roots
Modalities blocked	"Selective" block of pain conduction	Blockade of pain nerve fibers; can block sensory or motor fibers
Efficacy		
Surgical pain	Partial relief	Complete relief possible
Labor pain	Partial relief	Complete relief
Postoperative pain	Fair or good relief	Complete relief
Adverse effects	Nausea, vomiting, sedation, pruritus, constipation or ileus, urinary retention, respiratory depression	Hypotension, urinary retention, loss of sensation, loss of motor function (patient may not be able to bear weight and ambulate)

[a] Epidurally administered morphine and local anesthetics exert their effects mainly by a spinal mechanism of action; lipophilic opioids such as fentanyl and sufentanil achieve therapeutic plasma concentrations when administered epidurally and therefore exert their effects by a systemic mechanism of action.

[b] Other sites where opioid receptor binding sites are present.

TABLE 8-14
Adult Analgesic Dosing Recommendations for Epidural Infusion[115,122,123,125]

Drug Combination[a]	Infusion Concentration[b]	Usual Infusion Rate[b]
Morphine + bupivacaine	12.5–25 mcg/mL (M) 0.5–1.25 mg/mL (B)	4–10 mL/h
Hydromorphone + bupivacaine	3–10 mcg/mL (H) 0.5–1.25 mg/mL (B)	4–10 mL/h
Fentanyl + bupivacaine	2–5 mcg/mL (F) 0.5–1.25 mg/mL (B)	4–10 mL/h
Sufentanil + bupivacaine	1 mcg/mL (S) 0.5–1.25 mg/mL (B)	4–10 mL/h

[a] Use only preservative free products and preservative free 0.9% sodium chloride as the admixture solution.
[b] Exact concentrations and rates are institution specific. Initial concentration and rate often depend on the age and general condition of the patient and the location of the catheter.
B, bupivacaine; F, fentanyl; H, hydromorphone; M, morphine; S, sufentanil.

single dose), less dermatomal spread, and much greater systemic absorption. After several hours of epidural infusion, the dermatomal (regional) effect of fentanyl is lost, and analgesia is achieved because of a therapeutic plasma concentration. Morphine, which is relatively hydrophilic, has a slower onset of action, longer duration of action, greater dermatomal spread and migration to the brain, and less systemic absorption.[122,124] Morphine, unlike fentanyl, retains its spinal site of action.[122] The lipophilicity of hydromorphone is intermediate between fentanyl and morphine. Clinically, hydromorphone has a faster onset and shorter duration than morphine. Its site of action is likely in the spinal cord.[126] A comparison of the pharmacokinetic properties important to epidural opioids is found in Table 8-15.[115,116,124,125] T.M. should receive a combination of opioid and local anesthetic, such as hydromorphone and bupivacaine, as an epidural infusion for postoperative pain management.

CASE 8-15, QUESTION 3: Hydromorphone–bupivacaine is chosen for T.M. How should this be prepared, and what infusion rate should be chosen?

Hydromorphone and bupivacaine are commonly admixed in 0.9% sodium chloride (usual concentration ranges are found in Table 8-14). Concentrations are often institution-specific and depend on the rate of administration. Preservative free preparations of each drug should be used because neurologic effects are possible with inadvertent subdural administration of large amounts of benzyl alcohol or other preservatives. Strict aseptic technique should be used when admixing and administering an epidural solution.

The rate of administration is chosen empirically based on the anticipated analgesic response, the concentration of opioid in the admixture, and the potential for adverse effects. Usually, a rate of 4 to 10 mL/hour is adequate; the epidural space can safely handle up to approximately 20 mL/hour of fluid. An initial infusion rate of 8 mL/hour would be reasonable for T.M., with titration based on efficacy and adverse effects.

ADVERSE EFFECTS

CASE 8-15, QUESTION 4: Two hours after initiation of his hydromorphone–bupivacaine epidural infusion, T.M. experiences discomfort in the form of an itchy feeling on his nose, torso, and limbs. Is this related to his epidural infusion?

Adverse effects of the epidural infusion may be caused by the opioid or the local anesthetic. Pruritus has been associated with almost all opioids, with a significantly greater frequency when the opioid is administered as an epidural infusion rather than by IV administration.[127] This effect is usually seen within 2 hours and is probably dose-related. It generally subsides as the opioid effect wears off and can be more of a problem with continuous epidural administration of opioids or when opioids are administered via PCA. Although pruritus from opioids is probably mu-receptor mediated and not histamine mediated, antihistamines (e.g., diphenhydramine) are commonly used with equivocal effectiveness. A better approach is to administer very small doses of a mu-antagonist (e.g., naloxone 0.04 mg or nalbuphine 2.5 mg) to effectively reverse opioid adverse effects, such as pruritus, but not analgesia. Because of naloxone's short duration of action, nalbuphine is often preferred. Ondansetron has also shown some efficacy for managing itching from an intrathecal or epidural opioid.[128]

Other adverse effects possible with epidural opioids include nausea, vomiting, constipation, ileus, urinary retention, sedation, and respiratory depression. Although rare, respiratory depression from epidural opioids is the most dangerous adverse effect. Respiratory depression can occur as long as 12 to 24 hours after a single bolus of morphine[122,124] or within hours after beginning a continuous infusion of fentanyl–bupivacaine

TABLE 8-15
Pharmacokinetic Comparison of Common Epidural Opioid Analgesics[115,116,124,125]

Agent	Partition Coefficient[a]	Onset of Action of Bolus (minutes)	Duration of Action of Bolus (hours)	Dermatomal Spread
Fentanyl	955	5	2–4	Narrow
Hydromorphone	525	15	6–12	Intermediate
Morphine sulfate (Duramorph)	1	30	12–24	Wide
Sufentanil	1,737	5	2–4	Narrow

[a] Octanol–water partition coefficient; used to assess lipophilicity; higher numbers indicate greater lipophilicity.

or hydromorphone–bupivacaine. Sedation level, as well as respiratory rate and effort, must be assessed every hour for the first 12 hours, then every 2 hours for the next 12 hours, then if stable, every 4 hours until removal of the catheter.[129] As with parenteral opioids, particular attention must be paid to patients at high risk for respiratory depression from an opioid. These risk factors include age older than 65 years, obesity, pulmonary disease or other conditions that reduce ventilatory capacity, and known or suspected history of sleep apnea.[114] In a patient with known obstructive sleep apnea, for example, the anesthesia provider may prescribe an epidural analgesic solution containing bupivacaine only (no opioid).

Adverse effects of epidural local anesthetics include hypotension, urinary retention, lower limb paresthesias or numbness, and lower limb motor weakness. Depending on the degree of numbness and motor weakness, the patient may have difficulty ambulating. In a patient prone to hypotension or in whom motor weakness would be detrimental, for example, the anesthesia care provider may prescribe an epidural analgesic solution containing an opioid only (no local anesthetic). Monitoring for efficacy and adverse effects of epidural analgesia should include pain intensity and quality, response to treatment, number of on-demand requests (if epidural PCA is being used), analgesic consumption, BP, heart rate, respiratory rate and effort, level of sedation, urinary output, sensory and motor assessment (e.g., presence of numbness or tingling, inability to raise legs or flex knees or ankles), and a site and dressing check.

ADJUNCTIVE KETOROLAC USE

CASE 8-15, QUESTION 5: On the second postoperative day, T.M. is able to rest comfortably when undisturbed while receiving treatment with a lumbar epidural infusion of hydromorphone 10 mcg/mL and bupivacaine 1.25 mg/mL at a rate of 8 mL/hour. However, when he is moved at the change of each nursing shift, he complains of significant pain. Increasing the rate of his epidural infusion was tried, but caused unacceptable pruritus and sedation. How can T.M.'s intermittent pain needs be addressed?

The use of additional analgesics for breakthrough pain may be necessary in patients receiving continuous epidural infusion. T.M.'s intermittent pain could be managed by epidural PCA. Like IV PCA, patient-activated epidural boluses can be administered to control pain during movement. Alternatively, injectable ketorolac or acetaminophen may be considered for T.M.; these agents do not contribute to respiratory depression, sedation, or pruritus and can effectively treat moderate pain. The analgesic effects of acetaminophen and NSAIDs are additive with the opioids and can lower postoperative pain scores. Patient selection for ketorolac therapy should consider renal function, plasma volume and electrolyte status, GI disease, risk of bleeding, and concomitant drugs such as LMWH (which increases the risk for bleeding and epidural hematoma). Acetaminophen is contraindicated in patients with severe hepatic impairment, severe active liver disease, or known hypersensitivity to acetaminophen or any excipient in the formulation. Acetaminophen should be used with caution in patients with severe hypovolemia or severe renal impairment.[130]

ADJUNCTIVE ANTICOAGULANT ADMINISTRATION

CASE 8-15, QUESTION 6: The surgeon has determined that T.M. is at risk for developing postoperative venous thromboembolism. Enoxaparin 40 mg subcutaneously every day has been ordered postoperatively. What are the risks of enoxaparin in this situation? What are reasonable precautions?

Administration of an anticoagulant can increase the risk of epidural or spinal hematoma formation, which can lead to long-term or permanent paralysis. Administration of antiplatelet or anticoagulant drugs in combination with an anticoagulant (such as an LMWH) results in an even greater risk of hemorrhagic complications, including spinal hematoma. These findings have led to concern for the safety of epidural analgesia in patients receiving an LMWH. Important considerations for managing a patient being administered an LMWH and receiving continuous epidural analgesia are (a) the time of catheter placement and removal relative to the timing (and peak effect) of LMWH administration and (b) whether the anticoagulant dose is low (prophylactic dose) or high (treatment dose).[131] For T.M., the epidural catheter is already in place, and the LMWH is started postoperatively as a single daily low (prophylactic) dose. It is safe to leave the epidural catheter in place as long as the first dose of LMWH is administered 6 to 8 hours postoperatively. The second LMWH dose should be administered no sooner than 24 hours after the first dose. The timing of the catheter removal is of the utmost importance; it should be delayed for at least 12 hours after the last dose of LMWH, with subsequent LMWH dosing to occur a minimum of 2 hours after the catheter has been removed. The risk of spinal hematoma is even greater when treatment doses of LMWH are administered or if fondaparinux is selected as the anticoagulant for deep vein thrombosis prophylaxis. In these instances, the epidural catheter should be removed before the first dose of LMWH or fondaparinux, and the first dose given at least 2 hours after catheter removal. Because T.M. is receiving prophylactic daily enoxaparin, his catheter should be removed no earlier than 12 hours after his last dose of enoxaparin, with his next dose administered no earlier than 2 hours after catheter removal.

MULTIMODAL PAIN MANAGEMENT

CASE 8-16

QUESTION 1: W.W., a 36-year-old man, arrives at the ambulatory surgery center for an inguinal hernia repair. This procedure will be performed under local anesthesia, with sedation as needed, and is expected to be completed within

TABLE 8-16

Comparison of Select Opioids for Perioperative Pain Management[3,132–136]

Property	Intravenous Morphine	Intravenous Hydromorphone	Intravenous Fentanyl	Oral Hydrocodone	Oral Oxycodone
Onset	5 minutes	≤5 minutes	≤2 minutes	30–60 minutes	30–60 minutes
Peak effect	15–20 minutes	10–20 minutes	5–7 minutes	1–2 hours	1.5–2 hours
Duration	3–4 hours	2–3 hours	30–60 minutes	4–6 hours	3–4 hours
Approximate equianalgesic dose	2 mg	0.4 mg	25 mcg	5 mg	4 mg

TABLE 8-17
Commonly Used Analgesic Drugs and Nonpharmacologic Techniques for Postoperative Pain Management[105,106,132–136]

Type of Agent	Examples	Potential Adverse Effects
Local anesthetics	Tissue infiltration, wound instillation, peripheral nerve block, epidural	Tingling, numbness, motor weakness, hypotension, CNS and cardiac effects from systemic absorption
NSAIDs	Ketorolac (IV, IM, oral), ibuprofen (oral), naproxen (oral), celecoxib (oral)	GI upset, edema, hypertension, dizziness, drowsiness, GI bleeding, operative site bleeding (not celecoxib)
Other nonopioids	Acetaminophen (oral, intravenous, rectal)	GI upset, hepatotoxicity, hypotension (IV formulation)
Nonpharmacologic	Ice or cold therapy	Excessive vasoconstriction, skin irritation
	Distraction, music, deep breathing for relaxation	
Opioid combination products (oral)	Hydrocodone + acetaminophen, oxycodone + acetaminophen	Nausea, vomiting, pruritus, constipation, rash, sedation, respiratory depression
Opioids	Morphine (IV, epidural), hydromorphone (IV, epidural), fentanyl (IV, epidural), oxycodone (oral)	Nausea, vomiting, pruritus, constipation, rash, sedation, respiratory depression

CNS, central nervous system; GI, gastrointestinal; IM, intramuscular; IV, intravenous; NSAIDs, nonsteroidal anti-inflammatory drugs.

30 minutes. His medical and surgical histories are unremarkable. He is not currently taking any medication and reports no drug allergies. After discharge from the ambulatory surgery center, how should W.W.'s postoperative pain be managed?

In general, one expects that the greater the magnitude of the surgical trauma, the greater the patient's postoperative pain. For minor surgical procedures (e.g., inguinal hernia repair, breast biopsy), there is minimal surgical trauma, and the patient goes home shortly after surgery. For intermediate surgical procedures (e.g., total abdominal hysterectomy, laparoscopic cholecystectomy), short-term hospitalization is often necessary to observe the patient's recovery and to manage any pain. Patients undergoing major surgery (e.g., bowel resection, thoracotomy) experience a significant surgical stress response that can significantly increase postoperative morbidity. Effective pain management is essential, particularly in these patients.

If pain is mild in intensity, a nonopioid analgesic such as acetaminophen or an NSAID is appropriate. If pain is moderate or severe in intensity or not controlled with acetaminophen or an NSAID, an opioid is indicated. As previously discussed, the agent, dose, and route are determined by the clinical scenario. If the patient cannot take oral medications or a fast onset of action is required to control pain, an IV opioid is indicated. Administration of an oral opioid and nonopioid combination product will require a longer time before the patient will feel its analgesic effect. However, depending on the dose administered, the anticipated degree of analgesia it will produce can be greater than a lower dose of an IV opioid. One tablet of hydrocodone 10 mg plus acetaminophen 325 mg would be expected to provide greater and more long-lasting analgesia than one dose of morphine 2 mg IV (Table 8-16).[3,132–136] If a fixed combination of opioid and nonopioid is used, the total daily dose administered to the patient is limited by the maximum allowable daily dose of the nonopioid (e.g., acetaminophen, ibuprofen).

Multimodal or balanced analgesia is often used to provide postoperative analgesia. It can be difficult to optimize postoperative pain relief, to the point of achieving normal function, by using one drug or route of administration. By using two or more drugs that work at different points in the pain pathway, additive or synergistic analgesia can be achieved and adverse effects reduced because doses are lower and side effect profiles are different.

ONLINE CONTENT

For an illustration that shows the sites of action of the major drug classes used for pain management, go to http://thepoint.lwwcom/AT10e.

For perioperative pain management, combining acetaminophen with an NSAID provides superior analgesia than either agent alone.[137] Opioids are a mainstay of analgesic therapy for moderate to severe pain. However, opioids are often associated with intolerable adverse effects (e.g., nausea, vomiting, constipation, itching, sedation). Maximizing the use of nonopioid analgesics can result in less need for opioids and improved analgesia (Table 8-17).[105,106,136] When compared with morphine alone, the addition of an NSAID after major surgery reduces pain intensity and 24-hour morphine consumption, with a reduction in the incidence of morphine-related adverse effects of nausea, vomiting, and sedation.[133]

For W.W., the anticipated surgical trauma is minor, and he will recover at home. The surgeon will inject a long-acting local anesthetic (e.g., bupivacaine) into the tissues surrounding the surgical incision. This will provide intraoperative anesthesia at the surgical site and postoperative analgesia until the effects of the bupivacaine wear off. Then, W.W. will likely require acetaminophen or an NSAID for pain management. If his pain is not controlled, a less potent opioid (e.g., hydrocodone) plus acetaminophen may be used as a rescue analgesic.

KEY REFERENCES AND WEBSITES

A full list of references for this chapter can be found at **http://thepoint.lww.com/AT10e.** Below are the key references and websites for this chapter, with the corresponding reference number in this chapter found in parentheses after the reference.

Key References

American College of Cardiology/American Heart Association Task Force on Practice Guidelines et al. ACC/AHA focused update on perioperative beta-blockade. *J Am Coll Cardiol.* 2009; 54:2102. (5)

American Society of Anesthesiologists Task Force on Neuraxial Opioids et al. Practice guidelines for the prevention, detection, and management of respiratory depression associated with neuraxial opioid administration. *Anesthesiology*. 2009;110:218. (129)

Apfel CFC et al. A factorial trial of six interventions for prevention of postoperative nausea and vomiting. *N Engl J Med*. 2004;350:2441. (94)

Gan TJ et al. Society for Ambulatory Anesthesia guidelines for the management of postoperative nausea and vomiting. *Anesth Analg*. 2007;105:1615. (81)

Horlocker TT et al. Executive summary: regional anesthesia in the patient receiving antithrombotic or thrombolytic therapy: American Society of Regional Anesthesia and Pain Medicine Evidence-Based Guidelines (Third Edition). *Reg Anesth Pain Med*. 2010;35:102. (131)

McCaffery M, Pasero C. Pain Assessment and Pharmacologic Management. St. Louis, MO: Elsevier Mosby. 2011. (136)

Neal JM et al. ASRA Practice advisory on the treatment of local anesthetic systemic toxicity. *Reg Anesth Pain Med*. 2010;35:152. (43)

Pasero C. Assessment of sedation during opioid administration for pain management. *J Perianesth Nurs*. 2009;24:186. (110)

Weiskopf RB, Eger EI 2nd. Comparing the costs of inhaled anesthetics. *Anesthesiology*. 1993;79:1413.

Key Websites

Lipid Rescue Resuscitation for cardiac toxicity. **http://www.lipidrescue.org.**

Malignant Hyperthermia Association of the United States. **http://www.mhaus.org.**

San Diego Patient Safety Council. Tool Kit. Patient Controlled Analgesia (PCA) Guidelines of Care for the Opioid Naïve Patient. December 2009. **http://www.chpso.org/meds/pcatoolkit.pdf.** (114)

9

Acid–Base Disorders

Luis S. Gonzalez, III and Raymond W. Hammond

CORE PRINCIPLES

	CHAPTER CASES
1 Acid–base analysis should proceed in a stepwise approach to avoid missing complicated disorders that may not be readily apparent.	**Case 9-1 (Question 1)**
2 A normal anion gap metabolic acidosis is most commonly found in patients who have either diarrhea or are receiving large amounts of isotonic crystalloid infusions. A less common cause of a normal anion gap metabolic acidosis occurs with patients who present with one of several types of renal tubular acidoses.	**Case 9-1 (Questions 2–6)**
3 A metabolic acidosis with an elevated anion gap is created by a disease process that produces an acid, which is buffered by the major extracellular buffer, bicarbonate. It is important to include a calculation of the anion gap in the workup of all patients considered for acid–base analysis.	**Case 9-2 (Questions 1–4)**
4 Metabolic alkaloses can be classified according to a patient's volume status and responsiveness to the administration of chloride-containing solutions. A contraction alkalosis, also called chloride-responsive alkalosis, is generally caused by diuretic administration whereas a chloride-nonresponsive alkalosis may be caused by glucocorticoid administration.	**Case 9-3 (Questions 1–4)**
5 A respiratory acidosis can be acute, chronic, or acute-on-chronic. The best way to differentiate these disorders is with a careful patient history and review of previous blood gas values looking for elevated carbon dioxide levels when a patient is at his or her baseline.	**Case 9-4 (Questions 1–4)**
6 Unlike respiratory acidosis, most patients presenting with a respiratory alkalosis do so acutely. There are a relatively small number of conditions that cause an acute respiratory alkalosis, which can aid in the diagnosis when it is not apparent.	**Case 9-5 (Questions 1–4)**
7 Mixed metabolic and respiratory acid–base disorders occur commonly in acutely ill patients. Acid–base analysis can assist in the diagnosis of clinically difficult cases. Following a stepwise approach in the analysis of acid–base disorders should identify all clinically important abnormalities.	**Case 9-6 (Questions 1–3)**

Understanding the etiology of a clinically important acid–base disturbance is important because therapy generally should be directed at the underlying cause of the disturbance rather than merely the change in pH. Severe acid–base disorders can affect multiple organ systems, including cardiovascular (impaired contractility, arrhythmias), pulmonary (impaired oxygen delivery, respiratory muscle fatigue, dyspnea), renal (hypokalemia, nephrolithiasis), or neurologic (decreased cerebral blood flow, seizures, coma).

ACID–BASE PHYSIOLOGY

To protect body proteins, acid–base balance must be tightly controlled in an attempt to maintain a normal extracellular pH of 7.35 to 7.45 and an intracellular pH of approximately 7.0 to 7.3.[1] This narrow range is maintained by complex buffer systems, ventilation to expel carbon dioxide (CO_2), and renal elimination of acids and reabsorption of bicarbonate (HCO_3^-).[2] At rest, about 200 mL of CO_2, and even more during exercise, is transported

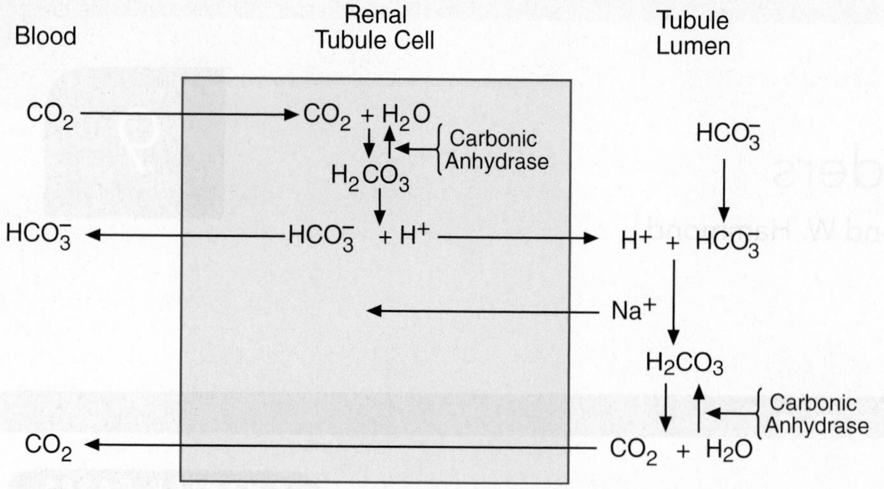

FIGURE 9-1 **Renal tubular bicarbonate reabsorption.**

from the tissues and excreted in the lungs.[3] Although HCO_3^- is responsible only for about 36% of intracellular buffering, it provides about 86% of the buffering activity in extracellular fluid (ECF).[1] Extracellular fluid contains approximately 350 mEq of HCO_3^-, which buffers generated H^+.

$$HCO_3^- + H^+ \Leftrightarrow H_2CO_3 \qquad \textit{(Eq. 9-1)}$$

Hydrogen ion (H^+) combines with HCO_3^- and shifts the equilibrium of Eq. 9-1 to the right. In the proximal renal tubule lumen, carbonic anhydrase catalyzes the dehydration of H_2CO_3 to CO_2 and H_2O, which are absorbed into the tubule cell, as illustrated in Eq. 9-2 and in Figure 9-1. Within the tubule cell, H_2O dissociates into H^+ and OH^-. The H^+ is then secreted into the lumen by a Na^+–H^+ exchanger. Carbonic anhydrase then catalyzes the combination of OH^- and CO_2 to HCO_3^-, which is carried into the circulation by a $Na^+HCO_3^-$ cotransporter.[4]

$$HCO_3^- + H^+ \Leftrightarrow H_2CO_3 \overset{CA}{\Leftrightarrow} CO_2\ (\text{dissolved}) + H_2O \qquad \textit{(Eq. 9-2)}$$

To maintain acid–base balance, the kidney must reclaim and regenerate all the filtered HCO_3^-. The daily amount that must be reabsorbed can be calculated by the product of the glomerular filtration rate (GFR) and the HCO_3^- concentration in ECF (180 L/day GFR × 24 mEq/L HCO_3^- = 4,320 mEq/day).[1] The proximal tubule reabsorbs about 85% of the filtered HCO_3^-. The loop of Henle and the distal tubule reabsorb about 10%.[5] Acid salts, such as HPO_4^- (pK_a of 6.8), that have a pK_a greater than the pH of the urine (titratable acids) can accept a proton and be excreted as the acid, thus regenerating an HCO_3^- anion.[5] Sulfuric acid and other acids with a pK_a less than 4.5 are not titratable. Protons from these acids must be combined with another buffer to be secreted. Glutamine deamination in proximal tubular cells forms NH_3, which accepts these protons. In the collecting tubule, the NH_4^+ produced is lipid insoluble, trapping it in the lumen and causing its excretion, eliminating the proton, and allowing for regeneration of HCO_3^-.[4–6] Figure 9-2 is a simplified illustration of the buffering of these acids.

The daily metabolism of carbohydrates and fats generates about 15,000 mmol of CO_2. Although CO_2 is not an acid, it reversibly combines with H_2O to form carbonic acid (i.e., H_2CO_3). Respiration prevents the accumulation of volatile acid through the exhalation of CO_2. Metabolism of proteins and fats results in several fixed acids and bases. Amino acids such as lysine and arginine have a net positive charge and serve as acids. Compounds such as glutamate, aspartate, and citrate have a negative charge. In general, animal proteins contain more sulfur and phosphates, producing an acidic diet. Vegetarian diets consist of more organic anions, resulting in a more alkaline diet.[7] Normally, fatty acids are metabolized to HCO_3^-; however, during starvation or diabetic ketoacidosis, they may be incompletely oxidized to acetoacetate and β-hydroxybutyric acid.[6] The typical diet generates a net nonvolatile acid load of about 70 to 100 mEq of H^+ (1.0–1.5 mEq/kg) per day.[1,8] Renal excretion of 70 mEq in 2 L of urine each day would require a pH of 1.5. Because the kidney cannot produce a pH less than 4.5, most of this fixed acid load must be buffered. The primary buffers for renal net acid excretion

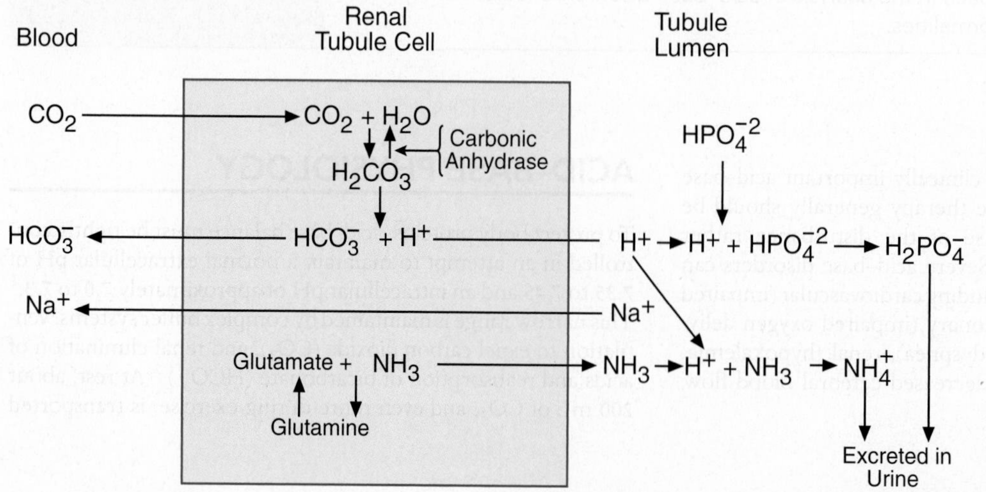

FIGURE 9-2 **Renal tubular hydrogen ion excretion.**

TABLE 9-1
Normal Arterial Blood Gas Values

ABGs	Normal Range
pH	7.36–7.44
Pao_2	90–100 mm Hg
$Paco_2$	35–45 mm Hg
HCO_3^-	22–26 mEq/L

ABG, arterial blood gas.

are NH_3^-/NH_4^+ and titratable buffers, such as $HPO_4^-/H_2PO_4^{2-}$, as mentioned earlier.[7] The correct assessment of acid–base disorders begins with an evaluation of appropriate laboratory data and an understanding of the physiologic mechanisms responsible for maintaining a normal pH.

Laboratory Assessment

Laboratory data used to evaluate acid–base status are arterial pH, arterial carbon dioxide tension ($Paco_2$), and serum bicarbonate (HCO_3^-).[9–11] These values are obtained routinely with an arterial blood gas (ABG) determination. Acid–base abnormalities occur when the concentration of $Paco_2$ (an acid) or HCO_3^- (a base) is altered. ABG measurements also include the arterial oxygen tension (Pao_2); however, this value does not directly influence decisions regarding acid–base abnormalities. Normal ABG values are listed in Table 9-1. When arterial pH is less than 7.35, the patient is considered acidemic, and the process that caused acid–base imbalance is called acidosis. Conversely, when the arterial pH is greater than 7.45, the patient is considered alkalemic, and the causative process is alkalosis. The process is further defined as respiratory in cases of an inappropriate elevation or depression of $Paco_2$ or metabolic with an inappropriate rise or fall in serum HCO_3^-.

Acid–base balance is normally maintained by the primary extracellular buffer system of HCO_3^-/CO_2. Components of this buffer system are measured routinely to assess acid–base status. Other extracellular buffers (e.g., serum proteins, inorganic phosphates) and intracellular buffers (e.g., hemoglobin, proteins, phosphates), however, also contribute significant buffering activity.[1,7–10] Serum electrolytes are obtained to calculate the anion gap, an estimate of the unmeasured cations and anions in serum. The anion gap helps determine the probable cause of a metabolic acidosis.[6,10,12–28] Urine pH, electrolytes, and osmolality help to further differentiate among the possible causes of metabolic acidosis.[10,29–33]

Acid–Base Balance, Carbon Dioxide Tension, and Respiratory Regulation

In aqueous solution, carbonic acid (i.e., H_2CO_3 formed through the reaction described in Eq. 9-1) reversibly dehydrates to form carbon dioxide (CO_2) and water (H_2O) as shown in Eq. 9-2.

The enzyme carbonic anhydrase (CA), present in red blood cells, renal tubular cells, and other tissues, catalyzes the interconversion of carbonic acid and carbon dioxide. Some of the carbon dioxide produced by dehydration of carbonic acid remains dissolved in plasma, but most exists as a volatile gas:

$$HCO_3^- + H^+ \Leftrightarrow H_2CO_3 \overset{CA}{\Leftrightarrow} CO_2\text{ (dissolved)} + H_2O \qquad \textit{(Eq. 9-3)}$$
$$\uparrow\downarrow$$
$$k \times CO_2\text{ (gas)}$$

In Eq. 9-3, k is a solubility constant that has a value of approximately 0.03 in plasma at body temperature.[2,33] Virtually all the carbonic acid in body fluids is in the form of carbon dioxide. The $Paco_2$, a measure of carbon dioxide gas, is therefore directly proportional to the amount of carbonic acid in the HCO_3^-/H_2CO_3 buffer system. The normal range for $Paco_2$ is 35 to 45 mm Hg.

The lungs can rapidly exhale large quantities of carbon dioxide and thereby contribute significantly to the maintenance of a normal pH. Carbon dioxide formed through the reaction described in Eq. 9-3 diffuses easily from tissues to capillary blood and from pulmonary capillary blood into the alveoli where it is exhaled from the body.[3] Pulmonary ventilation is regulated by peripheral chemoreceptors (located in the carotid arteries and the aorta) and central chemoreceptors (located in the medulla). The peripheral chemoreceptors are activated by arterial acidosis, hypercarbia (elevated $Paco_2$), and hypoxemia (decreased Pao_2). Central chemoreceptors are activated by cerebrospinal fluid (CSF) acidosis and by elevated carbon dioxide tension in the CSF.[3] Activation of these chemoreceptors stimulates the respiratory control center in the medulla to increase the rate and depth of ventilation, which results in increased exhalation of carbon dioxide.

BICARBONATE AND RENAL CONTROL

As described in the Acid–Base Physiology section, the kidneys are responsible for regulating the serum bicarbonate concentration. This is accomplished through two important and interrelated functions. First, they must reabsorb the bicarbonate that undergoes glomerular filtration and is present in the renal tubular fluid. Second, the kidneys must excrete hydrogen ions released from nonvolatile acids. Both functions are important in preventing systemic acidosis.

One mechanism of bicarbonate reabsorption in the proximal renal tubule is illustrated in Figure 9-1. Carbonic anhydrase catalyzes intracellular formation of carbonic acid (H_2CO_3) from carbon dioxide (CO_2) and water in the renal tubular cell. The carbonic acid then dissociates to form H^+ and HCO_3^-. The H^+ ion is secreted into the lumen of the tubule in exchange for a sodium ion (Na^+), and the bicarbonate from the renal tubule cell is reabsorbed into the capillary blood.

Inside the lumen, carbonic acid is re-formed from secreted H^+ and filtered HCO_3^-. Carbonic anhydrase present inside the lumen (on the brush border membrane of the cell) catalyzes conversion of carbonic acid to carbon dioxide, which can readily diffuse back into the blood. Thus, the net result is reabsorption of sodium and bicarbonate. Although a hydrogen ion is secreted into the lumen in this process, no net excretion of acid occurs because of the reabsorption of carbon dioxide.[4–6] Figure 9-2 illustrates H^+ excretion by the kidney. This process was also discussed in the Acid–Base Physiology section.

In clinical practice, the serum bicarbonate concentration usually is estimated from the total carbon dioxide content when the serum concentration of electrolytes are ordered on an electrolyte panel or calculated from the pH and $Paco_2$ on an ABG determination. These estimations of the serum bicarbonate concentration are more convenient than directly measuring serum bicarbonate. The total carbon dioxide content that is reported on serum electrolyte panels is determined by acidifying serum to convert all the bicarbonate to carbon dioxide and measuring the partial pressure of CO_2 gas. Approximately 95% of the total carbon dioxide content is bicarbonate. The serum bicarbonate concentration reported on ABG results is calculated from the patient's pH and $Paco_2$ using the Henderson–Hasselbalch equation (Eq. 9-4). This calculated bicarbonate concentration should be within 2 mEq/L of the measured total carbon dioxide. The normal range of serum bicarbonate using these methods is 22 to 26 mEq/L.[10]

BICARBONATE/CARBONIC ACID RATIO

The relationship between the pH and the concentrations of the acid–base pairs in buffer systems is described by the Henderson–Hasselbalch equation:

$$pH = pK + \log \frac{(\text{base})}{(\text{acid})} \qquad (Eq.\ 9\text{-}4)$$

The pK_a is the negative logarithm of the equilibrium constant for the buffer reaction. The pK for the carbonic acid–bicarbonate buffer system is 6.1. Because most of the carbonic acid in plasma is in the form of carbon dioxide gas, the concentration of acid (acid), can be estimated as $Paco_2$ multiplied by 0.03 (the solubility constant, k, in Eq. 9-3). The concentration of base (base) is equal to the serum bicarbonate concentration. Using these values, Eq. 9-4 can be rewritten as follows:

$$pH = 6.1 + \log \frac{(HCO_3^-)}{(0.03)(Paco_2)} \qquad (Eq.\ 9\text{-}5)$$

As shown by Equation 9-5, the arterial pH will be 7.40 when the ratio of HCO_3^-/H_2CO_3 is approximately 20:1. Note that it is the ratio of bicarbonate to the carbon dioxide tension and not the absolute concentration of these factors that determines the arterial pH. Therefore, if the serum bicarbonate concentration and the carbon dioxide tension are increased or decreased proportionately, the ratio remains fixed and the pH is not affected.[32–35]

EVALUATION OF ACID–BASE DISORDERS

Acid–base disorders should be evaluated using a stepwise approach.[31,32]

ONLINE CONTENT

For a narrated PowerPoint presentation that works through the following process, see http://thepoint.lww.com/AT10e.

1. Obtain a detailed patient history and clinical assessment.
2. Check the arterial blood gas, sodium, chloride, and HCO_3^-. Identify all abnormalities in pH, $Paco_2$, and HCO_3^-.
3. Determine which abnormalities are primary and which are compensatory based on pH.
   a. If the pH is less than 7.40, then a respiratory or metabolic acidosis is primary.
   b. If the pH is greater than 7.40, then a respiratory or metabolic alkalosis is primary.
   c. If the pH is normal (7.40) and there are abnormalities in $Paco_2$ and HCO_3^-, a mixed disorder is probably present because metabolic and respiratory compensations rarely return the pH to normal.
4. Always calculate the anion gap. If it is equal to or greater than 20, a clinically important metabolic acidosis is usually present even if the pH is within a normal range.[36]
5. If the anion gap is increased, calculate the excess anion gap (anion gap – 10). Add this value to the HCO_3^- to obtain corrected value.[37]
   a. If the corrected value is greater than 26, a metabolic alkalosis is also present.
   b. If the corrected value is less than 22, a nonanion gap metabolic acidosis is also present.
6. Consider other laboratory tests to further differentiate the cause of the disorder.
   a. If the anion gap is normal, consider calculating the urine anion gap.
   b. If the anion gap is high and a toxic ingestion is expected, calculate an osmolal gap.
   c. If the anion gap is high, measure serum ketones and lactate.
7. Compare the identified disorders to the patient history and begin patient-specific therapy.

METABOLIC ACIDOSIS

Metabolic acidosis is characterized by loss of bicarbonate from the body, decreased acid excretion by the kidney, or increased endogenous acid production. Two categories of simple metabolic acidosis (i.e., normal anion gap and increased anion gap) are listed in Table 9-2. The anion gap (AG) represents the concentration of unmeasured negatively charged substances (anions) in excess of the concentration of unmeasured positively charged substances (cations) in the extracellular fluid. The concentrations of total anions and cations in the body are equal because the body must remain electrically neutral. Most clinical laboratories, however, measure only a portion of these ions (i.e., sodium, chloride $[Cl^-]$, and bicarbonate). The concentrations of other negatively and positively charged substances, such as potassium (K^+), magnesium (Mg^+), calcium (Ca^{2+}), phosphates, and albumin, are measured less often. The concentration of unmeasured anions normally exceeds the concentration of unmeasured cations by 6 to 12 mEq/L, and the anion gap can be calculated as follows:

$$\text{Anion gap} = Na^+ - (Cl^- + HCO_3^-) \qquad (Eq.\ 9\text{-}6)$$

Of the unmeasured anions, albumin is perhaps the most important. In critically ill patients with hypoalbuminemia, the calculated AG should be adjusted using the following formula: adjusted AG = AG + 2.5 × (normal albumin − measured albumin in g/dL), where a normal albumin concentration is assumed to be 4.4 g/dL.[18–21] For example, a hypoalbuminemic patient (serum albumin, 2.4 g/dL) with early sepsis and lactic acidosis might have a calculated AG of 11 mEq/L; however, after the calculation is corrected for the effect of the abnormal serum albumin concentration, the presence of elevated AG acidosis is more prominent

TABLE 9-2
Common Causes of Metabolic Acidosis

Normal AG	Elevated AG
Hypokalemic	**Renal Failure**
Diarrhea	**Lactic Acidosis**
Fistulous disease	(see Table 9-4)
Ureteral diversions	**Ketoacidosis**
Type 1 RTA	Starvation
Type 2 RTA	Ethanol
Carbonic anhydrase inhibitors	Diabetes mellitus
Hyperkalemic	**Drug Intoxications**
Hypoaldosteronism	Ethylene glycol
Hydrochloric acid or precursor	Methanol
Type 4 RTA	Salicylates
Potassium-sparing diuretics	
Amiloride	
Spironolactone	
Triamterene	

AG, anion gap; RTA, renal tubular acidosis.

(the calculated AG is adjusted: $AG_{(adjusted)} = 11$ mEq/L + 2.5 × [normal albumin − measured albumin] = 16 mEq/L).

Metabolic acidosis with a normal AG (e.g., hyperchloremic metabolic acidosis) usually is caused by loss of bicarbonate and can be further characterized as hypokalemic or hyperkalemic.[5,30,33,38–49] Diarrhea can result in severe bicarbonate loss and a hyperchloremic metabolic acidosis. Elevated AG metabolic acidosis usually is associated with overproduction of organic acids or with decreased renal elimination of nonvolatile acids.[33,50–52] Increased production of organic acids (e.g., formic, lactic acids) is buffered by extracellular bicarbonate with resultant consumption of bicarbonate and appearance of an unmeasured anion (e.g., formate, lactate).[31,50,51] The decrement in serum bicarbonate approximates the increment in the AG, the latter being a good estimate of the circulating anion level. Prolonged hypoxia results in lactic acidosis. Uncontrolled diabetes mellitus or excessive alcohol intake with starvation can cause ketoacidosis. In the case of renal failure, the capacity for H^+ secretion diminishes, resulting in metabolic acidosis.[38] The accompanying increased AG results from decreased excretion of unmeasured anions such as sulfate and phosphate.[25]

Normal Anion Gap (Hyperchloremic) Metabolic Acidosis

EVALUATION

CASE 9-1

QUESTION 1: A.B., a 27-year-old, 60-kg woman, is hospitalized for evaluation of weakness. She has a history of bipolar affective disorder and reports recent ingestion of paint from the walls of her house. A.B.'s only current medication is lithium carbonate 300 mg three times a day (TID). On admission, she appears weak and apathetic and complains of anorexia. Laboratory tests reveal the following:

Serum Na, 143 mEq/L
K, 3.0 mEq/L
Cl, 121 mEq/L
Albumin, 4.4 g/dL
pH, 7.28
$Paco_2$, 26 mm Hg
HCO_3^-, 12 mEq/L
Urine pH, 5.5

A.B.'s urine pH after an ammonium chloride (NH_4Cl) 0.1 g/kg IV load is less than 5.1. A bicarbonate load of 1 mEq/kg infused intravenously (IV) for 1 hour induces bicarbonaturia (urinary pH, 7.0) and lowers the serum potassium to 2.0 mEq/L. Her blood pH only increased to 7.31. What type of acid–base disorder is present?

Using a stepwise approach, we see that A.B.'s history gives a clue to the cause for her acidosis. The low pH is consistent with a metabolic acidosis because her CO_2 and HCO_3^- are both reduced (Table 9-2). Alterations in pH resulting from a primary change in serum bicarbonate are metabolic acid–base disorders. Specifically, metabolic acidosis is associated with a decrease in serum HCO_3^- and decreased pH, whereas metabolic alkalosis is associated with an increase in serum HCO_3^- and increased pH. In respiratory disorders, the primary change occurs in the $Paco_2$. If A.B. had a decrease in pH and increase in $Paco_2$, a respiratory acidosis would be present. Because A.B. has a low $Paco_2$ and decreased serum HCO_3^-, she has a metabolic acidosis. In most cases of metabolic acidosis or alkalosis, the lungs compensate for the primary change in serum HCO_3^- concentration by increasing or decreasing ventilation. Most stepwise approaches would next suggest the evaluation of whether the decrease in $Paco_2$ of 14 mm Hg for A.B. is consistent with respiratory compensation (Table 9-3). A primary decrease in the serum bicarbonate to a level of 12 mEq/L should result in a compensatory decrease in the $Paco_2$ concentration by 12 to 17 mm Hg (Table 9-3). A.B.'s $Paco_2$ has fallen by 14 mm Hg (normal, 40 mm Hg; current, 26 mm Hg), confirming that normal respiratory compensation has occurred. When values for $Paco_2$ or serum HCO_3^- fall outside of normal compensatory ranges, either a mixed acid–base disorder, inadequate extent of compensation, or inadequate time for compensation should be suspected.

TABLE 9-3
Normal Compensation in Simple Acid–Base Disorders

Disorder	Compensation[a]
Metabolic acidosis	$\downarrow Paco_2$ (mm Hg) = 1.0 – 1.2 × HCO_3^- (mEq/L)
Metabolic alkalosis	$\uparrow Paco_2$ (mm Hg) = 0.5 – 0.7 × $\uparrow HCO_3^-$ (mEq/L)
Respiratory acidosis	
Acute	$\uparrow HCO_3^-$ (mEq/L) = 0.1 × $\uparrow Paco_2$ (mm Hg)
Chronic	$\uparrow HCO_3^-$ (mEq/L) = 0.4 × $\uparrow Paco_2$ (mm Hg)
Respiratory alkalosis	
Acute	$\downarrow HCO_3^-$ (mEq/L) = 0.2 × $\downarrow Paco_2$ (mm Hg)
Chronic	$\downarrow HCO_3^-$ (mEq/L) = 0.4 – 0.5 × $\downarrow Paco_2$ (mm Hg)

[a] Based on change from normal HCO_3^- = 24 mEq/L and $Paco_2$ = 40 mm Hg.

Nomograms, especially ones that are different for acute and chronic disorders, are inherently difficult to memorize, however, and are often not available to the clinician at the point of care. Following the stepwise approach advocated herein will enable clinicians to identify most clinically important disorders without needing to depend on tables or formulas.

CAUSES

CASE 9-1, QUESTION 2: What are potential causes of metabolic acidosis in A.B.?

Steps 4 to 7 of the stepwise approach in the evaluation of acid–base disorders are used to further determine the cause of the disorder. In patients with metabolic acidosis, calculation of the AG serves as a first step in classifying the metabolic acidosis and provides additional information about conditions that might be responsible. A.B.'s calculated AG is 10 mEq/L (Eq. 9-6). Thus, A.B. has hyperchloremic metabolic acidosis with a normal AG.

The common causes of metabolic acidosis are presented in Table 9-2.[5,10,50] Normal AG metabolic acidosis usually is caused by gastrointestinal loss of bicarbonate (diarrhea, fistulous disease, ureteral diversions); exogenous sources of chloride (normal saline infusions); or altered excretion of hydrogen ions (renal tubular acidosis). A.B. reports a history of both paint ingestion (perhaps lead-based paint) and chronic use of lithium. Both lead and lithium have been associated with the development of renal tubular acidosis.[30,53]

RENAL TUBULAR ACIDOSIS

CASE 9-1, QUESTION 3: How do the results of NH_4Cl and sodium bicarbonate ($NaHCO_3$) loading help identify the type of renal tubular acidosis in A.B.?

Renal tubular acidosis (RTA) is characterized by defective secretion of hydrogen ion in the renal tubule with essentially normal GFR. Many medical conditions and chemical substances have been associated with RTA (Table 9-4).[30,33] The recognized forms are type 1 (distal), type 2 (proximal), and type 4 (distal,

TABLE 9-4
Common Causes of Lactic Acidosis

Type A	Type B
Anemia	Diabetes mellitus
Carbon monoxide poisoning	Liver failure
Congestive heart failure	Renal failure
Shock	Seizure disorder
Sepsis	Leukemia
	Drugs
	Didanosine
	Ethanol
	Isoniazid
	Metformin
	Methanol
	Salicylates
	Zidovudine

hypoaldosterone). Type 1 RTA is caused by a defect in the distal tubule's ability to acidify the urine, type 2 by altered urinary bicarbonate reabsorption in the proximal tubule, and type 4 by hypoaldosteronism and impaired ammoniagenesis.[30,47]

Evaluation of bicarbonate reabsorption during bicarbonate loading and of response to acid loading by infusion of ammonium chloride is useful in distinguishing among the various types of RTA. In healthy subjects, approximately 10% to 15% of the filtered bicarbonate escapes reabsorption in the proximal tubule but is reabsorbed in more distal segments of the nephron. Urine bicarbonate excretion is therefore negligibly small, and urine pH is maintained between 5.5 and 6.5.

Type 2 RTA is associated with a decrease in proximal tubular bicarbonate reabsorption. The distal tubular cells partially compensate for this defect by increasing bicarbonate reabsorption, but urinary bicarbonate excretion still is increased. As occurred with A.B., serum HCO_3^- concentration in patients with type 2 RTA may acutely fall below a threshold of 15 but then stabilize around 15 mEq/L.[10,30] At this point, distal bicarbonate delivery no longer is excessive, allowing the distal nephron to acidify the urine appropriately and excrete acid in the form of titratable ammonia and phosphate.

In type 1 RTA, a defect in net hydrogen ion secretion results from a back-diffusion of H^+ from the tubule lumen to the tubule cell. Patients with type 1 RTA cannot reduce their urine pH below 5.5 even when systemic acidosis is severe.[47]

A.B.'s response to the acid (NH_4Cl) load demonstrates an ability to acidify the urine (i.e., pH <5.1), which helps rule out type 1 RTA. During bicarbonate loading in patients with type 2 RTA, serum bicarbonate concentration is increased, and abnormally large amounts of bicarbonate are again delivered to the distal tubule. Its hydrogen secretory processes are overwhelmed, resulting in bicarbonaturia. Administration of bicarbonate to A.B. produced bicarbonaturia and an elevation in urine pH (7.0), with low blood pH (7.31). These findings indicate that the reabsorption of bicarbonate in the proximal tubule is impaired, which is characteristic of type 2 RTA. Type 4 RTA is unlikely given her initial serum potassium of 3.0 mEq/L.

LEAD-INDUCED

CASE 9-1, QUESTION 4: What is the cause of A.B.'s proximal RTA?

The most likely cause of A.B.'s proximal RTA is her exposure to presumably lead-based paint. The pathogenesis of lead-induced type 2 RTA is unclear. Some studies suggest that carbonic anhydrase deficiency in the proximal tubule is the major factor, but these data are inconclusive.

CASE 9-1, QUESTION 5: Why is A.B. hypokalemic?

Bicarbonate wasting in proximal RTA is associated with sodium loss, extracellular fluid reduction, and activation of the renin-angiotensin-aldosterone axis. Aldosterone increases distal tubular sodium reabsorption and greatly augments potassium and hydrogen ion secretion. This results in potassium wasting, which explains A.B.'s hypokalemia.[54] When plasma bicarbonate achieves steady state, less bicarbonate reaches the distal tubule, and the stimulus for aldosterone release is removed. Therefore, A.B. experiences only a mild depletion of potassium body stores. When A.B. is exposed to bicarbonate loading, the renin-angiotensin-aldosterone axis is reactivated, and hypokalemia worsens. In addition, raising the concentration of bicarbonate in the blood drives potassium intercellularly and contributes to her hypokalemia.

TREATMENT

CASE 9-1, QUESTION 6: What treatment is indicated for A.B.?

Although it is rare for patients with type 2 RTA to develop severe acidosis and potassium depletion chronically, it is not uncommon in an acute situation such as this. A.B. has a bicarbonate deficit; thus, she should be treated with alkali replacement, and the offending agent, if confirmed to be lead, should be removed concurrently. Her serum potassium is also dangerously low, and bicarbonate correction could further decrease it. A.B. needs potassium supplementation. The clinician should obtain hourly blood samples for electrolytes until her potassium is greater than 3.5 mEq/L. In adults such as A.B., chronic treatment often is not needed because acidosis is self-limited. A.B., however, should be treated with sodium bicarbonate until proximal RTA resolves. Very large doses of bicarbonate (6–10 mEq/kg/day) would be required to increase serum bicarbonate to the normal range.[10] In adults with proximal RTA, however, the goal is to increase serum bicarbonate to no more than 18 mEq/L.[30] Bicarbonate can be provided as sodium bicarbonate tablets (8 mEq/600-mg tablet) or Shohl's solution. Shohl's solution, USP, contains 334 mg citric acid and 500 mg sodium citrate per 5 mL. Sodium citrate is metabolized to sodium bicarbonate in the liver. Shohl's solution provides 1 mEq of sodium and 1 mEq of bicarbonate per milliliter of solution. Therapy for A.B. should be initiated with 1 mEq/kg/day. The clinician should monitor A.B.'s lithium levels while she is receiving alkali therapy. Sodium ingestion might increase renal lithium excretion and exacerbate her bipolar disorder. Because of severe hypokalemia resulting from alkali administration, supplemental potassium as chloride, bicarbonate, acetate, or citrate salts also should be administered.

Metabolic Acidosis With Elevated Anion Gap

EVALUATION AND OSMOLAL GAP

CASE 9-2

QUESTION 1: G.D., a 34-year-old, 60-kg man, is brought to the emergency department (ED) by the police in a semicomatose state. He was found lying on the floor of his hotel room 30 minutes ago. G.D. has a long history of alcohol abuse. In the ED, supine blood pressure (BP) is

120/60 mm Hg, pulse is 100 beats/minute, and respiratory rate is 40 breaths/minute. G.D.'s pupils are reactive, and mild papilledema is noted. Laboratory tests reveal the following:

Serum Na, 140 mEq/L
K, 5.8 mEq/L
Cl, 103 mEq/L
Blood urea nitrogen (BUN), 25 mg/dL
Creatinine, 1.4 mg/dL
Fasting glucose, 150 mg/dL

ABG include pH, 7.16; $Paco_2$, 23 mm Hg; and HCO_3^-, 8 mEq/L. His toxicology screen is negative for alcohol, and his serum osmolality is 332 mOsm/kg. What acid–base disturbance is present in G.D., and what are possible causes of the disorder?

G.D. has an acidosis (pH, 7.16; HCO_3^-, 8 mEq/L) with a large AG (29 mEq/L). Subtracting 10 from the anion gap of 29 and adding this value to his serum bicarbonate concentration (see Step 5 in the section Evaluation of Acid–Base Disorders) yields a value of 27, suggesting no other metabolic abnormality is present.

An elevated AG metabolic acidosis often indicates lactic acidosis resulting from intoxications (e.g., salicylates, acetaminophen, methanol, ethylene glycol, paraldehyde, metformin) or ketoacidosis induced by diabetes mellitus, starvation, or alcohol.[14,28,32,38,51,55–60] Step 6 in the stepwise approach leads to the consideration of additional laboratory tests that may be helpful in the differential diagnosis of an elevated AG. These include serum ketones, glucose, lactate, BUN, creatinine, and plasma osmolal gap.[32] Osmolal gap is defined as the difference between measured serum osmolality (SO) and calculated SO using Eq. 9-7.

$$\text{Calculated SO (mOsm/kg)} = 2 \times \text{Na}^+(\text{mEq/L}) + \frac{\text{Glucose (mg/dL)}}{18} + \frac{\text{BUN (mg/dL)}}{2.8} \qquad \textit{(Eq. 9-7)}$$

When the difference between measured and calculated SO is greater than 10 mOsm/kg, the presence of an unmeasured osmotically active substance, such as ethanol, methanol, or ethylene glycol, should be considered.[32,61] G.D.'s calculated SO is 297 mOsm/kg, compared with the measured value of 332; therefore, his osmolal gap is 35 mOsm/kg. An increase in the anion gap and osmolal gap, without diabetic ketoacidosis or chronic renal failure, suggests the possibility of metabolic acidosis resulting from a toxic ingestion.[32] On the basis of G.D.'s presentation (papilledema, history of alcohol abuse, increased osmolal gap, increased AG metabolic acidosis), methanol intoxication should be considered.

CAUSES

METHANOL-INDUCED

CASE 9-2, QUESTION 2: How would G.D.'s methanol intake induce metabolic acidosis with an elevated anion AG?

Methanol intoxication results in the formation of two organic acids, formic and lactic acids, which consume bicarbonate with production of an AG metabolic acidosis. Alcohol dehydrogenase in the liver metabolizes methanol to formaldehyde and then to formic acid. The formic acid contributes to the metabolic acidosis and also is responsible for the retinal edema and blindness associated with methanol intoxication.[32,33,60]

TABLE 9-5
Classification of Metabolic Alkalosis

Saline-Responsive	Saline-Resistant
Diuretic therapy	Normotensive
Extracellular volume contraction	Potassium depletion
Gastric acid loss	Hypercalcemia
Vomiting	Hypertensive
Nasogastric suction	Mineralocorticoids
Exogenous alkali administration	Hyperaldosteronism
Blood transfusions	Hyperreninism
	Licorice

Serum lactic acid concentrations also are increased in patients with methanol intoxication.[32] Lactic acidosis classically has been divided into type A, which is associated with inadequate delivery of oxygen to the tissue, and type B, which is associated with defective oxygen utilization at the mitochondrial level (Table 9-5). Although these distinctions often are not clear, the lactic acidosis caused by methanol intoxication is most consistent with the type B variety.[62]

TREATMENT

CASE 9-2, QUESTION 3: How should G.D.'s methanol intoxication be managed acutely?

ANTIDOTES

Because G.D.'s mental status is impaired and his respiratory rate is 40 breaths/minute, his airway was secured via endotracheal intubation and he was placed on mechanical ventilatory support. Even though both ethanol and fomepizole compete with methanol for alcohol dehydrogenase binding sites and could be used to treat G.D., fomepizole is chosen because it is easier to dose and does not need serum level monitoring to ensure efficacy like ethanol.[33,60–64] Because ethanol and fomepizole have much greater affinity for alcohol dehydrogenase than methanol, these agents may reduce the conversion of methanol to its toxic metabolite, formic acid. The unmetabolized methanol then is excreted by the lungs and kidneys. Fomepizole can be given IV as a 15 mg/kg loading dose for 30 minutes, followed by bolus doses of 10 mg/kg every 12 hours. Because of induction of metabolism of fomepizole, doses should be increased to 15 mg/kg every 12 hours if therapy is required beyond 2 days.[60] Fomepizole is usually continued until the serum methanol concentration is less than 20 mg/dL (6.2 mmol/L). Adverse effects of fomepizole are relatively mild; G.D. should be monitored for headache, nausea, dizziness, agitation, metallic taste, abnormal smell, and rash. Because of its high cost and infrequent use, some hospitals might not have fomepizole readily available. In such cases, ethanol is an alternative. Administration of IV ethanol as an antidote can be technically difficult and may produce central nervous system (CNS) depression.[60,63] For G.D., an IV loading dose of 0.6 g/kg ethanol solution should be administered over the course of 30 minutes, followed by a continuous infusion of about 150 mg/kg/hour if the patient has been drinking, or 70 mg/kg/hour for nondrinkers if the patient was not drinking. Serum ethanol concentration should be maintained at more than 100 mg/dL.[33,62] Charcoal may be considered to bind other agents that may be coingested.[33,65]

When other low-molecular-weight toxins, such as ethanol or ethylene glycol, are not present, the serum methanol level can be estimated by multiplying the patient's osmolal gap by a standardized conversion factor of 2.6. G.D.'s osmolal gap of 35 mOsm/L, therefore, may reflect a methanol level of approximately 91 mg/dL (35 mOsm/L × 2.6). When methanol blood levels are higher than 50 mg/dL, hemodialysis is indicated to rapidly reduce concentrations of methanol and its toxic metabolite. The dosage of fomepizole or ethanol should be increased in patients receiving hemodialysis to account for the increased elimination of these antidotes.[33,62] Ethylene glycol poisoning can also be treated by using fomepizole or ethanol.

BICARBONATE

Severe acidosis causes reduced myocardial contractility, impaired response to catecholamines, and impaired oxygen delivery to tissues as a result of 2,3-diphosphoglycerate depletion. For this reason, some clinicians have judiciously administered IV sodium bicarbonate to patients with metabolic acidosis in an attempt to raise the arterial pH to about 7.20.[66–68] If IV sodium bicarbonate is given, the amount required to correct serum HCO_3^- and arterial pH can be estimated using Eq. 9-8 as follows:

$$\text{Bicarbonate dose (mEq)} = 0.5\ \text{(L/kg)} \times \text{Body weight (kg)} \times \text{Desired increase in serum } HCO_3^-\ \text{(mEq/L)} \qquad \textit{(Eq. 9-8)}$$

Bicarbonate distributes to approximately 50% of total body weight (thus, the factor of 0.5 L/kg in Eq. 9-8). To prevent overtreating, bicarbonate doses should only attempt to increase the bicarbonate concentration by 4 to 8 mEq/L (see Case 9-2, Question 4).[67] For G.D., the dose required to raise serum bicarbonate from 8 to 12 mEq/L amounts to 120 mEq of bicarbonate (0.5 L/kg × 60 kg × 4 mEq/L; Eq. 9-8). Clinical assessment of the effect of bicarbonate can be determined about 30 minutes after administration.[67] Arterial pH and serum bicarbonate concentrations should be obtained before any additional therapy.

RISKS OF BICARBONATE THERAPY

CASE 9-2, QUESTION 4: What are the risks of G.D.'s bicarbonate therapy?

Concerns about the risks of bicarbonate administration and the failure of studies to demonstrate significant short-term benefits have raised questions about the appropriateness of bicarbonate therapy in metabolic acidosis, particularly in ketoacidosis and lactic acidosis caused by cardiac arrest or other hypoxic events.[68–75] Bicarbonate administration can result in overalkalinization and a paradoxical transient intracellular acidosis. Whereas arterial pH can increase rapidly after bicarbonate administration, intracellular pH increases more slowly because of slow penetration of the negatively charged bicarbonate ion across cell membranes. The bicarbonate in plasma, however, is converted rapidly to carbonic acid, and the carbon dioxide tension increases as a result (Eq. 9-2). Because CO_2 diffuses into cells more rapidly than HCO_3^-, the intracellular HCO_3^-/CO_2 ratio decreases, resulting in a decrease in intracellular pH. This intracellular acidosis will persist as long as bicarbonate administration exceeds the CO_2 excretion; therefore, adequate tissue perfusion and ventilation must be provided in patients with diminished CO_2 excretion (e.g., cardiac or pulmonary failure).[70]

Overalkalinization also will cause a shift to the left in the oxygen–hemoglobin dissociation curve. This shift increases hemoglobin affinity for oxygen, decreases oxygen delivery to tissues, and potentially increases lactic acid production and accumulation.[33] Sodium bicarbonate administration also can cause hypernatremia, hyperosmolality, and volume overload; however, the excessive sodium and water retention usually can be avoided by the administration of loop diuretics.[33,61] Hypokalemia is another potential adverse effect of bicarbonate therapy. Acidosis stimulates movement of potassium from intracellular to extracellular fluid in exchange for hydrogen ions. When acidosis is corrected, potassium ions move intracellularly, and hypokalemia can occur. This translocation of potassium tends to reduce serum potassium levels by about 0.4 to 0.6 mEq/L for each 0.1 unit increase in pH, although wide interpatient variability in this relationship exists.[5,8] In G.D. and other patients with organic acid intoxications, raising extracellular pH helps to provide a gradient to shift the toxin from the CNS and "trap" it into the blood and urine, enhancing elimination. To prevent the risks of bicarbonate therapy, G.D.'s mental status, serum sodium and potassium levels, and ABG should be monitored.

ALTERNATIVE ALKALINIZING THERAPY

Although sodium bicarbonate is the most commonly used agent to raise arterial pH, alternative therapies are available. Sodium lactate and acetate have been used in select patients; however, these agents, which require metabolic conversion to bicarbonate, are associated with many of the same risks as sodium bicarbonate (i.e., sodium and fluid overload, overalkalinization, carbon dioxide production).[38]

Tromethamine acetate (THAM), a sodium-free organic amine with a pH of 8.6, is available commercially as a 0.3 mol/L (36 mg/mL) solution for IV administration. THAM can combine with hydrogen ions from carbonic acid and lactic, pyruvic, or other metabolic acids; however, its role in the management of metabolic acidosis needs clarification. THAM may produce hyperkalemia in patients with renal impairment and is contraindicated in anuric or uremic patients. Administration of THAM also has been associated with other serious side effects, including respiratory depression, increased coagulation times, and hypoglycemia.[76–79] Carbicarb and dichloroacetate have been used investigationally in the treatment of metabolic acidosis.[38,62,81] Carbicarb and THAM are better than bicarbonate at improving extracellular pH and bicarbonate and intracellular pH, while not increasing CO_2; however, neither has yet resulted in better patient outcomes.[5,24,71] Hemofiltration and continuous renal replacement therapies have been advocated for patients with lactic acidosis, especially in Europe; however, their roles need further study.

METABOLIC ALKALOSIS

Metabolic alkalosis is associated with an increase in serum bicarbonate concentration and a compensatory increase in $Paco_2$ (caused by hypoventilation). The two general classifications of metabolic alkalosis, saline-responsive and saline-resistant (Table 9-6), are usually distinguishable based on an assessment of the patient's volume status, BP, and urinary chloride concentration.

Saline-responsive metabolic alkalosis is associated with disorders that result in the loss of chloride-rich, bicarbonate-poor fluid from the body (e.g., vomiting, nasogastric suction, diuretic therapy, cystic fibrosis). Physical examination may reveal volume depletion (e.g., orthostatic hypotension, tachycardia, poor skin turgor), and the urinary chloride concentration often will be less than 10 to 20 mEq/L (although urine chloride levels may be >20 mEq/L in patients with recent diuretic use).[10,34,81]

Severe hypokalemia or excessive mineralocorticoid activity can result in a saline-resistant metabolic alkalosis, but this disorder is rare in comparison with saline-responsive metabolic alkalosis. Saline-resistant metabolic alkalosis should be suspected in alkalemic patients with evidence of increased ECF volume,

TABLE 9-6
Common Causes of Respiratory Acidosis

Airway Obstruction	Cardiopulmonary
Foreign body aspiration	Cardiac arrest
Asthma	Pulmonary edema or infiltration
COPD	Pulmonary embolism
Adrenergic blockers	Pulmonary fibrosis
CNS Disturbances	**Neuromuscular**
Cerebral vascular accident	Amyotrophic lateral sclerosis
Sleep apnea	Guillain-Barré syndrome
Tumor	Myasthenia gravis
CNS depressant drugs	Hypokalemia
Barbiturates	Hypophosphatemia
Benzodiazepines	Drugs
Opioids	Aminoglycosides
	Antiarrhythmics
	Lithium
	Phenytoin

CNS, central nervous system; COPD, chronic obstructive pulmonary disease.

hypertension, or high urinary chloride values (>20 mEq/L) without recent diuretic use.[10,81]

Evaluation

CASE 9-3

QUESTION 1: K.E., a 60-year-old, 50-kg woman, was admitted to the hospital 4 days ago with peripheral edema and pulmonary congestion consistent with a congestive heart failure exacerbation. Since admission, she has been treated aggressively with furosemide 80 to 120 mg IV daily, which has generated approximately 3 L of urine output each day. Her chest radiograph findings and peripheral edema now show considerable improvement with diuresis; however, she now complains of dizziness when she gets out of bed to go to the bathroom. Physical examination reveals a tachycardic (heart rate [HR], 100 beats/minute), thin elderly woman with poor skin turgor and slight muscle weakness. K.E.'s electrocardiogram shows flattened T waves and U waves. Laboratory tests reveal the following:

Serum Na, 138 mEq/L
K, 2.5 mEq/L
Cl, 92 mEq/L
Creatinine, 0.9 mg/dL
BUN, 28 mg/dL
pH, 7.49
$Paco_2$, 46 mm Hg
HCO_3^-, 34 mEq/L

Urine Cl concentration is 60 mEq/L. What acid–base disorder is present in K.E.?

Using the stepwise approach to the evaluation of acid–base disorders as previously described, K.E.'s elevated pH is consistent with alkalosis.

For a case that demonstrates how these steps would be worked through, see the narrated PowerPoint presentation at http://thepoint.lww.com/AT10e.

Furosemide-induced diuresis may be a clue to her acid–base disorder. The increased serum HCO_3^- and increased $Paco_2$ suggest primary metabolic alkalosis with respiratory compensation. K.E.'s anion gap is 12, suggesting no additional metabolic acid–base abnormalities are present. A $Paco_2$ of 46 mm Hg suggests normal respiratory compensation for metabolic alkalosis. Appropriate treatment of the metabolic alkalosis should return her $Paco_2$ to normal if there is no underlying pulmonary disease.

Causes

DIURETIC-INDUCED

CASE 9-3, QUESTION 2: What is the most likely cause of K.E.'s acid–base imbalance?

Common causes of metabolic alkalosis are listed in Table 9-5. The hypokalemic, hypochloremic, metabolic alkalosis in K.E. most likely is the result of diuretic-induced volume contraction. The incidence of this adverse effect is influenced by the type, dose, and dosing frequency of the diuretic.

Diuretics cause metabolic alkalosis (sometimes referred to as a "contraction alkalosis") by the following mechanisms. First, they enhance excretion of sodium chloride and water, resulting in extracellular volume contraction. Volume contraction alone will cause only a modest increase in plasma bicarbonate; however, volume contraction also stimulates aldosterone release. Aldosterone increases distal tubular sodium reabsorption and induces hydrogen ion and potassium secretion, resulting in alkalosis and hypokalemia. In addition, hypokalemia induced by diuretics will stimulate intracellular movement of hydrogen ions to replace cellular potassium, producing extracellular alkalosis. Hypochloremia also is important in sustaining metabolic alkalosis. In a hypochloremic state, sodium will be reabsorbed, accompanied by bicarbonate generated by secreted hydrogen (Fig. 9-1).[81–83]

Treatment

CASE 9-3, QUESTION 3: How should K.E.'s acid–base imbalance be corrected and monitored?

Treatment of metabolic alkalosis depends on removal of the cause. K.E.'s diuretic therapy should be temporarily discontinued until her volume status and electrolytes can be restored. The initial goal is to correct fluid deficits and replace chloride and potassium by infusing sodium and potassium chloride. As long as hypochloremia exists, renal bicarbonate excretion will not occur and the alkalosis will not be corrected.[82] The severity of alkalosis dictates how rapidly fluid and electrolytes should be administered. In patients with hepatic or renal failure or congestive heart failure, infusion of large volumes of sodium and potassium salts can produce fluid overload or hyperkalemia. Thus, fluid and electrolyte replacement should proceed cautiously, and these patients should be monitored closely for these complications.

Potassium chloride should be administered to correct K.E.'s hypokalemia. The amount of potassium required to replace total body stores is difficult to determine accurately because 98% of the potassium in the body is intracellular. Although wide variation exists, for each 1 mEq/L decrease in K^+ from an ECF concentration of 4 mEq/L, the total body K^+ deficit is about 4 to 5 mEq/kg.[10] K.E.'s serum potassium is 2.5 mEq/L, which correlates with a decrease of about 350 mEq in total body potassium stores. K.E. should be treated with the chloride salt to ensure potassium retention and correction of alkalosis. Potassium replacement can be achieved over the course of several days with supplements of 100 to 150 mEq/day given either orally in divided doses or as a constant IV infusion. K.E.'s laboratory tests for BUN, creatinine, chloride, sodium, and potassium should be monitored during sodium and potassium chloride therapy. As noted earlier, hypercapnia should disappear after correction of the alkalemia, and can be confirmed with an ABG, if clinically indicated.

CASE 9-3, QUESTION 4: What other agents are available to treat K.E.'s alkalosis if fluid and electrolyte replacement does not correct the arterial pH?

Patients unresponsive to sodium and potassium chloride therapy or those at risk for complications with these agents can be treated with acetazolamide, hydrochloric acid (HCl), or a hydrochloric acid precursor. The most commonly used agent is acetazolamide, a carbonic anhydrase inhibitor that blocks hydrogen ion secretion in the renal tubule, resulting in increased excretion of sodium and bicarbonate. Although the serum bicarbonate concentration often improves with acetazolamide, metabolic alkalosis may not completely resolve. Other concerns with the use of acetazolamide include its ability to promote kaliuresis and its relative lack of effect in patients with renal dysfunction.[81,84,85]

A solution of 0.1 N HCl may be administered to patients who require rapid correction of alkalemia. The dose of HCl is based on the bicarbonate excess using Eq. 9-9, where the factor 0.5 × body weight (kg) represents the estimated bicarbonate space.[10,81,82,84]

$$\text{Dose of HCl (mEq)} = 0.5 \times \text{Body weight (kg)} \times (\text{plasma bicarbonate} - 24) \quad \textit{(Eq. 9-9)}$$

Parenteral hydrochloric acid is prepared extemporaneously by adding the appropriate amount of 1 N HCl through a 0.22-μm filter into a glass bottle containing 5% dextrose or normal saline. The dilute solution should be administered through a central venous catheter in the superior vena cava to reduce the risk of extravasation and tissue damage. The infusion rate should not exceed 0.2 mEq/kg/hour.[84] ABG should be monitored at least every 4 hours during the infusion. HCl should not be added to total nutrient solutions.[85]

Precursors of hydrochloric acid, such as ammonium and arginine hydrochloride, are not recommended.[81] The adverse effect profile of these agents has significantly limited their role.[84] Ammonium hydrochloride is metabolized to HCl and NH_3 in the liver. Severe ammonia intoxication with CNS depression can occur during rapid infusion of ammonium hydrochloride or in patients with liver disease.[81] Arginine can cause rapid shifts in potassium from the intracellular to the extracellular space, resulting in dangerous hyperkalemia.[81]

RESPIRATORY ACIDOSIS

Respiratory acidosis occurs as a result of inadequate ventilation by the lungs. When the lungs do not excrete CO_2 effectively, the $Paco_2$ rises. This elevation in $Paco_2$ (a functional acid) causes a fall in pH (Eqs. 9-3 and 9-5). Common causes of respiratory acidosis are listed in Table 9-7. They generally can be categorized into conditions of airway obstruction, reduced stimulus for respiration from the CNS, failure of the heart or lungs, and disorders of the peripheral nerves or skeletal muscles required for ventilation.[86]

TABLE 9-7
Common Causes of Respiratory Alkalosis

CNS Disturbances	Pulmonary
Bacterial septicemia	Pneumonia
Cerebrovascular accident	Pulmonary edema
Fever	Pulmonary embolus
Hepatic cirrhosis	**Tissue Hypoxia**
Hyperventilation	High altitude
Anxiety-induced	Hypotension
Voluntary	CHF
Meningitis	**Other**
Pregnancy	Excessive mechanical ventilation
Trauma	Rapid correction of metabolic acidosis
Drugs	
Progesterone derivatives	
Respiratory stimulants	
Salicylate overdose	

CHF, congestive heart failure; CNS, central nervous system.

Evaluation

CASE 9-4

QUESTION 1: B.B., a 56-year-old man, is admitted to the hospital for treatment of an exacerbation of chronic obstructive pulmonary disease (COPD). He complains of worsening shortness of breath and increased production of sputum for the past 3 days. He has also noted a mild headache, a flushed feeling, and drowsiness within the past 24 hours. He has a history of COPD, hypertension, coronary artery disease, and low back pain. Current medications are ipratropium inhaler two puffs four times a day (QID), salmeterol dry powder inhaler one inhalation twice a day (BID), hydrochlorothiazide 25 mg daily, long-acting diltiazem 240 mg daily, and diazepam 5 mg TID as needed for back pain.

Vital signs include respiratory rate of 16 breaths/minute and HR of 90 beats/minute. Diffuse wheezes and rhonchi are heard on chest auscultation. Laboratory tests reveal the following:

Na, 140 mEq/L
K, 4.0 mEq/L
Cl, 100 mEq/L
pH, 7.32
$Paco_2$, 58 mm Hg
Pao_2, 58 mm Hg
HCO_3^-, 29 mEq/L

B.B's baseline ABG at the physician's office last month was pH, 7.35; $Paco_2$, 51 mm Hg; Pao_2, 62 mm Hg; and HCO_3^-, 28 mEq/L. Which of B.B.'s signs and symptoms are consistent with the diagnosis of respiratory acidosis?

A stepwise evaluation reveals a respiratory acidosis. A history of COPD and physical findings of dyspnea, headache, drowsiness, and flushing support the ABG evaluation. Respiratory acidosis also can cause more severe symptoms, including CNS effects, such as disorientation, confusion, delirium, hallucinations, and coma. These CNS abnormalities probably are partly caused by the direct effects of carbon dioxide. Hypoxemia (decreased Pao_2), which commonly accompanies respiratory acidosis, also contributes to these symptoms. Elevated $Paco_2$ causes cerebral vascular dilation, resulting in headache caused by increased blood flow and increased intracranial pressure. Cardiovascular effects typically include tachycardia, arrhythmias, and peripheral vasodilation.[87]

CASE 9-4, QUESTION 2: Is the respiratory acidosis present in B.B. consistent with an acute or a chronic disorder?

Following the stepwise approach, it is determined that B.B. has a respiratory acidosis. He has a normal AG. Comparing his current to previous values (e.g., pH, $Paco_2$, HCO_3^-), it appears B.B. has an acute-on-chronic respiratory acidosis because his baseline $Paco_2$ was 51 mm Hg with an acute worsening to 58 mm Hg. In respiratory acidosis, increased renal reabsorption of bicarbonate compensates for the increase in $Paco_2$; however, at least 48 to 72 hours are needed for this compensatory mechanism to become fully established.[10] Patients with COPD commonly present with an acute-on-chronic respiratory acidosis similar to B.B.

Causes

CASE 9-4, QUESTION 3: What potential causes of respiratory acidosis are present in B.B.?

Respiratory acidosis often is caused by airway obstruction, as shown in Table 9-7.[86,87] Chronic obstructive airway disease is a common cause of both acute and chronic respiratory acidosis. Upper respiratory tract infections, such as acute bronchitis, can worsen airway obstruction and produce acute respiratory acidosis.

DRUG-INDUCED

B.B.'s drug therapy also may be contributing to respiratory insufficiency. Many drugs (Table 9-7) decrease ventilation, but usually these drugs only significantly affect patients who are predisposed to respiratory problems because of underlying diseases. Because B.B. has COPD, he may be more sensitive to drugs affecting respiration. The benzodiazepines, barbiturates, and opioids minimally decrease respiration in normal subjects and in most patients with COPD when given in usual therapeutic doses. These drugs, however, can cause significant respiratory insufficiency when administered either in large doses or in combination with other respiratory depressant drugs.[87] B.B.'s diazepam may be contributing to hypoventilation and respiratory acidosis and should be withdrawn from his regimen. Nonselective adrenergic blocking drugs should not be used in patients with COPD.

Treatment

CASE 9-4, QUESTION 4: How should B.B.'s respiratory acidosis be treated?

As with most cases of respiratory acidosis, treatment primarily involves correction of the underlying cause of respiratory insufficiency. In this case, treatment of acute bronchospasm with ipratropium or a β-adrenergic agent, such as inhaled albuterol, is warranted. Corticosteroids, such as methylprednisolone (60–125 mg every 6–12 hours initially), are commonly used in hospitalized patients with acute exacerbations of COPD.[88] Antibiotic therapy with a β-lactam or β-lactamase inhibitor should be considered in hospitalized patients producing purulent, large-volume secretions.[89] B.B's respiratory status should be monitored closely during his hospitalization. If the acidosis, hypercarbia, or associated hypoxemia worsen, noninvasive positive-pressure ventilation or intubation with mechanical ventilation may be required.[67]

Treatment with IV sodium bicarbonate is not recommended in most cases of acute respiratory acidosis because of the risks associated with bicarbonate therapy (see Case 9-2, Question 4) and because an absolute deficiency of bicarbonate is not present. When the excess CO_2 is excreted, arterial pH should return to normal. Hypercapnia should not be overcorrected, because

TABLE 9-8

Laboratory Values in Simple Acid–Base Disorders

Disorder	Arterial pH	Primary Change	Compensatory Change
Metabolic acidosis	↓	↓HCO_3^-	↓$Paco_2$
Respiratory acidosis	↓	↑$Paco_2^-$	↑HCO_3^-
Metabolic alkalosis	↑	↑HCO_3^-	↑$Paco_2$
Respiratory alkalosis	↑	↓$Paco_2^-$	↓HCO_3^-

hypocapnia results in decreased lung compliance, increases dysfunctional surfactant production, and shifts the oxyhemoglobin dissociation curve to the left, restricting the release of oxygen to tissues.[74,75,90]

RESPIRATORY ALKALOSIS

Respiratory alkalosis usually is not a severe disorder. Excessive rate or depth of respiration results in increased excretion of carbon dioxide, a fall in $Paco_2$, and a rise in arterial pH. Common causes of respiratory alkalosis are presented in Table 9-8. Many conditions can cause respiratory alkalosis by stimulating respiratory drive in the CNS. In addition, pulmonary diseases can stimulate receptors in the lung to increase ventilation, and conditions that decrease oxygen delivery to tissues also can stimulate ventilation, causing respiratory alkalosis.[91,92]

Evaluation

CASE 9-5

QUESTION 1: S.P., a 35-year-old, 60-kg woman, is admitted for treatment of presumed bacterial pneumonia. She was in good health until 24 hours before presentation when she noted a fever; onset of a productive cough with thick, yellowish sputum; and chest pain on deep inspiration. She has taken aspirin 650 mg every 4 hours since the onset of fever, with mild relief. Since arriving in the ED, she has become anxious and lightheaded and has developed tingling in her hands, feet, and lips. Vital signs include the following: temperature, 38°C; respiratory rate, 24 breaths/minute; HR, 110 beats/minute; and BP, 135/70 mm Hg. Physical examination reveals dullness to percussion, rales, and decreased breath sounds over the left lower lung field.

Laboratory findings include the following:

Serum Na, 135 mEq/L
Cl, 105 mEq/L
pH, 7.49
$Paco_2$, 30 mm Hg
Pao_2, 90 mm Hg
HCO_3^-, 22 mEq/L

Gram stain of sputum reveals 25 white blood cells (WBC) per high-power field and many gram-positive diplococci. WBC count is 15,400 cells/μL with a left shift. A left lower lobe infiltrate is seen on chest radiograph. What acid–base disorder is present in S.P.?

Steps 1 to 3 in the evaluation of the ABG values, as described previously, indicate a respiratory alkalosis (increased pH, decreased $Paco_2$). The history and physical findings of deep, rapid breathing and tingling sensations are clues to the etiology. This disorder is most likely acute because her HCO_3^- concentration is normal. She does not have an AG. If a large AG were present, it would suggest she has a coexisiting metabolic acidosis, possibly caused by salicylate intoxication (see Case 9-5, Question 3).

CASE 9-5, QUESTION 2: Which of S.P.'s signs and symptoms are consistent with the diagnosis of acute respiratory alkalosis?

S.P.'s paresthesias of the extremities and perioral region, lightheadedness, tachycardia, and increased rate and depth of respiration are common signs and symptoms of respiratory alkalosis. Confusion and decreased mental acuity also may be evident.[5,6,10] Simple respiratory alkalosis rarely produces life-threatening abnormalities.

Causes

CASE 9-5, QUESTION 3: What is the cause of the acid–base disorder in S.P.?

Common causes of respiratory alkalosis are listed in Table 9-7.[5,6,10,91–93] Based on physical examination, laboratory findings, and chest radiograph, S.P. appears to have an acute bacterial pneumonia. Pneumonia and other pulmonary diseases can result in stimulation of ventilation and respiratory alkalosis, even with a normal Pao_2, as in this case. The anxiety S.P. is experiencing also may be contributing to respiratory alkalosis by producing the familiar anxiety-hyperventilation syndrome. Although salicylate intoxication is a potential cause of respiratory alkalosis because of the direct respiratory stimulant effect of salicylate,[93] S.P. displays few other symptoms of salicylate intoxication (e.g., nausea, vomiting, tinnitus, altered mental status, elevated AG metabolic acidosis). The total aspirin dose reportedly ingested (65 mg/kg in 24 hours) is not large enough to be associated with significant risk for toxicity.

Treatment

CASE 9-5, QUESTION 4: What is the appropriate treatment for S.P.'s respiratory alkalosis?

Similar to respiratory acidosis, treatment of respiratory alkalosis usually involves correcting the underlying disorder. Initiation of appropriate antibiotic therapy for a community-acquired pneumonia is indicated in this case (see Chapter 64, Respiratory Tract Infections). Simple respiratory alkalosis is unlikely to cause life-threatening symptoms, although mortality rates for critically ill patients with this disorder can be high.[87] The well-known remedy of rebreathing expired air from a paper bag for treatment of hyperventilation associated with anxiety appears to be effective for this cause of respiratory alkalosis and may be helpful for S.P.

MIXED ACID–BASE DISORDERS

Evaluation

CASE 9-6

QUESTION 1: B.L., a 58-year-old man who was transferred from a nursing home 2 days previously, is disorientated and lethargic. He was doing well until 1 week before admission, when the staff noted that he was somnolent. He progressively became more lethargic and could no longer remember the names of other persons. B.L. has a history of alcoholic cirrhosis, type 2 diabetes mellitus, and hypertension. Medications before admission were nadolol 80 mg daily, isosorbide mononitrate 20 mg BID, glyburide 10 mg daily, and spironolactone 50 mg BID. On admission, B.L. was disoriented to person, place, and time and was difficult to arouse. Vital signs include the following: temperature, 37°C; respirations, 16 breaths/minute; HR, 70 beats/minute; and BP, 154/92 mm Hg. Physical examination revealed asterixis and mild ascites. Laboratory studies included the following:

Na, 133 mEq/L	**Albumin, 3.2 g/dL**
K, 4.3 mEq/L	**Ammonia, 120 μmol/L**
Cl, 106 mEq/L	**pH, 7.43**
BUN, 5 mg/dL	**$Paco_2$, 30 mm Hg**
Creatinine, 0.7 mg/dL	**Pao_2, 90 mm Hg**
Fasting glucose, 150 mg/dL	**HCO_3^-, 19 mEq/L**

On admission, spironolactone was increased to 75 mg BID and lactulose 60 mL orally (PO) QID was started for treatment of hepatic encephalopathy. Within the first 24 hours of lactulose therapy, B.L. produced four loose, watery stools; however, his mental status worsened to the point of being unresponsive, his BP dropped to 100/60 mm Hg, and his breathing became labored and eventually required mechanical ventilation. At the time of intubation, his laboratory values were as follows:

Na, 136 mEq/L	**Arterial pH, 7.06**
K, 4.5 mEq/L	**$Paco_2$, 48 mm Hg**
Cl, 105 mEq/L	**Pao_2, 58 mm Hg**
BUN, 10 mg/dL	**HCO_3^-, 13 mEq/L**
Creatinine, 1.2 mg/dL	

Gram stain of peritoneal fluid revealed many WBC and gram-negative rods; the diagnosis of spontaneous bacterial peritonitis with possible septicemia is made. Describe B.L.'s acid–base status on admission and at the current time.

An evaluation of B.L.'s ABG using Steps 1 and 2 (in the section Evaluation of Acid–Base Disorders) reveals abnormal $Paco_2$ and serum bicarbonate values, suggesting the existence of an underlying acid–base abnormality. The direction of change in his $Paco_2$ and serum HCO_3^-, along with a pH of 7.43, suggests a respiratory alkalosis is the primary disorder. His calculated AG of 8 is not increased. Examination of the ranges of expected compensation in Table 9-3 reveals that these values are indeed consistent with chronic respiratory alkalosis (serum HCO_3^- decreased by 0.5 mEq/L for each 1 mm Hg drop in $Paco_2$). B.L.'s history of alcohol-induced liver disease is consistent with the diagnosis of chronic respiratory alkalosis (Table 9-8).[8,10]

The second set of ABG reveals severe acidosis. B.L.'s serum bicarbonate has fallen from 19 to 13 mEq/L, and his $Paco_2$ has increased acutely from 30 to 48 mm Hg. Because these values have changed in opposite directions, a mixed acid–base abnormality should be suspected.

The diagnosis of a mixed metabolic and respiratory acidosis can be confirmed by applying the stepwise approach outlined previously. If the acidosis were purely metabolic in nature, a serum HCO_3^- of 13 mEq/L should result in hyperventilation and a low $Paco_2$. B.L.'s $Paco_2$ of 48 mm Hg is high, which would be consistent with coexistent respiratory acidosis. The anion gap is 18, indicating an AG metabolic acidosis is present. The excess AG ($AG - 10 = 8$) added to B.L's gap of 18 yields a corrected HCO_3^- of 26, which is normal. This suggests no additional metabolic disturbances are present.

Causes

CASE 9-6, QUESTION 2: What are possible causes for the mixed acidosis in B.L.?

The AG should be calculated in all patients with a metabolic acidosis. B.L.'s calculated AG has increased from 8 to 18 mEq/L (11 and 21 mEq/L, respectively, after adjusting for hypoalbuminemia), suggesting that an elevated AG acidosis is now present. Septicemia from bacterial peritonitis can produce profound hypotension, which leads to tissue hypoperfusion, generation of lactic acid, and a subsequent elevation in the AG. Other causes of elevated AG metabolic acidosis can be excluded with additional laboratory data (e.g., serum ketones, glucose, osmolal gap).

Although diarrhea and spironolactone should be considered in the differential diagnosis, these are usually associated with hyperchloremic, normal AG metabolic acidosis (Table 9-2).[94] The coexisting respiratory acidosis is most likely the result of B.L.'s altered mental status and his diminished respiratory drive.

CASE 9-6, QUESTION 3: During the next 6 hours, B.L.'s hepatic encephalopathy, peritonitis, and acid–base disorders are aggressively treated with lactulose, antibiotics, fluids, and mechanical ventilation. His most recent ABG reveals the following:

pH, 7.45
$Paco_2$, 24 mm Hg
Pao_2, 90 mm Hg
HCO_3^-, 16 mEq/L

Ventilator settings are assist-control mode at 16 breaths/minute, tidal volume 700 mL, and inspired oxygen concentration 40%. B.L. is noted to be more awake, anxious, and initiating 25 to 30 breaths/minute. What is the current acid–base status and probable cause?

Evaluation of the ABG reveals a pH at the upper limit of normal with significant decreases in both $Paco_2$ and serum HCO_3^- concentration. This clinical scenario is most consistent with a mixed acute respiratory alkalosis and ongoing metabolic acidosis. The time frame in which B.L.'s $Paco_2$ decreased from 48 to 24 mm Hg is consistent with acute respiratory alkalosis. B.L.'s low serum HCO_3^- suggests ongoing metabolic acidosis as a result of his septicemia. The metabolic acidosis should improve with time, given adequate antibiotic therapy and supportive measures that maintain BP and increase oxygen delivery to the tissues.

The acute respiratory alkalosis in this case is most likely caused by the mechanical ventilator, B.L.'s anxiety, or sepsis. In the assist-control mode, any inspiratory effort by B.L. results in delivery of a full assisted breath by the ventilator.[95] B.L.'s anxiety and resultant tachypnea are stimulating the ventilator to hyperventilate him, producing excessive CO_2 excretion and respiratory alkalosis. Appropriate changes in therapy may include use of an anxiolytic, an analgesic if needed to treat pain, changing the ventilator mode, or probably a combination of these strategies.

KEY REFERENCES AND WEBSITES

A full list of references for this chapter can be found at http://thepoint.lww.com/AT10e. Below are the key references for this chapter, with the corresponding reference number in this chapter found in parentheses after the reference.

Key References

Adrogue HJ, Madias NE. Management of life-threatening acid–base disorders: first of two parts. *N Engl J Med.* 1998;338:26. (67)

Adrogue HJ, Madias NE. Management of life threatening acid–base disorders: second of two parts. *N Engl J Med.* 1998;338:107. (68)

Breen PH. Arterial blood gas and pH analysis: clinical approach and interpretation. *Anesthesiol Clin North Am.* 2001;19:885. (34)

Rose BD, Post TW. Metabolic alkalosis. In: Rose BD, Post TW, eds. *Clinical Physiology of Acid–Base and Electrolyte Disorders.* 5th ed. New York, NY: McGraw-Hill Medical; 2001:551. (2)

Rose BD, Post TW. Regulation of acid–base balance. In: Rose BD, Post TW, eds. *Clinical Physiology of Acid–Base and Electrolyte Disorders.* 5th ed. New York, NY: McGraw-Hill Medical; 2001: 325. (4)

Rose BD, Post TW. Introduction to simple and mixed acid–base disorders. In: Rose BD, Post TW, eds. *Clinical Physiology of Acid–Base and Electrolyte Disorders.* 5th ed. New York, NY: McGraw-Hill Medical; 2001:535. (8)

Rose BD, Post TW. Metabolic acidosis. In: Rose BD, Post TW, eds. *Clinical Physiology of Acid–Base and Electrolyte Disorders.* 5th ed. New York, NY: McGraw-Hill Medical; 2001:578. (33)

Rose BD, Post TW. Metabolic alkalosis. In: Rose BD, Post TW, eds. *Clinical Physiology of Acid–Base and Electrolyte Disorders.* 5th ed. New York, NY: McGraw-Hill Medical; 2001:551. (81)

Rose BD, Post TW. Respiratory acidosis. In: Rose BD, Post TW, eds. *Clinical Physiology of Acid–Base and Electrolyte Disorders.* 5th ed. New York, NY: McGraw-Hill Medical; 2001:647. (86)

Rose BD, Post TW. Respiratory alkalosis. In: Rose BD, Post TW, eds. *Clinical Physiology of Acid–Base and Electrolyte Disorders.* 5th ed. New York, NY: McGraw-Hill Medical; 2001:673. (93)

10 Fluid and Electrolyte Disorders

Alan H. Lau and Priscilla P. How

CORE PRINCIPLES

	CHAPTER CASES
FLUID AND SODIUM DISORDERS	
1 Plasma osmolality is maintained within normal limits through a delicate balance between water intake and excretion. Antidiuretic hormone (ADH) plays an important role in maintaining fluid balance in the body.	**Case 10-1 (Question 1)**
2 Signs of volume depletion include orthostatic hypotension, dry mucous membranes, and poor skin turgor. Because water and sodium are inherently linked, the assessment of volume status and selection of replacement fluid require examination of sodium concentration.	**Case 10-2 (Questions 1, 2)**
3 Aldosterone is the main regulatory hormone for sodium homeostasis. A patient may have hypotonic, isotonic, or hypertonic hyponatremia depending on the plasma osmolality.	**Cases 10-4 through 10-7**
4 Hypovolemic hypotonic hyponatremia can occur with volume depletion and decreased extracellular fluid. Calculation of sodium deficit will determine how much sodium replacement is required.	**Case 10-5 (Questions 1, 2)**
5 Hypervolemic, hypotonic hyponatremia is caused by a disproportionate accumulation of ingested water relative to sodium. It is also observed in patients with heart failure, liver and renal failure, and nephrotic syndrome. Management includes sodium and water restriction, as well as the use of diuretics.	**Case 10-6 (Question 1)**
6 Syndrome of inappropriate antidiuretic hormone is a common cause of normovolemic hypotonic hyponatremia. Persistent ADH secretion together with water ingestion results in hyponatremia.	**Case 10-7 (Question 1)**
7 Neurological symptoms may be manifested in acute or severe hyponatremia. Low plasma osmolality causes water to move into the brain resulting in cerebral edema, increased intracranial pressure, and central nervous system symptoms. Rapid or overly aggressive correction of hyponatremia can result in osmotic demyelination.	**Case 10-7 (Questions 3, 4)**
POTASSIUM DISORDERS	
1 The sodium-potassium adenosine triphosphatase pump plays a pivotal role in maintaining potassium homeostasis. Normal serum potassium concentration is 3.5 to 5.0 mEq/L. Clinical manifestations of hypokalemia include muscle weakness and electrocardiography (ECG) changes.	**Case 10-8 (Questions 1, 2)**
2 Potassium repletion should be guided by close monitoring of serum potassium. Oral supplementation is usually preferred. Patients who cannot tolerate oral potassium or who have severe/symptomatic hypokalemia can receive intravenous potassium. In general, the rate of potassium infusion should not exceed 10 mEq/hour, to prevent phlebitis.	**Case 10-8 (Question 3)**

continued

POTASSIUM DISORDERS *CONTINUED*	
3 Hyperkalemia can be caused by chronic kidney disease and medications that inhibit the renin-angiotensin-aldosterone system. Intravenous calcium is administered to antagonize the cardiac effects (ECG changes and ventricular arrhythmias) of hyperkalemia. Other treatment strategies include the use of insulin and glucose, β_2-agonists, sodium polystyrene sulfonate, sodium bicarbonate, and dialysis.	**Case 10-9 (Question 1), Case 10-10 (Questions 1, 2), Table 10-3**
CALCIUM DISORDERS	
1 Normal serum calcium is 8.5 to 10.5 mg/dL (corrected for serum albumin as calcium is protein-bound). Hypercalcemia can be caused by dehydration, malignancy, hyperparathyroidism, vitamin D intoxication, sarcoidosis, and other granulomatous disease. Clinical presentation of hypercalcemia includes signs and symptoms involving the neurologic, cardiovascular, pulmonary, renal, gastrointestinal, and musculoskeletal systems. First-line treatment for hypercalcemia is hydration and diuresis. Calcitonin and bisphosphonates are alternative agents used in the management of hypercalcemia.	**Case 10-11 (Questions 1–3), Table 10-4**
PHOSPHATE DISORDERS	
1 Hypophosphatemia can develop as a result of impaired intestinal phosphorus absorption, increased renal elimination, or shift of phosphorus from extracellular to intracellular compartments. Normal serum phosphorus concentration is 2.7 to 4.7 mg/dL.	**Case 10-12 (Questions 1, 2)**
2 Clinical effects of hypophosphatemia can involve multiple organ systems and are attributed to impaired cellular energy stores and tissue hypoxia secondary to ATP depletion. Phosphorus supplementation can be administered orally or intravenously, depending on the signs and symptoms, and severity of hypophosphatemia. Renal function, serum phosphorus, calcium, and magnesium need to be monitored closely. Diarrhea is a common dose-related side effect of oral phosphorus replacement.	**Case 10-12 (Questions 3, 4)**
MAGNESIUM DISORDERS	
1 Magnesium depletion (normal serum magnesium, 1.8–2.4 mEq/L) can result in abnormal function of the neurologic, neuromuscular, and cardiovascular systems. Typical findings include Chvostek and Trousseau signs, muscle fasciculation, tremors, muscle spasticity, convulsions, and possibly tetany. As serum magnesium does not reflect total body stores, symptoms are more important determinants of the urgency and aggressiveness of magnesium replacement.	**Case 10-13 (Questions 1, 2)**
2 Oral magnesium replacement is indicated in asymptomatic patients with mild depletion. Urinary excretion of magnesium increases during intravenous replacement. Thus, replenishment of magnesium stores usually takes several days. After intravenous magnesium administration, the patient should be monitored for hypotension, marked suppression of deep tendon reflexes, ECG and respiration changes, as well as hypermagnesemia.	**Case 10-13 (Questions 3, 4)**
3 A common cause of hypermagnesemia is the use of magnesium-containing laxatives and antacids by patients with renal impairment. Potentially life-threatening complications of severe hypermagnesemia include respiratory paralysis, hypotension, and complete heart block. Intravenous calcium should be administered to antagonize the respiratory and cardiac manifestations of magnesium. Diuretics may be given to patients with good renal function to enhance urinary magnesium excretion.	**Case 10-14 (Questions 1–3)**

Body Water Compartments and Electrolyte Composition

In newborns, approximately 75% to 85% of body weight is water. After puberty, the percentage of water per kilogram of weight decreases as the amount of adipose tissue increases with age.[1,2] Body water constitutes 50% to 60% of the lean body weight (LBW) in adult men but only 45% to 55% in women because of their greater proportion of adipose tissue. The water content per kilogram of body weight further decreases with advanced age. Total body water (TBW) is usually calculated as 0.6 × LBW in men, and 0.5 × LBW in women.

Two-thirds of the total body water resides in the cells (intracellular water). The extracellular water can be divided into different compartments—the interstitial fluid (12% LBW) and the plasma (5% LBW) are the two major compartments. Other compartments of the extracellular fluid include the connective tissues and bone water, the transcellular fluids (e.g., glandular secretions), and other fluids in sequestered spaces, such as the cerebrospinal fluid.[1]

The electrolyte composition differs between the intracellular and extracellular compartments. Potassium, magnesium, and phosphate are the major ions in the intracellular compartment, whereas sodium, chloride, and bicarbonate are predominant in the extracellular space.[2] Water travels freely across the cell membranes of most parts of the body. The cell membrane, however, is only selectively permeable to solutes. The impermeable solutes are osmotically active and can exert an osmotic pressure that dictates the distribution of water between fluid compartments. Water moves across the cell membrane from a region of low osmolality to one of high osmolality. Net water movement ceases when osmotic equilibrium occurs. Each fluid compartment contains a major osmotically active solute: potassium in the intracellular space and sodium in the extracellular fluid. The volumes of the two compartments reflect the asymmetrically larger number of solute particles or osmoles inside the cells.[2,3]

The capillary wall separates the interstitial fluid from plasma. Because sodium moves freely across the capillary wall, its concentration is identical across both sides of the wall. Therefore, no osmotic gradient is generated, and water distribution between these two spaces is not affected. Plasma proteins, which are confined in the vascular space, are the primary osmoles that affect water distribution between the interstitium and the plasma.[2] In contrast, urea, which traverses both the capillary walls and most cell membranes, is osmotically inactive.[2,3]

Plasma Osmolality

Osmolality is defined as the number of particles per kilogram of water (mOsm/kg). It is determined by the number of particles in solution and not by particle size or valence. Nondissociable solutes, such as glucose and albumin, generate 1 mOsm/mmol of particles; and dissociable salts, such as sodium chloride liberate two ions in solution to produce 2 mOsm/mmol of salt. The osmolality of body fluid is maintained between 280 and 295 mOsm/kg. Because all body fluid compartments are iso-osmotic, plasma osmolality reflects the osmolality of total body water. Plasma osmolality can be measured by the freezing point depression method, or estimated by the following equation, which takes into account the osmotic effect of sodium, glucose, and urea[2,3]:

$$P_{osm} = 2(\text{Na})(\text{mmol/L}) + \frac{\text{Glucose (mg/dL)}}{18} + \frac{\text{BUN (mg/dL)}}{2.8} \quad \textit{(Eq. 10-1)}$$

This equation predicts the measured plasma osmolality within 5 to 10 mOsm/kg. Although urea contributes to the measured osmolality, it is an ineffective osmole because it readily traverses cell membranes and, therefore, does not cause significant fluid shift within the body. Hence, the effective plasma osmolality (synonymous with tonicity, the portion of total osmolality that has the potential to induce transmembrane water movement) can be estimated by the following equation:

$$P_{osm} = 2(\text{Na})(\text{mmol/L}) + \frac{\text{Glucose (mg/dL)}}{18} \quad \textit{(Eq. 10-2)}$$

An osmolal gap exists when the measured and calculated values differ by greater than 10 mOsm/kg[4]; it signifies the presence of unidentified particles. When the individual solute has been identified, its contribution to the measured osmolality can be estimated by dividing its concentration (mg/dL) by one-tenth of its molecular weight. Calculating the osmolal gap is used to detect the presence of substances, such as ethanol, methanol, and ethylene glycol, that have high osmolality. Occasionally, the osmolal gap can also result from an artificial decrease in the serum sodium secondary to severe hyperlipidemia or hyperproteinemia.

CASE 10-1

QUESTION 1: J.F., a 31-year-old man, is admitted to the inpatient medicine service for methanol intoxication. Routine laboratory analysis reveals the following:

Sodium (Na), 145 mEq/L
Potassium (K), 3.4 mEq/L
Blood urea nitrogen (BUN), 10 mg/dL
Creatinine, 1.1 mg/dL
Glucose, 90 mg/dL

The blood methanol concentration was 108 mg/dL, and the measured plasma osmolality was 333 mOsm/kg. What is J.F.'s calculated osmolality? Are other unidentified osmoles present?

Using Equation 10-1, J.F.'s total calculated osmolality is

$$\begin{aligned} P_{osm} &= 2(145\ \text{mEq/L}) + \frac{90\ \text{mg/dL}}{18} + \frac{10\ \text{mg/dL}}{2.8} \\ &= 290 + 5 + 3.6 \\ &= 299\ \text{mOsm/kg} \end{aligned} \quad \textit{(Eq. 10-3)}$$

$$\begin{aligned} \text{Osmolal gap} &= 333\ \text{mOsm/kg} - 299\ \text{mOsm/kg} \\ &= 34\ \text{mOsm/kg} \end{aligned} \quad \textit{(Eq. 10-4)}$$

In J.F., the entire osmolal gap can be accounted for by the presence of the methanol (because 108 mg/dL of methanol will provide 108/3.2 = 33.7 mOsm/kg). It is unlikely, therefore, that other unmeasured osmoles are present (e.g., ethylene glycol, isopropanol, and ethanol). The laboratory determination of osmolality measures the total number of osmotically active particles but not their permeability across the cell membrane. Methanol increases plasma osmolality but not tonicity because the cell membrane is permeable to methanol. Therefore, no net water shift occurs between the intracellular and extracellular compartments. Conversely, mannitol, which is confined to the extracellular space, contributes to both plasma osmolality and tonicity.

Tubular Function of Nephron

The kidney plays an important role in maintaining a constant extracellular environment by regulating the excretion of water and various electrolytes. The volume and composition of fluid filtered across the glomerulus are modified as the fluid passes through the tubules of the nephron.

The renal tubule is composed of a series of segments with heterogeneous structures and functions: the proximal tubule, the medullary and cortical thick ascending limb of Henle's loop, the distal convoluted tubule, and the cortical and medullary collecting duct[2] (Fig. 10-1). The mechanism for sodium reabsorption is different for each nephron segment, but is generally mediated by carrier proteins or channels located on the luminal membrane of the tubule cell.[2] Na^+/K^+ ATPase (sodium-potassium adenosine triphosphatase) actively pumps sodium out of the renal tubule cell in exchange for potassium in a 3:2 ratio. Hence, the intracellular sodium concentration is kept at a low level. The potassium that is pumped into the cell leaks back out through potassium channels in the membrane, rendering the cell interior electronegative. The low intracellular sodium concentration and a negative intracellular potential produce a favorable gradient for passive sodium entry into the cell.[3] Na^+/K^+ ATPase also indirectly provides the energy for active sodium transport and the reabsorption and secretion of other solutes across the luminal membrane of the renal tubule. The distal segments are mainly involved in the reabsorption of sodium and chloride ions and the secretion of hydrogen and potassium ions.[2]

Iso-osmotic reabsorption of the glomerular filtrate occurs in the proximal tubule such that two-thirds of the filtered sodium and water and 90% of the filtered bicarbonate are reabsorbed. The Na^+/H^+ antiporter (exchanger) in the luminal membrane is instrumental in the reabsorption of sodium chloride, sodium bicarbonate, and water. The reabsorption of most nonelectrolyte solutes, such as glucose, amino acids, and phosphates, are coupled to sodium transport.[2,5]

Both the thick ascending limb of Henle's loop and the distal convoluted tubule serve as the diluting segments of the nephron because they are impermeable to water. Sodium chloride is extracted from the filtrate without water. Sodium transport in both of these segments is flow-dependent and varies with the amount of sodium ions delivered from the proximal segments of the nephron. Decreased sodium ions in the tubular fluid will limit sodium transport in the thick ascending limb of Henle's loop and the distal convoluted tubule.[2,6]

Reabsorption of sodium in the thick ascending limb of Henle's loop accounts for approximately 25% of the total sodium reabsorption. Sodium, chloride, and potassium are reabsorbed by

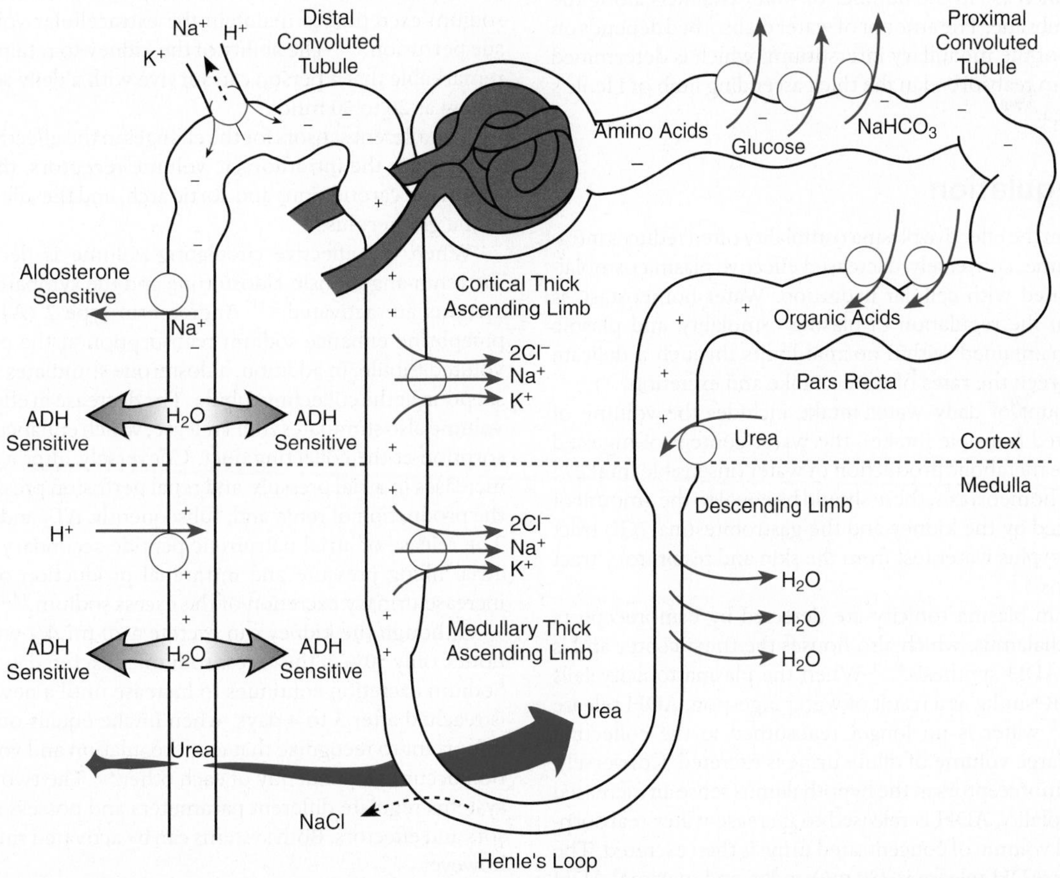

FIGURE 10-1 Sites of tubule salt and water absorption. Sodium is reabsorbed with inorganic anions, amino acids, and glucose in the proximal tubule against an electrical gradient that is lumen-negative. In the distal part of the proximal tubule (pars recta), sodium and water are reabsorbed to a lesser extent and organic acids (hippurate, urate) and urea are secreted into the urine. The electrical potential is lumen-positive in the pars recta. Water, but not salt, is removed from tubule fluid in the thin descending limb of Henle's loop, but in the ascending portion salt is reabsorbed without water, rendering the tubule fluid hyposmotic with respect to the interstitium. Sodium, chloride, and potassium are reabsorbed by the medullary and cortical portions of the ascending limb; the lumen potential is positive. Sodium is reabsorbed and potassium and hydrogen ions are secreted in the distal tubule and collecting ducts. Water absorption in these segments is regulated by antidiuretic hormone (ADH). The electrical potential is lumen-negative in the cortical sections and positive in the medullary segments. Urea is concentrated in the interstitium of the medulla and assists in the generation of maximally concentrated urine. (Reprinted with permission from Chonko AM et al. Treatment of edema states. In: Narins RG, ed. *Maxwell & Kleeman's Clinical Disorders of Fluid and Electrolyte Metabolism*. 5th ed. New York, NY: McGraw-Hill; 1994:545.)

the medullary and cortical portions of the ascending limb, but the leakage of reabsorbed potassium ions back into the tubular lumen, via potassium channels, makes the tubular lumen electropositive. This electrical gradient promotes the passive reabsorption of cations, such as sodium, calcium, and magnesium, in the distal convoluted tubules. Because the thick ascending limb of Henle's loop is impermeable to water, it contributes to the interstitial osmolality in the medulla. This high osmolality is key to the reabsorption of water by the medullary portion of the collecting duct under the influence of antidiuretic hormone (ADH, vasopressin). Therefore, the thick ascending limb of Henle's loop is important for both urinary concentration and dilution.[6]

Because, as noted previously, the distal convoluted tubule also is impermeable to water, the osmolality of the filtrate continues to decline as sodium is being reabsorbed. In the distal convoluted tubule and collecting duct, sodium is reabsorbed in exchange for hydrogen ions and potassium. When sodium ions are reabsorbed, the tubule lumen becomes electronegative, which promotes potassium secretion in the lumen via potassium channels. Aldosterone enhances sodium reabsorption in the collecting duct by increasing the number of opened sodium channels.[2,7]

The collecting duct is usually impermeable to water. Under the influence of ADH, however, water permeability is increased through an increase in the number of water channels along the luminal membrane. The amount of water reabsorbed depends on the tonicity of the medullary interstitium, which is determined by the sodium reabsorbed in the thick ascending limb of Henle's loop and urea.[2,7,8]

Osmoregulation

An increase in the effective plasma osmolality often reduces intracellular volume; conversely, decreased effective plasma osmolality is associated with cellular hydration. Water homeostasis is important in the regulation of plasma osmolality, and plasma tonicity is maintained within normal limits through a delicate balance between the rates of water intake and excretion.

The amount of daily water intake includes the volume of water ingested (sensible intake), the water content of ingested food, and the metabolic production of water (insensible intake).[2] To maintain homeostasis, these should be equal to the amount of water excreted by the kidney and the gastrointestinal (GI) tract (sensible loss) plus water lost from the skin and respiratory tract (insensible loss).[2,3]

Changes in plasma tonicity are detected by osmoreceptors in the hypothalamus, which also houses the thirst center and is the site for ADH synthesis.[9,10] When the plasma tonicity falls below 280 mOsm/kg as a result of water ingestion, ADH release is inhibited,[2] water is no longer reabsorbed in the collecting duct, and a large volume of dilute urine is excreted. Conversely, when the osmoreceptors in the hypothalamus sense an increased plasma osmolality, ADH is released to increase water reabsorption. A small volume of concentrated urine is then excreted. The threshold for ADH release is 280 mOsm/kg, and maximal ADH secretion occurs when the plasma osmolality is 295 mOsm/kg.[9] Thus, urine osmolality varies from 50 mOsm/kg in the absence of ADH to 1,200 mOsm/kg during maximal ADH release. The volume of urine produced depends on the solute load to be excreted, as well as the urine osmolality[2,3,9,10]:

$$\text{Urine volume (L)} = \left(\frac{\text{Solute load (mOsm)}}{\text{Urine osmolality (mOsm/kg)}}\right) \times \left(\frac{1}{\text{Density of water (kg/L)}}\right) \quad \textit{(Eq. 10-5)}$$

Therefore, for a typical daily solute load of 600 mOsm:

$$= \left(\frac{600\ \text{mOsm}}{50\ \text{mOsm/kg}}\right)\left(\frac{1}{1\ \text{kg/L}}\right) = 12\ \text{L (No ADH)} \quad \textit{(Eq. 10-6)}$$

$$= \left(\frac{600\ \text{mOsm}}{1{,}200\ \text{mOsm/kg}}\right)\left(\frac{1}{1\ \text{kg/L}}\right) = 0.5\ \text{L (Max ADH)} \quad \textit{(Eq. 10-7)}$$

Although the kidney has a remarkable ability to excrete free water, it is not as efficient in conserving water. ADH minimizes further water loss, but it cannot correct water deficits. Therefore, optimal osmoregulation requires increased water intake stimulated by thirst. Both ADH and thirst can be stimulated by nonosmotic stimuli. For example, volume depletion is such a strong nonosmotic stimulus for ADH release that it can override the response to changes in plasma osmolality. Nausea, pain, and hypoxia are also potent stimuli for ADH secretion.[11]

Volume Regulation

Sodium resides almost exclusively in the extracellular fluid; the amount of total body sodium, therefore, determines the extracellular volume.[2,11] Because daily sodium intake varies from 100 to 250 mEq, the body must rely on adjustments in urinary sodium excretion to maintain the extracellular volume and tissue perfusion.[2,11] The ability of the kidney to retain sodium is so remarkable that a person can survive with a daily sodium intake as low as 20 to 30 mEq.

The afferent sensors for the changes in the effective circulating volume are the intrathoracic volume receptors, the baroreceptors in the carotid sinus and aortic arch, and the afferent arteriole in the glomerulus.[11]

When the effective circulating volume is decreased, both the renin-angiotensin-aldosterone and the sympathetic nervous systems are activated.[2,11] Angiotensin type 2 (AT_2) and norepinephrine enhance sodium reabsorption at the proximal convoluted tubule. In addition, aldosterone stimulates sodium reabsorption at the collecting tubule. The decrease in effective arterial volume also stimulates ADH release, which enhances water reabsorption at the collecting duct. Conversely, after a salt load, the increases in atrial pressure and renal perfusion pressure suppress the production of renin and, subsequently, AT_2 and aldosterone. The release of atrial natriuretic peptide secondary to increased atrial filling pressure and intrarenal production of urodilators increase urinary excretion of the excess sodium.[12,13]

Although the kidney can excrete a 20-mL/kg water load in 4 hours, only 50% of the excess sodium is excreted in the first day.[3] Sodium excretion continues to increase until a new steady state is reached after 3 to 4 days, when intake equals output.[3,12] It is important to recognize that osmoregulation and volume regulation occur independently of each other.[2,3] The two homeostatic systems regulate different parameters and possess different sensors and effectors. Both systems can be activated simultaneously, however.

DISORDERS IN VOLUME REGULATION

Sodium Depletion

CASE 10-2

QUESTION 1: A.B., a 17-year-old girl, presented to the emergency department (ED) with complaints of anorexia, nausea, vomiting, and generalized weakness for the past

3 days. She denied other medical problems and had not used any medications. On examination, her supine blood pressure (BP) was 105/70 mm Hg, with a pulse of 80 beats/minute. Her standing BP was 85/60 mm Hg with a pulse of 100 beats/minute, and she complained of feeling dizzy when she stood up. Her mucous membranes were dry but her skin turgor was normal. The jugular vein was flat, and peripheral or sacral edema was not present. Laboratory blood tests showed the following:

Serum Na, 134 mEq/L
K, 3.5 mEq/L
Chloride (Cl), 95 mEq/L
Total CO_2 content, 35 mEq/L
BUN, 18 mg/dL
Creatinine, 0.8 mg/dL
Glucose, 70 mg/dL

Random urinary sodium was 40 mEq/L, potassium was 40 mEq/L, and chloride was less than 15 mEq/L. The hemoglobin was 14 g/dL, and white cell and platelet counts were normal. Based on the clinical and laboratory data in A.B., what is the most probable explanation for her presentation?

The signs and symptoms in A.B. are consistent with volume depletion. The loss of gastric fluid owing to vomiting and decreased oral intake secondary to anorexia led to moderate to severe volume depletion. She exhibits orthostatic changes in both her BP (a drop in systolic BP of 20 mm Hg) and pulse (an increase of 20 beats/minute). The dry mucous membranes, the flat jugular vein, and the absence of edema support volume depletion as well, and dizziness on standing indicates extracellular volume depletion.[14] Her hypochloremic metabolic alkalosis was probably initiated by loss of acidic gastric contents through vomiting. Her volume depletion increased renal bicarbonate reabsorption, perpetuating the metabolic alkalosis. The decreased renal perfusion brought about by volume depletion enhanced proximal tubular reabsorption of urea, resulting in an increased BUN to creatinine ratio (prerenal azotemia). When renal perfusion is decreased and the renin-angiotensin-aldosterone system is activated, the proximal reabsorption of sodium and chloride is increased. A.B.'s urinary sodium is, therefore, less than 10 mEq/L.[15] Excretion of the poorly permeable bicarbonate ions, however, results in obligatory urinary sodium loss to maintain luminal electroneutrality. A.B.'s urinary sodium was therefore elevated (40 mEq/L). In this situation, the urinary chloride remained low, and this is a better index of volume status.[15] Both urinary sodium and chloride are elevated, however, in patients using diuretics, in those undergoing osmotic diuresis, and in those with underlying renal disease or hypoaldosteronism, even in the face of volume depletion. Physical examination should therefore be conducted as part of the volume status assessment. A.B.'s volume depletion increased the concentration of red blood cells, which could explain her slightly elevated hemoglobin concentration of 14 g/dL.

CASE 10-2, QUESTION 2: How should A.B.'s volume depletion be managed?

The etiology of A.B.'s vomiting should be sought and the cause removed. Because the patient is neither hypernatremic nor hyponatremic, normal saline should be administered intravenously to replenish the extracellular volume and improve tissue perfusion.[2,14] If the patient is hypernatremic (having a greater deficit of water than solute), half-isotonic saline or dextrose solution, which contains more free water, should be administered. In contrast, hyponatremic hypovolemic patients have a greater deficit of solute than water; isotonic or hypertonic saline should then be given. The amount of volume deficit is often difficult to ascertain. Because A.B. was severely orthostatic, 1 or 2 L of fluid can be given over the course of 2 to 4 hours. The subsequent rate of infusion will depend on A.B.'s response and the prevailing symptoms. The clinician should monitor her body weight, skin turgor, supine and upright BP, jugular venous pressure, urine output, and urine chloride concentration to assess the adequacy of volume repletion. Because the treatment goal is to achieve a positive fluid balance, the infusion rate should be 50 or 100 mL/hour in excess of the sum of urine output, insensible losses, and other losses, such as emesis and diarrhea.[2]

Sodium Excess

CASE 10-3

QUESTION 1: L.J., a 45-year-old man, presented to the clinic with complaints of swollen legs and puffy eyelids. He also noticed that his urine had been foamy recently. On examination, his BP was 180/100 mm Hg and his pulse was 80 beats/minute. Bilateral periorbital edema and 2+ bilateral pitting edema up to the thigh were noted. On auscultation, his heart was normal and his lungs had bilateral crackles. His jugular venous pressure was elevated at 10 cm H_2O. Laboratory tests revealed the following:

Serum Na, 132 mEq/L
K, 3.8 mEq/L
Cl, 100 mEq/L
Bicarbonate, 26 mEq/L
BUN, 40 mg/dL
Creatinine, 2.5 mg/dL
Glucose, 120 mg/dL
Albumin, 2 g/dL
Serum cholesterol, 280 mg/dL,
Triglycerides, 300 mg/dL

The serum transaminases, alkaline phosphatase, and bilirubin were within normal limits. Urinalysis showed the following:

Specific gravity, 1.015
pH, 7.0
Protein, > 300 mg/dL
24-hour urinary protein excretion, 6 g
Creatinine clearance (CrCl), 40 mL/minute

Urinalysis also showed oval fat bodies and fatty casts. L.J. was taking no medications and he denied illicit drug use. Hepatitis B serology and human immunodeficiency virus (HIV) antibody were negative. The impression was anasarca (total body edema) secondary to nephrotic syndrome. What is nephrotic syndrome? What could be the cause of L.J.'s sodium excess state?

Nephrotic syndrome is characterized by hypoalbuminemia, urine protein excretion greater than 3.5 g/day, hyperlipidemia, lipiduria, and edema.[16,17] The heavy proteinuria is a result of damage to the selective barrier of the glomerulus. The causes of nephrotic syndrome are multiple and diverse.[16] The causes can be idiopathic (primary glomerular disease) or secondary to chronic systemic diseases (e.g., diabetes mellitus, amyloidosis, sickle cell anemia,[18] lupus), cancer (e.g., multiple myeloma, Hodgkin disease), infections (e.g., HIV,[19] hepatitis B, syphilis, malaria), intravenous (IV) drug abuse, and medications (e.g., gold, penicillamine, captopril, nonsteroidal anti-inflammatory drugs [NSAIDs][20]).

A heavy urinary protein loss results in various extrarenal complications.[16,17] Hypoalbuminemia reduces plasma oncotic pressure and contributes to the increased hepatic synthesis of both albumin and lipoproteins. This, coupled with the decreased catabolism of lipoproteins, resulted in L.J.'s hyperlipidemia.[16,21] Urinary loss of inhibitors of coagulation predispose these patients to thromboembolism.[16]

Specific therapy of nephrotic syndrome ranges from simple removal of the offending medication and treatment of the underlying infection to the use of immunosuppressive agents in specific glomerular diseases.

L.J.'s anasarca results from changes in both capillary hemodynamics and renal sodium and water retention.[22] The hypoalbuminemia (2 g/dL) and proteinuria (>300 mg/dL) produce an imbalance in the Starling forces across the capillary wall, namely, the hydrostatic and oncotic pressures in the capillary and interstitial compartments. The reduced capillary oncotic pressure favors movement of fluid from the vascular space into the interstitium.[23] This leads to contraction of the effective arterial blood volume, which in turn activates humoral, neural, and hemodynamic mechanisms that signal the kidney to retain sodium and water.[24,25] This underfill hypothesis has been challenged by data suggesting that hypoalbuminemia plays a minor role in nephrotic edema[26,27] and the observation that patients with nephrotic syndrome can have increased, normal, or decreased plasma volumes.[23]

A defect in the intrarenal sodium handling mechanism that causes inappropriate sodium retention also contributes to nephrotic edema.[23,26] According to this overflow hypothesis, proteinuric renal disease leads to increased sodium reabsorption in the distal nephron. The mechanism is not well defined but may be related to cellular resistance to atrial natriuretic peptide.[23] Thus, a sodium excess state occurs and edema results. It is likely that the interaction between the underfill and overflow mechanisms results in the production of nephrotic edema.[28] Patients with severe hypoalbuminemia (i.e., serum albumin level <1.5 g/dL) who have a severe reduction in plasma oncotic pressure are most likely to exhibit evidence of the underfill phenomenon.[22]

CASE 10-3, QUESTION 2: How should L.J.'s sodium excess state be managed?

The etiology of L.J.'s nephrotic syndrome should be identified for specific treatment. Although L.J.'s serum sodium concentration of 132 mEq/L is low, it reflects dilution secondary to fluid excess. Salt restriction is therefore important to control L.J.'s generalized edema.[23] For most nephrotic patients, modest dietary sodium restriction to approximately 50 mEq/day may be sufficient to maintain neutral sodium balance.[22,23] For nephrotic patients who are very sodium avid (urine sodium concentration <10 mEq/L), sufficient restriction is difficult to achieve. Thus, slowing the rate of edema formation rather than hastening its resolution should be the goal of therapy for these patients.[23] Bed rest reduces orthostatic stimulation of the renin-angiotensin-aldosterone and sympathetic systems, thereby favoring the movement of interstitial fluid into the vascular space.[23] The central blood volume is thus increased and natriuresis and diuresis are facilitated. Prolonged bed rest might, however, predispose these hypercoagulable patients to thromboembolism.[16] Similarly, use of support stockings may reduce the stimulation for sodium retention by redistributing blood volume to the central circulation.[23,29]

DIURETICS

Usually, loop diuretics are the mainstay of therapy in the management of nephrotic edema.[2,23] In most of these patients, the edema can be removed safely with rapid diuresis without compromising the systemic circulation, probably because of the rapid refilling of the plasma volume by interstitial fluid.[23] Nevertheless, as the edema resolves, the rate of fluid removal and weight loss should be decreased to avoid compromising the effective circulating volume. The patient should be monitored for the development of orthostatic hypotension.

Infusions of albumin can expand the plasma volume; however, it is expensive, the relief is temporary, and it should therefore be used only for resistant edema.[30] In patients who are resistant to the aforementioned measures, extracorporeal fluid removal, namely, ultrafiltration, may be necessary.[23,31]

L.J. was initially treated with IV furosemide 60 mg twice daily and placed on a low-sodium (50 mEq), low-fat, high–complex-carbohydrate diet that consisted of 0.8 g/kg protein of high biologic value with additional protein to match gram-per-gram of urinary protein loss. Fluid was restricted to 1,000 mL/day.[32] He had 5 L of diuresis in 2 days, with resolution of respiratory symptoms and a reduction in the anasarca. Parenteral furosemide was discontinued on the fifth day of hospitalization and oral furosemide 120 mg twice daily was started. After a total weight loss of 12 kg, he was then discharged with instructions to maintain the diet and oral furosemide.

DISORDERS IN OSMOREGULATION

Hyponatremia

Serum sodium concentration reflects the ratio of total body sodium to total body water and is not an accurate indicator of total body sodium. Both hyponatremia and hypernatremia can occur in the presence of a low, normal, or high total body sodium.[33,34]

ONLINE CONTENT

For an illustration of the effect of isotonic fluid volume deficit and excess and of hyponatremia and hypernatremia on extracellular (ECF) and intracellular fluid volume (ICF), go to http://thepoint.lww.com/AT10e.

Because the kidney can excrete greater than 12 to 16 L of free water daily, hyponatremia does not occur unless the water intake overwhelms the kidney's ability to excrete free water (e.g., psychogenic polydipsia),[35,36] or free-water excretion is impaired.[2,37]

Free water formation requires a normal glomerular filtration rate (GFR), the reabsorption of sodium chloride without water in the thick ascending limb of Henle's loop and the distal convoluting tubule, and the excretion of a dilute urine in the absence of ADH[37] (Fig. 10-1). Therefore, hyponatremia can occur when the kidney's diluting ability is exceeded or impaired owing to volume depletion and nonosmotic stimulation of ADH release or inappropriate stimulation of ADH production.[2,37]

Although plasma sodium is the primary determinant of plasma tonicity, hyponatremia does not always represent hypotonicity.[2,37] In patients with severe hyperlipidemia or hyperproteinemia (e.g., multiple myeloma), pseudohyponatremia can occur because the increased amounts of lipids and proteins displace plasma water, in which sodium ions dissolve, resulting in a lower concentration of sodium per unit volume of plasma.[34,37,38] Normally, water accounts for 93% of the plasma volume, and lipids and proteins make up the rest.[37] The increase in plasma lipid and protein contents expands plasma volume, displaces water, and increases the percentage of solids in plasma.[34,37] Because sodium is distributed only in the aqueous phase, the sodium content per liter of the newly recomposed plasma is thus decreased and the plasma sodium concentration is reduced.[34,37,38] The sodium concentration in plasma water remains the same, however. Because osmolality depends on the solute concentration in plasma water, serum osmolality remains unchanged.[34] Indeed, the measured osmolality is normal. Another example of isotonic hyponatremia can be found when a large volume of isotonic mannitol irrigant is used during prostate surgery.[34,37] Absorption of the irrigation solution can result in severe hyponatremia but normal osmolality. In contrast, use of large amounts of isotonic sorbitol and isotonic, or slightly hypotonic, glycine solutions during urologic surgery can cause the hypotonicity as a late complication.[34,37] Similar to mannitol, sorbitol and isotonic glycine initially distribute only in the extracellular space, resulting in hyponatremia without a change in osmolality.[37] Unlike mannitol, both sorbitol and glycine are later metabolized, leaving water behind to result in hypotonicity. The severe hypotonic hyponatremia, in conjunction with the neurotoxic effects of glycine and its metabolites, puts the patient at significant risk for severe neurologic symptoms (Table 10-1).[37,39]

CASE 10-4

QUESTION 1: T.T., a 63-year-old man with end-stage renal disease caused by diabetic nephropathy, is receiving chronic ambulatory peritoneal dialysis. Because of dietary and fluid noncompliance, T.T. complained of shortness of breath (SOB) and his dialysis prescription was adjusted to include six cycles of 2.5% peritoneal dialysis solutions. Today, his laboratory values are as follows:

Na, 128 mEq/L
K, 4 mEq/L
Cl, 98 mEq/L
Total CO_2, 24 mM
BUN, 50 mg/dL
Creatinine, 6 mg/dL
Glucose, 600 mg/dL

Evaluate T.T.'s plasma osmolality. What is the etiology of T.T.'s hyponatremia?

T.T.'s effective plasma osmolality is calculated to be 289 mOsm/L, of which 33 mOsm/L is contributed by the hyperglycemia. The slow utilization of glucose, because of the lack of insulin, causes water to move from the intracellular compartment into the plasma space because of the increased tonicity, thereby lowering the plasma sodium concentration.[34,37] Despite the lowered plasma sodium concentration, the plasma osmolality is normal because of hyperglycemia. Hence, no symptoms attributable to hypo-osmolality are observed. Indeed, when serum glucose is normalized with insulin and hydration, the serum sodium level will increase to approximately 136 mEq/L. For each 100-mg/dL increment in serum glucose, serum sodium decreases by 1.3 to 1.6 mEq/L.[34,37] Use of hypertonic mannitol or glycine solutions in patients with cerebral edema also results in a hyperosmolar hyponatremia.[34]

Hypotonic Hyponatremia With Decreased Extracellular Fluid

CASE 10-5

QUESTION 1: Q.B., a 30-year-old male athlete who has had multiple bouts of diarrhea for the last several days, has been drinking a sports drink to keep himself from getting dehydrated. His vital signs include supine BP, 145/80 mm Hg, and pulse, 70 beats/minute; standing BP, 128/68 mm Hg, and pulse, 90 beats/minute. Respiratory rate (RR) is 12 breaths/minute, and he is afebrile. His skin turgor is mildly decreased and laboratory data are the following:

Na, 128 mEq/L
K, 3.0 mEq/L
Cl, 100 mEq/L
Bicarbonate, 17 mEq/L
BUN, 27 mg/dL
Creatinine, 1.2 mg/dL

Urinary sodium and chloride were both less than 10 mEq/L. Assess Q.B.'s electrolyte and fluid status. What is the etiology of Q.B.'s hyponatremia?

Q.B. has true hypotonic hyponatremia with extracellular fluid depletion, suggesting that his total body sodium deficit is greater than that of total body water.[34] His poor skin turgor, orthostasis, prerenal azotemia, and low urinary sodium are consistent with volume depletion. The urinary sodium concentration helps distinguish between renal and nonrenal losses that result in the sodium and water deficits.[15,34,40] When the plasma volume is depleted, the urinary sodium concentration is less than 10 mEq/L, suggesting appropriate renal sodium conservation.[15] This is usually seen in patients such as Q.B. with GI fluid loss as in vomiting, diarrhea, or profuse sweating.[34,37,40]

Other causes of hypotonic hyponatremia are less likely in Q.B. They include surreptitious cathartic abuse and "third spacing," or accumulation of extracellular fluid in the abdominal cavity during acute pancreatitis, ileus, or pseudomembranous colitis.[37,40] If the urinary sodium is less than 20 mEq/L in the face of volume depletion, renal salt wastage should be considered.[15,37,40] The potential causes of this latter problem include diuretic use,[41–44] adrenal insufficiency,[44] and salt-wasting nephropathy[35] (e.g., chronic interstitial nephritis, medullary cystic disease, polycystic kidney disease, obstructive uropathy, and cisplatin toxicity[44,45]). In patients with renal insufficiency, neither the urinary sodium nor chloride concentration is a reliable index of volume status.[15]

Volume depletion leads to increased reabsorption of sodium and water in the proximal tubule and, thus, decreased sodium delivery to the diluting segments for free-water formation.[34,37,40] Decreased effective arterial volume is also a potent nonosmotic stimulus for ADH release.[9,10] These factors combine to dampen the ability of the kidney to form dilute urine and result in high urine osmolality despite a low serum sodium concentration.[34,37,40] Although the fluid lost in diarrhea is hypotonic, it is the replacement of fluid lost with an even more hypotonic fluid such as the sports drink or tap water that causes hyponatremia in patients such as Q.B.[37,40]

Q.B.'s diarrhea probably caused loss of potassium and bicarbonate through the GI tract, resulting in hypokalemia and hyperchloremic metabolic acidosis. The potassium depletion can sensitize ADH secretion in response to hypovolemic stimuli, and the hypokalemia also can lead to hyponatremia.[37] The cellular efflux of potassium causes cellular uptake of sodium, further reducing the serum sodium concentration.

CASE 10-5, QUESTION 2: How should Q.B.'s hyponatremia be treated?

The treatment of hypovolemic hyponatremia involves sodium replacement to correct the deficit. The sodium deficit can be

TABLE 10-1
Clinical Presentation and Treatment of Hyponatremia

Na^+ and H_2O Status	Clinical Presentation/Cause	Treatment
Edematous, Fluid Overload (Hypervolemic, Hypotonic)		
↑ Total body Na^+–↑↑ Total body H_2O	Cirrhosis/HF/nephrotic syndrome: A ↓ in renal blood flow activates renin angiotensin system. ↑ Aldosterone leads to ↑ Na^+, and ↑ ADH leads to free H_2O retention. Urine Na^+ is low (0–20 mEq/L) and urine osmolality ↓. Diuretics can induce paradoxical effects on urine Na^+ and osmolality. This form also can occur in patients with renal failure who drink excessive amounts of water. Patients have symptoms of fluid overload (ascites, distended neck veins, edema).	Fluid and Na^+ restriction. Correct underlying disorder (e.g., paracentesis for ascites). Diurese cautiously[a]; avoid ↓ ECF and accompanying ↓ tissue perfusion. ↑ BUN may indicate overly rapid diuresis. Conivaptan: Loading dose of 20 mg IV for 30 minutes, followed by 20 mg IV as continuous infusion for 24 hours for an additional 1 to 3 days; may titrate up to maximal dose of 40 mg/day; maximal duration is 4 days after the loading dose. Dedicated IV line recommended and site of peripheral IV lines should be changed every 24 hours. Caution if used together with fluid restriction. Tolvaptan: Start 15 mg PO once daily. Dose may be increased at intervals of at least 24 hours to 30 mg PO once daily and then to a maximum of 60 mg PO once daily as needed. Caution if used together with fluid restriction.
Nonedematous Hypovolemic (Hypotonic with ECF Depletion)		
↓↓ Total body Na^+ ↓ Total body H_2O	Occurs in GI fluid loss (e.g., diarrhea) with hypotonic electrolyte-poor fluid replacement, overdiuresis, "third spacing," Addison disease, renal tubular acidosis, osmotic diuresis. Replacement of fluid losses with solute-free fluid predisposes these patients to hyponatremia. Kidneys concentrate urine to conserve fluid (urine Na^+ <10 mEq/L). Symptoms: nonedematous; ECF depletion (collapsed neck veins, dehydration, orthostasis). Neurologic symptoms: (see Hyponatremia: Neurologic Manifestations in text).	Discontinue diuretics. Replace fluid and electrolyte (especially K^+) losses. 0.9% saline preferred unless Na^+ deficit[b] severe, then use 3%–5% saline.
Nonedematous, Normovolemic (Normovolemic, Hypotonic)		
↓ Total body Na^+ ↑ Total body H_2O	SIADH[a]: Hyponatremia, hypo-osmolality, renal Na^+ wasting (>40 mEq/L), absence of fluid depletion, $U_{osm} > P_{osm}$, normal renal and adrenal function. Free H_2O retained while Na^+ lost. *Causes:* (a) ADH production (infectious disease, vascular disease, cerebral neoplasm, cancer of lung, pancreas, duodenum); (b) exogenous ADH administration; (c) drugs; (d) psychogenic polydipsia.	See earlier for dosing of VRA (conivaptan and tolvaptan) Chronic treatment: Restrict fluids to less than urine loss. Demeclocycline (300–600 mg BID) induces reversible diabetes insipidus. Emergency treatment for unresponsive patients includes furosemide diuresis to achieve negative H_2O balance with careful replacement of Na^+ and K^+ using hypertonic saline solutions.[c]

[a] Remove estimated excess free water with IV furosemide (1 mg/kg). Repeat as necessary. Because furosemide generates a urine that resembles 0.5% NaCl, urine losses of sodium and potassium must be carefully measured and replaced hourly with hypertonic salt solutions. Correction rate: 1 to 2 mEq Na/h in symptomatic patients; 0.5 mEq/h in asymptomatic patients.

[b] Estimate sodium deficit: (mEq) = TBW (sodium desired – sodium observed). Rate of sodium and fluid repletion used depends on severity. Mild: replace with NS. First one-third for 6 to 12 hours at a rate of <0.5 mEq/L/h, remaining two-thirds for 24 to 48 hours. Severe (e.g., seizures): Use 3% to 5% saline, rate gauged by patient's ability to tolerate sodium and volume load. Monitor central nervous system function, skin turgor, blood pressure, urine sodium, signs of sodium or water overload, especially in patients with cardiovascular, renal, and pulmonary disease.

[c] Total body water (TBW) = 0.6 L/kg × weight in kg (for men) and 0.5 L/kg × weight in kg (for women).
TBW excess = TBW – [TBW (observed serum NA)/(desired serum NA)]

ADH, antidiuretic hormone; BID, twice daily; BUN, blood urea nitrogen; HF, heart failure; ECF, extracellular fluid; GI, gastrointestinal; IV, intravenous; NS, normal saline (0.9% Na); PO, orally; SIADH, syndrome of inappropriate ADH; TBW, total body weight.

estimated by the following formula:

$$\begin{aligned}\text{Na Deficit} &= \text{TBW} \times (\text{Desired} - \text{Current Na concentration})\\ &= 0.6\ \text{L/kg} \times 70\ \text{kg} \times (140 - 125\ \text{mEq/L})\\ &= 630\ \text{mEq}\end{aligned} \quad \textbf{(Eq. 10-8)}$$

Recall that TBW = 0.6 L/kg × weight in kg for men and 0.5 L/kg × weight in kg for women.

Approximately one-third of the deficit can be replaced over the course of the first 12 hours at a rate of less than 0.5 mEq/L/hour. The remaining amounts can be administered over the course of the next several days.

The use of isotonic sodium chloride solution is ideal for the treatment of hyponatremia associated with volume depletion. As renal perfusion is restored, free water will be excreted with appropriate retention of sodium.[40] Because Q.B. has only mild volume depletion, oral replacement fluids can be given. Oral solutions containing both electrolyte and glucose[46] or rice-based solutions[47] are ideal for the management of persistent fluid loss.

Glucose not only provides calories but also promotes the intestinal absorption of ingested sodium.[48] Because the rice-based solution provides more glucose and amino acids, both of which can promote intestinal sodium absorption, it is more effective than glucose alone.[2,48]

In patients with renal salt wasting, the ongoing daily sodium loss also should be taken into consideration when estimating the amount of replacement. Potassium should be given to correct hypokalemia, thereby reducing the hyponatremia as well. The serum sodium concentration may rise faster than expected because as tissue perfusion is restored, sodium delivery to the distal tubules will increase and ADH secretion will be suppressed appropriately.[34,37,40] In the absence of ADH, increased free-water excretion will improve the serum sodium concentration faster than initially estimated.

Hypervolemic Hypotonic Hyponatremia

CASE 10-6

QUESTION 1: T.W., a 55-year-old man with a longstanding history of alcoholic liver cirrhosis, is admitted to the hospital for worsening shortness of breath. His medical history includes portal hypertension, esophageal varices, and noncompliance with dietary restriction and medications. His BP is 120/60 mm Hg; pulse, 100 beats/minute; RR, 20 breaths/minute. He is afebrile. Physical examination reveals a jaundiced man in respiratory distress. His jugular vein is flat and lung examination reveals bilateral basal rales. Abdominal examination shows tense ascites with hepatomegaly and spider angiomas (telangiectasias resembling a spider). He has 1+ pedal edema bilaterally. Laboratory data on admission are as follows:

Na, 127 mEq/L
K, 3.4 mEq/L
Cl, 95 mEq/L
Total CO_2 content, 24 mEq/L
BUN, 10 mg/dL
Serum creatinine (SCr), 1.2 mg/dL
Albumin, 2.5 g/dL
Urine Na, <10 mEq/L
Osmolality, 380 mOsm/L

Identify the possible causes of hyponatremia in T.W. and discuss its pathophysiology. How should he be treated?

T.W. had no history of vomiting or diarrhea and had stopped using diuretics before admission. The physical findings of ascites and bilateral edema are not consistent with volume depletion but indicate a sodium-excess state. Both sodium and water retention occur, but the disproportionate accumulation of ingested water relative to sodium leads to hyponatremia.[34,37,40]

Cirrhotic patients who are susceptible to developing hyponatremia have a decreased effective arterial blood volume.[24,37,46,47] The low urinary sodium concentration suggests that the effective arterial blood volume was decreased.[15] The high urinary osmolality in the face of hypotonic hyponatremia suggests, however, that the release of ADH has been stimulated, impairing free-water excretion. Peripheral vasodilation causes decreases in systemic arterial BP despite a normal to high cardiac output. This, along with splanchnic venous pooling and decreased oncotic pressure secondary to hypoalbuminemia, decreases renal perfusion in patients with cirrhosis, such as T.W.[22,28,46] Decreased renal perfusion activates the renin-angiotensin-aldosterone system, the sympathetic nervous system, and the release of ADH. Reabsorption of sodium and water in the proximal tubules is enhanced, diminishing sodium and water delivery to the distal segments of the nephron. The diluting capacity of the kidney is thus impaired. Increased secretion of antidiuretic hormone also promotes free-water reabsorption at the collecting tubule and contributes to the hyperosmolality of urine and hyponatremia. The hypervolemic hyponatremia also is seen in patients with heart failure (HF) and nephrotic syndrome[24–28] and in patients with chronic renal disease who drink excessive amounts of water[37,40] (see Chapter 19, Heart Failure). As the GFR decreases, distal delivery of sodium is reduced and the ability to generate free water is impaired. In addition, the capacity to conserve sodium is impaired in these patients.[15]

Most patients who are edematous and hyponatremic are asymptomatic, but the degree of hyponatremia probably reflects the severity of the underlying disease.[46,47,49] Unless an acute decrease in serum sodium occurs, rapid therapeutic correction is not warranted.[37,40,46,47,50] Water restriction, the mainstay of therapy, is determined by the degree of hyponatremia and the severity of symptoms. Sodium restriction and judicious use of diuretics may help reduce the edematous state, but the patient must be monitored closely to avoid prerenal azotemia, which suggests overaggressive diuresis. Furthermore, diuretics can induce or worsen hyponatremia and volume depletion by impairing the diluting capacity of the kidney.[43–47]

T.W. had abdominal paracentesis to relieve respiratory discomfort with no sequelae. He was then prescribed a 1,000-mg-sodium diet, and water was restricted to 500 mL/day. Diuretic therapy was resumed.

Normovolemic Hypotonic Hyponatremia

CASE 10-7

QUESTION 1: C.C., a 50-year-old man who was diagnosed recently with small-cell lung carcinoma, was brought to the ED by his family because he had become progressively lethargic and stuporous during the past week. Laboratory data revealed the following:

Serum Na, 110 mEq/L
K, 3.6 mEq/L
Cl, 78 mEq/L
Bicarbonate, 22 mEq/L
BUN, 10 mg/dL
SCr, 0.9 mg/dL
Glucose, 90 mg/dL
Serum osmolality, 230 mOsm/kg
Urine osmolality, 616 mOsm/kg
Urine Na, 60 mEq/L

Arterial blood gas (ABG) examination at room air showed pH, 7.38; Pco_2, 38 mm Hg; and Po_2, 80 mm Hg. On physical examination, C.C. was normotensive, appeared to be euvolemic, and had no edema detected. Review of his medical records showed normal adrenal and thyroid function. C.C. was currently not using any medications. On admission to the ward, C.C. weighed 60 kg and was given 1 L of normal saline, after which his serum sodium concentration was 108 mEq/L. Identify the cause of hyponatremia in C.C. and describe its pathophysiology.

In a patient with hypo-osmolar hyponatremia with a volume status that is apparently normal, the differential diagnosis[40] includes hypothyroidism,[51] cortisol deficiency,[52] a reset osmostat,[53] psychogenic polydipsia,[36,38] and the syndrome of inappropriate antidiuretic hormone secretion (SIADH),[54–56] which is a diagnosis of exclusion. C.C.'s normal thyroid and adrenal function tests exclude hypothyroidism and cortisol insufficiency as causes of his hyponatremia. The inappropriately elevated urine osmolality (>100 mOsm/kg) is inconsistent with psychogenic polydipsia or a reset osmostat, because free-water excretion is usually not impaired in these disorders. These findings, in addition to a urine sodium concentration greater than 40 mEq/L and a normal acid–base and potassium balance, are consistent with SIADH.[37,55,56]

In SIADH, the ADH secretion is considered inappropriate because of its persistence in the absence of appropriate osmotic and hemodynamic stimuli. Water ingestion is essential to the development of hyponatremia in SIADH because persistent ADH activity impairs water excretion, resulting in expansion of body fluids and hypo-osmolar hyponatremia. Edema rarely is apparent because only one-third of the retained water resides in the extracellular space and the sodium homeostatic mechanisms are intact.[34,40] The extracellular fluid expansion activates volume receptors and results in natriuresis. At steady state, urinary sodium excretion reflects sodium intake and is usually greater than 40 mEq/L, as in C.C.'s case. Nonetheless, if sodium intake is reduced severely, the urinary sodium concentration may become less than 40 mEq/L.[37]

The causes of SIADH are diverse and are shown in Table 10-1. Four different patterns of inappropriate ADH release have been identified.[37] No correlation has been found between these patterns and the underlying causes of SIADH, however. Mechanisms for drug-induced SIADH include ADH-like action on the collecting tubule, central stimulation of ADH release, and potentiation of the ADH effect.[37,57] Small-cell lung carcinoma is the most likely cause of C.C.'s SIADH.

CASE 10-7, QUESTION 2: Why was C.C.'s serum sodium concentration lower after the saline infusion?

Isotonic sodium chloride solution (154 mEq/L each of sodium and chloride ions, or 308 mOsm/L) initially will increase the plasma sodium concentration because its osmolality is higher than C.C.'s.[58] C.C., however, has a relatively fixed urine osmolality of 616 mOsm/kg owing to persistent ADH activity; thus, he must excrete an osmolar load of 616 mOsm in a volume of 1,000 mL of urine at steady state. Because a total of 1 L of fluid containing 308 mOsm was administered, all the solutes were excreted in 500 mL of urine output, and 500 mL of free water was retained to cause a further dilution of sodium and a reduction in serum sodium concentration.[37,58]

Neurologic Manifestations

CASE 10-7, QUESTION 3: Why are C.C.'s neurologic manifestations characteristic of hyponatremia?

As the plasma osmolality declines, the osmotic gradient created across the blood–brain barrier favors the movement of water into the brain and other cells.[37,40] Water movement from the cerebrospinal fluid into the cerebral interstitium results in cerebral edema. Brain swelling is limited by the meninges and cranium, however, giving rise to increased intracranial pressure and neurologic symptoms. The degree of cerebral overhydration and the rapidity of its development appear to correlate with the severity of symptoms.[37,40]

When hyponatremia develops in less than 2 to 3 days or the rate of decline in serum sodium is greater than 0.5 mEq/L/hour, the situation is regarded as acute.[37,59,60] The patient often becomes symptomatic when serum sodium concentration falls to 125 mEq/L; early complaints include nausea, vomiting, and malaise.[37,61] Severe symptoms occur more commonly when the serum sodium falls to less than 120 mEq/L and the rate of decline is greater than 0.5 mEq/L/hour. The patient may present with headache, tremors, incoordination, delirium, lethargy, and obtundation. As the serum sodium drops less than 110 to 115 mEq/L, seizure and coma may result.[37,61] On occasion, severe brain edema leads to transtentorial herniation and eventually death. Women, especially those who are premenopausal, apparently are more susceptible to the development of severe neurologic symptoms and irreversible neurologic damage than are men.[62,63]

In contrast to acute hyponatremia, patients who are chronically hyponatremic are usually asymptomatic.[37,59] If present, symptoms are usually vague and nonspecific and tend to occur at lower serum sodium concentrations than those associated with symptomatic acute hyponatremia.[37,59,61] The patient may experience anorexia, nausea, vomiting, muscle weakness, and cramps. Irritability, hostility, confusion, and personality changes also may be seen. At extremely low sodium levels, stupor and, rarely, seizures have been reported.

Brain Adaptation to Hyponatremia

The difference in symptoms between acute and chronic hyponatremia is related to cerebral adaptation to hypotonicity. Two adaptive mechanisms are important in minimizing cerebral edema.[37,40,64,65] First, cerebral overhydration increases the hydrostatic pressure in the cerebral interstitium, which results in the movement of fluid from the cerebral interstitial space to the cerebrospinal fluid. Second, the extrusion of intracellular solutes reduces cellular osmolality, which in turn enhances water movement out of the cells. Sodium and potassium ions are the initial solutes extruded, followed over a period of hours to days by osmolytes such as inositol, glutamine, glutamate, and taurine.[64] Therefore, when the serum sodium concentration falls faster than the onset of brain osmotic adaptation processes, serious and permanent neurologic damage can occur.[37,40,64,65] On the other hand, when hyponatremia develops over the course of 2 to 3 days, symptoms are not usually seen unless the serum sodium concentration is reduced markedly.

It is often difficult to determine the acuity and chronicity of hyponatremia. Unless an obvious cause for acute hyponatremia is found, assume that the condition is chronic.[37,59,60,65] A rapid decline in serum sodium concentration usually suggests that hypotonic fluid was administered to a patient with a condition that overwhelms or impairs renal water excretion. These conditions include psychogenic polydipsia[35,36]; postoperative hyponatremia[62,63,66,67]; postprostatectomy syndrome[39]; and administration of thiazide diuretics,[41,42] parenteral cyclophosphamide,[68] oxytocin,[69] and arginine vasopressin or its analogs.[57] C.C.'s symptoms appear to have developed over the course of 7 days and are consistent with chronic hyponatremia.

Rate of Correction of Hyponatremia

CASE 10-7, QUESTION 4: How should C.C.'s hyponatremia be managed?

C.C.'s water excess should be calculated to estimate the amount of water that should be removed to achieve the desired sodium concentration.

$$\text{Water excess} = \text{TBW} - \text{TBW}\left(\frac{\text{Observed serum Na}}{\text{Desired serum Na}}\right)$$

$$= 36\text{ L} - 36\text{ L}\left(\frac{110\text{ mEq/L}}{120\text{ mEq/L}}\right)$$

$$= 3.0\text{ L} \qquad \textit{(Eq. 10-9)}$$

where

$$\text{TBW} = 0.6 \times 60 = 36\text{ L} \qquad \textit{(Eq. 10-10)}$$

The treatment of hyponatremia has been controversial. Severe hyponatremia is associated with high rates of morbidity and mortality, but its treatment can also result in morbidity. The rate of correction has been implicated as the main cause of complications.[59–61,65,70–72]

It takes time for the brain to lose osmolytes to reduce cerebral swelling during hyponatremia; conversely, the rate of reaccumulation of these osmolytes must keep pace with the rise in serum sodium concentration to avoid brain dehydration and damage. Indeed, rapid correction of hyponatremia can cause a constellation of neurologic findings known as osmotic demyelination syndrome (ODS).[71,72] Clinical manifestations usually are delayed and occur one to several days after the treatment has been started. Neurologic findings include transient behavioral changes, seizures, akinetic mutism in mild cases, and features of a pontine disorder in severe cases (pseudobulbar palsy, quadriparesis, and coma). In some patients, the damage is irreversible, and central pontine myelinolysis can be documented in fatal cases. Patients at greatest risk for osmotic demyelination are those with severe hyponatremia lasting greater than 2 days and those in whom the rate of correction of hyponatremia is greater than 12 mEq/L in any 24-hour period.[65,71,72] Hypokalemia, which was found in about 90% of patients with ODS associated with rapid hyponatremia correction, has been suspected as a predisposing factor in the development of ODS.[72] Because the etiology of this complication is unclear, it may be beneficial to correct the hypokalemia before correcting the severe hyponatremia.[72]

Retrospective reviews suggest that acute hyponatremia can be treated safely at a rate of 1 mEq/L/hour initially, until the serum sodium concentration reaches 120 mEq/L. Thereafter, the rate of correction should be reduced to less than or equal to 0.5 mEq/L/hour, such that an increment in sodium concentration does not exceed 12 mEq/L in the first 24 hours.[59,73] Slow correction is indicated for severe chronic hyponatremia. No neurologic complications were seen in patients with severe hyponatremia when the average rate of correction to serum sodium was less than 0.55 mEq/L/hour or when the increase in serum sodium was less than 12 mEq/L in 24 hours or less than 18 mEq/L in 48 hours.[73]

In C.C., the serum sodium concentration should be raised to approximately 120 mEq/L at a correction rate of approximately 0.5 mEq/L/hour, using hypertonic saline and furosemide. Serum sodium concentrations should be monitored closely because the equation for calculating water excess does not take into account insensible loss, which can increase the rate of sodium correction.

The use of normal saline is not useful in C.C. because he excretes salt normally (urine sodium, 60 mEq/L). C.C.'s sodium deficit is as follows:

$$(0.6\text{ L/kg})(60\text{ kg})(120 - 110\text{ mEq/L}) = 360\text{ mEq} \qquad \textit{(Eq. 10-11)}$$

Because 1 L of 3% sodium chloride solution contains 513 mEq of sodium, approximately 700 mL of 3% saline solution, which contains 360 mEq of sodium, will be required to correct the sodium deficit. The recommended serum sodium concentration correction rate is 0.5 mEq/L/hour; therefore, a minimum of 20 hours will be needed to raise the serum sodium concentration by 10 mEq/L (from 110 to 120 mEq/L). The amount of sodium replacement to safely increase the serum sodium concentration can be determined by the product of the rate of replacement (0.5 mEq/L/hour) and TBW (36 L, Eq. 10-10)—that is, 18 mEq/hour. The maximal rate of infusion of 3% saline, which contains 0.513 mEq/mL of sodium, is therefore 35 mL/hour (18 mEq/hour)/(0.513 mEq/mL). A rate of 30 mL/hour, therefore, is appropriate to safely replace C.C.'s sodium deficit.

Because calculations for water excess and sodium deficits are only approximations, the patient's serum osmolality, serum sodium, and clinical response must be monitored closely. Urinary losses can be replaced with 3% sodium chloride solution and appropriate amounts of potassium.

Chronic Management of the Syndrome of Inappropriate Antidiuretic Hormone Secretion

CASE 10-7, QUESTION 5: How should C.C.'s SIADH be managed chronically?

SIADH is usually transient if the underlying cause can be removed. Chronic SIADH can occur, however, as illustrated by C.C. Water restriction sufficient to create a negative water balance is the primary therapy and should be attempted first.[37,40] In general, all fluids, not just water, should be included in the restriction. Salt intake, however, should not be reduced or solute depletion can occur. The extent of fluid restriction depends on urine output, the amount of insensible water loss, and urine osmolality. For a given amount of solute excretion, patients with a high urine osmolality require a smaller volume of urine (i.e., more water retained) than those with a lower urine osmolality (i.e., less water retained). Hence, more stringent water restriction is required in patients with a high urine osmolality. Commonly, several days of restriction are needed before a significant increase in plasma osmolality is observed.

When fluid restriction fails to reverse the hypo-osmolar state or when the patient is unwilling or unable to comply with the severe fluid restriction, drugs that antagonize the effect of ADH can be used.[37,40] These include loop diuretics,[74,75] demeclocycline,[76] and lithium.[77] Furosemide (20–40 mg/day) reduces urine osmolality by blocking the concentrating ability of the kidney.[74] Demeclocycline and lithium directly impair the response to ADH at the collecting tubule, inducing nephrogenic diabetes insipidus.[76,77] Demeclocycline (300–600 mg twice daily) is usually better tolerated than lithium. Its effect on water excretion is delayed for a few days and it dissipates over a similar period of time after the drug is stopped. Nephrotoxicity has been reported with its use in patients with cirrhosis.[78] Limited data suggest that phenytoin may inhibit ADH secretion, but its effectiveness is questionable.[79] Urea can correct hypo-osmolality by increasing solute-free water excretion and reducing urinary sodium excretion.[80] It has been used effectively, at 30 to 60 g/day, both short term and long term, to reduce the need for fluid restriction.[81] An IV formulation of urea is available commercially; however, for oral administration, 30 g of urea crystals can be dissolved in 10 mL of aluminum-magnesium antacid and 100 mL of water. Orange juice or other strongly flavored liquids can be used to improve palatability.

VASOPRESSIN RECEPTOR ANTAGONISTS

Nonpeptide vasopressin receptor antagonists (VRAs), also known as the "vaptans" or "aquaretic agents," constitute a class of agents used for the treatment of hyponatremia. Arginine vasopressin (AVP), a neuropeptide hormone, plays an important role in maintaining serum osmolality, as well as circulatory and sodium homeostasis.[82] AVP exerts its physiologic effects by acting on V1A, V1B, and V2 receptors, causing effects such as vasoconstriction,[83,84] corticotropin release,[85] and water excretion,[86] respectively. V2 receptors are located in the renal collecting tubules and mediate the antidiuretic effects of AVP. Antagonism of the V2 receptors results in aquaresis, which is a unique solute-free and electrolyte-sparing (sodium and potassium) water excretion process in the kidneys. Because circulating levels of AVP are elevated in SIADH, cirrhosis, and HF, VRA can be beneficial in the management of hyponatremia associated with these conditions.

Conivaptan, a mixed V1A and V2 receptor antagonist, was the first VRA approved by the US Food and Drug Administration (FDA) for the treatment of euvolemic and hypervolemic hyponatremia in hospitalized patients.[82] Randomized, double-blind, placebo-controlled trials demonstrated its efficacy in increasing serum sodium concentrations in patients with euvolemic and hypervolemic hyponatremia associated with SIADH and heart failure, respectively.[87,88] It is administered as an IV infusion and its use is restricted to a short-term (4 days) inpatient use only. Close monitoring of serum sodium concentration is necessary to prevent overly rapid correction of hyponatremia and central pontine myelinolysis that may ensue. Because conivaptan is a potent inhibitor of the cytochrome P-450 3A4 (CYP3A4) enzyme, drug interactions with medications that undergo CYP3A4-mediated metabolism are possible.[82] In addition, patients may experience infusion-site reactions with conivaptan caused by the organic solvent, polypropylene glycol.

Tolvaptan, a selective oral VRA, was approved by the FDA in 2009 for the treatment of hypervolemic and euvolemic hyponatremia in patients with heart failure, cirrhosis, and SIADH. Because of its selectivity for the V2 receptor, tolvaptan increases urinary excretion of free water (aquaresis) and has less of a blood pressure–lowering effect. As such, it may be more suitable for use in patients with low to normal blood pressure, such as those with heart failure or cirrhosis. Tolvaptan has been shown to increase serum sodium concentration significantly and correct hyponatremia in patients with SIADH, chronic heart failure, or cirrhosis.[89] It has also been studied extensively in chronic heart failure where improvement in signs and symptoms such as reduction of edema and weight, as well as normalization of serum sodium concentrations, were shown.[90,91] However, the use of tolvaptan in heart failure had no effect on long-term cardiovascular mortality or hospitalization for heart failure.[92]

Lixivaptan and satavaptan are two other VRAs that are selective for the V2 receptor and are currently under investigation. Like tolvaptan, they are orally active and thus useful in patients who require chronic therapy or when oral therapy is preferred. Lixivaptan has been studied in patients with hyponatremia from HF, cirrhosis, and SIADH; the results showed significant increases in aquaresis and serum sodium concentrations.[93–95] When satavaptan was administered to patients with hyponatremia caused by SIADH, normalization of serum sodium concentrations or an increase by greater than or equal to 5 mEq/L was observed.[96]

Common adverse effects of VRAs include thirst, dry mouth, polyuria, and blood pressure reduction. Aquaretics increase thirst by increasing blood tonicity and urine volume; orthostatic hypotension has been reported.[97] These agents are thus contraindicated in hypovolemic hyponatremia. The risk of excessive correction of hyponatremia and the resultant neurological complications from osmotic demyelination exists with VRA, especially when used in combination with fluid restriction. These agents should therefore be initiated in the inpatient setting at the lowest possible dose and titrated slowly, with close monitoring of serum sodium concentrations and volume status. Additionally, the VRAs are substrates and inhibitors of the CYP3A4 enzyme. As a result, there is a potential for clinically significant drug interactions, particularly with concomitant administration of moderate or strong CYP3A4 inducers or inhibitors.

The VRAs should be used in hyponatremic patients with mild to moderately severe neurologic symptoms. Not only have they been shown to maintain normal serum sodium concentrations both short- and long-term but their aquaretic effect could also reduce or eliminate the need for fluid restriction normally required of patients.[89,98] The effectiveness of VRA to correct euvolemic and hypervolemic hyponatremia has now been shown. Their long-term safety with chronic use and their potential benefits on morbidity and mortality, however, need to be assessed.

Hypernatremia

Hypernatremia can occur under the following conditions: (a) normal total body sodium with pure water loss, (b) low total body sodium with hypotonic fluid loss, and (c) high total body sodium as a result of pure salt gain.[99] Therefore, as in hyponatremia, it is important to assess the volume status of the extracellular fluid when evaluating hypernatremia.

ONLINE CONTENT

For an illustration of the effect of isotonic fluid volume deficit and excess and of hyponatremia and hypernatremia on extracellular (ECF) and intracellular fluid volume (ICF), go to http://thepoint.lww.com/AT10e.

Pure water loss can result from the inability of the kidney to conserve water (diabetes insipidus) or from extrarenal water loss through the respiratory tract or the skin.[100] Usually, pure water loss does not cause hypernatremia unless the thirst center is damaged or access to free water is limited.[99]

Hypotonic fluid loss can occur renally as a result of osmotic diuresis, use of loop diuretics, postobstruction diuresis, or intrinsic renal disease. Extrarenally, hypotonic fluid loss can result from diarrhea, vomiting, burns, and excessive sweating.

Pure salt gain can result from the use of hypertonic saline during abortion, sodium bicarbonate administration during cardiopulmonary resuscitation, hypertonic feedings in infants, and, rarely, mineralocorticoid excess.

The management of hypernatremia includes correcting the underlying cause of the hypertonic state, replacing the water deficits, and administering adequate water to match ongoing losses.[99] The pure water deficit can be estimated as follows:

$$\text{Water deficit} = \text{TBW}\left(\frac{\text{Observed serum Na}}{\text{Desired serum Na}}\right) - \text{TBW}$$

$$= \text{TBW}\left(\frac{\text{Observed serum Na}}{\text{Desired serum Na}} - 1\right) \quad \textit{(Eq. 10-12)}$$

where desired serum sodium is usually 140 mEq/L.

The rate at which hypernatremia should be corrected depends on the severity of symptoms and degree of hypertonicity. Too-rapid correction can precipitate cerebral edema, seizures, and irreversible neurologic damage, and can be fatal. For asymptomatic patients, the rate of correction probably should not exceed changes of 0.5 mEq/L/hour in plasma sodium. A rule of thumb is to replace half the calculated deficit with hypotonic solutions over the course of 12 to 24 hours. Any ongoing water loss, including insensible loss, also should be replenished while carefully monitoring the patient's neurologic status. The remaining deficit can then be replaced during the ensuing 24 to 48 hours. Concomitant solute deficits and ongoing solute losses should also be replaced as appropriate. If hypernatremia is caused only by pure water loss, free water can be administered as 5% dextrose in water. Half-normal saline or quarter-normal saline is used if a sodium deficit is also present. In patients with hypotension or shock, the effective arterial blood volume should be restored with normal saline or colloids before the plasma tonicity is corrected.

CLINICAL USE OF DIURETICS

Diuretics reduce sodium and chloride reabsorption in the renal tubules, thereby increasing urine volume. Enhanced solute and fluid excretion can be initiated through osmotic diuresis or inhibition of transport in the kidney tubules. Diuretics are categorized according to the sites within the kidney tubules where they inhibit sodium reabsorption (see Chapter 14, Essential Hypertension, and Chapter 31, Chronic Kidney Diseases).

Loop Diuretics

The loop diuretics—furosemide, bumetanide, torsemide, and ethacrynic acid—are the most potent diuretics available. They are also known as high-ceiling diuretics because they can inhibit the reabsorption of up to 20% to 25% of the filtered sodium load. The loop diuretics act in the medullary and cortical portion of the thick ascending limb of Henle's loop. Sodium and chloride transport through the $Na^+/K^+/2Cl^-$ carrier in the luminal membrane is inhibited. Reabsorption of calcium and magnesium is reduced secondary to the reduction in sodium chloride transport. The loop diuretics also possess a vasodilatory effect that can contribute to their diuretic activity.

Thiazide Diuretics

The thiazide diuretics are a group of structurally similar compounds that share a common mechanism of action. Several other sulfonamide diuretics that differ chemically, such as chlorthalidone, indapamide, and metolazone, also have diuretic effects similar to the thiazides. The primary site of action of these diuretics is at the proximal portion of the distal tubule. Sodium reabsorption via the Na^+/Cl^- cotransporter is blocked through competition with the chloride site of the transporter. Some of these agents, such as chlorothiazide, may also reduce sodium transport in the proximal tubule. The contribution of this effect toward net diuresis is negligible, however, because the sodium ions that are not reabsorbed in the proximal tubule will subsequently be reabsorbed in Henle's loop. Thiazide diuretics can enhance the reabsorption of calcium ion through a direct action on the early distal tubule. Therefore, these agents are useful to reduce calciuria in patients with kidney stones. In contrast, magnesium excretion is increased by the thiazides, which may result in hypomagnesemia.

Potassium-Sparing Diuretics

SPIRONOLACTONE, TRIAMTERENE, AND AMILORIDE

Spironolactone, triamterene, and amiloride are potassium-sparing diuretics that inhibit sodium reabsorption in the cortical collecting tubules through different mechanisms. Spironolactone is a competitive receptor-site antagonist of aldosterone in the distal segment of the renal tubule and is indicated especially for patients with hyperaldosteronism secondary to decreased renal perfusion. Patients with hyperaldosteronism can be identified by urinary electrolyte screening, which shows high urine potassium excretion with concomitant diminished or absent urine sodium excretion. By serving as an aldosterone antagonist, spironolactone inhibits sodium reabsorption and decreases the excretion of potassium and hydrogen ions. Dosages as high as 200 to 400 mg/day may be needed to induce natriuresis in patients with hyperaldosteronism.

In contrast to spironolactone, triamterene and amiloride reduce the passage of sodium ions through the luminal membrane, independent of aldosterone activity, by directly acting on sodium and potassium transport processes in the distal renal tubular cells. Triamterene and amiloride offer the advantage of a more rapid onset of action than spironolactone.

The initial effects of spironolactone are usually delayed for 2 or 3 days, and several additional days are needed to attain maximal diuretic effect. This delay is caused partly by the formation of an active metabolite, canrenone, which accounts for approximately 70% of the antimineralocorticoid activity of spironolactone. The elimination half-life of canrenone is 13.5 to 24 hours in normal subjects and is prolonged in patients with chronic liver disease (59 hours [range, 32–105 hours]) or HF (37 hours [range, 19–48 hours]).[101] Although the elimination half-life of canrenone is prolonged in these patients, plasma canrenone concentrations do not differ significantly from those in normal subjects because assay methods for canrenone are nonspecific and include measurement of both active and inactive metabolites.[102,103]

Triamterene is absorbed incompletely from the GI tract. The drug has a short half-life of 1.5 to 2.5 hours. The total body clearance is high because of rapid and extensive hepatic metabolism. Both the parent compound and the metabolite undergo biliary and renal excretion. As with spironolactone, the hepatic metabolism of triamterene can be altered in patients with cirrhosis.[104] The diuretic effect of triamterene begins within 2 to 3 hours of administration, with a maximal duration of 12 to 16 hours.

Amiloride does not undergo hepatic metabolism; approximately 50% of amiloride is excreted in the urine unchanged and the remainder is recovered in the stool as unabsorbed drug or through biliary excretion. Serum amiloride concentrations peak 3 hours after oral ingestion, and the half-life is 6 hours. Although commonly administered doses are in the range of 2.5 to 10 mg, diuresis increases over a much greater range. The onset of action is 2 hours, with maximal effects at 4 to 6 hours. Duration of action is dose dependent and ranges from 10 to 24 hours. Amiloride does not undergo hepatic metabolism, and the drug can accumulate in patients with renal insufficiency.

The maximal amount of filtered sodium that can be excreted through the action of potassium-sparing diuretics is approximately 1% to 2%. Their natriuretic activity, therefore, is relatively limited compared with the thiazide and loop diuretics. These agents are often used concurrently with thiazide and loop diuretics to reduce potassium loss. Spironolactone is especially useful in patients with liver cirrhosis and ascites, who are likely to have high levels of aldosterone.

Acetazolamide

Acetazolamide inhibits carbonic anhydrase, an enzyme that mediates the excretion of sodium, bicarbonate, and chloride ions in the proximal tubule. Use of the drug will increase urine pH owing to the increased excretion of bicarbonate ion. The net diuretic and natriuretic effects are limited, similar to those of the potassium-sparing diuretics. Because of the drug's proximal site of action, the sodium ions that are not reabsorbed will subsequently be reclaimed in Henle's loop and the distal tubule. In addition, metabolic acidosis associated with the use of acetazolamide diminishes its diuretic effect.

Osmotic Diuretics

Osmotic diuretics are nonresorbable solutes in the kidney tubule. They act primarily in the proximal tubule, where the osmotic pressure they generate impedes the reabsorption of water and solutes. Unlike other diuretics, the amount of water loss exceeds the concurrent loss of sodium and potassium. Mannitol has been used in the early treatment of oliguric postischemic acute renal failure to increase urine output. Urea, another osmotic diuretic, and mannitol are used to reduce intracranial pressure through cellular dehydration.

Complications of Diuretic Therapy

Disturbances in fluid, electrolyte, and acid–base balance are common side effects associated with diuretic therapy. These side effects, including hypokalemia, are discussed in detail in Chapter 14, Essential Hypertension; Chapter 19, Heart Failure; and Chapter 45, Gout and Hyperuricemia. Two complications, hyponatremia and metabolic alkalosis and acidosis, are, however, discussed in the subsequent section because of their specific relevance to fluid balance.

HYPONATREMIA

Thiazides induce diuresis by inhibiting sodium and water reabsorption in the kidney tubule. Because both sodium and water are lost, overdiuresis per se is not expected to cause hyponatremia. Instead, hyponatremia represents a dilution of plasma sodium by excess free water caused by volume-depletion–induced ADH activity. The enhanced ADH secretion increases free-water reabsorption, resulting in hyponatremia. Large doses of diuretic, excessive water drinking, and severe sodium-intake restriction all will accentuate the hyponatremia. Elderly patients are particularly susceptible to this diuretic-induced complication due to the age-associated loss of nephrons and consequent impairment of sodium–potassium exchange.

METABOLIC ALKALOSIS AND ACIDOSIS

Metabolic alkalosis often occurs in conjunction with potassium depletion secondary to diuretic use. The diuretic-induced contraction of extracellular fluid volume stimulates the secretion of aldosterone, which promotes the absorption of sodium and the retention of hydrogen ions in the kidney tubule. The net urinary loss of hydrogen ions into the urine results in metabolic alkalosis. Generally, reducing the dose of the diuretic will restore the acid–base balance.

Acetazolamide causes metabolic acidosis by inhibiting carbonic anhydrase, which results in urinary excretion of sodium bicarbonate. Spironolactone, amiloride, and triamterene can cause hyperchloremic metabolic acidosis because of their ability to decrease potassium and hydrogen ion tubular secretion. Patients with renal dysfunction or those taking potassium supplements or angiotensin-converting enzyme inhibitors, which reduce aldosterone secretion, are at increased risk for developing hyperkalemia and metabolic acidosis.

POTASSIUM

Homeostasis

The total amount of potassium stored in the body is approximately 45 to 55 mEq/kg and varies with age, sex, and muscle mass. Lower total body potassium is found in older adults, females, and individuals with a low lean-body-mass to fat ratio. Potassium is distributed unevenly between the intracellular and extracellular compartments; 98% of the total body potassium resides in the intracellular compartment, predominantly the muscle, and only 2% is found in the extracellular space.[34,96,105] The disproportionate intracellular distribution of potassium is maintained by the Na^+/K^+ ATPase pump, which transports sodium out of the cell in exchange for potassium.[105–108] The cell membrane resting potential is determined by the ratio of intracellular/extracellular potassium concentrations. As this ratio increases, hyperpolarization of the cell membrane occurs. Conversely, cellular depolarization results when the ratio decreases. In both situations, generation of the action potential is impaired.

The plasma potassium concentration is maintained within a narrow range of 3.5 to 5.0 mEq/L. Although the plasma potassium concentration can be affected by the total body potassium store, total body potassium excess or deficit cannot be estimated accurately based solely on the plasma concentration. In fact, a normal plasma potassium concentration does not imply normal total body potassium because multiple factors affect the plasma potassium concentration independent of total body potassium.[106]

Potassium homeostasis is maintained by both renal and extrarenal processes. The renal process regulates total body potassium by matching potassium excretion to dietary intake (external balance),[109] whereas the extrarenal process regulates potassium distribution across cell membrane (internal potassium balance).[106,107]

The normal daily intake of potassium ranges between 50 and 100 mEq. Approximately 90% of the ingested potassium is eliminated by the kidneys and approximately 10% is eliminated via the GI tract.[109] Potassium is filtered freely through the glomerulus and then reabsorbed. By the time the filtrate reaches the distal convoluted tubule, greater than 90% of filtered potassium has already been reabsorbed. The amount of potassium excreted is determined by distal tubular potassium secretion in the principal cells of the cortical collecting duct, which is under the influence of aldosterone. Hyperkalemia, increased potassium load, and AT_2 can all stimulate aldosterone secretion.[106]

Factors that affect renal potassium excretion include tubular flow, sodium delivery to the distal segments of the nephron, the presence of poorly absorbable anions that increase luminal electronegativity, acid–base status, and aldosterone activity.[93] Potassium excretion increases during hyperkalemia and decreases during potassium depletion. Excretion of an acute potassium load is a slow process, with only half the potassium load excreted in the first 4 to 6 hours. Lethal hyperkalemia would ensue were it not for the extrarenal process that regulates intracellular/extracellular potassium distribution.[106]

The Na^+/K^+ ATPase pump, which extrudes sodium from the cell in exchange for potassium, is pivotal in maintaining internal potassium balance.[108] Different hormonal factors regulate the activity of the Na^+/K^+ ATPase pump, namely, insulin, catecholamines, and aldosterone. Insulin, the most important regulator, enhances potassium uptake by muscle, liver, and adipose tissue by stimulating Na^+/K^+ ATPase.[110] Indeed, basal insulin secretion is essential for potassium homeostasis.[106] Whereas β_2-adrenergic agonists activate the Na^+/K^+ ATPase pump via cyclic adenosine monophosphate and cause hypokalemia, α-adrenergic stimulation promotes hepatic potassium release and causes hyperkalemia.[111] Epinephrine, an α-agonist and β-agonist, causes a transient increase in plasma potassium (α-agonism) followed by a more sustained decrease in plasma potassium (β-agonism).[111,112] Besides its kaliuretic effect and enhanced potassium secretion in the colon, aldosterone also stimulates Na^+/K^+ ATPase.

Other factors that affect the transcellular distribution of potassium include systemic pH, plasma tonicity, and exercise.[106,108] The effect of acid–base balance on potassium distribution is not readily predictable and depends on both the nature and the direction of the underlying disorder. The concomitant effect of the acid–base disorder on renal potassium excretion further complicates the relationship between plasma potassium concentration and pH.[106,113] In acute inorganic acidosis, plasma potassium concentration increases by 0.2 to 1.7 mEq/L per 0.1-unit decrease in pH. Chronic inorganic metabolic acidosis usually is associated, however, with hypokalemia because of urinary potassium loss associated with both proximal (type 2) and distal (type 1) renal tubular acidosis.[106,113] In contrast, organic acidosis commonly has no effect on potassium distribution.[114]

Other associated factors in the organic acidosis may, however, affect cellular potassium distribution.[113] For example, hyperglycemia in diabetic ketoacidosis may increase the serum potassium concentration because of the hypertonic effect of glucose.[115] Hypertonicity causes cell shrinkage and increases the intracellular to extracellular fluid potassium gradient, favoring potassium egress. Acute metabolic alkalosis only modestly decreases the plasma potassium concentration: 0.3 mEq/L for each 0.1-unit pH increment.[106,113] As with chronic metabolic acidosis, chronic metabolic alkalosis causes profound renal potassium wasting and is associated with hypokalemia. Respiratory acid–base disorders usually are associated with less significant changes in plasma potassium concentration than are metabolic acid–base disorders.[113] Exercise often causes an increase in the serum potassium concentration to a degree that varies with the intensity of the exercise.[116]

Hypokalemia

ETIOLOGY

CASE 10-8

QUESTION 1: J.P., a 60-year-old woman, presents to the ED with complaints of malaise, generalized weakness, nausea, and vomiting for 3 days. Her medical history includes hypertension for 20 years. J.P.'s current medications include hydrochlorothiazide 25 mg/day and nifedipine XL 30 mg/day. She has not been able to take her medications in the past few days, however, because of vomiting. J.P. denies recent diarrhea or use of laxatives. Her BP is 130/70 mm Hg with a pulse of 80 beats/minute while sitting, and 120/70 mm Hg with a pulse of 95 beats/minute on standing. Physical examination reveals a thin, older woman with poor skin turgor, dry mucous membranes, and a flat jugular vein. T-wave flattening is noted on the electrocardiogram (ECG). Laboratory tests show the following:

Serum Na, 138 mEq/L
K, 2.1 mEq/L
Cl, 100 mEq/L
Bicarbonate, 32 mEq/L
BUN, 30 mg/dL
Creatinine, 1.2 mg/dL
Glucose, 100 mg/dL

ABG shows pH, 7.50; P_{CO_2}, 45 mm Hg; and P_{O_2}, 70 mm Hg at room air. Urine electrolytes are sodium, 30 mEq/L; potassium, 60 mEq/L; and chloride, less than 15 mEq/L. The patient's presentation is consistent with gastroenteritis. What are the causes of J.P.'s hypokalemia?

When evaluating hypokalemia, the clinician should determine whether the hypokalemia is a result of low intake, increased cellular uptake of potassium, or excessive loss of potassium via the kidneys, GI tract, or skin.[34,117] History and physical evidence of potassium depletion, medication history (including use of over-the-counter medicines), and assessment of the patient's BP, extracellular volume, and concurrent acid–base status can provide clues to the causes of hypokalemia.[34,117]

Because J.P. has been unable to eat for the past few days, decreased oral intake may have contributed to her hypokalemia. Because most foods are rich in potassium, however, inadequate intake rarely is the sole cause of potassium depletion unless inappropriate and continued renal or extrarenal losses occur, or potassium intake is severely restricted to less than 10 to 15 mEq/day.[117] Alkalosis,[113] insulin administration,[106] hypertonic solution administration, periodic paralysis,[118] β_2-agonists,[119] barium poisoning,[120] and treatment of megaloblastic anemia with vitamin B_{12}[121] all have been associated with increased cellular potassium uptake (Table 10-2). Although the relationship between the degree of hypokalemia and increase in blood pH varies widely,[113] J.P.'s metabolic alkalosis probably enhances the cellular uptake of potassium. The transcellular shift of potassium should not result in total body potassium depletion, however.

The GI tract is an important site of potassium loss, particularly through vomiting and diarrhea. Because the potassium content of gastric secretion (5–10 mEq/L) is much less than that of the intestinal secretion (up to 90 mEq/L),[117] loss of a large volume of gastric secretion is needed to produce substantial potassium depletion. Potassium deficit induced by vomiting, however, is commonly secondary to renal potassium loss, especially within the initial 24 to 48 hours.[122] The loss of hydrogen ion in gastric juice results in an elevated plasma bicarbonate concentration. The increased amount of bicarbonate ion, as a nonresorbable anion, increases water delivery to the distal nephron and enhances sodium reabsorption and potassium secretion, resulting in hypokalemia. The potassium wasting is often transient, because increased proximal reabsorption of sodium and bicarbonate will result in diminished bicarbonate delivery to the distal site. Reduced potassium excretion will ensue, commonly within 48 to 72 hours. Subsequent potassium loss will then be primarily consequent to gastric secretion removal.

The absence of diarrhea in J.P. excludes the GI tract as the source of potassium loss. Potassium loss through the skin also is unlikely in J.P. because the potassium concentration of sweat is less than 10 mEq/L. Therefore, profuse sweating, such as that induced by vigorous exercise in a hot, humid environment, or severe burns are needed to cause substantial loss.

J.P.'s inappropriately high urinary potassium concentration indicates that the kidney is the source of the potassium loss.[34,117] The urinary potassium concentration is a good marker for differentiating various hypokalemic syndromes. A urinary potassium excretion of less than 20 mEq/day suggests extrarenal potassium loss. Renal potassium wastage cannot be excluded, however, unless the low urinary potassium excretion is accompanied by a sodium intake of at least 100 mEq/day, because a low-sodium diet can reduce renal potassium excretion.[34] In J.P., the metabolic alkalosis and hypovolemia promote renal potassium wastage.[34,117] The distal delivery of a large sodium bicarbonate load and increased aldosterone activity (from hypovolemia) enhance potassium secretion and severely impair the kidney's ability to conserve potassium. The hydrochlorothiazide, which J.P. had been taking until 3 days before admission, could also have induced hypokalemia through volume depletion, hypochloremic metabolic alkalosis, and renal potassium wastage. The diuretic is unlikely, however, to be the cause for J.P.'s hypokalemia because she has stopped taking the medication, and this is reflected by the low urinary chloride concentration.[15] Bartter syndrome, which presents as normotension, hypokalemia, hypochloremic metabolic alkalosis, and renal potassium wastage, is characterized by impaired renal sodium and chloride reabsorption. The low urinary chloride concentration in J.P. can rule out Bartter syndrome. Other causes of hypokalemia are listed in Table 10-2.

TABLE 10-2
Drugs That Most Commonly Induce Hypokalemia

Drug	Mechanism	Predisposing Factors
Acetazolamide	Marked ↑ in renal K^+ loss	Most profound with short-term therapy
Amphotericin	Renal K^+ loss (renal tubular acidosis)	Concurrent piperacillin, ticarcillin
β_2-Agonists	Intracellular shift of K^+	
Cisplatin	Renal K^+ loss secondary to renal tubular damage	May be dose related but can occur after a single 50-mg/m^2 dose
Corticosteroids	Renal K^+ loss. Enhanced Na^+ reabsorption at distal tubule and collecting ducts in exchange for K^+ and H^+	Supraphysiologic doses of agents with moderate to strong mineralocorticoid activity (e.g., prednisone, hydrocortisone)
Insulin with glucose	Intracellular shift of K^+	Predictable effect when insulin administered to patients with diabetic ketoacidosis' combination used to treat hyperkalemia
Penicillins (piperacillin, ticarcillin)	High Na^+ load and nonresorbable anions can ↑ K^+ loss	Was more common with carbenicillin when it was available; newer penicillins are used in lower doses; less likely to produce hypokalemia
Thiazide and loop diuretics	Renal K^+ loss. ↑ Na^+ delivery to the late distal tubule, resulting in Na^+ resorption in exchange for K^+	Patients with hyperaldosteronism (e.g., cirrhosis, HF) predisposed; may be dose related

HF, heart failure.

In an asymptomatic hypokalemic patient with no apparent causes for potassium depletion or transcellular redistribution, pseudohypokalemia should be excluded before pursuing an intensive evaluation.[101] Spurious hypokalemia can occur in leukemic patients whose leukocyte count ranges from 100,000 to 250,000 cells/μL.[123] The potassium in serum is taken up by the large number of leukemic cells when the blood specimen is allowed to stand at room temperature.

CLINICAL MANIFESTATIONS

CASE 10-8, QUESTION 2: What clinical manifestations of hypokalemia are evident in J.P.?

The clinical presentation of hypokalemia, which depends on the severity of potassium depletion, is a result of changes in cell membrane polarization.[117] Patients are usually asymptomatic when the plasma potassium level is 3.0 to 3.5 mEq/L, but they may complain of malaise, weakness, fatigue, and myalgia. J.P.'s muscle weakness and ECG changes reflect the muscular and cardiac manifestations of hypokalemia, respectively.[124,125]

Potassium depletion can lead to hyperpolarization of myocardial cells and a prolonged refractory period. When serum potassium concentrations fall below 3 mEq/L, T-wave flattening, straight tubule segment depression, and prominent U waves are seen on the ECG.[125]

ONLINE CONTENT **For an illustration of ECG changes observed with hypokalemia and hyperkalemia, go to http://thepoint.lww.com/AT10e.**

Mild hypokalemia (potassium concentration of 3.0–3.5 mEq/L) is potentially arrhythmogenic in patients with underlying coronary artery disease. The incidence of ventricular arrhythmia increases with the degree of hypokalemia. Patients without underlying heart disease may be susceptible to these myocardial effects during exercise, especially if the patient's pre-exercise potassium concentration is less than 3.5 mEq/L, because the potassium concentration may drop to less than 3.0 mEq/L as a result of β_2-adrenergic receptor-mediated cellular potassium uptake.[117] Potassium depletion may also increase the BP,[118] which can be lowered with potassium supplementation.[126]

When the serum potassium concentration is less than 2.5 to 3.0 mEq/L, muscle weakness, cramps, general malaise, fatigue, restless leg syndrome, and paresthesia can occur, probably because potassium is necessary for vasodilation in skeletal muscle. In addition, severe potassium depletion (<2.5 mEq/L) can result in elevation of serum creatine phosphokinase, aldolase, and aspartate aminotransferase levels. Rhabdomyolysis can ensue when the serum potassium concentration falls below 2.0 mEq/L.[117,124]

Chronic potassium depletion can alter renal function and structure, which can manifest as decreased GFR and renal blood flow, disturbance in tubular sodium handling, impaired urinary concentrating ability with polydipsia, and ADH-resistant nephrogenic diabetes insipidus.[101,110] Reversible pathologic changes include renal hypertrophy and epithelial vacuolization of the proximal convoluted tubule. Interstitial scarring and tubular atrophy have been reported with prolonged potassium depletion.[117]

Other effects of hypokalemia and potassium depletion include decreased insulin secretion resulting in carbohydrate intolerance,[127] metabolic alkalosis, and increased renal ammoniagenesis, which may play a role in the development of hepatic encephalopathy.[128]

TREATMENT

CASE 10-8, QUESTION 3: How should J.P.'s hypokalemia be treated?

J.P.'s protracted vomiting should be corrected, and fluids and electrolytes (sodium, potassium, and chloride) should be replaced to correct the volume deficit, hypokalemia, and hypochloremic metabolic alkalosis. Hydrochlorothiazide should continue to be withheld.

The amount of potassium deficit and the rate of continued potassium loss should be determined to guide replacement therapy. It has been estimated that a 1-mEq/L fall in serum potassium from 4 to 3 mEq/L represents a total body deficit of approximately 200 mEq. When the serum potassium falls to less than 3 mEq/L, the total body deficit increases by 200 to 400 mEq for each 1 mEq/L reduction in serum concentration. Other data suggest that even greater degrees of potassium loss can occur—a deficit of 100 mEq per 0.27-mEq/L fall in the serum potassium concentration.[105] Transcellular redistribution of potassium may, however, significantly alter the relationship between serum concentration and total body deficit.[117] Therefore, potassium repletion should be guided by close monitoring of serum concentrations and analysis of J.P.'s urine for potassium content to help assess the need for additional replacement.

The route of potassium administration depends on the acuity and severity of hypokalemia,[129] but oral supplementation is usually preferred. The parenteral route is indicated for patients who cannot tolerate high dosages of oral potassium supplements and for those with severe or symptomatic hypokalemia. J.P.'s potassium deficit is estimated to be 300 to 500 mEq, but because she is only moderately symptomatic, aggressive therapy is not indicated. Potassium chloride can be added to her IV fluid in a concentration of 40 mEq/L and infused at a rate that does not exceed 10 mEq/hour. For patients with life-threatening, hypokalemia-induced arrhythmias or those with a serum potassium level less than 2.0 mEq/L, a more concentrated potassium solution (60 mEq/L) can be infused at a rate not exceeding 40 mEq/hour. A solution that is too concentrated or a rate of infusion that is too rapid would likely cause phlebitis in the peripheral veins and could cause arrhythmias, especially when administered through a central line. The potassium concentration should be monitored every 4 hours, more frequently in patients with severe potassium depletion or when a rapid infusion is given.[130] ECG monitoring is mandatory to identify life-threatening hyperkalemia that can result from over-correction.

Parenteral potassium can be given as chloride, acetate, or phosphate. The chloride salt is preferred in J.P., who has concurrent hypochloremic metabolic alkalosis. The acetate preparation is useful in cases of concomitant metabolic acidosis. Potassium phosphate is indicated if hypophosphatemia coexists. In the latter condition, the serum calcium concentration should also be monitored because hypocalcemia may ensue. Glucose solution should be avoided as the vehicle because glucose-induced insulin secretion will promote intracellular potassium uptake.[131]

Once J.P.'s potassium levels are replenished and she can take medicine by mouth, oral potassium chloride can be started (see Chapter 14, Essential Hypertension, and Chapter 19, Heart Failure).

Hyperkalemia

ETIOLOGY

CASE 10-9

QUESTION 1: A.B., a 25-year-old woman with type 1 diabetes and hypertension, returns to the clinic for follow-up. Her BP is 170/90 mm Hg with a pulse of 80 beats/minute, and her physical examination is remarkable for 2+ pedal edema. Laboratory tests show the following:

Plasma Na, 135 mEq/L
K, 5.8 mEq/L
Cl, 108 mEq/L
Total CO_2, 20 mEq/L
BUN, 28 mg/dL
Creatinine, 2 mg/dL
Glucose, 200 mg/dL

Current medications include oral captopril 25 mg three times daily, hydrochlorothiazide 25 mg/triamterene 37.5 mg one capsule daily, human isophane insulin 30 units subcutaneously (SC) every morning, and ibuprofen 200 mg as needed for menstrual cramps. She uses a salt substitute occasionally. What is the etiology of her hyperkalemia?

Before conducting any extensive evaluation to identify the etiology of hyperkalemia, the serum potassium concentration ought to be repeated to confirm the presence of hyperkalemia. Also to be ruled out are the different causes of spurious hyperkalemia, which can result from severe leukocytosis (>500,000/μL),[131] thrombocytosis (>750,000/μL),[132] or hemolysis within the blood collection tube.[133] Pseudohyperkalemia is a test-tube phenomenon that occurs when potassium is released from leukocytes, platelets, or erythrocytes during blood coagulation. These disorders can be confirmed easily by comparing serum (clotted) and plasma (unclotted) potassium concentrations from the same blood sample. The two values should agree within 0.2 to 0.3 mEq/L. Improper tourniquet technique, causing strangulation of the patient's arm before blood sampling, may also result in spurious hyperkalemia.[134]

Identifying the etiology of hyperkalemia can be approached systematically by considering possible disturbances in internal and external potassium balance. The former involves transcellular flux of potassium from the intracellular to the extracellular space, whereas the latter involves either increased intake, including increased endogenous potassium load (e.g., rhabdomyolysis,[135] tumor lysis syndrome[136]), or decreased elimination. A thorough medication history is important to identify drugs associated with hyperkalemia.[137–139] (Also see Chapter 31, Chronic Kidney Diseases, for additional information on hyperkalemia.)

A dietary history should ascertain whether A.B.'s consumption of potassium-rich foods, salt substitutes, or potassium supplements has increased. Dietary intake alone will not induce hyperkalemia unless renal excretion is impaired. Usually, the GFR must be less than 10 to 15 mL/minute, unless there is concurrent hypoaldosteronism or distal tubular potassium secretory defects.[1] A.B.'s renal insufficiency is mild, with an estimated CrCl of 40 mL/minute.

Conditions associated with low renin and aldosterone, which usually present as hyperkalemia and hyperchloremic metabolic acidosis, decrease potassium excretion by the kidneys. These include diabetes,[140] obstructive uropathy, sickle cell disease, lupus nephritis, and various tubulointerstitial diseases (e.g., gouty nephropathy, analgesic nephropathy). Adrenal insufficiency presents commonly with hyperkalemia because of mineralocorticoid deficiency.[141] A.B.'s hyperglycemia due to poorly controlled diabetes may cause movement of potassium-rich fluid from the intracellular space to the extracellular space because of the increased tonicity. Elevating the plasma tonicity by 15 to 20 mOsm/kg will increase the plasma potassium concentration by 0.8 mEq/L.[142] Patients with diabetes, mineralocorticoid deficiency, or end-stage renal failure, which commonly results in hyporeninemic hypoaldosteronism, are particularly susceptible.

A.B. is also taking several medications that may impair her ability to excrete potassium. Captopril indirectly decreases aldosterone secretion by decreasing the formation of AT_2.[143] Ibuprofen inhibits prostaglandin production as well as renin and aldosterone secretion.[144] Other drugs that cause hyperkalemia by impairing renin and aldosterone production include AT_2 receptor antagonists,[145] β-adrenergic blockers,[146] lithium,[147] heparin,[148–150] and pentamidine.[135] Triamterene, a component of her diuretic, inhibits tubular potassium secretion, as do amiloride, spironolactone, high-dose trimethoprim,[151,152] cyclosporine,[153] tacrolimus,[154] and digitalis preparations.[155] By inhibiting Na^+/K^+ ATPase, digitalis decreases tubular potassium secretion and reduces cellular potassium uptake. Arginine,[156] succinylcholine,[157] β-adrenergic blockers, α-adrenergic agonists, and hypertonic solutions also cause hyperkalemia by impairing transcellular potassium distribution into the intracellular space.

CASE 10-10

QUESTION 1: V.C., a 44-year-old woman with chronic renal failure, returns to the outpatient unit for routine hemodialysis with complaints of severe muscle weakness. Her vital signs are BP, 120/80 mm Hg; pulse, 90 beats/minute; RR, 20 breaths/minute; and temperature, 98°F. Laboratory data are as follows:

Serum K, 8.9 mEq/L
Total CO_2, 15 mM
BUN, 60 mg/dL
Creatinine, 9 mg/dL
Glucose, 100 mg/dL

The ECG reveals an increased PR interval and a widened QRS complex. What clinical manifestations of hyperkalemia are evident in V.C.?

Hyperkalemia decreases the intracellular/extracellular potassium ratio. Hence, the resting membrane potential becomes less negative and moves closer to the threshold excitation potential. Muscle weakness and flaccid paralysis result when the resting membrane potential approaches the threshold potential, rendering the excitable cells unable to sustain an action potential.

The cardiac toxicity of hyperkalemia is a major cause of morbidity and mortality, with ECG findings paralleling the degree of hyperkalemia. When plasma potassium is greater than 5.5 to 6.0 mEq/L, narrow, peaked T waves and a shortened QT interval are seen. As the plasma potassium concentration increases further, the QRS complex widens and the P-wave amplitude decreases. As the level reaches 8 mEq/L, the P wave disappears and the QRS complex continues to widen and merge with the T wave to form a sine wave pattern. If these ECG changes are not recognized and no treatment is initiated, ventricular fibrillation and asystole will ensue. Hyponatremia, hypocalcemia, and hypomagnesemia all reduce the threshold potential, thereby increasing the patient's susceptibility to the cardiac effects of hyperkalemia.[135] V.C.'s muscle weakness, ECG, chronic renal failure, and serum potassium concentration all are consistent with severe hyperkalemia.

TREATMENT

CASE 10-10, QUESTION 2: How should V.C.'s hyperkalemia be treated?

Hyperkalemia with ECG changes requires urgent treatment. Three therapeutic modalities are available: (a) agents that antagonize the cardiac effects of hyperkalemia, (b) agents that shift potassium from the extracellular into the intracellular space, and (c) agents that enhance potassium elimination. Considering V.C.'s severe ECG changes, calcium should be administered at a dose of 10 to 20 mL of 10% calcium gluconate IV over the course of 1 to 3 minutes. Calcium counteracts the depolarizing effect of hyperkalemia by increasing the threshold potential, thus making it less negative and moving it away from the resting potential. The onset of action occurs in a few minutes, but the effect is short-lived, lasting approximately 15 to 60 minutes. The dose can be repeated in 5 minutes if ECG changes do not resolve and as needed afterward for recurrence. With no response after the second dose, additional attempts, however, are not beneficial. When the hyperkalemia presents with a digitalis overdose, calcium should be used cautiously because it can worsen the cardiotoxic effects of digoxin.[135,158]

Because the serum potassium concentration is not affected by calcium administration, maneuvers should be used to shift potassium from plasma into the cells. Three modalities are available: insulin and glucose, β_2-agonists, and sodium bicarbonate.

Insulin rapidly shifts potassium into the cell in a dose-dependent fashion. The maximal effect occurs at insulin concentrations greater than 20 to 40 times the basal levels. Therefore, endogenous insulin secreted in response to dextrose administration is insufficient, and exogenous insulin must be administered.[106] Although high concentrations of dextrose may worsen hyperkalemia, particularly in diabetic patients because intracellular potassium may be shifted to the extracellular space owing to the elevated plasma tonicity,[159] it is always administered with insulin to prevent hypoglycemia. Regular insulin (5–10 units) can be given with 50 mL of 50% dextrose as IV boluses, followed by a continuous infusion of 10% dextrose at 50 mL/hour to prevent late hypoglycemia.[106] In dialysis patients susceptible to experiencing fasting hyperkalemia, 20 units of insulin can be added to 1 L of 10% dextrose and administered at a rate of 50 mL/hour to prevent the hyperkalemia.[160] The insulin–dextrose combination lowers serum potassium by direct stimulation of cellular potassium uptake and potentiates the potassium-lowering effect of β-adrenergic stimuation.[160] The reduction in potassium is apparent 15 to 30 minutes after the start of the therapy and persists for 4 to 6 hours.[135] In a diabetic patient who is both hyperkalemic and hyperglycemic, insulin alone may be insufficient. If the patient has end-stage renal disease, the insulin–glucose combination is more predictable in lowering plasma potassium concentrations than sodium bicarbonate.[105,158,160]

β_2-Agonists, by binding with the β_2-adrenoreceptor to activate adenylate cyclase, have an additive effect with the insulin–dextrose combination in decreasing serum potassium. When albuterol nebulization is used alone, the hypokalemic effect may be inconsistent.[161] Although side effects of albuterol nebulization are minimal, these agents can cause tachycardia and should be used cautiously in patients with underlying coronary artery disease.[162] Although not commercially available, IV albuterol has a faster onset of action (30 vs. 90 minutes).[163] In contrast, nebulization is easier to set up and is less likely to be associated with tachycardia, but multiple doses are often necessary to attain an adequate response. In conjunction with the insulin–dextrose combination, albuterol (20 mg dissolved in 4 mL of saline) can be administered by nebulization and inhaled over the course of 10 minutes to further decrease serum potassium, if necessary.[164]

Although sodium bicarbonate has long been recommended for the acute treatment of hyperkalemia, its efficacy in this setting has been questioned.[105,158] The usual dose, 44 to 50 mEq, is infused slowly over the course of 5 minutes and repeated in 30 minutes when necessary. Alternatively, it can be added to dextrose and saline solution to form an isotonic sodium bicarbonate infusion.[165] The hypokalemic effect is variable and may be delayed up to 4 hours, and it is reportedly ineffective in patients on maintenance hemodialysis. Although bicarbonate therapy is not a reliable option in the acute management of hyperkalemia, it may be beneficial in patients with severe metabolic acidosis (pH <7.20).[105] Potential complications of sodium bicarbonate therapy are volume overload and metabolic alkalosis.

The definitive treatment of hyperkalemia is removal of potassium from the body. Sodium polystyrene sulfonate (SPS) with sorbitol is an ion-exchange resin that binds potassium in the bowel and enhances its excretion in the stools.[166] Each gram of SPS exchanges 0.5 to 1.0 mmol of potassium for an equal amount of sodium. SPS can be administered orally or rectally; the latter route is preferred in the symptomatic hyperkalemic patient because intestinal potassium exchange occurs mainly in the ileum and colon. A dose of 50 g of SPS in sorbitol can be given

TABLE 10-3
Treatment of Hyperkalemia

Drug	Mechanism	Dose	Comment
Calcium gluconate	Reverse cardiotoxicity caused by K^+	10 to 20 mL 10% calcium gluconate IV over 1 to 3 minutes; may repeat once	*Onset:* 1 to 3 minutes *Duration:* 30 to 60 minutes. [K^+] remains unchanged
Insulin and glucose	Redistribution of K^+ intracellularly	5 to 10 units regular insulin with 50 mL 50% dextrose, then $D_{10}W$ infused at 50 mL/h[a]	*Onset:* 15 to 30 minutes *Duration:* several hours Watch for hypoglycemia and hypokalemia. Does not ↓ total body K^+
β_2-agonists (e.g., albuterol)	Redistribution of K^+ intracellularly	Oral: 2 or 4 mg TID–QID Inhalation: 20 mg in 4 mL saline via nebulizer	*Onset:* 30 to 60 minutes *Duration:* 2 hours
SPS	Cationic binding resin. 1 g of resin binds 0.5 to 1 mEq K^+ in exchange for Na^+	Oral: 15 to 20 g with 20 to 100 mL 70% sorbitol every 4 to 6 hours; PRN preferred Retention enema: 50 g in 50 mL (70% sorbitol and 150 mL H_2O). Retain 30 minutes and follow with nonsaline irrigation	*Onset:* Slow; 50 g will lower [K^+] by 0.5 to 1 mEq/L over 4 to 6 hours; watch for Na^+ overload (100 mg Na^+/1 g SPS)
$NaHCO_3$	Redistribution of K^+ intracellularly	50 mEq IV for 5 minutes. Repeat PRN	*Onset:* variable, ≈30 minutes May work best in acidosis Watch for Na^+ overload and hyperosmolar state No change in total body K^+
Dialysis	Removal of K^+		Use as last resort

[a] Glucose unnecessary in patients with high glucose concentrations.
BID, twice daily; IV, intravenous; PRN, as needed; QID, four times daily; SPS, sodium polystyrene sulfonate; TID, three times daily.

as an enema, retained for at least 30 to 60 minutes, at 4-hour to 6-hour intervals. For nonemergent removal of body potassium, 15 to 60 g of SPS with sorbitol suspension can be given orally, which can be repeated as needed. The onset of action is approximately 1 to 2 hours after administration. The major side effects are GI intolerance, including diarrhea and sodium overload, and, rarely, intestinal necrosis.[167]

Hemodialysis is the most efficient way to remove potassium; potassium clearance by peritoneal dialysis is lower than for hemodialysis.[168] The hypokalemic effect is immediate and lasts for the duration of dialysis[158]; however, the amount of potassium removed is variable.[169] Dialysis with a glucose-free dialysate will remove 30% more potassium than one containing 200 mg/dL of glucose.[170] Table 10-3 summarizes the treatment alternatives for hyperkalemia. Although V.C. is receiving chronic maintenance hemodialysis, the severe cardiac effects of hyperkalemia she experienced warrant immediate institution of the aforementioned measures while awaiting preparation for dialysis. Loop diuretics, which enhance kaliuresis, are rarely useful in managing severe hyperkalemia, especially in patients with renal dysfunction.

After V.C.'s condition stabilized, she admitted to eating a lot of fruits in the past few days. Because noncompliance with dietary potassium restriction is the most common cause for acute and chronic hyperkalemia in a dialysis patient, V.C. should be counseled to consume potassium-rich foods in moderation. Medications that impair V.C.'s extrarenal potassium handling should be avoided. If V.C. remains chronically hyperkalemic, SPS will then be needed, probably three or four times weekly. If hyperkalemia is associated with metabolic acidosis, however, an alkalinizing agent should be added to maintain a serum bicarbonate concentration of about 24 mEq/L.

CALCIUM

Homeostasis

Healthy adults have approximately 1,400 g of calcium in the body, of which greater than 99% is stored in bone. Nonetheless, the 0.1% of the total body calcium that is in the plasma and extravascular fluid plays a critical role in many physiologic and metabolic processes. Calcium is important in maintaining nerve tissue excitability and muscle contractility. It regulates the secretory activities of exocrine and endocrine glands and serves as a cofactor for enzyme systems and the coagulation cascade. It also is an essential component of bone metabolism.

Plasma calcium concentration is normally maintained within a relatively narrow range: 8.5 to 10.5 mg/dL. This is accomplished through a complex interaction between parathyroid hormone (PTH), vitamin D, and calcitonin, as well as the effect of these hormones on calcium metabolism in bone, the GI tract, and the kidneys.

Normally, about 40% of the plasma calcium is protein-bound, primarily to albumin, and is nondiffusible.[121] Of the 60% that is diffusible, about 13% is complexed to various small ligands: phosphate, citrate, and sulfate. The remaining 47% is ionized, free, and physiologically active. Changes in serum protein concentration will alter the concentrations of both protein-bound and total calcium. Therefore, the serum albumin concentration needs to be monitored to adequately interpret the total serum calcium concentration. Each 1-g/dL increase in serum albumin concentration is expected to increase the protein-bound calcium by 0.8 mg/dL, thus increasing the total serum calcium concentration by the same amount. The total serum calcium therefore can be corrected by the following equation:

$$\text{Correct Ca} = \text{Observed Ca} + 0.8\,(\text{Normal albumin} - \text{Observed albumin}) \quad \textit{(Eq. 10-13)}$$

where normal albumin = 4 g/dL.

Calcium is also bound to plasma globulins at the rate of 0.16 mg of calcium for each gram of globulin. When the total globulin concentration exceeds 6 g/dL, moderate hypercalcemia may be seen. Changes in pH have an effect on calcium protein-binding; acidosis decreases calcium binding, resulting in an increase in free-calcium fraction, whereas an increase in pH reduces the amount of ionized calcium. Changes in serum phosphate and sulfate concentrations are expected to alter the fraction of ionized calcium because of the formation of calcium complexes with these anions. The presence of abnormal plasma proteins with a high affinity for calcium-binding, as in patients with multiple myeloma, also affects the preceding equation for serum calcium concentration correction.[171]

Serum calcium concentration is regulated by the combined effect of GI absorption and secretion, renal reabsorption, and turnover of the skeletal calcium pool. Several hormones, such as PTH, 1,25-dihydroxyvitamin D_3, and calcitonin, have significant effects on these processes. Balanced diets generally contain 600 to 1,000 mg of calcium, although the minimum daily requirement is 400 to 500 mg. Calcium is primarily absorbed in the duodenum and jejunum via saturable and nonsaturable processes.[172] The nonsaturable process is diffusive in nature and varies with luminal calcium concentration. The saturable carrier-mediated component is stimulated by 1,25-dihydroxyvitamin D_3. Absorption of calcium is enhanced when the calcium intake is low and also when the demand is increased, such as in pregnancy and when total body calcium is depleted. Conversely, protein deficiency can reduce intestinal calcium absorption, presumably because of the reduced amount of specific calcium-binding protein.[173] Calcium also is secreted into the bowel lumen, which may account for the presence of a negative calcium balance when there is no oral calcium intake.[174]

The portion of plasma calcium that is not bound to protein is filtered by the glomerulus. Approximately 97% to 99.5% of the filtered calcium is reabsorbed: 60% in the proximal tubule, 20% in the ascending limb, 10% in the distal tubule, and 3% to 10% in the collecting duct. Approximately 20% of the calcium in the kidney tubule is ionized, whereas the remainder is bound to anions such as citrate, sulfate, phosphate, and gluconate. The extent of calcium reabsorption depends on the presence of specific anions and also on the urine pH, which affects the fraction of calcium bound to anions. Passive reabsorption at the proximal convoluted tubule is linked closely to sodium transport and is increased by extracellular fluid contraction and decreased by volume expansion. At the proximal straight tubule, the transport process is active and dissociable from sodium and water transport. PTH increases the calcium reabsorption at the distal tubule and also at the collecting duct independent of sodium reabsorption. Acidosis can also increase renal calcium excretion by inhibiting tubular reabsorption and by increasing the ultrafiltrable calcium through reduced binding of calcium to plasma proteins. Conversely, alkalosis promotes calcium protein binding, thus reducing the amount of ultrafiltrable calcium. It also induces hypocalciuria independent of PTH. Phosphorus administration reduces renal calcium excretion, whereas phosphorus depletion increases urinary calcium elimination. Normally, approximately 50 to 300 mg of calcium is excreted by the kidneys daily, but this can be increased to 600 mg/day.[175]

The other important factor regulating plasma calcium concentration is bone metabolism. The rate of bone turnover and calcium resorption is influenced by PTH, 1,25-dihydroxyvitamin D_3, and calcitonin.

Hypercalcemia

ETIOLOGY

CASE 10-11

QUESTION 1: A.C., a 62-year-old woman, is brought to the hospital by family members because she has become increasingly lethargic and unresponsive during the past several days. Approximately 4 years ago she underwent a radical mastectomy and node dissection followed by radiation and chemotherapy for breast carcinoma. Despite several courses of chemotherapy, she developed metastasis to the bone. About 1 week before this admission, A.C. complained of fatigue, muscle weakness, and anorexia. Since then, she has spent most of her time in bed and has had very limited oral intake. Medications taken before admission included hydrochlorothiazide, oral morphine sulfate, and tamoxifen. Physical examination reveals a dehydrated, cachectic woman responsive only to painful stimuli. Vital signs include BP, 100/60 mm Hg, and RR, 16 breaths/minute. Pertinent laboratory values are as follows:

Na, 138 mEq/L
K, 4.5 mEq/L
Cl, 99 mEq/L
CO_2, 33 mEq/L
BUN, 40 mg/dL
Creatinine, 1.2 mg/dL
Calcium, 19 mg/dL
Phosphate, 4.5 mg/dL
Albumin, 3.0 g/dL

The ECG revealed a shortened QT interval. What are the common causes of hypercalcemia? Which of these might be responsible for the hypercalcemia seen in A.C.?

MALIGNANCY

Malignancy and primary hyperparathyroidism are the most common causes of hypercalcemia. Hematologic malignancies, such as multiple myeloma, tend to be responsible for more hypercalcemia than are solid tumors. Cancer of the breast, lung, head and neck, and renal cell carcinoma are solid tumors commonly associated with hypercalcemia. Malignancy can cause paraneoplastic hypercalcemia secondary to bone metastasis, which results in increased bone resorption. Alternatively, patients may exhibit hypercalcemia in the absence of bone metastasis owing to the production of osteolytic humoral factors by the tumor. The mediators secreted may be PTH, PTH-like substances, prostaglandins, cytokines, transforming growth factor-α, and tumor necrosis factor.[176]

HYPERPARATHYROIDISM

Hyperparathyroidism is the other common cause of hypercalcemia. Although the etiology of primary hyperparathyroidism is unclear, women tend to experience the condition more frequently, especially in the fourth to sixth decades of life. Approximately 75% of patients have a single adenoma, whereas much smaller percentages of patients have multiglandular disease, hyperplasia, or carcinoma.[175] Other conditions that can result in hypercalcemia include postkidney transplantation, immobilization, vitamin A intoxication, hyperthyroidism, Addison disease, and pheochromocytoma. Hypercalcemia can also occur secondary to increased intestinal calcium absorption because of vitamin D intoxication, sarcoidosis, and other granulomatous diseases. Use of thiazide diuretics, lithium, estrogens, and tamoxifen, as well as excessive calcium ingestion together with alkali (milk-alkali syndrome), may result in hypercalcemia.

A.C.'s breast cancer bone metastasis, volume contraction, and use of hydrochlorothiazide and tamoxifen may all contribute to her hypercalcemia.

CLINICAL MANIFESTATIONS

CASE 10-11, QUESTION 2: How is hypercalcemia manifested in A.C.?

The clinical presentations of hypercalcemia vary substantially among patients, but the severity of the symptoms correlates well with free calcium concentrations.[177] The specific presentation depends on the rate of serum calcium concentration elevation, the presence of malignancy, the PTH concentration, and the patient's age. Concurrent electrolyte and metabolic abnormalities and underlying diseases also will have an effect. Because calcium is an important regulator of many cellular functions, hypercalcemia can produce abnormalities in the neurologic, cardiovascular, pulmonary, renal, GI, and musculoskeletal systems. As seen in A.C., the signs and symptoms can be nonspecific: fatigue, muscle weakness, anorexia, thirst, polyuria, dehydration, and a shortened QT interval on the ECG.

The effect of hypercalcemia on the central nervous system includes lethargy, somnolence, confusion, headache, seizures, cerebellar ataxia, altered personality, acute psychosis, depression, and memory impairment. The neuromuscular manifestations include weakness, myalgia, hyporeflexia or areflexia, and arthralgia.

Symptoms of impaired renal function include polyuria, nocturia, and polydipsia. These may reflect a defective concentrating ability, possibly because of resistance to the effects of ADH.[178] The GFR may be decreased because of afferent arteriolar vasoconstriction, and if hypercalcemia is prolonged, nephrolithiasis, nephrocalcinosis, chronic interstitial nephritis, and renal tubular acidosis may be present. Hypermagnesuria and metabolic alkalosis may also be observed.[175]

Calcium has a positive inotropic effect and reduces heart rate, similar to cardiac glycosides. ECG changes indicative of slow conduction, with prolonged PR and QRS intervals and shortened QT intervals, are commonly seen. In severe hypercalcemia, increased QT intervals, widened T waves, and arrhythmia may be present.[175,179]

The GI symptoms of hypercalcemia are related primarily to the depressive action of calcium on smooth muscle and nerve conduction. Constipation, anorexia, nausea, and vomiting result from reduced GI motility and delayed gastric emptying. Duodenal ulcer can occur because of increased acid and gastrin secretion. Pancreatitis can occur during acute hypercalcemia owing to the blockade of the pancreatic ducts caused by intraductal calcium deposits.[175] Proteolytic enzymes may also be activated by calcium to cause tissue damage. Both ulcer disease and pancreatitis are more common in hypercalcemia associated with primary hyperparathyroidism; they are less likely to be seen in patients with malignancy-induced hypercalcemia.[179]

Treatment

CASE 10-11, QUESTION 3: After vigorous fluid resuscitation with IV saline, combined saline and furosemide diuresis was instituted in A.C. Her serum calcium concentration declined very slowly, prompting the use of calcitonin. Despite initial success, the serum calcium concentration rose to pretreatment values within 24 hours. Higher dosages of calcitonin could have been attempted at this point; however, pamidronate was used instead. Her serum calcium concentration finally stabilized at 8 mg/dL after several days of therapy. What was the rationale for each of these regimens? What other agents are available for hypercalcemia treatment?

Several therapeutic approaches are used to lower serum calcium concentration: increasing urinary calcium excretion, inhibiting release of calcium from bone, reducing intestinal calcium absorption, and enhancing calcium complex formation with chelating agents. The underlying disease that causes the hypercalcemia should also be treated, if possible. The specific treatment used depends on the serum ionized calcium concentration, the presenting signs and symptoms, and the severity and duration of hypercalcemia. Immediate therapy was needed for A.C., who had symptoms consistent with severe hypercalcemia.

Specific interventions are described in the subsequent paragraphs, but as an overview, hydration and diuresis with furosemide generally are the first steps in the acute treatment of hypercalcemia. If these measures fail to reduce the serum calcium concentration adequately, several other agents can be added. Calcitonin provides a rapid onset of hypocalcemic effect, but its duration of action is relatively short. Thus, a bisphosphonate could be used to elicit a longer hypocalcemic response. Gallium nitrate is an alternative but it is not commonly used. Other agents, such as inorganic phosphates, glucocorticoids, and prostaglandin inhibitors, also have been used to treat hypercalcemia with varying success (Table 10-4).

HYDRATION AND DIURESIS

As noted, the first-line emergency treatment for hypercalcemia is hydration and volume expansion. Most patients with hypercalcemia are volume-depleted because of the accompanying polyuria, nausea, and vomiting. Normal saline 1 to 2 L is commonly given to correct the fluid deficit and to expand extracellular volume, which will increase urinary calcium excretion by increasing the GFR and inhibiting calcium reabsorption in the proximal tubule. Because both sodium and calcium are reabsorbed at the same site in the proximal tubule, saline hydration will reduce the reabsorption of both cations simultaneously. A.C. was hypotensive and appeared dehydrated; therefore, saline hydration was used initially to treat the hypercalcemia. In patients who have renal failure or HF, saline hydration and forced diuresis should be avoided.

After adequate volume repletion has been established, IV furosemide can be administered to augment calciuresis. Furosemide blocks the reabsorption of sodium, chloride, and calcium at the thick ascending limb of Henle's loop. Doses of 80 to 100 mg every 2 to 4 hours can be used until a sufficient decline of the serum calcium concentration is attained.[180] Smaller doses (20–40 mg) commonly are given to avoid the significant loss of fluid and electrolytes caused by the more aggressive regimen. Adequate amounts of sodium, potassium, magnesium, and fluid should be used to replace any therapy-induced electrolyte abnormalities. Fluid balance as well as serum and urine concentrations of these electrolytes must be monitored closely. Urine flow must be maintained and the renal loss of sodium chloride must be replaced to preserve the calciuric effect of furosemide.[181] In A.C., the decline of serum calcium concentration was slow, possibly because of inadequate restoration of plasma volume, replacement of renal sodium loss, or both. More aggressive hydration with adequate sodium replacement ensures that the efficacy of furosemide is not compromised.

CALCITONIN

Calcitonin can be used when saline hydration and furosemide diuresis fail to lower serum calcium concentration adequately or when their use is contraindicated. Calcitonin reduces serum calcium concentration by inhibiting osteoclastic bone resorption. It may also increase the renal excretion of calcium and phosphorus. Only the salmon-derived calcitonin product is available in the United States.

The serum calcium concentration is often reduced several hours after calcitonin is administered, and the response may last approximately 6 to 8 hours. The drug is relatively nontoxic compared with organic phosphates and may be used in patients

Hypermagnesemia

ETIOLOGY

CASE 10-14

QUESTION 1: J.O., a 63-year-old man with renal insufficiency, was admitted to the hospital because of increasing weakness during the past several days. J.O. began taking a magnesium–aluminum hydroxide antacid several times daily 2 weeks ago when he exhibited stomach upset. Physical examination reveals hypotension and depressed deep tendon reflexes. The ECG reveals prolonged PR and QRS intervals. The serum magnesium concentration is 6.5 mEq/dL. What is the most likely cause of hypermagnesemia in J.O.?

Because the kidney is the primary route of magnesium elimination, renal impairment is a virtual requisite for hypermagnesemia (see Chapter 31, Chronic Kidney Diseases). A common cause of hypermagnesemia is the use of magnesium-containing medications, such as antacids and laxatives, by patients with impaired renal function, including older adults. When a patient with renal failure, such as J.O., takes magnesium-containing medications, the serum magnesium concentration can increase substantially, resulting in toxicities. Hypermagnesemia may be seen when the creatinine clearance drops to less than 30 mL/minute; an inverse relationship is observed between the serum magnesium concentrations and the creatinine clearances.[274] Hypermagnesemia is also seen in patients with acute renal failure during the oliguric phase, but not the diuretic phase.[275] Other potential causes of hypermagnesemia include adrenal insufficiency,[224] hypothyroidism,[276] lithium,[276] magnesium citrate used as a cathartic for drug overdose,[277] and parenteral magnesium given for pre-eclampsia.[278]

CLINICAL MANIFESTATIONS

CASE 10-14, QUESTION 2: Describe the usual clinical presentation of a patient with hypermagnesemia.

An elevated magnesium serum concentration alters the normal function of the neurologic, neuromuscular, and cardiovascular systems. When the serum magnesium concentration is greater than 4 mEq/L, deep tendon reflexes are depressed; they are usually lost at greater than 6 mEq/L. Flaccid quadriplegia can develop when the concentration is greater than 8 to 10 mEq/L. Respiratory paralysis, hypotension, and difficulty in talking and swallowing may also be present. Changes in the ECG may include a prolonged PR interval and widening of the QRS complex. Complete heart block may be seen at concentrations of approximately 15 mEq/L. In mild hypomagnesemia, the patient may experience nausea and vomiting.

Drowsiness, lethargy, diaphoresis, and altered consciousness may be present at higher serum magnesium concentrations. J.O.'s increasing weakness, hypotension, depressed deep tendon reflexes, and ECG findings are consistent with hypermagnesemia.

TREATMENT

CASE 10-14, QUESTION 3: How should J.O.'s hypermagnesemia be treated?

If magnesium-containing medications are discontinued in patients with hypermagnesemia, the serum magnesium concentration will usually return to the normal range through renal elimination. When potentially life-threatening complications are present, as in J.O., 5 to 10 mEq of IV calcium should be administered to antagonize the respiratory and cardiac manifestations of magnesium.[278,279] The dose of the calcium can be repeated as necessary because its effect is short lived. In patients with good renal function without life-threatening complications, IV furosemide, plus 0.45% sodium chloride to replace lost urine volume, will enhance urinary magnesium excretion while preventing volume depletion. Hemodialysis or peritoneal dialysis is indicated for patients with significant renal function impairment and possibly for those with severe hypermagnesemia.

KEY REFERENCES AND WEBSITES

A full list of references for this chapter can be found at http://thepoint.lww.com/AT10e. Below are the key references for this chapter, with the corresponding reference number in this chapter found in parentheses after the reference.

Key References

Agus Z. Hypomagnesemia. *J Am Soc Nephrol.* 1999;10:1616. (267)

Alfrey AC. Normal and abnormal magnesium metabolism. In: Schrier RW, ed. *Renal and Electrolyte Disorders.* 6th ed. Philadelphia, PA: Lippincott Williams & Wilkins; 2003:278. (268)

Allon M. Hyperkalemia in end stage renal disease: mechanism and management. *J Am Soc Nephrol.* 1995;6:1134. (162)

Davidson TG. Conventional treatment of hypercalcemia of malignancy. *Am J Health Syst Pharm.* 2001;58(Suppl 3):S8. (181)

Decaux G et al. Non-peptide arginine-vasopressin antagonists: the vaptans. *Lancet.* 2008;371:1624. (97)

Gross P. Treatment of severe hyponatremia. *Kidney Int.* 2001; 60:2417. (61)

Morrison G et al. Hyperosmolal states. In: Narins RG, ed. *Maxwell & Kleeman's Clinical Disorders of Fluid and Electrolyte Metabolism.* 5th ed. New York, NY: McGraw-Hill; 1994:617. (99)

Rose BD. Introduction to disorders of osmolality. In: Rose BD et al, eds. *Clinical Physiology of Acid-Base and Electrolyte Disorders.* 5th ed. New York, NY: McGraw-Hill; 2000:682. (3)

Rose BD. Renal function and disorders of water and sodium balance. In: Rubenstein E, Federman DD, eds. *Scientific American Medicine.* New York, NY: Scientific American Inc., 1994; Section 10:1. (2)

Rubin MF, Narins RG. Hypophosphatemia: pathophysiological and practical aspects of its therapy. *Semin Nephrol.* 1990;10:536. (221)

Stanaszek WF, Romankiewicz JA. Current approaches to management of potassium deficiency. *Drug Intell Clin Pharm.* 1985;19:176. (129)

11

Vaccinations

Sherry Luedtke and Molly G. Minze

CORE PRINCIPLES

	CHAPTER CASES
GENERAL VACCINE PRINCIPLES	
1 **Adverse Effects:** Immunization adverse effects are in part dependent upon the type of vaccine preparation used. Adverse effects from live attenuated vaccines mimic the disease, but are less severe and occur 7 to 10 days postvaccination. Inactivated (killed whole virus) vaccination adverse effects include soreness at site of administration within 24 hours after vaccination. Vaccination adverse effects are significantly less severe than the disease itself.	**Case 11-1**
2 **Immunization Schedules:** Recommended immunization schedules are designed to optimize immune response, standardize regimens, and enhance immunization rates. Infant, child, adolescent, and adult immunization schedules are reviewed and updated annually.	**Case 11-2**
3 **Catch-up Immunization Schedules:** To catch up within an immunization series, it is not necessary to restart from the first dose of the schedule. A delay in receiving subsequent doses does not interfere with final immunity gained from the vaccination.	**Case 11-3**
INACTIVATED VACCINES	
1 **Hepatitis B:** Hepatitis B vaccination is effective for both pre-exposure and post-exposure prophylaxis. To prevent vertical transmission to an infant from a mother, it is key to provide vaccination within 12 hours of birth along with hepatitis B immunoglobulin for those mothers who test hepatitis-B–positive.	**Case 11-4 (Question 1)**
2 **Hepatitis B:** The highest incidence of hepatitis B infection occurs in young adults. Hepatitis B vaccination is recommended for adults who participate in high risk behaviors and those in close contact with the infected persons.	**Case 11-4 (Question 2)**
3 **Hepatitis A:** Hepatitis A immunization is targeted towards toddlers with the aim of preventing transmission to adolescents and adults.	**Case 11-5**
4 **Diphtheria, tetanus, and acellular pertussis/Pertussis booster:** Waning immunity against pertussis has resulted in outbreaks of pertussis in the United States. Adolescents and adults, particularly those with close contact with young infants, should receive a single dose of pertussis booster vaccine.	**Case 11-6**
5 **Haemophilus influenzae b:** Immunization recommendations for *Haemophilus influenzae* type b is age-dependent. The older an infant is at presentation, the fewer doses needed to elicit a response. A single vaccine dose may be considered in children and adults with underlying diseases that place them a risk for infection.	**Case 11-7**
6 **Polio:** Inactivated polio vaccine is recommended over the oral attenuated vaccine for polio vaccination in the United States because inactivated vaccine is associated with a lower incidence of vaccine-associated paralytic polio.	**Case 11-8**

continued

INACTIVATED VACCINES *CONTINUED*

7 **Polio:** Routine vaccination of adults against polio with inactivated poliovirus vaccine is not recommended unless individuals plan travel to endemic areas. Oral polio vaccine may be considered only in unique situations.	**Case 11-9**
8 **Meningococcal:** Vaccination is recommended within populations at increased for risk for contracting *Neisseria meningitidis,* including travelers to endemic areas, patients with specific immunodeficiencies, functional/anatomical asplenia, lab personnel dealing with meningococcus, and college students.	**Case 11-10**
9 **Human Papillomavirus:** This three-dose vaccination series is recommended for adolescent females for the prevention of cervical and anogenital cancers, anogenital warts, and recurrent respiratory papillomatosis. It is also recommended for males in the prevention of genital warts, but, unlike the female vaccine, has not proven cost-effective.	**Case 11-11**
10 **Pneumococcus:** *Streptococcus pneumoniae* mostly affects young children and the elderly. The conjugate vaccines protect against 80% (PCV 7) and 90% (PCV 13) of infectious strains that cause disease in children younger than 6 years old.	**Case 11-12 (Question 1)**
11 **Pneumococcus:** The polysaccharide vaccine does not elicit immune response in children younger than 2 years old, and protects against 23 strains of *S. pneumoniae* that typically cause adult disease.	**Case 11-12 (Question 2)**
12 **Influenza:** Vaccination is recommended for anyone older than 6 months of age who does not have a current contraindication. The inactivated vaccine is delivered intramuscularly, whereas the live attenuated vaccine is delivered as a nasal spray formulation.	**Case 11-13**

LIVE ATTENUATED VACCINES

1 **Rotavirus:** Infants vaccinated with the rotavirus vaccine shed the virus in the feces after immunization; however, the risk of transmission to an immunocompromised contact is relatively low with appropriate precautions.	**Case 11-14**
2 **Measles/Mumps/Rubella (MMR):** Parents are fearful of the risk of autism which has been falsely associated with the MMR vaccine. Pharmacists must provide counseling to overcome parental fears and ensure protection against measles.	**Case 11-15**
3 **Varicella:** Postexposure vaccination with the varicella vaccine is recommended within 5 days of exposure for those unvaccinated or who have not received a second dose of vaccine.	**Case 11-16 (Question 1)**
4 **Varicella:** Herpes zoster vaccination is recommended in adults older than 60 years of age to prevent reactivation of previously acquired wild-type varicella zoster infections. It is not recommended for anyone who previously received the varicella zoster vaccine.	**Case 11-16 (Question 2)**

IMMUNIZATION PRACTICES

1 **Vaccine Administration:** Intramuscular vaccinations are administered at a 90-degree angle into the muscle using a 1-inch needle. Subcutaneous vaccinations are administered at a 45-degree angle into the subcutaneous tissue by pinching this tissue up to prevent insertion into the muscle. When multiple injections are given at the same site, separate each injection by 1 inch.	**Case 11-17**
2 **Establishing Services:** Pharmacists must complete immunization training and adhere to guidelines and principles established by their state pharmacy practice act when administering immunizations to patients.	**Case 11-18**

The use of immunizations to control common infectious diseases is a major public health achievement. Children, adolescents, and adults are now routinely immunized against 17 infectious diseases.[1] Immunization rates are at an all-time high in the United States with more than 90% of children 3 years of age receiving all the recommended vaccines.[2] As a result, cases of diphtheria, tetanus, mumps, measles, rubella, polio, and *Haemophilus influenzae* type b are at record-low levels. Rates of immunization for adults against influenza and pneumococcus range from 33% to 69%, with higher coverage for individuals older than 65 years.[3] Unfortunately, despite overall high rates of immunization coverage, disparities still exist in vaccination coverage for the socioeconomically disadvantaged and by ethnicity. Clearly, there is room for improvement and an opportunity for all health professionals to have an impact.

The need for timely immunization administration is key to preventing disease resurgences.[4] As the incidence of vaccine-preventable disease continues to decrease, however, patients are becoming less aware of the significance and severity of the diseases that could be prevented. This, along with parental concerns regarding vaccine safety, may jeopardize previous vaccination achievements. Health care providers play a vital role in clarifying misconceptions and educating parents and other health professionals about the importance of proper and complete immunizations. Any contact with a patient represents an opportunity to promote immunization, and thus every medication history should include a review of immunization status to detect any deficiencies.[5–7]

VACCINE PRINCIPLES

General Principles

The principle of vaccination against disease is that the introduction of a small amount of the pathogen to the body produces protective immunologic memory (active immunity) and, if the pathogen is reintroduced at a later date, a greater immunologic response is elicited, but without inducing disease.[8] The ideal vaccine would present a nonvirulent form of a pathogen that produces a strong immunologic response once in the body.[9]

Current vaccines types include live attenuated, killed (inactivated) whole organism, subcellular/subunit, and DNA-based vaccines.[8] (See Table 11-1 for a listing of common vaccines and their formulation type.) Live attenuated vaccines contain weakened or inactivated forms of the pathogen, which causes replication within the host and ultimately elicits antibody and cell-mediated immunity within the body via B-cell and T-cell responses.[8,10] Live vaccine administration produces a mild, typically asymptomatic infection at the time of vaccination followed by long-lived immunity from a single immunization.[10,11]

Killed whole organism and subcellular/subunit vaccines do not replicate within the host, nor can they revert to pathogenicity, but often require adjuvants and/or multiple doses to increase the duration of immune response to the antigen.[8,9] Because the organisms in whole pathogen vaccines are inactivated (killed), their effectiveness may be impaired by circulating antibodies, maternal antibodies (in infants), or concomitant infections. Toxoids are a specific kind of inactivated vaccine formed by modifying a biological toxin (e.g., diphtheria and tetanus), usually by mixing it with formaldehyde.

Subunit vaccines contain either a protein or polysaccharide antigen within the vaccine and elicit less reaction than whole pathogen vaccines, thus immune responses are weaker and require multiple doses similar to inactivated vaccines.[8] Conjugated subunit vaccines, consisting of a polysaccharide-protein conjugate where the protein is the antigenic toxin, produce improved immune responses because of B-cell activation by the polysaccharide component and T-cell activation by protein component.[8] No recombinant DNA vaccines are currently marketed, but are in development for influenza, malaria, and cancer prevention.

Adverse Effects

CASE 11-1

QUESTION 1: H.P. is a 38-year-old woman concerned about the side effects of the annual influenza "shot." What information can be provided regarding expected adverse effects for H.P.?

Adverse reactions to inactivated vaccines include pain at the injection site and fever within 48 to 72 hours of administration. In contrast, adverse effects from live attenuated vaccines occur 7 to 10 days after immunization, after the virus has replicated and the immune system has responded. Adverse reactions to live attenuated vaccines mimic the symptoms of disease. Transient rash occurs in 5% of patients receiving measles, mumps, rubella (MMR) immunizations, and a mild varicellalike rash (median of five lesions) occurs in fewer than 5% of patients receiving the varicella vaccine. Syncope, usually occurring within 30 minutes of immunization, has been reported, with 70% of syncopal episodes occurring within 15 minutes of immunization, and occurs more commonly in female patients and adolescents.[12–14]

Although anaphylactic reactions to vaccines are rare, an allergic reaction may occur as a result of specific allergy to the vaccine itself or to trace components in the vaccine (e.g., preservatives, antibiotics).[15] Patients with egg allergy can receive vaccines produced in chick-embryo-fibroblast tissue culture (e.g., MMR) because the risk for serious reaction to these vaccines in egg-allergic individuals is very low.[16–18] MMR should be used cautiously in individuals with a history of a severe reaction to gelatin, which is a stabilizer in the MMR vaccine. Trace amounts of streptomycin, bacitracin, and neomycin are present in oral polio virus vaccine, inactivated polio vaccine, and MMR; therefore, these vaccines should not be administered to individuals with a history of an anaphylactic reaction to these antibiotics.[19]

Overall, vaccinations are safe, especially when compared with the risks of the diseases that these vaccines prevent, and the safety of immunizations are scrutinized continually. In response to concerns about vaccine safety, the National Vaccine Injury Compensation Act mandated an ongoing review of evidence regarding the possible adverse effects of vaccines and established a no-fault injury compensation program for selected vaccines.[19–21]

Contraindications

Misconceptions about contraindications and precautions for immunization often result in missed opportunities to provide needed immunizations. Acute, severe febrile illness; history of anaphylaxis to the vaccine or vaccine components; and history of a severe reaction to an immunization are clear contraindications to immunizations. Immunizations, however, should not be delayed in a patient who has a minor illness (e.g., upper respiratory tract infection, otitis media, diarrhea) even in the presence of a low-grade fever. A family history of seizures, allergies, and sudden infant death syndrome are not contraindications for immunizations. Immunization of a patient with a history of anaphylaxis to a vaccine or vaccine component should be withheld until he or she has undergone desensitization.[1] Preterm infants should begin to receive routine immunizations based on their

(Td) are for use in children older than 7 years of age and adults. Booster doses of tetanus (Td) should be administered every 10 years.[37]

Haemophilus Influenzae B

Haemophilus influenzae type b was the most common cause of bacterial meningitis and a leading cause of serious, systemic bacterial diseases in children younger than 5 years of age until an effective vaccine was added to the routine immunization schedule.[42–44] The mortality rate associated with Hib meningitis was approximately 5%, with neurologic sequelae observed in 25% to 35% of survivors.[45,46] Epiglottitis, cellulitis, septic arthritis, osteomyelitis, pericarditis, and pneumonia also were commonly caused by *H. influenzae.* Although *H. influenzae* is associated with otitis media and respiratory tract infections, type b strains account for only 5% to 10% of these infections.[47]

CASE 11-7

QUESTION 1: P.M. is a 12-month-old child who has not been immunized against Hib. His parents wish to enroll him in day care and are now trying to catch him up on his immunizations. How many doses of vaccine against Hib should he receive?

The Hib vaccine is a conjugate polysaccharide vaccine which is associated with a 95% reduction in the incidence of Hib disease in children younger than 5 years of age.[48] The four currently available Hib polysaccharide conjugate vaccines (HbCV or PRP) are as follows: Hib diphtheria toxoid conjugate vaccine or PRP-D (ProHIBiT), Hib meningococcal protein conjugate vaccine or PRP-OMP (PedvaxHIB), Hib tetanus toxoid conjugate vaccine or PRP-T (ActHIB, OmniHIB), and Hib diphtheria CRM197 protein conjugate vaccine or HbOC (HibTITER).[48] The immunogenicity of the conjugate vaccines are age-dependent (i.e., older children have an improved immune response).[49,50] The four conjugated vaccines are all approved for use in infants, the group at greatest risk for *H. influenzae* infection; however, they vary in their dosing regimens. The HbCV immunization series requires a priming series followed by a booster dose at 12 to 18 months. PRP-OMP's primary series is administered at 2 and 4 months of age in contrast to a schedule of 2, 4, and 6 months' primary series for the other vaccines.[1,24,51] Ideally, the primary series should be completed with the same HbCV; however, data support the interchangeability of the products for the priming and booster doses.[24,52] If PRP-OMP is used in a priming series with another HbCV, the number of doses necessary to complete the series for the other product should be administered.[52] Combination vaccines may also be used according to indications for each (see Table 11-2).[32,52]

The number of doses of HbCV vaccine needed in previously unimmunized older infants and children depends on their age at presentation. Children who begin HbCV at 7 to 11 months of age should receive a primary series of two doses of a vaccine containing HbOC, PRP-T, or PRP-OMP followed by a booster dose at 12 to 18 months of age administered at least 2 months after the previous dose.[24,52] Children ages 12 to 15 months should receive a primary series of one dose followed by a booster dose 2 months later. If a child reaches 15 months of age without receiving HbCV, only one dose is necessary.[24,52] HbCV is not routinely recommended in children younger than 5 years of age or adults. However, a single dose may be considered for those with sickle cell disease, leukemia, human immunodeficiency virus (HIV) infection, or who have had a splenectomy.[24,26,51,52] Because P.M. is 12 months of age, he should receive a single dose of vaccine followed by a booster dose 2 months later.

Polio

Polio, an infectious disease caused by a highly contagious enterovirus, can strike at any age, but primarily affects children younger than 3 years of age (>50% of cases). The three identified serotypes of poliovirus are transmitted person to person by direct fecal–oral contact or indirect exposure to infectious saliva, feces, or contaminated water.[53,54] After household exposure, 90% of susceptible contacts become infected.[53] The poliovirus enters through the mouth and then multiplies in the throat and intestines. Once established in the intestines, poliovirus can enter the bloodstream and invade the CNS, which may result in paralysis.[53–55]

Immunity to polio can be achieved after natural infection with poliovirus; however, infection by one serotype of the poliovirus does not protect an individual against infection from the other two serotypes.[53] Immunity can also be achieved through immunization, and the development of effective vaccines to prevent paralytic polio was one of the major medical breakthroughs of the 20th century. Since the advent of the trivalent oral polio vaccine (OPV) and inactivated polio vaccine (IPV), the incidence of paralytic poliomyelitis has been reduced dramatically.[55]

CASE 11-8

QUESTION 1: H.G. is the mother of a 2-month-old infant who is surprised when the nurse brings in a polio vaccine injection. She remembers that she received an oral form of the vaccine as a child. Why is H.G.'s infant receiving a different form of polio vaccine than she received?

Historically, the live attenuated oral polio vaccine (OPV or Sabin vaccine) was the formulation of choice in the United States. Its advantages include low cost, ease of administration, and induction of lifelong immunity.[53] In addition, OPV provides a high level of gastrointestinal immunity, thus preventing the carrier state. The fecal shedding of the attenuated OPV virus after vaccination is also an effective way to immunize or boost the pre-existing immunity in close contacts.[53,55] Despite these benefits, OPV carries the risk of vaccine-associated paralytic polio (VAPP), especially after the first dose in immunocompromised patients such as those with B-lymphocyte disorders (e.g., agammaglobulinemia, hypogammaglobulinemia).[54] In contrast to OPV, the enhanced IPV (IPOL, POLIOVAX), which is administered intramuscularly, has not been associated with VAPP or other reactions.[55,56] Although IPV provides similar systemic immunity as OPV, it induces less immunity in the gastrointestinal tract.[53,55] The risks of VAPP from OPV, despite its high efficacy, have resulted in the recommendation of IPV as the preferred dosage form for childhood immunization.[1,24,56]

As of 2000, the ACIP and AAP guidelines recommend that all children should receive four doses of IPV at ages 2 months, 4 months, 6 to 18 months, and 4 to 6 years. The first dose of vaccine should be administered no sooner than 6 weeks of life.[56] The last dose of the four-dose series should be administered after 4 years of age and at least 6 months after the previous dose.[23,24,56] Combination vaccines containing IPV are available and may be used to provide the initial four IPV doses. However, to ensure adequate immunity, it is recommended that an additional IPV booster be administered at 4 to 6 years, for a total of 5 doses[56] (see Table 11-2).

CASE 11-9

QUESTION 1: L.G. is a 28-year-old graduate student who is planning extensive travels through the African continent

and is concerned about polio because she had not been immunized as a child. What would be a prudent immunization schedule for her if her trip includes travel to a polio-endemic area?

Routine poliovirus vaccination of persons older than 18 years of age is not necessary in the United States because US residents are at minimal risk of exposure. Vaccination, however, should be considered for adults at high risk of polio exposure (e.g., travel to an area endemic for polio, close contact with children who will be receiving OPV, close contact with patients who may be excreting wild polioviruses, or work that requires handling poliovirus specimens).[55,56] IPV is the vaccine of choice because adults have a higher incidence of VAPP from OPV than children. Ideally, L.G. should receive two doses of IPV, administered 4 to 8 weeks apart, followed by a third dose 6 to 12 months later. If exposure is likely in less than 8 weeks, two doses of IPV should be administered at least 4 weeks apart.[55] If L.G.'s travel must be undertaken on short notice (<4 weeks) she should receive one dose of IPV with receipt of the remaining doses at a later date according to schedule.[55] Even if L.G. had been immunized as a child, a single dose of IPV may be considered for booster effect.[55]

Currently, OPV is recommended only in special circumstances, such as vaccination to control outbreaks of paralytic polio, unvaccinated infants traveling in less than 4 weeks to areas endemic for polio, and children of parents who reject the number of vaccine injections.[55,56] In parents who are concerned about the number of injections, OPV may be considered for the third and fourth vaccination after receiving systemic protection with IPV for the first two doses.[55] IPV is the only poliovirus vaccine that should be used in patients with an immunodeficiency disorder, those receiving immunosuppressive chemotherapy, or those living with a person who is known or suspected to have these conditions.[55,56]

Meningococcus

CASE 11-10

QUESTION 1: J.C. is a 12-year-old girl who presents for a check-up with her pediatrician. In discussion, it is found that her cousin attends a university where an outbreak of meningococcal disease recently occurred. Should she receive meningococcal vaccine?

After dramatic reductions of *Streptococcus pneumoniae* and *H. influenzae* type b strains of meningitis secondary to conjugate vaccines, *Neisseria meningitidis* has become a more prominent cause of bacterial meningitis. In 2005, the ACIP broadened the scope of population for which it recommends the meningococcal vaccine to include populations at increased risk, including travelers to endemic areas, those with certain immunodeficiencies (i.e., terminal complement deficiency), those with functional or anatomic asplenia, and laboratory personnel who may come in contact with aerosolized meningococcus. The ACIP also recommends its use for the control of meningococcal disease outbreaks.[57] These guidelines were updated and supplemented in 2010 to include a newly available third meningococcal vaccine. Other changes included the recommendation of routine vaccination plus a booster dose within the adolescent population; a two-dose primary series administered two months apart for persons aged 2 through 54 years with persistent complement component decifiency or functional or anatomical asplenia; and for adolescents with HIV.[58]

The three available meningococcal vaccine options include one polysaccharide preparation (MPS) and two different conjugated vaccines (MCV) covering serotypes A, C, Y, and W-135 of *N. meningitides*. The polysaccharide preparation (Menomune), or MPS4, is indicated for persons 2 to 10 years of age with the risk factors mentioned previously. It is important to note that polysaccharide vaccines such as this only stimulate B lymphocytes, not T lymphocytes, and thus do not produce a memory response. As a result, the effectiveness wanes over time. In addition, nasopharyngeal colonization of meningococcus is not reduced, so person-to-person transmission continues, blocking the development of herd immunity.[57]

Two conjugate vaccines available (Menactra and Menveo), both MCV4 conjugate vaccines, are indicated for individuals 11 to 55 years of age. The ACIP recommends administration of this vaccine to all persons at 11 to 12 years of age (or at high school entry if there is no history of vaccination) and to unvaccinated college freshmen residing in dormitories.[57,59] Additionally, as stated earlier, the ACIP recommends a booster dose around the age of 16 years, and a two-dose primary vaccination for patients with reduced response to a single dose.[58]

Adverse effects (e.g., fever, headache, chills, malaise, and arthralgias) from both vaccines are similar and relatively rare; however, in October 2006, the Centers for Disease Control and Prevention (CDC) and FDA issued a warning regarding the potential for increased risk of Guillain-Barré syndrome in patients receiving the Menactra conjugate vaccine.[60] Over the course of a 16-month period beginning in June 2005, 15 cases were reported in the 11- to 19-year age group, and 2 cases in those older than 20 years of age. All patients recovered. Despite this apparent small increased risk of Guillain-Barré syndrome, current recommendations remain the same, but monitoring of this development will continue.[60] Of note, no cases of Guillain-Barré syndrome have been reported with Menveo; however, surveillance is ongoing. At this time, J.C. should receive one of the two MCV4 vaccines and be advised to receive a booster dose at age 16.

Human Papillomavirus

CASE 11-11

QUESTION 1: J.S. is a 13-year-old girl who is healthy and not currently sexually active. Her mother and she would like background information including the role of the human papillomavirus (HPV) vaccine and recommendations for use of the vaccine in J.S.

HPV commonly infects the genital tract and is primarily transmitted by sexual contact. Infection with HPV has been associated with cervical cancer as well as other anogenital cancers, anogenital warts, and recurrent respiratory papillomatosis, and is estimated to be the most common sexually transmitted disease in the United States.[61,62] HPV affects both sexes with similar infection rates.[63] Acute HPV infections typically resolve without clinical complications within 1 year; however, 10% to 15% of infections remain persistent and pose a risk of invasive cervical carcinoma and other anogential carcinomas.[64] Although not all HPV infections cause cervical cancer, almost all (99%) cervical cancer in women is associated with a previous HPV infection.[62,64] The majority of disease associated with HPV is caused by the HPV types 6, 11, 16, and 18,[65] with HPV strains 16 and 18 accounting for approximately 70% of cervical cancers and approximately 50% of cervical cancer precursors.[66,67] In contrast, HPV strains 6 and 11 account for the cause of 90% of genital warts and most cases of recurrent respiratory papillomatosis.[65,68] Infection with one strain of HPV does not prevent infection from other strains; thus, repeated infections can occur through one's lifetime[64] and those with prior HPV infections benefit from immunization as well.

Two vaccines are available for the prevention of HPV infection: a quadravalent product (Gardasil) and a bivalent product (Cervarix). The quadravalent product is active against HPV strains 6, 11, 16, and 18 and is indicated for males and females ages 9 to 26 years of age, whereas the bivalent product is active against only HPV strains 16 and 18 and is indicated only for females ages 10 to 25 years old.[68] Gardasil is indicated for males for the purpose of prevention of genital warts.[68]

Routine vaccination with either HPV vaccine is recommended for female patients at 11 to 12 years of age.[68] Vaccination at this age attempts to achieve an immune response before the sexual debut[61] and involves a three-dose series administered at intervals of 0, 2, and 6 months.[68] Immunization against HPV is 90% effective in reducing persistent HPV infections and 100% effective in preventing HPV-related diseases such as genital warts or lesions.[65,68] The quadravalent vaccine may be given to males aged 9 to 26 years of age, although routine vaccination is not recommended for males.[68]

The mandatory requirement for immunization of adolescent girls against HPV is controversial and debated in many state legislatures because of ethical and social concerns. The CDC and AAP recommend immunization for adolescent girls, regardless of current sexual activity, to decrease the lifetime risk of cervical cancer and to protect against infection when the time comes that an individual chooses to become sexually active. Additionally, routine vaccination of males is not recommended by the CDC as the cost-effectiveness of vaccination in males is not as favorable as the cost-effectiveness of vaccination in females. The CDC currently suggests that improving vaccination rates in girls 11 to 12 years old may be more cost effective than adding vaccination requirements for males.[68] Based on the current recommendations, J.S. should receive the HPV vaccine.

Pneumococcus

CASE 11-12

QUESTION 1: M.T. is a 5-year-old boy with a history of asthma. His pediatrician recommends that he receive the pneumonia vaccine. What is the evidence behind this recommendation?

Streptococcus pneumoniae (pneumococcus) infection can cause meningitis, pneumonia, sinusitis, and otitis media, and is a major source of illness and death among children and adults.[69,70] Infants, young children, and older patients are at highest risk for exhibiting pneumococcal infections.[69] The risk for disseminated pneumococcal infections is increased by underlying medical conditions (heart failure, chronic obstructive pulmonary diseases), chronic liver disease (e.g., cirrhosis), functional or anatomic asplenia (e.g., sickle cell disease, splenectomy), and acquired or inherited immunosuppressive conditions (e.g., HIV, cancer, immunosuppressive therapy). *S. pneumoniae* is a common pathogen in children with HIV, often presenting as one of the first manifestations of HIV infection.[71]

Three pneumococcal vaccines are available: the original polysaccharide vaccine (Pneumovax) and two conjugate-pneumococcal vaccines (PCV 7 and PCV 13 [Prevnar]).[69,70] Pneumovax contains 23 of the most prevalent or invasive purified capsular-polysaccharide antigens types of *S. pneumoniae.* Antibody response to Pneumovax is inconsistent in children younger than 2 years of age partially because the antigens included in Pneumovax protect against strains that typically cause adult disease, but not childhood disease. In contrast, the conjugate pneumococcal vaccines (Prevnar 7 and Prevnar 13) improve immunogenicity and efficacy in infants and toddlers.[70] The PCV 7 vaccine provides protection against the seven pneumococcal strains that cause 80% of all pneumococcal invasive disease in children younger than 6 years of age, whereas PCV 13 protects against 13 (90%) of infectious serotypes.[72] ACIP recommends giving the conjugate 13 vaccine (PCV 13) to all children aged 2 to 59 months and children aged 60 to 71 months with underlying medical conditions that place them at high risk for experiencing pneumococcal disease or its complications.[70] Because M.T. has already passed the recommended age for vaccination and has asthma, he should receive the PCV 13 vaccine today.

Immunocompromised patients typically have an unreliable response to vaccines, but because of the potential benefits the pneumococcal vaccines should be administered. Some studies have found transient elevation of plasma HIV levels after pneumococcal vaccination, although this has not been associated with decreased patient survival.[73,74] To maintain immunity, revaccination with the 23-valent polysaccharide vaccine is recommended after 3 years in high-risk children younger than 10 years of age and after 5 years in older patients.

CASE 11-12, QUESTION 2: M.T.'s grandfather is a 68-year old who is a previous smoker and has cardiovascular disease. Should M.T.'s grandfather receive pneumococcal vaccine?

The adult population recommended to receive the 23-valent pneumococcal polysaccharide vaccine (Pneumovax) include patients age 65 years of age and older, and patients aged 19 to 64 with certain underlying medical conditions.[69] These underlying medical conditions include immunocompetent patients with chronic heart disease, chronic lung disease, diabetes mellitus, cerebrospinal fluid leaks, cochlear implants, alcoholism, chronic liver disease, and cigarette smoking. Specifically, adult patients with asthma and those who are cigarette smokers are proven to benefit from the pneumococcal vaccine. Patients with functional or anatomical asplenia and those adults who are immunocompromised are also recommended to receive the pneumococcal polysaccharide vaccine.[69] A second dose of the vaccine should be administered 5 years after the first dose in patients who received the initial pneumococcal vaccine prior to 65 years of age.[69] Patients who receive their primary vaccination at age 65 years or later in life should only receive one dose of the pneumococcal vaccine.[69] If a patient is uncertain as to the currency of their vaccination, or when they received it, they should not receive revaccination because of lack of clinical evidence regarding the benefit of revaccination safety and benefit.[69] M.T.'s grandfather (a previously unvaccinated 68-year-old man) should receive one dose of the 23-valent pneumococcal polysaccharide vaccine.

Influenza

Annual influenza vaccination is the most effective method for preventing influenza viral infections and its complications and sequelae.[75] Recommendations for influenza vaccination were recently expanded to include anyone older than 6 months of age who does not have a contraindication.[75] This wide age range for routine vaccination is supported by the AAP and clinical evidence confirms that annual influenza vaccination is a safe and effective preventative health measure with potential benefit for all ages of the population.[75,76] When vaccine supply is limited, priority for vaccination should be given to people who are[75]:

- 6 months old to 4 years old
- 50 or more years of age
- Residents of chronic care facilities
- Immunosuppressed via medication or human immunodeficiency virus

- Adults and children with chronic pulmonary or cardiovascular disorders, diabetes mellitus, renal dysfunction, hemoglobinopathies, or immunosuppression
- Children who are 6 months old to 18 years of age receiving aspirin therapy (because of an increased risk of Reye syndrome after influenza)
- Health care personnel
- Women who will be pregnant during the influenza season
- American Indian or Alaskan Natives
- Morbidly obese with body mass index greater than or equal to 40 kg/m^2
- Household members and care providers with medical conditions that put them at high risk for severe complications from influenza
- Household contacts and caregivers of children younger than 5 years old and adults older than 50 years old, with emphasis on vaccinating contacts of children younger than 6 months old

Each year, the influenza vaccine is formulated to contain three inactivated influenza virus strains (usually, two type A and one type B) predicted to be in circulation within the United States during the upcoming flu season. The vaccine is available as both an intramuscularly administered trivalent inactivated vaccine (TIV) and an intranasal live attenuated influenza vaccine (LAIV). The injectable TIV is indicated for use in children at least 6 months old to adults, including those with high-risk conditions. The LAIV (intranasal) is indicated for use in healthy nonpregnant patients ages 2 to 49 years old.[75]

Influenza vaccine should be administered annually for adequate protection. Children younger than 9 years of age require two doses of the vaccine administered 1 month apart to achieve adequate antibody response. If these children received only one dose of influenza vaccination in the preceding season, they should receive two doses of vaccine in the after influenza season. One dose of the vaccine is indicated for children 9 years of age and older. Influenza vaccine contains a small amount of egg protein and historically has been contraindicated in patients with a severe egg allergy. Evidence indicates, however, that even patients with severe egg allergies can safely receive the influenza vaccine.[76–78]

CASE 11-13

QUESTION 1: H.N. is a 72-year-old man inquiring about a new high-dose influenza vaccine. Is this a recommended vaccine for H.N.? Could he be given the LAIV instead?

A high-dose TIV (Fluzone High-Dose) came to market in the fall of 2010, and is indicated for patients aged 65 years and older. Standard-dose inactivated trivalent influenza vaccines contain a total of 45 mcg (15 mcg of each of the three recommended strains) of influenza virus hemagglutinin antigen per 0.5-mL dose. In contrast, Fluzone High-Dose has four times the activity and is formulated to contain a total of 180 mcg (60 mcg of each strain) of influenza virus hemagglutinin antigen in each 0.5-mL dose. The older than 65 population is targeted to receive the high-dose formulation because older patients respond with a lower antibody titer to the conventional TIV.[79] When antibody titers were measured after patients received the high-dose vaccine, significantly higher antibody titers for all three influenza strains were present.[80–82] However, it is unknown if there will be more robust protection against influenza infection observed among patients who receive the high-dose TIV.[79]

The LAIV (FluMist) is available for use in healthy, nonpregnant patients 2 to 49 years of age. After administration, recipients become infected with attenuated virus strains, which stimulates both local IgA and circulating IgG antibodies.[83–86] Because live attenuated influenza viral particles are present within the LAIV, recipients may experience mild signs or symptoms related to influenza infection, such as rhinorrhea, nasal congestion, fever, or sore throat.[75] Live vaccine may be especially useful for healthy individuals, including health care workers or during periods when the supply of inactivated vaccine may be low, potentially increasing availability of the inactivated product for those unable to receive the live vaccine. Individuals should not receive the live vaccine if any of the following apply[87]:

- Age younger than 2 years
- Hypersensitivity to eggs, egg proteins, gentamicin, gelatin, arginine, or previous life-threatening reactions to previous influenza vaccinations
- Moderate to severe illness
- Received another live vaccine within 4 weeks
- Pediatric and adolescent patients currently taking aspirin therapy
- Known or suspected immunodeficiency
- History of Guillain-Barré syndrome
- Asthma or reactive airway disease or other condition conferring high risk of severe influenza

Because of his age, HN should not be given the intranasal vaccine, but could receive either the standard or high-dose inactivated vaccine.

LIVE ATTENUATED VACCINES

Besides the live attenuated flu vaccine discussed previously, there are several other live attenuated vaccines currently available for use (Table 11-1).

Rotavirus

Rotavirus is a major cause of gastroenteritis and subsequent dehydration in the United States. Almost all children in the United States will experience rotavirus gastroenteritis within the first 5 years of their lives and up to 50% of hospitalizations secondary to gastroenteritis in children are caused by rotavirus infection.[88,89] The AAP and the CDC currently recommend routine immunization of infants with the rotavirus vaccine.[23,24] There are two oral, live attenuated rotavirus vaccines currently commercially available: Rotateq (RV5), a pentavalent vaccine, and Rotarix (RV1), a monovalent vaccine.[90] Both vaccines are believed to be equally effective despite lack of head-to-head comparison trials. The RV5 vaccine is administered in a three-dose series at 2, 4, and 6 months, whereas the RV1 vaccine follows a two-dose series at 2 and 4 months.[90] Initial vaccination should begin at a minimum of 6 weeks of age and the maximum age at which to administer the last dose is at 8 months of age.[90] It is preferred that all doses be administered with the same product, however if a combination of RV5 and RV1 is used, a total of three doses should be administered.[90] Although immunization against rotavirus does not prevent all future episodes of rotavirus infection, it can significantly reduce the severity of infections and reduce hospitalization rates.

CASE 11-14

QUESTION 1: J.M., a 24-year-old mother, presents her 2-month-old infant to receive immunizations. She is concerned about the administration of the rotavirus vaccine because the infant's grandmother is undergoing chemotherapy for breast cancer and she is concerned that the vaccine may put her mother at risk for infection as well as cause "bowel problems" for her baby.

Because the rotavirus vaccine is a live attenuated vaccine and infants can shed the virus after administration, the immunocompromised person (the grandmother) should avoid contact with the infant's feces and adhere to good handwashing procedures, particularly during the first week after vaccine administration.[88–90] Although an immunized infant can spread the rotavirus to an immunocompromised person, the risk is believed to be small relative to the benefits and risks to the immunocompromised individual. For example, if not immunized the infant may become infected with rotavirus and shed much higher amounts of the virus in their stool with a greater potential of spreading the illness to others. Thus, rotavirus immunization of infants under this circumstance still is strongly encouraged.[88]

The immunization of infants who themselves are immunocompromised is more controversial. Rotavirus immunization in this circumstance requires the medical practitioner to discuss risks and benefits with the infant's parents.

Despite being a live attenuated vaccine, the rotavirus vaccine may be administered at any time relative to the administration of blood products and antibody-containing products.[90] There appears to be no interference with the antibody response to the vaccine with the use of these products because much of the immune response is local within the gastrointestinal tract, which leads to protection from gastroenteritis.

Measles/Mumps/Rubella

CASE 11-15

QUESTION 1: J.C. is a 15-month-old girl who is scheduled to receive her MMR vaccination. J.C.'s mother is concerned about the risks of autism and other adverse effects from the vaccine. How should the mother be counseled?

Measles, historically a highly contagious and common disease of childhood, often is associated with symptoms such as high fever, rash, cough, rhinitis, and conjunctivitis.

ONLINE CONTENT **For two photos of children with measles, go to http://thepoint.lww.com/AT10e.**

Complications, although uncommon, include pneumonia and encephalitis. Live attenuated measles virus vaccine produces a benign infection that is thought to produce lifelong immunity. The United States is currently in its third attempt to eliminate measles infection. The most significant decrease in the incidence of measles occurred when American children were required to receive the vaccine before entering school.[91] During the 1985–1988 epidemic, most measles transmission occurred in areas with 95% immunization rates, indicating that some children fail to respond adequately to the initial vaccine dose.[92] In addition, up to 47% of reported cases of measles in the United States result from international importation; the remaining cases result from outbreaks in school-age children who did not receive a second dose of the vaccine.[93] Unfortunately, many parents are refusing immunization of their infants with the MMR vaccine due to media reports (now proven unfounded) about the risk of autism.

The concern regarding the risk from autism after vaccination with the MMR vaccine stems from a report by Wakefield et al. published in 1998. This report identified a causal relationship with the administration of the MMR vaccine and the subsequent development of autism in 12 children.[94] The results of this report became highly publicized and sparked fear in parents across the world. Further investigation revealed numerous counts of scientific misconduct for financial gains by Dr. Wakefield, which led to 10 of the 12 coinvestigators retracting their claims. The CDC has coordinated numerous investigations to uncover any relationship between the vaccine and autism, but despite years of research have been unable to find any association. Regrettably, efforts to counter the negative publicity for the MMR vaccine have not had success.

J.C.'s mother should be counseled regarding the lack of an association between autism and the MMR vaccine. If she still decides to refuse vaccination, appropriate forms for documenting such are available through the respective state's Department of Health.

The first dose of the MMR vaccine should be administered to children at 12 to 15 months of age, followed by a second dose at entrance to grade school (age 4 to 6 years).[1,94,95] Studies indicate that infants receiving the vaccine may be at higher risk of exhibiting a febrile seizure during the 2 weeks after vaccination when peak virus replication occurs.[95] The risk appears to be higher with the combination vaccine ProQuad. Because of this concern, the CDC recommends the preferential use of the MMR vaccine in children aged 12 to 47 months.[95] Although studies have not shown a benefit with the use of antipyretics for preventing febrile seizures from the vaccine, it is recommended that caregivers be counseled regarding the management of fever. No increased risk of febrile seizures has been noted with the second dose of the vaccine administered at 4 to 6 years of age,[95] thus the use of the combination vaccine is recommended at this age to reduce the number of injections and enhance compliance.[95]

Adult vaccination with MMR vaccine is also important to protect from epidemics. Adults should receive a second dose of MMR if they were born between 1963 and 1967, previously vaccinated with killed measles vaccine, are students in postsecondary institutions, work in health care facilities, travel internationally, or were recently exposed to a measles outbreak.[96] Persons born after 1968 should receive one dose of a measles-containing vaccine.[25,96] Health care workers must show documentation of having receipt of the appropriate number of doses or laboratory evidence of immunity to comply with infection control policies.[97]

Mumps and rubella antigens are combined with measles in the MMR vaccine in the United States. Mumps immunization remains controversial in childhood because mumps illness in children rarely produces complications. Meningoencephalitis generally is a benign meningitis, and postinfectious encephalitis, a serious complication, is extremely rare (1 of 6,000). Deafness, commonly considered a risk of mumps, occurs rarely (1 of 15,000) and is usually unilateral. Orchitis, another complication, affects adult men. Mumps vaccination at 12 to 15 months of age may not protect boys into their adult years.[96] Although administration of a second dose of MMR at age 4 to 6 years may provide longer protection, current immunization practices are aimed at eliminating the mumps virus from the pool of young children, thereby, minimizing the exposure of nonimmunized adults.[96]

The most significant consequences of rubella infection occur in pregnant women (e.g., spontaneous abortions, miscarriages, stillbirths, fetal anomalies), especially when infection occurs during the first trimester. Preventing congenital rubella through elimination of the viral pool is the primary objective of rubella immunization programs because about 10% to 20% of women of child-bearing age have not acquired natural immunity.[96] Immunization or rubella antibody titer screening of women at premarital examinations and post partum also is recommended. Women of childbearing age receiving the rubella vaccine should use contraception for at least 28 days after immunization.[98]

Varicella

CASE 11-16

QUESTION 1: J.T. is a 6-year-old girl who comes home from school with a note from the school nurse indicating that a child in her kindergarten class has been diagnosed with chickenpox. J.T.'s mother is quite concerned because J.T. has not been immunized with the varicella vaccine. She wants to know whether administration of the vaccine at this time will protect J.T. from becoming infected.

Varivax, a live attenuated vaccine against varicella-zoster (chickenpox), is the first herpesvirus vaccine to be widely tested in healthy and high-risk children and adults.[99–101] Chickenpox is a highly contagious, mild childhood disease in healthy children, but it can be severe and even fatal, especially in the immunocompromised patient.

For a photo of a patient with chickenpox, go to http://thepoint.lww.com/AT10e.

Unusual complications (e.g., severe bacterial superinfections, Reye syndrome, encephalopathies) are markedly reduced with an immunization program.[99] Before the vaccine was available, approximately 4 million cases of chickenpox were reported annually, with 4,000 to 9,000 hospitalizations and 100 deaths.[99] Historically, 55% of varicella-related deaths occured in adults, many of whom were infected by exposure to unvaccinated preschool-aged children with typical cases of varicella.[102]

Despite high vaccine coverage rates and 85% vaccine efficacy with the previous single dose vaccination, outbreaks of breakthrough varicella continued to occur in the United States.[103] As a result, current guidelines recommend a two-dose series for all children, adolescents, and adults without evidence of immunity.[1,23,103] The first varicella vaccine dose should be administered at 12 to 15 months of age, followed by the second dose at 4 to 6 years of age. For persons 7 to 13 years of age who have not received varicella vaccine, two doses of varicella vaccine should be administered at least 3 months apart. For persons older than 13 years of age, administer two doses of varicella vaccine at least 4 weeks apart.[103]

Postexposure varicella vaccination should be considered for J.T. Chickenpox infection can be prevented or symptoms reduced if varicella vaccine is administered within 3 days of exposure, and may provide some protection within 5 days.[101,103] If J.T. also needs MMR vaccination, the quadrivalent combination vaccine ProQuad containing measles, mumps, rubella, and varicella antigens may be considered. A second dose of varicella vaccine in 3 months should be recommended to ensure long term protection.

The most common adverse effect associated with varicella vaccine administration is rash. Transmission of the virus from the vaccine has been documented in only 3 of 15 million doses administered, all of which occurred in the presence of a vesicular rash after vaccination.[99] Caution should be used when patients exhibit a rash postvaccination to avoid contact with immunocompromised individuals until rash resolution.[103]

Although varicella vaccine might not entirely prevent the occurrence of chickenpox in an immunocompromised patient, it can modify the disease. In the National Institutes of Health's Collaborative Varicella Vaccine Study, a seroconversion rate of only 85% was observed after a single dose in adults, compared with 95% in healthy children and 90% in children with leukemia.[104] Varicella vaccine is generally not recommended in children who have cellular immunodeficiencies, but it can be used in those with impaired humoral immunity.[61] The vaccine should be avoided in children with symptomatic HIV, but may be considered in asymptomatic or mildly symptomatic patients.[99,103]

CASE 11-16, QUESTION 2: If the varicella vaccine is now universally recommended, what is the role of the herpes zoster vaccine?

After a primary infection with varicella, 15% to 30% of the population experiences a latent infection in the sensory nerve ganglia that reactivates, causing herpes zoster (HZ).[103,105] HZ typically occurs decades after initial varicella infection. This reactivation can result in postherpetic neuralgia or dissemination which results in skin eruptions ("shingles") and potential CNS, pulmonary, or hepatic complications.[103,105] Although some have theorized that universal varicella vaccination should eventually reduce the incidence of HZ because it prevents primary infection, others debate that the attenuated virus may have greater potential for becoming latent and reactiving.[103,105] Still others argue that with the elimination of wild-type virus in the community, the exposure of individuals with latent wild-type varicella to help boost immunity and prevent HZ is reduced. In this situation, the risk of HZ may be increased.[103,105] Routine varicella immunization began in 1995 and only long-term studies of vaccinated individuals will answer the questions about the impact of the varicella vaccination upon the incidence of HZ. However, currently the majority of adults are not immunized against varicella (unless required as a health care worker) and have previously acquired wild-type varicella infections. Therefore, most adults in the United States are at risk for exhibiting HZ as they age.

The zoster vaccine (Zostavax) is a live attenudated varicella zoster vaccine that uses the same strain and antigens as the varicella vaccines (Varivax and ProQuad); however, it is 14 times more potent and contains additional antigenic components. It was initially recommended for all individuals older than 60 years of age as a single subcutaneous injection to prevent HZ.[25,105] In 2011, FDA approval was given to use HZ vaccine in individuals 50 years of age or older. It may be given to patients with a previous history of HZ, but is not indicated to treat acute zoster or prevent further complications during an acute episode.[105] It is not recommended for routine immunization for anyone who has previously received the varicella vaccine. The zoster vaccine was shown in the Shingles Prevention Study to reduce the incidence of HZ by more than 50% and resulted in reductions in the severity and duration of pain, in addition to preventing the development of postherpetic neuralgia.[106]

ADMINISTRATION TECHNIQUES

Vaccines or other biological agents are typically administered as either an intramuscular (IM) or subcutaneous injection.

For videos of IM and subcutaneous injections, go to http://thepointlww.com. Note: The subcutaneous injection video actually discusses administration of a medication, rather than an immunization, but the same technique is used to administer an immunization subcutaneously.

Because appropriate administration by the correct route and technique is critical to the effectiveness of the specified vaccine, it is essential to consult the prescribing and administration

Hgb, 8.7 g/dL
Hct, 27%
MCV, 115 fL
MCH, 38 pg/cell
MCHC, 340 g/L
Reticulocytes, 0.4%
Poikilocytosis and anisocytosis on the blood smear
White blood cell (WBC) count, 4,000/μL
Platelets, 100,000/μL
Serum iron, 90 mcg/dL
TIBC, 350 g/dL
Ferritin, 140 ng/mL
RBC folate, 300 ng/mL
Serum vitamin B_{12}, 90 pg/mL
Intrinsic factor antibody, positive

What signs, symptoms, and laboratory findings in C.L. are typical of pernicious anemia?

C.L.'s signs and symptoms are classic for pernicious anemia. This disease occurs equally in both sexes (primarily in individuals of northern European descent), with an average onset of 60 years. Pernicious anemia develops from a lack of gastric intrinsic factor production, which causes vitamin B_{12} malabsorption and ultimately vitamin B_{12} deficiency. C.L.'s signs and symptoms of vitamin B_{12} deficiency include painful red tongue, loss of lower extremity vibratory sense, vertigo, and emotional instability.

The elevated MCV suggests megaloblastic anemia.

For an illustration of a peripheral blood smear in pernicious anemia, go to http://thepoint.lww.com/AT10e.

Folate and iron are two other factors that can affect the MCV and should be evaluated during the workup of a patient for anemia. In this case, C.L.'s folate and iron levels are normal, but his serum vitamin B_{12} level is low. The presence of poikilocytosis and anisocytosis observed in the blood smear represent ineffective erythropoiesis. Other cell lineages also may be affected in the bone marrow. Erythroid hypercellularity, along with a decrease in the myeloid cells (leukocytes and platelets), increases the erythroid to myeloid ratio in C.L. The patient's low Hgb, elevated MCV, low serum vitamin B_{12} levels, and presence of intrinsic factor antibodies are compatible with the diagnosis of pernicious anemia, which is often associated with atrophic body gastritis.[30] The Schilling test, which confirms intestinal malabsorption of vitamin B_{12}, is used less frequently in clinical practice owing to problems with the radioactive agents involved.

TREATMENT

CASE 12-2, QUESTION 2: How should C.L.'s pernicious anemia be treated? How soon can a response be expected?

C.L. should receive parenteral vitamin B_{12} in a dose sufficient to provide not only the daily requirement of approximately 2 mcg, but also the amount needed to replenish tissue stores (about 2,000 to 5,000 mcg; average, 4,000 mcg). To replete vitamin B_{12} stores, cyanocobalamin can be given IM in accordance with various regimens as shown in Table 12-7.[31] IM or deep subcutaneous administration provides sustained release of vitamin B_{12} with better utilization compared with rapid IV infusion. An oral tablet or intranasal cyanocobalamin gel is also available for maintenance therapy, after the patient has achieved hematologic remission.

Neurologic symptoms should begin to improve within 24 hours with adequate vitamin B_{12} therapy. However, with long-standing vitamin B_{12} deficiency, several months may pass before some symptoms are relieved; other symptoms may never resolve. Hematologic parameters should begin to improve within the first few days. The bone marrow becomes normoblastic within 48 hours, the reticulocyte count should peak around day 5 of therapy, and the Hct should return to normal in 1 to 2 months. Because the rapid production of RBCs can increase potassium demand, serum potassium should be monitored and potassium supplementation provided as necessary. Peripheral blood counts should be obtained every 3 to 6 months to evaluate the adequacy of therapy. If maintenance therapy is discontinued, pernicious anemia will recur within 5 years, making patient adherence vital to long-term success.

Oral Vitamin B_{12}

CASE 12-2, QUESTION 3: What factors affect the oral absorption of vitamin B_{12}? When is oral vitamin B_{12} therapy an effective alternative to parenteral therapy?

The amount of vitamin B_{12} that can be absorbed orally from a single dose or meal ranges from 1 to 5 mcg; approximately 5 mcg of vitamin B_{12} is absorbed daily from the average

TABLE 12-7
Cyanocobalamin (Vitamin B_{12}) Supplementation Regimens for Macrocytic Anemia[31]

	Initial Supplementation			Chronic Supplementation (lifelong)		
Patient Population	**Dose**	**Frequency**	**Route**	**Dose**	**Frequency**	**Route**
US regimens	100 mcg	Daily for 7 days, then on alternate days for 14 days, then q 3–4 days for 2–3 weeks	IM or SQ	100–200 mcg	Monthly	IM or SQ
				Up to 1,000 mcg[a]	Daily	Oral
				500 mcg	Weekly	Intranasal
	1,000 mcg	Weekly for 4–6 weeks	IM or SQ	1,000 mcg	Monthly	IM or SQ
	1,000–2,000 mcg	Daily for 1 month	Oral	125–500 mcg	Daily	Oral
UK regimen, without neurological involvement	250–1,000 mcg	On alternating days for 1–2 weeks, then 250 mcg weekly until counts normalize	IM or SQ	1,000 mcg	Monthly	IM or SQ
UK regimen, with neurological involvement	1,000 mcg	On alternating days as long as symptoms occur	IM or SQ			

[a]In patients with normal gastrointestinal absorption, doses of 1–25 mcg daily are considered sufficient as a dietary supplement.
IM, intramuscular; SQ, subcutaneous.

American diet. The percentage of vitamin B_{12} absorbed decreases with increasing doses. About 50% of a 1- to 2-mcg dose of vitamin B_{12} is absorbed, whereas only about 5% of a 20-mcg dose is absorbed.[32] Doses of more than 100 mcg must be ingested to absorb 5 mcg of vitamin B_{12}. Overall, oral vitamin B_{12} therapy is considered safe and effective,[33] although because of lack of long-term efficacy data, oral supplementation is not routinely used in the acute treatment of vitamin B_{12} deficiency.[29] Oral therapy for pernicious anemia using high dosages of oral cyanocobalamin (1,000 to 2,000 mcg) may be indicated in certain patients, especially those who refuse or cannot receive parenteral therapy.[29,34,35] Patients can be given 1,000 to 2,000 mcg/day for 1 month, followed by 125 to 500 mcg/day as maintenance treatment.[29,36] Issues of nonadherence or lack of response with oral therapy places the patient at substantial risk for significant neurologic damage. Patients receiving oral vitamin B_{12} therapy should be monitored more frequently to ensure adherence to therapy.

Anemias After Gastrectomy

CASE 12-3

QUESTION 1: F.M. has just undergone a total gastrectomy for recurrent nonhealing ulcers. What form(s) of anemia would be expected to develop in a patient after gastrectomy? Should F.M. receive prophylactic vitamin B_{12}?

Partial or total gastrectomy often results in anemia, particularly pernicious anemia, because the loss of intrinsic factor impairs oral vitamin B_{12} absorption. The hematologic and neurologic abnormalities associated with vitamin B_{12} deficiency do not develop until existing vitamin B_{12} stores are depleted (about 2 to 3 years). Nevertheless, prophylactic vitamin B_{12} should be administered to this patient after total gastrectomy. Because the vitamin B_{12} stores are not currently depleted, maintenance therapy, as discussed in Case 12-2, Question 2, should be adequate for F.M.

MALABSORPTION OF VITAMIN B_{12}

SIGNS AND SYMPTOMS

CASE 12-4

QUESTION 1: P.G., a 48-year-old man, began experiencing progressive confusion and lethargy 7 months ago. A CBC at that time revealed only mild leukocytosis. Today, he comes to the emergency department with a 4-week history of frequent (three to five per day) stools containing bright red blood. He reports continued lethargy, dizziness, ataxia, and paresthesias in his hands and feet.

Laboratory findings of interest include the following:

Hgb, 12 g/dL
MCV, 85 fL
Iron, 80 mcg/dL
Vitamin B_{12}, 87 pg/mL (normal, 200 to 1,000 pg/mL)
Folate, 19 ng/mL (normal, 7 to 25 ng/mL)
Hypersegmented PMNs
Bilirubin, 2.7 mg/dL
Lactate dehydrogenase (LDH), 550 U/L

A subsequent bone marrow aspirate demonstrates megaloblastic erythropoiesis, giant metamyelocytes, and a low stainable iron. A barium swallow and follow-through show numerous jejunal and duodenal diverticula. Jejunal and duodenal aspirates reveal aerobic and anaerobic bacterial overgrowth. What signs, symptoms, and laboratory findings are typical for vitamin B_{12} deficiency in P.G.?

The signs and symptoms in P.G. that are consistent with vitamin B_{12} deficiency include confusion, dizziness, ataxia, and paresthesias. Other signs and symptoms may be caused by other underlying conditions. For example, his lethargy may be the result of prolonged blood loss secondary to diverticulitis.

Notably, P.G. initially presented with a mild leukocytosis. Evaluation 9 months later shows a low Hgb, a low serum vitamin B_{12} level, and hypersegmented PMNs. The high LDH and bilirubin levels reflect intramedullary hemolysis of megaloblastic RBCs consistent with vitamin B_{12} deficiency, even though the MCV is within normal limits. The presence of megaloblastic erythropoiesis and giant metamyelocytes in the bone marrow also is consistent with vitamin B_{12} deficiency.

P.G.'s history of bloody stools and diverticula suggests substantial long-term blood loss, which increased demand for iron and vitamin B_{12} to replace RBCs. Concurrent iron deficiency can mask megaloblastic changes in RBCs, which explains the suspiciously normal MCV (dimorphic anemia). The serum folate concentration is also falsely normal. Although the RBC folate level is likely to be low, serum folate concentrations are normal because monoglutamated folates leak from cells into the serum in vitamin B_{12} deficient states.

TREATMENT

CASE 12-4, QUESTION 2: How should P.G.'s vitamin B_{12} deficiency be treated?

The cause of vitamin B_{12} malabsorption must be corrected before P.G. is given oral vitamin B_{12} therapy. The presence of diverticula is not the cause of vitamin B_{12} malabsorption because diverticula typically do not extend into the distal ileum. Instead, given P.G.'s medical history, the most likely cause of vitamin B_{12} malabsorption is bacterial usurpation of luminal vitamin B_{12}. P.G. should first be treated with a broad-spectrum antibiotic (e.g., tetracycline) or a sulfonamide for 7 to 10 days, then begin daily oral vitamin B_{12} supplementation to replenish his body stores. In this case, normal levels of intrinsic factor permit oral therapy. The recommended daily dose of vitamin B_{12} is 25 to 250 mcg. After antibiotic therapy, P.G. also should begin to absorb vitamin B_{12} in his diet.

Folic Acid Deficiency Anemia

FOLIC ACID METABOLISM

Folate is abundant in virtually all food sources, especially fresh green vegetables, fruits, yeast, and animal protein. As a result of food fortification, the average American diet provides 50 to 2,000 mcg of folate per day; however, excessive or prolonged cooking (>15 minutes) in large quantities of water destroys a high percentage of the folate that is contained in food.[37] Human requirements for folate vary with age and depend on the rate of metabolism and cell turnover but are generally 3 mcg/kg/day.[37] The minimal daily adult requirement of folate is 50 mcg, but because absorption from food is incomplete, a daily intake of 200 mcg is recommended. Folate requirements are increased in conditions in which the metabolic rate and rate of cellular division are increased (e.g., pregnancy, infancy, infection, malignancies, hemolytic anemia). The following are estimates of daily folate requirements based on age and growth demands: children, 80 to 400 mcg; infants, 65 mcg; pregnant or lactating women, 600 mcg.[38]

Dietary folic acid is in the polyglutamate form and must be enzymatically deconjugated in the GI tract to the monoglutamate form before it is absorbed. Once absorbed, the inactive deteriorating respiratory function, and should receive transfusions if his clinical status does not improve.

TREATMENT FOR FREQUENT VASO-OCCLUSIVE CRISES

CASE 12-7, QUESTION 4: What preventive therapies exist for J.T. that will reduce occurrences of vaso-occlusive crises?

Hgb F (HbF) has a protective effect against Hgb polymerization. Investigators have observed that patients with HbF levels greater than 20% experience a relatively mild or benign course with fewer vaso-occlusive crises.[42] Hydroxyurea has been found to increase HbF synthesis, which, in turn, may decrease RBC sickling and the occurrence of disease-related complications.[57–59] Hydroxyurea is used prophylactically in patients with recurrent moderate to severe vaso-occlusive crises, but not in treatment of the crises. The use of hydroxyurea in the sickle cell population should be carefully weighed for risk versus benefit, because it is a cytotoxic agent associated with bone marrow suppression. Patients taking hydroxyurea should have bone marrow studies performed before therapy and periodically during therapy. Other adverse effects of hydroxyurea include GI effects (nausea, vomiting, diarrhea), dermatologic effects (macular papular rash, pruritus), and potential risk of developing a secondary neoplasm (leukemia) with prolonged use. The treatment dose of hydroxyurea for sickle cell anemia is 15 to 35 mg/kg/day. After initiation of therapy, blood counts should be monitored closely and the dose adjusted accordingly. Several clinical trials evaluating hydroxyurea show improvement in the clinical course of patients with sickle cell anemia.[58,60] Other areas of potential promise for the treatment of sickle cell anemia include bone marrow transplantation and gene therapy.[61,62]

IRON CHELATION THERAPY

CASE 12-7, QUESTION 5: Despite optimal treatment with hydroxyurea, J.T. continues to experience exacerbations of his sickle cell disease requiring blood transfusions. J.T. estimates he has required six such transfusions in the last 2 years, and at least 25 units of blood in his lifetime. During a visit with his hematologist, J.T.'s serum ferritin is noted to be 1,050 mcg/L. What potential adverse effect of treatment is the hematologist's concern? What other tests may be performed to detect this?

Patients requiring chronic transfusions of PRBCs are at an increased risk for iron toxicity owing to iron overload.[63] Normally, plasma iron binds with transferrin; however, if transferrin becomes saturated, patients will have higher levels of toxic nontransferrin-bound iron. As nontransferrin-bound iron increases, it deposits in other organs, most frequently the liver. There, nontransferrin-bound iron produces free radicals, causing tissue damage and fibrosis.

Patients with sickle cell disease should be monitored for iron overload.[56,64] Obtaining a serum ferritin level is the most commonly used method of screening for iron overload, although the accuracy of this test is affected by inflammatory processes. Thus, serial serum ferritin values should be obtained when patients are not experiencing an acute crisis (i.e., steady-state values). More specific tests such as magnetic resonance imaging measure iron levels in organs such as the heart, liver, pancreas, and spleen, although owing to cost may not be routinely used.[63] The gold standard for assessing iron overload is liver iron concentration by biopsy, although this is an invasive procedure that should be performed by specialists.

Iron chelation therapy is one of the most commonly used treatments for iron overload. Another method of minimizing chronic iron burden is an exchange transfusion.[56] During this process, the patient's sickle RBCs are removed and replaced with normal RBCs. Although this process is more complex and requires experienced staff, this should be considered to minimize J.T.'s iron burden.

CASE 12-7, QUESTION 6: J.T. returns for continued assessment of iron overload. His repeat serum ferritin levels are 1,357 mcg/L and 1,500 mcg/L (3 months apart). Liver iron concentration is 7.8 mg/g dry weight. Does J.T. meet the criteria to receive iron chelation therapy? What options are available?

J.T. meets criteria for iron chelation therapy because of his steady-state serum ferritin levels being consistently more than 1,000 mcg/L and his liver iron concentration being greater than 7 mg/g dry weight.[56,64] Other considerations for a patient to receive iron chelation therapy include transfusion of approximately 100 mL/kg of PRBCs, or 20 units for a 40-kg or more patient.

There are two iron chelators currently approved for use in patients with sickle cell disease; their dosing and adverse effects are summarized in Table 12-8. These agents work by binding free iron present in circulation and tissues. The iron is then excreted in the urine and bile.

Deferoxamine (DFO) is the older of the two agents and has the most clinical experience. Both agents have been studied in patients with sickle cell disease who are as young as 2 years old. Because of its short half-life, DFO must be administered daily via continuous IV or subcutaneous infusion for 5 days. Deferasirox has a longer half-life, allowing for once-daily oral administration and enhanced patient convenience and adherence. A study of 195 patients with sickle cell disease observed similar reductions in iron levels between patients receiving DFO and patients receiving deferasirox at comparable doses.[65] Additionally, more patients in the deferasirox group reported their treatment was convenient.[63] DFO is associated with more dose-dependent oculotoxicity and audiotoxicity, although both agents may cause this.[66,67] Deferasirox has been associated with more nephrotoxicity, hepatotoxicity, and cytopenias.

The United Kingdom standards recommend either deferoxamine or deferasirox for first-line therapy, noting that deferasirox is especially useful in patients nonadherent to deferoxamine.[64] Revised US guidelines are anticipated in fall 2011 (**http://www.nhlbi.nih.gov/guidelines/scd**). Either DFO or deferasirox is appropriate for J.T. at this time. Patients receiving iron chelation therapy should also receive vitamin C supplementation, especially if they are noted to be deficient.

J.T. should also receive appropriate monitoring, consisting of serial serum ferritin levels and annual audiology and ophthalmology assessments. Some centers obtain liver biopsy every 2 years during treatment to assess efficacy.[56] Patients receiving deferasirox should have serum creatinine monitored weekly for the first month after initiation or a dose alteration, and monthly thereafter.[64] Monthly monitoring for proteinuria and assessment of liver function tests should also be initiated for patients receiving deferasirox.

Other Complications of Sickle Cell Disease

NEUROLOGIC COMPLICATIONS

Neurologic complications are age dependent. Stroke most commonly occurs in the first decade of life, whereas intracerebral

TABLE 12-8
FDA-Approved Iron Chelation Therapies

Medication	Dose	Frequency	Route	Common/Serious Adverse Effects	Notes
Deferoxamine (DFO, Desferal)	25–50 mg/kg/d, titrate to effect (Maximal dose 40 mg/kg for children)	Daily Monday–Friday	Subcutaneously for 8–12 hours	*Common:* headache, upper respiratory tract infection, abdominal pain, nausea, vomiting, pyrexia, pain, arthralgia, cough, nasopharyngitis, constipation, chest pain, injection site reactions, muscle spasms, viral infection *Serious:* audiotoxicity, hepatotoxicity, nephrotoxicity, ocular toxicity, hypotension, anaphylaxis, respiratory distress syndrome, growth retardation	Requires a syringe pump or balloon infuser Rotate sites to prevent scarring
Deferasirox (Exjade)	20 mg/kg/d, titrate to effect	Once daily	Oral drink	*Common:* headache, abdominal pain, nausea, pyrexia, vomiting, diarrhea, back pain, upper respiratory tract infection, arthralgia, pain, cough, nasopharyngitis, rash, constipation, chest pain *Serious:* nephrotoxicity, cytopenias, hepatic failure, GI hemorrhage, anaphylaxis, ocular disturbances	Should be dissolved in juice for administration

FDA, Food and Drug Administration; GI, gastrointestinal.

hemorrhage is a complication associated with adulthood. Primary prevention of stroke with RBC transfusions, targeted to maintain HbS level less than 30%, reduce the incidence of stroke in high-risk patients by 92%.[68] If a stroke occurs, approximately 50% of patients experience recurrent strokes within 3 years unless they are treated by chronic RBC transfusion therapy.[46] Preliminary evidence suggests that transitioning from RBC transfusions to chronic hydroxyurea might be an alternative option to prevent secondary stroke, and is being further investigated.[69,70]

RENAL AND GENITAL COMPLICATIONS

Renal and genital complications are common in sickle cell disease because the environment (hypoxic, acidotic, and hypertonic) predisposes the renal medulla or corpus cavernosum to infarction. As a result, patients might experience reduced potassium excretion, hyperuricemia, hematuria, hyposthenuria, and renal failure. Patients with renal disease generally have inappropriately low levels of EPO as well. Men experiencing occlusion of the corpus cavernosum can experience acute or chronic priapism. Conservative management includes IV fluid administration and pain control. Refractory cases may require surgery.[45,47]

MICROINFARCTIONS

Microinfarctions often produce ophthalmic, hepatic, orthopedic, and obstetric/gynecologic complications as well. Other references address these topics in more detail.[56,64]

ANEMIA OF CHRONIC DISEASE

Anemia of chronic disease (ACD) refers to a mild to moderate anemia that results from decreased RBC production that is associated with a number of disorders (e.g., autoimmune disorders, chronic infections, chronic renal failure, and neoplastic disease).[71] Because of the common occurrence of such conditions, ACD is encountered frequently and has been estimated to be the second most common anemia after iron deficiency. Most often, ACD is a normochromic, normocytic anemia, although RBCs may be hypochromic and microcytic in some patients. The availability of iron is altered and is not reliably reflected in iron indices. Additionally, the EPO response may be inappropriate for the degree of anemia because of a primary deficiency in EPO production.

Although the pathogenesis of ACD is not well understood, inflammatory cytokines are thought to play a major role in its development through multiple mechanisms.[72] Interferon-α, interferon-β, interferon-γ, tumor necrosis factor-α, and IL-1 inhibit RBC precursors, BFUe and CFUe, and decrease the number of EPO receptors, further contributing to the development of ACD. Interleukin-6 (IL-6) upregulates hepcidin, an acute-phase reactant produced in hepatocytes. Hepcidin alters iron hemostasis by decreasing duodenal iron absorption and inhibiting the release of iron stores, and high concentrations lead to hypoferremia and blunted erythrocyte production.[73]

Management of mild to moderate ACD usually focuses on the underlying disease process. ACD is not usually progressive or life threatening, although it generally affects a patient's quality of life. Patients may require blood transfusions for symptomatic anemia. Unless a concurrent deficiency of vitamin B_{12}, folate, or iron exists, administration of vitamin supplements is not of value. Recombinant human EPO (rhEPO), epoetin alfa, has been used successfully to treat ACD in patients with rheumatoid arthritis, acquired immunodeficiency syndrome (AIDS), some neoplastic diseases, and chronic kidney disease; however, medication costs can be significant and may outweigh benefits from the treatment of modest anemia.[71]

Human Recombinant Erythropoietin Therapy

Human recombinant erythropoietin therapy is indicated for use in anemia associated with end-stage renal disease, drug-induced anemia (chemotherapy and zidovudine therapy), and AIDS, and with autologous blood transfusions for elective surgery. Previously, blood transfusions temporarily deterred symptomatic ACD; however, transfusion therapy is associated with risks such as hepatitis, viral infections, iron overload, treatment-related acute lung injury, and immunogenic reactions. Response to rhEPO is dependent on both dose and the underlying cause of anemia. Variables that may predict patient response are both patient-specific and disease-specific and are not always reliable. For example, response to rhEPO in chronic renal failure is dose-related and can vary among patients with chronic renal failure, such that repeated dose modifications may be required during therapy until a desirable Hgb response is achieved.[74,75] Approximately 75% of patients with cancer respond to rhEPO.[76] Response in this population also is dose-related, and therapeutic doses are often higher in those patients than in those with renal failure. Lower rhEPO response rates are seen in patients who have received intensive chemotherapy or radiotherapy. In evaluating response to rhEPO, parameters such as increased serum ferritin, decreased transferrin saturation, increased corrected reticulocyte count, decreased transfusion requirements, and increased Hgb and Hct values have been used. Lack of response to rhEPO therapy in all patient populations is most commonly associated with iron deficiency. The ability of rhEPO to stimulate the production of erythrocytes normal in both size and Hgb concentration is highly dependent on the availability of functional iron.[77]

Darbepoetin alfa is an erythropoiesis-stimulating protein that differs from rhEPO by the addition of two carbohydrate chains. The significance of the additional carbohydrate chains is an increased sialic acid content that results in decreased clearance, and a serum half-life for darbepoetin alfa that is three times longer than that of rhEPO. These kinetic differences allow darbepoetin alfa to be administered less frequently than rhEPO. Similar to rhEPO, Hgb response to darbepoetin alfa is dose related. Most patients with chronic kidney disease[78,79] and cancer achieve the desired Hgb response with darbepoetin alfa treatment.[80] Table 12-9 illustrates current therapeutic uses of rhEPO and darbepoetin alfa.

Based on studies that have identified safety concerns with the use of epoetin alfa and darbepoetin alfa, the FDA has mandated a Risk Evaluation and Mitigation Strategy (REMS) program for the use of these agents. All patients treated with either of these medications for any indication must receive a medication guide and be educated on the risks and benefits of their use. Additionally, the APPRISE (Assisting Providers and Cancer Patients with Risk Information for the Safe Use of ESAs [erythropoiesis-stimulating agents]) program was instituted for those patients receiving these medications for an oncology indication.[81]

Renal Insufficiency-Related Anemia

CASE 12-8

QUESTION 1: K.S., a 35-year-old man with a 25-year history of diabetes mellitus, is diagnosed with renal failure and placed on hemodialysis three times weekly. One year later, K.S. is noted to have become increasingly transfusion-dependent for correction of his anemia. Significant laboratory values include the following:

Hgb, 7 g/dL
Hct, 26%
Ferritin, 360 ng/mL
Serum iron, 98 mcg/dL

In addition, K.S. complains of constant fatigue, poor appetite, and a low energy level. What treatments are available to correct K.S.'s anemia?

Unlike the anemia associated with most chronic diseases, the hematocrit of patients with chronic renal failure often is markedly reduced. The cause of the anemia is complex but involves reduced EPO production and a shortened RBC life span. Repeated transfusions are a possible treatment option but can cause complications, such as iron overload, infections, reactions to leukocyte antigens, or the development of cytotoxic antibodies.[82]

Because EPO is secreted in the kidney in response to anoxia and is responsible for normal differentiation of RBCs from other stem cells, rhEPO is used to treat anemia in patients with renal failure who are undergoing hemodialysis, and K.S. is a candidate for this therapy. A dose-dependent rise in Hct is observed in patients with end-stage renal disease at a usual dosage range of epoetin alfa 50 to 100 units/kg three times weekly or darbepoetin alfa 0.45 mcg/kg. Patients such as K.S. who have renal insufficiency appear to be predisposed to rhEPO-induced hypertension, and its use is contraindicated in patients with uncontrolled hypertension. Seizures also have been reported in approximately 5% of patients with end-stage renal disease. Other adverse events associated with use include thrombosis, cardiovascular events, and pure RBC aplasia (also see Chapter 31, Chronic Kidney Diseases). Targeting higher concentrations of Hgb (>13 g/dL) is associated with increased mortality and adverse effects, and the FDA-mandated black-box warning for these drugs states to individualize treatment to maintain an Hgb of 10 to 12 g/dL.[83–86] This target Hgb differs from the current National Kidney Foundation Kidney Disease Outcomes Quality Initiative guidelines.[87]

TABLE 12-9
Therapeutic Uses and Regimens for Recombinant Human Erythropoietin (rhEPO)[a]

	Epoetin Alfa		Darbepoetin Alfa		Time to Respond (weeks)	Overall Response Rate (%)
Anemia Pathogenesis	**Dose (units/kg)**	**Frequency**	**Dose (mcg/kg)**	**Frequency**		
HIV zidovudine therapy[b]	100	3×/wk			8–12	17–35
Chemotherapy-induced malignancy	150 or 40,000 units (total dose)	3×/wk or once a week, respectively	2.25 or 500 mcg (total dose)	Once a week or once every 3 weeks, respectively	2–8	32–61[c] 48–83[d]
Renal insufficiency	50–100	3×/wk	0.45	Once a week	2–8	90–97

[a]Adult dosing.
[b]Patients with AIDS with endogenous erythropoietin levels ≤500 units/L; zidovudine dose ≤4,200 mg/wk.
[c]Epoetin alfa.
[d]Darbepoetin alfa.

Malignancy-Related Anemia

CASE 12-9

QUESTION 1: T.K. is a 45 year-old woman who was diagnosed 2 months ago with non-Hodgkin lymphoma. She is being seen for her third of six cycles of chemotherapy. She reports shortness of breath and fatigue when she walks up stairs. The only medication T.K. takes is ibuprofen 200 mg as needed (PRN) for occasional headaches. Her CBC indicates the following:

Hgb, 9.7 g/dL
Hct, 29%
MCV, 90 fL
MCHC, 300 g/L
Serum erythropoietin, 29 U/L

The peripheral smear shows normochromic and normocytic RBCs. What is the most likely cause of T.K.'s anemia? What is the appropriate treatment?

T.K. appears to have malignancy-related anemia, which is often characterized as ACD or is chemotherapy-induced. This anemia is generally normocytic and normochromic and develops when a disease has persisted for more than 1 to 2 months. Generally, the anemia is mild or moderate, with a limited number of distinguishing characteristics. As with T.K., the anemia is often asymptomatic or mildly symptomatic (weakness, decreased exercise tolerance). Factors that can influence the incidence of chronic anemia in patients with cancer are the type of malignancy and the stage and duration of disease; the type, schedule, and intensity of treatment; and history of prior myelosuppressive chemotherapy or radiation. Although the prevalence of malignancy-related anemia is difficult to quantify, about 50% to 60% of patients with non-Hodgkin lymphoma, multiple myeloma, or treatment for ovarian and lung cancer experience anemia that requires blood transfusions. The myelosuppressive and anemia-inducing effects of platinum agents (e.g., cisplatin, carboplatin) are well known.[88] These and other myelosuppressive agents are widely used in the treatment of many malignancies, and patients receiving therapy should be appropriately monitored for the development of anemia. ACD does not respond to treatment with iron, vitamin B_{12}, or folic acid unless there is an associated vitamin deficiency. Therapy is directed at treatment of the underlying disease, if possible. Large, randomized, multicenter trials have failed to show a clinical benefit to using ESAs in anemia that is not chemotherapy-induced. Furthermore, mortality was either increased or trended in that direction in clinical trials of anemic patients with head and neck, breast, non–small cell lung, lymphoid, and cervical cancers receiving ESAs.[82] Because of these findings, a black-box warning was added to epoetin alfa and darbepoetin alfa product information to advise about increases in serious adverse events or disease progression for these patient populations. ESAs are recommended for anemic patients with cancer who are receiving myelosuppressive chemotherapy and the intent of treatment is not curative. Treatment cannot start until the Hgb is less than 10 g/dL, the lowest dose needed to avoid RBC transfusion should be given, and use should be discontinued at the end of chemotherapy treatment.[84,85]

In T.K.'s case, the clinician may choose from a number of anemia management options. For example, the current course of chemotherapy can be delayed to allow for hematologic recovery and resolution of anemia symptoms. Alternatively, an RBC transfusion can be given to relieve her symptoms and allow her to better tolerate chemotherapy. In addition, erythropoietic therapy with epoetin alfa or darbepoetin alfa also should be considered. Treatment with epoetin alfa or darbepoetin alfa increases Hct and Hgb, decreases the need for blood transfusions, and may improve quality of life. In clinical studies, response rates are 70% to 80%. Adverse events associated with therapy include cardiovascular events, thrombosis, increased mortality, and tumor progression, and to a lesser degree, hypertension, seizures, and pure RBC aplasia.[82,89–91]

If treatment with epoetin alfa is desired for T.K., therapy can be administered at an initial dose of 150 units/kg subcutaneously three times a week.[85] Alternative dosing regimens, such as 10,000 units three times a week or 40,000 units once a week, have proved to be safe and effective in terms of hematopoietic, quality of life, and transfusion effects.[89,92] Response can be assessed initially by monitoring the reticulocyte count, which should peak by day 10 of treatment. A positive rhEPO response also can be predicted by observation of an increased serum ferritin and decreased transferrin saturation. Epoetin alfa usually is administered for a minimum of 4 weeks, although an increase in Hgb and Hct values should be noted after 2 to 4 weeks. If no hematopoietic response (increase in Hgb by 1 to 2 g/dL) is noted by the fourth week, an additional 4 weeks of therapy should be considered at an increased dose. Common dose escalation schedules include 300 units/kg three times a week if initially treated with 150 units/kg three times a week or 60,000 units once a week if initially on 40,000 units once a week. A 25% dose reduction is made if there is a greater than 1 g/dL rise in the Hgb within 2 weeks. If no Hgb response is noted after 8 weeks of treatment or transfusions are still required, the drug should be discontinued.[85] The most common cause of nonresponse to erythropoietic therapy is iron deficiency. Iron studies should be evaluated before and during therapy with supplementation given if needed.

Darbepoetin alfa is also a treatment option for T.K. Initial dosing of darbepoetin alfa is 2.25 mcg/kg subcutaneously once a week.[80] Also, clinical studies of darbepoetin alfa 200 mcg administered every 2 weeks and 300 mcg or 500 mcg administered every 3 weeks have reported beneficial hematopoietic effects and decreased transfusion requirements.[89,90,93] A 40% dose reduction is made if there is a more than 1 g/dL rise in the Hgb within 2 weeks. If no Hgb response is noted after 6 weeks of treatment, the dose may be increased to 4.5 mcg/kg. Therapy initiation and response should be monitored in the same manner as epoetin alfa, with drug discontinuation after 8 weeks of therapy for nonresponders.[84]

AIDS-Related Anemia

CASE 12-10

QUESTION 1: J.M., a 37-year-old man, is currently calling his primary physician to report acute worsening of shortness of breath and pounding in his chest. J.M. has a known history of AIDS and has had recent episodes of *Pneumocystis carinii* pneumonia (PCP) and cytomegalovirus (CMV) esophagitis. J.M. also has experienced frequent diarrhea. Trimethoprim-sulfamethoxazole was given IV for treatment of PCP; however, J.M. experienced a fever while on maintenance therapy. J.M. is currently taking the following medications: dapsone 100 mg/day orally (PO) for PCP prophylaxis, ganciclovir 325 mg IV Monday through Friday for CMV prophylaxis, indinavir 800 mg PO every 8 hours, lamivudine 150 mg PO BID, zidovudine 300 mg PO BID, fluconazole 100 mg/day PO PRN for thrush, and loperamide liquid 5 mL PRN for diarrhea.

The only remarkable findings on physical examination include a respiratory rate of 24 breaths/minute and a heart

rate of 120 beats/minute. A chest examination reveals that J.M. is tachypneic and has bilateral dry rales. The Hickman catheter in the left subclavian vein appears dry and clean. Further workup of J.M.'s illness includes an unremarkable chest radiograph and negative cultures of the blood and sputum. The CBC includes normal WBC and platelet counts. Abnormal values include the RBC count of 3,300/μL, Hgb of 9.1 mg/dL, Hct of 28%, and a CD4 of 387 cells/mm^3 (normal, 440 to 1,600 cells/mm^3). The morphology of the RBC was moderately anisocytic, normochromic, and normocytic. What factors can contribute to J.M.'s anemia?

Anemia is a common finding in patients with AIDS and correlates with the severity of the clinical syndrome. In this patient population, anemia is a risk factor for early death.[94] Common symptoms such as fatigue, breathlessness, and difficulties in mental concentration may contribute to this patient population's decreased quality of life.[95] Anemia is multifactorial and is the result of three primary mechanisms: decreased RBC production, increased RBC destruction, and ineffective RBC production.[96] Anemia occurs more often in patients with infections (*Mycobacterium avium intracellulare, Cryptococcus neoformans,* and *Histoplasma capsulatum*), viruses (CMV, herpes simplex viruses type 1 and 2, and HPV B19), myelosuppressive drugs such as human immunodeficiency virus (HIV) drugs (e.g., zidovudine, zalcitabine, didanosine, lamivudine), other drugs often used to treat AIDS-associated illnesses (e.g., bone marrow suppressive chemotherapy, ganciclovir, trimethoprim-sulfamethoxazole, dapsone), or neoplasms.[97] Enhanced production of cytokines, such as tumor necrosis factor-α, also may be correlated with hematologic abnormalities. Kaposi's sarcoma and lymphoma, which impair normal bone marrow function, also can result in anemia in this population.

AIDS patients may be deficient in iron, vitamin B_{12} and folate. Vitamin B_{12} deficiency is a contributing cause to anemia in up to a third of these patients[98] and is correlated with progression to AIDS.[99] Vitamin B_{12} malabsorption can result from HIV-infected mononuclear cells within the ileum and altered gastric mucosal functioning caused by infection.[96] Alterations in the utilization of vitamin B_{12} and folate[98] can place a patient at risk for hematologic toxicity of drugs such as zidovudine and trimethoprim.

As illustrated by J.M., HIV-associated anemia has a characteristic RBC morphology, which is normochromic and normocytic. Mild anisocytosis and poikilocytosis also may be observed. Zidovudine-associated anemia is typically macrocytic.[100]

Erythropoiesis is often defective in patients with AIDS, as reflected by an inappropriately low reticulocyte count and an increased or blunted erythropoietic response for the degree of anemia. Treatment with rhEPO therapy increases the quality of life and Hgb in HIV-infected adult patients regardless of zidovudine use, CD4$^+$ count, or viral load.[94,96]

J.M. has many risk factors for ACD, including AIDS and its accompanying predisposition to malignancy and infection. He is also taking many medications (ganciclovir, zidovudine, and dapsone) that can induce anemia.

CASE 12-10, QUESTION 2: J.M.'s physician determines that J.M.'s endogenous EPO level is 421 units/L (normal, 4 to 26 units/L). Is J.M. a candidate for rhEPO? How can the best response to rhEPO be predicted? What would an appropriate starting dosing regimen be?

Patients taking zidovudine ($\leq$4,200 mg/week) who have baseline EPO levels less than 500 units/L experience a significantly higher rate of increase in Hct compared with patients with high baseline EPO levels.[101] A patient who has macrocytic anemia with moderate EPO response (<500 units/L) may require moderate transfusion support in response to zidovudine. A patient who has normocytic anemia with a high EPO response (>500 units/L) may have substantial transfusion requirements.[102] A significant reduction in transfusion requirements has been observed in those patients with macrocytic anemia with moderate EPO response who are given rhEPO 40,000 units subcutaneously once weekly. Therefore, rhEPO may be considered appropriate treatment for patients whose baseline EPO level is less than 500 units/L.

rhEPO therapy may be initiated at 100 units/kg three times weekly. RBC indices should be monitored weekly, and if response is noted, the dose may be decreased to the lowest dose necessary to prevent symptoms or RBC transfusion, and Hgb should not exceed 12 g/dL.[85] If J.M. has not responded after 8 weeks of therapy, the dose should be increased by 50 to 100 units/kg three times weekly with another dose escalation in 4 to 8 weeks to 300 units/kg three times weekly if there is still not response. If J.M. does not respond to 300 units/kg, it is unlikely that he will benefit from further rhEPO therapy.[85] Alternative once-weekly dosing with epoetin alfa has been evaluated at starting doses of 40,000 units.[103] The use of darbepoetin alfa has been assessed in HIV patients receiving hemodialysis and is as safe and effective as epoetin alfa for treating anemia.[104]

ACKNOWLEDGMENT

We gratefully acknowledge Kenneth Utz for his contributions to this chapter.

KEY REFERENCES AND WEBSITES

A full list of references for this chapter can be found at http://thepoint.lww.com/AT10e. Below are the key references and website for this chapter, with the corresponding reference number in this chapter found in parentheses after the reference.

Key References

Barbera L, Thomas G. Erythropoiesis stimulating agents, thrombosis and cancer. *Radiother Oncol.* 2010;95:269. (91)

Booth C et al. Infection in sickle cell disease: a review. *Int J Infect Dis.* 2010;14:e2. (50)

Dali-Youcef N, Andrès E. An update on cobalamin deficiency in adults. *QJM.* 2009;102:17. (29)

Fishbane S. The role of erythropoiesis-stimulating agents in the treatment of anemia. *Am J Manag Care.* 2010;16(Suppl):S67. (82)

Hurrell R, Egli I. Iron bioavailability and dietary reference values. *Am J Clin Nutr.* 2010;91:1461S. (17)

KDOQI. KDOQI Clinical Practice Guideline and Clinical Practice Recommendations for anemia in chronic kidney disease: 2007 update of hemoglobin target. *Am J Kidney Dis.* 2007;50:471. (87)

National Institutes of Health. National Heart, Lung, and Blood Institute Division of Blood Diseases and Resources. *The Management of Sickle Cell Disease.* Bethesda, MD: National Institutes of Health National Heart, Lung, and Blood Institute. NIH publication 02-2117; 2002. (56)

Redding-Lallinger R, Knoll C. Sickle cell disease—pathophysiology and treatment. *Curr Probl Pediatr Adolesc Health Care.* 2006;36:346. (47)

Snow CF. Laboratory diagnosis of vitamin B_{12} and folate deficiency: a guide for the primary care physician. *Arch Intern Med.* 1999;159:1289. (43)

Volberding PA et al. Anemia in HIV infection: clinical impact and evidence-based management strategies. *Clin Infect Dis.* 2004;38:1454. (96)

Zhu A et al. Evaluation and treatment of iron deficiency anemia: a gastroenterological perspective. *Dig Dis Sci.* 2010;55: 548. (4)

Key Websites

ESA Apprise Oncology Program. https://www.esa-apprise.com/ESAAppriseUI/ESAAppriseUI/default.jsp. Accessed November 30, 2010. (81)

Standards for the clinical care of adults with sickle cell disease in the UK. Sickle Cell Society. 2008. http://www.sicklecellsociety.org/pdf/carebook.pdf. Accessed November 22, 2010. (64)

SECTION EDITORS: JOSEPH J. SASEEN AND JEAN M. NAPPI

13 Dyslipidemias, Atherosclerosis, and Coronary Heart Disease

Matthew K. Ito

CORE PRINCIPLES

		CHAPTER CASES
1	The risk of atherosclerosis is directly related to increasing levels of serum cholesterol. Cholesterol, specifically lipoproteins, plays a central role in the pathogenesis of atherosclerosis. Thus, low-density lipoprotein cholesterol (LDL-C) is the primary target for intervention. The National Cholesterol Education Program Adult Treatment Panel III guidelines set the "optimal" level for LDL-C for all adults as less than 100 mg/dL.	**Case 13-1 (Question 1), Table 13-6**
2	Every new patient with dyslipidemia should be evaluated for four things in the following order: (a) secondary causes of the high cholesterol level, (b) familial disorders, (c) presence of coronary heart disease (CHD) and CHD equivalents, and (d) CHD risk factors.	**Case 13-1 (Question 2), Tables 13-2, 13-3, 13-6, 13-7**
3	LDL-C goals and the thresholds for instituting therapeutic lifestyle changes (TLC) and pharmacotherapy are guided by the presence of clinical atherosclerosis, the number of risk factors for CHD, and calculation of the 10-year risk of CHD.	**Case 13-1 (Questions 4, 5), Case 13-2 (Question 1), Case 13-3 (Question 1), Figure 13-7, Tables 13-4, 13-8, 13-10**
4	An adequate trial of TLC should be used in all patients, but pharmacotherapy should be instituted concurrently in high-risk patients or those with familial hypercholesterolemia.	**Case 13-1 (Question 6), Case 13-3 (Question 1), Tables 13-10, 13-11**
5	In most cases, statins are the medications of choice to treat high LDL-C because of their ability to substantially reduce LDL-C, ability to reduce morbidity and mortality from atherosclerotic disease, convenient once-daily dosing, and low risk of side effects.	**Case 13-2 (Question 1), Case 13-3 (Questions 1, 2), Tables 13-3, 13-12**
6	If statins or other drugs used to treat hyperlipidemia are prescribed, doses that reduce LDL-C by at least 30% to 40% should be recommended. In patients with CHD or acute coronary syndrome who have an optional LDL-C goal of less than 70 mg/dL, if it is not possible to attain LDL-C less than 70 mg/dL owing to a high baseline LDL-C, it is recommended to achieve an LDL-C reduction of at least 50%.	**Case 13-2 (Question 4), Case 13-1 (Question 9)**
7	Patients with a mixed dyslipidemia and the metabolic syndrome have an additional lipid parameter that needs to be assessed, namely non–high-density lipoprotein cholesterol (non–HDL-C, or total cholesterol minus high-density lipoprotein cholesterol [HDL-C]). The target for non–HDL-C is less than the patient's LDL-C target plus 30 mg/dL.	**Case 13-4 (Question 3), Tables 13-17, 13-18**
8	Combination drug therapy is often needed in patients with severe lipid abnormalities, higher-risk individuals with lower LDL-C goals, or patients with multiple lipid abnormalities such as those with the metabolic syndrome who have a secondary target of non–HDL-C.	**Case 13-3 (Questions 2–4), Case 13-4 (Questions 8–12), Table 13-12**

continued

		CHAPTER CASES
9	Patients with fasting triglycerides (TGs) greater than 500 mg/dL are at increased risk of acute pancreatitis. The primary goal in these individuals is to lower their TG levels with diet, exercise, weight reduction, and TG-lowering drugs such as nicotinic acid, fibrates, and omega-3 fatty acids.	**Case 13-4 (Questions 2, 3, 6, 8, 9), Case 13-6 (Question 1), Table 13-16**
10	To date, there is limited evidence demonstrating that adding a second or third drug to background statin therapy produces incremental benefit on the risk of CHD. Several clinical trials are ongoing to answer this question.	**Case 13-2 (Questions 2, 6), Case 13-4 (Questions 11, 12)**
11	Low HDL-C is associated with an increased risk of CHD. However, specific evidence from clinical trials that raising HDL-C reduces CHD is lacking. Patients with low HDL-C should be encouraged to exercise and maintain a healthy weight. If drug therapy is instituted for an elevated LDL-C, drugs that also significantly raise HDL-C can be considered.	**Case 13-1 (Question 8), Case 13-2 (Question 2), Case 13-4 (Question 8), Case 13-5 (Question 1), Table 13-19**

Dyslipidemias (one or more abnormalities of blood lipids) produce atherosclerosis, which in turn produces coronary heart disease (CHD) and coronary artery disease (CAD). Successful management of dyslipidemias alters the natural course of atherosclerosis and reduces CHD as well as other forms of atherosclerosis. This is the simple but profound notion behind the modern approach to reducing the incidence of the nation's number-one killer. The challenge for the clinician is to know how to assess the patient's CHD risk, to understand lipid-modulating therapies, to match the intensity of treatment with the patient's risk, and to implement treatments that meet and maintain treatment goals. The principal focus of this chapter is on providing the information required to meet this challenge.

Lipid Metabolism and Drug Effects

Dealing with this challenge begins with acquiring an understanding of how lipids are formed, transported, and used; how these processes can go awry; and how therapies alter these aberrant processes. At the center of these processes are cholesterol, triglycerides (TGs), and phospholipids. Of these three, cholesterol plays the central role in the pathogenesis of atherosclerosis. Cholesterol is a naturally occurring sterol that is essential for life. It is the precursor molecule for the formation of bile acids (which are required for absorption of nutrients), the synthesis of steroid hormones (which provide important modulating effects in the body), and the formation of cell membranes. TGs are an important source of stored energy in adipose tissue. TGs are synthesized from three molecules of fatty acids esterified to glycerol. Phospholipids are a class of lipids formed from fatty acids, a negatively charged phosphate group, nitrogen-containing alcohol, and a glycerol backbone. Phospholipids are essential for cellular function and the transport of lipids in the circulation by forming a membrane bilayer of lipoproteins (discussed subsequently), and they participate in the oxidation of lipoproteins in the arterial wall, which will be discussed later.

IN VIVO CHOLESTEROL SYNTHESIS

Cells derive cholesterol in two ways: by intracellular synthesis or by uptake from the systemic circulation. Within each cell, cholesterol is synthesized through a series of biochemical steps, many of which are catalyzed by enzymes (Fig. 13-1). One important and early step in its synthesis is the conversion of β-hydroxyl-β-methylglutaryl coenzyme A (HMG-CoA) to mevalonic acid. The enzyme HMG-CoA reductase catalyzes this step. One of the most effective therapies developed to date for managing dyslipidemias (i.e., HMG-CoA reductase inhibitors or statins) interferes with this enzyme and thereby reduces the cellular synthesis of cholesterol. Other catalytic enzymes involved in the biosynthesis of cholesterol, including HMG-CoA synthase and squalene synthase, have been targets in the search for therapies to reduce cholesterol synthesis, but thus far have been unsuccessful.

Intracellular cholesterol is stored in an esterified form. Free cholesterol is converted to this ester form through the action of the enzyme acetyl CoA acetyl transferase (ACAT). Two forms of ACAT have been identified. ACAT1 is present in many tissues, including inflammatory cells, whereas ACAT2 is present in intestinal mucosa cells and hepatocytes. ACAT2 is required for the esterification and absorption of dietary cholesterol from the gut. In theory, inhibition of this enzyme should reduce the absorption of dietary cholesterol, the secretion of cholesterol by the liver, and even the uptake and storage of circulating cholesterol in inflammatory cells in the arterial wall. Several inhibitors of ACAT have been developed. These inhibitors do not appear to reduce atherosclerosis, however.[1]

LIPOPROTEINS

The second way cells obtain cholesterol is by extracting it from the systemic circulation. The source of this cholesterol is the liver, where it is synthesized and secreted into the systemic circulation. Because cholesterol and other fatty substances are insoluble in water, they are formed into complexes (lipoprotein particles) in the hepatocyte and gut (enterocytes) before being secreted into the aqueous medium of the blood. These lipoproteins contain an oily inner lipid core made up of cholesterol esters and TGs and an outer hydrophilic coat made up of phospholipids and unesterified cholesterol (Fig. 13-2). The outer coat also contains at least one protein (apolipoproteins), which provides the ligand for interaction with receptors on cell surfaces, acts as cofactors for various enzymes, and adds structural integrity. The presence of a central lipid core and an outer protein gives rise to the name of these particles, *lipoproteins*.

The three major lipoproteins found in the blood of fasting (10–12 hours) patients are very-low-density lipoprotein (VLDL), low-density lipoprotein (LDL), and high-density lipoprotein (HDL).[2] These particles vary in size, composition, and accompanying proteins (Table 13-1).

VERY-LOW-DENSITY LIPOPROTEINS

VLDL particles are formed in the liver (Fig. 13-2). They normally contain 15% to 20% of the total blood cholesterol concentration and most of the total blood TG concentration. The concentration

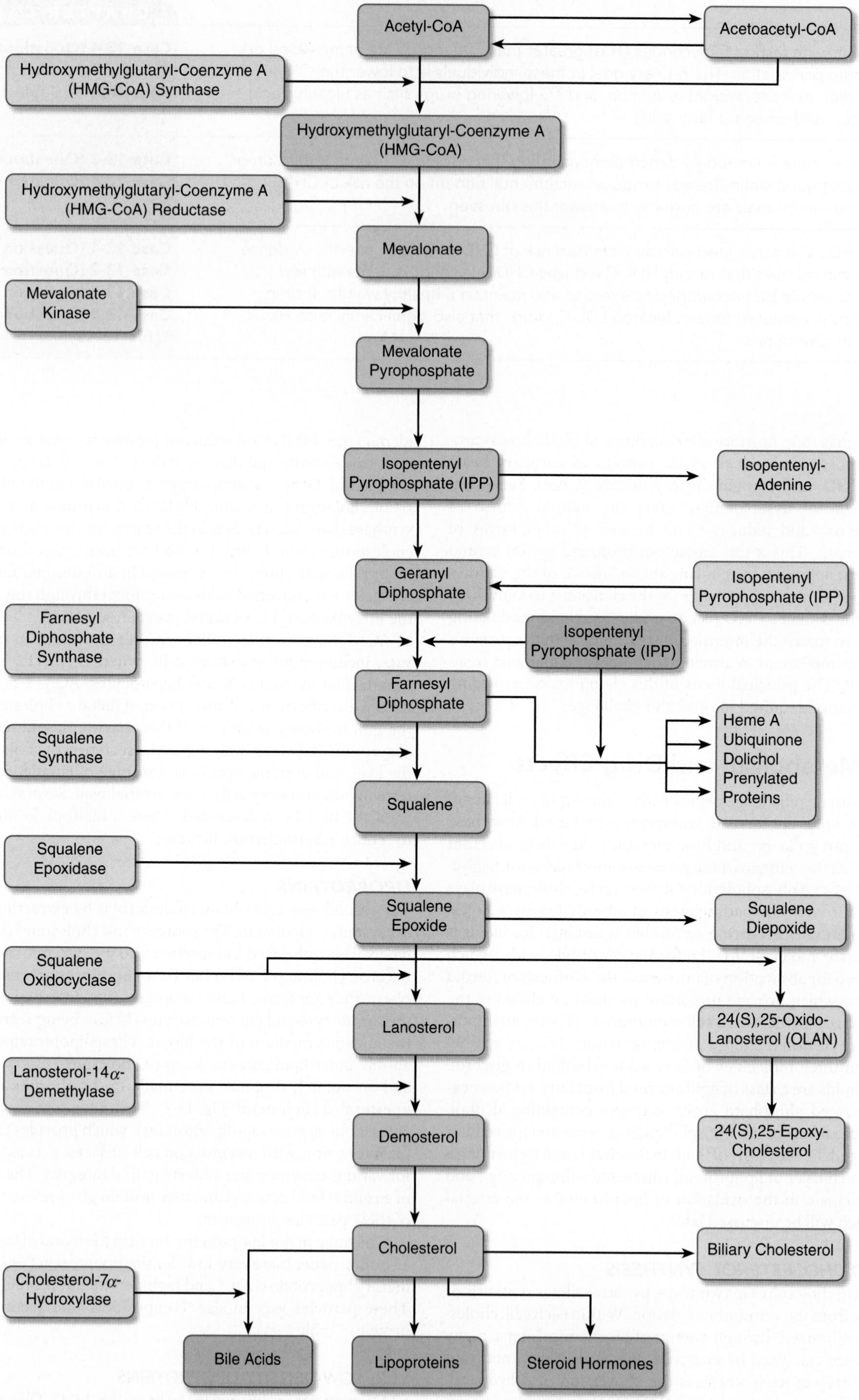

FIGURE 13-1 Biosynthetic pathway of cholesterol.

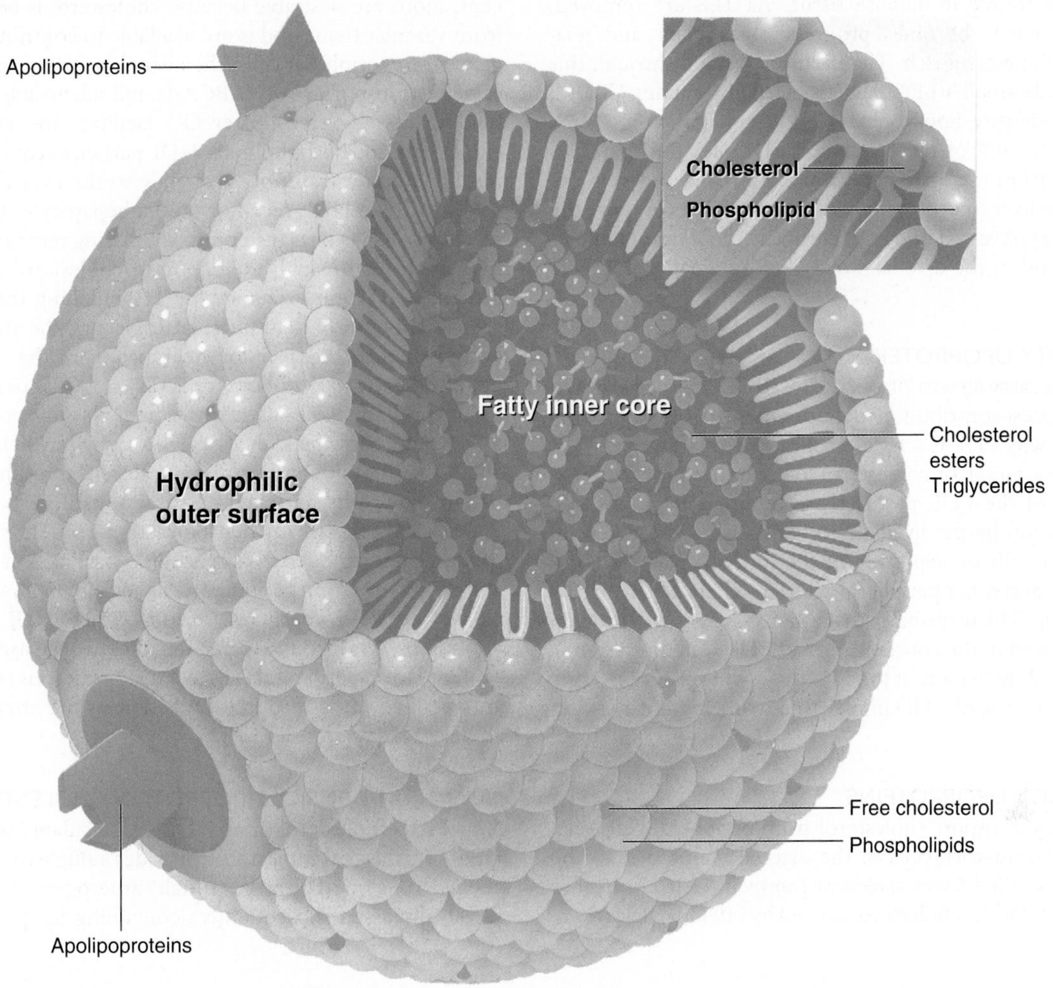

FIGURE 13-2 Basic structure of a lipoprotein. (Revised from Anatomical Chart Company, with permission.)

of cholesterol in these particles is approximately one-fifth of the total TG concentration; thus, if the total TG concentration is known, the VLDL-cholesterol (VLDL-C) level can be estimated by dividing total TGs by 5. VLDL particles are large (thus limiting their ability to migrate into the arterial wall) and appear to play only a small role in the pathogenesis of atherosclerosis.

VERY-LOW-DENSITY LIPOPROTEIN REMNANTS

As VLDL particles flow through capillaries, some of their TG content is removed through the action of the enzyme lipoprotein lipase (LPL). Drugs that enhance the activity of LPL (i.e., fibrates) increase the delipidization process and lower blood TG levels. The removed TGs are converted to fatty acids and stored

TABLE 13-1
Classification and Properties of Plasma Lipoproteins

	Chylomicron	VLDL	IDL	LDL	HDL
Density (g/mL)	<0.94	0.94–1.006	1.006–1.019	1.006–1.063	1.063–1.210
Composition (%)					
Protein	1–2	6–10	12–18	18–22	45–55
Triglyceride	85–95	50–65	20–50	4–8	2–7
Cholesterol	3–7	20–30	20–40	51–58	18–25
Phospholipid	3–6	15–20	15–25	18–24	26–32
Physiologic origin	Intestine	Intestine and liver	Produced from VLDL	Product of IDL catabolism	Liver and intestine
Physiologic function	Transport dietary CH and TG to liver	Transport endogenous TG and CH	Transport endogenous TG and CH	Transport endogenous CH to cells	Transport CH from cells to liver
Plasma appearance	Cream layer	Turbid	Clear	Clear	Clear
Electrophoretic mobility	Origin	Pre-β	Slow pre-β	β	α
Apolipoproteins	A-IV, B-48, C-I, C-II, C-III	B-100, C-I, C-III, C-III, E	B-100, C-I, C-II, C-III, E	B-100, (a)	A-I, A-II, A-IV

CH, cholesterol; HDL, high-density lipoprotein; IDL, intermediate-density lipoprotein; LDL, low-density lipoprotein; TG, triglyceride; VLDL, very-low-density lipoprotein.

as an energy source in adipose tissue. As TGs are removed, the VLDL particle becomes progressively smaller and relatively more cholesterol rich. The particles formed through this process include small VLDL particles (called remnant VLDL), intermediate-density lipoproteins (IDL), and LDL (Fig. 13-2). Approximately 50% of the remnant VLDL and IDL particles are removed from the systemic circulation by receptors on the surface of the liver (receptors called LDL or B-E receptors); the other 50% are converted into LDL particles. VLDL remnant particles are found in the arterial wall, albeit in smaller numbers than LDL.

LOW-DENSITY LIPOPROTEINS

LDL particles carry 60% to 70% of the total blood cholesterol and make the greatest contribution to the development of atherosclerosis. This is why LDL-C (cholesterol carried by LDL particles) is the primary target of cholesterol-lowering therapy. Approximately half of the LDL particles are removed from the systemic circulation by the liver; the other half may be taken up by peripheral cells or deposited in the intimal space of coronary, carotid, and other peripheral arteries, where atherosclerosis can develop. The probability that atherosclerosis will develop is directly related to the concentration of LDL-C in the systemic circulation and the length of time this level of exposure persists (the cumulative risk of CHD in men and women increases with age).

HIGH-DENSITY LIPOPROTEINS

HDL particles transport cholesterol from peripheral cells (i.e., lipid-rich inflammatory cells in the arterial wall) back to the liver, a process called *reverse cholesterol transport*.[3–5] In contrast to LDL-C, high HDL-C (cholesterol carried by HDL particles) concentrations are desirable because cholesterol is being removed from vascular tissue and is not available to contribute to atherogenesis. In peripheral cells, the adenosine triphosphate binding cassette transporter A-1 (ABCA-1) and adenosine triphosphate binding cassette transporter G-1 facilitate the efflux of both cholesterol and phospholipids. HDL particles acquire this cholesterol and either transport it directly to the liver through interaction with an HDL receptor on the hepatocyte (the scavenger receptor, SR-B1) or transfer it to circulating remnant VLDL and LDL particles through the action of cholesterol ester transfer protein (CETP) in exchange for TGs, making the HDL particle less cholesterol rich. If the latter occurs, the cholesterol can be returned to the liver for clearance from the circulation or delivered back to peripheral cells (Fig. 13-3). Patients who have a deficiency of CETP often have a high plasma concentration of HDL-C and a low incidence of CHD. Drugs are being developed and tested that inhibit this protein. Recent trials, however, have had mixed results, and their usefulness is still in question.[6,7]

HDL particles are further subfractionated. The smaller HDL_3 particle is converted to the larger HDL_2 particle as it acquires TGs and cholesterol from peripheral cells and circulating lipoproteins. Conversely, HDL_2 particles are converted to HDL_3 particles by lipolysis of TGs through the action of hepatic lipase. Cholesterol acquired from peripheral cells by HDL particles is converted into an esterified form through the action of the enzyme lecithin-cholesterol acyl transferase (LCAT).

NON–HIGH-DENSITY LIPOPROTEIN CHOLESTEROL

Non–HDL cholesterol (non–HDL-C), calculated by subtracting HDL-C from total cholesterol, provides a single measurement of cholesterol carried by all potentially atherogenic apolipoprotein B-100 (discussed subsequently)–containing lipoproteins, which

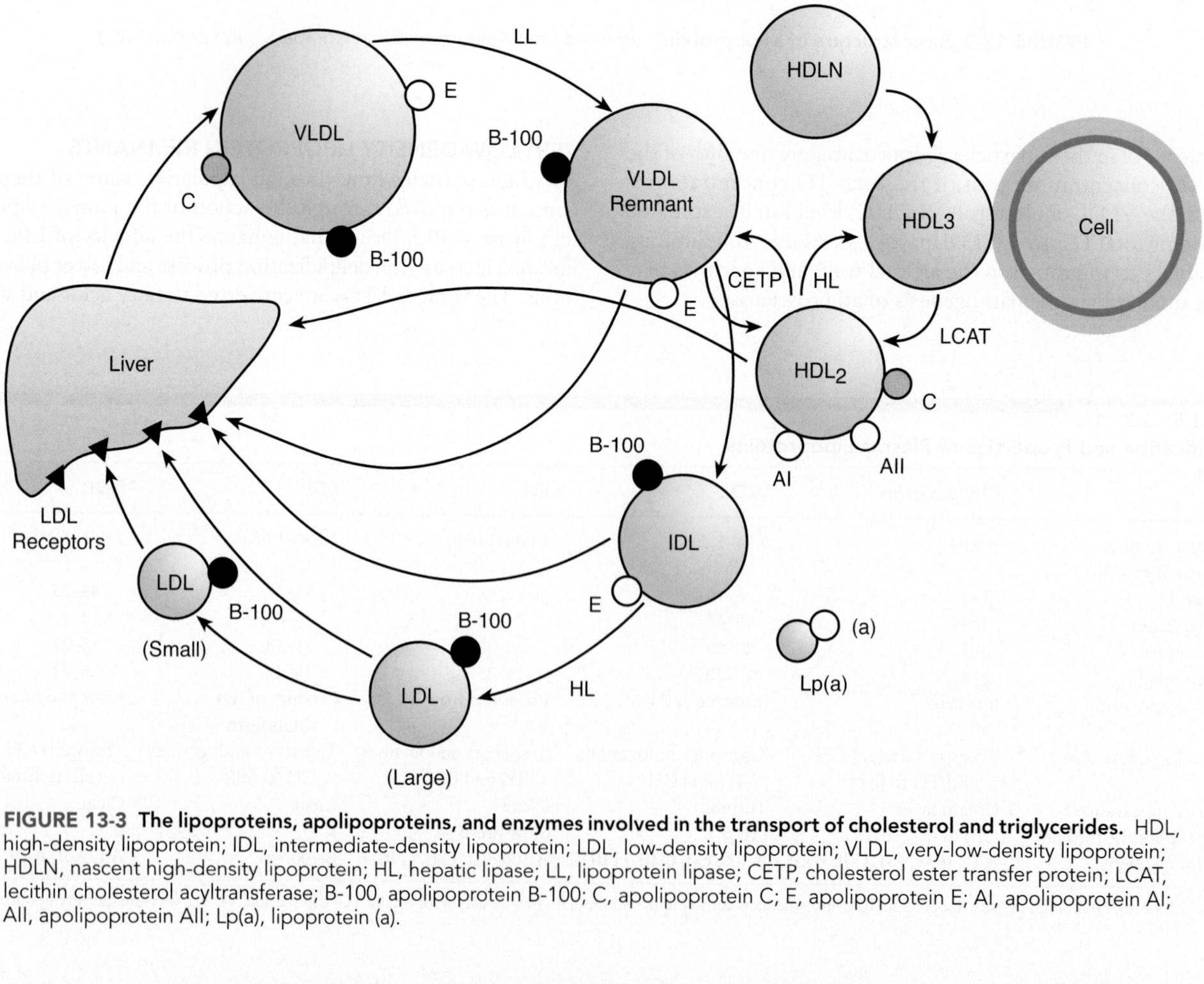

FIGURE 13-3 The lipoproteins, apolipoproteins, and enzymes involved in the transport of cholesterol and triglycerides. HDL, high-density lipoprotein; IDL, intermediate-density lipoprotein; LDL, low-density lipoprotein; VLDL, very-low-density lipoprotein; HDLN, nascent high-density lipoprotein; HL, hepatic lipase; LL, lipoprotein lipase; CETP, cholesterol ester transfer protein; LCAT, lecithin cholesterol acyltransferase; B-100, apolipoprotein B-100; C, apolipoprotein C; E, apolipoprotein E; AI, apolipoprotein AI; AII, apolipoprotein AII; Lp(a), lipoprotein (a).

include VLDL, VLDL remnants, IDL, and LDL particles. As indicated, more often an elevated LDL-C is observed, but in about 30% of cases, these other lipoproteins are concurrently elevated and the assessment of LDL-C alone may underestimate a patient's risk. In these cases, it is helpful to know how much cholesterol is being carried by all of these particles. Although apolipoprotein B-100 can be measured directly, measurement of non–HDL-C is more practical, reliable, and inexpensive and correlates well with apolipoprotein B-100.[8] Moreover, LDL-C can be incorrectly calculated in the presence of postprandial hypertriglyceridemia, whereas non–HDL-C is reliable when measured in the nonfasting state.

CHYLOMICRONS

Unlike the lipoproteins that transport cholesterol from the liver to peripheral cells and back (endogenous system), chylomicrons transport TGs and cholesterol derived from the diet or synthesized in the enterocytes from the gut to the liver (exogenous system) (Fig. 13-3, Table 13-1). Chylomicrons are large, TG-rich lipoproteins. As they pass through capillary beds on the way to the liver, some of the TG content is removed through the action of LPL in a manner similar to that described for TG removal from VLDL particles. In the rare individual who has an LPL deficiency, this removal process is faulty and TG levels in the blood become very high (e.g., 1,000 to 5,000 mg/dL).

After a fatty meal, the number of chylomicron particles (and therefore the concentration of TGs) is high. If the patient fasts for 10 to 12 hours, however, chylomicrons will have time to be removed from the blood. TG concentrations obtained during fasting reflect TG that is produced by the liver and carried in VLDL and other remnant particles (unless the patient has a rare chylomicron clearance disorder). This is why patients are asked to fast before a lipoprotein profile is obtained. A blood sample that is rich in chylomicrons (and to a lesser extent VLDL particles) appears turbid; the higher the TG level, the more turbid the sample. If the sample from a patient with hyperchylomicronemia is refrigerated, chylomicrons will float to the top and form a frothy white layer, whereas smaller VLDL stay suspended below.

APOLIPOPROTEINS

Each lipoprotein particle contains proteins on its outer surface called *apolipoproteins* (Fig. 13-3, Table 13-1). These proteins have three functions: (a) to provide structure to the lipoprotein, (b) to activate enzyme systems, and (c) to bind with cell receptors.[2] Abnormal metabolism of apolipoproteins, even in the face of seemingly normal blood cholesterol levels, can result in faulty enzyme activity or cholesterol transport and an increased risk of atherosclerosis. Because of this, clinicians often assess blood levels of apolipoproteins to evaluate dyslipidemic patients fully, especially those who have a family history of premature CHD. The five most clinically relevant apolipoproteins are A-I, A-II, B-100, C, and E.

VLDL particles contain apolipoproteins B-100, E, and C (Fig. 13-3). The B and E proteins are ligands for LDL receptors (also called *B-E receptors*) on the surface of hepatocytes and peripheral cells. Linkage allows the transfer of cholesterol from the circulating lipoprotein into the cell through absorptive endocytosis and cellular uptake of the particle. Defects in these proteins reduce their ability to bind with receptor proteins. This results in defective clearance of lipoproteins from the systemic circulation and increased levels of circulating cholesterol.

Apolipoprotein C-II is a cofactor for LPL. By activating LPL, Apolipoprotein C-II stimulates the hydrolysis of TGs from lipoprotein particles in the capillary beds. Deficiencies of apolipoprotein C-II result in faulty TG metabolism and ultimately in hypertriglyceridemia. Apolipoprotein C-III has become a marker of atherogenic dyslipidemia (described below) and thus an indicator for an increased risk of atherosclerosis. Apolipoprotein C-III downregulates LPL activity and interferes with the hepatic uptake of VLDL remnant particles. This leads to increased concentrations of small VLDL remnant particles, which are able to penetrate into the arterial wall and contribute to atherogenesis. In addition, prolonged residence of VLDL and LDL particles in the systemic circulation results in the formation of small, highly atherogenic LDL particles (see the Atherogenic Dyslipidemia section later in this chapter).[9]

Remnant VLDL particles retain apolipoproteins B-100 and E during the delipidization process; LDL particles contain only apolipoprotein B-100 (Fig. 13-3). Each VLDL, IDL, and LDL particle contains one apolipoprotein B-100. Thus, the blood concentration of apolipoprotein B-100 is an indication of the total number of VLDL, VLDL remnant, IDL, and LDL particles in the circulation. An increased number of lipoprotein particles (i.e., an increased apolipoprotein B-100 concentration) is a strong predictor of CHD risk. The ratio of non–HDL-C to apolipoprotein B-100 gives an estimate of the cholesterol contained in these atherogenic particles. Some patients have high levels of apolipoprotein B-100 (suggesting an increased number of atherogenic particles in the circulation), even though their cholesterol level is in the desirable range. These patients have an increased risk of atherosclerosis. An apolipoprotein B-100 to LDL-C ratio greater than 1 is also an indicator of the presence of small, dense LDL particles, which convey a higher CHD risk than larger LDL particles. Apolipoprotein B-100 is being considered as a recommended treatment target for inclusion in the next cholesterol guidelines.

HDL particles contain apolipoproteins A-I, A-II, and C. Apolipoprotein A-I activates LCAT, which catalyzes the esterification of free cholesterol in HDL particles. Levels of apolipoprotein A-I have a stronger inverse correlation with CHD risk than apolipoprotein A-II levels. HDL particles that contain only A-I apolipoproteins (LpA-I) are associated with a lower CHD risk than are HDL particles containing both A-I and A-II (LpA-I, A-II).[10]

LOW-DENSITY LIPOPROTEIN RECEPTOR

The uptake of cholesterol into peripheral and hepatic cells is accomplished by the binding of apolipoproteins B-100 and E on circulating lipoproteins to cell-surface LDL receptors. The synthesis of LDL receptors is stimulated by a low intracellular cholesterol concentration.[10] Conversely, LDL receptors can be degraded by another protein identified as proprotein convertase subtilisin/kexin type 9 (PCSK9), which is thought to influence the number of LDL receptor molecules expressed on the cell surface.[11] Within the cell, the receptor protein travels from the mitochondria (where it is synthesized) to the cell surface (where it migrates to an area called the *coated pits*). Once in this position, it is capable of binding with lipoproteins that contain apolipoprotein E or B-100, including VLDL, remnant VLDL, IDL, and LDL. Because remnant VLDL and IDL particles contain both B-100 and E proteins, they may have a higher affinity for LDL receptors than do LDL particles, which contain only the B protein. Furthermore, drugs that increase the synthesis of LDL receptors (e.g., statins) can increase the clearance of both VLDL remnant particles and LDL particles from the circulation. This would account for their ability to reduce serum TG levels as well as cholesterol levels. After these lipoproteins are bound, the lipoproteins undergo endocytosis and are taken up by lysosomes, where they are broken into elemental substances for use by the cell. The cholesterol is transferred into the intracellular cholesterol pool. The receptor protein may be returned to the cell surface, where it can bind with another circulating apolipoprotein

TABLE 13-2
Characteristics of Common Lipid Disorders

Disorder	Metabolic Defect	Lipid Effect	Main Lipid Parameter	Diagnostic Features
Polygenic hypercholesterolemia	↓LDL clearance	↑LDL-C	LDL-C: 130–250 mg/dL	None distinctive
Atherogenic dyslipidemia	↑VLDL secretion ↑ApoC-III synthesis ↓LPL activity ↓VLDL removal	↑TG ↑Remnant VLDL ↓HDL ↑Small, dense LDL	TG: 150–500 mg/dL HDL-C: <40 mg/dL	Frequently accompanied by central obesity or diabetes
Familial hypercholesterolemia Heterozygous	Reduction in functional LDL receptor	↑LDL-C	LDL-C: 250–450 mg/dL	Family history of premature CHD, tendon xanthomas, corneal arcus
Familial hypercholesterolemia Homozygous	Absent LDL receptors	↑LDL-C	LDL-C: >450 mg/dL	Family history of premature CHD, tendon xanthomas, corneal arcus; affected individuals exhibit CHD by second decade of life
Familial defective apoB-100	Defective apoB on LDL and VLDL	↑LDL-C	LDL-C: 250–450 mg/dL	Family history of CHD, tendon xanthomas
Dysbetalipoproteinemia (type III hyperlipidemia)	ApoE2:E2 phenotype, ↓VLDL remnant clearance	↑Remnant VLDL, ↑IDL	LDL-C: 300–600 mg/dL TGs: 400–800 mg/dL	Palmar xanthomas, tuberoeruptive xanthomas
Familial combined hyperlipidemia	↑ApoB and VLDL production	↑CH, TG, or both	LDL-C: 250–350 mg/dL TGs: 200–800 mg/dL	Family history, CHD Family history, hyperlipidemia
Familial hyperapobeta-lipoproteinemia	↑ApoB production	↑ApoB	ApoB: >125 mg/dL	None distinctive
Hypoalphalipoproteinemia	↑HDL catabolism	↓HDL-C	HDL-C: <40 mg/dL	None distinctive

ApoB, apolipoprotein B; ApoC-III, apolipoprotein C-III; ApoE, apolipoprotein E; CH, cholesterol; CHD, coronary heart disease; HDL, high-density lipoprotein; HDL-C, high-density lipoprotein cholesterol; IDL, intermediate-density lipoprotein; LDL, low-density lipoprotein; LDL-C, low-density lipoprotein cholesterol; TGs, triglycerides; VLDL, very-low-density lipoprotein.

E- or B-containing lipoprotein. Drugs that reduce the intracellular cholesterol concentration (e.g., bile acid resins, ezetimibe, and statins) cause the upregulation of LDL receptors and thereby increase the removal of cholesterol-carrying lipoproteins from the systemic circulation.

Abnormalities in Lipid Metabolism

As can be imagined from the above description of lipid synthesis and transport, literally hundreds of possible steps could malfunction and cause a lipid disorder. Only a few relatively common and important lipid disorders are seen, however. The first two described subsequently, polygenic hypercholesterolemia and atherogenic dyslipidemia, are largely the result of an interaction between genes and lifestyle choices; after these, several prominent, but rarer, familial lipid disorders are described. Table 13-2 summarizes the characteristics of the most common lipid disorders.

POLYGENIC HYPERCHOLESTEROLEMIA

Polygenic hypercholesterolemia, the most prevalent form of dyslipidemia, which is found in more than 25% of the US population, is caused by a combination of environmental (e.g., poor nutrition, sedentary lifestyle) and genetic factors (thus, the term "polygenic"). Saturated fatty acids in the diet of these patients can reduce LDL receptor activity, thus reducing the clearance of LDL particles from the systemic circulation. As a result, patients with polygenic hypercholesterolemia have mild to moderate LDL-C elevations (usually in the range of 130 to 250 mg/dL), but no unique physical findings are seen. Family history of premature CHD is present in approximately 20% of cases. These patients are effectively managed with dietary restriction of saturated fats and cholesterol and by drugs that lower LDL-C levels (i.e., statins, bile acid sequestrants, niacin, and ezetimibe).

ATHEROGENIC DYSLIPIDEMIA

Atherogenic dyslipidemia is found in about 25% of patients who have a lipid disorder. It is characterized by a moderate TG elevation (150 to 500 mg/dL, indicative of the increased presence of VLDL remnant particles), a low HDL-C level (<40 mg/dL), and a moderately high LDL-C level (including increased concentrations of small, dense LDL particles, non–HDL-C, and apolipoprotein B-100). Most commonly, these patients are either overweight or obese with increased waist circumference, hypertensive, and insulin resistant, manifesting as elevated fasting glucose or impaired fasting glucose, and are said to have *metabolic syndrome.*

Patients who have central obesity or have diabetes have an increased mobilization of fatty acids from adipose cells to the systemic circulation, which leads to increased TG synthesis and secretion of TG-rich VLDL particles by the liver. Often, these particles contain apolipoprotein C-III, which interferes with the action of LPL, thus retarding lipolysis of TGs from VLDL particles. This results in the formation of TG-rich VLDL remnant particles. TGs from these particles are exchanged with cholesterol esters from HDL under the influence of CETP, which means the VLDL remnant particles become enriched with cholesterol whereas HDL particles lose cholesterol (and gain TGs) (Fig. 13-3). TGs are also exchanged from VLDL remnant particles with cholesterol esters from LDL particles. Thus, VLDL remnants become even more cholesterol enriched and LDL becomes TG enriched. The cholesterol-enriched, small VLDL remnant particle is atherogenic. TG-rich LDL and HDL particles undergo lipolysis catalyzed by hepatic lipase to remove TGs, leaving small, cholesterol ester–deficient LDL particles (called *small dense LDL*) that are highly atherogenic and a reduction in HDL-C from the loss of apolipoprotein A-I by the kidneys.[12]

Patients with atherogenic dyslipidemia can often be effectively managed with weight reduction and increased physical activity.

If needed, drugs that enhance the removal of remnant VLDL and small dense LDL particles (i.e., statins) and that lower TG levels (i.e., niacin or fibrates) are effective in the management of these cases.

FAMILIAL HYPERCHOLESTEROLEMIA

Familial hypercholesterolemia (FH) is the classic lipid disorder of defective clearance. This autosomal dominant disorder is strongly associated with premature CHD.[13,14] Heterozygotes (1 of 500 people in the United States) of this disorder inherit one defective LDL receptor gene. Consequently, these persons possess approximately half the number of functioning LDL receptors and double the LDL-C level of unaffected patients (i.e., LDL-C ranging between 250 and 450 mg/dL).[15,16] Clinically, heterozygous FH patients may deposit cholesterol in the iris, leading to arcus senilis. Cholesterol also deposits in tendons, particularly the Achilles' tendon and extensor tendons of the hands, leading to tendon xanthomas observed on physical examination. The clinical diagnosis of FH is established by documenting a very high LDL-C level, a strong family history of premature CHD events, and the presence of tendon xanthomas. Untreated heterozygous FH patients have approximately a 5% chance of a myocardial infarction (MI) by age 30, a 50% chance by age 50, and an 85% chance by age 60. The mean age of death in untreated male heterozygotes is in the mid-50s; for untreated female heterozygotes, it is in the mid-60s.[17]

Homozygotes (1 of 1,000,000 people in the United States) for this disorder inherit a defective LDL receptor gene from both parents and generally have LDL-C levels greater than 500 mg/dL. This rare disorder results in CHD by age 10 to 20 years. Because these individuals have lost the ability to clear cholesterol-carrying lipoproteins from the circulation, LDL-apheresis (analogous to dialysis for the kidney failure patient) is required to help remove these atherogenic particles.

Familial defective apolipoprotein B-100 (FDB) is a genetic disorder clinically indistinguishable from heterozygous FH. These patients have normally functioning LDL receptors, but a defective apolipoprotein B-100, which results in reduced binding to LDL receptors and reduced clearance of LDL particles from the systemic circulation.[18,19] As with FH, LDL-C levels are usually 250 to 450 mg/dL.[18,20,21] Presumably, the apolipoprotein E and half of the apolipoprotein B in heterozygous FDB patients function normally, providing mechanisms for removal of these lipoproteins from the systemic circulation. Clinical diagnosis of FDB, as FH, is based on a very high LDL-C level, a family history of premature CHD, and tendon xanthomas. The definitive diagnosis requires molecular screening techniques.

ONLINE CONTENT

For a narrated PowerPoint presentation on familial hypercholesterolemia, go to http://thepoint.lww.com/AT10e.

FAMILIAL DYSBETALIPOPROTEINEMIA

Familial dysbetalipoproteinemia (also called *type III hyperlipidemia* and *remnant disease*) is caused by poor clearance of VLDL and chylomicron particles from the systemic circulation.[22] Apolipoprotein E is necessary for the normal clearance of these particles. It is inherited as an E2, E3, or E4 isoform from each parent. The E2 isoform has a low binding affinity for the LDL receptor. Thus, individuals with an apolipoprotein E2/E2 phenotype have delayed clearance of VLDL remnant (and possibly chylomicron) particles from the circulation and a reduced conversion of IDL to LDL particles. A lipid disorder, however, usually does not result unless triggered by other metabolic problems (e.g., diabetes, hypothyroidism, or obesity). Clinically, these patients have high cholesterol (owing to an enrichment of cholesterol esters in VLDL remnant particles), high TGs (usually in the range of 400 to 800 mg/dL), and a VLDL-C to TG ratio greater than 0.3.[23] Some patients have palmar xanthomas (yellow-orange discoloration in the creases of the palms and fingers) and tuberoeruptive xanthomas (small, raised lesions in areas of pressure, particularly the elbows and knees). A personal and family history of premature atherosclerotic vascular disease often is present. As noted above, these patients often have diabetes mellitus, hypertension, obesity, and hyperuricemia.

PROPROTEIN CONVERTASE SUBTILISIN/KEXIN TYPE 9

FH can be caused by various "gain-of-function" mutations in the gene encoding for PCSK9. The frequency of these mutations causing FH is unknown. When PCSK9 is secreted into the plasma, it binds to the cell-surface LDL receptors, leading to endocytosis, intracellular degradation, reduced number of LDL receptors, and increased LDL-C (to approximately 300 mg/dL).[11] Drugs targeting PCSK9 are under development.

FAMILIAL COMBINED HYPERLIPIDEMIA

Familial combined hyperlipidemia (FCHL) is the classic example of a dyslipidemia caused by increased production of lipoproteins. For reasons that are not clear, patients with FCHL overproduce apolipoprotein B–containing particles, VLDL, and LDL.[24–26] Many patients have an elevated apolipoprotein B-100 level.[27] As the name implies, patients with this disorder may have hypercholesterolemia (usually in the range of 250 to 350 mg/dL), hypertriglyceridemia (usually between 200 and 800 mg/dL), or a combination of both (usually with a low HDL-C level). First-degree relatives of these individuals frequently have a lipid disorder. A family history of premature CHD is often present as well. Patients with FCHL commonly are overweight and hypertensive and also may have diabetes or hyperuricemia. A diagnosis of FCHL is presumed in patients who have increased cholesterol or TG levels, a strong family history of premature CHD, and a family history of dyslipidemia.

FAMILIAL HYPERAPOBETALIPOPROTEINEMIA

Familial hyperapobetalipoproteinemia is a variant of FCHL. This disorder is characterized by increased hepatic production of apolipoprotein B in the absence of other lipid abnormalities.[28] These patients have acceptable LDL-C and TG levels and a family history of CHD. Their apolipoprotein B-100 concentration is usually greater than 125 mg/dL, indicating an increase in the number of cholesterol-carrying lipoprotein particles. It is likely that FCHL and hyperapobetalipoproteinemia are related disorders, both resulting from excessive secretion of apolipoprotein B-100–containing lipoproteins.[29]

HYPOALPHALIPOPROTEINEMIA

Low HDL-C (<40 mg/dL; hypoalphalipoproteinemia) without an increase in TG level is fairly uncommon, but it is associated with increased CHD risk.[30,31] Little, however, is known about the precise molecular defect causing this problem, although genetic influences undoubtedly are involved.[32] Recently, Tangier disease, which is characterized by low HDL-C, orange tonsils, and hepatosplenomegaly, has been linked to a defect in the ABCA-1 transporter responsible for the efflux of cholesterol from peripheral cells (i.e., inflammatory cells in the arterial wall). The inherited tendency to have low HDL-C is accentuated by lifestyle factors such as obesity, smoking, and lack of exercise. Despite strong epidemiologic evidence showing an inverse relationship between HDL-C and CHD, clinical trials demonstrating a benefit of raising isolated low HDL-C with drugs are lacking. What has been shown is that lowering LDL-C in patients with low HDL-C reduces CHD risk.[33] It is anticipated that therapies to raise HDL-C will become available and can be tested to see whether they reduce CHD risk also.

Rationale for Treating Dyslipidemia

Scientific data from animal studies, genetic studies, epidemiologic studies, and clinical trials support the link between cholesterol, atherosclerosis, and CHD. This collective body of knowledge resoundingly supports a critical role for cholesterol as the "root cause" in the pathogenesis of atherosclerosis.[34] Even more important, in clinical trials the lowering of blood cholesterol levels, specifically LDL-C, has been consistently associated with reduced CHD, whether the LDL-C was reduced by drug, diet, or surgical means. This is why LDL-C is identified as the primary target for intervention by the National Cholesterol Education Program Adult Treatment Panel III (NCEP ATP III) guidelines. Even the most vigorous cholesterol-lowering approach does not result in the complete amelioration of CHD, however, suggesting that other factors are in play. Some of the significant literature on the pathogenesis of atherosclerosis and clinical trials establishing the link between blood cholesterol and CHD is summarized next.

PATHOGENESIS OF ATHEROSCLEROSIS

Circulating cholesterol has a central role in the pathogenesis of atherosclerosis. Even the name *atherosclerosis* depicts this (from the Latin *athero* [porridgelike] and *sclerosis* [fibrouslike]. Atherosclerotic lesions begin with the accumulation and retention of lipoproteins in the subendothelium (Fig. 13-4).[34] This appears to be related to the level of circulating lipoproteins, subendothelial matrix molecules (such as chondroitin sulfate proteoglycans) that mediate retention, and the provocation by risk factors such as hypertension, smoking, diabetes, stress, and genetic predisposition. An important finding is that native LDL per se does not contribute to the development of atherosclerosis; instead, LDL must be modified (e.g., oxidized) before it becomes a factor in causing atherosclerosis.

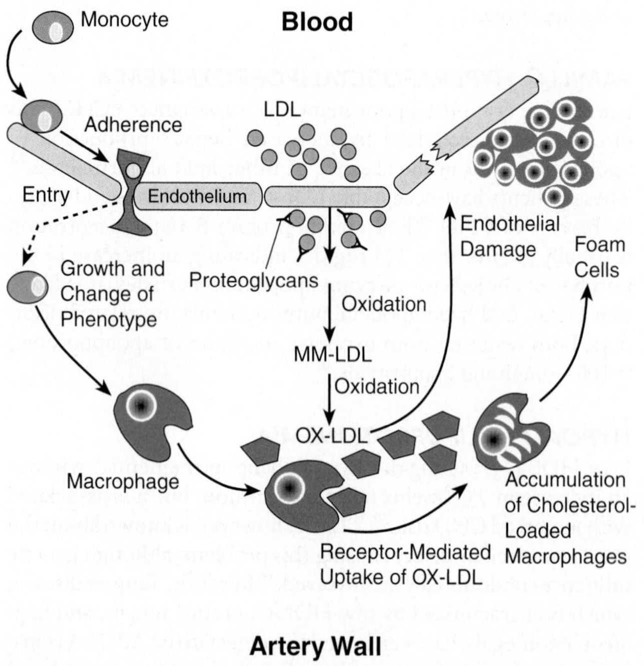

FIGURE 13-4 Some of the steps involved in the development of the fatty streak. LDL, low-density lipoprotein; MM-LDL, minimally oxidized low-density lipoprotein; OX-LDL, oxidized low-density lipoprotein.

Soon after taking up residence in the subendothelial space, lipoproteins are modified primarily by oxidation of phospholipids. Oxidized lipoproteins stimulate endothelial cells to release monocyte adhesion molecules on the surface of the lumen.[35,36] They cause circulating monocytes to attach to the intact endothelial surface, and then chemoattractants cause these monocytes to squeeze between endothelial cells into the intima (Fig. 13-4).[37] Thus, atherosclerosis is an inflammatory process in response to retained and modified lipoproteins. Once recruited, the monocytes are converted to macrophages, which begin to ingest oxidized lipoprotein particles. These modified particles are taken up by special scavenger or acetyl-LDL receptors on the surface of macrophage cells.[38] Modified lipoproteins serve as another chemoattractant for circulating monocytes, thus causing more monocytes from the systemic circulation to take up residence in the intima. Further engorgement with oxidized lipoproteins also inhibits the mobility of resident macrophage cells (blocking the egress of these cells from the intima); macrophage cells become a cytotoxic agent (causing damage to the endothelium).[35] As the uptake of modified lipoproteins into macrophage cells continues, the cells become laden with lipid, grow in size, and eventually become *foam cells* (Figs. 13-4, 13-5).

Early in the process, the monocellular layer surrounding the lumen (the endothelium) becomes dysfunctional. Notably, the release of nitric oxide from these cells is impaired, which results in vasoconstriction and ischemic symptoms. Regulation of blood cholesterol levels and management of other risk factors restore endothelial function, nitric oxide release, and the vasodilatory response.

The accumulation of foam cells in the intimal space below the endothelium eventually results in a raised lesion, the *fatty streak,* which is widely recognized as the precursor to atherosclerosis. Fatty streaks transform the once smooth endothelial surface of the artery into a lumpy, uneven surface. As this process continues, an atherosclerotic plaque is formed. In the initial stages, this plaque is characterized by a large lipid core made up of macrophage (foam) cells filled with cholesterol along the surface and at the shoulders of the lesion (Fig. 13-5).

During plaque growth, a number of cells (including macrophages, T cells, endothelial cells, platelets, and smooth muscle cells) secrete chemoattractant and growth factors, which cause smooth muscle cells from the media to migrate upward and proliferate near the luminal surface.[39] Collagen synthesis is increased. This leads to conversion of atherosclerotic lesions that initially are weak and unstable (because they contain a large lipid core surrounded by a thin fibrous cap) to become strong and hard (because they contain a small inner lipid core, much collagen, and matrix). At any given time, atherosclerosis at various stages of development can be found all along the arterial tree in high-risk patients (Fig. 13-4).

As atherosclerotic lesions grow, the coronary artery remodels. Lesions initially grow away from the lumen toward the media, thus preserving the luminal opening and ensuring normal blood flow. Late in the growth of the lesion, however, the luminal space is invaded and becomes progressively narrowed as the atherosclerotic lesion grows.

Similar to the stages of development, atherosclerotic lesions exist along a continuum from vulnerable lesions that can rupture and cause a thrombosis to older, rigid lesions that will not rupture. The younger lesions occupy only the intimal space, whereas

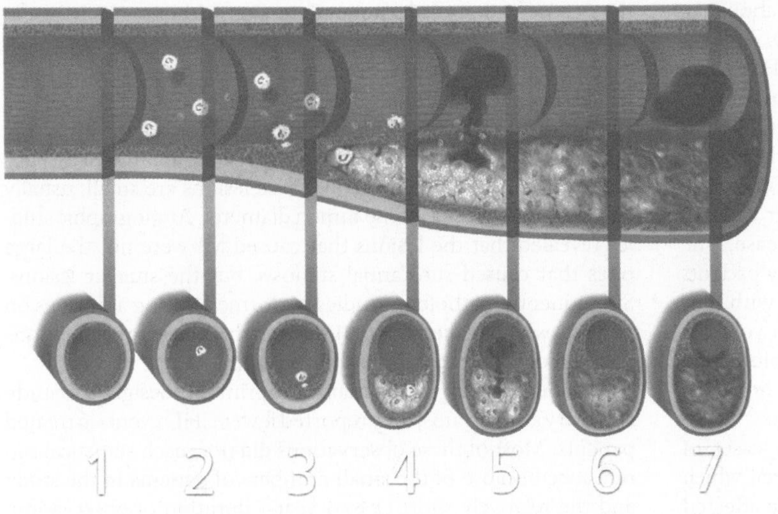

FIGURE 13-5 Initiation, progression, and complication of human coronary atherosclerotic plaque (numbers indicate order of progression).

the older lesions may protrude into the luminal space. In examining the coronary angiogram of a patient, evidence of stenosis (narrowing of the lumen) indicates the presence of older, more advanced lesions. When these lesions are seen, other lesions distal to the narrowing are likely to be present. They are younger and more susceptible to erosion or rupture, which can cause a thrombosis. In fact, the culprit lesion that results in an MI is usually not at the site of the greatest stenosis, but distal to it.[40]

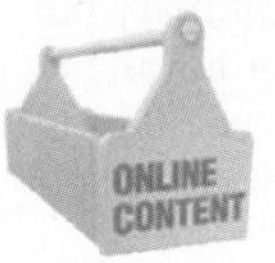

To view examples of coronary angiograms, go to http://thepoint.lww.com/AT10e.

A number of processes cause younger lesions to become unstable; most of these are a part of an active inflammatory and necrotic process. The uptake of cholesterol by activated macrophage cells is one of these processes. Chemoattractants, such as monocyte chemoattractant protein-1, adhesion molecules, and a family of T-cell substances, participate in the migration of monocytes into the intima. Macrophage colony-stimulating factor contributes to the differentiation of blood monocytes into macrophage cells. T cells elaborate inflammatory cytokines that stimulate macrophages, endothelial cells, and smooth muscle cells. Activated macrophage cells produce proteolytic enzymes that degrade collagen and weaken the fibrous cap.[41] The release of metalloproteinase enzymes causes the destruction of connective tissue and renders the atherosclerotic lesion vulnerable to rupture. Apoptosis (cell death) of smooth muscle cells in the shoulders of the atherosclerotic cap further weakens the lesion.[42–47] These processes increase the chance that the atherosclerotic lesion will rupture or erode, especially at the shoulders of the lesion, and expose the underlying tissue to circulating blood elements.[48] Collagen in the exposed plaque will trigger platelet activation, and tissue factor produced by macrophages and smooth muscle cells activates the coagulation cascade. Platelets may adhere, and microthrombi may form. The resultant clot can occlude blood flow entirely, causing an MI. More commonly, only partial occlusion of blood flow occurs, causing transient ischemic symptoms and unstable angina. The clot creates a barrier between the underlying tissue and circulating blood and allows healing to take place. Subsequently, as the atherosclerotic plaque grows further and again ruptures, a new clot can form to mend the lesion. This process of fissuring and rehealing appears to lead to the more complicated lesions of atherosclerosis.

In summary, the atherosclerotic lesions that result in sudden death or a nonfatal MI are not the large lesions that have formed over months and years and that appear prominently on a patient's coronary angiogram. Rather, they are the smaller, less stable lesions that have a large lipid core and a thin fibrous cap.[49] When shear forces, elevated blood pressure, or other toxic processes in the artery cause these plaques to fissure, erode, or rupture, a thrombosis can develop, leading to the occlusion of the affected vessel and a clinical event.

EPIDEMIOLOGIC STUDIES

During the past three decades, epidemiologic studies have established a direct relationship between blood cholesterol concentrations in a population and the incidence of CHD events.[50–52] For every 1% increase in blood cholesterol levels, a 1% to 2% increase exists in the incidence of CHD. HDL-C has an inverse relationship with CHD. For every 1% *decrease* in HDL-C levels, a 1% to 2% *increase* in the risk of CHD events occurs.[53]

Other epidemiologic trials have demonstrated the influence of environmental versus genetic factors on cholesterol levels and CHD incidence. One of the most revealing studies comes from the Honolulu Heart Study, which reported that Japanese individuals who had very low cholesterol levels and a low CHD death rate experienced a rise in cholesterol levels as well as the incidence of CHD when they migrated to Hawaii and subsequently to the west coast of the United States.[54] Similarly, Hispanics who live close to the US border have cholesterol levels and a CHD incidence that is similar to those of US residents, whereas those living in the southern part of Mexico have a lower cholesterol level and a lower incidence of CHD.

Sex differences have been the focus of other epidemiologic studies. Before menopause, the incidence of CHD in women is low,[55,56] but after menopause the rate of CHD in women parallels that of men. In fact, the prevalence of CHD in women is ultimately similar to that in men; it is just displaced by about 10 years.[52,57] Whereas men begin to experience CHD events in their 50s and 60s, women experience it in their 60s and 70s. Eventually, CHD causes nearly as many deaths in women as it does in men.[58] In fact, CHD is the cause of more deaths in women than all forms of cancer combined, including cancer of the breast, ovary, and cervix. Furthermore, the presence of diabetes in a woman with dyslipidemia negates whatever protection she may have had before menopause and is associated with a very high incidence of CHD events.[59,60] Conversely, a high HDL-C level may offer women more protection from CHD than a similar level offers a man.[53]

Finally, epidemiologic trials have taught us lessons about the influence of age on blood cholesterol levels and CHD. A direct relationship exists between blood cholesterol and CHD at all ages, to at least the mid-80s.[61] Because CHD risk increases with age, most CHD events occur among the elderly. In fact, CHD is the most common cause of death among the elderly.[62] Intravascular ultrasound studies that examine the inner walls of coronary arteries demonstrate that practically all patients older than 70 years have advanced and prevalent atherosclerotic disease. The relative risk of CHD is nearly twofold greater in elderly patients with elevated cholesterol levels compared with those with normal levels, but this risk level is less than that found in younger populations with similar cholesterol levels. The absolute rate of CHD deaths attributable to high blood cholesterol, however, increases in the elderly compared with younger patients.[62,63] An elevated blood cholesterol level contributes to more cases of CHD in the older patient population than in the younger, which is partly because of the sheer number of elderly people affected by the disease. Some authorities see age as a marker for plaque burden, suggesting that one way to identify patients with a high CHD risk is to use age as a surrogate for the presence of coronary artery plaque.[64] Because CHD is so prevalent in the elderly, it has been estimated that a mere 1% decline in mortality rates from CHD in the elderly would translate into 4,300 fewer deaths per year in the United States.[65]

CLINICAL TRIALS

ANGIOGRAPHIC REGRESSION TRIALS

Based on animal, epidemiologic, and genetic studies, the direct relationship between blood cholesterol levels and CHD events was established. The critical hypothesis that remained to be proven before cholesterol-lowering therapies could be widely recommended was that lowering blood cholesterol levels would reduce CHD risk. The proof for this hypothesis was ultimately demonstrated in clinical trials. The initial test of this hypothesis involved angiographic trials that sought to demonstrate that by lowering blood cholesterol levels, coronary stenosis visualized on coronary angiography would regress.[66–83] Much to the surprise of investigators, this did not occur. In fact, more commonly, cholesterol lowering seemed only to slow lesion progression.

Despite these disappointing results, angiographic trials taught many important lessons. They demonstrated that aggressive lipid lowering caused lesions to progress at a slower rate regardless of the vascular bed under study, including coronary,[67–75,78,79,81–83] carotid,[76,77,80] and femoral arteries.[72,80] They established that this effect was achieved regardless of the lipid-lowering therapy deployed: diet and other lifestyle modifications,[69] lipid-lowering drugs,[9,33,42–47,67,68,71,74–82] or ileal bypass surgery.[66] They also suggested that the more aggressive the lipid lowering, especially if it resulted in greater than 60% reduction in LDL-C, the greater the chance of plaque regression.[84,85]

The reason early angiographic studies failed to demonstrate lesion regression was not because this process did not occur, but because the methodology could not detect it. Angiograms outline the lesion from the outside of the coronary artery. Because atherosclerotic lesions initially remodel outward away from the lumen, as explained above, the lumen would appear normal until the late stage of atherosclerosis plaque development. Thus, lesions that were visible on a coronary angiogram were the older, more rigid lesions that were less likely to change with lipid-lowering therapy. Younger lesions, which were not visualized in a coronary angiogram, may well have regressed, however. Recent investigations of the contour of the inner lining of the lumen using intravascular ultrasound report that lipid lowering does cause widespread plaque regression without any change in lumen size.[86]

Angiographic studies were the first to suggest that lipid-modifying therapy could alter the composition of plaque. As summarized earlier, plaques are initially characterized by a large lipid core and a thin fibrous cap; these lesions are more susceptible to rupture.[37,48] Additionally, these lesions are small, usually less than 50% the size of the lumen diameter. Angiographic studies revealed that the lesions that caused MI were not the large ones that caused substantial stenosis, but the smaller lesions. Subsequently, pathology studies performed during autopsies on patients who had died after MI showed that these smaller lesions were lipid-laden and had thin fibrous caps.

Although angiographic trials were primarily designed to study coronary angiograms, they reported fewer CHD events in treated patients. Most of these observations did not reach statistical significance because of the small numbers of patients in the study and the relatively short (1 to 3 years) duration of observation. When these studies were combined, the message was clear, however: cholesterol lowering was associated with fewer CHD events.[49] These results set the stage for the larger clinical trials.

CHOLESTEROL-LOWERING CLINICAL TRIALS

Proof of whether LDL-C lowering reduces CHD events has been demonstrated by well-designed, large, placebo-controlled clinical trials. Since the early 1990s, the results of numerous major clinical trials have conclusively demonstrated the value of lipid-modifying therapy to prevent CHD events (Table 13-3).[87–104] Moreover, a recent meta-analysis of statin trials in primary prevention (in which 10% or less had a history of cardiovascular disease) of CHD events showed that statins reduced all-cause mortality, major vascular events, and revascularizations without an excess of cancers or muscle-related side effects.[105]

The first of these, the Lipid Research Clinics Coronary Primary Prevention Trial,[99] showed that a relatively modest 10% reduction in cholesterol levels with the bile acid resin cholestyramine compared with placebo for a 5-year period reduced CHD deaths and nonfatal MI by an impressive 19%. The results of this study launched the modern era of cholesterol management to reduce CHD risk.

Secondary Prevention

Beginning in the mid-1990s, the results of clinical trials with the more potent cholesterol-lowering statins were reported. Five of these (4S,[87] CARE,[89] LIPID,[88] TNT,[92] and IDEAL[93]) were secondary prevention trials (i.e., they were conducted in patients with known CHD). In 4S, CARE, and LIPID, CHD death and nonfatal MI occurred in 13% to 22% of placebo-treated patients in 5 years, compared with event rates of 10% to 14% with statin therapy. Total mortality was reduced significantly in two of these trials that were powered to assess total mortality. Fewer revascularization procedures were required in patients receiving statin therapy; also 31% fewer strokes occurred.[106] This important and unexpected finding suggests that the same mechanisms by which statins affect coronary atherosclerosis may be operable in extracranial carotid atherosclerosis. It also demonstrates that patients who have atherosclerosis in one vascular bed (e.g., the coronary vessels) are likely to have atherosclerosis in other vascular beds, and that cholesterol-lowering treatment can have beneficial effects throughout the vascular tree. Finally, these studies demonstrate that LDL-C–lowering therapy not only improves the quality of life (by preventing MI, strokes, and revascularization procedures) but also can prolong life (by delaying deaths from any cause). Most recently, the TNT and IDEAL trials demonstrated additional cardiovascular benefit for lowering LDL-C substantially to less than 100 mg/dL in patients

TABLE 13-3
Randomized End Point Trials With Cholesterol-Lowering Therapies

Trial	Intervention	LDL-C: Initial (on Rx)	LDL-C Changes (%)	Placebo CHD Rate (%)[a]	CHD Event Reduction (%)
CHD and CHD Risk Equivalent Patients					
4S[87]	Simvastatin 20–40 mg	188 (117)	↓35	21.8	↓34
LIPID[88]	Pravastatin 40 mg	150 (112)	↓25	15.9	↓24
CARE[89]	Pravastatin 40 mg	139 (98)	↓32	13.2	↓24
Post-CABG[83]	Lovastatin/resin	136 (98)	↓39	13.5	↓24
HPS[90]	Simvastatin 40 mg	131 (89)	↓32	11.8	↓24
PROSPER[91]	Pravastatin 40 mg	147 (97)	↓34	12.7	↓19
TNT[92]	Atorvastatin 80 mg	152 (77)	↓49	—	↓22
	Atorvastatin 10 mg	152 (98)	↓35	—	
IDEAL[93]	Atorvastatin 80 mg	121 (77)	↓33	—	↓20
	Simvastatin 20 mg	121 (104)	↓14	—	
ALLHAT[94]	Pravastatin 40 mg	146 (105)	↓28	—	↓9
	Usual care	146 (130)	↓11	—	
Acute Coronary Syndrome Patients					
MIRACL[95,96]	Atorvastatin 80 mg	124 (72)	↓42	—	↓26[b]
AVERT[97]	Atorvastatin 80 mg	145 (77)	↓42	—	↓36[b]
PROVE IT[98]	Atorvastatin 80 mg	106 (62)	↓51	—	↓16
	Pravastatin 40 mg	106 (95)	↓22		
Patients Without Evidence of CHD					
LRC-CPPT[99]	Resin	205 (175)	↓15	9.8	↓19
WOSCOPS[100]	Pravastatin 40 mg	192 (142)	↓26	14.9	↓31
AFCAPS/TexCAPS[101]	Lovastatin	150 (115)	↓25	3.0	↓40
ASCOT[102]	Atorvastatin 10 mg	132 (85)	↓31	4.7	↓50[c]
CARDS[103]	Atorvastatin 10 mg	117 (77)	↓34	5.5	↓37[d]
JUPITER[104]	Rosuvastatin 20 mg	108[e]	↓50	1.4	↓44

[a] Placebo CHD rate: nonfatal myocardial infarction and CHD death.
[b] Ischemic events.
[c] Estimated 5-year CHD risk reduction.
[d] Acute coronary events.
[e] Median.
CHD, coronary heart disease; LDL-C, low-density lipoprotein cholesterol; Rx, drug therapy.

with stable CHD. These two trials randomly assigned patients to receive either high-dose (atorvastatin 80 mg) statin therapy or moderate-dose (atorvastatin 10 mg or simvastatin 20 mg) statin therapy with an approximate follow-up period of 5 years. In both trials, more intensive lowering of LDL-C to significantly less than 100 mg/dL was associated with a reduction in CHD. The results of these two trials allowed the Writing Group for the cholesterol guidelines (see subsequently) to establish an "optional" target goal of LDL-C in patients with CHD to less than 70 mg/dL.[107,108] The further reductions in the incidence of heart attacks, revascularizations, and ischemic strokes with more-intensive lowering of LDL-C with statins compared with less-intensive statin regimens was verified in a recent meta-analysis of randomized trials. An additional 38.6-mg/dL reduction in LDL-C was associated with a 38% relative reduction in major vascular events ($p < 0.0001$). Cancer and nonvascular deaths were similar between statin-intensity groups.[109]

Similarly, the Heart Protection Study (HPS)[90] extended the results of the earlier statin trials (4S,[87] CARE,[89] LIPID[88]). The HPS included 20,536 patients with a history of CHD or cerebrovascular disease (stroke or transient ischemic attacks), peripheral vascular disease, or diabetes not considered by their general practitioner to have a clear indication for statin therapy because of relatively low baseline cholesterol levels (mean LDL-C was 131 mg/dL). Of note, with the exception of the patients with a history of CHD, this grouping of patients is designated by the NCEP ATP III as being a "CHD-equivalent population" because their risk of a CHD event is more than 20% in a 10-year period.[8] Treatment with simvastatin therapy for 5 years reduced LDL-C to 89 mg/dL and lowered the future risk of a CHD event in each of these populations by about 24% compared with placebo. By coincidence, the results of the HPS support the NCEP ATP III recommendation for aggressive management of cholesterol in patients at high risk for CHD events without established CHD. The CHD event reduction was achieved equally in men and women; in all age groups, including those ages 75 to 85 years; and regardless of the baseline LDL-C, including those with initial levels less than 100 mg/dL.

Trials carried out in patients with acute coronary syndromes have also demonstrated CHD risk reduction (Table 13-3). The MIRACL study randomly assigned patients presenting to the hospital with unstable angina or non–Q-wave MI to statin therapy or placebo for 4 months. This resulted in a 24% reduction in symptomatic ischemia requiring emergency hospitalization and a 60% reduction in nonfatal strokes in those receiving the statin.[95,96] The AVERT study evaluated statin-based medical management versus revascularization and usual medical care in patients who had stable CAD and were candidates for a revascularization procedure. After 18 months of therapy, the statin-treated group had 36% fewer cases of ischemia requiring hospitalization compared with placebo-treated patients.[97] These studies show that intervention with a statin in patients with acute coronary syndromes can have important effects on ischemic symptoms in a relatively brief time after beginning therapy. The CHD risk reductions reported in the 5-year clinical trial were evident within the first

1 to 2 years of statin therapy and were significantly different from placebo after 5 years of treatment. More recently, PROVE-IT[98] was designed to determine whether intensive LDL-C lowering with atorvastatin (80 mg) would reduce major coronary events to a greater extent compared with less-intensive LDL-C lowering with pravastatin (40 mg) in patients who had been hospitalized for an acute coronary syndrome. After 2 years of treatment, mean LDL-C levels in patients randomly assigned to receive atorvastatin (80 mg) and pravastatin (40 mg) were 62 mg/dL and 95 mg/dL, respectively. The composite cardiovascular end point (death from any cause, MI, documented unstable angina requiring rehospitalization, revascularization, and stroke) was significantly reduced by 16% with atorvastatin compared with pravastatin. Both treatments were well tolerated; however, elevations in alanine aminotransferase were threefold higher in patients treated with atorvastatin compared with pravastatin.

Primary Prevention

Six trials with statin therapy have been reported in patients without evident CHD (i.e., primary prevention) but with multiple CHD risk factors. WOSCOPS, which included men who had two or more CHD risk factors, found that CHD events and revascularization procedures were reduced by 31% and 37%, respectively, in those receiving statin therapy for 5 years; total mortality was reduced 22% ($p = 0.051$).[100] The ASCOT trial, which included men and women with hypertension and an average of 3.7 other CHD risk factors, reported that CHD events were reduced by 36% and strokes by 27% after only 3.3 years of statin treatment.[102]

Similarly, the ALLHAT trial enrolled 10,355 hypertensive patients with moderately elevated hypercholesterolemia with at least one additional CHD risk factor and randomly assigned them to nonblinded treatment with pravastatin or usual care for 4.8 years.[94] The results, however, were in contrast to those found in the ASCOT trial, likely because of the high use of nonstudy statin in the usual-care group (30%) and only a 77% adherence to pravastatin in the treatment group. This likely resulted in the total cholesterol difference between the two groups of only 9.6% and an insignificant reduction in CHD deaths and nonfatal MI of 9%.

The AFCAPS/TexCAPS trial was important because it included the lowest-risk population (without clinically evident atherosclerotic cardiovascular disease with average total cholesterol and LDL-C levels, but which did have below-average HDL-C levels), with an estimated 10-year CHD risk of only 6%. Despite this relatively low CHD risk, the composite end point (i.e., fatal and nonfatal MI, sudden cardiac death, and unstable angina) was reduced by 37%, fatal and nonfatal MI were reduced by 40%, and unstable angina was reduced by 32%, with 5 years of statin treatment.[101] Significant reductions in CHD events were seen in women, older patients, and diabetic patients, emphasizing the value of treatment in these populations. In a substudy of the AFCAPS/TexCAPS trial,[110] high-sensitivity C-reactive protein (hs-CRP) was measured to assess its prognostic utility. Plasma levels of hs-CRP appear to be a marker of inflammation (i.e., atherosclerosis) and is considered an emerging risk factor (to be discussed later). Plasma hs-CRP was measured at baseline and after 1 year in 5,742 patients who participated in the trial. Patients with the highest levels of hs-CRP had the highest rates of coronary events. Lovastatin reduced the event rate in patients with LDL-C lower than 149 mg/dL at baseline (levels below current target for lower-risk primary prevention) but elevated hs-CRP levels. However, lovastatin appeared not to benefit patients with both low baseline LDL-C and hs-CRP levels relative to placebo. This substudy suggested that hs-CRP may help guide primary prevention strategies and that statin therapy may benefit individuals with evidence of chronic inflammation, even if they do not have high cholesterol levels. This observation was then prospectively tested in the JUPITER trial.[104]

In JUPITER, primary prevention patients ($n = 17{,}802$) who would otherwise not be considered for statin therapy because of below average (<130 mg/dL) levels of LDL-C, but with hs-CRP levels of at least 2 mg/dL, were randomly assigned to rosuvastatin 20 mg daily or placebo and were followed for the occurrence of the combined primary end point of MI, stroke, arterial revascularization, hospitalization for unstable angina, or death from cardiovascular causes. The trial was stopped early owing to the benefits of rosuvastatin compared with placebo on the combined primary end point (hazard ratio for rosuvastatin, 0.56; 95% confidence interval, 0.46 to 0.69; $p < 0.00001$). The rate of occurrence of the primary end point per year was 0.77% in the rosuvastatin-treated patients and 1.36% in the placebo-treated patients. Thus, the absolute risk reduction for the combined primary end point during the approximately 2 years of the trial was only 1.2%, which was far less impressive than the relative risk reduction of 44%. An accepted method of determining clinical usefulness of an intervention is calculation of the numbers needed to treat (NNT) to prevent one adverse outcome. Based on the above absolute risk reduction, 83 patients would need to be treated for 2 years to prevent one adverse outcome. Rosuvastatin also significantly reduced deaths from any cause compared with placebo, and the absolute risk reduction was only 0.25%. Thus the NNT is 400 to prevent one death from any cause. This is a high number and will need to be carefully considered by those who are developing the next set of cholesterol treatment guidelines. The authors concluded that in apparently healthy persons without hyperlipidemia but with elevated hs-CRP levels, rosuvastatin significantly reduced the incidence of major cardiovascular events. However, since its publication, the JUPITER trial has received an avalanche of criticism for alleged study design flaws (i.e., prespecified early stopping rules were not detailed in the published description of the study protocol), stopping the trial early, and investigator bias by commercial interests, just to name a few. In the end, the final word on using hs-CRP as a therapeutic target requires further research, and a cost-effectiveness (the cost per quality-adjusted life-years saved) analysis from the JUPITER trial data will also need to be conducted.

Lowering LDL-C by other means also reduces CHD events.[66] For example, LDL-C lowering with ileal bypass surgery in the POSCH study resulted in a 40% reduction of CHD events compared with the groups not having this surgery.[66] These studies suggest that effective LDL-C lowering by any means can reduce CHD risk.

Taken together, the results of these trials demonstrate that LDL-C lowering reduces the risk of a CHD event in patients at practically any level of risk. In the aggregate, common CHD events, including sudden CHD deaths and nonfatal MI, were reduced by 25% to 40%. Revascularization procedures were reduced by 25% to 50%. Strokes were reduced by an average of 15% in primary prevention patients and 32% in secondary prevention patients.[106] In fact, essentially all known adverse consequences of atherosclerosis have been reduced with lipid-lowering therapy. In some of these studies, especially those in patients at very high risk for CHD, total mortality was significantly reduced. These trials show that aggressive lipid lowering improves the quality as well as the length of life. In addition, in patients with stable CHD and those who had an acute coronary event, aggressive lowering of LDL-C to less than 70 mg/dL provides further protection from CHD events. The protective effects are illustrated by a plot of the relative risk of CHD and LDL-C levels, which shows a log-linear relationship (Fig. 13-6),[108] which suggests the optimal level of LDL-C is far less than 70 mg/dL (the relative risk is set at 1.0 for LDL-C = 40 mg/dL). This log-linear relationship is

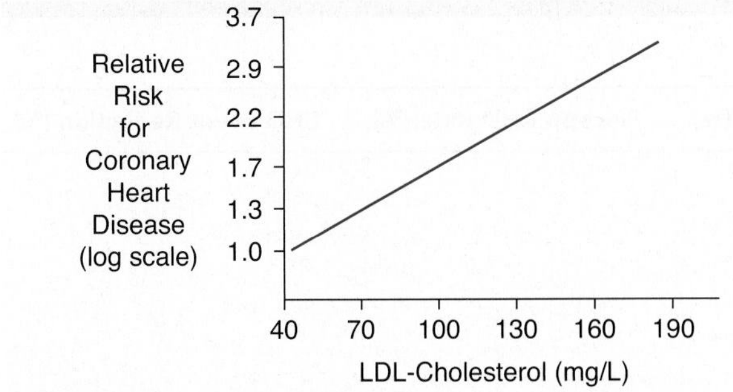

FIGURE 13-6 Log-linear relationship between low-density lipoprotein (LDL) cholesterol levels and relative risk for coronary heart disease. (Adapted with permission from Grundy SM et al. Implications of recent clinical trials for the National Cholesterol Education Program Adult Treatment Panel III guidelines. *Arterioscler Thromb Vasc Biol.* 2004;24:e149.)

consistent with epidemiologic data, clinical trials, and population data.[111] Evidence from hunter-gatherer populations (societies whose primary subsistence is based on hunting and foraging for food without resorting to domestication) who still follow their indigenous lifestyle shows no evidence for atherosclerosis into the seventh and eighth decades of life, and their estimated LDL-C levels are approximately 50 to 75 mg/dL. The above cumulative evidence has led the NCEP ATP III to define the "optimal" LDL-C level as less than 100 mg/dL and a reasonable goal of less than 70 mg/dL for all patients with CHD.[107,108]

Patients With Diabetes

Diabetic patients have a very high risk of macrovascular disease (i.e., CHD) as well as microvascular disease (e.g., retinopathy). Investigations have shown that diabetic patients with no history of CHD have the same risk of a future CHD event as do nondiabetic patients who have experienced an MI (approximately 20% risk in 7 years).[112] Because of this, NCEP ATP III and the American Diabetic Association considered patients with diabetes to be a CHD risk equivalent (>20% 10-year CHD risk) and recommended that these patients be treated with aggressive lipid-modifying therapy to an LDL-C goal of less than 100 mg/dL.[8] Findings from the prior clinical trials demonstrate that a reduction in CHD events with lipid-modifying therapy is of a similar or greater magnitude in diabetic patients compared with nondiabetic patients.[88,103] This supports the NCEP ATP III recommendation for aggressive management of diabetic patients.[8]

Close management of blood glucose levels appears to reduce microvascular disease, but not CHD.[113,114] However, recent analysis of the Action to Control Cardiovascular Risk in Diabetes (ACCORD) trial, which was designed to assess intensive therapy (targeting a glycated hemoglobin level <6.0%) or standard therapy (targeting a level of 7% to 7.9%) for glucose control in patients with type 2 diabetes and cardiovascular disease or additional cardiovascular risk factors, did show that intensive therapy significantly reduced nonfatal MI. Unfortunately, the trial was terminated early because of an increase in all-cause mortality in the intensive therapy group.[115]

GLOBAL CORONARY HEART DISEASE RISK IDENTIFICATION

The large number of clinical trials available illustrates the continuum of risk in patients with CHD (secondary prevention) and those without (primary prevention). In fact, the CHD risk in these two populations overlaps considerably. In secondary prevention patients, clinically significant atherosclerosis is known to be present and the risk of a subsequent event is great. In primary

TABLE 13-4

NCEP ATP III Major Risk Factors That Modify LDL-C Goals[8]

Positive Risk Factors (↑ Cardiovascular Risk)
Age: Man ≥45 years Woman ≥55 years Family history of a premature CHD (definite MI or sudden death before 55 years in father or other male first-degree relative or before 65 years in mother or other female first-degree relative) Current cigarette smoking Hypertension (≥140/90 mm Hg or on antihypertensive drugs) Low HDL-C (<40 mg/dL)
Negative Risk Factor (↓ Cardiovascular Risk, Protective)
High HDL-C (≥60 mg/dL)

Note: Presence of diabetes mellitus is considered a CHD risk equivalent (see Table 13-7). It is not included in counting the number of risk factors because its presence automatically qualifies the patient for aggressive treatment whether or not true CHD is manifest.
CHD, coronary heart disease; HDL-C, high-density lipoprotein cholesterol; LDL-C, low-density lipoprotein cholesterol; MI, myocardial infarction; NCEP ATP III, National Cholesterol Education Program Adult Treatment Panel III.

prevention patients with multiple risk factors, early atherosclerosis is likely present and increases the risk of a future CHD event. In fact, some primary prevention patients have so many risk factors that they reach the level of a "CHD risk equivalent" as defined by the NCEP ATP III guidelines, denoting a greater than 20% CHD risk in 10 years.[8] Others have only a few or no accompanying CHD risk factors and have a low to moderate future risk of a CHD event. Thus, the decision of how aggressively to treat patients begins with an assessment of their global CHD risk.

The first step is to identify patients who have two or more risk factors and no CHD and CHD risk equivalent history (Table 13-4). The next step is to assess their global CHD risk with an instrument such as that illustrated in the Framingham Heart Study (see online calculator at **http://hp2010.nhlbihin.net/atpiii/calculator.asp?usertype=prof**).[8] (It is not necessary to conduct a global risk assessment of CHD patients, as their risk is known to be >20% in 10 years or patients with fewer than two CHD risk factors because they generally have a risk of <10%.) Patients with a very high risk of a future CHD event (e.g., diabetic patients and those with a global risk of >20% in 10 years) can be considered a CHD equivalent and given aggressive LDL-C–lowering treatment with the same LDL-C goal as applied to patients who have experienced a CHD event (i.e., an LDL-C treatment goal of <100 mg/dL).[116] Those with less than 20% risk of a CHD event in 10 years can be given therapeutic lifestyle changes (TLC) and drug therapy, if needed, to reach an intermediate LDL-C goal (<130 mg/dL). This approach of assessing a patient's CHD risk and matching the intensity of treatment is illustrated in the cases that follow. One comment regarding the Framingham risk assessment calculator: although widely used by clinicians, it does not predict CHD risk in women as well as for men. The Reynolds Risk Score (**http://www.reynoldsriskscore.org/**) was developed and validated in 24,558 women based on a large panel of traditional and novel risk factors.[117] Two main differences are that the Reynolds Risk Score takes into account family history of CHD, and plasma levels of hs-CRP. This model seems to improve the accuracy of cardiovascular risk prediction compared with Framingham in women.

TRIGLYCERIDE-LOWERING CLINICAL TRIALS

Five large clinical trials have tested TG-lowering therapies (fibrates and niacin) in randomized end point trials involving

TABLE 13-5
Randomized End Point Trials With Triglyceride-Lowering Therapies

Trial	Intervention	Lipids: Initial (on Rx)	Lipid Changes (%)	Placebo CHD Rate (%)	CHD Event Reduction (%)
HHS[118]	Gemfibrozil	LDL-C: 189 (170	↓10		
		TG: 178 (116)	↓35	4	↓34
		HDL-C: 47 (52)	↑11		
VA-HIT[119]	Gemfibrozil	LDL-C: 111 (113)	0		
		TG: 161 (115)	↓31	22	↓22
		HDL-C: 32 (34)	↑6		
BIP[120]	Bezafibrate	LDL-C: 148 (138)	↓7		
		TG: 145 (115)	↓21	15	↓9.4
		HDL-C: 35 (41)	↑18		
FIELD[121]	Fenofibrate	LDL-C: 119 (94)	↓6		
		TG: 154 (130)	↓22	6	↓11
		HDL-C: 42 (44)	↑1		
ACCORD[122]	Fenofibrate + Simvastatin	LDL-C: 100 (30)	↓19	2.4	↓8
		TG: 164[a]	↓22		
		HDL-C: 38 (8)	↑8		
CDP[123]	Niacin	TC: 250 (235)	↓10	30	↓13
		TG: 480 (354)	↓26		

[a] Median.
CHD, coronary heart disease; HDL, high-density lipoprotein cholesterol; LDL-C, low-density lipoprotein cholesterol; Rx, drug therapy; TG, triglyceride.

patients who generally had baseline TG levels of 150 to 500 mg/dL and HDL-C levels less than 40 mg/dL (Table 13-5).[118–123] The Helsinki Heart Study studied 4,081 men without CHD and found a 34% reduction in CHD death and nonfatal MI after 5 years of gemfibrozil therapy compared with placebo.[118] Post hoc analysis of this study showed that the group of patients with TG levels greater than 200 mg/dL and an LDL to HDL ratio greater than 5.0 (generally with LDL-C >194 mg/dL and HDL-C <40 mg/dL) accounted for 71% of the CHD reduction achieved in the entire study, although this group represented only 10% of the total study population[124] (Table 13-5). The VA-HIT (HDL Intervention Trial) studied 2,531 men with a history of CHD and low HDL-C levels (mean HDL-C level, 32 mg/dL) and reported a 22% reduction in CHD events with gemfibrozil therapy. The authors reported that approximately 25% of this risk reduction resulted from the 6% increase in HDL-C.[125] The Bezafibrate Infarction Prevention (BIP) trial studied CHD patients with a lipid profile similar to the patients in the AFCAPS/TexCAPS trial (high LDL-C, low HDL-C, normal TGs) and reported an insignificant 9% reduction in CHD events associated with an 18% increase in HDL-C and a 21% reduction in TGs.[120] A post hoc analysis of this trial found that patients who had TG levels of greater than 175 and 200 mg/dL had significant CHD event reductions of 22% and 40%, respectively. The FIELD study investigated the effects of fenofibrate versus placebo with an average follow-up of 5 years on CHD events in patients with type 2 diabetes with a mean baseline LDL-C, HDL-C, and triglyceride level of 119 mg/dL, 42 mg/dL, and 153 mg/dL, respectively.[121] Similar to the BIP trial, this trial failed to demonstrate a significant reduction in major coronary events (11% reduction in risk; $p = 0.16$) in patients randomly assigned to receive fenofibrate. Because this trial allowed changes in therapy at the discretion of the patient's primary-care physician, significantly more patients receiving placebo (17%) compared with fenofibrate (8%) were taking nonstudy lipid-lowering agents. This may have partially accounted for the study results.

The current outcome evidence for fenofibrate and gemfibrozil (bezafibrate is not available in the United States) reasonably supports their use as second-line agents as an alternative to statin therapy when a statin is contraindicated or not tolerated in type 2 diabetes and secondary prevention with low HDL-C, respectively. In addition, post hoc analyses suggest that patients with atherogenic dyslipidemia obtain CHD risk reduction with fibrate therapy. Unlike statins, however, which have been associated with a reduction in total mortality,[87,88,90,105] fibrates appear not to reduce all-cause mortality.[126] The risk reduction in coronary events may be in line with that achieved with statins, although no head-to-head trials exist to refute or affirm this. This presents a dilemma for the clinician: When presented with a patient who has atherogenic dyslipidemia, which is the drug of choice, a statin or fibrate? Some guidance to this question will be provided during the case discussions that follow. Moreover, the question of the incremental CHD risk reduction benefits of adding a fibrate to background statin therapy in patients with mixed hyperlipidemia will be covered later.

Only one placebo-controlled end point study is available for niacin (Table 13-5). The study was completed in men who had a prior MI and mixed hyperlipidemia. After 5 years of niacin therapy, the CHD event rate was reduced by 13%.[123] Fifteen years after the start of the study, and 9 years after the study was terminated, the investigators reported that total mortality was 11% lower in the men in the niacin arm, suggesting that any period of lipid-modifying treatment may translate into a long-term benefit.[123] Combination therapy with niacin plus a statin has been studied in patients with CHD with low HDL-C and normal LDL-C.[127] Compared with a mean 3.9% progression in coronary stenosis with placebo, niacin–simvastatin therapy was associated with a mean regression of 0.4% ($p < 0.001$). The authors posited that event reduction with this combination should be equivalent to the sum of the LDL-C reduction and the HDL-C increase. In the study, LDL-C was reduced by 42% and HDL-C was increased by 26%, and the composite end point of death from coronary causes, MI, stroke, or revascularization for worsening ischemia was reduced 60% with the niacin–statin combination ($p = 0.02$). In addition, the results of the Arterial Biology for the Investigation of the Treatment Effects of Reducing Cholesterol (ARBITER-2) trial showed significant slowing of the progression of atherosclerosis by measuring carotid intima–media thickness in patients with known CHD treated with statin and niacin compared with those treated with a statin alone.[128]

Niacin has long been an intriguing drug to clinicians. It is one of the few drugs that positively affects each component of the lipid profile (LDL-C, TGs, and HDL-C). It is the best therapy available to raise HDL-C and one of the best at lowering TGs. It is logical to expect that these effects would translate into substantial CHD risk reduction. It is especially interesting to speculate on how these effects may combine to offer better risk reduction, especially when combined with one of the statins. This hypothesis is being evaluated in the ongoing AIM HIGH study and the HPS2-THRIVE study in combination with an investigational antiflushing drug Laropiprant.

Mechanisms of Coronary Heart Disease Risk Reduction

Given the consistent relationship between lowering blood cholesterol and reducing CHD events, the question arises, "what is the mechanism of this protection?" Scientists are offering many new and exciting answers to this question. At present, it appears that the reduction in CHD with lipid-altering therapy is mediated through, or at least tracked by, a reduction in cholesterol levels and serum lipoproteins. In addition to lowering blood cholesterol levels, statins and other lipid-altering therapies produce other, so-called pleiotropic effects that may partly explain their CHD-reducing capability.[129]

One way in which cholesterol lowering may reduce CHD is by changing atherosclerotic plaque from high-risk lesions with a large lipid core, thin fibrous cap, and many cholesterol-filled macrophage cells along the shoulders of the lesion to lower-risk lesions with a small lipid core and much connective tissue and smooth muscle matrix throughout. The lesion does not appear to change much in size, or at least not in ways that can be visualized on an arteriogram. The harder lesion created with lipid lowering is much less likely to rupture or erode, however, thus reducing the risk of forming an occluding clot and producing CHD events.

Lipid lowering may also affect endothelial function. Evidence indicates that high LDL-C levels cause endothelial dysfunction, as evidenced by a lowered ability of coronary arteries to dilate. Cholesterol lowering by practically any means restores endothelial function. Many studies have demonstrated improvement in brachial artery reactivity and coronary artery dilation when cholesterol levels are reduced.[130–135] Positron emission tomography scans demonstrate improved blood flow and reduced areas of ischemia throughout the myocardium in patients receiving lipid-altering therapy.[132,133] These effects may have important clinical benefits. In patients with CAD, cholesterol lowering reduces the number of ST-segment depressions recorded during a 48-hour electrocardiogram (ECG) Holter monitor study.[136,137] Therapy with a statin can also reduce ischemic events requiring acute management, a potential effect of restored endothelial function.[97]

Cholesterol lowering might also combat the inflammation that accompanies atherogenesis. Early in the development of plaques, monocyte-derived macrophages are recruited to engulf modified LDL particles, and in every stage of the disease, specific subtypes of T lymphocytes are present.[40,46] At various stages, cytokines, chemokines, and growth factors are released. Inflammatory processes may be especially active just before or after the plaque ruptures. Several investigators have attempted to identify markers of inflammation that may signal an increased risk of a CHD event. As discussed previously, one promising marker is hs-CRP. An elevated hs-CRP level predicts a high risk of future CHD events and appears to add to the risk predicted by LDL-C alone.[110,138] A subanalysis of the CARE trial reported that high levels of hs-CRP forecast CHD risk in patients on placebo, but this was attenuated and not significant in patients assigned to receive pravastatin, suggesting that statin treatment has an anti-inflammatory effect.[139] The American Heart Association (AHA),[140] alone and more recently in conjunction with the American College of Cardiology Foundation, continues to recommended that measurement of the hs-CRP level in asymptomatic adults (men ≥50 years and women ≥60 years) with LDL-C less than 130 mg/dL or in asymptomatic adults (men ≤50 years and women ≤60 years) who are intermediate-risk (generally those with two or more CHD risk factors) as a way to further characterize the patient's future CHD risk and detect candidates for drug therapy.[141] As mentioned previously, however, the role of hs-CRP as a therapeutic target has not been defined.

HYPERCHOLESTEROLEMIA

Evaluation of the Lipoprotein Profile

CASE 13-1

QUESTION 1: T.A., a 43-year-old premenopausal woman, is screened with a lipid profile during an annual medical evaluation. She has never taken cholesterol-lowering medication and currently takes only a multivitamin daily. She has had no symptoms of coronary, carotid, or peripheral vascular disease. She has a 20–pack-year history of smoking and exercises four times a week, without physical limitations. T.A. states that she follows a low-fat, low-cholesterol diet. Her father is alive and well at age 71, with a normal cholesterol level. Her mother had an MI at age 47 and died at age 57 from a second event. Her grandfather died of an MI at age 52; a sister has hypercholesterolemia and is taking simvastatin. Pertinent physical findings are weight, 125 pounds; height, 63 inches; blood pressure (BP), 120/82 mm Hg; pulse, 66 beats/minute and regular; carotid pulses symmetric bilaterally without bruits; no neck masses; no abdominal bruit; and no evidence of tendon xanthomas. Pertinent laboratory findings, obtained after a 12-hour fast, show the following results:

Total cholesterol, 290 mg/dL
TG, 55 mg/dL
HDL-C, 55 mg/dL
LDL-C, 224 mg/dL
Non–HDL-C, 235 mg/dL
Plasma glucose, 96 mg/dL
Thyroid-stimulating hormone (TSH), 0.92 international units/mL
Alanine aminotransferase (ALT), 11 units/L
Aspartate aminotransferase (AST), 8 units/L
Blood urea nitrogen, 12 mg/dL
Creatinine, 1.0 mg/dL
Urinalysis, negative

What is your assessment of T.A.'s lipid panel results?

T.A.'s LDL-C is considered very high (>190 mg/dL); NCEP defines the optimal LDL-C as less than 100 mg/dL.[8] Her HDL-C is right at the average HDL-C for a woman, and her TG is normal (<150 mg/dL) (Table 13-6). In most cases, it is wise to repeat the lipid profile to be sure the first results are not atypical. However, T.A.'s LDL-C is so high a repeat test is not likely to change the assessment. Thus, in this case, a second test is optional.

Although it is possible to measure LDL-C directly, it is common for many laboratories to calculate LDL-C. Total cholesterol, HDL-C, and TGs are measured directly and then the following formula (Friedewald equation) is applied to calculate LDL-C:

$$\text{LDL-C} = \text{Total Cholesterol} - (\text{HDL-C} + \text{VLDL-C}) \quad \textbf{\textit{(Eq. 13-1)}}$$

TABLE 13-6
NCEP ATP III Classifications of Blood Lipids[8]

LDL-Cholesterol	
<100 mg/dL	Optimal
100–129 mg/dL	Near optimal or above optimal
130–159 mg/dL	Borderline high
160–189 mg/dL	High
≥190 mg/dL	Very high
Total Cholesterol	
<200 mg/dL	Desirable
200–239 mg/dL	Borderline high
≥240 mg/dL	High
HDL-Cholesterol	
<40 mg/dL	Low
≥60 mg/dL	High
Triglycerides	
<150 mg/dL	Normal
150–199 mg/dL	Borderline high
200–499 mg/dL	High
>500 mg/dL	Very high

HDL, high-density lipoprotein; LDL, low-density lipoprotein; NCEP ATP III, National Cholesterol Education Program Adult Treatment Panel III.

Because the ratio of cholesterol to TGs in VLDL is 1:5, VLDL-C is estimated by dividing the total TG level by 5. Thus, the formula is rewritten as:

$$\text{LDL-C} = \text{Total Cholesterol} - (\text{HDL-C} + \text{TG}/5) \quad \textit{(Eq. 13-2)}$$

Applying the formula to T.A.'s lipid profile, the calculated LDL-C is 224 mg/dL.

$$\begin{aligned}\text{LDL-C} &= \text{Total Cholesterol} - (\text{HDL-C} + \text{TG}/5)\\ &= 290 - (55 + 55/5)\\ &= 224 \text{ mg/dL} \quad \textit{(Eq. 13-3)}\end{aligned}$$

If the TG level is greater than 400 mg/dL, the formula for estimating VLDL-C is not accurate and, therefore, LDL-C cannot be calculated. An accurate LDL-C measurement also requires that the patient fast for 10 to 12 hours. This provides sufficient time for exogenous TGs, carried by chylomicrons, to be cleared from the systemic circulation (provided the patient does not have hyperchylomicronemia). Most laboratories can measure LDL-C directly and should be asked to do so only when the TG is greater than 400 mg/dL or the patient has not fasted.

Non–HDL-C is calculated by the following formula:

$$\text{Non–HDL-C} = \text{Total Cholesterol} - \text{HDL-C} \quad \textit{(Eq. 13-4)}$$

For T.A.:

$$\begin{aligned}\text{Non-HDC-C} &= 290 \text{ mg/dL} - 55 \text{ mg/dL}\\ &= 235 \text{ mg/dL} \quad \textit{(Eq. 13-5)}\end{aligned}$$

As mentioned previously, non–HDL-C can be calculated regardless of whether a patient is fasting or not because VLDL-C does not need to be estimated. This provides the clinician information of a patient's CHD risk when LDL-C cannot reliably be calculated.

Secondary Causes of High Blood Cholesterol

CASE 13-1, QUESTION 2: Is there any evidence that T.A.'s elevated LDL-C is secondary to other conditions or concurrent drug therapy?

As a routine, every new patient with hypercholesterolemia should be evaluated for four things in the following order: (a) secondary causes of the high cholesterol level, (b) familial disorders, (c) presence of CHD and CHD equivalents, and (d) CHD risk factors.

Conditions that can produce lipid abnormalities (i.e., secondary causes) include diabetes mellitus, hypothyroidism, nephrotic syndrome, and obstructive liver disease. Selected drugs can also produce lipid abnormalities (Table 13-7). When one of these secondary causes is identified, it should be managed first (unless there is a compelling reason to use the medication implicated), as this may resolve or improve the lipid abnormality.

In T.A.'s case, no secondary causes are evident. Her blood glucose level does not indicate the presence of diabetes; her TSH level does not indicate hypothyroidism; her ALT and AST levels are within acceptable levels, suggesting normal liver function; and her blood urea nitrogen, creatinine, and urinalysis are acceptable, signifying normal renal function. She is not taking any drugs that could have contributed to her cholesterol elevation.

Familial Forms of Hypercholesterolemia

CASE 13-1, QUESTION 3: Could T.A. have an inherited form of hyperlipidemia?

T.A.'s history is consistent with polygenic hypercholesterolemia, the form of hypercholesterolemia that affects 98% of patients with hypercholesterolemia. As described previously, polygenic hypercholesterolemia is suspected when the patient's LDL-C is 130 to 250 mg/dL and no evidence is seen of tendon xanthomas (Table 13-2). A family history of CHD is present in approximately 18% of these patients and is a strong finding in T.A.'s case. Polygenic hypercholesterolemia is caused by a combination of nutritional and genetic factors that reduce the clearance of LDL particles from the plasma. It is impossible to determine which of these factors are causing hypercholesterolemia in a given patient by simply examining the lipoprotein profile. If the patient's blood lipids normalize with a low-fat diet, however, one can assume that the diet is a major etiologic factor for that person. Conversely, if little or no change is seen in blood cholesterol levels after dietary modification, genetics likely significantly influences the patient's elevated cholesterol. In most cases, a relatively equal contribution is made by genetic factors and environment on cholesterol elevations. When patients are identified with severely elevated LDL-C such as T.A., systematic family screening of relatives should be conducted to identify other individuals, including children, who might be affected and at high risk of CHD.

Coronary Heart Disease and Coronary Heart Disease Risk Equivalents

CASE 13-1, QUESTION 4: Does T.A. have evidence of CHD or a CHD risk equivalent?

A search for CHD starts with a good medical history of symptomatic CAD, but is quickly followed with a broader search for atherosclerotic disease in other artery beds, including the arteries of the limbs and carotid arteries[8] (Table 13-8). If detected in one site, atherosclerosis is likely to be present in all or most vessels, and it is associated with a fivefold to sevenfold higher risk of a major coronary event.[142–144]

The patient should be asked about a history of myocardial ischemia (exercise-induced angina), prior MI (i.e., severe angina

TABLE 13-7
Drug-Induced Hyperlipidemia

	Effect on Plasma Lipids			
	Cholesterol (%)	Triglycerides (%)	HDL-C (%)	Comments
Diuretics				
Thiazides	↑5–7 initially ↑0–3 later	↑30–50	↑1	Effects transient; monitor for long-term effects
Loop	No change	No change	↓ to 15	
Indapamide	No change	No change	No change	
Metolazone	No change	No change	No change	
Potassium-sparing	No change	No change	No change	
β-Blockers				
Nonselective	No change	↑20—50	↓10–15	Selective β-blockers have greater effects than nonselective; β-blockers with ISA or α-blocking effects are lipid neutral
Selective	No change	↑15–30	↓5–10	
α-Blocking	No change or ↓	No change	No change	
α-Agonists and Antagonists (e.g., prazosin and clonidine)	↓0–10	↓ 0–20	↑0–15	In general, drugs that affect α-receptors ↓cholesterol and ↑HDL-C
ACE Inhibitors	No change	No change	No change	
Calcium-Channel Blockers	No change	No change	No change	
Oral contraceptives				
α-Monophasics	↑5–20	↑10–45	↑15 to ↓15	Effects caused by reduced lipolytic activity or ↑VLDL synthesis; mainly caused by progestin component; estrogen alone protective
α-Triphasics	↑10–15	↑10–15	↑5–10	
Glucocorticoids	↑5–10	↑15–20		
Ethanol	No change	↑up to 50	↑	Marked elevations can occur in patients who are hypertriglyceridemic
Isotretinoin	↑5–20	↑50–60	↓10–15	Changes may reverse 8 weeks after stopping drug
Cyclosporine	↑15–20	No change	No change	

ACE, angiotensin-converting enzyme; HDL-C, high-density lipoprotein cholesterol; ISA, intrinsic sympathomimetic activity; VLDL, very-low-density lipoprotein.

with elevated cardiac creatine phosphokinase [CPK] or characteristic ECG changes), history of revascularizations (i.e., coronary artery bypass surgery, angioplasty with percutaneous transluminal coronary angioplasty or stent placement), or history of hospitalization because of unstable angina (see Table 13-8). The presence of any of these findings is associated with a very high (>20%) risk of a CHD death or nonfatal MI in the next 10 years; the risk approaches 40% if unstable angina and stroke are also considered. None of these signs are present in T.A.

TABLE 13-8
NCEP APT III Definitions of CHD and CHD Risk Equivalents[a,8]

Clinical CHD
Myocardial ischemia (angina)
Myocardial infarction
Coronary angioplasty and/or stent placement
Coronary bypass graft
Prior unstable angina
Carotid Artery Disease
Stroke history
Transient ischemic attack history
Carotid stenosis >50%
Peripheral Arterial Disease
Claudication
ABI >0.9
Abdominal Aortic Aneurysm
Diabetes Mellitus

[a] Estimated global CHD risk >20% in 10 years for any of the factors listed.
ABI, ankle-to-brachial blood pressure index; CHD, coronary heart disease; NCEP ATP III, National Cholesterol Education Program Adult Treatment Panel III.

The evaluation can stop here, but some would advocate continuing the search with noninvasive procedures, even if the patient has not experienced symptoms (Table 13-9). The case for pursuing these evaluations is more convincing in patients who have a high probability of atherosclerosis because of the presence of multiple risk factors or a strong family history of premature CHD events. One noninvasive evaluation is exercise testing with either ECG monitoring for signs of ischemia or pharmacologic perfusion imaging (e.g., exercise thallium). Because these tests are expensive and not widely available, they are reserved for selected use. Even if the results are found to be normal, atherosclerosis is not ruled out because both tests are designed to detect flow-limiting disease, and atherosclerosis can be present without causing obstructions in luminal blood flow.[8]

In recent years, electron beam computed tomography and spiral computed tomography have been used to detect calcium in coronary vessels. The presence of coronary calcium suggests the presence of old atherosclerotic plaque. If old disease is present, then it is likely that younger, more vulnerable plaques are also present. This test is simple, quick, and noninvasive, but it is relatively expensive, not widely available, and not typically covered by insurance plans. High coronary calcium volume scores

TABLE 13-9
Emerging CHD Risk Factors[8]

Noninvasive Evaluations for Subclinical Atherosclerosis	Blood Tests
Exercise ECG	Lipoprotein(a)
Myocardial perfusion imaging	Small, dense LDL
Stress echocardiography	Apolipoprotein B (particle concentration)
Carotid intimal-medial thickness (IMT)	High-sensitivity CRP (and other inflammatory markers)
Electron beam computed tomography (EBCT)	Homocysteine
	HDL subspecies
	Apolipoprotein A-I
	Apolipoprotein B:C-III
	Thrombogenic factors (e.g., fibrinogen, PAI-1, t-PA)
	LP-PLA$_2$

CHD, coronary heart disease; CRP, C-reactive protein; ECG, electrocardiogram; HDL, high-density lipoprotein cholesterol; LDL, low-density lipoprotein; LP-PLA$_2$, lipoprotein associated phospholipase A$_2$; PAI, plasminogen activator inhibitor; t-PA, tissue plasminogen activator.

can add to the prediction of future coronary events based on traditional risk factor assessment.[8] Use of these tests is particularly helpful in modifying the assessment of risk in patients with multiple risk factors. In T.A.'s case, her strong family history could support obtaining an electron beam computed tomography evaluation. If she has a significantly positive calcium volume score, more aggressive medical therapy could be considered.

A good history should also probe for evidence of atherosclerotic vascular disease in peripheral vessels. Patients with flow-limiting atherosclerosis in peripheral vessels often describe claudication (pain and weakness in the limb muscles) after walking a distance (see Chapter 15, Peripheral Vascular Disorders). NCEP recommends that patients older than 50 years of age be evaluated with an ankle-to-brachial index (ABI). This index is determined by measuring the systolic blood pressure of the brachial, posterior tibia, and dorsalis pedis arteries using a handheld Doppler device and dividing the higher of the two ankle systolic blood pressures by the higher of two systolic brachial pressures.[8] An ABI of less than 0.9 constitutes the diagnosis of peripheral vascular disease (PVD; also called peripheral arterial disease). Finding atherosclerosis in peripheral vessels probably means it is present in coronary arteries as well. In fact, most patients with PVD die of a CHD event. Furthermore, most patients with PVD have a very high (>20%) risk of a CHD event in the next 10 years, and so are said to have a CHD risk equivalent.

The clinician should also evaluate the patient for atherosclerosis in the carotid vessels by asking about signs and symptoms of transient ischemic attacks and strokes. On the physical examination, the carotid vessels should be evaluated for the presence of a bruit (indicative of a space-occupying lesion in the carotid vessel). If a bruit is present, further evaluation with carotid duplex imaging is indicated to detect stenotic lesions. Some authorities recommend performing carotid sonography to measure the carotid intimal-medial thickness (CIMT). This test is safe and simple but relatively expensive and not widely available. Intimal-medial thickness results correlate with the severity of coronary atherosclerosis. Patients who have experienced a stroke or transient ischemic attack have a more than 20% 10-year risk of experiencing a CHD event and so are also considered a CHD risk equivalent. Patients found to have a stenosis of greater than 50% in their carotid vessel, even if asymptomatic, have a more than 20% 10-year CHD risk and again can be considered a CHD risk equivalent. Patients found to have an increased intimal-medial thickness, suggesting the presence of subclinical atherosclerosis, may also have a high CHD risk and, therefore, are candidates for more aggressive medical therapy.[8]

Other conditions that confer a greater than 20% risk of a CHD event in the next 10 years, and thus are considered by NCEP to be CHD risk equivalents, include abdominal aortic aneurysm and the diagnosis of diabetes. More will be said about diabetes subsequently. T.A. does not have evidence of CHD or a CHD risk equivalent.

CORONARY HEART DISEASE RISK FACTORS

CASE 13-1, QUESTION 5: Does T.A. have CHD risk factors, and what is her global CHD risk?

Patients who are found to have CHD or CHD risk equivalent do not need a risk factor assessment to establish their LDL-C treatment goal; the presence of CHD or a CHD risk equivalent satisfies that. These patients, however, should have an appraisal of risk factors so that risk-factor modification can be incorporated in the overall treatment plan. For patients who do not have CHD or a CHD risk equivalent, risk-factor counting and global risk assessment is important to quantify baseline risk and to establish initial treatment goals and approaches.

Begin this process by counting the number of risk factors present (Table 13-4). Patients with either zero or one risk factor most likely have a low risk of a CHD event in the next 10 years and are assigned an LDL-C goal of less than 160 mg/dL. Patients with two or more risk factors have a moderate to high risk, depending on the number and type of risk factors present. NCEP recommends that patients who have two or more risk factors be further evaluated using the Framingham-based global risk assessment tool (**http://hp2010.nhlbihin.net/atpiii/calculator.asp?usertype=prof**) to define the 10-year risk. Patients with two or more risk factors have an LDL-C goal of at least less than 130 mg/dL. The clinician, however, has the option to treat these patients to reach less than 100 mg/dL depending on clinical judgment of the patient's absolute risk and potential benefit if that patient's Framingham calculated 10-year CHD risk is between 10% and 20%. If the patient's calculated risk is more than 20%, their risk is equivalent to someone with CHD and their LDL-C goal is less than 100 mg/dL. The presence of modifiable risk factors should become the target of any risk-reduction treatment program. It is important to note that the Framingham risk score is recommended to patient-specific baseline risk of a CHD event and baseline LDL-C goals. Although it is tempting to recalculate risk in primary prevention patients once risk factors have been modified, it is not the intent to use the Framingham risk score to guide therapy in a primary prevention patient with multiple major CV risk factors.

T.A. has two CHD risk factors: current cigarette smoking and a family history of premature CHD. She thus has an LDL-C treatment goal of less than 130 mg/dL (Table 13-10). T.A. is found to have a 5% 10-year CHD risk, which is several times greater than the average risk for women her age but below the threshold at which aggressive drug treatment is indicated (i.e., >10% CHD risk in 10 years). If she were not a smoker, her 10-year CHD risk estimate would be 1%, illustrating the prominent influence that smoking has on her future risk of a CHD event.

Based on this assessment and assuming that the noninvasive assessments performed on her, if any, were negative, T.A. should be counseled on diet and exercise and strongly advised to stop smoking. Because of its strong effect on her risk, smoking cessation (see Chapter 88, Tobacco Use and Dependence) should be a primary focus of her risk-reduction program. If these measures

TABLE 13-10
NCEP ATP III and AHA/ACC LDL-C Goals and Cut Points for Therapeutic Lifestyle Changes (TLC) and Drug Therapy[8,107,108]

Risk Category	LDL-C Goal	LDL-C at Which to Initiate TLC	LDL-C at Which to Consider Drug Therapy[a]
CHD or CHD risk equivalents (10-year risk >20%)	<100 mg/dL (Optional goal <70 mg/dL)[c]	>100 mg/dL	>100 mg/dL (<100 mg/dL; consider drug options)[b]
2+ risk factors (10-year risk 10% to 20%)	<130 mg/dL (Optional goal <100 mg/dL)	>130 mg/dL	>130 mg/dL (100–129 mg/dL; consider drug options)[d]
2+ risk factors (10-year risk <10%)	<130 mg/dL	>130 mg/dL	>160 mg/dL
<2 risk factors[e]	<160 mg/dL	>160 mg/dL	190 mg/dL (160–189 mg/dL; LDL-C–lowering drug therapy is optional)

[a] For all patients without CHD: LDL-C–lowering medications should be initiated at a dose that is consistent with at least a 30% to 40% reduction in LDL-C levels. The use of lower doses just to barely attain the LDL-C goal would not be a prudent use of medications.
[b] The clinician may select niacin or fibrate therapy if patient has high triglycerides or low HDL-C. The decision to lower LDL-C with drug therapy is optional based on available clinical trial evidence.
[c] All patients with CHD: When LDL-C <70 mg/dL is not achievable because of high baseline LDL-C levels, it generally is possible to achieve reductions of >50% by either statins or LDL-C–lowering drug combinations.
[d] The decision to lower LDL-C with drug therapy to achieve an LDL-C <100 mg/dL is optional based on available clinical trial evidence.
[e] Patients with fewer than two risk factors usually have a 10-year risk of <10%, and therefore do not need a 10-year risk assessment.
AHA/ACC, American Heart Association/American College of Cardiology; CHD, coronary heart disease; LDL-C, low-density lipoprotein cholesterol; NCEP ATP III, National Cholesterol Education Program Adult Treatment Panel III.

fail to bring her LDL-C to her treatment goal of less than 130 mg/dL and her LDL-C remains 160 mg/dL or more, drug therapy should be considered (Table 13-10). If she stopped smoking, however, she would have only one risk factor (family history), and her new LDL-C goal would be less than 160 mg/dL. In this case, drug therapy would be considered only if the LDL-C remains 190 mg/dL or more.

Therapy for Lowering Cholesterol Levels

DIET THERAPY

CASE 13-1, QUESTION 6: What lifestyle changes should be recommended to T.A.?

The centerpiece of treatment for high blood cholesterol is a diet low in saturated fat and cholesterol. The TLC diet recommended by NCEP restricts total fat intake to 25% to 35% of calories, saturated fats to less than 7% of calories, and dietary cholesterol to 200 mg/day (Table 13-11).[8] The TLC diet is aggressive and requires instruction by a dietitian, nurse, or other health professional well versed in nutrition counseling. The TLC diet is also flexible and allows for modification of carbohydrate and monounsaturated fat intake according to the individual patient's needs. The goals presented by the TLC diet are minimal goals, and some patients will want to exceed them, even to the point of following a vegetarian diet. This is permissible, as long as the diet is nutritionally balanced.

TABLE 13-11
NCEP ATP III Therapeutic Lifestyle Change Diet[8]

Nutrient	Recommended Intake
Total fat	25%–35% of total calories
Saturated fat	<7% of total calories
Polyunsaturated fat	Up to 10% of total calories
Monounsaturated fat	Up to 20% of total calories
Carbohydrate	50%–60% of total calories
Fiber	20–30 g/day
Cholesterol	<200 mg/d
Protein	Approx. 15% of total calories

When saturated fat is removed from the diet, it is important to understand what should be given in replacement. In the overweight or obese patient, it may be appropriate to do nothing, because a reduction in saturated fat is a good way to lower calories and encourage weight loss.

In individuals who are close to their ideal weight, such as T.A., replacing saturated fats with carbohydrates may not be the best choice. Increased intake of sugar and highly refined starches, as found in the many low-fat, high-calorie snack foods, may actually increase weight and reduce HDL-C as well as LDL-C.[145] More importantly, a low-fat, high-carbohydrate diet has not been shown to reduce the risk of CHD. Consumption of complex carbohydrates is recommended, however, and could be a replacement for saturated fat calories in a TLC diet.

Replacing saturated fat with unsaturated fats, especially monounsaturated fats (e.g., canola oil or olive oil products) and omega-3 polyunsaturated fats (e.g., fish oil sources), is highly desirable.[146] This is the diet of the Mediterranean people, who have a low incidence of CHD, and has the advantage of lowering LDL-C without affecting HDL-C. In fact, in a major randomized clinical trial in which the Mediterranean diet was compared with a "prudent Western-type diet," the Mediterranean diet was associated with a greater than 70% reduction in cardiovascular end points and total mortality, a result that exceeds that achieved by the best lipid-lowering drug trials.[147] This study alone illustrates how important it is to initiate a good diet in hyperlipidemic patients, even with the availability of very potent, highly efficacious, and safe drugs to lower serum cholesterol levels.

In Western society, diets high in protein and saturated fats and low in carbohydrates (e.g., Atkins diet) promise quick weight loss and other health effects. Although these diets can reduce lipid levels and cause weight loss, they are not nutritionally sound and may even be unhealthy. Patients should be advised to avoid them.

T.A. is likely to need help in translating the dietary recommendations of a TLC diet into practical terms and concepts that she can easily implement in her everyday life. Two approaches can be used to achieve this: (a) teach her to count calories or (b) provide general guidance in the selection of low-fat foods.

The more sophisticated patient may want to count calories or grams of total and saturated fat per day. The first step in teaching a patient to do this is to determine his or her daily caloric requirements, adjusted for his or her level of activity. The average caloric requirement for women is 1,800 calories/day; for men it is 2,500 calories/day. Based on this, T.A. should be instructed to keep her total fat intake to 450 to 630 calories/day (25% to 35% of calories) and saturated fat to less than 126 calories/day (<7% of total calories). Converting fat calories to grams (i.e., dividing calories by 9 cal/g), T.A. should be instructed to restrict her total fat intake to less than 50 to 70 g/day and saturated fat to less than 14 g/day.

Once these calculations have been made, the next step is to teach T.A. how to determine the grams of saturated and unsaturated fat contained in the foods she eats by reading food labels and referring to reference charts or books that list the nutritional content of foods. A good source for this nutrition information is the National Institutes of Health website on Therapeutic Lifestyle Change (**http://www.nhlbi.nih.gov/health/public/heart/index.htm**) under the Health Information icon. This site contains information on the TLC diet, a 10-year risk calculator, recipes, a virtual grocery store, a cyberkitchen, a fitness room, and a resource library. The AHA sites (**http://www.heart.org/HEARTORG/GettingHealthy/GettingHealthy_UCM_001078_SubHomePage.jsp** and **http://www.deliciousdecisions.org**) provide equally good information on risk assessment, a cholesterol tracker, low-fat recipes, and guidance for eating in restaurants, cooking, and fitness.

For patients who are not able or willing to count calories or grams, general instruction on how to select low-fat foods and control portion sizes of higher-fat foods would provide an alternative approach. Principles to teach include the following:

- Eat less high-fat food (especially food high in saturated fats).
- Replace saturated fats with polyunsaturated and monounsaturated fats and fish oils whenever possible.
- Eat less high-cholesterol food.
- Choose foods high in complex carbohydrates (starch and fiber).
- Attain and maintain an acceptable weight.

T.A. should be counseled to recognize and minimize the three main sources of saturated fats in her diet: meat products, dairy products, and oils used in processed foods and cooking.

All meat products, including beef, pork, and poultry, contain fat. Much of the fat is visible and should be trimmed off before consumption. The remaining fat is contained within the meat and can be limited by (a) selecting the leanest meat (e.g., lean beef, skinless chicken, fish), (b) limiting portion size to about the size of a deck of playing cards (no more than 6 ounces/day), and (c) cooking the meat in a manner that allows the fat to drip away from the meat (i.e., broiling, grilling).

High-fat dairy products are made with whole milk (~4% fat); low-fat alternatives are made with skim or 1% milk (which contain all of the nutrient value of whole-milk products). T.A. should be taught to substitute low-fat alternatives for high-fat products—for example, by choosing soft margarine (or no fatty spread at all) instead of stick butter (note that unsaturated fats exist normally in liquid form and saturated fats in solid form); nonfat creams rather than whole-milk creams; low-fat or nonfat soft cheese (e.g., cottage cheese) rather than natural or processed hard cheese (including cream cheese); skim milk rather than whole milk; light or nonfat sour cream rather than regular sour cream; and nonfat frozen yogurt rather than ice cream. She also should avoid or limit cream sauces on meats and vegetables and creamy soups.

Products prepared with coconut, palm, or palm kernel oils, as well as lard and bacon fat, contain a high concentration of saturated fats, and intake should be restricted. In their place, products made with monounsaturated fats (e.g., olive oil, canola oil) or polyunsaturated fats (especially oils that contain omega-3 fatty acids) may be substituted. Monounsaturated fats have little or no effect on blood lipids, and polyunsaturated fats actually may help reduce total cholesterol. Also, when the "good" (unsaturated) oils are partially hydrogenated (i.e., saturated to make them solid, as in some margarine products), they take on the character of saturated oils and may raise cholesterol levels. These are called *trans fatty acids*. Major sources of saturated and *trans* fatty acids include cakes, pies, cookies, chips, and crackers. T.A. should be advised to avoid or limit not only saturated fats, but also *trans* fatty acids by reading food labels.

It is best not to give the patient a list of foods to avoid; this aversive approach is likely to fail. Rather, good instruction about a low-fat diet should teach the patient how to make good selections. Any food, even a high-fat food, is not prohibited as long as portion size and frequency of use are controlled.

Another dietary approach to lowering blood cholesterol is to use dietary adjuncts. For example, adding 5 to 10 g of viscous fiber (e.g., guar, pectin, oat gum, psyllium) or other dietary sources of fiber (e.g., vegetables, legumes, whole grains, fruits) to the diet daily will aid in lowering blood cholesterol levels about 5% on average. Also, plant stanol and sterol esters have been made available in margarine and salad dressing products and can lower LDL-C 5% to 15% when the equivalent of one tablespoonful is ingested one to three times a day. They act by reducing the absorption of cholesterol in the intestine. The estimated cumulative percent reduction in LDL-C achievable through TLC is between 20% and 30%.

T.A. will need to follow a low-fat diet indefinitely to sustain its benefit. For this reason, it might be necessary to have T.A. work with a registered dietitian or other professional who understands low-fat, low-cholesterol diets and who can give her personalized instruction. Particularly important is instruction on how to shop for and prepare low-fat foods and how to select low-fat foods in restaurants.

EFFECT ON LOW-DENSITY LIPOPROTEIN CHOLESTEROL

CASE 13-1, QUESTION 7: What changes in T.A.'s LDL-C can be expected if she follows a TLC diet?

LDL-C is reported to be reduced by an average of 3% to 14% in men who restrict saturated fat to less than 10% of calories; a slightly smaller response is attained in women, perhaps because their intake of saturated fats is generally lower than that of men.[148–150] Patients who can restrict saturated fat intake to less than 7% of daily calories should experience an additional 3% to 7% average reduction. Most patients can attain at least a 5% reduction in cholesterol levels with a TLC diet, some patients much more. If dietary adjuncts are added, LDL-C may be lowered by an additional 5% to 15%.

Patients' response to a low-fat diet is variable. In some patients, blood cholesterol levels fall substantially, whereas in others practically no change occurs. Response to a low-fat diet depends on many factors, including the patient's dietary habits before implementing the low-fat diet, the patient's adherence with the diet, the degree to which the patient restricts fats and cholesterol, and the influence of genetic factors. The patient should not be discouraged if LDL-C levels do not change much or at all despite close adherence to the diet. The Mediterranean diet, for example, which is high in monounsaturated fats and fiber, has no appreciable effect on blood lipids, but can still reduce cardiovascular disease and mortality by 70%.[147] Patients who adhere to a low-fat diet might also respond to lower doses of lipid-lowering drugs.

Because T.A. is a woman and was following a low-fat diet before her diagnosis, a TLC diet is not likely to have a substantial effect on her blood cholesterol levels. It would be prudent to have her maintain a 3-day diary of everything she eats to allow a more objective view of her eating habits. If there are ways for her to improve her diet, this approach will reveal them.

OTHER LIFESTYLE CHANGES

CASE 13-1, QUESTION 8: What other modifications in behavior are prescribed in the TLC program?

Weight reduction in the overweight patient can reduce LDL-C and is a key component to the TLC plan. A 5- to 10-pound weight loss, for example, can up to double the LDL-C reduction achieved with a low saturated fat diet alone.[148] The predominant effect of weight loss is a reduction in serum TGs and a small increase in HDL-C, however.[151] In addition, weight reduction may offset the risk of developing hypertension and diabetes. The initial goal of a weight loss program is to reduce body weight by approximately 10% within about 6 months.[152] This is best achieved by restricting total daily energy consumption through a reduction in saturated and *trans* fatty acid intake and by increasing physical exercise. A normal weight is defined as a body mass index (BMI) between 18.5 and 24.9 kg/m^2, and a desirable waist circumference is less than 40 inches for male patients (<35 for Asian American men) and less than 35 inches for female patients (<31 for Asian American women).[152] Because T.A. has an acceptable weight, these considerations do not apply.

Smoking cessation substantially reduces the risk of CHD, pulmonary disease, and cancer and is a central component of a TLC program. This is an important consideration in T.A. The CHD risk she has from smoking is greater than the risk she has from her LDL-C elevation. By stopping smoking, T.A. will not only increase her HDL-C,[153] but will also substantially alter her risk profile. Because most patients gain weight when they stop smoking and because weight gain may worsen lipid levels, plans need to be made to alter her diet and increase physical activity to counter these effects.

Increasing physical activity should be a component of the treatment of any patient with any form of dyslipidemia. Regular physical exercise may reduce TG and VLDL-C levels, raise HDL-C levels slightly, promote weight loss or maintenance of desired weight, lower BP, and cause favorable changes in coronary blood flow.[154] Regular aerobic exercise (e.g., brisk walking, jogging, swimming, bicycling, and tennis) should be prescribed in terms of amount (e.g., walking 4 miles), intensity (e.g., walking 4 mph), and frequency (walking each day if possible, but at least three times a week). T.A. states that she is already physically active. The level of her activity should be documented and enhancements recommended if needed.

GOAL OF THERAPY

CASE 13-1, QUESTION 9: A fasting lipid profile obtained 12 weeks after T.A. initiated a TLC diet and exercise program and had stopped smoking revealed an LDL-C level of 195 mg/dL; HDL-C increased slightly and TG did not differ from baseline values. What is your assessment of the need for additional lipid-modifying treatment?

Based on her initial assessment, T.A.'s LDL-C goal is less than 130 mg/dL; drug therapy can be considered if her LDL-C is more than 160 mg/dL (Table 13-10). NCEP recommends that drugs be considered in patients with fewer than two risk factors if their LDL-C remains 160 mg/dL or more after implementing a TLC plan. Realistically, this is a therapeutic gray area in which clinical judgment must be exercised. T.A. has a relatively low risk of CHD (based on her Framingham score) despite her current LDL-C level. Her strong family history of premature CHD suggests, however, there is more to the story than LDL-C alone. NCEP also advises that when LDL-lowering drug therapy is used in high-risk or moderately high-risk persons, the intensity of therapy be sufficient to achieve at least a 30% to 40% reduction in LDL-C levels. In patients with an LDL-C goal of less than 70 mg/dL (patients with CHD or acute coronary syndrome), it may not be possible to attain such low levels of LDL-C because of high baseline levels. In such patients, LDL-C reductions of 50% or greater are recommended.[108]

EMERGING RISK FACTORS

CASE 13-1, QUESTION 10: To help determine whether to initiate lipid-lowering drug therapy in T.A., is there value in ordering additional laboratory tests to identify possible emerging risk factors?

As mentioned in Case 13-1, Question 4, noninvasive tests, such as ABI, CIMT, and electron beam computed tomography, can uncover evidence of subclinical atherosclerotic disease and help the clinician decide whether to pursue more aggressive therapy with lipid-lowering drugs. In addition, the clinician can measure several specialized laboratory tests of emerging risk factors to help with these decisions (Table 13-9). In T.A.'s case, a global risk assessment indicating about a 1% risk of a CHD event in 10 years and her strong family history for premature CHD events present conflicting information. Measuring one or more of the emerging risk factors may help focus the treatment decision in one direction or another.

Lipoprotein(a) (Lp(a), pronounced *el, pee, aye*) appears to be an independent risk factor for CHD, although this is not a universal finding.[155] This very small cholesterol-containing lipoprotein particle contains apolipoprotein a. Its structure suggests that it could be an important source of cholesterol for the formation of atherosclerosis as well as a stimulus for thrombogenic mechanisms. High Lp(a) levels suggest a high CHD risk and support a more aggressive approach to lowering LDL-C. Evidence has shown that lowering LDL-C aggressively can overcome the increased CHD risk predicted by an elevated Lp(a) level. The only drug that can lower Lp(a) is niacin, but no studies have shown that giving niacin to these patients reduces CHD risk.

Apolipoprotein B is a marker for the number of atherogenic lipoproteins (VLDL, VLDL remnants, IDL, Lp(a), and LDL) in the circulation. It is a strong predictor of CHD risk, at least as strong as LDL-C. It is a surrogate for LDL-C, but provides different information.[156] Some specialists prefer to use apolipoprotein B levels rather than, or in addition to, LDL-C in treating patients. Apolipoprotein B levels as well as non–HDL-C are usually disproportionately high in patients with high TGs, although they may also parallel LDL-C levels.

Severe elevations in homocysteine are positively correlated with CHD risk, especially in patients with inherited forms of hyperhomocysteinemia.[157] High levels of homocysteine are easily treated with B-complex vitamins pyridoxine (B_6), cobalamin (B_{12}), and folic acid; the recent fortification of foods with folic acid is predicted to substantially reduce homocysteine levels. However, several clinical trials have failed to demonstrate the benefits of treating hyperhomocysteinemia on CHD events. Thus, measuring homocysteine levels in T.A. would not be useful.

Atherosclerosis is a chronic low-grade inflammatory disease. Thus, markers of inflammation have been sought to measure arterial inflammation. As mentioned previously, hs-CRP has been well studied. Many observational studies have found that hs-CRP predicts a twofold to fourfold increase in CHD risk over what is predicted by LDL-C alone.[138] The AHA defined cut-off points for hs-CRP levels as follows: low risk (<1.0 mg/L), average risk

two or three divided doses daily) and slowly titrated as tolerated (e.g., daily doses increased by 250 mg every 3 to 7 days) to a maximum of 3,000 mg/day (Table 13-14). Higher doses have been used but are associated with unpleasant side effects. Niacin is also the only drug that lowers Lp(a), with reductions being as great as 30%.[174] Its metabolite, nicotinamide, has no effect on cholesterol and should not be used as a substitute to lower side effects. Herbal supplement products advertised as "flush-free" contain niacinamide or inositol hexanicotinate. These products do not cause flushing, but also contain minimal or no free, pharmacologically active niacin and thus lack lipid-altering effects.

Sustained-release (timed-release) dosage forms of niacin were developed to reduce the flushing side effects associated with crystalline niacin. These products are sold as a dietary supplement ostensibly for treating niacin deficiency, but are mistakenly purchased by patients to treat high blood cholesterol. These products may have slightly greater LDL-C–lowering efficacy at each dose level and slightly less HDL-C and TG effects compared with crystalline niacin, but they cannot be recommended because of a substantially increased risk of liver toxicity at higher dosages (see Adverse Effects section).

An extended-release dosage form of niacin, Niaspan, is available by prescription to treat elevated cholesterol and TG levels and appears to be better tolerated than either the crystalline or sustained-release forms. Extended-release niacin releases niacin for an 8- to 12-hour period, a feature that turns out to be important in improving its side effect profile, and it has the efficacy pattern of crystalline niacin. It lowers LDL-C by 10% to 15% and TGs by 20% to 30%, and it raises HDL-C by 15% to 25%, with daily doses between 1,000 and 2,000 mg. Daily doses of extended-release niacin should not exceed 2,000 mg/day to reduce the risk of liver side effects.

Mechanism of Action

Niacin inhibits the mobilization of free fatty acids from peripheral adipose tissue to the liver, which, either alone or together with other hepatic effects, results in reduced synthesis and secretion of VLDL particles by the liver.[175] This explains its effectiveness in lowering TG levels. Because LDL is a VLDL degradation product, reducing the secretion of VLDL particles secondarily lowers the LDL-C level. Niacin reduces the amount of apolipoprotein A-I extracted and catabolized from HDL during the hepatic uptake of cholesterol, thus preserving the structural and functional integrity of HDL particles.[176] As a result, cholesterol-deficient apolipoprotein A-I–containing HDL particles are recirculated from the liver to the peripheral cells, maintaining HDL levels and enhancing reverse cholesterol transport.[177]

Adverse Effects

The differences in release characteristics among various niacin products are important because they determine how the drug is metabolized, in turn influencing the side effect profile of the product. Niacin is metabolized through two separate metabolic pathways.[178] The nicotinamide (NAM) pathway is a high-affinity, low-capacity pathway. Crystalline niacin quickly saturates this pathway and is predominately metabolized through the high-capacity conjugation pathway. The flushing effect with crystalline niacin results from prostaglandin-mediated vasodilation associated with the formation of nicotinuric acid by the conjugation pathway. In contrast, sustained-release niacin is slowly absorbed and preferentially metabolized via the NAM pathway. Because of this, sustained-release niacin causes less flushing, but it can cause serious, dose-related hepatotoxicity because of the formation of toxic metabolites with the NAM pathway. Extended-release niacin, with its intermediate absorption rate, has a more balanced metabolism between the two pathways. The result is less flushing and less risk of hepatotoxicity, at least with daily doses of 2 g or less.

The main drawbacks to crystalline niacin therapy are frequent, bothersome vasodilation-related side effects: flushing, itching, and headache[161,173,179] (Table 13-15). The mechanism of cutaneous flushing is secondary to vasodilatory prostaglandins released from Langerhans cells in epidermis after nicotinic acid binds to the GPR109A receptor. These prostaglandins bind to prostaglandin D_2 type 1 receptors on vascular smooth muscle cells, causing relaxation and vasodilation.[180] A prostaglandin D_2 type 1 receptor antagonist is currently being evaluated in combination with extended-release niacin. Practically every patient will experience these side effects, at least transiently.[181] These symptoms can be reduced by having patients take doses with food and by taking 325 mg of aspirin 30 minutes before the morning dose of niacin (to inhibit prostaglandin synthesis, which is thought to mediate these side effects).[182] Use of extended-release niacin can further reduce these symptoms, and administering it once daily at bedtime can diminish the patient's awareness of flushing symptoms. Niacin also can cause fatigue and a variety of GI symptoms, including nausea, dyspepsia, and activation of peptic ulcer. As with flushing, GI side effects are minimized by taking the drug with food. Other less common, although potentially troublesome, side effects of niacin are hyperuricemia, gout, and transient worsening of glucose tolerance in some diabetic patients (Table 13-15).

The most worrisome side effect associated with niacin is hepatotoxicity, which is associated almost exclusively with the sustained-release forms of niacin.[161,183] Hepatotoxicity is detected by an increase in liver transaminase enzymes exceeding three times the upper limit of normal; in severe cases, this can be accompanied by symptoms such as fatigue, anorexia, malaise, and nausea. This side effect occurs when daily doses of sustained-release niacin exceed 1,500 mg. Hepatotoxicity has been reported to occur in up to half of the patients titrated to daily doses of 3,000 mg of sustained-release niacin; many of these patients had symptoms, as well as laboratory findings, consistent with toxicity.[161] Conversely, less than 1% of patients titrated up to 2,000 mg/day of extended-release niacin have elevated liver function tests. Rare cases of fulminant hepatitis have been reported with sustained-release niacin. Niacin-induced hepatotoxicity appears to be completely reversible when the drug is discontinued.

Because of the hepatotoxic effects of sustained-release niacin and the flushing side effects of crystalline niacin, extended-release niacin is the preferred form of niacin for general use. It can be safely used in a daily dose up to 2,000 mg. An estimated 30% of patients experience flushing symptoms that will cause them to discontinue therapy.

No apparent contraindications are seen to the use of niacin in L.W. Niacin, however, would not be expected to lower his LDL-C by the 35% to 50% required to reach his treatment goal of less than 130 mg/dL or less than 100 mg/dL (optional goal), respectively.

STATINS

Clinical Use

The group of drugs with the most potent cholesterol-lowering potential is the statins. They lower LDL-C by approximately 20% to 46% with initial doses and 35% to 60% with maximal doses[184,185] (Table 13-13). Statins also reduce TG levels by 15% to 45% and increase HDL-C modestly (5% to 8%; Table 13-16). The LDL-C lowering achieved is dose dependent and log linear. Low dosages produce substantial LDL-C–lowering effects, and with each doubling of the daily dose, LDL-C is lowered an additional 6% to 7% on average (Table 13-13).

TABLE 13-16

Average Effects of Selected Drugs on Lipoprotein Cholesterol and Triglycerides

Drug	LDL (%)	HDL (%)	TG (%)
Bile acid resin	–15 to –30	±3	+3 to –10
Ezetimibe	–18 to –22	0 to 2	0 to –5
Niacin	–15 to –30	20 to 35	–30 to –60
Statin	–25 to –60	5 to 15	–10 to –45
Fibrates	±10 to –25	10 to 30	–30 to –60

HDL, high-density lipoprotein; LDL, low-density lipoprotein; TG, triglycerides.

The currently available statins are atorvastatin, fluvastatin, lovastatin, pravastatin, rosuvastatin, pitavastatin, and simvastatin. Rosuvastatin provides the most substantial LDL-C lowering, followed by atorvastatin, simvastatin, pitavastatin, lovastatin, pravastatin, and fluvastatin in descending order. With clinical trial evidence that lower LDL-C levels are associated with less CHD, higher initial doses of these statins are being advocated, thus blurring these LDL-C differences. The efficacy of many statins is greater if administered in the evening to coincide with the nighttime upturn in endogenous cholesterol biosynthesis; atorvastatin, and rosuvastatin with a longer half-life and more potent LDL-C lowering, may be administered without regard to time of day. The LDL-C–lowering efficacy of twice-daily administration of statins is slightly greater (by 2% to 4%) than once-daily evening doses, but this difference is rarely sufficient to make a clinical difference. The bioavailability of lovastatin is improved by administration with food; thus, it is recommended for dosing with the evening meal. This, too, may not make much difference in the clinical setting.

The major statin trials described earlier in this chapter demonstrate that statins can significantly reduce CHD death and nonfatal MI, revascularization procedures, strokes, and total mortality. The complete mechanism for these beneficial outcomes is not fully known, but appears to be largely attributable to LDL-C reduction.[129] Most authorities believe that the CHD event reduction with statins is a class effect and can be accomplished with any of the available statins. This, coupled with their favorable safety profile and their potency in lowering LDL-C, supports the NCEP ATP III recommendation that statins are the drugs of first choice to lower cholesterol and reduce CHD risk.[8,186]

Mechanism of Action

Statins competitively inhibit the enzyme responsible for converting HMG-CoA to mevalonate in an early, rate-limiting step in the biosynthetic pathway of cholesterol (Fig. 13-1).[13] Reduction in hepatocellular cholesterol prompts an upregulation of LDL receptor proteins and thus increases the clearance of circulating LDL particles from the blood. The TG-lowering effects appear to be produced in two ways: by an increase in the clearance of VLDL and VLDL remnant particles from the systemic circulation (by the upregulation of LDL receptors) and by a reduced secretion of VLDL particles from the liver.[187–189] All statins have the ability to lower TG levels. Their TG-lowering efficacy is related, however, to their LDL-C–lowering effectiveness (thus, statins with greater LDL-C–lowering efficacy will have greater TG-lowering efficacy) and to the patient's baseline TG level (the higher the TG level, the greater the percentage of reduction produced by the statin).

Adverse Effects of Statins

CASE 13-2, QUESTION 3: L.W.'s provider decides to start therapy with 20 mg/day of simvastatin. Several days after starting the drug, he played tennis for the first time in several years. The next morning he experiences new leg and arm pain. He had been warned that statins can cause muscle damage. He does not complain of any other side effects since starting the drug. Could this be a side effect of simvastatin? Should he discontinue the therapy?

Statins are well tolerated by most patients. Headache, myalgias (without CPK changes), and GI symptoms, including dyspepsia, flatus, constipation, and abdominal pain, occasionally are experienced (Table 13-15).[184,190,191] These symptoms are usually mild and disappear with continued therapy. The statin side effects receiving the most attention include increases in liver function tests and myopathy. These two problems are described in detail next.

Statins can cause an elevation in transaminase enzyme levels of more than three times the upper limit of normal (ULN) in 1% to 1.5% of patients in a dose-dependent manner. The transaminase level can return to normal spontaneously even with continued statin therapy. Similarly, elevations in transaminase will return to normal if the statin is discontinued. Rechallenge with the same or a different statin after enzymes have returned to normal limits is acceptable. If the drug is tolerated on rechallenge, it can be continued; recurrence of transaminase elevation warrants further evaluation of other potential causes. The report of the National Lipid Association Statin Safety Task Force recommends if ALT or AST is one to three times the ULN during statin therapy, there is no need to discontinue the statin.[192] If ALT or AST exceeds three times the ULN during statin therapy, monitor the patient and repeat the transaminase measures. There is no need to discontinue the statin. If a patient's transaminase levels continue to rise or if there is further objective evidence (i.e., hepatomegaly, jaundice, elevated direct bilirubin, related symptoms) of liver injury, the statin should be discontinued. The estimated incidence of statin-associated liver failure is 1 per million person-years of use.[193] There is some evidence that patients with chronic liver disease, nonalcoholic fatty liver disease, or nonalcoholic steatohepatitis may safely receive statin therapy and may improve liver function tests.[194]

The potential for muscle toxicity is a different matter. Myositis, defined as the presence of muscle symptoms, including aches, soreness, or weakness, and an increase in serum CPK more than 10 times the ULN, occurs in approximately 0.1% to 1% of patients in a dose-dependent manner.[192] Myalgias (muscle ache or weakness without CPK elevations) occurs in approximately 5% of patients. Routine monitoring of CPK levels is unnecessary; rather, unexplained symptoms of muscle aches, weakness, or soreness should prompt a CPK evaluation. If myositis is present, a careful history is necessary to rule out usual causes (i.e., trauma, increased physical activity). If no explanation is present for the findings and the CPK is elevated (>10 times the ULN), the statin should be withdrawn until CPK levels return to normal. Occasionally, symptoms of myalgia are bothersome or intolerable to the patient, even with a normal CPK or one that is elevated but less than 10 times the ULN. In these cases, the statin should be discontinued. Once symptoms subside, statin therapy can be restarted at the same or reduced dose, or with a different statin. Alternate day and even once-weekly dosing of statins have been used in patients who have statin intolerance caused by myopathy.[195] Myositis is more likely to occur with high systemic concentrations of the statin and when there is a provocation for the event (e.g., hypothyroidism, trauma, or flulike syndromes). Myositis has also been reported more often when a statin is combined with gemfibrozil or when a drug is given concurrently that can increase blood levels of the statin, such as a macrolide antibiotic (e.g., erythromycin). Cases of rhabdomyolysis, myoglobinuria, and acute tubular necrosis have been reported in patients receiving statin therapy. Most of these cases have occurred with high doses, in patients with impaired renal or hepatic function, in older individuals, or when statins are used in combination with interacting drugs.

Drug interactions with statins that result in higher blood levels of the statin or an active metabolite can increase the risk of myositis. Statins that depend on the cytochrome P-450 (CYP) 3A4 enzyme system to be metabolized are most vulnerable to this interaction (i.e., lovastatin, simvastatin, and to a lesser extent atorvastatin). Fluvastatin is metabolized by the CYP2C9 system and, therefore, is more vulnerable to interactions with drugs that directly inhibit CYP2C9 or act as competitive inhibitors (substrates) for this alternative system. Rosuvastatin is metabolized minimally (i.e., about 10%) by CYP2C9 to less active metabolites. Pitavastatin is marginally metabolized by CYP2C9 and to a lesser extent by CYP2C8. The major metabolite in human plasma is the lactone, which is formed via glucuronidation by uridine 5′-diphospho-glucuronosyltransferases 1A3 and 2B7. Pravastatin undergoes isomerization in the gut to a relatively inactive metabolite. Variability of gastric metabolism has been shown to be associated with the LDL-C–lowering effects of pravastatin.[196] Some of the more commonly encountered drugs that inhibit the CYP3A4 enzyme system are azole antifungals (itraconazole, ketoconazole, and miconazole), certain calcium-channel blockers (diltiazem and verapamil), macrolide antibiotics (clarithromycin and erythromycin), protease inhibitors (e.g., ritonavir), and antidepressants (nefazodone). Drugs that are substrates for the CYP3A4 system include certain benzodiazepines (alprazolam, midazolam, triazolam), calcium-channel blockers (especially diltiazem), carbamazepine, cisapride, cyclosporine, estradiol, felodipine, loratadine, quinidine, and terfenadine. When these substrate drugs are used together with simvastatin or lovastatin (and to a lesser extent atorvastatin), systemic blood levels of the statin may be increased because of competitive inhibition of the CYP3A4 enzymes, and this may increase the risk for myositis. Inhibitors of CYP2C9 isoenzymes include alprenolol, diclofenac, hexobarbital, tolbutamide, and warfarin.

It is preferable to avoid the combined use of interacting drugs with statins. If the patient requires a short course of therapy with a potentially interacting drug (e.g., erythromycin), the statin should be discontinued during this period and restarted when the course has been completed. If an interacting drug must be used long term (e.g., cyclosporine) with a statin, the lowest effective dose of the statin should be selected, with careful monitoring of muscle symptoms. Moreover, cyclosporine-treated patients show several-fold higher systemic exposure for all statins, those metabolized by both CYP3A4 and CYP2C9. Therefore, the mechanism for this interaction does not seem to be solely caused by inhibition of CYP3A4 metabolism, but it is probably also a result of inhibition of statin transport (P-glycoprotein and organic anion-transporting polypeptide) in the liver. Finally, single-nucleotide polymorphisms located within the *SLCO1B1* gene that encodes the organic anion-transporting polypeptide have been identified that increase the risk of statin-induced myopathy. Genotyping these variants may help to identify patients at increased risk for statin-induced myopathy.[197] If myositis occurs, it is quickly reversible when the statin is discontinued.

Caution should also be exercised when adding gemfibrozil with a statin to treat patients with high blood cholesterol and TGs. Gemfibrozil interferes with the glucuronidation of statins, thereby interfering with their renal clearance. This interaction results in twofold to fourfold increases in systemic statin levels and has been demonstrated with all statins except fluvastatin. Because the interaction has not been reported to occur with fenofibrate, it is the preferred fibrate to add to a statin when treating patients with a mixed lipid disorder. Fenofibric acid (Trilipix) is the only fibrate medication that is FDA approved to be used in combination with a statin.

Hospitalizations and deaths caused by rhabdomyolysis led to the withdrawal of one statin, cerivastatin, from the market, punctuating the importance of this potential side effect. Cerivastatin at its top dosage of 0.8 mg daily caused a significantly higher incidence of myotoxicity than other currently marketed statins. Additionally, when interacting drugs or gemfibrozil were added to this dose of cerivastatin, many cases of severe muscle toxicity and rhabdomyolysis occurred. The FDA subsequently observed that factors that appeared to raise the risk of severe muscle toxicity and rhabdomyolysis with cerivastatin included older individuals (especially women), small body frame, reduced renal function, multiple organ diseases, and use of multiple concurrent medications, particularly those known to interact with statins. Currently, the FDA advises that the initial dose of 5 mg of rosuvastatin be considered in Asian patients because pharmacokinetics studies have demonstrated a twofold increase in systemic exposure in Asians compared with whites. The FDA also warned that risks of muscle injury are higher with simvastatin 80 mg compared with lower doses. Lower doses should be considered in patients with concomitant risk factors for myopathy and drugs known to inhibit simvastatin metabolism or in patients of Chinese descent taking niacin ($\geq$1 g/day). It is not known whether the increased risk for myopathy observed in these patients applies to other patients of Asian descent. The learner is encouraged to refer to the FDA Postmarket Drug Safety Information for Patients and Providers website for up-to-date warnings (**http://www.fda.gov/Drugs/DrugSafety/PostmarketDrugSafetyInformationforPatientsandProviders/ucm204882.htm**). Whenever these factors are present in a patient receiving a statin, it is advisable to use the lowest effective statin dose, to avoid or use interacting drugs with caution, and to monitor the patient carefully. It is also advisable not to unduly frighten the patient with dire warnings about the potential for this side effect; it occurs only rarely, especially when these drugs are used responsibly in the manner described.

As depicted in Figure 13-1, ubiquinone (also known as coenzyme Q10) is formed after the synthesis of mevalonate and upstream from the synthesis of cholesterol. Coenzyme Q10 is an isoprenoid that plays a unique role in cellular electron transport and energy synthesis. It is essential for the normal functioning of muscles. Statins have been shown to reduce blood levels of coenzyme Q10. The evidence of the value of supplementing coenzyme Q10 in patients experiencing statin-induced myopathy has been mainly anecdotal and is currently being evaluated in clinical trials (**http://clinicaltrials.gov/ct2/show/NCT01140308?term=Coenzyme+Q10&rank=2**).

There also has been interest in the possible relationship between statin myopathy and vitamin D deficiency. Vitamin D receptors are present in skeletal muscle, and vitamin D deficiency can cause myopathy. However, a recent systematic review concluded that it is presently premature to recommend vitamin D supplementation as treatment for statin-associated muscle complaints in the absence of low vitamin D levels.[198] Prospective randomized trials are needed to examine the potential role of vitamin D deficiency in statin myopathy.

Lovastatin and rosuvastatin may prolong the international normalized ratio in patients receiving warfarin anticoagulants concurrently; this effect is not caused by pravastatin. Statins should not be used in patients with active liver disease or those who are (or hope to become) pregnant because of potential hazards to the fetus.

Based on this information, it is unlikely that simvastatin is causing any serious side effects. His muscle pain is most likely the result of heavy exercise that is not part of his usual pattern of exercise. If the muscle soreness persists for more than the expected 2 to 3 days or worsens, he should report it to his doctor to determine whether measuring a CPK level is necessary.

CASE 13-2, QUESTION 4: Was simvastatin a good choice for L.W.? Was the dose appropriate?

A statin is the preferred drug for L.W. He is not receiving a potentially interacting drug and has no apparent contraindication to its use. Furthermore, it is more likely than a resin, ezetimibe, or niacin to help him reach his LDL-C goal. In selecting the specific statin for the patient, it is assumed, for reasons previously stated, that all statins are equally safe and have a similar potential to reduce CHD events. The characteristic that differentiates the statins is in the magnitude of their ability to lower LDL-C (Tables 13-13, 13-16). As mentioned earlier, when LDL-lowering drug therapy is used in high-risk or moderately high-risk persons such as L.W., the intensity of therapy should be sufficient to achieve at least a 30% to 40% reduction in LDL-C levels. In addition to the minimum of a 35% reduction required to achieve L.W.'s LDL-C goal, it would be preferable to select the statin with the greatest LDL-C–lowering potency, such as pitavastatin, simvastatin, atorvastatin, or rosuvastatin. At 2 mg/day of pitavastatin, 20 mg/day of simvastatin, 10 mg/day of atorvastatin, or 10 mg/day of rosuvastatin, LDL-C is reduced by an average of 39%, indicating that 50% of patients will experience at least this level of LDL-C reduction. Starting therapy with even higher doses (i.e., pitavastatin 4 mg, rosuvastatin 20 mg, simvastatin 40 mg, or atorvastatin 20 mg) will increase the chance of reaching L.W.'s minimal treatment goal of less than 130 mg/dL. Higher-potency statins, such as simvastatin, are available as generic medications, which reduces the total cost of therapy. For now the 20-mg starting dose of simvastatin given to L.W. is reasonable. He should be assessed for success in achieving his lipid goal in about 6 weeks.

FIBER

CASE 13-2, QUESTION 5: What role can supplemental fiber play in the treatment of L.W.?

Increasing fiber intake in the diet or adding supplemental fiber in the form of psyllium, oat bran, vegetable gum fiber, or other products might temporarily aid in LDL-C reduction. When given to a patient who is following a low-fat diet, the LDL-C reduction is modest (usually about 5%). A dietary supplement of fiber would make little overall contribution to L.W.'s treatment, although appropriate fiber intake in the form of fresh fruits, beans, and vegetables is highly advisable. Overuse of fiber is associated with bothersome GI symptoms, including flatulence and bloating.

FISH OILS

CASE 13-2, QUESTION 6: Is there a role for fish oil supplements in L.W.'s treatment?

Fish oils predominantly contain long-chain polyunsaturated (omega-3) fatty acids, eicosapentaenoic acid (EPA) and docosahexaenoic acid (DHA), which lower TG levels significantly (30% to 60%) but have variable effects on cholesterol levels. They do not provide LDL-C reduction, as is needed by L.W. As noted, however, under the discussion of diet, consumption of foods rich in omega-3 fatty acids (e.g., fish) several times a week has been associated with a reduced risk of heart disease, and they are recommended as part of a low-fat diet. Supplements of fish oils demonstrated a reduction in CHD in patients with a recent MI[199] and patients taking statins.[200] Recently, however, other trials have failed to demonstrate the benefits of omega-3 fatty acids in addition to standard cardiovascular drugs, such as statins, angiotensin-converting enzyme (ACE) inhibitors, β-blockers, and antiplatelet agents.[201] Commercial sources of fish oils vary in their content. The omega-3 fatty acids used in the GISSI study, which demonstrated a CHD risk reduction, contained 850 mg of combined EPA and DHA. Prescription-grade omega-3 fatty acid ethyl ester contains approximately 465 mg of EPA and 375 mg of DHA per 1-g capsule. It is FDA approved for treating TG levels greater than 500 mg/dL at a dose of 4 g/day. However, many health care organizations and third-party payers have limited prescription-grade omega-3 fatty acid ethyl esters to their nonformulary list of medications because of cost and advocate the use of dietary fish oil supplements for the treatment of hypertriglyceridemia. However, the amount of EPA and DHA per recommended serving in these products is highly variable, and clinicians should heighten their scrutiny in terms of selection of the appropriate product.[202]

Familial Hypercholesterolemia

CASE 13-3

QUESTION 1: D.E. is a 45-year-old man with no evidence of CHD. His father and grandfather both died suddenly of apparent heart attacks in their early 50s, but D.E. has no other CHD risk factors. He has no evidence of secondary causes of dyslipidemia. On physical examination, he is noted to have bilateral corneal arcus and bilateral Achilles' tendon xanthomas; the rest of his examination findings are normal. Likewise, his laboratory test results are within normal limits, except for the following lipid profile:

Total cholesterol, 440 mg/dL
TG, 55 mg/dL
HDL-C, 55 mg/dL
LDL-C, 374 mg/dL

What form of hypercholesterolemia does D.E. most likely have? Is he a candidate for drug therapy at this time?

The combination of a very high LDL-C, tendon xanthomas, corneal arcus, and a strong family history of premature CHD is consistent with a diagnosis of FH (Table 13-2). The risk of a CHD event in the next 10 years associated with FH is very high, well in excess of 20%. Thus, it is not necessary to conduct a global risk assessment because the diagnosis of the genetic disorder defines his risk. Although D.E. has bilateral tendon xanthomas, this finding would not necessarily be detected in all 45-year-old patients because it takes time for xanthomas to develop. With a strong family history and a very high LDL-C level independent of the presence or absence of xanthomas, however, it is still presumed that the person has either FH or severe polygenic hypercholesterolemia. Thus, he deserves aggressive lipid management (minimum of 50% reduction in LDL-C)[203,204] to reduce his high CHD risk. D.E. should be given therapy to lower his LDL-C to 130 mg/dL, lower if possible. To achieve this goal, D.E. will require a 65% LDL-C reduction, which almost assuredly will require combination drug therapy in addition to a low-fat diet. Because this is a genetically induced lipid abnormality, a low-fat diet alone will not correct the problem; in fact, diet may have little effect on his LDL-C. If D.E. is unable to reduce his LDL-C sufficiently or cannot tolerate maximal intensity therapy, LDL apheresis may be indicated.[204]

CASE 13-3, QUESTION 2: What cholesterol-lowering drugs should be combined to manage D.E.'s lipid disorder?

As stated previously, four drugs effectively reduce LDL-C: a statin, a resin, ezetimibe, and niacin (Table 13-12). When two or more of these are combined, an additive LDL-C–lowering effect is achieved. Combinations of niacin and resin result in LDL-C reductions of 32% to 43%,[67] a statin and a resin lower LDL-C by 45% to 55%,[68] and ezetimibe plus a statin reduces LDL-C by 46% to 70%.[165,205] LDL-C reductions of 50% to 60% are possible when the three-drug regimen of a statin plus resin plus niacin is used.[206,207]

The major limiting factor in combining drugs is side effects. Niacin and the older resins both cause bothersome side effects to the extent that 25% to 50% of patients cannot tolerate them. The use of extended-release niacin rather than crystalline niacin may reduce the vasodilatory side effects, however, and the use of colesevelam rather than one of the older resins should reduce GI intolerance.[208] The combination of a statin and niacin is said to be associated with an increased risk of myositis, although this risk appears to be very low.[209] The combination of a statin and ezetimibe is the one best tolerated and offers the most convenient once-a-day dosing of the possible combinations. This is the combination that was selected for D.E.

INITIATING THERAPY

CASE 13-3, QUESTION 3: How should combined therapy with a statin and ezetimibe be initiated in D.E.?

Given the amount of LDL-C lowering needed to reach D.E.'s LDL-C goal, it is reasonable to select one of the more-potent LDL-C–lowering statins (e.g., simvastatin, atorvastatin, pitavastatin, or rosuvastatin) and to start with a high daily dose (40 mg/day for simvastatin and atorvastatin, 4 mg/day for pitavastatin, 20 mg/day for rosuvastatin). Before therapy is initiated, baseline liver function tests and CPK levels should be obtained (Table 13-15). Renal function should be assessed because impaired renal clearance of the statin or its active metabolite could result in increased systemic levels, which might increase the risk of myopathy. LDL-C levels should be evaluated in about 6 weeks, when the maximal effect of the statin is anticipated. If the LDL-C is within 6% of D.E.'s goal, the dosage of the statin may be advanced to the maximal dose as this should be sufficient to achieve the goal. If the LDL-C is more than 6% above goal, however, ezetimibe (10 mg) daily should be added to the regimen. This should add an additional 15% to 20% LDL-C–lowering effect.[205] D.E. should be seen in another 6 weeks for further LDL-C evaluation. Alternatively, the patient can be started on a fixed combination product of simvastatin and ezetimibe (Table 13-14).

If D.E. does not achieve his goal with this two-drug combination, the addition of a third drug should be considered. Choices are to add a bile acid resin or niacin. This combination should be effective, but a limit may exist as to how much hepatic LDL receptors can be upregulated. Niacin has been successfully added as a third drug in a regimen and provides a 10% to 15% additional LDL-C–lowering effect when titrated to about 2,000 mg/day.

ADDING A THIRD LIPID-LOWERING DRUG TO THE REGIMEN

CASE 13-3, QUESTION 4: How should niacin be initiated in D.E., and what monitoring is required?

Before niacin therapy is started (and after its maximal dosage is reached), liver function tests should be evaluated (Table 13-15). Patients with uncontrolled diabetes or active peptic ulcer or liver disease should not receive niacin. Niacin should be used cautiously in patients with a history of gout. Niacin can increase glucose levels by 10% to 20% in some diabetic patients or patients with impaired fasting glucose levels, necessitating careful monitoring of glucose control. None of these issues is a factor in D.E.

The addition of niacin to D.E.'s statin and ezetimibe regimen should be initiated with low doses that are slowly titrated upward to allow tolerance to develop at each dosage level (Table 13-14). D.E. should be given as much control over niacin administration as possible. Extended-release niacin is initiated at 500 mg at bedtime with a low-fat snack and increased every 30 days to 1,000 mg, 1,500 mg, and 2,000 mg daily as tolerated by the patient. The herbal supplement sustained-release niacin dosage form is generally not recommended because of its increased risk of causing hepatotoxicity.

D.E. should be warned about the vasodilatory symptoms associated with niacin use (facial flushing, itching, rash) and reassured that these symptoms are not dangerous and that tolerance should develop after several weeks of therapy. He should be advised to take 325 mg of non–enteric-coated aspirin or another prostaglandin-inhibiting drug 30 minutes before the bedtime dose of extended-release niacin to decrease these symptoms. Taking each dose with food will help to reduce flushing and GI symptoms. D.E. should be advised not to take his extended-release niacin with hot or spicy food or alcohol. Avoiding hot showers after taking his extended-release niacin is good advice as well. Instruction can also be provided to reduce doses if necessary to manage bothersome symptoms. He should be encouraged to call his clinician whenever troublesome symptoms occur.

Several months after the 1,500-mg/day dosage is reached (Table 13-14), the patient should be evaluated for achievement of the LDL-C goal and side effects. If the LDL-C goal is not achieved with 1,500 mg/day, further increments can be made up to the 2,000 mg. In addition to a fasting lipid profile, laboratory tests of liver function, fasting glucose, and uric acid may be indicated.

MIXED HYPERLIPIDEMIA

Assessing the Patient With Mixed Hyperlipidemia

CASE 13-4

QUESTION 1: B.C., a 56-year-old man, experienced acute chest pain 3 months ago and was admitted to the local hospital with a diagnosis of unstable angina. His only known medical problem was hypertension treated with enalapril 10 mg every day. His lipid profile on admission was as follows:

Total cholesterol, 235 mg/dL
HDL-C, 30 mg/dL
LDL-C, 165 mg/dL
TG, 300 mg/dL

He underwent a cardiac catheterization, which revealed a 90% stenotic lesion in his left anterior ascending artery. A drug-eluting stent was placed without difficulty. He was subsequently discharged on simvastatin 40 mg every evening at bedtime, ezetimibe 10 mg every day, acetylsalicylic acid

TABLE 13-17

Treatment Targets for Patients Who Have Achieved Their LDL-C Goal and Have a Triglyceride Level > 200 mg/dL and Meet Criteria for the Metabolic Syndrome

Patient Category	LDL-C Treatment Target	Non–HDL-C Treatment Target	Apolipoprotein B Treatment Target[210]
CHD or CHD risk equivalent	<100 mg/dL	<130 mg/dL	<80 mg/dL
(Optional goal for patients with CHD)	<70 mg/dL	<100 mg/dL	<90 mg/dL
No CHD, >2 risk factors	<130 mg/dL	<160 mg/dL	Not specified
No CHD, <2 risk factors	<160 mg/dL	<190 mg/dL	Not specified

CHD, coronary heart disease; LDL-C, low-density lipoprotein cholesterol; non–HDL-C, non–high-density lipoprotein cholesterol.

325 mg every day, clopidogrel 75 mg every day, metoprolol 100 mg twice daily, and enalapril 10 mg every day.

Today, he weighs 220 pounds, is 6 feet tall (ideal body weight, 140 to 185 pounds), and has a waist circumference of 42 inches. He has lost 10 pounds since his diagnosis of unstable angina by following a low-fat diet and an exercise program. He swims 1 mile three times a week without symptoms of cardiac ischemia, and he drinks two glasses of wine each evening with dinner. His father died at age 58 of an MI (lipids unknown). He has never smoked. Pertinent physical findings include a BP of 148/90 mm Hg, heart rate that is 60 beats/minute and regular, arcus senilis, carotid pulses equal without bruits, and chest clear to auscultation without cardiomegaly. Laboratory tests disclose normal TSH levels, normal renal and liver function, and a fasting glucose level of 120 mg/dL. His urinalysis was normal. The lipid profile while taking the above regimen is as follows:

Total cholesterol, 143 mg/dL
TG, 210 mg/dL
HDL-C, 33 mg/dL
LDL-C, 68 mg/dL

What is your assessment of B.C.'s lipids and lipoprotein cholesterol concentrations?

According to NCEP guidelines, B.C. has reached the optional LDL-C treatment goal (<70 mg/dL) for a patient with a history of CHD (Table 13-10).[93,106] The LDL-C should be confirmed with a second lipid profile (because of biologic and analytical variability). According to NCEP guidelines, his TG level remains high (200–499 mg/dL) and his HDL-C is low (<40 mg/dL; Table 13-6). The lipid profile obtained during his hospitalization can be interpreted in a normal manner because it was drawn within 24 hours of his acute coronary event. Profiles drawn after 24 hours are generally lower, however, than pre-event levels and remain so for several weeks.

Based on his recent CHD event, B.C. has a greater than 20% chance of a recurrent CHD event in the next 10 years. He is therefore considered to be a very high-risk CHD patient. Additionally, B.C. has several risk factors for CHD that add to his risk: family history, man at least 45 years of age, high BP, and low HDL-C. His fasting blood glucose is defined as impaired fasting glucose (i.e., a fasting value 100 to 125 mg/dL). Some clinicians would consider him to be diabetic, given how close he is to the definition of diabetes (fasting blood sugar >125 mg/dL). Evaluation of glycosylated hemoglobin and a glucose tolerance test are indicated to further define B.C.'s diabetes state.

B.C. was appropriately treated with a statin (as well as antiplatelet, ACE inhibitor, and β-blocker therapy) and a TLC diet and exercise program to achieve an LDL-C less than 70 mg/dL. In such a high-risk patient, therapeutic interventions should not be delayed. Not only will the initiation of drug treatment in the hospital setting provide risk-reducing benefit, but the patient is more likely to relate this therapy to his acute event and adhere to it.[208]

Although B.C. has reached his LDL-C goal, the job of reducing his CHD risk is not complete. The next step is to evaluate the CHD risk associated with the high TG level and, if indicated, develop a plan to address it (Table 13-17).[210]

Relation of Triglycerides to Coronary Heart Disease

CASE 13-4, QUESTION 2: Does the increased TG level in B.C. indicate an increased CHD risk?

The exact role that TGs play in the pathogenesis of CHD is under intense investigation. Most epidemiologic studies have found that a high TG level is an independent risk factor for CHD when evaluated with univariate analysis. When other lipid abnormalities, such as increased LDL-C or low HDL-C are included in a multivariate analysis, TGs often lose their independent predictive power.[211] Part of the reason for this is the close interrelationship among lipids. Patients with high TG levels almost always have a low HDL-C, which also predicts CHD risk.[212,213] In addition, elevated TG levels are associated with increased levels of TG-rich lipoproteins (i.e., remnant VLDL particles) and small, dense LDL particles.[12,214] These particles are atherogenic and mediate a higher CHD risk than that associated with an elevated LDL-C alone.[215–218] When epidemiologic studies were combined, a meta-analysis found that TGs independently predicted CHD risk, even after adjustment for other lipid risk factors.[219] High TG levels are also found in certain familial disorders, including dysbetalipoproteinemia and FCHL, which carry increased CHD risk.[22,220] Additionally, hypertriglyceridemia is associated with a procoagulant state, which promotes coronary thrombosis.[214]

Paradoxically, very high TG levels (>500 mg/dL) are not commonly associated with an increased CHD risk, but do cause an increased risk of pancreatitis, especially when levels exceed 1,000 mg/dL. Often, a genetic defect in LPL is present in these cases that impairs the removal of TGs from TG-rich particles (VLDL and chylomicrons). These particles do not become enriched with cholesterol and, therefore, are not often atherogenic.[220,221] If the blood sample is stored in the refrigerator overnight, a thick creamy layer often appears on the surface, indicating the presence of chylomicrons. Although most patients with very high TGs remain free of CHD throughout their lives, some experience it.[221]

On the other hand, patients such as B.C., with TGs in the borderline to high range (150 to 500 mg/dL), have an increased CHD risk because they likely have atherogenic TG-rich lipoproteins (Table 13-6). Characteristically, B.C. has a high TG level and a low HDL-C and is likely to also have elevated remnant VLDL-C and small dense LDL levels. This is the profile of atherogenic dyslipidemia described earlier in this chapter, and it is linked to a high CHD risk. This is exemplified by the placebo groups in the HIT and BIP trials, two studies that included patients with mixed hyperlipidemia. Untreated subjects had CHD event rates of 15% to 22% in 5 to 6 years, respectively.[124,125]

Atherogenic Dyslipidemia

CASE 13-4, QUESTION 3: Why does atherogenic dyslipidemia occur? How should the clinician assess and treat atherogenic dyslipidemia?

Patients such as B.C. with borderline high or high TG levels (Table 13-6) secrete large numbers of TG-enriched VLDL particles from the liver. One reason for this is increased levels of nonesterified fatty acids in the systemic circulation that come from adipose cells (especially in patients with central obesity). The liver clears these fatty acids and is stimulated to increase the synthesis of TGs.[222]

A second reason for the increased secretion of VLDL particles is an upregulation of the gene expression for microsomal triglyceride transfer protein that is caused by the elevated insulin levels in these patients.[223] Microsomal triglyceride transfer protein is responsible for assembling VLDL particles in the hepatocyte. It brings together TGs, cholesterol, and apolipoproteins to form the VLDL particle. This mechanism suggests a molecular basis for the link between insulin resistance and increased VLDL secretion. One way to know that there are increased numbers of lipoprotein particles in the systemic circulation is to measure apolipoprotein B. One apolipoprotein B is attached to each VLDL and LDL particle. An increased apolipoprotein B level indicates an increased number of particles. Patients with a high apolipoprotein B level have a high risk of CHD.

With the increase in VLDL particles, plasma levels of apolipoprotein C-III also increase. Apolipoprotein C-III has two detrimental effects. It interferes with the normal removal of TGs from VLDL by reducing the action of LPL. This reduces lipolysis and increases the concentration of TGs in the VLDL particle. The second negative effect of apolipoprotein C-III is an interference with the normal removal of VLDL particles from the circulation via LDL receptors on the hepatocytes.[222]

TG-rich VLDL particles interact with other circulating lipoproteins through the action of CETP. Through this protein, a molecule of cholesterol ester is exchanged from circulating HDL and LDL particles for a molecule of TG from VLDL particles. With time, the HDL particles give up more than 50% of their cholesterol content and become enriched with TGs. This results in low HDL-C levels. VLDL becomes more enriched with cholesterol and simultaneously smaller in size, close to the size of LDL, and thus more atherogenic (both because of its smaller size and its higher cholesterol content). LDL particles take on more TGs than normal. Subsequently, under the influence of hepatic lipase, TG is removed from LDL particles, leaving a very small particle that is deficient in cholesterol and TGs, but is present in great numbers. Because of their small size and concentration, small, dense LDL particles are very atherogenic.

The net result of the above mechanisms is a high VLDL-C, low HDL-C, and increased small, dense LDL, a lipid triad termed *atherogenic dyslipidemia*. How does the clinician measure this in the clinical setting? VLDL-C and VLDL-TG levels are not available from most clinical laboratories. Several companies provide measurements of particle size, but these tests are expensive and do not yet relate to a reference standard; particle size measurements are best reserved for research purposes at present. The clinician can measure apolipoprotein B as an indicator of the number of atherogenic particles; these levels are available from most clinical laboratories. The American Diabetic Association and the American College of Cardiology recommend an apolipoprotein B treatment goal of less than 80 mg/dL (Table 13-17) in patients such as B.C.[210] A much easier, more accessible measure is non–HDL-C as discussed previously. Non–HDL-C is the product of VLDL-C and LDL-C and is determined by subtracting HDL-C from total cholesterol. NCEP recommends that non–HDL-C be determined in patients who have a TG in excess of 200 mg/dL after attaining their LDL-C goal.[8] Once the patient is at his or her LDL-C goal, any elevation in non–HDL-C will result from an increase in VLDL-C. Because VLDL-C levels are normally less than 30 mg/dL, non–HDL-C treatment goals are set 30 mg/dL greater than LDL-C treatment goals (Table 13-17). Included in this table are alternative apolipoprotein B treatment goals that have been recommended by authorities.[224] Note that non–HDL-C levels can be determined from a nonfasting sample measuring only total cholesterol and HDL-C, thus making it very convenient for the clinician to make these measurements any time of the day without regard to food intake.

SECONDARY CAUSES OF HYPERTRIGLYCERIDEMIA

CASE 13-4, QUESTION 4: In addition to an assessment of B.C.'s lipid profile, what other evaluations should be made?

One of the questions that should be answered routinely when evaluating patients with lipid disorders is whether there is a secondary cause of the patient's lipid disorder. Secondary causes of hypertriglyceridemia include chronic kidney disease, diabetes mellitus, alcohol use and abuse, a sedentary lifestyle, obesity, and the use of TG-raising drugs, including β-blockers, estrogens, and glucocorticoids (Table 13-7). B.C. has a normal TSH level, normal liver and renal function test results, and a normal urinalysis. His blood glucose is elevated into the impaired fasting glucose range, which can be associated with impaired TG metabolism, as described earlier. In addition, he is overweight, with abdominal obesity (i.e., a waist circumference >40 inches). Patients who have truncal obesity often overproduce TGs and oversecrete VLDL particles, thereby raising their TG level. The HDL-C is inversely reduced. This would appear to be an important factor affecting TG levels in B.C. A reduction in weight through an exercise program and a low-calorie, low–saturated fat, and low-carbohydrate diet would be one of the most effective ways to improve B.C.'s glucose level, raise his HDL-C, and lower his TG level.

Light to moderate alcohol intake, defined as up to two drinks per day for men and one drink per day for women (1 drink = 5 ounces of wine, 12 ounces of beer, or 1.5 ounces of 80-proof liquor), as practiced by B.C., has been associated with lower CHD rates. The observed reduction in CHD among light to moderate alcohol drinkers is consistently on the order of 40% to 60% in epidemiologic trials.[225,226] Available epidemiologic evidence supports arguments of causality.[227,228] It is problematic, however, to recommend alcohol consumption for CHD prevention. From a public health point of view, the adverse consequences of alcohol consumption are great and may outweigh the benefits gained. One known adverse consequence of alcohol consumption is hypertriglyceridemia, especially when alcohol is abused, but it may be seen with only moderate intake as well. Even though B.C.'s alcohol intake appears moderate, it may be contributing to his hypertriglyceridemia, so a period of abstinence is warranted to determine whether this is the case.

Use of a β-blocker could also raise TG levels (Table 13-7) and might be a contributing factor in B.C.'s lipid profile. He already had a high TG level on admission to the hospital before starting metoprolol therapy, however. In this case, the β-blocker is providing an important health benefit that probably outweighs the small risk posed by its effect of TG levels. More probably, B.C.'s weight and impaired fasting glucose are the key factors contributing to his increased TG level and are the logical places to start when attempting to correct secondary causes of elevated TG levels.

METABOLIC SYNDROME

CASE 13-4, QUESTION 5: B.C. has a combination of abdominal obesity, impaired fasting glucose, and hypertension, in addition to atherogenic dyslipidemia. What is the significance of this constellation of findings?

Not only does B.C. have CHD and a combination of lipid abnormalities that substantially raise his risk of CHD, but he also has a number of nonlipid risk factors that raise it as well.[213] These factors include abdominal obesity, impaired fasting glucose, and hypertension. Most of B.C.'s excess weight is concentrated around his waist. This central distribution of fat may reflect an excess of intra-abdominal fat, which in turn may influence the development of atherogenic dyslipidemia, as already described.[229] An increased outflow of fatty acids from intra-abdominal TG stores may provide the substrate for increased hepatic TG synthesis and VLDL secretion. This could explain B.C.'s elevated TG level.

Abdominal obesity also is strongly associated with insulin resistance.[217,230] Insulin resistance leads to mild hyperglycemia, and the pancreas responds by increasing insulin secretion; hyperinsulinemia results.[231,232] Some genetically predisposed patients are not able to secrete sufficient insulin to overcome this resistance, and they exhibit impaired glucose metabolism or diabetes. The presence of a fasting blood sugar between 100 and 125 mg/dL in B.C. suggests impaired glucose metabolism and probably insulin resistance (with hyperinsulinemia).[233]

B.C. has hypertension. The β-blocker and ACE inhibitor he is receiving to reduce his CHD risk also help lower his blood pressure. According to the most recent guidelines, B.C. still has stage 1 hypertension (systolic BP 140 to 159 mm Hg); his untreated BP may be higher.[234] Abdominal obesity and insulin resistance also are commonly associated with high BP and could be a factor in B.C.[235] The exact mechanisms for this remain speculative.

What emerges from the preceding discussion is the strong possibility that B.C.'s risk factors are not independent, but rather represent a constellation of medical problems that have a common pathway. This pathway may be related to insulin resistance.[235,236] NCEP called this constellation the *metabolic syndrome.*[8] Other names given the same problem in the literature are syndrome X, the deadly quadrangle, insulin resistance syndrome, and Reaven syndrome.[217,218,232,235–237] Metabolic syndrome is diagnosed when any three of the factors listed in Table 13-18 are present. The syndrome is associated with a substantial increase in CHD risk; the exact level of risk should be determined by using the risk-scoring calculator found at http://hp2010.nhlbihin.net/atpiii/calculator.asp?usertype=prof. B.C. has the metabolic syndrome by having met all five criteria in Table 13-18. Weight loss, especially loss of visceral abdominal adiposity, will be the centerpiece of his nondrug treatment program. The goal is for weight reduction to correct, or at least substantially improve, his blood glucose, TGs, and HDL-C levels and BP.

TABLE 13-18
Clinical Identification of the Metabolic Syndrome

Presence of any three of the following:	
• Waist circumference	
• Men	≥40 inches (>35 inches for Asian Americans)
• Women	≥35 inches (>31 inches for Asian Americans)
• Triglycerides	≥150 mg/dL (or on drug treatment for elevated triglycerides)
• High-density lipoprotein cholesterol (HDL-C)	
• Men	<40 mg/dL (or on drug treatment for reduced HDL-C)
• Women	<50 mg/dL (or on drug treatment for reduced HDL-C)
• Blood pressure (systolic/diastolic)	≥130/≥85 mm Hg (or on drug treatment for hypertension)
• Fasting glucose	>100 mg/dL (or on drug treatment for elevated glucose)

HYPERTENSION MANAGEMENT WITH ATHEROGENIC DYSLIPIDEMIA

CASE 13-4, QUESTION 6: If B.C.'s BP elevation persists after lifestyle changes are made, how should he be treated?

Consideration of antihypertensive therapy in a patient with dyslipidemia should take into account how BP-modifying drugs affect blood lipids. As noted above, the metoprolol B.C. is receiving can elevate TG levels, but the benefit in post-MI prophylaxis warrants its continued use.[234] Substitution of a β-blocker with intrinsic sympathomimetic activity (e.g., pindolol) or a mixed α,β-blocker (e.g., carvedilol) may have less adverse effect on lipids (Table 13-7), but a β-blocker with intrinsic sympathomimetic activity should never be used after MI.

The ACE inhibitor B.C. currently is receiving for his hypertension has a neutral effect on serum lipids. His BP is not under good control, however, so an adjustment to his antihypertensive regimen is in order. After maximizing the dose of ACE inhibitor and β-blocker, a thiazide diuretic maybe added in this type of patient.[234] Although thiazides can increase blood cholesterol levels (Table 13-7), these effects usually are small, especially with long-term use. The thiazide dose should be kept low (i.e., 12.5 mg/day) to minimize the effect on his blood lipids. Calcium-channel blockers are lipid neutral and are possible alternatives to a thiazide.

TREATMENT OF THE METABOLIC SYNDROME

CHOLESTEROL-LOWERING AND WEIGHT-LOSS DIET

CASE 13-4, QUESTION 7: What nondrug therapies should be implemented to help B.C. achieve his treatment goals?

B.C. needs to lose weight in addition to lowering his LDL-C and non–HDL-C levels. Effective weight loss and subsequent weight maintenance could substantially or fully correct his atherogenic dyslipidemia, lower his BP, reduce his waist circumference, and correct his blood glucose. He has already shown progress, having lost 10 pounds since his MI 3 months ago. He appears to be following a low-fat diet, which undoubtedly has helped him lose weight. He needs to lose more weight and needs to modify his lipids further, however. A more rigorous restriction of saturated fats might help him accomplish these goals. This will also substantially reduce total daily calories, because fats

in 6 to 8 weeks. A lower daily dose should be selected for patients with impaired renal function. As with all lipid-altering therapies, patients should be instructed on the purpose of the medication and its expected effects on blood lipids and on CHD risk reduction. They should be encouraged to remain adherent with the regimen to sustain its effects on serum lipids and, thereby, attain its CHD risk-reducing benefit. Discontinuing drug therapy, even after a long period of consistent cholesterol control, will likely result in a return of blood lipids to pretreatment levels. Patients should be counseled to call a health professional if they experience any untoward symptoms, especially muscle soreness or discomfort or a rash. A CPK level should be obtained whenever a patient experiences symptoms of myositis (muscle soreness and aches).

LOW HIGH-DENSITY LIPOPROTEIN CHOLESTEROL

CASE 13-5

QUESTION 1: J.M. is a 59-year-old man who has no history of CHD or a CHD risk equivalent. He has no known medical problems. He does not smoke. His mother had an ischemic episode at age 70 and subsequently had coronary artery bypass surgery. There is no other family history of CHD. J.M. eats a diet low in saturated fat and is sedentary. His physical examination is unremarkable: BP, 122/82 mm Hg, heart rate, 66 beats/minute and regular. He weighs 206 pounds and is 6 feet tall (BMI 28 kg/m^2). His laboratory values are as follows:

Fasting blood glucose, 80 mg/dL
Total cholesterol, 137 mg/dL
LDL-C, 84 mg/dL
TG, 120 mg/dL
HDL-C, 29 mg/dL

Should J.M. be treated for his low HDL-C?

J.M. has two CHD risk factors (age and low HDL) and an LDL-C goal of less than 130 mg/dL because his CHD risk is 6% in 10 years, mostly because of his age. His LDL-C is well within his treatment goal. His TGs are in the normal range. Epidemiologic studies clearly link low HDL-C with increased CHD events, especially in those older than 50 years of age. These studies show that a 1% decrease in HDL-C is associated with a 1% to 2% increase in CHD risk. Most commonly, low HDL-C is secondary to a number of lifestyle and medical conditions (Table 13-19). Of these conditions, being overweight, being physically inactive, and having a diet very low in fat may play a part in J.M.'s low HDL-C. Patients who substantially restrict saturated fats have lower HDL-C levels as well as LDL-C. A careful dietary history would be important to determine whether this is occurring with J.M. Vegetarians who have a low LDL-C and low BP have a low CHD risk despite having a low HDL-C. Increasing intake of monounsaturated fats and lowering carbohydrate intake is one maneuver to raise HDL-C. An obvious approach to improving J.M.'s HDL-C is to encourage him to increase his physical activity.

In addition to secondary causes, there are rare primary (genetic) causes of low HDL-C. Some are associated with increased CHD risk, whereas others are not. Tangier disease is associated with a reduction in the ABCA-1 transporter that moves cholesterol out of peripheral cells. Patients with Tangier disease have characteristic orange tonsils as well as splenomegaly and neuropathy. Fish-eye disease is characterized by corneal opacification and an HDL deficiency. About a third of patients with fish-eye disease have CHD. Patients with apolipoprotein A-I$_{Milano}$ have very low HDL-C levels, but live well into their 80s, apparently because their reverse cholesterol transport is very efficient. J.M. does not appear to have any of these disorders. Importantly, he also does not have a family history of premature CHD. This suggests that his low HDL-C is not caused by a genetic abnormality associated with an increased CHD risk.

TABLE 13-19
Factors Causing Low HDL-C

Secondary Causes
Hypertriglyceridemia
Obesity (visceral fat)
Physical inactivity
Type 2 diabetes
Smoking
Very-low-fat diet
Drugs
• β-Blockers
• Androgenic steroids
• Androgenic progestins
Primary (Genetic) Causes
Apo A-I
• Apo A-I mutations (e.g., ApoA-I$_{Milano}$)
LCAT
• Complete LCAT deficiency
• Partial LCAT deficiency (fish-eye disease)
ABCA-1
• Tangier disease
• Familial hypoalphalipoproteinemia (some families)
Unknown genetic etiology
• Familial hypoalphalipoproteinemia (most families)
• Familial combined hyperlipidemia with low HDL-C
• Metabolic syndrome

ABCA-1, adenosine triphosphate binding cassette A-1; Apo A, apolipoproteins; HDL-C, high-density lipoprotein cholesterol; LCAT, lecithin-cholesterol acyl transferase.

What makes cases of patients such as J.M. difficult to manage is that little clinical trial evidence indicates that raising low levels of HDL-C with diet or drugs will reduce CHD risk. Part of the problem is that no effective drugs substantially and specifically increase HDL-C. Niacin has the most substantial raising effect (mean increases of 25% to 35%). Fibrates also raise HDL-C by 10% to 20%, but they may also raise LDL-C in patients with hypertriglyceridemia. The available evidence indicates that aggressive LDL-C lowering is the most powerful way to reduce CHD risk in patients with low HDL-C. In fact, the lower the HDL-C level, the greater the CHD risk reduction with statin therapy.[256] Based on this evidence, NCEP recommended aggressive LDL-C lowering with a statin in patients with a low HDL-C.[8] In cases of isolated low HDL-C (without hypertriglyceridemia), NCEP recommended lifestyle modification with weight reduction and increased physical activity and the empiric use of HDL-C– raising drugs (niacin or a fibrate), if indicated, to reduce CHD risk.[8]

It would be prudent to encourage J.M. to lose weight and especially to adopt a more physically active lifestyle. This will help his overall well-being. Because he lacks a family history of premature CHD or associated CHD risk factors, his CHD risk would appear to be low and not supportive of an aggressive effort to raise his low HDL-C. If he did have a family history of premature CHD, a more aggressive approach, particularly with increased physical activity and possibly niacin therapy, would be advisable.

ANTIOXIDANT THERAPY

CASE 13-5, QUESTION 2: Should antioxidants, such as vitamin E or β-carotene, be considered in the management of hyperlipidemic patients, especially patients who have CHD?

TABLE 13-20

Randomized Clinical Trials of Vitamin E Supplementation and CHD Events

Investigator/Reference	Number of Subjects	Vitamin E Dose (units)	Population	Follow-Up (years)	Relative Risk
Rapola[262]	29,133	50	Men, no CHD	4.7	0.9 (NS)
Stephens[263]	2,002	400 and 800	Men and women, with CHD	1.4	0.53
Virtamo[264]	27,271	50	Men, no CHD	6.1	0.98 (NS)
GISSI[199]	2,830	300	Men and women, with CHD	3.5	0.95 (NS)
HOPE[265]	9,541	400	Men and women, high risk	4.5	1.05 (NS)
HPS[90]	20,536	600 (+ vitamin C and β-carotene)	Men and women, with CHD	5.0	1.02 (NS)

CHD, coronary heart disease; NS, not significant.

Only oxidized (or otherwise modified) lipoproteins are taken up by macrophage cells in the initial phase of atherogenesis. This observation has led to the supposition that drugs that have antioxidant properties might reduce or block the development of atherosclerosis. Vitamins E and C and β-carotene (the precursor of vitamin A) have antioxidant properties and have been variously recommended to prevent CHD.[257]

Studies in hypercholesterolemic animals have demonstrated that antioxidants, such as probucol, can reduce the development of atherosclerosis.[257,258] In humans, oxidized LDL has been detected in atheromatous lesions, and circulating antibodies to oxidized LDL have also been detected.[259,260] In epidemiologic studies, people who frequently used β-carotene and vitamin E had 35% to 50% fewer CHD events.[261] When the hypothesis that antioxidant therapy will prevent CHD events was tested in well-controlled, randomized clinical trials, however, no benefit was observed. For example, vitamin E, whether administered in low, moderate, or high daily doses, either as monotherapy or combined with other antioxidants, failed to demonstrate a CHD risk-reducing effect during clinical trials involving close to 100,000 patients (Table 13-20).[90,199,262–265] The latest, and one of the largest, of these trials, the Heart Protection Study, prescribed vitamin E (600 units) plus β-carotene or placebo daily for 5 years to 20,536 high-risk individuals. No demonstrable benefit was shown, whether measured as CHD death, nonfatal MI, stroke, or revascularization procedures and whether or not the study population had a history of CHD, stroke, PVD, or diabetes. Furthermore, no change was seen in the incidence of cancer, another claim of potential benefit for antioxidant therapy. These results effectively closed the door on the use of antioxidant therapy for the prevention of CHD events. Future randomized clinical trials will have to demonstrate a benefit before these products can be recommended.

HYPERCHYLOMICRONEMIA

CASE 13-6

QUESTION 1: M.B., an asymptomatic woman, is screened with a lipoprotein profile during an annual physical evaluation by her primary-care provider. She has type 2 diabetes, which is treated with 60 units/day of neutral protamine Hagedorn (NPH) insulin. M.B. is approximately 20% overweight. Her fasting lipoprotein profile and blood glucose is as follows:

Total cholesterol, 234 mg/dL
TG, 2,300 mg/dL
HDL-C, 24 mg/dL
LDL-C (directly measured), 160 mg/dL
Blood glucose, 290 mg/dL

What is the assessment of M.B.'s CHD risk, and what treatment, if any, should she be given?

Patients with fasting TGs in excess of 500 mg/dL have an increase in TG-rich chylomicron and VLDL particles. TG elevations of this magnitude typically increase the risk of pancreatitis, but usually not atherosclerosis and CHD. On the other hand, patients with type 2 diabetes have a high CHD risk. Thus, it is possible that M.B. has two lipid disorders, one causing hyperchylomicronemia and a second causing the typical pattern of atherogenic dyslipidemia. There is no way of knowing whether M.B. has atherogenic dyslipidemia until her TG levels are lowered. Because of the life-threatening nature of TG levels of this magnitude, the priority in treating this patient is to first lower her TGs to as close to normal as possible, then assess her LDL.

Most likely, she has an inherited deficiency of LPL, which is the most common cause of very high TG levels. TG levels this high can also be triggered by uncontrolled diabetes mellitus, alcohol abuse, obesity, or drugs, including estrogens, β-blockers, and steroids. Treatment of these patients should be aggressive. One of the first steps is to improve her diabetes control because this alone may normalize lipid levels. A TG-lowering diet (severe fat restriction) and avoiding alcohol are essential. Lovaza or niacin therapy could be initiated. Fibrate would generally be ineffective if she is LPL deficient. If the patient has symptoms of pancreatitis, she should be treated in the hospital. In the absence of symptoms, outpatient management is possible, but frequent follow-up and aggressive therapy are indicated. Once the TG level is reduced to less than 400 mg/dL, a calculated LDL-C can be determined; if it is greater than 100 mg/dL, therapy with a statin or other suitable lipid-modifying agent should be initiated to achieve an LDL-C level of less than 100 mg/dL.

KEY REFERENCES AND WEBSITES

A full list of references for this chapter can be found at http://thepoint.lww.com/AT10e. Below are the key references and website for this chapter, with the corresponding reference number in this chapter found in parentheses after the reference.

Key References

Brunzell JD et al. Lipoprotein management in patients with cardiometabolic risk: consensus conference report from the American Diabetes Association and the American College of Cardiology Foundation. *Diabetes Care*. 2008;31:811. (210)

Cholesterol Treatment Trialists' (CTT) Collaboration et al. Efficacy and safety of more intensive lowering of LDL cholesterol: a meta-analysis of data from 170,000 participants in 26 randomised trials. *Lancet*. 2010;376:1670. (109)

Expert Panel on Detection, Evaluation, and Treatment of High Blood Cholesterol in Adults. Executive Summary of the Third Report of the National Cholesterol Education Program (NCEP) Expert Panel on detection, evaluation, and treatment of high blood cholesterol in adults (Adult Treatment Panel III). *JAMA*. 2001;285:2486. (8)

Greenland P et al. 2010 ACCF/AHA guideline for assessment of cardiovascular risk in asymptomatic adults: a report of the American College of Cardiology Foundation/American Heart Association Task Force on Practice Guidelines. *J Am Coll Cardiol*. 2010;56:e50. (141)

Grundy SM et al. Implications of recent clinical trials for the National Cholesterol Education Program Adult Treatment Panel III guidelines. *Arterioscler Thromb Vasc Biol*. 2004;24:e149. (108)

Ito MK et al. Management of familial hypercholesterolemias in adult patients: recommendations from the National Lipid Association Expert Panel on Familial Hypercholesterolemia. *J Clin Lipidol*. 2011;5(3 Suppl):S38. (203)

O'Keefe JH Jr et al. Optimal low-density lipoprotein is 50 to 70 mg/dl: lower is better and physiologically normal. *J Am Coll Cardiol*. 2004;43:2142. (111)

Smith SC Jr et al. AHA/ACC; National Heart, Lung, and Blood Institute. AHA/ACC guidelines for secondary prevention for patients with coronary and other atherosclerotic vascular disease: 2006 update: endorsed by the National Heart, Lung, and Blood Institute [published correction appears in *Circulation*. 2006;113:e847]. *Circulation*. 2006;113:2363. (107)

Tabas I et al. Subendothelial lipoprotein retention as the initiating process in atherosclerosis: update and therapeutic implications. *Circulation*. 2007;116:1832. (34)

Taylor F, et al. Statins for the primary prevention of cardiovascular disease. *Cochrane Database Syst Rev*. 2011;(1):CD004816. (105)

Key Website

U.S. Food and Drug Administration. Postmarket Drug Safety Information for Patients and Providers. http://www.fda.gov/Drugs/DrugSafety/PostmarketDrugSafetyInformationforPatientsandProviders/default.htm. Accessed May 29, 2011.

14

Essential Hypertension

Joseph J. Saseen

CORE PRINCIPLES

	CHAPTER CASES
1 A diagnosis of hypertension is based on the mean of two or more properly measured seated blood pressure (BP) measurements taken on two or more occasions.	**Table 14-1, Case 14-1 (Question 1)**
2 Most patients with hypertension have a recommended BP goal of less than 140/90 mm Hg. Some patients with additional cardiovascular (CV) risk (e.g., diabetes) have a lower BP goal of less than 130/80 mm Hg.	**Figure 14-2, Case 14-1 (Question 6)**
3 Lifestyle modifications are the foundation for preventing hypertension, and they are an important component of first-line therapy in all patients treated with antihypertensive drug therapy.	**Table 14-6, Case 14-1 (Questions 11, 12)**
4 Evidence supports the use of an angiotensin-converting enzyme inhibitor, angiotensin receptor blocker, calcium-channel blocker, thiazide diuretic, or a two-drug combination as first-line therapy to prevent CV events.	**Figure 14-3, Case 14-1 (Questions 7, 9, 14, 15)**
5 Pharmacotherapy recommendations for patients with hypertension and compelling indications are specifically based on evidence demonstrating reduced risk of CV events.	**Figure 14-3, Case 14-2 (Questions 2–4)**
6 Elderly patients with hypertension should be managed using the same general treatment principles that apply to all patients with hypertension. However, to minimize adverse effects, only one antihypertensive agent should be started regardless of BP level in elderly patients (≥80 years).	**Case 14-2 (Questions 1–3), Case 14-3 (Question 6), Case 14-9 (Question 1)**
7 Most patients with hypertension need two or more drugs to attain goal BP values. Initial therapy using a two-drug regimen should be strongly considered in patients presenting with stage 2 hypertension. This is also an option for patients with stage 1 hypertension who have high CV risk.	**Figure 14-3, Case 14-1 (Question 16), Case 14-3 (Question 5), Case 14-4 (Question 10)**
8 Management of resistant hypertension should start by ensuring adherence to an optimal combination regimen that consists of three or more agents, ideally including appropriate diuretic therapy. Tests for specific secondary causes can be considered after ensuring other contributors (e.g., lifestyle factors, measurement errors) have been excluded.	**Case 14-11 (Questions 1–3)**
9 At commonly used low doses (12.5 to 25 mg daily), chlorthalidone is more effective in lowering BP than hydrochlorothiazide.	**Case 14-4 (Question 1)**

INTRODUCTION

More than 76 million Americans have hypertension, also called high blood pressure (BP).[1] It is estimated that approximately 30% of adult Americans have hypertension, making it the most frequently encountered chronic medical condition. It is also one of the most significant risk factors for cardiovascular (CV) morbidity and mortality resulting from target-organ damage to blood vessels in the heart, brain, kidney, and eyes. These complications can manifest as either atherosclerotic vascular disease or other forms of CV disease. The exact etiology of essential hypertension is unknown; however, lifelong management with lifestyle modifications and pharmacotherapy are usually needed.

Awareness, treatment, and control of hypertension have improved in the past decade, but are not optimal. Based on the most recent data from the National Health and Nutrition Examination Survey (NHANES), 2007–2008, approximately 81% of patients who truly have hypertension are diagnosed with this medical condition, leaving many patients undiagnosed.[2] Similarly, 73% of people with hypertension are receiving some form of treatment. Ultimately, only 50% of patients with hypertension, including those who are not treated, have controlled BP (defined as both systolic BP <140 mm Hg and diastolic BP <90 mm Hg).[2] When only those patients who are treated for hypertension are considered, 69% have controlled BP.[2] Although these numbers are improved from past estimates, they likely underestimate the magnitude of the problem because some patients may benefit from more aggressive BP control than a goal of less than 140/90 mm Hg. Considering the known risks of hypertension, continued improvements in diagnosing, treating, and overall management of hypertension remain essential to reducing the overall global burden of CV disease.

Blood Pressure

During systole, the left ventricle contracts, ejecting blood systemically into the arteries causing a sharp rise in arterial BP. This is the systolic BP (SBP). The left ventricle then relaxes during diastole, and arterial BP decreases to a trough value as blood returns to the heart from the venous system. This is the diastolic BP (DBP). When recording BP (e.g., 120/76 mm Hg), the numerator is the SBP and the denominator is the DBP. BP has a predictable diurnal rhythm, with fluctuations throughout the day. Values are lowest during the nighttime, sharply rise starting in the early morning, and peak in the late morning to early afternoon. These fluctuations are less pronounced in the black population and may be absent in patients with secondary hypertension.

Mean arterial pressure (MAP) is sometimes used to represent BP, especially in patients with hypertensive emergency. MAP collectively reflects both SBP and DBP, with one-third of the pressure from SBP and two-thirds from DBP. It is calculated using the following equation (Eq. 14-1):

$$\text{MAP} = (\text{SBP} \times 1/3) + (\text{DBP} \times 2/3) \qquad \textit{(Eq. 14-1)}$$

The Seventh Report of the Joint National Committee on Detection, Evaluation, and Treatment of High Blood Pressure (JNC-7), published in 2003, classified BP values and stages hypertension based on SBP and DBP values (Table 14-1).[3] Hypertension is defined as an elevated SBP, DBP, or both. A clinical diagnosis of hypertension is based on the mean of two or more properly measured seated BP measurements taken on two or more occasions. The JNC-7 classification includes normal BP, prehypertension, stage 1 hypertension, and stage 2 hypertension. Qualitative terms (e.g., mild, moderate, high-normal, severe) are not recommended and should not be used.

TABLE 14-1
Classification of Blood Pressure in Adults[3]

Classification[a]	SBP (mm Hg)	DBP (mm Hg)
Normal	<120	and <80
Prehypertension	120–149	or 80–89
Stage 1 hypertension	140–159	or 90–99
Stage 2 hypertension	≥160	or ≥100

[a] If SBP and DBP are in different categories, the overall classification is determined based on the higher of the two blood pressure categories.
DBP, diastolic blood pressure; SBP, systolic blood pressure.

PATHOPHYSIOLOGY OF BLOOD PRESSURE REGULATION

Various neural and humoral factors are known to influence and regulate BP.[4] These include the adrenergic nervous system (controls α- and β-adrenergic receptors), the renin-angiotensin-aldosterone system (RAAS) (regulates systemic and renal blood flow), renal function and renal blood flow (influences fluid and electrolyte balance), several hormonal factors (adrenal cortical hormones, vasopressin, thyroid hormone, insulin), and the vascular endothelium (regulates release of nitric oxide [NO], bradykinin, prostacyclin, endothelin). Knowledge of these mechanisms is important in understanding antihypertensive drug therapy. BP is normally regulated by compensatory mechanisms that respond to changes in cardiac demand. An increase in cardiac output (CO) normally results in a compensatory decrease in total peripheral resistance (TPR); likewise, an increase in TPR results in a decrease in CO. These events regulate MAP, as is represented in the following equation (Eq. 14-2):

$$\text{MAP} = \text{CO} \times \text{TPR} \qquad \textit{(Eq. 14-2)}$$

Adverse changes in BP can occur when these compensatory mechanisms are not functioning properly. It has been suggested that in hypertension an initial increase in fluid volume increases CO and arterial pressure. Eventually, with long-standing hypertension, it is believed that TPR increases so that CO returns to normal.

The kidney plays an important role in the regulation of arterial pressure, especially through the RAAS. Decreases in BP and renal blood flow, volume depletion or decreased sodium concentration, and an activation of the sympathetic nervous system can all trigger an increased secretion of the enzyme renin from the cells of the juxtaglomerular apparatus in the kidney. Renin acts on angiotensinogen to catalyze the formation of angiotensin I. Angiotensin-converting enzyme (ACE) converts angiotensin I to angiotensin II (see Figs. 19-2 and 19-6 in Chapter 19, Heart Failure). Angiotensin II is a potent vasoconstrictor that acts directly on arteriolar smooth muscle and also stimulates the production of aldosterone by the adrenal glands. Aldosterone causes sodium and water retention and the excretion of potassium. Several factors influence renin release, especially those that alter renal perfusion. The resultant increase in BP results in suppression of renin release through negative feedback.

Approximately 20% of patients with essential hypertension have lower-than-normal plasma renin activity (PRA), whereas approximately 15% have PRA concentrations that are higher than normal. Those with normal to high PRA (e.g., young, whites) should theoretically be more responsive to drug therapies that target the RAAS (e.g., ACE inhibitors, angiotensin receptor blockers [ARBs]). Patients with low PRA may be more responsive to diuretic therapy. However, routinely measuring PRA as a strategy to guide empiric drug selection has limited clinical utility, and does not generally result in an outcome superior to careful selection of antihypertensive drug therapy.

Arterial BP is also regulated by the adrenergic nervous system, which causes contraction and relaxation of vascular smooth muscle. Stimulation of α-adrenergic receptors in the central nervous system (CNS) results in a reflex decrease in sympathetic outflow, causing a decrease in BP. Stimulation of postsynaptic α_1-receptors in the periphery causes vasoconstriction. The α-receptors are regulated by a negative feedback system; as norepinephrine is released into the synaptic cleft and stimulates presynaptic α_2-receptors, further norepinephrine release is inhibited. This negative feedback results in a balance between vasoconstriction and vasodilatation. Stimulation of postsynaptic β_1-receptors located in the myocardium causes an increase in heart rate and contractility, whereas stimulation of postsynaptic β_2-receptors in blood vessels results in vasodilation.

A direct association exists between sodium and BP. Although there is a considerably high degree of patient variability in BP sensitivity to sodium (likely affected by heredity and interactions with other environmental exposures), patients with a high dietary sodium intake generally have a greater prevalence of hypertension than those with a low sodium intake. The mechanism by which excess sodium intake contributes to hypertension is uncertain, but it is believed to involve an undetermined natriuretic hormone (not the A- and B-type natriuretic peptides associated with heart failure) that may be induced as a consequence of impaired renal sodium excretion. This natriuretic hormone might also cause an increase in intracellular sodium and calcium, resulting in increased vascular tone and hypertension. The consequences of impaired sodium excretion may have an underlying evolutionary basis. Human physiology evolved in a "hunter-gatherer" society with diets characterized by low sodium and high potassium. The relatively recent shifts in diet patterns brought about by the advent of modern food processing, coupled with increased survival beyond reproductive years, may not have made it possible for modern humans to adapt successfully to high sodium exposure.

Epidemiologic evidence and clinical trials have demonstrated an inverse relationship between calcium and BP. One proposed mechanism for this relationship involves an alteration in the balance between intracellular and extracellular calcium. Increased intracellular calcium concentrations can increase peripheral vascular resistance, resulting in increased BP.

A decrease in dietary potassium has been associated with an increase in peripheral vascular resistance. In theory, diuretic-induced hypokalemia could counteract some of the antihypertensive effects of diuretic therapy, but this has not been seen in clinical trials. It is important, however, that potassium concentrations be maintained within the normal range because hypokalemia increases the risk of CV events, such as sudden death.

Insulin resistance and hyperinsulinemia also have been associated with hypertension. Kaplan[4] suggests that insulin resistance is responsible for the frequent coexistence of hyperglycemia, dyslipidemia, hypertension, and abdominal obesity (also called the *metabolic syndrome*).[5] Although the exact role of insulin resistance in the development of hypertension is still evolving, it is clear that these factors are intertwined and increase CV risk.

The vascular epithelium is a dynamic system in which vascular tone is regulated by numerous substances. As noted previously, angiotensin II promotes vasoconstriction of the vascular epithelium. However, several other substances regulate vascular tone. NO is produced in the endothelium and is a potent vasodilatory chemical that relaxes the vascular smooth muscle. The NO system has been firmly established as an important regulator of arterial BP. Hypothetically, some patients with hypertension have an intrinsic deficiency in NO release and inadequate vasodilation, which could contribute to hypertension and its vascular complications.

Factors that regulate BP are well understood and continue to evolve, but the cause of essential hypertension is still unknown. It is impossible to target therapy to specific abnormalities. Therefore, antihypertensive therapy should be selected based on evidence from clinical trials that have demonstrated reductions in hypertension-associated complications, as is discussed later in this chapter.

CARDIOVASCULAR RISK AND BLOOD PRESSURE

Direct correlations between BP values and risk of CV disease have been established based primarily on epidemiologic data. Beginning at a benchmark BP of 115/75 mm Hg, the risk of CV disease doubles with every increment of 20/10 mm Hg.[3,6] Clinically, it is important to note that incremental elevations in SBP are more predictive of CV disease than elevations in DBP, especially for patients older than 50 years of age. Therefore, SBP is the target of evaluation and intervention for most patients with hypertension. In younger patients with hypertension, elevated DBP may be the only BP abnormality present.

MEASURING BLOOD PRESSURE

AUSCULTATORY METHOD

The measurement of BP should be standardized to minimize variability in readings. The American Heart Association (AHA) technique for auscultatory BP measurement (Table 14-2)[7] should be used in most patients.[8]

TABLE 14-2
Auscultatory Method for Blood Pressure Measurement in Adults as Recommended by the American Heart Association[7]

1. **PATIENT:** Patient should be seated for 5 minutes with arm bared, unrestricted by clothing, and supported at heart level. Smoking or food ingestion should not have occurred within 30 minutes before the measurement.
2. **CUFF:** An appropriately sized cuff should be used. The internal inflatable bladder width should be at least 40% and the bladder length and cover at least 80% of the upper arm circumference. The cuff should be wrapped snugly around the arm with the center of the bladder over the brachial artery.
3. **MONITOR:** Measurements should be taken with a correctly calibrated mercury sphygmomanometer, an aneroid manometer, or a validated electronic device.
4. **PALPATORY METHOD:** SBP should be estimated using the palpatory method. The cuff is rapidly inflated in 10-mm Hg increments, while simultaneously palpating the radial pulse on the patient's wrist on the cuffed arm while observing the manometer. The pressure when the radial pulse is no longer palpable is the estimated SBP. The cuff is then deflated rapidly.
5. **KOROTKOFF SOUNDS:** The head of the stethoscope, ideally using the bell, should be placed over the brachial artery, with each earpiece in the clinician's ear. The cuff should then be rapidly inflated to 20 to 30 mm Hg above the estimated SBP from the palpatory method. The cuff is slowly deflated at a rate of 2 mm Hg per second while the clinician simultaneously listens for phase 1 (the first appearance of sounds) and phase 5 (the disappearance of sounds) Korotkoff sounds while also observing the manometer. When the pressure is 10 to 20 mm Hg below phase 5, the cuff can be rapidly deflated.
6. **DOCUMENTATION:** BP values should always be recorded. The BP values (SBP/DBP) should be recorded using even numbers (rounded up from an odd number)[a] along with the patient's position (seated, standing, or supine), arm used, cuff size, time, and date.
7. **REPEAT:** A second measurement should be taken after at least 1 minute in the same arm. If the readings differ by more than 5 mm Hg, additional measurements should be obtained. The mean of these values should be used to make clinical decisions. BP should be taken in both arms at the initial visit with the BP measured in the arm with the higher reading at subsequent visits.

[a] Terminal digit preference (i.e., tendency to report readings that end in 0 or 5) should be avoided.

BP, blood pressure; DBP, diastolic blood pressure; SBP, systolic blood pressure.

ONLINE CONTENT

For a video demonstrating the auscultatory method for blood pressure measurement in adults (Courtesy of the University of Colorado School of Pharmacy), go to http://thepoint.lww.com/AT10e.

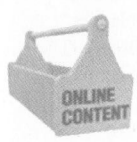

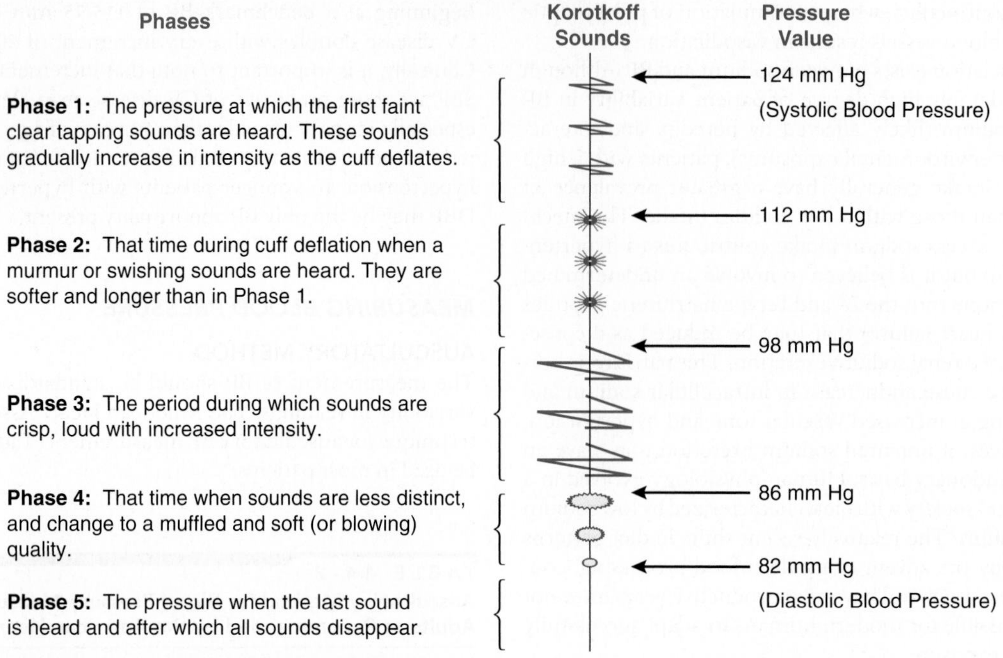

Phases
Korotkoff Sounds
Pressure Value
Phase 1: The pressure at which the first faint clear tapping sounds are heard. These sounds gradually increase in intensity as the cuff deflates.
124 mm Hg
(Systolic Blood Pressure)
Phase 2: That time during cuff deflation when a murmur or swishing sounds are heard. They are softer and longer than in Phase 1.
112 mm Hg
Phase 3: The period during which sounds are crisp, loud with increased intensity.
98 mm Hg
Phase 4: That time when sounds are less distinct, and change to a muffled and soft (or blowing) quality.
86 mm Hg
Phase 5: The pressure when the last sound is heard and after which all sounds disappear.
82 mm Hg
(Diastolic Blood Pressure)

FIGURE 14-1 Phases of the Korotkoff sounds heard when indirectly measuring blood pressure.

ONLINE CONTENT

For a video demonstrating the ascultatory method for blood pressure measurement in adults (Courtesy of the University of Colorado School of Pharmacy), go to http://thepoint.lww.com/AT10e.

Correct BP measurements require that the clinician listen through a stethoscope that is placed over the brachial artery for the appearance of the five phases of the Korotkoff sounds. Each sound has distinct features, which are depicted in Figure 14-1.[8] Examples of Korotkoff sounds can be found in the Thinklabs Medical Sound Library (http://www.thinklabsmedical.com/stethoscope_community/Sound_Library) under Blood Pressure—Korotkoff Sounds 1 and Blood Pressure—Korotkoff Sounds 2.

OUT-OF-OFFICE BLOOD PRESSURE MONITORING

Home BP measurements can provide information on response to therapy and may help improve adherence to therapy and goal BP achievement in some patients.[9,10] Devices for home measurement should be validated for accuracy according to established protocols from either the British Hypertension Society or the Association for Advancement of Medical Instrumentation. When placed in service, they should be routinely checked against office-based readings for accuracy, especially when readings between office and home are widely discrepant. Patients with average home BP values greater than 135/85 mm Hg are considered hypertensive.[7] Wrist or finger devices that measure BP are generally not accurate and should not be routinely used.

Ambulatory blood pressure monitoring (ABPM) typically measures BP every 15 to 30 minutes throughout the day and nighttime using a portable, noninvasive oscillometric device typically worn for 24 hours.[7] This form of specialized monitoring is indicated for patients with suspected white-coat hypertension, and also may be helpful in patients with apparent drug resistance, hypotensive symptoms while receiving antihypertensive therapy, episodic hypertension, and autonomic dysfunction.[7] Similar to self-BP measurements, ABPM values are typically lower than office-based measurements. As a comparison, the normal upper limit for BP in most patients is 140/90 mm Hg for office-based measurement, 130/80 mm Hg for ABPM (135/85 mm Hg while awake and 120/75 mm Hg while asleep), and 135/85 mm Hg for self-BP measurements.[7] Therefore, the threshold for normal versus abnormal is lower than that obtained during office-based measurements.

Evidence indicates that ABPM recordings can predict clinical outcomes more strongly than office-based BP measurements, most likely because the device factors in BP throughout nighttime hours, which provides a more accurate reflection of the overall average pressure load.[11] However, in clinical practice ABPM is not recommended for routine evaluation of responses to treatment for a number of reasons, including lack of widespread availability, cost, and intrusiveness of performing multiple ABPM sessions in the same patient.[7]

BP values measured outside the office should be considered in the overall treatment of patients with hypertension. However, it is important to acknowledge that office-based BP measurements have been the source used in the major clinical trials establishing that treatment of hypertension reduces morbidity and mortality rates. Therefore, they are still considered the standard values that should guide evaluation of response to antihypertensive drug therapy in most patients.

The reliability and accuracy of automated BP monitors, whether they are used in the office or out of the office can vary significantly. BP measurements that are used to make clinical decisions in the care of patients with hypertension should be obtained only from validated devices. For a summary of commercially available automatic monitors and whether they have passed validation protocols, please refer to the dabl Educational Trust website (http://www.dableducational.org). The use of BP measurements from automated machines commonly found in grocery stores and pharmacies may have questionable reliability. Measurements using these publically available machines should not be relied on to make clinical decisions, but should be used to direct patients for follow-up with their medical provider as a screening tool.

Types of Hypertension

ESSENTIAL HYPERTENSION

Most patients with hypertension have essential hypertension (also known as primary hypertension), in which there is no identifiable cause for their chronically elevated BP.

SECONDARY HYPERTENSION

Patients with secondary hypertension have a specific identified cause for elevated BP (Table 14-3). Although only 5% to 10% of those among the hypertensive population have causes that are purely secondary, further diagnostic evaluation should occur if physical or laboratory findings suggest the possibility of a secondary cause (Table 14-4).[3,12,13] Some secondary causes are potentially reversible and may normalize BP (e.g., coarctation of the aorta), whereas others are more often superimposed on and worsen an already elevated BP (e.g., obstructive sleep apnea). The distinction is important because treatment of an underlying cause may not always be expected to completely normalize BP and allow discontinuation of antihypertensive therapies. In patients who have resistant hypertension (see Resistant Hypertension section) or who have a sudden and significant increase in BP, further diagnostic workup for secondary causes should be considered.[3,4] Before proceeding with potentially expensive testing, adherence to existing antihypertensive regimen, and a thorough review of other prescription medications, nonprescription medications, and supplements should be conducted to rule out potential causes of BP elevations.[12]

PSEUDOHYPERTENSION

Although relatively rare, the possibility of pseudohypertension should be considered when measuring BP in elderly patients. In pseudohypertension, blood vessels become stiff and thick because of calcification and resist compression from the bladder of the inflatable BP cuff. Greater pressure is then needed to occlude the artery, and this can result in an overestimation of true SBP. Osler's maneuver is used to detect pseudohypertension. A BP cuff is inflated above the SBP while palpating the brachial or radial arteries to determine whether the pulseless artery is

TABLE 14-3
Secondary Causes of Hypertension[3,12]

Alcoholism
Chronic kidney disease
Chronic steroid therapy and Cushing syndrome
Coarctation of the aorta
Drug-induced or drug-related
- Amphetamines (amphetamine, dexmethylphenidate, dextroamphetamine, lisdexamfetamine, methylphenidate, phendimetrazine, and phentermine)
- Antidepressants (bupropion, desvenlafaxine, and venlafaxine)
- Antihypertensive agents that are abruptly stopped (only β-blockers and central α_2-agonists)
- Anabolic steroids (e.g., testosterone)
- Calcineurin inhibitors (cyclosporine and tacrolimus)
- Cocaine and other illicit drugs
- Corticosteroids (cortisone, dexamethasone, fludrocortisone, hydrocortisone, methylprednisolone, prednisolone, prednisone, and triamcinolone)
- Ephedra alkaloids
- Erythropoiesis-stimulating agents (darbepoetin-alfa and erythropoietin)
- Ergot alkaloids (ergonovine and methysergide)
- Estrogen-containing oral contraceptives (ethinyl estradiol)
- Licorice (including some chewing tobacco)
- Monoamine oxidase inhibitors (isocarboxazid, phenelzine, tranylcypromine sulfate) when given with tyramine-containing foods or with an interacting drug
- Nonsteroidal anti-inflammatory drugs (all types)
- Oral decongestants (e.g., pseudoephedrine)
- Phenylephrine (ocular administration)
- Vascular endothelial growth factor inhibitor (bevacizumab)
- Vascular endothelial growth factor receptor tyrosine kinase inhibitor (sorafenib and sunitinib)

Pheochromocytoma
Primary aldosteronism
Renovascular disease
Sleep apnea
Thyroid or parathyroid disease

TABLE 14-4
Clinical Findings Suggestive of Secondary Hypertension

Causes	Historical Findings	Physical Examination Findings	Laboratory Findings
Sleep apnea	Daytime fatigue and somnolence	Large neck circumference; overweight or obese	Abnormal sleep studies with frequent awakenings and anoxic episodes
Renovascular disease	Moderate or severe high BP before age 30 or after 55; rapidly progressive hypertension	Abdominal bruits; funduscopic hemorrhages	Suppressed or stimulated plasma renin activity; IVP (rapid sequence); digital subtraction angiography
Renoparenchymal disease	Dysuria, polyuria, nocturia; urinary tract infections; kidney stones; family history of polycystic or other types of kidney disease	Edema	Proteinuria; hematuria; bacteriuria
Coarctation of the aorta	Intermittent claudication	Diminished or absent femoral pulses compared with carotids; lower SBP in leg compared with arm	—
Pheochromocytoma	Paroxysmal headaches, palpitations, sweating, dizziness, and pallor	Nervousness, tremor, tachycardia, orthostatic hypotension	Clonidine suppression tests[a]; high urinary metanephrine or vanillylmandelic acid
Primary aldosteronism	Weakness, polyuria, polydipsia, intermittent paralysis	Orthostatic hypotension	Hypokalemia
Cushing syndrome	Menstrual irregularity	Moon face; truncal obesity; buffalo hump; hirsutism; violet striae	↑ serum glucose; ↑ plasma cortisol after suppression with dexamethasone

[a] Failure of plasma catecholamines to ↓ by 50% within 3 hours of administration of 0.3 mg clonidine highly suggests pheochromocytoma.
BP, blood pressure; IVP, intravenous pyelogram; SBP, systolic blood pressure.

palpable. If the artery is palpable, the patient might have pseudohypertension.

WHITE-COAT HYPERTENSION

White-coat hypertension describes patients who have consistently elevated BP values measured in a clinical environment in the presence of a health care professional (e.g., physician's office), yet when measured elsewhere or with 24-hour ambulatory monitoring, BP is not elevated.[7,8] Home BP monitoring or 24-hour ABPM is warranted in patients suspected of having white-coat hypertension to differentiate this from true hypertension.[7] The commonly used definition is a persistently elevated average office blood pressure of greater than 140/90 mm Hg and an average awake ambulatory reading of less than 135/85 mm Hg.[8] The label *white-coat hypertension* applies only to patients without target-organ disease who are not on antihypertensive therapy. It is estimated to be present in 15% to 20% of people with stage 1 hypertension.[8]

Significant controversies surround white-coat hypertension. Although this does not represent a clinical diagnosis, patients with white-coat hypertension are at risk for eventually developing essential hypertension. Moreover, patients with white-coat hypertension are at a higher risk for CV disease than normotensive patients.[14] The decision to treat or not treat white-coat hypertension is controversial. Many patients enrolled in the landmark clinical trials that demonstrated reductions in CV morbidity and mortality with antihypertensive therapy likely had white-coat hypertension because only office BP measurements were used for inclusion. At minimum, patients with white-coat hypertension should be treated with lifestyle modifications, and need to be closely monitored with a device that can measure BP outside the clinic environment if they are not treated with antihypertensive drug therapy.

HYPERTENSIVE CRISES

Hypertensive crises are situations in which measured BP values are markedly elevated, typically in the upper range of stage 2 hypertension (>180/110 mm Hg). They are classified as either a hypertensive emergency (with acute or progressive target-organ damage) or urgency (without acute or progressive target-organ damage).[4] Hypertensive emergencies require hospitalization for immediate BP lowering using intravenous (IV) medications and intra-arterial BP monitoring. Examples of acute target-organ damage include encephalopathy, myocardial infarction (MI), unstable angina, pulmonary edema, eclampsia, stroke, head trauma, life-threatening arterial bleeding, aortic dissection, severe retinopathy, or acute kidney failure. Hypertensive urgencies do not require immediate BP lowering; instead, BP should be slowly reduced within 24 hours (but not generally to goal BP so quickly) after drug therapy recommendations for stage 2 hypertension (see Chapter 21, Hypertensive Crises).

Hypertension Management

Hypertension is treated with both lifestyle modifications and pharmacotherapy. The JNC-7 is considered the "gold standard" consensus guidelines for the management of hypertension in the United States. The newest version of this guideline, the JNC-8, is expected to be published in 2012. The 2007 AHA scientific statement regarding the treatment of hypertension is another evidence-based guideline that is used by clinicians as a more aggressive option for managing hypertension.[15] In contrast to the JNC-7, the AHA 2007 guidelines provide more aggressive BP goals for several patient populations (Fig. 14-2), and update pharmacotherapy recommendations based on more recent evidence. Of note, the 2007 European Society of Hypertension/European Society of Cardiology also recommends more aggressive BP

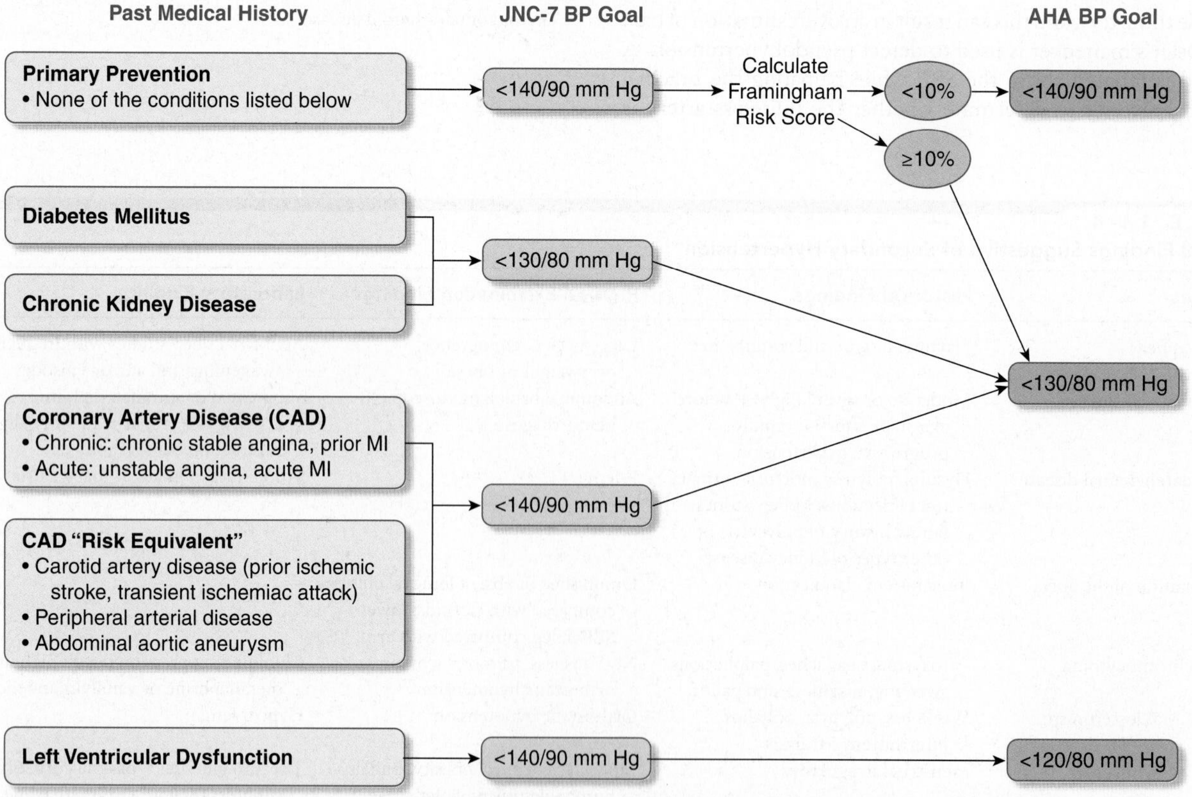

FIGURE 14-2 Goal blood pressure (BP) determination based on patient-specific history and cardiovascular risk assessment. AHA, American Heart Association; JNC-7, The Seventh Report of the Joint National Committee on Detection, Evaluation, and Treatment of High Blood Pressure.

TABLE 14-5
Hypertension-Associated Complications and Major Cardiovascular Risk Factors

Hypertension-Associated Complications

- Atherosclerotic vascular disease
  - Coronary artery disease (sometimes called coronary heart disease)
    - Myocardial infarction
    - Acute coronary syndromes
    - Chronic stable angina
  - Carotid artery disease:
    - Ischemic stroke
    - Transient ischemic attack
  - Peripheral arterial disease
  - Abdominal aortic aneurysm
- Other forms of CV disease
  - Left ventricular dysfunction (systolic heart failure)
  - Chronic kidney disease
  - Retinopathy

Major CV Risk Factors

- Advanced age (>55 years for men, >65 years for women)
- Cigarette smoking
- Diabetes mellitus
- Dyslipidemia
- Family history of premature atherosclerotic vascular disease (men <55 years or women <65 years) in primary relatives
- Hypertension
- Kidney disease (microalbuminuria or estimated GFR <60 mL/min/1.73 m^2)
- Obesity (BMI ≥30 kg/m^2)
- Physical inactivity

BMI, body mass index; CV, cardiovascular; GFR, glomerular infiltration rate.

goals, analogous to the AHA 2007 recommendations.[16] The overall principles common to these guidelines are to implement lifestyle modifications in addition to pharmacotherapy to control BP in patients with hypertension. The presence of specific complications of hypertension or comorbidities (referred to as "compelling indications") in any given patient should be considered when selecting specific pharmacotherapy to treat hypertension. These issues are discussed later in this chapter.

GOALS

The overarching goal of treating patients with hypertension is to reduce associated morbidity and mortality (also called CV events). These manifest as hypertension-associated complications (Table 14-5), which include atherosclerotic vascular disease and other forms of CV disease.

ONLINE CONTENT

For an animation that shows hypertension-associated complications, go to http://thepoint.lww.com/AT10e.

Clinical presentation of such complications can be an acute CV event (e.g., MI) or chronic medical condition (e.g., chronic kidney disease [CKD]). Hypertension-associated complications are the primary causes of death in patients with hypertension. There are several major CV risk factors that have been identified. These major CV risk factors increase the risk of developing hypertension-associated complications; they are not risk factors for the development of hypertension.

FRAMINGHAM RISK SCORING

Hypertension often occurs in tandem with other established CV risk factors, which in addition to elevated BP should be identified and managed in the overall treatment of patients with hypertension. Therefore, estimating individual risk for CV disease is essential for most patients with hypertension. In the United States, Framingham risk scoring (available online at **http://hp2010.nhlbihin.net/atpiii/calculator.asp?usertype=pub**) is considered an appropriate way to predict individual 10-year risk for coronary heart disease (CHD), also referred to as coronary artery disease (CAD). All patients with hypertension who do not have a history of hypertension-associated complications (Table 14-5) or diabetes (considered a CHD risk equivalent condition) should have Framingham risk scoring performed to assess their 10-year risk of developing hard CHD (non-fatal MI or fatal CHD). Patients with Framingham risk scores of 10% or greater are candidates for more-aggressive BP lowering according to the 2007 AHA guidelines.[15] For patients with hypertension-associated complications or diabetes, Framingham risk scoring is not needed because 10-year risk of CAD is assumed to be greater than 20%.

GOAL BLOOD PRESSURE VALUES

Achieving goal BP is an important step in the overall treatment of patients with hypertension. According to the JNC-7 guidelines, patients with hypertension have a BP goal of either less than 140/90 or less than 130/80 mm Hg (Fig. 14-2).[3] The 2007 AHA guidelines provide more-aggressive optional goals for certain patients with high CV risk by extending the less than 130/80 mm Hg goal to patients with CAD, patients with noncoronary atherosclerotic vascular disease, and patients with a Framingham score of 10% or greater, and recommends less than 120/80 mm Hg as a goal BP for patients with left ventricular dysfunction.[15]

The concept behind recommending more aggressive BP goals than the standard goal of less than 140/90 mm Hg is that certain patients, based on the presence of comorbid conditions or multiple major CV risk factors, are at higher risk for hypertension-associated complications. Therefore, further lowering BP may provide optimal reduction in risk of hypertension-associated complications. In patients with diabetes or CKD, some data from prospective clinical trials support this assumption.[17,18] However, more recent evidence has failed to show that more aggressive BP lowering below the standard goal of less than 140/90 mm Hg in diabetes or CKD provides additional clinical benefits.[19–23] In the Action to Control Cardiovascular Risk in Diabetes (ACCORD) trial, there was no difference in the primary end point of major CV events when patients with type 2 diabetes were treated to a SBP goal of less than 120 mm Hg compared with a SBP goal of less than 120 mm Hg after a mean of 4.7 years.[23] However, the incidence of stroke, a secondary end point, was lower in the group randomized to a SBP goal of less than 120 mm Hg.

The issue of whether aggressive BP goals (i.e., <130/80 or <120/80 mm Hg) result in better reductions in risk of CV events than the standard goal of less than 140/90 mm Hg remains an ongoing clinical controversy. Until newer clinical data and newer consensus guidelines are published, it is reasonable for clinicians to follow the BP goals recommended in the JNC-7, and to view the aggressive BP goals that are recommended by the AHA as therapeutic options. The Systolic Blood Pressure Intervention Trial (SPRINT) is a randomized, multicenter, clinical trial that is comparing intensive hypertension treatment (SBP goal <120 mm Hg) with standard treatment (SBP goal <140 mm Hg) in approximately 7,500 patients with hypertension and at least one other CV risk factor (patients with a history of diabetes or stroke are excluded). The SPRINT will not be completed until the year 2018 or later, but when completed will provide further evidence regarding goal BP values.

Another area of controversy is the BP goal value in the very elderly, commonly defined as those 80 years of age or older. Within this population, the only clear prospective data supporting antihypertensive therapy from the Hypertension in the Very Elderly Trial (HYVET) used a BP goal of less than 150/80 mm Hg.[24] Although applying the standard BP goals to the very elderly population is reasonable, it is an area where clinicians may disagree, and individual patient characteristics must be carefully considered. In a 2011 consensus document on hypertension in the elderly, the AHA in 2011 recommends that an achieved SBP of less than 140 mm Hg is appropriate for patients younger than 80 years of age.[25] However, based to some extent on the HYVET and expert opinion, they also recommend that a SBP between 140 and 145 mm Hg is acceptable for patients 80 years or older. It is important to note that BP goals among the elderly are based primarily on expert consensus.

Elevated SBP is more predictive of CV disease than DBP for most patients.[3] However, BP goal achievement requires reduction of both SBP and DBP to goal values. Control of SBP is imperative, and this usually results in control of DBP. Clinicians should appropriately implement and titrate therapy until the selected goal BP value is attained, despite the tendency to accept BP values that are close to, but not at, the goal. This has been referred to as "clinical inertia," when in the context of hypertension, an office visit at which no therapeutic move was made to lower BP in a patient with uncontrolled hypertension occurs.[26] Although clinical inertia is not the only reason why many patients with hypertension are not at their goal BP value, it is one that can be addressed through more intensive initiating, titrating, or changing of drug therapy.

LIFESTYLE MODIFICATIONS

Lifestyle modifications are the cornerstone of management for preventing and treating hypertension. AHA guidelines for lifestyle modifications recommend both diet and exercise.[27,28] These recommendations are summarized in Table 14-6. Engaging in these modifications is encouraged for all persons to prevent the development of hypertension; however, they are recommended as a component of first-line therapy in all patients with prehypertension, and in all patients with a diagnosis of hypertension regardless of whether their BP values are at goal or not (Table 14-1).[3] Independent of BP lowering, CV risk may also be reduced.

WEIGHT REDUCTION

Weight loss as small as 5% to 10% of body weight in overweight individuals may significantly lower CV risk. For most patients, an average weight loss of 10 kg can reduce SBP by 5 to 20 mm Hg, a reduction comparable to that achieved from the addition of an antihypertensive drug used as monotherapy.[3]

DASH EATING PLAN

The DASH (Dietary Approaches to Stop Hypertension) diet is rich in fruits, vegetables, and low-fat dairy foods, coupled with reduced saturated and total fat.[29] The patient education publication entitled "Your Guide to Lowering Your Blood Pressure with DASH" can be found at **http://www.nhlbi.nih.gov/health/public/heart/hbp/dash/index.htm**. The DASH diet can substantially reduce BP (8–14 mm Hg in SBP for most patients) and yield similar results to single-drug therapy. The low-fat component of this diet is important because weight loss is more readily achieved by a reduced-calorie diet (fats contribute more calories per gram than do either carbohydrates or protein) and lowered fat intake also reduces the risk of CV disease by lowering cholesterol.

DIETARY SODIUM RESTRICTION

The average American intake of sodium is more than 6 g/day. Restricting sodium should be encouraged for patients with prehypertension or hypertension, and the current recommendation to restrict daily sodium intake to no more than 1.5 g is lower than what has traditionally been suggested. Some clinicians may argue that the efficacy of implementing sodium restriction in patients with hypertension may vary. Evidence from clinical trials has shown, however, that sodium restriction provides mean reductions in BP of 5/2.7 mm Hg in patients with hypertension.[28] Excessive sodium ingestion also significantly contributes to resistant hypertension and poor response to antihypertensive drug therapy. Restricting sodium to less than 1.5 g daily has been shown to decrease SBP by more than 20 mm Hg in patients with resistant hypertension.[30] Some populations (diabetic patients, blacks, and elderly persons) respond better to sodium restriction than the general population, but all patients with hypertension should be instructed to reduce their sodium intake. They should be counseled not to add salt to foods, and to avoid or minimize ingestion of processed or packaged foods, foods with high sodium content, and nonprescription drugs containing sodium.

TABLE 14-6
Lifestyle Modifications to Prevent and Treat Hypertension[8,18,19]

Modification	Recommendation
Weight management	Lose weight if overweight or obese, ideally attaining a BMI <25 kg/m^2 Maintain a desirable BMI (18.5–24.9 kg/m^2) if not overweight or obese
Adopt DASH-type dietary patterns	Consume a diet that is rich in fruits and vegetables (8–10 servings/d), rich in low-fat dairy products (2–3 servings/d), but has reduced amounts of saturated fat and cholesterol
Reduced sodium intake	Reduce daily dietary sodium intake as much as possible; ideally to <65 mmol/d (equal to 1.5 g/d sodium, or 3.8 g/d sodium chloride)
Increased dietary potassium intake	Increase daily dietary potassium intake to 120 mmol/d (4.7 g/d), which is the amount provided in a DASH-type diet
Moderation of alcohol consumption	For patients who drink alcohol, limit consumption to no more than two drinks/d in men and no more than one drink/d in women and lighter-weight people.[a] Do not recommend alcohol consumption in patients who do not drink alcohol
Regular physical activity	Regular moderate-intensity aerobic physical activity; at least 30 minutes of continuous or intermittent 5 d/wk, but preferably daily

[a] Note: One drink is defined as 12 ounces of regular beer, 5 ounces of wine (12% alcohol), and 1.5 ounces of 80-proof distilled spirits.
BMI, body mass index; DASH, Dietary Approaches to Stop Hypertension.

INCREASED POTASSIUM INTAKE

Increasing dietary potassium intake is recommended, although it is not commonly identified by most patients as a dietary modification that will lower BP.[28] Adhering to a DASH eating plan will usually assure an intake of the recommended 4.7 g daily. Dietary supplementation should be the primary strategy to increase potassium. Implementing potassium supplementation outside of dietary sources for the sole purpose of lowering BP should be avoided because of potential harm from hyperkalemia. Moreover, potassium supplementation in patients with hypertension who are treated with a potassium-sparing diuretic, aldosterone antagonist, ACE inhibitor (ACEI), or an ARB may cause hyperkalemia. This can also occur in patients with hypertension and CKD who are treated with potassium supplementation. A diet that is low in sodium and high in potassium is believed to decrease the prevalence of hypertension and CV disease.[31]

MODERATE ALCOHOL CONSUMPTION

Explaining the need to limit alcohol consumption is complicated. Whereas data suggest that small daily doses of alcohol (e.g., one glass of red wine with dinner) are associated with lower CV risk, excessive alcohol intake can elevate BP, decrease the effectiveness of antihypertensive medications, and increase the risk of stroke. Patients who consume three to four drinks per day experience a 3- to 4-mm Hg increase in SBP and a 1- to 2-mm Hg increase in DBP compared with those who do not drink. These increases are even higher in patients who consume more alcohol. Moderate alcohol consumption of two or fewer drinks daily in men and one or fewer drinks daily in women or lighter-weight individuals can decrease SBP approximately 2 to 4 mm Hg. Patients should be instructed that one drink is equal to 1.5 ounces of 80-proof whiskey, 5 ounces of wine, or 12 ounces of beer.

PHYSICAL ACTIVITY

Regular physical activity can reduce SBP by 4 to 9 mm Hg in most patients.[3] Benefits include reducing the incidence of hypertension, assisting weight loss and weight loss maintenance, and improving overall CV fitness. Most patients with hypertension can safely increase their regular aerobic activity. Those with more severe forms of target-organ damage (e.g., angina, previous MI) may, however, need a medical evaluation before increasing their activity level. Physical activity should ideally occur for at least 30 minutes, at least 5 days of the week, but preferably daily. Walking, running, cycling, swimming, and cross-country skiing are examples of aerobic exercise that are recommended for physical activity.

PHARMACOTHERAPY

Numerous clinical trials have demonstrated that antihypertensive pharmacotherapy reduces the risk of hypertension-associated complications (e.g., CV morbidity and mortality).[3,15] This evidence is the foundation for the 2003 JNC-7 and 2007 AHA consensus guidelines, which recommend specific evidence-based pharmacotherapy recommendations based on patient-specific medical history and CV risk (Fig. 14-3).

As recommended in the 2007 AHA guidelines, evidence supports the use of an ACEI, ARB, calcium-channel blocker (CCB), thiazide diuretic, or a two-drug combination for first-line therapy for primary prevention patients.[15,32] This is in contrast to the 2003 JNC-7 guidelines that placed preference on using a thiazide diuretic over other agents for most patients, and also included a β-blocker as a potential first-line option.[3] Evidence obtained since the 2003 JNC-7 guidelines demonstrates, however, that for first-line treatment in primary prevention patients, β-blocker therapy is not as effective in reducing CV events compared with

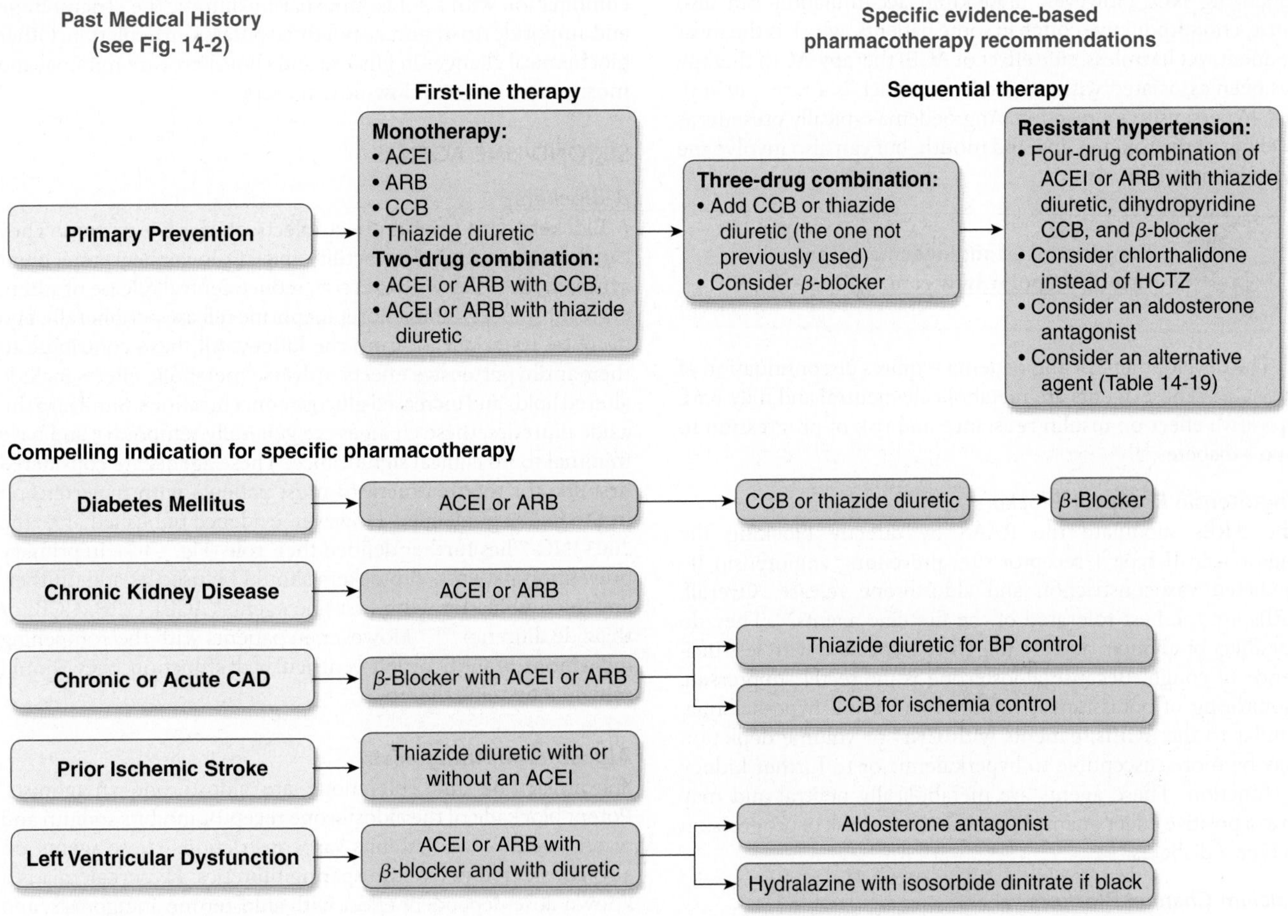

FIGURE 14-3 Recommended pharmacotherapy based on clinical trials evidence demonstrating long-term reductions in morbidity and mortality in patients with hypertension and specific comorbid conditions and cardiovascular risk. Combination therapy with two antihypertensive drugs is an option for patients with stage 1 hypertension (see Table 14-1) and is strongly recommended in patients with stage 2 hypertension. ACEI, angiotensin-converting enzyme inhibitor; ARB, angiotensin receptor blocker; CAD, coronary artery disease; CCB, calcium-channel blocker.

ACEI, ARB, CCB, or thiazide diuretic therapy.[33] Moreover, newer evidence also suggests that the reductions in CV events with ACEI, ARB, CCB, or thiazide diuretic are comparable, so that one agent is not automatically preferred over another.[32]

The selection of pharmacotherapy in patients with comorbid conditions that are considered compelling indications for specific pharmacotherapy is much more prescriptive than in primary prevention patients. Recommendations for patients with compelling indications for specific pharmacotherapy are outlined in Figure 14-3. These recommendations are based on evidence demonstrating reduced risk of CV events in patients with both hypertension and the compelling indication.

FIRST-LINE AGENTS

Angiotensin-Converting Enzyme Inhibitors

The ACEIs directly inhibit ACE, blocking the conversion of angiotensin I to angiotensin II. This action reduces angiotensin II–mediated vasoconstriction and aldosterone secretion, and ultimately lowers BP. Because additional pathways exist for the formation of angiotensin II, ACEIs do not completely block the production of angiotensin II. Aldosterone release is indirectly suppressed by ACEIs; thus, hyperkalemia is possible and potassium concentrations should be monitored. Patients with CKD or volume depletion may be more susceptible to hyperkalemia or to further kidney dysfunction owing to a higher dependence on the vasoconstriction provided by angiotensin II to support glomerular filtration rate (GFR) among these patients.

Inhibiting ACE also prevents the breakdown and inactivation of bradykinin, which may lead to additive vasodilation by enhancing NO. However, bradykinin accumulation can also cause a nonproductive cough in some patients, which is the most frequent, yet harmless, side effect of ACEI therapy. ACEI therapy has been associated with angioedema, which is a rare, but serious, hypersensitivity reaction. Angioedema typically presents as swelling of the tongue, lips, and mouth, but can also involve the eyes and upper airway.

ONLINE CONTENT

For pictures of angioedema, go to http://thepoint.lww.com/AT10e.

The development of angioedema requires discontinuation of the ACEI. These agents are metabolically neutral and may have a positive effect on insulin resistance and risk of progression to type 2 diabetes.[34]

Angiotensin Receptor Blockers

The ARBs modulate the RAAS by directly blocking the angiotensin II type 1 receptor site, preventing angiotensin II–mediated vasoconstriction and aldosterone release. Overall, ARBs are the best tolerated of the first-line agents.[35] They do not affect bradykinin and are therefore associated with less incidence of cough. Because aldosterone is indirectly suppressed, monitoring of potassium is important to avoid hyperkalemia. Similar to the ACEIs, patients with CKD or volume depletion may be more susceptible to hyperkalemia or to further kidney dysfunction. These agents are metabolically neutral and may have a positive effect on insulin resistance and risk of progression to type 2 diabetes.[34]

Calcium-Channel Blockers

The CCBs are pharmacologically complex. They reduce calcium entry into smooth muscles, which causes coronary and peripheral vasodilation and lowers BP. All decrease cardiac contractility (except amlodipine and felodipine). Dihydropyridine CCBs are primarily vasodilators that can cause a reflex tachycardia. This is in contrast to the nondihydropyridine CCBs (verapamil and diltiazem) that directly block the atrioventricular (AV) node, decrease heart rate, and decrease cardiac contraction, yet still have vasodilatory effects. Side effects depend on the type of CCB, but can include flushing, peripheral edema, tachycardia, bradycardia or heart block, and constipation.

Thiazide Diuretics

Diuretics, particularly thiazide and thiazidelike (e.g., chlorthalidone) diuretics, have been extensively studied in large landmark clinical trials for hypertension. When initially started, they induce a natriuresis that causes diuresis and decreases plasma volume and cardiac output. With chronic use, diuresis usually dissipates, and cardiac output gradually returns to near-normal levels. The long-term BP-lowering effect in the face of these changes suggests a sustained decrease in peripheral vascular resistance (PVR) as the primary mechanism responsible.

Overwhelming evidence from large outcome-based clinical trials indicates that diuretic therapy reduces CV morbidity and mortality rates.[32,36,37] Thiazide diuretics are generally well tolerated, and most can be given once daily. They are especially effective in lowering BP in elderly and black patients. Dose-related electrolyte and metabolic alterations (e.g., hypokalemia, hyperuricemia, hyperglycemia, hypercholesterolemia) can occur with thiazide diuretics. These effects were particularly problematic when high doses were used many years ago (e.g., hydrochlorothiazide [HCTZ] 100–200 mg/day), but are drastically minimized by using lower doses that are now considered the standard of care (e.g., HCTZ 12.5–25 mg/day).[37] Thiazide diuretics can be used in combination with a potassium-sparing diuretic (i.e., triamterene and amiloride) to minimize potential potassium depletion. Other biochemical changes in glucose and cholesterol are minimal and mostly transient with low-dose therapy.

SECOND-LINE AGENTS

β-Blockers

β-Blockers have several direct effects on the CV system. They can decrease cardiac contractility and CO, lower heart rate, blunt sympathetic reflex with exercise, reduce central release of adrenergic substances, inhibit norepinephrine release peripherally, and decrease renin release from the kidney. All these contribute to their antihypertensive effects. Adverse metabolic effects include altered lipids and increased glucose concentrations. Similar to thiazide diuretics, these changes are generally temporary and have minimal to no clinical significance. These agents are considered first-line for the treatment of most patients with hypertension in the JNC-7 guideline.[3] However, evidence published after the 2003 JNC-7 has further defined their role (Fig. 14-3). In primary prevention patients, β-blockers should be used as add-on therapy in combination with first-line agents (ACEI, ARB, CCB, or thiazide diuretic).[15,33] However, in patients with the compelling indications of CAD or left ventricular dysfunction, they should remain a first-line therapy.[15]

Aldosterone Antagonists

Spironolactone and eplerenone are aldosterone antagonists. Potent blockade of the aldosterone receptor inhibits sodium and water retention and inhibits vasoconstriction. These agents are also considered potassium-sparing diuretics. Hyperkalemia is a known dose-dependent effect with aldosterone antagonists, and is more prominent in patients with CKD or in patients taking a concurrent RAAS blocking agent (ACEI, ARB, or direct renin inhibitor). Gynecomastia is a side effect of spironolactone, usually more common with higher doses, that does not occur with eplerenone.

OTHER AGENTS

There are other antihypertensive drug classes, many of which are older agents, which should primarily be used to provide additional BP lowering only after first-line and second-line agents have been implemented.

Loop diuretics (e.g., furosemide, torsemide) can be used in some patients for hypertension.[37] When dosed appropriately, they can provide BP reductions similar to those seen with a thiazide diuretic. Because they are short-acting and subject to a significant postdose antinatriuretic effect, they should generally be reserved for patients with heart failure or severe CKD in whom their diuretic action remains prolonged. Significant edema usually accompanies these conditions, such that they generally require a loop diuretic instead of a thiazide diuretic for adequate diuresis and volume removal. Because they are more potent at inducing diuresis compared with thiazide diuretics, they can cause more electrolyte disturbances (e.g., hypokalemia).

Aliskiren, approved in 2007, is the only direct renin inhibitor. Similar to an ACEI or ARB, this agent is a RAAS blocker. It is approved for treatment of hypertension, and has been studied in combination with an ACEI, ARB, or thiazide diuretic. It is the newest antihypertensive drug class; therefore, its exact role will continue to evolve as additional clinical data are generated.

α-Blockers (e.g., doxazosin, prazosin, terazosin) attach to peripheral α_1-receptors, inhibiting the uptake of catecholamines in smooth muscle, and cause vasodilation. Although effective in lowering BP, they have more side effects than first-line or second-line agents. The most prominent side effect is hypotension, which is most evident after the first dose and with postural changes (arising from a lying position to a standing position).

Direct vasodilators (e.g., hydralazine, minoxidil) work on the arterial vasculature. They should be reserved for patients with specific conditions (e.g., severe CKD) or those with very difficult-to-control BP. Concomitant drug therapy with both a diuretic and an agent that lowers heart rate (a β-blocker, diltiazem, or verapamil) is usually needed to mitigate the associated fluid retention and reflex tachycardia that frequently occur.

Central α_2-agonists (e.g., clonidine, methyldopa) work in the vasomotor centers of the brain where they stimulate inhibitory neurons and decrease sympathetic outflow from the CNS. The resultant decrease in PVR and CO lowers BP. These agents commonly cause anticholinergic side effects (e.g., sedation, dizziness, dry mouth, fatigue) and possibly sexual dysfunction. Although α_2-agonists lower BP, they often cause fluid retention and should be used in combination with a diuretic.

Adrenergic antagonists (e.g., reserpine, guanadrel, guanethidine) are not frequently used to treat hypertension. Reserpine depletes catecholamines from storage granules to then decrease BP. High doses are associated with more side effects, but low-dose reserpine (0.05–0.1 mg/day), when used as an additive therapy, is well tolerated. Because of the potential for fluid retention, reserpine requires concurrent diuretic therapy. Guanadrel and guanethidine have numerous significant adverse effects and should be avoided.

CLINICAL EVALUATION

Patient Presentation

CASE 14-1

QUESTION 1: D.C. is a 44-year-old black man who presents to his primary care provider concerned about high BP. At an employee health screening last month he was told he had stage 1 hypertension. His medical history is significant for allergic rhinitis. His BP was 144/84 and 146/86 mm Hg last year during an employee health screening at work. D.C.'s father had hypertension and died of an MI at age 54. His mother had diabetes and hypertension and died of a stroke at age 68. D.C. smokes one pack per day of cigarettes and thinks his BP is high because of job-related stress. He does not believe that he really has hypertension. D.C. does not engage in any regular exercise and does not restrict his diet in any way, although he knows he should lose weight.

Physical examination shows he is 175 cm tall, weighs 108 kg (body mass index [BMI], 35.2 kg/m^2), BP is 148/88 mm Hg (left arm) and 146/86 mm Hg (right arm) while sitting, heart rate is 80 beats/minute. Six months ago, his BP values were 152/88 mm Hg and 150/84 mm Hg when he was seen by his primary-care provider for allergic rhinitis. Funduscopic examination reveals mild arterial narrowing and arteriovenous nicking, with no exudates or hemorrhages. The other physical examination findings are essentially normal.

D.C.'s fasting laboratory serum values are as follows:

Blood urea nitrogen (BUN), 24 mg/dL
Creatinine, 1.0 mg/dL
Glucose, 105 mg/dL
Potassium, 4.4 mEq/L
Uric acid, 6.5 mg/dL
Total cholesterol, 196 mg/dL
Low-density lipoprotein cholesterol (LDL-C), 141 mg/dL
High-density lipoprotein cholesterol (HDL-C), 32 mg/dL
Triglycerides, 170 mg/dL

An electrocardiogram (ECG) is normal except for left ventricular hypertrophy (LVH). What is the proper assessment of D.C.'s BP?

D.C. has uncontrolled stage 1 hypertension. He has had elevated BP values, measured in clinical environments, and meets the diagnostic criteria for hypertension because two or more of his BP measurements are elevated on separate days. SBP values are consistently stage 1, whereas DBP values are all in the prehypertension range. The higher of the two classifications is used to classify hypertension.[5]

CASE 14-1, QUESTION 2: Why does D.C. have hypertension?

D.C. has essential hypertension; therefore the exact cause is not known. He has several characteristics (e.g., family history of hypertension, obesity) that may have increased his chance of developing hypertension. Race and sex also influence the prevalence of hypertension. Across all age groups, blacks have a higher prevalence of hypertension than do whites and Hispanics.[1] Similar to other forms of CV disease, hypertension is more severe, more likely to include hypertension-associated complications, and occurs at an earlier age in black patients.

Patient Evaluation and Risk Assessment

The presence or absence of hypertension-associated complications as well as other major CV risk factors (Table 14-5) must be assessed in D.C. Also, secondary causes of hypertension (Table 14-3), if suggested by history and clinical examination findings, should be identified and managed accordingly. The presence of concomitant medical conditions (e.g., diabetes) should be assessed, and lifestyle habits should be evaluated so that they can be used to guide therapy.

CASE 14-1, QUESTION 3: Which hypertension-associated complications are present in D.C.?

A complete physical examination to evaluate hypertension-associated complications includes examination of the optic fundi; auscultation for carotid, abdominal, and femoral bruits; palpation of the thyroid gland; heart and lung examination; abdominal examination for enlarged kidney, masses, and abnormal aortic pulsation; lower extremity palpation for edema and pulses; and neurologic assessment. Routine laboratory assessment after diagnosis should include the following: ECG; urinalysis; fasting glucose; hematocrit; serum potassium, creatinine, and calcium; and a fasting lipid panel. Optional testing may include measurement of urinary albumin excretion or albumin-to-creatinine ratio, or additional tests specific for secondary causes if suspected.

D.C. does not yet have hypertension-associated complications. He is exhibiting early signs, however, based on his physical examination that, if left untreated, will likely develop into such complications. These early signs have likely evolved from his longstanding, poorly controlled hypertension. D.C.'s ECG revealed LVH, indicating early cardiac damage (Fig. 14-4). Although the gold standard for confirming LVH is echocardiography, this confirmatory procedure is not necessary unless symptoms are present indicating that LVH has progressed to left ventricular dysfunction (e.g., peripheral edema, shortness of breath). His funduscopic examination reveals mild arterial narrowing and arteriovenous nicking, which are early signs of retinopathy and atherosclerosis. D.C.'s serum creatinine is normal, ruling out overt CKD. Additional testing for microalbuminuria is needed, however, to confirm that he does not have early stage kidney disease.

CASE 14-1, QUESTION 4: What other forms of hypertension-associated complications is D.C. at risk for?

Hypertension adversely affects many organ systems, including the heart, brain, kidneys, peripheral circulation, and eyes. These are summarized in Table 14-5. Damage to these systems resulting from hypertension is termed *hypertension-associated complications, target-organ damage,* or *CV disease.* There are often misconceptions about the terms CV disease and CAD. CV disease encompasses the broad scope of all forms of hypertension-associated complications. CAD is simply a subset of CV disease

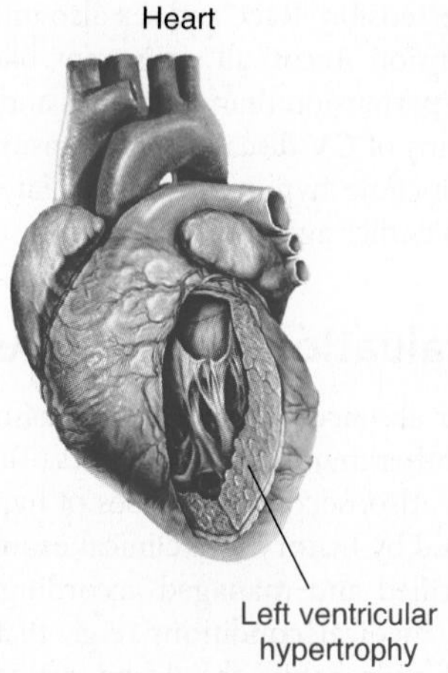

FIGURE 14-4 Left ventricular hypertrophy.

and refers specifically to disease related to the coronary vasculature, including ischemic heart disease and MI. Hypertension-associated complications and major risk factors for developing such complications should be assessed by a thorough patient history, a complete physical examination, and laboratory evaluation.

Hypertension can affect the heart either indirectly, by promoting atherosclerotic changes, or directly, via pressure-related effects. Hypertension can promote CV disease and increase the risk for *ischemic events,* such as angina and MI. Antihypertensive therapy has been shown to reduce the risk of these coronary events. Hypertension also promotes the development of LVH (Fig. 14-4), which is a myocardial (cellular) change, not an arterial change. These two conditions often coexist, however. It is commonly believed that LVH is a compensatory mechanism of the heart in response to the increased resistance caused by elevated BP. LVH is a strong and independent risk factor for CAD, left ventricular dysfunction, and arrhythmia. LVH does not indicate the presence of left ventricular dysfunction, but is a risk for progression to left ventricular dysfunction, which is considered a hypertension-associated complication. This may be caused by ischemia, excessive LVH, or pressure overload. Ultimately, left ventricular dysfunction results in a decreased ability to contract (systolic dysfunction).

Hypertension is one of the most frequent causes of cerebrovascular disease. Cerebrovascular signs can manifest as transient ischemic attacks, ischemic strokes, multiple cerebral infarcts, and hemorrhages. Residual functional deficits caused by stroke are among the most devastating forms of hypertension-associated complications. Clinical trials have demonstrated that antihypertensive therapy can significantly reduce the risk of both initial and recurrent stroke. A sudden, prolonged increase in BP also can cause hypertensive encephalopathy, which is classified as a hypertensive emergency.

The GFR is used to estimate kidney function, which declines with aging. This rate of decline is greatly accelerated by hypertension. Hypertension is associated with nephrosclerosis, which is caused by increased intraglomerular pressure. It is unknown whether a primary kidney lesion with ischemia causes systemic hypertension or whether systemic hypertension directly causes glomerular capillary damage by increasing intraglomerular pressure. Regardless, CKD, whether mild or severe, can progress to kidney failure (stage 5 CKD) and the need for dialysis. Studies have demonstrated that controlling hypertension is the most important strategy to slow the rate of kidney function decline,[38] but it may not be entirely effective in slowing the progression of renal impairment in all patients.

CKD is staged based on estimated GFR values.[38] Stage 3 CKD (moderate) is defined as a GFR 30 to 59 mL/minute/1.73 m^2, stage 4 CKD (severe) is 15 to 29 mL/minute/1.73 m^2, and stage 5 (kidney failure) is less than 15 mL/minute/1.73 m^2 or the requirement of dialysis. In hypertension, stage 3 CKD or worse is considered a hypertension-associated complication. An estimated GFR of less than 60 mL/minute/1.73 m^2 corresponds approximately to a serum creatinine concentration of greater than 1.5 mg/dL in an average man and greater than 1.3 mg/dL in an average woman. This level of kidney compromise lowers an individual's BP goal to less than 130/80 mm Hg according to multiple guidelines.[3,15,38] The presence of persistent albuminuria (>300 mg albumin in a 24-hour urine collection or 200 mg albumin/g creatinine on a spot urine measurement) also indicates significant CKD, for which achieving the more aggressive BP goal is a strategy to minimize the rate of progression to kidney failure. (Note: These definitions of the stages of kidney disease and albuminuria will be used throughout the remaining cases in this chapter.) Assessment of kidney function is discussed in Chapter 2, Interpretation of Clinical Laboratory Tests, and Chapter 31, Chronic Kidney Diseases.

Peripheral arterial disease, a noncoronary form of atherosclerotic vascular disease, is considered a hypertension-associated complication. It is equivalent in CV risk to CHD.[3] Risk factor reduction, BP control, and antiplatelet agent(s) are needed to decrease progression. Complications of peripheral arterial disease can include infection and necrosis, which in some cases require revascularization procedures or extremity amputation.

Hypertension causes retinopathies that can progress to blindness. Retinopathy is evaluated according to the Keith, Wagener, and Barker funduscopic classification system. Grade 1 is characterized by narrowing of the arterial diameter, indicating vasoconstriction. Arteriovenous nicking is the hallmark of grade 2, indicating atherosclerosis. Longstanding, untreated hypertension can cause cotton wool exudates and flame hemorrhages (grade 3). In severe cases (e.g., hypertensive emergency) papilledema occurs, and this is classified as grade 4.

MAJOR RISK FACTORS

CASE 14-1, QUESTION 5: Which major CV risk factors are present in D.C.?

Hypertension is one of nine major CV risk factors (Table 14-5). These are not risk factors for developing hypertension; rather, they increase the risk of hypertension-associated complications. D.C. has multiple CV risk factors: smoking, dyslipidemia, family history of premature CHD in a first-degree relative (father), hypertension, obesity, and physical inactivity.

CASE 14-1, QUESTION 6: What is D.C.'s BP goal and how can Framingham risk scoring influence BP goal determination?

D.C. is a primary prevention patient because he does not yet have any hypertension-associated complications (or compelling indications). He has multiple major CV risk factors, so controlling his BP is of paramount importance to reduce the risk of developing hypertension-associated complications. The JNC-7 guidelines, considered the gold standard for treatment, recommend a BP goal of less than 140/90 mm Hg for D.C. because he is a primary prevention patient without diabetes or CKD. However, some clinicians may choose to follow the more-aggressive AHA guidelines for selecting BP goals. For D.C., a Framingham risk score should be calculated to determine whether the optional AHA-recommended BP goal of less than 130/80 mm Hg is more appropriate (Fig. 14-2). This is accomplished by using the Framingham risk calculator (see **http://hp2010.nhlbihin.net/atpiii/calculator.asp?usertype=pub**). D.C.'s Framingham risk score is 8%, meaning that he has an 8% chance of experiencing CHD (or CAD) during the next 10 years.[15] Because this is less than 10%, D.C. is not currently in a higher CV risk group that would have the option of more aggressive therapy.

Many of D.C.'s risk factors are modifiable. He is a smoker and this significantly increases his CV risk and may reduce the efficacy of antihypertensive therapy. Smoking cessation may not independently lower D.C.'s BP, but it will decrease his overall risk of CV disease (see Chapter 88, Tobacco Use and Dependence). D.C. is obese based on his BMI. His lack of physical activity and dietary patterns have likely contributed to his obesity. A more focused patient interview on diet and exercise would be helpful to reinforce the assumption that he has a sedentary lifestyle. D.C.'s dyslipidemia (particularly his elevated LDL-C) increase his CV risk, and lipid-lowering therapy should be considered to further decrease the risk of CV disease (see Chapter 12, Dyslipidemias, Atherosclerosis, and Coronary Heart Disease).[39]

Advanced age is considered a major CV risk factor. Although CHD in the elderly is not considered premature, increasing age increases the risk of hypertension-associated complications. Premenopausal women are at low risk for CV disease. However, CV risk in women increases significantly after menopause, similar to the increased risk in men. Therefore, cutoff values for age as a risk factor in men and women are separated by 10 years (>55 years for men, >65 years for women). At age 50, D.C. does not yet have this risk factor according to JNC-7 guidelines.[3] Of note, in the context of treatment of dyslipidemia, the age cutoff points for CV risk are 45 years for men and 55 years for women.[39]

PRINCIPLES OF TREATMENT

Goals of Therapy

CASE 14-1, QUESTION 7: What are the goals of treating D.C.?

The overarching goal of treating hypertension is to lower hypertension-associated complications. Control of BP is the most feasible clinical end point to guide therapy and should be viewed as a surrogate for attaining this goal. D.C.'s goal BP is less than 140/90 mm Hg according to both the JNC-7 and AHA guidelines. Pharmacotherapy principles to achieve these goals include selecting a treatment regimen with antihypertensive agent(s) that reduces risk of CV events, complemented by appropriate lifestyle modifications (Table 14-6).

Health Beliefs and Patient Education

CASE 14-1, QUESTION 8: What patient education should be provided to D.C. regarding his hypertension?

Patient education is needed to ensure that D.C. understands his disease and its complications (Table 14-7). This should comprehensively include information on disease, treatment, adherence, and complications. Several approaches can be effective, but all methods should include direct communication between the clinician and the patient. Multidisciplinary approaches to disease-state management in hypertension can effectively use a team of different clinicians (e.g., physicians, nurse practitioners, physician assistants, pharmacists). Providing face-to-face education is most common, but the key components in patient education can be delivered via indirect interactions (e.g., telephone).

ONLINE CONTENT

For a video that shows multidisciplinary team-based approaches to managing hypertension (Courtesy of the University of Iowa), go to http://thepoint.lww.com/AT10e.

Education should be tailored to the patient's specific needs. For example, some patients are able to comprehend the importance of achieving controlled BP by reading written materials, whereas others understand this only after implementing self-BP monitoring. The patient education process must be continuous throughout the duration of therapy. Not all aspects need to be discussed during each clinical interaction. Careful selection of both written and verbal information should be considered so that patients are not overwhelmed or intimidated.

TABLE 14-7
Patient–Provider Interactions for Hypertension

Patient Education
• Assess patient's understanding and acceptance of the diagnosis of hypertension
• Discuss patient's concerns and clarify misunderstandings
• When measuring BP, inform the patient of the reading both verbally and in writing
• Assure patient understands his or her goal BP value
• Ask patient to rate (1–10) his or her chance of staying on treatment
• Inform patient about recommended treatment, including lifestyle modification. Provide specific written information using standard brochures when available
• Elicit concerns and questions and provide opportunities for patient to state specific behaviors to carry out treatment recommendations
• Emphasize: – the need to continue treatment – that control does not mean cure – that elevated BP is usually not accompanied by symptoms
Individualize Treatment Regimens
• Include the patient in decision making
• Simplify the regimen to once-daily dosing, whenever possible
• Incorporate treatment into patient's daily lifestyle
• Set realistic short-term objectives for specific components of the medication and lifestyle modification plan
• Encourage discussion of diet and physical activity, adverse drug effects, and concerns
• Encourage self-monitoring with validated BP devices
• Minimize the cost of therapy, when possible
• Discuss adherence at each clinical encounter
• Encourage gradual sustained weight loss

BP, blood pressure.

National Heart, Lung, and Blood Institute patient education materials are available at http://www.nhlbi.nih.gov/health/public/heart/index.htm#hbp. It is important that clinicians review all materials provided to patients to identify the source of information, assess ease of reading, and identify omitted information and sources of confusion or anxiety (e.g., drug side effects).

Patients such as D.C. often incorrectly explain BP elevation as stress related. Although certain patients (e.g., those with white-coat hypertension) may have BP that is more highly reactive, most patients with essential hypertension will have an elevated BP regardless of their stress level. D.C. should be informed about the cause of his disease and the lack of correlation between stress or symptoms and high BP. Importantly, D.C. needs to realize that elevated BP is almost always asymptomatic, but that it can cause serious long-term complications. It is essential that he understand the chronic nature of hypertension and the need for long-term therapy. Otherwise, he may adhere to his treatment only when he "feels his BP is high" or during stressful events.

Some patients believe they can control their BP by stress management rather than with antihypertensive drug therapy and lifestyle modifications. Controlled trials have not consistently proven that stress management is beneficial in treating hypertension.[40] It is important to determine the patient's health beliefs and attitudes and to provide education about the etiology and management of hypertension to promote BP control.

Another common myth patients believe is that treating hypertension commonly leads to fatigue, lethargy, and sexual dysfunction. This misconception can compromise adherence and be a limiting factor in appropriate management. Clinical trials have repeatedly reported that quality of life is better with active medication than with placebo.[41–44] Data have indicated that as many as 27% of men with hypertension have erectile dysfunction.[45] Although many patients believe this to be a medication-related side effect, and that incidence rates vary among antihypertensive agents and classes, erectile dysfunction is likely caused by penile arterial changes (probably atherosclerosis), which is related to uncontrolled or untreated hypertension.[45]

Benefits of Treatment

CASE 14-1, QUESTION 9: How can antihypertensive drug therapy reduce D.C.'s risk of hypertension-associated complications?

Without a doubt, antihypertensive therapy reduces the risk of CV disease and CV events in patients with hypertension. Numerous landmark placebo-controlled studies have clearly demonstrated these benefits. The first large-scale trial, published in 1967, was the Veterans Administration (VA) study in men with DBP between 115 and 129 mm Hg.[46] This study was prematurely stopped because benefits of treatment were so dramatic. Antihypertensive therapy significantly reduced cerebral hemorrhage, MI, left ventricular dysfunction, retinopathy, and kidney disease. Other landmark placebo-controlled studies have evaluated antihypertensive therapy in patients with less severe hypertension and have shown a reduced risk of CV events (stroke, ischemic heart disease, left ventricular dysfunction) and even CV death.[24,47–50] Placebo-controlled studies evaluating morbidity and mortality in hypertension are now not only unnecessary, but are considered unethical because of the well-established benefits of treatment. Even small reductions in BP have been associated with significant CV benefits. Based on prospective observational studies, a persistent 5 mm Hg reduction in DBP is associated with a 21% reduction in CHD and a 34% reduction in stroke.[51,52]

CASE 14-1, QUESTION 10: Will D.C.'s early signs of hypertension-associated complications improve or reverse with appropriate BP control?

Most antihypertensive drugs reduce LVH through varying mechanisms. It is logical that regression of LVH is desirable, but this remains unproved. Theoretically, myocardial function might be compromised if hypertrophied muscle regresses in size because of the increased ratio of collagen to muscle. Nonetheless, until proven otherwise, regression of LVH in D.C. is desirable.

Reductions in BP can reverse many of the changes associated with D.C.'s retinopathy. Studies have demonstrated that the risk of retinopathy in diabetes increases significantly when BP is elevated and that BP lowering can slow this progression. Although D.C. has an elevated fasting glucose, he does not have diabetes. Regardless, lowering BP is desirable for anticipated beneficial effects on his retinopathy.

HYPERTENSION MANAGEMENT

Lifestyle Modifications

CASE 14-1, QUESTION 11: Should D.C. start antihypertensive drug therapy, or are lifestyle modifications alone sufficient?

It is reasonable to assume that lifestyle modifications can partially help D.C. achieve his BP goal. Older JNC guidelines recommended lifestyle modifications for 6 to 12 months before starting drug therapy in patients with few or no risk factors, no hypertension-associated complications, and no compelling indications.[53] The 2007 European guidelines recommend lifestyle modifications alone to treat hypertension for only "several weeks" before starting drug therapy in patients with stage 1 hypertension who have "moderate" CV risk (i.e., one to two risk factors), and for "several months" in patients with stage 1 hypertension who are at "low" CV risk (i.e., no additional risk factors).[16] D.C. has multiple major CV risk factors and has early evidence of hypertension-associated complications. Lifestyle modifications are germane to the appropriate treatment of hypertension, but prospective clinical trials have not proven that this treatment approach prevents CV disease in patients with hypertension similar to what is proven antihypertensive drug therapy. Hence, initiation of drug therapy should not be delayed unnecessarily, especially for patients with CV risk factors.[3,15] Because D.C. has stage 1 hypertension with multiple risk factors, both lifestyle modifications and drug therapy should be implemented simultaneously.

MODALITIES THAT LOWER BP

CASE 14-1, QUESTION 12: Which lifestyle modifications can D.C. implement to lower his BP?

Weight reduction through dietary modifications and physical activity and sodium restriction are the most apparent lifestyle modifications for D.C to lower his BP. A thorough patient interview (diet history to quantify total calories, sodium, fat, and cholesterol, and social history to determine alcohol consumption and confirm cigarette use) should be obtained. Based on this interview, customized recommendations can be made.

The DASH diet should be strongly encouraged in D.C. based on proven benefits.[28,29] The role of supplementation with calcium and magnesium in hypertension is unclear and should not be routinely recommended in patients with hypertension for the purpose of lowering BP. Caffeine ingestion has been associated with an acute elevation in BP; however, these elevations appear to be transient. Limitations on caffeine intake are not recommended unless caffeine ingestion is detrimental for other medical reasons (e.g., cardiac arrhythmias, panic attacks).

D.C.'s BMI of 30 kg/m^2 or more classifies him as obese. As little as a 5% to 10% loss in weight (5–11 kg) will provide global health benefits. Strategies that increase his aerobic activity, in addition to diet, can augment weight loss.

OTHER CARDIOVASCULAR RISK-REDUCTION STRATEGIES

CASE 14-1, QUESTION 13: Aside from treating hypertension, which other CV risk reduction strategies should be recommended in D.C.?

SMOKING CESSATION

Smoking is an important modifiable major CV risk factor. Cigarette smoking has been shown to independently increase CV and overall mortality, and cessation can decrease the incidence of CV disease.[54] Although smoking does not chronically lower BP, smoking cessation is strongly recommended to improve overall health. Hypertensive smokers should be continually educated about the risks associated with cigarette smoking and directed to behavior-modification programs that can assist smoking cessation efforts (see Chapter 88, Tobacco Use and Dependence).

LOW-DOSE ASPIRIN

Low-dose aspirin therapy (81 mg daily) is recommended by the US Preventive Services Task Force (USPSTF) for the primary prevention of MI in certain men 45 to79 years old and ischemic stroke in certain women age 55 to 79 years old.[55] This recommendation is contingent on age and quantitative risk of CHD in men (e.g., Framingham risk scoring), and ischemic stroke in women. Low-dose aspirin is also recommended in patients who have a history of atherosclerotic vascular disease to reduce the risk of recurrent CV events or CV disease.[56] Patients with an absolute contraindication to aspirin therapy (e.g., aspirin allergy, gastrointestinal bleed, aspirin-induced bronchoconstriction) should not receive aspirin therapy. Severely elevated BP has been traditionally viewed as a contraindication for aspirin therapy because of an increased risk of hemorrhagic stroke. However, this should be considered when patients in the high end of stage 2 hypertension (e.g., SBP >180 mm Hg), perhaps even only in hypertensive emergency. Aspirin inhibits platelet aggregation, which provides the CV benefits, but can also increase risk of bleeding and is subject to many potential drug interactions. D.C. is not yet a candidate for low-dose aspirin based on his age.

CONTROLLING OTHER COMORBID DISEASES

In addition to treating hypertension and lowering BP to goal, controlling other comorbidities, which are themselves associated with increased CV risk, should be performed as part of a comprehensive CV risk reduction strategy. When present, dyslipidemia, diabetes mellitus, obesity, and any other forms of CV disease should be diligently treated and controlled. D.C. has dyslipidemia (elevated LDL-C, low HDL-C, and elevated triglycerides), and his CV risk would be reduced with better control of this condition (see Chapter 13, Dyslipidemias, Atherosclerosis, and Coronary Heart Disease).

Pharmacotherapy for Primary Prevention Patients

EVIDENCE-BASED RECOMMENDATIONS

CASE 14-1, QUESTION 14: Which treatment principles need to be considered when choosing an initial antihypertensive agent for D.C.?

Selecting an antihypertensive drug is complex. There are numerous choices, and all agents can effectively lower BP. Depending on the dose used, BP reductions are similar.[57] BP reduction, however, is only a surrogate end point of therapy and does not necessarily reflect overall effectiveness. Reducing hypertension-associated complications is the ultimate goal of treatment. Evidence-based medicine is the conscientious, explicit, and judicious use of current best evidence in making decisions about the care of individual patients.[58] Practicing evidence-based medicine in hypertension requires a balance between weighing the findings from outcome-based studies showing reduced hypertension-associated complications and considering specific drug therapies for each patient's individual situation.

CASE 14-1, QUESTION 15: Which antihypertensive agents are appropriate first-line treatments for D.C.?

The JNC-7 report from 2003, supplemented by more recent evidence in the AHA 2007 guidelines, outlines evidence-based pharmacotherapy recommendations accumulated from more than 50 years of clinical trials.[3,15] Although the JNC-7 recommended a thiazide diuretic alone or in combination with another agent as the initial drug choice for most patients, newer evidence demonstrates that either an ACEI, ARB, CCB, thiazide diuretic, or certain combinations of these agents is a reasonable first-line drug therapy option for primary prevention patients like D.C. (Fig. 14-3). This recommendation is based on the propensity of data showing reduced morbidity and mortality with these drug classes.[32,33,59] For patients with a compelling indication (Fig. 14-3), the choice of pharmacotherapy is more specific and is discussed later in this chapter.

Traditional landmark placebo-controlled hypertension studies (e.g., the Systolic Hypertension in the Elderly Program [SHEP],[47] Swedish Trial of Old Patients with Hypertension,[49] and Medical Research Council[48]) established that treating hypertension produces significant reductions in CV events (e.g., stroke, MI) and mortality. These traditional landmark trials used thiazide diuretic–based therapy, and thus thiazide diuretics have been the quintessential antihypertensive agent for most patients. Subsequently, several clinical trials evaluating newer agents (ACEI, ARB, and CCB) have provided additional evidence on CV event reduction.[17,50,60–80] Most of these trials do not include a placebo group (because it is unethical to use placebo in long-term studies); rather, they use an active antihypertensive agent as the comparator (often a thiazide diuretic or β-blocker or both). In those studies in which newer antihypertensive agents were compared with thiazide diuretics, very similar effects were seen. One of these studies was the Antihypertensive and Lipid-Lowering Treatment to Prevent Heart Attack Trial (ALLHAT).[62] In the ALLHAT, 33,357 patients with hypertension were randomly assigned in double-blind manner to thiazide diuretic (chlorthalidone), CCB (amlodipine), or ACEI (lisinopril)-based therapy. After a mean follow-up to 4.9 years, the incidence of the primary end point of fatal CHD or nonfatal MI was similar among all three treatment arms.

CASE 14-1, QUESTION 16: Should monotherapy or two-drug therapy be started in D.C. as his initial regimen?

A monotherapy approach is an option for D.C., because his BP is classified as stage 1 (Fig. 14-3). Monotherapy with an ACEI, ARB, CCB, or thiazide diuretic will likely reduce his BP to less than 140/90 mm Hg because his SBP is within 10 mm Hg of his goal value. For patients presenting with stage 2 hypertension, two antihypertensive agents are recommended from the start for initial treatment. Because CV risk is directly proportional to the degree of BP elevation, the more aggressive strategy in stage 2 patients is used as a means to obtain BP control more quickly and avoid clinical inertia. Low doses of two agents typically lower BP more effectively than high-dose monotherapy, and has the added advantage of fewer drug-related side effects compared with high-dose monotherapy.[81]

SPECIAL POPULATIONS

BLACK PATIENTS

CASE 14-1, QUESTION 17: How should D.C.'s race influence the selection of an antihypertensive regimen?

Black patients have a higher incidence of hypertension and hypertension-associated complications, and an increased need for combination therapy to achieve and maintain BP goals.[82] As monotherapy, it is well documented that a thiazide diuretic or a CCB is highly effective in lowering BP in black patients. This is likely because of the profile of low renin coupled with high plasma volume pattern of hypertension that is commonly seen in black patients with hypertension. Conversely, ACEI, ARB, or β-blocker monotherapy is less effective in lowering BP in blacks compared with white patients. However, when these agents are used in combination, especially with a thiazide diuretic, these race-based differences seen in BP lowering with monotherapy are abolished. This information may aid in selecting one drug option over another in a primary prevention patient, but does not apply to black patients with compelling indications, in whom choice of therapy follows an evidence-based approach to selection.

Treatment recommendations from the International Society on Hypertension in Blacks (ISHB) consensus statement are similar to the JNC-7 and 2007 AHA hypertension guidelines with respect to lifestyle modifications and pharmacotherapy.[3,15,82] The ISHB consensus statement highlights that attaining BP goal values is more challenging in blacks and usually requires more aggressive initiation of pharmacotherapy, and it recommends a BP goal of less than 135/85 mm Hg for most patients and less than 130/80 mm Hg for any black patient with hypertension-associated target-organ complications or compelling indications. These BP goals are more aggressive than what the JNC-7 recommends, and are not as widely accepted as the standard of care like the JNC-7 recommendations are. The ISHB also identifies that black patients are at higher risk of side effects with ACEI (both angioedema and cough) compared with whites.[82]

D.C. does not have any compelling indications for specific antihypertensive drug therapy. His first-line treatment options are an ACEI, ARB, CCB, or thiazide diuretic. Monotherapy with either a thiazide diuretic or a CCB would be very effective in BP lowering; either of these two drugs is an acceptable treatment option for him. A more aggressive approach using a two-drug combination of an ACEI or ARB with thiazide diuretic or an ACEI or ARB with CCB is also a reasonable two-drug combination and is considered additive for BP lowering.

VERY ELDERLY PATIENTS

CASE 14-2

QUESTION 1: B.D is an 83-year-old woman with a past medical history of hypertension, osteoporosis, and hypothyroidism. Her present medications are levothyroxine 100 mcg daily, alendronate 70 mg weekly, vitamin D 800 international units daily, and calcium carbonate 600 mg twice daily. She has been diagnosed with hypertension for 2 years, and it has been treated with lifestyle modifications (sodium restriction and exercise three times weekly). B.D. is 64 inches tall and weighs 55 kg. Her current BP is 160/78 mm Hg (160/80 mm Hg when repeated). All serum laboratory tests are normal. Her provider has been reluctant to start antihypertensive drug therapy because of B.D.'s age. How is treatment of B.D.'s hypertension different from that of a younger patient?

Older patients with hypertension (>65 years of age) have the lowest rates of BP control, and this rate decreases in even older populations.[1] Very elderly patients like B.D., similar to black patients, respond best to thiazides and CCBs and less to ACEIs, ARBs, and β-blockers when these are used as monotherapy. However, it is unclear whether these small differences in BP lowering among classes are clinically significant, so they should be viewed as medical myths rather than definitive realities.

Isolated Systolic Hypertension

B.D. has isolated systolic hypertension (ISH), which is defined as an elevated SBP (>140 mm Hg) with a normal DBP (<90 mm Hg).[3] This pattern of hypertension is most common in older patients and incurs a significant risk for CV disease. It was once thought that patients with ISH required high SBP to ensure normal perfusion of the heart and brain and that treating ISH would further lower DBP and worsen organ perfusion. Evidence clearly demonstrates, however, that treating ISH with antihypertensive drug therapy reduces the risk of CV events.[47,50,67] B.D.'s hypertension should be managed with drug therapy in addition to lifestyle modifications.

The care of patients with ISH, including the very elderly, should follow the same general hypertension care principles that apply to all patients, with two exceptions. The first exception is that lower doses should be used when first starting therapy. The second is that initial drug therapy, even with stage 2 hypertension, should only be started with monotherapy. Drug doses can be gradually increased as tolerated and combination therapy subsequently used to achieve recommended BP goals.[3] In earlier JNC recommendations, thiazide diuretics and long-acting dihydropyridine CCBs were preferred based on the evidence of reduced hypertension-associated complications. [47,49,50,67] The JNC-7 recommends that selection of pharmacotherapy in elderly patients be according to the same general treatment philosophies as for all patients with hypertension. These concepts are also recommended in the AHA expert consensus document on hypertension in the elderly.[25] Although lower starting doses may be needed, elderly patients eventually need standard treatment doses and often require combination therapy to reach and maintain BP goals.

CASE 14-2, QUESTION 2: What data support antihypertensive drug therapy in patients who are very elderly, similar to B.D.?

The very elderly (i.e., patients 80 years or older) have traditionally been underrepresented in landmark placebo-controlled clinical trials. However, the HYVET was a placebo-controlled, randomized trial evaluating the effect of antihypertensive pharmacotherapy (ACEI with or without a thiazidelike diuretic) in patients with hypertension age 80 years and older.[24] This trial was stopped prematurely, after 1.8 median years, owing to a significant reduction in overall mortality in the treatment arm. The HYVET provides compelling evidence that treatment of hypertension in the very elderly provides significant benefits. B.D. should be started on a low-dose thiazide diuretic or CCB for the treatment of her hypertension. For elderly patients with existing incontinence, diuretic therapy will be problematic. Under this circumstance, a CCB would be a more reasonable first-line option. Considering her advanced age, starting with monotherapy is appropriate to reduce her risk of orthostatic hypotension.

J-Curve Phenomenon

CASE 14-2, QUESTION 3: If B.D.'s BP is lowered too much, is she at risk for increased CV harm?

Data from observational studies generated concern that there is a "J-curve" phenomenon in which lowering BP too far may be harmful.[83,84] These data found that CAD events were decreased as expected when DBP was reduced to approximately 85 mm Hg. Below this level, however, the risk of events actually increased.

The J-curve phenomenon is a medical myth for patients who are relatively healthy. The data used to establish this phenomenon are observations from retrospective evaluations and, therefore, cannot establish cause and effect. The J-curve phenomenon has been associated only with CAD events, not stroke or kidney impairment. For stroke prevention and kidney impairment, data consistently suggest that the lower the BP, the better, unless BP reductions are too abrupt or are excessive. If the J-curve phenomenon has any validity, it would occur when BP is reduced much lower than the therapeutic range. Furthermore, patients with very low BP may have other illnesses that predispose them to coronary events (e.g., autonomic dysfunction, volume depletion).

Controlled evidence disputes the J-curve phenomenon. The Hypertension Optimal Treatment (HOT) trial was a prospective clinical trial designed to evaluate lower BP goals and CV events (challenging the J-curve phenomenon).[17] Patients (n = 18,790) were randomly assigned to goal DBP values of less than 90 mm Hg, less than 85 mm Hg, or less than 80 mm Hg. The risks for major CV disease events were the lowest when treatment BP was less than 149/83 mm Hg. The risk for cerebrovascular events was lowest at a treatment BP of less than 142/80 mm Hg. Only in patients with ischemic heart disease and diabetes did the lowest risk occur at a DBP less than 80 mm Hg. A significant increase in events was not seen in patients with lower BP values. Therefore, the HOT trial does not support the concept of a J-curve phenomenon. B.D. should start antihypertensive drug therapy without fear of exhibiting the J-curve phenomenon among the general population with hypertension.

CASE 14-2, QUESTION 4: If B.D. has a history of CAD, would she be at risk for increased CV harm if her BP was reduced to a value much lower than her BP goal?

Some data support a J-curve phenomenon in patients with established CAD. Within this population, it is possible that lowering BP too much may result in further compromise of coronary blood flow in the face of baseline abnormalities owing to coronary atherosclerosis. It is clear that lowering SBP to less than 140 mm Hg in patients with hypertension and CAD is associated with reduced CV risk.[85] However, subgroup analyses of patients with CAD have shown that low BP (e.g., <110–120/60–70 mm Hg) has been shown to portend an increased risk of CV events other than stroke.[86,87] If any case can be made for the presence of a J-curve phenomenon, it is among patients with CAD who are treated to achieve BP values that are much lower than 120/70 mm Hg.

ADDITIONAL CONSIDERATIONS

CASE 14-3

QUESTION 1: You are developing a collaborative drug therapy management (CDTM) protocol for treatment of hypertension that will be used by clinical pharmacists. In your CDTM protocol, you include multiple pharmacotherapy options (ACEIs, ARBs, CCBs, and thiazide diuretics) as equally recommended in primary prevention patients. However, you wish to include additional guidance on how to select an individual drug class to treat hypertension. What additional factors should be considered in your protocol when selecting a first-line agent for a specific primary prevention patient?

It cannot be emphasized enough that selecting pharmacotherapy should follow an evidence-based philosophy. In patients with compelling indications, certain antihypertensive drug classes are recommended in place of other options. In patients without compelling indications, factors such as concomitant diseases, medication costs, serum electrolytes, and prior medication intolerances should be considered (Table 14-8). These are helpful when selecting initial therapy for a primary prevention patient who has more than one acceptable drug class as a first-line option, or when selecting add-on therapy to further lower BP. These are discussed later in this chapter.

The costs of treating hypertension and related complications are substantial to patients and health systems.[88] With expanding

TABLE 14-8
Additional Considerations in Antihypertensive Drug Choice[a]

Antihypertensive Agent	Situations With Potentially Favorable Effects	Situations With Potentially Unfavorable Effects[b]	Avoid Use
ACEI	Low-normal potassium, elevated fasting glucose, microalbuminuria (with or without diabetes)	High-normal potassium or hyperkalemia	Pregnancy, bilateral renal artery stenosis, history of angioedema
ARB	Low-normal potassium, elevated fasting glucose, microalbuminuria (with or without diabetes)	High-normal potassium or hyperkalemia	Pregnancy, bilateral renal artery stenosis
CCB: dihydropyridine	Raynaud's phenomenon, elderly patients with isolated systolic hypertension, cyclosporine-induced hypertension	Peripheral edema, left ventricular dysfunction (all except amlodipine and felodipine), high-normal heart rate or tachycardia	
CCB: nondihydropyridine	Raynaud's phenomenon, migraine headache, supraventricular arrhythmias, high-normal heart rate or tachycardia	Peripheral edema, low-normal heart rate	Second- or third-degree heart block, left ventricular dysfunction
Thiazide diuretic	Osteoporosis or at increased risk for osteoporosis, high-normal potassium	Gout, hyponatremia, elevated fasting glucose (as monotherapy), low-normal potassium or sodium	

[a] These considerations should never replace drug recommendations for a compelling indication.
[b] May use but requires diligent monitoring.
High-normal refers to patients in the high end of the normal range, but not above the range.
Low-normal refers to patients in the low end of the normal range, but not below the range.
ACEI, angiotensin-converting enzyme inhibitor; ARB, angiotensin II receptor blocker; CCB, calcium-channel blocker.

availability of generic agents, costs attributed to drug acquisition are small in comparison to expenses for laboratory evaluations, office visits, and medical care for hypertension-associated complications. Whenever possible, affordable regimens that do not compromise efficacy should be designed. Generic antihypertensive products are equally effective and less expensive than brand-name products, and all first- and second-line antihypertensive classes have generic alternatives. The frequency of administration can influence treatment. Once-daily administration assists adherence; all major drug classes contain agents that are either naturally long-acting, or formulated in long-acting preparations,

Pharmacotherapy for Patients With Compelling Indications

Throughout the remainder of this chapter the term *compelling indications* will be used frequently. Compelling indications are defined as comorbid diseases for which specific antihypertensive classes are indicated based on evidence from clinical trials. Although these clinical trials may not have evaluated hypertension-related complications alone, they show significant benefits in reducing CV morbidity or mortality that warrants their use in a hypertensive patient with a given compelling indication (Fig. 14-3).

DIABETES

CASE 14-3, QUESTION 2: In your CDTM protocol, when should an ACEI or ARB be identified as first-line therapy ahead of other antihypertensive agents?

Kidney disease and CV disease are both long-term hypertension-associated complications that are at high risk of occurring in patients with diabetes. Evidence shows that treatment with antihypertensive agents (ACEIs, ARBs, CCBs, thiazide diuretics, and even β-blockers) in patients with diabetes reduces risk of CV events and progression of kidney disease.[89] When compared head to head, ACEIs are superior to dihydropyridine CCBs at reducing CV events.[70,71] Subgroup analyses of larger clinical trials further support CV event reduction with ACEIs and ARBs. Therefore, initial antihypertensive therapy for a patient with diabetes should ideally consist of an ACEI or ARB. Either a thiazide diuretic or CCB can be used as add-on agent, but strong data demonstrate that a CCB may be better at reducing CV events than a thiazide diuretic when used in combination with an ACEI.[90] Thereafter, a β-blocker would be another add-on therapy, if needed to provide additional BP lowering. Most patients with diabetes and hypertension require treatment with two or more antihypertensive drugs.[89,91]

The BP goal recommended in numerous guidelines of less than 130/80 mm Hg is considered the standard of care for this population.[3,15,82,89,91] For most patients with diabetes, this is probably a reasonable target. However, it should be acknowledged that evidence to support this recommendation is primarily based on a subgroup analysis of the HOT trial.[17] Recent prospective data evaluating hypertension control in patients with diabetes has failed to clearly demonstrate that lower BP goals are unequivocally better than standard BP goals. Specifically, a subrandomization within the ACCORD study compared CV event lowering in 4,733 patients with type 2 diabetes who were randomly assigned to standard BP goal (SBP <140 mm Hg) compared with intensive BP goal (SBP <120 mm Hg).[23] After 4.7 years, there was no difference in the primary composite end point of CV events between the groups. However, for the secondary outcome of stroke, there was a small difference in favor of the intensive arm. Although the main results of ACCORD-BP could be used to question the need for lower BP goals in patients with diabetes, those who advocate for lower BP goals in this population note that overall events were lower than expected in both groups, and that it may have been underpowered to find differences. Additionally, other residual CV risk factors (e.g., lipids, glucose) were aggressively managed within the study, which may have confounded the ability to isolate the specific additive benefit of a more intensive BP goal in this population.

CHRONIC KIDNEY DISEASE

It is common that CKD presents initially with microalbuminuria (30–299 mg albumin in a 24-hour urine collection) that can progress over the course of several years to overt kidney failure.[38] Progression is accelerated in the presence of both hypertension and diabetes. ACEI or ARB therapy should be used as first-line therapy in these patients because both have been shown to reduce the progression of CKD in type 1 diabetes,[92] in type 2 diabetes,[74,75] and in those without diabetes.[78,93] Recently, ARB therapy has also been shown to decrease risk of developing microalbuminuria in patients with diabetes.[94]

Although many of the long-term benefits of ACEI or ARB therapy may be from BP lowering, their evidence base is robust enough to support their first-line use in CKD.[95,96] After ACEI or ARB therapy has been implemented, data support a CCB as the second drug because this has been shown to reduce progression of CKD better than a thiazide diuretic as the second drug added based on the Avoiding Cardiovascular Events through Combination Therapy in Patients Living with Systolic Hypertension (ACCOMPLISH) trial.[97]

CASE 14-3, QUESTION 3: In your CDTM protocol, how should significant CKD be defined so that patients with this compelling indication can be identified and treated appropriately?

For hypertension management, patients have CKD sufficiently significant to be considered a compelling indication if they have one of the following three criteria: (a) an estimated GFR of less than 60 mL/minute/1.73 m^2 based on Modification of Diet in Renal Disease calculation (calculator available at: **http://www.kidney.org/professionals/KDOQI/gfr_calculator.cfm**); (b) a serum creatinine greater than 1.3 mg/dL in women or greater than 1.5 mg/dL in men because this roughly correlates to a GFR estimation of less than 60 mL/minute/1.73 m^2; or (c) albuminuria (>300 mg/day on a 24-hour urine collection or total protein to creatinine ratio >200 mg/g on a spot urinalysis).[3] These patients typically require three or more antihypertensive agents, among which an ACEI or ARB should be the foundation of the drug therapy regimen.[38]

The controversies surrounding BP goals in patients with CKD parallel the controversies in patients with diabetes. Consistently, guidelines have recommended a BP goal of less than 130/80 mm Hg in patients with CKD, either with or without diabetes.[3,15,38,91] It is reasonable to target a goal BP of less than 130/80 mm Hg in patients with CKD. Three clinical trials in nondiabetic patients with CKD generally support the BP goal of less than 130/80 mm Hg.[21,77,98,99] However, when they are considered together in a systematic review, it is somewhat inconclusive that a BP goal of less than 130/80 mm Hg improves clinical outcomes more than a goal of less than 140/90 mm Hg in adults with CKD.[100] It was suggested that a lower BP goal may be beneficial in patients with proteinuria greater than 300 to 1000 mg/day, as was seen in the Modification of Diet in Renal Disease Study.[99]

CHRONIC AND ACUTE CORONARY ARTERY DISEASE

CASE 14-3, QUESTION 4: In your CDTM protocol, when should β-blocker therapy be identified as the most appropriate first-line antihypertensive drug therapy?

The two most common forms of chronic CAD, post-MI and chronic stable angina, are compelling indications for specific pharmacotherapy.[3,15] Consistent with the JNC-7 and AHA hypertension guidelines, the American College of Cardiology (ACC)/AHA have guidelines for chronic CAD that recommend treatment with a β-blocker, followed shortly thereafter by the addition of an ACEI.[56,101] β-Blockers (those without intrinsic sympathomimetic activity [ISA]) decrease the risk of a subsequent MI or sudden cardiac death by decreasing the adrenergic burden on the heart, and progression of coronary atherosclerosis. ACEI therapy promotes cardiac remodeling, improves cardiac function, and reduces the risk of CV events. An ARB is an alternative in patients who do not tolerate an ACEI, because fewer data exist that assess the long-term impact of an ARB on CV events compared with an ACEI in chronic CAD.[102] A thiazide diuretic can be added to the core regimen of a β-blocker with an ACEI (or ARB) if additional BP reduction is needed. However, if an additional agent is needed to treat ischemic symptoms for patients with chronic stable angina, a dihydropyridine CCB can be added to this core regimen. If a β-blocker cannot be used because of intolerance or contraindication, a nondihydropyridine CCB can be used as an alternative to a β-blocker. Acute CAD, also called *acute coronary syndrome,* includes unstable angina, non–ST-segment elevation MI, and ST-segment elevation MI. The ACC/AHA guidelines for these conditions indicate a β-blocker as first-line pharmacotherapy.[103,104]

PRIOR STROKE

Prior ischemic stroke (the predominant etiology of most cases of stroke) is a compelling indication for specific antihypertensive pharmacotherapy to lower the risk of a recurrent stroke. Lowering BP to goal in patients with a history of stroke is beneficial once patients have stabilized after their acute event. Specifically, thiazide diuretic therapy with or without an ACEI reduces the incidence of recurrent stroke,[63,105] and is recommended as first-line therapy.[3,15,106] The role of ARB therapy, as an alternative to an ACEI, is unclear. Although ARB-based therapy has been shown to reduce the incidence of recurrent stroke more effectively than a dihydropyridine CCB-based treatment regimen,[80] when compared with placebo in patients with a history of a recent ischemic stroke there was no difference in recurrent stroke or CV event.[107]

LEFT VENTRICULAR DYSFUNCTION

Left ventricular dysfunction (sometimes called *systolic heart failure* or *chronic heart failure*) is a complication of hypertension in which cardiac contractility is compromised. According to the AHA guidelines, this compelling indication has the lowest BP goal of less than 120/80 mm Hg.[15] Although the JNC-7 guidelines recommend a BP goal of only less than 140/90 mm Hg in these patients, if left ventricular dysfunction is treated with the three-drug combination recommended by both the 2007 AHA hypertension guidelines and ACC/AHA heart failure guidelines, patients will likely attain the lower BP goal and experience maximal reduction in CV morbidity and mortality.[108]

Standard first-line therapy for left ventricular dysfunction should include a three-drug combination of an ACEI, a diuretic (either a thiazide or loop, depending on kidney function and need for diuresis), and a β-blocker. ACEIs have numerous landmark clinical trials showing reduced morbidity and mortality rates, whereas diuretics provide primarily symptomatic relief of edema.[108] As left ventricular dysfunction progresses, loop diuretics are almost always needed instead of a thiazide diuretic because they produce more pronounced diuresis. β-Blocker therapy is a component of standard first-line therapy for stable left ventricular dysfunction as numerous clinical trials have demonstrated reduced morbidity and mortality when it is added to the combination ACEI with diuretic regimen in well-compensated patients.[108]

According to evidence-based medicine principles, only metoprolol, carvedilol, and bisoprolol are indicated for left ventricular dysfunction. Other β-blockers (e.g., atenolol) should not be used in patients with left ventricular dysfunction because they do not have supporting data demonstrating they reduce CV event rates in these patients. Patients should be clinically euvolemic and hemodynamically stable before adding a β-blocker. As discussed in Chapter 19 (Heart Failure), it is important to start with very low doses of a β-blocker, then slowly titrate upward over the course of several weeks to the recommended dosing range for left ventricular dysfunction. An ARB can be used as an alternative to an ACEI.[108,109]

Additional antihypertensive agents reduce CV risk in this patient population in addition to the standard three-drug initial regimen. An aldosterone antagonist (spironolactone, eplerenone) can be added in patients with mild to severe symptoms of left ventricular dysfunction.[110–112] Potassium serum concentrations must be carefully monitored in this situation. Alternatively, the combination of hydralazine with isosorbide dinitrate can be added in black patients.[113]

Implementing Pharmacotherapy

MONOTHERAPY

Starting with one drug to treat hypertension is optimal when initial BP is close to goal values. When using a standard dose of first-line antihypertensive agents (an ACEI, ARB, CCB, or thiazide diuretic), and even with β-blockers, the average reduction in SBP/DBP is only 10/5 mm Hg.[81] This has been termed by some as the "10 over 5" rule.

There are two general approaches to monotherapy. In the stepped-care approach a single agent is initiated and the dose increased until BP is controlled, the maximal dose is reached, or dose-limiting toxicity occurs. If the goal BP is not achieved, a second drug from a different class is added. This process can be continued, if necessary, until three or even four drugs are used in combination. The VA Cooperative Studies Group on Antihypertensive Agents demonstrated that less than 60% of patients reach a DBP of less than 90 mm Hg with this approach when doses were titrated up to the maximal dosage.[41]

In the sequential therapy approach, a single agent is initiated and titrated to the maximal dose as needed. If goal BP is not achieved, another agent is selected to replace the first. Combination drug therapy is reserved for patients who do not achieve goal BP values after the second agent. Sequential therapy is most appropriate when the first drug is either poorly tolerated or results in minimal reduction in BP. The VA Cooperative Studies Group on Antihypertensive Agents also evaluated sequential therapy, and demonstrated that only an additional 49% of the nonresponders to the first agent achieved a DBP of less than 90 mm Hg when switched to a second drug.[114]

COMBINATION THERAPY

CASE 14-3, QUESTION 5: In your CDTM protocol, when should starting with initial two-drug therapy be recommended to treat hypertension in primary prevention patients?

Starting therapy with two drugs is an option for initial therapy. This approach is strongly encouraged for patients far from their BP goal (e.g., stage 2 hypertension) or in patients closer to their BP goal who have compelling indications for two drugs, or have BP goals of less than 130/80 mm Hg.[3,15,82] The average patient with hypertension will require two or more agents to achieve his or her goal BP value. In contrast to high-dose monotherapy, low-dose, two-drug combination therapy provides greater BP lowering with a lower risk of side effects.[81] Prospective clinical trials have demonstrated that goal attainment rates of more than 70% are achieved when initial two-drug combination therapy is used in patients with stage 2 hypertension.[115,116] Moreover, this approach achieves goal BP in a quicker, yet safe, time frame compared with the stepped-care approach to therapy.[116,117] As previously mentioned, elderly patients (age 80 years or older) should only have one antihypertensive agent started at a time to minimize risk of orthostatic hypotension.

PREFERRED COMBINATIONS

When treating patients with combination antihypertensive therapy, the presence of compelling indications should be used to guide selection of combination agents. In the absence of compelling indications (i.e., primary prevention patients), clinicians should use combinations that are additive in their ability to lower BP. This entails balancing a thorough understanding of the pathophysiology of hypertension along with the pharmacology of the drugs being used. Combinations of drugs from different drug classes with distinctly different mechanisms of action are ideal to provide the best reductions in BP. The American Society of Hypertension recommends the combination of an ACEI or ARB with a CCB or the combination of an ACEI or ARB with a diuretic as preferred combinations because they are highly effective in lowering BP.[118] Many patients can achieve a BP goal of less than 140/90 mm Hg with two drugs when appropriate combinations are used. It is not uncommon, however, to require three or more drugs to attain a goal BP of less than 130/80 mm Hg.

Diuretics, especially thiazide diuretics, provide additive effects in BP lowering when combined with most other antihypertensive agents.[3,37] This is especially true for any other antihypertensive drugs that block the RAAS (i.e., ACEI, ARB, direct renin inhibitor),[119] and to a lesser extent when diuretics are used in combination with CCBs.[120] In the case of the former, diuretics may "prime" the system because a compensatory increase in plasma renin usually occurs with the administration of diuretics. Diuretic therapy is also often used in combination with older alternative antihypertensive agents (e.g., direct arterial vasodilators, α_2-agonists) to mitigate compensatory fluid retention seen with many of these drugs.

ACCEPTABLE COMBINATIONS

Many combinations are recommended by the American Society of Hypertension as acceptable combinations. With these combinations, BP lowering is modest (but perhaps not as large as combinations identified as preferred) or these combinations have a synergistic effect of mitigating side effects. These combinations include a β-blocker or CCB with a diuretic, a dihydropyridine CCB with a β-blocker, a renin inhibitor with either a diuretic or ARB, or a thiazide diuretic with a potassium-sparing diuretic.[118]

LESS EFFECTIVE COMBINATONS

The American Society of hypertension recommends that several combinations as less effective in BP lowering. Most of these result from a lack of complementary pharmacologic actions. These less effective combinations include an ACEI with ARB, ACEI or ARB with a β-blocker, a nondihydropyridine CCB with a β-blocker, and a centrally acting agent with a β-blocker.[118]

The combination of an ACEI or ARB with a β-blocker is less effective in lowering BP as renin release is suppressed by β-blockade. When evaluating pure BP lowering, other combinations result in better reductions. However, this combination is certainly indicated when compelling indications for each agent coexist (e.g., CAD, left ventricular dysfunction) (Fig. 14-3).

The combination of an ACEI and ARB overall is not very beneficial. This combination should not be used specifically for the purpose of BP lowering, especially in primary prevention patients. When this combination was evaluated in the ONgoing Telmisartan Alone and in Combination With Ramipril Global Endpoint Trial (ONTARGET), the ACEI with ARB combination treatment arm provided only minimal additional reduction in

BP compared with either agent alone, and most importantly did not additionally lower risk of CV events.[121] Moreover, there was a higher risk of adverse events (e.g., kidney dysfunction, hypotension) with the combination arm.

The combination of an ACEI with ARB has been used in patients with left ventricular dysfunction based on promising data of a reduced risk of heart failure hospitalizations.[122,123] However, the overall clinical benefits of an ACEI with an ARB versus an ACEI without an ARB are very small; addition of an aldosterone antagonist is the preferred next step in patients with left ventricular dysfunction who are already treated with the standard regimen of a diuretic, ACEI, and a β-blocker.[108,124] One potential niche for the use of an ACEI with an ARB is in the setting of CKD with significant proteinuria (300 mg albumin/day or 500 mg protein/day or per gram of urinary creatinine), in which the combination of an ACEI with an ARB seems to reduce progression of proteinuria better than either drug alone.[96]

OTHER COMBINATIONS

Using two agents from the same drug class is almost always discouraged. However, there are two potential exceptions. The combination of two diuretics together from different subclasses is sometimes used in patients with resistant hypertension or nephrotic syndrome, but more often is done to minimize electrolyte depletion, especially hypokalemia and hypomagnesemia, which commonly occur with thiazide diuretics. The use of a dihydropyridine CCB with a nondihydropyridine CCB has marginal but additional benefits on BP lowering.[125,126] This combination may be helpful in patients with diabetes who are not responsive to more common three-drug combinations.[91]

ORTHOSTATIC HYPOTENSION

CASE 14-3, QUESTION 6: In your CDTM protocol, why should initial two-drug therapy never be recommended in elderly patients age 75 years or older?

Orthostatic hypotension occurs when standing upright results in a SBP decrease of more than 20 mm Hg (or a DBP decrease of more than 10 mm Hg) after 3 minutes of standing and is often accompanied by dizziness or fainting.[3,25] This is a risk of rapid BP lowering. Orthostatic hypotension is more frequent in elderly patients (especially those with ISH), diabetes, autonomic dysfunction, volume depletion, and in patients taking certain drugs (i.e., diuretics, nitrates, α-blockers, psychotropic agents, phosphodiesterase inhibitors). Combination therapy can still be used in these patients, but close monitoring and slow titration are needed. Dose increases should be gradual to minimize the risk of hypotension. Moreover, initial therapy with two drugs should be avoided in the elderly (age 80 years or older) owing to the increased risk of orthostatic hypotension.

MONITORING THERAPY

Four aspects of treatment must always be considered: (a) BP response to attain goal, (b) adherence with lifestyle modifications and pharmacotherapy, (c) progression to hypertension-associated complications, and (d) drug-related toxicity.

Reduction in BP should be evaluated 1 to 4 weeks after starting or modifying therapy for most patients. BP usually begins to decrease within 1 to 2 weeks of starting an agent, but steady-state antihypertensive effects can take up to 4 weeks. If patients are in hypertensive crisis, evaluation should occur sooner, within hours to days (see Chapter 21, Hypertensive Crises).

Two BP values separated by at least 1 minute should be measured during each clinical evaluation, with the average used to make a proper assessment. If dehydration or orthostatic hypotension is suspected, BP should be measured in both the seated and standing positions to detect orthostatic changes. For routine monitoring, measuring BP in the seated position is sufficient. Self-BP monitoring values should be considered if available. Normally, however, they are slightly lower (5 mm Hg) than clinic values even in patients without white-coat hypertension. For example, patients with a goal BP value of less than 140/90 mm Hg should have home measurements that are less than 135/85 mm Hg.[7]

All patients should be questioned in a nonthreatening manner regarding adherence with lifestyle modifications and drug therapy. This is especially important for complex regimens, when drug intolerance is likely, or when financial constraints hinder acquisition of medications. Evaluating hypertension-associated complications and drug side effects are essential. New hypertension-associated complications may necessitate changes to treat a compelling indication or attain a new BP goal. Drug-related side effects may similarly require therapy modifications.

CLINICAL SCENARIOS

Diuretics

CASE 14-4

QUESTION 1: B.A. is a 62-year-old woman who is postmenopausal, does not smoke, and never drinks alcohol. Since being diagnosed with hypertension, she has modified her diet, begun routine aerobic exercise, and has lost 10 kg in the past 18 months. She now weighs 72 kg and is 165 cm tall. Her BP is now 150/94 mm Hg (150/92 mm Hg when repeated) and has consistently remained near this value for the past year. Her BP when first diagnosed was 156/96 mm Hg. Physical examination shows no LVH and no retinopathy. Urinalysis is negative for protein. Other laboratory tests are normal, except for dyslipidemia. B.A. has no health insurance and is concerned about the cost of therapy. Her Framingham risk score is 22%. She takes over-the-counter calcium with vitamin D, and her provider wants to start HCTZ 25 mg/day. Is HCTZ an appropriate agent for B.A.?

B.A. is a primary prevention patient with uncontrolled hypertension. According to the JNC-7, her BP goal is less than 140/90 mm Hg, with an option of less than 130/80 mm Hg according to the AHA guidelines based on her Framingham risk score (Fig. 14-2).[3,15] Regardless of which BP goal is selected, initial monotherapy is reasonable because she is in the low end of stage 1 hypertension. Appropriate first-line treatment options include an ACEI, ARB, CCB, or thiazide diuretic. All of these drug classes have generic options, and should be easily affordable for B.A. A thiazide diuretic may also benefit her osteoporosis (Table 14-8) and is an appropriate choice. Several types of diuretics are used to manage hypertension (Table 14-9).[37] All lower BP, with differences being duration of action, potency of diuresis, and electrolyte abnormalities.

THIAZIDES

Thiazides are diuretics of choice for most patients with hypertension. Similar to loop diuretics, an initial diuresis is experienced. After approximately 4 to 6 weeks of thiazide diuretic therapy, diuresis dissipates, however, and is supplanted by a decrease in PVR, which is responsible for sustaining antihypertensive effects.

HYDROCHLOROTHIAZIDE VERSUS CHLORTHALIDONE

HCTZ and chlorthalidone have been used in several major outcome trials, although only chlorthalidone-based regimens have proven to be of benefit in the low doses commonly used in practice today.[47–49,62,68,115,127] Both agents are inexpensive and dosed

TABLE 14-9
Diuretics in Hypertension

Category	Selected Products	Usual Dosage Range (mg/d)	Dosing Frequency
Thiazide and thiazidelike	Chlorthalidone	12.5–25	Daily
	Hydrochlorothiazide	12.5–25	Daily
	Indapamide	1.25–5	Daily
	Metolazone	2.5–10	Daily
	Metolazone	0.5–1.0	Daily
Loop	Bumetanide	0.5–4	BID
	Furosemide	20–80	BID
	Torsemide	2.5–10	Daily
Potassium-sparing	Amiloride	5–10	Daily to BID
	Triamterene	50–100	Daily to BID
Potassium-sparing combination	Triamterene/HCTZ	37.5/25–75/50	Daily
	Spironolactone/HCTZ	25/25–50/50	Daily
	Amiloride/HCTZ	5–10/50–100	Daily
Aldosterone antagonist	Eplerenone	50–100	Daily to BID
	Spironolactone	12.5–50	Daily to BID

BID, twice daily; HCTZ, hydrochlorothiazide.

once daily, but HCTZ is most frequently used in the United States, and is more widely available in fixed-dose combination products. The usual starting dose of HCTZ or chlorthalidone is 12.5 mg once daily. A maintenance dose of 25 mg once daily can effectively lower BP and has a low incidence of side effects (e.g., hypokalemia, hyperuricemia) that can be managed with routine monitoring.[41,57,59]

To listen to a Capticast interview of Mike Ernst and Joseph Saseen by Nikki Hahn (on behalf of IForum) that focuses on the ACCOMPLISH trial and comments on hydrochlorothiazide and chlorthalidone, go to http://thepoint.lww.com/AT10e. To view the full IForum Capticast of the ACCOMPLISH trial, go to http://iforumrx.org/.

Significant controversy surrounds the comparative efficacy of HCTZ and chlorthalidone. Most clinicians, including the AHA, assume a class effect for these two drugs.[15] However, class effects can be legitimized only after assurance of equipotent dosing; for antihypertensives, when they are not directly compared in a CV event trial, it assumes that if two agents achieve similar BP lowering then both achieve similar reduction in CV events. With regard to HCTZ and chlorthalidone, this assumption is unproven. Chlorthalidone is more potent on a milligram per milligram basis and has a longer half-life than HCTZ (50–60 hours versus 9–10 hours).[128] Based on a comparative study using 24-hour ABPM, it appears that the equipotent dose of chlorthalidone 25 mg daily is HCTZ 50 mg daily, but this dose of HCTZ is unpopular because of increased side effects. Consequently, it is believed by some that the antihypertensive efficacy of chlorthalidone is greater than HCTZ when contemporary doses are used; the 12.5- to 25-mg doses of chlorthalidone do not appear to significantly increase the risk of hypokalemia more so than HCTZ.[129] Complicating this issue is evidence demonstrating that office BP tends to overestimate the response to HCTZ, and the 24-hour BP lowering with HCTZ is only comparable to other common agents (ACEI, ARB, CCB, and even β-blocker) when 50 mg daily is used.[130] Recently, data from the Multiple Risk Factor Intervention Trial indicate that chlorthalidone reduces CV events more than HCTZ.[131] Although chlorthalidone is the most optimal and evidence-based thiazide diuretic for B.A., HCTZ remains currently accepted in the clinical environment as a reasonable thiazide diuretic for hypertension assuming her BP goal can be readily achieved with its use.

LOOP DIURETICS

Loop diuretics produce a more potent diuresis, but a smaller decrease in PVR, and less vasodilation than thiazide diuretics. They are subject to a significant postdose antinatriuretic period, which offsets their antihypertensive effect. Therefore, a thiazide is more effective at lowering BP than loop diuretics in most patients. Loop diuretics are usually considered only for patients with severe CKD (estimated GFR <30 mL/minute/1.73 m^2), left ventricular dysfunction, or severe edema. In these patients potent diuresis is often needed. Furosemide has a short duration of effect and should be given twice daily when used in hypertension, whereas torsemide can be given once daily.

POTASSIUM-SPARING DIURETICS

Potassium-sparing diuretics (triamterene and amiloride) should be reserved for patients who experience hypokalemia while on a thiazide diuretic. With low-dose thiazide diuretics, less than 25% of patients develop hypokalemia, and most cases are not severe. Triamterene and amiloride usually do not provide significant additional BP lowering when added to a thiazide diuretic. Several fixed-dose products are available that include HCTZ with triamterene or amiloride. Empirically starting all patients with hypertension treated with a thiazide diuretic on triamterene or amiloride to avoid hypokalemia is not rational unless baseline serum potassium is in the low-normal range.

CASE 14-4, QUESTION 2: How should a thiazide diuretic be started in B.A.?

B.A. has stage 1 hypertension, and monotherapy with a thiazide diuretic is reasonable. A thiazide diuretic is a first-line option in primary prevention patients like B.A., and she has no contraindications (Table 14-10). Although B.A. has dyslipidemia, thiazide diuretics are unlikely to have a clinically significant effect on cholesterol when used in low doses.[132,133] An appropriate starting dose of HCTZ is 12.5 or 25 mg daily. B.A. has no additional risks for orthostatic hypotension, so starting at the higher 25-mg daily dose is safe, and will have a better chance of lowering her

TABLE 14-10

Side Effects and Contraindications of Antihypertensive Agents

	Side Effects			
	Innocuous but Sometimes Annoying	Potentially Harmful	Usually Requires Cessation of Therapy, at Least Temporarily	Contraindications
Thiazide diuretics	Increased urination (at onset of therapy), muscle cramps, hyperuricemia (without gout)	Hypokalemia,[a] hyponatremia, hyperglycemia, hypovolemia, pancreatitis, photosensitivity, hypercholesterolemia, hypertriglyceridemia, hyperuricemia with gout, orthostatic hypotension (more frequent in elderly)	Hypercalcemia, azotemia, skin rash (cross-reacts with only certain sulfonamide allergies), purpura, bone marrow depression, lithium toxicity in patients on lithium therapy, hyponatremia	Anuria, kidney failure
Loop diuretics	Increased urination, muscle cramps, hyperuricemia (less than with thiazides)	Hypokalemia,[a] hyperglycemia, hypovolemia, pancreatitis, hypercholesterolemia, hypertriglyceridemia, hearing loss with large IV doses, orthostatic hypotension (more pronounced in elderly)	Hyponatremia, hypocalcemia, azotemia, skin rash (cross-reacts with only certain sulfonamide allergies), photosensitivity, lithium toxicity in patients on lithium therapy	Anuria
ACEI	Dizziness, dry cough	Orthostatic hypotension (more pronounced in elderly treated with a diuretic), increased serum creatinine, increased potassium	Angioedema, severe hyperkalemia, increase in serum creatinine >35%	Bilateral renal artery stenosis, volume depletion, hyponatremia, pregnancy, history of angioedema
ARB	Dizziness	Orthostatic hypotension (more pronounced in elderly treated with a diuretic), increased serum creatinine, increased potassium	Severe hyperkalemia, increase in serum creatinine >35%	Bilateral renal artery stenosis, volume depletion, hyponatremia, pregnancy
CCB: dihydropyridines	Dizziness, headache, flushing	Peripheral edema, tachycardia	Significant peripheral edema	Left ventricular dysfunction (not with amlodipine or felodipine)
CCB: nondihydropyridines	Dizziness, headache, constipation	Bradycardia	Heart block, left ventricular dysfunction, interactions with certain drugs	Left ventricular dysfunction, second- or third-degree heart block, sick sinus syndrome
β-Blocker	Bradycardia, weakness, exercise intolerance	Masking the symptoms of hypoglycemia in diabetes, hyperglycemia, aggravation of peripheral arterial disease, erectile dysfunction, increased triglycerides, decreased HDL-C	Left ventricular dysfunction (not with carvedilol, metoprolol, bisoprolol), bronchospasm in patients with asthma or COPD (more pronounced with nonselective agents)	Severe asthma, second- or third-degree heart block, acute left ventricular dysfunction exacerbation, coronary artery disease for agents with intrinsic sympathomimetic activity
Aldosterone antagonist	Menstrual irregularities (spironolactone only) or gynecomastia (spironolactone only)	Increased potassium	Hyperkalemia, hyponatremia	Kidney failure. kidney impairment (for eplerenone: CrCl <50 mL/min, or type 2 diabetes with proteinuria, and creatinine >1.8 in women, >2.0 in men), hyperkalemia, hyponatremia

[a] Routine addition of potassium supplementation or empiric concurrent potassium-sparing diuretics should be discouraged unless hypokalemia is demonstrated, the patient is taking digoxin, or potassium is in the low-normal range.

ACEI, angiotensin-converting enzyme inhibitor; ARB, angiotensin II receptor blocker; CCB, calcium-channel blocker; COPD, chronic obstructive pulmonary disease; CrCl, creatinine clearance; HDL-C, high-density lipoprotein cholesterol; IV, intravenous.

BP to goal than the lower 12.5-mg dose because most antihypertensive agents provide a 10-mm Hg reduction in SBP and 5-mm Hg reduction in DBP with a standard starting dose.[81]

PATIENT EDUCATION

CASE 14-4, QUESTION 3: B.A. is prescribed HCTZ 25 mg daily. How should she be counseled regarding this therapy?

Several counseling points are summarized in Table 14-7. Some patients disregard lifestyle modifications when they start antihypertensive therapy, so B.A. must be encouraged to continue lifestyle modification to maximize her response to drug therapy. B.A. should be informed that diuretics lower both BP and risk of CV events and that taking her dose at about the same time each morning to minimize nocturia and provide consistent effects is recommended. B.A. should expect to experience increased urination when starting HCTZ, but should be informed that this diminishes with time. Inform B.A. that missed doses should be taken as soon as possible within the same day, but doubling doses the next day is not recommended. The potential for hypokalemia, which is easily identified and managed, and the need for routine monitoring of serum potassium should be reviewed. She should be counseled on the signs and symptoms of electrolyte abnormalities (e.g., leg cramps, muscle weakness) and encouraged to report these to her health care provider if they occur. Increasing dietary intake of potassium-rich foods to minimize electrolyte depletion is an option to minimize potassium loss. This should be encouraged only with thiazide and loop diuretics, but not with potassium-sparing agents.

CASE 14-4, QUESTION 4: After 4 weeks of HCTZ 25 mg daily, B.A. has no complaints and has not missed a dose. She is exercising and is following the DASH diet. Her BP values are 142/86 mm Hg (140/84 mm Hg when repeated). Her fasting laboratory values are as follows:

Serum potassium, 3.8 mEq/L
Uric acid, 7.3 mg/dL
Glucose, 99 mg/dL

All other values are unchanged. Last month, potassium was 4.0 mEq/L, uric acid was 6.8 mg/dL, and fasting glucose was 95 mg/dL. What is your assessment regarding the efficacy and toxicity of B.A.'s antihypertensive therapy?

Despite improvements with lifestyle modifications and reported adherence with HCTZ, B.A.'s goal BP of less than 140/90 mm Hg has not been met (her BP average is 141/83 mm Hg). No new signs of hypertension-associated complications are seen. She should be encouraged to continue with her current efforts, but other interventions are warranted.

POTASSIUM LOSS

Adverse reactions with low-dose thiazide diuretics (e.g., HCTZ 12.5–25 mg daily) are minimal compared with higher-dose therapy (HCTZ >25 mg daily). Moreover, side effects and tolerability with low-dose thiazide diuretic therapy are similar to other first-line drug therapy options and not much higher than what is seen with placebo.[41,43,44,57] Regardless, signs and symptoms of electrolyte and metabolic changes, such as hypokalemia, hyponatremia, hyperglycemia, or hyperuricemia, should be evaluated in all patients treated with thiazide diuretics. B.A. has experienced small changes in serum potassium and uric acid, which are typical thiazide-induced abnormalities. B.A. should be questioned about muscle cramps or weakness, which can be caused by decreased potassium.

CASE 14-4, QUESTION 5: Is B.A.'s potassium decrease concerning? If so, how should this be managed?

Most total body potassium is intracellular (~98%). Thiazide diuretics can cause potassium loss and can result in potassium serum concentrations in the low end of the normal range. However, with low-dose therapy overt hypokalemia is not common. HCTZ in doses of 12.5, 25, and 50 mg daily can decrease serum potassium by an average of 0.21, 0.34, and 0.5 mEq/L, respectively.[41,132,133] This is usually considered mild, with serum potassium concentrations reaching a nadir within the first month of therapy and remaining stable thereafter. Restriction of dietary sodium in patients receiving diuretic therapy has been shown to reduce the loss of potassium, and should be encouraged in B.A.[134]

SUBCLINICAL POTASSIUM DECREASES

The clinical significance of small potassium decreases when serum potassium concentrations are still in the normal range is controversial. B.A.'s potassium has dropped slightly, and her current serum concentration is in the low end of the normal range. Low serum potassium values have been cited as an independent predictor of development of diabetes.[135] Some data suggest that patients treated with a thiazide diuretic who experience the greatest decreases in potassium also experience the greatest increases in glucose values,[136] although this is not consistently demonstrated in other analyses.[137]

Large outcome trials have demonstrated that thiazide diuretic-based treatment results in a higher incidence of developing type 2 diabetes compared with other antihypertensive therapies.[34,138,139] Because of the possible association between potassium decreases and development of diabetes, some clinicians believe that it is optimal to maintain serum potassium in the middle to high end of the normal range (e.g., between 4.0 and 5.0 mEq/L) in patients treated with thiazide diuretics.[140] This may minimize the risk, albeit small, of increasing fasting glucose concentrations, and possibly development of type 2 diabetes. Although this is not necessarily a universally accepted recommendation to mitigate risk of developing type 2 diabetes in patients treated with thiazide diuretics, keeping serum potassium concentrations in the 4.0 to 5.0 mEq/L range can be accomplished by combining the thiazide diuretic with a potassium-sparing diuretic (including an aldosterone antagonist), or an ACEI, ARB. These strategies are particularly attractive when additional BP lowering is needed. Moreover, lifestyle modifications remain the best strategy to minimize risk of developing diabetes.[89]

The magnitude of fasting glucose increases with thiazide diuretics is variable and dose dependent. Patients with diabetes and high risk for diabetes because of elevated fasting glucose exhibit the greatest glucose increases, and patients without diabetes exhibit the smallest increases. When increases in serum glucose concentration occur in patients without diabetes, they are typically on average 3.6 to 6.7 mg/dL after multiple years of thiazide diuretic therapy.[41,133] It appears that these changes are not clinically relevant because CV events are reduced despite these changes. Moreover, diabetes is not a contraindication to diuretic use; it is a compelling indication (Fig. 14-3) because risk of CV events is reduced in patients with diabetes who are treated with a thiazide diuretic.[89,91]

B.A.'s fasting glucose concentration is still considered normal. Her fasting glucose values should be documented and monitored at least once a year to detect any increases. Adding either an ACEI or ARB is a reasonable option for B.A. She should be encouraged to continue dietary modifications, and response to therapy should be re-evaluated in 2 to 4 weeks.

HYPOKALEMIA

CASE 14-4, QUESTION 6: When is potassium correction needed to manage diuretic-induced hypokalemia?

B.A.'s potassium is within the normal range. Potassium replacement is not indicated. Diuretic-associated hypokalemia should be treated when serum concentrations are below normal regardless of whether symptoms (e.g., muscle cramps) are present. Serum potassium should be measured at baseline and 2 to 4 weeks after initiating therapy or increasing the diuretic dose.

Potassium-rich foods (e.g., dried fruit, bananas, potatoes, avocados) may help prevent small decreases in potassium, but they cannot be used as sole therapy to correct hypokalemia. For instance, one medium-size banana has only 11.5 mEq of potassium. The usual replacement dose of prescribed potassium chloride is 20 to 40 mEq/day but can range from 10 to more than 100 mEq/day. Potassium chloride, bicarbonate, gluconate, acetate, and citrate salts are available for potassium replacement therapy. Rather than supplement potassium, which does not effectively correct the underlying mechanisms responsible for hypokalemia, a more appropriate and effective strategy to manage diuretic-induced hypokalemia is to add a potassium-sparing diuretic. Hypomagnesemia often accompanies diuretic-induced hypokalemia, and must be normalized before hypokalemia can be effectively reversed.

OTHER METABOLIC ABNORMALITIES

CASE 14-4, QUESTION 7: How should the increase in B.A.'s uric acid be managed?

Thiazide diuretics can increase serum uric acid concentrations in a dose-dependent fashion. Uric acid increases also occur with loop diuretics, but to a lesser extent. Increased proximal tubular renal reabsorption, decreased tubular secretion, or increased postsecretory reabsorption of uric acid contribute to diuretic-induced hyperuricemia. Thiazide-induced hyperuricemia is usually small ($\leq$0.5 mg/dL) and is not clinically significant in patients without a history of gout.[133] For patients with a history of gout, diuretics are not contraindicated, but an increase in serum uric acid may require a decrease in dose or possibly discontinuation of the diuretic, especially for those not on preventive antihyperuricemic therapy (e.g., allopurinol, febuxostat). Acute gouty arthritis precipitated by diuretic therapy should be treated, and the diuretic should be discontinued, at least temporarily. Future use of the diuretic will depend on whether long-term antihyperuricemic therapy is to be added and the risk versus benefit for continuing the diuretic. B.A.'s serum uric acid concentration is elevated, but switching to a different agent or lowering the dose of HCTZ is unnecessary because she is not symptomatic of gout.

It should be noted that changes in parameters such as uric acid can be informative regarding dosing. When a given dose of a diuretic fails to lower BP, it is often unclear as to whether the failure is a result of mechanisms other than volume driving the hypertension, or a result of the diuretic dose being insufficient to achieve the desired physiologic effect. For example, the absence of an increase in uric acid suggests that the administered dose was insufficient, and that a higher dose merits consideration. In B.A.'s case, the increase in uric acid confirms that the given dose was sufficient to have had a physiologic effect, so adding an antihypertensive agent from a different drug class would be preferable to increasing the diuretic dose if further BP lowering is necessary.

CASE 14-4, QUESTION 8: How much will HCTZ alter B.A.'s cholesterol values?

Small increases in LDL-C and triglycerides are potential side effects of diuretic therapy. Dietary fat restrictions help minimize, but do not necessarily prevent, these effects. Contrary to other biochemical disturbances, diuretic-induced changes in the lipid profile are not dose related, and overall changes are small. Many clinical trials lasting more than 1 year have shown that these alterations with diuretic therapy are not sustained with prolonged use.[132,133] Even if these changes are persistent, they are very small and are not clinically significant. The presence of dyslipidemia should never be a reason to avoid diuretic therapy.

CASE 14-4, QUESTION 9: What other potential electrolyte abnormalities should be evaluated in B.A. because of her thiazide diuretic therapy?

Hyponatremia is a serious, yet infrequent, adverse effect of diuretics. Changes in sodium concentrations are usually small, and the majority of patients are usually asymptomatic. Frail, elderly women appear more susceptible to experiencing severe hyponatremia (<120 mEq/L) from diuretics, which rarely occurs, but definitely requires discontinuation of therapy. Attention should be paid to the presence of other medications that can contribute to hyponatremia (e.g., selective serotonin reuptake inhibitors, psychotropic drugs), and patients should be counseled to avoid excessive free water intake.

Hypomagnesemia is an often-overlooked metabolic complication of diuretic therapy. Both thiazide and loop diuretics increase urinary excretion of magnesium in a dose-dependent manner. Symptoms of significant hypomagnesemia include muscle weakness, muscle tremor or twitching, mental status changes, and cardiac arrhythmias. Presence of these symptoms would necessitate magnesium supplementation or use of a potassium-sparing agent as noted above if hypokalemia is also present.

Thiazide diuretics decrease urinary calcium excretion and can be used to prevent calcium-related kidney stones. The retention of calcium does not significantly increase serum calcium concentrations and does not place patients at risk for hypercalcemia. This effect, however, may be beneficial in women at risk for osteoporosis (e.g., postmenopausal) such as B.A. or in patients with osteoporosis. Conversely, loop diuretics increase renal clearance of calcium.

Reasons for Inadequate BP Control

CASE 14-4, QUESTION 10: What are common reasons for inadequate patient response to antihypertensive pharmacotherapy?

B.A. has been on her current dose of HCTZ for 4 weeks. The full antihypertensive effect of HCTZ has been achieved, but she still has uncontrolled hypertension. She has had a response, but it remains inadequate. Potential reasons for an inadequate response, or lack of attaining BP goal values, with an antihypertensive should be considered before modifying her drug therapy regimen (Table 14-11). A comprehensive medication history and medical evaluation is needed to rule out identifiable causes, in particular nonadherence to the prescribed regimen. Her BP reduction with HCTZ is typical. Her kidney function is good, and no evidence exists of edema, so volume overload is unlikely.

TABLE 14-11
Reasons for Not Attaining Goal Blood Pressure Despite Antihypertensive Pharmacotherapy

Drug Related	Health Condition or Lifestyle Related	Other
Nonadherence	Volume overload	Improper blood pressure measurement
Inadequate antihypertensive dose	Excess sodium intake	Resistant hypertension
Inappropriate antihypertensive combination therapy	Volume retention from chronic kidney disease	White-coat hypertension
Inadequate diuretic therapy	Secondary disease causes (Table 14-3)	Pseudohypertension
Secondary drug-induced causes (Table 14-3)	Obesity	
Clinician failure to intensify or augment therapy (i.e., clinical inertia)	Excessive alcohol intake	

There are no apparent secondary causes of elevated BP. It is reasonable to conclude that B.A. needs additional therapy to achieve her goal BP. It is very common that most patients require two or more agents to attain BP goal values.

Modifying Therapy

B.A.'s present dose of HCTZ is appropriate and should not be increased to the maximal recommended dose of 50 mg daily (considered high-dose therapy) because it may increase risk of electrolyte and metabolic side effects. B.A.'s potassium dropped to 3.8 mEq/L with HCTZ, and further dosage increases may produce hypokalemia (<3.5 mEq/L) requiring correction. Her hyperuricemia may also be worsened. The slightly increased antihypertensive response expected from increasing to 50 mg/day is therefore not justified.[130] Discontinuing HCTZ and starting a different agent is an option, but it is not prudent to abandon the HCTZ; she tolerated the treatment and experienced a reasonable BP response, and the HCTZ will augment the efficacy of nearly any other agent that may be added, and may benefit her osteoporosis.

TWO-DRUG REGIMENS

The role of two-drug regimens in the treatment of hypertension is very clear. Most patients require multiple agents for BP control, especially in populations with BP goals of less than 130/80 mm Hg. Consensus guidelines recommend two-drug regimens as initial therapy for patients in stage 2 hypertension, and list initial two-drug regimen as an option in stage 1 hypertension.[3,15,82,91]

Adding a second agent to B.A.'s regimen is needed to reduce BP to her goal. She is a primary prevention patient, so three potential add-on antihypertensive agents that are considered first-line include an ACEI, ARB, or CCB. Ideally, a combination of two drugs with different mechanisms of action should be selected to produce a complementary effect to lower BP.

Adding an ACEI or ARB to B.A.'s HCTZ will result in additive antihypertensive effects that are independent of reversing fluid retention. Diuretics reduce BP initially by decreasing fluid volume, but maintain their antihypertensive effects by lowering PVR. BP lowering, however, can stimulate renin release from the kidney and activate the RAAS. This compensatory mechanism is an in vivo attempt to neutralize BP changes and regulate fluid loss. An ACEI or an ARB blocks the RAAS, explaining why combinations of these agents with diuretics are additive. Data from the ACCOMPLISH trial support combination therapy for hypertension. In this randomized, double-blind trial, 11,506 patients with hypertension were randomly assigned to the combination of an ACEI with thiazide diuretic or an ACEI with CCB.[115] After a mean follow-up of 3 years, the risk of CV events was significantly lower with the ACEI with CCB combination. Switching B.A.'s HCTZ to an ACEI with CCB may be more effective in lowering CV events than adding an ACEI to her current HCTZ. This would be an acceptable modification. However, considering her response to HCTZ, simply adding an ACEI is also reasonable.

FIXED-DOSE COMBINATION PRODUCTS

Several fixed-dose combination products including two or three drugs are available.

ONLINE CONTENT

For tables showing fixed-dose combination products that include two or three drugs, see Online Tables 14-1 and 14-2 at http://thepoint.lww.com/AT10e.

Although individual dose titration is not simple with fixed-dose combination products, their use can reduce the number of tablets or capsules taken by patients. This has been demonstrated to improve adherence compared with using two separate single-drug products.[141] Improved adherence may increase the likelihood of achieving goal BP values.

Most fixed-dose combinations include a thiazide diuretic, and many are available generically. Other fixed-dose combination products combine a CCB with either an ACEI or ARB. These combinations, similar to a thiazide with an ACE or ARB, are highly effective in lowering BP. An economic advantage may even exist to using a fixed-dose combination if it allows the patient to receive two drugs for one medication copayment. The Simplified Treatment Intervention To Control Hypertension study demonstrated that initiating therapy with a fixed-dose combination product according to a treatment algorithm was superior in attaining goal BP values when compared with usual management according to national guidelines.[117] These data further support using a fixed-dose combination product for initial therapy.

B.A. is a candidate for fixed-dose combination product. If the combination of an ACEI with HCTZ is selected for her, many options exist. All of the products with an ACEI also include HCTZ at the dose she is currently on. If the combination of an ACEI with a CCB is selected, fewer options exist, but there are products that contain an ACEI with a dihydropyridine CCB or a nondihydropyridine CCB. Cost should be considered because this is a concern for B.A. Multiple ACEI with thiazide diuretic combinations are available generically, but there is only one generic ACEI with CCB combination.

Step-Down Therapy

CASE 14-5

QUESTION 1: T.J. is a 58-year-old man with a 10-year history of hypertension. He has been treated with lisinopril/hydrochlorothiazide 20/25 mg daily and amlodipine 10 mg daily for more than 2 years, and his BP has been well controlled during this time. His BP at an office visit today

is 128/74 and 130/72 mm Hg. He has no compelling indications and has no hypertension-associated complications, but he is a smoker. T.J. also has dyslipidemia, which is well controlled with simvastatin 40 mg daily. His Framingham risk score is 15%, and he denies dizziness or difficulties with his medications. Should T.J.'s antihypertensive therapy be changed to reduce his medication doses or possibly discontinue some of his medications?

Some patients with hypertension can have their BP medications slowly withdrawn, resulting in normal BP values for weeks or months after discontinuation of their medications. This is called *step-down therapy.* However, it is not a feasible option for most patients with hypertension. Primary prevention patients with no additional major CV risk factors who have very well-controlled BP for at least 1 year might be eligible for a trial of step-down therapy. This option should not be considered for patients with other major CV risk factors, a Framingham risk score of 10% or more, compelling indications, or hypertension-associated complications. Step-down therapy consists of attempting to gradually decrease the dosage, the number of antihypertensive drugs, or both without compromising BP control. Abrupt or large dosage reductions should be avoided because of the risk of rapid return of uncontrolled BP and even rebound surges in BP (as is seen with rapid withdrawal of a β-blocker or an α_2-agonist).

Step-down therapy is most often plausible for patients who have lost significant amounts of weight or have drastically changed their lifestyle. Any attempt at step-down therapy must be accompanied by scheduled follow-up evaluations because BP values can rise over the course of months to years after drug discontinuation, especially if lifestyle modifications are not maintained. With adherence to lifestyle modifications (weight loss, reduction in sodium and alcohol), nearly 70% of patients remained free of antihypertensives for up to 1 year after being withdrawn from thiazide-based therapy in the Hypertension Control Program.[142]

Step-down therapy in T.J. is not an option. Although he does not have compelling indications or hypertension-associated complications, he has multiple major CV risk factors and an elevated Framingham risk score that is greater than or equal to 10%.

Angiotensin-Converting Enzyme Inhibitor

CASE 14-6

QUESTION 1: A.R. is a 49-year-old black woman with type 2 diabetes. She started lisinopril 10 mg daily 2 weeks ago when her BP values were consistently in the stage 1 hypertension range (150/90 mm Hg). Since then, she has had weekly BP measurements, and her values have averaged 142/85 mm Hg despite strict adherence to her lifestyle modifications. Her BP today is 144/84 mm Hg (140/88 mm Hg when repeated), and her heart rate is 78 beats/minute. She is not a smoker, and her BMI is 29 kg/m². All her laboratory test results, including kidney function, are within normal limits, except that her spot urine albumin-to-creatinine ratio is 80 mg/g (2 weeks ago it was 90 mg/g). Is 2 weeks of lisinopril therapy long enough to assess her antihypertensive response?

Several ACEIs are available (Table 14-12). Most ACEIs are dosed once daily in hypertension (Table 14-12). In general, most ACEIs, if used in equivalent doses, are considered interchangeable.

TABLE 14-12
Angiotensin-Converting Enzyme Inhibitors in Hypertension

Drug	Usual Starting Dose (mg/d)[a]	Usual Dosage Range (mg/d)	Dosing Frequency
Benazepril	10	20–40	Daily to BID
Captopril	25	50–100	BID to TID
Enalapril	5	10–40	Daily to BID
Fosinopril	10	20–40	Daily
Lisinopril	10	20–40	Daily
Moexipril	7.5	7.5–30	Daily to BID
Perindopril	4	4–16	Daily
Quinapril	10	20–80	Daily to BID
Ramipril	2.5	2.5–20	Daily to BID
Trandolapril	1	2–4	Daily

[a] Starting dose may be decreased 50% if patient is volume depleted, in acute heart failure exacerbation, or very elderly (≥75 year).
BID, twice daily; TID, three times daily.

The time to reach steady-state BP conditions is similar to what is seen with other antihypertensive agents. It may take several weeks before the full antihypertensive effects of ACEIs are seen. Therefore, evaluating BP response 2 to 4 weeks after starting or changing the dose of an ACEI is appropriate. A.R. has been taking lisinopril for 2 weeks, and her present BP should be used to determine whether she has attained goal. Both her BP range during the past few weeks and today's average BP are above her goal of less than 130/80 mm Hg (because she has diabetes).

CASE 14-6, QUESTION 2: Why should A.R. have serum potassium and serum creatinine monitored while on lisinopril therapy?

Serum potassium can increase with ACEI therapy as a result of aldosterone reduction. Potassium increases with ACEI monotherapy are small (typically 0.1 to 0.2 mEq/L) and usually do not cause hyperkalemia. This risk is increased when ACEIs are used in patients with significant CKD (GFR <60 mL/minute/1.73 m²), or when they are used in combination with other drugs that can also raise potassium.

ACEI therapy can also cause a small increase in serum creatinine owing to decreased vasoconstriction of the efferent arteriole in the kidney. This results in a minor decrease in GFR that may be evidenced by a small increase in serum creatinine. A common mistake is to discontinue an ACEI in response to this rise in serum creatinine. Increases in serum creatinine of up to 30% from the baseline creatinine value are safe and anticipated. In these patients, the ACEI should be continued because a strong association exists between acute increases in serum creatinine of up to 30% that stabilize within the first 2 months of ACEI therapy and long-term preservation of renal function.[143] Patients with an increase in serum creatinine of greater than 30% should have their ACEI therapy temporarily discontinued, as this may indicate other medical problems. Some of these problems can be underlying renal disease (such as bilateral renal artery stenosis) or other situations that may be compromising renal blood flow (e.g., volume depletion, concomitant nonsteroidal anti-inflammatory drug therapy, heart failure). Serum potassium and serum creatinine, in addition to BP, should to be monitored in A.R. within 2 to 4 weeks after starting ACEI therapy or increasing the dose.

CASE 14-6, QUESTION 3: A.R.'s lisinopril dose is increased to 20 mg daily. Will this doubling of her dose place her at risk for significant hypotension?

The very elderly, patients with volume depletion, or patients with heart failure exacerbation may experience a significant first-dose response to an ACEI. This can manifest as orthostatic hypotension, dizziness, or syncope. The increased pretreatment activity of the RAAS, coupled with blockade of this system, explains this effect. These patients should initiate ACEI therapy at half the normal dose (Table 14-12), followed by slow titration to standard doses.

Concurrent diuretic therapy may predispose some patients to first-dose hypotension. When ACEIs were first approved, dosing guidelines recommended starting at half the standard dose of the ACEI, decreasing the dose of the diuretic, or stopping the diuretic before initiating the ACEI. This was owing to fear that BP would sharply and acutely drop. These dosing recommendations are not necessary unless the patient is hemodynamically unstable (volume depleted, hyponatremic, or poorly compensated heart failure) or very elderly. A.R. does not have any of these characteristics and can safely increase her dose of lisinopril.

CASE 14-6, QUESTION 4: Is an ACEI an effective therapy in a black patient such as A.R.?

ACEI monotherapy is generally more effective at lowering BP in white patients than in black or elderly patients. Elderly and black patients are more likely to have low renin hypertension, which may partially explain some of the differences in response. Nevertheless, many of these patients still respond to ACEIs as monotherapy. Combination therapy, especially with a thiazide diuretic, usually mitigates this race- and age-related difference in BP response.

When an antihypertensive agent is being selected as initial monotherapy in a black patient, an ACEI should generally not be chosen unless the patient has a compelling indication for an ACEI. A thiazide diuretic or CCB is otherwise preferred. If combination therapy is chosen initially, it should be an ACEI with either a thiazide or a CCB. Of note, black patients have a twofold to fourfold increased risk of angioedema and cough with ACEIs compared with white patients.[82] This does not preclude ACEI use in black patients unless there is a prior history of angioedema.

A.R. should not be treated as a primary prevention patient. She has type 2 diabetes, which is a compelling indication for an ACEI. She also has microalbuminuria, which further justifies ACEI use as a first-line therapy. A.R. is also above her goal BP of less than 130/80 mm Hg. Although an ACEI is ideal treatment, a monotherapy approach is not expected to get her to goal. She has had some BP reduction from lisinopril, and the dose could be increased to the maximum, but she will likely require the addition of a second agent, preferably a thiazide diuretic (Fig. 14-3).

COMPELLING INDICATIONS

For all compelling indications, ACEI therapy is recommended as a drug therapy that has been proven to reduce risk of CV events. Evidence has clearly demonstrated reduction in hypertension-associated complications in patients with these medical conditions.

DIABETES

ACEI therapy is first-line for management of hypertension in diabetes based on evidence showing reduced hypertension-associated complications, including CV events and kidney disease.[89,91] Multiple clinical trials of ACEIs in patients with diabetes have consistently demonstrated reductions in CV events and kidney disease progression.[69,89,144] These data further reinforce the role of ACEI in patients with diabetes and hypertension, and also the benefits of combination therapy in this population.

An added benefit of ACEIs in diabetes is that, unlike some other agents, they are metabolically neutral. Moreover, they may improve insulin resistance, which can result in a lower risk of progressing to type 2 diabetes for patients with hypertension who have impaired fasting glucose.[34]

CHRONIC KIDNEY DISEASE

The ACEIs protect the kidney from the unrelenting deterioration that occurs with CKD, hypertension, and diabetes. Therefore, these agents are recommended as first-line therapy in CKD. The increased intraglomerular pressure and mesangial cell proliferation that occurs in CKD leads to proteinuria and a progressive decline in kidney function. Reductions in renal blood flow cause the kidneys to increase renin release, thus activating the RAAS. This action constricts the efferent renal arteriole to preserve glomerular pressure, but may propagate renal impairment. ACEIs preferentially dilate the efferent arteriole, which relieves intraglomerular pressure. Data suggest that ACEIs may have unique renal preservation properties, making CKD a compelling indication for ACEI therapy. Some of the risk reduction is also related to systemic BP lowering.

Patients with diabetes are at high risk for nephropathy, especially those with type 1 diabetes. Evidence indicates that ACEI therapy reduces progression to severe CKD and kidney failure in patients with type 1 diabetes and proteinuria.[92] In type 2 diabetes, ACEI therapy has been proven to decrease initial development of microalbuminuria, and to reduce worsening of proteinuria, but evidence showing progression to severe CKD or failure is not available.[38,94] Nonetheless, both type 1 and type 2 diabetes are considered compelling indications for the use of ACEI therapy.

CHRONIC AND ACUTE CORONARY ARTERY DISEASE

ACEI therapy is a first-line treatment in patients with chronic CAD (post-MI, chronic stable angina) and acute CAD (non–ST-segment elevation MI, ST-segment elevation MI).[101,103,104] This should be in addition to β-blocker therapy. The benefit of ACEI therapy in patients with CAD is a reduced risk of CV events that is independent of both left ventricular function and BP. Patients with CAD who have controlled BP still appear to have reductions in CV events with the addition of ACEI therapy.[145] Because ACEI therapy will not provide anti-ischemic effects, the role of ACEI therapy in CAD is as an add-on to a β-blocker to reduce CV risk, not to treat underlying ischemic symptoms.

PRIOR STROKE

The perindopril protection against recurrent stroke study (PROGRESS) was a double-blind, placebo-controlled evaluation of an ACEI in combination with a thiazide diuretic for 4 years in 6,105 patients with a history of stroke or transient ischemic attack.[63] The incidence of stroke and total major vascular events were significantly reduced with the combination regimen, and reductions were seen regardless of baseline BP or reduction in BP. These data justify the compelling indication to use an ACEI (in combination with a thiazide diuretic) to reduce recurrence of stroke in patients who have had a stroke.

LEFT VENTRICULAR DYSFUNCTION

ACEIs reduce morbidity and mortality in patients with left ventricular dysfunction as a component of standard therapy (diuretic with an ACEI followed by the addition of a β-blocker).[108] In general, the CV benefits of ACEI therapy in left ventricular dysfunction are considered a class effect, and ACEIs are used interchangeably at equivalent dosages in these patients (see Chapter 19, Heart Failure).[15]

CASE 14-6, QUESTION 5: A.R. has microalbuminuria, and lisinopril may help preserve kidney function. However, is there a risk that lisinopril can cause acute renal dysfunction?

The ACEIs are effective in patients with hypertension-associated renal disease. They are contraindicated, however, in several situations, including bilateral renal artery stenosis, pregnancy, and volume depletion (Table 14-10). In the case of bilateral renal artery stenosis or volume depletion, high angiotensin concentrations maintain renal blood flow, and acute renal dysfunction can occur when an ACEI is started. Because it is often not known whether a patient has bilateral renal artery stenosis, problems with ACEI can be minimized by starting with recommended doses and careful monitoring of serum creatinine within 2 to 4 weeks of starting therapy. Modest elevations in serum creatinine that are less than 30% (for baseline creatinine values <3.0 mg/dL) do not warrant adjustment in therapy.[143] If greater increases occur, ACEI therapy should be stopped, and further medical evaluation should occur. Patients with elevated serum creatinine at baseline (up to 3.0 mg/dL) may particularly benefit from the vasodilatory effects of ACEIs in the kidney, but require careful drug initiation and close monitoring. A.R.'s serum creatinine was normal after 4 weeks of lisinopril therapy. She is not experiencing any kidney-related adverse effects from lisinopril.

CASE 14-6, QUESTION 6: What are the risks of using ACEIs in women of childbearing age?

Because ACEIs are teratogenic in the second and third trimester,[146] their use in pregnancy is contraindicated. Moreover, their use in women of childbearing potential is discouraged. If used in this population, patient education should be explicitly clear regarding risks to the fetus, which include potentially fatal hypotension, anuria, renal failure, and developmental deformities. A highly effective form of contraception should be strongly recommended.

Angiotensin Receptor Blockers

CASE 14-6, QUESTION 7: A.R.'s lisinopril is increased to 20 mg daily, then to 40 mg daily during a period of 8 weeks. Her current BP is 136/78 mm Hg (134/76 mm Hg when repeated) at an office visit today. Her serum potassium and creatinine are unchanged from previous values. However, she reports a persistent dry cough for the past few months. She has no additional signs suggesting upper respiratory infection or left ventricular dysfunction. How should A.R.'s therapy be modified?

A well-known side effect of ACEIs is a nonproductive, dry cough, which can occur in up to 15% of patients, with some estimates of cough prevalence being higher.[147] Patients may describe this as a tickling sensation in the back of the throat that commonly occurs late in the evening. This is distinctly different from the cough associated with left ventricular dysfunction, which might be associated with crackles and rales (on auscultation) indicating possible pulmonary edema. ACEI-related cough resolves with discontinuation. Many agents have been used to treat an ACEI cough with poor results. The best treatment option for a patient with an intolerable ACEI cough is to switch agents. For A.R., switching to an ARB would likely eliminate the cough and is an acceptable first-line treatment option for her considering her diabetes and microalbuminuria.[89,91] A.R. will also require the addition of a second agent, either a CCB or thiazide diuretic, because she has not achieved her goal BP of less than 130/80 mm Hg.

TABLE 14-13
Angiotensin Receptor Blockers in Hypertension

Drug	Starting Dose (mg/d)[a]	Usual Dosage Range (mg/d)	Dosing Frequency
Azilsartan medoxomil	80	80	Daily
Candesartan cilexetil	16	8–32	Daily to BID
Eprosartan mesylate	600	600–800	Daily to BID
Irbesartan	150	75–300	Daily
Losartan potassium	50	25–100	Daily to BID
Olmesartan medoxomil	20	20–40	Daily
Telmisartan	40	20–80	Daily
Valsartan	80–160	80–320	Daily

[a] Starting dose may be decreased 50% if patient is volume depleted, very elderly, or taking a diuretic.
BID, twice daily.

ARBs are first-line options for primary prevention patients and have data demonstrating reductions in CV events.[32,59] There are eight ARBs (Table 14-13), and many are available as two-drug fixed-dose combination products (Online Table 14-1), as well as two different three-drug fixed-dose combination products (Online Table 14-2).

PHARMACOLOGIC DIFFERENCES BETWEEN AN ANGIOTENSIN-CONVERTING ENZYME INHIBITOR AND AN ANGIOTENSIN RECEPTOR BLOCKER

CASE 14-6, QUESTION 8: How is an ARB different from an ACEI?

Unlike ACEIs, ARBs specifically bind to angiotensin II receptors in vascular smooth muscle, adrenal glands, and other tissues. Access of angiotensin II to its receptors is blocked, and angiotensin I–mediated vasoconstriction and aldosterone release is prevented, resulting in BP reduction. ARBs do not affect bradykinin; therefore dry cough does not occur.

Considerable investigation has focused on describing the pharmacologic differences between the angiotensin II type 1 and type 2 receptors. Stimulation of the type 1 receptor causes vasoconstriction, salt and water retention, and vascular remodeling. Other deleterious effects from type 1 receptor stimulation include myocyte and smooth muscle hypertrophy, fibroblast hyperplasia, cytotoxic effects in the myocardium, altered gene expression, and possible increased concentrations of plasminogen activator inhibitor. Stimulation of the type 2 receptor results in antiproliferative actions, cell differentiation, and tissue repair.

Theoretically, an ideal antihypertensive agent would block only type 1 and not type 2 receptors as is the case with ARBs. Therefore, it is possible that an ARB would be superior to an ACEI in reducing hypertension-associated complications because ACEIs ultimately decrease stimulation of both type 1 and type 2 receptors by decreasing production of angiotensin II. This argument is purely speculative and is not supported by clinical trial data. ONTARGET was a prospective, double-blind, randomized controlled trial that directly compared ARB-based therapy, ACEI-based therapy, and the combination of an ACEI with ARB.[121] After a median of 56 months, the incidence of CV events was no different among all three treatment groups. Therefore, ARB therapy is as effective as, but no more superior than, ACEI therapy in the overall management of hypertension.

CASE 14-6, QUESTION 9: Under what circumstances would an ARB be a more appropriate initial antihypertensive agent than an ACEI?

DIABETES

Patients with diabetes should be treated with either an ACEI or ARB. ARB-based treatment regimens, similar to ACEI-based treatment regimens, have been shown in clinical trials to reduce the progression of diabetic nephropathy among patients with type 2 diabetes and microalbuminuria.[89] ARB-based therapy is the only antihypertensive regimen for which evidence shows reduced kidney failure in patients with type 2 diabetes who have diabetic nephropathy with albuminuria (not microalbuminuria) and elevated serum creatinine.[73] Therefore, for patients with type 2 diabetes and advanced nephropathy, evidence supports ARB therapy, although ACEI therapy has not been studied in this population.

CHRONIC KIDNEY DISEASE

An ARB, similar to an ACEI, minimizes damage that occurs with CKD. Both ACEIs and ARBs preferentially dilate the efferent arteriole, which relieves intraglomerular pressure. Thus, CKD is a compelling indication for ARB therapy. For nondiabetic kidney disease, less evidence supports ARB use, and these agents should be reserved as alternatives to an ACEI.

CHRONIC AND ACUTE CORONARY ARTERY DISEASE

Angiotensin receptor blocker therapy is a reasonable alternative to ACEI therapy in patients with CAD although data are limited.

PRIOR STROKE

The role of ARB therapy in patients with a history of stroke is controversial. In the Morbidity and Mortality after Stroke Eprosartan Compared with Nitrendipine for Secondary Prevention study, ARB-based therapy reduced the incidence of recurrent stroke more than dihydropyridine CCB-based therapy in a large number of patients with cerebrovascular disease.[80] However, in the Prevention Regimen for Effectively Avoiding Second Strokes study 20,332 patients who recently had an ischemic stroke were randomly assigned to ARB therapy or placebo.[107] After a mean of 2.5 years, there was no difference in the incidence of the primary end point of recurrent stroke between the two groups. Therefore, it is unclear how well ARB therapy would work as an alternative to ACEI therapy in patients with a history of stroke.

LEFT VENTRICULAR DYSFUNCTION

Pharmacologic blockade of the RAAS in left ventricular dysfunction is of paramount importance. An ARB is a reasonable alternative in patients with hypertension and left ventricular dysfunction who cannot tolerate an ACEI (e.g., those who experience cough).[109] As sequential add-on therapy for patients with left ventricular dysfunction who are already treated with the standard regimen of a diuretic with an ACEI and β-blocker, ARB therapy has been proved to reduce risk of CV events.[122] However, the benefits are limited primarily to decreasing risk of heart failure hospitalizations. This is not similar to the reduction in mortality seen when adding an aldosterone antagonist. Aldosterone antagonists would be preferred over ARBs when considering sequential add-on therapy. Additionally, if an ARB is used with an ACEI, there is a significant increase in risk of side effects.[121]

CASE 14-6, QUESTION 10: If A.R. experienced angioedema from lisinopril, would treatment with an ARB be appropriate?

A history of ACEI-induced angioedema does not preclude the use of ARB therapy. The cross-reactivity between angioedema with an ACEI and ARB is not exactly known. The Candesartan in Heart Failure: Assessment of Reduction in Mortality and Morbidity Alternative study prospectively included patients with a history of ACEI intolerance who were randomly assigned, in a double-blind manner, to placebo or candesartan. Of the 2,028 patients enrolled, 39 had a history of ACEI angioedema, and only 1 of these patients experienced repeat angioedema that required discontinuation of the ARB.[109] In the Telmisartan Randomised Assessment Study in ACE Intolerant Subjects with Cardiovascular Disease trial, 5,926 patients with a history of ACEI intolerance were randomly assigned in this double-blind trial to an ARB or placebo for a median duration of 56 months.[148] A total of 75 patients had a history of ACEI angioedema, and none of those patients who were randomly assigned to the ARB treatment arm experienced repeat angioedema. Therefore, cross-reactivity in angioedema between ACEIs and ARBs appears possible, but unlikely and very small. ARBs are an alternative for patients who experience ACEI angioedema but should be reserved for patients with a compelling indication for an ACEI. Of note, the ACC/AHA guidelines recommend an ARB in patients who have experienced angioedema from an ACEI.[108]

Calcium-Channel Blockers

CCBs effectively lower BP. Elderly and black patients generally have greater BP reduction with a CCB than with other agents (β-blockers, ACEIs, ARBs). The addition of a diuretic to a CCB provides additive antihypertensive effects, but is not usually as effective as the combination of an ARB with a CCB. CCBs do not alter serum lipids, glucose, uric acid, or electrolytes.

All CCBs inhibit the movement of extracellular calcium, but there are two primary subtypes: dihydropyridines and nondihydropyridines (i.e., diltiazem and verapamil). Each has distinctly different pharmacologic effects.

ONLINE CONTENT

For a table that summarizes the pharmacologic effects of the two primary subtypes of CCBs, see Online Table 14-3 at http://thepoint.lww.com/AT10e.

DIHYDROPYRIDINE CALCIUM-CHANNEL BLOCKERS

Dihydropyridines are potent vasodilators of peripheral and coronary arteries. They do not block AV nodal conduction and do not treat arrhythmias. Moreover, the potent vasodilation associated with most dihydropyridines can induce a reflex tachycardia. With the exception of amlodipine and felodipine, dihydropyridines decrease cardiac contractility and should be avoided in patients with left ventricular dysfunction. Side effects of dihydropyridines are related to their potent vasodilatory effects (e.g., tachycardia, headache, peripheral edema).

NONDIHYDROPYRIDINE CALCIUM-CHANNEL BLOCKERS

The two nondihydropyridine CCBs, diltiazem and verapamil, are similar to each other. Relative to dihydropyridines, they are only moderately potent vasodilators, but they directly decrease AV nodal conduction and have greater decreases in cardiac contractility. The blockade of AV nodal conduction can slow heart

TABLE 14-14
Calcium-Channel Blockers in Hypertension[a]

Drug	Usual Dosage Range (mg/d)	Dosing Frequency
Nondihydropyridines[b]		
Diltiazem, sustained-release	120–480	Daily
Diltiazem, extended-release[c]	120–540	Daily
Verapamil, sustained-release	180–480	Daily to BID
Verapamil, controlled-onset extended-release[c]	180–480	QHS
Verapamil, chronotherapeutic oral drug absorption system[c]	100–400	QHS
Dihydropyridines		
Amlodipine	2.5–10	Daily
Felodipine, extended-release tablet	2.5–10	Daily
Isradipine, controlled-release tablet	5–20	Daily
Nicardipine, sustained-release capsule	60–120	BID
Nifedipine, sustained-release tablet[d]	30–90	Daily
Nisoldipine, extended-release tablet	17–34	Daily

[a] Immediate-release (IR) diltiazem, nifedipine, and verapamil should be avoided in hypertension.
[b] Many different long-acting products exist. Because their individual release characteristics vary, they are not exactly interchangeable using a milligram-per-milligram conversion.
[c] Chronotherapeutic agents are dosed primarily at bedtime and have a delayed drug release for a period of hours, followed by slow delivery of drug that starts just before morning, with no delivery during the early evening; because they use different delivery systems, they are not interchangeable products.
[d] Only sustained-release nifedipine is approved for hypertension. Immediate-release nifedipine should be avoided for the management of hypertension.
BID, twice daily; QHS, every night.

rate and is the basis for their use in controlling supraventricular tachycardias associated with certain arrhythmias (e.g., atrial fibrillation). Most patients only have a modest decrease in heart rate. However, heart block (first-, second-, or third-degree) is a potential adverse effect, especially with large doses. Both diltiazem and verapamil should be avoided in patients with an underlying second- or third-degree heart block. Under these circumstances, a dihydropyridine can be used if a CCB is needed. Verapamil and diltiazem should be avoided in patients with left ventricular dysfunction because they can significantly reduce cardiac contractility. Diltiazem may have a lower incidence of constipation than verapamil.

FORMULATIONS

Several CCBs are available for the treatment of hypertension. They are listed in Table 14-14. Immediate-release formulations should be avoided (see Chapter 21, Hypertensive Crises).[149]

SUSTAINED-RELEASE FORMULATIONS

CASE 14-7

QUESTION 1: C.F. is a 60-year-old man with hypertension, asthma, and type 2 diabetes. His hypertension is treated with HCTZ 25 mg daily and ramipril 20 mg daily for many years. Today his BP is 148/74 mm Hg (144/72 mm Hg when repeated), and his heart rate is 90 beats/minute. C.F.'s physician would like to add a CCB to his regimen to improve BP control. What are the differences between controlled-onset, extended-release verapamil and sustained-release verapamil? Are they interchangeable?

All CCBs have short half-lives, except amlodipine. Immediate-release forms require multiple daily doses to provide 24-hour effects. Sustained-released formulations are preferred when a CCB is used to treat hypertension. Various sustained-release delivery devices are available. Serum drug concentrations differ among sustained-release CCBs, but overall BP lowering is usually similar. Nonetheless, most of these products that include the same drug are not rated by the US Food and Drug Administration as equivalent and identical. Insurance formularies often encourage therapeutic substitution between these agents. Therapeutic interchange between modified-release drug delivery formulations that allow for once- or twice-daily dosing (e.g., sustained-release, extended-release, chronotherapeutic products), however, are not equivalent using a milligram-per-milligram conversion. Therapeutic substitution among these products may result in variable BP-lowering effects if not adjusted appropriately. BP and heart rate monitoring should occur within 2 weeks of interchanging sustained-release CCBs.

COMPELLING INDICATIONS

DIABETES

CASE 14-7, QUESTION 2: Why is diabetes a compelling indication for a CCB in C.F.?

CCBs have been shown to reduce risk of CV events in patients with diabetes,[3,91] although the evidence is not as convincing as that seen with an ACEI. The results of the Fosinopril versus Amlodipine Cardiovascular Events Randomized Trial and Appropriate Blood Pressure Control in Diabetes trial suggest that ACEIs have more CV protection than CCBs.[70,71]

The primary role of a CCB in the management of hypertension in diabetes is ideally as a component of sequential add-on therapy, after an ACEI or ARB. In a subgroup of 6,946 patients with diabetes from the ACCOMPLISH trial, patients on the combination of an ACEI with CCB had fewer CV events than patients on the combination of an ACEI with thiazide diuretic.[90] Therefore, these data support using a CCB ahead of a thiazide diuretic as the second drug added to an ACEI (or ARB as an alternative) for hypertension in diabetes. Because the BP goal in diabetes is less than 130/80 mm Hg, most patients with diabetes need three or more antihypertensive agents to achieve this goal. A CCB is frequently needed in this population.

Nondihydropyridine CCBs (particularly diltiazem) may slow the progression of CKD, although evidence is not as extensive or definitive as it is with an ACEI or ARB. The proposed mechanism is dilation of both the afferent and efferent arterioles, which would decrease intraglomerular pressure. Dihydropyridines have unclear effects on progression of kidney disease. The prevailing opinion is that the renal protective effects of an ACEI and ARB are superior to that of a CCB.

CHRONIC CORONARY ARTERY DISEASE

CASE 14-8

QUESTION 1: A.P. is a 71-year-old man with a BP of 168/90 mm Hg (170/90 mm Hg when repeated) and a heart rate of 88 beats/minute. He has a history of chronic stable angina that is treated with sublingual nitroglycerin as needed for ischemic symptoms. He also has severe chronic obstructive pulmonary disease that is worsened with β-blocker therapy. He currently has no ischemic symptoms. All laboratory results are normal, except his serum creatinine is 1.3 mg/dL. Is a CCB appropriate for A.P.? If yes, which type is preferred?

Chronic CAD (i.e., chronic stable angina) is a compelling indication for use of a CCB, but CCBs are an alternative to a β-blocker, or sequential add-on therapy to a β-blocker for patients who require additional anti-ischemic effects.[56,101] Alternatives to β-blockers are needed when contraindications or intolerances to β-blockers are present. Sustained-release CCB formulations or long-acting products (i.e., amlodipine) are always preferred. When used as an alternative to a β-blocker, a nondihydropyridine CCB is preferred because they decrease myocardial oxygen demand, improve myocardial blood flow, and have negative inotropic and chronotropic effects. All these may benefit patients with CAD. Dihydropyridine CCBs are similar, but do not lower heart rate, and have less negative inotropic effects. They can be used in patients with chronic CAD and possibly acute CAD, but verapamil and diltiazem are preferred when a CCB is used instead of a β-blocker.

Therapy with a CCB is preferred in A.P. because β-blockers worsened his severe chronic obstructive pulmonary disease. Verapamil will lower his elevated heart rate and BP as well as reduce episodes of ischemic symptoms (i.e., chest pain). Constipation, which is more prevalent in the elderly, is a common side effect with verapamil. This can be mitigated with dietary changes, bulk-forming laxatives, or the regular use of a stool softener. Similar to other antihypertensive agents, a low dose (120–180 mg daily) should be used initially and slowly titrated at 2- to 4-week intervals.

ADDITIONAL POPULATIONS

ISOLATED SYSTOLIC HYPERTENSION

CASE 14-9

QUESTION 1: T.C. is a 76-year-old woman with hypertension and dyslipidemia. She has been adherent with her regimen of chlorthalidone 25 mg daily for several years. Her BP values are 164/76 mm Hg (168/78 mm Hg when repeated). She has no other evidence of hypertension-associated complications, and no compelling indications. Her laboratory values and ECG are all normal. Amlodipine 5 mg daily is added to her regimen. What are the benefits of using a CCB to treat T.C.'s hypertension?

T.C. has ISH. This should be managed according to the general patient care principles for hypertension. Thiazide diuretics have traditionally been considered first-line therapy for this population based on historical data demonstrating CV event lowering in elderly patients with isolated systolic hypertension. The SHEP trial proved that treating ISH in the elderly is beneficial and established thiazide diuretic-based regimens as first-line agents.[47]

Long-acting dihydropyridine CCBs have been shown to reduce CV events in patients with ISH also. The Systolic Hypertension in Europe study was similar to the SHEP trial, but used a nitrendipine-based (a long-acting dihydropyridine CCB similar to long-acting nifedipine) regimen instead of a thiazide diuretic-based regimen.[50] Amlodipine is an appropriate add-on therapy for T.C. to control her BP and reduce her risk of CV events.

EDEMA FROM DIHYDROPYRIDINE CALCIUM-CHANNEL BLOCKERS

CASE 14-9, QUESTION 2: One month later, T.C.'s BP is down to 148/70 mm Hg (150/70 mm Hg when repeated). She is tolerating her amlodipine, except she has swelling in both ankles. T.C. has never had this problem before. A complete cardiovascular examination shows no signs of left ventricular dysfunction or other hypertension-associated complications that would explain this new peripheral edema. Her amlodipine therapy is identified as the cause of this edema. How should her edema be managed? Should chlorthalidone be changed to a loop diuretic, should amlodipine be stopped, or is there another option?

Peripheral edema with CCB therapy, especially a dihydropyridine CCB, is a dose-dependent side effect. It is a direct result of the potent peripheral arterial vasodilation. When there is not equal vasodilation in the venous vasculature, a risk exists for leaking though the capillaries in the legs and, thus, an increased risk of peripheral edema. The best way to manage this side effect is to reduce the dose of the dihydropyridine, or to add an agent that blocks the RAAS to decrease the effects of angiotensin II, which will result in a more balanced pressure gradient across her peripheral vasculature by providing vasodilation of both the arteries and veins. Adding either an ACEI or ARB can be used to accomplish this with the added benefit of further lowering BP. Clinicians should note that using diuretics for the primary purpose of treating peripheral edema that is secondary to CCB use is not recommended, and is not effective.

T.C.'s BP is not at her goal of less than 140/90 mm Hg, and additional drug therapy is needed. Her best option is to add an ACEI or ARB to minimize her edema. She has otherwise tolerated amlodipine, so no urgent need exists to discontinue this agent. Moreover, lowering the dose of amlodipine to 2.5 mg is an option, but BP lowering with this low dose is minimal, and she would still require the addition of another agent anyway.

ADDITIONAL POPULATIONS

Diltiazem and verapamil can also be used to treat atrial fibrillation, atrial flutter, and supraventricular arrhythmias owing to their ability to block the AV node and lower heart rate. Verapamil is effective in migraine prophylaxis. Patients with Raynaud's phenomenon can obtain symptomatic relief from the peripheral vasodilation associated with a dihydropyridine CCB. Lastly, CCBs are effective in treating cyclosporine-induced hypertension, but should be used cautiously because verapamil and diltiazem increase cyclosporine concentration.

OTHER CONSIDERATIONS

LEFT VENTRICULAR DYSFUNCTION

CASE 14-9, QUESTION 3: Why are nondihydropyridine CCBs contraindicated in left ventricular dysfunction (systolic heart failure)?

CCBs, especially nondihydropyridines, have negative inotropic effects that result in a decrease in cardiac contractility. This is most pronounced with verapamil, but is also present with diltiazem and with some dihydropyridines (Online Table 14-3). In left ventricular dysfunction, the primary physiologic problem is decreased cardiac contractility. Thus, using a CCB in this population can exacerbate left ventricular dysfunction, or potentially unmask left ventricular dysfunction that has not yet been diagnosed.

When patients with left ventricular dysfunction require a CCB to treat another condition (i.e., angina or hypertension), amlodipine or felodipine may be used. They are the only CCBs that have been safely used in clinical trials of patients with left ventricular dysfunction. Unlike many other antihypertensive agents, they do not, however, protect against left ventricular dysfunction-related mortality.

β-Blockers

CASE 14-10

QUESTION 1: E.K. is a 78-year-old black man with a history of hypertension. He was hospitalized for an acute MI 2 months ago and has been treated with metoprolol succinate 50 mg daily and lisinopril 20 mg daily since then. Today his BP readings are 148/92 and 146/90 mm Hg, and his heart rate is 80 beats/minute. He denies medication-related side effects. Because E.K. is black and elderly, will β-blocker therapy be effective?

β-Blockers reduce morbidity and mortality in patients with certain compelling indications.[3,15] These include left ventricular dysfunction, CAD, and diabetes. β-Blocker therapy should not be the primary antihypertensive agent for primary prevention patients, but is an effective alternative add-on agent for primary prevention patients to lower BP. Elderly and black patients may have less BP reduction than young or white patients. E.K. is elderly and might have more BP reduction with another agent (i.e., thiazide diuretic or CCB), but these points are moot in E.K. Age and race should never deter use of a β-blocker when a compelling indication is present. Because of E.K.'s previous MI, a β-blocker as first-line is compellingly indicated.

PHARMACOLOGIC DIFFERENCES

Many different β-blockers are available (Table 14-15). There is significant heterogeneity within the pharmacology of the class. These clinically important differences relate primarily to cardioselectivity, ISA, lipid solubility, and use in left ventricular dysfunction, and should be considered when selecting an agent.

CARDIOSELECTIVITY

CASE 14-10, QUESTION 2: What are the advantages of using a cardioselective β-blocker to treat E.K.'s hypertension?

β_1-Adrenergic receptors are primarily located in the heart, and β_2-adrenergic receptors are found in the lungs, kidneys, and peripheral arteriolar endothelium. Low-affinity β_1-receptors are also present in the lung, and low-affinity β_2-receptors are present in the heart. Some β-blockers (e.g., atenolol, metoprolol) demonstrate relative cardioselectivity with greater antagonism of cardiac β_1-receptors and less activity on β_2-receptors in the lung or bronchial tissue. Selectivity is not absolute, however, because it is dose-dependent. For instance, asthma has been precipitated even with cardioselective agents when they are used in higher doses, but not with low to moderate doses.

Nonselective β-blockers potentially have the disadvantage of blunting the symptoms of hypoglycemia in patients with diabetes. β_2-Blockade from nonselective β-blockers (e.g., propranolol) can lead to unopposed β_1-induced peripheral vasoconstriction. This may worsen Raynaud's phenomenon, peripheral arterial disease, or hypertension caused by catecholamine-producing tumors (pheochromocytoma). Despite these shortcomings, nonselective β-blockers are preferred in patients with non-CV indications for β-blocker therapy (e.g., migraine, essential tremor). Absent these reasons, cardioselective β-blockers are preferred. E.K. is taking metoprolol, which is a cardioselective agent and is appropriate therapy for E.K.

INTRINSIC SYMPATHOMIMETIC ACTIVITY

CASE 14-10, QUESTION 3: Why are acebutolol, carteolol, penbutolol, and pindolol contraindicated in E.K.?

Pure β-blockers occupy the β-receptor, inhibiting stimulatory catecholamine access while exerting no effect on their own. β-Blockers with ISA, such as acebutolol, carteolol, penbutolol, and pindolol, partially stimulate β-receptors while attached to this receptor, but much less so than a pure agonist. When given to a patient with a slow resting heart rate, ISA β-blockers can blunt the typical decrease in heart rate that is seen with other β-blockers.

β-Blockers with ISA are theoretically less likely to cause bradycardia, bronchospasm, reduced CO, and peripheral vasoconstriction than nonselective β-blockers. Nonetheless, these agents still

TABLE 14-15
Common β-Blockers in Hypertension

Drug	Usual Dosage Range (mg/d)	Dosing Frequency	Half-Life (hours)	β_1 Selectivity	Lipid Solubility
Atenolol	25–100	Daily to BID	6–7	++	Low
Bisoprolol	5–20	Daily	9–12	+++	High
Carvedilol	12.5–50	BID	6–10	0	High
Carvedilol	10–80	Daily	6–10	0	High
Labetalol	200–800	BID	6–8	0	Moderate
Metoprolol tartrate	100–400	BID	3–7	+	Moderate to high
Metoprolol succinate	25–400	Daily	3–7	+	Moderate to high
Nebivolol	5–10	Daily	12–19	+++	High
Propranolol	40–180	Daily (LA and XL) or BID	3–5	0	High

BID, twice daily.

TABLE 14-16
Alternative Antihypertensive Agents

Drugs/Mechanism of Action	Usual Dosage Range (mg/d)	Dosing Frequency
Aldosterone Antagonists (see Table 14-9)		
α_1-Blockers		
Doxazosin	1–8	Daily
Prazosin	2–20	BID to TID
Terazosin	1–20	Daily to BID
Direct Renin Inhibitor		
Aliskiren	150–300	Daily
α_2-Agonists (Central)		
Clonidine	0.1–0.8	BID
Clonidine	0.17–0.52	Daily
Clonidine transdermal	0.1–0.3	Once weekly
Methyldopa	250–1,000	BID
Arterial Vasodilators		
Hydralazine	25–100	BID to TID
Minoxidil	2.5–80	Daily to BID
Adrenergic Neuron Blockers		
Reserpine	0.05–0.25	Daily

BID, twice daily; TID, three times daily.

identifying occult volume expansion using serial hemodynamic measurements from noninvasive bioimpedance testing, followed by enhancing diuretic therapy, has been shown to reduce BP better than treatment selected by an experienced hypertension specialist.[152] Options to assure appropriate diuretic therapy include switching diuretic agents, switching diuretic classes, increasing the dose, or adding a different class of diuretic. Instead of increasing HCTZ to 50 mg daily, switching HCTZ to the more long-acting chlorthalidone is another possible option to enhance BP lowering. This is an option in R.R. Another option is switching HCTZ to a loop diuretic (e.g., furosemide or torsemide). This should be considered for patients with stage 4 or 5 CKD (GFR <30 mL/minute/1.73 m^2) or for those who need diuresis because of edema. This is not a reasonable treatment option for R.R. because he does not have CKD. Another option is to add an aldosterone antagonist, which is considered an alternative antihypertensive agent. Patients with resistant hypertension often require the use of an agent(s) (Table 14-16) that is not widely used as either a first- or second-line therapy. These therapies should not be used as monotherapy or a cornerstone of a multidrug regimen as there is less evidence to support their role in reducing CV events. It should be acknowledged, however, that some of these agents (e.g., reserpine, hydralazine) served as add-on agents to diuretics and β-blockers in early placebo-controlled, stepped-care approach trials in hypertension. R.R. has already failed to fully respond to, or tolerate, several drug classes that typically are associated with reductions in hypertension-associated complications. To attain his BP goal of less than 140/90 mm Hg, an alternative agent, other than clonidine, should be selected because he did not tolerate it in the past.

ALTERNATIVE ANTIHYPERTENSIVE AGENTS

CASE 14-11, QUESTION 2: How safe is it to use spironolactone 25 mg daily in R.R.?

ALDOSTERONE ANTAGONISTS

Spironolactone and eplerenone are aldosterone antagonists that are especially useful as an add-on therapy in patients with resistant hypertension and would be a reasonable addition to R.R.'s regimen.[13,153] Many patients with resistant hypertension have increased activation of the RAAS, which can result in increased aldosterone. Moreover, up to 20% of patients with resistant hypertension have primary aldosteronism.[13] These characteristics of patients with resistant hypertension make the addition of an aldosterone antagonist very effective in lowering BP in resistant hypertension.

R.R.'s potassium is in the normal range, but could increase after adding spironolactone. Therefore, it should be monitored 2 to 4 weeks after therapy is started to assure R.R. does not experience hyperkalemia. Eplerenone is more specific than spironolactone in aldosterone blockade, although some data suggest that spironolactone is more effective in primary aldosteronism.[154] Compared with spironolactone, gynecomastia is less frequent with eplerenone. The incidence of hyperkalemia may be greater with eplerenone, however. When used for hypertension, eplerenone is contraindicated in populations at high risk for hyperkalemia: patients with type 2 diabetes with microalbuminuria, an estimated creatinine clearance of less than 50 mL/minute, or elevated serum creatinine (>1.8 mg/dL in women and >2.0 mg/dL in men).

CASE 14-11, QUESTION 3: How beneficial would more intensive lifestyle modifications be in R.R.?

In addition to nonadherence with drug therapy, lifestyle factors (obesity, sodium ingestion, heavy alcohol intake) are a significant contributor to resistant hypertension.[13] Lifestyle modifications should continually be reinforced in patients, especially those with resistant hypertension. As previously discussed, these modifications should include dietary changes and physical activity. R.R should be instructed to restrict his daily sodium to less than 1.5 g because this has been shown to decrease SBP by more than 20 mm Hg in resistant hypertension.[30]

α-BLOCKERS

CASE 14-12

QUESTION 1: J.L. is a 64-year-old man with hypertension. His BP is 158/84 mm Hg (156/86 mm Hg when repeated). His current antihypertensive regimen is HCTZ 25 mg daily, irbesartan 300 mg daily, and nifedipine extended-release 60 mg daily. J.L. is not completely adherent with lifestyle modifications, but insists he is doing the best he can. He has been experiencing frequent nocturia, difficulty in starting urination, and a decrease in his urinary flow for the past several months and is diagnosed with benign prostatic hyperplasia (BPH). J.L.'s physician is considering changing one of his antihypertensive agents to an α-blocker. How do α-blockers compare with other agents in reducing CV events?

α-Blockers are not first-line agents in the management of hypertension. The ALLHAT trial originally included an α-blocker (doxazosin) treatment arm.[62] Interim results after a mean follow-up of 3.3 years revealed that doxazosin had a statistically higher risk of combined CV disease and heart failure when compared with chlorthalidone.[155] Therefore, the ALLHAT data show that chlorthalidone was more effective in lowering some hypertension-associated complications than doxazosin was. This study did not include a placebo group; therefore, to conclude that doxazosin is harmful is inaccurate. For J.L., discontinuing HCTZ, irbesartan, or nifedipine to start an α-blocker is not prudent. It may be appropriate, however, to add an α-blocker to his regimen because he has stage 1 hypertension and is already treated with three first-line agents. Adding a β-blocker would be a reasonable consideration, but an α-blocker will also have a benefit on his BPH (Table 14-8).

CASE 14-12, QUESTION 2: How can an α-blocker improve J.L.'s BPH?

The smooth muscle surrounding the prostate is innervated by α_1-receptors. By blocking these receptors, an α-blocker can improve the symptoms of BPH by reducing urethral tone and alleviating bladder outlet obstruction. Terazosin and doxazosin are both approved for the treatment of BPH. Prazosin should not be used because of the need for frequent dosing. Improvements in BPH symptoms with α-blockers are dose-related. A high dose is often needed, and this increases the risk of side effects, such as orthostatic hypotension. In J.L., an α-blocker will lower his BP and improve his urinary symptoms.

CASE 14-12, QUESTION 3: J.L. prefers to try doxazosin rather than undergo surgery to relieve his symptoms of BPH. How should this agent be started?

For J.L., it would be best to add a low dose of doxazosin to his present regimen. Based on his BP response and tolerance, the dose can be titrated up. One of his other antihypertensive agents can be decreased if he becomes hypotensive. The initial dose of doxazosin should not exceed 1 mg daily and it should be given at bedtime. This can minimize orthostatic hypotension, which is the most frequent side effect of α-blockers. This complication is most pronounced with the first dose, but can persist in some patients. Moreover, if an α-blocker is selected as add-on therapy in patients like J.L. with resistant hypertension, nighttime administration of an α-blocker has been shown to be effective in further lowering BP.[156]

CASE 14-12, QUESTION 4: How should J.L. be counseled regarding side effects of doxazosin?

α-Blockers are well tolerated if dosed appropriately. J.L. could experience side effects, such as drowsiness, headache, weakness, palpitations from reflex tachycardia, and nausea, but these do not occur in all patients. Patients starting an α-blocker should be instructed to take the initial dose at bedtime and to anticipate the first-dose effect of orthostatic hypotension. Specifically, patients should be counseled to rise more slowly from a seated or supine position.

Miscellaneous Agents

MIXED α/β-BLOCKERS

CASE 14-13

QUESTION 1: R.P. is a 68-year-old man with hypertension and a history of ischemic stroke (1 year ago). Two months ago, his BP values were 164/94 mm Hg (162/98 mm Hg when repeated), with a heart rate of 62 beats/minute while on atenolol 50 mg daily. He was started on benazepril/HCTZ 10/12.5 mg daily 2 months ago. His BP today is 142/82 mm Hg (144/82 mm Hg when repeated). All his laboratory values are normal except his serum creatinine, which is 1.9 mg/dL. J.L. has implemented lifestyle modification to the best of his ability. Could his atenolol be replaced with an agent such as labetalol and carvedilol?

Labetalol and carvedilol (Table 14-15) are nonselective β-blockers that also have α_1-receptor blocking activity. Their antihypertensive effects are only somewhat similar to a combination of a nonselective β-blocker with an α_1-antagonist.

These agents produce vasodilation because of the α-blocker effects. The only other β-blocker that provides vasodilation is nebivolol. However, nebivolol produces vasodilation without blockade of α-receptors. The same precautions and contraindications relevant to nonselective β-blockers apply to both carvedilol and labetalol because they block both β_1- and β_2-receptors (Table 14-10).

Carvedilol is approved for both hypertension and left ventricular dysfunction. Carvedilol has been shown to reduce morbidity and mortality in a wide range of patients with left ventricular dysfunction.[157,158] Labetalol and carvedilol have no clear advantage over other β-blockers in most patients with hypertension, with the exception that they offer a dual mechanism of action within a single drug formulation. In patients with type 2 diabetes, carvedilol has been shown to have no significant effect on glucose in comparison to metoprolol, which may slightly increase glucose.[159] However, R.P. does not have diabetes. If R.P. had the compelling indication of left ventricular dysfunction, switching to carvedilol would be reasonable. His heart rate is 62 beats/minute, so increasing the atenolol dose to 100 mg daily is possible but may induce heart block. Atenolol is renally eliminated, so his present dose is probably causing more BP lowering than usual doses based on his elevated serum creatinine. Increasing his ACEI will help to control both his BP and preserve his kidney function. This can be done without increasing his HCTZ by switching his fixed-dose combination product to benazepril/HCTZ 20/12.5 mg daily or simply increasing both the ACE and HCTZ by doubling his current dose.

DIRECT RENIN INHIBITORS

CASE 14-13, QUESTION 2: How is aliskiren different from an ACEI or ARB?

Aliskiren is a direct renin inhibitor. It inhibits the first step of the RAAS, which results in reduced PRA and BP lowering. This is different from the decreased production of angiotensin II with ACEIs and the blocked angiotensin II receptor effects with ARBs; however, BP-lowering effects are similar to those with ACEIs and ARBs. Aliskiren has a 24-hour half-life and, similar to most ACEIs and ARBs, is dosed once daily.

Some similarities and some differences exist among the side effects associated with aliskiren when compared with ACEIs and ARBs. Aliskiren should not be used in pregnancy because of the known teratogenic effects from blocking the RAAS system. Increases in serum creatinine and serum potassium have been associated with aliskiren. These are similar to ACEI and ARB therapy, and are mediated by the inhibition of angiotensin II vasoconstrictive effects on the efferent arterioles of the kidney and blocking of aldosterone. Monitoring of serum creatinine and serum potassium should be done in patients treated with aliskiren, particularly in those treated with the combination of aliskiren and an ACEI, ARB, potassium-sparing diuretic, or aldosterone antagonist. Angioedema has been also reported in patients treated with aliskiren.

CASE 14-13, QUESTION 3: What is the role of aliskiren in treating R.P.'s hypertension? Can aliskiren be added to his drug regimen considering he is on an ACEI?

The exact role of aliskiren in treatment of hypertension is unclear. It is approved as monotherapy or in combination therapy.

The BP reductions with aliskiren as monotherapy are similar to those seen with an ACEI, ARB, or CCB (specifically amlodipine). Aliskiren provides additive BP lowering when used in combination with HCTZ, ACEI, ARB, and CCB. Its efficacy in combination with maximal doses of ACEI is unknown, however. Aliskiren is an alternative antihypertensive agent at this time because of unknown long-term effects on CV events.

CENTRAL α_2-AGONISTS

The antihypertensive effects of α_2-agonists (Table 14-16) are attributed to their central α_2-agonist activity. Stimulation of α_2-receptors in the CNS inhibits sympathetic outflow (via negative feedback) to the heart, kidneys, and peripheral vasculature, resulting in peripheral vasodilation. Although the α_2-agonists effectively lower BP, they have many potential side effects and have not been evaluated in trials focused on CV events.

CLONIDINE

CASE 14-14

QUESTION 1: T.M. is a 43-year-old man. He is a truck driver with a 5-year history of hypertension. His Framingham risk score is less than 10%, and he does not have hypertension-associated complications or any compelling indications. Secondary causes have been ruled out. His regimen is losartan/HCTZ 100/25 mg daily and sustained-release diltiazem 240 mg daily. Other antihypertensive drugs have failed because of various side effects (captopril and lisinopril, dry cough; atenolol and carvedilol, fatigue; nifedipine and amlodipine, edema; terazosin, orthostasis). T.M. has been adherent with his present medications and lifestyle modification, but has been unable to quit smoking. His clinic values have been similar and averaged 150/95 mm Hg for the past 3 months. Clonidine 0.1 mg twice daily is added to his regimen. What problems might occur if T.M. is not adherent with clonidine therapy?

α_2-Agonists are most effective when used with a diuretic because they all can cause fluid retention. Ideally, they should be used with agents that have different mechanisms of action and with agents that do not affect other central adrenergic receptors. Clonidine can cause rebound hypertension when abruptly stopped. T.M.'s occupation may place him at risk for this complication if he misses doses because of unusual work hours or prolonged travel.

CASE 14-14, QUESTION 2: How should T.M.'s clonidine dose be titrated?

Clonidine should be started at a low dosage and gradually increased to achieve optimal BP lowering with minimal side effects. The immediate-release tablet is started as 0.1 mg twice daily, with 0.1- or 0.2-mg/day increases every 2 to 4 weeks until his BP goal is achieved or side effects appear. Clonidine also is available as an extended-release tablet and as a transdermal patch. The patch formulation releases drug at a controlled rate for 7 days and may have fewer side effects than the oral dosage form. The onset of initial BP effect may be delayed for 2 to 3 days after application; thus, rebound hypertension might occur when oral clonidine is switched to transdermal. To prevent this, an oral dose should be taken on the first day that the transdermal patch is used. Anticholinergic side effects, such as sedation and dry mouth, are the most frequent and bothersome side effects of clonidine. These are especially problematic in elderly patients.

CASE 14-14, QUESTION 3: After several months, T.M.'s BP is 148/84 mm Hg with clonidine 0.2 mg twice daily. However, he is now experiencing daytime somnolence and dry mouth. What other α_2-agonists are available?

METHYLDOPA

Methyldopa has been extensively evaluated and is considered safe in pregnancy. Therefore, it is recommended as a first-line agent when hypertension is first diagnosed during pregnancy.[160] Beyond that, little role exists for methyldopa in the management of hypertension. The usual initial dose is 250 mg administered twice daily up to 2,000 mg/day. Methyldopa causes side effects similar to those associated with clonidine, including sedation, lethargy, postural hypotension, dizziness, dry mouth, headache, and rebound hypertension. These may decrease with continued use. Other significant side effects include hemolytic anemia and hepatitis. Although these are both rare, they necessitate discontinuing the medication.

OTHERS

Guanfacine and guanabenz have a high incidence of side effects. These agents can cause dry mouth, sedation, dizziness, orthostatic hypotension, insomnia, constipation, and impotence. Guanfacine has a long half-life and may have less rebound hypertension than other α_2-agonists. The adverse effects of other α_2-agonists (methyldopa, guanfacine, and guanabenz) are nearly identical to those of clonidine. In general, patients who do not tolerate one α_2-agonist will not tolerate the others. An antihypertensive agent from a different class (aldosterone antagonist, aliskiren, reserpine, or an arterial vasodilator) should be chosen for T.M.

RESERPINE

CASE 14-14, QUESTION 4: Would reserpine be a reasonable option for T.M.?

Reserpine is one of the oldest antihypertensive agents currently available. It is extremely effective in lowering BP when added to a thiazide diuretic. Reserpine is inexpensive, and is dosed once daily. Several of the landmark trials that demonstrated reduced morbidity and mortality with BP lowering in hypertension used reserpine. The SHEP trial used reserpine as a second-step agent added to chlorthalidone in patients who could not take atenolol.[47]

Low-dose reserpine (0.05–0.1 mg once daily) is effective at lowering BP and has significantly fewer side effects compared with high doses. Reserpine can cause nasal stuffiness in many patients. Gastrointestinal ulcerations have been reported, but they are associated with either parenteral administration or very large doses. T.M. is a candidate for low-dose reserpine. He is already taking a thiazide diuretic, which should always be used with reserpine, and his therapeutic options are limited. Of all the agents remaining for T.M., other than aliskiren, reserpine has the most favorable side effect profile.

Many clinicians avoid reserpine because of the myth that it can cause depression. This fear was generated from case reports in the 1950s when high doses (0.5–1.0 mg/day) were used. Many of the patients described in these cases would not meet modern criteria for depression; rather, they would be considered oversedated. When reserpine is limited to a maximum of 0.25 mg daily, depression is no more frequent than with other antihypertensive agents.

ARTERIAL VASODILATORS

HYDRALAZINE

CASE 14-15

QUESTION 1: C.M. is a 56-year-old woman with a history of hypertension and severe CKD (estimated GFR of 14 mL/minute/1.73 m^2). Her antihypertensive regimen consists of torsemide 40 mg daily, amlodipine/olmesartan 10/40 mg daily, metoprolol succinate 200 mg daily, and lisinopril 40 mg daily. She started hydralazine 25 mg three times daily 4 weeks ago when her BP was 148/92 and 146/90 mm Hg. She has been very compliant, and her BP is now 146/88 mm Hg with a heart rate of 82 beats/minute. Her lung fields are clear, with 1+ bilateral pitting edema. Serum electrolytes are within normal limits. Why was hydralazine used in C.M.?

Hydralazine causes direct relaxation of arteriolar smooth muscle. Arterial vasodilators are infrequently used, except for patients with severe CKD. In this population, hypertension is difficult to control and often requires four or five agents. Severe CKD results in increased renin release and increased fluid retention. Potent vasodilation, in combination with diuresis, is often effective in lowering BP under these conditions. This vasodilation, however, stimulates the sympathetic nervous system and results in a reflex tachycardia, increased PRA, and fluid retention. Thus, the hypotensive effects of direct arterial vasodilators can quickly diminish with time when used as monotherapy. To prevent this, arterial vasodilators should always be used in combination with both a β-blocker to counteract reflex tachycardia, as well as a diuretic (often a loop diuretic if used in severe CKD) to minimize fluid retention.

CASE 14-15, QUESTION 2: After 18 months, C.M.'s hydralazine dose is 50 mg three times daily, and her BP is at goal. She now complains of joint pain in both her right and left hands, which extends to the wrists, and generalized weakness with frequent fevers. Laboratory findings for C.M. showed a positive antinuclear antibodies test (diffuse), a white blood cell count of 3,500/μL, and an erythrocyte sedimentation rate of 45 mm/hour, and she is diagnosed with drug-induced lupus. How should this be managed?

C.M.'s symptoms are consistent with drug-induced lupus (DIL). Hydralazine is one of the most common agents reported to cause DIL. Musculoskeletal pains are the most frequent symptoms, but systemic symptoms and rash may also occur. Hydralazine doses as low as 100 mg/day can cause DIL, and the risk significantly increases when greater than 200 mg/day is used.

Hydralazine should be discontinued. Symptoms should subside within days or weeks, and complete resolution can be expected.

MINOXIDIL

CASE 14-15, QUESTION 3: What alternatives to hydralazine are available for C.M.?

C.M.'s BP responded to hydralazine, so she would likely benefit from another arterial vasodilator. Minoxidil, a potent arterial vasodilator, is similar to hydralazine with regard to reflex tachycardia, increased CO, increased PRA, and fluid retention. Therefore, concomitant β-blocker and diuretic therapy is still needed. Minoxidil should be reserved for patients such as C.M. who have severe CKD or possibly for resistant hypertension.

CASE 14-15, QUESTION 4: How should C.M. be counseled if minoxidil is started?

Hypertrichosis is a common adverse effect of oral minoxidil, occurring in 80% to 100% of patients. The hair growth is not associated with an endocrine abnormality and begins within the first few weeks. It commonly occurs on the temples, between the eyebrows, on the cheeks, and on the pinna of the ear. Hair growth can extend to the back of the legs, arms, and scalp with continued use. Some patients, especially women, find the hypertrichosis so intolerable that they stop treatment. Topical minoxidil is an approved therapy for male pattern baldness, but topical administration does not provide BP-lowering effects.

Fluid retention with minoxidil is common, presenting as edema and weight gain. If adequate diuresis is not maintained during minoxidil therapy, left ventricular dysfunction may be precipitated or worsened. This also occurs with hydralazine. The compensatory reflex tachycardia with minoxidil also may precipitate angina in patients who have, or are at risk for, CAD.

KEY REFERENCES AND WEBSITES

A full list of references for this chapter can be found at http://thepoint.lww.com/AT10e. Below are the key references and websites for this chapter, with the corresponding reference number in this chapter found in parentheses after the citation.

Key References

ACCORD Study Group et al. Effects of intensive blood-pressure control in type 2 diabetes mellitus. *N Engl J Med*. 2010;362:1575. (23)

Arguedas JA et al. Treatment blood pressure targets for hypertension. *Cochrane Database Syst Rev*. 2009(3):CD004349. (19)

Beckett NS et al. Treatment of hypertension in patients 80 years of age or older. *N Engl J Med*. 2008;358:1887. (24)

Calhoun DA et al. Resistant hypertension: diagnosis, evaluation, and treatment: a scientific statement from the American Heart Association Professional Education Committee of the Council for High Blood Pressure Research. *Circulation*. 2008;117:e510. (13)

Chobanian AV et al. Seventh Report of the Joint National Committee on Prevention, Detection, Evaluation, and Treatment of High Blood Pressure. *Hypertension*. 2003;42:1206. (3)

Dorsch MP et al. Chlorthalidone reduces cardiovascular events compared with hydrochlorothiazide: a retrospective cohort analysis. *Hypertension*. 2011;57:689. (131)

Ernst ME, Moser M. Use of diuretics in patients with hypertension [published correction appears in *N Engl J Med*. 2010;363:1877]. N Engl J Med. 2009;361:2153. (37)

Flack JM et al. Management of high blood pressure in Blacks: an update of the International Society on Hypertension in Blacks consensus statement. *Hypertension*. 2010;56:780. (82)

Jamerson K et al. Benazepril plus amlodipine or hydrochlorothiazide for hypertension in high-risk patients. *N Engl J Med*. 2008; 359:2417. (115)

ONTARGET Investigators et al. Telmisartan, ramipril, or both in patients at high risk for vascular events. *N Engl J Med*. 2008; 358:1547. (121)

Rosendorff C et al. Treatment of hypertension in the prevention and management of ischemic heart disease: a scientific statement from the American Heart Association Council for High Blood Pressure Research and the Councils on Clinical Cardiology and Epidemiology and Prevention [published correction appears in *Circulation*. 2007;116:e121]. *Circulation*. 2007;115:2761. (15)

Key Websites

The American Heart Association. **http://my.americanheart.org**

National Cholesterol Education Program. Risk Assessment Tool for Estimating 10-year Risk of Developing Hard CHD (Myocardial Infarction and Coronary Death). **http://hp2010.nhlbihin.net/atpiii/calculator.asp?usertype=prof**

National Heart Lung and Blood Institute. The Seventh Report of the Joint National Committee on Prevention, Detection, Evaluation, and Treatment of High Blood Pressure (JNC 7). **http://www.nhlbi.nih.gov/guidelines/hypertension**

National Kidney Foundation. Calculators for Health Care Professionals. **http://www.kidney.org/professionals/KDOQI/gfr_calculator.cfm**

Peripheral Vascular Disorders

Patricia M. Schuler and C. Wayne Weart

15

CORE PRINCIPLES

	CHAPTER CASES
PERIPHERAL ARTERIAL DISEASE (PAD)	
1 PAD is a sometimes-painful complication from stenosis or occlusion in the peripheral arteries of the legs, usually caused by atherosclerosis. Intermittent claudication can be associated with PAD, and is described as aching, cramping, tightness, or weakness of the legs, which usually occurs during exertion.	Case 15-1 (Question 1)
2 Treatment for PAD should include therapeutic lifestyle changes and pharmacologic intervention based on risk factors present. Specific interventions may include smoking cessation; exercise; management of dyslipidemia, hypertension, and diabetes; antiplatelet therapy; and verapamil.	Case 15-1 (Questions 2–9)
RAYNAUD'S PHENOMENON (RP)	
1 RP is an exaggerated vasospastic response to cold or emotion, likely mediated through sympathetic response to the precipitating stimuli. RP is classified as primary or secondary, in which secondary causes include connective tissue diseases and occupational-related neural damage.	Case 15-2 (Question 1)
2 Treatment for RP should include therapeutic lifestyle changes and pharmacologic intervention based on clinical presentation and underlying etiology. First-line interventions may include avoidance of cold stimuli and medications associated with vasoconstriction, and treatment with calcium-channel blockers. Several other therapies may be emerging as possible therapeutic options, including renin-angiotensin-aldosterone inhibitors, topical nitroglycerin, statins, peripheral α-adrenergic blockers, intravenous prostanoids, endothelin antagonists, and oral phosphodiesterase inhibitors.	Case 15-2 (Questions 2–4)
NOCTURNAL LEG MUSCLE CRAMPS	
1 Nocturnal leg muscle cramps are idiopathic, involuntary contractions occurring at rest that cause a visible and palpable knot in the affected muscle, usually occurring in the early hours of sleeping.	Case 15-3 (Question 1)
2 The primary treatment goal of nocturnal leg muscle cramps is the prevention of episodes. Recommendations include stretching practices, alteration of sleeping position, and treatment of modifiable causes (i.e., electrolyte abnormalities).	Case 15-3 (Question 2)

PERIPHERAL ARTERIAL DISEASE

Peripheral arterial disease (PAD) is a common and sometimes painful complication from stenosis or occlusion in the peripheral arteries of the legs, usually caused by atherosclerosis. Some clinicians and patients have characterized claudication pain as "angina" of the legs. The association with coronary disease becomes clear when considering the risk factors and pathology of intermittent claudication (IC).

Intermittent claudication is described as aching, cramping, tightness, or weakness of the legs, which usually occurs during exertion. Claudication pain is relieved when the physical activity is discontinued. Moreover, tissue ischemia, marked by numbness or continuous pain in the toes or foot, may be present and can lead to ulceration. IC is a painful condition that can severely limit mobility and lead to tissue necrosis or amputation of the affected limb. Many patients with PAD, however, are asymptomatic or have atypical lower limb symptoms, such as leg fatigue, difficulty walking, or similar nonspecific complaints. Patients may not seek medical attention until the condition is advanced because of the gradual onset of symptoms associated with IC.

Epidemiology

Peripheral arterial disease is a relatively common condition that affects men and women equally, with a prevalence of 12%,[1] although men have a twofold increased prevalence of symptomatic IC.[2] The annual incidence of IC increases dramatically with age (Table 15-1). Most patients with PAD are largely asymptomatic, although their risk of developing symptoms of IC in the future is greatly increased. In a population with only a 2% prevalence of IC symptoms, 11.7% of patients had detectable large vessel atherosclerosis of the lower extremities.[3] This disparity between IC symptoms and the presence of PAD contributes to the observation that 50% to 90% of patients with IC do not mention the symptoms to their physician. Patients attribute the symptoms of IC to normal walking difficulties associated with aging, not a medical condition requiring treatment.[4] Public knowledge of the definition of PAD, risk factors for the development of the disease, associated symptoms and disease states, and amputation risk were evaluated in adults older than 50 years of age in a cross-sectional, population-based telephone survey. Unfortunately, only 25% of the population reported awareness of PAD; moreover, public awareness of PAD was lowest among respondents who were older, male, and nonwhite with a lower socioeconomic class and education level.[5]

Risk factors for developing occlusive PAD are similar to those for coronary artery disease. Longstanding diabetes is the most significant risk factor, with 30% of patients with diabetes affected by PAD.[6] PAD is five times more common in patients with diabetes than in patients without diabetes; in patients with diabetes, it develops at a younger age and progresses more rapidly. Each 1% increase in glycosylated hemoglobin is associated with a 28% risk of incident PAD.[7] Other atherosclerotic risk factors associated with PAD include cigarette smoking, hypertension, and dyslipidemia.[8] Hypertriglyceridemia is a more significant risk factor for PAD than for coronary artery disease, and this may partially explain the increased prevalence of PAD in patients with diabetes.[9]

Cigarette smoking has a higher correlation with the development of IC pain than any other risk factor, and the risk increases dramatically with the number of cigarettes smoked per day and the duration of smoking history.[10] In patients with other cardiovascular risk factors, including hypertension or diabetes, smoking further increases the rate of claudication development. Smoking confers a sevenfold increase in risk for PAD compared with not smoking. In contrast, the risk of coronary artery disease is only increased twofold in smokers. Thus, the mechanism by which cigarette smoking causes damage may be different for these two vascular diseases.[11]

TABLE 15-1
Annual Incidence of Intermittent Claudication by Age[3]

Age Group (years)	Annual Incidence (%)
40–49	2.0
50–59	4.2
60–69	6.8
70	9.2

TABLE 15-2
Long-Term Incidence of Outcomes in Patients With Intermittent Claudication[12,13]

Patient Population	Abrupt Limb Ischemia (%)	Amputation (%)
All patients	23	7
Diabetes	31	11
Smokers	35	21

Epidemiologic studies show that IC is nonprogressive in 75% of patients during a period of 4 to 9 years. The other 25% of patients with IC have worsening painful ischemic episodes during this period. Although rare, more serious complications can occur. Ischemic tissue changes, ulceration, and gangrene can accompany advanced peripheral atherosclerosis. Amputation of the affected limb may be necessary in up to 5% of patients with claudication.[12] The presence of two independent risk factors, such as diabetes and cigarette smoking, has an additive effect on the risk for the development of progressive IC and serious limb complications (Table 15-2). Finally, disease location in patients with severe disease may be associated with prognosis, such that proximal disease is associated with poor outcomes when compared with distal lesions; however, more epidemiological studies must be conducted to confirm these findings.[14]

During a relatively short 2-year follow-up of a population with IC, 3.6% of patients died, whereas 22% experienced a nonfatal cardiovascular event (defined as any cardiac, cerebral, or peripheral vascular event). Furthermore, 26% experienced a decline in their walking capability during the same time frame.[13,15] Although a relatively small fraction of patients died during the 2-year observation period, it is paramount to recognize that severe, short-term morbidity is highly likely in this patient population. IC clearly reflects generalized atherosclerosis and is associated with considerable morbidity.

Pathophysiology

Intermittent claudication, and its associated pain and impaired mobility, is the predominant complication of occlusive PAD. The major cause of occlusive PAD is arteriosclerosis obliterans, defined as the development of atherosclerotic plaques in the peripheral vasculature. These plaques develop as a result of endothelial activation associated with conditions such as dyslipidemia, diabetes mellitus, hypertension, and tobacco use. Plaques result in the proliferation of vascular smooth muscle, with subsequent damage to the vascular structure. The damaged endothelium of the vasculature has impaired vasodilatory capabilities because secretion of nitric oxide, also known as endothelium-derived relaxing factor, is decreased and secretion of vasoconstrictive substances, such as endothelin, are increased. Both defects impede blood flow to the extremities. In addition, growth of atherosclerotic lesions can physically limit blood flow. Exercise may induce IC symptoms in patients who have lesions with greater than 50% stenosis, whereas patients with lesions of greater than 80% stenosis can have pain at rest. The lesions themselves can be unstable and rupture, or adjacent smaller vessels experiencing high hemodynamic pressure caused by nearby plaques may rupture. Either situation can lead to acute vascular occlusion, analogous to unstable angina or acute myocardial infarction (MI) in coronary arteries.[16]

Figure 15-1 illustrates the common sites of atherosclerosis. Plaques that develop in central vessels (e.g., in the aorta and iliac artery) are primarily associated with buttock pain and erectile dysfunction. Those confined to the more distal femoral and

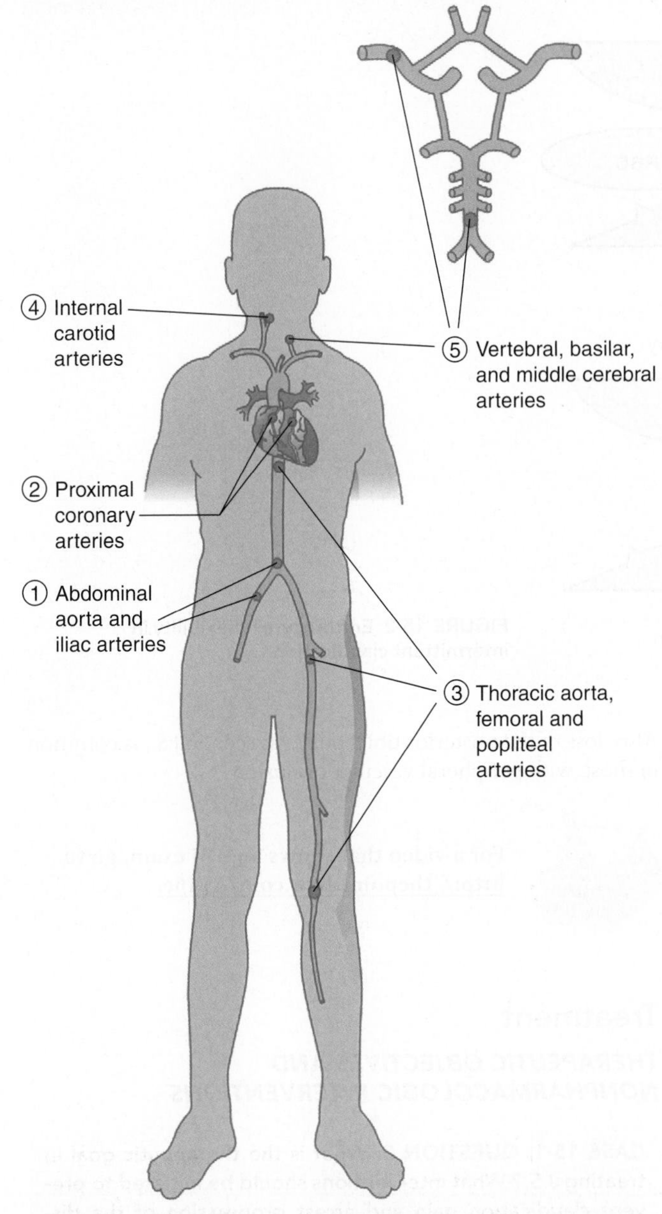

FIGURE 15-1 **Sites of severe atherosclerosis in order of frequency.** Adapted with permission from Rubin E, Farber JL. Pathology. 3rd ed. Philadelphia, PA: Lippincott-Raven; 1999:508.

popliteal arteries characteristically cause thigh and calf pain. Occlusion of the tibial arteries will produce claudication pain in the foot. When more than one arterial bed is affected by severe atherosclerosis, symptoms of IC will be diffuse. Symptoms of IC indicate an inadequate supply of arterial blood to peripheral muscles. Exercise, including walking, increases the metabolic demands of the muscles and can lead to claudication pain. Reduced blood supply to the muscles results from changes in perfusion pressures and vascular tone caused by atherosclerosis.

Atherosclerosis can impair the microcirculation of the peripheral muscles by altering the pressure gradient needed for perfusion of the capillaries. When obstruction develops, perfusion of tissue distal to the stenotic lesion relies on collateral blood flow. Collateral circulation consists of new blood vessels that develop to carry blood around the occluded area.

Erythrocyte deformability is an important factor for in vitro capillary perfusion.[17,18] In areas free of compromised blood flow, normal red blood cells (RBCs) have the ability to deform when passing through a small capillary. By aligning themselves in a planar manner, the RBCs also reduce the viscosity of the blood suspension, enabling them to pass smoothly through the capillary. In many patients with IC, RBCs have a marked decrease in this intrinsic ability to deform, which results in increased blood viscosity. This defect is promoted by chronic tissue ischemia and hypoxia caused by increased intracapillary leukocyte adherence, platelet aggregation, and activation of complement and clotting factors.[16] The vascular responses to hypoxia are detrimental because this sequence of events further inhibits blood flow and oxygen delivery to the tissues (Fig. 15-2).

Clinical Presentation

CASE 15-1

QUESTION 1: J.S. is a 54-year-old, 100-kg man with a history of type 2 diabetes mellitus, chronic stable angina, dyslipidemia, and tobacco use. His chief complaint today is right upper thigh pain while walking around the block. The pain has gradually increased during the past 12 months, but only recently has become intolerable. The pain is relieved within minutes after he stops walking. J.S. smokes 1.5 packs of cigarettes a day.

His most recent laboratory results are significant for the following results:

Total cholesterol, 290 mg/dL (SI units, 7.49 mmol/L)
Fasting triglycerides, 350 mg/dL (SI units, 3.95 mmol/L)
Low-density lipoproteins (LDL), 188 mg/dL (SI units, 4.86 mmol/L)
High-density lipoproteins (HDL), 32 mg/dL (SI units, 0.83 mmol/L)
Serum creatinine (SCr), 1.0 mg/dL (SI units, 60 mmol/L)
Blood urea nitrogen (BUN), 15 mg/dL (SI units, 0.3 mmol/L)
Hemoglobin (Hgb) A_{1c}, 10.0% (SI units, 0.1)
Fasting glucose, 150 mg/dL (SI units, 8.3 mmol/L)
Blood pressure (BP), 170/95 mm Hg
Heart rate (HR), 89 beats/minute

His posterior tibial artery pulse is not palpable. A Doppler ultrasound study is performed, and his ankle-to-brachial index is 0.7 (normal, >0.90).

J.S.'s medication list includes isosorbide dinitrate 20 mg three times daily (TID) (while awake), aspirin 325 mg every day, and enalapril 10 mg twice daily (BID). His insulin doses have progressively increased to neutral protamine Hagedorn (NPH) insulin 40 units in the morning and 35 units in the evening. What risk factors and elements of J.S.'s presentation are consistent with a diagnosis of IC?

J.S.'s medical history illustrates classic risk factors for vascular occlusion and IC, including dyslipidemia (specifically hypertriglyceridemia), diabetes, hypertension, and tobacco use. In particular, his diabetes is not adequately controlled based on elevated Hgb A_{1c} and fasting glucose levels, and he is obese. This constellation of disorders is known as the *metabolic syndrome.* These factors, along with smoking, are commonly seen together and have been linked with insulin resistance or hyperinsulinemia and accelerated atherosclerosis (Fig. 15-3).[19,20] The presence of angina indicates coronary artery disease, so it is not surprising that he has peripheral vascular occlusion as well.

The classic pain of IC described by J.S. is associated with exercise of the affected muscle group(s) and subsides with a few minutes of rest and reperfusion. IC pain also can occur at rest; however, this type of claudication pain is less common and is an indication of extensive disease. Other common symptoms of

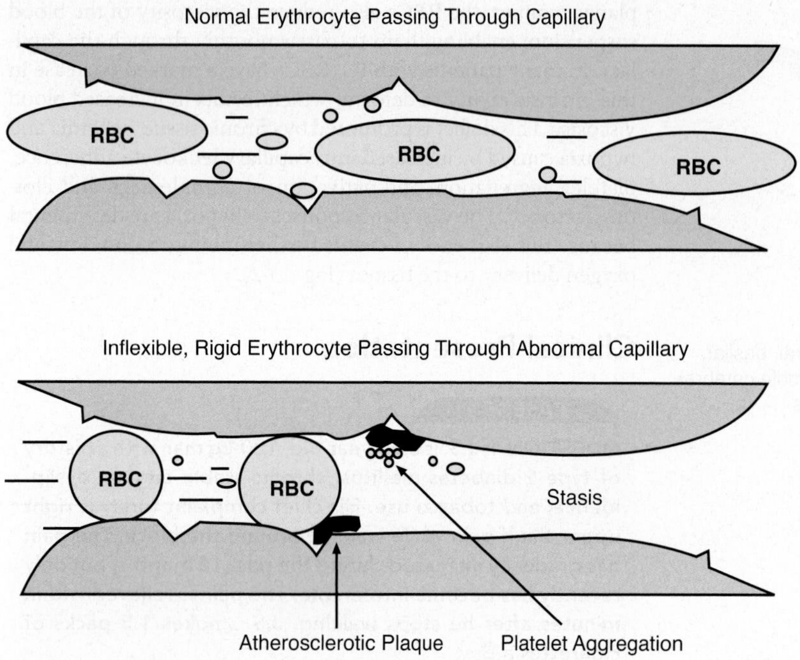

FIGURE 15-2 Erythrocyte inflexibility in intermittent claudication.

extensive atherosclerosis include cold feet and persistent aching of the feet during rest or sleep. Restricted blood flow to the feet along with pooling of blood secondary to inadequate pressure needed to propel blood back up the leg can lead to rubor (red or purple color of the foot). Other indicators of peripheral atherosclerosis are the loss of hair from the top of the feet, thickening of the toenails, and absence of sweating of the lower legs and feet, all caused by poor circulation.[16]

The results of objective studies performed on J.S. are consistent with IC. Doppler ultrasound of the spine is helpful in excluding pseudoclaudication caused by spinal stenosis and other neurogenic or musculoskeletal causes of leg pain. Ultrasound is also useful to measure BP of the lower extremities. An ankle-to-brachial index (ABI) of 0.7 means that the ankle systolic BP reading is only 70% of the systolic pressure in the brachial artery supplying blood to the arm. In patients with IC, this is caused by atherosclerotic obstruction of blood flow in the lower limbs and subsequent decreased perfusion pressures in the ankle compared with the arm (Table 15-3). The lower the ABI, the more blood flow to the extremities is compromised and the greater the severity of symptoms. An ABI less than 0.9 is diagnostic for PAD.

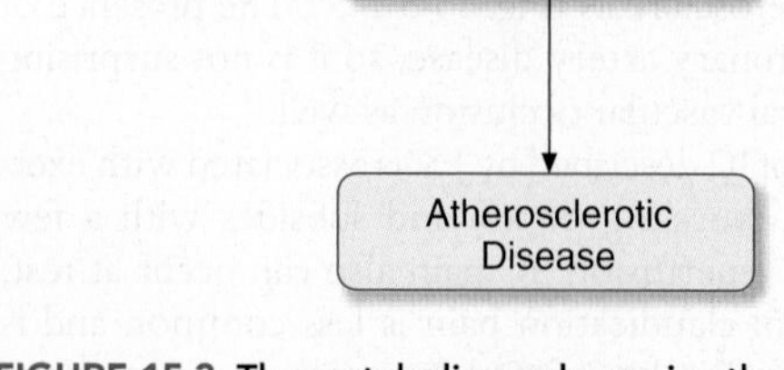

FIGURE 15-3 The metabolic syndrome in atherosclerosis.

Also, loss of the posterior tibial pulse, as seen in J.S., is common in those with peripheral vascular occlusion.

ONLINE CONTENT

For a video that shows an ABI exam, go to http://thepoint.lww.com/AT10e.

Treatment

THERAPEUTIC OBJECTIVES AND NONPHARMACOLOGIC INTERVENTIONS

CASE 15-1, QUESTION 2: What is the therapeutic goal in treating J.S.? What interventions should be initiated to prevent claudication pain and arrest progression of the disease?

The specific treatment goals for J.S. include preventing further claudication pain, lessening the current pain he experiences, arresting the progression of underlying disease, and decreasing his risk of cardiovascular events. Achieving these goals will provide J.S. with the best chance of avoiding further mobility impairment, amputation, and cardiovascular events such as stroke or MI. An important concept that should be stressed when explaining these treatment goals to J.S. is that all his diseases are closely

TABLE 15-3
Severity of Arterial Obstruction as Assessed by Ankle-to-Brachial Index[21]

Severity	Ankle-to-Brachial Index[a]
Normal	>0.90
Mild	0.70–0.89
Moderate	0.50–0.69
Severe	>0.50

[a]Ankle-to-brachial index is the systolic blood pressure in the ankle divided by the systolic blood pressure in the arm.

TABLE 15-4
Medical Treatment of Peripheral Arterial Disease and Expected Outcomes[8,22]

Intervention	Improve Leg Symptoms?	Prevent Systemic Complications?
Smoking cessation	Yes	Yes
Exercise	Yes	No
Cilostazol	Yes	No
Statin drugs	Yes	Yes
Angiotensin-converting enzyme inhibitors	Yes	Yes
Blood pressure control	No	Yes
Antiplatelet therapy[a]	No	Yes

[a]Aspirin or clopidogrel.

interrelated, and that a beneficial intervention for one disease is beneficial for all. Interventions that can be initiated include diet modification; exercise and weight loss; and attainment of goal blood pressure, lipids, Hgb A_{1c}, and fasting and postprandial blood glucose levels. The American College of Cardiology and American Heart Association have published guidelines that thoroughly evaluate the interventions and medications that have been used to treat IC and PAD.[8] Table 15-4 summarizes these recommendations. The two most important things that J.S. can do for his IC are summed up in five words: "Stop smoking and keep walking."[23]

SMOKING CESSATION

The importance of smoking cessation cannot be overemphasized to patients with IC. It is the most important modifiable factor in preventing the development of rest pain, prolonged limb ischemia, and the need for amputation, and in achieving an overall reduction in cardiovascular events. Several studies document improved survival and decreased amputation rates in patients with IC who stopped smoking compared with patients who continue to smoke.[24,25] Other benefits, such as improved treadmill walking distance, decreased progression to symptoms, and decreased complications after vascular reconstructive surgery, have been shown in patients who are able to quit smoking compared with patients who continue to smoke.[8,24,26–28] It is also the intervention that will decrease J.S.'s claudication pain most rapidly. If J.S. is able to stop smoking, his risk of developing rest pain or requiring limb amputation will be very low. He also will decrease his risk of MI and mortality by threefold and fivefold, respectively. Table 15-5 summarizes the risk of cigarette smoking and the value of smoking cessation on cardiovascular complications.

TABLE 15-5
Patient Outcomes Based on Smoking Status After Intermittent Claudication Diagnosis[12,24]

Outcome	Length of Follow-up (years)	Patient Population	
		Current Smokers (%)	Past Smokers[a]
Rest pain	7	16	0
Myocardial infarction	10	53	11
Amputation	5	11	0
Mortality	10	54	18

[a]Quit after intermittent claudication diagnosis.

Many pharmacologic products and strategies are available to aid patients such as J.S. to stop smoking (see Chapter 88, Tobacco Use and Dependence). Nicotine itself has harmful effects on the vasculature via catecholamine release and vasoconstriction, however, and it may play a role in endothelial damage and atherosclerosis progression.[29]

EXERCISE

An individualized and supervised exercise program has been endorsed for patients with PAD and will benefit J.S.'s other risk factors as well.[8] The pain associated with IC results in decreased mobility, and because of deconditioning from lack of exercise, patients with IC may slowly become dependent on others for activities of daily living. An exercise program is the most effective way to both preserve and increase mobility. It is more effective than the best pharmacologic therapy currently available.[30] The ideal exercise program consists of walking for a minimum of 30 to 45 minutes at least three times a week.[8] J.S. should walk as fast and far as he can until the pain becomes severe; he should then wait until the pain subsides, and then resume walking.[21] At first, J.S. may experience several painful episodes during each exercise session, but these should gradually decrease as the beneficial effects of exercise therapy begin to emerge. Studies have documented that this type of exercise program can more than double the pain-free distance a patient with IC is able to walk.[31] Additionally, lower extremity resistance training can provide improved functional performance measured by the following: quality of life, treadmill walking time, and ability to climb stairs.[32] Several surgical options are available for patients whose lifestyle and functional status are compromised after failing exercise and pharmacotherapeutic interventions, including surgical bypass of the affected arteries in addition to angioplasty and stenting.[8] An appropriate exercise program results in superior outcomes compared with angioplasty and stenting, and equal in terms of walking distance compared with surgery. Significant complications and mortality are associated with surgery, however, and when all outcomes are considered, an exercise program is far more advantageous than surgery.[31] For all patients able to walk, an exercise program should be supervised and individually designed, and the patient should understand the importance of exercise to his or her continued mobility.[30]

Rheologic abnormalities of increased blood viscosity, impaired RBC filterability, hyperaggregation, and polycythemia (elevated hematocrit) have been shown to return to normal in many patients with IC who participate in a regular exercise program.[33] Exercise may offset the need for pharmacologic intervention. The potential mechanisms by which exercise benefits patients with IC are listed in Table 15-6.

TABLE 15-6
Primary Mechanisms of Symptom Improvement With Exercise Therapy in Intermittent Claudication[30]

- Decrease of blood viscosity
- Metabolic changes in the muscle
  - Improved muscle metabolism
  - Improved oxygen extraction
- Improved endothelial function and microcirculation
- Decreased occurrence of ischemia and inflammation
- Atherosclerosis risk factors improved via:
  - Weight loss
  - Glycemic control
  - Blood pressure control
  - Increased high-density lipoprotein (HDL)
  - Decreased triglycerides
  - Decreased thrombotic tendency

CASE 15-1, QUESTION 3: Is lipid-lowering therapy indicated for J.S.?

Because IC is a consequence of atherosclerosis, arresting the progression of J.S.'s atherosclerotic disease is important (see Chapter 13, Dyslipidemias, Atherosclerosis, and Coronary Heart Disease). The initiation of the nutritional and exercise recommendations outlined in the National Cholesterol Education Program Adult Treatment Panel III and endorsed by the American Heart Association under therapeutic lifestyle changes,[34] as well as cholesterol-lowering agents, are the cornerstones for attaining this goal. Considerable data suggest that aggressive dietary and pharmacologic management of dyslipidemia, particularly lowering low-density lipoprotein cholesterol (LDL-C), leads to regression of atherosclerotic lesions in the coronary and carotid vasculature.[35–37] In contrast, relatively few prospective data exist about the effect of successful lipid-lowering therapy on the regression or stabilization of peripheral lesions, or on clinical events in patients with PAD. A post hoc analysis of a large lipid-lowering study in subjects with known coronary artery disease treated with simvastatin, however, demonstrated a significant decrease in new or worsening IC, suggesting that benefit is seen in the prevention of clinically symptomatic PAD in high-risk patients.[38] The Heart Protection Study randomly assigned patients with known arterial disease of various types to simvastatin 40 mg daily or placebo. After 5 years, a 15% decrease was found in noncardiac revascularizations, including amputations, among the patients receiving simvastatin.[39] Short-term outcomes (e.g., 6 months to 1 year), such as improved walking distance and walking time, have also been documented with simvastatin 40 mg/day.[40,41]

A meta-analysis of 10,049 subjects from several randomized trials using a variety of lipid-lowering therapies in patients with PAD demonstrated reduced severity of claudication and decreased disease progression as measured by angiography. A decrease in mortality did not reach statistical significance.[42] Limited data suggest high apolipoprotein [Lp(a)] concentrations may be particularly important in the development of PAD.[43]

All patients with evidence of atherosclerotic disease and an LDL cholesterol greater than 100 mg/dL (SI units, 2.6 mmol/L) are candidates for a lipid-lowering regimen according to the National Cholesterol Education Program.[34] J.S. has angina and lower extremity atherosclerosis, both of which indicate a need for aggressive lipid lowering. His LDL-C is 180 mg/dL, so a reduction of almost 50% is desired at a minimum. A clinician could argue for a more aggressive LDL goal of less than 70 mg/dL because of the following factors: presence of established cardiovascular disease risk equivalent in the form of PAD, diabetes, chronic stable angina, cigarette smoking, and metabolic syndrome.[44] Lowering non-HDL cholesterol is the secondary goals in J.S. and can be reassessed after his LDL goal has been reached and the effect of therapy on these parameters is measured. In addition to an aggressive dietary management program, a hydroxymethylglutaryl-coenzyme A (HMG-CoA) reductase inhibitor agent should be prescribed as initial therapy for J.S. HMG-CoA reductase inhibitors, exercise, and the American Heart Association diet will all improve his LDL-C level. They also have beneficial effects on triglycerides and HDL-C, and the need for additional therapy can be assessed after the impact of these measures is determined. There is a paucity of outcome data with many of the available agents for dyslipidemia; however, after the effect of a full-dose, high-potency HMG-CoA reductase inhibitor is realized, addition of omega-3 fatty acid, niacin, or fibric acid derivative may prove to be beneficial.[8,45]

MANAGEMENT OF HYPERTENSION

CASE 15-1, QUESTION 4: J.S.'s BP is elevated to 170/95 mm Hg despite enalapril therapy. Because he has angina, and his HR is 89, a β-adrenergic blocker is considered. Are there alternative antihypertensive therapies that might be preferable for J.S.?

J.S.'s hypertension has likely contributed to the development of his atherosclerosis and PAD. Hypertension (see Chapter 14, Essential Hypertension) has been associated with deficiencies in the synthesis of vasodilating substances, such as prostacyclin, bradykinin, and nitric oxide, by the endothelial cells lining the vasculature. Hypertension also increases concentrations of vasoconstricting substances, such as angiotensin II. An increase in vascular tone can alter local hemodynamics, especially in the presence of a stenotic lesion. Although it has not been determined whether normalization of BP has a positive effect on IC, it is well established that uncontrolled BP, as in J.S., results in vascular complications such as MI and stroke. In light of J.S.'s numerous risk factors for these complications, improved management of his hypertension is warranted.

β-Blockers are frequently cited as contraindicated in patients with IC owing to the potential for unopposed α-adrenergic–mediated vasoconstriction during peripheral β-blockade. Evidence to document worsening IC by β-blockade is lacking, however. Overall, controlled studies have been inconclusive, although a meta-analysis of placebo-controlled trials and studies with control groups concludes that β-blockers do not worsen claudication.[46,47]

Angiotensin-converting enzyme (ACE) inhibitors are first-line agents in patients with PAD.[8] Compared with other antihypertensive agents, the data available support their beneficial effects in this population. Compared with placebo, walking distance is increased with both perindopril and ramipril in patients with PAD.[48,49] The Heart Outcomes Prevention Evaluation (HOPE) study of the ACE inhibitor ramipril versus placebo included more than 4,000 patients with PAD, and this subgroup derived benefit in terms of decreased mortality, MI, and stroke.[50] There is an overall paucity of data associated with the use of angiotensin receptor blockers in PAD; however, the ONTARGET trial compared telmisartan, ramipril, and the combination of the two in patients with vascular disease or high-risk diabetes without heart failure for a composite end point of cardiovascular death, MI, stroke, or hospitalization for heart failure. The results indicate equivalency of telmisartan to ramipril for the primary end point and similar blood pressure reduction; however, the combination group experienced more adverse events without an increase in benefit. These results allow clinicians more freedom of choice when selecting a first-line agent for the treatment of PAD.[51]

Because J.S. has both hypertension and diabetes, his BP goal is less than 130/80 mm Hg.[52] He is already taking an ACE inhibitor, which is an excellent initial antihypertensive choice in a patient with diabetes and PAD. The dose of enalapril could be increased, or a low-dose diuretic, such as hydrochlorothiazide or chlorthalidone,[53,54] could be added; however, given his history of chronic stable angina, the addition of a calcium-channel blocker or a β-blocker would benefit him to a greater degree. The ACCOMPLISH trial compared the combination of benazepril–amlodipine with benazepril–hydrochlorothiazide, and found a reduction in cardiovascular events in patients with hypertension

TABLE 15-7
Effect of Diabetes Mellitus on Intermittent Claudication Outcomes After 5 Years[11]

	Patients With Diabetes (%)	Patients Without Diabetes (%)
Mortality	49	23
Major amputation	21	3
Deterioration	35	19

who were at high risk for such events in the benazepril-amlodipine group with similar BP control.[55]

MANAGEMENT OF DIABETES

CASE 15-1, QUESTION 5: Will improving J.S.'s diabetes control or slow the progression of his PAD? What changes in his diabetes management do you recommend?

Patients with type 2 diabetes mellitus (see Chapter 53, Diabetes Mellitus) are able to minimize macrovascular and microvascular complications of their disease with aggressive glucose control.[7,56,57] Insulin, sulfonylurea, or metformin therapies have a beneficial effect on slowing the development of the microvascular complications of diabetes, such as retinopathy and nephropathy. Metformin has specifically been shown to further reduce the occurrence of macrovascular complications such as stroke or MI compared with insulin or sulfonylureas in obese patients with type 2 diabetes.[56]

J.S.'s diabetes is a significant risk factor for progression to further ischemic events (Table 15-7). He has a twofold greater risk of death and a sevenfold greater risk of amputation compared with a patient without diabetes. Although a specific benefit for IC has not been demonstrated, it seems prudent to initiate or continue aggressive diabetes management in patients with type 2 diabetes mellitus and IC. The addition of metformin to J.S.'s therapy could improve his blood glucose control and decrease his risk of vascular complications. This agent will favorably affect hepatic glucose production and insulin sensitivity and could result in weight loss. It is hoped that J.S. can reach his Hgb A_{1c} goal of less than 7% and a fasting blood glucose of 70 to 130 mg/dL and 2-hour postprandial glucose of less than 180 mg/dL with diet, exercise, and metformin therapy, in addition to his BID NPH standing dose of insulin.[58,59] It may be prudent to educate J.S. on the utility of keeping a daily diary of his blood glucose results to enhance his care. These data will assist his clinicians in modifying his insulin regimen to improve outcomes.

J.S. also must take proper care of his feet to prevent ulcerative complications of IC. He should be encouraged to keep his feet warm, dry, and moisturized and to wear properly fitted shoes and perform daily foot inspections.[8] He should seek medical attention immediately for minor trauma to his feet or legs.[4] These measures can reduce the incidence of amputation in patients with diabetes.

PHARMACOLOGIC THERAPIES

ANTIPLATELET THERAPIES

CASE 15-1, QUESTION 6: Is the aspirin that J.S. is taking beneficial for preventing further complications of IC? Would an agent such as clopidogrel offer any advantage compared with aspirin?

Aspirin is one of several antiplatelet agents that may be considered for indefinite use in patients such as J.S. with IC. A paucity of studies has directly addressed the effects of aspirin on IC symptoms. For example, whether aspirin has any beneficial effects on walking distance or claudication pain in patients with IC has not been studied. Rather, most available data address the impact of aspirin on overall cardiovascular morbidity and mortality. Aspirin exerts its antiplatelet effect by irreversibly inhibiting cyclo-oxygenase. This enzyme is essential for the production of thromboxane A_2, a stimulus for platelet aggregation. Although aspirin has no direct effect on plaque regression, it does prevent and retard the role platelets play in the thrombogenic events that occur in the vicinity of atherosclerotic plaques.[60] Aspirin is an effective antithrombotic agent at dosages ranging from 50 to 1,500 mg daily. The minimal dosages proved to decrease cardiovascular events are 75 to 100 mg daily,[61] with the higher dosage showing benefit in active processes, such as acute ischemic stroke[62] and acute MI.[63] A dosage of 75 mg daily has demonstrated benefit in patients with hypertension[64] and stable angina.[65] No evidence indicates that these "low doses" are any more or any less effective than dosages of 900 to 1,500 mg daily.[66]

Aspirin is recommended in patients with vascular disease of any origin (this includes stroke, MI, PAD, and ischemic heart disease). At dosages of 75 to 162 mg/day, it decreases vascular death by approximately 15% and all serious vascular events (MI, stroke, or vascular death) by approximately 20% in high-risk patients, including those with PAD.[58,61,66] In patients with PAD, aspirin can delay the progression of established lesions as assessed by angiography. When used for primary prevention of cardiovascular disease in men, aspirin decreased the need for arterial reconstructive surgery needed because of PAD.[67] In a meta-analysis of 5,269 subjects with PAD, aspirin was associated with a significant reduction in nonfatal stroke with a statistically insignificant decrease of cardiovascular events.[68] However, in a recent large randomized, controlled trial in 3,350 patients 50 to 75 years of age without clinically evident cardiovascular disease but with a screening ABI of 0.95 or less, aspirin 100 mg/day was found to be no more effective than placebo in reducing the primary end point of fatal and nonfatal coronary events, stroke, or revascularization (13.7 events per 1,000 person-years in the aspirin group vs. 13.3 in the placebo group; hazard ratio, 1.03; 95% confidence interval, 0.84–1.27).[69]

Because all dosages of aspirin are similarly efficacious in decreasing vascular events in this patient population, side effects determine the dose chosen. Although few studies have directly compared varying doses, side effects appear to be dose related. Aspirin 30 mg daily results in less minor bleeding compared with approximately 300 mg daily,[70] and 300 mg daily results in fewer gastrointestinal (GI) side effects compared with 1,200 mg daily.[71] Therefore, J.S. should take the lowest effective dose of aspirin; 75 mg to 100 mg daily. Of note, J.S.'s hypertension should be controlled before initiating aspirin therapy to decrease the small increased incidence of cerebral hemorrhage associated with its use.[72]

Ticlopidine is a thienopyridine derivative that blocks adenosine 5′-diphosphate (ADP) receptors on platelets and decreases platelet-fibrinogen binding.[73] Several studies document its efficacy in patients with PAD on end points such as walking distance, cardiovascular death, and the need for revascularization surgery.[74,75] Diarrhea is a common side effect, however, and hematologic toxicities (neutropenia and, rarely, thrombotic thrombocytopenic purpura) further limit its use.[76,77]

Clopidogrel, an antiplatelet agent with the same mechanism of action as ticlopidine but with an improved safety profile, has largely replaced ticlopidine when thienopyridine therapy is desired. The effects of clopidogrel on specific PAD outcomes are not known, but it has been compared with aspirin in patients with known atherosclerotic disease. Dosages of 75 mg daily significantly reduced cardiovascular end points by approximately 25% compared with aspirin in this patient population.[78] In fact, the treatment effect was most pronounced in the subgroup that had PAD, leading to the suggestion that clopidogrel may be preferable in the patient population with PAD. No measure was taken of clopidogrel's effect on walking distance or claudication pain, however, nor have these results been replicated.

The combination of aspirin and clopidogrel was compared with aspirin alone in more than 15,000 patients at high risk of vascular events, of whom greater than 20% had a history of PAD and approximately 10% had IC.[79,80] In this large study that assessed cardiovascular end points, no benefit was found for dual antiplatelet therapy with aspirin and clopidogrel.[80] Thus, clopidogrel is an appropriate alternative to aspirin in patients unable to take aspirin therapy, perhaps owing to a serious allergy.[8] It should not be used in addition to aspirin, however, because the risk of bleeding and increased cost are not outweighed by any measurable vascular benefit.[80,81]

CILOSTAZOL

CASE 15-1, QUESTION 7: Are there any medications that can be used to increase the walking abilities of patients with IC?

Cilostazol is one of the few agents approved by the US Food and Drug Administration (FDA) specifically for the treatment of IC. Several studies have confirmed that a fixed dose of cilostazol 100 mg twice daily increases walking distance by approximately 50%,[82–85] and that discontinuation of cilostazol resulted in a decline in function.[86] This drug possesses antiplatelet and vasodilatory effects mediated by the inhibition of phosphodiesterase III.[87] Some in vitro observations suggest that these pharmacologic effects of cilostazol are particularly pronounced at the blood–vessel interface,[87] which may explain its particular efficacy in the patient population with PAD. Studies that included quality-of-life measurements have found that cilostazol improved overall quality of life in these patients.[82,88] Moreover, a small improvement was seen in ABI with chronic cilostazol therapy.[89] Two small studies indicate cilostazol is associated with a reduction in restenosis after endovascular therapy in femoropopliteal lesions.[90,91]

Despite these positive findings with cilostazol, several drawbacks exist to its use. It is contraindicated in patients with heart failure because other phosphodiesterase inhibitors cause excess mortality in patients with heart failure, presumably owing to increased arrhythmias.[92] Other common side effects include headache, occurring in up to one-third of patients, and loose stools or diarrhea.[83,93] Cilostazol is a cytochrome P-450 3A4 substrate; therefore, any inhibitor of this enzyme system may substantially increase cilostazol levels.

Cilostazol is an important advance in the treatment of IC. It is the first pharmacologic agent to demonstrate a consistent effect on a significant source of IC disability: walking and mobility measures. Although limited data address its impact on other important end points, such as amputation and revascularization procedures or cardiovascular events,[94] it should be added to J.S.'s existing medication regimen at a dosage of 100 mg twice daily to attenuate his symptoms of IC. It is hoped that its addition to smoking cessation, exercise, and optimal blood pressure and glycosylated hemoglobin attainment will result in good long-term symptomatic and vascular event outcomes.

RHEOLOGIC AGENTS

CASE 15-1, QUESTION 8: Has pentoxifylline been shown to be efficacious in patients such as J.S.? How does this drug benefit patients with IC?

Pentoxifylline, a methylxanthine derivative, is one of the few agents approved by the FDA for the treatment of IC. The exact mechanism of action is unclear; however, it appears to decrease blood viscosity by decreasing fibrinogen, improving the deformability of both red and white blood cells, and eliciting antiplatelet effects.[95] Although the theoretic and in vitro data on pentoxifylline are unique and positive, the data demonstrating clinical usefulness of this agent are controversial. In general, the improvements in walking distances from study to study are unpredictable, and the clinical importance of the sometimes minimal increases in walking distances is not clear (e.g., painfree walking of approximately 30 m greater than with placebo).[96] Some experts assert that these potential benefits of questionable clinical significance are not worth the expense of drug therapy or the GI side effects.[46,97] Because the therapy is of questionable benefit, the expense and potential for side effects are rarely justified.

Pentoxifylline's role in IC therapy is limited. It may have a role in patients who are unable to engage in exercise therapy or in patients with markedly reduced walking distances, in whom any small increase in walking distance would greatly improve the patient's level of activity.[98] It also may be tried in patients who have not gained the desired benefit from smoking cessation and exercise therapy, and in patients in whom contraindications to or failure of cilostazol therapy has occurred. A 2-month trial of pentoxifylline is adequate to determine whether the patient will benefit from the therapy.[21] J.S. is not severely debilitated, and the benefits of smoking cessation, exercise therapy, and cilostazol have not been fully realized. Therefore, pentoxifylline therapy should be withheld until his response to these well-proven therapies has been determined and the need for further improvement in walking distance is established.

VASODILATORS

CASE 15-1, QUESTION 9: J.S. is already taking isosorbide dinitrate for his angina. Because IC is made worse by vasoconstriction, should another vasodilating agent be added to treat both his hypertension and IC?

The use of vasodilators for J.S. would at first appear to be a logical pharmacologic intervention to prevent claudication pain. Vasodilators, including isosorbide dinitrate, directly or indirectly relax blood vessel walls and increase both skin and muscle blood flow as long as cardiac output is maintained. With obstructive arterial disease, however, vessels are sclerotic and unable to dilate any further. As a result, relatively healthy collateral vessels dilate to a greater extent than diseased vessels, and blood flow is redistributed (shunted) away from areas that have the greatest need. Blood pressure and perfusion paradoxically drop even further in the affected tissues. This process is known as the *steal phenomenon*.

Numerous vasodilators (i.e., prostaglandin E_1, prostacyclin, isoxsuprine, papaverine, ethaverine, cyclandelate, niacin derivatives, reserpine, guanethidine, methyldopa, tolazoline, nifedipine) have been used to treat IC. None, however, has convincingly or consistently improved exercise performance, despite earlier beliefs that they were effective.[99,100] Limited data suggest L-carnitine 1 g twice daily may have benefit in walking distance and initial claudication distance.[101] ACE inhibitors are the exception to this rule, as discussed above, and their beneficial effects are likely independent of their vasodilator properties. One small, controlled study demonstrated improvement in walking distance with verapamil, a calcium-channel blocker, compared with placebo in patients with IC.[102] Thus, although vasodilators have generally been eliminated from the treatment of IC and related obstructive vascular disorders,[16] verapamil may be an agent with vasodilating properties that is useful in patients with IC.

Smoking cessation, an exercise program, and cilostazol are the interventions that should reduce J.S.'s symptoms of IC to the greatest degree. After these three measures have been implemented and the impact of the modified BP regimen, which should definitely continue to include an ACE inhibitor, has been assessed, the addition of verapamil could be considered. Verapamil is a moderate cytochrome P-450 3A4 inhibitor, and would be expected to increase concentrations of cilostazol. The magnitude of this interaction has not been characterized, nor has its impact on efficacy and bleeding events been assessed. Based on the necessity of cilostazol therapy in J.S., the poorly characterized benefits of verapamil in IC, and the plethora of other antihypertensive and antianginal agents, avoidance of verapamil is prudent in this patient. If additional BP or antianginal effects are needed, β-blockade or amlodipine can be initiated.

OTHER THERAPEUTIC ALTERNATIVES

CASE 15-1, QUESTION 10: The sales clerk at a health-food store told J.S. that several nutritional supplements and herbal products would improve his circulation so that he could walk better. He is considering buying ginkgo biloba. Does ginkgo or any other herbals or vitamins really work?

Several herbs and vitamins have been used to treat IC, but most have not been rigorously studied. To complicate matters, many studies are published in foreign journals, making access and interpretation of the data challenging.

Ginkgo biloba is one of the few herbal therapies with double-blind, placebo-controlled trials to support its use. A meta-analysis of eight trials representing data from 385 patients reported a mean increase in painfree walking of 34 m (a 47% increase) with a median dosage of 160 mg daily for 6 months.[103] It has been proposed that ginkgo's therapeutic value is related to its antiplatelet properties.[104] Gingko is generally well tolerated with no major side effects, except for an increased risk of bleeding as would be expected with any platelet inhibitor.[105] Occasionally, mild GI upset or headache have been reported.[106] The treatment benefit is modest and consistent, and the side effects are minor; however, the clinical relevance remains in question.[107]

Vitamin E has been advocated for the treatment of IC for many years.[108] Only a few very small, poorly controlled studies, however, support its ability to improve blood flow and walking distance.[109,110] Vitamin E has not prevented cardiovascular events in patients with both established coronary artery disease and risk factors for cardiovascular disease.[110–112] A significant amount of data suggests dosages of greater than 400 international units/day of vitamin E are associated with an increase in all-cause mortality and are unlikely to offer any symptomatic relief or long-term protection from cardiovascular events to J.S.[113]

Moreover, a strong, graded association between low serum 25-hydroxyvitamin D [25(OH)D] levels and the prevalence of PAD was found in a cross-sectional subgroup analysis of the National Health and Nutritional Examination Survey. A paucity of mechanistic and prospective data exists with respect to pathophysiology of low serum 25(OH)D and the effect of vitamin D supplementation in PAD, respectively. Future studies are warranted to determine the potential benefit of this emerging possibility.[114]

Patients with IC have decreased intramuscular carnitine levels, and this impairs oxidative metabolism in skeletal muscle.[115,116] Exogenous propionyl-L-carnitine, 1 to 2 g/day, improves energy production in ischemic muscles. Small studies have demonstrated beneficial effects on walking distances[117,118] and quality of life[119] in patients with IC. Although it is not approved by the FDA, similar agents, such as levocarnitine, are available in the United States. Limited data suggest its effects are less than those seen with propionyl-L-carnitine.[118]

With the abundance of proven, therapeutic measures to be initiated in J.S., the use of relatively poorly studied and unsubstantiated alternative products is not warranted. J.S. should inform his doctors and pharmacist if he uses any of these agents so they can anticipate the inevitable drug interactions (e.g., ginkgo biloba plus antiplatelet drugs) and to allow for appropriate assessment and monitoring.

CASE 15-1, QUESTION 11: Three years have passed, and J.S. stopped smoking 6 months ago. His symptoms of IC have remained fairly stable until the recent development of a nonhealing ulcer on his toe. What options are there for J.S. if nonpharmacologic and pharmacologic interventions are not sufficient?

Surgical intervention eventually may be necessary for persistent and complicated disease. Because success rates for preventing amputation and postsurgical complications vary from institution to institution, surgery should be considered only for severely ischemic limbs and should be performed in a hospital with a good history of success.[120] Arterial bypass grafting and percutaneous transluminal angioplasty of the femoral or iliac arteries, similar to cardiac revascularization, are two procedures that can be performed. Angioplasty is beneficial in patients with localized disease, especially in the iliac or superficial femoral arteries, and should be considered in patients who truly are incapacitated by their activity limitations.[121] Angioplasty with or without stent deployment, atherectomy, and the use of drug-eluting stents in the peripheral arteries are all options.[8] The results obtained are based on several factors, including the vascular bed affected, the technique used, and the degree of occlusive disease. Interestingly, angioplasty has not decreased the number of amputations, yet costs for revascularization procedures have doubled.[122] The more invasive reconstructive arterial (bypass) surgery can be used if diffuse lesions preclude the use of localized angioplasty. The true benefits and pitfalls of these skilled interventions remain unclear.

Emergency surgical intervention may be required if acute, persistent ischemia develops. This is frequently owing to a thrombosis associated with advanced atherosclerosis, although other causes, such as cardiac emboli, cannot be excluded.[98] Both surgical thrombectomy and localized thrombolytic administration[123] with tissue-plasminogen activator or urokinase have equal success in alleviating acute limb-threatening ischemia.[124,125]

RAYNAUD'S PHENOMENON

Raynaud's disease, first described by Maurice Raynaud in 1862,[126] remains largely a medical enigma today. This disorder is essentially an exaggerated vasospastic response to cold or emotion. The digits initially turn white, indicating ischemia, then blue, signaling deoxygenation, and finally, digits appear red when reperfusion occurs.[127] It is usually limited to the skin of the hands and fingers, but can also occur in the feet. Between attacks, the digits may appear cool and moist or normal. This abrupt and discomforting phenomenon can be brought on by exposure to cold or emotional stress, both likely mediated through an exaggerated sympathetic response to the precipitating stimuli. Although both IC and Raynaud's phenomenon are disorders of the peripheral arterial circulation, they differ significantly in that IC results primarily from atherosclerotic obstruction, whereas Raynaud's disease is caused by vasospasm.

Diagnosis

This disorder can be separated into primary Raynaud's phenomenon, indicating an idiopathic origin, and secondary Raynaud's. Secondary Raynaud's consists of signs and symptoms of Raynaud's phenomenon in the presence of an associated disease or condition, most commonly a connective tissue disorder, such as scleroderma, rheumatoid arthritis, or systemic lupus erythematosus. Primary Raynaud's disease is diagnosed only when secondary causes have been excluded.[128] Common criteria for the diagnosis of primary Raynaud's phenomenon are listed in Table 15-8. The diagnosis is generally a subjective one, consisting of clinical signs and symptoms, and simply reflects cold hands, feet, or both without normal recovery after a cold stimulus or emotional stress.[130] In unaffected individuals, a cold provocation should result in some mottling and cyanotic changes in the hands, with recovery once the stimuli are removed. In patients with Raynaud's phenomenon, however, the same cold provocation causes closure of the digital arteries, which produces a sharply demarcated pallor and cyanosis of the digits that persists despite removal of the stimulus.[130] The most reliable objective method to measure artery closure during an attack is the finger systolic BP[131]; however, subjective diagnostic criteria are most commonly and easily used to diagnose Raynaud's phenomenon.

Epidemiology

In general, the prevalence of Raynaud's phenomenon is about 3% to 4% across several ethnic groups[128]; however, it may be as high as 20% in some geographically defined populations.[132] It is more common in women than men, tends to affect young patients, and has a higher prevalence in patients with family members who also experience Raynaud's phenomenon. An onset in the teenage years suggests primary Raynaud's phenomenon, whereas an onset after 30 years of age suggests a secondary cause.[129] Secondary Raynaud's phenomenon is usually associated with a connective tissue disorder, but several other conditions may predispose individuals to its development. These include occupational-related exposures to vibratory machinery (e.g., drills, grinders, chain saws) that cause neural damage,[133] vinyl chloride, or hand trauma.[134,135] The diagnosis of primary Raynaud's phenomenon is accurate approximately 85% of the time. The remaining 15% will manifest a connective tissue disorder during the next decade, and will most likely occur in individuals with serum antinuclear antibodies and thickened fingers.[136]

Raynaud's phenomenon can also be associated with medications, including β-adrenergic blocking agents, ergots, cytotoxic drugs, and interferon, all of which can induce vasoconstriction.[137,138] Although avoidance of β-adrenergic blocking agents in patients with Raynaud's phenomenon appears prudent, no discernible effect, as measured by skin temperature and blood flow, was found with the administration of both selective and nonselective β-blockers to patients with Raynaud's phenomenon.[139] Raynaud's phenomenon not associated with a connective tissue disorder is often transient, and does not interfere with daily activities.[139] The effect of smoking on Raynaud's phenomenon has yielded conflicting results. Overall, there appears to be a negligible effect of smoking on the prevalence of Raynaud's phenomenon, the incidence of attacks, and digital blood flow.[140,141]

TABLE 15-8
Criteria for Diagnosis of Primary Raynaud's Phenomenon[129]

Vasospastic attacks caused by cold or emotional stress
Symmetric attacks involving both hands
No evidence of digital ulcerations, pitting, or gangrene
Normal nailfold capillaries
No suggestion of a secondary cause
A negative antinuclear antibody test
A normal erythrocyte sedimentation rate

Pathophysiology

The blood vessels of the digital skin, which have a prime role in the regulation of body temperature, are supplied with vast amounts of sympathetic vasoconstricting nerves.[128] Cold-induced vasospastic attacks in patients with primary Raynaud's phenomenon involve a heightened vasoconstriction of these digital arteries that is mediated by α_2-adrenergic receptors.[142] The cause of this exaggerated response to cold stimuli is unknown; however, several plausible mechanisms involving peripheral α_2-adrenoreceptors could result in an intense vasoconstriction. These include an increased (a) number of α_2-adrenoreceptors, (b) temperature sensitivity of the α_2-adrenoreceptors, and (c) activity of the α_2-adrenergic intracellular signal-transduction pathway.[129]

The mechanism of secondary Raynaud's phenomenon is also not known, but it is thought to be similar to primary Raynaud's phenomenon. The α_2-adrenoreceptor aberrancy may be the result of arterial damage induced by an associated disease state, such as a connective tissue disorder.[129] It is also possible that serotonin receptors play a role in Raynaud's phenomenon. Serotonin agonists have caused decreased finger blood flow, and, conversely, antagonists have increased digital blood flow.[143]

Clinically, a patient with Raynaud's disease will present with a waxy pallor of one or more of the fingers after the sudden decrease of arterial blood flow. Hemoglobin desaturation occurs with static venous blood flow and causes the digit or digits to have a cyanotic appearance. The attack subsides with time, and the affected arteries vasodilate. As the skin temperature increases, classic rubor, or reddening of the afflicted area, will be seen. Many patients will be observed to have pallor only during the initial attack, in which the digits take on a white or yellow, sometimes patchy, appearance. In most cases, the ischemia produced by the phenomenon does not have important consequences; however, in severe cases, atrophy of the skin, irregular nail growth, and wasting of the tissue pads can occur.[128]

Clinical Presentation

CASE 15-2

QUESTION 1: F.K., a 39-year-old man, presents today with a 4-day history of left hand pain. He notes that the third digit of his left hand is "cold and somewhat blue," especially in the distal area. The other areas of his hand have recovered, but the distal portion of the digit remains cyanotic and numb. He has used acetaminophen and warm-water soaks without success. He is a construction worker who uses his hands "quite a bit" in his work. He has a history of gastroesophageal reflux and has no allergies. His social history is significant for smoking 1.5 packs of cigarettes a day for 19 years. On physical examination, his extremities reveal appropriate sensation of the forearm and hand. Some

blue areas are noted on the distal portion on the third phalanx, with no other signs and symptoms. When F.K.'s opposite hand was placed in cold water, several white splotches appeared, and he experienced tingling in this hand as a result of the cold-water exposure. He is diagnosed as having Raynaud's phenomenon. Does F.K. present with primary or secondary Raynaud's phenomenon?

F.K. presents with what is most likely secondary Raynaud's phenomenon owing to one of several potential underlying causes. His clinical presentation is classic for Raynaud's phenomenon, with vasospasm, pallor, and a cyanotic overtone. The diagnosis is confirmed by the cold-water test, which indicates that the vasospastic attack is precipitated by cold exposure. He has a work history that may easily include hand trauma and the use of vibrating machinery, and his age also suggests secondary Raynaud's phenomenon. Because of its association with connective tissue disorders, other laboratory tests such as an antinuclear antibody and erythrocyte sedimentation rate should be checked.

Treatment

NONPHARMACOLOGIC MANAGEMENT

CASE 15-2, QUESTION 2: What conservative measures can be taken with F.K. to prevent or decrease the painful vasospasm of Raynaud's disease?

Most patients with either primary or secondary Raynaud's phenomenon will respond to conservative management. Avoiding cold stimuli is the primary treatment. F.K. should be instructed to protect his hands and fingers from exposure by using mittens and insulated wrappers when handling cold drinks. Although protecting his hands is important, he must also protect other parts of the body from cold exposure to prevent a sympathetic response, which may trigger symptomatic vasoconstriction in his hands. This includes layering his clothing when working outside in cold weather. He should avoid medications that can induce vasoconstriction, particularly sympathomimetics, clonidine, serotonin receptor agonists, and ergot preparations.[129] He should be encouraged to stop smoking, which will avoid smoking-induced vasoconstriction and provide an overall positive health benefit. The impact of smoking cessation on Raynaud's phenomenon, however, actually appears to be negligible.[140,141]

F.K. has new-onset and relatively mild Raynaud's phenomenon. For others who have more severe symptoms and manifestations, especially patients with underlying connective tissue disorders, it is important to immediately and aggressively manage any ulcers that develop on the digits and to be extremely vigilant in detecting infected digits. Antibiotic therapy should be initiated if necessary.[144]

CALCIUM-CHANNEL BLOCKERS

CASE 15-2, QUESTION 3: Nifedipine extended-release 30 mg every day is ordered for F.K. What is the rationale for using a calcium-channel blocker in this case?

Drugs can be used to treat primary and secondary Raynaud's phenomenon if it interferes with the patient's ability to work or perform daily activities or if digital lesions develop. Most proposed treatments for Raynaud's are variably effective, and they introduce the risk for significant side effects. Nifedipine CR generic, the main calcium-channel blocker used in the treatment of patients with Raynaud's, is about $35 to $40/month.[145,146] Drug therapy should always be in addition to nonpharmacologic measures.

Calcium-channel blockers decrease calcium ion influx and prevent smooth muscle contraction, especially vascular responses evoked by cold exposure. Nifedipine and its two FDA-rated generic sustained-release formulations, a potent peripheral vasodilating calcium-channel blocker, has become the drug of choice in patients with Raynaud's disease not controlled by conservative measures. In primary Raynaud's phenomenon, ten or more episodes per week are common. Nifedipine therapy results in an approximate 50% decrease in the number of attacks, in addition to a decrease in severity by one-third.[146] Patients with secondary Raynaud's phenomenon experience a similar decrease in attack severity, and also achieve a decrease in number of attacks with nifedipine therapy. Because their baseline number of attacks per week often exceeds 20, the relative benefit is not as great as with primary Raynaud's phenomenon, averaging approximately a 25% decrease in weekly episodes.[147] Doses of 10 to 30 mg three times daily of immediate-release nifedipine are beneficial,[148,149] although higher doses, if tolerated, may be required for maximal benefit.[150] Most clinicians administer nifedipine as an extended-release formulation to increase convenience and decrease side effects such as dizziness, headache, facial flushing, and peripheral edema, which can occur in up to 50% of patients,[151] and this practice is supported by several clinical studies.[152–154] Even the extended-release preparation of nifedipine can cause bothersome edema owing to dilation of the precapillary bed.

Although less thoroughly studied than nifedipine, other vasoselective calcium-channel blockers (CCBs), such as amlodipine, felodipine, isradipine, and nisoldipine, decrease the frequency and severity of ischemic attacks.[155–158] Patients who do not benefit from nifedipine likely will not benefit by switching to another CCB. Patients who cannot tolerate the side effects of nifedipine (e.g., peripheral edema, headache) might benefit by switching to another CCB.

F.K. should be warned of the potential side effects with nifedipine therapy, especially dizziness associated with hypotension, and should return in 2 weeks for assessment. A 30-mg daily dose of extended-release nifedipine is a reasonable starting dose. He should be instructed to keep a diary documenting the number of attacks he experiences and details surrounding each attack, such as time course and precipitating factors. In addition to the usual side effects mentioned above, F.K. should be aware that his symptoms of gastroesophageal reflux could worsen with nifedipine therapy, which can cause a decreased lower esophageal sphincter pressure. This side effect should be specifically assessed at his follow-up appointment.

OTHER THERAPEUTIC AGENTS

CASE 15-2, QUESTION 4: What other drugs may be tried if F.K. cannot tolerate the calcium-channel blocker?

Other than CCBs, no proven therapy for Raynaud's phenomenon exists. Many agents, however, have been used on the basis of minimal data and anecdotal reports. The α_1-adrenergic antagonists are one such class of drugs. Prazosin, 1 mg three times a day, yielded moderate benefit in two-thirds of patients in two small studies.[159,160] Side effects of prazosin are significant at maximal doses and include dizziness, edema, fatigue, and orthostasis. The longer-acting α_1-adrenergic antagonist terazosin was evaluated in one small study, and it improved symptomatology as well as objective measures of blood flow.[161] No sufficient data with this class of drugs exist to routinely recommend their use in patients with Raynaud's phenomenon.

Several therapeutic approaches are being vigorously investigated, and show promise as future therapies for Raynaud's phenomenon. These include the intravenous prostanoids, iloprost and alprostadil, which enhance nitric oxide–mediated vasodilation[162]; endothelin antagonists, such as bosentan[163]; and oral phosphodiesterase inhibitors, such as sildenafil[164] and vardenafil,[165] which also promote vasodilation. Because of side effects, extreme cost, and administration difficulties, these agents are only being studied in the most severe cases of secondary Raynaud's phenomenon with digital ulcers or other systemic complications associated with connective tissue diseases. If benefit is proved, however, it will shed light on the pathogenesis of the disorder, and perhaps lead to therapies appropriate for the larger population with Raynaud's phenomenon.

Statins may have promise in severe cases resulting in digital ulcers secondary to systemic sclerosis (SSc). Pleiotropic effects of atorvastatin 40 mg/day on endothelial function compared with placebo were investigated in 84 SSc patients who fulfilled the American College of Rheumatology criteria for classification of SSc with secondary Raynaud's phenomenon despite ongoing vasodilator therapy. The study found a significant decrease in both new and the total number of digital ulcers in the atorvastatin group compared with placebo.[166]

The renin-angiotensin system mediators act as vasodilators and have been investigated in several small studies. ACE inhibitors and angiotensin receptor blockers, however, have yielded conflicting results with respect to beneficial effects in patients with Raynaud's phenomenon.[167–170] Small beneficial effects have been realized, specifically with captopril 25 mg three times a day and losartan 12.5 to 25 mg/day; however, no benefit has been found with enalapril 20 mg once daily.[169] Fluoxetine, a selective serotonin reuptake inhibitor, was shown in one study to reduce the symptoms of Raynaud's phenomenon.[171] It is hypothesized to exert its effect by depleting platelet serotonin, rendering the platelet unable to release a significant amount of the vasoconstrictive serotonin during activation and aggregation.

The application of nitroglycerin (NTG) ointment to the hands of patients with Raynaud's disease has been tried since the mid-1940s. High doses of NTG 0.2% ointment (3.5 inches) three times a day applied to the hands for 6 weeks resulted in fewer and less severe attacks.[172] Transdermal NTG patches also provide some benefit, although headaches may be a limiting factor.[173] The potential for tolerance developing to the nitrates for this indication has not been studied. Because the data supporting nitrate use in the management of Raynaud's phenomenon are sparse, these agents should be discontinued after 2 to 3 weeks if no benefit is observed.[144] Alternative therapies, such as ginkgo biloba and L-arginine, have also been studied in small trials with positive results; however, larger trials are needed to confirm the findings before these therapies can be recommended.[174–176]

All patients with Raynaud's phenomenon should be counseled regarding cold avoidance and other protective measures. A CCB, nifedipine if tolerated, should be initiated if conservative measures are ineffective and titrated to the highest tolerated dose and symptom resolution. Combination therapies have not been investigated, but another agent, such as an α_1-adrenergic antagonist, may be considered in addition to the CCB if symptom resolution is not satisfactory and side effects permit.

NOCTURNAL LEG MUSCLE CRAMPS

Nocturnal leg muscle cramps are idiopathic, involuntary contractions occurring at rest that cause a visible and palpable knot in the affected muscle. This type of muscle cramp usually afflicts middle-aged to elderly persons and is a distressing and painful condition. Its cause is unknown. The two primary hypotheses that attempt to explain the pathophysiology propose neurologic impairments. One involves a central nervous system impairment of γ-aminobutyric acid,[177] and the other, an impaired peripheral response to muscle lengthening.[178] Although the incidence of nocturnal cramps is unknown, some data indicate it is very common. In a survey of veterans (95% men averaging 60 years of age), 56% complained of leg cramps, with 12% having cramping nearly every night[179]; 36% of these veterans were also attempting some type of drug treatment for their symptoms. A survey of the general population revealed that the prevalence of nocturnal leg cramps was 37% in people older than 50 years of age, and increased to 54% in people older than 80 years of age. The prevalence in men and women is equal.[180] Nocturnal leg cramps are associated with lower extremity atherosclerosis, coronary artery disease, and peripheral neurologic deficits.[180,181]

Clinical Presentation

CASE 15-3

QUESTION 1: E.A., a 62-year-old woman, complains of cramps in her left calf that began last night around 10 PM. The cramping occurred several times throughout the night and has resolved slowly since she arose this morning. These nighttime cramping episodes occur frequently, are very painful, and cause her calf muscle to become "knotted." She denies any trauma, fever, or chills, has no other medical problems, and takes no medications. The pain is not associated with walking. The physical examination is unremarkable, and her vital signs are stable. An extended chemistry panel and thyroid function tests are within normal limits. E.A. works at an elementary school and walks up and down stairs throughout the day. Her physician associates the pain with nocturnal leg cramps. What characteristics differentiate E.A.'s nocturnal leg cramps from other pain syndromes?

Benign nocturnal leg cramps usually occur in the early hours of sleeping; they are asymmetric and are not exclusive to but primarily affect the calf muscle and small muscles of the foot. These cramps are not associated with exercise, specific electrolyte or laboratory abnormalities, or medication use. Nocturnal cramps occur with the further contraction of a muscle already in its most shortened position. For example, sleeping in the supine position may place the calf and ventral foot muscles in their most shortened and vulnerable position, predisposing these muscles to contract.[182]

For diagnosis and treatment, true muscle cramps first should be distinguished from other causes of muscle cramping, including drug-induced cramps (Table 15-9). The onset of cramps at rest is characteristic of ordinary leg cramps and is the primary symptom used for diagnosis. Clinical signs of sodium depletion, hyperthyroidism and hypothyroidism, tetany, and lower motor neuron disease should be evaluated. Laboratory measurements such as standard electrolytes and thyroid function tests can help rule out some of these other conditions.

Treatment

THERAPEUTIC OBJECTIVES AND NONPHARMACOLOGIC INTERVENTIONS

CASE 15-3, QUESTION 2: What are the therapeutic objectives in treating E.A.? What nonpharmacologic recommendations can be made?

TABLE 15-9
Other Causes of Muscle Cramps[182–184]

Drug-Induced Cramps	Biochemical Causes	Other
Alcohol	Dehydration	Contractures
Antipsychotics (dystonia)	Hemodialysis	Diabetes
β-Agonists (e.g., albuterol, terbutaline, salbutamol)	Hypocalcemia	Lower motor neuron disease
Cimetidine	Hypokalemia	Peripheral vascular disease
Clofibrate	Hypomagnesemia	Tetany
Diuretics	Hyponatremia	Thyroid disease
Lithium	Uremia	
Narcotic analgesics		
Nicotinic acid		
Nifedipine		
Penicillamine		
Statins		
Steroids		

The primary treatment goal is to prevent this uncomfortable condition. Sufferers of leg cramps are commonly advised to stretch out the afflicted muscle or perform dorsiflexion of the feet throughout the day and before bedtime, but this therapeutic modality has sparse, uncontrolled data in the literature and cannot be relied on to be helpful.[183] Patients are also warned to avoid plantar flexion while sleeping by hanging the feet over the edge of the bed when sleeping on the stomach. Once a cramp occurs, the goal is to relieve the cramp as quickly as possible. Acute therapy consists of dorsiflexion (grasping the toes and pulling them upward in the opposite direction of the cramp). This can be accomplished with the hands, by walking, or by leaning toward a wall while standing 2 feet away from it, maintaining the feet flat on the floor.[182]

QUININE

CASE 15-3, QUESTION 3: E.A. is amenable to the recommended stretching practices, and will avoid plantar flexion during sleep. She returns in 3 months, and reports a minor decrease in the attack frequency, but not severity. Her sleep is being affected 2 to 3 nights/week, and she feels it is affecting her performance as a teacher. She remembers her aunt taking a "pill" for her leg cramps. Is there any medication that may help relieve her symptoms?

Quinine is the most frequently prescribed medication for nocturnal leg cramps and was once a nonprescription product. In 1995, the FDA stated that quinine was not considered safe and effective for nocturnal leg cramps[185] and discontinued its over-the-counter status. Physicians can still prescribe quinine for the treatment of nocturnal leg cramps because it is commercially available and indicated for the treatment of malaria. The FDA, however, has clearly stated quinine should not be used for nocturnal leg cramps because of an unfavorable risk–benefit ratio.

Quinine has been used to treat nocturnal leg cramps since the 1940s, when four patients having leg cramps experienced marked improvement in symptoms after being treated with quinine.[186] When given placebo, their symptoms apparently worsened. Quinine may exert a beneficial effect by increasing the refractory period of skeletal muscle and by decreasing the excitability of the motor endplate. Despite its frequent use, significant controversy exists about its benefit. Only a few small controlled trials have been conducted, with mixed conclusions. A meta-analysis was published in 1998 that included both published and unpublished data addressing the efficacy of quinine in the treatment of leg cramps.[187] Pooled data from 659 patients indicated that quinine, at 200 to 325 mg/day, reduced the severity and average number of cramps experienced in a 4-week period from 17.1 to 13.5. Thus, the efficacy of quinine is proved; however, the magnitude of the benefit is rather small, and the risks associated with quinine therapy for a benign condition must also be considered. Of note, a recent study that randomly assigned patients to quinine cessation reported no effect on nocturnal leg cramp frequency (e.g., no worsening of symptoms).[188]

Before initiating quinine, prophylactic stretching and alteration of sleeping position should be tried and evaluated. Additionally, modifiable causes of cramps should be explored and addressed. If these measures do not result in adequate relief, therapy with quinine can be considered if the patient is fully aware of the risks, appreciates the small benefit she can expect, and has no medications or conditions that place her at increased risk of adverse effects.[189,190]

PRECAUTIONS WITH QUININE

CASE 15-3, QUESTION 4: What side effect information should both the physician and E.A. know about before initiation of quinine therapy? How long should therapy be continued?

If quinine therapy is successful, E.A. should see a decrease in the severity and frequency of her cramping attacks. Quinine is available in the United States only as the 324-mg sulfate salt, as the brand name Qualaquin. One tablet should be taken in the evening. Cinchonism, a syndrome that includes nausea, vomiting, blurred vision, tinnitus, and deafness, is a dose-related side effect of quinine.[182] Tinnitus alone occurs in up to 3% of patients.[187] With overdose, central nervous system manifestations, such as headache, confusion, and delirium, can occur. Self-limiting rashes that resolve with drug discontinuation have been described.[182] The unpredictable and life-threatening side effect of thrombocytopenia was the impetus for the FDA to ban the over-the-counter status of this preparation. Thrombocytopenia has been estimated to occur in up to 1 of 1,000 patients taking quinine.[185] Care should also be taken with the use of quinine because its clearance is decreased in the elderly,[191] and several drugs decrease its clearance, such as cimetidine, verapamil, amiodarone, and alkalinizing agents.[184] Each of these could increase the risk of quinine dose-related side effects, specifically the central nervous system manifestations. Quinine can also produce toxic levels of digoxin, phenobarbital, and carbamazepine[184] and is contraindicated in patients with glucose-6-phosphate dehydrogenase deficiency.

E.A. should be instructed to take the dose of quinine with food to minimize GI irritation. If a response is not seen within 2 weeks, it should be discontinued in light of the potentially serious side effects.[181] E.A. should be instructed to keep a diary documenting the frequency of the cramping episodes and possible adverse effects so that its efficacy can be objectively assessed.

OTHER THERAPIES

CASE 15-3, QUESTION 5: Are there other treatment options for E.A.?

Electrolyte replacement (e.g., sodium, potassium, calcium, magnesium) may be indicated if specific deficiencies are noted or if the onset of cramping is associated with a recent initiation or dosage increase of diuretic therapy. Prophylactic use of other pharmacologic agents has been attempted, but their use is mostly anecdotal. Diphenhydramine, riboflavin, carbamazepine, methocarbamol, and phenytoin have been used empirically,[182] but no data support their use in nocturnal leg cramps. Vitamin E has been recommended, but one controlled study with 800 international units/day of vitamin E showed no benefit.[192] Verapamil has been shown in an open-label trial of eight elderly patients to relieve quinine-resistant cramps. A dose of 120 mg of verapamil at bedtime was used, and relief was seen after 6 days of treatment.[193] Similar results were reported from a similar small study using diltiazem.[194] A small study found benefit associated with vitamin B complex administration for nocturnal leg cramps, but no quantification of a decrease in the number of cramps was provided.[195] Two small crossover studies suggested that chronic magnesium administration is not effective for the treatment of nocturnal leg cramps.[196,197]

Although nocturnal leg cramps are relatively benign, they do cause considerable discomfort. Nonpharmacologic measures should be maximized before drug therapy is contemplated. If drug therapy is warranted, quinine is the only agent with proven benefit, but the potential for side effects, especially in the elderly population, is very real. Careful patient selection, patient education, and vigilant monitoring for side effects should all be used to minimize the occurrence and progression of adverse effects from quinine.

KEY REFERENCES AND WEBSITES

A full list of references for this chapter can be found at **http://thepoint.lww.com/AT10e.** Below are the key references and websites for this chapter, with the corresponding reference number in this chapter found in parentheses after the reference.

Key References

Aung PP et al. Lipid-lowering for peripheral arterial disease of the lower limb. *Cochrane Database Syst Rev*. 2007;(4):CD000123. (42)

Chobanian A et al. The Seventh Report of the Joint National Committee on Prevention, Detection, Evaluation, and Treatment of High Blood Pressure: the JNC 7 report [published correction appears in *JAMA*. 2003;290:197]. *JAMA*. 2003;289:2560. (52)

Expert Panel on Detection, Evaluation, and Treatment of High Blood Cholesterol in Adults. Summary of the third report of the National Cholesterol Education Program (NCEP) Expert Panel on Detection, Evaluation, and Treatment of High Blood Cholesterol in Adults (Adult Treatment Panel III). *JAMA*. 2001;285:2486. (34)

Hirsch AT et al. ACC/AHA guidelines for the management of patients with peripheral arterial disease (lower extremity, renal, mesenteric and abdominal aorta): executive summary—a collaborative report from the American Association for Vascular Surgery/Society for Vascular Surgery, Society for Cardiovascular Angiography and Interventions, Society for Vascular Medicine and Biology, Society of Interventional Radiology, and the ACC/AHA Task Force on Practice Guidelines (Writing Committee to Develop Guidelines for the Management of Patients With Peripheral Arterial Disease) endorsed by the American Association of Cardiovascular and Pulmonary Rehabilitation; National Heart, Lung, and Blood Institute; Society for Vascular Nursing; TransAtlantic Inter-Society Consensus; and Vascular Disease Foundation. *J Am Coll Cardiol*. 2006;47:1239. (8)

Lane DA, Lip GY. Treatment of hypertension in peripheral arterial disease. *Cochrane Database Syst Rev*. 2009;(4):CD003075. (48)

Leng GC et al. Exercise for intermittent claudication. *Cochrane Database Syst Rev*. 2000;(2):CD000990. (31)

Robless P et al. Cilostazol for peripheral arterial disease. *Cochrane Database Syst Rev*. 2008;(1):CD003748. (85)

Sobel M et al. Antithrombotic therapy for peripheral artery occlusive disease: American College of Chest Physicians Evidenced-Based Clinical Practice Guidelines (8th Edition). *Chest*. 2008; 133(6 Suppl);815S. (61)

Key Websites

The Peripheral Arterial Disease Coalition (P.A.D. Coalition). **http://www.padcoalition.org.**

National Heart, Lung, and Blood Institute. Stay in Circulation. **http://www.nhlbi.nih.gov/health/public/heart/pad.**

Vascular Disease Foundation. **http://www.vdf.org.**

Thrombosis

16

Ann K. Wittkowsky and Edith A. Nutescu

CORE PRINCIPLES

		CHAPTER CASES
1	Venous thromboembolism (VTE), including deep venous thrombosis and pulmonary embolism, is caused by numerous additive risk factors, with diagnosis based on clinical findings and objective criteria.	Case 16-1 (Questions 1–3), Case 16-5 (Question 1)
2	VTE treatment includes initial injectable anticoagulants, followed by oral anticoagulation with warfarin.	Case 16-1 (Questions 4–6, 9), Case 16-5 (Questions 2, 3)
3	Unfractionated heparin is monitored with the activated partial thromboplastin time (aPTT) test; dosing adjustments are used to maintain the aPTT in therapeutic range, as well as monitoring for adverse effects, including thrombocytopenia and bleeding.	Case 16-1 (Questions 7, 8, 10–12), Case 16-2 (Question 1)
4	Outpatient treatment of VTE is possible with low-molecular-weight heparins (or fondaparinux).	Case 16-3 (Questions 1, 2)
5	Anticoagulation prophylaxis should be used in hospitalized patients at risk of VTE.	Case 16-4
6	Warfarin therapy is dosed and monitored according to therapeutic response as measured by the international normalized ratio. Monitoring for adverse effects including hemorrhage is also essential.	Case 16-5 (Questions 4–6), Case 16-6 (Questions 5, 6), Case 16-7
7	Warfarin therapy is influenced by multiple factors, and patients on warfarin require extensive and ongoing education to maintain safe and effective anticoagulation.	Case 16-6 (Questions 1–4), Cases 16-8, 16-14, 16-15, 16-16, 16-17
8	In addition to treatment of VTE, warfarin is used for stroke prevention in atrial fibrillation and artificial heart valve replacement.	Case 16-9 (Questions 1–3), Cases 16-10, 16-11
9	Pharmacists can play an important role in the management of anticoagulant therapy for invasive and dental procedures.	Cases 16-12, 16-13, 16-17

GENERAL PRINCIPLES

Thrombosis is the process involved in the formation of a fibrin blood clot. Platelets and a series of coagulant proteins (clotting factors) contribute to clot formation. An embolus is a small part of a clot that breaks off and is carried by blood flow to another part of the vascular system. Damage is caused when the embolus becomes trapped in a small vessel, causing occlusion and leading to ischemia or infarction of the surrounding tissue. Normal clot formation maintains the integrity of the vasculature in response to injury, but pathological clotting can occur in many clinical settings. Abnormal thrombotic events include venous thromboembolism (deep venous thrombosis [DVT] and its primary complication, pulmonary embolism [PE]), as well as stroke and other systemic manifestations of embolization of clots that form within the heart. Anticoagulant drug therapy is aimed at preventing pathological clot formation in patients at risk and at preventing clot extension and/or embolization in patients who have experienced thrombosis. This chapter emphasizes arterial and venous thromboembolic disease and the use of heparin, low-molecular-weight heparins, factor Xa inhibitors, direct thrombin inhibitors, and warfarin as anticoagulants. Chapter 13, Dyslipidemias, Atherosclerosis, and Coronary Artery Disease, Chapter 18, Acute Coronary Syndrome, and Chapter 59,

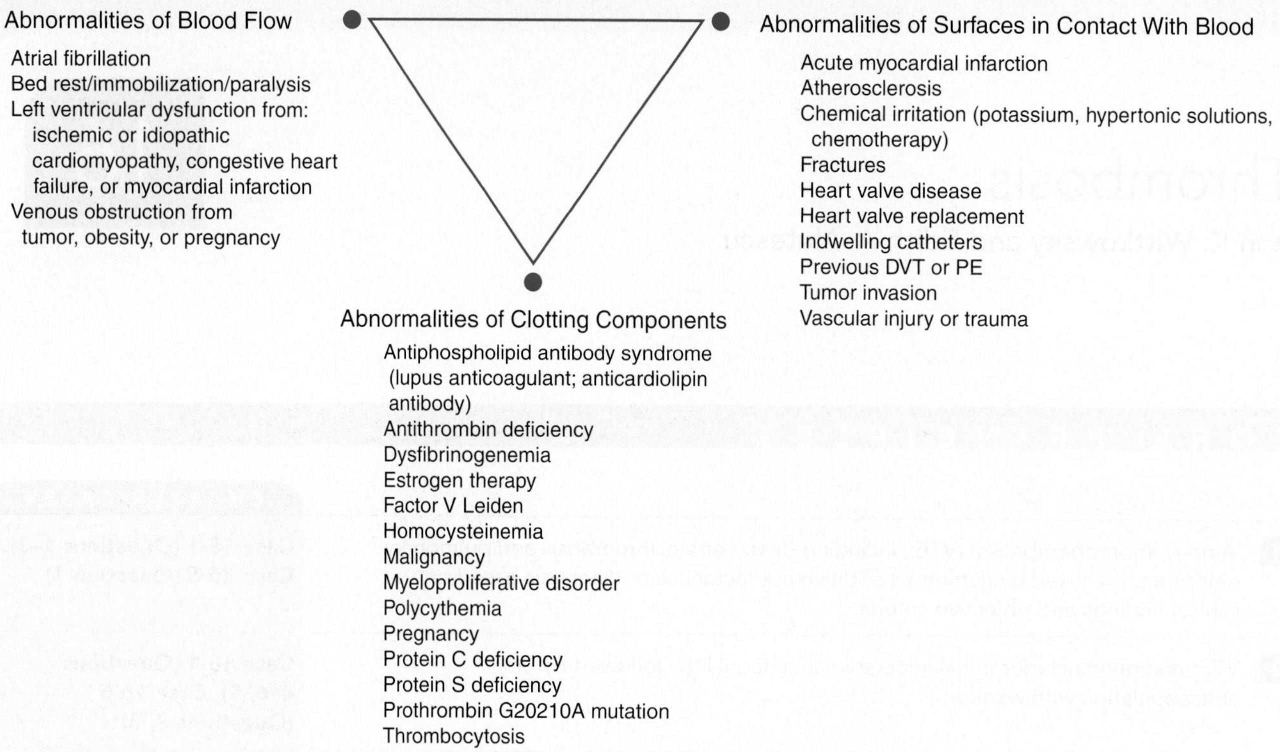

FIGURE 16-1 Risk factors for thromboembolism. DVT, deep venous thrombosis; PE, pulmonary embolism.

Cerebrovascular Disorders, provide more indepth discussions of thrombolytic agents and antiplatelet therapy.

Etiology of Thromboembolism

Three primary factors influence the formation of pathological clots and are described in a model referred to as Virchow's Triad (Fig. 16-1).[1] Abnormalities of blood flow that cause venous stasis can result in DVT, which can progress to PE if embolization occurs. Intracardiac stasis of blood can also result in clot formation within the heart chambers, and embolization of intracardiac thrombi may lead to stroke or other systemic manifestations. Abnormalities of blood vessel walls, such as those that occur in injury or trauma to the vasculature, are a second source of thrombus formation. The presence of foreign material within the vasculature, including artificial heart valves and central venous catheters, is also thrombogenic and, like vascular injury, represents the presence of an abnormal surface in contact with blood. Finally, hypercoagulability resulting from alterations in the availability or the integrity of blood-clotting components or naturally occurring anticoagulants also represents a significant risk factor for thromboembolic disease.[2]

Clot Formation

The intact endothelial lining of blood vessels normally repels platelets and inhibits clot formation through secretion of numerous inhibitory substances. Damage to the endothelium leads to exposure of circulating blood to subendothelial substances, and this results in a complex series of events, including platelet adhesion, activation, and aggregation, followed by activation of the clotting cascade. These events result in formation of a fibrin clot.[3]

ONLINE CONTENT **For an animation of hemostasis, go to http://thepoint.lww.com/AT10e.**

PLATELET ADHESION, ACTIVATION, AND AGGREGATION

Endothelial damage leads to exposure of blood to subendothelial collagen and phospholipids, resulting in platelet adhesion to the surface. Von Willebrand factor serves as the binding ligand for platelet adhesion, via the glycoprotein I (GPI) receptor on the platelet surface. Adhered platelets become activated and release numerous compounds, including adenosine diphosphate and thromboxane A2, which stimulate platelet aggregation. Fibrinogen serves as the binding ligand for platelet aggregation, via the GPIIb/IIIa receptor on the platelet surface.[4]

CLOTTING CASCADE

Transformation of the relatively unstable platelet plug (i.e., the aggregated platelets) to a stable fibrin clot occurs as a result of an imbalance between other procoagulant and anticoagulant factors. In addition to stimulating the platelet response, endothelial damage results in activation of the clotting cascade (Fig. 16-2). The extrinsic pathway of the clotting cascade is activated by the release of thromboplastin (tissue factor) from endothelial cells. Tissue factor converts factor VII to factor VIIa, which mediates the activation of factor X. The intrinsic pathway of the clotting cascade is activated by exposure of factor XII to subendothelial components exposed during vessel injury. The intrinsic pathway mediates factor X activation via a chain of events initiated by factor XI. The distinction between these pathways is primarily an in vitro phenomenon; in vivo, the two pathways are activated simultaneously.

Once stimulated, both the extrinsic and intrinsic pathways activate the common pathway of the clotting cascade via factor X. Activated forms of factors V and VIII serve independently to accelerate this process. The final steps include conversion of factor II (prothrombin) to factor IIa (thrombin), with eventual formation of a stable fibrin clot.

Naturally occurring inhibitors of clotting factors play a role in localizing fibrin formation to the sites of injury and in maintaining the fluidity of circulating blood. Table 16-1 outlines these

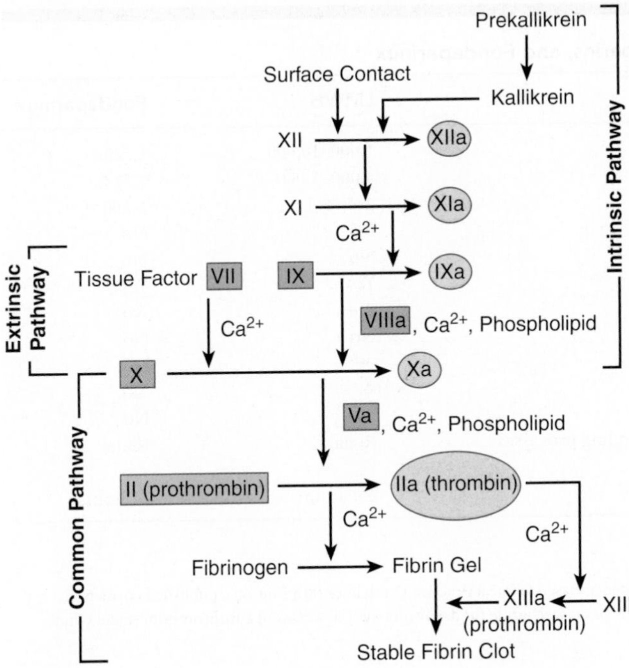

FIGURE 16-2 Simplified clotting cascade. Components in ovals are influenced by heparin; components in boxes are influenced by warfarin.

clotting inhibitors and their primary actions. In addition, the fibrinolytic system is involved in degradation of fibrin clots. The actions of both clotting inhibitors and the fibrinolytic system prevent excessive coagulation. Thus, the process of clot formation is dynamic and involves various factors that can stimulate, inhibit, and dissolve a fibrin clot.

PATHOLOGICAL THROMBI

Pathological thrombi are sometimes classified according to location and composition. Arterial thrombi are composed primarily of platelets, although they also contain fibrin and occasional leukocytes. Arterial thrombi generally occur in areas of rapid blood flow (i.e., arteries) and are typically initiated by spontaneous or mechanical rupture of atherosclerotic plaques followed by aggregation of platelets (see Chapter 13, Dyslipidemias, Atherosclerosis, and Coronary Heart Disease, and Chapter 18, Acute Coronary Syndrome). Venous thrombi are found primarily in the venous circulation and are composed almost entirely of fibrin and erythrocytes. Venous thrombi have a small platelet head and generally form in response to either venous stasis or vascular injury after surgery or trauma. The areas of stasis prevent dilution of activated coagulation factors by normal blood flow.

TABLE 16-1
Inhibitors of Clotting Mechanisms

Inhibitor	Target
Antithrombin	Inhibits factors IIa, IXa, and Xa
Protein S	Cofactor for activation of protein C
Protein C	Inactivates factors Va and VIIIa
Tissue factor pathway inhibitor	Inhibits activity of factor VIIa
Plasminogen	Converted to plasmin via tissue plasminogen activator
Plasmin	Lyses fibrin into fibrin degradation products

The selection of an antithrombotic agent is influenced by the type of thrombus to be treated. The anticoagulants heparin, low-molecular-weight heparins (LMWHs), factor Xa inhibitors, direct thrombin inhibitors and warfarin are used in the treatment and prevention of both arterial and venous thrombi. Drugs that alter platelet function (e.g., aspirin, clopidogrel), alone and/or in combination with anticoagulants, are used in the prevention of arterial thrombi. Fibrinolytic agents are used for rapid dissolution of thromboemboli, most notably during myocardial infarction (MI).

Pharmacology of Antithrombotic Agents

HEPARIN

Heparin is a rapid-acting anticoagulant that is administered parenterally. Standard heparin (unfractionated heparin [UFH]) is a heterogeneous mixture of glycosaminoglycans of varying molecular weights obtained from bovine lung or porcine intestinal mucosa (Table 16-2). The action of heparin is facilitated by its binding to the naturally circulating anticoagulant antithrombin (AT), a serine protease also referred to as heparin cofactor. Binding of heparin to AT accelerates the anticoagulant effect of AT. The heparin–AT complex attaches to and irreversibly inactivates factor IIa (thrombin) and factor Xa, as well as activated factors IX, XI, and XII.[5] Approximately one-third of the molecules present in UFH bind to AT and provide the anticoagulant properties of heparin. The remaining two-thirds of the heparin molecules bind to plasma proteins and to endothelial cells, saturable processes that contribute to the dose-dependent pharmacokinetic profile of the drug and limit its bioavailability. In addition to its anticoagulant effects, heparin inhibits platelet function and increases vascular permeability; these properties contribute to the hemorrhagic effects of heparin.

In cases of acute DVT or PE, the clotting cascade has been activated, generating abnormal quantities of thrombin and fibrin. In these situations, thrombin must be inactivated directly, a process that may require relatively large doses of heparin. However, when the clotting cascade is in a normal balance, it is possible to indirectly inactivate thrombin with smaller heparin doses by complexing factor Xa. Because of the amplification effect of the clotting cascade, inactivation of relatively small amounts of factor Xa indirectly prevents the production of large quantities of thrombin. This phenomenon is the basis for low-dose heparin prophylaxis after surgery or in cases of prolonged bed rest or immobilization.

Heparin may be administered intravenously (IV) by continuous infusion, or subcutaneously (SC), although its bioavailability is significantly reduced by SC administration. Intramuscular administration of heparin (as well as intramuscular administration of other drugs in patients who are anticoagulated) should be avoided because of the potential for hematoma formation.

After IV administration, the anticoagulant effect of heparin is noted immediately. During active thromboembolism, the high concentration of clotting factors necessitates a higher concentration of heparin to neutralize them. This increased dosing requirement may also be related to continuing thrombin formation on the surface of the thrombus. Once endothelialization (localization and incorporation of the clot into the vascular endothelium) of the clot begins and the concentration of clotting factors decreases, dosing requirements typically decrease. Considerable variability in dosing requirements among patients necessitates routine therapeutic monitoring to maintain an appropriate intensity of anticoagulation with heparin. The primary laboratory test for monitoring therapeutic heparinization is the activated partial thromboplastin time (aPTT) (see Tests Used to Monitor Antithrombotic Therapy section).

TABLE 16-2
Comparison of Unfractionated Heparin, Low-Molecular-Weight Heparins, and Fondaparinux

Property	UFH	LMWH	Fondaparinux
Molecular weight range[a]	3,000–30,000	1,000–10,000	1,728
Average molecular weight[a]	12,000–15,000	4,000–5,000	1,728
Anti-Xa : anti-IIa activity	1 : 1	2 : 1–4 : 1	>100 : 1
aPTT monitoring required	Yes	No	No
Inactivation by platelet factor 4	Yes	No	No
Capable of inactivation of platelet-bound factor Xa	No	Yes	Yes
Inhibition of platelet function	++++	++	No
Increases vascular permeability	Yes	No	No
Protein binding	++++	+	No
Endothelial cell binding	+++	+	No
Dose-dependent clearance	Yes	No	No
Primary route of elimination	1. Saturable binding processes 2. Renal	Renal	Renal
Elimination half-life	30–150 minutes	2–6 hours	17 hours

[a] Measured in daltons.
LMWH, low-molecular-weight heparin; UFH, unfractionated heparin.
Source: Hirsh J et al. Parenteral anticoagulants. American College of Chest Physicians Evidence-Based Clinical Practice Guidelines (8th Edition) [published correction appears in *Chest.* 2008;134:473]. *Chest.* 2008;133(Suppl 6):141S; Petitou M et al. The synthetic pentasaccharide fondaparinux: first in a class of antithrombotic agents that selectively inhibit coagulation factor Xa. *Semin Thromb Hemost.* 2002;28:393.

The plasma half-life of heparin varies from 30 to 150 minutes, but the half-life increases with increasing doses. Heparin is cleared by extensive binding to plasma proteins and endothelial cells, saturable processes that explain both its nonlinear kinetics and the variability in dosing requirements among patients. Additional clearance occurs by transfer to the reticuloendothelial system, with ultimate elimination controlled by the kidneys.

LOW-MOLECULAR-WEIGHT HEPARINS

By using chemical or enzymatic depolymerization techniques, UFH can be separated into fragments based on molecular weight.[6] Several LMWH molecules have been isolated and commercially marketed as anticoagulants. The LMWH products available in the United States are dalteparin, enoxaparin, and tinzaparin (Table 16-3). These products have replaced the use of UFH in many clinical situations. These compounds differ substantially from UFH with respect to molecular weight, antithrombotic and pharmacokinetic properties, adverse effect profiles, and monitoring requirements (Table 16-2).

To inactivate factor Xa, only the AT component of the heparin–AT complex is required to bind to factor Xa. Both the longer, high-molecular-weight fragments of UFH and the shorter, low-molecular-weight fragments of LMWHs are capable of inactivating factor Xa. However, to inactivate factor IIa (thrombin), both the heparin component and the AT component of the heparin–AT complex are required to bind to factor IIa. This binding requires heparin molecules of at least 18 saccharide units in length, which are less prevalent in LMWHs. Therefore, the anti-Xa properties of LMWHs are more significant than their anti-IIa properties. The resultant antithrombotic effect does not prolong the aPTT, meaning that these compounds do not require laboratory monitoring to ensure a therapeutic effect.

Additional advantages of LMWHs over UFH are explained by their reduced binding affinity for plasma proteins and endothelial cells. These compounds display improved bioavailability after SC injection, a predictable dose response, and a longer pharmacodynamic effect compared with UFH. In general, these compounds are administered subcutaneously every 12 to 24 hours at fixed doses. The LMWH products have been studied in the prevention and treatment of thromboembolic disease. They differ significantly in their molecular weight distributions, methods of preparation, and the ratio of anti-Xa : anti-IIa activities, as well as in their pharmacokinetic and pharmacodynamic characteristics (Table 16-3).

TABLE 16-3
Low-Molecular-Weight Heparin Products Available in the United States

Generic Name	Brand Name	Average Molecular Weight (range)[a]	Anti-Xa : Anti-IIa Activity
Dalteparin	Fragmin	5,000 (2,000–9,000)	2.0 : 1
Enoxaparin	Lovenox	4,500 (3,000–8,000)	2.7 : 1
Tinzaparin	Innohep	4,500 (3,000–6,000)	1.9 : 1

[a] Measured in daltons.

FONDAPARINUX

Fondaparinux is a selective indirect factor Xa inhibitor that is indicated for the prevention of venous thrombosis associated with orthopedic surgery and abdominal surgery, and for the treatment of deep vein thrombosis and pulmonary embolism.[6,7] It is a synthetic derivative of the five-residue saccharide sequence found in both UFH and LMWH that binds to AT to inactivate factor Xa with no direct impact on factor IIa. This agent has a long elimination half-life, allowing for once-daily SC administration at a fixed dose without the need for routine coagulation monitoring (Table 16-2).

DIRECT THROMBIN INHIBITORS

Argatroban, lepirudin, and bivalirudin are injectable direct thrombin inhibitors that are used as alternative anticoagulants in patients with heparin-induced thrombocytopenia.[8] (Table 16-4). Direct thrombin inhibitors bind to specific sites on the thrombin molecule to inhibit its activity, without acting through a cofactor like antithrombin. These agents are administered by continuous infusion and require aPTT monitoring for appropriate dosing adjustments. Bivalirudin is also used in patients with acute coronary syndrome, including those undergoing percutaneous

TABLE 16-4

Pharmacologic and Clinical Properties of Injectable Direct Thrombin Inhibitors

	Lepirudin	Bivalirudin	Argatroban
Route of administration	IV or SC (BID)	IV	IV
FDA-approved indication	Treatment of thrombosis in patients with HIT	Patients with UA undergoing PTCA; PCI with provisional use of GPI; patients with or at risk of HIT/HITTS undergoing PCI	Treatment of thrombosis in patients with HIT; patients at risk for HIT undergoing PCI
Binding to thrombin	Irreversible at catalytic site and exosite-1	Partially reversible at catalytic site and exosite-1	Reversible at catalytic site
Half-life in healthy subjects	1.3–2 hours	25 minutes	40–50 minutes
Monitoring	aPTT (IV) SCr/CrCl	aPTT/ACT SCr/CrCl	aPTT/ACT Liver function
Clearance	Renal	Enzymatic (80%) Renal (20%)	Hepatic
Antibody development	Antihirudin antibodies in up to 40%–60% of patients	May crossreact with antihirudin antibodies	No
Effect on INR	Slight increase	Slight increase	Increase
Initial dose for HIT	HITTS: Bolus[a]: 0.4 mg/kg, up to a maximum of 110 kg, given over 15 to 20 seconds Infusion: 0.15 mg/kg/h HIT: no bolus; 0.1 mg/kg/h infusion	No bolus Infusion: 0.15 mg/kg/h	No bolus Infusion: 2 mcg/kg/min[b] In critically ill patients: consider lower infusion rate of 0.5–1 mcg/kg/min
Initial dose for PCI	NA	Bolus: 0.75 mg/kg Infusion: 1.75 mg/kg/h	NA
Dosing in renal impairment	Bolus[a]: 0.2 mg/kg (bolus dose is best avoided in patients with renal impairment) Infusion: CrCl 45–60: 0.075 mg/kg/h CrCl 30–44: 0.045 mg/kg/h CrCl 15–29: 0.0225 mg/kg/h CrCl <15 mg/kg/h: no bolus; avoid or stop infusion HD: stop infusion and additional IV bolus doses of 0.1 mg/kg every other day should be considered if the aPTT ratio falls below 1.5	PCI: Bolus: no dose adjustment Infusion: CrCl <30: 1 mg/kg/h HD: 0.25 mg/kg/h HIT: No bolus Infusion: CrCl <30: 0.08 mg/kg/h HD: 0.02 mg/kg/h	CrCl <30 mg/kg/h: mean doses of 0.8 mcg/kg/min have been reported Note: Dose adjustment not required per product information but recent literature support dose adjustment as above
Dosing in hepatic impairment	Dose adjustment not required	Dose adjustment not required	Initiate at 0.5 mcg/kg/min then titrate to aPTT 1.5–3.0 × baseline

[a]Initial IV bolus ONLY recommended when life-threatening thrombosis is present.
[b]Recent reports indicate that lower initial infusion rates of ~1.5 mcg/kg/min may be more appropriate.
ACT, activated clotting time; aPTT, activated partial thromboplastin time; BID, twice daily; CrCl, creatinine clearance; GPI, glycoprotein IIb-IIIa inhibitor; HD, hemodialysis; HIT, heparin induced thrombocytopenia; HITTS, heparin induced thrombocytopenia and thrombosis syndrome; IV, intravenous; PCI, percutaneous coronary intervention; PTCA, percutaneous transluminal coronary angioplasty; SC, subcutaneous; SCr, serum creatinine; UA, unstable angina.

coronary intervention (see Chapter 18, Acute Coronary Syndrome).

Dabigatran is a new oral direct thrombin inhibitor, approved for stroke prevention in patients with atrial fibrillation.[9] It has also been investigated for prevention and treatment of venous thromboembolism. Unlike warfarin (see subsequent section), dabigatran is given at a fixed dose without the need for routine coagulation monitoring or dosing adjustments.[10] In patients with atrial fibrillation, a dose of 150 mg twice daily is used if creatinine clearance (CrCl) is >30 mL/minute, and lowered to 75 mg twice daily for CrCl 15 to 30 mL/minute. The drug is not recommended for use in patients with CrCl less than 15 mL/minute. Dabigatran is administered as a prodrug, dabigatran etexilate, which is rapidly converted to the active compound by hydrolysis, and then eliminated renally. Its elimination half-life is 14 hours in patients with normal renal function, and increases to greater than 27 hours in patients with severe renal impairment, due to its high degree of renal eliminination. The gastric absorption of dabigatran is moderated by P-glycoprotein (PGP), and thus inducers and inhibitors of PGP may respectively decrease and increase its serum concentrations. However, because dabigatran is not metabolized by cytochrome P-450 (CYP) enzymes, it is not susceptible to CYP-mediated drug interactions.

A number of other oral direct thrombin inhibitors are being investigated as alternative options to warfarin for stroke prevention in atrial fibrillation, prevention, and treatment of venous thromboembolism, acute coronary sydromes, and other indications. Should these agents, including rivaroxaban and apixaban, be approved by the US Food and Drug Administration (FDA), they will represent additional options for patient care, and many new opportunities for pharmacist involvement in drug selection, patient education, and long-term therapeutic management.

WARFARIN

Warfarin is an oral anticoagulant with a delayed onset of effect that acts as a vitamin K antagonist. Vitamin K is essential for the conversion (carboxylation) of precursors to clotting factors II, VII, IX, and X into inactive clotting factors and for the synthesis

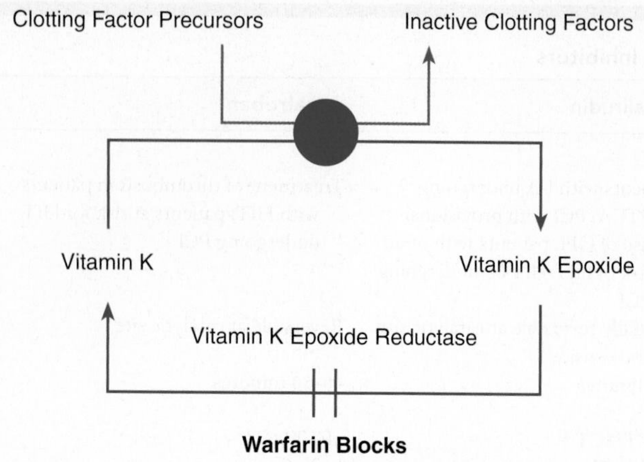

FIGURE 16-3 Mechanism of action of warfarin.

of the naturally occurring anticoagulants, protein C and protein S. During factor conversion, vitamin K is oxidized to inactive vitamin K epoxide (Fig. 16-3). In the nonanticoagulated patient, vitamin K epoxide is in reversible equilibrium with vitamin K, but this equilibrium is disrupted in patients taking oral vitamin K antagonists. Warfarin interferes with the hepatic recycling of vitamin K by inhibiting vitamin K epoxide reductase (VKOR), the enzyme that converts vitamin K epoxide to vitamin K.[11] The accumulation of vitamin K epoxide reduces the effective concentration of vitamin K and reduces the synthesis of coagulation factors. Concentrations of clotting factors II, VII, IX, and X are diminished gradually at rates commensurate with their elimination half-lives (Table 16-5). Thus, the onset of the anticoagulant effect of warfarin is delayed. It takes approximately 5 to 7 days to reach a steady state of anticoagulation after warfarin therapy is initiated or after dosing changes. Protein C and its cofactor protein S are also vitamin-K–dependent, and these proteins are depleted by warfarin at rates dependent on their elimination half-lives.

Warfarin is rapidly and completely absorbed in the upper gastrointestinal (GI) tract by passive diffusion, with nearly 100% bioavailability. Peak absorption of warfarin occurs in 60 to 120 minutes. It is approximately 99% bound to serum albumin. The volume of distribution for warfarin is 12.5% of body weight. This small volume of distribution is consistent with the extensive binding of warfarin to albumin. The primary laboratory test for monitoring warfarin therapy is the prothrombin time (PT). No correlation appears to exist between PT and the dose of warfarin, the total warfarin concentration, or the free warfarin concentration for any population of treated patients, although in individual patients an increasing dose of warfarin will increase the serum concentration (free and total) and the PT.

TABLE 16-5
Elimination Half-lives of Vitamin-K–Dependent Clotting Factors

Clotting Factor	Half-Life (hours)
II	42–72
VII	4–6
IX	21–30
X	27–48
Protein C	9
Protein S	60

Warfarin is administered orally as a racemic mixture containing equal parts of the enantiomers R(+)-warfarin and S(–)-warfarin. The S(–)-isomer is 2.7 to 3.8 times more potent as an anticoagulant than the R(+)-isomer, has a longer elimination half-life, and is primarily metabolized by CYP2C9. Comparatively, R(+)-warfarin is metabolized by primarily by CYP1A2 and CYP3A4. Many drugs interact with warfarin by stereoselectively inhibiting the metabolism of either the R(+)-isomer or the S(–)-isomer (see Drug Interactions section).

Genetic expression of CYP2C9 influences the rate of metabolism of warfarin and thus impacts dosing requirements to meet a particular therapeutic end point.[12] Variability in genetic expression of VKORC1 (the C1 subunit on the gene that codes for VKOR) also influences dosing requirements in patients taking warfarin. Genetic testing for CYP2C9 genotype and VKORC1 haplotype can be incorporated with clinical and demographic information to predict warfarin dose requirements in individual patients, using dosing algorithms that have been developed and investigated. A practical example is available online at **www.warfarindosing.org.**

Tests Used to Monitor Antithrombotic Therapy

Before the initiation of antithrombotic therapy, an assessment of baseline hemostatic status is necessary. The clinician should obtain a baseline platelet count and hemoglobin (Hgb) and/or hematocrit (Hct), as well as evaluate the baseline integrity of the extrinsic and intrinsic coagulation pathways with PT and aPTT, the tests used to monitor warfarin and heparin, respectively.

PROTHROMBIN TIME/INTERNATIONAL NORMALIZED RATIO

The PT is prolonged by deficiencies of clotting factors II, V, VII, and X, as well as by low levels of fibrinogen and very high levels of heparin. It reflects alterations in the extrinsic and common pathways of the clotting cascade, but not in the intrinsic system.[13] The PT is measured by adding calcium and tissue thromboplastin to a sample of plasma from which platelets have been removed by centrifugation. The time to clot formation is detected by automated instruments using light-scattering techniques that measure optical density. The mean normal PT, obtained by averaging a number of PT results from nonanticoagulated subjects, is approximately 12 seconds for most reagents.

The thromboplastins used in PT monitoring are extracted from various tissue sources by a number of techniques and prepared for commercial use as reagents. Unfortunately, thromboplastins are not standardized among manufacturers or among batches of reagent produced by the same manufacturer, leading to significant variability in PT results for anticoagulated patients. To standardize PT results, the World Health Organization developed a system by which all commercially available thromboplastins are compared with an international reference thromboplastin and then assigned an international sensitivity index (ISI). This value is used to mathematically convert PT to the international normalized ratio (INR) by exponentially multiplying the PT ratio to the power of the ISI of the thromboplastin being used in the laboratory to measure the test:

$$INR = (\text{PT patient}/\text{PT mean normal})^{ISI} \quad \textit{(Eq. 16-1)}$$

The ISI of the international reference thromboplastin is 1.0.

The INR is the internationally recognized standard for monitoring warfarin therapy.[14] Current recommendations for intensity of oral anticoagulation therapy for accepted clinical indications are summarized in Table 16-6. Regular-intensity therapy

TABLE 16-6
Optimal Therapeutic Range and Duration of Anticoagulation

Indication	Target INR (Range)	Duration	Comment
Atrial Fibrillation/Atrial Flutter			
Age ≤75 years with no risk factors[a]	None	Chronic	Use aspirin 81–325 mg daily alone
With 1 risk factor	2.5 (2.0–3.0)	Chronic	Or aspirin 81–325 mg daily
With 2 or more risk factors	2.5 (2.0–3.0)	Chronic	
With mitral stenosis or prosthetic heart valve	2.5 (2.0–3.0)	Chronic	Or higher valve-specific goal INR
With prior history of stroke/TIA/systemic embolism	2.5 (2.0–3.0)	Chronic	
After open heart surgery (in NSR)	2.5 (2.0–3.0)	4 weeks	
Precardioversion (AF or flutter >48 hours)	2.5 (2.0–3.0)	3 weeks	
Postcardioversion (in NSR)	2.5 (2.0–3.0)	4 weeks	
Ischemic Stroke			
Non-cardioembolic stroke or TIA	None	Chronic	Use antiplatelet therapy
Cardioembolic stroke or TIA	2.5 (2.0–3.0)	Chronic	
• With contraindications to warfarin	None	Chronic	Use ASA 81–235 mg daily
• Associated with aortic atherosclerotic lesions	None	Chronic	Use antiplatelet therapy
• Associated with mobile aortic arch thrombi	2.5 (2.0–3.0)	Chronic	Or antiplatelet therapy
• Associated with patent foramen ovale	None	Chronic	Use antiplatelet therapy
Myocardial Infarction			
After MI	2.5 (2.0–3.0)	Up to 4 years	And aspirin 81 mg daily; or INR 3–4 alone
After MI in high-risk[b] patients	2.5 (2.0–3.0)	At least 3 months	And aspirin 81 mg daily
THROMBOEMBOLISM (DVT, PE)	**(With concurrent UFH/LMWH/fondaparinux for at least 5 days and until INR >2 for 24 hours)** *(for DVT, add elastic compression stockings with 30–40 mm Hg at ankle for 2 years)*		
Treatment/prevention of recurrence **(including calf vein DVT, UE DVT, UE DVT associated with catheter use, and asymptomatic DVT/PE)**			
• Transient risk factors	2.5 (2.0–3.0)	3 months	
• Unprovoked/first event			
~ Proximal DVT or PE	2.5 (2.0–3.0)	Chronic	
~ Distal DVT	2.5 (2.0–3.0)	3 months	Consider chronic therapy
• Unprovoked/second event	2.5 (2.0–3.0)	Chronic	
• With malignancy	2.5 (2.0–3.0)	Chronic	Preceded by LMWH × 3–6 months
Chronic thromboembolic pulmonary hypertension	2.5 (2.0–3.0)	Chronic	
Cerebral venous sinus thrombosis	2.5 (2.0–3.0)	Up to 12 months	
Spontaneous superficial vein thrombosis	2.5 (2.0–3.0)	4 weeks	Or prophylactic LMWH
Valvular Disease			
Mitral valve prolapse			
• With TIAs or ischemic stroke	None	Chronic	Use aspirin 81 mg daily
• With recurrent TIA despite ASA therapy	2.5 (2.0–3.0)	Chronic	
Mitral annular calcification with AF	2.5 (2.0–3.0)	Chronic	
Rheumatic mitral valve disease:			
• With AF, hx systemic embolism, LA thrombus, or LA >55 mm	2.5 (2.0–3.0)	Chronic	
• s/p thromboembolic event despite anticoagulation	2.5 (2.0–3.0)	Chronic	Add aspirin 81 mg daily or INR 2.5–3.5
Valve Replacement, Bioprosthetic			
Aortic	None	Chronic	Aspirin 81 mg daily alone
Mitral	2.5 (2.0–3.0)	3 months	Followed by aspirin 81 mg daily
With LA thrombus	2.5 (2.0–3.0)	Until resolution	
With prior history systemic embolism	2.5 (2.0–3.0)	At least 3 months	
With additional risk factors[c] for thromboembolism	2.5 (2.0–3.0)	Chronic	Add aspirin 81 mg daily if low bleed risk
Valve Replacement, Mechanical			
Aortic			
• Bileaflet in NSR w/nl LA size	2.5 (2.0–3.0)	Chronic	
• Medronic Hall tilting disk in NSR w/nl LA size	2.5 (2.0–3.0)	Chronic	
• After prosthetic valve thrombosis	3.5 (3.0–4.0)	Chronic	Plus aspirin 81 mg daily
Mitral			
• Bileaflet or tilting disk	3.0 (2.5–3.5)	Chronic	
• After prosthetic valve thrombosis	4.0 (3.5 – 4.5)	Chronic	Plus aspirin 81 mg daily
Caged ball or caged disk (aortic or mitral)	3.0 (2.5 – 3.5)	Chronic	
With additional risk factors[d] for thromboembolism	3.0 (2.5 – 3.5)	Chronic	Add aspirin 81 mg daily if low bleed risk
With systemic embolism despite adequate anticoagulation	Increase INR goal	Chronic	Or add aspirin 81 mg daily

[a] Risk factors: age >75 years; history of hypertension; diabetes; congestive heart failure or moderate/severe left ventricular dysfunction.
[b] Risk factors: anterior MI, significant heart failure, intracardiac thrombus, history of thromboembolism.
[c] Risk factors: AF, hypercoagulable condition, low ejection fraction.
[d] Risk factors: AF, MI, LA enlargement, hypercoagulable condition, low ejection fraction.
AF, atrial fibrillation; ASA, aspirin; CHF, congestive heart failure; DVT, deep vein thrombosis; hx, history; INR, international normalized ratio; LA, left artium; LMWH, low molecular weight heparin; MI, myocardial infarction; nl, normal; NSR, normal sinus rhythm; PE, pulmonary embolism; s/p, status post; TIA, transient ischemic attack; UE, upper extremity; UFH, unfractionated heparin.

is defined as dosing warfarin to reach a goal INR of 2.5 (range, 2.0–3.0) and is appropriate for most settings that require the prevention and/or treatment of thromboembolic disease. High-intensity therapy is used in mechanical valve replacement and certain situations of thromboembolic recurrence, despite adequate anticoagulation, and is defined as dosing warfarin to reach a goal INR of 3.0 (range, 2.5–3.5).

ACTIVATED PARTIAL THROMBOPLASTIN TIME

The aPTT reflects alterations in the intrinsic pathway of the clotting cascade and is used to monitor heparin therapy.[13,14] The test is performed by adding a surface-activating agent (kaolin or micronized silica), a partial thromboplastin reagent (phospholipid; platelet substitute), and calcium to the plasma sample. Mean normal values vary among reagents, but typically fall between 24 and 36 seconds.

Like PT, the aPTT is a highly variable test based on differences among commercially available partial thromboplastin reagents. However, a system equivalent to the INR has not been developed for standardization of aPTT results. Heparinization to prolong the aPTT to 1.5 to 2.5 times the mean normal value historically was considered adequate to prevent propagation or extension of thrombus, but is no longer recommended because it is not appropriate for all reagents and testing systems. Instead, the aPTT should be calibrated for each reagent lot and coagulometer, and a reagent-specific therapeutic range in seconds determined that corresponds to therapeutic heparin levels of 0.3 to 0.7 international units/mL by factor Xa inhibition (anti-Xa activity).[6,14]

Hospital-based and independent clinical laboratories that offer aPTT monitoring will report the reagent-specific therapeutic range in seconds, and adjust it as new reagents are purchased and used clinically.

ANTI-FACTOR XA ACTIVITY

Although LMWHs do not require coagulation monitoring to ensure an appropriate antithrombotic effect or to adjust dosing, certain clinical situations may require assessment of the anti-factor Xa activity of LMWHs.[14] Because these agents are eliminated renally, patients with renal failure may accumulate LMWHs, leading to an increased risk of hemorrhagic complications. Evaluation of trough anti-factor Xa activity at the end of the dosing interval can assess this accumulation of effect. LMWHs are dosed according to total body weight, but clinical trials have included only limited numbers of obese patients. Therefore, it may be appropriate to monitor anti-factor Xa activity in patients who weigh more than 150 kg. Anti-factor Xa activity may also be evaluated in patients who experience unexpected bleeding complications secondary to anticoagulation with LMWHs, and in pregnant patients in whom LMWHs are used for treatment or prevention of thrombosis.

Anti-factor Xa activity is measured using a chromogenic assay that is expensive and of limited availability. If peak activity levels are used to assess dosing in obese and pregnant patients, they should be obtained approximately 4 hours after a SC dose of LMWH, with empiric dosing adjustments to maintain a level of roughly 0.5 to 1.0 international units/mL for therapeutic anticoagulation.[6,15] However, there is little correlation between peak anti-factor Xa activity and therapeutic effect, and thus monitoring is not recommended. Trough anti-factor Xa levels are expected to be less than 0.5 international units/mL at the end of the dosing interval. Like other measures of hemostasis, results vary considerably, requiring both instrument-specific and method-specific determination of therapeutic ranges.

DEEP VENOUS THROMBOSIS

Clinical Presentation

SIGNS AND SYMPTOMS

CASE 16-1

QUESTION 1: L.R., a 76-year-old, overweight (92 kg, 6-foot tall) man, was admitted to the hospital 3 days ago for management of recurrent angina. He was started on a nitroglycerin drip and confined to bed rest with gradual increases in his oral antianginal medications. On the third day of hospitalization, he noted progressive swelling and soreness of the right calf. He denied shortness of breath (SOB), cough, or chest pain. His medical history includes coronary artery disease, MI at ages 55 and 67, and hypercholesterolemia. His medications are diltiazem CD 360 mg/day orally (PO), isosorbide mononitrate 120 mg/day PO, atenolol 50 mg/day PO, aspirin 81 mg/day PO, and simvastatin 20 mg PO every evening. Initial laboratory values include:

Hct, 36.5%
PT, 10.8 seconds (INR, 1.0)
aPTT, 23.6 seconds
Platelet count, 255,000/μL

What signs and symptoms demonstrated by L.R. are consistent with DVT?

Patients with DVT typically present with unilateral leg swelling that often is accompanied by warmth and local tenderness or pain.[1] A tender, cordlike entity caused by venous obstruction can sometimes be palpated in the affected area. L.R. presented with the sudden onset of swelling along with soreness, but without evidence of a cord. Discoloration of the affected limb, including pallor from arterial spasm, cyanosis from venous obstruction, or a reddish color from perivascular inflammation, may also occur. The presence or absence of a positive Homans sign (pain behind the knee or calf on dorsiflexion of the foot) is rarely helpful in making the diagnosis because it is present in only about 30% of patients with DVT. Many patients (>50%) can present with asymptomatic disease, but even asymptomatic patients can have long-term complications such as recurrent DVT or postthrombotic syndrome. Because symptoms of DVT are nonspecific, the diagnosis must be confirmed by objective testing.[16]

RISK FACTORS

CASE 16-1, QUESTION 2: What risk factors does L.R. exhibit that are associated with DVT?

The diagnosis of DVT depends not only on the presenting signs and symptoms but also on the presence of risk factors (Fig. 16-1). L.R. has presented with obesity and immobilization (i.e., prolonged bed rest), two important risk factors for thromboembolism, as well as an acute medical illness. It is common for more than one risk factor to be present in patients who exhibit DVT, and these factors are cumulative in their effect.[17]

DIAGNOSIS

CASE 16-1, QUESTION 3: How should the final diagnosis of DVT be made in L.R.?

After evaluation of the signs and symptoms of DVT and consideration of risk factors for the development of thrombus, a

TABLE 16-7

Clinical Model for Evaluating the Pretest Probability of Deep Vein Thrombosis[a]

Clinical Characteristic	Score
Active cancer (cancer treatment within previous 6 months, or currently on palliative treatment)	1
Paralysis, paresis, or recent plaster immobilization of the lower extremities	1
Recently bedridden for ≥3 days, or major surgery within the previous 12 weeks requiring general or regional anesthesia	1
Localized tenderness along the distribution of the deep venous system	1
Entire leg swollen	1
Calf swelling at least 3 cm larger than that on the asymptomatic side (measured 10 cm below tibial tuberosity)	1
Pitting edema confined to the symptomatic leg	1
Collateral superficial veins (nonvaricose)	1
Previously documented deep vein thrombosis	1
Alternative diagnosis at least as likely as deep vein thrombosis	−2

[a] Clinical probability of deep vein thrombosis: low, <0; moderate, 1–2; high, >3. In patients with symptoms in both legs, the more symptomatic leg is used.
Source: Wells PS et al. Value of assessment of pretest probability of deep-vein thrombosis in clinical management. *Lancet*. 1997;350:1795.

definitive diagnosis should be made. Diagnostic strategies should include an assessment of pretest clinical probability (clinical suspicion), D-dimer assay (an evaluation of the presence of fibrin degradation products, indicative of clot formation; see Chapter 2, Interpretation of Clinical Laboratory Tests), and noninvasive imaging tests.[16,18]

Despite its limitations as a single diagnostic tool, clinical assessment can improve the diagnostic accuracy of noninvasive testing. A clinical prediction rule, such as the Wells criteria, takes into account signs, symptoms, and risk factors to categorize patients as being at low, intermediate, or high probability of having DVT (Table 16-7).[19] The D-dimer test can be used in conjunction with clinical evaluation or a clinical prediction rule to help "rule out" DVT in patients with a low clinical suspicion, and thus decrease the need for imaging tests in these patients.[20] A D-dimer should not be tested if the clinical suspicion is high because diagnostic imaging is indicated in these patients.

The most common noninvasive test is duplex scanning, which combines B-mode imaging or color flow imaging with Doppler ultrasonography to visualize veins and thrombi while investigating flow patterns. Other noninvasive testing options include ^{125}I-fibrinogen leg scanning (injection of radiolabeled fibrinogen followed by scanning to detect areas of accumulation corresponding to thrombosis), impedance plethysmography (use of pneumatic cuffs to detect leg blood volume changes associated with thrombosis), and Doppler ultrasonography alone (use of a transducer to audibly detect venous flow changes indicative of thrombosis). Each option differs with respect to sensitivity, specificity, and cost. Venography (radiographic visualization of the involved vessels with injection of radiocontrast material), an invasive diagnostic test, is the most sensitive and specific method for diagnosis of DVT, but exposes patients to the risks associated with contrast material.

Treatment

BASELINE INFORMATION

CASE 16-1, QUESTION 4: What additional baseline data should be obtained before administering anticoagulants to L.R.?

In addition to assessing the integrity of the clotting process with platelet count, Hgb/Hct, PT, and aPTT, the patient's baseline renal function should also be evaluated and documented because some anticoagulants are renally eliminated. Baseline values are used for comparison with the parameters that will be used in monitoring both therapeutic and adverse effects of anticoagulant therapy.

INITIATION OF THERAPY

CASE 16-1, QUESTION 5: Duplex scanning reveals clot formation in L.R.'s right calf extending to the right thigh. He does not exhibit signs of PE. What is the appropriate therapy for L.R., and how should it be initiated?

Prompt and optimal anticoagulant therapy is indicated to minimize thrombus extension and its vascular complications, as well as to prevent PE. Treatment options include IV UFH therapy initiated with a loading dose followed by a continuous infusion, adjusted-dose SC UFH, SC LMWH, or SC fondaparinux.[21] Because L.R. currently is hospitalized, IV UFH is selected for initial treatment of his DVT. Although pharmacoeconomic analysis suggests that the use of LMWHs for the treatment of acute venous thromboembolism (VTE) are more cost effective than UFH, many health care systems consider drug costs alone in determining inpatient treatment guidelines, and UFH is less expensive than LMWH.[22]

HEPARIN

LOADING DOSE

CASE 16-1, QUESTION 6: L.R.'s medical resident ordered a heparin bolus dose of 5,000 international units IV, to be followed by a continuous infusion of 1,000 units/hour. Is this heparin dosing regimen appropriate?

A loading dose of heparin is required for several reasons. Based on pharmacokinetic principles, a therapeutic serum level will be achieved more quickly; thus, pharmacodynamic and therapeutic responses to help prevent progression of clot will occur rapidly. Second, a relative resistance to anticoagulation exists during the active clotting process. Therefore, a larger initial dose generally is necessary to achieve a therapeutic effect.

Although standardized doses of heparin for initiation of therapy (e.g., 5,000 units loading dose; 1,000-units/hour maintenance dose) were used historically, this approach can result in significant delays in reaching a therapeutic intensity of anticoagulation. Body weight represents the most reliable predictor of heparin dosing requirement. For patients weighing less than 100 kg, the use of the actual body weight (ABW) is recommended to calculate the initial UFH dose. In patients who weigh more than 100 kg, the use of the ABW is controversial, and the use of an adjusted-dosing weight is recommended by some experts.[23] Options include two different "dosing weight" calculations:

$$\text{Ideal Body Weight (IBW)} + 0.3 \times (\text{ABW} - \text{IBW}) \qquad \textit{(Eq. 16-2)}$$

or

$$\text{IBW} + 0.4 \times (\text{ABW} - \text{IBW}) \qquad \textit{(Eq. 16-3)}$$

Compared with standardized dosing, weight-based dosing (80 units/kg loading dose; 18 units/kg/hour initial infusion rate) increases the frequency of therapeutic aPTT at 6 hours and at 24 hours, and decreases the risk of recurrent VTE.[24–26]

Initial heparin loading doses of 70 to 100 units/kg followed by an infusion rate of 15 to 25 units/kg/hour are commonly recommended. Selection of the lower or upper dosage range is guided by the severity of the patient's symptoms and his or her potential sensitivity to adverse effects. For this 92-kg patient, a midrange loading dose of 7,400 units (92 kg × 80 units/kg), followed by a continuous infusion of 1,700 units/hour (92 kg × 18 units/kg/hour), is recommended. Loading doses are typically rounded to the nearest 500 units and maintenance infusion rates to the nearest 100 units for convenience of administration.

DOSE ADJUSTMENTS

CASE 16-1, QUESTION 7: The orders for L.R. were rewritten by his attending physician. Based on the data shown subsequently, explain the variability in laboratory results. (At this institution, aPTT values of 60–100 seconds correspond with heparin plasma concentrations of 0.3–0.7 unitls/mL determined by anti-factor Xa assay.)

Time	aPTT (seconds)	Heparin Dosage Order
0800	31 (baseline)	7,400 units bolus followed by 1,700 units/h infusion
0900	130	Hold infusion for 30 minutes, then to 1,500 units/h
1500	40	Rebolus with 2,400 units, then to 1,700 units/h
2100	85	Continue at 1,700 units/h; recheck aPTT every morning

Although the aPTT drawn 1 hour after the initiation of the maintenance infusion (9 AM) demonstrates excessive prolongation of the aPTT (130 seconds), this value is most likely explained by inappropriate timing of the test. When aPTT values are drawn too soon after a heparin bolus dose (i.e., before the maintenance infusion has achieved a steady-state concentration in serum), they are predictably very high, but are not associated with a bleeding risk and do not accurately reflect the anticipated level of anticoagulation in the patient. To ensure accuracy, the clinician should obtain aPTT values no sooner than 6 hours after a bolus dose or any change in the infusion rate. Even results obtained at 6 hours may be excessively prolonged in some patients because of the dose-dependent pharmacokinetic characteristics of heparin.

L.R.'s heparin dose was decreased at 0900 based on this prolonged, yet inappropriately timed, value. A repeat aPTT at 3 PM was only 40 seconds. The decrease in the dosage to 1,500 units/hour and the repeat aPTT of 40 seconds reflect near steady-state conditions because 6 hours have elapsed since the dosage change. Because the aPTT was subtherapeutic at 3 PM (40 seconds), administration of a smaller repeat bolus dose (2,000 units) and an increase in the maintenance infusion to 1,700 units/hour was the correct course of action. Subsequent aPTT values reflected therapeutic anticoagulation.

Dosing nomograms or protocols have been recommended for adjustment of heparin dosing based on aPTT results.[6,27] Nomogram-based dosing reduces the time to reach therapeutic range compared with empiric dosing.[27] After initiation based on patient weight, dosing adjustments may also be weight-based or may simply be made in international units per hour. A heparin dosing nomogram specific for a reagent with a therapeutic aPTT range of 60 to 100 seconds (and used in the adjustment of heparin doses for L.R.) is illustrated in Table 16-8.

Responses to changes in infusion rates of heparin are not always linear, and to some extent, heparin doses are adjusted by trial and error. As the patient's condition improves after several days and endothelialization of the clot occurs, heparin dosing requirements may decrease.

THERAPEUTIC MONITORING

CASE 16-1, QUESTION 8: How should L.R.'s heparin therapy be monitored?

Once baseline clotting parameters have been established and a loading dose of heparin has been administered, the aPTT should

TABLE 16-8
Heparin Dosing Nomogram[a]

1. Suggested loading dose
   - Treatment of DVT/PE: 80 units/kg (rounded to nearest 500 units)
   - Prevention, including cardiovascular indications: 70 units/kg (rounded to nearest 500 units)
2. Suggested initial infusion
   - Treatment of DVT/PE: 18 units/kg/h (rounded to nearest 100 units)
   - Prevention, including cardiovascular indications: 15 units/kg/h (rounded to nearest 100 units)
3. First aPTT check: 6 hours after initiating therapy
4. Dosing adjustments: per this chart (rounded to nearest 100 units)

aPTT[b] (seconds)	Heparin Bolus	Infusion Hold Time	Infusion Rate Adjustment	Next aPTT
<50	4,000 units	0	Increase by 200 units/h	In 6 hours
50–59	2,000 units	0	Increase by 100 units/h	In 6 hours
60–100	0	0	None	Every AM
101–110	0	0	Decrease by 100 units/h	In 6 hours
111–120	0	0	Decrease by 200 units/h	In 6 hours
121–150	0	30 minutes	Decrease by 200 units/h	In 6 hours
151–199	0	60 minutes	Decrease by 200 units/h	In 6 hours
>200	0	PRN	Hold until aPTT <100	Every hour until <100

[a] University of Washington Medical Center.
[b] Based on aPTT reagent-specific therapeutic range of 60–100 seconds corresponding to a plasma heparin concentration of 0.3–0.7 units/mL determined by anti-factor Xa activity.
aPTT, activated partial thromboplastin time; DVT, deep vein thrombosis; PE, pulmonary embolism; PRN, as necessary.

be measured routinely to guide subsequent dosing adjustments. The aPTT should be evaluated no sooner than 6 hours after the loading dose or after any changes in infusion rate, as noted previously. If dosing is stable, the aPTT should be evaluated once daily (Table 16-8).

Additional monitoring parameters for heparin therapy include evaluation for potential adverse reactions and possible therapeutic failure. The Hgb and/or Hct and a platelet count should be checked every 1 to 2 days. L.R. should be examined for signs of bleeding, as well as for signs and symptoms associated with thrombus extension and PE. Finally, if unusual or unexpected aPTT results are reported, the clinician should consider the possible influence of solution preparation errors (see Chapter 2, Interpretation of Clinical Laboratory Tests), infusion pump failure, infusion interruption, and administration or charting errors in the assessment of L.R.'s heparin therapy.[28]

DURATION OF THERAPY

CASE 16-1, QUESTION 9: How long should heparin therapy be continued in L.R.?

Adherence of a thrombus to the vessel wall and subsequent endothelialization usually takes 7 to 10 days. However, anticoagulation therapy must generally continue for 3 months to prevent recurrent thrombosis.[21] Warfarin is preferred for this long-term anticoagulation because it can be administered orally, and it is generally initiated on the same day as heparin. The long elimination half-life of warfarin and the long elimination half-lives of clotting factors II and X necessitate a prolonged period of overlap between warfarin and heparin. Therefore, heparin is continued for a minimum of 5 days and until the INR is greater than 2 for 24 hours. Heparin therapy should not be discontinued before at least 5 days, even if the INR is therapeutic before then, because of the time required for adequate elimination of factors II and X by warfarin and the time required to reach its full antithrombotic potential. Shortening the duration of heparin therapy is associated with an increased risk of recurrent thrombosis.

ADVERSE EFFECTS

CASE 16-1, QUESTION 10: On day 2 of heparin therapy, L.R.'s complete blood count reveals a platelet count of 180,000/μL, decreased from 255,000/μL at baseline. What is a reasonable explanation for this thrombocytopenia, and how should it be managed?

Thrombocytopenia

Thrombocytopenia induced by heparin has two distinct presentations.[8] Heparin-associated thrombocytopenia (HAT) occurs as a direct effect of heparin on platelet function, causing transient platelet sequestration and clumping with reductions in platelet count, but usually remaining greater than 100,000/μL. This reversible form of thrombocytopenia occurs within the first several days of heparin therapy. Patients remain asymptomatic, and platelet counts return to normal even when heparin therapy is continued. L.R.'s reduction in platelet count is somewhat modest and likely represents HAT. His platelet count should be monitored daily, and heparin therapy should be continued.

Reductions in platelet count of greater than 50% from baseline suggest the development of heparin-induced thrombocytopenia (HIT), a more severe immune-mediated reaction with a typical delay in onset of 5 to 10 days after the initiation of heparin therapy. In contrast, "immediate-onset" HIT can occur rapidly (within 24 hours of UFH initiation) in patients previously exposed to heparin. In addition, delayed-onset HIT has also been reported, where the development of thrombocytopenia begins several days after heparin has been stopped in patients naive to UFH.[29]

In the immune-mediated reaction, heparin binds to an IgG antibody to form a heparin–antibody complex that then binds to platelets, leading to significant platelet aggregation. The observed thrombocytopenia is the result of drug-induced platelet aggregation as opposed to platelet destruction or bone marrow suppression as seen in other forms of drug-induced thrombocytopenia. The diagnosis of immune-mediated HIT is made based on clinical findings supplemented by laboratory tests confirming the presence of antibodies to heparin or platelet activation induced by heparin.[8] The 4-T score is a pretest probability test that can be used to estimate the likelihood of HIT based on extent and timing of platelet count reduction, the presence of thrombus, and the possibility of other causes of thrombocytopenia (Table 16-9).[30]

The overall incidence of HIT is less than 3% after 5 days of UFH use, but the cumulative incidence can be as high as 6% after 14 days of continuous heparin use. HIT occurs more frequently with bovine lung heparin than with heparin derived from

TABLE 16-9
The 4T Score: Pretest Probability of Heparin-Induced Thrombocytopenia

Category	2 Points	1 Point	0 Points
1. Thrombocytopenia	Platelet count fall >50% and platelet nadir ≥20 × 10^9 L−1	Platelet count fall 30%–50% or platelet nadir 10–19 × 10^9 L−1	Platelet count fall <30% or platelet nadir <10 × 10^9 L−1
2. Timing of platelet count fall	Clear onset between days 5 and 10 or platelet fall ≤1 day (prior heparin exposure within 30 days)	Consistent with days 5–10 fall, but not clear (e.g., missing platelet counts) or onset after day 10 or fall ≤1 day (prior heparin exposure 30–100 days ago)	Platelet count fall <4 days without recent heparin exposure
3. Thrombosis or other sequelae	New thrombosis (confirmed) or skin necrosis at heparin injection sites or acute systemic reaction after intravenous heparin bolus	Progressive or recurrent thrombosis or nonnecrotizing (erythematous) skin lesions or suspected thrombosis (not proven)	None
4. Other causes for thrombocytopenia	None apparent	Possible	Definite

TOTAL SCORE <3 = low probability of HIT 4–5 = intermediate probability of HIT >6 = high probability of HIT.
Source: Lo GK et al. Evaluation of pretest clinical score (4 T's) for the diagnosis of heparin-induced thrombocytopenia in two clinical settings. *J Thromb Haemost*. 2006;4:759.

porcine gut mucosa, and also with prolonged IV UFH use versus SC UFH.[8,29] Despite its low incidence, HIT is a life-threatening condition with high morbidity and mortality. Platelet aggregation secondary to HIT can lead to significant venous and arterial thrombosis, as well as thromboembolic stroke, acute MI, and skin necrosis. Amputation is necessary in up to 25% of patients, and mortality approaches 25% to 30%.

In patients who develop HIT, heparin therapy should be stopped immediately, and treatment with an alternative anticoagulant should be initiated.[8,29] Although associated with a lower risk of HIT (<1%) than UFH, LMWH products are contraindicated in patients with HIT because of a high incidence of immunologic cross-reactivity with heparin.[8] The future use of heparin in patients with HIT, especially in the first 3 months after the diagnosis, should be avoided. Treatment options include the direct thrombin inhibitors argatroban, lepirudin, and bivalirudin, although only the first two are approved for this indication by the FDA. The dose of lepirudin and argatroban should be titrated based on aPTT testing, and both are administered by IV infusion. Although some clinicians prefer argatroban because it has a shorter half-life and lower cost when compared to lepirudin, both agents are considered equally suitable for the initial treatment of HIT. Bivalirudin also appears to be a promising alternative for the treatment of HIT due to its short-half life, low immunogenicity, minimal effect on INR, and enzymatic metabolism. Various patient-related factors (such as the presence of renal or hepatic dysfunction; prior exposure to lepirudin; and drug availability, cost, and institutional preference) should be used to select the most appropriate agent[8,31] (Table 16-4).

CASE 16-1, QUESTION 11: On day 3 of heparin therapy, L.R.'s Hct has dropped from a baseline of 36.5% to 29%, and the patient noted blood in his commode after urination. Describe an approach to evaluate and interpret this event.

Hemorrhage

Bleeding is the most common adverse effect associated with heparin. A summary of eight studies reporting heparin-associated bleeding found the absolute frequency of fatal, major, and all (major or minor) bleeding to be 0.4%, 6%, and 16%, respectively.[32] The corresponding average daily frequencies were 0.05% for fatal bleeding, 0.8% for major bleeding, and 2% for major or minor bleeding; cumulative risk increased with the duration of therapy. The most common sites for heparin-associated bleeding are soft tissues, the GI and urinary tracts, the nose, and the oral pharynx. The use of different criteria to define major versus minor bleeding accounts for much of the variability in reported frequency of bleeding among studies.

In addition to length of therapy, many factors influence the risk of bleeding during heparinization, including advanced age, serious comorbid illnesses (heart disease, renal insufficiency, hepatic dysfunction, cerebrovascular disease, malignancy, and severe anemia), and concomitant antithrombotic therapy.[33] The incidence of UFH-associated bleeding complications is minimal with SC prophylactic doses, but higher (2%–4%) with therapeutic doses given via IV infusion. Soft tissue bleeding commonly occurs at sites of recent surgery or trauma. Previously undiagnosed abnormalities, including malignancy and infection, may be identified in some patients with GI or urinary tract bleeding associated with heparin therapy.

The influence of the intensity of heparinization on bleeding risk is controversial. Although an elevated aPTT has historically been considered a risk factor for bleeding complications, several investigators have been unable to substantiate a relationship between supratherapeutic aPTT values and hemorrhagic effects.[33] In addition, bleeding episodes can occur when coagulation test results are within the therapeutic range. These conflicting results may be explained in part by the influence of additional risk factors for bleeding and by the effect of heparin on platelet function and vascular permeability.

L.R. has developed hematuria despite an acceptable intensity of anticoagulation. He should be questioned and examined for the presence of nose bleeding (epistaxis), increased tendency to bruise (ecchymosis), bright red blood in the stool (hematochezia), black or tarry stool (melena), or coughing up of blood (hemoptysis). Blood pressure and pulse, both sitting and standing, should be obtained to determine whether orthostasis representing blood loss is present. A thorough evaluation of the urinary tract may reveal a previously unknown abnormality that will explain the bleeding episode. Although his concurrent low-dose aspirin therapy may increase the risk of minor bleeding complications, aspirin therapy would not be discontinued due to his history of coronary artery disease and MI.

CASE 16-1, QUESTION 12: What other side effects of heparin should be considered in L.R.?

Osteoporosis

The development of osteoporosis has been associated with administration of more than 20,000 international units/day of heparin for 6 months or longer.[34] Various mechanisms have been suggested, but the underlying pathophysiology of this rare adverse effect remains unclear. Affected patients may present with bone pain and/or radiographic findings suggestive of fractures. The possibility of osteoporosis should be considered in patients receiving long-term, high-dose heparin therapy such as pregnant patients, post-menopausal women, and elderly patients.

Hyperkalemia

Although rare, hyperkalemia has been attributed to heparin-induced inhibition of aldosterone synthesis. Hypoaldosteronism leading to hyperkalemia has been described with both high-dose and low-dose heparin therapy, may occur as quickly as within 7 days after initiation of heparin therapy, and appears to be reversible after discontinuation of heparin.[6] Patients with diabetes or chronic kidney disease may be at greatest risk.

Hypersensitivity Reactions

Other rarely occurring adverse effects associated with heparin include generalized hypersensitivity reactions, such as urticaria, chills, fever, rash, rhinitis, conjunctivitis, asthma, and angioedema, as well as priapism and a reversible temporal alopecia.[6]

REVERSAL OF EFFECT

CASE 16-2

QUESTION 1: P.B. is a 64-year-old woman with DVT. On day 4 of heparin therapy, she received 25,000 units of heparin during a 1-hour period as a result of an infusion pump malfunction. The infusion was stopped and within 30 minutes, she became diaphoretic and hypotensive. Bright red blood was evident on rectal examination, and a large retroperitoneal mass was noted. How should the excessive heparin effect be reversed?

P.B. has definite signs of hemorrhage from the GI tract, a site of bleeding associated with considerable mortality. Heparin should be discontinued immediately, and treatment should

TABLE 16-10
Dosing of Low-Molecular-Weight Heparin and Fondaparinux for the Treatment of Venous Thromboembolism

Dalteparin	Enoxaparin	Tinzaparin	Fondaparinux
100 international units/kg SC every 12 hours OR 200 international units/kg SC every 24 hours	1 mg/kg SC every 12 hours OR 1.5 mg/kg SC every 24 hours	175 international units/kg SC every 24 hours	5 mg SC every 24 hours if weight <50 kg 7.5 mg SC every 24 hours if weight 50–100 kg 10 mg SC every 24 hours if weight >100 kg

SC, subcutaneously.

include maintenance of fluid volume and replacement of clotting factors with whole blood, fresh frozen plasma, or clotting factor concentrates. If hemorrhage had not been present and the only manifestation of overdose had been a prolonged aPTT, administration of heparin simply could have been discontinued, permitting the effects to clear within a few hours.

Protamine can be used to neutralize heparin by forming an inactive protamine–heparin complex.[35] Protamine has a rapid onset of action, with effects lasting about 2 hours. Protamine sulfate is infused slowly over 3 to 5 minutes, as a 1% solution at a dose of 1 mg for each 100 international units of heparin administered, but only if it is given within 30 minutes of discontinuation of heparin administration. The maximum single recommended dose of protamine is 50 mg, but doses may be repeated if bleeding persists. If protamine therapy is delayed, dosing should be based on the estimated amount of heparin remaining, taking into consideration the elimination half-life of heparin. Response to protamine therapy can be assessed by a return of the aPTT to baseline. Adverse effects associated with protamine include systemic hypotension secondary to rapid administration; anaphylaxis characterized by edema, bronchospasm, and cardiovascular collapse; and catastrophic pulmonary vasoconstriction[36] (see Chapter 3, Anaphylaxis and Drug Allergies).

OUTPATIENT TREATMENT OF DVT

CASE 16-3

QUESTION 1: H.K. is a 44-year-old woman who presents to the emergency department (ED) complaining of right calf pain of 1 day's duration. She denies trauma to the calf, but reveals that she has just returned to the United States from Australia on a lengthy flight. She has no significant medical history, has no family history of clotting disorders, and takes no medications. A duplex ultrasound is positive for DVT, and immediate anticoagulation is indicated. What therapeutic alternative to hospitalization for IV UFH is available for this patient?

Historically, inpatient administration of UFH was the initial treatment of choice for acute DVT. However, LMWHs and fondaparinux have emerged as more convenient and practical treatment alternatives to UFH.[21] These agents, administered SC and without the need for routine coagulation monitoring, allow patients to be treated at home. In addition, meta-analysis data suggest that LMWH therapy for acute VTE results in fewer deaths, major hemorrhages, and recurrent VTE when compared to UFH.[37] Based on these advantages, outpatient use of LMWH has become the most common approach to treatment of uncomplicated DVT. Home treatment is safe and effective and improves the overall physical and social functioning of patients being treated for DVT.[38] The drug costs associated with LMWH treatment are much higher than the costs of IV UFH, but overall costs to health care systems are significantly reduced when patients can be treated at home rather than in the hospital.[39,40] Fondaparinux can also be considered as an alternative treatment as it has been shown to be as effective and safe as LMWH in the treatment of DVT.[41] Additionally, one study supports the efficacy of weight-based SC UFH (initial dose of 333 international units/kg followed by 250 international units/kg every 12 hours) without routine aPTT monitoring for the treatment of acute VTE.[42] The use of weight-based, unmonitored SC UFH has the potential to simplify the way acute VTE is treated and should be less costly than LMWHs. Vials of UFH at a concentration of 20,000 international units/mL are used by the pharmacy or the patient to draw up the weight-based dose. Although routine aPTT monitoring is not necessary, platelet count monitoring during the first two weeks is required to evaluate the possible development of HIT.

For H.K. to be treated at home with LMWH, she or a family member must be willing and able to administer SC injections, and she must be able to return for frequent follow-up visits, particularly during the first few weeks while warfarin therapy is initiated. In addition, her health care insurance should cover the cost of the drug, or she must be able to pay out of pocket. Contraindications to home treatment of DVT include a pre-existing condition that requires hospitalization, clinical symptoms of PE and/or hemodynamic instability, recent or active bleeding, and end-stage renal disease.

H.K. meets the eligibility requirements for home treatment and is interested in self-injection of LMWH at home for initial treatment of DVT. Possible treatment options and doses for H.K. are listed in Table 16-10. However, most institutional formularies carry only a single LMWH product, with formulary decisions based on FDA-approved indications and clinical data supporting use for treatment and prevention of thromboembolism in various settings, as well as cost. In this case, enoxaparin is the LMWH available for use. The usual dosing of enoxaparin for treatment of DVT is 1 mg/kg total body weight SC every 12 hours, rounded to the nearest 10-mg increment. Once-daily dosing, at 1.5 mg/kg SC every 24 hours is also an option, but this strategy is inferior to twice-daily dosing in patients with malignancy or obesity.[43]

Because LMWHs are eliminated renally, patients with significant renal impairment require dose reductions to prevent drug accumulation and to minimize the risk of bleeding complications.[44] The degree of drug accumulation can vary between the various LMWH preparations, thus specific guidelines for dose adjustments are agent-specific (Table 16-11).[45] Some experts suggest monitoring of anti-factor Xa activity to rule out accumulation of LMWHs in patients with renal impairment.[45,46] Fondaparinux is also renally excreted and is contraindicated in patients with creatinine clearance less than 30 mL/minute. Data with the use of LMWH and fondaparinux for the prevention and treatment of VTE in patients on hemodialysis are lacking; thus, UFH is the recommended treatment option in these patients.

TABLE 16-11

Dosing of Low-Molecular-Weight Heparins in Patients With Renal Impairment (CrCl < 30 mL/min)[a]

LMWH	Dalteparin	Enoxaparin	Tinzaparin
Product information recommendations	Use with caution	Prophylaxis—30 mg SC daily Treatment—1 mg/kg SC daily	Use with caution
Dosing suggestions based on agent-specific pharmacokinetic observations	CrCL <30[a] mL/min: no dose adjustment needed up to 1 week with prophylactic doses For use longer than 1 week, consider monitoring of anti-Xa activity and adjust dose if accumulation is noted CrCL 30–50 mL/min: no dose adjustment needed	CrCL <30[a] mL/min: Consider a 40%–50% dose decrease and subsequent monitoring of anti-Xa activity CrCL 30–50 mL/min: Consider a 15%–20% dose decrease with prolonged use (longer than 10–14 days) and subsequent monitoring of anti-Xa activity	CrCL <30[a] mL/min: consider a dose decrease of 20% and subsequent monitoring of anti-Xa activity CrCL 30–50 mL/min: no dose adjustment needed

[a] In patients with a CrCl <20 mL/min, data are very limited and use of unfractionated heparin is suggested.

CASE 16-3, QUESTION 2: What systems must be in place for H.K.'s home treatment to be successful? What is the role of the pharmacist or other caregiver in her therapy?

H.K. should be weighed to determine her dose of enoxaparin. Because she is not obese and does not have a malignancy, a 1.5 mg/kg dose once daily can be considered for convenience of administration. Dosing is typically rounded to the nearest 10 mg based on the availability of prefilled syringes. At 64 kg, H.K. will receive 100 mg SC every 24 hours. Warfarin therapy is initiated concurrently to expedite the conversion to oral treatment.

H.K. must be taught to self-administer enoxaparin by SC injection. Patient education resources, including videotaped instructions and written materials, should supplement hands-on instruction. H.K. will administer the first dose of enoxaparin in the ED with the assistance of a pharmacist. She should also be given prescriptions for enoxaparin and warfarin that must be filled immediately at the pharmacy of her choice.

For a video showing how to administer a subcutaneous injection, see http://thepoint.lww.com/AT10e. NOTE: Anticoagulants given by SC injection should be administered only into the abdomen; the thigh, upper arm, and other areas should not be used because of a high risk of bruising at these sites.

H.K. should be instructed regarding the potential adverse effects of LMWH therapy (bleeding, thrombocytopenia, pain and bruising at the injection site), required laboratory monitoring, and the expected duration of anticoagulation. At baseline, Hgb and/or Hct, INR, serum creatinine (SCr), and platelet count should be determined. Platelets will continue to be monitored at least every 2 to 3 days while the patient is receiving LMWH therapy, to a maximum of 10 to 14 days. H.K. can expect to continue enoxaparin therapy for a minimum of 5 days. If by day 5 her INR is therapeutic and stable, enoxaparin can be discontinued. Oral anticoagulation with warfarin should be continued for 3 months.[21]

To ensure the safety and efficacy of home treatment, H.K. should be provided with the names and telephone numbers of the health care providers who will assume responsibility for her care, including her primary physician and her anticoagulation management team. No patient should be sent home with LMWH without an adequate follow-up plan.

Prevention of Venous Thromboembolism

CASE 16-4

QUESTION 1: D.F., a 63-year-old obese woman, is to undergo elective abdominal surgery for treatment of diverticulitis. She has a medical history significant for hypertension, currently controlled by enalapril 10 mg daily (blood pressure, 135/85 mm Hg), and peripheral arterial disease. What therapeutic interventions might decrease the risk of DVT or PE in D.F.?

Surgical procedures represent a significant risk factor for DVT formation. However, all hospitalized patients, including both surgical and nonsurgical/medical patients, should be stratified for risk of VTE based on the presence of various factors.[17,47,48] Risk stratification is used to select the most appropriate therapeutic interventions to prevent DVT, and thereby reduce the risk of fatal PE. These interventions include both mechanical and pharmacologic strategies.

NONPHARMACOLOGIC MEASURES

Mechanical interventions aimed at preventing venous stasis and increasing venous return include the use of elastic compression stockings, as well as leg elevation, leg exercises, and early postoperative ambulation. Intermittent pneumatic compression (IPC) of the leg muscles, using inflatable cuffs applied to the calf and thigh, represents another alternative for the prevention of DVT.[17] Because it is generally less effective than pharmacologic prophylaxis, mechanical prophylaxis is most commonly used in patients at high risk of bleeding, or as an adjunct to pharmacologic prophylaxis in patients at very high risk for VTE.

PHARMACOLOGIC MEASURES

Fixed, low-dose unfractionated heparin (LDUFH), administered as 5,000 units SC every 8 to 12 hours depending on the indication, is an inexpensive and effective pharmacologic approach to DVT prevention in the setting of venous stasis in patients with acute medical illness, or after certain surgical procedures. Because LDUFH inactivates factor Xa without a direct effect on factor IIa, the aPTT is not prolonged, and therefore aPTT monitoring is unnecessary. Bleeding complications are minimized using this dosing regimen.

Fixed-dose SC LMWH and fondaparinux are alternative approaches for preventing DVT. Enoxaparin 30 mg SC every 12 hours or 40 mg SC once daily, dalteparin 2,500 to 5,000

TABLE 16-12
Prevention of Venous Thromboembolism[17]

General Surgery	
Low-risk patients undergoing minor procedures, with no additional risk factors	Early and frequent ambulation
Moderate-risk patients undergoing major procedures for benign disease	LMWM, LDUFH every 8–12 hours, or fondaparinux
Higher-risk patients undergoing major procedures for cancer	LMWH, LDUFH every 8 hours, or fondaparinux
High-risk patients with multiple risk factors	LMWH , LDUFH every 8 hours, or fondaparinux + GCS and/or IPC
Gynecologic Surgery	
Minor procedures, with no additional risk factors	Early and frequent ambulation
Laparoscopic surgery with additional VTE risk factors	LMWH, LDUFH every 8–12 hours, IPC or GCS
Major surgery for benign disease and no other risk factors	LMWH, LDUFH every 8–12 hours, or IPC
Major surgery for malignancy, or additional VTE risk factors	LMWH, LDUFH every 8 hours or IPC; or LDUFH/LMWH + IPC or GCS or fondaparinux
Urologic Surgery	
Low-risk procedures	Early and frequent ambulation
Major open procedures	LDUFH every 8–every 12 hours, GCS and/or IPC, LMWH, fondaparinux, or pharmacologic method + GCS and/or IPC
Orthopedic Surgery	
Hip replacement	LMWH daily OR BID, fondaparinux, or warfarin (INR 2–3)
Knee replacement	LMWH BID, fondaparinux, or warfarin (INR 2–3)
Hip fracture surgery	Fondaparinux, LMWH BID, or warfarin (INR 2–3)
Trauma	LMWH BID + IPC and/or GCS
Acute spinal cord injury	LMWH BID or LMWH/LDUFH + IPC/GCS
Neurosurgery	IPC/GCS ± LDUFH every 12 hours, or LMWH daily
Acutely medically ill	LDUFH every 8–12 hours or LMWH

BID, twice daily; GCS, graduated compression stockings; INR, international normalized ratio; IPC, intermittent pneumatic compression; LDUFH, low-dose unfractionated heparin (5,000 international units subcutaneously every 8–12 hours); LMWH, low-molecular-weight heparin (enoxaparin 40 mg subcutaneously daily or 30 mg SC every 12 hours; dalteparin 2,500–5,000 international units subcutaneously daily); fondaparinux (2.5 mg subcutaneously daily); VTE, venous thrombolembolism.

international units SC once daily, and fondaparinux 2.5 mg SC once daily are effective strategies, although enoxaparin has been studied for a larger number of indications. Current recommendations for prevention of VTE based on risk stratification are presented in Table 16-12.[17]

D.F. is at high risk for DVT and PE, not only because of general surgery but also because of her age (older than 40 years) and the presence of other risk factors for VTE (obesity, peripheral arterial disease, and probable postoperative immobilization). Options for DVT prevention include SC heparin at 5,000 international units every 8 hours or a LMWH (enoxaparin 40 mg SC daily, or dalteparin 2,500 international units initial dose followed by 5,000 international units SC daily). The first dose should be administered several hours preoperatively, and dosing should continue postoperatively until she is fully ambulatory. If bleeding risk is of concern, IPC could be used as an alternative. VTE prophylaxis is typically continued until hospital discharge, but may be continued for up to 30 days in certain high-risk populations, including patients with cancer, orthopedic surgery, bariatric surgery, or with a prior history of VTE.

PULMONARY EMBOLISM

Clinical Presentation

CASE 16-5

QUESTION 1: D.J. is a 38-year-old, 70-kg man. Several days ago, he developed a swollen left calf, which was painful and warm. This swelling gradually increased, affecting the entire left leg to the groin, and prompting him to seek medical attention. In the ED, he also notes the recent onset of right-sided pleuritic chest pain without SOB or hemoptysis. His medical history includes a gastric ulcer 4 years ago, treated with proton pump inhibitor therapy, that has not recurrured. Physical examination reveals an enlarged left leg and mild to moderate tenderness in the entire leg. Chest examination reveals a loud, pulmonary heart sound (P2). Vital signs include blood pressure, 150/85 mmHg; heart rate, 100 beats/minute; and respiratory rate, 28 breaths/minute and regular. Laboratory data include the following:

Hct, 26.7%
SCr 1.1 mg/dL
Arterial blood gases (on room air) Po_2, 72 mm Hg (normal, 75–100)
Pco_2, 30 mm Hg (normal, 35–45)
pH 7.48 (normal, 7.35–7.45)

The chest radiograph and lung scan (ventilation-perfusion [V/Q] scan) are highly suggestive of PE. An angiogram was not performed. The electrocardiogram (ECG) shows sinus tachycardia. The venogram is positive for defects in the ileofemoral vein. Coagulation test results include the following:

PT, 11.2 seconds (INR, 1.0)
aPTT, 28 seconds
Platelet count, 248,000/μL

What subjective and objective evidence in D.J. is consistent with PE?

SIGNS AND SYMPTOMS

The clinical diagnosis of PE is often difficult to make because of the nonspecificity of symptoms.[49] The most commonly observed subjective symptoms are dyspnea, pleuritic chest pain, apprehension (anxiety or a feeling of impending doom), and cough. Hemoptysis occurs occasionally. The objective signs most commonly observed are tachypnea at a rate of greater than or equal to 20 breaths/minute, tachycardia of greater than or equal to 100 beats/minute, accentuated pulmonary component of the second heart sound (P2), and rales. DVT precedes PE in 80% or more of patients. A combination of these signs and symptoms provides further evidence for acute PE. D.J. has presented with pleuritic chest pain, tachycardia, tachypnea, loud P2, and a decrease in Po_2; therefore, he may have developed PE.

DIAGNOSIS

Because the clinical signs and symptoms of PE are difficult to distinguish from many other medical conditions, further evaluation is necessary.[49,50] Chest radiograph, ECG, and arterial blood gas (alveolar-arterial oxygen gradient) abnormalities are often present in patients with PE, but like clinical signs and symptoms, they are somewhat nonspecific. Although pulmonary angiography has been considered the gold standard for diagnosis of PE, it is an invasive procedure that is expensive and technically difficult to perform. In addition, the contrast material used can be toxic or irritating, and some patients are unable to tolerate the procedure. Noninvasive tests such as V/Q lung scans, computed tomography (CT) and magnetic resonance imaging (MRI) scans are useful and the most frequently used diagnostic procedures to document the presence of PE. Lung scans that incorporate an assessment of perfusion, or regional distribution of pulmonary blood flow, and ventilation are referred to as V/Q scans; they involve both the injection and the inhalation of radiolabeled compounds. Test results are expressed as a high, intermediate, or low probability of PE. When ventilation (air movement) is normal over an area that shows abnormal perfusion (blood flow), a V/Q mismatch exists, and PE is highly probable. If a matched defect is noted (abnormal ventilation over an area of abnormal perfusion), another disease state, such as chronic obstructive airway disease, is more likely.

As in the case of DVT, clinical assessment can improve the diagnostic accuracy of noninvasive tests such as CT, MRI, or V/Q scanning. Validated assessment tools can be used to stratify patients into high, moderate, and low probability of a PE[50,51] (Table 16-13). In patients with a low clinical probability of PE, measuring a high-sensitivity D-dimer can be considered, and, if negative, PE can be ruled out eliminating the need of further imaging studies.[52] In patients with a moderate to high clinical probability of PE, diagnostic imaging studies should be performed.

A positive lung scan (D.J. had one highly suggestive of PE) or other test would confirm the presence of a PE. If the results of the clinical assessment and the noninvasive scan are discordant, pulmonary angiography can be performed to aid in making the definitive diagnosis. Nonetheless, when the diagnosis of PE is suspected, anticoagulation should be initiated immediately while awaiting results of more definitive diagnostic procedures. Mortality associated with PE has been documented to be as high as 17.5% over 3 months.[53]

TABLE 16-13

Clinical Model for Evaluating the Pretest Probability of Pulmonary Embolism[a]

Clinical Characteristic	Score
Cancer	+1
Hemoptysis	+1
Previous PE or DVT	+1.5
Heart rate >100 beats/min	+1.5
Recent surgery or immobilization	+1.5
Clinical signs of DVT	+3
Alternative diagnosis less likely than PE	+3

[a] Clinical probability of PE: low, 0–1; moderate, 2–6; high, ≥7.
DVT, deep vein thrombosis; PE, pulmonary embolism.
Source: Wells PS. Advances in the diagnosis of venous thromboembolism. *J Thromb Thrombolysis*. 2006;21:31.

Treatment

CASE 16-5, QUESTION 2: What anticoagulant strategy should be initiated for D.J.?

Treatment options for PE include IV UFH therapy initiated with a loading dose followed by a continuous infusion, or a LMWH or fondaparinux administered by SC injection.[21] UFH therapy could be started in D.J. with a loading dose of 5,600 units (80 international units/kg × 70 kg), followed by continuous infusion of 1,300 units/hour (18 units/kg/hour × 70 kg). Monitoring of the aPTT would be used to adjust dosing to maintain treatment within the therapeutic range (Table 16-8).

The alternative to UFH for treatment of PE is the use of a SC LMWH[21,54] or SC fondaparinux[21,55] (Table 16-10). D.J. could receive fixed-dose enoxaparin 70 mg SC every 12 hours (1 mg/kg every 12 hours × 70 kg) or dalteparin 15,000 international units SC every 24 hours (200 international units/kg, rounded to nearest syringe size). Generally, PE is not treated on an outpatient basis except in selected low-risk patients.[56] In this case, LMWH or fondaparinux would be used during the complete hospital course, or only for partial outpatient therapy in selected lower-risk and stable patients who may be discharged early.

The use of thrombolytic therapy should be reserved for patients with acute massive embolism, who are hemodynamically unstable (systolic blood pressure <90 mm Hg) and at low risk for bleeding.[21]

WARFARIN

TRANSITION FROM INJECTABLE ANTICOAGULANT THERAPY

CASE 16-5, QUESTION 3: When should warfarin be administered, and how should the transition from injectable anticoagulant therapy be accomplished?

As in the treatment of DVT, the use of heparin, LMWH, or fondaparinux therapy for PE should be continued for at least 5 days and until warfarin therapy is therapeutic for at least 24 hours. Warfarin should be started on the first day of hospitalization and continued for 3 months, or longer if indicated. However, a delay in the initiation of warfarin may be acceptable in the setting of an anticipated extended hospitalization, recent or anticipated surgery or other invasive procedures, or a medical condition with the potential for uncontrolled bleeding.[21]

There are several reasons to overlap heparin/LMWH/fondaparinux and warfarin therapy.[57] The onset of warfarin activity depends not only on its inherent pharmacokinetic characteristics (half-life >36 hours), but also on the rate of elimination of circulating clotting factors. Although warfarin inhibits production of the vitamin-K–dependent clotting factors, previously synthesized clotting factors must be eliminated at rates that correspond with their elimination half-lives (Table 16-5). Approximately four half-lives are required for these factors to reach a new steady state after their production is inhibited, so the effect of warfarin can be delayed for several days. Initial increases in the INR reflect only reductions in factor VII activity, but full anticoagulation with warfarin requires adequate suppression of factors II and X, which have significantly longer elimination half-lives. By overlapping a quick onset anticoagulant such as heparin or LMWH with warfarin therapy, adequate anticoagulation can be continued with heparin/LMWH/fondparinux until warfarin therapy reaches a therapeutic intensity.

In addition to suppressing the synthesis of the vitamin-K–dependent clotting factors, warfarin also inhibits the formation of the naturally occurring anticoagulant protein C and its cofactor, protein S. In patients with congenital protein C or protein S deficiency, initial warfarin therapy can suppress these proteins to concentrations that may result in hypercoagulability with possible thrombus extension, unless concurrent heparin therapy provides adequate anticoagulation. To prevent these complications, heparin/LMWH/fondaparinux and warfarin therapy should overlap.

Heparin therapy has been observed to prolong the INR,[58] and warfarin can prolong the aPTT by several seconds.[59] Thus, interference with laboratory tests should be considered in the evaluation of the intensity of anticoagulation during the overlap of heparin and warfarin therapy.

INITIATION OF WARFARIN THERAPY

CASE 16-5, QUESTION 4: In an effort to discharge D.J. from the hospital as soon as possible, an initial dose of warfarin 10 mg PO every evening for 3 days has been ordered. Is such a "loading dose" reasonable? What are more effective approaches to initiation therapy?

Initiation of warfarin dosing is complex because dosing requirements vary significantly among individuals. Daily doses as low as 0.5 mg and as high as 20 mg or more may be required in individual patients to reach a therapeutic INR.[60] Two primary methods for initiation of warfarin therapy are used.[61] The average daily dosing method relies on an understanding that although dosing requirements for warfarin vary significantly among patients, an average dosing requirement of 4 to 5 mg/day of warfarin is necessary to maintain an INR of 2.0 to 3.0 in most patients. When average daily dosing is used for initiation of warfarin therapy, patients are typically started at 4 to 5 mg daily, with dosing adjustments as necessary until the therapeutic goal is reached. However, patients who may be more sensitive to the effects of warfarin (Table 16-14) are expected to require lower dosages of warfarin. In these patients, therapy should be initiated at 1 to 3 mg daily, with subsequent dosing adjustments as necessary. Several dosing algorithms, using a 4-mg to 5-mg initiation dose, have been developed to aid with dosing decisions after the first few doses of warfarin have been administered.[62–64] Another popular dosing algorithm used a 10-mg initiation dose for the first 2 days, with the INR on day 3 used to guide dosing on days 3 and 4, and the INR on day 5 used to guide the next three doses[65] (Fig. 16-4). Although using this dosing algorithm helps

TABLE 16-14
Factors That Increase Sensitivity to Warfarin

Age older than 75 years
Clinical congestive heart failure
Clinical hyperthyroidism
Decreased oral intake
Diarrhea
Drug–drug interactions
Elevated baseline INR
End-stage renal disease
Fever
Hepatic disease
Hypoalbuminemia
Known CYP2C9 variant
Malignancy
Malnutrition
Postoperative status

INR, international normalized ratio.

Day-3 INR	Days/dose (mg) 3	4	Day-5 INR	Days/dose (mg) 5	6	7
<1.3	15	15	<2.0	15	15	15
1.3–1.4	10	10	2.0–3.0	7.5	5	7.5
			3.1–3.5	0	5	5
			>3.5	0	0	2.5
1.5–1.6	10	5	<2.0	7.5	7.5	7.5
1.7–1.9	5	5	2.0–3.0	5	5	5
			3.1–3.5	2.5	2.5	2.5
			>3.5	0	2.5	2.5
2.0–2.2	2.5	2.5	<2.0	15	5	5
2.3–3.0	0	2.5	2.0–3.0	2.5	5	2.5
			3.1–3.5	0	2.5	0
			>3.5	0	0	2.5
>3.0	0	0	<2.0	2.5	2.5	2.5
			2.0–3.0	2.5	0	2.5
			3.1–4.0	0	2.5	0
			>4.0	0	0	2.5

FIGURE 16-4 Warfarin initiation dosing algorithm based on starting with 10-mg doses on days 1 and 2. (Source: Kovacs MJ et al. Prospective assessment of a nomogram for the initiation of oral anticoagulant therapy for outpatient treatment of venous thromboembolism. *Pathophysiol Haemost Thromb.* 2002;32:131.)

achieve a therapeutic INR more quickly than using a 5-mg initial dose, these findings may not the generalizable to all patient populations because the patients evaluated were relatively healthy, young outpatients.[66] The 10-mg initiation dose may lead to overanticoagulation and heightened bleeding risk in elderly and ill patients with multiple medical problems.[67] Average daily dosing is often used to initiate therapy in ambulatory patients; in this case, the first INR should be evaluated within 3 to 5 days of initiation of warfarin therapy. In hospitalized patients, it is more common to evaluate the INR daily during initiation of therapy.

Flexible initiation of warfarin is an alternative approach for starting therapy that is based on evaluating the rate of increase in the INR and making daily dosing adjustments based on daily INR evaluation, with a goal of determining the eventual maintenance dosing requirement. A popular flexible initiation nomogram is presented in Table 16-15.[68,69] Using this nomogram, warfarin can be initiated with either a 10-mg or a 5-mg starting dose, with daily dosing adjustments based on the rate of increase in the INR. Flexible initiation does not necessarily shorten the time to reach the goal INR, and initiating therapy with a 10-mg dose as described in some protocols may be associated with an increased risk of early overanticoagulation in certain patients. Nonetheless, these methods offer a more individualized approach to initiation of therapy.

The baseline INR for D.J. was 1.0. Using the flexible initiation protocol presented in Table 16-15, the first dose of warfarin should be 10 mg administered in the evening on the first day of hospitalization. Subsequent INR values obtained daily will guide dosing requirements until a therapeutic INR is reached. The order for warfarin 10 mg orally every evening for three doses should be discontinued and replaced with daily orders for warfarin and INR monitoring.

INTENSITY AND DURATION OF THERAPY

CASE 16-5, QUESTION 5: What is the goal INR for D.J., and how long should anticoagulation be administered?

TABLE 16-15
Flexible Initiation Dosing Protocol for Warfarin Dosing, Including 10-mg and 5-mg Starting Dose Options

Day	INR	10-mg Initiation Dose (mg)	5-mg Initiation Dose (mg)
1		10	5
2	<1.5	7.5–10	5
	1.5–1.9	2.5	2.5
	2.0–2.5	1.0–2.5	1–2.5
	>2.5	0	0
3	<1.5	5–10	5–10
	1.5–1.9	2.5–5	2.5–5
	2.0–2.5	0–2.5	0–2.5
	2.5–3.0	0–2.5	0–2.5
	>3.0	0	0
4	<1.5	10	10
	1.5–1.9	5–7.5	5–7.5
	2.0–3.0	0–5	0–5
	>3.0	0	0
5	<1.5	10	10
	1.5–1.9	7.5–10	7.5–10
	2.0–3.0	0–5	0–5
	>3.0	0	0
6	<1.5	7.5–12.5	7.5–12.5
	1.5–1.9	5–10	5–10
	2.0–30	0–7.5	0–7.5
	>3.0	0	0

INR, international normalized ratio.
Source: Crowther MA et al. Warfarin: less may be better. *Ann Intern Med.* 1997;127:332.

In patients with DVT or PE, warfarin doses that prolong the PT to an INR of 2.0 to 3.0 are defined as regular intensity therapy. This therapeutic range is recommended to maximize the antithrombotic effect of warfarin while minimizing potential bleeding complications associated with excessive anticoagulation.[11]

Once formed, venous clots adhere to the blood vessel wall. Thus, the first step in resolution of a thrombus involves covering the clot with a layer of endothelial cells to prevent additional platelet aggregation at the site of vessel injury. This endothelialization process generally takes 7 to 10 days to be completed. Initial anticoagulant treatment is used to prevent clot extension while allowing adequate endothelialization to occur. Continued anticoagulation prevents further clotting.

The appropriate duration of warfarin therapy is based on the likelihood of a recurrent venous thromboembolic event and the risk of bleeding in each patient (Table 16-16). Patients with unprovoked (idiopathic) DVT or PE, as in the case of D.J., should be treated for at least 3 months, but considered for indefinite therapy as their likelihood of having a recurrent event can be as high as 30% over 5 years.[21] Patients with DVT or PE associated with transient or reversible risk factors (provoked VTE) are usually treated for 3 months, as the risk of recurrence is lower (approximately 10% over 5 years). Cancer-associated thrombosis is first treated with LMWH for 3 to 6 months, followed by long term oral anticoagulant therapy.

ADVERSE EFFECTS

CASE 16-5, QUESTION 6: What possible adverse effects from warfarin therapy should be considered in D.J., and how should they be monitored?

TABLE 16-16
Duration of Anticoagulation Therapy in Patients with Venous Thrombosis (Deep Vein Thrombosis and/or Pulmonary Embolism)

First Event	
Provoked	3 months
Unprovoked	At least 3 months; reevaluate risk–benefit at 3 months
Unprovoked with proximal presentation and low risk of bleeding	indefinite therapy
Cancer-associated	LMWH for 3–6 months, then indefinite therapy or until cancer is resolved
Recurrent Events	
Provoked	Indefinite therapy
Unprovoked	Indefinite therapy

Source: Kearon C et al. Antithrombotic therapy for venous thromboembolic disease: American College of Chest Physicians Evidence-Based Clinical Practice Guidelines (8th Edition) [published correction appears in *Chest.* 2008;134:892]. *Chest.* 2008;133(Suppl 6):454S.

Hemorrhage

Bleeding is the most common adverse effect associated with warfarin. A summary of experimental and observational inception cohort studies determined that the average annual frequency of fatal, major, and all (major or minor) bleeding in patients treated with warfarin was 0.6%, 3%, and 9.6%, respectively.[32] However, wide variation in bleeding frequencies has been reported, probably because of differences in patient characteristics, treatment protocols, and the definition and assessment of bleeding among trials.

Warfarin-associated bleeding most commonly occurs in the nose, oral pharynx, and soft tissues, followed by the GI and urinary tracts. Hemarthrosis (bleeding into joint spaces) and retroperitoneal and intraocular bleeding represent less common hemorrhagic complications of warfarin therapy.[33] As with heparin, GI and urinary tract bleeding associated with warfarin is often caused by previously undiagnosed lesions. Menstrual blood flow may be increased and prolonged in women taking anticoagulants. This problem may be clinically significant if there is an underlying pathological condition (ovarian cysts, uterine fibroids, or polyps) resulting in abnormal vaginal bleeding.

Although it is uncommon, intracranial bleeding resulting in hemorrhagic stroke represents the most common cause of fatal bleeding associated with warfarin therapy. Rates of intracranial hemorrhage associated with anticoagulants have been estimated to range from 0.3% to 2%, and up to 60% are fatal.[33]

Many factors influence the risk of hemorrhagic complications associated with warfarin. The frequency of bleeding is higher in the first 3 months of therapy than during subsequent months.[70] Unlike heparin, the intensity of anticoagulation with warfarin directly influences the risk of bleeding, including intracranial hemorrhage.[71] Other patient-specific variables that influence the risk of warfarin-associated bleeding include a history of GI bleeding; serious comorbid disease (including malignancy); and concomitant therapy with aspirin, clopidogrel, or nonsteroidal anti-inflammatory drugs (NSAIDs).[33]

The influence of age on bleeding risk is controversial. Older patients are known to require lower dosages of warfarin than younger patients to reach a therapeutic intensity of anticoagulation.[72] Inherent vitamin K deficiency or age-related differences in stereoisomeric disposition of warfarin may explain why older patients are more sensitive to the effects of warfarin and, therefore, require lower dosages than younger patients. This increased sensitivity to the effect of warfarin is not the result of differences in pharmacokinetic characteristics of warfarin between older and young patients, including protein binding and metabolism. It is also not related to sex, weight, underlying medical conditions, or the presence of interacting drugs.

Whether age alone is an independent risk factor for bleeding remains controversial.[72] In two studies in which comprehensive anticoagulation monitoring and follow-up were provided through anticoagulation management services, elderly patients did not experience an increased incidence of major bleeding.[73,74] However, other reports suggest that advanced age is linked to an increased risk of warfarin-related intracranial hemorrhage, even when patients are managed in an anticoagulation clinic setting.[71]

Hemorrhagic risk assessment can be used to predict bleeding risk during anticoagulant therapy. A popular bleeding index scoring system assigns level of risk based on the presence of age older than 65 years, history of GI bleeding, history of stroke, and one or more of four comorbid conditions: recent MI, anemia (Hct <30 mg/dL), renal insufficiency (SCr >1.5 mg/dL), and diabetes.[75] When validated prospectively in an anticoagulation clinic population, the risk of major bleeding low-risk, intermediate-risk, and high-risk patients was 0.8%/patient-years, 2.5%/patient-years, and 10.6%/patient-years, respectively.[76] The bleeding index can be useful in making decisions about management of drug interactions, overanticoagulation, bridge therapy for invasive procedures, and other issues that may present during anticoagulant therapy.

Bleeding complications in D.J. can be minimized by careful attention to the signs and symptoms of bleeding by the patient and his caregivers, maintenance of the INR within the therapeutic range, avoidance of therapy with concomitant drugs known to increase the risk of bleeding or to increase the INR, and routine outpatient follow-up for INR monitoring and clinical assessment.

Skin Necrosis

Warfarin-induced skin necrosis is a rare but serious adverse effect of oral anticoagulation, occurring in approximately 0.01% to 0.1% of patients treated with warfarin.[77] Patients present within 3 to 6 days of the initiation of warfarin therapy with painful discoloration of the breast, buttocks, thigh, or penis. The lesions progress to frank necrosis with blackening and eschar. Skin necrosis appears to be the result of extensive microvascular thrombosis within subcutaneous fat and has been associated with hypercoagulable conditions, including protein C or protein S deficiency. In these patients, rapid depletion of protein C before depletion of vitamin K–dependent clotting factors during early warfarin therapy can result in an imbalance between procoagulant and anticoagulant activity, leading to initial hypercoagulability and thrombosis. Adequate heparinization during initiation of warfarin can prevent the development of early hypercoagulability.

Warfarin therapy should be discontinued in patients who develop skin necrosis. However, subsequent warfarin therapy is not necessarily contraindicated if it is required for treatment or prevention of thromboembolic disease. In patients with protein C or protein S deficiency and a history of skin necrosis, warfarin therapy can be restarted at low dosages as long as therapeutic heparinization has been achieved. Therapy is maintained until the INR has been within the therapeutic range for 72 hours. Supplementation of protein C through administration of fresh frozen plasma also may be indicated.

Purple Toe Syndrome

Purple toe syndrome is a rarely reported adverse effect that typically occurs 3 to 8 weeks after the initiation of warfarin therapy and is unrelated to intensity of anticoagulation.[78] Patients initially present with painful discoloration of the toes that blanches with pressure and fades with elevation. The pathophysiology of this syndrome has been related to cholesterol microembolization from atherosclerotic plaques, leading to arterial obstruction. Because cholesterol microembolization has been associated with renal failure and death, warfarin therapy should be discontinued in patients who develop purple toe syndrome.

PATIENT EDUCATION

CASE 16-6

QUESTION 1: B.H. is a 30-year-old woman newly diagnosed with idiopathic DVT. Before anticoagulation is initiated, appropriate laboratory tests are drawn to evaluate the possibility of a hypercoagulable state. She will be treated as an outpatient with dalteparin 200 international units/kg SC daily and started on warfarin 4 mg PO daily using average daily dosing initiation. Her primary care physician would like her to receive follow-up care in the medical center's pharmacist-managed anticoagulation clinic. What are the benefits of formal anticoagulation management services?

One of the keys to successful oral anticoagulant therapy is appropriate outpatient management. In comparison with routine medical care, management of warfarin therapy by anticoagulation clinics is associated with significant reductions in bleeding and thromboembolic complications, with reductions in the rates of warfarin-related hospital admissions and ED visits, and with outcome-based cost savings for health care organizations.[79,80] Pharmacist-managed anticoagulation clinics offer many benefits for the management of anticoagulation therapy, including improved dosing regulation, continuous patient education, early identification of risk factors for adverse events, and timely intervention to avoid or minimize complications. B.H.'s referral to a pharmacist-managed anticoagulation clinic is likely to improve her overall satisfaction with care and to improve her clinical outcomes.

The availability of portable INR self-testing devices also allows the option of anticoagulation monitoring in the home setting. Patient self-testing of INRs has been shown to result in comparable outcomes to high-quality anticoagulation delivered via anticoagulation clinics.[11] For patients that may prefer this monitoring method, a structured education and follow-up program should be designed and integrated with the patient's provider or the anticoagulation management service.

CASE 16-6, QUESTION 2: At her initial visit to the anticoagulation clinic, B.H. will receive extensive education about her warfarin therapy. What information should be conveyed to her by her anticoagulation provider to ensure the safety and efficacy of warfarin therapy?

Successful warfarin therapy depends on the active participation of knowledgeable patients.[11] The anticoagulant effect of warfarin is influenced by various factors, and fluctuations in the intensity of the anticoagulant effect of warfarin can increase the risk of both hemorrhagic complications and recurrent thromboembolism. Pharmacists and other providers can improve adherence to the medication schedule, as well as ensure the safety and efficacy of warfarin therapy, by providing appropriate education to patients treated with this agent.

Key elements that form the basis of a thorough patient education program for warfarin therapy are listed in Table 16-17. This information may be conveyed through written teaching materials, videotaped instruction, individual or group discussion, or a combination of these approaches. Many useful educational tools

TABLE 16-17
Key Elements of Patient Education Regarding Warfarin

Identification of generic and brand names
Purpose of therapy
Expected duration of therapy
Dosing and administration
Visual recognition of drug and tablet strength
What to do if a dose is missed
Importance of prothrombin time/INR monitoring
Recognition of signs and symptoms of bleeding
Recognition of signs and symptoms of thromboembolism
What to do if bleeding or thromboembolism occurs
Recognition of signs and symptoms of disease states that influence warfarin dosing requirements
Potential for interactions with prescription and over-the-counter medications and natural/herbal products
Dietary considerations and use of alcohol
Avoidance of pregnancy
Significance of informing other health care providers that warfarin has been prescribed
When, where, and with whom follow-up will be provided

INR, international normalized ratio.

are available from the manufacturers of warfarin, and from other non-commercial sources.

B.H. should receive extensive education about warfarin therapy in an individual teaching session or an organized education program. A wallet card, medical bracelet, or alternative method of identifying her as a patient treated with warfarin should be provided. The health care provider who assumes responsibility for her outpatient warfarin therapy will need to provide continuing reinforcement of the essential elements of medication information at each follow-up visit.

FACTORS THAT INFLUENCE WARFARIN DOSING

CASE 16-6, QUESTION 3: After receiving 6 days of dalteparin therapy and six doses of warfarin 4 mg/day PO, B.H.'s INR is 2.4. Dalteparin is discontinued, and B.H. is instructed to continue her current dosage of warfarin. She is scheduled to return to the anticoagulation clinic in 1 week for re-evaluation. At that time, her INR is 1.7. What factors might account for this change in the intensity of anticoagulation?

Patients should always be questioned about their understanding of the prescribed dose and their adherence to the prescribed regimen. Questions might include, "What dose of the medication have you been taking?", "What time of the day do you take your medication?", and "How many times in the last week did you miss a dose of your medication?" If there is no evidence of misunderstanding of the correct dose or of noncompliance, numerous other factors should be considered that are known to influence warfarin dosing requirements in individual patients during both initiation and maintenance phases of therapy. Changes in dietary vitamin K intake, underlying disease states and clinical condition, alcohol ingestions, genetic factors, and concurrent medications can significantly change the intensity of therapy, resulting in the need for dosing adjustments to maintain the INR within the therapeutic range.

Dietary Vitamin K Intake

The two primary sources of vitamin K in humans are the biosynthesis of vitamin K_2 (menaquinone) by intestinal bacteria and dietary intake of vitamin K_1 (phytonadione). The US recommended daily allowance for vitamin K is 70 to 140 mcg/day, and the typical Western diet provides approximately 300 to 500 mcg/day.[81] Vitamin K is found in high concentrations in certain foods, including green leafy vegetables (asparagus, broccoli, Brussels sprouts, cabbage, cauliflower, chickpeas, collard greens, endive, kale, lettuce, parsley, spinach, and turnip greens), soy milk, certain oils, certain nutritional supplements, and multiple vitamin products. Green tea and chewing tobacco are other significant sources of vitamin K.

Variations in vitamin K intake have been linked to INR fluctuations in patients taking warfarin.[82,83] In addition, diets high in vitamin K content have been associated with acquired warfarin resistance, defined as excessive warfarin dosing requirements to reach a therapeutic INR range.[84] Numerous cases have also been reported in which patients previously stabilized with warfarin experienced elevations in INR with or without hemorrhagic complications when dietary sources of vitamin K were eliminated. Conversely, reductions in INR with or without thromboembolic complications have been reported in patients in whom dietary sources of vitamin K have been added.

These data illustrate the potential clinical significance of dietary changes in patients taking warfarin. To minimize these potential effects, B.H. should be counseled to maintain a consistent intake of dietary vitamin K.[85] Her final warfarin maintenance dose will be partially influenced by her typical diet. However, restriction of dietary vitamin K intake is unnecessary, except in cases of significant resistance to the anticoagulant effect of warfarin. B.H. should be aware of the types of foods and supplements that contain large quantities of vitamin K, and should be counseled to maintain a consistent diet, to avoid bingeing with foods high in vitamin K content, and to report significant dietary changes to her health care provider. Appropriate assessment and follow-up are essential to prevent hemorrhagic or thromboembolic complications that may arise from changes in INR resulting from dietary alterations.

Underlying Disease States and Clinical Conditions

The presence or exacerbation of various medical conditions can also influence anticoagulation status[61] (Table 16-18). Diarrhea-associated alterations in intestinal flora can reduce vitamin K absorption, resulting in elevations in INR. Fever enhances the catabolism of clotting factors and can increase INR. Heart failure, hepatic congestion, and liver disease can also cause significant elevations in INR because of a reduction in warfarin metabolism. End-stage renal disease is associated with decreased CYP2C9 activity, resulting in lower warfarin dose requirements.

Thyroid function can influence warfarin therapy significantly. Hypothyroidism decreases the catabolism of certain clotting factors, increasing their availability and producing a relative refractoriness to warfarin therapy. This results in the need for increased dosages to reach a therapeutic INR. The addition of thyroid supplementation in these patients reverses the influence of hypothyroidism and can lead to significant elevations in INR unless the warfarin dose is reduced. Conversely, hyperthyroidism increases the catabolism of clotting factors, leading to an increased sensitivity to warfarin. Frequent monitoring of and adjustments in warfarin therapy are necessary in patients with changing thyroid function.

Acute physical or psychological stress has been reported to increase INR. Increased physical activity has also been reported to increase the warfarin dosing requirement. Smoking can induce CYP1A2, which may increase warfarin metabolism in certain patients, resulting in increased dose requirements. Due to its high vitamin K content, chewing smokeless tobacco can suppress the INR response.

TABLE 16-18
Warfarin Interactions With Disease States and Clinical Conditions

Clinical Condition	Effect on Warfarin Therapy
Advanced age	Increased sensitivity to warfarin due to reduced vitamin K stores and/or lower plasma concentrations of vitamin K–dependent clotting factors
Pregnancy	Teratogenic; avoid exposure during pregnancy
Lactation	Not excreted in breast milk; can be used postpartum by nursing mothers
Alcoholism	• Acute ingestion: inhibits warfarin metabolism, with acute elevation in INR • Chronic ingestion: induces warfarin metabolism, with higher dose requirements
Liver disease	• May induce coagulopathy by decreased production of clotting factors, with baseline elevation in INR • May reduce clearance of warfarin
Renal disease	Reduced activity of CYP2C9, with lower warfarin dose requirements
Heart failure	Reduced warfarin metabolism due to hepatic congestion
Cardiac valve replacement	Enhanced sensitivity to warfarin postoperatively due to hypoalbuminemia, lower oral intake, decreased physical activity, and reduced clotting factor concentrations after cardiopulmonary bypass
Nutritional status	Changes in dietary vitamin K intake (intentional or as the result of disease, surgery, etc.) alter response to warfarin
Use of tube feedings	Decreased sensitivity to wafarin, possibly caused by changes in absorption or vitamin K content of nutritional supplements
Thyroid disease	• Hypothyroidism: decreased catabolism of clotting factors requiring increased dosing requirements • Hyperthyroidism: increased catabolism of clotting factors causing increased sensitivity to warfarin
Smoking and tobacco use	• Smoking: may induce CYP1A2, increasing warfarin dosing requirements. • Chewing tobacco: may contain vitamin K, increasing warfarin dosing requirements
Fever	Increased catabolism of clotting factors, causing acute increase in INR
Diarrhea	Reduction in secretion of vitamin K by gut flora, causing acute increase in INR
Acute infection/inflammation	Increased sensitivity to warfarin
Malignancy	Increased sensitivity to warfarin by multiple factors

INR, international normalized ratio.
Source: Wittkowsky AK. Warfarin. In: Murphy J (ed). *Clinical Pharmacokinetics* (5th ed). Bethesda, MD: American Society of Health System Pharmacists; 2011:345.

Thorough education of patients taking warfarin should include detailed attention to recognizing the signs and symptoms of changes in underlying disease states and clinical conditions that can influence warfarin dosing requirements. They should be instructed to contact their anticoagulation management program whenever changes occur that might influence INR and warfarin dose requirement.

Alcohol Ingestion

Chronic alcohol ingestion has been associated with induction of the hepatic enzyme systems that metabolize warfarin. Therefore, warfarin dosing requirements are sometimes higher in alcoholic patients. Conversely, acute ingestion of large amounts of alcohol can slow warfarin metabolism through competitive inhibition of metabolizing enzymes, leading to elevations in INR and an increased risk of bleeding complications.[85] Despite some reports linking low amounts of alcohol to an elevated INR,[86] in general it is believed that moderate intake of alcoholic beverages is not associated with alterations in the metabolism or the therapeutic effect of warfarin as measured by INR. Patients taking warfarin should be educated to limit their alcohol consumption to less than one to two alcoholic beverages per day. Chronic drinkers should be counseled to limit their drinking and maintain a regular pattern to avoid fluctuations in INR.[85] B.H. does not need to abstain from drinking alcoholic beverages in moderation, but she should be counseled to avoid the sporadic ingestion of large amounts of alcohol.

Conversely, alcoholic liver disease (i.e., cirrhosis) can alter multiple hemostatic mechanisms and reduces production of hepatic clotting factors. Decreased production and clearance of vitamin K–dependent clotting factors accounts for prolonged PT and INR often seen in these patients. Therefore, an increased response to warfarin would be expected in patients with liver impairment. Worsening liver function is also a predictor for bleeding complications and patients with end-stage liver disease are at increased risk of bleeding. Before instituting warfarin therapy in these patients, the risks of bleeding associated with both the underlying liver disease and warfarin therapy must be weighed against the benefit of preventing thromboembolic events. If warfarin is indicated, the best approach would be to use a cautious initiation and dose titration approach by starting with lower doses and titrate up slowly to goal. Small increases in dosage should be made, if indicated, recognizing that the full effect of any dose adjustment may be delayed in patients with severe liver dysfunction. Monitoring for bleeding complications is essential, even at goal INR ranges, when warfarin is used in patients with liver dysfunction.

Genetic Factors

CYP2C9 genotype[12,87] and VKORC1 haplotype[12,88] have been shown to correlate with the dose of warfarin required for effective anticoagulation. Dosing algorithms that incorporate CYP2C9 genotype and VKORC1 haplotype along with other patient characteristics to predict warfarin maintenance doses are being tested. A comparison of various dose prediction methods (empiric initiation, regression equation accounting for various clinical factors, suggested dosing from the warfarin package insert based on genomic information, mean dosing requirements based on genotype, and regression equation based on genomic and clinical factors) found that the percentage of patients whose predicted doses were within 20% of their stable therapeutic doses were 37%, 39%, 43%, 44%, and 52%, respectively.[89] The long-term utility of genetic-based warfarin dosing prediction methods is not yet clear. Importantly, these methods do not replace the need for routine coagulation monitoring with INR, and dose adjustments based on INR results.

CASE 16-6, QUESTION 4: How should B.H. be assessed and evaluated at this clinic appointment?

At each clinic visit, B.H. should be assessed for signs and symptoms of bleeding, and for signs and symptoms of clot progression and/or recurrence. Regardless of the INR result, all factors that

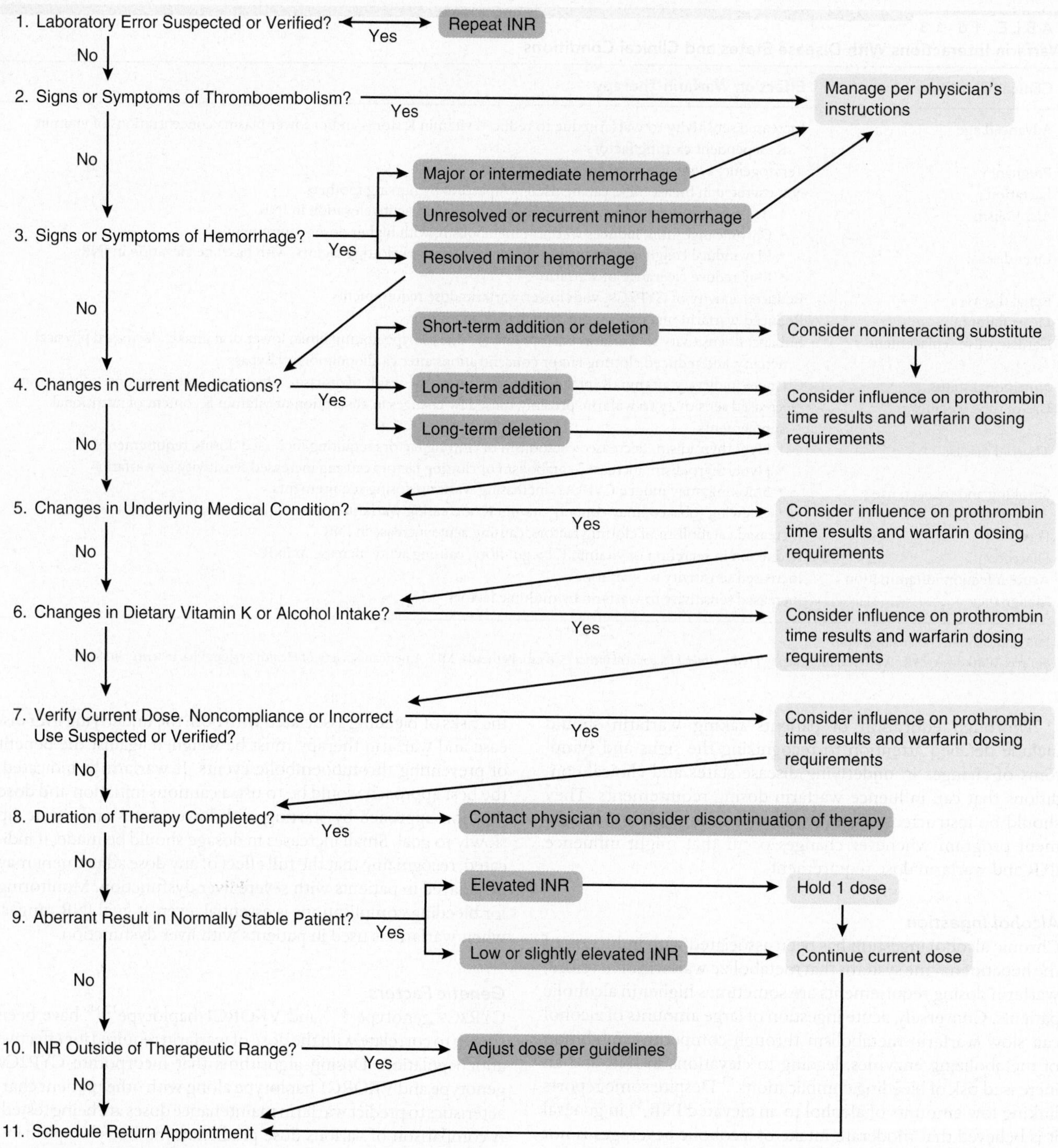

FIGURE 16-5 Assessment nomogram for patients taking warfarin.

may influence B.H.'s anticoagulation status should be evaluated carefully, including adherence with the warfarin dose schedule. A patient assessment nomogram (Fig. 16-5) is a helpful tool to assist with patient evaluation.

For a video that demonstrates how to assess a patient taking warfarin, go to http://thepoint.lww.com/AT10e.

ONLINE CONTENT

The accuracy and reliability of the INR test should be also considered. B.H. should be assessed thoroughly for signs and symptoms of thromboembolism and hemorrhage. Detailed questions should be asked to determine whether any changes in diet, alcohol intake, underlying disease states, concurrent medications, or other factors have occurred.

DOSING ADJUSTMENTS

CASE 16-6, QUESTION 5: After a thorough assessment, it is determined that B.H. has adhered to her prescribed warfarin dosage schedule and that there is no apparent explanation to account for her reduction in INR. How should her warfarin dosage be adjusted?

When overanticoagulation or underanticoagulation is verified, an adjustment in warfarin dosing may be necessary. Table 16-19 describes approaches to warfarin dosing adjustments for both regular-intensity and high-intensity maintenance therapy.

TABLE 16-19

Warfarin Dose Adjustment Nomogram for Maintenance Therapy[a]

For Goal INR 2–3	Adjustment	For Goal INR 2.5–3.5
INR <1.5	• Increase maintenance dose by 10%–20% • Consider a booster dose of 1.5–2 times daily maintenance dose • Consider resumption of prior maintenance dose if factor causing decreased INR is considered transient (e.g., missed warfarin dose[s])	INR <2.0
INR 1.5–1.8	• Increase maintenance dose by 5%–15% • Consider a booster dose of 1.5–2 times daily maintenance dose • Consider resumption of prior maintenance dose if factor causing decreased INR is considered transient (e.g., missed warfarin dose[s])	INR 2.0–2.3
INR 1.8–1.9	• No dosage adjustment may necessary if the last two INRs were in range, if there is no clear explanation for the INR to be out of range, and if in the judgment of the clinician the INR does not represent an increased risk of thromboembolism for the patient • If dosage adjustment is needed, increase by 5%–10% • Consider a booster dose of 1.5–2 times daily maintenance dose • Consider resumption of prior maintenance dose if factor causing decreased INR is considered transient (e.g., missed warfarin dose[s])	INR 2.3–2.4
INR 2.0–3.0	Desired range	INR 2.5–3.5
INR 3.1–3.2	• No dosage adjustment may necessary if the last two INRs were in range, if there is no clear explanation for the INR to be out of range, and if in the judgment of the clinician the INR does not represent an increased risk of hemorrhage for the patient • If dosage adjustment needed, decrease by 5%–10% • Consider resumption of prior maintenance dose if factor causing elevated INR is considered transient (e.g., acute alcohol ingestion)	INR 3.6–3.7
INR 3.3–3.4	• Decrease maintenance dose by 5%–10% • Consider resumption of prior maintenance dose if factor causing elevated INR is considered transient (e.g., acute alcohol ingestion)	INR 3.8–3.9
INR 3.5–3.9	• Consider holding one dose • Decrease maintenance dose by 5%–15% • Consider resumption of prior maintenance dose if factor causing elevated INR is considered transient (e.g., acute alcohol ingestion)	INR 4.0–4.4
INR >4.0	• Hold until INR < upper limit of therapeutic range • Consider use of minidose oral vitamin K • Decrease maintenance dose by 5%–20% • Consider resumption of prior maintenance dose if factor causing elevated INR is considered transient (e.g., acute alcohol ingestion)	INR >4.5

[a] University of Washington Medical Center.

INR, international normalized ratio.

Typically, dosing adjustments of 5% to 20% of the total daily dose (or the total weekly dose) are appropriate to reach the therapeutic range.[90] Because warfarin does not follow linear kinetics, small adjustments in dose can lead to large INR changes, thus large dose adjustments (i.e., greater than or less than 20% of the total weekly dose) are not recommended. These maintenance dosing guidelines should only be applied to patients who have reached a steady-state dose and not in the initiation phase of therapy.

Because B.H. is currently taking 4 mg daily, an adjustment of 10% would increase her dosage to approximately 4.5 mg/day. This dosing adjustment can be made by having her take one 4-mg tablet and half of a 1-mg tablet each day (same daily dosing) or by having her take 6 mg 2 days per week and 4 mg all other days of the week (alternate-day dosing). Patient preference and the likelihood of confusion about different tablet sizes versus different doses on different days of the week should be the primary considerations when selecting a dosing method.[91]

FREQUENCY OF FOLLOW-UP

CASE 16-6, QUESTION 6: B.H. agrees to increase her warfarin dosage to 4.5 mg/day. A new prescription for 1-mg tablets is written for her, and she is instructed about the use of these tablets. When should her INR be reassessed and her anticoagulation status, including physical assessment, be re-evaluated?

It will take several days for her warfarin level to reach a new steady state because of the long elimination half-lives of both warfarin and the vitamin K–dependent clotting factors. Her INR should be rechecked approximately 1 week after a dosing adjustment has been made. Once a stable dose has been reached, patient assessment and INR monitoring should occur every 4 to 6 weeks. However, if B.H. displays any signs of medical instability or nonadherence, a follow-up schedule of every 1 to 2 weeks is indicated (Table 16-20). Long term, should B.H. have difficulty maintaining her INR within the therapeutic range, the use of supplemental low-dose oral vitamin K (100–200 mcg daily) may be helpful if all other causes of INR variability have been excluded.[92]

MANAGEMENT OF OVERANTICOAGULATION

CASE 16-7

QUESTION 1: E.M., who has been taking warfarin for 6 months with good laboratory control, noted a slight pink color to his urine. In the ED, an INR of 5.6 was reported. His Hct and Hgb were both within normal limits, as were his vital signs. A stool guaiac test was negative, but urinalysis revealed more than 50 red blood cells per high-power field. How should this adverse effect of warfarin be treated in E.M.?

TABLE 16-20

Frequency of International Normalized Ratio Monitoring and Patient Assessment During Warfarin Therapy

Initiation Therapy	
Inpatient initiation	Daily
Outpatient flexible initiation method	Daily through day 4, then within 3–5 days
Outpatient average daily dosing method	Within 3–5 days, then within 1 week
After hospital discharge	If stable, within 3–5 days; If unstable, within 1–3 days
First month of therapy	Every 1–4 days until therapeutic, then weekly
Maintenance Therapy	
Medically stable inpatients	Every 1–3 days
Medically unstable inpatients	Daily
After hospital discharge	If stable, within 3–5 days If unstable, within 1–3 days In 1–2 days
Routine follow-up in medically stable and reliable patients	Every 4–6 weeks
Routine follow-up in medically unstable or unreliable patients	Every 1–2 weeks
Dose held today for significant overanticoagulation	In 1–2 days
Dosage change today	Within 1–2 weeks
Dosage change <2 weeks ago	Within 2–4 weeks

TABLE 16-21

Guidelines for Reversal of an Elevated International Normalized Ratio

INR	Recommendation
<5	Lower or hold dose.
5–8.9	Hold one or two doses, or hold dose and give vitamin K (1–2.5 mg orally). If more rapid reversal is required, give vitamin K (< 5 mg) orally. Repeat vitamin K (1–2 mg orally) if INR is still elevated at 24 hours.
≥9	Hold warfarin and give vitamin K (2.5–5 mg orally). Use additional vitamin K, if necessary.
Serious bleeding with high INR	Hold warfarin and give vitamin K (10 mg slow IV infusion) supplemented with fresh-frozen plasma, prothrombin complex concentrates, or recombinant factor VIIa. May repeat vitamin K every 12 hours, if necessary.
Life-threatening bleeding	Hold warfarin and give fresh-frozen plasma, prothrombin complex concentrates, or recombinant factor VIIa supplemented with vitamin K (10 mg slow IV infusion). Repeat as necessary.

Source: Hirsh J et al. Parenteral anticoagulants. American College of Chest Physicians Evidence-Based Clinical Practice Guidelines (8th Edition) [published correction appears in *Chest*. 2008;134:473]. *Chest*. 2008;133(Suppl 6):141S.
INR, international normalized ratio; IV, intravenously.

Management of overanticoagulation depends on the clinical presentation of the patient. In the case of an elevated INR without bleeding complications, interruption of warfarin therapy by holding one or two doses until the INR returns to the therapeutic range is usually sufficient.[93] Minor bleeding complications accompanied by an elevated INR can be also managed by withholding warfarin therapy for a short period until bleeding resolves. In either case, the patient should be questioned to determine a possible cause for overanticoagulation, including intake of extra doses of warfarin, changes in diet or alcohol intake, changes in underlying medical conditions, or the use of other medications. In some cases, no apparent explanation is identified. Depending on the cause, a reduction in the maintenance dosing of warfarin may be necessary.

The time required for INR to return to the therapeutic range after warfarin is withheld depends on several patient characteristics. Advanced age, lower warfarin maintenance dose requirements, and higher INR are associated with increased time for INR correction.[94] Other factors that can prolong the time for INR to return to the therapeutic range include decompensated heart failure, active malignancy, and recent use of medications known to potentiate warfarin.

To shorten the time to correction of overanticoagulation, an alternative approach is to withhold warfarin and administer a small dose of vitamin K (phytonadione)[11] (Table 16-21). An oral dose of 1 to 2.5 mg can correct overanticoagulation in 24 to 48 hours without causing prolonged resistance to warfarin therapy, a problem commonly seen with larger (10 mg) doses of vitamin K. Intramuscular administration is contraindicated due to the risk of hematoma formation, and SC administration of vitamin K is not recommended because of variable absorption.[95]

IV doses of 0.5 to 1 mg of vitamin K can correct overanticoagulation within 24 hours.[11] This approach is also useful for reversal of therapeutic anticoagulation before invasive procedures and can be used to correct overanticoagulation in high-risk cases. IV vitamin K should be diluted and administered by slow infusion over 30 to 60 minutes to prevent flushing, hypotension, and cardiovascular collapse.[96] Although these symptoms resemble anaphylaxis, the mechanism of this adverse response is unclear: It is not known if it is caused by phytonadione or by the vehicle in which phytonadione is formulated. If this adverse reaction occurs, administration of epinephrine may be indicated, as well as other standard measures to support blood pressure and maintain the airway.

Rapid reversal of warfarin therapy is indicated in the setting of major, life-threatening bleeding (e.g., severe gastrointestinal bleeding, intracranial hemorrhage). Fresh frozen plasma or factor concentrates to replace clotting factors will decrease the INR for 4 to 6 hours and should be administered as needed with careful monitoring of volume status. Supplementation with high-dose IV vitamin K (10 mg) may also be indicated. IV administration will reverse the effects of warfarin within 6 to 12 hours. However, if continued warfarin therapy is indicated when bleeding resolves, anticoagulation with heparin may be necessary for as long as 7 to 14 days until the effect of high-dose vitamin K is diminished and warfarin responsiveness returns.

Hematuria may be an early sign of more serious bleeding, but in many cases this condition is associated with only minor bleeding episodes. In a reliable patient, discontinuing warfarin until the INR returns to a therapeutic level usually suffices. A more rapid return to normal can be accomplished if low-dose vitamin K is administered. Because E.M. appears to be bleeding only into the urine and is hemodynamically stable, withholding warfarin and administering a low dose of oral vitamin K (1–2.5 mg) is appropriate. A thorough workup to evaluate the source of bleeding is indicated.

USE IN PREGNANCY

CASE 16-8

QUESTION 1: E.S., a 30-year-old woman, takes warfarin for chronic therapy of an unprovoked PE. She has just learned she is pregnant. What effects might warfarin have on the

TABLE 16-22
Recommendations for Anticoagulation During Pregnancy

Clinical Situation	Peripartum Options	Postpartum
1. Prophylaxis		
Known hypercoagulable state with no prior history of VTE	• Surveillance • Prophylactic UFH/LMWH	Warfarin to INR 2–3 for 4–6 weeks with UFH/LMWH overlap until INR >2.0
Single prior episode of VTE associated with transient risk factors, not receiving long-term anticoagulants	• Surveillance	Warfarin to INR 2–3 for 4–6 weeks with UFH/LMWH overlap until INR >2.0
Single prior episode of idiopathic or thrombophilia-related VTE, not receiving long-term anticoagulants	• Surveillance • Prophylactic UFH/LMWH • Intermediate-dose UFH/LMWH	Warfarin to INR 2–3 for 4–6 weeks with UFH/LMWH overlap until INR >2.0
Multiple prior episodes of VTE and/or receiving long-term oral anticoagulants for VTE	• Adjusted-dose UFH/LMWH • Intermediate-dose LMWH (or 75% of adjusted dose LMWH)	Long-term warfarin to INR 2–3 with UFH/LMWH overlap until INR >2.0
Long-term oral anticoagulants for mechanical valve replacement	• Adjusted-dose SC UFH • Adjusted-dose BID LMWH (adjusted to achieve manufacturer recommended 4-hour postdose peak anti-factor-Xa concentration)	Long-term warfarin to prior INR goal with UFH/LMWH overlap until INR above lower limit of therapeutic range
2. Treatment of VTE that occurs during pregnancy	• IV UFH for ≥5 days, followed by adjusted-dose SC UFH • Adjusted-dose LMWH	Warfarin to INR 2–3 for a minimum of 6 weeks with UFH/LMWH overlap until INR >2.0

Source: Bates SM et al. Venous thromboembolism, thrombophilia, antithrombotic therapy and pregnancy: American College of Chest Physicians Evidence-Based Practice Guidelines (8th Edition) *Chest*. 2008;133(Suppl 6):844.
BID, twice daily; INR, international normalized ratio; LMWH, low-molecular-weight heparin; SC, subcutaneous; UFH, unfractionated heparin; VTE, venous thromboembolic disease.
Prophylactic dose UFH: 5,000 international units SC every 12 hours.
Intermediate-dose UFH: adjusted to 0.1–0.3 international units/mL anti-Xa activity.
Adjusted-dose UFH: adjusted to maintain therapeutic aPTT at mid-dosing interval.
Prophylactic LMWH: enoxaparin 40 mg SC daily or dalteparin 5,000 units SC daily.
Intermediate-dose LMWH: enoxaparin 40 mg SC every 12 hours or dalteparin 5,000 units SC every 12 hours.
Adjusted-dose LMWH (weight-adjusted full treatment doses): enoxaparin 1 mg/kg SC every 12 hours or dalteparin 200 units/kg, or dalteparin 100 units/kg SC every 12 hours and adjusted throughout pregnancy to maintain 4-hour postinjection peak anti-Xa activity level of 0.5–1.2 units/mL (VTE) or greater then 1.0 units/mL (mechanical valves).

fetus? Are UFH or LMWHs safer alternatives in this situation?

Coumarin anticoagulants cross the placental barrier and may place the fetus at risk for hemorrhage and teratogenic effects.[97] Up to 30% of pregnancies that involve exposure to coumarin result in abnormal liveborn infants, and up to 30% in spontaneous abortion or stillbirth. Congenital abnormalities such as stippled calcifications and nasal cartilage hypoplasia primarily occurred in infants born to mothers receiving warfarin during the first trimester of pregnancy, with the highest risk during weeks 6 to 12. Other abnormalities, involving the central nervous system and eyes, are more likely to occur when the mother is taking warfarin later in the pregnancy. In addition, because warfarin crosses the placenta, fatal bleeding complications may occur.

Women of childbearing age who require anticoagulation should be counseled about options for contraception. Patients who become pregnant while receiving warfarin should be informed of the risks of continued anticoagulation to the fetus, as well as the risk to themselves of discontinuing anticoagulation.

Other options for pregnant women who require anticoagulation include UFH and LMWHs.[97] Because these agents do not cross the placenta, they are preferred over warfarin for use in pregnancy. UFH is typically recommended because it has been used extensively during pregnancy. However, many clinical trials have validated the safety and efficacy of LMWHs in the prevention and treatment of DVT and PE during pregnancy. These agents represent an alternative to UFH, with advantages as previously described. When used at full doses for the treatment of VTE during pregnancy, dosing must be adjusted throughout the pregnancy to account for the expected increase in the body weight of the mother and the reported increase in clearance of LMWH during pregnancy.[98] Current recommendations for use of anticoagulants in pregnancy are outlined in Table 16-22.

After being informed of the risks associated with warfarin, E.S. decided to continue her pregnancy and to begin anticoagulation with LMWH. Warfarin therapy should be discontinued immediately and LMWH initiated using SC treatment doses as previously described. Dosing adjustments may be required throughout pregnancy based on changes in body weight and clearance, possibly guided by anti-factor Xa monitoring. Potential adverse effects of LMWH use, including hemorrhage, thrombocytopenia, and osteoporosis, should be monitored appropriately.

Injections of LMWH should be discontinued 24 hours before elective induction of labor and resumed as soon as bleeding from delivery has been controlled. IV heparin should be discontinued 6 hours before delivery. Warfarin therapy can then be safely reinitiated. If spontaneous labor occurs, protamine can be used to reverse the effect of UFH, but will only partially reverses the effects of LMWHs. Warfarin is not secreted in breast milk; therefore, E.S. can safely breast-feed.

PREVENTION OF CARDIOGENIC THROMBOEMBOLISM

Atrial Fibrillation

ANTICOAGULATION BEFORE CARDIOVERSION

CASE 16-9

QUESTION 1: C.D., a 68-year-old woman with hypertension, presents to the cardiology clinic complaining of several

days of fatigue and a "racing heart." On physical examination, her pulse is irregularly irregular, and her heart rate is approximately 120 beats/minute. Using ECG, a diagnosis of atrial fibrillation is made and cardioversion planned. Should C.D. be anticoagulated before cardioversion?

In atrial fibrillation, compromised atrial activity and atrial enlargement causes stasis of blood within the atria and the left atrial appendage, often resulting in atrial thrombus formation. Atrial thrombus formation increases the risk of systemic embolization; clinical manifestations include arterial embolization of the extremities or embolization of the splenic, renal, or abdominal arteries. However, the most prevalent site of embolization is the cerebral arterial system, resulting in transient ischemic attack or stroke with potentially devastating neurologic and functional impairment.[99]

Both direct current cardioversion and pharmacologic cardioversion using antiarrhythmic drugs expose patients with atrial fibrillation to an initial short-term increase in stroke risk from embolization secondary to resumption of normal atrial mechanical activity (see Chapter 20, Cardiac Arrhythmias). Data from a prospective cohort study of 437 patients noted a stroke incidence of 5.3% in patients with atrial fibrillation who were cardioverted without prior anticoagulation, but a significant reduction in stroke incidence to 0.8% was noted if patients who had received cardioversion were anticoagulated.[100] In addition to preventing the development of new atrial thrombi, anticoagulation allows any thrombus that may be present to endothelialize and adhere to the atrial wall so that the thromboembolic risk is minimized. Based on the assumed time course of thrombus development, as well as the presumed time course of clot endothelialization, patients who have been in atrial fibrillation for 48 hours should receive 3 weeks of therapeutic anticoagulation with warfarin to a target INR of 2.5 (range, 2.0–3.0) before cardioversion is attempted.[99] Despite a lower risk of stroke than that associated with atrial fibrillation, patients with atrial flutter should be treated similarly.

Whether C.D. has been in atrial fibrillation for 48 hours is not known; therefore, she requires a 3-week course of therapeutic anticoagulation with a goal INR range of 2.0 to 3.0 before cardioversion is attempted. If C.D. cannot tolerate her heart symptoms despite control of the ventricular response rate, her medical team might consider immediate cardioversion without anticoagulation if transesophageal echocardiography (TEE) is used to rule out left atrial thrombi. TEE is much more sensitive than transthoracic echocardiography to visualize the left atrium and the left atrial appendage.

In a clinical trial, 1,222 patients with atrial fibrillation of more than 2 days' duration were randomly assigned to either treatment guided by TEE findings or to conventional precardioversion anticoagulation.[101] Patients assigned to conventional treatment and patients in the TEE group in whom thrombus was detected received a 3-week course of warfarin before cardioversion. Patients without detectable thrombus by TEE were cardioverted without precardioversion anticoagulation. All patients received 4 weeks of postcardioversion anticoagulation. Thromboembolic rates were identical between patients who received conventional treatment and those whose treatment was guided by TEE (0.5% vs. 0.8%, $p = 0.5$).

ANTICOAGULATION AFTER CARDIOVERSION

CASE 16-9, QUESTION 2: After 3 weeks of regular-intensity warfarin therapy, C.D. is successfully cardioverted. Should warfarin be discontinued?

Despite normalization of atrial electrical activity, restoration of effective atrial mechanical activity after cardioversion of atrial fibrillation can be delayed for up to 3 weeks. In addition, a significant number of patients with atrial fibrillation who initially are successfully cardioverted revert to atrial fibrillation during the first month. Both of these factors contribute to the recognized delay in stroke presentation after cardioversion in patients with atrial fibrillation. For these reasons, anticoagulation with warfarin should be continued after cardioversion for a minimum 4 weeks.

ANTICOAGULATION FOR PAROXYSMAL, PERMANENT, OR PERSISTENT ATRIAL FIBRILLATION

CASE 16-9, QUESTION 3: Two weeks after successful cardioversion, C.D. presents to the ED with chest palpitations and light-headedness. An ECG is evaluated, and atrial fibrillation is diagnosed again. What decisions regarding anticoagulation need to be made?

ANTICOAGULATION IN VALVULAR ATRIAL FIBRILLATION

Atrial fibrillation secondary to valvular heart disease has historically been recognized as a significant risk factor for stroke. Patients with atrial fibrillation who have a history of rheumatic mitral valve disease have a 17-fold higher incidence of stroke than in matched controls. Patients with valvular atrial fibrillation require long-term, regular-intensity anticoagulation to a target INR of 2.5 (range, 2.0–3.0) to prevent thromboembolism and stroke.[99,102]

ANTICOAGULATION IN NONVALVULAR ATRIAL FIBRILLATION

Nonvalvular heart disease is the most common cause of atrial fibrillation and, like valvular heart disease, represents a significant risk for stroke in patients with atrial fibrillation. Five clinical trials have substantiated the role of warfarin in the primary prevention of systemic embolization and stroke in chronic, nonvalvular atrial fibrillation.[99,102,103] All five trials compared warfarin with a placebo and were terminated before completion because of the substantial benefit of warfarin. In comparison with a placebo, warfarin significantly reduced the risk of stroke from approximately 5% per year to approximately 2% per year, with an average relative risk reduction of 67%. Based on the results of these trials, long-term anticoagulation with warfarin to a goal INR of 2.5 (range, 2.0–3.0) is recommended in patients like C.D., who have atrial fibrillation secondary to nonvalvular heart disease.[99,102,103]

Several clinical trials have attempted to define the comparative efficacy of warfarin versus aspirin in the prevention of stroke associated with atrial fibrillation.[99,102,104] Compared with a placebo or control, aspirin decreases the risk of stroke in patients with atrial fibrillation. However, that reduction is not as substantial as the reduction seen with warfarin. In clinical trials comparing warfarin and aspirin, the risk reduction associated with warfarin is significantly larger than that of aspirin. However, aspirin may be appropriate in certain patients at low risk for stroke associated with atrial fibrillation based on individualized risk assessment using the CHADS2 score (Table 16-6) (see Chapter 20, Cardiac Arrhythmias).

Subsequent trials have confirmed the superiority of warfarin over the combination of aspirin plus clopidogrel for stroke prevention in atrial fibrillation, and the increased risk of intracrantial hemorrhage when aspirin and clopidogrel are combined.[105,106] Recently, the RE-LY trial compared traditional warfarin for stroke prevention in atrial fibrillation to dabigatran, an oral direct thrombin inhibitor.[107] Dabigatran 150 mg twice daily was superior to warfarin for stroke prevention, with a comparable incidence of hemorrhagic complications. This agent offers a number of advantages as described in an earlier section of this chapter, and a recent update to previously published guidelines recommended it for use.[108]

The decision to continue long-term anticoagulation with warfarin in C.D. should be based on an evaluation of the likelihood that her atrial fibrillation will become chronic with a paroxysmal, persistent, or permanent presentation, as well as an assessment of her risk of stroke compared with her risk of warfarin-associated bleeding complications. Because of her age and history of hypertension, the appropriate strategy should be long-term warfarin therapy with a goal INR of 2.5 (range, 2.0–3.0).

Cardiac Valve Replacement

MECHANICAL PROSTHETIC VALVES

CASE 16-10

QUESTION 1: D.L., a 56-year-old woman with a history of rheumatic mitral valve disease, has undergone mitral valve replacement. A St. Jude (bileaflet mechanical) valve has been implanted, and heparin therapy is initiated postoperatively. Does D.L. require continued anticoagulation with warfarin?

Mechanical prosthetic valves confer a significant thromboembolic risk by providing a foreign surface in contact with blood components on which platelet aggregation and thrombus formation can occur. Valvular thrombosis can impair the integrity of valve function and can lead to embolization with systemic manifestations, including stroke.[109] The incidence of thromboembolic complications depends on the type of artificial valve (caged ball [Starr-Edwards] > tilting disk [Medtronic-Hall; Bjork-Shiley] > bileaflet [St. Jude]), as well as the anatomical position of the replacement (dual valve replacement > mitral > aortic).[110]

Long-term anticoagulation is required in patients with mechanical valve replacement because it significantly reduces the risk of stroke and other manifestations of systemic embolization (Table 16-6). Trials comparing different intensities of oral anticoagulation with warfarin in mechanical valve replacement helped identify the intensity of anticoagulation that protects against thromboembolic risk, while reducing the incidence of hemorrhagic complications.[111] Patients with a St. Jude bileaflet valve in the aortic position should receive long-term anticoagulant therapy with warfarin to a target INR of 2.5 (range, 2.0–3.0).[109,112] For all other mechanical valve types in the aortic position, and for any mechanical mitral valve replacement, chronic warfarin therapy with a target INR of 3.0 (range, 2.5–3.5) is recommended. The concurrent use of low-dose aspirin (81 mg daily) is recommended for patients with additional risk factors for systemic embolization (atrial fibrillation, left ventricular dysfunction, a history of prior systemic embolism, or a hypercoagulable condition), unless the patient has a significant risk for bleeding or a history of aspirin intolerance.

BIOPROSTHETIC VALVES

CASE 16-11

QUESTION 1: E.K., an 86-year-old woman with a history of symptomatic aortic stenosis, has received a bioprosthetic (mammalian) aortic valve replacement. Is anticoagulant therapy required in E.K.?

Prosthetic heart valves extracted from mammalian sources (porcine or bovine xenografts, homografts) are significantly less thrombogenic than mechanical prosthetic valves. The period of greatest thromboembolic risk appears to be during the first 3 months after implantation. Therefore, short-term, regular-intensity, preventive anticoagulation to an INR of 2.5 (range, 2.0–3.0) is recommended.[109,112] After this period, long-term aspirin therapy (minimum dose, 162 mg/day) is indicated. However, oral anticoagulation should be continued long term in patients with concurrent atrial fibrillation, a history of systemic embolism, or evidence of atrial thrombus at surgery.

BRIDGE THERAPY

Management of Anticoagulation Around Invasive Procedures

CASE 16-12

QUESTION 1: C.G. is a 43-year-old woman with a history of valvular heart disease associated with Marfan syndrome. She has a St. Jude mitral valve replacement and is anticoagulated with warfarin 7.5 mg once daily to a goal INR range of 2.5 to 3.5. Recently, she has complained of episodic rectal bleeding despite adequate anticoagulation. She is scheduled for colonoscopy in several weeks. Her gastroenterologist calls the anticoagulation clinic to determine the most appropriate plan for reversal of her warfarin before the procedure. What are the options?

When an invasive procedure is planned, it is often necessary to reverse the effects of warfarin to minimize the risk of bleeding complications associated with the procedure, which can be worsened by the presence of an anticoagulant. It can take several days for the anticoagulant effect of warfarin to be reversed after discontinuation of the drug, but in that period of time, a patient may be at risk for thromboembolic complications associated with underanticoagulation. Bridge therapy is the term that refers to the use of a relatively short-acting injectable anticoagulant (UFH, LMWH) as a substitute for warfarin before and immediately after an invasive procedure.[113] Because UFH and LMWH have shorter elimination half-lives than warfarin, they can be stopped just before the invasive procedure without increasing the risk of bleeding associated with the procedure. The last dose of LMWH and SC UFH is typically given 24 hours before the scheduled procedure, whereas IV UFH infusions are discontinued 6 hours before the procedure. Because of their shorter onsets of effect, these agents are resumed after invasive procedures to establish an immediate degree of anticoagulation. Warfarin is resumed simultaneously, and the bridging anticoagulant is continued until the INR reaches the therapeutic range.

Although bridge therapy has not been studied in randomized clinical trials, current guidelines for bridging are based on the results of case series, observational studies, and nonrandomized trials involving patients with various indications for anticoagulation, including valve replacement. The decision to use bridging depends on the risk of bleeding associated with continued anticoagulation for the surgery or procedure to be performed and on the risk of thromboembolism associated with underanticoagulation in the patient in question. Individualized risk assessment and bridge therapy planning are necessary for each patient who may require temporary discontinuation of warfarin. Current recommendations for risk stratification are outlined in Table 16-23. High-risk and moderate-risk patients typically receive bridge

lesions of 55% and 70% in the RCA and circumflex arteries, respectively; the LAD coronary artery is not involved. What is his prognosis?

The prognosis of patients with stable angina is variable and dependent on the presence of other factors and comorbid conditions. Developing a level of risk for a particular patient helps determine the appropriate treatment strategy. The extent of CAD, quantification of ventricular function, the response to stress testing, as well as the initial clinical evaluation all help to provide an estimate of risk in a given patient.

J.P.'s history and physical examination suggest he does not have HF; poor LV function would be an ominous concurrent finding. J.P. also does not have three-vessel disease or blockage of the LAD artery. J.P. does have type 2 diabetes, which elevates his risk for future cardiovascular events. The absence of other major comorbid conditions, myocardial dysfunction, along with the current extent of CAD indicate that J.P.'s prognosis at this time is favorable provided he initiate appropriate treatment strategies demonstrated to reduce morbidity and mortality in patients with CAD.[1,2,35]

Medical Management of Chronic Stable Angina

CASE 17-1, QUESTION 6: How should J.P. be managed at this time? Should he undergo revascularization with PCI or CABG, or be managed medically?

As previously discussed, goals for managing CAD and angina in J.P. include relief of symptoms and reduction of myocardial ischemia to improve quality of life, as well as prevention of major complications of CAD such as acute MI and death. Depending on the patient, both goals may be accomplished through surgical revascularization, medical management, or both. Regardless of the treatment strategy chosen to relieve ischemic symptoms, therapies that prevent death (vasculoprotective agents) should receive priority.

Presently, CABG is not the best option for J.P. because the usual indications for surgical therapy include presence of left main CAD, presence of three-vessel disease (especially if LV function is impaired), or ineffectiveness of medical therapy.[31,32] However, revascularization with PCI is a potential option along with medical management alone. Although PCI would offer no mortality advantage over medical therapy at this time, it has been shown to decrease the incidence of recurrent symptoms in the short term (1 year).[1] If J.P. can implement aggressive lifestyle modifications and control of risk factors, progression of CAD and control of ischemic symptoms will be similar to PCI within a 5-year time frame.[50] Both strategies, including the pros and cons of PCI or medical management alone, should be offered to J.P. so that an informed decision can be made in accord with his wishes. Overall, J.P. will probably do well with medical therapy. His life expectancy depends on progression of the disease and development of other complications of CHD (HF, MI, sudden cardiac death).

RISK FACTORS AND LIFESTYLE MODIFICATIONS

CASE 17-1, QUESTION 7: What independent risk factors for CAD are present in J.P.? Which of these may be altered?

The first step in the treatment of any patient with chronic stable angina or CAD should be the modification of any existing risk factors and the adoption of a healthy lifestyle. By addressing the underlying circumstances, which likely led to the development of CAD, a significant impact can be made at halting the progression of the disease and preventing complications of CAD. Current recommendations for the goals for risk factor management are listed in Table 17-3.[35,52] In addition to specific risk factor goals, attention should be paid to evidence that favors specific drug therapies that have evidence supporting reductions in morbidity and mortality. Examples would include the use of HMG-CoA reductase inhibitors in the treatment of hyperlipidemia,[1,2,35] as well as the use of ACE inhibitors for the treatment of hypertension.[52]

J.P. has several risk factors for CAD, some of which cannot be altered, such as middle age, male sex, and a strong family history of CAD. Risk factors, such as hypertension, obesity, hypercholesterolemia, smoking, and possibly stress, can potentially be modified to decrease the likelihood of adverse sequelae for J.P. His hypertension should be controlled and his serum cholesterol concentration should be tested and fractionated for LDL, high-density lipoprotein, and triglycerides (see Chapter 13, Dyslipidemias, Atherosclerosis, and Coronary Heart Disease). A fasting Hgb A_{1c} should be drawn with a goal of less than 7% (see Chapter 53, Diabetes Mellitus). Dietary modification and weight reduction for J.P. are mandatory, because they positively influence several risk factors. J.P., however, does not smoke cigarettes, which would significantly increase his cardiovascular risk.[1] J.P.'s active lifestyle may influence his prognosis favorably.[53]

CASE 17-1, QUESTION 8: Does glipizide represent the best option for diabetes management in J.P.?

Considerable attention has been directed not only at identifying whether tight glycemic control (targeting lower levels of Hgb A_{1c} than the currently recommended 7%) but also at whether different classes of antidiabetes medications have variable effects on long-term outcomes such as death and MI in patients with atherosclerotic vascular disease. Unfortunately, as is the case with the evidence supporting tighter glycemic control in CAD patients, there are few data that overwhelmingly suggests one class of agent to be superior at preventing hard CVD outcomes such as death, MI or hospitalizations. Of the available agents for diabetes management, metformin has the most promising support having one trial in obese patients where a reduction in CVD end points was observed (United Kingdom Prospective Diabetes Study, or UKPDS-39).[54] Recent attention had focused on the thiazolidinediones class with one agent being associated with worsening CVD outcomes (rosiglitazone), and another (pioglitazone) having one large randomized trial suggesting a reduction in CVD outcomes.[55,56] Additional considerations with thiazolidinediones are their association with increasing the risk of MI (particularly with rosiglitazone), and fluid retention that may precipitate heart failure. Lastly, J.P's diabetes is not currently at goal based on his Hgb A_{1c} value, although his current glipizide therapy has not been maximized as of yet. Several potential options are reasonable for J.P at this time considering his current therapy, current disease control, and known effects of diabetes medications on cardiovascular disease and outcomes. J.P could be maintained on glipizide with an increase in dose for better control. However, it would also be reasonable to alter his regimen from glipizide to metformin given his obesity, and based on UKPDS-39 he may derive an additional benefit of reduced CVD outcomes in conjunction with optimal glycemic control.

CASE 17-1, QUESTION 9: Is hydrochlorothiazide an optimal choice for hypertension control in J.P.?

Hydrochlorothiazide represents a first-line option, along with β-blockers, CCBs, and ACE inhibitors/ARBs in the primary management of hypertension. Currently J.P.'s blood pressure is above patients with hypertension and CAD,[81] acute MI,[11,12] and heart failure.[40] Although mortality benefits have not been demonstrated specifically in patients with chronic angina, the body of literature available supports the recommendation that all patients with angina should receive a β-blocker as initial therapy unless contraindicated.[52] J.P. at this time does not appear to have any contraindications to continuing his β-blocker therapy, and at this time his therapy should be optimized. (See Chapter 14, Essential Hypertension, and Chapter 19, Heart Failure, for more in-depth information on β-blocker product availability, dosage forms, pharmacology, and dosing.)

CASE 17-1, QUESTION 15: How should therapy with a β-blocker be optimized in J.P.?

All patients receiving antianginal drugs should be monitored for frequency of angina attacks and SL NTG consumption. Nevertheless, this provides only an estimate of therapeutic efficacy because the patient's exercise and stress levels change from day to day. Traditionally, clinicians have monitored the reduction in resting heart rate and have progressively increased the β-blocker dose until the resting heart rate was 55 or 60 beats/minute.[40] J.P. currently has a heart rate of 78 beats/minute, preserved blood pressure, and an increase in the dose of metoprolol is warranted at this time. A doubling of his dose to 100 mg once daily would be a reasonable increase, with close monitoring of heart rate and blood pressure. Additional goals with β-blocker therapy include a maximum heart rate of 100 beats/minute or less with exercise. Resting heart rates less than 50 beats/minute may be acceptable, provided the patient is asymptomatic and heart block is not present. Variations in resting heart rate are normal and subject to the influence of the endogenous sympathetic nervous system and other exogenous factors, such as drugs, tobacco, and caffeine-containing beverages. β-Blockers with intrinsic sympathomimetic activity (e.g., pindolol) will not reduce the resting heart rate as much as β-blockers lacking this activity.[39]

Exercise stress testing is probably the most accurate, but least practical, method of documenting the adequacy of β-blocker therapy. During an exercise tolerance test, metoprolol should substantially increase the time J.P. walks before developing angina. There also may be a reduction in ST-segment depression during exercise, indicating less myocardial ischemia. The rate–pressure product probably will be markedly lower, reflecting a decrease in both heart rate and systolic wall tension.[38] An alternative to conducting a formal stress test is to repeat the physical activity which produced angina during this hospitalization, namely, walking a few flights of stairs.

CASE 17-1, QUESTION 16: Would the decision to use β-blockers initially in J.P. be altered if he had a history of chronic obstructive pulmonary disease (COPD) or peripheral vascular disease (PVD)?

Although all β-blockers are equally effective in the treatment of angina, the addition of COPD or PVD to J.P.'s medical history would pose several relative contraindications to the use of some β-blockers. The concern directly relates to the potential for β-blockers to worsen either bronchoconstriction in the case of COPD by blunting β_2 receptors, or worsening vasoconstriction in the peripheral arteries, again, through blunting vasodilation through β_2 receptors. Although not absolute contraindications, the presence of these disease states warrants careful monitoring of β-blocker therapy during initiation and titration.[38] In the event that β-blocker therapy is not tolerated or considered too risky, initial therapy with a heart-rate–controlling CCB is the next best option, provided there is adequate heart rate and blood pressure to tolerate therapy. In patients who already have low heart rate and/or marginal blood pressure, ranolazine may be considered as an initial option. Long-acting nitrates are typically reserved for add-on therapy for reasons that will be subsequently discussed.

Cardioselective β-blockers are often considered in patients with COPD or PVD with the hope that β_2 receptors will be unaffected. J.P. is already receiving metoprolol, which would be a reasonable choice if COPD or PVD was present. In one meta-analysis, cardioselective β-blockers were not found to produce clinically significant adverse respiratory effects in patients who had mild to moderate reactive airway disease.[82] Cardioselective β-blockers also are less likely to inhibit β_2-mediated vasodilation in the peripheral arterioles. Therefore, cardioselective β-blockers are preferred over nonselective β-blockers for patients with peripheral vascular disease and Raynaud disease.

Unfortunately, cardioselectivity is not an all-or-none response; instead, it is a dose-dependent phenomenon. As the dose is increased, cardioselectivity is lost. The dose at which cardioselectivity will be lost in any given patient cannot be predicted, and even a very small dose (e.g., metoprolol 50–100 mg) could cause wheezing.[39,41] If β-blocker therapy is to be initiated in a patient with reactive airway disease or PVD, close monitoring for worsening of symptoms should occur and an alternative anti-ischemic medication should be used if symptoms worsen.

CASE 17-1, QUESTION 17: J.P. is being discharged from the hospital today with prescriptions for SL NTG 0.4 mg tablets, metoprolol succinate 100 mg once daily, metformin 500 mg BID, and lisinopril 20 mg once daily, and education regarding diet and exercise. Is there anything else J.P. should be receving for his chronic stable angina?

Antiplatelet therapy is a cornerstone in the management of a patient with athereosclerotic vascular disease. Antiplatelet therapy has been demonstrated to reduce the incidence of CVD events such as MI, stroke, and death. Although newer antiplatelet options are available, aspirin is still the first-line choice for patients with atherosclerotic vascular disease due to well-established efficacy and cost-effectiveness.

The mechanism of action for aspirin's antiplatelet effect is inhibition of cyclo-oxygenase (see Chapter 16, Thrombosis). By acetylating the active site of cyclo-oxygenase, aspirin blocks the formation of prostaglandin endoperoxides from arachidonic acid. This inhibits the formation of both thromboxane and prostacyclin. Thromboxane A_2 is a cyclo-oxygenase–catalyzed product of arachidonic acid metabolism and a potent vasoconstrictor and facilitates further activation of platelets. Prostacyclin (PGI_2), another arachidonic acid metabolite produced under the influence of cyclo-oxygenase, counterbalances the effect of thromboxane A_2. It is a potent inhibitor of platelet aggregation and a vasodilator. Researchers have tested various aspirin doses hoping to find a dose that inhibits thromboxane synthesis but does not inhibit formation of PGI_2. A single 100-mg aspirin dose virtually eliminates thromboxane A_2 production, whereas doses less than 100 mg result in a dose-dependent reduction in thromboxane A_2 synthesis. Therapeutic benefit has been demonstrated with doses as low as 30 mg/day.[83]

Recent research has attempted to determine the effect of aspirin doses on the thromboxane A_2 to PGI_2 balance. PGI_2 production recovers within hours of aspirin administration because the endothelial cell can resynthesize cyclo-oxygenase. In contrast, the inhibition of platelet cyclo-oxygenase is irreversible. Selective inhibition of platelet-generated thromboxane A_2 synthesis has been shown with 75 mg of controlled-release aspirin daily.[83–85] Theoretically, administration of 75 mg aspirin daily in a controlled-release formulation may selectively spare vascular endothelial PGI_2 production, but at the same time still inhibit platelet cyclo-oxygenase. Controlled clinical trials on this proposed aspirin dosage regimen are lacking, however. Therefore, the proposed biochemical selectivity of aspirin on platelet function versus the vascular endothelium is difficult to achieve clinically.

Because of the lack of precise understanding of the pharmacodynamic effect of aspirin, it is not surprising that controversy exists regarding the optimal dose to be used in patients with angina, as well as post MI and as secondary prevention of stroke. Although it has been theorized that higher doses of aspirin would produce a higher level of efficacy than low doses, all available literature indicates that low dosages of aspirin (75–325 mg/day) are as effective as higher dosages (625–1,300 mg/day) in the treatment of patients with angina.[85] Conversely, as the aspirin dosage increases, the incidence of adverse effects, especially gastrointestinal (GI) bleeding, increases as well. Therefore, current guidelines recommend a daily dosage of 75 to 162 mg orally for the prevention of MI and death in patients with CAD.[85] Given this information, J.P. should be advised to take aspirin at a dose of 81 mg/day to maintain efficacy but decrease the risk of adverse effects.

CASE 17-1, QUESTION 18: J.P. returns to the hospital 8 weeks after he was discharged from the hospital for recurrent angina. He mentioned he stopped his metoprolol 36 hours ago when he forgot to get his prescriptions refilled. He is transported to the hospital emergency department for treatment of angina unresponsive to 3 NTG tablets. How could J.P.'s situation have been avoided?

The β-blocker withdrawal syndrome places patients with CAD at high risk for adverse cardiovascular events, which may include acute MI and sudden cardiac death. After J.P.'s angina has been controlled with medications during this particular hospitalization and before reinstitution of β-blocker therapy, he should be warned not to precipitously discontinue his β-blockers in the future. Failure to renew prescriptions and financial hardship are common reasons for abrupt discontinuation, and clinicians need to have sufficient professional rapport with patients to understand when patients encounter difficulties in obtaining medications.

The β-blocker withdrawal syndrome is a rebound phenomenon resulting from heightened β-receptor density and sensitivity (i.e., upregulation) subsequent to receptor blockade. An "overshoot" in heart rate, as a consequence of sympathoadrenal activity from abrupt β-blocker withdrawal increases myocardial oxygen demand and platelet aggregation. Withdrawal syndromes may be less severe in patients taking β-blockers with partial agonist activity.[38–40]

If β-blockers are to be discontinued, a gradual tapering schedule (preferably for 1 to 2 weeks) should be used. Shorter periods for β-blocker withdrawal (e.g., 2–3 days) have been proposed, although the optimal strategy for discontinuation is not known. Ensuring that β-blockers are tapered and that the patient is reasonably monitored for adverse events for the duration of the taper is imperative. Patients should limit physical activity throughout the β-blocker withdrawal period and seek prompt medical attention when angina symptoms become apparent.

LONG-ACTING NITRATES

CASE 17-1, QUESTION 19: J.P. recovers quickly and is discharged from the hospital after 48 hours. He does well during the next several months, but he is still bothered by occasional angina episodes, ranging from two to four times per week. He was changed to the translingual spray form of NTG (0.4 mg/spray) because he had difficulty with storage of the tablets. The attacks usually are precipitated by strenuous work and are relieved by rest and two or three NTG sprays. The quality and location of the pain are unchanged, although the duration has increased by 1 or 2 minutes. He follows a low-cholesterol, no-added-salt diet.

Physical examination is unchanged except for a 20-pound weight loss. Vital signs include the following: supine BP, 119/76 mm Hg; heart rate, 60 beats/minute; and respiratory rate, 12 breaths/minute. J.P.'s cardiologist elected to start a long-acting prophylactic nitrate (isosorbide mononitrate) as well as continuing his metoprolol succinate (100 mg daily), lisinopril (20 mg daily), aspirin (81 mg daily), and metformin (500 mg twice daily). Is a long-acting nitrate the best add-on option for J.P.'s chronic stable angina?

Long-acting nitrates occupy a key role in the prevention of angina of all types. The goals of therapy are to decrease the number, severity, and duration of J.P.'s anginal attacks. A CCB could be prescribed for J.P. instead of isosorbide mononitrate because he has no contraindications to this class of drugs. A CCB would have been a good alternative if his BP had remained elevated, but for now, J.P.'s BP and pulse are within a desired range. Nitrates can also affect blood pressure, but will likely do so to a lesser extent that CCBs. Because sublingual nitrates were well tolerated by J.P., a long-acting nitrate would be acceptable. If a CCB is considered at this point, a dihydropyridine should be used because they have no effect on heart rate, unlike diltiazem or verapamil. Lastly, ranolazine would be an option for add-on therapy, especially if J.P. experiences any adverse hemodynamic effects from either a CCB or long-acting nitrate. Ultimately, the decision for additional therapy is based on the prescriber's personal choice and past experience, as well as the entire spectrum of the patient's disease complex.[86]

CASE 17-1, QUESTION 20: Will J.P. develop tolerance to the long-acting nitrate?

Early evidence for the development of nitrate tolerance and dependence came from the munitions industry. Workers in this industry were constantly exposed to NTG and ethylene glycol dinitrate, components of explosives.[87] Tolerance can develop in as few as 24 hours after continuous exposure to nitrate preparations, although the degree of tolerance may be variable in terms of percentage of efficacy lost. Importantly, tolerance can be limited by maintaining a nitratefree interval of about 10 to 12 hours daily. Nitrate dosing schedules should be arranged to permit a nitrate-free interval during which time the patient may receive angina protection from β-blockers, CCBs, or ranolazine. Most often, this nitrate-free interval is arranged during the night because angina is more likely to occur during the workday. Patients with nocturnal angina should arrange their nitrate-free interval during the day.[88] Because long-acting nitrates must be dosed intermittently to avoid tolerance, metoprolol therapy will provide J.P. with continuous protection, even during the nitratefree interval. Although J.P. uses a long-acting nitrate, he still will respond favorably to sublingual NTG. No evidence indicates that use of long-acting nitrates leads to resistance or tolerance to the effects of sublingual NTG.

CASE 17-1, QUESTION 21: What is the mechanism of action for nitrate tolerance?

Several mechanisms of nitrate tolerance have been proposed, including the depletion of sulfhydryl groups, which are necessary for the biotransformation of nitrate to NO; neurohormonal activation; plasma volume expansion; and abnormalities in NO signal transduction. More recent investigations, however, have identified that chronic nitrate administration produces a state of oxidative stress, leading to dysfunction of mitochondrial aldehyde dehydrogenase, which is the enzyme responsible for biotransformation of nitrates to NO.[89,90]

One potential consequence of this current theory is that long-term administration of organic nitrates, by producing neurohormonal activation and endothelial dysfunction, may have long-term detrimental effects. Further research is needed to confirm this hypothesis for nitrate tolerance and its long-term consequences on patient outcomes.[91]

CASE 17-1, QUESTION 22: Are all nitrate delivery systems capable of inducing nitrate tolerance? How can tolerance be minimized?

All organic nitrates exhibit similar hemodynamic effects through a common pharmacologic mechanism; yet, the differing pharmacokinetic profiles of the nitrate delivery systems lead to a variation in the development of tolerance.[42] Short-acting formulations (e.g., SL NTG, oral NTG spray, and SL isosorbide dinitrate) are not likely to induce tolerance given their rapid onset of action and short duration of effect. Oral nitrates and transdermal products, both having an extended duration of action, are likely to induce tolerance.

Intermittent application of transdermal NTG can limit tolerance development in patients with both chronic stable angina and HF. The effects of continuous (24 hours/day) and intermittent (16 hours/day) transdermal NTG (10 mg/day) were compared in 12 men with chronic stable angina who also were being treated with β-blockers or CCB.[92] Nitrate efficacy was maintained with intermittent treatment and an 8-hour nitratefree interval. Tolerance to the antianginal effects occurred, however, with continuous transdermal NTG treatment. Twelve-hour intermittent patch therapy also prevents tolerance.[93] The minimal time necessary for a nitratefree interval is unknown.

Despite the availability of nitrate preparations that can be dosed once or twice a day (isosorbide mononitrate), oral isosorbide dinitrate is still commonly used in a variety of settings for the treatment of angina. Isosorbide dinitrate needs to be dosed three times a day, and presents a challenge in ensuring patients have a nitratefree interval. If J.P. were to receive isosorbide dinitrate, he should take his oral nitrate at 7 AM, noon, and 5 PM because his exercise-induced angina is likely to occur during daylight hours. If he were to take isosorbide dinitrate on a more traditional three-times-a-day or every-8-hours schedule, he would be in danger of not having an adequate nitratefree interval.

CASE 17-1, QUESTION 23: Does isosorbide mononitrate offer any distinct advantages over other nitrate preparations for angina prophylaxis?

Isosorbide mononitrate is the primary metabolite of isosorbide dinitrate. In fact, most of the clinical activity of isosorbide dinitrate is due to the mononitrate. Therefore, both drugs share a similar pharmacology. Isosorbide mononitrate does not undergo first-pass metabolism and has no active metabolites. Its oral bioavailability is almost 100%, and its overall elimination half-life is about 5 hours.[42] Maximal serum concentrations are observed 30 to 60 minutes after a dose. To minimize the potential development of nitrate tolerance, isosorbide mononitrate should be used in a twice-daily, asymmetric dosing regimen in which the first dose is taken on awakening and the second dose about 7 hours later. Because of this unconventional dosing pattern and the availability of the extended-release product, which can be taken once a day, most use of isosorbide mononitrate is in the form of the extended-release preparation.

General precautions and adverse reactions for isosorbide mononitrate are similar to those for the other nitrates. Potential advantages for the clinical use of isosorbide mononitrate are less dosage fluctuation because of the absence of presystemic clearance and an effective once-daily or twice-daily dosing schedule, which could perhaps lead to improved patient adherence. Nevertheless, isosorbide dinitrate is effective clinically when administered two or three times a day and is a viable alternative.

CASE 17-1, QUESTION 24: J.P. likes the idea of using topical nitrates instead of an oral agent. Are the transdermal patches a viable alternative?

Transdermal NTG patches were originally designed to provide anti-ischemic protection with once-daily application. The concept of a compact, easy-to-apply transdermal NTG patch prompted pharmaceutical manufacturers to design a number of products, which the FDA subsequently approved based on plasma level data, not clinical efficacy studies. Subsquently, the shortcomings of plasma level data have become apparent and prompted numerous clinical efficacy studies.

Transdermal NTG therapy has been shown to increase exercise duration and maintain an anti-ischemic effect for 12 hours after patch application. These beneficial responses remained consistent throughout 30 days of therapy. No significant nitrate tolerance or rebound was noted when the patch was applied for not more than 12 of 24 hours.[42]

Although the various patches use different pharmaceutical delivery systems, clear-cut advantages of one over another are not apparent. Despite variations in surface area and NTG content, the most important common denominator of the transdermal NTG systems is the amount of drug released per hour expressed as the release rate (e.g., 0.2 mg/hour). Each product label includes this information. Low dosages (0.2 to 0.4 mg/hour) may not produce sufficient plasma and tissue concentrations to produce a clinically significant effect[3]; however, it is still recommended to start with a low-dose patch and titrate upward as needed. Because the skin is the major factor influencing NTG absorption rate, product release characteristics do not favor one system over another. Contact dermatitis has been reported with the transdermal patches. Patient instructions are included with the patches and should be reviewed with the patient, emphasizing the appropriate time for application of the patch, removal of the patch, as well as the appropriate sites on the body where the patch should be placed.

CALCIUM-CHANNEL BLOCKERS

CASE 17-2

QUESTION 1: B.N., a 56-year-old man, has just undergone cardiac catheterization which showed two-vessel coronary artery disease with obstructions of 55% and 65% in the right coronary and circumflex coronary arteries, respectively. Before catheterization he had a 2- to 3-month history of exertional angina for which his primary-care physician prescribed sublingual NTG tablets (0.4 mg) and oral isosorbide mononitrate (60 mg once daily). B.N. discontinued the use of isosorbide mononitrate after a few weeks due to intolerable headaches. His medical history includes asthma, hypertension, and hyperlipidemia. Currently his other medications include losartan 100 mg once daily, fluticasone inhaler two puffs twice daily, albuterol inhaler two puffs as needed, aspirin 81 mg daily, and atorvastatin

20 mg daily. Current vital signs include a resting heart rate of 75 beats/minute, BP of 125/80 mm Hg, and respiratory rate of 14 breaths/minute. His physician begins antianginal therapy with oral diltiazem 120 mg once daily. Is this a good option for B.N. and his chronic stable angina?

Calcium-channel blockers are effective in both vasospastic and classic exertional angina. These drugs relieve vasospasm of the large coronary arteries and, as a result, are effective in treating Prinzmetal variant angina. Their beneficial effect in chronic stable (effort-induced) angina is the result of multiple factors. Their vasodilatory effects in the coronary circulation increase myocardial oxygen supply, whereas dilation of the peripheral arterioles leads to a reduction in myocardial oxygen demand. Because coronary vasospasm can occur at the site of an atherosclerotic plaque, a CCB is particularly useful in patients who have a vasospastic component to their angina.[46,47]

Although β-blockers are considered the drugs of choice when instituting antianginal therapy, recent data indicate that the selection of a heart rate-lowering CCB may also be a reasonable first-line choice as well. Calcium-channel blockers and β-blockers appear to provide equivalent efficacy in head-to-head trials of chronic stable angina.[94,95] In addition, the available head-to-head trials with sufficient numbers also suggest that CCBs and β-blockers produce similar effects on cardiovascular outcomes and mortality in patients with chronic stable angina.[96,97] In addition, several recent trials in the setting of hypertension with CAD have demonstrated that CCBs can produce meaningful reductions in mortality.[98–100] It would appear that either a heart rate–lowering CCB, or a β-blocker, may be considered relatively equal options and initial therapy for chronic stable angina. The selection of a particular class will likely be dictated by patient characteristics.

In the case of B.N., his asthma may be worsened by the addition of a β-blocker. Although a cardioselective β-blocker could be tried to see if B.N. could tolerate it, a heart rate–lowering CCB is a good alternative to a β-blocker for the treatment of angina in this situation. The choice of a CCB as initial therapy in this patient is appropriate because of B.N.'s previous intolerance to nitrates and because nitrate therapy requires the scheduling of a nitrate-free period.[1]

Given B.N.'s current heart rate and BP, the selection of a heart rate–lowering CCB seems most appropriate. However, the distinct pharmacologic and adverse event profiles of the various classes may dictate agent selection from patient to patient. Some side effects of CCBs reflect an extension of their hemodynamic and electrophysiologic profiles and, therefore, are predictable (Table 17-6). Dihydropyridine-induced hypotension and dizziness occur in approximately 15% of patients. Patients also may complain of light-headedness, facial flushing, headache, and nausea. Swelling of the lower legs and ankles (peripheral edema) is related to the potent peripheral vasodilating effects of these agents. The non-dihydropyridines, verapamil and diltiazem, have similar side effect profiles, although diltiazem appears to be better tolerated. The lower incidence of side effects reported with diltiazem, compared with verapamil, may reflect a true difference or, perhaps, less aggressive dosing regimens. Both drugs can cause sinus bradycardia and worsen already existing conduction defects and heart block.[46,47] Neither should be used in patients with sick sinus syndrome or advanced degrees of heart block unless a functioning ventricular pacemaker is present. Patients should be monitored for signs of worsening HF, such as SOB, weight gain, and peripheral edema. Verapamil-induced constipation

TABLE 17-6
Calcium-Channel Blocker Hemodynamic and Electrophysiologic Profile

Effect	Dihydropyridine Derivatives[a]	Diltiazem	Verapamil
Peripheral vasodilation[b]	+++	++	++
Coronary vasodilation[b]	+++	+++	++
Negative inotropes[c]	±	++	+++
AV node suppression[c]	±	+	++
Heart rate	Increase (reflex)	Decrease or unchanged	Decrease or unchanged
Pharmacokinetics[d]			
Dosing[e]			
Side Effects			
Nausea, vomiting	+ (most)	+/1	±
Constipation	Not observed	±	+
Hypotension, dizziness[f]	++	+	+
Flushing, headache	++	+	+
Bradycardia, HF symptoms	±	+	++
Reflex tachycardia, angina	+[g]	Not observed	Not observed
Peripheral edema	+	±	±

See also Tables 13-15 and 13-16. [a] Dihydropyridine derivatives that are US Food and Drug Administration approved for angina: amlodipine (Norvasc), nicardipine (Cardene), and nifedipine (Adalat, Procardia). See Table 13-6 for others that are approved for hypertension but have been used clinically for angina. Investigational: nitrendipine (Baypress).

[b] Peripheral and coronary vasodilation helpful for angina, hypertension, and possibly HF, but peripheral dilation is the basis for side effects of flushing, headache, and hypotension.

[c] AV node suppression is helpful for controlling supraventricular arrhythmias, but this property plus the negative inotropic effect may worsen HF. Nifedipine has less negative inotropic effect than verapamil and diltiazem, but still may worsen HF. Amlodipine may have the least negative inotropic effect.

[d] All have poor bioavailability owing to high first-pass metabolism and all are eliminated primarily by hepatic metabolism; intradivisional and interindividual variability in bioavailability and metabolism is extensive. Diltiazem, nifedipine, nicardipine, and verapamil have a short half-life (<5 hours) requiring frequent dosing or use of sustained-release products. Amlodipine, isradipine (8 hours), and felodipine (10–20 hours) have longer half-lives.

[e] See Tables 13-6 and 13-16.

[f] Hypotension and reflex tachycardia most with immediate-release nifedipine, occasional with immediate-release diltiazem and verapamil, minimal with sustained-release products or intrinsically long-acting agents.

can be particularly troublesome to the elderly. Rare instances of fecal impaction requiring surgery illustrate the need for the aggressive use of stool-softening agents and, often, bulk-forming laxatives.

Generalized fatigue and nonspecific GI complaints can occur with any of the calcium channel blockers. In rare instances, elevations of hepatic enzymes and acute hepatic injury have occurred with CCBs. Appreciation for the individual side effect profiles helps determine preference for one CCB over another. B.N. is not likely to experience major side effects with either verapamil or diltiazem.

CASE 17-2, QUESTION 2: On questioning, B.N. does not report any previous adverse events or tolerance issues with an ACE inhibitor. Is an ARB appropriate to use in B.N, or should he be switched to an ACE inhibitor for his CAD?

As previously discussed, the totality of available evidence supports the role of ACE inhibitors in reducing total mortality, cardiovascular mortality, nonfatal MI, and stroke in patients with stable ischemic heart disease and preserved ventricular function. Although in theory ARBs should produce the same beneficial effects as ACE inhibitors in patients with atherosclerosis, there are far fewer clinical trials with ARBs. The best supporting evidence comes from the TRANSCEND and ONTARGET trials, both of which suggest ARBs produce similar benefits as ACE inhibitors in preventing CVD events.[101,102] Based on these trials, it would be reasonable to continue ARB therapy in B.N. at this time given he has demonstrated the ability to tolerate the medication. It would not be unreasonable though to discuss with B.N. the possibility of switching to an ACE inhibitor given the substantial body of evidence that exists for patients with CAD. The combination of an ACE inhibitor and ARB does not offer any increased benefit, but does increase the risk of hyperkalemia and renal insufficiency.[52]

CASE 17-2, QUESTION 3: Six months later B.N. returns to see his doctor. His current therapy consists of SL NTG 0.4 mg tablets, losartan 100 mg once daily, fluticasone inhaler two puffs twice daily, albuterol inhaler two puffs as needed, aspirin 81 mg daily, atorvastatin 20 mg daily, and diltiazem 180 mg once daily. Current vitals include a resting heart rate of 55 beats/minute, BP of 115/65 mm Hg, and respiratory rate of 10 breaths/minute. B.N. states he still is having roughly three to four anginal attacks per week when he exerts himself doing yard work. Would ranolazine be a therapeutic option for his chronic stable angina at this time?

Approved by the FDA in 2006, ranolazine was the first new antianginal agent to be marketed in nearly 20 years. The need for additional agents to modify and treat myocardial ischemia is illustrated by the fact that many patients have contraindications to one or more traditional antianginal agents, or may not tolerate larger therapeutic doses of a specific drug used as monotherapy. Others may have intolerance to the additive hemodynamic effects of combination therapy, as well as incomplete relief of symptoms from revascularization therapy. For example, despite the effectiveness of PCI at relieving symptoms of angina, 10% to 25% of patients still have angina and 60% to 80% require antianginal therapy 1 year after the procedure.[103,104] Therefore, a need clearly exists for new antianginal agents to complement existing pharmacologic and revascularization strategies.

Although higher doses of diltiazem could be used in B.N., his current heart rate and blood pressure would likely prevent further titrating of therapy. β-Blockers and/or nitrates are not good options due to the potential reductions in BP (β-blocker, nitrate) and heart rate (β-blocker) that may occur. Thus, ranolazine represents a good option for B.N. at this time. Several large, randomized studies with ranolazine have been conducted, all demonstrating it is effective at reducing ischemia and angina when added to existing therapy. The Monotherapy Assessment of Ranolazine in Stable Angina (MARISA) trial randomly assigned patients in a crossover fashion who had met screening exercise treadmill criteria to either escalating doses of ranolazine (500 mg BID, 1,000 mg BID, 1,500 mg BID) or placebo. All other antianginal agents, except for SL NTG, were discontinued before start of the study. Ranolazine significantly increased exercise duration, time to onset of angina, and 1-mm ST-segment depression during exercise treadmill testing.[105] Similar results were seen in the Combination Assessment of Ranolazine in Stable Angina (CARISA) trial in which ranolazine (500 mg BID, 750 mg BID, 1,000 mg BID) was added to antianginal monotherapy that consisted of either atenolol 50 mg/day, diltiazem 180 mg/day, or amlodopine 5 mg/day.[106] The Efficacy of Ranolazine in Chronic Angina (ERICA) trial assessed the effects of ranolazine added to the maximal dose of an existing antianginal agent, in this case amlodopine 10 mg/day. Importantly, up to one-half of the patients enrolled in ERICA were also on a long-acting nitrate. Patients were randomly assigned to either ranolazine 500 mg/day for 1 week and then had their dose increased to 1,000 mg/day for an additional 6 weeks, or placebo. Patients receiving 1,000 mg/day of ranolazine had a significant reduction in both the number of weekly anginal attacks, as well as the number of SL NTG tablets used on a weekly basis.[107] Ranolazine was well tolerated in the CARISA, MARISA, and ERICA trials with the most common side effects being dizziness, constipation, nausea, and headache. The incidence of adverse effects increased with increasing doses. No other significant adverse effects were noted, although it is important to note the duration of these trials was limited.[48]

Initial information regarding the safety of ranolazine in patients with longer drug exposure came from the Ranolazine Open Label Experience (ROLE) program,[108] which followed patients from the MARISA and CARISA trials who continued participation in an open-label extension program. A total of 746 patients initially entered the 6-year run-on safety program. At the time of publication, the mean duration of therapy was 2.82 years, with 23.3% of patients discontinuing therapy. One-half of the withdrawals were because of adverse events, but the incidence of common adverse effects did not seem to change from that seen in the randomized portions of the clinical trials. Mortality rates at both 1 year (2.8%) and 2 years (5.6%) indicate no adverse risk of ranolazine on overall mortality.

Additional safety data are now available from the Metabolic Efficiency with Ranolazine for Less Ischemia in Non–ST-Elevation Acute Coronary Syndrome (MERLIN)-TIMI 36 trial.[109] Patients in the MERLIN trial were randomly assigned to ranolazine or placebo in the setting of non–ST-segment elevation ACS. Ranolazine was administered as an intravenous (IV) infusion for 12 to 96 hours, then converted to 1,000 mg twice daily. Patients were assessed for clinical end points during the acute hospitalization, then every 4 months thereafter. Treatment was continued for a median of 348 days. The primary end point of the trial (cardiovascular death, MI, or recurrent ischemia) trended lower with patients on ranolazine, but was not statistically significant (23.5% placebo, 21.8% ranolazine, $p = 0.11$). The incidence of recurrent ischemia was significantly reduced, however, with ranolazine (4.2% vs. 5.9%, $p = 0.02$), providing additional support for the efficacy of ranolazine in treating chronic stable angina. Although ranolazine appeared to offer no benefit in the setting of ACS, significant long-term safety data were seen in the trial. Importantly, the risk of mortality, sudden cardiac death, or symptomatic arrhythmias was not increased with ranolazine versus

TABLE 17-7
Considerations for the Use of Ranolazine in Patients With Chronic Stable Angina[16,48,150]

Clinical Issue	Recommended Management Strategy
Renal insufficiency	Ranolazine plasma levels may increase up to 50%. Caution with dose titration to maximal recommended dose
Hepatic insufficiency	Ranolazine is contraindicated in patients with clinically significant hepatic impairment
Drug Interactions: Effects on Ranolazine	
Strong CYP3A4 inhibitors	Plasma concentrations of ranolazine are significantly elevated when combined with potent inhibitors of CYP3A4. Ranolazine is contraindicated in patients receiving strong CYP3A4 inhibitors (ketoconazole, clarithromycin, nelfinivir, etc.)
Moderate CYP3A4 inhibitors	Limit the dose of ranolazine to 500 mg twice daily in patients receiving moderate inhibitors of CYP3A4 (diltiazem, verapamil, erythromycin, fluconazole, etc.)
CYP3A4 inducers	Coadministration of ranolazine with CYP3A4 inducers is contraindicated and should be avoided
P-glycoprotein inhibitors	Caution should be exercised when coadministering ranolazine with P-glycoprotein inhibitors, and the dose of ranolazine may need to be lowered based on clinical response
Drug Interactions: Effects on Other Medications	
Simvastatin	Plasma levels of simvastatin are increased twofold with coadministration with ranolazine through CYP3A4 inhibition by ranolazine; closely monitor for adverse effects (e.g., myositis) from simvastatin
Digoxin	Ranolazine coadministration increases plasma concentrations of digoxin by 1.5 times. Adjust dose of digoxin accordingly to maintain desired therapeutic level and response.
CYP2D6 substrates	Ranolazine can inhibit the activity of CYP2D6, and plasma concentrations of 2D6 substrates (β-blockers, tricyclic antidepressants, antipsychotics) may be increased and lower doses of these agents may be required
QT prolongation	Caution is recommended if the patient is on other QT prolonging drugs, or has QT prolongation as baseline

placebo. In fact, the incidence of arrhythmias in the first 7 days as documented by Holter monitor was significantly lower with ranolazine than with placebo.[110] This was an important finding given ranolazine produces a dose-dependent increase in the QT interval.[16,48] As QT prolongation activity has been associated with proarrhythmia in other medications, results from the MERLIN trial are reassuring that ranolazine appears to be safe to use for chronic treatment of patients with stable angina.

B.N. is at goal heart rate, and his blood pressure is well controlled on his current regimen, but he continues to have anginal symptoms. Given the demonstrated efficacy in relieving anginal symptoms, as well as the safety profile in a patient like B.N., ranolazine would be an excellent option for him for additional angina control.

CASE 17-2, QUESTION 4: How should ranolazine be dosed in B.N.?

Initial investigations of ranolazine involved an immediate-release product that necessitated three times/day dosing. Because of the short half-life of the parent drug, the peak-to-trough ratios in clinical studies were suboptimal, with significant loss of therapeutic efficacy at the end of the dosing interval.[111–114] Consequently, ranolazine is marketed as an extended-release tablet formulation that should be dosed twice daily. Maximal plasma concentrations are observed 4 to 6 hours after administration of the extended-release formulation with a terminal half-life of 7 hours. With twice-daily dosing of the extended-release preparation, a more favorable peak-to-trough fluctuation of 1.6 is observed.[48] Steady-state is typically reached within 3 days and oral bioavailability is in the 30% to 55% range. Ranolazine is primarily metabolized by the liver through CYP3A4 (70%–85%), and CYP2D6 (10%–15%). Ranolazine also is a substrate for P-glycoprotein.[16,48] Patients should initially be started at an oral dose of 500 mg twice daily, which can be titrated up to a maximal dose of 1,000 mg twice daily.

Although ranolazine is an option in the treatment of chronic stable angina, careful patient selection is required for the drug to be used safely and effectively. Table 17-7 summarizes significant issues which should be evaluated when the drug is being considered for a patient. For B.N., the main issue is the drug–drug interaction with diltiazem, and the maximum dose that should be used in B.N. is 500 mg twice daily. B.N. should be monitored closely for possible increased adverse effects with ranolazine.

CASE 17-3

QUESTION 1: E.R. is a 58-year-old woman with a history of chronic stable angina for the last several years that has been managed primarily with medical therapy. Her current medications include oral isosorbide mononitrate 120 mg daily, oral metoprolol succinate 200 mg daily, ranolazine 1000 mg twice daily, fluticasone two puffs BID, albuterol two puffs as needed, NTG spray 0.4 mg as needed for chest pain, and enteric-coated aspirin 81 mg/day. Today she returns to your pharmacy to obtain refills of her medications. She mentions that a few years back she remembers that her mother was put on estrogen by her doctor to help control her heart disease and is wondering if she should be on estrogen replacement as well?

Epidemiologic evidence initially supported the notion that hormone-replacement therapy (HRT) in postmenopausal women would prevent cardiovascular events. When put to the test of a randomized, placebo-controlled trial, the benefits of

HRT on cardiovascular disease, however, were not seen and potential harm was noted.[115,116] One of these studies was the Women's Health Initiative, which sought to answer the question of whether administering estrogen alone (in women without a uterus) or estrogen plus progesterone (in women with a uterus) would prevent the development of CAD in healthy (without history of CAD) postmenopausal women. Unexpectedly, a 29% increase was found in the incidence of CAD in those women on estrogen plus progesterone compared with placebo after an average treatment duration of 5 years.[117] Although there is still some interest in clarifying the effects of HRT therapy based on the age and time from menopause for women, current guideline recommendations do not support HRT therapy for the primary and secondary prevention of heart disease in women.[118]

CASE 17-3, QUESTION 2: E.R. returns to the pharmacy 1 week later with her 64-year-old brother who wants to know if he should be taking an aspirin a day to prevent heart disease. His only medical history consists of hypertension for which he is taking oral hydrochlorothiazide 25 mg every day. Is primary prevention of CAD with aspirin appropriate for E.R.'s brother?

The question of whether aspirin is valuable in the primary prevention of cardiovascular events has been debated for more than 20 years. Older meta-analyses indicate that aspirin reduces the risk of a serious vascular event (nonfatal MI, nonfatal stroke, or death from vascular causes) by 25%; however, low-dose aspirin also doubles the risk of major extracranial bleeding (mostly GI), as well as hemorrhagic stroke.[119] As these proportional changes for both efficacy and safety typically apply to most categories of patients with vascular disease, the absolute risk–benefit ratio for aspirin in primary prevention will depend on the overall absolute risk of vascular ischemic events. More recent randomized trials have raised questions regarding the actual risks and benefits of aspirin for primary prevention, with a meta-analysis published in 2009 suggesting that any benefit for aspirin in reducing ischemic events is offset by an increase in bleeding, resulting in no net clinical benefit.[120]

Despite this controversy, in 2009 the US Preventative Services Task Force developed updated guidelines for aspirin use in primary prevention incorporating at the time the most recent published evidence.[121] Recommendations are differentiated initially by age and sex, recognizing that the ischemic benefit varies between men (reduction in nonfatal MI) and women (reduction in ischemic stroke). Aspirin for primary prevention may be considered for men aged 45 to 79 years, and in women aged 55 to 78 years. Because E.R.'s brother is 64 years of age, it is appropriate for him to consider the use of aspirin for primary prevention. The first step is to calculate what his risk is for developing cardiovascular disease. This can be done by using a validated risk assessment scoring system, such as the Framingham risk score (see Chapter 13, Dyslipidemias, Atherosclerosis, and Coronary Heart Disease).[111] Based on his age, if his 10-year risk of CVD is greater than 9%, the CVD benefit with aspirin will outweigh any potential bleeding harm according to the US Preventative Service Guidelines.[121] Recognizing the existing controversy surrounding the use of aspirin for primary prevention, a thorough review of the potential risk and benefits should take place with E.R.'s brother so that he may make the most informed decision possible.

CASE 17-3, QUESTION 3: During the discussion with E.R. regarding her brother, she buys a bottle of over-the-counter ibuprofen. On further questioning, you learn that E.R. suffers from occasional back and knee pain and uses ibuprofen three to five times a week for pain relief. How should E.R. be educated regarding the use of ibuprofen and aspirin concomitantly?

In 2006, the FDA released a warning statement on the concomitant use of both aspirin and ibuprofen. The impetus for the statement was the growing recognition that nonsteroidal anti-inflammatory drugs (NSAIDs), in particular ibuprofen, may attenuate the antiplatelet effects of low-dose aspirin. This FDA warning was then followed by an updated scientific statement from the AHA.[122] The mechanism behind this interaction is that both aspirin and nonselective NSAIDs bind to the same acetylation sites of the cyclo-oxygenase enzyme. Although aspirin does this in a nonreversible fashion, binding by an NSAID occurs in a reversible fashion. If an NSAID, such as ibuprofen, is present, aspirin will be unable to bind to its site of action, and will be rapidly cleared from the plasma. The result is the patient will not receive the antiplatelet benefit of aspirin.

E.R. should be counseled on the nature and consequences of the interaction between her low-dose aspirin and ibuprofen. Additionally, if she can avoid or at least minimize (both dose and duration) the use of ibuprofen, the effect on her cardiovascular health would be optimized. If occasional use of ibuprofen cannot be avoided, it should be administered in such a fashion as to minimize the potential for interacting with her low-dose aspirin. This would include taking ibuprofen at least 2 hours after her daily dose of aspirin, as well as taking her daily aspirin dose at least 8 hours after the last dose of ibuprofen. Although similar concerns exist for other nonselective NSAIDs (naproxen, diclofenac), no formal recommendations exist on how to manage concomitant use of these agents with aspirin.[122]

REVASCULARIZATION

Percutaneous Coronary Intervention

CASE 17-3, QUESTION 4: Nine months later E.R. returns to her cardiologist stating that her chronic angina has been worsening. She is experiencing chest pain more frequently and much sooner when she does any type of physical activity. Her current medications are the same as previously discussed and it is felt that her medical management has been optimized as much as possible. After discussions with her cardiologist, she elects to undergo revascularization with PCI for symptom relief. What is the current standard for prevention of acute complications during PCI?

Percutaneous coronary intervention, also known as angioplasty, involves the percutaneous insertion of a balloon catheter into the femoral artery in a similar fashion to angiography. The catheter is advanced up the aorta and into the coronary arteries at the coronary sinus. PCI, which was introduced in 1977, initially involved the inflation of a catheter-borne balloon that mechanically dilated a coronary artery obstruction through arterial intimal disruption, plaque fissuring, and stretching of the arterial wall. Balloon inflations were repeated until the plaque was compressed and coronary blood flow resumed. Since then, alternative devices have been developed, including rotational blades designed to remove atheromatous material, lasers to ablate plaques, and intracoronary stents that are designed to maintain the patency of the vessel after it is reopened.[123] Stents can be of the bare-metal (BMS) variety, or contain a drug impregnated on the surface of the stent to prevent restenosis (drug-eluting stent, DES). It is estimated that

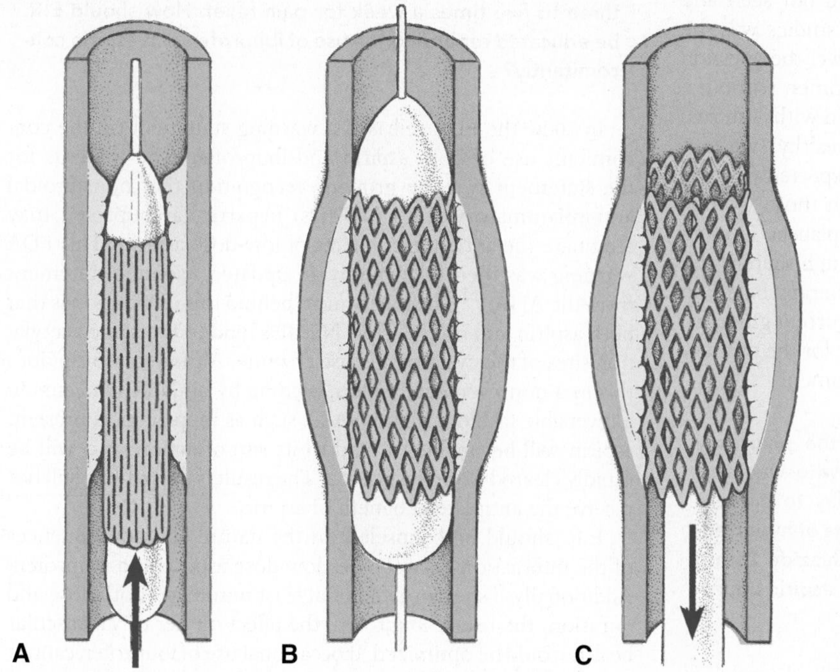

FIGURE 17-5 Vascular stent. A: A balloon catheter positions the stent at the site of arterial stenosis. **B:** Inflation of the balloon dilates the artery and expands the stent. **C:** The balloon is collapsed and withdrawn, leaving the expanded stent in position. (Illustration by Neil O. Hardy, Westpoint, CT.)

more than 1,265,000 PCI procedures are performed in the United States each year. An overwhelming majority of these procedures involve placement of a BMS or DES (Fig. 17-5). PCI is indicated in patients with single-vessel or multivessel disease and who are either symptomatic or asymptomatic.[123–125]

Because of mechanical disruption of the atherosclerotic plaques and exposure of plaque contents to the bloodstream during PCI, potent antiplatelet and antithrombotic strategies are needed to prevent acute thrombotic events such as MI and death. Initially, strategies involved the use of high-dose unfractionated heparin and aspirin. Current strategies in patients undergoing elective PCI involve the administration of aspirin, clopidogrel, an antithrombin agent, as well as a glycoprotein (GP) IIb/IIIa receptor antagonist in selected patients. Although prasugrel represents an alternative to clopidogrel in patients undergoing PCI, current ACC/AHA guidelines recommend its use only in patients undergoing PCI in setting of acute coronary syndromes. In patients not taking aspirin on a daily basis, 300 to 325 mg of aspirin should be given at least 2 hours before the procedure. Patients currently on daily aspirin therapy should receive 75 to 325 mg of aspirin before PCI is performed. A 600-mg loading dose of clopidogrel on or before the time of the procedure is currently recommended, producing an antiplatelet action within 2 hours.[11,124,125]

With the development of the GPIIb/IIIa receptor antagonists, significant improvements were made in patient outcomes during and after PCI.[125] Currently, three agents are available in the United States. Abciximab, a human-murine monoclonal antibody fragment, was the first agent available. Subsequently eptifibatide (cyclic heptapeptide) and tirofiban (nonpeptide mimetic) have become available.[125] These agents, when administered IV during PCI and for 12 to 24 hours afterward, significantly decrease the risk of death, acute MI, or need for repeat PCI. Major adverse effects include bleeding and thrombocytopenia. Therefore, hematocrit and platelet counts should be monitored appropriately. Clearance of both eptifibatide and tirofiban is renal, and dose adjustments should take place accordingly.[126]

In addition to appropriate use of the antiplatelet agents (aspirin, clopidogrel, and GPIIb/IIIa inhibitors), patients having PCI should also receive adequate antithrombin therapy during the procedure. Available options include unfractionated heparin, the low-molecular-weight heparin enoxaparin, and the direct thrombin inhibitor bivalirudin. Any of the available agents may be initiated at the time of the procedure, or may be continued with appropriate dose adjustment if administered to the patient before PCI. (See Chapter 18, Acute Coronary Syndrome, for information regarding appropriate dosing and management strategies for each agent.) Current guidelines do not specify a preference for any particular antithrombin agent during the course of PCI. Therefore, the choice of agent will likely depend on local practice variations.[125] Antithrombin agents are typically discontinued immediately after the PCI procedure unless a compelling separate indication exists for therapeutic anticoagulation. Of note, significant interest exists in using direct thrombin inhibitors, such as bivalirudin, in place of heparin during PCI. One advantage for this approach is that most patients receiving bivalirudin during PCI do not require a GPIIb/IIIa receptor antagonist. This strategy has the potential to reduce overall medication costs, as well as decrease the incidence of bleeding in association with PCI.[127]

CASE 17-3, QUESTION 5: E.R. undergoes PCI plus placement of a drug-eluting stent (sirolimus) to address a 75% lesion in her proximal left circumflex artery. What advantages and disadvantages are there in the decision to place a DES versus a BMS?

The overall success of any procedure is directly related to the experience of the operator, patient factors (such as LV function or number of vessels treated), and the equipment used. In patients receiving balloon angioplasty alone (without stent placement), repeat revascularization procedures (either repeat angioplasty or surgery) may be required in as many as 32% to 40% of cases because of lesion reoccurrence at the angioplasty site. The process is known as restenosis.[123] Many pharmacologic strategies have been studied in an attempt to reduce the risk of restenosis. The outcome with most methods has been disappointing. The only strategy that has been associated with a decrease in restenosis is the use of intraluminal stents.[123] Stents are essentially metal scaffolding devices placed into the vessel after balloon inflation has taken place. They provide a physical barrier to the reoccurrence of a significant stenosis at the site. One of the early drawbacks of the use of stents was the need for complicated anticoagulation regimens, including aspirin, heparin, dipyridamole, and warfarin, to prevent in-stent thrombosis. Dual antiplatelet therapy—a combination of a thienopyridine (clopidogrel or prasugrel) and aspirin—is effective at reducing in-stent thrombosis and is now recommended for use after stent placement.[124,125] The duration of dual antiplatelet therapy will depend on the type of stent used, as well as other clinical characteristics of the patient.

Recently, stents that elude antiproliferative agents such as sirolimus, paclitaxel, or everolimus have been shown in clinical trials to reduce the incidence of restenosis compared with BMS.[128,129] Restenosis rates in clinical trials with these DES were in the single-digit range, as compared to 15% to 20% with traditional BMS. Soon after their introduction to the US market, DES use grew to the point that greater than 90% of stent use was DES. This trend abruptly halted in the fall of 2006 when several reports indicated a higher than expected incidence of stent thrombosis a year or more after DES placement. Although late stent thrombosis had previously been reported with BMS usage, the incidence was rare.[129] Shortly after these initial reports, an explosion of scientific literature emerged on the topic. Many potential explanations exist for the occurrence of late stent thrombosis in a patient receiving a DES, but perhaps the most relevant from a pharmacotherapy standpoint is the delayed endothelialization seen with DES compared with BMS. After placement of an intracoronary stent, a healing process typically occurs resulting in growth of a protective layer of endothelial cells over the stent surface, removing the stent surface from blood exposure and drastically reducing the stimulus for thrombosis. In the case of DES coated with paclitaxel, sirolimus, or everolimus, cellular growth may be inhibited, significantly impairing endothelialization of the stent surface. In a small number of patients, endothelialization does not seem to occur at all. In this scenario, the stent structure remains continually exposed to flowing blood and is a potent stimulus for thrombosis.[130] Because of the concerns of late stent thrombosis, the usage of DES has decreased. Some use of DES is likely to continue, however, owing to the tangible benefits in reduction of revascularization procedures in some patients. Therefore, practitioners will need to continue to stay abreast of evolving information regarding appropriate strategies to prevent late stent thrombosis.

Although there has been speculation to the causes of late stent thrombosis with DES, one critical issue that has been identified is the premature discontinuation of dual antiplatelet therapy consisting of aspirin and clopidogrel. As such, considerations of whether the patient is likely to comply with thienopyridine therapy, or afford such therapy based on insurance status, has become a significant factor in the decision process between using a BMS or DES. Previous recommendations called for varying durations of combined therapy, depending on the type of stent used. Because of the recognition of a delayed healing response to DES, current guidelines recommend at least 1 year of dual antiplatelet therapy in patients receiving a DES if patients are not at an elevated risk of bleeding. For BMS placement, dual antiplatelet therapy should continue for a minimum of 1 month, and up to 1 year ideally, but this extended duration is not as critical as it is in the setting of DES placement. The dose of aspirin during dual antiplatelet therapy should be 162 to 325 mg/day, and then decreased to 81 mg/day once dual antiplatelet therapy is discontinued. When administered, the dose of clopidogrel should be 75 mg/day.[124,125]

For E.R. the decision of placing a DES versus a BMS will likely be a lower risk of needing a repeat revascularization for restenosis within 6 to 9 months. She will, however, need to take dual antiplatelet therapy for at least a year, significantly increasing the costs of her prescriptions as well as putting her at an increased risk of bleeding in the long run. Regardless, it is vital that E.R. be educated about the importance of maintaining her therapy with aspirin and clopidogrel to prevent complications. This discussion should commence before the PCI procedure to assess whether E.R. has the economic resources to comply with the needed therapy, or whether there may be any planned upcoming surgery necessitating the discontinuation of antiplatelet therapy.[131] If these present a problem for E.R., placement of a BMS is a viable option. E.R. should also be counseled to alert her cardiologist if another health care professional wishes to discontinue antiplatelet therapy for any reason.[132]

CASE 17-3, QUESTION 6: Would revascularization therapy with coronary artery bypass grafting have been a better option for E.R. than PCI and stent placement?

Coronary artery bypass grafting is a complicated surgical procedure during which an atherosclerotic vessel is bypassed using either a patient's saphenous vein or internal mammary artery (IMA; Fig. 17-6). The graft (i.e., the saphenous vein or IMA) then allows blood to flow past the obstruction in the native vessel. The goals of antianginal therapy, whether medical (pharmacologic) or revascularization, remain unchanged: (a) to prolong life, (b) to prevent MI, and (c) to improve the quality of life.

The outcomes of medical therapy, PCI, and revascularization with CABG have been compared, and current guidelines are available.[31,32] Of interest to practitioners and patients are the relative effects of each treatment modality on mortality, occurrence of symptoms, and quality of life. When compared with medical treatment in patients who would not be considered high

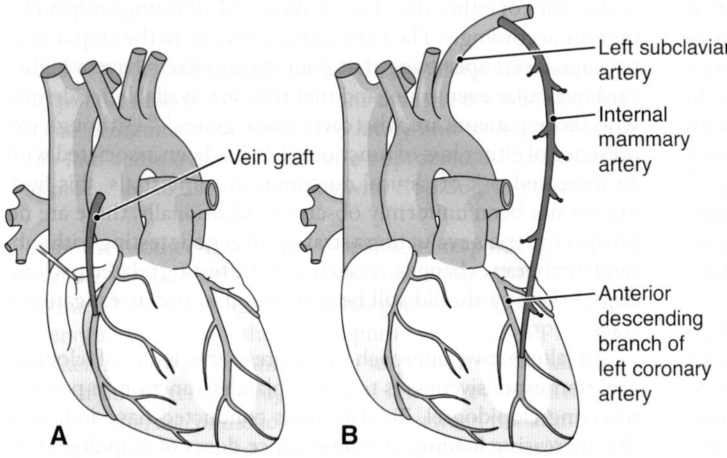

FIGURE 17-6 Coronary artery bypass graft (CABG). A: A segment of the saphenous vein carries blood from the aorta to a part of the right coronary artery that is distal to an occlusion. **B:** The mammary artery is used to bypass an obstruction in the left anterior descending (LAD) coronary artery. (Reprinted with permission from Cohen BJ. *Medical Terminology*. 4th ed. Philadelphia, PA: Lippincott Williams & Wilkins; 2003.)

LONG-TERM THERAPIES *CONTINUED*

2	Lifestyle modifications include smoking cessation, weight management through diet and exercise to reduce body weight by 10% if body mass index exceeds 25 kg/m^2, diabetic treatment to achieve a near normal hemoglobin A_{1c}, and serum lipid control to achieve an optimal low-density lipoprotein concentration of 70 mg/dL or less.	**Case 18-3 (Question 10)**

ACUTE CORONARY DISEASE

Despite advances in medical intervention and pharmacotherapy, cardiovascular disease continues to be a leading killer in the United States. Acute coronary syndrome (ACS) is an umbrella term that includes patients who present with either unstable angina (UA) or acute myocardial infarction (AMI) consisting of ST segment elevation myocardial infarction (STEMI) or non–ST segment myocardial infarction (NSTEMI). The etiology of ACS originates from the erosion or rupture of an unstable plaque within the coronary artery cascading to the formation of an occlusive or nonocclusive thrombus.[1–4] Although both UA,NSTEMI and STEMI lead to hospitalization, patients presenting with STEMI are considered medical emergencies and warrant immediate intervention. Until the 1980s, patients with AMI were treated symptomatically. Their pain was controlled; arrhythmic complications were treated; and bed rest, nitrates, and β-blockers minimized the amount of oxygen required by the heart. In 1980, an angiographic study by DeWood et al. found total occlusion in a coronary artery in 87% of patients who were examined by angiography within the first 4 hours of symptoms.[5] This study stimulated interest in using thrombolytic drugs to interrupt the progression of thrombus leading to myocardial necrosis. Today, the management of ACS is based on reperfusion and revascularization using a variety of strategies, including thrombolytic therapy, antiplatelet agents, anticoagulants, and nonpharmacological interventions such as percutaneous coronary intervention (PCI) and coronary artery bypass grafting (CABG).[2] A committee composed of representatives from the American College of Cardiology (ACC) and the American Heart Association (AHA) periodically review the literature and publish practice guidelines to aid health care practitioners in selecting the most effective treatments for patients with ACS.[1–4] These guidelines consist of graded recommendations based on the weight and quality of the evidence. Although there are most certainly local variations in practice, these guidelines serve as the foundation for care of patients with ACS.

Epidemiology

According to AHA statistics, 733,000 hospital discharges in the United States were attributable to ACS in 2006. Approximately 80% of these cases comprised either UA or NSTEMI, and about 20% were STEMI.[6] Financially, the impact of ACS is also exceedingly high, costing Americans more than $150 billion annually.[7] Nearly 20% of patients with ACS are rehospitalized within 1 year, and approximately 60% of the costs related to ACS are caused by rehospitalization.[8] Approximately one-third of STEMI patients die within 24 hours of onset of ischemia compared with 15% of patients with UA or NSTEMI who either die or experience a reinfarction within 30 days of hospitalization.[7] Although these numbers are substantial, the risk-standardized 30-day in-hospital mortality for Medicare beneficiaries admitted for AMI have significantly dropped during the past decade.[9] Additionally, a large population-based study suggests that age- and sex-adjusted incidence of AMI exhibited a 24% relative decrease between 1999 and 2008, and that the age- and sex-adjusted 30-day mortality after AMI decreased from 10.5% in 1999 to 7.8% in 2008 ($p < 0.001$).[10] These trends may be reflective of application of evidence-based guidelines as well as aggressive treatment of hypertension and hypercholesterolemia.[9]

Pathophysiology

The majority of ACS results from occlusion of a coronary artery secondary to thrombus formation overlying a lipid-rich atheromatous plaque that has undergone fissuring or rupture (Fig. 18-1). Plaques that are more susceptible to rupture are characterized by a thin fibrous cap, large fatty core, high content of inflammatory cells such as macrophages and lymphocytes, limited amounts of smooth muscle, and eccentric shape. Triggers such as surges in sympathetic activity with a sudden increase in blood pressure, pulse rate, myocardial contractility, and coronary blood flow can lead to erosion, fissuring, or rupture of the fragile fibrous cap surrounding the atheromatous plaque. Once ruptured, the thrombogenic components of the plaque consisting of collagen and tissue factor are exposed. This promotes activation of the platelet cascade, ultimately leading to the formation of a clot or thrombus as well as ischemia in the corresponding myocardial area. The extent of intracoronary thrombosis and distal embolization determines the type of ACS (Fig. 18-1). In patients with UA, the coronary lesion demonstrates severe stenosis or narrowing but with little thrombosis. In patients with NSTEMI, there exists partial thrombotic occlusion with or without distal embolization or severe stenosis. For STEMI, there exists total and persistent thrombotic occlusion.[11] It is important to highlight that 80% of patients presenting with ACS have two or more active plaques.[12]

Most infarctions are located in a specific region of the heart and are described as such (e.g., anterior, lateral, inferior). Some patients exhibit permanent electrocardiographic (ECG) abnormalities (Q waves) after an AMI. In the past, patients with Q-wave infarctions were generally believed to have more extensive necrosis and a higher in-hospital mortality rate. Patients with a non–Q-wave infarct were believed to have a greater likelihood of experiencing postinfarction angina and early reinfarction. More recently, however, these distinctions have come into question. Some cardiologists now believe there is no difference in prognosis. The terminology has changed because most patients who have STEMI are treated emergently, preventing the development of Q waves. An anterior wall infarction carries a worse prognosis than an inferior or lateral wall infarction because it is more commonly associated with development of left ventricular failure and cardiogenic shock.[1–3]

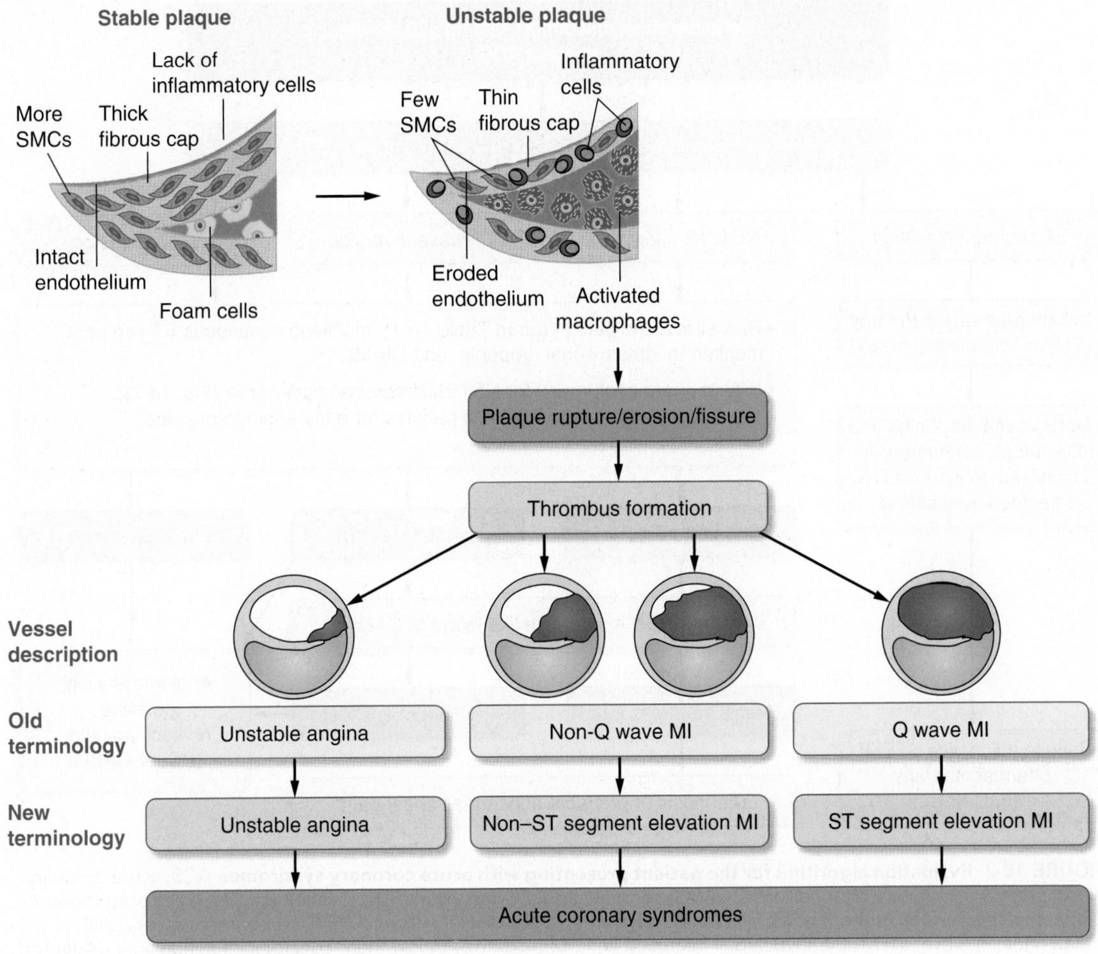

FIGURE 18-1 Thrombus formation and acute coronary syndrome definitions. MI, myocardial infarction; SMC, smooth muscle cells.

Clinical Presentation

One important part in establishing the diagnosis of ACS is obtaining the patient's "story" on admission, which can illicit crucial hallmark symptoms. Hallmark symptoms for ACS consist of increasing frequency of exertional angina or chest pain at rest, new-onset severe chest discomfort, or increasing angina with a duration exceeding 20 minutes. The pain is typically midline anterior chest discomfort that can radiate to the left arm, back, shoulder, or jaw and may be associated with diaphoresis, dyspnea, nausea, and vomiting as well as unexplained syncope.[1–4] Patients with STEMI will usually complain of unrelenting chest pain whereas patients with UA or NSTEMI will present with either angina at rest, new-onset (2 months or less) angina, or angina that increases in frequency, duration, or intensity. Presentation may differ by sex and age. Men commonly complain of chest pain, whereas women often present with nausea and diaphoresis.[1–4] Elderly patients may present with hypotension or cerebrovascular symptoms rather than chest pain. Additionally, onset of ACS does not occur at random, and many episodes appear to be triggered by external factors or conditions. Myocardial infarction occurs with increased frequency in the morning, particularly within the first hour after awakening; on Mondays; during winter months and on colder days the year around; and during emotional stress and vigorous exercise.

The physical examination may also be important in guiding initial therapy. Signs of severe left ventricular or right ventricular dysfunction may be present (see Chapter 19, Heart Failure). The patient may have severe hypertension as a result of pain or, conversely, may be hypotensive. Significant tachycardia (heart rate >120 beats/minute) suggests a large area of damage. On cardiac auscultation, a fourth heart sound (S_4) may be heard, denoting an ischemia-induced decrease in left ventricular compliance. New cardiac murmurs may be heard, resulting from papillary muscle dysfunction. The cerebral and peripheral vasculature should be assessed. Patients with a history of cerebrovascular disease may not be eligible for thrombolytic therapy. Peripheral pulses should be examined to assess perfusion and to obtain a baseline before invasive procedures are instituted.

Diagnosis

In addition to the patient's history and presentation, the diagnosis of ACS is based on the ECG and laboratory results from a cardiac injury profile. A 12-lead ECG should be obtained within 10 minutes of presenting to the emergency department (ED). The ECG is an indispensable tool in the diagnosis of ACS and has become the key point in the decision pathway (Fig. 18-2). Key findings on ECG consist of ST segment elevation, ST segment depression, or T-wave inversion.[1–3] By definition, STEMI consists of ST segment elevation in two or more contiguous leads and either exceeding 0.2 mV (2 mm) in leads V_1, V_2, and V_3 or 0.1 mV (1 mm) or greater in other leads (Fig. 18-3). NSTEMI consists of ST segment depression exceeding 0.1 mV in two or more contiguous leads or T-wave inversions exceeding 0.1 mV (mm).

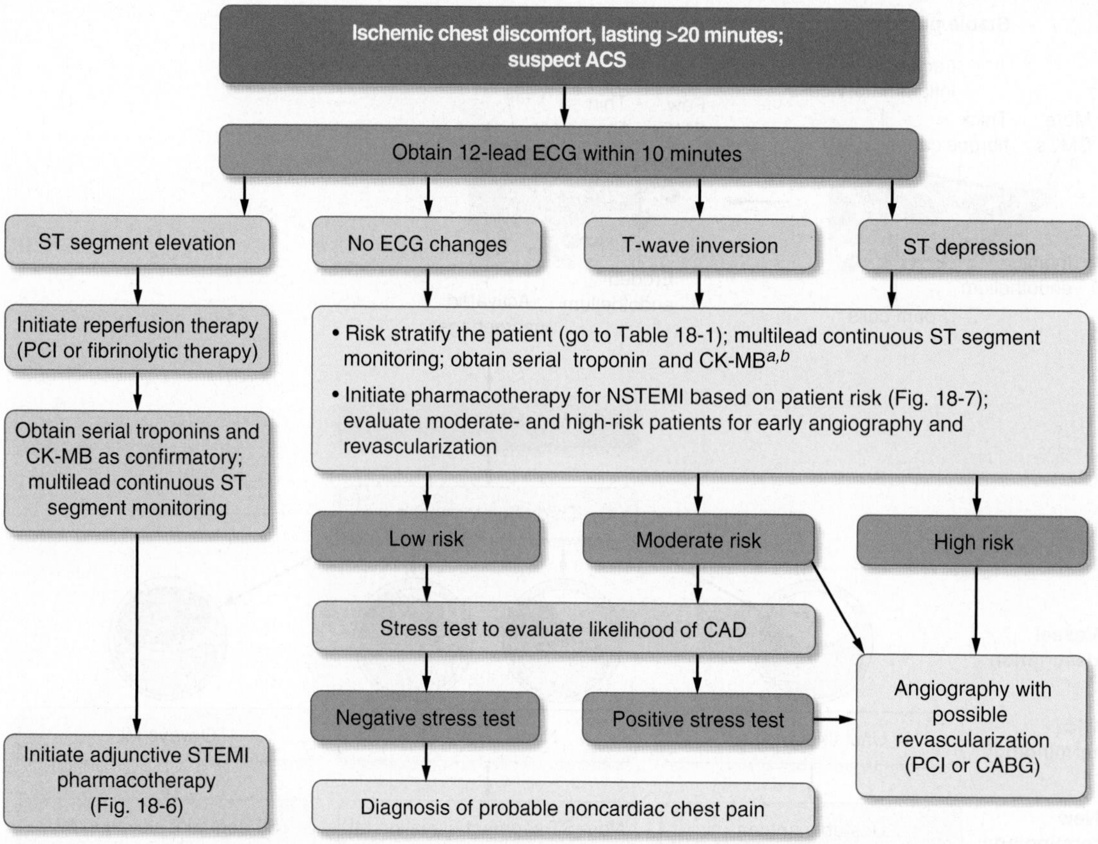

FIGURE 18-2 Evaluation algorithm for the patient presenting with acute coronary syndrome. ACS, acute coronary syndrome; CAD, coronary artery disease; CABG, coronary artery bypass graft; CK, creatinine; ECG, electrocardiogram; PCI, percutaneous intervention; NSTEMI, Non-ST segment myocardial infarction; STEMI, ST segment myocardial infarction. a: Positive, above the myocardial infarction limit; b: Negative, below the myocardial infarction limit. (Adapted with permission from Spinler SA. Evolution of Antithrombotic Therapy Used in Acute Coronary Syndromes. In: Richardson M, Chessman K, Chant C, Cheng J, Hemstreet B, Hume AI, eds. *Pharmacotherapy Self-Assessment Program*, 7th edition. Cardiology. Lenexa, KS: American College of Clinical Pharmacy; 2010.62.)

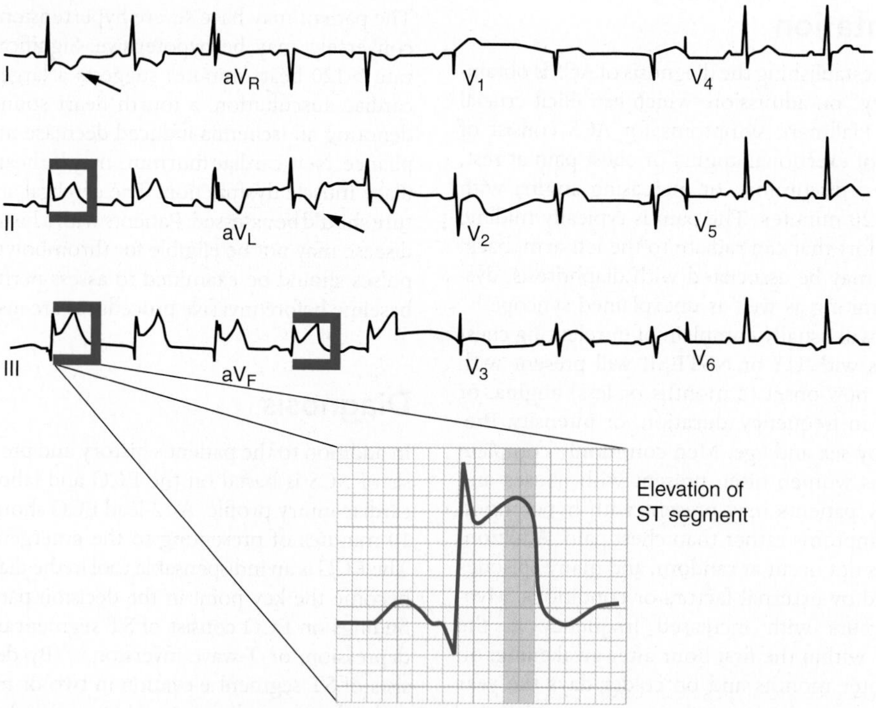

FIGURE 18-3 ECG changes related to STEMI. On this admission electrocardiogram (ECG), note the extensive ST segment elevation in leads II, III, and aV$_F$ (*brackets*), indicating an inferior wall acute myocardial infarction (AMI). The patient also displays reciprocal ST segment depression in leads I and aV$_L$ (*arrows*), which are the lateral ECG leads and are opposite the inferior leads.

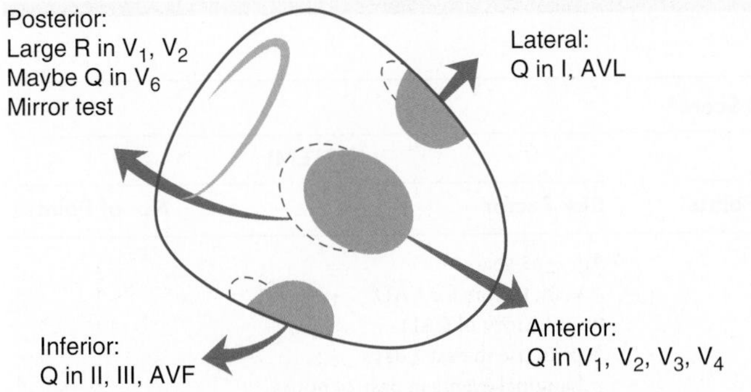

FIGURE 18-4 Location of an anterior, lateral, inferior, or posterior infarction based on the presence of Q waves in leads V_{1-6}. (Reprinted with permission from Dubin D. Infarction. In Dubin D, ed. *Rapid Interpretation of EKGs*. 6th ed. Tampa, FL: COVER Publishing Co; 2000:290.)

Additionally, the 12-lead ECG is helpful in determining the location of an infarct (Fig. 18-4).

Laboratory Changes

When a cardiac cell is injured, enzymes are released into the circulation. The measurement of these sensitive and specific enzymes (troponins T or I and creatine kinase [CK]) is routine in establishing the diagnosis of AMI (Fig. 18-5). There are three isoenzymes

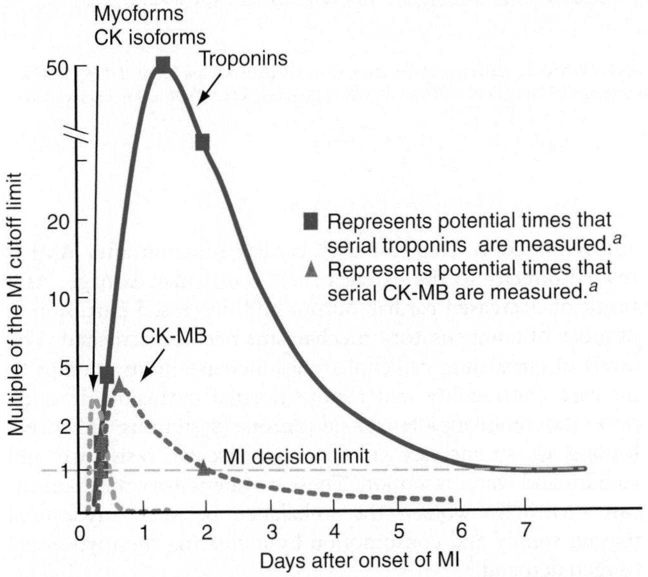

FIGURE 18-5 Cardiac biomarker elevation in acute coronary syndrome. CK, creatine kinase; MI, myocardial infarction. a. Serial troponins and CKMB are initially measured during first 12–24 hours of onset of chest pain and continued to be measured until the concentrations begin to decline. (Adapted with permission from Anderson JL, Adams CD, Antman EM, et al. ACC/AHA 2007 guidelines for the management of patients with unstable angina/non-ST-Elevation myocardial infarction: a report of the American College of Cardiology/American Heart Association Task Force on Practice Guidelines (Writing Committee to Revise the 2002 Guidelines for the Management of Patients With Unstable Angina/Non-ST-Elevation Myocardial Infarction) developed in collaboration with the American College of Emergency Physicians, the Society for Cardiovascular Angiography and Interventions, and the Society of Thoracic Surgeons endorsed by the American Association of Cardiovascular and Pulmonary Rehabilitation and the Society for Academic Emergency Medicine. *J Am Coll Cardiol.* 2007;50(7):e1–e157.)

of CK: the BB, MM, and MB bands. Of these, the CK-MB isoenzyme is the most specific for the myocardium. It can appear in the serum within 3 to 6 hours after myocardial damage, and levels generally peak in 12 to 24 hours and remain elevated for 2–3 days.[1–3] Unfortunately, several conditions other than AMI can elevate CK-MB, such as myositis, pericarditis, myocarditis, rhabdomyolysis, renal failure, hyperthermia, hypothermia, and renal failure (see Chapter 2, Interpretation of Clinical Laboratory Tests).[13]

Troponin has become the preferred biomarker for assessment of myocardial damage owing to its high cardiac specificity and sensitivity (90.7% and 90.2%, respectively) as well as the development of newer troponin assays.[14,15] Troponins T and I are detectable in blood within 4 to 12 hours after the onset of MI, and peak values are observed at 12 to 48 hours. Troponin levels may also stay elevated for 7 to 10 days after myocardial necrosis. As seen in Figure 18-5, the horizontal line depicts the upper reference limit (URL) for the cardiac biomarker in the clinical chemistry laboratory. The URL is that value representing the 99th percentile of a reference control group without MI. Because cardiac troponin I and T are not normally detected in the blood of healthy people, the definition of an abnormally increased level is a value that exceeds that of 99% of a reference control group. For the diagnosis of NSTEMI or STEMI, the patient should have one troponin value or two CK-MB values greater than the URL. Cardiac biomarkers are not typically elevated in patients with UA. Presently, no current marker is detectable immediately upon onset of MI, and therefore repeated measurements of cardiac enzymes after admission are warranted. Initially, enzymes will be measured every 4 to 6 hours on presentation for the first 12 to 24 hours and periodically thereafter.[1–3] If the patient presents with chest pain as well as elevated troponins and exhibits a reinfarction a few days later, CK-MB would be the preferred biomarker for diagnosis. Newer biomarkers that are being evaluated for diagnosis and risk stratification of patients consist of C-reactive protein and myeloperoxidase for inflammation and plaque destabilization as well as brain (B-type) natriuretic peptide (BNP) for detection of a left ventricular dysfunction (for additional information regarding BNP see Chapter 19, Heart Failure and Chapter 2, Interpretation of Laboratory Tests).[13]

Risk Stratification

The examination of a patient presenting with ACS begins with stratification for the risk of death and reinfarction, which takes into account the presenting signs and symptoms and past medical history, as well as ECG and cardiac biomarker changes. Patients can be stratified into low, medium, or high risk for mortality and the need for urgent coronary angiography and PCI (Fig. 18-2). The first risk stratification method was introduced in 1967 by Killip and Kimball[15] and was found to be a useful, convenient tool for early risk stratification for patients with STEMI. Higher Killip class was found to be associated with increased in-hospital and 1-year mortality (Table 18-1).[16] The Thrombolysis in Myocardial Infarction (TIMI) risk score was introduced in 2000 and can be used with either STEMI or UA/NSTEMI (Table 18-1).[17,18] For STEMI, the higher the risk score, the greater the 30-day mortality rate. However, patients with STEMI are at the highest risk of death and reinfarction, and initial treatment should proceed with revascularization without risk stratification. "Time is tissue," meaning that the sooner the thrombosed artery is opened, the lower the morality and greater amount of myocardium preserved. The ACC/AHA guidelines define a target time to initiate reperfusion for STEMI within 30 minutes of hospital presentation for thrombolytic therapy and within 90 minutes from presentation for PCI.

TABLE 18-1
Risk Stratifications Tools for Acute Coronary Syndrome

TIMI Risk Score[a]

STEMI Risk Factor	No. of Points	NSTEMI Risk Factor	No. of Points
Age 65–75 years	2	Age ≥65 years	1
Age ≥75 years	3	≥3 risk factors for CAD[b]	1
SBP <100 mm Hg	3	Prior history of CAD[c]	1
Heart rate >100 beats/min	2	Aspirin use in past 7 days	1
Killip class II–IV	2	≥2 anginal events in past 24 hours	1
Weight <67 kg	1	ST segment deviation ≥0.5 mm	1
History of HTN, diabetes, or angina	1	Elevation of cardiac markers[d]	1
Time to reperfusion therapy >4 hours	1		
Anterior ST segment elevation or left bundle branch block	1		

Killip Class[e]

Class	Symptoms	In-Hospital and 1-Year Mortality (%)
I	No heart failure	5
II	Mild heart failure, rales, S_3, congestion on chest radiograph	21
III	Pulmonary edema	35
IV	Cardiogenic shock	67

[a]TIMI risk score data from Antman EM et al. The TIMI risk score for unstable angina/non-ST elevation MI: A method for prognostication and therapeutic decision making. *JAMA.* 2000;284:835; Morrow DA et al. Application of the TIMI risk score for ST-elevation MI in the National Registry of Myocardial Infarction 3. *JAMA.* 2001;286:1356. A risk score is calculated by adding the total number of risk factors. Total points for STEMI are 0–14, in which risk scores of 0, 2, 4, 6, 7, and >8 correspond to a 30-day mortality rate of 0.8%, 2.2%, 7.3%, 16%, 23%, and 36%, respectively. Total points for NSTEMI are 0–7, in which scores of 0 or 1, 3, 5, and 7 correspond to a 3%, 5%, 12%, or 19% risk of death or repeat MI at 14 days, respectively.

[b]Risk factors include smoking, diabetes, hypertension, family history of coronary artery disease, and hypercholesterolemia.

[c]Defined as a prior coronary stenosis ≥50%; history of previous myocardial infarction, percutaneous coronary intervention, or coronary artery bypass graft; or chronic stable angina pectoris associated with a positive exercise tolerance test or pharmacologically induced nuclear imaging or echocardiographic changes (positive nuclear imaging or echocardiographic changes required if female).

[d]Either troponin I or T or creatine kinase-MB.

[e]Killip class data from Killip T 3rd, Kimball JT. Treatment of myocardial infarction in a coronary care unit. A two year experience with 250 patients. *Am J Cardiol.* 1967;20:457.

CAD, coronary artery disease; HTN, hypertension; NSTEMI, non–ST segment elevation myocardial infarction; SBP, systolic blood pressure; STEMI, ST segment elevation myocardial infarction; TIMI, Thrombolysis in Myocardial Infarction.

In the case of UA/NSTEMI, a TIMI risk score of 5 to 7, 3 to 4, and 0 to 2 reflect a high, medium, and low risk for death, MI, or need for urgent coronary artery revascularization, respectively (Table 18-1). A low-risk patient with negative cardiac biomarkers may undergo a stress test or be discharged from the ED with a diagnostic test scheduled for the near future. Moderate- to high-risk patients are often admitted to the hospital for pharmacologic treatment, further diagnostic tests, and angiography with possible intervention. Additional risk stratification tools such as the Platelet glycoprotein IIb/IIIa in Unstable angina: Receptor Suppression Using Integrilin Therapy (PURSUIT) risk score and Global Registry of Acute Cardiac Events (GRACE) risk score exist for in-hospital and 1-year morality.[19] Other risk scores are available to predict bleeding in patients with ACS.[20]

ONLINE CONTENT

For practice with using the TIMI risk score and other risk stratifying methods for ACS, please refer to the interactive multimedia case of RM at http://thepoint.lww.com/AT10e.

Complications

The primary complications of AMI can be divided into three major groups: pump failure, arrhythmias, and recurrent ischemia and reinfarction. Depression of cardiac function after AMI is related directly to the extent of left ventricular damage. As a result of decreased cardiac output and decreased perfusion, a number of compensatory mechanisms become activated. The levels of circulating catecholamines increase in an attempt to increase contractility and restore normal perfusion. In addition, the renin-angiotensin-aldosterone system is enhanced, leading to an increase in systemic vascular resistance and sodium and water retention. These compensatory mechanisms can eventually worsen the imbalance between myocardial oxygen supply and consumption by increasing the myocardial oxygen demand.[21]

Signs and symptoms of heart failure (HF) are common in patients who have abnormal wall motion affecting 20% to 25% of the left ventricle (LV). If 40% or more of the LV is damaged, cardiogenic shock and death may occur. In addition to systolic dysfunction, patients who have experienced an AMI may also have diastolic dysfunction. Scar formation after an AMI may lead to a decrease in ventricular compliance, resulting in abnormally high left ventricular filling pressures during diastole. (See Chapter 19, Heart Failure, for further discussion on systolic dysfunction versus diastolic dysfunction.)

Decreased contractility and a compensatory increase in left ventricular end-diastolic volume and pressure lead to increased wall stress within the LV. Left ventricular enlargement is an important determinant of mortality after AMI. During a period of days to months after an AMI, the infarcted area may expand as a result of dilatation and thinning of the left ventricular wall. These changes are known as *ventricular remodeling.* In addition, hypertrophy of the noninfarcted myocardium occurs. Administration of oral angiotensin-converting enzyme (ACE) inhibitors, angiotensin receptor blockers (ARBs), or aldosterone antagonists may limit remodeling and will attenuate the progression of left ventricular dilatation.[22]

During the peri-infarction period, the heart is irritable and subject to ventricular arrhythmias. The continuous monitoring of patients in a coronary care unit has reduced the in-hospital mortality rate related to ventricular arrhythmias. However, patients who have had an AMI have an increased risk of sudden cardiac death for 1 to 2 years after hospital discharge. The most important predictor for sudden cardiac death is an abnormal ejection fraction (EF). Other factors associated with an increased risk for sudden cardiac death are complex ventricular ectopy, frequent (>10/hour) premature ventricular complexes, and the identification of late potentials on a signal-averaged ECG.[21]

OVERVIEW OF DRUG AND NONDRUG THERAPY

Overlap exists regarding the pharmacotherapy for both STEMI and NSTEMI. According to the ACC/AHA guidelines, early therapies should consist of oxygen (if oxygen saturation is <90%), sublingual nitroglycerin, aspirin or clopidogrel, stool softener, β-blocker, statin, and anticoagulant. Adjunctive therapies such as analgesics and vasodilators can also be considered in selected patients. Table 18-2 summarizes the evidenced-based pharmacotherapies for both STEMI and UA or NSTEMI. Figure 18-6 provides an initial treatment algorithm for patients with STEMI, and Figure 18-7, for patients with NSTEMI. Administration of these pharmacotherapies serves as a performance measure for health systems to ensure effective, timely, safe, and efficient patient-centered care. The STEMI and UA or NSTEMI performance measures were recently revised by the ACC/AHA in 2008.[25]

ONLINE CONTENT

For greater detail regarding these performance measures, please refer to the PowerPoint presentation at http://thepoint.lww.com/AT10e.

Thrombolytic Drugs

Because the majority of STEMI cases result from the sudden occlusion of a coronary artery, the priority is to open the occluded artery as quickly as possible. This may be accomplished by administering a thrombolytic agent that enhances the body's own fibrinolytic system or by mechanically reducing the obstruction with PCI.[2]

Large clinical trials have proven that administration of a thrombolytic agent reduces mortality. Early mortality from STEMI has been reduced by approximately one-third (from 10%–15% to 6%–10%) with the advent of thrombolytic therapy.[26]

The thrombolytic drugs currently used for STEMI patients in the United States are streptokinase, alteplase (t-PA), reteplase (r-PA), and tenecteplase (TNK). Streptokinase is a polypeptide derived from β-hemolytic streptococcal cultures. It binds to plasminogen to form an active plasminogen–streptokinase complex that cleaves plasminogen to form plasmin. Plasmin, which is an active fibrinolytic enzyme, then acts on a fibrin clot to enhance its dissolution. Alteplase, or t-PA, is a naturally occurring enzyme produced by recombinant DNA technology. t-PA cleaves the same plasminogen peptide bond that urokinase cleaves. However, t-PA has a binding site for fibrin, which allows it to bind to a thrombus and preferentially lyse it instead of the circulating plasminogen. Reteplase is a genetically modified plasminogen activator that is similar to t-PA. Reteplase has a longer half-life, allowing it to be administered as two bolus injections 30 minutes apart, rather than as a bolus plus infusion. TNK is a genetically modified form of t-PA. Compared with t-PA, TNK has a longer plasma half-life, better fibrin specificity, and higher resistance to inhibition by plasminogen-activator inhibitor.[27] The pharmacologic properties and dosing of these agents are compared in Table 18-3.

Unfortunately, an ideal thrombolytic agent does not exist. Three problems common to all thrombolytic drugs are the inability to open 100% of coronary artery occlusions, inconsistent ability to maintain good blood flow in the infarcted artery after it is opened, and bleeding complications. When assessing coronary artery flow after reperfusion therapy, the TIMI flow grade is widely used. Flow in coronary arteries is classified as grade 0 (no flow), grade 1 (penetration without perfusion), grade 2 (partial perfusion), or grade 3 (complete perfusion).[28] When assessing an episode of bleeding, the TIMI criteria are also used. TIMI major bleeding consists of overt clinical bleeding or documented intracranial or retroperitoneal hemorrhage that is associated with a drop in hemoglobin of at least 5 g/dL or hematocrit of at least 15% (absolute). TIMI minor bleeding is defined as overt clinical bleeding associated with a fall in hemoglobin of 3 to 5 g/dL or in hematocrit of 9% to 15% (absolute).[29]

To minimize the risk of bleeding complications, contraindications to the use of thrombolytic agents must be evaluated before administration (Table 18-4). There are relatively few absolute contraindications to thrombolytic therapy, but each patient should be assessed carefully to ascertain whether the potential benefit outweighs the potential risk. Because of the serious nature of intracerebral hemorrhage associated with thrombolytic therapy, patients should be selected carefully before receiving these agents.[23] Generally, the diagnosis of STEMI must be ensured, with a history consistent with ischemia, and presence of ST segment elevation in two contiguous leads, or a new left bundle branch block on the ECG. Once the diagnosis is made, the thrombolytic agent should be administered immediately if there are no contraindications.[23]

The benefit derived from thrombolytic therapy is directly related to the time from the onset of chest pain to the time of administration. The 2004 guidelines recommend initiation of thrombolytic therapy within 12 hours from the onset of chest pain. However, data from clinical trials suggest that mortality reduction is greater when thrombolytic therapy is initiated within 0 to 2 hours of symptom onset compared with treatment initiated more than 2 hours after symptoms have begun (44% vs. 20%, respectively; $p = 0.001$).[24] The guidelines recommend a "door-to-needle time" of 30 minutes, meaning the diagnosis of STEMI and initiation of thrombolytic therapy should ideally take place within 30 minutes from the time the patient arrives at the hospital door.

In patients with UA or NSTEMI, thrombolytic agents are not recommended. Thrombi in this population are primarily platelet-rich rather than fibrin-rich, and thus are less responsive to thrombolytic therapy.[30] Additionally, data from the TIMI IIIB trials suggest that compared with placebo, alteplase was not associated with any improvement in death, MI, or failure of initial therapy at 6 weeks or 1 year and was associated with an increased incidence in fatal and nonfatal MI (4.9% vs. 7.4%, respectively; $p = 0.04$).[31–32]

TABLE 18-2
Evidenced-based Pharmacotherapies for Acute Coronary Syndromes[1–4,23]

Drug	Indication	Dose and Duration	Therapeutic End Points	Precautions	Comments
ACE inhibitors[a]	STEMI and NSTEMI within the first 24 hours of presentation for those with EF ≤40% or s/s of HF STEMI and NSTEMI for late hospital care for patients with hypertension, EF ≤40%, DM, or CKD STEMI and NSTEMI for indefinite use for all patients with EF ≤40%	Usual captopril dose 12–50 mg TID; then start longer-acting ACE inhibitor. Duration indefinite.	Titrate to usual doses and maintain systolic BP >90–110 mm Hg	Avoid IV therapy within 48 hours of infarct Avoid with SBP <100 mm Hg, pregnancy, acute renal failure, angioedema, bilateral renal stenosis, serum potassium ≥5.5 mEq/L	
Angiotensin receptor blockers[a]	STEMI and NSTEMI with ACE inhibitor intolerance	Usual doses of ARBs (see Chapter 19, Heart Failure). Continue indefinitely.	Same as for ACE inhibitors	Same as for ACE inhibitors	
Aldosterone antagonists[a]	STEMI and NSTEMI with EF ≤40% and either DM or HF symptoms already receiving therapeutic doses of an ACE inhibitor and β-blocker	Spironolactone 12.5–50 mg daily or eplerenone 25–50 mg daily. Duration indefinite.	Titrate to heart failure symptom control without evidence of hyperkalemia	Hyperkalemia, hypotension Avoid if potassium ≥5 mEq/L or SCr ≥2.5 mg/dL for men and 2.0 mg/dL for women or CrCl ≤30 mL/min	Dose can be increased every 4–8 weeks.
Aspirin[a]	STEMI and NSTEMI for all patients	162–325 mg during AMI, then 75–325 mg/d for an indefinite period.	No firm end point	Active bleeding, thrombocytopenia	Unless clear contraindication exists, aspirin should be given to all AMI patients. For contraindications see Chapter 17, Chronic Stable Angina.
β-Blockers[a]	STEMI and NSTEMI in all patients without contraindications	Variable; titrate to HR and BP. It is reasonable to administer an IV β-blocker at the time of presentation to STEMI patients who are hypertensive and who do not have any of the following: (a) signs of heart failure, (b) evidence of a low output state, (c) increased risk[c] for cardiogenic shock, or (d) other relative contraindications to β-blockade (PR interval >0.24 s, 2nd- or 3rd-degree heart block, active asthma, or reactive airway disease). Duration indefinite.	Titrate to resting HR approx. 60 beats/min, maintain systolic BP >100 mm Hg	Observe HR and BP closely when given IV Contraindicated in patients with HR <50 beats/min; PR ECG segment >0.24 s, 2nd- or 3rd-degree heart block, persistent hypotension, pulmonary edema, bronchospasm, risk of cardiogenic shock, severe reactive airway disease	Unless clear contraindication exists, β_1-selective agents such as metoprolol and atenolol should be given to all AMI patients. In patients with systolic dysfunction, metoprolol or carvedilol can be considered.

Bivalirudin[a]	STEMI and NSTEMI patients undergoing PCI who are at high risk of bleeding	<u>PCI</u>: 0.75 mg/kg IV bolus followed by 1.75 mg/kg/h infusion. If UFH given, discontinue UFH and wait 30 minutes before starting bivalirudin. Discontinue at the end of PCI or continue at 0.2 mg/kg/h if prolonged anticoagulation necessary. <u>Medical management before PCI</u>: 0.1 mg/kg IV bolus followed by 0.25 mg/kg/h infusion.		Avoid in patients with active bleeding	Reduce dose with renal dysfunction
Calcium-channel blockers	STEMI and NSTEMI for patients with ongoing ischemia who are receiving adequate doses of nitrates and β-blockers. Consider diltiazem or verapamil for patients with contraindication to β-blocker if EF normal	Usual doses of calcium-channel blockers are used. Duration dictated by clinical scenario.	Titrate to usual doses and maintain SBP >90 mm Hg	Usual calcium-channel blocker contraindications. Avoid nondihydropyridines in patients with pulmonary congestion or EF <40%	In patients with good EF, most calcium-channel blockers will exert beneficial effects. Some data support use of verapamil or diltiazem for non–Q-wave AMI, but not dihydropyridine types.
Clopidogrel[a]	STEMI and NSTEMI for patients allergic to aspirin	75 mg/d	No firm end point	Active bleeding, thrombotic thrombocytopenia purpura (rare)	
Clopidogrel + aspirin[a]	STEMI, before fibrinolytic therapy or before PCI after fibrinolytic therapy	<u>STEMI with fibrinolytic therapy without PCI:</u> 300–600 mg load followed by 75 mg daily and continue for 14 days to 1 year; aspirin 162–325 mg on first day, then 75–162 mg daily indefinitely. <u>STEMI with fibrinolytic therapy with PCI:</u> 300–600 mg load,[b] then no additional treatment; aspirin 162–325 mg on first day, then 75–162 mg daily indefinitely.	No firm end point	Active bleeding, thrombotic thrombocytopenia purpura (rare) Avoid loading dose in patients ≥75 years of age Discontinue at least 5 days for CABG	Whether administered before thrombolytic or PCI, clopidogrel + aspirin reduced CV death, MI, or ischemia at 30 days. The 600-mg load should be considered if a GP IIb/IIIa is not used. Clopidogrel + aspirin reduced death, reinfarction, or stroke through index hospitalization
	NSTEMI or STEMI before PCI	<u>STEMI or NSTEMI with PCI:</u> 300–600 mg load, followed by 75 mg daily or 150 mg daily for six days followed by 75 mg daily. If a coronary stent is deployed continue clopidogrel for 12–15 months. For a BMS, administer aspirin 162–325 mg daily for at least 1 month after PCI, then decrease to 75–162 mg indefinitely. For a DES, administer aspirin 162–325 mg daily for 3 months for a sirolimus-eluting stent and 6 months for a paclitaxel-eluting stent after PCI, then decrease to 75–162 mg daily indefinitely.			
	For NSTEMI and unstable angina patients	300–600 mg load, followed by 75 mg daily for 1–12 months; aspirin 75–325 mg daily.			

(continued)

TABLE 18-2
Evidenced-based Pharmacotherapies for Acute Coronary Syndromes[1–4,23] *(Continued)*

Drug	Indication	Dose and Duration	Therapeutic End Points	Precautions	Comments
Enoxaparin[a]	STEMI as an alternative for UFH or LMWH for patients receiving fibrinolytic therapy or for those not undergoing reperfusion therapy. NSTEMI for patients undergoing a conservative or invasive approach. For PCI, as an alternative for UFH or LMWH	STEMI or NSTEMI: 1 mg/kg SQ every 12 hours (CrCl >30 mL/min) 1 mg/kg SQ daily (CrCl 15–29 mL/min) NSTEMI undergoing PCI: A supplemental 0.3 mg/kg IV dose should be administered at the time of PCI if the last dose of SC enoxaparin was given 8–12 hours before PCI STEMI with fibrinolytic therapy: Age <75 years, administer 30 mg IV bolus followed by 1 mg/kg SQ every 12 hours (max dose of 100 mg for patients weighing ≥100 kg) Age ≥75, administer 0.75 mg/kg SQ every 12 hours (first two doses administer max dose of 75 mg for patients weighing ≥75 kg) For STEMI and NSTEMI continue throughout hospitalization or up to 8 days.	No firm end point	Avoid in patients with active bleeding, history of HIT, planned CABG, SCr ≥2.5 mg/dL in men and ≥2.0 mg/dL in women, or CrCl <15 mL/min	Reduce dose with renal dysfunction
Fibrinolytic therapy[a]	STEMI presenting within 12 hours after onset of symptoms, can be considered in patients presenting within 12–24 hours after onset of symptoms with continuing s/s of ischemia	See Table 18-3	Improved TIMI grade flow	See Table 18-4	
Fondaparinux[a]	STEMI as an alternative for UFH or LMWH for patients receiving fibrinolytic therapy or for those not undergoing reperfusion therapy NSTEMI as an alternative for UFH or LMWH for patients undergoing a conservative or invasive approach	STEMI and NSTEMI: 2.5 mg SQ daily starting on day 2 of hospitalization, continue for 8 days or discharge. NSTEMI: 2.5 mg SQ daily for 6 days.	No firm end point No firm end point	Avoid with active bleeding, SCr ≥3.0 mg/dL, or CrCl <30 mL/min	In STEMI, fondaparinux reduced mortality and reinfarction without increased bleeds or strokes compared with UFH, but only in patients not undergoing PCI. In NSTEMI, fondaparinux was at least as effective as enoxaparin but exhibited less bleeding. Can possibly be used in HIT.
GP IIb/IIIa inhibitors[a]	NSTEMI for patients undergoing PCI or those without high-risk features not undergoing PCI STEMI for patients undergoing PCI	See Table 18-5	No firm end point	Avoid with active bleeding, thrombocytopenia, prior stroke	

Heparin[a]	STEMI for patients undergoing PCI or for patients treated with fibrinolytic therapy NSTEMI in combination with antiplatelet therapy for conservative or invasive approach	STEMI with fibrinolytic therapy or NSTEMI: 60 units/kg IV bolus (max 4,000 units) followed by 12 units/kg/h (max 1,000 units/h) STEMI with PCI: 50–70 units/kg IV bolus if a GP IIb/IIIa inhibitor planned; or 70–100 units/kg IV bolus if no GP IIb/IIIa inhibitor Continue for 48 hours or until end of PCI	aPTT ratio 1.5–2.5 patient's control value, first aPTT should be obtained 4–6 hours if not treated with fibrinolytic therapy or PCI and within 3 hours if treated with fibrinolytic therapy	Avoid with active bleeding, thrombocytopenia, recent stroke	Unless clear contraindication exists, UFH should be given to all AMI patients who do not receive thrombolytic therapy.
Lidocaine	Treatment of VT, VF	Variable, 1.5 mg/kg loading dose, then 1–4 mg/min. Use for <48 hours.	Cessation of arrhythmia	Bradycardia. Observe for CNS toxicity.	Some data indicate increased mortality with routine use.
Morphine and other analgesics	STEMI and NSTEMI for patients whose symptoms not relieved by NTG or adequate anti-ischemic therapy	2–5 mg IV every 5–30 minutes PRN.	Decreased chest pain and HR	Avoid morphine with bradycardia, right ventricular infarct, hypotension, confusion	Has been associated with higher risk of death; discontinue nonselective NSAIDs and COX-2 selective agents
Prasugrel[a]	STEMI and NSTEMI added to aspirin for PCI	60 mg loading dose followed by 10 mg (if ≥60 kg) or 5 mg (if <60 kg). If a coronary stent is deployed continue prasugrel for 12–15 months. For a BMS, administer aspirin 162–325 mg daily for at least 1 month after PCI, then drop to 75–162 mg indefinitely; For a DES, administer aspirin 162–325 mg daily for 3–6 months after PCI, then drop to 75–162 mg daily indefinitely.	No firm end point	Avoid with active bleeding, prior stroke or TIA, age ≥75 years Do not start if urgent CABG needed; discontinue 7 days before elective CABG	
Nitrates[a]	STEMI and NSTEMI with persistent ischemia, hypertension, or control of pulmonary congestion	Variable; titrate to pain relief or SBP: 5–10 mcg/min titrated to 200 mcg/min typical regimen. Usually maintain IV therapy for 24–48 hours after infarct.	Titrate to pain relief or SBP >90 mm Hg	Avoid with SBP <90 mm Hg, right ventricular infarction, sildenafil or vardenafil within 24 hours or tadalafil within 48 hours	Use acetaminophen or narcotics for headache. NTG should be tapered gradually in ischemic heart disease patients. Topical patches or oral nitrates are acceptable alternatives for patients with refractory symptoms
Ticagrelor + Aspirin	STEMI, NSTEMI, Unstable Angina with or without PCI	STEMI, NSTEMI, or Unstable Angina: 180 mg load followed by 90 mg twice daily for at least 1 year; administer 325 mg load of aspirin followed by a maintenance dose of 75–100 mg daily indefinitely.	No firm endpoints	Avoid in patients with severe hepatic impairment or active bleeding. Maintenance doses of aspirin above 100 mg daily can decrease ticagrelor's effectiveness, Discontinue at least 5 days for CABG	Monitor closely for dyspnea
Warfarin	STEMI and NSTEMI for left ventricular thrombus or for patients with AF with CHAD2 score ≥2	Variable; titrate to INR 3. Duration usually for several months to indefinitely.	INR 2–3 times patient's control value	Usual warfarin problems such as noncompliance, bleeding, diatheses	May be useful in the presence of a left ventricular thrombus to prevent embolism.

[a]Indicates specific drug therapies that are known to reduce morbidity or mortality.

[b]For patients given fibrin- and nonfibrin-specific fibrinolytic drugs who are undergoing PCI within 24 hours, 300 mg should be used; for patients given a fibrin-specific fibrinolytic undergoing PCI after more than 24 hours, 300–600 mg should be used; for patients given a nonfibrin-specific fibrinolytic undergoing PCI between 24 and 48 hours, 300 mg should be used; for patients given a nonfibrin-specific fibrinolytic undergoing PCI after 48 hours, 300–600mg should be considered.

[c]Risk factors for cardiogenic shock (the greater the number of risk factors present, the higher the risk of developing cardiogenic shock) are age >70 years, SBP <120 mm Hg, sinus tachycardia >110 beats/min or HR <60 beats/min.

ACE, angiotensin-converting enzyme; AF, atrial fibrillation; AMI, acute myocardial infarction; aPTT, activated partial thromboplastin time; ARBs, angiotensin receptor blockers; BMS, bare-metal stent; CABG, coronary artery bypass graft; CHADS2, risk score for atrial fibrillation comprising congestive heart failure, hypertension, age, diabetes, and prior stroke; CKD, chronic kidney disease; CNS, central nervous system; COX-2, cyclo-oxygenase-2; CrCl, creatinine clearance; CV, cardiovascular; DES, drug-eluting stent; DM, diabetes mellitus; ECG, electrocardiogram; EF, ejection fraction; GP IIb/IIIa, glycoprotein IIb/IIIa inhibitor; HF, heart failure; HIT, heparin-induced thrombocytopenia; HR, heart rate; INR, international normalized ratio; IV, intravenously; LMWH, low-molecular-weight heparin; MI, myocardial infarction; NSAIDs, non-steroidal anti-inflammatory drugs; NSTEMI, non–ST segment elevation myocardial infarction; NTG, nitroglycerin; PCI, percutaneous coronary intervention; PRN, as needed; SBP, systolic blood pressure; SCr, serum creatinine; SQ, subcutaneously; s/s, signs and symptoms; STEMI, ST segment elevation myocardial infarction; TIA, transient ischemic attack; TID, three times a day; TIMI, Thrombolysis in Myocardial Infarction; UHF, unfractionated heparin; VF, ventricular fibrillation; VT, ventricular tachycardia.

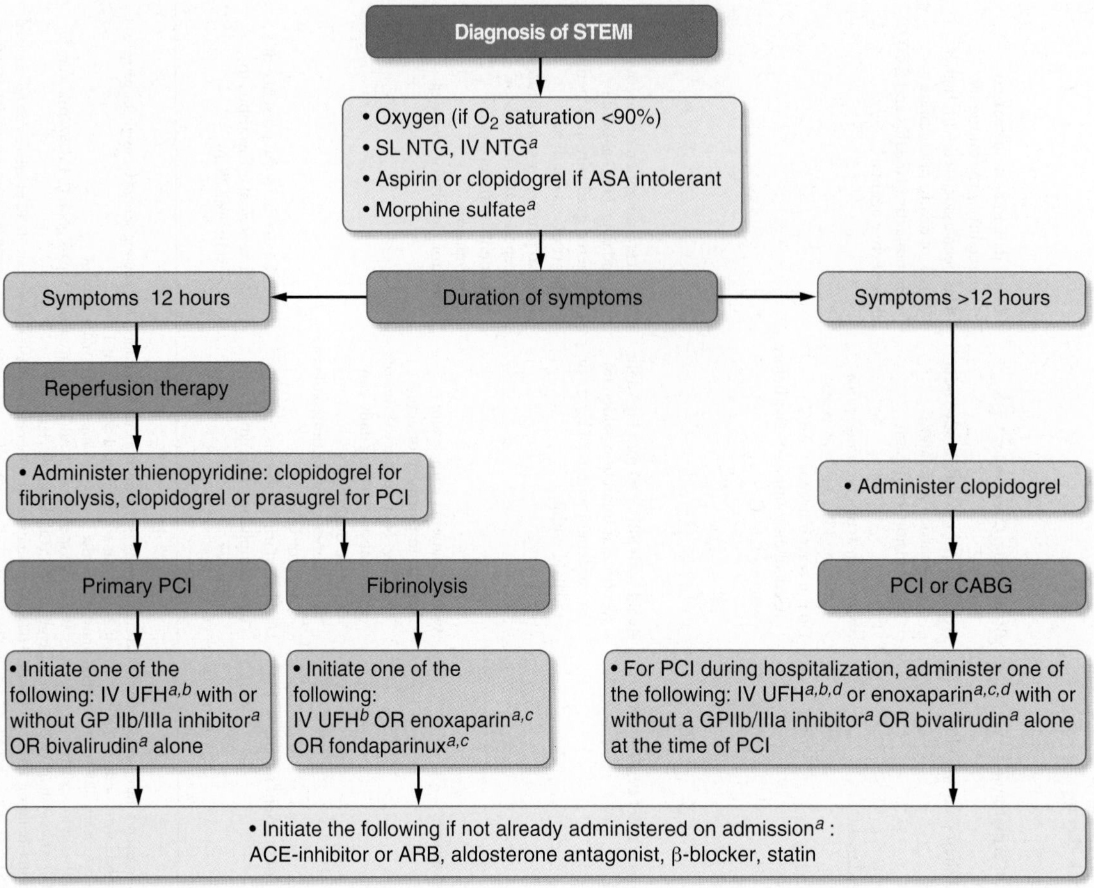

FIGURE 18-6 Initial treatment algorithm for STEMI. a: Refer to Table 18-2 for indications, dosing, and contraindications. b: For at least 48 hours. c: For the duration of the hospitalization, up to 8 days. d: Preferred therapy. ACE, angiotensin-converting enzyme; ARB, angiotensin receptor blocker; CABG, coronary artery bypass graft; GP IIB/IIIA, glycoprotein IIB/IIIA; NTG, nitroglycerin; O_2, oxygen; PCI, percutaneous coronary intervention; SL, sublingual; STEMI, ST segment elevation myocardial infarction; UFH, unfractionated heparin. (Source: Kushner FG et al. 2009 focused updates: ACC/AHA guidelines for the management of patients with ST-elevation myocardial infarction (updating the 2004 guideline and 2007 focused update) and ACC/AHA/SCAI guidelines on percutaneous coronary intervention (updating the 2005 guideline and 2007 focused update) a report of the American College of Cardiology Foundation/American Heart Association Task Force on Practice Guidelines [published corrections appear in *J Am Coll Cardiol.* 2010;55:612 (dosage error in article text); *J Am Coll Cardiol.* 2009;54:2464]. *J Am Coll Cardiol.* 2009;54:2205; Anderson JL et al. ACC/AHA 2007 guidelines for the management of patients with unstable angina/non-ST-Elevation myocardial infarction: a report of the American College of Cardiology/American Heart Association Task Force on Practice Guidelines (Writing Committee to Revise the 2002 Guidelines for the Management of Patients With Unstable Angina/Non-ST-Elevation Myocardial Infarction) developed in collaboration with the American College of Emergency Physicians, the Society for Cardiovascular Angiography and Interventions, and the Society of Thoracic Surgeons endorsed by the American Association of Cardiovascular and Pulmonary Rehabilitation and the Society for Academic Emergency Medicine [published correction appears in *J Am Coll Cardiol.* 2008;51:974]. *J Am Coll Cardiol.* 2007;50:e1).

Antiplatelet and Anticoagulant Drugs

When thrombolysis occurs, whether because of the administration of a thrombolytic agent or through activation of the body's own fibrinolytic system, the fibrin clot begins to disintegrate. As the clot dissolves, there is a paradoxical increase in local thrombin generation and enhanced platelet aggregability, which may lead to rethrombosis. Antiplatelet agents (aspirin, the thienopyridines clopidogrel or prasugrel, and the glycoprotein (GP) IIb/IIIa inhibitors), as well as parenteral anticoagulants (unfractionated heparin [UFH], low-molecular-weight heparins [LMWH] such as enoxaparin, and direct thrombin inhibitors [DTIs] such as bivalirudin), have been used to minimize repeat thrombosis. UFH has several limitations, including a highly variable anticoagulant effect necessitating frequent monitoring and development of heparin-induced thrombocytopenia (<0.2%). LMWH may offer advantages compared with heparin owing to its ease of administration, improved bioavailability, and need for less monitoring. Unlike UFH, the DTIs offer better protection against thrombin reactivation after therapy discontinuation. When used with early invasive treatment (<72 hours), DTIs appear to reduce the rate of death or reinfarction to a greater extent than UFH (9.50% vs. 13.86%, respectively; $p < 0.05$).[33]

Another class of agents being used is the GP IIb/IIIa inhibitors, which are tirofiban, eptifibatide, and abciximab. GP IIb/IIIa receptors are abundant on the platelet surface. Platelets become activated when patients are having an acute ischemic event or are undergoing PCI. With platelet activation, the GP IIb/IIIa receptor undergoes a conformational change that increases its affinity for binding fibrinogen. The binding of fibrinogen to receptors on platelets results in platelet aggregation, leading to thrombus formation. The GP IIb/IIIa receptor inhibitors prevent platelet aggregation by preventing fibrinogen from binding to GP IIb/IIIa receptor sites on activated platelets.[23]

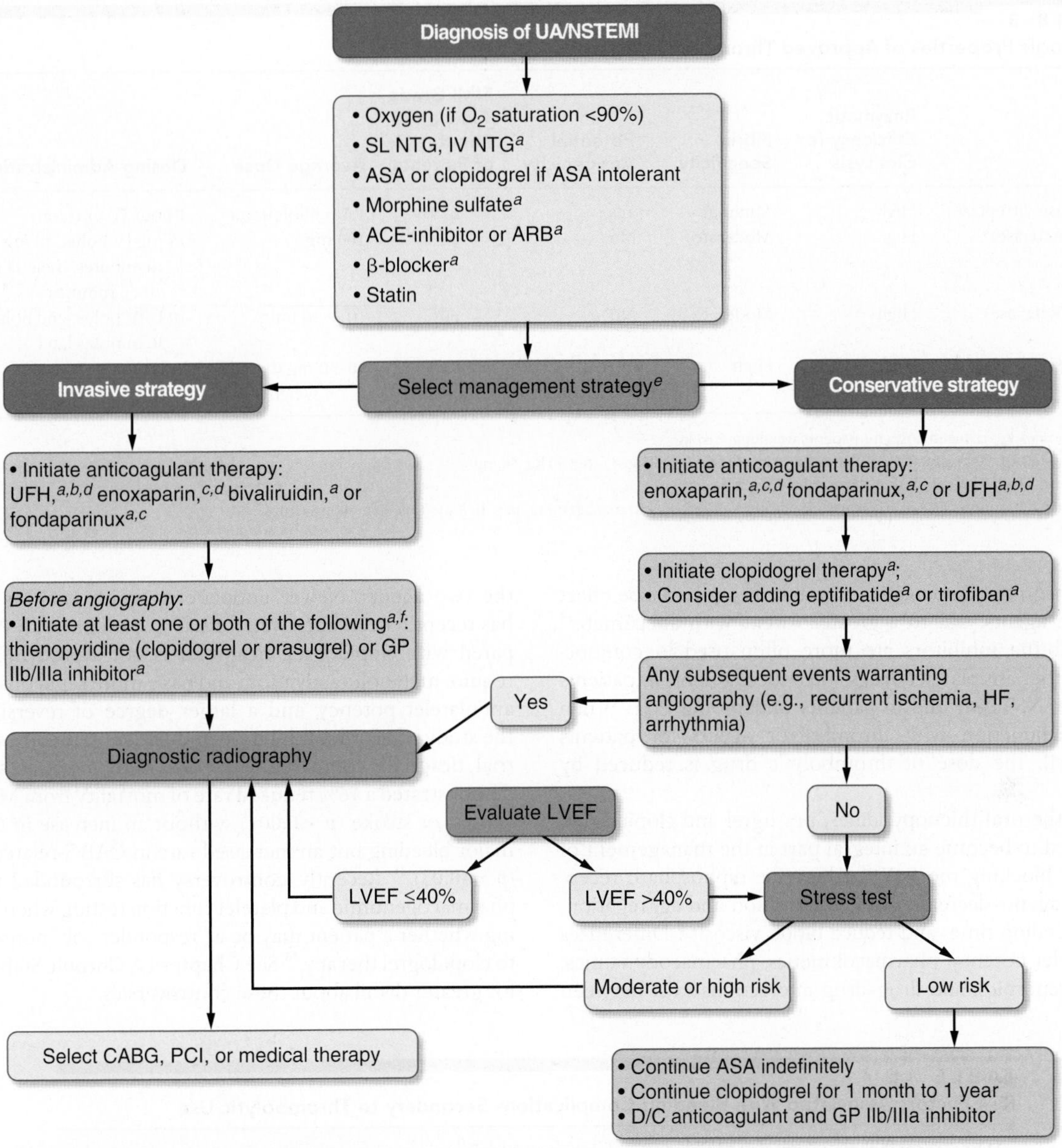

FIGURE 18-7 Initial treatment algorithm for NSTEMI. a: Refer to Table 18-2 for indications, dosing, and contraindications. b: For at least 48 hours. c: For the duration of the hospitalization, up to 8 days. d: Preferred therapy. e: An invasive strategy would be considered if one or more of the following occurs: recurrent angina or ischemia at rest, presence of elevated cardiac biomarkers, new or presumably new ST segment depression, signs or symptoms of heart failure (HF) or new worsening mitral regurgitation, hemodynamic instability, sustained ventricular tachycardia, percutaneous coronary intervention (PCI) within 6 months, prior coronary artery bypass graft (CABG), considered high risk per Thrombolysis in Myocardial Infarction (TIMI) risk score, left ventricular ejection fraction (LVEF) <40%. A conservative approach would be considered if the patient is classified as low-moderate risk per the TIMI risk score or if the patient or physician prefers a conservative approach in the absence of high-risk features. f: Factors favoring administration of both include delay to angiography, high-risk features, and early recurrent ischemia. ACE, angiotensin-converting enzyme; ARB, angiotensin receptor blocker; ASA, aspirin; CABG, coronary artery bypass graft; D/C, discontinue; LVEF, left ventricular ejection fraction; GP IIB/IIIA, glycoprotein IIB/IIIA; HF, heart failure; NSTEMI, non–ST segment elevation myocardial infarction; O_2, oxygen; PCI, percutaneous coronary intervention; TIMI, Thrombolysis in Myocardial Infarction; SL, sublingual; UFH, unfractionated heparin. (Adapted with permission from Anderson JL et al. ACC/AHA 2007 guidelines for the management of patients with unstable angina/non-ST-Elevation myocardial infarction: a report of the American College of Cardiology/American Heart Association Task Force on Practice Guidelines (Writing Committee to Revise the 2002 Guidelines for the Management of Patients With Unstable Angina/Non-ST-Elevation Myocardial Infarction) developed in collaboration with the American College of Emergency Physicians, the Society for Cardiovascular Angiography and Interventions, and the Society of Thoracic Surgeons endorsed by the American Association of Cardiovascular and Pulmonary Rehabilitation and the Society for Academic Emergency Medicine [published correction appears in *J Am Coll Cardiol.* 2008;51:974]. *J Am Coll Cardiol.* 2007;50:e1; and Wright SR, Anderson JL, Adams CD, et al. 2011 ACCF/AHA Focused update for the management of patients with unstable angina/non ST-elevation myocardial infarction, (updating the 2007 guideline): A report of the American College of Cardiology Foundation/ American Heart Association Task Force on practice guidelines. *J Am Coll Cardiol.* 2001;57:e1–e40.)

TABLE 18-3
Pharmacologic Properties of Approved Thrombolytic Agents

Drug	Enzymatic Efficiency for Clot Lysis	Fibrin Specificity	Potential Antigenicity	TIMI Grade Flow at 90 Minutes (% of Patients)	Average Dose	Dosing Administration	Cost
Streptokinase (Streptase)	High	Minimal	Yes	32%	1.5 million units	1 hour IV infusion	Low
Alteplase (Activase)	High	Moderate	No	54%	100 mg	15 mg IV bolus, 50 mg for 30 minutes, then 35 mg for 60 minutes[a]	High
Reteplase (Retavase)	High	Moderate	No	60%	10 + 10 units	10 U IV bolus, 2nd bolus 30 minutes later	High
Tenecteplase (TNK)	High	High	No	63%	30–50 mg (based on weight)[b]	Bolus for 5–10 seconds	High

[a] For patients = 65 kg; reduced doses for patients weighing <65 kg.
[b] For patients <60 kg, 30 mg; 60–69 kg, 35 mg; 70–79 kg, 40 mg; 80–89 kg, 45 mg; 90 kg, 50 mg.
IV, intravenous; TIMI, Thrombolysis in Myocardial Infarction.
Source: Kumar A, Cannon CP. Acute coronary syndromes: diagnosis and management, part II. *Mayo Clin Proc.* 2009;84:1021.

Acute thrombocytopenia is a rare but recognized side effect of all three agents, but to a greater extent with abciximab.[34] The GP IIb/IIIa inhibitors are more often used in conjunction with other antiplatelet drugs and anticoagulants in patients with UA or NSTEMI and in patients undergoing PCI. When used in conjunction with thrombolytic agents for patients with STEMI, the dose of thrombolytic drug is reduced by one-half.[23]

Finally, the oral thienopyridines, prasugrel and clopidogrel, have evolved to become an integral part in the management of ACS.[1–4] By blocking the P2Y12 adenosine diphosphate receptors, these agents decrease platelet activation and aggregation, increase bleeding time, and reduce blood viscosity. Differences in antiplatelet potency, pharmacokinetics, pharmacodynamics, pharmacogenomics, and drug–drug interactions exist between the two agents. Newer antiplatelet agents such as ticagrelor has recently been approved for use in patients with ACS. Compared with clopidogrel, ticagrelor is not a prodrug, does not require metabolic activation, and has a more rapid onset, greater antiplatelet potency, and a larger degree of reversibility.[35] In the study of Platelet Inhibition and Patient Outcomes (PLATO) trial, ticagrelor compared with clopidogrel in patients with ACS demonstrated a 16% reduced rate of mortality from MI, vascular causes, or stroke ($p < 0.001$) without an increase in the rate of major bleeding but an increased rate in CABG-related bleeding ($p = 0.03$).[35] Recently, controversy has surrounded the use of pharmacogenomic and platelet function testing when determining whether a patient may be a "responder" or "nonresponder" to clopidogrel therapy.[36] See Chapter 17, Chronic Stable Angina, for greater detail about these controversies.

TABLE 18-4
Risk Factors Associated With Bleeding Complications Secondary to Thrombolytic Use

Major (thrombolytic agents contraindicated)	Intracranial tumor (primary or metastatic)
	Prior intracranial hemorrhage
	Recent head or facial trauma within 3 months
	Suspected aortic dissection
	Ischemic stroke within 3 months, EXCEPT acute ischemic stroke within 3 hours
	Active internal bleeding or bleeding diathesis (excluding menses)
Important (relative contraindication)	Uncontrolled hypertension on presentation (SBP >180 mm Hg, DBP >110 mm Hg)
	Chronic, severe, poorly controlled hypertension
	Prior ischemic stroke >3 months, dementia, or known intracranial pathology
	Puncture of a noncompressible vessel
	Cardiopulmonary resuscitation for >10 minutes
	Major surgery (<3 weeks)
	Recent internal bleeding within 24 weeks
	Active peptic ulcer
	Current use of anticoagulants (the higher the INR, the greater the risk for bleeding)
	Pregnancy
	For streptokinase or anistreplase: prior exposure (>5 days) or prior allergic reaction

DBP, diastolic blood pressure; INR, international normalized ratio; SBP, systolic blood pressure.
Source: Antman EM et al. ACC/AHA guidelines for the management of patients with ST-elevation myocardial infarction—executive summary. A report of the American College of Cardiology/American Heart Association Task Force on Practice Guidelines (Writing Committee to revise the 1999 guidelines for the management of patients with acute myocardial infarction) [published correction appears in *J Am Coll Cardiol.* 2005;45:1376]. *J Am Coll Cardiol.* 2004;44:671.

β-Blockers

β-Blockers should be administered independently of the planned reperfusion strategy. β-Blockers reduce recurrent ischemia and reinfarction rates among patients receiving concomitant thrombolytic therapy.[23] In patients with ACS receiving either thrombolytic therapy or PCI, β-blockers significantly decreased the rates of cardiovascular mortality, recurrent nonfatal MI, and all-cause mortality.[1–3,23,37] The 2007 ACC/AHA guidelines recommend that oral β-blocker therapy be initiated within 24 hours after the onset of symptoms for all patients without contraindications. Both β-selective and nonselective agents have been evaluated; however, β-blockers with intrinsic sympathomimetic activity should be avoided as they have not been well studied and lack efficacy data. For patients with tachycardia or hypertension without signs of HF, IV β-blockers followed by oral administration can be considered.[1] Unless there are contraindications to their use, β-blocking agents should be prescribed for all patients after an AMI, and should be continued indefinitely.

Statins

β-Hydroxy-β-methylglutaryl-CoA (HMG-CoA) reductase inhibitors (statins) reduce long-term morbidity and mortality in patients with cardiovascular disease. What is less clear is whether statins provide short-term benefit when started immediately after AMI. Beyond their lipid-lowering properties, statins are believed to exhibit pleiotropic effects, which include plaque stabilization, anti-inflammation, antithrombogenicity, enhancement of arterial compliance, and modulation of endothelial function.[38] Data regarding early intensive statin therapy in patients with STEMI or NSTEMI exist with atorvastatin, simvastatin, pravastatin, rosuvastatin, and fluvastatin.[38–40] Debate continues to exist about which statin to initiate, the dosage, and the timing (see Chapter 13, Dyslipidemias, Atherosclerosis, and Coronary Heart Disease).[38]

Vasodilators

Other strategies for minimizing myocardial damage include the use of vasodilators in the peri-infarction period. Progressive left ventricular dilatation ("remodeling") occurs in some patients after an AMI and has become an important marker for prognosis. Vasodilators reduce oxygen demand and myocardial wall stress by reducing afterload or preload and can attenuate the remodeling process. Some vasodilators may increase the blood supply to the myocardium by enhancing coronary vasodilatation.[3,23]

ACE inhibitors have been assessed in a large number of clinical trials, and all trials using oral agents have demonstrated a reduction in mortality.[1,3] Intravenous ACE inhibitors should be avoided as they result in excessive hypotension and have not been shown to improve survival. The benefit of ACE inhibitors is greatest in patients with anterior infarction, signs of HF, tachycardia, or a history of previous infarction. Ideally, oral ACE inhibitors should be started within 24 hours of diagnosis, after blood pressure (BP) has stabilized. Initial doses should be low and then titrated as quickly as possible.[3,23] The ACC/AHA guidelines suggest that an ARB should be administered to patients with ACS who cannot tolerate ACE inhibitors.

Nitroglycerin has a vasodilatory effect on the coronary and peripheral vascular beds. Nitrates dilate venous capacitance vessels and peripheral arterioles. Their predominant effect is a decrease in preload, with a lesser effect on afterload. Consequently, nitrates lead to a decrease in both myocardial wall stress and oxygen demand. Pooled effects from several studies show a small but statistically significant benefit in reducing mortality in patients receiving nitrates.[3,23] Intravenous nitroglycerin should be used in patients who have refractory ischemic discomfort, and the dosage should be titrated to reduce systolic blood pressure to between 100 and 130 mm Hg and to maintain a heart rate less than 100 beats/minute.

Another class of vasodilators that has been investigated in the treatment of ACS is the calcium-channel blockers. There are several proposed mechanisms whereby a calcium-channel blocker might be beneficial. As a group, they dilate coronary and peripheral vessels. They also alleviate some of the coronary vasospasm present at the time of coronary thrombosis. In addition, they are effective anti-ischemic agents through their action in improving coronary blood supply and reducing myocardial oxygen demand.[3,23]

The ACC/AHA guidelines recommend calcium-channel blockers for patients with persistent or recurrent symptoms after treatment with full-dose nitrates and β-blockers, for patients with contraindications to β-blockade, and for patients with Prinzmetal or variant angina. For such patients, calcium-channel blockers that slow the heart rate (e.g., diltiazem or verapamil) are recommended. These nondihydropyridines should not be administered to patients with severe left ventricular dysfunction or pulmonary edema. The DAVIT (Danish Verapamil Infarction Trial) is the largest randomized trial to date to have evaluated the efficacy of a calcium-channel blocker for patients with ACS.[41] The study suggested a trend toward lower MI and mortality rates when verapamil was given to patients with suspected ACS. Similar reductions in MI and refractory angina rates have been demonstrated with diltiazem.[42] The dihydropyridine calcium antagonists amlodipine and felodipine have not been evaluated specifically for administration to patients with ACS, but trials involving normotensive patients with CAD or hypertensive patients with cardiovascular risk factors have demonstrated that these agents provide significant benefits.[43–44]

Analgesics

It is important to abolish the patient's pain as quickly as possible because the pain and anxiety associated with an AMI will contribute to increased myocardial oxygen demand. If the pain is not relieved by the thrombolytic or anti-ischemic medications (e.g., nitrates, β-blockers), then additional analgesia may be necessary. Morphine sulfate (2 to 4 mg IV with increments of 2 to 8 mg IV repeated at 5- to 15-minute intervals) is the analgesic of choice for management of pain associated with STEMI. In addition to diminishing pain and anxiety, morphine also has beneficial hemodynamic effects. By reducing pain and anxiety, the release of circulating catecholamines is diminished, possibly reducing the associated arrhythmias. Morphine also causes peripheral venous and arterial vasodilatation, which reduces preload and afterload and, consequently, the myocardial oxygen demand. However, retrospective studies have suggested the potential for increased mortality in patients with NSTEMI receiving morphine; thus the 2007 ACC/AHA guidelines have lowered their recommendation to Class IIa regarding morphine's use in this population.[3,45] The nonselective and cyclo-oxygenase (COX)-2–selective nonsteroidal anti-inflammatory drugs (NSAIDs) have been associated with an increased risk of mortality, reinfarction, hypertension, HF, and myocardial rupture. These agents should be discontinued at the time a patient presents with ACS.[1,3]

Stool Softeners

It is common to administer agents such as docusate to prevent constipation in AMI patients because straining causes undesirable stress on the cardiovascular system.[1,3]

Oxygen

Many patients are modestly hypoxemic during the initial hours of an AMI. Supplemental oxygen should be administered to patients with ACS with an arterial saturation less than 90%, respiratory distress, or other high-risk features for hypoxemia. Patients with severe hypoxemia or pulmonary edema may require intubation and mechanical ventilation.[1,3]

Antiarrhythmic Agents

Ventricular arrhythmias, including ventricular fibrillation, are common complications associated with myocardial ischemia and AMI as well as a major cause of death. More than half of the episodes of ventricular fibrillation that occur with an AMI are within 1 hour of the onset of symptoms. Lidocaine and amiodarone are the drugs of choice for the treatment of ventricular arrhythmias in the peri-infarction period. The routine use of prophylactic lidocaine or other antiarrhythmic agents to prevent ventricular tachycardia and ventricular fibrillation is not recommended. Although the routine use of lidocaine may reduce the number of episodes of ventricular fibrillation, it may contribute to an increased number of episodes of asystole.[23]

Suppression of ventricular ectopy after an AMI with the chronic use of oral antiarrhythmic agents is not recommended. Results of the Cardiac Arrhythmia Suppression Trial (CAST) -I and CAST-II demonstrated an increase in mortality in asymptomatic patients with ventricular ectopy after an AMI who were treated with flecainide, encainide, or moricizine (see Chapter 20, Cardiac Arrhythmias).[46,47]

Nondrug Therapy

For STEMI, PCI is an attractive alternative to thrombolytic therapy. The process and procedure associated with PCI as well as coronary stenting and CABG are discussed in Chapter 17, Chronic Stable Angina. Specific guidelines have been published by the ACC/AHA addressing PCI and stent use in AMI.[2]

PCI is preferred if a skilled interventional cardiologist and catheterization laboratory are available, if the procedure can be preformed within 90 minutes after initial medical contact (also referred to as "door-to-balloon time"), or if a contraindication for a thrombolytic agent exists.[2] This threshold is based on a multivariable analysis of patients undergoing PCI in which an increased door-to-balloon time exceeding 90 to 120 minutes was associated with a higher mortality rate.[48] Thrombolytic therapy should be given to patients who are unable to undergo PCI within 90 minutes of presentation, unless a contraindication is present.[1,2]

The disadvantages of PCI include the longer amount of time needed to mobilize the personnel needed to prepare the catheterization laboratory and its initial higher cost. A potential advantage of PCI is the greater ability to achieve TIMI grade 3 flow in the affected vessel (90% vs. 50%–60%, respectively).[23] Pooled data from major trials comparing PCI with thrombolysis have found PCI to be associated with fewer major adverse cardiac events, irrespective of patient presentation time. Unfortunately, many hospitals do not have the facilities or skilled personnel to complete this procedure in the necessary time frame.[23]

For NSTEMI, coronary angiography aids in defining the extent and location of coronary lesion and in directing the definitive care strategy (for example, PCI with stent placement, CABG, or medical management). However, because angiography is an invasive procedure, there is a small risk of serious complications. Therefore, coronary angiography should be used only in patients for whom the procedure's benefits outweigh its risks. With this principle in mind, two pathways of treatment for UA/NSTEMI patients have emerged: the early-invasive strategy (also called the invasive strategy) and the early-conservative strategy (also called the conservative strategy or ischemia-guided strategy) (Fig. 18-7). In the early-invasive strategy, all patients without contraindications undergo coronary angiography with the intent to perform revascularization within 4 to 24 hours of hospital admission. The early-conservative strategy consists of aggressive medical therapy for all patients and coronary angiography only for those with certain risk factors.

CLINICAL PRESENTATION OF ACS

CASE 18-1

QUESTION 1: P.H., a 68-year-old, 80-kg man, is being admitted to the ED after experiencing an episode of sustained chest pain while mowing his yard. After waiting 1 hour, he called 911 and was transported to the ED. Physical examination reveals a diaphoretic man who appears ashen. Heart rate and rhythm are regular, and no S_3 or S_4 sounds are present. Vital signs include BP 180/110 mm Hg, heart rate 105 beats/minute, and respiratory rate 32 breaths/minute. P.H.'s chest pain radiates to his left arm and jaw, and he describes the pain as "crushing" and "like an elephant sitting on my chest." He rates it as a "10/10" in intensity. Thus far, his pain has not responded to five sublingual (SL) nitroglycerin (NTG) tablets at home and three more in the ambulance. His ECG reveals a 3-mm ST segment elevation and Q waves in leads I and V_2 to V_4. Based on his history and physical examination, P.H. is diagnosed with an anterior infarction. Laboratory values include the following:

Sodium (Na), 141 mEq/L
Potassium (K), 3.9 mEq/L
Chloride (Cl), 100 mEq/L
CO_2, 20 mEq/L
Blood urea nitrogen (BUN), 19 mg/dL
Serum creatinine (SCr), 1.2 mg/dL
Glucose, 149 mg/dL
Magnesium (Mg), 1.3 mEq/L
CK, 1200 U/L, with a 12% CK-MB fraction (normal, 0%–5%)
Troponin I, 60 ng/mL (normal, <2)
Cholesterol, 259 mg/dL
Triglycerides, 300 mg/dL

P.H. has a prior history of coronary artery disease (CAD). A previous cardiac catheterization 2 years ago revealed lesions in his middle left anterior descending coronary artery (75% stenosis) and proximal left circumflex artery (30% stenosis). His echocardiogram at the time showed an EF of 58%. These lesions were deemed suitable for medical management. He also has a history of recurrent bouts of bronchitis associated with bronchospasm for 10 years, diabetes mellitus treated with insulin for 18 years with a hemoglobin A_{1c} of 6.8%, and stage 1 hypertension with blood pressures usually 140/85 mm Hg. His father died of an MI at age 70. His mother and siblings are all alive and well. P.H. has smoked one pack of cigarettes a day for 30 years, and he drinks approximately one six-pack of beer a week. He has no history of IV drug use. On admission, P.H.'s medications include insulin glargine 40 units daily; albuterol inhaler, as needed (PRN); hydrochlorothiazide, 25 mg daily; NTG patch, 0.2 mg/hour; and NTG SL, 0.4 mg PRN for chest

pain. What signs and symptoms does P.H. have that are consistent with the diagnosis of AMI?

P.H. described his pain as a pressure sensation, which is common with ischemic heart disease. The chest discomfort associated with ACS often is described as pressure or as a tight band around the chest rather than pain. Although P.H. was involved in physical exertion when his chest discomfort began, this is not always the case. It can begin at rest and, frequently, in the early morning hours. At least 20% of patients with AMI have no pain or discomfort; these episodes are described as "silent" MIs.[23] Presentations range from no symptoms to shortness of breath, hypotension, HF, syncope, or ventricular arrhythmias. Silent or atypical infarctions occur more commonly in people with diabetes or hypertension and in the elderly. P.H. is diaphoretic, a common finding, but other common symptoms such as nausea and anxiety are not present. He also describes his pain as "10/10" in intensity, or perhaps "the worst pain I've ever experienced," which is typical of an STEMI. The diagnosis primarily lies in the symptoms (e.g., the patient's "story"), the ECG, and the laboratory findings.

The history of diabetes, hypertension, smoking, and a positive family history in P.H. are all risk factors for coronary disease. His admission BP is high, which could indicate poor underlying control or anxiety and stress related to his ACS. The blood sugar of 149 mg/dL is high, again indicating either poor control or a stress response. Measurement of glycosylated hemoglobin is indicated during his hospitalization to better assess his diabetes control.

Laboratory Abnormalities

CASE 18-1, QUESTION 2: What laboratory abnormalities can you expect to see in P.H.?

P.H. demonstrates several laboratory abnormalities commonly seen with both STEMI and NSTEMI. Both his CK-MB and troponin are elevated, consistent with myocardial necrosis. With UA, cardiac biomarkers are not elevated. Several other nonspecific laboratory findings should be monitored in P.H. Hyperglycemia may develop because P.H. is a diabetic, but this can also occur in nondiabetic patients. ACS is also accompanied by an acute systemic inflammatory response manifested by fever, leukocytosis, and elevation of the erythrocyte sedimentation rate and C-reactive protein, as well as a drop in low-density lipoprotein (LDL), high-density lipoprotein (HDL), and total cholesterol. Specifically, these lipoprotein changes may begin to decrease within 24 to 48 hours after an ACS event, reaching a nadir within 1 week and then gradually recovering during the next 30 days.[49] Therefore, it is prudent to check serum lipid profiles within the first 24 to 48 hours of the AMI to get an accurate determination of the patient's lipid values.

ST Segment Elevation Myocardial Infarction Versus Non–ST Segment Elevation Myocardial Infarction

CASE 18-1, QUESTION 3: P.H. was noted to have "ST segment elevation and Q waves" on the ECG. What are the implications of an ST segment elevation versus non–ST segment elevation MI?

Perhaps the most important diagnostic test in someone suspected of having an AMI is the ECG. The ECG is an important tool because it is noninvasive, can be performed rapidly, is readily available in most clinical settings, and helps determine where the AMI is located (i.e., anterior, inferior, lateral; Fig. 18-4). P.H. has classic ECG changes (ST segment elevation and Q waves), and their presence in the anterior ECG leads (V_2–V_4) also points to the coronary artery that is likely to be blocked. P.H.'s previous left anterior descending lesion may have had a plaque rupture leading to thrombosis of the vessel.

The presence of ST segment elevation in two contiguous leads indicates severe ischemia and occlusion of the coronary artery. Every effort should be made to open the infarct-related artery as soon as possible, which could consist of PCI or thrombolytic therapy. If the ECG showed ST segment depression instead of elevation (e.g., NSTEMI), P.H. would not be eligible for thrombolytic therapy because the risks of thrombolytic therapy outweigh the benefits in NSTEMI; however, depending on the management strategy selected, P.H. could receive PCI.

Anterior Versus Inferior Infarction

CASE 18-1, QUESTION 4: What are the prognostic implications of an anterior versus an inferior MI?

Damage to the anterior section of the heart is more likely to be associated with increased morbidity (e.g., left ventricular dysfunction) and mortality. The patients at highest risk of death are those with an anterior ACS, left ventricular dysfunction, and complex ventricular ectopy. P.H. is at an increased risk because he has sustained an anterior infarction.

Risk Stratification

CASE 18-1, QUESTION 5: What is P.H.'s initial risk of mortality based on his presenting signs and symptoms?

Using the TIMI Risk Score for STEMI, P.H. has a TIMI risk score of 6 based on his age (2 points); history of angina, hypertension, and diabetes (1 point); heart rate (2 points); and location of his MI (1 point) (Table 18-1). P.H. has a 30-day mortality rate of 16%, thereby highlighting the serious nature of this event. If P.H. had experienced an NSTEMI with ST segment depression, he would have a TIMI risk score of 5 based on his age (1 point); at least 3 risk factors for CAD (1 point), prior CAD history (1 point), ST segment deviation (1 point), and elevated cardiac biomarkers (1 point). Based on this TIMI risk score, P.H. would be at high risk for death, MI, or need for urgent coronary artery revascularization within 30 days.

Therapeutic Objectives

CASE 18-1, QUESTION 6: What are the immediate and long-term therapeutic objectives in treating P.H.?

With both STEMI and NSTEMI, the immediate therapeutic objectives particularly as they apply to P.H. are to restore blood flow to the infarct-related artery, arrest infarct expansion, alleviate his symptoms, and prevent death. These objectives are achieved primarily by restoring coronary blood flow (administering a thrombolytic or performing a PCI for STEMI or performing PCI with NSTEMI) and lowering myocardial oxygen demand. Any life-threatening ventricular arrhythmias that develop must be treated. The long-term therapeutic objectives are to prevent or minimize recurrent ischemic symptoms, reinfarction, HF, and sudden cardiac death. As P.H. is experiencing a STEMI, the specific therapeutic regimens are discussed in the questions that follow.

TREATMENT FOR ST SEGMENT ELEVATION MYOCARDIAL INFARCTION

Thrombolytic Therapy

CASE 18-1, QUESTION 7: Is P.H. a candidate for thrombolytic therapy? Is any one agent preferred?

STEMI is a medical emergency, and rapid administration of drug therapy is crucial to save myocardial tissue. The results of several major trials have shown unequivocally that if used appropriately, thrombolytic agents can reduce the mortality associated with an AMI. Because mortality benefit is greatest when thrombolytic therapy is administered within 2 hours of symptom onset, many institutions are using early prehospital thrombolytic therapy, in which trained paramedics administer the thrombolytic in the field.[1,23] If PCI cannot be performed within 90 minutes, thrombolytic therapy should be given if no contraindications are present. Patients may benefit from thrombolytic therapy even if they receive the drug several hours after the onset of pain.

Controversy still exists about which thrombolytic should be used, the best dosing regimen, the most appropriate adjunctive therapy, and whether the risk outweighs the benefit in some subpopulations of patients (e.g., those with an inferior AMI). P.H. has a history of hypertension, and at presentation his BP is 180/110 mm Hg. A BP this high is a relative contraindication to thrombolytic therapy because of an increased risk of cerebral hemorrhage; however, P.H. has an anterior MI and is likely to benefit from thrombolytic therapy. In this case, he should receive IV NTG immediately because the onset of blood pressure control with this agent usually occurs within minutes. Once his systolic BP is less than 180 mm Hg and the diastolic is less than 110 mm Hg, a thrombolytic can be administered. The NTG will also reduce the workload on his heart and may provide pain relief.

Because P.H. has severe pain and ECG changes consistent with an anterior AMI, he is at great risk for substantial morbidity or mortality. Alteplase is a more rapid-acting and effective agent in restoring TIMI grade 3 blood flow than streptokinase; however, the slightly increased risk of stroke and the increase in cost with t-PA may outweigh its advantages. The argument for or against a specific thrombolytic is probably less important than the decision to use an agent and to administer the medication as soon as possible after the onset of symptoms. P.H. is fortunate because he has presented within 1 hour of the onset of chest pain. The newer fibrin-specific lytic agents have longer half-lives and can be administered as bolus agents; although these agents have demonstrated no further improvements in survival, they offer the convenience of easier administration and can be delivered more rapidly in the emergency department (Table 18-2).

The Global Utilization of Streptokinase and t-PA for Occluded Arteries (GUSTO) trial used this accelerated or front-loaded regimen for administration of t-PA. In this trial, t-PA was compared with streptokinase and a combination of streptokinase and t-PA.[50] The results showed that t-PA alone was the most effective in reducing mortality. The 30-day mortality rate for the accelerated t-PA group was 6.3% compared with 7.3% in the streptokinase group. In GUSTO, the t-PA regimen was also weight adjusted, such that after the 15-mg bolus dose, the infusion was 0.75 mg/kg for 30 minutes followed by 0.5 mg/kg for 60 minutes. The maximal dose received was 100 mg.

Most of the large trials with streptokinase have used an IV infusion of 1.5 million units administered for 60 minutes. There have been some trials in which the infusion was shortened to 30 minutes; however, there have been no large studies that have compared a 30-minute infusion with a 60-minute infusion.[23] Reteplase was compared with t-PA in the GUSTO-III trial.[51] Reteplase has a slower clearance from the body, allowing the drug to be given as a bolus without the need for a constant infusion. In the GUSTO-III trial, reteplase was administered in two bolus doses of 10 million units, given 30 minutes apart. The mortality rate and incidence of stroke were the same in the two groups of patients.

TNK was compared with t-PA in the Second Assessment of Safety and Efficacy of a New Thrombolytic (ASSENT-2) trial.[52] TNK was administered as a bolus of 30 to 50 mg for 5 to 10 seconds, based on body weight. No difference existed between TNK and t-PA in 30-day mortality and stroke. The 2004 ACC/AHA guidelines recommended t-PA or reteplase for patients who present early after onset of chest pain and for those with a large area of injury (e.g., anterior infarction) who have a low risk for an intracranial bleed.[23] These recommendations did not change with the 2007 and 2009 updates.[1,2] However, based on the ASSENT-2 trial, TNK appears to be just as effective as t-PA with fewer bleeding complications.[52] Compared with t-PA, both TNK and reteplase can be administered as bolus doses.

ADJUNCT THERAPY

CASE 18-1, QUESTION 8: Orders are written for an infusion of t-PA along with UFH 5,000 units IV bolus, followed by 1,000 units/hour by continuous infusion. Also prescribed is aspirin 325 mg stat. Are both UFH and aspirin agents necessary?

The Second International Study of Infarct Survival (ISIS-2) trial showed that aspirin 160 mg/day alone and in combination with streptokinase reduced mortality in patients with an AMI by 23% and 42%, respectively, when compared with a control group of patients who received neither aspirin nor streptokinase.[53] In doses of 162 mg or more, aspirin generates a prompt clinical antithrombotic effect as a result of its inhibition of thromboxane A_2 production. Thus, immediate administration of 162 to 325 mg of aspirin in all patients diagnosed with ACS is indicated. In the acute setting, aspirin should be chewed because it is absorbed more quickly. All patients should receive 75 to 162 mg of daily aspirin indefinitely after a diagnosis of ACS. If patients have a contraindication to aspirin, clopidogrel can be substituted.[3,23]

For more than 40 years, the use of UFH as adjunct therapy to prevent reocclusion has been evaluated in many studies.[23] Overall, it appears that UFH administration offers no benefit to patients receiving streptokinase or anistreplase.[23] However, because P.H. will receive t-PA, owing to his anterior wall infarct, an IV UFH bolus followed by a continuous infusion should be started before the end of the t-PA infusion. The 2007 ACC/AHA guidelines recommend an initial UFH bolus of 60 units/kg (maximum of 4000 units), followed by an initial infusion of 12 units/kg/hour (maximum of 1000 units/hour) for 48 hours after fibrinolysis, with a targeted activated partial thromboplastin time (aPTT) of 1.5 to 2 times the upper limit of normal. UFH should always be considered in patients at high risk for systemic or venous embolism.[1]

CASE 18-1, QUESTION 9: Would P.H. benefit from the addition of clopidogrel to his current drug regimen?

Two studies have defined the potential role of in-hospital clopidogrel as an integral part of thrombolytic therapy in patients with STEMI.[54,55] The Clopidogrel as Adjunctive Reperfusion Therapy–Thrombolysis in Myocardial Infarction 28 (CLARITY-TIMI 28) evaluated 3,497 patients with STEMI who received standard thrombolytic therapy, aspirin, and UFH, and were scheduled for angiography within 2 days.[55] Patients received either clopidogrel (300 mg loading dose, followed by 75 mg daily) or placebo within 10 minutes of thrombolytic administration. Clopidogrel was continued up to and including the day of angiography and stopped. The primary end point was the composite of an occluded infarct-related artery on predischarge angiography or death or an MI up to the start of coronary angiography. Compared with placebo, patients in the clopidogrel group demonstrated a 36% reduction in the primary end point ($p < 0.001$). By 30 days, the clopidogrel treatment group had a 20% reduction in cardiovascular death, recurrent MI, or recurrent ischemia ($p = 0.03$). No difference in the rate of major bleeding was seen between groups. In a substudy of patients proceeding to nonemergent PCI after thrombolytic therapy, patients receiving pretreatment with clopidogrel demonstrated a 66% reduction in 30-day mortality compared with those receiving placebo ($p = 0.034$).[56]

Finally, the Clopidogrel and Metoprolol in Myocardial Infarction Trial (COMMIT) evaluated the effect of administrating either clopidogrel 75 mg daily with no loading dose or placebo in 45,852 patients presenting with STEMI.[54] In the trial population, 93% had ST segment elevation or bundle branch block, 7% had ST segment depression, and 54% were treated with thrombolytic therapy. The initial clopidogrel dose was given within 24 hours of symptom onset and continued until hospital discharge or up to 4 weeks in the hospital. Compared with placebo, the allocation to clopidogrel was associated with a 9% reduction in death, reinfarction, or stroke ($p = 0.002$) and a 7% reduction in all-cause mortality ($p = 0.03$). No significant excess in bleeding was noted in the treatment group or in those who received concomitant thrombolytic therapy or who were younger than 70 years. On the basis of these two studies, P.H. should receive clopidogrel as an inpatient.

CASE 18-1, QUESTION 10: What dose of clopidogrel should be considered?

According to the 2007 ACC/AHA guidelines, clopidogrel should be added to aspirin in patients regardless of whether or not they undergo reperfusion with fibrinolytic therapy.[1] Based on the 2009 ACC/AHA guidelines, a loading dose of clopidogrel 300 to 600 mg can be administered with fibrinolytic therapy followed by 75 mg/day for maintenance if the patient is not proceeding to PCI. The maintenance dose should be continued for 14 days and up to 1 year.[2] This 1-year duration is extrapolated from experience with UA/NSTEMI.[1] It is important to note that there are no formal studies evaluating the 600-mg loading dose in patients with STEMI.[2] Additionally, uncertainty exists about the efficacy and safety of adding a loading dose of clopidogrel in adults 75 years of age and older, particularly when they receive a thrombolytic. Therefore in this population, a loading dose should be avoided. The 2009 ACC/AHA guidelines also recommend a single loading dose of 300 to 600 mg of clopidogrel in patients who receive any thrombolytic agent and are subsequently proceeding to PCI within 24 hours without a maintenance dose.[2] If the patient received a fibrin-specific thrombolytic and then proceeds to PCI after 24 hours has lapsed, then a loading dose of 300 to 600 mg can be considered. If at least 48 hours has elapsed after treatment with a nonfibrin-specific thrombolytic agent, then a dose of 300 to 600 mg can be considered.[2] For P.H., a loading dose of 300 mg of clopidogrel should be administered at the time of thrombolytic administration followed by 75 mg/day for 14 days to 1 year, if he does not proceed to PCI. Because P.H. has already received 325 mg of aspirin in the ED, he should continue either 81 or 162 mg of daily aspirin indefinitely.

CASE 18-1, QUESTION 11: What role do the other anticoagulant and antiplatelet agents have in P.H.'s management?

The replacement of UFH with an LMWH, factor Xa inhibitor, or the addition of an IV GP IIb/IIIa inhibitor to thrombolytic therapy have been evaluated in patients with STEMI.

In the Enoxaparin and Thrombolysis Reperfusion for Acute Myocardial Infarction Study-25 (ExTRACT-TIMI 25), 20,506 patients with STEMI scheduled for thrombolytic therapy were randomized to receive either enoxaparin or continuous infusion of UFH for 48 hours.[57] Enoxaparin was dosed according to age and renal function. For patients younger than 75 years, enoxaparin was given as a fixed 30 mg IV bolus followed 15 minutes later by 1 mg/kg subcutaneously (SQ) twice daily. For patients older than 75 years, the IV bolus was eliminated, and the dose reduced to 0.75 mg/kg SQ twice daily. If the creatinine clearance (using the Cockcroft-Gault formula) was less than 30 mL/minute, the dose was modified to 1 mg/kg SQ daily. UFH was dosed according to weight (60 units/kg bolus, followed by 12 units/kg/hour) and adjusted to achieve an aPTT 1.5 to 2.0 times control. The composite end point of death or nonfatal MI through 30 days occurred in 12.0% in the UFH group and 9.9% in the enoxaparin group, representing a 17% risk reduction ($p < 0.001$). Although no difference was noted in mortality between the two groups, treatment with enoxaparin did reduce the 30-day risk of nonfatal reoccurrence of AMI by 33% compared with UFH ($p < 0.001$). However, major bleeding was higher in the enoxaparin group compared with those receiving UFH (2.1% vs. 1.4%, respectively; $p < 0.001$).

The Organization for the Assessment of Strategies for Ischemic Syndromes (OASIS) 6 was a complex, randomized double-blind trial of 12,092 patients with STEMI designed to assess the effect of early initiation of fondaparinux with primary PCI and medical therapy.[58] The study compared the effects of fondaparinux (2.5 mg/day for up to 8 days) with two different control arms: stratum 1, in which placebo was used if UFH was not indicated (e.g., a nonfibrin-specific thrombolytic administered); and stratum 2, in which UFH was administered for up to 48 hours followed by placebo for up to 8 days. Each control group included a mix of the different treatment strategies, with essentially all primary PCI patients receiving UFH. Compared with the control group, those receiving fondaparinux had a significant reduction in the composite of death or reinfarction at 30 days (11.2% vs.. 9.7%, respectively; $p = 0.008$). Significant reductions in this end point were also observed at 9 days (7.4% for the fondaparinux group vs. 8.9% for controls; $p = 0.003$) and at the end of the study (13.4% vs. 14.8%; $p = 0.008$). Specifically, in stratum 1, fondaparinux reduced the incidence of death or MI compared with the control group (11.2% vs. 14.0%; $p < 0.05$), but in stratum 2 demonstrated no difference in this end point when compared with UFH. Fondaparinux did not appear to offer benefit in patients who were managed with primary PCI. Although the rates of death, MI, and severe bleeds did not differ in these patients, there was a higher rate of catheter thrombosis with fondaparinux.

The TIMI-14 trial demonstrated enhanced reperfusion (TIMI 3 flow) using reduced-dose t-PA combined with abciximab (0.25 mg/kg bolus, then 12-hour infusion of 0.125 mcg/kg/minute) compared with full-dose t-PA alone.[59] This improvement occurred without an increase in the risk of major bleeding. In the GUSTO-V trial, 16,588 patients with STEMI were randomly assigned to standard-dose reteplase or half-dose reteplase plus full-dose abciximab.[60] There was no difference in death rates between the groups at 30 days or 1 year. The combination group had less reinfarction and recurrent ischemia, but this benefit was offset by more episodes of moderate and severe bleeding, especially in the elderly. Similar rates of enhanced reperfusion have also been observed with the combination of double-bolus dose eptifibatide (180/90 mcg/kg, 10 minutes apart) with a 48-hour infusion (2 mcg/kg/minute) plus half-dose t-PA (50 mg).[61]

The ASSENT-3 trial randomly assigned 6,095 AMI patients to full-dose TNK plus enoxaparin, half-dose TNK plus UFH, and a 12-hour infusion of abciximab or full-dose TNK plus UFH.[62] The addition of either abciximab or enoxaparin to TNK reduced the composite end point of 30-day mortality, in-hospital reinfarction, or ischemia compared with UFH. More major bleeding complications were seen with abciximab compared with UFH.

In a meta-analysis of 11 trials involving 27,115 STEMI patients who received adjunctive abciximab in addition to either PCI or thrombolytic therapy, use of abciximab was associated with a significant reduction in 30-day ($p = 0.047$) and 1- to 6-month mortality ($p = 0.01$) in patients undergoing PCI but not in those receiving thrombolytic therapy.[63] Although both reperfusion strategies demonstrated a significant reduction in 30-day reinfarction ($p < 0.05$), only those patients receiving abciximab with a thrombolytic had an increased risk in major bleeding ($p < 0.001$).

Finally, in the HORIZONS-AMI (Harmonizing Outcomes With Revascularization and Stents in Acute Myocardial Infarction) trial, 3,602 patients with STEMI undergoing primary PCI were randomly assigned to bivalirudin (bolus 0.75 mg/kg, followed by 1.75 mg/kg/hour) or UFH plus a GP IIb/IIIa inhibitor.[64] The incidence of the primary end point of net adverse clinical events, defined as death, MI, ischemic target vessel revascularization, stroke, or major bleeding at 30 days, was 24% lower in the group treated with bivalirudin alone (9.2%) than in the group receiving UFH plus a GP IIb/IIIa inhibitor (12.1%; $p = 0.005$). This outcome was driven primarily by the 40% reduction in the rate of major bleeding in the bivalirudin group ($p < 0.001$).

Based on data from ExTRACT-TIMI 25 and OASIS-6, the 2007 ACC/AHA allow for substitution of UFH with either enoxaparin or fondaparinux.[1] However, whereas fondaparinux appeared to be superior to control therapy in the OASIS-6 trial, relative benefit compared with placebo and UFH separately cannot be reliably determined despite subgroup analyses discussed earlier.[1,65] For P.H., enoxaparin would be the more appropriate choice; however, he will have a higher risk for bleeding and will need to be monitored closely. Because P.H. is not undergoing PCI, he may not benefit from the addition of a GP IIb/IIIa at this time. If a GP IIb/IIIa inhibitor was to be used in conjunction with a thrombolytic agent for patients with STEMI, the dose of the thrombolytic agent is reduced by one-half.[23]

DETERMINATION OF REPERFUSION

CASE 18-1, QUESTION 12: How can you monitor for successful reperfusion in P.H. after he has received thrombolytic therapy?

It is important to determine whether thrombolysis has been successful because the prognosis of the patient is related to the presence or absence of an open infarct-related artery. If thrombolytic therapy fails to open the infarct-related artery, then the patient may benefit from PCI or a CABG. Although coronary angiography has been the standard for determining the success of reperfusion, this procedure is expensive and may be misleading, as some studies have suggested that microvascular perfusion may be impaired even when TIMI grade 3 flow has been achieved. A simple and readily available technique is evaluation of ECG ST segment resolution. A resolution of more than 50% of the ST segment elevation at 60 to 90 minutes after the initiation of thrombolytic therapy is a good indicator of improved myocardial perfusion.[1] The 2007 ACC/AHA guidelines recommend monitoring the pattern of ST segment elevation, cardiac rhythm, and clinical symptoms during the 60 to 180 minutes after thrombolytic therapy initiation.[1] Relief of symptoms, maintenance or restoration of hemodynamic or electrical stability or both, and a reduction of at least 50% in the initial ST segment elevation are all suggestive of adequate reperfusion.[1] P.H. should undergo a 12-lead ECG to evaluate reperfusion.

TIME FROM ONSET OF CHEST PAIN

CASE 18-1, QUESTION 13: If P.H.'s arrival at the hospital had been delayed more than 6 hours from the onset of his chest pain, should he still receive a thrombolytic?

Although efforts should be directed toward administering a thrombolytic as early as possible, many patients present several hours after the onset of chest pain. There are several theoretical reasons why the late administration of a thrombolytic may be helpful. Some patients present with a "stuttering" MI, which is chest pain that waxes and wanes for hours or days, presumably from recurrent or ongoing ischemia. These patients should be considered candidates for thrombolytic therapy or PCI. The magnitude of left ventricular dilatation may be diminished by reperfusion of the infarct-related artery, even if it is late. Another potential advantage of opening an infarct-related artery, even hours after an MI, is that the opened artery could become a source of collateral blood flow in the future.[23]

The ISIS-2 trial expanded patient enrollment to include patients admitted within 24 hours from the onset of chest pain. In that trial, there was a 17% reduction in vascular death at 5 weeks in the streptokinase group treated 5 to 24 hours from the onset of chest pain, compared with a 35% reduction in the group who received streptokinase within 4 hours from the onset of pain. Although the benefit was reduced, a statistically and clinically significant benefit was still present.[23,53]

Overall, there appears to be a statistically significant benefit associated with administering a thrombolytic up to 12 hours from the onset of chest pain and a trend toward benefit when given between 13 and 24 hours. Late administration may be most beneficial in patients at the highest risk for mortality.[23] This would include the elderly, patients with large infarctions, and those with continuing pain or hypotension. P.H. still may benefit from thrombolytic therapy if PCI is not available, even if he presents beyond the 6-hour time frame. If he is still having symptoms, he probably has viable myocardium at risk that may be salvaged.

READMINISTRATION OF THROMBOLYTIC AGENTS

CASE 18-1, QUESTION 14: This is P.H.'s first infarction. If he had a history of a previous MI that was treated with a thrombolytic agent, would he still be eligible for thrombolysis?

Many patients who are admitted to a hospital with an AMI have a history of a previous infarction. Both streptokinase and anistreplase are associated with the formation of neutralizing antibodies within several days after administration, and these antibodies remain up to 4 years with streptokinase. Unfortunately, the clinical significance of these antibodies on thrombolytic efficacy remains unknown. Based on observations made in ISIS-2, repeat doses of streptokinase were associated with allergic reactions (4.4% of individuals) consisting of shivering, pyrexia, or rashes, which were resistant to use of prophylactic corticosteroids.[66] If P.H. were presenting with a second infarction within a year and had received streptokinase for his first infarction, the thrombolytic drug of choice would be t-PA, TNK, or reteplase.

CASE 18-1, QUESTION 15: P.H. was stable initially after thrombolysis, but 48 hours later he experienced recurrent chest pain and ECG changes consistent with extension of his infarct. The attending cardiologist would like to readminister t-PA at this time. Is this a reasonable course of therapy?

Reocclusion of the infarct-related artery after initial successful thrombolysis is a major setback for this therapeutic strategy. If reocclusion occurs, mechanical intervention (e.g., PCI) is often attempted. Debate exists regarding whether to readminister the thrombolytic or refer the patient for PCI.[67] In a meta-analysis of eight trials composed of 1,177 patients with STEMI who failed thrombolytic therapy, patients receiving rescue PCI showed no significant reduction in all-cause mortality, but had a 27% risk reduction in HF ($p = 0.05$) and 42% reduction in reinfarction ($p = 0.04$) when compared with conservative treatment, defined as standard medical therapy for AMI without thrombolysis or PCI. Repeat fibrinolytic therapy was not associated with significant improvements in all-cause mortality or reinfarction. Both treatment strategies demonstrated a significant increase in minor bleeding, but PCI was associated with an increase in stroke.[68] Nonetheless, the 2009 ACC/AHA guidelines recommend that patients who have failed thrombolytic therapy should be moved expeditiously to the catheterization laboratory with appropriate antithrombotic therapy for catheterization if possible.[2] Those patients presenting to a non–PCI-capable facility should be triaged to undergo repeat thrombolytic therapy or immediate transfer for PCI. Patients best suited for transfer consist of those with high-risk features (i.e., cardiogenic shock, ≥75 years of age, hemodynamic or electrical instability, and persistent ischemic symptoms), those with high bleeding risk from thrombolytic therapy, and patients presenting late, that is, more than 4 hours after onset of symptoms.[2]

In the case of P.H., a repeat infusion with t-PA would probably be safe, but it may not be effective. As discussed in Case 18-1, Question 14, repeat doses of streptokinase should be avoided. If facilities for either PCI or surgery exist at the institution, most cardiologists would choose an invasive strategy at this time for P.H.

USE IN THE ELDERLY

CASE 18-1, QUESTION 16: If P.H. had been 85 years of age, should he have still received thrombolytic therapy?

Some of the early trials with thrombolytic therapy excluded the elderly. Although the elderly may have a higher prevalence of relative contraindications such as severe hypertension or history of stroke at presentation, they also have a higher incidence of mortality after an AMI. The 30-day mortality rate after an AMI is 19.6% for patients between 75 and 85 years of age and 30.3% for those who are 85 years of age.[69] In a trial using streptokinase, a higher incidence of bleeding in patients older than age 70 was reported. However, in the ISIS-2 trial, the greatest reduction in mortality occurred in the elderly subgroup. There are no controlled trials in which thrombolytic therapy has increased mortality in the elderly.[69] However, in a high-risk cohort of elderly female patients (older than 75 years, <67 kg), the ASSENT investigators demonstrated that compared with bolus and infusion of t-PA, TNK was associated with lower rates of major bleeding (15.15% versus 8.33%) and intracerebral hemorrhage (3.02% versus 1.14%).[69]

Percutaneous Coronary Intervention

ADJUNCT THERAPY

CASE 18-1, QUESTION 17: What if P.H. underwent PCI rather than receiving thrombolytic therapy for reperfusion? Would his initial oral antithrombotic therapy change?

As with thrombolytic therapy, the 2009 ACC/AHA guidelines recommend initiating dual antiplatelet therapy with aspirin (162–325 mg daily) and a thienopyridine, either clopidogrel or prasugrel.[2] Much of the data surrounding the use of clopidogrel with PCI has been evaluated with NSTEMI and will be discussed later. However, The PCI-CLARITY study was a planned subanalysis ($n = 1{,}863$) of the CLARITY-TIMI 28 study (see Case 18-1, Question 9) that evaluated the effects of pretreatment with aspirin plus clopidogrel, compared with aspirin plus placebo, in patients who went on to receive PCI with coronary artery stenting.[70] Compared with placebo, pretreatment with clopidogrel significantly reduced the incidence of cardiovascular death, MI, or stroke (6.2% versus 3.6%, respectively; $p = 0.008$) as well as the incidence of recurrent MI or stroke before PCI (6.2% versus. 4.0%, respectively; $p = 0.03$) with no significant excess in TIMI major or minor bleeding. These benefits were also demonstrated 30 days after PCI ($p = 0.001$).

Prasugrel has been evaluated in patients with ACS receiving PCI. In the Therapeutic Outcomes by Optimizing Platelet Inhibition with Prasugrel–Thrombolysis in Myocardial Infarction (TRITON-TIMI) 38 study, 13,608 patients with moderate to high-risk ACS, 26% of whom had STEMI, were randomly assigned to receive either prasugrel (60 mg loading dose followed by 10 mg daily) or clopidogrel (300 mg loading dose of clopidogrel followed by 75 mg daily).[71] All patients received aspirin (75–162 mg daily) within 24 hours of PCI. The primary outcome of death from cardiovascular causes, nonfatal MI, or nonfatal stroke occurred in 9.9% of patients receiving prasugrel and 12.1% of patients taking clopidogrel (hazard ratio [HR] for prasugrel versus clopidogrel, 0.81; 95% confidence interval [CI], 0.73–0.90; $p < 0.001$). In patients with STEMI, the primary outcome at 30 days was significantly reduced in patients receiving prasugrel compared with those receiving clopidogrel (6.5% vs. 9.5%, respectively; HR, 0.68; 95% CI, 0.54–0.87; $p = 0.0017$) and persisted to 15 months (HR, 0.79; 95% CI, 0.65–0.97; $p = 0.0221$).[72] In a post hoc analysis of patients with anterior MI, event rates at 15 months for the primary end point were lower with prasugrel compared with clopidogrel ($p = 0.0003$), whereas no difference was seen between groups in patients with a non–anterior wall MI ($p = 0.8749$).[72]

However, prasugrel was associated with a significant increase in TIMI major ($p = 0.03$), fatal ($p = 0.002$), and life-threatening bleeding ($p = 0.01$) when compared with clopidogrel. This bleeding risk was seen independently of type of ACS. A post hoc analysis suggested that three subgroups did not have a favorable net benefit from prasugrel exposure: patients with a history of stroke or TIA before enrollment, age at least 75 years, or body weight less than 60 kg. Patients with at least one of these risk factors exhibited a higher rate of bleeding.[71] The US Food and Drug Administration (FDA) recommends that the 5-mg rather than the 10-mg maintenance dose be considered for those patients weighing less than 60 kg, even though evidence supporting this dose is lacking.[2]

When compared with clopidogrel, prasugrel is more potent, exhibits a lower incidence of stent thrombosis, has fewer drug–drug interactions, and lacks variable response based on pharmacogenomics (refer to Chapter 17, Chronic Stable Angina, for additional details about responders and nonresponders to clopidogrel).[36,73] However, many providers have been concerned with the higher risk of bleeding. The guidelines do not explicitly endorse one thienopyridine versus another.[2] In the case of P.H., either clopidogrel or prasugrel should be added, as he does not have a contraindication to either drug.

CASE 18-1, QUESTION 18: It is decided that P.H. will receive clopidogrel. What loading dose should he receive and when should he receive it? What about his maintenance dose?

When considering an effective loading dose for clopidogrel for PCI in STEMI patients, the 2009 ACC/AHA guidelines recommend that at least 300 to 600 mg be administered as early as possible before the time of PCI followed by a maintenance dose of 75 mg.[2] The exact loading dose is controversial. Three to seven days is required for maximal platelet inhibition with the 75-mg daily dose of clopidogrel without a loading dose.

In a subanalysis of the HORIZONS-AMI trial (see Case 18-1, Question 11), patients with STEMI undergoing primary PCI were randomly assigned to receive bivalirudin or UFH plus a GP IIb/IIIa inhibitor but also were stratified according to clopidogrel loading dose: 300 mg (n = 1,153) or 600 mg (n = 2,158).[75] Compared with the 300-mg loading dose, those receiving 600 mg had significantly lower 30-day unadjusted rates of mortality (3.1% vs. 1.9%, respectively; $p = 0.03$), reinfarction (2.3% vs. 1.3%, respectively; $p = 0.02$), and definite or probable stent thrombosis (2.8% vs. 1.7%, respectively; $p = 0.04$), without higher bleeding rates. These findings were independent of the initial treatment strategy. In the multivariate analysis, the 600-mg loading dose was associated with an 18% lower rate of 30-day major adverse cardiac events ($p = 0.04$).

In the Clopidogrel Optimal Loading Dose Usage to Reduce Recurrent Events/Optimal Antiplatelet Strategy for Interventions trial (CURRENT OASIS-7), 8,560 patients with ACS proceeding to early PCI were randomly assigned to high-dose clopidogrel 600 mg loading dose on day 1 and then 150 mg once daily for the next 7 days, followed by 75 mg once daily until 30 days or to standard dosing.[76] Patients in the standard clopidogrel arm received a 300-mg loading dose on day 1, followed by 75 mg once daily until 30 days. Patients were also assigned in an open-label manner to 300 to 325 mg of aspirin once daily or 75 to 100 mg aspirin once daily. The primary end point was cardiovascular death, MI, or stroke at 30 days. Compared with the standard dose of clopidogrel, those receiving the high dose had a 14% reduced rate of the primary outcome ($p = 0.39$) and a significantly lower rate of stent thrombosis (1.3% vs. 0.7%, respectively; $p = 0.0001$), but a higher rate of major bleeding (1.1% vs. 1.6%, respectively; $p = 0.009$). No difference was seen in major bleeding or in the primary end point between the two aspirin groups.

Even after a loading dose, clopidogrel requires several hours to be metabolized to its active metabolite. The early timing of the loading dose is based on data from NSTEMI trials and the CLARITY-TIMI 28 study.[2] Studies in patients with NSTEMI suggest that the 300-mg loading dose should be given at least 15 hours before PCI whereas the European Guidelines recommend 6 hours.[77] With the 600-mg loading dose, pharmacodynamic studies suggest administering the dose least 2 hours before PCI.[77] Although increasing the dose to 900 mg has been associated with a marginal increase in the magnitude and speed of platelet inhibition, clinical efficacy and safety has not been established.[78]

After PCI with coronary stent deployment with either a drug-eluting or bare metal stent, clopidogrel 75 mg or prasugrel 5 to 10 mg should be administered for at least 12 months and up to 15 months.[2] This recommendation has changed from the previous guidelines, which recommended ideally 1 year of dual antiplatelet therapy for all coronary stents but a minimum of 1 month for a bare metal stent and 3 to 6 months for a drug-eluting stent.[1,22] It is important to highlight that clopidogrel and prasugrel should be discontinued for 5 and 7 days, respectively, if the patient is going to have surgery.[2] The dosing regimen of aspirin therapy is dependent on the type of coronary stent (see Table 18-2). As a rapid onset of action is needed, P.H. should receive a loading dose of 600 mg of clopidogrel as soon as possible, followed by 75 mg daily for at least 12 months. Aspirin should be continued indefinitely; however, the dosing regimen will depend on the type of coronary stent deployed (see Table 18-2).

CASE 18-1, QUESTION 19: In addition to his dual antiplatelet therapy of clopidogrel and aspirin, what specific anticoagulant should P.H. receive? Should a GP IIb/IIIa inhibitor be added?

If P.H. were to proceed to PCI, his anticoagulant therapy should consist of one of the following: IV UFH with or without a GP IIb/IIIa inhibitor or bivalirudin alone.

The advantages and dosing of UFH have been discussed earlier (Case 18-1, Question 8). Debate exists regarding the addition of a GP IIb/IIIa inhibitor to UFH. In the Value of Abciximab in Patients With Acute MI Undergoing PCI After High Dose Clopidogrel Pretreatment (BRAVE-3) trial, 800 patients presenting within 24 hours of an STEMI were pretreated with clopidogrel (600 mg), aspirin (500 mg), and heparin (60 U/kg) and then randomly assigned to receive wither abciximab or placebo before PCI. The primary end point was infarct size with a secondary end point of 30-day mortality, recurrent MI, stroke, or urgent revascularization. At study completion, no difference existed between groups in either the primary or secondary end points.[79] Similar findings have also been demonstrated in the Ongoing Tirofiban In Myocardial Infarction Evaluation 2 (ON-TIME 2) study, which evaluated 984 patients with STEMI who received either high-dose tirofiban or placebo along with aspirin (500 mg), clopidogrel (600 mg), and UFH (5000 U bolus) before PCI.[80] No difference was seen among groups in TIMI grade 3 flow ($p > 0.05$) or in 30-day mortality ($p = 0.051$). However, compared with placebo, major cardiac events at 30 days were significantly reduced in the tirofiban group (8.6% vs. 5.8%; $p = 0.043$).

Based on these studies, the 2009 ACC/AHA guidelines recommend that in the setting of dual-antiplatelet therapy used along with UFH, the adjunctive use of a GP IIb/IIIa inhibitor administered at the time of PCI cannot be recommended as routine therapy.[2] However, the guidelines do suggest that these agents may be beneficial in those with a large thrombus burden or who have not received adequate thienopyridine loading.[2]

Regarding the choice of GP IIb/IIIa, two meta-analyses comparing small-molecule GP IIb/IIIa inhibitors (tirofiban and eptifibatide) with abciximab in STEMI patients undergoing PCI showed no difference in 30-day mortality, reinfarction, or major TIMI bleeding.[81] No difference was seen in postprocedural TIMI

TABLE 18-5
Dosing of Glycoprotein IIb/IIIa in Acute Coronary Syndromes[2,4,24]

Medication	Dosing for STEMI PCI	Dose for NSTEMI With or Without PCI	Comments
Abciximab	0.25 mg/kg IV bolus followed by 0.125 mcg/kg/min infusion (max of 10 mcg/min), continue for 12 hours at the discretion of the physician	Not recommended	
Eptifibatide	180 mcg/kg IV bolus, then begin 2 mcg/kg/min infusion followed by second IV bolus of 180 mcg/kg 10 minutes after first bolus, continue infusion for 12–18 hours after PCI at the discretion of the physician	180 mcg/kg IV bolus, then begin 2 mcg/kg/min infusion, continue infusion for 12–18 hours Repeat bolus dose after 10 minutes for PCI	Reduce infusion by 50% in patients with CrCl <50 mL/min; not studied in patients with SCr >4.0 mg/dL
Tirofiban	25 mcg/kg IV bolus followed by an infusion of 0.1 mcg/kg/min, continue up to 18 hours at the discretion of the physician	0.4 mg/kg IV bolus administered for 30 minutes followed by an infusion of 0.1 mcg/kg/min for 12–24 hours	Reduce infusion by 50% in patients with CrCl <30 mL/min

CrCl, creatinine clearance; IV, intravenous; NSTEMI, non–ST segment elevation myocardial infarction; PCI, percutaneous coronary intervention; SCr, serum creatinine; STEMI, ST segment elevation myocardial infarction.

flow grade 3 or ST segment resolution. The 2009 ACC/AHA guidelines do not explicitly endorse one GP IIb/IIIa inhibitor versus another.[2] Table 18-5 describes the dosing of GP IIb/IIIa inhibitors in ACS.

Finally, in the HORIZONS-AMI trial (see Case 18-1, Questions 11 and 18), administration of bivalirudin alone compared with UFH with a GP IIb/IIIa inhibitor was found to exhibit a 24% lower incidence of the composite of 30-day mortality, MI, revascularization, stroke, or major bleeding ($p = 0.005$); 38% lower 30-day mortality rate from cardiovascular cause ($p = 0.03$); and 24% lower 30-day all-cause mortality ($p = 0.047$).[64] However, those receiving bivalirudin exhibited a 1% increased risk of acute stent thrombosis within 24 hours ($p < 0.001$) but not at 30 days. This risk appeared to be mitigated by the prior use of UFH and a loading dose of 600 mg of clopidogrel. Based on these data, the 2009 ACC/AHA guidelines consider bivalirudin alone useful for patients with STEMI undergoing PCI whether or not they received pretreatment with UFH, especially for patients who are at high risk of bleeding.[2] Dual antiplatelet therapy should be used when considering bivalirudin alone.

Because P.H. is not a high risk for bleeding, dual antiplatelet therapy in addition to UFH should be adequate therapy. If a large thrombus burden is demonstrated on angiography, a GP IIa/IIIb could be initiated during PCI.

Magnesium

CASE 18-1, QUESTION 20: Will the administration of IV magnesium be beneficial for P.H.? How is magnesium administered?

The use of magnesium in the setting of AMI has been widely debated. Suggested mechanisms for the benefits of magnesium include an antiarrhythmic effect, an antiplatelet effect, reversal of vasoconstriction, reduction of catecholamine secretion, and enhancement of adenosine triphosphate production.

In the Second Leicester Intravenous Magnesium Intervention Trial (LIMIT-2), a randomized, placebo-controlled, double-blind trial of 2,316 patients with suspected AMI, IV magnesium (2-g bolus followed by a 17-g infusion for 24 hours) was found to decrease mortality at 28 days by 24%.[82] However, these results were not reproduced in the MAGIC and ISIS-4 trials.[83,84] At this time, clinicians do not routinely administer IV magnesium to AMI patients unless there exists a documented magnesium deficit or patients exhibit torsades de pointes ventricular tachycardia.

Because P.H. has a low serum magnesium concentration (1.3 mEq/L), increasing P.H.'s serum magnesium concentration to 2 mEq/L could reduce his risk for arrhythmias.

β-Blockers

CASE 18-1, QUESTION 21: The physician wishes to write a prescription for a β-blocker. What are the benefits of administering a β-blocker to P.H.? Should it be given as IV therapy or started as oral therapy a few days after the infarction?

As with thrombolytic agents, β-blockers offer significant benefits to the MI patient as initial oral therapy during both the acute infarction period and several days later. Several large trials were designed to give IV β-blockers (up to 24 hours after symptom onset) followed by oral therapy; other studies used oral therapy alone beginning days after the infarction. Early IV administration appears to be most beneficial, with a reduction of mortality of about 25% in the first 2 days when the results of these trials are pooled. However, late oral therapy alone, up to 21 days after an MI in the β-Blocker in Heart Attack Trial, was also associated with a substantial reduction in mortality (around 10%).[1,23]

Propranolol, metoprolol, timolol, and atenolol have been studied extensively.[85–90] All have been given by early IV administration. Typically, metoprolol is used in the acute setting because of its β_1 selectivity, ease of dosing and administration, and weight of evidence. Oral carvedilol, a nonselective β- and α-blocker, has been used in the peri-infarction period, specifically in patients with left ventricular dysfunction. In the Carvedilol Post-Infarction Survival Control in Left Ventricular Dysfunction (CAPRICORN) trial, carvedilol 6.25 mg twice daily titrated to 25 mg twice daily reduced all-cause and cardiovascular mortality as well as recurrent nonfatal MI.[37]

In general, if a patient has transient cardiac decompensation (e.g., hypotension, bradycardia, or worsening symptoms of HF) during the acute infarction period, early IV β-blockers should be withheld. The patient's condition is then observed for a few days; if it stabilizes, oral therapy is initiated and titrated slowly. Data from COMMIT highlight the importance of tailored β-blockade therapy.[91] In this study, 45,852 patients were randomly assigned to receive placebo or metoprolol (up to 15 mg IV of metoprolol tartrate, then oral 200 mg metoprolol succinate daily) within 24 hours of AMI. Although metoprolol reduced reinfarction ($p < 0.001$) and ventricular fibrillation rates ($p < 0.001$) compared with placebo, the drug was also associated with a significant increase in episodes of cardiogenic shock ($p < 0.00001$). In a subgroup analysis, patients with hemodynamic instability at randomization appeared to be at greatest risk of early cardiogenic shock associated with metoprolol. The 2007 ACC/AHA guidelines provide specific dosing recommendations for the acute use of metoprolol in patients with STEMI. On hospital days 0 to 1, IV metoprolol tartrate (5 mg IV every 6–8 hours) can be considered in patients with hypertension without specific risk factors for cardiogenic shock (see Table 18-2). From hospital day 2 forward, metoprolol tartrate 25 to 50 mg orally every 6 hours should be initiated and eventually transitioned to an equivalent dose of metoprolol succinate. Doses should be titrated on the basis of BP and heart rate.[1]

In our case, P.H.'s acute situation is complicated by his history of intermittent pulmonary problems. In deciding whether to attempt use of β-blockers in patients with pulmonary disease, one must determine the nature of the pulmonary problem (i.e., reactive airways or restrictive lung disease). It also would be helpful to determine P.H.'s need for routine use of β-agonists to help quantify the severity of his disease. By history, P.H. does not use β-agonist bronchodilators routinely. No history is given regarding his pulmonary function tests or the degree of reversibility of his airway disease with bronchodilators. β_1-Selective antagonists are the drugs of choice in these patients, but at higher doses (e.g., metoprolol doses >100 mg/day), the relative β_1-selectivity may be lost. A patient would need to experience significant worsening of the pulmonary disease to justify avoiding β-blockers. A better history of P.H.'s pulmonary problems should be obtained. If they are minor and as he has experienced an uncomplicated MI, P.H may be a candidate for early IV therapy with metoprolol and low-dose oral therapy. A prescription for a β-blocker at hospital discharge is considered to be a quality performance measure.[25]

Nitroglycerin

CASE 18-1, QUESTION 22: On admission, P.H. was wearing a nitroglycerin patch; however, P.H. continues to have chest discomfort. Would he benefit from IV nitroglycerin?

As P.H. is exhibiting refractory ischemic discomfort despite receiving sublingual and topical nitrates, symptomatic management with IV NTG is indicated. NTG lowers the left ventricular filling pressure and systemic vascular resistance, thereby reducing myocardial oxygen consumption and myocardial ischemia. At lower doses (<50 mcg/minute), IV NTG preferentially dilates the venous capacitance vessels, which leads to a decrease in left ventricular filling pressure. For patients who have signs of pulmonary congestion, IV NTG is of particular value.

CASE 18-1, QUESTION 23: How should IV NTG be administered to P.H.? How should it be monitored?

A constant infusion is delivered in a controlled manner, starting with 5 to 10 mcg/minute, which is then increased by an additional 5 to 10 mcg/minute every 5 to 10 minutes. Many cardiologists routinely give patients an infusion of NTG for the first 24 to 48 hours after an AMI. Increasing doses may be required during this period to maintain the desired hemodynamic effect owing to tolerance that occurs from prolonged nitrate exposure. However, if more than 200 mcg/minute is needed to achieve the desired response, another vasodilator may be needed. NTG is typically administered in combination with thrombolytic agents in patients who require relief of myocardial ischemia.

Some patients, particularly those with an inferior or right ventricular infarct, may have a problem with increased sensitivity to NTG, evidenced by the development of hypotension (mean BP <80 mm Hg). P.H.'s BP should be monitored closely during this infusion. After starting NTG, we would expect to see his BP decline; the pulse rate may or may not increase. The NTG dose should be titrated to relieve pain while avoiding symptomatic hypotension. In patients with evidence of HF, NTG can reduce left ventricular filling pressure (preload), as well as improve orthopnea and pulmonary congestion. However, excessive doses of IV NTG can reduce left ventricular filling pressure to excess, and potentially decrease cardiac output, especially in patients like P.H. who do not have signs of HF. The systolic BP should be maintained to at least 90 mm Hg. Once P.H.'s chest pain is controlled, he may be transitioned to either an oral agent or a transdermal delivery system in which a nitrate-free interval should be used (see Chapter 17, Chronic Stable Angina.)

TREATMENT FOR UNSTABLE ANGINA OR NON–ST SEGMENT ELEVATION MYOCARDIAL INFARCTION

Invasive Versus Conservative Strategy

CASE 18-2

QUESTION 1: J.W. is a 65-year-old man who presents to the ED with chest tightness and shortness of breath. He gives a history of similar symptoms the previous day that lasted 20 minutes. He was given aspirin 325 mg, intranasal oxygen, IV metoprolol tartrate, and started on an IV NTG infusion, which was increased to 80 mcg/minute; at that time, his BP was 110/60 mm Hg, and his heart rate was 88. His ECG revealed segment depression in the anterior leads. His shortness of breath was relieved, but he still complained of chest tightness. His past medical history includes hypertension for which he takes hydrochlorothiazide 25 mg daily. He has smoked a pack of cigarettes per day for the past 30 years. Laboratory values include the following:

Na, 135 mEq/L
K, 4.0 mEq/L
Cl, 100 mEq/L
CO_2, 20 mEq/L
BUN, 15 mg/dL
SCr, 1.3 mg/dL
Glucose, 100 mg/dL
Mg, 2 mEq/L
CK-MB fraction, 1% (normal, 0%–5%)
Troponin I, 0.5 ng/mL (normal, <2)

Based on his symptoms and ECG, the diagnosis is presumed unstable angina. Should J.W. receive an invasive or conservative strategy for management of his UA?

Because J.W. has a TIMI risk score of 4 (e.g., moderate risk) with multiple negative biomarkers after 24 hours, he should receive a conservative approach to management (see Fig. 18-7), meaning that pharmacotherapy will be initiated followed by a noninvasive stress evaluation. If J.W. were to have elevated cardiac biomarkers during his presentation, then his diagnosis would change to NSTEMI. If during his hospitalization, J.W. were to experience any recurrent ischemia, arrhythmias, or signs and symptoms of HF, he would proceed directly to angiography and undergo possible PCI.

Anticoagulant Therapy

CASE 18-2, QUESTION 2: What anticoagulant regimen should J.W. receive?

The 2011 ACC/AHA guidelines recommend beginning anticoagulant therapy for all patients (without contraindications) with NSTEMI as soon as possible after presentation.[4] The guidelines recommend one of four agents as options: UFH, enoxaparin, fondaparinux, and bivalirudin (approved only for patients managed according to an invasive strategy). Table 18-2 summarizes the dosing and contraindications for each of these agents.

In UA/NSTEMI, UFH has been associated with lower rates of death or MI than aspirin alone.[92–94] Despite its limitations, UFH is the one of the preferred anticoagulants if the patient is to receive CABG or PCI because of its rapid clearance. For a conservative strategy, the 2011 ACC/AHA guidelines grant a higher level of evidence for enoxaparin and UFH over fondaparinux. If fondaparinux is to be considered, it should be administered with another anticoagulant with Factor IIa activity such as UFH.[3]

Data in support of LMWHs in this setting come from several studies. In the Efficacy and Safety of Subcutaneous Enoxaparin (ESSENCE) study, enoxaparin (1 mg/kg SQ twice daily) was compared with UFH (5,000 units IV bolus followed by continued infusion titrated to an aPTT of 55–86 seconds) administered for 48 hours to 8 days.[95] The composite outcome of death, MI, or recurrent angina at 14 days was 19.8% in the UFH group versus 16.6% in the enoxaparin group, a 20% relative risk reduction. This benefit was maintained for 1 year.

In the Superior Yield of the New Strategy of Enoxaparin, Revascularization and Glycoprotein IIb/IIIa Inhibitors (SYNERGY) trial, 9,978 high-risk NSTEMI patients were randomly assigned to receive either enoxaparin (1 mg/kg SQ twice daily) or weight-based UFH (60 units/kg bolus followed by 12 units/kg/hour adjusted to an aPTT 1.5 to 2 times control) before undergoing an early invasive strategy.[96] Enoxaparin was found to be as efficacious as UFH in reducing 30-day all-cause mortality or nonfatal MI but was associated with a significant risk of major bleeding ($p = 0.008$). Bleeding was especially problematic in those patients who crossed over from one treatment to the other during the trial.

In the TIMI-11B trial, enoxaparin (30 mg IV bolus followed by 1 mg/kg SQ twice daily for 8 days) compared with UFH (70 units/kg bolus followed by 15 units/kg/hour for 3–8 days) reduced the composite end point of death, MI, or need for urgent revascularization at 8 days ($p = 0.048$) and 43 days ($p = 0.048$).[97] Based on subanalyses of this study, the benefit of enoxaparin appears to be greatest for high-risk subgroups such as those with ST segment deviation, elevated troponins, and a high TIMI risk score.[16,97,98]

Finally, enoxaparin has been compared with fondaparinux. In the OASIS-5 trial, 20,078 NSTEMI patients were randomly assigned to receive either fondaparinux (2.5 mg SQ daily) or enoxaparin (1 mg/kg SQ twice daily) for a mean of 6 days and evaluated at 9 days for the primary end point of death, MI, or refractory ischemia.[99] No difference existed between groups for the primary end point; however, compared with enoxaparin, fondaparinux demonstrated a significantly lower incidence of major bleeding at 9 days ($p < 0.001$) and a greater reduction in mortality at 30 days ($p = 0.05$). Based on these data, the 2007 ACC/AHA guidelines give preference to fondaparinux compared with other anticoagulants for patients who are at an increased risk of bleeding and being treated with a conservative strategy.[1]

For an invasive strategy, the 2011ACC/AHA guidelines also give consideration for bivalirudin.[4] In the ACUITY (Acute Catheterization and Urgent Intervention Triage Strategy) trial, 13,819 patients with NSTEMI managed with an early invasive strategy were randomly assigned to receive either UFH (or enoxaparin) plus a GP IIb/IIIa inhibitor, bivalirudin plus a GP IIb/IIIa inhibitor, or bivalirudin alone.[100] No differences in the rates of the primary end point (composite of death, MI, unplanned revascularization for ischemia, and major bleeding at 30 days) were observed between the group receiving UFH plus a GP IIb/IIIa inhibitor and the group receiving bivalirudin plus a GP IIb/IIIa inhibitor. However, compared with those receiving UFH plus a GP IIb/IIIa inhibitor, the 30-day composite of ischemia or major bleeding was significantly lower for those receiving bivalirudin alone (11.7% vs. 10.1%, respectively; $p = 0.015$). This difference was attributable primarily to a substantially reduced rate of major bleeding in the UFH plus GP IIb/IIIA inhibitor ($p < 0.001$).

Because J.W. is receiving a conservative strategy for his UA and he has adequate renal function, either enoxaparin, UFH, orfondaparinux could be initiated and continued for the duration of the hospitalization or up to 8 days.

Antithrombotic Therapy

CASE 18-2, QUESTION 3: What oral antithrombotic medications should be considered for J.W.?

For both a conservative and invasive strategy, aspirin along with clopidogrel (loading with maintenance dose) should be added as soon as possible to anticoagulant therapy unless the patient is to proceed to CABG.[1] For an invasive strategy, prasugrel can be considered in lieu of clopidogrel based on the TRITON-TIMI 38 study (see Case 18-1, Question 17). The use of clopidogrel in UA or NSTEMI has been documented in two landmark studies.[101–102]

In the Clopidogrel in Unstable Angina to Prevent Recurrent Ischemic Events (CURE) trial, 12,562 patients with NSTEMI presenting within 24 hours were randomly assigned to receive placebo plus aspirin (75–325 mg) or clopidogrel (300 mg, immediately followed by 75 mg daily) plus aspirin.[101] After 9 months, cardiovascular death, MI, or stroke occurred in 11.5% of patients in the placebo group and in 9.3% of those receiving clopidogrel ($p < 0.001$). Clopidogrel was associated with reductions in severe ischemia and revascularization. Compared with placebo, an increase in major and minor bleeding was seen with clopidogrel. On the basis of these data, clopidogrel with aspirin should be administered immediately on admission and continued for at least 1 month and up to 1 year.[4]

In PCI-CURE, 2,658 patients from the CURE trial undergoing PCI were evaluated in a separate analysis.[102] Patients were treated before PCI with aspirin and study medication for a median of 10 days. After PCI, patients received open-label clopidogrel or ticlopidine for 2 to 4 weeks, after which the study drug was restarted for a mean of 8 months. In the clopidogrel group, there was a statistically significantly reduction in the composite of cardiovascular deaths, MIs, or urgent target-vessel revascularizations within 30 days of the PCI compared with placebo (4.5% vs. 6.4%, respectively; $p = 0.03$). Overall, patients receiving clopidogrel exhibited a 31% reduction in cardiovascular death or MI compared with those receiving placebo ($p = 0.002$).

The loading dose of clopidogrel (300–600 mg) remains controversial (see Case 18-1, Question 18). Nonetheless, for patients undergoing PCI, clopidogrel or prasugrel should be loaded before the procedure, followed by 75 mg daily for 12 to 15 months of additional treatment.[4] The 2011 ACC/AHA guidelines also allow for a maintenance dose of 150 mg daily for 6 days followed by 75 mg daily for 12–15 months.[4] Daily aspirin should be continued indefinitely; however, the dosage regimen will depend on the type of coronary stent deployed (Table 18-2). For a conservative strategy, as with J.W., patients should continue their dose of aspirin (75–162 mg/day) indefinitely and their clopidogrel (75 mg/day) for at least 1 month and ideally to up to 1 year.

CASE 18-2, QUESTION 4: Should J.W. receive an IV GP IIb/IIIa? If so, which one?

In patients with UA/NSTEMI, several large trials have demonstrated that the GP IIb/IIIa inhibitors are of benefit for patients considered high risk, those undergoing PCI, or both.[103] Analysis of GP IIb/IIIa studies suggest that those patients who obtain the greatest advantage from these agents are those who have elevated troponins, diabetes, ST segment changes,, or a TIMI risk score of 4 or higher at presentation.[4,104–109] The 2011 ACC/AHA guidelines recommend that for patients with UA or NSTEMI who will be treated initially according to an invasive strategy, either a GP IIb/IIIa inhibitor or clopidogrel should be added to aspirin and anticoagulant therapy before diagnostic angiography is performed.[4] The guidelines also state that considering both agents is reasonable. When used to treat patients medically, the GP IIb/IIIa inhibitors tirofiban or eptifibatide are generally given for 18 to 72 hours (Table 18-5).[4]

The GUSTO-IV-ACS trial enrolled 7,800 patients with UA/NSTEMI in whom early (<48 hours) revascularization was not intended. All patients received aspirin and either UFH or LMWH. They were randomly assigned to placebo, an abciximab bolus and 24-hour infusion, or an abciximab bolus and 48-hour infusion. At 30 days, death or MI occurred in 8.0% of patients taking placebo, 8.2% of patients receiving 24-hour abciximab, and 9.1% of patients receiving 48-hour abciximab (no significant difference). At 48 hours, death occurred in 0.3%, 0.7%, and 0.9% of patients in these groups, respectively (placebo vs. abciximab at 48 hours; $p = 0.008$).[110] Based on these findings and those of other studies, abciximab is indicated only if angiography will not be appreciably delayed and PCI is likely to be performed; otherwise, IV eptifibatide or tirofiban is the preferred choice (Fig. 18-7).[4]

J.W. has a TIMI risk score of 4; therefore, the addition of eptifibatide or tirofiban is a reasonable choice. Platelets and signs and symptoms of bleeding should be monitored closely.[111]

LONG-TERM THERAPY

Angiotensin-Converting Enzyme Inhibitors, Angiotensin Receptor Blockers, and Direct Renin Inhibitors

CASE 18-3

QUESTION 1: J.S. is 68-year-old man who presents with an STEMI along with signs and symptoms of HF. His past medical history includes hypertension treated with hydrochlorothiazide 25 mg daily and diabetes for which he takes glipizide 5 mg daily. He has smoked a pack of cigarettes per day for the past 40 years. On admission, his BP was 145/86 mm Hg, and his heart rate was 90 beats/minute. Laboratory values include the following:

Na, 139 mEq/L
K, 4.2 mEq/L
Cl, 100 mEq/L
CO_2, 20 mEq/L
BUN, 15 mg/dL
SCr, 1.3 mg/dL
Glucose, 130 mg/dL
Hemoglobin A_{1c}, 6.9%
Mg, 2 mEq/L
CK-MB fraction, 35% (normal, 0%–5%)
Troponin I, 10 ng/mL (normal, <2)

He is administered aspirin 325 mg, clopidogrel 300 mg load, IV NTG infusion, continuous infusion of UFH, and intranasal oxygen. J.S. is immediately sent to the catheterization laboratory in which he receives a drug-eluting stent (e.g., paclitaxel-eluting stent) in his left anterior descending artery. After stabilization of his HF symptoms, J.S. is started on oral metoprolol tartrate 25 mg every 6 hours. An echocardiogram is performed before discharge and shows an EF of 35% along with the appearance of a thrombus in the left ventricle. Is an ACE inhibitor appropriate for J.S.?

After an AMI, the heart undergoes processes that initially compensate for the loss of contractile function but may increase the long-term risk for development of HF. This is referred to as remodeling of the ventricle (see Chapter 19, Heart Failure). The increase in the number of survivors of AMI has led to an increase in the number of HF patients. A number of clinical trials with the use of ACE inhibitors have demonstrated reductions in HF symptoms and mortality after MI.[83,112–115]

For patients with ACS, oral ACE inhibitor therapy should be started within the first 24 hours of presentation for those with an EF of 40% or less (even if asymptomatic) or clinical evidence of HF. Additionally, ACE inhibitors should also be considered for patients with concomitant hypertension, diabetes, and chronic kidney disease.[3,23] The use of IV ACE inhibitor therapy is not recommended in the ACC/AHA guidelines.[3,23] Captopril could be given on postinfarction day 2 or 3, beginning with a test dose of 6.25 mg and then titrated to a maintenance dosage of 25 to 50 mg three times a day. The BP should be monitored closely, with systolic BP maintained greater than 90 mm Hg. Renal function and serum potassium levels should be monitored closely during the first few months of therapy. Once it is established that the patient can tolerate an ACE inhibitor, he or she can be switched to a longer-acting agent such as lisinopril or enalapril to simplify the regimen. Because J.S. presents with clinical symptoms of HF, he is a candidate for an ACE inhibitor. Additionally, as J.S. has HF with an EF of 40% or less, hypertension, and diabetes, the ACE inhibitor should be continued indefinitely (Table 18-2).

CASE 18-3, QUESTION 2: When should an ARB or direct renin antagonist be considered?

If the patient cannot tolerate an ACE inhibitor because of cough, an ARB may be an alternative. In the Optimal Therapy in Myocardial Infarction with the Angiotensin II Antagonist Losartan (OPTIMAAL) trial and Valsartan in Acute Myocardial Infarction Trial (VALIANT), losartan and valsartan demonstrated similar reductions in all-cause mortality compared with captopril, with an insignificant trend in favor of captopril.[116,117] Dual therapy of captopril with valsartan offered no additional benefits but increased side effects. Dual therapy with the direct rennin inhibitor aliskiren should not be considered. Preliminary data from the Aliskiren Study in Post-MI Patients to Reduce Remodeling (ASPIRE) trial suggest that the addition of aliskiren to and ACE inhibitor or ARB for patients after MI with an EF of 45% or less does not further protect against ventricular remodeling and may cause hypotension or hyperkalemia.[118] If J.S. does not tolerate his ACE inhibitor, then an ARB can be considered. Dual therapy with an ARB or aliskiren should not be used in J.S.

Aldosterone Antagonists

CASE 18-3, QUESTION 3: Should J.S. receive an aldosterone antagonist?

Like angiotensin II, aldosterone also plays an important role in left ventricular remodeling. Inhibiting aldosterone directly in addition to ACE inhibitor therapy was first evaluated in the HF patients in the Randomized Aldactone Evaluation Study (RALES) (see Chapter 19, Heart Failure). Another aldosterone antagonist, eplerenone, is a selective inhibitor of the mineralocorticoid receptor with fewer sexual side effects. In the Eplerenone Post Acute Myocardial Infarction Heart Failure Efficacy and Survival Study (EPHESUS), 6,600 patients with AMI and an EF less than 40% were allocated to optimal medical therapy with either eplerenone or placebo. After 16 months, a 15% risk reduction in mortality ($p = 0.008$), 13% reduction in sudden death ($p = 0.002$), and 21% reduction in cardiovascular death or hospitalization ($p = 0.02$) were seen in the eplerenone group compared with placebo.[119]

The ACC/AHA guidelines recommend an aldosterone antagonist in patients with UA/NSTEMI or STEMI without significant renal dysfunction (creatinine <2.5 mg/dL in men, <2.0 mg/dL in women, or creatinine clearance ≤30 mL/minute) or hyperkalemia (potassium <5 mEq/L) who are already receiving therapeutic doses of an ACE inhibitor, have an EF less than 40%, and have either symptomatic HF or diabetes.[3,23]

Because J.S. does have symptomatic HF with an EF less than 40% and diabetes, he is a candidate for aldosterone antagonism. Serum potassium and renal function need to be checked at 3 days and 1 week after therapy initiation and every month for the first 3 months. ACE inhibitor and potassium supplement doses may need to be adjusted.[120]

β-Blockers

CASE 18-3, QUESTION 4: Should J.S. receive a β-blocker on discharge?

The ACC/AHA guidelines recommend β-blocker therapy indefinitely for all patients after an ACS.[2,3] The benefits of β-blockers in reducing reinfarction and mortality outweigh the risk, even in patients with asthma, depression, insulin-dependent diabetes, severe peripheral vascular disease, first-degree heart block, and moderate left ventricular dysfunction. Propranolol, metoprolol tartrate, and metoprolol succinate, as well as atenolol, are available as generics, making any of them a cost-effective alternative. Metoprolol succinate and carvedilol are considered first-line choices in patients with HF, whereas atenolol, metoprolol tartrate, or metoprolol succinate should be considered in patients with stable asthma or bronchospastic pulmonary disorder. As J.S. has HF, he should be transitioned from oral metoprolol tartrate to metoprolol succinate or carvedilol, which should be continued indefinitely. Being prescribed a β-blocker at hospital discharge is also a quality performance measure.[25]

Lipid-Lowering Agents

CASE 18-3, QUESTION 5: Should J.S. be started on a lipid-lowering agent? When should it be initiated?

A complete fasting lipid profile would be helpful and should be completed within 24 hours of presenting with an AMI.[2,3] This is often overlooked or not done because the patient is not fasting. Most patients will require a low-cholesterol, low–saturated fat diet in addition to lipid-lowering therapy. The goal for J.S. will be to obtain an LDL of less than 100 mg/dL, with an ideal goal of less than 70 mg/dL, with a statin.[2,3] When triglycerides are at least 200 mg/dL, drug therapy with niacin or a fibrate is beneficial.[1,3]

The Myocardial Ischemia Reduction with Aggressive Cholesterol Lowering (MIRACL) trial, which enrolled NSTEMI patients, reported a 16% lower rate of death and nonfatal major cardiac events at 4 months' follow-up in patients receiving atorvastatin 80 mg/day within 24 to 96 hours of hospitalization when compared with placebo ($p = 0.048$).[121] In the Pravastatin or Atorvastatin Evaluation and Infection Therapy (PROVE-IT)-TIMI 22 trial, patients with ACS who received atorvastatin 80 mg/day for 10 days exhibited a 16% lower risk of death, MI, UA hospitalization, stroke, and revascularization when compared with pravastatin 40 mg/day ($p = 0.005$) after 2 years.[122] The A to Z trial showed a favorable trend toward major cardiovascular event reduction during 624 months of follow-up in AMI patients receiving an intensive simvastatin regimen (40 mg/day for 1 month followed by 80 mg/day thereafter) initiated within 12 hours of stabilization when compared with those receiving a less intensive regimen (placebo for 4 months followed by simvastatin 20 mg/day).[123] However, based on clinical trials, observational studies, adverse event reports, and prescription use data, the FDA warns that use of simvastatin 80 mg may be associated with increased muscle injury.[124]

In the case of J.S., a statin should be administered within 24 hours of his hospitalization and he should be discharged with a statin regardless of LDL cholesterol, which is a quality core performance measure.[1,3,25] Although not an FDA-approved starting dose, an evidenced-based approach would be to initiate a high-potency statin such as atorvastatin 80 mg/day.[38] Drug interactions, patient tolerability, and affordability should also be considered.

Antiplatelet Therapy

CASE 18-3, QUESTION 6: How long should J.S. continue his aspirin and clopidogrel?

Antiplatelet therapy with aspirin should be lifelong for J.S. because of its effects on secondary prevention of reinfarction. There appears to be no difference in efficacy for a wide range of aspirin doses (75–1,500 mg/day), although higher doses may increase the incidence of side effects. Much interest exists in using lower doses of aspirin for cardiovascular disease. Most clinicians use dosages of 81 to 325 mg daily. Dual antiplatelet therapy with clopidogrel and aspirin, compared with aspirin alone, reduces major cardiovascular events in patients with established ischemic heart disease, and it reduces coronary stent thrombosis.

Because J.S. proceeded to PCI and received a drug-eluting stent, his dose of aspirin will be 162 to 325mg daily for 6 months, then decreased to 75 to 162 mg daily indefinitely (Table 18-2).[1,3] He should continue his clopidogrel 75 mg daily for at least 1 year.[1,3] Aspirin should be prescribed at hospital discharge because it is a quality performance measure.[25]

Warfarin

CASE 18-3, QUESTION 7: Three days before J.S.'s anticipated discharge, the medical team is discussing the need to administer long-term warfarin in addition to his dual antiplatelet therapy with aspirin and clopidogrel. Is warfarin indicated for J.S. at this time?

Long-term warfarin may be beneficial in some patients, but clinical judgment is needed to decide whether the benefit is likely to exceed the risk. Data suggest that the incidence of a left ventricular thrombus is approximately 35% in patients who have an anterior infarction.[125] Although anticoagulation will decrease the incidence of stroke, less than 3% of patients will experience a cerebrovascular accident after an AMI if not anticoagulated. The ACC/AHA guidelines recommend warfarin for ACS patients at high risk for CAD and low bleeding risk who are unable to take aspirin or clopidogrel, patients with a left ventricular thrombus, and those with persistent atrial fibrillation.[2,3] Data have suggested that the use of high-intensity warfarin (international normalized ratio [INR], 3–4) or moderate-intensity warfarin (INR, 2–2.5) with low-dose aspirin (75–100 mg) may significantly reduce subsequent cardiovascular events and death after MI compared with aspirin (100–160 mg), but at the expense of major bleeding.[126] The 2007 ACC/AHA guidelines recommend that in patients receiving warfarin, clopidogrel, and aspirin, an INR of 2.0 to 2.5 is recommended with low-dose aspirin (75–81 mg daily) and with 75 mg of clopidogrel.[1] J.S. is probably a good candidate for 1 to 3 months of warfarin therapy titrated to an INR of 2 to 2.5 because of the presence of a left ventricular thrombus; however, his dose of aspirin could be decreased to 81 mg/daily if warfarin is prescribed.

CASE 18-3, QUESTION 8: Should J.S. receive a proton-pump inhibitor (PPI)?

The ACC/AHA/American College of Gastroenterology recommend using a PPI in patients receiving dual antiplatelet therapy with multiple risk factors for gastrointestinal bleeding such as advanced age; concomitant use of warfarin, steroids, or NSAIDs; or *Helicobacter pylori* infection.[127] However, controversy exists regarding the interaction between PPI and clopidogrel as well as which specific PPI to consider (see Chapter 17, Chronic Stable Angina, for greater detail). Presently, the FDA recommends against the use of omeprazole, as well as cimetidine, with clopidogrel because of the possible reduced effectiveness of clopidogrel.[128] These agents are known to inhibit the isoenzyme 2C19. As J.S. has two risk factors for a GI bleed, a PPI other than omeprazole should be considered.[127]

CASE 18-3, QUESTION 9: How would you summarize the long-term therapy needed by J.S. on discharge?

Appropriate discharge medications for J.S. include a β-blocker, aspirin 81 mg/day, an ACE inhibitor, clopidogrel, a PPI, and warfarin to achieve an INR of 2 to 2.5. He also should receive a prescription for sublingual NTG to carry with him for use as needed. Some clinicians also might choose to continue his chronic nitrate therapy. These agents should be continued long term except for the warfarin, which should be discontinued after a few months. J.S. should be started on a statin to achieve an LDL goal of less than 100 mg/dL, ideally 70 mg/dL. Routine liver function tests should be obtained before initiation of therapy and periodically thereafter. His previous hydrochlorothiazide may be discontinued because his hypertension will likely be controlled with the β-blocker and ACE inhibitor. His glipizide should be continued, and his blood glucose monitored closely. The goal is to achieve a state of β-blockade that will allow J.S. to maintain a systolic BP of more than 100 mm Hg; therefore, the clinician must balance the hypotensive effects of the ACE inhibitor and the β-blocker.

LIFESTYLE MODIFICATIONS

CASE 18-3, QUESTION 10: What types of lifestyle modifications should J.S. be encouraged to pursue to reduce his risk factors?

J.S. must be encouraged to stop smoking; this may be the most important intervention. In patients after an MI with an EF of 40% or less, smoking cessation was associated with a 40% lower risk of all-cause mortality and a 30% lower risk of death, recurrent MI, or HF hospitalization (see Chapter 88, Tobacco Use and Dependence).[129] For weight management, an initial goal of weight loss should be to reduce body weight by approximately 10% from baseline if body mass index exceeds 25 kg/m^2.[1] Other lifestyle modifications should be considered so that J.S. can achieve a hemoglobin A_{1c} less than 7.0%, a blood pressure goal of less than 130/80 mm Hg because J.S. has diabetes, and an optimal serum LDL less than 70 mg/dL.[1] (See Chapter 13, Dyslipidemias, Atherosclerosis, and Coronary Heart Disease, and Chapter 17, Chronic Stable Angina, for further information on lipid-lowering drugs and diet therapy.)

SUMMARY

Although mortality and incidence rates for ACS appear to be on the decline, ACS still remains a major cause of morbidity and mortality in the United States. Regarding STEMI, the use of PCI has significantly improved the survival of patients with STEMI. The major risk associated with thrombolysis is bleeding, especially intracerebral hemorrhage. Another problem associated with thrombolytic therapy is reocclusion of the artery that was initially opened. Coronary angioplasty is more effective than thrombolytic therapy; however, it is available only in hospitals with experienced invasive cardiologists, thereby limiting its availability to some patients.

Aspirin should be given to all patients with ACS; unless there is a contraindication, β-blockers and statins should be administered as well. Clopidogrel is often used in conjunction with aspirin, especially in patients receiving stents. ACE inhibitors, ARBs, and aldosterone antagonists have been shown to be beneficial in patients who have left ventricular dysfunction (EF $<40\%$) and are also recommended for secondary prevention. Nitrates are also useful, but care must be taken to maintain an adequate perfusion pressure. Secondary prevention emphasizing a healthy lifestyle and aggressive lipid lowering are important components to the overall treatment plan.

KEY REFERENCES AND WEBSITES

A full list of references for this chapter can be found at **http://thepoint.lww.com/AT10e.** Below are the key references and websites for this chapter, with the corresponding reference number in this chapter found in parentheses after the reference.

Key References

Abraham NS et al. ACCF/ACG/AHA 2010 Expert Consensus Document on the Concomitant Use of Proton Pump Inhibitors and Thienopyridines: A Focused Update of the ACCF/ACG/AHA 2008 Expert Consensus Document on Reducing the Gastrointestinal Risks of Antiplatelet Therapy and NSAID Use. *Circulation.* 2010;24:2619. (125)

Anderson JL et al. ACC/AHA 2007 guidelines for the management of patients with unstable angina/non-ST-Elevation myocardial infarction: a report of the American College of Cardiology/American Heart Association Task Force on Practice Guidelines [published correction appears in *J Am Coll Cardiol.* 2008;51:974]. *J Am Coll Cardiol.* 2007;50:e1. (3)

Antman EM et al. ACC/AHA guidelines for the management of patients with ST-elevation myocardial infarction–executive summary. A report of the American College of Cardiology/American Heart Association Task Force on Practice Guidelines [published correction appears in *J Am Coll Cardiol.* 2005;45:1376]. *J Am Coll Cardiol.* 2004;44:671. (23)

Antman EM et al. 2007 focused update of the ACC/AHA 2004 guidelines for the management of patients with ST-elevation myocardial infarction: a report of the American College of Cardiology/American Heart Association Task Force on Practice Guidelines [published correction appears in *J Am Coll Cardiol.* 2008;51:977]. *J Am Coll Cardiol.* 2008;51:210. (1)

Dangas G et al. Role of clopidogrel loading dose in patients with ST-segment elevation myocardial infarction undergoing primary angioplasty: results from the HORIZONS-AMI (harmonizing outcomes with revascularization and stents in acute myocardial infarction) trial. *J Am Coll Cardiol.* 2009;54:1438. (75)

De Luca G et al. Benefits from small molecule administration as compared with abciximab among patients with ST-segment elevation myocardial infarction treated with primary angioplasty: a meta-analysis. *J Am Coll Cardiol.* 2009;53:1668. (81)

Kushner FG et al. 2009 focused updates: ACC/AHA guidelines for the management of patients with ST-elevation myocardial infarction (updating the 2004 guideline and 2007 focused update) and ACC/AHA/SCAI guidelines on percutaneous coronary intervention (updating the 2005 guideline and 2007 focused update) a report of the American College of Cardiology Foundation/American Heart Association Task Force on Practice Guidelines [published corrections appear in *J Am Coll Cardiol.* 2010;55:612 (dosage error in article text); *J Am Coll Cardiol.* 2009;54:2464]. *J Am Coll Cardiol.* 2009;54:2205. (2)

Krumholz HM et al. ACC/AHA 2008 performance measures for adults with ST-elevation and non-ST-elevation myocardial infarction: a report of the American College of Cardiology/American Heart Association Task Force on Performance Measures (Writing Committee to develop performance measures for ST-elevation and non-ST-elevation myocardial infarction): developed in collaboration with the American Academy of Family Physicians and the American College of Emergency Physicians: endorsed by the American Association of Cardiovascular and Pulmonary Rehabilitation, Society for Cardiovascular Angiography and Interventions, and Society of Hospital Medicine. *Circulation.* 2008;118:2596. (25)

Montalescot G et al. Prasugrel compared with clopidogrel in patients undergoing percutaneous coronary intervention for ST-elevation myocardial infarction (TRITON-TIMI 38): double-blind, randomised controlled trial. *Lancet.* 2009;373:723. (72)

Mehta SR et al. Double-dose versus standard-dose clopidogrel and high-dose versus low-dose aspirin in individuals undergoing percutaneous coronary intervention for acute coronary syndromes (CURRENT-OASIS 7): a randomised factorial trial. *Lancet.* 2010;376:1233. (76)

Stone GW et al. Bivalirudin during primary PCI in acute myocardial infarction. *N Engl J Med.* 2008;358:2218. (64)

Wiviott SD et al. Prasugrel versus clopidogrel in patients with acute coronary syndromes. *N Engl J Med.* 2007;357:2001. (71)

Wright SR et al. 2011 ACCF/AHA Focused update for the management of patients with unstable angina/non ST-elevation myocardial infarction, (updating the 2007 guideline): A report of the American College of Cardiology Foundation/American Heart Association Task Force on practice guidelines. *J Am Coll Cardiol.* 2001;57:e1–e40. (4)

Yusuf S et al. Effects of fondaparinux on mortality and reinfarction in patients with acute ST-segment elevation myocardial infarction: the OASIS-6 randomized trial. *JAMA.* 2006;295:1519. (58)

Key Websites

American College of Cardiology. CardioSource. **http://www.cardiosource.org/acc.**

American Heart Association. **http://www.heart.org/HEARTORG/HealthcareResearch/Healthcare-Research_UCM_001093_SubHomePage.jsp.**

The TIMI Study Group. **http://www.timi.org/.**

U.S. Food and Drug Administration. Information for Healthcare Professionals: Update to the labeling of Clopidogrel Bisulfate (marketed as Plavix) to alert healthcare professionals about a drug interaction with omeprazole (marketed as Prilosec and Prilosec OTC). **http://www.fda.gov/Drugs/DrugSafety/PostmarketDrugSafetyInformationforPatientsandProviders/DrugSafetyInformationforHeathcareProfessionals/ucm190787.htm.** (128)

19 Heart Failure

Harleen Singh and Joel C. Marrs

CORE PRINCIPLES

	CHAPTER CASES
1 Heart failure (HF) "is a complex clinical syndrome that can result from any structural or functional cardiac disorder that impairs the ability of the ventricle to fill with or eject blood." This is further subdivided into HF with reduced left ventricular ejection fraction (LVEF) or HF with preserved LVEF (HFPEF), previously referred to as diastolic dysfunction.	**Case 19-1 (Question 1)**
2 HF symptoms, including limitations in activity, can be quantified with the use of the New York Heart Association functional classification system and the American College of Cardiology–American Heart Association classification of chronic heart failure. The cardinal signs and symptoms (e.g., peripheral edema, dyspnea, fatigue) of HF must be evaluated in light of the patient's medical history, physical examination, and results of additional testing.	**Case 19-1 (Questions 2, 3)**
3 Coexisting medical conditions that lead to HF (e.g., ischemic heart disease, hypertension, atrial fibrillation, diabetes mellitus, sleep apnea) or result from HF (e.g., atrial fibrillation, cachexia, depression) may influence the overall prognosis and treatment; therefore these should be assessed on a routine basis.	**Case 19-1 (Question 4), Case 19-2 (Question 7), Case 19-5 (Question 3)**
4 Several categories of medications (such as nonsteroidal anti-inflammatory drugs and glitazones) may exert unfavorable hemodynamic effects and may precipitate HF symptoms in patients with previously compensated HF. In some patients the occurrence of HF can be attributed to the cardiotoxic effect of a particular medication (anthracycline, cancer chemotherapeutic drugs).	**Case 19-1 (Question 5)**
5 Treatment goals are to improve symptoms, decrease hospitalizations, and prevent premature death in patients. The cornerstone of treatment for HF with reduced LVEF is to optimize life-prolonging therapies (e.g., angiotensin-converting enzyme inhibitors, angiotensin receptor blocking agents, β-blockers, aldosterone antagonists) and promote healthy lifestyle choices (e.g., sodium restriction, exercise training).	**Case 19-1 (Questions 6–20), Case 19-2 (Questions 1, 2, 4–6, 8, 9), Case 19-3 (Question 1)**
6 Prompt recognition of symptoms and appropriate treatment are critical in the management of acute decompensated heart failure. The mainstay of therapy in patients with volume overload is intravenous loop diuretics. Other therapies (e.g., inotropic drugs) have consistently failed to show long-term benefits in clinical trials.	**Case 19-4 (Questions 1–3), Case 19-5 (Questions 1, 2)**
7 An implantable cardioverter-defibrillator reduces the risk of sudden cardiac death in patients with reduced left ventricular function. Cardiac resynchronization therapy can be used in combination to improve symptoms and quality of life in patients with severe HF symptoms.	**Case 19-5 (Question 4), Case 19-6 (Questions 1, 2)**
8 There is little clinical trial evidence on which treatments are optimal to use in HFPEF.	**Case 19-7 (Question 1)**
9 Although controversial, certain patients may respond differently to drug therapy (e.g., African American patients, women).	**Case 19-2 (Question 3), Case 19-3 (Question 2)**

continued

10 HF is an extremely serious condition and requires careful diagnosis, ongoing monitoring, and the implementation of evidence-based therapy. Herbal remedies (e.g., hawthorn) have some evidence to support their role in improving symptoms of HF; however, they have no evidence demonstrating improvements in mortality. Herbals can also potentially interact with other heart medications.	**Case 19-8 (Question 1)**

Heart failure is "a complex clinical syndrome that can result from any structural or functional cardiac disorder that impairs the ability of the ventricle to fill with or eject blood."[1] As a consequence, the heart fails to pump sufficient blood to meet the body's metabolic needs. Congestive heart failure (CHF) is a specific subset of heart failure (HF) characterized by left ventricular (LV) systolic dysfunction and volume excess presenting as an enlarged, blood-congested heart. However, patients may lack symptoms of congestion and still have reduced cardiac output manifesting as fatigue and reduced exercise tolerance. Therefore, the term CHF has been replaced with HF.

The descriptive terminology, diagnostic techniques, and treatment of HF have undergone significant change in the past 15 to 20 years. Since 1994, a series of consensus and evidence-based practice guidelines have been published in an effort to standardize HF management. Several landmark clinical trials have led to new treatment options for HF. Guidelines from the Heart Failure Society of America,[2] American College of Cardiology (ACC), American Heart Association (AHA),[1] and the European Society of Cardiology[3] have been revised and updated to reflect ongoing changes in the management of HF. In 2009, the ACC/AHA guidelines were updated.[1] These revised guidelines continue to use the four disease stages of HF first assigned by the ACC/AHA 2001 guidelines (Fig. 19-1).[4] This classification promotes the early identification of risk factors that are associated with the development of LV dysfunction and HF symptoms. It emphasizes that appropriate therapeutic interventions in the early stages (stages A and B) can prevent progression to overt HF symptoms. It does not replace the New York Heart Association (NYHA) functional classification, but reinforces that they should be used in combination to classify patients.

Numerous programs and systems have been implemented during the years in an attempt to decrease the cost and length of hospital stay for HF. Thus, the updated guidelines included a new section on the management of hospitalized patients. It is highly recommended that practitioners look at least annually for the most recently published guidelines to be aware of the rapidly evolving treatment strategies for HF.

Incidence, Prevalence, and Epidemiology

It is estimated that there were 6 million people (1.5% to 2% of the population) with HF in the United States in 2006, and approximately 23 million people with HF worldwide.[5] The prevalence of HF continues to increase, with an estimated 772,000 new HF cases projected in the year 2040.[6] An analysis by an Olmstead County (Minnesota) epidemiologic group showed that although the prevalence of systolic HF did not change significantly, the recognition of diastolic HF has increased.[7] In the United States, the incidence of HF generally ranges from 2 to 5 per 1,000 person-years, depending on the cohort studied.[5] After age 65, HF incidence approaches 10 per 1,000 person-years and is the most common cause of hospitalizations in the elderly population in the United States.

The incidence of HF is greater in men and in the elderly; however, the incidence in black women is as high as that of white men. In women, coronary artery disease (CAD) and diabetes are considered the strongest risk factors for HF. African American individuals may present with HF at a younger age compared with white individuals. More aggressive treatment of hypertension may contribute to the lower incidence of HF in some populations; however, the 5-year survival for those with HF alone and HF with diabetes is still dismal (47% and 37%, respectively).[8] The high prevalence of risk factors such as chronic kidney disease, CAD, diabetes, and obesity are associated with increased HF incidence.

In 2004, approximately 1 million people were hospitalized for HF. In the United States, one in eight deaths has HF mentioned on the death certificate, 20% of which have HF as the primary cause of death. The mortality risk steadily increases with each year after the diagnosis of HF. The 6-month mortality rates are no different with patients with preserved or reduced LV ejection fraction (EF).[5] Direct and indirect health care costs of HF in 2010 were estimated to be $39.2 billion. HF is the number one discharge diagnosis in the Medicare population (70,000 hospitalized for HF).[8] In the 10-year period from 1996 to 2006, hospital

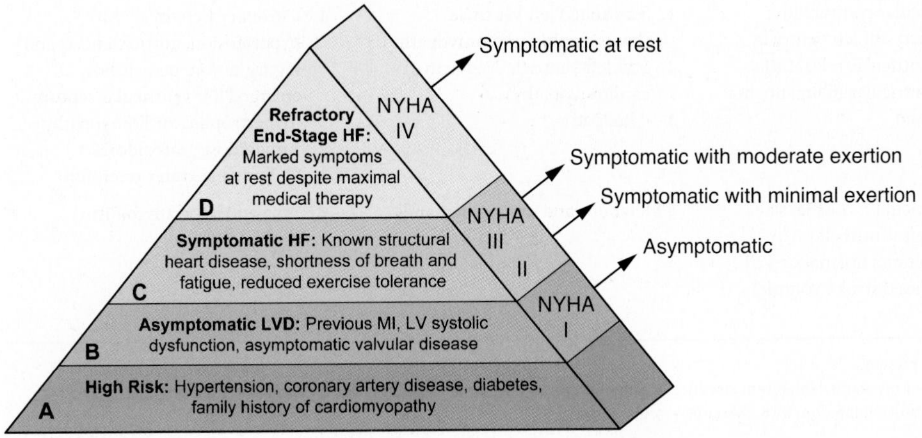

FIGURE 19-1 Staging and New York Heart Association (NYHA) classification of heart failure. Source: Hunt SA et al. ACC/AHA Guidelines for the Evaluation and Management of Chronic Heart Failure in the Adult: Executive Summary. A Report of the American College of Cardiology/American Heart Association Task Force on Practice Guidelines (Committee to Revise the 1995 Guidelines for the Evaluation and Management of Heart Failure): Developed in Collaboration With the International Society for Heart and Lung Transplantation; Endorsed by the Heart Failure Society of America. *Circulation*. 2001;104:2996.

discharges for HF increased by 26%.[8] In the year 2001, Medicare expended $5,912 per discharge for beneficiaries with HF.[9] As the size of the geriatric population increases, HF will likely become a more frequently encountered clinical entity. Furthermore, postdischarge mortality among patients with HF is 11% at 30 days and 37% at 1 year.[10] Thirty-day postdischarge HF readmission rates are now being considered as quality measures for HF management.

Currently, various risk prediction models have been developed to predict HF outcomes. Given the heterogeneous nature of the HF population (from ischemic to nonischemic, low to preserved EF), including multiple comorbid conditions, the validity of the risk prediction models may not be consistent in all HF populations. Therefore, it is very important to identify patients who are at high risk of HF and how various risks factors can predict outcomes.[11] Based on the strength of these associations, prevention measures need to be designed to decrease HF hospitalizations in targeted subpopulations.

Etiology

LOW-OUTPUT VERSUS HIGH-OUTPUT FAILURE

Traditionally, HF has been described as being either *low-output* or *high-output failure,* with a predominance (>90%) of cases being low-output failure (Table 19-1). In both types, the heart cannot provide adequate blood flow (tissue perfusion) to meet the body's metabolic demands, especially during exercise. The hallmark of classic low-output HF is a diminished volume of blood being pumped by a weakened heart in patients who have otherwise normal metabolic needs.

In high-output failure, the heart itself is healthy and pumps a normal or even higher than normal volume of blood. Because of high metabolic demands caused by other underlying medical disorders (e.g., hyperthyroidism, anemia), the heart becomes exhausted from the increased workload and eventually cannot keep up with demand. The primary treatment of high-output HF is amelioration of the underlying disease. Unless otherwise stated, this chapter focuses on the treatment of low-output HF.

LEFT VERSUS RIGHT VENTRICULAR DYSFUNCTION

Simple classification of HF as being low-output failure does not adequately describe the complex nature of this disorder. Consequently, low-output HF is further divided into left and right ventricular dysfunction, or a combination of the two (biventricular failure). Because the left ventricle is the major pumping chamber of the heart, it is not surprising that *left ventricular dysfunction* is the most common form of low-output HF and the major target for pharmacologic intervention. Right ventricular dysfunction may coexist with left ventricular HF if damage is sustained by both sides of the heart (e.g., after myocardial infarction [MI]) or as a delayed complication of progressive left-sided HF.

For an animation about congestive heart failure, see http://thepoint.lww.com/AT10e.

Isolated right-sided ventricular dysfunction, which is relatively uncommon, is usually caused by either primary or secondary *pulmonary arterial hypertension* and can subsequently lead to cor pulmonale. In these conditions, elevated pulmonary artery pressure impedes emptying of the right ventricle, thus increasing the workload on the right side of the heart.[12,13] Primary pulmonary arterial hypertension is idiopathic, caused by increased resistance of the pulmonary arterial vasculature of unknown etiology. Secondary causes include collagen vascular disorders, sarcoidosis, fibrosis, exposure to high altitude, and drug and chemical exposure. Drug-induced sources include opioid overdoses (especially heroin), 5-hydoxytryptamine-2B (5HT-2B) agonists (e.g., dexfenfluramine, fenfluramine, and pergolide), and pulmonary fibrosis caused by intravenous (IV) injection of poorly soluble forms of methylphenidate. Right-sided heart disease that occurs as a result of a primary pulmonary process is known as cor pulmonale, and often leads to right heart failure.

TABLE 19-1
Classification and Etiology of Left Ventricular Dysfunction

Type of Failure	Characteristics	Contributing Factors	Etiology
Low output, systolic dysfunction (dilated cardiomyopathy)[a]	Hypofunctioning left ventricle; enlarged heart (dilated left ventricle); ↑left ventricular end-diastolic volume; EF <40%; ↓stroke volume; ↓CO; S_3 heart sound present	1. ↓Contractility (cardiomyopathy) 2. ↑Afterload (elevated SVR)	1. Coronary ischemia,[b] MI, mitral valve stenosis or regurgitation, alcoholism, viral syndromes, nutritional deficiency, calcium and potassium depletion, drug induced, idiopathic 2. Hypertension, aortic stenosis, volume overload
Diastolic dysfunction	Normal left ventricular contractility; normal size heart; stiff left ventricle; impaired left ventricular relaxation; impaired left ventricular filling; normal EF; S_4 heart sound	1. Thickened left ventricle (hypertrophic cardiomyopathy) 2. Stiff left ventricle (restrictive cardiomyopathy) 3. ↑Preload	1. Coronary ischemia,[b] MI hypertension, aortic stenosis and regurgitation, pericarditis, enlarged left ventricular septum (hypertrophic cardiomyopathy) 2. Amyloidosis, sarcoidosis 3. Sodium and water retention
High-output failure (uncommon)	Normal or ↑contractility; normal size heart; normal left ventricular end-diastolic volume; normal or ↑EF; normal or increased stroke volume; ↑CO	↑Metabolic and oxygen demands	Anemia and hyperthyroidism

[a] Same as congestive heart failure if symptoms also present.
[b] Heart failure caused by coronary artery ischemia or myocardial infarction classified as ischemic etiology. All other types combined classified as nonischemic.
CO, cardiac output; EF, ejection fraction; MI, myocardial infarction; SVR, systemic vascular resistance.

SYSTOLIC VERSUS DIASTOLIC DYSFUNCTION; ISCHEMIC VERSUS NONISCHEMIC HEART FAILURE

Left ventricular dysfunction is further subdivided into systolic and diastolic dysfunction, with mixed disorders also being encountered (Table 19-1). In systolic dysfunction, the *stroke volume* (SV) (i.e., the volume of blood ejected by the heart with each systolic contraction; normal, 60–130 mL) and the subsequent 1-minute *cardiac output* (CO) (i.e., SV × heart rate; normal, 4 to 7 L/minute) are reduced. In diagnosing HF, a critical marker differentiating systolic from diastolic dysfunction is the *left ventricular ejection fraction,* defined as the percentage of LV end-diastolic volume expelled during each systolic contraction (normal, 60%–70%).

In *systolic dysfunction,* the LVEF is less than 40%, dropping to less than 20% in advanced HF. Thus, systolic dysfunction is synonymous with low EF heart failure and is almost always caused by factors causing the heart to fail as a pump (decreased myocardial muscle contractility). The heart dilates as it becomes congested with retained blood, leading to an enlarged hypokinetic left ventricle.

Heart failure caused by damage to heart muscle or valves because of chronic coronary ischemia or after MI is classified as *ischemic,* with all other types grouped as *nonischemic*. CAD is the cause of HF in approximately two-thirds of patients with LV systolic dysfunction. Other causes of LV pump failure include persistent arrhythmias, poststreptococcal rheumatic heart disease, chronic alcoholism (alcoholic cardiomyopathy), viral infections, or unidentified etiology (idiopathic dilated cardiomyopathy). Chronic hypertension, as well as certain cardiac valvular disorders (aortic or mitral stenosis), also precipitates systolic HF by increasing resistance to CO (i.e., a high afterload state). (Refer to the Afterload subsection of the Cardiac Workload section for more information.)

In contrast, LV diastolic dysfunction refers to impaired relaxation and increased stiffness of the left ventricle; the EF may or may not be abnormal, and the patient may or may not be symptomatic. The terms *diastolic dysfunction* and *diastolic heart failure* are not synonymous. Diastolic dysfunction is one diagnostic criterion for diastolic HF. Diastolic HF is defined as "a clinical syndrome of HF characterized by a normal EF and abnormal diastolic function."[14–18] In this form of HF, cardiac muscle function (contractility) is *not* impaired and, most importantly, the EF remains at or greater than 45%. The SV and CO are normal or decreased.[19] In simple terms, a high fraction of a low volume is ejected. Because diastolic dysfunction is difficult to measure, the term *heart failure with normal or preserved left ventricular ejection fraction (HF-PEF)* has been proposed instead of diastolic HF. Possible causes for diastolic failure include coronary ischemia, long-standing uncontrolled hypertension, LV wall scarring after an MI, ventricular wall hypertrophy, hypertrophic cardiomyopathy (formerly known as idiopathic hypertrophic subaortic stenosis), constrictive pericarditis, restrictive cardiomyopathy (e.g., amyloidosis and sarcoidosis), and valvular heart disease (mitral stenosis, acute aortic regurgitation, mitral regurgitation). These factors lead to LV wall stiffness (reduced wall compliance), an inability of the ventricle to relax during diastole, or both, which result in an elevated resting pressure within the ventricle despite a relatively low volume of blood in the chamber. In turn, the elevated pressure impedes LV filling during diastole that would normally occur by passive inflow against a low-resistance pressure gradient. Heart size is usually (but not always) normal. It is estimated that 20% to 60% of patients with HF may have normal LVEF and reduced ventricular compliance.[1,14–18,20,21] Because coronary ischemia, MI, and hypertension are contributors to both systolic and diastolic failure, many patients have symptoms of a combined disorder.

The pathology of systolic dysfunction most closely resembles what has historically been referred to as "congestive heart failure." Tremendous variability exists in the clinical presentation of both systolic and diastolic dysfunction, however, and both disorders can have essentially identical symptoms.[1,4,14] For example, some patients with either systolic or diastolic dysfunction exhibit exercise intolerance, but have little evidence of fluid retention. Others may have significant edema with few complaints of exercise intolerance or shortness of breath. It is also possible to have no symptoms in the early stages of both forms of HF. For all these reasons, it is best to avoid the abbreviation *CHF,* especially because CHF has also been used to denote chronic heart failure. In the meantime, clinicians are strongly encouraged to obtain an EF measurement in all patients. The diagnosis of HF should be based on a combination of typical symptoms and signs together with appropriate clinical tests.[1–3]

CARDIAC WORKLOAD

A common factor to all forms of HF is increased cardiac workload. Four major determinants contribute to LV workload: preload, afterload, contractility, and heart rate (HR).

PRELOAD

Preload describes forces acting on the *venous* side of the circulation to affect myocardial wall tension. The relationship is as follows: as venous return (i.e., blood flowing into the heart) increases, the volume of blood in the left ventricle increases. The volume is maximal when filling finishes at the end of diastole (LV end-diastolic volume). This increased volume raises the pressure within the ventricle (LV end-diastolic pressure), which in turn increases the "stretch," or wall tension, of the ventricle (see discussion of the Frank-Starling ventricular function curve in Cardiac Remodeling section). Peripheral venous dilation and decreased peripheral venous volume diminish preload, whereas peripheral venous constriction and increased peripheral venous volume increase preload.

Elevated preload can aggravate HF. For example, rapid administration of blood plasma expanders and osmotic diuretics or administration of large amounts of sodium or sodium-retaining agents can increase preload. A malfunctioning aortic valve (aortic insufficiency), resulting in regurgitation of blood back into the left ventricle, also can increase the volume of blood that must be pumped. A malfunctioning mitral valve (mitral regurgitation) can cause retrograde ejection of blood from the left ventricle back into the left atrium, with a resultant decrease in CO. In patients with systolic failure, ventricular blood is ejected less efficiently because of a hypofunctioning left ventricle; the volume of blood retained in the ventricle is thus increased, and preload becomes elevated. In diastolic failure with a stiffened left ventricle, relatively small increases in end-diastolic volume from sodium and water overload can lead to exaggerated increases in end-diastolic pressure, despite normal or even reduced end-diastolic volumes.

ONLINE CONTENT

For a narrated PowerPoint slide presentation regarding the pressure-volume loop (normal, HFPEF and LVSD), go to http://thepoint.lww.com/AT10e.

AFTERLOAD

Afterload is the tension developed in the ventricular wall as contraction (systole) occurs. The tension developed during contraction is affected by intraventricular pressure, ventricular diameter, and wall thickness. More simply, afterload is regulated by the systemic vascular resistance (SVR) or impedance against which the ventricle must pump during its ejection, and it is chiefly

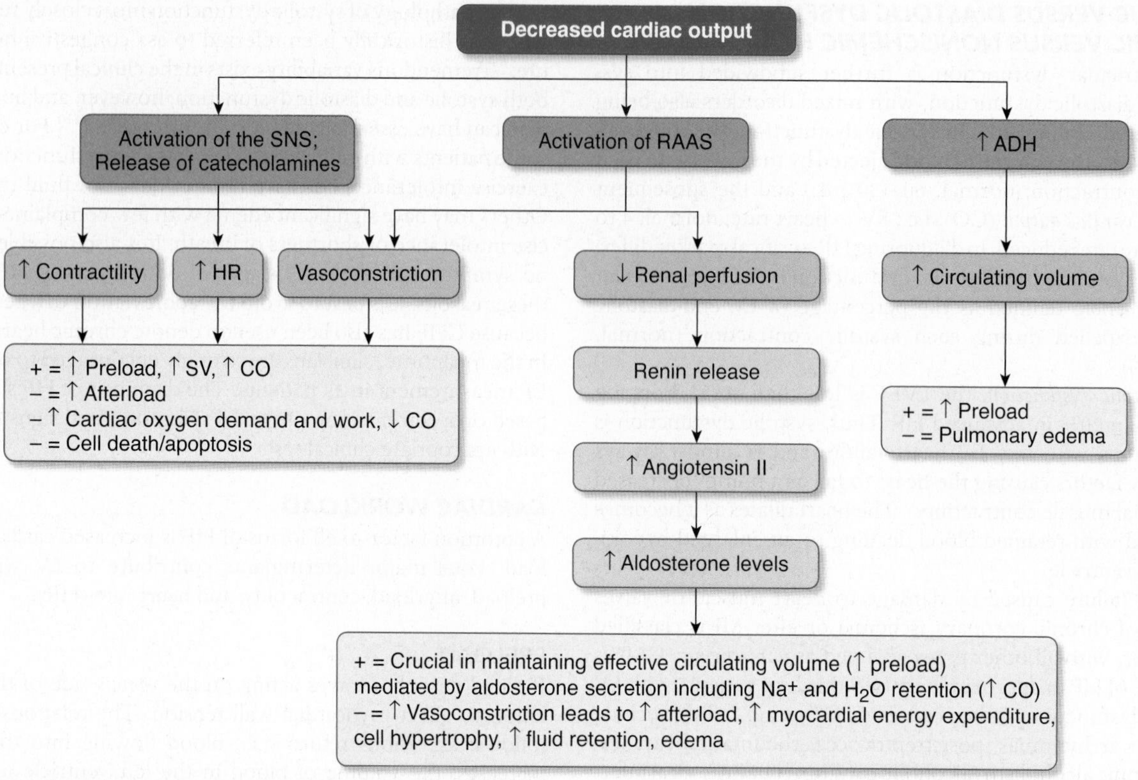

FIGURE 19-2 Adaptive mechanisms in systolic heart failure. +, beneficial results; –, negative (detrimental) effects; ADH, antidiuretic hormone; CO, cardiac output; HR, heart rate; H_2O, water; Na^+, sodium; RAAS, renin-angiotensin-aldosterone system; SNS, sympathetic nervous system; SV, stroke volume.

determined by arterial blood pressure (BP). Hypertension, atherosclerotic disease, or a narrowed aortic valve opening increases arterial impedance (afterload), thereby increasing the workload on the heart. Hypertension is a major etiologic factor in the development of both systolic and diastolic HF. The Framingham group found that 75% of patients who developed HF had a history of hypertension.[22,23] The risk of developing HF was six times greater for hypertensive than for normotensive patients.

CARDIAC CONTRACTILITY

The terms *contractility* and *inotropic state* are used synonymously to describe the myocardium's (cardiac muscle's) inherent ability to develop force and shorten its fibers independent of preload or afterload. Myocardial contractility is decreased when myocardial fibers are diminished or poorly functioning as may occur in patients with primary cardiomyopathy, valvular heart disease, coronary artery disease, or after an MI. Defects in contractility play a major role in systolic HF, but are not a component of pure diastolic dysfunction. Occasionally, drugs, such as nonselective β-adrenergic blockers or doxorubicin, induce HF by decreasing myocardial contractility.

HEART RATE

An increased heart rate is a reflex mechanism to improve CO as EF declines. As discussed subsequently, the sympathetic nervous system is the major mediator of this response. The workload and energy demands of a rapid heart rate ultimately place strain on the heart and can eventually worsen HF.

Pathophysiology

When the heart begins to fail, the body activates several complex compensatory mechanisms in an attempt to maintain CO and oxygenation of vital organs. These include increased sympathetic tone, activation of the renin-angiotensin-aldosterone system (RAAS), sodium and water retention, and other neurohormonal adaptations, which lead to cardiac "remodeling" (ventricular dilatation, cardiac hypertrophy, and changes in LV lumen shape). The long-term consequences of these adaptive mechanisms can create more harm than good (Fig. 19-2). The relative balance of each of these adaptive processes can vary depending on the type of HF (systolic versus diastolic dysfunction) and even from patient to patient with the same type of disorder. An understanding of the potential benefits and adverse consequences of these compensatory mechanisms is essential to understanding the signs, symptoms, and treatment of HF.[24]

SYMPATHETIC (ADRENERGIC) NERVOUS SYSTEM

The body's normal physiologic response to a decreased CO is generalized activation of the adrenergic (sympathetic) nervous system as evidenced by increased circulating levels of norepinephrine (NE) and other catecholamines. The inotropic (increased contractility) and chronotropic (increased HR) effects of NE initially maintain near-normal CO and preserve perfusion of vital organs such as the central nervous system (CNS) and myocardium. Other adverse consequences of NE activation include impaired sodium excretion by the kidneys, restricted ability of the coronary arteries to supply blood to the ventricular wall (myocardial ischemia), increased automaticity of cardiac tissue to provoke arrhythmias, hypokalemia, and oxidative stress to trigger programmed cell death (apoptosis).[4]

In the long-term, high levels of NE or its metabolites are potentially harmful to heart muscle because they decrease β_1-receptor sensitivity and reduce β_1-receptor density on the surface of myocardial cells by as much as 60% to 70% in severe HF.[24–30] The normal ratio of β_1- to β_2-receptors in the heart is 75 to 80 : 20 to 25. As a negative feedback response to overstimulation, this balance is shifted to a ratio of 60 to 70 : 30 to 40 in the failing myocardium by downregulation of β_1-subtype receptors. This selective downregulation of β_1-receptors is accompanied by a complex phenomenon of "uncoupling of the β_1- and β_2-receptor activity," whereby the number of β_2-receptors are unchanged and the responsiveness of these receptors in eliciting a response can be reduced by 30%.[25] Over time, this leaves the myocyte less responsive to adrenergic stimuli and further decreases contractile function. At the same time, the postsynaptic β_1-subtype is upregulated in the failing heart, resulting in cell growth (hypertrophy) and a positive inotropic effect. β_2-Receptors on the presynaptic side of the sympathetic nerve act to suppress NE release, providing a partial protective mechanism from adrenergic overstimulation.

Alterations in sympathetic adrenergic receptors in the heart during HF are complex and partially determined by genetic phenotype. Interestingly, among African American patients with HF, a disproportionately high incidence of polymorphisms for variants of the β_1-receptor that are associated with increased function is seen. Additionally, the combined presence of a variant of the β_1-receptor (β_1Arg389) and α_{2C}-adrenergic receptor (α_{2C}Del322-325) results in adrenergic overstimulation and increases the risk of HF in African Americans. These combined defects are found less often in whites, perhaps partially explaining a higher incidence of HF in African Americans. A better understanding of α- and β-receptor phenotyping may someday lead to improved prevention and treatment strategies for HF.[31]

RENAL FUNCTION AND THE RENIN-ANGIOTENSIN-ALDOSTERONE SYSTEM

The reduced CO in HF leads to the stimulation angiotensin II, which is a potent vasoconstrictor. Angiotensin II is also a potent stimulator of the sympathetic nervous system, which increases the SVR. This, in turn, sets off a complex chain of events leading to sodium and water retention and, eventually, increased blood volume. Renal vascular resistance is increased, and the glomerular filtration rate (GFR) is decreased. As the GFR decreases, more sodium is reabsorbed in the proximal tubule. Additionally, the glomerular filtrate may be preferentially shunted to nephrons with long loops of Henle, increasing the surface area for sodium reabsorption. A diminished effective circulating plasma volume and angiotensin II also stimulate release of antidiuretic hormone (ADH) from the pituitary, resulting in the retention of free water in the renal collecting ducts.

The kidney releases the enzyme renin when renal perfusion pressure is decreased. Renin acts to convert a substrate present in the blood called *angiotensinogen* into the inactive decapeptide, *angiotensin I*. Angiotensin I is further metabolized to the active decapeptide, *angiotensin II,* under the influence of circulating angiotensin-converting enzyme (ACE) (Fig. 19-2). Angiotensin II has multiple effects favoring sodium and water retention. Its vasoconstricting effects may further decrease GFR, and it stimulates the adrenal glands to secrete aldosterone, a hormone that increases sodium reabsorption in the distal tubule. Further, angiotensin II stimulates increased synthesis and release of vasopressin, thereby increasing free water retention and stimulation of thirst centers in the CNS. Finally, angiotensin II may directly stimulate NE release. The net result of the kidney and angiotensin II effects is detrimental. Increased sodium and water retention increase preload, whereas angiotensin II–induced vasoconstriction increases SVR and afterload.

Morphologic studies indicate that a chronic excess of aldosterone (plus salt loading), as occurs in HF, can cause fibrosis in the atria and ventricles, kidneys, and other organs in animals and humans.[32] Thus, aldosterone may promote the remodeling of organs and fibrosis independent of angiotensin II.

OTHER HORMONAL MEDIATORS

ENDOTHELINS

Several other regulatory hormones and cytokines have been identified as playing a role in the pathogenesis and adaptation to HF. The first of these are the endothelins, a family of 21–amino acid peptides.[33,34] Within this family, endothelin-1 (ET-1) is the most active. ET-1 was first isolated from vascular endothelial cells, but it is also synthesized by vascular and airway smooth muscle, cardiomyocytes, leukocytes, and macrophages. Serum concentrations of ET-1 are elevated in HF, pulmonary hypertension, MI, ischemia, and shock and are implicated in causing vasoconstriction, potentiation of cardiac remodeling, and decreased renal blood flow and glomerular filtration. Although these effects of ET-1 are detrimental in HF, its pharmacology is complex and dependent on the relative balance of two distinct G protein–coupled receptor subtypes referred to as ET_A and ET_B. As illustrated in Table 19-2, ET-1 can elicit opposing effects from each receptor, with the net effect being dependent on the relative density of the two receptors.

Synthesis of ET-I begins with a precursor protein called preproendothelin and involves several enzymatic steps and intermediates. Key enzymes in its synthesis are dibasic specific endopeptidase, carboxypeptidase, and endothelin-converting enzyme. Possible therapeutic implications of understanding this synthetic pathway are development of specific inhibitors of one or more of the enzymes to prevent activation of ET-1. Alternatively, selective inhibitors of ET_A receptors could shift responses toward the favorable aspects of ET_B receptor activation. Currently, no such drugs exist, but bosentan and tezosentan are investigational nonselective dual ET_A/ET_B antagonists. Bosentan has US Food and

TABLE 19-2
Biological Effects of Endothelin-1

Organ System	ET_A Receptor Effects	ET_B Receptor Effects	Other Effects
Blood vessels	Potent vasoconstrictor Collagen deposition	Vasodilation mediated through nitric oxide and prostacyclin release	
Heart	Hypertrophy and remodeling		↑ HR +/– inotropic effects
Lungs	Bronchoconstriction		
Kidney	Afferent and efferent vasoconstriction Decrease in RBF and GFR	Natriuresis and diuresis	
Neuroendocrine			Release of catecholamines, renin, aldosterone, and ANH

ANH, atrial natriuretic hormone; ET_A, endothelin A; ET_B, endothelin B; GFR, glomerular filtration rate; HR, heart rate; RBF, renal blood flow; +/–, positive/negative.
Source: Ergul A. Endothelin-1 and endothelin receptor antagonists as potential cardiovascular therapeutic agents. *Pharmacotherapy*. 2002;22:54.

Drug Administration (FDA) approval for the treatment of pulmonary hypertension and is being investigated for use in HF.[12,13]

NATRIURETIC PEPTIDES

Natriuretic peptides are a family of peptides containing a common 17–amino acid ring. A-type natriuretic peptide, previously referred to as either atrial natriuretic peptide or atrial natriuretic factor, is secreted by the atrial myocardium in response to dilatation and stretch. Similarly, B-type natriuretic peptide (BNP), formerly referred to as brain natriuretic peptide, is produced by the ventricular myocardium in response to elevations of end-diastolic pressure and volume. Type-C natriuretic peptide is secreted by lung, kidney, and vascular endothelium in response to shear stress. Collectively, the natriuretic peptides have been referred to as cardiac neurohormones and are generally considered to be a favorable form of neurohormonal activation. Among their positive attributes are antagonism of the renin-angiotensin system, inhibition of sympathetic outflow, and ET-1 antagonism. The net effect is peripheral and coronary vasodilation to decrease preload and afterload on the heart. As their name implies, they also have diuretic or natriuretic properties, with improved renal blood flow and glomerular filtration resulting from afferent arteriolar dilation and possibly efferent arteriolar constriction. Sodium reabsorption is blocked in the collecting duct by virtue of an indirect aldosterone inhibition. Natriuretic peptides also inhibit vasopressin secretion from the pituitary gland and block salt appetite and thirst centers in the CNS. Each of these CNS effects contributes further to diuresis. Of note, type-C natriuretic peptide has minimal diuretic properties.[35]

The BNP precursor is cleaved to produce the biologically active C-terminal fragment (BNP) and an inactive N-terminal fragment (NT-proBNP). Plasma level measurement of either BNP or NT-proBNP can be used as a biologic marker to differentiate HF-induced dyspnea from other causes of respiratory distress (e.g., chronic bronchitis).[36–38] BNP levels less than 100 pg/mL usually indicate absence of HF, whereas levels greater than 400 pg/mL are highly indicative of HF. However, the interpretation of BNP levels between 100 and 400 pg/mL can be challenging because elevated levels are also associated with renal failure, pulmonary embolism, pulmonary hypertension, and chronic hypoxia.[39] Higher concentrations correlate to severity of HF, with a mean plasma level of 241 pg/mL in NYHA class I patients and greater than 800 pg/mL in NYHA class IV HF. Similarly, clinical resolution of symptoms is often accompanied by a decline in BNP concentration.

Natriuretic hormone analogs or inhibitors of their metabolism have been investigated for drug therapy of HF. Nesiritide is a recombinantly produced human B-type natriuretic peptide approved by the FDA for IV management of acute HF exacerbations in hospitalized patients.[40,41] Downregulation of natriuretic peptide receptors, however, occurs during chronic HF, reducing the protective benefit of their actions and possibly limiting their usefulness as therapeutic entities.

VASOPRESSIN RECEPTOR ANTAGONISTS

To date, all standard therapies (such as loop diuretics) to relieve acute decompensated heart failure (ADHF) have had disappointing outcomes. These agents have either caused serious side effects or increased mortality in HF. Volume overload has been associated with increased hospitalizations. The potent vasoconstrictor antidiuretic hormone arginine vasopressin, which modulates volume homeostasis, is inappropriately elevated in HF. Early studies with tolvaptan (selective vasopressin subtype V2 receptor antagonist) demonstrated improvement in congestive symptoms of HF and overall hemodynamic profile but no improvement in long-term outcome.[42]

Publication of the findings in the EVEREST trial, which studied the efficacy of vasopressin antagonism in heart failure, provides evidence for another possible drug in the treatment armamentarium of HF.[43,44] Tolvaptan was tested in 4,133 patients with ADHF with NYHA class III or IV and LVEF of less than 40%. All patients also received standard therapy (ACE inhibitors, angiotensin receptor blockers [ARBs], β-blockers, diuretics, nitrates, and hydralazine). The patients were randomly assigned within 48 hours of hospitalization to 30 mg/day tolvaptan or placebo. The trial was a composite of three distinct analyses. The primary end point for the two identical short-term trials was to assess the change in global clinical status and body weight at day 7 or the day of discharge, whichever came earlier. The primary outcome for the long-term trial was all-cause mortality and cardiovascular (CV) death or HF hospitalizations. The results of the short-term trial showed only modest improvement in the global clinical score compared with placebo. The main clinical benefit was seen in change in body weight. The long-term trial failed to show any statistical significance between the study drug and placebo in achieving the primary end points. Common side effects that resulted in the discontinuation of tolvaptan were dry mouth and thirst. In a small number of patients, hyponatremia was corrected. Because long-term mortality benefits are lacking and the cost of the drug is very high, the use of tolvaptan should be restricted to patients who present with hypovolemic hyponatremia associated with severe HF despite fluid restriction and diuretic use.

CALCIUM SENSITIZERS

Calcium sensitizers represent another class of drugs investigated for the treatment of ADHF. They exert positive inotropic effects by stabilizing the calcium–troponin C complex and facilitating actin-myosin cross-bridging without increasing myocardial consumption of adenosine triphosphate.[45] Levosimendan, the prototype for this drug class, has a dual mechanism of action to increase myocardial contractibility and induce vasodilation. Unlike other inotropic agents, it does not affect the intracellular calcium concentrations and, therefore, has a lower potential for inducing proarrhythmias. The safety and efficacy of levosimendan in ADHF has been evaluated in placebo-controlled trials and in comparative trials with dobutamine. In patients with decompensated HF, levosimendan significantly reduced the incidence of worsening HF and improved hemodynamic indices.[46–48] In addition, mortality was lower in the levosimendan group. These trials, however, were not powered to show a difference in mortality as an end point. A recent trial comparing levosimendan with dobutamine in ADHF, designed to confirm the beneficial effects on morbidity and mortality, did not reduce all-cause mortality, which contrasts with earlier studies.[49] The most common adverse effects associated with levosimendan are headache and hypotension. Currently it is only approved in Europe for ADHF.

INFLAMMATORY CYTOKINES, INTERLEUKINS, TISSUE NECROSIS FACTOR, PROSTACYCLIN, AND NITRIC OXIDE

Vascular endothelial cells release various other proinflammatory cytokines and vasodilator and vasoconstrictor substances, including interleukin cytokines (IL-1β, IL-2, IL-6), tumor necrosis factor (TNF-α), prostacyclin, and nitric oxide (NO; also known as endothelium-derived relaxing factor).[50–52] The exact role of these mediators in the pathogenesis of HF is unclear. Recent studies have shown that patients with HF have elevated levels of the proinflammatory cytokines IL-1β, IL-6, and TNF-α that correlate with the severity of disease.[52–54] Initial enthusiasm for use of the TNF-α receptor antagonist etanercept as a treatment for HF has been abandoned after disappointing results in larger phase 2 and 3 clinical trials.[55] Of even greater concern, at least

47 spontaneous adverse event reports were made to the FDA describing new-onset HF or exacerbation of existing HF with etanercept and infliximab in patients being treated for either Crohn's disease or rheumatoid arthritis.[56]

Other investigators have tried using either NO or prostacyclin (epoprostenol) as therapeutic vasodilators with mixed success.[57–59] A particular concern with prostacyclin was a trend toward increased death rates despite an improved hemodynamic status in treated patients during the Flolan International Randomized Survival Trial (FIRST).[59]

CARDIAC REMODELING

Progression of HF results in a process referred to as *cardiac remodeling,* characterized by changes in the shape and mass of the ventricles in response to tissue injury.[60] The three primary manifestations of cardiac remodeling are chamber dilatation, LV cardiac muscle hypertrophy, and a resulting spherical shape of the LV chamber (Fig. 19-3). Cardiac remodeling, which starts months to years before the appearance of clinical symptoms, contributes to the progression of the disease despite treatment.

CARDIAC DILATATION

Cardiac dilatation results when the ventricles fail to pump an adequate volume of blood with each contraction. This is most evident in systolic dysfunction. If the rate at which blood is delivered to the heart (preload) remains the same, but the rate at which it is pumped to other tissues diminishes, residual blood will begin to accumulate in the ventricles. Thus, end-diastolic volume increases, myocardial fibers are stretched, and the ventricle(s) become dilated. In the healthy heart, the end-diastolic volume is about 110 to 120 mL. With an EF of 60%, the SV is approximately 70 mL, leaving an end-systolic residual volume in the ventricle of 40 to 50 mL. Early in HF, a near normal SV of 70 mL is maintained, although the EF may be low (e.g., 33%). With time, an enlarged heart will become evident on a chest radiograph, and the body cannot completely compensate. Cardiac dilatation is less evident in diastolic dysfunction because normal contractility is maintained and the stiffened left ventricle is resistant to filling and not likely to enlarge (Fig. 19-3).

FRANK–STARLING CURVE

The Frank-Starling ventricular function curve (Fig. 19-4) demonstrates a curvilinear relationship between LV myocardial muscle fiber "stretch" (wall tension) and myocardial work. As stretch increases, the volume of blood ejected with each systolic contraction (SV) increases. In systolic HF, the work capacity for any degree of stretch is diminished. A simple analogy is drawn using a balloon. The greater amount of air blown into a balloon, the

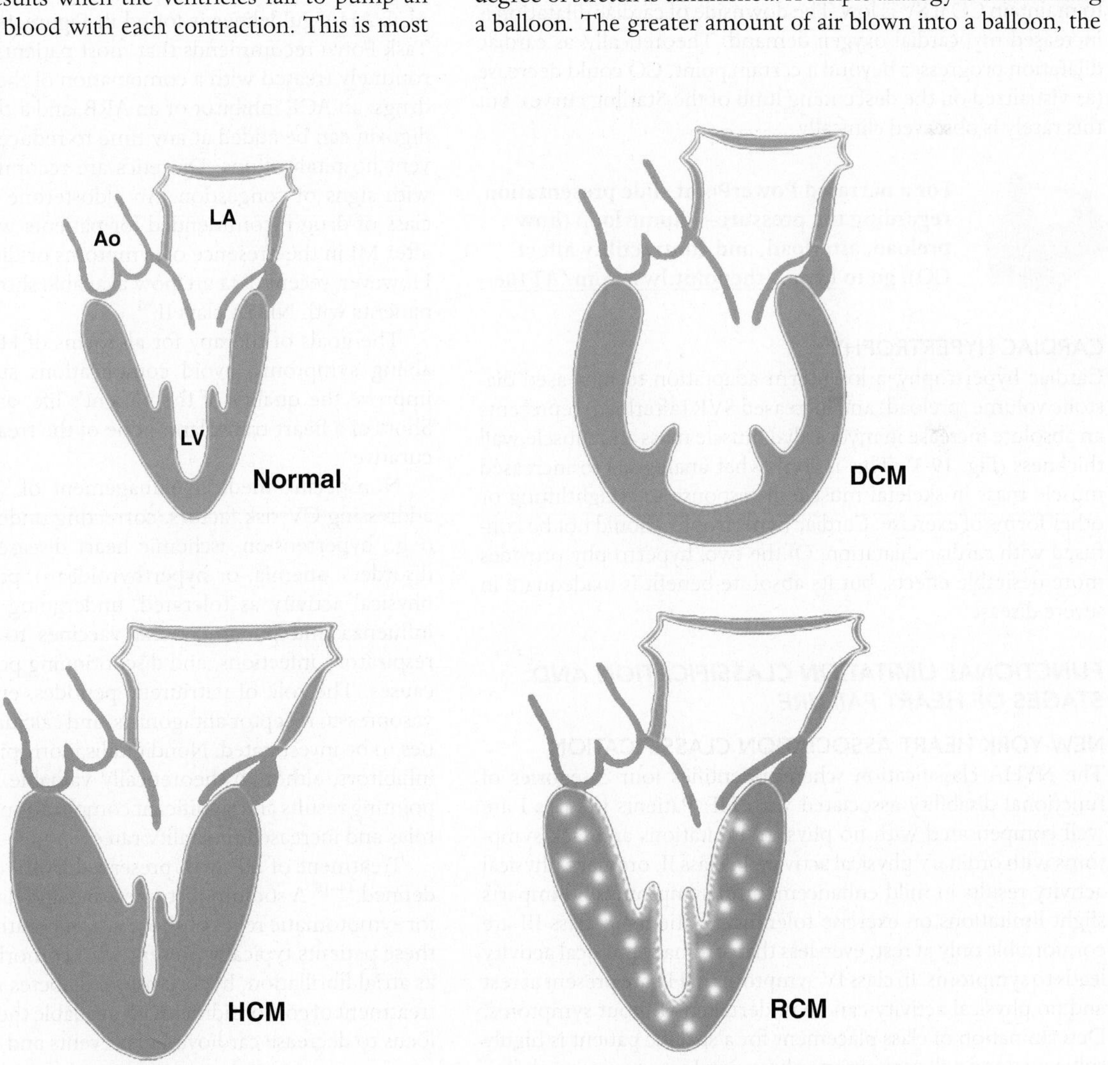

FIGURE 19-3 Cardiac remodeling. Dilated cardiomyopathy (DCM) results in thinning of the of the left ventricular walls and a decrease in systolic function; in hypertrophic cardiomyopathy (HCM), there is a marked thickening of the left ventricular walls leading to diastolic or systolic failure; and in restrictive cardiomyopathy (RCM), the left ventricular walls may be normal, hypertrophic, or slightly dilated, resulting in a decrease in diastolic compliance. Adapted with permission from Topol EJ et al, eds. *Textbook of Cardiovascular Medicine.* 3rd ed. Philadelphia, PA: Lippincott Williams & Wilkins; 2006.

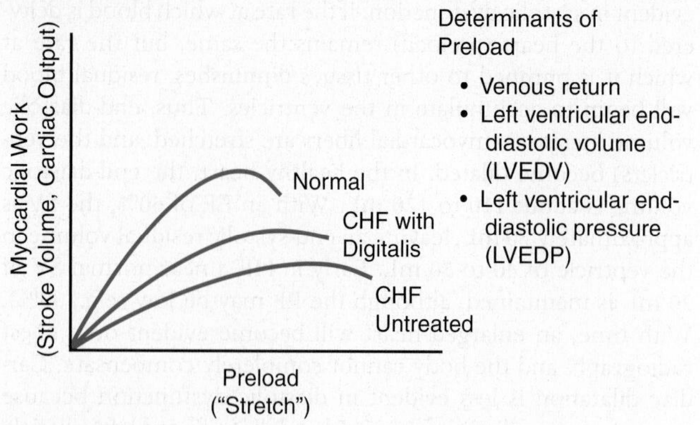

FIGURE 19-4 Representation of Frank-Starling ventricular function curve.

more it stretches and, if released, the farther it flies around a room. As the balloon gets old, it loses its elasticity and thus has less recoil when stretched. Similarly, dilatation of the ventricles initially may serve as an effective compensating mechanism in systolic failure, but it becomes inadequate as the elastic limits of the myocardial muscle fibers are reached. HR may also increase to maintain CO if SV is low. The downside of cardiac dilatation is increased myocardial oxygen demand. Theoretically, as cardiac dilatation progresses beyond a certain point, CO could decrease (as visualized on the descending limb of the Starling curve), but this rarely is observed clinically.

ONLINE CONTENT

For a narrated PowerPoint slide presentation regarding the pressure–volume loop (how preload, afterload, and contractility affect CO), go to http://thepoint.lww.com/AT10e.

CARDIAC HYPERTROPHY

Cardiac hypertrophy, a long-term adaptation to increased diastolic volume (preload) and increased SVR (afterload) represents an absolute increase in myocardial muscle mass and muscle wall thickness (Fig. 19-3). This is somewhat analogous to increased muscle mass in skeletal muscle in response to weightlifting or other forms of exercise. Cardiac hypertrophy should not be confused with cardiac dilatation. Of the two, hypertrophy provides more desirable effects, but its absolute benefit is inadequate in severe disease.

FUNCTIONAL LIMITATION CLASSIFICATION AND STAGES OF HEART FAILURE

NEW YORK HEART ASSOCIATION CLASSIFICATION

The NYHA classification scheme identifies four categories of functional disability associated with HF. Patients in class I are well compensated with no physical limitations and lack symptoms with ordinary physical activity. In class II, ordinary physical activity results in mild enhancement of symptoms and imparts slight limitations on exercise tolerance. Patients in class III are comfortable only at rest; even less than ordinary physical activity leads to symptoms. In class IV, symptoms of HF are present at rest and no physical activity can be undertaken without symptoms. Determination of class placement for a specific patient is highly subjective and will vary among observers. In some cases, subdivisions such as class III_A or III_B may be used to further individualize grading of severity.

A shortcoming of the NYHA classification scheme is that it does not include asymptomatic individuals who are at high risk for developing HF and who may benefit from pre-emptive lifestyle changes and drug therapy. In 2001 the ACC/AHA Practice Guidelines introduced a new staging algorithm that can be used in conjunction with the NYHA classifications.[4] Patients in stage A have hypertension, CAD, diabetes mellitus, or other conditions that, if left untreated, can result in the development of overt HF. HF symptoms or identifiable abnormalities of the myocardium or heart valves are absent in stage A. Patients in stage B remain asymptomatic but have structural defects within the heart (e.g., LV hypertrophy, dilatation, or valvular disease) that indicate the existence of impending HF. Patients in stage C exhibit varying degrees of HF symptoms corresponding to NYHA classes I through III along with structural changes in the heart consistent with systolic or diastolic HF. Stage D in the ACA/AHA scheme roughly correlates to NYHA class IV. Patients in this latter category are frequently hospitalized, dependent on IV therapy, and could be considered to have end-stage disease. Figure 19-1 summarizes these two classification schemes and how they overlap.

Overview of Treatment Principles

The 2005 and updated 2009 ACC/AHA Task Force Practice Guidelines serve as the primary basis for recommendations within this chapter.[1,21] A clinical algorithm reprinted from the ACC/AHA guidelines is found in Figure 19-5.[1] The ACC/AHA Task Force recommends that most patients with HF should be routinely treated with a combination of the following classes of drugs: an ACE inhibitor or an ARB, and a β-adrenergic blocker; digoxin can be added at any time to reduce symptoms and prevent hospitalizations. Diuretics are recommended for patients with signs of congestion. An aldosterone antagonist is a fifth class of drug recommended for patients with advanced HF or after MI in the presence of symptoms or diabetes and a low EF. However, recent data are now available showing a benefit in HF patients with NHYA class II.[61]

The goals of therapy for all forms of HF are to abolish disabling symptoms, avoid complications such as arrhythmias, improve the quality of the patient's life, and prolong survival. Short of a heart transplant, none of the treatment measures are curative.

Nonspecific medical management of systolic HF includes addressing CV risk factors, correcting underlying disease states (e.g., hypertension, ischemic heart disease, arrhythmias, lipid disorders, anemia, or hyperthyroidism), performing moderate physical activity as tolerated, undergoing immunization with influenza and pneumococcal vaccines to reduce the risk of respiratory infections, and discontinuing possible drug-induced causes. The role of natriuretic peptides, endothelin inhibitors, vasopressin receptor antagonists, and calcium sensitizers continues to be investigated. Nondigitalis inotropic agents and TNF-α inhibitors, although theoretically valuable, have yielded disappointing results and significant complications, including arrhythmias and increased mortality rates.

Treatment of HF with preserved LVEF (HFPEF) is less well defined.[14–18] A sodium-restricted diet and diuretics are indicated for symptomatic relief of shortness of breath or edema. Because these patients typically present with comorbid conditions (such as atrial fibrillation, hypertension, diabetes mellitus, and CAD), treatment of comorbidities with available therapies should be the focus to decrease cardiovascular events and improve survival.

PHYSICAL ACTIVITY

Patients should be encouraged to maximize their activities of daily life and exercise to maintain physical conditioning. Treatment goals in HF should not only include prolonging life but also improving the quality of life. The results of The Effects of

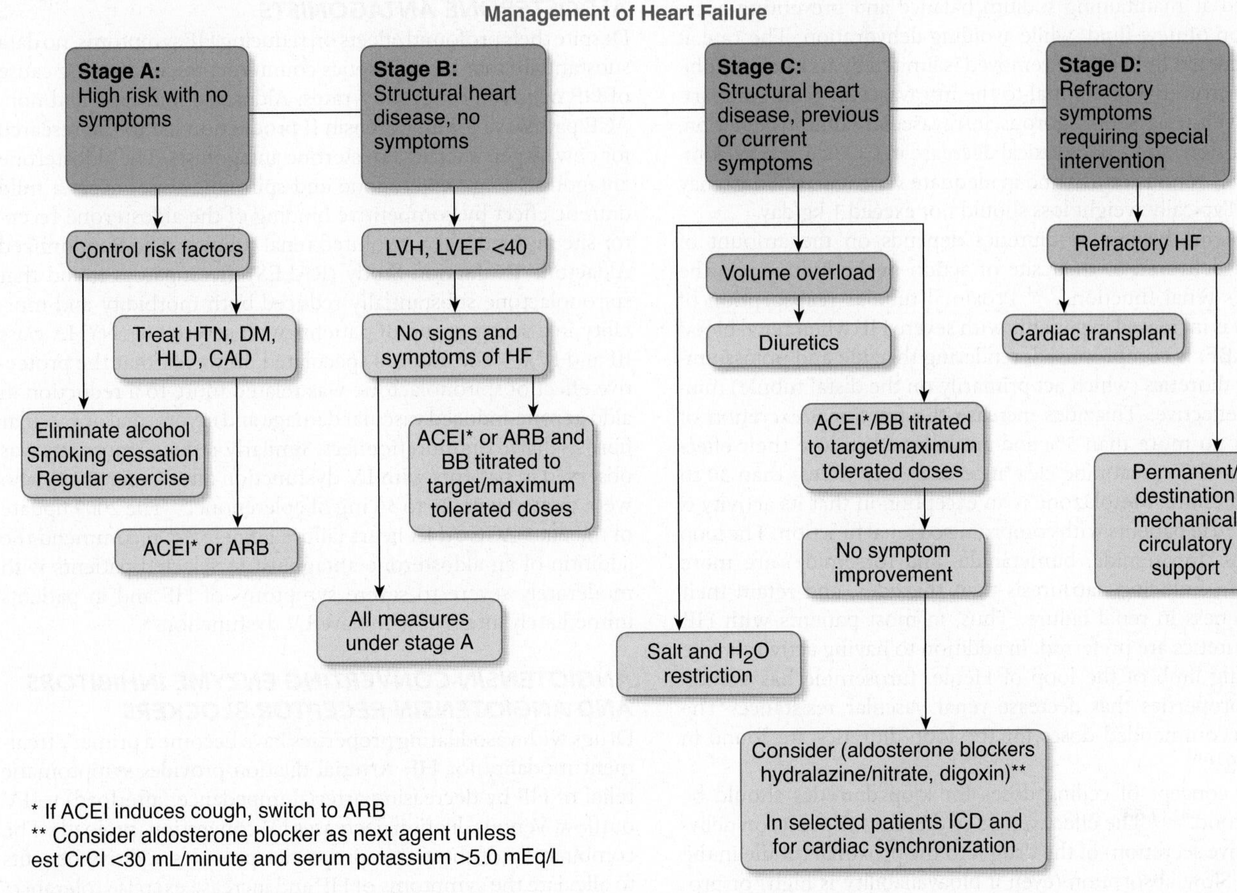

FIGURE 19-5 Stages in the development of heart failure and recommended therapy by stage. ACEI, angiotensin-converting enzyme inhibitors; ARB, angiotensin receptor blockers; BB, β-blockers; CAD, coronary artery disease; CrCl, creatinine clearance; DM, diabetes mellitus; EF, ejection fraction; HLD, hyperlipidemia; HTN, hypertension; ICD, implantable cardioverter-defibrillator; LVH, left ventricular hypertrophy.

Exercise Training on Health Status in Patients with Chronic Heart Failure (HF-ACTION)[62] trial showed that a highly structured exercise program in HF patients did not reduce all-cause mortality or all-cause hospitalization when compared with patients who were getting the usual care in which exercise was simply encouraged. However, according to the HF-ACTION substudy, the structured exercise training program improved the overall Kansas City Cardiomyopathy Questionnaire (KCCQ) score (health status was assessed using the KCCQ, a test that includes questions on physical limitations, symptoms, quality of life, and social limitations). The improvement occurred early on and was sustained for 3 years. The 2009 update of the 2005 ACC/AHA heart failure guidelines[1] recommends exercise training as an adjunctive therapy to improve clinical status in ambulatory patients with current or prior symptoms of HF and reduced EF. However, during acute exacerbations, bed rest and restricted physical activity decrease the metabolic demands of the failing heart and minimize gravitational forces contributing to the formation of edema. Renal perfusion is increased in the prone position, resulting in diuresis and eventual mobilization of edema fluid.

SODIUM-RESTRICTED DIET

Dietary indiscretion (i.e., high salt intake) is often cited as the cause of HF exacerbation and hospital admission. Consequently, the guidelines recommend that HF patients maintain a low-sodium diet, but acknowledge that the recommendation is based on consensus only.[1] Reduction of dietary salt is prudent in patients with hypertension or evidence of fluid retention. The effect of salt restriction in preventing HF in normotensive or asymptomatic patients has not been studied. In patients with clinically evident HF, moderate sodium restriction (<3 g/day sodium) may allow patients to use lower doses of diuretics by decreasing blood volume and offsetting abnormal retention of sodium by the kidneys. If the kidney's ability to excrete sodium is not severely compromised, it is possible to approach normal balance by restricting sodium intake to match excretion. Although less than 1 g of sodium chloride (NaCl) is required to meet physiologic needs, the average US diet contains 10 g. Dietary sodium can be reduced to 2 to 4 g of NaCl by eliminating cooking salt. This diet is more palatable and leads to better adherence than a severely salt-restricted diet.

DIURETICS

Only those points salient to the treatment of HF are included in this chapter. Diuretic use also is discussed in Chapter 14, Essential Hypertension. (See Chapter 10, Fluid and Electrolyte Disorders, for a thorough review of kidney physiology and the classification, mechanism of action, and side effects of diuretics.)

Diuretics are indicated in HF patients with congestion (pulmonary and peripheral edema) or cardiac dilatation (enlarged heart on chest radiograph). They produce symptomatic relief more rapidly than other drugs for HF. Because activation of the RAAS and sympathetic nervous system contributes to the progression of HF, diuretics should be combined with an ACE inhibitor and a β-blocker unless contraindications exist.[4,21]

Initially, the goal of diuretic therapy is symptomatic relief of HF by decreasing excess volume without causing intravascular volume depletion. Once excess volume is removed, therapy is aimed at maintaining sodium balance and preventing accumulation of new fluid, while avoiding dehydration. The rate at which edema fluid can be removed is limited by its rate of mobilization from the interstitial to the intravascular fluid compartment. If diuresis is too vigorous, intravascular volume depletion, hypotension, and a paradoxical decrease in CO (caused by compromised venous return and inadequate ventricular filling) may result. Typically weight loss should not exceed 1 kg/day.

The effectiveness of diuretics depends on the amount of sodium delivered to their site of action in the kidney and the patient's renal function.[63,64] Proximal tubular reabsorption of sodium is increased in patients with severe HF when renal blood flow (RBF) is compromised, rendering thiazide and potassium-sparing diuretics (which act primarily on the distal tubule) minimally effective. Thiazides increase the fractional excretion of sodium no more than 5% and are believed to lose their effectiveness when creatinine clearance decreases to less than 30 to 40 mL/minute. Metolazone is an exception in that its activity is preserved in patients with compromised renal function. The loop diuretics (furosemide, bumetanide, and torsemide) are more potent in inducing natriuresis than thiazides, and retain their effectiveness in renal failure. Thus, in most patients with HF, loop diuretics are preferred. In addition to having activity in the ascending limb of the loop of Henle, furosemide has vasodilating properties that decrease renal vascular resistance. The usual recommended doses for the loop diuretics are found in Table 19-3.[63]

The concept of ceiling doses for loop diuretics should be understood.[63,64] The effectiveness of diuretics depends on delivery (active secretion) of the drug into the proximal tubule in the kidney. Slow absorption (even if bioavailability is high) or protein binding impairs tubular delivery and compromises diuretic response. Once the drug is in the tubule and the threshold for diuresis is met, further drug delivery produces no greater diuresis. Increasing single doses beyond the ceiling dose produces no additional diuretic response. As an alternative, improved diuresis may be obtained by giving the drug more frequently.

As discussed later in this chapter, combinations of diuretics with different mechanisms (e.g., a loop diuretic and metolazone) are used in patients whose conditions are refractory to high-dose loop diuretics.[63,64] Diuretics are indicated in HFPEF, but pose a difficult challenge. This form of HF is highly volume dependent, becoming significantly worse in states of fluid overload, but responding with a rapid reduction in filling pressures and resolution of dyspnea after acute diuresis. Conversely, chronic diuresis eventually reduces the end-diastolic volume, resulting in a significant reduction of CO. Thus, an elevated filling pressure may be controlled at the expense of a greatly reduced SV such that the symptoms of dyspnea may be traded for those of fatigue and loss of exercise tolerance.[65]

ALDOSTERONE ANTAGONISTS

Despite their profound effects on reducing HF symptoms, no data substantiate that loop diuretics counteract the underlying cause of HF or modify mortality rates. Aldosterone escape and non-ACE pathways for angiotensin II production led to the research for new targets such as aldosterone antagonists. The aldosterone antagonists (e.g., eplerenone and spironolactone) exert a mild diuretic effect by competitive binding of the aldosterone receptor site in the distal convoluted renal tubules. The Randomized Aldactone Evaluation Study (RALES) investigators found that spironolactone substantially reduced both morbidity and mortality in a select group of patients with severe HF (NYHA class III and IV).[66] The authors speculated, however, that the protective effect of spironolactone was related more to a reduction in aldosterone-induced vascular damage and myocardial or vascular fibrosis than to its diuretic effect. Similarly, reduced mortality was observed in patients with LV dysfunction after a recent MI who were treated with 25 to 50 mg of eplerenone.[67] The 2009 update of the 2005 ACC/AHA heart failure guidelines[1] recommend the addition of an aldosterone antagonist in selected patients with moderately severe to severe symptoms of HF and in patients immediately after MI who have LV dysfunction.[67]

ANGIOTENSIN-CONVERTING ENZYME INHIBITORS AND ANGIOTENSIN RECEPTOR BLOCKERS

Drugs with vasodilating properties have become a primary treatment modality for HF. Arterial dilation provides symptomatic relief of HF by decreasing arterial impedance (afterload) to LV outflow. Venous dilation decreases LV congestion (preload). The combination of these two properties provides additive benefits to alleviate the symptoms of HF and increase exercise tolerance. The first vasodilator drugs to be studied were hydralazine (essentially a pure arterial dilator) and nitrates (predominately venous dilators). By combining these two drugs, significant reductions in HF symptoms can be achieved along with a modest reduction in mortality rates. With the advent of ACE inhibitors, the use of hydralazine and nitrates has been relegated to a secondary role.

Angiotensin-converting enzyme inhibitors possess both afterload- and preload-reducing properties (by blocking angiotensin II–mediated vasoconstriction) and volume-reducing potential (by inhibiting activation of aldosterone). They not only produce similar hemodynamic effects to the hydralazine–nitrate combination as a single agent but also favorably modify cardiac remodeling independent of vasodilation and have a more tolerable side effect profile. These advantages led to the recommendations that ACE inhibitors are the drugs of choice for initial therapy, even in patients with relatively mild LV systolic dysfunction.[1,2]

The ACC/AHA guidelines state that ACE inhibitors should be prescribed to all patients with HF caused by left ventricular

TABLE 19-3
Loop Diuretic Dosing[1]

	Furosemide	Bumetanide	Torsemide
IV loading doses	40 mg	1 mg	20 mg
Maximum total daily dose	600 mg	10 mg	200 mg
Ceiling dose			
Normal renal function	80–160 mg (PO/IV)	1–2 mg (PO/IV)	20–40 mg (PO/IV)
Cl_{cr}: 20–50 mL/min	160 mg (PO/IV)	2 mg (PO/IV)	40 mg (PO/IV)
Cl_{Cr}: <20 mL/min	200 mg (IV), 400 mg (PO)	8–10 mg (PO/IV)	100 mg (PO/IV)
Bioavailability	10%–100%	80%–90%	80%–100%
Duration of action	6–8 hours	4–6 hours	12–16 hours

Cl_{Cr}, creatinine clearance; IV, intravenous; PO, oral.

TABLE 19-4
ACE Inhibitor Dosing in Systolic Dysfunction[a]

Drug	Available Dosage Form	Initial Dose[b]	Maximal Dose
Captopril[c]	12.5, 25, 50, 100 mg tablets	6.25–12.5 mg TID	100 mg TID
Enalapril[d]	2.5, 5, 10, 20 mg tablets	2.5–5 mg every day	20 mg BID
Fosinopril	10, 20, 40 mg tablets	5–10 mg every day	40 mg every day
Lisinopril	2.5, 5, 10, 20, 40 mg tablets	2.5–5 mg every day	40 mg every day
Quinapril[d]	5, 10, 20, 40 mg tablets	5–10 mg every day	20 mg BID
Perindopril	2, 4, 8 mg tablets	2 mg every day	16 mg every day
Ramipril[d]	1.25, 2.5, 5, 10 mg capsules	1.25–2.5 mg every day	10 mg BID
Trandolapril	1, 2, 4 mg tablets	1 mg every day	8 mg every day

[a]Benazepril, cilazapril, moexipril, peridnopril, ramipril, trandolapril not labeled for use in heart failure.
[b]Start with lowest dose to avoid bradycardia, hypotension, or renal dysfunction. All but captopril given every day in the morning at starting doses. Increase dose slowly at 2- to 4-week intervals to assess full effect and tolerance.
[c]Captopril is short acting. Start with a 6.25- or 12.5-mg test dose, then 6.25 to 12.5 mg TID.
[d]Enalapril, quinapril, ramipril could possibly be given every day instead of BID based on half-life.
ACE, angiotensin-converting enzyme; BID, twice a day; TID, three times a day.

systolic dysfunction (LVSD) unless they have a contradiction to their use or have been shown to be unable to tolerate treatment with these drugs. In general, ACE inhibitors are used together with β-blockers. ACE inhibitors should be initiated at low doses, followed by increments in dose if lower doses have been well tolerated. Fluid retention can blunt the therapeutic effects, and fluid depletion can potentiate the adverse effects of ACE inhibitors. Clinicians should attempt to use doses that have been shown to reduce CV events in clinical trials, but they should not delay the initiation of β-blockers in patients because of a failure to reach target ACE inhibitor doses.[1]

The pharmacologic actions of all the ACE inhibitors are essentially identical, but some of them have not been extensively studied or received FDA approval for use in HF (Table19-4). Their value in diastolic failure or HFPEF still is being investigated. A related class of drugs is the ARBs.[68,69] ARBs offer theoretic advantages compared with ACE inhibitors by being more specific for angiotensin II blockade (preferentially bind to AT_1 receptors) and having a lower risk of drug-induced cough. On the other hand, indirect block of bradykinin, NE, or prostaglandins by some or all of the ACE inhibitors may offer an advantage compared with receptor inhibitors.

After the publication of the Candesartan in the Treatment of Heart Failure—Assessment of Reduction in Mortality and Morbidity (CHARM) trial, ARBs were shown to be as effective as ACE inhibitors in reducing morbidity and mortality in patients with HF. According to the 2005 ACC/AHA guidelines, ARBs can be used as an alternative to ACE inhibitors in patients who are intolerant of ACE inhibitors (e.g., angioedema or intractable cough). Also, ARBs might be considered as an add-on therapy in patients who continue to be symptomatic despite optimal conventional therapy, although the effectiveness of this approach is not well established. Currently, only candesartan and valsartan have FDA-approved labeling for the treatment of HF.

β-ADRENERGIC BLOCKING AGENTS

Until the mid-1990s, β-blockers were contraindicated in patients with systolic HF. This was based on the belief that sympathomimetic agonists and other positive inotropic drugs were the logical choices to counteract the hemodynamic defects of systolic failure and that negative inotropic drugs would exacerbate HF. A better understanding of the pathophysiology of HF led to a rethinking of this logic.[25–31] In combination with ACE inhibitors, β-blockers are considered first-line agents in patients with HF and LVSD. The 2005 and 2009 update ACC/AHA guidelines state that β-blockers should be prescribed to all patients with stable systolic HF unless they have a contraindication to their use or are unable to tolerate the treatment. Intolerance or resistance to other HF therapies should not preclude nor delay the initiation of β-blocker use in patients with HF.[1] Although some patients can initially have a temporary worsening of symptoms, continued use results in improved quality of life, fewer hospitalizations, and most importantly, a reduction in mortality by approximately 34% when added to other HF therapies that prolong life. Extended-release metoprolol succinate, carvedilol, and bisoprolol are FDA approved for use in HF. Metoprolol and bisoprolol are both partially selective β_1-blockers, and carvedilol is a mixed α_1- and nonselective β-blocking agent.

DIGITALIS GLYCOSIDES (DIGOXIN)

Digoxin has several pharmacologic actions on the heart. It binds to and inhibits sodium-potassium (Na^+/K^+) adenosine triphosphatase (ATPase) in cardiac cells, decreasing outward transport of sodium and increasing intracellular concentrations of calcium within the cells. Calcium binding to the sarcoplasmic reticulum causes an increase in the contractile state of the heart.

At one time, the primary benefit of digoxin in systolic HF was assumed to be an increase in the force of contraction (positive inotropic effect) of the failing heart to increase EF and CO. We now know that digoxin has beneficial neurohumoral and autonomic effects caused by reducing sympathetic tone and stimulating parasympathetic (vagal) responses at serum concentrations below those associated with positive inotropism.[1,70,71] Inhibition of Na^+/K^+ ATPase in vagal afferent fibers sensitizes cardiac baroreceptors, resulting in reduced sympathetic outflow from the CNS. Similarly, inhibition of Na^+/K^+ ATPase in renal cells reduces renal tubular reabsorption of sodium and indirectly suppresses renin secretion. This has led to the suggestion that the positive benefits of digoxin can be obtained with a lower risk of side effects by using small doses.[1] The optimal serum digoxin concentration for the treatment of systolic HF is 0.5 to 1 ng/mL.

In addition to effects on contractility, digoxin decreases the conduction velocity and prolongs the refractory period of the atrioventricular (AV) node. This AV node–blocking effect prolongs the PR interval and is the basis for use of digoxin in slowing the ventricular response rate in patients with AF and other supraventricular arrhythmias (see Chapter 20, Cardiac Arrhythmias).

Several studies have confirmed a clinical benefit for digoxin in reducing HF symptoms, independent of rhythm status, but there are no data that demonstrate a beneficial effect on survival. As a result, the guidelines state that digoxin is unlikely to benefit patients with stage A or stage B HF. In these patients, digoxin can be used for symptom management, only if they are treated with drug therapy shown to prolong survival (ACE inhibitors and β-blockers) or have not responded adequately to appropriate therapy. In symptomatic patients with stage C or stage D HF, digoxin can be beneficial in reducing HF-related hospitalizations.[1] Monotherapy with digoxin or in combination with only a diuretic is no longer recommended. Digoxin can also be considered in patients with HF who also have atrial fibrillation (AF), although β-blockers may be more effective than digoxin in controlling the ventricular response, especially during exercise. Further discussions of the controversies surrounding digoxin use and detailed dosing guidelines are found in the case studies.

OTHER VASODILATING DRUGS: HYDRALAZINE AND NITRATES

Although ACE inhibitors have become the vasodilator drug of choice, the first vasodilators used in patients with HF were hydralazine and nitrates. Hydralazine is a potent arterial dilating agent that provides symptomatic relief of HF by decreasing arterial impedance (afterload) to LV outflow. Nitrates (e.g., nitroglycerin [NTG], isosorbide dinitrate, isosorbide mononitrate) have venous dilating properties that decrease LV congestion (preload). Used in combination, these two agents have additive benefits in alleviating the symptoms of HF and increasing exercise tolerance. Importantly, the hydralazine–isosorbide dinitrate combination was the first treatment regimen to show improved survival in severe HF compared with placebo (while patients continued their previous diuretic or digitalis therapy). In the post hoc analysis of the hydralazine–isosorbide dinitrate combination trial, there appeared to be greater efficacy in the cohort of African American patients. The African American Heart Failure Trial (AHeFT)[72] confirms that the addition of hydralazine combined with isosorbide dinitrate to standard HF therapy with an ACE inhibitor or a β-blocker has added benefits of improving survival and HF hospitalizations. Based on the results of AHeFT, the FDA approved the combination product of hydralazine and isosorbide dinitrate (BiDil) for the treatment of HF as an adjunct to standard HF therapy in African American patients. The combination of hydralazine and a nitrate is reasonable in patients with current or prior HF symptoms and reduced LVEF who cannot tolerate ACE inhibitors or ARBs. The combination of hydralazine plus a nitrate is recommended to improve outcomes for patients self-described as African American with moderate to severe symptoms on optimal therapy with ACE inhibitors, β-blockers, and diuretics.[1] Intravenous NTG and nitroprusside (a mixed arterial and venous dilator) are also used in hospitalized patients with acute HF exacerbations. The role of these vasodilators in HFPEF is not well studied.

OTHER INOTROPIC AGENTS

Dopamine and dobutamine, both of which are sympathomimetics, are commonly used in acutely decompensated HF, but their use is limited by the need for IV administration (see Chapter 22, Shock, for a more detailed discussion of these drugs). Milrinone and other nonsympathomimetic inotropic agents (phosphodiesterase inhibitors) are associated with an increased incidence of mortality but are frequently used short-term. Both dobutamine and milrinone are used in some cases chronically in stage D patients.

Despite differing mechanisms of action responsible for their cardiac stimulatory effect (primarily sympathomimetics or phosphodiesterase inhibitors), and whether or not the drug also has vasodilating properties, initial positive hemodynamic effects during the first few weeks to months of therapy with these drugs are followed by increased mortality with continued therapy when compared with placebo. The explanation for these findings is related to an overall enhancement of sympathetic tone, overstimulation of an already fatigued heart, and proarrhythmic effects. All inotropic drugs are contraindicated in HFPEF.

CALCIUM-CHANNEL BLOCKERS

Amlodipine, felodipine, isradipine, nifedipine, and nicardipine are examples of dihydropyridine calcium antagonists with arterial vasodilating effects. Compared with the nondihydropyridine calcium-channel blockers (verapamil and diltiazem), they have minimal negative inotropic properties. Only amlodipine[73] and felodipine[74] have been documented to be safe in HF (i.e., do not make HF worse), but only a small subset of patients with nonischemic dilated cardiomyopathy actually had a beneficial effect of improved survival with amlodipine.[73] Until more data are available, calcium-channel blockers other than amlodipine and felodipine are contraindicated in patients with systolic dysfunction. On the other hand, verapamil and diltiazem are safe to use in HFPEF and may improve symptoms by reducing HR and allowing more time to fill the ventricle.

IMPLANTABLE CARDIOVERTER-DEFIBRILLATOR

Ventricular arrhythmias are common in patients with HF and cardiomyopathy (enlarged heart), ranging from asymptomatic ventricular premature beats to sustained ventricular tachycardia or ventricular fibrillation, which can lead to sudden cardiac death (SCD). SCD is highest in patients with severe HF symptoms, or stage D HF.[1] Patients with previous cardiac arrest or documented sustained ventricular arrhythmias have a higher risk of future events. In these patients, implantable cardioverter-defibrillator (ICD) implantation can reduce overall mortality. ICD implantation is indicated for secondary prevention of SCD in HF patients who have good clinical function and prognosis and low EF and experience syncope of unknown origin, as well as in a small subset of HF patients who are awaiting a planned cardiac transplant.[1] The ACC/AHA guidelines also recommend ICD for primary prevention of SCD in patients with nonischemic dilated cardiomyopathy or ischemic heart disease at least 40 days after MI, EF of 35% or less despite optimal drug therapy, with mild to moderate symptoms of HF and in whom survival with good functional capacity is otherwise anticipated to extend beyond 1 year (see Case 19-5, Question 4, for detailed discussion).

CARDIAC RESYNCHRONIZATION

Cardiac resynchronization therapy (CRT) is a therapeutic approach for treating patients with ventricular dyssynchrony (defined as a QRS duration of at least 120 milliseconds). Selected HF patients benefit from simultaneous pacing of both ventricles (biventricular pacing), or of one ventricle in patients with bundle branch block. The rationale for using CRT is that dyssynchrony causes ventricular remodeling and worsens HF, resulting in poor outcomes. CRT can be used alone or with an ICD device. Several clinical trials with CRT or CRT-D[75–78] (cardiac resynchronization defibrillator therapy) have demonstrated improvements in HF functional status, survival, and reduction in hospitalizations. The functional benefits were assessed by increased 6-minute walk distance, increased peak oxygen consumption, decreased hospitalizations for decompensated HF, and overall improvement in NYHA functional class. In addition, these improvements were accompanied by reverse remodeling. Current guidelines[1] support the use of CRT in patients with advanced HF (usually NYHA class III or IV), LVEF of 35% or less, and QRS interval of 120 milliseconds or longer with or without ICD. In 2010, the FDA expanded the approved indication for cardiac CRT-D to include patients with NYHA class II or ischemic class I HF, with an EF of less than 30% and a QRS duration of longer than 130 milliseconds, and left bundle branch block. These new indications were based on the results of the landmark trial,[76] which showed CRT-D is associated with a significant reduction in HF events among patients with mild HF symptoms when compared with ICD alone. These observations will result in the expansion of existing guideline recommendations for the use of CRT (see Case 19-6, Questions 1 and 2).

LEFT VENTRICULAR ASSIST DEVICES

A left ventricular assist device (LVAD) is a battery-operated, mechanical pump that is surgically implanted to maintain the pumping ability of the heart. Clinical trials using LVADs have shown improvement in survival and quality of life. For patients with end-stage heart failure, LVADs are used as a bridge to transplant or destination therapy, which is permanent device implantation for patients who are not candidates for a transplant.

The landmark trial REMATCH[79] (Randomized Evaluation of Mechanical Assistance for the Treatment of Congestive Heart Failure) found that end-stage HF patients who received an LVAD (HeartMate XVE) had a 52.1% chance of surviving 1 year, compared with a 24.7% survival rate for patients who received optimal medical therapy. At 2 years, the survival was 23% for the LVAD patients versus 8% for those receiving medical therapies. However, these survival rates were much lower than those seen with transplantation. Nonetheless, in 2003, the HeartMate XVE was approved for use as destination therapy. Advances in technology led to the introduction of the second-generation devices, notably HeartMate II, which was approved as a bridge to transplant in 2008.[80] In January of 2010 the HeartMate II (continuous flow), a smaller and inaudible device, was approved for destination therapy. In a head-to-head comparison with the first-generation HeartMate I device (pulsatile flow), 1- and 2-year survival rates were 68% and 58% with HeartMate II versus 55% and 24% with HeartMate XVE.[81] Adverse events were less frequent with the continuous-flow device. In addition, patients reported significant improvements in their quality of life. Recently, a new novel pump called HeartWare left ventricular assist device (HVAD) was tested in patients awaiting cardiac transplantation with refractory and advanced HF. The advantage of this device is that it is small in size and can be directly implanted into the pericardial sac. The multicenter nonrandomized ADVANCE trial[82] (Evaluation of the HVAD for the Treatment of Advanced Heart Failure) enrolled 140 patients who received HVAD and were compared with 499 patients who received a commercially available LVAD. The primary end points were survival and success rates between HVAD and control patients at 180 and 360 days after implantation. The study also evaluated the HVAD patient's functional capacity, quality of life, and adverse effects. At 180 days the survival was 92.0% for the HVAD group and 90.1% for the control group ($p < 0.001$). There was less bleeding and fewer infections reported with HVAD; however, the incidence of stroke was higher with HVAD. New clinical trials are being designed and conducted to evaluate adverse events between HVAD and HeartMate II. Until further improvements are implemented and demonstrated, cardiac transplantation remains the gold standard for the treatment of end-stage HF.

PATIENT EVALUATION

Signs and Symptoms

CASE 19-1

QUESTION 1: A.J., a 58-year-old man, is admitted with a chief complaint of increasing shortness of breath (SOB) and an 8-kg weight gain. Two weeks before admission, he noted the onset of dyspnea on exertion (DOE) after one flight of stairs, orthopnea, and ankle edema. Since then, his symptoms have worsened. He has also noted episodic bouts of paroxysmal nocturnal dyspnea (PND), and he has been able to sleep only in a sitting position. A.J. reports a productive cough, nocturia (two to three times a night), and edema.

A.J.'s other medical problems include a long history of heartburn, a 10-year history of osteoarthritis, depression, and hypertension, which has been poorly controlled. A strong family history of diabetes mellitus is also present.

Physical examination reveals dyspnea, cyanosis, and tachycardia. A.J. has the following vital signs: BP, 160/100 mm Hg; pulse, 90 beats/minute; and respiratory rate, 28 breaths/minute. He is 5 feet 11 inches tall and weighs 78 kg. His neck veins are distended. On cardiac examination, an S_3 gallop is heard; the point of maximal impulse is at the sixth intercostal space, 12 cm from the midsternal line. His liver is enlarged and tender to palpation, and a positive hepatojugular reflux is observed. He is noted to have 3+ pitting edema of the extremities and sacral edema. Chest examination reveals inspiratory rales and rhonchi bilaterally.

The medication history reveals the following current medications: hydrochlorothiazide (HCTZ) 25 mg every day, ibuprofen 600 mg four times a day (QID), ranitidine 150 mg every night at bedtime, and citalopram 20 mg every day. He has no allergies and no dietary restrictions.

Admitting laboratory values include the following:

Hematocrit, 41.1%
White blood cell count, 5,300/μL
Sodium (Na), 132 mEq/L
Potassium (K), 3.2 mEq/L
Chloride (Cl), 100 mEq/L
Bicarbonate, 30 mEq/L
Magnesium, 1.5 mEq/L
Fasting blood sugar, 100 mg/dL
Uric acid, 8 mg/dL
Blood urea nitrogen (BUN), 40 mg/dL
Serum creatinine (SCr), 0.8 mg/dL
Alkaline phosphatase, 44 units/L
Aspartate aminotransferase, 30 units/L
BNP, 364 pg/mL (normal <200 pg/mL)
Thyroid-stimulating hormone, 2.0 microunits/mL

The chest radiograph shows bilateral pleural effusions and cardiomegaly. What signs, symptoms, and laboratory abnormalities of HF does A.J. exhibit? Relate these clinical findings to the pathogenesis of the disease and to left-sided or right-sided HF.

Left-sided ventricular dysfunction primarily causes pulmonary symptoms because of a backing-up of fluid into the lungs, whereas right-sided ventricular dysfunction causes mostly signs of systemic venous congestion. Although LV failure usually develops first, most patients, including A.J., present with signs of biventricular failure. The signs and symptoms of both left-sided and right-sided ventricular dysfunction are summarized in Table 19-5.

LEFT-SIDED HEART FAILURE (LEFT VENTRICULAR DYSFUNCTION)

Weakness, fatigue, and cyanosis result from decreased CO and compromised tissue perfusion. If the left ventricle is not emptied completely, blood backs up into the pulmonary circulation. SOB, dyspnea (labored or uncomfortable breathing) on exertion, a productive cough, rales (crackles in the lung during auscultation), pleural effusions on chest radiograph, and cyanosis all result from

TABLE 19-5
Signs and Symptoms of Heart Failure

	Left Ventricular Failure	Right Ventricular Failure[a]
Subjective	DOE	
	SOB	
	Orthopnea (two to three pillows)	
	PND, cough	
	Weakness, fatigue, confusion	Peripheral edema
	Weakness, fatigue	
Objective	LVH	Weight gain (fluid retention)
	↓BP	
	EF <40%[b]	Neck vein distension
	Rales, S_3 gallop rhythm	Hepatomegaly
	Reflex tachycardia	Hepatojugular reflux
	↑BUN (poor renal perfusion)	

[a]Isolated right-sided failure occurs with long-standing pulmonary disease (cor pulmonale) or after pulmonary hypertension.
[b]Ejection fraction normal in patients with diastolic dysfunction.
BP, blood pressure; BUN, blood urea nitrogen; DOE, dyspnea on exertion; EF, ejection fraction; LVH, left ventricular hypertrophy; PND, paroxysmal nocturnal dyspnea; SOB, shortness of breath.

pulmonary congestion. Pulmonary symptoms are aggravated in the reclining position, which minimizes the gravitational effects on fluid in the extremities and improves venous return to the heart and lungs. SOB in the supine position (orthopnea) is quantified by the number of pillows the patient must lie on to sleep comfortably. A.J., for example, could sleep only sitting upright. PND, sometimes called cardiac asthma, is characterized by SOB that awakens the patient from sleep and is alleviated by an upright position.

Cardiac dilatation is caused by an increased end-diastolic volume (see Pathogenesis section) and is observed on chest radiography as an enlarged heart silhouette. The point of maximal impulse corresponds to the apex of the left ventricle and is visualized as an external pulsation on the left side of the chest. It is displaced laterally and downward from its normal location at the fifth intercostal space, less than 10 cm from the midsternal line. An S_3 gallop rhythm denotes a third heart sound often heard in close proximity to the second heart sound (closing of the aortic and pulmonary valves) in HF. Rapid filling of the ventricles causes the S_3 sound and, in an adult, usually indicates decreased ventricular compliance. In patients with mitral valve regurgitation, an S_3 heart sound is common and denotes systolic dysfunction and elevated filling pressure. Tachycardia is caused by compensatory increases in sympathetic tone.

Weight gain and edema reflect sodium and water retention resulting from decreased renal perfusion (see Pathogenesis section). As RBF and GFR decrease, a disproportionate amount of BUN may be retained. This phenomenon is termed *prerenal azotemia* and may be detected by an elevated BUN to SCr ratio of greater than 20:1. A.J. has a ratio of greater than 40:1. Prerenal azotemia also can be caused by dehydration and overuse of diuretics. Frequency of urination at night (nocturia) is caused by improved perfusion of the kidney when the patient is lying down.

RIGHT-SIDED HEART FAILURE (RIGHT VENTRICULAR DYSFUNCTION)

The signs and symptoms of right ventricular dysfunction are related either to hypervolemia, valvular disease, or pulmonary hypertension. The overall effect is elevation in central venous pressure.

Dependent pitting edema results from increased venous and capillary hydrostatic pressure, causing a redistribution of fluid from the intravascular to interstitial spaces. Ankle and pretibial edema are common findings after prolonged standing or sitting because fluid tends to localize in the dependent portions of the body secondary to gravitational forces. Sacral edema can be present in patients at bed rest. Edema is subjectively quantified on a 1+ (minimal) to 4+ (severe) scale. A.J. has 3+ pitting edema.

Hepatomegaly, hepatic tenderness, and ascites (fluid in the abdomen) arise from hepatic venous congestion and increased portal vein pressure. Metabolism of drugs highly dependent on the liver for body elimination can be notably impaired by both the retrograde venous congestion of the liver from right-sided heart failure and the decreased arterial perfusion of the liver from left-sided heart failure. Congestion of the gastrointestinal tract makes the patient anorectic.

Neck vein distension, primarily seen as internal jugular venous distension, denotes an elevated jugular venous pressure.

ONLINE CONTENT

For a video about jugular venous pressure, see http://thepoint.lww.com/AT10e.

How high the neck veins are distended while the patient is lying down and how much the patient's head has to be raised before the jugular venous distension disappears give the clinician a rough estimate of the patient's central venous pressure. Jugular distension in centimeters is measured as the vertical distance from the top of the venous pulsation down to the sternal angle. Neck vein distension of less than 4 cm when the patient is lying with the head elevated at a 45-degree angle is considered normal for an average, healthy adult. Applying pressure to the liver can cause further distension of the neck veins if hepatic venous congestion is present. This phenomenon is termed *hepatojugular reflux.*

EJECTION FRACTION MEASUREMENT

CASE 19-1, QUESTION 2: Does A.J. have LVSD?

Shortness of breath, crackles on auscultation, neck vein distension, edema, and nearly all of A.J.'s other signs and symptoms provide some important clues about the nature of the underlying cardiac abnormalities; however, they are limited in evaluating structural abnormalities. Some of these symptoms can be confused with other disorders, especially reduced exercise intolerance, which is often a gradual process that certain patients may fail to recognize and report to heath care providers. An enlarged heart on a chest radiograph increases the suspicion of LVSD, but this finding can be absent in some patients with LVSD and present in others with normal LV function. On the contrary, patients may be asymptomatic with structural abnormalities.

The most useful method to diagnose HF with LVSD is by measuring the LVEF. Thus, it is imperative that A.J., as with all patients with suspected HF, have an EF measured before beginning therapy because the treatment strategies between LVSD and HFPEF differ. Two-dimensional echocardiography coupled with Doppler flow studies (Doppler echocardiogram) is the diagnostic test of choice for measuring EF. This procedure uses sound waves, similar to sonar technology, to visualize and measure ventricular wall thickness, chamber size, valvular functioning, and pericardial thickness. EF is visually estimated based on changes in ventricular chamber size between diastole and systole. This method of EF measurement is not as technically accurate as that provided by ventriculography, but the procedure is more comfortable for the patient and the correlation of the measured EF to that of the other methods is acceptable.

Radionuclide left ventriculography (also called a multiple gated acquisition scan) uses radiolabeled technetium as a tracer to measure LV hemodynamics. Although this method is the most accurate measurement of EF, it is moderately invasive because it requires venipuncture and radiation exposure. In addition, radionuclide scanning does not provide information on the architecture of the left ventricle. Magnetic resonance imaging and computed tomography are useful in evaluating ventricular mass but do not provide EF data.

Subsequently, A.J. underwent an echocardiogram. The results were reported as left ventricular hypertrophy (LVH) with mild to moderate depression of EF, correlating approximately to an EF of 30% to 40%. Because he has the combination of systolic dysfunction and classic congestive signs, he fits the criteria for having true congestive HF.

STAGES OF HEART FAILURE AND NEW YORK HEART ASSOCIATION CLASSIFICATION

CASE 19-1, QUESTION 3: What stage of HF does A.J. exhibit according the ACC/AHA criteria? How severe is A.J.'s disability according to the NYHA functional classification of HF?

The ACC/AHA staging scheme and the NYHA functional classification are described in the Pathogenesis section of this chapter and are summarized in Figure 19-1.[4,27]

Because A.J. has active symptoms of HF and structural changes in cardiac architecture, he is in ACA/AHA stage C. On admission, A.J. is in NYHA functional class III as evidenced by a need to sleep upright and an inability to undertake even minimal physical activity. The staging does not imply that patients will progress through the stages in order. A patient with MI could move from stage A to stage C. Thus it is imperative to recognize that HF can progress very slowly in some patients and very rapidly in others.

PREDISPOSING FACTORS

CASE 19-1, QUESTION 4: What factors contributed to the cause of A.J.'s HF?

Several risk factors such as age, hypertension, MI, diabetes, tachycardia-induced cardiomyopathy, valvular heart disease, and obesity are well-established major risk factors associated with the development of HF. Other risk factors associated with HF are smoking, excessive intake of alcohol, dyslipidemia, anemia, and chronic kidney disease.[83] Recently there is interest in biochemical and genetic markers that are associated with HF. CAD, and in particular MI, is considered to be the most significant risk factor for HF in the elderly. During the past decades there has been an increase (74%) in the incidence of HF after MI. This increase has been attributed to the increased survival after MI as a result of therapeutic advancements in the management of MI.[84]

A.J.'s age of 58 puts him in a high-risk category for development of CV disease. He is especially vulnerable to HF because of his poorly controlled hypertension, which places an increased afterload on his left ventricle. Similar to MI, hypertension (HTN) can lead to myocyte hypertrophy, which is a compensatory response to increased afterload. Neurohormonal activation as a result of HTN leads to LVH. LVH is associated with a higher risk of HF, especially in younger individuals.[5] The lifetime risk for individuals developing HF with BP of at least 160/90 mm Hg is double that for those with BP less than 140/80 mm Hg.[8] In addition, the combined presence of HTN and HF is associated with worse outcomes; 5-year mortality after the onset of HF with HTN has been reported at 76% in men and 69% in women. Preventive strategies directed toward earlier and more aggressive BP control can reduce the incidence of HF by almost 50% and its associated mortality as well.[5]

NONSTEROIDAL ANTI-INFLAMMATORY DRUGS AND SODIUM CONTENT

Ibuprofen used for A.J.'s arthritis could contribute to sodium overload. All nonsteroidal anti-inflammatory drugs (NSAIDs; including cyclo-oxygenase-2 inhibitors) have well-documented, renally-mediated sodium-retaining properties, increasing the blood volume by up to 50% in some individuals (see Chapter 44, Rheumatoid Arthritis).[85] Published epidemiologic studies have indicated that NSAIDs can exacerbate HF symptoms, resulting in hospitalizations for HF.[86–88] This has been reported in patients with or without a previous diagnosis of HF.[89] Recent studies in two separate cohorts of patients with MI and HF showed a dose-related increase in the risk of death and rehospitalizations for MI and HF with all cyclo-oxygenase-2 inhibitors and some nonselective NSAIDs, including naproxen.[90,91] Interestingly, a rather small pilot study in the HF patients showed that once patients were educated that NSAIDs could potentially worsen HF, they would rather avoid taking them.[92] NSAIDs exert their anti-inflammatory effects by inhibiting prostaglandins (prostacyclin and thromboxane). Blocking prostaglandins leads to sodium reabsorption and counteracts the beneficial effects of diuretics and ACE inhibitors. Thus, ACC/AHA practice guidelines recommend avoiding NSAIDs whenever possible in patients with HF.[1]

Another potential source for sodium overload is in IV formulations. Sodium chloride is often used as a diluent for IV drug administration. Selected parenteral antibiotics, particularly nafcillin and ticarcillin, have a high sodium content, which should not be overlooked. Most prescription and nonprescription drug labels carry a disclosure of sodium content, however.

A.J.'s HTN and HF are both poorly controlled and he has gained 8 kg. His clinical presentation (orthopnea, dyspnea, SOB, lower extremity edema, elevated jugular venous pressure) clearly indicate fluid overload. This could be a result of high-dose ibuprofen use. His HCTZ should be replaced by a loop diuretic to enhance diuresis and resolve signs and symptoms of HF. Also, an ACE inhibitor should be added to the current regimen for BP control. Once he is euvolemic, the addition of a β-blocker before discharge should be considered. Lowering the dose or preferably discontinuing all NSAIDs might reduce sodium retention and edema and allow ACE inhibitor therapy to be more effective. Acetaminophen is an alternative for treating his osteoarthritis.

DIET

It is possible that A.J.'s diet contains a considerable excess of sodium from foods such as canned soups and vegetables, potato chips, or overuse of salt at mealtime. Dietary supplements (e.g., Ensure and Sustacal) and sports drinks (e.g., Gatorade) can also be rich sources of sodium. He should follow a controlled-sodium (e.g., 2–3 g/day) diet. If salt substitutes are used, he should be warned that they are high in potassium and could cause hyperkalemia if used concurrently with potassium supplements, an aldosterone inhibitor (spironolactone), or other potassium-sparing diuretics (amiloride, triamterene).

TABLE 19-6
Drugs That May Induce Heart Failure

Negative Inotropic Agents	
β-Blockers[a]	Most evident with propranolol or other nonselective agents
	Less with agents with intrinsic sympathomimetic activity (acebutolol, carteolol, pindolol); can also be caused by use of timolol eye drops
Calcium-channel blockers[a]	Verapamil has most negative inotropic and AV-blocking effects; amlodipine has least
Antiarrhythmics	Most with disopyramide; also quinidine
	Least with amiodarone
Direct Cardiotoxins	
Cocaine, amphetamines	Overdoses and long-term myopathy
Anthracycline cancer chemotherapeutic drugs	Daunorubicin and doxorubicin (Adriamycin); dose related; keep total cumulative dose <600 mg/m^2
Proarrhythmic Effects	
Class IA, Class III antiarrhythmic drugs	QT interval widening
	Probable torsades de pointes
	HF develops if disturbed rhythm compromises cardiac functioning
Nonantiarrhythmic drugs	Same mechanism as above
(See Crouch et al.[93] for a complete list)	Often associated with drug interactions that inhibit metabolism of the offending drug leading to higher than desired plasma levels
Expansion of Plasma Volume	
Antidiabetics	Metformin high dose may increase risk of lactic acidosis
	Na retention with pioglitazone (Actos) and rosiglitazone (Avandia)
NSAID	Prostaglandin inhibition; Na retention
Glucocorticoids, androgens, estrogens	Mineralocorticoid effect; Na retention
Licorice	Aldosteronelike effect; Na retention
Antihypertensive vasodilators (hydralazine, methyldopa, prazosin, minoxidil)	↓Renal blood flow, activation of renin-angiotensin system
Drugs high in Na$^+$	Selected IV cephalosporins and penicillins
	Effervescent or bicarbonate-containing antacids or analgesics
	Also liquid nutrition supplements
Unknown Mechanism	
Tumor necrosis factor antagonists	Multiple case reports of new-onset HF or exacerbation of prior HF with etanercept and infliximab in patients with Crohn's disease or rheumatoid arthritis

[a]β-Blockers and verapamil may be beneficial in diastolic HF. Carvedilol and metoprolol counteract autonomic hyperactivity in systolic dysfunction.
AV, atrioventricular; HF, heart failure; IV, intravenous; Na, sodium; NSAID, nonsteroidal anti-inflammatory drugs.

Drug-Induced Heart Failure

CASE 19-1, QUESTION 5: What are the basic mechanisms by which drugs can induce HF, and how can an understanding of these mechanisms be predictive of drugs to avoid in A.J.?

Drug-induced HF is mediated by three basic mechanisms: inhibition of myocardial contractility (negative inotropic agents and direct toxins), proarrhythmic effects, or expansion of plasma volume (Table 19-6). The latter category includes drugs that act primarily on the kidney (to either alter RBF or increase sodium retention) or those that increase total body sodium and water because of their high sodium content.

The most recognized negative inotropic agents are the β-blockers. Nonselective β-adrenergic blockers (e.g., propranolol) decrease myocardial contractility and slow the HR. Both of these factors can compromise the heart's ability to empty effectively. Other well-documented negative inotropic drugs include the calcium-channel blockers (CCB), most notably verapamil and diltiazem, and various antiarrhythmic agents, especially disopyramide, quinidine, flecainide, and dronedarone. The anthracyclines (daunorubicin and doxorubicin) have a direct, dose-related cardiotoxicity that can be minimized by limiting total cumulative doses to 500 to 600 mg/m^2.[94,95] (For a more detailed description of anthracycline toxicity see Chapter 90, Adverse Effects of Chemotherapy and Targeted Agents.) The final group of drugs gaining increased notoriety as cardiotoxins are cocaine and alcohol when used chronically in large quantities or after an overdose. Drugs that increase the QT interval induce proarrhythmic effects in some patients. Worsening of HF occurs if the disturbed rhythm compromises cardiac functioning.

Drugs that induce sodium and water retention are NSAIDs (via prostaglandin inhibition), certain antihypertensive drugs, glucocorticoids, androgens, estrogens, and licorice. Weight gain accompanied by peripheral and pulmonary edema has been observed in patients with stable HF given the thiazolidinedione antidiabetic drugs pioglitazone and rosiglitazone.[96] Worsening of HF appears to be dose-dependent and is presumed to be at least partly caused by fluid retention. As a consequence, the package insert for these two drugs recommend they not be administered to patients with NYHA class III or IV HF and that they be used cautiously in earlier stages of HF. Glucocorticoids and licorice (glycyrrhizic acid) cause sodium reabsorption.

TREATMENT

Therapeutic Objectives

CASE 19-1, QUESTION 6: What are the therapeutic goals in treating A.J.?

Cure is not a feasible therapeutic objective in patients with any form of HF, except patients who are candidates for cardiac transplantation or who have certain forms of dilated cardiomyopathy (e.g., viral, alcohol-induced, or tachycardia-induced). The immediate objective for A.J. is to provide symptomatic relief as assessed by a reduction in his complaints of SOB and PND, improved sleep quality, and increased exercise tolerance. During the next several days or weeks, the goal will be to get him back to his baseline status. Parameters used to measure success in meeting this objective include reduced peripheral and sacral edema, weight loss, slowing of the HR to less than 90 beats/minute, normalization of BP, reduction of the BUN back to baseline, a smaller heart size on chest radiograph, decreased neck vein distension, and loss of the S_3 heart sound. Long-range goals are to improve A.J.'s EF and quality of life including better tolerance of daily life activities, fewer future hospitalizations, avoidance of side effects of his therapy, and ultimately, an increased survival time. The achievement of these goals depends on the severity of A.J.'s disease, his understanding of his disease, and his adherence to prescribed interventions.

Diuretics

FUROSEMIDE AND OTHER LOOP DIURETICS

CASE 19-1, QUESTION 7: Bed rest and a 3-g sodium diet were ordered. The medical team decides to begin furosemide for A.J. What is the rationale for using diuretics and what route, dose, and dosing schedule should be used?

Excessive volume increases the workload of a compromised heart, and diuretics are an integral part of therapy. This is especially true if volume overload is symptomatic (e.g., pulmonary congestion) as it is in A.J. Diuretics produce symptomatic improvement more rapidly than any other drug for HF. They can relieve pulmonary and peripheral edema within hours or days, whereas the clinical effects of ACE inhibitors, β-blockers, and digoxin take weeks to months to be fully realized. Diuretics, however, should not be used alone in HF. Even when they are initially successful in controlling symptoms and reducing edema, they are ineffective in maintaining clinical stability for long periods without the addition of other drugs. More importantly, activation of the RAAS and sympathetic nervous system in response to diuresis could possibly lead to HF progression.

All current guidelines recommend diuretic therapy, both acutely and chronically, if clinical volume overload is evident, but further state that patients without peripheral or pulmonary edema can be treated either intermittently or without diuretics.[1] Diuretics used on an intermittent (as-needed) basis are titrated based on changes in weight gain, neck vein distension, peripheral edema, or SOB. Patients with a good understanding of their disease can be instructed to weigh themselves daily and start taking their medicine if they gain more than 1 to 2 pounds in 1 day or 5 pounds in 1 week or have leg or abdominal swelling. Diuretics can be withheld as long as patients are at their target weight. In other cases, diuretic-free intervals or weekends can be arranged. Even with these options, if the patient has experienced volume overload at some time during the course of his or her disease, either past or present, a diuretic should always be readily available.[1] Despite its remarkable initial benefits, vigorous diuretic therapy carries the risk of volume depletion, electrolyte abnormalities, and diminished CO. Abrupt worsening of renal function (increased BUN or SCr) or hypotension indicates the need to consider temporarily discontinuing diuretics.

The vast majority of patients with clinically evident HF require loop diuretics. A.J. has obvious signs of volume overload, indicating a need for more vigorous diuresis with a loop diuretic. His elevated BUN is worrisome and could worsen if he becomes dehydrated. The more likely outcome, however, is improved RBF as his HF symptoms resolve, and subsequently improved renal function tests.

ROUTE OF ADMINISTRATION

The pharmacology and dose comparison of loop diuretics is discussed in the Overview of Treatment Principles section of this chapter and in Table 19-3. Furosemide is the most commonly used loop diuretic for HF because of greater clinical experience and low cost. Bumetanide and torsemide are preferred in some settings because of more predictable absorption.[63,64,97,98] Ethacrynic acid, which is also a loop diuretic, is not the preferred diuretic in HF patients because of its ototoxic potential. However, unlike other loop diuretics, ethacrynic acid does not contain a sulfonamide moiety, and thus it is mainly reserved for patients with severe sulfonamide allergies to other loop diuretics.

According to one group of investigators, patients with HF treated with torsemide fare better than those receiving furosemide.[98] The authors hypothesized that because torsemide has more predictable absorption than furosemide, therefore better bioavailability, this should translate into a more-favorable outcome in HF patients. During a 1-year open-label trial of 234 subjects, patients receiving torsemide were less likely to be admitted to the hospital for HF (17% torsemide vs. 32% furosemide; $p = 0.01$). Admissions for all CV causes were also lower among patients taking torsemide (44%) than patients taking furosemide (59%). No differences were found in all-cause hospital admissions between the two groups (71% torsemide vs. 76% furosemide). Fatigue scores improved more in patients treated with torsemide, but no difference was found between groups in the rate of dyspnea score improvement. Generic torsemide is more expensive than generic furosemide, and this may be an issue for some patients.

Erratic responses to furosemide are more prevalent in persons with severe HF or diminished renal function. Some patients respond promptly and vigorously to small oral doses of furosemide, whereas others require large IV doses to achieve only minimal diuresis. Part of these differences can be explained by the drug's pharmacokinetics.[63,99] Loop diuretics are highly protein bound and have to be actively secreted into the proximal tubular lumen to elicit a response. Tubular secretion of loop diuretics can be compromised in the presence of increased levels of endogenous organic acids as a result of renal insufficiency and drugs (NSAIDs) that are competing for the same transporters. Also, oral absorption of furosemide is erratic and incomplete, averaging 50% to 60% in healthy subjects and 43% to 46% in those with renal failure. When taken with a meal, absorption is delayed because of slowed gastric emptying, but the total amount absorbed does not differ significantly from that in fasting states. There are claims that the absorption and, therefore, effectiveness of furosemide are further diminished in patients with HF attributable to edema of the bowel and decreased splanchnic blood flow. This has been partially refuted by one investigator, who noted an average furosemide bioavailability of 61% in patients with HF, the same as in normal patients.[100] Total absorption in patients with HF varies widely (34%–80%); however, both the rate of absorption and time to peak urinary excretion are delayed for furosemide and bumetanide.[63,64,100]

When interpreting these bioavailability data, another important factor must be considered. The rate and extent of absorption are not only different among individuals (as illustrated by the examples already given), but intraindividual variability also exists. Ingestion of the same brand of furosemide by the same individual on multiple occasions can show up to a threefold difference in bioavailability. These differences are evident whether considering the innovator's brand (Lasix) or one of several generic brands.[63,64,101,102] As with digoxin, these data on bioavailability differences are old and have not been verified or refuted by newer studies.

One might infer that IV therapy is the preferred route, giving a better response for any given dose. Surprisingly, this is not always the case. In both healthy volunteers and patients with HF, total daily fluid and electrolyte loss after oral therapy and parenteral therapy are comparable. The major difference is in the time course of response. During the first 2 hours, diuresis from the IV dose far exceeds that from the oral therapy, but by 4 to 6 hours, the total urinary output is equivalent.[100,103,104] Therefore, considering the significant cost differential between oral and parenteral furosemide, the clinical advantage in using IV therapy is small. Exceptions to the rule are those patients with severe pulmonary edema who need acute symptomatic relief and those patients who have failed to respond to an adequate oral challenge.

DOSING

Typically, a patient's treatment is initiated with 20 to 40 mg of oral or IV furosemide given as a single dose and monitored for responsiveness (Table 19-3). If the desired diuresis is not obtained, the dose can be increased in 40- to 80-mg increments to a total daily dose of 160 to 240 mg/day, usually divided into two or three doses. For torsemide, a usual starting dose is 10 to 20 mg/day, but a ceiling effect is noted in patients with HF at a dosage of 100 to 200 mg/day.[63,105] Equivalent doses of bumetanide are 0.5 to 1.0 mg once or twice daily, titrated to a maximum of 10 mg daily. Because A.J. is not in acute distress, it could be argued that oral therapy would suffice. The decision, however, is to give a single 40-mg IV dose of furosemide for immediate symptom control, followed by 40 mg each morning.

Opinions differ to whether furosemide should be given once daily, in multiple doses, or in continuous infusions. The drug's short half-life of 2 to 4 hours implies the need for multiple daily dosing. Nonetheless, equivalent daily diuresis has been observed after the same dose given in single or divided doses.[106] Another investigator found better effects from divided doses.[107] Because evening and nighttime doses of diuretics often disturb patients' sleep patterns (because of nocturnal diuresis), the total daily dose usually should be given as a single morning dose. For patients with symptomatic nocturnal dyspnea, two-thirds of the dose is given in the morning and one-third in the late afternoon or, if necessary, at night. Torsemide has a slightly longer half-life and generally can be given once daily.

Another alternative in hospitalized patients is to administer loop diuretics via continuous infusion. Multiple studies have demonstrated the benefits of continuous infusions compared with intermittent infusions.[108–110] However, the results of these studies have been questioned because of a lack of methodological rigor, and the studies have been underpowered to address the primary end points. Recently, the DOSE trial[111] (Diuretic Optimization Strategies Evaluation) showed no difference in efficacy or safety between intermittent IV bolus or continuous infusion. From a pharmacokinetic and pharmacodynamic perspective, there are potential benefits of continuous infusion when compared with intermittent bolus dosing. Bolus diuretic dosing can cause a higher rate of diuretic resistance owing to postdiuretic phenomenon. This phenomenon is typically attributable to subtherapeutic concentrations of diuretic administered during a 4- to 6-hour period, which results in sodium retention. In contrast, continuous IV infusion results in a constant delivery to the tubule, potentially reducing this phenomenon. Additionally, continuous infusions are also associated with lower incidence of ototoxicity owing to lower peak concentrations. Patients who are candidates for continuous IV infusion should receive a loading dose before infusion to reach steady-state concentrations faster. However, if the patient has received one or more IV boluses within the previous few hours, then an infusion can be started without a loading dose. In case of inadequate response, the loading dose should be repeated and the infusion rate increased. The rate of infusion depends on the patient's renal function.

ADVERSE EFFECTS

CASE 19-1, QUESTION 8: Examine A.J.'s laboratory values (see Question 1). Does A.J. have any abnormal values? What is the significance of these abnormalities?

More thorough discussions of diuretic-induced side effects are found in Chapter 10, Fluid and Electrolyte Disorders, and Chapter 14, Essential Hypertension. Those findings pertinent to A.J.'s case are discussed below.

AZOTEMIA

A.J. has an elevated BUN (40 mg/dL) but a normal SCr (0.8 mg/dL). Normally, a BUN-to-creatinine ratio of 10:1 to 15:1 is seen. Progressive renal failure is characterized by an elevation of both BUN and creatinine. A disproportionately elevated BUN relative to creatinine is indicative of prerenal azotemia, the major cause of which is dehydration (e.g., overdiuresis) or poor renal perfusion (e.g., HF). SCr will also rise in some patients with prerenal azotemia, but will quickly return to normal with rehydration.

A.J.'s laboratory values reflect prerenal azotemia, but his edematous state and elevated BP point to a cause other than dehydration. The most probable cause of his azotemia is decreased RBF secondary to decompensated HF. Diuretics should not be withheld and, in fact, judicious diuresis should improve his HF and help lower his BUN. Caution must be exercised because prolonged overdiuresis and dehydration can cause renal ischemia, leading to true renal damage. If this happens, the SCr also will begin to rise (see Case 19-1, Question 15).

HYPONATREMIA

A marginally low serum sodium of 132 mEq/L is noted. Low serum sodium, however, is not necessarily a sign of overdiuresis. Serum sodium reported by the laboratory is the concentration of sodium in the serum. A person may be significantly overdiuresed (dehydrated) with a large body deficit of sodium, but if that sodium is lost isotonically, the serum sodium concentration will be normal. Conversely, a person such as A.J. can be volume overloaded (edema and hypertension), indicating excessive body sodium, but the serum sodium concentration may be normal or even low as explained below.

Hyponatremia (low serum sodium concentration) reflects the dilutional effect of extra free water in the plasma on sodium concentration. The most common causes of dilutional hyponatremia are excess ADH production or excessive free water intake (i.e., electrolyte-free fluids). Individuals on severely sodium-restricted diets can experience hyponatremia. Likewise, patients given too much diuretic and who are then given salt-free fluids or who have compensatory ADH release by the body can become hyponatremic. Dilutional hyponatremia, resembling the syndrome of inappropriate antidiuretic hormone secretion, has been described after treatment with thiazide and loop diuretics. Patients with HF or hepatic cirrhosis are more likely to develop diuretic-induced dilutional hyponatremia because of pre-existing defects in free water excretion. The exact cause of hyponatremia in A.J. is unknown, but his marginally low serum sodium does not contraindicate continued diuretic therapy. In general, levels of serum sodium concentration less than 120 to 125 mEq/L are associated with adverse events in HF patients; chronic serum sodium concentrations of 130 mEq/L or less are associated with higher morbidity and mortality.[112] Asymptomatic hyponatremia can be treated with water restriction. In the setting of volume depletion, IV administration of normal saline may be effective. Vasopressin receptor antagonists can be used in patients with HF.

HYPOKALEMIA

A.J. has a serum potassium of 3.2 mEq/L. Hypokalemia reflecting total body potassium depletion is a well-described, but often overemphasized, side effect of thiazide and loop diuretics. Using a definition of hypokalemia as a serum potassium less than 3.5 mEq/L, the incidence is 15% to 40% in patients receiving 50 to 100 mg/day of HCTZ.[113,114] Lower doses of HCTZ (12.5–25 mg), however, can produce similar antihypertensive effects as higher doses, with little or no change in plasma concentrations of potassium.

Hypokalemia is associated with an increased incidence of ventricular arrhythmias. The development of arrhythmias may not be seen until the plasma concentration falls to 3.0 mEq/L or lower.[115] Some studies showed increased ectopic activity in persons with serum levels between 3.0 and 3.5 mEq/L.[116–118] These latter studies have been criticized for including patients at high risk for complications. Mild hypokalemia can escalate into life-threatening hypokalemia, however. The serum potassium concentration in patients before therapy should be taken into account as well as the actual degree of fall in serum potassium. It is estimated that the risk of arrhythmias increases by 27% with each 0.5 mEq/L reduction in the plasma potassium concentration less than 3.0 mEq/L.[119]

In chronic HF, potassium abnormalities are commonly seen, which is probably caused by the pathophysiologic alterations (renal dysfunction, activation of RAAS, and enhanced sympathetic tone) coupled with aggressive diuresis. Several investigators have reported sudden cardiac death related to low serum potassium levels.[120,121] The risk of sudden cardiac death in patients with HF may be lessened by using low doses of diuretics in combination with potassium-sparing agents, with the goal of maintaining serum potassium levels between 4.5 and 5.0 mEq/L.[122]

A.J.'s potassium is 3.2 mEq/L. A.J. will be receiving increased doses of diuretics for the next several days and, therefore, may need additional potassium supplementation to prevent life-threatening hypokalemia. In addition, if he needs digoxin therapy in the future, low serum potassium levels can predispose him to digitalis toxicity. Potassium replacement is warranted for A.J. at this time. Long-term potassium supplementation may not be necessary with concomitant administration of ACE inhibitors. If hypokalemia persists, A.J. can be started on an aldosterone antagonist.

HYPOMAGNESEMIA

A.J.'s serum magnesium level is 1.5 mEq/L. Severe hypomagnesemia can lead to somnolence, muscle spasms, a decreased seizure threshold, and cardiac arrhythmias, effects similar to those seen with hypokalemia. Some investigators have claimed that many of the arrhythmias previously ascribed to diuretic-induced hypokalemia were actually caused by diuretic-induced hypomagnesemia.[123] Concurrent hypokalemia and hypomagnesemia can be especially dangerous. A.J. should be given 1 g of magnesium sulfate IV and observed for changes in his magnesium level. If needed, he could be given chronic oral supplements of magnesium. A potential cause for magnesium wasting is aldosterone excess. Therefore, addition of an aldosterone antagonist can decrease this effect and diminish urinary magnesium losses.[124]

HYPERURICEMIA

Increases of 1 to 2 mg/dL in uric acid levels are common during thiazide administration. Rarely, 4- to 5-mg/dL elevations have been reported. A.J.'s uric acid level is 8 mg/dL, which is slightly elevated (normal range, 2–7 mg/dL). Most patients who exhibit elevated uric acid levels during treatment with diuretic agents remain asymptomatic and need not be treated, even though uric acid concentrations may exceed 15 mg/dL.[125,126] Because the elevations in plasma urate levels is primarily caused by the initial decrease in the rate of urate excretion, these patients are not at a risk of uric acid precipitation. It has been proposed that serum uric acid levels may be a valuable prognostic marker in HF patients. One study indicates a graded relationship between serum uric acid and HF survival.[127] In HF xanthine oxidase is upregulated, which can lead to endothelial dysfunction. Therefore treatment with allopurinol may improve endothelial function and promote reverse remodeling. The relationship between serum uric acid and CV disease is still controversial, and the guidelines do not recommend the use of xanthine oxidase inhibitors to treat hyperuricemia. In patients who experience symptomatic hyperuricemia, the addition of allopurinol should be considered (see also Chapter 45, Gout and Hyperuricemia).

BNP

A.J.'s BNP is elevated (365 pg/mL). Various studies evaluating the diagnostic accuracy of BNP and NT-proBNP have used different cut-offs to define abnormal values. The most commonly used plasma concentration to define the upper limit of normal for BNP is 100 pg/mL, with concentrations greater than 400 pg/mL being considered an indicator of HF. The age-related NT-proBNP diagnostic cut-off value is 125 pg/mL for patients younger than 75 years, and 450 pg/mL for patients older than 75 years of age. If the patient has a level below the cut-off for the respective assay used, then the symptoms are most likely attributable to causes other than HF. In patients with renal impairment, the clearance of these peptides is reduced; therefore, the upper limit of normal is 200 pg/mL for BNP and the corresponding value for NT-proBNP is 1,200 pg/mL.[128] Moreover, concentrations of these biomarkers are influenced by other factors such as age, sex, obesity, and other cardiac and noncardiac comorbidities. Asymptomatic patients with HF can also present with elevated BNP or NT-proBNP levels. This confounds the accurate interpretation of these markers and makes it challenging to integrate their usefulness into routine clinical practice. Elevated BNP and NT-proBNP have an established utility in ruling out HF in patients who present to the emergency department with shortness of breath.[129] Recently several natriuretic peptide–guided therapy trials have been published[130–132]; however, according to the ACC/AHA guidelines, the value of serial BNP measurements in guiding therapy for patients with HF is not well established.[1] A.J.'s elevated BNP level, along with his clinical presentation, is indicative of HF exacerbation.

POTASSIUM SUPPLEMENTATION

CASE 19-1, QUESTION 9: The physician gave A.J. one 1-g dose of magnesium sulfate and three 20-mEq doses of potassium chloride IV. This raised his serum magnesium to 2.0 mEq/L and his potassium to 3.9 mEq/L. Should he receive prophylactic magnesium or potassium supplementation? What is an appropriate dose?

At this time A.J. does not need further magnesium replacement, but his serum magnesium level should be measured again after he has received furosemide for a few days. If the level drops again, maintenance therapy with oral magnesium oxide tablets can be started.

A fall in serum potassium concentration can be seen within hours of the first dose of a diuretic, and the maximal fall usually is reached by the end of the first week of treatment. Potassium supplementation is not required in all patients receiving diuretics. They should be monitored frequently in the first few months of diuretic therapy to determine their potassium requirements. Similarly, when diuretics are stopped, it can take several weeks for serum potassium to return to normal. Therefore, it is possible that A.J.'s admitting potassium level of 3.2 mEq/L reflects the nadir of his response to HCTZ. His initial response to potassium supplementation shows that his hypokalemia will be easily controlled. It might be argued that he should be observed for a few days and not given further supplements; however, because his diuresis is to be increased and digitalis therapy may later be considered, potassium supplementation is warranted. Long-term potassium supplementation may not be necessary with concomitant administration of ACE inhibitors. If hypokalemia persists, A.J. should be started on an aldosterone antagonist.

DOSE REQUIREMENTS

It is difficult to predict the dose of potassium chloride that will be required to maintain proper potassium balance. Many patients do well with 20 mEq/day, but it is questionable how many patients need any supplement at all. People with well-documented hypokalemia can require anywhere from 20 to 120 mEq of potassium chloride per day.[113,114,133] Those patients with disease states associated with high circulating aldosterone levels require doses of potassium in excess of 60 mEq/day. In patients who need long-term potassium supplementation, efforts should be made to increase doses of ACE inhibitors to target doses or maximal tolerated doses. If hypokalemia persists, appropriate addition of an aldosterone antagonist should be considered. However, a few selected patients may still need to take potassium supplementation despite the addition of aldosterone blockers.

MONITORING

CASE 19-1, QUESTION 10: After a single 40-mg IV dose of furosemide, A.J. is begun on 40 mg of furosemide each morning and potassium chloride tablets 20 mEq BID. How should his therapy be monitored?

A.J. needs to be monitored for both an improvement in his HF and for side effects (Tables 19-5 and 19-7). Subjectively, the clinician should monitor for decreased pulmonary distress and an increased exercise tolerance, demonstrating control of HF. Objective monitoring parameters for disease control include weight loss (ideal, 0.5–1 kg/day until ideal dry weight is achieved), a decrease in edema, flattening of neck veins, and disappearance of the S_3 gallop and rales. Because A.J. has hypertension, his BP also requires monitoring with a goal to reduce it to <120/80 mm Hg.[134]

Patients are instructed to record their weight each day and are allowed to adjust their diuretic dose based on changes observed. If they are at their ideal "dry weight," they may reduce their dose of diuretic by 50% or even hold one or more doses. If weight increases more than 1 or 2 pounds in a day or 5 pounds per week, edema increases, or SOB returns, the dose of diuretic is temporarily increased.

Dizziness and weakness are subjective indices of volume depletion, hypotension, or potassium loss. Muscle cramps and abdominal pain could indicate rapid changes in electrolyte balance. Objectively, a lowering of BP, especially on standing, and a rising BUN (prerenal azotemia) signify overdiuresis. As discussed in Case 19-1 (Questions 8 and 9), serum sodium, potassium, and uric acid should be monitored routinely. Questioning the patient with regard to the onset of diuresis (relative to drug ingestion) and the duration of the diuretic effect helps develop the most convenient schedule for the patient.

TABLE 19-7
Monitoring Parameters with Diuretics

↓CHF symptoms (see Table 19-5)
Weight loss or gain; goal is 1- to 2-pound weight loss/day until "ideal weight" achieved[a]
Signs of volume depletion
Weakness
Hypotension, dizziness
Orthostatic changes in BP[b]
↓Urine output
↑BUN[c]
Serum potassium and magnesium (avoid hypokalemia and hypomagnesemia)
↑Uric acid
↑Glucose

[a] Weight loss may be greater during first few days when significant edema is present.
[b] A ↓ in systolic BP of 10–15 mm Hg or a ↓ in diastolic BP of 5–10 mm Hg.
[c] A rising BUN can be caused by either volume depletion from diuretics or poor renal blood flow from poorly controlled HF. Small boluses of 0.9% saline can be given cautiously to differentiate a rising BUN from volume depletion versus poor cardiac output. If volume depletion is present, saline will cause an ↑ in urine output and a ↓ in BUN. However, if the patient has severe HF, the saline could cause pulmonary edema.
BP, blood pressure; BUN, blood urea nitrogen; HF, heart failure.

REFRACTORY PATIENTS: COMBINATION THERAPY

CASE 19-1, QUESTION 11: If A.J.'s furosemide dose was increased to 80 mg twice a day (BID) without much response, what should be the next logical step?

As described in the discussion of the pharmacology of diuretics earlier in the chapter, all loop and thiazide diuretics must reach the tubular lumen to be effective. Because these drugs are highly bound to serum proteins and endogenous organic acids, they cannot enter the tubular lumen by glomerular filtration. For diuresis to begin, they must be transported into the proximal tubule by active secretion from the blood into the tubule. If this active transport is blocked, diuretics will not reach their site of action. This can lead to a diminished diuretic response in patients with either renal insufficiency or decreased RBF associated with uncompensated HF. In particular, patients with renal insufficiency or poor RBF often require large doses of diuretics to achieve a desired response. Endogenous organic acids also can accumulate during renal insufficiency, avidly binding the drug and preventing its access to the site of action.[63,64]

Both the total amount of drug delivered to the tubule and the rate of delivery of the drug to the tubule determine the magnitude of diuretic response elicited.[63,64] This explains why 80 mg of furosemide yields more diuresis than a 40-mg dose and why an IV injection provides a more rapid and vigorous diuresis than an oral dose. Once a threshold concentration (ceiling dose) is achieved within the tubule, higher concentrations produce no greater intensity of effect, but the duration of action may be prolonged. See Case 19-1, Question 7, for an expanded discussion about loop diuretic bioavailability and the concept of "gut wall edema."

In addition to these explainable causes, many patients exhibit a blunted diuretic response with continued therapy for unknown reasons. Generally, alternative treatment plans are pursued when the dose given approaches the ceiling doses for each drug listed in Table 19-3. Continuous infusions of furosemide (5–15 mg/hour), bumetanide (0.5–1 mg/hour), or torsemide (3 mg/hour) can be more efficacious than intermittent bolus doses in patients with severe HF or renal insufficiency.[63,64,135–137] Even higher doses have been recommended: 0.25 to 1 mg/kg/hour for furosemide, 0.1 mg/kg/hour for bumetanide, and 5 to 20 mg/hour for torsemide.[138] Another institution uses an aggressive protocol of a 100-mg IV bolus of furosemide followed by a continuous IV infusion at a rate of 20 to 40 mg/hour, which is doubled every 12 to 24 hours in unresponsive patients, to a maximal infusion rate of 160 mg/hour to attain a diuresis rate of 100 mL/hour or greater.[139]

In some instances, switching from one loop diuretic to another can overcome the problem.[64,67,138] For example, torsemide might work when furosemide fails because of more reliable absorption with torsemide.[97,98] If this maneuver fails, a combination of diuretics can be tried. The most effective regimens combine drugs that work at two different parts of the tubule.[64,67] For example, a loop diuretic that works on the ascending limb of the loop of Henle is used with metolazone, which blocks sodium reabsorption in the distal tubule. Various thiazide diuretics, including chlorthalidone, chlorothiazide, and HCTZ, have been reported to effectively enhance diuresis when combined with a loop diuretic, but it is unclear whether the responses are simply additive or truly synergistic. Triple-therapy regimens of metolazone, a loop diuretic, and an aldosterone antagonist are used to optimize diuresis and electrolyte control.

Most clinicians choose a combination of metolazone plus furosemide or bumetanide based on demonstrated value in the literature and clinical experience. A wide dose range of metolazone has been investigated,[140] leaving with no clear dosing recommendations. Typically a low dose of metolazone (2.5–5 mg) is first added to the furosemide therapy. In a minor group of patients who are well instructed, metolazone can be given intermittently to relieve congestion. The longer duration of action for metolazone can cause a greater than predicted diuresis and electrolyte loss when combined with a loop diuretic. Thus, careful monitoring of weight, urine output, BP, BUN, potassium, and SCr is required. Because no parenteral form of metolazone exists, chlorothiazide, at a dose of 500 to 1,000 mg once or twice daily, is the only option for a non–loop diuretic that can be given intravenously. Although A.J.'s furosemide dose could be increased, metolazone 2.5 mg daily should be added. A.J. may also require additional doses of potassium supplementation to avoid hypokalemia with the addition of metolazone.

Angiotensin-Converting Enzyme Inhibitors

AGENTS OF CHOICE

CASE 19-1, QUESTION 12: Along with furosemide, A.J. was started on 10 mg of lisinopril daily. Are there specific ACE inhibitors approved for use in HF patients?

As a general rule, formulary decisions are first based on comparative pharmacologic activity, efficacy, and drug safety. Other factors to consider are labeled (FDA approved) indications, convenience of dosing schedule, and—all else being equal—the cost to the pharmacy (or institution) and the patient (or insurance carrier). A confounding factor is that HTN is the primary labeled indication for all of the ACE inhibitors and was the initial basis for placing these drugs on formularies. The indication for HF was added after initial marketing and does not appear in the FDA-approved labeling for all of the drugs. Each of these factors is considered below.

The basic mechanism of action of all ACE inhibitors is the same and is described in the Pathogenesis section.[68,141,142] They inhibit ACE (also called kinase II), thereby reducing the activation of angiotensin II, a major contributor to the undesired hemodynamic responses to HF. Decreased circulating levels of NE, vasopressin, neurokinins, luteinizing hormone, prostacyclin, and NO also have been noted after administration of ACE inhibitors.

In addition, ACE is responsible for degradation of bradykinin, substance P, and possibly other vasodilatory substances unrelated to angiotensin II. Thus, part of the beneficial effects of ACE inhibitors is caused by the accumulation of bradykinin (Fig. 19-6). After attaching to bradykinin-2 (B_2) receptors, vasodilation is produced by stimulating the production of arachidonic acid metabolites, peroxidases, NO, and endothelium-derived hyperpolarizing factor in vascular endothelium. In the kidney, bradykinin causes natriuresis through direct tubular effects.

The net effect is that ACE inhibitors regulate the balance between the vasoconstrictive and salt-retentive properties of angiotensin II and the vasodilatory and natriuretic properties of bradykinin. The physiologic consequences of the pharmacologic effects of ACE inhibitors are reduced pulmonary capillary wedge pressure (preload) and lowered SVR and systolic wall stress (afterload). CO increases without an increase in HR. ACE inhibitors promote salt excretion by augmenting RBF and reducing the production of aldosterone and ADH. The beneficial effects on RBF, coupled with the drug's indirect inhibition of aldosterone, lead to a mild diuretic response, a distinct benefit compared with other vasodilator compounds such as hydralazine.

Vasodilation and diuresis are not the only value of ACE inhibitors in HF. Angiotensin II enhances vascular remodeling (referred to as trophic effects on cardiac myocytes), whereas bradykinin impedes this process.[68,143] In experimental models, ACE inhibitors impede ventricular remodeling by blocking the trophic effects of angiotensin II on cardiac myocytes. Evidence as to whether preserving bradykinin levels affects remodeling is inconclusive, although it might attenuate the progressive deposition of collagen during the chronic phase of post-MI cardiac remodeling.

Captopril, enalapril, fosinopril, lisinopril, quinapril, benazepril, and ramipril are all FDA-labeled with approval for treatment of HF (Table 19-4). Moexipril and trandolapril have FDA-labeled approval for the treatment of LV dysfunction after MI. There does not seem to be a significant difference in side effects among agents. Based on these factors, there is not a compelling reason to favor one ACE inhibitor over another.

Numerous placebo-controlled trials have documented the favorable effects of ACE inhibitor therapy on hemodynamic variables, clinical status, and symptoms of HF.[142,144] Multiple studies demonstrate a consistent 20% to 30% relative reduction in HF mortality that is superior to other vasodilator regimens, including the hydralazine–nitrate combination or ARBs. The benefits of ACE inhibitors are independent of the etiology of HF (ischemic vs. nonischemic) or the severity of symptoms (NYHA class I through class IV).

Table 19-8 provides a brief summary of the results of the key ACE inhibitor HF trials.[68,69,144–147,152,153,155–158] Of the five approved agents, the best evidence for improved survival is available for enalapril in both chronically symptomatic patients (NYHA classes II–IV) and asymptomatic patients (NYHA class I) with evidence of an impaired EF after an MI.[146,147,156–158] A 3-year follow-up to the Acute Infarction Ramipril Efficacy study

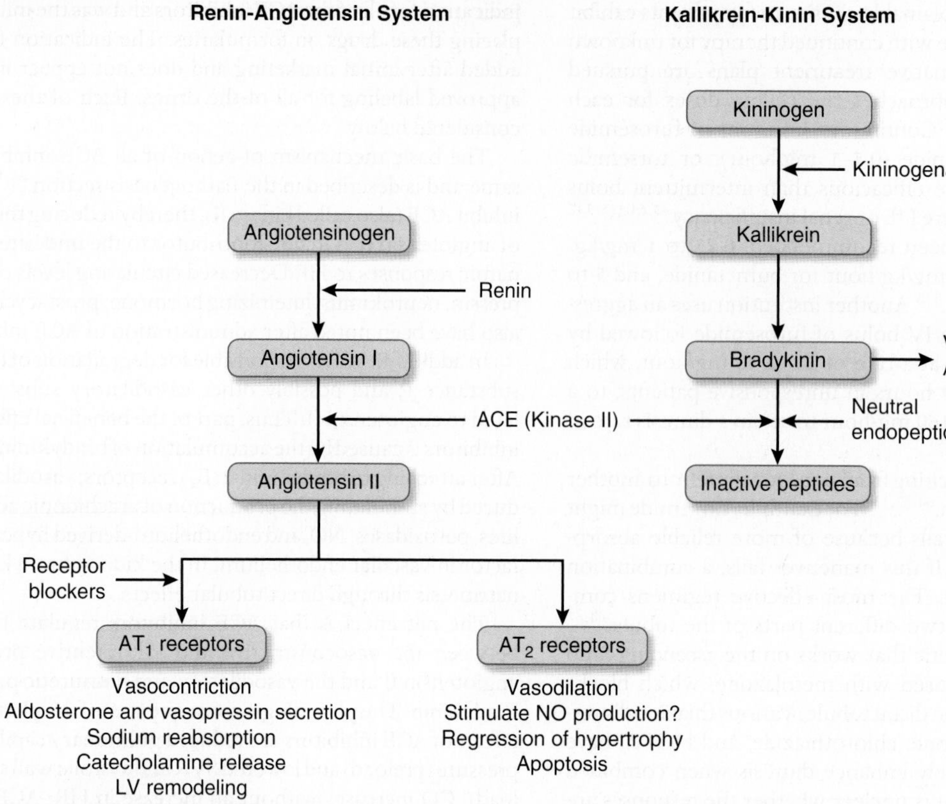

FIGURE 19-6 Angiotensin receptor blocker mechanism. ACE, angiotensin-converting enzyme; LV, left ventricular; NO, nitric oxide.

reported mortality rates of 27.5% in ramipril-treated subjects (target dose, 5 mg BID) compared with 38.9% with placebo, a 36% risk reduction.[159] Published data are also available for a positive effect on reducing short-term mortality with captopril, lisinopril, trandolapril, and zofenopril, primarily in relatively small populations of patients with chronic symptoms or in patients with new-onset HF symptoms after an MI.[141,154,160]

Direct comparison of different ACE inhibitors is limited to three trials. The first two comparing lisinopril (5–20 mg every day) with either captopril (12.5–50 mg daily in two divided

TABLE 19-8

Clinical Trials of ACE Inhibitors in Left Ventricular Dysfunction[141]

Study	Patient Population	ACE Inhibitor	Time Started After MI	Treatment Duration	Outcome
Studies in LV Dysfunction					
CONSENSUS[146]	NYHA IV (n = 253)	Enalapril vs. placebo		1 day–20 months	Decreased mortality and HF
SOLVD-Treatment[147]	NYHA II/III (n = 2,569)	Enalapril vs. placebo		22–55 months	Decreased mortality and HF
V-HeFT II[148]	NYHA II/III (n = 804)	Enalapril vs. hydralazine, isosorbide		0.5–5.7 years	Decreased mortality and sudden death
SOLVD-Prevention	Asymptomatic LV dysfunction (n = 4,228)	Enalapril vs. placebo		14.6–62 months	Decreased mortality and HF hospitalizations
Studies in LV Dysfunction after MI					
SAVE[149]	MI, decreased LV function (n = 2,331)	Captopril vs. placebo	3–16 days	24–60 months	Decreased mortality
CONSENSUS II[150]	MI (n = 6,090)	Enalaprilat/enalapril vs. placebo	24 hours	41–180 days	No change in survival; hypotension with enalaprilat
AIRE[151]	MI and HF (n = 2,006)	Ramipril vs. placebo	3–10 days	>6 months	Decreased mortality
ISIS-4[152]	MI (n >50,000)	Captopril vs. placebo	24 hours	28 days	Decreased mortality
GISSI-3[153]	MI (n = 19,394)	Lisinopril vs. placebo	24 hours	6 weeks	Decreased mortality
TRACE[154]	MI, decreased LV function (n = 1,749)	Trandolapril vs. placebo	3–7 days	24–50 months	Decreased mortality
SMILE[155]	MI (n = 1,556)	Zofenopril vs. placebo	24 hours	6 weeks	Decreased mortality

ACE, angiotensin-converting enzyme; HF, heart failure; LV, left ventricular; MI, myocardial infarction; NYHA, New York Heart Association.
Source: Brown NJ, Vaughan DE. Angiotensin-converting enzyme inhibitors. *Circulation*. 1998;97:1411.

doses)[161] or enalapril (5–20 mg daily)[162] were only 12 weeks in duration. Exercise duration improved significantly with all three drugs at weeks 6 and 12. No statistically significant differences were found between drugs for NYHA class changes, HF symptoms, or side effects, although a trend was noted toward greater exercise duration at week 12 with lisinopril compared with enalapril. In the third study, fosinopril (5–20 mg) was compared with enalapril (5–20 mg) daily for 1 year.[163] The fosinopril group had significantly fewer patients who were hospitalized for HF or who died (19.7%) than did the enalapril group (25%; $p = 0.028$). Nearly 60% of patients in the fosinopril group improved their NYHA class. The incidence of orthostatic hypotension was lower in the fosinopril group (1.6% vs. 7.6%; $p = 0.05$). No explanation was provided for why there might be a difference.

Based on the total body of data, it is difficult to designate an agent of choice. The ACC/AHA guidelines recommend selecting an ACE inhibitor that has shown reductions in both morbidity and mortality in clinical trials in either HF or in populations after MI. The following ACE inhibitors are considered first-line options based on clinical trials: captopril, enalapril, lisinopril, perindopril, ramipril, or trandolapril.[1]

Captopril and lisinopril are both active as the parent compound and do not have active metabolites. All other ACE inhibitors are inactive prodrugs that require enzymatic conversion by esterolytic enzymes to active metabolites (benazeprilat, enalaprilat, fosinoprilat, moexiprilat, perindoprilat, quinaprilat, ramiprilat, and trandolaprilat). The only clinical consequence of these differences is a slightly delayed onset of effect with the first dose (2–6 hours for captopril, 4–12 hours for the others). Of greater distinction, captopril has a relatively short half-life and duration of action, necessitating three to four times daily administration in most patients. Although this characteristic may be advantageous when initiating therapy by allowing closer assessment of early side effects, for chronic maintenance it is preferable to use a drug that can be given either once or twice daily. All other ACE inhibitors meet this criterion, either as the parent drug (lisinopril) or as the active metabolite (all others). Based solely on half-life data, there would be no expected difference among any of the longer-acting agents. Theoretically, they could all be administered once daily. Package insert labeling and common standards of practice, however, have led to twice-daily dosing, especially at higher doses, for enalapril, quinapril, and ramipril.

A.J.'s physician chooses to start lisinopril 5 mg daily based on evidence of clinical efficacy, improved survival, and availability as a generic medication. If there were concern about hypotension, then captopril would be preferred during the initial 1 to 2 days of initiation therapy to avoid dropping the patient's BP too quickly.

DOSE–RESPONSE RELATIONSHIPS

CASE 19-1, QUESTION 13: What is the target dose of lisinopril in A.J.? Do all patients need to be titrated to target doses?

Clinical trial evidence indicates a relationship between the degree of abatement in HF symptoms and the dose of drug given. Larger doses are more likely to improve the patient's quality of life and reduce the incidence of hospital stays, but the impact of larger doses on mortality is less clear. At the same time, higher doses are associated with a greater risk of side effects. Based on these principles, proposed recommended starting, target, and maximal doses for the ACE inhibitors are listed in Table 19-4.[21,145]

In general, the guidelines recommend that ACE inhibitors should be initiated at low doses, but titrated to the maximal tolerated target dose. Supporting this principle are the results of the Assessment of Treatment with Lisinopril and Survival trial.[164,165] Lisinopril was given to 3,164 patients hospitalized during the previous 6 months and with NYHA class II through IV HF and an LVEF less than 30%. Open-label lisinopril 2.5 to 5 mg was given for the first 2 weeks, then 12.5 to 15 mg for an additional 2 weeks. If the initial doses were tolerated, subjects were randomly assigned to daily therapy with lisinopril 2.5 to 5 mg (low dosage) or 32.5 to 35 mg (high dosage). All-cause mortality did not differ significantly between the two groups (8% lower in the highest dose group compared with the lowest dose; $p = 0.128$). In the high-dose group, hospitalizations and the combined end point of death and hospitalization were reduced by 24% ($p = 0.003$) and 12% ($p = 0.002$), respectively. The higher dose was tolerated by 90% of patients assigned this dose.

Despite these recommendations for using the highest tolerated doses, evidence also suggests that lower doses are beneficial. For example, the UK Heart Failure Network Study found that 10 mg of twice-daily enalapril was no more effective than 2.5 mg BID.[166] In this study, enalapril was given in low (2.5 mg BID), moderate (5 mg BID), and higher (10 mg BID) dosages to patients with NYHA class II or III HF. The primary combined end point (death, hospitalization from HF, and worsening HF incidence) occurred in 12.3%, 12.9%, and 14.7% of patients receiving low, moderate, and higher enalapril dosages, respectively. None of the differences among groups were statistically significant. Mortality, evaluated separately, was 4.2%, 3.3%, and 2.9%, respectively, and not significantly different. Further information on dosing, pharmacologic, and pharmacokinetic information regarding the ACE inhibitors is found in Chapter 14, Essential Hypertension.

For lisinopril, the recommended starting dosage is 2.5 to 5 mg/day. For older patients or those with other risk factors (i.e., systolic BP <100 mm Hg, those taking large doses of either loop diuretics or potassium-sparing diuretics, or those with preexisting hyponatremia, hyperkalemia, or renal insufficiency), the starting dose of 2.5 mg/day would be more appropriate. This dose, or an equivalent with one of the other drugs, should also be considered if the patient is being started directly on a long-acting drug without prior titration on captopril. For a patient such as A.J. who has already been treated with captopril for 2 days with no evidence of intolerance, a 5-mg dose is an appropriate recommendation.

The long-term target dosage of lisinopril for A.J. is 20 to 40 mg daily. No clear formula exists for deciding how quickly to titrate to this dose. It depends on several factors, including the degree of reduction in his HF symptoms and side effects, and his motivation to take the medicine. Whenever dosage adjustments are made, it may take as few as 24 hours for the patient to perceive symptom reduction, but generally full hemodynamic steady state is not reached for 1 to 2 months. On the other hand, hypotension and other side effects are more immediate. A.J. should have his dose reassessed in 1 to 2 weeks to determine whether he can tolerate a dosage increase to 20 mg daily. An SCr and potassium should be ordered at this time to assess the safety of titrating the ACE inhibitor. Thereafter, an extra 10 mg/day could be added every 2 to 4 weeks. Thus, it could take 3 months or more to titrate upward to 40 mg daily. If A.J.'s symptoms do not improve, but he has no side effects, titration can occur more quickly either by shortening the assessment periods (e.g., every week) or by using larger dose increments.

ONLINE CONTENT

For a narrated PowerPoint slide presentation regarding the challenges of initiating and titrating proven therapies in HF patients, go to http://thepoint.lww.com/AT10e.

TABLE 19-9
Clinical Trials of Angiotensin Receptor Blockers in Heart Failure

Trial	Patient Population	ARB	Treatment Duration	Outcome
ELITE[172]	NYHA II–IV (n = 722) EF ≤40%	Losartan (50 mg every day) or captopril (50 mg TID)	48 weeks	No significant difference observed for the primary end point (persistent renal dysfunction) or the secondary end point (composite of death/HF admissions). Losartan was associated with a lower mortality than captopril.
RESOLVD[174]	NYHA II–IV (n = 768) EF ≤40%	Candesartan (4, 8 or 16 mg), or candesartan (4 mg or 8 mg) + 20 mg enalapril, or 20 mg enalapril	43 weeks	Combination has greater benefits on LV remodeling. No difference in mortality. No difference in NYHA class, QOL, 6-minute walking distance.
ELITEII[173]	NYHA II–IV (n = 3,152) EF ≤40%	Losartan (50 mg every day) or captopril (50 mg TID)	48 weeks	Losartan was not superior to captopril in improving survival, but was significantly better tolerated. A subgroup analysis of ELITE II found a greater risk of death when losartan was used in addition to β-blockers.
Val-Heft[175]	NYHA II–IV (n = 5,010) EF <40%	Valsartan 160 mg BID or placebo BID	23 months	There was no difference in mortality between the two groups. In patients previously receiving both ACEI and a β-blocker (n = 1,610), the risk of death was increased with the addition of valsartan.
CHARM[176] Alternative	NYHA II–IV (n = 2,028) EF ≤40%	Candesartan (32 mg) vs. placebo	34 months	23% reduction in CV mortality or HF hospitalization favoring the candesartan group. More side effects in the candesartan group (hypotension, hyperkalemia, ↑ SCr) vs. placebo.
CHARM[177] Added	NYHA II–IV (n = 2,548) EF ≤40%	Candesartan (32 mg) + ACEI vs. placebo	41 months	15% risk reduction in CV mortality or HF admissions compared with placebo. However, more side effects in the candesartan group (hypotension, hyperkalemia, ↑ SCr) vs. placebo.
CHARM[178] Overall	NYHA II–IV (n = 7,599)	Candesartan (32 mg) vs. placebo	38 months	There was no overall difference in primary outcome of all-cause death.

ACEI, angiotensin-converting enzyme inhibitor; ARB, angiotensin receptor blocker; BID, twice a day; CV, cardiovascular; EF, ejection fraction; HF, heart failure; LV, left ventricular; NYHA, New York Heart Association; QOL, quality of life; SCr, serum creatinine; TID, three times a day.

ANGIOTENSIN RECEPTOR BLOCKERS

CASE 19-1, QUESTION 14: When should an ARB be used in A.J.?

Despite established life-saving therapies, many patients with HF remain at a high risk of CV death. Several clinical trials in HF have shown potential therapeutic benefit of the ARBs in modifying HF symptoms (Table 19-9).[167–174] Several of these trials were included in a meta-analysis that combined data on all-cause mortality and HF-related hospitalizations from a total of 17 clinical trials comparing an ARB with either placebo or an ACE inhibitor in patients with HF.[168] Most of the trials also assessed short-term clinical end points such as exercise tolerance and EF. In total, 12,469 patients were included and five ARBs (candesartan, eprosartan, irbesartan, losartan, and valsartan) were evaluated, assuming a class effect for all ARBs. ARBs favorably improved exercise tolerance and EF compared with placebo. They were not superior to ACE inhibitors in reducing all-cause mortality or hospitalizations for HF. The combination of an ARB and an ACE inhibitor was superior to ACE inhibitor monotherapy in reducing hospitalizations for HF but not in improving survival. In patients not receiving an ACE inhibitor (but receiving other HF drugs), an insignificant trend favored ARBs compared with placebo for both reductions in all-cause mortality and hospitalizations for HF.

The first major clinical trial comparing an ARB with an ACE inhibitor in patients with HF was the Evaluation of Losartan in the Elderly (ELITE) study.[172] Among the strengths of this trial are (a) a relatively large population (722 subjects) who were all ACE inhibitor–naïve, (b) comparison of the receptor antagonist with an ACE inhibitor (captopril), and (c) an adequate duration (48 weeks) to allow a preliminary outcome evaluation of frequency of hospitalizations and incidence of death. All subjects were 65 years of age or older with NYHA class II through IV HF, had an EF of 40% or less (mean, 31%), and were not previously treated with either an ACE inhibitor or an ARB. Diuretics were used by 75% of the subjects, with 55% taking digoxin and 40% taking a non–ACE inhibitor vasodilator. Losartan was started at 12.5 mg/day in 352 patients and titrated to a dose as high as 50 mg/day in 300 of them. The 370 subjects randomly assigned to receive captopril began therapy at 6.25 mg three times daily and were titrated to a maximal dose of 50 mg three times daily (n = 310). For the primary study end point, a sustained increase in renal function decline, the two drugs performed identically with 10.5% of subjects in each group having a greater than 0.3 mg/dL rise in SCr. Similarly, functional ability increases were equal in both groups, and only 5.7% of both groups were hospitalized for worsening HF. An unexpected finding was an insignificant trend toward more deaths from all causes in the captopril group (n = 32; 8.7%) compared with losartan (n = 17; 4.8%). Also, more subjects discontinued captopril than losartan because of adverse effects (20.8% vs. 12.2%). In particular, 3.8% of patients on captopril stopped the drug because of cough compared with none of those on losartan.

Several limitations of this study should be noted: (a) by design, the patients were all elderly; (b) 40% of the subjects were taking other vasodilators as a confounding variable; and (c) the primary end point was change in renal function, not hospitalization or death. Nonetheless, the study provided evidence that losartan was at least as effective as the reference ACE inhibitor (captopril) and that patients with HF have equal or fewer side effects with losartan, especially less cough.

The follow-up ELITE II Trial was specifically designed to test the hypothesis that losartan was superior to captopril in terms of reduction in mortality and morbidity in patients 60 years of age or older.[173] Inclusion criteria and the dosages of losartan and captopril were identical to those of the first ELITE Trial. By enrolling a larger number of subjects (n = 3,162), the study was powered to assess the primary end point of all-cause mortality. The intent was to continue the study until a combined total of 510 deaths occurred between the two treatment groups. After a mean follow-up of 1.5 years, no significance difference was seen in all-cause mortality (17.7% losartan vs. 15.9% captopril), sudden death (9% vs. 7.3%), or all-cause mortality plus hospitalization (47.7% vs. 44.9%) between the two treatment groups. Although ARB treatment was not clinically superior to ACE inhibitor therapy, it was better tolerated with a withdrawal rate of 9.4%, as compared with 14.5% with ACE inhibitor therapy ($p = 0.001$). Specifically, significantly fewer patients experienced cough with the ARB.

In the Randomized Evaluation of Strategies for Left Ventricular Dysfunction (RESOLVD)[174] study, 768 subjects were randomly assigned to receive enalapril (up to 20 mg/day), candesartan (up to 16 mg/day), or a combination of both drugs added to diuretics, digoxin, or both for an average of 43 weeks. Inclusion criteria included NYHA class II through IV HF, LVEF less than 40%, and a 6-minute walking distance less than 500 meters. As in the ELITE trials, all the subjects were ACE inhibitor naïve. The combination of candesartan and enalapril was more beneficial for preventing LV dilatation and suppressing neurohormonal activation than either candesartan or enalapril alone. No differences were found among any of the three treatment groups in either hospitalization or mortality rates. Although not powered as a mortality trial, mortality rates were higher in the subjects receiving candesartan alone (6.1%) or candesartan combined with enalapril (8.7%) than in the group that received enalapril alone (3.7%).

The Valsartan Heart Failure Trial (Val-HeFT) was a double-blind, placebo-controlled study to measure the morbidity and mortality in NYHA class II through IV HF patients given valsartan.[175] In contrast to the ELITE and RESOLVD studies, 93% of subjects were already taking an ACE inhibitor at the time of randomization, 35% were taking a β-blocker, and 30% were taking both drugs. Patients were randomly assigned to receive valsartan (n = 2,511) or placebo (n = 2,499) twice daily. The starting dose of valsartan was 40 mg BID, which was then titrated up to 160 mg BID by doubling the dose every 2 weeks. The target dose was achieved in 84% of patients taking the active drug. After a mean follow-up of 23 months (range, 0 to 38 months), no significant difference was observed in all-cause mortality between the valsartan group (19.7%) and the control group (19.4%). The combined end point of mortality and morbidity (including hospitalization from HF, cardiac arrest with resuscitation, and need for IV support) was significantly reduced among patients receiving valsartan (723 events, 28.8%) as compared with those receiving placebo (801 events, 32.1%), a 13% reduction ($p = 0.009$). Adverse events were low, leading to discontinuation of valsartan in 9.9% of subjects compared with 7.2% with placebo. Dizziness, hypotension, and renal impairment all occurred more frequently in those treated with valsartan.

Subgroup analysis of the Val-HeFT study data raises interesting questions. For example, the observed reduction in the combined end point of morbidity and mortality was most pronounced in the small subgroup of only 226 patients (7% of the total study population) not receiving an ACE inhibitor compared with patients on the combination of an ACE inhibitor and valsartan. Further post hoc analysis found that within the 35% of subjects (n = 1,610) taking the combination of an ACE inhibitor and a β-blocker at baseline, the addition of valsartan as a third drug was associated with a trend toward increased morbidity and a statistically significant increase in the combined end point of mortality and morbidity. The clinical significance of these findings is unknown.

The overall study results suggest that a combination of valsartan and an ACE inhibitor reduces morbidity, but not mortality. Despite the intriguing results of the subgroup analysis, it is difficult to determine the independent effect of valsartan (i.e., when not combined with an ACE inhibitor or β-blocker) on morbidity or mortality. More worrisome is the implication that the three-drug combination of valsartan, an ACE inhibitor, and a β-blocker adversely affects morbidity and mortality.

Subsequent trials were designed to determine whether a combination of neurohumoral agents provided additional benefits without causing harm in patients with HF. The Valsartan in Acute Myocardial Infarction Trial (VALIANT) of stable patients after MI with LV dysfunction was designed to test the hypothesis that valsartan alone and in combination with captopril (ACE inhibitor) would improve survival. In VALIANT, 70% of the patients were also receiving β-blockers. All-cause mortality, the primary end point, was identical in all groups. In addition, an increased rate of side effects was seen in the combination group. The failure to show a statistically significant difference in survival benefits could be owing to the trial design. The patients were simultaneously started on an ACE inhibitor and ARB, which is a variation from typical HF trials where patients are entered with an ACE inhibitor before the initiation of an ARB. Interestingly, among the subgroup of patients taking β-blockers, no evidence was found of harmful interaction with triple therapy.[179] As a result of the VALIANT trial, the FDA approved the use of valsartan in patients at high risk after a heart attack, and in those with HF, the drug is no longer only reserved for ACE inhibitor–intolerant patients.

The best evidence addressing the efficacy and safety of ARB in HF comes from a series of three investigations known collectively as the Candesartan in Heart Failure Assessment of Reduction in Morbidity and Mortality (CHARM) trial. The individual components of the CHARM Program are (a) CHARM-Alternative, (b) CHARM-Added, and (c) CHARM-Preserved.[176,177,180] All three investigations were randomized, double-blind, placebo-controlled trials that enrolled adult patients (>18 years of age) with at least a 4-week history of symptomatic (NYHA class II–IV) HF. Subjects randomly assigned to candesartan were started on 4 mg and titrated to 32 mg once daily, as tolerated. Standard therapy (diuretics, β-blockers, digoxin, and spironolactone) was continued. For all three trials, the primary end point was the combined incidence of CV death, HF hospitalizations, or both. The differences in admission criteria and outcomes among the individual trials are discussed in the sections below.

CHARM-Alternative enrolled 2,028 subjects who met all of the inclusion criteria defined above plus two additional criteria: an EF of 40% or less (i.e., systolic dysfunction) and intolerance of ACE inhibitors (cough, 72%; hypotension, 13%; renal dysfunction, 12%). Thus, subjects in this group received either an ARB alone (n = 1,013) or placebo (n = 1,015) without an ACE inhibitor, but this was not a head-to-head comparison of an ACE inhibitor with an ARB. After a median follow-up of 33.7 months, a 23% reduction was found in the primary outcome of CV death, hospital admission for HF, or both in the candesartan group (33%) compared with placebo (40%; $p = 0.004$). The overall incidence of drug discontinuations because of adverse

TABLE 19-10
Adverse Events That Lead to Permanent Drug Discontinuation

Trial	Outcomes	Candesartan	Placebo	p Value
CHARM-Alternative[176]	Any adverse event or laboratory abnormality	21.5%	19.3%	0.23
	Hypotension	3.7%	0.9%	<0.0001
	Increased creatinine	6.1%	2.7%	<0.0001
	Hyperkalemia	1.9%	0.3%	0.0005
CHARM-Added[177]	Any adverse event or laboratory abnormality			0.0003
	Hypotension	4.5%	3.5%	0.079
	Increased creatinine	7.8%	4.1%	0.0001
	Hyperkalemia	3.4%	0.7%	<0.0001
CHARM-Preserved[180]	Any adverse event or laboratory abnormality	17.8%	13.5%	0.001
	Hypotension	2.4%	1.1%	0.006
	Increased creatinine	4.8%	2.4%	<0.001
	Hyperkalemia	1.5%	0.6%	0.019
CHARM-Overall[178]	Any adverse event or laboratory abnormality	21%	16.7%	<0.001
	Hypotension	3.5%	1.7%	<0.0001
	Increased creatinine	6.2%	3.0%	<0.0001
	Hyperkalemia	2.2%	0.6%	<0.0001

events was not statistically different between candesartan (21%) and placebo (19%), but there were significantly more reports of symptomatic hypotension (3.7% vs. 0.9%), increased creatinine levels (6.1% vs. 2.7%), and hyperkalemia (1.9% vs. 0.3%) in those treated with candesartan. Of 39 patients who previously experienced angioedema when taking an ACE inhibitor, only 1 patient discontinued the study drug because of angioedema (Table 19-10). The authors concluded that candesartan was generally well tolerated and reduced CV morbidity and mortality in patients with symptomatic chronic HF who were not receiving ACE inhibitors because of intolerance.

The CHARM-Added trial attempted to determine whether the combination of an ACE-inhibitor plus an ARB offered any clinical advantages compared with an ACE inhibitor alone in patients with symptomatic HF with an EF of 40% or less (systolic dysfunction). Prior use of an ACE inhibitor was required for the 2,548 patients enrolled in this trial (96% were taking an ACE inhibitor dose comparable to that used in previous mortality trials). At baseline, 55% of the patients were treated with β-blockers and 17% were on spironolactone. After a median follow-up of 41 months, 483 (38%) of patients in the combination ACE inhibitor–candesartan-added group experienced the primary outcome of CV death, hospital admission for HF, or both compared with 538 (42%) in the placebo plus ACE inhibitor group (a 15% relative risk reduction; $p = 0.011$). Overall, the addition of candesartan to an ACE inhibitor and other usual HF treatments led to a further reduction in CV events in patients with chronic systolic HF. It is interesting to compare the result of the CHARM-Added trial with those of the Val-HeFT study. In Val-HeFT, 93% of the subjects receiving the ARB valsartan were concurrently receiving an ACE inhibitor. The combined end point of morbidity and mortality was significantly reduced with combination therapy in Val-HeFT, but mortality alone was not reduced. A trend toward more deaths in the small subgroup receiving the triple combination of a β-blocker with an ACE inhibitor and ARB was observed, whereas β-blocker use had no adverse effect in CHARM-Added.

The combined results of all three CHARM components (CHARM-Added, CHARM-Alternative, and CHARM-Preserved; see detailed discussion of CHARM-Preserved in Case 19-7, Question 1) were reported in the CHARM-Overall trial.[178] This composite analysis evaluates the benefits of candesartan in symptomatic patients with HF, regardless of LV systolic function. Overall, 3,803 patients were assigned to candesartan and 3,796 to placebo. A different primary end point was chosen for the CHARM-Overall analysis: all-cause death. Although the combined results failed to detect a clinically significant reduction in all-cause death between candesartan and placebo (9% reduction; $p = 0.32$), significant reductions were seen in CV death (12%), hospital admission for HF (21%), and combined CV death or hospital admission for HF (16%), which was the primary end point for the individual trials.

The collective results of the CHARM program further reinforce the conclusion that ARB can reduce morbidity and mortality in symptomatic patients with systolic HF, and they can be safely used in patients who are intolerant of ACE inhibitor therapy. Combination therapy (ACE inhibitor plus ARB) with concomitant use of β-blockers appears to be beneficial and safe, as long as patients are closely monitored for adverse effects. For symptomatic patients with HF with normal EF (diastolic dysfunction), addition of an ARB may be beneficial in reducing hospitalizations; however, the study did not show improved survival.

From this information, ARBs provide survival benefits in systolic HF when used in ACE inhibitor–intolerant patients or as an add-on therapy to ACE inhibitors and β-blockers. However, current guidelines do not recommend the routine use of triple therapy, and A.J. should not be started on an ARB in addition to his lisinopril. If A.J. develops a cough on lisinopril, he can be switched to an ARB such as candesartan. (See Chapter 14, Essential Hypertension, for further information on the mechanisms of action, metabolism, and dosing of ARBs.)

Side Effects

ANGIOTENSIN-CONVERTING ENZYME INHIBITOR–INDUCED COUGH

CASE 19-1, QUESTION 15: A.J. presents to the outpatient HF clinic with an annoying productive cough after 6 weeks of lisinopril therapy. His chest examination reveals no evidence of wheezing, with only a few crackles, his neck veins

are only minimally elevated over normal, his ankle edema is 1+, and his weight is stable. All laboratory values are normal. Could the cough be a symptom of his HF or is it ACE inhibitor–induced? What are the recommendations for an ACE inhibitor–induced cough?

Cough can be a sign of HF in patients with pulmonary congestion. In extreme cases, patients demonstrate "cardiac asthma" with severe air hunger, wheezing, and dyspnea. However, A.J.'s HF is much improved as evidenced by the objective data. The absence of wheezing and no prior history of asthma or smoking make an obstructive airways disease (asthma or chronic obstructive pulmonary disease) unlikely. It is possible that he does have bronchitis, but he does not report having a cold or other respiratory illness preceding the cough. Without other causes, an ACEI inhibitor–induced cough is most likely.

This side effect occurs with all ACE inhibitors.[181] Case reports indicate a possibly lower incidence with fosinopril, but this has not been confirmed under controlled conditions.[182] Cough is a well-established complication of ACE inhibitors and presents as dry and nonproductive; sometimes described as a "tickle in the back of the throat." This complication can arise within hours of the first dose, or it can present after weeks to months of treatment. Although resolution of the cough usually occurs within 1 to 4 weeks, in some patients it can persist up to 3 months after discontinuation of therapy.

Various case reports have found an incidence of cough in 5% to 35% of all patients. The incidence may be even lower, approximately about 3%, and is dose-independent.[183] One investigator found a 5% to 10% incidence in white patients of European descent that rose to nearly 50% in Chinese patients.[184] There may also be a higher incidence in women and black populations.[181]

Bradykinin accumulation within the upper airway and decreased metabolism of proinflammatory mediators such as substance P or prostaglandins are proposed mechanisms of ACE inhibitor–induced cough. These chemicals then act as irritant substances in the airways to increase bronchial reactivity and induce coughing. Bradykinin stimulates unmyelinated afferent sensory C fibers by type J receptors involved in the cough reflex.

Bradykinin is also a potent bronchoconstrictor, but pulmonary function remains unchanged, and persons with asthma are no more susceptible to the reaction than those who do not have asthma. Substance P, also degraded by ACE, has been implicated because it is a neurotransmitter for afferent sensory fibers, specifically C fibers. Because this is a pharmacologic effect rather than an allergic reaction, dose reduction or switching from one ACE inhibitor to another is generally not helpful. The only way to definitively diagnose the drug-induced cough is to discontinue therapy. Even then, false-positive results can occur if the patient had a mild case of bronchitis that spontaneously resolved at about the same time that the ACE inhibitor was discontinued. If the cough persists after drug discontinuation, other causes should be investigated such as coexisting gastroesophageal reflux disease or allergic rhinitis.

Because of the long-term survival benefits of ACE inhibitors, the AHA guidelines recommend continuing ACE inhibitors if the cough is not severe, even when other causes of cough have been excluded. In contrast, the American College of Chest Physicians evidence-based practice guidelines recommend discontinuation of therapy if ACE inhibitor–induced cough is even suggested.[183] After cessation of therapy, resolution of cough confirms the diagnosis. For patients with persistent cough, ARB or hydralazine-isosorbide are safe alternatives. Therefore, A.J. can continue taking lisinopril for another couple of weeks to determine whether the cough will resolve on its own. His symptoms of HF have abated since the initiation of ACE inhibitor therapy, and the cough may be no more than an annoyance. He is not at risk for experiencing asthma or other airway problems. If his cough persists, an ARB is probably the best alternative.

OTHER ANGIOTENSIN-CONVERTING ENZYME INHIBITOR AND ANGIOTENSIN RECEPTOR BLOCKER SIDE EFFECTS

HYPERKALEMIA

CASE 19-1, QUESTION 16: What are the other side effects of both ACE inhibitors and ARBs that need to be monitored? Does changing from an ACE inhibitor to an ARB reduce the risk of any of these side effects?

The ACE inhibitors, ARB, and nonselective β-blockers[185] have the potential to raise serum potassium concentrations via indirect aldosterone inhibition and other neurohormonal actions.[186,187] For most patients, the magnitude of increase in serum potassium concentration from ACE inhibitors and ARBs alone is relatively small, but the risk for developing hyperkalemia is greater if the patient has compromised renal function or advanced HF. Combination therapy of an ACE or ARB with potassium supplements, potassium-sparing diuretics, or β-blockers further accentuates the risk of hyperkalemia, regardless of the sequence of initiation of the individual drugs.

Several case reports and case series have reported hyperkalemia and hospitalizations induced by spironolactone in patients with HF. This became more evident as prescribing patterns for spironolactone dramatically changed after publication of the RALES study.[188] Not only was there a significant increase in the number of prescriptions for spironolactone for patients with HF, but doses higher than recommended by the clinical trials were often used, especially in patients with evidence of preexisting renal dysfunction. In addition, evidence indicated inadequate monitoring of serum potassium, renal function, and concomitant drug therapy. Although concurrent use of a potassium-wasting diuretic (e.g., a thiazide or loop diuretic) may counteract potassium retention from spironolactone or other drugs (ACE inhibitors, ARB, nonselective β-blockers), it is nearly impossible to predict who will exhibit hypokalemia or hyperkalemia or remain normokalemic.[189,190] Thus, each patient must be assessed individually for personal response to various drug combinations and to determine whether there is a need for potassium supplements or a reduction in their doses. Close monitoring of serum potassium is required; potassium levels and renal function should be checked in 3 days and at 1 week after initiation of therapy and at least monthly for the first 3 months (Table 19-11).

ANGIOEDEMA

Angioedema (angioneurotic edema) is a severe, potentially life-threatening complication of ACE inhibitor treatment.[191–193] Characterized by facial and neck swelling with obstruction to air flow by laryngeal and bronchial edema, this reaction resembles anaphylaxis. The mechanism of ACE inhibitor induction of angioedema is unknown, but is thought to be related to hypersensitivity to accumulated vasodilating kinins, similar to the cough reaction.

Some, but not all, persons with drug-induced angioedema have a history of familial angioedema associated with a genetic defect in their complement system. ACE inhibitors are contraindicated in this population. In one series of case reports, 22% of the reported angioedema reactions occurred within 1 month of starting therapy, with the remaining 77% arising from several months to years later.[192] Black patients and women may have a higher prevalence. Of concern is the observation that ACE inhibitor–induced angioedema is often misdiagnosed.[193] Several

TABLE 19-11
Various Causes of Hyperkalemia and Strategies to Minimize Risk

Cause	Mechanism	Strategies to Minimize Risk
Aldosterone blockers	Decreased levels of aldosterone and subsequent potassium retention.	GFR should be determined and aldosterone antagonist should be avoided if creatinine clearance is <30 mL/min and baseline serum potassium is >5.0 mEq/L. An initial dose of spironolactone 12.5 mg or eplerenone 25 mg is recommended, after which the dose may be increased to spironolactone 25 mg or eplerenone 50 mg if appropriate. Close monitoring of serum potassium is required; potassium levels and renal function should be checked in 3 days and at 1 week after initiation of therapy and at least monthly for the first 3 months.
RAAS blockade by ACE inhibitors and ARBs Note: risk increases at higher doses (enalapril or lisinopril ≥10 mg/d)	Inhibition of angiotensin II production or receptor binding reduces the delivery of sodium and water to the distal nephron, which, in combination with hypoaldosteronism, promotes hyperkalemia.	Doses of drugs should be decreased as appropriate.
NSAIDs	Inhibit renal prostaglandin synthesis (PGE_2 and PGI_2), resulting in hyporeninemic hypoaldosteronism. Decreased availability of sodium for exchange with potassium at distal tubular sites.	NSAIDs and cyclo-oxygenase-2 inhibitors should be avoided.
Potassium-sparing diuretics, cyclosporine, tacrolimus, trimethoprim, and heparin	Decreased excretion of potassium.	Close monitoring of serum potassium is required. Doses of drugs known to cause hyperkalemia should be decreased as appropriate.
Patients who have increased dietary potassium intake, use salt substitutes (a rich source of potassium), or take potassium supplements in combination with aldosterone antagonists	In the presence of renal insufficiency, decreased potassium excretion occurs.	Potassium supplements should be discontinued or reduced. Patients should be educated on foods rich in potassium and to avoid salt substitutes.
HF patients with diabetes taking aldosterone antagonists	Hyporeninemic hypoaldosteronism leading to decreased levels of aldosterone and subsequent potassium retention. Insulin deficiency can stimulate the shift of potassium to the extracellular space.	Hyperglycemia should be monitored and appropriate drug therapy should be determined to treat diabetes.
Advanced age, low muscle mass, or renal insufficiency (serum creatinine >1.6 mg/dL)	Impaired release of renin resulting in hypoaldosteronism. SCr may not accurately reflect GFR. Risk of hyperkalemia increases progressively as SCr rises.	GFR should be determined and doses adjusted accordingly.

ACE, angiotensin-converting enzyme; ARBs, angiotensin receptor blockers; GFR, glomerular filtration rate; HF, heart failure; NSAIDs, nonsteroidal anti-inflammatory drugs; PGE_2, prostaglandin E_2; PGI_2, prostaglandin I_2; RAAS, renin-angiotensin-aldosterone system.

of the patients described in one series had been treated again with the same or a different ACE inhibitor followed by a repeat episode of angioedema. It is prudent to avoid all ACE inhibitors in any patient with a history of angioedema from any cause.

Because the mechanism of ACE inhibitor–induced angioedema is thought to be caused by kinin accumulation, changing to an ARB might be an option.[194] Several case reports, however, have implicated candesartan, losartan, and valsartan as possible causative agents of angioedema.[191,195–198] In some cases, the subjects had previously experienced angioedema with an ACE inhibitor (indicating possible cross-reactivity), whereas others were ACE inhibitor–naïve. One author claims that ARB-induced angioedema usually manifests after long-term administration (late onset) and with milder symptoms compared with relatively earlier onset with ACE inhibitors. Similar findings showing a small but potential risk for ARB-induced angioedema in patients who are ACE inhibitor–intolerant comes from the CHARM-Alternative trial.[176] Of 39 patients with a history of angioedema while taking an ACE inhibitor, 3 experienced angioedema on candesartan, although only 1 of the 3 actually discontinued taking candesartan. For now, it is prudent to assess risk-benefit, and ARBs should be used cautiously in the management of patients who have angioedema from ACE inhibitors.

EFFECTS OF ANGIOTENSIN-CONVERTING ENZYME INHIBITORS AND ANGIOTENSIN RECEPTOR BLOCKERS ON KIDNEY FUNCTION

The effects of ACE inhibitors and ARBs on RBF and renal function are complex. As seen in Figure 19-7, glomerular filtration is optimal when intraglomerular pressure is maintained at normal pressures. The balance between afferent flow into the glomerulus and efferent flow exiting the glomerulus determines the intraglomerular pressure. A drop in afferent flow or pressure occurring as a result of hypotension, volume loss (e.g., blood loss or overdiuresis), hypoalbuminemia, decreased CO (e.g., HF), or obstructive lesions such as renal artery stenosis can significantly lower intraglomerular pressure and lead to impaired renal function. Similarly, long-standing HTN can damage glomerular basement membrane capillaries and cause renal insufficiency.

In the case of low-pressure or low-flow states, the RAAS is activated to maintain intraglomerular pressure. A key factor in preserving glomerular pressure is *efferent vasoconstriction*

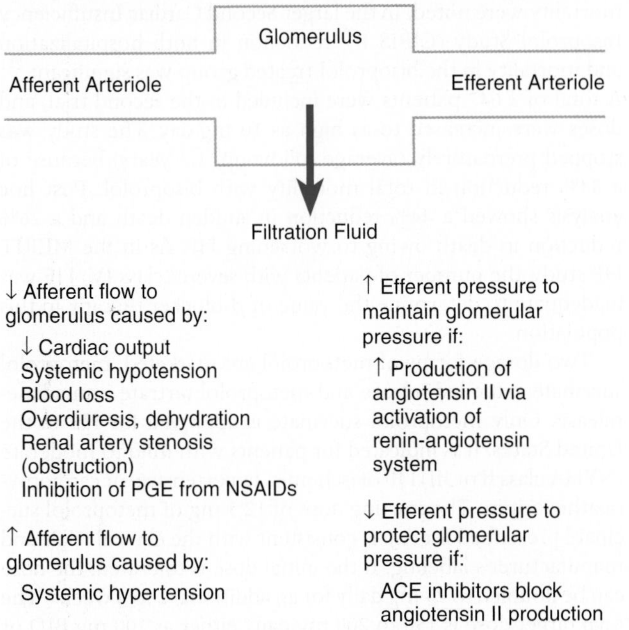

FIGURE 19-7 Factors affecting renal blood flow. Glomerular filtration is optimal when adequate hydrostatic pressure is maintained in the glomerulus. Governing factors include the blood flow rate to the glomerulus and the balance of afferent and efferent arteriole dilation and constriction. ACE, angiotensin-converting enzyme; NSAIDs, nonsteroidal anti-inflammatory drugs; PGE, prostaglandin E.

mediated by angiotensin II. Increased efferent pressure helps to maintain intraglomerular pressure by impeding blood flow out of the glomerulus. When patients with low-pressure states are given ACE inhibitors or ARBs, the protective mechanism of efferent vasoconstriction is inhibited and renal function can significantly and rapidly worsen. Conversely, in patients with hypertensive renal disease, glomerular function actually can improve because the ACE inhibitors lower afferent pressure and help protect the kidney. ACE inhibitors slow the progression of diabetic nephropathy and reduce proteinuria independent of their effect on BP (see Chapter 53, Diabetes Mellitus).

Patients with HF present with a complex picture. By decreasing afterload and preload, CO may improve after ACE inhibitor or ARB therapy, thus preserving or even enhancing RBF. If, however, starting ACE inhibitors or ARB leads to a rapid decrease in systemic BP that is not followed by an increase in CO, worsening renal function may ensue. It is impossible to predict which event will occur. Therefore, ACE inhibitor or ARB therapy needs to be started with low doses, and careful monitoring of the BP and renal function should occur as dosages are increased. Renal function and BP should be checked before and 1 to 2 weeks after initiation or dose increase. Patients with risk factors such as pre-existing renal insufficiency or concomitant treatment with NSAIDs or high-dose diuretics may require more frequent monitoring. Diuretics are not contraindicated, but the diuretic dosage may need to be reduced to avoid overly aggressive diuresis and the accompanying volume depletion and hypotension.

Use of β-Blockers in Systolic Heart Failure

CASE 19-1, QUESTION 17: After 3 days of furosemide and an ACE inhibitor, A.J.'s PND has resolved, but he still has difficulty walking without SOB and fatigue. His lower extremity edema has been significantly reduced. His current BP is 145/90 mm Hg, his pulse is 82 beats/minute, and his weight has dropped to 73 kg after diuresis. Repeat laboratory measurements include the following results:

Na, 139 mEq/L
K, 4.3 mEq/L
Cl, 98 mEq/L
CO_2, 27 mEq/L
BUN, 27 mg/dL
SCr, 0.6 mg/dL

The medical team has decided to discharge A.J. soon. You recommend that A.J. should be started on a β-blocker before discharge. What is your rationale?

The physiologic basis for the use of β-blockers in HF and the changes observed in receptor sensitivity are described in greater detail in the Pathophysiology section.[25–30] β-Blockers have been evaluated during randomized clinical trials in more than 20,000 patients with varying degrees of systolic HF.[25–30] Five meta-analyses have arrived at the same conclusions: the use of β-blockers (primarily bisoprolol, metoprolol succinate, or carvedilol) is associated with a consistent 30% reduction in mortality and a 40% reduction in hospitalizations in patients with HF.[199–203]

The ACC/AHA guidelines recommend bisoprolol, metoprolol succinate, or carvedilol for all patients with stable HF caused by LV systolic dysfunction, unless there is a contraindication to their use or the patient is unable to tolerate treatment with a β-blocker.[21] They should be a part of the primary treatment plan with an ACE inhibitor or ARB. Patients should receive a β-blocker to slow the rate of disease progression and reduce the risk of sudden death. Patients do not need to be taking high doses of ACE inhibitors before being considered for treatment with a β-blocker. To the contrary, in patients taking a low dose of an ACE inhibitor, the addition of a β-blocker produces a greater reduction in symptoms and in the risk of death than an increase in the dose of an ACE inhibitor. β-Blockers can be initiated before discharge for the vast majority of patients hospitalized for HF.[204] Only those clinically unstable patients who are hospitalized in an intensive care unit, require IV positive inotropic support, have severe fluid overload or depletion, have symptomatic bradycardia or advanced heart block (unless treated with a pacemaker), or have a history of poorly controlled reactive airways disease are not candidates for a β-blocker.[205]

Based on all these factors, there is no question that A.J. should be started on a β-blocker. Treatment with a β-blocker should be initiated at low doses, followed by gradual increments in dose every 1 to 2 weeks as tolerated by the patient. Transient bradycardia, hypotension, and fatigue are not uncommon during the first 24 to 48 hours when β-blockers are first started or during subsequent incremental increases in dosage. Thus, patients should be monitored daily for changes in vital signs (pulse and BP) and symptoms during this up-titration period. Bradycardia, heart block, and hypotension can be asymptomatic and require no intervention other than instructing the patient not to arise too quickly from a lying position to avoid postural changes. If either of these complications is accompanied by dizziness, lightheadedness, or blurred vision, it may be necessary to reduce the dose of β-blocker, the ACE inhibitor, or both or to slow the up-titration. The sense of lassitude generally resolves within several weeks without other intervention, but may be a reason to slow up-titration of the dose and, rarely, to reduce the dose or discontinue therapy. In patients in whom benefits are especially apparent, but bradycardia or heart block is a concern, insertion of a pacemaker should be considered.

Because initiation of β-blocker therapy can also cause fluid retention, patients should be instructed to weigh themselves daily and to adjust concomitantly administered diuretics as appropriate. Conversely, diuretic doses should be decreased temporarily when patients become hypotensive or their BUN begins to rise. Planned increments in the dose of a β-blocker should be delayed until any side effects observed with lower doses are tolerable or absent. In clinical trials, up to 85% of patients are able to tolerate short- and long-term treatment with these drugs and achieve the maximal planned dose.

METOPROLOL AND BISOPROLOL

CASE 19-1, QUESTION 18: Metoprolol succinate (12.5 mg) is prescribed for A.J. Is this a good choice of agent and starting dose? What other similar drugs have been used to treat HF?

Several clinical trials substantiate the clinical benefits of metoprolol, a relatively selective β_1-receptor blocker, in HF.[206–209] By blocking β_1 receptors in the myocardium, HR, contractility, and CO are reduced at rest and during exercise, without a compensatory increase in peripheral vascular resistance. The relative sparing of β_2-receptors in the peripheral vasculature and lungs reduces vasoconstrictive and bronchospastic complications. In contrast to bucindolol and carvedilol, metoprolol has been shown to upregulate myocardial β_2-receptors.[25]

In the Metoprolol in Dilated Cardiomyopathy (MDC) study, 383 patients with nonischemic dilated cardiomyopathy and class II or III HF were randomly assigned to immediate-release metoprolol tartrate (initiated at 5 mg BID and titrated to 100–150 mg/day in divided doses) or placebo.[209] All were continued on standard therapy with diuretics, vasodilators, and digoxin as tolerated. In this trial a trend toward decreased mortality and listing for heart transplantation in the active treatment group was noted.

The Metoprolol CR/XL Randomized Intervention Trial in Heart Failure (MERIT HF) showed a 35% reduction in all-cause mortality with sustained-release metoprolol succinate.[209] In this trial, 3,991 patients, most of whom had NYHA class II or III HF, were randomly assigned to receive metoprolol succinate controlled-release/extended-release (CR/XL) or placebo. The starting dose of metoprolol was 12.5 to 25 mg/day, which was gradually increased every 2 weeks to the target dose of 200 mg/day. Conventional therapy with diuretics, ACE inhibitors, and digoxin was continued. At the end of the trial, 64% of subjects assigned to active drug had reached the target dose. Planned follow-up was for 2 years, but the study was halted prematurely because of a statistically significant decrease in all-cause mortality in the metoprolol arm. Specifically, there was a 34% reduction in total mortality with a 38% decrease in CV mortality, 41% reduction in sudden death, and 49% reduction from death owing to worsening HF. All-cause hospitalization was also reduced by 18%, and hospitalization for worsening HF was decreased by 35%. Although the number of subjects was too small to detect a statistical difference, patients with severe (class IV) HF seemed to benefit as well. Up to 15% of subjects had clinical worsening of HF, even at low metoprolol doses.

Encouraging results have also been seen with another relatively β_1-selective drug, bisoprolol fumarate.[210,211] In the first Cardiac Insufficiency Bisoprolol Study (CIBIS I), 641 subjects with moderate to severe HF were randomly assigned to placebo or bisoprolol (starting dose, 1.25 mg/day; maximal dose, 5 mg/day) added to conventional therapy for an average of 23 months.[210] A statistically significant reduction in HF-associated hospitalization with the active drug and an insignificant trend toward reduced mortality were noted. In the larger Second Cardiac Insufficiency Bisoprolol Study (CIBIS II), reduction in both hospitalization and mortality in the bisoprolol-treated group was significant.[211] A total of 2,647 patients were included in the second trial, and doses were increased to as high as 10 mg/day. The study was stopped prematurely (average follow-up, 1.3 years) because of a 34% reduction in total mortality with bisoprolol. Post hoc analysis showed a 44% reduction in sudden death and a 26% reduction in death owing to worsening HF. As in the MERIT HF study, the number of patients with severe (class IV) HF was inadequate to determine the value of β-blocker therapy in this population.

Two dosage forms of metoprolol are marketed: metoprolol succinate extended-release and metoprolol tartrate immediate-release. Only metoprolol succinate is approved for HF in the United States. It is indicated for patients with mild to moderate (NYHA class II or III) HF of ischemic, hypertensive, or cardiomyopathic origin. The starting dose of 12.5 mg of metoprolol succinate prescribed for A.J. is consistent with the clinical trials and manufacturer's labeling. If the initial dose is tolerated, the dose can be doubled to 25 mg daily for an additional 2 to 4 weeks. The final target dose is 150 to 200 mg daily either as 100 mg BID or 200 mg once daily.

Even though it is not approved for this indication in the United States, immediate-release metoprolol tartrate is sometimes used. After a test dose of 12.5 mg, the starting dose is 12.5 mg twice daily for 1 or 2 weeks. The smallest immediate-release tablet size available is 25-mg tablets; therefore, during the initial 1 to 2 weeks of treatment, the tablets will have to be split in half to achieve the appropriate dosing regimen. Maintenance with a generic form of the immediate-release product is less expensive than the generic extended-release product.

When choosing among the various formulations of metoprolol, pharmacokinetic and bioavailability differences should be considered.[206,207] Metoprolol succinate is available as 25-, 50-, 100-, and 200-mg tablets. Each tablet contains many tiny metoprolol succinate pellets, each individually coated with an ethyl cellulose polymeric membrane. Gastrointestinal fluid penetrates the membrane of each pellet and slowly dissolves the drug. The saturated metoprolol solution is then released at a constant rate for 20 hours, consistent with zero-order kinetics, and provides β-blockade for 24 hours. The extended-release formulation retains its release characteristics even if the scored tablet is divided in half, but it should not be crushed or chewed. Having the ability to split tablets is useful in the titration of metoprolol succinate when the goal is to reach target doses and sometimes patients require slower titrations.

Metoprolol has several metabolic routes of elimination that can affect dosing and drug interactions. The major routes of elimination are via α-hydroxylation, *O*-demethylation, and *N*-dealkylation.[206,207] A smaller portion is metabolized by cytochrome P-450 2D6, and drugs that inhibit metabolism of that isoenzyme may affect the drug's plasma levels. Approximately 10% of patients are poor metabolizers, resulting in higher drug plasma concentrations in these patients.

A.J. should be advised that the beneficial clinical response to metoprolol is usually delayed and may require 2 to 3 months to become apparent. Even if symptoms do not abate, long-term treatment should be maintained to reduce the risk of major clinical events. Abrupt withdrawal of treatment with a β-blocker can lead to clinical deterioration and should be avoided.[212]

Bisoprolol is FDA approved for treatment of HF. Dosage size limitations, however, limit clinical use of this drug. For example, the starting dose of bisoprolol is 1.25 mg/day, whereas the smallest commercially available dose is a 5-mg scored tablet. Attempting to break the tablet into quarters is not clinically practical.

CARVEDILOL

CASE 19-1, QUESTION 19: Would carvedilol be a better alternative than metoprolol for A.J.? What would be an appropriate dose and dosing schedule?

Carvedilol, a mixed α- and β-blocker, was the first drug of this class to obtain FDA approval for management of HF.[213] It is also theorized to possess antioxidant effects, which can protect against loss of cardiac myocytes and scavenge oxygen free radicals that are thought to potentiate myocardial necrosis. The correlation of these findings to clinical outcome is unknown.

Two pivotal studies support the use of carvedilol. The first was the US Carvedilol Heart Failure Study.[214–218] Subjects were almost equally divided between NYHA class II and III HF and all had an EF of 35% or less (mean, 22%) despite diuretics (95%), digoxin (90%), and an ACE inhibitor (95%). Subjects with a major myocardial event in the previous 3 months were excluded. After an initial open-label period when all patients received 6.25 mg twice daily of carvedilol, subjects were stratified based on severity of their HF and then randomly assigned to receive either placebo ($n = 398$) or carvedilol ($n = 690$). The maximal dose given was 50 mg twice daily. Using an intention-to-treat analysis, 7.8% of deaths occurred in the placebo group during an average of 6.5 months compared with only 3.2% in the active treatment group, a statistically significant 65% risk reduction ($p = 0.001$). Most notably, death caused by progressive HF or sudden cardiac death was reduced. The patients treated with carvedilol also had fewer HF-related hospitalizations (19.6% vs. 14.1%). The most common side effect with carvedilol was dizziness, usually during the first few days of therapy, but more patients discontinued placebo for worsening HF or side effects than with carvedilol.

In the Australia/New Zealand Carvedilol Study, 415 patients with chronic, stable HF (NYHA class II or III, 85% taking concurrent ACE inhibitors, and average EF of 28%) were randomly assigned to receive placebo ($n = 208$) or carvedilol ($n = 207$).[219] As in the US study, those with severe symptoms were excluded, although 88% had a history of MI. Maintenance doses in subjects randomly assigned to receive carvedilol ranged from 6.25 to 25 mg twice daily with an average follow-up of 19 months. After 12 months, EF had increased by 5.3%, and heart size was reduced in the carvedilol group compared with essentially no change in the placebo group. No differences between groups were found in treadmill exercise time, change in NYHA classification, or HF symptom scores, however. Most (58% in both groups) had neither improvement nor worsening of symptoms.

At 19 months, the frequency of episodes of worsening HF was similar in the two groups. Total deaths in the carvedilol group ($n = 20$) were less than the placebo group ($n = 26$), but most of the difference in mortality was attributed to noncardiovascular deaths. No difference was found in death caused by HF or MI, or in total cardiac-related deaths. On a more positive note, there were 68% fewer hospital admissions for HF in the carvedilol group ($n = 23$) than for the placebo group ($n = 33$). Overall, these findings could be interpreted as evidence for safety with either no overall benefit or a modest improvement with carvedilol.

The original FDA-approved indication for carvedilol was to reduce the progression of HF in patients with mild to moderate (NYHA class II or III) HF of ischemic or cardiomyopathic origin and whose conditions had been stabilized with other drugs (digitalis, diuretics, and ACE inhibitors). In keeping with the exclusion of patients with an unstable condition from the study protocols, carvedilol was not approved for use in NYHA class IV decompensated cardiac failure. As discussed in Case 19-2, later studies confirmed the value of carvedilol in NYHA class IV HF. As with any β-blocker, carvedilol is not recommended for use in patients with asthma, chronic obstructive pulmonary disease, or poorly controlled diabetes.

The starting dose of carvedilol is 3.125 mg twice daily, with a doubling of the dose every 2 weeks as needed or tolerated up to a maximum of 25 mg twice daily in patients weighing less than 85 kg and 50 mg twice daily in larger patients. Hypotension, bradycardia, fluid retention, and worsening HF symptoms can occur in the first few weeks of therapy, necessitating additional diuretics, a reduction of dose, or discontinuation of carvedilol. Taking carvedilol with food slows the rate of absorption and reduces the incidence of orthostatic hypotension, which occurs in up to 10% of patients taking the drug. Carvedilol phosphate (Coreg CR), a once-a-day extended-release form of carvedilol, is marketed in the United States for HTN treatment, but currently it has not been studied in patients with HF.

Because carvedilol is metabolized by the cytochrome P-450 2D6 (CYP2D6) enzyme system, several potential drug interactions should be considered.[213,220] The best-documented ones are inhibition of metabolism by cimetidine and decreased carvedilol serum concentrations when taken with rifampin. Known inhibitors of CYP2D6 (e.g., quinidine, fluoxetine, paroxetine, and propafenone) can increase the risk of toxicity (especially hypotension), but substantiating data are lacking. Carvedilol has also been reported to increase serum digoxin levels by 15% by an unknown mechanism. Other sources of intrasubject variability in carvedilol response may be caused by differences in the extent or rate or absorption, stereospecific metabolism of the two isomers of the drug (carvedilol is a racemic mixture of $S[-]$ and $R[+]$ isomers), and impaired metabolism in the 10% of the population who lack CYP2D6 activity.[220]

CHOICE OF β-BLOCKER: METOPROLOL VERSUS CARVEDILOL

No consensus exists regarding the relative superiority of one β-blocker versus another. Although the additional properties of carvedilol (e.g., α_1-blockade and antioxidant properties) provide a theoretical basis for selecting carvedilol instead of metoprolol succinate or bisoprolol, the data from clinical trials provide conflicting conclusions. In one small head-to-head trial, carvedilol showed greater improvement in hemodynamic response during peak exercise and EF but no difference in symptom scores or exercise tolerance.[221] Another report studied 30 patients with HF with persistent symptoms, despite at least 1 year of combined metoprolol and an ACE inhibitor.[222] They were enrolled in an open-label, parallel trial and randomly assigned either to continue with metoprolol (mean dose, 142 ± 44 mg/day) or to cross over to maximal tolerated doses of carvedilol (mean dose, 74 ± 23 mg/day). At the end of 12 months, patients randomly assigned to carvedilol showed a greater decrease in end-diastolic volume, more improvement in LVEF, and fewer ectopic beats on electrocardiogram. No significant difference was seen in symptoms or quality-of-life measures.

One meta-analysis attempted a comparison of carvedilol with metoprolol using the surrogate end point of LVEF as a comparator.[223] Nineteen randomized, placebo- or active-controlled trials involving a total of 2,184 patients with impaired LVEF were reviewed. Patients received a mean dose of 58 mg of carvedilol or the equivalent of 162 mg of extended-release metoprolol. Combined results from the placebo-controlled trials showed that both drugs significantly improved LVEF, with carvedilol found to be significantly better than metoprolol. When compared with placebo, carvedilol increased LVEF by 6.5%, whereas metoprolol increased LVEF by 3.8%. These differences persisted when patients with ischemic HF were compared with those with nonischemic cardiomyopathy. In head-to-head comparative trials, carvedilol once again raised LVEF greater than metoprolol. No apparent difference, however, was noted between the two drugs based on improvements in symptom scores or exercise tolerance. The authors cautioned that EF is only one of several end points to be measured, and specific patient outcomes do not necessarily correlate well with EF.

After publication of the meta-analysis, the results of the Carvedilol or Metoprolol European Trial became available.[224] In this multicenter, double-blind trial, 3,029 patients with NYHA class II through IV HF and EF less than 35% were randomly assigned to receive either carvedilol (target dose, 25 mg BID) or metoprolol tartrate (target dose, 50 mg BID). Diuretics and ACE inhibitors were continued in all subjects if tolerated. All-cause mortality was 34% for carvedilol compared with 40% with metoprolol ($p = 0.0017$). The composite end point of mortality or all-cause hospital admissions was not significantly different between groups (74% carvedilol and 76% metoprolol). One major criticism of this study was use of metoprolol tartrate instead of the FDA-approved metoprolol succinate product. Comparable doses between the two study groups has been questioned because the target dose of carvedilol was 25 mg twice daily compared with the target dose of metoprolol tartrate being 50 mg twice daily. Also, the trial used resting HR to determine comparable β-blockade among study groups rather than HR response to exercise. Exercise-induced HR changes are considered a better indicator of β-blockade.

Side effects and patient tolerance are similar among β-blockers in most trials. One investigator observed that carvedilol caused more hypotension and dizziness than metoprolol or bisoprolol, possibly owing to α_1-blockade or more rapid absorption.[225] Thus, metoprolol or bisoprolol may be preferred in patients with hypotension or with complaints of dizziness. Conversely, carvedilol may be preferred in patients with inadequately controlled HTN.

Whether carvedilol is a better choice for A.J. cannot be definitely answered. A starting dosage of 3.125 mg twice daily of carvedilol could be used in place of metoprolol. In the past, metoprolol used to be the cheaper agent, but now that carvedilol has become generic in the past few years this has not been a determining factor between metoprolol and carvedilol. A.J.'s provider decided to continue metoprolol and reserve use of carvedilol if he has difficulty tolerating metoprolol.

β-Blockers in Severe Heart Failure

CASE 19-1, QUESTION 20: The original clinical trials of β-blockers excluded patients with severe (NYHA class IV) HF at the time of randomization. For this reason the FDA limited the original approval of carvedilol for use in NYHA class II and III HF. Likewise, the ACC/AHA guidelines strongly support the use of β-blockers in NYHA class II and III HF, but are less definitive about severe HF. If A.J. presented with NYHA class IV HF, what evidence supports or refutes the use of β-blockers in A.J.?

The COPERNICUS[226] study demonstrated clear benefit of carvedilol without undue side effects in patients with severe HF. Conversely, the β-Blocker Evaluation of Survival Trial (BEST) reported unimpressive results with another drug, bucindolol.[227] Details of these two trials are provided below.

The COPERNICUS study was a double-blind, placebo-controlled trial assessing the clinical benefits and risks of carvedilol in 2,289 patients with advanced HF (NYHA class IIIB or IV).[226] Subjects had symptoms of HF at rest or with minimal exertion and an EF of 25% or less despite diuretics (99%), ACE inhibitors (97%), and digoxin (67%). Subjects were excluded who required intensive care, had significant fluid retention, were hypotensive, had evidence of renal insufficiency, or were receiving IV vasodilators or positive inotropic drugs. The starting dose of carvedilol or matching placebo was 3.125 mg twice daily, which was increased every 2 weeks to a target dose of 25 mg twice daily. Of those in the carvedilol group, 65% achieved the target dose, with the mean dose being 37 mg at the end of the first 4 months of the trial. The trial was discontinued prematurely after an average patient follow-up of 10.4 months because of a significant survival benefit from carvedilol. There were 130 deaths in the carvedilol group and 190 deaths in the placebo group, with a 35% decrease in the risk of death with carvedilol (95% confidence interval [CI], 19% to 48%; $p = 0.0014$). For the secondary end point of all deaths and hospitalizations combined, there were 425 events with carvedilol compared with 507 in the placebo group, a 24% decrease (95% CI, 13% to 33%; $p = 0.001$). Fewer patients in the carvedilol group (14.8%) than in the placebo group (18.5%) withdrew because of adverse effects at 1 year ($p = 0.02$).

A concern about using β-blockers in patients with class IV HF is that they may be predisposed to more side effects during the initiation phase of therapy. One study retrospectively analyzed the outcomes of 63 patients who were NYHA class IV compared with 167 subjects ranging from class I through III.[228] Adverse events occurred more frequently in the class IV patients (43%) than in the other subjects (24%; $p = 0.0001$) and more often resulted in permanent withdrawal of the drug (25% vs. 13%). Conversely, more class IV patients treated with carvedilol improved by more than one NYHA functional class than in the less symptomatic group (59% vs. 37%). A reanalysis of the COPERNICUS study data did not confirm a higher rate of intolerance during the first 8 to 12 weeks of carvedilol compared with placebo.[229] No difference was found between carvedilol and placebo in terms of death, hospitalizations, or withdrawal because of adverse events during the first 8 weeks of therapy.

The BEST Investigators failed to demonstrate that bucindolol, a nonselective β-blocker with vasodilator properties, improved overall survival in patients with NYHA class III and IV HF.[227] They randomly assigned 2,708 patients to receive either bucindolol or placebo. Although the active drug yielded a significant decrease in NE levels and improvement in LV function, the study was stopped prematurely because of the low probability of showing any significant CV mortality benefit compared with placebo. A possible explanation is that bucindolol has intrinsic sympathomimetic activity that may counteract some of the benefits of β-blockade. Moreover, subgroup analysis suggested that black patients might have fared worse with bucindolol, raising concerns that β-blockers may not be effective therapy for black patients with advanced HF (see Case 19-3, Question 2, for further discussion of possible racial differences in drug response).

Controversy still remains about the safe and effective use of β-blockers in class IV HF. The best data to support safe and effective use exist for carvedilol. Bucindolol has not been approved by the FDA for treatment of HF. Clinically, the use of β-blockers is generally continued unless the ADHF patient requires inotropic therapy or a dose titration of the β-blockers was a cause of the ADHF. If the dose titration resulted in ADHF, then most patients are reduced back to their previous β-blocker dose, but some may require acutely holding the β-blockers and reinitiating once stabilized.

Aldosterone Antagonists

CASE 19-2

QUESTION 1: B.D. is a 65-year-old Caucasian man with an LVEF of less than 25% who presents to the heart failure

clinic today for follow-up of his recent HF hospitalization. His blood pressure is 120/85 mm Hg and his pulse is 70 beats/minute. His current medications include lisinopril 10 mg every day, metoprolol succinate 150 mg every day, and furosemide 20 mg every day. You have reviewed his chart and noted that these are the maximal tolerated doses of lisinopril and metoprolol owing to dizziness and near syncope with higher doses. Today his laboratory results show that his SCr is 0.9 mg/dL and his potassium level is 3.5 mEq/L. Is this patient a candidate for aldosterone antagonist therapy?

Aldosterone contributes to HF through the increased retention of sodium and the depletion of potassium. Likewise, the diuretic and potassium-sparing actions of spironolactone are attributed to inhibition of aldosterone.[230] Until recently, it was believed that optimal doses of ACE inhibitors fully suppressed the production of aldosterone because angiotensin II is a potent stimulus for aldosterone production. It is now recognized, however, that aldosterone levels can remain elevated through a combination of nonadrenal production and reduced hepatic clearance. In addition, it has become clear that both angiotensin II and aldosterone have other negative effects on the CV system, including myocardial and vascular fibrosis, direct vascular damage, endothelial dysfunction, oxidative stress, and prevention of NE uptake by the myocardium.[32,231] This led the Randomized Aldactone Evaluation Study (RALES) investigators to test the hypothesis that low doses of spironolactone might impart a cardioprotective effect in patients with severe HF independent of diuresis or potassium retention.[66] In this trial, 1,663 patients with a history of NYHA class IV HF within the previous 6 months (but in class III or IV on study entry), an EF of 35% or less, and continued treatment (unless contraindicated or not tolerated) with a loop diuretic (100%), an ACE inhibitor (94%), and digoxin (74%) were randomly assigned to receive either spironolactone 25 mg ($n = 822$) or placebo ($n = 841$). The dose of spironolactone could be increased to 50 mg if HF worsened without evidence of hyperkalemia.

The study was discontinued prematurely after a mean follow-up of 24 months when a statistically significant reduction in mortality was observed. There were 386 deaths in the placebo group (46%) compared with 284 (35%) in the spironolactone group. These differences were first evident at 2 to 3 months after starting treatment. The greatest reduction was in CV deaths. In addition, more subjects had symptomatic improvement (as evidenced by moving to a lower NYHA class) and fewer had symptomatic worsening with the active drug. Hospitalization rates were lower in the patients treated with spironolactone. SCr and potassium concentrations were somewhat higher with the active drug, but the changes were not considered clinically significant. Hyperkalemia developed in 2% of the patients on spironolactone and 1% of those on placebo. Gynecomastia was reported in 10% of men treated with spironolactone compared with only 1% of those receiving placebo.

It is important to emphasize that nearly all subjects had continuing HF symptoms despite maximal drug therapy with multiple drugs, including an ACE inhibitor. Although ACE inhibitors indirectly suppress aldosterone at therapeutic doses, the inhibition is not as complete as with spironolactone. Thus, this study provided the first clinical evidence that spironolactone protects against myocardial and vascular fibrosis and alters hemodynamic or hormonal mediators of HF.

Subsequently, the aldosterone receptor inhibitor eplerenone was studied in 6,632 patients with LV dysfunction after MI. In the Eplerenone Post-Acute Myocardial Infarction Heart Failure Efficacy and Survival Study (EPHESUS), subjects were randomly assigned to receive either eplerenone 25 mg every day initially, titrated to 50 mg every day, or placebo.[67] Concurrent therapy included diuretics (60%), ACE inhibitors (87%), β-blockers (75%), and aspirin (88%). During a mean follow-up of 16 months, there were 478 deaths (14.4%) in the active treatment group compared with 554 deaths (16.7%) with placebo (relative risk, 0.85; $p = 0.008$). Most deaths were attributable to CV causes. Similar to spironolactone, more subjects experienced hyperkalemia with eplerenone than with placebo. Because eplerenone does not block progesterone and androgen receptors, gynecomastia and sexual dysfunction may be less.[67,231] Eplerenone was initially approved by the FDA for HTN, and gained labeling for patients after MI in late 2003.

In 2011, the Eplerenone in Mild Patients Hospitalization and Survival Study in Heart Failure (EMPHASIS-HF) study was published. This study evaluated eplerenone in 2,737 patients with NYHA class II HF and an EF of less than 35%.[61] In the EMPHASIS study, subjects were randomly assigned to receive either eplerenone 25 mg every day initially, titrated to 50 mg every day, or placebo. Concurrent therapy included diuretics (85%), ACE inhibitors (78%), ARBs (19%), β-blockers (87%), digoxin (27%), and anticoagulant or antiplatelet therapy (88%). The primary outcome of the trial was death owing to CV causes or hospitalization for HF. During a median follow-up of 21 months, there were 249 primary outcome events (18.3%) in the active treatment group compared with 356 primary outcome events (25.9%) with placebo (hazard ratio, 0.63; $p < 0.001$). In the active treatment group there were 171 (12.5%) all-cause deaths compared with 213 (15.5%) with placebo (hazard ratio, 0.76; $p = 0.008$). Most deaths were attributable to CV causes in this study as was the case in the EPHESUS trial. This study further supports the role of aldosterone antagonists in systolic HF management and expands the known effectiveness to NYHA class II HF patients.

B.D. has NYHA class II HF based on his current symptom control and fits the profile of the subjects in the EMPHASIS-HF study, although he is on a low dose of ACE inhibitor. Starting B.D. on an aldosterone antagonist is appropriate because of his relative intolerance to increasing the dose of ACE inhibitor and β-blocker. An initial spironolactone dose of 25 mg per day should be chosen for B.D. based on the dose studied in the RALES trial. Spironolactone is chosen based on the likely class effects of aldosterone antagonists in HF treatment and the lower cost compared with eplerenone. This dose is safe based on his current potassium of 3.5 mEq/L and SCr of 0.9 mg/dL. He will need to be followed to determine whether a larger dose of spironolactone will be tolerated and safe after a measurement of his potassium and SCr 2 weeks after initiation. Specific monitoring parameters for the management of hyperkalemia in patients treated with aldosterone antagonists can be found in Table 19-11.

Digitalis Glycosides

CASE 19-2, QUESTION 2: B.D. has tolerated spironolactone 25 mg daily for 2 months. His laboratory test results today show that his potassium is 4.4 mEq/L and his SCr is 1.0 mg/dL. His blood pressure is 124/82 mm Hg and his pulse is 70 beats/minute. He has come to the clinic today for a follow-up appointment with his cardiologist who notes that B.D. has had four HF hospitalizations in the last year. B.D. also reports increased SOB, DOE, and PND, although his weight is stable and he takes all his medications as prescribed. The medical resident who is also staffing the clinic asks whether it would be appropriate to add digoxin to

B.D.'s medical treatment of HF. He was told by a colleague that in clinical trials digoxin reduced both HF symptoms and hospitalizations for HF. What would you recommend?

Debates raged for years about whether digitalis glycosides or vasodilators should be the drug(s) of first choice for treating HF. By the time the first ACC/AHA guidelines were published in 1994 to 1995, a clear consensus was evident. Vasodilators are first-line therapy, with digoxin being added for patients with either supraventricular arrhythmias, failure to achieve symptomatic relief with vasodilators alone, or intolerable side effects from vasodilators. ACE inhibitors are preferred compared with other vasodilators because of proven efficacy, convenience of dosing, and fewer side effects. By 1999, experts also recommended starting β-blocker therapy earlier in the treatment plan. Digoxin, however, continues to be widely debated.

CONTROVERSY ABOUT EFFICACY OF DIGOXIN

Correction of the underlying defect is a rational approach to the treatment of any disease. When considering HF solely as "pump failure" with a weakened myocardial muscle, then digitalis is the logical choice to improve cardiac contractility, CO, and renal perfusion. If focusing on symptom relief and increased exercise tolerance as markers of benefit, digoxin is effective. Critics, however, raised concerns that symptom relief was less in patients with normal sinus rhythm than in those with supraventricular arrhythmias. The most vocal critics claimed that the risk of digitalis toxicity did not warrant using this class of drugs in patients with normal sinus rhythm.

Using multivariate analysis, one group of investigators concluded that a third heart sound (S_3 gallop rhythm), an enlarged heart, and a low EF best predict those patients with normal sinus rhythm who will derive a beneficial response from digoxin.[232] Several other meta-analyses and critical reviews of the literature later concurred that many of the original trials were designed improperly or lacked proper controls and that digoxin therapy provides a beneficial effect, especially in patients with severe symptomatic ventricular systolic dysfunction.[233,234]

DIGOXIN WITHDRAWAL TRIALS

In 1993, two digoxin withdrawal trials, PROVED[235] and RADIANCE,[236] were published. Both attempted to determine whether patients with HF who were already treated with digoxin would show deterioration of control or remain stable after discontinuation of digoxin. In both studies, patients had documented systolic failure (LVEF <35%) and mild to moderate symptoms (NYHA class II or III), and they were in normal sinus rhythm and were stable for at least 3 months with a treatment regimen of a diuretic and digoxin (baseline digoxin level, 0.9–2.0 ng/mL). A significant difference was that patients in the RADIANCE trial were also stabilized on an ACE inhibitor in addition to the diuretic and digoxin.[235] A 12-week, double-blind, placebo-controlled treatment period followed initial stabilization in both studies. Patients in the active treatment groups continued digoxin at their previous dose. Those in the placebo groups were withdrawn from digoxin and given an identical-looking placebo.

In PROVED,[235] 42 subjects continued digoxin and 46 were given placebo. There were 29% treatment failures in the withdrawal group compared with only 19% in those still taking digoxin. Treatment failure was defined as worsening HF symptoms requiring a therapeutic intervention (e.g., increased diuretic dosage or addition of a new drug), an emergency department visit or hospitalization for HF, or death. Exercise tolerance worsened in more patients taking placebo. Those taking digoxin tended to maintain lower body weight and HR as well as higher EF.

In the RADIANCE study, 85 subjects continued digoxin therapy and 93 were switched to placebo.[236] During the 12-week follow-up period, only 4 of the subjects taking digoxin (4.7%) experienced worsening symptoms compared with 23 (24.7%) of the placebo-treated patients. More of the placebo-treated patients had worsening of EF and lower quality-of-life scores. The finding that deterioration in symptoms after discontinuing digoxin often was delayed for several weeks offers a possible explanation why earlier clinical trials using shorter observation periods failed to establish a benefit from digoxin. When comparing the two trials directly, fewer patients deteriorated in both arms in the RADIANCE study. Whether this is attributed to a greater benefit from combining an ACE inhibitor with a diuretic compared with using a diuretic alone (as in PROVED) cannot be established.

These studies establish a beneficial effect of digoxin, even in those patients receiving concurrent ACE inhibitors in RADIANCE. At least two factors, however, limit extrapolation to all patients with HF. First, the investigators only assessed the value of therapy indirectly by using a withdrawal design instead of initiating therapy in patients previously untreated with digoxin. Second, the patients had advanced disease as evidenced by NYHA class II or III symptoms despite triple-drug therapy. Thus, the benefit of digoxin as initial monotherapy in early disease remains an unanswered question.

EFFECT OF DIGOXIN ON MORTALITY

The seminal study to answer the question of whether treatment with digoxin improves survival in HF was the Digitalis Intervention Group (DIG) study.[237] In this study, 6,800 patients with HF from 302 centers in the United States and Canada were randomly assigned to receive either digoxin (n = 3,397) or placebo (n = 3,403). Eligibility requirements included an EF of 45% or less (mean, 28% in both treatment groups), normal sinus rhythm, and clinical evidence of HF. Most subjects were in NYHA class II or III HF, although a small number of both class I and class IV subjects were included. Concurrent therapies were diuretics (82%), ACE inhibitors (94%), and nitrates (42%). Of subjects in both groups, 44% were taking digoxin before randomization. The starting digoxin dose (or matching placebo) was based on age, weight, and renal function, with subsequent adjustments made according to plasma level measurements. Approximately 70% of subjects in both groups ended up taking 0.25 mg/day, compared with 17.5% taking 0.125 mg/day and 11% receiving dosages of 0.375 mg/day or higher. By 1 month, 88.3% of subjects on active drug had serum levels between 0.5 and 2.0 ng/mL, with a mean of 0.88 ng/mL. Patients were followed for an average of 37 months (range, 28 to 58 months).

For the primary outcome of total mortality from any cause, 34.8% of patients on digoxin and 35.1% of those on placebo died; corresponding CV deaths were 29.9% and 29.5%, respectively. Although neither of these differences is statistically different, a trend was seen toward fewer HF-associated deaths and statistically fewer hospitalizations (risk ratio, 0.72) with active treatment. As would be expected, cases of suspected digoxin toxicity were greater in the active treatment group (11.9% vs. 7.9%), but the incidence of true toxicity was low.

The DIG trial improves on the PROVED and RADIANCE trials because it added digoxin to other therapy as opposed to being a withdrawal study and also because of the larger study population. However, because nearly all patients were receiving concurrent vasodilator therapy, the value of digoxin as monotherapy on mortality rates remains unanswered.

As presented earlier in this chapter, the ACC/AHA guidelines indicate that patients with HF are unlikely to benefit from the addition of digoxin in stage A or stage B HF. In these patients, digoxin can be used for symptom management only if they are treated with drug therapy shown to prolong survival (ACE inhibitors and β-blockers) or have not responded adequately to appropriate therapy. In those patients who are stage C HF with current or prior symptoms of HF, despite receiving optimal doses of ACE inhibitors of β-blockers, digoxin can be beneficial to reduce HF hospitalizations.

Digoxin is also prescribed routinely in patients with HF and concurrent AF, but β-blockers may be more effective in controlling the ventricular response, especially during exercise. Digoxin should be avoided if the patient has significant sinus or AV block, unless the block is treated with a permanent pacemaker. Digoxin should be used cautiously in patients taking other drugs that can depress sinus or AV nodal function (e.g., amiodarone or β-blockers), although patients usually will tolerate this combination.

Despite being on maximal tolerated doses of lisinopril and metoprolol, B.D. continues to have HF symptoms. In patients with persistent HF symptoms, especially like B.D. who also presents with an EF less than 25%, digoxin can be used as an additional agent. However, digoxin is not indicated as primary therapy for stabilization of patients with acutely decompensated HF. Such patients should first receive appropriate treatment, including IV medications.

SEX DIFFERENCES IN RESPONSE TO DIGOXIN

CASE 19-2, QUESTION 3: If B.D. had been a woman, would it have made any difference in the determination to prescribe digoxin?

Until recently, nothing indicated that sex-based differences existed relative to the prognosis of HF or in response to drugs such as digoxin. Two interesting reports published in 2002 sparked interest in this topic. The first was an extension of the Framingham Heart Study.[233] It was observed that during the past five decades the incidence of HF has been constant in men, but has declined by 31% to 40% in women during the interval of the last decade. During the last decade, survival rates for patients with HF have improved in both men and women, although the mortality rate is higher in men than in women. The more aggressive use of drugs, such as ACE inhibitors and β-blockers, are likely contributors to the improved outcomes. The observed differences between men and women may reflect different causes of HF. For example, HTN is a predominate cause of HF among elderly women with preserved LVEF, whereas more men have prior MI as a contributor to HF.

The second report (a review article) more directly addresses the question of use of digoxin in men compared with women.[234] As previously discussed, the DIG Trial reported approximately equal mortality rates (35%) in subjects with HF randomly assigned to either placebo or digoxin, while continuing usual doses of diuretics and ACE inhibitors.[138] A 12% reduction was found in the rate of death attributable to HF in the digoxin group, but a corresponding increase was noted in death presumed to be caused by arrhythmias. The retrospective post hoc analysis of the DIG study data reported that women overall had a lower death rate from any cause than men (31.0% vs. 36.1%; $p = 0.001$), an absolute difference of 5.8%.[234] The death rate was also lower among women in the placebo group than among men taking placebo (28.9% vs. 36.9%; $p < 0.001$). Likewise, women taking digoxin had a lower death rate than men taking active drug (33.1% vs. 35.2%), but this difference was not statistically different ($p = 0.034$). A surprising finding was that women taking digoxin had a higher death rate than women taking placebo (33.1% vs. 28.9%), whereas death rates in men were essentially equal in both groups. The authors speculate that a possible mechanism for the increased risk of death among women taking digoxin is an interaction between hormone-replacement therapy and digoxin. Progesterone might increase serum digoxin levels by inhibiting P-glycoprotein (PGP), thus reducing digoxin renal tubular excretion. Consistent with this hypothesis, digoxin serum concentrations after 1 month of digoxin intervention were higher in women than in men. The study investigators, however, did not routinely gather data on estrogen and hormone-replacement therapy or consistently measure serum digoxin levels later in the trial. Because these observances are retrospective, it is difficult to establish the clinical significance of the data and it is premature to argue against the use of digoxin in women. Nonetheless, it is prudent to recommend keeping serum digoxin concentrations less than 1.2 ng/mL in all patients and avoid hormone-replacement therapy in women with HF when taking digoxin. More recently, Adams et al.[238] reanalyzed the DIG data and found that at lower serum concentrations (0.5–0.9 ng/mL) digoxin decreased the risk of hospitalizations and mortality in women. Serum concentrations greater than 1.2 ng/mL in the treatment group were associated with higher risk of death when compared with the placebo group. Thus, higher digoxin concentrations resulted in worse clinical outcomes both in men and women.

MAINTENANCE DOSE

CASE 19-2, QUESTION 4: What is the appropriate maintenance dose of digoxin for B.D.?

The usual maintenance doses of digoxin have traditionally ranged from 0.125 to 0.25 mg/day. With the increased emphasis on targeting lower serum concentrations, more patients are now empirically started at 0.125 mg/day. For example, because B.D. has essentially normal kidney function, he empirically would have been started on a 0.25-mg/day maintenance dose in the past. A 0.125-mg dose, however, is recommended for him now. It is safest to start with a conservative dose and assess his needs after 1 to 2 weeks.

In all cases, smaller doses of digoxin are given to patients with impaired excretion rates (e.g., those with renal failure, older patients) or small-framed individuals. For example, a totally anuric patient may receive only 0.0625 mg 3 or 4 days/week.

Loading doses of digoxin are rarely necessary. Slow initiation of therapy with maintenance doses of digoxin in lieu of a loading dose is the method of choice for ambulatory or nonacutely ill patients with normal renal function. Even in the acute-care setting, no indication exists for loading doses of digoxin for HF alone. The exception might be if the patient has AF and it is desired to control ventricular response as quickly as possible. Even then, alternative drugs are likely to be used (see Chapter 20, Cardiac Arrhythmias).

SERUM DRUG CONCENTRATIONS

CASE 19-2, QUESTION 5: What is the target serum digoxin concentration for B.D.?

The target therapeutic serum digoxin concentration is 0.5 to 1.0 ng/mL. Many older textbooks, review articles, and clinical trials contain the prior standard of targeting serum digoxin concentrations in the range of 0.8 to 2 ng/mL, or a mean of 1.0 ng/mL. These older recommendations should be abandoned. Factors driving this change are information suggesting that the positive hemodynamic and neurohormonal effects of digoxin can be achieved at lower serum concentrations than those needed to

Hyperkalemia can develop as a consequence of massive digitalis poisoning.[274] Toxic doses of digitalis severely poison the Na^+/K^+ ATPase system, causing inhibition of the uptake of potassium by the myocardium, skeletal muscle, and liver cells. The shift of potassium from inside to outside the cell can result in significant hyperkalemia, especially in patients with underlying renal insufficiency. These same patients also are likely to accumulate digoxin in the body because of decreased clearance of the drug.

Vague gastrointestinal symptoms characteristic of digitalis toxicity are difficult to evaluate because anorexia and nausea are also part of clinical picture seen in patients with congestion. During one prospective clinical study, an equal frequency of anorexia and nausea occurred in both toxic and nontoxic patients taking digoxin.[275] Anorexia may be the earliest symptom, followed in 2 to 3 days by nausea.

CNS symptoms of digitalis are common, possibly associated with potassium depletion in neural tissue. Chronic digitalis intoxication resulting from misformulation was observed in 179 patients.[275] Acute extreme fatigue or visual disturbances were a complaint in 95% of these patients. Approximately 80% experienced weakness of the arms and legs, and 65% had psychic disturbances in the form of nightmares, agitation, listlessness, and hallucinations. Hazy vision and difficulties in both reading and red–green color perception frequently were present. Other complaints included glitterings, dark or moving spots, photophobia, and yellow–green vision. Disturbances in color vision returned to normal 2 or 3 weeks after discontinuation of digitalis.

Interestingly, six elderly patients had apparent digitalis-induced visual disturbances at serum concentrations below those considered to be toxic (all <1.5 ng/mL; range, 0.2 to 1.5 ng/mL).[276] Five of the reactions were described as photopsia (seeing lights not present in the environment), and one person had decreased visual acuity. Color vision disturbances or seeing color lights, both well described with digitalis toxicity, were absent. The symptoms went away in all but one subject when digoxin was discontinued.

Some prospective studies have shown a good correlation between serum digoxin levels and toxicity,[275,277,278] whereas other investigators found a poor correlation.[279,280] In one study, 87% of digitalis-toxic patients had levels greater than 2 ng/mL and 90% of nontoxic patients had levels less than 2 ng/mL. Conversely, other investigators found that nearly 50% of subjects with a serum digoxin level greater than 3 ng/mL were clinically stable without signs of digitalis toxicity.[279] In the largest series studied to date, the average serum digoxin concentration in documented toxic patients (i.e., those with a suspected digitalis-induced arrhythmia that disappeared after drug withdrawal) was 2.9 ng/mL compared with 1.0 ng/mL in patients with suspected digitalis toxicity but in whom the arrhythmia persisted after drug withdrawal.[273] Approximately 38% of documented toxic patients, however, had serum digoxin concentrations less than 2 ng/mL. Once levels exceed 6 ng/mL, the risk of mortality greatly increases.[281]

Because a significant overlap between toxic and therapeutic levels exists, serum level determinations are currently most useful as an aid in confirming suspected digitalis toxicity and in individualizing dosing regimens so that toxicity might be avoided. In particular, subjects with low serum potassium concentrations can demonstrate digitalis toxicity at lower serum digoxin concentrations.[282]

For many patients without life-threatening arrhythmias or major electrolyte imbalances, simple withdrawal of digitalis is the only treatment required. As a general rule, potassium replacement should be considered in any patient with digitalis-induced ectopic beats who has low serum potassium levels. A more definitive treatment consists of administration of digoxin-specific antibodies that bind digoxin molecules, rendering them unavailable for binding at receptors in the heart and other areas of the body.[283–288] The use of digoxin Fab products is restricted to potentially life-threatening intoxications (severe arrhythmias or hyperkalemia) that are either refractory to more conservative therapy or associated with extremely high serum concentrations.

Non–Angiotensin-Converting Enzyme Inhibitor Vasodilator Therapy

CASE 19-3

QUESTION 1: T.R. is a 57-year-old African American man with an LVEF of 35% who presents to the heart failure clinic today for follow-up of his chronic HF. His BP is 130/79 mm Hg and his pulse is 65 beats/minute. His current medications include lisinopril 20 mg every day, metoprolol succinate 200 mg every day, spironolactone 25 mg every day, hydralazine 25 mg QID, and isosorbide dinitrate 20 mg three times a day. Why would the patient be on hydralazine and isosorbide? What other forms of nitrates can be used in place of the isosorbide? Is combination therapy rational?

T.R. has already been treated with an ACE inhibitor (lisinopril), a β-blocker, and spironolactone. Despite this therapy, he was still having HF symptoms. As noted in the case he was started on hydralazine and isosorbide dinitrate, which is a possible next step in treating a patient like T.R. with HF.

Hydralazine's predominate action is as an arteriolar dilator, making hydralazine the prototype afterload-reducing agent. Decreasing aortic impedance (afterload) is of little benefit in a normal or minimally diseased heart, but it may greatly improve severely compromised LV function. SVR is decreased predictably, and this, in turn, leads to an increase in CO (cardiac index).[148,158,289] Hydralazine is also a direct-acting smooth muscle relaxant with significant arteriolar dilating effects in the kidneys and limbs. It has essentially no effect on the venous system or on hepatic blood flow.

The reflex tachycardia and hypotension that frequently accompany hydralazine therapy when used in treating HTN are minimal or absent when it is used to treat HF. In patients with end-stage cardiomyopathy, however, significant hypotension can occur if the heart cannot respond appropriately by increasing CO. This pulmonary arteriolar dilating effect of hydralazine is generally less beneficial than the venodilating effects of drugs such as nitrates and nitroprusside. Because hydralazine is devoid of venous dilating properties, central venous pressure and pulmonary capillary wedge pressure (PCWP) are unchanged.[158,289]

The effect of a single dose of hydralazine occurs in about 30 minutes and lasts up to 6 hours. Larger doses than typically used for the treatment of HTN may be required for HF management. The average maintenance dose is 200 to 400 mg/day (50–100 mg every 6 hours). T.R. is only on an initial dose at this time and may warrant a higher dose in the future. Hydralazine used as monotherapy is not associated with long-term improvement in functional status, however.[289] Combination therapy of hydralazine with either nitrates or ACE inhibitors is highly effective.

Although tachyphylaxis generally is not a significant problem with prolonged courses of hydralazine, some patients require increased diuretic doses to counteract hydralazine-induced fluid retention. This latter response reflects activation of the renin-angiotensin system after vasodilation of the renal vasculature.

Other side effects accompanying hydralazine include transient nausea during the first few days of therapy; headache, flushing, or tachycardia; and a lupus syndrome associated with prolonged, high doses. (See Chapter 14, Essential Hypertension, for further discussion of hydralazine side effects and dosing.)

ORAL AND TOPICAL NITRATES

Nitrates have effects complementary to those of hydralazine.[148,158] They primarily dilate venous capacitance vessels, with minimal effects on selected arterial beds (coronary and pulmonary arteries). Venous dilation reduces preload, resulting in significant reductions in PCWP and right atrial pressure. They are especially effective in reducing the symptoms of pulmonary edema. The lack of significant arterial dilation accounts for the observations that SVR is minimally reduced and CO remains unchanged. Nitrate monotherapy is indicated for HF patients with valvular defects such as mitral or aortic regurgitation. In these patients, reduction of the ventricular filling pressure reduces LV congestion.

ISOSORBIDE DINITRATE

Because sublingual NTG has a short duration of response, more attention has been focused on sublingual and oral isosorbide dinitrate. Sublingual isosorbide is well absorbed and does not undergo first-pass metabolism. Its onset is rapid (approximately 5 minutes), but its effects are relatively short (1–3 hours). The usual starting dosage is 5 mg every 4 to 6 hours, but dosages may be titrated to 20 mg or more every 4 to 6 hours. These larger doses are associated with longer beneficial effects (approximately 3 hours), but also a high frequency of intolerable headaches and hypotension.

Previous claims of a poor response to orally administered isosorbide because of a large first-pass metabolic effect have been refuted. Large oral doses overwhelm the metabolic capacity of the liver and produce beneficial effects. Oral isosorbide has a slow onset (15–30 minutes), but the duration of activity is slightly longer than that associated with sublingual administration (4–6 hours). Oral doses of 5 mg are probably ineffective; 10 mg is the smallest effective starting dose, with further titration to dosages as high as 20 to 80 mg every 4 to 6 hours. The best dose for both sublingual and oral nitrates is that which provides the desired beneficial effect with the least side effects.

TRANSDERMAL NITROGLYCERIN

An innovative approach to NTG administration is transdermal patch systems. Topical application of these systems is believed to provide 24 hours of continuous cutaneous absorption with more convenience and less mess than NTG ointment. Although most published data on these dose forms are in patients with angina, several reports are on their use in HF.

The initial enthusiasm for transdermal NTG has been tempered by the suggestion that tolerance develops quickly, resulting in a benefit for much less than 24 hours after patch application. Considerable debate has arisen about this topic.[290–292] Some reviewers suggest abandoning this form of therapy, whereas others argue that the studies showing negative benefit were flawed. Removal of the patch during the night might lead to restoration of response the following day. It has been suggested that although the antianginal effects of NTG are attenuated with chronic therapy, the beneficial preload-reducing properties for HF are sustained. Large doses (20–40 mg/24 hours), however, may be required, necessitating the use of several patches per day and resulting in significant expense to the patient. (See Chapter 17, Chronic Stable Angina, for a more detailed discussion on the application and controversy surrounding NTG transdermal patches.)

HYDRALAZINE–NITRATE COMBINATION

Combined afterload and preload reduction is clearly of benefit both in improving symptoms and in enhancing long-term survival. Compared with ACE inhibitors, the hydralazine–isosorbide combination provides more significant improvement in exercise tolerance, but the side effect profile and survival statistics are better with ACE inhibitors.[156] With combination therapy, CO is greater for any given level of ventricular filling pressure. Generally, the use of the two drugs together is not accompanied by reflex tachycardia or hypotension, but it is important to be careful not to compromise coronary blood flow in patients with coexistent angina.

The most compelling argument for the use of combination hydralazine and nitrate vasodilator therapy comes from the results of the two Veterans Administration Cooperative Studies (V-HeFT I and V-HeFT II).[148,156,158] These two studies not only confirmed symptomatic relief and improved exercise tolerance with combination therapy, but they also showed improved survival. Also, see Case 19-3, Question 2, for the discussion of the unique place in therapy of the hydralazine–nitrate combination in African American patients.

In summary, nitrates alone are indicated for those patients with signs and symptoms of isolated pulmonary and venous congestion (i.e., dyspnea, increased pulmonary pressure, neck vein distension, edema). Conversely, use of an arterial dilator is more appropriate in a patient with high SVR, low CO, and normal PCWP. Most patients, such as T.R., exhibit symptoms of decreased CO and elevated venous pressure, making combination therapy the most attractive option. Although the hydralazine–isosorbide combination actually reduces symptoms slightly better than ACE inhibitors, the data on survival are more impressive with the ACE inhibitors, probably owing to better adherence. As illustrated by T.R.'s treatment regimen, a combination of an ACE inhibitor plus hydralazine, a nitrate, or both is common in patients with advanced disease.

Role of Race in the Pharmacotherapy of Heart Failure

CASE 19-3, QUESTION 2: Because T.R. is African American, would he be expected to respond any differently to ACE inhibitors or hydralazine–isosorbide dinitrate than a patient who is not African American?

In general, African American patients experience HF at an earlier age and are more likely to have HTN as a cause for HF. The rate of death caused by HF is higher for African American patients than for non–African American patients.

ANGIOTENSIN-CONVERTING ENZYME INHIBITORS AND HYDRALAZINE–ISOSORBIDE

Racial differences in response to drug therapy have been proposed, although this issue is far from resolved.[293–296] For example, a post hoc analysis of the V-HeFT trial data cited previously showed no difference in annual mortality between African American (n = 180) and non–African American patients (n = 450) in the placebo group (17.3% vs. 18.8%).[156,284] African American patients in the hydralazine–nitrate group had a significantly lower annual mortality rate (9.7%), however, than did African American subjects in the placebo group (17.3%), whereas non–African American subjects had no survival benefit from the drug combination (16.9% vs. 18.8%). This implies that African American patients, but not non–African American patients, derive benefit from the treatment with hydralazine–isosorbide. These same investigators then reanalyzed the V-HeFT II trial results for possible racial differences between response to enalapril and the hydralazine–nitrate combination.[158,294] The outcome is difficult to interpret because of the absence of a placebo group. The all-cause annual mortality rate for African American patients (n = 215) was identical in the two drug groups (12.8% with enalapril and 12.9% with hydralazine–isosorbide). In non–African American patients (n = 574), the corresponding mortality rates were 11% with enalapril and 14.9% with hydralazine–isosorbide. These data could be interpreted as either superior response to hydralazine–isosorbide in African American subjects or inferior activity of ACE inhibitors in African American patients. The latter interpretation is consistent with the hypothesis that ACE inhibitors might have a lesser BP-lowering effect in African American patients with HTN compared with non–African American patients. A similar reanalysis of the SOLVD Prevention and Treatment trials,[147] both of which compared enalapril with placebo in patients with recent MI, concluded that enalapril therapy is associated with a significant reduction in the risk for hospitalization for HF among white patients (44% reduction) with LV dysfunction, but not among similar African American patients. Confounding variables contributing to all of the analyses presented include disproportionately low numbers of African American subjects in the trials, and possibly more underlying risk factors (e.g., HTN) in the African American subjects.

To further address the effect of race on response to ACE inhibitors, a meta-analysis of the seven major ACE inhibitor studies, representing a total of 14,752 patients, was conducted.[295] The conclusion was that the relative risk for mortality when taking an ACE inhibitor compared with placebo was identical (0.89) for both African American and white patients. The authors of the meta-analysis urged that ACE inhibitors not be withheld from African American patients. One other consideration with ACE inhibitors is an observed higher rate, although still rare, of angioedema in black patients than in white patients. Until more data are available, ACE inhibitors should not be withheld from African American patients, but careful monitoring is required to assess response.

The African American Heart Failure Trial (AHeFT) was designed to determine possible superiority of combination hydralazine plus isosorbide dinitrate in African American patients.[72] AHeFT was a randomized comparison trial (n = 1,050) of hydralazine–isosorbide dinitrate and placebo in African American patients with NYHA class III or IV HF who were receiving standard HF therapy (94% diuretics, 87% β-blockers, 93% ACE inhibitors or ARB, 62% digoxin, and 39% aldosterone antagonists). The primary end point was a composite of all-cause death, first hospitalization for HF, and quality of life scores at 6 months with secondary end points being individual components of the primary end point. Reduction in the composite primary end point events was statistically significant in favor of the active drug combination. Importantly, all-cause mortality declined 43% in the hydralazine–isosorbide dinitrate arm versus that for the placebo group ($p = 0.012$). The study also reported a 39% reduction in first hospitalization for HF in the hydralazine–isosorbide dinitrate group versus placebo ($p < 0.001$). As a result, the 2009 ACC/AHA guideline recommendations state that the addition of hydralazine and isosorbide dinitrate to HF patients receiving ACE inhibitors and β-blockers is effective in African American patients with NYHA functional class III or IV HF.[1,21] The results of AHeFT were also the primary factor leading the FDA to approve the combination product of hydralazine and isosorbide dinitrate (BiDil) for adjunctive treatment of HF in self-identified African American patients already receiving standard therapy. Advantages of using BiDil in clinical practice include use of the same product studied in the clinical trial and potential improved compliance by using a combination tablet. Cost, however, may be lower when using generic hydralazine and isosorbide as separate drugs.

β-BLOCKERS

A possible racial difference in response to β-blocker drugs has also been hypothesized based on differential effects observed in patients with HTN.[293,295,296] A post hoc analysis of the various US Carvedilol Heart Failure trials[214–218] concluded, however, that the benefit of carvedilol was apparently of similar magnitude in both black (n = 217) and not black (n = 877) patients.[296] Using the combined end point of the risk of death as a result of any cause or hospitalization, the risk reduction of β-blockers compared with placebo was 48% in black patients and 30% in not black patients. Because fewer black patients were studied, these differences did not reach statistical significance. Also seen were a significant improvement in NYHA functional class, EF, and patient global symptom assessment with carvedilol in both black and not black patients.

Contradictory evidence comes from the BEST.[227] In this trial (also discussed in Case 19-1 Question 20), 2,708 patients with NYHA class III (92%) or IV (8%) HF were randomly assigned to either bucindolol or placebo. Bucindolol is a nonselective β-blocker with partial agonist activity that imparts weak vasodilation. A unique characteristic of this study was that a subgroup analysis for racial differences was planned from the start. Although there was a trend toward reductions in CV mortality and hospitalization with the active drug, the trial was terminated after 2 years when it was determined that there was no mortality benefit of active drug compared with placebo (33% mortality in placebo group vs. 30% with bucindolol). A subgroup analysis showed a mortality benefit in not black subjects, but none in black subjects. Subsequently, a meta-analysis of the five major β-blocker in HF studies was conducted, representing a total of 12,727 patients.[295] When the BEST was included in the meta-analysis, the relative risk for mortality when taking an ACE inhibitor compared with placebo was 0.69 in white subjects, but only 0.97 for black patients. When this trial was excluded, the relative risks were reduced in both groups to 0.63 and 0.67 in whites and blacks, respectively. The difference between the two groups was not statistically significant, although the 95% confidence interval for black patients was broader and included 1.0 (0.38–1.16). On the basis of all of these factors, it is likely that black patients will derive similar benefit from β-blockers as do white patients when given carvedilol, metoprolol, or bisoprolol. Bucindolol should be avoided depending on the pharmacogenomics of the patient, which happen to differ in black versus not black patients.

Critical Care Management of Heart Failure

CASE 19-4

QUESTION 1: L.M., a 62-year-old black man, was admitted several days ago with severe, progressive, and debilitating symptoms of HF. His family history is significant in that his father and two brothers died of heart attacks shortly after the age of 40. L.M. has a 5-year history of HF that is symptomatic despite treatment with furosemide 40 mg every day, lisinopril 10 mg every day, carvedilol 12.5 mg BID, digoxin 0.125 mg every day, and spironolactone 25 mg every day. His last echocardiogram showed an EF of 25%. He has a past medical history of HTN, CAD, and HF. During the last week, L.M.'s DOE became progressively worse, and he was mostly confined to bed because of

extreme fatigue. He wakes once or twice nightly with PND. Physical examination on this admission revealed significant jugular venous distension, bilateral rales, hepatomegaly, and 3+ peripheral edema. Chest radiograph revealed cardiomegaly and pulmonary congestion. His BP was 154/100 mm Hg and his pulse was 105 beats/minute.

Laboratory test results include the following:

Serum Na, 134 mg/dL
K, 4.3 mg/dL
BUN, 15 mg/dL
SCr, 1.3 mg/dL
Glucose, 90 mg/dL
BNP, 944 pg/mL

Hemoglobin, hematocrit, troponin, and liver enzymes were all within normal limits. L.M. was admitted to the hospital with ADHF. What factors are used to stratify risk for in-hospital mortality and morbidity?

ADHF is associated with high morbidity and mortality. It is the leading reason for hospitalizations among the elderly. Postdischarge mortality among patients with HF is 11% at 30 days and 37% at 1 year.[10] The most common precipitants of HF hospitalization are noncompliance (dietary or medication), acute myocardial ischemia, uncontrolled comorbidities (such as HTN, diabetes mellitus, chronic kidney disease, arrhythmias), and inappropriate prescribing (e.g., recent addition of negative inotropic agents or NSAIDs). Regardless of the precipitating event, the common pathophysiologic state that perpetuates the progression of HF is extremely complex. A cascade of hemodynamic and neurohormonal derangements provoke activation of adrenergic systems and RAAS, which get overwhelmed, leading to volume overload and hypoperfusion—classic symptoms of ADHF (see a detailed discussion in the Pathophysiology section). According to the ADHF National Registry, which is one of the largest multicenter, observational registries, nearly half of the patients who present with ADHF have preserved EF (>50%).[297] Because so few targeted therapies are available for HFPEF, ADHF in this subset of patients poses a unique challenge.

In-hospital mortality remains as high as 20% for patients who present with elevated BUN and creatinine, and low systolic BP (SCr >2.75 mg/dL, systolic BP <115 mm Hg, and BUN >43 mg/dL).[287] Patients presenting with hyponatremia, defined as a serum sodium level less than 135 mEq/L, have the worst outcomes and are more likely to receive inotropic agents. After discharge, patients who continue to be hyponatremic have an 8% risk of rehospitalization per 3 mEq/L decrease in serum sodium. Uric acid greater than 7 mg/dL in men and greater than 6 mg/dL in women is associated with a high admission rate for HF. Admission and discharge levels of BNP are also helpful in predicting rehospitalizations. According to some studies a greater than 30% to 40% reduction in BNP levels during hospitalization may result in improved outcomes. Other biomarkers such as cardiac troponin levels, C-reactive protein, and apolipoprotein A-I levels are all linked to HF readmissions.[11] Thus, all these factors can be used to stratify risk for in-hospital mortality.

Another approach to risk stratification and therapeutic decision making is based on hemodynamic profiles. Most patients with acute HF can be classified into one of four hemodynamic profiles using relatively simple assessment techniques (Fig. 19-8).[298–301] When using this scheme, patients are assessed

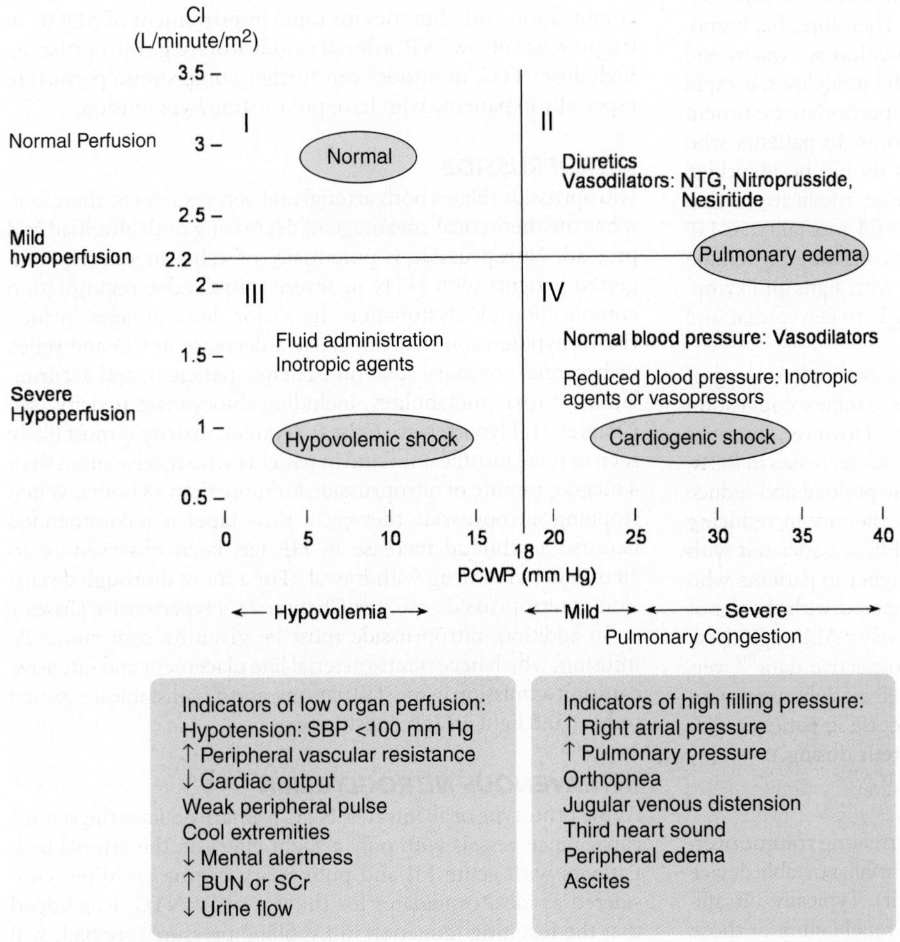

FIGURE 19-8 Hemodynamic profile of acute heart failure. BUN, blood area nitrogen; CI, cardiac index; NTG, nitroglycerin; PCWP, pulmonary capillary wedge pressure; SBP, systolic blood pressure; SCr, serum creatinine. Adapted with permission from Forrester JS et al. Correlative classification of clinical and hemodynamic function after acute myocardial infarction. *Am J Cardiol.* 1977;39:137.

for the presence or absence of elevated venous filling pressures ("wet" vs. "dry" patients) and adequacy of vital organ perfusion ("warm" vs. "cold" patients). Elevated filling pressure can be assessed at the patient's bedside by observing orthopnea, jugular venous distension, the presence of a third heart sound (S_3), peripheral edema, and ascites. Presence or absence of rales on auscultation is not considered a reliable indicator.[301] Hypotension, weak peripheral pulse, a narrow pulse pressure, cool forearms and legs, decreased mental alertness, and rising BUN and SCr are indicators of decreased organ perfusion. In one series, 67% of patients admitted to the hospital with a low LVEF and class IV HF symptoms were classified as "wet and warm," with 28% assessed as "cold and wet," and only 5% as "cold and dry."[298] Few, if any, patients were in the "warm and dry" category because this is the status the clinician is trying to achieve. Continuous BP, ECG, urine flow, and pulse oximetry measurements are standard noninvasive monitoring for all patients. Invasive hemodynamic monitoring is used in critically ill patients when more precise measurements of filling pressure (e.g., right atrial or pulmonary artery pressure), SVR, and CO or cardiac index are desired. The goals are to achieve a right atrial pressure of less than 5 to 8 mm Hg, pulmonary artery pressure of less than 25/10 mm Hg, pulmonary artery wedge pressure of 12 to 16 mm Hg or less, an SVR of 900 to 1,400 dyne · s/m^5 and a cardiac index of 2.8 to 4.2 L/minute/m^2 (see Chapter 22, Shock, for more detailed discussion of hemodynamic monitoring).

CASE 19-4, QUESTION 2: From his clinical presentation, what is L.M.'s hemodynamic profile? What are therapeutic goals for L.M.?

L.M.'s DOE, rales, peripheral edema, PND, and jugular venous pressure are consistent with ADHF and volume overload. L.M. does not have signs of hypoperfusion (does not have cool extremities and acute elevations in SCr). Therefore, his hemodynamic profile based on physical examination is "warm and wet" (subset II, Fig. 19-8). According to the guidelines, a rapid diagnosis of ADHF is necessary to initiate appropriate treatment and should be based on signs and symptoms. In patients who have established HF, precipitating factors should be identified and addressed. Also, at the time of discharge, medications that have been shown to decrease morbidity and mortality in HF should be optimized. BNP levels should be considered when the diagnosis is uncertain and, in conjunction with signs and symptoms of HF, can be helpful in differentiating between cardiac and noncardiac causes.

Because volume overload is central to the pathophysiology of most episodes of ADHF, the primary goal is to relieve congestion in patients in subset II (i.e., warm and wet). However, diuretics should be cautiously used in subset IV to avoid decreases in PCW less than 15 mm Hg as this can compromise preload and reduce CO. Despite diuretics being the mainstay therapy in reducing volume overload, their routine use in ADHF is associated with worsening mortality. Mortality rates are higher in patients who are receiving chronic diuretic therapy compared with those not receiving diuretics (3.3% vs. 2.7%, respectively). Although these findings are based on the analysis of retrospective data[302] versus prospective randomized trials, nevertheless, they suggest an association between mortality and diuretic use in patients with ADHF. (See Case 19-1, Question 7, for diuretic dosing.)

ULTRAFILTRATION

Ultrafiltration is an alternative approach for treating volume overload and congestion. It involves the use of a small, portable device to rapidly remove fluid (up to 500 mL/hour). Typically, ultrafiltration for HF is reserved for patients with renal failure or those unresponsive to diuretics. Small studies[303,304] in ADHF patients have shown that peripheral venovenous ultrafiltration results in greater weight loss and fluid removal, and reduced hospital length of stay and hospital readmissions compared with medical therapy. One study also reported significant reductions in neurohormonal activation and no significant changes in SCr or electrolytes with ultrafiltration.[305] The Ultrafiltration versus Intravenous Diuretics for Patients Hospitalized for Acute Decompensated Heart Failure (UNLOAD trial)[306] randomly assigned 200 patients to either ultrafiltration or aggressive IV diuretic therapy. The study showed that ultrafiltration compared with diuretics alone significantly improved weight loss at 48 hours (5.0 vs. 3.1 kg; $p < 0.001$), which decreased the need for vasoactive drugs (3% vs. 13%; $p = 0.02$) and reduced 90-day hospital readmission (18% vs. 32%; $p = 0.02$). Ultrafiltration is now a class IIa recommendation for patients with refractory HF not responsive to medical therapy. Patients with fluid overload and some degree of renal insufficiency and those refractory to diuretic therapy might make good candidates for ultrafiltration.[1,2]

Intravenous Vasodilators

CASE 19-4, QUESTION 3: L.M. received a 40-mg IV furosemide dose with no improvement in symptoms. Then he received an 80-mg IV dose with only marginal resolution of symptoms. The decision is made to start IV vasodilators. What is the role of vasodilator therapy in someone with ADHF such as L.M.?

The guidelines[1] recommend the addition of vasodilators in conjunction with diuretics to reduce congestion in patients with fluid overload. In the presence of asymptomatic hypotension, IV NTG, nitroprusside, or nesiritide may be considered cautiously in combination with diuretics for rapid improvement of ADHF. In the presence of low SVR, arterial vasodilators (e.g., nitroprusside, high-dose NTG, nesiritide) can further compromise perfusion, especially in patients who have pre-existing hypotension.

NITROPRUSSIDE

Nitroprusside dilates both arterial and venous vessels; therefore, it has the theoretical advantage of decreasing both afterload and preload. Nitroprusside is potentially of value in severely congested patients with HTN or severe mitral valve regurgitation complicating LV dysfunction. Its major disadvantages include risk of hypotension that can cause a decrease in CO and reflex tachycardia; coronary steal (in ischemic patients); and accumulation of toxic metabolites, including thiocyanate toxicity (see Chapter 21, Hypertensive Crises). Cyanide toxicity is most likely seen in renal insufficiency and in patients who receive more than 4 mcg/kg/minute of nitroprusside for more than 48 hours. When stopping nitroprusside therapy, a slow taper is recommended because a rebound increase in HF has been observed 10 to 30 minutes after drug withdrawal. (For a more thorough discussion of nitroprusside use, see Chapter 21, Hypertensive Crises.)

In addition, nitroprusside must be given by continuous IV infusion, which necessitates arterial line placement and intensive care unit admission in most situations, and it is unstable if exposed to heat and light after reconstitution.

INTRAVENOUS NITROGLYCERIN

As the prototype of all nitrates, NTG primarily dilates the venous capacitance vessels with only a slight effect on the arterial bed. Patients with acute MI and pulmonary edema are often considered as ideal candidates for the use of IV NTG. It is hoped that the resulting reduction in LV filling pressure (preload) will reduce PCWP to less than 18 mm Hg. Because nitrates have minimal or no effect on afterload, CO will likely remain unchanged or increase only slightly. NTG actually can decrease CO in some patients by reducing the LV filling pressure to less than 15 mm Hg. NTG is generally initiated at 10 mcg/minute and increased by increments of 10 to 20 mcg, until the patient's symptoms are improved or PCWP is less than 16 mm Hg. The most common side effect is headache, which can be treated with analgesics and often resolves after continuous therapy. Tachyphylaxis to NTG occurs as early as 1 to 2 hours after initiation of therapy. Approximately 20% of HF patients exhibit resistance to high doses of NTG.[1] Nitroprusside is a better choice for patients such as L.M. because he has elevated BP.

NESIRITIDE

Nesiritide is recombinantly produced human B-type natriuretic peptide containing the same 32 amino acids as native human BNP.[40,41] (The pharmacologic activity of the natriuretic peptides was reviewed in the Pathogenesis section.) BNP binds to guanylate cyclase receptors on vascular smooth muscle (the BNP receptor), leading to expression of cyclic guanosine monophosphate and subsequent vasodilation. Other actions include inhibition of ACE, sympathetic outflow, and ET-1. Peripheral and coronary dilation coupled with improved RBF and increased glomerular filtration all contribute to the beneficial effects of nesiritide. Metabolic clearance of nesiritide is by a combination of binding to cell surfaces with subsequent cellular internalization and lysosomal proteolysis as well as proteolytic cleavage by endopeptidase (e.g., neutral endopeptidase). It undergoes only minimal renal clearance. The mean elimination half-life is 8 to 22 minutes (mean, 18 minutes), necessitating a constant IV infusion.

In clinical trials of hospitalized patients with severe HF, nesiritide produced hemodynamic effects and reduction in dyspnea scores comparable to NTG when used in combination with IV diuretics and either dopamine or dobutamine.[40,41] Dose-dependent hypotension is the most common side effect with nesiritide, reported in 11% to 32% of patients. In some trials, nesiritide caused a higher incidence or longer duration of hypotension than NTG, whereas in other trials the incidence of hypotension was similar. The incidence of PVC and nonsustained ventricular tachycardia is less with nesiritide than with dopamine, dobutamine, or milrinone. Other side effects include headache, abdominal pain, nausea, anxiety, bradycardia, and leg cramps.

Because of high cost, the use of nesiritide is generally restricted to those patients with acute HF exacerbations who are fluid overloaded and have a PCWP greater than 18 to 20 mm Hg despite high doses of diuretics and IV NTG. In contrast to NTG, nesiritide has natriuretic properties that are additive to those of the loop diuretics. It should be avoided in patients with a systolic BP less than 90 to 100 mg Hg or in cases of cardiogenic shock. Dobutamine or milrinone should be added or substituted in hypotensive patients or those with a cardiac index of less than 2.2 L/minute/m^2.

The IV infusion of nesiritide is prepared by diluting the contents of a 1.5-mg vial to 6 mcg/mL in 250 mL of 5% dextrose or 0.9% NaCl. An initial loading dose of 2 mcg/kg is sometimes given intravenously for 60 seconds, followed by a continuous IV infusion at a rate of 0.01 mcg/kg/minute. The desired response is a reduction of PCWP of 5 to 10 mm Hg at 15 minutes. The dose can be increased in 0.005-mcg/kg/minute increments at 3-hour intervals to a maximum of 0.03 mcg/kg/minute. Dosage should be titrated to a PCWP less than 18 mm Hg and a systolic BP greater than 90 mm Hg.

Although nesiritide is indicated in the treatment of ADHF, concerns have been raised about its safety. A meta-analysis of randomized, controlled trials of nesiritide in ADHF suggests that nesiritide use may be associated with worsening renal function and increased mortality.[307,308] The conclusions of the meta-analysis have been criticized, however. For example, the Vasodilation in the Management of Acute Congestive Heart Failure (VMAC) study that was included in the meta-analysis was not designed to evaluate renal end points, and therefore the inclusion of the renal effects from this study may not be appropriate.[302,309] Also, differences in baseline characteristics of the treatment groups may have contributed to an increased risk of 30-day mortality seen in those patients treated with nesiritide.

The efficacy and safety of nesiritide have also been evaluated in the outpatient setting. The Follow-up Serial Infusions of Nesiritide (FUSION I) trial[310] was a pilot trial that included 202 patients with NYHA class III and IV who had been hospitalized for ADHF at least twice within the preceding year and once in the preceding month. Patients were randomly assigned to receive usual care with or without open-label nesiritide. A subgroup of patients was identified as high risk if they had at least four of the following: SCr greater than 2.0 mg/dL during the preceding month, NYHA class IV for the preceding 2 months, older than 65 years of age, a history of sustained ventricular tachycardia, ischemic HF etiology, diabetes, or use of nesiritide or inotropic agents as outpatients within the preceding 6 months. These patients at high risk experienced fewer HF exacerbations and renal adverse effects with nesiritide infusions.

This suggestion of potential benefit and safety in outpatients with severe HF was further explored in the Follow-Up Serial Infusions of Nesiritide for the Management of Patients With Heart Failure (FUSION II) trial.[311] This was a randomized, placebo-controlled, double-blind prospective trial of 911 subjects with advanced HF or chronic decompensated HF. Subjects were randomly assigned to receive a 2-mcg/kg nesiritide bolus followed by a 0.01-mcg/kg/minute infusion for 4 to 6 hours, or a matching placebo regimen, once or twice weekly for 12 weeks. Both groups also received optimal medical therapy and device therapy. Patients were entered only if their creatinine clearance was less than 60 mL/minute. No outpatient IV inotropic or vasodilator therapy was allowed during the 24-week study. After 24 weeks, no difference was noted in the primary end point of either death or hospitalization for cardiac or renal causes among patients in the nesiritide and placebo groups. Significantly more ($p < 0.001$) drug-related adverse events occurred in those in the nesiritide group (42.0%) compared with the placebo group (27.5%), mainly caused by hypotension. The incidence of worsening renal function, however, was significantly lower ($p = 0.046$) with nesiritide (32% in nesiritide group vs. 39% in the placebo group). There was no evidence that changes in SCr were associated with renal harm.

The results of these studies alleviated some concerns regarding the safety of nesiritide; however, a group of independent cardiologists designed an "Acute Study of Clinical Effectiveness of Nesiritide in Decompensated Heart Failure" (ASCEND-HF)[312,313] trial that would help to definitively answer the question of nesiritide safety and efficacy. This was a double-blind placebo trial, which enrolled 7,141 patients with ADHF in 30 countries. The participants were randomly assigned to receive IV bolus nesiritide (loading dose) of 2 mcg/kg or placebo (investigator's discretion for bolus), followed by continuous IV infusion of nesiritide 0.01 mcg/kg/minute or placebo for 7 days in addition to standard therapy. The coprimary end points were to assess a reduction in the rate of HF hospitalizations or all-cause mortality through day 30 and a significant improvement in self-assessed dyspnea at 6 or 24 hours using a 7-point Likert scale. Compared with placebo, nesiritide was not associated with a reduction in 30-day mortality or rehospitalization (10% vs. 9.4%; $p = 0.31$). Nesiritide improved dyspnea at 6 hours (15% vs. 13.4%; $p = 0.30$)

and at 24 hours compared with placebo (30.4% vs. 27.5%; $p = 0.007$), which is consistent with previous findings but did not meet the prespecified criteria or statistical significance at 6 or 24 hours. Also, nesiritide did not worsen renal function as had been suggested by prior meta-analysis. The proponents of nesiritide argue that even though the ASCEND-HF trial failed to show a major benefit, it is the only vasodilator that has been well studied. The controversy regarding the safety and survival of prescribing nesiritide can be put to rest; however, further analysis of the ASCEND-HF trial will provide better understanding of ADHF and patient profiles that may potentially benefit from nesiritide. The principal take-home message is that large clinical trials should be the norm before drugs are introduced into clinical practice.[288]

L.M. responded well to nitroprusside and needed no other therapy. However, IV NTG and IV nesiritide are alternatives to nitroprusside in patients with "wet and warm" acute HF. NTG or nesiritide can either be a substitute for nitroprusside or combined with nitroprusside. At the time of discharge, furosemide therapy should be continued, although the dose should be titrated to prevent DOE and peripheral edema. The dose of lisinopril and carvedilol should also be titrated to target or tolerated doses.

Inotropic Agents

CASE 19-5

QUESTION 1: B.J. is a 60-year-old man who presents to the emergency department with worsening DOE. He reports increased SOB during the last week. His medical history includes HTN, CAD, hyperlipidemia, and HF (EF 25%). His medications include metoprolol succinate 100 mg every day, enalapril 5 mg every day, furosemide 40 mg BID, aspirin 81 mg, and lovastatin 20 mg every night at bedtime. His vital signs on admission included BP of 92/70 mm Hg, HR of 92 beats/minute, respiratory rate of 18 breaths/minute, and O_2 saturation of 94% on room air. Laboratory values were BUN of 20 mg/dL and SCr of 1.4 mg/dL. Physical examination reveals pulmonary and peripheral edema. He is given 80 mg IV furosemide, and he does not respond adequately. His SCr has increased to 1.8 mg/dL. The decision is made to admit him to the coronary care unit where a pulmonary artery catheter (Swan–Ganz catheter) is placed, and the following hemodynamic variables are measured and calculated: PCWP, 21 mm Hg; cardiac index, 1.8 L/minute/m^2; SVR, 580 dyne · s/cm^5. Is B.J. a candidate for inotropic therapy? Why is milrinone preferred over inamrinone?

DOPAMINE AND DOBUTAMINE

The hemodynamic profile of B.J. is category IV (cold and wet) because of hypoperfusion and congestion. According to the ACC/AHA guidelines, IV inotropic agents (dobutamine, dopamine, milrinone, inamrinone) are indicated in symptomatic patients with reduced LVEF, low CO, or end-organ dysfunction (i.e., worsening renal function) and in patients who are intolerant to vasodilators.[1] They are also recommended for patients with cardiogenic shock or refractory symptoms, and may be used in patients requiring perioperative support after cardiac and noncardiac surgery or for those awaiting transplantation. Dobutamine should be the drug of choice in patients with low-output HF. Dobutamine improves CO, decreases PCWP, and decreases total SVR with little effect on HR or systemic arterial pressure when compared with dopamine.[314] (See Chapter 22, Shock, for further information on dopamine and dobutamine.)

PHOSPHODIESTERASE INHIBITORS: INAMRINONE AND MILRINONE

Although β-agonists, such as dobutamine, have been traditionally used in patients with ADHF, the phosphodiesterase inhibitors, inamrinone and milrinone, are alternatives to the catecholamines and vasodilators for the short-term parenteral treatment of severe congestive failure. These agents selectively inhibit phosphodiesterase III, the cyclic adenosine monophosphate (cAMP)-specific cardiac phosphodiesterase. They have direct cardiac-stimulating effects, but they are not sympathomimetics or inhibitors of Na^+/K^+ ATPase. Enzyme inhibition results in increased cAMP levels in myocardial cells and, thus, enhances contractility. Their activity is not blocked by β-blockers. Because they are phosphodiesterase inhibitors, they also act as vasodilators. It has been suggested that at low doses they act more as unloading agents rather than inotropic agents; others refute this viewpoint. Their overall hemodynamic effect probably results from a combination of positive inotropic action plus preload and afterload reduction.

Inamrinone is no longer used because of dose-dependent reversible thrombocytopenia (up to 20% of patients), drug fever, liver function abnormalities, and possibly drug-induced ventricular arrhythmias. Milrinone is structurally and pharmacologically similar to inamrinone.[315–317] Besides inhibiting phosphodiesterase, it also may increase calcium availability to myocardial muscle. It has both inotropic and vasodilating properties. HR increase and myocardial consumption may be less with milrinone than with dobutamine.[318,319] The half-life of milrinone is short (1.5–2.5 hours), with renal clearance accounting for approximately 80% to 90% of total body elimination. Although a loading dose of 50 mcg/kg administered during 10 minutes is in the product labeling, it is rarely given. Maintenance infusions are typically between 0.2 and 0.75 mcg/kg/minute. The infusion is adjusted according to hemodynamic and clinical responses and should be decreased in patients with renal insufficiency. The primary concern with the use of milrinone is induction of ventricular arrhythmias, reported in up to 12% of patients. Supraventricular arrhythmias, hypotension, headache, and chest pain also have been reported. Thrombocytopenia is rare, a distinct advantage compared with inamrinone. Overall, milrinone has become the drug of choice among the phosphodiesterase inhibitors.

The Outcomes of a Prospective Trial of Intravenous Milrinone for Chronic Heart Failure (OPTIME-CHF) trial assessed the in-hospital management of 951 patients with acute HF exacerbation (NYHA class III or IV, mean LVEF 23%) but not in cardiogenic shock.[318,319] In addition to standard diuretic and ACE inhibitor therapy, subjects were randomly assigned to receive either milrinone or placebo. The initial milrinone infusion rate was 0.5 mcg/kg/minute with no loading dose. For the primary end point of total numbers of days hospitalized for CV causes from the time of the start of study drug infusion to day 60, no difference was found between active drug and placebo (mean 12.3 days with milrinone and 12.5 days with placebo), nor was any difference seen in the mean number of days of hospitalization during the primary event. Death rates within 60 days were 10.3% with milrinone and 8.9% with placebo (not significant, $p = 0.41$).[318] Follow-up analysis categorized subjects by etiology of HF (ischemic vs. nonischemic).[319] Not unexpectedly, those with an ischemic cause did less well with hospital rates of 13.0 days for ischemic patients compared with 11.7 days for those without ischemia ($p = 0.2$). Corresponding death rates for 60 days were 11.6% and 7.5% ($p = 0.03$). Importantly, within the cohort of patients with ischemia ($n = 485$), milrinone-treated patients tended to have worse outcomes than those treated with placebo: 13.6 hospital days with milrinone versus 12.4 days with placebo. Death occurred in 13.3% of ischemic patients on milrinone compared with 10.0% of those on placebo. For the composite of patients dying or being rehospitalized, 42% of milrinone subjects had events compared with 36% with placebo ($p = 0.01$). In contrast, nonischemic patients ($n = 464$) had a trend toward better outcomes with milrinone than with placebo: 10.9 hospital days for milrinone versus 12.6 days with placebo, 7.3% deaths with milrinone compared with 7.7% with placebo, and the composite of death or hospitalization in 28% of subjects with milrinone versus 35% with placebo. From these data, it can be concluded that the benefits of milrinone in patients with acute exacerbations of HF are minimal and more likely to be seen in patients with a nonischemic etiology of HF. Worse outcomes may be seen in patients with ischemic HF. However, short-term infusions of milrinone were not associated with excess mortality.

Few trials have compared dobutamine with milrinone in ADHF patients. One small retrospective analysis evaluated 329 patients admitted for ADHF with an EF of less than 20% who either received IV dobutamine or milrinone.[320] Hemodynamic response, need for additional therapies, adverse effects, length of stay, and drug cost were evaluated. Patients in both groups were comparable in clinical presentation. Further, both groups had similar HR, BP, PCWP, and CO at baseline. The milrinone group, however, had higher mean pulmonary arterial pressure. A greater percentage of patients received dobutamine therapy (269, 81.7%) versus milrinone therapy (60, 18.3%.). Only 19% of patients were taking β-blockers before admission. Clinical outcomes in both groups were similar. There was no significant difference in the in-hospital mortality rate, adverse effects, ventilator use, or length of stay. More patients in the dobutamine group required nitroprusside to achieve optimal hemodynamic response. A slightly better hemodynamic response occurred in the milrinone group, which did not translate into a more beneficial short-term clinical outcome. The study concluded that both drugs have comparable efficacy.

Other factors to consider when deciding which inotropic agent should be used in ADHF are renal function, BP, and concomitant β-blocker use. Milrinone has a longer half-life than dobutamine, and accumulates in cases of renal dysfunction. Milrinone is also a vasodilator, which can limit its use in patients with hypotension. The concomitant use of β-blockers may antagonize the action of dobutamine.

B.J. has responded poorly to IV furosemide, his renal function has deteriorated, and his systolic BP is low. Patients with advanced HF, reduced BP, and normal or low SVR often will not tolerate vasodilator therapy. Inotropic agents may be necessary to maintain circulatory function in these patients. According to guidelines, IV inotropic drugs may be considered for patients who have symptomatic hypotension despite adequate filling pressure, who are unresponsive to diuretics and intolerant to vasodilators, or who have worsening renal function. Phosphodiesterase inhibitors are sometimes preferred instead of dobutamine for patients who are receiving concomitant β-blockers. For the above-mentioned reasons, B.J. is a candidate for milrinone therapy. Patients must be on telemetry because milrinone has the potential to cause arrhythmias. Vital signs, SCr, symptom relief, and urine output should be monitored. Once the patient's hemodynamic profile improves, milrinone should be discontinued, and oral furosemide therapy can be resumed. At discharge, the outpatient HF medications should be optimized.

Outpatient Inotropic Infusions

CASE 19-5, QUESTION 2: Are there any indications for using repeated intermittent infusions of inotropic agents as part of a home-care regimen?

The long-term safety and efficacy of inotropic therapy in general is regarded with skepticism. There are few studies assessing intermittent (e.g., weekly) infusions of dobutamine or milrinone. Nearly all the data on this therapeutic approach are from open-label and uncontrolled trials or studies that compare two inotropic agents without a placebo group.[321–325] It is unclear whether the benefit observed was the result of more intensive patient monitoring or an actual pharmacologic benefit. It is also speculated that long-term therapy may actually be cardiotoxic, as evidenced by an acute worsening of HF on withdrawal of the drug. The only placebo-controlled trial of intermittent infusion of dobutamine was terminated because of excess mortality in the treatment group.[322] Death occurred in 32% of 31 patients treated with dobutamine and only 14% of 29 treated with placebo. Whether this phenomenon was caused by progression of the underlying heart disease or continued drug therapy or was a true cardiotoxic effect remains unknown. No corresponding data exist for milrinone, although as cited previously, a placebo-controlled trial with milrinone failed to support the routine use of IV milrinone as an adjunct to standard therapy in the treatment of patients hospitalized for an acute exacerbation of chronic HF.[318,319] For this reason, the ACA/AHA guidelines explicitly indicate that intermittent infusions of dobutamine and milrinone in the long-term treatment of HF, even in advanced stages, should be avoided.[4] Dobutamine and milrinone are sometimes administered as long-term infusions in patients with refractory HF who are awaiting transplant. The lowest dose possible should be administered.

Ventricular Arrhythmias Complicating Heart Failure

AMIODARONE

CASE 19-5, QUESTION 3: B.J. was stabilized during the next several days and discharged home with furosemide 40 mg every day, enalapril 5 mg every day, metoprolol succinate 100 mg every day, aspirin 81 mg every day, and NTG 0.4 mg sublingual to be used as needed for chest pain. His EF was 23%. Laboratory values were all normal. ECG monitoring during B.J.'s hospital stay showed normal sinus rhythm, but he was having 15 to 20 asymptomatic PVCs/hour. At that time, it was decided not to treat his arrhythmia other than with metoprolol because he was asymptomatic. For the next several months, he continued to have frequent PVC during follow-up examinations in the cardiology clinic.

It has now been 5 months and he is still having up to 12 to 15 PVCs/hour. His exercise capacity is limited by SOB after walking about a block despite having his enalapril increased to 20 mg/day and metoprolol succinate to 200 mg/day and adding digoxin 0.25 mg every day. The furosemide is still at 40 mg/day because he has some edema. A repeat echocardiogram shows an EF of 20%. Is an antiarrhythmic agent indicated for B.J. at this time? What is the agent of choice, and what dose should be given?

PVCs and other arrhythmias are a common complication of LV dysfunction and may be present regardless of whether the patient has had an MI. Approximately 50% to 70% of patients with HF have episodes of nonsustained ventricular tachycardia on ambulatory monitoring.[4] This myocardial irritability may be a result of autonomic hyperactivity or ventricular remodeling that can accompany HF. It is not clear, however, whether these rhythm disturbances contribute to sudden death or simply reflect the underlying disease process. Recent studies suggest that bradyarrhythmia or electromechanical dissociation may be associated with sudden death in HF patients with nonischemic cardiomyopathy.[326,327] More importantly, suppression of ventricular ectopy in patients with HF has not been shown to lead to a reduction of sudden death in clinical trials. B.J.'s PVCs were first noted after his MI. As discussed in detail in Chapter 18, Acute Coronary Syndrome, and Chapter 20, Cardiac Arrhythmias, neither prophylactic antiarrhythmic therapy nor treatment of asymptomatic PVC after an MI has been proven to improve outcome or survival. In fact, because of concerns about proarrhythmic effects of most class IA (e.g., quinidine) and class IC (e.g., flecainide) drugs, as well as sotalol, treatment is considered contraindicated.

It is suggested that amiodarone has value in patients with HF with arrhythmias because it has both antiarrhythmic properties as well as coronary vasodilating effects and α- and β-blocking properties. Thus, it may offer a dual benefit to reduce myocardial irritability and improve the hemodynamics of HF.

One meta-analysis reviewed 13 randomized, controlled trials of prophylactic amiodarone in patients with either recent MI ($n = 8$) or HF ($n = 5$).[328] None of the individual trials were powered to detect a mortality reduction of less than 33%. Therefore, moderate reductions of mortality that still may be clinically relevant would not have been identified as statistically significant. After loading doses of 400 to 800 mg/day for 2 weeks, maintenance doses ranged from 200 to 400 mg/day. The authors concluded that prophylactic amiodarone reduces the rate of arrhythmic or sudden death in high-risk patients, and this effect results in an overall 13% reduction in total mortality. Because this analysis combined trials of both MI and HF patients, it is helpful to look at two of the key HF trials.

In the Grupo de Estudio de la Sobrevida en la Insuficiecia Cardiaca en Argentina (GESICA) study,[329] 516 patients with class II to IV HF symptoms (79% class III or IV), an average EF of 20%, and frequent PVCs on cardiac monitoring were randomly assigned to receive either standard treatment (diuretics, vasodilators, digoxin) or a fixed dose of amiodarone plus standard treatment. The dose of amiodarone was 600 mg daily for the first 2 weeks, then 300 mg/day for at least 1 year. Of 260 patients on amiodarone, 87 (33.5%) died during follow-up compared with 106 of 256 (41.4%) receiving standard treatment, a statistically significant difference in favor of amiodarone ($p = 0.02$). Similarly, the number of HF-related hospitalizations was reduced with amiodarone. No data were presented on changes in EF, but a trend toward more patients in the amiodarone group being judged to have a decrease of at least one stage in NYHA class was noted.

Somewhat different outcomes were noted by the investigators in the Veterans Administration (VA) Cooperative Survival Trial of Antiarrhythmic Therapy in Congestive Heart Failure (CHF-STAT) study.[330,331] Entry criteria to this trial were similar to the GESICA study, with a primary indicator being more than 10 asymptomatic PVCs per hour on 24-hour monitoring, but without sustained ventricular tachycardia. A higher dose of amiodarone was used, starting with 800 mg for the first 2 weeks, then 400 mg/day for 1 year. The dose was reduced to 300 mg/day after the first year, with the average follow-up being 45 months (4.5 years maximum). No difference between groups for either all-cause mortality (39% amiodarone vs. 42% placebo) or sudden cardiac death (15% amiodarone vs. 17% placebo) was found. Similarly, 2-year survival was 69.4% with amiodarone and 70.8% with placebo. Higher survival in the amiodarone group after the first 2 years was a noted trend, but the number of subjects observed for longer periods was not sufficiently large to establish significance. An encouraging finding in this study was that EF improved more in the patients treated with amiodarone, rising from a baseline average of 24.9% to posttreatment values of 33.7%. Corresponding change in the standard treatment group was from a baseline of 25.8% to 29.2% at follow-up. Despite the increase in EF, symptom scores did not differ between the two groups.

Together, these two studies still leave unclear the role of amiodarone in patients with HF with asymptomatic arrhythmias. The encouraging finding is that amiodarone does not seem to have a negative effect on mortality as seen with some of the other antiarrhythmic agents. On the other hand, the two studies cited have conflicting findings regarding value in improving survival and functional capacity of patients. In comparing the two studies, it has been noted that the patients in the GESICA study had more advanced disease (79% class III or IV; average EF 20%; 55% 2-year placebo mortality) than those in the VA study (43% class III or IV; average EF 25%; 29% 2-year placebo mortality); more patients had nonischemic cardiomyopathy in the GESICA study (60%) compared with 29% in the VA study; 99% of the VA subjects were men, whereas 19% of GESICA subjects were women; and the dose of amiodarone was lower in the GESICA study.[332] Further subgroup analysis suggests that those with more advanced disease, nonischemic cardiomyopathy, and female sex have better outcomes. Contradicting this speculation was a trend toward better outcomes in the small number of patients with class II symptoms in the GESICA study.[329] Other factors to consider are the potential for significant side effects with amiodarone (see Chapter 20, Cardiac Arrhythmias) and the risk that digoxin levels increase after the addition of amiodarone.

The ACC/AHA guidelines do not recommend routine ambulatory ECG monitoring to detect asymptomatic ventricular arrhythmias in patients with HF, and they also recommend against treatment if such arrhythmias are inadvertently detected.[21] If symptomatic ventricular arrhythmias should arise or there is determined to be a high risk for sudden death, one of the following should be considered: a β-blocking drug, amiodarone, or an ICD. As discussed extensively throughout this chapter, nearly all patients with HF should have a β-blocker as part of their regimen because these drugs reduce all-cause mortality, not just sudden death. B.J. continued to have ectopy despite continued use of a β-blocker. Nonetheless, it is decided not to use amiodarone because he has ischemic cardiomyopathy and is not bothered by his arrhythmia.

IMPLANTABLE CARDIOVERTER-DEFIBRILLATOR

CASE 19-5, QUESTION 4: Is B.J. a candidate for an ICD implantation?

Although amiodarone is the preferred antiarrhythmic agent in patients with HF with reduced EF to prevent recurrent AF and symptomatic ventricular arrhythmias, it has not improved survival benefits. Ventricular arrhythmias are associated with high frequency of SCD in patients with HF. Numerous trials have established the role of ICDs in primary and secondary prevention of SCD. The earliest of the primary prevention trials was the Multicenter Automatic Defibrillator Implantation Trial (MADIT).[333] This study was terminated early because of the survival benefit seen in the ICD group compared with conventional therapy (hazard ratio, 0.46; $p = 0.009$). There was no evidence that amiodarone, β-blockers, or any other antiarrhythmic therapy had a significant influence on the observed hazard ratio. Unlike MADIT, the MADIT II[334] study enrolled patients with no documented arrhythmias but with previous MI and LVEF less than 30%. Patients received either an ICD or conventional medical therapy. The primary end point was death from any cause. There was a 31% relative reduction in the risk of death and an absolute reduction of 6% in the ICD group compared with the medical group. This was the first trial to show mortality benefits of ICDs in patients with no documented history of abnormal heart rhythms.

The most recent trial, the Sudden Cardiac Death in Heart Failure trial (SCD-HeFT) evaluated the efficacy of amiodarone in patients with LV dysfunction (EF $\leq$35%).[332] The patients (NYHA class II–III) were randomly assigned to conventional therapy or placebo, conventional therapy plus amiodarone, or conventional therapy plus ICD. Amiodarone was no better than placebo, whereas ICD decreased mortality by 23% ($p = 0.007$) compared with conventional therapy. A subgroup analysis showed that patients with class II HF had a greater drop in mortality with ICD use than class III patients. Also, amiodarone decreased survival in class III HF. The role of amiodarone in patients with NYHA class III needs to be further evaluated before it is routinely used in patients with LV dysfunction.

The 2009 ACC/AHA guidelines recommend the use of ICDs in patients after MI with reduced LVEF and who have a history of ventricular arrhythmias. ICDs are also recommended for primary prevention in patients with nonischemic cardiomyopathy and ischemic heart disease who have an LVEF of 30% or less, those with with NYHA functional class II or III symptoms while on optimal standard oral therapy, and patients who have reasonable expected survival with a good functional status of 1 or more years. Patients with ischemic heart disease should be at least 40 days after MI to receive an ICD. B.J. is currently on optimal HF drug regimen, and his EF is 20%. According to guidelines, B.J. would benefit from ICD implantation.

CARDIAC RESYNCHRONIZATION THERAPY

CASE 19-6

QUESTION 1: C.M., a 49-year-old woman with a history of cardiomyopathy (EF 25%), presents to the HF clinic with NYHA class III symptoms. She reports increased SOB, chest pain, and fatigue. She has been optimized on drug therapy for 3 months. Her medications include metoprolol succinate 200 mg every day, furosemide 40 mg BID, lisinopril 20 mg every day, spironolactone 25 mg every day, and potassium chloride 40 mEq. An ECG showed sinus rhythm at a rate of 72 beats/minute and a QRS duration of 144 milliseconds. Is she a candidate for CRT?

Approximately one-third of the patients with advanced systolic HF exhibit intraventricular or interventricular conduction delays that cause the ventricles to beat asynchronously.[335] This ventricular dyssynchrony, which is often seen on the ECG as a wide QRS complex with a left bundle branch block, can lead to deleterious effects on cardiac function. Patients may present with reduced EF, decreased CO, and presence of NYHA class III or IV HF symptoms. These are all associated with increased mortality.

CRT is the use of cardiac pacing to coordinate the contraction of the left and right ventricles.[78] Initial randomized trials of CRT show reduced HF symptoms and improved exercise tolerance and quality of life, but they have not demonstrated conclusive mortality benefits. The Comparison of Medical Therapy, Pacing, and Defibrillator in Heart Failure (COMPANION) trial[78] enrolled 1,520 patients with NYHA class II or IV (ischemic or nonischemic cardiomyopathies, QRS interval of at least 120 milliseconds, and LVEF $\leq$35%) who were treated with optimal drug therapy (ACE inhibitors, diuretics, β-blockers, and spironolactone). Patients were randomly assigned to receive optimal drug therapy alone, optimal drug therapy and CRT with a pacemaker, or optimal drug therapy and CRT with ICD (CRT-D). The primary end point was a composite of all-cause mortality and hospitalization. Both CRT and CRT-D groups were associated with a decreased risk of primary end point ($p = 0.014$, $p = 0.01$, respectively) compared with optimal drug therapy alone. All-cause mortality at 1 year was decreased by 24% in the CRT group and 43% in the CRT-D group; however, it was not significantly reduced in the CRT group.

The results of the Cardiac Resynchronization in Heart Failure study (CARE-HF)[77] extended the landmark findings of the COMPANION trial. CARE-HF demonstrated a significant all-cause mortality reduction for CRT pacing without defibrillator backup (CRT) in patients with HF that was medically treated similarly. This study was conducted in a total of 813 patients. The inclusion criteria were NYHA class III or IV, EF of 35% or less, and QRS duration of 120 milliseconds or longer. Approximately 35% of patients had ischemic heart disease. The primary end point of all-cause deaths and hospitalizations for a major CV reason occurred in fewer patients in the CRT group compared with the optimal drug therapy group (39% vs. 55%; $p < 0.001$). Death or hospitalization for worsening HF was also significantly reduced in the CRT group.

Thus, the combined results of CARE-HF and COMPANION confirm the importance of CRT and CRT-D in improving ventricular function, HF symptoms, and exercise tolerance, while also reducing frequency of HF hospitalizations by 37% and death by 22%.[336] The role of CRT in patients with mild HF symptoms, narrow QRS, chronic AF, and right bundle branch block need to be explored.

According to the ACC/AHA guidelines,[1,21] patients with NYHA class III and ambulatory patients with class IV HF should receive CRT (unless contraindicated) if they meet the following criteria: LVEF of 35% or less, presence of electric asynchrony as shown by a wide QRS (>120 milliseconds), and receiving optimal HF standard medical therapy. Despite optimal doses of HF medications, C.M. continues to have HF symptoms. CRT therapy could provide incremental benefits beyond what is provided with neurohormonal therapy.

CASE 19-6, QUESTION 2: If C.M. presented with NYHA class I or II symptoms, would she be a candidate for CRT therapy? What is the evidence to support CRT in NYHA class I and II patients?

As mentioned in Case 19-7, Question 1, the CARE-HF and COMPANION trials provide strong evidence that CRT induces reverse modeling in patients with symptomatic NYHA class III and ambulatory class IV HF. The next logical step was to evaluate benefits of CRT therapy in HF patients with milder symptoms (asymptomatic or mildly symptomatic). The Multicenter InSynch ICD Randomized Clinical Evaluation (MIRACLE-ICDII)[337] trial was the first randomized trial to enroll only class II through IV HF patients but with separate specified end points for class II patients. In this trial, 186 patients with NYHA class II HF, an LVEF of less than 35%, and a QRS of more than 130 milliseconds received a CRT-ICD device. Subjects were randomly assigned to active CRT group (ICD activated, CRT on) or control group (ICD activated and CRT off). The primary end point was progression of HF, defined as all-cause mortality, hospitalizations for HF, and ventricular tachycardia or ventricular fibrillation requiring device intervention. A 15% reduction in HF progression was observed, but this was not statistically significant ($p = 0.35$). At 6 months patients within the active CRT group had improved exercise tolerance, but this was not significantly different from the control group. However, there was a significant decrease in ventricular end-systolic volume and increased LVEF after 6 months of therapy. Even though the study results did not translate into improved exercise tolerance, it helped to set the stage for future trials in patients with less symptomatic HF.

In 2008, the REVERSE trial[75] enrolled 610 participants from both the United States and Europe with NYHA class I or II HF,

LVEF less than 40%, and with a QRS duration of more than 120 milliseconds who received a CRT device (with or without ICD) in combination with optimal drug therapy. Similar to the MIRACLE ICD II trial, the patients in the active CRT group had significant improvement in LV end-systolic volume index, LV end-diastolic volume index, and LVEF ($p < 0.0001$, $p < 0.0001$, $p < 0.001$, respectively) compared with the control group, which are measures of reverse remodeling. Although the primary clinical end point (the percentage of patients with worsened clinical composite score) did not meet statistical significance at 12 months in the US cohort ($p = 0.1$), in the European cohort[338] statistical difference was seen at 24 months ($p = 0.01$). This difference was driven by increased time to first HF hospitalization. Significant differences were observed in several of the secondary end points. The aggregate data from these two clinical trials provided overwhelming evidence that linked CRT with substantial reverse remodeling in mild HF patients.

The question of whether CRT reduces progression of HF and reduces mortality in NYHA class I and II HF patients has also been studied. The MADIT-CRT[76] was the largest randomized trial designed to determine whether CRT-D therapy would reduce the primary end point (all-cause mortality or HF events, whichever occurred first) when compared with patients receiving ICD-only therapy. The study population involved cardiac patients in NYHA functional class I or II (no or mild symptoms) who had either ischemic or nonischemic heart disease with LVEF of 30% or less and QRS duration of more than 130 milliseconds on ECG. There was a 34% ($p < 0.001$) reduction in the primary end point, and a 44% ($p < 0.001$) reduction in HF events when compared with ICD therapy. Also, patients on CRT-D therapy showed an 11% improvement in LVEF after 1 year, compared with 3% improvement for ICD-alone patients. It is noteworthy that both MADIT-CRT and REVERSE excluded patients with AF. In addition, there were fewer asymptomatic patients, and some patients had NYHA class III symptoms before enrollment, but almost 80% of patients were classified as NYHA class II. Furthermore, both studies failed to show a benefit for CRT in patients with QRS duration less than 150 milliseconds.

In 2010, the Resynchronization/Defibrillation for Ambulatory Heart Failure Trial (RAFT),[339] confirmed the results of previous trials (including MADIT-CRT and REVERSE), showing that CRT had an increased benefit in patients with a QRS duration of 150 milliseconds or more and in those with left bundle branch block. RAFT investigators randomly assigned 1,798 patients from 34 centers with NYHA class II or III HF, LVEF of 30% or less, and a QRS duration of at least 120 milliseconds (or a paced QRS of at least 200 milliseconds) to either ICD therapy alone or an ICD with CRT (CRT-D). The mean follow-up time for all patients was 40 months. The primary outcome was a combination of total mortality and HF hospitalization. The secondary outcomes included death by any cause, death from a CV cause, and HF hospitalizations. The primary outcome was statistically significant in the ICD group compared with the ICD-CRT group (40% vs. 33%, respectively). These findings demonstrate that earlier intervention with CRT-D, in addition to guideline-recommended medical and ICD therapy, benefits this patient population.

HEART FAILURE WITH PRESERVED LEFT VENTRICULAR EJECTION FRACTION

CASE 19-7

QUESTION 1: D.F., a 72-year-old white woman, has a 5-year history of HF symptoms, including decreased exercise capacity, SOB, and distended neck veins. She has minimal peripheral edema. History is suggestive of rheumatic fever as a child, but she does not recall having any cardiac symptoms when she was younger, other than being told she had a murmur. Her symptoms are controlled with diuretics. She has history of HTN. She has no other medical problems, and all laboratory test findings are normal. Her BP is 155/85 mm Hg, and her HR is 90 beats/minute. Cardiac examination reveals a prominent S_4 heart sound. Noninvasive echocardiography reveals a normal EF of 50%. Prior treatment included furosemide, most recently at 40 mg BID. The physician is considering adding a β-blocker or CCB to control the BP. Why might this consideration be appropriate?

This case exemplifies a patient with HF with preserved LVEF (HFPEF), often referred to as diastolic HF. Risk factors for HFPEF include advanced age, female sex, HTN, and CAD. This diagnosis can be made on the basis of LVH, clinical evidence of HF, a normal EF, and Doppler tissue echocardiography findings. The ideal treatment strategies for HFPEF have not been extensively validated. A review of trials evaluating specific drug therapy in HFPEF is listed in Table 19-13. Also, no drug selectively enhances myocardial relaxation without having associated effects on LV contractility or on the peripheral vasculature.[14–18]

Factors affecting HF control, such as dietary sodium intake, fluid intake, compliance, and NSAID and herbal remedy use, should be appropriately managed along with drug therapy. Symptomatic LV diastolic HF is initially treated similarly to other forms of HF, by slow diuresis. Diuresis decreases preload and lessens passive congestion of the ventricles. Excessive lowering of venous and ventricular filling pressures, however, can worsen CO and cause hypotension.

The most common cause of diastolic HF and HFPEF is HTN that leads to LVH and decreased cardiac compliance.[353] Recent ACC/AHA guidelines recommend treating associated HTN in accordance with the national guidelines and lower BP targets for patients with diabetes and chronic kidney disease (<130/80 mm Hg).[21] Drugs that cause regression of LVH (e.g., ACE inhibitors, ARBs, β-blockers) may also slow or reverse structural abnormalities associated with diastolic HF.

Although ACE inhibitors have been used with success in some patients with HFPEF, the role of RAAS inhibition in HF with preserved LV function has not been rigorously studied. Several recent clinical trials have attempted to address this issue. In the Perindopril in Elderly patients with Chronic HF (PEP-CHF) trial,[342] the ACE inhibitor perindopril failed to reduce the incidence of the primary end point (all-cause mortality or HF hospitalizations), but did reduce symptoms and improved functional capacity in 2 years in patients with preserved LV function. The CHARM-preserved trial[180] also failed to show any difference in CV mortality, but fewer hospitalizations were seen in the candesartan group (see Case19-1, Question 13).

The Valsartan in Diastolic Dysfunction (VALIDD)[354] trial was the first large-scale, randomized trial comparing the effects of valsartan or placebo added to standard antihypertensive therapy (which included diuretics, β-blockers, CCBs, or α-blockers) in patients with mild HTN and diastolic HF. The hypothesis of this trial was that RAAS inhibition with an ARB would be associated with greater improvement in diastolic dysfunction, possibly because of a greater regression of LVH or myocardial fibrosis. Patients with a history of stage 1 or 2 essential HTN were randomly assigned to receive either valsartan 160 mg, titrated up to 320 mg, or matching placebo. Patients who did not achieve a target BP goal of less than 135/80 mm Hg received additional therapy starting with a diuretic followed by a CCB or a β-blocker,

TABLE 19-13

Clinical Trials of Pharmacotherapy in Heart Failure with Preserved Ejection Fraction

Study	Patient Population	Therapy Intervention	Outcome	Treatment Duration	Results
Aronow et al. (1993)[340]	NYHA III; Prior MI, EF >50%; (n = 21)	Enalapril vs. placebo	NYHA class, treadmill exercise time (seconds)	3 months	Enalapril: NYHA class from 3 ± 0 to 2.4 ± 0.5 ($p = 0.005$), exercise time from 224 ± 27 to 270 ± 44 ($p < 0.001$) vs. no difference in placebo
Lang et al. (1995)[341]	HF symptoms >3 months; EF >50%; (n = 12)	Lisinopril vs. placebo crossover	Dyspnea and fatigue	5 weeks for each treatment arm	No significant differences
Cleland et al. (2006)[342] PEP-CHF	Diastolic dysfunction; CV admission within 6 months; EF >40%; n = 850)	Perindopril vs. placebo	Primary: composite of all-cause mortality or hospitalization for HF	Mean 26.2 months	Primary: 23.6% in perindopril group vs. 25.1% in placebo (HR 0.92 [0.70–1.21], $p = 0.545$)
Zi et al. (2003)[343]	NYHA class II or III; EF ≥40%; (n = 74)	Quinapril vs. placebo	6-minute walk test, QoL, NYHA class	6 months	No significant differences
Yusuf et al. (2003)[180] CHARM-Preserved	NYHA II–IV; hospitalization for CV causes; EF >40%; (n = 3,023)	Candesartan vs. placebo	Primary: CV death or hospital admission for HF	Median 36.6 months	Primary: 22% in the candesartan group vs. 24% in the placebo group (adjusted HR 0.86 [0.74–1.00], $p = 0.051$).
Massie et al. (2008)[344] I-PRESERVE	NYHA II–IV; hospitalized for HF in last 6 months; EF ≥45%; (n = 4,122	Irbesartan vs. placebo	Primary: all-cause death or hospitalization for CV causes	Mean 49.5 months	Primary: 36% in the irbesartan group vs. 37% in the placebo group (HR 0.95 [95% CI 0.86–1.05], $p = 0.35$)
Yip et al. (2008)[345]	NYHA II–IV; history of HF in last 2 months; EF >45%; (n = 151)	Ramipril vs. irbesartan	QoL, 6-minute walk test, HF hospital admission	12 months	No significant differences
Warner et al. (1999)[346]	Diastolic dysfunction; DOE; EF >50%; SBP >150, <200 mm Hg (n = 20)	Losartan vs. placebo crossover	Exercise time, QoL	2 weeks for each treatment arm	Increase in exercise time (11.3 minutes at baseline, improved to 12.3 ± 2.6 minutes with losartan vs. 11.0 minutes with placebo, $p < 0.05$) and improvement in QoL (25 at baseline, improved to 18 with losartan vs. 22 with placebo); $p < 0.05$ for both end points
Parthasarathy et al. (2009)[347]	Diastolic dysfunction; DOE; EF >40%; (n = 152)	Valsartan vs. placebo	Primary: exercise time	14 weeks	No significant differences
Takeda et al. (2004)[348]	NYHA II–III and stage C heart failure; EF ≥45%	Carvedilol vs. placebo	Plasma BNP, NYHA class, exercise capacity	12 months	NYHA class improved by 0.77 (carvedilol) vs. 0.25 (placebo) ($p < 0.02$), exercise capacity in METs improved 0.69 (carvedilol) vs. worsened by 0.07 (placebo) ($p = 0.01$).
Flather et al. (2005)[349] SENIORS	HF hospital admission in last year; EF ≤35%; subgroup EF ≥35%	Nebivolol vs. placebo	Primary: composite of all-cause mortality or hospitalization for a cardiovascular cause	Mean 21 months	EF >35%, primary event rate 17.6% in nebivolol and 21.9% in placebo (HR 0.86 [95% CI 0.74–0.99], $p = 0.039$).
Aronow et al. (1997)[350]	NYHA II–III; prior Q-wave MI; EF >40%; n = 158)	Propranolol vs. placebo	All-cause mortality, all-cause mortality plus nonfatal MI	32 months	All-cause mortality (56% propranolol group vs. 76% placebo group, $p = 0.007$) and all-cause mortality plus nonfatal MI (59% propranolol vs. 82% placebo, $p = 0.002$).
Setaro et al. (1990)[351]	Abnormal diastolic filling; EF >45%; (n = 20)	Verapamil vs. placebo	Exercise capacity	2 weeks for each crossover	Exercise capacity (10.7 minutes at baseline, improved to 13.9 minutes with verapamil vs. 12.3 minutes with placebo, $p < 0.05$).
Ahmed et al. (2006)[352] DIG	NYHA I–IV; EF >45%; (n = 988)	Digoxin vs. placebo	Primary: composite of HF hospitalization or mortality	Mean 37 months	102 (21%) in the digoxin group vs. 119 (24%) in the placebo group (HR 0.82 [0.63–1.07], $p = 0.136$).

BNP, B-type natriuretic peptide; CV, cardiovascular; DOE, dyspnea on exertion; EF, ejection fraction; HF, heart failure; HR, hazard ratio; METs, metabolic equivalents; MI, myocardial infarction; NA, not available; NYHA, New York Heart Association; QoL; quality of life; SBP, systolic blood pressure.

then an α-blocker (excluding ARBs, ACE inhibitors, and aldosterone blockers). The primary end point was the change in diastolic myocardial relaxation velocity from baseline to 9 months with a secondary end point of change in LV mass. During the study, the placebo group received more concomitant antihypertensive therapy compared with the valsartan group. A small, but significant, increase was seen in diastolic relaxation velocity in both groups from baseline to follow-up ($p < 0.001$), but there was no significant difference between the treatment groups ($p = 0.29$). BPessure reduction at the end of the trial did not differ significantly between the two treatment groups (13 mm Hg reduction in valsartan vs. 10 mm Hg in placebo), which was associated with significant improvement in diastolic function. Thus, the authors concluded that aggressive BP control—even in mild HTN—was associated with improvement in diastolic dysfunction, irrespective of whether BP reduction was achieved with an RAAS inhibitor or other antihypertensive agents. Several other trials are in progress that may provide further insight into the role of RAAS inhibitors in HFPEF.

CHARM-Preserved[180] investigated the role of candesartan in patients with HFPEF. The trial enrolled 3,023 subjects who met the overall CHARM trial inclusion criteria defined previously plus one additional criterion: an EF of more than 40% (mean, 54%). Thus, subjects would be classified as having symptomatic HF with normal (preserved) EF. They received either an ARB alone (n = 1,514) or placebo; only 20% of subjects in both groups were taking an ACE inhibitor at randomization, 56% were on a β-blocker, and 11% were on spironolactone.[180] After a median follow-up of 36.6 months, an insignificant trend was noted toward reduction in the primary outcome of CV death or hospital admission for HF in the candesartan group (22%) compared with placebo (24.3%; $p = 0.118$). CV deaths (170 vs. 170) and all-cause mortality (244 vs. 237) were nearly identical in both groups, but the total number of hospitalizations for HF (402 vs. 566) was significantly reduced in the candesartan group ($p = 0.014$). Secondary outcomes consisting of composites of the primary outcomes plus MI, nonfatal stroke, and coronary revascularization also showed a not significant trend in favor of candesartan. The most common side effects with candesartan were hypotension (2.4%), increase in creatinine (4.8%), and hyperkalemia (1.5%). Discontinuation because of an adverse event occurred in 17.8% of those treated with candesartan compared with 13.5% of placebo recipients ($p = 0.001$) (Table 19-12). Overall, the conclusion is that in symptomatic patients with diastolic HF, no significant improvement in morbidity or mortality occurs with candesartan compared with placebo, other than a significant reduction in HF-related hospitalizations.

I-PRESERVE is the largest randomized controlled trial for the management of HFPEF performed at this time.[344] The study lasted for a mean of 49.5 months. The patient population included was 60 years of age or older with NYHA class II through IV symptoms, EF of at least 45%, and who were hospitalized for HF during the last 6 months or have persistent class III or IV symptoms (n = 4,128). Patients received irbesartan titrated to 300 mg daily or placebo. There was no difference in the primary end point between irbesartan (36%) and placebo (37%) (hazard ratio, 0.95; 95% CI, 0.86–1.05; $p = 0.35$). In addition, no significant difference in secondary outcomes (i.e., composite HF outcome, score on the Minnesota Living with HF scale at 6 months, composite vascular-event outcome, CV death) was noted. The irbesartan group had more patients experiencing hyperkalemia (>6 mmol/dL) than placebo. One possible reason for the neutral results of I-PRESERVE included the high rate of dual RAAS blockade at baseline (39% ACE inhibitor use in the irbesartan group and 40% in the placebo group; 28% spironolactone use in the irbesartan group and 29% in the placebo group). Based on this high use, the study is less likely to find benefit with ARBs in addition to other RAAS agents. Another potential limitation of the study included the high study discontinuation rate (34%). Overall, the study resulted in irbesartan showing no added benefit in reducing morbidity or mortality in HFPEF patients.

β-Blockers or nondihydropyridine CCBs are other classes of drugs of interest in HFPEF. Part of their value is to control HTN, a risk factor for all forms of HF. More specific to diastolic HF, β-blockers and CCBs (especially verapamil) possess negative inotropic properties that may favorably influence the pathophysiology of diastolic dysfunction by (a) slowing the HR to allow more time for complete ventricular filling (via more complete left atrial emptying), particularly during exercise; (b) reducing myocardial oxygen demand; and (c) controlling BP. In addition, negative inotropic agents decrease myocardial contractility and can assist in overcoming the mechanical obstruction below the aorta during systole in patients with hypertrophic cardiomyopathy. Both agents also are beneficial in decreasing ischemia in patients with CAD.

Previous HF trials of β-blockers demonstrating decreased morbidity and mortality have mainly focused on patients with reduced LVEF. The Study of the Effects of Nebivolol Intervention on Outcomes and Rehospitalization in Seniors with Heart Failure (SENIORS) study[349] is the first major trial to evaluate β-blocker use in elderly HF patients (70 years or older), irrespective of LV function. The trial randomly assigned patients to nebivolol (n = 1,067) or placebo (n = 1,061). Nebivolol is a selective β_1-adernergic receptor blocker with vasodilator properties that are mediated through NO release. This effect may be beneficial in elderly patients, who tend to have low reserves of endothelial vasodilation.

The primary end point of the study was the combination of all-cause mortality and CV hospital admissions. The end point was significantly reduced by 14% in the nebivolol group, regardless of the EF. Prospective subgroup analyses of the primary outcome by LVEF (≤35% or >35%), sex, or age (≤75 years or >75 years) showed benefits across all subgroups. Patients with EF greater than 35%, however, appeared to benefit a little more than those with low EF%, and all-cause mortality was lower in patients older than 75 years treated with nebivolol compared with placebo. The study reinforces the current recommendations that all HF patients with reduced EF should receive β-blockers. Only 35% of the patients had preserved LV function, however, and were mostly men. This is not typical of patients with HFPEF, who are generally women. Further studies are required to define the role of β-blockers in HFPEF.

No randomized controlled trials have demonstrated mortality benefits with CCBs in patients with preserved LV function. Nondihydropyridine CCBs can be used in patients who have a contraindication to β-blockers to control BP and HR. Nondihydropyridine CCBs should not be used in patients with impaired LV dysfunction.

The role of aldosterone antagonists in the management of patients with HFPEF has not been clearly defined. The Aldosterone Antagonist Therapy for Adults with Heart Failure and Preserved Systolic Function (TOPCAT)[355] study is expected to be completed in 2011. This trial is evaluating the impact of spironolactone versus placebo on CV morbidity and mortality during a 2-year study period in patients older than 50 years of age with an EF greater than 45%. Once completed, we will have a clearer answer on the role of aldosterone antagonists in the management of patients with HFPEF.

D.F. fulfills the criteria for having diastolic dysfunction, based on her history of long-standing HTN, which is been poorly controlled. Her BP is not at goal, and her HR is elevated. As already discussed, uncontrolled HTN can promote LVH and myocardial remodeling, and can adversely affect the diastolic function. Therefore, antihypertensive therapy is warranted. Tachycardia alone can compromise the ventricle filling time and cause myocardial ischemia. So far, no data support the use of one agent over another. β-Blockers and nondihydropyridine CCBs can each reduce BP and HR. Because more experience has accrued with β-blockers and there are some mortality data on their use with diastolic HF patients, D.F. can be started on a β-blocker such as metoprolol (25 mg BID).

Herbal Products and Nutritional Supplements

CASE 19-8

QUESTION 1: W.L., a 60-year-old man with HF recently diagnosed by his naturopath, is concerned about his decreasing exercise capacity and increasing SOB during his morning walks in the local mall. His blood pressure is 170/85 mm Hg, and he has 1 to 2+ ankle edema. He distrusts medical doctors and wants to treat his HF naturally. One time in the past he was given HCTZ for BP reduction, but stopped taking it after a few days because he did not tolerate the urinary urgency it caused. The naturopath has prescribed 200 mg/day of hawthorn leaf and 50 mg/day of coenzyme Q. How effective is this treatment plan likely to be?

HAWTHORN

Hawthorn extracts from the leaves and flowers of *Crataegus monogyna* and *Crataegus oxyacantha* have been reported to have beneficial effects in mild HF.[356,357] Oligomeric procyanidins and flavonoids are considered the key active ingredients. Hawthorn extracts have shown positive inotropic action, weak ACE inhibition, vasodilating properties, and increased coronary blood flow in vitro and in animal models. In short-term (8 weeks or less), placebo-controlled trials in patients with the equivalent of NYHA class II HF, modest improvements were noted in exercise tolerance and subjective symptoms as well as decreases in HR and BP. Patients with more advanced HF were excluded. A systematic review by Pittler et al. also concluded that hawthorn extract was efficacious in the treatment of HF on top of standard HF therapy.[358] Conversely, the results of the Hawthorne Extract Randomized Blinded Chronic Heart Failure (HERB-CHF) trial failed to provide any evidence that hawthorn was beneficial in patients with HF who were already receiving standard medical therapy.[359] In clinical trials, side effects of hawthorn include nausea, vomiting, diarrhea, palpitations, chest pain, and vertigo. These side effects are more common when doses exceed 900 mg/day, but in some trials they have not occurred more often than with placebo. The risks and benefits of using hawthorn and digoxin together, both of which have positive inotropic effects, are not known.

To further investigate the longer-term benefits of hawthorn, additive effects to conventional therapy and effect on mortality were tested in the Survival and Prognosis: Investigation of Crataegus Extract WS 1442 in Congestive Heart Failure (SPICE) trial.[360] The trial enrolled 2,681 patients with NYHA class II or III, LVEF of 35% or less, who were randomly assigned to hawthorn or placebo for 2 years. Although the study failed to show any clear cardioprotective benefits in the treatment of chronic HF, hawthorn was well tolerated and can be safely added to standard therapy.

COENZYME Q

Coenzyme Q, also known as ubiquinone and ubidecarenone, is an endogenously synthesized provitamin that is structurally similar to vitamin E, serves as a lipid-soluble electron transport carrier in mitochondria, and aids in the synthesis of adenosine triphosphate.[361,362] It may also have membrane-stabilizing properties, enhance the antioxidant effects of vitamin E, and stabilize calcium-dependent slow channels. In animal models, it has positive inotropic effects, although weaker than those from digoxin. More than 18 open-label and double-blind, randomized clinical trials have been conducted of coenzyme Q in patients with HF ranging from NYHA classes II to IV.[361] Doses varied from 50 to 200 mg/day. In contrast to hawthorn, the patients in many of these trials were also taking diuretics, ACE inhibitors, and digoxin. Different trials used different end point measurements. Positive effects on subjective symptoms, NYHA class improvement, EF, quality of life, and hospitalization rates have all been observed. Two trials, however, failed to demonstrate significant changes in EF, vascular resistance, or exercise tolerance. None of the trials had sufficiently large samples sizes or adequate duration of assessment to detect reduction in mortality. Side effects were consistently minimal, but included nausea, epigastric pain, diarrhea, heartburn, and appetite suppression. Mild increases in lactate dehydrogenase and hepatic enzymes have been rarely reported with coenzyme Q doses in excess of 300 mg/day.

It can be concluded that hawthorn and coenzyme Q are both safe in the treatment of HF and might provide symptomatic improvement, especially in patients with mild HF (NYHA class II). Only coenzyme Q has been shown to be of benefit as an adjunct to conventional therapies. It is unknown whether using hawthorn and coenzyme Q together, as prescribed for W.L., will have an additive effect. No conclusion can be drawn about their effects on mortality rates.

W.L. has poorly controlled systolic HTN and HF that is beginning to interfere with his activities of daily life. Although evidence indicates that patients with NYHA class II HF obtain symptomatic improvement with hawthorn and coenzyme Q, this does not address W.L.'s HTN. (As reviewed by Tran et al.,[361] conflicting data exist on the value of coenzyme Q in lowering BP.) Furthermore, the results of the SPICE trial did not demonstrate any mortality benefits. Also, no incremental benefits were seen when combined with standard therapy. Even if W.L. and his naturopath are both satisfied with his responses to hawthorn and coenzyme Q, significant concern still exists about what will happen when and if his disease progresses. Uncontrolled HTN in patients with HF can further lead to cardiac remodeling, resulting in worsening HF. Currently he is presenting with symptomatic HF; therefore he should be started on a diuretic to alleviate his symptoms. Starting with a 20-mg dose of furosemide and titrating slowly may be one approach. For all of the reasons cited throughout this chapter, one must also argue strongly for starting an ACE inhibitor to control his HTN. He should be counseled that the urinary frequency he experienced previously should diminish after a few days.

He is being started on both hawthorn and coenzyme Q simultaneously. If he does improve, it will be difficult to assess whether it is because of only one of the agents or the combination. With this in mind, it might be more logical to continue hawthorn alone at a dose of 450 mg BID. If no benefit is derived after 1 month, hawthorn should be stopped and coenzyme Q started at 100 mg/day.

The use of natural supplements is not routinely recommended by the guidelines.[2] The guidelines clearly state that natural products should not be used to treat symptomatic HF. Agents such as ephedra (which contain catecholamines), ephedrine metabolites, or imported Chinese herbs are contraindicated in HF because of increased risk of mortality and morbidity. Also no regulatory oversight, quality control, or regulations exist on the use of natural supplements.

KEY REFERENCES AND WEBSITES

A full list of references for this chapter can be found at **http://thepoint.lww.com/AT10e.** Below are the key references for this chapter, with the corresponding reference number in this chapter found in parentheses after the reference.

Key References

Bardy GH et al. Amiodarone or an implantable cardioverter-defibrillator for congestive heart failure [published correction appears in *N Engl J Med.* 2005;352:2146]. *N Engl J Med.* 2005;352:225. (332)

Barnes MM et al. Treatment of heart failure with preserved ejection fraction. *Pharmacotherapy.* 2011;31:312. (19)

Felker GM et al. Diuretic strategies in patients with acute decompensated heart failure. *N Engl J Med.* 2011;364:797. (111)

Granger CB et al. Effects of candesartan in patients with chronic heart failure and reduced left-ventricular systolic function intolerant to angiotensin-converting-enzyme inhibitors: the CHARM-Alternative trial. *Lancet.* 2003;362:772. (176)

Hunt SA et al. 2009 focused update incorporated into the ACC/AHA 2005 Guidelines for the Diagnosis and Management of Heart Failure in Adults: a report of the American College of Cardiology Foundation/American Heart Association Task Force on Practice Guidelines: developed in collaboration with the International Society for Heart and Lung Transplantation [published correction appears in *Circulation.* 2010;121:e258]. *Circulation.* 2009;119:e391. (1)

Lindenfeld J et al. HFSA 2010 Comprehensive Heart Failure Practice Guideline. *J Card Fail.* 2010;16:e1. (2)

[No authors listed]. Effect of metoprolol CR/XL in chronic heart failure: Metoprolol CR/XL Randomised Intervention Trial in Congestive Heart Failure (MERIT-HF). *Lancet.* 1999;353:2001. (209)

Packer M et al. Comparative effects of low and high doses of the angiotensin-converting enzyme inhibitor, lisinopril, on morbidity and mortality in chronic heart failure. ATLAS Study Group. *Circulation.* 1999;100:2312. (165)

Packer M et al. The effect of carvedilol on morbidity and mortality in patients with chronic heart failure. U.S. Carvedilol Heart Failure Study Group. *N Engl J Med.* 1996;334:1349. (214)

Pitt B et al. Eplerenone, a selective aldosterone blocker, in patients with left ventricular dysfunction after myocardial infarction [published correction appears in *N Engl J Med.* 2003;348:2271]. *N Engl J Med.* 2003;348:1309. (67)

Pitt B et al. The effect of spironolactone on morbidity and mortality in patients with severe heart failure. Randomized Aldactone Evaluation Study Investigators. *N Engl J Med.* 1999;341:709. (66)

Rathore SS et al. Association of serum digoxin concentration and outcomes in patients with heart failure. *JAMA.* 2003;289:871. (241)

Tang AS et al. Cardiac-resynchronization therapy for mild-to-moderate heart failure. *N Engl J Med.* 2010;363:2385. (339)

Zannad F et al. Eplerenone in patients with systolic heart failure and mild symptoms. *N Engl J Med.* 2011;364:11. (61)

Cardiac Arrhythmias

20

C. Michael White, Jessica C. Song, and James S. Kalus

CORE PRINCIPLES

	CHAPTER CASES
ATRIAL FIBRILLATION (AF)/FLUTTER	
1 Chest palpitations, lightheadedness, and reduced exercise tolerance are the most common symptoms of AF, but stroke is among the severe complications. The goals of therapy are to control the ventricular rate and reduce the risk of stroke.	**Case 20-1 (Questions 1, 2)**
2 Digoxin, β-blockers, and nondihydropyridine calcium-channel blockers are appropriate rate-controlling medications. Digoxin is usually adjunctive therapy. Antiarrhythmic drugs are recommended in patients with symptoms but not needed in asymptomatic patients (no symptoms other than palpitations).	**Case 20-1 (Questions 3–7)**
3 Before converting AF to sinus rhythm, assurance of a lack of clot is important but not required if someone is unconscious or cannot mentate. People with a $CHADS_2$ score of 2 or greater should receive chronic antithrombotic therapy with warfarin or dabigatran. Those with a score of 0 can receive aspirin, and those with a score of 1 can receive aspirin or antithrombotic therapy.	**Case 20-1 (Questions 8, 13)**
4 Antiarrhythmic drugs convert patients out of AF 50% of the time, whereas electrical shock is successful 90% of the time. To maintain sinus rhythm after conversion, class Ib agents cannot be used, class Ic agents cannot be used in patients with structural heart disease (left ventricular hypertrophy, myocardial infarction, or heart failure), and class Ia and III agents can increase the risk of torsades de pointes. Propafenone, sotalol, dronedarone, dofetilide, and amiodarone are commonly used antiarrhythmic agents for AF.	**Case 20-1 (Questions 9–12)**
5 Atrial flutter is less common than AF, but similar rate control and antiarrhythmic strategies can be tried. Radiofrequency ablation can be used to terminate atrial flutter.	**Case 20-2 (Question 1)**
6 A large percentage of patients exhibit AF after cardiac surgery. β-Blockers and amiodarone have been shown to decrease clinical manifestations of AF and reduce hospital length of stay. If AF occurs, it should be managed with rate control.	**Case 20-3 (Questions 1–3)**
PAROXYSMAL SUPRAVENTRICULAR TACHYCARDIA (PSVT)	
1 PSVT is caused by re-entry within the atrioventricular (AV) node. Palpitations and hypotension can occur. The Valsalva maneuver, adenosine, or nondihydropyridine calcium-channel blockers can be used to treat the arrhythmia.	**Case 20-4 (Questions 1–6)**
2 In Wolff-Parkinson-White syndrome patients with PSVT, the use of AV nodal blocking agents such as β-blockers, nondihydropyridine calcium-channel blockers, and digoxin can increase the risk of cardiac arrest. Ablation can destroy the bypass tract and cure the patient.	**Case 20-5 (Questions 1, 2)**

continued

accessory pathway tissue and can prevent recurrence of AF. All of these agents act by blocking potassium channels; however, sotalol also has additional β-blocking properties.[69,70] Both amiodarone and dronedarone block sodium channels and calcium channels, and have antiadrenergic effects in addition to potassium-channel blocking properties.[71]

Sotalol, Amiodarone, Dofetilide, and Dronedarone

The efficacy of sotalol in delaying the recurrence of AF was evaluated in a double-blind, placebo-controlled, multicenter, randomized trial that enrolled 253 patients with AF or atrial flutter.[72] The median times to recurrence were 27, 106, 229, and 175 days with placebo, sotalol 160 mg/day (divided in two doses), sotalol 240 mg/day (divided in two doses), and sotalol 320 mg/day (divided in two doses), respectively. Sotalol is contraindicated in patients with a creatinine clearance (CrCl) of less than 40 mL/minute because of the fact that the drug is largely renally cleared and can cause TdP in high concentrations. In a comparative study versus propafenone, sotalol was similarly effective in producing at least a 75% reduction in AF recurrence (79% of patients on propafenone vs. 76% on sotalol) and was similarly tolerated (4.8% of patients on propafenone had intolerable side effects vs. 10.5% on sotalol). Bradycardia, dizziness, and GI disturbances were the most common intolerable side effects.[73] Sotalol should not be used in patients with systolic heart failure owing to the negative inotropic effects of the drug. It may be useful as a first-line agent in patients with AF and concomitant underlying coronary artery disease or in patients with no cardiovascular disease.[11,12]

Amiodarone is more effective at maintaining sinus rhythm than sotalol[74] and propafenone.[75] The Canadian Trial of Atrial Fibrillation (CTAF) compared the ability of low-dose amiodarone (200 mg/day) versus propafenone (450 to 600 mg/day) and sotalol (160 to 320 mg/day) to prevent recurrence of AF in 403 patients with a recent episode of AF (within the preceding 6 months).[74] After a mean follow-up of 16 months, 35% of the amiodarone-treated patients had a recurrence of AF versus 63% in the combined group with sotalol and propafenone ($p = 0.001$). In view of its unusual pharmacokinetics and potential serious adverse effects (see Table 20-3 and Case 20-7, Question 2), amiodarone is only recommended as a first-line choice for patients with HF, for which it has specific safety data, or for patients with significant left ventricular hypertrophy.[11] Amiodarone could also be used when other agents such as sotalol, propafenone, or dofetilide have failed.[11,12]

Dofetilide has been shown to be an effective pharmacologic agent for conversion to, and maintenance of, normal sinus rhythm. Two clinical trials, EMERALD (European and Australian Multicenter Evaluative Research on Atrial Fibrillation Dofetilide)[76] and SAFIRE-D (Symptomatic Atrial Fibrillation Investigation and Randomized Evaluation of Dofetilide)[77] have shown conversion rates of 30% in patients with AF or atrial flutter receiving higher doses of dofetilide. Patients failing chemical conversion received electrical conversion. If this conversion succeeded, they were continued on dofetilide for 1 year. At 1 year, 60% of those converted were still in sinus rhythm with the 500-mcg dose. Also, dofetilide appears to exert neutral effects on mortality rates in HF and post-MI patients.[78,79]

Dofetilide dose is based on the patient's CrCl; the doses are 500, 250, and 125 mcg twice daily with CrCl greater than 60 mL/minute, 40 to 60 mL/minute, and 20 to 39 mL/minute, respectively. Drug interactions pose a significant problem with dofetilide. Cimetidine, ketoconazole, prochlorperazine, megestrol, and trimethoprim (including in combination with sulfamethoxazole) inhibit active tubular secretion of dofetilide and can elevate dofetilide plasma concentrations.[70,80] Because the incidence of TdP is directly related to dofetilide plasma concentrations, concomitant use with these agents is contraindicated.[80] Concomitant administration of dofetilide with verapamil or hydrochlorothiazide increases the incidence of TdP by an unclear mechanism and is contraindicated as well.[70] Concurrent use of agents that can prolong the QTc interval is not recommended with dofetilide.[80] Dofetilide also undergoes metabolism by the cytochrome P-450 CYP3A4 isoenzyme to a minor extent. Therefore, inhibitors of this isoenzyme (e.g., azole antifungal agents, protease inhibitors, serotonin reuptake inhibitors, amiodarone, diltiazem, nefazodone, zafirlukast) should be coadministered with caution with dofetilide. Other agents that can potentially increase dofetilide levels (through inhibition of tubular secretion) include metformin, triamterene, and amiloride. Hence, these agents should be cautiously coadministered with dofetilide.[80]

Dofetilide is considered a first-line agent for patients with heart failure or coronary artery disease, as the impact on mortality in this patient population is neutral.[78,79] Dofetilide can be considered as a second-line agent for patients without cardiovascular disease or left ventricular hypertrophy.[11,12]

Dronedarone is the newest antiarrhythmic drug approved in the United States. Dronedarone is structurally and pharmacologically similar to amiodarone; however, it lacks iodine, which gives dronedarone a much smaller volume of distribution than amiodarone. The lack of iodine also may make dronedarone less likely to cause thyroid-related or other adverse effects.[71] Dronedarone has been shown to have modest efficacy in maintaining sinus rhythm when compared with placebo. Rate of recurrence of AF at 1 year is approximately 40%, and the number of days to recurrence is nearly doubled with dronedarone.[81] The major clinical trial evaluating dronedarone was the ATHENA study. The primary end point of ATHENA was a composite of death or cardiovascular hospitalization, and patients received either dronedarone 400 mg twice daily or placebo for at least 1 year.[82] The primary composite end point was significantly reduced from 39.4% with placebo to 31.9% with dronedarone. This reduction in the composite was completely attributable to the reduction in cardiovascular hospitalizations, most of which were related to AF recurrence. Gastrointestinal events were the most common type of adverse effect with dronedarone in this study. It should be noted that patients with recent decompensated HF or New York Heart Association (NYHA) class IV heart failure were excluded from this trial. The exclusion of patients with severe or unstable heart failure was related to negative findings that led to the early discontinuation of the ANDROMEDA study.[83] ANDROMEDA was designed as a safety study, to evaluate the impact of dronedarone on mortality in patients with HF. Patients admitted with NYHA class III or IV systolic HF were included in this study. The study was stopped early because of an approximate doubling in the risk of death with dronedarone as compared with placebo. Therefore, dronedarone is contraindicated in a patient with severe or recently decompensated HF. Dronedarone has also been compared directly with amiodarone.[84] In this study, dronedarone was less effective than amiodarone, but was less likely than amiodarone to cause thyroid, neurological, skin, or ocular adverse effects. Gastrointestinal adverse effects were more common with dronedarone.[84] Dronedarone is appropriate as a first- or second-line agent for patients with AF and concomitant coronary artery disease, and possibly left ventricular hypertrophy or in patients with no cardiovascular disease. Dronedarone should not be used in a patient with severe HF symptoms or a recent hospitalization for HF, but may be used with mild, well-controlled HF.[12,32,83] It should also be noted that, at the time of this writing, the FDA has issued a warning regarding rare, but potentially serious hepatotoxicity associated with dronedarone use. As part of this warning, two cases of hepatic failure requiring transplantation and several less severe cases of hepatotoxicity were described (for more information, see **http://www.fda.gov/Drugs/DrugSafety/ucm240011.htm**).

In view of J.K.'s new onset of HF, sotalol, propafenone, and flecainide would not be indicated. Although dronedarone may be better tolerated than amiodarone, it would be contraindicated because J.K. was recently admitted with decompensated HF. Therefore, the only available options for J.K. would be either dofetilide or amiodarone, both of which have been proven safe in patients with HF. Selection between dofetilide and amiodarone could be based on renal function, the presence of any major drug interactions, or the desire to avoid adverse effects with amiodarone.

CASE 20-1, QUESTION 12: J.K. is to begin dofetilide today. As a precaution, he is admitted for dofetilide initiation. Why would J.K. need to be admitted for dofetilide initiation? Is it necessary to initiate all antiarrhythmic medications in the hospital?

Dofetilide was approved with the requirement for in-hospital initiation because of the relatively high risk of TdP. ECG monitoring is required for patients being initiated on dofetilide for a minimum of 3 days in a properly equipped facility. The initial regimen is determined by the patient's estimated creatinine clearance. The QTc interval must be measured (using a 12-lead ECG) 2 to 3 hours after the first dose and each subsequent dose while the patient is hospitalized. If the QTc interval increases by greater than 15% or if it surpasses 500 ms (550 ms in patients with ventricular conduction abnormalities) after the first dose, the dofetilide regimen should be reduced by 50%. If the QTc interval exceeds the above parameters any time after the second subsequent dose, dofetilide should be discontinued.[80]

Sotalol may also be arrhythmogenic in high doses, and the risk of inducing TdP has prompted its manufacturer to mandate a minimum of 3 days of ECG monitoring in a properly equipped facility during therapy initiation as well.[85] Further, during initiation and titration, QTc intervals should be monitored 2 to 4 hours after each dose. In fact, most antiarrhythmic agents for AF should probably be initiated in the inpatient setting, with the exception of amiodarone owing to the low risk of proarrhythmia with this drug.[11]

STROKE PREVENTION

ANTITHROMBOTIC THERAPY

CASE 20-1, QUESTION 13: J.K. is discharged from the hospital on dofetilide 500 mcg twice daily, which is appropriate given his CrCl of 92 mL/minute. He has been doing fine for 2 weeks after discharge. Should J.K. remain on warfarin therapy? Could any other antithrombotic options be considered?

Patients with nonvalvular and valvular AF have a 5- and 17-fold increased risk for stroke compared with patients without AF, respectively.[4,5] Stroke can lead to death or significant neurologic disability in up to 71% of patients, with an annual recurrence rate as high as 10%.[86] In three large, randomized trials, patients with nonvalvular AF benefited from antithrombotic therapy.[87–89] In the Stroke Prevention in Atrial Fibrillation (SPAF) study, both aspirin 325 mg/day and warfarin (titrated to an INR of 2.0 to 4.5) reduced the risk of stroke significantly with an acceptable level of hemorrhagic complications.[89] The results of SPAF II, a direct comparison of warfarin and aspirin, indicated that warfarin was more effective than aspirin in preventing stroke.[90] These results were verified by the Copenhagen AFASAK study, which found warfarin to be significantly better than aspirin and placebo at preventing cerebral emboli and overall vascular deaths (cerebral and cardiovascular).[87] More recently, clopidogrel plus aspirin has been studied for prevention of stroke in AF.[91,92] When clopidogrel plus aspirin was compared with warfarin, warfarin was more effective in stroke prevention and associated with a lower bleeding risk.[92] However, when clopidogrel plus aspirin was compared with aspirin alone in patients who were unable to take warfarin, the clopidogrel plus aspirin regimen was superior in efficacy but increased the risk of bleeding.[91]

Selection of an appropriate antithrombotic regimen for the patient with AF must be based on assessment of the underlying stroke and bleeding risk. Risk stratification in AF is performed with the use of the $CHADS_2$ scoring system. A $CHADS_2$ score is calculated by assigning one point each for the presence of congestive heart failure, hypertension, age older than 75 years, or diabetes and two points for a history of stroke. Points are totaled, and the subsequent score correlates with stroke risk.[42] Generally, patients with a $CHADS_2$ score of 2 or greater should receive warfarin (INR target 2–3) for stroke prophylaxis.[42] Warfarin is selected over aspirin because stroke risk is relatively high with a $CHADS_2$ score of 2 or greater and warfarin is superior to aspirin in prevention of stroke. Aspirin alone could be used with a $CHADS_2$ score of 0 or 1. The combination of clopidogrel plus aspirin may be considered in the patient who is unable to take warfarin because of practical issues (i.e., nonadherent with medications or unable to comply with frequent monitoring of INR). Although the combination of clopidogrel plus aspirin was more efficacious than aspirin alone, it was also associated with more bleeding.[91] Therefore, the combination should not be used in a patient who is unable to take warfarin as a result of perceived high bleeding risk.

Dabigatran, a new orally available direct thrombin inhibitor, was recently approved by the FDA to reduce the risk of stroke and systemic embolism in patients with nonvalvular AF.[93] In the Re-Ly trial, dabigatran 110 mg twice daily and 150 mg twice daily was compared with warfarin in patients with a $CHADS_2$ score of 1 or more (average $CHADS_2$ score of 2.1). The lower dose of dabigatran was not inferior to warfarin for stroke prevention but was associated with less bleeding. High-dose dabigatran was superior to warfarin for stroke prevention but comparable in bleeding.[94] The dabigatran 150-mg twice-daily dose was FDA-approved, as was a 75-mg twice-daily dose for those with a CrCl of 15 to 30 mL/minute. Dabigatran offers an alternative choice, does not require routine laboratory monitoring, does not have food interactions, and is not a substrate or inhibitor of the cytochrome P-450 system (see Chapter 16, Thrombosis, for more information).[93] Dabigatran is a P-glycoprotein substrate that interacts with rifampin (use with rifampin is contraindicated), but it does not appear to have clinically significant interactions with other P-glycoprotein inhibitors used commonly in AF (verapamil, quinidine, dronedarone, flecainide, propafenone). The capsules should not be chewed or opened. Dabigatran has no specific dosing recommendation for patients with a CrCl less than 15 mL/minute or those on dialysis. Numerous oral factor Xa inhibitors are being investigated, and some will likely be available in the future.

Even though J.K. is in normal sinus rhythm at this time, in the AFFIRM trial, only 73% and 63% of patients randomized to rhythm control remained in sinus rhythm at 3 and 5 years, respectively.[41] As such, the use of an antiarrhythmic drug does not eliminate the risk of stroke, and in fact, patients may return to AF and not be aware they are no longer in normal sinus rhythm. J.K. has a $CHADS_2$ score of 3 and does not appear to have any factors that would suggest a high bleeding risk (no recent history of GI bleeding, etc.). Therefore, he should continue to receive anticoagulation for stroke prophylaxis.

CASE 20-2

QUESTION 1: M.P. is a 38-year-old woman who has had chronic atrial flutter for the past 2 years. She has no other medical history and is taking metoprolol 50 mg twice daily. She does not want to take the drug any more because it reduces her exercise tolerance. Is there a nonpharmacologic therapy for atrial flutter? Does the treatment of atrial flutter differ from the treatment of AF? Is radiofrequency catheter ablation an acceptable nonpharmacologic option for M.P.?

Atrial flutter is an unstable rhythm that often reverts to sinus rhythm or progresses to AF. If atrial flutter is episodic, its underlying cause should be identified and treated if possible. If a patient remains in atrial flutter, the treatment goals (control of ventricular rate, return to normal sinus rhythm) are the same as those for AF. Similar agents and doses can be used to control the ventricular response. Chemical conversion, low-energy (<50 J) DC cardioversion, or rapid atrial pacing may acutely convert atrial flutter back to sinus rhythm, but the recurrence of atrial flutter is high.

Radiofrequency catheter ablation therapy could be used as a nonpharmacologic treatment for atrial flutter and, in some cases, AF. With both atrial flutter and AF, an electrophysiologic study is performed to identify whether ablation can be performed. Various sections of the atria and pulmonary veins (where they intersect with the atria) are probed with a catheter that delivers cardiac pacing. If an area is stimulated with pacing and an atrial ectopic or re-entrant focus is recognized, that area could be ablated. Ablation destroys tissue that is integral either to the initiation or to the maintenance of the arrhythmia by delivering electrical energy through electrodes on the catheter. If the focus of the arrhythmia is in the atrial tissue (typically for atrial flutter), then the focus itself is ablated. This procedure is successful in 75% to 90% of cases and can be recommended for patients with atrial flutter who are drug-resistant or drug-intolerant, or do not desire long-term therapy. In AF, an ectopic focus originating in the pulmonary veins can often initiate the arrhythmia. In this case, circumferential ablation, in which a circle of ablated tissue is made around the pulmonary veins, is performed. Circumferential ablation does not prevent the ectopic impulses from the pulmonary veins from occurring; however, it does prevent propagation of the impulse into the atria and may reduce the recurrence of AF.

Radiofrequency ablation therapy may be suitable for M.P. However, if exercise intolerance is her primary complaint, this might be relieved by switching M.P. to another drug, such as verapamil.[95,96]

ATRIAL FIBRILLATION AFTER BYPASS SURGERY

β-BLOCKERS AND AMIODARONE

CASE 20-3

QUESTION 1: H.L., a 55-year-old woman with triple-vessel disease, is scheduled for coronary artery bypass graft surgery (CABG) in 3 days. Her medical history includes exercise-induced angina treated with nitrates, metoprolol, and diltiazem. What is the incidence of AF after CABG surgery? Should H.L. be treated with a drug to prevent the postoperative occurrence of AF?

More than 750,000 CABG or heart valve surgeries (cardiothoracic surgery) are performed annually in the United States.[97] Without prophylaxis, AF develops in up to 65% of patients, and two-thirds of the cases occur on postoperative day 2 or 3.[98] The underlying mechanism is unknown, but may be related to sympathetic activation, pericarditis or inflammation, or atrial dilation from volume overload.[99–102] The arrhythmia usually converts spontaneously, but can result in temporary symptomatology (light-headedness), a higher risk of stroke, and a longer hospital stay.[102]

β-Blockers, amiodarone, sotalol, intravenous magnesium, and statins are proven prophylactic strategies to reduce the incidence of postcardiothoracic surgery AF.[100–102] Of these, β-blockers and amiodarone have been shown to reduce other clinical events and shorten length of stay.[97,100–102] In addition, both β-blockers and amiodarone can be used together in the same patient as a prophylactic strategy.[100,101] If a patient is receiving a β-blocker before surgery and cannot receive it after surgery, the risk of postcardiothoracic surgery AF is even higher than if they were never on the β-blocker (β-blocker withdrawal). So it is important to assure continuation of β-blockers after surgery if possible.[100,101]

Although many studies evaluating the use of amiodarone prophylaxis have been conducted, the Atrial Fibrillation Suppression Trial II (AFIST II) had a regimen that allowed for dosing patients with elective and emergent surgery, and the beneficial results were in addition to a high baseline utilization of β-blockers.[101] In AFIST II, a hybrid IV and oral amiodarone regimen was evaluated versus placebo. In this study, IV amiodarone (1,050 mg) was given for 24 hours after surgery and then oral drug (400 mg three times daily) was given for 4 postoperative days (equal to 7 g of oral drug given for 5 days). In this study, amiodarone reduced the 30-day risk of AF by 43% and symptomatic AF by 68%. Amiodarone regimens using only oral dosing have also been studied and showed similar benefits with similar delivered amiodarone doses.[100,102] H.L. is relatively young, does not have a history of AF or heart failure, and is not undergoing valve repair or replacement, so the risk of developing postoperative AF is probably not extremely high. Therefore, a prophylactic therapy may not be necessary.

CASE 20-3, QUESTION 2: H.L.'s metoprolol therapy is discontinued, and she is not treated prophylactically. She undergoes the surgery without complications. On postoperative day 2, she develops AF with a ventricular response rate of 142 beats/minute and a BP of 126/75 mm Hg. How should H.L. be managed?

The decision to treat H.L.'s AF depends on her heart rate and how well she tolerates the arrhythmia; antiarrhythmic agents are often not needed in the short-term management of this disorder. For many years, digoxin has been used to control the ventricular response. However, after surgery, patients have a high sympathetic tone, and digoxin often is ineffective. β-Blockers are effective and preferred if there are no contraindications.[103] They are especially preferred in patients like H.L. who have been taking β-blockers preoperatively because withdrawal of β-blockers can increase the occurrence of postoperative AF.[103,104]

H.L.'s rapid ventricular rate should be controlled. Propranolol 1 mg IV every 5 minutes (up to 0.1 mg/kg), metoprolol 5 mg IV repeated at 2-minute intervals (up to a total dose of 15 mg), and esmolol 0.5 mg/kg bolus followed by a continuous infusion at a rate of 50 to 300 mcg/kg per minute are all options for H.L., who appears to be hemodynamically stable. Verapamil 5 to 10 mg IV every 1 to 4 hours could be an option for most patients; however, this would be a therapeutic duplication because H.L. is already taking diltiazem. If one of these therapy choices is ineffective, a loading dose of digoxin can be administered IV as adjunctive therapy with the β-blocker or verapamil.

CASE 20-3, QUESTION 3: Metoprolol is started, and ventricular rate control is achieved 4 minutes after administering the second 5-mg dose. The patient receives 50 mg oral metoprolol therapy an hour later, converts to normal sinus rhythm spontaneously the next day, and is preparing for discharge. The metoprolol therapy is discontinued. Should an antiarrhythmic agent be initiated for H.L. to prevent recurrence of AF?

Using prophylactic antiarrhythmic agents after discharge in patients with AF within a few days of CABG surgery does not seem to protect against recurrent AF. In one trial, all patients with AF after CABG surgery were given verapamil, quinidine, amiodarone, or placebo at discharge and were then followed with Holter monitoring for 90 days. There was no difference in the occurrence of AF between the placebo group (3.3% incidence) and the other groups (6.7% incidence for each treatment group).[105] Because H.L. has coronary artery disease, it would be reasonable to resume the metoprolol.

Paroxysmal Supraventricular Tachycardia

CLINICAL PRESENTATION

CASE 20-4

QUESTION 1: B.J., a 32-year-old woman, presents to the emergency department (ED) complaining of fatigue and palpitations. She has had similar episodes approximately twice a year for the past 2 years, but has not sought medical attention for them. She is in no apparent distress and has a temperature of 98.0°F, heart rate of 185 beats/minute, BP of 95/60 mm Hg, and respiratory rate of 12 breaths/minute. Her ECG (Fig. 20-6) shows regular rhythm with a heart rate of 185. The P waves cannot be found, and the QRS complex is 110 ms (normal, <120 ms). The diagnosis is PSVT. What is the clinical presentation of PSVT, and what are the consequences of this arrhythmia?

PSVT often has a sudden onset and termination. At the time of PSVT, the heart rate is usually 180 to 200 beats/minute. As illustrated by B.J., patients experience palpitations and often nervousness and anxiety. In patients with a rapid ventricular rate, dizziness and syncope (near-fainting) can occur, and the rhythm may degenerate to other serious arrhythmias. Angina, HF, or shock may be precipitated depending on the patient's underlying degree of coronary atherosclerosis and left ventricular function. There is no evidence that patients with episodes of PSVT are at an increased risk of stroke.

ARRHYTHMOGENESIS AND RE-ENTRY

CASE 20-4, QUESTION 2: What is the arrhythmogenic mechanism of PSVT?

AV nodal re-entry is the most common mechanism of paroxysmal supraventricular arrhythmias (see Fig. 20-3). Under certain conditions, such as after an acute MI, atrial impulses will be blocked in one of the two AV nodal pathways in a unidirectional manner (antegrade block). After the impulse reaches the distal end of one pathway, it will conduct in a retrograde fashion through the other pathway, setting up a circular movement causing tachycardia. When AV nodal re-entry is the mechanism of the PSVT, it may be referred to as AV nodal re-entrant tachycardia or AVNRT. Reciprocating tachycardias occur when there is an accessory pathway for conduction of impulses between the atria and ventricles (also known as AVRT or atrioventricular re-entrant tachycardia). WPW syndrome is an example of a situation in which an accessory pathway exists and can produce PSVT (Fig. 20-7).

TREATMENT

CASE 20-4, QUESTION 3: B.J. tries the Valsalva maneuver, and her ventricular rate is reduced to 150 beats/minute; the other parameters are unchanged. She is given IV adenosine 6 mg, administered for 1 minute, with no effect on the PSVT rate. Another dose of adenosine 12 mg has no effect. No side effects are noted from therapy. What treatment options can be used if B.J. is hemodynamically unstable? What is the Valsalva maneuver? What is a probable reason for B.J.'s unresponsiveness to adenosine? Are there any drug interactions that might diminish adenosine's effect?

NONDRUG TREATMENT

Valsalva Maneuver

Although her BP is low at 95/60 mm Hg, B.J. is maintaining an adequate perfusion pressure, so vagal maneuvers should be attempted first. Two common vagal techniques are pressure over the bifurcation of the internal and external carotid arteries and the Valsalva maneuver (forcible exhalation against a closed glottis, similar to bearing down to have a bowel movement). The increase in pressure induced by these maneuvers is sensed by the baroreceptors, causing a reflex decrease in sympathetic tone and an increase in vagal tone. The increase in vagal tone will increase refractoriness and slow conduction in the AV node, thereby slowing the heart rate; the arrhythmia will terminate in 10% to 30% of cases.[96] If B.J. is hemodynamically unstable or becomes hemodynamically unstable, she should receive synchronized DC cardioversion.

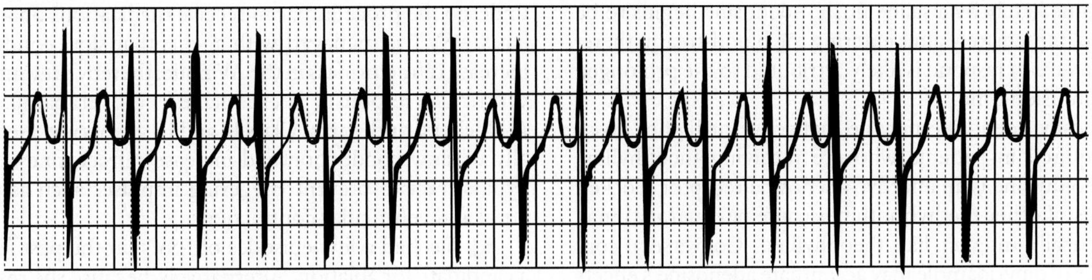

FIGURE 20-6 Supraventricular tachycardia. (Reproduced with permission from Stein E. *Rapid Analysis of Arrhythmias: A Self-Study Program.* 2nd ed. Philadelphia, PA: Lea & Febiger; 1992.)

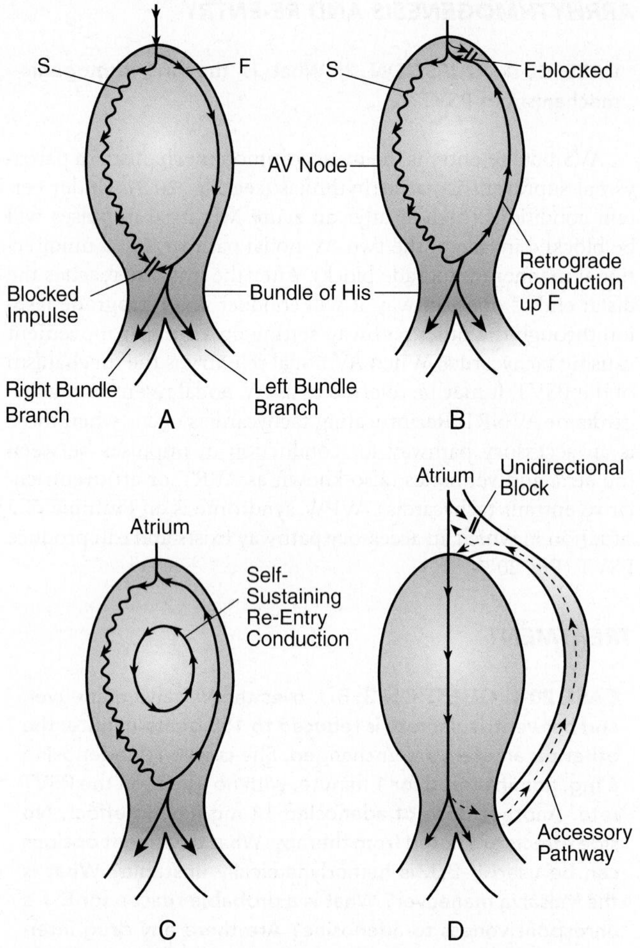

FIGURE 20-7 The atrioventricular (AV) node in paroxysmal supraventricular tachycardia and Wolff-Parkinson-White syndrome. **A:** A bifurcation of an impulse, one propagated fast and another slow. **B:** The slow impulse in **(A)** can send impulses in a retrograde fashion. **C:** The re-entry from **(A)** to **(B)** can be self-sustaining. **D:** Normal impulse conduction through the AV node, but abnormal retrograde conduction up an accessory pathway, as would be seen in a patient with Wolff-Parkinson-White syndrome.

DRUG THERAPY

Adenosine

Drug therapy for PSVT involves blocking the AV node, because most PSVT rhythms involve a re-entry circuit that includes this area. Adenosine, a purine nucleoside that exerts a transient negative chronotropic and dromotropic effect on cardiac pacemaker tissue,[106] is considered the drug of choice for the acute treatment of PSVT because of its rapid and brief effect. An initial 6-mg IV bolus is given; if this is unsuccessful within 2 minutes, it can be followed by one or two 12-mg IV boluses, up to a maximum of 30 mg. Because of its short half-life (9 seconds), adenosine should be administered as a rapid bolus (over 1 to 3 seconds), followed immediately by a saline flush. Adenosine begins to be metabolized immediately after entering the bloodstream; therefore, B.J.'s failure to respond is likely attributed to the prolonged (1-minute) infusion time.

Theoretically, adenosine may be ineffective or higher doses may be required in patients who are receiving theophylline because theophylline is an effective adenosine receptor blocker. Larger doses of other methylxanthines (caffeine, guarana) may also theoretically interact like theophylline. Conversely, concomitant use of dipyridamole may accentuate adenosine's effects because dipyridamole blocks the adenosine uptake (and subsequent clearance).

CASE 20-4, QUESTION 4: B.J. is given 12 mg adenosine IV during 2 seconds, followed by a 20-mL normal saline flush. Thirty seconds later, she complains of chest tightness and pressure. What is the explanation for these symptoms?

B.J. is experiencing a common side effect of adenosine. Patients receiving adenosine should be warned that they may feel transient chest heaviness, flushing, or a feeling of anxiety. Shortness of breath and wheezing may be observed in patients with asthma. The denervated heart of the patient who has undergone heart transplant is particularly sensitive to adenosine; therefore, lower doses of adenosine should be used.

Calcium-Channel Blockers

CASE 20-4, QUESTION 5: B.J. is still in PSVT. What other acute therapeutic options should be considered at this time?

Nondihydropyridine calcium-channel blockers, verapamil and diltiazem, can be used in patients with PSVT. Verapamil (2.5 to 5 mg IV given for 2 minutes) achieves peak therapeutic effects in 3 to 5 minutes after dosing and can be repeated at 10- to 15-minute intervals to a maximal dose of 20 mg if needed. The elderly should receive the verapamil infusion for 3 minutes to minimize the risk of adverse events. Diltiazem is given as a 0.25-mg/kg IV bolus for 2 minutes, and a second bolus of 0.35 mg/kg can be given 15 minutes later if the effect is inadequate. Both of these calcium-channel blockers have an 85% conversion rate.[107] However, verapamil should not be used in patients with wide complex tachycardia of unknown origin because it may lead to hemodynamic compromise and, potentially, VF. β-Blockers and digoxin can be used if calcium-channel blockers and adenosine fail.

CASE 20-4, QUESTION 6: B.J. is given 5 mg IV verapamil for 1 minute, followed by an additional 5 mg 10 minutes later. She converts to normal sinus rhythm 3 minutes after the second dose. Because she has experienced symptoms that could be attributed to PSVT in the past, she may be a candidate for chronic therapy to slow conduction and increase refractoriness at the AV node. Which agents have been evaluated for this indication? Is there a role for radiofrequency catheter ablation therapy for PSVT?

Radiofrequency catheter ablation is frequently used as a long-term treatment for PSVT. Electrophysiologic testing is used to determine the location of the re-entrant tract, which then can be ablated, thereby interrupting accessory pathways and re-entrant circuits. This treatment approach is potentially curative and is performed by a specially trained electrophysiologist. Patients who are not candidates for ablation, or who do not wish to undergo the procedure, can receive medications on a long-term basis. PSVT is managed with agents that slow conduction and increase refractoriness in the AV node, thereby preventing a rapid ventricular response. These include oral verapamil, diltiazem, β-blockers, or digoxin. Class Ic and III agents are used occasionally to slow conduction and increase refractoriness of the fast bypass tract to prevent triggering impulses such as premature atrial and ventricular contractions.

B.J. has had a few episodes of PSVT in the past and may be a candidate for ablation. Alternatively, because she responded to IV verapamil, oral SR verapamil could be prescribed at a dosage of 240 mg/day.

Wolff-Parkinson-White Syndrome

CASE 20-5

QUESTION 1: M.B., a 35-year-old man, presents to the ED with a chief complaint of chest palpitations for 4 hours. He relates a history of many similar self-terminating episodes since he was a teenager. He took an unknown medication 5 years ago that decreased the occurrence of the palpitations, but he stopped taking it because of side effects. M.B.'s vital signs are BP, 96/68 mm Hg; pulse, 226 beats/minute, irregular; respiratory rate, 15 breaths/minute; and temperature, 98.7°F. A rhythm strip confirms AF, with a QRS width varying from 0.08 to 0.14 seconds. To control the ventricular rate, 10 mg IV verapamil is administered for 2 minutes. Within 2 minutes of completing the infusion, VF is noted on the monitor. M.B. is defibrillated, and normal sinus rhythm is restored. A subsequent ECG demonstrates a P-R interval of 100 ms (normal, 120 to 200 ms) and delta waves, compatible with WPW. What is WPW syndrome?

WPW is a pre-excitation syndrome in which there is an accessory bypass tract (known as a Kent bundle) connecting the atria to the ventricles (Fig. 20-7). An impulse can travel down this pathway and excite the ventricle before the expected regular impulse through the AV node arrives (hence the term pre-excitation). If there is antegrade conduction over the bypass tract while the patient is in normal sinus rhythm, the ECG will demonstrate a short P-R interval (<100 ms), a delta wave that represents a fused complex from pre-excitation, and the regular QRS complex after AV conduction. WPW can occur in children and adults without overt cardiac disease. PSVT (specifically AVRT) and AF occur in these patients at a higher incidence than in the general population of the same age.[108] Similar to M.B., the rapid heart rate experienced during the tachycardia may cause palpitations, light-headedness, and fatigue. When patients with WPW develop AF, there is a danger that the rapid atrial impulses will be conducted directly to the ventricle through the bypass tract, causing a rapid ventricular rate that may evolve into VF.

CASE 20-5, QUESTION 2: Why did verapamil cause VF in M.B.? What drug or drugs would be appropriate for M.B., and what drugs should be avoided?

Verapamil can block AV conduction by increasing the effective refractory period, allowing all impulses from the atrial area to conduct down the bypass (Kent) tract. Because M.B. had AF, the rapid atrial impulses were conducted directly down the bypass tract to the ventricle, causing VF. In addition, verapamil may enhance conduction over the accessory pathway by shortening its effective refractory period. Also, peripheral vasodilation can induce a reflex sympathetic discharge that can, in turn, decrease the effective refractory period of the accessory pathway.[109,110]

The most common presentation of WPW syndrome involves normal antegrade conduction down the AV node and retrograde conduction back up through the accessory pathway. Thus, drugs that inhibit antegrade impulse conduction through the AV node (e.g., verapamil, digoxin) will terminate the re-entrant tachycardia and can be suitable in the absence of AF. The less common variety of WPW is antegrade conduction through the accessory pathway with retrograde transmission up through the AV node. Similarly, AV nodal blocking agents will terminate this type of re-entrant tachycardia. In some situations, such as that experienced by M.B., rapid AF with an accessory pathway occurs, which can lead to VF and cardiac arrest.

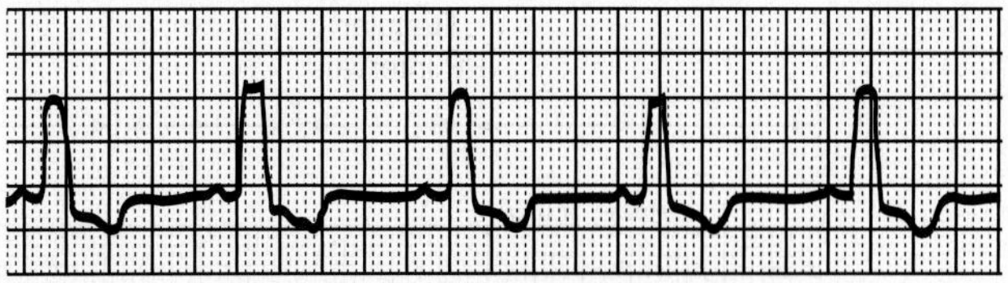

FIGURE 20-8 Bundle branch block. Note that the QRS interval is prolonged. A 12-lead electrocardiogram is required to make the diagnosis of left bundle branch block. (Reproduced with permission from Stein E. *Rapid Analysis of Arrhythmias: A Self-Study Program.* 2nd ed. Philadelphia, PA: Lea & Febiger; 1992.)

The antiarrhythmic drugs used to treat patients with AF who have an accessory pathway, such as M.B., include those that depress conduction and increase the effective refractory period of the fast sodium channel–dependent tissue of the accessory pathway. This includes most class I antiarrhythmic drugs, with the class Ib agents being least effective. Propafenone and flecainide are effective and may be preferred.[111–114] Amiodarone and sotalol may also be effective, but clinical experience is limited.[115–117] Radiofrequency ablation of the bypass tract is used more frequently for these patients to prevent VF.

Further therapy for M.B. may not be useful at this time. However, if he has recurrent AF or other symptomatology associated with WPW, radiofrequency catheter ablation or drug therapy as outlined previously could be indicated.

CONDUCTION BLOCKS

Various arrhythmias can result from blockage of impulse conduction. These can occur above the ventricle, such as first-, second-, and third-degree (complete) AV block. Others, such as right or left bundle branch block (RBBB or LBBB) and trifascicular block, originate below the bifurcation of the His bundle. Although conduction blocks can be classified as either supraventricular or ventricular arrhythmias, they are discussed as a separate group because their mechanism of arrhythmogenesis is similar and their treatment is different from other arrhythmias.

CASE 20-6

QUESTION 1: H.T., a 63-year-old man, was admitted to the coronary care unit (CCU) 12 hours ago with an acute inferior wall MI. He has remained stable. On admission, he had the rhythm strip shown in Figure 20-8 (left bundle branch block). Twelve hours later, it has changed to the rhythm strip shown in Figure 20-9 (Wenckebach or type I, second-degree AV block). Are these rhythms potentially hazardous to H.T.? How is second-degree AV block different from first- or third-degree AV block?

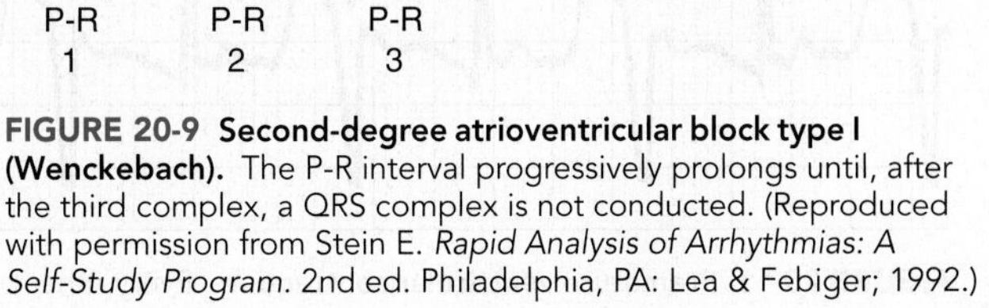

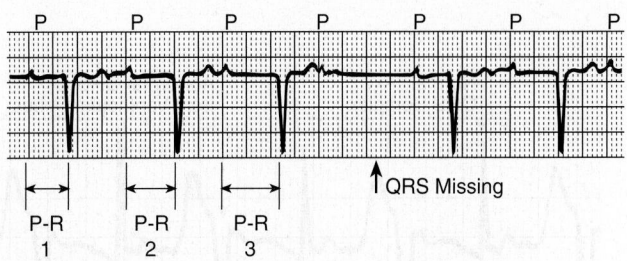

FIGURE 20-9 Second-degree atrioventricular block type I (Wenckebach). The P-R interval progressively prolongs until, after the third complex, a QRS complex is not conducted. (Reproduced with permission from Stein E. *Rapid Analysis of Arrhythmias: A Self-Study Program.* 2nd ed. Philadelphia, PA: Lea & Febiger; 1992.)

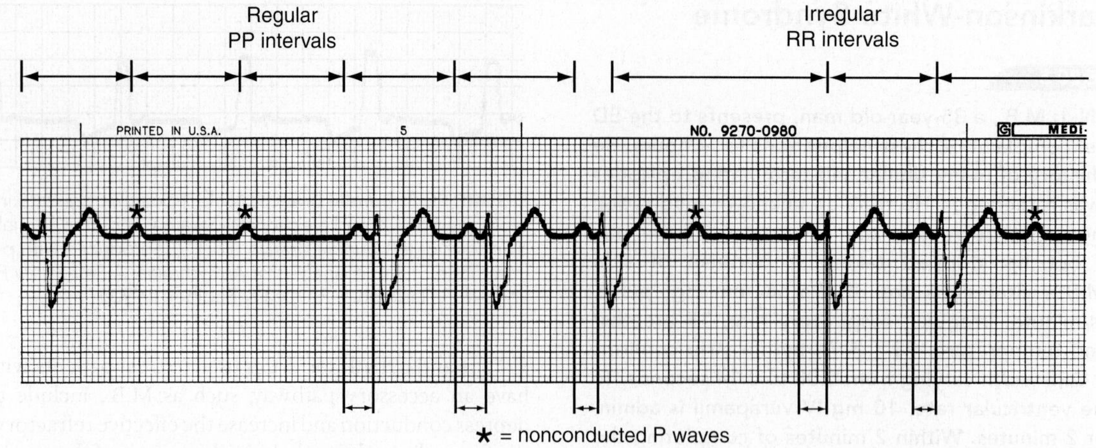

FIGURE 20-10 Sinus rhythm with second-degree AV block, Type II; note constant PR interval. (Reprinted with permission from Smeltzer SC, Bare BG. *Textbook of Medical-Surgical Nursing*. 9th Ed. Philadelphia: Lippincott Williams & Wilkins; 2000.)

H.T.'s rhythm strip revealed a diagnosis of LBBB. Bundle branch block occurs when the electrical impulse cannot be conducted along the left or right fascicle of the His-Purkinje system (see Fig. 20-1). In H.T., the impulse travels down the right bundle normally, and the right ventricle contracts at the normal time. The left bundle is blocked, and, therefore, the left side is depolarized from an impulse conducted from the right ventricle. This impulse must travel through atypical conduction tissues (with slower conduction), and hence the left side depolarizes later. This is revealed on the ECG by a widened QRS complex. Bundle branch blocks, particularly in the left fascicle, are associated with coronary artery disease, systemic hypertension, aortic valve stenosis, and cardiomyopathy.[118] Typically, they do not lead to clinical cardiac dysfunction on their own. Because H.T. has LBBB, he can develop complete heart block (third-degree block) if for any reason his right fascicle is damaged.

First-degree AV block usually is asymptomatic. The ECG will show P waves with a prolonged P-R interval (normal, <200 ms), but each P wave is followed by a normal QRS complex. First-degree AV block is a common finding in patients taking digoxin, verapamil, or other drugs that slow AV conduction.

Second-degree heart block consists of two types. Mobitz type I (Wenckebach) is characterized by progressive lengthening of the P-R interval with each beat and a corresponding shortening of the R-R interval until finally an impulse is not conducted; the cycle then starts over again. Mobitz type II (Fig. 20-10) impulse conduction is blocked in a fixed, regular pattern (e.g., 3:1 block, in which for every three P waves, only one is conducted).

Third-degree heart block (complete heart block) occurs when none of the impulses from the SA node are conducted to the ventricles. During third-degree block, the ventricle must develop its own pacemaker (escape rhythm), which may be too slow to provide adequate cardiac output, causing the patient to become symptomatic. A mechanical pacemaker is needed for treatment of third-degree AV block. AV blocks can be caused by drugs (β-blockers, calcium-channel blockers, digoxin), acute MI, amyloidosis, and congenital abnormalities.[119]

Atropine

CASE 20-6, QUESTION 2: How should H.T.'s heart block be treated?

H.T. is experiencing a Wenckebach rhythm, which often is transient after an inferior wall MI. As long as he is hemodynamically stable, he should be monitored closely. If his heart rate and BP drop, atropine 0.5 mg IV bolus (maximum 2 mg) can increase the heart rate. This is only a short-term therapy; if the hemodynamic compromise persists, a pacemaker must be inserted to initiate the impulse to control the heart rate.

VENTRICULAR ARRHYTHMIAS

Recognition and Definition

Ventricular arrhythmias arise from irritable ectopic foci within the ventricular myocardium. Impulses from these ectopic foci generate wide, bizarre-looking QRS complexes leading to PVCs (Fig. 20-11). PVCs can arise from the same ectopic site (unifocal) or can be multifocal in origin. They can be simple (e.g., isolated

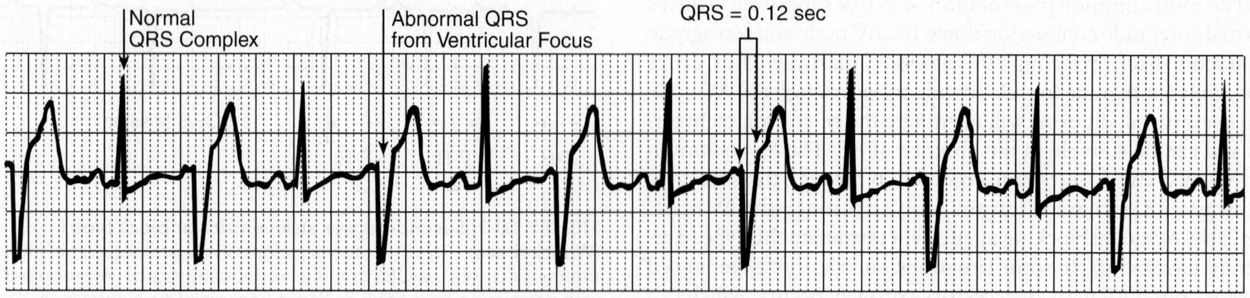

FIGURE 20-11 Premature ventricular contraction. Every other beat is a premature ventricular (ectopic) contraction.

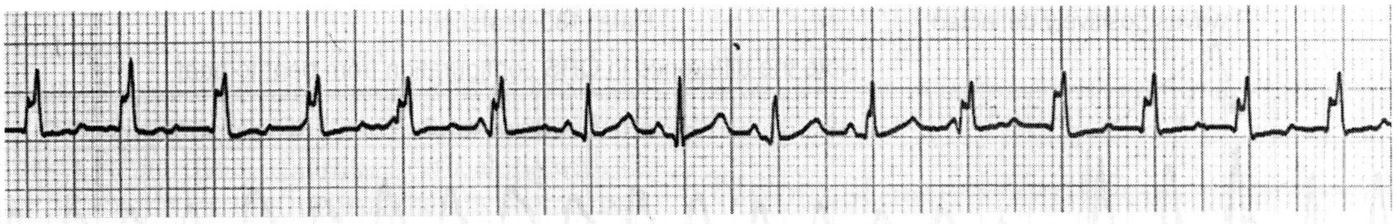

FIGURE 20-12 Nonsustained ventricular tachycardia. (Reprinted with permission from Mhairi G et al. *Avery's Neonatology Pathophysiology & Management of the Newborn.* 6th ed. Philadelphia: Lippincott Williams & Wilkins; 2005.)

or infrequent) or complex (e.g., R on T, in which the R wave of a PVC falls on top of a normal T wave). Other presentations include runs of two or more beats, bigeminy (every other beat is a PVC), or trigeminy (every third beat is a PVC). Three consecutive PVCs usually are defined as ventricular tachycardia (VT), which can be nonsustained or sustained. Ventricular flutter, VF, and TdP are other serious forms of ventricular arrhythmias. The presentation, etiology, treatment, and ion channels associated with TdP are discussed separately.

Nonsustained ventricular tachycardia (NSVT) (Fig. 20-12) commonly is defined as three or more consecutive PVCs lasting less than 30 seconds and terminating spontaneously. Sustained VT (SuVT) is defined as consecutive PVCs lasting more than 30 seconds, with a rate usually in the range of 150 to 200 beats/minute. P waves are lost in the QRS complex and are indiscernible. SuVT (Fig. 20-14) is a serious development because it can degenerate into VF. Ventricular flutter is characterized by sustained, rapid, regular ventricular beats (normal, >250 beats/minute) and usually degenerates into VF. VF (see Fig. 20-13) is characterized by irregular, disorganized, rapid beats with no identifiable P waves or QRS complexes. It is thought to be triggered by multiple re-entrant wavelets in the ventricle. There is no effective cardiac output in patients with VF.[118,119]

Etiology

Common factors that cause ventricular arrhythmias are ischemia, the presence of organic heart disease, exercise, metabolic or electrolyte imbalance (e.g., acidosis, hypokalemia or hyperkalemia, hypomagnesemia), or drugs (digitalis, sympathomimetic amines, antiarrhythmic drugs). It is essential to identify and remove any treatable cause (e.g., metabolic or electrolyte imbalance and proarrhythmic drugs) before initiating antiarrhythmic drug therapy.

Evaluation of Life-Threatening Ventricular Arrhythmias

An episode of life-threatening ventricular arrhythmia (i.e., SuVT, TdP, VF) carries a significant risk of morbidity and mortality. Adequate documentation of the arrhythmia and its suppression by either drugs or a mechanical device are essential. Patients suspected of having, or documented to have, symptoms of a life-threatening arrhythmia (e.g., syncope, out-of-hospital cardiac arrest) should be admitted to the hospital and evaluated. At present, the ACC/AHA/ESC practice guidelines recommend standard testing with a 12-lead ECG in all patients undergoing evaluation for ventricular arrhythmias. The writing group assigned a class I rating for exercise testing in two groups of patients with ventricular arrhythmias: (a) adults at intermediate risk of having coronary heart disease (CHD) by sex, age, and symptoms to induce ischemic changes or ventricular arrhythmias, and (b) patients with established or suspected exercise-induced ventricular arrhythmias, with the intent of provoking the arrhythmia, achieving a diagnosis, and assessing the patient's response to tachycardia. Pharmacological stress testing is preferred over exercise testing in patients with an intermediate probability of CHD if they are physically incapable of performing a symptom-limited exercise test. Two additional approaches are used to evaluate the arrhythmia and the effectiveness of therapy: ambulatory monitoring and electrophysiologic studies.[118]

AMBULATORY MONITORING

The frequency of suspected ventricular arrhythmias determines the ambulatory monitoring device indicated for patients.[119] For more frequent occurrences (once daily) of arrhythmias, Holter monitoring during a 24- to 48-hour period represents the first-line ambulatory monitoring device. The patient wears a portable ECG monitoring device in a purselike carrier, and electrodes connected to the monitor are taped to the patient's chest. The ECG is played back in the laboratory, correlating the presence of arrhythmias with a written patient activity and symptom log. In contrast, event recorders are selected for patients presenting with arrhythmias that occur less frequently.[119] The event recorder (or loop recorder) is worn constantly for up to 14 days (http://www.advmed.ca/ler.asp) and stores and saves data on instruction by the patient. Whenever a patient experiences symptoms, a switch on the recorder is depressed, resulting in storage of a record of the patient's heart rhythm at the time of the event. A telephone can transfer event recorder data for analysis.

ELECTROPHYSIOLOGIC STUDIES

Electrophysiologic (EP) studies represent another approach to evaluating ventricular arrhythmias, especially in patients with sporadic ventricular arrhythmias that may be missed by short-term monitoring.[118] EP testing serves as a diagnostic tool for evaluating drug effects, assessing the inducibility of VT, determining the risks of recurrent VT or sudden cardiac death (SCD), guiding ablation, and assessing the need for an ICD (implantable cardioverter-defibrillator).

Class I recommendations (per ACC/AHA/ESC) on the use of EP studies apply to the following patient subsets: (a) patients with

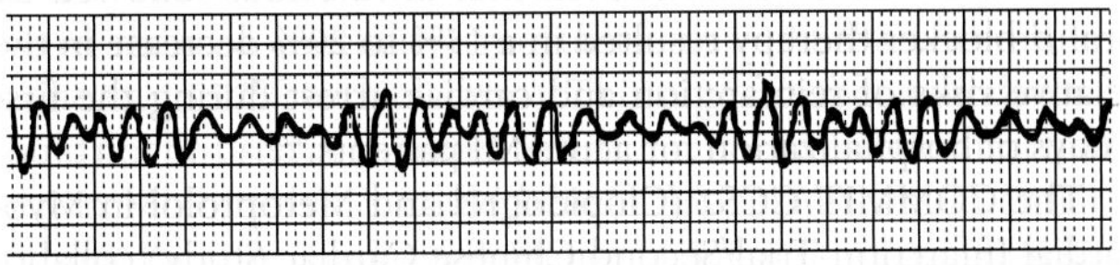

FIGURE 20-13 Ventricular fibrillation.

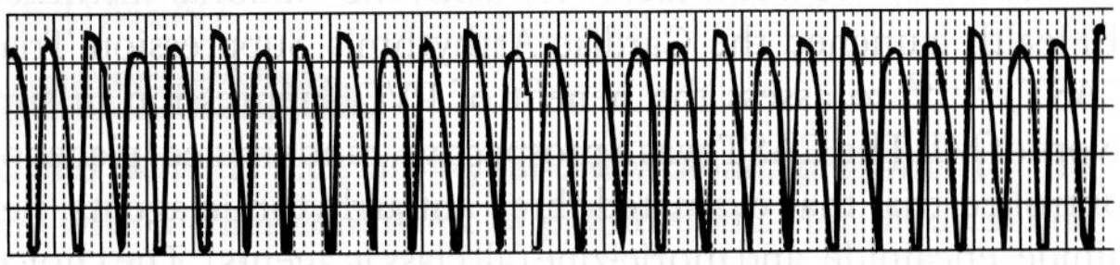

FIGURE 20-14 Sustained ventricular tachycardia.

inferior wall MI 6 months ago. She is pale and diaphoretic but able to respond to commands. Her vital signs are BP, 95/70 mm Hg; pulse, 145 beats/minute; and respiratory rate, 10 breaths/minute. When telemetry monitoring is established, S.L. is found to be in SuVT (Fig. 20-14). S.L.'s echocardiography (6 months earlier) revealed an LVEF of 35%. How should she be treated?

The acute treatment of patients with SuVT depends on their hemodynamic stability. If unstable, patients should receive synchronous cardioversion, which will decrease the chance of triggering VF. If the patient is conscious, a short-acting benzodiazepine (e.g., midazolam) should be administered before the procedure. The 2010 AHA guidelines for cardiopulmonary resuscitation (CPR) and emergency cardiovascular care addressed the potential efficacy of intravenous antiarrhythmic drugs in stable VT patients. A class IIa rating for the use of intravenous procainamide was recommended by the AHA guidelines, with amiodarone (class IIb) and sotalol (class IIb) representing alternative choices of antiarrhythmic therapy for wide-complex regular tachycardias.[137]

ANTIARRHYTHMIC AGENTS

Data from three observational studies[138–140] provided the basis for AHA recommendations on using amiodarone in terminating shock-resistant or drug-refractory VT. Moreover, one randomized parallel-group study demonstrated the superiority of amiodarone compared with lidocaine in the treatment of shock-resistant VT.[141] Amiodarone is primarily recommended for the treatment of patients presenting with hemodynamically stable VT, polymorphic VT with a normal QT interval, and wide-complex tachycardia of uncertain origin.[137] Intravenous amiodarone should be administered as a 150-mg dose for 10 minutes, followed by a 6-hour infusion at a rate of 1 mg/minute, and finally a 0.5-mg/minute infusion for 18 hours. For recurrent or resistant arrhythmias, supplemental infusions of 150 mg can be repeated every 10 minutes, up to a maximal total daily IV dose of 2.25 g. Commonly seen adverse effects associated with intravenous amiodarone include hypotension and bradycardia, which can be prevented by slowing the drug infusion rate.

Procainamide has been shown to be superior to lidocaine in abolishing spontaneously occurring VT[142] and may be considered for use in the treatment of patients with preserved ventricular function who present with stable monomorphic VT. The beneficial effect of this agent is likely the result of slowing conduction in myocardial tissue. An initial infusion of 20 to 50 mg/minute for VT can be administered until arrhythmia suppression occurs, hypotension ensues, achievement of 50% prolongation from baseline duration of the QRS complex occurs, or a cumulative dose of 17 mg/kg has been administered. The AHA writing group discouraged the practice of giving bolus doses of this drug to patients with VT because it increases the occurrence of toxic drug concentrations and hypotension. The maintenance infusion rate of procainamide hydrochloride ranges from 1 mg/minute to 4 mg/minute in patients with normal renal function, but should be lowered in the presence of renal dysfunction. The parent drug and the active metabolite, *N*-acetylprocainamide (NAPA) can accumulate. NAPA itself has class III antiarrhythmic activity and is eliminated entirely by the kidneys, but the clinical significance of NAPA as an antiarrhythmic has not been fully established.[143] Because of its potential to prolong QT intervals, this agent should be used with caution in patients receiving other QT-prolonging drugs. Continuous ECG and blood pressure monitoring should take place during administration of procainamide.[137]

Sotalol, like procainamide, represents another alternative to amiodarone therapy for termination of acute, monomorphic, sustained VT.[137] One randomized controlled trial demonstrated the superior efficacy of this agent compared with lidocaine for terminating acute sustained VT.[144] Similar to amiodarone, sotalol prolongs the duration of action potentials and increases cardiac tissue refractoriness. Per AHA 2010 recommendations, patients with monomorphic VT who receive intravenous sotalol should receive a 100-mg (1.5 mg/kg) dose infused for 5 minutes.[137] Intravenous sotalol is approximately dose-equivalent to the oral formulation, because an intravenous dose of 75 mg equals an 80-mg oral dose.[145] The manufacturer suggests diluting sotalol in 100 to 250 mL of 5% dextrose, normal saline, or lactated Ringer's solution, and administering the drug using a volumetric infusion pump for a 5-hour period. Common adverse effects associated with sotalol include bradycardia and hypotension. The propensity of this agent to induce TdP is covered later in this chapter. The mean elimination half-life of sotalol is 12 hours. Because it is cleared by the kidneys, its clearance is reduced and its half-life prolonged in patients with renal dysfunction. Consequently, patients receiving sotalol should receive continuous blood pressure, heart rate, and ECG monitoring. Patients who experience excessive QT prolongation while on sotalol should receive lower doses or the drug should be discontinued. Because S.L. appears to be relatively stable and she has an ejection fraction less than 40%, amiodarone is a suitable intravenous antiarrhythmic agent for terminating sustained VT.

Implantable Cardiac Defibrillators

CASE 20-9, QUESTION 2: On hospital day 2, S.L. experiences a run of VT lasting about 2 minutes. The cardiology consult service has recommended placement of an ICD. What is an ICD, and how does it work?

ICDs are devices implanted under the skin with wires or patches that are advanced or attached so they are in direct contact with the ventricular myocardium. The ICD is composed of a pulse generator, sensing and pacing electrodes, and defibrillation coils. The pulse generator consists of a microprocessor, a memory component capable of storing ECG data, a high-voltage capacitor, and a battery. The microprocessor controls the analysis of cardiac rhythm and delivery of therapy. An electrode is usually placed at the endocardium of the right ventricular apex, but in some rare cases, it is surgically placed on the epicardium. Patients with dual-chamber ICDs have a second electrode placed in the right atrial appendage. Biventricular ICDs have an additional electrode placed surgically on the epicardium of the left ventricle, or more commonly, placed transcutaneously in a branch off of the coronary sinus. Defibrillation coils are positioned on the right ventricular electrode at the level of the right ventricle and the superior vena cava. In most ICD systems, biphasic defibrillation current flows from the distal defibrillation coil to the pulse generator and to the proximal defibrillation coil.[146] ICDs can deliver multitiered therapy when a ventricular arrhythmia is detected, thereby reducing the need for high-energy defibrillation without compromising ICD efficacy. A typical multitiered program set for slow (160–180 beats/minute) ventricular tachycardia could start with antitachycardia pacing, followed by low-energy cardioversion (e.g., 5 J) and higher-energy defibrillation (e.g., 35 J). ICD programming for fast ventricular tachycardia (>180–200 beats/minute) usually starts with antitachycardia pacing and then proceeds directly to higher-energy defibrillation (e.g., 35 J). Programming for VF (>200 beats/minute) is characterized by multiple high-energy defibrillations (e.g., 35 J) delivered to the patient experiencing this type of arrhythmia.[146] Multiple clinical trials have proved the superiority of ICD treatment over antiarrhythmic therapy for the secondary prevention of SCD. On the basis of evidence from numerous clinical trials of primary and secondary prevention of SCD, the American College of Cardiology/American Heart Association/Heart Rhythm Society 2008 guidelines for device-based therapy of cardiac rhythm abnormalities assigned a class Ia-level evidence rating for ICD implantation in three groups of patients. ICD therapy is indicated for (a) survivors of cardiac arrest caused by VF or hemodynamically unstable sustained VT, (b) patients with LVEF equal to or less than 35% caused by a prior MI who are at least 40 days after the event and are in NYHA functional class II or III, and (c) patients with LVEF equal to or less than 30% caused by prior MI who are at least 40 days after the event and are in NYHA functional class I.[147]

Although ICDs have been shown to improve survival in select patient populations, the benefit may be offset by diminished quality of life associated with painful shocks, increased mortality compared with ICD patients who do not require shocks, and incomplete protection from the occurrence of SCD (5% of patients fail to respond).[148–150] In recent years, investigators have examined two different approaches to reducing the frequency of ICD shocks. Antiarrhythmic medications and prophylactic catheter ablation have been shown to reduce the incidence of ICD therapy. The OPTIC (Optimal Pharmacological Therapy in Cardioverter Defibrillator Patients) study enrolled 412 patients with St. Jude's Medical dual-chamber ICDs; LVEF of equal to or less than 40% who had inducible VT or VF by programmed ventricular stimulation; LVEF of equal to or less than 40% with a prior history of SuVT, VF, or cardiac arrest; or syncope of unknown cause with VF or VT.[148] The effect of amiodarone (mean dose range, 235–275 mg/day) plus β-blocker (metoprolol, carvedilol, or bisoprolol) compared with sotalol (mean dose range, 183–190 mg/day) or β-blocker alone (metoprolol, carvedilol, or bisoprolol) on the primary end point, first occurrence of any shock delivered by the ICD, was assessed for a median of 359 days (interquartile range, 236–367 days). One-year shock rates were 10.3%, 24.3%, and 38.5%, respectively, in amiodarone/β-blocker–treated patients, in sotalol-treated patients, and in β-blocker–treated patients. Patients receiving amiodarone combined with β-blocker had significantly lower risk of shock compared with patients receiving β-blocker monotherapy (hazard ratio, 0.27; 95% CI, 0.14–0.52; $p < 0.001$) and sotalol monotherapy (hazard ratio, 0.43; 95% CI, 0.22–0.85; $p = 0.02$). Of note, adverse effects such as pulmonary toxicity, thyroid effects, and symptomatic bradycardia contributed to an 18.2% discontinuation rate for amiodarone at 1 year.

The SMASH-VT (Substrate Mapping and Ablation in Sinus Rhythm to Halt Ventricular Tachycardia) study examined the effect of radiofrequency catheter ablation of arrhythmogenic ventricular tissue (ablation performed after ICD implantation in 87% of patients) on the incidence of ICD therapy (antitachycardia pacing or shocks).[149] This study investigated a population that consisted of 128 patients who were mostly male (87%) and generally in NYHA functional class I or II (77%–84%). VF accounted for 16% to 20% of index arrhythmias, and VT represented the most common index arrhythmia (47%–52%). Approximately half of the patients had an LEVF of equal to or less than 30%. Prophylactic catheter ablation resulted in a 65% reduction in ICD therapy compared with ICD only during a mean follow-up time of 22.5 ± 5.5 months (hazard ratio in ablation group, 0.35; 95% CI, 0.15–0.78; $p = 0.007$).

A few years later, results from the VTACH (Ventricular Tachycardia Ablation in Coronary Heart Disease) study extended the evidence that prophylactic catheter ablation may reduce the incidence of ICD therapy in patients with ICDs.[150] One hundred seven patients with stable VT, previous MI, and LVEF of 50% or less were enrolled in this study. Sixty percent of the patients had LVEF greater than 30%, and 2 in 3 patients had single-chamber ICDs. In this study, patients underwent ICD implantation a median of 3 days after ablation procedure or EP study. The primary end point, time from defibrillator implantation to recurrence of any SuVT or VF, occurred after a median of 5.9 months in the control group and 18.6 months in the ablation group ($p = 0.045$, log-rank test). In addition, a difference in recurrence rates of VT or VF was observed only in patients with LVEF exceeding 30%. The VTACH study investigators acknowledged that because this study did not compare the relative efficacies of ablation with antiarrhythmic drugs, the optimal approach for reducing ICD therapy has yet to be established.

Clearly, S.L. should have the device placed: It is her best chance for prolonging long-term survival. Depending on the number of times the machine discharges per month and the patient's response, adjunctive antiarrhythmic drugs or prophylactic ablation may be needed.

Amiodarone

CASE 20-9, QUESTION 3: S.L.'s cardiologist would like to start amiodarone as adjunctive therapy because S.L. has expressed concern about the number of ICD discharges that may occur after ICD placement. If S.L. is to be treated with amiodarone, how should it be initiated and monitored?

Amiodarone exhibits properties of classes I, II, III, and IV antiarrhythmic agents. Although it has class II effects on the heart, amiodarone is virtually devoid of antiadrenergic effects outside the heart and is not contraindicated in patients with asthma. The antiadrenergic effects arise from inhibition of adenylate cyclase, the enzyme that catalyzes production of the second-messenger product cyclic adenosine monophosphate. Amiodarone can also cause a reduction in β_1-receptor density.[151,152]

Because of the extremely long half-life of amiodarone, loading doses are used to accelerate the onset of drug effect. The OPTIC trial used a loading dose of oral amiodarone 400 mg, given twice daily for 2 weeks, followed by a daily dose of 400 mg for the next 4 weeks, and a daily maintenance dose of 200 mg thereafter.[148] Although a concentration-effect relationship is hard to determine for amiodarone, levels greater than 2.5 mg/L are associated with an increased incidence of adverse effects.[152]

Amiodarone has many serious adverse effects involving a variety of organ systems, the most serious and life-threatening of which is pulmonary toxicity. This historically occurred in 4% to 6% of patients, and the mechanism may involve two distinct pathways.[153] Direct toxicity may arise from lung parenchymal cell injury and a subsequent fibrotic response. The influx of inflammatory or immune effector cells to the lung could lead to indirect pulmonary toxicity in amiodarone-treated patients. Pulmonary toxicity consists of a variety of symptoms and conditions, such as exertional dyspnea, weight loss, nonproductive cough, occasionally low-grade fever, pneumonitis that culminates in pulmonary fibrosis, adult respiratory distress syndrome, respiratory failure, and death. Physical examination usually reveals bibasilar rales, with decreased breath sounds. Reticular infiltrates and patchy acinar infiltrates are commonly observed in chest radiographs of patients experiencing amiodarone-induced lung toxicity. Of note, amiodarone-associated pulmonary toxicity has been well documented in patients given chronic amiodarone doses of 375 to 685 mg/day, usually for a prolonged time.[153] However, a lower incidence of adverse pulmonary events was observed in patients receiving amiodarone doses of 100 to 420 mg/day.[154,155]

Despite the lower incidence of adverse pulmonary events observed in these studies, it is still necessary to monitor for the development of pulmonary fibrosis. A baseline chest radiograph and pulmonary function tests (diffusion capacity in particular) are recommended by the manufacturer.[156] The chest radiograph should be repeated at 3- to 6-month intervals, and patients should be specifically questioned about pulmonary symptoms because early detection can decrease the extent of lung damage.[156]

Liver toxicity can range from an asymptomatic elevation of transaminases (two to four times normal) to fulminant hepatitis. The mean latent period between the start of amiodarone therapy and evidence of liver injury is 10 months, but with rapid intravenous loading of amiodarone, a Reye's-like fulminant hepatitis can occur within a few days, most likely caused by the intravenous vehicle polysorbate-80. The precise mechanism of amiodarone-induced hepatotoxicity has not been fully elucidated. However, higher doses and prolonged drug use appear to place patients at higher risk of experiencing hepatotoxic effects of amiodarone. Thus liver enzymes should be monitored at baseline, 1 month, 3 months, 6 months, and semiannually afterward.[157] The most common gastrointestinal complaints are nausea, anorexia, and constipation, which occur in 25% of patients receiving amiodarone.[156]

Both hypothyroidism and hyperthyroidism have been reported, although hypothyroidism is more common. The thyroid complications are a consequence of amiodarone's large iodine content and its ability to block the peripheral conversion of thyroxine (T_4) to triiodothyronine (T_3). In addition, amiodarone and its metabolite, desethylamiodarone, appear to be directly cytotoxic to the thyroid gland.[158]

Other bothersome side effects are corneal deposits (usually asymptomatic), blue-gray skin discoloration in sun-exposed areas, photosensitivity, exacerbation of heart failure, and central nervous system effects that include ataxia, tremor, dizziness, and peripheral neuropathy. Other than eye examination and pulmonary function tests, which should be repeated when the patient is symptomatic, other blood tests should be repeated every 6 months for routine monitoring (after initial 6 months).[156] Amiodarone also blocks multiple cytochrome P-450 enzyme systems and P-glycoprotein pumps, resulting in clinically significant drug interactions.

Torsades de Pointes

PROARRHYTHMIC EFFECTS OF ANTIARRHYTHMIC DRUGS AND CLINICAL PRESENTATION

CASE 20-10

QUESTION 1: L.G. is a 69-year-old woman who is taking sotalol 80 mg twice daily for a previous episode of SuVT. L.G. was admitted to the hospital 3 days ago for altered mental status. She is also taking oral haloperidol 5 mg every morning and 10 mg every evening, along with paliperidone 3 mg twice daily for schizophrenia. At baseline, her QTc interval was 400 ms, and her CrCl was 50 mL/minute. Other laboratory values are as follows:

Sodium, 139 mmol/L
Chloride, 108 mmol/L
Potassium, 4.0 mmol/L
CO_2, 22 mmol/L
Blood urea nitrogen (BUN), 32 mg/dL
Serum creatinine, 1.5 mg/dL
Random glucose, 102 mg/dL
Calcium, 8.5 mg/dL
Albumin, 2.9 g/dL
Phosphorous, 3.3 mg/dL

Today, her ECG reveals a QT_c interval of 502 ms and TdP, with a ventricular rate of 110 beats/minute. What is QTc interval prolongation? Why does QTc interval prolongation indicate an increased risk of TdP? Could an antiarrhythmic agent such as sotalol cause this arrhythmia? How does creatinine clearance factor into this?

The QT interval denotes ventricular depolarization (the QRS complex in the cardiac cycle) and repolarization (from the end of the QRS complex to the end of the T wave). Certain ion channels in phases 2 and 3 of the action potential are vital in determining the QT interval (Fig. 20-1). An abnormal increase in ventricular repolarization increases the risk of TdP. TdP is defined as a rapid polymorphic VT preceded by QTc interval prolongation. TdP can degenerate into VF and as such can be life threatening (Fig. 20-15).[159]

Because there is tremendous variability in the QT interval resulting from changes in heart rate, the QT is frequently corrected for heart rate (QTc interval). Several correction formulas for the QT interval exist and give similar results at most heart rates. The most common correction formula uses QT and R-R intervals measured in seconds as follows: [$QTc = QT/(R\text{-}R^{0.5})$]. However, overcorrection of the QT interval may occur in persons with elevated heart rates (>85 beats/minute).[160,161] The Fridericia correction [$QT_c = QT/(R\text{-}R^{1/3})$] represents an alternative correction method for patients with heart rates exceeding 85 beats/minute.

The ACC and AHA recently addressed the issue of the prevention of TdP in hospital settings. They stated that each 10-ms increase in QT_c confers an additional 5% to 7% TdP risk in patients with congenital long-QT syndrome.[161] The International Conference on Harmonization (ICH) stated that prolongation of QT_c interval by more than 30 ms and in excess of 60 ms should be classified as a potential adverse effect and a definite adverse effect, respectively.[162]

Class Ia and class III antiarrhythmic agents have been shown to induce TdP in numerous literature reports.[163] Of note, class Ia antiarrhythmic agents do not exhibit dose-dependent association with TdP, whereas the incidence of TdP does appear to be dose-related with class III antiarrhythmic agents. QT prolongation associated with the use of class Ia antiarrhythmic agents is likely the result of blockade of outward potassium channels, but it is offset by concomitant blockade of inward sodium channels at increased drug concentrations.[163] TdP induced by class III antiarrhythmic agents arises from prolonged repolarization and cardiac refractoriness. With the exception of dronedarone, all class III antiarrhythmic agents have been implicated in cases of TdP. Amiodarone appears to have the lowest propensity for inducing TdP; one literature review of 17 uncontrolled studies (n = 2,878) showed an incidence of 0.7%.[164] The reason for the low propensity of amiodarone to cause TdP may be related to the fact that it blocks both the rapid and slow component of the delayed rectifier potassium channels. This provides less heterogeneity in ventricular repolarization and reduces the risk of TdP compared with agents that prolong QT_c interval solely by blocking the rapid component of the delayed rectifier potassium channel.

Class 1c antiarrhythmic agents do not exert significant effects on repolarization, and therefore have rarely been shown to induce TdP. To date, two cases of flecainide-induced TdP (with no associated triggering factor) have been published, along with one report of propafenone-associated TdP.[157,165,167]

Sotalol is known to cause QTc interval prolongation in a dose-dependent manner. Total daily doses of 160, 320, 480, and >640 mg gave patients a steady-state QTc interval of 463, 467, 483, and 512 milliseconds, and the incidence of TdP was 0.5%, 1.6%, 4.4%, and 5.8%, respectively.[167]

It is likely that L.G.'s reduced renal function put her at high risk for sotalol accumulation and accentuated QTc interval prolongation. In patients with a CrCl greater than 60 mL/minute, the sotalol dose of 80 mg twice daily is appropriate, but in patients like L.G. with a CrCl of less than 40 to 60 mL/minute, the starting dose should be 80 mg daily owing to sotalol's predominant renal clearance.

CASE 20-10, QUESTION 2: What transient conditions or other disorders can increase the risk of TdP in patients on class Ia or III antiarrhythmic agents?

Hypokalemia, hypomagnesemia, hypocalcemia (rare cases of TdP), concurrent use of more than one QT-prolonging drug, advanced age, female sex, heart disease (heart failure or myocardial infarction), treatment with diuretics, impaired hepatic drug metabolism, and bradycardia are important risk factors for TdP in hospitalized patients.[161] Hypokalemia may prolong QT interval by modifying the function of the inwardly rectifying potassium channel, resulting in heterogeneity and dispersion of repolarization. Prolonged ventricular cycle length can assume the form of complete AV block, sinus bradycardia, or a rhythm in which long cycles may progress to arrhythmogenic early afterdepolarizations.

Congenital long QT syndrome (LQTS) occurs in 1 in 2,500 individuals, and is a channelopathy associated with mutations identified in genes encoding voltage-gated sodium and potassium channels.[161] Since 1995, approximately 1,000 individual LQTS-causing mutations have been detected in 12 distinct LQTS-susceptibility genes. The LQTS-susceptibility genes *KCNQ1* (encoded I_{Ks} α-subunit), *KCNH2* (encoded I_{Kr} α-subunit), and *SCN5A* (encoded Nav1.5 α-subunit) account for nearly 75% of all congenital LQTS cases.

Because L.G. did not have a family history of hereditary long QT syndrome but was being treated with sotalol (an agent known to be associated with TdP) in renal dysfunction, it can be assumed that sotalol therapy was responsible for her arrhythmia.

PROARRHYTHMIC EFFECTS OF NONANTIARRHYTHMIC AGENTS

CASE 20-10, QUESTION 3: Which nonantiarrhythmic agents cause TdP? What is the mechanism of TdP initiation in this situation?

Nonantiarrhythmic agents can also exhibit potassium-channel inhibitory properties and can prolong the QTc interval. Most of these drugs, including erythromycin, clarithromycin, fluoroquinolones, azole antifungals, methadone, tricyclic antidepressants, and antipsychotics, cause QTc interval prolongation by inhibiting the inwardly rectifying potassium ion channel, just like quinidine and sotalol.[161,162,169–173] Moreover, toxic concentrations of nonantiarrhythmic drugs can induce TdP as a result of large doses, impaired kidney or liver function, or other drug therapy that interferes with metabolism of nonantiarrhythmic drugs.

Guidelines suggest that the risk of QTc prolongation is greater with certain antipsychotic agents, such as thioridazine, ziprasidone, and risperidone. To date, the risk for QTc prolongation with perphenazine, clozapine, olanzapine, quetiapine, aripiprazole, and haloperidol (except when given parenterally or in high doses in the critically ill) appears to be minimal relative to that with other antipsychotic agents.[174] In recent years, considerable controversy has been generated by the FDA recommendation of continuous ECG monitoring of patients receiving intravenous (off-label use in the United States) haloperidol. A review of 70 intravenous haloperidol-associated QT prolongation/TdP cases that were identified by searching PubMed, EMBASE, and Scopus databases, along with the FDA database, revealed 54 reports of TdP. Cumulative doses of 5 mg to 645 mg were administered to patients experiencing TdP, whereas cumulative doses ranging from 2 mg to 1,540 mg were administered to patients (n = 16) who experienced QTc prolongation (20–286 ms increase from baseline) without TdP. Forty-two patients experienced QTc prolongation followed by TdP and received cumulative doses of 2 mg to 1,700 mg. Ninety-seven percent of the 70 patients were determined to have additional risk factors for QTc prolongation or TdP, including electrolyte imbalance, underlying cardiac disease, concomitant proarrhythmic agents, and baseline QTc greater than 450 ms. The authors of the review concluded that patients with additional risk factors for developing QTc prolongation or TdP who receive cumulative doses of intravenous haloperidol in excess of 2 mg should have continuous ECG monitoring.[171] Cases of TdP associated with oral haloperidol have been reported to a lesser degree in the PubMed database, relative to intravenous haloperidol.[172]

During the past decade, multiple case reports of methadone-induced TdP have been published. Pearson et al. conducted a retrospective analysis of adverse events attributed to methadone that were reported to the FDA during a period of 33 years.[175] Forty-three patients (0.78%) experienced TdP, and 16 patients (0.29%) experienced QT prolongation. The mean daily dose of methadone was 410 mg (range, 29 mg to 1,680 mg), and 75% of the patients had other risk factors for cardiac arrhythmia, such as electrolyte imbalance, interacting medications, structural heart disease, and female sex. The recent emergence of methadone-associated TdP could be attributable to escalating doses used in recent years, given the preponderance of published cases of patients receiving very high doses of this agent.[173]

Currently, the utility of published cardiac risk data on anti-infective agents is limited, owing to underreporting, failure to completely eliminate contributory confounding variables (cardiac disease, electrolyte abnormalities, use of other QT-prolonging drugs), and the retrospective nature of some post-marketing studies.[162] However, the propensity of antimicrobial agents to induce QT prolongation appears to be especially marked with certain macrolide antibiotics (erythromycin, clarithromycin). All of the commercially available antifungal agents (ketoconazole, itraconazole, fluconazole, voriconazole, posaconazole) have been shown to induce TdP and QT prolongation.[176] Among the quinolones, ciprofloxacin appears to display the lowest potential for causing TdP.[169,170]

A list of nonantiarrhythmic agents implicated in causing QTc interval prolongation and known pharmacokinetic drug interaction increasing the blood concentrations of these drugs is given in Table 20-6.

Because L.G. was taking haloperidol in combination with sotalol, it is likely that QTc-prolonging effects resulting from concomitant use contributed to the development of TdP.

TREATMENT

CASE 20-10, QUESTION 4: How should TdP be treated? What treatments should be considered for L.G.?

If the patient is significantly hemodynamically compromised (frequently associated with a ventricular rate >150 beats/minute

TABLE 20-6
Nonantiarrhythmic Agents Implicated in QTc Interval Prolongation or Torsades de Pointes[a]

Drug Class	Agent	Drugs That Increase Blood Concentrations of These QTc Interval–Prolonging Drugs
Antianginal	Ranolazine	CYP3A4 inhibitors
Antibiotics: macrolides	Erythromycin (lactobionate and base)	CYP3A4 inhibitors
Antibiotics: fluoroquinolones	Gatifloxacin, grepafloxacin, lomefloxacin, moxifloxacin, sparfloxacin	
Antibiotics: other	Trimethoprim-sulfamethoxazole, pentamidine isethionate	
Antidepressants	Tricyclics, maprotiline	CYP1A2, 2D6, or 2C9 inhibitors
Antiemetics	Dolasetron	
Antimalarials	Mefloquine, quinine	Sodium bicarbonate, acetazolamide, cimetidine
Antipsychotics	Atypicals, butyrophenones, typicals	CYP1A2, 2D6, 2C9, 3A4 inhibitors
Calcium-channel blockers	Bepridil	
Dopaminergics	Amantadine	Hydrochlorothiazide, quinidine, quinine, trimethoprim-sulfamethoxazole
Narcotics	Methadone	CYP3A4 and 1A2 inhibitors
Sympathomimetics	Albuterol, ephedra, epinephrine, metaproterenol, terbutaline, salmeterol	Monoamine oxidase inhibitors
Other	Arsenic, organophosphates	

[a] An up-to-date list can be found at http://www.azcert.org

and unconsciousness) while in TdP, electrical cardioversion is the therapy of choice and should be given immediately. Stepwise increasing shocks of 100 to 200, 300, and 360 J (monophasic energy) can be tried if earlier shocks are unsuccessful.

MAGNESIUM

In a hemodynamically stable patient, magnesium is frequently considered the drug of choice to restore normal sinus rhythm. It benefits patients whether they have hypomagnesemia or normal serum magnesium levels. However, magnesium is not effective for patients with polymorphic VT without TdP and with normal QT intervals. Before administering magnesium, potassium levels should be supplemented to the high normal range of 4.5 to 5.0 mmol/L.[177,178] A common magnesium regimen is 2 g given for 60 seconds through the intravenous route, with a repeat dose administered 5 to 15 minutes later for refractory TdP. Some experts have recommended repeat doses every 6 hours if the QTc interval remains greater than 500 ms. Adult patients experiencing persistently refractory dysrhythmias have received continuous infusions of magnesium, with rates usually ranging from 3 to 10 mg/minute. The exact mechanism of action for magnesium in TdP is not known, but it reduces the occurrence of triggered activity such as early after-depolarizations. In addition, magnesium blocks L-type calcium channels in the membrane, and may stabilize the membrane gradient through activation of the sodium-potassium ATPase.[178]

OTHER TREATMENT OPTIONS FOR TDP

The second class of drugs used to abolish TdP is the class Ib antiarrhythmic agents (e.g., mexiletine, lidocaine). Unlike quinidine and the class III antiarrhythmic agents, the class Ib agents do not inhibit potassium outflow during phases 2 and 3.[178,179] In addition, blockade of inward sodium channels causes a shortening of the QT interval in some patients. Preliminary data suggest that class Ib antiarrhythmic agents have considerable benefit in patients with sodium channel–activated QT prolongation, but virtually no effect on patients with potassium channel blockade–induced QT prolongation.[180,181] In a landmark trial, mexiletine was given to patients who had hereditary long QT syndrome,[180] and the patients were analyzed by their genetic etiology of long QT. The group with a deficient gene for the potassium channel had no QT shortening, whereas those with a defective sodium gene had significant shortening of the QT interval. These divergent responses were confirmed in an in vitro study using mexiletine with either clofilium, a potassium-channel blocker, or almokalant, a pure sodium-channel activator.[181]

Cardioacceleration with isoproterenol (1–4 mcg/minute) or cardiac pacing has also been shown to be beneficial.[177,182,183] As previously described, sotalol, quinidine, and *N*-acetylprocainamide's ability to prolong the action potential duration is diminished at faster heart rates (reverse use dependence).[184] The more the inwardly rectifying potassium channels are activated, the less susceptible the channels are to inhibition by potassium-channel blocking drugs.

Transvenous pacing has been shown to be of some use in abolishing refractory TdP.[177] Before adjusting the ventricular rate to suppress ectopic ventricular beats, it is essential to ensure proper catheter placement and cardiac capture. In general, ventricular rates of 90 to 110 beats/minute can usually eliminate ventricular ectopy, but some patients may require rates as high as 140 beats/minute. Once control of TdP has been attained, the pacing rate can be gradually decreased to the lowest paced rate that suppresses further ectopy and dysrhythmia.

Because L.G. is hemodynamically stable, a bolus injection of 2 g of magnesium should be administered for 1 minute. In addition, she should receive potassium supplementation (infusion) to achieve a potassium level of 4.5 to 5.0 mmol/L. If it is not successful within 5 to 15 minutes after the first bolus dose, a repeat dose of magnesium 2 g should be administered to L.G. A continuous infusion of magnesium at a rate of 3 to 10 mg/minute should be given to L.G. if TdP persists after two bolus doses of magnesium. If the arrhythmia recurs, cardiac pacing should be used.

Naturopathic Therapy for Arrhythmias

CASE 20-10, QUESTION 5: L.G. is interested in natural products to replace her antiarrhythmic therapy, which she says is too expensive. Are there any herbal or natural agents that can prevent or treat arrhythmias?

HERBAL THERAPIES

Many herbal remedies have been touted as beneficial in "normalizing heart rhythm," but efficacy data from human studies are lacking for most agents.[185] Avoid using herbal products that contain cardiac glycosides such as lily of the valley, oleander, *Strophanthus hispidus* seeds, squill, dogbane, *Adonis vernalis,* ouabain, and *Thevetia peruviana.* Although the effects can mimic those of digoxin, there is no way to monitor blood concentrations, so they cannot be used safely.

FOOD SUPPLEMENTS AND MINERALS

Omega-3 polyunsaturated fatty acids (n-3 PUFAs), coenzyme Q_{10}, and L-carnitine are the best-studied alternative therapies for arrhythmias.[186–192]

The largest prospective randomized controlled trial to test the efficacy of n-3 PUFAs for secondary prevention of coronary heart disease was the Gruppo Italiano per lo Studio della Sopravvivenza nell'Infarto Miocardico (GISSI) prevention study.[187] In this trial, 11,324 patients with coronary heart disease were randomized to 300 mg of vitamin E, 850 mg of n-3 PUFAs (given as eicosapentaenoic acid [EPA] and docosahexaenoic acid [DHA] ethyl esters), both, or neither. After 3.5 years, the group given n-3 PUFAs had a 20% reduction in overall mortality and a 45% reduction in sudden death. Vitamin E was ineffective. Limitations to this study were that it was not placebo-controlled, and the dropout rate was 25%. Of note, the antiarrhythmic efficacy trials of PUFAs in patients with automatic ICDs have yielded inconsistent results, with one study suggesting a proarrhythmic effect associated with n-3 PUFAs. A meta-analysis of three trials of n-3 PUFA use in patients with automatic ICDs demonstrated an absence of overall antiarrhythmic effect.[188] To date, with the exception of one epidemiological study suggesting benefit from n-3 PUFA consumption in AF prevention, subsequent trials have not been confirmatory. A recent canine model study conducted by Sakabe et al. showed that consumption of oral n-3 PUFA supplements resulted in suppression of congestive heart failure–induced (triggered by ventricular tachypacing) atrial structural remodeling.[189]

Kowey et al. assessed the safety and efficacy of prescription omega-3 fatty acids (Lovaza) in a prospective, randomized, double-blind, placebo-controlled, parallel group study that included 542 patients with confirmed symptomatic PAF and 121 patients with persistent AF.[193] The primary outcome was symptomatic, first recurrence of AF in PAF patients. During the first week of the study, subjects received either placebo or a daily dose of 8 g of prescription omega-3 fatty acid. During weeks 2 through 24, patients received a maintenance dose of 4 g/day of prescription omega-3 fatty acid. After 24 weeks of treatment, the primary outcome occurred in 52% of prescription drug–treated patients and in 48% of placebo-treated patients (hazard ratio, 1.15; 95% CI, 0.90–1.46; $p = 0.26$). The investigators concluded that treatment of PAF patients (with no structural heart disease) with prescription omega-3 fatty acids did not lower the recurrence of symptomatic AF.

How is it possible to reconcile the potential proarrhythmic effect of n-3 PUFAs in patients with automatic ICDs with earlier studies suggesting protection from life-threatening ventricular arrhythmias? Differing mechanisms of arrhythmia generation may account for the conflicting findings reported within these study populations. n-3 PUFAs have been shown to exert a variety of cellular electrophysiological effects, such as slowing of impulse conduction and shortening of action potential duration. Patients who have experienced a recent MI are at heightened risk for arrhythmias caused by triggered activity. Consequently, the electrophysiological effects of n-3 PUFAs would have a beneficial reduction in arrhythmias in this population. However, patients with ischemic disease who have not experienced an MI may have arrhythmias initiated by re-entry. This population may therefore be at increased risk for arrhythmias associated with n-3 PUFAs.[186]

Coenzyme Q_{10}, a vitaminlike entity that is present in cardiac cells, serves as an electron carrier in oxidative phosphorylation. This supplement has been shown to enhance cell membrane stabilization in vitro, and by acting as a free radical scavenger, it exerts bioenergetic and antioxidant effects. Furthermore, coenzyme Q_{10} has demonstrated its ability to inhibit platelet aggregation and human vitronectin receptor expression.[190] Singh et al. performed a randomized, double-blind, placebo-controlled study that included 154 patients who experienced acute MI. Patients were randomly assigned to receive coenzyme Q_{10} (120 mg/day, divided in two doses) or placebo for 28 days. At 28 days' follow-up, 25.3% of placebo-treated patients experienced arrhythmias, compared with 9.5% of coenzyme Q_{10}–treated patients (relative risk, 0.37; 95% CI, 0.22–0.66; $p < 0.05$).[190]

Carnitine functions as a vital cofactor for the transport of fatty acyl groups from the cytoplasm to the mitochondrial matrix, where β-oxidation of the fatty acyl groups results in ATP production. Ventricular arrhythmias have been attributed to tissue fatty acid accumulation during myocardial ischemia; L-carnitine may be able to counteract the deleterious effect of high levels of free fatty acids.[191] Rizzon et al. conducted a double-blind, parallel group, placebo-controlled trial that included 56 patients who experienced acute MI. Patients underwent random allocation to receive placebo or carnitine dosed at 100 mg/kg every 12 hours for 36 hours. Carnitine treatment lowered the number of premature ventricular beats evaluated by Holter recording for 2 days.[192]

CARDIOPULMONARY ARREST

Cardiopulmonary Resuscitation

Cardiac arrest from VF, pulseless VT, pulseless electrical activity (PEA), and asystole are life-threatening emergencies. Table 20-7[137,194–200] reviews commonly used drugs for these indications, and Figure 20-16 highlights key features of the management of pulseless arrest in the 2010 AHA Guidelines. This section will review important aspects of therapy and will give clinical pearls, but the reader should also review the national consensus source document for these disorders, which includes more detail than can be given here.[194]

Treatment

CASE 20-11

QUESTION 1: M.N., a 52-year-old man, is visiting his wife, who is hospitalized for pneumonia. He goes into the bathroom and 2 minutes later his wife hears a dull thud. She calls out for her husband, but he does not respond. After an additional 2 minutes, health care workers open the bathroom door and find M.N. unresponsive and pulseless. CPR is initiated and a code blue is called. The ECG shows VF (Fig. 20-13), and there is no BP. In addition to CPR, what initial therapy is available?

Determining the underlying rhythm disturbance is important because it directs health care workers to follow the Advanced Cardiac Life Support (ACLS) algorithm for pulseless VT or VF (Fig. 20-16). This algorithm calls for electrical defibrillation first,

TABLE 20-7
Commonly Used Drugs in Cardiac Arrest

Drug	Formulation	Dosage/Administration	Rationale/Indications	Comments
Amiodarone	50 mg/mL Vials: 3, 9, 18 mL	300 mg diluted in 20–30 mL D5W or NS; additional 150 mg (diluted solution) can be given for recurrent or refractory VT or VF.	Exhibits antiadrenergic properties and blocks sodium, potassium, and calcium channels. First-line antiarrhythmic for pulseless VT and VF.	Excipients (polysorbate 80 and benzyl alcohol) can induce hypotension. Failing to dilute can induce phlebitis.
Epinephrine	0.1 mg/mL (1:10,000) or 1 mg/mL (1:1,000)	10 mL of a 1:10,000 solution of epinephrine (1 mg; dilute 1:1,000 solution in 0.9% sodium chloride) every 3–5 minutes.	Increases coronary sinus perfusion pressure through α_1 stimulation. Indicated in pulseless VT, VF, asystole, and PEA.	If administered through peripheral catheter, need to flush the line to get drug into the central compartment.
Vasopressin	20 units/mL Vials: 0.5, 1 mL, 10 mL	40-unit dose can be used to replace first or second dose of epinephrine	Increases coronary sinus perfusion pressure through vasopressin receptor stimulation. Indicated in pulseless VT, VF, asystole, and PEA.	Vasopressin is an acceptable alternative to epinephrine, may work better if time from cardiac arrest to ACLS is delayed.

ACLS, Advanced Cardiac Life Support; D5W, 5% dextrose in water; NS, normal saline; PEA, pulseless electrical activity; VF, ventricular fibrillation; VT, ventricular tachycardia.

but other clinicians should work to establish IV access in case defibrillation fails.[194]

EXTERNAL DEFIBRILLATION

Although commercially available manual defibrillators provide monophasic or biphasic waveform shocks, the biphasic defibrillator has become the preferred device owing to its high first-shock efficacy (>90% termination of VF at 5 seconds after shock).[194] Biphasic defibrillators deliver one of two waveforms, a truncated exponential waveform or a rectilinear waveform. Most commercially available biphasic defibrillators display the device-specific energy dose range that should be used. Respective initial selected energies of 150 J to 200 J and 120 J are reasonable choices for initial shocks delivered by truncated exponential waveform and rectilinear waveform defibrillators, respectively. However, if a health care provider operating a manual biphasic defibrillator is uncertain of the effective energy dose to terminate VF, using the maximal shock energy setting available is preferred. For second and subsequent shocks delivered by manual biphasic defibrillators, the same or higher energies should be used. For first and subsequent shocks, a shock of 360 J should be delivered if a monophasic defibrillator is used to terminate VF.

CASE 20-11, QUESTION 2: The initial shock fails to cause a return of spontaneous circulation in M.N. An IV catheter is established in a peripheral arm vein. The algorithm now calls for epinephrine or vasopressin, but which one should be used?

EPINEPHRINE AND VASOPRESSIN

Although epinephrine stimulates β_1-, β_2-, and α_1-adrenergic receptors, it is the α_1-adrenoceptor effects that are most closely associated with efficacy in VF or pulseless VT.[137,194] Applying α_1-adrenoceptor stimulation increases systemic vascular resistance (via vasoconstriction), which elevates coronary perfusion

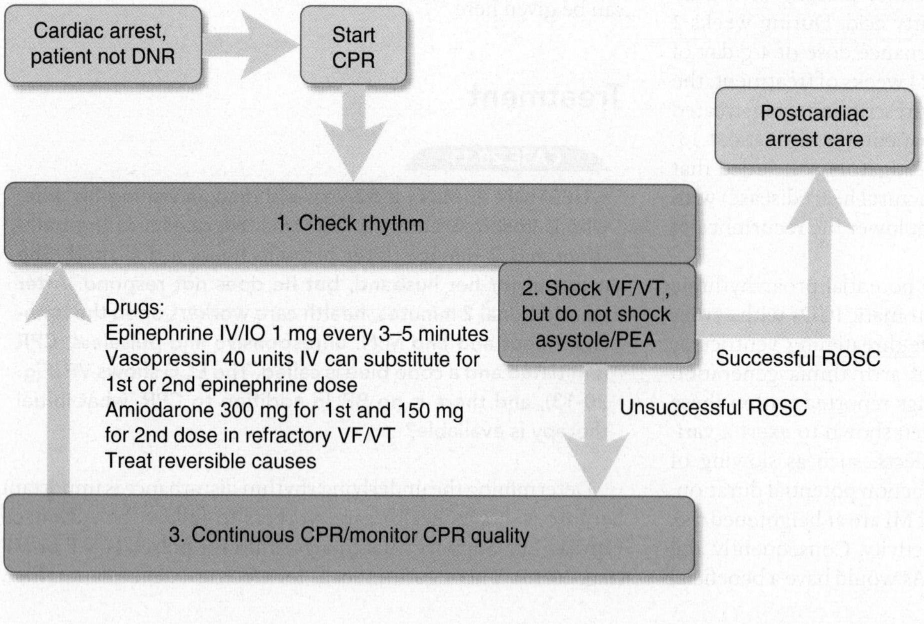

FIGURE 20-16 Cardiac arrest treatment algorithm. CPR, cardiopulmonary resuscitation; DNR, do not resuscitate; IO, intraosseous; IV, intravenous; PEA, pulseless electrical activity; ROSC, restoration of spontaneous circulation; VF, ventricular fibrillation; VT, ventricular tachycardia.

pressure. This increase in coronary perfusion pressure is most likely the key to enhancing the return of spontaneous circulation after subsequent electrical defibrillation. Epinephrine may convert fine VF to a coarse variety that may be more amenable to defibrillation.

The recommended dose of epinephrine is 1 mg (10 mL of a 1:10,000 dilution; refer to Table 20-7) given by IV push. The dosage can be repeated at 3- to 5-minute intervals during resuscitation. If the drug is given IV through a peripheral catheter, which in this case includes a peripherally inserted central catheter (PICC), then a 20-mL flush with normal saline is recommended to ensure delivery into the central compartment. Only chest compressions cause blood circulation in VF or pulseless VT, so movement of drugs from the periphery to the heart (where the benefit will occur) is severely impaired.

If intravenous access is unavailable, health care providers may attempt to establish intraosseous (IO) access in the patient. For IO injection of drugs, a cannula should be placed in a noncollapsible venous plexus; the onset and systemic drug concentrations achieved with IO administration are similar to that achieved by central venous access. Typical sites of intraosseous needle insertion include the anterior tibial bone marrow, the distal femur, medial malleolus, or the anterior superior iliac spine.[197]

Vasopressin is an exogenously administered antidiuretic hormone. In supraphysiologic doses, vasopressin stimulates V1 receptors and causes peripheral vasoconstriction. Vasopressin use during CPR causes intense vasoconstriction to the skin, skeletal muscle, intestine, and fat, with much less constriction of coronary vascular beds. Cerebral and renal vasodilation occurs as well.

The results of a prospective, randomized, controlled, multicenter study (n = 1,186) that enrolled out-of-hospital cardiac arrest patients who presented with VF, PEA, or asystole showed that administration of vasopressin as adjunctive therapy resulted in similar survival to hospital admission rates compared with adjunctive epinephrine therapy.[195] In this study, patients were randomly assigned to receive two ampules of 40 international units of vasopressin or two ampules of 1 mg of epinephrine. The second dose of vasopressor was injected if spontaneous restoration of circulation did not occur within 3 minutes after the first injection of the drug. If the absence of spontaneous circulation persisted, the physician administering CPR had the option of injecting epinephrine. The primary outcome measure of the study was overall survival to hospital admission. The reported survival rates were similar between the two treatment groups for both patients with PEA and those with VF. Of note, a post hoc analysis showed that survival to hospital admission rates were 29% and 20%, respectively, for vasopressin- and epinephrine-treated patients who presented with asystole requiring CPR ($p = 0.02$).

An in-hospital study of 200 cardiac arrest patients (initial rhythm: 16%–20% VF, 3% VT, 41%–54% PEA, 27%–34% asystole) showed no difference in 1-hour or hospital discharge survival for vasopressin 40 units versus epinephrine 1 mg.[196] Similarly, a meta-analysis of five randomized trials showed no survival advantage of vasopressin treatment versus epinephrine treatment at the times of hospital discharge or 24 hours after treatment.[197]

On the basis of these trials, it would be reasonable to use a single dose of vasopressin 40 units as an alternative to either the first or second dose of epinephrine 1 mg in the treatment of VF (or pulseless VT).

CASE 20-11, QUESTION 3: Because M.N. has an IV site and the time from cardiac arrest to ACLS was brief, epinephrine was chosen and a 1-mg bolus was given, followed with a 20-mL normal saline flush. The arm was elevated for 20 seconds to ensure adequate delivery. Thirty seconds after administration a 200-J shock is given (via biphasic manual defibrillator), but it fails to convert VF. What can be done now?

The most recently updated ACLS guideline calls for the use of amiodarone in cases of VF or pulseless VT that do not respond to CPR, shocks, and a vasopressor.[194]

IV AMIODARONE AND LIDOCAINE

Amiodarone's effect in VF or pulseless VT was studied in the ARREST (Amiodarone for Resuscitation of Refractory Sustained Ventricular Tachyarrhythmias) trial.[198] This study was conducted in patients who experienced cardiac arrest in an out-of-hospital situation with therapy given by paramedics in the field. Patients who failed three stacked shocks and one dose of epinephrine with an electrical countershock were randomly assigned to amiodarone 300 mg IV bolus or placebo. This was followed by other antiarrhythmic agents historically used in ACLS (2000 guidelines: lidocaine, procainamide, or bretylium) if the clinicians desired. Amiodarone significantly increased the chance of survival to hospital admission (44% vs. 34% of placebo group; $p = 0.03$), but survival to hospital discharge was not changed. Of note, 66% of patients received antiarrhythmic drug treatment for pulseless VT or VF after amiodarone administration. In addition, recipients of amiodarone were more likely to experience hypotension (59% vs. 48% of placebo; $p = 0.04$) or bradycardia (41% vs. 25% of placebo group; $p = 0.004$).

The occurrence of hypotension among amiodarone recipients has been attributed to the presence of two excipients, polysorbate 80 and benzyl alcohol. Of interest, a study conducted by Somberg et al.[199] showed that a new formulation of amiodarone (Amio-Aqueous) had a similar risk of hypotension as lidocaine after VT termination (1% in both groups).

The ALIVE (Amiodarone Versus Lidocaine in Ventricular Ectopy, n = 347) trial directly compared IV amiodarone 300 mg to lidocaine 1 to 1.5 mg/kg bolus.[199] In this trial, patients needed to fail three stacked shocks and epinephrine plus an additional shock to be eligible for randomization to either amiodarone or lidocaine. Amiodarone was given as an initial dose of 5 mg/kg followed by a shock. If unsuccessful, a dose of 2.5 mg/kg was given followed by a subsequent shock. Lidocaine was given as a 1.5 mg/kg bolus followed by a shock. If therapy failed, then a second bolus of 1.5 mg/kg was used with a subsequent shock. If the first antiarrhythmic drug failed, other routine antiarrhythmic drugs for cardiac arrest (per 2000 ACLS guidelines: e.g., procainamide, bretylium) could be tried. Patients given amiodarone were 90% more likely to experience the primary outcome, survival to hospital admission, than those given lidocaine ($p = 0.009$). Unfortunately, no significant advantage to hospital discharge occurred (5% vs. 3%).

On the basis of these findings, amiodarone is the only antiarrhythmic agent with proven ability to improve return of spontaneous circulation and short-term survival versus other antiarrhythmic therapy. However, it has not yet been shown to improve survival to hospital discharge.

CASE 20-11, QUESTION 4: Amiodarone 300 mg followed by electrical defibrillation fails to cause a return of spontaneous circulation in M.N. A subsequent 150-mg dose also fails. However, M.N. did convert to normal sinus rhythm for 9 seconds before going back into VF. Should resuscitation be discontinued?

M.N. is at serious risk of death as a result of VF. However, as long as M.N. remains in VF it is appropriate to continue active therapy. If M.N. degenerates into asystole after this long period of VF, then the resuscitation efforts should be discontinued. However, if a patient only had a brief period of VF before having asystole, it is prudent to apply active therapy.

Pulseless Electrical Activity

CASE 20-12

QUESTION 1: J.D. is an 80-year-old woman who experiences cardiac arrest in the hospital. A rhythm is noted on the monitor, but no femoral pulse is felt. M.N. is in pulseless electrical activity. How should she be treated?

The clinical situation in which there is organized electrical activity on the monitor without a palpable pulse is called PEA. Although electrical activity is present, it fails to stimulate the contractile process. Virtually all patients in true PEA die. However, not all patients who present with a rhythm and no pulse are in true PEA. Therefore, it is important to rule out treatable causes in patients who appear to be in PEA. The major treatable causes are hypovolemia, hypoxia, acidosis, hyperkalemia, hypokalemia, hypothermia, cardiac tamponade, pulmonary embolism, acute coronary syndrome, trauma, and drug overdose. In the absence of an identifiable cause, the focus of resuscitation is to administer high-quality CPR, and after the initial rhythm check, resume CPR during the establishment of IV or IO access.[194]

Once IV or IO access becomes available, administer epinephrine 1 mg every 3 to 5 minutes or give one dose of vasopressin 40 units in place of the first or second dose of epinephrine, as published studies have failed to demonstrate a survival advantage of either vasopressor for patients experiencing PEA.[194,196,197]

Asystole

CASE 20-13

QUESTION 1: K.K. is a 73-year-old man who experiences cardiac arrest. The ECG shows a flat line, and the patient is determined to be in asystole (Fig. 20-17). Is this rhythm treatable?

Lack of electrical activity or asystole, like PEA, carries a grave prognosis. Its development usually indicates a prolonged arrest, which may explain its poor response to treatment. However, a few patients will go directly from a sinus rhythm into asystole and may be resuscitated. Enhanced parasympathetic tone, possibly attributable to a vagal reaction, manipulation of the airway from intubation, suctioning or insertion of an oral airway, or chest compression, may play a role in inhibiting supraventricular and ventricular pacemakers.[137,194]

As described in K.K. a post hoc analysis performed by Wenzel et al.[194] demonstrated superior survival rates at the time of hospital admission in vasopressin-treated patients, compared with epinephrine-treated patients. However, no difference in intact neurologic survival was noted between the two vasopressor treatment groups. Consequently providers may choose to administer vasopressin 40 units IV (in place of the first or second dose of epinephrine) or epinephrine 1 mg IV every 3 to 5 minutes.

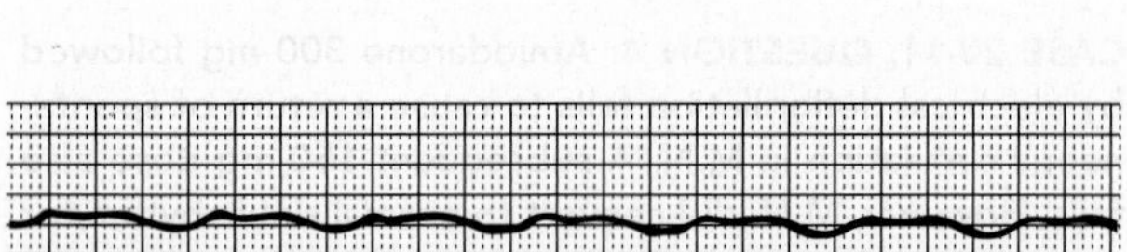

FIGURE 20-17 Asystole.

KEY REFERENCES AND WEBSITES

A full list of references for this chapter can be found at http://thepoint.lww.com/AT10e. Below are the key references and website for this chapter, with the corresponding reference number in this chapter found in parentheses after the reference.

Key References

Connolly SJ et al. Comparison of β-blockers, amiodarone plus β-blockers, or sotalol for prevention of shocks from implantable cardioverter defibrillators: the OPTIC study: a randomized trial. *JAMA*. 2006;295:165. (148)

Drew BJ et al. Prevention of torsade de pointes in hospital settings: a scientific statement from the American Heart Association and the American College of Cardiology Foundation [published correction appears in *Circulation*. 2010;122:e440]. *Circulation*. 2010;121:1047. (161)

Epstein AE et al. ACC/AHA/HRS 2008 Guidelines for Device-Based Therapy of Cardiac Rhythm Abnormalities: a report of the American College of Cardiology/American Heart Association Task Force on Practice Guidelines (Writing Committee to Revise the ACC/AHA/NASPE 2002 Guideline Update for Implantation of Cardiac Pacemakers and Antiarrhythmia Devices): developed in collaboration with the American Association for Thoracic Surgery and Society of Thoracic Surgeons [published correction appears in *Circulation*. 2009;120:e34]. *Circulation*. 2008;117:e350. (147)

Fuster V et al. ACC/AHA/ESC 2006 Guidelines for the Management of Patients with Atrial Fibrillation: a report of the American College of Cardiology/American Heart Association Task Force on Practice Guidelines and the European Society of Cardiology Committee for Practice Guidelines (Writing Committee to Revise the 2001 Guidelines for the Management of Patients With Atrial Fibrillation): developed in collaboration with the European Heart Rhythm Association and the Heart Rhythm Society [published correction appears in *Circulation*. 2007;116:e138]. *Circulation*. 2006;114:e257. (11)

Hazinski MF, ed. *Highlights of the 2010 American Heart Association Guidelines for CPR and ECC*. Dallas, TX: American Heart Association; 2010. (194)

Hohnloser SH et al. Effect of dronedarone on cardiovascular events in atrial fibrillation. *N Engl J Med*. 2009;360:668. (82)

Opolski G et al. Rate control vs. rhythm control in patients with nonvavular persistent atrial fibrillation. The results of the Polish How to Treat Chronic Atrial Fibrillation (HOT CAFÉ) Study. *Chest*. 2004;126:476. (36)

Roy D et al. Rhythm control versus rate control for atrial fibrillation and heart failure. *N Engl J Med*. 2008;358:2667. (38)

Singer DE et al. Antithrombotic therapy in atrial fibrillation: American College of Chest Physicians Evidence-Based Clinical Practice Guidelines (8th Edition). *Chest*. 2008;133(6 Suppl):546S. (42)

Wann LS et al. 2011 ACCF/AHA/HRS focused update on the management of patients with atrial fibrillation (updating the

2006 guideline): a report of the American College of Cardiology Foundation/American Heart Association Task Force on Practice Guidelines. *Heart Rhythm*. 2011;8:157. (32)

Zipes DP et al. ACC/AHA/ESC 2006 guidelines for management of patients with ventricular arrhythmias and the prevention of sudden cardiac death: a report of the American College of Cardiology/American Heart Association Task Force and the European Society of Cardiology Committee for Practice Guidelines (Writing Committee to Develop Guidelines for Management of Patients With Ventricular Arrhythmias and the Prevention of Sudden Cardiac Death). *Circulation*. 2006;114:e385. (118)

Key Websites

Blaufuss Medical Multimedia Laboratories ECG Tutorial. **http://www.blaufuss.org.**

21 Hypertensive Crises

Kristin Watson, Brian Watson, Kelly Summers, and Robert Michocki

CORE PRINCIPLES

		CHAPTER CASES
1	Hypertensive crisis is defined as a diastolic blood pressure greater than 120 mm Hg. This disorder can be further classified as hypertensive urgency or hypertensive emergency when there is evidence of acutely progressive end-organ damage.	**Case 21-1 (Question 1), Table 21-1**
2	Risk factors for the development of a hypertensive crisis include, but are not limited to, medication nonadherence, cocaine use, and drug–drug and drug–food interactions.	**Case 21-1 (Question 1), Case 21-7 (Question 1)**
3	Hypertensive urgency can be treated with oral antihypertensive agents including clonidine, labetalol, or captopril. Caution must be taken to prevent rapid reductions in blood pressure. The use of short-acting calcium-channel blockers are not recommended because of the risk of cardiovascular and cerebrovascular events seen with the use of immediate-release nifedipine.	**Case 21-1 (Question 2)**
4	The organs primarily affected as a result of a hypertensive emergency are the central nervous system, eyes, heart, and kidneys.	**Case 21-2 (Question 1)**
5	Parenteral therapy should be used to manage hypertensive emergencies, and therapeutic options are dictated by the affected organ(s) and other patient comorbidities. Mean arterial pressure should be reduced by no more than 25% initially, then subsequently reduced toward a goal of 160/100 mm Hg, for most patients, during the next 2 to 6 hours. Gradually reduce blood pressure to normal, for most patients, during the next 8 to 24 hours.	**Case 21-2 (Questions 2, 3, 5, 9–11), Case 21-3 (Questions 1, 2, 6), Case 21-4 (Questions 1, 2), Table 21-4**
6	Nitroprusside, a therapeutic option for hypertensive emergencies, has been associated with cyanide and thiocyanate toxicity, and monitoring is required to minimize the risk of these toxicities, especially in patients with renal impairment.	**Case 21-2 (Questions 6–8)**
7	The most commonly used agents for the management of postoperative hypertension are nicardipine, nitroglycerin, nitroprusside, and labetalol.	**Case 21-5 (Questions 1–2)**
8	Management of aortic dissection requires prompt control of blood pressure without increasing the force of cardiac contraction or heart rate.	**Case 21-6 (Question 1)**
9	The preferred treatment options for cocaine-induced hypertensive crisis are nicardipine, verapamil, or nitroglycerin in combination with a benzodiazepine. The use of β-blockers may lead to α-adrenergic vasoconstriction.	**Case 21-7 (Question 1)**

The term *hypertensive crisis* is arbitrarily defined as a severe elevation in blood pressure (BP), generally considered to be a diastolic blood pressure greater than 120 mm Hg.[1] If these disorders are not treated promptly, a high rate of morbidity and mortality will ensue.[2] However, even with effective therapy, the 5-year mortality for patients with a history of hypertensive crisis is 26%.[3] These disorders are divided into two general categories: *hypertensive emergencies* and *hypertensive urgencies* (Table 21-1).[4,5]

The distinction between *emergency* and *urgency* usually depends on the clinical assessment of the life-threatening nature of each episode. The term *hypertensive emergency* describes a clinical situation in which the elevated BP is immediately

TABLE 21-1
Hypertensive Emergencies Versus Urgencies

Emergencies	Urgencies
Severely elevated blood pressure (diastolic >120 mm Hg)[a]	Severely elevated blood pressure (diastolic >120 mm Hg)[a]
Potentially life-threatening	Not acutely life-threatening
End-organ damage acute or progressing	Chronic end-organ damage that is not progressing
CNS (dizziness, N/V, encephalopathy, confusion, weakness, intracranial or subarachnoid hemorrhage, stroke)	Optic disc edema
Eyes (ocular hemorrhage or funduscopic changes, blurred vision, loss of sight)	
Heart (left ventricular failure, pulmonary edema, MI, angina, aortic dissection)	
Renal failure or insufficiency	
Requires immediate pressure reduction	Treated for several hours to days
Requires IV therapy (Table 21-2)	Oral therapy (Table 21-3)

[a] Degree of blood pressure elevation less diagnostic than rate of pressure rise and presence of concurrent diseases or end-organ damage. See Chapter 14, Essential Hypertension, for staging of hypertension.
CNS, central nervous system; IV, intravenous; MI, myocardial infarction; N/V, nausea and vomiting.

life-threatening and needs to be lowered to a safe level (not necessarily to normal) within a matter of minutes to hours.[1,3] Hypertensive emergencies are associated with acutely progressive secondary organ damage (e.g., stroke or myocardial infarction). A *hypertensive urgency* is not immediately life-threatening, and a reduction of BP to a safe level can occur more slowly during 24 to 48 hours.[1,6]

Acute, potentially life-threatening elevations of BP can occur in previously normotensive individuals with acute glomerulonephritis, head injury, or severe burns; during pregnancy (eclampsia); and with use of recreational drugs such as cocaine. Other causes include abrupt medication withdrawal or medication nonadherence, drug–drug interactions (including herbal medications), erythropoietin administration, or drug–food interactions (i.e., patients receiving monoamine oxidase inhibitors who ingest foods rich in tyramine).[7–9] In addition, poor systolic blood pressure control has been identified as an independent risk factor for the development of hypertensive crisis.[10] Effective management of chronic hypertension has lowered the number of patients who present with hypertensive crisis to approximately 1%.[11]

CLINICAL PRESENTATION OF HYPERTENSIVE URGENCY

There are limited data describing the presentation and characteristics of those patients with a hypertensive urgency. In one study evaluating characteristics of patients presenting to the emergency room for hypertensive urgency, the most frequently reported symptoms included headache (42%) and dizziness (30%). Other symptoms include visual changes, chest discomfort, nausea, epistaxis, fatigue, and psychomotor agitation.[12] It should be noted that not all patients presenting with a hypertensive urgency will have symptoms. In this same study, 90% of patients had a history of hypertension, 16% of the patients reported running out of their medications, and 12% reported nonadherence to their antihypertensive regimens.

CLINICAL PRESENTATION OF HYPERTENSIVE EMERGENCY

Similar to hypertensive urgencies, hypertensive emergencies rarely develop in patients without a previous history of hypertension.[13] Most commonly, they complicate the accelerated phase of poorly controlled, chronic hypertension.[1] In several studies of patients with hypertensive emergency, a history of hypertension was previously diagnosed in more than 90% of the patients, suggesting that hypertensive emergencies are almost entirely preventable.[13,14] Hypertensive emergencies also tend to occur in patients with catecholamine-producing adrenal tumors (pheochromocytoma), or renal vascular disease. Additionally, hypertensive emergencies occur more often in African Americans than in Caucasians, among patients who have no primary-care physician, and among those who do not adhere to their treatment regimens.[13,15]

Symptoms associated with hypertensive emergency are highly variable and reflect the degree of damage to specific organ systems. Rapid, severe BP elevation is not always the hallmark of a hypertensive emergency. The primary sites of damage are the central nervous system, heart, kidneys, and eyes. Although hypertensive emergencies are much less common than hypertensive urgencies, without a thorough patient history it is often difficult to know whether end-organ dysfunction is new or has progressed.

In a study on the prevalence of end-organ complications in hypertensive crisis, central nervous system abnormalities were the most frequently reported. Cerebral infarctions were noted in 24%, encephalopathy in 16%, and intracranial or subarachnoid hemorrhage in 4% of patients. Central nervous system abnormalities were followed in incidence by cardiovascular complications, such as acute heart failure (HF) and pulmonary edema, which were seen in 36% of patients, and acute myocardial infarction (MI) and unstable angina, in 12% of patients. Acute dissection was noted in 2%, and eclampsia, in 4.5% of patients.[13]

Central Nervous System

Central nervous system damage can present solely as a severe headache or may be accompanied by dizziness, nausea, vomiting, and anorexia. Mental confusion with apprehension indicates more severe disease, as does nystagmus, localized weakness, or a positive Babinski sign (i.e., upward extension of the great toe and spreading of the smaller toes when moderate pressure is applied along a curve from the sole to the ball of the foot). Central nervous system damage may be rapidly progressive, resulting in coma or death. If a cerebrovascular accident has occurred, slurred speech or motor paralysis may be present.

Other Complications

Cardiac complications of hypertensive emergency include HF, acute pulmonary edema, angina pectoris, and acute coronary syndrome. Myocardial infarction can also be precipitated. Ocular symptoms of hypertensive emergency usually are related to changes in visual acuity. Complaints of blurred vision or loss of eyesight are often associated with funduscopic findings of hemorrhages, exudates (yellow deposits within the retina as a result of leaks from capillaries and microaneurysms), and occasionally papilledema (edema of the optic nerve). Acute kidney injury can also develop. Markers of renal dysfunction include hematuria, proteinuria, and elevated serum blood urea nitrogen (BUN) and serum creatinine levels.

OVERVIEW OF TREATMENT

Oral Versus Parenteral Therapy

Hypertensive urgency is not an indication for parenteral treatment. Oral antihypertensive regimens are more appropriate for the management of these urgent cases. Practitioners should exercise caution in the treatment of patients with elevated blood pressures in the absence of target organ damage. Aggressive dosing with oral medications to rapidly lower BP is not without risk and can lead to hypotension and subsequent morbidity. Some have suggested that the term *hypertensive urgency* leads to overly aggressive treatment and should be discarded in favor of a less ominous term such as *uncontrolled* blood pressure.[6] In contrast, hypertensive emergencies require immediate hospitalization, generally in an intensive care unit, and the administration of parenteral antihypertensive medications to reduce arterial pressure.[16] Effective therapy greatly improves the prognosis, reverses symptoms, and arrests the progression of end-organ damage. Treatment reverses the vascular changes in the eyes and slows or arrests the progressive deterioration in renal function. In those with acute kidney injury, renal function may gradually improve, after 2 to 3 months of adequate therapy, to the baseline renal insufficiency or to a new level, slightly deteriorated from the original baseline renal function. The time required for recovery of renal function ranges from 2 weeks to 2 years. A low serum creatinine level, in the absence of marked cardiomegaly or renal shrinkage, has been associated with a good chance for recovery of renal function.[17] In patients with mild encephalopathy, neurologic symptoms resolve within 24 hours after treatment.[18] Resolution of papilledema occurs in 2 to 3 weeks, whereas funduscopic exudates can require up to 12 weeks for complete resolution.[19] Whether treatment can completely reverse end-organ damage is related to two factors: how soon treatment is initiated and the extent of damage at the initiation of therapy.

There are two fundamental concepts in the management of hypertensive emergencies. First, immediate and intensive therapy is required and takes precedence over time-consuming diagnostic procedures. Second, the choice of drugs will depend on how their time course of action and hemodynamic and metabolic effects meet the needs of the emergent situation. If encephalopathy, acute left ventricular failure, dissecting aortic aneurysm, eclampsia, or other serious conditions are present, the BP should be lowered promptly with rapid-acting, parenteral antihypertensive medications such as clevidipine, esmolol, enalaprilat, fenoldopam, hydralazine, labetalol, nicardipine, nitroglycerin, or nitroprusside (Table 21-2).[1,3,4,20–24] If a slower BP reduction over the course of several hours or days is acceptable, as in the case of a hypertensive urgency, rapid-acting oral therapy using captopril, clonidine, labetalol, or minoxidil may be used (Table 21-3).[3,4,24–26] Figure 21-1 provides an overview of the management of a hypertensive crisis. A summary of treatment recommendations for acutely lowering BP for selected indications is listed in Table 21-4 on page 526.

Goals of Therapy

The rate of BP lowering must be individualized depending on whether the patient presents with a hypertensive urgency or emergency. Also, ischemic damage to the heart and brain can be provoked by a precipitous fall in BP.[26–30] As treatment is initiated, clinicians should recognize that the elderly and patients with severely defective autoregulatory mechanisms are at high risk for developing hypotensive complications. The latter group includes those with autonomic dysfunction or fixed sclerotic stenosis of cerebral or neck arteries.[31] In addition, patients who have chronically elevated BP are less likely to tolerate abrupt reductions in their BP, and the amount of reduction appropriate for those patients is somewhat less than for those whose BP is acutely elevated.

For hypertensive emergencies, it is recommended that the mean arterial pressure be reduced initially by no more than 25% (within minutes to 1 hour); then if stable, this should be followed by further reduction toward a goal of 160/100 mm Hg within 2 to 6 hours and gradual reduction to normal during the next 8 to 24 hours.[4] A diastolic pressure of 100 to 110 mm Hg is an appropriate initial therapeutic goal.[1] Lower pressures may be indicated for patients with aortic dissection. Another exception to this rule applies in patients with acute cerebrovascular accidents. Cerebral autoregulation is disrupted in this setting, and the use of antihypertensives may cause a reduction in cerebral blood flow and increasing morbidity.[32] Current guidelines recommend lowering BP after acute ischemic stroke if the systolic blood pressure (SBP) is greater than 220 mm Hg or the diastolic blood pressure (DBP) is greater than 120 mm Hg in patients ineligible for thrombolytic therapy, or if the SBP is greater than 185 mm Hg or DBP is greater than 110 mm Hg in those who are candidates for thrombolytics.[33] A lower BP in patients undergoing thrombolytic therapy reduces the risk of intracerebral bleeding. In the setting of an ischemic stroke, it is recommended to lower the BP by 15% to 25% within the first day.[33] Additionally, in those with hypertensive encephalopathy, cerebral hypoperfusion may occur if the mean BP is reduced by more than 40%.[34] Thus, in the presence of hypertensive encephalopathy it is suggested that within the first hour of treatment the mean pressure be lowered by no more than 20% or to a diastolic BP of 100 mm Hg, whichever is greater.[34,35]

HYPERTENSIVE URGENCIES

Patient Assessment

CASE 21-1

QUESTION 1: M.M. is a 60-year-old African American man with a long history of HF, poorly controlled hypertension believed to be caused by nonadherence, and a history of MI. He was referred from a community health center this morning for a thorough evaluation of his elevated BP. He has not taken his captopril, carvedilol, or hydrochlorothiazide for the past 7 days. M.M. is completely asymptomatic. Physical examination reveals a BP of 180/120 mm Hg and a pulse of 92 beats/minute. Funduscopic examination is pertinent for mild arteriolar narrowing, without hemorrhages or exudates. The discs are flat. His lungs are clear, and the cardiac examination is unremarkable. The electrocardiogram indicates normal sinus rhythm at a rate of 90 beats/minute with first-degree atrioventricular block. The chest radiograph is interpreted as mild cardiomegaly. Serum electrolytes, BUN, and serum creatinine are within normal limits. A urinalysis is significant for 2+ proteinuria. What is the therapeutic objective in treating M.M.? How quickly should his BP be lowered, and what therapeutic options are available?

TABLE 21-2

Parenteral Drugs Commonly Used in the Treatment of Hypertensive Emergencies

Drug (Brand Name)	Class of Drug	Dose/Route	Onset of Action	Duration of Action
Clevidipine (Cleviprex) 0.5 mg/mL	Arterial vasodilator (calcium-channel blocker)	Initial: 1–2 mg/h; titrate dose to desired BP or to a max of 16 mg/h	2–4 minutes	10–15 minutes after D/C
Enalaprilat[a] (Vasotec IV) 1.25 mg/mL, 2.5 mg/2 mL	ACE inhibitor	0.625–1.25 mg IV every 6 hours	15 minutes (max, 1–4 hours)	6–12 hours
Esmolol[b] (Brevibloc) 100 mg/10 mL, 2,500 mg/10 mL concentrate	β-adrenergic blocker	250–500 mcg/kg for 1 minute, then 50–300 mcg/kg/min	1–2 minutes	10–20 minutes
Fenoldopam (Corlopam) 10 mg/mL, 20 mg/2 mL, 50 mg/5 mL	Dopamine-1 agonist	0.1–0.3 mcg/kg/min	<5 minutes	30 minutes
Hydralazine[c] (generic) 20 mg/mL	Arterial vasodilator	10–20 mg IV	5–20 minutes	2–6 hours
Labetalol[d] (Normodyne) 20 mg/4 mL, 40 mg/8 mL, 100 mg/20 mL, 200 mg/20 mL	α- and β-adrenergic blocker	2 mg/min IV or 20–80 mg every 10 minutes up to 300 mg total dose	2–5 minutes	3–6 hours
Nicardipine[e] (Cardene IV) 25 mg/10 mL	Arterial vasodilator (calcium-channel blocker)	IV loading dose 5 mg/h increased by 2.5 mg/h every 5 minutes to desired BP or a max of 15 mg/h every 15 minutes, followed by maintenance infusion of 3 mg/h	2–10 minutes (max, 8–12 hours)	40–60 minutes after D/C infusion
Nitroglycerin[f] (Tridil, Nitro-Bid IV, Nitro-Stat IV) 5 mg/mL, 5 mg/10 mL, 25 mg/5 mL, 50 mg/10 mL, 100 mg/20 mL	Arterial and venous vasodilator	IV infusion pump 5–100 mcg/min	2–5 minutes	5–10 minutes after D/C infusion
Nitroprusside[g] (Nitropress), 50 mg/2 mL (most commonly used)	Arterial and venous vasodilator	IV infusion.[a] Start: 0.5 mcg/kg/min Usual: 2–5 mcg/kg/min Max: 8 mcg/kg/min	Seconds	3–5 minutes after D/C infusion
Phentolamine (Regitine)	α-adrenergic blocker	1–5 mg IV initially, repeat as needed	Immediate	10–15 minutes

Major Side Effects (All Can Cause Hypotension)	Avoid or Use Cautiously in Patients With These Conditions
Atrial fibrillation, nausea, vomiting, headache, acute renal failure, reflex tachycardia, MI	Allergy to soybeans, soy products, eggs or egg products, severe aortic stenosis, defective lipid metabolism, heart failure
Hyperkalemia	Hyperkalemia, renal failure in patients with dehydration or bilateral renal artery stenosis, pregnancy (teratogenic)
Nausea, thrombophlebitis, painful extravasation	Asthma, bradycardia, decompensated HF, advanced heart block
Tachycardia, headache, nausea, flushing	Glaucoma
Tachycardia, headache, angina	Angina pectoris, MI, aortic dissection
Abdominal pain, nausea, vomiting, diarrhea	Asthma, bradycardia, decompensated HF
Headache, flushing, nausea, vomiting, dizziness, tachycardia; local thrombophlebitis change infusion site after 12 hours	Angina pectoris, decompensated HF, increased intracranial pressure
Methemoglobinemia, headache, tachycardia, nausea, vomiting, flushing, tolerance with prolonged use	Pericardial tamponade, constrictive pericarditis, or increased intracranial pressure
Nausea, vomiting, diaphoresis, weakness, thiocyanate toxicity,[h] cyanide toxicity (rare)[i]	Renal failure (thiocyanate accumulation), pregnancy, increased intracranial pressure
Chest pain, nausea, vomiting, dizziness, headache, nasal congestion, arrhythmia	Angina pectoris, coronary insufficiency, MI or history of MI, hypersensitivity to mannitol

[a] Not approved by the U.S. Food and Drug Administration for treatment of acute hypertension.

[b] Approved for intraoperative and postoperative treatment of hypertension.

[c] Parenteral hydralazine is an intermediate treatment between oral agents and more aggressive therapies such as nitroprusside. It can be given IV or intramuscularly, but there is no appreciable difference in onset of action (20–40 minutes) between the two routes. This slow onset minimizes hypotension.

[d] Labetalol is contraindicated in acute decompensated heart failure because of its β-blocking properties. A solution for continuous infusion is prepared by adding two 100-mg ampules to 160 mL of IV fluid to give a final concentration of 1 mg/mL. Infusions start at 2 mg/min and are titrated until a satisfactory response or a cumulative dose of 300 mg is achieved.

[e] Indicated for short-term treatment of hypertension when the oral route is not feasible or desirable.

[f] Requires special delivery system owing to drug binding to polyvinyl chloride tubing. Also see Chapters 17, Chronic Stable Angina, and 18, Acute Coronary Syndromes, for further information regarding nitroglycerin.

[g] Nitroprusside is the drug of choice for acute hypertensive emergencies. It is supplied as 50 mg of lyophilized powder that is reconstituted with 2–3 mL of 5% dextrose in water (D_5W), yielding a red-brown solution. The contents of the vial are added to 250, 500, or 1,000 mL of D_5W to produce a solution for IV administration at a concentration of 200, 100, or 50 mcg/mL, respectively. The container should be wrapped with metal foil to prevent light-induced decompensation. Under these conditions, the solution is stable for 4 to 24 hours. A rising BP may indicate loss of potency. A change in color to yellow does not indicate effectiveness. The appearance of a dark brown, green, or blue color indicates loss in activity. The drug is more effective if the head of the bed is slightly raised. When changing to a new bag, the administration rate may require adjustment.

[h] Thiocyanate levels rise gradually in proportion to the dose and duration of administration. The half-life of thiocyanate is 2.7 days with normal renal function and 9 days in patients with renal failure. Toxicity occurs after 7 to 14 days in patients with normal renal function and 3 to 6 days in renal failure patients. Thiocyanate serum levels should be measured after 3 to 4 days of therapy, and the drug should be discontinued if levels exceed 10 to 12 mg/dL. Thiocyanate toxicity causes a neurotoxic syndrome of toxic psychosis, hyperreflexia, confusion, weakness, tinnitus, seizures, and coma.

[i] Signs of cyanide toxicity include lactic acidosis, hypoxemia, tachycardia, altered consciousness, seizures, and the smell of almonds on the breath. Concurrent administration of sodium thiosulfate or hydroxocobalamin may reduce the risk of cyanide toxicity in high-risk patients.

ACE, angiotensin-converting enzyme; BP, blood pressure; D/C, discontinued; HF, heart failure; IV, intravenous; MI, myocardial infarction.

TABLE 21-3
Oral Drugs Commonly Used in the Treatment of Hypertensive Urgencies

Drug[a] (Brand Name)	Dose/Route	Onset of Action	Duration of Action	Major Side Effects[a]	Mechanism of Action	Avoid or Use Cautiously in Patients With These Conditions
Captopril[b] (Capoten) 12.5-, 25-, 50-, 100-mg tablets	6.5–50 mg PO	15 minutes	4–6 hours	Hyperkalemia, angioedema, increased BUN if dehydrated, rash, pruritus, proteinuria, loss of taste	ACE inhibitor	Renal artery stenosis, hyperkalemia, dehydration, renal failure, pregnancy
Clonidine (Catapres) 0.1-, 0.2-, 0.3-mg tablets	0.1–0.2 mg PO initially, then 0.1 mg/h up to 0.8 mg total	0.5–2 hours	6–8 hours	Sedation, dry mouth, constipation	Central α_2-agonist	Altered mental status, severe carotid artery stenosis
Labetalol (Normodyne, Trandate) 100-, 200-, 300-mg tablets	200–400 mg PO repeated every 2–3 hours	30 minutes–2 hours	4 hours	Orthostatic hypotension, nausea, vomiting	α- and β-adrenergic blocker	Heart failure, asthma, bradycardia
Minoxidil (Loniten) 2.5-, 10-mg tablets	5–20 mg PO	30–60 minutes; maximum response in 2–4 hours	12–16 hours	Tachycardia, fluid retention	Arterial and venous vasodilator	Angina, heart failure

[a] All may cause hypotension, dizziness, and flushing.
[b] Other oral ACE inhibitors too slow in onset to be useful but should be used for maintenance therapy to improve adherence as captopril requires multiple daily doses
ACE, angiotensin-converting enzyme; BUN, blood urea nitrogen; PO, orally.

M.M. has stage 2 hypertension with a BP of 180/120 mm Hg.[4] However, the absolute magnitude of BP elevation does not in itself constitute a medical emergency requiring an acute reduction in BP. There is no evidence of encephalopathy, cardiac decompensation, chest pain, or rapid change in renal function. Therefore, no evidence exists to indicate a rapid deterioration in the function of target organs. One would classify M.M.'s case as a hypertensive urgency.

As is often the case, M.M.'s lack of BP control is related to medication nonadherence. M.M.'s clinical presentation requires that his BP be lowered during the next 12 to 24 to 48 hours while being careful not to induce hypotension. Rapid-acting oral agents can be used for this purpose; parenteral therapy is not warranted. A number of different oral regimens using clonidine, captopril, labetalol, or minoxidil are available. In M.M., restarting his medications in a controlled manner so as not to drop his BP too rapidly may also be a reasonable option for treatment. Later, he can be converted to a regimen designed to enhance adherence by selecting medications with once-daily dosing. For example, lisinopril or another long-acting angiotensin-converting enzyme (ACE) inhibitor would be preferred for maintenance instead of the captopril previously prescribed. Comprehensive patient counseling will help M.M. better understand the severity of his disease and the need to take his medications. One should also determine and address barriers to medication adherence with the patient including cost of therapy, lack of understanding of the benefits of therapy, misconceptions of the side effect profiles, and so forth. Timely follow-up within 1 week after treatment of hypertensive urgency is of paramount importance for the appropriate management of these patients.

Oral Drug Therapy

RAPIDLY ACTING CALCIUM-CHANNEL BLOCKERS

CASE 21-1, QUESTION 2: M.M.'s physician has ordered immediate-release nifedipine to be given 10 mg sublingually. Is this appropriate therapy to treat his hypertensive urgency?

Clonidine, labetalol, minoxidil, and captopril have all been used to lower BP acutely. These oral agents take several hours to adequately lower pressure and are therefore useful in treating hypertensive urgencies but not emergencies. Oral ACE inhibitors, other than captopril, are not useful for acutely lowering BP because their onset of action is too slow. The immediate-release calcium-channel blockers, including diltiazem, verapamil, and nicardipine, can rapidly lower BP; however, the most extensive experience is with nifedipine. Nifedipine, when given orally or by the "bite and swallow" method, was previously recommended as a rapid-acting alternative to parenteral therapy in the acute management of hypertension. However, its use has been associated with life-threatening adverse events related to ischemia, MI, and stroke.[26–30] The prompt absorption of rapidly acting dihydropyridine calcium-channel blockers is followed by a sudden and precipitous decrease in BP as a result of peripheral vasodilation. This reduces coronary perfusion, induces a reflex tachycardia, and increases myocardial oxygen consumption.[28,36] Decreased cerebral blood flow with sublingual nifedipine has also been reported.[37] Elderly patients with underlying coronary or cerebrovascular disease, volume depletion, or concurrent use of other antihypertensive drugs are at increased risk for significant adverse events. In addition, no outcome data are currently available to critically assess the efficacy of this therapeutic intervention. Therefore, until more data become available, administration of immediate-release nifedipine capsules or other rapidly acting calcium-channel blockers sublingually, by the "bite and chew" method, or by swallowing intact is not recommended.

The cavalier use of immediate-release nifedipine to acutely lower BP is potentially dangerous and should be discouraged in M.M. M.M.'s BP can be managed safely using other oral medications. Captopril, labetalol, or clonidine can be used to lower his BP, and he can be restarted on his oral maintenance regimen with appropriate follow-up care.

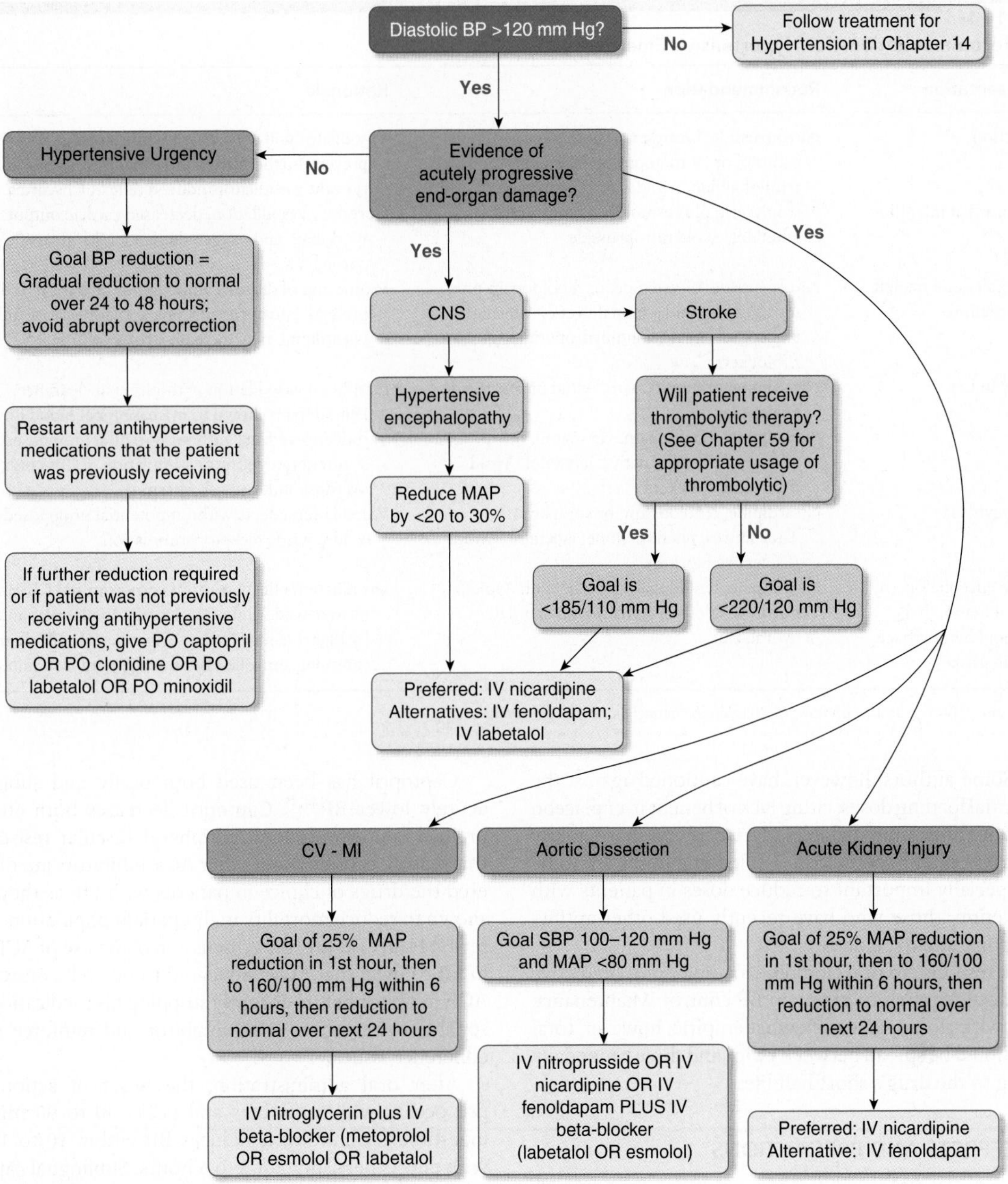
Diastolic BP >120 mm Hg?
No
Follow treatment for Hypertension in Chapter 14
Yes
Evidence of acutely progressive end-organ damage?
No
Hypertensive Urgency
Goal BP reduction = Gradual reduction to normal over 24 to 48 hours; avoid abrupt overcorrection
Restart any antihypertensive medications that the patient was previously receiving
If further reduction required or if patient was not previously receiving antihypertensive medications, give PO captopril OR PO clonidine OR PO labetalol OR PO minoxidil
Yes
CNS
Stroke
Hypertensive encephalopathy
Reduce MAP by <20 to 30%
Will patient receive thrombolytic therapy? (See Chapter 59 for appropriate usage of thrombolytic)
Yes
No
Goal is <185/110 mm Hg
Goal is <220/120 mm Hg
Preferred: IV nicardipine
Alternatives: IV fenoldapam; IV labetalol
Yes
CV - MI
Aortic Dissection
Acute Kidney Injury
Goal of 25% MAP reduction in 1st hour, then to 160/100 mm Hg within 6 hours, then reduction to normal over next 24 hours
IV nitroglycerin plus IV beta-blocker (metoprolol OR esmolol OR labetalol
Goal SBP 100–120 mm Hg and MAP <80 mm Hg
IV nitroprusside OR IV nicardipine OR IV fenoldapam PLUS IV beta-blocker (labetalol OR esmolol)
Goal of 25% MAP reduction in 1st hour, then to 160/100 mm Hg within 6 hours, then reduction to normal over next 24 hours
Preferred: IV nicardipine
Alternative: IV fenoldapam

FIGURE 21-1 Overview of management for a hypertensive crisis. BP, blood pressure; CNS, central nervous system; IV, intravenous; MAP, mean arterial pressure; MI, myocardial infarction; SBP, systolic blood pressure.

For an audio walk-through of this algorithm, go to http://thepoint.lww.com/AT10e.

CLONIDINE

CASE 21-1, QUESTION 3: A decision is made not to use nifedipine, but rather to give M.M. oral clonidine. What is an appropriate starting and maintenance dose?

Clonidine is considered a safe, effective first-line therapy for hypertensive urgency. It is a centrally acting, α_2-adrenergic agonist that inhibits sympathetic outflow from the central nervous system. After acute administration, clonidine reduces mean arterial pressure, cardiac output, stroke volume, and cardiac rate. There is little change in the total peripheral resistance or renal plasma flow. The initial reduction in cardiac output is caused by decreased venous return to the right side of the heart secondary to venodilation and bradycardia, not secondary to decreased contractility. Guanabenz has a similar mechanism of action, but documented efficacy in the treatment of hypertensive urgency is lacking.

BP can be lowered gradually over the course of several hours using oral clonidine. Traditional dosing regimens have included an initial oral loading dose (0.1–0.2 mg) followed by repeated doses of 0.1 mg/hour until the desired response is achieved or until a cumulative dose of 0.5 to 0.8 mg is reached.[38] A significant reduction in BP is first seen within 1 hour, and the mean arterial pressure decreases by 25% in most patients after several hours. Anderson et al. reported a 94% response rate to an oral loading dose.[38] Patients required a mean total dose of 0.45 mg, and the maximum response occurred 5 to 6 hours after the start

TABLE 21-4
Treatment Recommendations for Hypertensive Emergency

Clinical Presentation	Recommendation	Rationale
Aortic dissection	Nitroprusside, nicardipine, or fenoldopam plus esmolol or IV metoprolol; labetalol; trimethaphan. Avoid inotropic therapy.	Vasodilator will decrease pulsatile stress in aortic vessel to prevent further dissection expansion. β-blockers will prevent vasodilator-induced reflex tachycardia.
Angina, myocardial infarction	Nitroglycerin plus esmolol or metoprolol; labetalol. Avoid nitroprusside.	Coronary vasodilation, decreased cardiac output, myocardial workload, and oxygen demand. Nitroprusside may cause coronary steal.
Acute pulmonary edema, left ventricular failure	Nitroprusside, nicardipine, or fenoldopam plus nitroglycerin and a loop diuretic. Alternative: enalaprilat. Avoid nondihydropyridines, β-blockers.	Promotion of diuresis with venous dilatation to decrease preload. Nitroprusside, enalaprilat decrease afterload. Nicardipine may increase stroke volume.
Acute kidney injury	Nicardipine or fenoldopam. Avoid nitroprusside, enalaprilat.	Peripheral vasodilation without renal clearance. Fenoldopam shown to increase renal blood flow.
Cocaine overdose	Nicardipine, fenoldopam, verapamil, or nitroglycerin. Alternative: labetalol. Avoid β-selective blockers.	Vasodilation effects without potential unopposed α-adrenergic receptor stimulation. CCBs control overdose-induced vasospasm.
Pheochromocytoma	Nicardipine, fenoldopam, or verapamil. Alternatives: phentolamine, labetalol. Avoid β-selective blockers.	Vasodilation effects without potential unopposed α-adrenergic receptor stimulation.
Hypertensive encephalopathy, intracranial hemorrhage, subarachnoid hemorrhage, thrombotic stroke	Nicardipine, fenoldopam, or labetalol. Avoid nitroprusside, nitroglycerin, enalaprilat, hydralazine.	Vasodilation effects without compromised CBF induced by nitroprusside and nitroglycerin. Enalaprilat and hydralazine may lead to unpredictable BP changes when carefully controlled BP management is required.

BP, blood pressure; CBF, cerebral blood flow; CCB, calcium-channel blocker; IV, intravenous.

of therapy. Some authors, however, have cautioned against the use of sequential loading doses, citing lack of benefit over placebo and the potential for unpredictable adverse effects, particularly abrupt occurrences of hypotension.[39] If loading doses are to be used, it is especially important to reduce doses in patients with volume depletion, those who have recently used other antihypertensive drugs, and the elderly.[1,23,40]

The acute response to oral clonidine loading is not predictive of the daily dose required to maintain BP control. Maintenance oral therapy with clonidine is somewhat empiric; however, total daily doses should be spread between twice and three times daily dosing owing to the drug's short half-life.

ADVERSE EFFECTS AND PRECAUTIONS

CASE 21-1, QUESTION 4: What are the adverse effects and precautions that should be considered before recommending the use of clonidine?

Oral clonidine is generally well tolerated. Adverse effects include orthostatic hypotension, bradycardia, sedation, dry mouth, and dizziness. Clonidine can decrease cerebral blood flow by up to 28%; it should not be used in patients with severe cerebrovascular disease.[41] Clonidine also should be avoided in patients with HF, bradycardia, sick sinus syndrome, or cardiac conduction defects,[23] as well as patients at risk for medication nonadherence because of the rebound hypertension.[42,43]

OTHER ORAL DRUGS

CAPTOPRIL

CASE 21-1, QUESTION 5: M.M. has a history of HF and normal renal function. Based on these findings, would captopril be a reasonable choice for initial treatment? How should it be given? What if his BUN or serum creatinine were elevated?

Captopril has been used both orally and sublingually to acutely lower BP.[44,45] Captopril decreases both afterload and preload, and lowers total peripheral vascular resistance.[23] For this reason, captopril and other ACE inhibitors are often considered the drugs of choice in patients with HF as they have been shown to reduce mortality in this patient population. (See Chapter 19, Heart Failure, for a discussion of the use of ACE inhibitors in HF.) Given that M.M. appeared to be well controlled on his ACE inhibitor before abruptly stopping his medications, it is reasonable to restart an ACE inhibitor and reinforce medication adherence issues.

After oral administration, the onset of action of captopril occurs within minutes and peaks 30 to 90 minutes after ingestion.[46] Clinically, it reduces BP within 10 to 15 minutes, with effects persisting for 2 to 6 hours. Sublingual captopril is as effective as nifedipine but without reflex tachycardia in acutely reducing mean arterial pressure in both urgent and emergent conditions.[45–48]

Despite these beneficial effects, captopril, as well as all other ACE inhibitors, must be used with caution in patients with renal insufficiency or volume depletion. In most cases, an elevated BUN or serum creatinine will provide a clue to the existence of these conditions; however, captopril can also induce severe renal failure in patients with bilateral renal artery stenosis or renal artery stenosis in a solitary kidney. Such conditions may not be easy to detect in the context of an acute hypertensive emergency. Therefore, in patients in whom these conditions can be excluded, captopril can be considered for therapy. First-dose hypotension is a common limiting factor with captopril use. This complication is most likely to occur in the elderly and in patients with high renin levels such as those who are volume depleted or those receiving diuretics. Under these circumstances, initial doses should not exceed 12.5 mg, with repeat doses an hour or more later if necessary. Although he was not taking his diuretic, M.M. is still likely to have high renin levels as a result of his history of HF. Therefore, captopril would be a reasonable choice as initial therapy in M.M., which can later be replaced by a longer-acting ACE inhibitor.

CASE 21-1, QUESTION 6: What other oral agents are used in the treatment of hypertensive urgency?

Minoxidil, a potent oral vasodilator, has been used successfully in the treatment of hypertensive urgencies.[49,50] An oral loading dose of 10 to 20 mg produces a maximal BP response in 2 to 4 hours and can be followed by a dose of 5 to 20 mg every 4 hours if necessary. Unfortunately, its onset of action is slower than that of clonidine or captopril. Another complicating factor is that β-blockers and loop diuretics generally must be used concomitantly to counteract minoxidil-induced reflex tachycardia and fluid retention.[50] Because of this, minoxidil should only be prescribed by those who have experience with prescribing this agent and managing these adverse effects. These adverse effects make this agent a less than ideal choice in M.M. because of his history of HF. Minoxidil should be used only in patients presenting with hypertensive urgency who are not responding to other antihypertensive therapies or who have previously been taking this agent.

Oral labetalol, a combined α- and β-receptor antagonist, is an alternative to oral clonidine or captopril for the treatment of severe hypertension, but the most appropriate dosing regimen remains to be determined.[51–54] Initial doses of 100 to 300 mg may provide a sustained response for up to 4 hours.[52] Labetalol (200 mg given at hourly intervals to a maximum dose of 1,200 mg) was comparable to oral clonidine in reducing mean arterial pressure.[54] An alternative regimen using 300 mg initially followed by 100 mg at 2-hour intervals to a maximum of 500 mg was also successful in acutely lowering BP.[53] However, Wright et al.[55] were unable to achieve an adequate BP response in a small series of patients using a single loading dose of 200 to 400 mg. Because labetalol can cause profound orthostatic hypotension, patients should remain in the supine position and should be checked for orthostasis before ambulation. In addition, labetalol should be avoided in patients with asthma, bradycardia, or advanced heart block.

HYPERTENSIVE EMERGENCIES

Patient Assessment

CASE 21-2

QUESTION 1: M.R., a 55-year-old African American man, presents to the emergency department with a 3-day history of progressively increasing shortness of breath. During the past 2 days, he experienced a severe headache unrelieved by ibuprofen, as well as substernal chest pain, anorexia, and nausea. His medical history includes asthma and a 5-year history of angina, which resulted in hospitalization for an acute inferior MI 2 months before admission. He has been taking albuterol via metered-dose inhaler, furosemide, isosorbide dinitrate, felodipine, and lisinopril, but discontinued these medications on his own 3 weeks ago.

Physical examination reveals an anxious-appearing man who is alert, oriented, and in moderate respiratory distress. His vital signs include a pulse of 125 beats/minute, respiratory rate of 36 breaths/minute, BP of 220/145 mm Hg without orthostasis, and a normal body temperature. Funduscopic examination shows arteriolar narrowing and arteriovenous nicking without hemorrhages, exudates, or papilledema. There is no jugular venous distention, but bilateral carotid bruits are present. Chest examination reveals decreased breath sounds with bilateral rales extending to the tip of the scapula. M.R.'s heart is displaced 2 cm to the left of the midclavicular line with no thrills or heaves. The rhythm is regular with an S_3 and an S_4 gallop; no murmurs are noted. The remainder of M.R.'s examination is within normal limits.

Significant laboratory values include the following:

Sodium, 142 mEq/L
Potassium, 4.9 mEq/L
Chloride, 101 mEq/L
Bicarbonate, 23 mEq/L
BUN, 30 mg/dL
Serum creatinine, 1.2 mg/dL
Hematocrit, 38%
Hemoglobin, 13 g/dL
White blood cell count and differential, within normal limits

Urinalysis shows 1+ hemoglobin and 1+ protein. Microscopic examination of the urine reveals 5 to 10 red blood cells per high-power field and no casts. Pulse oximetry reveals an oxygen saturation of 88%. An electrocardiogram demonstrates sinus tachycardia and left ventricular hypertrophy. The chest radiograph shows moderate cardiomegaly and bilateral fluffy infiltrates.

What aspects of M.R.'s history and physical examination are characteristic of an emergent need to immediately lower his BP?

As discussed previously, hypertensive crisis occurs most often in African American men and individuals between the ages of 40 and 60. Furthermore, many patients who present with hypertensive crisis have a recent history of discontinuing the use of their antihypertensives,[13,15] as is the case with M.R. and M.M. in Case 21-1.

Recent-onset severe headache, nausea, and vomiting are consistent with central nervous system signs of severe hypertension, as are the acute onset of angina (substernal pain) and acute HF (shortness of breath, increased pulse and respiratory rate, cardiomegaly, S_3, and chest radiographic findings of pulmonary edema). The absence of signs of right-sided HF such as jugular venous distention or hepatomegaly suggests an acute onset of HF caused by hypertension as opposed to a gradual worsening of chronic HF. M.R.'s urinary sediment is relatively unimpressive at this time, especially in light of his history, and his ocular complications are minimal. M.R.'s presentation is considered hypertensive emergency because of the presence of HF symptoms; M.R. should be admitted to the hospital as intravenous (IV) antihypertensive therapy is warranted.

Parenteral Drug Therapy

NITROPRUSSIDE

CASE 21-2, QUESTION 2: M.R. is to be started on nitroprusside. Is this an appropriate choice of drug? What alternatives to nitroprusside are available?

M.R.'s arterial pressure should be lowered with parenteral medications, which have a rapid onset of action. Nitroprusside, fenoldopam, and IV nitroglycerin all decrease total peripheral resistance rapidly with minimal effect on myocardial oxygen consumption and heart rate. Of these agents, either nitroprusside or fenoldopam would be preferred in patients with hypertension accompanied by decompensated HF in the absence of MI. Parenteral nitroglycerin is similar to nitroprusside except that it has a relatively greater effect on the venous circulation and less effect on arterioles. It is most useful in patients with coronary insufficiency, ischemic heart disease, MI, or hypertension after coronary bypass surgery (also see Case 21-3, Question 6). In addition, nitroprusside and IV nitroglycerin may both decrease elevated left ventricular diastolic pressures in patients presenting with hypertensive emergency. Fenoldopam and nitroprusside are equally efficacious in acutely lowering BP.[56–59] Both drugs have an immediate onset, are easily titratable, have a short duration of action, and are relatively well tolerated. Fenoldopam may also increase renal blood flow, thereby reducing the risk for worsening renal function.[60–63] Unlike nitroprusside, fenoldopam does not cause cyanide or thiocyanate toxicity, but it is considerably more expensive than nitroprusside.

Therefore, in the absence of any significant renal or liver disease, nitroprusside is the preferred treatment for M.R.

HEMODYNAMIC EFFECTS

Nitroprusside has many pharmacologic effects that should improve M.R.'s condition. It dilates both venous and arterial vessels, thereby increasing venous capacitance and decreasing the venous return or preload on the heart (see Chapter 19, Heart Failure). A decrease in the pulmonary capillary wedge pressure and ventricular filling pressure will ultimately improve M.R.'s pulmonary edema. Afterload is also decreased as a result of arterial dilation. This action increases cardiac output, reduces arterial pressure, and increases tissue perfusion.

CONCURRENT USE OF DIURETICS

CASE 21-2, QUESTION 3: Should M.R. be given a diuretic before nitroprusside therapy is begun?

Administration of potent IV diuretics is relatively ineffective in the acute treatment of hypertensive crisis except in patients with concomitant volume overload or HF. Many patients with hypertensive emergencies are vasoconstricted and have normal or reduced plasma volumes; therefore, diuretics have little effect and may actually aggravate renal impairment or cause other adverse effects.[22,64] Furthermore, when diuretics are given acutely in combination with other antihypertensive agents, profound hypotension can occur.

The immediate value of diuretics in acute HF is related more to their hemodynamic effects (venodilation) than to diuresis. Venodilation after IV diuretic administration decreases right-sided cardiac filling pressures, decreases pulmonary artery and wedge pressures, and increases cardiac output before diuresis occurs.[65] The presence of HF and severely elevated BP in M.R. warrants the IV administration of a loop diuretic (e.g., furosemide 20 to 40 mg, torsemide [Demadex] 10 mg, or bumetanide [Bumex] 1 mg).

DOSING AND ADMINISTRATION

CASE 21-2, QUESTION 4: How should nitroprusside be prepared and administered? What dose should be used initially?

Because of its extreme potency, sodium nitroprusside must be prepared in exact concentrations and BP must be closely monitored. Sodium nitroprusside is supplied in units of 50 mg of lyophilized powder. The powder is reconstituted with 2 to 3 mL of 5% dextrose in water (D_5W) or sterile water for injection, shaking gently to dissolve.[66] The contents of the vial are then added to 250, 500, or 1,000 mL of D_5W to produce a solution for IV administration with a drug concentration containing 200, 100, or 50 mcg/mL. This solution should have a slight brownish tint.

Nitroprusside decomposes on exposure to light, so the solution should be shielded with an opaque sleeve. It is not necessary to protect the tubing from light. Reconstituted solutions are stable for 24 hours at room temperature. A change in the solution's color from light brown to dark brown, green, orange, or blue indicates a loss in activity, and the solution should be discarded.

Effective infusion rates range from 0.25 to 10 mcg/kg/minute.[67] For M.R., an infusion of nitroprusside should be initiated at a rate of 0.25 mcg/kg/minute. The dose should be increased slowly by 0.25 mcg/kg/minute every 5 minutes until the desired pressure is achieved. A maximum infusion rate of 10 mcg/kg/minute has been recommended. If adequate BP reduction is not achieved within 10 minutes after maximal dose infusion, nitroprusside should be discontinued.[4] The dosage must be individualized according to patient response using continuous intra-arterial BP recording and observing for signs or symptoms of toxicity.

THERAPEUTIC END POINT

CASE 21-2, QUESTION 5: A nitroprusside infusion of 0.25 mcg/kg/minute is started. What is the goal of therapy?

For most patients BP should be reduced by no more than 25% within the first minutes to hour, then if stable, therapy can be titrated to achieve a goal BP of 160/100 mm Hg during the next 2 to 6 hours. Blood pressures can be reduced to near-normal levels within 8 to 24 hours. However, because M.R. has cerebral occlusive disease (carotid bruits), excessive reduction of his BP should be avoided. Overly aggressive reduction of BP in the presence of major cerebral vessel stenosis may decrease cerebral blood flow and produce strokes or other neurologic complications.

Normal cerebral blood flow remains relatively constant over a wide range of systemic BP measurements through autoregulatory mechanisms.[40,68] The autoregulatory effects can prevent large alterations in cerebral blood flow from either slow or rapid changes in systemic arterial pressures. In addition, the arterial BP required to maintain cerebral perfusion is higher in hypertensive patients than in normotensive individuals. If M.R.'s BP is reduced excessively, cerebral blood flow may decrease sharply. Therefore, a diastolic BP of 100 to 105 mm Hg would be a reasonable initial therapeutic goal for him in the first 6 hours. If hypotension occurs, nitroprusside should be discontinued and M.R. should be placed in the Trendelenburg position, in which the head is kept lower than the trunk.

CYANIDE TOXICITY

CASE 21-2, QUESTION 6: M.R. is being treated with nitroprusside. However, during the last 36 hours, dose titration to 7 mcg/kg/minute has been necessary to control his BP. Is he at risk for developing cyanide toxicity? What indices of toxicity should be monitored? Are there agents available to prevent toxicity?

A major concern when using sodium nitroprusside is toxicity secondary to the accumulation of its metabolic byproducts, cyanide and thiocyanate. Sodium nitroprusside decomposes within a few minutes after IV infusion. Free cyanide, which represents 44% of nitroprusside by weight, is released into the bloodstream, producing prussic acid (hydrogen cyanide), which is responsible for the acute toxicity.[69] The amount of hydrogen cyanide released is directly proportional to the size of the dose.[70] Endogenous detoxification of cyanide occurs through a mitochondrial rhodanese system, which, in the presence of a sulfur donor such as thiosulfate, converts cyanide to thiocyanate.[69] Theoretically, cyanide can be expected to accumulate in the body when the rate of the sodium nitroprusside infusion exceeds 2 mcg/kg/minute for a prolonged period. The presence of hepatic or renal impairment may also predispose the patient to cyanide toxicity.[71,72]

It is generally stated that symptomatic cyanide toxicity occurs infrequently, although several deaths have been reported after the use of sodium nitroprusside.[73] Cyanide toxicity occurs most commonly when large doses (total dose 1.5 mg/kg) of nitroprusside are administered rapidly to patients undergoing a surgical procedure that requires induction of hypotension. However, cyanide toxicity and mortality associated with nitroprusside exceed 3,000 and 1,000 cases per year, respectively, according to two sources.[73,74] The product label warns that sodium nitroprusside administration increases the body's concentration of cyanide ion to toxic and potentially fatal levels, even when given within the range of recommended doses. The labeling further states that infusions at the maximum recommended dose can overwhelm the body's ability to buffer the cyanide within 1 hour.

Although concurrent sodium thiosulfate administration has been recommended in high-risk patients, no clinical data are available to indicate that it reduces overall mortality. Furthermore, this intervention may result in the accumulation of thiocyanate, particularly if sodium thiosulfate is given at high infusion rates or to patients with renal insufficiency. A 1-year retrospective review at a tertiary-care teaching hospital with a level 1 trauma center found that none of the patients receiving nitroprusside at infusion rates greater than 2 mcg/kg/minute were concurrently treated with sodium thiosulfate.[75] Hydroxocobalamin has also been used to reduce the risk of cyanide toxicity secondary to nitroprusside infusions, but its use is limited because of poor availability and cost considerations.[72] With the availability of safer alternatives (e.g., fenoldopam, IV labetalol, IV nicardipine) for use in high-risk patients, the use of hydroxocobalamin or thiosulfate is rarely required.

Cyanide toxicity can be detected early by monitoring M.R.'s metabolic status. Lactic acidosis is an early indicator of toxicity because the progressive inactivation of cytochrome oxidase by cyanide results in increased anaerobic glycolysis.[76] A low plasma bicarbonate concentration and low pH, accompanied by an increase in the blood lactate or lactate-to-pyruvate ratio, and an increase in the mixed venous blood oxygen tension could indicate cyanide toxicity.[77] Additional signs of cyanide intoxication include tachycardia, altered consciousness, coma, convulsions, and the occasional smell of almonds on the breath.[70,77] Hypoxemia resulting from pulmonary arterial shunting has also been reported during nitroprusside therapy. Measuring serum thiocyanate levels is of no value in detecting the onset of cyanide toxicity. If toxicity develops, the infusion should be stopped and appropriate therapy for cyanide intoxication instituted. The need for such a high-dose infusion of nitroprusside to maintain M.R.'s pressure may increase his risk for cyanide toxicity, warranting close monitoring of his acid–base balance.

THIOCYANATE TOXICITY

CASE 21-2, QUESTION 7: Explain the difference between cyanide toxicity and thiocyanate toxicity. What is M.R.'s risk for thiocyanate toxicity if he is continued on a dose of 7 mcg/kg/minute? Is monitoring of serum thiocyanate concentrations necessary?

Sodium nitroprusside is more likely to produce thiocyanate toxicity. Although this complication is also rare, patients with renal impairment who receive infusions beyond 72 hours are particularly susceptible. The cyanide released from nitroprusside is normally metabolized by thiosulfate in the liver to thiocyanate via sulfation. This conversion of cyanide to thiocyanate proceeds relatively slowly, and thiocyanate levels rise gradually in proportion to the dose and duration of sodium nitroprusside administration. The half-life of thiocyanate is 2.7 days with normal renal function and up to 9 days in patients with renal failure.[78] When sodium nitroprusside is infused for several days at moderate dosages (2–5 mcg/kg/minute), toxic levels of thiocyanate can occur within 7 to 14 days in patients with normal renal function and 3 to 6 days in patients with severe renal disease.[69]

Thiocyanate causes a neurotoxic syndrome manifested by psychosis, hyperreflexia, confusion, weakness, tinnitus, seizures, and coma.[71,78] Prolonged exposure to thiocyanate can suppress thyroid function through inhibition of iodine uptake and binding by the thyroid gland.[78] Routine measurement of blood levels of thiocyanate is unnecessary and is recommended only in patients with renal disease or when the duration of the nitroprusside infusion exceeds 3 or 4 days. Nitroprusside should be discontinued if serum thiocyanate levels exceed 10 to 12 mg/dL.[79,80] Life-threatening toxicity is of concern when blood thiocyanate levels exceed 20 mg/dL. In emergency cases, thiocyanate can be readily removed by hemodialysis.[78]

For M.R., the potential for thiocyanate toxicity is low because his renal function is normal and the anticipated infusion duration is relatively short. Therefore, measurement of thiocyanate levels is not indicated at this time.

Other side effects associated with nitroprusside therapy include nausea, vomiting, diaphoresis, nasal stuffiness, muscular twitching, dizziness, and weakness. These effects are usually acute and occur when nitroprusside is administered too rapidly. They can be reversed by decreasing the infusion rate.

CASE 21-2, QUESTION 8: M.R.'s serum chemistries and arterial blood gas values indicate a metabolic acidosis. Should the nitroprusside infusion be continued at 7 mcg/kg/minute? What alternative is available?

Although the duration of M.R.'s nitroprusside therapy has been short, tolerance to the antihypertensive effect requires the use of a high-dose infusion to maintain BP control. Thus, acidosis may represent toxicity as a result of cyanide accumulation. The nitroprusside infusion should be discontinued at this time, and another rapidly acting, easily titratable parenteral antihypertensive such as fenoldopam or IV nicardipine should be initiated.

FENOLDOPAM

CASE 21-2, QUESTION 9: What are the advantages and disadvantages of fenoldopam compared with sodium nitroprusside?

Fenoldopam is a parenteral, rapidly acting, peripheral dopamine-1 agonist used to manage hypertensive crisis when a rapid reduction of BP is required.[81–84] Stimulation of the dopamine-1 receptors vasodilates coronary, renal, mesenteric, and peripheral arteries.[85] Vasodilation of the renal vasculature increases renal blood flow in hypertensive patients,[60,61,63] a property that may be particularly advantageous in patients with impaired renal function.[62,86] However, no outcome data are available to document that this effect reduces morbidity and mortality in patients with hypertensive emergencies. Fenoldopam has also been used to control perioperative hypertension in patients undergoing cardiac bypass surgery because, relative to nitroprusside, it either maintains or increases urinary output.[87,88] Fenoldopam is as effective as sodium nitroprusside for treatment of hypertensive emergencies and does not cause either cyanide or thiocyanate toxicity.[57–59] Outcome studies will be required to assess the impact of fenoldopam on increasing renal blood flow and urine output in the management of patients with hypertensive emergencies. Until such time, it should be used only as an alternative to nitroprusside in patients such as M.R., who are at high risk for cyanide or thiocyanate toxicity.

CASE 21-2, QUESTION 10: If M.R. is converted to a continuous infusion of fenoldopam, what is the dose of this medication? What monitoring parameters should be followed?

Fenoldopam is administered as a continuous infusion (without a bolus dose) beginning at a rate of 0.1 mcg/kg/minute. It is then titrated upward, according to BP control, in increments of 0.05 to 0.1 mcg/kg/minute at 15-minute intervals. The maximum dose is 1.6 mcg/kg/minute, and has been studied for up to 48 hours of therapy. Clearance of fenoldopam is not altered by renal or liver disease. Like nitroprusside, fenoldopam also has a short duration of action, with an elimination half-life of approximately 5 minutes, thus allowing for easy titration. Once the target BP is achieved, fenoldopam can be gradually tapered as oral therapy is initiated, if rebound hypertension has not occurred.[83,89]

Fenoldopam is well tolerated and relatively free of side effects. BP and heart rate should be followed closely to avoid hypotension and dose-related tachycardia. The vasodilating effect may also cause flushing, dizziness, and headache. Serum electrolytes should be monitored, and in some cases, potassium supplementation is required. Fenoldopam should be used cautiously in patients with glaucoma or intraocular hypertension due to a dose-dependent increase in intraocular pressure.[90,91]

CASE 21-2, QUESTION 11: Which antihypertensive agents should be avoided in M.R.? Why?

Labetalol, a potent, rapidly acting antihypertensive with both α- and β-blocking activity, is very effective in the treatment of hypertensive emergencies,[91–98] but it should not be used in M.R. Hemodynamically, labetalol reduces peripheral vascular resistance (afterload), BP, and heart rate, with almost no change in the resting cardiac output or stroke volume.[99]

M.R. is experiencing chest pain, and he is tachycardic; these signs and symptoms are most likely caused by his severely elevated BP and the presence of acute left ventricular failure. Even though labetalol might improve M.R.'s angina, the negative inotropic action could acutely compromise his left ventricular dysfunction, an effect that outweighs the potential benefit of afterload reduction. In addition, even though labetalol is one of the safest blocking drugs when used in patients with asthma,[100] no β-blocker should be used as initial treatment in patients with asthma. Labetalol should be used only if alternative methods of reducing M.R.'s pressure fail.

LABETALOL

CASE 21-3

QUESTION 1: C.M., a 52-year-old Caucasian man, is admitted to the hospital with a 3-day history of increasing exertional substernal chest pain (without shortness of breath), diaphoresis, nausea, and vomiting. His history is significant for poorly controlled hypertension, glaucoma, and angina pectoris. Prior medications include dorzolamide ophthalmic drops, atenolol, hydrochlorothiazide, and oral nitrates. Physical examination reveals an anxious man who is alert and oriented. He has a BP of 210/146 mm Hg without orthostasis and a regular pulse of 115 beats/minute. Bilateral hemorrhages and exudates are present on funduscopic examination. The lungs are clear and the heart is enlarged, but there are no murmurs or gallops. Examination of the abdomen is unremarkable, and there is no peripheral edema. The neurologic examination is normal.

Significant laboratory values include the following:

Sodium, 140 mEq/L
Chloride, 109 mEq/L
Bicarbonate, 18 mEq/L
BUN, 49 mg/dL
Serum creatinine, 2.8 mg/dL

Renal function was previously noted to be within normal limits. Urinalysis shows proteinuria and hematuria. The electrocardiogram demonstrates sinus tachycardia with left-axis deviation, left ventricular hypertrophy, and nonspecific ST-T wave changes. The chest radiograph reveals mild cardiomegaly.

C.M. is given nitroglycerin sublingually and 1 inch of nitroglycerin ointment is applied topically. He is started on IV labetalol. Is this choice of treatment reasonable, considering C.M.'s angina and acute kidney injury?

The presence of chest pain, retinopathy, and new-onset renal disease, as well as the magnitude of the BP elevation in C.M., classifies his presentation as a hypertensive emergency that warrants a prompt reduction in BP. The combination of sublingual and topical nitroglycerin may help in acutely lowering his BP and relieving his chest pain while waiting for more definitive treatment to be implemented.

IV labetalol is a potent antihypertensive drug that has been used successfully in hypertensive emergencies.[92–98] Labetalol blocks both β- and α-adrenergic receptors and also may exert a direct vasodilator effect. The β-blockade is nonselective with β to α potency of 3:1 for oral and 7:1 for IV labetalol. Labetalol is particularly advantageous in C.M. because the immediate onset of action will reduce peripheral vascular resistance without causing reflex tachycardia. Myocardial oxygen demand will be reduced and coronary hemodynamics will be improved, making this agent an excellent choice for patients such as C.M., who have anginal symptoms or MI. In addition, IV labetalol does not significantly reduce cerebral blood flow; therefore, it may be useful in patients with cerebrovascular disease.[1,23]

Fenoldopam or nitroprusside could also be used to treat C.M. Fenoldopam could potentially benefit renal function by increasing renal blood flow, but C.M.'s history of glaucoma would preclude its use. In addition, fenoldopam would not be beneficial for C.M.'s anginal symptoms, and equally effective but less costly alternatives are available. Treatment with nitroprusside would expose C.M. to the potential risk of cyanide and thiocyanate toxicity with his new-onset renal failure. In contrast, labetalol has been used successfully in patients with renal disease without deleterious side effects.[101,102] Labetalol is eliminated by glucuronidation in the liver, with less than 5% of the dose being excreted unchanged in the urine. Therefore, labetalol may be better tolerated than nitroprusside by patients with hepatic failure because toxic nitroprusside metabolites also accumulate in this situation. The presence of renal disease in C.M. will not necessitate an alteration in the dose of labetalol.

CONTRAINDICATIONS AND PRECAUTIONS

CASE 21-3, QUESTION 2: What cautions should be exercised when using labetalol in C.M.?

Labetalol's disadvantages are primarily related to its β-blocking effects. Therefore, it should not be used in patients with asthma, heart block greater than first degree, or sinus bradycardia, and it should be used with caution in patients with decompensated HF[93,97,103] (see Case 21-2, Question 10). None of these are present in C.M. Like other β-blockers, labetalol may mask the symptoms of hypoglycemia in insulin-dependent diabetic patients; it should also be used with caution in patients with Raynaud's syndrome.[104] Labetalol has been effective in the treatment of hypertension associated with pheochromocytoma and excess catecholamine states as well as those with rebound hypertension from β-blocker withdrawal.[105] However, because labetalol is primarily a β-blocker, paradoxic hypertension may occur in patients with pheochromocytoma. These individuals have adrenal tumors that excrete high amounts of norepinephrine, which results in relatively unopposed α-receptor stimulation.[106] More clinical experience is required before labetalol can be recommended in patients with pheochromocytoma.[6,92]

There appears to be a positive correlation between age and response to labetalol. Older patients achieve a greater reduction in BP and, therefore, require smaller doses.[104,107] Failure to lower BP has also been observed.[108–110] This phenomenon is believed to be related to single-bolus administration or prior treatment with α- and β-blocking drugs.[103] However, subsequent studies have confirmed the effectiveness of labetalol in the management of hypertensive emergency in those pretreated with antihypertensives, including β-blockers.[111]

CASE 21-3, QUESTION 3: How should parenteral labetalol be given to C.M.?

For treatment of his hypertensive emergency, C.M. should be placed in the supine position. IV labetalol can be given by pulse administration or continuous infusion.[92–97] Small incremental bolus injections are administered, beginning with 20 mg given over 2 minutes, followed by 40 to 80 mg every 10 to 15 minutes until the desired response is achieved or a cumulative dose of 300 mg is reached. The desired response is usually achieved with a mean dose of 200 mg in 90% of patients.[93] After IV injection, the maximal effect occurs within 5 to 10 minutes,[95] and the antihypertensive response may persist for more than 6 hours.[111] Because the rate of BP reduction is accelerated with an increase in infusion rate,[95] a controlled continuous infusion may provide a more gradual reduction in arterial pressure with less frequent adverse effects.[97,112] A solution for continuous infusion (0.5–2.0 mg/minute) is prepared by adding two ampules (200 mg total) to 160 mL of IV fluid to give a final concentration of 1 mg/mL. The infusion can then be started at a rate of 2 mg/minute and titrated until a satisfactory response is achieved or until a cumulative dose of 300 mg is reached.

PARENTERAL TO ORAL CONVERSION

CASE 21-3, QUESTION 4: C.M. was treated with a labetalol infusion and required a cumulative dose of 180 mg to achieve a diastolic pressure of 100 mm Hg. His anginal symptoms resolved almost immediately, but 3 hours after the infusion, C.M. became faint and dizzy while ambulating. Should oral labetalol be withheld in C.M.?

Postural hypotension and dizziness are dose related and more commonly associated with the IV route of administration.[99,103] C.M. should remain in a supine position after the IV administration of labetalol, and his ability to tolerate an upright position should be established before permitting ambulation. Oral labetalol can be given to C.M. when his symptoms resolve. There is no correlation between the oral maintenance dose and the total initial IV dose. C.M. should be started on an empiric dose of 100 to 200 mg of oral labetalol twice daily, and this should be titrated as necessary.

CASE 21-3, QUESTION 5: What other side effects can occur with labetalol therapy?

Other side effects commonly associated with labetalol include nausea, vomiting, abdominal pain, and diarrhea in up to 15% of the patients.[103] Scalp tingling is an unusual side effect that has been reported in a few patients after IV administration; it tends to disappear with continued treatment. Other side effects include tiredness, weakness, muscle cramps, headache, ejaculation failure, and skin rashes.

NITROGLYCERIN

CASE 21-3, QUESTION 6: Would parenteral nitroglycerin be an acceptable alternative to labetalol for C.M.?

Hypertensive emergencies in the setting of unstable angina or MI requires an immediate reduction in BP. Nitroprusside has been used successfully, but IV nitroglycerin can have more favorable effects on collateral coronary flow in patients with ischemic heart disease.[113] By diminishing preload, nitroglycerin decreases left ventricular diastolic volume, diastolic pressure, and myocardial wall tension, thus reducing myocardial oxygen consumption.[114] These changes favor redistribution of coronary blood flow to the subendocardium, which is more vulnerable to ischemia. At high dosages, nitroglycerin dilates arteriolar smooth muscles, and this reduction in afterload also decreases myocardial wall tension and oxygen consumption.[115]

IV nitroglycerin has a rapid onset of action and a short duration, and is easily titratable. It is generally appropriate to begin IV nitroglycerin at dosages in the range of 5 to 10 mcg/minute, increased as needed to control pressure and symptoms. The usual dose is in the range of 40 to 100 mcg/minute. The major limiting side effects are headache and the development of tolerance. In general, IV nitroglycerin is well suited for use in patients such as C.M. who have angina or in patients who have hypertensive emergency associated with MI or coronary artery bypass surgery.

HYDRALAZINE

CASE 21-4

QUESTION 1: T.M., a 30-year-old Caucasian man with a history of chronic glomerulonephritis and poorly controlled hypertension, came to the emergency department complaining of early morning occipital headaches during the past week. He has no other complaints. He has not taken any BP medication in a month. Physical examination revealed an afebrile man in no acute distress with a BP of 160/120 mm Hg without orthostasis and a regular pulse of 90 beats/minute. Funduscopic examination revealed bilateral exudates without hemorrhages or papilledema. The lungs were clear. Cardiac examination was pertinent for cardiomegaly and an S_4 gallop. The remainder of the physical workup was normal.

Laboratory results include the following values:

Hematocrit, 32%
BUN, 40 mg/dL
Serum creatinine, 2.5 mg/dL (baseline serum creatinine 1.9 mg/dL)
Bicarbonate, 18 mEq/L

Urinalysis reveals 2+ protein, 2+ hemoglobin with 4 to 10 red blood cells per high-power field. The electrocardiogram demonstrates normal sinus rhythm with left ventricular hypertrophy. The chest radiograph is unremarkable.

T.M.'s presentation meets criteria for a hypertensive emergency (i.e., diastolic BP >120 mm Hg and presence of worsening renal function). Intravenous antihypertensive therapy is required for T.M. T.M. was given 20 mg hydralazine IV, and a repeat BP after 1 hour was 150/100 mm Hg. What are the advantages and disadvantages of parenteral hydralazine, and when should it be used to acutely lower BP?

Hydralazine is a direct vasodilator that reduces total peripheral resistance through relaxation of arterial smooth muscle. It is rarely used to treat hypertensive emergencies because its antihypertensive response is less predictable than that of other parenteral agents. Additionally, hydralazine has a prolonged half-life, which can be problematic if too fast correction or hypotension occurs.[22] It is not consistently effective in controlling crises associated with essential hypertension.

CONTRAINDICATIONS

Hydralazine should not be used in patients with coronary heart disease because the reflex tachycardia causes an increase in myocardial oxygen demand, which may result in the development or worsening of ischemic symptoms. In addition, hydralazine should be avoided in patients with aortic dissection because of its reflex cardiostimulating effect. In contrast, hydralazine can be useful in patients such as T.M., who have chronic renal failure because the reflex increase in cardiac output is accompanied by an increase in organ perfusion.[21]

DOSING AND ADMINISTRATION

Parenteral hydralazine should be considered an intermediate treatment between oral agents and more aggressive therapy with such agents as fenoldopam or nitroprusside. It can be given IV or intramuscularly. The onset of action develops slowly over 20 to 40 minutes, thus minimizing the risk of acute hypotension. Parenteral doses are considerably lower than oral doses because of increased bioavailability.

OTHER PARENTERAL DRUGS

CASE 21-4, QUESTION 2: Are there alternatives to hydralazine for parenteral treatment of hypertensive crisis?

INTRAVENOUS ENALAPRILAT

Enalaprilat, the active metabolite of the oral prodrug enalapril (Vasotec), is approved by the U.S. Food and Drug Administration for the treatment of hypertension when oral therapy is not feasible. However, enalaprilat has been used to treat severe hypertension.[116–121] The initial dose is 0.625 to 1.25 mg IV and can be repeated every 6 hours, if necessary. To minimize the risk of hypotension, the initial doses should not exceed 0.625 mg in patients receiving diuretics or in patients with clinical evidence of hypovolemia. The onset of action is within 15 minutes, but the maximal effect may take several hours. Because only 60% of the patients respond to BP reduction within 30 minutes, it cannot be reliably used to acutely lower pressure in hypertensive emergencies.[119] Although higher initial doses have been successfully used to achieve BP control,[120] some evidence indicates that doses greater than 0.625 mg do not significantly alter the magnitude of enalaprilat's antihypertensive effect.[118] Enalaprilat also is beneficial in patients with HF. Precautions for the use of enalaprilat are similar to those of captopril (see Case 21-1, Question 5). Because of the prolonged time required to achieve an adequate response, limited clinical experience, and variable response rates (especially in African Americans), enalaprilat cannot be recommended for the routine treatment of patients with hypertensive emergencies.[119,121]

INTRAVENOUS CALCIUM-CHANNEL BLOCKERS

CASE 21-5

QUESTION 1: H.C. is a 71-year-old Caucasian man undergoing urgent coronary artery bypass graft surgery after an MI. H.C. has a history of a cerebrovascular accident and chronic kidney disease (serum creatinine is stable at 1.6 mg/dL). Two hours after surgery H.C.'s systolic BP began to increase to 162 to 171 mm Hg with a diastolic BP of 121 to 133 mm Hg. H.C. was administered IV nicardipine postoperatively for BP control. Is nicardipine an appropriate choice for H.C.?

Nicardipine

Postoperative hypertension is typically short lived and is most commonly seen after neurosurgical, head and neck, vascular, and cardiothoracic procedures (as is the case with H.C.). Treatment is typically only required for 6 hours postoperatively, and up to 24 to 48 hours for some. Adequate control of BP postoperatively is necessary to minimize the risk of cardiovascular, neurological, or surgical-site complications such as bleeding.[122] When selecting an agent, one should consider therapies with a quick onset and short duration of action as well as established efficacy and safety in the postoperative setting.

Nicardipine is a potent cerebral and systemic vasodilator and a useful therapeutic option in the management of severe hypertension. Its onset of action is within 1 to 2 minutes, and its elimination half-life is 40 minutes.[123] Hemodynamic evaluations demonstrated that IV nicardipine significantly decreased mean arterial pressure and systemic vascular resistance and significantly increased cardiac index with little or no change in heart rate.[124] Titratable IV nicardipine has been studied extensively for use in controlling postoperative hypertension [124–127] and hypertensive emergencies [128–131]

In the treatment of postoperative hypertension,[124] IV nicardipine was administered as an infusion titrated in the following manner: 10 mg/hour for 5 minutes, 12.5 mg/hour for 5 minutes, and 15 mg/hour for 15 minutes, followed by a maintenance infusion of 3 mg/hour thereafter. The mean response time and infusion rate were 11.5 minutes and 12.8 mg/hour, respectively. Ninety-four percent of the patients responded, and adverse effects included hypotension (4.5%), tachycardia (2.7%), and nausea and vomiting (4.5%).

The efficacy and safety of IV nicardipine for the treatment of hypertensive crisis were documented in a double-blind, placebo-controlled multicenter trial of 123 patients.[128] Therapy of IV nicardipine was begun with dosages of 5 mg/hour and titrated up to 15 mg/hour as indicated until the therapeutic end point was achieved. The mean dosage of IV nicardipine at the end of maintenance therapy was 8.7 mg/hour. Ninety-one percent of patients on nicardipine achieved the prespecified BP target within a mean administration time of 77 minutes. In an open-label trial,[129] patients receiving nicardipine required significantly fewer dose adjustments per hour than patients receiving nitroprusside (1.7 vs. 3.3, respectively). Serious adverse effects reported in these trials were uncommon. The most commonly reported adverse effects included headache, hypotension, tachycardia, dizziness, and nausea.

When compared with sodium nitroprusside for patients with severe hypertension, IV nicardipine was as effective with fewer adverse effects.[129] In studies of patients receiving nicardipine versus nitroprusside for postoperative hypertension after cardiac endarterectomy and coronary artery bypass grafting, breakthrough BP was controlled more rapidly with nicardipine and required fewer overall dose titrations. In addition, nicardipine was well tolerated and did not lead to an increased risk of complications.[132,133]

Nicardipine is an appropriate choice of therapy for H.C. because this agent has a rapid onset of action, and provides sustained BP control during the infusion period. It is easily titratable, with a predictable response, and is relatively free of severe adverse effects, which is ideal in the postoperative setting. Therapy should be titrated to achieve a BP approximately 10% higher than the patient's baseline. In addition to nicardipine, nitroprusside, nitroglycerin, and labetalol are most commonly used to manage postoperative hypertension.[122] Finally, nicardipine may be useful in patients with cerebral insufficiency or peripheral vascular disease. Because of the potential for reflex tachycardia, it should be used with caution in patients with ongoing coronary ischemia.

CASE 21-5, QUESTION 2: What other IV forms of calcium-channel blockers are available? Would any of these agents be an appropriate choice of therapy for H.C.?

Nicardipine has been proven effective in multiple studies of populations with hypertensive emergencies, and, as a dihydropyridine, has less negative inotropic activity compared with nondihydropyridines. In contrast, the nondihydropyridines parenteral verapamil and diltiazem, although clinically effective for prompt lowering of BP, have not been extensively studied in patients with hypertensive emergencies. Clevidipine, a third-generation dihydropyridine, has been shown to be useful in controlling BP in hypertensive emergencies and in the perioperative setting.

Nondihydropyridines

IV verapamil (5–10 mg) produces a significant reduction in BP, which occurs within 15 minutes and persists for 6 to 8 hours. As a cardiovascular drug, it is primarily used as a rate-controlling agent in the treatment of supraventricular tachycardias.

IV diltiazem is approved for temporary control of the ventricular rate in atrial fibrillation or atrial flutter and for rapid conversion of paroxysmal supraventricular tachycardia.[134–136] Parenteral diltiazem has also been used to control hypertension that occurs intraoperatively and postoperatively[137,138] and in patients with acute coronary artery disease.[139,140] However, published experience with the use of IV diltiazem for the treatment of severe hypertension is limited. Onoyama et al.[141] administered a continuous infusion of diltiazem at a dosage of 5 to 40 mcg/kg/minute to a small group of patients with hypertensive crisis. A normotensive level was achieved within 6 hours without any signs of organ ischemia. In a follow-up study,[142] a continuous infusion of diltiazem averaging 11 mcg/kg/minute resulted in a 25% reduction in both systolic and diastolic BP measurements within 30 minutes. The magnitude of the decrease was directly correlated with the pretreatment BP level. Atrioventricular nodal conduction abnormalities were noted in both studies during drug infusion. Patients receiving IV diltiazem require continuous monitoring by electrocardiogram and frequent BP checks. This form of therapy should be avoided in patients with sick sinus syndrome or advanced degrees of heart block. Until additional information is available, caution should be exercised in using parenteral diltiazem to lower BP acutely. In addition, use of nondihydropyridines should be avoided when acutely treating any hypertensive patient with concomitant systolic HF owing to their negative inotropic effects.

Clevidipine

Clevidipine is another intravenous dihydropyridine calcium-channel blocker with arterial-selective vasodilation properties.[143] Clevidipine is quickly metabolized in extravascular tissue and blood by esterases, leading to a short elimination half-life of 1 minute[144] and complete resolution of hemodynamic effects within 10 minutes after the end of a 24-hour continuous infusion.[145] Clevidipine demonstrates a quick onset of action of 1 to 2 minutes.[146] These pharmacokinetic and pharmacodynamic properties make it an attractive agent for managing hypertensive emergencies. Clevidipine demonstrated efficacy in treatment of hypertension in both preoperative and postoperative cardiac surgery patients.[147,148] In this setting, therapy was initiated at a rate of 0.4 mcg/kg/minute. Target BP was a reduction of at least 15% from baseline. The dose was titrated every 90 seconds by doubling the dose up to an infusion rate of 3.2 mcg/kg/minute, then increasing the dose by 1.5 mcg/kg/minute to a maximum rate of 8 mcg/kg/minute. Clevidipine demonstrated a median time of effectiveness within 6 minutes in greater than 90% of the patients who received the study medication.

Clevidipine has been compared individually with nitroglycerin, nitroprusside, and nicardipine in management of perioperative hypertension in cardiac surgery patients.[143] This was a compilation of three parallel protocols that randomly assigned patients to clevidipine or the comparison agent. Outcomes were assessed by the occurrence of death, stroke, MI, or renal dysfunction from time of drug administration until postoperative day 30. There were no differences between clevidipine and the pooled comparison groups with regard to 30-day outcomes. Clevidipine was more effective in maintaining patients within a predefined BP target range when compared individually with nitroglycerin and nitroprusside, but this did not translate to differences in clinical outcomes. The incidence and severity of adverse events were similar among patients who received clevidipine and comparison agents.

A prospective, open-label study was conducted evaluating patients who presented in the emergency department or intensive care unit with systolic BP of greater than 180 mm Hg or diastolic BP greater than 115 mm Hg.[149] Patients were titrated on clevidipine to a patient-specific systolic BP range that was determined by the treating physician using criteria such as the patient's presenting condition, comorbidities, and baseline blood pressure. The initial infusion rate was 2 mg/hour for at least 3 minutes, then titrated every 3 minutes until the target BP was achieved or to a maximum rate of 32 mg/hour. If the target BP was achieved, the medication was continued for 18 to 96 hours. Overall, clevidipine demonstrated effectiveness in reaching the target BP in 88.9% of patients within a median time of 10.9 minutes. Only 7.7% of patients required concomitant intravenous antihypertensives during the entire study infusion. The majority (91.3%) of patients were able to effectively transition to oral antihypertensive therapy.

Based on the limited data, nondihydropyridines would not be an appropriate choice of therapy for H.C. Additionally, IV verapamil has a long duration of action, which is not an ideal characteristic in the setting of postoperative hypertension. Clevidipine, however, has a rapid onset of action and short duration of action. This agent has also been shown to be efficacious in controlling BP in the perioperative setting.

CASE 21-5, QUESTION 3: What factors should clinicians consider before recommending the use of clevidipine?

There are two attributes to the medication that should also be noted before initiation: reflexive tachycardia and formulation. It has been demonstrated that clevidipine infusions can increase heart rate by up to approximately 20 beats/minute.[145] Clevidipine is nearly water-insoluble; the medication is formulated in a 20% lipid emulsion. Because of this feature, patients with serum triglycerides greater than 400 mg/dL should not receive clevidipine, and any remaining drug should be discarded after 4 hours of use. Clevidipine is contraindicated in patients with allergies to soybeans, soy products, eggs, or egg products. This agent is also contraindicated in those with defective lipid metabolism or acute pancreatitis (if accompanied by hyperlipidemia), and in patients with severe aortic stenosis.[146]

INTRAVENOUS PHENTOLAMINE

IV phentolamine is primarily used in the management of hypertensive emergencies induced by catecholamine excess, as seen in pheochromocytoma or in those taking monoamine oxidase inhibitors who ingest excessive amounts of tyramine-containing foods. The mechanism of action is through nonselective competitive antagonist α-adrenergic receptors. Phentolamine is dosed in 1- to 5-mg boluses. The onset of action is almost immediate, and the duration of action is short (<15 minutes). IV infusions are not recommended owing to unpredictable drops in BP.

Cerebrovascular spasm, cerebrovascular occlusion, and MI have been reported after the administration of phentolamine. These adverse events are usually associated with significant hypotensive episodes. Tachycardia, arrhythmias, weakness, dizziness, flushing, and gastrointestinal effects have also been reported.[150]

Aortic Dissection

TREATMENT

CASE 21-6

QUESTION 1: B.S., a 68-year-old Caucasian man with a long history of hypertension and nonadherence, presents to the local emergency department complaining of the sudden onset of severe, sharp, diffuse chest pain that radiates to his back between his shoulder blades. Significant findings on physical examination include a pulse of 100 beats/minute, BP of 200/120 mm Hg, clear lungs, and an S_4 without murmurs. The laboratory data are unremarkable. The electrocardiogram results are interpreted as sinus tachycardia with left ventricular hypertrophy, but no acute changes are noted. The chest radiograph is significant for widening of the mediastinum. An emergency chest computed tomography scan reveals a dissection at the arch of the aorta. What antihypertensive medication(s) would be most appropriate for B.S., and why?

Dissection of the aorta occurs when the innermost layer of the aorta (the intima) is torn such that blood enters and separates its layers. The ultimate treatment for this type of hypertensive emergency depends on its location and severity; however, the first principle of therapy is to control any existing hypertension with agents that do not increase the force of cardiac contraction. This lessens the force that the cardiac impulse transmits to the dissecting aneurysm.

The aim of antihypertensive therapy in aortic dissection is to lessen the pulsatile load or aortic stress by lowering the BP. Reducing the force of left ventricular contractions, and consequently the rate of rise of aortic pressure, retards the propagation of the dissection and aortic rupture.[151,152] The treatment of choice for aortic dissection has classically been a vasodilatory agent such as sodium nitroprusside, fenoldopam, or nicardipine in combination with a β-blocker titrated to a heart rate of 55 to 65 beats/minute.[151,153] Labetalol monotherapy has been used as an alternative.[154] These drugs decrease BP, venous return, and cardiac contractility.

One common regimen is a combination of IV sodium nitroprusside (0.5–2 mcg/kg/minute) plus IV esmolol.[20,152] This combination can be used as initial therapy for B.S. The concurrent administration of a β-blocking agent with a vasodilator is desirable because the latter may induce reflex tachycardia in response to vasodilation.

Direct vasodilators such as hydralazine should be avoided because they increase stroke volume and left ventricular ejection rate. These effects augment the pulsatile flow and accentuate the sharpness of the pulse wave. This increases mechanical stress on the aortic wall and may lead to further dissection.[20]

Depending on the location of the dissection, surgical intervention may be required.[153,155] However, until a definitive diagnosis is made, the primary goal is to reduce the BP and myocardial contractility to the lowest level compatible with the maintenance of adequate renal, cerebral, and cardiac perfusion.[20] Aggressive BP control is warranted to minimize target organ damage and to prevent further dissection or hemorrhage.[152] For aortic dissection, it is suggested that the systolic BP should be lowered to 100 to 120 mm Hg or a mean arterial pressure of less than 80 mm Hg within 5 to 10 minutes.[20]

Patients presenting with an aortic dissection should be screened for tobacco, cocaine, and amphetamine use. Use of these substances has been shown to increase the risk of dissection. A population-based case-control study, after adjustment for other risk factors, revealed that amphetamine abuse or dependence in those aged 18 to 49 years of age was associated with a threefold increased risk of aortic dissection. A patient's lipid panel should be evaluated, and treatment should be initiated when appropriate (see Chapter 13, Dyslipidemias, Atherosclerosis, and Coronary Heart Disease). Long-term hypertension control is critical in this patient population. Connective tissue disorders, hereditary vascular disorders, trauma, and Turner syndrome (a chromosomal condition caused by a complete or partial absence of the second sex chromosome) are also presumed risk factors.[156]

CASE 21-6, QUESTION 2: What dose of esmolol should be administered to B.S.? And what adverse events can occur with esmolol therapy?

Esmolol is a parenteral cardioselective β_1-blocker with a rapid onset and short duration of action. For the management of hypertension, esmolol should be given as a loading dose of 250 to 500 mcg/kg for 1 minute, followed by a maintenance infusion of 50 to 300 mcg/kg/minute. Irritation, inflammation, and induration at the infusion site occur in 5% to 10% of patients.

Hypotension is the most commonly reported adverse event and is directly related to the duration of esmolol administration.[157] However, because of the short half-life, resolution of hypotension occurs within 30 minutes of discontinuing the infusion. Like other β-blockers, esmolol is contraindicated in patients with asthma, advanced heart block, or severe HF.

CASE 21-6, QUESTION 3: In which other patient populations may esmolol be indicated?

Esmolol has been used primarily in perioperative settings to control tachycardia induced by various surgical stimuli, including endotracheal intubation.[157] Esmolol has also been used to manage supraventricular tachyarrhythmias.[158–160] It has been particularly useful in treating postoperative hypertension, especially if associated with tachycardia. In a small series of patients undergoing cardiac bypass surgery, the antihypertensive effect of esmolol was comparable to that of nitroprusside.[161]

Cocaine-Induced Hypertensive Crisis

TREATMENT

CASE 21-7

QUESTION 1: B.K. is a 54-year-old Caucasian man who presents to the emergency department complaining of 8/10 chest pain associated with diaphoresis and nausea that began 2 hours ago. B.K. reports using cocaine about 1 hour before his chest pain began. His medical and social histories include hypertension for which he takes hydrochlorothiazide 25 mg daily. He also admits to using cocaine five to seven times per week for the past 21 years and smoking one and a half packs per day for the past 35 years. An electrocardiogram reveals ST segment elevations less than 1 mm in leads V_2 and V_3 and sinus tachycardia. The patient's blood was drawn to assess his cardiac enzymes; the first set is negative. His cardiac examination was unremarkable. His vital signs include a BP of 205/162 mm Hg, heart rate of 132 beats/minute, regular rate and rhythm, and respiratory rate of 24 breaths/minute, and he is afebrile. All laboratory values are within normal limits. Chest radiograph is unremarkable. What agents should be used to manage cocaine-induced hypertension? What agents should be avoided?

Cocaine, a sympathomimetic, can induce severe hypertension by inhibiting the reuptake of norepinephrine and dopamine and thereby increasing neurotransmitter concentrations in the synaptic cleft. This leads to pronounced vasoconstriction and tachycardia. This increase in heart rate or BP increases cardiac oxygen demand, leading to coronary vasospasm, and places the patient at risk for ischemia and acute coronary syndromes. Cocaine exerts its onset of action within seconds to minutes and has a serum half-life of 30 to 90 minutes.[162,163]

Management of cocaine-associated hypertensive emergencies should be controlled with nicardipine, verapamil, or nitroglycerin. Calcium-channel blockers and IV nitroglycerin are preferred in patients with active myocardial ischemia because they have both been shown to reverse cocaine-induced hypertension and vasoconstriction.[164,165] Benzodiazepines can also be used because they can attenuate the effect of cocaine on the cardiac system, decrease chest pain, and reduce heart rate.[162,166] Fenoldopam and nitroprusside can be used as alternative agents.[167,168]

The use of β-blockers should be avoided in patients who present with hypertension or myocardial ischemia or MI with recent cocaine use. β-blockers will result in unopposed α-adrenergic vasoconstriction, leading to further elevation in BP and heart rate.[167,168] Labetalol possesses both α- and β-blockade, and its use has been reported in cocaine-intoxicated patients.[169] Labetalol has been shown to increase seizure activity and mortality in animals with cocaine intoxication and does not alleviate cocaine-induced coronary vasoconstriction.[170,171] Labetalol has also been shown to worsen BP when α-stimulation has been left unopposed in patients with pheochromocytoma.[108,172] Therefore, caution should be used if labetalol is used in patients with recent cocaine use.

KEY REFERENCES AND WEBSITES

A full list of references for this chapter can be found at http://thepoint.lww.com/AT10e. Below are the key references for this chapter, with the corresponding reference number in this chapter found in parentheses after the reference.

Key References

Anderson RJ et al. Oral clonidine loading in hypertensive urgencies. *JAMA*. 1981;246:848. (38)

Curran MP et al. Intravenous nicardipine: its use in the short-term treatment of hypertension and various other indications. *Drugs*. 2006;66:1755. (131)

Devlin JW et al. Fenoldopam versus nitroprusside for the treatment of hypertensive emergency. *Ann Pharmacother*. 2004;38:755. (56)

Friederich JA, Butterworth JF 4th. Sodium nitroprusside: twenty years and counting. *Anesth Analg*. 1995;81:152. (71)

Gray RJ. Managing critically ill patients with esmolol. An ultrashort acting beta-adrenergic blocker. *Chest*. 1988;93;398. (157)

Grossman E et al. Should a moratorium be placed on sublingual nifedipine capsules given for hypertensive emergencies and pseudoemergencies? *JAMA*. 1996;276:1328. (36)

Haas CE, LeBlanc JM. Acute postoperative hypertension: a review of therapeutic options. *Am J Health-Syst Pharm*. 2004;61:1661. (122)

Khoynezhad A, Plestis KA. Managing emergency hypertension in aortic dissection and aortic aneurysm surgery. *J Card Surg*. 2006;21(Suppl 1):S3. (152)

Lebel M et al. Labetalol infusion in hypertensive emergencies. *Clin Pharmacol Ther*. 1985;37:615. (96)

Marik PE, Varon J. Hypertensive crises: challenges and management. *Chest*. 2007;131:1949. (20)

Murphy MB et al. Fenoldopam—a selective peripheral dopamine-receptor agonist for the treatment of severe hypertension. *N Engl J Med*. 2001;345:1548. (84)

Pollack CV et al. Clevidipine, an intravenous dihydropyridine calcium channel blocker, is safe and effective for the treatment of patients with acute severe hypertension. *Ann Emerg Med*. 2009;53:329. (149)

22 Shock

Andrew D. Barnes and Susan H. Lee

CORE PRINCIPLES

		CHAPTER CASES
1	Shock is a syndrome with multiple possible etiologies characterized by an impairment of tissue perfusion.	
2	The impairment of tissue perfusion, regardless of cause, can lead to cellular dysfunction, organ dysfunction or failure, and death.	
3	The diagnosis of shock is generally made by the findings of impaired tissue perfusion on physical examination, and hemodynamic and laboratory changes consistent with impaired perfusion. Hypotension may or may not be present. Hemodynamic monitoring is vital for the determination of the type of shock and assessment of response to interventions. Hypovolemic shock is caused by a reduction in intravascular volume, which then results in specific changes in the hemodynamic profile such as decreases in blood pressure, central venous pressure, pulmonary capillary wedge pressure, and cardiac output, and a compensatory increase in heart rate, systemic vascular resistance, and myocardial contractility.	**Case 22-1 (Question 1)**
4	Resuscitation is required to treat hypovolemic shock to maintain adequate tissue perfusion and oxygenation. This can be achieved by administration of intravenous fluids in the form of crystalloids, colloids, or blood.	**Case 22-1**
5	The physiologic response to fluid loss or gain is described by the Frank-Starling curve.	**Case 22-1 (Questions 10, 11)**
6	Cardiogenic shock results from a decrease in the heart's ability to maintain cardiac output that is unrelated to hypovolemia.	**Case 22-2 (Question 1)**
7	Treatment of patients in cardiogenic shock involves optimization of preload, increasing contractility, and reducing afterload if the blood pressure permits.	**Case 22-2, Case 22-3**
8	Septic shock is a type of distributive shock characterized by a profound vasodilatory response and resultant decrease in blood pressure.	**Case 22-4**
9	Treatment of septic shock involves stabilization with fluids, vasopressors, and inotropic agents and treatment of the underlying condition. Other therapies involve modification of the body's response to infection.	**Case 22-4 (Questions 3, 6–8)**
10	Patients with sepsis can experience disseminated intravascular coagulation, which can lead to hemorrhagic and thrombotic complications.	**Case 22-4 (Questions 9–12)**

INTRODUCTION

Shock is defined in simple terms as a syndrome of impaired tissue perfusion usually, but not always, accompanied by hypotension. This impairment of tissue perfusion eventually leads to cellular dysfunction, followed by organ damage and death if untreated.

The most common causes of shock are situations that result in a reduction of intravascular volume (hypovolemic shock), myocardial pump failure (cardiogenic shock), or increased vascular capacitance (distributive shock, sepsis). The type of treatment required depends on the etiology.

In recent years, medical support of patients with shock has improved because of better technologies for hemodynamic

TABLE 22-1
Classification of Shock and Precipitating Events

Hypovolemic Shock
Hemorrhagic
Gastrointestinal bleeding
Trauma
Internal bleeding: ruptured aortic aneurysm, retroperitoneal bleeding
Nonhemorrhagic
Dehydration: vomiting, diarrhea, diabetes mellitus, diabetes insipidus, overuse of diuretics
Sequestration: ascites, third-space accumulation
Cutaneous: burns, nonreplaced perspiration and insensible water losses
Cardiogenic Shock
Nonmechanical causes
Acute myocardial infarction
Low cardiac output syndrome
Right ventricular infarction
End-stage cardiomyopathy
Mechanical causes
Rupture of septum or free wall
Mitral or aortic insufficiency
Papillary muscle rupture or dysfunction
Critical aortic stenosis
Pericardial tamponade
Distributive Shock
Septic shock
Anaphylaxis
Neurogenic
Spinal injury, cerebral damage, severe dysautonomia
Drug-induced
Anesthesia, ganglionic and adrenergic blockers, overdoses of barbiturates and narcotics
Acute adrenal insufficiency

monitoring, recognition of the value of vigorous volume replacement, appropriate use of inotropic and vasoconstrictive agents, and the development of better ways to treat the underlying cause of the shock syndrome. Understanding the principles of shock should further enhance prompt recognition of patients at risk, rapid initiation of corrective measures, and development of innovative treatment regimens.

CAUSES

Table 22-1 outlines the classification of shock and precipitating events.[1] Recognition of the etiology and underlying pathology of the various forms of shock is essential for managing this condition. The distinctions among subtypes of shock only apply, however, in the relatively early stages. As the syndrome evolves and compensatory mechanisms are overwhelmed, it becomes increasingly difficult to determine the subtypes because the clinical and pathophysiologic features of advanced shock are the same for all. Also, different types of shock can occur at the same time (e.g., a patient with septic shock who is also hypovolemic).

PATHOPHYSIOLOGY

Tissue perfusion is a complex process of oxygen and nutrient delivery as well as waste removal. When perfusion is impaired, it sets up a cascade of events that can eventually end in death. Although the etiology of shock is varied, the eventual progression (if untreated) to cell death and subsequent organ dysfunction results from a common pathway of ischemia, endogenous inflammatory cytokine release, and the generation of oxygen radicals. When cells are subjected to a prolonged period of ischemia, anaerobic metabolism begins. This inefficient process results in a decrease of adenosine triphosphate stores and causes the buildup of lactic acid and other toxic substances that can alter mitochondrial function and eventually result in cell death. In the advanced stages of shock, irreversible cellular damage leads to multiple organ system failure, also known as multiple organ dysfunction syndrome.

Inflammatory cytokines are produced by the body in response to ischemia, injury, or infection. The phrase *systemic inflammatory response syndrome* (SIRS) is the recommended umbrella term to describe any acute, overwhelming inflammatory response, independent of the cause.[2] This syndrome has best been described in the sepsis literature; however, it can occur after a wide variety of insults, including hemorrhagic shock, infection (septic shock), pancreatitis, ischemia, multitrauma and tissue injury, and immune-mediated organ injury. SIRS is usually a late manifestation of hypovolemic forms of shock. It is uncommon in cardiogenic shock, but is the hallmark of septic shock. SIRS is clinically characterized by profound vasodilation, which impairs perfusion, and increased capillary permeability, which can lead to reduced intravascular volume.

CLINICAL PRESENTATION AND DIAGNOSIS

Independent of the pathophysiologic cause, the clinical syndrome of shock progresses through several stages. During each step, the body uses and exhausts various compensatory mechanisms to balance oxygen delivery ($\dot{D}O_2$) and oxygen consumption ($\dot{V}O_2$) in an effort to maintain perfusion of vital organs. Oxygen delivery is determined by the arterial concentration of oxygen multiplied by the blood flow (cardiac output [CO]) (Fig. 22-1 and Table 22-2). Normally, consumption is independent of supply, except at low rates of $\dot{D}O_2$. In some critically ill patients, however, consumption can depend on supply even in what would be considered "normal" $\dot{D}O_2$ ranges. When $\dot{V}O_2$ becomes dependent on the supply, it indicates an impairment of adequate perfusion.

For a more detailed discussion of hemodynamic principles, go to http://thepoint.lww.com/AT10e.

Although hypotension is often described as the hallmark of shock, it is not necessarily present in all patients.

The diagnosis of shock is based on the finding of impaired tissue perfusion on examination.[3] These findings may include the following:

- Systolic blood pressure (SBP) less than 90 mm Hg, or a greater than 40 mm Hg decrease from baseline in a hypertensive patient, or a mean arterial pressure (MAP) less than 65 mm Hg
- Tachycardia (heart rate [HR] >90 beats/minute)
- Tachypnea (respiratory rate [RR] >20 breaths/minute)
- Cutaneous vasoconstriction: cold, clammy, mottled skin (although not typical of distributive shock)
- Mental confusion (agitation, stupor, or coma)
- Oliguria: urine output less than 20 mL/hour

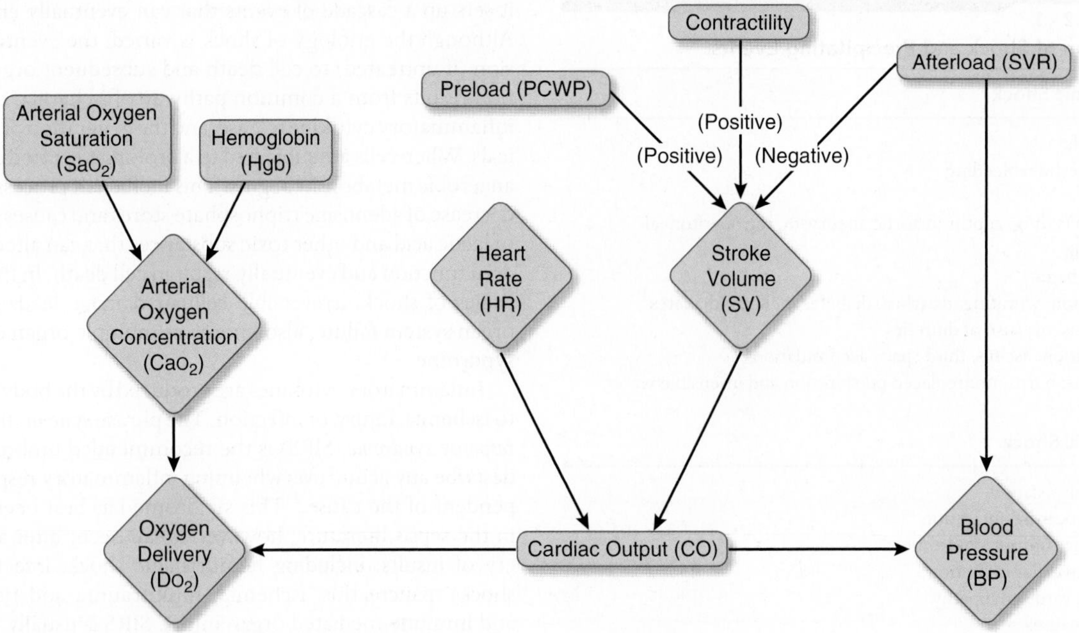

FIGURE 22-1 Determinants of blood pressure, cardiac output, and oxygen delivery.

- Elevated blood lactate level leading to metabolic acidosis
- Decreased venous oxygen saturation (mixed [SvO_2], central [$ScvO_2$]) (reflects increased $\dot{V}O_2$ or impaired oxygen supply)

Not all these described findings are encountered in every patient with shock, and considerable variability exists in both the rapidity and sequence of onset. This depends on the severity of the initiating event, the underlying mechanism, and the baseline condition of the patient, including medications that may alter the clinical presentation. Therefore, it is important to consider the patient's medical and pharmacologic history while closely monitoring for subtle clinical changes that may signal impending deterioration and necessitate immediate intervention.

TREATMENT OVERVIEW

The treatment of patients in shock requires both treatment of the underlying cause of shock, as well as early, aggressive measures to maintain adequate perfusion to vital organs. The general measures used are the restoration of adequate volume in hypovolemic patients, the use of vasopressors or inotropic agents when volume resuscitation is inadequate to maintain perfusion, and careful monitoring of the hemodynamic status of the patient. In sepsis, specific hemodynamic goals have been determined.[4] In other types of shock, specific goals have not been established; however, the principles of ensuring adequate tissue perfusion are the same.

HEMODYNAMIC MONITORING

Hemodynamic monitoring in the critically ill patient is mandatory to properly assess and manage various shock states. Both noninvasive and invasive monitoring techniques can be used to measure cardiovascular performance in patients and to differentiate the causes of various conditions that result in hypoperfusion and organ dysfunction. The values obtained with hemodynamic monitoring should always be used in conjunction with clinical judgment.

Noninvasive Monitoring

An important part of hemodynamic monitoring in the critically ill patient involves noninvasive measures. Clinical examination and vital signs (temperature, HR, blood pressure [BP], RR) provide valuable information regarding the cardiovascular system and organ perfusion. Other well-established noninvasive techniques for monitoring the hemodynamic status of patients include pulse oximetry (for measuring arterial oxygen saturation [SaO_2]) and transthoracic echocardiography, which can estimate the functional status of the heart and heart valves. Although important, noninvasive measures have limitations, and certain hemodynamic values important for the diagnosis and assessment of illness, as well as the patient's response to therapy, must be measured invasively at the present time.

Invasive Monitoring

ARTERIAL PRESSURE LINE

The arterial line is a common tool in the intensive care unit (ICU). It consists of a small catheter placed into an artery (usually the radial or femoral artery) and attached to a pressure transducer. This allows for continuous measurement of BP and also provides for easy access for arterial blood gas (ABG) samples to be drawn and analyzed. Arterial lines should never be used for medication administration.

CENTRAL VENOUS CATHETER

Common in the ICU, the central venous catheter consists of a large-bore catheter usually inserted into either a subclavian or jugular vein. It can be used for infusion of fluid and medications; when attached to a pressure transducer, it can be used to measure the central venous pressure (CVP), a reflection of right atrial pressure and the volume status of the patient. Central venous catheters that can continuously measure the central venous oxygen saturation ($ScvO_2$) have been developed and are becoming more common in the ICU. These catheters allow for the assessment and monitoring of tissue perfusion and the response to interventions. Low $ScvO_2$ has been associated with worse outcomes in several studies.[5,6] In patients with sepsis, guidelines call

TABLE 22-2
Normal Hemodynamic Values and Derived Indices

	Definition/Equation	Normal Value	Units
Directly Measured			
Blood pressure (BP) [systolic (SBP)/diastolic (DBP)]	Pressure in the central arterial bed, determined by cardiac output and systemic vascular resistance.	120–140/80–90	mm Hg
Cardiac output (CO)	Amount of blood ejected from the left ventricle per minute; determined by stroke volume and heart rate. $CO = SV \times HR$.	4–7	L/min
Central venous pressure (CVP)[a]	Measures mean pressure in right atrium and reflects right ventricular filling pressure and volume status. Primarily determined by venous return to the heart. The goal in most critically ill patients is 8–12 mm Hg.	2–6	mm Hg[a]
Heart rate (HR) (pulse)	Number of myocardial contractions per minute.	60–80	beats/min
Pulmonary artery pressure (PAP) systolic (SPAP)/ diastolic (DPAP)/mean (MPAP)	*Systolic* (SPAP): Measures pulmonary artery pressure during systole; reflects pressure generated by the contraction of the right ventricle. *Diastolic* (DPAP): Measures pulmonary artery pressure during diastole; reflects diastolic filling pressure in the left ventricle. May approximate pulmonary capillary wedge pressure (PCWP); normal gradient <5 mm Hg between DPAP and PCWP.	20–30/8–12	mm Hg
Pulmonary capillary wedge pressure (PCWP)	Measures pressure distal to the pulmonary artery; reflects left ventricular filling pressures (*preload*). Usually lower than or within 5 mm Hg of pulmonary artery diastolic pressure (DPAP).	5–12[c]	mm Hg
Central venous oxygen saturation ($Scvo_2$)	The oxygen saturation of blood returning to the heart.	>70	%
Mixed venous oxygen saturation (Svo_2)	The oxygen saturation of blood in the pulmonary artery.	>65	%
Derived Indices			
Cardiac index (CI)	Cardiac output per square meter of body surface area (BSA[d]). $CI = CO/BSA$	2.5–4.2	$L/min/m^2$
Left ventricular stroke work index (LVSWI)	Amount of work the left ventricle exerts during systole; adjusted for body surface area (BSA). A measure of *contractility*, the inotropic state of the myocardium. $LVSWI = (MAP - PCWP) \times SVI \times 0.0136$	35–85	g/m^2/beat
Mean arterial pressure (MAP)	$MAP = [(2 \times DBP) + SBP]/3$	80–100	mm Hg
Oxygen delivery ($\dot{D}o_2$)	The amount of oxygen delivered by the body per unit time. $\dot{D}o_2 = CO \times Cao_2$ where $Cao_2 = Hgb \times Sao_2 \times 13.9$	700–1,200	mL/min
Oxygen consumption ($\dot{V}o_2$)	The amount of oxygen consumed by the body per unit time. The product of cardiac output and the difference between the arterial and venous oxygen concentration. $\dot{V}o_2 = CO \times (Cao_2 - Cvo_2)$ where $Cvo_2 = Hgb \times Svo_2 \times 13.9$	200–400	mL/min
Perfusion pressure (PP)	The pressure gradient between the coronary arteries and the pressure in either the right atrium or left ventricle during diastole. A major determinant of coronary blood flow and oxygen supply to the heart. $PP = MAP - PCWP$	50	mm Hg
Pulmonary vascular resistance (PVR)	Primary determinant of right ventricular *afterload*. $PVR = [(MPAP - PCWP)/CO] \times 74$	20–120	$dynes \cdot s \cdot cm^{-5}$
Stroke volume (SV)	Amount of blood ejected from the ventricle with each systolic contraction. $SV = CO/HR$	60–130	mL/beat
Stroke volume index (SVI)	Stroke volume adjusted for body surface area. $SVI = SV/BSA$	30–75	$mL/beat/m^2$
Systemic vascular resistance (SVR)	Measure of impedance applied by systemic vascular system to systolic effort of left ventricle; determined by autonomic nervous system and condition of vessels. Determinant of left ventricular *afterload*. $SVR = [(MAP - CVP)/CO] \times 74$	800–1,440	$dyne \cdot s \cdot cm^{-5}$
Systemic vascular resistance index (SVRI)	SVR adjusted for body surface area. $SVRI = SVR \times BSA$	1,680–2,580	$dyne \cdot s \cdot cm^{-5} \cdot m^2$

[a]CVP is essentially synonymous with RAP.
[b]2–6 mm Hg = 3–6 cm H_2O (conversion: 1 mm Hg = 1.34 cm H_2O).
[c]May optimally ↑ PCWP to 16–18 mm Hg in critically ill patients.
[d]BSA, body surface area = 1.7 m^2 (average male).

for a goal CVP of 8 to 12 mm Hg and an $Scvo_2$ of more than 70%.[4]

PULMONARY ARTERY CATHETER

The introduction of flow-directed, balloon flotation pulmonary artery (PA) catheters by Swan and colleagues[7] (Swan-Ganz catheter) in the 1970s represented a major advance in invasive bedside hemodynamic monitoring. The PA catheter enables clinicians to assess both right and left intracardiac pressures, determine CO, and obtain mixed venous blood samples. These capabilities allow one to evaluate volume status and ventricular performance, derive hemodynamic indices, and determine systemic $\dot{D}o_2$ and $\dot{V}o_2$. There are several versions of the PA catheter. Some include additional lumens for intravenous (IV) infusions, temporary transvenous pacing, and continuous monitoring of Svo_2. Catheters are available that can measure CO on a continuous basis. The essential components for hemodynamic monitoring are incorporated in the standard quadruple-lumen catheter pictured in Figure 22-2. This catheter is composed of multiple lumens, each terminating at different points along the catheter. When properly positioned, the proximal port (C) terminates in the right atrium and is used to measure right atrial pressure, to inject fluid for CO determination, and to administer IV fluids. The distal port (B), which terminates at the tip of the catheter (E), is positioned in the pulmonary artery beyond the pulmonary valve and is used to measure pulmonary artery and pulmonary capillary wedge pressure (PCWP; described below) and to obtain mixed venous blood samples. Intermittent inflation of the balloon is accomplished by inserting 1.5 mL of air into the balloon inflation valve (D). The thermistor (A) contains a temperature probe and electrical leads that connect to a computer, which calculates CO by the thermodilution technique.

Although the PA catheter is confined to the pulmonary vasculature, left ventricular (LV) pressure can be ascertained from the PCWP. When the balloon is inflated, the PA catheter advances to a pulmonary artery branch of equal diameter and becomes lodged or "wedged" in this position. Because forward flow from the right ventricle ceases beyond the wedged PA segment, a static fluid column exists between the LV and PA catheter tip during diastole when the mitral valve is open. If no pressure gradients are present in the pulmonary vasculature beyond the balloon and if mitral valve function is normal, the PCWP then equilibrates with all distal pressures and thus indirectly reflects left ventricular end-diastolic pressure (LVEDP). Based on the relationship between pressure and volume, the LVEDP is equivalent to the left ventricular end-diastolic volume (LVEDV), which is also known as *preload*.

The use of PA catheters is not without potential complications. Arrhythmias, thrombotic events, infections, and, very rarely, PA rupture have been reported. Several recent trials have called into question the routine use of PA catheters. A meta-analysis of 13 randomized, controlled trials involving 5,051 patients found that the use of the PA catheter did not have a significant effect on mortality or number of days in the hospital.[8] The use of the catheter was associated with a higher use of inotropic agents and IV vasodilators. The trials included in the analysis excluded patients in whom the catheter was thought to be required for treatment. An international consensus conference recommends against the routine placement of the PA catheter in patients with shock.[3] More studies are needed to determine the value of PA catheter data–driven treatment protocols. Because hypotension alone is not required to define shock, the presence of inadequate tissue perfusion on physical examination is more important than the numbers obtained by invasive monitoring.[3] The use of PA catheters has been decreasing in the ICU as newer and less invasive technologies become available. In most situations, the PA catheter is reserved for those patients who specifically require the monitoring of PA pressures, such as patients with pulmonary hypertension or after cardiac surgery.[4]

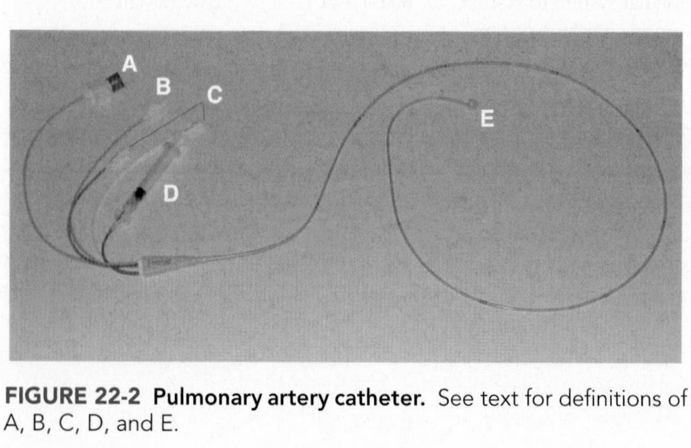

FIGURE 22-2 Pulmonary artery catheter. See text for definitions of A, B, C, D, and E.

OTHER MONITORING TOOLS

New technologies to monitor a patient's perfusion status are being developed. End-tidal carbon dioxide monitors are used to determine $\dot{V}o_2$ and help guide therapies designed to improve $\dot{D}o_2$ and $\dot{V}o_2$. New devices that can measure CO and tissue perfusion noninvasively (or minimally invasively), such as gastric tonometry, esophageal Doppler monitoring, thoracic bioimpedance, and others, have been developed,[9,10] Devices (PulseCO, PiCCO, LiDCO) that can measure CO by pulse wave analysis are seeing increased use in ICUs as an alternative to the PA catheter, which has been the standard for many years.[10,11]

The effective interpretation and management of hemodynamic parameters requires a thorough understanding of the physiologic determinants of CO and arterial pressure. Assuming oxygen content of blood is adequate, CO and systemic vascular resistance (SVR) are the ultimate determinants of $\dot{D}o_2$ and adequate arterial pressure, and thus overall tissue perfusion. As outlined in Figure 22-1, CO may be quantified as the product of stroke volume (SV) and HR. SV is determined by preload, afterload, and contractility. The effects of these factors on hemodynamic parameters are interrelated and complex and must be assessed carefully when selecting therapeutic interventions that will produce the desired response. A good review of the determinants of cardiac performance is found in Chapter 19, Heart Failure. Table 22-2 and the Glossary provide definitions of terms and normal hemodynamic indices.

ETIOLOGIC CLASSIFICATION OF SHOCK AND COMMON MECHANISMS

The most common clinical conditions associated with the major forms of shock are reviewed in the subsequent sections and detailed in Table 22-1. The pathogenesis, epidemiology, and clinical and hemodynamic manifestations for each classification are briefly discussed and further illustrated in case studies throughout the chapter. Table 22-3 describes the common hemodynamic findings for the various forms of shock.

HYPOVOLEMIC SHOCK

Shock secondary to a reduction in intravascular volume is referred to as *hypovolemic shock*. Whether the primary insult is the external loss of fluid volume (e.g., blood, plasma, or free

TABLE 22-3
Hemodynamic Findings in Various Shock States

	Hypovolemic	Cardiogenic	Distributive (Septic)
Heart rate	↑	↑	↑
Blood pressure[a]	↓	↑/↓	↓
Cardiac output	↓	↓	↓[b]
Preload (PCWP)	↓	↑	↑/↓
Afterload (SVR)	↑	↑	↓

[a]Patients may be in a state of compensated shock in which blood pressure is normal but clinical signs of hypoperfusion are evident.
[b]Cardiac output is increased early in sepsis but can be decreased in late or severe sepsis.
PCWP, pulmonary capillary wedge pressure; SVR, systemic vascular resistance.

water) or the internal sequestration of these fluids into body cavities (third spacing), the overall result is reduced venous return (decreases in CVP and PCWP) and decreased CO (Table 22-3). The severity of hypovolemic shock depends on the amount and rate of intravascular volume loss and each person's capacity for compensation. Although responses vary, a healthy person may tolerate an acute loss of as much as 30% of his or her intravascular volume with minimal clinical signs and symptoms.[12] Compensatory mechanisms such as increases in HR, myocardial contractility, and SVR are sufficiently effective for this loss in volume such that measurable falls in SBP are not detected. Losses in excess of 80% generally overwhelm compensatory mechanisms, and the patient's condition can deteriorate to overt shock with hypotension and signs of hypoperfusion. If restorative measures are not taken immediately, irreversible shock and death may result. The most common and dramatic cause of hypovolemic shock is hemorrhagic shock in which intravascular volume depletion occurs as a result of bleeding. Trauma is responsible for most cases of acute hemorrhagic shock; other significant causes are rupture of vascular aneurysms, acute gastrointestinal (GI) bleeding, ruptured ectopic pregnancy, and postoperative bleeding. Other mechanisms for hypovolemic shock are conditions associated with either excess fluid losses from GI or renal sources or plasma loss caused by burns or sequestration (also known as third-space accumulation).

Acute Hemorrhagic Shock

CASE 22-1

QUESTION 1: B.A. is a 55-year-old man brought to the emergency department (ED) after being stabbed in the abdomen; he had significant blood loss at the scene. On arrival, he is confused and oriented only to person. His skin is pale and cool, with vital signs showing an HR of 125 beats/minute, SBP of 85 mm Hg, and an RR of 30 breaths/minute. Describe the physiologic changes in B.A. in response to his injury. What are the goals of resuscitation in patients with hemorrhagic shock?

B.A. has lost a significant amount of intravascular fluid directly from his stab wound and also from traumatic tissue edema. He is hypotensive with a compensatory increase in both HR and RR. His pale, cool skin indicates shunting of blood from the periphery to maintain perfusion of vital organs. Based on his clinical presentation, B.A. is in decompensated shock.

The major hemodynamic abnormality in hypovolemic shock is decreased venous return (preload) to the heart, resulting in a decrease in CO. $\dot{D}O_2$ to the tissues is reduced from this and from the loss of oxygen-carrying hemoglobin. The physiologic response of the body to a sudden decrease in volume (preload) is a release of catecholamines (epinephrine, norepinephrine). The subsequent increase in HR and contractility help maintain CO. The peripheral vasoconstriction caused by the sympathomimetic response serves to maintain arterial pressure. In addition, fluid shifts from the interstitial spaces into the vasculature to increase preload. These responses are effective at maintaining BP in patients with a loss of up to approximately 30% of the total blood volume. B.A.'s increased HR and signs of peripheral vasoconstriction are consistent with these compensatory changes. His SBP is still low, however, and he has signs of decreased perfusion to his brain, manifested by confusion and disorientation. Given the severity of his condition, if intravascular losses are not rapidly replaced, myocardial dysfunction may ensue and lead to irreversible shock.

The goals of resuscitation of patients in hypovolemic shock are the correction of inadequate tissue perfusion and oxygenation, and limiting secondary insults. HR, BP, and urine output have been traditional markers for the adequacy of resuscitation, but reliance on these end points alone is acceptable only in the initial management of hemorrhagic shock. One concern is that patients may persist in a state of compensated shock even after these parameters are normalized.[13,14] Ongoing deficiencies in $\dot{D}O_2$ to vital organs may progress, and if left untreated, organ dysfunction and death may result. Measurement of base (bicarbonate) deficit and lactate levels can be used to assess the global adequacy of perfusion by tracking trends ensuring that the levels are decreasing. Metabolic acidosis can signal that resuscitation is incomplete despite normal vital signs.

TREATMENT

CHOICE OF FLUID IN HYPOVOLEMIC SHOCK

CASE 22-1, QUESTION 2: Is an IV saline solution adequate to compensate for B.A.'s blood loss? What other type of fluid might be better to resuscitate this patient?

Once an adequate airway is established and initial vital signs are obtained, the most important therapeutic intervention in hypovolemic shock is the infusion of IV fluids. Initially, crystalloids or colloids are used to restore blood volume as blood products may not be immediately available and are frequently unnecessary to manage mild shock (10%–20% blood loss).

CRYSTALLOIDS VERSUS COLLOIDS

Crystalloids are isotonic solutions that contain either saline (0.9% sodium chloride; "normal saline") or a saline equivalent (lactated Ringer's [LR] solution). *Colloidal solutions* contain large oncotically active molecules that are derived from natural products such as proteins (albumin), carbohydrates (dextrans, starches), and animal collagen (gelatin) (Table 22-4).

The choice of a crystalloid versus a colloid solution to restore blood volume in hemorrhagic shock is controversial. The controversy primarily involves the ultimate distribution of these fluids in the extracellular compartment, which, in turn, depends on their composition. Isotonic solutions (normal saline or LR solution) freely distribute within the extracellular fluid compartment, which is divided between the interstitial and intravascular spaces at a ratio of 3:1. This distribution is determined by the net forces of colloid oncotic pressure (COP) and hydrostatic pressure, both inside and outside the capillary vascular space. Consequently, large volumes of crystalloid fluid are required to expand the intravascular space during resuscitation. In contrast, intact capillary membranes are relatively impermeable to colloids and, therefore, colloids effectively expand the intravascular space with

TABLE 22-4
Composition and Properties of Crystalloids

Solution	Sodium (mEq/L)	Chloride (mEq/L)	Potassium (mEq/L)	Calcium (mEq/L)	Magnesium (mEq/L)	Lactate (mEq/L)	Tonicity Relative to Plasma	Osmolarity (mosm/L)
5% Dextrose	0	0	0	0	0	0	Isotonic	253
0.9% Sodium chloride	154	154	0	0	0	0	Isotonic	308
Plasma-Lyte (Baxter)	140	103	10	5	3	8	Isotonic	312
Lactated Ringer's	130	109	4	3	0	28	Isotonic	273
7.5% Sodium chloride	1,283	1,283	0	0	0	0	Hypertonic	2,567

little loss into the interstitium. Comparatively smaller volumes of colloids than of crystalloids are thus required for resuscitation, and because these large molecules persist intravascularly, their duration of action is longer. It is often thought that three to four times as much volume of crystalloid is necessary to provide the same degree of volume expansion as obtained from a colloid. Many of the colloidal agents, however, can cause allergic or hypersensitivity reactions as well as coagulopathic effects, and colloids are much more expensive than crystalloids.

Proponents of crystalloids argue that both intravascular and interstitial fluids are depleted in hypovolemic shock because of the rapid shifts between the extracellular compartments. Volume replacement of both fluid spaces is best accomplished by using crystalloids. In addition, loss of capillary integrity in shock can cause the leak of larger molecules (e.g., the colloidal proteins) into the interstitium. This increase in the oncotic pressure in the interstitium would favor fluid movement out of the vascular space into the tissues, with resultant edema.

Proponents of colloids contend that resuscitation with these solutions more rapidly and effectively restores intravascular volume after acute hemorrhage. For a given infusion volume, colloidal solutions (e.g., albumin) will expand the intravascular space two to four times more than crystalloids. Because a larger volume of crystalloid would have to be infused to restore the vascular space, the risk of developing pulmonary edema may be higher. It is also argued that large volumes of crystalloids will further dilute the plasma proteins, resulting in a decrease in the COP, which can also promote the development of pulmonary edema. This concept is based on Starling's law of capillary forces governing fluid movement, which in the pulmonary vessel wall is determined by the COP–PCWP gradient (i.e., the net force generated by the colloid oncotic pressure minus the pulmonary hydrostatic pressure [PCWP]). The normal COP is 25 mm Hg and an average PCWP is 12 mm Hg; thus, a net intravascular force of 13 mm Hg favors fluid retention in the vascular space. In critically ill patients, a COP–PCWP gradient less than 6 mm Hg is thought to be associated with a higher incidence of pulmonary edema. Despite these theoretical differences, clinical studies comparing colloids with crystalloids have failed to show any differences in the development of pulmonary edema. Research suggests that certain subgroups may be at greater risk for the development of pulmonary edema, but considerable variance remains because of differences in physiologic end points, criteria for assessing pulmonary edema, and the extent of shock.

In an effort to find a consensus among the results of divergent clinical trials, numerous meta-analyses have been performed comparing resuscitation with crystalloids or colloids. Two earlier meta-analyses concluded that resuscitation of burn and trauma patients with colloids result in increased mortality.[15,16] The explanation offered for the detrimental effect of colloids is that trauma and burns cause an increase in pulmonary capillary and vascular permeability, resulting in extravasation of the colloid into the interstitium, which further worsens the effective vascular volume and pulmonary edema. The Cochrane Database analysis found that albumin was associated with an overall higher risk of death, whereas the most recent meta-analysis funded by the Plasma Protein Therapeutics Association did not find an increase in mortality in any patient group, including trauma.[17,18] It is important to recognize that several limitations to these meta-analyses exist because of differences in study inclusion criteria (heterogeneity), differences in fluid management, and dosages of albumin used. What is known is the difference in cost per therapy. One study determined the secondary cost-effectiveness analysis per therapy, which revealed that the cost of using crystalloids was $43.13 per life saved, as opposed to $1,493.60 per life saved with colloid.[17] These estimates were based on an average per-patient intake of 6.57 L of fluid for the crystalloid group, at a cost of $5.95/L, and an average of 230 g of albumin in the colloid group, at a cost of $5.00/g.

Recent evidence supports the idea that albumin may not be as detrimental as once thought. The SAFE trial is the largest randomized, prospective trial to evaluate albumin versus normal saline solution resuscitation in the critically ill.[19] The primary end point was 28-day mortality, which was not statistically different for albumin compared with normal saline solution. Also, no statistical differences were identified in any of the predetermined subgroups (trauma, adult respiratory distress syndrome [ARDS], severe sepsis), although a trend was seen toward increased mortality in the trauma patients who received albumin, most specifically in patients with head trauma. Because resuscitation with albumin was not found to be better than saline solution, this landmark trial will most likely alter perceptions of albumin; whether or not this trial will have an impact on albumin prescribing practices remains to be determined.

Given the lack of evidence for a significant clinical difference between crystalloids and colloids and the greater expense of using albumin, the guidelines for the use of resuscitation fluids developed by the University Hospital Consortium, a nonprofit alliance of US academic medical centers, remain unchanged.[20] For the resuscitation of hemorrhagic shock, crystalloids should be the initial fluid of choice. The American College of Surgeons Advanced Trauma Life Support course[12] also recommends the rapid infusion of isotonic crystalloids for the initial fluid resuscitation of trauma patients. Thus, use of either normal saline or LR solution would be appropriate for B.A. Albumin is not needed and blood should only be used if there is ongoing blood loss demonstrated by a decreasing hematocrit or hemoglobin.

CRYSTALLOIDS

CASE 22-1, QUESTION 3: A large-bore IV catheter is inserted into B.A.'s arm and STAT blood samples are sent for type and crossmatch, complete blood count (CBC), prothrombin time (PT), partial thromboplastin time (PTT), and serum chemistry (blood urea nitrogen [BUN], creatinine [SCr], Na, K, Cl, and bicarbonate). Warmed LR solution (2 L) is infused rapidly, and the operating room is notified. B.A.'s

SBP has increased to 90 mm Hg, but the bleeding has not stopped. A Foley catheter is inserted to measure urine output. LR is continued, with 500- to 1,000-mL boluses ordered to be given to maintain hemodynamic stability while waiting for fully crossmatched blood. Are the doses of LR given to B.A. appropriate? What clinical and objective parameters should be monitored to determine the success of fluid replacement?

Volume Requirements

Isotonic crystalloids equilibrate rapidly between the interstitial and intravascular spaces at a ratio of 3:1. For every liter of fluid infused, approximately 750 mL will pass into the interstitium, whereas 250 mL will remain in the plasma. Based on estimated blood loss, the "three-to-one rule" may be applied as a general guideline: for each 1 mL of blood loss, 3 mL of crystalloid is infused. Because this determination of blood loss is based solely on clinical assessment and not on quantitative measurements, treatment is best directed by the response to initial therapy rather than the initial classification. Close observation of hemodynamic status with consideration of the patient's age, particular injury, and prehospital fluid therapy is essential to avoid inadequate or excessive fluid administration.

A safe and effective approach for using crystalloids in the resuscitation of patients in hemorrhagic shock is to give 1 to 2 L of fluid as an initial bolus as rapidly as possible for an adult or 20 mL/kg for a pediatric patient.[12] Additional fluid boluses may be necessary, depending on the patient's response. Between boluses, fluids are slowed to maintenance rates (150–200 mL/hour), with ongoing evaluation of the patient's physiologic response for signs of continued blood loss or inadequate perfusion that would indicate the need for additional volume replacement. The fluid boluses given to B.A. are an appropriate initial measure, then assessment of his level of perfusion is vital to determining the need for additional boluses.

Indications that circulation is improving include normalization of BP, pulse pressure, and HR. Signs that actual organ perfusion is normalizing and that fluid resuscitation is adequate include improvements in mental status, warmth and color of skin, improved acid–base balance, and increased urinary output. The minimal acceptable urine output for a patient is 0.5 mL/kg. Persistent metabolic acidosis in a normothermic shock patient usually indicates the need for additional fluid resuscitation; sodium bicarbonate is not recommended unless the pH is less than 7.2.[12] Serum lactate and base deficit are important values to monitor to determine that the patient is receiving adequate resuscitation. As perfusion improves, lactate and base deficit will decrease; thus, the actual values are not as important as the trend. It is important to note that resuscitation is not defined by just one value or number, such as BP, but the constellation of indicators of overall perfusion.

LACTATED RINGER'S VERSUS NORMAL SALINE

CASE 22-1, QUESTION 4: Is there an advantage to using LR solution versus normal saline solution?

The American College of Surgeons Committee on Trauma recommends LR solution as the fluid of choice for the initial resuscitation of trauma patients and normal saline solution as the second choice.[12] Because normal saline solution has a high chloride content (45 mEq more than LR), it can cause hyperchloremic acidosis, thereby worsening the tissue acidosis that occurs in the setting of hypovolemic shock. This likelihood is increased with impaired renal function. LR, in contrast, is a buffered solution designed to simulate the intravascular plasma electrolyte concentration. It contains 28 mEq/L of lactate, which is metabolized to bicarbonate in patients with normal circulation and intact liver function. In situations in which hepatic perfusion is reduced (20% of normal) or hepatocellular damage is present, lactate clearance may be significantly decreased, particularly in combination with hypoxia (Sao_2 50% of normal).[21] In patients with shock and those having cardiopulmonary bypass during surgery, the half-life of lactate, normally 20 minutes, increases to 4 to 6 hours and 8 hours, respectively. Because unmetabolized lactate can be converted to lactic acid, prolonged infusion of LR could cause tissue acidosis in predisposed patients. In actuality, however, no differences in serum pH, electrolytes, lactate, or survival have been found in patients with hemorrhagic trauma who have received either LR or normal saline solution. In practice, normal saline and LR solutions typically are used interchangeably because neither solution appears to be superior to the other.

Hypertonic Saline

CASE 22-1, QUESTION 5: What is the role of hypertonic saline (HS) solution in the setting of hemorrhagic shock?

The use of HS solution (with and without dextran) for resuscitation in hemorrhagic shock has been studied extensively in animal models,[22–24] and has been the focus of clinical research.[25–27] The advantage of HS solution as a resuscitative fluid is the smaller volume of fluid required to expand the intravascular compartment compared with isotonic solutions. This could be a particular advantage in the prehospital setting (e.g., field rescue by emergency medical technicians) given the large volumes of fluids necessary to keep up with ongoing blood loss.

With a high concentration of sodium, HS solution exerts an osmotic effect, translocating fluid from the interstitial and cellular compartments to the intravascular space. Consequently, plasma volume is rapidly expanded to a greater extent than similar volumes of crystalloid solutions, and systemic BP, CO, and $\dot{D}o_2$ are readily increased. HS solution also improves myocardial contractility, causes peripheral vasodilation, and redistributes blood flow preferentially to the splanchnic and renal circulations. In addition, intracranial pressure is reduced, which may be a potential advantage in trauma patients with concomitant head injury.[22–27]

Hypertonic saline–dextran (7.5% sodium chloride in 6% dextran 70 [HSD]) solution was compared with isotonic crystalloid solution for prehospital resuscitation in a multicenter trial of hypotensive trauma patients.[26] Patients were randomly assigned to receive 250 mL of either HSD or a standard isotonic solution, after which fluids were given as necessary to achieve stabilization. No differences in overall survival were noted; however, a significant survival advantage was seen in the HSD group requiring surgery. Fewer complications occurred in the HSD group, including a lower incidence of ARDS, renal failure, and coagulopathy. Although serum sodium levels were significantly higher in the HSD group, no adverse clinical symptoms of hypernatremia were seen.

In a similar trial, the effects of resuscitation with 250-mL volumes of HS (7.5%), HSD, or normal saline solution were compared in trauma patients admitted to the ED in hypovolemic shock.[27] Differences in overall mortality or complication rates in the three groups were not significant. In comparison with isotonic saline solution, however, the hypertonic solutions significantly improved MAP and significantly decreased the volume of fluid required to restore SBP.

Studies with HS solution suggest that it may help to reduce multiple organ system failure and infections after traumatic injury. The mechanism has yet to be fully elucidated, but in animal models, HS solution reduces neutrophil margination,[28] which may play a role in the development of lung injury, ARDS, and reperfusion injury. In another study, the use of HS solution resulted in a decreased susceptibility to sepsis and improved survival in a murine model of hemorrhagic shock.[29]

These clinical trials suggest that HS solution may be safe and effective for the initial resuscitation of hemorrhagic shock and may help prevent the development of posttraumatic multiple system organ failure and sepsis. Despite these positive findings, HS solutions are not widely used.

BLOOD REPLACEMENT

CASE 22-1, QUESTION 6: B.A. has received 3 L of LR solution to maintain hemodynamic stability. His current vital signs are BP, 92/60 mm Hg; HR, 115 beats/minute; and RR, 28 breaths/minute. He is still confused and is becoming more agitated and combative. Urine output has been only 10 mL in the past 30 minutes. Laboratory results include the following:

Hematocrit, 23% (down from 27%)
Hemoglobin, 7.6 g/dL (down from 9 g/dL)
pH, 7.18
P_{CO_2}, 35 mm Hg
P_{O_2}, 110 mm Hg
HCO_3^-, 17 mEq/L

Two units of packed red blood cells (PRBCs) are now available, and B.A. is being prepared for the operating room. Describe the current status of B.A.'s resuscitation and the need for blood products.

B.A. is still exhibiting signs of inadequate tissue perfusion. Although his BP has improved and his HR has decreased, his mental status has declined, urine output has been negligible, and his ABG indicates metabolic acidosis. B.A. has not been adequately resuscitated from his hemorrhage, is still actively bleeding, and should receive available blood at this point.

The prior conventional approach to the transfusion of critically ill patients was to maintain the hemoglobin greater than 10 g/dL or the hematocrit greater than 30%. This transfusion trigger was found to be detrimental in a population of mixed medical-surgical ICU patients compared with a group of patients who were maintained at a lower hemoglobin of 7 g/dL and therefore received fewer transfusions. This lower hemoglobin level may be appropriate for critically ill patients who are in an ICU and have decreased hematocrit values because of fluid resuscitation and daily blood draws, but not for a patient who is actively bleeding as evidenced by the falling hemoglobin and hematocrit and signs of underperfusion. In acute hemorrhage, the actual degree of blood loss is not accurately reflected by the hemoglobin and hematocrit values, and it also does not take into account the body's ability to compensate for the loss of oxygen-carrying capacity. Because it takes at least 24 hours for all fluid compartments to come to equilibrium, a normal hematocrit (or hemoglobin concentration) in the setting of hemorrhagic shock does not rule out significant blood loss or indicate adequacy of transfusion. Only when equilibrium has been reached can these measures be used reliably to gauge blood loss. On the other hand, if cardiopulmonary function is normal and if volume status is maintained, an increase in CO can compensate for a reduction in hemoglobin (O_2 content) to a certain degree (Fig. 22-1).

Because inadequacy of tissue perfusion, and hence $\dot{D}o_2$, is the primary abnormality in shock, the need for transfusion therapy is more accurately determined by the patient's oxygen demand, rather than an arbitrary hematocrit or hemoglobin value. Calculation of $\dot{D}o_2$ and $\dot{V}o_2$ can be used to determine the adequacy of perfusion. Although these values can be determined by use of a PA catheter and arterial and venous blood samples, for practical purposes, the patient's response to initial fluid resuscitation and clinical signs of inadequate tissue perfusion are the primary determinants for blood transfusion. Patients who are not acutely bleeding and who do not respond to initial volume resuscitation or who transiently respond but remain tachycardic, tachypneic, and oliguric clearly are underperfused and will likely require blood transfusion. Trauma patients who have acute bleeding issues or who demonstrate signs of underperfusion should be considered for transfusion much sooner; thus, B.A. should receive a transfusion.

ADVERSE EFFECTS OF TRANSFUSION

CASE 22-1, QUESTION 7: After the transfusion, B.A. has a serum potassium concentration of 4.8 mEq/L compared with 4.5 mEq/L before the transfusion. Could this be a result of the blood product? Is B.A. also at risk for contracting human immunodeficiency virus or viral hepatitis from his transfusion of PRBCs?

Possible risks of blood transfusions include electrolyte abnormalities, hemolytic reactions, transmission of infectious disease, coagulopathies, and immunosuppression. Banked blood is stored with a citrate anticoagulant additive. With multiple transfusions, the large amount of citrate can cause hypocalcemia and acid–base abnormalities. Hyperkalemia also can occur because transfusion of stored blood causes the release of potassium from hemolyzed (ruptured) red blood cells. Hemolytic transfusion reactions are the most common cause of acute fatalities from blood transfusions. Astute recognition of the signs and symptoms of a transfusion reaction, such as anxiety, pain at infusion site, fever, hypotension, tachycardia, hemolysis, and hemoglobinuria, can prevent unnecessary morbidity and mortality. Transfusions can also cause acute lung injury owing to recipient neutrophil priming by reactive lipid products from the red blood cell membrane, which causes capillary endothelial damage in the lungs. The increase in serum potassium observed in B.A. may be from the blood product or it may simply reflect hemolysis of blood cells in the test tube after the blood draw. In either case, the measured serum concentration of 4.8 mEq/L is not sufficiently high to be of concern. It is unlikely that a true hemolytic reaction is occurring.

Blood products and donors are screened for disease; thus, transmission of viral illness is a small risk. It is estimated that the transmission of hepatitis C is 1:1,149,000, and human immunodeficiency virus is 1:1,467,000.[30] Hemostatic abnormalities, specifically coagulopathies and thrombocytopenia, may be transiently related to dilution from administration of large volumes of crystalloids, colloids, or banked blood, but are more likely caused by the extent of injury and the development of disseminated intravascular coagulopathy (DIC). Banked whole blood contains sufficient coagulation factors (including labile factors V and VIII) to maintain hemostasis during the life span of the unit; however, it does not contain platelets because they do not survive the temperatures required for red blood cell storage.

Immunosuppression has also been associated with blood transfusions as evidenced by enhanced graft survival in renal transplant recipients, tumor recurrence in patients with colorectal carcinoma, and postoperative infections. The immunosuppression from transfusion is multifactorial, but it is most likely caused by the infusion of donor white blood cells (WBCs), which create a competition between the donor and recipient leukocytes. This mechanism is not, however, the only cause because immunosuppression is associated with autologous blood transfusions as well as the infusion of plasma alone.

Because of the limited supply and potential adverse effects associated with blood, research is under way to develop blood substitutes. The ideal agent would have a longer shelf life, a reduced risk of disease transmission, and less risk of transfusion reactions. The agents in various stages of clinical research include the modified hemoglobins and the perfluorocarbons. The exact role the blood substitutes would play in transfusions is unclear, and problems have occurred, such as short half-life and vasoconstriction associated with some of the products thus far. No agents have yet been approved, but research is continuing.

Postoperative Hypovolemia

HYPOVOLEMIA VERSUS PUMP FAILURE

CASE 22-1, QUESTION 8: B.A. goes to the operating room, and his surgeons find several colonic tears that require a colon resection. He has been admitted to the ICU after surgery, and is intubated and receiving 60% oxygen. His ABGs are adequate, and he is receiving 150 mL/hour of LR solution IV. His initial postoperative and 2-hour postoperative hemodynamic profiles are as follows (initial parameters in parentheses):

BP (S/D [diastolic]/MAP), 90/50/63 mm Hg (110/70/68 mm Hg)
Pulse, 90 beats/minute (84 beats/minute)
CO, 3 L/minute (4.5 L/minute)
CVP, 6 mm Hg (10 mm Hg)
Urine output, 25 mL/hour (70 mL/hour)
Temperature, 37.9°C (35°C)
Hematocrit, 32% (30%)

From the hemodynamic profile, determine whether B.A. is hypovolemic or experiencing pump failure after his surgery.

Most of B.A.'s hemodynamic changes are consistent with hypovolemia. These include a drop in BP, CVP, CO, and urine output. The decrease in CVP suggests that preload is reduced, resulting in a lower CO. Urine output has declined and probably reflects a compensatory drop in renal perfusion to preserve intravascular volume. The pulse pressure is narrowed, suggesting blood flow has decreased. (Changes in pulse pressure correlate with changes in SV in individual patients; that is, as SV decreases pulse pressure narrows.) B.A.'s HR did not increase by that much, but it is unclear whether he was taking any medications before his injury, such as a β-blocker. As the body temperature rises postoperatively, vasodilation decreases SVR and increases the intravascular space. If intravascular volume is inadequate and increased sympathetic tone cannot generate a sufficient CO, mean BP falls. The most likely explanation for the hemodynamic change in B.A. is hypovolemia, although he also should be evaluated for the occurrence of a perioperative cardiac event. His ABG should be checked to assess oxygen requirements.

CAUSES

CASE 22-1, QUESTION 9: What are the most likely causes of hypovolemia in B.A.?

Common causes of hypovolemia in surgical patients are postoperative bleeding, third spacing, and temperature-related vasodilation. Postoperative bleeding can produce hypovolemia; however, B.A.'s initial and 2-hour postoperative hematocrit of 30% and 32%, respectively, do not support bleeding as a cause.

After major vascular or bowel surgery, it is not unusual for patients to third space significant amounts of intravascular volume. The bowel walls and interstitial space can sequester large amounts of fluids, and this can produce a state of relative hypovolemia as is occurring with B.A. This is especially apparent for the first 12 to 24 hours after the surgical procedure. B.A. is receiving 150 mL/hour of LR solution, but this is apparently not sufficient to maintain his intravascular volume.

Mild hypothermia is common during operative procedures. As patients warm up postoperatively, vasodilation occurs, expanding the intravascular space. If the amounts of IV fluids administered are insufficient to compensate for the increased venous capacitance, BP and CO will decline during the rewarming phase, which can range from 1 to 6 hours. B.A. has rewarmed from 34°C to 37°C in 2 hours, which is not unusual after a major operative procedure. His temperature could conceivably rise to as high as 38°C to 38.5°C during the first 12 to 24 hours after surgery.

Other considerations include inadequate fluid administration during the operative procedure and the effects of drugs given in the operating room or in the immediate postoperative period (e.g., morphine sulfate and other narcotics) that have systemic vasodilatory properties.

VOLUME REPLACEMENT AND VENTRICULAR FUNCTION

CASE 22-1, QUESTION 10: How will volume replacement improve B.A.'s CO and perfusion pressure?

The Frank-Starling mechanism indicates that the volume of blood returned to the heart is the main determinant of volume pumped by the heart. Therefore, as venous return is increased, the CO also will increase within physiologic limits (Fig. 22-1). As B.A. does not have a PA catheter to measure PCWP, the best indicator of preload, the CVP, which provides an estimate of volume status, can be used to assess venous return and volume status.

A ventricular function curve can be constructed by plotting a measure of cardiac pumping action (CO, SV, or LV stroke work index) against a measure of preload. A change in preload moves the ventricular output upward or downward along a given curve (Fig. 22-3). Two hours after surgery, B.A.'s CVP has fallen from 10 to 6 mm Hg and his CO has fallen from 4.5 to 3 L/minute. Therefore, additional volume replacement is warranted.

CASE 22-1, QUESTION 11: B.A. is given a 500-mL bolus of normal saline solution in 10 minutes, and this results in the following hemodynamic profile:

BP (S/D/M), 96/60/71 mm Hg
Pulse, 84 beats/minute
CO, 3.5 L/minute
CVP, 10 mm Hg

Assess B.A.'s response to the fluid challenge (see Table 22-2 for normal values).

According to the Frank-Starling curve, a small change in preload in response to a volume challenge with a minimal change in CO represents a ventricle on the flat portion of the ventricular function curve (Fig. 22-3). Additional fluid therapy given to these patients can increase their risk for pulmonary edema

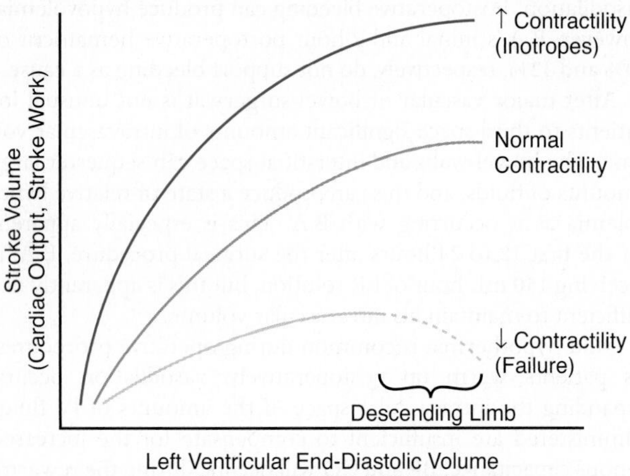

FIGURE 22-3 Ventricular function (Frank-Starling) curve. In the normal heart, as preload (left ventricular end-diastolic pressure [LVEDP]), measured clinically by pulmonary capillary wedge pressure (PCWP), increases, stroke volume (cardiac output, stroke work) increases until the contractile fibers reach their capacity, at which point the curve flattens. A change in contractility causes the heart to perform on a different curve. If the contractile fibers exceed their capacity, as with severe heart failure, the heart will operate on the descending limb of the curve.

without improving CO. In contrast, a large change in preload in response to a fluid challenge with a significant increase in CO represents a ventricle on the steep portion of the curve. In B.A., the change in CVP from 6 to 10 mm Hg and the increase in CO show that he is still responsive to fluid; thus, it is reasonable to administer more fluid to enhance CO and renal perfusion.

FLUID CHALLENGE

CASE 22-1, QUESTION 12: One hour after the 500-mL normal saline solution bolus, B.A.'s hemodynamic profile returns to his postoperative state. ABGs are acceptable, and LR solution is being infused at 200 mL/hour. B.A. is continuing to third space intravascular volume. Based on this information, develop guidelines for additional fluid challenges in B.A.

Acceptable guidelines for administering additional fluid challenges to hypovolemic patients are based on the direction and degree of change in the various hemodynamic parameters in response to a fluid load rather than to their absolute values. These include the CVP (PCWP if available), CO, and BP. Using the CVP as a guide, an increase in the CVP of 5 mm Hg after a 250- to 500-mL fluid challenge in 10 minutes implies the LV is still functioning on the steep portion of the volume–pressure curve. If the CVP rises abruptly as fluid is given, with a small change in CO, the flat portion of the ventricular function curve has been reached and the IV infusion rate should be slowed. If signs and symptoms of inadequate tissue perfusion fail to improve or worsen and if the CVP remains greater than 10 to 14 mm Hg, fluid challenges should be stopped and inotropic therapy initiated.

Generally, most critically ill patients require a cardiac index (CI) of more than 2.5 L/minute/m^2 and a PCWP of 10 to 18 mm Hg, or a CVP of 8 to 14 mm Hg to maintain an acceptable MAP of 65 to 75 mm Hg. A downward trend in the lactate and base deficit and the change in hemodynamic parameters as well as vital signs and urine output should serve as appropriate indicators for whether additional fluid is required.

ALBUMIN AND HETASTARCH

CASE 22-1, QUESTION 13: B.A. has received a total of 3.5 L of normal saline solution in boluses during the past 6 hours and remains hemodynamically unchanged. His urine output has averaged 25 mL/hour for the past 4 hours, indicating volume replacement is inadequate. Given his age and the lack of response to initial crystalloid administration, the decision is made to infuse a colloid solution. How does hetastarch compare with human serum albumin as a volume expander for B.A., and which agent should be used?

Albumin, the predominant protein in the plasma, accounts for approximately 80% of the COP,[31] the force that maintains fluid in the intravascular space. Human serum albumin is the colloidal agent against which all others are compared for volume-expanding properties. It is prepared commercially from pooled donor plasma that is heat-treated to eliminate the potential for disease transmission. On infusion, 5% albumin increases plasma volume by approximately half the volume infused, with an initial duration of action of 16 hours.[31] Substantial side effects primarily involve transient clotting abnormalities and anaphylactic reactions (0.5%), both of which are rare.[23] The anaphylactoid reaction is caused by the pasteurization process, causing albumin to polymerize, which produces an antigenic macromolecule. Albumin solutions also contain citrate, which can lower serum calcium concentrations, which in turn could theoretically lead to decreased LV function. It is now generally believed that the effects on coagulation and serum calcium are related to the volume of fluid infused rather than albumin administration.[31] Albumin is available as a 5% solution that is isotonic with the plasma and a 25% solution that is hypertonic. The 5% solution is generally preferred for routine volume expansion, whereas the 25% solution is most useful in correcting hypoproteinemia or intravascular hypovolemia in patients with excess interstitial water.

Hetastarch or hydroxyethyl starch (HES) is a synthetic colloid made from amylopectin, which closely resembles human serum albumin, but is considerably less expensive. Available as a 6% solution in normal saline solution, HES expands the plasma volume by an amount greater than the volume infused because the high oncotic pressure draws water from the interstitial spaces. HES solutions are composed of a wide range of molecular weights, which explains its complex pharmacokinetics as it has an average molecular weight of 69,000 daltons with a range of 10,000 units to greater than 1 million units. Dose-related reductions in platelet count and transient increases in PT and PTT have been reported with moderate infusions of HES (<1,500 mL/day) and are significant with larger volumes.[32] HES causes factor VIII levels to be lowered beyond that which can be attributed to hemodilution and also increases fibrinolysis. This places patients with von Willebrand disease at greater risk of bleeding.

Numerous clinical studies have compared albumin and hetastarch for fluid resuscitation in patients with and without shock. One study reported that HES was as effective as albumin in restoring hemodynamic stability and improving $\dot{D}O_2$ in patients who were given comparable amounts of either fluid for 24 hours.[33] Other studies in hypovolemic patients have reported no difference in hemodynamic parameters when similar volumes of either HES or albumin were given as serial boluses to maintain CO and ventricular filling pressures.[34,35] In postoperative cardiac surgery patients, HES and albumin were found to be equally efficacious in restoring volume status and maintaining hemodynamic stability.[36,37] Although there is evidence to prove HES has comparable efficacy to albumin, controversy exists regarding the use of HES owing to adverse effects associated with its use. These adverse effects include renal dysfunction, severe pruritus, and coagulopathy. The renal dysfunction was associated with increasing doses of HES and was observed in patients with severe sepsis.[38] Experts argue that HES should not be used because of the potential adverse effects and that other alternatives are available.[39] For this reason, it is decided to use albumin for further volume expansion in B.A.

CARDIOGENIC SHOCK

A shock state arising primarily from an abnormality of cardiac function constitutes cardiogenic shock. The causes of cardiogenic shock can be separated largely into mechanical and nonmechanical (Table 22-1), although occasionally patients may have a combination of causes. Regardless of the source, the underlying problem in cardiogenic shock is a decrease in CO that is not caused by a reduction in circulating blood volume. This decrease in CO results in the syndrome of shock: hypotension with a decrease in arterial BP, and hypoperfusion as the delivery of oxygenated blood to the tissues is reduced. Eventually, organ dysfunction and death result if measures to restore perfusion are not successful.

The most common cause of cardiogenic shock is LV dysfunction and necrosis as a result of acute myocardial infarction (AMI) (see Chapter 18, Acute Coronary Syndrome). Necrosis of the left ventricle can be the result of a single massive myocardial infarction (MI), or it may follow numerous smaller events. Increases in sympathetic tone—seen clinically as increased HR and peripheral vasoconstriction—initially serve to increase CO and maintain central arterial pressure. When LV necrosis exceeds approximately 40% of the contractile mass of the heart, normal compensatory responses can no longer maintain CO, and hypotension and hypoperfusion result. In addition to decreased perfusion to vital tissues and organs, the decrease in CO leads to a reduction in the flow of blood through the coronary arteries, which can lead to infarct extension and a further worsening of cardiac performance.

The incidence of cardiogenic shock after AMI has remained relatively stable. A registry of 2,496 patients admitted for ST-elevation MI from 1987 to 2004 found an incidence of 7.6%.[40] The in-hospital mortality for those patients experiencing shock has decreased somewhat during this time frame, most likely because of coronary reperfusion strategies. The overall mortality rate, however, has remained high, with most series reporting an average of 60% to 80%.[41,42]

Nonmechanical origins of cardiogenic shock involve a decrease in the function of the heart muscle itself. MI involving the right ventricle (RV) can cause cardiogenic shock, even with normal LV systolic function. In this situation, the volume of blood reaching the LV (preload) is reduced because of the inability of the RV to move blood to the left side of the heart. In most patients with cardiogenic shock and RV infarction, significant LV dysfunction is present as well.

Cardiogenic shock caused by mechanical problems occurs relatively infrequently. In this setting, the systolic function (contractile ability) of the heart may be normal, but other defects render the heart unable to eject a normal volume of blood. Pericardial tamponade (bleeding into the pericardial sac) and tension pneumothorax (air leakage from the lung into the chest) cause cardiogenic shock by compressing the heart and decreasing the diastolic filling. Acute valvular insufficiency or stenosis prevents the normal ejection of blood. Ventricular septal or free wall rupture can occur, often in the setting of AMI, with the reduction in CO related to the inability of the LV to eject a normal volume of blood during systole.

Patients with chronic heart failure (HF) (see Chapter 19, Heart Failure) usually can compensate for their poor cardiac function, but acute exacerbations can cause cardiogenic shock with hypotension, hypoperfusion, and organ dysfunction. Cardiac dysfunction occasionally can be seen with severe sepsis because of increases in the production of inflammatory cytokines that have a depressant effect on the myocardium. A similar picture also can be seen after cardiopulmonary bypass during heart surgery, which activates the inflammatory cascade.

The symptoms of cardiogenic shock are largely the same as for other types of shock. Hypotension and signs of inadequate tissue perfusion, such as confusion, oliguria, tachycardia, and cutaneous vasoconstriction, are present in many patients. Differentiating cardiogenic shock from distributive or hypovolemic shock requires further examination. A history of coronary artery disease or symptoms of MI are important findings. Hypovolemia occurs in up to 20% of patients in cardiogenic shock, but patients frequently have signs of volume overload because the heart cannot move blood through the circulation. Peripheral edema can be seen in the extremities; lung sounds are diminished, and rales may be present as pulmonary edema develops. These findings are particularly evident in patients with severe HF.

Because the distinction between cardiogenic and other forms of shock can be difficult to make based on physical examination alone, further testing with invasive hemodynamic monitoring may be required to establish the diagnosis and guide therapy. Table 22-5 lists the common laboratory, electrocardiogram (ECG), and chest radiograph findings, and Table 22-3 lists the common hemodynamic findings in cardiogenic shock.

TABLE 22-5
Typical Findings of Early Cardiogenic Shock

- Arterial blood gas (ABG)
  - Hypoxemia secondary to pulmonary congestion with ventilation–perfusion abnormalities
  - Metabolic acidosis with a compensatory respiratory alkalosis
- Elevated blood lactate levels (which contributes to the acidosis)
- Complete blood count (CBC)
  - Leukocytosis
  - Thrombocytopenia (if disseminated intravascular coagulation is present)
- Elevated cardiac enzymes if myocardial infarction is present
- Electrocardiogram (ECG)–one or more of the following
  - T-wave changes indicating infarction
  - Left bundle branch block
  - Sinus tachycardia
  - Arrhythmia
- Chest radiograph
  - Pulmonary edema or evidence of adult respiratory distress syndrome (ARDS)
- Echocardiography
  - Valvular or mechanical problems if present
  - Normal or decreased ejection fraction

Hemodynamic monitoring—one or more of the following:
  - Reduced cardiac output
  - Arterial hypotension
  - Elevated pulmonary capillary wedge pressure (PCWP) and pulmonary artery pressure (PAP)
  - Elevated systemic vascular resistance (SVR)

Postoperative Cardiac Failure

ASSESSMENT BY HEMODYNAMIC PROFILE

CASE 22-2

QUESTION 1: R.G. is a 68-year-old man who is admitted to the ICU after undergoing coronary artery bypass grafting. He has a long history of ischemic heart disease with

two previous MIs. His preoperative ejection fraction was 45%. He also has a history of hypertension and hypercholesterolemia. His home medications are aspirin, lisinopril, metoprolol, and simvastatin. He is sedated, intubated, and receiving mechanical ventilation with 60% inspired oxygen, and he has a PA catheter in place. One hour after admission to the ICU, his BP and urine output have fallen. Urine output has dropped from 80 mL/hour initially to 15 mL/hour. Chest tube output has been stable at 40 mL/hour. His ECG shows no signs of ischemia. Laboratory values show the following:

pH, 7.32
$Paco_2$, 28 mm Hg
Pao_2, 110 mm Hg
HCO_3^-, 20 mEq/L
Hematocrit, 34%

His current hemodynamic profile is as follows:

BP (S/D/M), 92/45/61 mm Hg
Pulse, 105 beats/minute
CO, 2.8 L/minute
CI, 1.4 L/minute/m^2
CVP, 12 mm Hg
PA pressure (S/D), 35/22 mm Hg
PCWP, 22 mm Hg
SVR, 1,400 dyne · s · cm^{-5}

What is your assessment of R.G.'s clinical status and hemodynamics?

Clinically, R.G. has signs of hypoperfusion manifested by low urine output and metabolic acidosis. Evaluation of his hemodynamics will help determine a potential cause for his hypoperfusion and assist with the decision about appropriate therapeutic interventions to prevent his condition from worsening to serious organ dysfunction and death.

Possible causes of shock in cardiac surgery patients include hypovolemia from operative and postoperative bleeding, excessive vasodilation from medications, the effects of cardiopulmonary bypass on the inflammatory cascade, reperfusion injury, tamponade, or perioperative MI. Another concern is "stunning" of the myocardium caused by surgical trauma, which can take from hours to days to resolve.

Hypovolemia should always be evaluated first when assessing hemodynamic profiles. Using vasopressor or inotropic agents in the setting of hypovolemia is rarely effective and can lead to serious adverse effects (e.g., cardiac arrhythmias). Also, correction of hypovolemia is relatively straightforward and can be accomplished rapidly. R.G.'s tachycardia, low urine output, low BP, and low CO could indicate volume depletion. However, his hematocrit is adequate, and the data from his PA catheter show an elevated CVP and PCWP, suggesting that preload is not the problem.

Excessive vasodilation is also unlikely in R.G., given that his calculated SVR (afterload) is in the high normal range. Cardiac tamponade should always be considered after cardiac surgery, and is usually manifested by very high CVP, PCWP, and PA pressures, with significant decreases in CO and BP. R.G.'s CVP and PCWP are not as high as would be expected in pericardial tamponade, and his chest tube output has remained consistent, suggesting that blood is not accumulating.

Based on this hemodynamic profile, it appears that R.G. is in shock because of acute HF, most likely from postoperative myocardial dysfunction, although he should also be evaluated for myocardial ischemia or infarction and to rule out early cardiac tamponade. This evaluation should not delay the initiation of therapy. His severely depressed CO should be treated immediately to prevent further decompensation.

THERAPEUTIC INTERVENTIONS

CASE 22-2, QUESTION 2: The chest radiograph shows mild pulmonary edema, and fine rales were heard throughout the lower half of the lung fields on auscultation. Tamponade is not evident on the radiograph. The ECG shows ST-T wave changes, but no indication is seen of an AMI. Cardiac enzymes are pending. BP and CO need to be improved to increase perfusion to vital organs. Three therapeutic interventions are available: fluid challenge, vasodilators, and inotropic agents. How would these choices affect R.G.'s ventricular function?

FLUID CHALLENGE (INCREASE PRELOAD)

Augmentation of preload with a fluid challenge to improve CO is the first option. However, R.G.'s PCWP is 22 mm Hg and increasing this value above 18 to 20 mm Hg usually does not result in further benefit.[43,44] Furthermore, R.G. has signs of pulmonary edema on chest radiograph, and his Pao_2 is 110 mm Hg on 60% inspired oxygen. Therefore, elevation of intravascular volume might increase the pulmonary vascular hydrostatic pressure and worsen his pulmonary edema. If a fluid challenge is attempted to enhance preload, no more than 100 mL of normal saline solution should be given without repeating the hemodynamic measurements. If the PCWP rises but the CO does not improve, fluid challenges should be discontinued. Elevating the preload without appreciably improving CO also can increase LV wall tension, which is a major determinant of myocardial $\dot{V}o_2$; consequently, myocardial ischemia could develop. Although R.G. has signs of pulmonary edema, diuretics to reduce his volume overload can be detrimental to his CO and BP and should not be used until R.G.'s hemodynamics and signs of hypoperfusion have improved.

VASODILATORS (PRELOAD AND AFTERLOAD REDUCTION)

A peripheral vasodilator also could be used. This will decrease pulmonary venous congestion by reducing preload (PCWP), and thus pulmonary vascular hydrostatic pressure. It will improve CO by decreasing the resistance to ventricular ejection (afterload) as well. With myocardial ischemia, a reduction of the LV filling pressure may improve subendocardial blood flow, reduce the myocardial wall tension, and reduce the LV radius. The resultant decrease in myocardial $\dot{V}o_2$ will help prevent further depression of cardiac function.

In patients with LV failure, arterial resistance is also elevated because of a reflex increase in sympathetic tone in response to a fall in systemic arterial pressure. In LV failure, CO is inversely related to resistance to outflow from the LV. Lowering an elevated SVR will shift the ventricular function curve up and to the left, depending on whether an arterial, venous, or mixed vasodilator is used, thereby improving cardiac performance at a lower filling pressure (Fig. 22-4).

R.G. appears to have LV failure with elevations in PCWP and SVR. Vasodilator therapy in this setting will likely improve his CO and, therefore, increase the $\dot{D}o_2$ to the tissues and prevent organ dysfunction. The major risk of vasodilator therapy in R.G., however, is further reduction of an already low MAP. Although the reduction in BP may be offset by an increase in CO, a significant drop in arterial BP could occur, which could reduce coronary perfusion pressure and thereby exacerbate or produce

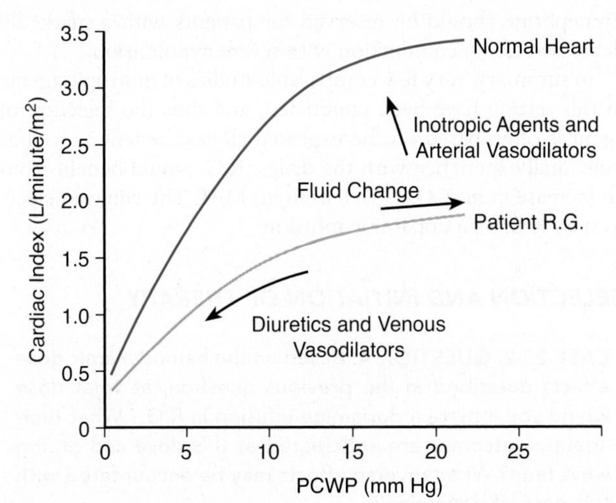

FIGURE 22-4 Ventricular function curve for R.G. PCWP, pulmonary capillary wedge pressure.

myocardial ischemia in addition to decreasing perfusion to other vital organ systems. Vasodilator therapy should be reserved for situations in which hemodynamic monitoring shows the patient to have LV failure with elevations in PCWP and SVR, and a systolic BP greater than 90 mm Hg.

INOTROPIC SUPPORT

A rapid-acting inotropic agent (e.g., dopamine, dobutamine, epinephrine) also can be used to increase myocardial contractility and CO. This intervention shifts the ventricular function curve upward and slightly to the left (Fig. 22-4). The disadvantage of this intervention is that improved CO is accompanied by an increased myocardial oxygen demand. Depending on the agent selected, three of the determinants of myocardial $\dot{V}O_2$ could be elevated: HR, contractility, and ventricular wall tension. Therefore, inotropic support is directed at establishing or maintaining a reasonable arterial pressure and ensuring adequate tissue perfusion by improving the CO.

In summary, the most appropriate therapeutic intervention for R.G. at this time would be inotropic support. The PCWP is elevated, suggesting that the preload has been maximized; therefore, fluid boluses may worsen R.G.'s pulmonary edema. Although R.G.'s SVR is slightly elevated (1,400 dyne · s · cm^{-5}), his BP is low; therefore, initial use of a peripheral vasodilator could jeopardize perfusion. Thus, an acceptable initial therapeutic intervention to improve CO and tissue perfusion is inotropic support. After a reasonable BP has been established, addition of a peripheral vasodilator could be considered to further enhance CO if needed, and diuretics added to reduce his pulmonary edema.

INOTROPIC AGENTS

CASE 22-2, QUESTION 3: Which inotropic agent is the best choice for R.G.?

DOPAMINE

Dopamine, a precursor of norepinephrine, has inotropic, chronotropic, and vasoactive properties, all of which are dose dependent (Table 22-6). At 0.5 to 2 mcg/kg/minute, dopamine stimulates dopaminergic receptors primarily in the splanchnic, renal, and coronary vascular beds. The effect on dopaminergic receptors is not blocked by β-blockers, but is antagonized by dopaminergic-blocking agents such as the butyrophenones and phenothiazines. Depending on the clinical state of the patient, low dosages of dopamine may slightly increase myocardial contractility, but usually will not alter HR or SVR significantly.

At 2 to 5 mcg/kg/minute, the improved cardiac performance produced by dopamine is through direct stimulation of β_1-adrenergic receptors and indirectly through release of norepinephrine from nerve terminals. Increased β_1-adrenergic

TABLE 22-6
Inotropic Agents and Vasopressors

		Receptor Sensitivity			Pharmacologic Effect			
Drug	**Usual Dose**	**α**	**β1**	**β2**	**VD**	**VC**	**INT**	**CHT**
Dobutamine	2.5–15 mcg/kg/min	+	+++	++	++	−−	+++[a]	+
Dopamine	0.5–2 mcg/kg/min[b] (renal)	−−	−−	−−	−−[b]	+	+	+
	2–5 mcg/kg/min	−−	+	−−	−−[b]	+	+	+
	5–10 mcg/kg/min	+	++	−−	++	++	++	++
	15–20 mcg/kg/min	+++	++	−−	−−[b]	+++	++	++
Epinephrine[c]	0.01–0.1 mcg/kg/min	+	+++	++	+	−	+++	++
	0.1 mcg/kg/min	+++	++	++	−−	+++	++	++
Isoproterenol	0.01–0.1 mcg/kg/min	−−	++++	+++	+++	−−	+++	+++
Milrinone	50 mcg/kg bolus, then 0.375–0.75 mcg/kg/min	−−	−−	−−	+++	−−	++	−−
Norepinephrine	0.05–0.5 mcg/kg/min Highly variable, titrate to desired MAP	++++	++	−−	−−	+++	+[d]	+
Phenylephrine	0.5–5 mcg/kg/min Highly variable, titrate to desired MAP	+++	−−	−−	−−	+++	−−	−−
Vasopressin[e]	0.04 units/min[f]	−−	−−	−−	−−	+++	−−	−−

[a]Dobutamine and milrinone have more inotropic effect than dopamine.
[b]Dopamine at 0.5–2 mcg/kg/min stimulates dopaminergic receptors, causing vasodilation in the splanchnic and renal vasculature.
[c]Epinephrine has predominant inotropic effects; norepinephrine has predominant vasoconstrictive effect. Epinephrine may vasodilate at low dosages, vasoconstrict at high dosages.
[d]Cardiac output unchanged or may decline because of vagal reflex responses that slow the heart.
[e]Vasopressin stimulates V_1 receptors to cause vasoconstriction in the periphery.
[f]Dosing for sepsis; in other vasodilatory conditions, may be titrated from 0.01 to 0.1 units/min.
CHT, chronotropic; INT, inotropic; MAP, mean arterial pressure; VC, peripheral vascular vasoconstriction; VD, peripheral vascular vasodilation.

receptor stimulation increases SV (inotropic effect), HR (chronotropic effect), and consequently CO. These cardiac effects can be blocked by β-blockers.

At infusion rates of 5 to 10 mcg/kg/minute, the α-adrenergic receptors are activated. At this dosage, the vasoactive effects on peripheral blood vessels are unpredictable and depend on the net effect of β_1-adrenergic stimulation, α-adrenergic stimulation, and reflex mechanisms. MAP and PCWP usually will rise.

At doses greater than 15 to 20 mcg/kg/minute, dopamine primarily stimulates peripheral α-adrenergic receptors. SVR increases, splanchnic and renal blood flow decreases, and LV filling pressure is raised. Cardiac irritability is a potential complication, and the overall myocardial $\dot{V}o_2$ is increased. The increase in SVR limits CO; thus, infusion rates should be limited to less than 10 to 15 mcg/kg/minute in patients with cardiac failure.

DOBUTAMINE

Dobutamine, a synthetic catecholamine, is a potent positive inotropic agent with predominant direct β_1-agonist effects and weak β_2- and α_1-adrenergic effects. With greater β_2-vasodilatory than α_1-vasoconstrictive actions, dobutamine can produce reductions in systemic and pulmonary vascular resistance. The reduction in SVR also may be caused by a reflex decrease in vasoconstriction secondary to enhanced CO. Phenoxybenzamine blocks the α-adrenergic response and propranolol blocks the β-adrenergic response. Unlike dopamine, dobutamine does not release endogenous norepinephrine or stimulate renal dopaminergic receptors.[45]

Studies assessing dobutamine in cardiac failure demonstrate consistent increases in CO and SV, with reductions in PCWP and SVR. The reduction in filling pressures, as indicated by a lowered PCWP, results in a decrease in LV wall tension and myocardial $\dot{V}o_2$. Consequently, coronary perfusion pressure, a major determinant of coronary blood flow, improves, and thus the oxygen supply to the heart is improved.

Compared with dopamine, dobutamine has equal or greater inotropic action. Dobutamine lowers PCWP and SVR with increasing doses, whereas dopamine may increase PCWP and SVR with increasing doses.[46] The effect on HR is variable; however, evidence suggests that dobutamine is less chronotropic than dopamine at lower infusion rates. In the clinical setting, dobutamine may be preferred in patients with depressed CO, elevated PCWP, and increased SVR with mild hypotension. The increase in CO may not be sufficient to raise the BP in a patient who initially is moderately to severely hypotensive. Thus, dopamine may be preferred in patients with depressed CO, normal or moderately elevated PCWP, and moderate or severe hypotension.

EPINEPHRINE

Similar to dopamine, epinephrine has dose-dependent hemodynamic effects (Table 22-6). At lower infusion ranges (0.01–0.1 mcg/kg/minute) epinephrine stimulates β_1-adrenergic receptors, causing increases in HR and contractility. As the dose increases, more α_1-receptor stimulation occurs, resulting in vasoconstriction and corresponding increases in SVR.

Epinephrine is frequently used in the cardiac surgery setting, despite a lack of comparative evidence. A survey from Germany found that epinephrine was the first agent chosen for low CO by 41.8% of physicians, compared with dobutamine by 30.9%.[47] The favorable hemodynamic effects (increased CO and BP) make it an attractive option for R.G.; however, epinephrine can induce hyperglycemia through gluconeogenesis and has been shown to increase lactate levels compared with other vasopressors and inotropic agents.[48] R.G. already has signs of acidosis (pH, 7.32; HCO_3^-, 20 mEq/L), and increased lactic acid production by epinephrine could be detrimental to his organ function. Epinephrine should be reserved for patients with a markedly depressed CO in conjunction with severe hypotension.

In summary, very few comparable studies of inotropic agents in this setting have been conducted, and thus the selection of agent is often based on the expected clinical benefit as well as individual experience with the drugs. R.G. would benefit from an increase in his CO, as well as in his MAP. The clinician elects to start R.G. on a dopamine infusion.

SELECTION AND INITIATION OF THERAPY

CASE 22-2, QUESTION 4: Based on the hemodynamic dose effects described in the previous question, at what dose would you initiate a dopamine infusion in R.G.? What therapeutic outcomes are anticipated at this dose and during what time? What adverse effects may be encountered with this dose of dopamine?

R.G. has an MAP of 61 mm Hg, a CI of 1.4 L/minute/m^2, a PCWP of 22 mm Hg, and an HR of 105 beats/minute. The goal of therapy is to increase the CI to at least 2.5 L/minute/m^2, maintain an MAP of at least 70 mm Hg (preferably closer to 80 mm Hg, depending on clinical signs of hypoperfusion), reduce the PCWP, and maintain an HR of less than 125 beats/minute. A urine output of at least 0.5 mL/kg/hour (37 mL/hour in R.G.) is desirable. A reasonable initial infusion rate would be 3 mcg/kg/minute. This dose should increase cardiac contraction and CO, resulting in an increase in renal blood flow. Because the onset of action is within minutes, the patient can be re-evaluated and the infusion rate can be titrated upward by 1 to 2 mcg/kg/minute every 10 minutes, depending on the hemodynamic data obtained. The hemodynamic response to dopamine is highly variable among patients; thus, careful titration using the lowest effective infusion rate is advised.

Adverse effects encountered with dopamine infusion include increased HR, anginal pain, arrhythmias, headache, hypertension, vasoconstriction, nausea, and vomiting. Extravasation of large amounts of dopamine during infusion can cause ischemic necrosis and sloughing. At higher dosages, α_1-adrenergic effects are more prominent, causing peripheral arterial vasoconstriction and an increase in venous pressure that leads to increases in afterload, preload, and myocardial oxygen demand as well as ischemia.

CASE 22-2, QUESTION 5: Dopamine is initiated at 3 mcg/kg/minute in R.G. and titrated to 8 mcg/kg/minute during the next 2 hours. A repeat chest radiograph shows slight worsening of pulmonary edema. The following hemodynamic profile is obtained (previous values are in parentheses):

BP (S/D/M), 115/62/80 mm Hg (92/45/61 mm Hg)
Pulse, 140 beats/minute (105 beats/minute)
CO, 3.8 L/minute (2.8 L/minute)
CI, 2.2 L/minute/m^2 (1.4 L/minute/m^2)
CVP, 10 mm Hg (12 mm Hg)
PCWP, 20 mm Hg (22 mm Hg)
SVR, 1,473 dyne · s · cm^{-5} (1,400 dyne · s · cm^{-5})
Urine output, 30 mL/hour (15 mL/hour)
Hematocrit, 36% (34%)

Do these data indicate a favorable or adverse hemodynamic effect from dopamine in R.G.?

Dopamine at 8 mcg/kg/minute has established a trend in the desired direction for CI; however, the HR has increased significantly. The SVR and PCWP have not changed appreciably, and the urine flow has increased. Further analysis reveals that the SV (CO/HR) has only increased from 25 mL/beat to 27 mL/beat; thus, the major increase in CO has resulted from the chronotropic rather than the inotropic effect of dopamine. As a net response, the dopamine has most likely affected the myocardial oxygen supply to demand ratio adversely; however, this cannot be established definitively. R.G. should be monitored closely for signs of myocardial ischemia.

CHANGING THERAPY

CASE 22-2, QUESTION 6: The clinician decides that an HR of 140 beats/minute is unacceptable in R.G., who has a history of MI. Subsequent attempts to taper the dopamine to lessen the induced tachycardia without dropping the CI and perfusion pressure are unsuccessful. Dobutamine is suggested as an alternative to dopamine. What hemodynamic changes would you expect with dobutamine in R.G.? Does dobutamine offer any advantages compared with dopamine?

As mentioned above, dobutamine has equivalent or greater inotropic action than dopamine with less tachycardia. The major difference between the two agents is the effect of dopamine on α_1-receptors. With dobutamine's absence of clinical effect on α_1-receptors, patients may experience a decrease in the SVR resulting from the unopposed β_2-receptor effects. In R.G., there should be an increase in CI from the inotropic effect and perhaps a decrease in SVR, which would further improve his CI. R.G. will have to be monitored carefully as his MAP is still relatively low, and any major reduction in SVR could lead to further reduction in his BP.

CASE 22-2, QUESTION 7: How would you initiate therapy with dobutamine and reduce the dopamine?

Dobutamine should be started at a low dosage (i.e., 2.5 mcg/kg/minute). The onset of effect is rapid and the half-life short (approximately 2 minutes), with steady-state conditions generally achieved within 10 minutes of initiation of therapy. This allows dose titration every 10 minutes based on patient tolerance. The rate of infusion required to increase CO typically is between 2.5 and 10 mcg/kg/minute, although higher infusion rates are sometimes required (up to 20 mcg/kg/minute). Once the dobutamine has been started, a reduction in the dose of dopamine should be attempted. A decrease of 20% of the current infusion rate every 10 to 15 minutes is reasonable.

CASE 22-2, QUESTION 8: What are the adverse effects associated with dobutamine?

Adverse effects that can occur during dobutamine administration are arrhythmias, nausea, anxiety, and tremors. The increases in contractility and HR caused by dobutamine can cause an increase in myocardial $\dot{V}O_2$ and can lead to ischemia in patients with coronary artery disease. Another limiting factor to dobutamine is tolerance to its hemodynamic effects with long-term continuous use. A decline in CO and HR has been seen after prolonged infusion and is most likely caused by downregulation of β_1-receptors. Of concern, evidence suggests that inotropic agents can be associated with an increased risk of mortality in patients with HF despite the improvement of symptoms and hemodynamic indices.[49]

CASE 22-2, QUESTION 9: Dobutamine is initiated and titrated up to 7.5 mcg/kg/minute. Concurrently, the dopamine is tapered down to 2 mcg/kg/minute, resulting in the following hemodynamic profile (previous values in parentheses):

BP (S/D/M), 122/60/80 mm Hg (115/62/80 mm Hg)
Pulse, 115 beats/minute (140 beats/minute)
CO, 4.2 L/minute (3.8 L/minute)
CI, 2.5 L/minute/m^2 (2.2 L/minute/m^2)
CVP, 10 mm Hg (10 mm Hg)
PCWP, 16 mm Hg (20 mm Hg)
SVR, 1,333 dyne · s · cm^{-5} (1,473 dyne · s · cm^{-5})
PaO_2, 115 mm Hg (110 mm Hg)
$PaCO_2$, 38 mm Hg (28 mm Hg)
pH, 7.41 (7.32)
HCO_3^-, 24 mEq/L (20 mEq/L)
Urine output, 60 mL/hour (30 mL/hour)

Assess the improvement in hemodynamic change and urine output with the addition of dobutamine and decreased infusion rate of dopamine.

The CI has continued to increase and the PCWP and SVR have fallen. The increase in perfusion pressure in conjunction with the fall in afterload, preload, and HR will favorably affect the myocardial oxygen supply to demand ratio. The fall in HR with the increase in CO indicates that the SV has increased significantly from 27 to 36 mL/beat. Other signs of improved systemic perfusion include the reversal of the acidosis observed initially and improved urine output.

The improved urine output can be attributed to the combined effects of dobutamine on the CO and subsequent improvement in the perfusion to the kidney and perhaps to the renal effects of dopamine, although the latter effects are controversial and have been debated vigorously. Traditionally, it was thought that the effects of low-dose dopamine on the dopaminergic receptors in the renal vasculature improved kidney blood flow and, consequently, renal function. Randomized, controlled trials have demonstrated increases in urine output with low-dose dopamine,[50] but they have not been able to show a reduction in incidence or degree of renal dysfunction.[51,52] Despite the lack of convincing evidence for benefit, low-dose dopamine is widely used in critical care units.

TAPERING INOTROPIC SUPPORT

CASE 22-2, QUESTION 10: R.G. has remained stable with dobutamine 7.5 mcg/kg/minute and dopamine 2.0 mcg/kg/minute for the past 4 hours. Urine output continues to be adequate. How would you taper the inotropic agents, and what parameters would you monitor?

An acceptable method frequently used is to taper dobutamine by 2 mcg/kg/minute every 30 to 60 minutes and discontinue the dopamine. At such a low infusion rate, the effect of dopamine on R.G.'s hemodynamics is probably negligible, and there is no need to titrate down at this level. Dobutamine has an elimination half-life of approximately 2.5 minutes; thus, steady-state plasma levels will occur in a short period. When tapering vasoactive agents, it is prudent, however, to let the patient stabilize hemodynamically at new infusion rates for a period that exceeds the time to achieve a new steady-state plasma concentration. After each reduction in the infusion rate, hemodynamic data can be assessed. Reasonable guidelines would be to keep the MAP at 75 to 80 mm Hg, HR at less than 110 beats/minute, PCWP at 12 to 18 mm Hg, and CI at more than 2.5 L/minute/m^2. After the dobutamine is discontinued, R.G. should be evaluated for reinstitution of the medications he was receiving before surgery.

Acute Myocardial Infarction

IMMEDIATE GOALS OF THERAPY AND GENERAL CONSIDERATIONS

CASE 22-3

QUESTION 1: M.J., a 57-year-old woman, is brought to the ED complaining of severe chest pain and difficulty breathing. On physical examination, M.J. has a BP of 80/40 mm Hg (by cuff) with a weak pulse of 115 beats/minute. Her RR is 24 breaths/minute, and her breathing is shallow. Heart sounds include S_3/S_4 gallops, but no murmurs are heard. The jugular venous pulse is normal. She has diffuse rales over the lower lung fields with moderate wheezing. M.J. is cold and clammy to touch; however, her temperature is normal. She is restless, anxious, and confused about time and date. ABG measurements on 2 L/minute oxygen via nasal prongs are Pao_2, 65 mm Hg; $Paco_2$, 44 mm Hg; pH, 7.22; and HCO_3^-, 18 mEq/L. The ECG shows ST segment elevation in the anterior lateral leads and 6 to 10 premature ventricular contractions per minute. Serum potassium is normal. A Foley catheter is inserted to monitor urine output. Cardiac enzymes are pending. M.J. has no known history of cardiac disease and takes no medication. What immediate goals of therapy are necessary to stabilize and treat M.J.?

M.J. has signs of cardiogenic shock with decreased systemic perfusion. Her BP is low, her HR is elevated, and her respiratory status is compromised. M.J. is restless, anxious, and confused, indicating poor cerebral perfusion. Her ABG results indicate a component of metabolic acidosis secondary to poor systemic perfusion. The ST elevation on the ECG is consistent with an acute anterior MI.

As discussed in Chapter 18, Acute Coronary Syndrome, most patients presenting with MI are routinely treated with aspirin, a β-blocker, and immediate percutaneous coronary intervention (PCI) if available or, if not, thrombolytic therapy (unless contraindicated). The presence of cardiogenic shock can alter the interventional strategy, however. Patients presenting in cardiogenic shock after MI may progress rapidly to irreversible organ system dysfunction as the compensatory mechanisms fail to maintain tissue perfusion. Treatment of these critically ill patients involves two components: stabilization and definitive treatment. Initial stabilization of the patient must be attained before further evaluation and treatment of the cause of cardiogenic shock can proceed. The goals are to maintain adequate $\dot{D}o_2$ to the tissues and to prevent further hemodynamic compromise. Stabilization includes (a) establishing ventilation and oxygenation (arterial Po_2 should be greater than 70 mm Hg); (b) restoring central arterial BP and CO with vasopressors and inotropic agents, if needed; (c) infusing fluids, if hypovolemic; and (d) treating pain, arrhythmias, and acid–base abnormalities, if present.

Administration of oxygen by mechanical ventilation enhances the myocardial oxygen supply and may contribute to improved ventricular performance. Mechanical ventilation is indicated when arterial oxygen saturation cannot be maintained above 85% to 90% despite 100% oxygen per face mask. Once the patient is intubated, maximal sedation should be provided to alleviate anxiety and discomfort.

The arterial pressure must be increased to provide adequate coronary and systemic perfusion to meet oxygen requirements. Some areas of ischemia in the infarct zone may be depressed but viable, provided myocardial oxygen supply exceeds demand. If the myocardial oxygen demands are not met, however, myocardial tissue necrosis will expand into the area of ischemia. This results in further hemodynamic impairment and initiates a vicious feedback cycle that can lead to intractable pump failure and irreversible shock. To be effective, treatment of cardiogenic shock should favorably influence the balance between oxygen supply and demand in the ischemic zone.

Optimizing preload to improve CO and systemic perfusion is crucial, especially in patients with RV infarction. In patients with severe LV impairment caused by cardiogenic shock, increasing intravascular volume can worsen pulmonary congestion. M.J. currently has signs of pulmonary congestion and RV infarction is not immediately evident; thus, a fluid challenge must be administered cautiously or withheld until hemodynamic monitoring can be established.

Inotropic agents or vasopressors should be used to increase systemic BP and re-establish coronary perfusion in patients with cardiogenic shock and hypotension. The use of vasoactive agents is not without risk, however, because they can exacerbate ventricular arrhythmias and increase $\dot{V}o_2$ in ischemic myocardium. Therefore, the minimal dose that will provide adequate perfusion pressure should be used. Achieving an MAP of 65 to 70 mm Hg is the immediate goal of therapy. Elevation of the MAP to more than 80 mm Hg is unnecessary because at this level, coronary blood flow is not significantly changed, but energy expenditure is high.

Correction of metabolic acidosis is best accomplished by treating the underlying cause. Improving tissue perfusion by optimizing oxygen content and increasing CO can eventually restore aerobic metabolism and eliminate lactic acid production. The use of sodium bicarbonate to correct lactic acidosis in cardiogenic shock and other critically ill patients is controversial. Sodium bicarbonate can have numerous adverse effects, such as hypernatremia, paradoxical intracellular acidosis, and hypercapnia; conclusive data on its efficacy are lacking. Bicarbonate therapy, therefore, warrants caution and is recommended only, if at all, when severe acidemia (pH <7.2 or HCO_3^- <10 to 12 mEq/L) is present.

Inotropic agents and vasoconstrictors can increase myocardial $\dot{V}o_2$ and potentially extend the area of necrosis in patients with infarct-induced cardiogenic shock; thus, the careful selection and titration of agents that will best preserve myocardium while sustaining systemic arterial pressure and tissue perfusion is essential. Although correction of volume deficits and early pharmacologic support may prevent the extension of myocardial damage, it must be emphasized that exclusive use of these measures does not improve survival. Therefore, drug therapy must be considered only an interim maneuver to preserve myocardial and systemic integrity while further therapeutic interventions and definitive therapy are being considered.

As mentioned, cardiogenic shock after AMI occurs in only a small percentage of patients, but carries a high mortality rate. Reperfusion of the occluded artery is of paramount importance in these patients. Two options are available for restoring patency of the artery: thrombolytic therapy and PCI (see Chapter 18, Acute Coronary Syndrome).

Thrombolytic therapy in AMI may reduce the incidence of subsequent cardiogenic shock, but its value may be limited in patients who have already experienced shock.[53] The effectiveness of thrombolytics is reduced in this setting, possibly because of reduced delivery of the agent to the coronary artery thrombus as a result of hypotension.[54] The use of an intra-aortic balloon pump (IABP) to augment coronary artery blood flow may improve the efficacy of thrombolytic agents.[55] In settings in which interventional cardiac procedures such as percutaneous transluminal coronary angioplasty or stenting are not readily available, insertion of an IABP and thrombolytic agents should not be delayed if indicated.

Early PCI may be of more benefit than thrombolytic agents in patients with cardiogenic shock complicating AMI. In a subset of patients with cardiogenic shock in the GUSTO-1 trial, angioplasty resulted in a reduction in 30-day mortality rate from 61% to 43%.[56] Numerous other trials have demonstrated improved outcomes with PCI in patients with shock compared with historical controls. However, problems with subgroup analysis and nonrandomized trials include the potential for selection bias. Operator skill also is a consideration in this setting, and larger centers with greater experience may have better outcomes than smaller centers.

An early revascularization strategy with angioplasty or bypass surgery was compared with medical management of these patients, including thrombolytic therapy and intra-aortic balloon counterpulsation.[57] No significant difference was found in mortality rate at 30 days; however, at 6 months, the mortality rate in the revascularization group was 50.3% versus 63.1% for the medical therapy group. Follow-up at 1 year also demonstrated a significant increase in survival.[58]

ASSESSMENT BY HEMODYNAMIC PROFILE

CASE 22-3, QUESTION 2: M.J. has a history of cerebrovascular disease and is thus ineligible for thrombolytic therapy. Therefore, she will require revascularization in the form of PCI or coronary artery bypass surgery to improve her chances of survival. Meanwhile, she is given dopamine at 5 mcg/kg/minute to stabilize her hemodynamically before revascularization procedures are initiated. Oxygen administration is changed to 100% via face mask. Morphine sulfate, 2 mg IV, is given for chest pain. IV nitroglycerin was initiated at 0.25 mcg/kg/minute for myocardial ischemia, but had to be discontinued because intolerable hypotension developed. M.J. is admitted to the ICU, where an arterial line and PA line are placed, revealing the following hemodynamic profile (previous values in parentheses):

BP (S/D/M), 92/46/61 mm Hg (80/40 mm Hg by cuff)
Pulse, 122 beats/minute (115 beats/minute)
CO, 2.8 L/minute
CI, 1.5 L/minute/m^2
Svo_2, 48%
CVP, 16 mm Hg
PCWP, 26 mm Hg
SVR, 1,314 dyne · s · cm^{-5}
Pao_2, 70 mm Hg (65 mm Hg)
$Paco_2$, 48 mm Hg (44 mm Hg)
pH, 7.24 (7.22)
HCO_3^-, 21 mEq/L (18 mEq/L)
Urine output, 10 mL/hour

M.J. weighs 82 kg and has a body surface area of 1.9 m^2. The chest radiograph shows evidence of pulmonary edema. Assess M.J.'s hemodynamic profile and response to dopamine therapy.

M.J.'s clinical and hemodynamic parameters confirm the diagnosis of cardiogenic shock. She is clearly not hypovolemic, as manifested by an elevated CVP and PCWP. Although her SBP is slightly improved, her CI (<1.8 L/minute/m^2), PCWP (>18 mm Hg), and low urine output (<25 mL/hour) are all characteristic findings with this form of shock. Her decreased Svo_2 shows that she has impaired perfusion owing to her low $\dot{D}o_2$. Patients with cardiogenic shock from an acute event (such as an MI) are usually in a much more critical clinical situation than patients who have an acute exacerbation of chronic HF. Patients with HF have compensated with time for the increases in preload and reduced CO, but patients such as M.J. have not had time to develop compensatory mechanisms.

Dopamine, at an infusion rate of 5 to 10 mcg/kg/minute, has made M.J. more tachycardic and has not substantially enhanced CO, and the MAP is less than optimal for coronary perfusion. M.J. has signs of pulmonary edema that are consistent with the elevated PCWP. The Pao_2 of 70 mm Hg is marginally acceptable considering she is on 100% oxygen per face mask.

THERAPEUTIC INTERVENTIONS

FLUID THERAPY VERSUS INOTROPIC SUPPORT

CASE 22-3, QUESTION 3: The decision is made to intubate M.J. Would a fluid challenge or additional doses of dopamine improve M.J.'s status?

In M.J., a fluid challenge could exacerbate the pulmonary edema because after an AMI, ventricular compliance is decreased and a small change in LVEDV could result in a disproportionately large increase in PCWP. Thus, in patients with an AMI, the benefits of a fluid challenge must be balanced against the risk of aggravating pulmonary edema. M.J. has an elevated CVP and PCWP, indicating that she has at least adequate, if not excessive, preload. If a fluid challenge is going to be administered, no more than 100 mL of normal saline solution should be infused without further evaluation of hemodynamic and clinical data.

Increasing the dopamine infusion rate might improve CO and perfusion pressure, but at the expense of increasing the HR even further. The increased HR, along with the elevated PCWP, could adversely affect the myocardial oxygen supply to demand ratio. However, it is hoped the increase in coronary blood flow (caused by the rise in arterial pressure) and the decrease in LV chamber size (associated with the increase in contractility) would tend to offset the increase in myocardial oxygen requirements.

It is not entirely clear which patients in cardiogenic shock will respond to dopamine. One trial of 24 patients in cardiogenic shock found that a mean infusion rate of 9.1 mcg/kg/minute was required to produce beneficial effects on CO, urine output, HR, and PCWP in survivors.[59] Nonsurvivors had no change in MAP, PCWP, or HR at an average infusion rate of 17.1 mcg/kg/minute.

COMBINATION INOTROPIC THERAPY

CASE 22-3, QUESTION 4: Occasionally, a patient's hemodynamic status improves with the combined use of inotropic agents. Would the addition of dobutamine or a phosphodiesterase inhibitor to treat M.J.'s cardiogenic shock be beneficial?

The combination of dobutamine and dopamine was studied in eight cardiogenic shock patients requiring mechanical ventilation.[60] None of the patients had experienced an MI within the preceding 7 days. Each patient received three infusions in a randomly assigned order: dopamine at 15 mcg/kg/minute; dobutamine at 15 mcg/kg/minute; and a combination of dopamine and dobutamine each at 7.5 mcg/kg/minute. All three regimens increased CI, stroke index, LV stroke work index, and HR similarly. MAP increased with the dopamine and the dobutamine–dopamine combination, but did not change with dobutamine alone. SVR was significantly lower with dobutamine alone compared with the other two regimens. PCWP was elevated most with the dopamine infusion alone as was myocardial $\dot{V}O_2$. The combination regimen offered hemodynamic superiority compared with either agent alone in this group of patients.

Given M.J.'s significantly low arterial BP, the addition of a phosphodiesterase inhibitor, such as milrinone, would be problematic. These agents tend to have more vasodilating properties than dobutamine, and their long half-lives can present difficulties in management if hypotension does develop. Until M.J.'s BP is improved, phosphodiesterase inhibitors should be avoided.

In summary, further inotropic support with dopamine or the addition of dobutamine would be indicated in M.J. at this time. The dopamine could be increased to 12.5 mcg/kg/minute or dobutamine could be initiated at 5 mcg/kg/minute. Neither maneuver is without risk. Dobutamine could lower the MAP, adversely affecting coronary perfusion pressure. Dopamine might elevate the PCWP. The addition of dobutamine or an increase in dopamine dose could increase HR even more. Any of these would adversely affect the myocardial oxygen supply to demand ratio and could further extend the area of ischemia or necrosis.

CASE 22-3, QUESTION 5: Despite the addition of dobutamine at a rate of 5 to 7.5 mcg/kg/minute and initiation of ventilatory support by tracheal intubation, M.J. continues to show signs of deterioration, with progressive obtundation and loss of bowel sounds. Her systemic arterial pressure has continued to decline, and her dopamine is now up to 18 mcg/kg/minute. Preload reduction was attempted previously with nitroglycerin; however, the drop in BP was intolerable. A repeat hemodynamic profile shows the following values (previous values in parentheses):

BP (S/D/M), 86/40/55 mm Hg (92/46/61 mm Hg)
Pulse, 132 beats/minute (122 beats/minute)
CO, 3.0 L/minute (2.8 L/minute)
CI, 1.6 L/minute/m^2 (1.5 L/minute/m^2)
SvO_2, 40% (48%)
CVP, 18 mm Hg (16 mm Hg)
PCWP, 24 mm Hg (26 mm Hg)
SVR, 986 dyne · s · cm^{-5} (1,314 dyne · s · cm^{-5})
Urine output, 8 mL/hour (10 mL/hour)
PaO_2, 75 mm Hg (70 mm Hg)
$PaCO_2$, 42 mm Hg (48 mm Hg)
pH, 7.26 (7.24)
HCO_3^-, 19 mEq/L (21 mEq/L)

The ECG shows atrial tachycardia with occasional premature ventricular contractions. What therapeutic alternatives can be considered at this time?

M.J. is still in severe cardiogenic shock, and her tissue perfusion continues to deteriorate as evidenced by a further reduction in urine output, a loss in bowel sounds, continuing acidosis, and central nervous system obtundation. Because her systemic arterial pressure and tissue perfusion have declined despite the addition of dobutamine and maximal doses of dopamine, additional support with a potent vasopressor and the insertion of an IABP or other percutaneous ventricular assist device are indicated.

NOREPINEPHRINE

Norepinephrine is a potent α-adrenergic agonist that vasoconstricts arterioles at all infusion rates, thereby increasing SVR. Thus, systemic arterial and coronary perfusion pressures both rise. Norepinephrine also stimulates β_1-adrenergic receptors to a lesser extent, resulting in increased contractility and stroke volume. However, HR and CO usually remain constant, or may even decrease secondary to the increased afterload and reflex baroreceptor activation. Although coronary perfusion pressure is enhanced as a result of the elevation in diastolic pressure, myocardial $\dot{V}O_2$ also is increased. Consequently, myocardial ischemia and arrhythmias may be exacerbated and LV function further compromised.

Infusions of norepinephrine are begun at 0.01 to 0.05 mcg/kg/minute and titrated upward to achieve an SBP of 90 to 100 mm Hg. Administration should be through a central IV line because local subcutaneous necrosis can result from peripheral IV extravasation. Prolonged infusion of larger doses will transiently exert a beneficial effect by diverting blood flow from the peripheral and splanchnic vasculature to the heart and brain; however, this ultimately can compromise capillary perfusion to the extent that end-organ failure, particularly renal failure, ensues.

To reduce the potential risk of end-organ damage, a reasonable approach is to add norepinephrine to the infusion of dobutamine, and reduce the dopamine infusion rate to 0.5 to 2 mcg/kg/minute. This will theoretically support renal and splanchnic perfusion, although this effect is controversial, as discussed above. In addition, any deficits in plasma volume should be corrected when identified by hemodynamic monitoring.

Adverse effects of norepinephrine are related mostly to excessive vasoconstriction and compromise of organ perfusion. Worsening of ventricular function can occur because of increased afterload, and tissue necrosis and sloughing can develop if extravasation occurs. Cardiac arrhythmias can emerge and HR can increase; however, in some cases the HR may slow secondary to baroreceptor-mediated reflex increases in vagal tone.

Again, it must be emphasized that pharmacologic support for M.J., particularly the use of norepinephrine, is only an interim maneuver to temporarily maintain hemodynamic function while revascularization procedures are being considered. Patients who cannot be stabilized with pharmacologic intervention, and in whom systemic or myocardial perfusion is becoming compromised, may require further support through insertion of a mechanical circulatory assist device.

MECHANICAL CIRCULATORY SUPPORT

When drug therapy is ineffective at stabilizing patients in cardiogenic shock, mechanical intervention should be considered. Mechanical interventions can rapidly stabilize patients with cardiogenic shock, especially those with global myocardial ischemia or infarction complicated by mechanical defects, such as papillary muscle rupture or ventricular septal rupture. Intra-aortic balloon counterpulsation augments coronary arterial perfusion pressure during diastole and reduces LV impedance during systole. Sometimes combined inotropic support and intra-aortic balloon counterpulsation are required to maintain an acceptable BP (SBP $>$90 mm Hg) and CI ($>$2.2 L/minute/m^2).

The IABP or intra-aortic counterpulsation has been in use for more than 30 years and remains the most commonly used mechanical assist device. It is designed to improve coronary perfusion and reduce afterload, thus providing short-term reperfusion of the ischemic myocardium. A 30- to 40-mL balloon catheter is inserted into an artery (usually femoral) and advanced to just below the arch of the aorta. Balloon inflation and deflation are synchronized with the ECG to inflate during diastole (after the aortic valve closes) and deflate at the onset of systole. The inflated balloon in diastole increases coronary perfusion by elevating the mean aortic pressure. The rapid deflation of the balloon at the onset of systole decreases SBP, thus reducing afterload and modestly improving CO. The enhanced myocardial perfusion provided by IABP may reduce vasopressor requirements, thereby further decreasing myocardial $\dot{V}O_2$. Occasionally, IABP augmentation is sufficient to allow the institution of vasodilators (e.g., nitroprusside) or inodilators (e.g., milrinone). Complications of IABP include thrombocytopenia from the mechanical destruction of platelets and the potential for limb ischemia because of reduced blood flow in the artery into which the IABP catheter is inserted. Heparin anticoagulation is usually used with IABP because the device has a large surface area that can be thrombogenic. A review of clinical studies supporting the use of the IABP has found no differences in 30-day mortality and an increase in the risk of bleeding complications and stroke.[61] Despite the lack of evidence, this device is still commonly used to support patients with cardiogenic shock.

Newer devices have been developed (TandemHeart, Impella) that augment CO directly and decrease the load on the LV.[62] These small pumps are placed percutaneously in the cardiac catheterization laboratory, so do not require major cardiac surgery. They are best used for temporary circulatory support until more definitive therapy is available. Systemic anticoagulation is required with these devices, and adverse effects include bleeding and thrombosis.

Advanced circulatory assist devices (HeartMate, Novacor, Abiomed) have been developed and are available in centers with access to cardiac surgical procedures. Mechanical assistance with these devices is used for patients with cardiogenic shock who need support while awaiting definitive, corrective therapy or as a bridging mechanism before cardiac transplantation.[63] Long-term use of some of these devices has been investigated in patients with severe cardiac failure who are not transplant candidates.[64] Implantation of an LV assist device was compared with medical management in patients with severe HF. Survival at 1 year was 52% in the LV assist device group, compared with 25% in the medical management group. The high cost of these devices will undoubtedly limit their use to only the most severely ill patients.

In summary, M.J.'s condition has continued to deteriorate since her admission to the ICU. Attempts at stabilizing her hemodynamic parameters with dopamine, dobutamine, and norepinephrine have failed. This is evidenced by inadequate tissue perfusion, which is reflected clinically by her continued lactic acidosis, decreased urine output, reduced bowel sounds, and central nervous system obtundation. M.J.'s best chance of survival is to have early revascularization of her ischemic myocardium with either coronary bypass surgery or PCI. Meanwhile, the addition of norepinephrine and intra-aortic counterpulsation can provide temporary support for M.J. before her procedure.

SEPTIC SHOCK

Distributive Shock

Distributive shock is characterized by an overt loss of vascular tone, causing acute tissue hypoperfusion. Although numerous events such as anaphylaxis or neurogenic causes can initiate distributive shock, most cases are readily reversed by supportive measures and treatment or elimination of the underlying cause.

SEPTIC SHOCK

Distributive shock secondary to sepsis, or septic shock, is associated with a high mortality rate, reflecting the limited therapeutic options available at this time. Approximately 500,000 cases of sepsis syndrome are seen annually, with mortality rates ranging from about 30% at 1 month to 50% at 5 months. Epidemiology studies show that approximately 25% of cases of sepsis syndrome eventually result in septic shock. Septic shock is the number one cause of death in the noncoronary ICU and the 13th most common cause of death in the United States. It has been projected that the incidence of sepsis will increase 1.5% per year mainly because of the disproportionate growth of the elderly in the US population.[65–68]

The consensus conference of the American College of Chest Physicians and the Society of Critical Care Medicine defines sepsis syndrome as a systemic inflammatory response resulting from infection.[2] When associated organ dysfunction, hypoperfusion, or hypotension is present, it is termed *severe sepsis;* when hypotension persists despite adequate fluid resuscitation and requires inotropic or vasopressor support, it is termed *septic shock* (see Table 22-7 for definitions). More than half the cases of septic syndrome occur in the ICU, one-third occur in other currently hospitalized patients, and 10% to 15% of cases are present on admission to the ED.[19] Progression to septic shock occurs in about half of patients who have septic syndrome within 1 month of onset, as defined by hypotension. Persons most at risk for septic shock are those who are immunocompromised or have underlying conditions that render them susceptible to bloodstream invasion. Groups at risk include neonates, the elderly, patients with acquired immune deficiency syndrome, alcoholics, childbearing women, and those undergoing surgery or who have experienced trauma. Other predisposing factors include coexisting diseases such as diabetes mellitus, malignancies, chronic hepatic or renal failure, and hyposplenism; exposure to immunosuppressant drugs and cancer chemotherapy; and procedures such as insertion of urinary catheters, endotracheal tubes, and IV lines.

Septic shock is characterized initially by a normal or high CO and a low SVR (Table 22-3). Hypotension is caused by the low SVR as well as alterations in macrovascular and microvascular tone, which result in maldistribution of blood flow and volume. Changes in the microvasculature can lead to loss of normal microvascular autoregulatory mechanisms, resulting in constriction of capillaries, changes in cellular rheology, fibrin deposition, and neutrophil adherence. This causes vascular "sludging" and, in some cases, arteriovenous shunts that bypass capillary beds. Loss of intravascular fluid caused by increased vascular permeability and third spacing of fluid further adds to hypovolemia. In an effort to compensate for the changes in volume and SVR, the body goes into a hyperdynamic state and increases CO. Most patients exhibit myocardial dysfunction as manifested by decreased myocardial compliance, reduced contractility, and ventricular dilation, but maintain a normal CO because of tachycardia and cardiac dilatation which increases or maintains preload. Although the cause of, and mechanism for, this abnormality is not fully understood, it is not believed to be attributable to myocardial ischemia. Rather, it is thought to be caused by one or more circulating inflammatory mediators, such as cytokines, tumor necrosis factor-α (TNF-α), platelet activating factor, arachidonic acid, nitric oxide (NO), and reactive oxygen species. In late septic shock, the body is no longer able to compensate because of the cardiac effects of the inflammatory mediators and resultant myocardial edema, thus resulting in a decreased CO. The end product of this complicated pathway is cellular ischemia, dysfunction, and eventually cellular death unless the chain of events is interrupted.

The pathogenesis of sepsis is more fully understood now, but the exact mechanisms are still not completely clear. It is known that the changes that take place during sepsis are caused by the immunologic host response to infection, which involves inflammatory and immunodepressive (anti-inflammatory) phases. It is unknown, however, whether these phases are sequential (inflammatory then immunodepressive) or whether immunosuppression is a primary response to sepsis rather than a compensatory response.

The inflammatory stage of sepsis is initiated by an infection with a microorganism, most commonly bacterial. Organisms can either enter the bloodstream directly (producing positive blood cultures) or may indirectly elicit a systemic inflammatory response by locally releasing their toxins or structural

TABLE 22-7
ACCP/SCCM Consensus Conference Definitions

Infection	Microbial phenomenon characterized by an inflammatory response to the presence of microorganisms or the invasion of normally sterile host tissue by those organisms.
Bacteremia	The presence of viable bacteria in the blood.
Systemic inflammatory response syndrome (SIRS)	The systemic inflammatory response to a variety of severe clinical insults. The response is manifested by two or more of the following conditions: Temperature >38°C or <36°C Heart rate >90 beats/min Respiratory rate >20 breaths/min or $PaCO_2$ <32 mm Hg (<4.3 kPa) WBC >12,000 cells/μL, <4,000 cell/μL, or >10% immature (bands) forms
Sepsis	The systemic response to infection. The systemic response is manifested by two or more of the following conditions as a result of infection: Temperature >38°C or <36°C Heart rate >90 beats/min Respiratory rate >20 breaths/min or $PaCO_2$ <32 mm Hg (<4.3 kPa) WBC >12,000 cells/μL, <4,000 cell/μL, or >10% immature (band) forms
Severe sepsis	Sepsis associated with organ dysfunction, hypoperfusion, or hypotension. Hypoperfusion and perfusion abnormalities may include, but are not limited to, lactic acidosis, oliguria, or an acute alteration in mental status.
Septic shock	Sepsis with hypotension, despite adequate fluid resuscitation, along with perfusion abnormalities that may include, but are not limited to, lactic acidosis, oliguria, or an acute alteration in mental status. Patients who are on inotropic or vasopressor agents may not be hypotensive at the time that perfusion abnormalities are measured.
Hypotension	A systolic BP of <90 mm Hg or a reduction of >40 mm Hg from baseline in the absence of other causes for hypotension.
Multiple organ dysfunction syndrome	Presence of altered organ function in an acutely ill patient such that homeostasis cannot be maintained without intervention.

BP, blood pressure; WBC, white blood cells.
Reprinted with permission from American College of Chest Physicians (ACCP)/Society of Critical Care Medicine (SCCM) Consensus Conference: definitions for sepsis and organ failure and guidelines for the use of innovative therapies in sepsis. *Crit Care Med.* 1992;20:864.

components at the site of infection. The lipopolysaccharide endotoxin of gram-negative bacteria is the most potent soluble product of bacteria that can initiate a response and is the most studied, but other bacterial products can initiate the response, including exotoxins, enterotoxins, peptidoglycans, and lipoteichoic acid from gram-positive organisms. The binding of these toxins to cell receptors promotes proinflammatory cytokine production, primarily TNF-α and interleukin-1 (IL-1). These toxins stimulate the production and release of numerous endogenous mediators that are responsible for the inflammatory consequences of sepsis. The cytokines act synergistically to directly affect organ function and stimulate the release of other proinflammatory cytokines, such as IL-6, IL-8, platelet activating factor, complement, thromboxanes, leukotrienes, prostaglandins, NO, and others.[69]

The presence of these cytokines promotes inflammation and vascular endothelial injury, but also causes an overwhelming activation in coagulation. Thrombin has potent proinflammatory and procoagulant activities, and its production is increased in sepsis. The human body normally counteracts these effects by increasing fibrinolysis, but the homeostatic mechanisms in the septic patient are dysfunctional. There are decreases in the levels of protein C, plasminogen, and antithrombin III as well as increased activity of plasminogen activator inhibitor-1 and thrombin-activatable fibrinolysis inhibitor, endogenous agents that inhibit fibrinolysis.[70] The patient is in a coagulopathic state, which promotes formation of microvascular thrombi leading to hypoperfusion, ischemia, and, ultimately, organ failure. Multiple organ failure is responsible for about half the deaths caused by septic shock.[71]

The clinical features of septic shock are fever, chills, nausea, vomiting, and diarrhea. Characteristic laboratory findings include leukocytosis or leukopenia, thrombocytopenia with or without coagulation abnormalities, and, often, hyperbilirubinemia. These features are usually readily detectable and occur within 24 hours after bacteremia develops, particularly if the bacteremia is caused by gram-negative organisms. In the extremes of age (very young or very old) or in debilitated patients, hypothermia can be present, however, and positive findings may be limited to unexplained hypotension, mental confusion, and hyperventilation.

Persons dying of septic shock often have a normal or elevated CO. Death within the first week after the onset of sepsis occurs as a result of intractable arterial hypotension that is secondary to a significantly depressed SVR. This causes extensive maldistribution of blood flow in the microvasculature, with subsequent tissue hypoxia and the development of lactic acidosis. Death occurring beyond the first week usually is caused by multiple organ failure that began during the acute circulatory failure. Severe, unresponsive hypotension as a result of a decreased CO does occur in a subpopulation of patients with septic shock; cardiogenic shock becomes superimposed on the distributive shock of sepsis, but this is not the most common cause of death.[72]

Clinical and Hemodynamic Features

CASE 22-4

QUESTION 1: M.K., a 56-year-old man, was admitted 5 days ago with a chief complaint of acute abdominal pain of 3 days' duration associated with bloody diarrhea, fever, tachypnea, and hypotension. The diagnosis was superior mesenteric artery occlusion with necrotic bowel and he subsequently underwent surgery to remove necrotic bowel

tissue. During postoperative days 1 through 4, his SCr increased to 1.5 mg/dL, and he could not be weaned completely from ventilatory support. Vital signs were stable. Antibiotic therapy included ciprofloxacin and metronidazole in appropriate doses.

M.K. has a history of coronary artery disease with stable angina pectoris that has been treated with lisinopril, simvastatin, and nitroglycerin. He had no other medical problems before admission.

On the morning of postoperative day 5, M.K. has a spiking fever to 39.4°C. Physical findings include a BP of 98/60 mm Hg, pulse 128 beats/minute, and an RR of 28 breaths/minute. His urine output has dropped to 25 mL/hour, and bowel sounds are absent. The chest radiograph shows an enlarged heart with bilateral pulmonary infiltrates and right lower lobe atelectasis. M.K. has become confused and disoriented. ABG on an inspiratory oxygen concentration of 40% are as follows:

Pao_2, 76 mm Hg
$Paco_2$, 34 mm Hg
HCO_3^-, 15 mEq/L
pH, 7.31

M.K. has had increased bronchial secretions for the past 2 days. Pertinent laboratory values are as follows:

SCr, 1.8 mg/dL
BUN, 32 mg/dL
WBC count, 18,000 cells/μL

Urine, sputum, and blood samples are sent for culture and sensitivity. A fluid bolus of 1,000 mL of normal saline solution is given. Arterial and pulmonary artery catheters are inserted, revealing the following hemodynamic profile:

BP (S/D/M), 90/50/63 mm Hg
Pulse, 122 beats/minute
CO, 6 L/minute
CI, 3.5 L/minute/m^2
PCWP, 12 mm Hg
SVR, 720 dyne · s · cm^{-5}

M.K. weighs 70 kg and has a body surface area of 1.7 m^2. What hemodynamic and clinical features of M.K. are consistent with septic shock?

Hemodynamic signs consistent with septic shock include hypotension, tachycardia, elevated CO, low SVR, and a low PCWP. Although the absolute value for CO is high or at the upper limits of the normal range, in septic shock it is inadequate to maintain a BP that will perfuse the essential organs in the face of a decreased SVR, evidenced by the low $\dot{D}o_2$ and $\dot{V}o_2$. M.K. has a metabolic acidosis (pH of 7.31 with a $Paco_2$ of 30 mm Hg and HCO_3^- of 15 mEq/L), indicating anaerobic metabolism most likely caused by decreased perfusion causing lactic acidosis, and a CO that is inadequate to meet the oxygen requirements of the tissues.

Other features consistent with septic shock in M.K. include worsening pulmonary function as indicated by his ABG measurement; declining urine output and altered sensorium, indicating decreased renal and cerebral perfusion; a rising WBC count; and a spiking fever.

Therapeutic Approach

The management of septic shock is directed toward three primary areas: (a) eradication of the source of infection, (b) hemodynamic support and control of tissue hypoxia, and (c) inhibition or attenuation of the initiators and mediators of sepsis.

ERADICATING THE SOURCE OF INFECTION

CASE 22-4, QUESTION 2: What factors should be considered in determining antimicrobial therapy in septic shock? What are the potential sources of infection in M.K.?

Systemic infection caused by either aerobic or anaerobic bacteria is the leading cause of septic shock. Fungal, mycobacterial, rickettsial, protozoal, or viral infections can also be encountered. Among sepsis syndromes caused by aerobic bacteria, gram-negative organisms (e.g., *Enterobacteriaceae, Pseudomonas,* and *Haemophilus,* in decreasing order of frequency) are implicated slightly more often than gram-positive bacteria (e.g., *Staphylococcus aureus, Staphylococcus* coagulase negative, *Streptococcus,* and *Enterococcus,* from highest to lowest frequency). Even these trends vary, however, depending on the infection site. For example, when an organism can actually be cultured in the blood, slightly more gram-positive infections (35%–40%) than gram-negative infections (30%–35%) are found. In nonbloodstream infections (e.g., respiratory tract, genitourinary system, and the abdomen, in descending order of frequency) 40% to 45% can be attributed to gram-negative organisms, and 20% to 25% are caused by gram-positive organisms.[67] Polymicrobial infections make up the next largest group, followed by fungi, anaerobes, and others. In 10% to 30% of sepsis syndrome cases, no organisms can be isolated. Careful consideration of the patient's history and clinical presentation often reveals the most likely cause.

Eradicating the source of infection involves the early administration of antimicrobial therapy, and, if indicated, surgical drainage. The use of an appropriate antibiotic regimen is associated with a significant increase in survival. In one large retrospective study, shock and mortality rates were reduced by 50%.[73] The selection of antibiotics should take into account the presumed site of infection; whether the infection is community or health care associated; recent invasive procedures, manipulations, or surgery; any predisposing conditions; and the likelihood of drug resistance. Ideally, the primary source of the infection can be determined and therapy specifically tailored to the most likely organisms. If the source of infection is unclear, however, early institution of broad-spectrum antibiotics is generally recommended while awaiting culture results. Empiric therapy is indicated, given a greater than 50% mortality rate caused by gram-negative sepsis within the first 2 days of illness and the increasing frequency of polymicrobial infections.[73] Recommended empiric regimens typically include an antipseudomonal penicillin or third- or fourth-generation cephalosporin plus vancomycin or a similar broad-spectrum agent to cover for gram-positive cocci, aerobic gram-negative bacilli, and anaerobes (also see Chapter 60, Principles of Infectious Diseases).

M.K. has several potential sources of sepsis. The first is hospital-acquired pneumonia. M.K. has been intubated for 5 days, infiltrates appear on chest radiograph, and sputum production has increased during the past 2 days. Abdominal abscess or recurrent bowel ischemia also should be considered because bowel sounds are absent. Although no complaints of abdominal tenderness have been elicited, surgical exploration may be necessary. Other potential sources for infection include the urinary tract because M.K. has had an indwelling Foley catheter in place since admission. All IV catheters should be changed if possible.

Ciprofloxacin and metronidazole should be discontinued and imipenem and vancomycin added to broaden M.K.'s antibiotic coverage. Imipenem should adequately cover nosocomial gram-negative pathogens such as *Pseudomonas aeruginosa* and

Acinetobacter baumannii as well as abdominal anaerobic organisms. Vancomycin will cover *S. aureus* from possible IV contamination as well as potential staphylococcal pneumonia. Antimicrobial therapy should be adjusted once cultures are finalized.

INITIAL STABILIZATION

CASE 22-4, QUESTION 3: What are the immediate goals of therapy in M.K.? How can they be achieved and assessed?

The goals in treating septic shock, in addition to eradicating the precipitating infection, are to optimize $\dot{D}O_2$ to the tissues and to control abnormal use of oxygen and anaerobic metabolism by reducing the tissue oxygen demand. Tissue injury is widespread during sepsis, most likely because of vascular endothelial injury with fluid extravasation and microthromboses, which decrease oxygen and substrate utilization by the affected tissues. The mainstay of therapy is volume expansion to increase intravascular volume, enhance CO, and ultimately delay associated development of refractory tissue hypoxia. The therapeutic goals used for hemodynamic resuscitation are controversial. The issue is whether therapy should be directed to physiologic end points of tissue perfusion or clinical end points, such as BP and urine output. The physiologic end points include clearance of blood lactate concentrations, base deficit, SvO_2, and increased CO. Although definitive evidence is lacking, a combination of these physiologic and clinical end points should be used to guide therapy.

Fluids are the mainstay of treatment because increasing CO will improve capillary circulation and tissue oxygenation by maintaining sufficient intravascular volume. If fluids do not correct the hypoxia or if filling pressures are increased, the sequential addition of vasopressors and inotropic agents is indicated. Blood transfusions should be used if the hematocrit is less than 21% unless there is an active source of bleeding or a history of cardiac disease, in which case the hematocrit value would be maintained at a higher value. Crystalloids (with electrolytes to correct imbalances) should be initiated to maintain the CI goal as well as an MAP of 65 mm Hg or an SBP of 90 mm Hg. The MAP is a better reflection of systemic arterial pressure because it considers the diastolic pressure, which is an essential component of blood flow. Although MAP and BP are not absolute measures of blood flow to all vital organs, these pressures are considered the therapeutic end points that will sustain myocardial and cerebral perfusion. After optimization with fluid therapy, vasopressor and inotropic agents are indicated if the patient remains hypotensive with a low CI and if signs of inadequate tissue perfusion persist.

One study has shown that early goal-directed therapy in the treatment of severe sepsis and septic shock leads to improved survival.[74] This approach to patient care integrates both physiologic and clinical end points of resuscitation as early as possible to maintain perfusion during the early stages of sepsis. This study randomly assigned patients admitted to an ED to standard therapy versus goal-directed therapy, which consisted of at least 6 hours of continuous care in the ED where they received a central venous catheter capable of measuring $ScvO_2$. The treatment group maintained a CVP of 8 to 12 mm Hg with continued fluid boluses and a nMAP greater than 65 mm Hg with vasopressor treatment initiated if necessary. If the $ScvO_2$ was less than 70%, red blood cells were transfused to achieve a hematocrit of at least 30%. If the CVP, MAP, and hematocrit were optimized and the $ScvO_2$ was still less than 70%, dobutamine was administered to improve the $\dot{D}O_2$ to the tissues. The primary efficacy end point was in-hospital mortality, which was statistically significantly lower in the early goal-directed group. The results of this study have prompted many institutions to develop "sepsis bundles" that incorporate these same variables and end points of therapy as early as possible in the treatment of sepsis. Sepsis bundles often include many additional issues addressed in the Surviving Sepsis Campaign Guidelines,[4] such as ventilatory support, initial choice of antibiotics, glucose control, and stress ulcer prophylaxis.

M.K should receive fluid boluses to maintain perfusion with an MAP greater than 65 mm Hg and a CVP in the 8- to 12-mm Hg range, and ideally receive a central line to monitor his SvO_2. Continued, excessive fluid challenges to increase preload in M.K. must be approached cautiously, however, because he has a history of ischemic heart disease and ongoing evidence suggestive of pneumonia, both of which could be made worse by overly aggressive fluid boluses. In addition, patients in septic shock are susceptible to experiencing noncardiogenic pulmonary edema or ARDS, which can cause severe deterioration in pulmonary function. Therefore, fluid boluses should be given with ongoing monitoring to determine the CVP and PCWP at which CO is maximal. This approach will avoid excessive CVP and PCWP beyond which CO is no longer increased, thereby reducing the potential formation of pulmonary edema.

In summary, the immediate goal of therapy is to maximize $\dot{D}O_2$ to the tissues. Fluid resuscitation is the mainstay of therapy and improves $\dot{D}O_2$ by increasing CO; however, inotropic and vasopressor agents are often required for additional cardiovascular support. A favorable response to immediate resuscitative efforts will be reflected by a reversal or halt in the progression of the metabolic acidosis, improved sensorium, and increased urine output. In M.K., surgical evaluation for an ongoing or new abdominal process and selection of appropriate antibiotics while maintaining hemodynamic support are the clinical goals of therapy.

HEMODYNAMIC MANAGEMENT

FLUID THERAPY VERSUS INOTROPIC SUPPORT

CASE 22-4, QUESTION 4: M.K. is given two 1,000-mL fluid boluses, and norepinephrine is begun at a rate of 0.05 mcg/kg/minute. During the next 2 hours, he receives 3 L of fluid in boluses, and the norepinephrine is increased to 0.3 mcg/kg/minute to maintain his BP. Signs of pulmonary edema have become more prominent. M.K. has the following hemodynamic profile (previous values in parentheses):

BP (S/D/M), 94/46/62 mm Hg (90/50/63 mm Hg)
Pulse, 124 beats/minute (122 beats/minute)
CO, 7.0 L/minute (6 L/minute)
CI, 3.2 L/minute/m^2 (3.5 L/minute/m^2)
CVP, 13 mm Hg (8 mm Hg)
PCWP, 18 mm Hg (12 mm Hg)
SVR, 560 dyne · s · cm^{-5} (733 dyne · s · cm^{-5})
Urine output, 15 mL/hour
PaO_2, 62 mm Hg (76 mm Hg)
$PaCO_2$, 38 mm Hg (34 mm Hg)
HCO_3^-, 19 mEq/L (15 mEq/L)
pH, 7.30 (7.31)
$\dot{D}O_2$, 445 mL/minute (438 mL/minute)
$\dot{V}O_2$, 118 mL/minute (114 mL/minute)
Positive end-expiratory pressure, 10 cm H_2O

Which of the following therapeutic considerations would be reasonable for M.K. at this time: additional fluid boluses, an increase in the norepinephrine infusion rate, or initiation of a different vasopressor?

M.K. continues to be hypotensive despite a PCWP of 18 mm Hg and a norepinephrine infusion rate of 0.3 mcg/kg/minute. The goals of therapy remain the same (i.e., maximize arterial oxygen content and $\dot{D}o_2$ to reverse cellular anaerobic metabolism).

M.K.'s Pao_2 of 62 mm Hg correlates with an oxygen–hemoglobin saturation of approximately 90%, which should provide an adequate arterial oxygen content. However, $\dot{D}o_2$ still may be inadequate because the CI is less than 3.5 L/minute/m^2, and $\dot{D}o_2$ and $\dot{V}o_2$ have not reached normal levels. In addition, decreased oxygen use can contribute to the continued acidosis. Thus, further attempts to enhance the CI and, hence, $\dot{D}o_2$ are appropriate. However, M.K. has worsening signs of pulmonary edema and a history of cardiovascular disease that will influence the choice of therapeutic options.

Although fluid administration is the mainstay of therapy in septic shock, the elevation of M.K.'s PCWP to 18 mm Hg without a significant increase in CO suggests that an optimal PCWP has been reached. Therefore, additional fluid therapy to maintain his BP may worsen his pulmonary edema and further compromise his pulmonary gas exchange. A plot of CO versus the PCWP (ventricular function curve) would provide a more accurate assessment of the PCWP at which CO is maximal. Additional fluid boluses at this time should be used only to maintain the current level of intravascular volume status.

VASOPRESSORS

NOREPINEPHRINE

When fluid therapy fails to maintain a satisfactory MAP despite an elevated CO, the use of a vasopressor should be considered. Norepinephrine is predominantly an α-adrenergic agonist (Table 22-6) and is frequently used as an adjunct to therapy when inotropic agents alone are unsuccessful. Because concern exists that excessive vasoconstriction might cause reflex decreases in CO and hypoperfusion of vital organs, the use of norepinephrine has often been limited to end-stage shock. However, studies indicate that norepinephrine alone or in combination with inotropic agents can be beneficial in the management of septic shock.[75]

Martin et al. compared the ability of dopamine and norepinephrine to reverse hemodynamic and metabolic abnormalities of hyperdynamic shock.[76] They prospectively randomly assigned 32 volume-resuscitated patients with hyperdynamic sepsis to receive either dopamine or norepinephrine with the goal of achieving and maintaining normal hemodynamic and oxygen transport parameters for at least 6 hours. If goals were not achieved with one agent, the other agent was added. With the use of dopamine, 31% of patients met the predefined therapeutic goals. In contrast, 93% of patients treated with norepinephrine met the predefined goals. Of the patients who did not respond to dopamine, 91% achieved the goals with the addition of norepinephrine. In this study, norepinephrine was found to be superior to dopamine, with improvement in arterial BP, urine flow, $\dot{D}o_2$, $\dot{V}o_2$, and lactate levels.

In a similar study of patients in whom previous therapy with plasma volume expansion and dopamine or dobutamine had failed, norepinephrine reversed hypotension and significantly increased MAP, SVR, and urine output.[75] The CI was increased, albeit insignificantly, in 7 of 10 patients, presumably because of stimulation of cardiac β-receptors. By limiting the indexed SVR to 700 dyne · s · cm^{-5}/m^2, the investigators were able to prevent excessive vasoconstriction and promote an increased perfusion pressure to vital organs as reflected by an improved urine flow. $\dot{D}o_2$ and $\dot{V}o_2$ were measured in 6 of 10 patients with variable results. Although no patient died of refractory hypotension, 4 of 10 patients died of progressive hypoxia, leading the authors to conclude that regardless of the catecholamines used, the ultimate goal of therapy should be to maximize $\dot{D}o_2$ and $\dot{V}o_2$.

PHENYLEPHRINE

Occasionally, patients will respond to epinephrine or phenylephrine when other catecholamines have failed, although neither of these agents is considered to be first-line therapy. Epinephrine stimulates α-, β_1-, and β_2-adrenergic receptors (Table 22-6). CO is augmented via increased contractility and HR, with the contribution of each being highly variable. Blood vessels in the kidney, skin, and mucosa constrict in response to α-adrenergic stimulation, whereas vessels in the skeletal muscle vasodilate because of β_2 effects. A biphasic response in SVR is observed with increasing doses as β_2-receptors are activated at the lower range, and α_1-receptors are stimulated at higher levels. The improvement in CO, therefore, may be negated by an increase in afterload at higher dosages.

Phenylephrine is a pure α-adrenergic agonist (Table 22-6) and, thus, increases systolic, diastolic, and mean arterial pressures through vasoconstriction. Reflex bradycardia can occur secondarily because of the absence of β-adrenergic effects. The increase in afterload, while increasing myocardial $\dot{V}o_2$, correspondingly increases coronary blood flow because of increased perfusion pressure and autoregulation. Therefore, in patients with myocardial hypoxia, or in those experiencing atrial or ventricular arrhythmias, phenylephrine can be beneficial because it has minimal direct cardiac effects. In situations in which the CO is decreased, however, phenylephrine can be detrimental. Preload is reduced as plasma fluid is lost owing to increased capillary hydrostatic pressure, forcing water and solutes from the vascular space into the interstitial spaces. This response, in addition to the reflex bradycardia, may significantly impair CO (Table 22-6).

VASOPRESSIN

Catecholamines have been the mainstay of treatment to support BP in septic patients once adequate fluid resuscitation has been achieved. Sepsis, however, can cause a decrease in responsiveness to catecholamines resulting in refractory hypotension, possibly because of downregulation of adrenergic receptors. Thus, other avenues of supportive treatment have been researched. Septic patients exhibit an increased sensitivity to vasopressin. Vasopressin is an endogenous hormone that has very little effect on BP under normal conditions, but becomes very important in maintaining BP when the baroreceptor reflex is impaired, such as in shock states. Vasopressin's direct vasoconstricting actions are mediated by the vascular V_1 receptors coupled to phospholipase C.[77,78] When these receptors are activated, calcium is released from the sarcoplasmic reticulum in smooth muscle cells, leading to vasoconstriction. One study found that vasopressin levels were very low in septic patients, whereas patients in cardiogenic shock displayed an appropriate increase in vasopressin release for the degree of hypotension.[79] The same investigators showed that a low-dose, continuous IV infusion of vasopressin at 0.04 units/minute in septic shock caused a statistically significant increase in vasopressin levels, systolic arterial pressure, and SVR when added to pre-existing catecholamine treatment, with several patients maintaining BP on vasopressin alone. It is presumed that vasopressin secretion is impaired as opposed to enhanced vasopressin metabolism, but it is not entirely clear why this occurs. Most likely it is a combination of a deficient baroreceptor reflex–mediated secretion of vasopressin, impaired sympathetic function, and potentially depletion of the secretory stores of vasopressin.

Until recently, it was unknown whether the addition of vasopressin affected mortality. The VASST study compared norepinephrine to vasopressin in patients with septic shock unresponsive to fluids and on vasopressor therapy and looked at mortality at 28 days as the primary end point.[80] Vasopressin was initiated and then titrated to a maximal dose of 0.03 units/minute.

Vasopressin therapy significantly decreased the amount of norepinephrine required; however, there was no statistical difference in mortality between the treatment groups except when the patients were stratified according to severity of sepsis. The patients with less severe septic shock benefited from vasopressin therapy. This study evaluated vasopressin as a catecholamine-sparing drug rather than as rescue therapy for catecholamine-unresponsive shock, which was how it was studied in previous trials.

M.K. has decreased MAP despite the addition and increased titration of norepinephrine. Because patients in septic shock have decreased endogenous levels of vasopressin, it would be reasonable to add vasopressin at 0.03 units/minute to the norepinephrine infusion to increase the MAP and renal perfusion.

INOTROPIC AGENTS

Although the use of inotropic agents is well established, controlled comparative studies have not clearly determined which agent, or combination of agents, is most useful in the management of septic shock. Because differences among the inotropic agents are significant, however, selection of the most appropriate drug should be guided by careful consideration of the patient's hemodynamic status.

DOPAMINE

Dopamine has frequently been the initial pharmacologic agent chosen for the treatment of septic shock. If the MAP is low with a depressed CO and a low SVR, dopamine is an appropriate choice because its combined α-adrenergic vasoconstrictive actions and β-adrenergic inotropic effects will increase SVR and CO, thereby effectively raising it. In situations in which the PCWP is elevated or in patients with decreased ventricular compliance, the use of dopamine may be limited because it significantly increases venous return and ventricular filling pressure. In addition, dopamine increases shunting of pulmonary blood flow, leading to a decline in Pa_{O_2}. This effect may worsen hypoxemia in patients with pneumonia or ARDS.

DOBUTAMINE

Dobutamine is often advocated as the secondary inotropic agent in the management of septic shock, particularly in patients with low CO and high filling pressures. Dobutamine produces a greater increase in CO than dopamine, but also lowers SVR. In contrast to dopamine, dobutamine lowers PCWP, and causes less pulmonary shunting. Because dobutamine can lower ventricular filling pressure, volume status must be monitored closely to avoid the development of hypotension and reduced MAP. Fluids should be administered as needed to maintain the PCWP at maximal tolerated levels of 16 to 18 mm Hg. With the administration of greater amounts of fluid, CO, $\dot{D}_{O_2}$, and systemic $\dot{V}_{O_2}$ are significantly increased. Dobutamine does increase $\dot{D}_{O_2}$ and CI when given concurrently with or after volume resuscitation. Decreases in Pa_{O_2} and increases in venous P_{O_2}, as well as adverse effects on myocardium, may be evident at higher dosages (>6 mcg/kg/minute).[81]

Combinations of vasopressors and inotropic agents can also be used to achieve desired hemodynamic parameters. Because GI perfusion can be compromised owing to the vasoconstricting effects of catecholamines and may play a role in the pathogenesis of multiple organ dysfunction, the combination of norepinephrine and dobutamine has been studied to determine whether an advantage exists to using norepinephrine alone, epinephrine alone, or a combination.[82,83] One prospective study randomly assigned patients with an MAP less than 60 mm Hg despite adequate fluid resuscitation and treatment with high-dose dopamine to either dobutamine plus norepinephrine or epinephrine monotherapy titrated to an MAP greater than 80 mm Hg.[82] The variables were the MAP, metabolic effects as evidenced by lactate and pyruvate concentrations, and splanchnic perfusion measured by the gap between gastric pH and P_{CO_2}. This study showed that both therapies, norepinephrine plus dobutamine and epinephrine monotherapy, were equally effective at achieving hemodynamic goals, but that treatment with epinephrine alone could worsen splanchnic oxygen utilization and potentially lead to ischemic injury. Currently, it is unknown whether a specific catecholamine regimen provides a significant benefit over others. There are conflicting data about which vasopressor can increase gastric perfusion and whether this increase can alter progression to organ dysfunction.

CASE 22-4, QUESTION 5: Given M.K.'s history of cardiovascular disease, what factors should you consider before initiating a vasopressor agent? Outline an overall approach to maintaining adequate hemodynamic status.

M.K. has a history of coronary artery disease and is susceptible to myocardial ischemia. Therefore, a careful balance must be achieved between myocardial $\dot{V}_{O_2}$ and coronary perfusion pressure. Further attempts to optimize MAP and CI with norepinephrine alone could increase myocardial $\dot{V}_{O_2}$ and precipitate ischemia. Evidence suggests that the goal of therapy in treating patients with septic shock, or any form of shock for that matter, is not to simply normalize BP, but to optimize $\dot{D}_{O_2}$ and $\dot{V}_{O_2}$. Once anemia and hypoxia have been corrected, CO becomes the remaining parameter that can be adjusted to increase oxygen supply, but raising arterial BP and CO with inotropic agents or vasopressors before restoring adequate blood volume actually can worsen tissue perfusion. Therefore, the selection of an inotropic agent must take into consideration the patient's current hemodynamic status and the individual properties of those agents that will most effectively maintain or increase the MAP and CO. In many instances, because of individual variability and response, more than one inotropic agent or addition of a vasopressor is required to achieve these end points. These interventions must be made with strict monitoring of the patients' response to the interventions to prevent any adverse consequences, especially in those patients who are predisposed to an adverse event such as M.K.

It is important to realize that the response to exogenous catecholamines in patients with septic shock is highly variable and a successful regimen in one patient may be unsuccessful in another. In addition, septic patients often require infusion rates in the moderate-to-high range. Therefore, the goal is to use one or more agents at the dosages necessary to achieve the desired end points without unduly compromising the patient's status. The use of catecholamines, however, is only a stabilizing measure. Strict attention to all other physiologic parameters—as well as nutritional support, antibiotic modification, and ongoing surgical intervention—cannot be overemphasized.

OTHER THERAPIES

Therapies directed against the initiators and mediators of sepsis are currently the focus of intense investigation. As previously discussed, numerous exogenous and endogenous substances are involved in the pathogenesis of sepsis. Strategies under development include antioxidants and free radical scavengers; antiendotoxin therapy; and inhibition of leukocytes, secondary mediators (i.e., TNF-α, IL-1, cytokine pathway), coagulation and arachidonic acid metabolites, complement, and NO. Although several experimental therapies hold considerable promise for the future, controlled human data are still lacking.

CORTICOSTEROIDS

CASE 22-4, QUESTION 6: What is the rationale for the use of glucocorticosteroids in the treatment of septic shock, and is there evidence to support their use for this indication in M.K.?

The use of corticosteroids in sepsis and septic shock has been a controversial topic for many years. Corticosteroids were originally proposed as a treatment option because of their anti-inflammatory properties with the hope of attenuating the body's response to infection. More recently it has been shown that critically ill patients exhibit impaired cortisol secretion because of a relative adrenocortical insufficiency, and it is suspected that these patients display a glucocorticoid peripheral resistance syndrome. Almost 50% of patients with septic shock exhibit relative adrenal insufficiency defined as a maximal change in cortisol level of less than 9 mcg/dL after a 250-mcg IV dose of corticotropin.[84]

Several clinical trials have been performed during the past few decades with varying results, and meta-analyses have recommended discontinuation of high-dose corticosteroid therapy because of detrimental outcomes.[85,86] End points that have been studied include time to reversal of septic shock (defined by cessation of vasopressor support) and mortality. Older trials used different definitions of septic shock, however, and the timing and dosing of steroids were highly variable. Two recent trials have shown that corticosteroid therapy may be beneficial in severe septic shock at lower, physiologic doses. The trial by Annane et al.[87] showed a mortality benefit with the use of low doses of hydrocortisone and fludrocortisones in patients with severe septic shock who exhibited a relative adrenocortical insufficiency. On the other hand, the CORTICUS[88] trial showed a faster resolution of shock for those patients on hydrocortisone as evidenced by faster time to weaning from vasopressors; however, those patients also had a higher incidence of superinfection and new episodes of sepsis or septic shock. There was also no mortality benefit seen with the use of corticosteroids. The CORTICUS trial included patients with septic shock, whereas the study by Annane et al. only enrolled patients with severe septic shock unresponsive to vasopressor therapy. The results of these studies demonstrate that corticosteroid therapy may not have a role in the general population of patients with septic shock; however, it may be beneficial for those patients unresponsive to vasopressors who are treated early.

Because M.K. is refractory to increasing doses of norepinephrine and is in severe sepsis, it was decided to start hydrocortisone 50 mg IV every 6 hours.

STATINS

CASE 22-4, QUESTION 7: Is there any significance to the fact that M.K. was on statin therapy before his episode of sepsis? Should his statin therapy be continued?

Aside from their well-described lipid-lowering effects, statins appear to have immunomodulatory and anti-inflammatory effects. Statin therapy lowers C-reactive protein levels, inhibits endothelial cell dysfunction, causes upregulation of endothelial NO synthase, and blocks immune cell receptors.[89] A growing body of evidence shows that patients who are on a statin before the inciting septic event may have a decreased likelihood of developing sepsis, and a mortality benefit may exist for those with sepsis or multiple organ dysfunction. All studies in humans thus far have been retrospective and in patients who were previously on a statin. One trial showed a significant survival benefit associated with continuing statin therapy in patients who were bacteremic compared with those who were never on statin therapy.[90] Potentially more important is that the highest mortality was seen in those patients who had been on statin therapy, but had been discontinued (result not statistically significant). These results may lend credence to the idea of a rebound phenomenon that could be detrimental if statins are not continued. Statins are often discontinued in septic patients because of concern for adverse effects and further organ dysfunction. Presently, it is not clear whether statins should always be continued in septic patients, and it is unknown whether statins should be initiated in patients who develop sepsis. Further evidence by means of prospective, randomized trials is needed to further define the role of statins in sepsis.

DROTRECOGIN ALFA

CASE 22-4, QUESTION 8: What is the rationale for recombinant activated protein C in septic shock?

Activated protein C (APC) is an endogenous protein that acts as one of the regulators of the coagulation cascade and also interrupts the amplification cycle of inflammation.[68] Protein C is the inactive precursor to APC, and conversion to the active form requires thrombin to complex with thrombomodulin. APC enhances fibrinolysis and has potent inhibitory effects on thrombin, which possesses thrombotic as well as inflammatory effects. Other anti-inflammatory effects of APC stem from suppression of TNF-α, IL-6, and IL-1production.

Patients in septic shock exhibit microvascular thrombosis, which leads to organ hypoperfusion, cell dysfunction, multiple organ dysfunction, and death. The systemic response to infection activates the coagulation pathway, leading to the generation of thrombin and deposition of fibrin as well as initiating an inflammatory reaction via activation of cytokines. Adult and pediatric septic patients have low levels of protein C, and a poor outcome is expected for those patients with the lowest levels.[91] The deficiency in protein C is probably caused by enhanced degradation as well as impaired synthesis of protein C. It is also apparent that patients in septic shock exhibit lower levels of thrombomodulin, the protein necessary for the conversion of protein C to APC. Thus, the use of APC would counter the anticoagulant deficiency as well as suppress the inflammatory reaction that would normally take place owing to the infection.

The Protein C Worldwide Evaluation in Severe Sepsis (PROWESS)[69] trial was a phase III clinical trial to evaluate the safety and efficacy of drotrecogin alfa (recombinant APC). It was a randomized, double-blind, placebo-controlled, multicenter trial that was stopped early because of the statistically significant difference in the primary end point, 28-day all-cause mortality, before enrollment was complete. Included in the study were patients with a known or suspected infection plus three or more signs of systemic inflammation and at least one organ system dysfunction caused by sepsis. Patients also had to begin treatment of drotrecogin alfa at 24 mcg/kg/hour for 96 hours within 24 hours of meeting inclusion criteria. The list of exclusion criteria was extensive to ensure that patients who were at higher risk for bleeding did not participate in the trial. No standardized protocol was established for the critical care provided to the patient (e.g., antibiotics, vasopressors, inotropes). Treatment with drotrecogin alfa reduced D-dimer and IL-6 levels, indicating attenuation of the procoagulant and inflammatory effects of sepsis. Treatment with drotrecogin alfa was associated with a 6.1% absolute reduction in mortality at 28 days after the start of infusion. The incidence of serious bleeding was higher in the APC group, almost reaching statistical significance ($p = 0.06$). A

ASTHMA

According to the National Institutes of Health (NIH) Expert Panel Report 3 (EPR-3), Guidelines for the Diagnosis and Management of Asthma,[1] *asthma* is defined as a chronic inflammatory disorder of the airways in which many cells and cellular elements play a role, in particular, mast cells, eosinophils, T lymphocytes, neutrophils, and epithelial cells. In susceptible persons, this inflammation causes recurrent episodes of wheezing, breathlessness, chest tightness, and cough, particularly at night and in the early morning. These episodes are usually associated with widespread but variable airflow obstruction that is often reversible either spontaneously or with treatment. The inflammation also causes an increase in the existing bronchial hyperresponsiveness to a variety of stimuli.[2] This definition of asthma is the same as the 1997 NIH guidelines[2] and has evolved from earlier national and international guidelines.[3–6]

At least 22 million Americans have asthma.[1] It is an underdiagnosed and undertreated condition that is estimated to have overall costs exceeding $12 billion annually in the United States.[7] Asthma is the leading cause of lost school days in children and is a common cause of lost workdays among adults.

Mortality from asthma has decreased in the 21st century, from 4,657 deaths in 1999 to 3,447 deaths in 2007 in the United States according to the Centers for Disease Control and Prevention,[8,9] but morbidity and mortality are still unacceptably high, especially in inner-city minority populations. This chapter emphasizes the 2007 NIH EPR-3 guidelines.[1] Application of the principles of these recent guidelines by clinicians and patients is vital to further reducing asthma morbidity and mortality.

Etiology

Childhood-onset asthma is usually associated with atopy, which is the genetic predisposition for the development of immunoglobulin E (IgE)–mediated response to common aeroallergens. Atopy is the strongest predisposing factor in the development of asthma.[1] A very common presentation of asthma is a child with a positive family history of asthma and allergy to tree and grass pollen, house dust mites, household pets, and molds.

Adult-onset asthma may also be associated with atopy, but many adults with asthma have a negative family history and negative skin tests to common aeroallergens. Some of these patients may have nasal polyps, aspirin sensitivity, and sinusitis. In the British 1958 birth cohort study, participants were monitored for wheezing and asthma at periodic intervals from birth into their mid-forties.[10] In the subset of patients who were seemingly asymptomatic during late adolescence and early adulthood, the presence of asthma at 42 years of age was significantly higher in those patients who had a history of wheezing in childhood. Exposure to factors (e.g., wood dust, chemicals) at the workplace that may cause airway inflammation is also important in many adults. Inflammatory mechanisms are similar, but not the same, as in atopic asthma. Some clinicians may still refer to *intrinsic asthma* when referring to these patients and *extrinsic asthma* when discussing atopic asthma.

In addition to atopy and exposure to occupational chemical sensitizers being major risk factors for the development of asthma, several contributing factors may increase the susceptibility to the development of the disease in predisposed individuals.[1,5] These factors include viral infections, small size at birth, diet, exposure to tobacco smoke, and environmental pollutants.[1,5]

Recent literature has focused on the "hygiene hypothesis," an imbalance of T_H2 and T_H1 type T lymphocytes, to explain the marked increase in asthma in westernized countries.[1,5,8] Infants who have older siblings, early exposure to day care, and typical childhood infections are more likely to activate T_H1 responses (protective immunity), resulting in an appropriate balance of T_H1 to T_H2 cells and the cytokines that they produce. On the other hand, if the immune response is predominately from T_H2 cells (which produce cytokines that mediate allergic inflammation), development of diseases such as asthma is more likely. Examples of factors favoring this imbalance include the common use of antimicrobial agents, urban environment, and Western lifestyle. Further insights into the pathogenesis of asthma continue to be discovered.[1,7,11,12]

Pathophysiology

Asthma is caused by a complex interaction between inflammatory cells and mediators. As noted in the definition of asthma, mast cells, eosinophils, T lymphocytes, neutrophils, and epithelial cells are of central importance. The bronchial epithelium in asthmatic patients has been described as fragile, with various abnormalities including destruction of ciliated cells and overexpression of epidermal growth factors.[13] Figure 23-1 depicts the complex interaction of cells and mediators associated with airway inflammation.

After exposure to an asthma-precipitating factor (e.g., aeroallergen), inflammatory mediators are released from bronchial mast cells, macrophages, T lymphocytes, and epithelial cells. These mediators direct the migration and activation of other inflammatory cells, most notably eosinophils, to the airways.[1,11,12] Eosinophils release biochemicals (e.g., major basic protein and eosinophil cationic protein) that cause airway injury, including epithelial damage, mucus hypersecretion, and increased reactivity of smooth muscle.[1,7,11]

Research continues to determine the role of a subpopulation of T lymphocytes (T_H2) in asthmatic airway inflammation.[1,11] T_H2 lymphocytes release cytokines (e.g., interleukin [IL] 4 and IL-5) that at least partially control the activation and enhanced survival of eosinophils.[1,4,11] The complexity of airway inflammation is indicated by the fact that at least 27 cytokines may have a role in the pathophysiology of asthma.[11] In addition, at least 18 chemokines (e.g., eotaxins) have been identified that are important in delivery of eosinophils to the airways.[11] One biomarker of airway inflammation is exhaled nitric oxide (NO), which has been used as a treatment guide in chronic asthma.[1] Bronchial NO has been found to be elevated during periods of exacerbations and is measurably decreased with administration of inhaled steroids but not β_2-agonists.[1,14] Failure to adequately minimize severe and long-term airway inflammation in asthma may result in airway remodeling in some patients. Airway remodeling refers to structural changes, including an alteration in the amount and composition of the extracellular matrix in the airway wall, leading to airflow obstruction that eventually may become only partially reversible.[1,15]

Hyperreactivity (defined as an exaggerated response of bronchial smooth muscles to trigger stimuli) of the airways to physical, chemical, immunologic, and pharmacologic stimuli is pathognomonic of asthma.[2] Examples of these stimuli include inhaled allergens; respiratory viral infection; cold, dry air; smoke; other pollutants; and methacholine. Endogenous stimuli that can worsen asthma include poorly controlled rhinitis, sinusitis, and gastroesophageal reflux disease.[1] In addition, premenstrual asthma has been reported, but the exact hormonal mechanism is not known.[16]

Although patients with allergic rhinitis, chronic bronchitis, and cystic fibrosis also experience bronchial hyperreactivity, these patients do not experience bronchiolar constriction as severely as do patients with asthma. The degree of bronchial

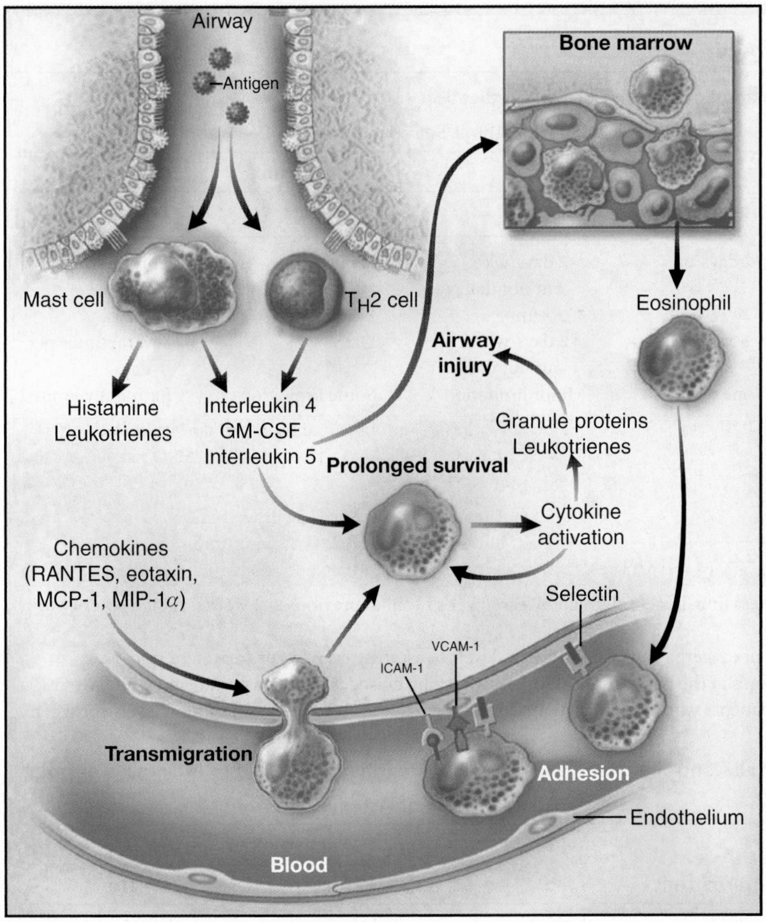

FIGURE 23-1 Airway inflammation. Inhaled antigen activates mast cells and T_H2 cells in the airway. They in turn induce the production of mediators of inflammation (such as histamine and leukotrienes) and cytokines including interleukin 4 and interleukin 5. Interleukin 5 travels to the bone marrow and causes terminal differentiation of eosinophils. Circulating eosinophils enter the area of allergic inflammation and begin migrating to the lung by rolling, through interactions with selectins, and eventually adhering to endothelium through the binding of integrins to members of the immunoglobulin superfamily of adhesion proteins: vascular-cell adhesion molecule 1 (VCAM-1) and intercellular adhesion molecule 1 (ICAM-1). As the eosinophils enter the matrix of the airway through the influence of various chemokines and cytokines, their survival is prolonged by interleukin 4 and granulocyte-macrophage colony-stimulating factor (GM-CSF). On activation, the eosinophil releases inflammatory mediators, such as leukotrienes and granule proteins, to injure airway tissues. In addition, eosinophils can generate GM-CSF to prolong and potentiate their survival and contribution to persistent airway inflammation. MCP-1, monocyte chemotactic protein; MIP-1α, macrophage inflammatory protein; RANTES, chemokine ligand 5. Adapted with permission from Busse WW, Lemanske RF Jr. Asthma. *N Engl J Med.* 2001;344:350.

hyperreactivity of asthmatic patients correlates with the clinical course of their disease, which is characterized by periods of remissions and exacerbations. During times of remission, a more intense stimulus is required to produce bronchospasm than during times of increased symptoms. Numerous theories have been proposed to explain the bronchial hyperreactivity found in asthma, yet none fully explains the phenomenon. Inflammation appears to be the primary process in the pathogenesis of bronchial hyperreactivity; however, neurogenic imbalances in the airways also may play a significant role.[5] Inflamed airways are hyperreactive (i.e., irritable). Hyperreactivity can be measured in the physician's office by having the patient inhale small concentrations of nebulized methacholine or histamine or by exercise (e.g., treadmill). The concentration of aerosolized methacholine or histamine that decreases the forced expiratory volume in 1 second (FEV_1) by 20% is referred to as the PD_{20} or the PC_{20} (provocative dose or concentration that decreases the FEV_1 by 20%).[2] An indicator of optimal anti-inflammatory therapy is an increase in the PD_{20} with time as the airways become less inflamed and therefore less hyperreactive.

Another concept related to inflammation is "late-phase" versus "early-phase" asthma (Fig. 23-2). The inhalation of specific allergens in atopic asthmatic patients produces immediate bronchoconstriction (measured by a drop in peak expiratory flow [PEF] or FEV_1) that spontaneously improves in an hour or is reversed easily by inhalation of a β_2-agonist. Although this early asthmatic response (EAR) is blocked by the preadministration of β_2-agonists, cromolyn, or theophylline, a second bronchoconstrictive response often occurs 4 to 12 hours later. This late asthmatic response (LAR) often is more severe, more prolonged, and more difficult to reverse with bronchodilators than is the EAR. The LAR is associated with the influx of inflammatory cells and mediators as described previously. Bronchodilators do not block the LAR to allergen challenge; corticosteroids block the LAR but do not affect the EAR; and cromolyn blocks both.[2]

Pathologic changes found at autopsy performed on asthmatic patients include (a) marked hypertrophy and hyperplasia of the bronchial smooth muscle, (b) mucous gland hypertrophy and excessive mucus secretion, and (c) denuded epithelium and mucosal edema owing to an exudative inflammatory reaction and inflammatory cell infiltration.[1] Hyperinflation of the lungs from air trapping with extensive mucous plugging is found at

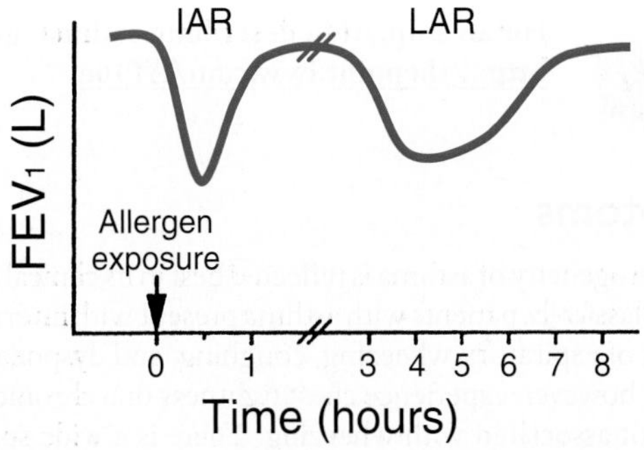

FIGURE 23-2 Typical immediate and late asthmatic responses seen after exposure to relevant allergen. Immediate asthmatic response (IAR) occurs within minutes, whereas late asthmatic response (LAR) occurs several hours after exposure. Patients may demonstrate isolated IAR, isolated LAR, or dual responses. FEV_1, forced expiratory volume in 1 second. Adapted with permission from Herfindal ET, Gourley DR, eds. *Textbook of Therapeutics Drug and Disease Management.* 7th ed. Baltimore, MD: Lippincott Williams & Wilkins; 2003.

TABLE 23-1
Classifying Asthma Severity in Children 0 to 4 Years of Age

Classifying Severity in Children who are not Currently Taking Long-term Control Medication

Components of Severity		Classification of Asthma Severity (Children 0–4 Years of Age)			
			Persistent		
		Intermittent	Mild	Moderate	Severe
Impairment	Symptoms	≤2 days/wk	>2 days/wk but not daily	Daily	Throughout the day
	Nighttime awakenings	0	1–2×/mo	3–4×/mo	>1×/wk
	SABA use for symptom control (not prevention of EIB)	≤2 days/wk	>2 days/wk but not daily	Daily	Several times per day
	Interference with normal activity	None	Minor limitation	Some limitation	Extremely limited
Risk	Exacerbations requiring oral systemic corticosteroids	0–1/y	≥2 exacerbation in 6 months requiring oral corticosteroids or ≥4 wheezing episodes in 1 year lasting >1 day AND risk factors for persistent asthma		
		Consider severity and interval since last exacerbation. ← Frequency and severity may fluctuate with time. → Exacerbations of any severity may occur in patients in any severity category.			

Level of severity is determined by both impairment and risk. Assess impairment domain by caregiver's recall of previous 2–4 weeks. Assign severity to the most severe category in which any feature occurs.

At present, there are inadequate data to correspond frequencies of exacerbations with different levels of asthma severity. For treatment purposes, patients who had ≥2 exacerbations requiring oral corticosteroids in the past 6 months, or ≥4 wheezing episodes in the past year, and who have risk factors for persistent asthma may be considered the same as patients who have persistent asthma, even in the absence of impairment levels consistent with persistent asthma.

Classifying Severity in Patients After Asthma Becomes Well Controlled, by Lowest Level of Treatment Required to Maintain Control

	Classification of Asthma Severity			
		Persistent		
	Intermittent	Mild	Moderate	Severe
Lowest level of treatment required to maintain control (See Fig. 23-7 for treatment steps.)	Step 1	Step 2	Step 3 or 4	Step 5 or 6

EIB, exercise-induced bronchospasm; SABA, short-acting inhaled β_2-agonist.
Reprinted from National Institutes of Health. *Expert Panel Report 3: Guidelines for the Diagnosis and Management of Asthma.* Bethesda, MD: National Heart, Lung, and Blood Institute; 2007. NIH publication 07-4051.

autopsy in patients who have died of acute asthma attacks, but these changes also are seen at autopsy in asthmatic patients dying of other causes. The bronchial smooth muscle hypertrophy and mucus hypersecretion are secondary to the chronic inflammatory response.[17]

ONLINE CONTENT

For an animation describing asthma, go to http://thepoint.lww.com/AT10e.

Symptoms

The heterogeneity of asthma is reflected best in its clinical presentation. Classically, patients with asthma present with intermittent episodes of expiratory wheezing, coughing, and dyspnea. Some patients, however, experience chest tightness or a chronic cough that is not associated with wheezing. There is a wide spectrum of disease severity, ranging from patients with occasional, mild bouts of breathlessness to patients who wheeze daily despite continuous high dosages of medication. In addition, the severity of asthma may be influenced by environmental factors (e.g., specific seasonal allergens). Symptoms often are associated with exercise and sleep (refer to Case 23-11, Case 23-12, and Case 23-14).

Classification of asthma severity is of major importance in defining initial long-term treatment. Within three age groups, EPR-3 uses the classifications of intermittent, mild persistent, moderate persistent, and severe persistent asthma (Tables 23-1–23-3). The frequency of symptoms is a key component of asthma classification.[1] For example, mild persistent asthma is defined as symptoms more than two times per week or nocturnal symptoms (including early morning chest tightness) more than two times per month. Many clinicians are unaware that this level of symptoms is defined as persistent asthma. This classification is of major significance when selecting long-term drug therapy in that daily use of anti-inflammatory agents is an essential part of management for persistent asthma.[1]

Diagnosis and Monitoring

HISTORY

The diagnosis of asthma is based primarily on a detailed history of intermittent symptoms of wheezing, chest tightness, shortness of breath, and coughing. These episodes may be worse seasonally (e.g., springtime or late summer and early fall) or in association with exercise. History of nocturnal symptoms with awakening in the early morning is a critical component to assess. In addition, history of symptoms after exposure to other common triggers (e.g., cats, perfume, secondhand tobacco smoke) is typical (Table 23-4). A positive family history and the presence of rhinitis or atopic dermatitis also are significant. After a careful history is obtained, skin testing may be useful in identifying triggering

TABLE 23-2
Classifying Asthma Severity in Children 5 to 11 Years of Age

Classifying Severity in Children who are not Currently Taking Long-term Control Medication

Components of Severity		Classification of Asthma Severity (Children 5–11 Years of Age): Intermittent	Persistent: Mild	Persistent: Moderate	Persistent: Severe
Impairment	Symptoms	≤2 days/wk	>2 days/wk but not daily	Daily	Throughout the day
	Nighttime awakenings	≤2×/mo	3–4×/mo	>1×/wk but not nightly	Often 7×/wk
	SABA use for symptom control (not prevention of EIB)	≤2 days/wk	>2 days/wk but not daily	Daily	Several times per day
	Interference with normal activity	None	Minor limitation	Some limitation	Extremely limited
	Lung function	• Normal FEV_1 between exacerbations • FEV_1 >80% predicted • FEV_1/FVC >85%	• FEV_1 >80% predicted • FEV_1/FVC >80%	• FEV_1 = 60%–80% predicted • FEV_1/FVC 75%–80%	• FEV_1 <60% predicted • FEV_1/FVC <75%
Risk	Exacerbations requiring oral systemic corticosteroids	0–1 in 1 year (see note)	≥2 in 1 year (see note) →		
		Consider severity and interval since last exacerbation. Frequency and severity may fluctuate with time for patients in any severity category. Relative annual risk of exacerbations may be related to FEV_1.			

Level of severity is determined by both impairment and risk. Assess impairment domain by patient's or caregiver's recall of the previous 2–4 weeks and spirometry. Assign severity to the most severe category in which any feature occurs.

At present, there are inadequate data to correspond frequencies of exacerbations with different levels of asthma severity. In general, more frequent and intense exacerbations (e.g., requiring urgent, unscheduled care, hospitalization, or ICU admission indicate greater underlying disease severity. For treatment purposes, patients who had ≥2 exacerbations requiring oral systemic corticosteroids in the past year may be considered the same as patients who have persistent asthma, even in the absence of impairment levels consistent with persistent asthma.

Classifying Severity in Patients After Asthma Becomes Well Controlled, by Lowest Level of Treatment Required to Maintain Control

	Classification of Asthma Severity: Intermittent	Persistent: Mild	Persistent: Moderate	Persistent: Severe
Lowest level of treatment required to maintain control **(See Fig. 23-8 for treatment steps.)**	Step 1	Step 2	Step 3 or 4	Step 5 or 6

EIB, exercise-induced bronchospasm; FEV_1, forced expiratory volume in 1 second; FVC, forced vital capacity; ICU, intensive care unit; SABA, short-acting β_2-agonist.
Reprinted from National Institutes of Health. *Expert Panel Report 3: Guidelines for the Diagnosis and Management of Asthma.* Bethesda, MD: National Heart, Lung, and Blood Institute; 2007. NIH publication 07-4051.

allergens, but it is only of supportive value in the diagnosis of asthma.

PULMONARY FUNCTION TESTS

The diagnosis of asthma is based in part on demonstration of reversible airway obstruction. A brief discussion of tests to detect reversibility of airway obstruction is important. Furthermore, a short summary of arterial blood gases (ABGs) is pertinent here in assessing the severity of asthma exacerbations.

SPIROMETRY

Lung volumes often are measured to obtain information about the size of the patient's lungs because pulmonary diseases can affect the volume of air that can be inhaled and exhaled. The tidal volume is the volume of air inspired or expired during normal breathing. The volume of air blown off after maximal inspiration to full expiration is defined as the vital capacity (VC). The residual volume (RV) is the volume of air left in the lung after maximal expiration. The volume of air left after a normal expiration is the functional residual capacity (FRC). Total lung capacity (TLC) is the VC plus the RV. Patients with obstructive lung disease have difficulty with expiration; therefore, they tend to have a decreased VC, an increased RV, and a normal TLC. Classic restrictive lung diseases (e.g., sarcoidosis, idiopathic pulmonary fibrosis) present with decrements in all lung volumes.[18] Patients also may have mixed lesion diseases, in which case the classic findings are not apparent until the disease has advanced considerably.

The spirometer also can be used to evaluate the performance of the patient's lungs, thorax, and respiratory muscles in moving air into and out of the lungs. Forced expiratory maneuvers amplify the ventilation abnormalities produced. The single most useful test for ventilatory dysfunction is the forced expiratory volume (FEV). The FEV is measured by having the patient exhale into the spirometer as forcefully and completely as possible after maximal inspiration. The resulting volume curve is plotted against time (Fig. 23-3) so that expiratory flow can be

TABLE 23-3
Classifying Asthma Severity in Youths ≥12 Years of Age and Adults

Classifying Severity in Patients who are not Currently Taking Long-term Control Medication

Components of Severity		Classification of Asthma Severity (Youths ≥12 Years of Age and Adults): Intermittent	Persistent: Mild	Persistent: Moderate	Persistent: Severe
Impairment	Symptoms	≤2 days/wk	>2 days/wk but not daily	Daily	Throughout the day
	Nighttime awakenings	≤2×/mo	3–4×/mo	>1×/wk but not nightly	Often 7×/wk
	SABA use for symptom control (not prevention of EIB)	≤2 days/wk	>2 days/wk but not >1×/day	Daily	Several times per day
Normal FEV_1/FVC: 8–19 years, 85%; 20–39 years, 80%; 40–59 years, 75%; 60–80 years, 70%	Interference with normal activity	None	Minor limitation	Some limitation	Extremely limited
	Lung function	• Normal FEV_1 between exacerbations • FEV_1 >80% predicted • FEV_1/FVC normal	• FEV_1 ≥80% predicted • FEV_1/FVC normal	• FEV_1 >60% but <80% predicted • FEV_1/FVC reduced 5%	• FEV_1 <60% predicted • FEV_1/FVC reduced >5%
Risk	Exacerbations requiring oral systemic corticosteroids	0–1 in 1 year (see note)	≥2 in 1 year (see note) →		
		← Consider severity and interval since last exacerbation. Frequency and severity may fluctuate with time for patients in any severity category. → Relative annual risk of exacerbations may be related to FEV_1.			

Level of severity is determined by assessment of both impairment and risk. Assess impairment domain by patient's or caregiver's recall of previous 2–4 weeks and spirometry. Assign severity to the most severe category in which any feature occurs.

At present, there are inadequate data to correspond frequencies of exacerbations with different levels of asthma severity. In general, more frequent and intense exacerbations (e.g., requiring urgent, unscheduled care, hospitalization, or ICU admission) indicate greater underlying disease severity. For treatment purposes, patients who had ≥2 exacerbations requiring oral systemic corticosteroids in the past year may be considered the same as patients who have persistent asthma, even in the absence of impairment levels consistent with persistent asthma.

Classifying Severity in Patients After Asthma Becomes Well Controlled, by Lowest Level of Treatment Required to Maintain Control

	Classification of Asthma Severity: Intermittent	Persistent: Mild	Persistent: Moderate	Persistent: Severe
Lowest level of treatment required to maintain control (See Fig. 23-9 for treatment steps.)	Step 1	Step 2	Step 3 or 4	Step 5 or 6

[a] EIB, exercise-induced bronchospasm; FEV_1, forced expiratory volume in 1 second: FVC, forced vital capacity; ICU, intensive care unit; SABA, short-acting β_2-agonist.
Reprinted from National Institutes of Health. *Expert Panel Report 3: Guidelines for the Diagnosis and Management of Asthma*. Bethesda, MD: National Heart, Lung, and Blood Institute; 2007. NIH publication 07-4051.

estimated. For a video that shows how to take a lung function test, see **http://www.european-lung-foundation.org/index.php?id=15411**.

Standard spirometers contain pneumotachographs in the mouthpieces that can measure airflow directly. A number of important measures of lung function are made from the resulting flow–volume curves (Fig. 23-4). The advantages of this technique include a display of simultaneous flows at any lung volume, visual estimation of patient effort and cooperation, high reproducibility within as well as across individuals, and an analysis of the distribution of flow limitation.[18,19] The FEV_1 of the forced vital capacity (FVC, the maximal volume of air exhaled with maximally forced effort from a position of maximal inspiration) commonly is measured to determine the dynamic performance of the lung in moving air. The FEV_1 usually is expressed as a percentage of the total volume of air exhaled and is reported as the FEV_1 to FVC ratio. Healthy persons generally can exhale at least 75% to 80% of their VC in 1 second and almost all of it in 3 seconds. Thus, the FEV_1 normally is 80% of the FVC. The patient's breathing ability is compared against "predicted normal" values for patients with similar physiologic characteristics because lung volumes depend on age, race, sex, height, and weight. For example, an average-sized young adult man may have an FVC of 4 to 5 L and a corresponding FEV_1 of 3.2 to 4 L. The FEV_1 and the FVC are the most reproducible of the pulmonary function tests.

PEAK EXPIRATORY FLOW

The PEF is the maximal flow that can be produced during the forced expiration. The PEF can be measured easily with various handheld peak flow meters and commonly is used in emergency departments (EDs) and clinics to quickly and objectively assess the effectiveness of bronchodilators in the treatment of acute asthma attacks. Peak flow meters also can be used at home by patients with asthma to assess chronic therapy. The changes in PEF generally parallel those of the FEV_1; however, the PEF is a less reproducible measure than the FEV_1.[5] A healthy,

TABLE 23-4
Sample Questions for the Diagnosis and Initial Assessment of Asthma[a]

A "yes" answer to any question suggests that an asthma diagnosis is likely.

In the past 12 months . . .

- Have you had a sudden severe episode or recurrent episodes of coughing, wheezing (high-pitched whistling sounds when breathing out), chest tightness, or shortness of breath?
- Have you had colds that "go to the chest" or take more than 10 days to get over?
- Have you had coughing, wheezing, or shortness of breath during a particular season or time of the year?
- Have you had coughing, wheezing, or shortness of breath in certain places or when exposed to certain things (e.g., animals, tobacco smoke, perfumes)?
- Have you used any medications that help you breathe better? How often?
- Are your symptoms relieved when the medications are used?

In the past 4 weeks, have you had coughing, wheezing, or shortness of breath . . .

- At night that has awakened you?
- On awakening?
- After running, moderate exercise, or other physical activity?

[a] These questions are examples and do not represent a standardized assessment or diagnostic instrument. The validity and reliability of these questions have not been assessed.

Reprinted from National Institutes of Health. *Expert Panel Report 3: Guidelines for the Diagnosis and Management of Asthma*. Bethesda, MD: National Heart, Lung, and Blood Institute; 2007. NIH publication 07-4051.

average-sized young adult man typically has a PEF of 550 to 700 L/minute. Commercial peak flow meters come with a chart for patients to determine their predicted normal PEFs based on their sex, age, and height.

OBSTRUCTIVE VERSUS RESTRICTIVE AIRWAY DISEASE

Generally, pulmonary disorders fall into two categories: those that restrict the lungs and thorax and those that obstruct them.

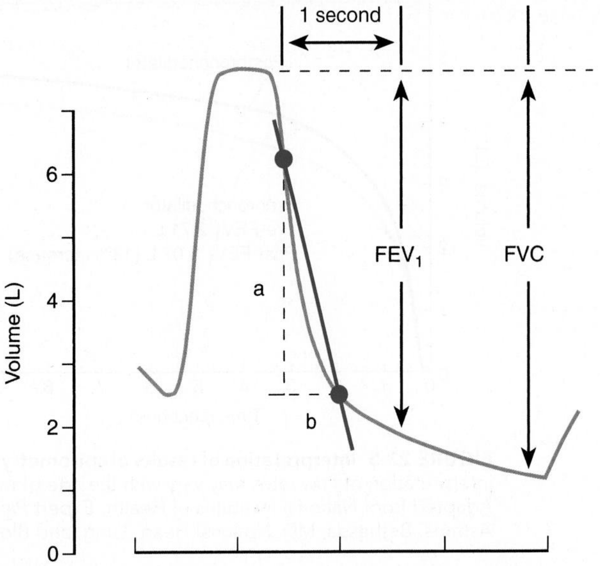

FIGURE 23-3 Volume–time curve from a forced expiratory maneuver. FEV_1, forced expiratory volume in 1 second; FVC, forced vital capacity.

In simplest terms, restrictive disease limits airflow during inspiration, and obstructive disease limits airflow during expiration. Restrictive disease results from a loss of elasticity (e.g., fibrosis, pneumonia) or physical deformities of the chest (e.g., kyphoscoliosis), with a consequent inability to expand the lung and a reduced TLC. Therefore, a typical flow–volume curve (Fig. 23-4C) for a patient with restrictive disease shows markedly depressed volumes with increased flow rates (when corrected for the volume).

Whereas restrictive airway diseases limit lung expansion, obstructive airway diseases (e.g., bronchitis, asthma) narrow air passages, create air turbulence, and increase resistance to airflow. In obstructive diseases, maximal expiration may begin at higher-than-normal lung volumes, and the expiratory flow is depressed (Fig. 23-4B). Resistance to flow is increased at lower lung

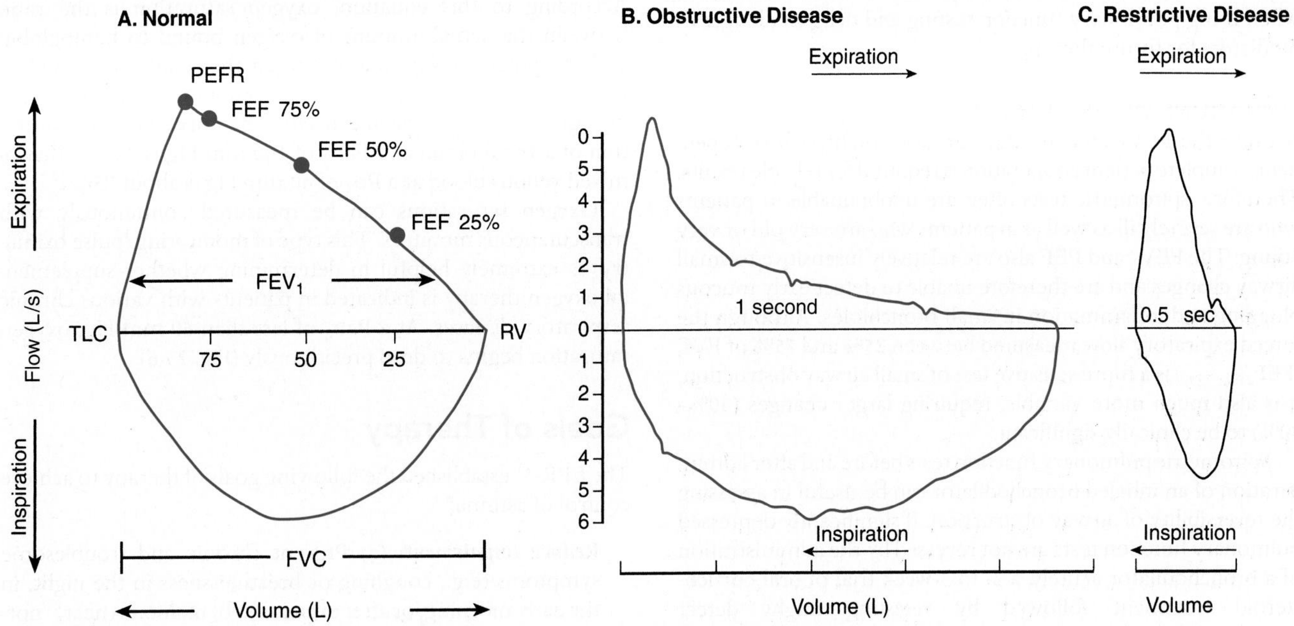

FIGURE 23-4 Flow–volume curves resulting from a forced expiratory maneuver. A: Normal flow–volume curve. **B:** Typical pattern for obstructive disease. **C:** Typical pattern for restrictive disease. FEF 25%, 50%, 75%, forced expiratory flow at 25%, 50%, and 75% of FVC; FEV_1, forced expiratory volume in 1 second; FVC, forced vital capacity; PEFR, peak expiratory flow rate; RV, residual volume; TLC, total lung capacity.

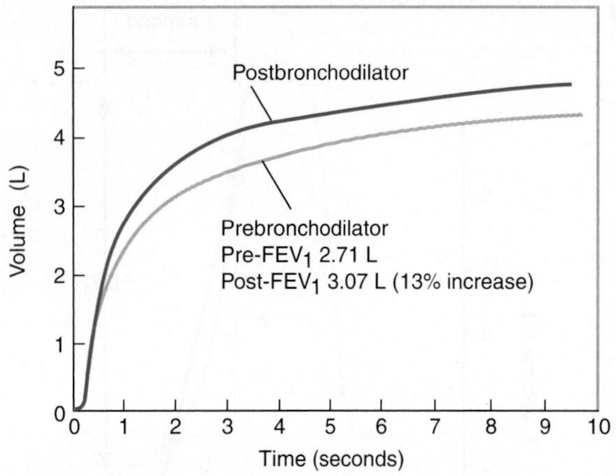

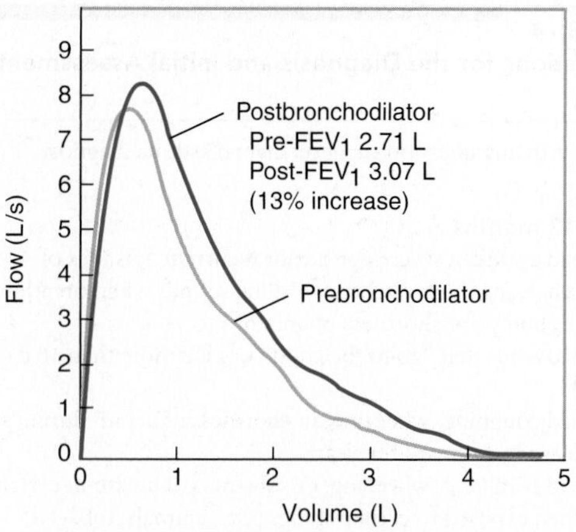

FIGURE 23-5 Interpretation of results of spirometry. The graphs depicted are for illustration only. The interpretation of flow rates may vary with the age of the patient. FEV_1, forced expiratory volume in 1 second. Adapted from National Institutes of Health. *Expert Panel Report 2. Guidelines for the Diagnosis and Management of Asthma.* Bethesda, MD: National Heart, Lung, and Blood Institute; 1997. NIH publication 97-4051.

volumes, giving the characteristic scooped-out appearance of the obstructive flow–volume curve (Fig. 23-4B).

REVERSIBLE AIRWAY OBSTRUCTION

Spirometry often is used to determine the reversibility of airway disease. Although many generally associate reversibility with bronchospasm, therapy can improve airflow by reversing any of the causative pathologic processes of asthma described previously. Significant clinical reversibility produced from bronchodilators is determined by the tests outlined in Figure 23-5. The FEV_1 is considered the gold standard test for determining reversibility of airway disease and bronchodilator efficacy. Significant clinical reversibility is defined as a 12% improvement in FEV_1 after administration of a short-acting bronchodilator.[1] An improvement of 20% in FEV_1 provides noticeable subjective relief of respiratory symptoms in most patients. For patients with a very low baseline FEV_1 (e.g., <1 L), an absolute improvement of 250 mL sometimes is considered a better indicator of therapeutic benefit than assessing percentage of change. In either case, the patient's subjective clinical impression also should be considered when using pulmonary function testing and drug challenges as predictors for future therapy.

LIMITATIONS OF SPIROMETRY

Because the FEV_1 and the PEF are both highly effort dependent, complete patient cooperation is required for reliable results. Therefore, spirometric tests often are unobtainable in patients who are severely ill as well as in patients who are very old or very young. The FEV_1 and PEF also are relatively insensitive to small airway changes and are therefore unable to detect early mucous plugging and inflammation in small bronchioles. Although the forced expiratory flow measured between 25% and 75% of FVC ($FEF_{25\%-75\%}$) is a more sensitive test of small airway obstruction, it is also much more variable, requiring larger changes (30%–40%) to be clinically significant.

Spirometric pulmonary function tests before and after administration of an inhaled bronchodilator can be useful in assessing the reversibility of airway obstruction. If significantly depressed pulmonary function tests are not reversed by the administration of a bronchodilator acutely, a 2- to 3-week trial of oral corticosteroid treatment followed by retesting might detect reversibility.[1]

If pulmonary function is normal or near normal at the time of spirometric assessment, the patient can be challenged by exercise or drugs that are known to produce bronchospasm in asthmatic patients (e.g., aerosolized methacholine).

BLOOD GAS MEASUREMENTS

The best indicators of overall lung function (ventilation and diffusion) are the ABGs (i.e., arterial partial pressure of oxygen [Pa_{O_2}], arterial partial pressure of carbon dioxide [Pa_{CO_2}], and pH). Although ABG measurements also are dependent on the patient's cardiovascular status, they are indispensable in assessing both acute and chronic changes in pulmonary patients. (See Chapter 9, Acid–Base Disorders, for a review of ABGs.) Another means of assessing the patient's ability to oxygenate tissues adequately is to measure oxygen saturation, which is described by the following equation:

$$O_2 \text{ saturation} = \frac{\text{Quantity of } O_2 \text{ actually bound to hemoglobin}}{\text{Quantity of } O_2 \text{ that can be bound to hemoglobin}} \times 100 \qquad \textit{(Eq. 23-1)}$$

According to this equation, oxygen saturation is the ratio between the actual amount of oxygen bound to hemoglobin and the potential amount of oxygen that could be bound to hemoglobin at a given pressure. The denominator in the preceding equation is the oxygen capacity. The normal oxygen saturation of arterial blood at a Pa_{O_2} of 100 mm Hg is 97.5%; that of mixed venous blood at a P_{O_2} of 40 mm Hg is about 75%.[18]

Oxygen saturations can be measured continuously with transcutaneous monitors. This type of monitoring (pulse oximetry) is extremely helpful in determining whether supplemental oxygen therapy is indicated in patients with various chronic respiratory diseases. At a Pa_{O_2} of less than 60 mm Hg, oxygen saturation begins to drop precipitously (Fig. 23-6).

Goals of Therapy

The EPR-3[1] established the following goals of therapy to achieve control of asthma:

Reduce Impairment: (a) Prevent chronic and troublesome symptoms (e.g., coughing or breathlessness in the night, in the early morning, or after exertion); (b) maintain (near) "normal" pulmonary function; (c) maintain normal activity levels (including exercise, other physical activities, and attendance at work or school); (d) require infrequent use of short-acting

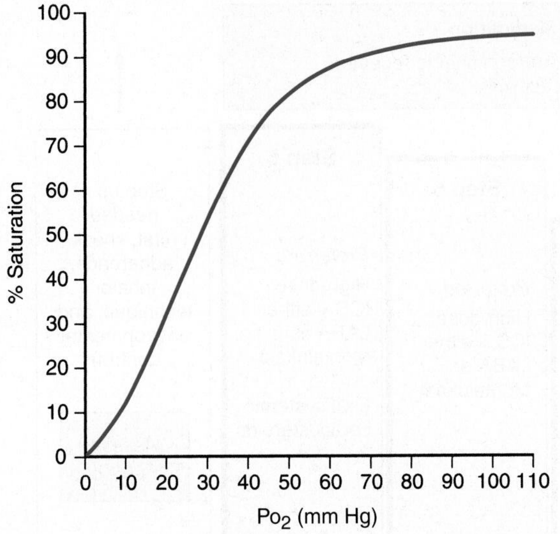

FIGURE 23-6 The oxygen dissociation curve reveals that the percent saturation of hemoglobin increases almost linearly with increases in the arterial O_2 tension until a partial pressure of arterial oxygen (PaO_2) of 55 to 65 mm Hg is reached. At PaO_2 values above this, the increase in hemoglobin saturation becomes proportionately less, and relatively little additional oxygen is added to the hemoglobin despite large increases in PaO_2. Adapted with permission from Guenther CA, Welch MH. *Pulmonary Medicine*. 2nd ed. Philadelphia, PA: JB Lippincott; 1982.

inhaled β_2-agonists ([SABAs], $\leq$2 days a week for quick relief of symptoms); and (e) meet patients' and families' expectations of and satisfaction with asthma care.

Reduce Risk: (a) Prevent recurrent exacerbations of asthma and minimize the need for ED visits or hospitalizations; (b) prevent progressive loss of lung function—for children, prevent reduced lung growth; and (c) provide optimal pharmacotherapy with minimal or no adverse effects.

MAJOR COMPONENTS OF LONG-TERM MANAGEMENT

To achieve these goals of therapy, EPR-3[1] also outlines some general treatment principles. Asthma management has four major components, including (a) measures of asthma assessment and monitoring, (b) education for a partnership in asthma care, (c) control of environmental factors and comorbid conditions that affect asthma, and (d) medications. Optimal long-term management requires a continuous care approach, including each of these four major components, to prevent exacerbations and decrease airway inflammation. Early therapeutic interventions in managing acute exacerbations are very important in decreasing the chance of severe narrowing of the airways. Achieving the goals of asthma therapy also involves individualizing each patient's therapy. In addition, optimal care involves establishing a "partnership" between the patient, the patient's family, and the clinician.

For most patients with asthma, the condition can be well controlled by using the step–care approach recommended by EPR-3[1] (Figs. 23-7, 23-8, 23-9). A concerted effort in patient education as an integral part of state-of-the-art long-term management has been demonstrated to improve outcomes, including quality of life in patients with asthma. Because of the excellent outcomes associated with optimal long-term management, if a patient requires an ED visit or hospitalization, great care should be given to determining how the acute-care visit could have been prevented.

ACUTE ASTHMA

Assessment

SIGNS AND SYMPTOMS

CASE 23-1

QUESTION 1: Q.C., a 6-year-old, 20-kg girl, presents to the ED with complaints of dyspnea and coughing that have progressively worsened during the past 2 days. These symptoms were preceded by 3 days of symptoms of a viral upper respiratory tract infection (sore throat, rhinorrhea, and coughing). She has experienced several bouts of bronchitis in the last 2 years and was hospitalized for pneumonia 3 months ago. Q.C. is not being treated with any medications at present. Physical examination reveals an anxious-appearing young girl in moderate respiratory distress with audible expiratory wheezes; occasional coughing; a prolonged expiratory phase; a hyperinflated chest; and suprasternal, supraclavicular, and intercostal retractions. Bilateral inspiratory and expiratory wheezes with decreased breath sounds on the left side are heard on auscultation. Q.C.'s vital signs are as follows: respiratory rate (RR), 30 breaths/minute; blood pressure (BP), 110/83 mm Hg; heart rate, 130 beats/minute; temperature, 37.8°C; and pulsus paradoxus, 18 mm Hg. Her arterial oxygen saturation (SaO_2) by pulse oximetry is 90%. Q.C. is given O_2 to maintain SaO_2 greater than 90% and 2.5 mg of albuterol by nebulizer every 20 minutes for three doses. After the initial treatment, Q.C. claims some subjective improvement and appears to be more comfortable; however, wheezing on auscultation becomes louder. What signs and symptoms in Q.C. are consistent with acute bronchial obstruction? Does increased wheezing after albuterol indicate failure of the medication?

Asthma is an obstructive lung disease; therefore, the primary limitation to airflow occurs during expiration. This outflow obstruction leads to the classic findings of dyspnea, expiratory wheezes, and a prolonged expiratory phase during the ventilatory cycle.[1] Wheezing is a whistling sound produced by turbulent airflow through a constricted opening and usually is more prominent on expiration. Thus, the audible expiratory wheezing in Q.C. is compatible with bronchial obstruction. In fact, Q.C.'s obstruction is so severe that even inspiratory wheezes and decreased air movement were detected on auscultation. It is important to realize that the classic symptom of wheezing requires turbulent airflow; therefore, effective therapy of acute asthma actually may result in increased wheezing initially as airflow increases throughout the lung. As a result, Q.C.'s increased wheezing on auscultation is compatible with her clinical improvement after the albuterol nebulizer treatments.

The coughing experienced by Q.C. is another common finding associated with acute asthma attacks. The coughing may caused by stimulation of "irritant receptors" in the bronchi by the chemical mediators of inflammation (e.g., leukotrienes) that are released from mast cells or from the mechanics of smooth muscle contraction.

In the progression of an asthma attack, the small airways become completely occluded during expiration, and air can be trapped behind the occlusion; therefore, the patient has to breathe at higher-than-normal lung volumes.[1] Consequently, the thoracic cavity becomes hyperexpanded, and the diaphragm is lowered. As a result, the patient must use the accessory muscles of respiration to expand the chest wall. Q.C.'s hyperinflated chest and her use of suprasternal, supraclavicular, and intercostal

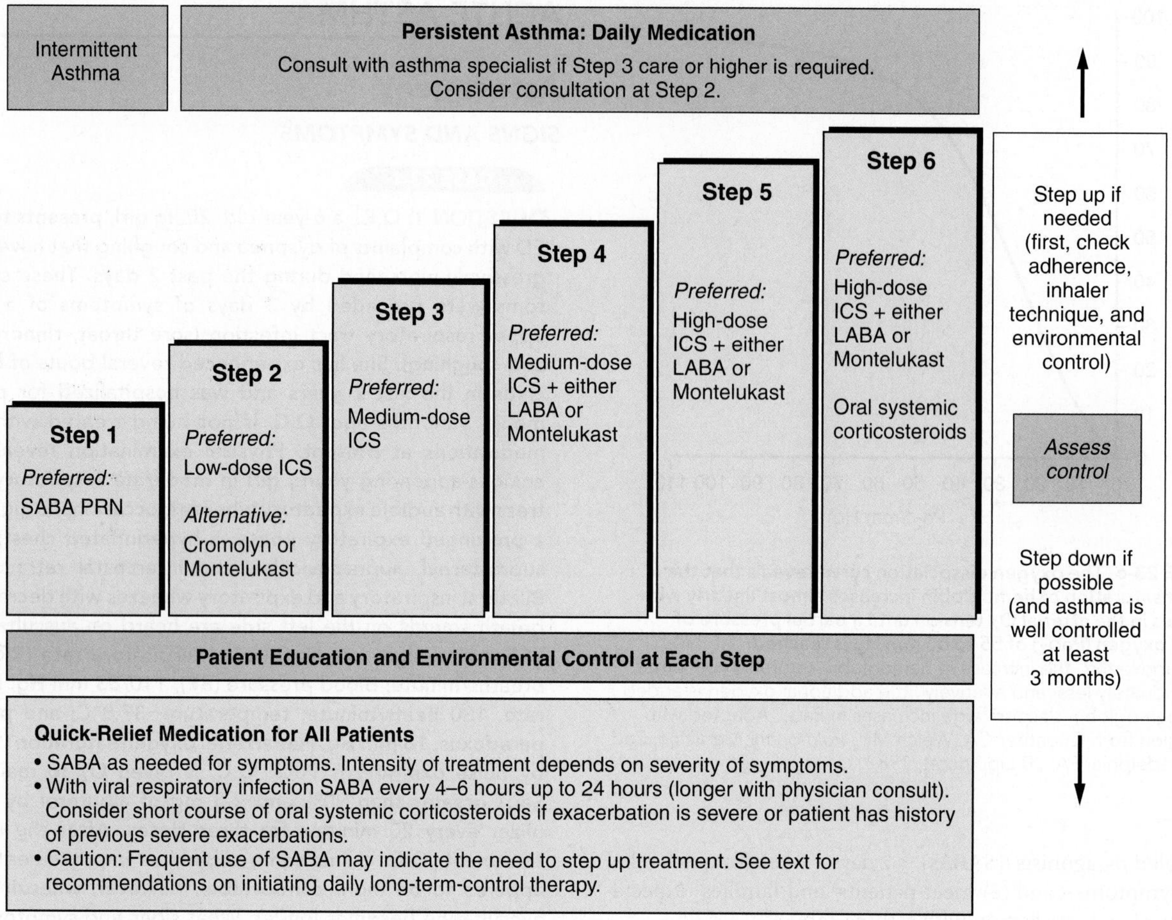

Key: **Alphabetical order is used when more than one treatment option is listed within either preferred or alternative therapy.** ICS, inhaled corticosteroid; LABA, inhaled long-acting β_2-agonist; SABA, inhaled short-acting β_2-agonist.

Notes:

- The stepwise approach is meant to assist, not replace, the clinical decision-making required to meet individual patient needs.
- If alternative treatment is used and response is inadequate, discontinue it and use the preferred treatment before stepping up.
- If clear benefit is not observed within 4–6 weeks and patient/family medication technique and adherence are satisfactory, consider adjusting therapy or alternative diagnosis.
- Studies on children 0–4 years of age are limited. Step 2 preferred therapy is based on Evidence A. All other recommendations are based on expert opinion and extrapolation from studies in older children.

FIGURE 23-7 Stepwise approach for managing asthma in children 0 to 4 years of age. Reprinted from National Institutes of Health. *Expert Panel Report 3: Guidelines for the Diagnosis and Management of Asthma.* Bethesda, MD: National Heart, Lung, and Blood Institute; 2007. NIH publication 07-4051.

muscles to assist in breathing also are compatible with obstructive airway diseases.

Occlusion of the small airways, air trapping, and resorption of air distal to the obstruction can lead to atelectasis (incomplete expansion or collapse of pulmonary alveoli or of a segment of a lobe of the lung). Localized areas of atelectasis often are difficult to distinguish from infiltrates on a chest radiograph, and atelectasis can be mistaken for pneumonia.

Q.C.'s history of multiple bouts of "bronchitis" is significant and typical of many young asthmatic patients. In any patient with recurring episodes of bronchial symptoms (i.e., bronchitis, pneumonia), the possible diagnosis of asthma should be investigated.

The increased pulse, RR, and anxiety experienced by Q.C. can be attributed both to hypoxemia and the feeling of suffocation. The hypoxemia in acute asthma is caused principally by an imbalance between alveolar ventilation and pulmonary capillary blood flow, also known as ventilation–perfusion ($\dot{V}/\dot{Q}$) mismatching.[20] Each alveolus of the lung is supplied with capillaries from the pulmonary artery for gas exchange. When ventilation is decreased to an area of the lung, the alveoli in that area become hypoxic, and the pulmonary artery to that region constricts as a normal physiologic response. As a result, blood flow is shunted to the well-ventilated portions of the lung because of the need to preserve adequate oxygenation of the blood. The pulmonary arteries, however, are not constricted completely, and when a small amount of blood flows to the poorly ventilated alveoli, mismatching is the result. Conditions of diffuse bronchial obstruction (i.e., acute asthma) increase the amount of mismatching. In addition, some mediators of acute bronchospasm (e.g., histamine) further worsen mismatching by constricting bronchial smooth muscle while concurrently relaxing vascular smooth muscle.

Q.C. also demonstrated a significant pulsus paradoxus. *Pulsus paradoxus* is defined as a drop in systolic BP of more than 10 mm Hg with inspiration. In general, pulsus paradoxus correlates with the severity of bronchial obstruction; however, it is not always present.[20]

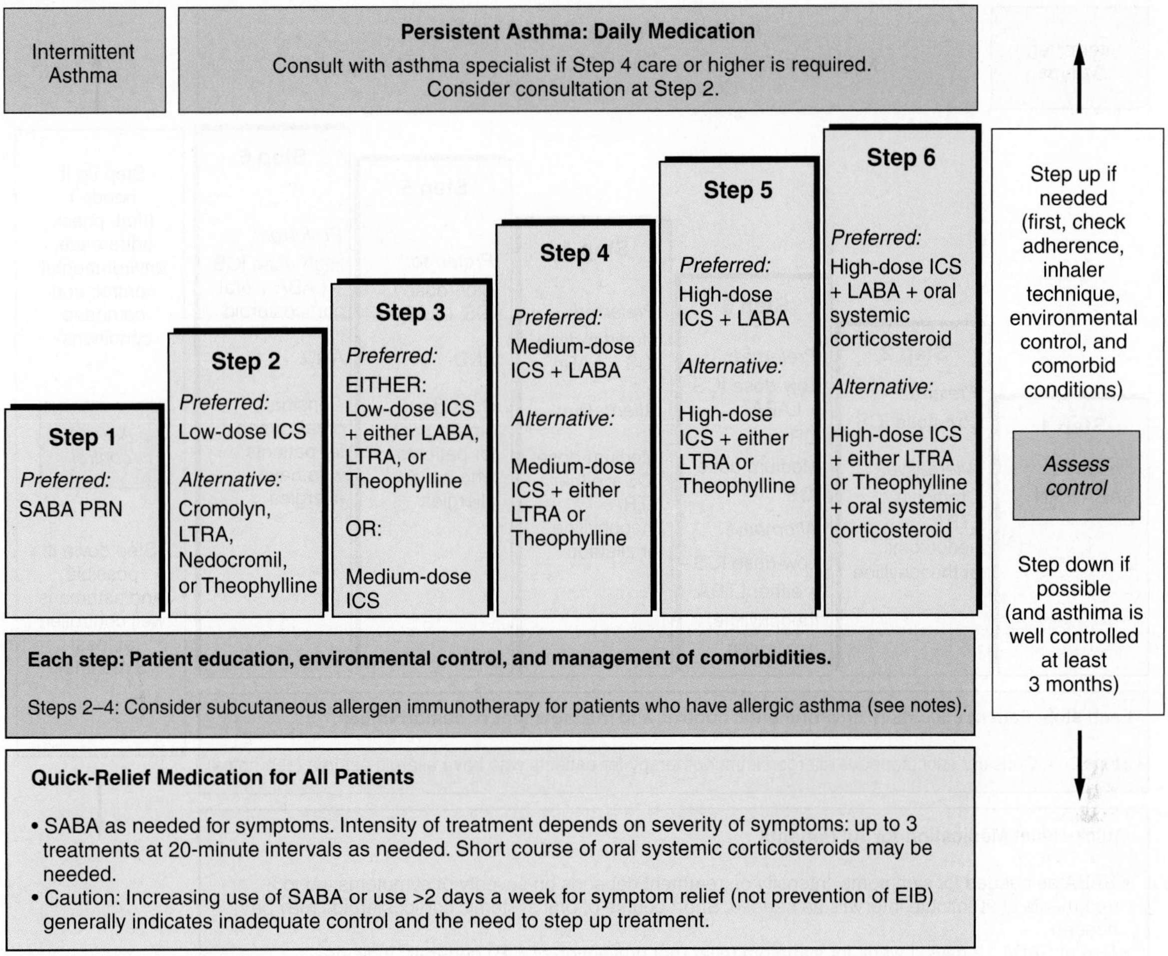

Intermittent Asthma
Persistent Asthma: Daily Medication
Consult with asthma specialist if Step 4 care or higher is required.
Consider consultation at Step 2.
Step 1
Preferred:
SABA PRN
Step 2
Preferred:
Low-dose ICS
Alternative:
Cromolyn, LTRA, Nedocromil, or Theophylline
Step 3
Preferred:
EITHER:
Low-dose ICS + either LABA, LTRA, or Theophylline
OR:
Medium-dose ICS
Step 4
Preferred:
Medium-dose ICS + LABA
Alternative:
Medium-dose ICS + either LTRA or Theophylline
Step 5
Preferred:
High-dose ICS + LABA
Alternative:
High-dose ICS + either LTRA or Theophylline
Step 6
Preferred:
High-dose ICS + LABA + oral systemic corticosteroid
Alternative:
High-dose ICS + either LTRA or Theophylline + oral systemic corticosteroid
Step up if needed (first, check adherence, inhaler technique, environmental control, and comorbid conditions)
Assess control
Step down if possible (and asthima is well controlled at least 3 months)
Each step: Patient education, environmental control, and management of comorbidities.
Steps 2–4: Consider subcutaneous allergen immunotherapy for patients who have allergic asthma (see notes).
Quick-Relief Medication for All Patients
• SABA as needed for symptoms. Intensity of treatment depends on severity of symptoms: up to 3 treatments at 20-minute intervals as needed. Short course of oral systemic corticosteroids may be needed.
• Caution: Increasing use of SABA or use >2 days a week for symptom relief (not prevention of EIB) generally indicates inadequate control and the need to step up treatment.

Key: **Alphabetical order is used when more than one treatment option is listed within either preferred or alternative therapy.** ICS, inhaled corticosteroid; LABA, inhaled long-acting β_2-agonist; LTRA, leukotriene receptor antagonist; SABA, inhaled short-acting β_2-agonist.

Notes:

- The stepwise approach is meant to assist, not replace, the clinical decision-making required to meet individual patient needs.
- If alternative treatment is used and response is inadequate, discontinue it and use the preferred treatment before stepping up.
- Theophylline is a less desirable alternative because of the need to monitor serum concentration levels.

FIGURE 23-8 Stepwise approach for managing asthma in children 5 to 11 years of age. Reprinted from National Institutes of Health. *Expert Panel Report 3: Guidelines for the Diagnosis and Management of Asthma.* Bethesda, MD: National Heart, Lung, and Blood Institute; 2007. NIH publication 07-4051.

EXTENT OF OBSTRUCTION

CASE 23-1, QUESTION 2: What additional tests would be helpful in assessing the extent of pulmonary obstruction in Q.C.?

Chest radiographs are not recommended routinely but should be obtained in patients who are suspected of having a complication (e.g., pneumonia).[1] Hyperinflated lungs and areas of atelectasis can be seen on a chest x-ray film; however, chest x-ray studies usually are negative and of little value in evaluating acute asthma attacks. The finding of a local decrease in breath sounds in Q.C.'s left lung may justify the need for a chest x-ray study, particularly if a significant differential in air movement persists after initial therapy. A local decrease in breath sounds may indicate pneumonia, aspiration of a foreign object, pneumothorax, or merely thickened mucous plugging of a large bronchus.

Pulmonary function testing (e.g., FEV_1, PEF) provides objective measurement of the degree of airway obstruction. Peak flow meters are helpful in the ED for assessing both the severity of airway obstruction and the response to bronchodilator therapy. Unfortunately, infants and many young children do not have the cognitive or motor skills necessary to perform pulmonary function tests. EPR-3 points out that in one study, only 65% of children 5 to 16 years of age could complete either FEV_1 or PEF during an acute exacerbation. Because of Q.C.'s initial anxiety, the PEF should be measured after bronchodilator therapy has been initiated when she may be calmer. One disadvantage of pulmonary function tests in acute asthma is that the forced expiratory maneuver commonly triggers coughing. ABG measurements are the gold standard for assessing very severe airway obstruction.[21] EPR-3[1] suggests ABGs for evaluation of $Paco_2$ in patients who have suspected hypoventilation, severe distress, or FEV_1 or PEF less than 25% of predicted after initial treatment. However, in less severe exacerbations, ABG measurements are unnecessary if other objective measures of airway obstruction (e.g., pulmonary function tests) have been monitored.[1] In acute asthma, ABG determinations usually indicate hypoxemia because of mismatching and hypocapnia with respiratory alkalosis because of hyperventilation.[21] The degree of hypoxemia

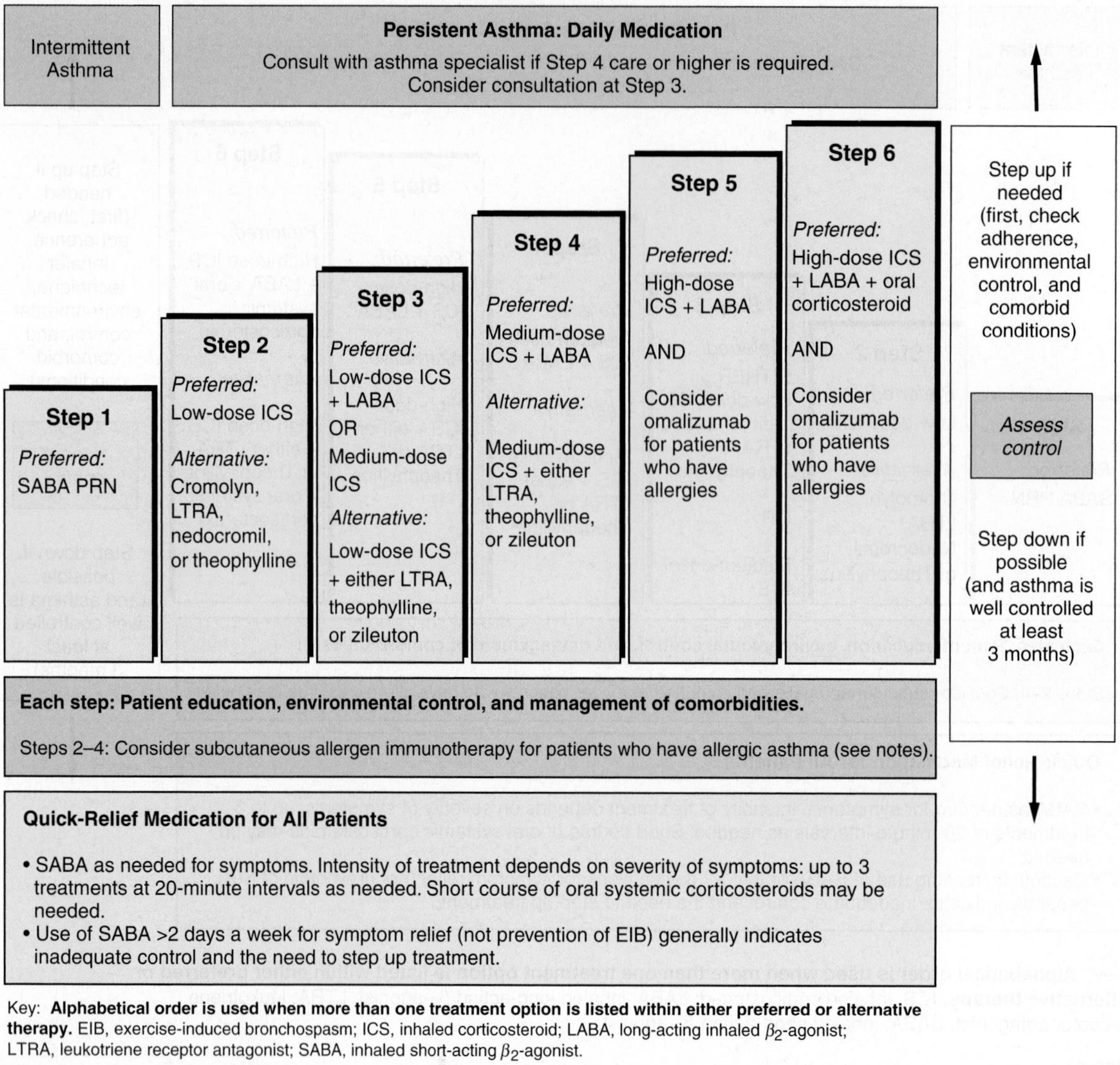

Notes:

- The stepwise approach is meant to assist, not replace, the clinical decision-making required to meet individual patient needs.
- If alternative treatment is used and response is inadequate, discontinue it and use the preferred treatment before stepping up.
- Zileuton is a less desirable alternative because of limited studies as adjunctive therapy and the need to monitor liver function. Theophylline requires monitoring of serum concentration levels.
- In step 6, before oral systemic corticosteroids are introduced, a trial of high-dose ICS + LABA + either LTRA, theophylline, or zileuton may be considered, although this approach has not been studied in clinical trials.

FIGURE 23-9 Stepwise approach for managing asthma in youth 12 years of age or older and adults. Reprinted from National Institutes of Health. *Expert Panel Report 3: Guidelines for the Diagnosis and Management of Asthma*. Bethesda, MD: National Heart, Lung, and Blood Institute; 2007. NIH publication 07-4051.

correlates with the severity of obstruction. Severe hypoxemia ($Pa{O_2}$ <50 mm Hg) that is associated with an FEV_1 less than 15% of predicted represents very severe airway obstruction.[20,21] Likewise, when the FEV_1 is less than 25% of the predicted value, carbon dioxide increasingly is retained and the $Pa{CO_2}$ begins to rise into the usual normal range.[1] Because of mismatching and the ease of correction of hypoxemia with oxygen therapy, the $Pa{CO_2}$ is the more sensitive indicator of ventilation abnormalities in acute asthma with prolonged or chronic airway obstruction; carbon dioxide retention (hypercapnia) and respiratory acidosis are prominent. ABG measurements are indicated in patients who fail to respond adequately to initial therapy or in patients requiring hospitalization; they are not indicated at this time for Q.C. A repeat pulse oximetry at 1 hour after treatment initiation is warranted in Q.C. to ensure adequate arterial oxygen saturation.

NEED FOR HOSPITALIZATION

CASE 23-1, QUESTION 3: Q.C. may require hospitalization. Which clinical test is predictive of the need for admission or whether Q.C. will relapse if sent home from the ED? Are Q.C.'s signs and symptoms predictive of whether she will relapse and return to the ED if not hospitalized?

The most useful predictive tool is the FEV_1 or PEF response to initial treatment. Patients who do not improve to at least 40% of predicted FEV_1 or PEF after initial intensive therapy are more likely to require hospitalization.[1] Although Q.C. is not able to perform spirometry, she is able to execute the PEF maneuver, and the plan is to check her PEF after 1 hour of therapy. Signs and symptom scores alone are not adequate to predict outcome

school, and she has used a variety of medications intermittently (clemastine, fexofenadine, beclomethasone nasal, ketotifen ophthalmic) over the years. C.L. is a competitive runner but has been unable to run as far or as often as usual due to bothersome symptoms. She is also reluctant to use medications as they may be prohibited by her race sponsors. A running partner mentioned that she could control her allergy symptoms with diet, exercise, and herbal remedies purchased at a local nutritional supplement shop. What, if any, alternative treatments have been shown to be efficacious in allergic rhinitis?

Alternative treatments are common among adults with rhinitis and should be taken into account by health care providers. A survey of 300 adults indicated that herbal agents, caffeine-containing products, homeopathy, acupuncture, aromatherapy, reflexology, and massage were common alternative treatments for respiratory conditions.[127] Still, because allergic rhinitis is largely a self-managed disease, it is likely that reported use of these agents is underestimated. For these reasons, patients should always be questioned specifically about the use of alternative therapies during the patient interview. Although some alternative approaches have been deemed to be safe, efficacy for many modalities has not been clearly established.[23,40] In addition, some complementary therapies have been associated with side effects and potential drug interactions.[128–130] Because of C.L's reluctance to use medications, other strategies are appropriate to consider to help her manage her rhinitis symptoms.

LIFESTYLE CHANGES

Some reports have indicated that patients with allergic rhinitis may benefit from hydration and a diet low in sodium, omega-6 fatty acids, and transfatty acids, but high in omega-3 fatty acids (e.g., fish, almonds, walnuts, pumpkin, and flax seeds), and at least five servings of fruits and vegetables per day.[131] These recommendations are not without merit, because they may be beneficial for the population at large, but insufficient evidence exists to support specific value for allergic rhinitis symptoms.

PHYSICAL TECHNIQUES

For the motivated patient, mind–body interventions, such as yoga, hypnosis, and biofeedback-assisted relaxation and breathing exercises, are beneficial for stress reduction in general which may improve the quality of life associated with rhinitis symptoms and treatment.[128] Acupuncture has been shown to have an attributive effect in inflammatory diseases such as rhinitis; however, data are not sufficient to recommend this therapy at this time.[132]

Menthol-delivered rubs have been shown to have an ameliorating effect on nasal congestion; however, the effects are short-lived.[133] Other forms of aromatherapy suggested to relieve nasal congestion include massaging the essential oils of lavender and niaouli around the sinuses, or inhaling eucalyptus and peppermint oils.[134] Data are also lacking about the efficacy of these treatments.

Phototherapy for allergic rhinitis has been investigated with positive results[135] but simpler methods are needed for this to be useful outside of the research arena.[23] Saline nasal irrigation (e.g., neti pot) is simple, inexpensive and has been shown to have some efficacy.[23,61]

HERBAL MEDICINES

It has been suggested that herbs that support improved immune function could also help to ease symptoms of allergy.[136] With this in mind, echinacea has become one of the top-selling herbal products in the United States. Echinacea, however, is closely related to sunflowers, daisies, and ragweed—all members of the Compositae (Asteraceae) family.[137] The possibility that cross-sensitivity between echinacea and other environmental allergens may trigger allergic reactions is supported by an Australian review of all adverse drug reports, including cases of anaphylaxis, associated with echinacea.[137] Patients with known allergy to these plants should be cautioned regarding the use of echinacea products.

A few herbal therapies, including butterbur[138–140] and spirulina,[141] potentially hold some promise but more investigation is needed before they can be included in recommended treatment algorithms.[23] No good clinical data are available on the efficacy of supplements containing vitamin C, grapeseed extract, bee pollen and honey, probiotics, burdock, ginger, freeze-dried stinging nettle leaves, or quercetin (a bioflavonoid found in apples, buckwheat, grapes, red onions, red wine, and white grapefruit).[40]

OTHER

Reports regarding the use of intranasal zinc for upper respiratory symptoms, particularly those associated with the common cold, have been conflicting. Although zinc gels and sprays are popular OTC products, they have been shown to be ineffective in a double-blind, placebo-controlled clinical trial[142] and have been associated in zinc-induced anosmia syndrome, particularly when the products are sniffed deeply.[143] Some products have been removed from the market because of this problem.

Some studies have shown that patients with allergic rhinitis who received homeopathic dilutions of allergens had significantly better nasal air flow than those in the placebo group, but overall no difference was seen in subjective measurement on a visual analog scale.[144] Further investigation is needed before homeopathy can be recommended for allergic rhinitis.

Although a variety of alternative remedies are widely available and used frequently in self-treatment, based on evaluation of these data, there is no firm recommendation for C.L. regarding the use of alternative therapies in allergic rhinitis.[40,130] C.L. should be advised to consult with the specific regulating agency that governs her sporting activities (e.g., the World Anti-Doping Agency for Olympic events) to gain a clear understanding of medicines that are banned in all cases as compared to those that may be used with medical exemptions or used outside of the competitive window. This may allow her to use many conventional treatments (e.g., intransal steroids) with confidence. Saline irrigation would also be a safe, noncontroversial option that may offer some efficacy.

Immunotherapy

EFFICACY

CASE 25-6

QUESTION 1: R.C. is a 25-year-old schoolteacher who has experienced allergic symptoms since childhood, but noticed a worsening after she graduated from college and moved to a new area of the country. Although she has mild symptoms year-round, she has severe exacerbations during April through June and August through October each year. During these periods, she feels that exposure to cut grass and weeds provoke profound nasal symptoms. She also notes that when she spends more time outdoors in spring and early fall, her regular therapy, fluticasone nasal spray (2 sprays per nostril once daily), is less effective. She has added loratadine (10 mg daily) during this time, but is frustrated by having to take so many medications while continuing to experience symptoms. R.C. asks your opinion about allergy shots, remarking that she started them as

a child with some relief, but moved after a year and never resumed treatment. Is allergen immunotherapy effective for reducing symptoms of allergic rhinitis?

Allergen-specific immunotherapy has long-term efficacy, induces clinical and immunologic tolerance, and may prevent progression of allergic disease.[145,146] This process usually involves subcutaneous injection (sometimes called "allergy shots") of dilute solutions of allergen extracts to increase tolerance to allergens so that the threshold for symptoms is increased (i.e., subsequent exposure elicits no or mild symptoms).

Immunotherapy administered via SIT has been used empirically since the early 1900s, and its efficacy has been documented in many controlled trials.[147] A meta-analysis of 51 published studies involving 2,871 patients concluded that SIT is effective in the treatment of allergic rhinitis.[54] In addition, studies of immunotherapy for allergic rhinitis in children suggest that immunotherapy may prevent the onset of asthma.[148,149] Taken together, these studies show that SIT should be considered a supplement to drug therapy in specific patients and possibly be used earlier in the course of allergic disease to achieve maximal benefit.[2]

ALLERGEN TESTING

CASE 25-6, QUESTION 2: How can the clinician determine R.C.'s specific sensitivities?

Skin testing using the modified prick test method or a prick-puncture method is used to confirm the diagnosis of allergic rhinitis and to determine specific allergen sensitivities. Skin testing is a highly sensitive and a relatively inexpensive objective measurement of allergen sensitivity. Small quantities of allergen are introduced into the skin by pricking or puncturing the skin in the immediate presence of the diluted allergen extract. Fifteen to 35 tests are placed on the upper portion of the back or the palmar surface of the forearms. A positive skin test produces a wheal and flare at the site within 15 to 30 minutes of application. An experienced clinician, usually an allergist, should conduct skin testing using high-quality allergen extracts and should interpret the results.[150]

The allergens tested vary with geographic location, emphasizing the most common offending plant species that generate airborne particles. Pollen, the primary particle, is produced by trees, grasses, and weeds. Each of these plant groups generally pollinate at about the same time each year: trees in the spring, grasses from early to midsummer, and weeds from late summer into fall before the first killing frost. The onset and potency of the pollen season varies with geographic location and weather, particularly with respect to temperature and moisture. Seasonality can be misleading, however, because settled pollen particles from a previous season may be resuspended in the air following the spring snow melt or periods of heavy winds.

Mold spores also are common airborne allergens. The outdoor molds release their spores from early spring through late fall. Within this long season, spore counts increase and decrease, depending on the presence of local flora on which these molds grow (e.g., grain and other crops, forests, and orchards). Some perennial allergens (e.g., house dust mites, insect and animal dander, and some indoor molds) occur consistently across all geographic distributions. In each case, skin test results must be correlated with the patient's clinical history.[145]

R.C.'s perennial symptoms with seasonal exacerbations indicate sensitivity to the common perennial allergens with a particular sensitivity to seasonal allergens such as tree, grass, and weed pollen, but these subjective relationships should be confirmed with skin testing.

An alternative to skin testing is the radioallergosorbent test (RAST), in which the patient's serum is tested for allergen-specific IgE antibodies. However, this test is less sensitive and more expensive than skin testing.[151] It is indicated only in selected clinical situations: when a patient consistently reacts positively to the negative control skin test (dermatographism), when antihistamine therapy cannot be discontinued, or when the patient has extensive atopic dermatitis or other skin lesions. Blood eosinophil counts and total serum IgE antibody measurements are neither sensitive nor sufficiently specific to be useful in the diagnosis of allergic rhinitis.[1]

CASE 25-6, QUESTION 3: R.C. is currently using medications (fluticasone nasal spray and loratadine) for her symptoms. Should these be discontinued before skin testing?

Antihistamines blunt the wheal-and-flare reaction by blocking the effects of histamine on capillaries. Different antihistamines vary in the extent to which they can inhibit wheal formation and in the duration of the inhibitory effect (Table 25-7). Depending on the agent selected, antihistamines must be discontinued from 24 hours to 10 days before skin testing, and even then considerable interpatient variability exists in blocking effects.[152,153] For best

TABLE 25-7
Effects of Antihistamines on Allergen Skin Tests[1,23,109,147,149,150,151,153,154]

Drug	Extent of Suppression[a]	Half-Life (hours)[b]	Duration of Suppression (days)
Azelastine (intranasal)	+/–	22	0
Brompheniramine	+	24.9	1–4
Cetirizine	+++	7.4–11 (7)	3–10
Chlorpheniramine	+	24.4 (11)	1–4
Clemastine	++	21.3	1–10
Cyproheptadine	+/–	16	1–4
Desloratadine	+/++	27 (27)	3–10
Diphenhydramine	+/–	4–9	1–4
Fexofenadine	++	14 (18)	3–10
Hydroxyzine	++	20 (7.1)	1–10
Loratadine	+/++	11–24 (3.1)	3–10
Promethazine	+	12	1–4

[a]+++, extensive; ++ moderate; +, mild; +/–, minimal to none.
[b]Parenthetical numbers indicate half-life in children.
Adapted with permission from Facts & Comparisons eAnswers. http://online.factsandcomparisons.com/index.aspx?. Accessed December 15, 2010.

TABLE 25-8
General Recommendations for Discontinuation of Antihistamines Before Allergen Skin Testing

1. Remind patient that allergic symptoms may return during the antihistaminefree period, but that reliable skin tests cannot be performed in a patient taking antihistamines.
2. Discontinue any short-acting antihistamine (i.e., those in Table 25-7 with a duration of suppression ≤4 days) 4 days before skin testing.
3. Discontinue longer-acting antihistamines (i.e., those in Table 25-7 with a duration of suppression >4 days) at an interval appropriate to their duration of effect (e.g., hydroxyzine should be discontinued 10 days before skin testing).
4. Before applying the full battery of skin tests, apply histamine (positive) control and glycerinated diluent (negative) control tests. Application of a 1 mg/mL histamine base equivalent should yield wheal-and-flare diameters of 2–7 mm and 4.5–32.5 mm, respectively, to be considered a normal histamine reaction. A normal cutaneous reaction to histamine control suggests that accurate skin testing can be performed.

Source: Bousquet J et al. Allergic rhinitis and its impact on asthma (ARIA) 2008 update (in collaboration with the World Health Organization, GA[2]LEN and AllerGen). *Allergy*. 2008;63(Suppl 86):8.

results, R.C.'s loratadine should be discontinued 10 days before her skin testing.

Other allergy medications, including cromolyn and nasal corticosteroids, have no effect on skin tests. Likewise, most asthma medications, including leukotriene modifiers, inhaled β_2-agonists, cromolyn, theophylline, and inhaled and short-course systemic (burst) corticosteroids have no effect on skin tests.[23,150,154] R.C. can continue the use of fluticasone nasal spray while she waits to be skin tested.

Other medications can interfere with skin testing by blocking the cutaneous wheal and flare reactions or increasing skin reactivity. These include: oral β_2-agonists, long-term systemic corticosteroids, and high-potency topical corticosteroids (applied to the skin testing sites), tricyclic antidepressants, phenothiazine-type antipsychotics and antiemetics.[23,150] Depending on the indication for drug therapy, however, discontinuation of these drugs before skin testing is not always advisable. Recommendations for discontinuing antihistamines before allergen skin testing are listed in Table 25-8.

CASE 25-6, QUESTION 4: Is R.C. a candidate for immunotherapy injections?

Immunotherapy via SCIT is indicated for patients with evidence of sustained, clinically relevant IgE-mediated disease and a limited spectrum of allergies (i.e., one or two clinically relevant allergens) and in whom pharmacotherapy and avoidance measures are insufficient.[155] Further considerations are the patient's attitude to available treatment modalities, costs of treatment, and the quality of allergen vaccines available for treatment.[145] In the case of R.C., she has year-round symptoms with seasonal exacerbations, she has not experienced symptom relief when using appropriate therapies, and she is motivated to try immunotherapy. In addition, a previous trial in childhood was beneficial. For these reasons, skin testing and a trial of immunotherapy with specific allergens are reasonable.

LENGTH OF THERAPY

CASE 25-6, QUESTION 5: If R.C. decides to proceed with immunotherapy, how long should her therapy continue and how long will the effects last?

After identifying the offending allergens via skin testing, subcutaneous immunotherapy is generally administered in two phases. During the build-up phase, increasing doses of allergen are given once or twice a week until a predetermined target or maintenance dose is achieved. This usually takes 3 to 4 months (e.g., 16–18 injections). Once this maintenance dose is reached, shots are usually administered every 2 to 3 weeks for the ensuing several years of treatment. Clinical improvement with immunotherapy usually occurs in the first year. In a small percentage of patients, there is no improvement and immunotherapy is discontinued. If symptoms are reduced, however, injections are usually continued for 4 to 5 years of maintenance therapy.[145]

Although immunotherapy can lead to long-term remission of symptoms, one drawback is the lengthy treatment period. Preliminary data involving a 2-year study of 19 patients allergic to ragweed who underwent one allergy shot per week for 6 weeks before the ragweed season suggest that significant relief can be obtained from a shorter term of treatment.[156] SIT alters the natural course of disease and evidence suggests that efficacy persists long after therapy ends.[157]

RISKS

CASE 25-6, QUESTION 6: R.C. is interested in proceeding but concerned about the time commitment associated with the office visits required for immunotherapy. She inquires whether it would be safe to have her boyfriend (who is studying to be an accupuncturist) administer the injections. How should you respond to R.C.'s query?

Local adverse reactions (i.e., redness, swelling) to immunotherapy can be common, but the risk of severe reaction (i.e., anaphylaxis) is low. A classification system for grading systemic reactions has been proposed, which categorizes these into immediate (occurring within 30 minutes) and late (occurring after 30 minutes).[145] In addition, pretreatment with antihistamines during immunotherapy induction has been shown to reduce the incidence of such adverse events. In view of the occasional occurrence of systemic side effects, it is important that R.C.'s injections be administered by personnel who are fully trained and experienced in the early recognition and treatment of such reactions.[54]

DRUG-INDUCED NASAL CONGESTION: RHINITIS MEDICAMENTOSA

CASE 25-7

QUESTION 1: L.K. is a 27-year-old man who has suffered intermittent symptoms of allergic rhinitis for several years. He reports that his symptoms are most bothersome in the spring and associated with blooming of various grasses. During these periods, he has typically used oral chlorpheniramine (4 mg every 6 hours), which relieves his symptoms but makes him drowsy at work. This season, he reports that his symptoms have been more severe, with sneezing, runny nose, and extreme itching in his nose. He tried oral loratadine (10 mg daily) with partial relief of symptoms. He also states that nasal congestion has been more of an issue with this episode and to address this he has used xylometazoline nasal spray (0.1% solution) for the past 3 weeks. Despite increasing the use of nasal spray from two sprays per nostril twice daily to three sprays per nostril four times

a day, however, he reports that the congestion is getting worse. What might be an explanation for L.K.'s increasing need for nasal decongestant?

Selected medications and some drugs of abuse can cause nasal congestion through a variety of mechanisms.[10] Table 25-9 lists agents associated with drug-induced nasal symptoms. In this case, L.K. is likely experiencing rebound nasal congestion as a result of a specific form of drug-induced rhinitis called rhinitis medicamentosa (RM).

ONLINE CONTENT

For a visual of rhinitis medicamentosa, go to http://thepoint.lww.com/AT10e.

TABLE 25-9
Drugs Capable of Causing Nasal Symptoms

Local Inflammatory Mechanisms
Aspirin
Nonsteroidal anti-inflammatory drugs
Neurogenic Mechanisms
Centrally Acting Sympatholytics
Clonidine
Methyldopa
Reserpine
Peripherally Acting Sympatholytics
Prazosin
Guanethidine
Doxazosin
Phentolamine
Vasodilators
Sildenafil
Tadalafil
Vardenafil
Idiopathic Mechanisms
Antihypertensives
Amiloride
Angiotensin-converting enzyme inhibitor class
β-Blocker class
Calcium-channel blockers
Chlorothiazide
Hydralazine
Hydrochlorothiazide
Hormonal Products
Exogenous estrogens
Oral contraceptives
Neuropsychotherapeutic Agents
Alprazolam
Amitriptyline
Chlordiazepoxide
Chlorpromazine
Gabapentin
Risperidone
Perphenazine
Thioridazine

Source: Dykewicz MS et al. Diagnosis and management of rhinitis: complete guidelines of the Joint Task Force on Practice Parameters in Allergy, Asthma and Immunology. American Academy of Allergy, Asthma, and Immunology. *Ann Allergy Asthma Immunol.* 1998;81(5 Pt 2):478; Ramey JT et al. Rhinitis medicamentosa. *J Investig Allergol Clin Immunol.* 2006;16:148; Varghese M et al. Drug-induced rhinitis. *Clin Exper Allergy.* 2010;40:381.

Topical decongestants are indicated for short-term use. When used acutely, sympathomimetic (adrenergic) agents stimulate α-adrenergic receptors on blood vessels, resulting in vasoconstriction (which serves to relieve nasal congestion associated with edematous, congested blood vessels). But when these agents are used chronically, this can result in (a) overstimulation of α-adrenergic receptors leading to tachyphylaxis, (b) stimulation of β-adrenergic receptors causing vasodilation, and (c) decreased production of endogenous norepinephrine through a negative feedback mechanism.[158–160] RM has also been associated with the presence of BKC as a preservative in some nasal products.[159,160]

When RM occurs, many patients will attempt to treat the rebound congestion by using the offending topical decongestant more frequently and/or at increased doses, creating a vicious cycle. L.K.'s description of using the xylometazoline for an extended period of time (3 weeks), more frequently (from twice daily to four times daily) and at high doses (from two sprays per nostril to three sprays per nostril) support the diagnosis of RM.

Strategies for Resolution

CASE 25-7, QUESTION 2: How should L.K.'s rhinitis medicamentosa be managed?

The best strategy for managing RM is prevention, by limiting the duration of topical decongestant use to fewer than 5 days. When these medications must be used for longer than 5 days, the patient should be advised to take a 1- to 2-day holiday during which the topical agent is not used before resuming treatment. Patients should be counseled about this whenever topical decongestants are recommended or purchased. When preventative strategies fail, several options for treatment exist.[158]

The first step is to discontinue the offending topical decongestant and, if necessary, substitute another therapy that will not cause nasal symptoms.[10] Because abrupt discontinuation of an agent that has been used long-term may cause the patient considerable discomfort for up to 7 days, it is recommended to add an intranasal corticosteroid or a short course of an oral decongestant (e.g., pseudoephedrine 120 mg twice daily for one week).[10,159] Saline nose drops or spray can be added to moisturize and alleviate any nasal irritation. In refractory cases, a short course of systemic corticosteroids may be necessary.[10] Note that if the patient has used the topical decongestant continuously for many months or even years, the nasal mucosa may have undergone irreversible changes.

An alternative to abrupt cessation of the topical decongestant is to recommend that the patient discontinue use of the topical decongestant in a stepwise manner (i.e., one nostril at a time). For example, have the patient substitute normal saline nasal spray for decongestant spray in the right nostril every other dose. Later, use saline twice for each decongestant dose. Eventually, the decongestant is discontinued totally in the right nostril and saline is substituted. Repeat the process for the left nostril. Saline can be used as often as needed throughout this process and after the topical decongestant is completely withdrawn. This method has been suggested in several reviews, although no prospective trial results are available to support it.[10,160] Thus, this method should be combined with careful patient education, support, and frequent follow-up.

In the case of L.K., because he not only needs treatment for the RM but also for the original symptoms (sneezing, runny and itchy nose) that occur seasonally, a reasonable option would be to discontinue the xylometazoline, and begin treatment with mometasone nasal spray (2 sprays in each nostril daily) with as needed saline nasal spray.

IDIOPATHIC RHINITIS

Diagnosis

CASE 25-8

QUESTION 1: M.S., a 29-year-old man, complains of profuse watery rhinorrhea that has been a chronic and progressively worsening problem for the past 5 years. He also experiences some nasal congestion with the rhinorrhea, but denies nasal itching or sneezing. Although the symptoms tend to remit and exacerbate, they do not occur in any definable seasonal pattern. His symptoms are worsened by exposure to tobacco smoke, strong fumes such as paint or ammonia, and cold air. These often are associated with headaches. M.S. has no other medical problems and no family history of allergies. He does not smoke and rarely drinks alcohol. His only medication, mometasone (50 mcg/spray, two sprays in each nostril once daily as needed), only partially relieves the symptoms. M.S. sniffs and blows his nose several times during the medical history taking. Physical examination reveals a mildly erythematous nasal mucosa and a minimally edematous inferior turbinate. Copious nasal discharge is clear and watery and air movement through the nose is relatively good. There is no sinus tenderness. The remainder of his physical examination is normal. Microscopic examination of a nasal smear demonstrates only a few neutrophils and no eosinophils. What information about M.S. supports the diagnosis of idiopathic rhinitis?

Idiopathic rhinitis is a diagnosis of exclusion encompassing those patients with nasal mucous membrane inflammation with no proved immunologic, microbiologic, pharmacologic, hormonal, or occupational cause.[8,12] The syndrome is sometimes called "vasomotor rhinitis", but using this terminology can be confusing because the cause of the symptoms has still not been clearly identified.[1,4,161] The prevailing theory holds that an imbalance in the autonomic nervous system exists in which the cholinergic parasympathetic activity exceeds the α-adrenergic activity in the nasal mucosa.[8] Theoretically, this is the reason that stimuli that normally increase parasympathetic activity in the nose, such as cold air and inhaled irritants, aggravate symptoms.[161] Still, substantial debate exists over whether idiopathic rhinitis represents a localized allergic response in the absence of systemic atopic markers[162] as well as the evidence for inflammatory pathophysiology in the disease.[163]

The symptoms of idiopathic rhinitis are variable. Most patients experience perennial nasal obstruction accompanied by profuse, watery nasal and postnasal discharge. Many patients complain of nasal obstruction as the primary symptom, whereas for others it is rhinorrhea. Sneezing is usually not a prominent symptom and nasal itching is uncommon.[8,12] Headache may occur and usually is frontal or localized over the bridge of the nose. In patients with chronic nasal obstruction, chronic sinusitis and significant morbidity can result. In contrast to allergic rhinitis, the onset of symptoms in patients with idiopathic rhinitis usually occurs in adulthood.[4]

Patients report worsening of their symptoms when exposed to nonspecific irritants, including tobacco smoke, industrial pollutants, strong odors and perfumes, newsprint, and chemical fumes; cold, dry air; changes in humidity; and ingestion of very cold or very hot beverages or spicy foods. Most patients have no history or evidence of atopy.[4]

The appearance of the nasal mucosa also is variable. The turbinates are usually erythematous and, during an exacerbation, considerable quantities of nasal secretions usually are present. Mast cells may be present in the nasal smear; however, by definition, nasal eosinophilia is not present. Skin tests are usually negative.[8]

M.S.'s symptoms of bothersome watery rhinorrhea, nasal congestion, and headache without itching or sneezing are typical. His complaint of worsening symptoms with exposure to noxious inhalants, cold air, and hot beverages supports the diagnosis of idiopathic rhinitis. The nasal smear, which notably lacks large numbers of eosinophils, initially differentiates this disease from NARES.

Choice of Therapeutic Agent

CASE 25-8, QUESTION 2: M.S. asks what causes idiopathic rhinitis and what can be done to alleviate his symptoms. What nonpharmacologic and pharmacologic treatments are appropriate to manage M.S.'s idiopathic rhinitis?

Nasal symptoms in patients with idiopathic rhinitis have been shown to be influenced by psychological factors. Some therapeutic benefit may be realized by establishing an ongoing, trusting relationship between the health care provider and the patient. This should include a thorough explanation of the disease state and the realistic outcomes of therapy for most patients. Psychotherapy is helpful in some cases. In addition, patients should be instructed to avoid as many aggravating factors as possible, such as smoking, exposure to smoke or other irritants, and very cold or very hot beverages. Saline irrigation is valuable as a general soothing and moisturizing treatment. Exercise may be particularly helpful for patients with idiopathic rhinitis because it increases sympathetic tone.[8]

Pharmacotherapy for idiopathic rhinitis should be directed toward the predominant symptoms of the individual patient.[8,12] For patients with predominant nasal congestion and minimal rhinorrhea, the intranasal corticosteroids may be helpful. The addition of oral decongestants may improve nasal obstruction in some patients with idiopathic rhinitis, but objective measures of improvement are affected variably and side effects can be problematic.

M.S.'s case is typical of the often frustrating course in treating idiopathic rhinitis.[8,12] Commonly, multiple therapeutic plans fail, and M.S. has responded incompletely and unsatisfactorily to intranasal corticosteroids. There is some older evidence suggesting topical nasal capsaicin may be effective, but this option has not garnered widespread support.[12] Surgical treatments have been attempted for patients in whom medical management fails, although recent clinical evidence is limited primarily to case reports.[164]

In patients such as M.S., who have rhinorrhea as their predominant symptom, FGAs may be helpful because of their anticholinergic drying effects. In general, however, FGAs are less effective in the treatment of idiopathic rhinitis than for allergic rhinitis, and patients may have difficulty adhering to therapy because of side effects.[165] Of note, the nonsedating SGAs have little value in idiopathic rhinitis because they lack anticholinergic properties. Another option for decreasing nasal secretions is nasal ipratropium bromide, a topically active congener of atropine.[8] Ipratropium bromide's quaternary ammonium structure makes it lipophobic; therefore, it is absorbed poorly from the nasal mucosa and gastrointestinal tract and does not cross the blood–brain barrier. It significantly reduces rhinorrhea (as measured by the number of nose-blowing episodes or daily number of tissues used), but has no effect on sneezing or nasal obstruction.[165]

The recommended dose of ipratropium bromide is two sprays of the 0.03% nasal solution (42 mcg) in each nostril two to three times per day, but dosage individualization (from 168 to 1,600 mcg/day) is often required to achieve symptomatic relief.[110] A 0.06% nasal formulation is also available, but its use is typically reserved for short-term treatment of common cold symptoms. Table 25-5 includes information about intranasal ipratropium dosing and availability.

In general, intranasal ipratropium bromide is well tolerated, although its use is associated with dose-related side effects.[1] The most common side effects are nasal dryness, nasal burning, bloody nasal discharge (epistaxis), dry or sore throat, and dry mouth.[110] Theoretically, elderly men with BPH may experience difficulty in urinating, but the risk is low because of negligible systemic absorption. No significant adverse cardiovascular or blood pressure effects have been observed.

In the case of M.S., because he has been comfortable using an intranasal product (mometasone) in the past, it would be reasonable to initiate a trial of ipratropium bromide 0.03% two sprays in each nostril three times daily. Once the rhinorrhea is controlled, he should be advised to reduce the dosage to twice daily. Nasal saline can also be used as needed if excessive dryness occurs during dosage optimization.

MIXED ALLERGIC–NONALLERGIC RHINITIS

CASE 25-9

QUESTION 1: D.W. is a 56-year-old woman with a long-standing history of allergic rhinitis related to triggers with seasonal ragweed. Her primary symptoms are rhinorrhea and sneezing, which she has relieved by using various oral anthistamines (clemastine 1.34 mg daily and, more recently, cetirizine 10 mg daily) which she takes several weeks each autumn. Recently (during winter), she has experienced new rhinitis symptoms associated with the weather and various odors that were not a problem in the past, specifically, perfumes and food spices. When she encounters these, she exhibits watery rhinorrhea and profound congestion. She has tried a combination of cetirizine with pseudoephedrine for these episodes, but reports that it "doesn't seem to help much and it makes me feel jumpy." Are D.W.'s new symptoms the result of breakthrough (uncontrolled) allergic rhinitis or do they represent something new?

Distinguishing between allergic rhinitis and nonallergic rhinitis may be difficult in clinical practice, and the presence of concomitant allergic and nonallergic rhinitis in some patients confounds the diagnosis further.[33,34] A careful history should be gathered from the patient and an assessment made of the temporal nature of the symptoms and various exposures. The Clinical Presentation and Assessment of Rhinitis section in this chapter includes diagnostic criteria that can be used to distinguish between allergic and nonallergic causes of rhinitis. When a patient presents with characteristics suggestive of both types, especially in the case of new symptoms or triggers despite optimized therapy, mixed rhinitis should be considered.

Although D.W. has a confirmed history of ragweed pollen sensitivity (supporting the allergic rhinitis diagnosis), the timing of the more recent symptoms and the new triggers (i.e., odors) suggest that she may have developed sensitivities of a nonallergic (non–IgE-based) nature. The patient's age also is consistent with the development of vasomotor rhinitis (nonallergic) which can present around the time of menopause. This, combined with the lack of efficacy from a previously successful therapy (i.e., oral antihistamine), suggest that D.W. may be exhibiting a mixed allergic–nonallergic rhinitis presentation.

CASE 25-9, QUESTION 2: How should D.W.'s mixed rhinitis be treated? How is this different from the management of allergic rhinitis?

The high prevalence and importance of nonallergic causes of rhinitis has been recognized in recent years. A recent study suggests that knowledge and opinions about the prevalence and relative importance of nonallergic rhinitis varies among physicians.[166] Among those who had an allergy specialist in their practice, there was a greater awareness that treatment approaches might vary between allergic and nonallergic triggers as compared to physicians who did not also have an allergist resource.

The important point about nonallergic triggers, or new onset triggers such as those present in D.W., is that oral anthistamines and other therapies directed primarily at allergic responses may be ineffective in relieving symptoms. Good clinical evidence suggests that intranasal steroids are an effective option, and some limited evidence suggests that these patients may benefit from intranasal antihistamine therapy.[23] Avoidance or minimization of exposure to the triggers is also an important strategy. For D.W., a 4-week therapeutic trial of a BKC-free intranasal steroid (e.g., ciclesonide 2 sprays in each nostril once daily) with counseling about appropriate administration is warranted. Intransal steroid therapy may improve the response to both allergic and nonallergic triggers.

SUMMARY

The initial management of rhinitis should be directed at preventing symptoms, which can be achieved through a variety of pharmacologic and nonpharmacologic methods. Treatment plans for allergic rhinitis, the most common subtype, should include patient education, allergen or irritant avoidance, and the appropriate medications, including immunotherapy, if indicated. Control of the disease process is the expected outcome, so that patients are able to live their lives comfortably without symptoms or impairment. Customizing therapy for each patient based on symptom history and response to treatments is important. Rhinitis can be controlled and effective management can greatly improve the quality of patients' lives.

ACKNOWLEDGMENTS

The authors acknowledge the assistance of Margrit B. Rosado-Duroisin and Caroline A.R. Lindsay in the preparation of this chapter.

KEY REFERENCES AND WEBSITES

A full list of references for this chapter can be found at **http://thepoint.lww.com/AT10e**. Below are the key references for this chapter, with the corresponding reference number in this chapter found in parentheses after the reference.

Key References

Bousquet J et al. Allergic rhinitis and its impact on asthma (ARIA) 2008 update (in collaboration with the World Health Organization, GA(2)LEN and AllerGen). *Allergy*. 2008;63(Suppl 86):8. (23)

Brozek JL et al. Allergic rhinitis and its impact on asthma (ARIA) guidelines: 2010 revision. *J Allergy Clin Immunol.* 2010;126:466. (41)

Church MK et al. Risk of first generation H(1)-antihistamines: a GA(2)LEN position paper. *Allergy*. 2010;65:459. (73)

Dykewicz MS, Hamilos DL. Rhinitis and sinusitis. *J Allergy Clin Immunol.* 2010;125:S103. (6)

Meltzer EO et al. Physican perceptions of the treatment and management of allergic and nonallergic rhinitis. *Allergy Asthma Proc.* 2009;30:75. (166)

ARIA in the pharmacy: management of allergic rhinitis symptoms in the pharmacy. Allergic rhinitis and its impact on asthma. *Allergy*. 2004;59:373. (39)

Pattanaik D et al. Vasomotor rhinitis. *Curr Allergy Asthma Rep.* 2010;10:84. (12)

Varghese M et al. Drug-induced rhinitis. *Clin Exper Allergy*. 2010; 40:381. (159)

Wallace DV et al. The diagnosis and management of rhinitis: an updated practice parameter [published correction appears in *J Allergy Clin Immunol.* 2008;122:1237]. *J Allergy Clin Immunol.* 2008;122:S1. (3)

26 Cystic Fibrosis

Paul M. Beringer and Michelle Condren

CORE PRINCIPLES

	CHAPTER CASES
1 Cystic fibrosis (CF) is a genetic disorder affecting approximately 30,000 individuals in the United States that is caused by a defect in the cystic fibrosis transmembrane conductance regulator protein, which is a chloride channel that regulates fluid and electrolyte transport within secretory epithelial cells throughout the body.	**Case 26-1 (Question 1)**
2 The principal manifestations of CF include malnutrition secondary to pancreatic insufficiency and pulmonary dysfunction resulting from chronic airway obstruction, infection, and inflammation.	**Case 26-1 (Question 1)**
3 Diagnosis of CF is based on newborn screening or presence of the typical signs and symptoms of the disease, and either documented abnormalities in ion transport or identification of two CF mutations.	**Case 26-1 (Questions 1, 2)**
4 Administration of pancreatic enzymes and fat-soluble vitamins are prescribed to correct malabsorption and vitamin deficiencies and improve nutritional status.	**Case 26-1 (Question 2)**
5 Key therapies for management of CF pulmonary disease include inhaled dornase alfa and hypertonic saline in combination with mechanical airway clearance techniques to combat airway obstruction, inhaled antibiotics to combat airway infection, and oral azithromycin for airway inflammation.	**Case 26-2 (Questions 1–3), Case 26-3 (Question 3)**
6 Periodically patients will experience acute pulmonary exacerbations characterized by increased pulmonary symptoms, acute loss of lung function, and loss of weight, which require intensification of airway clearance, administration of systemic antibiotics, and nutritional supplements.	**Case 26-3 (Questions 1, 2, 4)**
7 Key monitoring parameters in patients with CF include trends in pulmonary function tests to determine response to therapies and identify possible acute pulmonary exacerbations, and body mass index to assess nutritional status.	**Case 26-1 (Question 3)**
8 Therapy for patients with CF should include attention to complications including cystic fibrosis–related diabetes mellitus, osteoporosis, and depression. Future therapies directed against the basic defect offer a potential cure for CF.	**Case 26-3 (Question 5)**

Cystic fibrosis (CF) is a severe, complex, hereditary disease that affects 1 of every 3,200 live births, or approximately 30,000 children and adults in the United States. One in 31 Americans carries the autosomal recessive gene for CF, which arises from a mutation in coding for the cystic fibrosis transmembrane regulator protein (CFTR). This genetic mutational error results in the complex, multisystem disease of CF, which is characterized by malabsorption and a state of chronic lung obstruction, inflammation, and infection.

The course and severity of CF are variable and unpredictable. The median life expectancy (i.e., about 40 years) for a child born with CF in 1990 was about double what would have been expected for a child diagnosed with CF 20 years earlier because of advances in the management of this disorder.[1] Although current therapy continues to rely on treatment of symptoms, several compounds in clinical development are directed at the basic defect and offer a potential cure. In the meantime, aggressive treatment with existing therapies can decrease the morbidity of this disease and increase the life expectancy of the patient.[2]

GENETIC BASIS

CF is caused by mutations in the *CFTR* gene, which is a member of the ATP binding cassette family. CFTR is dependent on cyclic adenosine monophosphate for chloride transport: defective coding for CFTR inhibits the normal regulation of ion transport in and out of the cell on the apical surface of secretory epithelial cells.[3] CFTR also regulates the transport of bicarbonate and sodium ions, mucous rheology, pulmonary inflammation, and bacterial adherence.[4–8]

CF is an autosomal recessive disorder, which means there is a 25% chance of inheriting the malfunctioning genes from both parents and developing the disease, a 50% chance of inheriting one abnormal gene (i.e., carrier), and a 25% chance of inheriting two normal genes. Approximately 5% of whites are asymptomatic carriers of the CF mutation. The high frequency of this mutation has been attributed to a heterozygote-selective advantage that presumably protected the carrier against dehydration from cholera, or other enteric infections.[9,10] More than two decades have passed since the identification and cloning of the gene responsible for CF, and greater than 1,800 new *CFTR* mutations have been discovered (**http://www.genet.sickkids.on.ca/cftr/app**). These mutations have been grouped into five major classes according to the functional consequence of the defect (Fig. 26-1).[11,12] The most common variant is ΔF508, representing 66% of all mutations. Approximately 90% of all patients with CF have at least one copy of this mutation.

The importance of identifying the gene mutation relates to potential new therapies currently in various stages of clinical development. The greatest excitement and anticipation involves new therapies directed at the basic defect that offer a potential cure for CF. Replacement of the defective gene or repair of the dysfunctional CFTR protein are two approaches actively being pursued.

Cystic Fibrosis Transmembrane Conductance Regulator Modulation

These therapies are designed to correct the function of the defective CFTR protein made by the *CFTR* gene, allowing normal chloride and sodium transport across epithelial cells lining the lungs and other organs. As demonstrated in Figure 26-1, several compounds are currently in clinical drug development for patients with different CFTR mutations, demonstrating a pharmacogenomic approach to CF treatment that is likely to be realized in the near future.

VX-770 AND VX-809

VX-770, known as a CFTR potentiator, aims to increase the function of defective CFTR proteins by increasing the gating activity, or ability to transport ions across the cell membrane, of CFTR at the cell surface. In people with the G551D mutation, CFTR proteins do not function normally at the cell surface (Fig. 26-1). A phase 2 trial of VX-770 in CF patients with at least one copy of a G551D mutation demonstrated improvements in biological measures of CFTR function (nasal potential difference and sweat chloride) and pulmonary function (forced expiratory volume in 1 second [FEV_1]).[13] Phase 3 trials of VX-770 recently were completed, and a New Drug Application is expected to be submitted in 2011.

VX-809, known as a CFTR corrector, aims to increase CFTR function by increasing the trafficking, or movement, of CFTR to the cell surface. In people with the ΔF508 mutation, there is improper folding of the CFTR protein, leading to proteosomal degradation and failure of the CFTR protein to reach the cell surface in normal amounts (Fig. 26-1). In addition, the small amount of protein that does make it to the cell surface fails to activate properly. A phase 2 study is currently evaluating multiple combinations of VX-770 and VX-809 in people with two copies of the ΔF508 mutation. The primary goals of the trial are to evaluate the safety, tolerability, and effect on CFTR function as measured by sweat chloride.

ATALUREN

Ataluren is a novel, small-molecule compound that promotes the readthrough of premature truncation codons in the CFTR mRNA. It aims to treat CF patients with nonsense mutations (nmCF). A nonsense mutation is an alteration in the genetic code that prematurely halts the synthesis of an essential protein (Fig. 26-1). Data from a phase 2 clinical trial of ataluren in pediatric and adult patients with nmCF demonstrated ataluren results in production of functional CFTR and statistically significant improvements in CFTR chloride channel function in the airways.[14] A phase 3, 48-week study of ataluren in people with

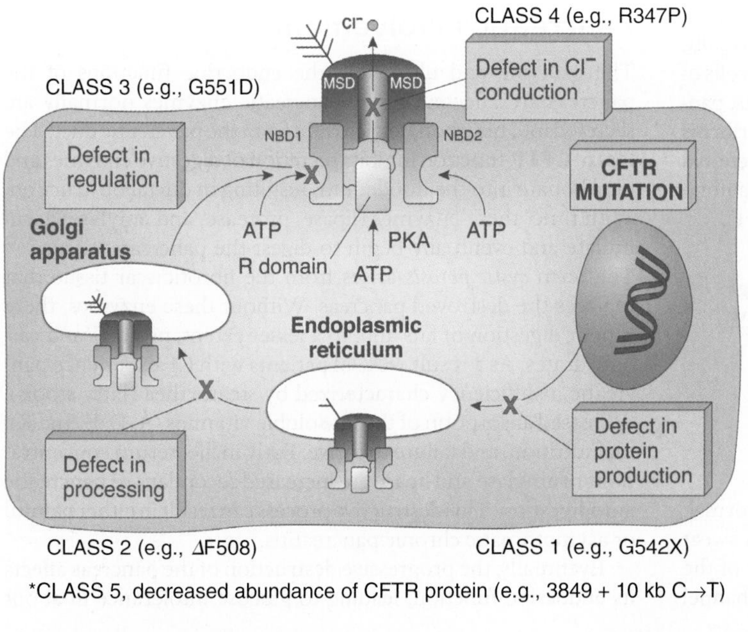

FIGURE 26-1 Classification of mutations. Class I mutations include those in which the production of the cystic fibrosis transmembrane regulator (CFTR) protein is blocked owing to *stop mutations.* Defective protein processing is responsible for the class II mutations. In this class, the protein is made, but it is unable to make its way from the endoplasmic reticulum to the apical membrane, where it is needed for proper operation. This includes the most common mutation, ΔF508, which is caused by improper folding of the protein. Class III mutations cause the disruption of the channel to open properly. Class IV mutations are unable to achieve proper ion conduction. Class V is a milder form of class I mutations and includes mutations that cause reduced production of functional CFTR. (Adapted with permission from Rubin E MD and Farber JL MD. *Pathology*, 3rd Edition. Philadelphia: Lippincott Williams & Wilkins, 1999.)

CF age 6 and older completed enrollment in fall 2010. The main goal of the trial is to determine whether ataluren can improve lung function in patients with CF.

Gene Therapy

Since the discovery of the *CFTR* gene in 1989 there has been hope that a gene therapy treatment would soon be available as a potential cure to CF. Initial attempts at gene therapy using viral vectors were hampered by low transfer efficiency and short retention within the airways as a result of host immunogenicity. Recently, investigators have reported a novel approach using directed evolution of the adeno-associated virus to select viral variants with enhanced infection of human airway epithelium.[15] Using the modified virus the investigators demonstrated more than 100-fold improvement in gene transfer and correction of the CF epithelial chloride transport defect. Studies in animal models of CF are currently under way.

A second approach uses plasmid DNA encapsulated within cationic liposomes to deliver the gene to the airways. Potential advantages of nonviral approaches are that they are noninfectious and relatively nonimmunogenic, can accommodate a large DNA plasmid, and may be produced simply on a large scale. A single-dose phase 1 clinical trial of PGM169/GL67A is currently being conducted by the UK Gene Therapy Consortium.[16]

Interestingly, even among individuals with identical genotypes, a broad spectrum of disease severity is seen.[17,18] The contribution of genetic factors other than the misfunctioning CFTR can have a great influence on disease severity.[19–26] For example, mutations in the transforming growth factor β-1 gene enhance the modulatory effect of mannose binding lectin on the age of first bacterial infection and the rate of decline of pulmonary function.[27] Another potentially important gene modifier is interferon-related developmental regulator 1, deficiency of which causes reduced neutrophil function, resulting in an anti-inflammatory response.[28] Screening for genetic modifiers is currently a research tool that will hopefully lead to the development of new potential therapies.[29,30]

CLINICAL MANIFESTATIONS

Genotype, environmental factors, and modifier gene status all contribute to the highly variable clinical course of CF. The linking of the loss of CFTR function to clinical manifestations of the disease, however, has been central to gaining an understanding of the disease and in the discovery of new therapies. Normally, CFTR is highly expressed on the membranes of epithelial cells of the lungs, sweat glands, salivary glands, male genital ducts, pancreas, kidney tubules, and digestive tract. The CFTR performs different functions in specific tissues; therefore, a dysfunctional or absent CFTR has different effects on different organs, resulting in the multiorgan clinical manifestations of CF (Table 26-1).

ONLINE CONTENT

For an illustration of the systemic changes in cystic fibrosis, go to http://thepoint.lww.com/AT10e.

TABLE 26-1
Clinical Manifestations of Cystic Fibrosis

Manifestation	Approximate Incidence (%) Children (Infants)	Adults
Pancreatic		
Insufficiency	85 (80–85)	90
Pancreatitis	1–2	2–4
Abnormal glucose tolerance	38	75
Diabetes mellitus	14	40–50
Hepatobiliary		
Biliary cirrhosis	10–20	>20
Cholelithiasis	5	5–10
Biliary obstruction	1–2	5
Intestinal		
Meconium ileus	20	
Meconium ileus equivalent	1–5	10–20
Rectal prolapse	10–15	1–2
Intussusception	1–5	1–2
Gastroesophageal reflux	1–5	>10
Appendiceal abscess	0–1	1–2
Respiratory		
Nasal polyps	4–10 (<1)	15–20
Pansinusitis		90–100
Bronchiectasis	30–50	>90
Pneumothorax	1–2	10–15
Hemoptysis	5–15	50–60
Reproductive		
Delayed puberty		85
Infertility		
Males		98
Females		70–80

Sweat Glands

Fluid secreted by the sweat glands in patients with CF is normal, but a defect in the reabsorption of electrolytes leads to sweat with a high salt content. CFTR, in the apical membrane of the resorptive area of the sweat gland, functions as an ion channel for chloride transport and also activates an associated epithelial sodium channel.[31] Normally, these channels efficiently reabsorb sodium chloride from sweat. In patients with CF, loss of these functioning channels blocks the ability of the sweat ducts to reabsorb salt, leading to elevated sweat sodium chloride concentrations (Fig. 26-2). The loss of these sodium and chloride ion channels serves as the basis for the diagnostic sweat chloride test.

Pancreatic Involvement

The exocrine and ultimately the endocrine functions of the pancreas are affected in CF. Pancreatic enzymes normally are secreted into bicarbonate-rich fluid from the pancreatic duct. The loss of CFTR function inhibits secretion of digestive enzymes and bicarbonate into the duodenum, resulting in ductal obstruction. With time, these enzymes (lipase, protease, and amylase) accumulate and eventually begin to digest the pancreatic tissue.[8,32] The term *cystic fibrosis* arises from the fibrotic scar tissue that replaces the destroyed pancreas. Without these enzymes, there is poor digestion of fats and, to a lesser extent, proteins and carbohydrates. As a result, 90% of patients with CF experience pancreatic insufficiency characterized by steatorrhea (fatty stools), decreased absorption of the fat-soluble vitamins (A, D, E, and K), malnutrition, and failure to thrive. Early in life, serum concentrations of amylase and lipase are increased secondary to pancreatic autodigestion. This destructive process can result in either painful or asymptomatic chronic pancreatitis.

Eventually, the progressive destruction of the pancreas affects its endocrine function, leading to glucose intolerance in about

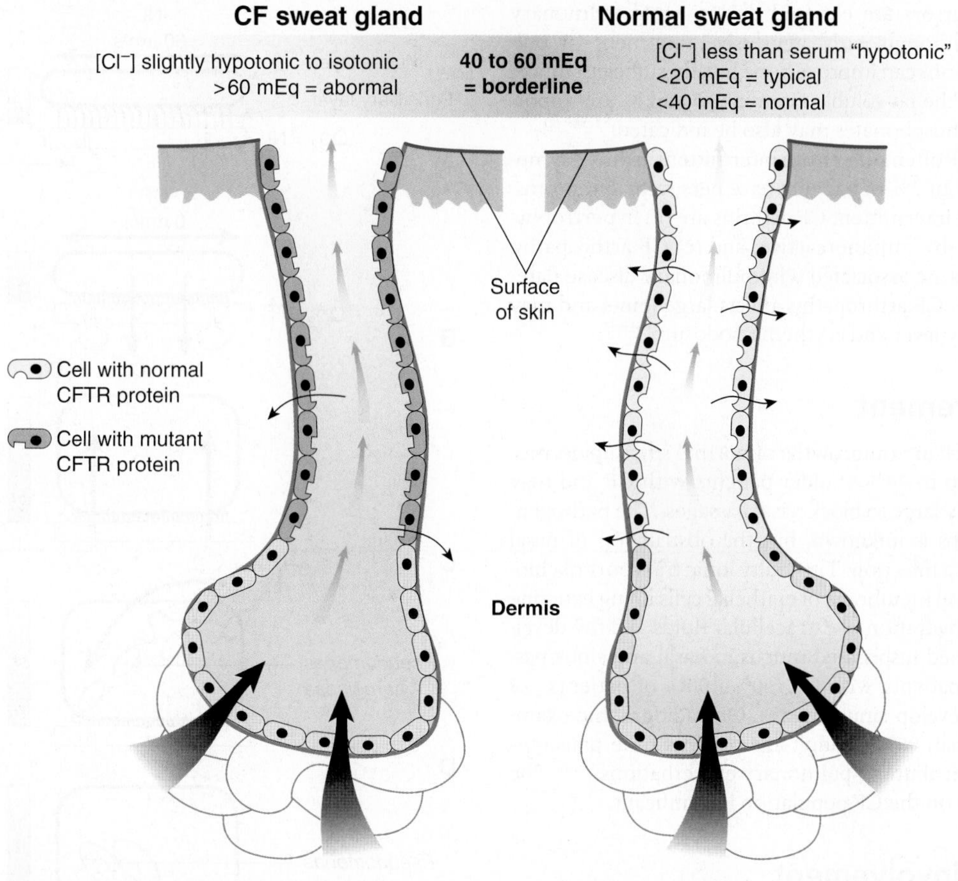

FIGURE 26-2 Chloride transport in sweat glands of normal and cystic fibrosis individuals. (Source: Lyczak JB, et al. Lung infections associated with cystic fibrosis. *Clinical Microbiology Reviews.* 2002; 15(2):194–222.)

17% of children and 75% of adults.[33,34] Diabetes mellitus occurs in approximately 40% to 50% of adult patients with CF.[35] The additional diagnosis of diabetes in CF is associated with significantly increased morbidity and mortality,[36,37] and a decrease in insulin sensitivity is associated with pulmonary exacerbations.[38] Early aggressive insulin therapy can result in improved clinical outcomes.[39]

Gastrointestinal Involvement

Meconium ileus, an intestinal obstruction at birth, occurring in 20% of newborns with CF, is an inheritable trait of this disease.[40] Outside the neonatal period, distal intestinal obstruction syndrome (DIOS, also called *meconium ileus equivalent*) can occur at any age and results from the complete or partial obstruction of the intestine. Intestinal obstruction occurs in 10% to 20% of patients and results from the inspissation of intestinal secretions and incompletely digested intestinal contents. A right lower quadrant mass, abdominal distension, failure to pass stools, and vomiting can accompany DIOS.

Gastroesophageal reflux disease (GERD) is common in both children and adults with CF.[41–43] Children with CF should be screened for GERD and treated, if diagnosed. Other intestinal complications include rectal prolapse, intussusception, and appendiceal abscesses.

Hepatic Involvement

Located on the apical surfaces of the cells lining the intrahepatic and extrahepatic bile ducts and the gallbladder, CFTR functions to facilitate ion transport.[44] In patients with CF, the abnormal chloride efflux across the cells results in the reduction in water and sodium movement into the bile. The resulting decrease in the volume and flow of bile leads to stasis and obstruction of the biliary tree. With chronic obstruction, there is inflammation, giving rise to the characteristic lesion of focal biliary cirrhosis.[45]

Liver disease develops in the first decade of life. Significant liver disease is seen in 13% to 25% of children with CF.[46–48] Prevalence rates may be underestimated. Progressive cirrhosis is associated with portal hypertension, hypersplenism, esophageal varices, ascites, and, in a small number of patients, complete hepatic failure requiring transplantation. Approximately 30% of adult patients with CF have abnormal gallbladder function and size (absent or small gallbladder) with 5% to 10% of patients forming gallstones.[49]

Genitourinary Involvement

Approximately 98% of male patients with CF are infertile secondary to in utero obstruction of the vas deferens or related structures. Hormonal secretion and secondary sexual characteristics are normal. In a small number of patients, infertility can be the only manifestation of disease, and CF may go undiagnosed until fertility testing is performed. The prevalence of infertility is higher in women with CF and hypothesized to be related to the production of thick and tenacious cervical mucus. Hundreds of pregnancies have been carried successfully to term, but these are not without risk, especially for patients with moderate to severe pulmonary disease.[50]

Bone and Joint Involvement

Patients with CF have low bone mineral density, slower rate of bone formation, accelerated rate of bone loss, and arthritis.[51,52]

Osteoclastic precursors are elevated during acute pulmonary exacerbation.[53] Although early, aggressive treatment of pulmonary exacerbations can improve bone health, sufficient intake and absorption of the fat-soluble vitamins, D and K, are important, and oral bisphosphonates may also be indicated.[52,54–60]

Patients with CF often suffer from intermittent arthritis symptoms, but only about 2% of patients have persistent symptoms. The three types of intermittent CF arthritis are (a) hypertrophic osteoarthropathy, (b) immunoreactive, and (c) CF arthropathy. The first two types are associated with pulmonary disease flare-up. The third type, CF arthropathy, affects large joints and may be accompanied by fever and erythema nodosum.[61–65]

Sinus Involvement

Nasal polyps, which are outgrowths of normal sinus epidermis, can be found in up to 20% of older patients with CF and may become sufficiently large to block nasal passages. The pathogenesis of these polyps is unknown, but the obstruction of nasal passages can lead to infection. The faulty ionic transport of chloride across the apical membrane of epithelial cells lining exocrine glands leads to dehydration of extracellular fluids and the development of thickened inspissated mucus in nasal and sinus passages. Nearly all patients with CF (90%–100% of patients >8 months of age) develop sinus disease. On radiographic examination, greater than 90% of adult-age patients have pansinusitis, which can contribute to pulmonary exacerbations.[66,67] The impact of sinusitis on the CF population is significant.

Pulmonary Involvement

Respiratory disease is of major importance in patients with CF because it is the principal cause of repeated hospitalizations, decline in pulmonary function, and death. Although the exact pathophysiological mechanisms leading from the CFTR cellular defect to the development of bronchiectasis and loss of pulmonary function are not currently known, research in the past two decades since the discovery of the genetic defect has greatly expanded our understanding of this process.

AIRWAY OBSTRUCTION, INFECTION, AND INFLAMMATION

ONLINE CONTENT

For animations depicting the effect of CFTR function on airway clearance, courtesy of the CF Foundation, go to http://thepoint.lww.com/AT10e.

One of the leading theories regarding the pathogenesis of airway disease in CF is depicted in Figure 26-3.[68] The lower airways of a normal lung are maintained free of pathogens through various lung defense mechanisms. For example, a thin film of liquid on the airway surfaces called the *airway surface layer* (ASL) contains antimicrobials, antioxidants, proteases, and other substances that work to eliminate pathogens. In addition, the ASL can remove invading microbes from the lung by moving a mucous gel toward the mouth through ciliary motion. Mucociliary clearance of microbes and debris is aided by the cough reflex to keep the airways clear. Because coughing is an important defense mechanism, cough suppressants should not be used in patients with CF.

In patients with CF, the CFTR defect reduces the ASL, resulting in markedly thickened mucus and impaired mucociliary clearance. Continued mucus hypersecretion leads to mucus plugging and airway obstruction. Additionally, the CFTR defect causes alkalinization of intracellular organelles and accumulation of ceramide, resulting in increased susceptibility to infection with *Pseudomonas aeruginosa*.[69] Accelerated ion transport increases oxygen consumption, leading to hypoxic gradients within the mucus. *P. aeruginosa* adapts to the anaerobic environment by increasing alginate production and through the formation of biofilms. In response to infection, proinflammatory

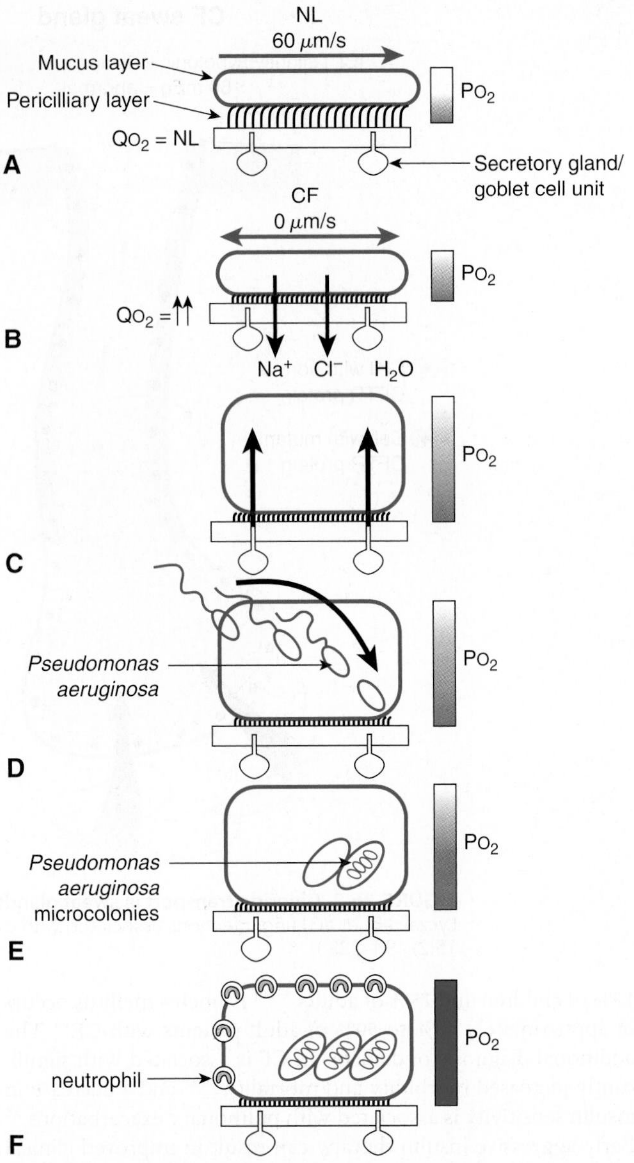

FIGURE 26-3 Pathophysiology of cystic fibrosis lung disease. Treatments in italics are investigational. **A:** Normal airway epithelia with functional CFTR demonstrates normal mucociliary clearance. **B:** CFTR defect leads to reduced periciliary liquid and loss of mucociliary clearance. Accelerated ion transport (sodium reabsorption) leads to increased oxygen consumption (QO_2) and hypoxic gradients (pO_2) in the airways. **C:** Impaired mucociliary clearance leads to accumulation of mucous within the airways causing airway obstruction. **D:** Retained secretions provide an optimal environment for initial infection. **E:** Chronic *Pseudomonas aeruginosa* infections form microcolonies (i.e., biofilms) which resist host defenses as well as antibiotics. **F:** A chronic inflammatory response mediated by neutrophil recruitment to the airways leads to release of reactive oxygen species and proteases which damage the airways. (Reprinted with permission from Worlitzsch D et al. Effects of reduced mucus oxygen concentration in airway *Pseudomonas* infections of cystic fibrosis patients. *J Clin Invest.* 2002;109:317.)

cytokines (e.g., tumor necrosis factor-α, interleukin [IL] 1), chemokines (e.g., IL-8), and other inflammatory mediators (e.g., leukotriene B_4) are released from airway epithelial cells and alveolar macrophages, resulting in neutrophil recruitment into the airways. As the neutrophils undergo apoptosis, they release their DNA, which accumulates and contributes to airway obstruction. In the normal host, proteases (e.g., neutrophil elastase) are released in response to an infectious insult and digest the bacteria, while lung tissue is protected by the presence of antiproteases. In patients with CF the intense neutrophilic infiltration in response to IL-8 results in an imbalance between airway proteases and antiproteases.[70] The excess proteases cause degradation of elastin, a structural component of the airways. In addition, recent data demonstrate that airway proteases degrade the cell surface receptor CXCR1 from neutrophils, leading to impaired bactericidal activity accounting for the persistence of *P. aeruginosa* within the airways despite a robust inflammatory response.[71] The chronic cycle of airway obstruction, infection, and inflammation leads to bronchiectasis, progressive loss of lung function with eventual respiratory failure, and death.

MICROBIOLOGY

The microbiology of airways in patients with CF changes as a function of age. In infants and toddlers, the principal organisms include nontypeable *Haemophilus influenzae* and *Staphylococcus aureus*. The prevalence of methicillin resistant *S. aureus* has increased dramatically in the last 5 years and has been associated with a more-rapid decline in pulmonary function and increased mortality.[72,73] In older children and adults, *P. aeruginosa* becomes the predominant pathogen. Other unique pathogens in CF include *Burkholderia cepacia* and *Aspergillus fumigatus*.

PSEUDOMONAS AERUGINOSA

Infections with *P. aeruginosa* occur in three distinct phases. First, the patient acquires the organism and presents with an initial infection. Treatment often leads to eradication; however, reinfection eventually occurs and leads to chronic infection. Under pressure from hypoxic gradients within the mucus, *P. aeruginosa* within the airways converts to the mucoid phenotype. Observational studies have noted significant structural as well as functional changes within the lung in patients with sputum cultures that grow mucoid *P. aeruginosa* when compared with patients with nonmucoid strains or who are not infected with *P. aeruginosa*. Specifically, when compared with patients with nonmucoid *P. aeruginosa*, those with mucoid *P. aeruginosa* had significant abrupt declines in percentage of predicted FEV_1.[74] The median time to acquisition of nonmucoid and mucoid strains is 1 and 13 years, respectively; however, there is tremendous variability in the initial acquisition and development of chronic infection. Some patients avoid acquisition of *P. aeruginosa* until their adolescent years, whereas others acquire mucoid *P. aeruginosa* early in childhood (e.g., 5–6 years of age). Patients with delayed acquisition of *P. aeruginosa* typically have minimal lung disease and few hospital admissions when compared with children who acquire *P. aeruginosa* (in particular mucoid *P. aeruginosa*) earlier in life. The relatively long period between nonmucoid and mucoid *P. aeruginosa* offers an opportunity for intervention with pharmacologic therapy designed to eradicate the organism from the airways. The mucoid strains create a significant therapeutic challenge because they can develop into biofilms. A biofilm is a community of bacteria that adheres to tissues (e.g., airway epithelial cells) and secretes a slimy coating (mucoid exopolysaccharide), which protects it from the hostile environment within which it resides. *P. aeruginosa* biofilms create a therapeutic challenge when compared with their planktonic (freely motile) bacterial counterparts because they evade local defense mechanisms, are slow growing, and can sequester β-lactamase.

BURKHOLDERIA CEPACIA

Occasionally infections involve atypical organisms, including *B. cepacia* (2.8%). *B. cepacia* is actually a complex consisting of several distinct species. *Burkholderia cenocepacia* is the most frequently isolated and clinically relevant species in patients with CF. *B. cepacia* is easily transmitted via inhalation or contact with a reservoir of *B. cepacia,* including other patients with CF, health care professionals, or contaminated medical instruments. Colonization with *B. cepacia* can manifest as chronic asymptomatic carriage, progressive deterioration of lung function, or fatal decline during a short interval often associated with septicemia (known as *B. cepacia* syndrome), and is associated with a 50% reduction in life expectancy.[75] *B. cepacia* is intrinsically resistant to many antibiotics, including aminoglycosides and β-lactams, which limits treatment options. Because of the adverse health outcomes and limited treatment options, chronic infection with *B. cenocepacia* is a relative contraindication to lung transplantation at many centers, emphasizing the importance of preventing acquisition of this organism through active infection control measures.

ASPERGILLUS FUMIGATUS

Aspergillus species present a unique challenge in patients with CF. The presence of this organism often ignites an immunologic response characterized by an increase in serum immunoglobulin E and eosinophilic infiltration of the alveoli. This syndrome is referred to as allergic bronchopulmonary aspergillosis. The typical symptoms of this syndrome include wheezing, shortness of breath, low-grade fever, and production of thick, brownish, or bloody sputum. This disease is not invasive; however, chronic eosinophilic infiltration can lead to bronchiectasis and lung scarring. Allergic bronchopulmonary aspergillosis is present in approximately 10% of patients with CF and accounts for 10% of acute pulmonary exacerbations. The diagnosis of allergic bronchopulmonary aspergillosis can be challenging owing to the overlap in clinical features with acute pulmonary exacerbations. A consensus conference sponsored by the Cystic Fibrosis Foundation in 2001 provided guidelines for diagnosis and treatment of allergic bronchopulmonary aspergillosis in patients with CF.[76] The minimal diagnostic criteria include clinical deterioration, elevated total serum immunoglobulin E (greater than 500 international units/mL), positive immediate *A. fumigatus* skin test or serum immunoglobulin E antibodies, and *A. fumigatus* serum precipitins or immunoglobulin G antibodies or radiographic changes. Annual screening of serum immunoglobulin E concentrations is recommended for patients with CF older than 6 years of age.

DIAGNOSIS

The diagnosis of CF can be made soon after birth through newborn screening or later in life based on the presentation of symptoms. As of December 2010, all states in the United States use newborn screening for early diagnosis of CF. However, those born before the implementation of newborn screening in their birth state may be diagnosed later in life once symptoms appear. The newborn screening test is based on measurement of trypsinogen concentrations in blood. Trypsinogen is normally produced in the pancreas and is carried to the small intestine, where it changes from an inactive proenzyme to the active enzyme trypsin, which is used in digestion of proteins. In infants with CF, mucus can block the ducts from the pancreas into the small intestine. The mucus prevents trypsinogen from reaching the intestines, resulting in accumulation in the blood. This process can be detected and measured because immunoreactive trypsin (IRT) levels increase in the blood of the infant. The IRT testing is a screening test; confirmatory testing including a sweat chloride test and DNA analysis for CF mutations should be performed in infants with a positive IRT.[77]

When the pilocarpine iontophoresis test (i.e., sweat chloride test) is conducted at a certified CF center and is positive ($\geq$60 mM), the diagnosis of CF can be applied. In infants younger than 6 months of age, a sweat chloride value of 30 to 59 mM indicates possible CF and should be repeated in conjunction with DNA analysis.[77] In those older than 6 months of age, a value of 40 to 59 mM indicates possible CF and should be repeated in conjunction with DNA analysis.[77]

DNA analysis is recommended and is expected to identify 90% of CFTR mutations.[77] The DNA analysis used for population screening is not as sensitive at detecting CFTR mutations in non-white populations. Prenatal screening for the presence of a CF carrier state in the parents is recommended by the American College of Medical Genetics and the American College of Obstetrics and Gynecology.[78]

Symptoms Suggestive of Cystic Fibrosis

For those in whom CF may not have been detected by newborn screening, the suspicion for CF is raised by clinical symptoms. Infants born with meconium ileus, an intestinal obstruction attributable to thickened meconium, at birth are highly likely to have CF. Other clinical symptoms that require further diagnostic testing are listed in Table 26-2. Presence of these symptoms warrants obtaining a sweat chloride and DNA analysis.

CASE 26-1

QUESTION 1: K.M. is a 1-week-old girl weighing 2.9 kg who presents for routine follow-up. Her birth weight was 2.7 kg. She is growing well on breast milk every 3 hours. A review of systems reveals no abnormalities. K.M.'s newborn screening panel has returned with an elevated IRT concentration.

What further testing is recommended to determine whether this infant has CF?

At this time, it is recommended that K.M. have a sweat chloride test and DNA analysis performed. If K.M. has a positive sweat chloride, additional testing is recommended to determine whether she has pancreatic insufficiency. The preferred testing method is the fecal elastase, which is measured in a single stool sample. Fecal elastase is not degraded during intestinal transit and has been shown to correlate well with duodenal lipase, amylase, trypsin, and bicarbonate concentrations. A low value indicates the presence of pancreatic insufficiency necessitating enzyme supplementation. Although 25% of infants with CF are pancreatic sufficient at the time of diagnosis, most will become pancreatic insufficient in the first year of life.[77] For those at least 8 years of age, a serum trypsinogen may be used to assess pancreatic function.[77]

TABLE 26-2
Phenotypic Features Consistent With Diagnosis of Cystic Fibrosis (CF)

Persistent colonization or infection with typical CF pathogens (e.g., *Staphylococcus aureus,* nontypeable *Haemophilus influenzae, Pseudomonas aeruginosa,* and *Burkholderia cepacia*
Chronic cough and sputum production
Persistent chest radiograph abnormalities
Airway obstruction manifested by wheezing and air trapping
Nasal polyps; radiographic or computed tomographic abnormalities of paranasal sinuses
Digital clubbing
Meconium ileus, distal intestinal obstruction syndrome, rectal prolapse
Pancreatic insufficiency, recurrent pancreatitis
Chronic hepatic disease
Failure to thrive, hypoproteinemia and edema, complications secondary to fat-soluble vitamin deficiency
Salt loss syndromes: acute salt depletion, chronic metabolic alkalosis
Male urogenital abnormalities resulting in obstructive azoospermia (CBAVD)

CBAVD, congenital bilateral absence of the vas deferens.
Reprinted with permission from Farrell PM et al. Guidelines for diagnosis of cystic fibrosis in newborns through older adults: Cystic Fibrosis Foundation consensus report. *J Pediatr.* 2008;153:S4.

EARLY INTERVENTIONS AND THERAPY

CASE 26-1, QUESTION 2: K.M. returns to the clinic 2 weeks later. Testing has revealed a sweat chloride of 84 mM and the presence of homozygous ΔF508 mutations. Fecal elastase is low, and the diagnosis of pancreatic insufficiency is made. What therapy should be initiated at this time?

K.M. now meets the diagnostic criteria for CF with pancreatic insufficiency. Early nutritional therapy to ensure appropriate growth is essential as good nutritional status has been associated with improved pulmonary outcomes.[79] CF patients are hypermetabolic and do not absorb fats and proteins normally. Therefore, the CF diet must be high in calories, fat, and protein. It is recommended that those with CF have an energy intake of 110% to 200% of that recommended for the general population.[80] If K.M. has difficulty gaining weight, the frequency of breastfeeding may need to increase or she will need to be changed to a high-calorie infant formula.

Vitamin and Mineral Supplementation

The malabsorption of fats in patients with CF with pancreatic insufficiency also results in decreased gastrointestinal absorption of the fat-soluble vitamins (A, D, E, and K). Approximately 45% of the CF population is deficient in one of these vitamins, even when pancreatic enzymes are being used appropriately.[81] The current recommendations for replacement therapy are listed in Table 26-3.[82] Concerns about inadequate supplementation of vitamins D and K resulting in poor bone health have arisen.[56,57,83–85] Calcium supplementation will be needed for those receiving inadequate calcium in their diet. Iron supplements might also be needed if iron deficiency anemia occurs.

K.M. should be started on a liquid multivitamin preparation at a dose of 1 mL once daily. Additional vitamins may be supplemented if laboratory monitoring reveals an abnormality. Additionally, K.M. should receive 1/8 teaspoon of table salt per day to account for sodium loss in sweat.[86] At 6 months of age, the dose increases to 1/4 teaspoon. For bottle-fed infants, a small amount of salt is added to each feeding. For K.M., who is breast-fed, the parents should attempt pumping and bottle-feeding with breast milk twice a day to add salt. If K.M. does not tolerate bottle-feeding, the salt is not supplemented, and they should ensure K.M. is not exposed to warm conditions for a prolonged time.

TABLE 26-3
Daily Recommended Doses of Fat-Soluble Vitamins for Patients With Cystic Fibrosis and Vitamin Content in Specialty Vitamin Formulations

Age	Vitamin A (international units)	Vitamin E (international units)	Vitamin D (international units)	Vitamin K (mg)
0–12 months	1,500	40–50	400	0.3–0.5
1–3 years	5,000	80–150	400–800	0.3–0.5
4–8 years	5,000–10,000	100–200	400–800	0.3–0.5
>8 years	10,000	200–400	400–800	0.3–0.5
Vitamin Content				
AquaDEK chewable tablet	9,083 (87% as β carotene)	50	400	0.35
Vitamax chewable tablet	5,000 (50% as β carotene)	200	400	0.2
SourceCF chewable tablet	16,000 (88% as β carotene)	200	1,000	0.8
Vitamax liquid (per 1 mL)	3,170	50	400	0.3
SourceCF liquid (per 1 mL)	4,627 (75% as β carotene)	50	500	0.4
AquADEK liquid (per 1 mL)	5,751 (87% as β carotene)	50	400	0.4
AquADEK softgel capsules	18,167 (92% as β carotene)	150	800	0.7
SourceCF softgel capsules	16,000 (88% as β carotene)	200	1,000	0.8

Enzyme Supplementation

The mainstay of treatment for pancreatic insufficiency is exogenous replacement of pancreatic digestive enzymes. The goals of pancreatic enzyme supplementation are to (a) improve weight gain, (b) minimize steatorrhea, and (c) eliminate abdominal cramping and bloating. Supplementation with currently available therapies does not fully restore fat absorption, and the absorption of sufficient fat-soluble vitamins continues to be problematic.[87] The digestive enzymes (lipase, protease, and amylase) are available in a mixture of approximately one part amylase to three parts protease and three parts amylase in capsules that contain enteric-coated microspheres of these enzymes (Table 26-4). The enteric coating protects these enzymes from gastric acid. Because the breakdown of fat is the most important function of these enzymes, dosing is based on the lipase content, and the dose varies according to weight, age, dietary fat intake, and symptom severity. The initial dose for infants is 2,000 to 5,000 units of lipase per breast-feeding or per 120 mL of bottle-feeding. Infants eating solid food begin at a dose of 1,000 units/kg/meal.[86] For children older than 4 years of age, 500 units of lipase/kg/meal is the initial dose for enzyme supplementation.[80] A full dose is taken with meals, and half the prescribed dose is taken with snacks. Subsequent dosing adjustments are titrated to response. Lack of weight gain, smelly, greasy stools, and abdominal pain or bloating might be indicative of insufficient enzyme supplementation.[88,89]

TABLE 26-4
Pancreatic Enzyme Formulations

Product[a]	Microencapsulated Enzymes: Lipase	Protease	Amylase
Creon 3	3,000	9,500	15,000
Creon 6	6,000	19,000	30,000
Creon 12	12,000	38,000	60,000
Creon 24	24,000	76,000	120,000
Pancreaze	4,200	10,000	17,500
Pancreaze	10,500	25,000	43,750
Pancreaze	16,800	40,000	70,000
Pancreaze	21,000	37,000	61,000
Zenpep 3	3,000	10,000	16,000
Zenpep 5	5,000	17,000	27,000
Zenpep 10	10,000	34,000	55,000
Zenpep 15	15,000	51,000	82,000
Zenpep 20	20,000	68,000	109,000
Zenpep 25	25,000	85,000	136,000

[a] Dosing and comparison of products based on lipase content.

High-strength pancreatic enzymes have been associated with colonic strictures, which are accompanied by symptoms similar to that of DIOS. Although cause and effect have not been firmly established, doses greater than 6,500 units of lipase/kg/meal have been associated with stricture formation. As a result, most recommend that the daily dose of lipase not exceed 10,000 units of lipase/kg or 2,500 units of lipase/kg/meal.[80]

When patients require unusually high doses of enzyme supplements, it sometimes can be attributable to high gastric acidity. The enteric coating on the pancreatic enzyme microspheres dissolves at a pH of 5.8, and the enzymes are destroyed at a pH of 4.0. Patients with CF have longer postprandial periods when the pH is less than 4.0 in the bowel and also have significantly less time when the pH is greater than 5.8. Because enzymes may be less effective when the bowel pH is very low,[90,91] adding a histamine type H_2 antagonist or a proton-pump inhibitor to increase gastric pH might help lower the enzyme dosing requirement.[92–94]

K.M. should receive a pancreatic enzyme supplement of 2,000 to 5,000 units per feeding. Even though K.M. is not yet eating solid food, the capsule may be opened and the contents sprinkled on a small amount (e.g., a baby's spoonful) of rice cereal, baby food, or applesauce and given before each feeding. K.M.'s caregivers should ensure that no beads are left in her mouth after the feeding is complete.

Pulmonary Interventions

Although data on the benefits of airway clearance and bronchodilator therapy in infants are sparse, these interventions are recommended by the Cystic Fibrosis Foundation.[86] Generally, albuterol may be administered before percussion and postural drainage (see Treatment of Cystic Fibrosis Airway Disease: Mechanical Methods section) once daily in infants with CF. The frequency of treatments may be increased if symptoms become evident. Respiratory syncytial virus affects most infants and may more adversely affect those with CF. Therefore, palivizumab is recommended in those with CF who are younger than 2 years of age.[86] K.M. should receive albuterol by nebulizer or metered-dose inhaler and spacer once daily before airway clearance. She should also receive palivizumab 15 mg/kg intramuscularly once a month during respiratory syncytial virus season.

CASE 26-1, QUESTION 3: What monitoring is recommended for K.M.?

K.M.'s head circumference, height, and weight should be plotted on standard growth charts every month for the first year. The goal is for her to have a weight-for-length status of the 50th percentile.[80] After the first year, quarterly growth evaluations are recommended. From 2 to 20 years of age, the goal for growth is to achieve at least the 50th percentile for body mass index. An experienced, knowledgeable registered dietitian should meet with the family to help them understand the importance of appropriate nutrition and help develop a plan for K.M. Fasting blood glucose, liver function tests, albumin, serum electrolytes, complete blood count, prothrombin time, and vitamins A, D, and E levels should be determined now, at 1 year of age, and at least annually. An abdominal examination should be done to determine liver and spleen size and consistency at each office visit.

Pulmonary status is monitored based on clinical symptoms, auscultation of the chest, and chest radiographs until about 5 years of age, when pulmonary function testing may be performed. Oropharyngeal cultures are recommended at least quarterly to detect the presence of pathogenic bacteria.

Those with CF are at risk for CF-related diabetes, warranting annual oral glucose tolerance testing starting at 10 years of age. They are also at increased risk for osteoporosis and should be assessed annually for risk factors. Bone densitometry is recommended for all adults and starting at 8 years of age in those with risk factors including low vitamin D, FEV_1 less than 50%, oral corticosteroid use greater than 90 days in a year, diabetes, delayed puberty, and body mass index less than the 25th percentile. K.M. currently does not have any known risk factors for osteoporosis and is too young for bone densitometry. Her risk should be re-evaluated annually starting at 8 years of age.

Treatment of Cystic Fibrosis Airway Disease

Treatment of CF airway disease involves the use of medications and techniques to mobilize pulmonary secretions, antibiotics to manage infection, and anti-inflammatory agents to reduce airway inflammation. A summary of the current evidence for specific therapies is depicted in Table 26-5.[95]

MUCOCILIARY CLEARANCE

Sputum in patients with CF is difficult to mobilize because pulmonary secretions are thick as a result of the CFTR defect, the large amounts of viscous DNA from the breakdown of white blood cells, and the bacterial debris left over from chronic infections. Mechanical clearance methods, inhaled mucolytics, and airway hydration therapies can be helpful in mobilizing pulmonary secretions.

TABLE 26-5
Evidence-Based Review of Pulmonary Medications for Cystic Fibrosis

Treatment Question	Type of Review	Studies	Total (n)	Strength of Evidence	Estimate of Net Benefit	Recommendation
Inhaled tobramycin						
Moderate-severe lung disease	S	3 RCT; 1 RCO; 2 one-arm trials	679	Good	Substantial	A
	C					
Asymptomatic-mild disease	S	2 RCT	202	Fair	Moderate	B
Other inhaled antibiotics (colistin, gentamicin, ceftazidime)	S	2 RCT, 2 RCO	206	Poor	Small	I
Dornase alfa						
Moderate to severe lung disease	S	10 RCT; 3 crossover; 6 trials without comparison groups	3,140	Good	Substantial	A
	C					
Asymptomatic-mild lung disease	S	3 RCT; 1 crossover	520	Fair	Moderate	B
Hypertonic saline	S	2 RCT; 2 RCO (compared with dornase alfa)	284	Fair	Moderate	B
	C					
Inhaled corticosteroids	S	5 RCT; 2 RCO	388	Fair	None	D
	C					
Oral corticosteroids						
Age, 6–18 years	S	3 RCT	354	Good	Negative	D
	C					
Age, >18 years	S	1 crossover	20	Poor	None	I
Oral nonsteroidal anti-inflammatory drugs	S	3 RCT	145	Fair	Moderate	B
	C					
Leukotriene modifiers	M	2 RCO; 1 controlled trial	64	Poor	None	I
Cromolyn	M	2 RCT; 1 clinical trial	44	Poor	None	I
Macrolide antibiotics	S	2 RCT; 1 crossover; 1 clinical trial	296	Fair	Substantial	B
	C					
Antistaphylococcal antibiotics	M	3 RCT; 1 crossover	306	Fair	Negative	D
	C					
Inhaled β_2-adrenergic receptor agonists	C	14 RCO: nebulized and metered dose	257	Good	Moderate	B
Inhaled anticholinergics	C	5 RCO	79	Poor	None/small	I
Oral *N*-acetylcysteine	M	1 phase 1 trial; 1 RCO; 1 controlled trial; 2 crossover	145	Poor	None	I

C, Cochrane; M, modified systematic; RCO, randomized crossover; RCT, randomized, controlled trial; S, systematic.

Reprinted with permission from Flume PA et al. Cystic fibrosis pulmonary guidelines: chronic medications for maintenance of lung health. *Am J Respir Crit Care Med.* 2007;176:957.

MECHANICAL METHODS

Methods used to mechanically break up and mobilize mucus in the pulmonary tree include traditional hand percussion and postural drainage (P&PD), oscillating positive-end pressure (OPEP) with the flutter valve, high-frequency chest-wall oscillation (HFCWO), intrapulmonary percussive ventilation, and autogenic drainage (a technique of deep-breathing exercises). (For a video of how one of the HFCWO options, the Vest, works, see the last chapter at **http://www.thevest.com/resources/videos.asp.**)

ONLINE CONTENT

For an illustration of postural drainage, go to http://thepoint.lww.com/AT10e.

These mechanical approaches for mobilizing mucus are about equal in efficacy, and the selection of the most appropriate one for a patient depends on the ability, motivation, preference, and resources of the patient.[96] When the traditional P&PD was compared with HFCWO and OPEP, clinical efficacy and safety were comparable, but 50% of patients preferred the HFCWO, 37% preferred OPEP, and 13% preferred P&PD.[97]

DORNASE ALFA

Dornase alfa is an inhaled recombinant form of human deoxyribonuclease I, which breaks up the extracellular DNA formed by apoptotic neutrophils that contributes to airway obstruction in patients with CF. The pivotal clinical trial demonstrated improvement in pulmonary function (FEV_1 5.8% vs. placebo, $p < 0.01$) and a reduction in exacerbation frequency (28% vs. placebo, $p = 0.04$) in patients receiving dornase alfa.[98] Based on these benefits, the use of dornase alfa is recommended in all patients 6 years of age and older.[95] Dornase alfa is very expensive, with costs averaging about $2,300/month, and the cost–benefit ratio for its use continues to be debated.[99–101] A reasonable approach is to provide a brief trial of dornase alfa (1–2 months) to determine whether there is improvement in pulmonary function and the medication is well tolerated. A longer trial (up to 1 year) may be necessary to assess its effect on hospitalization rate.

Dornase alfa is available in 2.5-mg vials and is administered once daily via a vented jet nebulizer. The drug must be stored in the refrigerator and protected from light. Patients should be instructed in the proper use and maintenance of the nebulizer and compressor system. In addition, patients should be instructed not to dilute or mix dornase alfa with other drugs in the nebulizer.

AIRWAY HYDRATION THERAPIES

Hypertonic Saline

Inhalation of hypertonic saline (IHS) improves mucociliary clearance.[102] Hypertonic saline rehydrates the airways through osmotic flow of water. When twice-daily inhaled normal saline was compared with 7% (hypertonic) sodium chloride, no difference was noted in the primary outcome, which was the linear rate of pulmonary function decline during the 48-week study period.[103] However, patients randomly assigned to receive IHS experienced a significant reduction in exacerbations (56% decrease vs. placebo, $p = 0.02$). In two small, randomized, crossover trials, dornase alfa provided a greater improvement in lung function, albeit at a much higher financial cost than IHS ($70/month). One approach is to consider the use of IHS in patients who are intolerant or do not respond to a trial of dornase alfa. In addition, IHS should be considered as add-on therapy in patients with airway congestion despite optimal standard therapy (i.e., dornase alfa and chest physiotherapy). A short-acting β_2-agonist should be given before IHS treatment because IHS has been associated with bronchospasm.[104] IHS is available commercially, and its use is recommended to improve lung function and reduce exacerbations in all patients 6 years of age or older.[95]

Dry Powder Mannitol

Inhalation of a dry powder formulation of mannitol (Bronchitol) is designed to rehydrate the airways through osmotic effects. Dry powder mannitol has completed phase 3 studies and is currently undergoing marketing review in multiple countries. Results of the trials demonstrated significant improvement in pulmonary function (FEV_1 8.2%, $p = 0.001$) during the 6-month trial period when compared with baseline. The most common adverse effects associated with inhalation of dry powder mannitol include cough (8.8%), hemoptysis (5.7%), and headache (4.2%). The inhalation of dry powder mannitol has not been directly compared with IHS. Although its place in therapy is currently not known, the addition of dry powder mannitol would provide an alternative to hypertonic saline for those intolerant to IHS.

BRONCHODILATION

The chronic use of inhaled β_2-agonists improves lung function in patients with bronchial hyperresponsiveness or a positive bronchodilator response, and is recommended for use.[95] In addition, they may assist in airway clearance when administered before chest physiotherapy. No clear consensus exists for the use of other bronchodilators. Studies in support of inhaled anticholinergic medications for the treatment of CF also are limited, and the results have been mixed.[105]

CASE 26-2

QUESTION 1: J.P. is a 12-year-old girl who was seen for a routine quarterly visit at the CF center. J.P. was diagnosed with CF at age 7 months as a result of failure to thrive. Genotyping revealed she is homozygous for ΔF508. At this visit she has complaints of increased cough and chest congestion when compared with her visit 3 months ago. She has a history of hemoptysis, but has not had an episode recently. She has had no pulmonary exacerbations in the last 12 months. Her current medications include pancreatic enzymes (approximately 2000 units of lipase/kg/meal) with all meals, a fat-soluble vitamin supplement, two puffs of albuterol inhaler before airway clearance treatment once daily, dornase alfa 2.5 mg via nebulization once daily, and fluticasone 44 mcg inhaler two puffs daily. She performs airway clearance using HFCWO for 30 minutes once daily and reports she is tolerating this therapy well. Microbiological cultures of her oropharyngeal tract grow *S. aureus*; she has not grown *P. aeruginosa* in the past. J.P.'s body mass index is in the 60th percentile (stable from last visit), and her lung function tests show an FEV_1 of 1.99 L (89% predicted), which is down from her baseline of 2.05 L (92% predicted). A recent chest computed tomography revealed mild bronchiectatic changes in all lobes as well as mucus plugging and air trapping. What steps should be taken to improve J.P.'s airway clearance?

Methods of mechanical assistance to remove pulmonary secretions are all equally effective, and the decision about which device to use should be individualized. J.P. is currently using HFCWO and appears to be tolerating this well. One advantage to this treatment is the independence it provides when compared with manual percussion and drainage, which requires the assistance of another individual. It also is efficient as the patient can perform some nebulization treatments while on the therapy vest (e.g., dornase alfa, hypertonic saline).[95] This is especially an important consideration to improve adherence. The typical frequency and duration of treatment with HFCWO is 30 minutes twice daily. J.P. is currently using the therapy vest only once daily and could benefit from increasing the frequency of treatment to twice daily.

Dornase alfa improves sputum viscosity in patients with CF and provides benefit early in the course of the lung disease.[106] In the Pulmozyme Early Intervention Trial, the risk of pulmonary exacerbations was reduced by 34% in young patients with mild lung function abnormalities, and pulmonary function tests improved even in patients with close to normal pulmonary function. J.P. is currently receiving dornase alfa and should continue on this therapy to improve pulmonary function and reduce the risk of pulmonary exacerbations.

Hypertonic saline (7%) twice daily should also be considered for J.P. to enhance the mucociliary clearance and improve pulmonary function. The albuterol should be increased to twice daily to provide bronchodilation to prevent potential bronchospasm from the hypertonic saline. The recommended sequence of the treatments is albuterol for bronchodilation, hypertonic saline to hydrate the airways, and dornase alfa to liquefy the mucus, followed by airway clearance therapy to clear the mucus.[95] If adherence is an issue, the dornase alfa and hypertonic saline can be administered during airway clearance treatment.

Control of Inflammation

The inflammatory response in CF airways contributes significantly to destruction of the airways and eventual pulmonary function decline. Pharmacological intervention to block the intense neutrophilic inflammatory response is a key strategy to reducing pulmonary disease progression. Corticosteroids, nonsteroidal anti-inflammatory drugs, and macrolides have all been used to control the inflammation seen in CF lung disease. Although leukotriene modifiers have improved lung function in small studies, the overall data are insufficient to support a recommendation for their use.[107] Cromolyn use also is not routinely recommended because of limited evidence of positive outcomes with this drug.[95]

CASE 26-2, QUESTION 2: Is J.P. a candidate for anti-inflammatory therapy?

CORTICOSTEROIDS

Oral corticosteroids are not recommended in the treatment of CF. Although prednisone 1 to 2 mg/kg every other day demonstrated a significant reduction in decline of lung function and decreased pulmonary exacerbations in patients with *Pseudomonas* infections, long-term use was associated with unacceptable adverse effects including cataracts, glucose intolerance, osteoporosis, and persistent growth retardation.[108–110] Although inhaled corticosteroids are widely prescribed to patients with CF, there are limited data supporting their use in this population. In particular, a randomized, controlled trial of withdrawal of inhaled corticosteroids demonstrated no change in pulmonary function after discontinuation; therefore, they are not recommended for routine use in patients with CF.[95,111] Fluticasone should be discontinued in J.P., and pulmonary function testing should be performed at the next clinic visit. In addition, J.P. should be questioned about wheezing or shortness of breath.

NONSTEROIDAL ANTI-INFLAMMATORY DRUGS

Nonsteroidal anti-inflammatory drugs have been used to slow lung function decline. High-dose ibuprofen (20–30 mg/kg twice daily with doses titrated to a peak concentration of 50–100 mg/L) can significantly slow the annual rate of FEV_1 decline in children between 5 and 13 years of age.[112] Ibuprofen serum concentrations must be measured and monitored closely to stay in the therapeutic range because lower concentrations can paradoxically increase neutrophil infiltration. Because these doses are much higher than the recommended doses to treat pain or fever, concerns about long-term side effects, including gastrointestinal bleeding and renal toxicity, together with the need for frequent blood draws have not made this method of treatment common. Less than 5% of the CF population is using ibuprofen.[101,113] For patients at least 6 years of age with an FEV_1 greater than 60% of predicted, chronic oral ibuprofen is recommended to reduce the loss of lung function.[95] Considering J.P.'s history of hemoptysis, the use of high-dose ibuprofen is not recommended.

AZITHROMYCIN

Azithromycin is an antibiotic with anti-inflammatory properties. Although its use is established in patients with CF with chronic *P. aeruginosa* infection (see Case 26-3, Question 3), a recent study conducted in children and young adults who were not infected with *P. aeruginosa* demonstrated a significant reduction in exacerbation frequency (50%) and increased weight (0.58 kg) during the 24-week study period; however, no improvement in pulmonary function was noted.[114] Because J.P. has not experienced any pulmonary exacerbations during the past year, there would be little advantage to adding azithromycin at this point.

ANTIBIOTIC THERAPY

Treatment of pulmonary infections in patients with CF has undoubtedly contributed to the improved survival observed in patients with CF in the past 30 years. Antibiotics are indicated in patients with CF for (a) early eradication of *P. aeruginosa* at the time of first detection with the intent to prevent or delay chronic infection, (b) treatment of acute pulmonary exacerbations, and (c) chronic maintenance therapy with inhaled antibiotics to control the bacterial burden within the airways with the goal of slowing the progression of pulmonary function decline.

EARLY ERADICATION OF *PSEUDOMONAS AERUGINOSA*

CASE 26-2, QUESTION 3: J.P. returns to clinic 6 weeks later for a follow-up visit to evaluate pulmonary function and response to the hypertonic saline and the increased airway clearance therapy. Subjectively she reports less chest congestion and cough. Spirometry demonstrates her FEV_1 has returned to baseline. A throat culture is obtained and reveals *P. aeruginosa*. Should J.P. be started on antibiotics for treatment of *P. aeruginosa*?

Because of the increased rate of pulmonary function decline and shortened survival in patients chronically infected with *P. aeruginosa*, early treatment with the goal of eradication is recommended.[95] Results of two recent studies provide guidance on the optimal treatment approach. The Early Inhaled Tobramycin for Eradication trial demonstrated that treatment with inhaled tobramycin 300 mg twice daily for 28 or 56 days was similar in terms of eradication at 1 month (93% vs. 92%) and time to recurrence of *P. aeruginosa* (66% vs. 69% culture free at 27 months).[115] The recently completed Early Pseudomonas Infection Control trial demonstrated that therapy (inhaled tobramycin 300 mg twice daily for 28 days with or without ciprofloxacin twice daily for 14 days) initiated when quarterly respiratory cultures are positive for *P. aeruginosa* was not different in eradication or recurrence when compared with a similar antibiotic regimen cycled for 28 days followed by 56 days off for a period of six quarterly cycles.[116] Based on the results of these two studies, it would be appropriate to start J.P. on inhaled tobramycin 300 mg twice daily for 28 days. Cultures should be obtained on completion of the therapy to confirm eradication and quarterly thereafter to monitor for recurrence of *P. aeruginosa*.

Acute Pulmonary Exacerbation

Acute pulmonary exacerbations are an inevitable consequence of pulmonary disease in most patients with CF. A pulmonary exacerbation is defined as a change in respiratory signs and symptoms from the patient's baseline that necessitates treatment with antibiotics and augmented airway clearance. Key indicators include increased cough or sputum production, decreased exercise tolerance, loss of weight or appetite, decrease in FEV_1 or forced vital capacity (FVC) by more than 10%, or onset of new or increased crackles.[117] Approximately one-third of patients experience at least one pulmonary exacerbation annually; however, the onset and frequency varies widely in the population. The frequency of exacerbations is correlated with severity of pulmonary disease. Traditional management for an acute CF exacerbation includes nutritional repletion, antibiotics, and chest physiotherapy.[118] For mild exacerbations the patient can typically be managed in the outpatient setting using oral antibiotics and an intensification of airway clearance and nutritional therapies. For moderate to severe exacerbations, patients are typically hospitalized and receive a 14-day course of intravenous (IV) antibiotics, as well as airway clearance and nutrition therapies. If the patient demonstrates a significant improvement in signs and symptoms he or she may be a candidate to complete treatment at home before completion of the 14-day course.[119]

ANTIBIOTIC DRUG SELECTION

Antibiotic drug selection is based on sputum or throat culture and susceptibility data. Combination therapy with two antibiotics with different mechanisms of action is often prescribed for treating acute pulmonary exacerbations involving *P. aeruginosa* to prevent the development of resistance and provide potential synergistic activity. Therefore, the combination of an antipseudomonal β-lactam and an aminoglycoside or fluoroquinolone is frequently used. Results of a controlled trial comparing β-lactam monotherapy versus β-lactam plus an aminoglycoside demonstrated similar improvement in pulmonary function, but greater reduction in bacterial density in sputum and a longer duration before readmission for a new pulmonary exacerbation in the patients receiving combination therapy.[120] Multidrug-resistant strains, defined as resistance to all agents within two of the three major classes of antipseudomonal therapies (e.g., β-lactams, aminoglycosides, and fluoroquinolones), are reported in 15% to 20% of patients. Treatment of infections involving these organisms may require the use of IV colistimethate. The use of IV colistin requires close monitoring as this drug exhibits both neurotoxic and nephrotoxic effects.

ANTIBIOTIC DOSING

The antibiotics used most commonly to treat acute pulmonary exacerbations and their dosage ranges are listed in Table 26-6. Typical dosage regimens used in other populations may not be adequate in patients with CF owing to reduced lung penetration, decreased activity in sputum, presence of bacteria within biofilms, heavy inocula, and reduced susceptibility. Altered pharmacokinetics of drugs in patients with CF is also frequently cited in the published literature. In particular, both the volume of distribution and clearance of a number of antibiotics (e.g., β-lactams and aminoglycosides) are reported to be higher in patients with CF when compared with healthy control subjects. As many of the β-lactam antibiotics are cleared renally, it has been hypothesized that the enhanced renal clearance observed in patients with CF might be related to a higher tubular clearance as a result of upregulation of organic anion and cation transporters as a compensatory response to the CFTR defect.[121] However, subsequent controlled trials failed to confirm this hypothesis.[122,123] A more unifying explanation of the observed differences in pharmacokinetics in CF is related to differences in body composition.

TABLE 26-6
Antibiotic Doses for Cystic Fibrosis

Systemic Antibiotics			
Drug	**Daily Dosage (mg/kg)**	**Frequency**	**Maximal Individual Dose (mg)**
Amikacin	30	Every 24 hours	TDM
Ceftazidime	150–225	Divided every 6–8 hours	2,000
Cefuroxime	150–225	Divided every 8 hours	1,500
Ciprofloxacin IV	30	Divided every 8 hours	400
Ciprofloxacin PO	40	Divided every 12 hours	1,000
Colistimethate	5	Divided every 8 hours	150
Gentamicin	10	Every 24 hours	TDM
Imipenem	40–80	Divided every 6 hours	1,000
Meropenem	50–100	Divided every 6–8 hours	2,000
Oxacillin	200	Divided every 4–6 hours	2,000
Piperacillin	200–400	Divided every 4–6 hours	4,000
Ticarcillin/clavulanate	200–400	Divided every 4–6 hours	3,100
Tobramycin	10	Every 24 hours	TDM
TMP/SMZ	10–15	Divided every 8–12 hours	800

Inhaled Antibiotics			
Drug	**Dosage (mg)**	**Interval**	**Comments**
Aztreonam	75	TID	
TOBI	300	BID	28 days on, 28 days off
Colistin	37.5–75	BID	

BID, twice daily; TDM, therapeutic drug monitoring (gentamicin/tobramycin desired maximal concentration is 20–30 mg/L once-daily dosing); TID, three times daily; TMP/SMZ, trimethoprim/sulfamethoxazole; TOBI, tobramycin for inhalation.

older than 6 years who are colonized with *P. aeruginosa*.[95] Based on the pivotal trial, the dose of azithromycin is 500 mg three times/week for patients weighing more than 40 kg and 250 mg three times weekly for patients weighing less than 40 kg. One contraindication to treatment with azithromycin is colonization with mycobacteria because of the potential for development of resistance.

CASE 26-3, QUESTION 3: B.W. comes to the outpatient clinic 2 weeks after hospital discharge for a follow-up visit and reports a significant reduction in cough and sputum production, and no shortness of breath. Spirometry reveals an FEV_1 of 85% of predicted. He has resumed his outpatient treatment regimen, which includes one multiple vitamin every day, two microencapsulated pancreatic enzyme capsules (16,000 units of lipase/capsule) with meals, and one or two capsules with snacks as needed, and dornase alfa 2.5 mg nebulized daily. What changes, if any, should be made to B.W.'s treatment regimen?

Because B.W. has had two exacerbations in the last 6 months, he would benefit from the addition of medications to reduce the frequency of exacerbations. In addition to the disruption to his life, frequent exacerbations are associated with more rapid decline in pulmonary function and reduced survival.[133] Key pharmacological therapies demonstrated to improve pulmonary function and reduce the frequency of pulmonary exacerbations include dornase alfa, inhaled tobramycin, IHS, and azithromycin. B.W. is already receiving dornase alfa, but is not on inhaled tobramycin, IHS, or azithromycin. One important consideration when adding new therapies is the treatment burden, particularly with inhaled therapies. Inhaled tobramycin 300 mg twice daily cycled for 28 days on and 28 days off and oral azithromycin 500 mg every Monday, Wednesday, and Friday would be appropriate additions to the treatment regimen because B.W. is chronically infected with *P. aeruginosa,* and these particular agents demonstrated the greatest improvement in pulmonary function when compared with IHS. In addition, azithromycin has a minimal effect on treatment burden as it can be administered orally 3 days a week. IHS would also be of benefit by reducing exacerbation frequency; however, it could be added in the future if B.W. demonstrates a decline in pulmonary function or increased frequency of exacerbations despite the new additions.

ORAL ANTIBIOTICS

CASE 26-3, QUESTION 4: One year later, B.W. returns to the clinic exhibiting signs and symptoms of a mild exacerbation, but refuses IV antibiotics or hospitalization because he is in the middle of final examinations. What alternative to IV therapy is available to treat B.W.?

The quinolone family of antibiotics is currently the only option for oral treatment of *P. aeruginosa*. Emergence of resistant strains of *Staphylococcus* and *Pseudomonas* species have led the CF medical community to restrict the use of quinolones to the treatment of acute CF exacerbations.[134,135] Oral fluoroquinolones (e.g., ciprofloxacin) have become widely used in patients with CF because they are less expensive, easy to administer, and as effective as IV therapy in an acute exacerbation.[136,137]

Because of the past sensitivities of B.W.'s organisms and his refusal to be admitted to the hospital, ciprofloxacin 1,000 mg orally twice daily for 1 week can be initiated in addition to the aerosolized tobramycin and oral azithromycin.[138] After 1 week of the combined aerosol and oral therapies, B.W. should be reevaluated for hospital admission if his condition worsens, or his therapy can be continued if his condition improves.

CASE 26-3, QUESTION 5: B.W. returns to the outpatient clinic 3 months later for his annual comprehensive visit. Results of laboratory studies, dual-emission x-ray absorptiometry (DXA) scan, spirometry, and an oral glucose tolerance test (OGTT) are as follows:

BUN, 10 mg/dL
Creatinine, 0.6 mg/dL
Urine microalbumin/creatinine, 12 mcg/mg
2-hour OGTT plasma glucose, 220 mg/dL
Glycosylated hemoglobin, 7.8%
DXA Z-score, −2.1 (pelvis)
FEV_1, 83% of predicted

How should these laboratory studies be interpreted and what new therapies would you recommend?

The elevated 2-hour OGTT plasma glucose indicates B.W. has CF-related diabetes mellitus. This is confirmed by the elevated glycosylated hemoglobin. The urine microalbumin testing indicates that B.W. is not spilling protein into the urine as a result of the CF-related diabetes mellitus. Treatment with insulin should be initiated in B.W. to improve nutritional status and prevent microvascular complications. The DXA scan results indicate B.W. has osteopenia and should be initiated on calcium 500 mg orally twice daily and his vitamin D status should be determined. Treatment of osteopenia is recommended to prevent progression to osteoporosis, which would put the patient at risk for fractures. In addition, osteoporosis is a relative contraindication for lung transplantation because of the risk for fractures after transplantation that may impair adequate recovery.

B.W.'s spirometry results indicate that his pulmonary function is stable and his current pharmacotherapeutic regimen should be continued.

LUNG TRANSPLANTATION

Pulmonary disease progression leading to eventual respiratory failure is an inevitable consequence of the chronic cycle of airway obstruction, infection, and inflammation. End-stage lung disease (defined by an FEV_1 of <30% of predicted) significantly affects the quality of life for patients with CF as a result of reduced exercise tolerance, heavy treatment burden, need for oxygen therapy, and frequent hospitalizations for pulmonary exacerbations. Lung transplantation is a potential therapeutic option for CF patients with end-stage lung disease.[139] The optimal time to refer a patient for lung transplantation is not precisely defined; however, patients are typically referred when their FEV_1 is approximately 40% to maximize the chances of obtaining new lungs before the patient experiences respiratory failure. Transplant evaluation includes assessments of pulmonary disease severity, patient adherence to therapies, and concomitant illnesses. Once accepted into the program, the patient is placed on the transplant list awaiting availability of potential organs. The waiting time to receive a lung transplant is highly variable and depends on the Lung Allocation Score, a score that distributes organs on the basis of model-predicted benefit from transplantation. The mean survival after lung transplantation is approximately 50% at 5 years. Importantly, the quality of life for many lung transplant recipients improves significantly.

KEY REFERENCES AND WEBSITES

A full list of references for this chapter can be found at **http://thepoint.lww.com/AT10e.** Below are the key references and websites for this chapter, with the corresponding reference number in this chapter found in parentheses after the reference.

Key References

Flume PA et al. Cystic fibrosis pulmonary guidelines: chronic medications for maintenance of lung health. *Am J Respir Crit Care Med*. 2007;176:957. (95)

Stallings VA et al. Evidence-based practice recommendations for nutrition-related management of children and adults with cystic fibrosis and pancreatic insufficiency: results of a systematic review. *J Am Diet Assoc*. 2008;108:832. (80)

Key Websites

Cystic Fibrosis Foundation. Drug Development Pipeline. **http://www.cff.org/research/DrugDevelopmentPipeline/.**

Cystic Fibrosis Mutation Database. **http://www.genet.sickkids.on.ca/cftr/app.**

Johns Hopkins Cystic Fibrosis Center. **http://www.hopkinscf.org/main/whatiscf/index.html.**

27 Upper Gastrointestinal Disorders

Randolph V. Fugit and Rosemary R. Berardi

CORE PRINCIPLES

PEPTIC ULCER DISEASE	CHAPTER CASES
1 Chronic peptic ulcer disease (PUD) is causally linked to *Helicobacter pylori* (*H. pylori*) infection or the use of nonsteroidal anti-inflammatory drugs (NSAIDs) and is usually characterized by epigastric pain or discomfort, sometimes accompanied by heartburn, bloating, and belching.	**Case 27-1 (Questions 1, 2), Case 27-2 (Question 1)**
2 Treatment for PUD is aimed at relieving ulcer symptoms, healing the ulcer, eradicating *H. pylori* (if positive), preventing ulcer recurrence, and reducing ulcer-related complications; eradication is recommended for all patients with an *H. pylori*–positive active ulcer or a history of a previous ulcer or ulcer-related complication; proton-pump inhibitors (PPIs) are the drugs of choice for healing and reducing the risk of an NSAID ulcer; patients with a peptic ulcer should stop or reduce cigarette smoking and NSAID use, reduce psychological stress, and avoid foods and beverages that trigger symptoms.	**Case 27-1 (Questions 3–10), Case 27-2 (Questions 2–10)**
3 Treatment of an *H. pylori* ulcer should be initiated with a PPI-based three-drug eradication regimen; the regimen should be effective, well-tolerated, easy to comply with, cost-effective, and should take into consideration antibiotic resistance; if a second course of therapy is necessary, it should contain different antibiotics.	**Case 27-1 (Questions 3, 4, 6–10)**
4 PPIs are preferred to histamine-2 receptor antagonists (H_2RAs) and sucralfate for healing an *H. pylori*–negative NSAID ulcer as they accelerate ulcer healing and provide more effective symptom relief; the duration of treatment should be extended if the NSAID is continued; if the patient is *H. pylori*–positive, a PPI-based three-drug regimen should be used.	**Case 27-2 (Questions 2, 3, 10)**
5 Prophylactic risk reduction therapy with a PPI or misoprostol or switching to an NSAID with greater cyclo-oxygenase-2 (COX-2) selectivity is recommended for patients at risk of exhibiting an ulcer or ulcer-related complication; when selecting a PPI, its gastrointestinal benefits must be weighed against the cardiovascular risks associated with COX-2 inhibitors and concomitant antiplatelet therapy.	**Case 27-2 (Questions 4–7)**
6 Patients receiving an *H. pylori* eradication regimen, those undergoing treatment for an active NSAID ulcer, and individuals receiving prophylactic risk reduction therapy require patient education regarding ulcer risk, potential ulcer complications, and drug therapy.	**Case 27-1 (Question 5), Case 27-2 (Questions 8, 9)**

continued

GASTROESOPHAGEAL REFLUX DISEASE

1	The classic symptoms associated with gastroesophageal reflux disease (GERD) are usually very specific and include heartburn and acid regurgitation, however, not all patients will present with these typical symptoms and may present with more serious "alarm symptoms" or extra esophageal manifestations warranting referral for further evaluation.	**Case 27-3 (Question 1)**
2	Appropriate management for the patient with GERD is focused on relieving symptoms, promotion of healing of the esophageal mucosa, and prevention of relapse or the development of complicated disease. This is accomplished with lifestyle modification and pharmacotherapy directed at reducing esophageal mucosal exposure to gastric acid.	**Case 27-3 (Questions 2–4)**
3	Diagnostic testing strategies for patients with more severe GERD include empiric acid suppression test, upper endoscopy and biopsy, 24-hour continuous pH monitoring, radiologic testing, and esophageal manometry.	**Case 27-4 (Question 1)**
4	Mild to moderate GERD can be managed acceptably with antacids, sucralfate, and H_2RAs, however for more severe, frequent, or complicated GERD, the drugs of choice are PPIs, which have demonstrated superiority over these other agents in terms of symptom relief and esophageal healing.	**Case 27-4 (Question 2)**
5	GERD can be associated with numerous manifestations that occur outside of the esophagus, including noncardiac chest pain, asthma, hoarseness, laryngitis, and chronic cough.	**Case 27-5 (Question 1)**

UPPER GASTROINTESTINAL BLEEDING

1	Stress-related mucosal bleeding (SRMB) is a serious complication that can occur in critically ill patients under severe physiologic stress. Appropriate prophylactic management includes identification of risk factors for SRMB, such as mechanical ventilation and coagulopathy, and then implementation of an appropriate pharmacotherapy strategy (e.g., PPIs, H_2RAs, sucralfate) aimed at reducing the risk of exhibiting SRMB.	**Case 27-6 (Questions 1–4)**

UPPER GASTROINESTINAL DISORDERS

Upper gastrointestinal (GI) disorders include a wide spectrum of maladies that range in importance from simple discomfort to life-threatening illness and include dyspepsia, peptic ulcer disease (PUD), gastroesophageal reflux disease (GERD), and upper GI bleeding. The majority of upper GI disorders are acid-related diseases in which gastric acid plays an important role in their development, progression, and treatment. In the United States, more than $97 billion in direct costs are spent yearly treating GI disorders, with more than $10 billion of this amount spent on proton-pump inhibitors (PPIs), a primary pharmacotherapeutic option used to reduce gastric acid secretion.[1,2] These diseases place a substantial burden on both patients and the health care system. It has been estimated that in 2004, more than 18 million outpatient clinic visits were for patients evaluated for a diagnosis of GERD, and an additional 1.5 million were seen for issues related to PUD.[2] Between 250,000 and 300,000 patients are hospitalized each year for upper GI bleeding, resulting in 15,000 to 30,000 deaths, and despite numerous advances in diagnostic techniques and management strategies, mortality rates of approximately 10% to 15% are reported with more than $2.5 billion spent each year to manage these patients.[3–5]

The introductory section of this chapter includes a brief discussion of the physiology of the upper GI tract and the pharmacotherapy of drugs used to treat upper GI disorders in adults. This section highlights the most important aspects associated with these topics. A more in-depth and comprehensive review can be found in GI textbooks or journal articles that discuss upper GI physiology and the pharmacology, pharmacokinetics, interactions, and side effects of the drugs.

PHYSIOLOGY OF THE UPPER GASTROINTESTINAL TRACT

The upper GI tract consists of the mouth, esophagus, stomach, and the duodenum (Fig. 27-1). Ingested food or liquids pass from the mouth through the esophagus and into the stomach. As these substances enter into the esophagus, the lower esophageal sphincter (LES), an area of smooth muscle near the distal end of the esophagus, relaxes to allow their entry into the stomach. The LES usually remains contracted to prevent the reflux of gastric contents into the esophagus. However, peristaltic contractions of the esophageal muscles allows the LES to remain open until all food has entered the stomach.[6] Although the LES is the

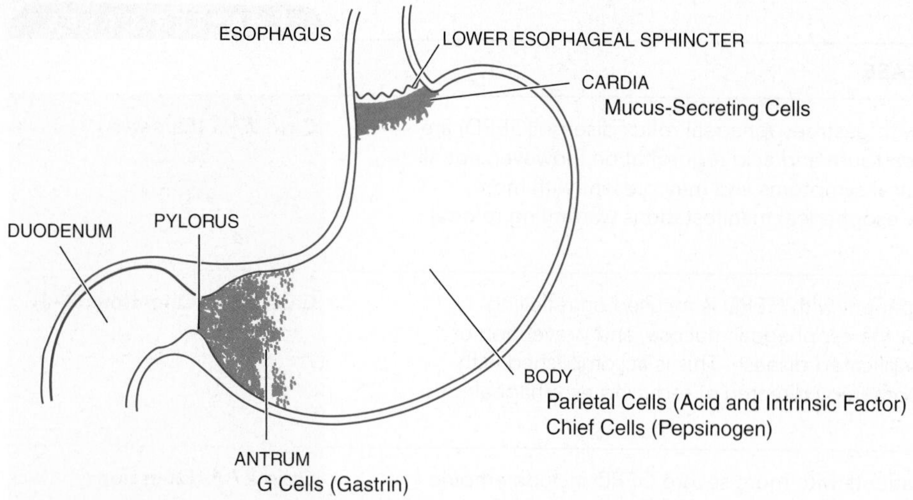

FIGURE 27-1 Gastrointestinal anatomic regions.

primary barrier for the prevention of gastric refluxate entering the esophagus, healthy individuals reflux throughout the day and night without clinical consequences.[7]

The stomach consists of three distinct anatomical regions, each responsible for a variety of specialized functional processes (Fig. 27-1). The cardia (~5% of stomach surface area), which is the uppermost portion of the stomach at the junction between the esophagus and stomach, is responsible for the mucus secretion that protects against the acid milieu of the stomach. The body, which makes up the majority of the surface area (80%–90%) of the stomach, contains the parietal cells, which are responsible for gastric acid and intrinsic factor (required for vitamin B_{12} absorption) secretion. The body also contains the peptic (chief) cells, which secrete pepsinogen (a precursor to pepsin). Pepsinogen, under acidic conditions in the stomach, is converted to pepsin (a proteolytic enzyme), which is responsible for breaking down protein. The antrum makes up the final 10% to 20% of the stomach. It contains the G cells, which secrete the hormone gastrin, which through a feedback mechanism stimulates acid secretion by the parietal cell. The final portion of the upper GI tract is the duodenum, which begins just after the pylorus and extends to ligament of Treitz. At this point, the jejunum begins the first portion of the lower GI tract.

The parietal cell is responsible for secreting gastric acid (Fig. 27-2). Three stimuli (neurologic, physical, and hormonal) trigger the parietal cell to secrete acid. Neurologic impulses, from the central nervous system (CNS) and initiated by the sight, smell, and taste of food, travel along cholinergic pathways to stimulate the release of acetylcholine, which arrives via nerve endings and activates the muscarinic receptor on the parietal cell.[8] Ingested food causes gastric distension, which triggers the release of acetylcholine and also stimulates G cells within the antrum to produce gastrin. Elevated intragastric pH also stimulates the production of gastrin. Gastrin works via a feedback mechanism that, although produced in response to elevated pH, can be inhibited by low gastric pH. The stomach is protected from overproduction of gastric acid by the release of somatostatin from antral D cells, which signal the G cell to stop the production of gastrin.[8,9] Gastrin enters the blood and arrives at the parietal cell, where it binds to the gastrin receptor. Acetylcholine and gastrin promote the release of histamine from the mast cell or enterochromaffinlike (ECL) cells, which then bind to the histamine H_2 receptor on the parietal cell. Histamine release is associated with both postprandial and nocturnal acid secretion. The gastrin, histamine H_2, and muscarinic receptors are located on the basolateral membrane of the parietal cell (Fig. 27-2). Binding of any of these receptors leads to a cascade of events that stimulates gastric acid secretion. Calcium influxes into the parietal cell, leading to increased intracellular levels of calcium. Levels of cyclic adenosine monophosphate also increase and activate intracellular protein phosphokinases. This in turn activates the hydrogen-potassium adenosine triphosphatase (H^+/K^+-ATPase) or proton pump to move into position in the secretory canaliculus located in the apical membrane of the parietal cell. The proton pump is an ion transport pathway that transports hydrogen ions out of the cytoplasm and into the

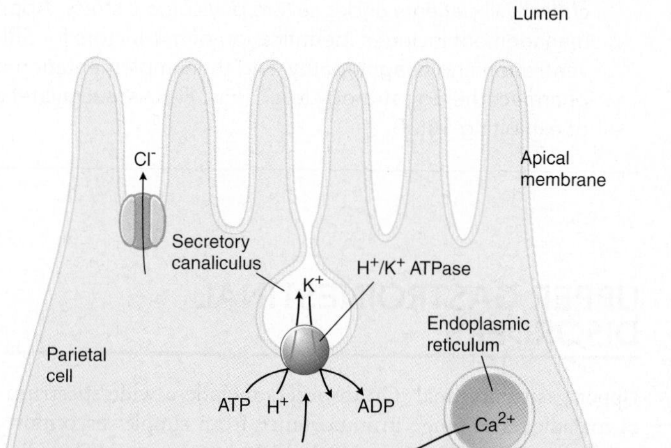

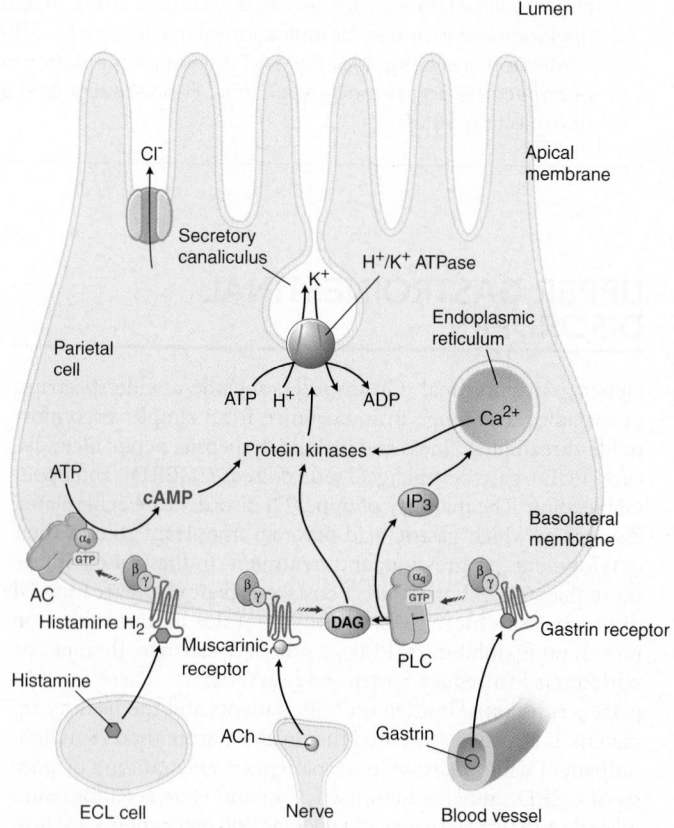

FIGURE 27-2 Parietal cell. (Adapted with permission from Golan DE, et al. *Principles of Pharmacology: The Pathophysiologic Basis of Drug Therapy*, 2nd Edition. Baltimore: Wolters Kluwer Health, 2008.)

secretory canaliculus, where they are exchanged for potassium ions that enter the parietal cell via the opposite ion channel. In the secretory canaliculus, hydrogen ions combines with chloride from the blood to form hydrochloric acid, which is then released into the gastric acid lumen.[8] The proton pump is the final common pathway for gastric acid secretion.[8]

PHARMACOTHERAPY OF DRUGS USED TO TREAT ACID-RELATED DISORDERS

The following section briefly reviews the pharmacotherapy of drugs used to treat acid-related disorders (Table 27-1). Their therapeutic use is discussed under each specific GI disorder.

Antacids and Alginic Acid

Antacids are widely used to relieve mild and infrequent symptoms associated with acid-related diseases. They act by neutralizing gastric acid and thus increasing intragastric pH.[10] The elevation of intragastric pH is dose-dependent and usually requires a substantial dose to raise the intragastric pH above 4 or 5.[10,11] Antacids are very quick acting and modestly elevate intragastric pH within minutes, but their duration of action is short (about 30 minutes on an empty stomach). The duration of action can be extended to 3 hours when given with or within 1 hour after a meal.[10] Antacids are available as individual salts or as combination of salts of magnesium, aluminum, calcium, or sodium. Aluminum-containing and magnesium-containing salts are also able to bind bile salts.[10] Aluminum salts may enhance mucosal protection by increasing mucosal prostaglandins, stimulating mucus and bicarbonate secretion, and enhancing microvascular blood flow. Antacids may also inhibit the action of pepsin. These findings suggest that in addition to their acid neutralizing capacity, antacids have other mechanisms by which they act. This helps to explain their many pharmacotherapeutic benefits.[10] A review of specific antacid products and their acid-neutralizing capacity is discussed elsewhere.[10] Antacids can also be combined with alginic acid. Alginic acid, however, is not an acid-neutralizing agent. It acts by forming a viscous solution that floats on top of the gastric contents and theoretically protects the esophageal mucosa from the potent acid refluxate.[12]

Antacids are generally well tolerated. The magnesium-containing antacids may cause a dose-related osmotic diarrhea, but combining it with aluminum salts (which can cause constipation when used alone) can offset this side effect. When higher doses of combination magnesium/aluminum antacids are used, the predominating side effect is diarrhea.[10,13] Small amounts of aluminum and magnesium are absorbed systemically and have the potential to accumulate in patients with renal insufficiency and lead to toxicity. Thus, magnesium-containing antacids should be avoided in patients with a creatinine clearance less than 30 mL/minute, and chronic use of aluminum-containing antacids in patients with renal failure should be avoided.[10,13] Hypercalcemia has been described in patients taking prolonged courses of large doses of calcium carbonate (>20 g/day in patients with normal renal function and >4 g/day in patients with renal failure).[10] This issue is especially important when considering that many well-known over-the-counter (OTC) antacid products that did not originally contain calcium, have been reformulated recently to include the addition of calcium, or have replaced another antacid salt with calcium, yet retained a similar trade-name.[13] High-dose regimens of calcium (4–8 g/day) in combination with alkalinizing agents (sodium bicarbonate) can produce the milk-alkali syndrome (i.e., hypercalcemic nephropathy with alkalosis).[10,13] Aluminum-containing antacids (with the exception of aluminum phosphate) binds to dietary phosphate within the GI tract to form insoluble salts that are excreted in feces. High-dose or frequent administration may lead to hypophosphatemia.[10,13] Sodium bicarbonate should not be used for long periods of time (especially in the renally impaired patient) because systemic alkalosis can result from the accumulation of bicarbonate. Additionally, the high sodium content (274 mg sodium/g sodium bicarbonate) has been associated with sodium retention and may pose a problem in patients with hypertension, ascites, severe renal dysfunction, or heart failure.[10,13]

Antacids may interfere with the absorption of many orally administered drugs (e.g., digoxin, phenytoin, isoniazid, ketoconazole, itraconazole, iron preparations) that require an acidic environment for dissolution and absorption.[10,12,14] This may lead to potential therapeutic failures with these medications. Antacids containing calcium, aluminum, or magnesium can bind to concomitantly administered drugs and interfere with the absorption of drugs that are susceptible to complexation with these salts. Tetracyclines and the fluoroquinolones are susceptible to this interaction, as they bind to divalent and trivalent cations.[13] The bioavailability of ciprofloxacin, for example, is reduced by more than 50% when concomitantly administered with an antacid, because aluminum and magnesium ions chelate with the antibiotic to form an insoluble and inactive complex. The administration of ciprofloxacin 2 hours before an antacid increases ciprofloxacin bioavailability more than when administered 2 hours after the antacid.[15] An increase in gastric pH may also result in the premature dissolution and altered absorption of enteric-coated dosage forms as the enteric coating is usually designed to dissolve at a pH greater than 6.0.[14] Urinary alkalinization may result in increased urinary excretion (salicylates) or decreased excretion (amphetamines and quinidine) leading to decreased or increased blood concentrations, respectively.[10,13] The majority of these drug interactions can be avoided by separating the antacid from the interacting drug by a minimum of 2 hours.[13]

Histamine-2 Receptor Antagonists

There are currently four H_2-receptor antagonists (H_2RAs) approved for use in the United States. These include cimetidine, ranitidine, famotidine, and nizatidine. All four agents are available in prescription and OTC dosage forms, as well as oral and parenteral formulations (nizatidine is not available parenterally in the United States). H_2RAs competitively and selectively inhibit the action of histamine on the H_2 receptors of the parietal cells, thus reducing both basal and stimulated gastric acid secretion (Fig. 27-2). Although the relative antisecretory potency on a milligram-per-milligram basis differs (famotidine has the greatest potency, followed by nizatidine, ranitidine, and cimetidine), this is not an important factor, as standard oral dosages of the four H_2RAs have been adjusted accordingly to have an equipotent antisecretory effect (Table 27-1).[16] Oral absorption from the small intestine is rapid, and peak drug concentrations usually are achieved within 1 to 3 hours after administration.[16] The bioavailability is lower for cimetidine, famotidine, and ranitidine because they are absorbed incompletely and undergo first-pass metabolism resulting in 40% to 65% bioavailability. The bioavailability of nizatidine is considered near 100% because this agent does not undergo first-pass metabolism.[16,17] Parenteral H_2RAs given by the intravenous (IV) route have 90% to 100% bioavailability. All four drugs are eliminated by a combination of hepatic metabolism, glomerular filtration, and tubular secretion.[16] Hepatic metabolism is the principal pathway for the elimination of cimetidine, famotidine, and ranitidine, whereas renal excretion

TABLE 27-1
Oral Medications Used to Treat Upper Gastrointestinal Disorders

	Gastric and Duodenal Ulcer Healing	Maintenance of Gastric and Duodenal Ulcer Healing	Reduction of Gastric Ulcer Risk Associated with NSAIDs	Relief of Heartburn and Indigestion (OTC Use)	Relief of GERD Symptoms (Rx Use)	Esophageal Healing[a]	Maintenance of Esophageal Healing[a]	Hypersecretory Diseases[a,b]
H_2 Receptor Antagonists								
Cimetidine	300 mg QID 400 mg BID 800 mg daily	400–800 mg HS	Not indicated	200 mg BID PRN	300 mg QID	400 mg QID 800 mg BID	400–800 mg HS	[a]
Famotidine	20 mg BID 40 mg HS	20–40 mg HS	Not indicated	10 mg BID PRN 20 mg BID PRN	20 mg BID	40 mg BID	20–40 mg BID	[a]
Nizatidine	150 mg BID 300 mg HS	150–300 mg HS	Not indicated	75 mg BID PRN	150 mg BID	300 mg BID	150–300 mg BID	[a]
Ranitidine	150 mg BID 300 mg HS	150–300 mg HS	Not indicated	75 mg BID PRN 150 mg BID PRN	150 mg BID	300 mg BID	150–300 mg BID	[a]
Proton-Pump Inhibitors								
Esomeprazole	20–40 mg daily	20 mg daily	20 mg daily	Not indicated	20 mg daily	20–40 mg daily	20 mg daily	60 mg daily
Dexlansoprazole	Not indicated	Not indicated	Not indicated	Not indicated	30 mg daily	60 mg daily	30 mg daily	Not indicated
Lansoprazole	15–30 mg daily	15–30 mg daily	15–30 mg daily	15 mg daily[c]	15–30 mg daily	30 mg daily	15–30 mg daily	60 mg daily
Omeprazole	20 mg daily	20 mg daily	20 mg daily	20 mg daily[c]	20 mg daily	20–40 mg daily	20 mg daily	60 mg daily
Pantoprazole	40 mg daily	40 mg daily	40 mg daily	Not indicated	20 mg daily	40 mg daily	40 mg daily	80 mg daily
Rabeprazole	20 mg daily	20 mg daily	20 mg daily	Not indicated	20 mg daily	20 mg daily	20 mg daily	60 mg daily
Rabeprazole ER[d]	Not indicated	Not indicated	Not indicated	Not indicated	Unknown	50 mg daily	Unknown	Not indicated
Other Agents								
Sucralfate	1 g QID 2 g BID	Not indicated	Not indicated	Not indicated	Not indicated	Not indicated	Not indicated	Not indicated
Misoprostol	Not indicated	Not indicated	200 mcg TID–QID	Not indicated	Not indicated	Not indicated	Not indicated	Not indicated

[a] Although FDA-labeled for this indication, H_2RAs are not recommended even in higher dosages because they are not as effective as the PPIs.
[b] Initial starting dose; daily dosage must be titrated to gastric acid secretory response.
[c] Duration of treatment should not exceed 14 consecutive days; if needed, repeat 14-day treatment every 4 months.
[d] Not FDA approved at time of publication.
BID twice a day; GERD, gastroesophageal reflux disease; HS, at bedtime; NSAID, nonsteroidal anti-inflammatory drug; OTC, over-the counter; PRN, as needed; QD, every day; QID, four times a day; Rx, prescription; TID, three times a day.

is the major route for elimination of nizatidine.[16–20] For each of these agents, the elimination half-life is increased, the total body clearance is decreased, and dosage reduction is recommended for patients with moderate to severe renal insufficiency. The pharmacokinetics appear to be unaffected by hepatic dysfunction; however, in patients with combined hepatic failure and renal insufficiency, dosage reduction is likely necessary.[18]

H_2RAs are remarkably safe, and the frequency of severe adverse effects is low for all four drugs.[21] A meta-analysis of randomized placebo-controlled trials reported no difference in the incidence of adverse events of cimetidine versus placebo.[22] The most common adverse effects include GI discomfort (e.g., diarrhea, constipation), CNS effects (e.g., headache, dizziness, drowsiness, lethargy, confusion, psychosis, and hallucinations), and dermatologic effects (e.g., rashes).[21] The most frequent hematologic adverse effect is thrombocytopenia, which occurs in about 1% of patients but is reversible on discontinuation of the H_2RA.[23] Although thrombocytopenia is more commonly reported with IV administration, it is likely that the overall incidence of H_2RA-associated thrombocytopenia is overestimated.[24] Hepatotoxicity, although uncommon, has been described primarily in patients receiving IV H_2RAs.[25] Cimetidine has demonstrated weak antiandrogenic effects, and its use in high doses (hypersecretory conditions) has been associated with gynecomastia and impotence in men. This effect is reversible with discontinuation of the medication or by switching to another H_2RA.[21,26] Patients at highest risk of experiencing any of these adverse effects include the elderly, those requiring higher doses (usually parenteral), and those with altered renal function.[26,27]

All four H_2RAs can potentially alter the absorption and reduce the bioavailability of drugs that require an acidic environment for absorption. The most important of these interactions is with ketoconazole, which requires an acidic pH for dissolution and absorption. Concomitant administration of a H_2RA and ketoconazole may lead to therapeutic failure of the antifungal.[14] Cimetidine has the greatest potential to cause drug interactions because of its ability to inhibit several hepatic cytochrome P-450 (CYP450) isoenzymes. The greatest concern is with those agents that have a relatively narrow therapeutic window (e.g., theophylline, lidocaine, phenytoin, quinidine, and warfarin).[14] Although ranitidine is more potent on a molar basis, it binds less intensely to the CYP450 isoenzyme system than cimetidine. Thus, when used in equipotent doses, there is less potential for interactions. Famotidine and nizatidine do not bind appreciably to the CYP450 system and do not interact with drugs that are metabolized through this hepatic system.[14] Because H_2RAs undergo renal tubular excretion, there is a potential for competition with other medications.[28] Cimetidine and ranitidine inhibit the tubular secretion of procainamide by as much as 44%, but famotidine does not have this effect.[29] Tachyphylaxis or tolerance has been described with all H_2RAs because of up-regulation of the H_2 receptor site. It appears to occur more frequently with high-dose parenteral formulations, but has also been described with oral therapy.[30,31] Tolerance to the antisecretory effect may develop after several days of regularly scheduled (continuous) use but can be avoided by taking the H_2RA only when needed.

Proton-Pump Inhibitors

PPIs are highly specific inhibitors of gastric acid secretion and include omeprazole, lansoprazole, rabeprazole, pantoprazole, esomeprazole, and dexlansoprazole. These agents are substituted benzimidazoles and act by irreversibly binding to the H^+/K^+-ATPase (proton pump). PPIs are the most potent inhibitors of gastric acid secretion in that they inhibit the terminal step in the acid production cycle.[32–34] They inhibit both basal and stimulated gastric acid secretion in a dose-dependent and sustained fashion.[33] PPIs are prodrugs and require an acidic environment for conversion to the active sulfonamide. They are absorbed in the small intestine (protected from the acidic milieu of the stomach by enteric coating) and taken via the bloodstream to the acidic secretory canaliculus of the parietal cell for protonation to the active form (Fig. 27-2).[32,34] This conversion requires an actively secreting proton pump, and hence, these agents are most efficacious when taken 30 to 60 minutes before a meal on an empty stomach.[34] The most recent PPIs, dexlansoprazole MR (modified-release) and rabeprazole extended-release, differ from others in this class in that they use dual delayed-release technology which extends the duration of their antisecretory effect. Dexlansoprazole MR contains two different pH-dependent granules. The first of these is initially released in the proximal duodenum similar to the other PPIs, followed by a second release of drug in the distal small intestine about 4 hours later. Given this broadened duration of drug exposure, dexlansoprazole MR may also be taken without regard to meal times.[35] Rabeprazole extended-release, currently under investigation, is a new formulation which uses two different releasing mechanisms. Despite the short plasma elimination half-lives (~1–2 hours) of the other PPIs, the duration of their antisecretory effect is 48 to 72 hours because of covalent (irreversible) binding to the proton pump.[34,36] PPIs have similar acid-inhibitory effects and healing rates when used in equivalent doses (Table 27-1).[37–42] PPIs are superior to H_2RAs in reducing gastric acid secretion and mucosal healing.[36,42,43] A dosage reduction is not required in patients with renal insufficiency, but is recommended for patients with severe hepatic impairment.[44]

The oral PPIs are formulated as delayed-release enteric-coated granules within capsules (omeprazole, lansoprazole, esomeprazole, dexlansoprazole MR, rabeprazole extended-release), delayed-release enteric-coated tablets (pantoprazole, rabeprazole, OTC omeprazole), a rapidly disintegrating tablet (lansoprazole), delayed-release oral suspension (lansoprazole), and an immediate-release formulation (omeprazole and sodium bicarbonate capsules and powder for oral suspension).[32] IV formulations in the United States include pantoprazole and esomeprazole. Various methods of administration, specific dosage forms, and compounding options for patients with special needs (e.g., dysphagia, gastric tubes) will be discussed later in this chapter (see Upper Gastrointestinal Bleeding section).

The short-term adverse effects of PPIs are relatively infrequent and comparable to H_2RAs or placebo. The most common side effects include GI discomfort (e.g., nausea, diarrhea, abdominal pain), CNS effects (e.g., headache, dizziness), and rare isolated reactions (e.g., skin rash, increased liver enzymes).[32,45] The immediate-release formulation of omeprazole contains sodium bicarbonate, and care should be taken in sodium-restricted patient populations, as discussed in the Antacids and Alginic Acid subsection of the Pharmacotherapy of Drugs Used to Treat Acid-Related Disorders section of this chapter. All PPIs are metabolized by the hepatic CYP450 microenzyme system. Omeprazole and esomeprazole have been described as inhibiting CYP2C19 and decreasing the clearance of diazepam, phenytoin, and R-warfarin, whereas lansoprazole increases the metabolism of theophylline by inducing CYP1A.[34,46] Although the clinical importance of these interactions is thought to be negligible, care should be taken when combining these agents to prevent possible toxicity or therapeutic failure.

The potential CYP2C19 interaction with PPIs and the thienopyridine antiplatelet drug clopidogrel has generated a substantial amount of interest and debate. In 2008, consensus guidelines developed by the American College of Cardiology, the

American Heart Association, and American College of Gastroenterology recommended the prophylactic use of PPIs in patients receiving concomitant dual antiplatelet therapy with aspirin and clopidogrel to reduce the risk of upper GI bleeding.[47] Since the publication of this document, there have been numerous reports suggesting an interaction between PPIs and clopidogrel which attenuates the antiplatelet effects of clopidogrel and potentially increases the risk of adverse cardiovascular outcomes.[48–52] The hypothesis for this interaction is based on the requirement of clopidogrel to undergo biotransformation through CYP2C19 for conversion from prodrug to active metabolite. Because PPIs also require this metabolic pathway for metabolism, it has been suggested in pharmacokinetic and pharmacodynamic studies that concurrent use of PPIs may inhibit or compete for this enzyme, leading to a reduction in the conversion of clopidogrel to its active metabolite and, therefore, a reduction in its efficacy toward platelet inhibition.[49–52] Cardiovascular outcomes studies involving a plethora of investigational designs have produced conflicting results.[52] To date, only a single randomized, prospective, controlled trial evaluating this drug interaction has been published.[53] Although the trial was stopped early because of financial reasons, the results demonstrated no significant difference in adverse cardiovascular outcomes between subjects presenting with an acute coronary syndrome or undergoing a percutaneous coronary intervention randomly assigned to treatment with aspirin and a combination of omeprazole and clopidogrel or clopidogrel alone. However, adverse GI outcomes were reduced significantly in the group receiving concomitant PPI pharmacotherapy.[53]

One important confounding variable involved in the evaluation of this interaction is the role played by genetic polymorphisms in CYP2C19—these can result in loss of function alleles, which has been related to decreased clopidogrel effectiveness as a result of reduced ability to convert clopidogrel to the active metabolite responsible for platelet inhibition.[54] Upon review of this body of evidence, the US Food and Drug Administration (FDA) issued a labeling change for clopidogrel and a safety warning recommending providers to avoid the coadministration of omeprazole, omeprazole/sodium bicarbonate, or esomeprazole with clopidogrel.[55] An update to the 2008 consensus document has attempted to critically evaluate the evidence regarding the interaction and give direction for health care providers.[56] Although this document has taken a more cautious approach, suggesting that a likely interaction may exist especially between clopidogrel and omeprazole, there are few data to support definitive adverse clinical outcomes as a result of the interaction. Also, the consensus document suggests there is no evidence to suggest switching from one PPI to another or that separating the timing of doses has any clear benefit on reducing the magnitude of the interaction.[56] Until more comprehensive evidence becomes available, the most important aspects to consider are to ensure that patients have an appropriate indication for the use of a PPI, to determine that the benefit outweighs risk on a case by case basis, and, if possible, to avoid concomitant use of omeprazole or esomeprazole with clopidogrel unless absolutely necessary.

An increase in intragastric pH may increase the bioavailability of orally administered medications (e.g., digoxin, nifedipine) leading to the possibility of toxicity, or it may decrease the absorption of ketoconazole and cefpodoxime, increasing the possibility of therapeutic failure.[34,46]

PPIs have been associated with a number of adverse effects when used long term and in high dosages.[57,58] However, in most cases, there is insufficient evidence to support a causal relationship between the PPI and the effect. There is evidence to suggest a relationship between elevated serum gastrin concentrations and ECL hyperplasia as a result of the PPIs' profound ability to inhibit gastric acid secretion. It has been hypothesized that this can progress to gastric carcinoid tumors (a precursor of gastric cancer). Although ECL hyperplasia has been described with the use of PPIs, there is no clinical evidence to suggest that long-term (>10 years) therapy progresses to a higher grade of hyperplasia or gastric ECL carcinoid.[59] Atrophic gastritis has been observed in gastric corpus biopsies from patients treated long term with omeprazole and positive for *Helicobacter pylori*. However, review of the data by the FDA has been inconclusive and not able to show causality between long-term use of PPIs, *H. pylori*, and atrophic gastritis.[57–59]

PPIs have been associated with an increased risk of infections (e.g., pneumonias, enteric infections) possibly owing to the ability of the microorganisms ability to survive in a less acidic environment.[57–61] Acute nosocomial infections (pneumonia) associated with critically ill patients will be described later when discussing high-dose oral and parenteral PPI therapy (see Upper Gastrointestinal Bleeding section). The risk of development of community-acquired pneumonia in patients treated with PPIs has also been evaluated in numerous retrospective studies, however causality has been very difficult to establish and remains controversial.[58] Enteric infections and cancer have also been described as a result of potential bacterial overgrowth. The most common pathogens are *Clostridium difficile, Salmonella typhimurium, and Campylobacter jejuni*; however, data suggest that they rarely lead to illness.[60–61] A retrospective database study of PPI use describes a near threefold increase in the risk of *C. difficile*–associated diarrhea in patients receiving PPIs versus patients not on a PPI, but the overall risk remains low and should not be considered a contraindication to therapy.[61] Bacterial overgrowth (secondary to PPI treatment) has been hypothesized to increase the risk of gastric cancer, because bacteria in the stomach responsible for conversion of dietary nitrates to nitrites can flourish at a higher pH and increase the development of *N*-nitrosamines (a carcinogenic by-product). Presently, there are no convincing studies to support the increased production of *N*-nitrosamines in humans with prolonged PPI therapy.[59,60]

Long-term PPI use in older patients on high dosages has also been associated with an increased risk of hip fractures through the presumed inhibition of calcium absorption by PPI induced hypochlorhydria or through inhibition of proton pumps within the osteoclastic vacuole resulting in decreased bone resorption.[57,62] Although the overall risk was low and was statistically significant, data from previous studies reported normal calcium absorption in patients on PPIs for at least 4 years.[63] Long-term PPI use has also been modestly associated with fractures of the spine, forearm, and wrist.[64] Additional studies are required to confirm a causal relationship between long-term PPIs and bone fractures and at this time additional bone density testing and calcium supplementation are not suggested beyond age-related recommendations.[65]

A decrease in vitamin B12 (cyanocobalamin) has been described in patients with long-term PPI use and may occur because gastric acid is required to liberate the vitamin from dietary sources.[57–59] This may only be problematic in the elderly, vegetarians, and patients with chronic alcohol ingestion. Hypomagnesemia may occur in adults taking PPIs for longer than 1 year, but cases have been reported after 3 months of treatment.[66] The exact mechanism by which PPIs increase the risk of hypomagnesemia is uncertain, but may be associated with altered intestinal absorption of magnesium. Malabsorption of iron secondary to long-term gastric acid suppression has been suggested, but has not been confirmed in clinical trials.[57,58] PPIs have been associated with interstitial nephritis, but this is an extremely rare finding.[58,67] Although the long-term effects associated with PPIs are uncommon, the benefit of long-term use must always be weighed against potential risks in each individual patient.

Sucralfate

Sucralfate (an aluminum salt of a sulfated disaccharide) promotes gastric mucosal protection by shielding ulcerated tissue from aggressive factors such as acid, pepsin, and bile salts.[68] At a pH of 2.0 to 2.5, sucralfate binds to damaged and ulcerated mucosa, forming a physical barrier against injury from these aggressive factors. The drug has minimal systemic absorption and does not possess antisecretory activity. Sucralfate may also have other protective actions related to the stimulation of mucosal prostaglandins.[68] The most common side effect associated with sucralfate is constipation, which occurs in about 1% to 3% of patients.[68] This is most likely attributable to the aluminum content of the compound. Because aluminum toxicity has occurred secondary to accumulation in patients with renal insufficiency, long-term use should be avoided.[68] Because aluminum salts can bind with dietary phosphate in the GI tract, the potential for hypophosphatemia exists (see the Antacids and Alginic Acid subsection of the Pharmacotherapy of Drugs used to Treat Acid-Related Disorders section). Sucralfate tablets are large, and some patients, particularly the elderly, may have difficulty swallowing them. Gastric bezoar formation has also been described.[68] A liquid formulation is available for patients with swallowing difficulties. The bioavailability of oral fluoroquinolones, warfarin, phenytoin, levothyroxine, quinidine, ketoconazole, amitriptyline, and theophylline may be reduced when concomitantly administered with sucralfate.[14] The mechanism of these interactions is thought to be caused by binding of the medication with sucralfate in the GI tract, thus limiting their absorption. Because of these interactions, sucralfate should be given at least 2 hours after these medications.

Misoprostol

Misoprostol, a synthetic prostaglandin E_1 analog, is the only prostaglandin analog approved for use in the United States. Misoprostol acts primarily by enhancing mucosal defense mechanisms.[69] It produces cytoprotective effects by stimulating the production of mucus and bicarbonate, improving mucosal blood flow, and reducing mucosal cell turnover similar to the effects of endogenous prostaglandin.[69] Misoprostol also produces a dose-dependent inhibition of gastric acid, but even at high doses, the inhibition is less than that of H_2RAs. The use of misoprostol is limited because of its potential to cause dose-dependent diarrhea (in up to 30% of patients) and abdominal cramping.[69] Taking the drug with meals may help to reduce the diarrhea. Decreasing the daily dose may reduce the diarrhea, but efficacy may be compromised[70] (see Peptic Ulcer Disease section). Other troublesome side effects include nausea, flatulence, and headaches. Misoprostol is excreted primarily as metabolites in the urine, but a dose reduction is not required in patients with renal insufficiency. Misoprostol is an abortifacient because of its uterotrophic effects. Thus, it is contraindicated in women who are pregnant who take it for a GI indication.[69,71] Use in women in their childbearing years requires a negative serum pregnancy test and adequate contraception.

Bismuth Salts

Bismuth subsalicylate has been used for years as an OTC option for many GI aliments. Although its mechanism of action is not completely understood, bismuth is thought to work by binding to and protecting mucosal lesions and enhancing cellular protective mechanisms. Bismuth also has an antimicrobial effect, primarily against *H. pylori*.[72] Bismuth salts have no acid-inhibitory effects. Bismuth-containing products have few side effects, but patients with renal impairment may have a decreased elimination of the bismuth. Bismuth subsalicylate should be used with caution in patients on concomitant salicylates, as the potential exists for salicylate toxicity or increased risk of bleeding. Patients with salicylate allergies or sensitivities should also be warned of the salicylate component. Long-term use is also not advised. Bismuth salts are associated with a harmless black coloring of the stools owing to colonic conversion of bismuth to bismuth sulfide and a potential black discoloration of the tongue with liquid dosage forms.[13] Bismuth subcitrate potassium (biskalcitrate) is only available as a combination product with metronidazole and tetracycline for the treatment of *H. pylori*[73] (see Peptic Ulcer Disease section). Although side effects are similar to bismuth subsalicylate, it has the advantage of not containing salicylate.

DYSPEPSIA

The term *dyspepsia* is derived from the Greek words that mean "hard or difficult digestion" and refers to a subjective feeling of pain or discomfort located primarily in the upper abdomen.[74,75] Although the symptom complex and duration may vary, most patients complain of acute dyspeptic symptoms (indigestion) that are often, but not necessarily restricted to, food or alcohol consumption; medications such as nonsteroidal anti-inflammatory drugs (NSAIDs), antibiotics such as erythromycin and tetracycline, iron and potassium supplements, digoxin, theophylline, and bisphosphonates; and smoking or a stressful lifestyle (Fig. 27-3). Chronic dyspepsia is defined as recurrent symptoms that include one or more of the following: epigastric pain, burning, abdominal boating, belching, nausea, vomiting, and early satiety (early sense of fullness with meals). Patients usually have intermittent symptoms during a long time despite periods of remission. Heartburn may coexist with dyspepsia, but is usually suggestive of GERD.

Patients who have not undergone diagnostic testing are referred to as having "uninvestigated" dyspepsia, whereas those who have undergone testing (usually upper endoscopy) are said to have "investigated" dyspepsia (Fig. 27-3). Major causes of investigated dyspepsia include disorders such as chronic PUD, GERD with or without esophagitis, malignancy, and functional or idiopathic dyspepsia. Functional dyspepsia is a clinical syndrome in which there is no evidence of mucosal damage related to PUD, GERD, or malignancy found at endoscopy. Specific types of functional dyspepsia include nonulcer dyspepsia (NUD), which describes "ulcerlike" symptoms, and nonerosive reflux disease (NERD), which describes "GERD-like" symptoms in an endoscopy-negative patient.

Epidemiology

Dyspepsia is a common problem that occurs in about 25% of the US population when patients with typical GERD symptoms are excluded.[74] When all patients with heartburn or regurgitation are excluded, the prevalence is lower. The prevalence remains stable, as the numbers who exhibit dyspepsia are similar to the numbers who no longer complain of symptoms.

Pathophysiology

Acute, infrequent dyspepsia is most often related to food, alcohol, smoking, or stress. Chronic dyspepsia may be related to an underlying cause such as PUD, GERD, or malignancy or may not have any known cause (endoscopy-negative, functional, idiopathic dyspepsia). About 40% of patients with functional dyspepsia have pathophysiological disturbances that involve delayed

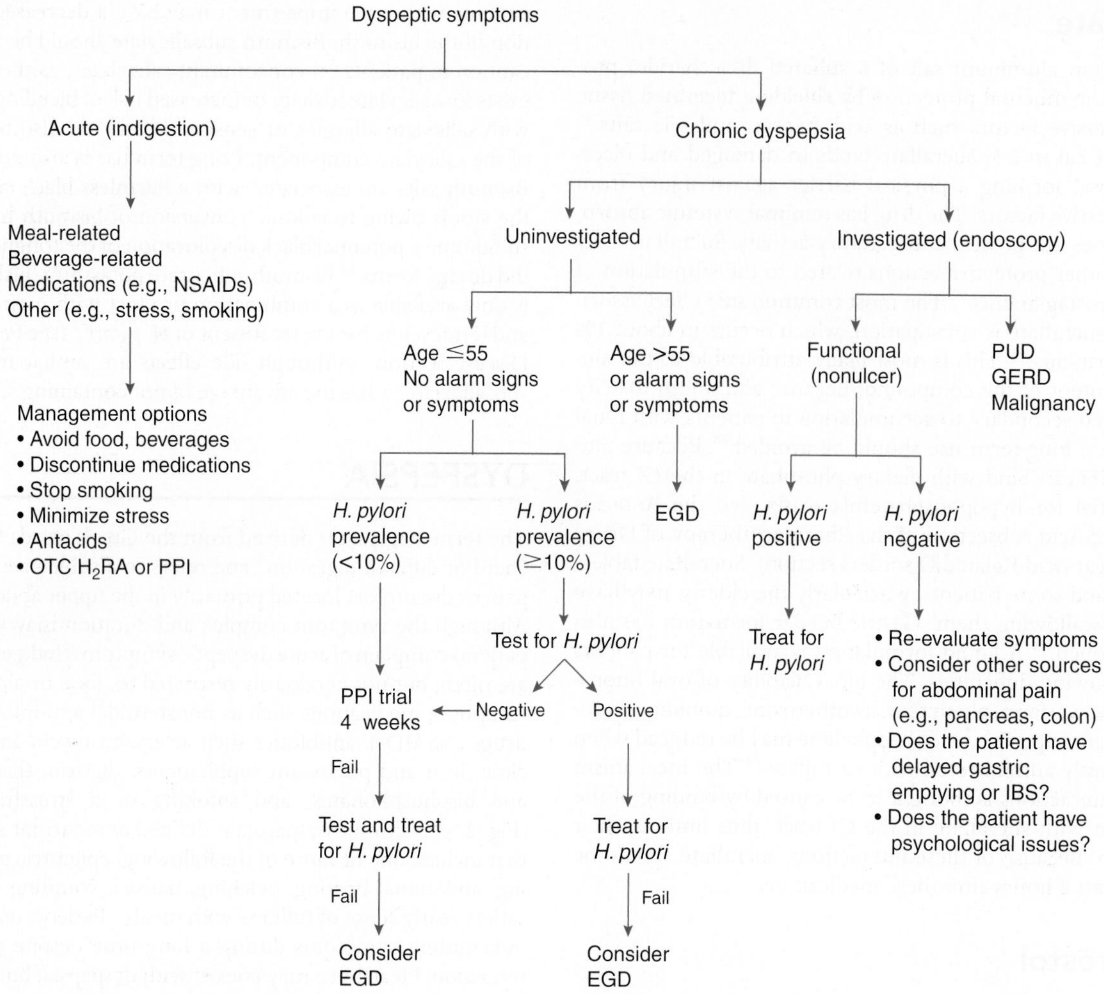

FIGURE 27-3 Management of dyspeptic symptoms. EGD, esophagogastroduodenoscopy; GERD, gastroesophageal reflux disease; *H. pylori*, *Helicobacter pylori*; H_2RA, H_2 receptor antagonist; IBS, irritable bowel syndrome; NSAID, nonsteroidal anti-inflammatory drug; OTC, over-the-counter; PPI, proton-pump inhibitor; PUD, peptic ulcer disease.

gastric emptying.[75] There is also evidence that the esophagus, stomach, duodenum, and other regions of the GI tract are hypersensitive and may be associated with irritable bowel syndrome, especially in women.[75] Others have failed to find a pathological association between functional dyspepsia and gastroduodenal motility, hypersensitivity, or any other GI abnormality, and suggest that psychological disturbances are an important contributing factor. Although *H. pylori* infection has been identified in 20% to 60% of patients with functional dyspepsia, its pathophysiological relevance remains uncertain.[74]

Clinical Assessment and Diagnosis

Acute, infrequent dyspepsia is usually self-limiting and generally requires no further investigation. Chronic dyspeptic symptoms cannot be used to predict endoscopic findings of PUD, GERD, or malignancy in patients with uninvestigated dyspepsia.[75–77] In addition, individual symptoms or symptom subgroups such as PUD-like, GERD-like, or dysmotilitylike dyspepsia are not useful in distinguishing organic disease from functional dyspepsia, nor does it appear to aid in management. This is because there is considerable overlap of symptoms among patients with PUD, GERD, malignancy, and functional dyspepsia.

The clinical assessment of uninvestigated dyspeptia in patients younger than or 55 years of age with no alarm signs or symptoms includes a test-and-treat *H. pylori* option, which is preferable in geographic areas of moderate to high prevalence of *H. pylori* infection (≥10%)[75] (Fig. 27-3). *H. pylori* testing should be conducted by using a nonendoscopic-validated test (see Tests for Detecting *Helicobacter pylori* section). New-onset dyspepsia in an older individual is considered an independent risk factor for an underlying malignancy such as gastric cancer.[75] Dyspeptic patients older than 55 years of age or those with alarm signs or symptoms should undergo upper endoscopy (Fig. 27-3). Other alarm features that assist in identifying serious underlying diseases, especially malignancy, include early satiety, anorexia, worsening dysphagia or odynophagia, unexplained weight loss (>10% body weight), vomiting, anemia, GI bleeding, lymphadenopathy, jaundice, a history of PUD, a family history of upper GI tract cancer, previous gastric surgery, or malignancy.[75] Although a symptom duration threshold has not been established, a long history of symptoms or antisecretory drug use may suggest a serious underlying condition.

Treatment

The recommended strategies for managing dyspepsia in adults are presented in Figure 27-3. Individuals with acute dyspepsia (indigestion) can be effectively treated with self-directed therapy using antacids or OTC antisecretory drugs if they are unable or unwilling to avoid offending foods and beverages, stop smoking, or discontinue troublesome medications. The initial management of patients 55 years of age or younger with uninvestigated chronic dyspepsia and no alarm features depends on the

TABLE 27-2
Indications for Testing and Treating *Helicobacter pylori* Infection

Recommended (evidence established)
• Uninvestigated dyspepsia (depending on *H. pylori* prevalence)
• PUD (active gastric or duodenal ulcer)
• History of PUD (confirmed ulcer not previously treated for *H. pylori*)
• Gastric MALT lymphoma
• After resection of early gastric cancer
• Reduce the risk of recurrent bleeding from gastroduodenal ulcer
Controversial (evidence not well established)
• NUD
• Individuals using NSAIDs (no signs/symptoms of peptic ulcer)
• GERD
• Individuals at risk for gastric cancer
• Individuals with unexplained iron deficiency anemia

GERD, gastroesophageal reflux disease; MALT, mucosa-associated lymphoid tissue; NUD, nonulcer dyspepsia; NSAID, nonsteroidal anti-inflammatory drug; PUD, peptic ulcer disease.
Source: Talley NJ, Holtmann G. Approach to the patient with dyspepsia and related functional gastrointestinal complaints. In: Yamada T et al, eds. *Principles of Clinical Gastroenterology.* 5th ed. Hoboken, NJ: Wiley-Blackwell; 2008:38; Chey WD et al. American College of Gastroenterology guideline on the management of *Helicobacter pylori* infection. *Am J Gastroenterol.* 2007;102:1808; De Vries AC, Kuipers EF. *Helicobacter pylori* infection and nonmalignant diseases. *Helicobacter.* 2010;15(Suppl 1):29; Figura N et al. Extragastric manifestations of *Helicobacter pylori* infection. *Helicobacter.* 2010;15(Suppl 1):60.

prevalence of *H. pylori* and whether the patient is *H. pylori*–positive or *H. pylori*–negative (Table 27-2). Empiric therapy with a PPI for 4 weeks is considered first-line treatment and cost effective in areas with a low prevalence of *H. pylori* and in patients who are *H. pylori*–negative.[75–77] PPIs should be discontinued after 1 month if the patient's symptoms respond to treatment. If symptoms recur, then longer-term PPI therapy may be considered, but the need for a PPI should be evaluated every 6 to 12 months.[74] Endoscopy is advocated for patients who fail to respond to an initial 4 to 8 weeks of empiric PPI therapy and those whose symptoms continue to recur after stopping the PPI (Fig 27-3). Prokinetics are not recommended as first-line therapy for uninvestigated dyspepsia in the United States.[74,75] Patients who are *H. pylori*–positive should receive a PPI-based eradication regimen[74–77] (see *Helicobacter pylori*–Related Ulcers section).

Early endoscopy with biopsy for *H. pylori* is recommended for patients older than 55 years of age with uninvestigated chronic dyspepsia and those with alarm features. In the event that an abnormality (such as PUD, GERD, or malignancy) is found, it should be treated accordingly. The medical management of functional dyspepsia (e.g., NUD) is challenging and, when possible, should take into consideration the cost-effectiveness of treatment.[75–77] Although pharmacotherapy is considered for most patients, evidence of benefit is limited because of the lack of well-designed studies and an incomplete understanding of the disorder. Meta-analyses have demonstrated the efficacy of H_2RAs and PPIs, but there is no evidence to support the use of antacids, sucralfate, and misoprostol.[78] There appears to be no difference in efficacy between full-dose or double-dose PPIs.[78] An economic review suggests that PPIs are cost-effective for functional dyspepsia in the United States.[79] The impact of *H. pylori* eradication in functional dyspepsia remains limited, in part, because of the lack of short-term symptomatic benefit and because of the steadily declining prevalence of *H. pylori* in the United States.[76] An updated meta-analysis, however, reports a small therapeutic gain with eradication when compared with placebo at 12 months of follow-up.[80] Although the benefit of prokinetics have been reported, most studies were conducted with cisapride, which was withdrawn from the US market.[78] The use of available prokinetics (metoclopramide, erythromycin) should be reserved for difficult-to-treat patients because of their limited efficacy and side effects.[75,77] Antidepressants, especially the tricyclics, are often prescribed in functional dyspepsia and may have some benefit, however, the mechanism for this finding is unclear, and published clinical trials are small and of poor quality resulting in uncertain efficacy.[75,77,78] Alternative therapies, including herbal products, remain unproven.[75] Patients with persistent dyspepsia despite a negative endoscopy in whom PPI therapy and *H. pylori* eradication fails should have their diagnosis reevaluated.

PEPTIC ULCER DISEASE

PUD is one of the most common gastroenterologic diseases affecting the upper GI tract.[81] Chronic peptic ulcers are defects in the gastric (gastric ulcer) or duodenal (duodenal ulcer) mucosa that require gastric acid for their formation. Chronic peptic ulcers differ from erosions and gastritis in that the ulcer extends deeper into the muscularis mucosa.[81,82]

ONLINE CONTENT

For an illustration of peptic ulcer disease, go to <u>http://thepoint.lww.com/AT10e</u>.

Stress ulcer is an acute form of peptic ulcer, but it occurs primarily in critically ill patients and differs in its underlying pathogenesis (see Stress-Related Mucosal Bleeding section).

Epidemiology

It is difficult to estimate the epidemiology of PUD because of the different methods used to diagnose peptic ulcers (e.g., symptom-based, ulcer-related complications, radiology or endoscopy) as well as differences in NSAID use, *H. pylori* prevalence, and cigarette smoking. Improved medical treatment, changes in the criteria and coding for hospitalizations and mortality, and the evolution from hospital-based to ambulatory care has also altered the epidemiology of PUD.[81] Current data suggest a shift in the prevalence of PUD in the United States from predominantly men to a comparable rate in men and women.[81] A declining ulcer rate in younger individuals and an increasing rate for older adults reflect a decline in *H. pylori* infection and an increased use of NSAIDs in the United States. Office visits, hospitalizations, and deaths have modestly declined during the last four decades, but deaths among older patients (>75 years) has increased and is most likely related to NSAID use.[81]

Etiology and Risk Factors

H. pylori and NSAIDs are the two most common causes of chronic PUD and influence the chronicity of the disease.[81] Less common causes include hypersecretory states such as Zollinger-Ellison syndrome (ZES) (see Zollinger-Ellison Syndrome section), viral infections (e.g., cytomegalovirus), radiation, and chemotherapy (e.g., hepatic artery infusion).[81] Factors that may increase the risk of a peptic ulcer include alcohol ingestion, cigarette smoking, psychological stress; corticosteroids; and chronic diseases such as renal failure, cirrhosis, pancreatitis, obstructive pulmonary disease, Crohn disease, or organ transplantation.[81]

HELICOBACTER PYLORI–*RELATED ULCERS*

H. pylori infection is causally linked to chronic gastritis, PUD, mucosa-associated lymphoid tissue (MALT) lymphoma, and gastric cancer (Table 27-2).[81–86] The lifetime risk of exhibiting an endoscopic ulcer in *H. pylori*–positive individuals is 10% to 20% and the risk for developing gastric cancer is 1% to 2%.[81,82,86] Differences in strain variability and host-specific factors account for the variable pathogenesis of the organism.[82,85] Although it has been suggested that *H. pylori* may play a causal role in dyspepsia, GERD, diabetes mellitus, and cardiovascular, respiratory, neurological, hepatobiliary and gynecological diseases, there is insufficient evidence at this time to support such claims.[75,87,88] There is increasing evidence that iron deficiency anemia and idiopathic thrombocytopenia are associated with *H. pylori* infection, but cause and effect remain unproven.[83,88] The association between *H. pylori* and PUD bleeding remains unclear, but *H. pylori* eradication decreases recurrent bleeding[83] (see Upper Gastrointestinal Bleeding section).

The prevalence of *H. pylori* varies by geographic location, socioeconomic status, ethnicity, and age, and is more common in developing countries than in industrialized nations.[82] The overall prevalence in the United States is estimated to be 30% to 40% but is higher in older individuals (50%–60%) than in children (10%–15%).[82] The higher prevalence among older adults reflects acquisition during infancy and early childhood. However, infection rates in the United States have been declining in children because of improved socioeconomic conditions.[82,83]

Transmission occurs usually during childhood from the infected person by either the gastro–oral (vomitus) or fecal–oral (diarrhea) route or from fecal-contaminated water or food.[82,84] Individuals living in the same household with an *H. pylori*–positive person, especially when there is household crowding (intrafamilial clustering), are at increased risk for acquiring the infection.[82,84] *H. pylori* can also be transmitted through the use of inadequately sterilized endoscopes.

Nonsteroidal Anti-Inflammatory Drug–Induced Ulcers

There is considerable evidence linking the chronic use of NSAIDs with GI injury.[81,89–92] Endoscopically confirmed gastric and duodenal ulcers develop in 15% to 30% of chronic NSAID users, and 2% to 4% experience ulcer-related bleeding or perforation.[89,90] Gastric ulcer is most common and develops primarily in the antrum. NSAIDs may also cause ulcers in the esophagus and the colon, but these ulcers occur less frequently and differ in their underlying pathogenesis.[89,92] It is estimated that NSAIDs account for about 100,000 hospitalizations and 7,000 to 10,000 deaths annually in the United States, but mortality may be overstated because of the recent decline in hospitalizations.[90] A national prescription audit in the United States revealed an annual NSAID cost of $4.9 billion, with additional nonprescription NSAID sales of $3 billion.[93] The risk factors for NSAID-induced ulcers and upper GI complications are listed in Table 27-3. Combinations of factors confer an additive risk.

TABLE 27-3
Risk Factors for Nonsteroidal Anti-Inflammatory Drug–Induced Ulcer and Ulcer-Related Upper Gastrointestinal Complications

Established

- Confirmed prior ulcer or ulcer-related complication
- Age >65 years
- Multiple or high-dose NSAID use
- Concomitant use of aspirin (including low cardioprotective dosages, e.g., 81 mg)
- Concomitant use of an anticoagulant, corticosteroid, bisphosphonate, clopidogrel, or SSRI
- Selection of NSAID (selectivity of COX-1 vs. COX-2)

Controversial

- *H. pylori*
- Alcohol consumption
- Cigarette smoking

COX-1, cyclo-oxygenase-1; COX-2, cyclo-oxygenase-2; NSAID, nonsteroidal anti-inflammatory drug; SSRI, selective serotonin reuptake inhibitor.
Source: Soll AH, Graham DY. Peptic ulcer disease. In: Yamada T et al, eds. *Textbook of Gastroenterology.* 5th ed. Hoboken, NJ: Wiley-Blackwell; 2009:936; Chey WD et al. American College of Gastroenterology guideline on the management of *Helicobacter pylori* infection. *Am J Gastroenterol.* 2007;102:1808; Scarpignato C, Hunt RH. Nonsteroidal antiinflammatory drug-related injury to the gastrointestinal tract: clinical picture, pathogenesis and prevention. *Gastroenterol Clin North Am.* 2010;39:433; Lanza FL et al. Guidelines for prevention of NSAID-related ulcer complications. *Am J Gastroenterol.* 2009;104:728; Malfertheiner P et al. Peptic ulcer disease. *Lancet.* 2009:374:1449; Vonkeman H et al. Risk management of risk management: combining proton pump inhibitors with low-dose aspirin. *Drug Healthc Patient Saf.* 2010;2:191; Targownik LE et al. Selective serotonin reuptake inhibitors are associated with a modest increase in the risk of upper gastrointestinal bleeding. *Am J Gastroenterol.* 2009;104:1475; Dall M et al. There is an association between selective serotonin reuptake inhibitor use and uncomplicated peptic ulcers: a population-based case-control study. *Aliment Pharmacol Ther.* 2010;32:1383; Andrade C et al. Serotonin reuptake inhibitor antidepressants and abnormal bleeding: a review of clinicians and a reconsideration of mechanisms. *J Clin Psychiatry.* 2010;71:1565.

Pathophysiology

A physiological balance exists in healthy individuals between gastric acid secretion and gastroduodenal mucosal defense. Peptic ulcers occur when the balance between aggressive factors (gastric acid, pepsin, bile salts, *H. pylori,* and NSAIDs) and mucosal defensive mechanisms (mucosal blood flow, mucus, mucosal bicarbonate secretion, mucosal cell restitution, and epithelial cell renewal) are disrupted.[81,91] Increased acid secretion may occur in patients with duodenal ulcer, but most patients with gastric ulcer have normal or reduced rates of acid secretion.[8] Pepsin is an important cofactor that plays a role in the proteolytic activity involved in ulcer formation. Mucosal defense and repair mechanisms protect the gastroduodenal mucosa from noxious endogenous and exogenous substances.[81] The viscous nature and near-neutral pH of the mucus-bicarbonate barrier protect the stomach from the acidic contents in the gastric lumen. The maintenance of mucosal integrity and repair is mediated by the production of endogenous prostaglandins. When aggressive factors alter mucosal defense mechanisms, back diffusion of hydrogen ions occurs with subsequent mucosal injury. *H. pylori* and NSAIDs cause alterations in mucosal defense by different mechanisms and are important factors in the formation of peptic ulcers.

HELICOBACTER PYLORI–*RELATED ULCERS*

H. pylori is a gram-negative, spiral-shaped bacillus that thrives in a microaerophilic environment. The bacterium resides between the mucus layer and surface epithelial cells in the stomach or any location where gastric-type epithelium is found.[82,] Flagella enable it to move from the lumen of the stomach, where the pH is low, to the mucus layer, where the pH is neutral. Acute infection is accompanied by transient hypochlorhydria, which enables the organism to survive the acidic gastric juice. Although the exact method by which *H. pylori* induces hypochlorhydria is uncertain, it is hypothesized that its urease-producing ability hydrolyzes urea in the gastric juice and converts it to ammonia and carbon dioxide, which creates a neutral microenvironment that surrounds the bacterium.[82,91] Adherence pedestals attach to gastric-type epithelium and prevent the bacterium from being shed during cell turnover and mucus secretion.

Disease outcome depends on the patterns of *H. pylori* colonization and inflammation within the stomach.[82,91] Colonization of the antrum and acid-secreting body (corpus) of the stomach is associated with gastric ulcer and gastric adenocarcinoma and is typically accompanied by gastric atrophy and decreased acid secretion. When *H. pylori* colonizes the antrum and the body of the stomach is spared, the risk for duodenal ulcer is increased and gastric acid is normal or slightly increased. Ulcers in the duodenum arise from the colonization by antral organisms of gastric-type epithelium that develops in the duodenum in response to changes in duodenal pH.[82]

Direct mucosal damage is produced by virulence factors (e.g., cytotoxin-associated gene, vacuolating cytotoxin), elaborating bacterial enzymes (e.g., urease, lipases, proteases) and adherence.[82,91,94] Cytotoxin-associated gene A (CagA) protein occurs in about 60% of *H. pylori* strains in the United States and is associated with severe gastritis, peptic ulcers, and gastric cancer when compared with CagA-negative strains.[82,91,94] Although vacuolating cytotoxin A (VacA) is present in almost all *H. pylori* strains, differences in cytotoxic activity are related to variations in the *VacA* gene structure and are associated with an increased risk for PUD and possibly gastric cancer.[82,94] *H. pylori* infection may also cause alterations in the host immune response.[82,94] Host polymorphisms related to interleukin (IL)-1β and its receptor antagonist, tumor necrosis factor α (TNF-α), and IL-10, may be associated with increased gastric acid secretion and duodenal ulcer or acid suppression and gastric cancer.[82,94]

Nonsteroidal Anti-Inflammatory Drug–Induced Ulcers

Nonselective NSAIDs (Table 27-4), including aspirin, cause peptic ulcers and upper GI complications by systemically inhibiting protective prostaglandins in the gastric mucosa.[81,89,91] NSAIDs inhibit cyclo-oxygenase (COX), the rate-limiting enzyme in the conversion of arachidonic acid to prostaglandins. There are two COX isoforms: cyclo-oxygenase-1 (COX-1), which is found in the stomach, kidney, intestine, and platelets, and cyclo-oxygenase-2 (COX-2), which is induced with acute inflammation.[81,89] The inhibition of COX-1 is associated with upper GI and renal toxicity, and the inhibition of COX-2 is related to anti-inflammatory effects.[81,89] Nonselective NSAIDs, including aspirin, inhibit both COX-1 and COX-2 to varying degrees and decrease platelet aggregation, which may increase the risk for upper GI bleeding.[81,89]

TABLE 27-4
Selected Nonsteroidal Anti-Inflammatory Drugs

Salicylates
Acetylated: aspirin Nonacetylated: trisalicylate, salsalate
Nonsalicylates[a]
Nonselective (traditional) NSAIDs: ibuprofen, naproxen, tolmetin, fenoprofen, sulindac, indomethacin, ketoprofen, ketorolac, flurbiprofen, piroxicam Partially selective NSAIDs: etodolac, diclofenac, meloxicam, nabumetone Selective COX-2 inhibitors: celecoxib[b], rofecoxib[c], valdecoxib[c]

[a] Based on COX-1/COX-2 selectivity ratio in vitro.
[b] Initially marketed as a COX-2 inhibitor, but current FDA labeling is consistent with nonselective and partially selective NSAIDs.
[c] Withdrawn from the US market.
COX-2, cyclo-oxygenase-2; NSAID, nonsteroidal anti-inflammatory drug.

The coadministration of selected NSAIDs (e.g., ibuprofen) with aspirin also reduces the antiplatelet effects of aspirin.[47] Although prostaglandin inhibition is regarded as the major cause of gastric ulcers, diversion of arachidonate through the lipoxygenase pathway enhances leukotriene synthesis and results in vasoconstriction and release of oxygenfree radicals which may also contribute to impairment of mucosal defense.[89] There is increasing evidence that NSAIDs may cause gastric damage by interfering with the mucosal synthesis of nitric oxide and hydrogen sulfide, important mediators in maintaining gastric mucosal intergrity.[89]

The relative COX selectivity among NSAIDs varies and is thought to be an important factor in determining the propensity for ulcer formation.[81,89] Thus, certain NSAIDs may be more COX-1–sparing than others (e.g., the partially selective NSAIDs; Table 27-4) and may be associated with less GI toxicity, but there are few controlled trials to support this claim.[81,89,95,96] COX-2 inhibitors such as rofecoxib and valdecoxib (Table 27-4) do not inhibit gastric mucosal prostaglandin synthesis or serum thromboxane A_2, which accounts for their improved GI safety.[89,96] In contrast to the nonselective NSAIDs, the COX-2 inhibitors do not inhibit platelet aggregation and alter bleeding time. Unfortunately, both rofecoxib and valdecoxib were withdrawn from the US market in 2004 because of concerns about cardiovascular safety.[81] Celecoxib, an NSAID initially marketed as a COX-2 inhibitor, currently remains available in the United States despite similar concerns about cardiovascular risk, especially at higher dosages.[81] However, the benefit of celecoxib in reducing the risk of gastric ulcer and upper GI complications may be lower than with rofecoxib and valdecoxib (Table 27-4).

Aspirin and nonaspirin NSAIDs also have a topical (direct) irritating effect on the gastric mucosa, but the resulting inflammation and erosions usually heal within a few days. Gastric damage is associated with the acidic properties of aspirin and nonaspirin NSAIDs and their ability to decrease the hydrophobicity of the mucous gel layer in the gastric mucosa.[89,97] Thus, direct mucosal injury appears to correlate with the pK_a of a compound—suggesting the lower the acidity of the drug, the less the short-term topical damage.[89] Formulations such as enteric-coated aspirin, buffered aspirin, NSAID prodrugs, and parenteral or rectal preparations may spare topical effects on the gastric mucosa, but all have the potential to cause a gastric ulcer because of their systemic inhibition of endogenous prostaglandins.[81,98] Clopidogrel does not cause ulcers, but may impair the healing of gastric erosions.[99]

Clinical Presentation

SIGNS AND SYMPTOMS

The signs and symptoms associated with a peptic ulcer range from mild epigastric pain to life-threatening upper GI complications.[81,91] A change in the character of the pain may indicate an ulcer-related complication. The absence of epigastric pain, especially in older adults who are taking NSAIDs, does not exclude the presence of an ulcer or related complications. Although the reasons for this are unclear, they may be related to the analgesic effect of the NSAID. There is no one sign or symptom that differentiates an *H. pylori*–related ulcer from an NSAID-induced ulcer. Ulcerlike symptoms may occur in the absence of peptic ulceration in association with *H. pylori*–related gastritis or duodenitis.

COMPLICATIONS

The most serious life-threatening complications associated with chronic PUD are upper GI bleeding, perforation into the abdominal cavity or penetration into an adjacent structure (e.g., pancreas, liver, or biliary tract), and obstruction.[81,91,100]

Ulcer-related bleeding is the most frequent complication and occurs with all types of ulcers (see Upper Gastrointestinal Bleeding section). The incidence of ulcer-related upper GI bleeding and perforation is highest in individuals taking NSAIDs who are older than 60 years of age.[89,91] The bleeding may be occult (hidden), present as melena (black-colored stools), or hematemesis (vomiting of blood). Mortality is higher in patients who continue to bleed or who rebleed after the initial bleeding has stopped and in patients with a perforated ulcer.[4,5] The pain associated with perforation is typically sudden, sharp, and severe, beginning in the epigastric area but quickly spreading throughout the upper abdominal area. Gastric outlet obstruction, the least frequent complication, is caused by previous ulcer healing and scarring or edema of the pylorus or duodenal bulb and can lead to symptoms of gastric retention, including early satiety, bloating, anorexia, nausea, vomiting, and weight loss.

Clinical Assessment and Diagnosis

TESTS FOR DETECTING HELICOBACTER PYLORI

The detection of *H. pylori* infection can be made by using gastric mucosal biopsies in patients undergoing upper endoscopy or by nonendoscopic tests (Table 27-5).[82,83,101] The selection of a specific method is influenced by the clinical circumstance and the availability and cost of the individual test. The endoscopic tests require a mucosal biopsy for the rapid urease test, histology, or culture. Medications that reduce urease activity or the density of *H. pylori* may decrease the sensitivity of the rapid urease test by up to 25%.[83] For this reason, when possible, antibiotics and bismuth salts should be withheld for 4 weeks, and H_2RAs and PPIs for 1 to 2 weeks before endoscopic testing. Patients who are taking these medications at endoscopy will require histology in addition to the rapid urease test. At least three biopsies are taken from different areas of the stomach because patchy distribution of *H. pylori* can result in false-negative results. Acute ulcer bleeding at the time of testing is likely to decrease the sensitivity of the rapid urease test and histology and increase the likelihood of false-negative results.[83,102]

Nonendoscopic tests either identify active infection or detect antibodies to *H. pylori*.[82,83,101] If endoscopy is not planned, these tests are a reasonable choice to determine *H. pylori* status as they are noninvasive, more convenient, and less expensive than the endoscopic tests. Testing should only be undertaken if eradication is planned in light of positive results. The urea breath test (UBT), the most accurate noninvasive test, detects active *H. pylori* infection and is also effective after eradiation treatment.[82,83,101] The ^{13}carbon (nonradioactive isotope) and ^{14}carbon (radioactive isotope) tests require that the patient ingest radiolabeled urea, which is then hydrolyzed by *H. pylori* (if present in the stomach) to ammonia and radiolabeled bicarbonate. The radiolabeled bicarbonate is absorbed in the blood and detected in expired breath. The in-office and laboratory antibody tests are a cost-effective method to initially diagnose *H. pylori* infection, but because they do not differentiate between active infection and previously eradicated *H. pylori,* they should not be used to confirm eradication.[82,83,101] The fecal antigen test identifies *H. pylori* antigens in the stool and is less expensive and easier to perform than the UBT.[82,83,101] Although usually comparable to the UBT in the initial detection of *H. pylori,* the fecal antigen test may be less accurate when used to document eradication posttreatment. Salivary and urine antibody tests are under investigation.[101]

LABORATORY TESTS, RADIOGRAPHY, AND ENDOSCOPY

Generally, laboratory tests are not helpful in the diagnosis of PUD. Fasting serum gastrin concentrations are only recommended for patients unresponsive to therapy or those suspected of having a hypersecretory disease. Serum hematocrit (Hct) and hemoglobin (Hgb) and guaiac fecal occult blood tests assist in the evaluation of ulcer-related bleeding.

Gastric acid secretory studies are not routinely performed for patients suspected of having an uncomplicated peptic ulcer. However, measurements of acid secretion are instrumental in the evaluation of patients with severe, recurrent PUD that is unresponsive to standard drug therapy. Acid secretion is expressed as basal acid output (BAO), in response to a meal (meal-stimulated acid secretion), or as maximal acid output (MAO).[8] These tests estimate the acid-secretory response under various circumstances and are measured by inserting a nasogastric tube into the stomach and aspirating the gastric contents.[8] The aspirate is estimated by titration with a basic solution of known concentration and expressed as milliequivalents of H^+ per hour. Results obtained for an individual patient is then compared with standard ranges for each test. The BAO, meal-stimulated acid secretion, and MAO vary according to age, sex, health, and time of day. The BAO follows a circadian rhythm, with the highest acid secretion occurring at night and the lowest in the morning. An increase in the BAO/MAO ratio suggests a basal hypersecretory state such as ZES.

Confirmation of a peptic ulcer requires visualizing the ulcer either by GI radiography or upper endoscopy.[81] Radiography is sometimes the initial diagnostic procedure because it is less expensive than endoscopy and more widely available, but small ulcers are often difficult to detect and false-positives may result from trapped barium.[81] Fiberoptic upper endoscopy (esophagogastroduodenoscopy [EGD]) is the gold standard, as it detects greater than 90% of peptic ulcers and permits direct inspection, biopsy, visualization of superficial erosions, and sites of active bleeding. Upper endoscopy is preferred if complications are suspected or if an accurate diagnosis is required. If a gastric ulcer is found on radiography, malignancy should be excluded by direct endoscopic visualization and histology.

Clinical Course and Prognosis

The natural history of PUD is characterized by periods of exacerbations and remissions unless the underlying cause is removed.[81] *H. pylori* and NSAIDs are the two most important risk factors for the development of peptic ulcer.[81] Successful eradication of *H. pylori* heals ulcers and dramatically decreases ulcer recurrence and GI complications.[81] The risk for NSAID-induced ulcer and life-threatening GI complications is greatest in the elderly and those with a history of PUD. Prophylactic cotherapy or the use of a selective COX-2 inhibitor markedly decreases ulcer risk and complications.[89,90] Gastric cancer in *H. pylori*–infected individuals develops slowly during 20 to 40 years and is associated with a slightly higher lifetime risk than that in patients with duodenal ulcer or in the general population.[82,85,86]

Treatment

THERAPEUTIC GOALS

The therapeutic goals for treating PUD in adults depend on whether the ulcer is related to *H. pylori* or associated with an NSAID. Treatment goals may differ depending on whether the ulcer is initial or recurrent and whether complications have occurred. Treatment is aimed at relieving ulcer symptoms, healing the ulcer, preventing ulcer recurrence, and reducing ulcer-related complications. When possible, the most cost-effective drug regimen should be utilized.

TABLE 27-5
Diagnostic Tests for *Helicobacter pylori* Infection

Tests Using Gastric Mucosal Biopsy in Patients Undergoing Endoscopy

Rapid Urease Test

- Tests for active *H. pylori* infection; >90% sensitivity and specificity.
- In the presence of *H. pylori* urease, urea is metabolized to ammonia and bicarbonate resulting in an increase in pH, which changes the color of a pH-sensitive indicator.
- Results are rapid (within 24 hours), and test is less expensive than histology or culture.
- Withhold H_2RAs and PPIs 1 to 2 weeks before testing and antibiotics and bismuth salts 4 weeks before testing to reduce the risk of false-negatives.

Histology

- "Gold standard" for detection of active *H. pylori* infection; >95% sensitive and specific.
- Permits further histologic analysis and evaluation of infected tissue (e.g., gastritis, ulceration, adenocarcinoma); tests for active *H. pylori* infection.
- Results are not immediate; not recommended for initial diagnosis; more expensive than rapid urease test.

Culture

- Permits sensitivity testing to determine antibiotic choice or resistance; 100% specific; tests for active *H. pylori* infection.
- Use usually limited to patients who fail initial course of eradication therapy.

Polymerase Chain Reaction

- Detects *H. pylori* DNA in gastric tissue; highly specific and sensitive.
- High rate of false-positives and false-negatives; positive DNA does not correlate directly with presence of the organism; used primarily for research.

Nonendoscopic Tests That Do Not Use Gastric Mucosal Biopsy

Urea Breath Test

- Tests for active *H. pylori* infection; >95% sensitive and specific.
- Radiolabeled urea with either C^{13} or C^{14} is given orally; urease secreted by *H. pylori* in the stomach (if present) hydrolyzes radiolabeled urea to produce radiolabeled CO_2, which is exhaled and then quantified from the expired breath; radiation exposure is minimal.
- Withhold H_2RAs and PPIs 1 to 2 weeks before testing and antibiotics and bismuth salts 4 weeks before testing to reduce the risk of false-negatives.
- Used to detect *H. pylori* before treatment and to document posttreatment eradication.
- Results usually take about 2 days; less expensive than tests that utilize gastric mucosal biopsy but more expensive than serologic tests; availability and reimbursement is inconsistent.

Antibody Detection (In-Office or Near Patient)

- Qualitative test; detects IgG antibodies to *H. pylori* in whole blood or fingerstick.
- Effective for primary diagnosis, but not of benefit in confirming eradication because antibodies to *H. pylori* remain positive for years after successful eradication of the infection.
- Results obtained quickly (usually within 15 minutes) but reduced sensitivity and specificity compared with laboratory-based tests; widely available and inexpensive.
- Results not affected by H_2RAs, PPIs, or bismuth; antibiotics given for other indications may result in a positive antibody test.

Antibody Detection (Laboratory)

- Quantitative test; detects IgG antibodies to *H. pylori* in serum using laboratory-based ELISA tests and latex agglutination techniques.
- More accurate than in-office tests; similar sensitivity and specificity to rapid urease biopsy and urea breath tests.
- Unable to determine if antibody is related to active or cured infection; antibody titers vary between individuals and take up to 6 months to 1 year to return to the uninfected state.
- Results not affected by H_2RAs, PPIs, or bismuth; antibiotics given for other indications may result in a positive antibody test.

Fecal Antigen Test

- An enzymatic immunoassay test that identifies *H. pylori* antigen in stool; sensitivity and specificity comparable to the UBT for initial diagnosis.
- H_2RAs, PPIs, antibiotics, and bismuth may cause false-negative results but to a lesser extent than the UBT.
- Considered an alterative to detecting *H. pylori* before treatment and documenting posttreatment eradication; patients may have a reluctance to obtain stool samples.

ELISA, enzyme-linked immunosorbent assay; H_2RA, H_2 receptor antagonist; IgG, immunoglobulin G; PPI, proton-pump inhibitor; UBT, urea breath test.
Source: Washington MK, Peek RM. Gastritis and gastropathy. In: Yamada T et al, eds. *Textbook of Gastroenterology.* 5th ed. Hoboken, NJ: Wiley-Blackwell; 2009:1005; Chey WD et al. American College of Gastroenterology guideline on the management of *Helicobacter pylori* infection. *Am J Gastroenterol.* 2007;102:1808; Calvet X et al. Diagnosis of *Helicobacter pylori* infection. *Helicobacter.* 2010;15(Suppl 1):7.

NONPHARMACOLOGIC THERAPY

Patients with PUD should discontinue NSAIDs (including aspirin) if possible. Patients unable to tolerate certain foods and beverages (e.g., spicy foods, caffeine, and alcohol) may benefit from dietary modifications. Lifestyle modifications including reducing stress and decreasing or stopping cigarette smoking is encouraged.

Probiotics, especially strains of lactic acid–producing bacteria such as *Lactobacillus* and *Bifidobacterium,* lactoferrin, and foodstuffs (e.g., cranberry juice, ginger, chili, oregano, some milk proteins) have been used to supplement *H. pylori* eradication.[81,103–105] Animal and in vitro data have shown that probiotics have both bactericidal and protective effects, but meta-analyses of clinical trials suggest only a slight improvement in eradication

TABLE 27-6

Oral Drug Regimens Used to Eradicate *Helicobacter pylori* Infection

Drug Regimen	Dose	Frequency	Duration
Proton-Pump Inhibitor–Based Three-Drug Regimens			
PPI	Standard dose[a]	BID[a]	14 days[b]
Clarithromycin	500 mg	BID	14 days[b]
Amoxicillin[c]	1 g	BID	14 days[b]
Or			
PPI	Standard dose[a]	BID[a]	14 days[b]
Clarithromycin	500 mg	BID	14 days[b]
Metronidazole[c]	500 mg	BID	14 days[b]
Bismuth-Based Four-Drug Regimens			
Bismuth subsalicylate[d]	525 mg	QID	10–14 days
Metronidazole	250–500 mg	QID	10–14 days
Tetracycline plus	500 mg	QID	10–14 days
PPI	Standard dose[a]	Daily or BID[a]	10–14 days
Or			
H_2RA[e]	Standard dose[e]	BID[e]	4–6 weeks
Sequential Therapy[f]			
PPI	Standard dose[a]	BID[a]	Days 1–10
Amoxicillin	1 g	BID	Days 1–5
Clarithromycin	250–500 mg	BID	Days 6–10
Metronidazole	250–500 mg	BID	Days 6–10
Secondary or Rescue Therapy			
Bismuth subsalicylate[d]	525 mg	QID	10–14 days
Metronidazole	500 mg	QID	10–14 days
Tetracycline	500 mg	QID	10–14 days
PPI	Standard dose[a]	Daily or BID[a]	10–14 days
Or			
PPI	Standard dose[a]	BID[a]	10–14 days
Amoxicillin	1 g	BID	10–14 days
Levofloxacin	500 mg	Daily	10–14 days

[a] Omeprazole 20 mg BID; lansoprazole 30 mg BID; pantoprazole 40 mg BID; rabeprazole 20 mg daily or BID; esomeprazole 20 mg BID or 40 mg daily.
[b] Although 7–10 day regimens may provide acceptable eradication rates, the preferred treatment duration in the United States is 14 days.
[c] Use amoxicillin in non–penicillin-allergic individuals; substitute metronidazole for amoxicillin in penicillin-allergic patients.
[d] Pylera, a prepackaged *H. pylori* regimen, contains bismuth subcitrate potassium (biskalcitrate) 140 mg as the bismuth salt in place of bismuth subsalicylate, metronidazole 125 mg, and tetracycline 125 mg per capsule. The patient is directed to take three capsules/dose with each meal and at bedtime. A standard dose of a PPI is added to the regimen and taken twice daily. All medications are taken for a 10-day period.
[e] See Table 27-1 for standard peptic ulcer healing dosage regimens.
[f] Requires validation in the United States.
BID, twice a day; H_2RA, H_2 receptor antagonist; PPI, proton-pump inhibitor; QID, four times a day.
Source: Soll AH, Graham DY. Peptic ulcer disease. In: Yamada T et al, eds. *Textbook of Gastroenterology.* 5th ed. Hoboken, NJ: Wiley-Blackwell; 2009:936; Washington MK, Peek RM. Gastritis and gastropathy. In: Yamada T et al, eds. *Textbook of Gastroenterology.* 5th ed. Hoboken, NJ: Wiley-Blackwell; 2009:1005; Malfertheiner P et al. Peptic ulcer disease. *Lancet.* 2009:374:1449; Gisbert JP et al. Sequential therapy for *Helicobacter pylori* eradication: a critical review. *J Clin Gastroenterol.* 2010;44:313; Gisbert JP et al. *Helicobacter pylori* first-line treatment and rescue options in patients allergic to penicillin. *Aliment Pharmacol Ther.* 2005;22:1041; Gisbert JP et al. *Helicobacter pylori* first-line treatment and rescue option containing levofloxacin in patients allergic to penicillin. *Dig Liver Dis.* 2010;42:287; Vergara M et al. Meta-analysis: comparative efficacy of different proton-pump inhibitors in triple therapy for *Helicobacter pylori* eradication. *Aliment Pharmacol Ther.* 2003;18:647; Gisbert JP et al. Meta-analysis: proton pump inhibitors vs. H_2-receptor antagonists—their efficacy with antibiotics in *Helicobacter pylori* eradication. *Aliment Pharmacol Ther.* 2003;18:757; Gisbert JP. Review: Second-line rescue therapy of *Helicobacter pylori* infection. *Therap Adv Gastroenterol.* 2009;2:331.

rates.[81,103,104] Lactoferrin, a member of the transferrin family, has been reported to inhibit *H. pylori* attachment to gastric epithelial cells.[105] Although certain strains of *Lactobacillus* and *Bifidobacterium* or lactoferrin may enhance eradication, they are not effective as single agents. Additional clinical trials are necessary before probiotics or lactoferrin are routinely recommended as supplements to *H. pylori* regimens.

Patients with ulcer-related complications may require surgery for bleeding, perforation, or obstruction.[100] Surgery for medical treatment failures (e.g., vagotomy with pyloroplasty or vagotomy with antrectomy) are rarely performed because of effective medical management. However, patients may present with postoperative consequences (e.g., postvagotomy diarrhea, dumping syndrome, anemia) associated with these procedures.

PHARMACOTHERAPY

Drug regimens used to eradicate *H. pylori* are identified in Table 27-6. Recommended first-line treatment in the United States includes PPI-based three-drug regimens or a bismuth-based four-drug regimen (Fig. 27-4). However, there is controversy as to whether sequential therapy should replace the standard PPI-based triple drug regimen as first-line treatment. If initial eradication fails, a second course of therapy should be based on the selection of antibiotics that have not been previously used. Successful treatment eradicates the infection and heals the ulcer. Treatment of *H. pylori*–positive patients with a conventional antiulcer drug or combining an antisecretory drug with sucralfate is not recommended because of high rates of ulcer recurrence and complications. Maintenance therapy with a PPI or H_2RA

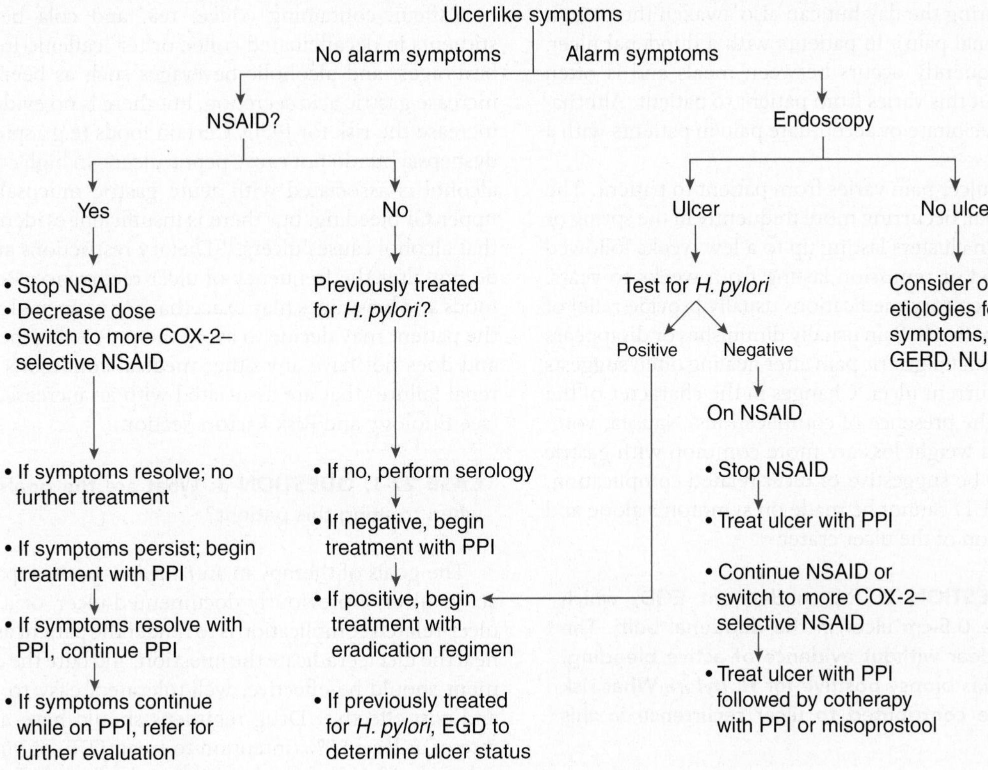

FIGURE 27-4 Management of peptic ulcer disease. COX-2, cyclo-oxygenase-2; EGD, esophagogastroduodenoscopy; GERD, gastroesophageal reflux disease; *H. pylori, Helicobacter pylori;* NSAID, nonsteroidal anti-inflammatory drug; NUD, nonulcer dyspepsia; PPI, proton-pump inhibitor.

(Table 27-1) should only be necessary in high-risk patients with a history of ulcer complications, those with *H. pylori*–negative ulcers, and patients with other concomitant acid-related diseases (e.g., GERD).

Drug regimens used to treat and prevent NSAID-induced ulcers are identified in Table 27-1. Patients with NSAID-induced ulcers should be tested to determine their *H. pylori* status. *H. pylori*–positive patients should be initially treated with a PPI-based three-drug eradication regimen (Fig. 27-4). If the patient is *H. pylori*–negative, the NSAID should be discontinued and treatment should be initiated with antiulcer medications. The duration of treatment should be extended if the NSAID is continued. Prophylactic cotherapy with a PPI or misoprostol or switching to an NSAID with greater COX-2 selectivity is recommended for patients at risk of exhibiting ulcer-related upper GI complications.

HELICOBACTER PYLORI–RELATED PEPTIC ULCER

CASE 27-1

QUESTION 1: R.L. is an otherwise healthy 45-year-old man who works in a high-stress job as an air traffic controller at a major airport. He complains of a 2-week history of "burning stomach pain" sometimes accompanied by "indigestion and bloating." The pain initially occurred several times a day, usually between meals, and sometimes awakened him at night, but it has increased in frequency during the last week. Initially, the pain was temporarily reduced by food or antacids. Last week, R.L. tried an OTC H_2 receptor antagonist that "lasted longer" but did not provide adequate symptom relief. R.L. states that he experienced a similar type of pain about 12 years ago when he was treated with omeprazole for a suspected peptic ulcer. He has smoked one pack of cigarettes daily for the past 20 years, has an occasional glass of red wine with dinner, and usually drinks 4 to 6 cups of caffeinated coffee throughout the day. R.L. takes acetaminophen when needed for occasional headaches and a daily multivitamin but denies the use of any other OTC or prescription medications, including NSAIDs and the previous use of clarithromycin or metronidazole. He denies nausea, vomiting, anorexia, weight loss, and changes in stool consistency or color. A review of other body systems is noncontributory. He has no known food or drug allergies.

Physical examination is normal except for epigastric tenderness on palpation of the upper abdomen. Vital signs include a temperature of 98.8°F, blood pressure of 132/80 mm Hg, and a heart rate of 78 beats/minute. Pertinent laboratory values include the following:

Hgb, 14.0 g/dL
Hct, 44%
Stool guaiac test, negative

All other laboratory values are within normal limits. What signs and symptoms are suggestive of a recurrent peptic ulcer?

Most patients with PUD present with abdominal pain that is epigastric and often described as burning or gnawing, whereas others complain of abdominal discomfort, fullness, or cramping. Epigastric pain, however, does not necessarily correlate with an ulcer, as patients with ulcerlike symptoms may have NUD and asymptomatic patients may have an NSAID-induced ulcer. Heartburn, bloating, and belching may accompany the pain. Ulcer pain typically occurs during the day but can also awaken the patient from sleep (nocturnal pain). In patients with a duodenal ulcer, epigastric pain frequently occurs between meals and is often relieved by food, but this varies from patient to patient. Alternatively, food may precipitate or accentuate pain in patients with a gastric ulcer.

The severity of ulcer pain varies from patient to patient. The pain may be seasonal, occurring more frequently in the spring or fall and occurring in clusters lasting up to a few weeks followed by a painfree period or remission lasting from weeks to years. Antacids and antisecretory medications usually provide relief of ulcer pain in most patients. Pain usually diminishes or disappears during treatment, but epigastric pain after healing often suggests an unhealed or recurrent ulcer. Changes in the character of the pain may suggest the presence of complications. Nausea, vomiting, anorexia, and weight loss are more common with gastric ulcer but may also be suggestive of ulcer-related complication. The diagnosis of PUD cannot be made on symptoms alone and requires visualization of the ulcer crater.

CASE 27-1, QUESTION 2: R.L. underwent EGD, which revealed a single 0.5-cm ulcer in the duodenal bulb. The ulcer base was clear without evidence of active bleeding. Antral gastritis was biopsy positive for *H. pylori*. What risk factors may have contributed to ulcer recurrence in this patient?

R.L. indicates that he had a similar type of abdominal pain about 12 years ago, when he was treated with omeprazole for a suspected peptic ulcer. When conventional antiulcer therapy (e.g., PPI) is discontinued after ulcer healing, the ulcer tends to recur. The most important etiologic factors that influence ulcer recurrence are *H. pylori* infection and NSAID use. It is not known whether R.L. underwent testing for *H. pylori* 12 years ago. The patient denies the use of OTC and prescription NSAIDs. The long-term use of maintenance therapy (Table 27-1) to maintain remission after initial ulcer healing with a conventional antiulcer medication was standard practice for years and may have been an option for this patient at the time.[91] However, successful eradication of *H. pylori* (in an *H. pylori*–positive patient) cures the infection, heals the ulcer, and eliminates the need for long-term maintenance therapy in most patients.[83,91]

Other factors such as cigarette smoking, psychological stress, and diet may have contributed to ulcer recurrence in this patient. There is strong epidemiologic evidence indicating that cigarette smoking is a major risk factor for PUD and that the risk is proportional to the number of cigarettes smoked per day.[81] Several mechanisms have been postulated, including delayed gastric emptying, inhibition of pancreatic bicarbonate secretion, promotion of duodenogastric reflux, reduction in mucosal prostaglandin production, and increased gastric acid secretion. Although cigarette smoking exacerbates PUD, there is insufficient evidence to conclude that it causes a peptic ulcer. However, cigarette smoking, nicotine, or other components of smoke may provide a favorable milieu for *H. pylori* infection.

R.L. works as an air traffic controller, which is a high-stress job. The importance of psychological stress and how it affects PUD is complex and multifactorial. Results from controlled trials are conflicting and have failed to demonstrate a cause-and-effect relationship.[81,91] However, the clinical observation of ulcer patients with high-stress jobs and a stressful lifestyle suggest that they are adversely affected. In addition, emotional stress may induce behavioral risks such as cigarette smoking and the use of NSAIDs or alter the inflammatory response or resistance to *H. pylori* infection.

Caffeine-containing coffee, tea, and cola beverages, constituents in decaffeinated coffee or tea, caffeine-free carbonated beverages, and alcoholic beverages such as beer and wine all increase gastric acid secretion, but there is no evidence that they increase the risk for PUD. Certain foods (e.g., spicy) may cause dyspepsia but do not cause peptic ulcers. In high concentrations, alcohol is associated with acute gastric mucosal damage and upper GI bleeding, but there is insufficient evidence to confirm that alcohol causes ulcers.[81] Dietary restrictions and bland diets do not alter the frequency of ulcer recurrence. Because certain foods and beverages may exacerbate or worsen ulcer symptoms, the patient may decide to avoid them. R.L. is otherwise healthy and does not have any other medical conditions (e.g., chronic renal failure) that are associated with an increased risk of PUD (see Etiology and Risk Factors section).

CASE 27-1, QUESTION 3: What are the goals of therapy when treating this patient?

The goals of therapy in an *H. pylori*–positive patient with an active ulcer, a previously documented ulcer, or a history of an ulcer-related complication is to render the patient asymptomatic, heal the ulcer, eradicate the infection, and cure the disease. Treatment should be effective, well-tolerated, easy to comply with, and cost-effective. Drug regimens should have an eradication rate of at least 80% (intention-to-treat, ITT) or 90% (per protocol analysis) and should minimize the potential for antimicrobial resistance.[106] The use of a single antibiotic, bismuth salt, or antiulcer drug does not achieve this goal. Two-drug regimens (PPI and amoxicillin or clarithromycin) are not recommended in the United States because of low and variable eradication rates and because of the inclusion of only one antibiotic.

Primary Treatment of *Helicobacter pylori* Infection

CASE 27-1, QUESTION 4: What factors should be taken into consideration when selecting a first-line eradication regimen? What are the therapeutic options for first-line *H. pylori* eradication in the United States? Which is the preferred *H. pylori* eradication regimen for R.L.?

The selection of a first-line *H. pylori* eradication regimen should be based on proven effectiveness and should take into consideration antibiotic combinations that permit second-line treatment (if necessary) with different antibiotics, treatment duration, the likelihood of antibiotic resistance, and the ability to adhere to the drug regimen. The antibiotics that have been most extensively studied in the United States and found to be effective in various combinations include clarithromycin, amoxicillin, metronidazole, and tetracycline.[81,83,91]

Current treatment guidelines in the United States and Europe recommend two first-line eradication therapies for patients with an *H. pylori*–positive peptic ulcer: standard PPI-based three-drug regimens or a PPI or H_2RA bismuth-based four-drug regimen (Table 27-6).[83,106] Despite these recommendations, there are recent concerns about the efficacy of these regimens because of declining eradication rates thought to be related to antibiotic resistance, particularly with clarithromycin, and the potential for nonadherence, especially with bismuth quadruple therapy (see Case 27-1, Question 8).[83,107–110] Controversy exists as to whether standard PPI triple therapy, in its present form, should remain as first-line treatment in the United States.[83,107–110] Some clinicians believe that sequential therapy (Table 27-6) should replace the standard PPI-based three-drug regimens because of superior eradication rates or that the bismuth-based four-drug regimen should be used exclusively as first-line treatment.[107,110] Others believe that more robust clinical trials involving a broader range of patients is needed before sequential therapy replaces the standard PPI three-drug regimens in the United States and that medication adherence remains problematic with bismuth quadruple therapy.[83,108,109]

The most recommended treatment of *H. pylori* infection in the United States has been the standard PPI-based three-drug regimen (Table 27-6). When combined with a PPI and clarithromycin, the inclusion of amoxicillin or metronidazole provides similar eradication rates.[83] Amoxicillin is usually preferred initially because it is associated with little or no bacterial resistance, has fewer adverse effects, and leaves metronidazole as an option for second-line therapies.[81] However, recent data suggest that eradication rates with PPI triple therapy have been declining during the last decade from greater than 90% to less than 80% ITT, which is considered less acceptable.[107,108] Various strategies have been undertaken to enhance eradication rates, including lengthening treatment duration and increasing the antibiotic or antisecretory drug dosages. The recommended duration of treatment in the United States is 14 days, even though international guidelines recommend 7 to 10 days.[83] The superiority of the 14-day regimen over a 7-day or 10-day treatment course has been confirmed and is less likely to be associated with antimicrobial resistance.[83] A treatment duration of less than 7 days is associated with unacceptable eradication rates and is not recommended.[83] Increasing the antibiotic daily dose or extending antibiotic treatment beyond 14 days (Table 27-6) usually does not improve eradication rates. The PPI may be extended to 28 days if needed for ulcer healing. Twice-daily dosing of the PPI appears to be more effective than a single daily dose.[111] Pretreatment with a PPI before initiating *H. pylori* eradication does not decrease eradication.[112]

Bismuth-based quadruple therapy containing a bismuth salt, metronidazole, tetracycline, and either a PPI or H_2RA (Table 27-6) has been advocated as first-line treatment because it usually yields satisfactory eradication rates despite increased resistance to clarithromycin.[83,110] The complexity of this regimen and the potential for increased side effects often relegates it to preferred second-line status if not previously used. However, eradication rates, tolerability, and medication adherence were reported to be similar to PPI triple therapy when used as first-line treatment, although both regimens yielded eradication rates of less than 80% ITT.[113] Using a PPI instead of an H_2RA permits a shorter duration of treatment (10 days vs. 14 days) and may provide increased efficacy in patients with metronidazole-resistant strains of *H. pylori*.[83] Increasing the duration of quadruple therapy to 1 month does not substantially increase eradication although the antisecretory drug may be continued for an additional 2 weeks (PPI) or 4 weeks (H_2RA) in patients with an active ulcer. Comparable eradication rates are achieved when bismuth subcitrate potassium (biskalcitrate) is used in place of bismuth subsalicylate (Table 27-6), but the 10-day package makes it difficult to provide 14 days of treatment.[114]

Sequential therapy with a PPI and amoxicillin for 5 days followed by a PPI, clarithromycin, and an imidazole for an additional 5 days (Table 27-6) has achieved eradication rates (>80% ITT) that appear to be superior to the standard PPI-based three-drug regimens containing clarithromycin.[83,107–110,115–117] An increased efficacy has also been reported with sequential therapy in patients with clarithromycin-resistant *H. pylori* strains.[107,115,118] The rationale for sequential therapy is to initially treat the patient with antibiotics that rarely promote resistance (e.g., amoxicillin) in order to reduce the bacterial load and pre-existing resistant organisms and then to follow with different antibiotics to kill the remaining organisms. Although the precise mechanism for the success of sequential therapy is uncertain, the increased efficacy may be related to the number of antibiotics (amoxicillin, metronidazole, and clarithromycin) to which the organism is exposed.

The higher eradication rates make a case for switching to sequential therapy as the preferred first-line treatment in the United States.[107,110,115,116] However, the majority of studies are small and were conducted primarily in Italy.[107–109] Most importantly, many of the clinical trials and their respective meta-analyses are thought to be of suboptimal quality and may overestimate the effect of treatment.[108,109,119] In addition, sequential therapy is more complex than standard PPI triple therapy as it requires a mid-course change in medications. Lastly, sequential therapy has not been adequately compared with standard triple therapy containing a PPI-clarithromycin-metronidazole or bismuth-based quadruple therapy in the United States.

The therapeutic options available for the eradication of *H. pylori* should be carefully considered in each individual patient. The PPI-amoxicillin-clarithromycin regimen is an acceptable first-line management strategy for R.L., as he has not previously received clarithromycin (see Case 27-1, Question 8) and has no known allergies to penicillin (see Case 27-1, Question 6). Recommendations based on current treatment guidelines allow for a successful cure in a number of patients even though eradication rates in some clinical trials and meta-analyses appear unsatisfactory. Posttreatment testing should be considered, but may not be necessary if R.L. remains asymptomatic (see Case 27-1, Question 9). A 10-day to 14-day regimen of bismuth-metronidazole-tetracycline-PPI would have been a logical first-line treatment if R.L. were allergic to penicillin or had been previously treated with clarithromycin. Although sequential therapy may overcome clarithromycin resistance and have a role as first-line treatment, it is unclear, at this time, whether it would provide any increased benefit in this patient.

Patient Education

CASE 27-1, QUESTION 5: R.L. is prescribed a 14-day PPI-based three-drug eradication regimen containing amoxicillin and clarithromycin. What instructions would you provide R.L. regarding his medications?

R.L. should be informed of the importance of taking his medications as prescribed to minimize treatment failure and the development of antibiotic resistance. He should be advised that the PPI is an integral part of the three-drug regimen and should be taken twice daily 30 to 60 minutes before breakfast and dinner (see Pharmacotherapy, Proton-Pump Inhibitors section) along with amoxicillin and clarithromycin (Table 27-6). If R.L. was placed on bismuth quadruple therapy containing a PPI, he should take all medications except the PPI four times a day, with meals and at bedtime. If prescribed once daily, the PPI should be taken 30 to 60 minutes before breakfast; if twice daily, the second dose should be taken 30 to 60 minutes before dinner.

R.L. should also be informed of the most common side effects associated with his treatment regimen. All antibiotics included in the *H. pylori* eradication regimens are usually associated with mild side effects including nausea, abdominal pain, and diarrhea. *C. difficile*–associated diarrhea, a serious antibiotic-related complication, occurs occasionally. Oral thrush and vaginal candidiasis (in women) may also occur. Clarithromycin and metronidazole may cause taste disturbances. If R.L.'s medications included metronidazole, tetracycline, or a bismuth salt, he should be provided additional information on these medications. Metronidazole-containing regimens increase the frequency of side effects (especially when the dose is >1 g/day) and may be associated with a disulfiramlike reaction in patients who consume alcohol. Tetracycline may cause photosensitivity and should not be used in children because it may cause tooth discoloration. Bismuth salts may cause darkening of the tongue and stool.

R.L., as well as all other patients receiving *H. pylori* eradication therapy, should be advised of the risk for clinically important drug–drug interactions that may occur with the medications included in their eradication regimen. Special attention should be given to metronidazole and clarithromycin (inhibitors of CYP3A4), as well substrates of CYP2C9 (inhibited by metronidazole).[120] Drug–drug interactions may also occur with H_2RAs and PPIs (see Pharmacotherapy of Drugs Used to Treat Acid-Related Disorders section).

Regimens for the Management of *Helicobacter pylori* Infection in Patients With Penicillin Allergies

CASE 27-1, QUESTION 6: What would have been the preferred initial *H. pylori* eradication regimen if R.L. had a documented allergy to penicillin?

There are two first-line treatment options if R.L. had a documented allergy to penicillin. Metronidazole can be substituted for amoxicillin in the PPI-based three-drug regimen, as similar eradication rates are achieved (Table 27-6).[83,121] Bismuth-based quadruple therapy may also be used, as it provides similar eradication rates to the PPI-based three-drug regimens.[83,113] Regimens which substitute levofloxacin for amoxicillin in PPI triple therapy have been used with success, but there are fewer studies to supporting their efficacy.[122] The most common sequential therapy contains amoxicillin and therefore is not suitable for a penicillin-allergic patient.

CASE 27-1, QUESTION 7: What drug substitutions are acceptable in the standard PPI-based three-drug and bismuth-based four-drug eradiation regimens?

Substitution of one PPI for another is acceptable and does not enhance or diminish eradication rates in either the three-drug or four-drug regimens.[83,112,123] A PPI may be substituted for an H_2RA in the bismuth-based four-drug regimen (Table 27-6). However, an H_2RA should not be substituted for a PPI in the three-drug regimens unless the patient is unable to tolerate the PPI.[124,125] There are insufficient data to support the substitution of ampicillin for amoxicillin, doxycycline for tetracycline, and azithromycin or erythromycin for clarithromycin.

Substitution of clarithromycin 250 to 500 mg four times a day for tetracycline in the bismuth-based four-drug regimen (Table 27-6) yields similar results, but substitution of amoxicillin for tetracycline lowers the eradication rate and is not recommended.[81,91]

CASE 27-1, QUESTION 8: What are the most important predictors of *H. pylori* treatment outcomes, and how may they alter R.L.'s response to treatment?

The two most important factors in predicting *H. pylori* treatment outcomes are antibiotic resistance and medication adherence.[83,107,108,110] The major factors which influence antibiotic resistance are prior exposure to the antibiotic, nonadherence to the drug regimen, and the indiscriminate use of antibiotics.[83,107,108] Antibiotic resistance rates are highly variable throughout the United States and the world and thus are difficult to compare.[83,108,110] However, there is evidence that clarithromycin resistance is increasing in North America and Europe and is thought to be the most important reason for the decreasing efficacy of clarithromycin-containing eradication regimens.[83,107,108,110] Because treatment with clarithromycin may increase the likelihood of *H. pylori* resistance, clinicians should ask about previous macrolide use when deciding upon an eradication regimen.[83]

The clinical importance of metronidazole resistance is unclear, as higher metronidazole doses and the synergistic effect of combining metronidazole with other antibiotics appears to render resistance to metronidazole more relative.[83,108,110,120] Resistance to amoxicillin and tetracycline is uncommon. Levofloxacin is emerging as a component of eradication therapy, but there are recent reports of increasing resistance to fluroquinolones.[107,108,110,120] Resistance to bismuth has not been reported.

Medication adherence decreases with multiple medications, increased frequency of administration, increased duration of treatment, intolerable adverse effects, and costly drug regimens.[83,107] Although most eradication studies report greater than 95% adherence to medications, this high rate must be questioned as it is very difficult to accurately assess the level of compliance in clinical trials where patients take their own medications.[107] Additionally, medication adherence is usually more problematic in clinical practice. A longer treatment duration may contribute to nonadherence, but missed doses in a shorter regimen may also lead to failed eradication. Most bismuth-based four-drug regimens require the patient to take medications four times a day and as many as 18 tablets/capsules per day. The complexity of this regimen as well as a mid-treatment change in medications with sequential therapy should be considered when selecting an eradication regimen. Although mild side effects are common with all of the eradication regimens, some patients will experience clinically important effects that lead to discontinuation of a specific drug or of the entire regimen.

Other factors that may contribute to treatment failure include the high bacterial load, the specific *H. pylori* strain (e.g., CagA), low intragastric pH, and genetic polymorphism (e.g., CYP2C19 polymorphism) when PPIs are used as part of the eradication regimen.[83,108,110,120,126,127] There are limited data to suggest that smoking, alcohol consumption, and diet may negatively affect eradication.

CASE 27-1, QUESTION 9: What parameters should be monitored to determine R.L.'s response to treatment?

Posttreatment testing to confirm eradication is recommended for patients with an *H. pylori*–related ulcer, persistent dyspeptic symptoms, MALT lymphoma, or early gastric cancer.[83] However, posttreatment testing is neither practical nor cost-effective for all patients with an *H. pylori*–positive peptic ulcer.[83] When endoscopy follow-up is not necessary, the UBT (Table 27-5) is the preferred test to confirm eradication of *H. pylori*. To avoid confusing bacterial suppression with eradication, the UBT must be delayed at least 4 weeks after the completion of treatment. The term eradication or cure is used when posttreatment tests conducted 4 weeks after the end of treatment do not detect the organism. Antibody tests should be avoided posttreatment, because antibody titers remain elevated for a long period of time (up to 1 year) before they return to the uninfected range after successful eradication.[82,83] If performed posttreatment, only a negative test is considered to be reliable.

Upper endoscopy should only be used to confirm eradication and ulcer healing if indicated (e.g., severe or frequent recurrent symptoms, current or previous ulcer complication), as the procedure is costly and invasive. When endoscopic follow-up is necessary, testing to prove eradication includes a biopsy for the rapid urease test and histology (Table 27-5). Ulcer healing can also be confirmed at that time.

In clinical practice, the need for confirmation of ulcer healing and eradication in light of the declining success with the most commonly recommended eradication regimens must be weighed against the need, feasibility, availability, and cost of tests and procedures. Although posttreatment testing to confirm *H. pylori* eradication is recommended, patients like R.L., who present with an uncomplicated *H. pylori*–positive ulcer, are usually monitored for symptomatic recurrence 1 to 2 weeks after completion of drug therapy.[83] The absence of symptoms is considered a surrogate marker for successful ulcer healing and eradication. The persistence, or recurrence, of symptoms within 2 weeks after the end of treatment suggests failure of ulcer healing or eradication or an alternative diagnosis such as GERD.

Secondary or Rescue Therapy for *Helicobacter pylori* Infection

CASE 27-1, QUESTION 10: What other drug regimens can be used if R.L. fails initial eradication therapy with a PPI-amoxicillin-clarithromycin regimen? What regimens can be used when secondary treatment fails?

All initial eradication regimens require that there be an effective second-line treatment. Eradicating *H. pylori* is more difficult after initial treatment fails and attempts to eradicate the organism are extremely variable.[83] Second-line regimens should (a) avoid using antibiotics that were used during initial therapy, (b) use antibiotics that have less problems with resistance, (c) use drugs that have a topical effect (e.g., bismuth), and (d) use a 10-day to 14-day treatment duration.[83,107,110,128] If R.L. was not successfully eradicated initially with the PPI-amoxicillin-clarithromycin, he should receive second-line therapy with bismuth subsalicylate, metronidazole, tetracycline, and a PPI for 10 to 14 days.[83,107,110,128,129]

Bismuth-based regimens are the most frequently used second-line treatments in the United States when standard PPI-based three-drug regimens fail (Table 27-6).[83] A number of alternatives have been evaluated in small studies utilizing fluoroquinolone, rifabutin (an antibiotic used to treat tuberculosis), or furazolidone (no longer marketed in the United States).[83,107] The results from the levofloxacin-based clinical trials look promising and suggest that these regimens may be an alternative to second-line bismuth quadruple therapy, especially for patients who have no prior use of a fluoroquinolone.[83,107,122,128] However, increasing fluoroquinolone resistance, which appears to be easily acquired, is of concern and may limit the use of these agents for *H. pylori* eradication.[128] Various rifabutin-based regimens are effective in treating patients with *H. pylori* strains resistant to clarithromycin or metronidazole.[83,128] Regimens which include rifabutin should be the last option and only used for patients with multiple eradication failures as the drug is very expensive and there are concerns about major hematologic side effects and the possibility of resistance.[128]

NONSTEROIDAL ANTI-INFLAMMATORY DRUG–INDUCED PEPTIC ULCER

CASE 27-2

QUESTION 1: A.D. is a 70-year-old woman who retired from teaching 5 years ago. A few days ago, she noticed black "tarry" stools and was hospitalized for an upper GI bleed most likely secondary to NSAID use. She complains of "feeling tired" and occasionally dizzy for about 1 week. A.D. presents with a 5-year history of osteoarthritis for which she takes naproxen 250 mg in the morning and 500 mg in the evening. When questioned, she denies the use of corticosteroids, bisphosphonates, anticoagulants, clopidogrel, or a selective serotonin reuptake inhibitor (SSRI). She did not have a history of a previous ulcer or related complication. Other medications include hydrochlorothiazide 25 mg daily and lisinopril 20 mg daily for hypertension, self-directed treatment with enteric-coated aspirin 81 mg daily, calcium carbonate, and a multivitamin. A.D. does not use tobacco or drink caffeinated beverages but does have an occasional glass of wine. She denies epigastric pain, nausea, vomiting, anorexia, and weight loss but notes a recent change in stool color. A review of other body systems are noncontributory other than previously indicated. There are no known food or drug allergies.

Physical examination reveals a well-developed weak woman in no acute distress. The abdomen was normal with no pain on palpation. Bowel sounds were normal with no guarding, masses, hepatomegaly, or splenomegaly. The rectum was normal but with guaiac-positive stool. Vital signs include a temperature of 98.9°F, blood pressure of 100/65 mm Hg, and a heart rate of 90 beats/minute. Pertinent laboratory values include:

Hgb,11.0 g/dL
Hct, 35%
Blood urea nitrogen (BUN), 40
Serum creatinine (SCr), 1.5 mg/dL

All other laboratory values are within normal limits. What factors placed A.D. at increased risk for experiencing an NSAID-induced ulcer and related upper GI bleeding?

Risk factors for NSAID ulcers and related complications are presented in Table 27-3. The use of a nonselective NSAIDs (e.g., naproxen) is linked to a threefold to fourfold increase in upper GI complications, and there is a twofold to threefold increase with COX-2 inhibitors when partially and highly selective agents are evaluated as a group (Table 27-4).[96] The risk for upper GI events are dose-related, occur at any dosage, including low doses of OTC NSAIDs,[130] and can occur at any time during treatment.[89–91] A.D.'s self-treatment with cardioprotective dosages (81–325 mg/day) of aspirin in combination with an NSAID (naproxen) increases her risk of upper GI events to a greater extent than the use of either drug alone.[89–91] The use of buffered or enteric-coated aspirin confers no added protection from ulcer or upper GI complications.[90,98,131] A.D.'s age (70 years) is an independent risk factor for NSAID-induced ulcers, as risk increases with the age of the patient (Table 27-3).[89,90] The increased incidence in older patients may be explained by age-related changes in gastric mucosal defense. Although A.D. did not have a history of an ulcer or ulcer-related complication before admission, a history of an NSAID-related upper GI event further increases the risk of NSAID-related GI injury.[89–91]

Corticosteroids do not increase the ulcer risk when used alone, but the risk is increased twofold in corticosteroid users who are also taking concurrent NSAIDs.[89–91] The risk of upper GI bleeding is markedly increased when NSAIDs are taken with anticoagulants, antiplatelet medications such as clopidogrel, or bisphosphonates.[56,89–91,96] SSRIs independently increase the risk of upper GI bleeding, and although the magnitude of the risk is variable, it is increased in patients taking NSAIDs.[132–134] The pharmacologic mechanism underlying this adverse effect is thought to be related to SSRI inhibition of platelet aggregation which may interfere with ulcer healing, but it remains unknown if SSRIs have a direct ulcerogenic effect.[132–134] It is uncertain whether *H. pylori* is a risk factor for NSAID-induced ulcers, but a higher incidence of PUD in *H. pylori*–positive patients taking NSAIDs suggests an additive effect which may increase the risk of NSAID-related GI complications.[83,89–91] A.D.'s multiple risk factors convey an increased risk for an NSAID-related upper GI event (see Case 27-2, Question 4).

CASE 27-2, QUESTION 2: A.D. was admitted for further evaluation and treatment. An EGD revealed two bleeding antral ulcers (0.2 and 0.4 cm) and endoscopic hemostasis was performed. An antral biopsy was reported to be *H. pylori*–negative. All medications were discontinued before endoscopy. Oral oxycodone was instituted after endoscopy at 5 mg every 6 hours when needed to control A.D.'s arthritic pain while she was hospitalized. Consideration was given to decreasing the naproxen dose and switching to acetaminophen, a nonacetylated salicylate, or a partially selective NSAID (Table 27-4), but none of these options were satisfactory for this patient. Treatment was initiated with a continuous infusion of IV pantoprazole for 3 days and then switched to oral pantoprazole 40 mg twice a day (BID). A.D. was discharged on pantoprazole 40 mg daily and naproxen 250 mg in the morning and 500 mg in the evening. Hydrochlorothiazide, lisinopril, calcium carbonate, and the multivitamin were reinstituted upon discharge from the hospital. Will A.D.'s gastric ulcer heal if she continues to take the naproxen?

The naproxen should be discontinued, if possible, in the presence of an active ulcer.[81,91] If the NSAID was discontinued and A.D.'s treatment was continued with alternative therapy such as oxycodone, a PPI is the preferred treatment to heal the ulcer as it provides a more rapid rate of ulcer healing (4 weeks) and symptom relief than an H_2RA or sucralfate (6–8 weeks).[81,89,91] Because the naproxen was reinstituted at discharge in the presence of an active ulcer, a PPI is the drug of choice, as potent acid suppression is required to heal the ulcer and relieve the symptoms.[81,89,91] The duration of PPI therapy should be extended from 4 weeks to 8 to 12 weeks as continuing the NSAID, aspirin or a COX-2 inhibitor, will interfere with ulcer healing.[81,91] Cardiovascular risk and the need for low-dose aspirin must be determined by the patient's primary-care physician or cardiologist and if not needed, the aspirin should be discontinued. However, low-dose aspirin should be continued after endoscopic hemostasis in patients at cardiovascular risk.[81,135] Clopidogrel should not be substituted for low-dose aspirin in order to reduce GI bleeding.[56,90]

CASE 27-2, QUESTION 3: Which ulcer-healing regimen would be recommended if A.D. were reported to be *H. pylori*–positive?

All patients with NSAID-induced GI events should be tested for *H. pylori* (Figure 27-4). A PPI-based eradication regimen is recommended in an *H. pylori*–positive patient with an active ulcer who is also taking an NSAID. One reason for this is that it is not possible to determine whether the *H. pylori*, the NSAID, or both actually caused the ulcer. If an individual is tested and found to be *H. pylori*–positive, he or she should be offered eradication therapy whether or not there is a documented ulcer. The selection of a specific regimen (Table 27-6) depends on a number of factors, including whether the individual is allergic to penicillin.

Strategies to Reduce the Risk of Nonsteroidal Anti-Inflammatory Drug–Induced Peptic Ulcers

CASE 27-2, QUESTION 4: Three months later, A.D. returned to her gastroenterologist for a follow-up EGD, which confirmed that the gastric ulcers were healed. On return to her primary-care physician, the pantoprazole was changed to ranitidine 150 mg BID and the patient was advised to discontinue low-dose aspirin. Current medications include naproxen 250 mg in the morning and 500 mg in the evening, hydrochlorothiazide 25 mg daily, lisinopril 20 mg daily, calcium carbonate, and multivitamins. What pharmacological options are available to reduce the risk of an NSAID ulcer now that A.D.'s initial ulcer is healed and she continues to take the naproxen?

Strategies to reduce the risk of NSAID (including aspirin) ulcers and upper GI complications include cotherapy with a PPI or misoprostol, the use of a COX-2 inhibitor, or various combinations of a PPI, misoprostol, and a COX-2 inhibitor.[47,81,89–91,93,99] All PPIs, when used in standard dosages (Table 27-1), are effective for this indication.[90] Standard H_2RA dosages (Table 27-1) should not be recommended as prophylactic cotherapy to reduce the risk of NSAID ulcers as they are not effective in reducing the risk of gastric ulcer, which is the most common ulcer associated with NSAIDs.[90,91] Higher H_2RA dosages (e.g., famotidine 40 mg twice daily) reduce the risk of gastric and duodenal ulcer, but are less effective than a PPI.[89,90] Famotidine 20 mg twice daily may be an alternative to a PPI in patients at risk who are taking low-dose aspirin,[136] but comparative trials with PPIs are needed to support the use of standard dose H_2RAs for this indication. There are no studies that have evaluated the use of H_2RAs in reducing the risk of ulcer-related upper GI complications. H_2RAs may be used when necessary to relieve NSAID-related dyspepsia.

Misoprostol reduces the risk of NSAID-induced gastric and duodenal ulcers,[89–91] as well as the risk of upper GI complications in high-risk patients.[137] Initially, the recommended dosage was 200 mcg four times a day, but diarrhea and abdominal cramping limited its use. A lower daily dosage of 600 mcg/day should be used as it reduces GI side effects and is comparable in efficacy.[90,91] Dosage reductions to 400 mcg/day or less minimize GI side effects but compromise gastroprotective effects. When used as cotherapy, misoprostol and PPIs have a similar efficacy in preventing gastric ulcer, but PPIs have few side effects.[90,91] A fixed dosage form containing misoprostol 200 mcg and diclofenac (50 mg or 75 mg) is available, but flexibility to individualize dosage is lost.

Two large randomized, placebo-controlled, multicenter, clinical trials compared the GI safety of COX-2 inhibitors to nonselective and partially selective NSAIDs and reported a reduction of 50% to 60% in upper GI events with the COX-2 inhibitors.[138,139] A 6-month trial (CLASS) of celecoxib in patients who were not taking low-dose aspirin revealed a statistically lower rate of ulcer complications when compared with ibuprofen or diclofenac,[138] but evaluation at 1 year found no GI safety advantage among those taking celecoxib.[90] This explains why celecoxib contains the same GI warnings as the nonselective and partially selective NSAIDs (Table 27-4).[140] In addition, a post hoc analysis at 6 months indicated that patients taking celecoxib and concomitant cardioprotective doses of aspirin had a similar rate of upper GI events as those taking either diclofenac or ibuprofen, thus negating the beneficial effects of celecoxib.[138] Low-dose aspirin appears to have similar effects on other COX-2 inhibitors. Unlike the CLASS study, the rofecoxib (VIGOR) trial excluded aspirin users. Results from this trial indicated that ulcers and related complications were lower with rofecoxib than with naproxen.[139]

A.D. remains at high risk for another NSAID-related complication even though gastric ulcer healing was confirmed, as she continues to take naproxen. Cotherapy with a PPI or misoprostol is preferred for this patient because both are effective in reducing the risk of NSAID-related UGI events. A.D.'s osteoarthritis is well controlled with naproxen so there is no need to switch her to celecoxib or another more costly NSAID. Combining a PPI with misoprostol is not necessary, but some physicians prefer to use combination therapy for older patients with multiple risk factors. Standard H_2RA dosages (e.g., ranitidine 150 mg BID) should not be used as prophylactic cotherapy for A.D. as they are not effective in reducing the risk of NSAID-related gastric ulcer. Although higher H_2RA dosages (e.g., ranitidine 300 mg BID) reduce the risk of gastric ulcer they are less effective than a PPI. The ranitidine should be discontinued and prophylaxis should be instituted with a standard dose of a PPI (e.g., pantoprazole 40 mg daily). All PPIs, when used in standard dosages, are effective for this indication, but A.D.'s out-of-pocket cost should be taken into consideration when selecting a PPI.

Cyclo-Oxygenase-2 Inhibitors and Cardiovascular Toxicity

CASE 27-2, QUESTION 5: What is the concern regarding the use of COX-2 inhibitors and the risk for cardiovascular toxicity?

The risk for cardiovascular events in patients taking COX-2 inhibitors increases with a number of factors, including increased COX-2 selectivity, higher dosages, a longer duration of treatment, and preexisting cardiovascular risk.[90,91,140–142] Although ulcers and related GI complications were less likely with rofecoxib than with naproxen in the VIGOR trial, the number of myocardial infarctions and thrombotic strokes were increased with rofecoxib.[139] Similar cardiothrombotic events were observed in other rofecoxib studies of longer duration.[143] In 2004, rofecoxib was withdrawn from the US market and soon thereafter valdecoxib was withdrawn amid concerns about cardiovascular risk.[90]

The cardiovascular safety of celecoxib has been evaluated, but the risk of myocardial infarction and thrombotic stroke is less certain.[90] Although there was no difference in cardiovascular events when celecoxib was compared with diclofenac and ibuprofen in the CLASS trial,[138] cardiovascular events were significantly higher in a clinical trial where patients were taking higher dosages of celecoxib (400 mg twice daily).[144] Celecoxib remains available in the United States, but the underlying cardiovascular risk of the patient must be assessed when considering the use of this drug. The lowest effective celecoxib dose should always be used for the shortest duration of time.[140]

The risk for cardiovascular events is also increased in patients taking nonselective and partially selective NSAIDs, with the possible exception of naproxen.[90,91,145] Naproxen is usually the preferred NSAID, especially in patients with increased cardiovascular risk.[90,91] NSAIDs and COX-2 inhibitors should be avoided in patients at very high GI and cardiovascular risk.[90] Consideration should be given to using less risky therapeutic options including acetaminophen, tramadol, or narcotics.[146] Thus, the selection of a drug regimen to reduce the risk of NSAID ulcers and GI complications should not only be based on the GI safety of the NSAID or COX-2 inhibitor but must be weighed against the cardiovascular risk for each patient.[90,91,145]

CASE 27-2, QUESTION 6: How does a COX-2 inhibitor compare with a PPI and a non- or partially-selective NSAID when used to decrease ulcer risk and related complications? Have any studies evaluated GI safety in patients taking a COX-2 inhibitor plus a PPI?

There have been several small non–placebo-controlled trials in *H. pylori*–negative patients at high risk for NSAID-related complications that compared celecoxib with a PPI plus a nonselective or partially-selective NSAID.[90,147,148] Results from these trials suggest that in high-risk, *H. pylori*–negative patients, a COX-2 inhibitor may be as beneficial as a nonselective NSAID plus a PPI in reducing NSAID-related ulcer complications. However, neither the COX-2 inhibitor nor the NSAID plus a PPI appears to eliminate the risk of ulcer recurrence or upper GI bleeding in high-risk patients.[90,148] Combining a COX-2 inhibitor with a PPI may be considered in very high-risk patients, but this regimen is likely to be of modest benefit.[90,148]

CASE 27-2, QUESTION 7: What factors should be considered when evaluating management strategies for patients at risk of experiencing an NSAID-induced ulcer? What risk reduction strategies are considered acceptable for A.D.?

Strategies to reduce the risk of NSAID ulcers and related complications depend on the assessment of upper GI (Table 27-3) and cardiovascular risks. Although there are no universally accepted definitions, the levels of risk can be arbitrarily stratified into low, moderate, and high GI risk and low or high cardiovascular risk.[90,91] High cardiovascular risk implies a physician-recommended requirement for low-dose aspirin to prevent serious cardiothrombotic events.[90] In general, individuals younger than 65 years of age, and those taking NSAIDs in the short term, who do not require low-dose aspirin, are considered to be at low GI and cardiovascular risk and usually do not require GI risk-reduction therapy.[90,91]

Patients at moderate risk GI risk typically have one to two risk factors which include age older than 65 years, a history of a prior uncomplicated ulcer, treatment with high-dose NSAIDs, or the concurrent use of aspirin (including low-dose), corticosteroids, or anticoagulants (Table 27-3). The recommended risk reduction strategy in this group is cotherapy with either a PPI or misoprostol, but misoprostol is usually considered a secondary option because of the dose-dependent diarrhea and abdominal cramps and the need for more frequent daily dosing.[90,91] If the patient requires low-dose aspirin, naproxen is the NSAID of choice. Although a COX-2 inhibitor provides similar gastroprotective effects as a nonselective or partially-selective NSAID plus a PPI or misoprostol, the use of COX-2 inhibitors (including celecoxib) has declined dramatically as they are typically more costly than the NSAID plus PPI and because of the concerns related to myocardial infarction and thrombotic events.[90]

Patients at very high GI risk include those with a prior history of an ulcer-related complication or multiple (>2) risk factors.[90,91] If cardiovascular risk is low, alternative therapies such as oxycodone are preferred, but a COX-2 inhibitor plus a PPI or misoprostol may be used.[90] Although it is best to avoid an NSAID if the patient had a complicated ulcer, some physicians will continue the same NSAID that provided the most effective anti-inflammatory effect. This should be done with extreme caution and with maximally effective cotherapy. NSAIDs and COX-inhibitors should be avoided in patients at high GI risk and high cardiovascular risk and alternative therapy should be used.[90,91]

Patients like A.D., who have a history of a recent ulcer and related upper GI bleed, are at high risk for future NSAID-related ulcers and complications and require an effective risk-reduction strategy. Additionally, A.D. has other factors that contribute to her high-risk status, including her age (70 years) and the continued use of a nonselective NSAID (naproxen). Ranitidine should be discontinued immediately, and A.D. should be switched to an evidence-based risk-reduction regimen. If celecoxib is used, the risk of cardiovascular effects must be weighed against the gastroprotective benefits, especially because A.D. has a history of hypertension. If A.D. had renal dysfunction (creatinine clearance <30 mL/minute), NSAIDs and COX-2 inhibitors should be avoided and the patient treated with other analgesics (e.g., tramadol, narcotics), keeping in mind that NSAIDs and COX-2 inhibitors are associated with fluid retention, hypertension, and renal failure. Although switching naproxen to celecoxib plus a PPI or continuing the oxycodone may be preferred by some, the selection of the optimal strategy for a high-risk patient like A.D. is debatable, and should take into consideration the risks, benefits, patient preferences, and cost of treatment. Cotherapy with a PPI or misoprostol is an acceptable risk-reduction strategy given A.D.'s GI and cardiovascular risk.

CASE 27-2, QUESTION 8: What information should be conveyed to A.D. regarding the combined use of OTC aspirin and NSAIDs?

Remind A.D. that her physician has recommended that she discontinue taking the enteric-coated aspirin and that she should not restart it without his/her consent. Explain to A.D. that enteric-coated aspirin may protect against the topical mucosal damage in the stomach and minimize dyspepsia, but the enteric coating does not prevent an ulcer. Even low-dose aspirin (e.g., 81 mg/day) is capable of causing an ulcer, especially when used in conjunction with an NSAID (naproxen). Buffered aspirin may cause less dyspepsia, but buffering does not prevent ulcers. Taking food, milk, or an antacid with aspirin or NSAIDs may minimize dyspepsia but does not prevent an ulcer. Inform A.D. that she should not take OTC NSAIDs in conjunction with her naproxen unless advised to do so by her physician, as combining NSAIDs will increase the risk for ulcers and GI bleeding. Advise A.D. that even though NSAIDs available for self-treatment may have different generic names (e.g., ibuprofen, naproxen) or brand names (e.g., Advil, Aleve), they all belong to the same drug class and have similar side effects.

CASE 27-2, QUESTION 9: A.D.'s physician decides to maintain her on naproxen but changes the ranitidine to lansoprazole 30 mg daily. What instructions should you provide A.D. regarding her medications?

A.D. should be advised of the major signs and symptoms of upper GI bleeding and cardiovascular disease and what action should be taken if these signs or symptoms develop. She should be instructed to take the lansoprazole every day 30 to 60 minutes before breakfast and continue taking naproxen twice daily. The importance of adhering to PPI cotherapy must be stressed, especially because A.D. may not have accompanying dyspeptic or ulcerlike symptoms. There is a strong relationship between the level of adherence to gastroprotective medication and the risk for ulcers and serious GI complications in patients like A.D. who are high-risk NSAID users.[149] Older patients, like A.D., who are at risk for osteoporosis and hip fractures and who require long-term PPI therapy should be counseled to take age-related recommended dosages of a calcium salt and vitamin D and have periodic bone density examinations (see Pharmacotherapy of Drugs Used to Treat Acid-Related Disorders section).

CASE 27-2, QUESTION 10: What parameters should be monitored to determine A.D.'s response to treatment?

High-risk patients like A.D. who continue to take an NSAID should be closely monitored for upper abdominal pain and signs or symptoms associated with bleeding, obstruction, or perforation. The presence of upper abdominal pain or a change in the severity of the pain may suggest an upper GI complication. Every effort should be made to monitor A.D.'s compliance to her PPI regimen because of the strong relationship between nonadherence and the risk of upper GI complications in high-risk NSAID users.

ZOLLINGER-ELLISON SYNDROME

Zollinger-Ellison Syndrome (ZES) is an uncommon gastric acid hypersecretory disease characterized by severe recurrent peptic ulcers that result from a gastrin-producing tumor (gastrinoma).[129,150] The primary tumor is usually located in the duodenum or pancreas, but other locations (e.g., mesenteric lymph nodes, spleen, stomach, liver) have been described.[129,150] Although most gastrinomas occur sporadically, about 25% occur in association with multiple endocrine neoplasia type 1 (MEN 1), which is an autosomal dominant inherited syndrome.[150] Most gastrinomas are malignant and tend to be slow-growing, but a small number grow and metastasize rapidly to the regional lymph nodes, liver, and bone. Abdominal pain is the most predominant symptom and is usually related to persistent peptic ulcers, which are less responsive to antisecretory therapy. Duodenal ulcers occur most often, but ulcers may also occur in the stomach or jejunum. Diarrhea, which is present in more than half of patients, may precede ulcer symptoms and results from massive gastric acid hypersecretion, which activates pepsinogen and contributes to mucosal damage.[129,150] Steatorrhea may also occur and results from inactivation of pancreatic lipase by low duodenal pH resulting from excessive acid load.[150] This leads to the precipitation of bile acids, which in turn reduces micelle formation necessary for fatty acid absorption. Vitamin B_{12} deficiency may develop secondary to malabsorption related to reduced intrinsic factor activity. GERD often occurs and is complicated by esophageal ulcers and strictures. Other symptoms include nausea, vomiting, upper GI bleeding, and weight loss. Upper GI bleeding is related to duodenal ulceration and may be the presenting symptom.

Epidemiology

The incidence of ZES in the United States is 0.1% to 1.0% among patients with duodenal ulcer.[150] The majority of patients are diagnosed between the age of 30 and 50 years, with men being slightly more affected than women.[150] The morbidity and mortality of ZES has decreased because of improved medical and surgical management.

Pathophysiology

The pathophysiology of ZES is related to a non-β islet cell gastrin-secreting tumor that stimulates the parietal cells of the stomach to hypersecrete gastric acid.[129,150] Large amounts of gastrin are produced by the gastrinoma cells, usually resulting in a profound hypergastrinemia. The gastric parietal cell mass is expanded in response to the trophic effects of hypergastrinemia and causes an increase in basal and stimulated acid output. Hypersecretion of gastric acid results in severe mucosal ulceration, diarrhea, and malabsorption, and is responsible for the signs and symptoms associated with ZES.

Clinical Assessment and Diagnosis

The diagnosis of ZES is established when the fasting serum gastrin is greater than 1,000 pg/mL and the BAO is greater than 15 mEq/hour in patients with an intact stomach (or >5 mEq/hour in the postgastric surgery patient) or when hypergastrinemia is associated with a gastric pH value less than 2.[150] When serum gastrin is between 100 and 1,000 pg/mL and gastric pH is less than 2, a provocative test (secretin or calcium) is recommended to assist in the diagnosis. Imaging techniques are performed to localize the tumor and are useful in evaluating metastatic disease. Upper endoscopy is performed to confirm mucosal ulcerations. The use of PPIs may mask the clinical presentation and complicate the diagnosis.[129]

Treatment

The goal of treatment for ZES is to pharmacologically control gastric acid secretion and to surgically resect the tumor, if possible. The oral PPIs are the drugs of choice for controlling acid secretion because of their potent and prolonged antisecretory effect. Treatment should be initiated with omeprazole 60 mg/day or an equivalent oral dose of lansoprazole, pantoprazole, esomeprazole, or rabeprazole (Table 27-1) and should be titrated to maintain a BAO less than 10 mEq/hour (1 hour before next dose) in uncomplicated patients or less than 5 mEq/hour in patients with complicated disease.[150] Once adequate control of acid secretion has been achieved, the daily PPI dose should be gradually reduced and administered every 8 to 12 hours. In most patients, an omeprazole dose of 60 to 80 mg/day reduces the BAO to target levels. IV PPIs should be reserved for those patients who are not able to take oral medications. H_2RAs are no longer used to treat ZES, even though they were initially proven to be effective (Table 27-1).

Somatostatin analogues are used with varying success to treat gastrinomas, but they are only available parenterally and rarely used as first-line treatment.[150] Octreotide, a synthetic somatostatin analogue, inhibits gastric acid secretion and decreases serum gastrin concentrations, but its subcutaneous route of administration, frequent dosing, and side effect profile (abdominal pain, diarrhea, gallstones, and pain at the injection site) make it less desirable for use in treating ZES. The long-acting depot formation of octreotide acetate for injection suspension can be administered less frequently and may be useful in controlling temporal growth. Patients with metastatic gastrinomas can be treated with chemotherapeutic agents to inhibit tumor growth or may require resection of the tumor. Localization and surgical removal of the gastrinoma should be considered in all patients unless widespread metastases exist.

GASTROESOPHAGEAL REFLUX DISEASE

GERD is a common acid-related GI disorder associated with a wide array of symptoms, the most frequent of which is heartburn and acid regurgitation. Gastroesophageal reflux (GER) is defined as the retrograde passage of gastric contents from the stomach into the esophagus. It is primarily the result of transient relaxation of the LES. When the LES is relaxed, the esophagus is exposed to small amounts of acidic stomach contents. This normal physiological event occurs many times throughout the day in healthy individuals.[7,151,152] Protective mechanisms such as esophageal peristalsis and bicarbonate-rich saliva quickly return the acidic pH to normal. GERD develops when alterations in reflux result in symptoms, mucosal injury, or both.[65,153] Esophageal injury occurs with continued exposure of the mucosa to gastric acid and results in inflammation that can progress to ulceration (erosive esophagitis).[7,154] Complications associated with long-standing GERD include esophageal strictures, Barrett metaplasia (replacement of normal esophageal squamous epithelium by specialized intestinal-like columnar epithelium), and adenocarcinoma of the esophagus.[7]

ONLINE CONTENT

For an illustration of Gastroesophageal Reflux Disease, go to http://thepoint.lww.com/AT10e.

Epidemiology

GERD is a chronic disease that affects patients across all age groups with equal distribution between men and women.[7] The prevalence of GERD appears to be greater in the Western population with patients presenting with more clinically important disease and complications than in Eastern countries (especially Asian populations) where GERD is uncommon. However, recent studies suggest that GERD may be emerging in the Eastern populations and that its increasing prevalence may someday match Western populations.[155] When considering the symptoms of GERD, such as heartburn and acid regurgitation, the overall prevalence in the United States is approximately 45%.[7] In Western populations, 25% of patients report heartburn monthly, 12% weekly, and 5% describe daily symptoms.[156] It has also been estimated that 7% of the US population have complicated GERD associated with erosive esophagitis; however, this finding is difficult to validate, as most patients do not undergo diagnostic esophageal endoscopy.[7] Many patients with erosive esophagitis are asymptomatic on diagnosis, which suggests that symptoms do not correlate with the degree of esophageal injury. Up to 75% of patients who undergo endoscopic procedures as a result of symptoms associated with GERD have normal esophageal findings.[157] These patients are identified as having functional heartburn, NERD, or endoscopy-negative reflux disease (ENRD). Other patients with GERD have symptoms that occur outside of the esophagus which are considered atypical or extraesophageal manifestations of GERD. Extraesophageal manifestations may be present with or without accompanying typical symptoms (e.g., heartburn). Extraesophageal manifestations have been estimated to occur in about 80% of patients with at least weekly symptoms of GERD (see Extraesophageal Manifestations section).[158]

Childhood GERD appears to continue into adolescence and adulthood. Although most infants exhibit physiological regurgitation, or spitting up, the majority (95%) will have abatement of symptoms by 1 year of age.[159] However, infants with persisting symptoms beyond 2 years of age are at risk of exhibiting complicated GERD.[160,161] One prospective study evaluated children with a prior diagnosis of complicated GERD (erosive esophagitis) made at about 5 years of age and then reevaluated the subjects 15 years later. This study revealed that 80% of the children reported monthly symptoms of heartburn and regurgitation, and 23% described weekly symptoms. In addition, 30%

still required antisecretory therapy, and 24% underwent antireflux surgery[162] (see Chapter 99, Common Pediatric Illnesses). Pregnancy has also been associated with an increased incidence of GERD, with 30% to 50% of pregnant women complaining of heartburn, especially in the second and third trimesters; however, in individuals without a previous diagnosis of GERD, the symptoms resolve when the child is born.[7] The mechanisms for GERD in pregnancy are related to the hormonal effects of progesterone and estrogen, which lower LES pressure, and increasing intra-abdominal pressure[7,163] (see Chapter 49, Obstetric Drug Therapy, for complete discussion related to the management, as well as the risks and benefits associated with treating GERD in the pregnant patient).

Complications associated with GERD include esophageal erosions (5%), strictures (4%–20%), and Barrett metaplasia (8%–20%).[7] Male sex and advancing age (men and women) are associated with an increase in the prevalence of esophageal complications, presumably as a result of refluxed acidic contents damaging the mucosa over time.[7] Patients with GERD may have a decrease in quality of life. When comparing quality of life in patients with GERD to those with other chronic medical diseases, the quality of life in GERD patients was between patients with psychiatric disorders and patients with mild heart failure.[164]

Etiology and Risk Factors

The causes of GERD are associated with factors that increase the frequency or duration of GER leading to increased contact of the acidic refluxate with the esophageal mucosa. Risk factors associated with GERD include dietary and lifestyle factors, drugs, and certain medical and surgical conditions[7,13,151–154,165,166] (Table 27-7). These factors may precipitate or worsen GERD symptoms by lowering the LES pressure (e.g., nitrates, progesterone, foods high in fat, mint, chocolate) or having a direct irritating effect on the esophageal mucosa (e.g., citrus, tomatoes, bisphosphonates).

TABLE 27-7
Risk Factors Associated with Gastroesophageal Reflux Disease[7,13,151–154,165,166]

Drugs	Dietary
α-Adrenergic agonists	Foods high in fat
Anticholinergics	Spicy foods
Aspirin	Carminatives (peppermint, spearmint)
Barbiturates	Chocolate
Benzodiazepines	Caffeine (coffee, tea, colas)
β_2-Adrenergic agonists	Garlic or onions
Bisphosphonates	Citrus fruits and juices
Calcium-channel blockers	Tomatoes and juice
Dopamine	Carbonated beverages
Estrogen	
Isoproterenol	**Lifestyle**
Iron	Cigarette/cigar smoke
Narcotics	Obesity
Nitrates	Supine body position
NSAIDs	Tight-fitting clothing
Progesterone	Heavy exercise
Potassium	
Prostaglandins	**Medical/Surgical Conditions**
Quinidine	Pregnancy
Tetracycline	Scleroderma
Theophylline	ZES
Tricyclic antidepressants	Gastroparesis
Zidovudine	Nasogastric tube intubation

NSAID, nonsteroidal anti-inflammatory drug; ZES, Zollinger-Ellison syndrome.

Stress reflux from increased intra-abdominal pressure has been associated with overeating, coughing, and bending or straining to lift heavy objects, as well as tight-fitting clothing.[7,13] Certain medical and surgical conditions such as gastroparesis, scleroderma, ZES, and long-term placement of nasogastric tubes may also be associated with GERD.[7] Although it has been suggested that the eradication of *H. pylori* infection may increase the risk of GERD symptoms and esophagitis, additional information is needed to confirm this association.[83,167,168]

Pathophysiology

The pathophysiology of GERD is associated with defects in transient relaxations of the LES, esophageal acid clearance and buffering capabilities, anatomy, gastric emptying, mucosal resistance, and with exposure of the esophageal mucosa to aggressive factors (gastric acid, pepsin, and bile salts) leading to esophageal damage.

TRANSIENT RELAXATIONS OF THE LOWER ESOPHAGEAL SPHINCTER

The LES, when in a resting state, remains at a high pressure (10–30 mmHg) to prevent the gastric contents from entering into the esophagus.[7] Pressures are lowest during the day and with meals and highest at night.[7] Transient relaxations of the LES are short periods of sphincter relaxation that are different from those that occur with swallowing or peristalsis.[8,169,170] They occur as a result of vagal stimulation in response to gastric distension from meals (most common), gas, stress, vomiting, or coughing and can persist for more than 10 seconds.[8] These transient relaxations of the LES are associated with virtually all GER events in healthy individuals but account for 50% to 80% of occurrences in patients with pathogenic GERD.[8] Thus, not all transient relaxations of the LES are associated with GERD.

A small percentage of patients may also have a continuously weak and hypotensive LES (decreased LES resting tone). Stress reflux increases intra-abdominal pressure and may blow open the hypotensive LES.[8] When LES pressures remain constantly low, the risk for serious complications (e.g., erosive esophagitis) increase dramatically. Scleroderma, which is related to fibrosis of smooth muscle, may reduce LES tone and increase the potential for GERD.[171]

ESOPHAGEAL ACID CLEARANCE AND BUFFERING CAPABILITIES

Although the number of reflux events and quantity of refluxate are notable, it is the duration of time the mucosa is in contact with these noxious substances that determines esophageal damage and complications. More than 50% of patients diagnosed with severe esophagitis have decreased acid clearance from the esophagus.[7] Peristalsis is the primary mechanism by which acid refluxate is removed from the esophagus. Other mechanisms include swallowing, esophageal distension in response to refluxate, and gravity (which is only effective when the patient is in an upright position).

Saliva plays an important role in the neutralization of gastric acid within the esophagus. Its bicarbonate-rich content buffers the residual acid that remains in the esophagus after peristalsis.[7] However, saliva is only effective on small amounts of gastric acid, as patients with larger volumes of acid refluxate may not have the neutralizing capacity in saliva necessary to protect the esophagus.[7] Swallowing increases the rate of saliva production and esophageal acid clearance. The reduction of swallowing that occurs during sleep is associated with nocturnal GERD. Patients with decreased saliva production (e.g., elderly, patients taking medication with anticholinergic effects, and those with certain medical conditions such as xerostomia or Sjögren syndrome) may also be at increased risk of experiencing GERD.[7,172]

ANATOMIC ABNORMALITIES

Hiatal hernia (protrusion of the upper portion of the stomach into the thoracic cavity because of weakening in the diaphragmatic muscles) is frequently described as a cause of GERD, but its causal relationship remains uncertain.[7] Although hiatal hernia is associated with a greater degree of esophagitis, strictures, and Barrett metaplasia, not all patients with hiatal hernia exhibit symptoms or complications. This may be related to the size of the hiatal hernia and its effect on LES pressure.[7] An increase in the size of the hernia may decrease its ability to remain below the diaphragm during swallowing and thus reduces LES pressure. Hypotensive LES in combination with hiatal hernia increases the likelihood of reflux and complicated disease.[7]

GASTRIC EMPTYING

Delayed gastric emptying increases the volume of gastric fluid remaining within the stomach that is available for reflux and is associated with gastric distension.[7] Although delayed gastric emptying is present in up to 15% of patients with GERD, a causal relationship has not been established.[7,173] Because some patients such as those with diabetic gastroparesis also have GERD, the association between delayed gastric emptying and GERD cannot be overlooked.[7]

MUCOSAL RESISTANCE

The capability of the esophageal mucosa to endure contact with and withstand injury from gastric refluxate (acid and pepsin) is a substantial determinate for the development of GERD. When considering the mucosal resistance within the esophagus compared with that of the stomach and duodenum, the esophagus is less resistant to damage from gastric acid.[7] However, mucosal resistance in the esophagus is composed of many defensive factors working in tandem to prevent esophageal injury. An increase in mucosal cell thickness and intracellular junctional complexes prevents the diffusion of hydrogen ions from penetrating into the esophageal epithelium and leading to cell death.[7] The esophagus also secretes a protective mucous layer and bicarbonate.[7,174] Enhanced blood flow in response to an acidic environment within the esophagus improves tissue oxygenation, provides nutrients, and helps to maintain a normal acid–base balance.[7] Esophageal injury also occurs when the concentration of acid and pepsin exceed the protection afforded by mucosal resistance mechanisms.

AGGRESSIVE FACTORS ASSOCIATED WITH ESOPHAGEAL DAMAGE

The gastric refluxate, which is composed primarily of gastric acid and pepsin, is the primary aggressive factor associated with GERD. The development and degree of mucosal damage is dependent on the pH and contents of the refluxate as well as the total exposure time of refluxate with the esophageal mucosa. A pH less than 4 is usually required to produce injury to the esophageal mucosa, but as the refluxate becomes more acidic, the mucosal damage is accelerated.[7] The addition of pepsin (which is converted from secreted pepsinogen in an acidic pH) to the acidic refluxate will markedly increase the propensity of the refluxate to compromise mucosal resistance and increases the potential for esophageal bleeding.[7,173,175] Duodenogastric reflux or alkaline reflux containing bile acids and pancreatic juices may also contribute to esophagitis.[7] Because gastric and duodenogastric reflux are often concomitantly present, their actions may be additive in causing esophageal damage. The duration of total exposure time of the esophagus to the refluxate is the primary mechanism involved in the development of GERD and its complications. The longer the duration of exposure time, the greater the possibility of severe disease, including progression to Barrett metaplasia.

ERADICATION OF HELICOBACTER PYLORI

The relationship between *H. pylori* infection and GERD remains controversial.[167] Early studies suggest that *H. pylori* eradication is associated with increased gastric acidity and subsequent development of erosive esophagitis.[83,167] Within this context, it appeared that *H. pylori* may actually be protective against GERD symptoms and related complications.[83,167] This is presumably caused by the microorganisms ability to decrease the acidity of the refluxate, as it does not appear to affect the functional defense mechanisms of the esophagus.[167,168] However, based on a systematic review of the literature, current guidelines for the eradication of *H. pylori* do not support this hypothesis, and although *H. pylori* testing in patients with GERD is not standard practice, if the patient is tested and found to be *H. pylori*–positive, eradication is recommended[83] (see Primary Treatment of *Helicobacter pylori* section).

Clinical Presentation

SIGNS AND SYMPTOMS

CASE 27-3

QUESTION 1: W.J. is a 39-year-old, 130-kg, 170-cm-tall man who presents with complaints of indigestion. He describes a burning sensation behind his breastbone and some belching that is often associated with an acid taste in the back of his mouth. He indicates that his symptoms began a few months ago, and they only occur a few times a month, especially after eating large or spicy meals. Also, if he eats too close to his bedtime, the burning keeps him up at night. He has used liquid antacids in the past for these symptoms and states they work fairly well, but he has to take frequent doses, as the symptoms return quickly. He does not take any other medications. Which of W.J.'s symptoms are consistent with GERD?

Symptoms that are typically associated with GERD include heartburn, pyrosis (a retrosternal burning that occurs in the upper esophagus and travels up through the throat), regurgitation of gastric contents into the throat, or in many patients, the presence of both.[7,65,153,176] These symptoms may be episodic or meal-related and are often alleviated by antacids.[7,153] Heartburn, the most frequent typical symptom, is caused by the contact of acidic refluxate with nerve endings within esophageal mucosa.[7] Other symptoms include water brash (salty or sour fluid occurring abruptly within the mouth), early satiety, belching, hiccups, nausea, and vomiting.[7] Worrisome symptoms (alarm signs or symptoms) include dysphagia (trouble swallowing), odynophagia (painful swallowing), vomiting of blood, bloody or tarry stools, unexplained weight loss, and anemia.[7,65,153] These symptoms suggest complicated disease such as erosive esophagitis, esophageal stricture, malignancy, or GI bleeding and require immediate evaluation by a health care professional. Some patients, such as the elderly, may not have typical GERD symptoms, but present initially with alarm symptoms.[7,177] This is attributable in part to older patients having a reduced pain perception and a possible reduction in the acidity of the refluxate.[7] Other patients may present with only extraesophageal or atypical symptoms (see Treatment of the Extraesophageal Manifestations of Gastroesophageal Reflux Disease section). Despite the lack of esophageal symptoms, the potential for serious esophageal damage exists, as there is no correlation between symptoms and

TABLE 27-8

Dietary and Lifestyle Modifications Used to Manage Gastroesophageal Reflux Symptoms[13,65,153,166,176,179]

Dietary	Medication	Lifestyle
Avoid foods listed in Table 26-7	Avoid medications with a potential to relax the lower esophageal sphincter or that have a direct irritant effect on the esophageal mucosa (Table 27-7)	Stop or decrease smoking/tobacco
Avoid eating large meals	Medications with the potential to irritate the esophagus should be taken with a full glass of water	Avoid alcohol
Avoid eating within 3 hours of bedtime		Lose weight[a] Elevate the head of bed 6–8 inches or use a foam wedge[a] Sleep in the left lateral decubitus position[a]

[a] Sufficient evidence exists to support lifestyle modification.

the degree of esophageal injury.[7] W.J.'s symptoms of a burning sensation (heartburn), regurgitation soon after eating spicy or large meals, and the association of symptoms with eating a meal near his bedtime are all consistent with GERD. The fact that his symptoms are relieved by his use of antacids is also suggestive of GERD.

Treatment

THERAPEUTIC GOALS

CASE 27-3, QUESTION 2: What are the therapeutic goals for the treatment of W.J.'s GERD?

The therapeutic goals for the management of GERD are to alleviate symptoms, promote esophageal healing, prevent recurrence, provide cost-effective pharmacotherapy, and avoid long-term complications.[7] One long-term consequence is Barrett esophagus, or Barrett metaplasia, which is identified in 10% to 15% of GERD patients on endoscopic evaluation.[7,178] This premalignant condition may predispose the patient to esophageal adenocarcinoma. Patients with Barrett esophagus have a risk of exhibiting esophageal cancer that is 30 to 40 times higher than patients without this disorder.[178] GERD is a chronic disease that carries the potential for serious complications.

NONPHARMACOLOGIC MEASURES AND SELF-DIRECTED TREATMENT

CASE 27-3, QUESTION 3: What lifestyle and dietary changes may potentially reduce W.J.'s GERD symptoms?

Lifestyle and dietary modifications comprise the initial step in managing patients with GERD[13,65,153,166,176,179] (Table 27-8). Strategies should be discussed with the patient and tailored to his or her specific needs. The paucity of evidence to date suggests that although many patients may benefit from these modifications, they are unlikely to completely alleviate symptoms in most patients.[65,153,176,179] Lifestyle modifications are aimed at reducing acid exposure within the esophagus by increasing LES pressure, decreasing intragastric pressure, improving esophageal acid clearance, and avoiding specific agents that irritate the esophageal mucosa. There is evidence to support several modifications that reduce esophageal gastric acid exposure and symptoms.[65,153,179] These include raising the head of the bed 6 to 8 inches by using blocks underneath the legs of the bed or using a foam wedge instead of traditional pillows; sleeping in a left lateral decubitus position; and weight loss, which also decreases intra-gastric pressure.[65,153,179] Avoiding large meals within 3 hours of bedtime or lying down in the supine position may also decrease symptoms.

Patients with GERD symptoms should avoid foods and beverages known to trigger symptoms (Table 27-7). However, the evidence suggesting benefit remains uncertain.[65,153,176,179] It is likely that most GERD patients have tried many of the dietary and lifestyle modifications without obtaining satisfactory relief of their symptoms and that others will not be amenable to making these changes in their life. However, individualized lifestyle and dietary modifications should be recommended to all patients with GERD symptoms. When appropriate, OTC or prescription medications should be recommended.[13]

W.J. should be counseled to lose weight, wear loose-fitting clothing, and avoid eating spicy meals that he knows will exacerbate his symptoms. Recommend that he avoids eating at least 3 hours before bedtime and that he considers raising the head of his bed 6 to 8 inches with wooden blocks. W.J. should be asked to keep a journal in order to track symptoms in relationship to diet and lifestyle and to record the effect of any lifestyle and dietary modifications. The health care practitioner should review the journal and discuss with W.J. which dietary and lifestyle factors trigger symptoms and which measures are most effective in relieving his symptoms.

CASE 27-3, QUESTION 4: Which OTC treatment options (if any) would you recommend for W.J.?

Many patients with mild, infrequent symptoms can be managed with OTC medications[7,13,180–182] (Fig. 27-5). First, a determination must be made as to the suitability of the patient for self-treatment. If the patient does not meet the criteria for self-treatment as described subsequently, he or she should be referred for further medical evaluation.[7,13,181,182] It is important to ensure that the following are not present: alarm signs or symptoms, severe or frequent (2 or more days a week) heartburn lasting greater than 3 months, presence of extraesophageal manifestations (see Question 27-5), or symptoms that persist despite appropriate drug therapy. OTC antacids and H_2RAs are the drugs of choice for patients with mild, infrequent heartburn. The nonprescription PPIs (omeprazole, immediate-release omeprazole with sodium bicarbonate, and lansoprazole) should be reserved for patients who experience frequent heartburn.[13]

Antacids remain an effective option for treating mild, infrequent heartburn, as they rapidly (within minutes) relieve symptoms, but the duration of symptom relief only lasts about 30 minutes when taken on an empty stomach.[7,13,181] The duration can be extended for several hours if taken within 1 hour after a meal.[13] Antacids are available in tablet and liquid form and are usually interchangeable when used in recommended dosages.[13] The dose can be repeated every 1 to 2 hours as needed, but the maximum recommended daily dose should not be exceeded. The addition of alginic acid to the antacid may improve

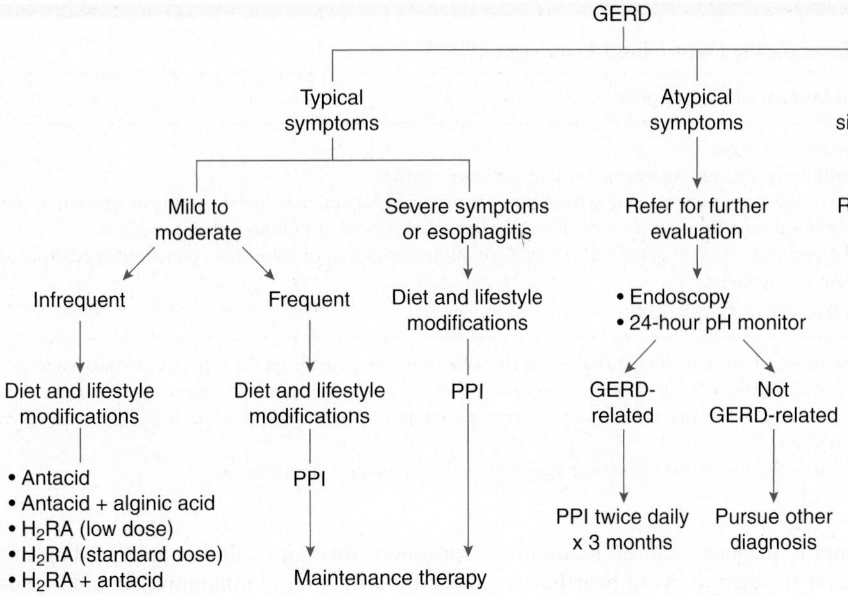

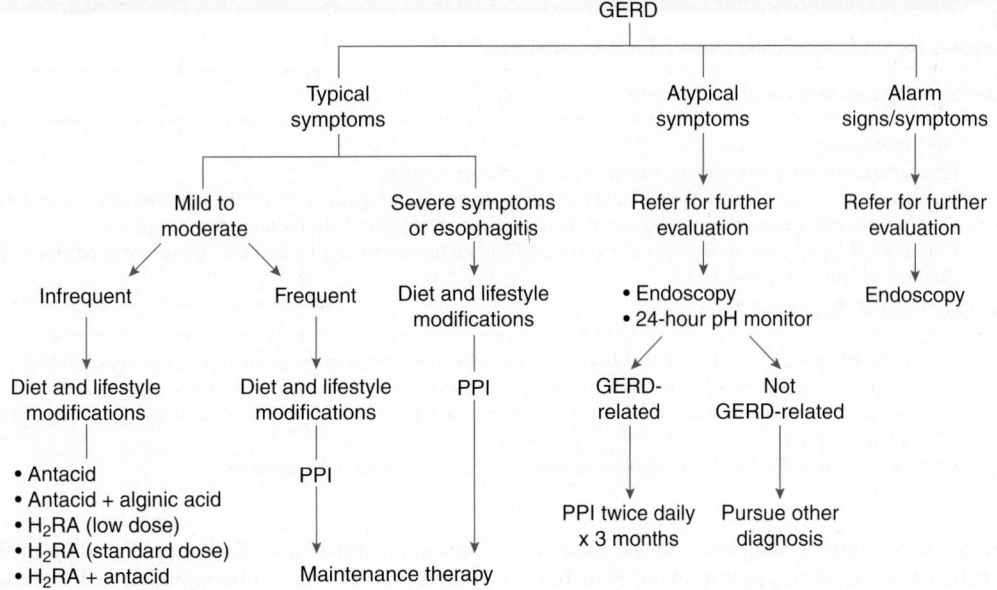

FIGURE 27-5 Management of gastroesophageal reflux disease. H_2RA, H_2 receptor antagonist; PPI, proton-pump inhibitor.

symptom relief for some patients.[8,13,180] Patients requiring frequent or regular antacid use for more than 2 weeks should be reevaluated, as an OTC H_2RA or PPI may be needed.[13,181,182] About 20% of patients will achieve symptom relief with the use of antacids.[7] Antacids are not effective in healing erosive esophagitis.[7]

The OTC H_2RAs are indicated for mild to moderate infrequent GERD symptoms.[13,181] When compared with antacids, their onset of symptom relief occurs within 30 to 45 minutes, and they have a longer duration of action (up to 10 hours).[7,13] One benefit of the H_2RAs is that they can be taken before eating a heavy or spicy meal as prophylaxis for postprandial GERD symptoms.[7,13] They also have a beneficial effect on reducing nocturnal acid secretion.[13] Tachyphylaxis (tolerance) has been reported with continued use of H_2RAs, but this effect can be overcome with intermittent or as-needed use.[13] OTC H_2RAs are available in one-half the original prescription low dose and as the full prescription doses. Patients should use the lower OTC dose twice daily for mild, intermittent symptoms and the higher dose twice daily for moderate symptoms[13] (Table 27-1). The four OTC H_2RAs (cimetidine, famotidine, ranitidine, nizatidine) are interchangeable when used in recommended dosages.[13] Patients should avoid cimetidine if the potential for a clinically important drug interaction exists with drugs metabolized by the hepatic CYP450 enzyme system. When used for self-treatment, the H_2RA dose should not exceed two doses per day, and the treatment duration should not exceed 2 weeks. Use beyond 2 weeks should be under the care of a health care provider.[7,13]

Omeprazole magnesium is available OTC in the original prescription strength as a 20.6-mg tablet (metabolized to 20 mg omeprazole) and as an immediate-release formulation capsule consisting of omeprazole 20 mg and sodium bicarbonate 1100 mg. Lansoprazole is also available OTC as a 15-mg capsule. These potent inhibitors of gastric acid are indicated for use in patients with frequent heartburn (2 or more days a week).[13] The onset of symptom relief is slower (2 to 3 hours) than with H_2RAs, and complete relief may require up to 4 days after initiating therapy. PPIs are superior to H_2RAs with regard to symptom relief and duration of acid suppression.[13] Patients should take the OTC PPIs 30 to 60 minutes before a meal (breakfast is preferable) and not take more than one dose daily for up to 2 weeks. Another course of therapy should not be taken more than every 4 months unless directed by a health care provider, as this may indicate more serious disease.[7,13,181,182]

W.J. is an appropriate candidate for self-treatment because his symptoms are mild and occur infrequently, and he has no alarm symptoms. Although antacids are an acceptable option for W.J., he has tried these and is unhappy with the frequency of dosing needed to relieve his heartburn. Because W.J. has requested a medication to specifically "prevent" meal-related symptoms, he should take an H_2RA 30 to 60 minutes before eating or drinking. If symptoms remain infrequent but are unrelated to meals, the use of an OTC H_2RA as needed for symptoms may be required. He can increase the dose to twice daily if symptom relief is not optimal and may consider an OTC PPI if symptoms occur more than 2 days a week. If he continues to have symptoms beyond 2 weeks, the symptoms become more severe, or they are accompanied by alarm symptoms, he should be referred for further evaluation.

SEVERE DISEASE WITH COMPLICATIONS

CASE 27-4

QUESTION 1: L.F. is a 48-year-old woman who presents to her primary-care provider complaining of recurrent heartburn occurring daily for the past 6 weeks. She states that the heartburn occurs frequently after meals and often wakens her at night. Lately, she has been experiencing difficulty swallowing solid foods. L.F. currently smokes two packs of cigarettes per day and likes to have two glasses of wine each night with her dinner. She states that she occasionally uses OTC ranitidine 150 mg orally up to twice daily, which temporarily relieves her symptoms. What diagnostic modalities are available for the evaluation of her GERD?

Clinical Assessment and Diagnosis

Numerous diagnostic options exist for the evaluation of the patient with presumed GERD. The medical history should include the identification of specific symptoms and an assessment of symptom frequency, severity, and duration as well as

TABLE 27-9

Classification Systems for Endoscopically Determined Esophagitis[186–188]

The Savary Miller Classification System of Esophagitis	
Grade 0	Normal esophageal mucosa
Grade 1	Erythema or diffusely red mucosa, edema causing accentuated folds
Grade 2	Isolated round or linear erosions extending from the gastroesophageal junction upward, not involving entire circumference
Grade 3	Confluent erosions extending around entire circumference or superficial ulceration without erosions
Grade 4	Complicated cases; erosions as in grade 3 plus deep ulcerations, strictures, or columnar epithelium-lined esophagus
Grade 5	Presence of Barrett metaplasia
The Los Angeles Classification System of Esophagitis	
Grade A	One (or more) mucosal break no longer that 5 mm that does not extend between the tops of two mucosal folds
Grade B	One (or more) mucosal break more that 5 mm long that does not extend between the tops of two mucosal folds
Grade C	One (or more) mucosal break that is continuous between the tops of two or more mucosal folds but that involves <75% of the circumference
Grade D	One (or more) mucosal break that involves at least 75% of the esophageal circumference

risk factors or triggers. An empiric diagnosis can be made in the majority of patients based on the symptoms of heartburn and regurgitation. However, patients who present with severe symptoms, alarm symptoms, or long-standing GERD or who do not respond to empiric therapy warrant further diagnostic evaluation.

ACID SUPPRESSION EMPIRIC TEST

A trial of a PPI is commonly used to empirically diagnose typical GERD-like symptoms in patients without alarm symptoms or symptoms of complicated disease. Doses used in clinical trials range from 20 mg to 80 mg omeprazole (or equivalent) once daily for up to 4 weeks.[7,183] If symptoms are relieved after a short trial of a PPI (7 to 14 days), an empiric diagnosis of GERD may be made and other invasive and costly diagnostic methods may be avoided.[7,151,153,180,183,184] However, this methodology is not without its limitations. The test cannot differentiate between other acid-related disorders such as PUD, and studies evaluating its ability to detect GERD versus other diagnostic options have been equivocal.[7,153,183,184] Despite these shortcomings, guidelines suggest that an empiric trial of a PPI is appropriate in selected patients given its ease of use and reduced cost.[153] The empiric use of a PPI may also be beneficial in identifying patients with extraesophageal manifestations of GERD[7] (see Treatment of Extraesophageal Manifestations of Gastroesophageal Reflux Disease section). Further diagnostic evaluation is warranted in patients who do not respond to acid suppressive therapy, who present with alarm symptoms or symptoms suggestive of complicated disease, or who have long-standing GERD where the possibility of Barrett esophagus exists.

UPPER ENDOSCOPY AND BIOPSY

Upper endoscopy is the primary diagnostic method for evaluating the esophageal mucosa for injury or cellular changes. (To view a video of severe esophagitis, go to **http://www.gastrointestinalatlas.com/English/Esophagus/Esophagitis/esophagitis.html.**) This test is highly specific, yet only moderately sensitive for the diagnosis of GERD, because many patients present with nonerosive disease. There are four primary reasons why endoscopy is performed in patients suspected of having GERD[7,185]: (a) to rule out significant disease (e.g., adenocarcinoma of the esophagus) or complications (e.g., stricture); (b) to screen for Barrett metaplasia; (c) to evaluate and grade the severity of esophagitis; (d) to allow the provider to optimize treatment and predict the long-term course of the disease. The endoscope can be fitted with surgical instruments to allow the operator to perform procedures or obtain tissue specimens for biopsy. Endoscopic grading of the esophagus is based on the level of inflammation and mucosal damage. Two endoscopic classification systems are used for the grading of esophagitis[186,187] (Table 27-9). The Savary-Miller classification categorizes patients from grade 0 to grade 4 based on the severity of mucosal erosions of the esophagus.[186] The addition of a grade 5 was added to include the diagnosis of Barrett esophagus.[188] Although this classification system is no longer recommended in the United States, it is still used in many practices, as well as in Europe. The Los Angeles classification is preferred because it is more specific and categorizes patients from grades A to D based on the number of mucosal breaks, their size, and the amount of surface area with esophagitis involvement.[187] There is no classification for normal esophagus with this system and symptomatic patients are often classified with NERD.

Biopsy of the esophageal mucosa is performed during endoscopy, and tissue samples are evaluated by microscopy for evidence of Barrett metaplasia or neoplastic disease.[8] In patients with suspected Barrett metaplasia, the biopsy is obtained after the esophagus has healed to prevent misinterpretation of the inflammatory markers for dysplastic syndrome. Mucosal biopsy for inflammatory markers in nonerosive disease remains debatable.

24-HOUR CONTINUOUS AMBULATORY pH MONITORING

Ambulatory pH monitoring is a valuable diagnostic test for evaluating GERD. It is especially helpful in patients who have not responded adequately to reasonable pharmacotherapy, in patients with nonerosive disease, and when there is the need to correlate reflux events with symptoms. A small (2–3 mm diameter) pH electrode is threaded through the patient's nostril (similar to placing a nasogastric tube), past the patient's larynx, to approximately 5 cm above the LES in the distal esophagus.[7] Once it is connected to a logging device, which documents pH measurements every few seconds, it allows for the determination of reflux events (defined as esophageal pH <4), duration of reflux events, and percentage of time within a 24-hour period that the patient's pH is less than 4. The patient is asked to keep a diary to record symptomatic events that can be correlated with a decrease in esophageal pH. This is especially important when correlating extraesophageal manifestations with reflux events.

RADIOLOGIC TESTING

The barium esophagram (barium swallow) is used primarily to identify suspected esophageal abnormalities such as strictures, narrowing, and hiatal hernia and to determine peristalsis disorders.[7] The procedure is relatively noninvasive and inexpensive when compared with endoscopy.

ESOPHAGEAL MANOMETRY

Esophageal manometry is used to evaluate the patient's LES pressure and esophageal peristalsis.[8] This procedure does not have a specific role in the diagnosis of GERD, as it does not detect the presence of acid within the esophagus. It is used primarily to evaluate patients before 24-hour continuous ambulatory pH monitoring and antireflux surgical procedures (e.g., Nissen fundoplication) to determine the location of the LES.[8,189]

CASE 27-4, QUESTION 2: L.F.'s frequent severe symptoms continue despite OTC famotidine 20 mg orally twice daily and the presence of warning signs warranted that she undergo endoscopy, which revealed moderate esophagitis (Los Angeles grade C), the presence of an esophageal stricture, and no evidence of Barrett metaplasia. Esophageal dilation was performed during the procedure to widen the lumen of the esophagus. What treatment options exist for L.F.?

Pharmacotherapy

ANTACIDS

Antacids are useful only in the relief of mild symptoms associated with GERD (see Nonpharmacologic Measures and Self-Directed Treatment section). Because of their short duration of action and inability to heal erosive esophagitis, they are not an option for treating moderate to severe GERD.[7,13]

HISTAMINE-2 RECEPTOR ANTAGONISTS

H_2RAs are effective in treating patients with mild to moderate GERD, but response rates vary with the severity of disease, the dose of the drug, and the duration of therapy. H_2RAs are considered equally effective when used in equipotent doses for symptomatic relief and esophageal healing (Table 27-1). They are effective in reducing nocturnal symptoms but only modestly effective in relieving meal-related symptoms, as they only block one mechanism of parietal cell activation (the H_2 receptor).[7] H_2RAs relieve symptoms in about 50% to 60% of patients treated after 12 weeks of continuous therapy and are superior to placebo.[153,190] Increasing the H_2RA dose may not improve symptoms in some patients.[191] Esophageal healing requires higher doses (e.g., famotidine 40 mg BID) compared with those used for symptom relief (Table 27-1). Esophageal healing rates with H_2RAs are reported to be about 50% after 8 to 12 weeks of treatment, but rates will vary depending on the degree of esophagitis.[153,176,190] For example, endoscopic healing rates in trials with high-dose H_2RAs were approximately 60% to 90% in patients with grades 1 and 2 esophagitis but were only 30% to 50% in patients with more severe disease (grades 3 and 4 esophagitis).[7,190] Some investigators have attributed inadequate esophageal healing to the development of tachyphylaxis.[180]

PROTON-PUMP INHIBITORS

PPIs are the drugs of choice for patients with frequent moderate to severe GERD symptoms and esophagitis because they provide more rapid relief of symptoms and esophageal healing than do H_2RAs. When used in recommended dosages, all of the PPIs provide similar rates of symptom relief and esophageal healing (Table 27-1). Their superior efficacy, when compared with H_2RAs, is related to their ability to maintain an intragastric pH less than 4 for a long duration time (up to 24 hours/day vs. up to 10 hours with a H_2RA).[13,192] Typically, PPIs are taken once daily 30 to 60 minutes before breakfast, but if a second dose is required, it should be taken before the evening meal.

A large meta-analysis of 16 trials confirms that PPIs are superior to H_2RAs for achieving rapid and complete relief of GERD symptoms. Complete symptom relief (within 4–12 weeks) was achieved in 77.4% of patients taking a PPI versus 47.6% of those taking an H_2RA ($p < 0.0001$).[190] PPIs have also been shown to heal esophagitis more quickly and effectively than H_2RAs. In the same meta-analysis, which evaluated 43 double-blinded or single-blinded, randomized studies (including patients with severe esophagitis), PPIs (83.6%) were more effective than H_2RAs (51.9%) at healing erosive esophagitis at 12 weeks.[190] Healing also occurred more quickly with PPI therapy in that by week 2, 63.4% of patients had healed with the PPI, whereas it took 12 weeks with the H_2RAs for 60.2% of patients to heal.[190] Another large meta-analysis, which evaluated more than 33 randomized trials, demonstrated similar results with 81.7% of patients healed at 8 weeks with a PPI versus 52.0% with an H_2RA.[43]

Esophageal healing among PPIs appears to be equivalent, as about 85% to 90% of patients achieve complete healing at 8 weeks in numerous head-to-head trials with equivalent doses.[38–41] One meta-analysis, which compared esophageal healing rates among omeprazole 20 mg, lansoprazole 30 mg, pantoprazole 40 mg, and rabeprazole 20 mg (each given once daily), reported no statistical difference.[37] However, all of the PPIs were superior to ranitidine 300 to 600 mg/day. Esomeprazole 40 mg once daily has been reported to be superior to omeprazole 20 mg once daily, both at 4 and 8 weeks, when used to heal erosive esophagitis.[193] However, the esomeprazole 40 mg and omeprazole 20 mg dosages are not equipotent, and this study has been heavily criticized based on this fact. Another study, which compared equipotent doses of esomeprazole (40 mg) and lansoprazole (30 mg), also suggests that esomeprazole has statistically significant greater healing rates (92.6% vs. 88.8%, respectively, $p = 0.0001$).[40] In contrast, a similar study comparing lansoprazole 30 mg with esomeprazole 40 mg showed no statistical difference in esophageal healing, albeit with a smaller population.[41] Dexlansoprazole MR 60 mg once daily has been compared with lansoprazole 30 mg once daily in randomized, double-blind clinical trials to assess healing of erosive esophagitis.[194] The results using life-table analysis reveal similar healing rates with dexlansoprazole MR 60 mg and lansoprazole 30 mg (92%–93% vs. 86%–92%, respectively), but the results were not statistically significant.[194] A higher dose of dexlansoprazole MR (90 mg daily) was superior to lansoprazole (30 mg daily) in patients with more severe disease (Los Angeles Classification grades C and D), but these are not equipotent doses. In spite of the lack of supportive evidence, some clinicians prefer to use esomeprazole 40 mg/day or dexlansoprazole MR 60 mg/day for patients with severe erosive esophagitis.

The ability of a high-dose PPI to reverse Barrett metaplasia remains controversial.[7,195] Although studies have demonstrated islands of normal squamous epithelium returning, no data have determined that this is associated with a risk reduction in adenocarcinoma.[7,195] In fact, others have suggested that this return of normal mucosa may actually mask carcinogenic changes occurring deeper in the gastric mucosa.[196]

Improvement of quality of life has also been evaluated in patients receiving PPI therapy in the management of GERD. A recent study comparing esomeprazole with ranitidine during a period of 6 months showed a significant improvement in both physical functioning and sleep with the PPI therapy.[197]

PROKINETIC AGENTS

Two prokinetic agents, metoclopramide and bethanechol, may be effective in the management of GERD. Both drugs increase LES pressure and stimulate the motility of the upper GI tract without altering gastric acid secretion.[7] Although these drugs may provide relief of symptoms, they are ineffective in healing erosive esophagitis unless they are combined with an H_2RA or PPI. Prokinetics are not widely used to treat GERD because they are not as effective as other treatments and are associated with numerous side effects (sedation, anxiety, extrapyramidal symptoms, etc.).[7,153] Prokinetics are reserved for patients who are refractory to other available treatment options or who have delayed gastric emptying.

SUCRALFATE

Sucralfate appears to be effective in treating mild cases of GERD and possibly mild esophagitis but is not effective in the management of severe disease.[198] Given more effective options at this time, sucralfate is rarely used in the management of GERD.

PPIs are considered the drugs of choice for patients with frequent or severe GERD symptoms, or who have complicated disease, because of their potent inhibition of gastric acid secretion[65,151,153,176,180–182] (Fig. 27-5). In this case, L.F., who presents with severe esophagitis (Los Angeles grade C), will require a PPI taken once daily in order to relieve her symptoms and heal the esophagus (Table 27-1). A reasonable option for L.F. would be lansoprazole 30 mg daily to be taken 30 to 60 minutes before breakfast each morning for the next 8 weeks; however, if the cost of therapy is an issue, generic omeprazole 40 mg daily would also be an acceptable alternative. L.F. should also be counseled regarding lifestyle and dietary modifications, including smoking cessation and abstinence from alcohol. She should avoid eating large meals before bedtime and may wish to elevate the head of her bed by 6 to 8 inches with wooden blocks.

Maintenance Therapy

CASE 27-4, QUESTION 3: L.F.'s symptoms resolved in about 2 weeks after starting PPI therapy, and she remained asymptomatic after 8 weeks. She then underwent endoscopy again, which revealed that the esophagus had healed completely. Her primary-care physician then stopped the PPI. Now, 2 weeks later, she is experiencing mild heartburn. Is L.F. a candidate for long-term maintenance therapy?

GERD is chronic disease. Up to 80% of patients with severe esophagitis and 15% to 30% with less severe disease have a symptomatic relapse within 6 months after discontinuing treatment.[7] The goal of maintenance therapy is to keep the patient symptom-free and prevent potentially life-threatening complications. Continuous maintenance therapy with a daily PPI is more effective than an H_2RA, with reported relapse rates of 25% and 50%, respectively.[7] Thus, PPIs are the drugs of choice for maintaining remission in patients with healed esophagitis. An H_2RA may be considered for patients with mild nonerosive disease. Although one-half of the PPI dose used for esophageal healing has been suggested, guidelines indicate that the recommended maintenance dose should be the dose that is required to render the patient asymptomatic.[65,153,180] Maintenance therapy, to reduce the risk of morbidity associated with chronic, relapsing disease, should be initiated with lansoprazole 15 mg to 30 mg once daily given the severity of L.F.'s esophagitis and symptomatic recurrence after discontinuing the PPI.

On-Demand Pharmacotherapy

The use of intermittent (on-demand) courses of PPI therapy (2–4 weeks) has been suggested as being potentially beneficial in patients with GERD.[199–204] One trial, which compared continuous maintenance therapy with esomeprazole 20 mg daily versus on-demand therapy with the same drug and dose in patients with healed erosive esophagitis, reported that continuous therapy was superior to on-demand therapy (81% vs. 58%, respectively) in maintaining endoscopic remission at 6 months.[204] The ability to maintain remission with on-demand therapy was reduced as the severity in esophagitis increased. Although numerous studies with a variety of PPIs have demonstrated patient satisfaction with on-demand therapy,[200–203] a systemic review of 17 trials evaluating the use of on-demand therapy indicates that intermittent therapy should only be considered in patients with mild, nonerosive disease.[199]

Combination of a Proton-Pump Inhibitor and Histamine-2 Receptor Antagonists

The addition of an H_2RA at bedtime to a once or twice daily PPI regimen is sometimes used for patients who continue to have nocturnal symptoms, although the evidence to support this combination remains inconclusive and current guidelines do not endorse this type of antisecretory management strategy at this time.[65,153] The rational for this practice is based on evidence that suggests a period of nocturnal acid breakthrough (defined as intragastric pH <4 for longer than 1 hour during the night) in a significant number of patients despite twice-daily PPI therapy, suggesting that histamine release may have an important function in nocturnal acid secretion.[205] One study suggests that the addition of an H_2RA to a twice-daily PPI regimen resulted in a statistically significant reduction in nocturnal acid breakthrough during the sleeping hours.[205] This trial, however, evaluated only a single bedtime dose of an H_2RA and did not consider the tachyphylaxis that can occur with continuous use. A subsequent trial using a twice-daily PPI regimen with continuous use of an H_2RA for 4 weeks demonstrated no difference in nocturnal acid suppression, suggesting that tolerance does play an important role in the use of H_2RAs for this indication.[31] It has been theorized that one way to possibly avoid this occurrence is to use the H_2RA on only an as-needed basis when lifestyle and dietary modifications are not effective for preventing nocturnal symptoms.[7]

Nonerosive Reflux Disease

Up to 75% patients with typical GERD symptoms who undergo endoscopy will not have evidence of esophagitis or complicated disease.[206] These patients are described as having functional heartburn, NERD or ENRD, and often undergo 24-hour ambulatory pH monitoring to determine whether abnormal reflux is present despite a negative endoscopy. A trial of a PPI is usually indicated despite no esophageal findings, as many patients will respond to this therapy.[206] Further medical evaluation is required if a patient does not respond to PPI therapy despite a doubling of the daily dose.

Extraesophageal Manifestations

CASE 27-5

QUESTION 1: S.P. is a 71-year-old retired man who was eating dinner with his wife when he experienced a sudden onset of chest pain described as crushing, burning, and squeezing. His wife notified emergency personnel, who transported S.P. to the emergency department. His past medical history reveals some cardiovascular risk factors, including age, hypertension, hyperlipidemia, and a sedentary lifestyle. His medications before admission include

Section 4 Gastrointestinal Disorders

aspirin 81 mg daily, hydrochlorothiazide 25 mg daily, and atorvastatin 40 mg at bedtime. He also takes OTC famotidine 20 mg daily as needed for dyspepsia. On examination, he complains of substernal crushing chest pain that has lasted more than 1 hour. He is diaphoretic and extremely anxious. He denies any shortness of breath, pain radiating to upper extremities or jaw, or cough. His vital signs include a temperature of 99.1°F, blood pressure of 155/95 mm Hg, and heart rate of 115 beats/minute. Pertinent laboratory results at this time are:

White blood cell (WBC) count, 7,700/μL
Hgb,14.2 g/dL
Hct, 45%
Platelets, 270,000/μL
SCr, 1.1 mg/dL
BUN, 11 mg/dL
Total cholesterol, 161 mg/dL
Low-density lipoprotein, 96 mg/dL
High-density lipoprotein, 30 mg/dL
Triglycerides, 190 mg/dL
Sodium, 141 mEq/L
Potassium, 4.1 mEq/L
Troponin I, 0.3 ng/mL

Electrocardiogram reveals sinus tachycardia with no evidence of ST-segment elevation, depression, or T-wave inversion or new left bundle branch block. Because of S.P.'s cardiovascular risk factors and indeterminate troponin, he underwent immediate diagnostic cardiac catheterization, which showed normal coronary angiography and an ejection fraction of 65%. S.P. was diagnosed with noncardiac chest pain (NCCP). Could S.P.'s chest pain be associated with an extraesophageal manifestation of GERD?

Extraesophageal (atypical) manifestations of GERD are those signs and symptoms that occur outside of the esophagus yet are presumed to be associated with GERD. The extraesophageal manifestations of GERD include NCCP; pulmonary symptoms; and complaints related to the ear, nose, and throat; as well as hypersalivation and dental erosions (Table 27-10). Interestingly, these symptoms are often the only complaint that a patient has when he or she presents to the health care provider.[7,207]

NONCARDIAC CHEST PAIN

About 30% of patients with anginalike chest pain have normal coronary arteries or minimal microvascular disease as demonstrated by cardiac angiography.[208] Up to 60% of these patients will have concomitant GERD as demonstrated by an abnormal esophageal endoscopy or ambulatory pH monitoring.[7,208] The symptoms associated with NCCP are very similar to those associated with cardiac angina. The chest pain is usually described as crushing, squeezing, or burning; retrosternal in location; and with or without lateral radiation to the upper extremities, back, neck, or jaw. The pain is often temporary related to a meal or occurs nocturnally, usually awakening the patient and continuing for hours. The onset of pain may coincide with a reflux episode, and symptoms are often relieved by oral antacid therapy.[7,208] Numerous trials have evaluated the use of acid suppression as a means to treat NCCP once cardiac etiology has been ruled out through appropriate evaluation.[208–210] Meta-analysis and guidelines have suggested the PPI test, in which a short course (4 weeks) of high-dose (twice-daily) PPI is used, is an effective diagnostic tool and is associated with a reduction in costs compared with other diagnostic methods of GERD.[65,209,210] An appropriate workup for coronary artery disease must be performed in all patients presenting with chest pain before considering a GI cause or trial of antireflux therapy.[65,208] This is especially important in women, the elderly, and diabetic patients, as their initial presentation may be similar to GI complaints when in fact an acute coronary syndrome is present.

TABLE 27-10
Atypical Manifestations of Gastroesophageal Reflux Disease[7,207]

Noncardiac Chest Pain	**Pulmonary**
Ear, Nose, and Throat	Chronic cough
Laryngitis/Pharyngitis	Nonallergic, nonseasonal asthma
Hoarseness	Aspiration
Globus sensation	Bronchiectasis/bronchitis
Laryngeal cancer	Sleep apnea
Sinusitis	Idiopathic pulmonary fibrosis
Otitis	Pneumonia
Other	
Hypersalivation	
Dental erosions	

ASTHMA AND GASTROESOPHAGEAL REFLUX DISEASE

GERD may play a role in the pathophysiology of asthma. Reports suggest that concomitant GERD occurs in up to 80% of the asthmatic population.[211] Two theoretical mechanisms exist as to how GERD can potentially exacerbate asthma symptoms. The reflex theory proposes that symptoms result from the direct irritation of the vagus nerve when refluxate comes into contact with the esophageal mucosa, resulting in reflex bronchospasm.[212,213] In contrast, the reflux theory proposes that aspiration of refluxed acid into the lungs causes caustic injury of tissue within the bronchial tree, resulting in asthmatic symptoms.[213,214] Significant controversy exists regarding the benefit of antireflux pharmacotherapy in patients with asthma, especially in those patients who do not endorse typical GERD symptoms. An important meta-analysis of trials that evaluated the effects of antireflux therapy on patients with asthma indicates that asthma symptoms improved in 69% of patients, that the use of asthma medications was reduced by 62%, and that only 26% of the subjects showed improvement in evening peak expiratory flow rate. All other pulmonary function tests showed little or no change with antireflux therapy.[215] However, this meta-analysis only evaluated studies of up to 8 weeks in duration. A more recent trial with esomeprazole 40 mg daily for 3 months demonstrated improvements in pulmonary function tests and a decreased use of short-acting rescue bronchodilators in asthmatics with GERD compared with asthmatics without GERD. One-third of the patients in the GERD group were also able reduce their dose of inhaled corticosteroid and remained stable.[216] Current National Institutes of Health guidelines for the management of asthma suggest that GERD and antireflux therapy be considered in patients with poorly controlled asthma, even if they do not have typical symptoms of GERD.[217] These data have led to the empiric use of PPIs in difficult-to-manage asthmatic patients.[65] However, a large randomized, double-blind trial evaluated esomeprazole 40 mg twice daily versus placebo for 6 months in patients with poorly controlled asthma managed with inhaled corticosteroids, who lacked typical GERD symptoms. Results revealed no benefit in asthma control with the addition of a PPI, despite 40% of the subjects demonstrating GERD by ambulatory pH monitoring.[218] The American Gastroenterological Association position statement accepts the use of an empiric trial of twice-daily PPI for two months in asthmatic patients with a concomitant GERD diagnosis, with the caveat that, if the treatments fails, other causes be explored.[65]

OTOLARYNGOLOGY SYMPTOMS AND GASTROESOPHAGEAL REFLUX DISEASE

GERD is the most common etiologic factor in 60% of patients with chronic laryngitis[219] and in 25% to 50% of patients with a globus sensation (the feeling that something is caught in the throat).[219] Symptoms relating to GERD are responsible for up to 10% of the patients seen by otolaryngologists.[219] The most likely mechanism for the pathophysiology of GERD-related laryngitis is that damage and inflammation occurs at night while the patient is sleeping. It is during this time when upper esophageal sphincter pressures are especially low and the protective or neutralizing mechanisms of cough and salivation are suppressed.[220] This damage may be in addition to injury or laryngeal inflammation sustained from other causes such as excessive voice usage, smoking, chronic throat clearing or cough, vomiting, or injury from endotracheal tubes.[207,221] The extent of injury in GERD-related hoarseness is directly related to the exposure time of the pharyngeal mucosa to the refluxate as well as the pH. Patients with GERD-related hoarseness usually do not have any other GERD-related symptoms.[207] The diagnostic procedure of choice is laryngoscopy and should be considered in all patients presenting with GERD-related hoarseness. Once the diagnosis of GERD-related hoarseness or laryngitis is established, the patient will likely require extended high-dose PPI therapy with the understanding that the majority of patients will relapse within 6 weeks once therapy is discontinued.[222]

TREATMENT OF THE EXTRAESOPHAGEAL MANIFESTATIONS OF GASTROESOPHAGEAL REFLUX DISEASE

Experts suggest that treatment should be initiated with a high-dose (twice-daily) PPI for at least 3 months before considering drug therapy to be ineffective; however, data are lacking to support this recommendation with the exception of noncardiac chest pain.[65] Recent guidelines suggest this empiric strategy is acceptable if concurrent typical GERD symptoms are present.[65] Alternatively, it is possible that GERD may not be the cause of the patient's symptoms.

S.P.'s chest pain is not of cardiac origin based on angiographic findings. Therefore, it is reasonable to presume that he is having an extraesophageal manifestation of GERD. S.P.'s symptoms were meal-related, and he has a history of dyspepsia for which he takes an OTC H_2RA. The H_2RA should be discontinued, and S.P. should be given a trial of empiric twice-daily PPI therapy for a period of 2 to 4 weeks. If symptoms are severe, the use of endoscopy (to determine if esophageal damage is present) or 24-hour esophageal pH monitoring (to correlate reflux events with symptomatic chest pain) is appropriate.

Antireflux Surgery

CASE 27-5, QUESTION 2: S.P. responded well to the trial of omeprazole 40 mg orally twice daily and has not had chest pain in 2 months. He has heard that surgical options exist that may eliminate his need for medications, as they are very expensive for him. Is S.P. a candidate for antireflux surgery?

Numerous surgical and endoscopic procedures exist for patients with GERD. These include, but are not limited to, Nissen fundoplication, Toupet partial fundoplication, Belsey Mark IV repair, and the Hill posterior gastropexy repair, as well as newer endoscopic techniques.[7] The primary goal of these procedures is to restore LES pressure by repairing a hiatal hernia or diaphragmatic hiatus. Appropriate candidates include patients who are in a good health and request another treatment option as a result of poor medication adherence, patients who are unable to afford their medication, patients who suffer from side effects or worry about risks with long-term therapy, patients with extraesophageal symptoms who have responded well to antireflux therapy, or patients experiencing volume regurgitation and aspiration of gastric contents who have not responded to PPI therapy.[7,65,153,189] Despite the availability of these surgical options, the consideration of antireflux surgery is one in which the benefits should be heavily weighed against the risks of such an invasive approach, as these procedures are not without potential complications. The effectiveness of these procedures has been questioned, as many patients will still require drug therapy.[7,65] S.P. has responded well to high-dose PPI therapy for his NCCP, but he describes some financial difficulties with affording his medications. Alternatively, he is 64 years of age, which may increase the risk associated with surgery. S.P. should be referred for further medical evaluation to determine whether he is a candidate for antireflux surgery.

UPPER GASTROINTESTINAL BLEEDING

Upper GI bleeding is a common medical emergency that occurs in up to 160 cases per 100,000 adults annually and is associated with increased morbidity and mortality as well as substantial costs to the health care system.[223,224] Despite advances in endoscopic hemostatic therapy and pharmacotherapy, the mortality rate associated with upper GI bleeding remains at 5% to 15%, which is the same as it has been for the last 20 to 40 years.[3,4,223,224] Upper GI bleeding can be categorized as either variceal or nonvariceal bleeding (see Chapter 29, Complications of End-Stage Liver Disease). Nonvariceal bleeding describes bleeding associated with PUD or stress-related mucosal bleeding (SRMB). Other causes include erosive esophagitis, Mallory-Weiss tear (a tear near the gastroesophageal junction associated with retching or coughing), and malignancy.[5] Although PUD and SRMB are both acid-related disorders, their presentation and pathophysiology differ.

Peptic Ulcer Bleeding

EPIDEMIOLOGY

The majority of upper, nonvariceal GI bleeding is caused by PUD.[4,5,223,224] Bleeding ulcers account for more than 400,000 hospitalizations in the United States each year.[224] As mentioned, the mortality rate for peptic ulcer bleeding can be as high as 15%. It has been suggested that an older presenting patient population (>60 years of age) with a greater number of comorbidities may account for this continued high mortality rate.[3,223–225] Fortunately, the vast majority (80%) of upper GI bleeding events are self-limited and require only minimal intervention.[3] Length of stay has been dramatically reduced in the majority of patients who receive early endoscopy (within 24 hours of admission).[223,224] However, in the 20% to 25% of patients who continue to bleed or rebleed after appropriate intervention, mortality increases to nearly 40%.[5,226]

PATHOPHYSIOLOGY

The most common causes of upper GI bleeding in patients with PUD are NSAID use and *H. pylori* infection.[81] Bleeding occurs when an ulcer extends deeper into the mucosa and erodes the wall of a blood vessel.[227] The incidence of *H. pylori* infection in bleeding ulcers is 15% to 20% lower than in patients with nonbleeding ulcers.[227] Bleeding associated with PUD is generally not caused by the hypersecretion of gastric acid, with the exception of patients with ZES.[227] The pathophysiology and risk factors associated with PUD are described earlier in this chapter (see Peptic Ulcer Disease section).

CLINICAL ASSESSMENT AND DIAGNOSIS

The clinical presentation of a patient with a bleeding peptic ulcer usually includes the presence of melena (dark, tarry stools), which occurs in 20% of patients, hematemesis (vomiting of blood) in 30%, and both in about 50% of patients. Up to 5% of patients present with hematochezia (bloody diarrhea) indicative of rapid and substantial blood loss.[227] The primary step in evaluating the patient is to assess the degree of urgency for rapid medical management.[227] Two validated prognostic scales exist for early risk stratification into high-risk or low-risk for patients presenting with upper GI bleeding. The pre-endoscopy Rockall score and Glasgow-Blatchford score utilize laboratory and clinical characteristics of the patient to assist the clinician in determination of need for and emergent nature of endoscopy in the individual patient.[5,223,224] The complete Rockall score, which includes data from the endoscopy, is used to predict the likelihood of rebleeding after endoscopy and mortality.[5,223,224] Hypovolemia owing to substantial blood loss can rapidly lead to shock. The initial management of these patients should focus on volume resuscitation and improving the patient's hemodynamic status. Clinical features suggestive of high-risk for rebleeding or mortality include patients older than 65 years of age, serious comorbidities (e.g., hepatic or renal dysfunction, cardiac or pulmonary disease), hemodynamic instability (e.g., hypotension, tachycardia), shock, poor health, continued bleeding, mental status changes, and prolonged prothrombin/activated partial thromboplastin time (aPTT) (or elevated international normalized ratio [INR]).[3,5,223,225–229] These patients should immediately be transferred to an intensive care setting.

Most patients should receive early diagnostic endoscopic evaluation within 24 hours of presentation to determine the source of the bleeding, to predict the risk for rebleeding, and, when required, to perform endoscopic interventions directed at stopping the bleeding ulcer and restoring hemostasis.[223,224] Risk of rebleeding may be predicted based on the presenting lesion(s) identified on endoscopy.[5,227] The most common ulcer identified on endoscopy is a clean-base ulcer found in about 42% of patients. This ulcer has a very low risk of rebleeding (5%), and the patient can usually be discharged immediately after recovery from the endoscopy and managed with appropriate antisecretory therapy. Intermediate stigmata of bleeding include lesions identified as flat-spot ulcers and/or adherent clots, which have a risk of rebleeding of 10% and 22%, respectively. Although endoscopic procedures are not usually necessary with flat-spot ulcers, adherent clots remain an area of controversy and usually require the endoscopist to attempt to remove the clot and manage the underlying lesion.[223] Patients identified with high-risk ulceration (nonbleeding visible vessel or active bleeding) will require endoscopic intervention and have a high risk of rebleeding (43% and 55%, respectively) despite intervention. Nonbleeding visible vessel and active bleeding are associated with an 11% mortality on initial presentation.[227] Ulcer size is also predictive of mortality and rebleeding, as ulcers greater than 1 or 2 cm in diameter confer greater risk.[227] Despite appropriate endoscopic hemostasis, approximately 20% of patients with peptic ulcer bleeding will rebleed within 48 to 72 hours after treatment.[5,223,226,227] Mortality associated with rebleeding is about 30% to 37%.[226] Patients undergoing endoscopy should be tested for *H. pylori* infection with biopsy (rapid urease test), as infection with this organism is associated with an increased risk of rebleeding.[223,224] Because false-negatives can occur in the presence of active bleeding, all *H. pylori*–negative patients should have a confirmatory follow-up test with serologic antibody testing on discharge to ensure that the patient is not infected.[223]

TREATMENT

Patients with upper GI bleeding require rapid risk stratification based on the presenting signs and symptoms. Patients with hemodynamic instability require immediate institution of resuscitative measures.[5,223,224,230] IV access should be obtained with two large-bore (e.g., 16 to 18 gauge) catheters to facilitate the administration of fluids and blood products.[5,224] Intravascular volume should initially be replenished with normal saline to prevent the patient from going into hypovolemic shock. During this time, blood can be typed and crossed in the event a transfusion is required. Guidelines recommend the transfusion of packed red blood cells for patients with a hemoglobin level of less than 7 g/dL; however, consideration is warranted in the patient with tachycardia or hypotension and a hemoglobin level of 10 g/dL.[223,224] A nasogastric tube should be placed to allow for lavage and determination of the upper GI tract as the source of the bleed and evaluation of continued bleeding.[5,223,224,230]

Endoscopic evaluation with hemostatic techniques (when required) should be performed as soon as safely possible.[223,224] Endoscopic hemostasis is the cornerstone of management for patients with serious bleeding ulcers, as it reduces the incidence of rebleeding, the need for surgery, and mortality when compared with placebo or drug therapy.[223,224] Endoscopic procedures include thermocoagulation, laser therapy, injection therapy (epinephrine, ethanol, or saline), injection with sclerosing agent, or placement of endoscopic clips. Combining thermocoagulation with injection therapy is superior to either therapy alone and hemoclipping alone in patients with serious ulcer bleeding.[5,223–225] Despite initial hemostasis, however, the potential for rebleeding remains high, especially in patients with high-risk lesions.[5,223–227]

Improvements in hemostatic parameters (e.g., platelet aggregation, inactivation of pepsin, and correction of coagulation) leading to clot stabilization correlate directly with an intragastric pH greater than 6.[224,225,228] Therefore, treatment with an antisecretory drug is beneficial in patients after endoscopy to promote healing of the lesion. After the acute phase, the patient should be placed on appropriate drug therapy to continue healing and prevent ulcer recurrence (see Peptic Ulcer Disease section). Patients who are *H. pylori*–positive should receive appropriate eradication pharmacotherapy and confirmation of eradication at a later time.[223]

HISTAMINE-2 RECEPTOR ANTAGONISTS

Once widely used to manage upper GI bleeding, H_2RAs are now considered inferior to PPIs for reducing the incidence of rebleeding and the need for surgery.[223–225] This is likely related to the inability of H_2RAs to achieve an intragastric pH greater than or equal to 6 (even with continuous IV administration) and the rapid development of tachyphylaxis (especially with high IV doses).[223,225,228,231] Thus, H_2RAs are no longer recommended for the prevention of rebleeding associated with a peptic ulcer.[223,224]

PROTON-PUMP INHIBITORS

PPIs are the drugs of choice to reduce the incidence of PUD-related rebleeding and the need for surgical intervention.[5,223,224,232–234] However, no clinical trials were able to show a mortality benefit with PPIs when entire treatment cohorts were evaluated.[232–234] A Cochrane Collaboration meta-analysis of 24 studies evaluating randomized, controlled trials that compared IV or orally administered PPIs with H_2RAs or placebo showed similar results with a reduction in rebleeding, surgery, and required repeat endoscopic treatment.[232] A more recent update of this meta-analysis with seven additional studies reaffirmed these outcomes.[233] Based on these available data, PPI therapy for peptic ulcer bleeding is superior to H_2RAs and placebo.[223] Although no reduction in the number of deaths were identified when all patients were considered, PPI treatment of patients at the highest risk of mortality, as evidenced by endoscopically determined active bleeding or nonbleeding visible vessel, did impart a mortality benefit.[233] All-cause mortality was also reduced in Asian trials, with a concomitant greater reduction in the incidence of rebleeding and need for surgery than in trials performed elsewhere in the world. This may be explained by the inclusion of a younger patient population, more potent acid suppression because of genetic polymorphism in CYP450 metabolism leading to a slower clearance of PPIs, a lower parietal cell mass, and a greater incidence of *H. pylori* infection.[232]

Despite the data, important questions remain as to the most appropriate dose and route of administration for PPIs in patients with peptic ulcer bleeding. Evidence suggests that most patients with low-to-intermediate risk lesions (clean-base or flat-spot ulcers) and who are hemodynamically stable may be treated with oral PPIs and immediately discharged after endoscopy, as rebleeding is infrequent in this population.[223,232,235] Patients with an adherent clot present a perplexing dilemma for practitioners in that risk of rebleeding and appropriate pharmacotherapy is based on the underlying lesion.[223] However, in patients with higher-risk endoscopic stigmata (e.g., nonbleeding visible vessel or active bleeding), a parenteral PPI should be administered after the endoscopic procedure.[223,224,232–234] Current guidelines suggest an initial IV bolus equivalent to 80 mg of omeprazole followed by a continuous IV infusion of 8 mg/hour of the omeprazole equivalent for 72 hours (although no head-to-head trials of omeprazole equivalence have been performed with pantoprazole or esomeprazole, most clinicians consider them equivalent on a milligram-per-milligram basis).[223–225,228,232–236] Rebleeding is highest during this first 72 hours and is the reason for such high-dose therapy.[223–225,227] However, a systematic review and meta-analysis evaluating seven trials comparing this high-dose strategy versus non-high dose regimens (including both parenteral and oral dosing) failed to demonstrate a statistically significant difference in outcomes related to rebleeding rates, surgical requirements, or mortality after endoscopic management.[237] Despite this data, high-dose IV PPIs remains the recommended treatment of choice in high-risk patients given that the cost of therapy is lower than the incremental expense of managing an extra rebleeding event.[223] Finally, one meta-analysis has also suggested that PPI therapy is associated with reduced blood transfusion requirements.[238] Some patients may be switched to an oral PPI if rapid stabilization occurs, but careful clinical assessment should be performed to ensure the patient is stable.[235] Early initiation of a PPI bolus infusion before endoscopy has been shown to reduce the proportion of patients with active bleeding once endoscopy is performed, reduce the requirements for endoscopy, and reduce hospital stay.[239] However, this strategy should not replace early endoscopic management in high-risk patients, as combination PPI therapy with endoscopic maneuvers have been proven to be more effective than monotherapy with an IV PPI.[223,224,240]

Once the high-risk patient has stabilized and is considered safe for discharge after endoscopy and 72 hours of IV PPI, the patient should be discharged with a prescription for at least once-daily PPI pharmacotherapy for continued healing of the lesion and further prevention of rebleeding.[223] The actual dose and duration, however, should be decided based on the patients severity of disease and identified complications, with more severe disease warranting consideration of twice daily therapy.[223] Patients who are required to remain on cardioprotective aspirin or NSAID therapy may require long-term secondary prophylaxis in an attempt to prevent future upper GI bleeding events.[223]

OTHER AGENTS

The use of somatostatin or octreotide is not recommended for the treatment of patients with nonvariceal upper GI bleeding, as there is no evidence of benefit to support their use.[223,224] However, these agents are commonly used in the management of variceal bleeding (see Chapter 29, Complications of End-Stage Liver Disease).

Stress-Related Mucosal Bleeding

Acute SRMD is a type of erosive gastritis that occurs in critically ill patients with severe physiological stress (e.g., surgery, trauma, organ failure, sepsis, severe burns, neurologic injuries).[236,241–244] The term stress ulcer is a misnomer in that SRMD may range from numerous diffuse superficial erosive mucosal lesions (those that do not penetrate the muscularis mucosa) to major deep ulceration (penetration of the muscularis mucosa and potentially submucosa).[245–246] Initial lesions occur early (<24 hours) and appear as subepithelial petechiae that can develop into superficial erosions and ulcerations.[244,245] Early stress-related mucosal lesions are multiple, usually asymptomatic, without perforation, and commonly bleed from superficial mucosal capillaries.[243,245] The gastric fundus is the most likely anatomical region of the stomach to be involved. Distal lesions involving the gastric antrum and duodenum have also been described, but tend to appear later in the hospital course and are often deeper and associated with a greater probability for bleeding.[245] SRMB from these lesions may be categorized into three distinct types based on clinical presentation.[243–246] Occult (hidden) bleeding is defined as aspirated gastric fluid or stool that is guaiac-positive for the presence of occult blood and without other signs or symptoms. Overt bleeding is defined as frank hemorrhage identified by hematemesis (bloody vomitus or the appearance of coffee grounds in gastric aspirates or vomitus), hematochezia (bloody diarrhea), or melenic stools. Clinically important bleeding or life-threatening bleeding is the presence of overt bleeding that is associated with hemodynamic changes (tachycardia, hypotension, orthostatic changes, or hemoglobin concentration decline of >2 g/dL) and the requirement of transfusion of blood products. Endoscopic therapy is generally not a viable option because of the extensive distribution of lesions associated with SMBD.[241]

EPIDEMIOLOGY

The majority (>75%) of critically ill patients admitted to intensive care units (ICUs) will exhibit mucosal lesions consistent with SRMD within 24 hours of admission.[241,243–246] Only a small percentage (up to 6%) of these patients will progress to clinically important GI bleeding.[243–246] Clinically important SRMB has been associated with an increased length of stay in the ICU by up to 11 days and results in substantial increases in the cost of health care.[241,243–245,247] The mortality of clinically important SRMB approaches 50%, but mortality may also be associated with underlying comorbidities related to the critical illness.[236,244]

PATHOPHYSIOLOGY

Numerous factors have been identified in the pathogenesis of SRMD and resultant bleeding. These include gastric acid and pepsin secretion, disruptions to the normal homeostatic mechanisms that protect the gastric mucosa against the highly acidic environment (decreases in prostaglandin, bicarbonate, and GI mucus formation as well as impaired turnover of gastric epithelium), GI motility disturbances, and mucosal ischemia resulting from decreased blood flow.[241,243,244,246] Gastric acid is likely the central factor associated with development of SRMD.[241,245] Because of the absence of protective defenses, substantial amounts of acid are not required for the formation of lesions, but some acid is required for damage to occur.[246] Although some patients may have increased acid secretion (e.g., sepsis, CNS injuries, small bowel resections), the majority of critically ill patients have normal or decreased acid secretion.[242,245,246] Pepsin secretion is associated with the lysis of clots owing to its proteolytic action on fibrin.[241,248] Gastric prostaglandins play a key role in the cellular defense against gastric acid.[241,246] These prostaglandins are responsible for maintaining the integrity of the mucosal barrier by stimulating mucus and bicarbonate production; regulating blood flow; and, to some degree, inhibition of acid production. Mucosal ischemia secondary to splanchnic hypoperfusion also plays a large role in the pathogenesis of SRMD.[241,243,246] Mucosal ischemia is associated with reduced ability to neutralize hydrogen ions leading to intracellular acidosis within the mucosa and subsequent cell death. These factors all contribute to an imbalance by increasing injurious factors and reducing the protective mechanisms within the gastric fundus.

RISK FACTORS

CASE 27-6

QUESTION 1: J.S., a 58-year-old, 110-kg man was admitted to the medical ICU for severe necrotizing pancreatitis identified on abdominal computed tomography. The patient was immediately made "nothing by mouth" and started on imipenem/cilastatin 1,000 mg IV piggyback (IVPB) every 8 hours. He was given hydromorphone 1 mg IV every 3 hours as needed for pain. He subsequently exhibited shortness of breath on his third day after admission. He required intubation and was placed on a ventilator. A chest x-ray showed a left lower lobe infiltrate suggestive of hospital-acquired pneumonia. Antibiotic coverage was increased with the addition of ciprofloxacin 400 mg IVPB every 12 hours and linezolid 600 mg IV every 12 hours. He has a temperature of 103.5°F, heart rate of 115 beats/minute, and blood pressure of 70/40 mm Hg. Pertinent laboratory results at this time include:

WBC count, 38,000/μL
Hgb, 13.6 g/dL
Hct, 40%
Platelets, 150,000/μL
SCr, 1.3 mg/dL
BUN, 24 mg/dL
INR, 1.0
aPTT, 39 seconds
Aspartate aminotransferase, 292 units/L
Alanine aminotransferase, 305 units/L
Amylase, 508 units/L
Lipase, 624 units/L

In addition to the antimicrobials and initiation of fluid resuscitation, the critical care team is considering stress ulcer prophylaxis. What risk factors does J.S. have (if any) for SRMB, and is he a candidate for stress ulcer prophylaxis?

Numerous risk factors have been associated with SRMB[241–245] (Table 27-11). However, a large landmark, multicenter, prospective study involving more than 2,200 critically ill patients admitted to a medical ICU identified only the requirement of mechanical ventilation (respiratory failure) or coagulopathy as independent risk factors for development of clinically important bleeding.[249] Considering the cost associated with the reduction of risk related to SRMB, the authors concluded that only these two risk factors warrant the use of prophylactic therapy. Because not all risk factors impose the same level of risk, clinical guidelines and most practitioners recommend prophylaxis only when the patient is mechanically ventilated, has a coagulopathy, or when two or more of the remaining risk factors are present[241,242,244] (Table 27-11). J.S.'s risk factors include septic shock as evidenced by hemodynamic instability and mechanical ventilation. Therefore, a prophylactic regimen to reduce the risk of SRMB is appropriate.

TABLE 27-11
Risk Factors for Stress-Related Mucosal Bleeding[241–245]

- Respiratory failure
- Coagulopathy
- Hypotension
- Sepsis
- Hepatic failure
- Acute renal failure
- Enteral feeding
- High-dose corticosteroids[a]
- Organ transplant
- Anticoagulants
- Severe burns (>35% of body surface area)
- Head injury
- Intensive care unit stay >7 days
- History of previous GI hemorrhage

[a] Greater than 250 mg/day hydrocortisone or equivalent.

TREATMENT

CASE 27-6, QUESTION 2: What options exist to prevent SRMB in J.S.?

Not all patients admitted to the critical care unit will require prophylaxis for SRMB. However, because mortality can be high in patients when bleeding occurs, evaluation of risk is of absolute importance to ensure that protective pharmacotherapy is initiated in appropriate patients.[241–246] Because acid is required for mucosal injury, the inhibition of gastric acid is the primary target when pharmacotherapy is used to reduce the risk of SRMB. An intragastric pH greater than 4 is the recommended goal of therapy.[241,236,242–246] Therapeutic options include the use of antacids, sucralfate, H_2RAs, and PPIs (Table 27-12).

ANTACIDS

The use of aggressive antacid therapy is superior to placebo in reducing clinically important SRMB when an intragastric pH greater than 3.5 is maintained.[241,243,244] Although antacids are effective in preventing SRMB, their use has fallen out of favor because of difficult administration regimens (every 1–2 hours) with the continuous requirement of intragastric pH monitoring for dose titration, electrolyte abnormalities (especially in patients with renal dysfunction), diarrhea, constipation, and the potential risk of aspiration pneumonia.[241,243–245] These issues, coupled with the fact that potent acid suppression is available in far more convenient dosage forms have all but eliminated the use of antacids as SRMB prophylaxis.[241]

SUCRALFATE

Sucralfate is effective in preventing SRMB but does not have an important effect on intragastric pH.[250,251] Despite the fact

TABLE 27-12
Stress-Related Mucosal Bleeding Prevention: Regimens and Doses

Agent	Dose and Frequency of Administration	FDA Approval[a]
Antacid	30 mL PO/NG every 1–2 hours	No
Cimetidine	300 mg IV every 6–8 hours or	No
	300 mg IV loading dose, then 50 mg/h continuous IV infusion	Yes
Famotidine	20 mg IV every 12 hours or	No
	1.7 mg/h continuous infusion	No
Ranitidine	50 mg IV every 6–8 hours or	No
	6.25 mg/h continuous infusion	No
Sucralfate	1 g PO/NG every 6 hours	No
Omeprazole	20–40 mg PO/NG[b] every 12–24 hours	No
Omeprazole/sodium bicarbonate powder for oral suspension	40 mg PO/NG initially, followed by 40 mg in 6–8 hours as a loading dose, then 40 mg PO/NG every 24 hours	Yes
Lansoprazole	30 mg PO/NG[b,c] every 12–24 hours	No
Pantoprazole	40 mg IV/PO/NG[b] every12–24 hours	No
Esomeprazole	40 mg IV every 12–24 hours	No

[a] For prevention of stress-related mucosal bleeding.
[b] Extemporaneously compounded in sodium bicarbonate.
[c] Oral disintegrating tablet.
IV, intravenous; NG, by nasogastric tube; PO, by mouth.

that antisecretory therapy is preferred, sucralfate remains an available therapeutic option. Early studies suggested a reduction in nosocomial pneumonia with sucralfate when compared with ranitidine or antacids. However, a subsequent randomized trial involving 1,200 mechanically ventilated patients revealed no increase in pneumonia with H_2RAs when compared with sucralfate or antacids.[252] The usual dose of 1 g four times daily can present problems within the critical care setting because of multiple daily dosing, binding of other drugs, and occlusion of nasogastric tubes (may be reduced with available suspension). Other potential issues include the potential for aluminum toxicity in patients with renal failure, constipation, and electrolyte imbalances. The concomitant use of sucralfate with antisecretory therapy may reduce the effectiveness of sucralfate as an intragastric pH less than 4 is needed for conversion to its active form, which binds to the gastric mucosa.[244]

HISTAMINE-2 RECEPTOR ANTAGONISTS

H_2RAs are effective in preventing SRMB and are the most widely used for this indication.[253,254] Although only cimetidine continuous infusion has been FDA-labeled for the prevention of SRMB, continuous or intermittent infusions of ranitidine and famotidine are most often used for this indication.[241,228,243] Continuous infusions have been suggested as being more effective in maintaining a pH greater than 4, but there are no data comparing these two treatment options with respect to clinical outcomes.[241,245] Despite this, intermittent dosing is used more commonly than continuous infusions for the prophylaxis of SRMB.[228,243,253,254]

Numerous meta-analyses have evaluated the effectiveness of H_2RAs for prophylaxis of SRMB.[255,256] Cook et al. reviewed 63 randomized trials and determined that prophylaxis with H_2RAs was associated with a statistically significant reduction in overt and clinically important upper GI bleeding when compared with no therapy and a significant reduction in overt bleeding when compared with antacids.[255] A trend toward reduced clinically important bleeding was identified when H_2RAs were compared with sucralfate, but this was not statistically significant. In another meta-analysis, ranitidine was shown to be of no benefit in preventing SRMB and increased the risk of pneumonia.[256] However, neither of these meta-analyses included the large study involving 1,200 mechanically ventilated patients that compared sucralfate, ranitidine, and placebo.[252] Despite these conflicting results, H_2RAs remain a recommended option for the prophylaxis of SMRB.[253,254] One shortcoming of H_2RAs is that tolerance may develop (within 72 hours) and thus theoretically lead to potential prophylaxis failure.[231] H_2RAs are eliminated renally, and dosage reductions may be required in patients with renal failure.

PROTON-PUMP INHIBITORS

PPIs, because of their profound ability to inhibit gastric acid secretion and lack of tolerance to their antisecretory effect, would appear to be the preferred option for preventing SRMB. However, there is very little evidence to confirm their clinical superiority to H_2RAs for this indication. Numerous studies have compared PPIs with H_2RAs or placebo in critically ill patients in small populations using varied predetermined end points.[244,257] These studies suggest that PPIs provide greater acid suppression compared with H_2RAs and are likely to be as effective in preventing SRMB.[244,257] One study in 359 critically ill patients evaluated the use of immediate-release omeprazole suspension in bicarbonate given via nasogastric tube at a dose of 40 mg for two doses, then 40 mg/day versus IV cimetidine given as a 300 mg bolus and then infused at 50 mg/hour (dosing was adjusted for patients with renal dysfunction).[258] The results indicate that the PPI-bicarbonate suspension was associated with a greater mean time of intragastric pH greater than 4 than the cimetidine infusion but that the rate of clinically important bleeding did not differ between cimetidine (6.8%) and omeprazole (4.5%). The FDA considered the immediate-release omeprazole-bicarbonate suspension to be noninferior to cimetidine for the prevention of SRMB.[259] An extremely important analysis aimed at identifying the most appropriate dose for IV PPIs in SMRB prophylaxis was performed in more than 200 critically ill patients.[260] This analysis included five different dosing approaches of IV pantoprazole intermittent infusions (40 mg given every 8, 12, or 24 hours or 80 mg given every 12 or 24 hours) compared with cimetidine given as a 300-mg IV bolus immediately followed by a 50 mg/hour continuous infusion. The patients received a minimum of 48 hours of therapy with a maximum of 7 days. In all the study arms, pH control was achieved (defined as intragastric pH ≥4), however in all the pantoprazole arms pH control continued

TABLE 27-13
Alternative Proton-Pump Inhibitor Administration Options[244,259,262]

	Omeprazole	Lansoprazole	Pantoprazole	Esomeprazole	Rabeprazole	Dexlansoprazole
Capsule granules sprinkled on selected soft foods (i.e., applesauce)		✓[a]		✓[a]		✓[a]
Capsule granules mixed in water and flushed down NG tube				✓		
Capsule granules mixed in juice (can be administered via NG tube if required)	✓[a]	✓[a]		✓[a]		
Extemporaneous compound of PPI in bicarbonate for NG tube	✓	✓	✓			
Package for oral suspension	✓[a,b]	✓[a,c]				
Oral disintegrating tablet		✓[a]				
IV formulation	Not available in the United States	Removed from US market	✓[a]	✓[a]		

[a] Labeled by the FDA for this administration option.
[b] Omeprazole suspensions available in 20-mg and 40-mg packets with bicarbonate (1680 mg); both contain same amount of bicarbonate, and two 20-mg packets cannot be substituted for one 40-mg packet.
[c] Not to be administered via NG tube, as occlusion of tube is possible.
IV, intravenous; NG, nasogastric; PPI, proton-pump inhibitor.

to improve from day 1 to 2, whereas a decline was noted in the cimetidine group, suggesting the occurrence of tachyphylaxis. No upper GI bleeding was noted in any patient during the trial regardless of treatment group assigned. The conclusions of this study demonstrate that patients may have adequate pH control with an initial IV dose of pantoprazole 80 mg followed by 40 mg IV every 12 hours. Finally, a recent meta-analysis that included seven studies evaluating the efficacy and safety of PPIs compared with H_2RAs demonstrated no statistically significant difference between the two options with respect to the important endpoints of overt or clinically important bleeding, mortality or incidence of pneumonia.[257]

The incidence of nosocomial pneumonia in patients receiving PPI therapy in the critical care setting has been evaluated. A 22-month observational study in 80 patients receiving either omeprazole or ranitidine did not find a difference in the rates of nosocomial pneumonia between the two groups, thus suggesting rates may be equivalent.[261] Numerous alternative administration options exist for patients in the critical care setting who cannot take medications by mouth, have nasogastric tubes in place, or have difficulty swallowing[244,259,262] (Table 27-13). PPIs are becoming first-line therapy for the prevention of SRMB, but additional studies are needed to confirm the most effective dose and route of administration in order to obtain optimal clinical outcomes in patients at risk of SRMB.[243,253] The use of early enteral tube nutrition that is initiated within 48 hours of admission to the ICU has also been evaluated as a means of prophylaxis against SMRB.[263] This was demonstrated in a meta-analysis of 17 studies which suggested that patients who require enteral tube feedings may not require additional forms of SRMB prophylaxis and may also have a reduced risk of pneumonia or death when compared with patients receiving an H_2RA-based SMRB prophylaxis regimen.[263] This meta-analysis, however, was only hypothesis-generating and should be interpreted with care until a large controlled study is available to confirm these findings.

MONITORING

CASE 27-6, QUESTION 3: J.S. has been started on famotidine 20 mg IV every 12 hours. How should this pharmacotherapy be monitored for safety and efficacy?

The famotidine dose should be adjusted to maintain an intragastric pH greater than 4 and should be based on severity of the patient's illness, renal function, and intragastric pH measurements. The intragastric pH can be determined with an indwelling probe or by measuring the pH of nasogastric aspirates. The patient should be monitored for signs of bleeding (e.g., presence of blood or coffee-ground material in nasogastric aspirates, hematemesis, hematochezia, or melena), hypotension, reductions in hemoglobin or hematocrit, and thrombocytopenia.

CASE 27-6, QUESTION 4: During the next 6 days, J.S. improves and is subsequently removed from mechanical ventilation and transferred to the medical ward. He is now able to eat normally. Should J.S. be continued on SRMD prophylaxis?

Patients receiving prophylaxis for SRMB should be evaluated for the continued presence of risk factors. As the patient improves, the risk factors should in turn be reversed, and the need for SMRB prophylaxis should diminish. Factors such as extubation, correction of coagulopathies, discharge from the intensive care setting, and the ability to take oral feeding advocate the discontinuation of prophylaxis. Numerous studies have suggested that up to 54% of patients were ordered SRMD prophylaxis outside the ICU setting and without a compelling indication.[264] Erstad and colleagues surveyed 153 institutions within the United States and found that in 65% of the hospitals, more than 25% of patients remained on SRMB prophylaxis after discharge from the ICU.[265] This can lead to increased costs, the potential of the patient being discharged on medication for which there is no indication, and future potential adverse effects from the medication.[264] Because J.S. does not possess any risk factors for SRMB, the famotidine should be discontinued at this time.

KEY REFERENCES

A full list of references for this chapter can be found at http://thepoint.lww.com/AT10e. Below are the key references for this chapter, with the corresponding reference number in this chapter found in parentheses after the reference.

Key References

Abraham NS et al. ACCF/ACG/AHA 2010 expert consensus document on the concomitant use of proton pump inhibitors and thienopyridines: a focused update of the ACCF/ACG/AHA 2008 expert consensus document on reducing the gastrointestinal risks of antiplatelet therapy and NSAID use: a report of the American College of Cardiology Foundation Task Force on Expert Consensus Documents. *Am J Gastroenterol*. 2010;105:2533. (56)

Ali T, Harty RF. Stress-induced ulcer bleeding in critically ill patients. *Gastroenterol Clin N Am*. 2009;38:245. (241)

Armstrong D, Sifrim D. New pharmacologic approaches in gastroesophageal reflux disease. *Gastroenterol Clin N Am*. 2010;39:393. (152)

Barkun AN et al. International consensus recommendations on the management of patients with nonvariceal upper gastrointestinal bleeding. *Ann Intern Med*. 2010;152:101. (223)

Chey WD et al. American College of Gastroenterology guideline on the management of *Helicobacter pylori* infection. *Am J Gastroenterol*. 2007;102:1808. (83)

DeVault KR et al. Updated guidelines for the diagnosis and treatment of gastroesophageal reflux disease. *Am J Gastroenterol* 2005;100:190. (153)

Gisbert JP et al. Sequential therapy for *Helicobacter pylori* eradication: a critical review. *J Clin Gastroenterol*. 2010;44:313. (108)

Kahrilas PJ et al. American Gastroenterological Association Medical Position Statement on Management of gastroesophageal reflux disease. *Gastroenterology*. 2008;135:1383. (65)

Lanza FL et al. Guidelines for prevention of NSAID-related ulcer complications. *Am J Gastroenterol*. 2009;104:728. (90)

Napolitano L. Refractory peptic ulcer disease. *Gastroenterol Clin N Am*. 2009;38:267. (129)

[No authors listed]. ASHP therapeutic guidelines on stress ulcer prophylaxis. ASHP Commission on Therapeutics and approved by the ASHP Board of Directors on November 14, 1998. *Am J Health Syst Pharm*. 1999;56:347. (242)

O'Connor A et al. Treatment of *Helicobacter pylori* infection 2010. *Helicobacter*. 2010;15(Suppl 1):46. (107)

Scarpignato C, Hunt RH. Nonsteroidal antiinflammatory drug-related injury to the gastrointestinal tract: clinical picture, pathogenesis and prevention. *Gastroenterol Clin N Am*. 2010;39:433. (89)

Tytgat GN et al. New algorithm for the treatment of gastro-oesophageal reflux disease. *Aliment Pharmacol Ther*. 2008;27:249. (180)

Yang YX, Metz DC. Safety of proton pump inhibitor exposure. *Gastroenterology*. 2010;139:1115. (58)

Lower Gastrointestinal Disorders

28

Geoffrey C. Wall

CORE PRINCIPLES

	CHAPTER CASES
INFLAMMATORY BOWEL DISEASE	
1 Inflammatory bowel disease (IBD) is a generic classification for a group of chronic, idiopathic, relapsing inflammatory disorders of the gastrointestinal tract. Symptoms of IBD are thought to result from dysregulation of the mucosal immune system. By convention, IBD is divided into two major disorders, ulcerative colitis (UC) and Crohn's disease (CD).	**Cases 28-1, 28-2, 28-3**
2 Ulcerative colitis (UC) is an inflammatory condition of the large intestine, but it can cause disturbances in other organ systems. It is typified by abdominal pain, chronic loose bloody stools, and fatigue.	**Case 28-1 (Question 1)**
3 Crohn's disease usually causes significant diarrhea without frank blood, abdominal pain, and weight loss. Extraintestinal symptoms such as skin lesions, arthralgias, and ocular inflammation occur more commonly with CD than UC. CD can affect any part of the gastrointestinal tract, but small and large bowel involvement is most common.	**Case 28-3 (Question 1)**
4 Treatment for both UC and CD are divided into two areas: induction treatment, which controls symptoms, and maintenance treatment, which prevents recurrences. Specific agents used for induction in UC depend on the extent of disease, but corticosteroids are often used for this purpose.	**Case 28-1 (Question 3)**
5 Topically applied agents (suppositories, foams, enemas), specifically mesalamine products (5-aminosalicylic acid), are effective for induction in UC confined to the rectum (proctitis) or the distal colon.	**Case 28-1 (Question 6)**
6 Long-term use of corticosteroids for treatment of both UC and CD is not effective and can result in serious adverse effects; thus, other agents should be used for maintenance of remission.	**Case 28-1 (Questions 7, 12)**
7 Corticosteroids are used most often for induction in CD patients. Agents such as azathioprine, infliximab, or other agents are used to maintain remission.	**Case 28-3 (Questions 2, 3)**
8 Tumor necrosis factor blocking agents such as infliximab are used in patients who do not respond to less aggressive therapy, including azathioprine. These agents have a high acquisition cost and carry significant risks for developing infections. However, clinical trials have shown that they are generally more effective than other therapies.	**Case 28-3 (Question 6)**
IRRITABLE BOWEL SYNDROME	
1 Irritable bowel syndrome (IBS) is a common and often debilitating condition that involves abdominal pain and bloating associated with a change in bowel habits (usually constipation or diarrhea). It does not significantly affect patient mortality but is often associated with significant morbidity.	**Case 28-4 (Question 1)**

continued

IRRITABLE BOWEL SYNDROME *CONTINUED*

2	Treatment for IBS is based on the predominant symptoms of the patient. For constipation-predominant symptoms (IBS-C), an increase in dietary fiber is recommended, followed by laxatives and then lubiprostone.	**Case 28-4 (Questions 3, 4)**
3	Treatment for diarrhea-predominant IBS (IBS-D) includes antimotility agents such as loperamide. Pain and bloating associated with IBS (mixed IBS or IBS-M) may respond to antispasmodic agents such as hyoscyamine, low-dose tricyclic antidepressants, or selective serotonin reuptake inhibitors.	**Case 28-5 (Questions 1, 2)**

OVERVIEW OF INFLAMMATORY BOWEL DISEASE

Definition and Epidemiology

Inflammatory bowel disease (IBD) is a generic classification for a group of chronic, idiopathic, relapsing inflammatory disorders of the gastrointestinal (GI) tract. IBD is common in developed countries.[1] It is estimated that more than 1.4 million persons in the United States have IBD, and the prevalence of these disorders ranges from 20 to 200 per 100,000 people; however, the prevalence of IBD may actually be greater because many affected patients may be asymptomatic or have mild symptoms for which they do not seek medical attention.[2] By convention, IBD is divided into two major disorders: ulcerative colitis (UC) and Crohn's disease (CD).[1,3]

For visuals of the bowel changes in Crohn's disease and the mucosal changes in ulcerative colitis, see http://thepoint.lww.com/AT10e.

However, approximately 10% to 15% of patients with IBD have symptoms that defy this schema.[4] Both UC and CD frequently affect a similar group of patients (Table 28-1).[2,5] Whites appear to have a higher incidence of IBD compared with Asians or blacks. In particular, Jews of European descent may have up to a fourfold increase in the incidence of IBD. Studies have found trends toward an increased incidence of IBD in urban compared with rural communities. Hypotheses for this trend include overcrowding, exposure to infectious agents, and lifestyle differences. Although both UC and CD are generally considered diseases of the young, with peak incidences from ages 20 to 40 years, about 15% of IBD cases are diagnosed in patients older than 60 years.[6] There seems to be no significant sex preference for IBD.

TABLE 28-1
Population Characteristics of Patients at High Risk for Inflammatory Bowel Disease Development[25]

Peaks between ages of 15 and 30 years
European ancestry
Urban greater than rural dwellers
Caucasian race greater than non-Caucasians
Jewish patients living in Europe and North America greater than non-Jewish patients
Occurs in familial clusters
NOD-2 gene

Etiology

The true cause of IBD is unclear; however, hypotheses for these disorders include a combination of genetic abnormalities, chronic infection, environmental factors (bacterial, viral, and dietary antigens), host or intestinal microbiome interactions, and other abnormalities of immunoregulatory mechanisms.[1] Whatever the mechanism, it is now generally agreed that the symptoms of IBD result from dysregulation of the mucosal immune system. The role of genetics has been strongly supported by epidemiologic studies, showing familial aggregation, consistent ethnic differences, and an increased concordance rate in monozygotic twins. Patients with a first-degree relative with IBD are at an increased risk of developing the disorder, with a frequency of up to 40%. Detailed mapping of the Human Genome Project has led to genetic studies showing a number of associations with IBD, including the *NOD2/CARD15* gene, and an increased susceptibility to ileal and ileocolonic disease in CD.[7] Other gene abnormalities associated with IBD include *ATG16L1*, the immunity-related guanosine triphosphate hydrolase M protein (IRGM), and chemokine receptor 6 (CCR6).[5] The presence of these genetic markers is associated with a variety of complex immune system functions, including alterations in mucosal T-cell and B-cell function and deregulation of cytokine release. Some genetic associations are more specific for CD than for UC, but using genetic testing as an aid to diagnosing patients with indeterminate colitis is not currently recommended. A number of environmental exposures have been associated with IBD. Smoking has been the most consistent and most studied environmental factor associated with IBD. Interestingly, the effects of smoking are different between UC and CD, with smokers having a decreased risk of developing UC but an increased risk for CD.[8] Use of nonsteroidal anti-inflammatory drugs (NSAIDs) has been associated with exacerbation of IBD, and use of these drugs is usually not recommended in patients with active disease.[9]

Debated for decades, the theory of an infectious etiology for IBD remains appealing. Murine models of colitis have shown a decreased development of IBD in a microbefree environment.[1] Repeated exposure of the GI tract to a particular micro-organism may trigger the immune dysregulation evident in this disease. However, some investigators believe that normal intestinal flora may be a catalyst for IBD. As mentioned previously, patients may be genetically predisposed to mucosal immune dysregulation, and either normal flora or bacterial pathogens may trigger the inflammatory response that leads to IBD. At various times, common intestinal organisms such as *Escherichia coli* and unusual bacteria such as *Mycobacterium paratuberculosis* have been investigated as causes of IBD, but no causal relationship has yet been found.[10] Clinically, antibiotics have a minor role in the treatment of IBD.

Pathogenesis

Under normal conditions, the mucosal immune system interacts with luminal antigens and mucosal bacteria on a continuous basis to maintain a state of controlled inflammation. As might be expected, the GI tract is exposed to an extremely high number of antigenic substances daily, including commensal flora, and a delicate balance must exist for the system to operate properly. In IBD, genetic predisposition leads to immune response dysfunction, and an autoimmune cascade occurs. Thus, proinflammatory cytokines in the gut trigger an "attack" on the colonic mucosa by leukocytes and other factors, leading to edema, ulceration, and destruction of the tissue. Normal immune regulators fail to halt this process, and the disease progresses. This can be attributable to a lack of regulatory or suppressor cells, an enhanced numbers of T cells, or both. For example, the T-cell immune response is Th1 dominated, which is manifested by an increased production of interferon and tumor necrosis factor, which promotes macrophage activation and development of delayed-type hypersensitivity response. Recently, Th17 cells were identified as a new subset of T-helper cells that may play a role in the autoimmune dysregulation associated with UC.[11] Studies have demonstrated that this increase of proinflammatory cytokines, chemokines, prostaglandin, and reactive oxygen species leads to increased inflammation and tissue destruction.[1]

TABLE 28-2

Pathophysiological Differences Between Ulcerative Colitis and Crohn's Disease[1–3,14,16]

Characteristic	Ulcerative Colitis	Crohn's Disease
Incidence (per year)	6–12/100,000	5–7/100,000
Anatomical location	Colon and rectum	Mouth to anus
Distribution	Continuous, diffuse, mucosal	Segmental, focal, transmural
Bowel wall	Shortened, loss of haustral markings, generally not thickened	Rigid, thick, edematous, and fibrotic
Gross rectal bleeding	Common	Infrequent
Crypt abscesses	Common	Infrequent
Fissuring with sinus formation	Absent	Common
Noncaseating granulomas	Absent	Common
Strictures	Absent	Common
Abdominal mass	Absent	Common
Abdominal pain	Infrequent	Common
Toxic megacolon	Occasional	Rare
Bowel carcinoma	Greatly increased	Slightly increased

Clinical Presentation

ULCERATIVE COLITIS

UC usually presents as a shallow, continuous inflammation of the colon ranging from limited forms of proctitis (rectal involvement only) to disease involving the entire colon. Crypt abscesses consisting of accumulations of polymorphonuclear neutrophil (PMN) cells, necrosis of the epithelium, edema, hemorrhage, and surrounding accumulations of chronic inflammatory cells are typical in UC.[12] Fistulas, fissures, abscesses, and small bowel involvement are not present. The inflammation is limited to the mucosa, which presents as friable, granular, and erythematous, with or without ulceration. Most patients with UC experience a chronic, intermittent course of disease. Chronic, loose, bloody stools are the most common symptom of UC.[3,12] Other common complaints include tenesmus (urge to defecate) and abdominal pain. Patients with pancolitis usually have more severe symptoms than those with disease limited to the rectum. Mild UC is defined as fewer than four stools a day, no systemic signs of toxicity, and a normal erythrocyte sedimentation rate (ESR). Moderate disease is characterized by more than four stools a day but minimal evidence of systemic toxicity. Severe disease is defined as more than six bloody stools a day, fever, tachycardia, anemia, or an ESR greater than 30.[13,14] Proctitis is usually considered a separate type of UC for treatment purposes. Constipation can occasionally be the presenting symptom with proctitis. Relapses and remissions are common in UC, with up to 70% of patients with active disease relapsing within 1 year after induction treatment.

CROHN'S DISEASE

CD is a chronic, transmural, patchy, granulomatous, inflammatory disease that can involve the entire GI tract, from mouth to anus, with discontinuous ulceration (so-called skip lesions), fistula formation, and perianal involvement. The degree of colonic involvement is variable; however, the terminal ileum is most commonly affected. Intestinal involvement is characteristically segmented and can be interrupted by areas of normal tissue. Unlike UC, the severity of the disease does not correlate directly with the extent of bowel involvement. Patients usually present with one of three patterns of disease: predominantly inflammatory, stricturing, or fistulizing. These patterns are the primary determinants of the disease course and the nature of complications.[13] The inflammatory infiltrate is made up of T and B lymphocytes, macrophages, and plasma cells.

The disease course of CD is variable. Years of frequent relapses may be followed by complete remission. Patients with IBD often require surgery to control symptoms. For patients with UC, surgery is often curative. In contrast, in patients with CD, the frequency of recurrent disease after surgery is high and anatomically correlates with the original pattern of the disease.[15]

Patients usually present with abdominal pain and chronic, often nocturnal, diarrhea.[16] Weight loss, low-grade fever, and fatigue are also common. Features such as abdominal masses or abscesses and fistulae (abnormal communications between two organs) can make management of CD difficult and often require surgical intervention. Fistulizing disease is particularly difficult to treat and is the source of significant morbidity in CD patients. Enterocutaneous and enterorectal fistulae are common, but other types, such as enterovaginal, can occur. Fistulae can be excruciatingly painful, can be a source of infection, and can also exert significant psychosocial distress. Other similarities and differences in the pathophysiology of these disease states are outlined in Table 28-2.[1,3,13] Extraintestinal manifestations of IBD that can cause significant morbidity include reactive arthritis, uveitis, ankylosing spondylitis, pyoderma gangrenosum, and primary sclerosing cholangitis. Although their incidence varies, many of the extraintestinal manifestations of UC and CD are similar, as summarized in Table 28-3.[17] A careful patient history, physical examination, and endoscopic and radiologic studies are necessary to determine the severity of IBD. Laboratory studies such as an increased ESR or C-reactive protein can also aid in the diagnosis, but no single marker is pathognomic. Recently, researchers have examined the utility of certain serologic markers (usually antibodies to flora such as *Saccharomyces cerevisiae* or glycans such as laminaribioside) that seem to have a fairly high specificity for either UC or CD.[18] Some experts have advocated routine use of such markers to aid in diagnosis of UC or CD, to help classify patients with indeterminate endoscopic or histologic findings, or to predict disease course.[19] However, such testing is not yet considered standard of care, and its actual role remains largely undefined in management guidelines. Defining the

TABLE 28-3
Extraintestinal Complications of Ulcerative Colitis and Crohn's Disease

Manifestation	Ulcerative Colitis (%)	Crohn's Disease (%)
Acute arthropathy		
Type 1: Associated with flare of gastrointestinal symptoms	35	29
Type 2: Independent of gastrointestinal symptoms	24	20
Erythema nodosum	20	20
Pyoderma gangrenosum	1	2–3
Iritis/uveitis	4–12	4–12
Ankylosing spondylitis	1–3	3–5
Sacroiliitis	9–11	9–11
Primary sclerosing cholangitis	5–10	1
Metabolic bone disease	20–40	30–50

Source: Ardizzone S et al. Extraintestinal manifestations of inflammatory bowel disease. *Dig Liver Dis.* 2008;40(Suppl 2):S253.

severity of CD is a difficult, yet important, step in successful treatment. Current guidelines from the American College of Gastroenterology define mild-to-moderate CD as ambulatory patients who are able to tolerate oral feeding without signs of systemic toxicity. Moderate-to-severe disease is defined as patients with symptoms of fever, weight loss, abdominal pain, nausea and vomiting, or significant anemia. Severe fulminant disease refers to patients with persistent symptoms despite standard induction regimens or those with signs of severe systemic toxicity.[16]

Treatment

When considering IBD therapy, one must appreciate that the cause of the disease is unknown and, therefore, precludes definitive therapy. In addition, specific therapy depends on the anatomical location of the disease. Other factors to take into consideration are coexisting medical conditions, patient perception of quality of life, medication adherence behavior, lifestyle (e.g., smoking), dietary factors, and patient's knowledge of the disease.

With the advent of newer treatments for IBD, aggressive goals of therapy should be considered. These would include (a) complete relief from symptoms (induction and maintenance of remission); (b) improving quality of life; (c) maintaining adequate nutritional status; (d) relieving intestinal inflammation, dysfunction, and the development of cancer; and (e) reducing the need for surgery or chronic corticosteroid use.[20] Additionally, with the advent of biologic therapy, many experts believe that complete mucosal healing is an attainable goal in IBD that has been correlated with improvement in clinical status.

Most drug therapies for IBD have been tested for both UC and CD (Table 28-4). It is important to differentiate therapy used for acute exacerbations from those used to maintain remission.

AMINOSALICYLATES

Aminosalicylates were the first class of drugs to show benefits in IBD. The prototypical agent is sulfasalazine, which is composed of sulfapyridine (a sulfonamide antibiotic) linked by an azo bond to 5-aminosalicylic acid (5-ASA). The former moiety acts as a carrier to transport 5-ASA past its primary absorption site in the upper intestine. Later, cleavage of the azo bond by lower intestinal bacteria releases 5-ASA (the active moiety) for localized action in the colon. Systemic absorption of the sulfapyridine is responsible for most of the drug's adverse effects, but contributes nothing to the therapeutic benefit.

A significant number of patients discontinue this medication because of dose-dependent adverse effects, including nausea, vomiting, headache, alopecia, and anorexia. Other idiosyncratic adverse effects include hypersensitivity rash, hemolytic anemia, hepatitis, agranulocytosis, pancreatitis, and male infertility. This poor adverse effect profile has led to the development of safer sulfafree compounds that contain only 5-ASA. Techniques to decrease systemic absorption and maximize local delivery of 5-ASA to the lower bowel include creating pH-dependent materials to delay drug dissolution and developing hybrid or dimer molecules of 5-ASA that are activated by gut bacteria (Table 28-5). Various synonyms and generic names have been assigned to these 5-ASA derivatives, including aminosalicylate, mesalamine, and mesalazine (in Europe). Mesalamine products have been developed for both oral and rectal administration. Administration of mesalamine by retention enemas or suppositories is significantly more effective in the treatment of active distal colitis than placebo and is recommended as the preferred treatment of ulcerative proctitis.[21] Significant efficacy advantages of any 5-ASA drug versus another have not been demonstrated. Combination oral and rectal therapy for ulcerative proctitis may be superior to either modality alone.[21] 5-ASA suppositories are indicated for proctitis, whereas enema formulations can be useful in IBD confined to the distal colon. With the exception of abdominal pain, cramps, and discomfort, rectally administered mesalamine is well tolerated. Enemas or suppositories should be administered in the evening. The oral 5-ASA agents are effective in inducing remission in mild-to-moderate UC and for maintaining remission in UC and perhaps for mild CD confined to the colon. Recent studies have confirmed that higher doses rather than proprietary delivery system of mesalamine are associated with improved response.[22] One study examined a 6-week course of high-dose (4.8 g daily) Asacol tablets versus standard-dose therapy (2.4 g daily).[23] The primary efficacy outcome was overall improvement defined as complete remission or response to therapy from baseline to week 6. This outcome was achieved by 57% of patients taking 2.4 g/day and 72% of patients given 4.8 g/day ($p = 0.0384$). Both regimens were well tolerated. The primary problems with achieving a higher dose of 5-ASA are the cost and the significant pill burden, which makes adherence difficult. New higher-dose formulations of 5-ASA (e.g., Lialda®) decrease the daily pill burden but are expensive. Adverse effects of the oral 5-ASA compounds include diarrhea, headache, arthralgias, abdominal pain, and nausea. Interstitial nephritis has rarely been reported with chronic use of mesalamine, but the association remains controversial. An important drug interaction is the possibility of increasing 6-mercaptopurine levels in patients receiving balsalazide.[24]

CORTICOSTEROIDS

Corticosteroids are the most commonly used agents in the treatment of acute flares in patients with moderate-to-severe IBD.[25] The anti-inflammatory actions of corticosteroids are well known, but how these translate into their full mechanism of controlling IBD is not completely understood. First-line treatment for moderate-to-severe active IBD includes doses of corticosteroid equivalent to 40 to 60 mg of prednisone.[26] Data are insufficient to demonstrate any difference between single versus divided oral doses or continuous versus intermittent bolus intravenous (IV) administration. IV doses should be equivalent to hydrocortisone 300 mg/day or methylprednisolone 40 to 60 mg/day. Although corticosteroids are effective for inducing remission in many cases of IBD, up to 50% of patients may not respond (steroid resistant)

TABLE 28-4
Pharmacotherapy for Inflammatory Bowel Disease[12–14,16]

Drug	Indication	Dose	Adverse Reactions	Comment
Sulfasalazine	UC: mild-to-moderate maintenance CD: limited role	See Table 28-5	N/V, diarrhea, HA, rash, myelosuppression	High ADR rate has caused use to decline
Mesalamine	UC: mild-to-moderate induction/maintenance CD: limited role	See Table 28-5	N/V, diarrhea, HA, abdominal pain	Topical forms effective for proctitis and distal UC
Olsalazine	As above	See Table 28-5	As above, diarrhea common	
Balsalazide	As above	See Table 28-5	As above	
Corticosteroids	UC: mild-to-severe induction CD: mild-to-severe induction	Various	Hyperglycemia, CNS excitation, immunosuppression, osteoporosis, cataracts	Goal should be avoiding chronic use in UC and CD
Budesonide	UC: limited role CD: mild-to-moderate induction/maintenance	9 mg daily	As above for corticosteroids, probably less short-term effects	Long-term use may still cause chronic corticosteroid ADRs
6-MP/azathioprine	UC: mild-to-severe maintenance CD: mild-to-severe maintenance	6-MP: 0.75–1.5 mg/kg/d Azathioprine: 1.5–2.5 mg/kg/d	N/V, diarrhea, HA, rash, myelosuppression (esp. neutropenia), pancreatitis	Pharmacogenomic guided testing now commonly performed prior to initiating drug
Methotrexate	UC: limited role CD: mild-to-moderate induction/maintenance	25 mg IM/SQ weekly induction dose, then 15 mg weekly for maintenance	N/V, stomatitis, hepatotoxicity, pulmonary fibrosis	Usually reserved for patients who have failed 6-MP/azathioprine
Infliximab	UC: moderate-to-severe induction/maintenance CD: moderate-to-severe induction/maintenance (fistulizing disease)	5 mg/kg IV at weeks 0, 2, and 6, then every 8 weeks thereafter	Infusion reactions (acute and delayed), immunosuppression, reactivation of latent infection (TB, hepatitis B, histoplasmosis), may worsen neuromuscular disease and congestive heart failure	Probable small increase in lymphoma Scheduled treatment preferred to episodic treatment to maintain response and decrease delayed infusion reactions
Adalimumab	CD: moderate-to-severe induction/maintenance Loss of response to infliximab	160 mg SQ day 1, 80 mg SQ day 14, then 40 mg SQ every other week	As with infliximab, injection site reactions	Can be self-administered by patients, often used if infliximab is not effective or well tolerated
Certolizumab	CD: moderate-to-severe induction/maintenance	400 mg at weeks 0, 2, and 4. If response occurs, follow with 400 mg every 4 weeks	As with infliximab, injection site reactions	Not approved for patient self-administration

ADR, adverse drug reaction; CD, Crohn's disease; CNS, central nervous system; HA, headache; IM, intramuscularly; IV, intravenously; N/V, nausea/vomiting; 6-MP, 6-mercaptopurine; SQ, subcutaneously; TB, tuberculosis; UC, ulcerative colitis.

or will be steroid-dependent at 1 year.[25] Additionally, rates of mucosal healing with these drugs are less than those with other modalities.[27] This combined with the significant adverse effects of corticosteroids argue against their long-term use in IBD, and practice guidelines reflect this recommendation.[14,16]

Topical steroids (enemas, foams, and suppositories) are beneficial for distal colitis and can serve as an adjunct in patients with rectal disease who also have more proximal disease and have failed topical 5-ASA therapy.[21] Selection of dosage form is based on extent of disease similarly to topical 5-ASA therapy. Corticosteroids are absorbed to a significant extent from the rectum and, with long-term use, can cause adrenal suppression. Oral enteric-coated budesonide is approved for the treatment of CD. Budesonide possesses a high degree of topical anti-inflammatory activity with low systemic bioavailability.[28] The Entocort EC formulation of budesonide delivers drug primarily to the ileum and ascending colon. It was believed that these factors would make budesonide more effective than traditional corticosteroids, while decreasing systemic side effects. Current data suggest that budesonide may be as effective as or slightly less effective than traditional corticosteroids in active CD.[29] Short-term corticosteroid-associated adverse effects may be less than with traditional agents, and its use up to 1 year seems to be well tolerated.[30] Compared with traditional corticosteroids, budesonide has a number of potential drug interactions owing to its metabolism via the cytochrome P-450–3A4 system.[31] Studies suggest that budesonide is as effective as traditional corticosteroids for the treatment of mild-to-moderate CD localized to the right colon or ileum, and recent guidelines identify budesonide as the preferred agent in this situation.[32]

IMMUNOMODULATORS

Azathioprine (AZA) and 6-mercaptopurine (6-MP) are commonly used for the management of corticosteroid-dependent and quiescent IBD. AZA is converted to 6-MP, which is then metabolized to thioinosinic acid, the active agent that inhibits purine ribonucleotide synthesis and cell proliferation. It also alters the immune response by inhibiting natural killer cell activity and suppressing cytotoxic T-cell function. AZA (2–2.5 mg/kg/day) and 6-MP (1–1.5 mg/kg/day) are used in the treatment of active UC and CD in patients whose conditions have not responded to systemic steroids.[14,16] These drugs are also used as maintenance therapy for both UC and CD and may be used as "steroid-sparing" agents in patients unable to be weaned from corticosteroids.[33] Because of the long onset of action of 6-MP and AZA, many clinicians prefer to induce remission with corticosteroids and

TABLE 28-5
Comparison of Aminosalicylate Compounds

Generic (Trade)	Delivery System	Intestinal Site of Release	Usual Dose and Frequency
Balsalazide (Colazal)	Bacterial cleavage of azo bond	Colon	750 mg PO TID
Mesalamine (Apriso)	Polymer matrix/enteric coating that dissolves at pH 6	Ileum (distal), colon	1,500 mg PO every day
Mesalamine (Asacol, Asacol HD)	pH-dependent coating (Eudragit S) dissolves at pH ≥7	Ileum (distal), colon	800 mg PO TID
Mesalamine (Lialda)	Multi-matrix (pH-sensitive coating and delayed-release)	Ileum (distal), colon	2.4–4.8 g PO every day
Mesalamine (Pentasa)	Controlled-release microspheres	Duodenum, jejunum, ileum, colon	1 g PO QID
Mesalamine (Rowasa)	Direct topical therapy	Rectum (supp)	500 mg PR every day–BID
		Descending colon/rectum (enema)	4 g/60 mL enema PR at bedtime
Olsalazine (Dipentum)	Bacterial cleavage of azo bond	Colon	500 mg PO BID
Sulfasalazine (Azulfidine)	Bacterial cleavage of azo bond	Colon	Initially 500 mg PO BID; increase to 1 g PO TID–QID

BID, twice daily; PO, orally; PR, per rectum; QID, four times daily; TID, three times daily; supp, suppository.
Reprinted with permission from Fernandez-Becker NQ, Moss AC. Improving delivery of aminosalicylates in ulcerative colitis: effect on patient outcomes. *Drugs.* 2008;68:1089; *Drug Facts and Comparisons.* Drug Facts and Comparisons 4.0 [on-line] 2010. Available from Wolters Kluwer Health Inc. Accessed January 27, 2011.

use these agents for maintaining remission. Adverse effects of 6-MP and AZA include rash, nausea, pancreatitis, and diarrhea. Myelosuppression, especially neutropenia, may have a delayed onset, and clinicians should monitor the complete blood count monthly for the first 3 months of treatment, then every 3 months thereafter. Neutropenia necessitating discontinuation of therapy occurs in approximately 10% of patients. Pharmacogenomic testing of these drugs to avoid the development of serious adverse effects is gaining popularity with clinicians despite a lack of controlled data supporting its use (see below). Despite previous concerns, it appears these agents do not increase the risk of developing lymphoma.[34]

Methotrexate (MTX), a folate antagonist, impairs DNA synthesis. MTX appears to be ineffective for induction or maintenance of UC.[35] However, data suggest that MTX (15–25 mg intramuscular [IM] weekly) may have a role for both initial and chronic treatment of CD. The onset and degree of effect is comparable to that with 6-MP and AZA.[36] Most experts and recent guidelines suggest reserving MTX use for patients with CD intolerant of, or refractory to, 6-MP or AZA treatment.[16] Adverse effects with MTX include stomatitis, neutropenia, nausea, hypersensitivity pneumonitis, alopecia, and hepatotoxicity. MTX-induced nausea and stomatitis may be prevented by the addition of folic acid 1 mg orally (PO) daily. Some data suggest that even the risk of hepatotoxicity may be ameliorated by folate use.[37]

Cyclosporine (CSA), which selectively inhibits T-cell–mediated responses, has been used to treat severe, acute UC.[38] Because of serious adverse effects, CSA is usually reserved for patients with severe UC refractory to corticosteroids. A randomized controlled trial found equal efficacy (about 85% response) with a 2-mg/kg daily IV dose compared with the standard 4-mg/kg dose.[39] The emergence of the tumor necrosis factor drugs for IBD has caused CSA use for this indication to decline. Current guidelines do recommend this drug as a second-line medical therapy for severe colitis not responding to corticosteroids, but warn of its numerous adverse effects.

ANTI-TUMOR NECROSIS FACTOR AGENTS

INFLIXIMAB

Infliximab is a recombinant chimeric monoclonal antibody that binds to human tumor necrosis factor (TNF) α and neutralizes its biological activity by binding with high affinity to both soluble cell receptors and free TNF-α in the blood. Infliximab is indicated for a broad spectrum of IBD patients. This includes inducing and maintaining remission in patients with moderate-to-severe active CD.[40]

Infliximab is also largely the only effective medical therapy for healing CD fistulae, with data showing that chronic treatment can maintain fistula closure and decrease the need for surgery.[41] Infliximab received an indication for the induction and maintenance of moderate-to-severe UC refractory to other treatments.[42] For all indications, infliximab is given as a 5-mg/kg IV infusion for 2 hours. An induction regimen, administered at 0, 2, and 6 weeks, is followed by a maintenance infusion every 8 weeks. Some clinicians will increase the dose to 10 mg/kg in patients experiencing a loss of response. The response to infliximab is usually rapid, often occurring within several days, and can be dramatic in up to 60% of patients. However, loss of effectiveness is particularly problematic in some patients, and research is ongoing to determine its cause and prevention.[43] Because infliximab is a monoclonal antibody, a number of immunologic-mediated adverse effects are associated with therapy. Antibodies to infliximab have been detected in up to 60% of CD patients using the drug, and emerging data suggest that patients who develop these antibodies may be at more risk not only for infusion reactions but also for reduced efficacy with time.[44] Immediate infusion-related reactions such as fever, chills, pruritus, urticaria, and (rarely) severe cardiopulmonary symptoms can occur in about 1% of patients. Delayed hypersensitivity reactions resembling serum sickness and severe pulmonary symptoms are rarely reported and are more common in patients receiving episodic (rather than scheduled maintenance) treatment.[45] Infectious complications, including pneumonia, cellulitis, sepsis, cholecystitis, endophthalmitis, furunculosis, and reactivation of tuberculosis and histoplasmosis, have also been reported in 2% to 6% of patients.[46] Tubercular infections, including reactivation of latent disease, are a particular concern with infliximab, and patients should be appropriately screened for latent disease before starting infliximab treatment.[47] Patients who have latent tuberculosis (usually identified by a positive tuberculin test) must start antitubercular treatment before use of infliximab can be considered. Patients with active tuberculosis should not receive the drug. Numerous case reports of reactivation of hepatitis B have also been published, and some experts recommend a serum hepatitis screen before therapy with infliximab begins.[48] Lupuslike symptoms, such as arthralgias, have been seen rarely and usually resolve after discontinuation of the drug. Patients with serious active infections, a history of chronic infections, a history of a neural demyelinating disorder, or severe heart failure should avoid infliximab treatment.[16] The latter two cautions are because of previous reports of exacerbations of multiple sclerosis and heart failure when patients with those diseases received anti-TNF-α therapy.

OTHER BIOLOGICAL THERAPIES

Success with infliximab in IBD has led scientists to develop and test other biological therapies designed to either block proinflammatory mediators or enhance anti-inflammatory mediators in the gut. To date, three other biologic agents are approved in the United States for the treatment of moderate-to-severe CD: the humanized α4-integrin antibody natalizumab, the fully humanized anti-TNF-α antibody adalimumab, and pegylated humanized Fab′ fragments against TNF-α (certolizumab pegol). Two randomized controlled trials have found that natalizumab may be beneficial for induction and maintenance of remission in a small subset of patients, but at the increased risk of developing progressive multifocal leukoencephalopathy, a potentially fatal adverse effect.[49] Natalizumab is approved for inducing and maintaining remission in adults with moderate-to-severe CD who have had an inadequate response to or are unable to tolerate conventional therapies. Patients should not be on concomitant immunosuppressive therapies and need to be enrolled in a mandatory patient registry to receive the drug. Adalimumab is approved for the treatment of moderate-to-severe CD and may be particularly useful in patients with an attenuated response to infliximab.[50] Clinical studies have suggested a roughly equivalent symptom response between adalimumab and infliximab, and because the former drug is also a potent TNF-α blocker, similar safety concerns and adverse effects have been shown between the two agents.[40] One potential advantage of adalimumab is its ability to be self-administered subcutaneously by patients. Certolizumab contains only the antibody receptor for TNF-α bound to polyethylene glycol to increase its duration in the body. Like the other biologic agents discussed, it is effective in both inducing and maintaining remission in CD.[51] Infectious and other adverse effects have been reported in clinical trials that are similar to other TNF-α blockers. The precise place in therapy of the newer biologic agents for CD is controversial. Most experts consider infliximab the biologic agent of first choice with the other agents reserved for a loss or lack of efficacy or adverse effects.[52] Recent data highlight the controversy surrounding the placement of biologic agents in the treatment algorithm of CD. One trial found that initial therapy with infliximab with or without AZA therapy was superior to AZA alone in inducing remission as well as causing mucosal healing.[53] Findings such as these have prompted experts to advocate initial therapy with biologic drugs in high-risk patients with moderate-to-severe CD ("top-down" therapy) rather than initiation after other agents have failed.

ANTIBIOTICS

Because an infectious etiology has been proposed for IBD, it stands to reason that antibiotics may have some utility.[3] However, most studies evaluating antibiotics have shown little benefit with the exception of metronidazole in perianal or perhaps postoperative CD.[54] Adverse effects with chronic, high-dose metronidazole include metallic taste and peripheral neuropathy, which is common. Metronidazole may also be used for gastrointestinal infections, particularly *Clostridium difficile* associated disease.[55]

NUTRITIONAL THERAPIES

Nutritional therapies for IBD have been used because dietary intraluminal antigens may stimulate a mucosal immune response.[3] Patients with active CD respond to bowel rest, total parenteral nutrition (TPN), or total enteral nutrition. Enteral nutrition, with elemental or peptide-based preparation, appears to be as efficacious as TPN, without its associated complications. Unfortunately, poor compliance often limits this modality. Such therapy is used more commonly in the pediatric population with mild-to-moderate CD.[56]

SUPPORTIVE THERAPY

Symptomatic management of IBD is important to the patient's quality of life. This includes pain relief and diarrhea control. Loperamide or diphenoxylate-atropine may be used to treat mild symptoms provided obstruction or toxicity is not evident.[57] Severe worsening of symptoms and abdominal distension may indicate toxic megacolon caused by the inability to empty rapidly produced secretory products of the bowel. Patients should be monitored for iron and vitamin B_{12} deficiencies, especially if ileal involvement is extensive or resection has been performed.

SURGERY

Surgery is indicated in the treatment of UC when the patient (a) fails to respond to medical management acutely or chronically, (b) experiences uncontrollable drug-related complications, (c) experiences impaired quality of life from the disease or its drug therapy, (d) has complications of a severe attack (perforation, acute dilation), (e) fails to grow and develop at a normal rate, or (f) exhibits carcinoma of the rectum or colon.[14,58]

In addition, patients who have had UC for longer than 10 years or who demonstrate premalignant changes on rectal biopsy may be managed surgically as a prophylactic measure against colonic carcinoma.

Generally accepted indications for surgical intervention in patients with CD include failure of medical management, incapacitation because of the disease or its drug therapy, retarded growth and development in children, intestinal obstruction, fistula formation, abscess formation, toxic megacolon, perforation and hemorrhage, and carcinoma.[16] Despite advances in medical treatment of CD, surgical intervention is common in these patients.

ULCERATIVE COLITIS

Pathophysiology and Clinical Presentation

CASE 28-1

QUESTION 1: C.M., a 25-year-old female college student, has had episodic, watery diarrhea and colicky abdominal pain relieved by defecation for the past 9 months. Eight weeks before admission, the diarrhea increased to 3 to 5 semiformed stools daily. The frequency of the stools gradually increased to 5 to 10 times a day 1 week ago. At that time, C.M. noted bright red blood in the stools. Stool frequency has now increased to 10 to 15 per day, although the volume of each stool is estimated to be only "one-half cupful." She feels a great urgency to defecate, even though the volume is small. She has not traveled outside the United States, has not been camping, and has not taken any antibiotics within the past 6 months. She has no known medication allergies, and takes only occasional over-the-counter acetaminophen for body aches or headaches.

C.M. complains of anorexia and a 10-pound weight loss during the past 2 months. For the past 4 months, she has had intermittent swelling, warmth, and tenderness of the

left knee, which is unassociated with trauma. She denies any skin rashes or any difficulties with her vision. A review of other body systems and social and family history are largely noncontributory; however, her mother does have a history of postmenopausal osteoporosis.

C.M. appears to be a slightly anxious and tired young woman of normal body habitus. She is 158 cm tall and weighs 51 kg. Her temperature is 100°F; her pulse rate is 100 beats/minute and regular. Physical examination is normal, except for evidence of acute arthritis of the left knee and tenderness of the left lower abdomen to palpation.

Stool examination shows a watery effluent that contains numerous red and white cells with no trophozoites. Stool cultures and an amebiasis indirect hemagglutination test are negative. Other laboratory values include the following results:

Hematocrit (Hct), 32%
Hemoglobin (Hgb), 8.5 g/dL
White blood cell (WBC) count, 15,000/μL with 82% PMNs
ESR, 70 mm/hour
Serum albumin, 2.4 g/dL
Alanine aminotransferase (ALT), 35 U/mL

Sigmoidoscopy showed evidence of granular, edematous, and friable mucosa with continuous ulcerations extending from the anus throughout the colon. What is the most likely cause of C.M.'s diarrheal illness, and what is the evidence for this?

C.M.'s presentation is typical of a patient with new-onset UC. Drug-induced (pseudomembranous colitis) and infectious (parasitic) causes of diarrhea have been ruled out by history (no travel outside the United States, no recent camping, no antibiotic use) and stool examination. As discussed previously, UC is an inflammation of the mucosal layer of the colon and rectum.[1] Characteristically, the inflammation does not extend beyond the submucosa, and transmural ulcers are rare. On examination, the mucosa appears erythematous and is friable. Differentiation from CD is made by endoscopic and radiologic evidence of continuous distribution of pathologic disease (as opposed to segmental), as well as the anatomical location (confined to colon and rectum).

C.M. presents with the classic triad of UC clinical symptoms: chronic diarrhea, rectal bleeding, and abdominal pain. The diarrhea is secondary to the decreased colonic absorption of water and electrolytes and diminished colonic segmental contractions that normally serve to decrease the flow of bowel content. A good indication of the severity of the patient's disease is the volume of stool passed per day.[14] As the severity of the disease increases, incontinence and nocturnal diarrhea commonly occur. Diarrhea can vary in severity from three to four bowel movements daily to one to two bowel movements per hour. The stools are usually soft, mushy, formed, and often contain small amounts of mucus mixed with blood, although in patients with mild, early involvement, blood and mucus may be totally absent. In addition to the diarrhea, the malabsorption of water and electrolytes causes dehydration, weight loss (as observed in C.M.), and electrolyte disturbances.

C.M.'s rectal bleeding is secondary to colonic mucosal erosions and occurs in most patients with UC. Generally, bright red blood mixed in the stools indicates a colonic origin, whereas blood-streaked stools indicate an anal or rectal origin. The anemia associated with UC is generally secondary to this rectal bleeding. It presents as a hemorrhagic or iron-deficiency anemia, depending on the acuteness of the bleeding. Hemoglobin and hematocrit laboratory values often are decreased as in C.M.'s case. Chronic inflammatory disease–induced hypoalbuminemia is often exacerbated by malnutrition.

C.M.'s abdominal pain and cramping are caused by spasm of the irritated and inflamed colon. This abdominal pain is commonly associated with urgency to defecate. As illustrated by C.M., the pain is usually relieved with defecation, even though the stool volume may be small.

C.M.'s arthritis and elevated ALT are indicative of the extraintestinal manifestations that occur in IBD (Table 28-3).[59] Her nonspecific symptoms (i.e., anorexia, fatigue, weight loss, anxiety, tachycardia) could become profound during an exacerbation of UC. Fever, leukocytosis, and increased ESR are also systemic manifestations of an inflammatory disease. Rehydration is important to assure fluid balance and maintain good renal function. Given her anemia (Hgb of 8.5%), tachycardia, and elevated ESR, and her having more than six bloody stools daily, C.M.'s disease would be classified as severe.

CASE 28-1, QUESTION 2: How should C.M.'s diarrhea be managed?

Treatment of the diarrhea associated with UC is often difficult. In patients with mild-to-moderate disease, antidiarrheals, such as loperamide or diphenoxylate with atropine, may help minimize chronic diarrhea. Extreme caution must be used, however, especially in patients with severe disease because of the chance of inducing toxic megacolon, a life-threatening condition and medical emergency. For this reason, antidiarrheals are best avoided in patients with severe active disease and, if used, should be titrated according to the volume of stool produced. Bulk-forming agents, such as psyllium, may be helpful for patients suffering from constipation caused by ulcerative proctitis.[60] Given the risk of toxic megacolon, standard antidiarrheals should be avoided at this time, and C.M. should be treated with anti-inflammatory agents aimed at symptom remission.

Remission Induction

CORTICOSTEROIDS

CASE 28-1, QUESTION 3: What agents can be used to induce disease remission in C.M.?

Corticosteroids are the most effective agents to induce remission of acute, severe exacerbations of UC. Clinical improvement or remission occurs in 45% to 90% of patients taking 15 to 60 mg/day of prednisone, with an increased response at 40 to 60 mg/day.[25] However, corticosteroids are not beneficial for maintaining remission. One strategy to minimize adverse effects of therapy with corticosteroids includes well-defined tapering regimens. Once improvement has occurred, prednisone is tapered by 5 to 10 mg/week until the dose is 15 to 20 mg/day. The dosage is then tapered by 2.5 to 5 mg/week until the drug is discontinued. Unfortunately, a subset of patients will experience a disease flare if the corticosteroid dosage is decreased or tapered too quickly. IV corticosteroids are an important option, especially in patients who have poor oral intake. Patients with active distal disease can be treated with hydrocortisone enemas; however, 5-ASA topical therapy is equivalent or more effective. Other medications that could be considered for induction of remission would include cyclosporine and infliximab. Because of cost and safety issues with these agents, they should probably be considered only in fulminant disease or in those who have failed corticosteroids.[61]

CASE 28-1, QUESTION 4: Methylprednisolone at a dosage of 40 mg IV every 6 hours is ordered. What are the treatment goals for C.M.?

The goal of parenteral corticosteroid therapy for C.M. should be to achieve a rapid therapeutic response as measured by decreased frequency of stools, decreased pain, and decreased fever and heart rate. This goal may be attained with a high initial dose followed by a gradual dosage reduction to minimize the development of corticosteroid adverse reactions. The initial dose, as well as the rate of a subsequent dosage reduction, should be individualized on the basis of the severity of the patient's signs, symptoms, and disease course.

Poorly nourished patients in whom oral intake is expected to be absent for more than 7 days should receive parenteral nutrition, and treatment should be continued until oral feeding is tolerated.[62] An adequate response is defined as resolution of fever, improved patient well-being, no tachycardia, and less abdominal tenderness on palpation. Diarrhea is usually considered to be resolved with four or fewer bowel movements daily. Stools are rarely formed at this stage, but macroscopic bleeding has stopped. Patients can then receive oral prednisone, a 5-ASA drug, and a light diet. If the patient does not respond within 72 hours of starting high-dose corticosteroids, infliximab or surgery may be indicated. Once C.M.'s symptoms are controlled, the goal should be to switch to oral corticosteroids and discharge her from the hospital.

ORAL ADMINISTRATION

CASE 28-1, QUESTION 5: C.M. is responding well to methylprednisolone. She is afebrile, her abdominal pain is reduced (to a score of 5 on a 1–10 scale), and her diarrhea is decreasing. When is the oral route of corticosteroid administration indicated in UC? What are the most appropriate dosages?

Oral corticosteroids are effective for the initial treatment of mild-to-moderate acute UC.[26] In addition, they should be substituted for parenteral corticosteroids once a satisfactory initial response of more severe exacerbations has been achieved. Forty milligrams daily of prednisone was significantly more efficacious than 20 mg/day in controlling ambulatory patients with moderately severe acute UC, but prednisone doses of 60 mg/day had no additional therapeutic value, while causing more adverse effects.[14] In addition, a single 40-mg morning dose of prednisone was as effective as and more convenient than an equivalent divided dose (10 mg four times a day [QID]). Therefore, the initial dose of corticosteroid for a patient with moderately severe acute UC is 40 mg of prednisone or its equivalent administered once daily in the morning.

TOPICAL ADMINISTRATION

CASE 28-1, QUESTION 6: What if C.M.'s UC was limited to the distal colon or rectum? Would topical corticosteroids be indicated? When should other topical agents be considered for C.M.?

Topically administered 5-ASA and corticosteroids, in the form of suppositories, foams, and retention enemas, are effective in the management of acute, mild-to-moderate UC that is limited to the distal colon and rectum.[21] To justify the use of such a difficult route of administration, a clear-cut advantage of either increased efficacy or decreased side effects compared with other administration routes for these agents must be demonstrated.

Theoretically, 5-ASA and corticosteroids administered via this topical route provide a higher concentration of drug to the diseased mucosal area, exerting a local anti-inflammatory effect while minimizing systemic side effects. Unfortunately, variable but significant systemic absorption (up to 90%) and adrenal suppression occur from the topical administration of corticosteroid to the rectum and distal colon.[63] Therefore, the beneficial effects produced by topical use of these agents may accrue from both systemic and local effects. The apparent and relatively low incidence of corticosteroid side effects associated with topical administration may be related to the low doses used and to the infrequent administration (daily to twice daily) needed to control mild acute UC.

5-ASA suppositories and enemas are preferred over topical corticosteroids for the treatment of distal UC and proctitis because they produce higher remission rates in proctitis and effectively maintain remission of distal UC.[64] For distal UC, therapy is initiated with a nightly enema (4 g of mesalamine), and the response should be evaluated in 3 to 4 weeks. If remission is attained, therapy can be tapered to one enema every third night. Simultaneous therapy with oral plus topical mesalamine showed greater efficacy than either alone in achieving remission of distal UC.[21] Administrating one suppository of 5-ASA twice daily for 3 to 6 weeks is generally sufficient to induce disease remission in patients with mild acute proctitis. Improvement should be seen in 2 to 3 weeks, and therapy should be maintained until complete remission is achieved. Therapy can then be tapered to one suppository or enema, two to three times weekly. If topical corticosteroids are to be used to manage mild, acute UC, the corticosteroid of choice would be the one with the lowest absorptive characteristics. Unfortunately, no trials have compared the absorption characteristics of all corticosteroids available for administration by this route. Assuming C.M. did have severe distal colitis, systemic corticosteroids (methylprednisolone 40 mg IV every 6 hours or, if tolerated, prednisone 40 mg daily, for 7 to 10 days) would be a reasonable induction agent with topical 5-ASA agents for maintenance of remission.

ADVERSE EFFECTS

CASE 28-1, QUESTION 7: What particular corticosteroid adverse effects should the clinician monitor in C.M.?

Corticosteroid side effects and precautions for use often limit the therapeutic effectiveness of these agents and should never be overlooked.[25] Certain glucocorticoid adverse effects are of particular importance in patients with IBD in that they may mimic, mask, or intensify symptoms and complications of this disease. For example, the symptoms of one of the major complications of intestinal perforation, peritonitis, may be masked by corticosteroids. Other deleterious effects of corticosteroids include hyperglycemia, avascular necrosis, cataract formation, and central nervous system effects, including mood disorders, insomnia, psychoses, and euphoria.

Patients with IBD are at risk for decreased bone mineral density, which is exacerbated by prolonged use of corticosteroids.[65] This is an often-overlooked side effect of these drugs. One study suggested that even budesonide, with its low overall bioavailability, causes this adverse effect.[66] Thus, calcium, vitamin D supplements, and possibly bisphosphonates (e.g., alendronate 35 mg weekly) are recommended to minimize metabolic demineralization in all IBD patients taking corticosteroids for longer than 3 months.[67] Given the patient's family history (a mother with osteoporosis) and given her high risk of bone loss, the alendronate regimen listed above with 1,500 mg daily of calcium and 800 international units of vitamin D intake should be initiated.

receive the seasonal influenza vaccine as well as the 23-valent pneumococcal polysaccharide vaccine and the hepatitis B vaccine. Many patients with IBD would also be candidates for the human papilloma virus vaccine, and given the increased incidence of abnormal Papanicolaou tests in this population, this would be a reasonable strategy.[84]

Surgical Intervention

CASE 28-2

QUESTION 1: J.K. is a 49-year-old man who has had UC for 22 years. His disease is fairly well controlled with mesalamine tablets 800 mg PO TID. He has not had any UC flares for more than 5 years. He underwent a colonoscopy 1 week ago for routine cancer screening. Pathology results from this procedure indicate premetaplastic lesions in several areas of his colon. What are C.K.'s medical and surgical options for treatment of these lesions?

Of the various therapeutic modalities available for the management of UC, surgery is the most definitive form of therapy in that it is curative in most instances.[85] Because the lesions in UC are generally localized and continuous, colectomy will remove the primary focus of the disease. It will also eliminate both extraintestinal and local complications of UC in most patients. In addition, patients may require further surgery for anastomotic leaks, intraperitoneal abscesses, adhesions, obstruction, stomal ileitis, and mechanical problems associated with the ileostomy. Patient acceptability of ileostomies is poor, and major psychological adjustments are required of patients and their families.[86] Patients must be given support and educated with regard to the care of their ileostomies; this includes the prevention and management of common skin problems as well as control of odor and leakage of the effluent. In certain cases, an alternative to the presence of a stoma is an ileal pouch–anal anastomosis (IPAA). The IPAA procedure involves removal of the entire colon and rectum with preservation of the anus and sphincter muscles. A pouch from the end of the small intestine is formed surgically and is attached directly to the anus. This procedure is becoming increasingly common in UC patients requiring total colectomy.[87] Although it preserves some semblance of normal bowel function, the IPAA procedure has its own complications, in particular, pouchitis (inflammation of the pouch), which can cause symptoms very much like an UC flare.[88] Therefore, even though UC can be cured by surgery, it is indicated only after all reasonable nonsurgical forms of therapy have been exhausted. Considering the degree of inflammatory damage that occurs in colonic tissue, it is probably not surprising that the risk for colon cancer is elevated in patients with UC. Surveillance colonoscopies are recommended on a regular basis (usually every 1–2 years after the patient has had the disease 10 years) to screen for precancerous lesions.[66] If dysplastic lesions are detected, as they have been in J.K., surgical resection is usually considered the treatment of choice. Thus, even in patients with well-controlled UC, surgery may be required for cancer prevention.

CROHN'S DISEASE

Pathophysiology and Clinical Presentation

CASE 28-3

QUESTION 1: J.P., a 30-year-old man, was well until 18 days ago when he experienced crampy right lower quadrant abdominal pain associated with an increased frequency of semiformed stools (four to five per day). The pain was episodic at first, exacerbated by meals, and somewhat relieved by defecation. During this time, J.P. experienced anorexia and a 10-pound weight loss. He denied any change in vision, joint pain, or the appearance of skin rashes. He has not traveled outside the United States or taken antibiotics recently.

Physical examination is essentially normal, except for soft, loose, watery stools that are streaked with fat and positive for occult blood. The abdomen is tender on palpation of the right lower quadrant. Vital signs include a temperature of 37.8°C, pulse of 100 beats/minute, and blood pressure of 135/75 mm Hg. He is 180 cm and weighs 80 kg. Pertinent laboratory values include the following:

Hct, 28%
Hgb, 9 g/dL
WBC count, 14.0 × 10^9/L
ESR, 60 mm/hour

Results of sigmoidoscopy and rectal biopsy are negative. Stool cultures and toxin studies for *C. difficile* are negative, as is the examination for signs of trophozoites. A barium enema shows an edematous ileocecal valve and a terminal ileum that has a nodular irregularity of the mucosa. Follow-up colonoscopy reveals a cobblestone-appearing terminal ileum with areas of normal tissue separated by diseased mucosa. Which of J.P.'s signs, symptoms, and laboratory data are consistent with CD? Describe the pathophysiological basis for J.P.'s clinical presentation.

J.P., like most patients with CD, presents with the classic symptom triad of abdominal pain, diarrhea, and weight loss.[16] His most frequent symptom is right lower quadrant abdominal pain, which is secondary to an indolent inflammatory process in the ileocecal area. Diarrhea is also a characteristic symptom; however, in contrast to UC, the stools are usually partly formed, and gross blood is generally not visible. If the disease is limited to the colon, the diarrhea may be of the same quality and quantity as that associated with UC. If the disease is limited to the ileum, as it appears to be with J.P., the diarrhea is generally moderate, with four to six stools daily. If ileal involvement is significant, bile salt malabsorption may occur, resulting in steatorrhea. Weight loss may be pronounced in patients with long-standing CD because of anorexia and malabsorption. Additionally, vitamin deficiencies, including vitamin B_{12} and vitamin D, are more common in CD patients than control subjects.[89]

Rectal bleeding often occurs in patients with CD, particularly those with colonic involvement, although it is not as common as that associated with UC. Slow blood loss may occur in patients with disease limited to the small intestine, which may cause occult blood-positive feces and, eventually, anemia, as illustrated by J.P. Massive hemorrhage is usually a late complication of CD and is generally caused by transmural ulceration and subsequent erosion into a major blood vessel.

J.P.'s leukocytosis and increased ESR demonstrate that, like UC, CD is a systemic disease. Extraintestinal manifestations such as arthritis, liver disease, and skin rash occur in CD with the same frequency as UC. However, some types of extraintestinal disease appear to be more common in UC (e.g., primary biliary cirrhosis) than CD (e.g., pyoderma gangrenosum).[90]

Most patients with CD have recurrent, symptomatic episodes of pain and diarrhea with gradual progression of their disease to shorter and shorter asymptomatic periods. Although the clinical course is generally progressive, 10% of patients will remain essentially asymptomatic after a few acute episodes.[91] Other patients may only manifest a slight fever for years until a late complication of the disease, such as fistula formation, develops. Alternatively, CD may be rapidly progressive.

Remission Induction

CASE 28-3, QUESTION 2: What agents can be used to induce a remission of J.P.'s CD?

Because the clinical course of CD varies among patients, the management of this disease must be individualized. The anatomical location of the disease is also an important determinant of therapy. Most investigations evaluating the treatment of acute symptomatic CD have ignored this factor and are therefore difficult to assess or compare.

CORTICOSTEROIDS

Corticosteroids are the most widely used therapeutic agents for the treatment of active, symptomatic CD.[16,25] A systematic review of the literature confirms that steroids have a valuable role in remission induction.[63] Landmark studies have demonstrated that approximately 60% to 80% of patients with active CD will respond to a course of corticosteroids.[25] These agents seem to be particularly effective in ileal and ileocolonic disease and can induce remission in even moderate-to-severe CD. Budesonide is recommended in current CD guidelines for active mild-to-moderate ileocolonic CD.[16]

5-AMINOSALICYLIC ACID

Although previously used extensively for mild-to-moderate CD, current trial data and expert opinion have limited the role of 5-ASA drugs to mild active colonic CD. A large meta-analysis comparing 5-ASA (Pentasa) versus placebo found a small and probably clinically insignificant treatment benefit.[92]

OTHER INDUCTION AGENTS

The immunomodulators AZA, 6-MP, and MTX have an onset of action of weeks to months and are not usually appropriate therapy alone for treatment of a CD flare. Infliximab is effective as a treatment for both active and quiescent disease. It can be used alone owing to its rapid onset. A recent landmark study found that early aggressive use of infliximab, with or without AZA, was associated with both corticosteroidfree clinical remission as well as mucosal healing in patients with moderate-to-severe CD.[53] This general approach to treatment (known as a "top-down" strategy) is currently being debated by experts in IBD. Certainly the added expense and risk of using biologics earlier in this population needs to be weighed against the possibility of longer periods of remission and avoidance of surgery. An additional concern is reports of hepatosplenic T-cell lymphoma in young men receiving both AZA or 6-MP with or without concomitant infliximab, which is usually fatal.[93] An algorithm for the treatment of CD is depicted in Figure 28-2.

Remission Maintenance

CASE 28-3, QUESTION 3: After 4 weeks of prednisone 40 mg daily, J.P. experienced fewer symptoms of CD; he has one to two well-formed stools a day, increased appetite and weight, decreased abdominal pain and tenderness, and normal body temperatures. Should prednisone be discontinued? What agents are effective in maintaining remission of symptoms in patients with CD?

CORTICOSTEROIDS

Once prednisone has induced remission of active symptomatic CD, attempts should be made to taper the drug.[16] The tapering schedule is usually fairly slow (typically, a dose reduction of 5%–10% per week), taking several weeks to months to complete. Several studies have demonstrated that corticosteroids are ineffective in maintaining remission in CD, and many patients continue to have active disease while receiving therapy. However, a significant subset of patients (25%) with CD requires chronic administration of corticosteroids to prevent recurrence of symptoms (termed steroid-dependent CD).[94] Given the poor long-term adverse effect profile of steroids, many clinicians attempt treatment with other modalities to maintain remission.

6-MERCAPTOPURINE OR AZATHIOPRINE

Evidence suggests that both 6-MP and AZA have a major role in maintenance treatment of CD.[95] In addition, these agents are often used as a steroid-sparing strategy. Recent guidelines recommend the use of 6-MP and AZA in most relapsing cases of CD, regardless of anatomical site, and for both severe and steroid-dependent disease. Provided patients are appropriately monitored, these agents are safe with a favorable risk-benefit ratio. Both 6-MP and AZA are the first-line immunomodulators used in CD. Should these agents be ineffective or not tolerated, either MTX or infliximab can be used to maintain remission.[16] As mentioned above, the top-down strategy of starting TNF blockers earlier in the course of disease is currently under debate.[96] Some experts believe that infliximab should be used earlier in the course of relapsing disease, especially in patients with fistulae.[97]

In summary, J.P.'s prednisone should be tapered as suggested previously and then discontinued if possible. As the tapering regimen is begun, J.P. should start 6-MP 120 mg (approximately 1.5 mg/kg/day) or AZA 200 mg (approximately 2.5 mg/kg/day). This is because of the long onset of effect for the latter drugs (usually 3–6 months). J.P.'s WBC counts should be monitored regularly, and he should be counseled regarding the signs and symptoms of severe infection (e.g., fever, sore throat, or chills) and pancreatitis (e.g., severe epigastric pain and nausea).

Adverse Effects

CASE 28-3, QUESTION 4: Six weeks after starting to taper J.P.'s prednisone dosage (currently, 10 mg/day) and the initiation of AZA, he returns to the clinic for routine laboratory monitoring. His WBC count is 1,800/μL with an absolute neutrophil count of 1,100/μL. He is afebrile and without complaint. His physical examination is negative for any sign of infection. Why is J.P. experiencing leukopenia? What is the treatment for this side effect?

6-MERCAPTOPURINE AND AZATHIOPRINE MONITORING

AZA is a prodrug that is converted to the active moiety, 6-MP, in the liver. 6-MP is then metabolized by xanthine oxidase, hypoxanthine-guanine phosphoribosyltransferase, or thiopurine-*S*-methyltransferase (TPMT). Genetic polymorphism determines the extent of TPMT activity. In approximately 90% of whites, TPMT activity is considered high, but the remainder of the population has either intermediate or low TPMT activity.[98] These patients are predisposed to 6-MPor AZA myelosuppression because diminished TPMT activity leads to the metabolism of these compounds being shunted to the other enzymatic pathways. Accumulation of the 6-thioguanine byproducts is correlated with leukopenia. Pharmacogenomic testing

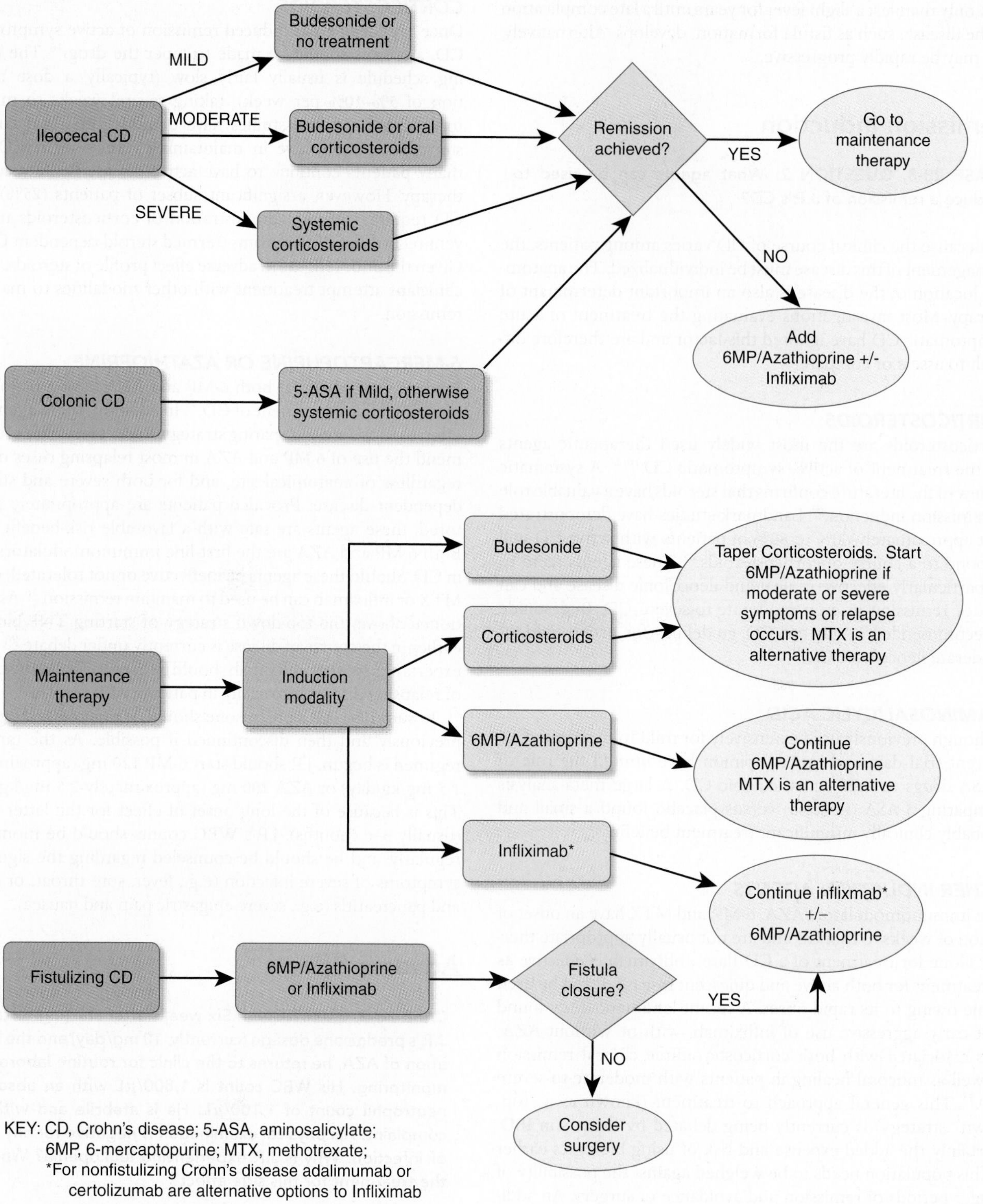

FIGURE 28-2 Treatment algorithm for Crohn's disease.

to assess TPMT activity has been developed and found to be effective in guiding therapy with AZA or 6-MP, while minimizing the incidence of bone marrow suppression.[99] The CD guidelines note that no randomized controlled trials have compared pharmacogenomic guided dosing to usual care dosing in patients receiving AZA or 6-MP. However, the US Food and Drug Administration recommends such testing before initiating these medications.[100] Additionally, several retrospective studies have assessed the clinical utility of measuring AZA and 6-MP metabolites such as 6-thioguanine and 6-methylmercaptopurine.[101] Although some experts have used these data to suggest a therapeutic level for these metabolites (for example 6-thioguanine levels of 250–400 pmol/8 $\times$ 10^8 red blood cells have been considered optimal), the CD guidelines do not recommend their routine use.[16] The optimal role for these tests remains to be fully determined, and data in this area are rapidly evolving.

In patients who have experienced neutropenia from AZA therapy, as J.P. has, the primary treatment is to discontinue AZA. In most cases, the WBC count will normalize over the course of several days to weeks. In extreme cases, the use of granulocyte colony-stimulating factor may be considered.[102] J.P. should be monitored for signs and symptoms of infection, and the AZA should be withheld. Frequent, probably daily, WBC determinations should be made until the count is greater than 3,000/μL.

OTHER AGENTS

CASE 28-3, QUESTION 5: J.P.'s leukocyte count returned to normal after 2 weeks. Unfortunately, he experienced a flare of his CD symptoms, specifically, an increase in diarrhea and abdominal pain that J.P. has noted during the past 5 days. What other agents should be considered to maintain remission in J.P.?

A number of other immunosuppressive drugs have been examined in CD. MTX produces and maintains remission in patients with refractory disease. Clinical improvement or reduction in corticosteroid dosages have been observed with 15 mg/week oral MTX or 25 mg/week of intramuscular or subcutaneous MTX in roughly 40% of patients who had active bowel disease.[103] In clinical studies, GI toxicity was the most common reason for discontinuing treatment, but neutropenia and liver enzyme elevations were also reported.[104] Current guidelines recommend reserving MTX for patients who have failed or are intolerant of 6-MP or AZA. Some experts consider MTX to be inferior to 6-MP or AZA in CD, but no comparison studies have been published to date.

METRONIDAZOLE

Recent guidelines recommend that antibiotics have little role in the maintenance of remission in CD, but they may be helpful in fistulizing disease or in patients with abscesses. Taste disturbances and peripheral neuropathy are the most commonly reported adverse effects associated with metronidazole treatment. Given an apparent therapeutic failure with 6-MP, a reasonable approach would be a short course of corticosteroids (prednisone 40 mg daily with a taper for 6 to 8 weeks) and MTX 25 mg weekly. Folic acid 1 mg daily should be initiated in patients started with the MTX. Alternatively, biologic therapy could also be considered.

INFLIXIMAB

CASE 28-3, QUESTION 6: J.P. has developed an enterocutaneous fistula with his latest disease exacerbation, and nothing is helping him achieve remission. What alternatives are appropriate for J.P.?

Infliximab is now firmly established as an important therapy in the treatment of CD, especially fistulizing disease. However, a number of concerns regarding this agent must be discussed with the patient before initiation of therapy. It is an expensive therapy (about $15,000/year), although it may be cost effective in CD.[105] Fistulizing disease seems to respond particularly well to infliximab, and its use may avert the need for surgery.[106] Acute and delayed hypersensitivity reactions can occur and are occasionally life threatening. Some clinicians premedicate patients with a combination of diphenhydramine, acetaminophen, or corticosteroids before an infusion; however, the most effective strategy to avoid a serious reaction is to regularly monitor vital signs during infliximab infusion and slow the rate or stop the infusion if any symptoms develop. The majority of reactions consist of headache, flushing, itching, and dizziness, with anaphylactic reactions rarely occurring. Also of concern is the development of human antichimeric antibodies in some patients receiving infliximab, which may lead to either loss of response or immunologic adverse reactions.

Infliximab should be avoided in patients who have a serious active infection. Because of reports that infliximab treatment may reactivate tuberculosis, all patients considered for treatment must receive a tuberculin skin test to rule out the disease (see Chapter 65, Tuberculosis). If this test is negative and because J.P. does not appear to have any other contraindications, he would seem to be an appropriate candidate for infliximab. If latent tuberculosis is found, antitubercular treatment must be initiated before infliximab can be considered, although even patients with treated latent tuberculosis still have an increased risk of active disease.[107] In addition, screening for hepatitis B (and probably hepatitis C) is reasonable owing to the number of cases describing reactivation of these viral infections. Current data concerning a link between TNF-α blockers use and malignancy are conflicting.[108] To date, the balance of data suggests a small but real risk of developing lymphoma in CD patients using TNF-α blockers, but despite this, its use is associated with an increase in quality-adjusted years of life.[109] Another problem commonly faced by clinicians and patients is loss of effectiveness in patients receiving TNF-α blockers. This may occur months or years after initiation of therapy. Common strategies to regain response may include increasing the dose of infliximab to 10 mg/kg per dose or switching to another TNF-α blocker. The success of these strategies is variable, and often comes with significantly increased treatment costs.[110] A recent paper has shed light on the possible causes of this loss of efficacy.[44] In 155 patients receiving infliximab who had declining response to the drug, both trough serum infliximab levels as well as human anticlonal antibodies (HACA) were measured. The authors found that in patients with subtherapeutic trough infliximab levels, increasing the dose of the drug was a successful strategy to regain response, whereas those patients who were HACA-positive benefited more from changing to another TNF-α blocker. This paper brings up the possibility that such laboratory markers could be routinely used to assess the effect of infliximab, but more data on this issue are needed to make such a recommendation.

Surgery in Crohn's Disease

CASE 28-3, QUESTION 7: J.P. initiated infliximab 400 mg IV every 8 weeks, and it was successful at keeping him symptomfree. However, after 2 years of remission, J.P. is hospitalized for an acute exacerbation of right lower quadrant pain associated with abdominal distension, lack of bowel movements, and vomiting during the past 24 hours. Radiographic studies indicate partial small bowel obstruction at the terminal ileum. Is surgery indicated at this time?

Because medical therapy of CD is often inadequate, 78% of patients with this disease will require surgery within 20 years of symptom onset.[3] In contrast to UC, surgical removal of the involved bowel in CD is not a definitive form of therapy. CD can recur even after extensive resections.[91] Various investigations have determined that cumulative recurrence rates after surgery for this disease are as high as 80%, depending on the surgical procedure and disease location. Therefore, multiple operations and their attendant risks are often necessary during the life of the CD patient. Depending on the amount and site of the bowel removed during surgery, specific malabsorption syndromes can occur (e.g., vitamin B_{12} malabsorption with removal of the terminal ileum). If an ileostomy is part of the surgical procedure, the patient will have to undergo significant psychological adjustments. Therefore, surgery is indicated only for specific complications that are unresponsive to medical therapy, and it should be avoided if possible.

IRRITABLE BOWEL SYNDROME

Irritable bowel syndrome (IBS) is one of the most common chronic disorders causing patients to seek medical treatment. It exerts a significant economic burden and is responsible for considerable morbidity in Western countries. Until recently, little was understood about the pathophysiology or etiology of this disorder. Indeed, some controversy exists today as to whether IBS is a distinct syndrome or a grouping of several chronic GI disorders. Still, investigators have made strides in understanding IBS, particularly the role of the enteric nervous system in the etiology of this disorder. As a result, new pharmacotherapeutic options are emerging for patients experiencing this often-bewildering condition.

IBS can be defined as "a functional bowel disorder characterized by abdominal pain associated with a change of bowel habit."[111] The incidence of IBS has been reported to be 3% to 20% in Western countries.[112] It is the most common disorder seen by gastroenterologists and is commonly seen by primary-care clinicians as well.[113] Prevalence rates are dependent on IBS diagnostic criteria, which have varied over the years. A female sex predominance of about 3:1 is evident in most epidemiologic studies of IBS.[112] Some studies have demonstrated a white predominance in IBS, whereas other studies have found no such association. Many patients with IBS never seek medical attention, and those who do tend to see their physician frequently.[114]

Many of these patients also have other functional disorders, such as fibromyalgia and interstitial cystitis, and psychiatric disorders, such as major depression and generalized anxiety disorder. As mentioned previously, the economic costs associated with IBS are considerable; it is estimated that IBS accounts for $33 billion in direct and indirect costs in the United States annually.[115]

ONLINE CONTENT

For a visual of the effects of irritable bowel syndrome, see http://thepoint.lww.com/AT10e.

Pathophysiology

Although knowledge of the cause of IBS remains incomplete, several theories have emerged to explain the underlying pathophysiology of this disorder. Previously, the primary cause of IBS was believed to be psychiatric or psychosomatic. This picture was at least partially validated by the finding that many IBS patients had psychiatric comorbidities. Today, it is believed that factors such as psychological stress may exacerbate the disease, but they are not the cause of IBS.[116] It has long been known that IBS patients tend to exhibit visceral hypersensitivity to colonic stimulation or manipulation. Although concomitant anxiety and hypervigilance undoubtedly played a role in such observations, it is now believed that the reaction to visceral stimuli in these patients results in the perception of abdominal pain, whereas patients without IBS would have no symptoms. The etiology of this hypersensitivity is the focus of intense research efforts. Theories have emerged suggesting that the activation of silent gut nociceptors owing to ischemia or infection may lead to increased abdominal pain in IBS.[116] Other experts propose that an increase in the excitability of neurons in the dorsal horn of the spinal cord lead to gut hyperalgesia. An abnormality in the processing of ascending signals from the dorsal horn may be responsible for a lower pain threshold in IBS patients. Similarly, findings suggest that neurotransmitter abnormalities may cause the symptoms of IBS. Of particular interest is the role of serotonin (5-HT) in the etiology of this disorder. Greater than 95% of the body's 5-HT is located in the GI tract and is stored in many cells, such as enterochromaffin cells, neurons, and smooth muscle cells. When released, this 5-HT can trigger both GI smooth muscle contraction and relaxation, as well as mediate GI sensory function.[117] Different 5-HT receptor subtypes may be responsible for these differing actions. A study examining rectal biopsy specimens in patients with IBS found defects in 5-HT signaling, supporting the theory of neurotransmitter abnormalities.[118] The primary 5-HT subtypes in the GI tract are 5-HT_3 and 5-HT_4. Some data suggest that IBS patients may have higher levels of 5-HT in the colon compared with control subjects.[119] Thus, these receptors have become the target of pharmacotherapeutic manipulation for IBS.

Another proposed pathological mechanism of IBS is altered colonic motility. Diarrhea, constipation, and abdominal bloating are common features of IBS. Patients with IBS are often categorized as having either diarrhea-predominant or constipation-predominant disease.[111] About one-half of patients with IBS report increased symptoms postprandially, and patients with diarrhea-predominant IBS (IBS-D) have been shown to have an exaggerated response to cholecystokinin after eating, leading to increased colonic propulsions.[120] However, constipation-predominant IBS (IBS-C) patients tend to have fewer colonic propulsions postprandially. Patients in whom bloating is the primary symptom of IBS may have gas production from poor fermentation of carbohydrates.[121] This has led investigators to search for a link between bacterial overgrowth of the small bowel (leading to an increase of gas production and pain and bloating symptoms) and IBS.

Etiology

The pathogenesis of IBS is poorly understood, although consensus theories are emerging. Some investigators believe that inflammation of the GI mucosa associated with infection may be the triggering factor that results in IBS.[114] The fact that symptoms associated with IBS can appear in up to 30% of patients who had an episode of bacterial gastroenteritis in the recent past lend credence to an infectious etiology.[122] Recent studies have also determined that a percentage of patients diagnosed with IBS may in fact have small intestinal bacterial overgrowth.[123] Diagnosis of the latter disorder is particularly important as treatment may involve a simple course of antibacterials. Also controversial is the possible association of a history of physical or sexual abuse and the development of IBS.[124] Most IBS patients under emotional or psychological stress will report an exacerbation of their symptoms, but this is not surprising considering that such stressors affect non-IBS patients' GI function as well.[125] Familial clustering of IBS patients suggests that both genetics and formative environments may play a role in the pathogenesis of this disorder.[126] Finally, food intolerances (e.g., lactose intolerance) may be involved in the etiology of IBS or may be misdiagnosed as IBS.

Diagnosis

One of the more challenging and frustrating aspects of IBS is its lack of biochemical or physical markers that are pathognomic for the disorder. Thus, the diagnosis of IBS is usually symptom based, with the newest guidelines for treatment suggesting that a simplified approach to diagnosis (without extensive imaging studies) be adopted.[111] Unfortunately, this lack of "objective" criteria for diagnosis can propagate the notion that IBS is a psychological or psychosomatic disorder. Many patients express frustration with the traditional medical establishment and individual providers.[127]

TABLE 28-6
Alarm Symptoms Requiring Gastroenterology Consultation

Weight loss
Gastrointestinal bleeding
Anemia
Fever
Frequent nocturnal symptoms

Source: Theis VS, Rhodes JM. Review article: minimizing tuberculosis during anti-tumour necrosis factor-alpha treatment of inflammatory bowel disease. *Aliment Pharmacol Ther.* 2008;27:19.

Patients and providers often want expensive laboratory or imaging tests to rule out other diseases; however, guidelines suggest that extensive testing in IBS patients is usually unnecessary provided that patients are younger than 50 years and do not present with any so-called alarm symptoms (Table 28-6). Although several symptom-driven criteria have been published, including the different Rome Foundation systems and the Manning criteria, it is important to realize that most such systems have rarely been validated in IBS patients and their use to confirm or exclude the disorder is controversial.[128] This may be why newer guidelines have focused on a simple and practical definition for IBS: abdominal pain or discomfort that is accompanied by a change in bowel habit for at least 3 months (without alarm symptoms).[111] Once IBS is diagnosed, it should be further differentiated by symptom pattern into IBS-D, IBS-C, or mixed IBS (IBS-M). As mentioned above, small intestinal bacterial overgrowth or celiac sprue may be tested for in selected patients, but routine screening in not currently recommended. Because there is no known cure for IBS, it is logical to use these subgroups to help direct symptomatic therapy. In most cases, the primary-care clinician can successfully manage the IBS patient using the treatment algorithm depicted in Figure 28-3. However, the presence of alarm symptoms or an unusual finding on routine examination (e.g., thyroid abnormality) may prompt further referrals and testing.

There are limited data concerning the natural history of IBS. IBS is generally considered a benign disease with a good prognosis.[129] Patients' symptoms often wax and wane, and, in some cases, the syndrome resolves spontaneously.

Management

PATIENT EDUCATION

CASE 28-4

QUESTION 1: V.H. is a 33-year-old woman who presents with complaints of severe abdominal pain (rated 6 on a scale of 1–10), bloating, and the passage of hard pelletlike stools about every 3 days. This has gone on for about 6 months, and V.H. notices that an "attack" occurs usually after a large meal. Her past medical history is significant for a generalized anxiety disorder. Her current medications include buspirone and Yaz (drospirenone and ethinyl estradiol). Her immediate family is alive and well, except for a brother with depression. She drinks socially and does not smoke or use illicit drugs. V.H. is concerned that her symptoms are indicative of cancer. How should the clinician respond to V.H.'s concerns?

Clinicians must reassure patients with IBS that their symptoms are real. Furthermore, patients should be thoroughly counseled concerning the prognosis of IBS. Many patients are fearful that their symptoms are indicative of severe pathology such as cancer. Reassurance and education are vital to assuage fears and to reinforce the generally benign nature of this disorder. Involving patients at the earliest stages in their treatment plan is vital for patient acceptance and to avoid "doctor shopping." Further, some patients exhibit a phenomenon known as *somatization*. This is defined as a tendency to experience and communicate somatic distress in response to psychosocial stress and is a factor in how often IBS patients seek health care for their condition.[130] Educational sessions and psychologic techniques are thought to decrease the risk of developing somatization, but data to date are limited concerning these interventions.[131] Unfortunately, psychological disorders are present in a large segment of IBS patients. The clinician should again reinforce the notion that IBS is not "all in the patient's head." However, treatment of comorbid disorders, including the discovery of a history of physical or sexual abuse (and possible posttraumatic stress disorder), is an important component in successfully treating IBS.[129] Thus, the initial intervention with patients of IBS should include an interactive patient education session emphasizing the points above and earning the patient's trust.

DIET

CASE 28-4, QUESTION 2: After a discussion concerning IBS, V.H. seems less worried. She relates her concern that her dietary habits are responsible for the symptoms she is experiencing. She wonders if changing her diet will "cure" her of IBS. What is the role of diet in the treatment of IBS? Will V.H. be relieved of her IBS symptoms if she changes her diet?

Food intolerance may cause symptoms similar to those associated with IBS. Patients with lactose intolerance can experience pain, bloating, and diarrhea after ingesting milk-based products. A dietary and symptom diary may reveal such an intolerance, and avoidance of the implicated foods would constitute effective treatment. Unfortunately, most patients with IBS have difficulty complying with exclusion diets or will not achieve significant relief with them. Patients with IBS-C may benefit from increased dietary consumption of fiber, with a recent study finding that psyllium significantly improved IBS symptoms during 3 months of treatment compared with placebo.[132] Treatment guidelines conditionally recommend an increase in dietary fiber (e.g., wheat bran up to 20 g daily) as a reasonable first-line treatment for IBD-C, but also note the lack of high-quality evidence to support this modality.[111] Patients should be counseled that large doses of fiber can lead to abdominal gas and bloating, and overall objective long-term evidence of benefit in IBS is lacking.

Pharmacotherapy for Constipation-Predominant IBS

CASE 28-4, QUESTION 3: V.H. has gradually increased her dietary fiber during the past 6 weeks. The frequency of her stools has improved slightly, but she often still feels constipated. In addition, new symptoms of abdominal bloating have occurred in the past week. What is a reasonable strategy to treat V.H.'s IBS-C?

In patients with IBS-C in whom fiber therapy fails, other standard laxatives may be tried for symptomatic relief. These may include milk of magnesia, lactulose, senna, or polyethylene glycol without electrolytes (Miralax®). This last agent was shown to improve the number of bowel movements in a cohort of adolescents with IBS-C, but had no effect on abdominal pain or bloating.[133] Few well-designed trials looking at any laxative for IBS have been published. These agents are usually well tolerated, although they can occasionally cause abdominal bloating.

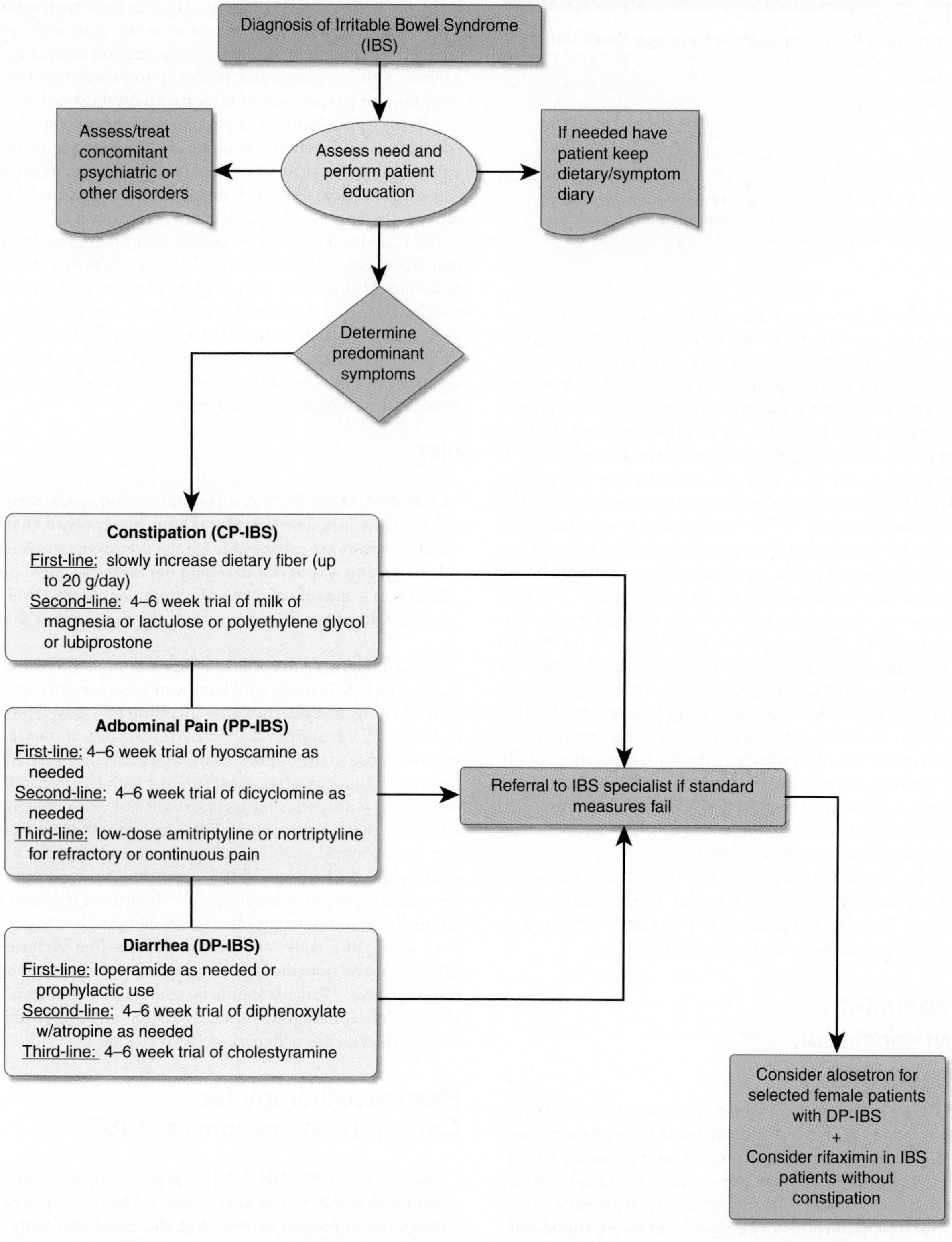

FIGURE 28-3 Treatment algorithm for irritable bowel syndrome. (Source: American College of Gastroenterology Task Force on Irritable Bowel Syndrome et al. An evidence-based position statement on the management of irritable bowel syndrome. *Am J Gastroenterol.* 2009;104(Suppl 1):S1; Pimentel M et al. Rifaximin therapy for patients with irritable bowel syndrome without constipation. *N Engl J Med.* 2011;364:22.)

Other adverse effects of the osmotic laxatives include diarrhea, taste disturbances, and hypermagnesemia (especially in patients with renal impairment). Although laxatives may provide relief of constipation, they will not effectively treat abdominal pain. Thus, other treatments will be required in many patients. Given its low cost and the lack of contraindications in this patient, milk of magnesia 15 mL daily is a reasonable first treatment.

CASE 28-4, QUESTION 4: Several months have passed since V.H. was first diagnosed with IBS-C. She has had therapeutic trials of several agents that were either poorly tolerated (poor palatability of propylene glycol) or lacked effectiveness. What other options are available for treating V.H.'s IBS-C?

TEGASEROD

Stimulation of the 5-HT_4 receptor accelerates colonic transit and has been exploited as a target for pharmacotherapy of IBS-C. The first of these agents, tegaserod, was originally approved in the United States for women with IBS-C. Tegaserod is a specific 5-HT_4 partial agonist that was evaluated in women with at least a 3-month history of IBS-C symptoms.[134] Clinical studies demonstrated a modest but significant benefit with tegaserod. Unfortunately, postmarketing analysis by the US Food and Drug Administration found an increased incidence of heart attack, stroke, and unstable angina in patients receiving the drug, and in April 2008, the manufacturer of tegaserod halted all sales and marketing of this agent.

LUBIPROSTONE

Lubiprostone, a GI chloride-channel activator (ClC-2 channels) that enhances intestinal fluid secretion and acts as a laxative, was approved in the United States for IBS-C in women older than 18 years of age. The drug has several actions on GI function including increasing small and large bowel transit time and decreased gastric emptying.[135] The dose of lubiprostone for IBS-C is 8 mcg orally twice daily, which is a lower dose than used for chronic idiopathic constipation. A recent analysis of two randomized controlled studies of lubiprostone versus placebo in women with IBS-C found that the drug was moderately effective in improving patient perception of constipation symptoms (17.9% vs. 10.1% of placebo groups responded; $p = 0.001$).[136] Primary adverse effects of lubiprostone include nausea and vomiting, but the effects are less likely at the dose of the drug approved for IBS-C and can be somewhat ameliorated by taking the medication with food.[135] Too few men with IBS-C were enrolled in the clinical trials with lubiprostone to draw any conclusions about its effectiveness in this population. Because the drug is associated with teratogenic effects in animals, the manufacturer recommends that women who could become pregnant have a negative pregnancy test before beginning therapy and be able to comply with effective contraceptive measures during therapy.[137] The drug is significantly more expensive than traditional laxatives, and should generally be reserved for patients who have failed other therapy for IBS-C. Because in this case V.H. has exhausted numerous other therapies, a trial of lubiprostone 8 mcg orally twice daily would be reasonable.

Irritable Bowel Syndrome–Associated Pain and Bloating

CASE 28-5

QUESTION 1: L.K. is a 38-year-old woman who has a long history of abdominal pain and episodic diarrhea. L.K. works as a sales representative for a major software vendor and is called on periodically to make formal presentations. She finds that just before these presentations she experiences "attacks" of abdominal pain and diarrhea. Her past medical history is significant for fibromyalgia, which manifests as chronic tiredness and fatigue. She has no other medical problems and takes no medications. She has no known drug allergies. She does not drink, smoke, or use illicit drugs. She has undergone an extensive workup, including colonoscopy, upper GI endoscopy with small bowel follow-through, computed tomography abdominal scans, serum electrolytes, thyroid function tests, and stool studies. These procedures and tests were negative, and L.K.'s gastroenterologist has diagnosed her with IBS. L.K. currently has one to two loose stools daily. They are not greasy appearing or foul smelling. She has bouts of abdominal pain (severity of 7 on a 1–10 scale) with or without diarrhea several times daily. She describes the pain as "stabbing" and "cramping." She has not noted any temporal relationship to meals or that certain foods exacerbate her condition. What pharmacologic options are available for L.K.'s abdominal pain? What adverse effects are associated with these medications?

ANTISPASMODICS

Drugs that possess smooth muscle relaxation properties, usually by anticholinergic pathways, have long been used to treat IBS. In the United States, the two most commonly prescribed antispasmodics are hyoscyamine and dicyclomine, both of which possess significant anticholinergic properties.[114] Clinical trials that have examined the use of these agents in IBS have been plagued by small numbers and methodologic problems, and recently several meta-analyses have been conducted to provide insight in this area. In general these systematic reviews have found that, as a class, smooth muscle relaxants were superior to placebo in improving abdominal pain, although they are less effective at treating other IBS symptoms.[138] Unfortunately there seems to be significant heterogeneity when looking at the efficacy of single agents in this class. Additionally, many agents studied in clinical trials are not available in the United States. Current treatment guidelines list antispasmodics as options for antispasmodic drugs for pain or bloating associated with IBS. If prescribed, an as-needed strategy of use has been advocated by some experts as opposed to continuous dosing owing to anticholinergic adverse effects.[125] Peppermint oil capsules also have smooth muscle relaxation properties and have been shown to be beneficial in IBS-related pain and cramping in several studies.[139]

ANTIDEPRESSANTS

Current treatment guidelines recommend the use of either tricyclic antidepressants or selective serotonin reuptake inhibitors (SSRIs) for patients with severe or continuous abdominal pain.[111] The analgesic effects of these agents are well known, and it is believed that these agents may work by a similar mechanism in IBS-associated pain and bloating as well as global well-being. One recent meta-analysis examined the class as a whole in IBS patients and found low-dose tricyclic antidepressants significantly improved pain, bloating, and IBS symptoms compared with placebo.[140] A dose–response relationship was not noted, and low doses of tricyclic antidepressants (e.g., amitriptyline 10–25 mg at bedtime) are often effective in relieving abdominal pain and diarrhea. A 3-month trial at a target dose of a drug (e.g., amitriptyline 50 mg) should be attempted before therapeutic failure is confirmed. Secondary amine tricyclic antidepressants (nortriptyline, desipramine) are better tolerated by many patients than tertiary amines (amitriptyline, imipramine) owing to decreased anticholinergic adverse effects such as sedation, dry mouth and eyes, urinary retention, and weight gain. SSRI use is more controversial in IBS patients as conclusive evidence of efficacy is lacking.[141] Still, practice guidelines note that these agents are also reasonable agents to consider in patients with pain or bloating associated with IBS. Information on other antidepressants for IBS symptoms is limited. A recent pilot study suggested that duloxetine may improve pain and diarrhea in IBS patients, but more data are needed before this drug can be recommended.[142] Nortriptyline 10 mg orally at bedtime should be initiated with titration to symptom relief and lack of adverse effects.

Diarrhea-Predominant Irritable Bowel Syndrome

CASE 28-5, QUESTION 2: Two weeks after L.K. starts nortriptyline 25 mg at bedtime, she reports significant relief from both her abdominal pain and fatigue. She reports that she is sleeping better, and she now rates her pain as a 2 on a 1–10 scale. Her diarrhea has improved somewhat; however, she still suffers from a "diarrhea attack" before each presentation. What other treatments are available for IBS-D? What are the risks and benefits of these treatments?

STANDARD ANTIDIARRHEALS

Small bowel and colonic transit is accelerated in patients with IBS-D; thus, drugs that slow this process should be effective in relieving diarrhea.[143] Loperamide, an opioid agonist that penetrates poorly into the central nervous system, is the preferred agent for IBS-D. Meta-analyses have found loperamide to be an effective agent for improving diarrhea and, in some cases, improving patients' global well-being.[144] As with the antispasmodics, as-needed treatment is preferred to scheduled dosing (e.g., 2–4 mg PO up to four times daily as needed). Prophylactic dosing before a stressful situation or an event during which bathroom access is limited is particularly effective. Diphenoxylate with atropine is generally considered a second-line agent because of its increased risk of anticholinergic adverse effects. Finally, cholestyramine is occasionally used in refractory cases of IBS-D, especially when bile acid malabsorption is suspected or confirmed.[145] This agent is often poorly tolerated as a result of palatability problems. Cholestyramine also has a significant number of drug interactions of which the clinician must be aware.

ALOSETRON

Alosetron is a highly potent 5-HT_3 receptor antagonist that slows colonic transit time, increases intraluminal sodium absorption, and decreases small intestinal secretions.[146] Constipation is the most frequently reported adverse effect in clinical studies (approximately 30% of alosetron patients), with approximately 10% of patients withdrawing from studies for this reason. Postmarketing reports of severe constipation with cases of bowel obstructions and ischemic colitis were reported.[147] Bowel perforation and, rarely, death were also reported with alosetron use, and the drug was voluntarily withdrawn from the market in November 2000. After extensive lobbying by several patient groups, alosetron was reintroduced to the US market in June 2002, with restricted conditions for use. Prescribers must be registered with the drug manufacturer, and patients must sign a patient–physician agreement and be provided with a written medication guide. The new starting dose and regimen for alosetron is 0.5 mg BID for 1 month. If, after 4 weeks, this is well tolerated but does not adequately control IBS symptoms, then the dosage can be increased to 1 mg BID.[148] It is imperative that patients not start alosetron if they have a history of problems with constipation, bowel obstruction or ischemic colitis, IBD, or a thromboembolic disorder. Patients must immediately discontinue alosetron if they become constipated or have symptoms of ischemic colitis, such as new or worsening abdominal pain, bloody diarrhea, or blood in the stool. A recent review of the mandatory postmarketing surveillance system designed to monitor the safety of the drug found an overall low rate of ischemic colitis.[149]

EMERGING THERAPIES

Currently, numerous agents are being investigated for all types of IBS.[150] Newer generation serotonergic agonists and antagonists, including prucalopride and velusetrag, which have much higher affinity for gut serotonergic receptors (5-HT_4), have shown some efficacy in small trials and are undergoing further examination. Higher specificity to these receptors is thought to retain the efficacy of these medications and improve their safety profile. As mentioned earlier, some evidence exists concerning a possible association of bacterial GI infection and IBS symptoms. This has prompted some investigators to postulate that small bowel flora overgrowth may be responsible for or contribute to IBS symptoms. The nonabsorbable antibiotic rifaximin had been shown in two small studies to improve global symptoms in IBS for up to 10 weeks.[151,152] More recently a report of two randomized, double-blind, placebo-controlled trials of rifaximin in IBS (without constipation) was published.[153] In this trial a 14-day course of rifaximin 550 mg TID was found to significantly improve relief of global IBS symptoms during the first 4 weeks after treatment compared with placebo. The magnitude of improvement was small but considered clinically relevant. Treatment guidelines suggest that a course of rifaximin (400 mg BID for 10 days) may be reasonable in IBS patients, particularly those with IBS-D. Probiotic agents such as *Lactobacillus plantarum and Bifidobacterium infantis,* which may alter colonic inflammation, have shown some efficacy in a small study, but treatment guidelines note the wide variability of different probiotic compounds and do not strongly recommend their use for IBS.[154] In L.K.'s case, initiation of loperamide 2 mg as needed before a stressful situation would be a cost-effective approach to her symptoms. Should her symptoms worsen or her current regimen lose effectiveness, a course of rifaximin would be considered an alternative strategy, primarily owing to its expense.

KEY REFERENCES AND WEBSITES

A full list of references for this chapter can be found at **http://thepoint.lww.com/AT10e**. Below are the key references and websites for this chapter, with the corresponding reference number in this chapter found in parentheses after the reference.

Key References

Afif W et al. Clinical utility of measuring infliximab and human anti-chimeric antibody concentrations in patients with inflammatory bowel disease. *Am J Gastroenterol.* 2010;105:1133. (44)

American College of Gastroenterology Task Force on Irritable Bowel Syndrome et al. An evidence-based position statement on the management of irritable bowel syndrome. *Am J Gastroenterol.* 2009;104(Suppl 1):S1. (111)

Colombel JF et al. Infliximab, azathioprine, or combination therapy for Crohn's disease. *N Engl J Med.* 2010;362:1383. (53)

Kornbluth A et al. Ulcerative colitis practice guidelines in adults: American College of Gastroenterology, Practice Parameters Committee. *Am J Gastroenterol.* 2010;105:501. (14)

Lichtenstein GR et al. American Gastroenterological Association Institute technical review on corticosteroids, immunomodulators, and infliximab in inflammatory bowel disease. *Gastroenterology.* 2006;130:940. (26)

Lichtenstein GR et al. Management of Crohn's disease in adults. *Am J Gastroenterol.* 2009;104:465. (16)

Pimentel M et al. Rifaximin therapy for patients with irritable bowel syndrome without constipation. *N Engl J Med.* 2011;364:22. (153)

Regueiro M et al. Clinical guidelines for the medical management of left-sided ulcerative colitis and ulcerative proctitis: summary statement. *Inflamm Bowel Dis.* 2006;12:972. (21)

Key Websites

Crohn's and Colitis Foundation of America. **http://www.ccfa.org**

Irritable Bowel Syndrome Self Help and Support Group. **http://www.ibsgroup.org/ibsassociation**

29 Complications of End-Stage Liver Disease

Yasar O. Tasnif and Mary F. Hebert

CORE PRINCIPLES

	CHAPTER CASES
ASCITES	
1 Cirrhosis is defined as the fibrosis of the hepatic parenchyma resulting in altered hepatic function, restricted venous outflow, and portal hypertension. Cirrhosis results in an overall vasodilated state, activation of the renin-angiotensin-aldosterone system, altered hepatic synthetic function, and development of complications such as ascites and other complications of cirrhosis.	**Case 29-1 (Question 2)**
2 Physical findings of ascites can include the presence of an enlarged fluid-filled abdomen, increased abdominal girth, a positive fluid wave, increased body weight, and is often accompanied by peripheral edema. The goals of treatment for ascites are to mobilize ascitic fluid, diminish abdominal discomfort, as well as to prevent complications such as bacterial peritonitis and respiratory distress.	**Case 29-1 (Questions 1, 3)**
3 The treatment for ascites involves sodium restriction (2 g/day), water restriction for severe dilutional hyponatremia, and the use of spironolactone and furosemide (100:40 mg ratio). Management and monitoring of ascites includes ensuring adequate weight loss, maintaining electrolyte balance, and preventing complications of diuretic therapy.	**Case 29-1 (Questions 4–8)**
4 In cases of refractory ascites (diuretic-resistant), large-volume abdominal paracentesis along with albumin replacement is often indicated. Transjugular intrahepatic portosystemic shunt (TIPS), surgical shunts, or liver transplantation are options for the treatment of refractory ascites when paracentesis is deemed ineffective, or in patients who are intolerant or who have a contraindication to paracentesis.	**Case 29-1 (Questions 9–11)**
5 Spontaneous bacterial peritonitis (SBP) is a common complication of ascites. Prophylactic regimens include the long-term administration of oral antibiotics such as fluoroquinolones (norfloxacin), or trimethoprim-sulfamethoxazole to prevent the recurrence of SBP. Recommendations also include the administration of antibiotic prophylaxis for prevention of SBP in patients with variceal hemorrhage.	**Case 29-1 (Question 12), Case 29-2 (Question 4)**
ESOPHAGEAL VARICES	
1 Because esophageal varices are directly related to the severity of portal hypertension, the treatment is aimed at primary prevention of bleeding by reduction of portal pressure with the use of non-selective β-blockers, and/or elimination of the varices with endoscopic variceal ligation (EVL). Treatment approaches depend on the size of the varices and the risk of hemmorhage.	**Case 29-2 (Question 5)**
2 Secondary prophylaxis to prevent recurrent bleeding episodes include the combination of non-selective β-blockers and EVL. TIPS may be an option in patients who experience recurrent variceal hemorrhage despite combination pharmacological and endoscopic therapy.	**Case 29-2 (Question 6)**

continued

ESOPHAGEAL VARICES *CONTINUED*

3 Acute variceal bleeding is considered a medical emergency and should be treated immediately. Treatment goals include volume resuscitation, acute treatment of bleeding, and prevention of recurrence of variceal bleeding. For the control and management of acute hemorrhage, the combination of pharmacologic therapy and variceal ligation is the preferred approach. In cases of acute variceal bleeding uncontrolled by pharmacologic and endoscopic therapy, TIPS can be an effective option.	**Case 29-2 (Questions 1–3)**

HEPATIC ENCEPHALOPATHY

1 Hepatic encephalopathy is a metabolic disorder of the central nervous system that occurs in patients with either advanced cirrhosis or fulminate hepatic failure. The clinical features include altered mental state, asterixis, and fetor hepaticus. Several theories exist about the pathogenesis of hepatic encephalopathy; however, the pathogenesis of hepatic encephalopathy is likely multifactorial. Precipitating causes can include GI bleeding, diuretic-induced hypovolemia and/or electrolyte abnormalities, metabolic alkalosis, as well as sedating drugs.	**Case 29-3 (Questions 1–3)**
2 After identifying and removing precipitating causes of hepatic encephalpathy, therapeutic management is aimed primarily at reducing the amount of ammonia or nitrogenous products in the circulatory system by limiting protein intake and by the use of lactulose. Other therapeutic options include rifaximin and neomycin.	**Case 29-3 (Questions 4, 5)**
3 Monotherapy with lactulose should be tried first. If satisfactory results do not occur, switching to another option (neomycin or rifamixin) or combination therapy should be considered.	**Case 29-3 (Question 6)**

HEPATORENAL SYNDROME

1 Hepatorenal syndrome (HRS) is a complication of advanced cirrhosis, and is diagnosed by exclusion of other known causes of kidney disease. The definitive treatment for type 1 and type 2 HRS is liver transplantation, which is the only treatment that assures long-term survival. The main goal of pharmacologic therapy is to reverse HRS sufficiently so that appropriate candidates for liver transplantation can survive until suitable donor organs can be procured.	**Case 29-3 (Questions 7, 8)**

OVERVIEW

According to the National Vital Statistics Report published by the Centers for Disease Control and Prevention, chronic liver disease and cirrhosis is the 12th leading cause of death in the United States, accounting for approximately 29,165 deaths each year.[1] Cirrhosis, or end-stage liver disease, can be defined as fibrosis of the hepatic parenchyma resulting in nodule formation and altered hepatic function, which results from a sustained wound-healing response to chronic or acute liver injury from a variety of causes. Although there are other common causes of cirrhosis, most cases of cirrhosis worldwide result from chronic viral hepatitis, or liver injury associated with chronic alcohol consumption.[2] This chapter describes the pathogenesis of cirrhosis and the associated complications of portal hypertension (esophageal varices, gastric varices, ascites, spontaneous bacterial peritonitis, hepatic encephalopathy, and hepatorenal syndrome), the clinical symptoms of these complications, and the pharmacologic approach to their treatment.

PATHOGENESIS OF CIRRHOSIS

The liver consists of the hepatic parenchyma (hepatocytes) and a large proportion of nonparenchymal cells, including sinusoidal endothelial cells, Ito cells, and macrophages also known as Kupffer cells. Most of the liver's role in detoxification (phase I and phase II metabolism) takes place within the hepatocytes, whereas the nonparenchymal cell population provides physical and biochemical structure to the liver as well as active transport of substances into the bile.[3] Although the liver has a strong capacity to regenerate, this ability can be impaired by toxic or viral agents, such as ethanol and hepatitis viruses.[4]

Stress on the liver, such as chronic ethanol abuse in humans, leads to liver injury and over time cirrhosis and a disruption of hepatic function. Fatty liver or steatosis from ethanol, the first stage of liver injury, is characterized by lipid deposition in the hepatocytes. Steatosis is followed by liver inflammation (steatohepatitis), hepatocyte death, and collagen deposition leading to fibrosis. The specific mechanisms by which chronic ethanol-induced liver injury is initiated and progresses are not completely understood.[5] Research into the causes of alcohol-related liver injury has primarily focused on the role of ethanol-induced oxidative stress on the liver. Multiple pathways leading to oxidative stress have been described, and many systems likely contribute to the ability of ethanol to induce a state of oxidative stress. It is important to note that not all heavy drinkers experience liver cirrhosis.[6] Factors such as sex, genetic predisposition, and chronic viral infection play a role in the development and progression of ethanol-induced liver disease.[7]

Hepatitis C virus (HCV) affects millions of people worldwide, with approximately 20% of infections progressing to cirrhosis.[8] The progression of liver disease in patients with HCV is dependent on both patient and viral factors. Although the mechanisms by which HCV causes liver damage are not well known, a few proposed mechanisms for liver injury associated with HCV infection include diminished immune clearance of HCV, oxidative stress, hepatic steatosis, increased iron stores, and increased rate of hepatocyte apoptosis.[9] Because not all patients infected with HCV experience cirrhosis, factors other than viral clearance, such as the individual's immune response to the virus, age at the time of infection, sex, hepatic iron content, and HCV genotype are all implicated as cofactors in the development of cirrhosis.[10]

Among other causes, autoimmune hepatitis, primary biliary cirrhosis, primary sclerosing cholangitis, biliary atresia, metabolic disorders (e.g., Wilson disease and hemochromatosis), chronic inflammatory conditions (e.g., sarcoidosis), and vascular derangements can lead to hepatic fibrosis and cirrhosis.[2] Although not common, end-stage liver disease can also stem from problems related to obesity. An estimated 20% of Americans have nonalcoholic fatty liver disease (NAFLD), a condition that in most cases has no symptoms, but is occasionally characterized by symptoms of upper abdominal discomfort and right upper quadrant fullness. The most common physical examination findings are obesity and occasionally hepatomegaly, with biopsy results showing macrovesicular steatosis or fatty liver. Risk factors commonly associated with the development of NAFLD include obesity, hyperlipidemia, and diabetes. Although corticosteroids cause fatty liver, NAFLD diagnosis excludes corticosteroids and other causes of fatty liver such as hepatitis B, hepatitis C, autoimmune hepatitis, and Wilson disease. Nonalcoholic steatohepatitis (NASH) is a more serious form of NAFLD. Most patients generally tolerate NAFLD well, whereas NASH can lead to cirrhosis. Current evidence suggests that insulin resistance and lipid peroxidation play a role in the pathogenesis of this condition.[11,12] Regardless of the cause of end-stage liver disease, the most frequent complications of portal hypertension are esophageal or gastric varices, ascites with or without spontaneous bacterial peritonitis, hepatic encephalopathy, and hepatorenal syndrome.[13]

COMPLICATIONS OF CIRRHOSIS

Portal Hypertension

The portal vein begins as a confluence of the splenic, superior mesenteric, inferior mesenteric, and gastric veins, and ends in the sinusoids of the liver (Fig. 29-1). Blood in the portal vein contains substances absorbed from the intestine, and delivers these substances to the liver to be metabolized before entering the systemic circulation. Once the portal blood reaches the liver, it crosses through a high-resistance capillary system within the hepatic sinusoids.

Portal pressure is a function of flow and resistance to that flow across the hepatic vasculature, and described mathematically by Ohm's law (Pressure = Flow × Resistance). In cirrhosis, increased intrahepatic resistance results from intrahepatic vasoconstriction that is hypothesized to be caused by a deficiency in intrahepatic nitric oxide (NO).[14] Increased intrahepatic resistance also results from an enhanced activity of vasoconstrictors, and by structural changes within the liver owing to liver regeneration, sinusoidal compression, and fibrosis.

Portal hypertension results from both an increase in resistance to portal flow and also an increase in portal venous inflow, which is hypothesized to be caused by splanchnic vasodilatation that, in turn, is secondary to increasing NO production in the extrahepatic circulation leading to vasodilation and increased in-flow.[15]

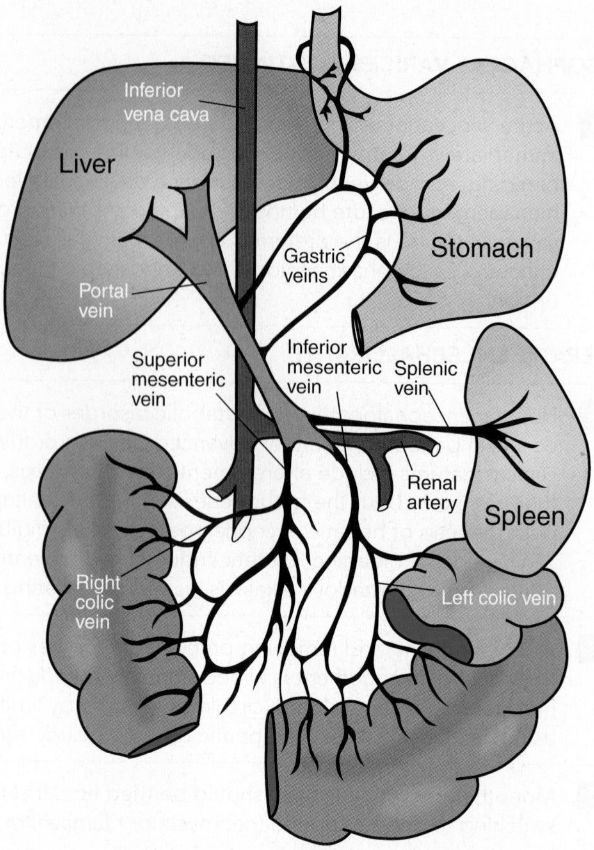

FIGURE 29-1 Schematic diagram of the portal venous system.

Portal pressure can be assessed by the use of surgical procedures, which are invasive and not routinely performed. The hepatic venous pressure gradient (HVPG), which reflects the gradient between the portal vein and vena cava pressure, is another accurate, safe, and less-invasive procedure that has been widely accepted as a measurement of the portal venous pressure gradient.[16–18] Normal portal pressure is generally below 6 mm Hg, and in cirrhotic patients may increase to 7 to 9 mm Hg. Clinically significant portal hypertension develops, however, when the portal pressure increases to greater than 10 to 12 mm Hg, the threshold for complications of portal hypertension, such as esophageal varices and ascites.[17,19] Portal hypertension can be further classified as prehepatic, intrahepatic, or posthepatic portal hypertension (Table 29-1).[20–22] Persistent portal hypertension may (a) change both blood flow as well as the lymphatic circulation and lead to ascites formation; (b) increase pressure in the vessels that branch off the portal vein, such as the coronary veins, leading to the formation of esophageal varices; and (c) lead to the development of increased abdominal collateral circulation. Hepatic encephalopathy and hepatorenal syndrome are other complications associated with advanced cirrhosis and portal hypertension.[20–22] The American Association for the Study of Liver Diseases and European Association for the Study of the Liver Single-Topic Conference in 2008 classified cirrhosis into two main categories, compensated and decompensated. Patients can be cirrhotic with a portal pressure less than 10 mm Hg and an absence of the complications of cirrhosis (e.g., ascites, variceal hemorrhage, or encephalopathy) and thus would be considered to be compensated. This is in contrast to a patient presenting with ascites, esophageal hemorrhage, hepatic encephalopathy, or

TABLE 29-1
Classification and Etiologies of Portal Hypertension

Classification	Prehepatic	Intrahepatic	Posthepatic
Etiologies	Splenic vein thrombosis Portal vein thrombosis	Hepatic cirrhosis Hepatic fibrosis Nodular regeneration (with distortion of hepatic veins)	Hepatic vein obstruction (Budd-Chiari syndrome) Inferior vena cava obstruction Right-sided heart failure

hepatorenal syndrome, which are complications of decompensated cirrhosis.[23] Patients with compensated cirrhosis are managed by treatment of the underlying cause of the cirrhosis, prevention (primary prophylaxis), as well as early diagnosis of the complications of cirrhosis. For patients with decompensated cirrhosis, the aim is to treat the complications of cirrhosis and prevent sequela (secondary prevention).[24]

LABORATORY FINDINGS

Laboratory evaluations may not reflect the extent of the parenchymal necrosis, cellular regeneration, and fibrotic nodular scarring in cirrhotic liver disease. Conventional liver "function" tests, such as the serum aminotransferases (aspartate aminotransferase [AST, formerly known as SGOT], alanine aminotransferase [ALT, formerly known as SGPT]), and alkaline phosphatase, are actually better characterized as liver "injury" tests and are modestly helpful to the clinician for screening hepatobiliary disease and after liver injury progression. These tests, however, do not quantitatively measure the functional capacity of the liver. The aminotransferases are released during the normal turnover of liver cells (see Chapter 2, Interpretation of Clinical Laboratory Tests). High serum concentrations of aminotransferases suggest release of these enzymes from injured hepatocytes. The serum concentrations of AST and ALT may initially rise very high with acute liver injury and then fall when the cause for liver injury is removed or when necrosis is so severe that few hepatocytes remain.

Because alkaline phosphatase is present in high concentrations in biliary canaliculi (as well as bone, intestines, kidneys, placenta, and white blood cells [WBCs]), an increase in the serum concentration of alkaline phosphatase is greater with biliary injury rather than during a parenchymal injury. High serum concentrations of gamma glutamyl transpeptidase and bilirubin are also suggestive of biliary injury. Increases in serum concentrations of alkaline phosphatase, AST, and/or ALT may suggest hepatic injury, but because they are also found intracellularly in other places in the body their elevation is not diagnostic for liver disease.[25,26]

Serum concentrations of proteins such as albumin, or factor V and factor VIII, as well as coagulation tests such as the prothrombin time (PT) and international normalized ratio (INR), can provide insight into the functional capacity of the liver. The hepatic parenchymal cells exclusively synthesize albumin, therefore albumin concentrations can provide some indication of hepatocellular function. Changes in albumin concentration are nonspecific, however, and can be influenced by other factors, including poor nutrition, renal wasting (proteinuria), and gastrointestinal (GI) losses. Prolongation of PT owing to vitamin K deficiency is often a result of poor nutrition, malabsorption of fat-soluble vitamins, or biliary tract obstruction.[27] Usually a 10-mg subcutaneous or oral dose of vitamin K improves coagulopathy due to vitamin K deficiency within 24 hours. A prolonged PT owing to poor hepatic synthetic function is not responsive to vitamin K administration.[27] If the INR requires rapid correction because of bleeding or a planned invasive procedure, fresh frozen plasma should be transfused.[27]

A number of the factors just described have been incorporated into the Child-Turcotte-Pugh classification of liver disease severity (Table 29-2).[28,29] This classification yields a scoring system to help clinicians grade disease severity, and predict the long-term risk of mortality and quality of life. A person with Child-Turcotte-Pugh class A cirrhosis may survive as long as 15 to 20 years, whereas those with class C cirrhosis may survive only 1 to 3 years.[30] The main limitation of the Child-Turcotte-Pugh classification is the use of subjective measures, such as ascites and hepatic encephalopathy, which are subject to clinical interpretation and may be altered by therapy.[31,32] As a general guide, and not a rule, class A patients are considered to be compensated, and classes B and C decompensated.[24]

An alternative method for assessing short-term survival in patients with liver disease is the Model for End-Stage Liver Disease (MELD) score that utilizes laboratory values, and is used to predict short-term (3-month) mortality associated with liver disease. The MELD score is calculated by the formula[32]:

$$\text{MELD score} = (0.957 \times \ln[\text{creatinine mg/dL}] + 0.378 \times \ln[\text{total bilirubin mg/dL}] + 1.120 \times \ln[\text{INR}] + 0.643) \times 10 \qquad \textbf{(Eq. 29-1)}$$

Because of the good correlation between the MELD score and short-term mortality as well as the objective nature of the MELD scoring system, it has replaced the Child-Turcotte-Pugh score in the United Network for Organ Sharing (UNOS) prioritization of organ allocation of cadaveric livers for transplantation.[33–35] MELD scores range from 6 (less ill) to 40 (gravely ill), with an added category of Status 1 patients (acute and severe onset of liver failure) who have a life expectancy of hours to a few days without liver transplantation. A high MELD score is strongly associated with early pretransplantation wait-list mortality. Therefore, patients with the highest MELD score are given priority by UNOS in terms of organ allocation; the only exception being Status 1 patients who are given the highest priority.[36]

TABLE 29-2
Child-Turcotte-Pugh Classification of Severity of Liver Disease

	Score[a]		
	1 Point	2 Points	3 Points
Bilirubin (mg/dL)	<2	2–3	>3
Albumin (mg/dL)	>3.5	2.8–3.5	<2.8
INR	<1.7	1.7–2.3	>2.3
Ascites	None	Mild to moderate	Severe
Encephalopathy (grade)	None	Mild to moderate (1 and 2)	Severe (3 and 4)

[a]Class A, 5–6 points; class B, 7–9 points; class C, 10–15 points.
INR, international normalized ratio.

CASE 29-1

QUESTION 1: R.W. is a 54-year-old man with a 2-week history of nausea, vomiting, and lower abdominal cramps without diarrhea. Despite chronic anorexia, he has managed to drink a fifth of vodka (750 mL) and eat about two meals a day for the past 2 years. During this time, he experienced a 30-lb weight loss. He began drinking 9 years ago when his wife became disabled after diagnosis of a brain tumor. Two years ago, his alcohol consumption increased from one pint to a fifth daily. Recently, he has noted bilateral edema of his legs, an increased tenseness and girth of his abdomen, jaundice, and scleral icterus. His medical history is noncontributory, other than a history of spontaneous bacterial peritonitis (SBP) 6 months ago. He is not taking any medications and has no known drug allergies.

Physical examination reveals an afebrile, jaundiced, and cachectic male in moderate distress. Spider angiomas were found on his face and upper chest. In addition, palmar erythema was noted.

ONLINE CONTENT

For photos of spider angiomas and palmar erythema, go to http://thepoint.lww.com/AT10e.

Abdominal examination reveals prominent veins on a very tense abdomen. The liver edge is percussed below the right costal margin and ascites is noted by shifting dullness and a fluid wave. The spleen is not palpable. On neurologic examination, R.W. is awake and oriented to person, place, and time. Cranial nerves II to XII are grossly intact, but a decrease in vibratory sensation of the lower extremities is noted bilaterally. Admission laboratory data are as follows:

Sodium, 135 mEq/L
Chloride, 95 mEq/L
Potassium, 3.8 mEq/L
Bicarbonate, 25 mEq/L
Blood urea nitrogen (BUN), 15 mg/dL
Serum creatinine (SCr), 1.4 mg/dL
Glucose, 136 mg/dL
Hemoglobin (Hgb), 11.2 g/dL
Hematocrit (Hct), 33.4%
AST, 212 international units
Alkaline phosphatase, 954 international units
PT, 13.5 (INR, 1.1)
Total/direct bilirubin, 18.8/10.7 mg/dL
Albumin, 2.3 g/dL
Guaiac positive stools

On admission to the hospital, the impression is alcoholic cirrhosis, ascites, and heme-positive stools.

What subjective and objective evidence are compatible with alcoholic cirrhosis in R.W.?

R.W.'s liver function tests (elevated AST, alkaline phosphatase, and bilirubin) and physical findings (an enlarged, palpable liver edge; jaundice; spider angiomas on his face and upper chest; palmar erythema; and cachexia) are all consistent with advanced alcoholic cirrhosis in a patient with a history of chronic alcohol abuse. The prolonged PT and hypoalbuminemia suggest impaired hepatic synthesis of both albumin and vitamin K–dependent clotting factors. The low albumin contributes to both the ascites and edema. The bilirubin of 18.8 mg/dL suggests that vitamin K absorption may be a factor in the prolonged PT. The presence of ascites (an enlarged fluid-filled abdomen) and prominent abdominal veins are suggestive of portal hypertension. A biopsy of the liver may confirm or establish the presence and severity of cirrhosis. R.W.'s prolonged PT, however, will increase the risk of bleeding from a liver biopsy. R.W.'s positive guaiac finding could be indicative of bleeding esophageal varices but could also be explained by bleeding from another GI source. This needs to be confirmed by endoscopy. He is oriented to person, place and time, but needs to be fully tested for hepatic encephalopathy. R.W.'s calculated MELD score is 22, which predicts a 90-day mortality of approximately 20%.[33] A patient's MELD score may increase or decrease for a period of time depending on the patient's clinical status and treatment. A number of MELD scores will be calculated during the course of R.W.'s treatment if the patient is listed as a transplantation candidate to determine his status for organ allocation.[36] Muscle wasting and poor nutrition are the most common causes of weight loss in patients with alcoholic cirrhosis (see Chapter 87, Alcohol Use Disorders).

ASCITES

Pathogenesis of Ascites

CASE 29-1, QUESTION 2: What physiologic mechanism predisposes R.W. to fluid accumulation in the peritoneal cavity?

Ascites, or accumulation of fluid in the peritoneal cavity, is the most commonly encountered clinical symptom of cirrhosis.[37] This complication can be detected during the physical examination when more than 3 L of fluid has accumulated. In addition to an obviously enlarged abdomen, R.W. was found to have a positive fluid wave and shifting dullness, indicating that the abdominal enlargement is not simply obesity. The fluid wave can be observed by having the patient lie on his or her back. While supporting one side of the abdomen with one hand, use the second hand to tap the opposite side of the abdomen. A wave of fluid moving across the abdomen can be felt by the hand on the opposite side. Dullness can be determined during percussion of the abdomen. This sound denotes the presence of free peritoneal fluid. As the patient is turned from one side to another, if dullness continues to be percussed, the patient is determined to have shifting dullness. If the diagnosis is in doubt, which sometimes occurs in obese patients, ascites can be confirmed with ultrasound. Generally speaking, in obesity the abdomen enlarges over time (months to years), in contrast to ascites where abdominal enlargement can occur over a few weeks.[38] Once ascites develops, the 1-year patient survival rate decreases to about 50%.[37]

In cirrhosis, hepatic venous outflow is restricted, resulting in an increase in the portal vein back-pressure. High hepatic venous pressure leads to high intrasinusoidal pressure and development of ascites across the hepatic capsule. Portal hypertension from cirrhosis is associated with splanchnic dilatation and increased splanchnic blood flow. This increase in splanchnic blood flow is associated with an upregulation of endothelial nitric oxide synthase and increased production of a potent vasodilator, NO. This increase in NO has been proposed as a major mediator of the arterial dilatation and hyperdynamic circulation in cirrhosis.[39] NO leads to an overall vasodilated state. The systemic compensation to this vasodilation is an increase in cardiac output and sodium retention and water retention in the kidneys as a result of activation of the renin-angiotensin-aldosterone system (RAAS).[40]

The activation of RAAS, in addition to R.W.'s hypoalbuminemia (2.3 g/dL) leads to worsening of the ascites. Exudation of fluid from the splanchnic capillary bed and the liver surface when the drainage capacity of the lymphatic system is exceeded, and decreased ability of fluid to be contained within the vascular space owing to impaired hepatic albumin synthesis, contributes to the development of ascites.

Goals of Therapy

CASE 29-1, QUESTION 3: What are the therapeutic goals in the treatment of R.W.'s ascites?

The goals of treatment for R.W.'s ascites are to treat the cause of cirrhosis by ceasing alcohol consumption; mobilize ascitic fluid; diminish abdominal discomfort, back pain, and difficulty in ambulation; as well as to prevent complications (e.g., bacterial peritonitis, hernias, pleural effusions, hepatorenal syndrome, and respiratory distress).[38] The goal is a weight loss of 0.5 to 1 kg/day, which corresponds to a net fluid volume loss of about 0.5 to 1 L/day. Treatment of ascites in R.W. should be undertaken cautiously and gradually because acid–base imbalances, hypokalemia, or intravascular volume depletion caused by overly aggressive therapy can lead to compromised renal function, hepatic encephalopathy, and death.[41,42] The initial medical management of ascites involves restriction of sodium intake and the use of diuretics to promote salt and water excretion.[38]

Fluid and Electrolyte Balance

URINARY NA:K RATIO

CASE 29-1, QUESTION 4: The 24-hour urinary electrolytes for R.W. were as follows:

Na, 10 mEq/L
K, 28 mEq/L

Why would sodium or water restriction be appropriate (or inappropriate) for R.W.?

Normally, the urine concentration of electrolytes mirrors the serum concentration of electrolytes (i.e., sodium concentration is greater than that of potassium). A reversal of this pattern (i.e., potassium excretion exceeding sodium excretion) may indicate a relative hyperaldosteronism secondary to diminished renal blood flow and low oncotic pressure. A study by Trevisani et al.[43] evaluated renal sodium and potassium handling and plasma aldosterone in a 24-hour period in cirrhotic patients without ascites ($n = 7$), with ascites ($n = 8$), and healthy controls ($n = 7$). Plasma aldosterone was significantly higher in patients with ascites, resulting in reduced renal sodium excretion, and more than doubling renal potassium excretion in comparison to healthy controls.[43] For urine electrolyte monitoring to be meaningful, the first sample must be obtained before initiating diuretic therapy.[44,45]

SODIUM RESTRICTION

Although serum sodium in patients with ascites is often low, they are total body sodium overloaded. Sodium restriction has been shown to enhance mobilization of ascites, because fluid loss and weight change are directly related to sodium balance in patients with portal-hypertension–related ascites.[46] This finding has been incorporated into the American Association for the Study of Liver Diseases (AASLD) guidelines for the treatment of ascites. The AASLD recommends that dietary sodium should be restricted to 2,000 mg/day (88 mmol/day) and R.W. should be advised to limit his sodium intake accordingly.[38] Due to previous thought that upright posture activates sodium-retaining systems, bedrest has been advocated. However, no controlled trials support this practice.[38,42]

WATER RESTRICTION

A large prospective, observational study ($n = 997$) by Angeli et al.[47] evaluated the prevalence of low serum sodium concentration and the association between serum sodium levels with severity of ascites and complications of cirrhosis. The results indicated that low serum sodium levels are a common feature in patients with cirrhosis, and that serum sodium concentrations less than 135 mEq/L are associated with a poor control of ascites as well as a greater frequency of hepatic encephalopathy, hepatorenal syndrome, and spontaneous bacterial peritonitis compared with patients with serum sodium concentrations within the normal range (135–145 mEq/L).[47] In addition, very low serum sodium concentrations (<120 mEq/L) are independent predictors of 3-month to 6-month mortality from the MELD score in patients with end-stage liver disease. The AASLD recommends that water restriction should be implemented in cirrhotic patients who have severe dilutional hyponatremia (serum Na <120–125 mEq/L).[38] For R.W., water restriction is not indicated at this time because his serum sodium concentration is within normal limits (135 mEq/L).

VASOPRESSIN RECEPTOR ANTAGONISTS

Vasopressin (V2) receptor antagonists are a class of drugs that act by selectively antagonizing the V2 vasopressin receptors located in the principal cells of the collecting ducts in the kidney and are being used in the treatment of hyponatremia.[48] Due to the effect of vasopressin in causing reabsorption of solute-free water in the kidney, the administration of V2 antagonists also known as "vaptans" (e.g., satavaptan, conivaptan, tolvaptan) is associated with a marked increase in solute-free water excretion and reduction in urine osmolality, resulting in an increase in urine volume.[49] Currently, these agents are not available in the United States and the AASLD guidelines do not recommend the use of vaptans due to the lack of clinical trials in patients with cirrhosis, side effects, as well as the low cost-effectiveness of these medications.[38] However, a recent prospective, multicenter, randomized, double-blind, placebo-controlled study by Gines et al.[48] has shown that satavaptan (a selective V2 receptor oral vaptan) improved ascites control and increased serum sodium levels in patients with cirrhosis, ascites, and hyponatremia. Satavaptan is still undergoing clinical trials for ascites due to cirrhosis, and is not US Food and Drug Administration (FDA)–approved. It is possible that with more evidence from clinical trials, this class of medications may find a niche in the treatment of hyponatremia in cirrhotic patients.

Diuretic Therapy

CHOICE OF AGENT

CASE 29-1, QUESTION 5: R.W. was prescribed sodium restriction after initial evaluation. Spironolactone 100 mg/day and furosemide 40 mg/day were ordered to induce diuresis. Why is spironolactone preferred over other diuretics in the treatment of ascites?

Most patients with cirrhosis have elevated plasma concentrations of aldosterone.[50] High serum concentrations of aldosterone may be attributed to both increased production and decreased excretion of the hormone. Increased portal pressure, ascites, depletion of intravascular volume, and decreased renal perfusion can lead to activation of the RAAS.[51] In addition, hepatic shunting also increases aldosterone production by decreasing renal blood flow.[52] The liver metabolizes aldosterone, and hepatic impairment prolongs the physiologic half-life of aldosterone.[53] The AASLD consensus guidelines recommend the use of spironolactone as the initial diuretic of choice in the treatment of ascites.[38] Although no large comparative studies have evaluated different diuretics as first-line treatment of ascites, spironolactone is a rational diuretic choice for R.W. based on its aldosterone antagonist activity. Perez-Ayuso et al.[54] conducted a small randomized trial to study the efficacy of furosemide versus spironolactone in nonazotemic cirrhotic patients ($n = 40$) with ascites. They found that spironolactone was more effective than furosemide, and that the activity of the renin-aldosterone system influences the diuretic response to furosemide and spironolactone in patients with cirrhosis. In the study, patients were treated with furosemide (initial doses of 80 mg/day, maximal dose of 160 mg/day) or spironolactone (initial dose 150 mg/day, maximal dose of 300 mg/day). Patients not responding to furosemide or spironolactone were later converted to the alternate therapy. The results showed a higher response to spironolactone than furosemide (18/19 vs. 11/21; $p < 0.01$). Of the 10 non-responders to furosemide, 9 responded to spironolactone when therapy was switched. The authors also found that patients with higher renin and aldosterone levels did not respond to furosemide and required higher doses of spironolactone to achieve a diuretic response.[54]

Some clinicians may initiate spironolactone at a dose of 25 mg once daily or twice daily (BID); however, much larger doses (100–400 mg/day) are generally necessary to antagonize the high circulating levels of aldosterone present in patients with ascites.[38] The diuretic effect is enhanced when spironolactone is combined with sodium restriction (0.5–2 g/day).[42] In addition, furosemide can be started to minimize the risk of hyperkalemia and enhance diuresis. The AASLD guidelines recommend starting spironolactone 100 mg and furosemide 40 mg simultaneously and maintaining a 100:40 mg ratio. The doses of both oral diuretics can be increased simultaneously every 3 to 5 days (maintaining the ratio) to achieve adequate response. Usual maximal doses are 400 mg/day of spironolactone and 160 mg/day of furosemide.[38] In controlled clinical trials, sodium restriction and diuretic therapy are effective in 90% of patients without renal failure.[55–57]

Triamterene and amiloride can be used as alternatives to spironolactone if intolerable side effects (e.g., gynecomastia) occur with spironolactone.[58,59] In a small trial conducted by Angeli et al.,[60] cirrhotic patients were randomly assigned to receive amiloride ($n = 20$) or potassium canrenoate (an active metabolite of spironolactone not available in the United States; $n = 20$) to study the efficacy of each drug in nonazotemic cirrhotic patients with ascites. The initial doses of amiloride and potassium canrenoate were 20 and 150 mg, respectively, and were increased (up to 60 and 500 mg/day) if no response occurred.

Nonresponders to the highest doses of each drug were later converted to the alternate agent. A higher response rate was seen in the canrenoate group versus the amiloride group (14/20 vs. 7/20; $p < 0.025$). The authors also assessed plasma aldosterone activity and found that all responders to amiloride had normal plasma aldosterone concentrations, and all nonresponders to amiloride who later responded to potassium canrenoate had increased levels of plasma aldosterone.[60]

Eplerenone (a selective aldosterone blocker, more specific for the aldosterone receptor with a lower affinity for progesterone and androgen receptors than spironolactone) has been studied in patients with heart failure, hypertension, and renal disease.[61,62] The usual dose for eplerenone is 25 to 50 mg/day.[63] No dosage adjustment is needed with mild to moderate liver disease, but severe liver disease has not been studied.[64] Approximately 10% of patients treated with spironolactone exhibit gynecomastia or breast pain, with 2% requiring drug discontinuation.[65] In contrast, gynecomastia occurs at a similar rate with eplerenone as with placebo (0.5%).[66,67] Eplerenone is also much more expensive than spironolactone.[67] The lower risk of gynecomastia with eplerenone may make it a useful alternative to spironolactone. However, given its higher cost and the lack of data in the treatment of ascites and patients with severe liver disease, its role in ascites treatment remains unclear.

R.W. should receive spironolactone 100 mg and furosemide 40 mg simultaneously (and maintaining a 100:40 mg ratio) as recommended by the AASLD.[38] This approach to therapy may be taken, as long as the patient is carefully monitored for diuretic complications and a clinical response to diuresis (see Case 29-1, Questions 6–8).

MONITORING

CLINICAL RESPONSES

CASE 29-1, QUESTION 6: What clinical responses should be monitored to ensure the therapeutic effectiveness of spironolactone therapy for R.W.?

Because ascitic fluid is slow to re-equilibrate with vascular fluid, diuresis greater than 0.5 to 1 kg/day (>0.5–1 L) may be associated with volume depletion, hypotension, and compromised renal function.[38] Patients may tolerate a faster diuresis if peripheral edema is present. Once edema has resolved, a scaled-back weight loss, not to exceed 0.5 kg/day, can be used as a rule of thumb to minimize the risk of renal insufficiency induced by plasma volume contraction and other diuretic-induced complications.[38,68] Monitoring body weight and abdominal girth are routinely performed in both the inpatient and outpatient settings. Monitoring fluid intake and urine output are performed primarily for inpatients, owing to practical constraints in the outpatient setting. Ideally, urine output should exceed fluid intake by about 300 to 1,000 mL/day. These measurements do not account for nonrenal fluid losses; therefore, total fluid loss will be somewhat higher. Abdominal girth measurement (circumference around the abdomen) is subject to error, because of its dependence on patient position and measurement location on the abdomen.[69] Attempts should be made to standardize patient position (e.g., sitting at a 45-degree angle) and location of measurement (level of umbilicus) to minimize variability in abdominal girth measurements.

LABORATORY PARAMETERS

CASE 29-1, QUESTION 7: What laboratory parameters could be monitored to assess the therapeutic efficacy of R.W.'s spironolactone treatment?

Serum concentrations of creatinine and urine chemistries (sodium and potassium) can be monitored to define and guide the need for increasing dosage of spironolactone. A low baseline urine Na:K ratio (<1.0) suggests high intrinsic aldosterone activity and that larger dosages of spironolactone may be needed, as is the case for R.W. If necessary, the dosage of adjunctive diuretic therapy may be doubled after a few days.[51] AASLD recommends increasing both spironolactone and furosemide simultaneously every 3 to 5 days (maintaining a 100:40 mg ratio) to achieve adequate diuresis and maintain a normal serum potassium.[38]

DIURETIC COMPLICATIONS AND MANAGEMENT

CASE 29-1, QUESTION 8: The spironolactone and furosemide dosages were increased to 200 mg/day and 80 mg/day (maintaining a 100:40 mg ratio). What potential complications from the diuretic therapy might arise in R.W. and how can they be minimized?

ELECTROLYTE AND ACID–BASE DISTURBANCES

Hyponatremia, hyperkalemia, metabolic alkalosis, and, uncommonly, hypokalemia occur as side effects of diuretic therapy in patients with ascites. Hyponatremia results from a reduction in filtered sodium, an increase in sodium reabsorption, and a reduction in free water clearance (dilutional hyponatremia). Diuresis exacerbates hyponatremia by causing volume depletion and antidiuretic hormone (ADH) release. Hyponatremia, if present, usually can be corrected by temporary withdrawal of diuretics and free water restriction.[55,70–72] Although serum sodium may be low, these patients are total body sodium overloaded. Hyperkalemia is common in patients with refractory ascites and impaired renal function requiring high doses of diuretics such as spironolactone. Hyperkalemia can be approached in multiple ways, depending on the clinical situation (see Chapter 10, Fluid and Electrolyte Disorders). Furosemide is added to the therapeutic regimen to maintain normal serum potassium.[38] Decreasing or holding spironolactone may be appropriate depending on the patient's renal function and serum potassium.[24] Metabolic alkalosis, another acid–base disorder found in cirrhotic patients as a result of loop diuretics, occurs because of increased urinary hydrogen loss from enhanced distal hydrogen secretion. Hypokalemia often accompanies metabolic alkalosis owing to loop diuretics.[71] Furosemide can be temporarily withheld in patients presenting with hypokalemia.[38] R.W. has some degree of renal impairment (SCr 1.4 mg/dL) and is receiving spironolactone and furosemide. Therefore, his electrolytes and renal function tests should be monitored daily while hospitalized. After hospital discharge, monitoring will be dictated by the stability of the patient and need for diuretic dosage adjustments. For example, outpatients may need electrolytes and renal function monitoring once or twice weekly early after hospital discharge to as infrequently as every 3 months for the very stable patient.[38]

PRERENAL AZOTEMIA

Prerenal azotemia usually results from overdiuresis with subsequent compromise of intravascular volume and decreased renal perfusion. In addition to looking for clinical signs of hypovolemia, such as dizziness, orthostatic hypotension, and increased heart rate, frequent measurements of BUN and serum creatinine concentrations provide a relatively simple means of assessing the intravascular volume. A gradual rise in serum creatinine, BUN, as well as the BUN:serum creatinine ratio can serve as a warning to slow the rate of diuresis.[73] In a small study conducted by Pockros et al.,[68] serial measurements of plasma volume and ascites volume were made during treatment with diuretics in patients with cirrhosis ($n = 14$). Patients with ascites and no edema were able to mobilize more than 1 L/day during rapid diuresis, but at the expense of plasma volume contraction and renal insufficiency. Patients with peripheral edema appear to be somewhat protected from these effects and may safely undergo diuresis at a more rapid rate (>2 kg/day) until edema resolves.[68] Others suggest, however, that the maximal daily fluid loss should not exceed more than 0.5 L/day (>0.5 kg/day) for patients with ascites alone or more than 1 L/day (>1 kg/day) for those with both ascites and edema to prevent plasma volume depletion and decreased renal perfusion. If faster removal of ascites is required because of respiratory distress, large-volume paracentesis may be more effective than rapid diuresis (see Case 29-1, Question 9).[38,45,74,75]

Because R.W. presented with both edema and ascites, an initial fluid loss of up to 1 L/day would be reasonable. The rate of weight loss should be slowed not to exceed more than 0.5 L/day when the edema resolves. Gradual diuresis avoids diuretic-induced depletion of intravascular fluid volume by permitting ascitic fluid to equilibrate with intravascular fluid. Long-term management of ascites is done in the outpatient setting. Severe cases with respiratory distress or impaired ambulation as well as patients with spontaneous bacterial peritonitis require hospitalization. If outpatient therapy is an option, a weekly evaluation initially would be prudent to prevent overdiuresis and electrolyte disturbances.[38]

Refractory Ascites

CASE 29-1, QUESTION 9: Over the next several days, R.W.'s spironolactone dosage was increased to 400 mg/day. Furosemide was simultaneously increased to 80 mg BID without major improvement in his diuresis. Laboratory data revealed that R.W.'s SCr had increased to 3.2 mg/dL (estimated creatinine clearance: 26 mL/minute) and his BUN had increased to 45 mg/dL. Serum electrolytes were as follows:

K, 3.1 mEq/L
Na, 130 mEq/L
Cl, 88 mEq/L
Bicarbonate, 32 mEq/L

R.W. became progressively short of breath because of restricted diaphragmatic movement secondary to his significantly enlarged abdomen. What therapeutic measures are appropriate for R.W.'s refractory (diuretic-resistant) ascites?

Because of the increase in SCr and respiratory distress, R.W.'s ascites treatment needs modification. Patients with cirrhosis experiencing respiratory distress despite diuretic therapy and sodium restriction warrant more aggressive second-line treatment, including large volume paracentesis, shunting procedures, or both.[38] Paracentesis involves the removal of ascitic fluid from the abdominal cavity with a needle or a catheter. Although paracentesis can remove large amounts of ascitic fluid (e.g., 10 L), removal of as little as 1 L of fluid may provide considerable relief from the painful stretching of skin and the respiratory distress that occurs with massive ascites. The ascitic fluid often reaccumulates rapidly after paracentesis owing to transudation of fluid from the interstitial and plasma compartments into the peritoneal cavity. The major complications of overly aggressive, large-volume paracentesis include hypotension, shock, oliguria, encephalopathy, and renal insufficiency. Other potential complications of paracentesis are hemorrhage, perforation of the abdominal viscera, infection, and protein depletion.[38]

ALBUMIN

CASE 29-1, QUESTION 10: R.W. continues to reaccumulate ascitic fluid and is exhibiting signs of declining renal function. A 6-L paracentesis coupled with a 50-g albumin infusion is ordered. Why are albumin infusions used in conjunction with paracentesis?

Large volume (>4 L) paracentesis should be performed for patients with tense ascites resulting in respiratory distress or impaired ambulation. However, large volume paracentesis alone is associated with paracentesis-induced circulatory dysfunction (PICD). This dysfuction is characterized by a reduction in

or ciprofloxacin IV (400 mg BID) when oral administration is not possible. Ceftriaxone IV (1 g/day) may be a preferable option in centers with a high prevalence of quinolone-resistant organisms.[38,109] C.V. should be treated with norfloxacin 400 mg orally once daily (dose adjusted for creatinine clearance of 30 mL/minute), or ceftriaxone 1 g/day for 7 days to prevent SBP.

PRIMARY PROPHYLAXIS

CASE 29-2, QUESTION 5: All variceal hemorrhage interventions up to this point were aimed at terminating the acute bleeding episode. Could drug therapy have helped prevent the first episode of bleeding from C.V.'s esophageal varices?

Preventing the initial occurrence of variceal bleeding is referred to as primary prevention or primary prophylaxis. Pharmacologic prophylaxis is aimed at reducing the HVPG to less than or equal to 12 mm Hg, or a decrease from baseline of greater than or equal to 20%.[146,147] In a small study by Vorobioff et al.,[146] none of the patients with HVPG less than or equal to 12 mm Hg ($n = 6$) bled from portal hypertensive-related causes as compared to 42% in the HVPG greater than 12 mm Hg group ($n = 24$). In addition, only 1 of the 6 patients with an HVPG less than or equal to 12 mm Hg as compared with 16 (of 24) in the HVPG greater than 12 mm Hg group died during the study period ($p < 0.06$).[146] This study suggests that patients with an HVPG less than or equal to 12 mm Hg may have a better prognosis than those with HVPG greater than 12 mm Hg. Escorsell et al.[147] has shown that a fall of HVPG by 20% or more from baseline was associated with a decreased risk of variceal bleeding (6% vs. 45%; $p = 0.004$).

β-BLOCKERS

Nonselective β-adrenergic blockers decrease portal pressure through a reduction in portal venous inflow as a result of a decrease in cardiac output (β_1-adrenergic blockade) and splanchnic blood flow (β_2-adrenergic blockade). They are the most frequently studied drug class for primary prevention of bleeding. Only nonselective β-blockers have an adrenergic dilatory effect in mesenteric arterioles resulting in a decrease in portal blood circulation and pressure. Nonselective β-blockers have been studied in comparison with other modalities of treatment, such as endoscopic variceal ligation, for the primary prevention of variceal hemorrhage in patients with existing varices in a number of randomized trials.[148,149] Usual starting dosages of propranolol are 10 mg three times a day, or nadolol 20 mg daily. Selective β-blockers (e.g., atenolol and metoprolol) have little effect on mesenteric arterioles and have not been shown to be effective in primary prophylaxis.[150]

Propranolol or nadolol, given in dosages to reduce the resting heart rate to 55 to 60 beats/minute or by 25%, have been shown to prevent or delay the first episode of variceal bleeding.[15] Nonselective β-blockers are considered first-line drug therapy in the prevention of variceal hemorrhage based on numerous randomized, placebo-controlled trials and meta-analyses.[127,151] For example, Pascal et al.[152] conducted a prospective, randomized, multicenter, single-blinded trial of propranolol compared with placebo in the prevention of bleeding in patients with large esophageal varices without previous bleeding. Patients received either propranolol ($n = 118$) or placebo ($n = 112$), with the endpoints of the study being bleeding and death. The dosage of propranolol was progressively increased to decrease the heart rate by 20% to 25%. The cumulative percentages of patients free of bleeding 2 years after inclusion in the study (74% vs. 39%; $p < 0.05$) and cumulative 2-year survival (72% vs. 51%; $p < 0.05$) were higher in the propranolol group versus the placebo group.[152]

The role of propranolol added to EVL in the prevention of first variceal bleeding has also been compared with EVL alone as primary prophylaxis. Sarin et al.[153] conducted a prospective, randomized, controlled trial comparing EVL with propranolol ($n = 72$) with EVL alone ($n = 72$) in the prevention of first variceal bleeding among patients with high-risk varices. The mean duration of follow-up for both groups was about 12.2 months ($\pm$ 10.7 months). EVL was performed at 2-week intervals until obliteration of varices. Propranolol was administered at a dosage sufficient to reduce heart rate to 55 beats/minute or 25% reduction from baseline, and continued after obliteration of varices. No significant differences were seen in the rates of bleeding and survival between groups, although more patients in the EVL alone group had recurrence of varices ($p = 0.03$).[153]

Treatment with a β-blocker must be continued indefinitely. A study by Abraczinskas et al.[154] reported the outcomes of patients in whom β-blocker therapy was discontinued. Patients completing a prospective, randomized, double-blind, placebo-controlled trial of propranolol for the primary prevention of variceal hemorrhage were tapered off of propranolol and placebo and followed prospectively for subsequent events. The authors found that when propranolol was withdrawn, the risk of variceal hemorrhage increased from 4% (while on propranolol therapy) to 24% (after propranolol withdrawal), and was comparable to the risk of bleeding in an untreated population (22% in the placebo group from the previous study). The authors suggested that the protective effect of propranolol against variceal hemorrhage was no longer present. Also, patients who discontinued β-blockers experienced increased mortality compared with the untreated population (48% vs. 21%; $p < 0.05$).[154] Therefore, avoiding sudden discontinuation of β-blockers in this population is essential.

The AASLD/ACG guidelines recommend nonselective β-blockers for primary prophylaxis in patients with small varices that have not bled, but are at increased risk of hemorrhage (Child-Turcotte-Pugh class B or C or presence of red wale marks on varices). Patients with medium or large varices that have not bled but are at a high risk of hemorrhage (Child-Turcotte-Pugh class B or C or variceal red wale markings on endoscopy), nonselective β-blockers or EVL may be recommended. In contrast, patients with medium or large varices that have not bled and are not at the highest risk of hemorrhage (Child-Turcotte-Pugh class A patients and no red signs), nonselective β-blockers are preferred and EVL should be considered in patients with contraindications, intolerance or noncompliance to β-blockers. The β-blocker should be titrated to the maximal tolerated dose.[109]

ISOSORBIDE-5-MONONITRATE

Isosorbide-5-mononitrate has been evaluated as primary prophylaxis for variceal hemorrhage as monotherapy in patients intolerant or refractory to β-blockers and in combination with β-blockers in a number of trials.[155] When studied for primary prevention of bleeding in patients with cirrhosis, isosorbide-5-mononitrate in combination with β-blockers has had mixed success. In addition, its use as monotherapy has not proven to be effective.[155,156] Garcia-Pagan et al.[156] conducted a prospective, multicenter, double-blind, randomized, controlled trial evaluating whether isosorbide-5-mononitrate prevented variceal bleeding in cirrhotic patients ($n = 133$) with gastroesophageal varices, who had contraindications or could not tolerate β-blockers. Patient received isosorbide-5-mononitrate ($n = 67$) or placebo ($n = 66$). No significant differences were noted in the 1-year and

2-year actuarial probability of bleeding or survival between the two treatment groups.[156]

When combined with a β-blocker, isosorbide-5-mononitrate causes a greater reduction in the hepatic venous pressure gradient than propranolol alone.[157] Merkel et al.[158] examined the value of combining nadolol and isosorbide-5-mononitrate for primary prevention of variceal bleeding. Patients in the nadolol monotherapy group ($n = 74$) received between 40 and 160 mg/day titrated to achieve a 20% to 25% decrease in resting heart rate. Patients receiving both drugs ($n = 72$) received nadolol and isosorbide-5-mononitrate 10 to 20 mg orally BID. The overall risk of variceal bleeding was 18% in the nadolol group compared with 7.5% in the combined treatment group ($p = 0.03$). However, a higher number of patients had to be withdrawn from the combination therapy group compared with the nadolol monotherapy group (8 vs. 4 patients) due to side effects.[158] The AASLD and ACG guidelines suggest that nitrates (either alone or in combination with β-blockers), shunt therapy, or sclerotherapy should not be used in the primary prophylaxis of variceal hemorrhage.[109]

SECONDARY PROPHYLAXIS

CASE 29-2, QUESTION 6: C.V.'s hepatologist would like to start treatment to prevent further variceal hemorrhage. What are the long-term objectives for the treatment of C.V.? What treatment approaches can be used to prevent a recurrence of bleeding (secondary prevention)?

Secondary prevention or secondary prophylaxis is the terminology used to describe therapy to prevent rebleeding once it has occurred. All patients who survive a variceal bleeding episode should receive therapy to prevent recurrent episodes. It is important that the initiation of β-blockers be delayed until after recovery of the initial variceal hemorrhage. Initiation of a β-blocker during the treatment of an acute bleed would block the patient's acute tachycardia in response to his or her hypotension, which may adversely impact survival. The benefit of nonselective β-blockers in the prevention of rebleeding episodes has been demonstrated by a number of trials.[130,159,160] For example, a trial by Colombo et al.[159] studied the efficacy of β-blockers in preventing rebleeding in cirrhotic patients. Patients were randomly assigned to propranolol ($n = 32$), atenolol ($n = 32$), or placebo ($n = 30$). Randomization was made at least 15 days after the bleeding episode. Propranolol was given orally and titrated until the resting pulse rate was reduced by approximately 25%, and atenolol was given at a fixed dose of 100 mg daily. The incidence of rebleeding was significantly lower in patients receiving propranolol than in those on placebo ($p = 0.01$). Bleeding-free survival was better for patients on active drugs than for those on placebo (propranolol vs. placebo, $p = 0.01$; atenolol vs. placebo, $p = 0.05$).[159]

Eradication of varices by endoscopic procedures is also effective in preventing recurrent variceal bleeding.[15,160] A study by de la Pena et al.[160] showed that nadolol plus EVL ($n = 43$) reduced the incidence of variceal rebleeding compared with EVL alone ($n = 37$). Variceal bleeding recurrence rate was 14% in the EVL plus nadolol group and 38% in the EVL alone group ($p = 0.006$). Mortality was similar in both groups and the actuarial probability of variceal recurrence at 1 year was lower in the EVL plus nadolol group than in the EVL alone group (54% vs. 77%; $p = 0.06$). The adverse effects in the β-blocker group were higher, and led to the withdrawal of 20% to 30% of the patients.[160] Interestingly, Gonzalez-Suarez et al.[161] conducted a study to compare the occurrence of SBP in cirrhotic patients treated with nadolol plus isosorbide mononitrate ($n = 115$) versus sclerotherapy or endoscopic variceal ligation ($n = 115$) for the prevention of rebleeding. They found that the probability of SBP was lower in the medication group at 1 year (6% vs. 12%; $p = 0.08$) and at 5 years (22% vs. 36%; $p = 0.08$). The probability of survival was similar in both groups.[161]

TIPS may be an option for those patients who fail both EVL and prophylaxis with β-blocker therapy. Escorsell et al.[162] studied 91 Child-Turcotte-Pugh class B or class C cirrhotic patients surviving their first episode of variceal bleeding. Subjects were randomly assigned to TIPS ($n = 47$) or combination therapy with propranolol and isosorbide-5-mononitrate ($n = 44$) to prevent variceal rebleeding. Rebleeding occurred in a lower percentage of patients treated with TIPS versus those treated with drug (13% vs. 39%; $p = 0.007$). The 2-year rebleeding probability was lower in the TIPS group (13% vs. 49%; $p = 0.01$). Encephalopathy was more frequent in TIPS than in patients treated with drug (38% vs. 14%, $p = 0.007$). Child-Turcotte-Pugh class improved more frequently in those treated with drug than with TIPS (72% vs. 45%; $p = 0.04$). The 2-year survival probability was identical (72%). The cost of therapy was doubled for patients treated with TIPS as compared to those treated with drug therapy. In high-risk cirrhotic patients, drug therapy was less effective than TIPS in preventing rebleeding; however, drug therapy caused less encephalopathy, had identical survival, and more frequent improvement in Child-Turcotte-Pugh class at lower costs.[162]

The AASLD/ACG guidelines suggest the use of a combination of nonselective β-blockers plus EVL for secondary prophylaxis. TIPS should be considered in patients who are Child-Turcotte-Pugh class A or B who experience recurrent variceal hemorrhage despite combination pharmacological and endoscopic therapy.[90,109]

Depending on the size of C.V.'s varices on endoscopy and the risk of hemorrhage, C.V. should have been given nonselective β-blockers (propranolol or nadolol) or EVL to prevent or delay the first episode of variceal bleeding. Because C.V. has a history of recurrent upper GI bleeding, the best option to prevent further bleeding is to initiate a nonselective β-blocker and begin EVL. The β-blocker should be titrated to reduce the resting heart rate to 55 to 60 beats/minute or by 25%. EVL should be repeated every 1 to 2 weeks until obliteration with a repeat endoscopy performed 1 to 3 months after obliteration and then every 6 to 12 months to check for variceal recurrence.[109] If this combination fails to prevent variceal hemorrhage, then TIPS would be considered as a therapeutic option.[90]

HEPATIC ENCEPHALOPATHY

CASE 29-3

QUESTION 1: R.C., a 57-year-old man, was admitted to the hospital because of nausea, vomiting, and abdominal pain. He had a long history of alcohol abuse, with multiple hospital admissions for alcoholic gastritis and alcohol withdrawal. Physical examination revealed a cachectic male patient (weighing 55 kg) with clouded mentation who was not responsive to questions about name and place. Tense ascites and edema were noted, and the liver was percussed at 9 cm below the right costal margin. The spleen was not palpated, and no active bowel sounds were heard. Laboratory results on admission included the following:

Na, 132 mEq/L
K, 3.7 mEq/L

Cl, 98 mEq/L
Bicarbonate, 27 mEq/L
BUN, 24 mg/dL
SCr, 1.4 mg/dL
Hgb, 9.2 g/dL
Hct, 24.1%
AST, 520 international units
Alkaline phosphatase, 218 international units
Lactate dehydrogenase (LDH), 305 international units
Total bilirubin, 3.5 mg/dL
PT, 22 seconds (INR 1.8)

A 70-g protein, 2,000-kcal diet was ordered. Furosemide 40 mg IV every 12 hours was ordered in an attempt to reduce the edema and ascites. Morphine sulfate and prochlorperazine were ordered for his abdominal pain and nausea, respectively. Two days after admission, R.C. had an episode of hematemesis. He became mentally confused and at times nonresponsive to verbal command. An NG tube was inserted and coffee-ground material was produced on continuous suctioning. Saline lavage was continued until the aspirate became clear. The next morning, R.C. was still in a confused mental state. He demonstrated prominent asterixis, and fetor hepaticus was noted on his breath. On the second day of his hospitalization, laboratory data were as follows:

Hgb, 7.4 g/dL
Hct, 21.2%
K, 3.1 mEq/L
SCr, 1.4 mg/dL
BUN, 36 mg/dL
PT, 22 seconds (INR 1.8)
Guaiac positive stool

Hepatic encephalopathy and upper GI bleeding were added to the problem list.

What aspects of R.C.'s history are compatible with a diagnosis of hepatic encephalopathy?

Hepatic coma or encephalopathy is a metabolic disorder of the central nervous system (CNS), which occurs in patients with either advanced cirrhosis or fulminate hepatic failure. It is commonly accompanied by portal systemic shunting of blood. The clinical features (as seen in R.C.) include altered mental state, asterixis, and fetor hepaticus. During the early phase of encephalopathy, the altered mental state may present as a slight derangement of judgment and personality, and change in sleep pattern or mood. Drowsiness and confusion become more prominent as the encephalopathy progresses. Finally, unresponsiveness to arousal and deep coma ensue.

Asterixis, or flapping tremor, is the most characteristic neurologic abnormality in hepatic encephalopathy.

ONLINE CONTENT

For a photo that shows the method to detect asterixis, go to http://thepoint.lww.com/AT10e.

This tremor can be demonstrated by having the patient hyperextend his or her wrist with the forearms outstretched and fingers separated. It is characterized by bilateral, but synchronous, repetitive arrhythmic motions occurring in bursts of one flap (twitch) every 1 to 2 seconds. Asterixis is not specific for hepatic encephalopathy and may also be present in uremia, hypokalemia, heart failure, ketoacidosis, respiratory failure, and sedative overdose.

Fetor hepaticus, a peculiar sweetish, musty, pungent odor to the breath, is believed to be caused by circulating unmetabolized mercaptans. A staging scheme for grading the severity of hepatic encephalopathy is found in Table 29-4.[163,164] As discussed in the questions that follow, the pharmacologic management of encephalopathy is guided by both an understanding of the pathogenesis of this disorder and the stage of severity demonstrated by the individual patient. In most cases, hepatic encephalopathy is fully reversible; therefore, it is likely a metabolic or neurophysiologic rather than an organic disorder.[163] Severe, progressive hepatic encephalopathy can lead to irreversible brain damage (caused by increased intracranial pressure), brain herniations, and death.[165,166]

Pathogenesis

CASE 29-3, QUESTION 2: What is the pathogenesis of hepatic encephalopathy?

Several theories exist about the pathogenesis of hepatic encephalopathy. The most widely referenced theories involve abnormal ammonia metabolism; altered ratio of branched chain to aromatic amino acids; imbalance in brain neurotransmitters, such as γ-aminobutyric acid (GABA) and serotonin; derangement in the blood brain–barrier; and exposure of the brain to accumulated "toxins."[167] None of these are considered to be a single cause, and the pathogenesis of hepatic encephalopathy is likely multifactorial.

TABLE 29-4
Stages of Encephalopathy

Physical Sign	Stage I Prodrome	Stage II Impending Coma	Stage III Stupor	Stage IV Coma	Stage V Coma
Mental status	Alert; slow mentation; euphoria, occasional depression, confusion; sleep pattern reversal	Stage I signs amplified; lethargic, sleepy	Arousable, but generally asleep; significant confusion	Unarousable or responds only to pain	Unarousable
Behavior	Restless, irritable, disordered speech	Combative, sullen, loss of sphincter control	Sleeping, confusion, incoherent speech	None	None
Spontaneous motor activity	Uncoordinated with tremor	Yawning, grimacing, blinking	Decreased, severe tremor	Absent	None
Asterixis	Absent	Present	Present	Absent	Absent
Reflexes	Normal	Hyperactive	Hyperactive + Babinski	Hyperactive + Babinski	Absent

TABLE 29-5
Factors That May Precipitate Hepatic Encephalopathy

Excess Nitrogen Load	Fluid and Electrolyte Abnormalities	Drug-Induced Central Nervous System Depression
Bleeding from gastric and esophageal varices	Hypokalemia	Sedatives
Peptic ulcer	Alkalosis	Tranquilizers
Excess dietary protein	Hypovolemia	Narcotic analgesics
Azotemia or kidney failure	Excessive diarrhea	
Deteriorating hepatic function	Overdiuresis	
Infection: tissue catabolism		
Constipation	Excessive vomiting	

AMMONIA

Ammonia is a byproduct of protein metabolism, and a large portion is derived from dietary ingestion of proteins or presentation of protein-rich blood into the GI tract (e.g., from bleeding esophageal varices). Bacteria present in the GI tract digest protein into polypeptides, amino acids, and ammonia. These substances are then absorbed across the intestinal mucosa, where they are either further metabolized, stored for later use, or used for production of new proteins. Ammonia is readily metabolized in the liver to urea, which is then renally eliminated. When blood flow and hepatic metabolism are impaired by cirrhosis, serum and CNS concentrations of ammonia are increased. The ammonia that enters the CNS combines with α-ketoglutarate to form glutamine, an aromatic amino acid. Ammonia has been considered central to the pathogenesis of hepatic encephalopathy. An increased ammonia level raises the amount of glutamine within astrocytes, causing an osmotic imbalance resulting in cell swelling and ultimately brain edema. Although high serum ammonia and cerebrospinal glutamine concentrations are characteristic of encephalopathy, they may not be the actual cause of this syndrome.[166,168]

AMINO ACID BALANCE

Body stores of branched chain and aromatic amino acids are affected by their rate of synthesis from protein metabolism (both in the GI tract and in the liver), their utilization in the resynthesis of new proteins within the liver, and their utilization by various tissues for energy. In both acute and chronic liver failure, the serum concentrations of aromatic amino acids significantly increase and as a result the ratio of the branched chain to aromatic amino acids is altered. The utilization of branched chain amino acids for skeletal muscle metabolism during liver failure can decrease branched chain amino acids.[167] At the same time, the blood–brain barrier appears to be more permeable to aromatic amino acid uptake into the cerebrospinal fluid (CSF). Once in the CSF, some aromatic compounds can be metabolized to produce "false neurotransmitters" (e.g., tyrosine conversion to octopamine) that disrupt normal CSF neurotransmitter balance, and compete with norepinephrine for normal CNS function.[168]

γ-AMINOBUTYRIC ACID

Schafer et al.[169] proposed that in liver disease, gut-derived GABA escapes hepatic metabolism, crosses the blood–brain barrier, binds to its postsynaptic receptor sites, and causes the neurologic abnormalities associated with hepatic encephalopathy. Others hypothesize that endogenous benzodiazepinelike substances, via their agonist properties, contribute to the pathogenesis of hepatic encephalopathy by enhancing GABA-ergic neurotransmission. The role of GABA and endogenous benzodiazepines in hepatic encephalopathy is still not clearly defined and requires further clarification.[170,171]

Of all the toxins suspected to cause hepatic coma, ammonia and certain aromatic amino acids are most commonly studied. Other precipitating factors (Table 29-5) increase the serum ammonia or produce excessive somnolence in patients with impending hepatic coma. Excess nitrogen load and metabolic abnormalities may increase ammonia levels and precipitate an exacerbation of hepatic encephalopathy.[172,173]

CASE 29-3, QUESTION 3: What are the probable precipitating causes of hepatic encephalopathy in R.C.?

The main precipitating cause of the encephalopathy in R.C. was the sudden onset of upper GI bleeding. The bacterial degradation of blood in the gut results in absorption of large amounts of ammonia and possibly other toxins into the portal system. Other important contributory factors in this case are diuretic-induced hypovolemia (BUN:SCr ratio, >20), hypokalemia (potassium, 3.1 mEq/L), and potentially metabolic alkalosis (continuous NG suctioning and furosemide). Overzealous diuretic therapy enhances hepatic encephalopathy by inducing prerenal azotemia, hypokalemia, and metabolic alkalosis. Alkalosis promotes diffusion of nonionic ammonia and other amines into the CNS. The associated intracellular acidosis "traps" the ammonia by converting it back to ammonium ion (NH_4^+).[174,175]

Sedating drugs can also precipitate hepatic encephalopathy. Drugs that have been associated with hepatic encephalopathy are opioids (e.g., morphine, methadone, meperidine, codeine), sedatives (e.g., benzodiazepines, barbiturates, chloral hydrate), and tranquilizers (e.g., phenothiazines). Encephalopathy precipitated by most drugs can be explained by increased CNS sensitivity and decreased hepatic clearance with subsequent drug and, in some cases, active metabolite accumulation. In addition, the effects of some highly protein-bound drugs such as chlorpromazine, and diazepam might be increased in liver disease because of decreased plasma protein binding. In this case, the morphine and prochlorperazine might have contributed to the worsening of his hepatic encephalopathy. Although not applicable to R.C., excessive dietary protein, infections, and constipation can contribute to excess nitrogen load and the genesis of hepatic coma as well (Table 29-5).

Treatment and General Management

CASE 29-3, QUESTION 4: What non-drug steps should be taken to manage R.C.'s hepatic encephalopathy?

After identifying and removing precipitating causes of hepatic coma, therapeutic management is aimed primarily at reducing the amount of ammonia or nitrogenous products in the circulatory system. In general, the 2006 European Society for Clinical Nutrition and Metabolism (ESPEN) recommends an energy intake of 35 to 40 kcal/kg of body weight/day and a protein intake of 1.2 to 1.5 g/kg of body weight/day for cirrhotic patients and those awaiting liver transplantation surgeries.[176–179] A study conducted by Cordoba et al.[180] assessed the effects of the amount of protein in the diet on the evolution of hepatic encephalopathy.

Cirrhotic patients admitted to the hospital for encephalopathy ($n = 30$) were randomly assigned to two dietary groups, in addition to standard measures to treat hepatic encephalopathy, for 14 days. The first group followed a progressive increase in the dose of protein in the diet, and received 0 g of protein for the first 3 days, then the amount of protein was increased progressively every 3 days (12, 24, and 48 g) up to 1.2 g/kg/day for the last 2 days. The second group received 1.2 g/kg/day from the first day. Results showed that the course of hepatic encephalopathy was not significantly different between both dietary protein restriction groups. The patients in the first group, however, experienced a higher degree of protein breakdown.[180]

R.C. is a chachectic male, and care should be taken in refeeding malnourished patients. However, the 70-g protein, 2,000-kcal diet ordered for R.C. is appropriate because it falls within the recommended weight-based ranges established by the ESPEN guidelines.[176,177]

CASE 29-3, QUESTION 5: Which pharmacologic interventions are appropriate to manage R.C.'s hepatic encephalopathy?

LACTULOSE

Lactulose is broken down by GI bacteria to form lactic, acetic, and formic acids. It is believed that acidification of colonic contents converts ammonia into the less readily absorbed ammonium ion. Back diffusion of ammonia from the plasma into the GI tract can also occur. The net result is a lower plasma ammonia concentration. The absorption of other protein breakdown products (e.g., aromatic amino acids) may also be reduced. Lactulose-induced osmotic diarrhea may also decrease the intestinal transit time available for ammonia production and absorption, and may help clear the GI tract of blood. Lactulose syrup (10 g/15 mL) has been used successfully in both acute and chronic hepatic encephalopathy. For acute encephalopathy, lactulose 30 to 45 mL is administered every hour until evacuation occurs. The dosage is then titrated to two to four soft bowel movements per day and clear mentation. When the oral route of administration is not possible, as in the treatment of a comatose patient, it may be necessary to administer the drug through an NG tube. Alternatively, a rectal retention enema compounded with 300 mL of lactulose in 700 mL water can be prepared. The lactulose water mixture (125 mL) is retained for 30 to 60 minutes, although this is difficult in patients with altered mental status. The beneficial clinical effect of lactulose occurs within 12 to 48 hours. Patients may need long-term administration of lactulose as maintenance therapy, especially in patients with recurring encephalopathy. For chronic encephalopathy, oral dosing of lactulose should be administered daily to four times daily titrating to two to four soft stools per day and clear mentation. The chronic administration of lactulose permits better dietary protein tolerance and is well tolerated if dosages are kept sufficiently low to avoid diarrhea.[181]

Although lactulose has been the mainstay of hepatic encephalopathy treatment,[182] very limited data exist evaluating the efficacy of lactulose for the treatment of hepatic encephalopathy. Care should be taken not to induce excessive diarrhea that could lead to dehydration and hypokalemia, both of which have been associated with exacerbation of hepatic encephalopathy. Although lactulose is generally well tolerated, 20% of patients may complain of gaseous distention, flatulence, or belching. Dilution with fruit juice, carbonated beverages, or water can reduce the excessive sweetness of the syrup.[164]

RIFAXIMIN

Rifaximin is a synthetic antibiotic structurally related to rifamycin. It displays a wide spectrum of antibacterial activity against gram-negative and gram-positive bacteria, both aerobic and anaerobic, and has very limited systemic absorption.[183] It has been available for enteric bacterial conditions for more than a decade in several countries outside the United States, and was introduced in the United States for the treatment of travelers' diarrhea.[184] It has recently gained an indication for use in hepatic encephalopathy.[185] The dosages used in trials have ranged from 550 mg twice daily to 400 mg every 8 hours[186,187]; the 550 mg twice daily regimen is the FDA approved dose for hepatic encephalopathy.[185]

Rifaximin is well tolerated, although reported adverse effects seen with rifaximin therapy include flatulence, nausea, and vomiting. It is considered relatively safe due to its limited systemic absorption. Some urticarial skin reactions have been reported with prolonged use.[188] The manufacturer notes that its use may result in bacterial superinfections (*C. difficile*—associated diarrhea) in patients being treated with rifaximin for more than 2 months. Of note, 96.6% of the drug is recovered in the feces as unchanged drug, and what is absorbed undergoes metabolism with minimal renal excretion of unchanged drug.[185,189]

NEOMYCIN

Neomycin, at dosages of 500 mg to 1 g orally four times daily, or as a 1% solution (125 mL) given as a retention enema (retained for 30–60 minutes) four times daily, is effective in reducing plasma ammonia concentrations (presumably by decreasing protein-metabolizing bacteria in the GI tract). Approximately 1% to 3% of the neomycin dose is absorbed. Chronic use in patients with severe renal insufficiency can cause ototoxicity or nephrotoxicity. Routine monitoring of the serum creatinine, the presence of protein in the urine, and estimation of creatinine clearance are advisable for patients receiving high dosages for more than 2 weeks.[181] Neomycin therapy can also produce a reversible malabsorption syndrome that not only suppresses the absorption of fat, nitrogen, carotene, iron, vitamin B_{12}, xylose, and glucose but also decreases the absorption of some drugs, such as digoxin, penicillin, and vitamin K.[164]

FLUMAZENIL

Based on the theory of accumulation of endogenous benzodiazepinelike substances in hepatic encephalopathy, flumazenil, a benzodiazepine antagonist, has been evaluated for its role in the treatment of hepatic encephalopathy. Several trials have demonstrated both clinical and electrophysiologic improvement in patients with hepatic encephalopathy.[190] However an IV product with modest benefits in the treatment of hepatic encephalopathy is not an ideal treatment option.

COMPARATIVE EFFICACY

Due to the availability of options for the treatment of hepatic encephalopathy, most recently with the approval of rifaximin, several trials have been conducted evaluating their comparative efficacy.

LACTULOSE VERSUS RIFAXIMIN

An extensive review of rifaximin for the treatment of hepatic encephalopathy conducted by Lawrence et al.[191] examined the literature published from 1966 to 2007 and found that rifaximin was equally effective, and in some studies superior, to lactulose in mild to moderate hepatic encephalopathy. The authors also noted that patients treated with rifaximin required less hospitalization, had shorter duration of hospitalization, and lower hospital charges compared with lactulose-treated patients.[191]

Bucci et al.[192] evaluated the use of rifaximin in a double-blind study comparing rifaximin and lactulose in patients ($n = 58$) with moderate to severe hepatic encephalopathy. Rifaximin was administered at a dose of 1,200 mg/day, and lactulose was administered at a dose of 30 g/day, both for 15 days. At the end of the treatment period, cognitive function test scores improved in both groups. In addition, concentrations of ammonia normalized after 7 days of treatment in both groups. Rifaximin therapy was better tolerated.[192] Although the data reported from these and other trials suggest a benefit with rifaximin for the treatment of hepatic encephalopathy, larger trials must be conducted to determine its superiority over lactulose. In addition, the current cost of rifaximin is considerably higher than both lactulose and neomycin (lactulose [60–100 g daily] ~$120–200/month; neomycin [500 mg four times daily] ~$160/month; and rifaximin [550 mg twice daily] ~$1300/month; price data per drugstore.com).

RIFAXIMIN VERSUS NEOMYCIN

Miglio et al.[193] conducted a randomized, controlled, double-blind study to evaluate the efficacy and tolerability of rifaximin (400 mg three times daily) in comparison to neomycin (1 g three times daily) treatment for 14 days each month for 6 months ($n = 49$). During the study, blood ammonia concentrations in both the rifaximin and in the neomycin groups decreased a similar amount.[193] A study conducted by Pedretti et al.[194] comparing rifaximin 400 mg every 8 hours versus neomycin 1 g every 8 hours in patients with cirrhosis ($n = 30$) showed a higher rate of adverse events (increases in BUN, plasma creatinine [$n = 4$]; nausea, abdominal pain, and vomiting [$n = 5$]) in the neomycin group after 21 days of therapy. A significant decrease in blood ammonia levels was observed at the end of the treatment period in both groups. However, rifaximin produced an earlier reduction of blood ammonia levels.[194] Due to the lower adverse-effect profile and considerable efficacy, rifaximin has taken over as second-line therapy for hepatic encephalopathy over neomycin at many institutions.

LACTULOSE VERSUS NEOMYCIN

A study conducted by Orlandi found that lactulose and neomycin appear to have similar efficacy for the acute treatment of hepatic encephalopathy.[195] In the treatment of an acute exacerbation, particularly in an acute GI bleed, lactulose may, however, produce a faster response than neomycin. In the past, neomycin has been used in patients who do not respond to lactulose.[181]

Interestingly, although lactose therapy is considered the standard of practice in both acute and chronic hepatic encephalopathy, a meta-analysis evaluating the efficacy of lactulose in patients with hepatic encephalopathy questions its benefit.[196] Large randomized, controlled trials are needed to determine the optimal treatment for hepatic encephalopathy management.[166]

Lactulose would be the preferred option to treat R.C.'s encephalopathy because it would shorten the time to clear the blood from his GI tract and, it is hoped, lead to a rapid resolution of his encephalopathy. Although neomycin is not contraindicated for R.C., the potential for worsening of his coagulopathy (by interfering with vitamin K absorption) and risk of nephrotoxicity (SCr, 1.4 mg/dL) make this a less optimal choice. If R.C.'s renal function continues to decline, neomycin may become contraindicated. Lactulose can be initiated at 30 mL every hour until diarrhea occurs; the dose can then be reduced to maintain two to four soft stools per day and improved mental status. R.C. may receive lactulose by NG tube if necessary in the early treatment period. Rifaximin 550 mg twice daily may be an option if lactulose therapy fails, because it can be used in renal insufficiency.

COMBINATION THERAPY WITH LACTULOSE

CASE 29-3, QUESTION 6: Would combination therapy provide any additive beneficial effect for R.C.?

A recent randomized, double-blind, placebo-controlled trial by Bass et al.[186] compared rifaximin versus placebo in the prevention of hepatic encephalopathy, and hospitalization in patients recovering from recurrent hepatic encephalopathy (≥2 episodes within the previous 6 months). Patients were assigned to either rifaximin at a dose of 550 mg twice daily ($n = 140$) or placebo ($n = 159$) for 6 months. The study allowed the use of lactulose (approximately 90% of patients received concomitant therapy). The results of the study showed that a breakthrough episode of hepatic encephalopathy occurred in 22.1% of patients in the rifaximin group, as compared with 45.9% of patients in the placebo group, and that rifaximin significantly reduced the risk of an episode of hepatic encephalopathy as compared with placebo for a 6-month period (58% risk reduction; $p < 0.001$). A total of 13.6% of the patients in the rifaximin group had a hospitalization involving hepatic encephalopathy, as compared with 22.6% of patients in the placebo group (50% risk reduction; $p = 0.01$). Adverse events were similar among the two groups (rifaximin was continued in all cases).[186]

The ACG guidelines state that combination therapy of lactulose and neomycin may be reasonable in patients who do not respond to monotherapy. Although the mechanism of additive effects is unclear, theoretically it may be that either degradation of lactulose may not be essential for reduction of ammonia level or there are other unknown mechanisms for the activity of lactulose. However, lactulose alone may be more desirable for long-term use because it is potentially less toxic in patients with renal impairment. The guidelines state that lactulose should be tried first, and if satisfactory results do not occur, neomycin alone should be given a trial. If both agents fail when used as monotherapy, the two agents can then be tried in combination.[181]

However, due to recent trial data, such as the Bass et al.[186] study, after treatment failure with monotherapy rifaximin is being used in some centers in combination with lactulose rather than neomycin, due to the efficacy and tolerability of rifaximin. The major issue limiting the use of rifaximin is cost.[197] R.C. would not benefit from combination therapy at this time.

HEPATORENAL SYNDROME

CASE 29-3, QUESTION 7: Lactulose treatment was initiated at 30 mL every hour and titrated to effect with some improvement in R.C.'s mental status. A few days after resolution of his GI bleeding, his serum creatinine increased from 1.4 to 2.7 mg/dL and he became progressively oliguric. His BP was 85/65 mm Hg, pulse rate was 70 beats/minute, and respiratory rate was 16 breaths/minute. Furosemide was discontinued, and R.C. was treated with albumin infusions to allow volume expansion and improve urine output. A renal ultrasound did not reveal any specific abnormalities.

Minimal improvement occurred in his blood pressure and urine output. Laboratory results included the following:

Na, 123 mEq/L
K, 3.6 mEq/L
Cl, 98 mEq/L
Bicarbonate, 25 mEq/L
BUN, 96 mg/dL
SCr, 2.7 mg/dL
Hgb, 8.4 g/dL
Hct, 27.1%
AST, 640 international units
Alkaline phosphatase, 304 international units
LDH, 315 international units
Total bilirubin, 4.1 mg/dL
PT, 22 seconds (INR 1.8)

A 24-hour urinalysis showed the following:

Protein, 50 mg/day
Red blood cells, 1 to 2 per high power field
Negative for WBC, glucose, and ketones

After exclusion of other possible causes of kidney disease, R.C. is diagnosed with hepatorenal syndrome. What are potential treatment options for R.C.'s hepatorenal syndrome?

Pathogenesis

Hepatorenal syndrome (HRS) is a complication of advanced cirrhosis. It is characterized by an intense renal vasoconstriction, which leads to a very low renal perfusion and glomerular filtration rate, as well as a severe reduction in the ability to excrete sodium and free water.[198] Cardenas et al.[199] have summarized the pathogenesis and the precipitating factors of HRS (Fig. 29-3). HRS is diagnosed by exclusion of other known causes of kidney disease in the absence of parenchymal disease. The revised criteria for the diagnosis of HRS as defined by the International Ascites Club (IAC) are listed in Table 29-6.[200,201]

Hepatorenal syndrome can be classified into two categories. Type 1 HRS is characterized by an acute and progressive kidney failure defined by doubling of the initial serum creatinine concentrations to a level greater than 2.5 mg/dL in less than 2 weeks. Type 1 HRS is precipitated by factors such as SBP or large volume paracentesis, but can occur without a precipitating event. This usually occurs within the setting of an acute deterioration of circulatory function characterized by hypotension and activation of endogenous vasoconstrictor systems. It may be associated with impaired cardiac and liver functions as well as encephalopathy. The prognosis of patients exhibiting type 1 HRS is very poor.[201,202] In contrast, type 2 HRS is a progressive deterioration of kidney function with a serum creatinine from 1.5 to 2.5 mg/dL. It is often associated with refractory ascites,

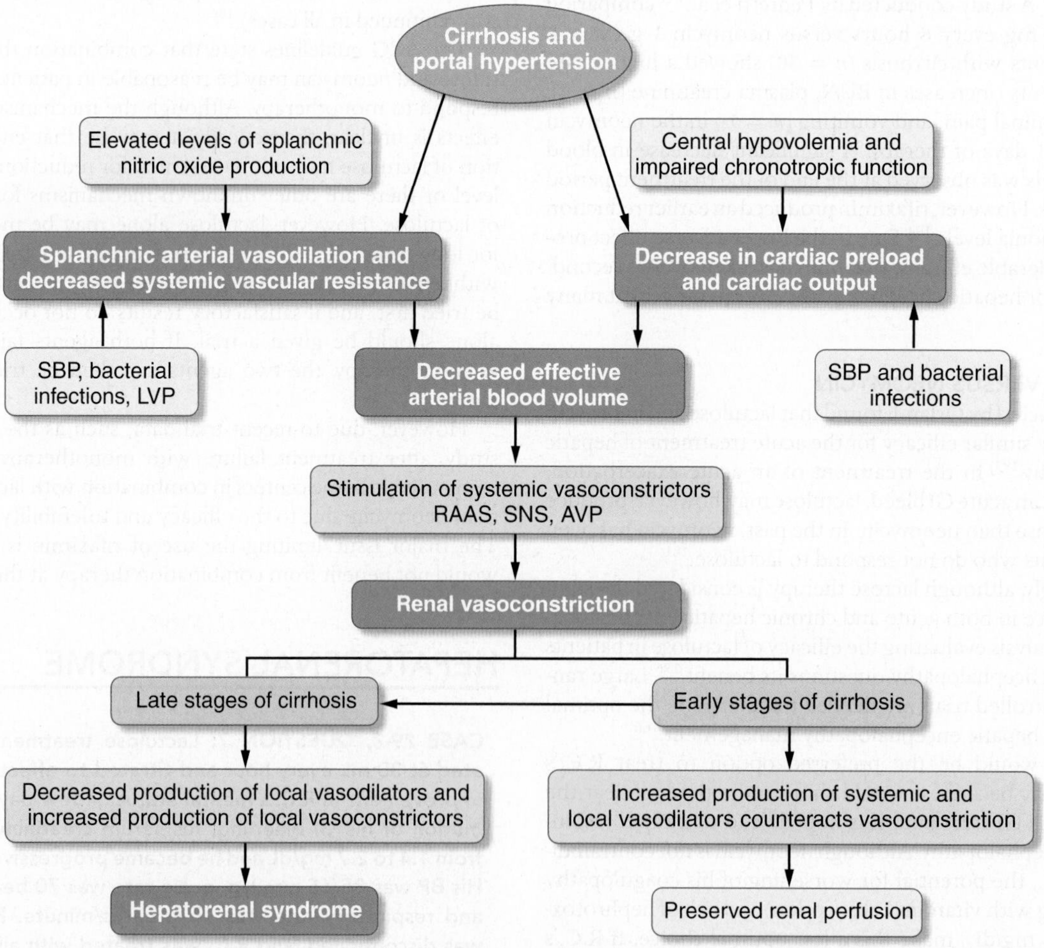

FIGURE 29-3 Pathogenesis of hepatorenal syndrome and its precipitating factors. AVP, arginine vasopressin; LVP, large-volume paracentesis; RAAS, renin-angiotensin-aldosterone system; SBP, spontaneous bacterial peritonitis; SNS, sympathetic nervous system. Reproduced with permission from Cárdenas A, Ginès P. Therapy insight: management of hepatorenal syndrome. *Nat Clin Pract Gastroenterol Hepatol.* 2006;3:338.

TABLE 29-6

Diagnostic Criteria for Hepatorenal Syndrome in Cirrhosis

1. Cirrhotic patients with ascites
2. Serum creatinine >133 μmol/L (1.5 mg/dL)
3. No improvement of serum creatinine (↓ to a level of ≤133 μmol/L) after at least 2 days along with
   a. Diuretic withdrawal and
   b. Volume expansion with albumin (1 g/kg of body weight per day up to a maximum of 100 g/d)
4. The absence of shock
5. No current or recent treatment with nephrotoxic drugs
6. The absence of parenchymal kidney disease as indicated by
   a. Proteinuria >500 mg/d
   b. Microhematuria (>50 red blood cells per high-power field)
   c. And/or abnormal renal ultrasonography

Reprinted with permission from Salerno F et al. Diagnosis, prevention and treatment of the hepatorenal syndrome in cirrhosis. A consensus workshop of the international ascites club. *Gut.* 2007;56:1310.

and has a better survival rate than that of patients with type 1 HRS.[199–201]

Treatment

Treatments for HRS are still investigational. HRS is associated with a high mortality rate (within 2 weeks of diagnosis of type 1 HRS and within 6 months of type 2 HRS). The definitive treatment for type 1 and type 2 HRS is liver transplantation, which is the only treatment that assures long-term survival.[72] The main goal of pharmacologic therapy is to reverse HRS sufficiently so that appropriate candidates for liver transplantation can survive until suitable donor organs can be procured.[200,201] Diuretic therapy must be stopped because this can worsen the kidney disease.[199]

A small randomized study by Solanki et al.[203] showed that vasoconstrictor therapy using terlipressin, in conjunction with albumin, was an effective treatment for patients with type 1 HRS. Patients were randomly assigned to treatment with IV terlipressin 1 mg at 12-hour intervals ($n = 12$) or placebo at 12-hour intervals ($n = 12$). Urine output, creatinine clearance, and mean arterial pressures significantly increased in patients treated with terlipressin compared with the placebo group ($p < 0.05$). Survival was significantly higher in the terlipressin group compared with placebo (42% vs. 0%; $p < 0.05$). All survivors in the terlipressin group had a reversal of HRS.[203]

Sanyal et al.[204] conducted a prospective, randomized, double-blind, placebo-controlled clinical trial where subjects with type 1 HRS were randomly assigned to terlipressin (1 mg intravenously every 6 hours; $n = 56$) or placebo ($n = 56$). If, after 3 days of therapy, the SCr level had not decreased by at least 30% from the baseline value, the dose of the study drug was increased to 2 mg every 6 hours. All patients in this study received albumin 100 g on day 1 and 25 g daily until the end of treatment. The primary end point (treatment success) at day 14 was defined as a SCr level less than or equal to 1.5 mg/dL on two occasions at least 48 hours apart, without dialysis, death, or recurrence of HRS type 1 on or prior to day 14. The terlipressin group was twice as likely as the placebo group to achieve the primary end point (25% vs. 12.5%; $p = 0.093$), although this did not reach statistical significance. In addition, terlipressin did not improve survival. However, terlipressin was superior to placebo for HRS reversal as defined by decrease in SCr level to less than 1.5 mg/dL (34% vs. 13%; $p = 0.008$). The total adverse event rate was similar to placebo.[204] In 2009, the FDA accepted the final section of the New Drug Application seeking marketing approval for terlipressin for the treatment of type 1 HRS, and granted priority review and fast-track designation.

Other nonrandomized studies suggest that vasoconstrictor therapy with norepinephrine (combined with albumin and furosemide) or midodrine (combined with octreotide and albumin) improve renal function in patients with type 1 HRS.[205–207] Esralian et al.[208] conducted a retrospective chart review of type 1 HRS patients ($n = 60$) who received a combination of octreotide, midodrine, and albumin compared to untreated controls ($n = 21$) who received albumin only. Octreotide administration started at 100 mcg subcutaneously TID, with the goal to increase the dose to 200 mcg subcutaneous TID. Midodrine administration started at 5, 7.5, or 10 mg TID orally, with the goal to increase the dose to 12.5 or 15 mg if necessary. Adjustment in medication doses was based on a goal of increasing the mean arterial pressure by at least 15 mm Hg from baseline. All patients received intravenous expansion of plasma volume with 1.5 L of saline combined with an average of 120 g of human albumin after diuretic withdrawal. The authors found that at 30 days, 40% of treated patients had a sustained reduction in serum creatinine, compared with 10% of the concurrent untreated controls ($p = 0.01$). In that same time period, 43% of patients in the treatment group had died, compared with 71% of controls ($p = 0.03$).[208]

Duvoux et al.[207] conducted a pilot study describing the efficacy and safety of norepinephrine in combination with IV albumin and furosemide in patients ($n = 12$) with type 1 HRS. Norepinephrine was given for 10 plus or minus 3 days, at a mean dosage of 0.8 plus or minus 0.3 mg/hour. Reversal of HRS was observed in 83% of patients after a median of 7 days, with a reduction in serum creatinine (358 ± 161 to 145 ± 78 μmol/L; $p < 0.001$), a rise in creatinine clearance (13 ± 9 to 40 ± 15 mL/minute; $p = 0.003$), an increase in mean arterial pressure (65 ± 7 to 73 ± 9 mm Hg, $p = 0.01$) and a marked reduction in active renin and aldosterone plasma concentrations ($p < 0.05$).[207] The IAC guidelines recommend that vasoconstrictors and albumin are to used as a first line treatment for type 1 HRS. They advocate for the use of terlipressin (2–12 mg/day) in combination with albumin (20–40 g/day after 1 g/kg on the first day), and mention that about 60% of renal failure cases recover with this therapy. The IAC recommends midodrine (in addition to octreotide) and norepinephrine as two possible alternatives to terlipressin.[201] In contrast to the statement by the IAC, the latest recommendation of the AASLD is to consider the use of albumin infusion plus octreotide and midodrine (largely due to the lack of availability of terlipressin in the United States).[38] The impact of vasoconstrictor therapy in terms of efficacy (i.e., improvement of kidney function and survival) and safety needs to be evaluated in large, randomized clinical trials.[205–207] Type 2 HRS manifests itself as a progressive disease and, therefore, patients do not present acutely with deterioration in kidney function. No particular treatment exists for type 2 HRS. The main clinical problem in type 2 HRS is refractory ascites, which can be controlled by large volume paracentesis along with IV albumin or TIPS.[199,205,209] Studies are needed to determine the place in therapy for vasoconstrictors and other potential treatments (e.g., TIPS) in patients with type 2 HRS.[201]

Because of the poor prognosis associated with hepatorenal syndrome, R.C. should be evaluated for transplantation. It might be beneficial to enroll R.C. in an investigational research study evaluating the use of vasoconstrictor therapy in conjunction with albumin while awaiting transplantation.

CASE 29-3, QUESTION 8: Why should liver transplantation be considered in patients with end-stage liver disease such as R.C.?

Liver transplantation for appropriate candidates may be the best option for end-stage liver disease and its complications. Transplantation is generally considered in patients with refractory ascites, severe hepatic encephalopathy, esophageal or gastric varices, and hepatorenal syndrome.[210] Because of the shortage of organs available and significant complications associated with transplantation, therapeutic alternatives should be considered to avoid the necessity for transplantation. For patients such as R.C. who are candidates for transplantation, therapeutic strategies to improve outcomes after transplantation should be considered in therapeutic decision-making before transplantation (see Chapter 34, Kidney and Liver Transplantation, for further information on the indications for liver transplantation).[209]

KEY REFERENCES AND WEBSITES

A full list of references for this chapter can be found at **http://thepoint.lww.com/AT10e**. Below are the key references for this chapter, with the corresponding reference number in this chapter found in parentheses after the reference.

Key References

Blei AT et al. Hepatic encephalopathy. *Am J Gastroenterol.* 2001; 96:1968. (181)

Boyer et al. The Role of Transjugular Intrahepatic Portosystemic Shunt (TIPS) in the Management of Portal Hypertension: update 2009. *Hepatology.* 2010;51(1):306. (90)

Garcia-Tsao G et al. Prevention and management of gastroesophageal varices and variceal hemorrhage in cirrhosis [published correction appears in *Am J Gastroenterol.* 2007;102: 2868]. *Am J Gastroenterol.* 2007;102:2086. (109)

Plauth M et al. ESPEN guidelines for nutrition in liver disease and transplantation. *Clin Nutr.* 1997;16:43. (177)

Runyon BA et al. AASLD Practice Guidelines Committee: Management of adult patients with ascites due to cirrhosis: an update. *Hepatology.* 2009;49:2088. (38)

Salerno F et al. Diagnosis, prevention and treatment of the hepatorenal syndrome in cirrhosis. A consensus workshop of the international ascites club. *Gut.* 2007;56:1310. (201)

SECTION EDITOR: MYRNA Y. MUNAR

30

Acute Kidney Injury

Myrna Y. Munar and Donald F. Brophy

CORE PRINCIPLES

	CHAPTER CASES
1 Acute kidney injury (AKI) is characterized clinically by an abrupt decrease in renal function over a period of hours to days, resulting in the accumulation of nitrogenous waste products (azotemia) and the inability to maintain and regulate fluid, electrolyte, and acid–base balance.	**Case 30-1 (Question 1)**
2 Risk factors for the development of AKI include older age, higher baseline serum creatinine (SCr), chronic kidney disease (CKD), diabetes, chronic respiratory illness, underlying cardiovascular disease, prior heart surgery, dehydration resulting in oliguria, acute infection, and exposure to nephrotoxins.	**Case 30-1 (Question 1), Case 30-2 (Questions 1, 2), Case 30-5 (Question 2), Case 30-6 (Question 1)**
3 The clinical course of AKI has three distinct phases: the oliguric phase—a progressive decrease in urine production after kidney injury; the diuretic phase—initial repair of the kidney insult with resultant diuresis of accumulated uremic toxins, waste products, and fluid; and the recovery phase—return of kidney function depending on the severity of injury.	**Case 30-1, Equations 30-1–30-5**
4 AKI is classified according to the physiologic event leading to AKI: prerenal azotemia—decreased renal blood flow; functional—impairment of glomerular ultrafiltrate production or intraglomerular hydrostatic pressure; intrinsic—damage to the kidneys; and postrenal—outflow obstruction in the urinary tract.	**Case 30-1 (Question 1), Case 30-2 (Question 1), Case 30-3 (Question 1), Case 30-5 (Question 1), Case 30-6 (Question 1), Case 30-7 (Question 1), Case 30-8 (Question 1), Table 30-1**
5 The urinalysis is an important diagnostic tool for differentiating AKI into prerenal azotemia, intrinsic, or obstructive AKI. Urinary chemistries are used to differentiate between prerenal azotemia and intrinsic AKI.	**Case 30-1 (Question 2), Case 30-3 (Question 1), Case 30-6 (Question 1), Case 30-7 (Question 1), Case 30-8 (Question 1), Tables 30-2, 30-3**
6 Many equations exist for calculating creatinine clearance (ClCr) or estimated glomerular filtration rate (eGFR). The Modification of Diet in Renal Disease (MDRD) equation is used to quantify glomerular filtration rate, to detect or stage the degree of CKD, and to follow progression. The Cockcroft and Gault (CG) equation is used to adjust the doses of medications that are eliminated by the kidneys.	**Equations 30-1–30-5**

continued

TABLE 30-5
Risk Factors for Developing Aminoglycoside Nephrotoxicity

Patient Factors
Elderly
Underlying renal disease
Dehydration
Hypotension and shock syndromes
Hepatorenal syndrome
Aminoglycoside Factors
Aminoglycoside choice: gentamicin > tobramycin > amikacin
Therapy >3 days
Multiple daily dosing
Serum trough >2 mg/L
Recent aminoglycoside therapy
Concomitant Drug Therapy
Amphotericin B
Cisplatinum
Cyclosporine
Foscarnet
Furosemide
Radiocontrast media
Vancomycin

laboratory indices are consistent with those listed for ATN in Table 30-2.

The mechanism of aminoglycoside-induced ATN is complex. Approximately 5% of filtered aminoglycoside is actively reabsorbed by the proximal tubule cells. These agents are polycationic and bind to the negatively charged brush-border cells within the tubule lumen. Once attached, these agents undergo pinocytosis and enter the intracellular space, setting off complex biochemical events that result in the formation of myeloid bodies. With continued formation of myeloid bodies, the brush-border cells swell and burst, releasing large concentrations of aminoglycoside and lysosomal enzymes into the tubule lumen, thereby beginning a cascade of further tubular destruction.[56,58] The following rank order of nephrotoxicity has been collated from human and animal data: neomycin > gentamicin = tobramycin = amikacin = netilmicin > streptomycin.[57]

EXTENDED-INTERVAL DOSING

CASE 30-6, QUESTION 3: Is "extended-interval" aminoglycoside dosing less nephrotoxic than multiple daily dosing regimens?

Extended-interval aminoglycoside dosing entails the administration of one large daily aminoglycoside dose. This dosing scheme takes advantage of the concentration-dependent killing activity and postantibiotic effect observed with aminoglycosides while minimizing time-dependent toxicity. The net effect of this dosing scheme, purportedly, is greater efficacy with reduced toxicity. Aminoglycoside nephrotoxicity is a function of drug exposure, and it might be minimized with extended-interval dosing because of saturable uptake kinetics in the proximal tubule. That is, only a maximal amount of aminoglycoside is transported into the tubule cell, no matter how much aminoglycoside is present in the tubule. Consequently, once saturation occurs, the remaining aminoglycoside concentration passes through the proximal tubule without being absorbed, and is excreted in the urine. Accumulation is therefore averted.[59] This concept is supported by studies demonstrating that continuous-rate gentamicin infusions, which produce sustained low plasma concentrations, result in greater proximal tubule uptake and nephrotoxicity than extended-interval regimens. This is probably because the achieved drug concentrations are well below those required to saturate the uptake mechanism. Extended-interval dosing results in very high peak concentrations to improve efficacy and generally undetectable trough concentrations before the next dose, thus minimizing accumulation. Numerous clinical trials and meta-analyses have compared the efficacy and toxicity of extended-interval aminoglycoside dosing with conventional multiple daily dosing regimens. Many of these meta-analyses concluded that less nephrotoxicity was associated with extended-interval aminoglycoside dosing. Given the inherent biases of meta-analyses, these results, however, must be interpreted cautiously. For example, meta-analyses combine results from different clinical trials, which can differ in terms of patient population, severity of illness scores, degree of underlying renal dysfunction, dosing regimen, and duration of therapy. Most of the clinical trials did not show a clinically or statistically significant difference in efficacy or toxicity between regimens. Contemporary practice suggests that patients should receive extended-interval aminoglycoside dosing unless they have specific contraindications.

In summary, extended-interval aminoglycoside dosing appears to result in similar or greater efficacy, with similar or reduced toxicity. This dosing schedule is also less costly when considering therapeutic drug monitoring, preparation, and administration costs. Although the typical extended interval in patients with normal renal function is dosing every 24 hours, the interval may have to be prolonged to several days in patients with renal failure.

Drug-Induced Acute Interstitial Nephritis

Drug-induced AIN accounts for approximately 1% to 3% of all AKI cases. A variety of antibiotics, such as penicillins, cephalosporins, quinolones, sulfonamides, and rifampin, as well as NSAIDs have been implicated as major causes of drug-induced AIN. The pathophysiology of this reaction is not well understood; it is suspected that either humoral or cell-mediated immune mechanisms or both are involved.[60] Humoral immune reactions occur within minutes to hours of drug exposure and involve the drug or its metabolite acting as a hapten that binds to host proteins, making them antigenic. The drug–protein antigens become lodged in the renal tubules, which initiate the inflammatory cascade. Cell-mediated injury can occur days to weeks after drug exposure and is identified by the presence of mononuclear inflammation and the lack of detectable immune complexes. This suggests a delayed hypersensitivity rather than a direct cytotoxic effect from a given drug. Both immune mechanisms probably contribute to the development of drug-induced AIN.

PENICILLIN-INDUCED ACUTE INTERSTITIAL NEPHRITIS

CASE 30-7

QUESTION 1: J.S. is a 50-year-old Hispanic woman (height = 5 feet, 3 inches; weight = 160 pounds) who exhibited a cellulitis 3 days after a car door was closed on her right hand. She was admitted to the hospital, where blood and wound cultures were found to be positive for methicillin-sensitive *Staphylococcus aureus*. She received two full days of nafcillin 2 g IV every 4 hours before being discharged to complete a 14-day course with dicloxacillin 500 mg PO four times daily (QID). Ten days after discharge, J.S. returned to

the emergency department complaining of malaise, fever, diffuse rash, hematuria, and reduced urine output. The following laboratory values were significant:

BUN, 39 mg/dL
SCr, 2.3 mg/dL
WBC count, 18,500 cells/μL with 18% eosinophils

The urinalysis was positive for elevated specific gravity, WBC, RBC, eosinophiluria, and an FE_{Na} of 3%. What objective data suggest drug-induced AIN?

J.S.'s onset of symptoms suggests drug-induced AIN. As illustrated by this case, the median onset of penicillin-induced AIN generally occurs 6 to 10 days after drug exposure. Hallmark symptoms of AIN include fever, macular rash, and malaise. Fever is present in nearly all patients with AIN, and rash occurs in 25% to 50% of patients. J.S.'s objective laboratory data that suggest AIN include azotemia, elevated SCr, proteinuria, cellular urinary sediment, eosinophilia, and eosinophiluria. Her FE_{Na} of 3% suggests intrinsic renal disease, and her eosinophiluria and eosinophilia indicate an immune-mediated allergic reaction. Drug-induced AIN is generally nonoliguric, but oliguria can develop in severe cases of AIN.

CASE 30-7, QUESTION 2: How should J.S.'s drug-induced AIN be treated?

The dicloxacillin should be stopped immediately because most patients recover normal kidney function once the offending agent is discontinued. General supportive measures that maintain fluid and electrolyte balance are necessary. Corticosteroids have been used with variable results to shorten the duration of AKI, but no clinical guidelines have been developed to delineate when to administer them and for how long. Some administer prednisone 1 mg/kg for 7 days and then gradually taper the dose during the next several weeks. The response to corticosteroids may be delayed or absent in some patients. Dialysis may be needed in patients who are oliguric, but it is usually not required for those who are nonoliguric. The clinician should document J.S.'s allergic reaction to penicillins because repeated exposure is likely to result in similar reactions.

POSTRENAL ACUTE KIDNEY INJURY

Any condition that results in the obstruction of urine flow at any level of the urinary tract is termed postrenal AKI. Common causes of postrenal AKI are stone formation, underlying malignancies of the prostate or cervix, prostatic hypertrophy, or bilateral ureter strictures. Conditions that result in bladder outlet obstruction (e.g., prostatic hypertrophy) are the most common causes of postrenal AKI. The onset of signs and symptoms is generally gradual; it often presents as decreased force of urine stream, dribbling, or polyuria. Drugs can also result in insoluble crystal formation in the urine and should be included in the differential diagnosis.

Nephrolithiasis

Kidney stones are relatively common and affect approximately 13% of men and 7% of women at least once in their lifetime.[61,62] The increasing prevalence of kidney stones is related to rising rates of obesity, diabetes, metabolic syndrome, hypertension, and CKD. A strong genetic predisposition appears to exist in this population. Epidemiologic data have found that men with stones were three times more likely to have parents or siblings with a history significant for stones.[63] In addition to genetics, other underlying risk factors exist for stone development (Table 30-6). White patients are twice as likely as black patients to develop stones. Kidney stones generally consist of uric acid, cystine, struvite (also called magnesium ammonium phosphate or triple phosphate nephrolithiasis), and calcium salts. Of these, calcium stones are by far the most prevalent.

TABLE 30-6
Risk Factors for Nephrolithiasis

Low urine volume
Hypercalciuria
Hyperoxaluria
Hyperuricosuria
Hypercitruria
Chronically low or high urinary pH

CALCIUM STONES

Calcium nephrolithiasis constitutes approximately 70% to 80% of all kidney stones,[63] with calcium oxalate and calcium phosphate stones making up most of these. Genetic factors appear to play an important role in the development of calcium nephrolithiasis; the stereotypical patient is a man in his third to fifth decade of life. Other risk factors for developing calcium nephrolithiasis are low urine output, inadequate hydration (e.g., living in a hot climate and not drinking adequate fluids), hypercalciuria, hyperoxaluria, hypocitraturia, hyperuricosuria, and distal renal tubular acidosis. Generally, more than one of these conditions is present simultaneously.

STRUVITE STONES

Magnesium ammonium phosphate crystallization, termed struvite stones, represents the second most common type of nephrolithiasis (~2%–20% of cases). Struvite stones can result in significantly high morbidity and mortality because they tend to recur and can result in irreversible kidney damage.[64] These stones often fill the renal collecting ducts and assume a "staghorn" appearance. Struvite stones generally result when existing stones are colonized with urease-producing bacteria (*Proteus* species, *Haemophilus* species, *Klebsiella* species, and *Ureaplasma urealyticum*). Urease is an enzyme that hydrolyzes urea and alkalinizes the urine. The alkaline environment promotes the formation of insoluble crystals of ammonium, calcium, and phosphate. In vitro, simply alkalinizing the urine results in the immediate precipitation of amorphous struvite stones. Populations at risk for developing struvite stones include obese women, patients with frequent urinary tract infections or pyelonephritis, and patients with genitourinary tract abnormalities that promote bacterial colonization or make eradication of infection difficult. The most problematic form of stone disease develops in paralyzed patients with indwelling Foley catheters. Recurrent nephrolithiasis is one of the most common causes of death in patients with spinal cord injury. Treatment of struvite stones can consist of surgical intervention; prolonged courses of broad-spectrum antibiotics; administration of acetohydroxamic acid, which inhibits bacterial urease; or shock-wave lithotripsy.[64]

URIC ACID STONES

Uric acid stones commonly occur in patients whose uric acid metabolism is altered because of various medical conditions. In particular, patients with gout and those receiving chemotherapy are susceptible to these stones. This topic is discussed further in Chapter 45, Gout and Hyperuricemia.

CYSTINE STONES

Cystinuria is a rare autosomal-recessive hereditary disorder of amino acid transport in the renal tubules that results in the urinary excretion of large amounts of cystine. These stones form when the cystine excretion rate exceeds the urinary solubility limit. The calculi form staghorns in the renal tubules and can cause urinary obstruction, infection, and AKI. Therapy of cystine stones is targeted at reducing the urinary cystine excretion while increasing its urinary solubility. This can be accomplished by diet modification, increased fluid intake, urine alkalization, and drug therapy. Low-sodium diets decrease cystine excretion, and restriction of methionine, a cystine precursor, may reduce cystine excretion. It may also result in depletion of other important amino acids, however. To decrease the urinary cystine concentrations, urine volume should be increased by maintaining a fluid intake of more than 4 L/day. The solubility of cystine in urine also can be increased by alkalinizing the urine. Pharmacologic therapy is indicated when these nondrug measures have failed. Drug therapy is targeted at increasing the urinary solubility of cystine, which can be achieved by forming a thiol–cysteine disulfide bond. D-penicillamine and tiopronin are the most commonly used drugs, although tiopronin appears to be better tolerated than D-penicillamine.

PRESENTATION AND TREATMENT

CASE 30-8

QUESTION 1: T.C., a 48-year-old Asian man (height = 5 feet, 5 inches; weight = 140 pounds), presents to the emergency department complaining of sharp flank pain radiating to the groin, gross hematuria, and dysuria. He states that these symptoms have been present for 4 hours and that they are similar to previous episodes of calcium nephrolithiasis he has experienced. Serum chemistries are ordered and are significant only for a BUN of 34 mg/dL and an SCr of 1.5 mg/dL, which are up from his baseline values of 15 and 0.9 mg/dL, respectively. A urine sample was obtained and visualized with microscopy. It was determined that T.C. passed a kidney stone, based on the large amount of calcium oxalate crystals found in the urinary sediment. On questioning, he admits that he has not been drinking much fluid during the past week owing to a busy work schedule, and his urine volume has been markedly lower than usual. What are the common subjective and objective data that suggest nephrolithiasis, and how can this be prevented from occurring in the future?

T.C. illustrates the classic presentation of nephrolithiasis: acute, severe flank pain that radiates to the groin. It is usually accompanied by gross or microscopic hematuria, dysuria, or frequency. Kidney stones entering the ureters can cause moderate to severe colic. For most patients, analgesics are paramount for pain relief. Opiates (e.g., morphine sulfate) or NSAIDs can be used short term alone or in combination for pain management.[61,62] Among the NSAIDs, diclofenac (Voltaren) has been the most studied. Ketorolac provides effective pain relief with less sedation. Meperidine should be avoided in patients with decreased kidney function. In most cases, pain resolves after passing the stone, obviating the need for pain medication.

Of symptomatic calculi, 90% pass spontaneously, as in T.C.'s case, and invasive surgical treatment is rarely necessary.[65] After passing the stone, renal function rapidly reverts to normal. The risk factors that predispose T.C. to stone recurrence include a previous episode of nephrolithiasis, age within the fourth decade, and decreased fluid intake and urine output.

T.C. should take preventive measures to reduce the likelihood of stone recurrence. Many randomized trials have demonstrated that nondrug and pharmacologic mechanisms can prevent stone formation. The most cost-effective way to prevent stone formation is to increase fluid intake. A classic 5-year randomized study compared a high fluid intake group (>2 L/day) with one that had normal daily fluid intake (~1 L/day). The results demonstrated a significantly longer time to stone recurrence (39 vs. 25 months) in the high fluid intake group.[66] Dietary modifications remain controversial. Although it appears that limiting protein, calcium, and sodium intake should decrease the likelihood of recurrent nephrolithiasis, the data are conflicting.[67] Dietary calcium restriction reduces calcium binding to dietary oxalate, leading to more unbound oxalate absorption in the colon, eventual urinary excretion, and increased likelihood of stone formation.[62] In summary, a high calcium intake probably increases the risk of nephrolithiasis but only in patients with absorptive hypercalciuria and not in normal subjects.

Pharmacologic control of calcium oxalate stones has been tried with thiazide diuretics.[68] Thiazide diuretics promote calcium reabsorption in the distal tubule, which decreases the concentration in the lumen. Thiazides also may decrease intestinal calcium absorption in patients with absorptive hypercalciuria, although this remains unclear. Patients receiving thiazide diuretics should restrict their sodium because excessive sodium intake negates their hypocalciuric effect. Allopurinol has been used successfully to prevent recurrent calcium oxalate nephrolithiasis, presumably by inhibiting purine and uric acid metabolism.[68] Alkalization of the urine with potassium citrate and potassium-magnesium citrate also prevents recurrent calcium oxalate nephrolithiasis.

T.C. should be instructed to drink at least 2 L of fluid (~eight 8-ounce glasses) daily. Given his busy work schedule, a thiazide diuretic probably is not the most convenient option for T.C., and noncompliance is likely. Allopurinol 200 mg orally once daily is probably the most convenient preventive strategy for T.C., and data suggest it is effective in preventing recurrent nephrolithiasis. Alternatively, urinary alkalinization with potassium citrate or potassium-magnesium citrate is likely to benefit T.C., but it may be less convenient because it needs to be administered two to four times daily.

DRUG-INDUCED NEPHROLITHIASIS

CASE 30-8, QUESTION 2: Can drugs crystallize in the urine and cause AKI?

Many commonly prescribed drugs are insoluble in urine and crystallize in the distal tubule (Table 30-7). Risk factors that predispose patients to crystalluria include severe volume contraction, underlying renal dysfunction, or acidotic or alkalotic urinary pH. In conditions of renal hypoperfusion, high concentrations of drug become stagnant in the tubule lumen. Drugs that are weak acids (e.g., methotrexate, sulfonamides) precipitate in acidic urine; drugs that are weak bases (e.g., indinavir, other protease inhibitors) precipitate in alkaline urine. Prevention of crystal-induced AKI is targeted at dosage adjustment for

TABLE 30-7
Commonly Used Drugs That Cause Crystal-Induced Acute Kidney Injury

Acyclovir
Indinavir
Methotrexate
Sulfonamides
Triamterene

patients with underlying renal dysfunction, volume expansion to increase urinary output, and urine alkalization to enhance renal elimination of drugs that are weak acids. Similarly, for established crystal-induced AKI, the same general supportive measures should be performed. Dialysis may be necessary in a small percentage of patients. With appropriate pharmacotherapy, crystal-induced AKI is usually reversible without long-term complications.

SUPPORTIVE MANAGEMENT OF ACUTE KIDNEY INJURY

CASE 30-9

QUESTION 1: J.W. is a 75-year-old Native American man (height = 6 feet, 2 inches; weight = 200 pounds) who presents to the emergency room with shortness of breath and progressive worsening edema in both lower extremities. His medical history includes nephrotic syndrome secondary to diabetic nephrosclerosis, type 1 diabetes, hypertension, and chronic obstructive pulmonary disease. His surgical history includes a right-sided nephrectomy many years ago. His chronic medications are furosemide 80 mg PO twice a day, metolazone 10 mg PO once a day, lisinopril 5 mg PO once a day, diltiazem extended-release 120 mg PO once a day, albuterol, and 20 units insulin glargine at bedtime and insulin aspart before meals. Vital signs are temperature 36.3°C, pulse 77 beats/minute, respirations 16 breaths/minute, and BP 179/86 mm Hg. Physical examination reveals periorbital edema, jugular venous distension at a 45-degree angle to the jaw, dullness to percussion halfway up the lungs bilaterally, and 4+ pitting edema. Admitting laboratory tests reveal the following:

Sodium, 140 mEq/L
Potassium, 5.5 mEq/L
Chloride, 103 mEq/L
Bicarbonate, 19 mEq/L
Glucose, 249 mg/dL
BUN, 67 mg/dL
SCr, 5.2 mg/dL
Serum albumin, 2.0 g/dL
Spot urine protein:creatinine ratio, 350 mg/g

Baseline renal function tests 1 month ago are BUN 45 mg/dL and SCr 3.0 mg/dL. J.W. is oliguric with a urine output of 10 mL/hour. The nephrologist wants to use supportive management of AKI by first optimizing diuretic therapy. If no increase in urine output occurs during the next several hours, then the patient will undergo RRT. What is supportive management of AKI?

Despite years of study, no pharmacologic "cure" for AKI exists. Supportive management is therefore directed at preventing its morbidity and mortality. This is achieved by close patient monitoring; strict fluid, electrolyte, and nutritional management; treatment of life-threatening conditions such as pulmonary edema, hyperkalemia, and metabolic acidosis; avoidance of nephrotoxic drugs; and the initiation of dialysis or CRRT.

As discussed earlier, diuretics currently have no role in preventing AKI progression or reducing mortality, but they can prevent complications, such as pulmonary edema. For edema, intravenous furosemide (e.g., 80 to 120 mg) is preferred because of its potency and pulmonary vasodilation properties. Oral furosemide therapy should be avoided because gut edema may limit its bioavailability. Torsemide, another loop diuretic, has excellent oral bioavailability and is unaffected by gut edema. Previously, torsemide was reserved for patients with demonstrated bioavailability problems with furosemide because of cost concerns, but a generic version of torsemide is now available. The dosage of diuretic needed is highly patient specific, especially in those with frank proteinuria, glomerulonephritis, or the nephrotic syndrome. Low serum albumin limits drug transport to the kidneys and thus limits diuretic effectiveness. In addition, furosemide is highly protein bound, and thus binds to filtered protein, which negates its pharmacologic effect on the kidneys. Combinations of loop and thiazide diuretics may be needed in patients with AKI if they become diuretic resistant. This combination acts synergistically to block sodium and water reabsorption in both Henle's loop and the distal convoluted tubule. Other alternatives include continuous loop diuretic infusions, such as furosemide 1 mg/kg/hour. The infusion rate should not exceed 4 mg/minute because these rates are associated with ototoxicity, especially when given in combination with aminoglycoside antibiotics. Close monitoring of potassium, magnesium, and calcium is necessary when giving large doses of loop diuretics. Dietary sodium restriction of 2 to 2.5 g/day should be instituted.

Hyperkalemia commonly occurs in patients with AKI because the kidneys regulate potassium homeostasis. J.W. is mildly hyperkalemic, but his serum potassium may decrease after furosemide therapy. Management of hyperkalemia is discussed in Chapter 10, Fluid and Electrolyte Disorders. In cases of severe hyperkalemia in which conventional pharmacologic treatment is not feasible, emergency hemodialysis should be performed.

Metabolic acidosis is a common manifestation of AKI because the kidneys are responsible for excreting organic acids. As GFR declines to less than 30 mL/minute, organic acids accumulate and clinical symptoms can occur. J.W.'s serum bicarbonate concentration reveals slight academia that does not require correction at this time. Severe metabolic acidosis should be corrected with dialysis, but early initiation of oral bicarbonate may prolong or obviate the need for dialysis.

Clinicians should closely monitor patient vital signs (e.g., weight, temperature, BP, pulse, and respirations) several times per day. Diuresis should aim for a weight loss of 0.5 to 1.0 kg per day. The patient's volume status should be assessed daily, and all fluids should be adjusted based on laboratory chemistries to detect fluid and electrolyte abnormalities, urine output, and gastrointestinal and insensible losses. The patient's medication profile should be reviewed daily to assess for appropriate dosage adjustment in renal dysfunction. Because estimation of creatinine clearance is difficult in patients with changing renal function, therapeutic drug monitoring should be performed when using drugs with narrow therapeutic indices. When possible, nephrotoxic drugs should be avoided, but this may be difficult in patients who are septic or hypotensive and require nephrotoxic antibiotics and vasopressors. Preventive measures to reduce the likelihood of AKI should be used, such as monitoring volume status to ensure adequate renal perfusion, using dosing strategies or products that are associated with less nephrotoxicity, and avoiding drug therapy combinations that enhance nephrotoxicity (e.g., NSAID, aminoglycosides).

Extracorporeal Continuous Renal Replacement Therapy

Renal replacement therapy is not always indicated in AKI. It is reserved for patients with severe acid–base disorders, fluid overload, hyperkalemia, symptomatic uremia, or drug intoxications. RRT can be divided into intermittent hemodialysis or CRRT, such as continuous peritoneal dialysis or extracorporeal CRRT.

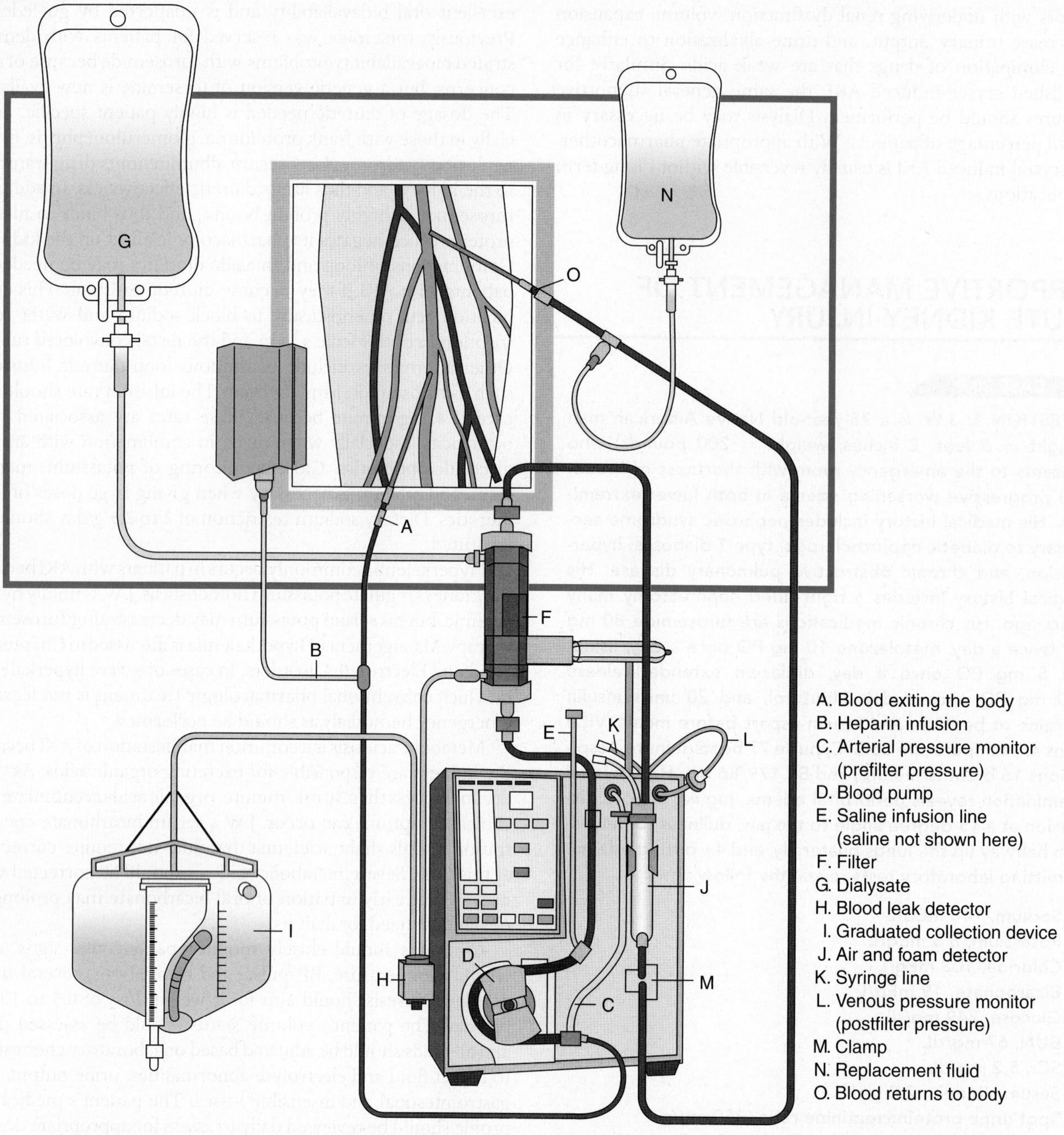

FIGURE 30-6 Schematic of continuous venovenous hemofiltration (CVVH). Blood is accessed by a dual-lumen catheter in a central vein and is pumped through the extracorporeal circuit by a roller blood pump. The blood pump maintains a constant hydrostatic pressure to create ultrafiltration, even in hypotensive conditions. Patients receiving CVVH are most often in the intensive care unit and often receive concomitant parenteral nutrition.

The decision to use one versus the other is most often decided by the nephrologist's experience and comfort level. Extracorporeal CRRT differs from peritoneal and hemodialysis in its mechanism of solute removal; dialysis modalities rely primarily on solute diffusion across a semipermeable membrane, whereas CRRT relies primarily on convective ultrafiltrate production. This discussion will be limited to extracorporeal (hemofilter membrane is outside of the body) CRRT therapies (see Chapter 32, Renal Dialysis, for a complete overview of peritoneal and hemodialysis).

Not all extracorporeal CRRT is alike[69]; many variations exist and include modalities such as continuous arteriovenous hemofiltration (now obsolete), continuous venovenous hemofiltration (CVVH; Fig. 30-6), continuous venovenous hemodialysis, and continuous venovenous hemodiafiltration (CVVHDF). Differences among these modalities are illustrated in Table 30-8. Drug dosing can be difficult in patients receiving these therapies, especially in those who are undergoing both dialysis and hemofiltration modalities (i.e., CVVHDF).

ONLINE CONTENT **For a narrated PowerPoint presentation on continuous renal replacement modalities, go to http://thepoint.lww.com/AT10e.**

Estimating Drug Removal

CASE 30-9, QUESTION 2: Are there ways to calculate drug removal in extracorporeal CRRT modalities?

TABLE 30-8

Comparison of Extracorporeal Continuous Renal Replacement Therapies

Parameter	Continuous Venovenous Hemofiltration (CVVH)	Continuous Arteriovenous Hemofiltration (CAVH)	Continuous Venovenous Hemodialysis (CVVHD)	Continuous Venovenous Hemodiafiltration (CVVHDF)
Volume control in hypotensive patients	Good	Variable	Good	Good
Solute control in highly catabolic patients	Adequate	Inadequate	Adequate	Adequate
Blood flow rates in hypotensive patients	Adequate	Poor	Adequate	Adequate
Ease of drug dosing	Published recommendations	Difficult	Difficult	Difficult
Dialytic solute clearance	None	None	Moderate	Moderate
Convective solute clearance	Good	Good	Minimal	Moderate
Corresponding GFR (mL/min)	15–17	10–15	17–21	25–26
Blood pump required	Yes	No	Yes	Yes
Replacement fluid required	Yes	Yes	Yes	Yes
Pharmacy expense	High	High	High	High

GFR, glomerular filtration rate.

Recent reviews provide an excellent background on dosing drugs in patients receiving CRRT.[70–72] The principles for drug removal in hemofiltration are basically identical with those for removal in hemodialysis. For example, drugs with a small volume of distribution and low protein binding are removed readily by these modalities. The sieving coefficient (SC) of a drug is the non–protein-bound fraction of the drug that is in plasma. For example, an SC of 0.8 means that 80% of the drug is unbound in plasma. Drug SC can be obtained from the literature or by measuring concentrations simultaneously in the prefilter blood and ultrafiltrate. The ratio of the ultrafiltrate concentration to plasma concentration is the SC. Drug clearance can be calculated by multiplying the SC by the ultrafiltration rate. For example, if a patient is receiving CVVH at an ultrafiltration rate of 1 L/hour, and he or she is receiving vancomycin (which has an SC of 0.8) 1 g/day, the vancomycin clearance while receiving CVVH is $0.8 \times 1{,}000$ mL/hour = 800 mL/hour or 13 mL/minute.

Calculating drug clearance is much more difficult in hemodiafiltration modalities (CVVHDF) because both convection and diffusion account for drug clearance and it is difficult to predict drug clearance precisely. The use of SC can be useful for small-molecular-weight drugs, but the accuracy declines with larger drug molecules, such as vancomycin. When possible, therapeutic drug monitoring should be performed to maintain therapeutic concentrations and to maximize drug therapy.

KEY REFERENCES AND WEBSITES

A full list of references for this chapter can be found at http://thepoint.lww.com/AT10e. Below are the key references and websites for this chapter, with the corresponding reference number in this chapter found in parentheses after the reference.

Key References

Cerda J et al. Modalities of continuous renal replacement therapy: technical and clinical considerations. *Semin Dial.* 2009;22:114. (69)

Churchwell MD et al. Drug dosing during continuous renal replacement therapy. *Semin Dial.* 2009;22:185. (70)

Goldfarb DS. In the clinic. Nephrolithiasis. *Ann Intern Med.* 2009;151:ITC2. (61)

Heintz BH et al. Antimicrobial dosing concepts and recommendations for critically ill adult patients receiving continuous renal replacement therapy or intermittent hemodialysis. *Pharmacotherapy.* 2009;29:562. (71)

Lafrance JP et al. Selective and non-selective non-steroidal anti-inflammatory drugs and the risk of acute kidney injury. *Pharmacoepidemiol Drug Saf.* 2009;18:923. (35)

Levey AS et al. A more accurate method to estimate glomerular filtration rate from serum creatinine: a new prediction equation. Modification of Diet in Renal Disease Study Group. *Ann Intern Med.* 1999;130:461. (22)

Levey AS et al. A new equation to estimate glomerular filtration rate. *Ann Intern Med.* 2009;150:604. (26)

Levey AS et al. Using standardized serum creatinine values in the modification of diet in renal disease study equation for estimating glomerular filtration rate. *Ann Intern Med.* 2006;145:247. (24)

Massicotte A. Contrast medium-induced nephropathy: strategies for prevention. *Pharmacotherapy.* 2008;28:1140.

Mehta RL et al. Acute Kidney Injury Network: report of an initiative to improve outcomes in acute kidney injury. *Crit Care.* 2007;11:R31. (3)

Rodriguez-Iturbe B et al. The current state of poststreptococcal glomerulonephritis. *J Am Soc Nephrol.* 2008;19:1855. (40)

Key Website

K/DOQI clinical practice guidelines for chronic kidney disease: evaluation, classification, and stratification. *Am J Kidney Dis.* 2002;39(2 Suppl 1):S1. http://www.kidney.org/professionals/KDOQI/guidelines_ckd/toc.htm. (23)

31 Chronic Kidney Disease

Darius L. Mason and Magdalene M. Assimon

CORE PRINCIPLES

	CHAPTER CASES
1 Chronic kidney disease (CKD) is progressive, irreversible kidney damage characterized by decreased estimated glomerular filtration rate (eGFR) or evidence of kidney damage for at least 3 months.	**Case 31-1 (Question 1)**
2 Staging of CKD should be determined on the basis of kidney function, defined by the National Kidney Foundation Kidney Disease Outcomes Quality Initiative (NKF K/DOQI) Guidelines. Each stage is associated with certain action plans.	**Case 31-1 (Question 1)**
3 Diabetes is the number one cause of CKD in the United States. Optimal control of blood glucose levels is essential to slow the progression of CKD and reduce morbidity and mortality.	**Case 31-1 (Questions 2–4)**
4 Fluid accumulation and electrolyte abnormalities secondary to CKD often complicate the treatment of hypertension and can have cardiotoxic effects.	**Case 31-1 (Questions 5–9)**
5 Metabolic acidosis presents in late stages of CKD from reduced hydrogen ion excretion and bicarbonate production. Metabolic acidosis can worsen bone disease and other metabolic processes.	**Case 31-1 (Question 8)**
6 Treating anemia of CKD is essential to reducing cardiovascular disease (CVD) complications and decreased quality of life. Management of anemia includes administration of erythropoiesis-stimulating agents and iron supplementation.	**Case 31-1 (Questions 10–12)**
7 CVD is the number one cause of morbidity and mortality in CKD. Cardioprotective measures should be addressed at all stages.	**Case 31-2 (Question 1)**
8 Hypertension is the second leading cause of CKD in the United States. Treating hypertension to target goals is necessary to slow the progression of CKD and reduce mortality.	**Case 31-2 (Question 2)**
9 CKD increases the risk for atherosclerosis progression. Cholesterol management is essential to reduce the morbidity from atherosclerosis.	**Case 31-2 (Question 3)**
10 Mineral and bone disorders (MBD) become more common as CKD progresses. Mineral abnormalities lead to the development of vascular calcifications and increase the risk for cardiovascular mortality.	**Case 31-3 (Questions 1, 2)**
11 Hyperphosphatemia is managed with various phosphate-binding agents, including calcium salts (carbonate and acetate), sevelamer, lanthanum carbonate, aluminum salts, and magnesium salts.	**Case 31-3 (Question 2)**
12 Activated forms of vitamin D (calcitriol, paricalcitol, and doxercalciferol) or a calcimimetic agent (cinacalcet) may be necessary to achieve proper calcium and bone metabolism.	**Case 31-3 (Question 2)**

continued

	CHAPTER CASES
13 Uremic neuropathies are a collection of central nervous system disorders that can affect dialysis patients' quality of life and morbidity.	**Case 31-4 (Question 1)**
14 Glomerulonephropathies (GN) are a collection of glomerular diseases caused by a variety of immunologic mechanisms and the third leading cause of CKD. Patients with GN may present with nephrotic syndrome and require treatment with immunosuppressant therapy.	**Case 31-5 (Questions 1, 2), Case 31-6 (Questions 1, 2), Case 31-7 (Question 1)**

INTRODUCTION

Chronic kidney disease (CKD) describes the continuum of kidney dysfunction from early to late-stage disease. Estimated glomerular filtration rates (eGFR) range from 90 mL/minute/1.73 m^2 in the early stages to less than 15 mL/minute/1.73 m^2 in the late stages of disease. The most severe stage of CKD, known as end-stage renal disease (ESRD), occurs when eGFR is less than 15 mL/minute/1.73 m^2 or when chronic renal replacement therapy in the form of dialysis or kidney transplantation is necessary to sustain life.[1] Complications associated with CKD that increase the complexity of this condition include fluid and electrolyte abnormalities, anemia, cardiovascular disease, mineral and bone disorders, and malnutrition. Optimal treatment of patients with CKD is best achieved using a multidisciplinary approach to address the concurrent medical problems and complex pharmacotherapeutic regimens. Alterations in drug disposition that occur with kidney impairment and the subsequent need for dosage adjustments are additional considerations when determining rational pharmacotherapy in this population.

ONLINE CONTENT

For a diagram of the pathophysiologic changes that take place in chronic kidney disease, go to http://thepoint.lww.com/AT10e.

Implementation of clinical practice guidelines leads to improved patient outcomes and reduced variability in patient care.[2] As a result many countries have developed evidence-based clinical practice guidelines for the treatment of kidney disease. In the United States, the National Kidney Foundation (NKF) established the Kidney Disease Outcomes Quality Initiative (K/DOQI) to provide evidence-based treatment guidelines for all stages of kidney disease and related conditions. However, because kidney disease is a worldwide public health issue and the problems faced by kidney disease around the world are universal, the Kidney Disease: Improving Global Outcomes (KDIGO) was established in 2003. The mission of KDIGO is to improve the care and outcomes of kidney disease patients worldwide by promoting coordination, collaboration, and integration of initiatives. KDIGO is managed by the NKF. Contact information for K/DOQI and KDIGO and corresponding web addresses for clinical practice guidelines can be found in Table 31-1.

TABLE 31-1
Resources for Kidney Disease Clinical Practice Guidelines

National Kidney Foundation Kidney Disease Outcomes Quality Initiative 30 East 33rd Street New York, New York 10016 Phone: 1-800-622–9010 Website: http://www.kidney.org/professionals/KDOQI/index.cfm
Kidney Disease: Improving Global Outcomes 30 East 33rd Street, Suite 900 New York, New York 10016 Phone: 212-889-2210 x288 Website: **http://www.kdigo.org/clinical_practice_guidelines/index.php**

Definitions

Chronic kidney disease is characterized by a progressive deterioration in kidney function with time characterized by irreversible structural damage to existing nephrons. A staging system is used to classify kidney disease according to the eGFR, which is estimated clinically using creatinine clearance (CrCl) (Table 31-2). Specifically, CKD is defined as kidney damage with normal or a mildly decreased eGFR (stages 1 and 2) or an eGFR less than 60 mL/minute/1.73 m^2 for at least 3 months with or without evidence of kidney damage (stages 3 to 4). Kidney damage is indicated by pathologic abnormalities of the kidneys or markers of kidney injury, including abnormalities in blood or urine tests and imaging studies.[1] The presence of protein in the urine (defined as *proteinuria, albuminuria,* or *microalbuminuria* based on protein type and amount) is an early and sensitive marker of kidney damage (Table 31-3).

A substantial decline in kidney function also leads to *azotemia,* the accumulation of nitrogenous wastes such as urea in the plasma, and an increased risk for developing complications of CKD. Uremic signs and symptoms from accumulation of nitrogenous wastes and other toxins manifests clinically as an elevated blood urea nitrogen (BUN) and leads to a myriad of complications affecting most major organ systems. Laboratory abnormalities include azotemia, hyperphosphatemia, hypocalcemia, hyperkalemia, metabolic acidosis, and worsening anemia.

TABLE 31-2
Staging of Chronic Kidney Disease Based on eGFR

Stage	Description	eGFR (mL/min/1.73 m^2)
–	At increased risk	≥90 (with CKD risk factors)
1	Kidney damage with normal or ↑ eGFR	≥90
2	Kidney damage with mild ↓ eGFR	60–89
3	Moderate ↓ eGFR	30–59
4	Severe ↓ eGFR	15–29
5	Kidney failure	<15 (or need for renal replacement therapy)

CKD, chronic kidney disease; eGFR, effective glomerular filtration rate.
Adapted with permission from the National Kidney Foundation. K/DOQI Clinical Practice Guidelines for Chronic Kidney Disease: Evaluation, Classification, and Stratification. *Am J Kidney Dis.* 2002;39:S1.

TABLE 31-3
Diagnostic Criteria for Proteinuria and Albuminuria

	Total Protein			Albumin		
	24-hour Collection (mg/d)	Spot Urine Dipstick (mg/dL)	Spot Urine Protein-SCr Ratio (mg/g)	24-hour Collection (mg/d)	Spot Urine Dipstick (mg/dL)	Spot Urine Albumin-SCr Ratio (mg/g)
Normal	<300	<30	<200	<30	<3	<17 (men) <25 (women)
Microalbuminuria	NA	NA	NA	30–300	>3	17–250 (men) 25–355 (women)
Albuminuria or clinical proteinuria	>300	>30	>200	>300	NA	>250 (men) >355 (women)

SCr, serum creatinine.
Adapted with permission from National Kidney Foundation. K/DOQI Clinical Practice Guidelines for Chronic Kidney Disease: Evaluation, Classification, and Stratification. *Am J Kidney Dis*. 2002;39:S1.

Clinical signs of CKD and its associated complications, including hypertension, uremic symptoms (e.g., nausea, anorexia), and bleeding, are observed as the disease advances to stages 3 through 5. Interventions to slow the progression of kidney disease are critical. Patients who reach an eGFR of less than 30 mL/minute/1.73 m^2 (stage 4), in general, will ultimately progress to ESRD.

Epidemiology of Chronic Kidney Disease

INCIDENCE AND PREVALENCE

The National Health and Nutrition Examination Survey (NHANES) 1999–2004 was a national cross-sectional study of more than 13,000 adults 20 years of age or older conducted from 1999 through 2004 to provide information on the stages and characteristics of those with CKD in the United States.[3] From these data, it is estimated that approximately 10.1 million Americans are at risk for developing CKD or have a mild decrease in kidney function (CKD stages 1 or 2), and roughly 16.2 million Americans have CKD stages 3 to 4.[3]

Data describing the ESRD population are made available annually by the US Renal Data System (USRDS). These reports characterize the development, treatment, morbidity, and mortality associated with ESRD in the United States and include data from patients who received kidney transplants. Based on the most recent data from the USRDS, more than 381,000 ESRD patients received chronic dialysis therapy at the end of 2008. Of this prevalent dialysis population, 101,033 patients began hemodialysis (HD) therapy, and 6,455 patients began peritoneal dialysis (PD) during 2008.[4] CKD has been identified as one of the focus areas for the Healthy People 2010 national health initiative; one of the specific CKD-related objectives is to reduce the number of new cases of ESRD.[5] From 2007 to 2008, the rate of new ESRD cases decreased by 1.1% to 351 cases per 1 million population. Despite the decrease in new ESRD cases, this number remains well above the Healthy People 2010 target of 221cases per 1 million population.[4]

In 2008, a higher proportion of the ESRD population were male (56%), and the majority of ESRD patients were 45 to 64 years of age (45%).[4] However, the age groups with the highest incidence of ESRD were those aged 65 years or older (49%). Approximately 61% of ESRD patients were white, 32% were African American, 5% were Asian, and 1% were Native American. Furthermore, 85% of prevalent ESRD patients were of a non-Hispanic ethnicity. African Americans and Native Americans had a 3.6 and 1.8 times greater incidence rate of kidney failure, respectively, compared with white individuals, and the incidence rate of ESRD in the Hispanic population was 1.5 times higher than that of non-Hispanics, which may be indicative of racial and ethnic disparities.[4]

ETIOLOGY

In CKD, the progressive loss or damage to functioning nephrons as a function of time is the result of a primary disorder or disease of the kidney, a secondary complication of certain systemic diseases (e.g., diabetes mellitus or hypertension), or an acute injury to the kidney that results in irreversible kidney damage. In 2008, the leading causes of ESRD in newly diagnosed American patients were diabetes mellitus (44%), hypertension (28%), and chronic glomerulonephritis (7%).[4] The remaining cases of ESRD can be attributed to a variety of other pathologies; examples include polycystic kidney disease, congenital malformations of the kidneys, nephrolithiasis, interstitial nephritis, renal artery stenosis, renal carcinoma, and human immunodeficiency virus–associated nephropathy.

ONLINE CONTENT

For a visual of a polycystic kidney, go to http://thepoint.lww.com/AT10e.

RISK FACTORS

A variety of risk factors associated with development, initiation, and progression of CKD have been identified. Initiation factors are medical conditions that directly cause kidney damage. Risk factors for the progression of CKD exacerbate kidney damage and are related to an accelerated decline in kidney function with time. The majority of susceptibility factors are not modifiable, but may identify people who are at high risk for developing CKD. In contrast, pharmacotherapy and lifestyle interventions have been shown to modify CKD-related initiation and progression factors (see Prevention and Diabetic Nephropathy section). A summary of risk factors associated with CKD can be found in Table 31-4.

MORBIDITY AND MORTALITY

Rates of hospitalizations and mortality are much greater in those with kidney disease compared with the non-CKD population. Not surprisingly, in 2008 the mortality rate of non-dialysis patients with stages 3 to 5 CKD was 40% higher compared with those without CKD, and the adjusted rates of all-cause mortality were 6.4 to 7.8 times higher for dialysis patients compared

TABLE 31-4
Risk Factors for Chronic Kidney Disease

Susceptibility	Initiation	Progression
Advanced age	Diabetes mellitus	Glycemia
Reduced kidney mass	Hypertension	Hypertension
Low birth weight	Glomerulonephritis	Proteinuria
Racial/ethnic minority	Drug induced or toxicity	Smoking
Family history	Smoking	Obesity
Low income or education	Obesity	
Systemic inflammation		
Dyslipidemia		

Reprinted from US Department of Health and Human Services. *Healthy People 2010*. Washington, DC: US Government Printing Office; 2000.

with the general population.[4,6] However, the mortality rates for patients with renal transplants approached that of the general population, only 1.2 to 1.5 times higher.

Advances in dialysis and transplantation have improved patient care, and as a result mortality in the first year of HD treatment has begun to decline.[4] Cardiovascular-related events, particularly cardiac arrest and myocardial infarction, remain the leading causes of hospitalizations and death in both the non–dialysis CKD and ESRD populations. This is not surprising given the high prevalence of coexisting cardiac disorders in patients with kidney disease and the elevated risk for mortality associated with these conditions. However, since 1999 the overall rate of cardiovascular mortality in the ESRD population has continued to decline. In 2008, the rate fell by 5.9% to 64.1 deaths per 1,000 patient-years, nearing the Healthy People 2010 goal of 62.1 deaths per 1,000 patient-years.[4]

After cardiovascular disease, infection (predominantly septicemia) is a substantial contributor to overall morbidity and mortality in patients with ESRD. Since 1994 the rates of hospitalizations for infection among the HD population has increased by 45.8%. Furthermore, infection remains one of the leading causes of death among dialysis patients during their first year of renal replacement therapy.[4]

Medication Use

Data regarding medication use in the kidney disease population reveal non–dialysis CKD patients are prescribed an average of 6 to 8 medications and HD patients are prescribed approximately 12 medications (10 home medications and 2 in-center medications).[7,8] These patterns of medication use are reflective of the higher prevalence of complications and comorbidities in the latter stages of CKD, which require additional drug therapies. The extent of medication use and the complexity of prescribed drug regimens contribute to nonadherence and medication-related problems (MRPs) in the ESRD population.[8]

To manage MRPs, some dialysis units use a clinical pharmacist as part of the multidisciplinary health care team to provide pharmaceutical care to ESRD patients. Services provided by a clinical pharmacist have been shown to be cost-effective and associated with maintenance of health-related quality of life.[9,10] Additionally, a randomized study of 104 ESRD patients investigated the impact of pharmaceutical care (individualized drug therapy reviews conducted by a clinical pharmacist) to standard care (brief drug therapy reviews conducted by a nurse) on drug use, drug costs, hospitalization rates, and MRPs.[11] After a 2-year follow-up, patients who received pharmaceutical care were taking fewer medications and had fewer all-cause hospitalizations compared with those receiving standard care.

Economics

The cost of treating both non–dialysis CKD patients and ESRD patients is substantial. In 2008, the overall per person per year cost of medical treatment for Medicare non–dialysis CKD patients was more than $19,000 and the cost of medical care for those with stages 3 to 4 CKD was 14.2% higher than those with CKD stages 1 to 2.[6] Furthermore, the majority of the costs of medical care provided to those with ESRD are paid by the federal government. In 2008, the cost for ESRD was $26.8 billion dollars, corresponding to 5.9% of the Medicare budget, including Medicare Part D.[4] This amount reflects a consistent increase from prior years and an increase in the percentage of the Medicare budget dedicated to ESRD care. The increase is most likely associated with the higher prevalence of ESRD, changes in the standard of care, reimbursement structure, and types of patients being treated (e.g., diabetic patients versus nondiabetic patients).

The continually growing costs of ESRD care require careful attention, given the implementation of the Centers for Medicare and Medicaid Services' new bundled payment system that changed how Medicare pays for dialysis services. Under the new system, Medicare provides a single payment to ESRD facilities to cover all dialysis-related services for each dialysis treatment.[12] In the prior reimbursement system, Medicare paid a composite rate to dialysis units to cover the costs of an individual's dialysis treatment, certain routine medications (e.g., heparin), laboratory tests, and supplies. In addition to the composite rate, Medicare was billed separately for other related dialysis services and billable items (e.g., erythropoietin-stimulating agents).[12] The bundled payment system is likely to reduce the government reimbursement for dialysis services, but may increase barriers to care for some ESRD patients (e.g., patients may have to pick up medications at the pharmacy that were previously administered at the dialysis unit).

Pathophysiology

Progression of kidney disease to ESRD generally occurs over the course of months to years and is assessed by the rate of eGFR decline. Each kidney contains approximately 1 million nephrons (the functional units of the kidney), and every nephron maintains its own single-nephron eGFR. In the face of nephron loss, the remaining functional nephrons maintain renal function by increasing their single-nephron eGFR via compensatory glomerular hemodynamic changes.[13] With time, this compensatory increase in single-nephron eGFRs eventually leads to hypertrophy and an irreversible loss of nephron function from sustained increases in glomerular pressure. Furthermore, glomerulosclerosis (glomerular arteriolar damage) develops from prolonged elevation of glomerular capillary pressure and increased glomerular plasma flow, resulting in a continuous cycle of nephron destruction. Regardless of the cause, a predictable and continuous decrease in kidney function occurs in patients when the eGFR drops below a critical value, approximately one-half of normal.[14] Usually, the rate of decline in renal function remains fairly constant for an individual, but can vary substantially among patients and disease states. An accelerated rate of decline in kidney function has been associated with black race, lower baseline eGFR, male sex, older age, and smoking.[1] Compared with hypertensive kidney disease, conditions associated with a more rapid progression include diabetic kidney disease, glomerular diseases, and polycystic kidney disease.[1] Progressive kidney disease is typically identified by persistent proteinuria, decreasing kidney function, and the development of glomerulosclerosis. Although early changes in kidney function can be detected through routine laboratory monitoring (e.g., serum creatinine [SCr]), most patients do not develop signs and symptoms of uremia until they have reached the more severe stages of the disease (stage 4 CKD and ESRD).

As the leading causes of ESRD in the United States, diabetes mellitus, hypertension, and glomerular diseases have been the focus of research to identify their associated mechanisms of kidney damage. In the case of diabetes mellitus, excess filtration of glucose and contact with glomerular and tubular cells leads to increased cellular osmotic pressure and thickening of the capillary basement membrane. The resulting glomerulopathy may or may not result in proteinuria. Systemic hypertension is a potent stimulus for the development and progression of kidney disease caused by the association with increased single-nephron eGFRs.[13,15] Hypertension, whether the primary cause of kidney disease or a coexisting disease in the presence of other etiologies, can promote kidney damage through transmission of elevated systemic pressure to glomeruli. The result is glomerular capillary hyperperfusion and hypertension leading to progressive kidney damage as nephron destruction continues. Glomerular ischemia induced by damage to the preglomerular arteries and arterioles also occurs. People with coexistent diabetes mellitus and hypertension increase the risk of developing ESRD by fivefold to sixfold compared with those with hypertension alone.[16] Most glomerular diseases are mediated by immune mechanisms. The deposition and formation of immune complexes in the glomerulus cause injury, resulting in increased glomerular permeability to macromolecules (e.g., proteins).[17]

Proteinuria, one of the initial diagnostic signs of kidney disease, can also contribute to the progressive decline in renal function. A faster rate of progression has been associated with higher protein excretion.[18] Immunologic and hemodynamic mechanisms have been identified to explain the glomerular injury. Increases in renal plasma flow are associated with proteinuria and high protein intake. Inflammatory cytokines may be responsible for fibrosis and renal scarring, ultimately resulting in loss of nephron function.

Dyslipidemias, common in patients with CKD, are often observed concurrently with proteinuria. Increased low-density lipoprotein (LDL) cholesterol, total cholesterol, and apolipoprotein B, as well as decreased high-density lipoprotein (HDL) cholesterol, have been observed in patients with progressive kidney disease.[19] Hypercholesterolemia has been associated with loss of kidney function in patients with and without diabetes.[20–22] Accumulation of apolipoproteins in glomerular mesangial cells contributes to cytokine production and infiltration of macrophages and has been implicated in the progression of CKD, primarily in the presence of previous kidney disease or other risk factors such as hypertension.[21] LDL is thought to promote glomerular damage by initiating a series of cellular events in mesangial cells and through oxidation to a more cytotoxic derivative once within these cells. Although serum total cholesterol, triglycerides, and apolipoprotein B all correlate with the rate of decline in eGFR, it is not clear that they directly increase the rate of progression of kidney disease, particularly when present with concomitant conditions that also cause kidney damage. Some evidence, however, suggests that treatment of hypercholesterolemia with statin therapy in patients with CKD may reduce proteinuria and progression of CKD.[23]

Drug-Induced Causes of Chronic Kidney Disease

ANALGESIC NEPHROPATHY

Analgesic nephropathy results from habitual ingestion of analgesics for many years. Particularly, agents containing at least two antipyretic analgesics and usually caffeine or codeine are commonly associated with the development of this disease. It is a tubulointerstitial kidney disease characterized by renal papillary necrosis as a primary lesion and chronic interstitial nephritis as a secondary lesion.[24] Analgesic nephropathy is a slowly progressive disease, and the clinical signs and symptoms are similar to the nonspecific presentation of CKD attributable to any other etiology. Phenacetin, an acetaminophen prodrug, was the first agent to be identified as causing this syndrome.

Currently in the United States, most cases are caused by long-term use or misuse of compound analgesics containing acetaminophen and aspirin along with caffeine or codeine.[24] Similar findings in terms of the effect on kidney function have also been observed with chronic nonsteroidal anti-inflammatory drug (NSAID) therapy.[25] The uses of acetaminophen, aspirin, and NSAIDs have been associated with the progression of renal disease in CKD patients in a dose-dependent manner.[26] The cumulative amount (at least 1 to 2 kg of acetaminophen), rather than the duration of analgesic intake, is a primary risk factor for developing chronic analgesic nephropathy.[27] Thus, analgesics should be used with caution in the CKD population, and chronic analgesic therapy should be discouraged. Recommendations made by the NKF on analgesic use have been published.[24]

Analgesic nephropathy is more prevalent in female patients, with a female to male ratio of 5:1 to 7:1. The peak incidence occurs between the fourth and fifth decades of life.[24,27] Patients usually have a history or complaint of chronic pain syndromes. Often, patients who develop analgesic nephropathy are dependent on analgesic therapy and may exhibit psychiatric manifestations indicative of an addictive behavior. At presentation, patients may have a reduced eGFR and findings consistent with CKD, such as elevated SCr, BUN, and proteinuria. However, during acute necrosis, patients may experience flank pain, pyuria, and hematuria. As necrosis progresses, cellular debris may cause ureteral obstruction. Kidney dysfunction is characterized as a salt-wasting nephropathy, with a substantial reduction in urine-concentrating and urine-acidifying capabilities. The exact mechanism for kidney damage is uncertain, but it is thought that because acetaminophen accumulates in the renal medulla, its oxidative metabolite produced by the medullary cytochrome P-450 enzyme system may bind to macromolecules, causing cellular necrosis. Although the reduced form of glutathione in the medulla can prevent this process, agents that reduce medullary glutathione content (e.g., aspirin) may promote kidney damage. This mechanism may explain a lack of analgesic nephropathy associated with acetaminophen alone. NSAIDs, which attenuate prostaglandin-mediated vasodilatation, may induce an ischemic state within the renal medulla, leading to papillary necrosis.[25]

Data on the chronic renal effects of selective cyclo-oxygenase-2 (COX-2) inhibitors are limited and less clear. A meta-analysis of 114 randomized, double-blind clinical trials evaluated the adverse renal events of COX-2 inhibitors. The authors reported that, of the six agents evaluated, only rofecoxib was associated with adverse renal effects, defined as significant changes in urea or creatinine levels, clinically diagnosed kidney disease, or renal failure. In contrast, celecoxib was associated with a lower risk of renal dysfunction.[28] A cohort study of 19,163 newly diagnosed CKD patients examined the association between analgesic use and the risk of progression to ESRD. Among the COX-2 inhibitors, only rofecoxib use was significantly associated with an increased risk of progression to ESRD.[26] However, rofecoxib was voluntarily withdrawn from the market in 2004 because of increased concern about cardiovascular events.

The long-term management of analgesic nephropathy is generally supportive and primarily involves discontinuation of the offending agent and subsequent abstinence from the use of

NSAIDs and combination analgesics. If patients develop CKD or ESRD, treatment of kidney disease-related comorbidities should be treated in the same manner as those with kidney disease owing to any other cause. For patients requiring analgesics, aspirin taken alone may be a reasonable alternative. Acetaminophen as a single agent may be safe, although habitual use can contribute to progression of kidney disease as well as to liver toxicity.[27] Patients requiring chronic analgesic therapy should use the lowest dose to control pain, avoid combination products when possible, and maintain adequate hydration.

LITHIUM NEPHROPATHY

Lithium use has been associated with alterations in kidney function secondary to acute functional and histological changes and has been associated with the development of chronic pathologic changes to the kidneys (e.g., chronic interstitial nephritis). The role of lithium as a causative agent in the development of CKD has been controversial, but has been clarified by a variety of epidemiologic, clinical, and histopathological studies.[29] The concentrating ability within the kidney and eGFR have been shown to decline with long-term lithium use.[30] Lithium-induced chronic renal disease has a slow progression (average latency between onset of lithium use and ESRD is 20 years) in which the rate of progression is related to the duration of lithium therapy.[31]

Patients with lithium nephropathy are generally asymptomatic. They typically present with an insidious decline in renal function over the course of many years, and proteinuria is usually absent or minimal.[29] In patients taking chronic lithium therapy, close monitoring of serum lithium concentrations is advised, and regular measurements of SCr should be obtained to detect changes in kidney function. Current clinical practice guidelines recommend monitoring SCr every 2 to 3 months during the first 6 months of chronic lithium therapy, followed by yearly measurements thereafter.[29] If patients develop CKD or ESRD, management of kidney disease–related comorbidities should be treated in the same manner as those with kidney disease owing to any other cause. The decision to discontinue lithium and to initiate another mood stabilizer should be a mutual decision made by the psychiatrist, the nephrologist, and the patient.[29]

Clinical Assessment

EVALUATION OF RENAL FUNCTION AND STAGING OF CHRONIC KIDNEY DISEASE

Laboratory parameters and indices used in the clinical setting to evaluate kidney function and to monitor disease progression time include SCr, CrCl, and eGFR. Specifics regarding the equations and methods used to calculate CrCl and eGFR can be found in Chapter 30, Acute Kidney Injury. Estimated glomerular filtration rate and CrCl hold different places in clinical practice. The Modification of Diet in Renal Disease (MDRD) equation is used to calculate eGFR to stage CKD, and the Cockcroft-Gault equation is used to determine drug dosing of medications cleared by the kidneys in patients with impaired kidney function (see Chapter 33, Dosing of Drugs in Renal Failure).

Historically the term *chronic renal insufficiency* was used to describe patients with decreased kidney function not requiring dialysis. This included a broad range of patients from the earlier stages of the disease, with eGFR greater than 60 mL/minute/1.73 m^2, as well as those patients with more severe disease, with eGFR less than 30 mL/minute/1.73 m^2. Failure to distinguish patients at these differing levels of kidney function resulted in failure to recognize differences in management approaches required at varying levels of eGFR. A staging system was developed to promote a more consistent dialogue when referring to patients with kidney dysfunction. Kidney disease is classified into five stages on the basis of the eGFR (Table 31-2).[1] Patients with stage 1 or 2 CKD would have some pathologic abnormality indicative of kidney damage (see Definitions section), although their eGFR is relatively normal. Continued screening and interventions to delay progression are essential at these stages. Patients with stages 3 to 4 CKD are diagnosed with the disease on the basis of eGFR alone (eGFR <60 mL/minute/1.73 m^2). At these stages, management of CKD-related complications and comorbidities becomes a standard of care. Stage 5 CKD, also known as ESRD, is the most severe stage. ESRD occurs when eGFR is less than 15 mL/minute/1.73 m^2 or when chronic renal replacement therapy (e.g., dialysis or transplantation) is necessary for survival.

PROTEINURIA

Normally, proteins are not filtered at the glomerulus because of their relatively large molecular size. Thus, only trace amounts of protein are present in the urine in patients without kidney disease. However, with glomerular damage, proteinuria is commonly observed and may precede elevations in SCr. The amount of protein present in the urine has been shown to be a predictor of kidney disease progression. As a result, protein excretion should be monitored in patients at risk for kidney disease as well as those with existing kidney disease at routine checkups.

Microalbuminuria is defined as an albumin excretion rate of 20 to 200 mcg/minute or 30 to 300 mg/24 hours. Specific assays with increased sensitivity relative to standard assays are required for detecting quantities of protein in the range defined as microalbuminuria. *Proteinuria* is defined as a total protein excretion rate >200 mcg/min or >300 mg/24 hr (referred to as *albuminuria* if albumin is the only protein measured). Measurement of total protein includes quantification of albumin plus other proteins, such as low molecular weight globulins and apoproteins. Assessment of albuminuria is a better indicator of early kidney disease because it is primarily indicative of glomerular damage as opposed to total protein, which is not specific for glomerular damage. Other tests, including urinalysis, radiographic procedures, and biopsy, may also be valuable in further assessing kidney function.

Determination of albuminuria can be done using timed urine samples. Typically, a 24-hour collection period is used, although a timed sample collected overnight may be more reliable because protein excretion can vary throughout the day and with postural changes (i.e., orthostatic proteinuria). Untimed or "spot" urine samples for measurement of protein- or albumin-to-creatinine ratios are more convenient. As opposed to measuring protein or albumin in a timed collection, this method corrects for variations in hydration status and may be more accurate because protein excretion is normalized to glomerular filtration. The albumin and creatinine concentrations in the urine are measured from a spot urine sample, preferably from first morning urine sample, because it correlates best with 24-hour protein excretion. If a first morning urine sample is not available, a random sample is acceptable. Factors associated with proteinuria, such as ingestion of a high-protein meal and vigorous exercise, must be considered when evaluating urinary protein. Measuring urinary protein after exercise will result in a falsely elevated urine protein level as a consequence of an increase in the membrane permeability of the glomeruli to protein and a saturation of the tubular reabsorption process of filtered protein. To minimize this risk, it is recommended to wait approximately 4 hours after exercise to test for proteinuria.[32] Screening for albuminuria can also be done using urine dipstick testing of a spot urine sample. Reagent strips are available from several commercial vendors and differ with regard to the specified testing procedure and the sensitivity and specificity for detecting albuminuria. Patients with a positive dipstick screening test should have a subsequent quantitative assessment of the protein- or albumin-to-creatinine ratio to confirm proteinuria. The NKF K/DOQI Guidelines for CKD provide criteria for diagnosis of proteinuria and albuminuria based on testing method and sex (Table 31-3).[1]

COMPLICATIONS OF CHRONIC KIDNEY DISEASE

Complications specific to CKD begin to develop as kidney disease progresses, most often when patients reach stage 3 disease (eGFR <60 mL/minute/1.73 m^2). These complications include fluid and electrolyte abnormalities, metabolic acidosis, anemia, mineral and bone disorder, cardiovascular complications, and poor nutritional status. Often, these complications go unrecognized or are inadequately managed during the earlier stages of CKD, leading to poor outcomes by the time a patient is in need of dialysis therapy. Hypoalbuminemia and anemia were identified in more than 50% of a population of patients new to dialysis therapy, and these findings were associated with a decreased quality of life.[33] Late referral to a nephrologist to manage CKD and its associated complications has also been associated with increased mortality in the ESRD population.[34] These and similar reports underscore the need for early and aggressive therapy to manage complications of CKD. Complications of CKD will be presented in more detail throughout this chapter, and complications associated with dialysis therapy are discussed in Chapter 32, Renal Dialysis.

Prevention

Appropriate management of CKD includes measures to slow progression of the disease and regular evaluation of kidney function to assess changes in disease severity and to monitor therapy. This includes aggressive strategies to manage the disorders that cause kidney disease or are known to accelerate the disease process, such as diabetes mellitus, hypertension, high protein intake, and dyslipidemias (see Chapter 13, Dyslipidemias, Atherosclerosis, and Coronary Heart Disease; Chapter 14, Essential Hypertension; and Chapter 53, Diabetes Mellitus).

DIETARY PROTEIN RESTRICTION

Proteinuria was identified as the most significant predictor of ESRD in patients with type 2 diabetes and early CKD.[35] Increases in protein ingestion are associated with a rise in eGFR, possibly as a result of structural changes of the glomerulus and changes in renal plasma flow with an increased protein load.[36] Evidence such as this has led to the investigation of methods to reduce the degree of proteinuria. In addition to controlling the primary causes of kidney disease (e.g., diabetes, hypertension, and glomerulopathies) and using angiotensin-converting enzyme (ACE) inhibitor and angiotensin receptor blocker (ARB) therapy, dietary protein restriction has been evaluated as a strategy for reducing proteinuria and delaying progression of kidney disease.

A number of studies have investigated the effect of protein restriction on disease progression with varying results.[37,38] These conflicting conclusions may be attributable to differences in study design, patient populations, methods to assess kidney function, degrees of protein restriction, and dietary compliance. The MDRD study evaluated the effects of protein restriction and strict blood pressure (BP) control on the progression of kidney disease. There was no difference in renal function deterioration comparing patients who received a normal protein diet (1.3 g/kg/day) with those receiving a low-protein (0.58 g/kg/day) diet.[37] In contrast, patients receiving a low-protein diet (0.58 g/kg/day) compared with those receiving a very low protein diet (0.28 g/kg/day plus keto and amino acid supplementation) had a faster decline in renal function. A secondary analysis of the MDRD study, which accounted for dietary compliance, suggested that patients with severe kidney disease (eGFR <25 mL/minute/1.73 m^2) could benefit from protein restriction of 0.6 g/kg/day.[38] However, a follow-up analysis of the MDRD study found no significant benefit.

The potential benefits of protein restriction in patients with CKD must be weighed against the potentially adverse effect on overall nutritional status. Malnutrition is prevalent in patients with CKD starting dialysis and is a predictor of mortality in this population.[39] The decision to restrict protein should be done with referral to a dietitian and frequent monitoring of nutritional status.

ANTIHYPERTENSIVE THERAPY

Antihypertensive therapy prevents kidney damage and slows the rate of progression of CKD in both diabetic and nondiabetic patients.[40,41] In addition, the added benefit of reduced cardiovascular mortality further supports the use of antihypertensive therapy in patients at risk for progressive CKD. Despite what is known about the beneficial effects of BP control in patients with CKD, rates of hypertension control in the predialysis population remain suboptimal.[42]

The target BP for patients with or at risk for kidney disease differs from that recommended for the general population. Evidence now exists to support lowering BP beyond the generally advocated target of less than 140/90 mm Hg. According to the Seventh Report of the Joint National Committee on Prevention, Detection, Evaluation, and Treatment of High Blood Pressure (JNC-7) and recommendations from the NKF K/DOQI Hypertension and Diabetes Executive Committee, the goal BP for individuals with CKD or diabetes is less than 130/80 mm Hg.[43,44] Furthermore, results from the MDRD study showed that further lowering of BP to less than 125/75 mm Hg (or a mean arterial pressure <92 mm Hg) was more beneficial than usual BP control in patients with higher rates of urinary protein excretion (>1 g protein/day).[18,40] This benefit was maintained for 7 years after the end of randomization.[40] The effects of more aggressive BP control on progression of kidney disease was also studied in the African American Study of Kidney Disease and Hypertension (AASK) trial.[45] African Americans aged 18 to 70 years with hypertensive renal disease (eGFR 20 to 65 mL/minute/1.73m^2) were included in this study. Changes in eGFR during a 4-year evaluation period did not differ significantly between patients with a higher BP goal (mean arterial pressure of 102 to 107 mm Hg) and those with a lower BP goal (mean arterial pressure ≤92 mm Hg).[45] A post hoc analysis of the AASK trial found that patients with proteinuria greater than 1 g/day assigned to the low BP target had slower progression to ESRD.[46] Clearly, BP control is important to delay progression of kidney disease, and with the expanding data supporting more aggressive BP lowering in patients with more severe proteinuria, the importance of BP control in this patient population is pivotal in slowing progression of CKD.

Among the available classes of antihypertensive agents, ACE inhibitors (e.g., enalapril, captopril, lisinopril) and ARBs (e.g., losartan, irbesartan, candesartan) may afford additional benefits in preserving kidney function. As a result, ACE inhibitors and ARBs are recommended by JNC-7 as first-line treatment options for hypertension in those with CKD and those at risk for CKD (e.g., diabetics).[43] In conditions of decreased eGFR, angiotensin II primarily causes compensatory vasoconstriction of the efferent arteriole, thereby increasing glomerular capillary pressure (P_{GC}) and eGFR (Fig. 31-1). This effect is beneficial in conditions of acute renal failure; however, sustained increases in P_{GC} cause hypertrophy of individual nephrons and progressive kidney disease. ACE inhibitor and ARB therapy prevents the chronic increase in glomerular pressure mediated by angiotensin II. Benefits of ACE inhibitors have been demonstrated in patients with diabetes with some degree of proteinuria, suggesting that

bicarbo
prepara
Each 65
sodium
contain
to prov
be used
sodium
carbon
loaded,
exacerb
sible alt
patients
alumint
ing alur
do not
bonate
The use
day, usu
used to
bicarbo
metabo
Onc
ease, int
ate or ci
At this
metabo
bicarbo
delivere
into the
apy is ir
supplen

Othe
Distu

CASE
metab

G.B.
eliminat
detailed
lines fo
dietary
adequat
and ene
ciated w
The
mon fin
tion of
the kidr
nesium
1.73 m²
rarely
nausea,
reflexes
conduct
avoiding
use of r
requirin
G.B.
uricemi
owing t
of a hist
uricemi

DIABETIC NEPHROPATHY

CASE 31-1

QUESTION 1: G.B. is a 44-year-old, African Am woman (weight, 175 pounds; height, 5′5″) with a 2 history of type 2 diabetes mellitus. She presents to t betes clinic for her quarterly checkup. She has bee compliant with regular appointments, and her bloc cose has generally remained greater than 200 mg prior evaluations, with a hemoglobin A_{1c} of 10.1% <7%) 2 months ago. Lately G.B. complains of gener sea, malaise, and poor appetite. She has been treat peptic ulcer disease for the past 6 months. The w reveals the following pertinent laboratory values:

Serum sodium (Na), 143 mEq/L
Potassium (K), 5.3 mEq/L
Chloride (Cl), 106 mEq/L
CO_2 content, 18 mEq/L
SCr, 2.9 mg/dL
BUN, 63 mg/dL
Random blood glucose, 289 mg/dL

Physical examination reveals a BP of 160/102 m 2+ pedal edema, and mild pulmonary congestion, 10-pound weight gain. Additional laboratory studies the following results:

Serum phosphate, 6.6 mg/dL
Calcium (Ca), 8.8 mg/dL
Albumin (Alb) 3.6 g/dL
Magnesium (Mg), 2.8 mEq/L
Uric acid, 8.8 mg/dL

Hematologic studies show the following results:

Hematocrit (Hct), 28%
Hemoglobin (Hgb), 9.3 g/dL
White blood cell (WBC) count, 9,600/μL
Platelet count, 155,000/μL

Red blood cell (RBC) indices are normal. G.B.'s locyte count is 0.5%. Her urinalysis (UA) showed 4- teinuria, later quantified as a urinary albumin of 700 hours. What subjective and objective data in G.B. ar sistent with a diagnosis of advanced kidney disease?

G.B.'s abnormal values for SCr, BUN, serum potassiu nesium, phosphate, uric acid, CO_2 content, hemoglob hematocrit are all consistent with kidney disease and its ated complications. Assuming relatively stable kidney f (i.e., no acute changes in kidney function), her eGFR is imately 21 mL/minute/1.73 m² based on the MDRD ec placing her in stage 4 CKD (eGFR 15 to 29 mL/minute/1. (See Chapter 30, Acute Kidney Injury, for definition of the equation.) As the eGFR declines to the degree observed normal regulation of fluids and electrolytes is impaired tions in SCr, BUN, sodium, potassium, magnesium, phc and uric acid as well as signs of fluid accumulation are ob Although potassium is mildly elevated in G.B., overall po balance is usually maintained within the normal range un severe kidney disease develops (i.e., eGFR <10 mL/minu m²). The substantial degree of proteinuria observed in consistent with advanced glomerular damage. Volume o from continued intake and decreased sodium and wate tion leads to weight gain, hypertension, and edema. Me acidosis results from impaired synthesis of ammonia by

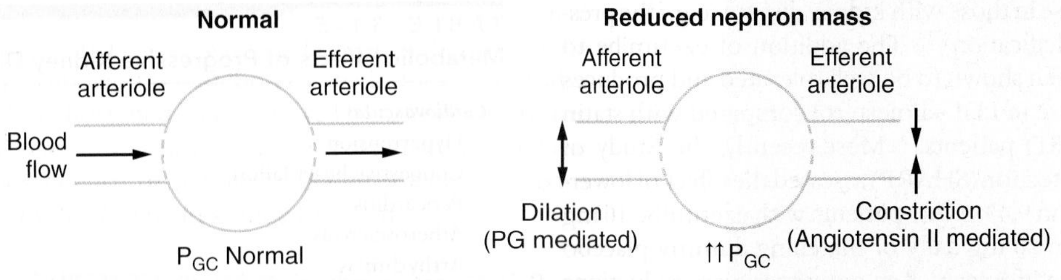

FIGURE 31-1 Renal hemodynamics are dependent on afferent and efferent arteriolar tone and glomerular capillary pressure (P_{GC}). With reduced nephron mass, afferent arteriolar vasodilation (mediated primarily by prostaglandins [PG] I_2 and E_2) and efferent arteriolar constriction (mediated primarily by angiotensin II) occur within remaining functioning nephrons to compensate. This leads to an increase in blood flow, intraglomerular capillary filtration pressure (P_{GC}), and hyperfiltration (increased single-nephron effective glomerular filtration rate). Sustained increases in plasma flow and hydrostatic pressure lead to hyperfiltration injury and glomerular sclerosis. With time, these changes contribute to continued loss of nephron function (i.e., progression of kidney disease). Angiotensin-converting enzyme inhibitors and angiotensin receptor blockers prevent vasoconstriction of the efferent arteriole and reduce the P_{GC}.

ACE inhibitor use be considered in this population regardless of BP.[41,47–49] In patients without diabetes, ACE inhibitors have been shown to reduce BP, decrease proteinuria, and slow the progression of kidney disease when compared with other agents.[45,50–52] An initial and mild decrease in eGFR is expected with ACE inhibitor therapy; therefore, an increase in SCr of approximately 30% within the first 2 months of therapy is acceptable.[53] Hypotension, acute kidney failure, and severe hyperkalemia are reasons to consider discontinuing therapy (also see Chapter 19, Heart Failure).

Angiotensin II receptor blockers offer similar benefits to ACE inhibitors on the basis of their ability to decrease efferent arteriolar resistance by blockade of the angiotensin type 1 (AT_1) receptor. In patients with type 2 diabetes mellitus, losartan decreased the incidence of a doubling of SCr by 25% and of ESRD by 28% when compared with placebo after a mean of 3.4 years of therapy.[35,54] Similar effects were observed in the Irbesartan Diabetic Nephropathy Trial (IDNT), with a 23% decreased risk of ESRD observed in patients treated with irbesartan.[55] In both studies, these beneficial effects were independent of reduction in BP. Reduction in the degree of proteinuria has also been demonstrated with candesartan and valsartan.[56,57] Combination therapy with an ARB and ACE inhibitor is controversial.[58] Further studies are needed to further ascertain the effect of combination therapy on proteinuria and kidney disease progression (see Antihypertensive Therapy section).

Aliskiren is the first available agent in a new class of antihypertensive drugs that target the renin-angiotensin-aldosterone system (RAAS) by directly inhibiting renin. The advantages of renin inhibition include inhibition of the rate-limiting step of angiotensin II formation, preventing compensatory RAAS activation by ACE inhibitor or ARB therapy, and possible synergistic effects with other antihypertensive regimens. In patients with diabetes mellitus, hypertension, and diabetic nephropathy, treatment with aliskiren and losartan compared with patients taking losartan and placebo resulted in significant reduction in albuminuria, indicating that aliskiren may have renoprotective effects.[59]

Calcium-channel blockers have been considered for preventing progression of kidney disease owing to their effects on renal hemodynamics and cytoprotective and antiproliferative properties (prevention of mesangial expansion and renal scarring). The nondihydropyridine agents (e.g., diltiazem and verapamil) have been beneficial in reducing proteinuria when compared with dihydropyridines (e.g., amlodipine), which have been found to worsen proteinuria.[60] The NKF K/DOQI guidelines suggest that dihydropyridine calcium-channel blockers should not be used alone in nondiabetic or diabetic kidney disease with proteinuria, but can be used safely in combination with an ACE inhibitor or ARB. Combination therapy with an ACE inhibitor and nondihydropyridine agents has resulted in greater reductions in proteinuria in patients with diabetes than with either agent alone, suggesting that it may be rational to use multiple agents in this population.[61]

β-Blockers may offer benefits in the treatment of diabetic nephropathy as demonstrated by the United Kingdom Prospective Diabetes Study, which showed similar effects of atenolol and captopril on decreasing the incidence of albuminuria in patients with diabetes.[62]

TREATMENT OF DYSLIPIDEMIA

The role of antihyperlipidemic drug therapy in preventing progression of CKD is uncertain. A meta-analysis of trials, predominantly in patients with diabetes and CKD, showed that lipid-lowering therapy slowed the rate of decline in eGFR.[63] Some studies have demonstrated an association of statin use with decreased proteinuria and preservation of eGFR, whereas others have found that statins are no different than placebo.[64–67] Additionally, treatment with fibrates does not seem to have an effect on the progression of CKD.[68,69] Despite uncertainty of therapy with regard to delaying progression, dyslipidemia should be treated in the kidney disease population. Abnormal lipid metabolism is present in these patients, which predisposes them to the development of atherosclerotic disease. The question of whether strategies used to prevent and treat hyperlipidemia in the general population should be extrapolated to the population with kidney disease was addressed by the NKF Task Force on Cardiovascular Disease.[70] This group supported application of the National Cholesterol Education Program (NCEP ATP III) guidelines to the population with kidney disease and classified these patients in the highest risk group.[71] Guidelines for management of dyslipidemias in patients with CKD are available (NKF K/DOQI guidelines).[72] These guidelines support classifying patients with CKD as coronary heart disease risk equivalents, the highest risk category for cardiovascular disease.

The choice of the specific antihyperlipidemic agent should be based on the individual lipid profile. In general, NCEP guidelines should be followed, with particular consideration of the effect of such interventions on patients with CKD, such as dietary restrictions and cautious use of agents that are eliminated by the kidney. Statin therapy has been shown to be safe and effective in those with kidney diseases.[73] However, the cardiovascular benefits of statin use observed in the general population have not consistently been demonstrated in the CKD and dialysis populations, possibly owing to the multifactorial pathogenic process of

cardiovascular disease in those with kidney disease
ence of vascular calcification).[74] The addition o
statin therapy has been shown to be well toleratec
an additional decrease in LDL cholesterol compa
therapy alone in CKD patients.[75] Most recently
Heart and Renal Protection (SHARP) assessed the
ing LDL cholesterol in 9,438 CKD patients with ez
daily and simvastatin 20 mg daily or matching du
tablets for an average of 5 years. Key outcomes w
of major atherosclerotic events and kidney diseas
SHARP results showed a 25% risk reduction on ma
rotic events. However, there was no effect on the
kidney disease.[76] Fibrates should be used cautiou
with CKD; all agents in this class are metabolized
and are eliminated primarily via the kidney, whic
an increased risk of rhabdomyolysis. Small studie
excretion of gemfibrozil in renal insufficiency to b
compromised; therefore, the NKF K/DOQI recom
brozil as the fibrate of choice in patients with CK
triglyceridemia (see Chapter 13, Dyslipidemias, A
and Coronary Heart Disease).[72]

END-STAGE RENAL DISEASE (STAGE 5 CHRONIC KIDNEY D

Clinical Signs and Symptoms

During stages 4 and 5, patients may develop the mo
and symptoms associated with advanced kidney
referred to as *uremic syndrome*. The manifestations
consequences of advanced kidney disease are listed
These manifestations certainly may develop in the
of CKD, underscoring the importance of early int
they become more prominent as the disease worse
genesis of these disorders has been attributed, i
accumulation of uremic toxins. The search for ure
led to the identification of nitrogenous compound
sistently observed in the serum of patients with kid
cause-and-effect relationship between these comp
clinical manifestations of uremia has not been clear
however.[77]

Treatment

DIALYSIS AND TRANSPLANTATION

As ESRD becomes inevitable, the appropriate dia
must be selected on the basis of patient preference a
vascular access for HD or peritoneal access for PD.
for dialysis therapy and timely initiation may lowe
bidity and mortality. (Indications for dialysis and c
in selection of modality are discussed in Chapter 32
sis.) Kidney transplantation is an option for all patie
without specified contraindications if a suitable o
available (see Chapter 34, Kidney and Liver Trans

PHARMACOTHERAPY

Pharmacotherapy in patients with ESRD requires
to manage comorbid conditions and secondary co
CKD. The extent of medication use, including m
ministered during dialysis therapy, contributes to
for drug interactions, adverse reactions, and non
therapy.[78] The effect of decreased kidney functio
tion, distribution, metabolism, and elimination of p
agents, in addition to the contribution of dialysis to

is not well defined. Some clinicians have suggested, however, that plasma levels of 80 mg/L or more may correlate with auditory dysfunction.

Vancomycin has an elimination half-life of 3 to 9 hours in patients with normal renal function.[100] This increases to 129 to 189 hours in patients with ESRD.[101–103] Using pharmacokinetic principles and considering that the plasma clearance of vancomycin is approximately 60% to 70% of CrCl[98] and the Vd averages 0.7 L/kg,[98,100,104] the estimated Vd_{vanco} and Cl_{vanco} can be calculated using the following equation:

$$Cr_{Cl} = 30.5 \text{ mL/minute (calculated from Eq. 33-5)}$$

$$\begin{aligned} Cl_{vanco} &= (0.65)(CrCl) \\ &= (0.65)(30.5 \text{ mL/minute}) \\ &= 19.8 \text{ mL/min } \textit{or} \text{ rounded off to } 1.2 \text{ L/hour} \end{aligned} \quad \textit{(Eq. 33-28)}$$

$$\begin{aligned} Vd_{vanco} &= (0.7 \text{ L/kg})(\text{body weight}) \\ &= (0.7 \text{ L/kg})(70 \text{ kg}) \\ &= 49 \text{ L} \end{aligned} \quad \textit{(Eq. 33-29)}$$

Based on estimated values for Cl_{vanco} and Vd_{vanco}, the elimination rate constant can be calculated using the following equation:

$$\begin{aligned} Kd &= \frac{Cl_{vanco}}{Vd_{vanco}} \\ &= \frac{1.2 \text{ L/hour}}{49 \text{ L}} \\ &= 0.024 \text{ hour}^{-1} \end{aligned} \quad \textit{(Eq. 33-30)}$$

$$\begin{aligned} Cp &= \frac{\dfrac{Dose}{Vd_{vanco}}}{1 - e^{-Kdt}} \\ &= \frac{\dfrac{500 \text{ mg}}{49 \text{ L}}}{1 - e^{-(0.024 \text{ hour}^{-1})(24 \text{ hours})}} \\ &= 23 \text{ mg/L} \end{aligned} \quad \textit{(Eq. 33-31)}$$

$$\begin{aligned} Cp_{trough} &= Cp_{peak}(e^{-Kdt}) \\ &= 23 \text{ mg/L}(e^{-(0.024/\text{hour}^{-1})(24 \text{ hours})}) \\ &= 13 \text{ mg/L} \end{aligned} \quad \textit{(Eq. 33-32)}$$

Because M.H.'s estimated peak concentration is less than 40 mg/L and her trough falls within the range of 10 to 15 mg/L, the starting dose of 500 mg every 24 hours is appropriate for M.H.

Routine monitoring of plasma vancomycin concentrations in patients with normal renal function is controversial because the likelihood that toxicity will develop in this group is relatively low. However, in patients with renal failure, such as M.H., it is advisable to measure vancomycin levels several days after initiation of therapy to ensure that they are within an acceptable range.[100,102,103,105] This is prudent if an extended course of therapy is anticipated. Vancomycin is usually infused over the course of 60 minutes.

HEMODIALYSIS OF VANCOMYCIN

CASE 33-5, QUESTION 3: M.H.'s renal function begins to deteriorate to the point where she requires hemodialysis. How should her regimen now be altered?

Patients with ESRD may have measurable vancomycin levels for up to 3 weeks after a single dose despite conventional hemodialysis.[103] This suggests that the ability of these patients to eliminate vancomycin is minimal and that little of the drug is removed by conventional hemodialysis. The elimination half-life for vancomycin in these individuals averages 5 to 7 days, which is consistent with a residual vancomycin clearance of 3 to 4 mL/minute.[101–103] Only about 5% of vancomycin is metabolized hepatically in patients with normal renal function.

Conventional hemodialysis removes about 7% of vancomycin during a typical 4-hour dialysis run.[106] The elimination half-life on and off dialysis and plasma levels of the drug before and after hemodialysis do not differ significantly. The poor removal of vancomycin by conventional hemodialysis is attributable to its large MW of 1,400.

Patients receiving conventional hemodialysis are typically given a single, 1-g dose every 7 to 10 days.[100,103,105] Based on M.H.'s estimated Vd of 49 L, this dose will produce an initial peak plasma level of approximately 20 mg/L. If vancomycin is administered weekly, steady-state peak and trough levels of 40 and 16 mg/L, respectively, would be predicted.

Vancomycin is removed to a greater extent by high-flux hemodialysis than by conventional hemodialysis. As a result, more frequent dosing is necessary to maintain therapeutic vancomycin concentrations. High-flux dialysis clearance of vancomycin using the Fresenius polysulfone dialyzer is 45 to 160 mL/minute and varies with membrane surface area.[60,107] Up to 50% of a dose of vancomycin is removed in 4 hours by high-flux hemodialysis compared with 6.9% using conventional dialysis. A rebound phenomenon after dialysis suggests that the total amount of drug removed may be less than initially reported.[108,109] In any case, the efficiency of high-flux procedures in removing vancomycin is greater than that of conventional dialysis. Therefore, plasma levels should be monitored carefully in these patients, and the necessity for postdialysis replacement doses of around 500 mg (~10–15 mg/kg) should be anticipated.

Amphotericin

DOSING

CASE 33-5, QUESTION 4: M.H. continues to be febrile despite her triple antimicrobial regimen. Amphotericin therapy is started empirically for a potential fungal infection. In addition, pentamidine is begun to cover *Pneumocystis jiroveci* pneumonia. How should amphotericin be administered in patients such as M.H. with renal dysfunction?

Amphotericin is an antifungal agent used to treat serious infections, such as invasive aspergillosis and cryptococcal meningitis. The exact mechanism of elimination for this drug is unclear, but it may involve hepatic metabolism or inactivation in body tissues. Small amounts of amphotericin are gradually excreted in the urine for several weeks after its discontinuation.[110] This slow elimination may be because of extensive distribution of amphotericin into peripheral tissue and its large Vd (4 L/kg).[110,111] The drug appears to bind to cholesterol-containing cytoplasmic membranes of various tissues, resulting in a very long elimination half-life of 15 days. Pharmacokinetic studies report no significant change in the disposition of amphotericin in patients with renal or liver disease. Therefore, no dosage adjustments are required in patients with renal dysfunction.

Amphotericin is associated with acute tubular necrosis, which is believed to be dose dependent.[112–114] To prevent exacerbation of nephrotoxicity, lower doses often are administered to patients with decreased renal function. Administration of amphotericin every other day often is suggested for patients with renal failure. In addition to conventional amphotericin, a liposomal (liposomal

bicarbonate levels of at least 22 mEq/L. Treatment includes use of preparations containing sodium bicarbonate or sodium citrate. Each 650-mg tablet of sodium bicarbonate provides 8 mEq of sodium and 8 mEq of bicarbonate. Shohl's solution and Bicitra contain 1 mEq of sodium and the amount of citrate or citric acid to provide 1 mEq of bicarbonate/mL. These latter agents may be used in patients who experience excessive GI distress with sodium bicarbonate because of production and elimination of carbon dioxide. If a patient such as G.B. is sodium and fluid overloaded, it is important to consider that sodium bicarbonate can exacerbate this problem. Polycitra, or potassium citrate, is a possible alternative; however, the potassium content limits its use in patients with more severe kidney disease. Citrate also promotes aluminum absorption and should not be used in patients taking aluminum-containing agents. The NKF K/DOQI guidelines do not give an exact recommendation of the amount of bicarbonate supplementation to achieve a bicarbonate of 22 mEq/L. The use of two to four 650-mg sodium bicarbonate tablets per day, usually divided into two to three doses, is a typical regimen used to correct metabolic acidosis. Equations based on the serum bicarbonate level are available if an immediate correction of the metabolic acidosis is warranted.[97]

Once dialysis therapy is initiated in patients with kidney disease, intravenous (IV) and oral supplementation with bicarbonate or citrate or citric acid preparations is generally not required. At this point, dialysis therapy is used to chronically manage metabolic acidosis through use of dialysate baths containing bicarbonate. Bicarbonate is added to the dialysate solution and is delivered through the process of diffusion from the dialysate bath into the plasma (see Chapter 32, Renal Dialysis). If dialysis therapy is initiated in G.B., the continued need for oral bicarbonate supplementation should be reassessed.

Other Electrolyte and Metabolic Disturbances of Chronic Kidney Disease

CASE 31-1, QUESTION 9: What other electrolyte and metabolic disturbances are exhibited by G.B.?

G.B.'s hyperphosphatemia is a result of decreased phosphorus elimination by the kidneys (see Case 31-3, Question 2, for a more detailed discussion of hyperphosphatemia). The KDIGO guidelines for metabolism and bone disorder recommend reducing dietary phosphorus to 800 to 1,000 mg/day while maintaining adequate nutritional needs.[98] Phosphorus-containing laxatives and enemas should also be avoided. Hyperphosphatemia is associated with low serum calcium concentrations.

The mild degree of hypermagnesemia seen in G.B. is a common finding in patients with CKD owing to decreased elimination of magnesium by the kidney. Magnesium is eliminated by the kidney to the extent required to achieve normal serum magnesium concentrations until eGFR is less than 30 mL/minute/1.73 m^2. Serum magnesium concentrations less than 5 mEq/L rarely cause symptoms. Higher concentrations can lead to nausea, vomiting, lethargy, confusion, and diminished tendon reflexes, whereas severe hypermagnesemia may depress cardiac conduction. The risk of hypermagnesemia can be reduced by avoiding magnesium-containing antacids and laxatives and by use of magnesium-free dialysate in patients with stage 5 CKD requiring dialysis.

G.B. also has mild hyperuricemia. Asymptomatic hyperuricemia frequently develops in patients with kidney disease owing to diminished urinary excretion of uric acid. In the absence of a history of gout or urate nephropathy, asymptomatic hyperuricemia does not require treatment.

ANEMIA OF CHRONIC KIDNEY DISEASE

CASE 31-1, QUESTION 10: What findings in G.B. are consistent with the diagnosis of anemia of CKD, and what is the etiology of this disorder?

G.B.'s hemoglobin of 9.3 g/dL and hematocrit of 28% are substantially lower than the normal range for premenopausal females, indicating that she has anemia.[99] Her normal RBC indices suggest her red cells are of normal size, but the absence of an elevated reticulocyte count suggests an impaired bone marrow response for her degree of anemia. Her recent history of peptic ulcer disease may also have contributed to the observed drop in hemoglobin and hematocrit as a result of blood loss. Her complaint of general malaise is consistent with the symptoms of anemia.

Characteristics and Etiology

Anemia, which affects most patients with CKD, is caused by a decreased production of erythropoietin (EPO), a glycoprotein that stimulates red blood cell production in the bone marrow and is released in response to hypoxia. Approximately 90% of the total EPO is produced in the peritubular cells of the kidney; the remainder is produced by the liver. EPO concentrations in patients with kidney failure are lower than in individuals with normal kidney function who have the same degree of anemia and, therefore, the same stimulus for EPO production and release.[99]

Anemia appears as early as stage 3 CKD and is characterized by normochromic (normal color) and normocytic (normal size) red blood cells unless a concomitant iron, folate, or vitamin B_{12} deficiency exists. A direct correlation between eGFR and hematocrit has been demonstrated, with a 3.1% decrease in hematocrit for every 10 mL/minute/1.73 m^2 decline in eGFR.[100] A higher prevalence of anemia occurs in the population with an eGFR less than 60 mL/minute/1.73 m^2.[1] Pallor and fatigue are the earliest clinical signs, with other manifestations developing as anemia progresses with declining kidney function. A significant consequence of anemia is development of left ventricular hypertrophy (LVH), further contributing to cardiovascular complications and mortality in patients with CKD. LVH has been observed in approximately 30% of patients with eGFR 50 to 75 mL/minute/1.73 m^2 (stages 2 and 3 CKD) and in up to 74% of patients at the start of dialysis (stage 5 CKD).[101] These findings support the need for early and aggressive treatment of anemia of CKD before the development of stage 5 CKD.

A more complete workup for anemia of CKD is recommended for patients with an eGFR of less than 60 mL/minute/1.73 m^2.[1,99] This workup includes monitoring of hemoglobin and hematocrit, assessment of iron indices with correction if iron deficiency is present, and evaluation for sources of blood loss, such as bleeding from the GI tract. This workup should be done regularly as CKD progresses because of the association between anemia and the progressive decline in eGFR.

The availability of recombinant human EPO to directly stimulate erythrocyte production revolutionized the treatment of CKD-associated anemia. However, iron deficiency is the leading cause of erythropoiesis-stimulating agent (ESA) hyporesponsiveness and must be corrected before ESA therapy is initiated. Iron deficiency can develop as a result of increased requirements for RBC production with ESA administration and from chronic blood loss owing to bleeding or HD. Identification and management of iron deficiency through regular follow-up testing and iron supplementation is essential for adequate RBC production (see Case 31-1, Question 12, for Iron Therapy, and also Chapter 12, Anemias).[99]

Other factors that contribute to anemia include a shortened RBC life span secondary to uremia, blood loss from frequent phlebotomy and HD, GI bleeding, severe hyperparathyroidism, protein malnutrition, aluminum accumulation, severe infections, and inflammatory conditions.[99] Substances present in the plasma of patients with CKD, collectively termed *uremic toxins,* may inhibit the production of EPO, the bone marrow response to EPO, and the synthesis of heme. The negative effects of these substances on RBC production are supported by improvement in erythropoiesis with dialysis, which removes these uremic toxins. This uremic environment also causes a decrease in the RBC life span, from a normal life span of 120 days to approximately 60 days in patients with severe CKD. A shortened RBC life span has been observed in uremic patients transfused with RBCs from individuals with normal kidney function, whereas RBCs from uremic individuals maintain a normal survival time when transfused into patients without kidney failure.[102]

Blood loss also contributes to anemia of CKD, particularly in patients requiring HD. With each HD session, generally performed three times per week, blood loss occurs. In addition, these patients are usually administered heparin during dialysis or antiplatelet drugs to prevent vascular access clotting, which further increases the risk of bleeding. Although a stool guaiac test was not performed in G.B., many patients with uremia and CKD will have a positive guaiac reaction because of the risk of bleeding from uremia itself. G.B. also has a peptic ulcer, which increases her potential for blood loss.

Other deficiencies can contribute to anemia of CKD. Deficiency of folic acid, as evidenced by low serum folate concentrations and macrocytosis, is relatively uncommon in patients with early kidney disease, but occurs most often in patients on dialysis because folic acid is removed by dialysis. Therefore, the daily prophylactic administration of the water-soluble vitamins, including 1 mg of folic acid, is recommended. Routine use of fat-soluble vitamin A is discouraged, because hypervitaminosis A may develop, contributing to anemia.[103] Several multivitamin preparations devoid of vitamin A (e.g., Nephrocaps) are available for patients with kidney failure. Pyridoxine (vitamin B_6) deficiency can also occur in both dialyzed and nondialyzed patients with CKD. Significant similarities are seen between this deficiency and the symptoms of uremia, which include skin hyperpigmentation and peripheral neuropathy. Current multivitamin products for patients with stage 5 CKD contain adequate amounts of pyridoxine to prevent deficiency.

Goals of Therapy

CASE 31-1, QUESTION 11: What are the goals of therapy for anemia of CKD in G.B.?

TARGET HEMOGLOBIN

NKF K/DOQI guidelines recommend a target of 11 to12 g/dL for hemoglobin in patients with CKD receiving ESA therapy.[99] It is at these targets that benefits such as increased survival, exercise capacity, quality of life, cardiac output, cognitive function, and decreased risk of LVH were observed in the CKD population.[99] Routine maintenance of hemoglobin levels of 13 g/dL or more is not recommended for patients being treated with ESA because of the increased risk for serious cerebrovascular or cardiovascular events and mortality. Three trials have evaluated the efficacy and safety of hemoglobin targets in patients with CKD not on HD. In each study, the higher target hemoglobin groups (hemoglobin ≥13 g/dL) experienced increased cardiovascular events, stroke, or mortality rates.[104–106] These results have had an impact on the nephrologist community with many clinicians lowering their threshold to the US Food and Drug Administration (FDA)–recommended ESA therapy initiation and hemoglobin target ranges (i.e., hemoglobin level 10–12 g/dL).

Hemoglobin, rather than hematocrit, should be used to evaluate anemia in this population for several reasons. Hematocrit is dependent on volume status, which can be problematic for patients with fluctuations in plasma water (e.g., dialysis, volume overload). In addition, a number of variables can affect the hematocrit value including temperature, hyperglycemia, the size of the red blood cell, and the counters used for the test. These variables do not significantly affect hemoglobin, making it the preferred test for anemia.[99]

G.B.'s iron status should be evaluated first, and corrected if necessary. If achieving an adequate iron status does not improve anemia management, ESA therapy may be started (see Treatment section, and also Chapter 12, Anemias).

IRON STATUS

Iron deficiency is the primary cause of ESA hyporesponsiveness; thus, iron status assessment is essential before initiating erythropoietic therapy. The two tests that best evaluate iron status are the transferrin saturation percent (TSAT) and serum ferritin.[99] Transferrin is a carrier protein, and its concentration depends on nutritional status. The TSAT indicates the saturation of the protein transferrin with iron and is determined as follows:

$$\%\ \text{TSAT} = \frac{\text{serum iron}\left[\frac{\text{mcg}}{\text{dL}}\right]}{\text{TIBC}\left[\frac{\text{mcg}}{\text{dL}}\right]} \times 100 \qquad \textit{(Eq. 31-1)}$$

where TIBC is the total iron-binding capacity of the transferrin protein. The TSAT is considered iron readily available for RBC production. Serum ferritin is a marker for iron reserves, which are stored primarily in the reticuloendothelial system (e.g., liver, spleen). The goal of iron replacement therapy is to maintain the TSAT greater than 20% and a serum ferritin greater than 100 ng/mL for CKD stages 2 through 4 and greater than 200 ng/mL for CKD stage 5 to provide sufficient iron for erythrocyte production.[99] Values below these targets are indicative of absolute iron deficiency. A functional iron deficiency may exist when ferritin is greater than 500 ng/mL, TSAT is less than 20%, and anemia persists despite appropriate ESA therapy. In these cases, iron supplementation may lead to improved erythropoiesis. Other tests, including the percentage of hypochromic red blood cells, reticulocyte hemoglobin content, serum transferrin receptor, red blood cell ferritin, and zinc protoporphyrin, have been proposed as indicators of iron status.[99] Although some of these markers have demonstrated predictive value in assessing iron status, either alone or in conjunction with other laboratory data, further investigation is warranted to determine their utility and to make such testing procedures readily available.

Treatment

CASE 31-1, QUESTION 12: Describe the options available to treat anemia of CKD and achieve the goals of therapy in G.B.

IRON THERAPY

Before initiating ESA therapy, G.B.'s iron indices should be determined. If G.B. is iron deficient, as indicated by the TSAT and serum ferritin and other supporting laboratory data (see Chapter 12, Anemias), supplemental iron therapy should be administered. If iron deficiency is the cause of anemia, G.B. may benefit from iron supplementation alone (i.e., without erythropoietic therapy) to increase hemoglobin. Peptic ulcer disease will need to be evaluated as a source of blood loss. Given the poor bioavailability of oral iron and patient noncompliance, oral iron is usually inadequate for repletion of iron in patients receiving HD who experience chronic blood loss.[107] For the population with early CKD and for patients receiving PD, an initial trial of oral iron may correct the deficiency because these patients do not have the same degree of blood loss. However, IV therapy will be required to replenish iron and meet the increased demands once erythropoiesis is stimulated with ESA therapy. Administration of IV iron requires IV access and frequent outpatient visits, which are drawbacks to therapy with IV iron in CKD stages 3 and 4. A recent trial examined an accelerated dosing regimen (500 mg given on two consecutive days) of IV iron sucrose to address these issues. This regimen was adequate to restore iron stores with only two patients experiencing hypotension related to iron therapy.[108]

Common infusion-related effects associated with IV iron include hypotension, myalgias, and arthralgias. Despite the controversy about the best strategy for iron supplementation in patients with early CKD, current recommendations support reserving IV iron for patients in whom oral iron has failed.[109] Therefore, a trial of oral iron is reasonable for G.B. Oral iron supplementation with 200 mg/day of elemental iron should be started to address iron deficiency, if present, and this regimen should be continued to maintain sufficient iron status while receiving ESA therapy. Many oral iron preparations are available, and their iron content varies as will the number of tablets or capsules that must be taken per day to provide the required elemental iron (Table 31-6). Some oral formulations include ascorbic acid to enhance iron absorption. A heme iron product, Proferrin-ES, has recently been approved. Heme iron is more readily absorbed; however, a large number of tablets are required to supply the required 200 mg of elemental iron (Table 31-6). G.B. should be advised to take oral iron on an empty stomach to maximize absorption, unless side effects prevent this strategy. She also should be counseled on potential drug interactions with oral iron (e.g., antacids, quinolones) and GI side effects (e.g., nausea, abdominal pain, diarrhea, constipation, dark stools). Noncompliance with therapy as a result of side effects is a common cause of therapeutic failure with oral iron. An acidic environment is needed for adequate iron absorption, and acid-suppression therapies (e.g., proton-pump inhibitors) may limit the absorption of oral iron. Oral iron is a mucosal toxin, and her previous history of peptic ulcer disease requires caution with the use of oral iron.

If G.B.'s condition does not respond to oral therapy, as indicated by either persistent iron deficiency based on iron indices or inadequate response to what is considered an adequate dose and duration of erythropoietic therapy, IV iron is necessary. The IV iron preparations currently available are iron dextran (INFeD, DexFerrum), sodium ferric gluconate complex in sucrose (Ferrlecit), iron sucrose (Venofer), and ferumoxytol (Feraheme). The dextran products have caused anaphylactic reactions and, as a result, have an FDA-mandated black-box warning that requires administration of a 25-mg test dose followed by a 1-hour observation period before the total dose of iron is infused.[110] The dextran component is believed to be the cause of such reactions. The dose of IV iron recommended to correct absolute iron deficiency is a total dose of 1 g administered in divided doses or for a prolonged period to minimize the risk of adverse effects.[99] For iron dextran, the approved dose is 100-mg increments, administered during 10 dialysis sessions for patients on HD to provide a total of 1 g.[110] Larger doses of 500 mg up to the total 1-g dose have been safely administered during a longer infusion period of 4 to 6 hours.[99,109]

Sodium ferric gluconate and iron sucrose are the most widely used iron products in the CKD population. Both the ferric gluconate and iron sucrose products have been used successfully in patients who have experienced allergic reactions to the dextran products, and evidence indicates that they are safer: 8.7 adverse events per million doses for dextran versus 3.3 adverse events for gluconate.[111] To provide the recommended total dose of 1 g, ferric gluconate is administered as 125 mg (10 mL) during eight consecutive dialysis sessions for patients on HD. The dose can be administered as a slow IV injection at a rate of up to 12.5 mg/minute or diluted in 100 mL of normal saline and infused for 1 hour.[112] Administration of 125 mg for 10 minutes (without a test dose) was determined to be a safer alternative to dextran preparations in patients on HD and is an approved dosing strategy.[112,113] Doses up to 250 mg for 1 hour have been administered safely.[114] The flexibility of administering larger doses of iron is an important factor in achieving efficiencies in the outpatient setting for patients with early CKD and those receiving PD.

Iron sucrose (Venofer) is a polynuclear iron hydroxide sucrose complex. The recommended dose of iron sucrose is 100 mg (5 mL) during 10 consecutive HD sessions to provide the total dose of 1 g.[115] The dose can be administered by a slow IV injection for 5 minutes or diluted in 100 mL of normal saline and infused for at least 15 minutes. As with sodium ferric gluconate, a test dose is not required. Iron sucrose doses of 250 to 300 mg have been safely administered for 1 hour and found to be as effective as sodium ferric gluconate administration in maintaining hemoglobin in patients receiving epoetin.[116]

Smaller doses of IV iron, in increments of 25 to 200 mg, can be administered on a weekly, every 2-week, or monthly basis, to patients without absolute iron deficiency. These doses will sustain adequate iron stores, maintain target hemoglobin values, and potentially reduce the required dose of the erythropoietic agent.[99] This regimen is most convenient for patients on HD

TABLE 31-6
Oral Iron Preparations

Preparation	Common Brand Names	Commonly Prescribed Unit Size (Amount Elemental Iron in mg)[a]	Number of Units/Da to Yield 200 mg Elemental Iron
Ferrous sulfate	Slow FE, Fer-In-Sol	325 (65)	3 tablets
Ferrous gluconate	Feratab	325 (36)	5 tablets
Ferrous fumarate	Femiron, Feostat	200 (66)	3 capsules
Iron polysaccharide	Niferex, Nu-Iron	150 (150)	2 capsules
Heme iron polypeptide	Proferrin-ES Proferrin-Forte	12 (12)	17 tablets

[a] Unit size reflects common tablet or capsule sizes prescribed and not necessarily that of the brand names listed.

who have regular IV access and increased iron needs because of chronic blood loss. Maintenance iron therapy replaces these losses and minimizes the need for the more aggressive 1-g total doses of IV iron required for absolute iron deficiency. If G.B. starts on HD in the future, regular dosing of IV iron during dialysis is the most reasonable way to maintain adequate iron required for sustained erythropoiesis. Iron indices should be monitored at least every 3 months to guide IV iron therapy. Targeting a ferritin of at least 500 ng/mL is not routinely recommended because of the lack of evidence available.[99] A recent study evaluating the response to iron therapy in patients with elevated ferritin (500 to 1,200 ng/mL) and a low TSAT ($\leq$25%) found that administration of IV iron resulted in a statistically significant increase in hemoglobin levels and a faster hemoglobin response in patients receiving ESA therapy.[117] This strategy, however, could lead to increased exposure to free iron, which may place the patient at an increased risk of adverse effects (e.g., inflammation, oxidative stress).[118]

Ferumoxytol (Feraheme) is a semisynthetic carbohydrate-coated, superparamagnetic iron oxide nanoparticle recently approved in the treatment of iron-deficiency anemia of CKD. The small content of free iron in the formulation allows for doses of 510 mg to be administered safely for 17 seconds, followed by a second 510-mg IV injection 3 to 8 days later. Contrary to previous IV iron formulations, a 1-g repletion regimen of ferumoxytol can be completed in two settings. Prospective, randomized studies in patients with CKD (stages 1–5) demonstrated the superior effectiveness of ferumoxytol in increasing hemoglobin levels in CKD patients compared with oral iron.[119] The carbohydrate coating of ferumoxytol is suggested to reduce immunologic sensitivity, potentially resulting in less risk for anaphylactic type reactions compared with the other available high molecular weight IV iron products (e.g., iron dextran).[120] However, since approval there has been an adverse drug event rate of 0.2%.[121] Although the ease of administration of ferumoxytol and suggested lower adverse effects make it an ideal candidate for anemia, comparison studies of ferumoxytol to other IV iron formulations are needed to confirm these benefits. Ferumoxytol presents the same side effect profile as other IV iron preparations (i.e., hypotension or hypersensitivity reactions, including anaphylaxis or anaphylactoid reactions). Additionally, ferumoxytol can affect the diagnostic ability of magnetic resonance imaging (MRI) for up to 3 months after the last dose.[122]

ERYTHROPOIESIS-STIMULATING AGENT THERAPY

Recombinant human EPO should be initiated for anemia of CKD in G.B. if there is no response in her hemoglobin to IV iron. Regular dialysis may improve an anemic condition, but it will not restore the hemoglobin concentrations to normal because the primary cause of anemia is reduced EPO production by the kidneys. Although blood transfusions were once the mainstay of treatment, they are now avoided, if possible, because they are associated with a risk for viral diseases (hepatitis, human immunodeficiency virus [HIV]), iron overload, and further suppression of erythropoiesis. Transfusions may be required in certain patients with substantially low oxygen-carrying capacity or substantial blood loss, and in those patients exhibiting persistent symptoms of anemia (e.g., fatigue, dyspnea on exertion, tachycardia). Currently, G.B. is not a candidate for transfusions based on her hemoglobin of 9.3 g/dL and the absence of significant symptoms on presentation. Androgens raise EPO concentrations and were previously used to treat the anemia of CKD. However, inconsistent erythropoietic response, many adverse effects, and the availability of recombinant EPO have terminated the use of androgens as a treatment of anemia.

HUMAN ERYTHROPOETIN-EPOETIN ALFA

Human erythropoietin or epoetin, the exogenous form of EPO, is produced using recombinant technology. Epoetin alfa is available in the United States, whereas epoetin beta is available primarily outside the United States. Since it became available in 1989, epoetin alfa (Epogen, Procrit) has provided an effective treatment option for anemia and has substantially decreased the need for RBC transfusions. Epoetin alfa stimulates the proliferation and differentiation of erythroid progenitor cells, increases hemoglobin synthesis, and accelerates the release of reticulocytes from the bone marrow.

For patients such as G.B. who do not yet require dialysis and for patients receiving PD, epoetin alfa is generally administered by subcutaneous (SC) injection. However, HD patients often receive epoetin alfa by IV administration because easy IV access is established. According to the NKF K/DOQI guidelines for anemia management, SC administration is preferred because lower doses can be administered less frequently and cost is lower than with IV administration.[78,123] Starting doses for epoetin alfa administration are 50 to 100 units/kg three times weekly.[124] For patients being converted from IV to SC administration (half-life of epoetin alfa is 8.5 hours IV vs. 24.4 hours SC) whose hemoglobin is within the target range, the SC dose is usually two-thirds the IV dose.[78] For patients not yet at the target hemoglobin, an SC dose equivalent to the IV dose is recommended. Patients receiving epoetin alfa SC should be instructed on the appropriate administration technique, which includes rotating the sites for injection (e.g., upper arm, thigh, abdomen).

Extended dosing intervals for SC administration of epoetin alfa have been evaluated in patients with CKD who are not on dialysis.[125] Doses of 10,000 units once weekly to 40,000 units once every 4 weeks have been shown to maintain target hemoglobin values for those patients with CKD not on dialysis.[126] Such dosing strategies may provide more convenient therapy for these patients who are not yet on dialysis but must come to the clinic for erythropoietic therapy.

DARBEPOETIN ALFA

Darbepoetin alfa (Aranesp) was approved in 2001 for the treatment of anemia of CKD, whether or not the patient requires dialysis. Darbepoetin is a hyperglycosylated analog of epoetin alfa that stimulates erythropoiesis by the same mechanism. Instead of the three *N*-linked carbohydrate chains on epoetin alfa, darbepoetin has five, which increase the capacity for sialic acid residue binding on the protein. The increased protein binding slows total body clearance and increases the terminal half-life to 25.3 hours and 48.8 hours after IV and SC administration, respectively. Darbepoetin alfa's longer half-life relative to epoetin alfa offers the potential advantage of less frequent dosing to maintain target hemoglobin values.

Studies in patients with early CKD (stages 3 and 4) determined that starting SC doses of 0.45 mcg/kg administered once per week and 0.75 mcg/kg once every other week were effective in achieving target hemoglobin and hematocrit values in patients who had not previously received erythropoietic therapy.[127] In patients on dialysis converted from epoetin alfa to darbepoetin alfa (IV and SC), darbepoetin maintained target hemoglobin values when administered less frequently (i.e., one dose every week in patients previously receiving epoetin alfa three times per week, and one dose every other week in patients previously receiving epoetin once weekly).[128,129]

The approved starting dose of darbepoetin alfa in patients who have not previously received epoetin therapy is 0.45 mcg/kg given either IV or SC once weekly.[130] Patients who are already receiving epoetin therapy may be converted to darbepoetin alfa based on the current total weekly epoetin dose (Table 31-7).[130] For patients

TABLE 31-7
Estimated Darbepoetin Alfa Starting Doses Based on Previous Epoetin Alfa Dose

Previous Weekly Epoetin Alfa Dosage (units/wk)	Weekly Starting Darbepoetin Alfa Dosage (mcg/wk)	
	Adults	Children
<1,500	6.25	[a]
1,500–2,499	6.25	6.25
2,500–4,999	12.5	10
5,000–10,999	25	20
11,000–17,999	40	40
18,000–33,999	60	60
34,000–89,999	100	100
≥90,000	20	200

Reprinted with permission from Facts & Comparisons eAnswers.
[a] For children receiving a weekly epoetin alfa dosage of <1,500 units/week, the available data are insufficient to determine a darbepoetin alfa conversion dosage http://online.factsandcomparisons.com/MonoDisp.aspx?monoid=fandc-hcp12341&book=DFC&search=193833&pipe;5&isStemmed=True&asbooks=#fandc-hcp12341.ad-section.5. Accessed November 13, 2010.

currently receiving epoetin alfa two to three times per week, darbepoetin alfa may be administered once weekly. Patients who are receiving epoetin alfa once weekly should receive darbepoetin alfa once every 2 weeks. To calculate the once every 2-week darbepoetin dose, the weekly epoetin alfa dose should be multiplied by 2 and that value used in column 1 of Table 31-5 to find the corresponding darbepoetin dose from column 2 in Table 31-7. For example, a patient receiving epoetin 6,000 units/week should receive 40 mcg of darbepoetin alfa once every 2 weeks (6,000 units epoetin × 2 = 12,000 units, which corresponds to a weekly darbepoetin dose of 40 mcg).[130]

Epoetin alfa and darbepoetin alfa are generally well tolerated, with hypertension being the most common adverse event reported. Although elevated BP is not uniformly considered a contraindication to therapy, BP should be monitored closely so that changes in antihypertensive therapy and the dialysis prescription are made, if justified. Failure to elicit a response to erythropoietic therapy requires evaluation of factors that cause resistance, such as iron deficiency, infection, inflammation, chronic blood loss, aluminum toxicity, malnutrition, and hyperparathyroidism. Resistance to erythropoietic therapy has been observed in patients receiving ACE inhibitors, although data are conflicting.[131] Rare cases of antibody formation to epoetin therapy have been reported.[132] Neutralizing anti-EPO antibodies were identified in 13 patients with pure red blood cell aplasia who required blood transfusions after a course of therapy with epoetin alfa or beta.[132] Similar cases have been reported, primarily with one epoetin alfa product manufactured outside the United States, Eprex. Some evidence supports cross-reactivity of these antibodies with darbepoetin, although the information is currently limited.[133] Although the clinical implications of antibody formation in patients receiving erythropoietic therapy are uncertain, clinicians should be aware of these reports when evaluating response to therapy.

Treatment of G.B.'s anemia must be initiated, given the chronic nature of her kidney disease and her current hemoglobin. Patients with hemoglobin values less than 10 g/dL, such as G.B., are the best candidates for erythropoietic therapy. It is also important to identify and correct any iron or folate deficiency and perform a stool guaiac test to rule out active GI bleeding. Iron supplementation is indicated, not only if G.B. is iron deficient but also to maintain iron status while receiving erythropoietic therapy (see Iron Therapy section). Although administration of iron alone may improve her anemia, epoetin alfa or darbepoetin alfa will likely be required, based on the severity of her anemia and the progressive nature of her kidney disease. G.B. may start epoetin alfa at a dose of 6,000 units (~100 units/kg) administered SC once per week or divided into two weekly doses of 3,000 units, assuming her iron status is appropriate (see Iron Status section). Another option would be darbepoetin alfa administered at a dose of 25 mcg (0.45 mcg/kg) SC once per week. She also should be instructed on how to administer SC epoetin alfa or darbepoetin alfa. Dose adjustments should not be made more frequently than once every 4 to 6 weeks for either agent because of the time course for response (i.e., the pharmacodynamic effects on RBC homeostasis). The time it takes to reach a new steady state, when RBC production is equal to RBC destruction, depends on the life span of the red blood cell, which is approximately 60 days in patients with kidney failure. Therefore, it will take approximately 2 to 3 months to reach a plateau in measured hemoglobin. Dose adjustments should be made on the basis of G.B.'s hemoglobin, which should be monitored every 1 to 2 weeks after initiation of therapy or after a dose change. If a rapid increase in hemoglobin is observed (hemoglobin >1.0 g/dL during a 1- to 2-week period) or the target hemoglobin is exceeded, then doses of either agent should be decreased by approximately 25%. If response is inadequate (hemoglobin increase <1 g/dL in 2 to 4 weeks), then the doses should be increased by approximately 50% for epoetin alfa and 25% for darbepoetin alfa.[99,130] Once stable, the hemoglobin should be monitored every 2 to 4 weeks. If a response is not observed despite appropriate dose titration, G.B. should be evaluated for possible reasons for nonresponse (i.e., iron deficiency, bleeding, aluminum intoxication, hyperparathyroidism, infection).

In early 2007, an FDA-mandated black-box warning was added to the safety labeling for all ESA products, which states that use of ESA therapy may increase the risk for death and for serious cardiovascular events when administered to achieve a hemoglobin greater than 12 g/dL. This came as a result of four recently completed cancer trials that evaluated new dosing regimens, use of ESA in a new patient population, and use of new unapproved ESA. Since then, two trials in patients with CKD have shown that targeting hemoglobin levels to greater than 13 g/dL results in increased mortality and morbidity; thus, observing these black-box warnings in CKD is warranted.[104,105]

OTHER ESA AGENTS

Continuous Erythropoietin Receptor Activator (CERA)

Continuous erythropoietin receptor activator (Mircera) is a long-acting ESA not currently available in the United States. CERA is twice the molecular weight of EPO from the addition of a single 30-kDa polymer chain into the erythropoietin molecule that results in a considerably longer elimination half-life compared with EPO (130 hours vs. 4 to 28 hours). This allows for extended-interval dosing of biweekly and once monthly. It has an efficacy and safety profile comparable to other available ESAs. Extended-interval dosing agents, such as CERA, have several advantages in patients with CKD stages 3 and 4, including improved patient compliance, less administration costs, reduced burden on patient from fewer injections given, and fewer outpatient visits to receive IV administration.[134]

Peginesatide

Peginesatide (Hematide) is a synthetic erythropoietin-mimetic peptide currently in phase III studies for anemia of CKD. Peginesatide is dosed monthly and can correct anemia in patients with pure red blood cell aplasia.[135] If approved, Hematide will provide health care professionals with a new option to correct anemia of CKD.

CARDIOVASCULAR COMPLICATIONS

CASE 31-2

QUESTION 1: H.B. is a 65-year-old white man with stage 5 CKD who has just started chronic HD. He comes in today for his third HD session (dialysis scheduled three times per week, 4-hour duration). He has a history of hypertension, which has been poorly controlled during the past 4 months (BP ranges 150–190/85–105 mm Hg), and has experienced shortness of breath and a significant weight gain during the past month. His pertinent medical history includes hypertension for the past 14 years. H.B.'s current medications include metoprolol tartrate 50 mg BID, furosemide 80 mg BID, calcium carbonate 500 mg TID with meals, and Nephrocaps 1 by mouth (PO) every day. H.B.'s most recent predialysis BP was 175/98 mm Hg, and his postdialysis BP was 158/90 mm Hg. A recent ECG showed evidence of LVH.

Predialysis laboratory values were as follows:

Serum sodium (Na), 140 mEq/L
Potassium (K), 5.1 mEq/L
Chloride (Cl), 101 mEq/L
CO_2 content, 23 mEq/L
SCr, 8.8 mg/dL
BUN, 84 mg/dL
Phosphate, 6.5 mg/dL
Calcium, 8.6 mg/dL
Serum albumin, 3.0 g/dL
Cholesterol (nonfasting), 345 mg/dL
Triglycerides, 285 mg/dL
TSAT, 18%
Ferritin, 250 ng/mL
Hct, 27%
Hgb, 9.0 g/dL

H.B. has a urine output of 50 mL/day. What conditions evident in H.B. put him at increased risk of cardiovascular complications and mortality?

H.B. has uncontrolled hypertension that is not adequately managed with his current drug therapy or HD. Hypertension is associated with LVH, ischemic heart disease, and heart failure, all of which are contributing factors to overall mortality in patients with stage 5 CKD who are undergoing dialysis.[4] H.B.'s ECG evidence of LVH should trigger additional evaluation to determine the extent of cardiac involvement and diagnosis of heart failure, which is associated with increased mortality in both diabetic and nondiabetic patients (see Chapter 19, Heart Failure). LVH develops early in the course of CKD and progresses as kidney disease progresses.[101] H.B. is in the most severe stage of CKD and has greatest likelihood of developing LVH. Anemia contributes substantially to the development of LVH and heart failure as well. H.B.'s hemoglobin of 9.0 g/dL is below the target value and requires treatment based on evaluation of his iron indices (see Anemia section).

Additional factors that increase the risk of cardiovascular complications and mortality in H.B. include elevated cholesterol and triglycerides levels as well as hypoalbuminemia (serum albumin, 3.0 g/dL). Increased levels of homocysteine are common in patients with kidney failure and have been associated with increased risk of coronary artery disease (CAD).[136] Because elevated concentrations of homocysteine have been observed in conjunction with decreased folate and vitamin B_{12} levels, more aggressive supplementation of these vitamins in this population has been suggested. Because H.B.'s total corrected calcium (corrected for hypoalbuminemia; see Case 31-3, Question 2, for an explanation of this correction) is 9.1 mg/dL, his calcium and use of a calcium-containing phosphate binder will need to be monitored frequently. Cardiac calcification is common in patients with kidney disease and also is associated with cardiovascular complications. It has been reported that up to 80% of patients with ESRD have detectable coronary artery calcification.[137]

Cardiovascular disease and complications continue to be the leading cause of mortality in patients with kidney failure. According to data from a large population of patients on dialysis, cardiovascular disease increases the risk of all-cause mortality fivefold when compared with the general Medicare population without kidney disease.[4] All-cause death rates are almost four times greater in patients age 65 and older who are on dialysis, such as H.B., than in the general Medicare population.[4]

Hypertension

CASE 31-2, QUESTION 2: What options are available to treat H.B.'s hypertension considering his other cardiac complications and BP goal?

DIALYSIS

Hypertension is common in patients with CKD with a prevalence that varies depending on the cause of CKD and residual kidney function. Prevalence of hypertension has been estimated to be 80% in HD and 50% in PD populations.[94] Multiple factors are involved in the development of hypertension in the CKD population, including extracellular volume expansion from salt and water retention and activation of the renin-angiotensin-aldosterone system.[131]

Because H.B. is just beginning dialysis therapy, it is difficult to assess the degree to which volume removal will ultimately affect his BP. To control BP related to volume changes, dialysis therapy should be adjusted as needed to achieve H.B.'s *dry weight*, the postdialysis weight at which symptoms of hypervolemia and hypovolemia are absent (i.e., normovolemia and free from edema). H.B. has had recent findings consistent with worsening volume status (shortness of breath, weight gain) that should be considered when modifying his dialysis prescription; further workup is needed to determine whether H.B. has systolic or diastolic heart failure. It is also important to counsel H.B. on the importance of salt and fluid intake restriction between HD sessions to minimize weight gain, volume expansion, and hypertension. Restriction of salt intake to less than 2.4 g/day and fluid to 1 L/day is appropriate and will require regular follow-up by a dietitian.

ANTIHYPERTENSIVE THERAPY

Antihypertensive therapy should be used in conjunction with dialysis therapy in H.B. to target a BP of less than 140/90 mm Hg before HD and less than 130/80 mm Hg after HD.[94] For some patients, initiation of dialysis alone may achieve this goal, and antihypertensive therapy may be withdrawn. The aim of the BP goal in patients with stage 5 CKD is to minimize cardiovascular complications, but it should not increase the risk for hypotension and its associated complications during dialysis. The choice of an agent is based on the patient's comorbid conditions because no single agent has a proven mortality benefit in patients on HD. The complexity of managing hypertension in patients on HD is enhanced by the apparent U-shaped relationship between BP and mortality. A study of patients on HD found an increased risk of cardiac-related death at a systolic BP less than 110 mm Hg and at a systolic BP greater than 180 mm Hg.[138] The mortality risk with a low pre-HD BP may be indicative of severe cardiac disease at the initiation of HD. If patients experience hypotensive symptoms during HD, the goal BP can be increased, but they also should be evaluated for other cardiovascular disorders. Because the BP between dialysis sessions varies owing to volume changes, the ideal time to measure BP relative to dialysis (i.e., predialysis versus postdialysis) is unclear, but predialysis BP has been favored.

Diuretics are commonly used in patients in the early stages of CKD. As previously discussed, the effectiveness of diuretics depends on the amount of sodium delivered to their site of action in the kidney tubule and on the patient's kidney function. For example, a decrease in the eGFR from 125 to 25 mL/minute/1.73 m^2, theoretically, could result in an approximate 80% decrease in the amount of sodium filtered. Early in the course of kidney failure, thiazides or thiazidelike diuretics are effective antihypertensive agents. As eGFR is further reduced (eGFR <30 mL/minute/1.73 m^2), the thiazide diuretics become essentially ineffective. Potassium-sparing diuretics are also ineffective and may increase the risk of hyperkalemia. Loop diuretics (e.g., furosemide), which function more proximally, are indicated in patients with stage 4 CKD (eGFR 15 to 29 mL/minute/1.73 m^2).[139] These drugs can be effective for BP and volume control in patients with advanced kidney disease if residual kidney function is substantial (urine output >100 mL/day). Their effect must be frequently reevaluated on the basis of urine output and any effect on volume control. H.B.'s urine output should be assessed to determine the rationale for continued use of furosemide, and the current dose should be assessed because doses higher than his current dose of 80 mg BID are often required in patients with this degree of kidney dysfunction. It is likely that furosemide will need to be discontinued as H.B.'s residual kidney function declines.

Given the role of the renin-angiotensin system in the development of hypertension in patients with CKD, ACE inhibitors are a logical choice for antihypertensive therapy. ACE inhibitors are effective antihypertensive agents in patients with CKD and have been shown to reverse LVH.[140] ACE inhibitors are underused in this population. Response must be assessed individually to determine whether renin-angiotensin-aldosterone activity is a predominant etiology of hypertension. Initiating therapy with low doses is prudent to evaluate patient response and tolerance. Use of these agents in combination with other antihypertensives is often required for adequate BP control. Most of these agents can be administered once daily; however, because of the kidney elimination of the parent drug or active metabolite, dosage adjustments are necessary in patients with CKD. Fosinopril is the exception because it undergoes substantial hepatic elimination. ACE inhibitors use should be avoided in patients undergoing dialysis with the polyacrylonitrile (AN69) membranes. The AN69 dialyzer increases bradykinin production, whereas ACE inhibitors decrease the breakdown of bradykinin, predisposing patients to systemic or immune-mediated reactions that can lead to anaphylactic reactions.

Although ARBs effectively lower BP and reverse LVH in patients without kidney disease,[141] less is known about their effectiveness in patients with kidney failure. These agents may offer an alternative to ACE inhibitors in patients experiencing kinin-mediated adverse effects; however, similar side effects have been reported with ARBs. The combined use of an ARB with other antihypertensive agents may be rational when patients are unresponsive to other regimens.

Beta-adrenergic blockers (β-blockers) inhibit release of renin and may be useful in hypertension associated with CKD. β-Blockers can counteract the elevated sympathetic activity observed in dialysis patients, lower the risk of sudden cardiac death, and improve survival in heart failure.[142] Unfortunately, they are underutilized, and the mentioned benefits are understudied in the dialysis population.[143] Risk versus benefit should be evaluated when β-blockade is considered in conjunction with other comorbid conditions such as asthma, heart failure, and lipid abnormalities. Dosage adjustment is required for the less lipophilic agents (i.e., atenolol, nadolol).

Calcium-channel blockers are effective antihypertensive agents in patients with CKD. Because the nondihydropyridine agents (i.e., diltiazem, verapamil) have negative chronotropic and inotropic effects, they should be used with care in patients with heart disease. Generally, dosage adjustment is not required in patients with kidney disease.

Other agents used to treat hypertension in the CKD population include centrally acting agents (e.g., clonidine, methyldopa), vasodilators (e.g., minoxidil, hydralazine), and α_1-adrenergic blockers (prazosin, terazosin, doxazosin).

H.B. is currently taking the β-blocker metoprolol and the loop diuretic furosemide. It is likely that his diuretic will need to be discontinued as his residual kidney function decreases and response to therapy is inadequate. If changes imposed in H.B.'s HD prescription are able to improve volume control and achieve his dry weight but do not reduce his BP, another antihypertensive regimen should be selected. A reasonable antihypertensive regimen would include an ACE inhibitor (e.g., ramipril). The selection will depend substantially on follow-up results of his cardiac disease, BP control with HD, and the development of adverse effects (see Chapter 14, Essential Hypertension, and Chapter 19, Heart Failure).

Dyslipidemia

CASE 31-2, QUESTION 3: How should H.B.'s lipid abnormalities be treated?

H.B. has elevated serum cholesterol and triglyceride concentrations, a common finding in patients with CKD. Dyslipidemia and increased oxidative stress contribute to premature atherogenesis in these patients. Several atherogenic factors in patients with CKD have been postulated, including arterial wall injury, platelet activation and adherence, smooth muscle cell proliferation, and intra-arterial accumulation of cholesterol. Whether lowering of serum lipids will improve long-term morbidity and mortality remains to be determined, but treatment should be consistent with NCEP ATP III guidelines and the NKF K/DOQI guidelines for treatment of dyslipidemias (see Chapter 13, Dyslipidemias, Atherosclerosis, and Coronary Heart Disease).[71,72] Dietary intervention successfully reduces triglyceride and cholesterol concentrations, and many drugs are available to treat lipid abnormalities in patients with stage 5 CKD.

MINERAL AND BONE DISORDERS

CASE 31-3

QUESTION 1: W.K. is a 24-year-old Hispanic woman who has an 18-year history of type 1 diabetes mellitus with complications of diabetic nephropathy, retinopathy, and neuropathy. She was diagnosed with stage 5 CKD 2 years ago. She started PD at that time. Her current medications include metoclopramide (Reglan) 10 mg TID before meals, insulin aspart 10 units with meals, insulin glargine 25 units

nightly, docusate 100 mg every day, Os-Cal 500 mg PO TID with meals, EPO 5,000 units IV twice weekly, iron sucrose 100 mg IV three times per week, paricalcitol 1 mcg IV three times weekly, and Nephrocaps 1 capsule every day. At a recent clinic visit, findings on physical examination included a BP of 128/84 mm Hg, abnormal bone biospy, diabetic retinopathic changes with laser scars bilaterally, and diminished sensation bilaterally below the knees. Her laboratory values were as follows:

Normal serum electrolytes
Random blood glucose, 250 mg/dL
BUN, 45 mg/dL
SCr, 8.9 mg/dL
Hgb, 10 g/dL
WBC count, 6,200/μL
Calcium, 8.5 mg/dL
Phosphate, 6.8 mg/dL
Intact parathyroid hormone (iPTH), 750 pg/mL
Total serum protein, 5.0 g/dL
Serum albumin, 3.1 g/dL
Uric acid, 8.9 mg/dL

Describe the etiology of W.K.'s abnormal bone, calcium, phosphorus, and parathyroid hormone (PTH) findings.

Etiology

Mineral and bone disorder of CKD (CKD-MBD) is the term used to collectively describe the mineral (e.g., phosphorus, calcium, parathyroid hormone), bone (osteodystrophy), and soft-tissue calcification abnormalities that develop as a complication of CKD. The older collective term of kidney osteodystrophy failed to adequately illustrate the broader clinical complications associated with the biomarker abnormalities and calcification, and is now only used to describe, specifically, the bone pathology.[98] The 2003 K/DOQI mineral and bone disease guidelines have traditionally set the target goals for management of mineral and bone disease (i.e., phosphorous, calcium, and parathyroid hormone).[144] In 2009, KDIGO published guidelines for the management of CKD-MBD. Although KDIGO are the new guidelines, many clinicians have not totally adopted them into practice, and current clinical performance measurements that dictate reimbursement schemes are still determined by the K/DOQI CKD-MBD guidelines.[145] Until reimbursement schemes are consistent with the KDIGO guidelines, most clinicians will continue to manage patients according to the K/DOQI guidelines.

Hyperphosphatemia, hypocalcemia, hyperparathyroidism, decreased production of active vitamin D, and resistance to vitamin D therapy are all frequent problems in CKD that can lead to the secondary complications of CKD-MBD. Although the interrelationships among phosphorus, calcium, vitamin D, and PTH have been reviewed extensively, fibroblast growth factor 23 (FGF23), a phosphaturic hormone discovered within the last decade, has added some new insight.[146] Increased dietary phosphorus intake stimulates FGF23 secretion. FGF23 increases phosphorus excretion via the proximal tubules, inhibits vitamin D activation, increases activated vitamin D catabolism, and is associated with kidney disease progression.[147]

The "trade-off" hypothesis best describes the events leading to changes in bone metabolism. As eGFR decreases, phosphorus excretion by the kidney decreases, resulting in hyperphosphatemia. Hyperphosphatemic conditions lead to a corresponding decrease in ionized calcium concentration, a primary stimulus for release of PTH from the parathyroid gland. Higher concentrations of PTH decrease kidney tubular reabsorption of phosphorus and promote its excretion. Both serum phosphorus and calcium concentrations are corrected depending on the degree of remaining kidney function, but this occurs at the expense of an elevated PTH concentration (the trade-off). As kidney disease becomes more severe (eGFR <30 mL/minute/1.73 m^2), the phosphaturic response to PTH diminishes, and sustained hyperphosphatemia, elevated FGF23, and hypocalcemia develop. In response to hypocalcemia, calcium is mobilized from the bone, a mechanism largely controlled by PTH. Retention of phosphorus and secondary hyperparathyroidism (sHPT) play a major role in the development of osteitis fibrosa or high-turnover bone disease. Virtually all patients with kidney failure develop sHPT. Decreased PTH degradation by the kidney may also contribute to the hyperparathyroid state in patients with kidney disease.

The kidney is the principal organ responsible for vitamin D production, and, as such, vitamin D metabolism is altered in the presence of uremia. The discovery of FGF23 has required an update in this trade-off hypothesis, providing a mechanism for the declining vitamin D level that develops as CKD progresses. Persistent hyperphosphatemia stimulates the release of excessive FGF23, which inhibits the normal conversion of 25-hydroxyvitamin D_3 to its biologically active metabolite, 1,25-dihydroxyvitamin D_3, by the enzyme 1-α-hydroxylase (Fig. 31-2). This enzyme is present in proximal tubular cells of the kidney and is necessary for conversion of vitamin D to the active form. This active form of vitamin D, also known as *calcitriol,* increases gut absorption of calcium and interacts with vitamin D receptors on the parathyroid gland to suppress PTH release. As a result of decreased calcitriol production, the absorption of dietary calcium in the gut is diminished. Decreased suppression of PTH release by vitamin D in conjunction with hypocalcemia promotes continued stimulus for mobilization of calcium from bone. Furthermore, uremic patients require a higher extracellular calcium concentration to suppress secretion of PTH. This is also described as an increase in the calcium "set point" or the concentration of calcium required to inhibit 50% of maximal PTH secretion.[148]

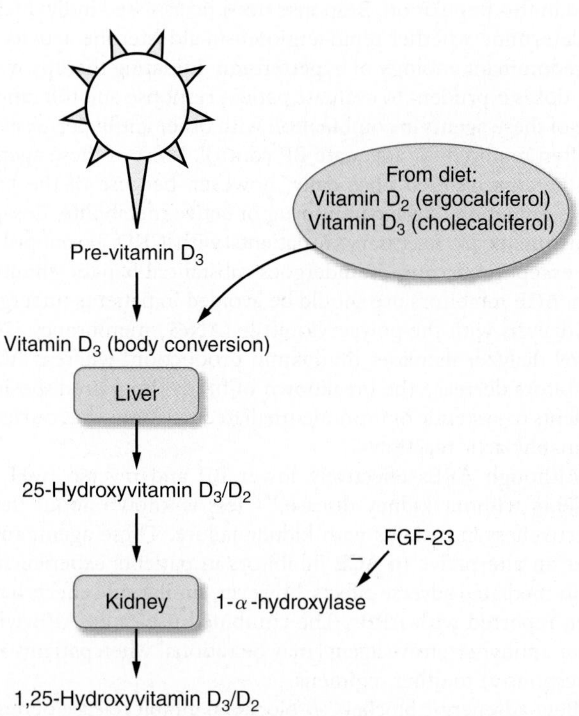

FIGURE 31-2 Vitamin D biotransformation.

The chronic effects of hyperparathyroidism on the skeleton lead to bone pain, fractures, and myopathy. In children, these effects may be particularly severe and usually retard growth. The metabolic acidosis of kidney disease also contributes to a negative calcium balance in the bone.

W.K.'s presentation is consistent with CKD-MBD based on the observed changes in bone architecture and abnormalities in serum phosphorus, calcium, and PTH; all can be attributed to her kidney disease.

Vitamin D levels (i.e., 25-hydroxyvitamin D) should be checked in stage 3 CKD. Insufficient (<30 ng/mL) and deficient (<15 ng/mL) vitamin D levels are prevalent in the majority of CKD and ESRD patients. Several studies have linked depressed vitamin D levels to increased vascular calcification, cardiovascular disease, and mortality.[149]

Treatment

CASE 31-3, QUESTION 2: What are the goals of therapy for W.K.'s calcium, phosphorus, and PTH abnormalities? What options are available to treat these disorders?

The management objectives for W.K. are to (a) manage serum calcium and phosphorus concentrations, (b) prevent or manage secondary hyperparathyroidism, and (c) restore normal skeletal development without inducing adynamic bone disease (or low bone turnover). These goals are best achieved with dietary phosphorus restriction, appropriate use of phosphate-binding agents, vitamin D therapy, calcimimetics, and dialysis.

DIETARY RESTRICTION OF PHOSPHORUS

In general, serum phosphorus should be lowered toward near normal levels. KDIGO recommends normal levels for all stages of CKD, whereas K/DOQI allows a more liberal phosphorus management in stage 5 of 3.5 to 5.5 mg/dL.[98,144] Dietary phosphorus restriction can prevent hyperphosphatemia and maintain target phosphorus concentrations. Dietary phosphorus should not exceed 800 to 1,000 mg/day.[98] Predominate sources of phosphorus are protein-rich foods, which presents a challenge in tailoring a diet that lowers dietary phosphorus intake while providing adequate nutrition. However, efforts should be made to distinguish between organic (e.g., plant seeds, nuts, legumes, and meats) and inorganic phosphorus (e.g., preservatives and additive salts found in processed foods) sources. Inorganic phosphorus sources are absorbed to a greater extent than organic phosphorus (90% vs. 50%, respectively) and should be minimized in the diet.[150] Dark carbonated beverages are a common culprit for elevated phosphorus levels; their consumption should be discouraged, and the beverages should be removed from vending machines in dialysis clinics. Although phosphorus is removed to some extent by dialysis, neither HD nor PD removes adequate amounts to warrant complete liberalization of phosphorus in the diet. Regular dietary counseling by a kidney specialist dietitian is necessary to reinforce the importance of phosphorus restriction and other dietary recommendations.

PHOSPHATE-BINDING AGENTS

A significant reduction of serum phosphorus is difficult to achieve with dietary intervention alone, particularly in patients with more advanced kidney disease (eGFR <30 mL/minute/1.73 m^2). For these patients, phosphate-binding agents used in conjunction with dietary restriction are necessary. Phosphate-binding agents limit phosphorus absorption from the GI tract by binding with the phosphorus present from dietary sources. Therefore, these agents must be administered with meals. Available binders include products that contain calcium, lanthanum, aluminum, or magnesium cations or the polymer-based agent, sevelamer.

CALCIUM-CONTAINING PREPARATIONS

Calcium-containing preparations, especially calcium carbonate and calcium acetate, are frequently used to prevent hyperphosphatemia in patients with kidney disease. The many preparations available vary in their calcium content (Table 31-8). Correction of hypocalcemia is an added beneficial effect of the calcium-containing preparations; however, a risk exists of hypercalcemia and cardiac calcification associated with the prolonged use of these agents.[151] Calcium citrate is a calcium salt with a phosphate-binding capacity similar to that of calcium carbonate; however, because it also increases aluminum absorption from the GI tract, its use is not recommended in patients with kidney disease.

Although calcium-containing binders have an added benefit of correcting hypocalcemia, the potential for hypercalcemia must be frequently evaluated in patients receiving these agents chronically. Simultaneous administration of vitamin D preparations and calcium also increases the risk of hypercalcemia. A corrected serum calcium should be determined before therapy is started and at regular intervals thereafter.

Calculating corrected calcium adjusts for the change in the ratio of free (unbound) versus protein-bound calcium owing to reduced serum albumin concentrations (Eq. 31-2). K/DOQI recommends a corrected total calcium toward normal levels for stage 3 and 4 CKD and a corrected total calcium range of 8.4 to 9.5 mg/dL for stage 5.[144]

$$\begin{aligned}&\text{Corrected calcium [mg/dL]}\\&\quad = \text{measured Ca [mg/dL]}\\&\qquad + 0.8 \times (4\ \text{g/dL} - \text{measured albumin [g/dL]}) \quad \textit{(Eq. 31-2)}\end{aligned}$$

Traditionally, the calculated calcium–phosphorus product (Ca × P) value is used as an indication as to when calcium and phosphate may precipitate and deposit into soft tissue, leading to calcific uremic arteriolopathy (CUA). CUA, or calciphylaxis, is characterized by calcification of the arterioles and small arteries with intimal proliferation and endovascular fibrosis and manifests visually as necrosis of the skin. K/DOQI guidelines set a target goal of the Ca × P to be less than 55 mg^2/dL^2, whereas a Ca × P greater than 60 to 70 mg^2/dL^2 suggests an increased risk of CUA.[152] However, KDIGO suggests the Ca × P provides no additional clinical information than the individual values of calcium and phosphorus and is not recommended for guiding therapy.[98]

If the patient experiences hypercalcemia or evidence of advance calcification, the patient should be switched to a non–calcium-based phosphate binder. Alternatives include sevelamer and cations, such as lanthanum carbonate or magnesium preparations. For patients requiring dialysis, reducing the calcium concentration of the dialysate bath may decrease the risk of hypercalcemia. Although avoiding hypercalcemia should reduce the risk of cardiac calcification, calcifications still can occur because of other contributing factors in the CKD population (e.g., hyperphosphatemia).

Nausea, diarrhea, and constipation are other side effects of calcium-containing products. Because calcium-containing phosphate binders may interact with other drugs, timing of their administration relative to other agents must be considered. Fluoroquinolones and oral iron, for example, should be taken at least 1 or 2 hours before calcium-containing phosphate binders. Importantly, if the calcium products are being used as supplementation to treat hypocalcemia or osteoporosis, they should be taken between meals to enhance intestinal absorption. This is

TABLE 31-8
Phosphate-Binding Agents

Product	Select Available Agents[a]	Content of Compound	Starting Dose
Calcium carbonate (40% calcium)	Tums	200, 300, 400 mg	0.8–2 g elemental Ca with meals
	Os-Cal-500	500 mg	
	Nephro-Calci	600 mg	
	Caltrate 600	600 mg	
	Calcarb HD (powder)	2,400 mg/packet	
	$CaCO_3$ (multiple preparations)	200–600 mg	
Calcium acetate (25% calcium)	Phos-Lo 667 mg	169 mg	2–3 tablets with meals
Sevelamer hydrochloride	Renagel (tablet, capsule)	400, 800 mg (tablet)	800–1,600 mg with meals
Sevelamer carbonate (polymer-based)	Renvela (tablet, powder)	800 mg (tablet), 0.8 g (powder)	
Lanthanum carbonate aluminum	Fosrenol	250, 500, 750, 1,000 mg	250–500 mg with meals
hydroxide[b]	AlternaGel (suspension)	600 mg/5 mL	300–600 mg with meals
	Amphojel (tablet and suspension)	300, 600 mg (tablet) 320 mg/5 mL (suspension)	
	Alu-Cap (capsule)	400 mg	
	Alu-Tab	500 mg	
	Basaljel (tablet, capsule, and suspension)	500 mg (tablet, capsule) 400 mg/mL (suspension)	
Magnesium carbonate[b]	Mag-Carb (capsule)	70 mg	70 mg with meals
Magnesium hydroxide[b]	Milk of Magnesia (tablet and suspension)	300, 600 mg (tablet) 400, 800 mg/5 mL (suspension)	300–400 mg with meals

[a] Tablet unless noted otherwise.
[b] Not first-line choice as a phosphate binder for chronic use.

in contrast to their administration with meals if they are being used as phosphate binders. Starting doses of common calcium-containing phosphate binders are listed in Table 31-8.

SEVELAMER

Sevelamer hydrochloride (Renagel) or carbonate (Renvela) is a nonabsorbed, polymer-based product that binds phosphorus in the GI tract.[153,154] The benefit of lowering phosphorus without significantly affecting serum calcium has led to the increased use of sevelamer in patients with CKD. Sevelamer also lowers LDL and total serum cholesterol, a benefit considering the increased risk of cardiovascular events in this population.[98]

Sevelamer has a potential benefit of attenuating the progression of coronary calcification, which may be related to its LDL and total serum cholesterol-lowering effects and a benefit from reduced calcium loading. The actual benefit of sevelamer on mortality is controversial. The post hoc analysis of the Renagel in New Dialysis (RIND) trial showed a survival advantage with sevelamer compared with calcium acetate; however, the Dialysis Clinical Outcomes Revisited (DCOR) trial failed to show a difference in mortality between the two agents.[155] One explanation for the disparity in these results may be the difference in the population of patients on HD between the two trials. The RIND trial included incident patients on HD, whereas the DCOR trial included prevalent HD patients who likely would have advanced cardiovascular disease.

Sevelamer hydrochloride is available as 400-mg and 800-mg tablets. Sevelamer carbonate is available as 800-mg tablets and 0.8-g powder packets. The phosphorus-binding capacity remains equipotent between the two formulations. The starting dose is variable and depends on the baseline serum phosphorus concentration (800 mg TID with meals if serum phosphorus is <7.5 mg/dL; 1,600 mg TID with meals if serum phosphorus is >7.5 mg/dL).[153,154] Gradual adjustments can be made at 2-week intervals, based on serum phosphorus levels. Dosing guidelines for sevelamer are also available for patients being converted from calcium acetate. On the basis of studies showing similar reductions in serum phosphorus, 800 mg of sevelamer is considered equivalent to 667 mg of calcium acetate (169 mg of elemental calcium).[154]

The administration of sevelamer hydrochloride to patients on HD is associated with a lowering of serum bicarbonate; this effect should be taken into account when using this agent. Sevelamer carbonate avoids the metabolic acidosis seen with the hydrochloride formulation and raises the serum bicarbonate level.[156] Adverse reports of fecal impaction, ileus, intestinal obstruction, and perforation should caution the use in patients with gastrointestinal disease.[154]

Data regarding drug interactions with sevelamer are limited; however, in recent evaluations, no drug interactions with digoxin, warfarin, metoprolol, and enalapril were observed. The current prescribing information recommends administering sevelamer 1 hour before or 3 hours after administration of other agents with narrow therapeutic indices.[154]

LANTHANUM CARBONATE

Lanthanum carbonate (Fosrenol) is a newly approved phosphate binder that offers another option for a noncalcium, nonaluminum preparation. When ingested, it dissociates into a trivalent cation with similar binding capacity as aluminum salts, and lanthanum also has been found to be as effective and tolerable as standard treatment. Both calcium and iPTH were lower in the lanthanum group.[157] Lanthanum is mainly excreted via the biliary route, with minimal kidney elimination.

Studies have evaluated the deposition and toxicity of lanthanum in the bone, liver, and brain because of concerns of lanthanum accumulation. Although lanthanum accumulates in lysosomes in the liver, this has not been correlated with increased liver enzymes or hepatobiliary adverse events in patients receiving lanthanum for up to 6 years.[158] This is likely an excretory process through the biliary tract similar to that for iron and copper. A prospective trial of patients on HD receiving lanthanum for 1 year found minimal deposition of lanthanum within the bone and less likelihood of adynamic bone histology compared with patients receiving calcium carbonate.[159] During a 2-year period, patients receiving lanthanum were not found to accelerate the natural deterioration in cognitive function seen in patients on HD.[160]

Lanthanum is supplied as chewable tablets for oral administration in four strengths: 250, 500, 750, and 1,000 mg. The recommended initial total daily dose is 750 to 1,500 mg given with meals, and dosage titration up to a maximal dosage of 3,000 mg daily should be based on serum phosphate levels. Lanthanum retains the same phosphorus-binding capabilities whether it is chewed or crushed into a powder.[161] Drug interactions with lanthanum include a reduction in the bioavailability of ciprofloxacin (~50% reduction) and levothyroxine. The most frequent adverse events reported in clinical trials are nausea and vomiting.[162]

OTHER PHOSPHATE BINDERS

Aluminum preparations are very potent dietary phosphorus binders. Although these products were once used as first-line agents to decrease phosphorus, aluminum accumulation and toxicities in patients with CKD have restricted their use. Aluminum toxicity occurs in dialysis patients because absorbed aluminum is not removed by the diseased kidney and enters various tissues where it binds to tissue and plasma proteins. Aluminum accumulation in the bone, brain, and other organs leads to toxicities such as osteomalacia (aluminum-related bone disease), microcytic anemia, and a fatal neurologic syndrome referred to as *dialysis encephalopathy*.[98] Treatment of aluminum toxicity requires chelation with deferoxamine. Aluminum-containing agents should only be considered on a short-term basis (up to 4 weeks) for patients with a severely elevated phosphorus[98]; however, high-dose lanthanum may generally be preferred in these situations. Sucralfate, used primarily for the treatment of ulcers, also contains aluminum and should be used cautiously in patients with kidney disease.

Magnesium agents (magnesium hydroxide, magnesium carbonate) may be beneficial, but as with aluminum, their use should be limited because at the high doses required to control serum phosphorus concentrations, severe diarrhea and hypermagnesemia invariably result. Magnesium might, however, be considered in patients whose serum phosphorus concentrations cannot be controlled adequately by other phosphate-binding agents. In this instance, a magnesium-containing phosphate binder may be added in conjunction with a reduction in the dialysate magnesium concentration (in the dialysis population). These agents should not be considered first-line therapy for control of phosphorus, and careful monitoring of magnesium is warranted if therapy is started.

W.K.'s corrected calcium is approximately 9.2 mg/dL. More aggressive control of serum phosphorus is needed to lower serum phosphorus toward normal levels. Currently she is receiving 1,500 mg of elemental calcium. Although presumably much of this calcium will be bound to phosphorus in the GI tract, a potential exists for calcium absorption. The total dose of elemental calcium provided by binders should not exceed 1,500 mg/day (or 2,000 mg/day from binders and diet). Sevelamer should be started to limit her calcium exposure and decrease her phosphorus levels. The recommended starting dose is 800 mg TID with meals, titrated based on follow-up phosphorus values. Adjustments should also be considered in conjunction with vitamin D therapy (see Vitamin D section). W.K. should be instructed to take her phosphate binder with meals. This regimen should be implemented in conjunction with a restricted-phosphorus diet. Regular reinforcement of the importance of compliance is necessary because nonadherence with prescribed dietary phosphorus restriction and drug therapy is one of the most significant factors associated with treatment failure. Use of a low-calcium dialysate may also help decrease her risk of hypercalcemia.

VITAMIN D

NATIVE VITAMIN D

Vitamin D occurs naturally as ergocalciferol (vitamin D_2) obtained from dietary sources and as cholecalciferol (vitamin D_3) obtained from dietary sources and activated in the skin by sunlight in mammals, both of which are inactive precursors of active forms of vitamin D. An intermediate activation step (25-hydroxylation) occurs in the liver to produce 25-hydroxy vitamin D (25-hydroxycalciferol), which is also relatively inactive (Fig. 31-2). Final activation (1-hydroxylation) occurs in the kidney, yielding calcitriol (1,25-dihydroxycholecalciferol), the active form of vitamin D. Thus, the response to vitamins D_2 and D_3 in patients with compromised kidney function can vary, depending on the degree of kidney dysfunction and the ability of the kidney to metabolize 25-hydroxyvitamin D to calcitriol. Decreased levels of 25-hydroxyvitamin D occur in the early stages of CKD, reducing substrate for producing calcitriol.[163] Altered vitamin D metabolism that occurs in this population warrants measurement of 25-hydroxyvitamin D and supplementation with vitamin D precursors, such as ergocalciferol or cholecalciferol.[98] Oral therapy with active vitamin D (oral calcitriol) or an analog (oral doxercalciferol) is likely warranted only when PTH remains elevated despite normal 25-hydroxyvitamin D levels.[98,163] As the final, active metabolite of vitamin D, calcitriol (or another activated form of vitamin D) is usually required in patients with more severe kidney disease (stage 5 CKD).

Several studies have shown that native vitamin D (i.e., ergocalciferol or cholecalciferol) administration benefits extend beyond bone and mineral metabolism. Reduction in ESA doses, improved glycemic control, reduced activated vitamin D administration, and inflammation modulation are benefits observed from native vitamin D supplementation in dialysis patients.[164,165] Although some effects have been repeated in different studies, randomized control trials are needed to confirm these benefits.

ACTIVATED VITAMIN D

Calcitriol

Administration of active vitamin D, in conjunction with control of serum phosphorus and calcium, is necessary in many patients with CKD to manage CKD-MBD. Calcitriol interacts with the vitamin D receptor (VDR) located in the parathyroid gland, intestines, bone, and kidney. It is thought to decrease PTH messenger RNA (mRNA), resulting in decreased PTH secretion. It also lowers the calcium set point for PTH release in patients with CKD with sHPT, most likely through a direct effect on calcium receptors within the parathyroid gland.[148] In addition, calcitriol stimulates calcium absorption from the GI tract to correct hypocalcemia and prevent sHPT. To avoid hypercalcemia, the lowest effective dose should be used, and the patient's serum calcium should be monitored at least every 2 weeks for 1 month and then monthly thereafter. Furthermore, control of serum phosphorus is critical before calcitriol is initiated, as vitamin D increases GI phosphorus absorption.

Calcitriol is available as an oral formulation (Rocaltrol) or IV formulation (Calcijex). Administration of calcitriol by either the oral or IV route may be based on conventional dosing (usually 0.25 to 0.5 mcg/day) or pulse dosing (intermittent dosing of 0.5 to 2.0 mcg two to three times per week). Higher doses (e.g., 4 mcg three times per week) are generally required to reduce PTH secretion in more severe sHPT (PTH >1,000 pg/mL). Daily dosing of 0.25 to 0.5 mcg may be preferred in patients with hypocalcemia because this regimen primarily works to stimulate calcium absorption from the GI tract. Intermittent dosing of IV calcitriol is routine in the HD population because administration is coordinated with dialysis. In contrast, oral dosing is more convenient in patients with CKD who are not having dialysis and the PD population. Intact PTH and serum calcium concentrations are used to determine starting doses and dosing adjustments for calcitriol.

Intact PTH (1–84 PTH) is the 84–amino acid biologically active form of this hormone. It is metabolized into smaller, less-active fragments (e.g., 7–84 PTH) with activity that is not well characterized. These fragments are cleared from the circulation by the kidney and may accumulate in patients with CKD. Assays used for iPTH measure the intact structure as well as the biologically active and inactive PTH fragments. Thus, proposed ranges for iPTH in current guidelines are based on these assays. Recently, assays that measure only the biologically active form (1–84 biPTH) have become available. When iPTH is measured using both methods, there is roughly a 2:1 ratio between the nonspecific and specific assay results. An iPTH of 150 pg/mL would correspond to a biPTH 75 pg/mL. These newer assays have not yet been adopted for most of the CKD population; however, they are being used in some clinical settings.[143] Clearly, the clinician must know which assay has been used to appropriately interpret the results, establish the desired PTH range, and correctly adjust therapy.

K/DOQI guidelines recommend maintaining the iPTH level to within 35 to 70 pg/mL in stage 3; 70 to 110 pg/mL in stage 4; and 150 to 300 pg/mL in stage 5.[144] After reviewing the current literature, the KDIGO workgroup thought that the data surrounding the current K/DOQI iPTH ranges were inadequate for extrapolating to all CKD patients. Thus, the KDIGO guidelines vary as they recommend iPTH levels to be maintained within the normal limits in stages 3 and 4 CKD. However, the stage 5 CKD iPTH target range is two to nine times the upper normal limits.[98]

Dose adjustments of calcitriol are generally made in 0.5- to 1.0-mcg increments every 2 to 4 weeks in the early stages of therapy until iPTH and serum calcium are maintained at target levels. If hypercalcemia develops, the decision to withhold therapy or to switch to a vitamin D analog (see Vitamin D Analogs section) must be made. Serum iPTH should be monitored every 3 to 6 months, and adjustments of calcitriol doses made to maintain the goal iPTH and to prevent hypercalcemia and hyperphosphatemia.

Paricalcitol

The unique interactions of vitamin D with the VDR have led to the development of newer vitamin D analogs, which vary in their affinity for the VDR. In the case of treatment for sHPT, some were developed to retain the suppressive effect on PTH release while decreasing the potential for hypercalcemia relative to calcitriol. Currently approved agents for managing sHPT in the United States are paricalcitol (Zemplar), also referred to as 19-nor-1,25-dihydroxyvitamin D_2, and doxercalciferol (Hectorol), or 1-α-hydroxyvitamin D_2. Doxercalciferol requires conversion to the active form (1-α-,25-dihydroxyvitamin D_2) by the liver.

In patients with sHPT, paricalcitol significantly decreases iPTH without significantly increasing calcium or phosphorus. Paricalcitol is approximately 10-fold less hypercalcemic and hyperphosphatemic than calcitriol.[166,167] The initial dose of IV paricalcitol is 0.04 mcg/kg to 0.1 mcg/kg (2.8–7 mcg) administered with each dialysis session or every other day.[168] Oral paricalcitol capsules are available in three strengths (1, 2, and 4 mcg) administered daily or three times weekly. The starting dose should be 1 mcg daily or 2 mcg three times weekly if the baseline iPTH level is 500 pg/mL or less, and 2 mcg daily or 4 mcg three times weekly if the iPTH is greater than 500 pg/mL. Some data have also suggested paricalcitol dosing based on initial PTH levels (paricalcitol dose = PTH/80) rather than weight as a reasonable dosing strategy.[168] Doses can be titrated every 2 to 4 weeks based on iPTH values.

The recommended conversion ratio for calcitriol to paricalcitol is 1:4 (i.e., for every 1 mcg of calcitriol, 4 mcg of paricalcitol should be administered). This information is based on similar efficacy observed when patients treated for secondary hyperparathyroidism with calcitriol were switched to paricalcitol using this dosing strategy.[166,167] A lower ratio of 1:3 also has been proposed in patients resistant to therapy with calcitriol.[169]

Doxercalciferol

Doxercalciferol, another vitamin D analog, is an alternative to calcitriol and has been studied in patients with stage 5 CKD on dialysis.[149,170] Doxercalciferol has similar effects on PTH as the other vitamin D analogs; however, it increases phosphorus and calcium to a greater degree than paricalcitol.[171] Doxercalciferol is available as a capsule and IV injection. The doses were 4 mcg IV or 10 mcg orally three times per week with HD. Oral and IV therapy are both effective in reducing iPTH levels in patients with sHPT; however, some evidence indicated that intermittent IV therapy may result in less hypercalcemia and hyperphosphatemia than oral intermittent therapy.[170] The recommended starting dose of doxercalciferol for patients on dialysis is 4 mcg IV or 10 mcg orally administered three times per week with dosing titration based on changes in iPTH.[172,173]

Vitamin D analogs offer an alternative for patients in whom persistent hypercalcemia develops with calcitriol therapy. Use of these agents is increasing in clinical practice because of the concerns of hypercalcemia and its adverse consequences. Repeated observational reports indicate lower overall and cardiovascular-related mortality rates with activated vitamin D therapy, regardless of the agent received, than in those not receiving vitamin D therapy.[149] Two trials also examined the survival advantages among the different forms of vitamin D in patients on HD. One report indicated that receiving paricalcitol for 36 months conferred a survival advantage starting at 12 months from initiation of therapy and increased with time compared with those receiving calcitriol. Another study reported that patients taking either paricalcitol or doxercalciferol had a significantly lower mortality rate than patients receiving calcitriol, although when adjusted for laboratory values and clinic standardized mortality, no difference was found between the products.[149]

Possible biologic reasons for vitamin D improving outcomes include its role in downregulating the RAAS and immunomodulatory properties. A prospective trial would be required to confirm a survival advantage associated with vitamin D therapy.

CALCIMIMETICS

Calcimimetic agents increase the sensitivity of the calcium-sensing receptors (CaSR) to extracellular calcium ions and inhibit the release of PTH, lowering PTH levels within hours after administration. The discovery of extracellular CaSR prompted research with calcimimetic agents that allosterically modulate CaSR. CaSR have been identified in the parathyroid gland, thyroid, nephron, brain, intestine, bone, lung, and other tissues. The calcimimetic cinacalcet is the first agent in this class to be approved by the FDA to treat secondary hyperparathyroidism in end-stage kidney disease. Cinacalcet has been demonstrated to be an effective agent at reducing and sustaining iPTH within target concentrations in HD patients.[174] No data are found on survival rates for patients receiving cinacalcet versus those treated with vitamin D. However, cinacalcet offers an additional choice of agent to lower PTH when vitamin D cannot be increased because of elevated calcium or phosphorus. Current studies are also examining the role of combined therapy with cinacalcet and vitamin D therapy to improve bone metabolism and achievement of disease targets.[175] Cinacalcet is not FDA approved for use in CKD patients not receiving dialysis because it is associated with frequent hypocalcemic episodes.[176]

Appropriate treatment for W.K. should be based on assessment of her serum calcium, phosphorus, and PTH values. She currently has an elevated PTH, phosphorus, and calcium–phosphorus product; therefore, cinacalcet should be started in conjunction with her dietary phosphorus restriction, phosphate-binder regimen, and vitamin D therapy. Cinacalcet should be initiated at a dose of 30 mg daily, with dosage titrations occurring every 2 to 4 weeks to 60, 90, 120, or a maximum of 180 mg daily to achieve target iPTH levels. Serum calcium and phosphorous levels should be drawn within 1 week after initiation or dosage increase, and plasma PTH levels drawn within 4 weeks after initiation of therapy or dosage adjustment. Nausea and vomiting are the most common adverse events associated with cinacalcet. In phase III trials, 66% of patients receiving cinacalcet experienced at least one episode of hypocalcemia (serum calcium <8.4 mg/dL), although less than 1% of patients discontinued treatment.[177] The high incidence of hypocalcemia is not solely caused by lowered PTH activity but is also attributed to the mechanism of action of cinacalcet. It is thought that activation of CaSR in bone, intestine, and other tissues may contribute to hypocalcemia.[178] Most episodes of hypocalcemia occur during the initiation of cinacalcet therapy, and slowly titrating the dose reduces the risk. However, seizures caused by hypocalcemia have been reported. Vitamin D or calcium-based phosphate binders can be used to increase serum calcium levels between 7.5 and 8.4 mg/dL. If serum calcium falls below 7.5 mg/dL and is associated with symptoms of hypocalcemia and vitamin D cannot be increased further, cinacalcet should be withheld until serum calcium is 8.0 mg/dL or the patient is asymptomatic.[177] Cinacalcet is a strong in vitro inhibitor of cytochrome P-450 isoenzyme CYP2D6; therefore, dose adjustments of concomitant medications that are predominantly metabolized by CYP2D6 may be required. Cinacalcet is also a substrate of CYP3A4, and ketoconazole, a potent inhibitor of CYP3A4, has been shown to increase the area under the curve of cinacalcet 2.3 times. Thus, other inhibitors of the CYP3A4 isoenzyme should be used in caution in patients receiving cinacalcet.[177]

PARATHYROIDECTOMY

The parathyroid glands enlarge as a compensatory response to disturbances of phosphorus, calcium, and calcitriol metabolism in patients with CKD. Timely administration of vitamin D therapy to prevent parathyroid hyperplasia is crucial because treatment with vitamin D cannot adequately reverse established hyperplasia.[179] Under circumstances in which severe sHPT cannot be controlled by dietary phosphorus restriction and drug therapy, parathyroidectomy is considered. Parathyroidectomy can be subtotal, total, or total with autotransplantation. One of the major complications of parathyroidectomy is the early development of postsurgical hypocalcemia. Clinical symptoms of hypocalcemia include muscle irritability, fatigue, depression, and memory loss. Patients should be monitored closely after parathyroidectomy, and all patients with signs or symptoms of hypocalcemia should be treated with calcium supplementation (see Chapter 10, Fluid and Electrolyte Disorders). In patients who have had subtotal parathyroidectomy, the remaining parathyroid tissues will start functioning adequately, so the acute hypocalcemia is transient, lasting only a few days. With total parathyroidectomy, however, hypocalcemia is permanent, necessitating long-term treatment with calcitriol and oral calcium supplements (1 to 1.5 g/day of elemental calcium).

OTHER COMPLICATIONS OF CKD

Endocrine Abnormalities Caused by Uremia

CASE 31-3, QUESTION 3: Does W.K.'s hypothyroidism have any relationship to her CKD? What other endocrine abnormalities are associated with uremia?

Disturbances in thyroid function are frequently encountered in patients with CKD because the kidney is involved in all aspects of peripheral thyroid hormone metabolism. Common laboratory abnormalities include reduced serum concentrations of total thyroxine (T_4) and 3,5,3′-triiodothyronine (T_3) and a low free thyroxine index (FTI). The thyroid-stimulating hormone (TSH) concentration is usually normal, but peripheral conversion of T_4 to T_3 is reduced in uremic patients.[180] Despite these abnormalities, clinical hypothyroidism does not occur solely as a result of kidney disease, probably because the amount of free (unbound to protein) thyroid hormone in serum remains normal. Hypothyroidism in patients with kidney failure should be confirmed by the presence of an elevated serum TSH concentration and a low serum concentration of free T_4.

Other endocrine abnormalities that have been observed in patients with CKD include gonadal dysfunction leading to impotence, diminished testicular size, menstrual abnormalities, and cessation of ovulation.[181] Decreased libido and infertility occur in both sexes. Uremic women of childbearing age should be counseled on the risk of becoming pregnant because of the multiple complications of pregnancy in ESRD, including high termination rates. In children with kidney disease, growth retardation occurs despite normal or elevated growth hormone. Hyperprolactinemia and altered vasoactive hormone activity are other endocrine disturbances that can occur in patients with CKD.[180]

Altered Glucose and Insulin Metabolism

CASE 31-3, QUESTION 4: Other than the obvious effect of W.K.'s diabetes mellitus on blood glucose, are there any effects of kidney disease itself on glucose metabolism?

Uremia often is associated with glucose intolerance early in the course of kidney disease in nondiabetic patients, and this may be referred to as *pseudodiabetes*. Specifically, patients with CKD often exhibit an abnormal response to an oral glucose challenge and have sustained hyperinsulinemia.[182] The fasting blood glucose is typically within normal limits. Diminished tissue sensitivity to the action of insulin is also observed. Although their exact role is unclear, several uremic toxins, including urea, creatinine, guanidinosuccinic acid, and methylguanidine, have been implicated as causes for insulin resistance. Elevated concentrations of growth hormone, PTH, and glucagon also may contribute to glucose intolerance. Most nondiabetic patients with kidney disease do not require therapy for hyperglycemia, and dialysis can correct these abnormalities in glucose metabolism.[180]

Patients with diabetes mellitus and advanced kidney disease may experience improved glucose control and decreased insulin requirements. This is because the kidney is responsible for a substantial amount of daily insulin degradation and, as the disease progresses, less insulin is cleared and its metabolic half-life is increased. A decreased clearance of insulin by muscle tissue also can occur in patients with uremia.[180] Thus, in diabetic patients with progressive kidney disease, blood glucose concentrations should be monitored and insulin doses adjusted to avoid hypoglycemia. W.K. has stage 5 CKD and is receiving her insulin in the peritoneal dialysate solution. Hyperglycemia is also a concern in W.K. because the glucose present in her continuous ambulatory peritoneal dialysis (CAPD) fluid to promote fluid removal will be absorbed systemically. Insulin dosage adjustments should be made on the basis of repeated home blood glucose measurements, changes in the CAPD prescription, and glycosylated hemoglobin determinations.

Gastrointestinal Complications

CASE 31-3, QUESTION 5: One month before her current clinic visit, W.K. complained of nausea and vomiting of partially digested food. Metoclopramide (Reglan) was begun at that time. Could W.K.'s nausea and vomiting have been caused by her kidney failure? Was the appropriate therapy selected?

Gastrointestinal abnormalities are extremely common in patients with CKD and include anorexia, nausea, vomiting, hiccups, abdominal pain, GI bleeding, diarrhea, and constipation. Diminished gastric motility can occur from uremia; however, this problem may improve with adequate HD. Dyspeptic complaints and gastroparesis may be more prevalent in the PD population than in the HD population and in the earlier stages of CKD.[183] W.K. has diabetes and diabetic neuropathy, which also contributes to the delayed gastric emptying (diabetic gastroparesis) and retention of food in the upper intestinal tract. This frequently causes distension, nausea, and vomiting. Metoclopramide is recommended to relieve these symptoms, although the risk for extrapyramidal side effects should be considered. A lower dose of 5 mg before meals may be warranted for W.K.

Severe uremia also causes nausea and vomiting, and these can be initial presenting symptoms of kidney failure. At this stage of clinical presentation, dialysis is the preferred therapy. Drug-induced nausea and vomiting always should be considered because patients with CKD often take multiple drugs and are at risk for drug toxicity because of diminished kidney function (e.g., digitalis intoxication).

BLEEDING

CASE 31-3, QUESTION 6: During her clinic visit, W.K. reports that her bowel movements have become black and tarry in appearance. A rectal examination reveals guaiac-positive stools. Is GI bleeding related to kidney failure?

W.K. should be evaluated for peptic ulcer disease and lower GI bleeding. Uremic patients are at risk for bleeding from mucosal surfaces such as the stomach. W.K.'s hemoglobin is below the target values (10 to 12 g/dL for hemoglobin), despite therapy with epoetin, and it is likely that bleeding is contributing to poor responsiveness to therapy. Angiodysplasia of the stomach and duodenum, as well as erosive esophagitis, are the most common causes of bleeding in patients with CKD.[184] Treatment of upper GI bleeding in uremic patients usually consists of cautious use of antacid therapy and H_2-receptor antagonists, which should be given in reduced doses according to the degree of kidney function. Proton-pump inhibitors are primarily eliminated by nonkidney routes and can be administered at standard doses (see Chapter 27, Upper Gastrointestinal Disorders). Use of H_2-receptor antagonists has generally replaced chronic antacid use for treatment of dyspepsia in patients with CKD.

Neurologic Complications

CASE 31-4

QUESTION 1: V.D. is a 69-year-old, 72-kg, black man, receiving HD for the past 15 years. His general complaints during the past few weeks include weakness, nausea, lethargy, decreased exercise tolerance, and general malaise. His medical history is unremarkable, except he recalls recent memory lapses. His medications include amlodipine 10 mg daily, clonidine 0.1 mg twice daily, and Nephrovite capsules once daily. An examination by his primary-care physician reveals a BP of 168/92 mm Hg, and funduscopic examination showed grade III hypertensive changes. On neurologic examination, V.D. is slightly confused, appears somnolent, and has diminished sensation to pinprick in both lower extremities; asterixis is present. Examination of the skin shows pallor and excoriations across the abdomen, legs, and arms. Pertinent laboratory values are as follows:

Hct, 20%
Hgb, 10.7 g/dL
WBC count, 9,100/μL
Serum Na, 135 mEq/L
K, 5.8 mEq/L
Cl, 109 mEq/L
CO_2 content, 16 mEq/L
Random blood glucose, 119 mg/dL
BUN, 76 mg/dL
SCr, 5.6 mg/dL
Ca, 8.5 mg/dL
Phosphate, 7.0 mg/dL
Intact PTH, 830 pg/mL
Uric acid, 11.9 mg/dL
Albumin, 3.0 g/dL

What is the likely explanation for V.D.'s altered mental status? What treatment, if any, is indicated for his neurologic findings?

Disorders of the central nervous system (CNS) that occur in patients receiving dialysis are referred to collectively as *uremic neuropathy*. Accumulation of uremic toxins, vascular dementia, cerebral hypoperfusion, and repeated silent strokes predispose dialysis patients to several neurologic complications. Symptoms are prevalent in 60% to 90% of the dialysis population. V.D.'s altered neurologic complications are likely a function of his extensive dialysis history, age, and uncontrolled hypertension; a careful drug history should exclude the possibility of drug effects. Symptoms of uremic neuropathy include alterations in cognitive dysfunction, restless legs syndrome, autonomic neuropathy, carpal tunnel syndrome, and uremic myopathy. Patients or their family members may note fatigue, daytime drowsiness, insomnia, diminished cognitive abilities, slurred speech, vomiting, and emotional volatility.[185,186]

Uremic toxins can play a role in this disorder, possibly having a neurotoxic effect. Elevated calcium and phosphorus enhance the entry of calcium into the brain and peripheral nerves, are directly neurotoxic, and increase the rate of cerebral calcification. The peripheral nervous system also shows abnormal function in many patients with advanced CKD, as illustrated by V.D., who has loss of sensation in his legs by pinprick examination. Typically, the peripheral neuropathy will be slowly progressive, distal, and symmetric, usually first involving sensory function. The abnormalities seen usually are indistinguishable from other types of neuropathy, especially diabetic neuropathy. Nerve conduction studies often reveal abnormalities preceding clinical symptoms. Treatment generally consists of measures to alleviate symptoms with agents, such as tricyclic antidepressants (e.g., amitriptyline) and anticonvulsants (e.g., phenytoin, gabapentin). Increasing the intensity of dialysis does not affect the neuropathy; however, successful kidney transplantation may ameliorate nerve dysfunction.

Abnormalities of the autonomic nervous system also have been observed in patients with kidney failure and present as postural hypotension, impotence, impaired sweating, and alterations in gastric motility. HD may be more likely to correct autonomic dysfunction in nondiabetic patients.

Dermatologic Complications

CASE 31-4, QUESTION 2: Why does V.D. have excoriations on his skin? What therapy would be useful?

Several dermal abnormalities have been observed in patients with CKD, including hyperpigmentation, abnormal perspiration, skin dryness, and persistent pruritus. Of these, *uremic pruritus* can be the most bothersome for the patient and may lead to repeated scratching and skin excoriation. Hyperparathyroidism, hypervitaminosis A, and dermal mast cell proliferation with subsequent histamine release have been suggested as causes of pruritus.[187]

Treatment of pruritus often is a frustrating experience for the patient and clinician. Although many therapies have been advocated, few have provided sustained benefit. A trial-and-error approach is recommended. Efficient dialysis therapy relieves pruritus in some patients and pharmacologic therapy may be avoided.[187] When necessary, initial pharmacologic treatment usually consists of oral antihistamines (e.g., hydroxyzine). Topical emollients or topical steroids may provide benefit if antihistamine therapy is not completely successful. If pruritus is still present, other treatment options can be tried. These include cholestyramine, ultraviolet B (UVB) phototherapy, and oral administration of activated charcoal. Control of calcium, phosphorus (V.D. is hyperphosphatemic), and PTH concentrations are also advocated to reduce pruritus in patients with CKD.

GLOMERULAR DISEASE

Glomerular diseases lead to many complications that result from disruption of normal glomerular structure and function. Several clinical syndromes of glomerular disease exist; however, glomerulonephritis, characterized as proliferation and inflammation of the glomerulus, is observed most frequently. According to the most recent USRDS report, glomerulonephritis as a broad category remains the third leading cause of ESRD in the United States.[4] In developing countries, ESRD caused by glomerulonephritis is more common as a result of various infectious processes causing kidney failure.

Nephrotic Syndrome

Nephrotic syndrome is characterized by proteinuria greater than 3.5 g/day, hypoalbuminemia, edema, and hyperlipidemia. In more severe conditions, hypercoagulable conditions are increased from a loss of hemostasis control proteins, including antithrombin III, protein S, and protein C. This syndrome can occur with or without a change in glomerular filtration rate. Nephrotic syndrome may be caused by a primary disease, such as membranous glomerulopathy, which is characterized by deposition of immune complexes, or other systemic diseases including diabetic glomerulosclerosis and amyloidosis. Elevated serum cholesterol and triglycerides are observed in patients with this degree of proteinuria (>3.5 g/day). This hyperlipidemic condition also predisposes patients with nephrotic syndrome to accelerated atherosclerosis. Hyperlipidemia itself can also contribute to progression of kidney disease. Because nephrotic syndrome is associated with numerous causes, further evaluation of the patient for systemic causes is required to then determine the course of therapy and prognosis.

Chronic Glomerulopathies

Glomerulonephritis can occur as a primary disease that is idiopathic in origin (e.g., focal segmental glomerulosclerosis [FSGS]) or as a secondary manifestation of other systemic disease (e.g., lupus nephritis [LN], Wegener's granulomatosis). Kidney biopsy is often required for definitive diagnosis. Glomerular lesions associated with glomerulopathies are characterized as diffuse, focal, or segmental, depending on the extent of involvement of individual glomeruli. Pathologic changes are characterized as proliferative, membranous, and sclerotic based on the pattern observed. Proliferative changes usually involve an overgrowth of the epithelium or mesangium, whereas membranous changes are typically described as a thickening of the glomerular basement membrane. Signs and symptoms of glomerulonephritis include hematuria, proteinuria, and decreased kidney function. An autoimmune reaction is the predominant pathogenic process leading to most forms of primary and secondary glomerulonephritis. Although a number of autoantibodies are associated with glomerulonephritis, their exact role in the pathogenesis of glomerulonephritis is still unclear. Nonetheless, analysis of autoantibodies in the clinical setting can aid in early diagnosis of glomerulonephritis.[188]

Glomerular damage generally occurs in two phases: acute and chronic. During the acute phase, immune reactions occur within glomeruli that stimulate the complement cascade, ultimately resulting in glomerular damage. Nonimmune mechanisms that occur in response to loss of nephron function and hyperfiltration of remaining nephrons are characteristic of the chronic phase.

Glomerulonephritis often causes acute kidney failure. Patients with damage to more than 50% of glomeruli in the presence of rapid loss in kidney function (over the course of days to weeks) are classified as having rapidly progressive glomerulonephritis (RPGN).[188] If kidney involvement is severe, signs and symptoms of uremia may develop. RPGN may be classified based on the immunopathogenic etiology of the glomerular damage: (a) immune complex deposition (e.g., LN), (b) nonimmune deposit-mediated mechanism (e.g., Wegener's granulomatosis), and (c) sclerotic lesions of the glomerulus (e.g., FSGS).[188] This chapter focuses on the treatment of the more common forms of chronic glomerulonephritis (i.e., LN, Wegener's granulomatosis, FSGS). (See also Chapter 30, Acute Kidney Injury.)

LUPUS NEPHRITIS

Systemic lupus erythematosus (SLE) is a multisystem autoimmune disease characterized by abnormalities in cell-mediated immunity, such as B-cell hyperresponsiveness and defective T-cell–mediated suppressor activity. In certain predisposed individuals, SLE can lead to the development of lupus nephritis, a secondary form of glomerulonephritis. LN is the prototypical immune complex–mediated kidney disease, characterized by deposition or in situ formation of autoantibody–antigen complexes along the glomerular capillary network. LN remains an important cause of mortality. Up to 60% of adults with SLE have some degree of kidney involvement later in the course of their disease, discernible from clinical evidence of kidney damage: heavy proteinuria, hematuria, decreased eGFR, and hypertension. Early in the disease, laboratory abnormalities indicative of kidney involvement are seen in approximately 25% to 50% of patients.

CASE 31-5

QUESTION 1: S.L., a 34-year-old black woman with a 7-year history of SLE, presents to the nephrology clinic for follow-up of LN. Pertinent laboratory values are as follows:

Serum Na, 146 mEq/L
K, 4.2 mEq/L
Cl, 100 mEq/L
CO_2 content, 25 mEq/L
SCr, 2.0 mg/dL
BUN, 20 mg/dL
WBC count, 9,600/μL

RBC indices are normal. Platelet count is 175,000/μL. Her 24-hour urine contains 2.3 g of albumin (normal, <30 mg/day), and her urine analysis shows 12 RBCs/high-power field (HPF) (normal, 0 to 3). Compared with her visit of a week ago, S.L.'s kidney function and urinary indices (proteinuria, hematuria) show substantial worsening of her nephritis. S.L. was hospitalized, and a kidney biopsy showed inflammation of 40% of the glomeruli. What subjective and objective data in S.L. are consistent with a diagnosis of LN, and what is the stage of her nephritis?

S.L. has clinical evidence of kidney damage as demonstrated by her proteinuria, hematuria, and a slightly increased SCr concentration. Glomerular damage is most evident by the presence of RBC or red cell casts in the urine, a finding observed in S.L.

CLASSIFICATIONS

The International Society of Nephrology and the Renal Pathology Society (ISN/RPS) classification system was developed in 2003 to replace the previous classification system published by the World Health Organization (Table 31-9).[189] This classification scheme provides a reasonable correlation among histopathology, outcome, and response to treatment. S.L. has proteinuria, hematuria, and inflammation of less than 50% of her glomeruli, and she is diagnosed as having class III/A (focal proliferative) glomerulonephritis.

TREATMENT

CASE 31-5, QUESTION 2: Should S.L.'s LN be treated?

Unlike nonkidney manifestations of SLE, serologic markers of disease correlate poorly with LN. Therefore, elevations in SCr and worsening of proteinuria and hematuria, as seen in S.L., are used as primary markers of disease activity.

Treatment of LN must address both management of the acute disease process and maintenance therapy for the more stable chronic disease process. A general consensus is that patients, such as S.L., who present with focal or diffuse proliferative glomerulonephritis (class III or IV) should be treated aggressively, with the primary goal of preventing irreversible kidney damage. The prognosis of kidney function in patients with SLE has improved. The likelihood of developing ESRD or dying within 10 years of diagnosis has decreased from more than 80% to less than 20%; however, the prognosis is worse in blacks when compared with the white population treated for SLE.[190] Elevated serum creatinine, heavy proteinuria, anemia, and disease onset during childhood or in those older than 60 years of age are other predictors of a worse prognosis. Advances in pharmacologic therapy (i.e., safer immunosuppressive regimens, and antihypertensives) have improved the prognosis for the population as a whole.

The treatment of LN is primarily empiric but is based, to some extent, on histological findings. Although appropriate treatment can improve patient outcomes, vigorous attempts to suppress SLE activity may lead to serious drug-related complications. The primary strategy in the treatment of LN involves suppression of the immune system with corticosteroids and cytotoxic agents, such as cyclophosphamide (CYC), azathioprine (AZA), and mycophenolate mofetil (MMF). Clinicians need to be aware of the potential complications associated with these therapies and carefully monitor patients to determine the indication for treatment and improved prognosis. Toxicities associated with immunosuppressive agents depend on both the dose and the duration of therapy. Abnormalities in hematopoiesis, such as neutropenia and thrombocytopenia, are the most common adverse effects associated with cytotoxic agents. Immunosuppression, in general, increases a patient's susceptibility to a vast array of infections and to lymphocytic malignancies. In addition, the alkylating agent cyclophosphamide can cause nausea and vomiting, gonadal toxicity, hemorrhagic cystitis, and alopecia. The risk versus benefit of CYC use has to be seriously weighed in young women

TABLE 31-9
2003 International Society of Nephrology/Renal Pathology Society Classification of Lupus Nephritis

Class	Histologic Characterization	Usual Clinical Presentation
I	Minimal mesangial lupus nephritis	Mild proteinuria
II	Mesangial proliferative glomerulonephritis	Mild proteinuria and urine sediment abnormalities
III	Focal and segmental proliferative glomerulonephritis A: Active lesions; A/C: active and chronic lesions; C: chronic lesions	Proteinuria and hematuria
IV	Diffuse proliferative segmental (S) or global (G) glomerulonephritis A: Active lesions; A/C: active and chronic lesions; C: chronic lesions	Heavy proteinuria; active sediment; hypertension; renal failure
V	Membranous glomerulonephritis	Proteinuria; often nephrotic syndrome
VI	Advanced sclerosing glomerulonephritis	Proteinuria; renal failure; nephrotic syndrome

Data from the 2003 International Society of Nephrology/Renal Pathology Society Classification of Lupus Nephritis Lazar E et al. Long-term outcomes of cinacalcet and paricalcitol titration protocol for treatment of secondary hyperparathyroidism. *Am J Nephrol.* 2007;27:274.

who are considering pregnancy in the future. The antimetabolite AZA can cause pancreatitis and abnormalities in liver function. The selective inhibitor of inosine monophosphate dehydrogenase, MMF, although relatively benign compared with the other agents, can cause GI disturbances.

Induction Therapy

Therapy for LN is usually not indicated in patients with normal kidney function and proteinuria less than 2 g, regardless of class, because these patients have a good prognosis. Corticosteroids represent the cornerstone of therapy in patients with a mild form of LN. Low-dose prednisone should be initiated for patients with stable LN. In patients with a more severe form (class III and IV), prednisone 1 to 2 mg/kg/day for 4 to 8 weeks, as a single morning dose, may be initiated. Gradual tapering of prednisone to a low-dose regimen of 0.2 to 0.4 mg/kg/day must be attempted once glomerulonephritis has stabilized. For the treatment of acute exacerbations of LN, high-dose pulse therapy with methylprednisolone may be warranted. Given that S.L.'s LN has worsened, she should receive pulse methylprednisolone (0.5 to 1 g IV, not to exceed 1 g) for 3 days in an attempt to reduce the degree of proteinuria and improve kidney function.[190] Although generally well tolerated, rapid methylprednisolone injections can cause transient tremor, flushing, and altered taste sensation. To reduce the risk of adverse effects associated with the rate of injection, S.L. should receive methylprednisolone for 30 minutes. After a course of pulse methylprednisolone therapy, oral prednisone at a dose 10 to 20 mg daily may be initiated.[190] Suppression of S.L.'s active LN should be demonstrated by a reduction in proteinuria and hematuria and an increase in her eGFR.

The addition of cytotoxic agents is reserved for patients who do not respond to corticosteroids alone, or those who have unacceptable toxicity to corticosteroids, worsening kidney function, severe proliferative lesions, or evidence of sclerosis on kidney biopsy. Induction therapy with six monthly pulse doses of IV CYC (0.5 to 1 g/m^2) or six doses of CYC given every 2 weeks at a dose of 0.5 g/m^2 along with steroid therapy was shown to have improved kidney outcomes with fewer flares and relapses.[191] Before and for 24 hours after initiating IV CYC, the patient must be well hydrated to prevent bladder toxicity. Recently, MMF (2,000 to 3,000 mg/day times 6 months) has been proven to be as effective as CYC in the induction treatment for LN.[192] Given the significant toxicities associated with CYC (e.g., gonadal toxicity, hemorrhagic cystitis), the anti-inflammatory properties of MMF resulting in a possible retardation of atherosclerosis, and the lower side effect profile with MMF, the option to use MMF as an alternative agent in LN seems promising, but its use in LN is still unclear. Studies are currently ongoing to determine the optimal dosing and duration of therapy with MMF, as well as which patient population would benefit the most from this therapy in the induction therapy for LN.

Maintenance Therapy

Once the acute flare resolves (generally in up to 12 weeks), low-dose, maintenance steroid therapy with 5 to 15 mg/day of prednisone can be initiated in combination with cytotoxic therapy, if indicated, based on severity of LN. In a meta-analysis assessing the efficacy of therapeutic agents used to treat LN, improved outcomes (total mortality and ESRD) were associated with use of oral prednisone in combination with IV CYC. As a result, the National Institutes of Health recommends the use of IV CYC pulse therapy (0.5 to 1 g/m^2) every 3 months for up to 2 years for maintenance therapy of LN.[193] An additional benefit of combination therapy with immunosuppressive agents is their steroid-sparing effect and, potentially, lower risk of steroid toxicity.

Studies have evaluated other immunosuppressive agents (AZA, MMF) for maintenance therapy in light of the toxicities associated with CYC. The most recent trial compared maintenance therapy with AZA (1 to 3 mg/day) and MMF (500 to 3,000 mg/day) with CYC along with steroids after induction with CYC in patients with severe LN. Patients receiving AZA had a lower mortality rate than those treated with CYC, and the MMF treatment group had fewer relapses than the CYC treatment group.[194] Until results from long-term trials with AZA and MMF are available, CYC is still considered first-line therapy for most classes of LN. MMF and AZA may be indicated in patients resistant to CYC therapy or with a more severe type of LN (class III and IV). The addition of CYC, AZA, and MMF, along with corticosteroid therapy, should be considered in S.L. once the acute lupus flare resolves. Once suppression of S.L.'s LN is documented, initiation of either AZA or MMF and steroids is indicated because of the severity of her LN (class III). The duration of therapy is dictated by the individual's response, but typically patients will require up to 2 years of maintenance therapy.

Alternative Agents

Exploration of alternative therapies for LN are also being studied. Rituximab, a monoclonal antibody that inhibits B-cell production, is being studied because B-cell hyperactivity is one of the major pathophysiologic mechanisms of LN. Small studies in patients with LN resistant to therapy have shown rituximab to be of benefit.[193] Cyclosporine, in doses of 5 mg/kg/day, may also provide an alternative therapy to treat lupus in the maintenance phase in patients unresponsive to treatment.[190]

WEGENER'S GRANULOMATOSIS

CASE 31-6

QUESTION 1: J.M. is a 42-year-old white man who presents to the clinic with a 1-month history of cough, nasal congestion, facial pain with headache, fever, and lethargy. During the past week, he has noted bright red blood in his phlegm, which has worsened in the past 3 days. Pertinent laboratory values are as follows:

Serum Na, 143 mEq/L
K, 5.1 mEq/L
Cl, 102 mEq/L
CO_2 content, 24 mEq/L
SCr, 2.8 mg/dL
BUN, 41 mg/dL

This compares with last year's physical checkup visit when his SCr and BUN were within the normal range. Hematologic studies reveal an Hct of 35%, an Hgb of 11.7 g/dL, a mean corpuscular volume (MCV) of 69 μL, a mean corpuscular Hgb (MCH) concentration of 24%, and a reticulocyte count of 1.8%. RBC indices are normal, and the platelet count is 175,000/μL. His 24-hour urine contains 3.8 g of albumin (normal, <30 mg), and his eGFR is calculated to be 27 mL/minute/1.73 m^2. His urine also contains many RBC casts and 16 RBCs/HPF (normal, 0 to 3 RBCs/HPF). Chest radiograph shows alveolar shadowing spreading from the hilar region. The result of J.M.'s cytoplasmic-staining, antineutrophil cytoplasmic antibody (c-ANCA) is positive. On the basis of his subjective and objective data, which of the chronic glomerulopathies is J.M. likely to have?

Wegener granulomatosis is a primary systemic vasculitis characterized by granulomatous inflammation of the upper and lower respiratory tract and secondary glomerulonephritis.

Primary systemic vasculitic syndromes, such as Wegener granulomatosis, often cause glomerulonephritis. Although vasculitis involves inflammation of blood vessels of any size, the small- and medium-size vessels are most commonly affected.[195] The etiology of Wegener granulomatosis is unclear; however, an autoimmune response is suspected for two reasons. First, Wegener granulomatosis is a systemic inflammatory disease without a known infectious etiology. Second, good treatment response can be obtained with immunosuppressive therapy.

The clinical features of Wegener granulomatosis include upper airway disease, such as sinusitis, epistaxis, and nasopharyngitis, as well as otitis media caused by blockage of the eustachian tube. Constitutional symptoms include fever, night sweats, arthralgia, anorexia, and malaise. After a few months, weakness may progress, severely limiting physical activity. Although the lungs are invariably affected, most patients remain asymptomatic; however, cough and hemoptysis may be present. J.M.'s presenting symptoms are consistent with the above clinical features. The laboratory signs also are nonspecific and indicate the presence of a systemic inflammatory process. They include an elevated erythrocyte sedimentation rate in virtually all patients, anemia of chronic disease, and thrombocytosis.[195] Hematuria and proteinuria can be prominent features of Wegener granulomatosis and are present on initial presentation in 80% of patients. The presence of severely diminished kidney function, seen in approximately 10% of patients, is an ominous sign, with nearly one-third of these patients progressing to ESRD. All patients with Wegener granulomatosis are at risk for developing irreversible, rapidly progressive kidney failure. Kidney histological findings are nonspecific, with most patients exhibiting necrotizing crescentic glomerulonephritis.[195]

Wegener granulomatosis is diagnosed primarily by the presenting signs and symptoms. According to the American College of Rheumatology 1990 classification, a person is diagnosed with Wegener granulomatosis if any two of the following four criteria are present: (a) nasal or oral inflammation, (b) abnormal chest radiograph, (c) microhematuria (>5 RBCs/HPF) or RBC casts in the urine sediment, or (d) granulomatous inflammation on biopsy.[195] J.M. has satisfied three of the four criteria for diagnosing Wegener granulomatosis.

TREATMENT

CASE 31-6, QUESTION 2: How should J.M.'s Wegener granulomatosis be treated?

The discovery of c-ANCA and its strong association with Wegener granulomatosis has permitted a more certain diagnosis. Because of the substantial rise in titer that commonly precedes relapse of Wegener granulomatosis, the c-ANCA test is best used to follow the course of disease activity and guide induction of therapy. Treatment with CYC and corticosteroids results in improvement in kidney function in approximately 80% to 85% of patients, versus 75% with pulse steroids alone.[196] The main predictive factors for treatment success are the extent of kidney damage before therapy starts and how long therapy is delayed after symptoms develop.

Cyclophosphamide

Because Wegener granulomatosis is considered an autoimmune inflammatory disease, immunosuppressive therapy is the mainstay of treatment. Therapy is generally indicated for 6 months if remission occurs and up to 12 months in resistant cases.[196] J.M. should be started on oral CYC 2 mg/kg/day, as a single morning dose, to prevent irreversible glomerular scarring. With a more fulminant form of the disease, higher doses (4 to 5 mg/kg/day) may be used, although the potential for toxicities must be carefully considered. High fluid intake (>3 L/day) and Mesna reduces the risk of hemorrhagic cystitis. Regular urinalysis should be performed (every 3 to 6 months) to detect hematuria caused by hemorrhagic cystitis.

Induction treatment with pulse IV boluses of CYC is associated with high relapse rates. However, the two conditions for which IV CYC may be considered are (a) patients whose conditions have not responded to conventional treatment and (b) patients in whom severe kidney dysfunction developed initially, including those requiring dialysis. In the former, IV CYC 1 g/m^2 in 150 mL of saline can be administered for 60 minutes. The dose must be reduced by 25% in patients with an eGFR of less than 10 mL/minute/1.73 m^2. This regimen may be administered monthly for 6 months, after which a dosage reduction may be attempted.[197]

Corticosteroids

The main role of corticosteroids is to induce remission of the disease. J.M. should receive prednisone 1 mg/kg/day in addition to CYC. The combined regimen should be continued for 2 to 4 weeks until the immunosuppressive effect of CYC becomes evident. Then, during the next 2 months, the prednisone dose can be tapered to 60 mg every other day to reduce the risk of infection. Then, the dose can be tapered by 5 mg/week to discontinue prednisone over the course of 3 to 6 months. For patients with a more fulminant form of the disease, pulse methylprednisolone 1 g/m^2/day for three doses is administered. The dose can be repeated in 1 to 2 weeks if disease progression is uncontrolled.

Azathioprine and Mycophenolate Mofetil

Azathioprine and MMF are effective as maintenance therapy once remission has been achieved with CYC. However, a comparative study demonstrated mycophenolate to be less effective at maintaining remissions compared with azathioprine.[198]

Alternative Agents

Methotrexate may be beneficial for patients with milder disease, although one study demonstrated high relapse rates in patients treated initially with weekly methotrexate and daily prednisone; disease was controlled in only select patients.[199] Use of trimethoprim-sulfamethoxazole for 1 year was evaluated for patients in remission or after treatment with CYC and prednisolone. A reduction in relapse rate was demonstrated compared with placebo; however, trimethoprim-sulfamethoxazole use is not supported.[199] Tumor necrosis factor alpha blockade with infliximab and etanercept has demonstrated activity with a reduced time to remission and early tapering of steroids. Greater benefits are seen with infliximab. B-cell depletion from rituximab therapy has had successful results with 70% to 100% remission rates from anecdotal reports and small studies.[195]

FOCAL SEGMENTAL GLOMERULOSCLEROSIS

CASE 31-7

QUESTION 1: A.G. is a 37-year-old morbidly obese (body mass index, 40 kg/m^2), black woman who presents to the clinic with complaints of increased swelling in her extremities for the last 2 weeks, decreased urine output, and pink-colored urine. Her medical history is significant only for hypertension, which is well controlled with amlodipine 5 mg PO every day. She takes no other prescription or

over-the-counter medications. Pertinent laboratory values are as follows

SCr, 2.1 mg/dL (normal, 0.6 to 1.2 mg/dL)
Spot albumin-to-creatinine ratio, 1,200 mg/g (normal < 30 mg/g)
UA, 18 RBCs/HPF (normal, 0 to 3)
eGFR, 34 mL/minute/1.73 m^2

The nephrologist schedules a biopsy to obtain a definitive diagnosis for her new-onset kidney disease. Biopsy results are as follows: light micrograph shows a moderately large segmental area of sclerosis with capillary collapse on the upper left side of the glomerular tuft; the lower right segment is relatively normal. Electron micrograph shows diffuse epithelial cell foot process fusion with occasional loss of the epithelial cells. The other major finding is massive subendothelial hyaline deposits under the glomerular basement membrane. The pathologist's impression is FSGS. What is the relevance of FSGS, and what are the management strategies for FSGS?

Focal segmental glomerulosclerosis is characterized by sclerotic lesions of the glomerulus, which can be either focal or segmental in nature. The development of FSGS may be idiopathic (primary) or secondary to other diseases (i.e., morbid obesity, sickle cell disease, congenital heart disease, AIDS). Currently, FSGS is the leading cause of idiopathic nephrotic syndrome and accounts for 15% to 20% of the cases. Black patients are two to four times more likely to experience idiopathic FSGS than white patients, and they have a higher incidence of ESRD caused by FSGS.[200] Genetic variants of the *MYH9* gene predominate in patients of African ancestry and have been identified as a major risk factor.[201,202]

Most patients with FSGS will present with proteinuria, but only about half of them will initially present with nephrotic syndrome. Patients with nephrotic syndrome will also likely present with hypertension, increased serum creatinine levels, and hematuria. During the early stages of FSGS, the symptoms may be indistinguishable from minimal-change nephropathy, a glomerulopathy characterized by similar lesions within the glomeruli. A kidney biopsy is necessary for diagnosis. Predictors of increased risk of progression to ESRD include massive proteinuria (>10 g/day), higher serum creatinine level (>1.3 mg/dL), and black race.[200,201]

TREATMENT

Corticosteroids

A.G. should be placed on steroids, in addition to an ACE inhibitor or ARB and a loop diuretic, because she has FSGS and nephrotic syndrome.[203] A course of high-dose steroids (1 to 2 mg/kg) for 3 to 4 months with tapering of the dose over the course of 3 months is recommended. The lower remission rates associated with this high-dose regimen compared with low-dose regimens have led to this recommendation. The median time to remission is 3 to 4 months, with most patients achieving complete remission by 5 to 9 months. Patients whose proteinuria does not respond after a 4-month trial of therapy should be considered resistant to steroids and be rapidly tapered off over the course of 4 weeks.[201]

Cytotoxic Agents

The addition of cytotoxic agents (CYC, AZA, chlorambucil) may be considered for A.G. if she is steroid resistant, intolerant of long-term steroid therapy, severely nephrotic, frequently relapsing, or steroid dependent. The data supporting the use of these agents in FSGS are limited. Retrospective studies have shown that use of cytotoxic drugs can produce complete remission in 50% of cases. Length of therapy of these agents may predict the remission rates of FSGS. Recent prospective studies support a longer duration of therapy. Patients who received either chlorambucil or CYC up to 75 weeks obtained a higher complete remission rate (30% to 47%). The duration of use of these agents is limited by their toxicities (gonadal toxicity, malignancies). Cumulative doses of 300 mg/kg of CYC and 10 mg/kg of chlorambucil have been shown to increase the risk of developing these toxicities; thus, limiting the exposure to these agents is important.[201]

Calcineurin Inhibitors

Evidence supporting the efficacy and safety of calcineurin inhibitors (cyclosporine, tacrolimus, and sirolimus) in FSGS is growing. Calcineurin inhibitors provide a steroid-sparing effect in FSGS steroid-sensitive patients. Cyclosporine studies are the most prevalent of the three calcineurin inhibitors. Cyclosporine response is highly dependent on the previous steroid response. Complete remission rates of 73% can be seen with cyclosporine in steroid-sensitive patients.[201] Conversely, therapy with cyclosporine doses of 5 mg/kg/day for 6 to 12 months has been found to be effective and can result in remission rates of up to 69% in patients resistant to steroids.[204,205] Limitations of cyclosporine therapy include high relapse rate (23% to 100%), side effect profile (nephrotoxicity, hypertension), and resistance to therapy. The exact dose and duration of cyclosporine therapy should be determined by the response of the patient's proteinuria and serum creatinine. Studies evaluating tacrolimus as a treatment option for FSGS are few and conflicting but with promising results. Tacrolimus has a similar side effect profile to that of cyclosporine.[201] Further studies are needed to determine the role cyclosporine (i.e., appropriate dosing) and tacrolimus (i.e., efficacy) therapy has in certain types of patients with FSGS. Sirolimus is associated with nephrotoxicity in FSGS and is not recommended for treatment.

Mycophenolate Mofetil

Mycophenolate mofetil has the potential for a steroid-sparing effect; however, relapses are common. A small study of patients with FSGS resistant to steroids, cytotoxic agents, or both and cyclosporine received MMF for 6 months. At the end of 6 months, 44% of patients had improved proteinuria, but no patient achieved complete remission.[206] Other studies examining MMF therapy at doses of 1,500 to 2,000 mg/day have found no clinically significant effect on remission rates. More than half the patients in one study that enrolled 22 FSGS patients achieved a moderate decrease in proteinuria. Kidney function largely influenced the response rate to MMF in this trial.[201] Treatment with MMF in FSGS is limited, and well-designed, prospective, randomized trials are necessary to determine its role, if any, in FSGS.

KEY REFERENCES AND WEBSITES

A full list of references for this chapter can be found at http://thepoint.lww.com/AT10e. Below are the key references and websites for this chapter, with the corresponding reference number in this chapter found in parentheses after the reference.

Key References

Block GA et al. Mortality effect of coronary calcification and phosphate binder choice in incident hemodialysis patients. *Kidney Int.* 2007;71:438. (155)

Coyne DW et al. Ferric gluconate is highly efficacious in anemic hemodialysis patients with high serum ferritin and low transferrin saturation: results of the Dialysis Patients' Response to IV Iron with Elevated Ferritin (DRIVE) study. *J Am Soc Nephrol.* 2007;18:975. (117)

Gutiérrez OM. Fibroblast growth factor 23 and disordered vitamin D metabolism in chronic kidney disease: updating the "trade-off" hypothesis. *Clin J Am Soc Nephrol.* 2010;5:1710. (146)

Kalantar-Zadeh K, Kovesdy CP. Clinical outcomes with active versus nutritional vitamin D compounds in chronic kidney disease. *Clin J Am Soc Nephrol.* 2009;4:1529. (149)

Kidney Disease: Improving Global Outcomes (KDIGO) CKD-MBD Work Group. KDIGO Clinical Practice Guideline for the Diagnosis, Evaluation, Prevention, and Treatment of Chronic Kidney Disease–Mineral and Bone Disorder (CKD-MBD). *Kidney Int Suppl.* 2009;(113):S1. (98)

Kidney Disease Outcomes Quality Initiative (K/DOQI). K/DOQI Clinical Practice Guidelines on Hypertension and Antihypertensive Agents in Chronic Kidney Disease. *Am J Kidney Dis.* 2004;43(Suppl 1):S1. (94)

Murray AM. Cognitive impairment in the aging dialysis and chronic kidney disease populations: an occult burden. *Adv Chronic Kidney Dis.* 2008;15:123. (186)

National Kidney Foundation. K/DOQI Clinical Practice Guidelines and Clinical Practice Recommendations for Anemia of Chronic Kidney Disease [published correction appears in *Am J Kidney Dis.* 2006;48:518]. *Am J Kidney Dis.* 2006;47(5 Suppl 3):S11. (99)

National Kidney Foundation. K/DOQI Clinical Practice Guidelines and Clinical Practice Recommendations for Diabetes for Chronic Kidney Disease. *Am J Kidney Dis.* 2007;49(2 Suppl 2):S12. (78)

National Kidney Foundation. K/DOQI Clinical Practice Guidelines for Bone Metabolism and Disease in Chronic Kidney Disease. *Am J Kidney Dis.* 2003;42(4 Suppl 3):S1. (144)

National Kidney Foundation. K/DOQI Clinical Practice Guidelines for Chronic Kidney Disease: Evaluation, Classification, and Stratification. *Am J Kidney Dis.* 2002;39(2 Suppl 1):S1. (1)

National Kidney Foundation. K/DOQI Clinical Practice Guidelines on Managing Dyslipidemias in Chronic Kidney Disease. *Am J Kidney Dis.* 2003;41(4 Suppl 3):S1. (72)

Pfeffer MA et al. A trial of darbepoetin alfa in type 2 diabetes and chronic kidney disease. *N Engl J Med.* 2009;361:2019. (106)

US Renal Data System. *USRDS 2010 Annual Data Report: Atlas of End-Stage Renal Disease in the United States.* Bethesda, MD: National Institutes of Health, National Institute of Diabetes and Digestive and Kidney Diseases; 2010. (4)

Key Websites

KDIGO Clinical Practice Guideline for the Diagnosis, Evaluation, Prevention, and Treatment of Chronic Kidney Disease–Mineral and Bone Disorder (CKD-MBD). **http://www.kdigo.org/clinical_practice_guidelines/kdigo_guideline_for_ckd-mbd.php.**

Kidney Disease Outcomes Quality Initiative (K/DOQI). K/DOQI Clinical Practice Guidelines on Hypertension and Antihypertensive Agents in Chronic Kidney Disease. **http://www.kidney.org/professionals/KDOQI/guidelines_bp/index.htm.**

National Kidney Foundation. K/DOQI Clinical Practice Guidelines and Clinical Practice Recommendations for Anemia of Chronic Kidney Disease (2006). **http://www.kidney.org/professionals/KDOQI/guidelines_anemia/index.htm.**

National Kidney Foundation. K/DOQI Clinical Practice Guidelines and Clinical Practice Recommendations for Diabetes for Chronic Kidney Disease. **http://www.kidney.org/professionals/KDOQI/guideline_diabetes/.**

National Kidney Foundation. K/DOQI Clinical Practice Guidelines for Bone Metabolism and Disease in Chronic Kidney Disease. **http://www.kidney.org/professionals/KDOQI/guidelines_bone/index.htm.**

National Kidney Foundation. K/DOQI Clinical Practice Guidelines for Chronic Kidney Disease. **http://www.kidney.org/professionals/KDOQI/guidelines_ckd/toc.htm.**

National Kidney Foundation. K/DOQI Clinical Practice Guidelines on Managing Dyslipidemias in Chronic Kidney Disease. **http://www.kidney.org/professionals/KDOQI/guidelines_lipids/toc.htm.**

US Renal Data System. **http://www.usrds.org/.**

Renal Dialysis

Myrna Y. Munar

32

CORE PRINCIPLES

	CHAPTER CASES
1 End-stage renal disease (ESRD) occurs when there is progressive loss of kidney function over a period of months to years to the point where the kidneys can no longer remove wastes; concentrate urine; maintain acid–base homeostasis; and regulate fluid, electrolytes, and other important body functions.	**Case 32-1 (Question 1)**
2 Dialysis is a process that facilitates the removal of excess water and solutes from the body, both of which accumulate as a result of inadequate kidney function. Solutes from the blood are removed through diffusion and convection. Accumulated water is removed by ultrafiltration.	**Case 32-1 (Question 1)**
3 The ability of a dialyzer to remove solutes and water is determined by its composition, pore size, surface area, and configuration.	**Case 32-1 (Question 1)**
4 Dialysate is an electrolyte solution that simulates plasma. The concentration of electrolytes in dialysate can be manipulated to control the diffusion of electrolytes from the blood into dialysate to maintain homeostasis. Metabolic acidosis is controlled with the addition of bicarbonate to dialysate.	**Case 32-1 (Question 1)**
5 Different types of vascular access are available: arteriovenous (AV) fistula, AV graft, double-lumen or tunneled catheters, and catheters with subcutaneously implanted access ports. An AV fistula is preferred because of its longer survival rates and its low rates of complications.	**Case 32-1 (Question 2)**
6 Anticoagulation is necessary during hemodialysis (HD) to prevent blood from clotting in the extracorporeal circuit. Several methods have been used to provide adequate anticoagulation without increasing the risk of bleeding.	**Case 32-1 (Question 3)**
7 Complications can arise during HD. The most common complications are hypotension and muscle cramps. Graft thrombosis and graft infection are common chronic complications.	**Case 32-1 (Questions 4–7)**
8 Continuous ambulatory peritoneal dialysis is performed by instilling sterile dialysate into the peritoneal cavity through a surgically placed resident catheter. The solution dwells within the cavity for 4 to 8 hours, and then is drained and replaced with a fresh solution. This process of fill, dwell, and drain is performed three to four times during the day, with a longer dwell overnight.	**Case 32-2 (Question 1)**
9 The process of peritoneal dialysis (PD) is similar to HD; in this process, however, the peritoneal membrane covering the abdominal contents serves as an endogenous dialysis membrane, and the vasculature embedded in the peritoneum serves as the blood supply. Fluid is removed by manipulating the dextrose concentration in dialysate to control the osmotic pressure gradient for fluid removal.	**Case 32-2 (Question 1)**
10 The most significant complication among patients having PD is peritonitis. Empiric antibiotics can be administered by the intraperitoneal (IP) route and must cover both gram-positive and gram-negative organisms.	**Case 32-2 (Questions 2, 4)**

continued

		CHAPTER CASES
11	Other medications can be administered IP. Heparin can be added to dialysate to prevent fibrin clots from forming and obstructing outflow from the peritoneal cavity. Regular insulin can be administered IP to patients with diabetes.	**Case 32-2 (Questions 3, 7)**
12	Prevention of catheter exit-site infections (and thus peritonitis) is the primary goal of exit-site care. Routine care consists of handwashing with antibacterial soap before touching the exit site, washing the exit site daily with antibacterial soap, and use of antimicrobial creams around the exit site.	**Case 32-2 (Questions 5, 6)**

End-stage renal disease (ESRD) occurs when there is progressive loss of kidney function over a period of months to years to the point where the kidneys can no longer remove wastes, concentrate urine, maintain acid–base homeostasis, and regulate fluid and electrolytes and other important body functions. ESRD is classified under stage 5 chronic kidney disease (CKD), which refers to patients with an estimated glomerular filtration rate (eGFR) less than 15 mL/minute/1.73 m^2, or those requiring dialysis or transplantation.[1] Demographic characteristics of ESRD population are based primarily on data from the Centers for Medicare and Medicaid Services, because patients with ESRD are eligible for Medicare benefits. Coverage for ESRD began in 1972, when Congress enacted the End-Stage Renal Disease Program as an amendment to Medicare. Data from the ESRD program are reported annually by the United States Renal Data System. According to the 2009 Annual Report, diabetes and hypertension continue to be leading causes of ESRD.[2] Racial differences in the prevalence of ESRD persist with rates of new cases in the African American and Native American populations that are 3.7 and 1.8 times greater, respectively, than the prevalence rate among the white population. Patients aged 45 to 64 years account for the largest segment of the ESRD population.

The prevalence of ESRD in the United States in 2007 was 1,665 per million population. Of these, 341,264 patients were treated by hemodialysis (HD), 26,340 were on peritoneal dialysis (PD), and 158,739 received a kidney transplant.[2] The rise in the prevalence rate of HD has slowed from 8.7% in 1997 to 3.8% in 2007, whereas the prevalence rate of PD has remained stable. The greatest growth has occurred in kidney transplantation, with a 5% to 6% increase each year since 2001. The shortage of donor kidneys and the existence of patients with ESRD who are unacceptable transplant recipients sustain the demand for dialysis. Kidney transplantation is further discussed in Chapter 34, Kidney and Liver Transplantation.

The two primary modes of dialysis therapy are HD and PD. Both HD and PD were developed as methods for the removal of metabolic waste products across a semipermeable membrane.

ONLINE CONTENT

For a narrated PowerPoint presentation on renal dialysis, go to http://thepoint.lww.com/AT10e.

HD is an extracorporeal (dialysis membrane is outside of the body) process, whereas PD uses the patient's peritoneal membrane for the clearance of water and solutes. Variations of PD include continuous ambulatory peritoneal dialysis (CAPD) and automated peritoneal dialysis (APD), an increasingly common modality that permits greater patient flexibility with dialysis. Among the nearly 367,600 dialysis patients in the United States, 93% undergo HD.[2] Most of these patients receive dialysis three times a week in a center designed primarily for stable, ambulatory patients at either a hospital-based or a free-standing dialysis facility. Home HD accounts for less than 1% of dialysis patients. Patients having PD also are managed through dialysis centers for routine care, although less often than patients on HD. Several factors are considered in the selection of the type of dialysis for each patient. Often, the overriding consideration is the suitability of the procedure for the patient's lifestyle. A patient who needs flexibility and freedom from a rigid schedule may prefer PD versus HD to avoid the necessity of being at a dialysis center three times weekly for a 3-hour to 4-hour dialysis treatment. Other considerations include the availability of a vascular access site for HD, or a patient's ability to perform self-care for dialysate exchanges with PD.

Without dialysis or transplantation, patients with ESRD will die of the metabolic complications of their renal failure. Patient characteristics and comorbid conditions influence the death rate, including age (increased with increased age), race (increased in black patients), and primary cause of ESRD (increased with diabetes and hypertension compared with glomerulonephritis).[3] Since 1980, mortality rates have fallen across all renal replacement modalities and lengths of therapy, with a first-time decline in first-year death rates reported in 2007.[2] However, all-cause mortality rates are 6.7 to 8.5 times higher for dialysis patients than in the general population, and highest in the third month of dialysis. Mortality rates among transplant patients are 1.3 to 1.6 times greater than patients without ESRD. The length of time on dialysis influences the mortality rate. In 2007, mortality for patients on dialysis for 5 years or longer was 20.6% greater than the rate among dialysis patients newer to therapy.[2] Last of all, the initial modality appears to influence mortality rates depending on age and comorbidities. Patients expected to live longer (e.g., <65 years, without cardiovascular disease, without diabetes) had 8% lower mortality when initiated on peritoneal dialysis than on hemodialysis.[4]

The rapid growth of the number of patients having dialysis calls attention to the need for practitioners who understand the processes and therapies for these patients. This chapter addresses the fundamental clinical aspects of both HD and PD, including principles, complications, and management. Throughout the chapter, reference will be made, when appropriate, to the clinical practice guidelines developed by the National Kidney Foundation, originally published in 1997, and updated in 2000 and 2006.[5–8] The initial guidelines focused on dialysis issues, the Dialysis Outcomes Quality Initiative (DOQI), and included four workgroups: Hemodialysis Adequacy,[9] Peritoneal Dialysis Adequacy,[10] Vascular Access,[11] and Anemia.[12] The updated clinical practice guidelines have been renamed the Kidney Disease Outcomes Quality Initiative (K/DOQI) to reflect the broader nature and impact of renal impairment. Additional clinical practice guidelines developed under K/DOQI include Nutrition of Chronic Renal Failure[13] and Chronic Kidney Disease: Evaluation,

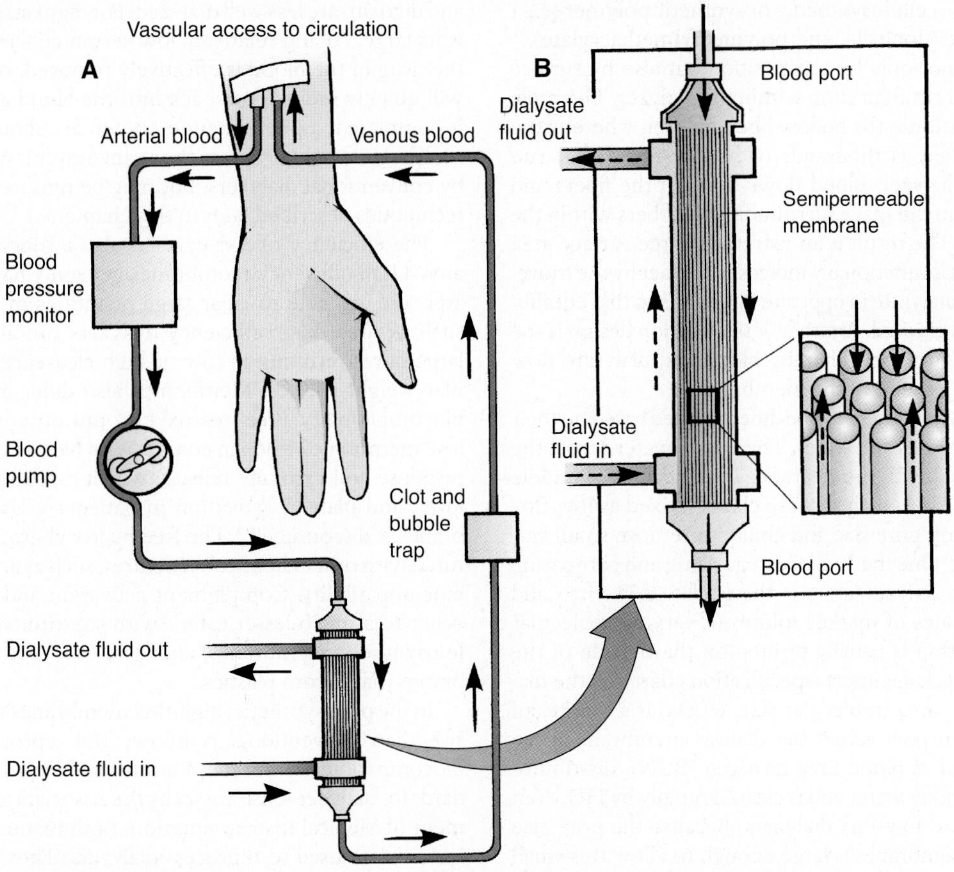

FIGURE 32-1 Hemodialysis system. (A) Blood from an artery is pumped into **(B)**, a dialyzer where it flows through the cellophane tubes, which act as the semipermeable membrane (inset). The dialysate, which has the same chemical composition as the blood except for urea and waste products, flows in around the tubules. The waste products in the blood diffuse through the semipermeable membrane into the dialysate. Adapted with permission from Smeltzer SC, Bare BG. *Textbook of Medical-Surgical Nursing*. 9th ed. Philadelphia, PA: Lippincott Williams & Wilkins; 2000.

Classification, and Stratification.[1] The latter guideline is addressed in Chapter 31, Chronic Kidney Diseases.

HEMODIALYSIS

Principles and Transport Processes

Dialysis is a process that facilitates the removal of excess water and toxins from the body, both of which accumulate as a result of inadequate kidney function. During HD, a patient's anticoagulated blood (circulated to the dialyzer from a vein in the arm) and an electrolyte solution that simulates plasma (dialysate) are simultaneously perfused through a dialyzer (artificial kidney) on opposite sides of a semipermeable membrane. Solutes (e.g., metabolic waste products, toxins, potassium, and other electrolytes) are removed from the patient's blood by diffusing across concentration gradients into the dialysate. The rate of removal of various solutes from the blood is a function of blood and dialysate flow rates through the dialyzer, relative concentration of each solute in the blood and dialysis solution (thus determining their concentration gradients across the membrane), physical characteristics of the dialysis membrane (e.g., total available surface area, thickness, and pore size), and properties of the solute being removed (e.g., molecular size in daltons, molecular weight, volume of distribution, and protein binding). Because blood and dialysate flow in opposite directions through the dialyzer, the concentration gradient for each solute across the membrane is amplified (Fig. 32-1). This principle is defined in greater detail in the Dialyzer Characteristics section.

Solutes from the blood are removed through diffusion and convection. Diffusion is the process whereby the molecule moves across its concentration gradient by passing through pores in the dialysis membrane.[14] Once the concentration of a solute reaches equilibrium on both sides of the membrane, the net movement is zero because the rate of movement from the blood to dialysate compartment is equal to the rate from the dialysate to the blood compartment. For most substances, equilibrium is not achieved, either because the blood and dialysate flow rates are too rapid or the molecule is too large to easily move through the pores.

Accumulated water is removed by the process of ultrafiltration. A controlled pressure difference across the semipermeable membrane permits water movement through the membrane pores, which carries with it solute into the dialysate, thereby further enhancing solute removal. Flux is the rate of water transfer across the dialyzer. Convection is the process that removes toxins and other dissolved solutes during dialysis through the ultrafiltration of plasma water from the blood compartment.[14] The removal of solutes by convection during ultrafiltration generally is small relative to their elimination through diffusion.

DIALYZER CHARACTERISTICS

Dialyzers are characterized by many factors, such as membrane composition, size, and ability to clear solutes. Their primary component is the dialysis membrane, made of cellulose (e.g., cuprammonium cellulose), substituted cellulose (e.g., cellulose acetate, cellulose triacetate), cellulosynthetic, or synthetic polymer (e.g., polysulfone, polyacrylonitrile, and polymethylmethacrylate).[15] Membranes differ not only by composition but also by surface area, thickness, and configuration within the dialyzer. The most common configuration is the hollow fiber dialyzer, whereby the membrane is formed as thousands of hollow fibers that run the length of the dialyzer. Blood flows through the fibers and the dialysate flows in the space surrounding the fibers within the dialyzer cartridge. The result is an extremely large surface area for diffusion, which is functionally increased further by the movement of blood and dialysate in opposite directions so that equilibrium is never fully achieved. Another, less-common design is the parallel-plate configuration, whereby blood and dialysate flow between alternating sheets of the membrane.

Functionally, dialysis filters can be differentiated based on their ability to remove solutes and water. The flux of water across the dialyzer is correlated with the clearance of molecules of middle molecular weight. Thus, dialyzers are characterized as low-flux or high-flux based on pore size and ability to remove small versus large molecules. One method of categorizing and comparing efficiency (flux) of dialyzer units is their relative in vitro and in vivo clearance rates of marker solutes of varying molecular size. This information is usually printed on the outside of the dialyzer or in the package insert (specification chart) for the dialyzer. For example, urea (molecular size, 60 Da) is a marker of small-molecule transport across the dialysis membrane. Urea (found in the blood as blood urea nitrogen [BUN]) distributes freely throughout body water and is cleared rapidly by HD, even when using standard low flux dialyzers. Because the pore size of most dialyzer membranes is large enough to allow this small molecule to freely diffuse, the rate-limiting step for the removal of urea is blood flow through the dialyzer. A larger molecule, vitamin B_{12} (molecular size, 1,355 Da), also has been used as a measure of dialysis efficiency. Because vitamin B_{12} is too large to easily cross through the pores of conventional dialysis membranes, its dialysis clearance is less dependent on blood flow than urea. Instead, the overall removal of vitamin B_{12} depends more on the type of membrane (i.e., thickness and pore size) and the duration of dialysis. The clearance of β_2-microglobulin, an even larger molecule than vitamin B_{12} (molecular size, 11,800 Da), has been used to characterize the flux of a dialyzer.[5,15] High-flux dialyzers are defined as providing β_2-microglobulin clearances of at least 20 mL/minute.[5] High-flux membranes have larger pores and are able to clear larger molecules (e.g., middle molecules such as β_2-microglobulin and leptin) and drugs (e.g., vancomycin or vitamin B_{12}, with molecular weights in the range of 1,000–5,000 Da) more effectively than low-flux membranes with smaller pores. High-flux membranes also have a greater permeability to water, as reflected in a KUf value (to be defined later) of more than 10 mL/hour/mm Hg. Importantly, β_2-microglobulin is not only a surrogate marker for middle molecule dialysis clearance but its plasma levels have also been found to be predictive of mortality.[16] It also plays a role in the pathogenesis of amyloidosis (see the Amyloidosis section for further discussion). β_2-microglobulin clearance, however, is not consistently reported in all dialyzer specification charts.

Similarly, molecular weight of drugs is a predictor of dialysis clearance. At a molecular weight of less than 500 Da (e.g., aminoglycosides and theophylline), dialyzability is expected to be high. For these drugs, the actual amount dialyzed will vary based on protein binding (i.e., amount of unbound drug available to cross the dialysis membrane), volume of distribution (Vd) (i.e., a large Vd indicates a relatively small amount of drug will be available in the blood for dialysis), blood flow rate through the dialyzer, dialysis flow rate, and dialyzer surface area. Drugs with a molecular weight between 500 and 1000 Da (e.g., morphine and digoxin) are less well dialyzed. For digoxin, a greater problem is its large Vd and relatively low serum concentrations. Even if the drug in the blood is effectively removed, tissue-bound drug will quickly redistribute back into the blood as soon as dialysis is completed, a phenomenon known as rebound. Finally, large molecular weight drugs, such as vancomycin, are poorly dialyzed by conventional dialyzers, but may be removed using high-flux techniques described later in this chapter.

The efficiency of a dialyzer is also a function of its surface area. High-efficiency membranes generally have a large surface area and are able to clear large quantities of small molecules, such as urea. High-efficiency dialyzers can also have small or large pores resulting in low or high clearance of larger molecular weight solutes. Membranes also differ in their degree of biocompatibility. Free hydroxyl groups on unsubstituted cellulose membranes when in contact with blood evoke complement response and cytokine release, which can lead to hypotension, fever, and platelet activation in patients.[17] Use of these membranes is discouraged.[5] The free hydroxyl groups can be substituted with other chemical structures, such as acetate, to improve biocompatibility. Complement activation and cytokine release occur to a much lesser extent with substituted cellulose or cellulosynthetic membranes, and least of all with synthetic membranes made from plastics.

In the past, synthetic, high-flux membranes were more expensive than conventional cellulose, and reprocessing high-flux, biocompatible membranes for reuse reduced these costs.[18] Standards for dialyzer reuse are set by the Association for the Advancement of Medical Instrumentation. Both manual and automated systems are used to reprocess dialyzers. These systems include rinsing of blood and clots from the dialyzer, cleaning with agents such as dilute sodium hypochlorite (bleach), testing of dialyzer performance, and sterilization. The average number of times a dialyzer is reused depends on quality control standards within the dialysis center, but generally it is ten or more times for a patient. Universal precautions should be used to handle dialyzers, and reused dialyzers should never be shared between patients. Controversial issues regarding reuse programs include safety of disinfectants, dialyzer efficiency after processing, contamination and risk of infection, and pyrogenic reactions. As a result of declining prices, and the decision of a major dialysis manufacturer to discontinue reuse, single use disposable dialyzers are now more commonplace.[5]

A typical package insert for a dialyzer will provide information on the clearance of various molecules (e.g., urea, creatinine, phosphate, and vitamin B_{12}). Urea clearance has become a common measure of comparison for membranes; however, clearance also depends on other factors, such as blood and dialysate flow rates. A more standard measure for comparison is KoA_{urea}, the mass transfer area coefficient for urea. Based on the urea clearance data from the package insert, KoA_{urea} can be estimated based on blood flow. Using this information, the dialysis prescription can be individualized to provide a specified dose of dialysis for the patient.

Patients having chronic HD typically are dialyzed for 3 to 4 hours, three times a week, either Monday-Wednesday-Friday or Tuesday-Thursday-Saturday. During the interdialytic period, fluids ingested and produced through metabolic processes are retained in the patient. Although patients generally are on fluid-restricted diets, accumulation of 1 to 5 L of fluid (translating into 1- to 5-kg weight gain) between sessions is common and must be removed during the dialysis treatment.

BLOOD AND DIALYSATE FLOW

Although small-molecule clearance is highly dependent on blood flow, the relationship is not strictly linear. Increased blood flow yields a less than proportional response in urea clearance.[19] This is likely because of an insufficient time for equilibration to occur between the blood and dialysate compartments as well as a greater membrane resistance to diffusion from an increased stagnant layer. A typical blood flow rate for dialysis is 400 to 500 mL/minute but is dependent on the vascular access site and the cardiovascular status of the patient. Some patients are not able to tolerate this rate, and a lower blood flow rate may be necessary. Dialysate flow rates generally are 500 mL/minute and can be increased to 800 mL/minute for high-flux dialysis, which will increase urea clearance by approximately 10%.[20]

CASE 32-1

QUESTION 1: R.W., a 55-year-old man with a 25-year history of hypertension and stage 4 CKD, presents to the renal clinic for reassessment of his kidney function. He is 70 inches tall and weighs 70 kg. Since his last visit 3 months ago, his creatinine clearance (ClCr) has decreased from 22 to 12 mL/minute and the BUN has increased to 89 mg/dL. The serum potassium (K) is 4.5 mEq/L and HCO_3 is 17 mEq/L. He has selected HD as his form of therapy until a suitable donor kidney is available and is expected to begin dialysis within the next 1 to 3 months. When he begins dialysis, he will be dialyzed three times a week for 4 hours each treatment, using a Fresenius F-60S dialyzer, with blood and dialysate flows of 400 and 500 mL/minute, respectively, and bicarbonate-containing dialysate. What characteristics of the Fresenius F-60S dialyzer make it a good choice for R.W.? What determines the composition of the dialysate?

The Fresenius dialyzer is a high-flux dialyzer as described in the introduction. This polysulfone membrane is a synthetic membrane with larger pore sizes than conventional cellulose membranes. The F-60S has a KUf (the ultrafiltration coefficient [volume of water removed/mm Hg across the membrane per hour of dialysis]) of 40 mL/mm Hg/hour, indicating a high ultrafiltration capability; an in vitro KoA_{urea} of 709, a measure of dialyzer efficiency for urea removal; urea clearance of 185 mL/minute at a blood flow of 200 mL/minute; and a surface area of 1.3 m^2. This information can be located in the product literature from the manufacturer or summary tables from common dialysis references.[15] These data are used to individualize the dialysis prescription for a patient.

DIALYSATE COMPOSITION

Dialysate composition usually is standardized within certain limits of electrolyte content, yet allows for individualization as necessary. Water is obtained through the public water system, which then undergoes treatment by reverse osmosis, followed by ion exchange with activated charcoal to remove contaminants, such as aluminum, copper, and chloramines, as well as bacteria and endotoxins.[21] The dialysate solution does not require sterilization because the dialysis membrane separates the blood and dialysate compartments. Nevertheless, pyrogen reactions may occur, and a greater risk may exist with high-flux membranes because of the increased pore size.

The final dialysate solution is prepared in the dialysis machine by proportioning a dialysate concentrate with the purified water, resulting in a final product, which typically contains those elements listed in Table 32-1. By adjusting electrolyte concentration in the dialysate, the efficiency of dialysis for particular chemicals can be manipulated. For example, if the patient is hyperkalemic, the dialysate contains a low concentration of potassium for diffusion of potassium from blood into dialysate. On the other hand, if the patient is normokalemic at the start of dialysis, the potassium concentration of the dialysate is set at a normal physiologic concentration to minimize flux of this electrolyte across the membrane. If the concentration of a solute is higher in the dialysate than in the blood, the net movement will be into the blood, not out.

TABLE 32-1
Electrolyte Composition of Hemodialysis and CAPD Dialysate Solutions

Solute	Hemodialysis (mEq/L)	CAPD (mEq/L)
Sodium	135–145	132
Potassium	0–4	0
Calcium	2.5–3.5	3.5
Magnesium	0.5–1.0	1.5
Chloride	100–124	102
Bicarbonate	30–38	
Lactate		35
pH	7.1–7.3	5.5

CAPD, continuous ambulatory peritoneal dialysis.

Before delivery, the dialysate is heated to 37°C to maintain body temperature and avoid hemolysis, which can occur with excessive heating. Metabolic acidosis, which is associated with ESRD because of an inability to excrete the daily obligatory load of acid, is controlled with the addition of bicarbonate buffer to the dialysate solution. Precipitation of calcium carbonate previously was a problem with the addition of bicarbonate to the dialysate, which led to the use of acetate to control acidemia instead. Acetate enters the blood compartment by diffusion from the dialysate and is metabolized to bicarbonate in vivo. Acetate, however, is associated with hypotension and cardiac instability during HD and is no longer used.[14] Improvements in delivery systems that provide for special mixing methods prevent precipitation and allow for the resumption of bicarbonate dialysis. Liquid bicarbonate concentrate and reconstituted bicarbonate-containing dialysate, however, can support the growth of gram-negative bacteria, filamentous fungi, and yeast.[22] Use of dry bicarbonate cartridges or membrane filters at the point where the dialysate leaves the machine before entering the patient's dialyzer obviates the problem of bacterial growth and contamination of the final dialysate solutions.[21,22]

Vascular Access

CASE 32-1, QUESTION 2: To achieve a sufficient blood flow for dialysis, R.W. must have a vascular site for chronic access. What are the options for chronic vascular access in R.W.?

A permanent vascular access site provides easy access to high blood flow, which cannot be achieved through routine venipuncture of superficial veins. Different types of vascular access are available: arteriovenous (AV) fistula, AV graft composed of expanded polytetrafluoroethylene, double-lumen or tunneled catheters, and catheters with subcutaneously implanted access ports. AV fistulas and grafts are placed in the nondominant arm. Ideal vascular access delivers blood flow rates necessary for chronic HD, has a long period of use, and has a low rate of complications (e.g., infection, stenosis, thrombosis, aneurysm, and limb ischemia).

An AV fistula is preferred because of its longer survival of approximately 75% at 3 years (compared with 30% for the AV graft) and low rates of complications.[23] An AV fistula is created surgically by subcutaneous anastomosis of an artery to an adjacent vein. The AV fistula may not be suitable for patients with poor vasculature, such as elderly patients or those with diabetes, atherosclerosis, or small vessels. The K/DOQI guidelines for vascular access advocate placement of a fistula at the location of the wrist (radial-cephalic), or secondarily the elbow (brachial-cephalic), as the preferred vascular access sites. If neither of these is feasible for the patient, insertion of an arteriovenous graft or creation of a transposed brachial basilica vein fistula is recommended. Once created, vascular access requires time to mature before it can be used for HD. The fistula should preferably be created 3 to 4 months before its intended use to allow the vein to mature. The graft can be used soon after insertion, although 2 weeks will allow for healing at the anastomosis sites and may prolong patency. AV fistulas fail to mature at a higher rate than grafts; however, grafts require fourfold higher interventions per year (elective angioplasty, thrombectomy, or surgical revision) to maintain long-term patency for HD.[24] Central venous catheters are discouraged for chronic vascular access.

During the dialysis procedure, one needle or catheter is placed into the fistula site to deliver blood to the dialyzer. This is often referred to as the "arterial line" to the dialyzer. Blood exiting the dialyzer is returned back to the patient's fistula site through a second catheter and needle, referred to as the "venous line" from the dialyzer.

If R.W. has adequate vasculature, a fistula should be created for chronic access. Vascular access is critical for chronic HD and often has been labeled the Achilles' heel of dialysis therapy. Complications associated with vascular access are a significant problem in patients having chronic HD. The most common is thrombosis, usually the result of venous stenosis.[7] If not treated, thromboses will result in loss of the access. Access-related complications are a major cause of hospitalization and, therefore, attention to these problems is important both clinically and economically.

ANTICOAGULATION

CASE 32-1, QUESTION 3: Recommend a reasonable anticoagulation regimen for R.W. with the initiation of his HD. What are alternatives for patients at high risk for bleeding?

Most patients having HD are anticoagulated with IV heparin during the dialysis treatment. Anticoagulation is necessary to prevent blood from clotting in the extracorporeal circuit. Several methods have been used in an attempt to provide adequate anticoagulation without increasing the risk of bleeding. Approaches include the administration of heparin in adequate quantities to anticoagulate the patient during the dialysis procedure either by intermittent bolus injections or an initial bolus followed by a continuous infusion.[25] Modern HD delivery systems have incorporated heparin infusion devices that can be programmed to provide the desired infusion rate during dialysis.

With no evidence of a bleeding disorder, recent surgery, or other risk factors for heparin anticoagulation, therapy should be initiated with a 2,000-unit bolus of IV heparin 3 to 5 minutes before initiation of dialysis, followed by an infusion of 1,200 units/hour.[25] The target activated clotting time (ACT) is 40% to 80% above the average baseline for the dialysis unit (e.g., 200–250 seconds, for normal values of 120–150 seconds). The clinician should monitor for signs of bleeding and measure the ACT at 1-hour intervals during dialysis. Heparin should be discontinued 1 hour before the end of dialysis to prevent excessive bleeding after dialysis. Using these standard doses, the estimated elimination half-life for heparin is approximately 50 minutes and it should have a linear dose–response relationship within the target ACT.[25]

Patients at increased risk of bleeding include those who have had recent surgery, retinopathy, gastrointestinal bleeding, and cerebrovascular bleeding. For these patients, the goal is to prevent clot formation within the dialysis circuit as well as to minimize the risk of active bleeding. This may be accomplished by using "minimal-dose" heparin (tight ACT control), or even heparin-free anticoagulation. The minimal-dose heparin approach individualizes therapy to achieve ACT values 40% above baseline after an initial bolus of 750 units.[25,26] The ACT is measured 3 minutes after the bolus dose, which should allow for vascular distribution of the heparin to be complete. If the goal ACT level is not achieved, repeat bolus doses of heparin can be administered at a dose that is adjusted based on the expectation of a linear response. For example, if the first dose of 750 units reaches 75% of the ACT goal, an additional 250 units would be appropriate for the second dose. Similarly, the initial heparin maintenance infusion rate of 600 units/hour can be modified by monitoring the ACT at 30-minute intervals. Adjustments in the infusion rate should be proportionate to the bolus dose needed to maintain the ACT at 40% above baseline. Samples collected for determination of ACT should be obtained from the arterial line into the dialyzer, before the infusion of heparin, to reflect systemic anticoagulation effects.

Heparin-free dialysis is an alternative to heparinization for hemodialysis patients who are at a moderate to high risk of bleeding or who are actively bleeding.[25,27] This approach requires priming the hemodialysis circuit and dialyzer with heparin 3,000 units/L in normal saline to coat the extracorporeal surfaces. The heparin-containing priming fluid is allowed to drain by filling the circuit with either the patient's blood or normal saline alone at the outset of dialysis. Next, hemodialysis is set at a high blood flow rate of 400 mL/minute, if tolerated. During dialysis, the dialyzer is flushed with normal saline every 15 to 30 minutes to rinse away microclots that may have formed. The incidence of clotting with this approach is approximately 5%.

Enoxaparin, dalteparin, and tinzaparin are low-molecular-weight heparins (LMWH) that are commercially available, but not yet approved by the US Food and Drug Administration (FDA) for hemodialysis. In a meta-analysis of 11 randomized trials, LMWH was compared with unfractionated heparin in ESRD patients undergoing either hemodialysis or hemofiltration. LMWH did not significantly affect the number of bleeding events (relative risk [RR], 0.96; 95% confidence interval [CI], 0.27–3.43) or extracorporeal circuit thrombosis (RR, 1.15; 95% CI, 0.70–1.91) compared with unfractionated heparin.[28] In a randomized, crossover study comparing the safety and efficacy of enoxaparin with standard heparin, a dose of 1.0 mg/kg body weight of enoxaparin produced less minor fibrin or clot formation in the dialyzer, but more frequent minor hemorrhage between dialyses. Dosage reduction of enoxaparin to 0.75 mg/kg body weight resulted in similar efficacy and eliminated the minor hemorrhage.[29] Differences in body weight were found to influence maximal concentrations of dalteparin. Therefore, weight-based dosing of dalteparin in patients on hemodialysis is under investigation.[30] Tinzaparin also has been shown to be effective as an anticoagulant during HD, using a weight-based IV dose of 75 international units/kg or a fixed IV dose of 2,500 international units just before dialysis.[31,32]

Although LMWH can be used to prevent clotting during HD, several factors need to be taken into account when considering LMWH for prevention and treatment of venous thromboembolism in HD patients. Because LMWH undergoes renal elimination, dose adjustments are necessary in patients with ESRD, accompanied by careful patient monitoring. Although LMWH inhibits factor X_a, factor XII_a, and kallikrein, measurement of antifactor X_a activity is the only available laboratory monitoring parameter for these factors; because active heparin metabolites that are not detected by the factor X_a assay can accumulate in dialysis patients, the clinical utility of this test is unclear.[33–35]

Another concern with LMWH is that patients on dialysis exhibit greater sensitivity to its effect than healthy volunteers.[35] Furthermore, LMWH administered at fixed-weight doses and without monitoring shows unpredictable anticoagulant effects in patients with stage 4 and 5 CKD. In a case series of patients on HD treated with LMWH for acute coronary syndrome, two patients who received as few as two to three doses of LMWH exhibited dialysis–access site bleeding, hematuria, and massive melena. Another subject who received 10 doses experienced hemorrhagic pericardial effusion resulting in death. Only one patient in the series, who received a total of five doses, did not have hemorrhagic complications.[36] Based on these findings, it is recommended that unfractionated heparin, rather than LMWH, be used in patients on dialysis for prophylaxis and treatment of thromboembolic disease.[37]

Another class of agents with potential use in patients requiring anticoagulation during HD is the direct thrombin inhibitors, argatroban and lepirudin. Their use is especially attractive in individuals who experience heparin-induced thrombocytopenia (HIT). This complication is reported to occur in 0% to 12% of patients on HD receiving heparin for anticoagulation. Argatroban is a synthetic derivative of L-arginine, which is approved by the FDA for use in patients susceptible to thrombosis who also have a history of HIT. Most dosage regimens for argatroban consist of an initial bolus dose at the start of HD followed by a continuous infusion during dialysis.[38] Because it is eliminated by nonrenal routes, argatroban dosing in patients with renal failure is the same as for patients with normal kidney function.[39] Murray et al.[40] evaluated three argatroban regimens in patients having high-flux hemodialysis. Anticoagulation was more consistently achieved (ACT >140% of baseline) when a continuous infusion of 2 mcg/kg/minute with or without a bolus of 250 mcg/kg was used. The infusion was discontinued 1 hour before the end of the HD session. Approximately 20% of argatroban was removed during HD. Argatroban therapy provided adequate, safe anticoagulation throughout HD. No thrombosis, bleeding, or other serious adverse events occurred.[40]

Another antithrombin product, lepirudin, is produced through recombinant DNA technology. It is biologically similar to hirudin, which is isolated from the saliva of leeches. Unlike argatroban, lepirudin is significantly cleared by the kidneys and infusions should be avoided or stopped in HD patients. Patients with HIT who need anticoagulation to prevent clotting during dialysis require individualized dosage adjustment based on residual renal function.[39,41] No established dosage regimens exist, because elimination is substantially delayed; monitoring should be performed using a target activated partial thromboplastin time of 2.0 to 2.5 times baseline.

Two heparinoids, danaparoid and fondaparinux, are also available for anticoagulation in patients with HIT. Danaparoid has a prolonged half-life in renal failure, therefore monitoring with anti-X_a assays is recommended.[25] Cross-reactivity with HIT antibodies has been reported in 10% of cases.[25,42] A review of 122 published outcomes of danaparoid anticoagulation in HD found that danaparoid prevented clotting in 95% of cases.[42] However, four cases of nonfatal major bleeds were reported, and four deaths (3 cases as a result of mesenteric vein thrombosis and 1 case because of pulmonary embolism) occurred in HIT patients within 48 hours of danaparoid treatment initiation. A preliminary study found that fondaparinux can be used as an anticoagulant only in patients using low-flux polysulfone dialyzers.[43] An increased risk of thrombosis occurred with high-flux dialyzers attributed to increased removal of fondaparinux resulting in inadequate anticoagulation. Further studies are necessary to define the role of these newer agents in patients on chronic HD.

The regional administration of trisodium citrate through the arterial line is an alternative to systemic anticoagulation. It binds free calcium, which is necessary for the coagulation process. The calcium citrate complex is removed by the dialysate and, based on plasma calcium values, calcium chloride is administered on the venous side to replace the citrate-bound calcium to prevent hypocalcemia or hypercalcemia. Some of the administered citrate is returned to the patient and is metabolized to bicarbonate, leading to metabolic alkalosis in some cases. Regional citrate anticoagulation is reserved for patients who are at risk for bleeding and requires additional monitoring to adjust the dual infusions.[25] In a prospective study of 1,009 consecutive high-flux dialysis procedures in 59 patients, long-term citrate anticoagulation achieved excellent anticoagulation (99.6%) with rare (0.2%) adverse effects on ionized calcium levels, electrolytes, and acid–base balance.[44]

Complications

HYPOTENSION

CASE 32-1, QUESTION 4: The dry weight for R.W. is 69.1 kg. During his most recent dialysis session, he complained of nausea and light-headedness 3 hours into the procedure. His diastolic pressure had dropped from 85 to 60 mm Hg. Ultrafiltration was discontinued, and he recovered without further event. His postdialysis weight was 69.9 kg. What are possible etiologies for his hypotension?

In addition to solute removal, the artificial kidney must be used to maintain fluid balance in the patient without renal function. Most patients will become anuric once stabilized on HD, requiring control of ingested fluids between treatment sessions. Fluid removal during dialysis then is necessary to achieve the "dry weight," or weight below which the patient could become symptomatic from volume depletion. Achieving the dry weight is accomplished by ultrafiltration, through adjustment of the transmembrane pressure. The dry weight for R.W. has been set at 69.1 kg. Below this weight, R.W. exhibited symptoms of orthostasis.

Intradialytic hypotension (IDH) can produce a variety of clinical signs and symptoms, including nausea and vomiting, dizziness, muscle cramps, and headache. The reported incidence of hypotension is 10% to 30%, and even higher in patients with specific risk factors, such as autonomic dysfunction associated with diabetes and cardiac disease. It primarily is caused by excessive fluid removal from the vascular compartment at a rate exceeding mobilization of fluid stores.[45] As a consequence, patients with an inadequate hemodynamic response to intravascular volume depletion will exhibit a decrease in blood pressure and other symptoms. An ultrafiltration rate greater than 10 mL/hour/kg was found to be associated with higher odds of IDH (odds ratio = 1.30; $p = 0.045$) and a higher risk of mortality (RR, 1.02; $p = 0.02$).[46] It may be necessary to adjust the dry weight upward if the patient is volume-depleted and symptomatic after dialysis.

Other causes of hypotension relate to rises in core body temperature.[47] Sympathetic nervous system activity increases in response to ultrafiltration leading to vasoconstriction of the dermal circulation and impaired heat dissipation. Increased central heat production can occur during the dialysis procedure. The increase in core body temperature can overcome peripheral vasoconstriction resulting in hypotension. Excessive heating of dialysate can also produce vasodilation. Cooling of the dialysate to slightly below body temperature may correct this problem, although many patients are uncomfortable and do not tolerate the cooling effect. The use of acetate as the buffer in the dialysate has been associated with hypotension because of its direct vasodilating effects, but it is no longer used. Antihypertensive therapy before dialysis may exacerbate hypotensive episodes as well; in some patients, these drugs may need to be withheld until after the dialysis session. Immediate treatment of the hypotensive episode can be accomplished by placing the patient in the Trendelenburg position (bed positioned with legs raised and head lowered), administering a small (100 mL) bolus of normal saline into the venous blood line, and reducing the ultrafiltration rate.

Several pharmacologic agents have been proposed for the management of IDH, including ephedrine, fludrocortisone, caffeine, vasopressin, L-carnitine, sertraline, and midodrine. Perazella[48] reviewed these agents for their potential use in the treatment of IDH and concluded that only midodrine, sertraline, and L-carnitine show potential benefit in patients. Midodrine is an oral prodrug that is converted to desglymidodrine, a selective α_1-agonist. Doses of 10 to 20 mg, 30 minutes before dialysis are effective for most patients, but the presence of active myocardial ischemia is a major contraindication.[48] Sertraline is a selective serotonin reuptake inhibitor that has shown promise in IDH at daily doses of 50 to 100 mg/day. The mechanism is proposed to be through attenuation of paradoxical sympathetic withdrawal. L-Carnitine has also been tried for treatment of IDH with IV doses of 20 mg/kg at dialysis. Its mechanism of action is not known, but it may be related to improvements in vascular smooth muscle and cardiac functioning.[48] However, a meta-analysis of five studies examining the role of L-carnitine supplementration for IDH failed to confirm a benefit.[49]

Because the volume status of R.W. is associated with his weight, another consideration is a change in his lean mass. R.W. has noted an improvement in his appetite lately and, as a result, added a few extra pounds. It is important to consider "real" weight changes when assessing the dry weight and volume status. Without appropriately increasing the dry weight goal to compensate for his real weight gain, R.W. became volume depleted and hypotensive. His dry weight should be adjusted upward to the point at which he no longer is symptomatic (to ~70 kg).

CASE 32-1, QUESTION 5: What other hemodialysis-related complications must be watched for and how can they be treated?

MUSCLE CRAMPS

Perhaps also related to fluid shifts, muscle cramps experienced during dialysis may be induced by excessive ultrafiltration resulting in altered perfusion of the affected tissues. Several treatments have been attempted, including reduced ultrafiltration and infusion of hypertonic saline or glucose to improve circulation.[50,51] Exercise and stretching of the affected limbs also may be beneficial. Long-term therapy may be directed at prevention with the use of vitamin E 400 international units at bedtime.[52] Vitamin E in combination with vitamin C 250 mg daily has been found to be more effective than either therapy alone.[53] Vitamin C therapy, however, is known to produce hyperoxaluria, oxalate-containing urinary stones, and renal damage. Therefore, the long-term safety of vitamin C in hemodialysis patients needs to be evaluated. Quinine sulfate is no longer available for use in leg cramps. It is associated with a number of serious adverse events, some of which are potentially fatal. In the mid-1990s, the FDA banned over-the-counter availability of quinine, and in February 2007 the FDA banned prescription quinine products for leg cramps.

HYPERSENSITIVITY

Reports of anaphylactic reactions to dialyzer membranes, particularly on initial exposure, may be directly related to the membrane itself, or to ethylene oxide, which is commonly used to sterilize the dialyzer.[54,55] Membranes most commonly responsible for reactions are unsubstituted cellulose membranes (bioincompatible) or the high-flux polyacrylonitrile membrane when used in conjunction with angiotensin-converting enzyme inhibitors.[56] This latter reaction is thought to be related to the inhibition of bradykinin metabolism by angiotensin-converting enzyme inhibitors, resulting in an anaphylactoid reaction.

DIALYSIS DISEQUILIBRIUM

Dialysis disequilibrium is a syndrome that has been recognized since the initiation of HD more than 30 years ago. Its etiology is related to cerebral edema, and patients new to HD are at a greater risk because of the accumulation of urea.[57] Rapid removal of urea from the extracellular space lowers plasma osmolality, thereby leading to a shift of free water into the brain. Lowering of intracellular pH, as can occur during dialysis, has also been suggested as a cause. Clinical manifestations occur during or shortly after dialysis and include central nervous system effects, such as headache, nausea, altered vision, and in some cases, seizures and coma. Treatment is aimed at prevention by initiating dialysis gradually by using shorter treatment times at lower blood flow rates in new patients. Direct therapy can be provided in the form of IV hypertonic saline or mannitol.[57]

THROMBOSIS

CASE 32-1, QUESTION 6: R.W.'s physician is considering use of a twice daily combination product containing extended-release dipyridamole 200 mg/aspirin 25 mg to prevent platelet clots in R.W.'s HD access site and to reduce the risk of stroke. Is this an appropriate choice of treatment?

Dialysis access loss is most often the result of thrombosis, which is usually a consequence of venous stenosis. Prospective monitoring of access function (e.g., intra-access flow; static or dynamic venous pressures; measurement of access recirculation; and physical findings, such as swelling of the arm, clotting of the graft, prolonged bleeding after needle removal, or altered character of the pulse or thrill) is paramount to the prevention of thrombosis. Fistula patency generally is much greater than synthetic graft patency, although thrombosis and loss of function may occur in both.[7,24] The stenosis may be corrected by percutaneous transluminal angioplasty or, if necessary, surgical revision of the access site. Successful correction is effective as a means to prevent thrombosis. Once it occurs, thrombosis is managed by surgical thrombectomy or with pharmacomechanical or mechanical thrombolysis.[24]

If clotting occurs, a number of thrombolytic protocols exist, and selection is determined by the degree of catheter malfunction.[58] Alteplase and reteplase appear to be effective for thrombomechanical lysis of the vascular access site.[59,60] Life-threatening adverse events have been associated with streptokinase, and urokinase was withdrawn from the US market because of viral contamination. Thrombolytic therapy should be avoided in those patients with an increased risk of bleeding.

Anticoagulants and antiplatelet agents have been evaluated in the prevention of graft thrombosis. A large, multicenter, randomized, placebo-controlled trial found a modest effect of extended-release dipyridamole and low-dose aspirin in reducing HD graft stenosis during the period immediately after graft placement, and improving patency duration by 6 weeks.[61] Bleeding occurred at a similar rate (12%) in the treatment and placebo groups. In two separate randomized, placebo-controlled trials, therapy with low-dose warfarin to achieve a target international normalized ratio of 1.4 to 1.9 or combination therapy with clopidogrel and aspirin in patients with polytetrafluoroethylene grafts showed no benefit in the prevention of thrombosis or prolongation of graft survival.[62,63] In both studies, patients receiving active treatment experienced a significantly increased risk of bleeding. A small single-center, randomized, placebo-controlled clinical trial found that fish oil reduced graft thrombosis,[64] and a larger, multicenter trial is underway.[65]

Based on these studies, extended-release dipyridamole 200 mg–aspirin 25 mg is not an appropriate therapy for R.W. Although short term use of this regimen after initial placement of the HD graft may reduce graft thrombosis and improve patency, there is no indication for continued use as prophylaxis after the graft has matured and dialysis has begun. Use for stroke prevention is only for patients with a history of prior transient ischemic attacks or strokes.

INFECTION

CASE 32-1, QUESTION 7: Should R.W. be given prophylactic antibiotics (e.g., cefazolin with each dialysis) to avoid graft infection?

Access infections, usually involving grafts to a greater extent than a native fistula, are predominantly caused by *Staphylococcus aureus* or *Staphylococcus epidermidis*. Infections with gram-negative organisms as well as *Enterococcus* species occur with a lower frequency.[7] Access infections can lead to bacteremia and sepsis with or without local signs of infection.

There is no evidence that prophylactic antibiotics are of value; to the contrary, indiscriminate use of antibiotics could lead to colonization with resistant organisms. Thus, R.W. should not receive a prophylactic antibiotic. However, if evidence of infection is present, a prompt response is important. Treatment usually is initiated with vancomycin, administered as a single, 1-g dose, repeated as necessary, depending on the type of dialysis being used, or cefazolin 20 mg/kg three times weekly, and gentamicin 2 mg/kg with appropriate serum concentration monitoring.[66] High-flux dialysis results in greater removal of vancomycin than conventional dialysis and, therefore, more than a single dose may be necessary for adequate treatment.[67,68] Vancomycin can be given either during or after high-flux dialysis. A vancomycin post-dialysis dosing algorithm using fewer plasma vancomycin concentration measurements for patients receiving thrice-weekly high-flux dialysis was developed by Pai et al.[69] The algorithm achieved predialysis vancomycin concentrations comparable to those found with more frequent monitoring. Cost savings was realized because of a 70% reduction in the number of drug concentration measurements. Intradialytic dosing of vancomycin is a convenient mode of drug administration in patients receiving high-flux dialysis. It avoids the need for additional intravenous access, longer stays in the hemodialysis unit, or home antibiotic administration. Two studies have shown that vancomycin dosing in the last 1 to 2 hours of high-flux hemodialysis achieves adequate predialysis plasma concentrations of 5 to 20 mcg/mL depending on the administered dose.[70,71] K/DOQI clinical practice guidelines for vascular access also advocate surgical incision and resection of infected grafts. Fistula infections are rare and should be treated as subacute bacterial endocarditis with 6 weeks of antibiotic therapy.[7]

Other long-term complications associated with HD include aluminum toxicity, amyloidosis, and malnutrition.

ALUMINUM TOXICITY

Aluminum accumulation in patients having HD was a significant problem before water sources were adequately treated to remove aluminum. Major complications of aluminum toxicity include dementia, aluminum bone disease, and anemia. Aluminum accumulation still occurs in patients treated with aluminum-containing antacids as binding agents for phosphate in the gastrointestinal tract, although not to the degree associated with water supplies.[72] (See Chapter 31, Chronic Kidney Diseases, for further discussion.) Aluminum toxicity is diagnosed by clinical signs and symptoms associated with the aforementioned conditions, and a serum aluminum concentration of greater than 200 ng/mL or a deferoxamine-stimulated serum aluminum concentration increase of greater than 200 ng/mL.[73] Deferoxamine chelates with serum aluminum and the shift in equilibrium results in movement of aluminum from tissue storage sites. The complex can be removed by dialysis (600 Da), and high-flux membranes are capable of removing the complexed aluminum in a single dialysis session, minimizing systemic exposure to deferoxamine and its potential adverse effects. The latter include mucormycosis, a fungal infection caused by a rhizopus that grows avidly in iron media, as well as ocular, auditory, and neurologic toxicity.[74,75] Deferoxamine generally is continued until the stimulated aluminum concentration is less than 50 ng/mL, which may require 1 year of therapy.[76]

AMYLOIDOSIS

Amyloidosis is caused by the deposition of β_2-microglobulin–containing amyloid in joints and soft tissues over prolonged periods.[77] The incidence of amyloidosis is approximately 50% after 12 years of dialysis and nearly 100% after 20 years. β_2-Microglobulin (molecular weight, 11,800 Da) normally is eliminated by filtration and metabolism in the intact nephron. Renal failure leads to reduced elimination and accumulation of this substance even during dialysis. High-flux membranes are more effective than conventional membranes for the removal of β_2-microglobulin. Carpal tunnel syndrome, manifested as weakness and soreness in the thumb from pressure on the median nerve, is the most common symptom. Bone cysts also appear along with joint deposition of amyloid, which can lead to substantial disability as a result of chronic arthralgias and joint immobility.[77] The type of membrane used for dialysis also has been implicated in increasing the rate of production of β_2-microglobulin, in that some types seem to cause more rapid amyloid deposition. Biocompatible membranes are proposed to stimulate production to a lesser degree, but prospective studies demonstrating their long-term benefit have not been conducted.[78]

MALNUTRITION

Chronic kidney disease produces a catabolic state in patients and, along with the multifactorial complications of ESRD, leads to malnutrition. Serum albumin concentrations less than 3.0 g/dL are associated with an increased mortality rate compared with higher values. Inadequate dietary intake and losses of amino acids by dialysis contribute to protein malnutrition, which in turn can lead to additional complications, such as impaired wound healing, susceptibility to infection, and others (see Chapter 31, Chronic Kidney Diseases, for further discussion).

L-CARNITINE

L-Carnitine supplementation has been advocated in patients with ESRD to relieve intradialytic symptoms. It is a metabolic cofactor that facilitates transport of long-chain fatty acids into the mitochondria for energy production. This cofactor is found in both plasma and tissue as free carnitine, the active component, or bound to fatty acids as acylcarnitine. The primary source of carnitine is dietary intake, primarily from red meat and dairy products. Patients with renal failure may have what appear to be normal or elevated total carnitine concentrations but low levels of free carnitine. Accumulation of acylcarnitine, decreased carnitine synthesis, reduced dietary intake, and dialytic losses may account for the normal to elevated total concentrations in this population.[79,80]

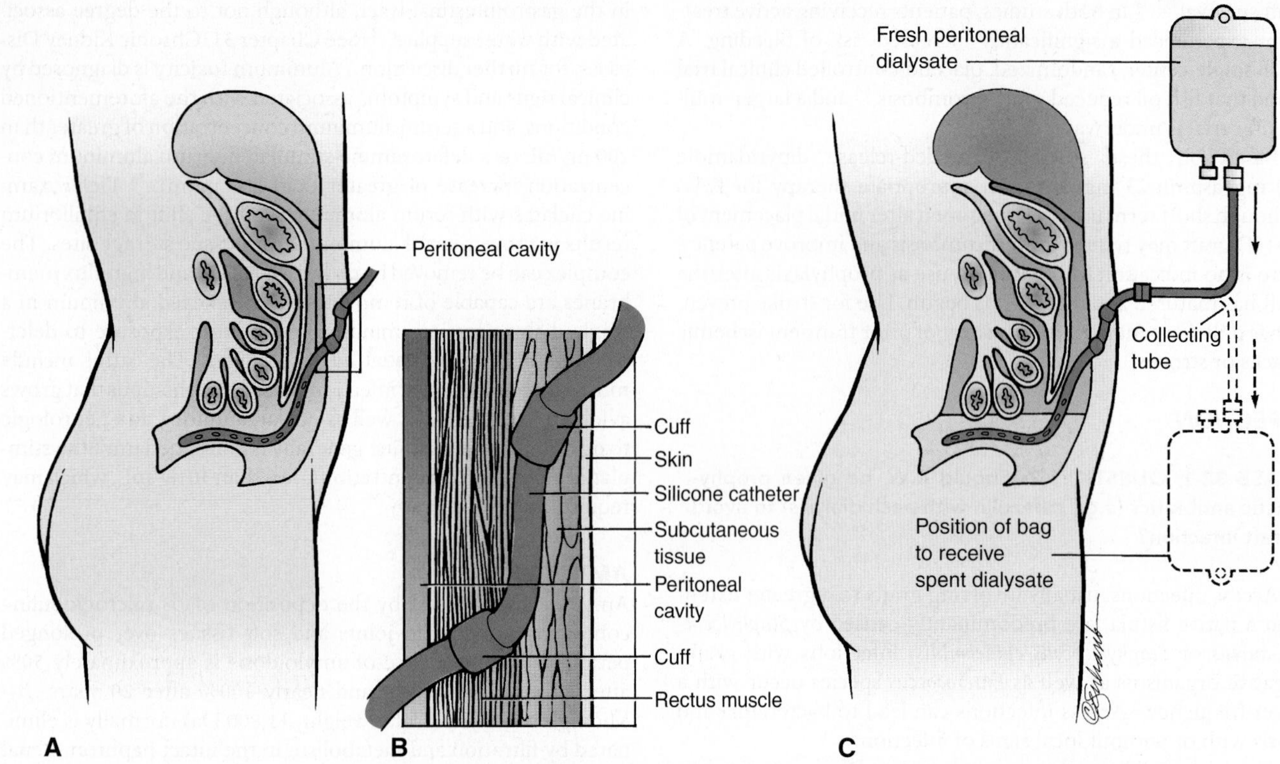

FIGURE 32-2 Continuous ambulatory peritoneal dialysis. (A) The peritoneal catheter is implanted through the abdominal wall. **(B)** Dacron cuffs and a subcutaneous tunnel provide protection against bacterial infection. **(C)** Dialysate flows by gravity through the peritoneal catheter into the peritoneal cavity. After a prescribed period of time, the fluid is drained by gravity and discarded. New solution is then infused into the peritoneal cavity until the next drainage period. Dialysis thus continues on a 24-hour-a-day basis during which the patient is free to move around and engage in his or her usual activities. Adapted with permission from Smeltzer SC, Bare BG. *Textbook of Medical-Surgical Nursing*. 9th ed. Philadelphia, PA: Lippincott Williams & Wilkins; 2000.

Carnitine is a small water-soluble molecule that is freely dialyzed, thus its levels are reduced in hemodialysis. The potential benefits of correcting this relative carnitine deficiency have been primarily studied in patients having chronic HD. Recommended doses of carnitine are 10 to 20 mg/kg IV after each HD treatment. Although some have suggested that carnitine supplementation benefits muscle cramps and hypotension during dialysis (as well as minimizing fatigue, skeletal muscle weakness, cardiomyopathy, and anemia resistant to large doses of erythropoietic therapy), no evidence supports its routine use in patients undergoing chronic HD.[13,49,81]

PERITONEAL DIALYSIS

Peritoneal dialysis is performed using several different modalities, including the most common, CAPD. Development of specialized devices to facilitate the exchange process and improve patient convenience has led to processes referred to as APD, including continuous cycling peritoneal dialysis (CCPD) and nocturnal intermittent dialysis (NIPD). CAPD is the most common method for chronic PD, but the APD methods are rapidly growing in popularity. Although lower rates of peritonitis are observed in APD compared with CAPD,[82] other outcomes measures, such as need for transition to HD and mortality, are similar between the two modalities.[83]

Principles and Transport Processes

Continuous ambulatory peritoneal dialysis is performed by the instillation of 2 to 3 L of sterile dialysate solution into the peritoneal cavity through a surgically placed resident catheter. The solution dwells within the cavity for 4 to 8 hours, and then is drained and replaced with a fresh solution. This process of fill, dwell, and drain is performed three to four times during the day, with an overnight dwell by the patient in his or her normal home or work environment (Fig. 32-2). Conceptually, the process is similar to HD in that uremic toxins are removed by diffusion down a concentration gradient across a membrane into the dialysate solution. In this case, the peritoneal membrane covering the abdominal contents serves as an endogenous dialysis membrane, and the vasculature embedded in the peritoneum serves as the blood supply to equilibrate with the dialysate. A primary difference is that because the dialysate solution is resident, the result is a very slow dialysate flow rate of approximately 7 mL/minute when 10 L of fluid is drained per day. Solute loss occurs by diffusion for small molecules, and through convection for larger, middle molecules.

BLOOD AND DIALYSATE FLOW

Hemodialysis provides constant perfusion of fresh dialysate, thereby maintaining a large concentration gradient across the dialysis membrane throughout the dialysis treatment. During a typical dwell period for CAPD, urea and other substances increase in the dialysate relative to unbound plasma concentrations. For a daytime dwell period of 4 hours, urea achieves nearly equal concentrations with plasma; therefore, the rate of elimination can become very small (Fig. 32-3). Instillation of fresh dialysate solution will re-establish the diffusion gradient leading to an increased rate of urea removal. For a patient making four exchanges of 2 L each per day, assuming the urea dialysate concentration equals the plasma concentration, and 2 L are removed by ultrafiltration, the urea clearance would be approximately 7 mL/minute. This is substantially lower than urea

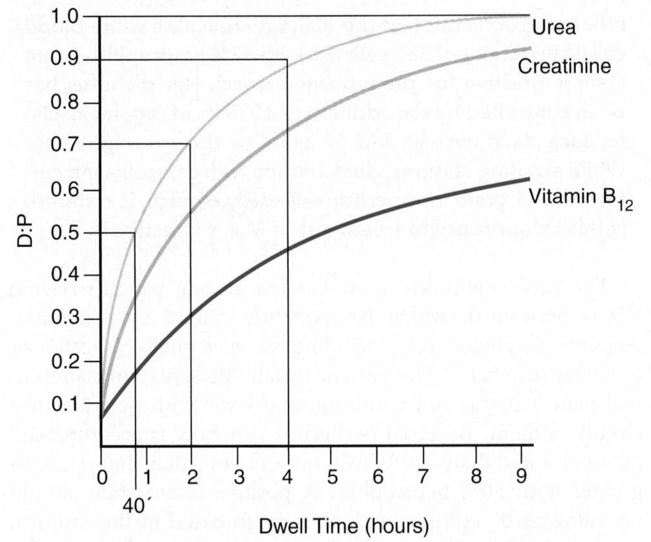

FIGURE 32-3 Rate of entry into peritoneal dialysate of urea, creatinine, and vitamin B_{12}. The *y*-axis indicates the ratio of dialysate to plasma concentration (D:P). Reprinted with permission from Blake PG et al. Physiology of peritoneal dialysis. In: Daugirdas JT et al, eds. *Handbook of Dialysis*. 4th ed. Philadelphia, PA: Lippincott Williams & Wilkins; 2007:332.

clearances achieved with HD; therefore, CAPD must be performed continually (daily) throughout the week to achieve adequate urea removal. Clearance depends on blood flow; dialysate flow; and peritoneal membrane characteristics such as size, permeability, and thickness. Dialysate flow, the only easily adjusted variable to alter clearance, has been used effectively in acute PD to achieve relatively high clearances with 30-minute to 60-minute dwell periods in a cycling system. CCPD uses this concept of shorter dwell periods during the sleeping hours with automatic fill, dwell, and drain periods, leaving a high-dextrose dialysate in the peritoneal cavity throughout the day until the next cycling session. NIPD is similar, with nightly exchanges, but the peritoneum is left unfilled, or dry, during the daytime. As a result, urea clearance is lower with NIPD, but may be suitable for many patients, and preferable to the volume load in the peritoneal cavity throughout the day with CCPD.[84] Electrolyte concentrations in the dialysate solution are near physiologic concentrations to prevent substantial shifts in serum electrolyte levels (Table 32-1). A potential advantage of PD compared with HD is the continuous dialysis of larger, middle molecules that have been implicated as a possible source of toxic effects. These molecules are cleared through convection and follow water as it is removed through ultrafiltration. Clearance of these molecules depends less on flow and more on duration of dialysis. The continuous process of PD, albeit associated with low clearance values, provides for a more physiologic condition in patients, rather than the intermittent treatment provided with HD.

FLUID REMOVAL

Fluid is removed by ultrafiltration through adjustment of the transmembrane pressure during HD. Because this pressure is not easily adjusted in PD, fluid is removed by altering the osmotic pressure within the dialysate. This is accomplished by the addition of dextrose monohydrate to the dialysate in varying concentrations, depending on the degree of fluid removal necessary in the patient. Concentrations of dextrose in commercially available solutions include 1.5%, 2.5%, and 4.25%, with net fluid losses during a 4-hour dwell period of 200 mL and 400 mL for the 1.5% and 2.5% solutions, respectively, and approximately 700 mL for the 4.25% solution after an overnight dwell.[85] As the dwell time persists, the dextrose is absorbed and is diluted by the movement of fluid from the vascular space, so that most ultrafiltration occurs early during the dwell period.

Acid–base balance is achieved through the absorption of lactate from the dialysate, which subsequently is metabolized to bicarbonate in vivo. Bicarbonate is not compatible with the calcium and magnesium in the dialysate and can lead to precipitation.

Access

Delivery of dialysate into the peritoneal cavity is accomplished through an indwelling catheter inserted through the abdominal wall. The most common design is the Tenckhoff catheter, made of silicone rubber or polyurethane; it consists of a tube, straight or curled, with many holes in the distal end for fluid inflow and outflow.[86] The catheter also has a single or double cuff, which serves to anchor it to the internal and external attachment sites by promoting fibrous tissue growth; this also serves as a barrier to bacterial migration. Several modifications to the original catheter have appeared on the market, mostly in an attempt to overcome problems related to outflow of dialysate. Maintaining an unobstructed outlet port is essential for successful PD.

Delivery of dialysate through the catheter is accomplished in several modes. A straight transfer set uses tubing attached to the catheter at one end, and to the bag of dialysate at the other, via a spike. The transfer set usually is changed every 1 to 2 months in the dialysis clinic. For each dialysate exchange, the patient attaches a bag of fresh dialysate, warmed to body temperature, to the transfer set and infuses the solution. The tubing is clamped and rolled up with the attached bag and placed into a pouch carried on the patient. The primary purpose for maintaining the connection is to prevent contamination and the development of peritonitis. After the dwell period, the patient unrolls the bag and tubing, places it on the floor, unclamps the tubing and awaits drainage of the fluid, usually 5 to 15 minutes. Using aseptic technique, the patient changes the dialysate bag and infuses fresh solution to repeat the process. This process is used rarely today and has been replaced by Y sets and double-bag systems. The Y transfer set uses three limbs, with fresh dialysate attached to the upper arm of the Y, an empty bag to the lower arm, and the stem connected to the catheter.[86] Clamping the inflow arm and opening the stem and outflow arm allow dialysate to drain from the peritoneum into the empty bag. Reversing the clamps then permits infusion of the fresh dialysate solution after a small rinse of the line is performed with the fresh solution. Clamping of the catheter allows removal of the Y transfer set and bags from the patient. The double-bag system uses preattached bags to both limbs and the patient and makes only a single connection to the catheter. Use of the Y transfer set has reduced episodes of peritonitis from approximately one for every 9 to 12 patient-months to one for every 24 to 36 patient-months.[87] PD performed with the cycler involves only two disconnections of the system, compared with four for CAPD.

Dialysis Prescription

CASE 32-2

QUESTION 1: M.J., a 27-year-old woman, has a 14-year history of insulin-dependent diabetes mellitus. She is 5 feet, 5 inches tall and weighs 60 kg. One complication of her diabetes is ESRD necessitating dialysis. She has been

undergoing CAPD for 1 year and, until now, has done well without any complications. Her dialysis prescription consists of three exchanges with 1.5% dextrose during the day and a fourth, overnight exchange with 4.25% dextrose. She has a double-cuff Tenckhoff catheter and uses a Y transfer set for her exchanges. Her blood pressure is controlled and she shows no evidence of edema. She has no residual renal function. What is the purpose of the addition of 1.5% dextrose to M.J.'s dialysate? Why would the concentration of dextrose be increased to as high as 4.25% in some situations?

The initial CAPD prescription for most patients consists of three exchanges during the day with 1.5% dextrose and a fourth, overnight, exchange with 4.25% dextrose. This would be expected to achieve fluid removal of approximately 1,300 mL, based on 200 mL from each daytime exchange and 700 mL overnight. Based on assessment of the patient's fluid status, it may be necessary to increase or decrease the dialysate prescription to achieve fluid balance. Fluid retention is solved by increasing the dextrose content of the daytime exchanges, beginning with 2.5% in place of one of the 1.5% solutions. This is expected to result in an additional removal of 200 mL, and therapy can be further adjusted as necessary. For patients with excessive fluid removal, it may be possible to decrease the number of exchanges per day as long as adequate solute removal is present. If four exchanges are needed, the fluid intake can be liberalized to maintain adequate hydration.

Cycler machines automatically cycle dialysate into and out of the peritoneal cavity. Patients having CCPD will generally need three to five exchanges, each lasting approximately 2 hours, using a cycler while the patient sleeps. During the daytime hours, the patient maintains a reservoir of dialysate in the peritoneal cavity resulting in a long dwell. The cycler process repeats at night. Six to eight exchanges are performed every night for patients having NIPD. The peritoneum is left dry and patients do not continue dialysis during the day. Nightly dwell times are generally 1 to 2 hours for each exchange, resulting in a higher clearance for small molecules because of the increased dialysate flow rate.[84]

Dextrose is the dextrorotatory form of glucose. Glucose is a small molecule that rapidly diffuses across the peritoneal membrane. As glucose is absorbed, the osmotic gradient of the dwell progressively dissipates, reducing ultrafiltration. Toward the end of the long dwell, more dialysate fluid may be absorbed than ultrafiltered, resulting in a negative net ultrafiltration volume where the drained volume is less than the infused volume. A negative net ultrafiltration volume is undesirable. Greater ultrafiltration and fluid management are predictors of survival.[88]

An alternative to dextrose as the osmotic agent in the dialysate solution is icodextrin, a starch-derived, water-soluble, glucose polymer that is approximately 40% absorbed and subsequently metabolized to maltose oligosaccharides. Icodextrin is approved for use in the United States in patients having CAPD or APD during the long dwell period. Unlike glucose, icodextrin does not readily diffuse across the peritoneal membrane, but is slowly removed from the peritoneal cavity via convective uptake into the peritoneal lymphatics.[89] It is superior to 1.5%, 2.5%, and 4.25% dextrose solutions for ultrafiltration.[90,91] Its use may be most beneficial in those patients characterized as high average to high transporters.

PERITONITIS

CASE 32-2, QUESTION 2: M.J. now presents to the dialysis clinic with complaints of abdominal tenderness and cloudy effluent. Examination of the dialysate reveals a white blood cell (WBC) count of 330 cells/μL with 62% neutrophils. Gram stain is positive for gram-positive cocci. Her diabetes has been controlled by the addition of 10 units of regular insulin to each daytime bag and 15 units to the overnight bag. While awaiting cultures, dual therapy with cefazolin and ceftazidime, 1 gram intraperitoneally daily of each, is ordered. Is this an appropriate treatment of M.J.'s infection?

The most significant complication among patients having PD is peritonitis, which is frequently caused by coagulase-negative staphylococci, including *S. epidermidis* (39.9%) or *S. aureus* (21.6%).[92] The patient usually presents with abdominal pain, nausea, and vomiting, and fever with or without a cloudy effluent. Bacterial peritonitis generally is accompanied by an elevated dialysate WBC count greater than 100/μL with greater than 50% neutrophils. A positive Gram stain should be followed by culture, with therapy initiated in the interim. For lower cell counts or negative Gram stain, a culture should be obtained followed by treatment for positive cultures and continued observation for negative results. Specific consensus recommendations of the Advisory Committee on Peritonitis Management of the International Society for Peritoneal Dialysis are located at http://www.ispd.org.[93] These guidelines were first published in 1983 and revised in 1989, 1993, 1996, 2000, and 2005. The initial focus of the International Society for Peritoneal Dialysis recommendations was the treatment of peritonitis and exit-site infections. The most recent guidelines stress the importance of prevention.

Empiric antibiotics must cover both gram-positive and gram-negative organisms.[93] The increasing prevalence of vancomycin-resistant organisms has resulted in a shift in empiric therapy away from vancomycin, toward first-generation cephalosporins (cefazolin or cephalothin). Without a Gram stain, therapy should be initiated with a combination of cefazolin or cephalothin (to cover gram-positive organisms) and ceftazidime (to cover gram-negative organisms), coadministered in the same dialysate solution at a dose of 1 g/bag for both drugs, once daily, given intraperitoneally.[94] Separate syringes must be used to add the antibiotics to dialysis solutions. An aminoglycoside can be used in place of ceftazidime, but it is not recommended initially, in an attempt to preserve residual renal function. Gentamicin, tobramycin, or netilmicin are given at doses of 0.6 mg/kg/bag, once daily, and for amikacin, 2 mg/kg/bag once daily. Antibiotics should be allowed to dwell for at least 6 hours.[93] In addition to antibiotics, heparin 500 to 1,000 units/L may be added to each exchange to prevent the formation of fibrin clots, which can result in catheter failure.[94] Subsequent antibiotic therapy should be based on culture and sensitivity results, incorporating specific dosage regimens based on the treatment guidelines.[94]

This is M.J.'s first episode of peritonitis. The most likely pathogen, a *Staphylococcus* species, is consistent with the positive Gram stain. Her treatment should consist of monotherapy with cefazolin (or cephalothin) one gram daily intraperitoneally as ordered. Ceftazadime should be discontinued. Vancomycin should not be used for empiric therapy. Instead, it should be reserved for methicillin-resistant *S. aureus* infections or methicillin-resistant *S. epidermidis* if M.J. does not respond to empiric therapy.

CASE 32-2, QUESTION 3: A new order is written to add heparin to M.J.'s dialysate fluid. What is the reason for this? She is also receiving insulin intraperitoneally. Is this appropriate or should she be switched to subcutaneous insulin?

Heparin 1,000 units/L should be added to the dialysate to prevent fibrin clots from forming and obstructing outflow from the peritoneal cavity. Her blood glucose should be monitored, because infection causes insulin resistance and peritonitis will increase glucose and insulin absorption. Inability to control the blood glucose concentration may require temporary discontinuation of the intraperitoneal (IP) insulin and administration by another route. Also see Case 32-2, Question 7, for other considerations regarding insulin dosing.

CASE 32-2, QUESTION 4: If M.J. was receiving APD instead of CAPD, would the treatment of her infection be different?

For patients having APD, the choice of first-line antibiotics is the same as for CAPD because the likely organisms are similar. Drug dosage regimens, however, can differ because patients having CCPD or NIPD undergo PD only during the nighttime hours, and those having NIPD do not have residual peritoneal fluid during the day. For aminoglycoside antibiotics, once-daily dosing is preferred for the foregoing reasons, as well as their longer duration of action because of the postantibiotic effect (see Chapter 31, Chronic Kidney Diseases). Vancomycin and other glycopeptides can be administered intermittently because of their prolonged elimination half-life in patients with ESRD. Because of the lack of clinical trials with other antibiotics in patients having APD, extrapolation from the CAPD literature may be necessary. A review addresses the current knowledge and issues surrounding the pharmacokinetics of antibiotics in patients with peritonitis undergoing APD.[95]

EXIT-SITE INFECTION: PROPHYLAXIS

CASE 32-2, QUESTION 5: Catheter site exit infections are a significant risk factor for developing peritonitis. Would it be appropriate to incorporate mupirocin cream into M.J.'s catheter care routine? Would gentamicin cream be a better alternative?

Prevention of catheter exit-site infections (and thus peritonitis) is the primary goal of exit-site care.[93] Several preventative measures are important: adequate catheter placement, dedicated postoperative catheter care, and routine daily care of the exit site. Dressing changes of a newly placed catheter are done by a dialysis nurse using sterile technique until the exit site is well healed, which can take up to 2 weeks. Once the exit site is well healed, the patient is educated and trained to do routine exit-site care. Routine care consists of thorough handwashing with antibacterial soap before touching the exit site. Antiseptics that contain at least 60% ethanol or isopropyl alcohol can be used to augment handwashing.[96] The exit site is then washed daily with antibacterial soap, although use of an antiseptic (e.g., povidone iodine or chlorhexidine) is a reasonable option.[93] Hydrogen peroxide should be avoided as a routine antiseptic because it causes drying. After daily cleansing, antimicrobial creams (e.g., mupirocin, gentamicin) are applied around the catheter exit site using a cotton swab. Mupirocin ointment, not the cream, can cause structural damage to polyurethane catheters, and should be avoided in patients with these catheters.[93]

Catheter exit-site infections are most often caused by *S. aureus* and *Pseudomonas* species.[97] In a randomized, double-blind trial, gentamicin sulfate 0.1% cream was found to be as effective as mupirocin 2% cream in preventing *S. aureus* infections.[98] Gentamicin cream was also highly effective in reducing *Pseudomonas aeruginosa* and other gram-negative catheter infections, whereas mupirocin cream was not. A longer time to first catheter infection and a reduction in peritonitis, particularly gram-negative organisms, was also seen with gentamicin use. For these reasons, daily gentamicin cream at the exit site is considered to be the prophylaxis of choice in patients having PD and would be the preferred treatment for M.J.[98] Finally, the catheter should be immobilized with a small gauze dressing and tape to prevent pulling and trauma to the exit site, which may lead to infection.

EXIT-SITE INFECTION: TREATMENT

CASE 32-2, QUESTION 6: If M.J. were to exhibit an exit-site infection despite appropriate cathether care, could oral therapy be used or is intraperitonal therapy required?

Empiric therapy for exit-site infections may be started immediately, and should always cover *S. aureus*. Oral antibiotic therapy has been shown to be as effective as IP therapy.[93] Local erythema alone can be treated with topical agents, whereas purulent drainage indicates more significant infection and the need for systemic antibiotics.[94] Hypertonic saline dressings, as well as oral antibiotic therapy, can be used for especially severe exit-site infections.[93] Hypertonic saline is prepared by adding 1 tablespoon of salt to 1 pint (500 mL) of sterile water. The solution is then applied to gauze and wrapped around the catheter exit site for 15 minutes, once or twice a day. Gram-positive organisms are treated with first-generation oral cephalosporins, a penicillinase-resistant penicillin, or trimethoprim-sulfamethoxazole. A 1-week course of rifampin may be added at 600 mg/day orally (in single or split dose) for nonresponding infections with positive cultures after 1 week of appropriate therapy. Rifampin monotherapy treatment of *S. aureus* should be avoided. In areas where tuberculosis is endemic, rifampin should also be avoided in the treatment of *S. aureus* to reserve this drug for treatment of tuberculosis.[93] Oral quinolone antibiotics are recommended as first-line agents in the treatment of *P. aeruginosa* exit-site infections. *P. aeruginosa* infections are difficult to treat and often require prolonged therapy with two antibiotics.[93] If the infection is slow to resolve or if in cases of a recurrence, a second antipseudomonal drug can be added (e.g., ceftazidime IP). Gram-negative organisms can be treated with ciprofloxacin 500 mg orally twice daily.[94] Scheduling of the quinolone dose is important so that coadministration with foods or other drug therapies that may chelate the quinolone in the gut is avoided. Potentially chelating agents include calcium products, iron, multivitamins, antacids, zinc, sucralfate, and dairy products. Antibiotic therapy should be continued for a minimum of 2 weeks until the exit site appears entirely normal.

WEIGHT GAIN

CASE 32-2, QUESTION 7: M.J. is noted to have gained weight since starting peritoneal dialysis. Besides fluid retention, what other possible cause is there for the weight gain? How might this affect her insulin requirements?

Dextrose is present in dialysate solutions primarily to serve as an osmotic agent for the removal of fluid during each exchange. Higher concentrations are expected to result in greater fluid removal. Approximately 500 to 1,000 kcal/day are absorbed as glucose from PD solutions, which can lead to weight gain in patients. Some patients may require modification of oral caloric intake to avoid excessive weight gain. Insulin requirements generally are increased in patients with diabetes as a result of the additional calories and, when administered IP, usually are two to three times the normal subcutaneous dose because of their reduced bioavailability of 20% to 50% by this route. Also see Case 32-2, Question 3, for other considerations regarding insulin dosing.

KEY REFERENCES AND WEBSITES

A full list of references for this chapter can be found at **http://thepoint.lww.com/AT10e.** Below are the key references and websites for this chapter, with the corresponding reference number in this chapter found in parentheses after the reference.

Key References

[No authors listed]. NKF-K/DOQI Clinical Practice Guidelines for Chronic Kidney Disease: Evaluation, Classification, and Stratification. *Am J Kidney Dis*. 2002;39:S1. (1)

[No authors listed]. NKF-K/DOQI Clinical Practice Guidelines for Hemodialysis Adequacy: Update 2006. *Am J Kidney Dis*. 2006;48(Suppl 1):S2. (5)

[No authors listed]. NKF-K/DOQI Clinical Practice Guidelines for Peritoneal Dialysis Adequacy: Update 2006. *Am J Kidney Dis*. 2006;48(Suppl 1):S91. (6)

[No authors listed]. NKF-K/DOQI Clinical Practice Guidelines for Vascular Access. *Am J Kidney Dis*. 2006;48(Suppl 1):S176. (7)

Ahmad S et al. Hemodialysis apparatus. In: Daugirdas JT et al, eds. *Handbook of Dialysis*. Philadelphia, PA: Lippincott, Williams & Wilkins; 2007:59. (15)

Blake PG. Adequacy of peritoneal dialysis and chronic peritoneal dialysis prescription. In: Daugirdas JT et al, eds. *Handbook of Dialysis*. Philadelphia, PA: Lippincott, Williams & Wilkins; 2007:387. (85)

Davenport A et al. Anticoagulation. In: Daugirdas JT et al, eds. *Handbook of Dialysis*. Philadelphia, PA: Lippincott, Williams & Wilkins; 2007:204. (25)

Leehey DJ et al. Infections. In: Daugirdas JT et al, eds. *Handbook of Dialysis*. Philadelphia, PA: Lippincott, Williams & Wilkins; 2007:542. (66)

Piraino B et al. ISPD Guidelines/recommendations. Peritoneal dialysis-related infections recommendations: 2005 update. *Perit Dial Int*. 2005;25:107. (93)

Ward RA et al. Product water and hemodialysis solution preparation. In: Daugirdas JT et al, eds. *Handbook of Dialysis*. Philadelphia, PA: Lippincott, Williams & Wilkins; 2007:79. (21)

Key Websites

NFK KDOQI Guidelines. **http://www.kidney.org/professionals/KDOQI/guideline_upHD_PD_VA/index.htm** (1, 5, 6, 7)

33

Dosing of Drugs in Renal Failure

David J. Quan and Francesca T. Aweeka

CORE PRINCIPLES

		CHAPTER CASES
1	The pharmacokinetics and pharmacodynamics of many drugs are altered in patients with impaired renal function (e.g., declining glomerular filtration rate) or who are on hemodialysis.	Case 33-1 (Questions 1, 2), Case 33-2 (Question 1), Case 33-3 (Questions 1, 3), Case 33-4 (Questions 1, 2), Case 33-5 (Questions 1, 4), Case 33-8 (Questions 1–4), Case 33-9 (Question 1)
2	Clinicians should be aware of drugs that require dosage adjustment in the setting of renal dysfunction to avoid adverse drug events and poor patient outcomes.	Case 33-1 (Questions 1, 2), Case 33-3 (Questions 1, 3), Case 33-4 (Question 1), Case 33-5 (Questions 1, 4), Case 33-9 (Question 1)
3	Dosages of drugs that are cleared by the kidneys should be adjusted according to the patient's renal function (e.g., creatinine clearance). The initial dose can be determined using the manufacturer's prescribing information, published guidelines, or published literature.	Case 33-1 (Question 1), Case 33-3 (Question 3), Case 33-4 (Question 1), Case 33-5 (Questions 1, 4), Case 33-9 (Question 1)
4	Many drugs have a narrow therapeutic window (range of drug concentrations that will achieve the desired effect), for which there may be lack of efficacy with subtherapeutic levels and adverse events associated with elevated levels. Serum drug concentration monitoring should be performed to achieve the desired target concentration.	Case 33-1 (Questions 2, 3), Case 33-5 (Question 2), Case 33-7 (Question 1), Case 33-8 (Question 3)
5	Renal replacement therapy (e.g., hemodialysis, continuous venovenous hemofiltration) can have a significant influence on the extracorporeal removal of drug. Clinicians should be aware of the method of renal replacement therapy and its impact on drug dosing.	Case 33-1 (Questions 5–8), Case 33-2 (Questions 1, 2), Case 33-3 (Questions 1, 4), Case 33-5 (Questions 3, 4), Case 33-6 (Question 1)
6	Biotransformation of drugs may be altered in patients with renal failure. Active or toxic metabolites may accumulate in patients with renal failure, leading to adverse effects. Excipients such as diluents can also accumulate in the setting of renal failure, resulting in toxicity.	Case 33-3 (Question 2), Case 33-8 (Questions 1–3)

BASIC PRINCIPLES

It is important to design specific pharmacotherapeutic regimens for patients with renal impairment. Without careful dosing and therapeutic drug monitoring for select medications in these patients, accumulation of drugs or toxic metabolites can occur, resulting in serious adverse effects. Many patients are treated with multiple medications, which may require even greater attention to dosage adjustment.

In addition to altered drug elimination, numerous other factors associated with kidney disease predispose patients to potential drug toxicity by altering pharmacokinetic disposition and the pharmacodynamic effects of drugs. For example, the physiologic changes associated with uremia can change drug absorption, protein binding, distribution, or elimination. These physiologic affects can alter drug concentrations in the plasma or blood, and at the targeted tissue site of activity, thereby affecting drug efficacy and toxicity.

Less is known about the effect of renal disease on drug pharmacodynamics, i.e., the pharmacologic or toxicologic effects produced relative to the drug concentration. Patients with renal disease can be more sensitive to some drugs, and experience an increased frequency of adverse drug reactions.

Effect of Renal Failure on Drug Disposition

BIOAVAILABILITY

Although several factors can potentially affect drug absorption in patients with kidney disease, limited data are available describing altered bioavailability. For example, drug absorption could be impaired in uremia by nausea, vomiting, diarrhea, gastritis, and edema of the gastrointestinal (GI) tract, the latter condition being a complication of nephrotic syndrome. Gastric and intestinal motility, as well as gastric emptying time, can be altered by the neuropathy associated with uremia. Uremia also can increase gastric ammonia, leading to an increased gastric pH, which may affect bioavailability of ferrous sulfate or other drugs that require an acidic environment for absorption.[1] Similarly, calcium-containing antacids used by patients with renal failure for GI symptoms and hyperphosphatemia neutralize hydrochloric acid in the stomach and increase gastric pH. Patients with end-stage renal disease often take oral phosphate binders, such as sevelamer and lanthanum carbonate, which can impair the absorption of other medications.[2,3]

The bioavailability of orally administered drugs also depends on the extent to which the drug is eliminated by first-pass (presystemic) metabolism. The first-pass hepatic metabolism of oral propranolol was found to be reduced in patients with renal disease, leading to increased bioavailability.[4] Subsequent studies, however, attributed the observed increased concentrations of propranolol in renal failure to a significant increase in the blood to plasma ratio.[5] Intestinal P-glycoprotein activity may be decreased as well.[6] Other drugs exhibiting increased bioavailability in renal disease include cloxacillin, propoxyphene, dihydrocodeine, encainide, and zidovudine (AZT). For example, the area under the concentration–time curve of dihydrocodeine is increased by 70% in those patients with impaired renal function.[7]

PROTEIN BINDING AND VOLUME OF DISTRIBUTION

The extent to which a drug exerts its pharmacologic effects is related to the amount of free or unbound drug available for distribution to target tissues. Patients with renal failure often have alterations in plasma protein binding, which can increase the amount of unbound drug.[8] Clinically, this is most important for highly protein-bound acidic drugs (>80%), whereas the binding of basic drugs is usually unchanged or possibly decreased in renal disease. Decreased protein binding of affected drugs results in increases in the free fraction of drug, an increase in the apparent volume of distribution (Vd), and higher plasma clearance (Cl) for drugs with a low-extraction ratio. However, the simultaneous increase in both the Vd and clearance results in little or no change in the elimination half-life ($t_{1/2}$) of these drugs. Alternatively, the Vd of high-extraction ratio drugs can increase without a concomitant change in clearance. In this situation, the $t_{1/2}$ would increase, based on the following relationships, where Kd is the elimination rate constant of the drug:

$$Kd = Cl/Vd \quad \textit{(Eq. 33-1)}$$

$$t_{1/2} = 0.693 \times Vd/Cl \quad \textit{(Eq. 33-2)}$$

In patients with renal failure, the accumulation of uremic toxins may also alter protein binding. When the free fraction of drugs that are highly protein bound changes, the interpretation of the total drug concentration must also be considered. That is, with an increase in the free fraction, the total drug concentration necessary to exert the desired pharmacologic effect is lower than that needed under normal conditions.

TABLE 33-1
Plasma Protein Binding (%) of Acidic Drugs in Renal Failure

Drug	Normal	Renal Failure
Cefazolin	85	69
Cefoxitin	73	25
Clofibrate	97	91
Diazoxide	94	84
Furosemide	96	94
Pentobarbital	66	59
Phenytoin	88–93	74–84
Salicylate	87–97	74–84
Sulfamethoxazole	66	42
Valproic acid	92	77
Warfarin	99	98

Hypoalbuminemia is a common complication of renal failure. Because acidic rather than basic drugs are bound to albumin, their protein binding tends to be altered in patients with renal failure (Table 33-1).[9] Patients with uremia accumulate acidic byproducts that may inhibit binding or displace acidic drugs from albumin binding sites. This is supported by the observed improvement in protein binding after removal of uremic byproducts by hemodialysis. Finally, the structural conformation of albumin is altered in renal disease, which may reduce the number or affinity of binding sites for drugs. Studies have demonstrated differences in the amino acid composition of albumin between healthy people and patients with uremia.[10] The anticonvulsant, phenytoin, is a classic example of a drug whose protein binding is altered in renal disease.[11] This is discussed in more detail later in this chapter.

Renal disease can change the Vd of various drugs. The Vd or "apparent volume of distribution" is the "volume" or size of a compartment necessary to account for the total amount of drug in the body if it were present throughout the body at the same concentration as that found in plasma. A decrease in the plasma protein binding of highly protein-bound drugs, such as phenytoin, leads to an increase in the apparent Vd.

Drugs that are not highly protein bound (e.g., gentamicin, isoniazid) have little change in their Vd in renal disease. Digoxin is a unique exception in that its Vd is decreased in renal disease. This is attributed to a decrease in myocardial tissue uptake of digoxin, leading to a decrease in the myocardial or tissue to serum concentration ratio.[12]

ELIMINATION

The extent to which renal disease affects the elimination of a drug depends on the amount of drug normally excreted unchanged in the urine and the degree of renal impairment. As kidney disease progresses, the kidney's ability to excrete uremic toxins diminishes. Consequently, the ability to eliminate certain drugs that are renally excreted also decreases. If the dose of these drugs is not modified for the patient's degree of renal dysfunction, these drugs will accumulate, potentially leading to an increase in the pharmacologic effect and toxicity.

The kidney eliminates drugs primarily by filtration or active secretion. Characteristics of a drug that determine its ability to be filtered include its affinity for protein binding and its molecular weight. Drugs with low protein binding or those that are displaced from proteins in the setting of renal disease (e.g., phenytoin) are filtered more readily. Molecules with a high molecular weight (>20,000 Da) are not readily filtered because of their large size. The reasons for how renal disease selectively alters the process of glomerular filtration or tubular secretion of specific drugs are not well understood. The elimination of drugs by the kidneys in patients with renal disease usually can be estimated by measuring the ability of the kidney to eliminate substances such as creatinine (i.e., creatinine clearance [CrCl]) (see Chapter 30, Acute Kidney Injury).

Organic anion transporters (OATs) are predominantly found in the basolateral membrane of the renal tubules. OATs facilitate the uptake of small organic anions into renal tubular cells. Decreased OAT activity as a result of acute kidney injury can decrease the renal secretion of various drugs such as methotrexate, nonsteroidal anti-inflammatory drugs, and acetylsalicylic acid.[13]

Renal disease can also have an important impact on the elimination of drugs that are primarily metabolized by the liver.[14] Metabolic processes, such as hydroxylation and glucuronidation, often produce inactive, more polar compounds that can be eliminated by the kidney. The metabolites of some drugs (e.g., meperidine, morphine, procainamide) are pharmacologically active or toxic. In patients with renal disease, these metabolites may accumulate, leading to an increase in pharmacologic activity and adverse effects.[15,16] For example, the central nervous system (CNS) toxicity observed in renal disease has been attributed to accumulation of the morphine metabolite, morphine-6-glucuronide. Therefore, careful dosing modifications or avoidance of these drugs are warranted in patients with renal impairment. Metabolic enzymes have been found within renal tissue, and may play a role in the metabolism of some of these drugs.[17,18] For example, the nonrenal clearance of drugs (e.g., acyclovir) decreases in patients with renal impairment, and is believed to be caused by a decrease in "renal" metabolism.[19]

Excipients used to formulate medications should also be considered. For example, the pharmacokinetics of itraconazole and voriconazole are not significantly altered in the setting of renal dysfunction. However, the parenteral formulations of itraconazole and voriconazole contain the solubilizing agent, β-cyclodextrin, which is normally rapidly eliminated by glomerular filtration but can accumulate in patients with renal impairment, causing GI disturbances.[20]

Drug Removal by Dialysis

The effect of dialysis on the removal of a specific drug must be considered when using medications in patients undergoing dialysis. Patients may need supplemental doses of a medication after a dialysis session or alteration in their dosage to maintain therapeutic drug concentrations. Dialysis also can be initiated to hasten drug removal from the body in some cases of drug overdose.

When using dialysis to manage a drug overdose, patients may respond clinically to factors unrelated to dialysis of the drug. For example, declining plasma concentrations may be caused by concurrent drug elimination by hepatic metabolism or renal excretion, which is independent of the dialysis procedure itself. Furthermore, clinical improvement may result from removal of active metabolites by dialysis rather than the parent compound.

The primary literature should be used to determine whether any information is available about the ability of dialysis to remove the drug. The application of data from the literature to a specific clinical situation often is difficult, however, and information pertaining to the dialysis of a specific drug may be limited. Anecdotal case reports in the primary literature seldom provide quantitative information. The effectiveness of dialysis is often based on a positive clinical outcome rather than on objective measurements of drug concentrations in the plasma and dialysate.

When applying information from the primary literature to a specific patient, the specifics of the dialyzer (e.g., type of machine, membrane surface area, pore size, and blood and dialysis flow rates) must be considered (see Chapter 32, Renal Dialysis). Furthermore, patient-specific information (e.g., time of drug ingestion, liver and renal function) from case reports in the literature also should be evaluated appropriately. The method used to calculate dialysis clearance also should be considered. In addition, clinical investigators often use predialysis and postdialysis serum drug concentrations for estimating drug dialyzability without considering the contributing effects of drug metabolism and excretion on drug elimination.

DRUG-SPECIFIC PROPERTIES

The physical and chemical characteristics of drugs can be used to predict the effectiveness of dialysis on drug removal.[21–23] Low-molecular-weight (MW) compounds are more readily dialyzed by conventional hemodialysis procedures because they can pass with greater ease across the dialysis membrane. Using cuprophane dialysis membranes, compounds with an MW of 500 or less are more likely to be significantly dialyzed than compounds with a high MW (e.g., vancomycin, MW approximately 1,400). Newer high-flux dialyzers using polysulfone membranes more effectively remove large chemical compounds (see High-Flux Hemodialysis section, and Chapter 32, Renal Dialysis). In addition, water-soluble drugs are removed more readily by dialysis than are lipid-soluble compounds.

Pharmacokinetic characteristics (e.g., Vd, protein binding) also can affect drug dialyzability. A drug with a large Vd that distributes widely into the peripheral tissues resides minimally in the plasma and, therefore, is not substantially removed by dialysis. This is particularly true for highly lipid-soluble drugs such as digoxin (Vd = 300–500 L), and amiodarone (Vd = 60 L/kg). In addition, drugs that are highly protein bound, such as warfarin (99%) and ceftriaxone (83%–96%), are not significantly removed by dialysis because the large protein–drug complex is unable to pass through the dialysis membrane.

Because clearance values are additive, the hepatic and other nonrenal plasma clearance of a drug should be considered in relation to the dialysis clearance. Only when dialysis clearance contributes a substantially additive effect to the patient's own clearance is drug elimination enhanced. For example, AZT has a large nonrenal plasma clearance in patients with severe renal disease (approximately 1,200 mL/minute). Therefore, despite a hemodialysis clearance of 63 mL/minute, the contribution of dialysis to total AZT removal is negligible.

HIGH-FLUX HEMODIALYSIS

High-flux hemodialysis uses higher blood and dialysate flow rates compared with conventional methods. The enhanced efficiency of high-flux dialysis and the larger pore size of the polysulfone membranes allow for small- and mid-MW compounds (e.g., vancomycin) to be partially removed. Drugs such as gentamicin and foscarnet, which are removed by conventional dialysis, are also efficiently removed by high-flux hemodialysis.[24,25] In many cases, the net amount of drug removed during a high-flux dialysis session is greater than the amount removed during conventional dialysis because of the use of higher blood flow rates. The principal difference is the greater efficiency and the ability to clear drugs of larger MW compared with conventional dialysis.

CONTINUOUS AMBULATORY PERITONEAL DIALYSIS

Continuous ambulatory peritoneal dialysis (CAPD) uses the patient's peritoneum as the dialysis membrane. Patients maintained with CAPD undergo infusion of a dialysate solution via a catheter inserted into the peritoneal cavity; the solution is allowed to dwell in the cavity for several hours. The accumulated fluid and uremic byproducts diffuse from the blood into the dialysate solution, which is exchanged every 4 to 8 hours (see Chapter 32, Renal Dialysis).

Some drugs, such as antibiotics, can be administered intraperitoneally in patients on CAPD by directly adding them to the dialysate solution. This is particularly useful for patients with peritonitis who require high intraperitoneal concentrations of antimicrobial agents to treat this infection. After intraperitoneal administration of drugs, such as the aminoglycosides, plasma and intraperitoneal drug concentrations will eventually reach equilibrium. Despite systemic absorption of these drugs from the peritoneal fluid, peritoneal dialysis (PD) usually is inefficient at removing drugs from the plasma.[26] Because CAPD contributes little to the overall elimination of most drugs, dosage modifications are not always necessary in patients having this procedure.

CONTINUOUS RENAL REPLACEMENT THERAPIES

ONLINE CONTENT

For a narrated PowerPoint presentation on continuous renal replacement modalities, go to http://thepoint.lww.com/AT10e.

Continuous venovenous hemofiltration (CVVH) is a form of continuous renal replacement therapy (CRRT) used in the critically ill patient with renal failure. CRRT is typically reserved for patients who are unable to tolerate hemodialysis because of hemodynamic instability. As with hemodialysis, this procedure removes fluid, electrolytes, and low- and mid-MW molecules from the blood. Using a hollow fiber that is made of a semipermeable membrane, water and solutes are filtered by hydrostatic pressure. A countercurrent dialysate can be added to the circuit to improve solute removal (continuous venovenous hemodialysis with filtration).

Limited data are available on the effect of CVVH on the removal of drugs. Drugs that have a high sieving coefficient (permeability of a drug through a semipermeable membrane), such as the aminoglycosides, ceftazidime, vancomycin, and procainamide, are readily removed by CVVH.[27–29] Data concerning the removal of drugs by hemodialysis cannot be extrapolated to CVVH because of differences in the membranes used, blood flow rates, ultrafiltration rate, dialysate flow rate, and the continuous nature of the procedure compared with intermittent hemodialysis. CVVH clearance can be estimated to determine the appropriate dosage regimen based on the pharmacologic characteristics of a specific drug (see Case 33-1, Question 8).

HEMOPERFUSION

Hemoperfusion is another method of drug removal that may be used to facilitate the elimination of a drug in the setting of an overdose.[30,31] During the hemoperfusion procedure, blood is passed through a column of adsorbent material (e.g., activated charcoal or resin) to bind toxins and drugs. Hemoperfusion can be particularly useful for removing large-MW compounds or highly protein-bound drugs that are not removed efficiently by hemodialysis. Large compounds and drug–protein complexes are adsorbed onto the high-surface-area resin as blood passes through the adsorbent column. Hemoperfusion can also be used to remove lipid-soluble drugs not easily removed by hemodialysis. Lipid-soluble drugs often have a large Vd. Removal of drugs by hemoperfusion is of limited value because a significant amount of these lipophilic compounds reside in peripheral tissues.

Pharmacodynamics and Renal Disease

Few studies have investigated the pharmacodynamics of drugs in patients with renal disease. Clinical observations report that patients with renal disease are more sensitive to various drugs. For example, morphine has been associated with increased neurologic depression in patients with renal failure.[32,33] The ability of morphine to potentiate the CNS depressant effects of uremia may result from an alteration in the permeability of the blood–brain barrier that results in higher CNS levels of morphine and morphine-6-glucuronide.

Another example of altered drug response in uremia is that of nifedipine, which at similar unbound plasma concentrations has an increased antihypertensive effect in patients with renal disease.[34] The mean maximal effect change in diastolic blood pressure values in the control group and in patients with severe renal failure were 12% and 29%, respectively. Therefore, the dose of nifedipine needs to be adjusted in patients with renal disease because of changes in drug effects rather than pharmacokinetic alterations.

The pharmacokinetics of warfarin is not significantly altered in renal failure. However, patients with renal failure who are prescribed warfarin have a higher incidence of hemorrhagic complications, likely because of platelet dysfunction from uremia, and drug–drug interactions from concomitant medications.[35,36]

PHARMACOKINETICS AND PHARMACODYNAMICS OF SPECIFIC DRUGS IN RENAL FAILURE

Ceftazidime

DOSAGE MODIFICATION: FACTORS TO CONSIDER

CASE 33-1

QUESTION 1: G.G., a 31-year-old, 70-kg woman with a 3-year history of systemic lupus erythematosus, presents to the emergency department (ED) with a 5-day history of fatigue, weakness, and nausea as well, as worsening of her facial rash and a fever of 40°C. Her systemic lupus erythematosus had been moderately controlled until this acute flare. Her admission laboratory workup now reveals the following pertinent values:

Potassium (K), 6.0 mEq/L
Sodium (Na), 142 mEq/L
Serum creatinine (SCr), 3.4 mg/dL
Blood urea nitrogen (BUN), 38 mg/dL

Complete blood count reveals a hematocrit of 32% and a hemoglobin of 9.2 g/dL. The platelet count is 50,000/μL, and her erythrocyte sedimentation rate is 35 mm/hour. Physical examination is significant for a blood pressure of 136/92 mm Hg and 2+ pedal edema. Prednisone is started at a dose of 1.5 mg/kg/day.

Two weeks into her hospital course, G.G.'s condition worsens and signs of sepsis develop. *Pseudomonas aeruginosa* is cultured from her urine. Therapy with ceftazidime is initiated at a dose of 1 g every 8 hours, a dose commonly used for patients with good renal function. Considering that G.G.'s renal function has remained stable and that she has an estimated CrCl of 27 mL/minute, what factors should be considered before modifying her dose? What would be an appropriate dose of ceftazidime for G.G.?

Before modifying the dose of any drug, its route of elimination should be established. As a general rule, the degree to which renal impairment affects elimination depends on the percentage of unchanged drug that is excreted by the kidney. Thus, the elimination of most drugs that are primarily cleared by the kidneys will be decreased in the setting of renal impairment. For many drugs dependent on the kidney for elimination, relationships between some measurement of renal function (e.g., CrCl) and some parameter of drug elimination (e.g., plasma clearance or half-life) have been established to help clinicians determine the appropriate dosing modifications in patients with renal disease.

In contrast, the clearance of drugs that are eliminated primarily by nonrenal mechanisms (e.g., hepatic metabolism) is not altered significantly in patients with renal disease. However, some drugs have water-soluble metabolites that have either pharmacologic activity or potential toxicity and that may accumulate with renal dysfunction, warranting dosage adjustment or avoidance of the drug entirely (e.g., meperidine; see Case 33-8, Question 1).

Enzymes with metabolic capacity have also been found within renal tissue, which can result in the kidneys playing a limited role in the metabolism of certain drugs (see Case 33-3, Question 2). The clinical importance of this elimination pathway is unclear.

Another important factor to consider is the "therapeutic window" for a given drug, i.e., the range of drug concentrations thought to be most effective. Drug concentrations below this range are usually subtherapeutic, whereas concentrations above this range can lead to a greater incidence of adverse effects. For drugs with a wide therapeutic window, the difference between toxic and therapeutic concentrations is large. Although many drugs that are cleared primarily by the kidney may require dosing modifications in patients with renal dysfunction, aggressive dose reduction may not be necessary for drugs with a large therapeutic window, particularly if the adverse effects of the drug (e.g., fluconazole) are relatively mild. This is in contrast to drugs (e.g., aminoglycosides, vancomycin, or foscarnet) that are eliminated primarily by the kidney and have narrow therapeutic windows. For these drugs, the toxic plasma concentrations are very close to the therapeutic drug concentrations, with little room for dosing error.

Ceftazidime is a cephalosporin that has excellent activity against most strains of *Pseudomonas* species. As with most cephalosporins, ceftazidime primarily is cleared by the kidneys, with little nonrenal or hepatic elimination. The correlation between the clearance of ceftazidime and CrCl in mL/minute is represented by the following equation[37]:

$$Cl_{ceftaz}(\text{mL/minute}) = (0.95)(\text{CrCl}) + 6.59 \quad \textit{(Eq. 33-3)}$$

Using Equation 33-3, the clearance of ceftazidime in G.G. is estimated to be 32 mL/minute compared with an average normal clearance of approximately 100 mL/minute. Because her drug clearance is approximately one-third of normal, she would require about one-third of the normal daily dose (i.e., 1 g every 24 hours). As with other cephalosporins, ceftazidime has a large therapeutic window.[38] Failure to reduce the dose from a normal dose of 1 g every 8 hours, although likely safe, might lead to accumulation of ceftazidime, predisposing G.G. to seizures and other adverse effects associated with toxic β-lactam antibiotic plasma levels.[39,40] This is in contrast to the aminoglycosides, which must be dosed based on specific pharmacokinetic calculations. Therefore, more generalized or empirical dosage modifications can be made with ceftazidime.

Aminoglycosides

CASE 33-1, QUESTION 2: G.G.'s medical team decides that the addition of an aminoglycoside antibiotic is necessary to treat her infection. Considering that her renal function has remained stable, how should gentamicin be dosed in G.G.? Is it best to alter the dose or the dosing interval for this drug?

ALTERATION OF DOSE VERSUS DOSING INTERVAL

The aminoglycosides (e.g., tobramycin, gentamicin, amikacin) are effective in the treatment of serious systemic infections caused by gram-negative organisms such as *Pseudomonas* species. Unlike the cephalosporins and penicillins, however, the aminoglycosides have a relatively narrow therapeutic window. Using pharmacokinetic principles, a dose regimen can be designed to produce specific peak and trough serum concentrations. Peak serum concentrations (Cp_{peak}) (e.g., gentamicin or tobramycin 5–8 mg/L) correlate best with therapeutic efficacy, whereas toxicity tends to correlate with elevated trough levels (Cp_{trough}), which reflects prolonged exposure to high drug concentrations. To minimize the risk of toxicity, trough levels of less than 2 mg/L should be maintained. In patients with normal renal function, these target serum aminoglycoside concentrations are usually obtained after standard doses (e.g., 1.5 mg/kg) administered every 8 hours. Peak and trough levels are typically measured once steady state is achieved, which is typically within 24 hours.[41–44]

Many clinicians now use once-daily dosing of the aminoglycosides (e.g., 5 mg/kg every 24 hours) for patients with normal renal function in an attempt to minimize aminoglycoside accumulation and nephrotoxicity. The rationale for this regimen is based on the aminoglycosides' concentration-dependent killing and postantibiotic effect. This approach is not recommended for patients with advanced renal impairment, however. When once-daily dosing is used, peak concentrations are less helpful; however, trough concentrations should be monitored with a target of being below the limit of analytic detection (<1 mg/L). The discussion regarding aminoglycoside dosing in renal impairment that follows is based on the traditional every 8 hours dosing regimen.

Aminoglycosides are almost completely eliminated by the kidneys; thus, the clearance of these drugs essentially is equal to the glomerular filtration rate (GFR). The pharmacokinetic properties of gentamicin and tobramycin are similar. A close correlation also exists between CrCl (a surrogate for GFR) and gentamicin total body clearance. As renal function deteriorates, aminoglycoside doses must be modified to achieve the desired peak and trough plasma concentrations. Failure to appropriately adjust the dosage of aminoglycosides in renal insufficiency can lead to high drug plasma levels that can result in ototoxicity and nephrotoxicity.

In many cases, the aminoglycoside dose can be modified by extending the dosing interval rather than simply reducing the dose. This permits maintenance of adequate peak plasma concentrations to ensure efficacy, while allowing for sufficient elimination between doses to produce trough levels less than 2 mg/L. The advantages and disadvantages of adjusting the dosing interval versus reducing the dose are summarized in Table 33-2.

Figure 33-1 illustrates the effect of increasing the dosing interval in a patient such as G.G. with renal function that is 30% of normal. Although this is the preferred method for adjusting the dose of aminoglycosides, for many other drugs requiring dose adjustments in renal disease, simple dosage reduction is sufficient. Commonly used drug references such as Facts and Comparisons can be used for dosing guidelines for drugs used in patients with renal failure.[45]

DETERMINATION OF APPROPRIATE DOSE

A number of methods have been developed to determine the appropriate aminoglycoside dose for patients.[46] One method is

TABLE 33-2
Advantages and Disadvantages of General Approaches to Dosing Adjustments in Renal Disease

Method	Advantages	Disadvantages
Variable Frequency		
Use the same dose but ↑ the dosing interval	Same Cp_{ave}, Cp_{max}, Cp_{min} Normal dose	Levels may remain subtherapeutic for prolonged periods in patients requiring dosing intervals >24 hr
Variable Dose With Fixed Cp_{ave}		
↓ Dose to maintain a target Cp_{ave}; keep the dosing interval the same	Same Cp_{ave} Normal dosing interval	↓ Peak levels, which may ↑ be subtherapeutic; ↑ trough levels, which may ↑ be potential for toxicity

Cp_{ave}, average plasma concentration; Cp_{max}, maximum plasma concentration; Cp_{min}, minimum plasma concentration.

Bayesian forecasting, in which pharmacokinetic data obtained in the individual patient are integrated with population parameters. Initially, a dose is used that is based on population parameter values adjusted for characteristics such as increased SCr. Drug concentrations for the individual patient are measured at specific times (e.g., peak and trough measurements), and these are compared with the expected values from the population data. Individualized pharmacokinetic parameter estimates are subsequently derived using Bayes' theorem to calculate a more patient-specific dosing regimen.[47]

Because of the wide interpatient variability in aminoglycoside pharmacokinetic parameters and the narrow therapeutic index for these drugs, doses should be adjusted based on pharmacokinetic principles (e.g., Bayesian calculations or methods described later in this chapter) and plasma concentrations that are specific for this patient.

PATIENT-SPECIFIC METHODS

Sawchuk et al. developed a method to derive patient-specific estimates of Vd and clearance based on the patient's size and estimated CrCl.[43] These parameters can be used to calculate a specific dose for G.G. that will produce the desired gentamicin peak and trough concentrations. If steady-state serum concentrations of gentamicin are known, they can be used to calculate even more-specific parameters. To initiate gentamicin therapy,

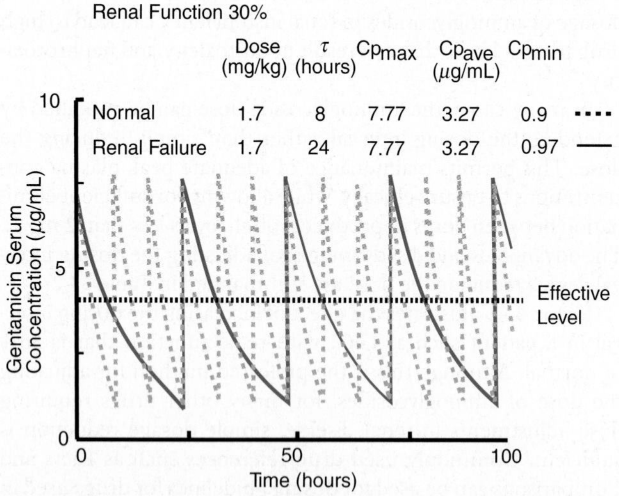

FIGURE 33-1 Serum concentration versus time profile for a patient with renal function 30% of normal in whom the interval of drug administration has been extended for dose adjustment. Advantages to this method are summarized in Table 33-2. (Reprinted with permission from Brater DC. *Drug Use in Renal Disease*. Sydney: ADIS Health Science Press; 1983.)

pharmacokinetic parameters should first be estimated from population values.

The clearance of gentamicin (Cl_{gent}) can be calculated based on G.G.'s CrCl. Using the Cockcroft and Gault equation,[48] the CrCl can be estimated as follows:

$$\text{CrCl (males)} = \frac{(140 - \text{age})(\text{IBW})}{(\text{SCr})(72)} \quad \textbf{(Eq. 33-4)}$$

$$\text{CrCl (females)} = \frac{(140 - \text{age})(\text{IBW})}{(\text{SCr})(72)}(0.85) \quad \textbf{(Eq. 33-5)}$$

where IBW is ideal body weight in kilograms, age is measured in years, and SCr is serum creatinine in mg/dL.

With a SCr of 3.4 mg/dL, an ideal body weight of 70 kg, and an age of 31 years, G.G.'s estimated CrCl, is 27 mL/minute.

For practical purposes, Cl_{gent} is usually considered equivalent to CrCl. Therefore, Cl_{gent} also is approximately 27 mL/minute or 1.6 L/hour. The Vd of gentamicin (Vd_{gent}) is approximately 0.25 L/kg in patients with normal or impaired renal function.[43,48,49]

The Vd_{gent} will be different in obese patients or those who have fluid overload. Although G.G. does have some fluid retention, this is minimal and should not affect her Vd_{gent} significantly. Therefore, the Vd_{gent} for G.G. is as follows:

$$\begin{aligned} Vd_{gent} &= (0.25\ \text{L/kg})(\text{body weight}) \\ &= (0.25\ \text{L/kg})(70\ \text{kg}) \\ &= 17.5\ \text{L} \end{aligned} \quad \textbf{(Eq. 33-6)}$$

The loading dose of gentamicin (LD_{gent}) can be determined using the following equation:

$$LD_{gent} = (Vd_{gent})(\text{desired } Cp_{peak}) \quad \textbf{(Eq. 33-7)}$$

For treatment of infections caused by *Pseudomonas* species, a peak level of approximately 6 to 8 mg/L is desired:

$$\begin{aligned} LD_{gent} &= (17.5\ \text{L})(7\ \text{mg/L}) \\ &= 122.5\ \text{mg or round off to 120 mg} \end{aligned} \quad \textbf{(Eq. 33-8)}$$

Using Cl_{gent} and Vd_{gent}, the elimination rate constant (Kd) and half-life for gentamicin can be estimated as follows:

$$\begin{aligned} Kd &= \frac{Cl_{gent}}{Vd_{gent}} \\ &= \frac{1.6\ \text{L/hour}}{17.5\ \text{L}} \\ &= 0.091\ \text{hour}^{-1} \end{aligned} \quad \textbf{(Eq. 33-9)}$$

$$\begin{aligned} t_{1/2} &= \frac{0.693}{Kd} \\ &= \frac{0.693}{0.091\ \text{hour}^{-1}} \\ &= 7.6\ \text{hours} \end{aligned} \quad \textbf{(Eq. 33-10)}$$

For the aminoglycosides, the dosing interval (τ) is determined by doubling the half-life because by the end of two half-lives, 75% of the drug will have been eliminated. This will usually lead to a desired trough level of less than 2 mg/L. Therefore, gentamicin should be administered at least every 16 hours. For convenience, an interval of 24 hours can be used, which also will achieve the desired trough concentration.

Gentamicin is usually infused for 30 minutes. To determine the peak gentamicin concentration, serum samples are drawn 30 minutes after the infusion has been completed. Because the estimated elimination half-life of gentamicin in G.G. (7.6 hours) is much longer than the infusion time (0.5 hours), the intravenous bolus model can be used to calculate an appropriate maintenance dose.

To achieve the peak concentration of 7 mg/L, the following equation can be used:

$$\begin{aligned}\text{Dose} &= \frac{(\text{Cp}_{\text{peak}})(1 - e^{-\text{Kdt}})(\text{Vd}_{\text{gent}})}{(e^{-\text{Kdt}_{\text{sample}}})}\\ &= \frac{(7\text{ mg/L})(1 - e^{-(0.091\text{ hour}^{-1})(24\text{ hour})})(17.5\text{ L})}{(e^{-(0.091\text{ hour}^{-1})(1\text{ hour})})}\\ &= 119.2\text{ mg}\\ &= \text{or round off to }120\text{ mg}\end{aligned} \quad \textit{(Eq. 33-11)}$$

where t_{sample} usually equals 1 hour (30 minutes after a 30-minute infusion).

The expected trough level in G.G. can now be estimated by the following equation:

$$\begin{aligned}\text{Cp}_{\text{trough}} &= (\text{Cp}_{\text{peak}})(e^{-\text{Kdt}_{\text{sample}}})\\ &= (7\text{ mg/L})(e^{-(0.091\text{ hour}^{-1})(24\text{ hours})})\\ &= 0.8\text{ mg/L}\end{aligned} \quad \textit{(Eq. 33-12)}$$

Although not the case for G.G., patients with normal renal function may eliminate a significant amount of gentamicin during the 30-minute infusion. In these patients, the intermittent infusion model should be used to account for this loss of drug, where t_{in} is the duration of the infusion:

$$\text{Dose} = \frac{(\text{Cl}_{\text{gent}})(\text{Cp}_{\text{peak}})(1 - e^{-\text{Kdt}})(t_{\text{in}})}{(1 - e^{-\text{Kdt}_{\text{in}}})(e^{-\text{Kd}\tau})} \quad \textit{(Eq. 33-13)}$$

REVISED PARAMETERS

CASE 33-1, QUESTION 3: After 72 hours of gentamicin therapy, G.G.'s peak and trough levels are 7.6 and 2.6 mg/L, respectively. Her physician attributes this to a gradual decline in renal function. (Her most recent SCr is 4.8 mg/dL.) How would you revise G.G.'s dosing regimen based on these levels?

A gentamicin trough level of more than 2 mg/L suggests that G.G.'s dosing interval is too short. Although her peak concentration is within the normal range of 5 to 8 mg/L, her trough concentration indicates that she is at a potentially toxic level. Her pharmacokinetic parameters can be revised based on these values, and a new Kd can be estimated from the following equation:

$$\text{Kd} = \frac{\ln\left(\dfrac{\text{CP}_1}{\text{CP}_2}\right)}{\Delta t} = \frac{\ln\left(\dfrac{7.6\text{ mg/L}}{2.6\text{ mg/L}}\right)}{23\text{ hours}} = 0.047\text{ hour}^{-1} \quad \textit{(Eq. 33-14)}$$

Because little change in G.G.'s Vd_{gent} is expected, a new Cl_{gent} ($\text{Cl}_{\text{revised}}$) can be estimated from her revised elimination constant (if necessary, a revised Vd_{gent} could be calculated, keeping Cl_{gent} constant, although the clearance is more likely to change than the volume of distribution):

$$\begin{aligned}\text{Cl}_{\text{revised}} &= (\text{Vd}_{\text{gent}})(\text{Kd})\\ &= (17.5\text{ L})(0.047\text{ hour}^{-1})\\ &= 0.82\text{ L/hour}\end{aligned} \quad \textit{(Eq. 33-15)}$$

These revised values for Kd and Cl can now be used to calculate a revised maintenance dose to maintain the $\text{Cp}_{\text{trough}}$ at less than 2 mg/L using Equation 33-11:

$$\begin{aligned}\text{Dose} &= \frac{(7\text{ mg/L})(1 - e^{-(0.047\text{ hour}^{-1})(48\text{ hours})})(17.5\text{ L})}{e^{-(0.047\text{ hour}^{-1})(1\text{ hour})}}\\ &= 115\text{ mg}\end{aligned} \quad \textit{(Eq. 33-16)}$$

$$\begin{aligned}\text{Cp}_{\text{trough}} &= (7\text{ mg/L})(e^{-(0.047\text{ hour}^{-1})(48\text{ hours})})\\ &= 0.73\text{ mg/L}\end{aligned}$$

The revised dose is now 115 mg (or ~110 mg) every 48 hours.

CASE 33-1, QUESTION 4: What are some limitations in calculating G.G.'s CrCl based on her SCr? Can this estimate safely be used to predict gentamicin clearance?

See Chapter 30, Acute Kidney Injury, for information about equations used to calculate CrCl and estimate GFR. For patients with stable renal function, CrCl can be estimated from SCr using the Cockcroft and Gault equation (see Eqs. 33-4 and 33-5). In a patient such as G.G., however, whose renal function continues to decline during the hospital course, estimation of renal function based on her increasing SCr becomes more difficult. Because her SCr does not reflect a steady-state level, the previous equations can no longer be used to accurately estimate her renal function. Because G.G.'s SCr has increased rapidly from 3.4 to 4.8 mg/dL during the past few days, her CrCl is probably much lower than that estimated using the Cockcroft and Gault method. A rising SCr may represent a decline in renal function manifesting as an accumulation of creatinine.

Although prediction equations such as the Modification of Diet in Renal Disease (MDRD) equations are a good measure of GFR,[50] they have not been validated for the dosing of most drugs in the setting of renal dysfunction.[51,52] There can be significant differences in drug dosing regimens when the MDRD and Cockcroft and Gault methods are used to estimate renal function.[53,54] The manufacturer's prescribing information and available literature should be evaluated to determine the appropriate dosage regimen.

ONLINE CONTENT

For spreadsheets and exercises used to illustrate creatinine clearance and estimated glomerular filtration rate calculations, go to http://the point.lww.com/AT10e.

Effect of Hemodialysis

CONVENTIONAL DIALYSIS

GENTAMICIN

CASE 33-1, QUESTION 5: G.G.'s renal function continues to deteriorate to the extent that she requires hemodialysis. What additional alterations in her gentamicin dosing regimen are necessary when she is having dialysis?

For a narrated PowerPoint presentation on renal dialysis, go to http://thepoint.lww.com/AT10e.

Gentamicin has a molecular weight of about 500 and a relatively low Vd (averaging 0.25 L/kg), and is about 10% bound to proteins, all favoring effective removal by conventional hemodialysis.[44] For a given patient, the observed dialysis clearance of gentamicin using conventional methods also depends on factors such as the physical properties of the dialysis filter, the blood and dialysate flow rates, and the length of dialysis. Studies indicate that dialysis clearance of gentamicin averages 45 mL/minute compared with an average plasma clearance of 5 mL/minute in patients with end-stage renal disease (ESRD).[55,56] Therefore, G.G.'s gentamicin dose must be adjusted to compensate for the amount of drug that will be removed by dialysis. Because drug removal represents a combination of drug elimination by the body and dialysis, the following equation can be used:

$$Cl_{total} = Cl_{dial} + Cl \qquad \textit{(Eq. 33-17)}$$

where Cl_{total} is the total clearance of the drug during dialysis, Cl_{dial} is the clearance by dialysis, and Cl is plasma clearance. If dialysis clearance is high relative to plasma clearance, drug removal will be enhanced by the dialysis procedure. The total clearance of gentamicin in a patient with severe renal dysfunction during dialysis is 50 mL/minute (45 mL/minute + 5 mL/minute) or 10 times the clearance while off dialysis. Plasma clearance and dialysis clearance are related to the elimination half-life by the following equation:

$$t_{1/2} = \frac{(0.693)(Vd)}{Cl_{dial} + Cl} \qquad \textit{(Eq. 33-18)}$$

Thus, assuming a constant Vd of 17.5 L (i.e., 0.25 L/kg × 70 kg), the elimination half-life on dialysis is approximately 4 hours compared with 40 hours off dialysis. In addition, the extent (fraction) of drug removal (FD) during a timed dialysis run can be predicted from the following equation:

$$FD = 1 - e^{-(Cl+Cl_{dial})(t/Vd)} \qquad \textit{(Eq. 33-19)}$$

where t is the duration of dialysis. Therefore, the fraction of gentamicin removed (FD) during a 4-hour conventional dialysis procedure is approximately 50%. If specific data are not available for dialysis and plasma clearance, the following equation will predict fraction removed using the elimination half-life data alone obtained during dialysis:

$$FD = 1 - e^{-(0.693/t_{1/2on})(t)} \qquad \textit{(Eq. 33-20)}$$

The estimated value of 50% removal is consistent with literature values indicating that 50% to 70% of a dose of gentamicin is removed during a 4-hour dialysis procedure. A limitation of this equation, however, is that it does not consider the redistribution of drug from the tissues back into the plasma after the dialysis procedure.

It generally is difficult to calculate an appropriate maintenance dose for patients having hemodialysis that will maintain peak and trough concentrations similar to patients with normal renal function, in part because of the large variability found in aminoglycoside pharmacokinetic parameters.[56,57] Sustained plasma concentrations greater than 2 mg/L can increase the risk of toxicity; however, dosing gentamicin to achieve trough concentrations of less than 2 mg/L may lead to prolonged periods of subtherapeutic peak concentrations because one would have to use smaller doses with lower peak concentrations to allow the troughs to drop before the next dose. Another practical consideration is that unless one expects the patient to recover renal function in the future, renal toxicity of the drug is less of a concern. As a compromise in patients receiving hemodialysis, gentamicin doses are given to achieve a predialysis trough concentration of approximately 3 mg/L. This can generally be achieved with a loading dose of 2 mg/kg, followed by a maintenance dose of 1 mg/kg after each dialysis session.

CEFTAZIDIME

CASE 33-1, QUESTION 6: Why does the dose of ceftazidime in G.G. have to be adjusted because of her hemodialysis when this drug has such a large therapeutic window?

Because only 21% of ceftazidime is protein bound and its Vd is 0.2 L/kg, it should be readily removed by hemodialysis. The mean dialysis clearance of ceftazidime is 55 mL/minute, with 55% of the drug removed during 4 hours of conventional hemodialysis.[58] A supplemental dose of ceftazidime should be given to G.G. after each hemodialysis session to maintain a therapeutic concentration. Half of the daily ceftazidime dose should be administered after each dialysis session.

HIGH-FLUX HEMODIALYSIS

CASE 33-1, QUESTION 7: G.G.'s physician is considering changing her from a conventional dialysis system to a high-flux system that uses high-efficiency polysulfone membranes. How does the dialyzability of gentamicin and ceftazidime differ with high-flux hemodialysis compared with conventional hemodialysis?

High-flux hemodialysis is more effective than conventional dialysis at removing certain pharmacologic agents (see Chapter 32, Renal Dialysis) because the membranes are more efficient and the blood flow through the dialyzer is increased. Although limited data are available, a greater fraction of drugs, such as aminoglycosides, ceftazidime, and vancomycin, are removed by high-flux versus conventional hemodialysis.[59,60] Approximately 50% to 70% of gentamicin is removed during a 2.5-hour, high-flux dialysis session.[24,61] The clearance of ceftazidime by high-flux dialysis is 75 to 240 mL/minute compared with 55 mL/minute for conventional hemodialysis.[59] Thus, further dosage adjustments for gentamicin and ceftazidime may be necessary if G.G. is converted from conventional hemodialysis to high-flux hemodialysis.

CONTINUOUS VENOVENOUS HEMOFILTRATION

CASE 33-1, QUESTION 8: What changes would be necessary in G.G.'s gentamicin dosing if she were to start a CRRT such as CVVH?

Because of the continuous nature of CVVH, the extent of drug eliminated by CRRTs will differ from intermittent modes such as hemodialysis. The clearance of a drug in a patient receiving CVVH can be described in a fashion similar to Equation 33-17, where Cl_{dial} is replaced with Cl_{cvvh}.

$$Cl_{total} = Cl + Cl_{cvvh} \qquad \textit{(Eq. 33-21)}$$

In G.G., the $Cl_{revised}$ from Equation 33-15 can be used for the plasma clearance (Cl). The clearance by CVVH can be described by the following equation:

$$Cl_{cvvh} = Fu \times UFR \quad \text{(Eq. 33-22)}$$

where Fu is the fraction of drug unbound, and UFR is the ultrafiltration rate. Gentamicin exhibits low plasma protein binding (Fu = 0.95). Typical ultrafiltration rates for CVVH are approximately 1 L/hour, but can vary.

$$\begin{aligned} Cl_{cvvh} &= Fu \times UFR \\ &= 0.95 \times 1 \text{ L/hour} \quad \text{(Eq. 33-23)} \\ &= 0.95 \text{ L/hour} \end{aligned}$$

$$\begin{aligned} Cl_{total} &= Cl_{revised} + Cl_{cvvh} \\ &= 0.82 \text{ L/hour} + 0.95 \text{ L/hour} \\ &= 1.77 \text{ L/hour} \quad \text{(Eq. 33-24)} \\ &= 29.5 \text{ ml/minute} \end{aligned}$$

Because the clearance of gentamicin approximates that of CrCl, G.G.'s total clearance is approximately one-third the normal clearance of 100 mL/minute. Therefore, the gentamicin dose should be approximately one-third of the normal dose. G.G. should be given 1.5 mg/kg/day or 100 mg of gentamicin as a single daily dose (normal dose is approximately 5 mg/kg/day). Gentamicin trough concentrations should be monitored, and her dose adjusted to maintain a trough concentration of less than 2 mg/L.

CONTINUOUS AMBULATORY PERITONEAL DIALYSIS

CASE 33-2

QUESTION 1: J.J., a 24-year-old man with ESRD, is maintained with CAPD. He presents to the ED with a fever of 38.2°C and complains of severe abdominal pain. He also reports that his peritoneal dialysate has become cloudy in the past few days. All these symptoms are consistent with peritonitis, a frequent complication of CAPD. His culture results reveal *Escherichia coli*, sensitive to gentamicin. How should gentamicin be dosed in this patient?

Management of dialysis-related peritonitis can vary from one institution to another. Antibiotics often are administered intraperitoneally (IP) with or without systemic antibiotic therapy. For less severe cases, IP administration is often considered sufficient. With IP administration, the goal is to deliver a concentration of drug similar to the desired plasma concentration for the treatment of systemic infections. Therefore, 8 mg of gentamicin into each liter of dialysate (or 16 mg into a 2-L bag of dialysate) is recommended. Once equilibrium or steady state is achieved, the dialysate concentration will be comparable to the concentration of gentamicin in the plasma. Despite a more rapid transfer of drug into the plasma because of increased permeability of the peritoneal membrane in patients with peritonitis, there will still be a substantial lag time before steady state is reached. For more serious cases of peritonitis, concomitant systemic antibiotics should be given.

CASE 33-2, QUESTION 2: Is gentamicin eliminated by CAPD?

In general, most drugs are not well removed via CAPD. This is particularly true for drugs that are highly protein bound or for drugs with a large Vd. Gentamicin and other aminoglycosides, on the other hand, are effectively removed by CAPD because they have low protein binding and a small Vd. It is estimated that 10% to 50% of gentamicin is removed by CAPD.[62]

Acyclovir

RENAL CLEARANCE

CASE 33-3

QUESTION 1: D.M., a 28-year-old man with acquired immune deficiency syndrome, presents with a severe herpetic infection requiring intravenous (IV) acyclovir. Because of other complications associated with his human immunodeficiency virus (HIV) infection, D.M. has developed renal insufficiency during his hospital course. His SCr is 4.5 mg/dL, and his CrCl is 20 mL/minute. What are important considerations for dosing acyclovir in D.M. now, and also if he requires dialysis?

Acyclovir is used to prevent or treat a variety of viral infections, such as those caused by herpes simplex and varicella zoster viruses.[63] It is cleared primarily by the kidneys, with approximately 70% to 80% excreted unchanged in the urine. Dosage adjustment is necessary in patients with renal disease.[19,64] Renal tubular secretion in addition to filtration contributes to the elimination of acyclovir, which explains why the renal clearance of acyclovir is about three times greater than the estimated CrCl.

Acyclovir also can precipitate in the renal tubules and exacerbate D.M.'s renal failure. This is more likely to occur when high doses are infused too rapidly to patients with renal dysfunction.[64] To minimize nephrotoxicity, the patient should be adequately hydrated to maintain good urine flow, and the acyclovir dose should be infused over the course of 1 hour. Nephrotoxicity is usually reversible on discontinuation of the drug or reduction of the dose. In addition, acyclovir-associated neurotoxicity correlates with elevated plasma concentrations, and further underscores the need for adequate dosage adjustments in patients with renal dysfunction.[65]

The clearance of acyclovir correlates with the CrCl according to the following relationship:

$$\begin{aligned} &Cl_{acyclovir} \text{ in mL/minute/1.73 m}^2 \quad \text{(Eq. 33-25)} \\ &= (3.4)(\text{CrCl in mL/minute/1.73 m}^2) + 28.7) \end{aligned}$$

In patients with normal renal function, the clearance of acyclovir ranges from 210 to 330 mL/minute; in patients with ESRD, the clearance is 29 to 34 mL/minute.[19,64,66] Although this change in clearance primarily results from decreased renal clearance of the drug, nonrenal clearance of acyclovir also decreases in these patients.[19,66] As a result, the elimination half-life increases significantly from approximately 3 hours in patients with normal kidney function to 20 hours in patients with ESRD. Therefore, doses should be reduced proportionately from a normal daily dose of 15 mg/kg body weight (5 mg/kg given every 8 hours) for serious herpes simplex infections to doses as low as 2.5 mg/kg/day (given as a single daily dose) in patients with ESRD.[67] Because D.M. has a CrCl of 20 mL/minute and an estimated $Cl_{acyclovir}$ of 97 mL/minute (approximately one-third of normal), a single daily dose of 5 mg/kg (one-third of normal) would be appropriate to treat this infection.

DIALYSIS

Acyclovir is moderately removed by conventional hemodialysis, with plasma concentrations decreasing by 60% after 6 hours of dialysis.[68] The elimination half-life on and off dialysis is 6 and 20 hours, respectively, whereas the dialysis clearance averages 80 mL/minute. Therefore, a supplemental dose of 2.5 mg/kg after dialysis is recommended to replace the amount of drug removed by hemodialysis. No data are available on the removal of acyclovir by high-flux hemodialysis.

CASE 33-3, QUESTION 2: Does D.M.'s renal dysfunction affect the metabolism of acyclovir? Are there other drugs that are affected similarly?

Approximately 20% of acyclovir is cleared by nonrenal mechanisms.[19,66] The only significant metabolite that has been isolated is 9-carboxymethoxymethylguanine, which accounts for 9% to 14% of an administered dose. It is believed that this metabolite is a product of hepatic metabolism; however, the kidney may also play an important role.[19] Whether renal dysfunction alters hepatic metabolism or metabolic enzymes are present within the kidney is unclear. Renal tissue contains many of the same metabolic enzymes found in the liver. Mixed-function oxidases have been found in segments of the proximal tubule, whereas other metabolic processes, such as glucuronidation, acetylation, and hydrolysis, also occur within the kidney.[17,18,69]

Several studies have examined the effect of renal failure on hepatic metabolic enzyme activity.[70,71] Most of these investigations were carried out in animals that had diminished microsomal, mitochondrial, and cytosolic enzyme activities. Renal dysfunction substantially alters the nonrenal clearance of certain cephalosporins, such as ceftizoxime and cefotaxime,[72–75] as well as the benzodiazepines, diazepam and desmethyldiazepam.[76,77]

Zidovudine

DOSAGE ADJUSTMENT

CASE 33-3, QUESTION 3: D.M. also is being treated with AZT for his HIV disease. Will his AZT doses need to be adjusted?

AZT was the first drug approved for treatment of HIV infection and is still used as part of combination antiretroviral regimens. Because it has potent bone marrow–suppressive effects,[78] the dose of AZT may require adjustment based on the patient's clinical response and the development of toxicity.

AZT is metabolized primarily by the liver to the inactive glucuronide metabolite (GAZT), which is eliminated by the kidneys. Only 18% of AZT is eliminated unchanged by the kidneys. Little change in AZT clearance and elimination half-life occurs in patients with renal failure. Two studies report only slight increases in the elimination half-life (from 1.0 to 1.4 hours, and from 1.4 to 1.9 hours in patients with renal failure),[79,80] whereas another case report measured a half-life of 2.9 hours in a single patient with renal impairment.[81] Although GAZT accumulates in renal disease, this is not clinically important.[79]

Despite little change in AZT plasma levels, patients with renal failure are predisposed to bone marrow suppression because their kidneys produce less erythropoietin. In addition, their white blood cell (WBC) counts are also decreased. Therefore, AZT should be used more cautiously in these patients (see Chapter 73, Pharmacotherapy of Human Immunodeficiency Virus Infection).

HEMODIALYSIS

CASE 33-3, QUESTION 4: Is AZT significantly removed by dialysis?

A number of reports describe the removal of AZT by dialysis.[79–81] Based on the chemical characteristics, AZT would be expected to be dialyzable: it has a low MW of 267, a relatively small Vd (1–2.2 L/kg), and low protein binding (34%–38%). The dialysis clearance of AZT is minimal, however, when compared with its plasma clearance (primarily nonrenal) in patients with renal failure. Clearance by dialysis averages 63 mL/minute compared with a plasma clearance (after oral administration) of approximately 1,200 mL/minute. Little change occurs in the AZT plasma levels during dialysis; however, the elimination of GAZT may be enhanced.[79]

Penicillin

DOSAGE ADJUSTMENT

CASE 33-4

QUESTION 1: T.H., a 57-year-old, 85-kg man with chronic kidney disease secondary to poorly controlled hypertension, presents to the ED with a 24-hour history of fever (39°C), altered mental status, nausea, and vomiting. On physical examination he is found to have nuchal rigidity and a positive Brudzinski sign. Laboratory analysis reveals the following:

WBC count, 22,000/μL with 89% neutrophils
BUN, 45 mg/dL
SCr, 4.4 mg/dL

A lumbar puncture yields cerebrospinal fluid (CSF) with a WBC count of 2,000/μL (90% polymorphonuclear neutrophils), a glucose concentration of 36 mg/dL, and a protein concentration of 280 mg/dL. Gram-positive diplococci are seen on CSF smear. A diagnosis of meningococcal meningitis is made, and potassium penicillin G is ordered. What dose should be used?

Meningococcal meningitis can be treated with 20 to 24 million units of IV penicillin G in patients with normal renal function. As with many β-lactam antibiotics, penicillin is primarily excreted unchanged in the urine with little or no evidence of hepatic metabolism. Thus, the elimination half-life, which averages less than 1 hour in patients with normal kidney function, increases to 4 to 10 hours in patients with ESRD.[82–84]

Methods to modify the dose of penicillin in renal insufficiency have been developed by numerous investigators. The clearance of penicillin correlates closely to CrCl according to the following equation[84]:

$$Cl_{pen} \text{ in mL/minute} = 35.5 + 3.35 \text{ CrCl in mL/minute} \quad \textit{(Eq. 33-26)}$$

This correlation is based on data from patients with varying degrees of renal impairment.

An equation to estimate the total daily dose for patients with renal failure to achieve serum levels similar to those produced by high-dose penicillin (20–24 million units/day) in patients with normal renal function has been developed for patients with an estimated CrCl of less than 40 mL/minute. The dose for T.H. should be given in equal divided doses at 6- or 8-hour intervals:

$$Dose_{pen} \text{ in million units/day} = 3.2 + (CrCl/7) \quad \textit{(Eq. 33-27)}$$

Using the Cockcroft and Gault method, T.H.'s CrCl is approximately 20 mL/minute. Therefore, his daily dose of penicillin should be 6 million units. A dose of 2 million units every 8 hours would be appropriate for T.H. Penicillin G is often given as the potassium salt (penicillin G potassium), which contains approximately 1.7 mEq of potassium per 1 million units of penicillin. Accumulation of potassium owing to renal impairment may lead to hyperkalemia. Penicillin G sodium is an alternative formulation that would be appropriate.

As is true for many agents, these dosing recommendations are empiric and based on pharmacokinetic principles for patients in renal failure. These recommendations have not been subjected to carefully designed clinical trials that establish therapeutic efficacy. Therefore, other factors that can influence host response also should be considered when designing an individualized therapeutic regimen. These include the host's immune status, the presence of other medical conditions, microbial sensitivity patterns, and changes in pharmacokinetic disposition (e.g., concomitant liver disease, fluid overload, dehydration).

PENICILLIN-INDUCED NEUROTOXICITY

CASE 33-4, QUESTION 2: The prescriber fails to consider T.H.'s renal dysfunction when he orders penicillin, and begins a dose of 4 million units every 4 hours. Four days later, T.H. is encephalopathic (confused, disoriented, and difficult to arouse), with some twitching noted on the right side of his face. Are these toxic symptoms associated with high-dose penicillin? What predisposing factors may contribute to this neurotoxicity?

T.H. is experiencing signs of neurotoxicity that are consistent with elevated penicillin concentrations in the plasma and CSF. Penicillin usually produces few serious adverse effects. When large doses are used in patients with renal impairment, toxic symptoms such as those exhibited by T.H. can result. Signs and symptoms of penicillin-induced CNS toxicity include myoclonus, complex or generalized seizure activity, and encephalopathy progressing to coma.[39,40]

PREDISPOSING FACTORS

T.H.'s renal dysfunction predisposes him to penicillin-induced neurotoxicity. In a review of 46 cases of penicillin-associated neurotoxicity, decreased renal function was present in 35 patients.[40] Several possible explanations for this observation exist. Penicillin accumulates in patients with renal failure. The binding of acidic drugs (such as penicillin) to albumin is decreased, resulting in an increased fraction of free or active drug that can pass into the CSF. Alterations in the blood–brain barrier have been observed in uremic patients, which can lead to further increases in CSF drug levels.[39] High plasma concentrations of penicillin per se may contribute to changes in the blood–brain barrier permeability of this drug.[39] All these factors, together with the increased sensitivity of patients with renal failure to centrally acting agents, make CNS toxicity more likely. Previous neurotrauma, history of seizures, elderly age, and concurrent drugs that lower the seizure threshold can also contribute to neurotoxicity. As with penicillin, the carbapenem antibiotic combination, imipenem–cilastatin, is associated with a higher incidence of seizures in patients with renal dysfunction.[85,86] Other β-lactam antibiotics such as ceftazidime, cefepime, and piperacillin/tazobactam have been associated with seizures.[87,88]

Antipseudomonal Penicillins

PIPERACILLIN

CASE 33-5

QUESTION 1: M.H., a 44-year-old, 70-kg woman with acute nonlymphocytic leukemia, was admitted to the oncology ward for placement of a Hickman catheter for her chemotherapy. Seven days after treatment with cytarabine and daunorubicin, her temperature spiked to 39.4°C. Other physical findings consistent with sepsis included a blood pressure of 102/68 mm Hg, pulse rate of 112 beats/minute, and a respiratory rate of 27 breaths/minute. M.H. is neutropenic with a WBC count of 1,400/μL (3% polymorphonuclear leukocytes, 70% lymphocytes, and 22% monocytes). Her platelet count is 16,000/μL. M.H. also has renal dysfunction as reflected by an SCr and BUN of 2.6 and 38 mg/dL, respectively. Empiric therapy for sepsis is started with tobramycin, piperacillin/tazobactam, and vancomycin. How should piperacillin/tazobactam be dosed in M.H.?

Piperacillin is an antipseudomonal penicillin that is often used with an aminoglycoside to treat serious infections caused by gram-negative organisms.[89] Piperacillin is commonly given as a combination with tazobactam, a β-lactamase inhibitor.[90] In patients with normal renal function, piperacillin is primarily excreted unchanged by the kidney with a clearance of 2.6 mL/minute/kg, and a half-life of approximately 1 hour.[91,92] Doses of piperacillin/tazobactam can be as high as 4.5 g every 6 hours for the treatment of serious *Pseudomonas* species infections. In patients with ESRD, mean piperacillin clearance and half-life values are 0.7 mL/minute/kg and 3.3 hours, respectively.[91–93] Although these parameters are significantly different, they are less than those expected for a drug primarily cleared by the kidneys, suggesting that some other compensatory mechanism for elimination must be present. Piperacillin is partially cleared by biliary excretion, a route of elimination that is increased in patients with renal failure.[93,94] Therefore, aggressive dosage reductions in M.H. are unnecessary. An appropriate dose of piperacillin/tazobactam for M.H. would be 3.375 g every 8 hours. Widely used drug references such as Facts and Comparisons can be used for dosing guidelines for drugs commonly used in patients with renal failure.[45]

Vancomycin

PHARMACOKINETIC DOSAGE CALCULATIONS

CASE 33-5, QUESTION 2: In addition to the aforementioned regimen for M.H., vancomycin therapy is initiated at 500 mg every 24 hours to cover the possibility of an infection resistant to antistaphylococcal penicillins, such as nafcillin. Is this an appropriate dosing regimen for M.H.?

Vancomycin is a bactericidal antibiotic with excellent activity against most gram-positive organisms such as methicillin-resistant *Staphylococcus aureus* and *Streptococcus* species, including some isolates of *Enterococcus* species. It is used empirically in febrile neutropenic patients because the incidence of infection secondary to resistant organisms is much greater in this patient population. However, cases of vancomycin-resistant enterococci have emerged at rates as high as 50%, raising concern and reducing its empiric use.[95]

Vancomycin is poorly absorbed by the oral route and must be administered IV when used to treat systemic infections. As with many other antibiotics, vancomycin primarily is cleared by the kidneys.[96] Significant toxicities have been associated with elevated serum concentrations, making careful dosing modification in renal failure necessary.[97]

As with the aminoglycosides, pharmacokinetic calculations can be used to individualize a dosing regimen to produce the desired peak and trough plasma levels. Unlike the aminoglycosides, the therapeutic range for vancomycin is less clear. Normally, doses are designed to achieve peak levels of 25 to 40 mg/L and trough levels of 10 to 15 mg/L.[98,99] The correlation between vancomycin toxicity (e.g., ototoxicity) and plasma levels is not well defined. Some clinicians have suggested, however, that plasma levels of 80 mg/L or more may correlate with auditory dysfunction.

Vancomycin has an elimination half-life of 3 to 9 hours in patients with normal renal function.[100] This increases to 129 to 189 hours in patients with ESRD.[101–103] Using pharmacokinetic principles and considering that the plasma clearance of vancomycin is approximately 60% to 70% of CrCl[98] and the Vd averages 0.7 L/kg,[98,100,104] the estimated Vd_{vanco} and Cl_{vanco} can be calculated using the following equation:

$$Cr_{Cl} = 30.5 \text{ mL/minute (calculated from Eq. 33-5)}$$

$$\begin{aligned} Cl_{vanco} &= (0.65)(CrCl) \\ &= (0.65)(30.5 \text{ mL/minute}) \qquad \textit{(Eq. 33-28)} \\ &= 19.8 \text{ mL/min } \textit{or} \text{ rounded off to } 1.2 \text{ L/hour} \end{aligned}$$

$$\begin{aligned} Vd_{vanco} &= (0.7 \text{ L/kg})(\text{body weight}) \\ &= (0.7 \text{ L/kg})(70 \text{ kg}) \qquad \textit{(Eq. 33-29)} \\ &= 49 \text{ L} \end{aligned}$$

Based on estimated values for Cl_{vanco} and Vd_{vanco}, the elimination rate constant can be calculated using the following equation:

$$\begin{aligned} Kd &= \frac{Cl_{vanco}}{Vd_{vanco}} \\ &= \frac{1.2 \text{ L/hour}}{49 \text{ L}} \qquad \textit{(Eq. 33-30)} \\ &= 0.024 \text{ hour}^{-1} \end{aligned}$$

$$\begin{aligned} Cp &= \frac{\dfrac{Dose}{Vd_{vanco}}}{1 - e^{-Kdt}} \\ &= \frac{\dfrac{500 \text{ mg}}{49 \text{ L}}}{1 - e^{-(0.024 \text{ hour}^{-1})(24 \text{ hours})}} \qquad \textit{(Eq. 33-31)} \\ &= 23 \text{ mg/L} \end{aligned}$$

$$\begin{aligned} Cp_{trough} &= Cp_{peak}(e^{-Kdt}) \\ &= 23 \text{ mg/L}(e^{-(0.024/\text{hour}^{-1})(24 \text{ hours})}) \qquad \textit{(Eq. 33-32)} \\ &= 13 \text{ mg/L} \end{aligned}$$

Because M.H.'s estimated peak concentration is less than 40 mg/L and her trough falls within the range of 10 to 15 mg/L, the starting dose of 500 mg every 24 hours is appropriate for M.H.

Routine monitoring of plasma vancomycin concentrations in patients with normal renal function is controversial because the likelihood that toxicity will develop in this group is relatively low. However, in patients with renal failure, such as M.H., it is advisable to measure vancomycin levels several days after initiation of therapy to ensure that they are within an acceptable range.[100,102,103,105] This is prudent if an extended course of therapy is anticipated. Vancomycin is usually infused over the course of 60 minutes.

HEMODIALYSIS OF VANCOMYCIN

CASE 33-5, QUESTION 3: M.H.'s renal function begins to deteriorate to the point where she requires hemodialysis. How should her regimen now be altered?

Patients with ESRD may have measurable vancomycin levels for up to 3 weeks after a single dose despite conventional hemodialysis.[103] This suggests that the ability of these patients to eliminate vancomycin is minimal and that little of the drug is removed by conventional hemodialysis. The elimination half-life for vancomycin in these individuals averages 5 to 7 days, which is consistent with a residual vancomycin clearance of 3 to 4 mL/minute.[101–103] Only about 5% of vancomycin is metabolized hepatically in patients with normal renal function.

Conventional hemodialysis removes about 7% of vancomycin during a typical 4-hour dialysis run.[106] The elimination half-life on and off dialysis and plasma levels of the drug before and after hemodialysis do not differ significantly. The poor removal of vancomycin by conventional hemodialysis is attributable to its large MW of 1,400.

Patients receiving conventional hemodialysis are typically given a single, 1-g dose every 7 to 10 days.[100,103,105] Based on M.H.'s estimated Vd of 49 L, this dose will produce an initial peak plasma level of approximately 20 mg/L. If vancomycin is administered weekly, steady-state peak and trough levels of 40 and 16 mg/L, respectively, would be predicted.

Vancomycin is removed to a greater extent by high-flux hemodialysis than by conventional hemodialysis. As a result, more frequent dosing is necessary to maintain therapeutic vancomycin concentrations. High-flux dialysis clearance of vancomycin using the Fresenius polysulfone dialyzer is 45 to 160 mL/minute and varies with membrane surface area.[60,107] Up to 50% of a dose of vancomycin is removed in 4 hours by high-flux hemodialysis compared with 6.9% using conventional dialysis. A rebound phenomenon after dialysis suggests that the total amount of drug removed may be less than initially reported.[108,109] In any case, the efficiency of high-flux procedures in removing vancomycin is greater than that of conventional dialysis. Therefore, plasma levels should be monitored carefully in these patients, and the necessity for postdialysis replacement doses of around 500 mg (~10–15 mg/kg) should be anticipated.

Amphotericin

DOSING

CASE 33-5, QUESTION 4: M.H. continues to be febrile despite her triple antimicrobial regimen. Amphotericin therapy is started empirically for a potential fungal infection. In addition, pentamidine is begun to cover *Pneumocystis jiroveci* pneumonia. How should amphotericin be administered in patients such as M.H. with renal dysfunction?

Amphotericin is an antifungal agent used to treat serious infections, such as invasive aspergillosis and cryptococcal meningitis. The exact mechanism of elimination for this drug is unclear, but it may involve hepatic metabolism or inactivation in body tissues. Small amounts of amphotericin are gradually excreted in the urine for several weeks after its discontinuation.[110] This slow elimination may be because of extensive distribution of amphotericin into peripheral tissue and its large Vd (4 L/kg).[110,111] The drug appears to bind to cholesterol-containing cytoplasmic membranes of various tissues, resulting in a very long elimination half-life of 15 days. Pharmacokinetic studies report no significant change in the disposition of amphotericin in patients with renal or liver disease. Therefore, no dosage adjustments are required in patients with renal dysfunction.

Amphotericin is associated with acute tubular necrosis, which is believed to be dose dependent.[112–114] To prevent exacerbation of nephrotoxicity, lower doses often are administered to patients with decreased renal function. Administration of amphotericin every other day often is suggested for patients with renal failure. In addition to conventional amphotericin, a liposomal (liposomal amphotericin) or lipid-based formulation is available.[21] Lipid-based formulations have reduced distribution to the kidneys, and are associated with a lower incidence of nephrotoxicity.[115] Triazole antifungal agents (e.g., fluconazole, posaconazole, voriconazole) or an echinocandin class (e.g., anidulafungin, caspofungin, micafungin) are alternative choices that are not potentially nephrotoxic, nor do they need to be dose adjusted in the setting of renal dysfunction (with the exception of fluconazole). The oral formulation of voriconazole should be used in renal dysfunction or for patients with a CrCl of less than 50 mL/minute to prevent accumulation of sulfobutyl ether β-cyclodextrin, the solvent vehicle found in the IV formulation.[116]

HEMODIALYSIS OF AMPHOTERICIN

Amphotericin is not removed significantly by hemodialysis because it is a very large compound and distributes widely into peripheral tissues. Therefore, little drug remains in the plasma to be removed by dialysis. Studies have found that less than 5% of amphotericin is removed during a 4-hour conventional hemodialysis period.

Cefazolin

PERITONEAL DIALYSIS

CASE 33-6

QUESTION 1: M.J. is a 65-year-old woman with chronic kidney disease awaiting a kidney transplant. She has been managed with PD for the past 8 years. She presents with a cloudy effluent and abdominal pain. Analysis of the effluent reveals a WBC count of 323/μL and gram-positive cocci and clusters on Gram stain. The patient has a history of *S. aureus* peritonitis that was readily treated with cefazolin 2 years ago. The patient has no allergies, and weighs 52 kg. How should M.J.'s PD-related infection be managed?

Gram-positive cocci such as *S. aureus* are common causes of PD-related infections. The selection of empiric antibiotics should be made based on the patient's and program's history of microorganisms and sensitivities. A first-generation cephalosporin such as cefazolin would be a reasonable choice for M.J. Programs with a high rate of methicillin-resistant organisms should use vancomycin.

IP antibiotics can be given with each exchange (continuous dosing). In this situation, a single 500-mg/L loading dose of cefazolin is given followed by a maintenance dose of 125 mg/L with subsequent exchanges. Antibiotics can also be given intermittently (once daily per exchange). With intermittent dosing, the antibiotic-containing dialysis solution should dwell for at least 6 hours to allow for adequate absorption. Cefazolin 15 mg/kg (rounded off to 750 mg) is typically given in one exchange. For patients on automated PD, the dose of cefazolin is 20 mg/kg every day in a long-day dwell. The management of PD-related infections and dosing of various antibiotics is discussed in the International Society for Peritoneal Dialysis guidelines.[117]

Phenytoin

PROTEIN BINDING

CASE 33-7

QUESTION 1: R.S., a 24-year-old man with ESRD from rapidly progressive glomerulonephritis, is treated by hemodialysis three times weekly. He has a 7-year history of generalized tonic-clonic seizures and has been treated with phenytoin. He presents to the ED after having had a seizure lasting about 5 minutes. His mother states that he ran out of phenytoin 4 weeks ago. Because his plasma phenytoin concentration on admission was less than 2.5 mg/L, R.S. is given an IV loading dose of phenytoin: 15 mg/kg in 30 minutes. Additional admission laboratory work includes the following:

SCr, 8.6 mg/dL
BUN, 110 mg/dL
Potassium, 5.4 mEq/L
Calcium, 9 mg/dL
Albumin, 2.9 g/dL

Eight hours after administration of phenytoin, his level is 5 mg/L. Is this level subtherapeutic?

R.S. has severe renal disease, which will affect the total (bound plus free) phenytoin concentration achieved and how this concentration is interpreted. Decreased plasma protein binding will result in lower measured total phenytoin concentrations, and the calculated apparent Vd may increase. In patients with normal renal function, approximately 90% of the measured phenytoin is bound to albumin, and 10% is free. The free fraction of phenytoin is increased to about 20% to 25% in patients with uremia.[11,118–122] Because the free fraction for phenytoin is increased in patients with uremia, lower plasma concentrations will produce therapeutic effects that will be equivalent to those produced by higher phenytoin concentrations in patients with normal renal function.[8,123] Phenytoin is an acidic drug that is bound primarily to albumin. A number of mechanisms have been proposed that account for the decreased binding, including (a) decreased albumin concentration, (b) accumulation of uremic byproducts that displace acidic drugs from their binding sites, and (c) alteration in the conformation or structure of albumin in uremic patients, resulting in a reduced number of binding sites or decreased affinity for drugs (see Chapter 58, Seizure Disorders). Other acidic drugs with altered protein binding in renal disease are listed in Table 33-1.

Figure 33-2 illustrates changes in phenytoin levels when uremic and nonuremic patients are given equivalent doses.[124]

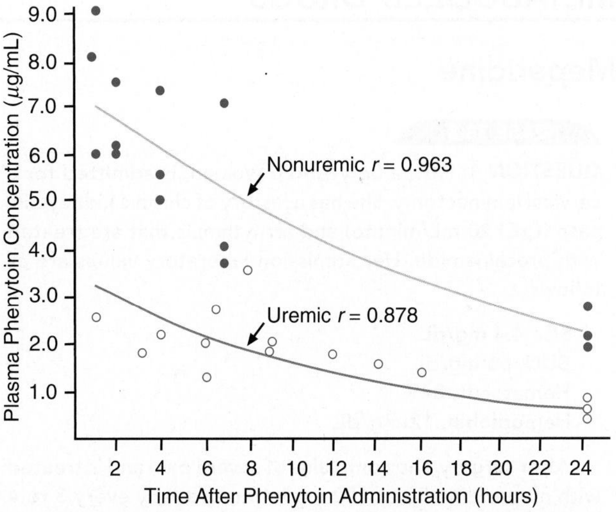

FIGURE 33-2 **Plasma phenytoin concentrations in uremic (○) and nonuremic (●) patients after 250 mg of intravenous (IV) phenytoin.** (Reprinted with permission from Letteri JM et al. Diphenylhydantoin metabolism in uremia. *N Engl J Med.* 1971;285:648. Copyright © 2001 Massachusetts Medical Society. All rights reserved.)

The following equation should be used to correct for R.S.'s altered binding owing to his renal dysfunction and hypoalbuminemia[121]:

$$Cp_{\text{Normal Binding}} = \frac{Cp'}{(0.48)(1-\alpha)\left(\frac{P'}{P_{NL}}\right)+\alpha} \qquad \text{(Eq. 33-33)}$$

where Cp' is the measured plasma concentration reported by the laboratory, and $Cp_{\text{Normal Binding}}$ is the corrected plasma concentration that would be seen if the patient had normal renal function and normal albumin. Alpha (α) is the normal free fraction (0.1), P' is the patient's serum albumin, and P_{NL} is normal albumin (4.4 g/dL). The factor 0.48 was derived from patients on hemodialysis and represents the decreased affinity of phenytoin for albumin.

For R.S., a total plasma phenytoin concentration of 5 mg/L is comparable to 13 mg/L in a patient without renal failure. Because this falls within the phenytoin's therapeutic range of 10 to 20 mg/L, his measured level is not subtherapeutic.

The factor 0.48 should be used only to estimate changes in protein binding for patients with ESRD receiving hemodialysis. Data for patients with moderate renal disease are limited, and it is unclear what changes exist in the binding of phenytoin to albumin.[119] For patients with normal or moderate renal impairment, the following equation should be used only if the serum albumin is low; the factor 0.48 should be omitted:

$$Cp_{\text{Normal Binding}} = \frac{Cp'}{(1-\alpha)\left(\frac{P'}{P_{NL}}\right)+\alpha} \qquad \text{(Eq. 33-34)}$$

Fosphenytoin, a prodrug of phenytoin, does not need to be dissolved in propylene glycol, and therefore can be administered more quickly. This offers an important advantage for seizures that must be controlled quickly. In patients with renal failure, the conversion of fosphenytoin to phenytoin was equally efficient in patients with renal disease and healthy subjects.[125] Once fosphenytoin is converted to phenytoin, the impact of renal disease on protein binding is expected to be similar to that seen with phenytoin and thus the same considerations should be made for patients with renal failure.

EFFECT OF RENAL FAILURE ON METABOLIZED DRUGS

Meperidine

CASE 33-8

QUESTION 1: F.G., a 56-year-old woman, is admitted for a cervical laminectomy. She has a history of chronic kidney disease (CrCl 20 mL/minute) and arrhythmias that are treated with procainamide. Her admission laboratory values are as follows:

SCr, 4.4 mg/dL
BUN, 66 mg/dL
Hematocrit, 34%
Hemoglobin, 12.6 g/dL

After surgery, she complains of severe pain and is treated with meperidine 50 to 100 mg intramuscularly every 3 to 4 hours. Three days postoperatively, F.G. experiences a generalized tonic-clonic seizure. She has no history of seizures. What might be responsible for this sudden event?

TABLE 33-3
Drugs With Active or Toxic Metabolites Excreted by the Kidney

Drug	Metabolite
Acetohexamide	Hydroxyhexamide
Allopurinol	Oxypurinol
Bupropion	Threo/erythro-hydrobupropion
Cefotaxime	Desacetylcefotaxime
Chlorpropamide	Hydroxy metabolites
Clofibrate	Chlorphenoxyisobutyrate
Cyclophosphamide	4-Ketocyclophosphamide
Daunorubicin	Daunorubicinol
Meperidine	Normeperidine
Methyldopa	Methyl-*O*-sulfate-α-methyldopamine
Midazolam	α-Hydroxymidazolam
Morphine	Morphine-3-glucuronide Morphine-6-glucuronide
Phenylbutazone	Oxyphenbutazone
Primidone	Phenobarbital
Procainamide	*N*-acetylprocainamide (NAPA)
Propoxyphene	Norpropoxyphene
Rifampicin	Desacetylated metabolites
Sodium nitroprusside	Thiocyanate
Sulfonamides	Acetylated metabolites
Tramadol	*O*-Demethyl-*N*-demethyltramadol

Meperidine is a narcotic analgesic commonly used to control acute pain. It is metabolized hepatically via *N*-demethylation to normeperidine, a metabolite known to accumulate in renal insufficiency.[15,126] Although meperidine has both CNS excitatory and depressant properties, normeperidine is a very potent CNS stimulant that can cause seizures in patients with renal failure who are receiving multiple doses of the parent drug.[127] In a study of 67 cancer patients treated with meperidine, 48 experienced neurologic adverse effects; 14 of these 48 patients had renal dysfunction defined as a BUN greater than 20 mg/dL.[127] Because the renal clearance of normeperidine correlates significantly with CrCl, renal dysfunction can lead to its accumulation, resulting in neurologic toxicity. In another study, the normeperidine to meperidine plasma concentration ratio was consistently higher in patients with renal failure, averaging 2.0 compared with a mean of 0.6 for patients with good renal function.[127] Table 33-3 lists examples of additional drugs that have active or toxic metabolites that may accumulate in renal disease.

Narcotic Analgesics

CASE 33-8, QUESTION 2: Are the pharmacokinetics or pharmacodynamics of other narcotic analgesics altered in patients with renal insufficiency?

MORPHINE

The pharmacokinetic disposition of morphine does not appear to be altered in patients with renal failure[128]; however, its active metabolite, morphine-6-glucuronide, as well as its principal metabolite, morphine-3-glucuronide, do accumulate in renal disease. The elimination half-life of morphine-6-glucuronide increases from 3 to 4 hours in normal subjects to 89 to 136 hours in subjects with renal failure.[129] This metabolite penetrates the blood–brain barrier more readily, has a greater affinity for CNS receptors, and has analgesic activity that is 3.7 times greater than morphine.[130] Therefore, accumulation of morphine-6-glucuronide may be responsible for the morphine-induced narcosis reported in patients with severe renal disease.[32,33]

CODEINE

Other analgesics that have been associated with CNS toxicity in patients with renal failure include codeine, propoxyphene, and dihydrocodeine.[126] The disposition of orally administered codeine does not appear to be altered in renal failure; however, there have been case reports of codeine-induced narcosis.[131] Although the dose of codeine did not exceed 120 mg/day, CNS and respiratory depression persisted for up to 4 days after discontinuing codeine and initiating naloxone administration. The elimination half-life of codeine is prolonged in patients on chronic hemodialysis. Although the Vd of codeine was twice as large, the total clearance was not significantly decreased.[132] A lower initial dose should be used because codeine is metabolized to morphine.

HYDROMORPHONE

Hydromorphone is metabolized in the liver to hydromorphone-3-glucuronide, dihydroisomorphone, dihydromorphine, and small amounts of hydromorphone-3-sulfate, norhydromorphone, and nordihydroisomorphone.[133] All metabolites that are eliminated are excreted by the kidneys. Hydromorphone can be used in patients with renal failure; however, smaller initial doses may be warranted.[132]

Procainamide

CASE 33-8, QUESTION 3: F.G.'s procainamide level is 9 mg/L (normal, 4–8 mg/L) and her *N*-acetylprocainamide (NAPA) level is 34 mg/L (normal, 10–20 mg/L). How is the disposition of procainamide affected in patients with renal disease?

The pharmacokinetics of procainamide in patients with renal insufficiency is complex. Of the parent drug, 50% to 70% is excreted unchanged in the urine, and it can accumulate in patients with renal disease because plasma clearance values are reduced by as much as 70%.[134] Procainamide is also partially acetylated to NAPA, which has antiarrhythmic properties similar to procainamide and is primarily excreted by the kidneys.[135,136] Figure 33-3 summarizes the elimination of procainamide and NAPA. The half-life of NAPA is longer, especially in patients with renal impairment, increasing from 6 hours in control subjects to as long as 40 hours in patients with ESRD.[134,135] Because significant cardiac toxicity has occurred in some patients with NAPA levels greater than 30 mg/L, plasma level monitoring of both NAPA and procainamide is recommended. When procainamide is used in patients with renal failure, appropriate dosage reduction of procainamide may be necessary. It also is important to realize that the time required to reach steady state for NAPA in patients with renal failure may be as long as 5 days. Therefore, plasma levels measured early in therapy must be interpreted carefully, because these concentrations may be considerably lower than those that will be achieved under steady-state conditions.

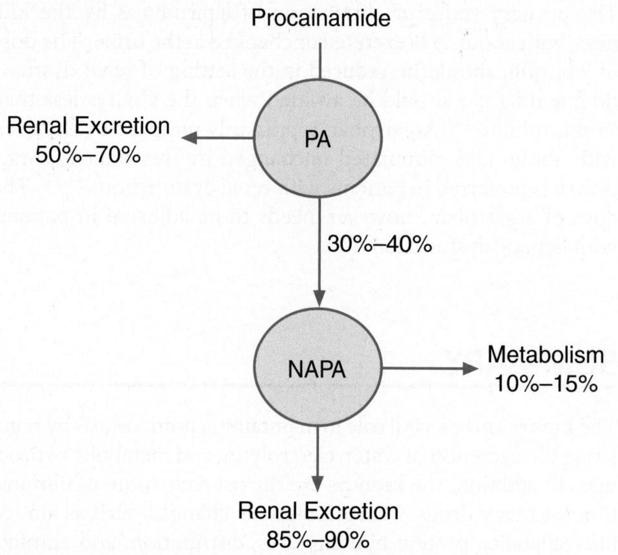

FIGURE 33-3 **Elimination of procainamide (PA) and *N*-acetylprocainamide (NAPA) in subjects with normal renal and liver function.**

Enoxaparin

CASE 33-8, QUESTION 4: Because F.G. is not ambulating well after her surgery, her physician would like to initiate deep vein thrombosis prophylaxis with enoxaparin. Are there any dosing considerations for enoxaparin in this patient?

Enoxaparin is a low-molecular-weight heparin that is used to prevent and treat various thromboembolic disorders, such as deep venous thrombosis, unstable angina, and non–Q wave myocardial infarction. The kidneys play a major role in the clearance of enoxaparin,[137] and a higher incidence of bleeding complications is associated with the use of enoxaparin in patients with renal dysfunction.[138] The elimination half-life of enoxaparin is prolonged in patients with ESRD, although the other pharmacokinetic parameters are similar to those in healthy subjects.[139,140] The increased incidence of bleeding complications cannot be completely attributed to pharmacokinetic changes, but may also be related to the effects of enoxaparin on antifactor IIa and antithrombin III, as well as the effects of uremia on hemostasis.[141]

Enoxaparin should be used cautiously in patients with a CrCl less than 30 mL/minute, with a recommended lower dosage of 30 mg subcutaneously daily. Although monitoring of the anticoagulant effect by anti-Xa activity is not necessary in clinically stable patients, it may be warranted in patients with renal dysfunction as well as those who have other factors that may increase the risk of bleeding complications.

Direct Thrombin Inhibitors

CASE 33-9

QUESTION 1: A.H. is a 55-year-old woman with a history of chronic kidney disease (SCr 3.7 mg/dL) who is diagnosed with a pulmonary embolus. While being administered anticoagulation with a heparin infusion, her platelet count drops from a baseline of 135 × $10^3/\mu L$ to 40 × $10^3/\mu L$. A positive heparin-platelet factor 4 antibody result confirms the diagnosis of heparin-induced thrombocytopenia. What options are available for the therapeutic anticoagulation of A.H. in the setting of heparin-induced thrombocytopenia?

Argatroban and lepirudin are direct thrombin inhibitors that are US Food and Drug Administration approved for the management of heparin-induced thrombocytopenia.[142] Lepirudin is a recombinant hirudin that inhibits the catalytic site of thrombin.

The primary route of elimination of lepirudin is by the kidneys, with about 35% excreted unchanged in the urine. The dose of lepirudin should be reduced in the setting of renal dysfunction, and its use should be avoided when the CrCl is less than 15 mL/minute.[143] Argatroban is primarily removed by the liver, with about 15% eliminated unchanged by the kidneys. Argatroban is preferred in patients with renal dysfunction.[144,145] The dose of argatroban, however, needs to be adjusted in patients with hepatic dysfunction.[146]

SUMMARY

The kidneys play a vital role in maintaining homeostasis by regulating the excretion of water, electrolytes, and metabolic byproducts. In addition, the kidneys are the primary route of elimination for many drugs. Pharmacokinetic changes, such as altered bioavailability, protein binding, drug distribution, and elimination, can occur with many drugs in patients with renal failure. Pharmacodynamic changes, such as altered sensitivity or response to medications, can also occur in this patient population. Renal replacement therapies, such as hemodialysis, CAPD, and CVVH, will aid in the removal of fluid, electrolytes, and metabolic byproducts in drugs as well. Data from clinical trials provide valuable information about the disposition of drugs in patients with renal failure. Pharmacokinetic principles should be applied when appropriate to determine the optimal dose of drugs for patients with renal failure.

KEY REFERENCES AND WEBSITES

A full list of references for this chapter can be found at **http://thepoint.lww.com/AT10e.** Below are the key references and websites for this chapter, with the corresponding reference number in this chapter found in parentheses after the reference.

Key References

Aronoff GR et al. *Drug Prescribing in Renal Failure*. 5th ed. Philadelphia, PA: American College of Physicians; 2007. (91)

Heintz BH, Matzke GR, Dager WE. Antimicrobial dosing concepts and recommendations for critically ill adult patients receiving continuous renal replacement therapy or intermittent hemodialysis. *Pharmacotherapy*. 2009;29:562.

Winter ME. *Basic Clinical Pharmacokinetics*. 5th ed. Baltimore, MD: Lippincott Williams & Wilkins; 2010.

Key Websites

Cockroft-Gault Calculator. **http://www.nephron.com/cgi-bin/CGSI.cgi.**

Renal Drug Handbook Online version. **http://www.radcliffe-oxford.com/electronic/E24_Renal_Drug_Handbook_3e_%28online%29/default.asp.**

2010 Dialysis of Drugs. **http://www.ckdinsights.com/downloads/DialysisDrugs2010.pdf.**

Kidney and Liver Transplantation

34

David J. Taber and Robert E. Dupuis

CORE PRINCIPLES

		CHAPTER CASES
1	Successful kidney transplantation involves rigorous evaluation of both donor and recipient. This results in immunologic categorization as either a high-risk or low-risk transplant and determines the immunosuppressive regimen an individual recipient should receive. The majority of these patients will receive combination therapy which includes a calcineurin inhibitor, an antiproliferative agent, and a corticosteroid.	**Case 34-1 (Questions 1–3)**
2	Induction therapy is used in most kidney transplant cases. Rabbit antithymocyte globulin, alemtuzumab, or basiliximab are common agents. Differences among these agents include dosing regimen and side effect profile. Rabbit antithymocyte globulin or alemtuzumab are often used in high-risk patients, including those with delayed graft function, whereas basiliximab is frequently used in low-risk recipients.	**Case 34-1 (Questions 4–8)**
3	Immunosuppressive therapy is directed at prevention of rejection. Acute rejection can be either T cell–mediated or B cell–mediated. T cell–mediated rejection can be successfully treated whereas B cell–mediated rejection is much more resistant. Despite success in reducing acute rejections, chronic rejection and chronic graft dysfunction are major causes of graft loss.	**Case 34-1 (Questions 9–10)**
4	Cyclosporine is a calcineurin inhibitor with a complex pharmacokinetic profile associated with multiple adverse effects and requires therapeutic drug monitoring (TDM). Its use has declined since the introduction of tacrolimus.	**Case 34-2 (Questions 1–3)**
5	The mTor inhibitors, sirolimus and everolimus, have complex pharmacokinetic profiles, significant adverse effects, and require TDM. These agents appear to be most useful in minimizing the use of calcineurin inhibitors or other agents.	**Case 34-2 (Question 4)**
6	The calcineurin inhibitors cyclosporine and tacrolimus and steroids have significant toxicity profiles, particularly with chronic long-term use. Calcineurin inhibitor–induced nephrotoxicity is a major problem. Steroids have a negative impact on the cardiovascular, bone, and endocrine system. Several strategies have been developed in an attempt to either avoid or minimize these adverse effects.	**Case 34-3 (Questions 1, 2), Case 34-4 (Question 1)**
7	BK polyomavirus is almost exclusively seen in kidney transplantation and is associated with graft loss. The best approach to reducing its occurrence is viral surveillance. If it is present, then reduction of immunosuppression appears to be the most effective treatment.	**Case 34-5 (Questions 1–3)**
8	Cardiovascular complications, including hypertension, hyperlipidemia, and diabetes, are prevalent among kidney transplant recipients. These contribute to poor patient survival and graft loss. Other complications such osteoporosis are frequently observed. Monitoring and treatment of these complications, which may be drug-induced, are part of the posttransplant care plan.	**Case 34-6 (Questions 1–3)**

continued

		CHAPTER CASES
9	Liver transplantation is considered the treatment of choice for patient with end-stage liver disease. Common early posttransplant complications include surgical (biliary leaks and bleeding), neurologic (continued hepatic encephalopathy, drug toxicity), and infectious (pneumonias, urinary tract infections, and biliary bacteremias).	**Case 34-7 (Questions 1, 2)**
10	Tacrolimus is considered the cornerstone of the immunosuppressant regimen for the vast majority of solid organ transplant recipients. It has complex pharmacokinetics, and therefore requires close TDM for optimal use. Tacrolimus is a potent agent that has significantly reduced acute rejection rates; additionally, compared to cyclosporine, tacrolimus has fewer cosmetic side effects (hirsutism, gingival hyperplasia), fewer effects on serum lipoproteins and blood pressure, but has more severe effects on serum glucose levels and more pronounced neurotoxicities.	**Case 34-7 (Questions 3–6)**
11	Acute rejection of the transplanted liver is a common, but usually reversible, consequence after this surgery. It is usually asymptomatic, but can be identified early through serial monitoring of serum transaminases and bilirubin, and definitively diagnosed only through liver biopsy. Treatment usually consists of pulse dose corticosteroids, followed by a taper, or the use of rabbit antithymocyte globulin for more severe rejections or those refractory to steroid therapy.	**Case 34-7 (Questions 7, 8)**
12	Mycophenolate is considered the adjuvant agent of choice in solid organ transplantation, and is used to reduce calcineurin inhibitor exposure or augment immunosuppressant regimen potency. TDM is not common and has yet to prove effective in optimizing therapy. Common side effects with this agent include gastrointestinal issues (nausea, vomiting, diarrhea) and cytopenias (leukopenia and thrombocytopenia).	**Case 34-7 (Question 9)**
13	Drug interactions with immunosuppressants are numerous and are commonly encountered clinical dilemmas in the transplant recipient. Pharmacists should prospectively screen for these interactions, and, depending on their magnitude, may need to prospectively adjust medication regimens. Closer TDM or clinical monitoring is always warranted when adding or removing an interacting medication to a patient on immunosuppression.	**Case 34-8 (Question 1)**
14	Infections, including opportunistic infections, are common complications after transplant. Prophylaxis with antimicrobial agents is critical for the most common and severe pathogens. Hepatitis B and C are problematic after liver transplant, and require immunoprophylaxis or treatment in certain circumstances.	**Case 34-9 (Question 1)**
15	Cytomegalovirus is the most common and debilitating opportunistic infection after solid organ transplantation. Reactivation or new infection with this virus can lead to severe tissue invasive disease and potentially death. Indirect effects include acute rejection, chronic rejection, graft loss, and potentially, lymphoma. Prophylaxis with potent antivirals (ganciclovir or valganciclovir) is the cornerstone of prevention. Treatment involves a long course of antiviral therapy usually in conjunction with reductions in immunosuppression.	**Case 34-10 (Questions 1–4)**
16	Posttransplant lymphoproliferative disorder (PTLD), which is usually a B-cell lymphoma, is the most common cancer encountered after organ transplant. Early PTLD is generally responsive to reductions in immunosuppression; advanced PTLD is usually not responsive to this nor to traditional chemotherapy. The use of rituximab, a monoclonal antibody directed against B cells, has shown promise for treatment of this disease.	**Case 34-11 (Questions 1, 2)**

INTRODUCTION TO TRANSPLANTATION

Solid organ transplantation is an established therapeutic option for patients with end-stage kidney, liver, heart, and lung disease. For many of these patients, it is the only option. One-year patient survival for these major organs is between 85% and 98%. One-year graft survival approaches these figures as well.[1] Pancreas or combined pancreas–kidney transplantation is available as a treatment for diabetic patients with end-stage renal failure. Intestinal transplantation is performed, but in a limited number of patients. Pediatric and elderly patients are transplant candidates, increasing the pool of potential recipients. Surgical techniques involving multiorgan transplantation (e.g., heart with lung, liver, kidney); pancreatic islet cell and liver cell transplantation; intestinal transplantation; living-related, unrelated, and segmental human organ transplantation (e.g., kidney, liver, lung, pancreas); domino heart and heart–lung transplantation; along with improvements in mechanical assist devices (e.g., for heart transplant candidates) have made the transplantation of organs an increasingly viable treatment option. Research continues in overcoming the immunologic barriers associated with xenotransplantation (animal to human).

Despite these approaches, many more patients are in need of transplantation than there are organs available. In 2008, about 27,000 organ transplants were performed, whereas 100,000 people were waiting for organs. Consequently, a significant number of candidates die while waiting for a transplant.[1]

During the 1960s, drugs such as azathioprine, prednisone, antilymphocyte serum, and antilymphocyte globulin made the success of kidney transplantation possible. In the late 1970s, the introduction of cyclosporine created a new era in solid organ transplantation, and in the 1980s the first monoclonal antibody approved for human use, OKT3, was introduced, but is no longer available.

Since the mid-1990s, a number of new agents have been approved. These include tacrolimus, mycophenolate mofetil, mycophenolate sodium, and sirolimus (formerly rapamycin); monoclonal antibodies, such as daclizumab and basiliximab; a polyclonal antibody, anti-thymocyte globulin (rabbit) (rabbit antithymocyte globulin); and everolimus. More recently, several agents, such as intravenous immunoglobulins (IVIG), alemtuzumab, and rituximab, have also been incorporated into transplant protocols. Several new agents are undergoing investigation. These provide more individualized, specific, and selective therapies for solid organ transplant recipients.

Although transplantation has had a significant positive impact on the quality of life in most patients with end-stage disease, issues such as retransplantation because of graft failure or disease recurrence, donation source (living-related and unrelated organs), and costs to individuals, insurers, and society continue to be discussed vigorously. Costs during the initial transplantation period range from $50,000 for kidney transplants up to $250,000 for heart, liver, or lung transplants. In addition, routine follow-up monitoring and drug therapy for the first year can cost $10,000 to $60,000. The ability of transplant recipients to pay for their medications or insurance denial or termination of coverage is a major issue. Also, the cost-effectiveness and adverse effects of immunosuppressive agents are important issues.

The goal of immunosuppressive therapy is to prevent organ rejection, prolong graft and patient survival, and improve quality of life. Short-term (i.e., 1–2 years) survival after transplantation has improved dramatically. Long-term survival also has improved, but not to the same degree.[2] The current immunosuppressive regimens do not produce a permanent state of tolerance (i.e., when the transplanted organ is seen as "self"). Limited data suggest that some selected patients may not require lifetime immunosuppression; these are in a minority, and more definitive studies must be done. As patients live longer after transplantation, the focus of therapy has shifted to survival and management of long-term complications. Immunosuppressive agents are associated with significant long-term complications. These include nephrotoxicity, hypertension, hyperlipidemia, osteoporosis, and diabetes, as well as graft loss secondary to infection, malignancy, recurrence of primary disease, and nonadherence. Although acute rejection rates are significantly lower, this remains a problem, along with chronic rejection and/or chronic graft dysfunction. The search for safer and more effective immunosuppressive regimens continues, along with a better understanding of optimal long-term immunosuppression. This chapter addresses the immunology of transplantation and rejection, indications for solid organ transplantation, appropriate use of immunosuppressive agents, and the management of postoperative and long-term complications in the patient who receives a solid organ transplant. Many of these issues are similar for the various types of solid organ transplantations, but there can be significant differences. This chapter addresses some of these issues as they relate to kidney and liver transplantation.

TRANSPLANTATION IMMUNOLOGY

Successful organ transplantation has come from a greater understanding and application of pharmacology, microbiology, molecular and cellular biochemistry and biology, genetics, and immunology. Suppression of the host's immune system and prevention of rejection are vital for host acceptance of the transplanted organ. The ultimate goal is permanent acceptance or tolerance, a situation in which the new organ is seen as "self" by the host's immune system. In general, the currently used immunosuppressive drugs provide a nonpermanent form of tolerance and lifelong immunosuppression is required. A basic understanding of the immune system and the mechanisms of rejection is key to the effective use of immunosuppressive drugs in organ transplantation.

Major Histocompatibility Complex and Human Leukocyte Antigen

The degree to which allogeneic grafting (i.e., a transplanted organ from a genetically different donor of the same species) is successful depends on the genetic similarities or differences between the organ of the donor and the immune system of the recipient. The recipient recognizes the transplanted graft as either self or foreign. This recognition is based on the host's reaction to alloantigens or antigens (i.e., substances that initiate an immune response that can lead to rejection of the transplanted organ). These substances, also known as histocompatibility antigens, play a very important role in organ transplantation. The ABO blood group system of red blood cells are also important and in most cases, the donor and recipient should be ABO-compatible; otherwise, immediate graft destruction can occur because of antibodies directed against the ABO antigens.

Histocompatibility antigens are glycoproteins that are located on the surface of cell membranes. These are encoded by the major histocompatibility complex (MHC) genes located on the short arm of chromosome 6. In humans, the MHC is called the human leukocyte antigen (HLA). The gene products encoded on the HLA are divided into classes I, II, and III based on their tissue distribution, antigen structure, and function. Class I antigens (HLA-A, HLA-B, and HLA-C) are present on all nucleated cell surfaces and are the primary targets for cytotoxic T-lymphocyte reactions against transplanted cells and tissues. The three class II antigens (HLA-DR, HLA-DQ, HLA-DP) have a more limited distribution and are found on macrophages, B lymphocytes, monocytes, activated T lymphocytes, dendritic cells, and some endothelial cells, all of which can act as antigen-presenting cells (APCs). Individual HLA loci are extensively polymorphic. Each one possesses two A, B, and DR antigens, one from each parent. This is called a haplotype. Recognition of these polymorphic loci by host T lymphocytes appears to account for rejection events seen in vivo. Class III antigens (C4, C2, and Bf) are part of the complement system and do not play a specific role in the graft rejection process.

Rejection of a transplanted organ is the outcome of the natural response of the immune system to a foreign substance, or antigen, and is a complex process, the understanding of which continues to evolve. This process involves an array of interactions between foreign antigens, T lymphocytes, macrophages, cytokines (soluble mediators secreted by lymphocytes, also called lymphokines [the interleukins]), adhesion molecules (also referred to as costimulatory molecules), and membrane proteins expressed on a wide variety of cells that enhance binding of T and B lymphocytes. This process of organ rejection ultimately can involve all elements of the immune response, but it is predominantly T cell–mediated. This process can be divided into several important steps, which include antigen presentation, T-cell recognition, activation, proliferation, and differentiation of the various components of the immune response (Fig. 34-1).[3]

For foreign antigens to interact with recipient T cells and B cells, they must be prepared for presentation by APCs. These

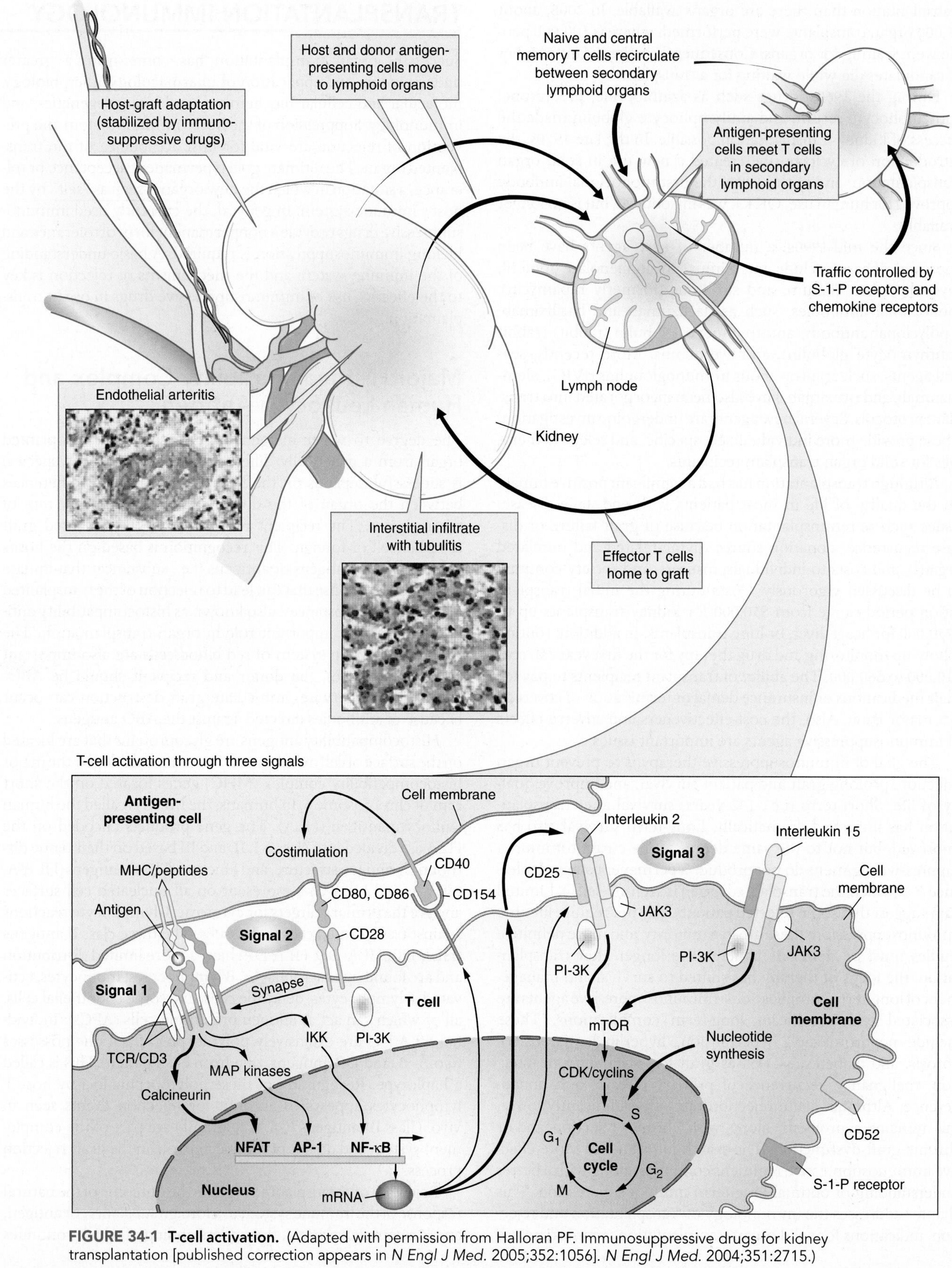

FIGURE 34-1 T-cell activation. (Adapted with permission from Halloran PF. Immunosuppressive drugs for kidney transplantation [published correction appears in *N Engl J Med.* 2005;352:1056]. *N Engl J Med.* 2004;351:2715.)

APCs (Fig. 34-1) usually are recipient macrophages (indirect pathway of allorecognition), although donor cells—referred to as dendritic cells or passenger leukocytes and graft endothelial cells—also can serve as APCs (direct pathway of allorecognition). This phase takes place within the blood, lymph nodes, spleen, and the transplanted organ.

The next step (signal one) involves T-cell recognition of the HLA molecules presented on the surface of the APC. The primary site for this to occur is at the CD3–T-cell receptor complex (TCR) on recipient T lymphocytes. This step involves the binding of the antigen, MHC, and TCR for T-cell activation. These T lymphocytes also express other molecules (clusters of differentiation [CD]) on their surfaces that, along with CD3, recognize and respond to different types of antigens. These T cells are known as $CD4^+$ cells (T_H, helper or inducer T cells) and $CD8^+$ cells (T_C, cytotoxic or suppressor T cells). $CD4^+$ cells interact with class II antigens. $CD8^+$ cells interact with class I antigens.

In addition, proteins known as adhesion molecules or costimulatory molecules promote T-cell signaling and activation (signal two). For T-cell activation to occur, binding of these costimulatory molecules as well as binding of the TCR with the presented antigen and MHC is required. Examples of these molecules include intercellular adhesion molecule (ICAM)-1 on APC, which bind with lymphocyte function-associated antigen expressed on the surface of T cells; ICAM-1 and -3 on APC with CD2 on T cells; B7 (now called CD80 and CD86) on APC with either CD28 or CTLA4 on T cells; and CD40 on APC with CD40 ligand (now called CD154) on T cells.

The binding of costimulatory molecules are critical to T-cell activation. Without this costimulation, T cells undergo abortive activation or programmed T cell death (apoptosis). These costimulatory molecules have become important targets for investigational drugs (e.g., CTLA4Ig, anti-CD40, anti-CD154) designed to try to prevent acute and chronic rejection and to promote long-term tolerance with minimal immunosuppression or none at all.

Once recognition occurs, T-cell activation and proliferation are initiated. After interacting with class II antigens and stimulation from IL-1 secreted from macrophages, T_H cells produce and secrete cytokines (e.g., interleukin [IL]-2 and interferon [INF]-γ). T_H cells are classified according to their cytokine-secretion pattern into either T_{H1} or T_{H2} cells. T_{H1} cells secrete IL-2, INF, and tumor necrosis factor (TNF), which stimulate cytotoxic T cells (T_C). T_{H2} cells secrete IL-4, IL-5, IL-6, IL-10, and IL-13, which stimulate B cells. T_H cells, along with T_C cells, are stimulated to express cell-surface IL-2 receptors (IL-2R) and other cytokines. Once the T_C cells express IL-2R, they bind to IL-2 and other cytokines, which leads to signal transduction that results in proliferation, division, and stimulation of T cells (signal 3). These committed T_C cells bind directly to allogeneic cells and produce cell lysis. T_H-secreted cytokines recruit other T cells, which results in further cytotoxicity. During this process, T_H cells also produce cytokines that trigger a cascade of events involving B cells and antibody production, complement fixation, increased macrophage infiltration, neutrophil involvement, fibrin deposition, platelet activation and release, prostaglandin release, and inflammatory response at the graft site. These delayed-type hypersensitivity and humoral responses occur in conjunction with one another and are not mutually exclusive. This results in cellular and tissue graft destruction (Fig. 34-1).

The antibodies produced by plasma cells, which are transformed B cells under the influence of cytokines, bind to the target antigenic cells. This leads to local deposition of complement and results in immune complexation and injury to the graft (complement-mediated cell lysis). The newly formed antibodies cause a series of interactions to occur with T cells, which lead to cytotoxicity (antibody-dependent, cell-mediated cytotoxicity). These cell-mediated and humoral immunologic events can impair organ function so significantly that without therapeutic intervention, complete organ graft dysfunction may occur. Under certain circumstances, which are not clear, the T_C cells, known as suppressor T cells, can actually downregulate the immune response to alloantigen.[3,4]

Human Leukocyte Antigen Typing

The genetic compatibility between donor and recipient can have an impact on acute rejection, chronic rejection, graft survival, and patient survival. For example, in kidney transplantation, the closer the HLA matching is between recipient and donor, the better the outcome, particularly over the long term. To determine this compatibility, a number of laboratory tests, including serologic, flow cytometric, genetic-DNA–based, and cellular assessments of donor and recipient serum and lymphocytes, are performed before organ transplantation. This process is referred to as tissue typing.[5] Lymphocytes are typed for HLA-A, HLA-B, and HLA-DR. Typing for HLA is performed using the donor and recipient lymphocytes for serology-based techniques or tissue or fluid containing nucleated cells.

The panel reactive antibodies (PRA) test is commonly used to assess organ compatibility because recipients may have HLA antibodies from previous exposure to antigenic stimuli (e.g., blood transfusions, previous transplantation, pregnancy). In this test, the recipient's serum is tested against a cell panel of known HLA specificities that are representative of possible donors in the general population. The percentage of cell reactions (recipient with donor) determines a recipient's PRA.[5] It is done periodically on patients on the waiting list to determine their immunologic reactivity. The potential recipient with a higher percentage of PRA ($>$20%–50%) is at higher risk for rejection and will generally have longer wait time for a kidney than patients with PRA less than 20%.

A lymphocyte cross-match is also performed prior to transplantation. In this case, the potential recipient's serum is cross-matched to determine whether preformed antibodies to the donor's lymphocytes are present. A positive cross-match indicates the presence of recipient cytotoxic IgG antibodies to the donor. In kidney transplantation, a positive cross-match is considered a strong contraindication, although in some HLA highly sensitized kidney transplants IVIG, plasmapheresis, and rituximab may be given to the recipient before and after transplant to overcome the antibody reactions.[6] In liver transplantation, a positive cross-match is not an absolute contraindication because the need is urgent and because the liver appears to be more resistant immunologically to this type of reaction. These liver transplant recipients can, however, experience significant complications and experience early acute rejection.

ABO blood typing is one of the most critical of all evaluations when determining the genetic compatibility for all solid organ transplants. Transplantation of an organ with ABO incompatibility typically results in a hyperacute rejection and destruction of the graft, although in kidney transplant newer therapeutic approaches to overcome ABO incompatibility have been successful.[7]

IMMUNOSUPPRESSIVE AGENTS

Immunosuppressives, based on an improved understanding of their mechanisms of action and the mechanisms of rejection, have had the most significant impact on patient and graft survival. The currently used immunosuppressives are shown in Table 34-1, and a significant number of newly developed, more selective, and potentially less toxic immunosuppressive agents are under

TABLE 34-1
Currently Used Immunosuppressive Agents

Drug (Brand Name)	Usual Dose (How Supplied)	Therapeutic Use(s)	Adverse Effects
Alemtuzumab (Campath-H1)	0.3 mg/kg or 30 mg × 1 dose (30-mg vial for injection)	Prevention of acute rejection; steroid-free protocols	Lymphopenia, leukopenia, infection
Azathioprine (Imuran)	1–3 mg/kg/d (50-mg tablet; 100-mg vial for injection)	As maintenance agent to prevent acute rejection	Leukopenia, thrombocytopenia, hepatotoxicity, nausea and vomiting, diarrhea, pancreatitis, infection
Antithymocyte globulin, equine (Atgam)	10–20 mg/kg/d (250 mg/5 mL ampule for injection)	Treat acute rejection (including severe or steroid-resistant forms); as induction agent in high-risk patient to prevent acute rejection	Anemia, leukopenia, thrombocytopenia, arthralgia, myalgias, nausea and vomiting, diarrhea, fevers, chills, hypotension, tachycardia, anaphylaxis, infection
Antithymocyte globulin, rabbit (Thymoglobulin)	1.5 mg/kg/d given daily for 4–10 days (25 mg/5 mL vial for injection)	Treat acute rejection (including severe or steroid-resistant forms); as induction agent in high-risk patient to prevent acute rejection	Fever, chills, nausea and vomiting, hypotension, neutropenia, flushing, rash, itching, joint pain, myalgias, thrombocytopenia, infection
Basiliximab (Simulect)	20 mg; 2 doses 10 mg; 2 doses for children if <35 kg (10-mg and 20-mg vial for injection)	As induction agent to prevent acute rejection	Abdominal pain, dizziness, insomnia, hypersensitivity reaction (rare)
Cyclosporine (Sandimmune)	Oral 5–10 mg/kg/dose BID IV 1.5–2.5 mg/kg/dose (100 mg/mL oral solution; 25- and 100-mg capsule; 250 mg/5 mL ampule for injection)	As maintenance agent to prevent acute rejection	Nephrotoxicity, hypertension, neurotoxicity, hair growth, gingival hyperplasia, hyperglycemia, hyperkalemia, dyslipidemia, hypomagnesemia, infection, neoplasm
Cyclosporine (Neoral, Gengraf, various others)	4–8 mg/kg/d BID (100-mg oral solution; 25-, 50-, and 100-mg capsule)	As maintenance agent to prevent acute rejection; conversion agent from tacrolimus in patients with intolerance or inefficacy	Same as above
Everolimus (Zortress)	0.5 to 1.5 mg PO BID (0.25-mg, 0.5-mg, 0.75-mg tablets	As maintenance agent to prevent acute rejection; conversion agent from CNI in patients with intolerance or inefficacy	Dyslipidemia, thrombocytopenia, neutropenia, impaired healing, mouth ulcers, proteinuria, pneumonitis (rare)
Methylprednisolone sodium succinate (Solu-Medrol, various others)	10–1,000 mg/dose (40-mg, 125-mg, 250-mg, 500-mg, 1,000-mg, and 2,000-mg vial for injection)	As induction and maintenance agent to prevent acute rejection; to treat acute rejection	Hyperglycemia, psychosis, euphoria, impaired wound healing, osteoporosis, acne, peptic ulcers, gastritis, fluid, electrolyte disturbances, hypertension, dyslipidemia, leukocytosis, cataracts, cushingoid state, infection, insomnia, irritability
Mycophenolate mofetil (CellCept)	1.5–3.0 g/d BID IV/PO (250-mg capsule; 500-mg tablet; 200 mg/mL oral suspension; 500-mg vial for injection)	As maintenance agent to prevent acute rejection; conversion agent from azathioprine and sirolimus in patients with intolerance or poor response	Diarrhea, nausea and vomiting, neutropenia, dyspepsia, ulcers, infection, thrombocytopenia, anemia
Mycophenolate sodium (Myfortic)	360–720 mg BID PO	As maintenance agent to prevent acute rejection. Alternative to MMF	Similar side effect profile as MMF
Prednisone (Deltasone, others)	5–20 mg/d (1-mg, 2.5-mg, 5-mg, 10-mg, 20-mg, 50-mg, and 100-mg tablet)	As maintenance agent to prevent acute rejection	See methylprednisolone
Sirolimus (Rapamune)	2–10 mg/d (1-mg and 2-mg tablet; 1 mg/mL oral solution)	As maintenance agent to prevent acute rejection; conversion agent from CNI or mycophenolate or azathioprine in patients with intolerance or poor response	Dyslipidemia, thrombocytopenia, neutropenia, anemia, diarrhea, impaired healing, mouth ulcers, proteinuria, pneumonitis (rare)
Tacrolimus (Prograf)	Oral 0.15–0.3 mg/kg/d BID IV 0.025–0.05 mg/kg/d as continuous infusion (0.5-mg, 1-mg, and 5-mg capsule; 5 mg/mL ampule for injection)	As maintenance agent to prevent acute rejection; conversion agent from cyclosporine in patients with intolerance	Nephrotoxicity, hypertension, neurotoxicity, alopecia, hyperglycemia, hyperkalemia, dyslipidemia, hypomagnesemia, infection, neoplasm

BID, twice daily; CNI, calcineurin inhibitor; IV, intravenous; MMF, mycophenolate mofetil; PO, orally.

investigation. Sites of action of the currently used agents, along with some of the investigational agents, are represented in Figure 34-2.[8]

Azathioprine

Azathioprine is a prodrug of 6-mercaptopurine (6-MP). Azathioprine and 6-MP are purine antagonist antimetabolites. The introduction of cyclosporine, tacrolimus, mycophenolate, and sirolimus has led to a significant reduction of azathioprine use or its elimination altogether in immunosuppressive protocols, especially in the United States. It may be useful in some cases, however, because it is available generically, or in patients who cannot tolerate other agents. It continues to be used in other countries.

Azathioprine, a nonspecific antimetabolite immunosuppressive agent, affects both cell-mediated (i.e., T cell) and antibody-mediated (i.e., B cell) immune responses. Because it inhibits the early stages of cell differentiation and proliferation, azathioprine is useful for preventing rejection, but it is ineffective for the treatment of acute rejection. 6-MP, an active metabolite, is incorporated into DNA and RNA, thereby interfering with the intracellular formation of thioguanine nucleotides (TGN). 6-MP is intracellularly converted by hypoxanthine phosphoribosyl transferase to thioinosinic acid and then to thioguanine nucleotides. 6-MP may have two separate immunosuppressive effects: inhibition of cellular proliferation and cytotoxicity. A decrease in the levels of intracellular purine ribonucleotides decreases cellular proliferation, and incorporation of TGN into DNA mediates cytotoxicity.[9]

Azathioprine can be given intravenously (IV) or orally. Oral absorption is rapid but incomplete. The usual dose is 1 to 3 mg/kg/day. Although the mean bioavailability of azathioprine in renal transplant recipients is approximately 50%, oral doses usually are converted from IV with a 1:1 ratio.

The half-lives for azathioprine and 6-MP are estimated to be 10 to 12 minutes and 40 to 60 minutes, respectively. Major metabolic conversion of azathioprine to 6-MP is via nucleophilic attack by glutathione. The liver and red blood cells are thought to be major tissue sites for this metabolic conversion. The 6-MP formed by this reaction can be metabolized further to thiopurine ribonucleosides and ribonucleotides such as 6-thioguanine nucleotide. These active metabolites, which have longer half-lives, are responsible for immunosuppressive activity. Azathioprine pharmacokinetics are not affected by renal dysfunction, but 6-TGN metabolite concentrations can accumulate in this situation.[10]

The most common adverse effect of azathioprine is bone marrow suppression, which presents as leukopenia or, less commonly, as thrombocytopenia and megaloblastic anemia. Myelosuppression is dose-dependent and typically observed after 7 to 14 days of therapy. Bone marrow suppression may be related to a genetic deficiency of the enzyme, thiopurine methyltransferase. Low activity of this enzyme is rare but in some individuals it leads to greater availability of 6-MP, elevated 6-thioguanine levels, and susceptibility to myelosuppression. Low levels of thiopurine methyltransferase and specific genetic polymorphisms of this enzyme have been associated with severe azathioprine myelotoxicity and reduced efficacy in some transplant recipients; testing for this polymorphism has been advocated.[11] However, few centers perform genetic testing prior to use. Hepatitis, cholestasis, and reversible and irreversible liver damage have been reported with azathioprine use. The irreversible liver damage appears histologically compatible with central vein phlebitis and occlusion, fibrosis, lobular necrosis, and biliary stasis.[12]

The white blood cell (WBC) count should be maintained at greater than 5,000/μL. If it decreases to 3,000 cells/μL to 5,000 cells/μL, the azathioprine dosage should be reduced by 50%. If the dose reduction fails to keep the WBC count above 3,000 cells/μL, azathioprine should be discontinued and reinstituted at the lower dose when the leukopenia is resolved, if needed. A similar approach should be taken if thrombocytopenia or anemia occurs. If hepatotoxicity or other serious side effects occur, azathioprine is discontinued.

Pancreatitis has been associated with azathioprine. Long-term azathioprine administration also has been associated with the occurrence of non-Hodgkin lymphoma, squamous cell skin cancer, primary hepatic tumors, fever, rigors, rash, headache, myalgia, tachycardia, hypotension, polyarthritis, and acute hypersensitivity reactions. Anorexia, nausea, and vomiting also occur.

Mycophenolate Mofetil and Mycophenolate Sodium

As a result of several multicenter comparative registry trials in kidney transplant recipients, mycophenolate mofetil (MMF, CellCept) has replaced azathioprine in many transplant protocols, especially in the United States. Studies in other transplant populations have shown positive results as well. MMF is used as adjunctive therapy in combination with cyclosporine or tacrolimus, prednisone, sirolimus, and monoclonal and polyclonal antibodies to prevent acute rejection. It is also used as rescue therapy when patients have not responded to, or cannot tolerate, the side effects of other immunosuppressive agents.[13]

MMF, as with azathioprine, is an antiproliferative antimetabolite that also inhibits purine synthesis, but in a more selective manner. Unlike azathioprine, MMF interferes with the de novo pathway for purine synthesis. MMF is the morpholinoethyl ester prodrug of mycophenolic acid (MPA), which is the active component. MPA selectively, noncompetitively, and reversibly blocks an enzyme known as inosine monophosphate dehydrogenase (IMPDH) found primarily in actively proliferating T and B lymphocytes. T and B lymphocytes rely on this enzyme and the de novo purine pathway to produce purine nucleotides for DNA and RNA synthesis. Thus, MPA interferes with T-cell and B-cell proliferation. MPA also may affect cytokine production. Other secondary effects include inhibition of B-lymphocyte antibody production, decreased adhesion molecule expression, decreased smooth muscle proliferation and recruitment, and infiltration of neutrophils.[14,15] (MMF pharmacokinetics are complex and discussed in detail in Case 34-7, Question 9.)

Another oral formulation of MPA, enteric-coated mycophenolate sodium (Myfortic), is also approved by the US Food and Drug Administration (FDA) to prevent rejection in kidney transplantation, when used in combination with a calcineurin inhibitor (CNI) and corticosteroids. The original purpose of designing the enteric-coated formulation was to reduce or prevent the gastrointestinal (GI) side effects commonly seen with MMF. However, most data suggest that the efficacy rates and side-effect profiles of MMF and mycophenolate sodium are nearly identical. These two agents are not bioequivalent: A 1-gram dose of MMF is equivalent to 720 mg of mycophenolate sodium.[16]

More recently, two issues have emerged with mycophenolate. These include approved generic products and the role of therapeutic drug monitoring, which will be addressed later in the chapter (Case 34-7, Question 9).

Corticosteroids

Prednisone, methylprednisolone, and prednisolone—all synthetic analogs of hydrocortisone—are the primary corticosteroids used to prevent and treat rejection of transplanted organs.

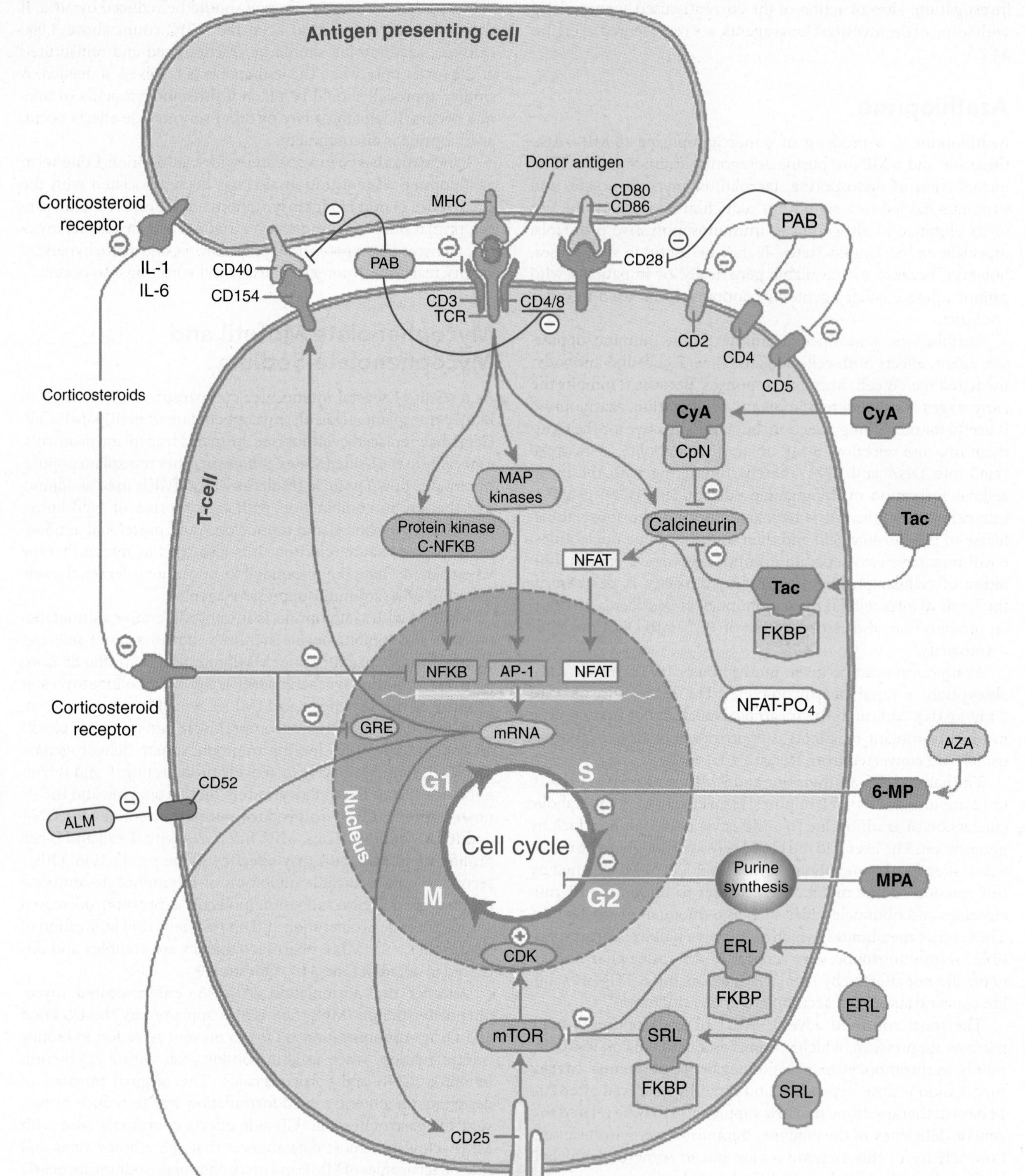

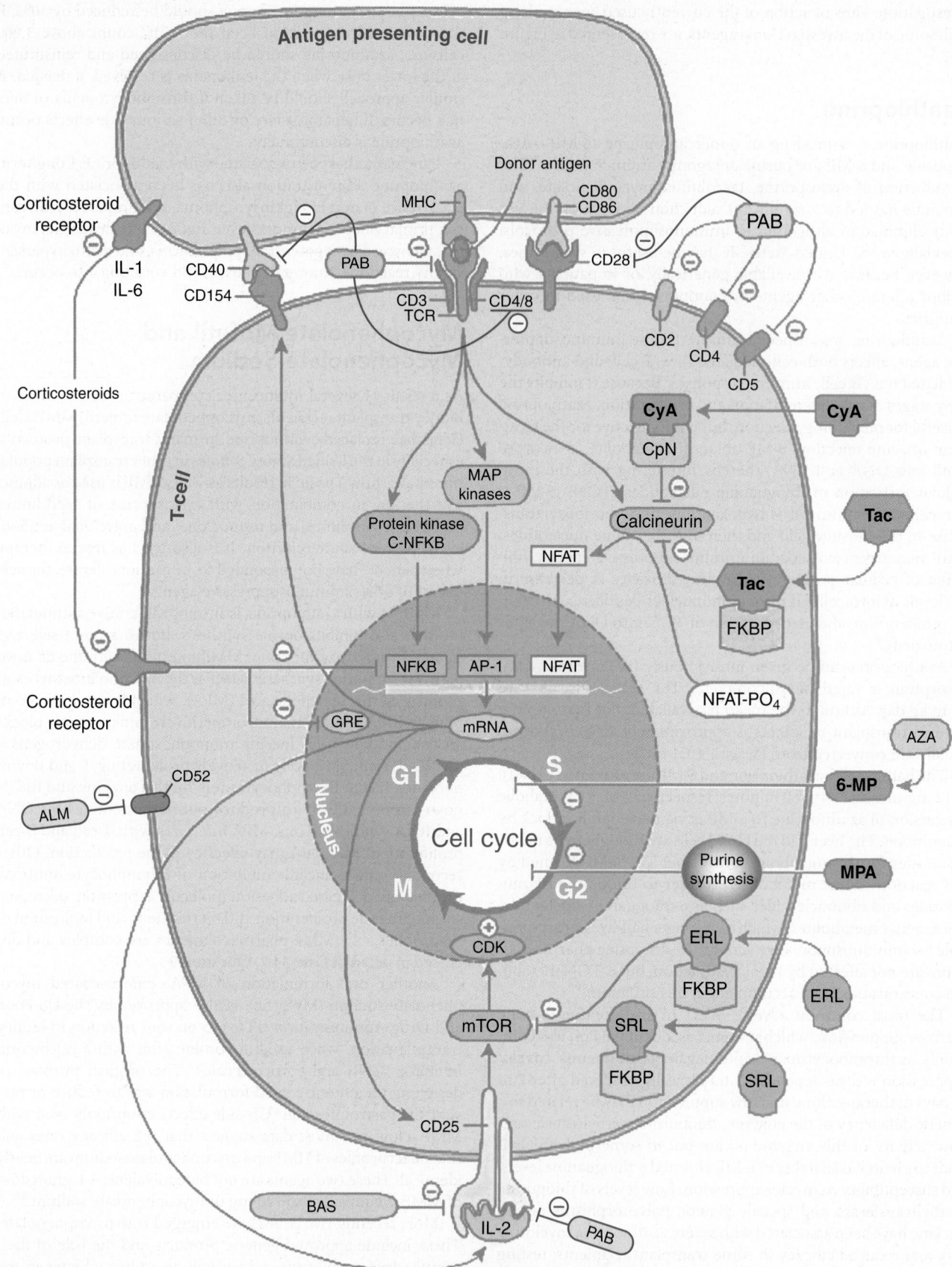

FIGURE 34-2 Schematic representation summarizing the mechanisms of action of approved and investigational immunosuppressive agents. ALM, alemtuzumab; AZA, azathioprine; BAS, basiliximab; CyA, cyclosporine; DAC, daclizumab; IL, interleukin; MPA, mycophenolic acid; PAB, polyclonal antibodies; SIR, sirolimus; TAC, tacrolimus; ERL, everolimus.
(Adapted with permission from Topol EJ et al, eds. *Textbook of Cardiovascular Medicine*. 3rd ed. Philadelphia, PA: Lippincott Williams & Wilkins; 2006.)

Although they are an important part of immunosuppression, a goal of most transplantation programs is to minimize, eliminate, or avoid corticosteroid use because of their numerous and significant side effects.[17]

Corticosteroids have multiple effects on most cells and tissues of the body, but it is their anti-inflammatory and, more importantly, their immunosuppressive properties that serve as the basis for their use in organ transplant recipients. These effects are exerted through specific intracellular glucocorticoid receptors. The corticosteroids bind with these receptors and interfere with RNA and DNA synthesis as well as transcription of specific genes. Cell function is altered, resulting in suppression or activation of gene transcription. Corticosteroids also affect RNA translation, protein synthesis, cytokine production and secretion, and protein and cytokine receptor expression.

Even after a single dose, corticosteroids cause marked lymphocytopenia by redistribution of circulating lymphocytes to other lymphoid tissues, such as the bone marrow, rather than by cell lysis; however, they also transiently increase the number of peripherally circulating neutrophils. Corticosteroids inhibit IL-1 and IL-6 production from APC, a number of events associated with T-cell activation, and IL-2 and IFN-γ production. They interfere with the action of IL-2 and IL-2R on activated T cells, resulting in the inhibition of T_{H1} function. They can enhance IL-10 regulatory function and enhance T_{H2} cell function. Moderate-dose to high-dose corticosteroids also inhibit cytotoxic T-cell function by inhibiting cytokine production and lysis of T cells. They can inhibit early proliferation of B cells but have a minimal effect on activated B cells and immunoglobulin-secreting plasma cells. The corticosteroids affect most cells and substances associated with acute allograft rejection and inflammatory reactions. They inhibit accumulation of leukocytes at sites of inflammation; inhibit macrophage functions, including migration and phagocytosis; inhibit expression of class II MHC antigens induced by INF-γ; block release of IL-1, IL-6, and TNF; inhibit the upregulation and expression of costimulatory molecules and neutrophil adhesion to endothelial cells; inhibit secretion of complement protein C3; inhibit phospholipase A_2 activity; and decrease production of prostaglandins.[18]

The plasma half-lives of prednisone and methylprednisolone are much shorter than their biologic half-lives. Prednisone is a prodrug that is rapidly converted to its active form, prednisolone. Bioavailability in transplant recipients is rapid and complete and similar to healthy subjects. In transplant recipients, plasma half-lives are approximately 2.5 to 4 hours for prednisolone and methylprednisolone. Prednisolone is metabolized extensively. Prednisolone and methylprednisolone are 70% to 90% protein bound. Clearance of the unbound fraction is reduced in kidney and liver transplant recipients. These agents usually are given in fixed doses or dosing is based on body weight (mg/kg) despite the pharmacokinetic differences.[19,20]

Calcineurin Inhibitors

CYCLOSPORINE

The introduction of cyclosporine as an immunosuppressive agent has been the single most important factor in the current success of organ transplantation. Its use increased patient and graft survival, reduced morbidity associated with rejection and infection, and extended the types and numbers of organ transplantations performed. Cyclosporine or tacrolimus are the primary agents used in almost all transplant recipients. In contrast to azathioprine and mycophenolate, cyclosporine has relatively nonmyelotoxic immunosuppressive effects.

Cyclosporine is an 11-amino acid undecapeptide metabolite extracted from a soil fungus, *Tolypocladium inflatum Gams.* The activity of cyclosporine is mediated through a reversible inhibition of T-cell function, particularly T_H cells. Its major effect is inhibiting the production of IL-2 and other cytokines, including INF-γ. These actions result in an inhibition of the early events of T-cell activation, sensitization, and proliferation. Cyclosporine has little effect on activated mature cytotoxic T cells. Therefore, it has little usefulness in the treatment of acute rejection. Its site of action is within the cytoplasm of T cells after antigenic recognition and signaling occurs. Cyclosporine binds to an intracellular protein (immunophilin) called cyclophilin. Although binding to cyclophilin is required, it alone is not sufficient for immunosuppression. This cyclosporine–cyclophilin complex then binds to a protein phosphatase, calcineurin. This is thought to prevent activation of nuclear factors involved in the gene transcription for IL-2 and other cytokines, including IFN.[21] Also, because of this inhibition, cyclosporine indirectly impairs the activity of other cells, macrophages, monocytes, and B cells in the immune response. Cyclosporine has no effect on hematopoietic cells or neutrophils. Cyclosporine is metabolized extensively in the liver to more than 25 metabolites. Two of these metabolites, AM1 (formerly M17) and AM9 (formerly M1), can elicit an immunosuppressive effect in vitro, but they have much lower activity than cyclosporine. The role of these metabolites in the development of toxicity with cyclosporine is unclear. The pharmacokinetics and therapeutic drug monitoring (TDM) of cyclosporine are described in Case 34-2, Questions 1 and 3.

TACROLIMUS

Tacrolimus (formerly FK506) is isolated from a soil fungus, *Streptomyces tsukubaensis.* It is a macrolide with a different molecular structure than cyclosporine. Tacrolimus is as effective as cyclosporine in liver and kidney transplant recipients as the primary immunosuppressant in combination with corticosteroids or mycophenolate, azathioprine, sirolimus, and antibodies. It also is effective in some patients as rescue treatment in liver and kidney recipients experiencing acute or chronic rejection resulting from failure of standard immunosuppressive therapy. Although they appear to be equally effective, tacrolimus is the preferred CNI over cyclosporine in most transplant centers.

The activity of tacrolimus is similar to that of cyclosporine, but the concentrations of tacrolimus needed to inhibit production of IL-2, are 10 to 100 times lower than those of cyclosporine. Tacrolimus also inhibits production of other cytokines, including IL-3, IL-4, and INF-γ, TNF, and granulocyte-macrophage colony-stimulating factor. It has variable effects on B-cell response and also has anti-inflammatory effects. The action of tacrolimus on T cells is more difficult to reverse than cyclosporine. As with cyclosporine, tacrolimus binds to an intracellular, although different, protein: FK binding protein 12. This protein, which interacts with calcineurin, inhibits gene transcription of cytokines and interferes with T-cell activation.[22] The pharmacokinetics and TDM of tacrolimus are described in Case 34-7, Question 3.

mTOR Inhibitors

Sirolimus, formerly known as rapamycin, is an FDA-approved agent for prevention of acute rejection and for withdrawal of cyclosporine in kidney transplantation. It was isolated from soil samples on Rapa Nui (Easter Island) and is a macrolide, structurally related to tacrolimus. In multicenter clinical trials, sirolimus combined with cyclosporine and prednisone significantly reduced acute rejection episodes in kidney transplant recipients when compared with a combined regimen of cyclosporine, azathioprine, and prednisone. The rejection rate was decreased from approximately 30% to 40% to less than 20%.

Positive results for sirolimus also have been observed in other transplantation populations; in situations in which it is used in combination with other agents, including antibodies, tacrolimus, and mycophenolate; and when it has been used for rescue therapy. Its major use is in CNI avoidance, withdrawal, or minimization protocols.[23]

Unlike CNIs, which work earlier in the T-cell activation cycle and inhibit cytokine production, sirolimus is an inhibitor of late T-cell activation. It does not block cytokine production; rather, it inhibits signal transduction, which blocks the response of T cells and B cells to cytokines such as IL-2. Sirolimus binds to the same immunophilin bound by tacrolimus, FK binding protein. This complex interferes with the action of certain enzymes or proteins involved in cell proliferation signaling. Both cyclosporine and tacrolimus inhibit calcineurin, whereas sirolimus influences a protein called the mammalian target of rapamycin (mTOR). Sirolimus also inhibits an enzyme called P7056 protein kinase, which is involved in microsomal protein synthesis. These effects result in cell-cycle arrest, blockage of messenger RNA production, and blockage of cell proliferation. Early in its development, in vitro studies indicated that tacrolimus and sirolimus were antagonistic. Clinical studies indicate that this is not true. Sirolimus and cyclosporine or tacrolimus appear to work synergistically. Sirolimus also inhibits proliferation of smooth muscle cells and may, although it is too early to tell, reduce the development of chronic rejection and, potentially, cancer.[23]

Everolimus is the newest FDA-approved mTOR inhibitor for use in kidney transplantation. Its mechanism of action is similar to sirolimus. Everolimus is hepatically metabolized through the cytochrome P-450 3A4 but has a shorter half-life and different dose and frequency schedule than sirolimus. Similar to sirolimus, it requires monitoring of trough blood concentrations, although the target range is different from sirolimus. Its role in transplantation remains to be determined, particularly compared to sirolimus.[24] Metabolism, pharmacokinetics, and TDM are discussed in Case 34-2, Question 4.

Antithymocyte Globulins

Polyclonal antibody products have been used for decades to prevent and treat acute rejection. Polyclonal products used today are administered IV and include equine (lymphoglobulin) and rabbit antithymocyte globulin, which is considered the polyclonal antibody of choice.

Antithymocyte globulin (ATG) preparations have also been made in goats and sheep for investigational study. However, the following discussion is limited to the products produced in horses and rabbits. Regardless of the species from which they are produced, all ATG products have similar pharmacologic effects. Their potency and antibody specificity vary, however, from batch to batch and between products.[25] The production of polyclonal equine or rabbit antibody begins with the injection of homogenized human spleen or thymus preparations into the animals. This injection induces an immune response in the animals directed against human T lymphocytes; serum containing antibodies to T cells is collected from the animals and purified. Other antibodies to human cells are produced as well, however. These antibodies bind to all normal blood mononuclear cells in addition to T lymphocytes and B lymphocytes, resulting in depletion of lymphocytes, platelets, and leukocytes from the peripheral circulation. The mechanism of action of these agents is thought to be linked to lysis of peripheral lymphocytes, uptake of lymphocytes by the reticuloendothelial system, masking of lymphocyte receptors, apoptosis, and immunomodulation. These agents contain antibodies to a number of cell-surface markers on lymphocytes, including CD2, CD3, CD4, CD8, CD11a, CD25, CD44, CD45, HLA-DR, and HLA class I antigens. They also interfere with leukocyte adhesion and trafficking and also have effects against $CD20^+$ B cells. ATG preparations can produce a rapid and profound depletion of circulating T cells, often within 24 hours of the initial dose. The duration of the effect can last several weeks after a course of therapy, particularly with rabbit antithymocyte globulin. Antibodies can be produced to these products as well. This, however, does not appear to influence clinical outcomes.[26]

Monoclonal Antibodies

BASILIXIMAB

Basiliximab is an IL-2R antagonist, monoclonal antibody approved for use in combination with other immunosuppressives to prevent acute cellular rejection in kidney transplantation. Daclizumab, another monoclonal antibody, was also approved but has been recently taken off the market due to decreased market demand. Basiliximab is a chimeric antibody that contains both murine and human antibody sequences.[27] This agent prevents episodes of acute rejection in kidney transplant recipients. It has been used, although not as frequently, in liver transplants. Comparative studies between basiliximab and other antibodies, such as rabbit antithymocyte globulin, have been conducted. Advantages over these other agents include ease of administration, minimal side effects, low immunogenicity, no greater infections or malignancy rates, and fewer required doses. It is well tolerated, although there are rare reports of anaphylaxis. Basiliximab appears to be most effective in immunologically low-risk patients, whereas in high-risk patients, its use may be limited. As with other antibodies, it is expensive. Basiliximab is given as a 20-mg dose on days 0 and 4 after transplantation. It binds to the α-subunit of the IL-2R, also known as CD25 or the TAC subunit, which is expressed only on the surface of activated T cells; this subunit is critical to IL-2 activation of T cells in the acute rejection process. Basiliximab prevents the IL-2R from binding with IL-2, thereby blocking T-cell activation.[27]

Basiliximab has a terminal half-life of 4 to 14 days, therefore only a few doses are administered. Basiliximab, with the two-dose regimen, saturates the receptor for approximately 36 days in kidney transplants. Duration of IL-2 saturation was a found to be shorter in liver transplant recipients than that reported in kidney transplant recipients. The half-life and clearance of basiliximab has been shown to be shorter and faster, respectively, in liver transplant recipients than kidney recipients.[28]

ALEMTUZUMAB

Alemtuzumab is a humanized monoclonal antibody against CD52 proteins on the surface of T cells and B cells, natural killer cells, macrophages, and monocytes. It is approved for use in certain types of leukemias, but not in organ transplant. Because it causes a profound reduction or depletion in lymphocytes, especially T_H lymphocytes, a number of studies have evaluated its effect as induction therapy to prevent acute rejection after kidney transplant. Several studies have investigated its use in steroid avoidance or withdrawal regimens and CNI avoidance or withdrawal regimens. Short-term studies have indicated a role for this agent in these situations. It is rarely used in liver transplantation. Most protocols with this agent give a single 30-mg IV dose in the operating room. With this dose, significant neutropenia and lymphopenia may occur, lasting for months to years in some patients. This single dose regimen has been successful in reducing the incidence of fungal and viral infections as compared with multiple dose regimens.[29]

Investigational Agents

A number of agents are in various stages of development. These include belatacept, CP-690550, ISA247, alefacept, eculizumab, and AEB-071. These agents have more specific activity directed at T-cell and B-cell function and some interfere with costimulatory proteins.[30] Belatacept is a CTL4-Ig, which blocks the co-stimulatory pathway of CD28 or CTL-A4:CD80/CD86 binding interactions. CTLA4-Ig binds to CD80/CD86 to a greater degree than CD28, resulting in inhibition of costimulation and T-cell activation. Belatacept, which is given IV, once every few weeks in combination with other agents, is currently undergoing phase III trials as a replacement for CNI.[31] ISA247 is a cyclosporine derivative, with a less toxic profile. AEB071 (sotrastaurin) is a protein kinase C inhibitor, whereas CP690550 is a JAK3 inhibitor. In addition, a number of monoclonal antibodies and peptides such as alefacept (approved for psoriasis) and eculizumab are undergoing investigation. The targets of these antibodies and peptides are antigen-binding sites, receptors, and adhesion molecules.[30]

KIDNEY TRANSPLANTATION

Indications and Evaluation

CASE 34-1

QUESTION 1: G.P. is a 52-year-old, 72-kg African American man with end-stage renal disease (ESRD) secondary to non–insulin-dependent diabetes mellitus, hypertension, and hyperlipidemia. He has been undergoing hemodialysis three times a week for 4 years. Other medical problems include anemia, hypocalcemia, and hyperphosphatemia. G.P.'s medications include amlodipine 10 mg daily, ramipril 10 mg twice daily (BID), Lipitor 20 mg daily, Tums two tablets with meals and at bedtime, sevelamer 800 mg with meals, NPH insulin 30 international units BID, regular insulin 8 international units BID, and erythropoietin 8,000 international units IV three times weekly. He has been on the kidney transplant waiting list for 2 years. He is called by the transplant coordinator and admitted for a possible deceased donor (formerly called cadaveric) kidney transplant. G.P. has the same blood type as the donor. His most recent PRA is 10%. Cross-match is negative, and HLA typing reveals a three-antigen match (A1, A2, B35) between donor and recipient. On admission to the hospital, his laboratory values are as follows:

Na, 141 mEq/L
Potassium (K), 4.7 mEq/L
Cl, 102 mEq/L
Bicarbonate (HCO_3), 23 mEq/L
Blood urea nitrogen (BUN), 44 mg/dL
Serum creatinine (SCr), 13.9 mg/dL
Calcium (Ca), 7.8 mEq/L
Phosphorus, 6.2 mg/dL
Glucose, 225 mg/dL
WBC count, 8.4 cells/μL
Hemoglobin (Hgb), 10.8 g/dL
Hematocrit (Hct), 32%

His serology is negative for HIV, hepatitis B surface antigen (HbsAg), hepatitis C, and cytomegalovirus (CMV), and is positive for antibody to the surface antigen of hepatitis B (anti-Hbs). What are the indications for and potential benefits of kidney transplantation in G.P.?

All patients with ESRD are potential candidates for kidney transplantation unless contraindicated. The contraindications (absolute or relative) are determined by the individual transplant center. Absolute contraindications include current malignancy, active infection, active liver disease, HbsAg-positive, severe or symptomatic cardiac or pulmonary disease, specific renal diseases with an accelerated recurrence rate, substance abuse, and abnormal psychosocial and noncompliant behavior. Relative contraindications for the recipient of a kidney transplant include chronic liver disease, active infection, positive for hepatitis C, human immunodeficiency virus (HIV)–positive, morbid obesity, current positive cross-match, and age greater than 70 years.[32] The relative contraindication for the elderly with ESRD is controversial because approximately 40% of the ESRD population is older than 65 years and an increasing number of these patients are undergoing kidney transplantation. Patients with ESRD need not wait until they are receiving dialysis before being considered for a kidney transplant because early transplantation is associated with lower cost, better quality of life, and longer survival than patients on dialysis awaiting transplantation. The primary diseases leading to ESRD and transplant are diabetes, hypertension, glomerulonephritis, and polycystic kidney disease.

In G.P., diabetes and hypertension would be the most likely causes of his ESRD. For G.P., a kidney transplant should return his renal function to near normal (i.e., a glomerular filtration rate between 50 and 80 mL/minute), improve his quality of life, and correct the complications of ESRD such as anemia, hypocalcemia, and hyperphosphatemia, but not diabetes, hypertension, or hyperlipidemia.

The risk-benefit ratio must be considered when evaluating a patient for any organ transplantation. In general, kidney transplants are performed to improve the quality of life and avoid the complications and outcomes associated with dialysis and renal failure. It is also more cost effective than dialysis. On the other hand, patients who are candidates for liver transplantation will die if the transplanted liver fails. Therefore, the criteria established for organ transplantation must be evaluated carefully before it is offered to any patient.

Donor and Recipient Matching

CASE 34-1, QUESTION 2: What criteria are important in determining a good match between the donor and G.P.?

G.P. had a series of serologic tests to determine his genetic compatibility with the donor. He had a negative cross-match and low PRA of 10%, indicating that he is not already sensitized to this donor's antigens, which should result in a more favorable posttransplantation course. HLA matching also indicated a three-antigen match between G.P. and the donor. Matching of donor and recipient at the HLA-A, HLA-B, and HLA-DR loci is associated with better graft survival and longer half-lives for both living-related and deceased donor kidney transplants. A six-antigen match is ideal, whereas a zero antigen match is less favorable. The half-life refers to the time it takes for half of the grafts that survive the first year to fail. Organ half-lives are longer with living donors (average 15 years) compared with deceased donors (average 8 years). For kidney recipients with a match similar to G.P., the 1-year and 3-year graft survival for a first deceased donor transplant is projected to be greater than 90% and greater than 80%, respectively. These positive factors may be offset, however, by his ethnicity. Patient and graft survival after kidney transplantation is reduced in the African American population compared with others because of immunologic, medical, pharmacologic, pharmacokinetic, pharmacogenomic, and socioeconomic reasons.[33] Along with African American race, other risk factors associated with decreased survival include advanced donor age, recipient age less than 15 years and greater than 50 years, retransplantation, a high PRA (>20%–50%), and delayed graft function. Recipients who fall into these categories are referred to as high-risk patients.[34]

Because of a limited number of donors, this pool has been expanded to include what are called expanded criteria donors. These are deceased donors who either are older than the standard-criteria deceased donor or have evidence of some preexisting hypertension, higher serum creatinine, or death caused by cerebrovascular disease. Survival appears to somewhat lower in recipients of organs from extended donor criteria. G.P.'s donor was a standard-criteria deceased donor.

Immunosuppressive Therapy

CASE 34-1, QUESTION 3: Before the transplant procedure, G.P. receives MMF 1 g orally (PO) and cefazolin 1 g IV. During surgery, just before reperfusion of his new kidney, he received methylprednisolone 500 mg IV and rabbit antithymocyte globulin 100 mg IV. He is also given furosemide 100 mg IV after the kidney has been transplanted. Methylprednisolone 250 mg IV is to be given on the day after surgery. The methylprednisolone dose is to be decreased to 100 mg IV on the second postoperative day for one dose. Prednisone 60 mg (1 mg/kg/day) PO is to be given on the subsequent day for one dose and tapered by 0.3 mg/kg/day to 20 mg daily by day 7 after surgery and further tapered to 5 mg daily within a month. Tacrolimus nasogastric (NG) or PO 0.1 mg/kg/day or 3 mg every 12 hours will be started within 12 hours after surgery if renal function improves. The dosage will be adjusted according to tacrolimus whole blood trough concentrations. MMF will be continued at 1 g PO BID. He will also continue with antibody induction with rabbit antithymocyte globulin 100 mg IV on days 1 and 3 after surgery. Why is G.P. being treated with this immunosuppressive regimen?

The major goal of immunosuppressive therapy is to prevent rejection and infection with minimal adverse effects and to ensure long-term patient and graft survival. Overall acute rejection rates are 10% to 20% during the first year after kidney transplantation. Most of these episodes respond to acute antirejection therapy.

No consensus exists on the best induction and maintenance immunosuppressive regimen, and selection primarily depends on the program and the specific organ to be transplanted. Although studies have evaluated the various regimens, comparisons are influenced by differences in donor selection and condition, organ preservation and procurement, organ ischemic (cold and warm) time, recipient's pretransplant conditions, comorbid and high-risk or low-risk factors, surgical procedures and individual surgical techniques, postoperative management and monitoring, and length of follow-up. Another important consideration is that many of the newer agents show significant effects during the first year, but fail to show a significant impact on long-term effects such as chronic rejection and graft survival.[4] The choice of a particular regimen generally depends on the risk factors present at the time of transplantation. During this early time period, because the risk of acute rejection is highest in the first few weeks to months, the number of agents, doses, and target drug concentrations are higher than later on after transplantation.

Most initial immunosuppressive drug regimens rely on three to four agents, although monotherapy or dual therapy has been used, depending on organ type and risk factors. Common combination regimens include a CNI (cyclosporine or tacrolimus) with MMF or sirolimus, and prednisone. Regimens may also include a monoclonal antibody (alemtuzumab, basiliximab) or a polyclonal antibody (rabbit antithymocyte globulin) in patients requiring additional immunosuppression. Regimens that avoid the use of steroids and CNIs, or use a short course in the early transplantation period, or are withdrawn some time (usually several months) after transplantation in an attempt to avoid the long-term side effects of these agents are also commonly used.[35]

With deceased donor kidney transplants, quadruple or triple therapy is used because they are at higher risk of rejection. The most commonly used regimen is one that contains an antibody with tacrolimus, MMF, and prednisone. Cyclosporine or tacrolimus are the foundation of this type of regimen, however, tacrolimus is used in more than 70% of new kidney transplant recipients.[22] In HLA-identical, living-related kidney transplants, conventional dual therapy (e.g., tacrolimus or mycophenolate and prednisone) gives excellent results; however, acute rejection may still occur. Combination therapy is used to take advantage of different mechanisms of action and to reduce drug toxicity by using sequential therapy and smaller doses of multiple agents rather than larger doses of any agent used alone. These multidrug combinations can lead, however, to increased drug costs, compliance issues, a higher incidence of infection and malignancy, and difficulty in assessing adverse effects.

G.P. is receiving a deceased donor transplant and triple or quadruple therapy would be used. In many centers, an antibody such as rabbit antithymocyte globulin, alemtuzumab, or basiliximab would be added, because G.P. is considered a high-risk recipient (he is African American).

After the first 6 months, drug dosages are reduced over time and maintained at a stable dose for 6 months to 1 year. In G.P., MMF or the corticosteroid may be discontinued. Although the discontinuation of a drug may reduce adverse effects, it must be counterbalanced against the risk of rejection and graft loss. Monotherapy, generally with tacrolimus or cyclosporine, may be achieved in low-risk kidney, liver, and heart transplant recipients at some time after transplantation. Most patients, however, require lifetime immunosuppression.

CASE 34-1, QUESTION 4: What is induction therapy?

Induction therapy after transplantation refers to the use of an antibody, typically at time of transplant and during the first week after transplant. Delayed graft function and acute rejection occur in the early transplant period. Both of these have a negative impact on graft survival. Antibody induction reduces the incidence of acute rejection and delayed graft function and has typically been used in immunologically high-risk patients. Their use in patients at low to moderate risk is increasing, however, often as a means of reducing or avoiding the use of CNI and steroids. The newer antibodies (e.g., basiliximab and alemtuzumab) are playing a bigger role in these situations because they are easier to administer.[27,29] Recent data indicate that about 80% of all kidney transplants received induction therapy, with rabbit antithymocyte globulin making up about 60%.[36]

Thymoglobulin and Antithymocyte Globulin

DOSING AND ADMINISTRATION

CASE 34-1, QUESTION 5: How would rabbit antithymocyte globulin be administered and monitored in G.P.?

Both rabbit antithymocyte globulin and ATG are effective as induction therapy or as treatment of acute rejection. In general, rabbit antithymocyte globulin appears to be more effective than ATG and is the antibody of choice. rabbit antithymocyte globulin, when used for induction, results in reduced acute rejection, improved survival, and manageable side-effect profile.[37] The dose of rabbit antithymocyte globulin is 1.5 mg/kg/day, and the dose of ATG is 10 to 20 mg/kg/day. These drugs can be diluted in 0.9% NaCl for injection and administered for 4 to 6 hours. Both are usually infused into a high-flow central vein to reduce pain, erythema, and phlebitis at the injection site. Peripheral administration has been used successfully with rabbit antithymocyte globulin by adding heparin and hydrocortisone to the IV solution.[26] Skin testing is recommended before horse-derived ATG use, but not rabbit-derived rabbit antithymocyte globulin. Patients previously sensitized to horse serum are at risk for an anaphylactoid reaction, but the prevalence of anaphylaxis has diminished with improved purification of this product. Patients with a positive pretherapy skin test could undergo desensitization, but alternatives, such as rabbit antithymocyte globulin, may be substituted.

DOSE REGIMEN AND DURATION OF THERAPY

The first dose of rabbit antithymocyte globulin is usually given intraoperatively. Intraoperative administration of rabbit antithymocyte globulin reduces the incidence and severity of delayed graft function as compared with postoperative adminstration.[37] Duration of therapy with rabbit antithymocyte globulin or ATG is 3 to 10 days for induction therapy. Protocols used to treat rejection commonly use a 7-day to 10-day course of therapy.[26] In patients such as G.P., a three-dose prophylactic regimen has been shown to be as effective as a longer regimen.[38]

ADVERSE EFFECTS

A number of adverse effects have been related to the use of rabbit antithymocyte globulin or ATG. Local phlebitis and pain usually can occur. Anaphylaxis is rare. Chills and fever, erythema, rash, hives, pruritus, headache, leukopenia, and thrombocytopenia are commonly encountered. Fever, chills, nausea, and vomiting may be caused by the release of cytokines, such as TNF and IL-6, from lysed lymphocytes. These symptoms can be minimized by premedication with acetaminophen and diphenhydramine before each dose. Methylprednisolone, up to 500 mg, is given 1 hour before rabbit antithymocyte globulin for the first two doses to minimize infusion reactions. Serum sickness leading to acute glomerulonephritis, hypotension, and acute respiratory distress also has been associated with these agents. It may not be evident until the seventh day of therapy or within 2 weeks of discontinuation.[39] Opportunistic viral (CMV and Epstein-Barr virus [EBV]) and fungal infections are the predominant delayed side effect. Susceptibility to malignancy, such as posttransplantation lymphoproliferative disease (PTLD) is also a concern. Because of the increased risk of CMV infection, patients are often given oral valganciclovir or IV ganciclovir during therapy and then oral valganciclovir, which is continued up to several months after induction.

MONITORING

Vital signs should be monitored hourly during infusion, and WBC and platelet counts should be monitored daily. If the patient's WBC count drops to less than 3,000 cells/μL or if the platelet count drops to less than 100,000 cells/μL, the dose of drug is decreased by 50% or held entirely until the counts return to desired levels. G.P. is receiving rabbit antithymocyte globulin for induction and it is unlikely that a dose would be held based on counts, because his regimen is limited to two doses. Patients who receive rabbit antithymocyte globulin for the treatment of acute rejection may have doses held or decreased based on the degree of thrombocytopenia and leucopenia; however, the response to therapy would be carefully considered in this decision.

Dosages also can be adjusted based on absolute lymphocyte counts or lymphocyte subsets as a way of maximizing efficacy and minimizing infectious complications. For example, the dose can be adjusted by using a target absolute T-lymphocyte count (CD2 or CD3) of less than 25 to 50 cells/μL, particularly if used for treatment of acute rejection. It is less common to adjust doses based on CD2 of CD3 counts when used for induction as in G.P.'s case. Using CD2 and CD3 counts results in a lower dose, less frequent dosing (e.g., every other day instead of daily), lower costs, and a lower rate of viral infection. rabbit antithymocyte globulin produces a more profound and longer duration of effect on lymphocytes than antithymocyte globulin; however, it does not result in a greater risk for infection and malignancy.[26]

CASE 34-1, QUESTION 6: Could basiliximab be used as an alternative to rabbit antithymocyte globulin?

Basiliximab is approved for use as induction therapy in kidney transplantation; however, it is also used in other organ transplant recipients. It is administered in combination with cyclosporine or tacrolimus and steroids with or without MMF or sirolimus. It has a limited role in high-risk populations such as G.P., or patients with high PRA or long ischemic times, delayed graft function, patients who have received a previous transplant, and children. In these patients, induction with polyclonal antibodies is used in most centers. The large initial trials with this IL-2R antibody included very few high-risk patients or excluded them altogether. More potent agents, such as rabbit antithymocyte globulin, are still preferred in high-risk patients. A prospective study comparing rabbit antithymocyte globulin with basiliximab in high-risk kidney transplants demonstrated that acute rejection rates were lower in patients receiving rabbit antithymocyte globulin.[34] Basiliximab can be used for low-risk to intermediate-risk patients and in patients where CNI minimization or steroid avoidance is implemented.[26]

Postoperative Course and Delayed Graft Function

CASE 34-1, QUESTION 7: G.P. is admitted to the transplant ward for initial posttransplantation management. His urine output during the next 3 hours has decreased from 300 to 40 mL/hour. He is receiving IV fluids at a rate equivalent to his urine output. He received 3 L of fluids in the operating room. His blood pressure is 140/83 mm Hg, heart rate is 87 beats/minute, and temperature 36.9°C; he has no signs of dehydration. His BUN is 56 mg/dL and his SCr is 12.8 mg/dL. Another dose of furosemide 100 mg IV increased his urine output to 140 mL/hour, but his urine output returned to less than 40 mL/hour in a few hours. Fluids and IV furosemide were given again with similar results. Renal ultrasound indicates no urine leaks, fluid collections, or ureteral obstruction. A diethylenetriamine penta-acetic acid renal scan indicates good perfusion, but decreased accumulation and clearance. During the next 2 days, G.P.'s BP is 150/93 mm Hg, weight is 76 kg (4 kg higher than pretransplantation), urine output has fallen to less than 200 mL/day, and relevant laboratory values are as follows:

BUN, 85 mg/dL
SCr, 13.2 mg/dL
K, 5.8 mEq/L

The decision is made to institute hemodialysis. What has happened to G.P.'s renal function? What is the most likely diagnosis?

After kidney transplantation, recipients require management and monitoring for fluid and electrolyte imbalance (potassium, magnesium, phosphorous, and calcium), BP and blood glucose changes, surgical complications, GI complications, infection, rejection, immunosuppressive dosing and toxicity, and, most important, kidney function. If all goes well, recipients should be discharged from the hospital within 3 to 5 days after transplantation. The initial renal function after kidney transplantation can reflect excellent, moderate, or slow graft function or delayed graft function. In recipients with excellent function, a good diuresis begins immediately and continues; the serum creatinine rapidly declines to less than 2.5 mg/dL within the first few days after transplantation. Most living-related transplants and between 30% and 50% of deceased donor transplants generally experience this excellent graft function pattern. Kidney transplant recipients with moderate or slow graft function usually experience a slower decline in serum creatinine, which stabilizes within the first week. Recipients with delayed graft function usually experience anuria or oliguria, require dialysis in the early period, and take days to weeks to recover. Delayed graft function is most common in recipients of organs from deceased transplant donors, occurring in between 2% and 50% of cases.[40]

The diagnosis of delayed graft function is based on clinical, laboratory, and diagnostic criteria that may vary among centers. Delayed graft function has been defined as the need for dialysis in the first 7 to 14 days posttransplant, whereas at others, the definition may be based on both a lack of improvement in the serum creatinine (e.g., it does not fall below 2.5–4 mg/dL or by 25%–30% from pretransplantation) and the presence of anuria or oliguria within the first 6 to 24 hours after other causes of acute tubular necrosis are ruled out. Slow graft function is another term that has been used to describe a lag in improvement and does not involve dialysis. Delayed graft function is influenced by the donor (age, condition of organ, prolonged ischemic time), intraoperative conditions (hypotension, fluid imbalance, ischemia or reperfusion injury), and recipient characteristics such as prior transplantation, postoperative hypovolemia or hypotension, and use of nephrotoxic drugs.[40]

In G.P., poor urine output in the first hours after transplantation and subsequent oliguria, the exclusion of other causes of acute tubular necrosis, the results of the renal scan, the lack of improvement in BUN and serum creatinine, and the need for dialysis are indicative of delayed graft function. Delayed graft function reduces kidney long-term graft survival, increases the risk of acute rejection, and influences a patient's early management by requiring dialysis, increasing the length of hospital stay, and increasing the costs of therapy. It also may make the assessment of acute rejection more difficult because the patient already has impaired renal function. In delayed graft function, a renal biopsy may be obtained if no improvement in serum creatinine is seen by day 7.[40]

CASE 34-1, QUESTION 8: What adjustments should be made in G.P.'s immunosuppressive regimen at this time?

The adverse renal effects of CNIs may contribute to the onset of delayed graft function as well as prolong its duration. Therefore, tacrolimus should be discontinued temporarily or its dose significantly reduced. Because of this effect, some protocols do not include CNIs, use them only in low doses for the first week, or delay their use until kidney function improves. These protocols often include antibodies and provide more intense immunosuppression early after transplantation when the risk of delayed graft function and acute rejection is highest. Rabbit antithymocyte globulin is sometimes used in patients with delayed graft function because it may shorten the duration of delayed graft function and the need for dialysis when compared with the CNI. Another potential option would be to use basiliximab, which has been shown to reduce acute rejection rates and extend the time to first rejection. Its use in high-risk patients (African Americans, retransplantations, high PRA, prolonged ischemic time, delayed graft function) is based primarily on single-center and retrospective studies with encouraging results, but its effectiveness in prospective studies in preventing acute rejection has not always been equal to other antibodies such as rabbit antithymocyte globulin.[41] Another concern with use of basiliximab is that a CNI may be required sooner than with rabbit antithymocyte globulin because this agent does not provide as long a duration of protection from rejection.

In G.P., rabbit antithymocyte globulin would be administered for 5 to 10 days, depending on improvement in his SCr and urine output, along with his current regimen of prednisone and mycophenolate. Typical dose would be 1.5 mg/kg/day or every other day, depending on his $CD3^+$ level, and WBC and platelet counts. Tacrolimus will not be started until his SCr decreases.

Rejection

CASE 34-1, QUESTION 9: G.P. was started on rabbit antithymocyte globulin 1.5 mg/kg as a 6-hour IV infusion on days 0, 1, and 3 for induction, but because of his delayed graft function, he received an additional dose on day 5. He received this along with his prednisone taper and MMF. Tacrolimus PO 3 mg BID was initiated on day 5 after transplant. G.P.'s urine output has increased gradually to ~1,600 mL/day after stopping rabbit antithymocyte globulin. His weight has decreased to 73 kg, and the following is recorded:

BP, 142/84 mm Hg
Heart rate, 82 beats/minute
Temperature, 36.7°C
BUN, 23 mg/dL
SCr, 2.3 mg/dL
K, 4.6 mEq/L

He is on a regular diet and taking all oral medications. His current medications include MMF 500 mg BID, prednisone 10 mg daily, tacrolimus 5 mg BID, ranitidine 150 mg at bedtime, dioctyl sodium sulfosuccinate 100 mg BID, amlodipine 10 mg daily, metoprolol 50 mg PO BID, NPH insulin 28 international units BID, regular insulin 10 international units BID, valganciclovir 450 mg daily, and trimethoprim-sulfamethoxazole (TMP-SMX) double strength, one tablet on Mondays, Wednesdays, and Fridays. Sixty days after stopping rabbit antithymocyte globulin, G.P.'s weight increased to 74.6 kg, and we note the following:

BP, 160/94 mm Hg
Heart rate, 98 beats/minute
Temperature, 37.6°C
BUN, 30 mg/dL
SCr, 3.4 mg/dL
K, 4.8 mEq/L
Trough whole blood tacrolimus concentration, 5 ng/mL
Urine output decreased during the last 24 hours to 850 mL

He feels tired and has a decreased appetite, but his fluid intake has been adequate during the past day. What evidence is consistent with rejection in G.P.?

Although significant improvements in reduction in acute rejection and improved graft survival have occurred over the past decade, certain types of acute rejection and chronic rejection continue to be a major reason for graft loss in kidney transplants. Rejection episodes can be categorized as hyperacute, accelerated, acute, antibody-mediated, chronic, or chronic allograft nephropathy. Kidney biopsy is considered the gold standard for making the diagnosis of rejection after kidney transplant. Approved criteria are used to classify and grade the type of rejection.[42]

HYPERACUTE REJECTION

Hyperacute rejection, which occurs within minutes to hours after transplantation of the allograft, is the result of preformed cytotoxic antibodies against donor-specific class I antigens. This type of rejection is rare because of ABO matching and improved HLA typing before transplant, but it remains associated with a poor prognosis. Clinically, the patient presents with anuria, hyperkalemia, hypertension, metabolic acidosis, pulmonary edema and, in some cases, disseminated intravascular coagulopathy. A perfusion scan of the kidney would indicate no uptake. If other causes of anuria are excluded and this diagnosis is made, then the transplanted kidney must be removed.

ACCELERATED REJECTION

Accelerated rejection usually occurs within a few days after organ transplantation. This is a result of prior sensitization to antigens that are similar to those of the donor and newly developed donor-specific antibodies. Accelerated rejections of transplanted kidneys occur primarily in recipients who have had prior transplantation, multiple pregnancies, or blood transfusions. These patients usually maintain good renal function for a few days before developing acute renal failure. Accelerated organ rejections generally are more resistant to pharmacologic therapy.

ACUTE REJECTION

Acute rejection is the most common type of kidney rejection in transplant recipients and most episodes respond to therapy. Most episodes of acute rejection are T cell–mediated (cellular), although some can be B cell (antibody or humoral)–mediated, and others are a combination of both. Acute rejection of a transplanted kidney significantly reduces the half-life and survival of both living-donor and deceased-donor transplants. Acute rejection can occur in the first week to months after kidney transplantation. The prophylactic use of antibody induction may, however, delay the onset for several weeks, as illustrated by G.P.'s case. If acute rejection occurs, its onset is almost always within the first year, with most episodes occurring within the first 60 days after transplantation. Acute rejection can, however, also occur at any time after transplant and can be a result of patient nonadherence (also called noncompliance) to medications and monitoring. The clinical presentation of patients with acute rejection of a kidney ranges from an asymptomatic patient with mild renal dysfunction as indicated by an elevated serum creatinine, which is common, to patients presenting with a flulike illness and acute oliguric renal failure.[43]

G.P. presents with subjective complaints of malaise or tiredness and lack of appetite. Such nonspecific complaints occur often in patients with rejection and can be accompanied by myalgias as well as pain and tenderness at the graft site. Objectively, G.P.'s increased weight, hypertension, decreased urine output, and increase in serum creatinine are consistent with acute kidney rejection. In addition, the tacrolimus trough concentration and mycophenolate doses are low, suggesting inadequate immunosuppression. Acute rejection of a transplanted kidney must be distinguished from CNI nephrotoxicity, and infections (e.g., pyelonephritis, CMV polyoma) also must be ruled out. Although the clinical evidence in G.P. probably represents an acute cellular rejection, a kidney biopsy is the gold standard for establishing the diagnosis. Biopsy results usually are available within 6 to 8 hours. If there is acute rejection, the biopsy will show an interstitial infiltration of mononuclear cells with tubulitis or intimal arteritis in more severe cases. The severity of acute rejection will be classified and graded according to standardized pathologic criteria and is important in determining treatment. Less severe grades will receive high-dose steroids, whereas more severe grades will often receive rabbit antithymocyte globulin.[43]

ANTIBODY-MEDIATED REJECTION

Antibody-mediated (also called humoral) rejection can be either acute or chronic rejection mediated by antibodies. It differs histologically from acute cellular rejection in that there is no lymphocyte infiltration on biopsy. Presence of positive staining for the complement component C4d suggests antibody-mediated rejection. Humoral rejection can occur hours to years after transplantation. Antibody-mediated rejection often is associated with hemodynamic compromise and is more resistant to drug therapy. In addition to standard therapy such as steroids and rabbit antithymocyte globulin, plasmapheresis, IVIG, and rituximab may be required to treat acute antibody-mediated rejection.[44] Other agents, not currently approved for transplantation, are being studied as treatment for antibody-mediated rejection and include bortezomib and ecluzimab.[44]

CHRONIC REJECTION

Chronic rejection is a major cause of long-term kidney graft loss after the first year. It can be either cellularly or humorally mediated. It occurs slowly in most cases over several years. The characteristic signs of chronic rejection are hypertension, proteinuria, and a progressive decline in renal function leading to renal failure. Because no specific treatment exists, therapy is supportive (e.g., dialysis in the case of kidney transplantation). Ultimately, retransplantation is needed. Some data suggest that some patients may benefit from some of the newer agents, such as mycophenolate and sirolimus, that are considered nonnephrotoxic, but this requires further study. The diagnosis of chronic rejection is determined by clinical signs and biopsy findings indicative of obliterative fibrosis of hollow structures and vessels within the graft. The chronic rejection of a kidney must be distinguished from chronic CNI nephrotoxicity, chronic infection, and recurrence of the original kidney disease.[45]

CHRONIC ALLOGRAFT NEPHROPATHY

Chronic allograft nephropathy (CAN) is a term that has been used, generally, as a diagnosis of exclusion that indicates a slow deterioration of renal function over months to years after kidney transplant, where the exact cause is unknown. Immunologic and nonimmunologic mechanisms play a role in CAN. Immunologic factors that increase the likelihood of CAN include a history of acute rejection, inadequate immunosuppression, noncompliance with immunosuppressive therapy, and previous infection, such as CMV. Nonimmunologic factors are donor-related (age, hypertension, diabetes), increased ischemic times, recipient hypertension, hyperlipidemia, CNI nephrotoxicity, and elevated body mass index. Another term, chronic allograft dysfunction (CAD) is the functional result of CAN. It is a slow, insidious process that usually manifests as an increase in serum creatinine after about 1 year, although it can occur as early as 3 months after transplantation. CAD is irreversible and unaffected by increased immunosuppressive therapy. Most recently, it has been recommended that the term CAN be eliminated from the pathologic diagnostic criteria for renal dysfunction because it is nonspecific and the end result of a number of different processes.[45]

Acute Rejection Treatment

CASE 34-1, QUESTION 10: A biopsy of G.P.'s transplanted kidney shows grade 1A, moderate acute rejection. G.P. is started on methylprednisolone 500 mg daily IV for three doses. His maintenance oral prednisone is discontinued, but his other medications are maintained. He will be placed on a high-dose oral prednisone tapering regimen after his IV doses. Why is methylprednisolone therapy of G.P.'s first acute episode of rejection appropriate?

High-dose or "pulse" IV methylprednisolone, IV rabbit antithymocyte globulin, IV antithymocyte globulin, or oral prednisone are options to treat acute rejection in all types of solid organ transplants. A high-dose corticosteroid (usually IV methylprednisolone) is considered first-line therapy because it works very quickly in decreasing lymphocyte responsiveness, is easy to administer, and reverses at least 75% of acute rejection episodes. rabbit antithymocyte globulin is usually reserved for steroid-resistant rejection or more severe grades of rejection. IVIG has also been used as an alternative for resistant rejection.[46] The ideal corticosteroid dosage, route, and regimen are unknown, and the number of corticosteroid protocols is as varied as the number of transplantation programs. IV methylprednisolone and oral prednisone are equally effective in reversing rejection, but oral corticosteroids are given for a longer period and have been associated with a higher incidence of adverse effects. Even though 50 mg of IV methylprednisolone has a similar lymphocyte suppressive effect as a 1-gram IV dose most programs use methylprednisolone 250 to 1,000 mg (most commonly 500 mg) IV every day for three doses and adjust the prerejection oral prednisone regimen accordingly. An example of an oral prednisone regimen is 100 to 200 mg/day tapered for 1 to 3 weeks to baseline maintenance dose.[47]

For G.P., IV methylprednisolone is appropriate because corticosteroids are considered first-line therapy for acute rejection of a transplanted kidney, and first rejection episodes (such as G.P.'s) are very responsive. In addition, G.P. has received a prophylactic course of rabbit antithymocyte globulin recently and additional doses should be avoided, if possible. Rabbit antithymocyte globulin is associated with a higher risk of CMV infection and malignancy; it is more difficult to administer, requires more intensive monitoring, is more expensive, and usually is held in reserve for corticosteroid-resistant or more severe forms of rejection.

Nevertheless, high-dose corticosteroids are not without risk. They increase the risk of infection, and long-term therapy can induce ocular, bone, cardiovascular, and endocrine abnormalities. Although G.P. will be receiving high-dose IV methylprednisolone for only 3 days, because he is diabetic he should be monitored for hyperglycemia and a change in his insulin requirements should be anticipated because corticosteroids can alter glucose metabolism. Short-course methylprednisolone also can mask signs of infection (e.g., fever, changes in WBC counts, pain associated with inflammation) and delay the diagnosis. Insomnia, nervousness, euphoria, mood shifts, acute psychosis, and mania also can occur with short-term corticosteroid use. If the methylprednisolone regimen is effective in reversing G.P.'s acute rejection, his serum creatinine concentration should decline within 2 to 5 days and his urine output increase.

In addition, it would be appropriate to increase G.P.'s tacrolimus dosage to 7 mg twice a day because the concentration is low (5 ng/mL) and low trough have been associated with a higher risk of acute rejection. Because small changes in tacrolimus dose can increase levels disproportionately, a trough whole blood concentration should be re-evaluated in 2 to 3 days. The mycophenolate dose could be increased to 1 g BID and up to 1.5 g BID, because this dose in combination with a CNI has reduced acute rejection in African American patients. If G.P. had been on cyclosporine, another option would be to change cyclosporine to tacrolimus, which has been shown to reduce future episodes of acute rejection. Another important aspect for prevention of future rejection would be to assess G.P.'s adherence with, and understanding of, his medication regimen. Nonadherence is a cause of acute rejection and graft loss.[48]

Cyclosporine

PHARMACOKINETICS

CASE 34-2

QUESTION 1: B.B. is a 27-year-old, 60-kg African American man who received a deceased donor kidney transplant. Within 12 hours of the transplantation, his immunosuppression consisted of modified cyclosporine (Neoral) 300 mg PO BID, MMF 1.5 g PO BID, and prednisone. He was taking other medicines for hypertension and infection prophylaxis. Describe the pharmacokinetic characteristics of cyclosporine. Based on this information, is B.B.'s cyclosporine regimen appropriate?

Cyclosporine pharmacokinetic parameters (e.g., absorption, distribution, and metabolism) exhibit significant intrapatient and interpatient variability. A number of factors are known to influence its pharmacokinetic behavior. These include age, transplant type, underlying disease, time after transplantation, GI metabolism and motility; biliary and liver function; metabolism, body weight, cholesterol, albumin, red blood cell mass; and drug interactions and formulation.[49] These factors can change cyclosporine's pharmacokinetics and can influence therapeutic concentrations and, ultimately, outcomes.[50,51] For example, children, African Americans, and patients with cystic fibrosis tend to have reduced absorption, increased clearance of cyclosporine, or both. Patients who are obese or who have decreased liver function will have reduced clearance. Oral absorption of cyclosporine, which has been characterized as slow, incomplete, and highly variable, is the parameter that is most significantly affected. Absorption can depend on the type of transplant, time after transplantation, presence of food and its composition, intestinal function (e.g., diarrhea, ileus), small bowel length, and presence or absence of external bile drainage. Bioavailability ranges from less than 5% to 90%.[51] In most transplant recipients, cyclosporine absorption increases over time.

DOSING

Because the original cyclosporine (Sandimmune) absorption was so poor and erratic, the IV route was used for the first few days after transplantation, particularly after liver transplantation. Cyclosporine can be given IV as a continuous infusion (2–3 mg/kg/day) or intermittently (2.5 mg/kg/day) over 2 to 6 hours divided into two equal doses. Sandimmune is used in very few patients today.

B.B. was given modified cyclosporine (Neoral), a readily absorbed cyclosporine formulation in a solubilized microemulsified state. Neoral's bioavailability is better than that of Sandimmune. Furthermore, Neoral absorption is much less dependent on bile and thus can be used in most liver transplant recipients early after transplant without the need for IV administration. However the doses used are initially higher (10–15 mg/kg/day) than those used after kidney transplant.[51]

Neoral and Sandimmune are not bioequivalent and, therefore, not interchangeable. Neoral produces a higher maximum concentration (C_{max}), shorter time to C_{max} (T_{max}), and higher area under the concentration-time curve (AUC) than Sandimmune. It has significantly less intrasubject and intersubject pharmacokinetic variability, and a better correlation exists between single doses and trough concentrations and AUC than Sandimmune. The bioavailability of Neoral is approximately 20% higher than that of Sandimmune (absolute bioavailability is 10%–89%). In patients converted from one formulation to another, trough concentrations are obtained within 4 to 7 days of conversion, and dosage adjustments are made accordingly. Most patients tolerate conversion well, although some experience concentration-related headaches, tremors, or elevated serum creatinine levels that resolve with dose adjustment. In most patients, the Neoral dose is 10% to 20% lower than the Sandimmune dose, but as much as a 50% difference can be seen in patients taking large doses (>10 mg/kg/day) of Sandimmune.[51]

The first generic cyclosporine, SangCya, is no longer available. SangCya was bioequivalent to Neoral but not Sandimmune. Several other generic capsules are now available, which are AB-rated bioequivalent to Neoral (Gengraf from Abbott and modified cyclosporine from Eon and Sidmak). Neoral and Sandimmune are available as both capsule and liquid.

Cyclosporine is extensively distributed into red blood cells (about 60%) whereas in plasma it is highly bound to lipoproteins (about 90%). It is extensively metabolized by both the gut and liver cytochrome P-450 3A4 enzymes and transported by P-glycoprotein. The average half-life is about 15 to 20 hours.[49–51]

B.B. was started on Neoral 10 mg/kg/day BID. Because he is African American, he may require even higher doses, because the absorption of cyclosporine has been reported to be reduced in this population.[51] His trough concentration will be monitored closely and adjusted if necessary. He should be watched closely for signs of rejection and toxicity.

ADVERSE EFFECTS

CASE 34-2, QUESTION 2: What are some of the adverse effects associated with cyclosporine?

Cyclosporine can cause a number of adverse effects, of which acute or chronic nephrotoxicity is the most frequent and worrisome. Other major effects include hypertension, hyperlipidemia, tremors, headaches, seizures, paresthesias, hypomagnesemia, hypokalemia or hyperkalemia, hyperuricemia, hyperglycemia, gout, gingival hyperplasia, hirsutism, hemolytic-uremic syndrome, and hepatotoxicity. If these occur, they generally respond to a reduction in dose, although some cases require discontinuation of cyclosporine.[52]

THERAPEUTIC DRUG MONITORING

CASE 34-2, QUESTION 3: B.B.'s cyclosporine levels are measured by whole blood liquid chromatography–tandem mass spectrometry. How should cyclosporine levels be used to optimize his therapy?

Cyclosporine concentrations are monitored to prevent toxicity, optimize efficacy, and assess patient compliance to the prescribed regimen. Most institutions monitor trough cyclosporine levels. During the early postoperative period, cyclosporine levels should be measured daily, keeping in mind that these may not reflect steady-state concentrations, and that dosage changes should be made every few days. Once B.B. is home, cyclosporine monitoring is necessary less frequently and eventually only every 1 to 2 months. The target trough therapeutic concentration of cyclosporine during the first 2 months posttransplant is 150 to 300 ng/mL with most whole blood assays. About 1 to 6 months after transplantation, the cyclosporine trough concentration target is lowered to 150 to 250 ng/mL. After 6 months, the targeted cyclosporine trough concentration is lowered even further to 50 to 150 ng/mL. These ranges differ among institutions and depend on the transplant type, time after transplantation, and other agents used. The range is reduced over time, given that less immunosuppression is required after transplantation and that the pharmacokinetics change over time.[49,50]

A number of assay methods are used to measure cyclosporine concentrations, and most institutions use the method that is most familiar to their transplant physicians. The type of cyclosporine assay used by a particular institution influences interpretation of results because there are significant differences between methodologies that may change the target trough. These issues have contributed to the debate on the value of monitoring cyclosporine concentrations. The pharmacologic effects of cyclosporine metabolites and whether the concentrations of these metabolites should be monitored individually are controversial.[53]

Assays currently in use include high-performance liquid chromatography (HPLC), radioimmunoassay with polyclonal or monoclonal antibodies, enzyme immunoassay (EMIT), and fluorescence polarization immunoassay (TDX). The most commonly used assay is the whole blood monoclonal assay.[53]

More recently, a number of centers have moved away from immunoassays to liquid chromatography–tandem mass spectrometry because of cost, specificity, sensitivity, improved turnaround time, and ability to measure several immunosuppressives simultaneously.[54] No assay appears to be superior in its ability to correlate cyclosporine trough levels with clinical events. Although many studies have attempted to correlate acute rejection or nephrotoxicity to trough concentrations of cyclosporine, results from these studies are conflicting. It may be that the ability to correlate a single blood level during the course of a day with a clinical event that takes place over a longer time period is influenced by too many other variables (e.g., other immunosuppressives, time since transplant, dosage regimen, route, transplant type, assay method, sample matrix, compliance, donor–recipient interaction). Nevertheless, most transplant programs, if not all, use cyclosporine concentrations to guide therapy decisions.

Cyclosporine troughs are poorly correlated with AUC; therefore, some programs use a more intensive sampling procedure (e.g., 6–10 samples collected during 12–24 hours) when cyclosporine concentrations are expected to be at steady state. The AUC and average steady-state concentrations are calculated and used to guide cyclosporine dosage adjustments. A more limited sampling strategy involving one to three samples (1–4 hours after a dose at steady state) to calculate AUC collected over a dosing interval has also been advocated.[55–57] In studies, conducted in kidney and liver transplant recipients, a Neoral AUC 0 to 4 hours was better correlated with an AUC 0 to 12 hours than any single time point, including a C0 or trough level. A number of studies have advocated the use of what is known as C2 monitoring. This level is obtained 2 hours after the Neoral dose. Some studies indicate that C2 level is a more sensitive predictor of acute rejection and toxicity than C0 or trough levels.[56] The limitations to this approach are (a) it requires training and education of staff and patients, (b) it requires potentially more personnel, (c) it necessitates modification of procedures, and (d) there are potential errors in accurate timing of dose and sampling. Therapeutic levels are different for kidney and liver transplant recipients with this approach.[57]

As in all cases, pharmacokinetic data must be interpreted in conjunction with the patient's clinical condition. In addition, deference always must be given to trends established by multiple cyclosporine levels rather than reacting to a single level. Single levels may be erroneous because of variability in dose administration, incorrect sampling time or techniques, or assay error.

Sirolimus

PHARMACOKINETICS

CASE 34-2, QUESTION 4: B.B. developed GI intolerance, nausea, vomiting, and diarrhea, to both mycophenolate products (MMF and Myfortic) and cannot take either one anymore. A decision is made to use sirolimus instead. Describe the pharmacokinetic characteristics of sirolimus. What would be the appropriate regimen and monitoring parameters for this agent?

Pharmacokinetic data for sirolimus are derived primarily from kidney transplant studies. Sirolimus exhibits significant pharmacokinetic variability. It is rapidly absorbed after oral administration of the liquid from with a median T_{max} of about 1 hour. Its average bioavailability is 15%; C_{max} and AUC are linear over a wide range of doses. Sirolimus is extensively distributed, with a mean apparent volume of distribution of 12 L/kg. It distributes primarily into red blood cells and is highly plasma-protein–bound, approximately 92%. It also binds to lipoproteins. Sirolimus is extensively metabolized in the gut and liver by cytochrome P-450 3A4 isoenzymes, and it is a substrate for P-glycoprotein. Its drug interaction profile is similar to that of cyclosporine and tacrolimus. Renal elimination accounts for 2% of a dose. The terminal half-life is approximately 57 to 63 hours and the time to steady state is 10 to 14 days. In children, it can be shorter.[58]

DOSING

Sirolimus can be used in the immediate posttransplant period although impaired wound healing and lymphocele development in kidney transplantation have limited its used in the early period. In the case of liver transplantation, its use is contraindicated in the early posttransplantation period because of hepatic artery thrombosis. Sirolimus may be added later, as is the practice in many centers, as replacement for or minimization of cyclosporine, tacrolimus, steroids, or mycophenolate.[59] Early experience advocated an initial loading dose followed by a once-daily maintenance dose; however, because of its adverse effect profile, not all centers use loading doses. The starting maintenance dose is 2 to 5 mg. The typical loading dose is 6 mg followed by 2 mg every day. In high-risk patients, such as African Americans, a 15-mg loading dose and 5-mg daily dose is recommended along with cyclosporine. Other centers have used loading doses of 10 to 15 mg, followed by 5 to 10 mg/day for the first week with target troughs of 10 to 15 ng/mL for the first month, and 5 to 10 ng/mL thereafter when used with tacrolimus.[60] Sirolimus is often given 4 hours after the morning dose of cyclosporine. If administered at the same time as cyclosporine, sirolimus concentrations are on average 40% higher.[61]

ADVERSE EFFECTS

As with other immunosuppressives, sirolimus is associated with a number of side effects, including oral ulcerations, diarrhea, arthralgias, epistaxis, rash, acne, leukopenia, thrombocytopenia, nausea and vomiting, lymphocele, hypokalemia, anemia, hypertension, pneumonitis, and infection. The most concerning side effects are dose-related hypertriglyceridemia and hypercholesterolemia. This occurs within the first few weeks of therapy and is sufficiently significant to require intervention with lipid-lowering agents, although it will respond to dosage reduction to some degree.[59] There are also reports of sirolimus causing proteinuria in kidney transplant recipients. The exact mechanism is unknown, but many transplant centers are now routinely monitoring for proteinuria in patients on sirolimus therapy and may avoid its use in patients with pre-existing proteinuria.[62]

THERAPEUTIC DRUG MONITORING

Monitoring of blood concentrations plays an important role in the dosing of sirolimus. Trough concentrations are obtained and correlate well with sirolimus AUC; therefore, trough monitoring is conducted. Because it has a longer half-life than the CNI, concentrations are obtained less frequently and only 5 to 7 days after a dose change. The target trough is usually 5 and 15 ng/mL; however, this continues to be refined with more experience. Early studies achieved concentrations greater than15 ng/mL, especially when used without a CNI, which were associated with a greater immunosuppression and adverse events. Because sirolimus is synergistic with CNIs, the target concentrations of the CNIs are also reduced when these agents are used together. Target tacrolimus trough targets are 5 to 10 ng/mL, and the cyclosporine trough targets are 75 to 100 ng/mL when used with sirolimus.[59]

B.B. could be started on sirolimus at 2 mg daily. Sirolimus blood trough concentration should be obtained 5 to 7 days after initiation. B.B.'s cyclosporine may need to be reduced if concentrations exceed 100 ng/mL. Monitoring parameters should include a fasting lipid panel, complete blood count, chemistries, and electrolytes.

Calcineurin Inhibitor–Induced Nephrotoxicity

CASE 34-3

QUESTION 1: C.C. is a 60-year-old man who received a deceased-donor kidney transplant 3 years ago. His serum creatinine at 1 year after transplant was 1.8 mg/dL; at 2 years, it was 2.0 mg/dL; now it is 2.3 mg/dL. He says he feels fine. His BP is well controlled and urinalysis is negative for protein. A kidney biopsy conducted at this time indicates that he has no signs of acute or chronic rejection, but has evidence of CNI nephrotoxicity. His current regimen is cyclosporine 275 mg BID, MMF 500 mg BID, and prednisone 5 mg daily. After the biopsy results, prednisone was reinstituted at 20 mg daily. His current labs show the following:

Cyclosporine blood trough, 220 ng/mL (target 100–150 ng/mL)
K, 5.5 mEq/L
Mg, 2.3 mg/dL
Uric acid 8.0 mg/dL

Why does C.C. have CNI nephrotoxicity?

CNI nephrotoxicity is one of the most common adverse effects and occurs to some degree in all patients. The rise in the serum creatinine concentration is more gradual than and not as high as that seen with rejection. CNI concentrations may be elevated, although some patients may experience CNI nephrotoxicity even with levels below or within the targeted therapeutic range. Two forms of CNI nephrotoxicity have been identified: functional or acute renal dysfunction and chronic nephrotoxicity.[63]

Acute CNI nephrotoxicity is more likely to occur in the first months after transplantation because CNI doses and levels are highest at this time. Functional renal dysfunction or acute nephrotoxicity, the most common form of renal dysfunction, is characterized by rapid reversal when the CNI dose is held or reduced. This syndrome typically is not associated with histopathologic abnormalities, which suggests that it is related to severe vasoconstriction of the renal afferent arterioles. Repeated episodes of transient acute renal dysfunction can result in protracted acute renal dysfunction. Recovery of renal function after repeated episodes usually is not complete even if the CNI is withdrawn. Protracted acute renal dysfunction can be associated with the development of thrombosis of glomerular arterioles or diffuse, interstitial fibrosis.

The other syndrome is a chronic, usually irreversible, nephrotoxicity, which is associated with mild proteinuria and tubular dysfunction. Renal biopsies in allograft patients with chronic CNI-related nephropathy show tubulointerstitial abnormalities, sometimes with focal glomerular sclerosis. Chronic nephrotoxicity is usually seen after 6 months of therapy, and may be irreversible. In this situation, renal function progressively declines to a point that dialysis or retransplant is required.[63]

The pathophysiology of cyclosporine or tacrolimus-induced transient acute renal failure is not understood completely, but seems to be related to its effects on renal vessels. For example, CNI can induce glomerular hypoperfusion secondary to vasoconstriction of the afferent glomerular arteriole, thereby reducing glomerular filtration. One possible explanation for these effects is that cyclosporine alters the balance of prostacyclin and thromboxane A_2 in renal cortical tissue. Increased thromboxane A_2 results in renal vasoconstriction. Endothelin release from renal vascular cells stimulated by CNI also may contribute to this acute effect through its potent vasoconstrictive properties. Activation of the renin-angiotensin-aldosterone system may also play a significant role. CNI also can cause a reversible decrease in tubular function. The alterations in tubular function reduce magnesium reabsorption and decrease potassium and uric acid secretion. This may be a result of direct tubular toxicity and possibly the result of thromboxane A_2 stimulation of platelet activation and aggregation.

Concern for chronic nephrotoxicity has led to the development of cyclosporine or tacrolimus withdrawal or substitution protocols, using agents, such as mycophenolate or sirolimus, or protocols using low doses of cyclosporine or tacrolimus.[64] C.C.'s rise in serum creatinine and hypertension in conjunction with a high cyclosporine level suggests acute cyclosporine toxicity as the most likely cause of his findings. In this case, the total cyclosporine dose should be lowered by approximately 25% to 225 mg twice a day, and C.C. should be monitored closely for resolution of the symptoms or worsening if rejection results from lowering the dose. His elevated potassium and, uric acid and low magnesium should correct themselves with this dose reduction if it is acute CNI toxicity. In any case, magnesium should be replaced to maintain a level greater than 1.5 mEq/L. If the nephrotoxicity is caused by cyclosporine, a decrease in the serum creatinine may be evident when the cyclosporine dose is reduced. If no such reduction occurs or if the serum concentration of creatinine continues to increase, then a renal biopsy is needed to rule out rejection, nephrotoxicity, or other causes.

Calcineurin Inhibitor Avoidance, Withdrawal, or Minimization

CASE 34-3, QUESTION 2: Would it be appropriate to withdraw cyclosporine in C.C.? If attempted, how could this be accomplished?

Cyclosporine and tacrolimus are associated with a number of metabolic, cardiovascular, neurologic, and cosmetic side effects but the most concerning is nephrotoxicity, which is a major contributor to graft loss. The potential benefit of withdrawing cyclosporine would be to reduce toxicity, but this has to be weighed against the risk for rejection, graft loss, and toxicities of replacement agents.

Basiliximab, sirolimus, and mycophenolate, which are not associated with nephrotoxicity, have been evaluated in protocols that attempt to avoid, minimize, or withdraw CNI. Protocols completely avoiding CNIs usually contain combinations of sirolimus, mycophenolate, steroids and an antibody. Studies, which were usually done in low-risk populations, observed lower serum creatinine levels and fewer CNI-induced toxicities, but were associated with higher rates of acute rejection (30%–50%). More recent trials in small numbers of patients that compared combinations of rabbit antithymocyte globulin or basiliximab, sirolimus, mycophenolate, and steroids with either cyclosporine or tacrolimus avoidance, withdrawal, or minimization protocols have shown equal effectiveness with acute rejection rates of less than 15%.[65]

In the case of early cyclosporine withdrawal, there is a 10% to 20% increased risk of acute rejection, but no change in graft survival. Protocols are used that withdraw the CNI or at least reduce the dose to a minimal level. Many attempt this within the first 3 to 12 months after transplantation in the hope that the nephrotoxic effects can be reversed before significant chronic damage occurs. These approaches add mycophenolate, sirolimus, or both as the CNI is withdrawn or reduced in dose, but they have been primarily tested in low-risk patients.[65] Data with sirolimus suggest that patients without proteinuria and an estimated glomerular filtration rate greater than 40 mL/minute in the first year had a lesser decline in renal function. Whether this applies to other agents remains to be determined.[66] Usually, when sirolimus is added to the CNI regimen the CNI dose is reduced by 50% initially and in some cases slowly withdrawn altogether during several weeks to months. Improvement in serum creatinine may be seen initially, which may be attributed to the diminution of the CNI vasoconstrictive effects.

CNI minimization or withdrawal may not reverse the nephrotoxicity observed in C.C.'s biopsy, but it may slow the rate of deterioration of his renal function. Because C.C. is currently receiving mycophenolate, one approach would be to continue to reduce his cyclosporine, increase his mycophenolate, and maintain steroids. Another approach would be to replace the mycophenolate with sirolimus, maintain steroids, and reduce or withdraw the cyclosporine. The best regimen for someone such as C.C. has not been established, because the long-term consequences of these changes are not known. If this approach is attempted, C.C. should be watched carefully for acute rejection, and side effects of these agents and infections should be closely monitored. In addition, BP control as well as control of hyperlipidemia and hyperglycemia could improve with reduction or withdrawal of cyclosporine and could also be important in minimizing renal injury.

STEROID AVOIDANCE OR WITHDRAWAL

CASE 34-4

QUESTION 1: D.T., a 60-year-old white woman, will receive a deceased-donor kidney transplant today because she has a negative cross-match to this donor and her previous PRA was less than 10%. She will be given one dose of alemtuzumab 30 mg IV and 1 dose of methylprednisolone 500 mg IV intraoperatively. After transplant, she will be started on tacrolimus 0.025 mg/kg BID, adjusted to trough levels of 8 to 12 ng/mL for the first 3 months, along with MMF 750 mg BID. Methylprednisolone IV will be given as 250 mg IV on postoperative day 1, 125 mg IV on postoperative days 2

and 3, and then discontinued. Is D.T. a good candidate for steroid avoidance or withdrawal?

Another important issue after kidney transplantation is the role of short-term and long-term steroid use. Most transplant protocols incorporate steroid therapy, although an increasing number of protocols use steroids only in the early postoperative period. The concept of either avoiding or discontinuing corticosteroids is appealing because they cause significant adverse effects such as diabetes, cataracts, infection, hypertension, hyperlipidemia, osteoporosis, and avascular necrosis, and have psychiatric, neurologic, and cosmetic effects. Steroid withdrawal or avoidance, however, may increase the risk of acute rejection, compromise long-term graft function, and necessitate higher doses of the other immunosuppressives.[17]

Steroid avoidance is defined as either no steroid use or steroid use only for the first few days after transplant. Preliminary studies suggest no adverse impact on short-term graft survival exists and no need is seen for higher doses of other immunosuppressives when corticosteroids are not included in maintenance regimens. These protocols have included regimens such as alemtuzumab; daclizumab, basiliximab, or rabbit antithymocyte globulin; mycophenolate or sirolimus; and cyclosporine or tacrolimus.

Steroid withdrawal is the complete discontinuation of prednisone posttransplant. In the era of cyclosporine (Sandimmune) and azathioprine-based regimens withdrawal was associated with a high rate of acute rejection and late graft loss. With the introduction of newer agents, steroid avoidance or withdrawal has been viewed with renewed interest. Steroid withdrawal has been successful in at least 50% of kidney transplant recipients—resulting in reductions in blood pressure and lipid levels. Some protocols withdraw corticosteroids within the first few days to weeks after the initial transplantation period, whereas others withdraw them 3 to 6 months or later after transplantation. The rate of success depends not only on the immunosuppressives used but on the population (high-risk vs. low-risk) and timing of withdrawal. Regimens that appear most successful include an antibody with cyclosporine or tacrolimus, mycophenolate, or sirolimus. African Americans, pediatric patients, patients who have retransplants, highly sensitized patients, patients with a high serum creatinine (>2.5 mg/dL), and those who have had a recent rejection episode are more difficult to withdraw from steroids. This is particularly true early (<3 months) after transplantation. Withdrawal in these cases is associated with a higher rate of rejection. Later withdrawal may be attempted, but the benefits in terms of side-effect profile may not be as great. Low-risk populations are candidates for steroid avoidance or early withdrawal. First-time transplantation, living-donor, well-matched transplantation, older age, and stable graft function without rejection are factors associated with a positive benefit to steroid withdrawal.[17]

D.T. would be considered a low-risk patient because of her low immunologic activity evidenced by a low PRA, her age, and ethnicity. Therefore a steroid avoidance protocol, such as the one indicated here, would be appropriate. As with other transplant recipients, she must be closely monitored for rejection and adverse effects.

BK Polyomavirus Infection

CASE 34-5

QUESTION 1: K.T., a 45-year-old white man, is now 16 months posttransplant. His posttransplant course has been complicated by two rejection episodes. The first was severe and required rabbit antithymocyte globulin therapy; the second was a mild rejection several weeks later that was adequately treated with three pulse-doses of 500 mg IV methylprednisolone. His current immunosuppressant regimen consists of tacrolimus 8 mg PO BID, MMF 1 g PO BID, and prednisone 10 mg PO daily. In addition, he is receiving amlodipine 10 mg PO daily, benazepril 10 mg PO daily, pravastatin 40 mg PO at bedtime, and calcium with vitamin D 500 mg PO BID. Today, he is in the transplant clinic for a routine follow-up visit. He has no complaints and says he has been feeling "great," although he has noticed some blood in his urine during the past couple of weeks. Because of this, a urinalysis is ordered in addition to the standard laboratory values. The results are as follows:

Na, 145 mEq/L
K, 4.2 mEq/L
Cl, 104 mEq/L
HCO_3, 26 mEq/L
BUN, 32 mg/dL
SCr, 2.7 mg/dL
Ca, 10.1 mEq/L
Phosphorus, 4.5 mg/dL
Glucose, 110 mg/dL
Amylase, 50 international units/L
Lipase, 32 international units/L
WBC count, 7.7 cells/μL
Hgb, 10.4 g/dL
Hct, 31%
Tacrolimus trough, 9 ng/mL
Urinalysis, color yellow
Specific gravity, 1.013
pH, 7.0
Protein, 100 mg/dL
Glucose, negative
Ketones, negative
Bilirubin, negative
Blood, moderate
Nitrite, negative
Leukocyte, negative
Squamous epithelial cells, 3 cells/high-power field
Bacteria, negative

Urinalysis revealed "decoy" cells and plasma BK virus PCR was greater than 10^4. Because of the increasing serum creatinine, a percutaneous kidney biopsy is performed. The pathologist reviews the histology of the tissue sample and determines that it is consistent with BK virus nephritis. What is BK polyomavirus? How is it diagnosed and what are its clinical manifestations?

BK virus is a human polyomavirus, first isolated in 1971. Polyomaviruses are small, nonenveloped viruses with a closed, circular, double-stranded DNA sequence. Little is known about the transmission or about the primary infection of BK virus. It is believed that viremia during the initial exposure results in systemic seeding and subsequently becomes a latent infection. The kidney is the main site of BK virus latency in healthy people. More than 50% of the general population express BK virus antibodies by age 3 years. Immunosuppression after transplantation probably leads to the reactivation of the virus, but other factors, such as organ ischemia and coinfection with other pathogens, may contribute to reactivation. Reactivation inevitably leads to viruria or viral shedding into the urine. Asymptomatic viruria occurs in approximately 10% to 45% of kidney transplant recipients.[67]

Diagnosis of BK virus nephritis is made by careful review of clinical, laboratory, and histologic findings. Patients are often asymptomatic, although hematuria has been noted in some patients. Clinically, BK virus nephritis mimics acute rejection and increases in serum creatinine often lead to a tissue biopsy. Tissue histology is similar to cases of acute rejection and BK virus nephritis, with mononuclear infiltration as the predominant finding. The abundance of plasma cells, prominent tubular cell apoptosis, collecting duct destruction, and absence of endarteritis are features that may distinguish BK virus nephritis from acute cellular rejection. Although BK virus has been implicated in up to 5% of all cases of interstitial nephritis (of which 30% go on to graft failure), it is still unclear whether asymptomatic biopsy findings in the kidney transplant recipient is a prognostic indicator. Decoy cells in the urine and BK virus–PCR in blood are used as screening tools. Blood or plasma BK virus–PCR is a more sensitive and stable test and correlates better with renal dysfunction than decoy cells.

Most cases of BK nephritis occur within the first 3 months after transplantation, although a number of cases have been reported as long as 2 years after transplantation. The major risk factor for the development of BK nephritis and subsequent graft dysfunction or loss is the degree of immunosuppression. In addition, accelerated graft loss has been demonstrated in patients who received antilymphocyte antibodies in the presence of BK virus nephritis misdiagnosed as an acute rejection episode. K.T., like many patients with BK virus, is asymptomatic with an elevated serum creatinine. Because K.T. has received higher doses of immunosuppression recently to treat two acute rejection episodes, he is at higher risk for developing BK virus nephritis.

TREATMENT

CASE 34-5, QUESTION 2: K.T. is told to stop taking MMF and to reduce his tacrolimus dose to 4 mg PO BID with target trough levels less than 6 ng/mL. Why was K.T.'s immunosuppressive regimen significantly reduced?

Because BK virus reactivation and BK nephritis are strongly associated with the degree of immunosuppression, reduction in, or removal of, immunosuppressant agents is considered first-line therapy and most effective approach. Beneficial clinical responses have been demonstrated in some patients when the dose of CNI is reduced and/or other agents removed. Not all patients, however, respond to this maneuver. In addition, reduction in immunosuppression puts patients at higher risk for an acute rejection episode. Close clinical follow-up after reduction of immunosuppression is important to ensure adequate response and to make sure the patient does not experience an acute rejection episode. In K.T.'s case, an improvement of renal function can be expected, as seen by a reduction in serum creatinine over time. Also, monitoring viral loads both from the urine and serum have been shown to correlate with clinical disease.[68]

ANTIVIRAL THERAPY

CASE 34-5, QUESTION 3: During the next 2 weeks, K.T.'s serum creatinine remains unchanged, and his serum and urine viral loads also remain approximately the same. Are there any additional treatment options for K.T.'s BK nephritis at this time?

Cidofovir, an antiviral agent indicated for the treatment of CMV retinitis, inhibits polyomavirus replication in vitro; however, to date, no well-conducted clinical trials have proved this agent to be effective in treating or preventing BK virus nephritis in the transplant population. In a small number of case reports and case-series, this agent was beneficial, but the appropriate dose and frequency are still undetermined. Most reports have used very small doses (0.25–1.0 mg/kg/dose) to minimize nephrotoxicity. It is given IV either weekly or every other week and usually continued until renal dysfunction is resolved and a decrease in the viral load occurs.

Cidofovir is associated with a high incidence of nephrotoxicity, especially at much higher doses; therefore, patients usually receive predose and postdose hydration with 0.9% NaCl boluses. Close clinical monitoring of the patient is advised if this treatment option is used. Because the doses of cidofovir currently used are approximately 5% to 10% of the standard dose used to treat CMV (5 mg/kg/dose), use of probenecid as a premedication to prevent high-dose cidofovir-induced nephrotoxicity is not advocated. Other therapies that have been tried with mixed success are IVIG and leflunomide in place of the discontinued antimetabolite, such as mycophenolate, and the addition of ciprofloxacin (which has some anti–BK virus activity). Retransplantation has also been conducted with some success.[68]

New Onset Diabetes After Transplant

CASE 34-6

QUESTION 1: J.F. is a 28-year-old African American man who received a kidney transplant 6 weeks ago secondary to focal segmental glomerulosclerosis. His medical history is significant for hypertension and nephrotic syndrome. Before the transplant, he was taking lisinopril 20 mg PO daily, amlodipine 10 mg PO daily, and valsartan 160 mg PO daily. After the transplant, amlodipine 10 mg PO daily was continued. J.F. was started on tacrolimus 12 mg PO BID, MMF 1 g PO BID, and a corticosteroid taper. He also receives 10 mg prednisone PO BID, and will be tapered down during the next 6 weeks to 5 mg PO daily. J.F.'s tacrolimus trough concentrations have been between 10 ng/L and 14 ng/L. During the next 12 weeks, he will be maintained on a dose of tacrolimus to achieve trough concentrations between 8 ng/L and 12 ng/L. J.F. currently weighs 108 kg and is 6 feet tall. His body mass index (BMI) is 32 kg/m^2. After transplant, he has required a sliding-scale regular insulin regimen to maintain a blood glucose level between 120 mg/dL and 180 mg/dL. His BP readings during the past two weeks have ranged between 145–155/90–95. Fasting lipid panel is a total cholesterol, 261 mg/dL; LDL, 161 mg/dL; HDL, 40 mg/dL; and triglycerides, 200 mg/dL. What posttransplant complications are common and what is J.F. at risk of developing?

Posttransplantation diabetes mellitus, or now more commonly referred to in the transplant literature as new onset diabetes after transplant (NODAT), is another common problem that appears to be on the increase in transplant recipients, similar to the increase in diabetes mellitus in the general population. Diabetes significantly affects morbidity and mortality in transplant recipients. It is often a pre-existing condition in renal transplant recipients and a cause of ESRD. In recipients of other organs, such as livers, diabetes is common as well, both as a pre-existing condition and as a posttransplantation complication. The definition of NODAT varies among studies. It has been based on symptoms and plasma glucose, oral glucose challenge results, or the need for insulin or oral antidiabetic drugs after transplantation. Reported rates are 3% to greater than 40%, with most cases of NODAT occurring within the first year after transplantation. Risk factors, besides pretransplantation diabetes, include advanced age, family history, CMV infection, certain HLA phenotypes, race (African American or Hispanic), increased BMI, and infection with hepatitis C in the liver transplant population.[69]

One of the most critical factors in the development of NODAT is the immunosuppressive regimen. Cyclosporine, tacrolimus, and prednisone are all associated with NODAT. The CNI appear to have a direct toxic effect on the pancreatic beta cells leading to decreased insulin synthesis and secretion; this effect seems to be dose-related and generally reversible. Although still debated by a few clinicians, the literature now clearly suggests that tacrolimus is more likely to cause NODAT than cyclosporine. Additionally, conversion from tacrolimus to cyclosporine has been useful in some patients with NODAT. Other risk factors, such as CNI drug concentrations, steroid doses, African American race, transplant type, and time lapsed after transplantation, must also be considered.[69]

As with diabetes in the general population, a similar intensive approach in controlling blood glucose should be undertaken. Also, other conditions (e.g., hypertension and hyperlipidemia) should be managed aggressively.[70] Reducing or withdrawing diabetes-inducing immunosuppression as much as possible without jeopardizing graft function or using agents that are nondiabetogenic (such as mycophenolate) may be beneficial. One important aspect of posttransplant diabetes management is to realize the differences in pharmacologic management in this population, as compared with patients who are not transplant recipients. Often, in the immediate posttransplant period, because of the rapidly changing organ function and the dramatic tapering of corticosteroids, a patient's antidiabetic medicines may need frequent adjustment. During the first 3 to 4 weeks posttransplant, insulin is the agent of choice owing to the ability of the clinician to use sliding-scales, the availability of several insulin products, and the ease in changing doses. Once patients are stabilized on their immunosuppressant regimen, and their organ function has also, the use of oral antidiabetic agents can be introduced or restarted. Because of metformin's contraindications, particularly with liver and renal function, it is usually not recommended for use in transplant recipients.

J.F. was not diabetic pretransplant but is now requiring insulin. By some clinicians' definitions, he would be classified as having NODAT. Others would wait to see if J.F. still required insulin after his immunosuppressant regimen was tapered to lower levels. In either regard, because J.F. is obese and is African American, he is considered at high risk for the development of NODAT. At this point, J.F.'s diabetes should continue to be controlled on a sliding-scale insulin regimen. Once J.F.'s immunosuppression regimen is stable, he can be switched to oral antidiabetic agents if needed. J.F. should be counseled on diet and exercise to help control his blood glucose level. Other pharmacologic interventions that may help prevent long-term diabetes in J.F. is changing his tacrolimus to cyclosporine and reducing or withdrawing his prednisone. The risks and benefits of changing immunosuppressant regimens must always be weighed. For instance, changing his tacrolimus to cyclosporine, or reducing or removing J.F.'s steroids, may reduce his blood glucose level and may prevent NODAT, but it also will put J.F. at higher risk of developing acute rejection.

Posttransplant Hypertension

CASE 34-6, QUESTION 2: What pharmacologic options would be used for J.F.'s hypertenstion?

Cardiovascular disease is very common in patients with ESRD and after kidney transplantation. Cardiovascular disease after transplant is associated with graft loss and lower patient survival. In those recipients who die with a functioning graft, 40% die secondary to a cardiovascular event.[71] Some immunosuppressives, including cyclosporine, tacrolimus, and steroids contribute to the development of hypertension. Some studies have indicated that blood pressure is higher and more difficult to manage in patients on cyclosporine compared with tacrolimus.[72]

The appropriate blood pressure goals are similar to those in the general population, that is, less than 140/90 mm Hg in patients without proteinuria, as seen in this case. Nonpharmacologic therapies should be implemented; however, in transplant recipients pharmacologic management is key, often requiring multiple antihypertensives.

Pharmacologic agents used in transplant recipients are the same as those used in the general population. In the transplant recipient, one must consider the drug interaction profile and comorbidities. For example, nondihydropyridine calcium-channel blockers (CCBs), such as amlodipine, are less likely to interact with CNIs than diltiazem or verapamil. CCBs may also ameliorate some of the vasoconstrictive effects produced by the CNIs. In many programs, CCBs are considered first-line therapy. β-Blockers such as metoprolol are also frequently used in transplant recipients. Many recipients have or are at risk for coronary artery disease and these agents can be effective in these situations. Angiotensin-converting enzyme (ACE) inhibitors and angiotensin receptor blockers (ARBs) can be used in transplant recipients. Historically these agents were avoided, because of concern for their association with impaired kidney function. However, these have significant cardiovascular and renal benefits in patients with comorbidities such as diabetes, proteinuria, and congestive heart failure. Their use in transplant recipients has increased and are introduced shortly after transplant to months after transplant when renal function is more stable. Certainly if an ACE inhibitor or ARB is used, SCr and potassium levels must be monitored closely. Diuretics are useful in patients with evidence of fluid overload. In refractory patients, agents such as clonidine, hydralazine, and minoxidil may be required.[73] In J.F.'s case, because he is already on amlodipine, a second agent such as lisinopril or metoprolol would be appropriate at this time with close monitoring and follow-up.

Posttransplant Hyperlipidemia

CASE 34-6, QUESTION 3: What would be an appropriate lipid lowering therapy for J.F.'s hyperlipidemia?

Hyperlipidemia is another cardiovascular issue that must be addressed in transplant recipients. As with hypertension, it is fairly common pretransplant and posttransplant. It is associated with negative cardiac outcomes and reduced graft and patient survival in transplant recipients.[70] Immunosuppressives including cyclosporine, tacrolimus, steroids, sirolimus, and everolimus can cause elevations in total cholesterol, LDL, and triglycerides and also reduce HDL.[72] Goals of treatment are based on the Kidney Disease Outcomes Quality Initiative/Kidney Disease: Improving Global Outcomes guidelines (http://www.kdigo.org/clinical_practice_guidelines/pdf/KITxpGL_summary.pdf) and primarily based on targeting and LDL of less than 100 mg/dL.[70] Treatment involves diet, which alone appears to have minimal effect; therefore, pharmacologic treatment is usually required. Agents utilized in the nontransplant population are effective in reducing lipids in transplant recipients. Considerations in selecting treatments for hyperlipidemia include drug interactions with the immunosuppressives and the side effect profile. Statins are considered first-line treatment and have substantial evidence to support their use.[74] Cyclosporine can increase concentrations of simvastatin and rosuvastatin, therefore limiting their doses. Atorvastatin is often used and appears to be safe and effective in this population. Fibrates, ezetimibe, bile acid binders, and niacin are considered second line agents. In J.F., atorvastatin would be an appropriate choice.

Posttransplant Osteoporosis

Rapid bone loss with the subsequent development of osteopenia or osteoporosis is another common posttransplantation disorder that must be evaluated, prevented, and treated. Osteoporosis, a silent disease, is characterized by low bone mass and microarchitectural deterioration of bone tissue, which increases bone fragility and eventually leads to fracture. Various epidemiologic and cross-sectional studies estimate that 7% to 11% of nondiabetic kidney transplant recipients, 45% of diabetic kidney transplant recipients, and 24% to 65% of liver transplant recipients exhibit atraumatic fractures resulting from osteoporosis in the posttransplantation period.[75]

RISK FACTORS

Osteoporosis risk factors for transplant recipients, which are similar to those in the general population, include menopausal status, family history, smoking, alcohol use, lack of physical activity, poor nutritional status, and use of various medications such as corticosteroids, phenytoin, thyroxine, heparin, warfarin, and loop diuretics. Additional factors responsible for bone loss in organ transplant recipients depend on the underlying disease state and the particular organ system transplanted. For example, patients with ESRD commonly have at least some evidence of renal osteodystrophy, which includes hyperparathyroidism, osteomalacia, osteosclerosis, and adynamic or aplastic bone disease. Hypogonadism can also be present. Many kidney transplant recipients have already been exposed to medications that can affect bone and mineral metabolism, such as corticosteroids, cyclosporine for immune complex disease, loop diuretics, or aluminum-containing phosphate binders.

Drugs used to prevent organ rejection predispose patients to osteoporosis, especially the corticosteroids. As noted, efforts are underway among transplant centers to develop corticosteroid-free or rapid-taper corticosteroid immunosuppressant regimens to prevent post-transplant bone disease. Corticosteroids reduce net intestinal calcium absorption, increase urinary calcium excretion, increase parathyroid hormone, decrease production of skeletal growth factors, and decrease androgen and estrogen synthesis in the gonads and adrenal gland. They also decrease bone formation by osteoblasts and increase bone resorption.[76] The most dramatic reduction in bone loss after transplantation occurs within the first 3 to 6 months, when high doses of steroids are tapered to prednisone doses equivalent to 7.5 to 10 mg every day. Areas of the skeleton rich in trabecular or cancellous bone, such as the ribs, vertebrae, distal ends of long bones, and the cortical rim of the vertebral body, are most at risk for osteoporotic fracture because (a) a greater degree of bone remodeling or bone turnover occurs in these areas and (b) this is a target of corticosteroid activity. Most studies suggest a minor effect of CNI on bone. Other currently used agents appear to have little or no effect.[77]

TREATMENT

Because rapid bone loss and fractures can occur during the first few months postoperatively, strategies to prevent bone loss and fractures should be initiated immediately after transplantation and if possible before transplantation. Most recommendations are based on the American College of Rheumatology's guidelines for the prevention and treatment of corticosteroid-induced osteoporosis.[76] These recommendations focus on providing calcium and vitamin D (variable dosing depending on kidney and liver functions) to patients who will be receiving continuous corticosteroid therapy. If patients are diagnosed with low bone mineral density (osteopenia) or even osteoporosis with bone mineral density scans using dual-energy x-ray absorptiometry (DXA) scans, calcium and vitamin D analogs are recommended in conjunction with either a bisphosphonate or calcitonin.[76,77]

Clinical trials have demonstrated that bisphosphonates and vitamin D analogs are effective in preventing and treating posttransplant bone disease. However, these studies have failed to show a significant improvement in bone fracture rates, bone pain, or immobility owing to bone disease. Most studies show that these agents can minimize the loss of bone posttransplant, as demonstrated by stabilization of DXA scans.[77]

Although J.F. is young and likely does not have severe bone disease, a DXA scan should still be performed, and he could be given calcium and vitamin D because he is receiving steroids (unless he has a contraindication to this therapy, such as hypercalcemia). Based on the results of J.F.'s DXA scan, he may need to receive either a bisphosphonate or an activated vitamin D analog, such as calcitriol, and possibly calcium supplementation. A repeat DXA scan should be performed in 1 to 2 years. J.F. should be carefully counseled on how to take his medicine correctly to minimize adverse effects and he should be monitored for hypocalcemia or hypercalcemia.

LIVER TRANSPLANTATION

Indications

CASE 34-7

QUESTION 1: E.P., a 58-year-old, 78-kg man with an 18-year history of chronic liver disease secondary to hepatitis C infection arrives at the emergency room with a 2-day history of confusion, fever up to 102.2°F, and worsening jaundice, with scleral icterus. Because the patient has severe abdominal distention, a paracentesis is performed, and 7 L of fluid is drained from his peritoneal cavity. A diagnosis of spontaneous bacterial peritonitis is made.

E.P.'s clinical status during the next several days gradually worsens, and he is moved to the intensive care unit for closer monitoring and better supportive care. E.P. continues to be severely jaundiced, with worsening liver function tests (LFTs). He becomes progressively more confused, and eventually comatose, requiring intubation. Within 3 days of admission into the intensive care unit, a suitable liver donor, matched for size and ABO blood group, is found, and E.P. receives an orthotopic liver transplant with a choledochocholedochostomy (duct-to-duct anastomosis). CMV serology for E.P. is negative, and the donor liver is CMV-positive.

After the transplantation, E.P. is started on fluid maintenance with 0.45% normal saline; tacrolimus 2 mg NG/PO BID; and high-dose methylprednisolone with a rapid taper: 50 mg IV every 6 hours for four doses, 40 mg IV every 6 hours for four doses, 30 mg IV every 6 hours for four doses, 20 mg IV every 6 hours for four doses, 20 mg IV every 12 hours for two doses, then 20 mg IV daily; famotidine 20 mg IV every 12 hours; and ganciclovir 150 mg IV daily. Piperacillin tazobactam 3.5 g IV every 6 hours for 48 hours was begun in the operating room. An order also is written to limit all pain medications and sedatives. E.P. returned from surgery with three abdominal Jackson-Pratt

concluded that oral ganciclovir is more effective than oral acyclovir. Ganciclovir prophylaxis seems most effective when used in D+/R– patients.[124]

When ganciclovir prophylaxis, either oral or IV, is used in high-risk kidney transplant recipients, it appears to reduce the incidence of CMV disease.[124] As in the liver transplantation population, ganciclovir is superior to oral acyclovir. In most studies, prophylaxis is continued for approximately 12 weeks after transplantation.

VALGANCICLOVIR

Valganciclovir was developed because oral ganciclovir has a very low bioavailability (<10%). Valganciclovir is the L-valyl ester of ganciclovir, which is a prodrug that is rapidly and completely converted into ganciclovir by hepatic and intestinal esterases once absorbed across the GI tract. The absolute bioavailability of valganciclovir is approximately 60%, so that a 900-mg single PO dose given with food is an AUC equivalent to a 5 mg/kg IV dose of ganciclovir. This is roughly twice the AUC achieved by 1,000 mg of ganciclovir given orally TID.[125] Valganciclovir is currently FDA-approved for the treatment of HIV-associated CMV retinitis, and to prevent CMV disease in heart, lung, kidney, and pancreas transplantation.[126,127] Valganciclovir is not FDA-approved for prevention of CMV disease in liver transplantation, although it is often used in such cases.[124] Several small studies have demonstrated that valganciclovir is effective in treating CMV infection pre-emptively and potentially preventing CMV disease.[126,127]

Because valganciclovir is very expensive and has a high potential for causing hematologic toxicities, several studies have been conducted using reduced dosing strategies. Most use half the recommended dose of 900 mg PO daily in patients with good renal function and have shown equivalent clinical outcomes with the potential of reducing cost and toxicities. These studies were conducted in kidney transplant patients, and the dosing of this agent is transplant center–specific based on institutional protocols.

ACYCLOVIR

Acyclovir is ineffective in the treatment of established CMV disease, but it does appear to have a modest beneficial preventive role. Since the introduction of oral ganciclovir, several trials have compared the prophylactic efficacy of high-dose acyclovir (800 mg PO 5×/day) with oral ganciclovir.[128,129] As already noted, oral ganciclovir appears to be more effective in preventing CMV disease, especially in the D+/R– subgroup. Because of this, most consider oral acyclovir to be second-line therapy to IV or oral ganciclovir or valganciclovir as a CMV prophylactic agent.

VALACYCLOVIR

One published meta-analysis of 12 trials that included 1,574 patients evaluated valacyclovir as a prophylactic agent in transplant recipients.[130] Valacyclovir was found to be more effective than acyclovir in preventing herpes viruses, including CMV. Most transplantation centers, however, do not use valacyclovir for routine prophylaxis of CMV, and still consider valganciclovir first-line.

CYTOMEGALOVIRUS HYPERIMMUNE GLOBULIN

The role of CMV hyperimmune globulin in preventing CMV disease is controversial. Many studies have combined this agent with either oral acyclovir or ganciclovir, but because of its high cost and IV route, its use as a prophylactic agent has decreased. In addition, in patients who are D+/R–, results have been mixed.[123]

CASE 34-10, QUESTION 4: Should A.A. have received prophylactic therapy and, if so, which agent should be used?

A.A. has several risk factors that predispose him to developing CMV disease. At the time of transplantation, A.A. was CMV D+/R–, which means that he has about an 80% chance of developing CMV infection and a 40% chance of developing CMV disease. In addition, A.A. had an early acute rejection episode, which means he received higher doses of immunosuppression, also putting him at higher risk for developing CMV disease. Because of these risk factors, A.A. should have (and did) receive CMV prophylaxis for at least 3 months after transplantation. Some centers may extend prophylaxis to 6 months posttransplant in patients like A.A. A.A. developed CMV disease and is being treated with ganciclovir 190 mg every 12 hours IV. Once A.A. is tolerating oral medications, he can start receiving oral valganciclovir at a dose of 900 mg daily with food. Because A.A. has renal insufficiency, his oral valganciclovir dose will be adjusted to 450 mg daily.[131]

ONLINE CONTENT

To reference a chart that specifies valcyte dosing based on estimated creatinine clearance for CMV prophylaxis, go to http://thepoint.lww.com/AT10e.

As illustrated by A.A.'s case, a patient who has received prophylactic therapy does not preclude the development of CMV disease after the prophylaxis is withdrawn or, in rare instances, during prophylactic therapy. The incidence of CMV disease while receiving valganciclovir is significantly lower when compared to oral ganciclovir, probably because drug exposure is approximately two times higher.[126,127]

PRE-EMPTIVE THERAPY

Because of recent advances in the laboratory tests used to identify and quantify CMV; because prophylactic therapy is not always effective; and because it is often toxic and very expensive, pre-emptive therapy has also been used to prevent CMV disease. The technique involves withholding prophylactic therapy and monitoring laboratory tests to identify presymptomatic CMV viremia, usually by using serum CMV DNA PCR. Once a patient develops viremia (CMV PCR viral load >2,000 copies/mL), he or she receives treatment with IV ganciclovir or oral valganciclovir. This strategy has been prospectively studied and is as effective as universal prophylaxis, with some potential cost advantages.[132] However, a few recent studies have demonstrated a higher incidence of the indirect effects of CMV in the pre-emptive group—most-concerning in one study, graft loss. Thus, the pre-emptive therapy role is controversial, with many centers still using universal CMV prophylaxis in all solid organ transplant recipients.[133]

Posttransplantation Lymphoproliferative Disorder

RISK FACTORS

CASE 34-11

QUESTION 1: A.L., a 16-year-old, 42-kg girl, underwent liver transplant 1 year ago secondary to biliary atresia with a failed Kasai procedure. She now presents with low-grade fever, malaise, pain, and a 1-week history of decreased appetite. She has experienced two episodes of rejection that were treated with 1 to 2 g of methylprednisolone each time, with the last rejection episode requiring rabbit antithymocyte globulin therapy. She received tacrolimus and prednisone after transplantation and had MMF added to her immunosuppressant regimen after the second rejection episode. She has just finished a course of IV ganciclovir

(4 weeks) for CMV infection. The donor was CMV-positive and she is CMV-positive. Her EBV DNA PCR is now 18,000 copies/mL (normal, <500 copies/mL); this value was negative at the time of transplant, but since her last rejection episode has been increasing in value. On physical examination, she was noted to have mediastinal adenopathy. She denies chills, sweats, nausea, vomiting, or diarrhea. A chest computed tomography scan revealed a mediastinal mass. Vital signs and all laboratory tests are within normal limits. Her tacrolimus trough is 9.8 ng/mL. Seven days after admission, a biopsy of this mass shows a thoracic lymphoproliferative lesion identified as a thoracic immunoblastic lymphoma adherent to the right side of the heart. Ten days later, she developed tachy/brady syndrome and a pacemaker was implanted. Given the location of her lymphoma and symptoms, surgery and radiation therapy are not viable options, and chemotherapy is started the next day. What clinical signs and risk factors in A.L. are associated with lymphoma?

A.L. has developed a PTLD, one of many types of malignancies that have been reported after solid organ transplantation. The exact etiology of this condition is unclear and probably multifactorial. The presentation of PTLD varies significantly. Patients can present asymptomatically, with mild mononucleosislike symptoms or with multiorgan failure. A.L. presents with fever, lymphadenopathy, malaise, and lack of appetite. Although these symptoms are consistent with PTLD, they also are consistent with infection. Because PTLD can involve various organ systems, patients can present with organ-specific symptoms (e.g., acute abdominal pain, perforation, obstruction, bleeding if a tumor is in the GI tract). Depending on its location, a tumor can impinge on the function of other organs, as seen in A.L.[134]

Besides immunosuppression, two factors that have been strongly associated with PTLD are the presence of EBV and the age of the patient. Children have a higher incidence of PTLD.[135] A.L. developed EBV DNA viremia, indicating that she had been exposed to this virus at the time of transplantation or afterward. EBV also can be transmitted from the donor liver and/or blood products. Also, EBV-positive recipients at the time of transplantation can experience reactivation of this virus as a result of immunosuppression.

A.L. received a significant amount of immunosuppression. This could lead to an inability to suppress an active viral infection by cytotoxic T cells and result in uncontrolled B-cell proliferation and polyclonal and monoclonal expansion. In addition to this T-cell defect, an imbalance or alteration in cytokine production in response to EBV, which infects B lymphocytes, may contribute to the exaggerated B-cell expansion and transformation; most are classified as non-Hodgkin lymphomas primarily of B-cell origin. Small percentages are of T-cell origin, however, and are harder to treat.[136]

The incidence and detection of PTLD has increased. Newer, more potent immunosuppressive agents used in different combinations, increased numbers of transplantation procedures, and closer monitoring contributes to this phenomenon. When cyclosporine-based regimens were compared with azathioprine or cyclophosphamide-based regimens, lymphomas made up 26% and 11% of all cancers, respectively. The lymphomas occurred, on average, within 15 months after transplant in the cyclosporine group versus 48 months in the azathioprine group. One-third of these malignancies occurred in the first 4 months in the cyclosporine group compared with only 11% in the latter group.[136]

The incidence of PTLD increases with rabbit antithymocyte globulin therapy and appears to be related to a cumulative dose and multiple courses. PTLD is not caused by any single agent but probably reflects the intensity of immunosuppression with multiple agents. Chronic antigenic stimulation by foreign antigens, repeated infections, genetic predisposition, and indirect or direct damage to DNA are other variables that might affect the development of PTLD.[137] A.L. had a recent CMV infection, which also could have contributed to this process.

As a percentage of all malignancies, PTLD occurs more commonly in thoracic than in other types of solid organ transplants and is even more common in children.[135] Lymphomas develop in about 1% of kidney transplantations and 2% of liver transplantations. These tumors often appear early and progress rapidly. The overall prevalence of malignancies in the transplantation population averages about 6%, and the risk of cancer increases with time after a transplantation. Major organ transplant recipients are 100 times more likely to have cancer than the general population.[137] Furthermore, the most common types of cancer observed in transplant recipients (e.g., lymphomas, cancer of the skin and lips) are uncommon in the general population. The development of skin and lip cancers in the transplant population has been attributed partially to exposure to sunlight and sensitization of skin to sunlight by an azathioprine metabolite, methylnitrothioimidazole.[137]

TREATMENT AND OUTCOMES

CASE 34-11, QUESTION 2: What are the therapeutic maneuvers and outcomes that would be expected in A.L.?

Treatment of a PTLD depends on timing, presentation, symptoms, extent of involvement, histologic type, and transplant type. Early experiences with PTLD indicated that reduction or discontinuation of immunosuppression led to regression of the cancer. Therefore, the first step in treating PTLD is to consider the discontinuation of all immunosuppressives, with the potential exception of the corticosteroids. This course of action is not feasible for A.L., however, because her transplanted liver is essential for her life. Immunosuppressive drugs can be discontinued in kidney recipients because dialysis can be reinstituted. A.L. will need chemotherapy for her cancer. Therefore, her MMF probably should be discontinued to minimize the potential for severe bone marrow toxicity. Additionally, A.L. will likely have a small reduction in her tacrolimus doses, with the goal of achieving trough concentrations on the lower end of her therapeutic range (6 to 12 ng/mL); her prednisone should also be reduced to the lowest dose possible. If her immunosuppressive drug therapy is diminished, she should be monitored closely for rejection.[138]

Antiviral therapy with IV acyclovir or ganciclovir has been used to inhibit EBV replication in an effort to treat PTLD. Response is variable and may depend on the type and extent of PTLD. A.L. already has received ganciclovir for 4 weeks during which time she presented with PTLD. Surgery, radiation therapy, and chemotherapy are used to treat PTLD depending on the situation. Interferon and immunoglobulin have been effective in a few cases that appeared unresponsive to other therapies. Monoclonal or immunoblastic, disseminated, rapidly progressive PTLD responds poorly to traditional therapy and has a mortality rate as high as 70%.[138] Rituximab (an anti–B-cell, anti-CD20 antibody) is considered first-line therapy for CD20-postive B-cell PTLD along with reduction or withdrawal of immunosuppression if possible. Patients usually get 375 mg/m^2 weekly for 4 weeks; some groups have used prolonged therapy. Patients may have relapse or disease progression that may respond to chemotherapy regimens such as cyclophosphamide, adriamycin, vincristine, prednisone, or dexamethasone (CHOP); CHOP plus rituximab (CHOP-R); and cyclophosphamide, doxorubicin, etopside, prednisone, cytarbine, bleomycin, vincristine, and methotrexate (PROMACE-cytaBOM).[134,138] Transplant recipients have a higher risk of myelotoxic side effects, depending on their maintenance immunosuppression. A.L.'s prognosis is poor given the type and extent of her PTLD, which would have been more responsive to therapy if it had been diagnosed early before it had metastasized. Polyclonal PTLD responds well to reduction or discontinuation of immunosuppression and high-dose acyclovir or ganciclovir therapy for several weeks to months. The roles of prophylactic antivirals, immunoglobulins, and EBV PCR monitoring in the prevention of PTLD is currently controversial, with mixed results in current literature.[138]

KEY REFERENCES AND WEBSITES

A full list of references for this chapter can be found at **http://thepoint.lww.com/AT10e.** Below are the key references for this chapter, with the corresponding reference number in this chapter found in parentheses after the reference.

Key References

Avery RK et al. Update on immunizations in solid organ transplant recipients: what clinicians need to know. *Am J Transpl.* 2008;8:9.

Fishman JA. Infection in solid-organ transplant recipients. *N Engl J Med.* 2007;357:2601. (108)

Kidney Disease: Improving Global Outcomes (KDIGO) Transplant Work Group. KDIGO clinical practice guideline for the care of kidney transplant recipients. *Am J Transplant.* 2009;9 (Suppl 3):S1. (70)

Manitpisitkul W et al. Drug interactions in transplant patients: what everyone should know. *Curr Opin Nephrol Hypertens.* 2009; 18:404. (104)

Marcen R et al. Immunosuppressive drugs in kidney transplant. Impact on patient survival, and incidence of cardiovascular disease, malignancy, and infection. *Drugs.* 2009;69:2227. (72)

Naesens M et al. Calcineurin inhibitor nephrotoxicity. *Clin J Am Soc Nephrol.* 2009;4:481. (63)

Nankivell BJ, Alexander SI. Rejection of the kidney allograft. *N Engl J Med.* 2010;363:1451. (3)

Neuberger J. Developments in liver transplantation. *Gut.* 2004;53: 759. (80)

Parker A et al. Management of post-transplant lymphoproliferative disorder in adult solid organ transplant recipients—BCSH and BTS Guidelines. *Br J Haematol.* 2010;149:693. (138)

Srinivas TR, Meier-Kriesche HU. Minimizing immunosuppression, an alternative approach to reducing side effects: objectives and interim results. *Clin J Am Soc Nephrol.* 2008;3(Suppl 2):S101. (64)

Wolfe RA et al. Trends in organ donation and transplantation in the United States, 1999–2008. *Am J Transplant.* 2010;(4 Part 2):961. (1)

Key Websites

www.ustransplant.org

www.srtr.org

35

Basics of Nutrition and Patient Assessment

Jeff F. Binkley

CORE PRINCIPLES

		CHAPTER CASES
1	A complete nutritional assessment of the patient is imperative before specialized nutrition is initiated. Parameters to consider are nutrition and weight history, physical examination, anthropometric and biochemical measurements, and malnutrition risk.	Case 35-1 (Question 1)
2	The nutritional status of a patient can be assessed using the Subjective Global Assessment (SGA) technique, which has been found to be highly predictive of outcome, as the SGA correlates strongly with other subjective and objective measures of nutrition.	Case 35-1 (Question 1)
3	Patients who cannot meet their nutritional needs by consuming food orally should be considered for specialized nutrition support, which is the provision of parenteral or enteral nutrients.	Case 35-1 (Question 2)
4	Protein and calorie goals are assessed on the basis of the disease status and body weight of the patient.	Case 35-1 (Question 3)
5	Nutritional support regimens should be tailored on the basis of the requirements, response, and tolerance of the patient. Patients with inflammatory bowel disease are particularly at risk for developing vitamin and other micronutrient deficiencies, and therefore supplementation is warranted.	Case 35-1 (Question 4)
6	The fluid needs of a patient are determined by the following: (a) need to correct fluid imbalances, (b) maintenance fluid requirements, and (c) replacement of ongoing fluid losses.	Case 35-1 (Question 5)
7	Continued success of a nutrition support regimen can be accomplished by appropriate nutrition assessment after the initiation of therapy. Consider parameters such as patient weight trends, nitrogen balance, and prealbumin when determining the need to adjust therapy.	Case 35-1 (Question 6)
8	Overfeeding should be avoided in patients, and a gradual and conservative approach to instituting nutrition support should be used to prevent potential metabolic abnormalities.	Case 35-1 (Question 7)

Recognition of the importance of adequate and appropriate nutrition is paramount to the maintenance of optimal health. When an imbalance exists between the supply and demand for sources of nutrients and energy by the body, a nutritional disorder can occur. Years of research and clinical experience have led to the creation of various screening tools, assessment techniques, and guidelines to aid practitioners in their quest to delay or prevent patients from developing dangerous sequelae associated with deviations from optimal nutrition.[1] Despite many advances in nutritional science, impaired nutritional status in developing nations continues to be a main cause of morbidity and mortality, especially in young children.

NUTRITION BASICS

Adequate levels of energy sources and essential nutrients are critical for retaining the structural and biochemical integrity of the human body. Energy is provided in the diet by macronutrients such as carbohydrates, protein, and lipid. Essential nutrients, none of which offer any caloric value, are supplied to the body in the form of water, electrolytes, vitamins, and minerals.

Macronutrients

Humans need to consume food to sustain life. The unique structure and function of our cellular architecture allow human beings to convert the chemical free energy contained within the diet into high-energy, biologically active compounds. This transformation of food energy into forms of viable free energy through cellular respiration is an extremely inefficient process. Close examination of the distribution of food energy within the human body reveals that approximately 50% is lost as heat, 45% is available to the body in the form of adenosine triphosphate, and the remaining 5% is thermodynamically required for the conversion to heat because the entropy of the final products is greater than the initial substrates. Ultimately, all of the energy derived from food is expended in the form of external work or heat.

In nutritional contexts, the energy available from food is expressed in terms of the calorie. A calorie is technically defined by the amount of heat required to raise the temperature of 1 g of water by 1°C. This unit, however, is too small from a dietary perspective. A food calorie (sometimes written as *Calorie* with a large *C*, although this convention is not strictly followed) is equivalent to 1,000 calories or one kilocalorie (kcal). One food calorie is also equal to 4.184 kilojoules.[2] It is not uncommon for a single kilocalorie to be referred to as a calorie when communicating the energy content of food. This ambiguity must be understood by practicing clinicians to communicate properly not only to colleagues, but to patients and the general public who may not have an appreciation for this subtlety and remain confused when reading calories on nutrition labels yet, seeing kilocalories in textbooks, scientific publications, patient records, and the Internet.

CARBOHYDRATES

Carbohydrates, also known as saccharides, are organic compounds that are chemically the hydrates of carbon. There are four main types of carbohydrates: monosaccharides, disaccharides, oligosaccharides, and polysaccharides. Dieticians frequently classify carbohydrates as either simple (monosaccharides and disaccharides) or complex (oligosaccharides and polysaccharides), yet the exact delineation of these categories is often not clear. Although carbohydrates serve as a common source of energy for living organisms, these compounds also function as structural components and building blocks for complex genetic molecules.

Monosaccharides (e.g., glucose) are the simplest of carbohydrates and cannot be hydrolyzed into smaller saccharide molecules. They are the major sources of fuel, as glucose serves as a nearly universal and accessible reservoir of calories. In the context of food science, monosaccharides, collectively along with disaccharides, are commonly referred to as sugars and are found in foods such as candy and desserts. Natural sources of monosaccharides include fruits and vegetables, but these compounds are also found in commercially manufactured products such as high-fructose corn syrup. The latter is a common replacement for table sugar in processed foods composed of a high proportion of fructose relative to glucose.

Oligosaccharides are short chains of monosaccharides typically composed of three to ten molecules linked through glycosidic bonds. These molecules are typically found connected to proteins or lipids functioning as chemical markers for cellular recognition. An example is their important role in the classification of blood groups. Polymeric carbohydrate structures are referred to as polysaccharides and function either as storage forms of energy, such as glycogen in animals or starch in plants, or as a structural component, such as cellulose in plants. In humans, dietary polysaccharides must be catabolized to their constituent monosaccharides before absorption can occur.[3]

Dietary carbohydrates are composed of approximately 60% polysaccharides, mainly starch, and the disaccharides sucrose and lactose, which represent 30% and 10%, respectively. All carbohydrates provide 4 kcal of energy per gram. Although the exact amount of dietary carbohydrates sufficient for good health is not known, a mixed-fuel diet in which carbohydrates constitute 45% to 65% of the total energy intake is considered an acceptable distribution range.[4]

PROTEIN

Polypeptides are linear chains of amino acids. These polypeptides can twist and fold alone or together into three-dimensional globular or fibrous structures, generating a biochemical compound known as the protein. Proteins are crucial to all living organisms and participate in a wide spectrum of processes. Many proteins function as enzymes, which serve as catalysts to biochemical reactions and are important for metabolism. Additionally, proteins can play a role in structure and function, such as actin and myosin in muscle—the largest source of protein in higher animals. Some proteins stabilize blood by giving it the appropriate viscosity and osmolarity, and yet other proteins participate in cell signaling and immune responses.

Protein is the second largest store of energy in the body after adipose tissue.[5] Although protein differs from the other two primary dietary energy sources because of its inclusion of nitrogen, the amino acid residues from proteins can be converted to glucose via gluconeogenesis to supply a continuous source of glucose for the body after the depletion of glycogen. Like carbohydrates, each gram of protein supplies 4 kcal of energy. The loss of more than 30% of body protein, however, can compromise muscle strength, affect respiratory function, and negatively influence the immune system, all of which ultimately lead to organ dysfunction and death. It should be noted that protein and energy requirements of the body are intimately connected. During times of infection or injury, metabolic rates rise and body protein is suddenly oxidized into amino acids and mobilized for fuel utilization. In most instances, the injuries that patients experience are minimal and self-limiting; however, patients with chronic illnesses or those with complicating factors that result in a long-term hypermetabolic state can subsequently experience a dangerous loss of body nitrogen.

LIPIDS

Lipids comprise a broad spectrum of molecular species ranging from hydrophobic triglycerides and sterol esters to hydrophilic phospholipids and cardiolipins, as well as dietary cholesterol and phytosterols. Biological lipids function as a form of energy storage, serve as the structural components of cell membranes, and participate as messengers in the vital process of cellular signaling.

In a nutritional context, fats that exist as liquids at room temperature are typically called oils, whereas fats that remain solid at room temperature are labeled as fats. Although the term lipid is frequently used synonymously for fat, fats are actually a subgroup of lipids also known as triglycerides. Triglycerides are synthesized by chemically combining glycerol with three fatty acid molecules. These fatty acids are generally nonbranched hydrocarbons containing an even number of carbon atoms ranging from 4 to 26 carbons. Adipose tissue is composed of fatty acids in varying lengths.

An unsaturated fat is a fatty acid that includes at least one double bond within the fatty acid chain, and therefore a saturated fat is one that contains no double bonds. Unsaturated fatty acids result in less energy after the oxidation process of cellular metabolism compared with an equivalent amount of saturated fatty acids. Commercial manufacturers of processed food favor saturated fats because they are less vulnerable to rancidity (lipid peroxidation) and remain solid at room temperature. Foods containing unsaturated fats include avocado, nuts, and vegetable oils such as canola and olive oils. Meat products contain both saturated and unsaturated fats.

Importantly, each gram of fat yields 9 kcal of energy, twice that of either carbohydrate or protein. Approximately 35% to 40% of the total daily calories consumed by the average human being are lipids. Higher-fat diets can contribute to more rapid weight gain, a positive attribute if the individual is malnourished or underweight, but a negative attribute if trying to achieve weight loss.[6] Triglycerides make up by far the largest proportion of dietary lipids consumed by humans. Although humans possess the biological pathways to synthesize lipids, there are two essential lipids that must originate from the diet to prevent essential fatty acid deficiency—linoleic acid and α-linolenic acid.

Essential Nutrients—Water

Water plays a critical role in nearly every biological function necessary for life. The total body water in an adult male without fluid and electrolyte disorders is approximately 50% to 60% of the lean body weight.[7] Infants and children possess a much higher fractional water content, which then decreases progressively with age. Individuals with a greater percentage of body fat, such as women or obese patients, also tend to have less water for a given weight.

The total aqueous volume in the body can be divided into the intracellular and extracellular compartments. Because the intracellular fluid is the site of major metabolic activity, homeostatic mechanisms are therefore in constant execution to provide an environment of optimal ionic strength. The primary function of the extracellular fluid is to serve as a conduit between cells and between organs. Substantial ionic alterations within extracellular fluid can occur without a clinically significant impact on body function. This extracellular compartment can be further divided into three fractions: the interstitial volume, plasma volume, and transcellular water volume. Interstitial fluid flows around cells, allowing the total surface area of a cell to serve as an area of exchange. Plasma is the route for rapid transit within the body. Transcellular water is the smallest component of extracellular fluid and is the portion of total body water that can be found contained within epithelial-lined spaces. Transcellular water includes the luminal fluid of the gastrointestinal (GI) tract, the fluids of the central nervous system, and the fluid in the eye, as well as the lubricating fluids at serous surfaces.

The basal requirement for water in a given individual is dependent on the sensible (urinary) and insensible losses of water. Urine osmolality and the total amount of solute excreted from the body dictate the volume of water comprising urine. Fever can promote dehydration by increasing one's basal metabolic rate in addition to raising the vapor pressure of expired air and sweat—resulting in higher respiratory and skin water losses, respectively. In the absence of fever and sweating, water loss through the skin is relatively fixed; however, urinary water excretion can vary greatly.

Essential Nutrients—Micronutrients

ELECTROLYTES

A subtle and complex balance of electrolytes exists between the intracellular and extracellular milieu. The precise maintenance of these electrolyte gradients is critical as such gradients regulate hydration and pH and ultimately have an impact on nerve and muscle function. Sodium, chloride, and bicarbonate are the main solutes in the extracellular fluid, whereas potassium, magnesium, phosphate, and proteins are the dominant solutes inside the cell.

Although water can freely travel across the membrane of a cell, the cell membrane itself is only selectively permeable to solutes. Osmotically active solutes are those that are impermeable and thereby exert an osmotic pressure by which the distribution of water between fluid compartments is determined.

Electrolyte balance is traditionally maintained by the oral intake of substances containing electrolytes. Foods such as fruit juices, sports drinks, milk, and many fruits and vegetables are replete with electrolytes. In oral rehydration therapy, electrolyte drinks containing sodium and potassium salts replenish the water and electrolyte levels in the body after dehydration caused by exercise, excessive alcohol consumption, diaphoresis, diarrhea, vomiting, intoxication, or starvation. Hormones, such as antidiuretic hormone, aldosterone, and parathyroid hormone, regulate electrolytes once in the body, and the kidneys function to flush out those ions in excess.

VITAMINS

Vitamins are organic compounds that cannot be biologically synthesized in sufficient quantities by human beings yet remain a vital requirement for the sustainment of life. The biochemical functions of vitamins are diverse. Some vitamins assist in the regulation of electrolyte metabolism, whereas others participate in the control of cell and tissue growth and differentiation. Most vitamins function as cofactors, which are molecules that bind to enzymes to promote their catalytic activities.

Vitamins are classified by their biological and chemical activity. Vitamins are designated as either water-soluble or fat-soluble. There are four fat-soluble vitamins (A, D, E, and K) and nine water-soluble vitamins (eight B vitamins and vitamin C) in humans. Water-soluble vitamins are used by the body quite rapidly, and amounts in excess are readily excreted from the body in urine. The fat-soluble vitamins are absorbed by the body using processes that closely parallel the absorption of lipids. Fat-soluble vitamins are more likely to lead to toxicity, or hypervitaminosis. Fat-soluble vitamin regulation is also of particular significance in cystic fibrosis.

Vitamins are procured through the diet or supplements. The body can manufacture only three vitamins from nondietary sources: vitamins D, K, and the B vitamin biotin. Critically ill patients experiencing metabolic stress possess vitamin needs that may increase dramatically. Many disease states such as inflammatory bowel disease, liver and renal disease, short-bowel syndrome, cancer, and acquired immunodeficiency syndrome–associated wasting can also result in a higher demand for vitamins. A parenteral formulation of multivitamins combining both fat- and water-soluble vitamins into an aqueous solution designed for incorporation into intravenous infusions is available for these classes of patients.

TRACE ELEMENTS

Appropriate intake levels of certain dietary minerals have been demonstrated to be required in small amounts to maintain optimal health. These dietary minerals are known as trace elements or ultratrace elements. Iron, zinc, copper, manganese, and fluoride are classified as trace elements. These minerals are required in amounts between 1 and 100 mg/day by adults. Ultratrace elements, or those dietary minerals that are required in quantities less than 1 mg/day, include arsenic, boron, chromium, iodine, selenium, silicon, nickel, and vanadium.

Consuming specific foods rich with the dietary mineral of interest is the recommended method for satisfying these micronutrient requirements. Many trace elements are naturally present in foods; however, some are added to foods to prevent nutrient deficiencies—such as fortifying salt with iodine to prevent development of hypothyroidism and goiter. When dietary intake is insufficient to meet the daily nutrient requirements of an individual or when chronic or acute deficiencies arise from pathology and injury, dietary supplements remain a viable option. Supplements can be formulated to include multiple trace elements, a combination of vitamins, or a single trace element.

MALNUTRITION

Malnutrition may occur when there is any disruption of nutrition status, including disorders resulting from overfeeding or underfeeding or through impaired nutrient metabolism. Clinically, a more useful definition of malnutrition is the state induced by alterations in dietary intake, which results in subcellular, cellular, or organ function changes that expose the individual to increased risks of morbidity and mortality and can be reversed by adequate nutritional intervention.[8] An incidence of malnutrition as high as 55% has been reported among hospitalized patients.[9,10] In these hospitalized patients, the risk of acute malnutrition development is greater because nutrient intake is often inadequate, nutrient stores can be depleted, or the patients may experience concurrent injury or stress (e.g., trauma, infection, major surgery). The presence of acute stress or injury increases energy requirements to repair tissues. Breakdown of skeletal muscle to release amino acids for energy production by conversion to glucose occurs if exogenous energy is not provided to stressed patients. Even patients who were well nourished before the stressful event may quickly become at risk for this type of iatrogenic malnutrition. Usually conditional, acute malnutrition resolves once the illness or injury improves and normal nutrient intake is resumed.

In stark contrast to stress-induced malnutrition, patients in starvation or semistarvation states adapt slowly to inadequate nutrient intake. In this scenario, endogenous fat stores are used for energy and a slow loss of muscle proteins ensues. Nevertheless, energy and protein stores are not unlimited, and death occurs in previously normal-weight individuals after about 60 to 70 days of starvation.[11,12] Patients with a history of chronic malnutrition who are faced with stress or injury are at the greatest risk of developing malnutrition.

The most common type of nutrition deficiency in hospitalized patients is protein-calorie malnutrition, which includes depletion of both tissue energy stores and body proteins. Complications develop more frequently for hospitalized patients who are malnourished as a result of organ wasting and functional impairments. These complications may include weakness, decreased wound healing, altered hepatic metabolism of drugs, increased respiratory failure, decreased cardiac contractility, and infections such as pneumonia and abscesses. Complications often increase the length of hospital stay and costs of care, and may even ultimately reduce reimbursement for institutions.[13–15]

Malnutrition or its risk may occur in patients with inadequate intake for 7 to 14 days or in patients with an unintentional weight loss of 10% before their illness. For these patients, nutritional intervention is appropriate and should be considered.[16,17] Patients who cannot meet their nutritional needs by consuming enough food orally should be considered for an alternative nutrition mechanism. Specialized nutrition support is the provision of parenteral or enteral nutrients, which are specifically formulated or delivered to maintain or restore nutrition status.[18] For those who cannot eat by mouth but who have a functional GI tract, the first line of nutrition intervention to be considered should be enteral feeding through an appropriate access device (see Chapter 37, Adult Enteral Nutrition, and Chapter 38, Adult Parenteral Nutrition).

To mimic the normal physiologic state when possible, the GI tract should be used for providing nutrients. Enteral nutrients may be more beneficial and are generally less costly than those provided by the parenteral route.[19] Enteral nutrients stimulate the intestine, thus maintaining the mucosal barrier structure and function. This has been associated with decreased infectious morbidity in critically ill patients compared with those receiving nutrients parenterally.[20–24] Parenteral nutrition is therefore reserved for patients whose GI tracts are not functional or cannot be accessed, or who do not absorb enough nutrients to maintain adequate nutrition status.[16]

ONLINE CONTENT

For a diagram that shows the classification of malnutrition, go to http://thepoint.lww.com/AT10e.

NUTRITION SCREENING

According to the Joint Commission Accreditation Standards (http://www.jointcommission.org), hospitals are required to screen patients within 24 hours of admission to determine whether they are malnourished or at risk for developing malnutrition. The nutrition screening process identifies needs for further nutrition intervention or monitoring based on nutrition risk. The information collected in the screening process is dependent on the patient population, the health care setting, and individual institution policy. A number of screening tools have been described in the literature with varying reliability, specificity, and sensitivity. Some parameters included in nutrition screening may have wider applicability in the outpatient setting than in inpatient arenas.[1,9]

Patient Assessment

Nutrition assessment of a patient incorporates a collection of historical data, analysis of body composition, and evaluation of physiological function. Proper patient assessment should include the examination of multiple factors and should not rely on any one parameter. This assessment serves to identify the presence and severity of malnutrition or the risk of developing malnutrition. A complete patient assessment performed by a trained practitioner can help determine the goals of therapy and specify the need for specialized nutrition support. Goals of therapy may be maintenance of existing nutrition status, repletion of fat and lean body mass, and prevention of complications associated with malnutrition.

NUTRITION HISTORY

A nutrition history is crucial in an effective nutrition assessment. Practitioners may gain valuable information by interviewing the patient or the patient's family and by reviewing the medical record to identify factors that can contribute to malnutrition or increase the risk of developing malnutrition.

Multiple factors can contribute to the development of malnutrition, including the patient's underlying disease states, past

TABLE 35-1
Components of a Nutrition History

Medical history
Chronic illnesses
Surgical history
Psychosocial history
Socioeconomic status
History of gastrointestinal problems (nausea, vomiting, or diarrhea)
Diet history, including diets for weight gain or loss
Food preferences and intolerances
Medications
Weight history
Increase or decrease
Intentional or unintentional
Time period for weight change
Functional capacity

medical history, and socioeconomic circumstances. Medications can adversely affect nutrition status by decreasing the synthesis of nutrients, minimizing food intake through alteration of appetite and taste, changing the absorption or metabolism of nutrients, or increasing nutrient requirements. A complete evaluation of present and past body weight habits contributes significantly to an appropriate nutrition history.

The components of a nutrition history are summarized in Table 35-1, some of which are expanded on subsequently.

WEIGHT HISTORY

Weight history and influences are important in evaluating nutrition status. Weight loss is a sign of negative energy and negative protein balance and is often associated with poor outcome in hospitalized patients.[9,25] A patient's current weight often is compared with a standard for ideal body weight (IBW). Percentage of IBW[9] is determined as shown in Equation 35-1:

$$\%\,\text{IBW} = \frac{\text{Current weight (100)}}{\text{IBW}} \qquad \textit{(Eq. 35-1)}$$

The primary limitation of this method of assessing weight is that the patient's weight is compared with a population standard rather than using the individual as the reference point. For example, a patient who is significantly overweight but has lost large amounts of weight may still be more than 100% of IBW and therefore not considered at risk for developing malnutrition. A more patient-specific method of evaluating weight is to compare current weight with the patient's usual weight. This can be determined using Equation 35-2:

$$\%\,\text{Usual body weight} = \frac{\text{Current weight (100)}}{\text{Usual body weight}} \qquad \textit{(Eq. 35-2)}$$

Using this method, the obese patient who has lost weight may be determined to be less than 90% of usual weight and therefore nutritionally at risk. It is also important to assess over what time period the change has occurred. Involuntary weight loss is considered severe if loss exceeds 5% of usual weight within 1 month, or 10% of usual weight within 6 months. A nonvolitional weight loss of more than 10% is considered significant for malnutrition.[18] Patterns of weight loss must be evaluated to determine whether the loss is stabilizing or continual, the latter being a more serious concern. Weight gain after a significant weight loss may be considered a positive sign.

PHYSICAL EXAMINATION

Nutrition deficiencies may be identified on physical examination, and these findings may require further evaluation. Muscle and fat wasting (often noticed in the temporal area), loss of subcutaneous fat and muscle in the shoulders, and loss of subcutaneous fat in the interosseous and palmar areas of the hands are readily identifiable. Other physical parameters that may be less obvious are assessment of hair for color changes and sparseness; skin for turgor, pigmentation, and dermatitis; mouth for glossitis, gingivitis, cheilosis, and color of the tongue; nails for friability and lines; and abdomen for signs of ascites or enlarged liver.

ANTHROPOMETRICS

Anthropometry is the science of body composition based on measurement of weight, stature, body circumferences, and subcutaneous fat thickness. Physical examination may include measurement of subcutaneous fat and skeletal muscle mass. Assessment of fat stores provides information about fat loss or gain and assumes fat is gained or lost proportionally throughout the entire body. The subcutaneous compartment contains approximately 50% of body fat. Triceps skinfold and subscapular skinfold thickness measurements are methods used to assess subcutaneous fat, allowing associated estimations of total body fat.

Reference standards[26] are used to compare against values obtained in the examination. Somatic protein mass or skeletal muscle mass can be estimated by measuring mid-arm circumference and then calculating arm muscle circumference. These values are also compared with standards, and the amount of muscle mass is then estimated.

Anthropometric measurements accurately reflect total body fat and skeletal muscle mass when used for the long-term comparisons of large, nutritionally stable populations. However, anthropometric measurements of hospitalized patients are of little value. Changes experienced during acute illness and stress may result in errors of interpretation of subcutaneous fat and weight assessments, and peripheral edema can result in inflated values for skinfold thickness and mid-arm circumference.[9,25]

Biochemical Assessment

Biochemical assessment of nutrition status includes the examination of protein status. No single test or group of tests can be recommended as a routine or reliable indicator of protein status. It is a combination of measures—biochemical, anthropometric, dietary, and clinical findings—that produce a more complete picture of protein status.

The protein composition of the human body can be viewed as a two-compartment model—somatic and visceral proteins. Somatic proteins are those proteins constituting skeletal muscle; they account for approximately 75% of total body protein. The remaining 25% of total body protein are visceral proteins, which are found in the internal organs and serum. Albumin, prealbumin, transferrin, and retinol-binding protein are the most common visceral proteins used to assess nutrition status. These proteins are produced by the liver and often reflect hepatic synthetic capability. When hepatic insufficiency develops or when intake of substrates is inadequate for synthesis of proteins, the serum concentration of visceral proteins decreases. During stress or injury, inflammatory cytokines are released and substrates are shunted away from the synthesis of these proteins to synthesize other acute-phase proteins such as C-reactive protein, haptoglobin, fibrinogen, and others.[27] Serum protein concentrations are altered during acute stress or inflammatory states and chronic starvation.[25,27]

Albumin is the classic visceral protein used to evaluate nutrition status and is a prognostic indicator. Serum concentrations of less than 3 g/dL correlate with poor outcome and an increased length of stay of hospitalized patients.[28] Albumin serves as a carrier protein for fatty acids, hormones, minerals, and drugs, and is necessary for maintaining oncotic pressure. Albumin has

available. S.P.'s visceral proteins are also in low-normal ranges, indicating both short-term (prealbumin) and longer-term (albumin) malnutrition. Consideration of these factors leads one to conclude that S.P. is severely malnourished. This assessment can be further validated by using other tools such as the SGA.[29]

Because nutrition assessment can often be difficult, a clinician may choose to use the SGA to appropriately categorize their patients. Application of the SGA technique classifies patients into three areas: class A (the well-nourished patient), with less than 5% weight loss or more than 5% total weight loss but recent gains and improvements in appetite; class B (moderately malnourished), identified by those patients with 5% to 10% weight loss without recent stabilization or gain, poor dietary intake, and mild loss of subcutaneous tissue; and class C (severely malnourished), with an ongoing weight loss of more than 10% with severe subcutaneous tissue loss and muscle wasting, often with edema. The utility of the SGA is its simplicity for implementation and strong correlation with other subjective and objective measures of nutrition.

Clinicians place patients into one of the three categories on the basis of their subjective rating of two broad factors: history and physical examination. There are four elements to the history: (a) weight loss in the 6 months before the examination, expressed as a proportionate loss from previous weight, (b) dietary intake in relation to the patient's usual pattern, (c) presence of significant GI symptoms, and (d) functional capacity or energy of the patient, ranging from full capacity to bedridden. Applying these four elements to S.P., one first finds that S.P. is reporting a 25% weight loss during the past 6 months. It is also important to recognize the pattern of weight loss. Querying a patient regarding recent weight loss (in conjunction with the weight change in 6 months), often in the past 2 weeks, can help establish a pattern of chronic weight loss. In S.P.'s case, she reports increasing weight loss in the past 3 months, which confirms a progression. It is also recommended that clinicians explore weight history by asking for the patient's maximal weight at specific times, such as 1 year ago, 6 months ago, 1 month ago, and at the present time. Confirmation of weight history can be conducted by having the patient discuss his or her change in clothing size or how his or her clothes fit.

With respect to the second element regarding dietary intake, S.P. says she has a poor appetite, and attempts to consume supplements have been unsuccessful. Using the SGA, patients are classified as having either normal or abnormal intake in the weeks to months before the examination. In this case, S.P. clearly is experiencing abnormal intake; however, one can also ask S.P. certain questions such as "How has the amount of food you have consumed over the past several weeks to months changed?" or "Are there certain kinds of foods that you no longer can eat?" and "Give me an example of a typical meal" to establish eating patterns. It is also important to determine why a patient is eating less—intentional reduction or unintentional reduction. S.P. is not communicating any intention of wanting to lose weight, and her change in consumption is related to her chronic pathology.

In terms of the third element of the history, significant GI symptoms are those that have persisted on virtually a daily basis for a period longer than 2 weeks. Given the presentation of S.P. to the hospital with her history of 3 months of vomiting, it is highly likely that she satisfies the definition for possessing significant GI symptoms. However, a clinician can always clarify this by asking S.P. more specific questions.

The final element of S.P.'s history, functional capacity, is one that should be explored further, yet it is not likely to have an impact on the final nutritional assessment given the prior objective findings of the patient. Patients who cannot eat will often complain of weakness and fatigue—many times to the point of which they are bedridden. Observation of the activity levels of patients, their overall mood, skeletal muscle function, and their respiratory movements can all provide clues to the clinician regarding functional impairment. Given the joint pain and squared-off appearance of her shoulders from the combination of muscle and subcutaneous tissue loss, functional capacity of S.P. is likely to be diminished.

Having completed the history component of the SGA, the clinician moves to the second component of the SGA, or the physical. This section of the SGA essentially asks the clinician to look for physical signs of malnutrition such as loss of subcutaneous fat in the triceps and chest region, muscle wasting in areas like the quadriceps and deltoids, presence of ankle or sacral edema, and finally any presence of ascites. For each of the traits, the clinician should consider the severity, if any are present. In the case of S.P., there is definite muscle wasting. Given the history and physical components of the SGA, S.P. would be classified as severely malnourished (class C) as there are obvious signs of malnutrition such as subcutaneous tissue loss and muscle wasting in the presence of a clear and convincing pattern of ongoing weight loss greater than 10%.

CASE 35-1, QUESTION 2: Is S.P. a candidate for specialized nutrition support therapy?

The fundamental goal of specialized nutritional support therapy is to meet the energy requirements of metabolic processes, to support the hypermetabolism associated with critical illness, and to minimize protein catabolism. Crohn's disease is a form of inflammatory bowel disease that is associated with potentially great nutritional insult. Nutritional abnormalities can arise in Crohn's disease patients from malabsorption, decreased food intake, medications, and intestinal losses. Disease location along the GI tract, symptomatology, and dietary restrictions all contribute to the development of protein energy malnutrition with specific nutritional deficiencies. S.P. is admitted to the hospital for tests to evaluate her Crohn's disease, weight loss, and associated symptoms. The subjective and objective evidence points to a nonfunctioning GI tract. If the diagnosis of advanced Crohn's exacerbation is accurate, S.P. may require parenteral nutrition therapy until enteral therapy can be established (see Chapter 38, Adult Parenteral Nutrition). In addition, previous attempts at enteral nutrition were unsuccessful with continued increased retching and vomiting, indicating decreased GI motility. With her malnourished state, continued inadequate nutrition in the hospital will result in further deterioration of her nutrition status. Specialized nutrition support intervention should be implemented.

Goals of Therapy

CASE 35-1, QUESTION 3: Calculate calorie and protein goals for S.P.

Nutritional support begins with an estimation of the patient's caloric requirements.[30,31] Accurate determination of caloric needs is essential to obtaining the full benefits of nutritional therapy and aids in preventing the problems associated with underfeeding as well as overfeeding. The Harris-Benedict equation is one of the most commonly used methods for estimating caloric needs or BEE; however, there is still controversy regarding the best method to accurately estimate the caloric needs of a patient. The Harris-Benedict equation may overestimate or underestimate resting energy expenditure in certain critically ill patients, particularly when clinical conditions are changing and when body weight fluctuates because of changes in fluid status. The most common approach is based on body weight in kilograms. The energy requirements are standardized and are determined by the metabolic condition of the patient. S.P.'s initial calorie goals are to meet her current energy expenditure needed for basal metabolism and activity of ambulating. S.P. would fall into the category of "moderate stress, malnourished" requiring 25 to 30 kcal/kg/day. For this calculation, S.P.'s actual weight of 92 pounds (41.8 kg) should be used because her metabolism and current energy expenditure reflect this decrease in body mass. Using usual weight or IBW in patients who have severe weight loss may result in overfeeding. For S.P., the caloric goal should be 1,045 to 1,255 kcal/day.

Protein is the building block of life. Once hepatic glycogen stores are depleted, muscle protein is degraded to provide three-carbon backbones for hepatic gluconeogenesis. Initially, protein catabolism is resistant to the administration of exogenous amino acids, and it can sometimes take weeks until a patient is found to be in a state of positive nitrogen balance. In addition to protein catabolism, exogenous protein is required for wound healing and to replace protein lost in wounds and fistulae. Protein goals are estimated based on weight, degree of stress, and disease state. The goal is to minimize the loss of lean body mass, and as a general rule this requires anywhere from 1.0 to 1.5 g/kg/day of protein depending on the degree of illness and injury. Because S.P. has not had surgery and her stress is minimal, her protein goal should be based on the desire to maintain her current protein status. Using the guidelines provided in Table 35-4, S.P.'s protein dose is 1.2 to 1.5 g/kg/day, or 50 to 63 g/day. As with energy expenditure, calculations of protein needs are only estimates; the patient's clinical course should be monitored, and the protein dose adjusted accordingly. If S.P. requires surgery, her energy or calorie goals should be reassessed to include an additional stress factor.

Micronutrients

CASE 35-1, QUESTION 4: What vitamin and mineral deficiencies would you expect to find in S.P.? What options are available to the clinician to address them?

The therapeutic effects of specialized nutrition support accrue through the combined provision of macronutrients and micronutrients. These elements support vital cellular and organ functions, immunity, tissue repair, protein synthesis, and capacity of skeletal, cardiac, and respiratory muscles. As with any medical therapy, a nutritional support regimen should be adjusted based on the requirements, response, and tolerance of the patient. Patients who have inflammatory bowel disease are particularly at risk for developing altered levels of vitamins and other micronutrients. The etiology of these micronutrient losses is multifactorial and encompasses decreased oral intake, increased losses secondary to diarrhea, and malabsorption. In particular, deficiencies in vitamin D, folate, vitamin B_{12}, calcium, magnesium, and zinc are common to this patient population.

Given the prevalence of these deficiencies, S.P. should be prescribed a daily multivitamin and mineral supplement. If it is determined that S.P. has significant fat malabsorption, a water-miscible fat-soluble vitamin formulation can be considered. There is an increased incidence of osteoporosis in patients with Crohn's disease (with or without corticosteroid use), and therefore S.P. should be assessed to ensure that her calcium and vitamin D intake is normal. Recommended daily oral calcium requirements are 800 to 1,500 mg/day, but increase to 1,500 to 2,000 mg/day when replacement is needed for a deficiency. S.P. should be consuming a daily amount of 400 international units of vitamin D orally; however, if serum 25-hydroxyvitamin D levels are subtherapeutic, greater amounts will be required and doses based on the specific disease progression and functionality of S.P.'s GI tract.

Medications such as methotrexate (a folate antagonist) and sulfasalazine (which blocks folate absorption) can be used to treat inflammatory bowel disease and, therefore, increase folate requirements for patients. Daily folate supplementation at a dose of 1 mg orally can be beneficial to S.P. if she is prescribed either of these medications.

Patients with surgical resection of the stomach or terminal ileum are at risk of developing vitamin B_{12} deficiency given the locations of intrinsic factor production and site of absorption, respectively. Given that S.P. has had no surgical intervention to date, it is wise to monitor her vitamin B_{12} status and look for signs of deficiency (i.e., megaloblastic anemia) before instituting aggressive supplementation.

Magnesium deficiency can be a concern in patients with increased intestinal losses, as is the case with many individuals who have inflammatory bowel disease. When considering enteral magnesium supplementation, the change in pH along the GI tract, GI transit time, and fat content of a meal can all affect magnesium absorption. Large doses of enteral magnesium can result in diarrhea; therefore, administering smaller doses throughout the day can lead to improved tolerance and therapeutic efficacy. Choosing a magnesium supplement that can deliver 150 mg of elemental magnesium and dosing it four times a day is the recommended oral replacement regimen for patients.

Inflammatory bowel disease patients can experience excessive stool losses resulting in a zinc deficiency. S.P. should receive an oral zinc supplement that delivers 50 mg of elemental zinc daily.

Maintenance Fluids

CASE 35-1, QUESTION 5: Determine the daily fluid requirements for S.P. while she receives specialized nutrition support.

When determining the fluid needs of a patient, the clinician should consider the following: (a) correction of fluid imbalances, (b) maintenance fluid requirements, and (c) replacement of ongoing fluid losses.

The extended periods of diarrhea, vomiting, or both that occur with inflammatory bowel disease may lead to dehydration. Dehydration results in a loss of body weight, decreased urine output, dry mouth, and progressive thirst. Hypotension, tachycardia, and poor skin turgor are all clinical signs of dehydration. Apathy, stupor, coma, and death will follow if fluid replacement is not undertaken. Fluid deficits should be estimated from the clinical appearance of the patient, recent weight loss, and serum sodium and blood urea nitrogen concentrations, and replaced by giving half the estimated deficit intravenously over the course of 8 hours. After 8 hours, a new assessment of fluid status should be made, and half of the new estimated deficit should be replaced during the next 8 hours. This process should be repeated until normal hydration is achieved (see Chapter 10, Fluid and Electrolyte Disorders).

Maintenance fluid is that volume of daily fluid intake that replaces the insensible losses and at the same time allows excretion of the daily production of excess solute load in a volume of urine that is of an osmolarity similar to plasma. Maintenance fluid needs can be estimated using several methods. The simplest method uses 30 to 35 mL/kg/day as the basis. Another method is to provide 1,500 mL for the first 20 kg of body weight plus an additional 20 mL/kg for actual weight beyond the initial 20 kg. Both methods provide estimates of fluid needs for basic maintenance. S.P.'s fluid needs are estimated as follows:

$$\begin{aligned} \text{mL/day} &= 1{,}500\ \text{mL} + [(20\ \text{mL/kg})(41.8\ \text{kg} - 20\ \text{kg})] \\ &= 1{,}500\ \text{mL} + (20\ \text{mL/kg})(21.8\ \text{kg}) \qquad \textit{(Eq. 35-3)} \\ &= 1{,}500\ \text{mL} + 436\ \text{mL} \\ &= 1{,}936\ \text{mL} \end{aligned}$$

If S.P. experiences vomiting, nasogastric tube output, diarrhea, or other significant fluid losses, additional fluid must be provided. Some losses are measurable and can be directly replaced milliliter for milliliter on a regular basis. Others, however, are not measurable and can only be estimated. The electrolyte composition of the lost fluid is an important consideration for the clinician and dictates the ultimate choice of the replacement fluid.

Evaluating Specialized Nutrition Support Effectiveness

CASE 35-1, QUESTION 6: What parameters should be examined to determine the effectiveness of S.P.'s nutrition support regimen?

Implementing a successful nutrition support regimen begins with proper nutrition assessment of the patient. Nutritional goals that identify macronutrient, micronutrient, and fluid requirements are then established. Follow-up support and monitoring of the patient once nutrition support has been instituted is important to maintain the integrity and efficacy of the therapy.

To minimize the risk of refeeding syndrome in S.P. (a metabolic and electrolyte disturbance that occurs as a result of supplying nutrition to patients who are severely malnourished), all electrolyte abnormalities must be corrected before any nutrition is initiated. Because S.P.'s electrolytes are within normal ranges, no adjustments are necessary. Nutrition should then be implemented slowly, and vitamins administered routinely. Electrolytes, including phosphorus, potassium, magnesium, and glucose, should be monitored at least daily during the first week. Although electrolyte and mineral abnormalities may not be avoided, careful recognition of and close monitoring for refeeding syndrome will prevent serious complications.[32,33]

Although it can sometimes be difficult to obtain a reliable weight for a patient, weight can be an important parameter to help assess not only fluid balance but also the long-term appropriateness of caloric intake. Most patients should gain or lose no more than 1 kilogram per week when receiving nutrition support (assuming normal fluid status). However, clinicians must be aware of the impact that fluids have on the weight of a patient. Large intake or loss of fluids can influence weight measurements and mask the trends of body mass. Having S.P. record daily weights, in addition to fluid intake and output, and monitoring trends can serve as one, but not the only, key in determining the effectiveness of her regimen.

Nitrogen balance is another parameter that can help determine the degree of catabolism and protein requirements in a patient. Nitrogen balance is the difference between nitrogen intake and nitrogen excretion. It is estimated by the nitrogen intake along with collecting a 24-hour urine urea nitrogen sample from the patient. Positive nitrogen balance is a reasonable goal during nutrition support therapy for recovery of a patient, but may also require increasing caloric loads on a periodic basis. If a nitrogen balance study is ordered for S.P., increasing protein intake should be considered if results indicate a negative nitrogen balance; however, a negative nitrogen may be unavoidable during high-stress states, regardless of the amount of nutrients provided.

Finally, prealbumin levels for S.P. should also be monitored once a week as a marker for short-term gross adequacy of calorie and protein intake. A lack of prealbumin increase is an indicator of poor patient outcomes. With adequate feeding, prealbumin can increase more than 4 mg/dL per week. It should be noted that in the case of S.P. who is suffering from Crohn's disease and may likely be receiving either oral or parenteral corticosteroids as treatment, administration of corticosteroids can falsely elevate prealbumin levels, making S.P. appear to be at a lower nutritional risk.

CASE 35-1, QUESTION 7: Members of the medical team are anxious to have S.P. gain weight and are concerned by her malnourished appearance. Therefore, there is a desire to increase the calories provided to S.P. What potential complications could result from overfeeding S.P.?

Overfeeding should be avoided in all patients because of a plethora of potential complications, especially those with respiratory concerns.[34] Although restoration and maintenance of body cell mass is the goal of nutrition support therapy, a gradual and conservative approach yields fewer metabolic abnormalities. Supplying an abundance of calories to a patient in need of nutrition support increases the metabolic rate, which in turn places greater demands for cardiopulmonary effort and oxygenation. Overfeeding with carbohydrates is particularly detrimental because of the amount of carbon dioxide produced relative to the amount of oxygen consumed. This results in carbon dioxide retention that may lead to acid–base disturbances. Hyperglycemia is also a common metabolic abnormality secondary to excessive carbohydrate administration that can lead to osmotic diuresis and immune dysfunction.

ACKNOWLEDGMENTS

The author acknowledges contributions from previous chapter authors: Jane M. Gervasio, Jennifer L. Ash, Carol J. Rollins, and Yvonne Huckleberry.

KEY REFERENCES AND WEBSITES

A full list of references for this chapter can be found at http://thepoint.lww.com/AT10e. Below are the key references and websites for this chapter, with the corresponding reference number in this chapter found in parentheses after the reference. The following key references and websites may be used as guideline tools for clinicians who manage patients' nutrition interventions.

Key References

ASPEN Board of Directors and the Clinical Guidelines Task Force. Guidelines for the use of parenteral and enteral nutrition in adult and pediatric patients [published correction appears in *JPEN J Parenter Enteral Nutr.* 2002;26:144]. *JPEN J Parenter Enteral Nutr.* 2002;26(1 Suppl):1SA. (16)

Brooks MJ, Melnik G. The refeeding syndrome: an approach to understanding its complications and preventing its occurrence. *Pharmacotherapy.* 1995;15:713. (33)

Section 7 Nutrition Issues

Detsky AS et al. What is subjective global assessment of nutritional status? *JPEN J Parenter Enteral Nutr*. 1987;11:8. (28)

Mueller C et al. A.S.P.E.N. Clinical guidelines: nutrition screening, assessment, and intervention in adults. *JPEN J Parenter Enteral Nutr*. 2011;35:16. (1)

Key Websites

American Society for Parenteral and Enteral Nutrition. http://www.nutritioncare.org.

USDA Food and Nutrition Information Center. http://fnic.nal.usda.gov/nal_display/index.php?info_center=4&tax_level=1.

36 Obesity

Maria Ballod

CORE PRINCIPLES

	CHAPTER CASES
1 Patients should be assessed for obesity and the risk for related comorbid conditions.	**Case 36-1 (Questions 1, 3)**
2 An understanding of body composition is essential when evaluating the health status of a patient with regard to body fat.	**Case 36-1 (Question 1)**
3 Management and treatment of obesity can include a combination of diet and behavioral modifications along with increased physical activity.	**Case 36-1 (Questions 4–6)**
4 Nonprescription dietary supplements may assist some individuals with weight loss by encouraging proper dietary intake.	**Case 36-1 (Question 6)**
5 Medication to treat obesity should be considered for patients with a body mass index greater than 30 kg/m^2 without risk factors or greater than 27 kg/m^2 with an obesity-related risk factor.	**Case 36-1 (Question 7)**
6 Medications used to treat obesity include amphetamines and other sympathomimetic agents, antidepressants (selective serotonin reuptake inhibitors and bupropion), and gastrointestinal lipase inhibitors (orlistat). Nonprescription orlistat is available at half the dose of the prescription product.	**Case 36-1 (Questions 7–10)**
7 Antiepileptic drugs (topiramate and zonisamide) and a selective serotonin type 2C receptor agonist (lorcaserin) are being investigated as weight-loss drugs.	**Case 36-1 (Question 10)**
8 Alteration of gastrointestinal tract and stomach size after bariatric surgery can alter drug pharmacokinetics and place patients at risk for adverse events associated with some medications.	**Case 36-1 (Question 11)**

Maintenance of normal body weight is a common problem in our society, both in the United States and worldwide. Despite the public and medical pressure to "stay fit," the prevalence of obesity has become an epidemic, including more than 30% of the US adult population[1] and more than 400 million people worldwide.[2] It is recognized by the World Health Organization (WHO) and US Federal Government as a growing problem that is burdening our health care organizations and economy. Analyses estimate the total annual US economic costs associated with obesity are in excess of $215 billion.[3] Healthy People 2020, a US initiative to improve the health of the American population, maintains its goal to reduce chronic disease risk through the consumption of healthful diets and to achieve and maintain healthy body weight, with a specific objective to reduce the proportion of adults who are obese.[4]

DEFINITIONS

Obesity is characterized by an excessive accumulation of fat in the body. It is a chronic metabolic disorder that is determined by multiple biological and environmental factors, a sedentary lifestyle, and a genetic predisposition. The current worldwide epidemic of obesity may be secondary to overconsumption of high-fat, energy-rich foods; unhealthy snacking between meals; more food choices at restaurants, snack bars, and grocery stores; readily available inexpensive food 24 hours a day; larger-sized portions of food and drinks; increased advertising of high-fat or high-carbohydrate foods and drinks; and lack of physical activity and sleep. The addition of 20 to 30 kcal/day over a number of years can lead to significant weight gain; thus, energy intake and energy output through physical activity must be balanced for weight control.[5] The increase in the prevalence of obesity and negative health outcomes (diabetes, hyperlipidemia, cardiovascular disease) are major public health problems throughout the world.[2]

Weight measurement is commonly used to assess a patient's body composition status, especially in regard to fat accumulation. People are often grouped into weight-range categories of underweight, normal weight, overweight, and obese.[2] Overweight individuals weigh more than comparative standards for their given height and have extra body weight from muscle, bone, fat, or water. If excess weight is from fat as opposed to muscle, they are considered to have more fat accumulation than is optimally healthy. However, a person may also be considered "overweight" if muscle mass is great enough to significantly contribute to total weight. On the other hand, a patient may be considered "normal weight" while having excess fat accumulation and decreased muscle mass. Obese individuals have an excessive amount of fat accumulation that significantly impairs health status. Weight measurement in either the overweight or obese range estimate fat status in regard to overall health.[6,7]

An understanding of body composition is essential when evaluating a person's health status in regard to body fat. Use of other means to evaluate fat distribution is particularly useful in situations in which a patient may be considered normal weight but has excess abdominal fat accumulation. We frequently use weight measurements to guide our treatment decisions; however, we must take into consideration body composition and fat distribution to determine overall health risk. Accurate assessment of body fat mass or fat distribution can be obtained using medical imaging and testing such as computed tomography, magnetic resonance imaging, dual-energy x-ray absorptiometry, underwater body weighing, air displacement, total body water measurement, and bioelectric impedance and conductivity. However, these techniques are time-consuming, often very expensive or unavailable, and unnecessary for clinical evaluation to determine health risk. Anthropometric measurements of skinfold thickness, weight, and waist and limb circumference are easier to obtain and provide accurate estimates of body fat composition that can be obtained during a routine physical examination.

Obesity and weight can be defined by using body mass index (BMI), a measure of weight in relation to height, and used to classify underweight, normal weight, overweight, and obese. This classification scheme is accepted by the WHO and National Institutes of Health (NIH) and is closely correlated with body fat percentage.[2,6,8] BMI is calculated as weight (in kg) divided by height (in meters) squared (Table 36-1). Normal weight is defined as a BMI of 18.5 to 24.9 kg/m^2. Obesity is defined as a BMI greater than or equal to 30 kg/m^2 and is correlated to an estimated 50% to 100% increased mortality rate compared with nonobese individuals with BMI in the range of 20 to 25 kg/m^2 (Table 36-1).[9–13] Obesity is further divided into class I (BMI 30–34.5 kg/m^2), class II (BMI 35–39.9 kg/m^2), and class III (BMI >40 kg/m^2). People with a BMI range of 25 to 29.9 kg/m^2 are considered overweight and those with BMI greater than 28 have an increased risk of experiencing chronic illnesses (e.g., musculoskeletal disorders, cardiovascular disease, and diabetes).[2,6]

Fat distribution in the abdominal region has been linked to many of the metabolic consequences of obesity including hypertension, hypercholesterolemia, insulin sensitivity, and coronary heart disease. Measurement of waist circumference (WC) is used to assess for increased abdominal fat accumulation and to determine health risk. Waist circumference measurements greater than 102 cm (40 in) in men and 88 cm (35 in) in women have been proposed by the NIH as markers for increased risk of metabolic diseases.[2] Increased WC, independent of BMI classification, has been shown to predict obesity-related diseases such as diabetes, hypertension, dyslipidemia, and cardiovascular disease.[14–17] Therefore, WC measurement is useful in identifying individuals that are normal weight or overweight with health risk due to increased abdominal fat accumulation.[2]

TABLE 36-1
Body Mass Index and Guidelines for Weight Classes

Weight Status	BMI[a]	Obesity Class
Underweight	<18.5	
Normal	18.5–24.9	
Overweight	25.0–29.9	
Obesity	30.0–34.9	I
	35.0–39.9	II
Extreme, morbid, or severe obesity	≥40	III

[a] Metric conversion formula using kilograms and meters:

$$\text{BMI} = \frac{\text{Weight in kilograms}}{\text{Height in meters}^2}$$

Nonmetric conversion formula using pounds and inches:

$$\text{BMI} = \frac{\text{Weight in pounds}}{\text{Height in inches}^2} \times 703$$

BMI, body mass index.
Source: Clinical guidelines on the identification, evaluation, and treatment of overweight and obesity in adults: executive summary. Expert Panel on the Identification, Evaluation, and Treatment of Overweight in Adults. *Am J Clin Nutr.* 1998;68:899.

EPIDEMIOLOGY

Obesity is a major public health concern worldwide and is the leading cause of numerous medical conditions (e.g., cardiovascular disease, hypertension, dyslipidemia, diabetes, sleep apnea) and premature death.[9,12,18] According to the WHO, there were approximately 1.6 billion overweight and 400 million obese adults globally in 2005. WHO further projects that by 2015, approximately 2.3 billion adults will be overweight and more than 700 million will be obese.[6] In the United States, the prevalence of obesity has been examined as part of the National Health and Nutrition Examination Survey (NHANES). The most recent NHANES data, evaluated from 2007 to 2008, showed the prevalence of obesity was 32.2% among adult men and 35.5% among adult women.[1] Adult obesity usually results from a steady weight gain from the mid-20s to between ages 40 and 59, when the prevalence of obesity peaks.[1,19] The increased prevalence of obesity with increasing age may be secondary to continued consumption of calories that are not expended because of reduction in daily exercise, reduction in the amount of energy the body needs for daily functions, and smoking cessation.[19]

Obesity is more common in women (with higher rates in low socioeconomic status groups).[20] The most recent NHANES data report obesity and overweight were more prevalent among non-Hispanic black and Mexican American women, consistent with previous years.[1,19] The rate of extreme obesity (BMI ≥40) was also highest among non-Hispanic black women (14.2% vs. 5.7% among all US adults).[1] Despite the striking increases in obesity prevalence in the 1980s and 1990s, current NHANES data suggest that obesity prevalence may be stabilizing, showing nonsignificant increases compared with the 2003 to 2004 NHANES data.[1,21]

Obesity is also a significant problem among children and adolescents, with alarmingly high prevalence rates. The WHO estimates that greater than 42 million children under age 5 are overweight. NHANES data from 2007 to 2008 reported that approximately 10% of infants and toddlers (<2 years of age) were at or above the 95th percentile of the weight-for-recumbent-length growth charts. For children and adolescents (age 2–19 years), 16.9% were considered obese, being at or above the 95th percentile. As with adults, the trend in obesity increase may have begun to stabilize, with no significant change in obesity prevalence compared with the 1999 to 2000 NHANES data.[1,12] However, as this prevalence rate has remained alarmingly high, childhood obesity must be addressed because of the health consequences the obese child takes on into adulthood. Studies have shown that an elevated BMI in childhood and adolescence is correlated with an increase of adult coronary heart disease, cardiovascular disease, cancer, and premature mortality.[22–25] Childhood and adolescent obesity is also an increased risk for adult overweight and obesity.[26,27]

ETIOLOGY AND PATHOPHYSIOLOGY

Obesity results from an imbalance of energy intake and energy expenditure. Body fat accumulation will occur when an individual consumes more calories than are burned. This can easily occur with very small differences over long periods of time. For example, an excess of 100 kcal/day over the course of a year will result in an approximate weight gain of approximately 5 kg. If this continues over many years, it is easy for individuals to gain enough excess weight to place them in the obese category.[2,7]

The exact cause of obesity is difficult to identify and is likely a mixture of genetic, environmental, and behavioral factors. Investigators have tried to understand the origin of this disease by studying the influences of society, culture, socioeconomic status, medical conditions such as hypothyroidism, medications that stimulate appetite, parental weight, and hereditary traits on dietary habits and physical activity.[12,28] Some have concluded that genetic factors are important in determining susceptibility to obesity whereas environmental and behavioral influences are responsible for triggering the increased prevalence of the disorder.[29] Recently, there have been several association studies linking short sleep duration and metabolic changes such as obesity, insulin resistance, and diabetes.[30] One study showed that children aged 30 months and younger who lacked sleep were at risk of exhibiting obesity at 7 years.[31] Alteration of the hypothalamic regulation of appetite and energy expenditure owing to sleep loss is one possible explanation. Normally, when a person has eaten an adequate amount of food, neurotransmitters or peptides in the brain signal the satiety centers in the hypothalamus and there is a reduced desire to eat. Sleep loss has also been shown to be associated with low leptin levels and high ghrelin levels; both factors contribute to signaling of energy deficit and hunger, which may contribute to overeating and obesity.[32] Each potential cause of obesity continues to be investigated as a possible target for treatment and prevention of this disease.

Genetic Features

There is a clear link between genetics and obesity, both in childhood and adulthood, shown mostly through twin and adoption studies.[29,33–38] One study by Wardle et al. demonstrated a heritability estimate of 77% for BMI and 76% for waist circumference.[34] Other genetic studies show that 80% of children with two obese parents are obese compared with 40% of children with one obese parent, and 10% of children with two normal-weight parents.[28] Recently, investigators found a variant in the fat mass and obesity-associated gene that may be linked to BMI and obesity.[39] However, genetic studies have identified hundreds of other genes that may be associated as well.[29] In animal models, mutations of genes including the *ob* (obesity) gene encoding leptin and the *db* (diabetes) gene cause mice to become obese.[40]

HYPOTHALAMUS DYSREGULATION

Neurobiological theories of eating disorders have focused on dysregulation of the hypothalamic-pituitary-adrenal, hypothalamic-pituitary-gonadal, and hypothalamic-pituitary-thyroid axes as well as dysregulation of neurotransmitters, neuropeptides, endogenous opioids, growth hormone, insulin, and leptin.[5,28,41,42] Alterations in hypothalamic functioning are associated with appetite changes, mood disorders, and neuroendocrine disturbances.[5,40,41] The hypothalamus is the major appetite and eating control center in the brain and is sensitive to a variety of facilitatory and inhibitory neurotransmitters and polypeptide neurohormones from the brain and gastrointestinal (GI) tract.[5,28] Disruption of the ventromedial hypothalamus produces hyperphagia and obesity, whereas lesions of the lateral hypothalamus cause hypophagia and weight loss. This suggests that there is a ventromedial "satiety" and lateral "feeding" center in the hypothalamus. The hypothalamus receives input from peripheral satiety sites (e.g., gastric and pancreatic peptides released secondary to food passing through the GI tract), from leptin that is produced by fat cells, and from the catecholamine and indoleamine neurotransmitter system in the brain.[5,40,41,43]

NEUROTRANSMITTER DYSREGULATION

SEROTONIN

Serotonin plays an important role in postprandial satiety, anxiety, sleep, mood, obsessive–compulsive, and impulse control disorders.[5,41] Serotonin is synthesized from the essential amino acid L-tryptophan, which must come from the diet.[44] Under the influence of darkness, serotonin is metabolized in the pineal gland to melatonin, a major neuromodulator of sleep and reproductive function. Serotonin activity in the region of the medial hypothalamus has an inhibitory effect on appetite and is responsible for satiety or the feeling of fullness after food intake.[44–46] Pharmacologic treatments that increase intrasynaptic serotonin or those that directly activate serotonin receptors cause satiety and reduce food consumption.[46] Physical exertion increases central serotonin synthesis and turnover, which perpetuates reduced food intake and body weight.

Diminished serotonin activity (either by tryptophan depletion or serotonin antagonists) can contribute to increased food intake and carbohydrate craving.[45,47] Dietary restriction of tryptophan has been shown to reduce brain serotonin synthesis, causing a deficiency state. The reduction in serotonin activity may upregulate the appetite or satiety centers in the brain, thereby increasing the amount of food a person wants to eat. Agents that block postsynaptic serotonin activity (e.g., clozapine, cyproheptadine, mirtazapine, olanzapine, risperidone, and quetiapine) can stimulate appetite and may cause weight gain.

DOPAMINE

Agents that increase dopamine activity (e.g., apomorphine, a dopamine agonist; levodopa, a metabolic precursor of dopamine; and amphetamine, a stimulator of release of dopamine from presynaptic stores) have been shown to have anorexic effects.[48] Dopamine agonists increase dopaminergic transmission and motor activity, which causes loss of appetite and hyperactivity. At higher doses, these agents may cause psychosis (hallucinations and delusions) and repetitive or stereotypical behaviors.[48] The central nervous system (CNS) effects of dopaminergic agents occur in the cerebral cortex, in the reticular-activating system, and in the hypothalamic feeding center. The mesolimbic–mesocortical dopaminergic circuits are important for behavior reward and reinforcement, and are involved with "addictive" behaviors.[48] Dopamine-augmenting agents such as amphetamines are used for the treatment of exogenous obesity and may produce tolerance, dependence, and withdrawal reactions. Conversely, dopamine receptor antagonists such as chlorpromazine, clozapine, and pimozide may cause dysphoria and are often associated with weight gain.

NOREPINEPHRINE

The hypothalamus is innervated by noradrenergic pathways; thus, norepinephrine is involved in the regulation of eating behavior, the hypothalamic control of thyrotropin-releasing hormone secretion, corticotropin-releasing hormone (CRH) release, and gonadotropin secretion.[48] D-Amphetamine, which inhibits the reuptake of norepinephrine, decreases hunger sensations and food intake. Abnormalities in leptin and β_3-adrenergic activity have been associated with obesity and diabetes.[18,49] The human β_3-adrenoceptor is involved in a feedback loop with leptin to regulate energy balance, lipolysis in adipocytes, serum insulin levels, and food intake.[50] People with hereditary obesity or non–insulin-dependent diabetes mellitus may have abnormalities in the β_3-adrenoceptor or in leptin activity, signaling, or receptors.[49] A genetic variant of the β_3-adrenoceptor in humans has been associated with morbid obesity and non–insulin-dependent diabetes. It is possible that some cases of obesity may be secondary to failure of the β_3-adrenoreceptor on brown adipocytes to respond appropriately to leptin-induced sympathetic activity.[51] β_3-Adrenergic receptor agonists are being studied to induce thermogenic activity and promote weight loss when combined with a calorie-restricted diet.[50]

NEUROPEPTIDE AND LEPTIN DYSREGULATION

LEPTIN

Leptin is a 167–amino-acid protein synthesized by adipocytes in white adipose tissue as well as in brown adipose tissue, gastric chief cells, skeletal muscle, and other organs. It acts on receptors of the hypothalamus to act as an afferent satiety signal in the brain to regulate body fat mass.[5,40,52,53] Leptin reduces food intake, decreases serum glucose and insulin levels, increases metabolic rate, and reduces body fat mass and weight by reducing neuropeptide Y (NPY) activity (a potent feeding stimulant secreted by the hypothalamus and cells in the gut).[52,54] Leptin serum levels are highly correlated with BMI and body fat,[53] and its secretion has a circadian rhythm and an oscillatory pattern similar to other hormones.[49,55]

Leptin is supposed to signal the brain to reduce the desire to eat, but the signal may not get through properly in some overweight people.[52] It has been postulated that some obese individuals may have partially resistant hypothalamic receptors or that there is a defect in the blood–brain barrier transport system for bringing leptin into the brain.[40,52,55,56] Cerebrospinal fluid leptin levels in some obese humans have been found to be much lower than expected compared with serum leptin levels, which suggests that the uptake of leptin into the brain may be defective.[5,40] Other studies suggest that obese individuals may have a dysregulation of leptin in response to overfeeding, with a lack of serum increase. Compared with lean individuals, this may indicate that the obese individuals lacks a protective mechanism of increase in serum leptin levels in response to increased caloric intake to prevent weight gain.[57] It has been demonstrated that elevated baseline serum leptin levels are associated with inability to maintain weight loss.[58] Another potential mechanism may be reduced leptin receptor protein expression found in skeletal muscle of obese patients that could lead to leptin resistance in the presence of elevated leptin serum levels.[59] Leptin and leptinlike products have been investigated for promotion of weight loss, but no agents have been successfully developed.[52,60]

NEUROPEPTIDES

The pancreatic polypeptides NPY, found in the central and peripheral nervous system, and peptide YY (PYY), found in the gut, are chemically related, 36–amino-acid peptides and are two of the most potent stimulators of appetite.[5,45] Both enhance food intake in animals, possibly by causing hunger.[61] PYY is three times more potent in stimulating food intake than NPY.[41] Injection of NPY into the brain causes all of the features of leptin deficiency (e.g., hyperphagia and obesity).[56] Many of leptin's effects on food intake and energy expenditure are centrally mediated in the hypothalamus by neurotransmitters such as NPY.[40,52,54] A study of 497 obese patients showed that NPY Y5 receptor antagonism did not produce increased weight loss when added to 6 months of either orlistat or sibutramine therapy.[62] Early studies of experimental PYY administration have found an intranasal formulation to be ineffective for weight reduction and poorly tolerated in obese patients.[63] A small dose escalation study of subcutaneous injections of two forms of PYY, PYY_{1-36} and PYY_{3-36}, found some positive results on inducing lower subjective hunger and thirst ratings and higher satiety ratings with PPY_{3-36} administration.[64] Another evaluation of subcutaneous PPY_{3-36} in combination with another postprandial hormone, oxyntomodulin, showed additive effects on food intake in overweight and obese patients.[65]

MISCELLANEOUS NEUROHORMONES AND PEPTIDES

Food intake and gastric emptying are regulated by the peripheral release of GI peptides such as cholecystokinin, glucagon, calcitonin, bombesin, and somatostatin, all of which inhibit feeding.[5,66] Other hormones, neurotransmitters, and peptides involved in the regulation of hunger and satiety (e.g., histamine, oxytocin, vasopressin, galanin, CRH, melanocyte-stimulating hormone, hypocretin, and orexin) and lipotic action (e.g., growth hormone and dehydroepiandrosterone) are being investigated. Histamine is involved in the regulation of appetite, and histamine-1–blocking agents (e.g., tricyclic antidepressants, antipsychotics, antihistamines) cause sedation and increased appetite in animals and humans.[67] Growth hormone, a lipolytic hormone that acts at adipose tissue, reduces and redistributes body fat by releasing glycerol and free fatty acids into the circulation.[68] Growth hormone secretion is significantly lower in obese individuals and lipolysis is, therefore, reduced. As people age, the secretion of growth hormone declines (it is estimated that 50% of people >65 years have growth-hormone deficit).[68] Replacement doses of growth hormone have been suggested to treat obesity and to reverse body changes associated with aging.

Environmental Influences and Behavioral Factors

Despite the known genetic influences predisposing certain individuals to obesity, environmental influences play a role by providing exposure to a lifestyle promoting energy imbalance.[7] Modern society provides an overabundance of calorie-dense food. Aggressive and sophisticated food marketing, availability of easily accessible food 24 hours a day, and large portion sizes encourage increased caloric intake. Many of our sociocultural traditions also promote overeating. Decreased energy expenditure due to a sedentary lifestyle has become common, often supported by less-active daily rituals. Many individuals spend most of their waking hours sitting, whether it is in front of a computer, in traffic, or watching television.[2]

A review of twin and adoption studies by Silventoinen et al. clearly demonstrated that environmental factors affect BMI variation in childhood, but the effect of common environment disappears in adolescence.[33] These results portray a stronger influence of genetics in the incidence of obesity in adulthood. In the current obesity-promoting environment, individuals often have negative attitudes toward a healthy lifestyle consisting of a balanced diet and adequate physical activity. This, combined with genetic predisposition, seems to be triggering an increased prevalence of obesity.[40]

Medical Conditions and Medications

Although less common, certain congenital genetic syndromes may be the primary cause of obesity such as Prader-Willi syndrome. Some neuroendocrine causes of overweight and obesity that are more common include hypothyroidism, polycystic ovarian syndrome, Cushing syndrome, and growth hormone deficiency. Hypothalamic injury is rare in humans, but also a known neuroendocrine cause.[69] Individuals with mental illness are especially prone to exhibiting obesity, and treatment with psychotropic medications including chlorpromazine, clozapine, risperidone, and olanzapine cause significant weight gain.[69,70] Of patients with severe chronic mental illness, 40% to 62% are overweight before initiation of medication.[71]

Several other medications besides the psychotropic agents are associated with significant weight gain. These include steroids, thiazolidinediones, sulfonylureas, insulin, anticonvulsants, and antidepressants.[69,72] If medications can be identified as possible sources of weight gain, substitution with possible alternatives should be attempted. Table 36-2 provides a list of medications and medical conditions that may cause weight gain.

TABLE 36-2
Medications and Medical Conditions That May Cause Weight Gain

Medications
α-Blockers and β-blockers (e.g., terazosin, atenolol, propranolol)
Antidepressants (e.g., mirtazapine, paroxetine, phenelzine, trazodone, tricyclic antidepressants)
Antidiabetics (e.g., insulin, sulfonylureas, thiazolidinediones)
Antiepileptic drugs (e.g., carbamazepine, gabapentin, pregabalin, valproic acid)
Antihistamines (e.g., diphenhydramine, cyproheptadine, histamine-2 blockers)
Antipsychotics (e.g., most typicals, clozapine, olanzapine, risperidone, quetiapine)
Glucocorticoids (e.g., prednisone)
Mood stabilizers (e.g., lithium)
Progestin-containing hormones (e.g., medroxyprogesterone)
Protease inhibitors (e.g., ritonavir, indinavir)
Medical Conditions
Chronic heart failure
Cushing syndrome
Depression (e.g., seasonal affective disorder, premenstrual dysphoric disorder)
Diabetes mellitus type 2
Hypothyroidism
Polycystic ovarian syndrome
Schizophrenia

Source: Yager J, Powers PS, eds. *Clinical Manual of Eating Disorders.* Washington, DC: American Psychiatric Publishing; 2007.

CLINICAL FEATURES

CASE 36-1

QUESTION 1: S.B. is a 48-year-old woman with a past medical history of hypertension, sleep apnea, osteoarthritis, and depression. She has struggled with her weight since her teenage years and has progressively gained approximately 2 kg per year since her 20s. Her height is 168 cm, current weight is 98 kg, and WC is 96 cm. She presents to her primary physician for a routine physical examination. She complains of dissatisfaction with her weight and reports having tried multiple diets during the past 20 years, but has had little success with weight loss and always regains any weight she manages to lose. S.B. expresses a desire to attempt medication therapy for weight loss. Her current medications include hydrochlorothiazide, metoprolol, naproxen, and tramadol. Her blood pressure is currently 162/98 mm Hg and she is complaining of daytime fatigue due to sleep apnea. How is obesity defined and assessed in a patient like S.B., and what should her physician do to manage her risk of experiencing new obesity-related conditions?

Initial Assessment

The NIH recommends a two-step process of assessment and management for the proper treatment of obesity. Assessment involves a physical exam and patient interview to classify the degree of obesity and determination of risk for obesity-related morbidity and mortality. Calculation of BMI and measurement of WC will classify the degree of obesity and indicate relative risk and the need to initiate treatment.[2] The best method to determine the degree of overweight or obesity is to measure the BMI, which is associated with total body fat content.[12] Measurement of WC is also useful in identifying normal weight and overweight patients at risk for obesity-related diseases as it is an independent predictor of morbidity in all patients and correlates to abdominal fat content.[9,12] High relative health risks are seen in patients with waist circumference greater than 102 cm (40 inches) in men and greater than 88 cm (35 inches) in women compared with patients with normal weight. Fat deposited around the waist seems to be more likely than fat on the hips or thighs to lead to health risks such as cardiovascular disease, insulin resistance, type 2 diabetes, hyperlipidemia, and increased blood pressure. The waist circumference may not be as useful in terms of risk prediction in patients with BMI greater than 35 kg/m^2 and height less than 5 feet.[12]

Waist to hip ratio indicates regional fat distribution and increased health risk is seen in patients with high intra-abdominal fat (waist to hip ratio >1 in men and >0.8 in women).[9] Skinfold thickness can be used to assess body fat at various sites, but measurements may vary between observers and it does not provide information about intramuscular or abdominal fat.[9] S.B.'s BMI is 34.7 (98 kg $\div$ [1.68 m]^2), which is in obesity class I. Her waist circumference is greater than 88 cm, indicating abdominal obesity that puts her at additional risk for increased morbidity and mortality.

To determine absolute risk and need for treatment of overweight or obesity, clinicians should be familiar with related diseases and other risk factors (Table 36-3). Evaluation for existing comorbidities including coronary heart disease, atherosclerosis, and diabetes indicate high absolute risk and the need for intense management. Specific cardiovascular risk factors in the presence of obesity put a patient at high absolute risk and

TABLE 36-3
Conditions That Increase the Risk Status in Overweight or Obese Patients

Disease Conditions	Risk for Disease Complications, Mortality
Coronary heart disease Atherosclerotic disease Type 2 diabetes mellitus Sleep apnea Other obesity-related diseases	Very high
Gynecologic abnormalities Osteoarthritis Gallstones and complications Stress incontinence Cardiovascular risk factors	High
Cigarette smoking Hypertension Increased LDL cholesterol Low HDL cholesterol Impaired fasting blood glucose Family history of premature CHD Age (men >45, women >55 or postmenopausal) Physical inactivity High serum triglycerides	Very high if ≥2 risk factors

CHD, coronary heart disease; HDL, high-density lipoprotein; LDL, low-density lipoprotein.
Source: Clinical guidelines on the identification, evaluation, and treatment of overweight and obesity in adults: executive summary. Expert Panel on the Identification, Evaluation, and Treatment of Overweight in Adults. *Am J Clin Nutr.* 1998;68:899.

indicate the need for intense blood pressure and cholesterol management per the guidelines published by the National Cholesterol Education Program[73] and the Joint National Committee on Prevention, Detection, Evaluation and Treatment of High Blood Pressure.[74] Risks include cigarette smoking, hypertension, high low-density lipoprotein (LDL) cholesterol, low high-density lipoprotein (HDL) cholesterol, impaired fasting blood glucose, family history of premature coronary heart disease, and age.[2,73,74] Other obesity-associated risk factors that should be considered include lack of physical activity and elevated triglycerides.[2] S.B. already has hypertension that is not well controlled by her current medications. She should be questioned about her adherence to her diuretic and β-blocker and then her antihypertensive regimen should be optimized. Naproxen may also be contributing to her continued hypertension and could be replaced with acetaminophen.

During the patient interview, information should be obtained regarding the patient's eating habits and physical activity. It is important to establish baseline data so that response to changes in diet and exercise are noted throughout treatment. Successful weight loss involves a change in energy balance through reduced caloric intake or increased energy expenditure. This can necessitate active and sometimes very difficult changes to a patient's diet and exercise habits.[2] In S.B.'s case, she has tried multiple diets in the past with little success on her own, so it may be beneficial for her to receive professional dietary counseling. Patients should also be screened for medical conditions or medications that can increase the risk for obesity, and these underlying factors should be corrected before recommending treatment. S.B.'s past medical history does not indicate any medical causes of obesity and her current medications are not associated with weight gain. It would be appropriate to check thyroid function to rule out hypothyroidism—a common condition in women that can contribute to unexplained weight gain or inability to lose weight.

It is also important to evaluate a patient's "weight-loss readiness" or self-motivation before initiation of therapy. A patient's motivation to lose weight is a significant predictor of success or failure in the weight management program. S.B. has expressed desire to lose weight and her willingness to make significant lifestyle changes in order to achieve this should be evaluated. Patients who lack motivation may not be good candidates for therapeutic intervention. Achievement of weight loss involves an investment of time and effort by both the patient and practitioner. The willingness to participate in a regimen may depend on types of diets tried in the past, social support at home and workplace, patient's understanding of the illness, time, and financial burden.[12] Poor outcomes of weight-loss therapy have been observed in those unmotivated to engage in lifestyle changes necessary to produce results and those who do not feel that these lifestyle changes will help them to lose weight. Practitioners should take an active role to encourage obese patients to lose weight and make them highly motivated to do so.[2,75,76] Unmotivated obese patients, as well as overweight patients with one risk factor or less, should be encouraged to prevent further weight gain and manage obesity-related risk factors. It is essential to provide optimal therapy for hypertension, dyslipidemia, impaired fasting blood glucose, and smoking cessation.[2]

Obesity is considered a chronic medical condition because it causes multiple physical complications.[9] The greater the degree of obesity, the harder it is for a person to lose weight permanently without medical and behavioral interventions. Major depressive disorder, anxiety disorders, and low self-esteem are common in obese patients owing to social prejudice and discrimination in the work force.[77]

Course and Prognosis

CASE 36-1, QUESTION 2: S.B. reports that she has never received dietary counseling from a medical professional and has always dieted on her own by restricting fat intake. Although she has not attempted to lose weight recently, S.B. expresses desire to try a program for weight loss and start an exercise regimen. After review of her medical, social, and dietary history with her physician, primary causes of obesity are ruled out and a plan for weight loss is initiated. What is the typical course and prognosis of obesity?

Obesity is a chronic disease that can begin in childhood or adolescence and can be characterized by a slow and steady increase in body weight during adult life. Most obese patients battle with weight loss and regain throughout their entire lives. This includes struggling with various diets or exercise programs to attempt to lose or maintain loss. The other issues obese patients must deal with throughout life are prevention and management of the medical complications of obesity. It is known that weight loss will improve obesity-associated morbidity and mortality, but successful weight loss or maintenance is not easy to achieve.[2,7] In S.B.'s case, she expresses motivation and an understanding about the significance of lifestyle changes to improving her overall health. Maintaining weight loss, however, is key to long-term management of obesity. More than 80% of people who lose weight gradually regain it; patients who continue on weight maintenance programs consisting of dietary, physical, and behavioral therapy have a better chance of not regaining weight than those who discontinue weight maintenance programs.[12] S.B. should be encouraged to commit to the behavioral modification program and surround herself with supportive individuals that can continue to motivate her to achieve her weight-loss goals.

Medical Complications

CASE 36-1, QUESTION 3: S.B. understands that she already has hypertension, sleep apnea, and osteoarthritis, which are comorbidities that increase her risk of mortality. She is also at risk for experiencing additional obesity-associated medical comorbidities if she does not lose or continues to gain weight. What are the other common medical conditions associated with obesity?

Obesity is associated with an increased risk of morbidity and mortality. Some obesity-associated diseases that are generally not life-threatening include gynecological abnormalities, osteoarthritis, gallstones and their complications, and stress incontinence.[2] Other obesity-related conditions have a tremendous impact on physiologic functioning and medical illnesses. Obese people tend to die young, and the more abdominal body fat, the greater the mortality.[78] Obesity is linked to many disabling diseases such as diabetes mellitus (non–insulin-dependent and insulin-resistant), pulmonary impairment (hypoventilation, hypoxia, hypercapnia, and sleep apnea), gallbladder disease (gallstones and cholecystitis), cancers (colorectal, prostate, breast, cervical, endometrial, uterine, and ovarian), osteoarthritis (hips, knees, and back), gout, cardiac disease (hypertension, stroke, congestive heart failure, and coronary heart disease), increased cholesterol and triglycerides (TG) (increased low-density lipoproteins and decreased high-density lipoproteins), dermatologic problems (intertrigo and stretching of skin), and menstrual irregularities.[12,28] The Nurses Health Study showed that the risk of developing diabetes in women with BMI greater than 35 was 60 times higher than the lowest risk group (BMI <22 kg/m^2).[79] It is estimated that greater than 60% of type 2 diabetes mellitus cases are due to obesity.[80] Weight loss helps to control diseases associated with obesity and may even help prevent development of these diseases. Weight loss has been shown to be beneficial in lowering blood pressure, total cholesterol, LDL, TG, and blood glucose in patients with diabetes mellitus type 2, and in increasing HDL.[12] In S.B.'s case, weight loss through diet and exercise could help her decrease or eliminate medications needed to control her hypertension, alleviate pain associated with osteoarthritis, decrease symptoms of sleep apnea, and reduce her BMI and WC, therefore improving her morbidity and mortality risk. In the meantime, her hypertension should be aggressively managed per the current guidelines.

MANAGEMENT AND TREATMENT

Obesity is a chronic disease that requires lifelong effort for successful treatment.[2] Treatment may involve a multidisciplinary approach including the expertise of a general practitioner, dietician, pharmacist, psychiatrist, or surgeon depending on the specific needs of the individual. Guidelines for the management and treatment of obesity have been published by the National Institutes of Health and the American Gastroenterological Association.[2,7] These guidelines recommend a thorough assessment of the degree of obesity and risk factors, management of weight via decrease in energy intake or increase in energy expenditure, and treatment of risk factors. The goals of therapy involve weight loss or weight maintenance to improve or eliminate obesity-related medical complications.[7]

Medical Management

CASE 36-1, QUESTION 4: The physician recommends that S.B. reduce her weight during the next 12 months to help improve the quality of her life, reduce the associated morbidity from related medical conditions, and prolong her life. What would be appropriate goals for weight loss? What type of nutritional and exercise plan should be recommended?

According to the National Heart, Lung, and Blood Institute guidelines, weight-loss treatment should be initiated for patients who are overweight, who have increased waist circumference plus two or more risk factors, or are obese (BMI ≥ 30).[12] The general goals of weight loss and management are to prevent weight gain, reduce body weight, and maintain weight loss over a long period.[12] Treatment options to facilitate weight loss include moderate caloric restriction, medications (e.g., appetite suppressants, lipase inhibitors), physical activity, and behavior therapy. Obese patients (like S.B.) should strive to lose 10% of baseline weight at a rate of 1 to 2 pounds/week with an energy deficit of 500 kcal/day for 6 months. Overweight patients should ideally lose 0.5 pounds/week with an energy deficit of 300 to 500 kcal/day for 6 months. A low-calorie diet consistent with National Cholesterol Education Program Step 1 or Step 2 diet has been shown to be most effective. A low-fat diet does not decrease weight unless total caloric intake is decreased. Total fat intake should account for 30% or less of total calories consumed per day.[12] Drastic caloric restriction is difficult to maintain and may lead to reduced metabolism and overeating due to hunger. Severe caloric restriction and rapid weight loss can be harmful and result in rebound binge-eating behavior and weight gain.[81]

Increased physical activity can facilitate weight loss and is essential in preventing weight gain. Overweight children and adults should have at least 30 minutes of moderate-intensity physical exercise daily (with a gradual increment of increasing exercise by several minutes each day up to 30 minutes per day). It has recently been shown that moderate exercise (e.g., 4 kcal/g per week) can improve physiologic variables.[82] Modest weight loss is beneficial, because even a small amount of weight loss, as little as 5%, is associated with significant improvements in health status.

Nonpharmacologic Therapy

CASE 36-1, QUESTION 5: S.B. agrees to be evaluated and enrolled in a behavior modification program in which she will meet with a dietician on a regular basis and participate in exercise classes for obese patients. The program will provide weekly social support meetings and teach S.B. more desirable behaviors for self-monitoring her diet and exercise. What types of nonpharmacologic therapies or programs are available for weight reduction and relapse prevention?

Behavioral modification programs using support groups, a balanced diet, and exercise are most effective for mild obesity (20%–40% overweight).[28] Behavioral modification programs (e.g., nutritional education, exercise, cognitive restructuring, self-monitoring) are the most effective for overweight children and help to motivate parents and children to alter their lifestyles.[12] Supportive family therapy is desirable, particularly for obese children. Obesity may be related to cultural attitudes, family eating behaviors, and social events involving food. Relapse prevention should identify high-risk situations or events that may cause weight gain so that the person can learn new coping strategies to avoid overeating.

Because of the high demand by consumers, there are numerous types of weight-loss programs, diets, and products that may or may not be effective. Individuals who want to lose weight frequently seek out popular structured programs (e.g., Jenny Craig, Weight Watchers). Other weight-loss programs include low-fat, low-sodium, vegetarian, soy, Atkins, and Zone diets. Regardless of which weight-loss program is chosen, patients should select a program that emphasizes the following: (a) counseling for lifestyle changes, (b) trained staff, (c) coping strategies for stressful times, (d) weight-loss maintenance, and (e) flexible and appropriate food choices and cost.[83]

Overall, a combination of low-calorie diet, behavioral modifications, and increased physical activity are most effective for reducing and maintaining weight loss. S.B. questioned her physician about weight-loss medications, but she has never made an effort to lose weight through a structured weight-loss program. These measures must be attempted and maintained for at least 6 months before considering pharmacotherapy.[12]

NONPRESCRIPTION DIET AIDS

CASE 36-1, QUESTION 6: Are diet aids such as Ultra Slim Fast effective as weight-loss agents?

Weight loss occurs when caloric intake is less than caloric expenditure for a sustained period of time. Products like Slim Fast, Ultra Slim Fast, and other branded or "house generics" are low-fat dietary supplements that clearly label the caloric, fat, carbohydrate, and protein content per "dosage unit" to assist in counting daily calorie intake. An important added ingredient is hydrophilic colloids and fiber (listed on the product label as grams of fiber per dosage unit), which absorb water and give a feeling of satiety (fullness). These products come in a variety of forms to fit the dieter's lifestyle including powders to mix with milk, breakfast bars, waferlike cookies, and tablets to swallow. Using Slim Fast and Ultra Slim Fast powder as examples, the dieter places one measuring scoop of the product in eight ounces of reduced fat milk to produce a "shake" that is drunk in the morning for breakfast and again in the afternoon for lunch. For dinner, the package inserts encourage the dieter to eat a healthy, normal meal. According to the package labels, both products provide 18 to 19 g of carbohydrate, 5 g of protein, less than 1 g of fat, 110 mg of sodium, and 240 mg of potassium per scoop. Depending on the type of milk used, an additional 90 to 130 calories and 0.5 to 5 g of fat are consumed in each feeding from nonfat (skim) and 2% milk, respectively. Thus, less than 500 calories are ingested during the first two meals of the day combined allowing up to an additional 500 to 1,500 calories for dinner or snacks. The greater the adherence to reduced caloric intake, the faster weight loss will occur. The only other difference is that Slim Fast provides 90 calories and 2 g of fiber compared with 100 calories and 5 g of fiber per scoop in Ultra Slim Fast. The larger amount of fiber in the "Ultra" formula theoretically reduces the sensation of hunger between meals. Perhaps the most useful attribute of these products is the detailed package inserts that provide excellent information on healthy eating. For example, the inserts recommend eating raw vegetables (low-calorie and high-fiber) for between-meal snacks; using low-fat dairy products; and avoiding cakes, cookies, candy, sugared soft drinks, and large amounts of fruit juices. Guidance on portion size and healthy content for the dinner meal is also provided. In short, these products can produce significant weight loss if used correctly for a period of several months, but will fail if the person continues to consume too many calories from other sources or is not exercising properly. Substituting instant breakfast drinks mixed with milk or breakfast bars is another option, but typically they have higher calorie content (250 to 300 calories), more sugar and fat, and the absence of significant amounts of fiber. After learning proper dietary habits, the same goal can be accomplished without these products by eating correctly. Limitations include taste fatigue (only three flavors available: vanilla, chocolate, strawberry); dislike of the taste or gritty texture of the product; and continuing hunger between meals, especially during the first few days of use.

Pharmacologic Therapy

AMPHETAMINES AND SYMPATHOMIMETICS

CASE 36-1, QUESTION 7: S.B. returns to her physician for follow-up 1 year later. She has managed to lose 14 kg and at a weight of 84 kg, her BMI is now 29.8 kg/m^2. Although she has lost a significant amount of weight and is now considered overweight as opposed to obese, S.B. still wants to lose additional weight. Her hypertension remains controlled. She again asks the physician about medications that can help with weight loss. Would a sympathomimetic type agent be a good choice for S.B.? What are their mechanisms of action, efficacy, and potential adverse effects?

A comprehensive treatment approach to obesity includes a weight-loss diet, exercise, supportive psychotherapy, and behavioral modification techniques. If indicated, medications such as an anorectic agent (to suppress hunger and appetite) or a GI lipase inhibitor (to reduce fat absorption) may be prescribed.[84] Weight loss is possible for most patients, but the main problem is that the vast majority of people regain the weight with time.[70] Obesity is a chronic, lifelong illness that may require long-term medication therapy. Medication should be considered only for patients with a BMI greater than 30 kg/m^2 without risk factors or greater than 27 kg/m^2 with an obesity-related risk factor (Table 36-3).[12] In S.B.'s case, she would be a candidate for pharmacotherapy as her BMI is 29.8 kg/m^2 with obesity-related risk factors of hypertension, sleep apnea, and osteoarthritis. She has been successful with behavioral modification therapy, but would still benefit from additional weight loss. Anorectic medications or lipase inhibitors should not be considered a replacement for diet, behavioral modification, and exercise, but rather as add-on therapy.

Medications used for the treatment of obesity in the United States are listed in Table 36-4. Although there are many medications with varying mechanisms of action that have been theorized to be effective for weight loss, currently marketed drugs for weight loss do so by suppressing the appetite or decreasing the absorption of fat.[84] However, the development of safe and efficacious pharmacologic agents for weight loss is at a standstill, due to the withdrawal of most agents due to postmarketing discovery of serious adverse effects.[85] According to recent meta-analyses and critical reviews, orlistat has been shown to have consistent and sustained, albeit modest, weight-loss effects over other pharmacologic classes of drugs for up to 1 year.[86,87]

Amphetamines, dextroamphetamine, and sympathomimetics have been used as appetite suppressants and thermogenic agents for several decades.[88] The enhancement of dopaminergic activity is believed to be responsible for amphetamine's rewarding, reinforcing, and addictive properties.[89] Because of their euphoric properties and risks of drug abuse, amphetamines are schedule II controlled agents and are not routinely used for weight loss.[90] They have been associated with increased cardiovascular events and labeling now contains a black-box warning

TABLE 36-4
Medications Marketed or Used for the Treatment of Obesity

Generic Name	Trade Name	Dosage	DEA Schedule or Class
Amphetamine or dextroamphetamine	Adderall	5–30 mg/d	II[a]
Benzphetamine hydrochloride	Didrex	25–50 mg one to three times daily	III
Dextroamphetamine			
Immediate release	Dexedrine	5–10 mg before meals	II[a]
Extended release	Dexedrine	10–30 mg	II[a]
Diethylpropion hydrochloride			
Immediate release	Tenuate	25 mg TID; 75 mg AM	IV
Controlled release	Tenuate Dospan	75 mg AM	IV
Methamphetamine hydrochloride			
Immediate release	Desoxyn	2.5–5 mg before meals	II[a]
Orlistat	Xenical, Alli	120 mg TID, 60 mg TID	Prescription, OTC
Phendimetrazine tartrate	Bontril, Prelu-2	35 mg TID; 105 mg AM	III
Phentermine			
Hydrochloride	Adipex-P	8 mg TID; 30–37.5 mg AM	IV

[a] High abuse potential, not recommended for routine or long-term use.
BID, twice a day; DEA, Drug Enforcement Administration; OTC, over the counter; TID, three times a day.
Source: Campfield LA et al. Strategies and potential molecular targets for obesity treatment. *Science.* 1998;280:1383; DeWald T et al. Pharmacological and surgical treatments for obesity. *Am Heart J.* 2006;151:604.

regarding this risk. Additional concerns with sympathomimetics are the potential for rebound binge-eating, weight gain, lethargy, and depression when the medication is discontinued.[28] Other centrally active appetite suppressants that augment catecholamines (e.g., phentermine, mazindol, phendimetrazine, and diethylpropion) were developed for the treatment of obesity and may have a lower incidence and severity of CNS side effects compared with amphetamines.[88]

Although amphetamines and sympathomimetics may be quite effective for weight loss, they are not without significant risks. Fenfluramine and dexfenfluramine were voluntarily removed from the US market in 1997 due to studies linking their usage to valvular heart disease and primary pulmonary hypertension.[91] Phentermine, a similarly structured agent to fenfluramine, is still available as monotherapy for the short-term (<12 weeks) treatment of obesity as an adjunct to exercise, behavioral modification, and caloric restriction. This is a schedule IV agent that stimulates the secretion of noradrenalin in the central nervous system and suppresses the appetite. Phentermine is approved for use in patients older than 16 years of age, at a dosage of 18.75 to 37.5 mg taken 2 hours after breakfast. Dosing may also be divided into two 18.75-mg doses, but should not be administered late in the day due to insomnia.[92] Phentermine was commonly used with fenfluramine in the combination product Fen-Phen until the removal of fenfluramine from the market. Phentermine has been associated with cardiovascular adverse events itself, including case reports of pulmonary hypertension.[93]

Diethylpropion, another schedule IV amphetaminelike compound with minor sympathomimetic properties has been shown to produce weight loss in obesity. Although currently recommended for short-term administration, diethylpropion use has been studied up to 1 year. Results showed clinically significant weight loss that was maintained throughout treatment. Cardiovascular safety was evaluated and found to be similar to placebo, with no significant increases in mean systolic and diastolic blood pressure or electrocardiogram changes.[94] Diethylpropion can be administered as immediate-release 25-mg tablets three times daily 1 hour before meals or as extended-release 75-mg tablets once daily in the morning. Adverse reactions include insomnia and dry mouth. Cardiovascular parameters including blood pressure and heart rate should be monitored during therapy.[94] Even though S.B. is a candidate for medication therapy, use of an amphetamine or sympathomimetic agent is not the most appropriate choice. Her history of uncontrolled hypertension and continued issue of sleep disturbances from sleep apnea may be exacerbated by the stimulant effects of these medications.

CASE 36-1, QUESTION 8: Are there any nonprescription stimulant-type weight-loss drugs available?

As of April 2004, the US Food and Drug Administration (FDA) has prohibited the sale of dietary supplements containing ephedrine alkaloids (ephedra) owing to the many reports of serious adverse effects (e.g., stroke, seizures, arrhythmias, and death).[95] Ephedrine (found in ephedra and ma huang) was included in many over-the-counter (OTC) and herbal products that promoted their ability to increase energy expenditure, thus causing weight loss.[72] Phenylpropanolamine (PPA), a popular synthetic catecholamine that was widely found in OTC weight-loss products and decongestants, was also voluntarily withdrawn in 2000.[96] PPA increased satiety by stimulating norepinephrine and dopamine release in the hypothalamic feeding center, but studies found an increased risk of hemorrhagic stroke in women who took appetite suppressants containing more than 32 mg/day PPA.[97] Most recently, sibutramine, a prescription medication structurally related to amphetamines (β-phenylethylamine) was removed from marketing in Europe, the United States, and Canada due to its association with a high risk of nonfatal myocardial infarction and nonfatal stroke.[85,98,99] Current OTC weight-loss products contain stimulant compounds such as caffeine or the herbal product guarana. Because of significant adverse effects of sympathomimetics, these agents are no longer recommended for weight loss.

ANTIDEPRESSANTS

CASE 36-1, QUESTION 9: How effective are antidepressants compared with stimulants for achieving weight loss? Would one of these agents be appropriate for S.B.?

Serotonin-augmenting or norepinephrine-augmenting agents (e.g., serotonin or norepinephrine reuptake inhibitors) are the most effective agents for suppressing appetite drive and reducing weight. For obese binge-eating patients, selective serotonin reuptake inhibitor (SSRI) antidepressants such as fluoxetine have been used successfully to reduce binge-eating behavior, but this is not always associated with weight loss. The reason for the weight regain is unclear, but may relate to the development of tolerance or the lack of frequent follow-up visits.[100] In a recent meta-analysis, high-dose fluoxetine was shown to produce a pooled weight loss of 4.74 kg at 6 months and 3.15 kg at 12 months.[87] A comparison of fluoxetine and sertraline in obese patients with binge-eating disorder showed moderate but comparable results regarding weight loss and decrease of binge-eating symptoms.[101] Use of SSRIs in depressed, obese patients may be useful and may be considered as a conjunctive therapy for S.B., as she is currently not receiving any medical therapy for depression. Dosing for these agents is generally higher than the initial dosing for major depressive disorder. In this patient population, fluoxetine is generally administered at 40 to 80 mg and sertraline at 100 to 200 mg.[87,101] Studies with other SSRIs are either lacking, limited by small sample size, or have shown nonsignificant results.[87]

Bupropion, an antidepressant that inhibits dopamine and norepinephrine reuptake, has a known side effect of weight loss when used for the treatment of depression and smoking cessation.[102] As a result, there has been investigation of bupropion as a potential weight-loss therapy for obese patients. As drug monotherapy, it has been shown to produce some weight-loss (2.77 kg) effects at 6 and 12 months when combined with other weight-loss measures (diet, exercise).[87] It is thought that the weight-loss effects of bupropion occur as a result of stimulation of pro-opiomelanocortin (POMC) neurons in the hypothalamus causing release of α-melanocyte-stimulating hormone, an anorexiant. However, these weight-loss effects are possibly attenuated by a β-endorphin-mediated autoinhibitory feedback loop activated by opioid receptors on POMC neurons as a compensatory mechanism.[102,103] This has led to the investigation of bupropion as combination therapy with the opioid antagonist naltrexone. Naltrexone may impede this negative feedback loop by blocking the opioid receptors on the POMC neurons that release β-endorphin, and therefore results in continued weight loss or improved weight-loss maintenance.[102]

Trials have been completed comparing various dosage combinations and dosage forms of bupropion and naltrexone to monotherapy and placebo. Bupropion sustained-release has been studied in dosages of 360 to 400 mg daily with naltrexone sustained-release or immediate-release in dosages of 16 to 48 mg daily. A large phase III, randomized, double-blind, placebo-controlled trial evaluated use of this combination for 56 weeks. Results showed that when combined with diet and exercise, bupropion–naltrexone is generally well tolerated and can produce sustained weight loss of greater than 5% baseline body weight when used long term.[104] The effects on weight loss seem to be additive, as weight reduction was significantly greater with combination therapy in comparison to monotherapy and placebo.[104,105] Nausea, insomnia, headache, dizziness, and dry mouth have been reported as the most common side effects.[104,106] Because S.B. has a history of depression, either an SSRI or bupropion should be considered. However, her depression is not currently a problem and she would like to avoid this class of drugs.

LIPASE INHIBITORS

CASE 36-1, QUESTION 10: S.B. is concerned about the side effects of both the stimulant drugs and antidepressants, including how they may influence her blood pressure and cognitive ability. Thus her physician recommends that she start on orlistat 120 mg three times a day. Is this a good choice for S.B.? What is the mechanism of action of orlistat and the most common side effects that S.B. should be counseled about?

Orlistat (Xenical), an FDA-approved weight-loss medication, works to reduce dietary fat absorption by inhibiting GI (stomach and pancreatic) lipase activity.[107,108] Given S.B.'s concerns about CNS-acting drugs, this is a good choice for her. In February 2007, the FDA approved the OTC marketing of orlistat under the trade name, Alli at a 50% reduced dosage compared with the prescription product.[109] Orlistat is a hydrogenated derivative of lipstatin (a naturally occurring lipase inhibitor produced by *Streptomyces toxytricini*) that is a potent inhibitor of lipases and weak inhibitor of other intestinal hydrolases.[108] Gastric and pancreatic lipase are enzymes that play a pivotal role in the digestion of dietary fat (TG). Before digestion and absorption of dietary fat is possible, each TG molecule must be hydrolyzed by lipase enzymes into absorbable products—two fatty acid molecules and one 2-monoacylglycerol molecule. Orlistat inhibits lipase by binding to and inactivating the enzyme. Subsequently, TG cannot be absorbed, and approximately 30% of ingested fat is excreted in the feces.[108] The therapeutic activity of orlistat takes place in the stomach and small intestine and effects are seen as soon as 24 to 48 hours after dosing.

Orlistat does not exert appetite suppressant effects, has no CNS effects, and has no systemic absorption.[108] It is most effective if combined with a reduced fat and calorie diet[110] and is indicated to reduce the risk of weight regain after prior weight loss. It also is indicated for obese patients with an initial BMI greater than or equal to 30 kg/m^2, or greater than 27 kg/m^2 in the presence of other obesity-related risk factors. Orlistat is an appropriate addition to S.B.'s current diet and exercise program to promote additional weight gain. In a meta-analysis, orlistat was shown to produce average weight loss of 2.9 kg; orlistat also improved blood pressure and LDL and HDL concentrations.[86] GI adverse events were common, although there was no report of vitamin deficiencies. Orlistat may also reduce the risk of related diseases; in a 4-year study, orlistat plus lifestyle changes was associated with a 37% risk reduction of diabetes in greater than 3,300 obese patients.[111] Use of orlistat in combination with a low-fat diet is comparable to a low-carbohydrate ketogenic diet for improvements in metabolic parameters such as fasting serum lipid profiles and C-reactive protein.[112,113]

The most common adverse effects associated with orlistat include GI problems (loose stools, oily spotting, flatus with discharge, fecal urgency, fatty or oily stools, increased defecation, fecal incontinence, bloating, and cramping).[110] The most common adverse events reported are fatty or oily stool, fecal urgency, and oily spotting. The most common non-GI adverse effect was headache (6%). Side effects usually develop early in treatment and persist for 1 to 4 weeks, but occasionally last longer than 6 months. Because GI adverse effects are worse with a high-fat diet, orlistat may enhance dietary compliance with a low-fat diet. Side effects that continue to be problematic have been associated with nonadherence to orlistat therapy and therefore variability in patient outcomes.[114]

Orlistat may reduce the absorption of fat-soluble vitamins (A, D, E, and K) and patients should take a multivitamin supplement that contains these vitamins.[110] The supplement should be taken once a day at least 2 hours before or after the administration of orlistat, such as at bedtime. It may be appropriate to check vitamin D serum levels before starting therapy, and periodically throughout, due to high rates of vitamin D deficiency in the general population as well as the obese. Supplementation with higher doses of vitamin D may be necessary to prevent metabolic bone disease.[72] Orlistat may interfere with vitamin K absorption and potentiate the bleeding effects of warfarin. Orlistat may also reduce the absorption of amiodarone and cyclosporine. When used in diabetic patients, weight loss may be accompanied by improved control of diabetes, which requires a reduction in doses of diabetic medications, including insulin. Orlistat has additive effects when combined with lipid (cholesterol)-lowering agents such as pravastatin; thus, the dose of statins may be reduced.[108] The dosage of prescription orlistat in adults is 120 mg three times daily (OTC dose is 60 mg three times daily), during (or up to 1 hour after) each main meal containing fat. If a meal occasionally is missed or contains no fat, the dose may be omitted. Dosages exceeding 120 mg three times daily do not provide additional benefit. S.B. should be counseled on a low-fat diet to decrease side effects related to fat malabsorption and be instructed to take a fat-soluble supplement daily.

ANTIEPILEPTICS

Topiramate is a second-generation antiepileptic agent also approved for the treatment of migraines, which acts as an agonist at γ-aminobutyric acid ($GABA_A$) receptors and as an antagonist at non–*N*-methyl-D-aspartic acid glutamate receptors. It has been shown to produce a dose-dependent weight loss between 1 and 8 kg and may also produce weight loss in patients with bipolar affective disorder.[115] In a pooled analysis of six studies with a wide range of dosages, topiramate produced a 6.5% weight loss compared with placebo at 6 months.[87] A long-term study evaluating topiramate use for 2 years showed dose-dependent weight loss up to 9.7% with topiramate 256 mg/day.[116] Paresthesia, CNS, and GI effects were commonly seen at higher doses.[87,116]

The mechanism by which weight loss occurs with topiramate is unclear, but may be related to a direct action on adipose tissue.[117] This has led to investigation of the effects of topiramate on improving metabolic parameters in obese patients with diabetes mellitus type 2. Parameters of fasting plasma glucose levels, glycosylated hemoglobin (Hgb A_{1c}), and blood pressure improved with topiramate use compared with placebo. However, the incidence of CNS and psychiatric events including paresthesia, dizziness, and difficulty with memory and concentration seem to preclude its use.[117–119] Topiramate was also studied with phentermine, but the FDA voted against this weight-loss combination due to its significant side effects including depression, anxiety, sleep disorders, other cognitive disorders, metabolic acidosis, increased heart rate, and teratogenicity.

Zonisamide has been studied in randomized controlled trials for weight loss in obese patients with and without binge eating.[120,121] It is thought to have activity-enhancing effects on serotonin and dopamine.[122] One double-blind, placebo-controlled study showed that the active treatment group lost an average of 6% of baseline body weight compared with the placebo group at the end of 4 months.[120] In the binge-eating population, tolerability was low for zonisamide and resulted in a 20% dropout rate.[121] More recently, a preliminary open-label investigation evaluated the effects of the combination of zonisamide at a target dose of 400 mg daily with bupropion 200 mg daily on weight loss in obese women, predicting that the effects of the two agents together on dopamine, norepinephrine, and serotonin may lead to greater weight loss than either agent alone and possibly reduce the seizure risk associated with bupropion. The zonisamide–bupropion group lost an average of 7.2 kg over the 12-week study, which was statistically greater than the average 2.9-kg weight loss with zonisamide alone. Adverse events reported with the combination therapy included anxiety, dry mouth, memory problems, difficulty concentrating, language and speech difficulty, irritability, lightheadedness, nausea, and constipation.[122] Further evaluation through large double-blind, placebo-controlled trials are necessary for recommendation of zonisamide for weight loss in obese patients.

INVESTIGATIONAL AGENTS

Lorcaserin, a selective serotonin type 2C receptor agonist, is one of the newest agents being investigated for weight loss and under review by the FDA. It is thought that specific selective affinity for this receptor 15 times that of the serotonin type 2A receptor and 100 times that for the serotonin type 2B receptor will promote weight loss through mechanisms similar to the nonselective serotonin agonists withdrawn from the market (fenfluramine and dexfenfluramine) without the cardiac adverse event profile.[123,124] Activation of the serotonin type 2C receptor helps to promote feelings of satiety as they are located in the hypothalamus, a major center for hunger and food intake regulation.[124] The serotonin type 2B receptor has been associated with cardiovascular adverse effects including valvulopathy of the nonselective agents as it is expressed on cardiac valvular interstitial cells, but not in the brain.[123]

Results from a multicenter, placebo-controlled, phase III trial randomly assigned patients with a BMI of 30 to 45 kg/m^2 or a BMI of 27 to 45 kg/m^2 with at least one coexisting condition (hypertension, dyslipidemia, cardiovascular disease, impaired glucose tolerance, or sleep apnea) to receive lorcaserin 10 mg or placebo twice daily. Lifestyle modification counseling to promote moderate exercise and caloric restriction was provided. After 1 year of treatment, the lorcaserin group was more successful with 47.5% of patients losing 5% or more of their baseline body weight versus 20.3% of the placebo group ($p < 0.05$).[123] Average weight loss in the lorcaserin group was 5.8% of baseline body weight at 1 year. The trial continued on for a second year where patients receiving active therapy were randomly assigned to continue lorcaserin or change to placebo. Results demonstrated maintained weight loss in 67.9% of patients that remained on lorcaserin therapy and had lost 5% of their body weight during the first year compared with 50.3% that were reassigned to receive placebo ($p < 0.05$). Therapy with lorcaserin was also associated with significant decreases in waist circumference, fasting glucose, Hgb A_{1c}, total cholesterol, LDL cholesterol, and triglycerides at year 1, but tended to increase in year 2.[123]

Adverse event profiles were carefully evaluated and no significant differences in valvulopathy were found with lorcaserin (2.7%) compared with placebo (2.3%, $p = 0.70$) at year 1. The incidence of valvulopathy was essentially the same in the placebo group (2.7%) at year 2 compared with the lorcaserin group (2.6%). The most common adverse events that have been reported with lorcaserin include headache and nausea, which tend to be mild and dissipate with time.[123,124]

Tesofensine, an investigational agent that inhibits noradrenalin, dopamine, and serotonin reuptake, was initially developed to treat neurodegenerative disease and found to produce weight loss in obese patients with Parkinson or Alzheimer disease.[105,125] Early results evaluating this agent for weight loss in combination with caloric restriction have shown dose-dependent reductions in weight up to 10.6% of baseline body weight after 24 weeks of therapy. Adverse reactions associated with tesofensine included nausea, constipation, diarrhea, insomnia, and dry mouth. Heart rate was significantly increased at all doses compared with placebo as was systolic heart rate at the highest dose of tesofensine. As with all currently available weight-loss medications, discontinuation of therapy was associated with weight regain.[125] Further studies are needed to evaluate the safety and efficacy profile of tesofensine in larger patient populations and for long-term use.

CASE 36-1, QUESTION 11: S.B. returns to her physician 2 years later. She has gained 21 kg and her BMI is now 37.2 kg/m^2. She reports discontinuing therapy with orlistat due to intolerable GI side effects and inability to maintain her weight with diet and exercise therapy after completion of the behavioral modification program in which she was participating. Laboratory tests provide the following results:

Blood pressure, 154/92 mm Hg
Fasting blood glucose, 162 mg/dL
TG, 354 mg/dL
Total cholesterol, 227 mg/dL
HDL, 35 mg/dL
LDL, 182 mg/dL

Her physician recommends S.B. be referred to a bariatric clinic for evaluation for surgical intervention for weight loss. How could a bariatric surgical procedure affect medication administration in S.B. postoperatively?

Surgery

Surgery should be used only for morbidly obese individuals (BMI $\geq$40, or $\geq$35 kg/m^2 with comorbid conditions) in whom behavioral or pharmacologic treatments have failed.[126] For severely obese patients (>100% more than normal weight), the most effective treatment is a surgical procedure to reduce the size of the stomach. Bariatric surgical procedures either reduce the absorptive surface of the GI tract resulting in malabsorption, or reduce the stomach volume so that the person feels full after a smaller meal. According to recent guidelines, gastric banding, vertical banded gastroplasty, Roux-en-Y gastric bypass, and biliopancreatic diversion are effective options, although the degree of weight loss and complications may differ.[127] Gastric bypass has been shown to produce a greater weight loss compared with gastroplasty procedures.[128] In addition, laparoscopic (vs. open surgical approaches) may be preferred for reducing postoperative complications and hospital stay.[127]

ONLINE CONTENT

For an illustration showing four surgical procedures for morbid obesity, go to http://thepoint.lww.com/AT10e.

The mortality rate from bariatric surgery is estimated to be 0.3% to 1.9% and literature has shown that centers that perform surgeries at high volume have better outcomes.[84] S.B. may be a potential candidate for a bariatric intervention as she has failed both behavioral and pharmacological interventions. Although she has successfully lost weight in the past, she has failed to maintain weight loss and continued to experience obesity-related conditions including diabetes mellitus type 2 and dyslipidemia. These comorbidities should be aggressively managed, as they are increasing her absolute risk of morbidity and mortality.

Some of the complications of bariatric surgery include nausea, stomach ulceration, stenosis, anemia, and cholelithiasis. Postsurgical precautions include careful evaluation of meal sizes and timing along with meal content, especially immediately after surgery. Patients should be aware that they will not be able to resume their normal eating habits, and they should be properly educated on lifestyle modifications for maintenance of weight loss. In addition, medications and adequate intake of necessary nutrients are important considerations after surgery. Medications such as nonsteroidal anti-inflammatory drugs, salicylates, and bisphosphonates may cause ulcerations, and medications that are delayed-release or extended-release may not be absorbed owing to changes in gastric size.[129] Medications may need to be administered using liquid formulation and other dosage routes. Transdermal formulations need to be carefully dosed to account for changes in body surface area postsurgically.[129]

KEY REFERENCES AND WEBSITES

A full list of references for this chapter can be found at http://thepoint.lww.com/AT10e. Below are the key references and websites for this chapter, with the corresponding reference number in this chapter found in parentheses after the reference.

Key References

Kaplan LM. Pharmacologic therapies for obesity. *Gastroenterol Clin N Am.* 2010;39:69. (72)

Miller AD, Smith KM. Medication and nutrient administration considerations after bariatric surgery. *Am J Health Syst Pharm.* 2006;63:1852. (129)

National Institutes of Health. The Practical Guide. Identification, Evaluation, and Treatment of Overweight and Obesity in Adults. NIH Publication No. 02-4084. Bethesda, MD: National Heart, Lung, and Blood Institute, National Institutes of Health, US Department of Health and Human Services; 2000. (2)

Key Websites

Centers for Disease Control and Prevention. Division of Nutrition, Physical Activity, and Obesity (DNPAO). http://www.cdc.gov/obesity/. Accessed June 24, 2011.

US Department of Health and Human Services. Healthy People 2020: summary of objectives. http://www.healthypeople.gov/2020/topicsobjectives2020/pdfs/NutritionandWeight.pdf. Accessed November 15, 2010. (4)

US Department of Health and Human Services. National Institute of Diabetes and Digestive and Kidney Diseases (NIDDK). Weight-Control Information Network. http://win.niddk.nih.gov/. Accessed June 24, 2011.

37

Adult Enteral Nutrition

Carol J. Rollins and Jennifer H. Baggs

CORE PRINCIPLES

		CHAPTER CASES
1	Patients should be assessed for the appropriate timing and route for nutrition support.	Case 37-1 (Questions 1, 2)
2	The type of tube placement and site of formula delivery is determined by several factors.	Case 37-2 (Question 1)
3	Formula selection is based on nutrient requirements, fluid restrictions, and the extent of impaired digestion and absorption.	Case 37-2 (Questions 2–5)
4	The administration regimen for feeding is influenced by the feeding route, formula selected, and duration of feeding.	Case 37-2 (Questions 6–8)
5	While the preferred route for nutrition intervention in critical illness is enteral, the ideal formula composition remains unresolved.	Case 37-3 (Questions 1–4)
6	Macronutrient content should be considered when selecting an enteral formula for patients with diabetes.	Case 37-4 (Question 1)
7	Appropriate monitoring is essential to recognize and prevent complications associated with enteral nutrition.	Case 37-4 (Question 2)
8	Medication administration through a feeding tube requires selection of appropriate dosage forms and proper preparation.	Case 37-4 (Question 3)
9	Feeding tube occlusion is a common problem influenced by medication-related and non–medication-related factors.	Case 37-4 (Question 4)
10	Patients must meet strict criteria for Medicare coverage of home enteral nutrition.	Case 37-5 (Question 1)
11	Diarrhea in patients receiving enteral nutrition is multifactorial, including both tube-feeding–related and non–tube-feeding-related causes.	Case 37-6 (Question 1)

Enteral nutrition refers to nutrition provided via the gastrointestinal (GI) tract. However, as the term is commonly used, enteral nutrition (EN) is synonymous with delivery of nutrients into the GI tract by tube (e.g., nasogastric or jejunostomy feeding). Tube feeding allows continued use of the GI tract when one or more steps in the normal process of obtaining nutrients from oral intake are disrupted. Table 37-1 lists functional anatomic units of the GI tract along with major steps occurring in preparing nutrients for absorption and examples of conditions potentially impairing each region. Chewing or swallowing may be completely disrupted, but some digestive and absorptive function must remain for tube feeding to be a viable option.

Patient Selection and Route of Feeding

CASE 37-1

QUESTION 1: O.D., a 44-year-old woman, 5 feet 4 inches tall, 100 kg, was brought to the emergency department (ED) last night complaining of severe left-sided upper abdominal pain. Tests performed in the ED were consistent with acute pancreatitis. O.D. was admitted to the hospital and has "nothing by mouth" (NPO) orders in her chart. The gastroenterology service was consulted; endoscopic retrograde cholangiopancreatography (ERCP) is scheduled for tomorrow. A nutrition support consult was ordered. O.D. is

TABLE 37-1
Functional Units of the Gastrointestinal Tract

Functional Unit	Major Steps	Conditions/Diseases Disrupting Function
Mouth and oropharynx	Chew and lubricate food; swallow; taste	Amyotrophic lateral sclerosis, muscular dystrophy, severe RA, CVA, end-stage Parkinson disease, paralysis, coma. Anorexia due to other disease: cardiac or cancer cachexia, renal failure and uremia, liver failure, neurologic disease.
Esophagus	Transport food to the stomach	Esophageal ulcer, cancer, obstruction, or fistula; esophagectomy; CVA.
Stomach	Hold food for mixing and grinding; add acid and enzymes; release chyme to small bowel; osmoregulation	Severe gastritis or ulceration, gastroparesis, gastric outlet obstruction, gastric cancer, severe gastroesophageal reflux.
Duodenum	Osmoregulation; neutralize stomach acid	Severe duodenal ulcer or fistula; cancer: gastric or pancreatic; surgical resection or bypass of the duodenum: Whipple-type procedures.
Small bowel: jejunum and ileum	Digestion; absorption	Enterocutaneous fistula, severe enteric infection, malnutrition, malabsorption, Crohn's disease, celiac disease, ileus and dysmotility syndrome.
Pancreas	Secretion of digestive enzymes	Pancreatitis, pancreatic cancer, pancreatic injury, pancreatic fistula.
Colon	Absorb fluid; ferment soluble fiber and unabsorbed carbohydrate; absorb water	Ulcerative colitis, Crohn's disease, colon cancer, colocutaneous fistula, colovaginal fistula, diverticulitis, colitis of any etiology, colon surgery.

CVA, cerebrovascular accident; RA, rheumatoid arthritis.

currently receiving intravenous (IV) 5% dextrose/0.9% sodium chloride with KCl 20 mEq/L at 150 mL/hour. She is also receiving hydromorphone via a patient-controlled analgesia (PCA) pump.

O.D. has been having crampy upper right quadrant pain on and off for about a month and saw her primary care physician two weeks ago. She is allergic (rash) to sulfa. She was told that her problem was most likely her gallbladder and she might need surgery if her symptoms continued or the pain worsened. In addition, her doctor said blood pressure and glucose control "needed improvement" and mentioned it might be because her weight was up 10 pounds. She does not smoke; she occasionally drinks a glass of wine with dinner.

Laboratory values this morning are as follows:

Sodium, 137 mEq/L
Potassium, 3.9 mEq/L
Blood urea nitrogen (BUN), 7 mg/dL
Serum creatinine (SCr), 0.9 mg/dL
Glucose, 175 mg/dL
Albumin, 3.7 g/dL
Amylase, 625 units/L (down from 906 units/L in the ED)
Lipase, 749 units/L (down from 1,014 in the ED
Triglycerides, 192 mg/dL
White blood cells (WBC), 12.7 × $10^3/\mu L$
Hemoglobin (Hgb), 12.1 g/dL
Hematocrit (Hct), 36.2%

Does O.D. require nutritional intervention at this time? When should nutrition intervention be considered for O.D.?

Patients generally are considered at risk for nutrient depletion and associated increased morbidity and mortality when intake is inadequate to meet nutritional requirements for 5 to 7 days or when weight loss exceeds 10% of pre-illness weight within a 6-month period.[1,2] For adequately nourished patients, specialized nutrition support is generally not warranted when support will be needed for fewer than 7 to 10 days.[3] Undernourished patients require nutritional intervention sooner. See Chapter 35, Basics of Nutrition and Patient Assessment, for further information on malnutrition. O.D. was adequately nourished before admission based on her weight for height and serum albumin. She has weight gain per the clinic visit and has been NPO for less than 24 hours. Nutrition support is not warranted at this time. However, once the ERCP has been completed, the need for nutrition intervention should be reassessed. If O.D. must remain NPO for a week or more, nutritional intervention would be warranted. Obesity does not preclude the need for nutritional intervention.

CASE 37-1, QUESTION 2: What route of nutrition intervention would be most appropriate for O.D. if she cannot restart her diet in a timely manner?

Routes of nutrition intervention may include modified oral diet, including oral supplements or altered consistency diets (e.g., thickened liquids, pureed foods), EN by tube, or parenteral nutrition (PN). Tube feeding is considered the route of choice in patients with a functional GI tract in whom oral nutrient intake is contraindicated or is insufficient to meet estimated needs.[1,3] Other than potential "gallstone" pancreatitis, O.D. is expected to have a functional GI tract. The ERCP and pain symptoms will help determine whether O.D. will remain NPO or have a diet started. It appears her pancreatitis is improving based on decreasing amylase and lipase values. For patients with severe acute pancreatitis, Society of Critical Care Medicine (SCCM) and American Society for Parenteral and Enteral Nutrition (ASPEN) Critical Care (SACC) guidelines recommend initiation of EN as soon as volume resuscitation is complete.[4] For patients such as O.D. with mild to moderate acute pancreatitis, symptoms typically resolve before nutrition intervention is necessary. When symptoms are prolonged and nutrition support is required, EN is the preferred route of nutrition support because EN may reduce the inflammatory response and decrease complications.[4–6]

EN may be appropriate for patients with the disorders listed in Table 37-1, depending on the extent to which normal intake, transport, digestion, and absorption of nutrients is impaired. Clinical circumstances, not specific diagnoses, should be the determining factor for initiating tube feeding. EN should be used with caution in patients with severe necrotizing or hemorrhagic pancreatitis, distal high-output enterocutaneous fistulae, hypotension with significant inotropic support, GI ischemia, and partial bowel obstruction.[1,3,4] Contraindications to EN generally include diffuse peritonitis, complete bowel obstruction, severe paralytic ileus, intractable vomiting or diarrhea, severe malabsorption, severe GI bleed, inability to access the GI tract, and when aggressive intervention is not warranted or desired.

Frequent reassessment is recommended because patients may become candidates for EN as the condition improves or resolves.

Feeding Tube Placement and Site of Formula Delivery

CASE 37-2

QUESTION 1: B.A., a 78-year-old man, was hospitalized 5 days ago after collapsing while at the bank. He was diagnosed with ischemic stroke and his condition has changed little since admission. B.A. is estimated to be 5 feet 11 inches tall; his weight is 62 kg. His maintenance IV drip is 5% dextrose/0.45% sodium chloride with KCl 10 mEq/L at 80 mL/hour. Laboratory evaluation today shows the following:

Sodium, 140 mEq/L
Potassium, 3.6 mEq/L
Chloride, 104 mEq/L
Glucose, 89 mg/dL
SCr, 0.8 mg/dL
Serum albumin, 3.1 g/dL

Due to failing his swallow study today, B.A. will remain NPO for at least 4 weeks until after a repeat swallow study is done. Nutrition support via tube feeding is ordered.

What is the most appropriate type of feeding tube placement and site for formula delivery?

The type of tube placement and site of formula delivery for EN are determined by the anticipated duration of tube feeding, disrupted region or process in the GI tract, and the risk of aspiration. Figure 37-1 illustrates the two basic types of tube placement—nasal versus ostomy—and the sites available for formula delivery (i.e., gastric, duodenal, or jejunal). The name of the feeding route usually includes both the type of tube placement and the site of formula delivery. For example, nasogastric (NG) indicates nasal placement with gastric delivery of formula, whereas gastrostomy indicates ostomy placement with gastric delivery of formula.

Nasal tube placement is preferred for short-term use in patients expected to resume oral feeding and without obstruction of nasal, pharyngeal, or esophageal passages. The tube is secured to the nose or cheek after placement to prevent the tube from being displaced.

ONLINE CONTENT **For an illustration of an NG tube, go to http://thepoint.lww.com/AT10e.**

Clinically evident injury from nasal intubation is very low, but patients may suffer mucosal trauma in the nasopharynx.[7–9] Pharyngitis, sinusitis, otitis media, and incompetence of the lower esophageal sphincter are associated with nasal tubes, especially large-bore tubes. The incidence of inadvertent pulmonary placement of small-bore feeding tubes is 4% or less.[7] Radiographic confirmation of tube placement is mandatory to rule out pleural perforation and pulmonary intubation in unconscious patients and remains the standard to ensure correct tube placement in all patients. Tube displacement is a potential complication occurring in 25% to 41% of cases.[7]

Feeding ostomies (tube enterostomies) generally are reserved for long-term EN, interpreted as anywhere from 4 weeks to 6 months, depending on clinical circumstances and the type of tube enterostomy placed. Access for enterostomies can be achieved through open surgery, laparoscopy, or via percutaneous access. Percutaneous access is usually performed under local anesthesia or conscious sedation by endoscope (percutaneous endoscopic gastrostomy [PEG] or jejunostomy [PEJ]) or by radiography (percutaneous radiologic gastrostomy [PRG] or jejunostomy), including fluoroscopy, ultrasound, or computed tomography.[7,10,11] The major advantage of radiologic compared with endoscopic placement is reduced contamination of the puncture site by oral pharyngeal microorganisms, which are implicated in the 5.4% to 30% incidence of site infections.[9] Most patients requiring long-term EN receive either a PEG or PRG.

ONLINE CONTENT **For an illustration of a PEG, go to http://thepoint.lww.com/AT10e.**

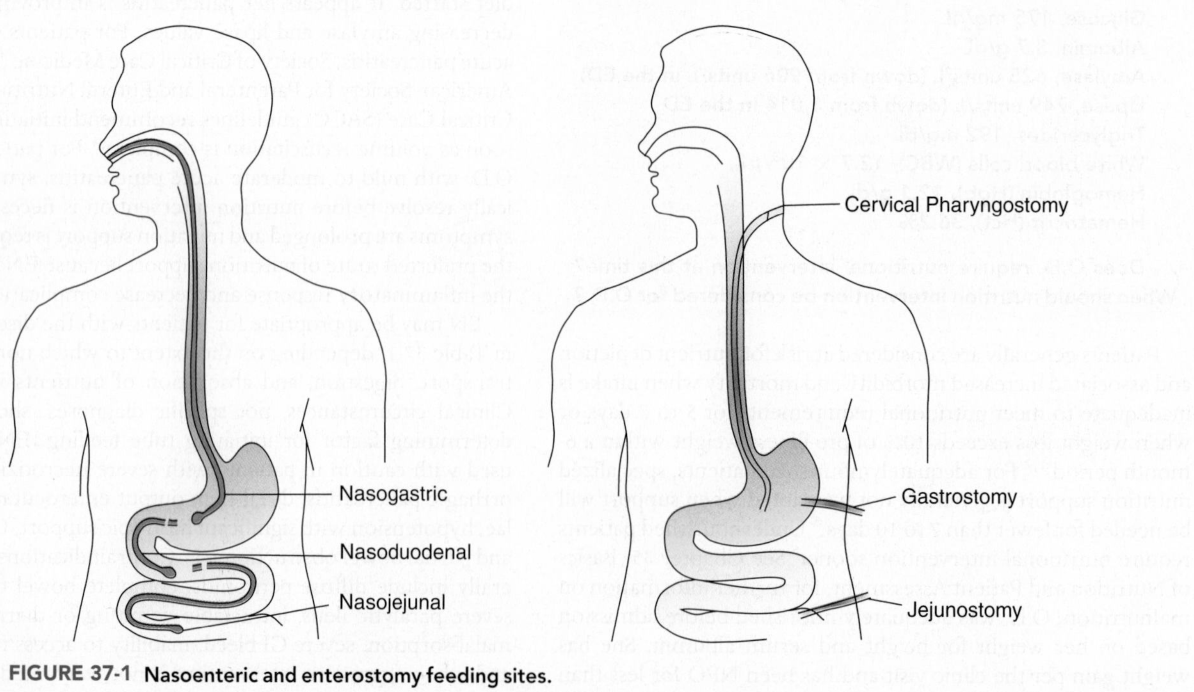

FIGURE 37-1 Nasoenteric and enterostomy feeding sites.

The 2006 Nationwide Inpatient Sample database, which represents 20% of nonfederal discharges within the United States, included 187,597 discharges in which a PEG or a PEG with combined gastric and jejeunal access (PEGJ or G-J tube) was performed, and of those, 96% were PEGs.[12]

Endoscopic placement is contraindicated when obstruction prevents passage of the endoscope, but radiographic placement may be possible in such cases. Relative contraindications to percutaneous feeding tube placement include inability to see the endoscopic light through the abdominal wall (e.g., morbid obesity, massive ascites), peritoneal dialysis, coagulopathy, gastric varices, portal hypertension, hepatomegaly, and neoplastic or infiltrative disease of the gastric or jejunal wall.[7–11,13] Prior total or subtotal gastrectomy prevents percutaneous gastrostomy placement, but percutaneous jejunostomy may be possible. Major advantages of percutaneous access are shorter procedure time and lower cost; morbidity and mortality appear to be similar to surgical feeding tube access.[8,13] Major complications, such as aspiration, peritonitis, hemorrhage, gastrocutaneous fistula formation, necrotizing fasciitis, gastric perforation, and migration of the tube through the gastric wall are generally low but have been reported in up to 2.5% of patients.[7,14]

Formula delivery into the stomach is preferred when feasible because it is the most physiologically normal feeding site. Stimulation of normal digestive processes and hormonal responses associated with eating occur with gastric feeding. The stomach serves as a reservoir, typically allowing tolerance of bolus, and intermittent or continuous feeding. Gastric feeding requires adequate gastric motility to prevent accumulation of formula in the stomach. Patients with gastric outlet obstruction, gastroparesis, gastric distension, or gastroesophageal reflux are poor candidates for gastric feeding.

Transpyloric feeding into the duodenum or jejunum may be appropriate when gastric dysfunction or disease is present, for early postoperative feeding when gastric emptying may be impaired, when pancreatic stimulation is to be avoided, or when risk of aspiration is high. Critically ill patients are at risk for aspiration and ventilator-associated pneumonia, with a 25% to 40% incidence of aspiration in patients with long-term nasoenteric feeding.[15,16] However, evidence of reduced aspiration and improved outcomes with postpyloric feeding remains controversial.[4] Poor differentiation between aspiration of oral secretions and aspiration of feedings may result in erroneously high rates being reported for aspiration of postpyloric feedings. Tube placement beyond the ligament of Treitz may be best for patients at risk of tube migration and aspiration; however, studies are not conclusive, and either gastric or small bowel feeding is considered acceptable in the intensive care unit (ICU) setting.

B.A. will require EN for at least 4 weeks and may require longer-term EN depending on the results of the repeat swallow study. A feeding ostomy is appropriate for him. Because there does not appear to be a contraindication to feeding into the stomach, a gastrostomy is appropriate. He will likely have a PEG or PRG placed to avoid the need for surgery.

FORMULA SELECTION

CASE 37-2, QUESTION 2: What factors should be considered in selecting an enteral formula for B.A.?

Enteral formula selection is based on nutrient requirements, fluid restrictions, and the extent of impaired digestion and absorption. Many enteral formulas are available, but because of similarities between products, institutional formularies are generally limited but still provide an adequate selection to meet a variety of patient needs. Categorizing formulas as listed in Table 37-2 simplifies the formula selection process. There are three major categories of enteral formulas: (a) polymeric formulas, (b) oligomeric formulas, and (c) specialized formulas.

Polymeric Formulas

Polymeric formulas are designed for patients with full digestive capability and are used most often. Osmolality is decreased and palatability increased in these formulas by use of relatively intact nutrients, including whole (i.e., intact) proteins. Administration of approximately 1.5 to 2 L of most polymeric formulas provides 100% of Dietary Reference Intakes (DRI) for vitamins and minerals; thus, these formulas sometimes are called "complete" formulas.[17] As indicated in Table 37-2, the relative cost for polymeric formulas tends to be less than that of oligomeric or specialized formulas, although prices can vary considerably based on specific nutrient content (e.g., omega-3 fatty acids [ω-3FAs], fiber).

Oligomeric Formulas

Oligomeric formulas, also called predigested, monomeric, or chemically defined formulas, are designed for patients with reduced digestive function. Pancreatic enzyme activity is required for digestion of oligosaccharides (carbohydrates) and fats. Brush-border disaccharidase activity also is required. Minimal digestion is required, however, for the hydrolyzed protein and medium-chain triglyceride (MCT) components. These formulas can be used for patients with pancreatic insufficiency, reduced mucosal absorption, or reduced hydrolytic capability. Patients most likely to benefit from oligomeric formulas are those with severe pancreatic insufficiency or short bowel syndrome.[1] Although the Canadian Clinical Practice (CCP) guidelines noted patients with these and other GI complications may benefit from oligomeric formulas, insufficient data were available to make recommendations regarding use of such formulas.[18,19] Pancreatic enzyme supplementation combined with polymeric formulas may be tried before oligomeric formulas for some patients with pancreatic insufficiency (e.g., cystic fibrosis, chronic pancreatitis).

Two subgroups of oligomeric formulas can be differentiated based on the protein source. True "elemental" formulas contain free amino acids, whereas "peptide-based" formulas contain oligopeptides plus dipeptides, tripeptides, and free amino acids from hydrolysis of protein. Amino acids require no digestion, but the sodium-dependent active transport mechanism appears to be somewhat slow and inefficient with only about one-third of dietary protein absorbed as free amino acids; the remaining two-thirds are absorbed as dipeptides and tripeptides.[20,21] Specific carriers for absorption of dipeptides and tripeptides, located in small bowel mucosa, do not compete with the free–amino-acid transport system. Peptides longer than three amino acids require further hydrolysis within the lumen of the small bowel before they are absorbed. Most peptide-based formulas contain a significant portion of peptides that require hydrolysis before absorption. No well-designed, randomized, controlled trials have clearly delineated clinical differences in elemental (free amino acid) versus peptide-based formulas. Elemental formulas generally have the lowest fat content (10% or less of calories from fat). Peptide formulas typically contain one-fourth to one-third of calories from fat, but provide 20% to 70% of the fat as MCT to minimize the risk of malabsorption.

Oligomeric formulas are typically hypertonic owing to their partially digested nature, although peptide-containing formulas tend to be less hypertonic than free–amino-acid products. Osmotic diarrhea can occur because of the hyperosmolality;

TABLE 37-2

Generic Groups and Subgroups of Enteral Formulas with Relative Costs[a]

Type of Formula	Relative Cost[b]	Examples
Polymeric Formulas[c]		
STANDARD CALORIC DENSITY, STANDARD (OR HIGH NITROGEN[d]) CONTENT WITH VARIED fiber CONTENT		
Fiber free for oral supplement or tube feeding	$	Ensure; Nutren 1.0
Low fiber (from 1 up to 9 g /1,000 kcal)	$	Nutren Probalance[d]
Moderate fiber (>9 to <14 g/1,000 kcal)	$	Ensure with fiber; Fibersource HN[d]
High fiber (≥14 g/1,000 kcal)	$	Glucerna; Jevity 1.2 Cal[d]; Nutren 1.0 with fiber
STANDARD NITROGEN CONTENT, fiber-FREE (OR LOW fiber[e]) WITH VARIED CALORIC DENSITY		
Standard caloric density (1–1.2 kcal/mL)	$	Ensure; Nutren 1.0
Moderate density (1.5 kcal/mL)	$	Boost Plus; Ensure Plus; Isosource 1.5 Cal[e]; Nutren 1.5
Calorically dense (1.8–2 kcal/mL)	$	Nutren 2.0
STANDARD CALORIC DENSITY, fiber-FREE WITH VARIED NITROGEN (PROTEIN) CONTENT		
Low nitrogen (6%–10% of kcal as protein)	$	Resource Breeze
Standard nitrogen (11%–16% of kcal as protein)	$	Ensure; Nutren 1.0
High nitrogen (17%–20% of kcal as protein)	$	Isosource HN; Osmolite 1.2 Cal
Very high nitrogen (>20% of kcal as protein)	$$	Boost High Protein; Promote; Replete
Oligomeric Formulas		
Elemental (free amino acids)[f]	&&	f.a.a.; Tolerex; Vivonex T.E.N.
PEPTIDE-BASED		
Standard protein	&	Peptamen; Peptamen with Prebio
High protein	&	Peptamen 1.5
Very high protein (NPC:N <100:1; >20% calories as protein)	&&	Crucial; Peptamen AF; Peptamen VHP
Specialized Formulas		
RENAL FAILURE		
Essential amino acid enriched[f]	&&&&	Renalcal
Polymeric, low electrolyte (less than standard potassium, phosphorus, and magnesium)	$$$$	
• Low nitrogen		Suplena
• Standard nitrogen		Novasource Renal
• High nitrogen (for dialysis)		Nepro
Hepatic failure (high BCAA, low AAA[f])	&&&&	Nutrihep
STRESS OR CRITICALLY ILL		
Branched-chain enriched	&&&	
High nitrogen plus conditionally essential nutrients	$$	
Immune modulating	&&	Oxepa
Pulmonary disease (standard; not IMP)	$$	Nutren Pulmonary; Pulmocare
Glucose control	$$$$	Diabetisource AC; Glucerna; Nutren Glytrol

[a] Based on average cost per 1,000 calories for equivalent formulas on University of Arizona Medical Center contract from 2008–2010.
[b] Index product is a standard caloric density, standard nitrogen content, fiber-free formula. Cost is indicated relative to an index product given a value of 1:
$ = same cost as index product, up to 1.5 times that cost per 1,000 calories
$$ = cost is 1.6 to 2.5 times the cost of the index product per 1,000 calories
$$$ = cost is 2.6 to 3.5 times the cost of the index product per 1,000 calories
$$$$ = cost is 3.6 to 4.5 times the cost of the index product per 1,000 calories
& = cost is 11 to 15 times the cost of the index product per 1,000 calories
&& = cost is 16 to 20 times the cost of the index product per 1,000 calories
&&& = cost is 20 to 24 times the cost of the index product per 1,000 calories
&&&& = cost is 25 to 30 times the cost of the index product per 1,000 calories
[c] All products listed in the table are lactosefree.
[d] High nitrogen.
[e] Low fiber.
[f] Special order, not on formulary used for price calculations.
AAA, aromatic amino acids; BCAA, branched-chain amino acids; IMP, immune-modulating pulmonary; NPC:N, nonprotein calorie to nitrogen ratio.

however, the CCP guidelines meta-analysis found no difference in diarrhea occurrence between patients receiving intact protein and those receiving peptide-rich formulas.[18,20] Taste and cost are disadvantages of oligomeric formulas. Flavoring packets are available and newer formulas may be better accepted, but patients commonly complain of a bitter taste when these formulas are taken orally. In general, patients do not tolerate adequate oral consumption of an oligomeric formula to meet daily requirements. As shown in Table 37-2, the cost of oligomeric formulas tends to be greater than ten times the cost of polymeric formulas.

Specialized Formulas

Specialized formulas are designed for specific disease states or conditions; however, clinical benefits are often controversial. Formulas generally have a good theoretic basis for use, yet many lack conclusive clinical evidence of improved efficacy compared with standard formulas. Well-designed studies showing a difference in outcome between specialized and standard enteral formulas providing equal nitrogen and equal calories are limited for most types of specialized formulas. As shown in Table 37-2, there are several different types of specialized formulas; costs and evidence for use vary greatly among them.

B.A. requires EN because he cannot adequately protect his airway when swallowing. There is no evidence presented to suggest he has problems with digestion or absorption. One of the polymeric formulas on the hospital EN formulary should be selected for B.A. The choice of polymeric formula can be narrowed by several factors, including requirements for calories, protein, fluid and fiber, as well as potential nutrient intolerances.

CASE 37-2, QUESTION 3: What are B.A.'s requirements for calories, protein, and fluid? Does he have any special nutrient requirements?

B.A.'s nutrient requirements must be assessed before proceeding in the selection of enteral formula. Based on his weight–height ratio and serum albumin concentration, B.A. has mild to moderate malnutrition. Low serum albumin in the elderly is a risk factor for malnutrition, sarcopenia, and mortality.[22] Mild visceral protein depletion may have resulted from metabolic stress associated with his stroke. Weight loss to 82% of ideal body weight ([IBW], 75.3 kg) most likely is owing to chronic deficiency in total energy intake, but may also be associated with significant loss of lean mass, especially in older men.[23]

Because B.A. has an IBW less than the ideal for his height, his actual weight should be used to estimate energy and protein requirements. Use of IBW to estimate requirements for undernourished patients may result in fluid and electrolyte imbalance. Once the patient is stabilized on nutrition support, calories can be increased, if necessary, to achieve weight gain.

B.A.'s level of metabolic stress is relatively low. He has no surgical wounds, fractures or skeletal trauma, burns, or major infections. Therefore, caloric requirements are only slightly higher than basal needs. Although the term calorie is used interchangeably with kilocalorie (kcal) in nutrition literature, the large "Calorie" or kilocalorie technically is correct and energy requirements generally are listed as kcal/day or kcal/kg body weight when specific numbers are given for a patient. See Chapter 35, Basics of Nutrition and Patient Assessment, for methods of determining nutrient requirements. An estimation of 20 to 25 kcal/kg actual weight can be used based on B.A.'s low level of metabolic stress, but higher caloric intake (25 to 30 kcal/kg/day) may be needed for weight gain after he is stable.

Protein requirements for healthy elderly people are estimated to be to be 1 g/kg/day, which is slightly higher than the DRI of 0.8 g/kg/day.[17,24] Mild visceral protein depletion and metabolic stress are expected to increase B.A.'s protein needs to at least 1 to 1.2 g/kg actual weight per day. Renal function appears adequate for B.A. to tolerate up to 1.2 g/kg/day without experiencing azotemia. SCr, however, may provide a poor estimate of renal function in underweight patients owing to less-than-normal muscle mass.

Daily fluid requirements for geriatric patients can be estimated at 30 to 35 mL/kg, with a minimum of 1,500 mL daily, plus replacement of excess losses from hyperthermia, vomiting, or diarrhea.[1,24] Baseline requirements of 1,500 mL for the first 20 kg plus 20 mL per each additional kilogram of body weight also can be used to estimate fluid requirements. Based on caloric intake, fluid requirements can be estimated as 1 mL/kcal ingested.[1] B.A. does not appear to have any excess fluid losses at this time; therefore, calculation of baseline fluid requirements should provide adequate fluids.

B.A.'s estimated daily requirements are approximately 1,240 to 1,550 total calories, 62 to 74 g protein, and 1,860 to 2,168 mL of fluid. These are estimated requirements that should be adjusted based on frequent reassessment of B.A.'s response to therapy and changes in his clinical situation. Additional calories and protein may be needed for repletion of weight and protein status.

B.A.'s apparently suboptimal nutrition before hospitalization increases his risk for vitamin deficiencies (see Chapter 35, Basics of Nutrition and Patient Assessment). Medical, medication, and dietary histories should be evaluated to determine nutritional risks associated with specific conditions. B.A.'s age, along with his acute illness and mild to moderate mixed protein-calorie malnutrition, increase his risk of vitamin deficiencies, and it is likely that he has at least some subclinical deficiencies. He should receive at least 100% of the DRI for vitamins and minerals daily.[17] If actual deficiencies are identified, B.A. will require higher, therapeutic doses for the specific vitamins that are deficient.

B.A. may be at risk of refeeding syndrome. His weight is low (82% of IBW), although his body mass index is acceptable at 18.9 kg/m^2. Chronic malnutrition can lead to intracellular depletion of potassium, phosphorus, and magnesium, while serum concentrations are maintained. When specialized nutrition support begins, refeeding syndrome may develop as these electrolytes move from the extracellular space into the cells, causing a decrease in serum concentrations during the first few days of feeding.[25] Failure to monitor the patient and replace electrolytes as necessary can result in serious electrolyte abnormalities. Knowing B.A.'s weight history, particularly recent weight loss, and his diet history could help assess his potential for clinically significant electrolyte and fluid abnormalities associated with refeeding syndrome.

CASE 37-2, QUESTION 4: Which category of polymeric formulas would be most appropriate for B.A. based on his estimated nutritional requirements?

Polymeric formulas can be divided into several categories based on nutrient sources, caloric density, and protein content. Each category should be evaluated because formula characteristics overlap between the categories.

NUTRIENT SOURCE

Polymeric formulas can be subgrouped based on lactose content. Hospitalized patients are presumed to be lactose intolerant due to reduced disaccharidase production during fasting, malnutrition, and various GI tract diseases.[26,27] In addition, most ethnic groups, except northern Europeans, have reduced lactase production in adulthood, leading to lactose intolerance. Lactose ingestion can cause bloating, flatulence, abdominal cramps, and watery diarrhea in patients with permanent or transient lactose intolerance. Lactosefree formulas are the standard for tube-fed adults. Most enteral products are lactosefree, except the powdered products reconstituted with milk and generally intended for oral consumption. Proteins, even those derived from milk, do not contribute to lactose content because lactose is a carbohydrate. The majority of enteral formulas are also glutenfree to avoid GI symptoms associated with celiac disease.

CALORIC DENSITY

Caloric density influences the volume of formula needed to meet nutrient requirements. Standard caloric density is 1 to 1.2 kcal/mL. Table 37-3 lists the general descriptions for caloric density and macronutrient quantities in enteral formulas. Increased caloric density increases formula osmolality. Gastric emptying can be reduced when osmolality exceeds 800 mOsm/kg and this may result in feeding intolerance.[28] GI intolerance (e.g., nausea, flatulence, abdominal discomfort) also can occur if the capacity of intestinal enzymes is overwhelmed by infusion of a calorically dense formula.

TABLE 37-3

General Descriptions of Macronutrient Quantity in Enteral Formulas

	Caloric Density (kcal/mL)	Free Water (%)	Nitrogen (Protein) Content (% kcal as protein)	NPC:N	Fiber Content (g/1,000 kcal)
Low	<1	>85%	6%–10%	>220:1	1–9
Standard	1–1.2	80%–85%	11%–16%	200:1–130:1	None
Moderate	1.5	75%–80%			>9 to <14
High	1.8–2	65%–75%	17%–20%	125:1–100:1	≥14
Very high			>20%	<100:1	

NPC:N, nonprotein calorie to nitrogen ratio.

Caloric density reflects the free-water content of EN formulas. Risk of dehydration increases with increasing caloric density; however, standard caloric density formulas can result in fluid overload in patients with congestive heart failure, renal failure, or other fluid-sensitive conditions. Calculation of water provided by EN helps determine the volume of additional fluid that must be provided to meet daily fluid requirements. Free-water content is generally 80% to 85% (800 mL to 850 mL per liter of formula) for formulas with 1 to 1.2 kcal/mL. Table 37-3 lists free-water content associated with other caloric densities. The available history for B.A. does not suggest a need for fluid restriction; therefore, it would be reasonable to initiate feedings with a standard caloric density product (1 to 1.2 kcal/mL).

PROTEIN CONTENT

Protein needs increase disproportionately to caloric needs during injury and critical illness, whereas protein tolerance may limit protein provision in other conditions. To meet the need for varying ratios between calories and protein, polymeric formulas are available with a range from low to very high protein content. Either percentage of calories from protein or nonprotein calories to nitrogen (NPC:N) ratio can be used to define protein content. Table 37-3 lists the general descriptions for protein content. High-nitrogen enteral formulas are designed for patients with an increased protein requirement without a proportional increase in caloric needs. Formulas providing greater than 20% of calories as protein or with an NPC:N under 100:1 may be referred to as very-high-nitrogen formulas and are generally intended for critically ill patients or those with large wounds to heal. Low-nitrogen formulas are available for patients requiring protein restriction. Some low-nitrogen formulas are designed for patients with reduced renal function and can be classified as specialized formulas.

B.A. could obtain adequate protein from a formula with standard protein content. A formula with slightly higher protein content (17%–18% of calories) would also be acceptable. A high-nitrogen formula that meets B.A.'s calorie needs will provide protein at the upper end of the estimated requirement (1.2 g/kg/day), whereas a standard nitrogen formula will provide between 0.8 and 1 g/kg/day. A high-nitrogen formula may replete B.A.'s somatic and visceral protein status sooner but it may not provide adequate calories for weight gain. The decision to use a high-nitrogen versus standard-nitrogen formula depends on the exact nutrient composition of product formulations on the EN formulary.

CASE 37-2, QUESTION 5: Should the EN product selected for B.A. contain fiber and if so, what type and amount?

Fiber has potential physiologic benefits, including increased fecal bulk, decreased bowel transit time in patients susceptible to constipation, increased transit time in patients with diarrhea, reduction of serum cholesterol, and improved glycemic control in patients with diabetes. Recommended daily fiber intake for healthy Americans is 21 to 25 g for women and 30 to 38 g for men, with the lower end of these amounts for people 51 years of age or older.[29,30] Adequate intake is determined by calorie intake and fiber intake observed to protect against coronary artery disease (14 g/1,000 calories). Optimal fiber intake for ill persons has not been determined. Fiber-supplemented formulas vary considerably in fiber content. There is no standardized terminology for low-fiber, moderate-fiber, and high-fiber content; however, the amounts listed in Table 37-3 can serve as a general guideline.

Enteral formulas may contain either insoluble or soluble fiber, or both. Insoluble fiber is associated with changes in fecal bulk and transit time, whereas soluble fiber tends to be responsible for effects on cholesterol and glycemic control. Soluble fibers, such as pectin, psyllium, and certain gums, tend to form gels and are used as a single fiber source only for low-fiber formulas. Fructo-oligosaccharides (FOS) are naturally occurring sugars that are added to some enteral formulas for soluble fiber benefits with better formulation characteristics (i.e., less gelling). Soluble fibers and FOS can be fermented to short-chain fatty acids by *Bifidobacterium* in the colon.[31,32] Short chain fatty acids stimulate colonic blood flow, enhance fluid and electrolyte absorption, and provide a trophic effect in the colon.

The most common fiber source for enteral formulas is soy polysaccharide, or soy fiber. Although soy polysaccharide demonstrates beneficial effects associated with both soluble and insoluble fibers in healthy subjects and non–critically ill patients, studies do not provide clear evidence of improved bowel function in critically ill patients.[31] Given the current data, stable patients on long-term EN appear most likely to benefit from fiber-supplemented formulas. Some patients on short-term EN without GI pathology who experience altered stool consistency may benefit from fiber supplementation.

Addition of fiber to enteral formulas creates some potential problems. Fiber-containing formulas often require a pump for administration through feeding tubes due to increased viscosity compared to fiberfree formulas. GI symptoms from fiber can include increased gas production and abdominal discomfort.[27,31] Improvement in constipation has been noted with FOS administration; however, intake of greater than 45 g/day may cause diarrhea.[33] Flatulence and bloating can limit tolerance to FOS for some patients. Gradual introduction of fiber may help reduce these symptoms. Bezoar formation also has been reported in a patient receiving fiber-containing tube feedings and medications that suppressed GI motility.[31] Caution is advised for the use of fiber-containing formulas in patients with poor GI motility and underlying GI dysfunction. Insoluble fiber should be avoided in critically ill patients, and patients at high risk of bowel ischemia or severe dysmotility should not receive either soluble or insoluble fiber.[4] Inadequate fluid intake may also contribute to the risk of bezoar formation and intestinal blockage with fiber; therefore, fluid provision should be carefully monitored.

B.A. is not critically ill and does not appear to have bowel pathology that would preclude use of a fiber containing formula. He will require EN for a moderate duration of time and potentially long-term. It would be reasonable to provide a formula with at least moderate fiber content. However, B.A. could experience GI symptoms from the fiber, especially if his diet has previously been of low-fiber content. If necessary, a low-fiber formula could be used initially and then transitioned to higher fiber once symptoms of bloating and gas improve.

CASE 37-2, QUESTION 6: What is an appropriate administration regimen for B.A.'s tube feeding?

The feeding route, formula selected, and anticipated duration of feeding influence the administration regimen. Patient location (e.g., hospital, nursing facility, home) and cost also are considered when developing the regimen, including the rate for initiating and advancing feedings, and the administration method (i.e., syringe, gravity drip, pump).

ONLINE CONTENT

For an illustration of the pump and tube set up for a patient receiving nasogastric feeding, go to http://thepoint.lww.com/AT10e.

Limited scientific data exist regarding EN administration regimens; thus, expert opinion plays an important role and different regimens can be used in various settings, all of which appear to meet the needs of the patients and personnel. The administration regimen should be adjusted as necessary for feeding intolerance. Four basic schedules for formula delivery are available to provide the daily volume of formula: (a) continuous infusion, (b) cyclic infusion, (c) intermittent infusion, and (d) bolus delivery of formula.

Continuous Infusion

Continuous infusion provides formula at a continuous rate for 24 hours/day and can be used with any route of feeding. Intragastric continuous infusion is most commonly used for hospitalized patients, although small bowel feeding may be more appropriate in certain settings (e.g., ICU).[18,19] Risks of gastric distension and aspiration may decrease with continuous infusion compared with intermittent gastric infusion.[16] In addition, the slower infusion rate associated with continuous infusion may be better tolerated as judged by stool frequency and time to attain full nutrition support, especially in the elderly and in metabolically unstable patients.[34–37] However, data were considered insufficient to include a recommendation for continuous infusion versus other administration methods for critically ill patients in the CCP guidelines.[18,19] Feeding into the duodenum or jejunum is best initiated with continuous infusion because rapid infusion of large formula volumes into the small bowel can result in symptoms consistent with a dumping syndrome, including sweating, lightheadedness, abdominal distension, cramping, hyperperistalsis, and watery diarrhea. With time, the jejunum may adapt to larger volumes over a shorter time allowing cyclic or longer intermittent infusions.

Cyclic Feeding

Cyclic feeding provides formula at a continuous rate for less than 24 hours daily. This method is most commonly used for patients who need supplemental nutrition because of an inability to consume adequate oral nutrients, during transition to an oral diet, and for long-term home EN patients. Infusions are typically given at night for 8 to 12 hours to minimize interference with oral intake during the day and normal activities such as work or school, although cycles can be as long as 20 hours. Most patients do not start on a cyclic regimen; rather, they transition from continuous feeding. Formula volume and osmolality can limit tolerance to cyclic feedings, especially jejunal feedings, and transition from continuous to cyclic infusion may require several days to weeks depending on the cycle length and patient tolerance. For gastric feeding, the transition usually takes only a few days.

Intermittent and Bolus Feedings

Formula is provided in three to eight gastric feedings daily for intermittent and bolus administration. Intermittent infusion occurs for 30 to 60 minutes using a feeding container or bag, with or without an enteral pump, and bolus feedings are for about 15 minutes using gravity administration via a syringe.[35–39] The stomach's reservoir capacity allows administration of relatively large volumes on an intermittent or bolus schedule. This is more physiologic than continuous feeding and more convenient for patients in nursing facilities and ambulatory patients at home on EN.

Initiation of Feedings

The regimen for initiating EN primarily depends on the site of feeding and condition of the patient's GI tract. Use of full-strength (i.e., undiluted) formula is recommended for initiation of feedings.[35–39] Dilution delays delivery of adequate nutrients without significantly affecting the incidence of GI intolerance. Hypertonic formulas are diluted rapidly in the GI tract, reaching isotonicity before or shortly beyond the ligament of Treitz (distal end of duodenum).[40] Continuous feedings are commonly initiated at a rate of 10 to 40 mL/hour with advancement by 10 to 20 mL/hour every 8 to 12 hours as tolerated, although stable patients may tolerate initiation of EN at goal rate.[35,37] For critically ill patients, those with abnormal GI function, patients without use of the GI tract for a prolonged time, those at risk of refeeding syndrome, and when calorically dense or high-osmolality formulas are used, starting at the lower rate and advancing at the slower rate (i.e., start at 10 to 20 mL/hour and advance by 10 to 15 mL/hour every 12 hours) may be preferable, although this is based on consensus rather than evidence from well-designed studies.[25,34–38]

Patients are typically started on continuous infusion feedings, then transition to intermittent infusions, and eventually to the shorter administration time of bolus feedings, if desired. Bolus feedings are administered for at least 15 minutes to avoid bloating, cramping, nausea, and diarrhea. A rate of less than 60 mL/minute is suggested to minimize symptoms of GI intolerance with bolus feedings.[38,39] For intermittent feeding, rates of 200 to 300 mL every 4 to 6 hours are generally tolerated; volumes up to 750 mL may be tolerated.[34,38,39] Initiation of feedings at goal rate may be tolerated by some patients, although starting slower is appropriate for most patients.

B.A. receives gastric feeds; therefore, continuous infusion, intermittent infusion, or bolus feedings could all be used. Continuous infusion most commonly is used for hospitalized patients despite no clearly established difference in tolerance compared with intermittent infusion. Full-strength formula should be used to initiate feedings. The goal volume of enteral nutrition for B.A. is 1,440 mL/day of a standard caloric density formula

(1.06 kcal/mL, 0.44 g protein/mL, 83.5% free water), or 60 mL/hour continuous infusion. The infusion could be started at 30 mL/hour (half goal rate); however, given B.A.'s risk for refeeding syndrome, it is preferable to start slower. Starting at 15 mL/hour for 12 hours, then increasing by 15 mL/hour every 12 hours would achieve the goal rate of 60 mL/hour within 48 hours. If B.A. experiences diarrhea or abdominal distension, the feeding may be held at 15 mL/hour for 24 hours, then increased by only 10 mL/hour every 12 to 24 hour as tolerated. Extra care must be taken to ensure he receives an adequate fluid intake until the formula is at goal rate.

Continuous infusion enteral feeding can be administered by gravity drip or by enteral pump. With gravity drip, the infusion rate must be adjusted frequently to maintain a consistent flow rate, and the formula flow must be checked regularly to ensure that the flow has not stopped because of kinked administration tubing or an empty delivery container. Gravity infusion has no alarms to alert nurses to these problems. Enteral pumps provide a consistent flow rate and alarms to alert nurses if there are problems with the infusion, but they are more expensive than gravity drips. Pumps often are used for hospitalized patients to help maintain delivery of the prescribed volume of enteral formula. Either gravity drip or an enteral pump could be used for B.A., depending on the hospital's protocol for enteral feeding. To prevent inadvertent IV infusion of enteral formula when an enteral pump is used, the connector at the distal (patient) end of the delivery set should not be compatible with IV devices.[35,37,41]

Transition From Continuous to Intermittent/Bolus Feeding

CASE 37-2, QUESTION 7: B.A. has received EN for 8 days. He has tolerated his continuous tube feeding without problems and has not required electrolyte replacements for the past 3 days. The plan is to transfer B.A. to a skilled nursing facility (SNF) in the next few days. The SNF requests that B.A. be on an intermittent/bolus feeding regimen before transfer to the SNF. How should B.A. be changed from continuous infusion to intermittent or bolus feeding?

Many nursing facilities do not routinely use enteral pumps because of increased cost. Without a pump, delivery of the prescribed volume of formula at a consistent rate may not be reliable and increased nursing time may be required to prevent tube occlusion and ensure adequate volume of formula is delivered. B.A. is currently receiving continuous infusion feedings. The transition to intermittent delivery of formula can be accomplished by various methods. An overlapping regimen of gradually decreasing the continuous infusion rate and increasing the intermittent volume appears to be an economical and efficient method of changing the feeding regimen.[34] For B.A., decrease the continuous rate from 60 mL/hour down to 40 mL/hour and add four intermittent feedings of 120 mL for 60 minutes every 6 hours initially. If tolerated, decrease continuous infusion to 20 mL/hour and increase intermittent feeding to 240 mL. Finally, stop the continuous feeding and increase intermittent feedings to 360 mL, or add a fifth feeding to keep the intermittent volume at 285 to 300 mL. To keep the feeding volume in a more convenient increment of 120 mL (half of an 8-ounce can), B.A. could receive two feedings of 360 mL and three feedings of 240 mL if five daily feedings are needed.

Another transition method is to stop the continuous feedings and restart feedings with a regimen for initiating intermittent feedings. Starting volume is typically 60 to 120 mL for the first two or three feedings when initiating intermittent feedings, and feeding intervals are often every 4 hours. Volume is increased by 60 to 120 mL every 8 to 12 hours, as tolerated, until at goal volume.[37] Feeding intervals can be increased once goal volume is reached. B.A. could start with 120 mL for 60 minutes every 4 hours for two feedings, then advance to 240 mL per feeding. If tolerated, the volume per feeding could increase to 360 mL to allow feedings every 6 hours. Once at the desired number of feedings per day, the infusion time could be decreased based on tolerance. If feeding for 30 minutes is well tolerated, B.A. could be changed to bolus administration for 15 to 20 minutes.

The discharge EN prescription should state clearly the desired caloric density, protein content, fiber content per 1,000 kcal, and formula volume, or the daily calories, protein, fiber, and fluid, to be provided. The brand name may be included, but the SNF may not carry the same brand of formula. Any special considerations for the feeding schedule also should be communicated (e.g., B.A. does not tolerate feeding after 9 PM; raise the head of the bed to 45 degrees for 3 hours after the last daily feeding to avoid regurgitation).

Fluid Provision

CASE 37-2, QUESTION 8: How much additional fluid must be included in the feeding regimen to meet B.A.'s estimated daily fluid requirements?

The free-water content of EN must be calculated to determine the volume of additional fluid that must be provided. As noted previously, standard caloric density formulas generally contain 80% to 85% free water. The formula selected for B.A. contains 83.5% free water; therefore, at his goal volume of 1,440 mL/day (six cans) the formula provides approximately 1,200 mL of free water daily. Using 1,860 mL daily (30 mL/kg/day × 62 kg) as B.A.'s fluid requirement (see Case 37-2, Question 5), he will need 660 mL/day in addition to the enteral formula. If 2,168 mL (35 mL/kg/day × 62 kg) is used for fluid requirements, B.A. needs about 970 mL of additional fluid. The additional fluid is typically provided with medications and tube irrigation (flushes). Feeding tubes should be irrigated with 30 mL of fluid every 4 hours during continuous feeding, or before and after each intermittent or bolus feeding.[35,37] The tube should be flushed with a minimum of 15 mL of water before and after medication administration through the tube, as well as with 15 mL between each medication.[35–39] Fluid also is required for diluting medications before administration through the tube. The flush volume and/or number of flushes will need to be increased to provide B.A. with adequate fluid because 30 mL every 4 hours plus fluid for medication administration will not provide the 660 mL to 970 mL fluid needed in addition to his EN. Because B.A. is receiving gastric feedings, hypotonic fluid is of less concern than in the jejunum.[40,42] Increasing flush volumes to between 100 mL and 150 mL should meet B.A.'s daily fluid requirement, depending on the amount needed for medication administration. Diluting the formula itself to increase fluid provision is not recommended because this increases the risk of error and contamination.

Nutrition in Critical Illness

Nutrition support is an important component of care in critical illness where patients are typically in a catabolic stress state and metabolism may be altered. Multiorgan dysfunction, as well as fluid and electrolyte imbalances, add to the complexity of this population and confound attempts to provide proper nutrition. The preferred route for nutrition support is generally EN, although the ideal formula composition remains unresolved.

CASE 37-3

QUESTION 1: R.S., a 65-year-old man with a past medical history of osteoarthritis and hypertension, presents to the ED with complaints of shortness of breath, productive cough, wheezing, and fever. R.S. subsequently requires intubation and is transferred to the ICU with a diagnosis of pneumonia. During the next 24 hours, his respiratory status further declines, and he is diagnosed with acute respiratory distress syndrome (ARDS). In anticipation of a prolonged course of mechanical ventilation, a feeding tube is placed into the small bowel. The chart indicates a height of 70 inches and an admission weight of 75 kg.

Laboratory evaluation today includes the following:

Sodium, 139 mEq/L
Potassium, 3.8 mEq/L
Chloride, 108 mEq/L
Carbon dioxide content, 22 mM
BUN, 15 mg/dL
SCr, 0.9 mg/dL
Glucose, 115 mg/dL
Albumin, 3.5 g/dL
Aspartate aminotransferase, 32 international units/L
Alanine aminotransferase, 37 international units/L
Alkaline phosphatase, 64 international units/L
Total bilirubin, 0.7 mg/dL
WBC, 14.7 × $10^3/\mu L$
Hgb, 13.4 g/dL
Hct, 39.9%

Should a specialized critical care formula be used for initiation of EN in R.S.?

R.S. is critically ill and several types of EN formulas have been developed for critically ill patients. However, the role of specialized EN formulas, and certain components in particular, remains controversial in critical illness. Table 37-4 includes many of the formulas marketed for critical illness and lists the components which are altered compared to standard polymeric formulas. Due to the catabolic nature of critical illness, formulas are generally high protein. Many formulas contain an NPC:N ratio of less than 100:1 (i.e., high or very high protein content). Other formulas containing slightly lower protein content (i.e., NPC:N ratio between 100:1 and 125:1) target the inflammatory element of critical illness with addition of components designed to mitigate the inflammatory response. Formulas designed for critical illness are typically fiberfree; none contain insoluble fiber, although a few formulas include small amounts of soluble fiber. Supplementation of specific amino acids, including branched-chain amino acids (BCAAs), glutamine, and arginine, in EN for critical illness remains an unsettled issue.

ENHANCED BRANCHED-CHAIN AMINO ACID CONTENT

Formulas containing greater than 35% of protein content as BCAAs were among the first specialized formulas marketed for critical illness. Standard EN formulas contain 15% to 20% of protein as BCAAs and hepatic failure formulas contain 45% to 50%, along with lower-than-normal concentrations of aromatic amino acids (AAAs), especially phenylalanine. Theoretically, increasing BCAAs and decreasing AAAs improves hepatic encephalopathy by reducing inhibitory and false neurotransmitter formation.[26,43,44] Most studies have not shown a clear advantage for hepatic failure formulas, especially with respect to mortality, and most patients with liver disease tolerate formulas with standard protein sources.[1,26,43,44] High-BCAA stress/critical care formulas are not therapeutically interchangeable with hepatic formulas as the BCAA content is typically lower and the AAA content is not reduced in stress formulas.

The theory behind high BCAA content in stress formulas is as follows: BCAAs are used preferentially for energy production in skeletal muscle of critically ill patients and exogenous BCAA reduces skeletal muscle breakdown and improves protein synthesis.[26,43,44] Studies evaluating the effectiveness of BCAA in stressed patients have primarily involved parenteral BCAA, although results for both parenteral and enteral administration are conflicting and controversial, with no significant improvement in clinical outcome, including morbidity and mortality. Objective criteria for defining critical illness and determining entry into studies may contribute to the inconclusive and controversial results when these studies are viewed as a group. Depending on the protein source, EN formulas for critical illness may contain higher BCAA content than standard polymeric formulas; however, this is seldom used today as a marketing point. High to very high protein is currently emphasized over BCAA content.

GLUTAMINE

The proposed role of glutamine in critical illness is enhanced neutrophil function and maintenance of intestinal barrier function, thereby preventing translocation of bacteria and endotoxins from the GI tract into systemic circulation and reducing bacteremia.[45–47] Glutamine potentially reduces the inflammatory response, lowers the risk of insulin resistance, and maintains acid–base balance. As a nonessential amino acid, glutamine is synthesized in sufficient quantities for its roles in transamination, as an intermediate in numerous metabolic pathways, such as gluconeogenesis and renal ammoniagenesis, as a fuel source for rapidly dividing lymphocytes and enterocytes, and in the synthesis of glutathione. However, glutamine may be considered conditionally essential during metabolic stress, as endogenous synthesis may become inadequate. Large, abrupt drops in plasma and muscular glutamine concentrations, which appear to correlate with increased mortality, have been reported in patients who are critically ill or septic.[45,48] Although this observation does not necessarily indicate depletion, it is a basis for supplementation of glutamine in certain patient populations.

A number of benefits have been attributed to provision of glutamine; however, study results are often conflicting. Glutamine supplementation has been associated with improvements in protein catabolic rate and immune function indicators in critically ill patients, yet improvements in nitrogen balance and visceral protein status are rarely noted. Garrel et al. reported decreased blood infections and mortality in burn patients receiving enteral glutamine.[49] Less pneumonia, bacteremia, and septic events in other critically ill patients receiving enteral glutamine supplementation have also been reported, although this has not translated into reduced mortality.[46] Parenteral, high-dose glutamine may be linked more closely with decreased complications and mortality rates than enteral supplementation. Data from a meta-analysis support the concept that beneficial effects of glutamine in the critically ill may be very dependent on dose and route of administration.[46]

Protein-bound glutamine is present in all enteral formulas. Free glutamine is unstable in ready-to-use formulas, however, and is generally administered separately from the formula. Glutamate is stable in water and functions in many roles attributed to glutamine. Additional research is needed to determine whether physiologic effects are equivalent for glutamate, protein-bound glutamine, and free glutamine. Until such questions are answered, supplementation of free glutamine separately from the formula is likely to continue despite its uncertain role in many patient populations and suggestions that it is not

TABLE 37-4

Selected High-Protein Enteral Formulas With Altered Protein or Fat Sources[a]

Formula[b,c]	kcal/mL (mOsm/kg)	Free Water (%)	Protein g/L (% kcal)	NPC:N	Protein Source	ARG g/L[d]	GLN g/L[d]	Fat g/L (% kcal)	Fat Sources	Fat kcal as MCT (%)	Ratio of -6FA to -3FA[d]	Fiber g/L[d]
Crucial[c]	1.5 (490)	77	94 (25)	67:1	Hydrolyzed casein; L-arginine	15	–	67.6 (39)	MCT oil; fish oil (<2%); soybean oil; lecithin	50	1.5:1	–
f.a.a[c]	1.0 (850)	85	50 (20)	100:1	Crystalline amino acids	–	–	11.2 (10)	Soybean oil; MCT	25	–	–
Impact[c]	1.0 (375)	85	56 (22)	71:1	Sodium and calcium caseinates; L-arginine	12.5	–	28 (25)	Palm kernel oil; menhaden oil	–	1.4:1	–
Impact with Fiber[c]	1.0 (375)	87	56 (22)	71:1	Sodium and calcium caseinates; L-arginine	12.5	–	28 (25)	Palm kernel oil; menhaden oil	–	1.4:1	10
Impact 1.5[c]	1.5 (550)	78	84 (22)	71:1	Sodium and calcium caseinates; L-arginine	18.7	–	69 (40)	MCT; palm kernel oil; menhaden oil	33	1.4:1	–
Impact Glutamine[c]	1.3 (630)	81	78 (24)	62:1	Whey protein hydrolysate; free amino acids; sodium caseinates; L-arginine	16.3	15	43 (30)	Palm kernel oil; menhaden oil	–	1.4:1	10
Optimental[b]	1.0 (540)	83.2	51 (20.5)	97:1	Soy protein hydrolysate; partially hydrolyzed sodium caseinate; L-arginine	5.5	–	28.4 (25)	Structured lipid (interesterified sardine oil [EPA, DHA] and MCT); canola oil; soy oil	NA	–	5 FOS
Osmolite 1.2 Cal[b]	1.2 (360)	82	55.5 (18.5)	110:1	Sodium and calcium caseinate	–	–	39 (29)	High-oleic safflower oil; canola oil; MCT oil; lecithin	20	–	–
Osmolite 1.5[b]	1.5 (525)	76	62.7 (16.7)	125:1	Sodium and calcium caseinates; soy protein isolates	–	–	49 (29)	High-oleic safflower oil; canola oil; MCT oil; lecithin	20	–	–
Oxepa[b]	1.5 (535)	78.5	62.5 (16.7)	125:1	Sodium and calcium caseinates	–	–	93.8 (55)	Canola oil; MCT oil; sardine oil; borage oil	25	–	–
Peptamen VHP[c]	1.0 (270–380)	84	62.4 (25)	75:1	Hydrolyzed whey protein	–	–	39 (33)	MCT oil; soybean oil (<2%); lecithin	70	7.4:1	–
Peptamen AF[c]	1.2 (390)	81	75.6 (21)	76:1	Hydrolyzed whey protein	–	–	54.8 (39)	MCT oil; soybean oil (<2%); fish oil (<2%); lecithin	50	1.8:1	5.2 (FOS and other fibers)
Perative[b]	1.3 (460)	79	66.6 (20.5)	97:1	Partially hydrolyzed sodium caseinate; whey protein hydrolysate; L-arginine	6.5	–	37.4 (25)	Canola oil; MCT oil; corn oil	40	–	6.5 FOS
Pivot 1.5 Cal[b]	1.5 (595)	75.9	93.8 (25)	75:1	Partially hydrolyzed sodium caseinate; whey protein hydrolysate	13	6.5	50.8 (30)	Structured lipid (interesterified sardine oil [EPA, DHA] and MCT); soy oil; canola oil	20	–	7.5 FOS

[a] Changes periodically occur in nutrient sources and content; use this table as a general reference only and not for specific patient care issues.
[b] Abbott (Ross) product.
[c] Nestle product.
[d] None or unknown indicated by "–".
AF, advanced formula; ARG, arginine; DHA, docosahexaenoic acid; EPA, eicosapentaenoic acid; FOS, fructo-oligosaccharides; GLN, glutamine; MCT, medium-chain triglycerides; NPC:N, nonprotein calorie to nitrogen; ω-3FA, ω-3 fatty acids; ω-6FA, ω-6 fatty acids; VHP, very high protein.

necessary.[50] The currently recommended maximal dose of glutamine is 0.57 g/kg/day, although lower doses are used in most studies and greater than 0.2 g/kg/day was adequate to see benefit in one meta-analysis.[51,52] Doses of enteral glutamine used in studies reviewed for the CCP guidelines varied from 0.16 to 0.5 g/kg/day, and the CCP guidelines committee decided a reasonable dose would be 0.3 to 0.5 g/kg/day.[18,53] The SACC guidelines concur with this glutamine dose.[4]

Available data do not indicate a harmful effect of glutamine; however, theoretic concerns are associated with providing a large quantity of one amino acid that shares transport systems with other amino acids in the body and that has a role in ammoniagenesis. Glutamine supplementation should be avoided in patients with total bilirubin greater than 10 mg/dL or creatinine clearance less than 30 mL/minute because ammonia excretion could be impared.[54] Monitoring for potential complications with glutamine supplementation is advised given these theoretic concerns.

ARGININE

Arginine is a nonessential amino acid synthesized by the urea cycle during detoxification of ammonia and is normally available in sufficient quantities for growth and tissue repair. In times of metabolic stress, however, endogenous synthesis may become inadequate, making arginine conditionally essential. The postulated benefit of arginine in critical illness is related to enhanced protein synthesis, cellular growth, and immune system support. In contrast, several mechanisms have been proposed that suggest potential adverse effects with arginine supplementation, including one in which arginine is used as a substrate in the synthesis of nitric oxide (NO), a potent vasodilating agent, which may also have implications in mitochondria damage, organ dysfunction, and increased gut barrier permeability.[55] Although synthesis of NO increases during sepsis (thereby creating a negative arginine balance), the exact role of this effector molecule remains controversial. Many believe that excess NO is part of an adaptive response directed toward limiting infection, ischemia, coagulation, inflammation, and tissue injury. Additional studies with well-defined patient populations are necessary to determine appropriate arginine doses and the effects of arginine alone or in combinations of immune-modulating components. Few studies with surgery and critically ill patients have used arginine alone, and results with arginine plus other immune-modulating components, most commonly ω-3FAs, nucleotides, glutamine, and antioxidants, are controversial.

Immune-Modulating Formulas

Several formulas included in Table 37-4 have an NPC:N ratio of less than or equal to 125:1 and also contain supplemental arginine, glutamine, or nucleic acids, or a modified fat component. Such formulas are often referred to as "immune-modulating" formulas based on their proposed beneficial modulation of biologic responses to stress. Study formulas frequently contain varying portions of two or more potentially immune-modifying components, making it difficult to determine the effect of any given component.

The results of clinical trials examining the effects of immune-modulating enteral formulations on mortality, hospital length of stay (LOS), ICU days, incidence of nosocomial infection, duration of mechanical ventilation, and GI complications are conflicting.[4,18,19,45–56] Several meta-analyses have shown benefit on clinical outcomes (e.g., infectious complications, ventilator days, LOS); however, no mortality benefit has ever been found in critically ill patients receiving immunonutrition versus standard EN.[50,57] Difficulty in isolating effects of immunonutrition from other effects of critical illness may contribute to inconsistent results. Differences in study design, patient population, enteral formulation (varying combinations of immune-modulating components and doses), time to EN commencement, and volume of formula received, also make it difficult to reliably compare study results. Nonetheless, various analytical techniques have been applied to study data to allow some guidance on use of immune-modulating EN.

Based on subgroup analysis, particular subsets within the major immune-modulating EN studies may be at greater risk from use of certain immune-modulating components whereas other subgroups exhibit better outcomes. Arginine is the most controversial immune-modulating component, and it has been identified as potentially causing adverse effects in certain subpopulations, specifically in septic patients. Subgroup analysis of higher quality studies reveals that arginine supplementation in the critically ill patient population may be detrimental owing to an enhanced systemic inflammatory response and hemodynamic instability.[4,18,19] On the other hand, septic patients, mostly with pneumonia, receiving a high arginine-containing (>12 g/L), immune-enhancing formula had significant decreases in the incidence of bacteremia, and decreased mortality was reported in another study.[4] Such conflicting results leave considerable uncertainty regarding use of arginine supplemented EN in critically ill patients.

The population which appears to have better outcomes with immune-modulating EN is patients undergoing major elective surgery, particularly surgery for upper GI malignancy. A recent meta-analysis showed reduced infection risk and shorter length of stay in high-risk elective surgery patients receiving immunonutrition with EN supplemented with both arginine and fish oil.[56] The majority of studies included in this analysis enrolled patients with upper GI malignancy, which supports the use of immune-modulating formulations in this patient population. The SACC guidelines recommend use of an immune-modulating EN formula in patients undergoing major elective surgery.[4]

Additional studies with well-defined patient populations are necessary to determine the effects of combinations of immune-modulating components (arginine, glutamine, nucleic acids, ω-3FAs), optimal component and dose combinations, and the most beneficial timing for administration of immune-modulating components. Continued research is necessary to further refine the knowledge of patient populations likely to benefit from arginine supplemented immune-modulating EN and those in whom it should be avoided. Until such information is available, the immune-modulating formulas containing arginine must be used with caution and after careful evaluation of each patient for potential risks versus benefits. Guidelines, consensus statements, and recommendations have been developed to help the clinician provide evidence-based nutrition therapy; however, many barriers to implementation exist.[1,4,18,19,58,59]

Use of arginine-containing, immune-enhancing diets is not recommended for critically ill patients in the CCP guidelines because higher-quality studies indicated no effect on mortality with these formulas and increased mortality was reported for septic patients in some studies.[18] The more recently published SACC guidelines appear to conflict with the CCP guidelines by recommending use of immune-modulating formulations in the appropriate patient populations, including those undergoing major elective surgery, trauma, burns, head and neck cancer, and mechanically ventilated critically ill patients without severe sepsis.[4] Per the guidelines, patients not meeting these criteria should receive a standard EN formula. On closer scrutiny, it is evident that neither the CCP guidelines nor the SACC guidelines recommend use of an arginine-supplemented immune-modulating formula for patients with severe sepsis.[4,18,19]

Altered Fat Components

Stress or critical care and immune-modulating formulas contain different sources of fat to alter the type of fatty acids provided. Fat sources commonly include MCTs, along with predominantly canola oil, high oleic oils, or fish oils as long-chain fatty acids. Enteral formulas often contain MCTs to improve fat absorption. MCT absorption is relatively independent of pancreatic enzymes and bile salts; thus, they can be absorbed in patients experiencing malabsorption of the long-chain triglycerides. Rapid, carnitine-independent metabolism occurs with MCT, whereas long-chain triglycerides require carnitine for metabolism. Therefore, use of long-chain triglycerides is compromised when carnitine deficiency occurs, but MCT metabolism is unaffected. Formulas containing a relatively large percentage of fat calories as MCTs are frequently marketed for critically ill patients with malabsorption.

Canola oil contains approximately two-thirds monounsaturated fatty acids (MUFAs), compared with less than half this amount in polyunsaturated vegetable oils. High-oleic safflower and sunflower oils also have high MUFA content. MUFAs have been popularized by reports of low cardiovascular disease in populations using olive oil, but further research is needed to determine the role of these fatty acids in ill patients. The combination of canola oil and high-oleic oil does increase the content of linolenic acid. Usual polyunsaturated vegetable oils (i.e., corn, soy, and safflower oils) are avoided or provided in relatively small quantities in critical care formulas to limit omega-6 fatty acids (ω-6FAs), which are precursors to arachidonic acid and therefore to dienoic or "2" series prostaglandins, prostacyclins, and thromboxanes, and to "4" series leukotrienes. These "2" and "4" series compounds, taken as a whole, are potent inflammatory, vasoconstrictive, and platelet-aggregating agents.[60,61] The source of ω-6FAs may, however, also influence the type of prostaglandins produced.[62] Dietary α-linolenic acid is converted to γ-linolenic acid (GLA), then to dihomo-GLA, and subsequently to arachidonic acid. As a dietary supplement, GLA is converted to dihomo-GLA, which effectively competes with arachidonic acid in the pathways for prostaglandin synthesis rather than being elongated to arachidonic acid. The resulting "1" series prostaglandins have lower proinflammatory effects, similar to "3" series prostaglandins. Small amounts of ω-6FAs are required in the diet to prevent deficiency of linolenic acid, an essential fatty acid not provided by MCT and fish oils.

Fish oils, including menhaden oil, provide fatty acids primarily from the ω-3 family, with the very-long-chain fatty acids eicosapentaenoic acid and docosahexaenoic acid predominating. The proposed role of ω-3FAs in critical illness is to reduce infectious complications and death in selected patient populations. The ω-3FAs are precursors to the "3" series prostaglandins, prostacyclins, and thromboxanes and "5" series leukotrienes. In total, these compounds are less inflammatory and more vasodilatory than compounds from ω-6FA.[60–62]

Few data are available evaluating effects of only fat modification in EN for critical illness, and combinations of immune-modulating components may produce different effects than single nutrients. Improved clinical outcomes for postsurgical and critically ill patients have been associated with EN-containing ω-3FAs, usually in conjunction with other immune-modulating components, although the effects remain controversial.[4,18,26] A recent meta-analysis examined the clinical impact of several enteral formulas with varying supplements of arginine, glutamine, and fish oil and found no overall effect on mortality with the use of the immune-modulating formulas in general.[63] However, when EN was supplemented with fish oil only, benefit was seen as lower rates of secondary infections, LOS, and mortality. This benefit was lost in patients receiving EN formulas supplemented with both arginine and fish oil, suggesting that arginine may counteract the benefit of fish oil.[63]

Studies suggest a minimum of 5 to 7 days of supplementation with immune-modulating components, including ω-3FAs, is necessary to see beneficial effects on postoperative outcomes.[58] Incorporation of ω-3FAs into cell membranes may be required to see benefits; this has been demonstrated in humans with supplementation for 5 days.[64] Decreased wound infections and reduced mortality have been demonstrated in burn patients with low-fat diets containing 50% of fat as fish oil.[65] Other studies, however, have shown no benefit in this population.[60] Fat modification to provide high ω-3FA content also has been studied in ARDS and acute lung injury (as discussed in the Pulmonary Disease section).[56]

Further research is needed to elucidate effects of ω-3FAs alone and to determine their safety and efficacy in various disease states. Effects of ω-3FAs on antioxidant levels, especially vitamin E, and the need for supplementation require study. Appropriate quantities of ω-3FAs and the most beneficial ratios of ω-6FA to ω-3FA also must be determined before routine supplementation with ω-3FAs can be recommended beyond modifying the diet to include foods rich in ω-3FAs (i.e., fish, such as salmon). Current ratios of ω-6FA to ω-3FA in diets range from about 4:1 in Japan to 16:1 in the United States, although a specific intake amount resulting in adverse effects has not been determined for either ω-6FAs or ω-3FAs.[60–62] No data exist regarding appropriate ratios of ω-6FA to ω-3FA in various illnesses, although studies have attempted to elucidate effects of ω-3FA supplements on various inflammatory disease states.

The question of whether to initiate EN in R.S. with an immune-modulating formula does not have a clear-cut answer. The data provided for R.S. do not indicate sepsis; thus, he would be a candidate for an immune-modulating formula using the SACC guidelines.[4] The more conservative CCP guidelines would not recommend an arginine-containing immune-modulating formula.[18] The decision of whether to use the immune-modulating formula would likely depend on practices within the hospital and the immune-modulating formulas available. Because R.S. was admitted with pneumonia and now has ARDS, the other consideration would be whether a specialized pulmonary formula would be more appropriate for his EN.

Pulmonary Disease

CASE 37-3, QUESTION 2: How do pulmonary formulas differ from standard polymeric formulas? If R.S. receives a specialized pulmonary formula, what nutrient modifications should the formula contain?

There are two types of EN formulas intended for patients with pulmonary conditions. Both have a moderate caloric density (1.5 kcal/mL) and the percentage of calories from fat is relatively high (40%–55%), although the types of fats differ. The premise for higher fat content is that fat metabolism produces less carbon dioxide (CO_2) than carbohydrate metabolism, thereby reducing the work load of the lungs. Early studies comparing isocaloric, high-fat, low-carbohydrate diets with higher carbohydrate diets showed improved respiratory parameters in ambulatory patients with chronic obstructive pulmonary disease (COPD) as well as reduced time on the ventilator and decreased arterial CO_2 concentrations in mechanically ventilated patients.[26,43,44] Caloric intake in these studies ranged from 1.7 to 2.25 times the measured energy expenditure, which is excessive by current standards. Excess calories contribute to higher CO_2 production; thus, the early studies are of questionable relevance, and in practice, preventing overfeeding is as important for control of CO_2 as high-fat, low-carbohydrate diets.[26,27] In addition, improved respiratory parameters with a high-fat EN product are unlikely to be seen in patients without excess CO_2 production or retention. A more recent study in 60 malnourished, underweight patients with COPD does suggest respiratory status in this population is more likely to benefit from a high-fat, low-carbohydrate (28% of calories) formula compared with a high-carbohydrate (60%–70% of calories) formula.[66,67] Although the percent of calories from fat (55%) in the high-fat formula was similar to traditional pulmonary formulas, fat distribution was considerably different with 20% of fat as MCTs and a predominance of MUFAs. Currently marketed pulmonary formulas contain 20% to 40% of fat calories as MCTs and fat sources providing higher MUFAs. During a period of overfeeding for weight gain, pulmonary formulas may be reasonable; however, they are not warranted for routine use in most patients.

The second type of pulmonary EN formula is an immune-modulating pulmonary (IMP) formula with an anti-inflammatory lipid profile (fish oils rich in ω-3FAs, borage oil rich in GLAs), antioxidants (vitamins C and E, beta carotene), and no supplemental arginine, which has been studied in patients with ARDS and acute pulmonary injury.[68] Three studies comparing this formula with a typical high-fat pulmonary formula with elevated ω-6FA content were included in a recent meta-analysis by Pontes-Arruda et al. and showed a significant reduction in new organ failures, time receiving mechanical ventilation, ICU LOS, and mortality.[69]

Based on the one study available at the time the CCP guidelines were published, the committee concluded that the use of IMP formulas with a combination of fish oils, borage oil, and antioxidants should be considered in patients with ARDS.[18] Evaluation of all three studies was included for the updated CCP and the SACC guidelines, which recommend that patients with acute lung injury or ARDS be placed on an IMP formula.[4,18] However, the choice of control formula in these otherwise high-quality studies has been questioned because there is some evidence of harmful effects from administration of ω-6FA-rich fats in critically ill patients.[18,19]

R.S. was diagnosed with ARDS; therefore he is a candidate for an IMP formula based on both the CCP and SACC guidelines.[4,18,19] The formula should contain fish oils to provide a high ω-3FA content, borage oil to provide GLA, and increased antioxidant vitamin content. Delayed gastric emptying is associated with high-fat diets, and must be considered when evaluating possible benefits and adverse effects of high-fat EN. This applies to both IMP and routine pulmonary formulas. Abdominal distension, increased gastric residuals, nausea, and vomiting can result from delayed gastric emptying. R.S. has his feeding tube placed in the small bowel, so delayed gastric emptying from the high fat content is not a concern. However, the potential to overwhelm pancreatic lipase activity resulting in fat malabsorption should be considered when a high-fat load, especially long-chain triglycerides, is delivered into the small bowel. Continuous infusion is more likely to be tolerated than other, more rapid delivery methods in most patients. As shown in Table 37-2, the cost of routine pulmonary formulas is slightly higher than for standard polymeric formulas and IMP formulas are significantly more expensive.

RENAL FAILURE

CASE 37-3, QUESTION 3: R.S. has been in the ICU for 10 days. His ARDS has improved; however, he now has acute kidney injury and hemodialysis will start today. Morning laboratory results include the following:

Sodium, 133 mEq/L
Potassium, 5.6 mEq/L
BUN, 78 mg/dL
SCr, 3.6 mg/dL
Glucose, 105 mg/dL on an insulin drip
Magnesium, 2.8 mg/dL
Phosphorus, 5.4 mg/dL
WBC, 9.7 × $10^3/\mu L$
Hgb, 11.4 g/dL
Hct, 34.3%

An EN formula for renal failure is ordered. How do the nutrient components in renal formulas differ from standard polymeric EN formulas? Is a renal formula appropriate for R.S.?

Two types of EN formulas for renal disease/injury are available and both are calorically dense (1.8 to 2 kcal/mL) to limit fluid provision. Highly specialized formulas with enriched essential amino acid content are based on the theory that recycling of urea nitrogen for nonessential amino acid synthesis reduces the accumulation of BUN.[26,43,44] Clinically significant recycling of nitrogen and incorporation into nonessential amino acids does not appear to occur, however. Essential amino acid formulas may be appropriate for patients with chronic renal failure with glomerular filtration rates less than 25 mL/minute/1.73 m^2 who are receiving very-low-protein diets and for whom dialysis is not an option.[1,43] Use should be limited to no more than 2 to 3 weeks, because hyperammonemia and metabolic encephalopathy have been associated with longer use. These formulas are not appropriate for patients with acute kidney injury, such as R.S., or for those receiving dialysis. The NPC:N ratio is approximately 300:1 in these formulas. Water-soluble vitamins are typically included in currently available high essential amino acid formulas; however, vitamin content should be reviewed as some essential amino acid formulas do not contained vitamins. Renalcal contains higher-than-normal essential amino acids with about two-thirds essential combined with one-third nonessential amino acids.

Polymeric enteral formulas designed for renal failure or renal insufficiency are the standard for hospitalized patients with impaired renal function. These formulas contain a balanced amino acid profile and are not enriched with essential amino acids. The NPC:N ratio varies from about 130:1 (for patients with increased nitrogen losses from dialysis) to 230:1 (typically used for nondialyzed patients). Lower-than-normal concentrations of potassium, phosphorus, and magnesium are used in these formulas to minimize electrolyte problems. Many critically ill patients receiving dialysis for acute kidney injury tolerate a nonrenal formula; however, those with elevated potassium, phosphorus, or magnesium generally require a renal formula to control electrolyte levels. Based on his electrolytes, R.S. will require a renal formula. A polymeric formula with a lower NPC:N ration (i.e., 140:1; moderate protein content) would be appropriate given the plan for dialysis. Polymeric renal formulas meet 100% of the DRI with less than 2,000 mL/day.

Modular Components

CASE 37-3, QUESTION 4: After several days on the renal formula (NPC:N ratio, 140:1), there are indications that R.S.'s protein intake should be higher. Serum electrolytes today include the following:

Sodium, 137 mEq/L
Potassium, 5.2 mEq/L
Phosphorus, 4.4 mg/dL
Magnesium, 2.5 mg/dL.

What are the options for increasing protein provision?

R.S. is receiving a renal formula with moderately high protein content based on the NPC:N ratio of 140:1. There are no very-high-protein formulas with low potassium, phosphorus, and magnesium on the market; therefore, a very high protein formula will provide significantly more of these electrolytes than R.S. currently receives. His current serum levels of the renally eliminated electrolytes are near the upper end of normal, and would likely rise above the normal range if the EN is changed to a nonrenal formula. Using a lower potassium concentration in the dialysis bath might keep serum potassium within normal range. Addition of a phosphate binder to the medication regimen could be considered; however, the risk of tube occlusion may be increased with a phosphate binder. A better option is to provide additional protein from a modular protein component, although this can also increase the risk of tube occlusion if not administered properly.

Modular components are individual nutrient substrates, or combinations of two substrates, designed for addition to oral diets or enteral formulas. They provide only the macronutrient(s) without electrolytes or vitamins, and should only be used to supplement a diet or EN, not as a sole source of nutrition. Protein modules are powders containing 3 to 5 g protein/tablespoon. Most protein modules are intact protein. Arginine and glutamine are available as individual packets to allow supplementation as a single amino acid. Glucose polymers are used to supplement calories as carbohydrate. They do not increase osmolality or alter food or formula flavor. Powdered carbohydrate modules contain 20 to 30 kcal/tablespoon, whereas liquids contain 2 kcal/mL. Protein and carbohydrate modular components typically are mixed with water and administered through the feeding tube rather than being mixed directly into the formula. Additional fat can be provided as 50% safflower oil emulsion (Microlipid) or as MCT oil. A modular fiber product containing soluble fiber in the form of partially hydrolyzed guar gum is also available.

Glucose Control Formulas

CASE 37-4

QUESTION 1: J.K., a 66-year-old man, is admitted to the hospital secondary to dehydration and for a GI workup related to a 50-pound unintentional weight loss during the past 2 months. He states he has been unable to eat for at least a week due to continual nausea, although he reports no vomiting. J.K. received IV fluids in the ED and currently has 0.9% sodium chloride infusing at 125 mL/hour. Past medical history includes hypertension, hyperlipidemia, gastric reflux, and diabetes mellitus type 2. J.K. is 5 feet 9 inches tall and his admit weight is 115 kg. Laboratory values from this morning show the following results:

Glucose, 229 mg/dL
BUN, 18 mg/dL, down from 27 mg/dL in the ED
SCr, 1.2 mg/dL, down from 2.1 mg/dL in the ED
Sodium, 139 mEq/L
Potassium, 4.1 mEq/L
Chloride, 103 mEq/L

His small bowel follow-through study indicates severely delayed gastric emptying. A feeding tube is to be placed into the small bowel for a trial of enteral feeding.

Should a "glucose control" or "diabetic" formula be used for initiating tube feedings in J.K.? How do formulas for glucose control differ from standard polymeric EN formulas?

Formulas for hyperglycemic patients, known as diabetic formulas, are higher protein formulas and have caloric distributions of 31% to 40% carbohydrate, 42% to 49% fat, and 16% to 20% protein. The carbohydrate content is lower and fat content is higher than in most high protein polymeric formulas. High MUFA sources predominate to provide greater than 60% of fat as MUFAs. The source and type of carbohydrates in diabetic formulas varies, with a predominance of more complex carbohydrates (i.e., oligosaccharides, cornstarch, fiber) and insulin-independent sugars (i.e., fructose) despite total carbohydrate content probably being more important than carbohydrate type.[26,70] Fiber sources associated with improved glycemic control, mainly soluble fibers but also soy polysaccharide, are included in these formulas to help minimize postprandial hyperglycemia. Fiber content ranges from 14 to 21 g/L and formulas are 1 kcal/mL; thus, the recommended fiber intake of 25 to 38 g daily generally can be achieved with less than 2,000 kcal/day.[29,30]

Multiple studies comparing diabetic formulas to standard EN formulas providing equal calories and protein have been conducted. A large meta-analysis included 23 studies, of which 19 were randomized controlled trials. Patients predominantly had type 2 diabetes.[71] Short-term, single-meal trials generally used the EN formulas as an oral supplement in healthy volunteers, whereas the 7 longer-term trials (6 days to 3 months follow-up) included in the meta-analysis tended to provide formula to patients by feeding tube. Results of the meta-analysis favor the diabetic formulas for glucose control. Postprandial increases in glucose were significantly reduced with the diabetic formulas, as were glucose area under the curve and peak blood glucose concentrations. However, the diabetic formulas showed no significant effects on total cholesterol, high density lipoprotein, or triglyceride concentrations. Overall complication rates were not significantly different between formulas in the two randomized controlled trials reporting this parameter for tube-fed patients. Also, mortality differences were not found in the single 2-week trial reporting mortality for critically ill patients.

J.K. could receive either a diabetic formula or a standard formula. The meta-analysis discussed previously would suggest glucose control may be better with a diabetic formula; however either choice would be appropriate based on available guidelines.[71] The American Diabetes Association suggests either a standard formula with 50% carbohydrate or a formula containing 33% to 40% carbohydrate for tube feeding.[72] Practice guidelines for nutrition support suggest no changes in macronutrients compared with the standard diet recommendations for diabetes, including 45% to 65% of calories from carbohydrate.[1] Problems with delayed gastric emptying or fat malabsorption must be weighed against possible benefits of improved glucose control with diabetic formulas. These problems are of minimal concern for J.K. as he is being fed into the small bowel and his history does not suggest fat malabsorption. Treatment goals for EN in patients with diabetes mellitus should include individualization of macronutrient composition, avoidance of excess calories, and maintenance of euglycemia.[1] J.K. may benefit from a treatment plan that includes gradual weight loss and this may influence the decision of whether to use a diabetic formula or a very high protein formula that would permit lower total calories while still providing adequate protein.

MONITORING ENTERAL NUTRITION SUPPORT

CASE 37-4, QUESTION 2: What types of complications can occur with tube feeding? What steps can be taken to prevent complications in J.K., and how should he be monitored for complications?

Appropriate monitoring of patients receiving EN is essential to recognize and prevent complications. Complications can be divided into three groups: mechanical, metabolic and GI (Table 37-5).

Mechanical Complications

The major mechanical complications are tube occlusion and aspiration. Mechanical complications often can be avoided with good nursing technique and careful observation of feeding tolerance. Adequate tube flushing is essential to prevent tube occlusion. Flushing with 30 mL of water every 4 hours during continuous feeding or before and after intermittent feedings is recommended.[35,37] Flushing must also occur before and after medication administration and after withdrawal of gastric contents. J.K.'s tube should be flushed using these guidelines. Frequent assessment of tube placement by auscultation, location of markings on the tube, and withdrawal of gastric contents is important to prevent pulmonary aspiration of the formula secondary to displacement of the tube into the esophagus or pharynx. Tube placement should be evaluated every 4 to 6 hours with continuous feeding, or before each intermittent or bolus feeding.[35,38–40,42,44]

Withdrawal of gastric contents through a gastric tube using a syringe allows evaluation of volume in the stomach (gastric residual volume [GRV]). Endogenous secretions from saliva and gastric fluids, about 4,500 mL/day in normal adults receiving food, contribute to GRV when gastric emptying is impaired.[40] Variations in GRV also occur based on the volume and timing of previous feeds, especially for intermittent or bolus feeds, feeding tube characteristics, and patient position and activity.[38–40] Gastrostomy tubes may yield less volume than NG tubes because of their more anterior position in the stomach. Soft, small-bore feeding tubes may collapse when GRV is checked, resulting in falsely low GRV. GRV is not usually checked through tubes placed in the postpyloric region because (a) problems with tube collapse have been reported and (b) the small bowel does not serve as a reservoir for residuals. J.K. has a jejunal feeding tube; thus, GRV is not reliable when checked through his feeding tube. If J.K. has an NG tube in addition to a small bowel feeding tube, GRV can be checked through the NG tube to assess whether formula is "backing-up" or refluxing into the stomach. Previously, methylene blue or blue food coloring was added to the formula to evaluate reflux; however, reports of mortality associated with this practice resulted in its abandonment.[4,16,35,37,73] The use of glucose oxidase test strips to detect the presence of enteral formula in tracheobronchial secretions lacks sensitivity and specificity, and the results have not been shown to correlate with aspiration; thus, it is not a recommended practice.[34,35,37,38] Current practice recommendations are to hold feeding for GRV greater than 500 mL and consider jejunal placement of the feeding tube when GRV is consistently greater than 500 mL.[37] In addition, use of a promotility agent should be considered when GRV is greater than 250 mL after a second check. These agents may improve feeding tolerance and formula delivery, and the risk of aspiration may be decreased, although the benefit of these agents has been questioned. If the feeding is held because of a high GRV, hourly evaluation of the GRV is recommended until the volume is less than 200 to 250 mL and the feeding is restarted. The fluid withdrawn for GRV assessment may be infused through the tube back into the stomach to minimize electrolyte imbalances. Elevating the head of the bed to 30 to 45 degrees, with 45 degrees preferred in critically ill patients, during and after feedings also is recommended to reduce the risk of aspiration.[19,37,42]

Metabolic Complications

Major metabolic complications of EN include hyperglycemia, electrolyte abnormalities, and fluid imbalance. Although rigorous studies evaluating monitoring frequency are lacking, regular biochemical determinations similar to those used for PN are recommended to identify and correct metabolic abnormalities before severe abnormalities occur. Baseline values for serum glucose, SCr, BUN, and electrolytes should be available to guide selection of the enteral formula. The few baseline laboratory results available for J.K. may be adequate as a baseline, but additional laboratory parameters will be necessary as part of the monitoring regimen once EN starts.

Fingerstick glucose measurements every 6 hours or an insulin protocol are recommended before EN starts in diabetic or hyperglycemic patients or if hyperglycemia is anticipated. Given J.K.'s history of diabetes and a baseline glucose greater than 200 mg/dL, diligent monitoring and treatment of his hyperglycemia is warranted even before EN starts. J.K. will require long-term glucose monitoring; however, routine glucose monitoring in nondiabetic patients can be stopped once a stable euglycemic state is established with EN at the goal volume and infusion regimen.

A basic metabolic panel ([BMP]; serum glucose, sodium, potassium, chloride, bicarbonate, calcium, BUN, and SCr) is generally checked daily after feeding starts in critically ill patients and those at risk of electrolyte abnormalities or renal dysfunction. More stable patients may have serum glucose and electrolytes (sodium, potassium, chloride, bicarbonate) monitored rather than a BMP. During the first week of EN, whether initiated in the hospital or alternate site (SNF or at home), a BMP, phosphorus, and magnesium should be monitored a minimum of two to three times weekly in patients with weight loss; once or twice weekly may be adequate if there is no weight loss. Monitoring frequency can be reduced once tolerance to tube feeding is established and there are no metabolic abnormalities. Daily BMP for a minimum of 4 to 5 days is probably best for J.K. considering his recent dehydration. Daily phosphorus and magnesium also should be considered for a few days in J.K. because of his significant weight loss and risk of refeeding syndrome. Despite being obese, J.K. is at risk of electrolyte abnormalities associated with refeeding syndrome.[25] Failure to monitor J.K. and replace electrolytes as necessary could result in serious electrolyte abnormalities. Once J.K.'s BMP, phosphorus, and magnesium are stable, the frequency of monitoring could be reduced to once or twice weekly. Critically ill patients generally require daily or every other day monitoring while in the ICU. For patients receiving long-term EN, the frequency of laboratory monitoring gradually is decreased. Laboratory monitoring should be done once or twice yearly in stable patients without significant medical problems. Patients who have medical problems that can affect nutrient, electrolyte, or trace element requirements or tolerances should be monitored as appropriate to the medical condition.

Weight and fluid status are important parameters to monitor throughout EN therapy, especially in patients with unusual losses, an inability to recognize thirst, or inability to voluntarily adjust their oral fluid intake. For hospitalized patients, weight is primarily a reflection of fluid status and increasing weight for 3 or 4 consecutive days may be an indication fluid intake needs

TABLE 37-5
Complications of Tube Feeding

Complication	Cause/Contributing Factor	Treatment/Prevention
Mechanical Complications		
Aspiration	Deflated tracheostomy cuff	Inflate tracheostomy cuff before feeding; keep inflated 1 hour after feeding; consider small-bore feeding tube placed past the ligament of Treitz
	Displaced feeding tube	Reinsert tube, check placement; consider hand restraints or feeding tube bridle
	Reduced gastric emptying	Check residuals every 4–6 hours for gastric tube; raise head of bed 30–45 degrees; use lower-fat formula; use prokinetic medication; use small bowel feeding tube
	Lack of gag reflex; coma	Place feeding tube into jejunum; keep head of bed elevated to 45 degrees; provide continuous feeding
Nasal or pharyngeal irritation or necrosis; esophageal erosion; otitis media	Large-bore, polyvinyl chloride tube for long periods of time	Reposition tube daily, change tape; use smaller-bore tube; position tube to avoid pressure on tissues; moisten mouth and nose several times daily
Tube obstruction	Poorly crushed medications	Crush medications thoroughly, dissolve in water; use liquid medications whenever possible; check compatibility of medication with tube and formula
	Inadequate flushing after medications or thick formula	Flush tube with 50–150 mL water after medications or thick formula and every 4–6 hours with 20 mL minimum
	Poorly dissolved or mixed formula	Use blender to mix powdered formula (check manufacturer's mixing guidelines); use ready-to-use formula
	Formula mixed with low pH substance	Avoid checking gastric residuals when safe to do so; use larger-diameter tubes when checking residuals; avoid administering acidic medications through small-diameter tubes; consider a nonacidic therapeutic alternative; flush with a minimum of 30 mL water before and immediately after medication administration
Gastrointestinal Complications		
Nausea, vomiting, distension, cramping	Too rapid administration	Slow administration rate; change bolus to intermittent infusion
	Osmolarity too high; intolerance to volume of formula	Change hypertonic formula to isotonic formula; increase the number of bolus or intermittent feedings so the volume per feeding is reduced, or change to continuous infusion; change to a more calorically dense formula if volume is the major problem (osmolarity will likely increase with higher caloric density)
	Gastric retention; poor GI motility	Place feeding tube distal to the pylorus; consider a promotility agent, such as metoclopramide; evaluate medications and change those possibly contributing to gastric dysmotility, if possible
Dumping syndrome (weakness, diaphoresis, palpitations)	Hyperosmolar load bolused or infused rapidly into the small bowel	Do not bolus into the small bowel; temporarily decrease continuous infusion rate and gradually increase rate after symptoms subside; use an isotonic formula
	Rate or volume of feeding increased too fast	Temporarily decrease continuous infusion rate or volume of intermittent or bolus feeding, and gradually increase rate after symptoms subside
Diarrhea	Atrophy of microvilli; malabsorption related to a disease process (e.g., pancreatitis, short bowel syndrome, Crohn's disease)	Use a oligomeric formula until absorption improves; use a relatively isotonic and advance slowly; use a formula low in long-chain fatty acids when fat is malabsorbed and/or consider pancreatic enzymes
	Hypertonic formula	Change to a lower osmolarity formula
	Dumping syndrome	See Dumping syndrome entry in this table
	Rapid advancement of formula volume	Temporarily reduce rate or volume, then advance slowly; consider enteral pump for better control of administration rate
	Lactose intolerance	Change to lactosefree formula if previously using lactose-containing formula; evaluate lactose content of medications and supplemental foods, if patient is not strict NPO
	Contaminated formula	Hang fresh formula every 4 to 6 hours when using an open administration system; do not add fresh formula to volume remaining in the feeding container; change the formula container and tubing daily; follow clean/aseptic technique when working with the formula or feeding tube; minimize manipulation of the feeding tube; consider changing to a closed enteral system; avoid powdered formulas requiring reconstitution

(continued)

TABLE 37-5
Complications of Tube Feeding

Complication	Cause/Contributing Factor	Treatment/Prevention
Gastrointestinal Complications (*Continued*)		
	Medications; antibiotics; magnesium-containing antacid; high-osmolarity liquid dosage forms	Check stool for *C. difficile* and treat if present; consider probiotic agent; administer antidiarrheal if not contraindicated; consider alternate therapy such as histamine-2 blocking agent or proton pump inhibitor; use calcium-based antacid; reduce dose or divide dose into 3—4/day, when feasible to do so; dilute medication with water before administrations; consider alternate dosage form (transdermal, IV); change to crushed tablet and use appropriate precautions to avoid tube occlusion
Constipation	Inadequate fluid or free water intake	Increase volume and/or frequency of tube flushes to increase fluid intake; change to a formula with lower caloric density, if possible
	Inadequate fiber intake	Change to a formula with fiber or with a higher fiber content; administer fruit juice or bulk-forming laxative (e.g., psyllium) using caution to prevent tube occlusion
	Fecal impaction	Administer stool softener daily using caution to prevent tube occlusion if administered via the tube
	Poor gastric/GI motility	Encourage ambulation; consider promotility agent
	Medications, especially narcotics and anticholinergics	Use lowest effective dose of medication and transition to an alternate medication with fewer constipating effects, if possible
Metabolic Complications		
Hyperglycemia, glycosuria (can lead to dehydration, coma, or death)	Stress response; diabetes mellitus	Monitor fingerstick glucose every 6 hours, use sliding scale insulin plus appropriate routine insulin (e.g., insulin drip in critically ill)
	High-carbohydrate formula	Change formula
	Drug therapy (steroids)	Monitor intake and output accurately
Excess CO_2 production (high RQ)	High percentage of carbohydrate calories or excess calories from any source	Reduce total calories to avoid overfeeding; consider formula with higher fat calories
Hyponatremia	Dilutional (fluid excess, SIADH); inadequate sodium intake; excess GI losses	Use full-strength formula or change to 1.5–2 kcal/mL formula; add salt to tube feeding (1 tsp = 2 g Na = 90 mEq); use diuretics if appropriate; replace GI losses
Hypernatremia	Inadequate free-water intake	Use 1 kcal/mL formula; monitor intake and output accurately; temperature and weight daily; increase flush volume
	Excess water losses (diabetes insipidus, osmotic diuresis from hyperglycemia, fever)	Correct hyperglycemia and the cause of fever or diabetes insipidus
Hypokalemia	Medications (diuretics, antipseudomonal penicillins, amphotericin B)	Monitor serum potassium; give PO or IV potassium replacement PRN
	Intracellular or extracellular shifts (insulin therapy, acidosis)	Correct underlying problem
	Excess GI losses (NG suction, small bowel fistula, diarrhea)	Routinely provide potassium in replacement fluid
Hyperkalemia	Potassium-sparing medications (triamterene, amiloride, spironolactone, ACE inhibitors); potassium-containing medications (penicillin G potassium)	Monitor serum potassium; change to medications without potassium-sparing effect or without potassium salts
	Renal failure	Monitor renal function; change to formula with lower potassium content
Hypercoagulability	Warfarin antagonism due to formula	Hold formula 1–2 hours before and after warfarin dose; monitor coagulation status; check vitamin K content and change to lower vitamin K, if appropriate (most EN formulas are not high in vitamin K)

ACE, angiotensin-converting enzyme; EN, enteral nutrition; GI, gastrointestinal; IV, intravenous; NG, nasogastric; NPO, nothing by mouth; PO, oral; PRN, as needed; RQ, respiratory quotient; SIADH, syndrome of inappropriate antidiuretic hormone secretion.

to be reduced, whereas decreasing weight may indicate a need for increased fluid unless the patient had been fluid overloaded. Generally, total fluid can be adjusted by the number of times the feeding tube is flushed daily and the volume of each flush. In long-term patients, fluid is an important parameter for adequacy of caloric intake. Consistent increases or decreases from the required enteral formula volume can have significant effects on weight. For example, a weight loss of 12.5 pounds over the course of a year can be expected if the daily intake of a 1-kcal/mL formula is 120 mL less than required. Changing caloric density of the formula may be a potential option to help manage fluid when altering the number or volume of flushes is not adequate for fluid control. For patients with a stable fluid status, the week-to-week weight change can be used as an indicator of appropriate caloric intake. An upward trend in weight (e.g., ≥3 consecutive weeks with an increase) may indicate a need for fewer calories unless weight gain is a goal. A downward trend may indicate a need to increase caloric intake, unless weight loss is desired. A plan that includes gradual weight loss is appropriate for J.K. based on his obesity.

Respiratory status should be evaluated every 8 hours in hospitalized patients, to help recognize pulmonary edema and pulmonary aspiration. Auscultation with a stethoscope should be conducted at least two times per week, but simple observation of the patient's breathing pattern is adequate at other times unless altered respirations are noted. Coughing or respiratory distress may be indications of aspiration or other developing respiratory problems. Vital signs also may provide clues to aspiration or other problems, such as dehydration, fluid overload, or infection.

In addition to monitoring for complications, monitoring for response to EN and changes in nutritional status is recommended. This should occur routinely in patients receiving either short-term or long-term EN. Chapter 35, Basic Nutrition and Patient Assessment, discusses parameters used for nutrition assessment and on-going monitoring of nutritional status.

Gastrointestinal Complications

Assessment of GI symptoms is important for determining EN tolerance because GI complications are frequently associated with tube feeding. Abdominal distension and bloating should be evaluated at least every 8 hours while J.K. is hospitalized. Abdominal distension may be an indication of accumulating formula. The possibility of falsely low GRV due to malposition or collapse of the tube during withdrawal of gastric fluid should be considered if abdominal distension occurs when GRV is low. Gas formation secondary to lactose intolerance or rapid increases in fiber intake, and poor gastric emptying secondary to a high-fat formula, medications, recent surgery, critical illness, or an underlying disease such as diabetes are among the conditions associated with distension. When considerable distension is present, the formula should be held temporarily, and the patient evaluated further to rule out a contraindication to EN.

Nausea, vomiting, abdominal cramping, diarrhea, and constipation are other GI symptoms monitored as indicators of EN tolerance. J.K. has some of these symptoms associated with his gastroparesis, and disease associated symptoms should not be confused with feeding intolerance. Vomiting creates the most immediate concern because tube displacement and pulmonary aspiration can occur. Nausea and vomiting commonly occur with a high GRV, severe gastric distension, poor gastric emptying during gastric feeding, GI tract obstruction, or poor GI motility. Diarrhea occurs in 2% to 70% of patients, depending on the definition used, and is one of the most difficult problems for patients and caregivers to address.[35–40,74] Predisposing illnesses, including diabetes mellitus, GI infections, pancreatic insufficiency, and malabsorption syndromes, are more likely to cause diarrhea in patients receiving EN than the formula itself.[34,38,75] J.K. has type 2 diabetes; however, at this time, diarrhea has not been reported as a problem.

Formula-related GI infections could occur from contamination of an opened can or package. Sources of contamination include the water used for reconstitution or dilution, transfer to the delivery bag, formula kept in the delivery bag for a prolonged period, and poorly cleaned feeding bags or administration sets. Water used to flush the tube can also be a source of contamination; therefore, current practice recommendations are to use sterile water as the flush solution for immunocompromised patients.[37] Closed enteral feeding systems using ready-to-hang bags of formula decrease contamination by reducing manipulation of the bag and formula, and are commonly used in the hospital setting. Concurrent drug therapy (e.g., antibiotics) is another major contributor to diarrhea in tube-fed patients, potentially accounting for 61% of diarrhea cases.[38]

Bolus feeding into the jejunum can lead to diarrhea and abdominal cramping, as well as nausea and vomiting. Because J.K. is being fed into the jejunum, he should remain on a continuous infusion protocol. Initiation of EN with a hypertonic formula, a rapid rate of infusion or a large volume, and use of formula at refrigerator temperature are other factors often cited as causing GI symptoms. Although controlled studies have not supported these factors as significant contributors to GI intolerance, subjective evidence suggests they are important. Constipation is most likely to occur with long-term tube feeding in nonambulatory patients. Inadequate fluid intake and lack of fiber may be factors associated with constipation. Diabetic EN formulas contain fiber. However, if the decision is to use a very-high-protein formula for J.K., a fiber-containing formula would be reasonable to use based on his known history.

MEDICATIONS AND ENTERAL NUTRITION BY TUBE

CASE 37-4, QUESTION 3: J.K. has been receiving EN for 4 days and has been at goal rate for 2 days. Laboratory evaluation today shows the following:

Sodium, 135 mEq/L
Potassium, 2.7 mEq/L (decreased from 3.5 mEq/L yesterday, 3.9 mEq/L the previous day, and 4.6 mEq/L when tube feeding started)
Chloride, 95 mEq/L
Calcium, 7.9 mg/dL
Magnesium, 1.4 mEq/L (decreased from 2.5 mEq/L 2 days ago)
Phosphorus, 2.8 mg/dL (decreased from 4.4 mg/dL 2 days ago)
Albumin, 2.4 g/dL

Micro-K (8 mEq KCl/capsule) has been ordered as six capsules via feeding tube along with calcium carbonate (260 mg elemental calcium/tablet) as two tablets twice daily via feeding tube. Orders were also placed in the chart for J.K. to begin warfarin. He was placed on a heparin drip yesterday for a newly diagnosed deep vein thrombosis (DVT) in his left leg, despite prophylactic heparin therapy since admission. Home medications are to be restarted, including enteric-coated aspirin, 81 mg daily; famotidine tablet, 20 mg twice daily; simvastatin tablet, 20 mg daily; metoprolol succinate tablet, 95 mg daily; and verapamil capsule, 240 mg daily. How should J.K.'s medications be administered when he is receiving EN?

Patients receiving EN often receive medications through the same tube. Feeding tube occlusion, adverse effects caused by changes in pharmaceutical dosage forms, and alteration of medication pharmacokinetics and pharmacodynamics are among the potential problems.[76–79] Interactions related to pharmacologic or physiologic effects of medications or enteral nutrients also may occur. For this reason, oral medication administration should be considered unless a strict NPO status is required. J.K. has severe gastroparesis, a diagnosis not requiring a strict NPO status; however, the medical team is concerned that medications administered by mouth may have erratic absorption and poor efficacy due to delayed gastric emptying. Medications are ordered to be administered through J.K.'s feeding tube.

Medication Selection

Solid dosage forms are a challenge to administer by feeding tube. Crushing a medication and mixing the powder in water results in an altered pharmaceutical dosage form, and this may affect its efficacy or patient tolerance. Liquid dosage forms are generally recommended for administration through a feeding tube, but they are not without problems, and a liquid dosage form may not always be the best choice. Liquids should be diluted at a minimum of 1:1 with water before administration to avoid coating the tube interior. High viscosity liquids, such as suspensions, should be diluted 3:1 with water. Pharmaceutical syrups with a pH of 4 or less must be used with caution because immediate clumping and tackiness of formulas mixed with the syrups have been reported.[76,77] For medications not available in liquid form, a therapeutically equivalent medication in a liquid form can be considered. Extemporaneous preparation of a liquid also may be considered, but can increase cost significantly. Medications in a soft gelatin capsule are best avoided for administration through a feeding tube. If there is no alternative, the capsule can be dissolved in warm water. Undissolved gelatin should not be administered, because this may occlude the tube. The safety and efficacy of simple compressed tablets are not affected by crushing and dissolving in water immediately before use. Simple compressed tablets can be crushed to a fine powder, then dissolved or suspended in water for administration. Powder in hard gelatin capsules can be poured into water and mixed thoroughly before administration through a feeding tube. Failure to adequately suspend or thoroughly dissolve any of these dosage forms in water before administration through the tube can result in occlusion. Some medications appear to be particularly troublesome for administration through a feeding tube. Calcium salts, iron salts, lansoprazole, omeprazole, multivitamins, pentoxifylline, potassium chloride, phenytoin, protein supplements, sucralfate, and zinc salts were identified by nurses as the products most frequently contributing to feeding tube occlusion.[74,78] J.K. has both calcium and potassium ordered today.

Calcium carbonate is a simple compressed tablet that can be crushed, suspended in 30 mL of water, and administered through the feeding tube. Risk of tube occlusion from an inadequately crushed tablet may be decreased by use of calcium carbonate suspension (500 mg calcium/5 mL), if available. Administration of either crushed and suspended tablets or commercial suspension requires flushing the tube with 15 mL of water before and after medication administration.[37] Diluting the suspension at least 1:1 with water, preferably 3:1, and flushing with 75 to 100 mL may be advisable because suspensions may otherwise coat the tube. The appropriateness of calcium supplementation should be questioned, however, because J.K.'s serum calcium concentration is within normal limits after correction for his low serum albumin concentration, and the ionized calcium concentration would likely be within normal limits. Administering any medication via the feeding tube may occlude the tube; therefore, administering an unneeded medication through the feeding tube is an unwarranted risk. Alternative dosage forms for electrolytes are limited to IV forms so the easiest and most cost effective route is via feeding tube if J.K. cannot take oral medications.

Potassium supplementation is ordered today for J.K.'s low serum potassium. Potassium should have been considered yesterday because the serum level has been decreasing since tube feeding began. The selected potassium supplement is inappropriate for administration by tube because Micro-K is a slow-release product. Crushing any type of slow-release or sustained-release product destroys slow-release mechanisms, resulting in the immediate release of several hours worth of the medication at one time. An exaggerated therapeutic response may be seen initially, followed by a loss of response part way through the dosing interval. Deaths have occurred when sustained-release or long-acting products are crushed before administrations; therefore, these dosage forms should not be crushed.[80] Instead, an immediate-release dosage form should be used, with appropriate adjustment of dose and dosing interval, or an alternate administration route (e.g., intravenous, suppository, transdermal patch) may be available. Potassium chloride powder for solution (three packets with 15 mEq KCl/packet) or liquid (10% KCl 35 mL, 15% KCl 25 mL, or 20% KCl 15–20 mL) should be ordered rather than the slow-release product. Dividing the potassium dose into two or three smaller doses and diluting each dose with 60 mL of water may be better tolerated. Giving 45 to 50 mEq of potassium as a single dose may cause nausea, vomiting, abdominal discomfort, or diarrhea. These symptoms might be mistaken as intolerance to EN, resulting in the tube feeding being stopped temporarily. The larger fluid volume for administration also may help reduce the GI irritation associated with potassium doses.

Potassium supplementation could also be partially accomplished by changing part of the potassium ordered to potassium phosphate, which is available as a 250 mg capsule that provides 8.1 mmol of phosphate and 14.2 mEq of potassium. J.K. appears to have a mild refeeding syndrome, with phosphorus and magnesium slightly less than the normal range and having decreased significantly during the past 2 days.[25] Supplements should be started today so that smaller daily quantities can be used before electrolytes are critically low. This may decrease the risk of diarrhea and GI upset caused by the administration of oral phosphate or magnesium. Contents of each potassium phosphate capsule are designed to be dissolved in 75 mL of water for administration, so dissolution is not a concern. One potassium phosphate capsule twice a day plus KCl liquid to provide 20 mEq potassium is the same potassium dose as is ordered currently. The liquid KCl dose should be separated from the potassium phosphate to minimize GI effects.

Magnesium supplementation could be accomplished with a magnesium oxide tablet (400 or 500 mg) administered two to four times daily. These are simple compressed tablets that can be crushed and suspended for administration via feeding tube. An alternative would be magnesium hydroxide suspension 5 mL two to four times daily. Magnesium doses are distributed through the day to reduce the risk of diarrhea. The feeding tube must be flushed adequately before and after each dose of electrolyte replacement. The flush volume should be a minimum of 15 mL, although 75 to 100 mL after the magnesium dose may be better to ensure the electrolyte preparation is out of the tube. The volume of other tube flushes can be adjusted to limit the total fluid intake to the estimated requirements. It can be difficult to provide large quantities of potassium, phosphate, and magnesium via feeding tube secondary to the GI intolerance they cause. Therefore, IV electrolyte replacement may be necessary if intracellular depletion is extensive and J.K. does not tolerate oral electrolyte replacement.

Famotidine is a simple compressed tablet that can be crushed. However, both the verapamil and metoprolol dosage forms ordered for J.K. contain multiple doses intended to be slowly released. The once-daily dosing schedule helps identify these two medications as slow-release products and, for metoprolol, the succinate salt is also a clue as this is different than other dosage forms of metoprolol. Both verapamil and metoprolol should be changed to immediate-release dosage forms if J.K. cannot take them by mouth. The dose and frequency of dosing will need to be adjusted to reflect the immediate release dosage form.

Enteric-coated tablets are designed to release medication in the small bowel because the medication is either acid labile or irritates the stomach. Protection for the medication or stomach is lost when enteric-coated tablets are crushed and delivered via feeding tube into the stomach, resulting in decreased efficacy of the medication or increased gastric irritation. When an irritating medication must be given by tube into the stomach, diluting the medication in at least 60 mL of water is recommended.[76] J.K. has enteric-coated aspirin ordered for administration into a jejunal feeding tube. The enteric coating is designed to dissolve in the small bowel and could be dissolved with bicarbonate solution before administration into the small bowel. However, it would be better to use a noncoated tablet for his aspirin dose. If enteric-coated beads, such as those found in several proton pump inhibitor dosage forms, are to be administered through a feeding tube, use of an acidic liquid (e.g., fruit juice) helps prevent the enteric coating from becoming sticky and adhering to the inside of the feeding tube. This should only be considered for a large-bore feeding tube, such as a gastrostomy, or the beads will occlude the tube. Film-coated tablets also cause problems when crushed because the coating does not crush well and becomes sticky in water. J.K.'s simvastatin has a film coating and may be a problem to crush and administer through the feeding tube.

Administering buccal or sublingual dosage forms via feeding tube may result in altered absorption or destruction of the medication by stomach acid. Therefore, therapeutically equivalent medications (e.g., isosorbide dinitrate rather than sublingual nitroglycerin) or an alternate route of administration (e.g., nitroglycerin ointment or transdermal system rather than sublingual nitroglycerin) should be used. A listing of medications that should not be crushed is available at http://www.ismp.org/Tools/DoNotCrush.pdf.[81] Carcinogens, teratogens, or cytotoxic agents that should not be crushed are included in the list.

Pharmacokinetic parameters can be altered when medications are administered by feeding tube. J.K. has a jejunal tube and delivering medication into the jejunum could affect bioavailability, although few studies address this issue. Medications taken orally are delivered to the stomach, where dissolution occurs for most dosage forms and hydrolysis of some medications may occur. Delivery into the small bowel may alter these processes, thereby affecting bioavailability. For instance, recovery of digoxin from intrajejunal dosing is higher than with oral administration, primarily because of reduced intragastric hydrolysis.[28,76] Bioavailability of medications also can be affected by the presence of enteral formula in the GI tract. Medications affected by the presence of food are expected to be affected in a similar manner by the presence of formula.[77,79] For example, administration of tetracycline with formula present is expected to reduce tetracycline bioavailability because of interactions with divalent cations. A similar interaction is expected between ciprofloxacin and enteral formula, although some evidence suggests a mechanism other than binding with divalent cations is responsible for reduced ciprofloxacin concentrations with enteral feeding.[28]

Phenytoin is particularly troublesome to manage in patients receiving EN, with reduced phenytoin concentrations reported in numerous case reports and small studies. Methods suggested for management include using a meat-based formula, administering phenytoin capsules rather than the suspension, and stopping formula delivery for 1 to 2 hours before and after the phenytoin dose.[76,82] Holding formula administration before and after phenytoin dosing is often recommended, although others claim that adequate dilution will reduce loss of the medication. None of these methods, however, clearly prevents low phenytoin concentrations; thus, monitoring of serum concentrations is important whenever EN is started or altered. Large-scale, controlled trials are needed to determine the most appropriate method for managing the phenytoin–EN interaction.

Warfarin can also be troublesome to manage in patients with a feeding tube, and J.K. is to start warfarin for a newly diagnosed DVT. Reversal of warfarin anticoagulation by vitamin K included in enteral formulas is an important pharmacologic interaction.[28] The vitamin K content of most enteral formulas today is about the same as found in a mixed diet and is unlikely to interfere with anticoagulation, but should be evaluated if adequate anticoagulation is difficult to achieve. In addition, binding of warfarin to a component of enteral formulas, likely protein, has been proposed to explain warfarin resistance with formulas containing low vitamin K content.[28] Stopping formula administration for an hour before and after warfarin administration appears to prevent this type of interaction. Unfortunately, rigorous, randomized studies to provide evidenced based guidance for the management of this potential interaction are lacking.

Liquid dosage forms are often hypertonic. Diarrhea is a potential problem related to physiologic effects of hypertonic medications. Diluting hypertonic medications (e.g., potassium chloride) with 30 to 60 mL of water before administration is suggested. Dividing the medication dose and separating doses by about 2 hours also decrease GI effects of hypertonic medications. In addition, selection of brands and dosage forms with minimal sorbitol can reduce the risk of diarrhea. Sorbitol is a nonabsorbed sugar alcohol found in many liquid dosage forms. Cumulative sorbitol doses greater than 5 g can cause bloating and flatulence, whereas larger doses may act as a cathartic.[37,76,77]

Tube Occlusion

CASE 37-4, QUESTION 4: J.K.'s feeding tube has occluded (clogged). What are the causes of feeding tube occlusion and how can occlusions be managed? What can be done to avoid occluding J.K.'s tube in the future?

The incidence of feeding tube occlusion is 1.6% to 66%.[9,35,37,78] Pump malfunction, lack of periodic tube flushing, formula characteristics, and tube characteristics are non–medication-related factors affecting tube occlusion. Important tube characteristics include the inner diameter (bore size), tube material, and the arrangement and number of delivery holes (ports) at the distal end. The most important formula characteristic appears to be the protein source. In vitro studies suggest formulas with intact protein, particularly caseinates or soy, coagulate and clump when exposed to an acidic pH, whereas formulas with hydrolyzed protein do not.[28,76]

Medication-related factors influencing feeding tube occlusion include the administration method, dosage form, pH, and viscosity. Medications must be crushed to a fine powder, mixed with water to form a smooth slurry, and adequately diluted before administration. Medications admixed with formula have the greatest potential for occluding tubes owing to alteration of the texture, viscosity, or physical form of the medication or formula. Therefore, medications should not be admixed directly with formula. The enteral formula infusion should be stopped, the tube flushed with a minimum of 15 mL water before and after medication administration, and with 15 mL between each medication.[35,37,38,42,76] Contact between medications and formula within the tube lumen should be limited to decrease the risk of occlusion. Each medication should be administered separately to reduce the risk of interactions.

When a feeding tube occludes, it must be replaced unless patency can be restored. Frequent tube replacement disrupts nutrient delivery and increases patient discomfort as well as the cost of care. The initial treatment for tube occlusion is to flush the tube with warm water using a large syringe, at least 20 mL but preferably 50 mL, to avoid generation of excessive pressure that could rupture the tube. When a specific cause for occlusion can be identified (e.g., a specific medication) and physiochemical characteristics of the responsible product are known (e.g., solubility, pH), it may be possible to select a more appropriate flush preparation than water. In most cases, however, use of an acidic or basic flush preparation could worsen the occlusion. Acidic liquids (e.g., cranberry juice, diet soda, regular soda) may perpetuate or extend the occlusion, especially when coagulated proteins are the cause.[76,77] When water fails to restore patency, activated pancreatic enzymes may be effective. Previously, one crushed pancrelipase tablet and one sodium bicarbonate tablet (324 mg) were dissolved in 5 mL of warm water just before instillation into the occluded tube.[38,76] A commercial product containing multiple enzymes, buffers, and antibacterial agents in a powder form (Clog Zapper) is now available. Adherence to flush protocols and proper medication administration techniques are essential to maintain patency once tube patency is restored.

Transfer to Home on Enteral Nutrition

CASE 37-5

QUESTION 1: B.A., a 78-year-old man, was admitted 2 days ago from an SNF for evaluation of a hematoma on his left lower extremity and possible bone fracture due to a fall. He receives intermittent feedings through his PEG. The volume is 1,680 mL (seven cans) daily. B.A.'s history indicates he was hospitalized approximately 5 weeks ago with an ischemic stroke and was discharged to an SNF (see Case 37-2). B.A.'s tube-feeding volume has increased from 1,440 mL on discharge, but the formula remains the same (1.06 kcal/mL, 0.044 g protein/mL, 15 g fiber/1,000 kcal polymeric formula). His weight has increased 2 kg since hospital discharge and his overall status has improved. Bone fracture is ruled out and B.A. is able to participate in physical therapy (PT). The PT consult indicates B.A. can ambulate safely with a walker and is able to transfer from bed to chair and to the bedside commode with minimal assistance. He is deemed appropriate for outpatient PT after hospital discharge. The swallow study performed this morning indicates B.A. must continue NPO for at least another 6 months when the swallow study will be repeated again. B.A.'s daughter has made arrangements for him to move in with her family. She is concerned about insurance coverage for the EN therapy and states B.A. has Medicare insurance, including a Part D prescription plan. Will Medicare cover EN?

Before addressing the coverage of EN therapy in the home, it should be determined whether B.A. is an appropriate candidate for home versus return to the SNF. Based on the PT assessment, it is likely B.A. is appropriate for discharge home, providing he will have some supervision and assistance available. Typically, a case manager or social worker is involved in arranging appropriate discharge facilities; however, the health care professional managing nutrition support in the hospital setting should facilitate the nutrition support portion of discharge, as necessary. The pharmacist should review the medication regimen to assure it is appropriate for administration through the feeding tube.

Strict guidelines exist for home EN coverage. Medicare Part B (not Part D) will cover 80% of the cost if criteria are met.[83–85] EN must be medically necessary to "maintain weight and strength commensurate with overall health status" and there must be a functional disability of the GI tract (e.g., dysphagia, swallowing disorder) that is expected to be "permanent."[86,87] The formula must be delivered by feeding tube (i.e., not oral supplements) and must provide most of the patient's nutritional requirements (i.e., not supplemental nutrition). Approval is on an individual basis, requires a physician's written order, and sufficient documentation must be available to support the need for EN. Calories less than 20 kcal/kg/day or greater than 35 kcal/kg/day require additional documentation. The duration of therapy must be 90 days or more to meet the test of permanence. B.A.'s therapy falls within these guidelines. In addition, the formula B.A. receives is in a category that does not require him to meet additional eligibility criteria related to the formula itself. Additional documentation would be needed to justify a pump if B.A. was receiving EN via pump.

Enteral formulas are divided into five categories for reimbursement purposes by Medicare Part B (Table 37-6). Formula manufacturers typically list the Medicare category on the product label. Medicare intermediaries may also list formula categories.[88] Most polymeric formulas containing intact (whole) protein and 1 to 1.2 kcal/mL are in category I. These products have the lowest reimbursement rate and do not require documentation of medical necessity for the specific formula itself, but still require documentation of the need for EN. Clear documentation of medical need for formulas in specific categories (e.g., categories III and IV) is required for their higher reimbursement rates. Appropriate forms available from the Centers for Medicare and Medicaid must be completed for Medicare reimbursement of any EN therapy.[89]

Evaluation of Tube Feeding Intolerance

CASE 37-6

QUESTION 1: S.D., a 29-year-old woman, was admitted to the hospital 65 days ago after a motor vehicle crash. She sustained multiple traumatic injuries and exhibited multiple complications. S.D. has undergone several exploratory laparotomies and has been treated for multiple infections, including pneumonia, sepsis, and wound infection. She has been treated for *Clostridium difficile* diarrhea but has not had diarrhea since therapy was completed 3 weeks ago. Lysis of adhesions, closure of an enterocutaneous fistula, and placement of a feeding jejunostomy tube (J tube) were done during the last laparotomy 8 days ago. Enteral feedings were started through her J tube 3 days ago and advanced to the goal rate of 80 mL/hour within 36 hours. The EN provides 35 kcal/kg/day and 1.75 g protein/kg/day, which is less than her protein requirement based on nitrogen balance. She has received PN for nutrition support during most of her hospitalization and the PN rate was decreased as EN increased. S.D. now has diarrhea, which started approximately 18 hours after her EN was increased to goal rate. What is the likely cause of the diarrhea? What other information related to the EN regimen would be helpful to determine if the EN should be stopped and the parenteral nutrition formulation restarted?

Diarrhea affects 15% to 30% of patients in the ICU.[90] In patients receiving EN, diarrhea is multifactorial. Factors associated with diarrhea, but not related to EN, include medications, partial small bowel obstruction or fecal impaction, bile salt malabsorption, intestinal atrophy, hypoalbuminemia, malnutrition, infections such as *C. difficile,* and underlying conditions affecting the GI tract.[38,39,42,75–77,90] Tube feeding-related causes of diarrhea include high fat content, lactose content, and bacterial contamination. Formula temperature, caloric density, osmolality, formula strength, lack of fiber content, and method of delivery also have been associated with diarrhea, although a cause-and-effect relationship is not clear.

TABLE 37-6
Medicare Categories for Enteral Formulas

Category and Code[a]	Description	Examples (Partial Listing)
Category I B4150	Semisynthetic intact protein or protein isolates (general purpose formulas)	Boost, EnsurePowder, Isosource HN, Jevity 1.0 Cal, Nutren1.0 Fiber, Osmolite 1.2 Cal *Disease-specific formulas:* Glytrol
Category II B4152	Intact protein or protein isolates; calorically dense	Boost Plus, Carnation Instant Breakfast Lactose Free VHC, Ensure Plus, Ensure Plus HN, Isosource 1.5 Cal, Jevity 1.5 Cal, Nutren 1.5, Nutren 2.0, Resource 2.0
Category III[b] B4153	Hydrolyzed protein or amino acids	Optimental, Peptamen 1.5, Peptamen AF, Perative, Vital HN Documentation that may provide justification for use: dumping syndrome, uncontrolled diarrhea, evidence of malabsorption on appropriate semisynthetic formulas (e.g., isotonic, low long-chain fat content, lactosefree) that resolves with an oligomeric formula or documentation of the disease process causing malabsorption
Category IV[b] B4154	Defined formula for special metabolic need (i.e., disease-specific formulas)	Advera, Alitraq, Glucena 1.0, Glucerna 1.5, Glucerna Shake, NutriHep, Nepro with Carb Steady, Nutren Renal, Oxepa, Peptamen, Peptamen VHP, Pulmocare, Renalcal, Suplena with Carb Steady Documentation that may provide justification for use: evidence of inability to meet nutritional goals with category I or II products without compromising patient safety and documentation of the specific diagnosis for which a formula is intended
Category V[b] B4155	Modular components for protein, fat, and carbohydrate	*Protein:* Complete amino acid mix, ProMod Liquid Protein *Carbohydrate:* Moducal, Polycal, Polycose *Fat:* MCT oil Documentation that may provide justification for use: inability to meet specific nutrient requirements (i.e., protein, carbohydrate, or fat) with a commercially available formula

[a] Code refers to the Health Care Procedure Code System (HCPCS) billing code used by providers billing the Center for Medicare and Medicaid.
[b] Failure to provide adequate documentation of medical necessity for the specific formula will likely result in denial of claim or payment at the lower category I rate for Medicare Part B insurance coverage.
MCT, medium-chain triglyceride.

S.D.'s hospitalization has been unusually long and complicated. Many factors could contribute to her diarrhea; however, the diarrhea coincides relatively closely with initiation and advancement of tube feeding. She may have intestinal atrophy and impaired absorptive function because of her prolonged period without GI tract stimulation. She has had multiple surgeries, including GI surgeries, and may have reduced absorptive capacity, bile salt malabsorption, dumping syndrome, or reduced pancreatic enzyme availability related to her complications and surgeries. At least theoretically, an oligomeric formula would be better absorbed if any of these conditions exist. Some practice-based publications suggest consideration of an oligomeric formula for patients whose GI tract has not been used for more than 7 days.[1,91,92] The CCP guidelines recommend initiation of EN with a polymeric formula.[18,19] The SACC guidelines recommend a standard formulation for those not meeting guidelines for an immune-modulating product.[4] Only four studies comparing oligomeric with polymeric formulas in critically ill patients were found for the CCP guidelines, and none met the criteria for the highest level of study. Available data did not indicate a clinically important benefit for oligomeric formulas; however, these studies did not evaluate patients without use of the GI tract for weeks before EN initiation. Formula selection is often determined by physician preference and the calorie, protein, and fat content of formulas on the institution's formulary. Because S.D. had been more than 2 months without significant use of the GI tract, she was started on an oligomeric formula which is lactosefree and fiberfree.

The EN formula selected for S.D. is only slightly more than isotonic at 460 mOsm/kg. Risk of diarrhea from fat malabsorption should be minimal because the formula contains only 15% of calories from a 50% MCT–50% long-chain triglycerides fat mix. Increasing EN to goal rate within 36 hours may have contributed to diarrhea. Initiation at 10 to 20 mL/hour and advancement by 10 mL every 8 to 12 hours to reach goal in 48 to 72 hours would have been appropriate for S.D. because she had not used her GI tract for about 2 months.[34–40] The jejunum adapts slowly to changes in volume or concentration, and formula volume was increased less than 24 hours before diarrhea started. Also, an enteral infusion pump should be used to maintain consistent flow. Changing back to the previous volume or slightly less should decrease stool output within 24 hours if the volume change was responsible. If S.D. does not respond to decreasing formula volume, the formula may be held for 24 hours to assess whether diarrhea decreases or stops. Diarrhea related directly to EN usually is an osmotic diarrhea that stops within 24 hours of stopping the formula.[42] A more objective approach than stopping the formula is to measure stool osmolality. Enteral-formula–induced diarrhea is associated with a large osmotic gap, whereas secretory diarrhea (e.g., infectious diarrhea) is associated with a low or negative osmotic gap.[42]

The selected oligomeric formula is ready-to-use; therefore, bacterial contamination from mixing technique is not of concern. Cleanliness during formula transfer to the delivery bag, the period of time formula is in the bag, and methods of cleaning the delivery bag may contribute to bacterial contamination of formula. S.D. is receiving her formula from a closed enteral system (i.e., ready-to-hang formula-filled containers), and this virtually eliminates transfer-related contamination when proper technique is used. Any addition (e.g., medication, carbohydrate, fat or protein module, MCT oil) to the prefilled container before hanging can contaminate the system, and guidelines (e.g., hang-time, set changes) for an open enteral system then apply. Even when administered separately from the formula, modular components are a potential contributor to diarrhea due to their osmolarity and potential contamination during preparation and administration. The selected formula does not meet S.D.'s protein requirement; therefore, a modular protein is needed to supplement the enteral formula. In addition, the SACC guidelines recommend consideration of enteral glutamine administration in two or three divided doses to 0.3 to 0.5 g/kg/day.[4] The nutrition plan includes both enteral glutamine and addition of a modular protein component; however, on review of the medication administration record, neither of these has been started.

Medications are a major contributor to diarrhea in tube-fed patients.[38] S.D. currently receives antibiotics and has for some time. However, study results implicating antibiotic therapy in diarrhea have been questioned because of failure to report stool frequency and consistency as well as lack of a clear definition of diarrhea.[93] *C. difficile* may have relapsed after her previous treatment. Stool specimens should be sent for culture and/or *C. difficile* toxin. Evaluation of S.D.'s medications may reveal medications associated with diarrhea (e.g., sorbitol-containing products, antacids, oral magnesium, potassium chloride, phosphate supplements, H_2 receptor antagonists) for which therapeutic alternatives or different routes of administration could be considered.[38] High osmolality liquid medications should be diluted before administration to reduce GI side effects.[35,37,76,77]

S.D.'s GI tract should continue to be used to the extent possible. EN appears to be better than PN for maintaining the GI tract barrier and host immunologic function.[1,4,18,19,58,59,64,91,92,94] Both the CCP and SACC guidelines strongly recommend use of EN over PN in critically ill patients.[4,18,18] Both guidelines also recognize the need for PN at some point when EN cannot meet the patient's nutritional requirements; however, neither guideline addresses patients with long-term, chronic critical illness such as S.D. The risk of sepsis increases without enteral stimulation of the GI tract. Whether this occurs through bacterial translocation, an unproved process in humans in which enteric bacteria or endotoxin cross the GI mucosa into mesenteric lymph nodes and portal circulation, or through another mechanism is unclear. In addition, the GI tract serves an immune function, especially with respect to IgA secretion. Respiratory tract infections, such as pneumonia, may increase without proper stimulation of the GI tract, owing to less-effective protection from IgA. Compared with PN, EN attenuates catabolism in highly stressed patients, although initiation of feedings soon after the stressing event may be required to obtain this response. Before a decision is made to stop S.D.'s EN, all possible causes of diarrhea should be investigated. Possible benefits of improved fluid and electrolyte balance from stopping EN should be weighed against the potential benefits of reduced infections from continued use of the GI tract. Combined EN plus PN can also be considered, especially if S.D. tolerates partial EN but cannot advance to goal rate. Full PN should be provided if EN is stopped for more than 1 or 2 days.

KEY REFERENCES AND WEBSITES

A full list of references for this chapter can be found at http://thepoint.lww.com/AT10e. Below are the key references and websites for this chapter, with the corresponding reference number in this chapter found in parentheses after the reference.

Key References

Bankhead R et al. Enteral nutrition practice recommendations. *JPEN J Parenter Enteral Nutr*. 2009;33:122. (37)

Gottschlich MM et al, eds. *A.S.P.E.N. Nutrition Support Core Curriculum: A Case-Based Approach—The Adult Patient*. Silver Spring, MD: American Society for Parenteral and Enteral Nutrition; 2007. (2, 3, 7)

Marik PE, Zaloga GP. Immunonutrition in critically ill patients: a systematic review and analysis of the literature. *Intensive Care Med*. 2008;34:1980. (63)

Marik PE, Zaloga GP. Immunonutrition in high-risk surgical patients: a systematic review and analysis of the literature. *JPEN J Parenter Enteral Nutr*. 2010;34:378. (56)

Merritt R et al, eds. *A.S.P.E.N. Nutrition Support Practice Manual*. 2nd ed. Silver Spring, MD: American Society for Parenteral and Enteral Nutrition; 2005. (8)

Key Websites

American Society for Parenteral and Enteral Nutrition. http://www.nutritioncare.org and http://www.nutritioncare.org/library.asps to access content for:

- ASPEN Board of Directors and the Clinical Guidelines Task Force. Guidelines for the use of parenteral and enteral nutrition in adult and pediatric patients [published correction appears in *JPEN J Parenter Enteral Nutr.* 2002;26:144]. *JPEN J Parenter Enteral Nutr.* 2002;26(Suppl 1):1SA. (1)
- McClave SA et al. Guidelines for the Provision and Assessment of Nutrition Support Therapy in the Adult Critically Ill Patient: Society of Critical Care Medicine (SCCM) and American Society for Parenteral and Enteral Nutrition (A.S.P.E.N.). *JPEN J Parenter Enteral Nutr.* 2009;33:277. (4)

Heyland DK et al. Canadian Critical Care Nutrition Clinical Guidelines. Summary of topics and recommendations. Critical Care Nutrition. http://www.criticalcarenutrition.com/index.php?option=com_content&review=article&id=18&Itemid=10. Accessed November 28, 2010. (19)

Institute for Safe Medication Practices (ISMP). Oral dosage forms that should not be crushed. http://www.ismp.org/Tools/DoNotCrush.pdf. Accessed January 17, 2011. (81)

38 Adult Parenteral Nutrition

Jane M. Gervasio and Jennifer L. Ash

CORE PRINCIPLES

		CHAPTER CASES
1	Parenteral nutrition (PN) is indicated in patients with a nonfunctioning gastrointestinal tract. Patients should be assessed for appropriate indications of the use of PN.	Case 38-1 (Question 2), Case 38-2 (Question 1)
2	Fluid requirements as well as caloric and protein goals are based on the patient's individual needs. Macronutrient and micronutrient needs must also be determined based on the patient's history, presentation, and nutrient requirements.	Case 38-1 (Questions 3, 5, 7), Case 38-2 (Question 3)
3	Before specialized nutrition support is initiated, the practitioner must be aware of potential metabolic and respiratory complications including refeeding syndrome, increased carbon dioxide production, and hyperglycemia, some of the more commonly observed complications associated with specialized nutrition support delivery. Appropriate fluid, macronutrient, and micronutrient adjustments to specialized nutrition support must be implemented to avoid or diminish the expected problems.	Case 38-1 (Questions 8, 9)
4	In the acute-care setting, daily monitoring of the patient's vital signs, body weight, temperature, serum chemistries, hematologic indices, nutrition intake, and fluid intake and output must be performed to avoid adverse complications. Weekly assessments of the patient's prealbumin and hepatic function tests are warranted to determine success of PN delivery or necessary changes.	Case 38-2 (Question 16)
5	Advancements in the delivery of home PN have increased patients' acceptance and willingness to participate in the process. The practitioner must have an understanding of the patient's fluid and nutrient needs for optimal delivery of home PN, thereby offering the best quality of life for the patient.	Case 38-3 (Questions 1, 2)
6	Practitioners should be aware of the additional complications associated with home (or long-term) delivery of PN including liver enzyme elevation and steps to initiate to avoid or resolve this complication.	Case 38-3 (Question 3)
7	Fluid requirements, macronutrient selections, electrolyte quantities, and vitamin and mineral alterations may be warranted in patients presenting with hepatic or renal failure, short bowel syndrome, obesity, diabetes, pancreatitis, and respiratory failure.	Cases 38-4–38-6

Since the mid-1600s, efforts have been made to provide nutrients intravenously. Cannulas were introduced into peripheral veins, and various feeding solutions, including salt water, cow's milk, and glucose, were administered. Unfortunately, peripheral venous access necessitated the administration of large volumes (up to 5 L/day) of solutions with low nutrient content to provide sufficient calories to a patient. This method of feeding often resulted in thrombophlebitis or fluid overload.

It was not until the 1960s that Dudrick et al.[1] introduced the technique of placing an intravenous (IV) catheter into the superior vena cava, a large vessel with rapid blood flow. Hemodilution of fluids administered into this vessel allowed delivery of small volumes of solutions with high concentrations of nutrients.[1]

Since then, many advances in the techniques for IV cannulation and formulation of IV nutrient solutions have been made. Today, the IV provision of complex mixtures of nutrients, known as parenteral nutrition, is an integral part of the medical management of patients, both hospitalized and at home, who cannot eat or ingest nutrients by the gastrointestinal (GI) tract.

VENOUS ACCESS SITES

When parenteral nutrition is necessary, the type of venous access must be selected. Parenteral nutrient formulations may be administered via peripheral veins or central veins, depending on the anticipated duration of parenteral nutrition therapy, nutrient requirements, and availability of venous access.[2]

Peripheral

Peripheral administration may be considered when parenteral nutrition is expected to be necessary for more than 10 days and when the patient has fairly low energy and protein needs owing to minimal stress. Candidates for peripheral parenteral nutrition must have good peripheral venous access and must be able to tolerate large volumes of fluids.[3]

Parenteral nutrient formulations for administration via peripheral veins have traditionally contained relatively low concentrations of dextrose (5%–10%) and amino acids (3%–5%), providing less than 1 kcal/mL. Therefore, several liters may be needed daily to meet energy and protein needs. Even though partially diluted with nutrients, the osmolarity of these formulations is still 600 to 900 mOsm/L (normal 280–300 mOsm/L). These hypertonic formulations are irritating to peripheral veins and can cause thrombophlebitis. This necessitates frequent site rotations (at least every 48–72 hours), which may quickly exhaust venous access sites. Caloric density can be increased with only a modest increase in osmolarity by administering IV lipids concurrently or by adding lipids to the dextrose and amino acid mixtures. Lipids may also protect the vein against irritation through dilution and a buffering effect.[4,5]

Central

Administration of parenteral nutrient formulations through a central vein is preferred for patients whose GI tracts are nonfunctional or should be at rest for more than 7 days, who have limited peripheral venous access, or who have energy and protein needs that cannot be met with peripheral nutrient formulations.[2,3,6]

Traditionally, the central venous catheter is percutaneously inserted into the subclavian vein and threaded through the vein so the tip rests in the upper portion of the superior vena cava (SVC) just above the right atrium. A newer catheter technique involves the use of a peripherally inserted central catheter (PICC) that is inserted in the antecubital vein and advanced until the end of the catheter reaches the upper SVC.[6,7] The internal and external jugular veins may also be used to thread a catheter into the SVC. However, maintaining a sterile dressing on these sites is more difficult than with the subclavian approach or PICC. The SVC is an area of rapid blood flow, which quickly dilutes concentrated parenteral nutrient formulations, thereby minimizing phlebitis or thrombosis. Some patients are not candidates for placement of catheters in the SVC and require a femoral vein insertion with the tip of the catheter in the inferior vena cava. There may be a greater risk for infection with catheters placed using this technique.[6]

ONLINE CONTENT

For an illustration of a peripherally inserted central catheter, go to http://thepoint.lww.com/AT10e.

Central venous catheters can have single or multiple lumens. Multilumen catheters permit the administration of several therapies through the same IV site. Unlike peripheral venous sites, the central venous access site does not require frequent rotation. In fact, some patients requiring parenteral nutrition for months to years have permanently placed central venous catheters.[8] Parenteral nutrient formulations designed for administration through central veins can contain relatively high concentrations of dextrose (20%–35%), amino acids (5%–10%), and lipids providing a caloric density of greater than 1 kcal/mL in a solution with an osmolarity of greater than 2,000 mOsm/L.

COMPONENTS OF PARENTERAL NUTRIENT FORMULATIONS

Parenteral nutrient formulations are very complex mixtures containing carbohydrate, protein, lipid, water, electrolytes, vitamins, and trace minerals. These admixtures must be prepared under aseptic conditions as described by the American Society of Health-System Pharmacists and US Pharmacopeia standards.[9,10] Although parenteral feeding is an important adjuvant therapy for patients with many disease states, errors have occurred in managing this complex therapy, resulting in patient harm and death. Guidelines for safe practices have been developed for the situations in which inconsistent practices have the potential to cause harm. Pharmaceutical problem areas that are addressed in the Safe Practices for Parenteral Nutrition Formulations are compounding, formulas, labeling, stability, and filtering of parenteral nutrient formulations.[11]

The three macronutrients used in parenteral nutrient formulations (carbohydrate, fat, and protein) are available from various manufacturers. Water, as sterile water for injection, is also used to dilute the macronutrients to achieve the prescribed final concentrations of dextrose, amino acids, and lipids, as well as the final volume of the parenteral nutrient formulation.

Carbohydrate

Dextrose in water is the most common carbohydrate for IV use. It is available commercially in concentrations ranging from 2.5% to 70%. These dextrose solutions are mixed with other components of the parenteral nutrient formulation and diluted to various final concentrations. From these concentrations of dextrose, all parenteral nutrient formulations can be compounded. IV dextrose is monohydrated and provides 3.4 kcal/g, in comparison with dietary carbohydrate, which has a caloric density of 4 kcal/g.

Glycerol, a sugar alcohol with a caloric density of 4.3 kcal/g, is also available (as a 3% mixture with 3% amino acids) for administration as a peripheral parenteral nutrient formulation. Unfortunately, because of the dilute formulations needed to reduce osmolarity that allow peripheral administration, large volumes of solution may be necessary to meet the patient's caloric requirements, limiting the usefulness of the formulation. Other carbohydrates such as fructose, sorbitol, and invert sugar have been used investigationally in parenteral nutrient formulations, but are associated with adverse effects and are not available commercially.

Lipid

Lipid for IV use is supplied as emulsions of either soybean oil or a 50:50 physical mixture of soybean and safflower oils that provide long-chain fatty acids (>16 carbon length). Soybean emulsion is available in three concentrations: 10%, 20%, and 30%. The soybean/safflower oil emulsion is available as 10% and 20%. The 10% and 20% IV lipid emulsions may be administered concurrently (IV piggyback) with dextrose/amino acid solutions or admixed with dextrose and amino acids. The 30% IV lipid emulsion should not be used for IV piggyback administration. It is used exclusively for compounding formulations that combine dextrose, amino acids, and lipid in the same container.

Although lipid has a caloric density of 9 kcal/g, the caloric density of the IV lipid emulsions is increased to approximately 10 kcal/g by the addition of glycerol, which is added to adjust the osmolarity. Egg phospholipids are also added as emulsifiers. The phospholipids are derived from egg yolks; therefore, IV lipids are contraindicated in patients with severe egg allergies, especially egg yolk allergies. Phospholipids also contribute approximately 15 mmol/L of phosphorus.

Medium-chain triglycerides (MCTs) are used investigationally. MCTs are 6 to 12 carbons in length and provide 8.3 kcal/g. Physical mixtures of soybean oil and MCTs are being evaluated for potential use in the United States and are already commercially available in other countries.[12]

Research investigating the use of lipid formulations enhanced with omega-3 fatty acids is also being performed, with results showing improved patient outcomes (decreased length of hospital stay, decreased infections).[13] However, similar to the MCT mixtures, commercially available products are not available in the United States at this time.

Amino Acids

Protein for parenteral administration is available as synthetic amino acids and serves as the source of nitrogen. Nitrogen is the building block of cell structure and is used to produce enzymes, peptide hormones, and serum proteins. Amino acid concentrations of 3.5% to 20% are available commercially and vary slightly from one product to another in the specific amounts of each amino acid, electrolyte content, and pH. Generally, amino acid products are characterized as standard mixtures, which provide a balanced mix of essential, nonessential, and semiessential amino acids, or specialty mixtures, which are modified for specific disease states. For example, the specialty amino acid mixture for use in patients with hepatic failure contains increased amounts of the branched-chain amino acids and decreased amounts of the aromatic amino acids. Protein formulations designed for critically ill patients are supplemented with branched-chain amino acids, but have normal amounts of the other amino acids. Amino acid products for patients experiencing renal failure have increased amounts of the essential amino acids or provide only essential amino acids.[14] Amino acid products designed to meet the special needs of neonates also are available.

Protein or amino acids have a caloric density of 4 kcal/g. Protein calories have not always been included in the calculation of energy needs for patients receiving parenteral nutrient formulations. Ideally, protein is used to stimulate protein synthesis and tissue repair and is not oxidized for energy; however, the human body cannot compartmentalize energy metabolism this way. Today, the conventional wisdom is to include the protein calories in the total calorie calculations. Table 38-1 summarizes available nutrients and their caloric density.

Premixed parenteral nutrition solutions are available commercially in different percentages of dextrose and amino acid preparations. Premixed parenteral nutrition solutions are sterile products and have a longer shelf life; however, formulation customization in patients is limited.

Micronutrients

Micronutrients are electrolytes, vitamins, and trace minerals needed for metabolism. These nutrients are available from various manufacturers as either single entities or in combinations. For example, the trace element zinc is available commercially as a single trace element product or as a combination product with copper, chromium, manganese, and selenium. It is important to be aware of the specific products available in each institution to avoid providing inadequate or excessive amounts of various micronutrients.

TABLE 38-1
Caloric Density of Intravenous Nutrients

Nutrient	kcal/g	kcal/mL
Amino acids	4	
Amino acids 5%		0.2
Amino acids 10%		0.4
Dextrose	3.4	
Dextrose 10%		0.34
Dextrose 50%		1.7
Dextrose 70%		2.38
Fat	10	
Fat emulsion 10%		1.1
Fat emulsion 20%		2
Fat emulsion 30%		3
Glycerol	4.3	
Glycerol 3%		0.129
Medium-Chain Triglycerides	8.3	

PARENTERAL NUTRITION

Patient Assessment: No Acute Stress

CASE 38-1

QUESTION 1: S.D., a 39-year-old cachectic woman, is admitted to the hospital with shortness of breath and pleuritic chest pain. She has a history of moderate scleroderma (fibrosis of the skin, blood vessels, and visceral organs) diagnosed 3 years ago. She presents to the hospital with an increasing weight loss during the past 3 months accompanied with regurgitation, vomiting, and poor appetite. Approximately 3 months ago, S.D. weighed 130 pounds. Her weight today is 98 pounds; her height is 64 inches. Past medical history is also significant for hypertension. Physical examination reveals a thin woman with wasting of subcutaneous fat in the temporal area and squared-appearing shoulders. Attempts at enteral nutrition with tube feeds have resulted in sustained gastric residual volumes of greater than 400 mL.

Admission laboratory values are as follows:

Sodium (Na), 135 mEq/L
Potassium (K), 4.0 mEq/L
Chloride (Cl), 100 mEq/L
Bicarbonate (HCO_3^-), 25 mEq/L
Blood urea nitrogen (BUN), 4 mg/dL
Creatinine, 0.6 mg/dL
Glucose, 87 mg/dL
Calcium (Ca), 8.2 mg/dL
Magnesium (Mg), 2.0 mg/dL
Phosphorus (P), 3.0 mg/dL
Total protein, 6.0 g/dL
Albumin, 3.5 g/dL
Prealbumin, 15 mg/dL
White blood cell (WBC) count, 6,800/μL

Based on history and physical findings, S.D.'s working diagnosis includes aspiration pneumonia and advanced scleroderma with cutaneous, joint, and GI involvement. Assess her nutrition status.

Assessment of nutrition status requires evaluation of multiple factors. S.D.'s nutrition history indicates that she is unable to eat because of the gastroparesis, and the scleroderma diagnosis raises the question of nutrient malabsorption. Most striking about S.D.'s history is her weight loss of 30 pounds in 3 months, or about 2.5 pounds/week. S.D. is now 75% of her usual weight (see Eq. 35-2 in Chapter 35, Basics of Nutrition and Patient Assessment). Another way of analyzing this is that she has lost 25% of her original weight, which is a severe weight loss. S.D.'s physical findings of cachectic appearance, temporal wasting, and loss of subcutaneous fat and muscle in her shoulders are significant. No anthropometric measurements are available. S.D.'s visceral proteins are also in low-normal ranges, indicating both short-term (prealbumin) and longer-term (albumin) malnutrition. See Chapter 35, Basics of Nutrition and Patient Assessment, for a more detailed description of evaluation of patients with nutritional deficiencies. The principles from Chapter 35 will be applied to this and all others cases throughout this chapter.

Consideration of these factors leads one to conclude that S.D. is severely malnourished. Her cachectic appearance with loss of subcutaneous fat and muscle, but normal visceral proteins, would be best classified as marasmus malnutrition (see Chapter 35, Basics of Nutrition and Patient Assessment). If S.D. were to be faced with stress or injury (e.g., major surgery, infection) necessitating use of visceral proteins for energy production, she would likely exhibit characteristics of both marasmus and kwashiorkor, or mixed protein-calorie malnutrition in which fat, muscle, and visceral proteins are all depleted.

CASE 38-1, QUESTION 2: S.D. is admitted to the hospital for tests to evaluate her scleroderma, weight loss, and aspiration pneumonia. Why is S.D. a candidate for parenteral nutrition therapy?

Many of the expected diagnostic tests will require that S.D. remain NPO (nothing by mouth.) The subjective and objective evidence points to a nonfunctioning GI tract. If the diagnosis of advanced GI scleroderma is accurate, S.D. may require long-term parenteral nutrition therapy. In addition, attempts at enteral nutrition were unsuccessful, with continued increased gastric residual volumes, indicating decreased GI motility. With her malnourished state, continued inadequate nutrition in the hospital will result in further deterioration of her nutrition status. Parenteral nutrition should be implemented.

GOALS OF THERAPY

CALORIE AND PROTEIN GOALS

CASE 38-1, QUESTION 3: Calculate calorie and protein goals for S.D.

S.D.'s initial calorie goals are to meet her current energy expenditure needed for basal metabolism and activity of ambulating. S.D. would fall into the category of "moderate stress, malnourished" requiring 25 to 30 kcal/kg/day (see Table 35-3 in Chapter 35, Basics of Nutrition and Patient Assessment). For this calculation, S.D.'s actual weight of 98 pounds (44.5 kg) should be used because her metabolism and current energy expenditure have causes a decrease in body mass. Using usual weight or ideal body weight in patients who have severe weight loss may result in overfeeding. For S.D., the caloric goal should be 1,112 to 1,335 kcal/day.

Protein goals are estimated based on weight, degree of stress, and disease state. Because S.D. has not had surgery and her stress is minimal, her protein goal should be based on the desire to maintain her current protein status. Using the guidelines provided in Table 35-4 (Chapter 35, Basics of Nutrition and Patient Assessment), S.D.'s protein dose is 1.2 to 1.5 g/kg/day, or 53.4 to 66.7 g/day. As with energy expenditure, calculations of protein needs are only estimates; the patient's clinical course should be monitored, and the protein dose adjusted accordingly. The protein source for parenteral nutrition is synthetic amino acids. Generally, 1 g of protein is equivalent to 1 g of amino acids. S.D. will need 53.4 to 66.7 g/day of amino acids. If S.D. requires parenteral nutrition after a surgery, her energy or calorie goals should be reassessed to include a stress factor.

ACCESS

CASE 38-1, QUESTION 4: S.D. has a peripheral IV catheter, and her peripheral access appears to be adequate. Is she a candidate for using a peripheral parenteral nutrition formulation?

With good peripheral access, S.D. meets one of the criteria for peripheral parenteral nutrition. Furthermore, she should be able to tolerate the volume of a peripheral parenteral nutrition formulation necessary to meet her goals. A common complication (up to 70%) of peripheral parenteral nutrition is phlebitis, which occurs within 72 hours.[4,15] Phlebitis is usually attributed to the acidic pH or hyperosmolarity of the nutrient formulation. The osmolarity of typical peripheral parenteral feedings ranges from 600 to 900 mOsm/L compared with an osmolarity of 280 to 300 mOsm/L of plasma. Osmolarity of a dextrose/amino acid formulation can be approximated quickly by multiplying the percent dextrose concentration by 50 and the percent amino acid concentration by 100. Alternatively, the osmolarity can be estimated by multiplying the number of grams of dextrose by 5 and the number of grams of amino acids by 10, then dividing by the total volume in liters. Approximately 150 mOsm/L should be added to account for the contribution of electrolytes, vitamins, and trace elements. Although the concurrent administration of fat emulsions (up to 60% of nonprotein calories) decreases osmolarity, buffers the pH, and improves peripheral vein tolerance, it does not eliminate the risk of thrombophlebitis.[16]

Because parenteral nutrition is anticipated to be a long-term therapy for S.D., it would be most appropriate to obtain central venous access. Central access allows for longer-term administration and more-concentrated solutions, and has no osmolarity restrictions.

FORMULATION DESIGN

Macronutrients and Micronutrients

CASE 38-1, QUESTION 5: Design a parenteral nutrient base formulation for S.D. based on the caloric and protein goals determined previously.

S.D.'s caloric and protein goals are determined to be approximately 1,300 kcal/day and 60 g protein/day. Giving 60 g of protein per day will provide 240 kcal/day (1 g protein = 4 kcal). Subtracting these protein calories from total desired calories results in the amount of nonprotein calories needed (to be provided by carbohydrates and fat). For S.D., this would be 1,300 total calories minus 240 protein calories, or 1,060 nonprotein calories needed.

Typically, dextrose should account for 60% to 70% of nonprotein calories, and lipids would account for the remaining 30% to 40% of nonprotein calories. Providing S.D. with 742 kcal of dextrose (approximately 218 g of dextrose; 1 g dextrose = 3.4 kcal) will supply 70% of nonprotein calories as dextrose. The remaining 30% of nonprotein calories will be provided by lipids at 318 kcal (31.8 g of lipids; 1 g of IV lipids = 10 kcal).

As with any medical therapy, the parenteral nutrition formula should be adjusted based on patient response and tolerance. If S.D. develops complications of hyperglycemia, the dextrose component can be reduced with a subsequent increase in the lipid proportion of nonprotein calories. If hypertriglyceridemia occurs, the lipid component should be reduced with a subsequent increase in dextrose.

S.D.'s nutrient formulation should also contain standard amounts of electrolytes, as well as a daily dose of IV multivitamins and trace elements.

CASE 38-1, QUESTION 6: The pharmacy has the following stock solutions available for compounding the parenteral nutrition formula: dextrose 70%, amino acids 10%, and IV lipids 20%. How much of each stock solution is needed to compound the parenteral nutrition formula determined previously?

For dextrose, a 70% stock solution provides 70 g of dextrose/100 mL. To obtain 218 g of dextrose, 311 mL of the stock solution is needed:

$$\text{mL} = \frac{218\text{ g dextrose} \times 100\text{ mL}}{70\text{ g dextrose}}$$
$$= 311.4\text{ mL} \qquad \textit{(Eq. 38-1)}$$

Similarly, the volume necessary to provide 60 g of amino acids is 600 mL. IV lipids at 20% provide 20 kcal/mL or 20 g/100 mL. Using this stock solution, 159 mL would provide 31.8 g of lipids. The total volume of the compounded solution would be 1,070 mL/day.

Fluids

CASE 38-1, QUESTION 7: The institution uses a total nutrient admixture (TNA) system, and S.D.'s parenteral nutrient formulation is provided in 1,070 mL/day. Will this meet S.D.'s maintenance fluid requirements?

Maintenance fluid needs can be estimated using several methods. The simplest method uses 30 to 35 mL/kg/day as the basis. Another method is to provide 1,500 mL for the first 20 kg body weight plus an additional 20 mL/kg for actual weight beyond the initial 20 kg. Both methods provide estimates of fluid needs for basic maintenance, and additional fluid must be provided for increased losses such as vomiting, nasogastric (NG) tube output, diarrhea, or large open wounds. S.D.'s fluid needs are estimated as follows:

$$\text{mL/day} = 1{,}500\text{ mL} + [(20\text{ mL/kg})(44.5\text{ kg} - 20\text{ kg})]$$
$$= 1{,}500\text{ mL} + (20\text{ mL/kg})(24.5\text{ kg})$$
$$= 1{,}500\text{ mL} + 490\text{ mL}$$
$$= 1{,}990\text{ mL} \qquad \textit{(Eq. 38-2)}$$

The peripheral parenteral nutrient formulation will not meet S.D.'s needs of 1,990 mL/day. Thus the parenteral nutrition formula can be supplemented with sterile water to make the final formula 1,990 mL. Another option would be to provide the additional fluids via a separate IV line. It is important to not supply fluids in excess. The extra fluid intake may put patients at risk for becoming fluid overloaded, manifesting as hypervolemic, hypotonic hyponatremia. Therefore, S.D. should be monitored for signs of fluid overload, including peripheral edema, shortness of breath, daily intake exceeding daily output, hyponatremia, and rapidly increasing weight.

MONITORING AND MANAGEMENT OF COMPLICATIONS

CASE 38-1, QUESTION 8: What metabolic complication is a potential concern owing to S.D.'s malnutrition?

Refeeding syndrome is the term used to define the severe hypophosphatemia and associated metabolic complications that occur when malnourished patients receive a concentrated source of calories via parenteral or enteral nutrition. This phenomenon was first reported when the Holocaust victims and prisoners of war in World War II were rescued and given normal food and liquid intake. Complications coinciding with refeeding these individuals included hypertension, cardiac insufficiency, seizures, coma, and death. These complications were reported later in the 1970s and 1980s, with the introduction of parenteral nutrition in chronically ill, essentially starved hospitalized patients.

Metabolic complications from refeeding are associated primarily with severe hypophosphatemia, but hypokalemia, hypomagnesemia, vitamin deficiencies, fluid intolerance, and glucose alterations may occur. In a starved, depleted individual, there is a loss of lean body mass, water, and minerals. Individuals may preserve some intracellular electrolytes, including phosphorus. When these individuals are given a concentrated source of calories, the carbohydrates are converted to glucose. Glucose, in turn, results in the secretion of insulin. The release of insulin enhances the uptake of glucose, water, phosphorus, and other intracellular electrolytes. The combination of phosphorus depletion and intracellular uptake causes severe hypophosphatemia.

To minimize the risk of refeeding syndrome in S.D., all electrolyte abnormalities must be corrected before any nutrition is initiated. Because S.D.'s electrolytes are within normal range, no adjustments are necessary. Nutrition should then be implemented slowly and vitamins administered routinely. Laboratory values including phosphorus, potassium, magnesium, and glucose should be monitored at least daily for the first week. Although electrolyte and mineral abnormalities may not be avoided, careful recognition of and close monitoring for refeeding syndrome will prevent serious complications.[17,18]

CASE 38-1, QUESTION 9: Members of the medical team are anxious to have S.D. gain weight and are concerned by her malnourished appearance. Therefore, there is a desire to increase the calories provided to S.D. What potential complications could result from overfeeding S.D.?

Overfeeding should be avoided in all patients, especially those with respiratory concerns (i.e., mechanically ventilated, chronic obstructive airway disease). Overfeeding with carbohydrates is particularly detrimental because of the amount of carbon dioxide produced relative to the amount of oxygen consumed. This results in carbon dioxide retention that may lead to acid–base disturbance (or disturbances). Complete oxidation of carbohydrate is demonstrated at dextrose infusions of 4 to 5 mg/kg/minute. Infusions exceeding this rate increase carbon dioxide production and may cause respiratory distress. In designing a parenteral nutrient formulation for S.D., it is important to provide a moderate calorie dose and to limit her dextrose dose to less than 4 mg/kg/minute.[19,20] S.D.'s current parenteral nutrition formulation provides 3.4 mg/kg/minute of dextrose.

For adults, the daily lipid intake should not exceed 2.5 g/kg/day. However, current literature supports a maximum of 1 g/kg/day. S.D.'s formulation provides approximately 32 g of lipid daily, or 0.72 g/kg/day. It is also important to monitor serum triglyceride levels to assess tolerance to this dose of IV lipid. If the blood sample is obtained while the triglycerides are infusing, as with the TNA formulation, a serum triglyceride concentration of 400 mg/dL, although elevated, is acceptable.[21] Hypertriglyceridemia can sometimes be noted quickly by gross observation of turbidity in the blood sample.

Patient Assessment: Moderate Stress

CASE 38-2

QUESTION 1: D.C., a 38-year-old man with a 12-year history of Crohn's disease, is admitted to the hospital after being evaluated in the clinic for a complaint of increasing abdominal pain, nausea, and vomiting for 9 days, and no stool output for 5 days. Questioning reveals that over the past week he has been drinking only liquids secondary to nausea and vomiting, and his weight has decreased 10 pounds during that time. D.C.'s medical history is significant for frequent exacerbations of his Crohn's disease during the past 2 years. His surgical history includes an exploratory laparotomy 6 months ago for resection of 10 cm of ileum. Family and social histories are noncontributory. His current medications include mesalamine 1,000 mg orally (PO) four times a day (QID) and prednisone 10 mg PO every day. Review of systems is positive for severe abdominal pain. On physical examination, D.C. appears thin, and his abdomen is distended. Vital signs are notable for a temperature of 38.3°C, heart rate of 98 beats/minute, and a blood pressure of 108/71 mm Hg. He is 6 feet tall and weighs 60.5 kg. His medical record indicates that 1 month ago he weighed 64 kg, and 6 months ago, his weight was 70 kg. Abdominal radiographs are consistent with a small bowel obstruction.

Admission laboratory values are as follows:

Na, 131 mEq/L
K, 3.2 mEq/L
Cl, 98 mEq/L
HCO_3^-, 28 mEq/L
BUN, 19 mg/dL
Creatinine, 0.9 mg/dL
Glucose, 105 mg/dL
Albumin, 3.2 g/dL
WBC count, 10,900/μL
Hematocrit, 46%
Alanine aminotransferase, 29 units/L
Aspartate aminotransferase, 25 units/L
Alkaline phosphatase, 45 units/L
Total bilirubin, 0.5 mg/dL

D.C. is admitted with a diagnosis of a small bowel obstruction secondary to a stricture or narrowed area in his small intestine. The plan is to manage him with IV fluids, bowel rest, decompression, and possible surgery. Why is D.C. a candidate for parenteral nutrition?

Parenteral nutrition should be considered when the patient's nutrient intake has been inadequate for 7 days or longer and the GI tract is not functioning. D.C. has eaten little in the past week, and his 5% decrease in weight is of concern. Furthermore, his weight has decreased by more than 10% during the past 6 months, which is considered a severe weight loss. D.C. is not expected to resume oral intake because his small bowel obstruction is being managed conservatively with bowel rest and decompression.

Assessment of weight loss should include evaluation of hydration status, especially because D.C.'s vomiting and minimal oral intake for the past week place him at risk of dehydration. Loss of lean body mass is probably less than that reflected by the decrease in weight. Although D.C. may be dehydrated, he also may have significant loss of muscle resulting from his chronic intake of prednisone, which stimulates gluconeogenesis and muscle breakdown for amino acids. In addition, D.C.'s admission serum albumin concentration is low at 3.2 g/dL. His hydration status should be considered when evaluating this visceral protein, since D.C.'s serum albumin concentration will probably decrease further after he is rehydrated.

One factor contributing to his low serum albumin is the loss of proteins from the GI tract (protein-losing enteropathy) during exacerbations of his Crohn's disease. Continued inadequate nutrient intake increases his risk of malnutrition. Some type of specialized nutrition support should be initiated, and because D.C.'s GI tract is not functioning, parenteral nutrition is indicated.

CASE 38-2, QUESTION 2: What type of malnutrition does D.C. have?

At this point, D.C. exhibits some loss of fat and muscle, as well as depletion of visceral proteins. He has components of both marasmus and kwashiorkor malnutrition; therefore, he would be considered to have mixed protein-calorie malnutrition (see Chapter 35, Basics of Nutrition and Patient Assessment).

CALORIE AND PROTEIN GOALS

CASE 38-2, QUESTION 3: After hydration with IV fluids, D.C.'s weight is 62.5 kg. Parenteral nutrition therapy was delayed because within 24 hours after admission, D.C. experienced severe abdominal pain and distension and required surgery. An exploratory laparotomy was performed, and 25 cm of ileum was resected to remove an area of bowel with severe disease and a stricture that was causing the obstruction. A small abscess near his colon was also drained. His postoperative medications include hydrocortisone 100 mg IV every 8 hours and piperacillin-tazobactam 4.5 g IV every 6 hours. Bowel sounds are absent. He has a right subclavian triple-lumen central venous catheter and an NG tube output of 1,800 mL/day. His urine output is 1,400 mL/day. Parenteral nutrition is to begin on postoperative day 1. Calculate energy and protein goals for D.C.

Using the Harris-Benedict equation for men (see Table 35-3 in Chapter 35, Basics of Nutrition and Patient Assessment) and his current weight of 62.5 kg, height of 182.9 cm, and age of 38 years, D.C.'s basal energy expenditure (BEE) is 1,583 kcal/day. To estimate his total energy expenditure, the BEE should be modified with an activity factor of 1.2 for being confined to bed and a stress factor of 1.2 for surgery. These modifications result in an estimated energy expenditure of 40% greater than his BEE, or 2,216 kcal/day. Using the simpler method for moderate stress (27 kcal/kg/day) results in an estimated energy expenditure of 1,875 kcal/day. Therefore, an energy goal of 2,000 kcal/day is reasonable. In a similar manner, his protein goal (see Table 35-4 in Chapter 35, Basics of Nutrition and Patient Assessment) for moderate stress is 75 to 94 g/day of protein (1.2–1.5 g/kg/day).

CASE 38-2, QUESTION 4: Design a single daily bag, TNA parenteral nutrient formulation for D.C. that provides 2,200 kcal and 90 g of amino acids with a nonprotein calorie distribution of 75% carbohydrate and 25% lipid. The macronutrients available on the formulary for compounding the parenteral nutrient formulations are 70% dextrose, 30% lipid emulsion, and 10% amino acids.

1. Amino acids calculation

$$\text{Calories from amino acids (protein)} = 90 \text{ g} \times 4.0 \text{ kcal/g} = 360 \text{ kcal}$$

$$\text{mL of 10\% amino acids} = \frac{90 \text{ g}}{0.1 \text{ g/ml}} = 900 \text{ mL} \quad \textit{(Eq. 38-3)}$$

2. Dextrose calculation

$$\text{Calories from dextrose} = (2{,}200 - 360)(0.75) = 1{,}380 \text{ kcal}$$

$$\text{g of dextrose} = \frac{1{,}380 \text{ kcal}}{3.4 \text{ kcal/g}} = 406 \text{ g}$$

$$\text{mL of 70\% dextrose} = \frac{406 \text{ g}}{0.7 \text{ g/mL}} = 580 \text{ mL} \quad \textit{(Eq. 38-4)}$$

3. Lipid emulsion calculation

$$\text{Calories from lipid} = (2{,}200 - 360)(0.25) \text{ or } (1{,}840 - 1{,}380) = 460 \text{ kcal}$$

$$\text{mL of 30\% lipid emulsion} = \frac{406 \text{ kcal}}{3.0 \text{ kcal/mL}} = 153 \text{ mL} \quad \textit{(Eq. 38-5)}$$

4. Calculation of final volume

900 mL amino acids 10%
580 mL dextrose 70%
153 mL lipid emulsion 30%
1,633 mL total volume *(Eq. 38-6)*

Other additives such as electrolytes, vitamins, and trace elements are included in the parenteral nutrient formulation and slightly increase the final volume to 1,800 mL/day. The infusion rate for this formulation can be calculated as follows:

$$\text{Hourly infusion rate (mL/hour)} = \frac{1{,}800 \text{ mL/day}}{24 \text{ hours/day}} = 75 \text{ mL/hour} \quad \textit{(Eq. 38-7)}$$

D.C.'s parenteral nutrient formulation of 1,800 mL/day will not meet his maintenance fluid needs of 2,350 mL/day (see Case 38-2, Question 7). He will require extra fluid to meet the remainder of his basic fluid needs plus additional fluid to replace the fluid loss from his NG tube. These additional fluids should be provided through another IV.

MONITORING AND MANAGEMENT OF COMPLICATIONS

METABOLIC COMPLICATIONS: ESSENTIAL FATTY ACID DEFICIENCY

CASE 38-2, QUESTION 5: What consequences are associated with providing only dextrose and amino acids to meet D.C.'s nutrient needs?

A small amount of lipid is necessary to prevent essential fatty acid deficiency (EFAD). The essential fatty acids, linoleic and α-linolenic, are those that cannot be synthesized by humans. Of these, linoleic acid appears to be the only one required by adults. The continuous infusion of hypertonic dextrose from the parenteral nutrition is associated with high circulating concentrations of insulin. Because insulin promotes lipogenesis rather than lipolysis, linoleic acid cannot be released from adipose tissue.[22]

Clinical symptoms of EFAD are dry, thickened, scaly skin, hair loss, poor wound healing, and thrombocytopenia, which may be observed after a few weeks to months of lipidfree parenteral feedings.[23] Biochemical evidence of EFAD, determined by a triene to tetraene ratio of greater than 0.4, may be seen after 1 week of lipidfree parenteral feedings and is characterized by a decrease in the serum concentrations of linoleic and arachidonic acids and an increase in the concentration of 5,8,11-eicosatrienoic acid.[22] The requirement for essential fatty acids is 1% to 4% of total caloric intake and can usually be met by the administration of 500 mL of a 10% lipid emulsion twice weekly or 500 mL of a 20% lipid emulsion once a week to patients receiving a dextrose/amino acid parenteral nutrient formulation.[2,22] The lipid emulsions should be infused at a rate of less than 0.11 g/kg/hour to prevent adverse effects, which include impaired hepatic, pulmonary, immune, and platelet function.[12]

METABOLIC CONSEQUENCES OF EXCESSIVE DEXTROSE ADMINISTRATION

CASE 38-2, QUESTION 6: What are the benefits of using a mixed-fuel system, combining dextrose and fat to meet energy needs?

Providing a portion of nonprotein calories as fat may reduce the metabolic consequences of excessive dextrose administration. The maximal rate of dextrose metabolism in humans is 5 to 7 mg/kg/minute, or approximately 7 g/kg/day. In doses of greater than 7 g/kg/day, dextrose is used inefficiently and is converted to fat.[23] The conversion to fat may be associated with respiratory compromise and hepatic dysfunction.[24–26] Hyperglycemia, another complication of excessive dextrose infusion, is associated with electrolyte and acid–base disturbances, osmotic diuresis, increased risk of infections (especially *Candida albicans*), and altered phagocyte and complement function. Furthermore, using a mixed-fuel system allows the administration of a small amount of IV lipid daily and avoids the need for larger boluses of lipid twice weekly to prevent EFAD. Rapid administration of IV lipids has been associated with alterations in the reticuloendothelial system that are not observed with continuous administration of small doses.[27] Typically, a mixed-fuel system provides 15% to 30% of nonprotein calories as fat, 70% to 85% as carbohydrate.

TOTAL NUTRIENT ADMIXTURES

CASE 38-2, QUESTION 7: What are the advantages of combining the dextrose, fat, and amino acids in one container?

The system of providing one container per day offers the advantage of convenience to pharmacy staff, nursing personnel, and the patient. The pharmacy department usually prepares TNA only once per day and, therefore, requires fewer supplies and inventory; waste of unused feeding formulations is minimized as well. Nursing time to administer TNAs is decreased because only one bag is hung per day, minimizing venous catheter interruptions and avoiding the need to manipulate a secondary infusion of lipid emulsions, as well as avoiding additional IV tubing and an infusion pump.[28]

Although there are many practical benefits to using TNA parenteral feeding formulations, this system is not without concerns. These formulations must be mixed in plastic containers constructed with ethyl vinyl acetate. Containers with diethylhexyl phthalate should be avoided because this toxic material may be extracted by the lipid and may harm patients. The addition of lipid to the traditional mixture of dextrose and amino acids converts the mixture into a complex emulsion formulation with physiologic differences that alter the stability of the product.[29] These differences must be considered in the compounding of TNA parenteral feeding formulations.

STABILITY

CASE 38-2, QUESTION 8: How stable are the TNA parenteral feeding formulations? Why is the use of an infusion filter necessary?

IV lipid emulsions alone gradually deteriorate with time because of increased formation of free fatty acids and a resultant decrease in pH. When lipids are mixed with dextrose and amino acids, this process is accelerated. IV lipid products commercially available in the United States use an anionic egg yolk phosphatide emulsifier, which stabilizes the lipid droplets of the dispersed phase with the aqueous external phase and maintains the integrity of the dispersion. Because the emulsifier is anionic, the addition of any substance with cationic properties can neutralize the negative charge of the emulsifier and alter the emulsion's stability. When the emulsion becomes unstable or breaks down, the fat particles begin to aggregate and the particle size increases.

Destabilization of the emulsion occurs in steps that begin with creaming and end with the coalescence of the lipid particles, or "cracking" of the emulsion. A decrease in pH and the addition of divalent cations (Mg^{2+}, Ca^{2+}) increase fat particle size. Although dextrose decreases the pH, the addition of amino acids provides an adequate buffer for this variable. The amount of divalent cations added to TNAs should be limited to minimize the risk of emulsion instability. Trivalent cations such as iron should never be added to a TNA parenteral nutrient formulation. Nutrient formulations containing lipid must be assessed visually for signs of phase separation, in which the instability of the emulsion is manifested by "oiling out," indicated by a continuous layer of oil or individual fat droplets. Fat emulsion particles have an average size of 0.5 μm. A destabilized emulsion is not visibly apparent until the lipid particles are 40 to 50 μm. Fat particles as small as 5 μm may occlude pulmonary capillaries.[28,29] Therefore, the use of a 1.2-μm filter is recommended to protect against the infusion of enlarged lipid particles.[11,28]

Using dual-chamber bags may extend the shelf life of TNAs because they allow the lipid to be physically separated from the dextrose, amino acids, and other additives until it is time to administer the feeding. The use of dual-chamber bags has the greatest advantage for the home care setting, where up to a week's supply of parenteral feedings are prepared at one time.[28]

After preparation, TNAs should be refrigerated (4°C) to preserve stability. Once the bag is removed from the refrigerator, it may be warmed to room temperature and the contents mixed well before administration. Mixing is best accomplished by gently inverting the container up and down to ensure top-to-bottom transfer of the fluid. Vigorous shaking should be avoided because it introduces air, which can destabilize the emulsion.[28,29]

MICROBIAL GROWTH

CASE 38-2, QUESTION 9: How does the microbial growth in TNAs compare with that of dextrose/amino acid formulations?

Dextrose/amino acid parenteral nutrient formulations are not conducive to growth of most organisms because of their high osmolarity (>2,000 mOsm/L) and acidic pH. Lipid emulsions alone, however, are isotonic and have a physiologic pH, providing an optimal growth medium. Combining these three substrates in a TNA provides a formulation with a microbial growth potential that is intermediate between these two.[28,29] The number of central venous catheter violations or manipulations correlates strongly with the incidence of catheter-related infections. From an infection-control perspective, the use of a single daily bag TNA system limits the number of manipulations of the central venous catheter to one per day, thereby minimizing touch contamination. The Centers for Disease Control and Prevention guidelines allow TNA or dextrose/amino acid formulations to hang for up to 24 hours. However, because of concerns about the potential of lipid emulsions to support microbial growth, the hang time for lipids when administered alone is 12 hours.[28]

MICRONUTRIENTS

Electrolytes

CASE 38-2, QUESTION 10: D.C.'s current laboratory values are as follows:

Na, 137 mEq/L	Glucose, 148 mg/dL
K, 4.5 mEq/L	Ca, 8.9 mg/dL
Cl, 102 mEq/L	Mg, 1.9 mg/dL
HCO_3^-, 26 mEq/L	P, 2.8 mg/dL
BUN, 9 mg/dL	Albumin, 3.0 mg/dL
Creatinine, 0.8 mg/dL	

Which electrolytes should be included in D.C.'s parenteral nutrient formulation?

Electrolytes added are sodium, potassium, chloride, acetate (which is metabolized to bicarbonate), magnesium, calcium, and phosphate. Electrolytes should be added to the parenteral nutrient formulation based on the individual patient's needs. However, patients without significant fluid and electrolyte losses, hepatic or renal dysfunction, or acid–base disturbances do well with maintenance doses of electrolytes. Electrolytes may be added individually or as commercially available combination products of maintenance doses, but the electrolyte content of the amino acid solution should be considered. General guidelines for electrolyte requirements for parenteral feedings are included in Table 38-2.

Vitamins and Trace Elements

CASE 38-2, QUESTION 11: What doses of multiple vitamins and trace elements should D.C. receive in his parenteral nutrient formulation?

Vitamins and trace elements are essential for normal metabolism and should be included in a patient's daily parenteral

TABLE 38-2
Guidelines for Daily Electrolyte Requirements

Electrolyte	Amount
Sodium	80–100 mEq
Potassium	60–80 mEq
Chloride	50–100 mEq[a]
Acetate	50–100 mEq[a]
Magnesium	8–20 mEq
Calcium	10–15 mEq
Phosphorus (phosphate)	20–40 mmol

[a] As needed to maintain acid–base balance.

nutrition regimen. Guidelines for the 13 essential vitamins have been established by the Nutrition Advisory Group of the American Medical Association[30] (Table 38-3).

Guidelines for daily doses of the trace elements, chromium, copper, manganese, and zinc have also been developed.[31] In addition to these trace elements, many practitioners provide selenium on a daily basis. Recommended doses of the trace elements are listed in Table 38-4. As with vitamins, trace elements are available as single entities or combination products. Molybdenum and iodine are also available commercially.

CASE 38-2, QUESTION 12: D.C.'s daily parenteral nutrient formulation of 1,800 mL provides 2,200 calories (75% non-protein calories as carbohydrate, 25% as fat) and 90 g of amino acids with the following additives per daily volume: NaCl, 75 mEq; K acetate, 70 mEq; phosphate as Na salt, 27 mmol; $MgSO_4$, 16 mEq; calcium gluconate, 10 mEq; and standard doses of adult multivitamins and multiple trace elements providing chromium, copper, manganese, selenium, and zinc. The infusion is initiated at a rate of 40 mL/hour. Why is this slow infusion rate selected?

Standard practice for administering parenteral nutrient formulations containing hypertonic dextrose is to begin at a slow infusion rate of less than 250 g during the first 24 hours for most patients and less than 150 g for patients with known diabetes

TABLE 38-3
Recommended Adult Daily Doses of Parenteral Vitamins

Vitamins	Dose
Fat-Soluble Vitamins	
A	3,300 international units (990 retinol equivalents)
D	200 international units (5 mg cholecalciferol)
E	10 international units (6.7 mg/dL-α-tocopherol)
K	150 mcg
Water-Soluble Vitamins	
Thiamine (B_1)	6 mg
Riboflavin (B_2)	3.6 mg
Niacin (B_3)	40 mg
Pyridoxine (B_6)	6 mg
Cyanocobalamin (B_{12})	5 mcg
Folic acid	600 mg
Pantothenic acid	15 mg
Biotin	60 mcg
Ascorbic acid (C)	200 mg

TABLE 38-4
Recommended Daily Adult Doses of Parenteral Trace Elements

Trace Element	Dose
Chromium	10–15 mcg
Copper	0.3–0.5 mg
Manganese	60–100 mcg
Selenium	20–60 mcg
Zinc	2.5–5 mg

mellitus or hyperglycemia. The infusion is increased slowly during the next 24 to 48 hours to the goal infusion rate. This initial period allows the clinician to assess the patient's ability to tolerate the nutrient formulation components and to avoid metabolic complications, primarily hyperglycemia.[22] If D.C.'s serum glucose level remains less than 150 mg/dL, the parenteral nutrient formulation infusion rate can be increased to his goal rate of 75 mL/hour.

MONITORING AND MANAGEMENT OF COMPLICATIONS

METABOLIC COMPLICATIONS

Parenteral nutrition therapy may be associated with multiple metabolic complications. The most common abnormalities are hypokalemia, hypomagnesemia, hypophosphatemia, and hyperglycemia. The plan for parenteral nutrition therapy should include routine monitoring of these serum chemistries to identify complications early and institute methods to manage or prevent complications.

CASE 38-2, QUESTION 13: During the next 24 hours, D.C.'s infusion rate is increased to the goal rate of 75 mL/hour. A comparison of his intake and output reveals an overall negative fluid balance because a high volume of gastric fluid is being removed via the NG tube. Laboratory values at this time are the following:

Na, 138 mEq/L	**Glucose, 279 mg/dL**
K, 3.1 mEq/L	**Ca, 7.8 mg/dL**
Cl, 91 mEq/L	**Mg, 1.4 mg/dL**
HCO_3^-, 33 mEq/L	**P, 1.8 mg/dL**
BUN, 28 mg/dL	**Albumin, 2.8 g/dL**
Creatinine, 0.9 mg/dL	

Arterial blood gas (ABG) results are pH, 7.46; PO_2, 98 mm Hg; PCO_2, 47 mm Hg; and HCO_3^-, 31 mEq/L. What factors contribute to these metabolic abnormalities?

Hypokalemia

Hypokalemia, a common metabolic abnormality associated with the initiation of parenteral nutrition, usually occurs within 24 to 48 hours. Potassium moves, along with dextrose, from the extracellular to the intracellular space. Furthermore, building lean body mass (i.e., anabolism) requires approximately 3 mEq of potassium per gram of nitrogen provided by the amino acids. Administering dextrose promotes repletion of glycogen stores, which also requires potassium.[18,22,32]

D.C.'s decreased serum potassium concentration is compounded by metabolic alkalosis caused by his loss of gastric secretions through the NG tube and the administration of hydrocortisone. With this type of metabolic alkalosis, the renal excretion of potassium is increased. Additional potassium should be administered and can be provided in D.C.'s parenteral feeding or through another IV.

Hypomagnesemia

Magnesium, like potassium, is primarily an intracellular cation and is considered an anabolic electrolyte. It is common to observe decreases in magnesium serum concentrations during the administration of parenteral nutrient formulations. Synthesis of lean tissue requires 0.5 mEq magnesium per gram of nitrogen.[18,22,32] Additional magnesium can be added to the parenteral nutrient formulation. However, when a TNA formulation is used, the amount of magnesium must stay within the guidelines for the cation content to maintain the stability of the lipid emulsion.

Hypophosphatemia

Hypophosphatemia occurs when phosphorus moves into the cells for the synthesis of adenosine triphosphate (ATP), an important energy carrier. Phosphorus is depleted quickly with the administration of hypertonic dextrose, especially in malnourished patients (see Case 38-2, Question 8, for discussion of refeeding syndrome). The phosphorus is used for ATP synthesis, primarily in the liver and skeletal muscle. Alkalosis also decreases phosphate stores by stimulating the phosphorylation of carbohydrates. As a component of 2,3-diphosphoglycerate, found in red blood cells (RBCs), phosphorus is necessary for the disassociation of oxygen from hemoglobin.[32]

Clinical signs and symptoms of hypophosphatemia usually occur when serum concentrations fall to less than 1.0 mg/dL. They include lethargy, muscle weakness, impaired WBC function, glucose intolerance, rhabdomyolysis, seizures, hemolytic anemia, reduced diaphragmatic contractility, and death. Moderate to severe, complicated hypophosphatemia can be managed by administering up to 0.625 mmol/kg of phosphate IV.[18,32–34] Although D.C.'s serum phosphorus is not less than 1.0 mg/dL, it is low (1.8 mg/dL), and he should receive 15 to 30 mmol of phosphate in the parenteral nutrient formulation per day. Additional supplements may be necessary to replete his phosphorus stores.[33]

Metabolic Alkalosis

D.C. has evidence of a metabolic alkalosis based on his ABG results, hypochloremia, and elevated bicarbonate level. The continued loss of fluid and HCl from the NG tube is the most probable cause of his metabolic alkalosis. Management of this type of metabolic alkalosis is to replace the fluid and chloride through another IV. Because acetate is converted to bicarbonate and can further contribute to the alkalosis, the acetate salts in the parenteral nutrient formulation can be changed to chloride salts.[32] Nevertheless, the parenteral nutrient formulation is not the primary vehicle for adjusting and supplementing electrolytes and fluids. Instead, the fluid and electrolyte balance should be adjusted with maintenance IV fluid and electrolyte supplements.

Hyperglycemia

Hyperglycemia is a common metabolic complication of parenteral nutrition therapy, especially in stressed patients. Stress alone increases gluconeogenesis, and the administration of hypertonic dextrose compounds the potential for hyperglycemia.[35] D.C. is at particular risk for hyperglycemia because he is recovering from surgery and is receiving steroids, which increase gluconeogenesis.

Persistent hyperglycemia leads to glucosuria and an osmotic diuresis, resulting in dehydration and concomitant electrolyte abnormalities. It also compromises the immune response by causing abnormalities in chemotaxis and phagocytosis and by impairing complement function. Hyperglycemia is associated with an increased risk of infections, especially *C. albicans.* In extreme cases, hyperglycemia progresses to hyperosmolar, nonketotic acidosis and coma, a condition associated with 40% mortality.

Hyperglycemia can be minimized by limiting the dextrose infusion rate to less than 4 mg/kg/minute.[36] (D.C.'s parenteral nutrient formulation provides 4 mg/kg/minute.) Other measures that will minimize the risk of hyperglycemia include gradually increasing the parenteral nutrient formulation infusion rate, frequently monitoring capillary blood glucose concentrations, and advancing therapy only when the serum glucose is consistently less than 150 mg/dL for stable patients and less than 120 mg/dL for critically ill patients. Insulin therapy should be considered if serum glucose concentrations exceed these parameters and can be administered subcutaneously according to a sliding scale, IV by continuous infusion, or by adding insulin to the parenteral nutrient formulation.[37,38] Only regular insulin can be added to a parenteral nutrient formulation. A reasonable strategy for adding insulin to the parenteral nutrient formulation is to begin with 0.1 units of regular insulin per gram of dextrose. This dosage is adjusted depending on serum glucose concentrations.[37] Clinical evidence suggests that treatment of hyperglycemia and maintenance of euglycemia may reduce morbidity and mortality, length of stay, and hospital costs.[38–42]

Formulation Design

COMPATIBILITY

CASE 38-2, QUESTION 14: In response to these serum chemistries, the electrolytes in D.C.'s parenteral nutrient formulation are changed to the following per liter: NaCl, 160 mEq; KCl, 140 mEq; phosphate as K salt, 60 mmol; $MgSO_4$, 54 mEq; and calcium gluconate, 30 mEq. How do the doses of calcium and phosphate compare with maintenance doses? What calcium and phosphate incompatibilities should be anticipated? Will the calcium and magnesium content alter the lipid stability?

The dose of calcium ordered for D.C. is more than three times the usual maintenance dose (Table 38-2). This amount of calcium is not necessary because the observed hypocalcemia merely reflects D.C.'s low serum albumin concentration; therefore, less calcium is bound to albumin. D.C. probably does not have true hypocalcemia because his free (or ionized) calcium, which is critical for physiological function, has not changed. If available, obtaining an ionized calcium concentration is advised. However, some laboratories do not have this test available. In this situation, a "corrected" calcium formulation may be used. For every 1-g/dL decrease in serum albumin concentration, there will be about a 0.8-mg/dL reduction in the serum calcium concentration.[43] For D.C., a serum calcium of 7.8 mg/dL will correct to a serum concentration of 8.8 mg/dL ([4.0–2.8 g/dL albumin][0.8] + 7.8 mg/dL calcium).

The amount of phosphate prescribed for D.C. at this time exceeds the usual recommended dose of 15 to 30 mmol/day (Table 38-2). Although D.C. has a low serum phosphorus concentration and needs additional phosphate, increasing the dosage in the parenteral nutrient formulation to 60 mmol/day may be incompatible with the calcium content, resulting in calcium phosphate precipitation. Administering a parenteral nutrient formulation containing calcium phosphate crystals may occlude blood flow, especially in the lungs, and has been associated with adverse events, such as respiratory distress and death.[11,44]

It is important to consider the factors that affect calcium phosphate solubility and to take measures that ensure the solubility limits are not exceeded when preparing parenteral nutrient formulations. The in vitro precipitation of calcium phosphate depends on multiple factors, including the calcium salt, concentrations of calcium and phosphate, amino acid concentration, temperature, pH of the formulation, and infusion time. Using calcium gluconate rather than the chloride salt can enhance calcium phosphate solubility. In solution at equimolar concentrations, calcium chloride dissociates more than calcium gluconate, thereby increasing the yield of free calcium available for binding with phosphate.

The amounts of calcium and phosphorus in the formulation are critical. Multiple investigators have varied the calcium and phosphate concentrations in parenteral nutrient formulations and have developed precipitation curves to assist practitioners in determining the amounts of calcium and phosphate that can be added safely to nutrient formulations. These guidelines help predict the points at which calcium phosphate precipitation is likely to occur. However, extrapolating these data to parenteral nutrient formulations different from those described is difficult because these mixtures are extremely complex, and numerous variables affect the interrelationship between calcium and phosphate.

The solubility of calcium and phosphate must be determined based on the volume of the formulation at the time the calcium and phosphate are mixed together, not the final volume. For example, if the electrolytes including calcium and phosphate are added to 1,000 mL of a dextrose/amino acid mixture and then 300 mL of IV fat is added, the calcium phosphate solubility is based on the 1,000 mL, not the final 1,300 mL volume. In addition, some amino acid products contain phosphate ions, and these should be considered when determining calcium phosphate solubility.[11]

Last, calcium and phosphate should not be added to the parenteral nutrient formulation in close sequence. It is recommended to add phosphate first and calcium last, thereby taking advantage of the maximal parenteral volume. Also, during preparation, the parenteral nutrient formulation should be agitated periodically and inspected for precipitates.[45] Other guidelines for improving the solubility of calcium are a final amino acid concentration of greater than 2.5% and a pH less than 6. Temperature is a critical variable, and an increase in the ambient temperature can facilitate the precipitation of calcium phosphate. Formulations should be infused within 24 hours after compounding if stored at room temperature; if refrigerated, they should be infused within 24 hours after rewarming. Furthermore, slow infusions may decrease solubility. Increasing temperature and slow infusions may result in precipitation in the IV catheter, even if precipitation has not occurred in the infusion container.[11]

The amount of divalent cations, calcium (20 mEq) and magnesium (30 mEq), exceeds the general guidelines for maximal amounts that can be added safely to a TNA without disrupting the stability of the lipid emulsion. A limit of 20 divalent cations per liter is a general guideline. The amount prescribed for D.C.'s regimen is excessive because it provides 50 divalent cations in 1.8 L (28 divalent cations/L) and may result in a potentially unstable admixture.

Last, a 1.2-μm air-eliminating filter should be used when infusing TNA parenteral nutrient formulations, and a 0.22-μm air-eliminating filter should be used for non–lipid-containing admixtures.[11]

MEDICATION ADDITIVES

CASE 38-2, QUESTION 15: In addition to his parenteral nutrient formulation, D.C. is receiving ranitidine 50 mg IV every 8 hours and hydrocortisone 100 mg IV every 8 hours, and now he needs insulin. Can these medications be mixed with his parenteral nutrient formulation to simplify his medication regimen?

Patients receiving parenteral nutrition therapy often require concomitant drug therapy. Most patients have adequate venous access or have multiple-lumen central venous catheters, so that mixing medications with the parenteral nutrient formulation is not an issue. However, for some patients with limited venous access, directly added medications or piggybacking medications via a secondary infusion may be considered.

The stability of medications when mixed with parenteral nutrient formulations is a complex issue. Some medications may be added directly to the parenteral nutrient formulation, whereas others should be administered via a secondary infusion set (piggybacked). Many medications have been studied for physical compatibility, but few have been evaluated for pharmacologic activity. Furthermore, the study conditions vary, and different nutrient formulations have been used; therefore, interpretation and application of data from a particular scientific study to a specific nutrient formulation may be difficult. This area of knowledge is growing rapidly, and current information regarding compatibility and stability is available in standard references such as Trissel's *Handbook of Injectable Drugs*.[46]

Although insulin, antibiotics, chemotherapeutic agents, histamine type 2 (H_2)-receptor antagonists, and heparin have been considered for addition to parenteral nutrient formulations in some specific circumstances, the routine addition of medications to parenteral nutrient formulations is discouraged. The addition of insulin to parenteral nutrient formulations may be an option, as described in Case 38-2, Question 13, and Case 38-6, Question 2.

MONITORING PARAMETERS

CASE 38-2, QUESTION 16: Design a plan to monitor the adequacy of D.C.'s specialized nutrition support and to identify and prevent adverse complications.

Routine evaluation of patients receiving nutrition support should include an assessment of nutrition and the metabolic effects of therapy. Goals for nutrition therapy are estimates of a patient's needs; therefore, the adequacy of therapy to meet these needs must be evaluated. Daily monitoring parameters must include vital signs, body weight, temperature, serum chemistries, hematologic indices, nutrition intake, and fluid intake and output.

The adequacy of nutrition therapy should be assessed weekly. This may include measuring serum concentrations of visceral proteins (see Table 35-2 in Chapter 35, Basics of Nutrition and Patient Assessment). Because prealbumin has a half-life of only 2 to 3 days, serum concentrations of this protein should increase with adequate nutrition and improving clinical status. Albumin, with a much longer half-life, may not change for several weeks to months despite provision of adequate nutrients. In addition, it is reasonable to perform indirect calorimetry to reassess energy expenditure.

Another method to assess the adequacy of protein intake is to evaluate nitrogen balance. This test is designed to estimate the amount of nitrogen retained by comparing the amount of nitrogen administered to the amount of nitrogen excreted (amount "in" vs. amount "out"). The nitrogen "in" is provided by the amino acid (AA) component of the parenteral nutrient formulation and other sources from tube feeding or an oral diet. Each commercially available amino acid formulation has a slightly different amount of nitrogen per gram of amino acids, and the manufacturer's product information should be consulted to obtain this value. An average value is 6.2 g of nitrogen per gram of amino acids.

Most of the nitrogen is excreted as byproducts of protein breakdown for energy. This nitrogen is excreted in the urine as urea nitrogen, which increases with increasing stress. To determine this value, urine must be collected for 24 hours and the amount of urea nitrogen (UUN) measured. Some laboratories have the capability of measuring total urine nitrogen, which measures all nitrogen entities in the urine. In addition, some nitrogen lost via skin, respiration, and stool is not measurable but is estimated to be 2 to 4 g/day.

$$\begin{aligned}\text{Nitrogen balance} &= \text{Nitrogen in} - \text{Nitrogen out}\\ &= \frac{\text{AA (g)}}{6.2} - [\text{UUN (g)} + 3\ \text{g}]\\ &= \text{g} \qquad \textit{(Eq. 38-8)}\end{aligned}$$

Achieving a positive nitrogen balance is difficult, if not impossible, in critically ill patients; therefore, the calculation may result in a negative number or zero. For convalescing patients, a nitrogen balance of plus 2 to 4 g is acceptable. A negative nitrogen balance prompts a re-evaluation of the amount of protein and energy a patient is receiving. For patients with a negative nitrogen balance, it may be helpful to increase intake of both calories and protein.

As with all tests, assessment should include monitoring several parameters, including the patient's clinical status. Most important is the identification of trends that may alert one to impending complications. A suggested schedule for monitoring is provided in Table 38-5.

TABLE 38-5
Routine Monitoring Parameters for Parenteral Nutrition

Before Initiating Therapy
Body weight
Serum electrolytes (Na, K, Cl, HCO_3^-, BUN, creatinine)
Glucose
Ca, Mg, P
Albumin, transthyretin
Triglycerides
CBC
Liver-associated tests (AST, ALT, alkaline phosphatase, bilirubin)
INR, prothrombin time
Daily
Body weight
Vital signs (pulse, respirations, temperature)
Fluid intake
Nutritional intake
Output (urine, other losses)
Serum electrolytes (Na, K, Cl, HCO_3^-, BUN, creatinine)
Glucose
Two or Three Times a Week
CBC
Ca, Mg, P
Weekly
Albumin, transthyretin
Liver-associated tests (AST, ALT, alkaline phosphatase, bilirubin)
INR, prothrombin time
Nitrogen balance

ALT, alanine aminotransferase; AST, aspartate aminotransferase; BUN, blood urea nitrogen; Ca, calcium; CBC, complete blood count; Cl, chloride; HCO_3^-, bicarbonate; INR, international normalized ratio; K, potassium; Mg, magnesium; Na, sodium; P, phosphorus.

Home Therapy

ENTEROCUTANEOUS FISTULAS

CASE 38-3

QUESTION 1: S.A. is a 24-year-old woman hospitalized after an abdominal trauma injury requiring abdominal surgery to repair a small bowel perforation. On hospital day 10, she presents with a fever and green, purulent fluid draining from a small hole in her abdominal incision site. She is diagnosed with an enterocutaneous fistula, which is a communication between her intestine and the skin. The fluid loss from S.A.'s fistula is about 1,300 mL/day. Management will include NPO and parenteral nutrition for 4 to 6 weeks in anticipation that the fistula will heal and further surgery can be avoided. The physician would like to begin parenteral nutrition therapy in the hospital with the plan to discharge S.A. home in a few days. S.A. is 5 feet 4 inches and weighs 54 kg. Design an appropriate home peripheral nutrition formula for S.A.

Parenteral nutrition therapy in the home has allowed patients such as S.A. to be discharged after a much-shortened hospital stay. Candidates for home therapy must be physically and medically stable, have a strong support network in the home setting to assist with care, and have an appropriate home environment; they must be educated regarding the prescribed therapy.[47]

The first step in designing a parenteral nutrition regimen is to estimate energy and protein needs (see Chapter 35, Basics of Nutrition and Patient Assessment). S.A. is 10 days after injury, and her estimated requirements would be 25 to 30 kcal/kg/day or 1,550 to 1,620 kcal/day. Protein goals must include adequate nitrogen (protein) for wound healing and replacement for losses from the enterocutaneous fistula. A goal of 1.5 to 1.8 g/kg/day (81–97 g) is reasonable.

To simplify her nutrition and fluid regimen, all of S.A.'s fluids, including parenteral nutrients, electrolytes, vitamins, trace minerals, and water, should be provided in one container per day. S.A.'s home parenteral nutrient formulation can be provided in 3,000 mL/day to meet maintenance requirements (30–35 mL/kg/day) and to replace losses from her enterocutaneous fistula (1,300 mL/day). Nutrients provided include 95 g of amino acids (390 kcal); 217 g of dextrose (750 kcal); 38 g of lipid (375 kcal); and electrolytes, vitamins, and minerals to maintain normal serum chemistries. Initially, daily intake and output must be monitored; therapy should be adjusted based on this information and S.A.'s clinical status.

Adjustments in fluids and electrolytes may be needed. The fluids secreted by the GI tract are rich in electrolytes, including sodium, potassium, chloride, and bicarbonate. Measurement of the electrolyte content of the fistula fluid will determine those that must be replaced, and in what quantities. Both fluid and electrolytes should be replaced to prevent dehydration and electrolyte and acid–base imbalances.

In addition to losses of fluids and electrolytes, the trace element zinc is lost in fluid from the small intestine. Approximately 12 mg of zinc is lost in each liter of small bowel fluid, and should be replaced to prevent zinc deficiency. Furthermore, zinc may play a role in wound healing.[47] Management of enterocutaneous fistulas may include octreotide 50 to 100 mg given subcutaneously two or three times daily or added to the parenteral nutrient formulation to decrease fistula output.[48]

A home infusion pharmacy will be responsible for preparing S.A.'s parenteral nutrient formulations. Typically, nutrient formulations for 7 days are prepared and delivered to the patient's home. These formulations must be refrigerated until administration; however, formulations should be warmed to room temperature and visually inspected for particulate matter before being administered. Because some additives such as multivitamins are not stable for long periods, the patient or caregiver must add these to the parenteral nutrient formulation just before administration.

Patients and caregivers preparing for home parenteral nutrition therapy must be taught how to manage home therapy. This includes assessment of fluid status, care of a central venous catheter, infection, and the technical aspects of administering parenteral feeding formulations.[49]

Preparation for home parenteral nutrition includes placement of a central venous access device. Various devices are available for long-term therapy.[6,8] However, because the duration of S.A.'s therapy is expected to be 4 to 6 weeks, she may be a good candidate for a PICC.

CYCLIC THERAPY

CASE 38-3, QUESTION 2: What other measures can be used to simplify S.A.'s parenteral feeding regimen and encourage ambulation?

After S.A.'s daily nutrient and fluid needs are consolidated and she is stable on that regimen, her parenteral nutrient regimen can be cycled. *Cycling* means infusing the parenteral nutrient formulation for less than 24 hours so there is some time free from therapy. Cycling is usually done gradually and depends on the patient's ability to tolerate the changes in fluid and dextrose intake. Initially, the infusion period is decreased by 2 to 6 hours, and the infusion rate is increased to compensate for the shorter infusion period. For example, a 24-hour infusion at 100 mL/hour would be changed to a 20-hour infusion at 120 mL/hour. This gradual adjustment is more likely to ensure that all nutrients are infused and well tolerated. With each incremental decrease in time, the infusion rate should be increased.

Vital signs, fluid intake and output, and serum electrolytes and glucose concentrations should be monitored during this period. The serum glucose concentration should be evaluated 30 minutes after the infusion is completed to be sure that hypoglycemia does not occur as the result of the rapid cessation of the nutrient formulation. If hypoglycemia occurs, the infusion rate can be tapered at the end of the infusion because a gradual decrease in glucose intake should minimize the potential for hypoglycemia. Furthermore, the infusion can be gradually increased to minimize sudden hyperglycemia at the beginning of the infusion. Infusion management devices used at home can automatically make these adjustments in the infusion rate. Eventually, the nutrient formulation can be infused for 10 to 12 hours during the night, leaving S.A. free from her infusion bag during the day.

METABOLIC COMPLICATIONS: ELEVATED LIVER-ASSOCIATED ENZYMES

CASE 38-3, QUESTION 3: After receiving home parenteral nutrition for 3 weeks, S.A.'s liver function tests are found to be elevated. Current values are as follows:

Bilirubin, 0.8 mg/dL
Aspartate aminotransferase, 70 units/L
Alanine aminotransferase, 90 units/L
Alkaline phosphatase, 100 units/L

Could her parenteral nutrition be contributing to these abnormalities?

Elevations in liver function tests are common in adults receiving long-term parenteral nutrition therapy and may be noted as early as 2 to 3 weeks after beginning therapy. The abnormalities are usually mild and transient and do not progress to significant liver dysfunction in adults. The predominant type of hepatobiliary dysfunction is steatosis (fatty liver), whereas other patients develop cholestasis or cholelithiasis (biliary obstruction). Liver-associated enzyme elevations usually resolve when parenteral nutrition therapy is discontinued. Rarely does this dysfunction proceed to hepatic failure.[50,51]

Although parenteral nutrition-associated liver abnormalities were first noted more than 30 years ago, a cause-and-effect relationship has been difficult to establish because patients have many confounding factors that can also cause liver dysfunction, including medications, inflammatory bowel disease, and sepsis. Other contributing factors are overfeeding with parenteral nutrient formulations containing high amounts of carbohydrate, amino acid deficiencies, excess fat, EFAD, carnitine deficiency, choline deficiency, toxic effects of the amino acid degradation products, bacterial overgrowth in the small intestine, and lack of stimulation of the GI tract.[50,51] Other than avoiding overfeeding with carbohydrate and lipid, there are few options to prevent or manage parenteral nutrition-associated liver abnormalities. Potential treatments include metronidazole and supplements of ursodeoxycholic acid, choline, and carnitine. Patients with progressive liver disease may be candidates for liver and small bowel transplantation.[51]

The elevations in S.A.'s liver enzymes are not of concern at this time because they are less than three times normal. However, they should be monitored weekly for continued increases. Because she may not need lifelong parenteral nutrition therapy, the mild elevations are likely to resolve.

USE OF PARENTERAL NUTRITION IN SPECIAL DISEASE STATES

Hepatic Failure

CASE 38-4

QUESTION 1: V.G. is a 42-year-old woman with a 15-year history of alcohol abuse, cirrhosis, ascites, and esophageal varices who was admitted to the hospital 5 days ago with an upper GI bleed after a weekend drinking binge. She was supported initially with IV fluids, packed RBCs, and fresh frozen plasma. Endoscopic examination showed bleeding esophageal varices, which were banded. V.G.'s hospital course is now complicated by primary bacterial peritonitis causing a paralytic ileus. On physical examination, V.G. is cachectic, with a large protuberant abdomen and ascites; bowel sounds are absent. She is alert, oriented, and without evidence of encephalopathy. V.G. has a central venous catheter. The plan is to begin parenteral nutrition because she has not eaten in 8 days and is not expected to eat for several more days after her peritonitis resolves. Is V.G. a candidate for a specialty amino acid product specifically designed for use in hepatic failure?

AROMATIC AMINO ACIDS AND BRANCHED-CHAIN AMINO ACIDS

Patients with chronic hepatic failure, especially those with alcohol-induced disease, are malnourished and prone to complications such as GI bleeding and infection. The metabolism of glucose, fat, and protein is altered in liver disease. Amino acid metabolism is particularly affected because blood is shunted around the liver.

TABLE 38-6
Amino Acid Product Comparison

Description	Product Name	Available Concentrations (%)
Standard Formulations		
Contain essential[a] and nonessential[b] amino acids, some available with electrolytes[c]	Aminosyn, Aminosyn II	3.5,[c] 5, 7,[c] 8.5,[c] 10,[c] 15
	FreAmine III	3, 8.5, 10
	Novamine	15
	ProSol	20
	Travasol	3.5,[c] 5.5,[c] 8.5,[c] 10
Hepatic Failure Formulations		
Contain essential and nonessential amino acids with a proportion of branched-chain amino acids (leucine, isoleucine, valine)	HepatAmine	8
	HepAtasol	8
Renal Failure Formulations		
Contain primarily essential amino acids; RenAmin also contains a complement of nonessential amino acids	Aminess	5.2
	Aminosyn-RF	5.2
	NephrAmine	5.4
	RenAmin	6.5
Stress Formulations		
Contain percentages of leucine, isoleucine, and valine, as well as all essential and nonessential amino acids	Aminosyn HBC	7
	FreAmine HBC	6.9
Supplements		
Contain only branched-chain amino acids (isoleucine, leucine, valine); must be used with a general formulation	BranchAmin	4

[a]Essential amino acids: isoleucine, leucine, lysine, methionine, phenylalanine, thionine, tryptophan, valine, histidine.
[b]Nonessential amino acids: cysteine, arginine, alanine, proline, glycine, glutamine, aspartate serine, tyrosine.
[c]These concentrations are available with or without electrolytes.
Source: Zerr KJ et al. Glucose control lowers the risk of wound infection in diabetics after open heart operations. *Ann Thorac Surg*. 1997;63:356; Rose BD. *Clinical Physiology of Acid–Base and Electrolyte Disorders*. 4th ed. New York, NY: McGraw-Hill; 1994:891.

In patients with hepatic insufficiency, adequate protein must be provided to support regeneration of the liver and other vital functions such as the immune system. However, administration of protein may result in hepatic encephalopathy, a severe complication of hepatic failure. Encephalopathy is characterized by progressive depression and impaired neurologic function. The pathogenesis of encephalopathy is controversial, although several theories have been proposed. It is probably caused by the inability of the diseased liver to remove neurotoxins, which accumulate in the brain, resulting in abnormal neurotransmitters (see Chapter 29, Complications of End-Stage Liver Disease).

Cirrhosis and chronic hepatic failure are associated with significant protein breakdown. The branched-chain amino acids (BCAAs) (e.g., leucine, isoleucine, valine) are used in the muscle as an energy source rather than being released into the circulation. Although the BCAAs are used for energy, the aromatic amino acids (AAAs; phenylalanine, tyrosine, and free tryptophan) are released, increasing circulating concentrations of these amino acids. This results in increased plasma concentrations of the AAAs and methionine and subnormal concentrations of the BCAAs. Both AAAs and BCAAs share a common pathway across the blood–brain barrier and compete for entry into the cerebrospinal fluid. The "false neurotransmitter" theory proposes that because the concentration of AAAs is greater, more are transported across the blood–brain barrier, where they accumulate and form "false neurotransmitters" such as octopamine and serotonin, an inhibitory neurotransmitter. These compete with normal neurotransmitters for binding sites and impair normal neurotransmission and brain activity.[52]

Based on these theories, an amino acid mixture was designed to provide adequate protein for anabolism while also treating hepatic encephalopathy. To normalize the amino acid profile in the brain, specially designed products with increased amounts of BCAAs and decreased amounts of both AAAs and methionine are available (Table 38-6). Controversy exists with regard to the ability of this special amino acid mixture to improve encephalopathy by altering the amino acid profile of the cerebrospinal fluid.[52–54] Generally, this amino acid mixture is reserved for patients with significant hepatic encephalopathy.

Because V.G. is alert, oriented, and without signs of encephalopathy, use of this product is not warranted at this time. Furthermore, protein restriction is not necessary. She should receive 1 to 1.2 g/kg/day of a standard amino acid product, and she should be monitored for signs of encephalopathy. Should she exhibit hepatic encephalopathy while receiving the standard amino acids, temporary protein restriction of 0.6 to 0.8 g/kg/day is reasonable while the etiology of the encephalopathy is determined and treated. The use of the increased BCAA–decreased AAA mixture may be appropriate for patients with chronic encephalopathy who are unresponsive to pharmacotherapy.[2]

CASE 38-4, QUESTION 2: What other amino acid mixtures are enriched with BCAAs?

BCAAs have metabolic properties that are considered beneficial during physiological stress (multiple trauma, sepsis, and major surgery). BCAAs can be used as an alternative energy source by the heart, brain, and skeletal muscle. The BCAAs can increase protein synthesis in muscle and liver, decrease excessive proteolysis in muscle, and normalize abnormal plasma amino acid profiles. These unique properties led to the design of commercially available amino acid mixtures that provide about 45%

of the amino acids as BCAAs. In comparison, most standard amino acid mixtures contain 19% to 25% BCAAs.

Multiple trials have evaluated the effects of BCAA-enriched amino acid formulations in critically ill patients. Although most evidence suggests that these formulations may improve nitrogen retention, they do not appear to improve clinical outcome.[55,56] It is important to appreciate the differences between the amino acid composition of the mixtures for hepatic failure and those designed for stress. They are not therapeutically equivalent, and one should not be substituted for the other.

Renal Failure

CASE 38-5

QUESTION 1: O.M. is a 75-year-old man with a long history of hypertension, coronary artery disease, and peripheral vascular disease. Four days ago, he was admitted to the hospital complaining of severe abdominal pain and was diagnosed with a ruptured abdominal aortic aneurysm, which was repaired surgically. Hypotension and hemodynamic instability requiring pressors, respiratory distress necessitating endotracheal intubation and mechanical ventilation, and renal failure with oliguria have complicated his postoperative course. Furthermore, there is concern that O.M. has an ischemic bowel, which precludes using his GI tract for enteral feeding. Serum chemistries are as follows:

Na, 130 mEq/L	**Glucose, 143 mg/dL**
K, 5.2 mEq/L	**Ca, 7.9 mg/dL**
Cl, 99 mEq/L	**Mg, 2.4 mg/dL**
HCO_3^-, 15 mEq/L	**P, 5.8 mg/dL**
BUN, 79 mg/dL	**Albumin, 2.7 g/dL**
Creatinine, 4.0 mg/dL	

The decision is made to initiate parenteral nutrition therapy via a central venous catheter. In view of O.M.'s acute renal failure, what adjustments should be made in the amount and type of protein (amino acid) provided in the parenteral feeding formulation?

The protein dose in acute renal failure should be reduced to 0.6 to 1 g/kg/day because the kidneys have a limited ability to excrete nitrogenous byproducts of protein metabolism.[57] The use of essential amino acids (EAAs) orally has been demonstrated to improve uremic symptoms. Based on this experience, parenteral amino acid mixtures containing only EAAs were investigated. These studies compared parenteral feedings containing dextrose and EAAs to the administration of only dextrose with the observation of an improved rate of recovery in the group that received the EAA and dextrose. Subsequent studies comparing parenteral nutrient formulations containing a standard mix of both EAAs and nonessential amino acids with those containing EAAs alone have not demonstrated any difference in urea appearance or nitrogen balance.[57,58] It is concluded that the use of EAAs alone in parenteral nutrient formulations for patients with acute renal failure offers no clinical advantage over formulations providing a balanced mixture of EAAs and nonessential amino acids.

CASE 38-5, QUESTION 2: What other adjustments should be made in formulating a parenteral nutrient formulation for O.M.?

O.M.'s nutrient needs should be provided in the least amount of fluid possible. This can be accomplished by using the most concentrated macronutrients of 70% dextrose, 20% amino acids, and 30% lipid. Using these substrates, a patient's entire needs can often be provided in less than 1,200 mL/day. Electrolytes should also be adjusted. Initially, patients with acute renal failure may not require potassium, magnesium, and phosphorus because they cannot excrete them. However, once parenteral feedings begin and an anabolic state occurs, these patients commonly experience decreases in the serum concentrations of these minerals and will require small daily doses to maintain normal serum concentrations.

RENAL REPLACEMENT THERAPIES

CASE 38-5, QUESTION 3: O.M.'s renal failure progresses, and he requires renal replacement therapy. Because of his hemodynamic instability, continuous venovenous hemodialysis (CVVHD) is initiated. How should his nutrition therapy be altered?

Continuous renal replacement therapies (CRRTs), including CVVHD, continuous arteriovenous hemodialysis, continuous venovenous hemofiltration, continuous venovenous hemodiafiltration, and slow continuous ultrafiltration delivery provide a means to remove large volumes of water, nitrogenous byproducts, and electrolytes (see Chapter 30, Acute Kidney Injury, and Chapter 32, Renal Dialysis). Consequently, the delivery of unlimited quantities of fluids, nutrients, and electrolytes is possible. Several factors must be considered in the nutritional management of a patient requiring these therapies. First, a dialysate solution of 1.5% to 2.5% dextrose may be used. If so, some dextrose is absorbed during the process and contributes to the caloric intake. A solution with a 1.5% dextrose concentration at a rate of 1 L/hour delivers approximately 5.8 g of glucose per hour. Increasing the dextrose concentration of the dialysate solution to 2.5% increases the glucose delivery to 11.5 g/hour. The amount of glucose absorbed (550–700 kcal/day) must be considered when designing the amount of calories that will be provided in the parenteral nutrient formulation.[57–62]

The second nutritional consideration is the loss of amino acids across the dialysis filter, which can range from 20 to 28 g of nitrogen per day. Sufficient amino acids should be provided to compensate for this daily loss of 120 to 175 g of amino acids (approximately 6.25 g of amino acids per gram of nitrogen).[57,59,61,62] Protein requirements for patients on CRRT may be as high as 2.5 g/kg/day to promote positive nitrogen balance.[63]

Last, the rapid loss of electrolytes must be considered. Patients may experience dramatic decreases in potassium, magnesium, and phosphorus once CRRT is initiated. This requires frequent monitoring and replacement of these electrolytes, usually as IV supplements rather than as additions to the parenteral feeding formulation.

CASE 38-5, QUESTION 4: After several days of CVVHD, O.M. is changed to intermittent (three times a week) hemodialysis. What alterations in his parenteral nutrition are necessary?

Hemodialysis also allows the passage of amino acids through a semipermeable membrane. The loss is approximately 1 g of amino acids for each hour of hemodialysis with a glucose-free dialysate. This loss is reduced by 50% when a glucose-containing dialysate solution is used. These losses should be considered when determining the dosage of protein that will be provided by the parenteral nutrient formulation. The recommended protein dosage for patients requiring hemodialysis is 1.2 to 1.3 g/kg/day,[57,61,62] but dosages up to 1.8 g/kg/day have been reported.[57,64] In addition, hemodialysis can increase energy expenditure by increasing oxygen consumption and gluconeogenesis; therefore, energy goals should range between 25 and 35 kcal/kg/day.[57] Patients requiring chronic hemodialysis may require protein doses of 1.2 to 1.4 g/kg/day to maintain a positive nitrogen balance and prevent protein malnutrition. Patients requiring peritoneal dialysis have higher losses of protein through the peritoneal cavity and may need 1.2 to 1.5 g/kg/day of protein. In contrast to patients on hemodialysis, those on peritoneal dialysis require fewer calories provided by parenteral feedings because 600 to 800 kcal/day may be absorbed through the peritoneal membrane from the glucose-containing dialysate.[57,61,62]

Diabetes, Obesity, and Short Bowel Syndrome

CASE 38-6

QUESTION 1: F.L., a 51-year-old man with a history of diabetes mellitus, is hospitalized after receiving a gunshot wound to the abdomen. His injuries include a lacerated spleen, requiring a splenectomy, and several tears in his small and large intestine, necessitating resection of these areas. A feeding jejunostomy tube was placed at the time of surgery, and enteral tube feedings were begun on postoperative day 2. Five days later, F.L. is noted to have a temperature of 39.6°C, a WBC count of 18,900/μL, and a distended, tender abdomen. He requires surgery for a small bowel perforation at the site of the feeding jejunostomy and peritonitis. The jejunostomy tube is removed, but F.L. is not expected to have return of bowel function for 7 to 10 days. Parenteral nutrition is to be initiated. F.L. is 5 feet 8 inches tall, and his usual weight is 215 pounds. What adjustments should be made in determining F.L.'s energy goals?

First, F.L. is considered obese, and an adjusted body weight should be calculated and used in nutrition calculations. Obesity is defined as weight exceeding 120% of ideal body weight or a body mass index (BMI) of greater than 27 kg/m^2. F.L. weighs 215 pounds, or 98 kg, which is 142% of his ideal body weight of 69 kg minus 10%. BMI is determined as shown by Equation 38-9.

$$\begin{aligned} \text{BMI} &= \frac{\text{W (kg)}}{\text{Height (m)}^2} \\ &= \frac{98 \text{ kg}}{(1.73 \text{ m})^2} \\ &= 32.7 \text{kg/m}^2 \end{aligned} \qquad \textit{(Eq. 38-9)}$$

Obese patients should have their weight adjusted because adipose tissue is not metabolically active. However, about one-fourth of the adipose tissue is composed of some supporting tissue that is metabolically active. Adjusted weight for obesity is calculated using Equation 38-10.[65]

$$\begin{aligned} \text{Adjusted weight} &= (0.25)(\text{Actual weight} - \text{IBW}) + \text{IBW} \\ &= (0.25)(98 - 69) + 69 \\ &= 76 \text{ kg} \end{aligned} \qquad \textit{(Eq. 38-10)}$$

Using an adjusted weight will decrease the risk of overfeeding, which can further increase adipose tissue and complicate glucose management, especially in a patient with a history of diabetes mellitus. Another approach is to use the Ireton-Jones predictive equation that includes a factor for obesity. Using indirect calorimetry to obtain an measured energy expenditure (MEE) may more accurately assess energy expenditure and avoid overfeeding.

CASE 38-6, QUESTION 2: What special considerations should be addressed in designing a parenteral nutrient regimen for F.L.?

Patients without a history of diabetes mellitus may exhibit hyperglycemia under conditions of stress. Even greater derangements in glucose metabolism may be observed in patients with diabetes mellitus during a critical illness. Dextrose should be limited to 150 g during the first 24 hours of therapy, and the amount of dextrose should not be increased until serum glucose concentrations are consistently less than 150 mg/dL. It can be anticipated that F.L. will need supplemental insulin when his parenteral nutrient regimen is infused. Insulin may be added to the parenteral nutrient formulation. Initial insulin therapy of 0.1 units of regular insulin per gram of dextrose is a good starting point and should be adjusted to achieve serum glucose levels between 80 and 120 mg/dL. Alternatively, a separate insulin infusion may be used. Frequent capillary glucose monitoring is required in these patients, and it may be necessary to provide additional subcutaneous insulin.[39,40,66] (See Case 38-2, Question 13, for additional discussion on management of hyperglycemia.)

CASE 38-6, QUESTION 3: F.L. has a prolonged hospital course complicated by multiple intra-abdominal abscesses, poor wound healing, and necrotic bowel, requiring removal of all but 55 cm of his small intestine but leaving his colon intact. F.L. is given a diagnosis of short bowel syndrome (SBS). What issues should be addressed in the nutrition and metabolic management of this patient?

SBS is characterized by maldigestion, malabsorption, dehydration, and both macronutrient and micronutrient abnormalities (see Chapter 28, Lower Gastrointestinal Disorders). Severe malnutrition will develop without adequate nutrition support. To maintain adequate nutrition status, F.L. will require parenteral nutrition until his remaining intestine begins to adapt. This adaptive period may take several weeks to months to years. Adaptation is enhanced by stimulation of the enterocytes with nutrients, which is best provided by small, frequent oral meals or tube feeding.[2,67,68]

First, F.L. should be continued on parenteral nutrition support, including therapy at home, to meet his nutrient and fluid requirements. After extensive small bowel resection, F.L. may experience severe diarrhea. This increase in GI losses may lead to dehydration and electrolyte abnormalities, including hyponatremia, hypokalemia, hypomagnesemia, hypocalcemia, and metabolic acidosis.[68] F.L.'s fluid status must be monitored and evaluated daily for clinical signs of dehydration or fluid overload.

Medication therapy plays an important role in managing fluid and electrolyte imbalances secondary to excessive GI fluid losses. H_2-receptor antagonists are useful in decreasing gastric secretion, thereby reducing fluid and electrolyte losses and enhancing absorption. Antimotility agents should be used to decrease diarrhea. Octreotide also may have a role in decreasing diarrhea in patients with SBS. Patients with extensive small bowel resections and an intact colon, such as F.L., may experience diarrhea as a result of bile salt depletion.[2,67,68]

Patients with SBS are at risk for having vitamin deficiencies, especially folate and vitamin B_{12}. These patients should receive supplemental vitamin B_{12} and IV parenteral or oral liquid multivitamin supplements. GI losses of trace minerals, particularly zinc and selenium, are increased in SBS, and these minerals should be supplemented.[67,68]

Pancreatitis and Respiratory Failure

CASE 38-7

QUESTION 1: K.R., a 59-year-old woman, is admitted to the hospital complaining of increasing abdominal pain and vomiting. She is diagnosed with pancreatitis. This is her third admission for acute pancreatitis during the past year. Her past medical history is significant for ethanol abuse and chronic obstructive pulmonary disease. An NG tube is inserted, and she is to be NPO. IV fluids are begun for hydration. During the next 5 days, K.R.'s abdominal pain subsides, her pancreatitis resolves, and she is started on an oral diet. Two days after beginning an oral diet, K.R. complains of severe abdominal pain and is vomiting. She is febrile, her WBC count has increased to 21,000/μL, and she is hypotensive, requiring large volumes of IV fluids. Furthermore, she experiences respiratory distress and requires endotracheal intubation and mechanical ventilation. Her most recent ABG is notable for pH, 7.36; Pco_2, 51 mm Hg; Po_2, 88 mm Hg; and HCO_3^-, 28 mEq/L. This clinical presentation is consistent with severe pancreatic necrosis. A small-bore nasojejunal feeding tube is placed, and enteral nutrition therapy is begun. However, K.R. experiences severe abdominal pain and distension, and bowel sounds are absent, so the enteral feeding is discontinued. The decision is made to begin parenteral nutrition because K.R. is not expected to have a functional GI tract in the near future and her nutrient intake has been inadequate during her hospitalization. What special considerations should be addressed in designing a parenteral feeding formulation for K.R.? Is the use of fat contraindicated in patients with pancreatitis?

Several observations have caused concern about the use of IV lipid emulsions in patients with pancreatitis. The oral ingestion of fats may stimulate pancreatic exocrine function and should be restricted in patients with pancreatitis. Although hyperlipidemia has been well described in patients with alcohol-induced pancreatitis, it is unlikely that it is primarily responsible for initiating the pancreatitis. Hypertriglyceridemia associated with acute pancreatitis is most often seen in patients with hereditary or acquired defects in lipid metabolism. Furthermore, pancreatitis alone may be associated with hypertriglyceridemia.[69]

Several investigators have evaluated the effects of parenteral nutrient formulations containing fat emulsions in patients with acute pancreatitis and have found no stimulation of pancreatic exocrine function. Furthermore, IV lipids did not result in abdominal pain or relapse in patients with a history of pancreatitis. Available data suggest that IV lipid emulsions are a safe and efficacious form of calories for patients with pancreatitis.[69]

Monitoring serum triglyceride concentrations should be part of routine management for patients with pancreatitis and those receiving parenteral nutrient formulations containing lipids. Serum triglyceride concentrations should be maintained at less than 400 mg/dL with a continuous infusion of lipids and less than 250 mg/dL when checked 4 hours after the infusion for patients receiving intermittent lipid infusions.[2,21,69] If serum concentrations exceed these parameters, consideration must be given to decreasing or eliminating the IV lipid from the parenteral nutrient regimen.

CASE 38-7, QUESTION 2: K.R. is recovering from her pancreatitis, and the small-bore nasojejunal enteral feeding tube is reinserted. Tube feeding is considered because she cannot eat by mouth because of the endotracheal tube and mechanical ventilation. How should she be transitioned from parenteral to enteral feedings?

Tube feedings can begin with a full-strength isotonic enteral feeding formulation at a slow infusion rate (25 mL/hour) (see Chapter 37, Adult Enteral Nutrition). Concurrently, the parenteral nutrient formulation should be decreased to avoid fluid overload and to keep the calorie and protein intake constant. It can be anticipated that K.R. can transition from parenteral to enteral feedings in 24 to 48 hours.

KEY REFERENCES AND WEBSITES

A full list of references for this chapter can be found at http://thepoint.lww.com/AT10e. Below are the key references and websites for this chapter, with the corresponding reference number in this chapter found in parentheses after the reference.

Key References

Driscoll DF. Intravenous lipid emulsions: 2001. *Nutr Clin Pract*. 2001;16:215. (12)

Gottschlich MM et al, ed. *The Science and Practice of Nutrition Support: A Case-Based Core Curriculum*. Dubuque, IA: Kendall/Hunt Publishing; 2001. (3,22,28,49,52,68,69)

Kearns LR et al. Update on parenteral amino acids. *Nutr Clin Pract*. 2001;16:219. (14)

Mirtallo J et al. Safe practices for parenteral nutrition [published correction appears in *JPEN J Parenter Enteral Nutr*. 2006;30:177]. *JPEN J Parenter Enteral Nutr*. 2004;28:S39. (11)

Key Websites

American Society for Parenteral and Enteral Nutrition. http://www.nutritioncare.org. http://www.nutritioncare.org/Library.aspx to access content for:

- ASPEN Board of Directors and the Clinical Guidelines Task Force. Guidelines for the use of parenteral and enteral nutrition in adult and pediatric patients. *JPEN J Parent Enteral Nutr*. 2002;26(Suppl 1):1SA. (2)
- McClave SA et al. Guidelines for the provision and assessment of nutrition support therapy in the adult critically ill patient: Society of Critical Care Medicine (SCCM) and American Society for Parenteral and Enteral Nutrition (A.S.P.E.N.). *JPEN J Parent Enteral Nutr*. 2009;33:277.

SECTION EDITOR: TIMOTHY J. IVES

Dermatotherapy and Drug-Induced Skin Disorders

39

Richard N. Herrier

CORE PRINCIPLES

		CHAPTER CASES
1	The accurate assessment of dermatological conditions is primarily based on the appearance and location of the skin lesion, plus age, sex, symptoms, current and past personal and family history.	Case 39-1 (Question 1)
2	Atopic dermatitis is a common dermatological condition characterized by eczematous lesions and intense pruritus. Most patients have a family or personal history of other atopic disorders such as asthma and allergic rhinitis. Atopic dermatitis is primarily treated with topical corticosteroids and emollients.	Case 39-2 (Questions 1–4)
3	The selection of topical corticosteroid is based on the nature of the lesion (wet vs. dry), the concentration of the corticosteroid, the nature of the vehicle, the corticosteroid potency, the location of the lesion, and the thickness of the epidermis.	Case 39-2 (Questions 2–4)
4	Topical corticosteroids can cause a variety of side effects and adverse reactions that may require adjustment of therapy including changing products or discontinuing their use.	Case 39-2 (Questions 5–10), Case 39-3 (Question 1)
5	Dry skin is a common condition that may occur alone or with a variety of dermatological disorders and requires appropriate treatment depending on geographic location.	Case 39-4 (Question 1)
6	Medications are a common cause of a variety of dermatological disorders. Timing relative to medication ingestion and principles of dermatological assessment are important to identify potential life-threatening adverse reactions.	Case 39-1 (Question 1), Case 39-5 (Question 1)
7	Allergic contact dermatitis is one of the most common dermatologic conditions seen by pharmacists. Drugs (neomycin), plants (*Rhus*), chemicals, detergents, metals (nickel), and organic products (latex) are common causes. Treatment consists of removal of the antigen and use of topical or systemic corticosteroids.	Case 39-6 (Question 1), Case 39-7 (Questions 1–3)

ANATOMY AND PHYSIOLOGY OF THE SKIN

The skin is the largest organ in the body and constitutes, on average, 17% of a person's body weight. The skin's thickness ranges from 3 to 5 mm. Figure 39-1 shows a cross section of the anatomy of human skin. The major function of the skin is to protect underlying structures from trauma, temperature variations, harmful penetrations, moisture, humidity, radiation, and invasion of micro-organisms. There are three layers of skin: epidermis, dermis, and subcutaneous tissue.[1–6]

Epidermis

The epidermis consists of four distinct layers: stratum corneum, stratum lucidum, stratum spinosum, and stratum germinativum. The major function of the epidermis is to serve as a barrier. This layer keeps chemicals and other substances from penetrating into the body and prevents the loss of water from the skin and underlying tissues. The maturation of keratinocytes from the stratum germinativum to the stratum corneum is critical for this barrier function. As keratinocytes migrate to the skin surface, they change from living cells to dead, thick-walled, nonnucleated cells containing keratin, a hard fibrous protein. It normally takes

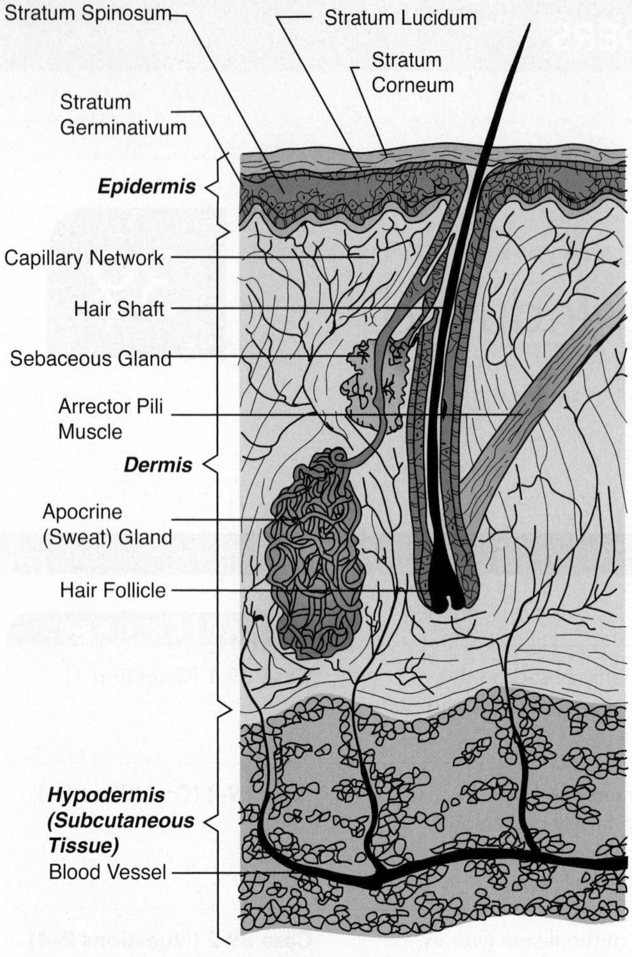

FIGURE 39-1 Cross section of the anatomy of human skin.

26 to 28 days for a keratinocyte to divide, differentiate, move up to the stratum corneum, and be sloughed off.

The *stratum corneum,* which is composed of the dead cells, provides the greatest resistance to the percutaneous absorption of chemicals and drugs. It behaves as a semipermeable membrane through which drugs are absorbed by passive diffusion. Factors that can affect drug absorption are hydration of the skin and damage to the stratum corneum. In general, the greater the damage to the stratum corneum, the greater is the absorption of topically applied drugs. Skin diseases affecting only the epidermis heal without scarring.[1–6]

Dermis

The dermis, which ranges in thickness from 1 to 4 mm, is composed of collagen fibers, elastic fibers, and an extrafibrillar gel of mucopolysaccharides called *glycosaminoglycans* (formally called *ground substances*). The major function of the dermis is to protect the body from mechanical injury and to support the dermal appendages (i.e., apocrine and eccrine sweat glands, sebaceous glands, hair follicles) and the epidermis. It also provides capillary, lymphatic, and nerve supply to the skin and its appendages. The capillary network plays a major role in temperature regulation and provides nutrition to the epidermis. The nerves transmit sensations of touch and pain. Finally, the dermis contains large amounts of water, thus serving as a water storage organ. All but the most superficial injuries to the dermis generally result in scarring as the wound heals.[1–6]

Drugs passing through the epidermis penetrate directly into the dermis and may be absorbed into the general circulation through the capillary network. Generally, only small amounts of topically applied drugs enter the dermis via the sweat glands or the pilosebaceous units.

Subcutaneous Layer

The subcutaneous layer supports the dermis and epidermis and serves as a fat storage area. This layer helps regulate temperature, provide nutritional support, and cushion the outer skin layers.[1–6]

INFLAMMATORY LESIONS

One of the dermatologic axioms regarding therapy is particularly useful in selecting dosage forms: "If it's wet, dry it; if it's dry, wet it." Paradoxically, wet dressings are most useful in drying acute, inflamed lesions because they draw out fluid as they evaporate. Ointment-type bases are most useful for chronic, lichenified, scaling lesions. The choice of vehicle for chronic lesions is often based on what the patient has found to work best or is willing to use. Frequently, patients with chronic dermatologic conditions use multiple types of vehicles concomitantly (e.g., cream bases [which are drying]) during the day, as they are cosmetically acceptable, and ointment bases at night (greasy, but better emollients).

Acute Lesions

Acute inflammatory lesions can be characterized by vesiculation, erythema, swelling, warmth, pruritus, oozing, or weeping. Generally, the more severe the dermatitis, the milder is the initial topical therapy. For instance, cool water in the form of an aqueous vehicle, preferably a wet dressing, soak, or bath, is more effective as the initial therapeutic agent than a potent topical corticosteroid applied to a warm, erythematous, weeping dermatitis. The specific approach depends on the part(s) of the body involved.

Subacute and Chronic Lesions

Subacute lesions are characterized by decreasing vesiculation and oozing and are often covered with crusts. They still require cleaning and drying with aqueous preparations, but for a shorter duration than with acute lesions. Chronic inflammatory lesions are characterized by erythema, scaling, lichenification, dryness, and pruritus. There are no absolute rules for treating chronic lesions. If the lesion is dry, an oleaginous or occlusive base should be used, perhaps with a keratolytic agent.

DERMATOLOGIC DRUG DELIVERY SYSTEMS

A range of dermatologic formulations is available: solutions, suspensions or shake lotions, powders, lotions, emulsions, gels, creams, ointments, and aerosols. Each dermatologic delivery vehicle has specific characteristics and uses based on the type, relative acuteness, and location of the lesion.

Solutions

Solutions provide evaporative cooling and vasoconstriction, with resultant mild antipruritic effects. They soothe and cool inflamed

TABLE 39-1
Solutions for Wet Dressings or Drying Weeping Lesions

Agent[a]	Strength	Preparation (H_2O)	Germicidal Activity	Astringent Activity	Comments
Normal saline	0.9% NaCl	1 tsp NaCl per pint H_2O	None	None	Inexpensive; easy to prepare
Aluminum acetate (Burow solution) (Domeboro packets/tablets)	5%	Dilute to 1 : 10–1 : 40 (0.5%–0.125%) One packet or tablet to a pint of water yields a 1 : 40 solution; two packets or tablets yields a 1 : 20 solution	Mild	+	
Potassium permanganate	65- and 330-mg tablets	Dilute to 1 : 4,000–1 : 16,000; 65-mg tablet to 250–1,000 mL; 330-mg tablet to 1,500–5,000 mL	Moderate	None	Stains skin, clothing
Silver nitrate	0.1%–0.5%	1 tsp of 50% stock solution to 1,000 mL will yield a 0.25% solution	Good	+	Stains; can cause pain
Acetic acid[b]	1%	Dilute 1 pint of standard 5% household vinegar with 5 parts H_2O	Good	+	Unpleasant odor; can be irritating

[a] Although many substances are added to wet dressings, the cleansing and drying effect of the water is the major benefit.
[b] Used primarily for *Pseudomonas aeruginosa* infections.
Source: Arndt KA, Hsu JHS, eds. *Manual of Dermatologic Therapies: With Essentials of Diagnosis*. 7th ed. Philadelphia, PA: Lippincott Williams & Wilkins; 2006.

skin, dry oozing lesions, soften crusts, aid in cleaning wounds, and assist in the drainage of purulent wounds. Aqueous solutions are most useful for acutely inflamed, oozing lesions; erosions; and ulcers. In most instances, solutions should be the sole therapy until the oozing or weeping subsides. If other topical medications are applied to oozing or weeping lesions, they will be washed away and will not provide the desired effect. The most commonly used solutions are normal (0.9%) saline and aluminum acetate 5% solution (Burow solution) diluted 1 : 10 to 1 : 40. Solutions are often applied as wet dressings.

The most important component of a solution is water. Although active or inert substances may be added to solutions, the cleansing, drying, and cooling effect of water provides the major therapeutic benefit. Some of the products (e.g., Burow solution) also have *astringent* properties that alter the skin surface and interstitial spaces to cause contraction and wrinkling. Water penetration is reduced to minimize edema, inflammation, and exudation. Table 39-1 lists the most commonly used solutions. Boric acid should not be used as a topical agent because it can be absorbed through the skin, causing systemic toxicity.[7]

Depending on the affected area and its size, a patient may soak the affected area directly in the solution for 15 to 30 minutes three to six times per day. If larger areas are involved or if the affected area cannot be easily soaked (e.g., a shoulder), a clean towel or cloth soaked in the solution (lightly wrung out) is directly applied to the lesion(s) as a wet dressing. The soaked cloth should be left in place for 5 to 10 minutes, then resoaked in the solution and reapplied. The patient may repeat this procedure for 15 to 30 minutes three times daily. Solutions applied with a cloth should have the cloth material wrapped around the lesions several times, if possible. If large areas are involved, the patient may draw a bath, add appropriate amounts of medications, and soak for 15 to 30 minutes three to six times per day. It is impractical to prepare a Burow solution bath at the 1 : 10 to 1 : 40 concentration. Again, the concentration of the Burow solution is probably insignificant because the major effect of the solution is produced by the water. In general, no more than one-third of the body should be soaked in this manner at any time. One should be aware that evaporation can concentrate solutions, potentially making them too irritating to use. Small volumes of a 1 : 40 concentration of Burow solution left standing open at room temperature after 30 to 60 minutes may yield a 1 : 10 solution. This problem is not as significant with larger volumes or if the solution is stored in a closed container. For this reason, wet dressings should always be freshly prepared (i.e., within 24 hours), kept in closed containers, and never reused. Wet dressings are most comfortable if they are slightly cool or warm, depending on the patient's preference. When drying the affected area after a wet dressing has been used, care must be taken not to irritate the inflamed skin by rubbing it with a towel. The proper technique for drying the skin is to pat the area gently with a soft, clean towel.[7]

Baths

In addition to wet dressings and soaks, topical solutions can be applied to large areas of the body through bathing. In using this type of treatment, the bath should be about half full. Soothing and antipruritic colloidal bath additives may be used to treat widespread eruptions such as lichen planus, pityriasis rosea, urticaria, and other weeping or crusting dermatoses. Colloidal oatmeal (1 cup of oatmeal [Aveeno] mixed with 2 cups of cold tap water and poured into 6 inches of a lukewarm bath) produces a pleasing and soothing bath. Alternatively, a starch bath using 2 cups of hydrolyzed starch (Linit) or cornstarch mixed with 4 cups of tap water and added to a bath may be used. A mixture of equal parts baking soda and starch may also be used. Epsom salt baths, made by dissolving 3 cups of magnesium sulfate in 6 inches of lukewarm water in a tub, are useful in treating pyodermas, furuncles, and necrotic acne (especially when the back, shoulders, and buttocks are affected). Water-soluble coal tar preparations applied via a bath for the treatment of psoriasis may be the most acceptable way to apply this medication. Ointments or creams containing coal tar are malodorous and have a tendency to stain materials on contact.

A variety of bath oils are available: Alpha-Keri, Domol, Lubriderm, and Nutraderm. Adding bath oil directly to the bath is not recommended because it makes the tub slippery and potentially dangerous. The concentration of the oil in the water becomes almost insignificant anyway (5–10 mL in 20–40 gallons). Five to 10 mL of bath oil may be applied directly to wet skin on leaving a bath and patted dry with a towel for a more significant effect. This is most useful in preventing and treating mild cases of xerosis (dry skin). With moderate to severe cases of xerosis, additional topical oleaginous products are generally required to improve the condition. Patients may make their own bath oil by adding 2 ounces of olive oil or Nivea oil to a cup of milk and applying it after a bath.[7]

Powders

Powders are drying and cooling; they absorb moisture and create more surface area for evaporation. They are used mainly in intertriginous areas (e.g., groin, under the breasts, or in skin folds) to decrease friction, which can cause mechanical irritation. They also are useful in the treatment of chafing, tinea pedis (athlete's foot), tinea cruris (jock itch), and diaper dermatitis (diaper rash). Occasionally, powders are applied on top of ointments to protect clothing from the ointment. The liberal use of powders on bedridden patients helps prevent pressure ulcers (bed sores).

Powders can be applied with a cotton puff or shaker. Care should be taken to minimize breathing the powder because this can lead to respiratory tract irritation, particularly in infants. Powders that contain starch or cellulose should be washed off before reapplication, as continued buildup can produce mechanical irritation. Corn starch–containing powders should not be used for intertrigo (inflammation of body folds—thighs, armpits, under breasts or enlarged abdomen; aggravated by heat, moisture, and maceration) because starch can serve as a substrate for *Candida albicans*. Powders should not be applied to oozing lesions because they tend to cake into hard granules, making them difficult and painful to remove and promoting maceration. Concerns regarding the association of routine cosmetic talc use and ovarian cancer and granulomatous lung changes are without convincing evidence.[8] The most commonly used powder is talc.

Lotions

Lotions are suspensions or solutions of powder in a water vehicle. They are usually cooling and drying, but may provide some lubrication, depending on the formulation. Lotions are used to treat superficial dermatoses, especially if there is slight oozing. They are useful if large or intertriginous areas are affected, and they are especially advantageous in the treatment of conditions characterized by significant inflammation and tenderness. In these situations, creams or ointments may cause pain on application. Sunburn, acute contact dermatitis, and poison ivy or poison oak are examples of conditions in which this principle may apply. Also, lotions are useful for hairy areas of the body and scalp. Generally, lotions are applied three or four times daily, with each fresh application placed over previous application, unless there is significant oozing present, which could promote caking of dried solid ingredients. If this is the case, the area should be cleansed before repeat application. Because many lotions are suspensions, it is advisable to shake the lotion well before application. Generally, 6 ounces of lotion covers the entire body of an average adult.[7]

Emulsions

Emulsions are solid or liquid and can be divided into two classes: *oil-in-water* and *water-in-oil* emulsions. Cream preparations are generally oil-in-water emulsions, whereas ointment preparations are water-in-oil emulsions. As the amount of oil increases, the viscosity of the emulsion will also increase.

The indications for liquid oil-in-water emulsions are similar to those for lotions and creams, except that this dosage form provides greater occlusion and is more useful in conditions in which dry skin predominates. Liquid water-in-oil emulsions have similar indications to ointments, except they can be applied more easily than ointments. Water-in-oil emulsions are most useful in conditions in which dry skin predominates; application to hairy or intertriginous areas should be avoided. As with lotions, 6 ounces of a liquid emulsion will cover all exposed skin on an average adult.[7]

TABLE 39-2
Commercially Available Emulsion Bases

Oil-in-Water	Water-in-Oil
Acid mantle cream	Aquaphor
Aquaphilic	Eucerin
Cetaphil	Lubriderm
Dermabase	Nivea Cream
Dermovan	Nutraderm
Hydrophilic ointment USP	Polysorb
Keri Lotion	Vanicream
Lanaphilic	Velvachol
Unibase	

Adapted with permission from Arndt KA, Hsu JHS, eds. *Manual of Dermatologic Therapies: With Essentials of Diagnosis*. 7th ed. Philadelphia, PA: Lippincott Williams & Wilkins; 2006.

Table 39-2 lists some commercially available oil-in-water and water-in-oil emulsion bases.

Gels

Gels are a form of ointment (semisolid emulsion) that contain propylene glycol and carboxypolymethylene. They are clear, nongreasy, nonstaining, nonocclusive, and quick drying. They are thixotropic (i.e., become thinner with rubbing and may sting on application). Gels are most useful when applied to hairy areas or other areas such as the face or scalp, where it is considered cosmetically unacceptable to have the residue of a vehicle remain on the skin. Because of their ingredients, gels tend to be more drying.

Creams

Creams are the most commonly used vehicle in dermatology. Most are oil-in-water emulsions and are intended to be rubbed in well until they vanish (vanishing creams). Because creams do not provide much occlusiveness, they are most often recommended for subacute lesions and occasionally for chronic lesions without significant lichenification. The most common mistake made by patients when applying creams is that they use too much or do not rub them in fully. Generally, if the cream can be seen on the skin after application, the patient has made one or both of these application mistakes. Ultimately, they are wasting the preparation or are not getting the full therapeutic benefits. One gram of cream should cover 100 cm^2 of surface area. Table 39-3 lists the approximate amount of cream required for application to various parts of the body.[7]

Ointments

Ointments are made of inert bases such as petrolatum or may consist of droplets of water suspended in a continuous phase of oleaginous material (water-in-oil emulsions). Ointments are most useful on chronic lesions, relieving dryness, brittleness, and protecting fissures owing to their occlusive properties. They should not be used on acutely inflamed lesions. Ointments should not be applied to intertriginous or hairy areas because they tend to trap heat and promote maceration. Ointments are greasy and may be cosmetically unacceptable.

TABLE 39-3
Amount of Topical Medication Needed for Various Dosage Regimens

Area Treated	Single Application (g)	BID for 1 Week (g)	BID for 1 Month (g)
Hands, head, face, anogenital area	2	28	120
On arm, anterior or posterior trunk	3	42	180
One leg	4	56	240
Entire body	30–60	420–840 kg (14–28 oz)	1.8–3.6 kg (60–120 oz)

BID, twice a day.
Source: Arndt KA, Hsu JHS, eds. *Manual of Dermatologic Therapies: With Essentials of Diagnosis*. 7th ed. Philadelphia, PA: Lippincott Williams & Wilkins; 2006.

TABLE 39-4
Appropriate Dermatologic Vehicle Selection Across the Range of Dermatologic Lesions

Range of Lesions	Range of Vehicles
Acute inflammation: Oozing, weeping, vesication, edema, pruritus	Aqueous vehicles and water, and then powder solutions, lotions, sprays, and aerosols
↓	↓
Subacute inflammation: Crusting, less oozing, pruritus	Creams, gels
↓	↓
Chronic inflammation: Lichenification, dryness, erythema, pruritus, scaling	Ointments

Aerosols

Aerosols are the most expensive and inefficient way to apply dermatologic medications. Their only advantage over other dosage forms is that they do not require direct mechanical contact with the skin and may be useful if application causes intolerable pain for the patient. If an aerosol is used, it should be shaken well before use, and the patient should be cautioned not to spray the product around the face where it could get into the eyes or nose or could be inhaled. Generally, aerosols should be sprayed from approximately 6 inches above the skin in bursts of 1 to 3 seconds. Aerosols are also useful for application to hairy areas if a special application nozzle is used. Aerosols have a drying effect and should not be used for a long period of time.

Other Delivery Systems

The addition of solvents, such as dimethyl sulfoxide, may enhance dermal absorption, allowing the delivery of many drugs directly through the skin. Skin patch delivery systems have also been designed to deliver drugs directly through the skin. Examples include scopolamine, nitroglycerin, clonidine, nicotine, opioids, and various hormones. These dermatologic drug delivery systems, or similar ones, offer great potential for the sustained delivery of pharmaceuticals for extended periods.

Selection of a Delivery System

Dermatologic vehicles should be matched to the type of lesion for which they will be used. Acute lesions require aqueous vehicles until the lesions become dry. Subacute lesions also benefit from aqueous vehicles, but for shorter periods before switching to creams or gels. Chronic lesions usually require ointments because of their dry, lichenified characteristics. Although there are exceptions, these principles are depicted in Table 39-4.

ASSESSING THE DERMATOLOGIC PATIENT

CASE 39-1

QUESTION 1: C.B., a 23-year-old, 66-kg woman, complains of a rash. What types of questions should C.B. be asked to help determine the appropriate diagnosis and treatment?

The diagnosis of dermatologic conditions can be simplified by considering six primary factors: morphology (what the lesions look like, pattern of the lesions); location or distribution of the lesions on the body; symptoms, both local and systemic; history of the present condition as well as related conditions; age of the patient; and patient sex. These six factors are discussed in the following sections, along with their significant qualifying characteristics. Direct observation of the skin lesion, plus C.B.'s responses to questions about these factors, will allow an appropriate diagnosis and treatment plan.

Morphology

Table 39-5 provides a listing of common dermatologic lesions, their respective definitions, and some well-known clinical examples. Lesions may also be classified as either primary or secondary. Primary lesions are lesions as they first appear on the skin, whereas secondary lesions develop from primary lesions. A papule (primary lesion) might progress to a pustule (secondary lesion). A pustule may also be a primary lesion if it originally developed as a pustule. The ability to recognize and describe specific lesions is critical to a successful diagnosis and communication regarding response to therapy.

In addition, many lesions present in a particular distribution or pattern. Poison ivy lesions are commonly distributed linearly. Herpetic lesions are so typical that the term herpetiform is used for lesions caused by other conditions that have a herpeslike distribution. The specific size of the lesion is also important in assessing a patient's condition. Dermatologic terms related to lesion distribution or pattern are shown in Table 39-6. The lesion's consistency (firm vs. soft), borders, and color are also important diagnostic considerations.

Location

"Location, location, location" is another axiom of dermatology. Simply put, certain lesions or conditions almost always occur in certain body locations. Table 39-7 provides a list of anatomic sites with common dermatoses occurring in those locations. For example, diseases of the sebaceous glands (e.g., acne, seborrheic dermatitis, rosacea) occur only in sites with high concentrations of sebaceous glands, such as the scalp, head, neck, chest, and umbilicus. Atopic dermatitis shows a predilection for the flexor surfaces of the body (i.e., antecubital and popliteal fossae).

Symptoms

Most skin conditions have only localized symptoms with the most common symptom being pruritus. Occasionally, localized burning or pain is the predominant symptom.

TABLE 39-5
Dermatologic Lesions, Definitions, and Clinical Examples

Name	Definition	Examples
Primary Lesions		
Macule	Nonpalpable, flat, change in color, <1 cm	Freckles, flat moles
Patch	Nonpalpable, flat, change in color, >1 cm	Vitiligo, café au lait spots, chloasma
Papule	Palpable, solid mass, may have change in color, <1 cm	Verrucae, noninflammatory acne (comedone), raised nevus
Nodule	Palpable, solid mass, most often below the plane of the skin, 1–2 cm	Erythema nodosum, severe acne
Tumor	Palpable, solid mass, >2 cm, most often above and below the plane of the skin	Neoplasms
Plaque	Flat, elevated, superficial papule with surface area greater than height, >1 cm	Psoriasis, seborrheic keratosis
Wheal	Superficial area of cutaneous edema, fluid not confined to cavity	Urticaria (hives), insect bite
Vesicle	Palpable, fluid-filled cavity, <1 cm, filled with serous fluid (blister)	Herpes simples, herpes zoster, contact dermatitis
Bulla	Palpable, fluid-filled cavity, >1 cm, filled with serous fluid (blister)	Pemphigus vulgaris, second-degree burn
Pustule	Similar to vesicle, but filled with purulent fluid	Acne, impetigo, folliculitis
Special Primary Lesions		
Comedone	Plugged opening of sebaceous gland	Acne, blackhead, whitehead
Cyst	Palpable lesion filled with semiliquid material or fluid	Sebaceous cyst
Abscess	Accumulation of purulent material in dermis or subcutaneous layers of skin; purulent material not visible on surface of skin	
Furuncle	Inflammatory nodule involving a hair follicle, following an episode of folliculitis	Small boil
Carbuncle	A coalescence of several furuncles	Large boil
Secondary Lesions		
Erosion	Loss of part or all the epidermis	Ecthyma
Ulcer	Loss of epidermis and dermis	Stasis ulcer
Fissure	Linear crack from epidermis into dermis	Tinea pedis
Excoriation	Self-induced linear, traumatized area caused by intense scratching	Atopic dermatitis, extreme pruritus
Atrophy	Thinning of skin with loss of dermal tissue	Striae
Crusts	Dried residue of pus, serum, or blood from a wound, pustule, or vesicle	Impetigo, scabs
Lichenification	Thickening of epidermis, accentuated skin markings, usually induced by scratching or chronic inflammation	Atopic dermatitis, allergic contact dermatitis

TABLE 39-6
Descriptive Dermatologic Terms

Term	Characteristics	Examples
Annular	Ring shaped	Tinea
Acneiform	Acnelike	Acne vulgaris
Arcuate	Shaped like an arc	Syphilis
Circinate	Circular	Tinea
Confluent	Lesions run together	Psoriasis, tinea
Discrete	Lesions remain separate	Psoriasis, tinea
Eczematous	General term for dry, red flaky or lichenified skin without clear border	Chronic allergic contact dermatitis, atopic dermatitis
Geographic	Shaped like islands or continents; maplike	Generalized psoriasis
Grouped	Lesions clustered together	Herpes
Herpetiform	Appears like herpes simplex	Herpes simplex
Intertrigo	Irritant dermatitis in skin folds	Diaper dermatitis
Iris	Looks like a bull's eye, lesion within a lesion, target lesion	Erythema multiforme
Keratotic	Horny thickening	Psoriasis, corn, callus
Linear	Shaped in lines	Poison ivy
Multiform	More than one type or shape of lesion	Erythema multiforme
Papulosquamous	Papules with desquamation	Psoriasis
Serpiginous	Snakelike lesions	Cutaneous larva migrans
Zosteriform	Appears like herpes zoster	Herpes zoster

TABLE 39-7
Common Skin Diseases by Body Location

Location	Skin Diseases
Scalp	Seborrheic dermatitis, dandruff
Face	Acne, rosacea, seborrheic dermatitis, perioral dermatitis, impetigo, herpes simplex, atopic dermatitis
Ears	Seborrheic dermatitis
Chest or abdomen	Tinea versicolor, tinea corporis, pityriasis rosea, acne, herpes zoster
Back	Tinea versicolor, tinea corporis, pityriasis rosea
Genital area	Tinea cruris, scabies, pediculosis, condyloma acuminate (venereal warts)
Extremities	Atopic dermatitis (cubital and popliteal fossa)
Hands	Tinea manuum, scabies, primary irritant contact dermatitis, warts
Feet	Tinea pedis, contact dermatitis, onychomycosis
Generalized or localized	Primary irritant or contact dermatitis, photodermatitis

History

Although a diagnosis may often be made from morphology, location, and symptoms, the patient history provides useful diagnostic and therapeutic information. Similar to the historical information obtained for any acute medical problem, the following questions should always be asked:

1. When and how did the problem start?
2. How has it progressed or changed since its onset? How have the lesions changed in size, color, appearance, or severity?
3. What is the patient's past and current medical history? What other symptoms might indicate that this is a dermatologic manifestation of a systemic disease?
4. What are the patient's symptoms?
5. What kind of allergies does the patient have?
6. What makes the condition worse or better?
7. What events or happenings have occurred with the onset or worsening of the condition (e.g., increased stress, exposure to new products, recent travel, changes in climate)?
8. What have you used to treat the condition, and how have the treatments worked?
9. How did the patient use any previous therapy, and for how long did they use it?

Age

Many conditions occur predominantly in certain age groups, such as acne in neonates and those ages 11 to 20 years, seborrheic dermatitis in neonates and those ages 11 to 12 years, rosacea in those older than 30 years, and atopic dermatitis primarily in children younger than 6 years. In fact, atopic dermatitis begins and ends before 6 years of age in 95% of patients. It is equally important to realize that many conditions, such as primary irritant and allergic contact dermatitis, occur independent of age. In addition, the skin of children and patients older than 65 years is more penetrable, thus more responsive and more susceptible to adverse effects from therapy with topical agents. Topical therapeutic agent potency and delivery systems must be carefully evaluated before usage.

Sex

Although most dermatologic conditions occur in both sexes, sometimes frequency and severity are sex dependent. Rosacea occurs more frequently in women, but is often more serious in men.

TOPICAL CORTICOSTEROIDS

General Principles of Therapy

Table 39-8 lists the most common topical corticosteroid preparations by their degree of potency. The following principles are used to guide the choice of agent and application technique.

- Topical corticosteroids should be applied no more than twice daily. Increasing the application from twice daily to four times daily does not produce superior responses, is more expensive, and may lead to increased frequency of topical and systemic adverse effects.[9]
- Preparations should be rubbed in thoroughly and, when possible, applied while the skin is moist (e.g., after bathing).[7] Hydration of the skin increases percutaneous absorption and the resultant therapeutic effect of topical steroids.
- Appropriate-strength preparations should be used to control the condition. For maintenance, most dermatologic conditions requiring topical corticosteroids can be managed with medium- or low-strength corticosteroid preparations (i.e., 1% hydrocortisone or a low-strength fluorinated corticosteroid such as triamcinolone acetonide 0.025%).[9,10]
- Occluded areas and certain, thin-skinned areas of the body, such as the face and flexures, are more prone to the development of side effects.[9,11] If corticosteroids must be used on the face or flexures, hydrocortisone or other nonfluorinated topical steroids should be used to reduce the probability of side effects.
- Children, elderly patients, and patients with liver failure are at risk for systemic corticosteroid toxicities. In addition, patients who use the highest-potency preparations for longer than 2 weeks are susceptible to percutaneous absorption and systemic toxicity.[9–11]
- With chronic conditions such as atopic eczema or allergic contact dermatitis, it is best to discontinue therapy gradually. This reduces the potential for rebound flares of topical lesions.[7]

Indications

A topical corticosteroid is often the drug of choice for inflammatory and pruritic eruptions. In addition, topical corticosteroids are useful with hyperplastic and infiltrative disorders. The following conditions generally respond well to topical corticosteroids: primary irritant and allergic contact dermatitis, alopecia areata, atopic eczema, discoid lupus erythematosus, granuloma annulare, hypertrophic scars and keloids, lichen planus, lichen simplex, lichen striatus, various nail disorders, pretibial myxedema, psoriasis, sarcoidosis, and seborrheic dermatitis.

Contraindications

The following conditions (predominantly infectious etiologies) are worsened by topical corticosteroids: acne vulgaris, ulcers, scabies, warts, molluscum contagiosum, fungal infections, viral infections, and balanitis. However, during the acute phase, topical corticosteroids are sometimes combined with other active ingredients (e.g., antifungal agents) for a few days if marked inflammation is present.

Side Effects

Although relatively infrequent, both localized (i.e., at the application site) and systemic side effects (from percutaneous absorption) can be caused by topical corticosteroids. The risks for

TABLE 39-8

Topical Corticosteroid Preparations by Stoughton–Cornell Classification of Potency

Corticosteroid	Brand Name(s)	Vehicle
1 (Most Potent) no More than 2 weeks' use		
Betamethasone dipropionate	Diprolene 0.05%	Ointment, optimized vehicle
Clobetasol propionate	Temovate 0.05%	Cream, ointment, optimized vehicle
Diflorasone diacetate	Psorcon 0.05%	Ointment
Halobetasol propionate	Ultravate 0.05%	Cream, ointment
2		
Amcinonide	Cyclocort 0.1%	Cream, lotion, ointment
Betamethasone dipropionate	Diprolene AF 0.05%	Cream
Betamethasone dipropionate	Diprosone 0.05%	Ointment
Desoximetasone	Topicort 0.25%	Cream, ointment
Desoximetasone	Topicort 0.05%	Gel
Diflorasone diacetate	Florone, Maxiflor 0.05%	Ointment
Fluocinonide	Lidex 0.05%	Cream, ointment, gel
Halcinonide	Halog 0.1%	Cream
Mometasone furoate[a]	Elocon 0.1%	Ointment
Triamcinolone acetonide	Kenalog 0.5%	Cream, ointment
3		
Amcinonide	Cyclocort 0.1%	Cream, lotion
Betamethasone	Benisone, Uticort 0.025%	Gel
Betamethasone benzoate	Topicort LP 0.05%	Cream (emollient)
Betamethasone dipropionate	Diprosone 0.05%	Cream
Betamethasone valerate	Valisone 0.1%	Ointment
Diflorasone diacetate	Florone, Maxiflor 0.05%	Cream
Fluocinonide	Cutivate 0.005%	Ointment
Fluticasone propionate	Lidex E 0.05%	Cream
Halcinonide	Halog 0.1%	Ointment
Triamcinolone acetate	Aristocort A 0.1%	Ointment
Triamcinolone acetate	Aristocort HP 0.5%	Cream
4		
Betamethasone benzoate	Benisone, Uticort 0.025%	Ointment
Betamethasone valerate	Valisone 0.1%	Lotion
Desoximetasone	Topicort-LP 0.05%	Cream
Fluocinolone acetonide	Synalar-HP 0.2%	Cream
Fluocinolone acetonide	Synalar 0.025%	Ointment
Flurandrenolide	Cordran 0.05%	Ointment
Halcinonide	Halog 0.25%	Cream
Hydrocortisone valerate[a]	Westcort 0.2%	Ointment
Mometasone furoate[a]	Elocon 0.1%	Cream
Triamcinolone acetonide	Aristocort, Kenalog 0.1%	Ointment
5		
Betamethasone benzoate	Benisone, Uticort 0.025%	Cream
Betamethasone dipropionate	Diprosone 0.02%	Lotion
Betamethasone valerate	Valisone 0.1%	Cream
Clocortolone	Cloderm 0.1%	Cream
Fluocinolone acetonide	Synalar 0.025%	Cream
Flurandrenolide	Cordran 0.05%	Cream
Fluticasone propionate	Cutivate 0.05%	Cream
Hydrocortisone buryrate[a]	Locoid 0.1%	Cream
Hydrocortisone valerate[a]	Westcort 0.2%	Cream
Prednicarbate	Dermatop 0.1%	Cream
Triamcinolone acetonide	Aristocort 0.25%	Cream
6		
Alclometasone dipropionate	Aclovate 0.05%	Ointment
Betamethasone valerate	Valisone 0.1%	Lotion
Desonide[a]	Tridesilon 0.05%	Cream
Fluocinolone acetonide	Synalar 0.01%	Solution
Triamcinolone acetonide	Kenalog 0.1%	Cream, lotion
7 (Least Potent)		
Hydrocortisone[a]	Generic 0.5%, 1.0%, 2.5%	Cream, ointment
Dexamethasone	Decadron 0.1%	Cream

[a] Nonfluorinated corticosteroid.

adverse reactions are influenced by the potency of preparation used, frequency of application, duration of use, anatomical site of application, and individual patient factors. Any of the previously discussed factors that increase potency, such as inflammation and occlusion, increase the chances of side effects.[9]

Epidermal and dermal atrophy (thinning of the skin), telangiectasia, localized fine hair growth, bruising, hypopigmentation, and striae can result from repeated application of topical corticosteroids.[11] Epidermal changes consisting of a reduction in cell size may begin within several days of therapy and are generally reversible after therapy is stopped.[9] Exposed areas (face) and thin-skinned areas (groin) are most vulnerable to epidermal atrophy.

Dermal atrophy generally takes several weeks to occur and is usually reversible, depending on how long the patient has used the corticosteroid, and on individual host factors such as skin age. Inguinal, genital, and perianal areas are most vulnerable to dermal atrophy. Many cases of dermal atrophy are reversible within 2 months after stopping the corticosteroid.[11]

Telangiectasia, which occurs most often on the face, neck, groin, and upper chest, may not be reversible after stopping corticosteroid therapy. Striae, which occur most commonly in the cubital and popliteal fossa, groin, axillary, and inner thigh areas, are usually permanent.[11] Fine hair growth may be particularly bothersome to female patients using corticosteroid preparations on the face. This problem is generally reversible after stopping therapy. Hypopigmentation, predominantly a problem of dark-skinned patients, is generally reversible after therapy is discontinued.[11]

Prolonged (several weeks or months) application of high-potency steroids to large areas of the body, especially if occlusion is used, can lead to systemic absorption and subsequent adrenal suppression. Rarely, typical Cushingoid features are observed.

Atopic Dermatitis

CASE 39-2

QUESTION 1: P.K., a 17-year-old boy, presents to a dermatology clinic with 30% of his body covered with a pruritic, eczematous rash. There is extensive involvement of popliteal and cubital fossae bilaterally. There is evidence of excoriation with cosmetic disfigurement in the antecubital fossae, around the neck, and on his forehead. P.K.'s mother and aunt have asthma. One sister (L.K.), age 15, has seasonal allergic rhinitis and eczema. His father and younger brother, age 11, appear to have no atopic manifestations. A rash was first noted 1 month after birth. The scalp, face, and neck were the only areas affected, and the rash continued with varying degrees of severity until age 2 years, when it spontaneously resolved. A similar rash reappeared at age 12, was diagnosed as atopic dermatitis, and has not disappeared since that time. P.K. experienced seasonal allergic rhinitis at age 6 years and has had occasional attacks of asthma (last attack, age 15). He has had a difficult time trying to follow provided nondrug recommendations for eczema. He has used over-the-counter topical hydrocortisone cream to treat flare-ups during the years. He reports a variable course; clearing in the summer and during periods of little stress, and worsening during the winter and periods of stress.

On physical examination, P.K. is a well-nourished, well-developed, adolescent boy with no abnormal physical findings other than marked allergic shiners, pale boggy nasal mucosa, and Dennie-Morgan folds noted near the eyes, plus extensive skin lesions. Oozing, crusted, excoriated areas caused by scratching, erythematous, eczematous, lichenified, maculopapular, and fine papulovesicular eruptions are on his face, neck, flexor aspects of both arms and legs, hands, and chest. There is some evidence of secondary bacterial infection in both cubital fossae and on portions of the left leg. Identify the presenting history, symptoms, and signs characteristic of eczema.

Atopic dermatitis, a form of eczema, can be acute or subacute, but is more commonly a chronic pruritic inflammation of the epidermis and dermis. Roughly two-thirds of the patients have a personal or family history of allergic rhinitis, eczema, or asthma. Atopic dermatitis in infants may be a prelude to the development of other atopic disorders later in life (i.e., allergic rhinitis or asthma). Presence of these disorders many times is the key to differential diagnosis. About 80% of patients with atopic dermatitis have a type I (immunoglobulin E [IgE] mediated) hypersensitivity reaction occurring as a result of the release of vasoactive substances from both mast cells and basophils that have been sensitized by the interaction of the antigen with IgE. An allergy workup is rarely helpful in determining the allergen. The disorder affects 0.5% to 1.0% of the general population, although its prevalence in children is 5% to 10%. In infants and young children, the dermatitis often occurs on the scalp, face, and extensor surfaces. In older children and adults, it tends to localize to the flexural areas, especially the cubital and popliteal fossae and the neck. In addition, the rash may affect the dorsal surface of the hands and feet, sometimes in the absence of eczema elsewhere.

ONLINE CONTENT

For a photo of atopic dermatitis, go to http://thepoint.lww.com/AT10e.

Most patients become afflicted between infancy and 12 years of age, with 60% being affected by the first year; another 30% are seen for the first time by 5 years of age, with the final 10% experiencing atopic dermatitis between 6 and 20 years of age.

Pruritus is the hallmark of atopic dermatitis. The constant scratching leads to a vicious cycle of itch-scratch-rash-itch, with the rash consisting primarily of lichenification of the skin. Atopic dermatitis has been described as "the itch that rashes, rather than the rash that itches." In other words, the itching precedes the rash. Wool, detergents, soaps, a change in room temperature, and mental or physical stress can precipitate itching. Patients tend to have dry skin (xerosis) all over the body. This is attributable to a reduced water-binding capacity and a higher transdermal water loss. Xerosis is worsened during periods of low humidity, such as winter in northern latitudes. Treating the xerosis can prevent or control the disease in milder or episodic cases.

P.K.'s family and medical history are classic for atopic dermatitis. His family history is significant for asthma, allergic rhinitis, and atopic dermatitis. He had his initial outbreak at the age of 1 month and then experienced seasonal allergic rhinitis and asthma. His skin examination reveals findings of both acute and chronic atopic eczema, with typical lesion location and description.

CASE 39-2, QUESTION 2: What are the relevant biopharmaceutic considerations for selecting a topical corticosteroid for P.K.?

Topical corticosteroids are classified into potency categories (Table 39-8). The relative potency assigned to a topical corticosteroid is determined by the ability of the preparation to penetrate the skin after release from the vehicle, the intrinsic activity of the corticosteroid at the receptor, and the rate of clearance from the receptor. Activity of corticosteroids may be enhanced by the use of a more occlusive vehicle, the addition of penetration-enhancing substances (i.e., petrolatum, propylene glycol), and modifications of the steroid molecule. Hydrocortisone was the initial local corticosteroid discovered, and since then, the molecule has been modified in several ways. The addition of a fluorine atom at the 9 position protects the steroid ring from metabolic conversion, resulting in more potent activity. The introduction of an acetonide bond or lipophilic ester groups increases skin penetration. Many newer topical corticosteroids have incorporated one or more of these molecular changes, resulting in increased-potency agents and a growing armamentarium of agents.

It is believed that topical corticosteroids penetrate into the stratum corneum by passive diffusion, which varies considerably, depending on the part of the body to which the preparation is applied. When a standard hydrocortisone preparation was applied to various parts of the body, absorption was found to be 0.14% on the plantar surface of the foot, 1% on the forearm, 4% on the scalp, 7% on the forehead, 13% on the cheeks, and 36% on the scrotum. Because penetration is high in the groin, axillae, and face, lower-potency nonfluorinated topical preparations such as hydrocortisone 0.5% to 1% should be used on these areas.[9,10] In areas where penetration is poor, owing to thickening of the stratum corneum, such as the elbows, knees, palms, or soles, higher-potency preparations should be used.[9]

For P.K., a 1% hydrocortisone cream or nonfluorinated corticosteroid, e.g., mometasone, should be used on his face and other areas of high penetrability to reduce the possibility of complications.[9] A high-potency cream (intermediate- or higher-potency classification as listed by Stoughton–Cornell class of corticosteroid potency in Table 39-8) should be used initially on acutely inflamed areas or where high penetration is not a problem. This will "cool down" these lesions quickly and dry them out. Once the acute phase is controlled, the cream should be converted to the ointment for its emollient properties.

When equal amounts of a corticosteroid are incorporated into ointments, gels, creams, and lotion bases, the gel and ointment preparations are generally more active than creams and lotions.[9,10] However, with the increased use of optimized vehicles, that rule is not as true as in the past. The addition of certain substances enhances penetration and potency. Using these principles, pharmaceutical manufacturers have increasingly developed optimized vehicles that maximize diffusion of individual corticosteroids into the stratum corneum. Therefore, for new products, the only reliable way to ascertain potency is to consult the manufacturer's literature for its Stoughton classification. Increasing the concentration of a corticosteroid in a preparation also increases its potency, but not in a linear fashion. Because P.K. has some fine papulovesicular eruption, a cream should be used initially to facilitate drying. However, patients often express a preference (e.g., cream or gel), and this should be considered.

Occlusion

CASE 39-2, QUESTION 3: It has been some time since P.K.'s atopic eczema has been aggressively treated. He has many acute, inflamed lesions. Should occlusive therapy be used? What complications could develop from occlusion? How should the use of occlusion be explained to P.K.?

As discussed previously (see Dermatologic Drug Delivery Systems section), occlusion traps heat and promotes maceration. This same mechanism increases the hydration of the skin and resultant absorption of corticosteroid preparations, thus producing a heightened therapeutic effect. As a general rule, occlusion enhances the potency of corticosteroids by a factor of 10. Occlusion can be accomplished by one of three methods: (a) selecting an ointment-based corticosteroid, (b) applying a nonmedicated ointment base over another corticosteroid preparation (gel, cream, lotion, or aerosol), or (c) by enveloping the medicated area with plastic (e.g., plastic wrap, gloves, or plastic suit).[5,7,9,11] Because several hours of occlusion are all that are necessary to increase potency, these relatively short periods of occlusion can be clinically useful. Occlusion can be uncomfortable, and can lead to sweat retention and an increased risk of bacterial and candidal infections. To reduce these problems and the chances of systemic side effects, occlusion should not be maintained for more than 12 hours in a 24-hour period. Occlusion should not be used for acute lesions, which already have increased absorptive capability and need the vasoconstrictive effects of cooling first. Occlusion is best used for chronic lesions that are thick and scaly, in which drug absorption is impaired. Most patients with atopic dermatitis do not tolerate occlusion because their itch threshold is low, and heat, sweat retention, and maceration increase pruritus. The long-term benefit of occlusion in a patient with atopic dermatitis is reduced by the increased pruritus, which may lead to nonadherence. When using occlusion in patients with eczema, care should be taken not to occlude unaffected skin (because of the low itch threshold). For other chronic dermatologic conditions (e.g., psoriasis) that are not associated with severe pruritus, occlusion could be used for prolonged periods if necessary. Increasing the hydration of the skin (after a shower or bath) also increases the effects of medications immediately applied after the bath or shower, which would be an appropriate recommendation for P.K.

Product Selection

PHARMACOKINETIC CONSIDERATIONS

CASE 39-2, QUESTION 4: P.K. received a prescription for halcinonide 0.25% cream, 30 g, to be applied at bedtime to nonfacial areas and mometasone furoate cream 0.1%, 30 g, twice daily to the facial lesions. Based on pertinent biopharmaceutical considerations, why is this prescription appropriate for P.K.?

Corticosteroids tend to penetrate human skin very slowly, leading to a reservoir effect. With low-potency preparations, this reservoir effect persists for several days, and with the most potent preparations under occlusion, the effects may persist for up to 14 days.[9,10] The clinical implication of this reservoir effect on chronic conditions is a cumulative effect with repeated application of topical corticosteroids. As a result, the number of applications per day can be reduced, and less-potent preparations can be used after the acute inflammatory process has been brought under control. Results from P.K.'s treatment regimen might be improved by providing more frequent (twice-daily) application or a more potent preparation for twice-daily administration to control inflamed lesions. Once the weeping is stopped, a less-potent preparation in the ointment form should be used for maintenance and the number of applications may be reduced. Because of the reservoir effect, control can be maintained in many cases with intermittent regimens such as once daily, every other day, or every third day use of topical corticosteroids. In addition, intermittent regimens can involve alternating corticosteroids and agents such as topical pimecrolimus or tacrolimus to maintain control and minimize adverse effects of either agent.

Side Effects

ACNE

CASE 39-2, QUESTION 5: After several months of continuous corticosteroid therapy in a maintenance format using 2.5% hydrocortisone ointment, P.K. presents with four pustules and two closed comedones on his forehead and multiple pustules on both cheeks. What problems from the use of topical corticosteroid therapy on the face does this represent?

The face is particularly vulnerable to corticosteroid side effects because of enhanced penetration.[11] Acne, acne rosacea, and perioral dermatitis can develop after several weeks to months of application. Corticosteroid-induced conditions can generally be distinguished from naturally occurring disorders. Corticosteroid-induced acne lesions are uniformly at the same level of development throughout the affected area and are present only in areas treated with the corticosteroid. Generally, steroid acne, acne rosacea, and perioral dermatitis resolve after discontinuing the drug. Application of corticosteroid preparations (particularly the potent preparations) to areas around the eye can lead to increased intraocular pressure, glaucoma, cataracts, increased risk of ocular mycotic infections, and exacerbation of pre-existing herpes simplex infections.[11] Hydrocortisone or nonfluorinated topical corticosteroids such as mometasone are the agents of choice for facial lesions.

P.K.'s acneiform lesions may get worse after the application of topical corticosteroids. He should be instructed to apply the corticosteroid preparation only to the atopic eczema and to avoid areas where acne exists. If the atopic dermatitis and acne lesions are in the same area and his acne gets worse after using the topical corticosteroid, switching to tacrolimus or pimecrolimus for a brief period would be indicated. Some improvement in corticosteroid-exacerbated acne may be achieved by decreasing the strength of the topical product applied to the face and reducing the frequency of application. An alternative to this approach, if P.K.'s acne is severe, would be to continue topical corticosteroid therapy, but treat the acne systemically.[5,6] (See Chapter 40, Acne, for a more extensive discussion.)

ADRENAL AXIS SUPPRESSION AND RISK OF INFECTION

CASE 39-2, QUESTION 6: P.K. recently sustained a knee injury, and corrective surgery is being considered. Should he receive a systemic corticosteroid during the perioperative period as a precaution against adrenal insufficiency? Should he wear a Medic-Alert tag while using long-term topical corticosteroids? Is he at risk for experiencing an infection after surgery?

Systemic adrenal axis suppression from topically applied corticosteroids appears to be more of a theoretic risk than a clinical entity in adults, except when the highest-potency preparations are used[12] or other risk factors are present (Table 39-9). Although suppression has been reported with use of mild to moderately potent agents, these cases can be attributed to excessive use or to application of corticosteroids over large areas of the body for prolonged periods under occlusion. If suppression does occur, it reverses within 2 to 4 weeks after application is stopped. Patients using more than 45 g/week of a high-potency corticosteroid are at risk for adrenal axis suppression.[12] Therefore, the use of preparations such as clobetasol should be limited to no more than 45 g/week for 2 weeks or less. In addition, these preparations should not be used under occlusion and should be reserved for dermatoses that are unresponsive to less potent preparations.

TABLE 39-9
Risk Factors for Systemic Side Effects From Topical Corticosteroids

Duration of application
Prolonged application (>3–4 weeks)
Potency of corticosteroid
Weak or moderately strong, 100 g/wk without occlusion
Very potent, >45 g/wk without occlusion
Application location
Thin stratum corneum results in easier penetration (eyelids, forehead, cheeks, armpits, groin, and genitals)
Age of patient
Very young children and elderly people have very thin epidermis
Manner of application
Occlusion
Presence of penetration-enhancing substances
Propylene glycol
Salicylic acid
Urea
Condition of the skin
General factors
Compromised liver function

Because young children absorb corticosteroids to a greater extent, they have a greater risk of developing adrenal axis suppression and other systemic side effects.[12] To reduce this risk, hydrocortisone topical preparations should be used in children, and their use should be limited to short periods. Patients whose corticosteroid clearance is impaired (e.g., liver failure) should also use hydrocortisone and be monitored closely for signs of systemic toxicity.[11]

The risk of developing an addisonian crisis during surgery or at other times of stress secondary to adrenal suppression from topical steroids is extremely low. Patients who have used potent topical corticosteroids over large areas of their bodies (>30%) or those who have used occlusion are at greater risk (see previous discussion) and are often given systemic hydrocortisone prophylactically before surgery. Because P.K. is not likely to require such supplementation, a Medic-Alert tag is unnecessary.

Infection secondary to topically administered corticosteroids is also a theoretic risk, but is uncommon. Although anecdotal reports of secondary bacterial infections appear in the literature, there is scant evidence to suggest that they occur with any frequency. Topical corticosteroids do not alter normal skin flora.[13]

Topical Antibiotics with Corticosteroids

CASE 39-2, QUESTION 7: P.K.'s atopic dermatitis presentation is complicated with areas of erythematous, honey-colored, crusted lesions on his forehead, arm, and leg. Can a corticosteroid and an antibiotic preparation be used together? What are the risks associated with topical antibiotics?

It is determined that P.K. has impetigo superimposed on his atopic dermatitis. Because impetigo can be treated with topical antibiotics such as mupirocin, combination therapy with a corticosteroid–antibiotic preparation appears to be a logical choice. The corticosteroid suppresses the clinical signs of infection and helps re-establish the normal skin barrier function. This, in combination with an appropriate antibiotic, allows the skin's normal defense mechanisms to ward off the infection. However, because staphylococci toxins act as superantigens, eliciting the

TABLE 39-10
Spectrum of Activity of Antibiotics Available for Topical Use

Bacitracin
Effective against all anaerobic cocci, most strains of streptococci, staphylococci, and pneumococci. Not effective against most gram-negative organisms.

Gentamicin
Effective against most gram-negative organisms (similar to neomycin), including *Pseudomonas* and many strains of *Staphylococcus aureus*.

Mupirocin
Very effective against *S. aureus* and does not interfere with wound healing. Currently, the only topical antibiotic that has been proved to be more effective than the vehicle based on US Food and Drug Administration guidelines.

Gramicidin
Effective against most gram-positive organisms. Not effective against most gram-negative organisms.

Neomycin
Effective against most gram-negative organisms (except *Pseudomonas*) and some gram-positive organisms. Group A streptococci are resistant.

Polymyxin B
Effective against most gram-negative organisms (including *Pseudomonas*). Most strains of *Proteus, Serratia,* and gram-positive organisms are resistant.

Retapamulin
Effective against *Streptococcus pyogenes* and methicillin-sensitive strains of *S. aureus*.

production of IgE, thus worsening the atopic dermatitis, almost all clinicians treat atopic dermatitis–associated impetigo with oral antibiotics such as dicloxacillin, macrolides, or cephalexin, in combination with topical corticosteroids for the eczema.[14–16] Oral antibiotics reduce the bacterial counts faster and have a lower incidence of recurrent impetigo compared with topical agents. In areas in which community methicillin-resistant *Staphylococcus aureus* rates are high, other more effective antibiotic therapy might be indicated.

Table 39-10 describes the spectrum of activity of common topical antibiotics. Although mupirocin may be an appropriate alternative for some topical dermatologic infections, the current over-the-counter topical antibiotics (bacitracin, neomycin, and polymyxin) are ineffective for most dermatologic infections and are indicated only for the prophylaxis of skin infections. Mupirocin resistance occurs with overuse.[17]

P.K. would most likely benefit from a treatment course of an oral antibiotic plus a topical corticosteroid preparation.

SIDE EFFECTS

There have been many reports of contact dermatitis caused by topical antimicrobials, particularly neomycin.[18] Neomycin sensitivity has been reported in 4% of the general population by patch testing and in 40% of patients with a history of allergic contact dermatitis or a history of recurrent use of topical antibiotics.[18,19] The corticosteroid contained in many neomycin preparations does not prevent these allergic reactions, although it may decrease the severity of the reaction.

Pruritus

CASE 39-2, QUESTION 8: As stated in Case 39-2, Question 2, one of P.K.'s complaints is pruritus. What could you recommend for relief of pruritus?

TABLE 39-11
Systemic Diseases Associated With Pruritus

Brain abscesses
Carcinoid syndrome
Carcinoma of the breast, lung, or stomach
Central nervous system infarct
Diabetes mellitus
Gout
Hodgkin disease and other lymphomas
Hypertension
Iron-deficiency anemia
Multiple myeloma
Multiple sclerosis
Mycosis fungoides
Obstructive biliary disease
Polycythemia vera
Pregnancy (first trimester)
Thyroid disease (both hyperthyroidism and hypothyroidism)
Uremia

Pruritus (itching) is the most common cutaneous symptom. It has many different causes and has been associated with a variety of systemic diseases, several of which are listed in Table 39-11.[5,7,20] In the absence of a cutaneous manifestation, a careful history and physical examination should be performed to rule out one of the systemic causes of pruritus. In addition, a chest radiograph, stool examination for occult blood, complete blood count with differential, thyroid panel, blood urea nitrogen, creatinine, liver function panel, glucose, and urinalysis may be necessary to help screen for the aforementioned systemic diseases.[20]

Scratching, which can damage or fatigue receptor nerve endings, is the most common method of relieving pruritus. One would, therefore, expect topically applied local anesthetics or antihistamines to be effective in dulling the sensation. However, this approach is often disappointing, probably because the intact epidermis poorly absorbs the salt forms of these drugs. Also, low concentrations are used in many over-the-counter preparations. If adequate concentrations of local anesthetics are used (lidocaine 3%–4%), pruritus or pain may be reduced for up to 45 minutes. These agents are most useful for relieving pruritus or pain for short periods (e.g., when trying to go to sleep at night).[20] A drawback to the use of benzocaine and topical antihistamine preparations are their propensity to induce allergic contact dermatitis.[21–23]

P.K. could also try cold water or ice cubes, which effectively relieve pruritus via vasoconstriction, as do products containing aluminum acetate (Burow solution), tannic acid, or calamine. A cool bath may be useful for the relief of pruritus from dermatologic lesions if they are widespread.

Moisturizing mixtures such as Eucerin, Nivea, Lubriderm, or, simply, mineral or baby oil are useful in the treatment of pruritus caused by dry skin. This problem is often encountered in the elderly and others during the winter months. Bathing should be restricted to avoid washing away normal body oils, the drying effect of water, the irritant effect of alkaline soaps, and the trauma of toweling.[7]

Topical corticosteroid applications can be very effective if dermatological lesions exist. They reduce inflammation, which helps soothe the affected area.

Systemic antihistamines are effective antipruritics, although their major beneficial effect may be attributable to sedation. The newer, nonsedating antihistamines are notably ineffective at relieving itch, with the exception of cetirizine.[24] There is disagreement over which antihistamine or antiserotonin agents are

TABLE 39-12
Nondrug Recommendations for Patients with Atopic Dermatitis or Other Irritant Dermatoses

- Clothing should be soft and light. Cotton or corduroy is preferred. Wools and coarse, heavy synthetics should be avoided.
- Heat should be avoided because it often makes eczema worse. The environment should be well ventilated, cool, and low in humidity (30%–50%). Rapid changes in ambient temperature should be avoided.
- Bathing should be kept to a minimum (no longer than 5 minutes), and the patient should use a nonirritating soap (e.g., Basis soap). A colloid bath or the use of appropriate amounts of bath oil may be useful.
- The skin should be kept moist with frequent applications of emollients (e.g., Lubriderm, Nivea, Aquaphor, Eucerin, or petrolatum).
- Primary irritants such as paints, cleansers, solvents, and chemical sprays should be avoided.

most effective for treatment of pruritus.[20,24,25] Many practitioners consider hydroxyzine to be the antihistamine of choice; doses of 10 to 25 mg three to four times a day are commonly used. Other practitioners favor cyproheptadine. There is little evidence that antihistamines are effective in treating non–histamine-mediated pruritus, except that their inherent sedative effect may be somewhat beneficial in all pruritic conditions. Doxepin, a tricyclic antidepressant with potent H_1-blocking properties, is valuable as a second-line antihistamine topically or systemically if others fail.[26] Because P.K.'s pruritus is worse at night, as is typical with atopic dermatitis, the use of any of the three H_1-blockers mentioned at bedtime would be appropriate.[27]

Nondrug Recommendations for Atopic Dermatitis

CASE 39-2, QUESTION 9: In addition to prescriptions for topical corticosteroids, a systemic antibiotic (cephalexin 500 mg four times daily for 7–10 days), and an oral antihistamine (hydroxyzine 25 mg, one to two tablets at bedtime as needed), what nondrug interventions should be suggested for P.K.?

The general goals of therapy for atopic dermatitis are to decrease pruritus, suppress inflammation, lubricate the skin, and reduce anxiety. The nondrug recommendations shown in Table 39-12 are useful adjuncts and mainstays for use between disease flares for patients such as P.K. with atopic dermatitis or any other irritant dermatitis. Often careful attention to nonpharmacologic measures can markedly reduce the incidence of disease flare. Because even nonlesional skin in patients with atopic dermatitis has reduced moisture, the use of emollients should include all skin surfaces.

P.K. should be warned to avoid people with active herpes simplex infections because severe disseminated infections can occur. Similarly, based on the anthrax bioterrorism attack in October 2001, debate has emerged on the advisability of reinitiating routine vaccination against smallpox. Vaccinia virus was the live poxvirus used throughout the world as the vaccine against smallpox. Because of the increased risk for eczema vaccinatum, vaccinia vaccine should not be administered to persons with eczema of any degree, those with a past history of eczema, household contacts who have active eczema, or household contacts who have a history of eczema.[25,28]

Tachyphylaxis, Specialized Corticosteroid Dosage Forms, and Antihistamines

CASE 39-2, QUESTION 10: P.K. responded well to the previous treatment plan and is given a prescription for hydrocortisone ointment 2.5% as maintenance therapy. The bacterial superinfected areas have cleared. Without informing anyone, he continues to have problems with his fingers. He been applying an old prescription for betamethasone dipropionate to his hands five to six times daily for the past 2 weeks without any noticeable improvement. Halcinonide and mometasone creams resolved the rash on other areas of his body. Other than occasional sedation early on from the hydroxyzine and when he uses it intermittently, he has not had any other adverse effects. As P.K. continues to follow other nondrug recommendations, he inquires whether anything else could be done for his hands. Assess P.K.'s use and response to the corticosteroids.

P.K. is overusing the potent topical corticosteroid and may have developed tachyphylaxis. Tachyphylaxis can occur within 1 week of therapy, but generally takes several weeks to a month to occur.[29] To treat this problem, P.K. should stop applying the betamethasone preparation for 4 to 7 days and then restart therapy in a more appropriate manner (i.e., twice daily). Alternatively, patients may be switched to topical tacrolimus or pimecrolimus. Limited courses of treatment separated by short periods of rest may be more effective than continuous treatment. However, clinicians commonly misdiagnose tachyphylaxis. Failure of topical corticosteroids to clear difficult atopic dermatitis after an initial improvement may give the false impression of tachyphylaxis when the actual problem is a primary failure of the treatment.[30] This could be caused by either inappropriate application technique by the patient or the choice of a product with inadequate potency.

Flurandrenolide 4 mg/cm^2 tape (Cordran) may be useful after P.K. stops his other corticosteroids for 4 to 7 days. Although this product is expensive, it is effective for small areas because the tape serves as a protectant and provides occlusion. It is a good choice for use on the hands, particularly the fingers, where P.K. is having problems, because other vehicles are often quite messy when applied to the hands. When using flurandrenolide tape, the general principles previously outlined for occlusion should be followed.

Topical tacrolimus or pimecrolimus are effective alternatives to topical corticosteroids and are safe for use in children.[31,32] In addition to its inhibitory effect on cytokine production, topical tacrolimus has been shown to cause alterations in epidermal antigen-presenting dendritic cells that may result in decreased immunologic response to antigens. Transient burning, erythema, and pruritus are the most common adverse effects. Pimecrolimus cream 1% is an immunomodulatory agent with properties similar to those of cyclosporine and tacrolimus, but it does not appear to affect the systemic immune response and might, therefore, be better tolerated for long-term therapy.[33] Neither pimecrolimus nor tacrolimus causes skin atrophy, making them attractive alternatives for patients with lesions on the face and neck. Recently, issues regarding the long-term safety of these products has led the US Food and Drug Administration to place a black-box warning in the manufacturer's literature regarding a potential increased cancer risk.

CASE 39-3

QUESTION 1: P.K.'s sister, L.K., who also has atopic dermatitis, started using a new topical corticosteroid preparation (halcinonide) 10 days ago. She has been complaining of a burning sensation lasting for 1 hour after every application of this product. She stopped using the product 2 days ago because of this. Is it possible that she has developed an allergy to a corticosteroid-containing medication?

Cortisol is endogenously secreted by the adrenal gland and is essential to life. As a result, allergic reactions to topical corticosteroid preparations are rare. When allergic symptoms do occur, they are generally not caused by the corticosteroid, but rather the preservatives (e.g., paraben) or other ingredients in the formulation or the base (e.g., lanolin). Allergic sensitization can occur within 2 weeks of therapy, but may be difficult to diagnose because the corticosteroid can modify the allergic reaction.[34] One should suspect an allergic reaction if lesions change appearance after starting therapy, if healing does not occur within the expected time, or if the condition improves and then abruptly gets worse. Most case reports of allergic reactions (dryness, itching, burning, or irritation) to topical corticosteroids are nonspecific and are seen in patients with atopic dermatitis.[34] However, because the skin is very dry in atopic dermatitis, rather than representing an allergic reaction, the use of creams or gels may cause excessive dryness, burning, and irritation. Switching to an ointment can alleviate those symptoms. Atopic individuals are more likely to react to the vehicle base than the active corticosteroid ingredient.

Because of the time course of the burning sensation in L.K. (starting the first day and lasting only 1 hour), it is doubtful that she is actually allergic to this product and points to the cream being the cause. However, atopic dermatitis patients often have sensitive skin that reacts idiosyncratically to a variety of topical preparations.[34] To remedy this situation, L.K. should be given another topical corticosteroid preparation with an ointment. If the reaction continues with a new product, an allergy workup may be necessary and patch testing could be considered.

XEROSIS

CASE 39-4

QUESTION 1: C.R., a 64-year-old woman, requests something for dry skin on her arms and back. She has had this problem for a number of years. It is generally not a problem in the summer, with most symptoms troubling her in the winter. She has no other medical conditions and only takes an occasional aspirin for "arthritis." How would you advise C.R. to manage this condition?

C.R.'s complaints represent a common problem of the elderly, xerosis (dry skin). The seasonal cycle described is frequently called "winter itch." Most cases of dry skin are caused by dehydration of the stratum corneum.[35] Table 39-13 gives general recommendations for the treatment of dry skin.

However, before recommending therapy, the following differential diagnosis should be considered: ichthyosis vulgaris (familial history usually present), atopic dermatitis, psoriasis, contact dermatitis, and hypothyroidism. Usually, simple questioning can rule out these conditions.

TABLE 39-13

General Recommendations for Treatment of Dry Skin

1. Use room humidifiers.
2. Keep room temperature as low as comfortable to prevent sweating and water loss from the skin.
3. Keep bathing to a minimum (every 1–2 days) with warm, but not hot, water. After bathing, the patient should immediately apply an emollient (Table 39-2). When the skin is soaked for 5 to 10 minutes, the stratum corneum can absorb as much as six times its weight in water. Application of an emollient immediately after bathing will trap the water in the skin and reduce dryness.
4. Eliminate exposure to solvents, drying chemicals, harsh soaps, and cleaners. These substances remove oils from the skin and reduce its barrier function. As the barrier function is lost, water loss from the skin is increased up to 75 times higher than normal. Exposure to cold, dry winds will also enhance water loss.
5. Apply emollients (Table 39-2) three to six times a day, especially after bathing to help retain moisture in the skin from bathing.
6. The selection of emollients depends on the atmospheric moisture content of the region. In dry parts of the western United States where humidity is very low, water-in-oil emollients such as Lubriderm, Eucerin, or Nivea are preferred because the high oil content prevents the loss of moisture from the skin. In those areas, a general rule is to avoid products in which glycerin is one of the top four ingredients on the label because glycerin is hygroscopic and in low humidity will pull moisture out of the dermis, leading to drier, cracked skin. In areas with higher humidity such as the eastern United States, glycerin in both types of emollients pulls moisture from the atmosphere into the skin. Regardless of region, if application of an emollient appears to be ineffective, switching to a product with less glycerin and more oil may resolve the dryness.
7. If scaling is a problem, a keratolytic (Lac-Hydrin, AmLactin) or a higher-strength, urea-containing preparation (20%) may be useful.

DRUG ERUPTIONS

Clinically recognizable adverse drug reactions are manifested on the skin more often than any other organ or organ system.[36,37] An estimated 1% to 5% of hospitalized patients experience a drug eruption.[37] Outpatient statistics are more difficult to obtain, but are probably within the same range. There is no correlation between age, diagnosis, or severity of illness and the likelihood of developing a drug eruption. Women appear to be twice as likely as men to experience a drug eruption.

The most common type of eruption encountered in clinical practice, and probably the one most often overlooked, is the exanthematic (bursting out) eruption. This type of reaction comprises both morbilliform (measleslike) and scarlatiniform (scarlet fever–like) eruptions. Stevens-Johnson syndrome (SJS), toxic epidermal necrolysis, drug hypersensitivity syndrome, vasculitis, serum sickness, coagulant-induced skin necrosis, and angioedema are the most important severe reactions and require immediate attention and management. Many of the common dermatologic reactions that can be induced by drugs have other causes as well, so a complete workup must include other nondrug etiologies. Viral, fungal, and bacterial infections, as well as certain systemic diseases and foods, have been identified as causes for common reactions such as urticaria, erythema multiforme, and erythema nodosum. The diagnosis of drug eruptions is best made by identifying the type of lesions observed and associating the lesions with specific drug therapy. The most important diagnostic criterion is an accurate assessment of the skin lesions. With this critical information, the clinician can then refer to a drug information source to associate any current or past drug therapy with the specific lesions observed.

Acneiform Eruptions

Acneiform eruptions appear very much like common acne. They may be distinguished from acne by their sudden occurrence, the absence of comedones, uniform appearance (i.e., all at the same stage of development), and the fact that they may occur on any part of the body. Cysts and scarring are rarely associated with drug-induced acne. Eruptions can also occur during any period of the patient's life; thus, drug-induced acne should be suspected when the lesions appear in persons outside the typical age bracket for acne. Drugs implicated include adrenocorticotropic hormone, anabolic steroids, azathioprine, danazol, glucocorticoids, halogens (iodides, bromides), isoniazid, lithium, gefitinib, erlotinib. lapatinib, and oral contraceptives. For patients with acne vulgaris, these drugs may worsen existing lesions (see Chapter 40, Acne).

Photosensitivity Reactions

Photosensitivity eruptions require the presence of both a drug (or chemical) and a light source of appropriate wavelength. These eruptions are divided into two subtypes: phototoxic and photoallergic. *Phototoxic* reactions, the most common drug-induced photodermatosis, manifest themselves as an exaggerated sunburn or increased sensitivity to sunburn. The ultraviolet A (UVA) light source alters the drug to a toxic form, resulting in tissue damage independent of any allergic response, and occurs in everyone who gets high enough skin levels of the offending drug. This eruption can occur on first exposure to a drug, is dose related, and will continue as long as the skin concentration of the drug exceeds the threshold level for the reaction to occur. *Photoallergic* reactions, which are very uncommon, may appear as a variety of lesions, including urticaria, bullae, and sunburn. UVA light alters the drug so it becomes an antigen or acts as a hapten. Photoallergic eruptions require previous contact with the offending drug, are not dose related, exhibit cross-sensitivity with chemically related compounds, and are secondary to the use of topical agents. Unfortunately, outside light through a window and fluorescent lighting permit passage of or can emit UVA light. In addition, until recently there were inadequate topical preparations that provide protection against UVA light. Avobenzone, although covering much of the UVA spectrum, is photolabile, losing 60% of its effectiveness in less than 1 hour. However, many products now solve that problem by adding agents such as octocrylene, which stabilize avobenzone's photolability and are usually labeled "stabilized UVA protection." New products containing ecamsule appear to offer an advance in protection against lower spectrum UVA rays. In some instances, a drug may produce both photoallergic and phototoxic reactions. Most phototoxic and photoallergic reactions occur fairly soon after exposure to light. Implicated drugs are numerous, including, among others, antibiotics (tetracyclines, fluoroquinolones, and sulfonamides), antidepressants (tricyclics), antihypertensives (hydrochlorothiazide, β-blockers), hypoglycemics (sulfonylureas), nonsteroidal anti-inflammatory drugs, sunscreens (p-aminobenzoic acid [PABA]), oral contraceptives, and antipsychotics (phenothiazines) (see Chapter 42, Photosensitivity, Photoaging, and Burns).

Allergic Contact Dermatitis

Topical administration of a sensitizing agent produces localized papulovesicular lesions. These lesions are limited only to areas that come in contact with the topical product. Neomycin, benzocaine, and diphenhydramine are well-known topical sensitizers (Table 39-14). Systemic administration of a drug to a patient previously sensitized to the drug by topical application can provoke widespread dermatitis. Implicated systemically or topically administered drugs that reactivate allergic contact dermatitis include procaine or benzocaine, radiographic contrast media or iodine, and streptomycin and gentamicin or neomycin, among others.

TABLE 39-14
Frequent Contact Sensitizers

Substance	Found In
Ammonia	Soaps, chemicals, hair dyes
Antihistamines	Topical anti-itch creams and ointments
Balsam of Peru	Cosmetics
Benzyl alcohol	Medications, cosmetics
"Caine" anesthetics	Medications (e.g., over-the-counter benzocaine products)
Carba	Rubber
Chromium	Jewelry
Epoxy resin	Glue
Ethylenediamine	Stabilizer in topical products (e.g., aminophylline)
Formaldehyde	Shoes, clothing, soaps, insulations
Mercaptobenzothiazole	Rubber
Naphthyl	Rubber
Neomycin	Topical medications (e.g., Neosporin)
Nickel sulfate	Jewelry, fasteners
Paraben	Preservative in many topical products
Paraphenylenediamine	Hair dyes, leather
Potassium dichromate	Shoes, leather
Thiomersal	Preservatives, contact lens products
Thiram	Rubber products
Turpentine	Paint products
Wool alcohols	Lanolin-containing products, clothes

Erythema Multiforme

As the name implies, erythema multiforme (EM) eruptions take on a varied spectrum of morphologic forms, ranging from the mildest with tiny maculovesicular lesions to more severe forms such as SJS and toxic epidermal necrolysis syndrome (TENS) with extensive bullous lesions and routine involvement of mucous membranes. Although all forms have been reported to have oral lesions, they are much more severe in SJS and TENS, in which genital, nasal, and ocular mucosae are also involved. Target lesions are usually present in all forms of the disorder, which characteristically are erythematous, iris-shaped papules and vesiculobullous lesions typically involving the extremities (especially the palms and soles) in EM and the torso in SJS and TENS. The lesions take on the appearance of a circular target with a bull's-eye in the middle, thus the term target lesion. However, questions have recently been raised about the shared pathological nature of these forms of EM.[38] EM in its mildest forms, EM minor and EM major, is more common in children and young adults, and is self-limited in nature with only transient hypopigmentation or hyperpigmentation as complications. Sometimes malaise, a low-grade fever, and itching or burning may accompany this type of eruption. Etiologic factors associated with EM include drugs, mycoplasma and herpes infections, radiation therapy, foods, and sometimes neoplasms. Allopurinol, barbiturates, phenothiazine, and sulfonamides are the drugs most often implicated in EM eruptions.

Stevens-Johnson Syndrome

SJS is probably the most common type of severe drug eruption. The syndrome is usually a moderate mucocutaneous and systemic reaction. Blisters and atypical target lesions involve less than 10% of body surface area, with some epidermal detachment, which can cause scarring in some cases.

ONLINE CONTENT

For a photo of Stevens-Johnson syndrome, go to http://thepoint.lww.com/AT10e.

With more extensive involvement, clinical findings are almost indistinguishable from toxic epidermal necrolysis. The skin can become hemorrhagic, and pneumonia and joint pains may occur. Serious ocular involvement is common and can culminate in partial or complete blindness. Besides drugs, this syndrome has been associated with infections, pregnancy, foods, deep radiographic therapy, and neoplasms. Mortality is estimated to be in the range of 5% to 18%. The duration of the syndrome is usually 4 to 6 weeks. The long-acting sulfonamides are most often implicated. Allopurinol, carbamazepine, fluoroquinolones, hydantoin, phenylbutazone, and piroxicam are also possible causative agents.

Toxic Epidermal Necrolysis Syndrome

Epidermal necrolysis, a severe, life-threatening mucocutaneous and systemic reaction, may be preceded by a prodrome characterized by malaise, lethargy, fever, and occasionally throat or mucous membrane soreness. Epidermal changes follow and consist of erythema and massive bullae formations that easily rupture and peel, giving the skin a scalded appearance.

ONLINE CONTENT

For a photo of toxic epidermal necrolysis syndrome, go to http://thepoint.lww.com/AT10e.

Hairy parts of the body are usually not affected, but mucous membrane involvement is common. Blisters cover more than 30% of body surface area, with extensive epidermal detachment that can result in scarring. Approximately 30% of patients with TENS succumb, often within 8 days after bullae appear. The usual cause of death is infection complicated by massive fluid and electrolyte loss, similar to patients with extensive burns. Although the skin takes on a grave appearance, healing occurs within 2 weeks in approximately 70% of patients, with some potential for scarring. In addition to drugs, certain bacterial infections and foods are believed to cause this type of eruption. Most causes of TENS in children are owing to infection (e.g., *S. aureus*). A higher incidence of this type of drug eruption appears to occur in HIV-positive patients. Drugs most frequently implicated include allopurinol, aminopenicillins, carbamazepine, hydantoin, phenylbutazone, piroxicam, and sulfa drugs.

Erythema Nodosum

Erythema nodosum eruptions appear as red, indurated, inflammatory nodules on the shins and knees.

ONLINE CONTENT

For a photo of erythema nodosum, go to http://thepoint.lww.com/AT10e.

In addition to the unusual distribution, the lesions are tender when palpated. Occasionally, these lesions are accompanied by mild constitutional symptoms, but there is usually no mucous membrane involvement. Etiologic factors associated with the development of erythema nodosum include drugs, female sex, rheumatic fever, sarcoidosis, leprosy, certain bacterial infections (e.g., tuberculosis), and systemic fungal infections such as coccidioidomycosis. Usually, the lesions heal slowly over the course of several weeks after the offending agent is removed. Oral contraceptives are the most frequently implicated drug with this type of eruption. Other implicated drugs include sulfonamides and analgesics.

Drug Hypersensitivity Syndrome

This severe systemic reaction is also known as anticonvulsant hypersensitivity syndrome and as a drug reaction with eosinophilia and systemic symptoms (DRESS). Symptoms begin with a high fever followed by widespread maculopapular-pustular rash on the trunk, arms, and legs that may lead to exfoliative dermatitis with large areas of skin sloughing. Hair and nails are sometimes lost. Eosinophilia occurs in greater than 50% of cases, 30% have abnormal lymphocytosis, and 20% have lymphadenopathy. Internal organ damage appears late in the syndrome with elevations of liver function or renal function laboratory values. These may be accompanied by other general systemic symptoms such as headache and malaise. Secondary bacterial infections can occur. Approximately 10% of patients die, many because of infection. If exfoliative dermatitis occurs, it can take weeks or months to resolve, even after withdrawal of the offending agent. The most commonly implicated drugs are sulfonamides, antimalarials, anticonvulsants, and penicillin. Although rarely reported in the literature, its broad range of symptoms, confusing nomenclature, and symptom overlap with other drug-related adverse effects may lead to underdiagnosis and reporting.

Fixed Drug Eruptions

Fixed drug eruptions, unlike the previously mentioned reactions, are caused exclusively by drugs. The lesions are erythematous and sharply bordered, and have a tendency to be darker than the surrounding, unaffected skin. Eruptions can be eczematous, urticarial, vesicular, bullous, or nodular.

ONLINE CONTENT

For a photo of fixed drug eruption, go to http://thepoint.lww.com/AT10e.

Lesions appear 30 minutes to 8 hours after readministration in sensitized individuals. Because these lesions have a marked propensity to recur at the same location with each drug exposure, the word *fixed* is applied. The face and genitalia are common sites for this type of drug eruption. Although the eruptions heal after withdrawal of the causative drug, there is usually a marked hyperpigmentation of the area that may take months to resolve. The mechanism by which fixed drug eruptions occur has not been elucidated, but it is believed to be allergic in nature. It can be described figuratively as islands of hypersensitivity, with one area of the skin having the ability to evoke an allergic response and other areas lacking this ability. Commonly implicated drugs include antimicrobial agents (tetracycline, sulfonamides, metronidazole, nystatin), anti-inflammatory drugs (salicylates, nonsteroidal anti-inflammatory drugs), barbiturates, oral contraceptives, and phenolphthalein-containing laxatives.

Maculopapular Eruptions

Maculopapular eruptions are subdivided into two groups: scarlatiniform and morbilliform. Most drug eruptions fall within one of these two groups. *Scarlatiniform* eruptions are erythematous and usually involve extensive areas of the body. They are differentiated from streptococcal-induced scarlet fever by the lack of other diagnostic signs and laboratory studies. *Morbilliform* eruptions usually begin as discrete, reddish-brown maculae that may coalesce to form a diffuse rash. These eruptions are differentiated from measles by the lack of fever and other typical clinical signs. In either type of maculopapular eruption, pruritus may or may not be present. Generally, this type of eruption appears within 1 week after the causative drug (with penicillins, 2 or more weeks) has been started and completely clears within 7 to 14 days after stopping it. Morbilliform eruptions commonly are caused by ampicillin, amoxicillin, and allopurinol.

Urticaria

Urticarial eruptions are immediate hypersensitivity reactions (IgE-mediated) and usually appear as sharply circumscribed (raised), edematous, and erythematous lesions (wheals) with an abrupt onset.

ONLINE CONTENT

For a photo of urticaria, go to http://thepoint.lww.com/AT10e.

In most cases, individual lesions disappear within 24 hours and are replaced with new lesions elsewhere until the offending allergen is cleared from the body. Urticarial lesions are associated with an intense itching, stinging, or prickling sensation. Commonly called *hives*, urticarial eruptions are frequently associated with certain drugs, foods, psychic upsets, and serum sickness. Rarely, parasites or neoplasms can precipitate hives. The most frequently implicated drugs with this type of reaction are aspirin, penicillin, and blood products. Patients who exhibit urticaria attributable to a drug are at increased risk of anaphylaxis if re-exposed to the same medication in the future.

Angioneurotic Edema

Angioneurotic edema (also called angioedema) is a more severe form of urticaria in which giant hives penetrate more deeply into surrounding tissues.

ONLINE CONTENT

For a photo of angioedema, go to http://thepoint.lww.com/AT10e.

Lips, mouth, tongue, and eyelids are common locations. Extensive involvement of the tongue, throat, or larynx can be fatal.

Angiotensin-converting enzyme inhibitors (ACEIs) are the most common drug cause of angioedema. Patients taking ACEIs should be warned to look out for any unusual swelling in the facial or oral area and, if present, should go immediately to the nearest emergency room for treatment. Although it usually occurs within the first several months of treatment, cases have been reported up to as long as 3 years after initiation of ACEI therapy (see Chapter 19, Heart Failure).

CASE 39-5

QUESTION 1: D.Z., a 42-year-old man with a chronic seizure disorder and long-standing anxiety, was recently given a prescription for penicillin V 250 mg four times daily for a group A, α-hemolytic streptococcal-positive pharyngitis. Chronic medications include carbamazepine 200 mg three times daily and clonazepam 2 mg twice daily. One week later, D.Z. presents with urticarial lesions on his chest and arms. Is this a typical time of onset for a drug-induced dermatologic reaction? How should the drug eruption in D.Z. be managed?

Although most drug eruptions occur within 1 to 2 weeks after starting therapy, it may take 3 to 4 weeks after an initial exposure to a medication for the reaction to occur. Repeated exposure to the same offending agent can reduce the time of onset of the reaction to a few days or even within hours of ingestion. Because D.Z. has been taking clonazepam and carbamazepine chronically and penicillin for only 8 days, the temporal relationship would logically lead to the conclusion that penicillin is a highly probable cause. Almost all cases of urticaria are associated with extensive eosinophilia; however, it is not specific for any particular antigen. However, before labeling penicillin as the cause of his drug eruption, a thorough history to rule out other common nondrug causes should be taken.

For D.Z., a different antibiotic should be substituted for penicillin (to complete the 10-day course of therapy). The individual lesions should begin to clear in 24 hours of eruption (if the penicillin is the cause of the urticaria). If the urticaria does not begin to clear in a few days, another cause should be investigated.

Treatment is primarily supportive, and use of an oral antihistamine (e.g., diphenhydramine 25–50 mg four times daily) for several days would be recommended. If the reaction is severe, a 1- to 2-week course of prednisone 40 to 60 mg/day will control most symptoms within 48 hours.

ALLERGIC CONTACT DERMATITIS: POISON IVY, POISON OAK, OR POISON SUMAC

Poison ivy (*Rhus*) dermatitis is the major cause of allergic contact dermatitis in the United States, exceeding all other causes combined. It is estimated that 50% to 95% of the population is sensitive to the plant to some degree. The severity of the condition varies from mild discomfort to an extremely painful, debilitating condition. *Rhus* dermatitis is caused by sensitization to an allergic substance in the leaves, stems, and roots of poison ivy, poison oak, and poison sumac plants. All three plants contain the same sensitizing oleoresin, urushiol oil, which contains pentadecacatechol, the actual sensitizing agent. Therefore, the dermatitis caused by the three different plants is identical.

Direct contact with the plant is unnecessary for the rash to occur. Highly sensitive persons may develop severe dermatitis merely from exposure to *Rhus* oleoresin carried by pollen or by smoke from burning leaves. The oleoresin may remain active for months on clothing, shoes, tools, and sporting equipment. Once the toxic substance comes in contact with the skin, it can be spread by the hands to other areas of the body (e.g., genitals or eyes) or to people who may come into close contact with the exposed person. Although washing with soap and water will not prevent the dermatitis, even if it is done within 15 minutes of exposure, it will prevent spread of the oleoresin to other parts of the body.

Rhus dermatitis can be contracted throughout the year, even in winter, by contact with the roots of the plant. The virulence of the leaf sap varies little during the foliage period. The incidence of poison ivy is higher during the spring because the leaves are tender and bruise easily, and people spend more time outdoors. Sensitive individuals should be instructed to avoid contact with the offending plant. If contact is inevitable, every effort should be made to shield exposed areas of the skin with appropriate clothing, and bentoquatam (Ivy Block), a topical organoclay compound, should be considered. A 5% lotion applied to the skin 15 minutes before exposure and reapplied every 4 hours has reduced or prevented contact dermatitis induced by experimental challenge with urushiol in sensitive individuals. Cost may limit its routine use.

Exposed individuals should bathe or shower as soon as they come in from outdoors and should wash their clothes. A nonprescription topical cleanser called Tecnu Extreme claims to remove urushiol oil embedded in the skin through the action of microfine scrubbing beads and surfactants, thus possibly preventing the rash or limiting spread. It also contains the homeopathic agent grindelia as an antipruritic. It is formulated as a thick, creamy gel that is applied to exposed areas of the skin, followed by vigorous scrubbing, and rinsed off after application.

After an initial incubation period of 5 to 21 days, a patient would be expected to react to the oleoresin in 12 to 48 hours after re-exposure. A mild exposure to these plants in a sensitized person results in a typical erythematous, vesicular, linear, and sometimes, oozing rash after 2 to 3 days; complete clearing occurs in 1 to 3 weeks.

ONLINE CONTENT

For a photo of allergic contact dermatitis, go to http://thepoint.lww.com/AT10e.

If a large area is exposed, lesions appear within 6 to 12 hours and may appear blistered and eroded; in some cases, ulcers may appear. Healing occurs more slowly, often requiring 2 to 3 weeks for complete resolution. The following factors contribute to the development of poison ivy, poison oak, or poison sumac dermatitis: the concentration of the oleoresin to which the skin is exposed, area of exposure (i.e., the thickness of the stratum corneum), duration of exposure, site of exposure, genetic factors, and immune tolerance. It is important to determine the areas of the body that are affected. If the eyes, genital areas, mouth, respiratory tract, or more than 15% of the body is affected, the patient should receive a course of systemic corticosteroids.

Because different sites of the body differ in their sensitivity to the oleoresin and because patients spread the *Rhus* oleoresin to different parts of their bodies over time, lesions often erupt for a period of several days. A common misconception many people have is that the fluid from the *Rhus*-induced vesicles will spread the disease to unaffected areas. A more likely explanation is the presence of residual resin underneath poorly washed fingernails, soiled clothes (including gloves used in yard work), and pet fur.

Treatment

CASE 39-6

QUESTION 1: K.P., a 27-year-old woman, has recently returned from an outing in the woods. She now has vesicular eruptions that appear in a linear pattern on one arm and hand. She believes that she has had a poison oak reaction and requests therapy. What should be recommended at this point? What should be recommended if the condition becomes more severe?

Weeping lesions should be treated with aqueous vehicles (e.g., Burow solution or saline) as outlined in the beginning of this chapter. Lesions that are not wet or weeping should be treated with calamine lotion applied two to four times daily. The zinc oxide in calamine lotion may act as a mild astringent, although some people find this preparation to be unacceptable because of its pink color, which can stain clothes. Alternatively, a topical corticosteroid appropriate for the body part affected could be used. If K.P.'s poison oak reaction becomes more severe, additional treatment with prednisone 1 mg/kg/day for at least 2 or 3 weeks will be required; such therapy should be withdrawn slowly (1–2 weeks) to prevent recurrence of the lesions.

SYSTEMIC THERAPY

CASE 39-7

QUESTION 1: Z.T., a 19-year-old man, has just returned from a fishing trip and now has an erythematous, linear, dry eruption on his leg and arm, and a generalized eruption on his hands and face. He has been in areas that have dense poison ivy growth, and he may have burned some in the campfire. Z.T. has washed himself and his clothes thoroughly. How should he be treated?

The fact that Z.T.'s facial rash is not linear (as one would expect if he had just contacted the plant) suggests that he may have contacted the smoke of a burning poison ivy plant. This can be quite serious because the oleoresin can be carried in smoke and, if inhaled, can cause severe respiratory problems. Z.T. should be observed for signs of respiratory difficulties and should be treated with a course of systemic corticosteroids.

RELAPSE

CASE 39-7, QUESTION 2: Z.T.'s physician prescribed prednisone for his rash. He was instructed to take 80 mg/day for 14 days and to decrease the dose by 5 mg/day each day thereafter. Calamine lotion (three times daily to affected areas) also was prescribed. After 12 days, Z.T. complains that the lesions seem to be getting worse. The lesions had cleared after 8 days of treatment, and he began rapidly tapering the prednisone at that time. Why is he experiencing a relapse?

Two weeks is the minimum course of treatment when systemic corticosteroids are used for severe cases of poison ivy, poison oak, or poison sumac. The oleoresin remains fixed in the skin, and if the systemic corticosteroid is withdrawn too soon, the lesions return. This is probably the most common reason for treatment failure with systemic corticosteroids. Alternatively, systemic corticosteroids can be discontinued before 2 weeks of treatment and a moderate-potency topical hydrocortisone preparation can be started 24 hours before discontinuation of systemic corticosteroids to prevent relapse.

Drug-Induced Allergic Contact Dermatitis

CASE 39-7, QUESTION 3: Z.T.'s corticosteroid therapy was reinstated. After 3 weeks, most of the lesions had disappeared, and the prednisone therapy was discontinued. However, Z.T. continued to complain of a rash on his hands. Further questioning revealed that he was continuing to apply an over-the-counter topical calamine lotion containing diphenhydramine. What is a potential drug-related cause of this persistent rash?

Topical application of diphenhydramine and other antihistamines may cause allergic contact dermatitis.[23] Z.T. should stop using this product to see whether his rash clears. A list of common contact sensitizers is found in Table 39-14.

The treatment for sensitivity reactions is basically the same as that outlined for poison ivy, poison oak, or poison sumac.

KEY REFERENCES AND WEBSITES

A full list of references for this chapter can be found at **http://thepoint.lww.com/AT10e.** Below are the key references for this chapter, with the corresponding reference number in this chapter found in parentheses after the reference.

Key References

Arndt KA, Hsu JHS. *Manual of Dermatologic Therapies: With Essentials of Diagnosis*. 7th ed. Philadelphia, PA: Lippincott Williams & Wilkins; 2006. (7)

Buddenkotte J, Steinhoff M. Pathophysiology and therapy of pruritus in allergic and atopic diseases. *Allergy*. 2010;65:805.

Carbone A et al. Pediatric atopic dermatitis: a review of the medical literature. *Ann Pharmacother*. 2010;44:1448.

Darsaw U et al. ETFAD/EADV eczema task force 2009 position paper on diagnosis and treatment of atopic dermatitis. *J Eur Acad Dermatol Venereol*. 2010;24:317. (27)

Freedberg IM et al, eds. *Fitzpatrick's Dermatology in General Medicine*. 6th ed. New York, NY: McGraw-Hill; 2003. (5)

Lee NP, Arriola ER. Topical corticosteroids: back to basics. *West J Med*. 1999;171:351. (9)

James WD et al, eds. *Andrews' Diseases of the Skin: Clinical Dermatology.* 11th ed. Philadelphia, PA: WB Saunders; 2011. (3)

Pracash AV, Davis MDP. Contact dermatitis in older adults: a review of the literature. *Am J Clin Dermatol*. 2010;11:373.

Tadicherla S et al. Topical corticosteroids in dermatology. *J Drugs Dermatol*. 2009;8:1093.

Wasserbauer N, Ballow M. Atopic dermatitis. *Am J Med*. 2009; 122:121.

40 Acne

Ellen R. DeGrasse and Jamie J. Cavanaugh

CORE PRINCIPLES

		CHAPTER CASES
1	Acne vulgaris is a condition in which androgen-mediated excess sebum production leads to inflammatory changes and abnormal desquamation of keratinocytes lining the pilosebaceous units of the skin, plugging and distending the pores. *Propionibacterium acnes* overgrowth also contributes to inflammation. Uninflamed clogged pores, or comedones, become pustules, papules, or nodules depending on the depth and extent of inflammation.	**Case 40-1 (Question 1), Case 40-2 (Question 1), Case 40-3 (Question 1), Case 40-4 (Question 1)**
2	Usually beginning during adolescence, acne persists for years and cannot be cured, only controlled. After a drug regimen achieves control, treatment must continue with a maintenance regimen, usually less intense, for months to years. Early, aggressive therapy prevents scarring and psychosocial sequelae.	**Case 40-1 (Questions 1, 7), Case 40-2 (Question 3)**
3	Acne severity relates to the number and severity of lesions.	**Case 40-1 (Question 1), Case 40-2 (Question 1), Case 40-3 (Question 1)**
4	Drug therapies work by reducing sebum production, normalizing keratinization in the pilosebaceous units, reducing *P. acnes*, or reducing inflammation.	**Case 40-1 (Question 2), Case 40-2 (Question 1), Case 40-3 (Question 1)**
5	Patients must be counseled that pharmacotherapy works best to prevent future lesions, not to resolve current ones. Therefore, they must apply topical therapies regularly to the entire acne-prone area(s), not just to lesions, and expect to wait weeks to months, depending on the therapy, to see the full treatment effect.	**Case 40-1 (Questions 5, 7), Case 40-2 (Question 3)**
6	Appropriate choice of vehicle ensures efficacy and tolerability of topical therapy. Noncomedogenic moisturizers are important adjuncts because many topical acne agents can dry and irritate. Moisturizers may also contain the sunscreen patients must use with the majority of acne therapies. Excessive irritation can aggravate problems with postinflammatory hyperpigmentation, a problem increasingly common the darker a patient's skin color.	**Case 40-1 (Questions 5, 7), Case 40-4 (Question 1)**
7	Topical retinoids are first-line monotherapy for mild acne in guidelines, although benzoyl peroxide is a popular alternative because it is inexpensive and available over-the-counter. Topical retinoids are also key components of combination therapies in more severe acne, and preferred agents to continue for maintenance therapy once acne is under control.	**Case 40-1 (Questions 2–5, 7), Case 40-2 (Questions 1, 3), Case 40-4 (Question 1)**
8	Initial treatment of moderate acne calls for a topical retinoid in combination with antibiotics. Topical or oral antibiotics are chosen based on the severity and distribution of lesions. Benzoyl peroxide may also be included to minimize the development of antibiotic resistance. Antibiotic duration should be limited to the period needed to obtain control of acne; then the retinoid, with or without benzoyl peroxide, is continued as maintenance therapy.	**Case 40-1 (Question 7), Case 40-2**

continued

CHAPTER CASES

9	Antiandrogenic therapies, such as combined oral contraceptives or spironolactone, are useful alternatives in nonpregnant women.	Case 40-2 (Question 1)
10	Severe acne, or treatment-resistant moderate acne, warrants oral isotretinoin monotherapy. Extremely effective, isotretinoin can induce lengthy remission of acne, but its adverse effect profile and need for laboratory monitoring preclude its use in milder acne. The iPLEDGE risk-management program controls isotretinoin distribution to prevent accidental prescription of this severe teratogen to pregnant women.	Case 40-3

Definition and Epidemiology

The term *acne* usually refers to acne vulgaris, a condition in which the pilosebaceous units of the skin become plugged and distended. Acne vulgaris is characterized by chronic inflammatory dermatosis, appearing as comedones and inflammatory lesions such as papules, pustules, or nodules.[1] Comedones, plugged follicular openings, are noninflammatory lesions that may be closed ("whiteheads") or open ("blackheads").[2,3]

ONLINE CONTENT

For photos of acne lesions (closed comedones, open comedones, papules and pustules, and nodules), go to http://thepoint.lww.com/AT10e.

Inflammatory lesions are typically erythematous and can include papules (raised, solid lesions up to several millimeters in diameter), pustules (raised, superficial, pus-filled lesions), and nodules (like papules but larger and deeper in the skin). In severe cases (acne conglobata), multiple lesions coalesce into abscesses with draining sinus tracts. Acne lesions generally appear on the face, but the chest, back, or upper arms may also be affected. Unless otherwise stated, all references to acne in this chapter refer to acne vulgaris.

Acne affects more than 50 million people in the United States,[4] including greater than 90% of all adolescents.[5] Although it occurs in people of all ages, it primarily afflicts teenagers and young adults. Acne often begins when sebaceous gland activity increases in association with puberty. Accordingly, the age of onset of acne, like that of puberty, has decreased during the last several years and is now seen as early as age 8 to 9.[6,7] Although acne affects both sexes equally, females typically develop acne at a younger age and have milder cases than males.[8] Most cases resolve by the mid-20s, but acne persists into later life in 7% to 17% of patients, more often in women than in men.[8] Acne may be slightly less common in people with darker skin, but prevalence research may be confounded by poorer access to health care among people of color; most studies find that acne is the top dermatologic complaint in patients of all skin tones.[9] Severe nodular acne is more common in light-skinned individuals, but those with dark skin show more inflammation at the histologic level than light-skinned people with similar clinical lesion severity. Dark-skinned individuals are also more likely to contend with postinflammatory hyperpigmentation and keloid scar formation in the wake of acne lesions.[9,10]

Ample treatment information resources are available for individuals with acne. Tables 40-1 and 40-2 provide a list of valuable acne websites and organizational contact information.

TABLE 40-1
Patient Information Resources

Medline Plus Acne website. Available at: http://www.nlm.nih.gov/medlineplus/acne.html
Mayo Clinic Acne website. Available at: http://www.mayoclinic.com/health/acne/DS00169
Nemours Foundation Acne website. Available at: http://kidshealth.org/kid/grow/body_stuff/acne.html
U.S. Food and Drug Administration Acne website. Available at: http://www.fda.gov/ForConsumers/ConsumerUpdates/ucm174521.htm

Pathophysiology

Studies suggest that acne is primarily an inherited disorder with environmental factors playing a secondary role.[11] Acne results when increased sebum production causes inflammatory changes in pilosebaceous follicles and changes in their bacterial colonization.

TABLE 40-2
Acne Professional Organizations

American Academy of Dermatology P.O. Box 4014 Schaumburg, IL 60168 (866) 503-SKIN Website: http://www.aad.org/
American Skin Association 346 Park Avenue South, 4th Floor New York, NY 10010 (800) 499-SKIN Website:http://www.americanskin.org
American Society for Dermatologic Surgery 5550 Meadowbrook Drive, Suite 120 Rolling Meadows, IL 60008 (847) 956-0900 Website: http://www.asds.net/
National Institute of Arthritis and Musculoskeletal and Skin Diseases (NIAMS) 1 AMS Circle Bethesda, MD20892–3675 (877) 22-NIAMS Website: http://www.niams.nih.gov/
American Academy of Family Physicians P.O. Box 11210 Shawnee Mission, KS 66207–1210 (800) 274-2237 Website: http://www.aafp.org/

For a diagram of comedogenesis, go to http://thepoint.lww.com/AT10e.

Androgens such as dehydroepiandrosterone sulfate (DHEAS) are metabolized in the skin to dihydrotestosterone (DHT), which in turn stimulates sebum biosynthesis. DHEAS levels rise before puberty and begin to decline in early adulthood.[12] Increased sebum production dilutes the availability of linoleic acid and increases the production of interleukin 1-α.[13,14] Keratinocytes in the follicular epithelial lining respond by proliferating and undergoing changes in cellular differentiation. Keratinization of the follicular lining increases, which in turn increases cell-to-cell adhesion, interfering with normal desquamation. Cellular debris and sebum accumulate to plug sebaceous follicles and form clinically undetectable microcomedones.

If the superficial portion of the follicular opening dilates from the pressure of the impaction, an open comedo ("blackhead") forms. The dark color of open comedones is caused by light refraction, not dirt; comedo contents are white when expressed.[14] Such lesions rarely become further inflamed because as pressure builds from further sebum production and cellular accumulation, follicular contents can escape to the skin surface.[13] If the follicular opening remains narrow and a closed comedo ("whitehead") forms, increased pressure can rupture the follicular wall, with infiltration of foreign matter into the dermis inciting a marked local inflammatory response. The depth and extent of this occurrence determine whether a papule, pustule, or nodule results.[15]

Increased sebum production also creates a lipid-rich, microaerobic environment favorable to *Propionibacterium acnes.* This gram-positive rod stimulates upregulation of cytokines and releases proteases, hyaluronidases, lipases, and chemotactic factors that attract neutrophils, T-cells, and macrophages.[16] Hydrolytic enzymes released by macrophages may contribute to weakening of the follicular wall, hastening rupture and the resulting progression of comedo to inflammatory lesion.[13] Inflammatory mediators traverse the follicular wall into the dermis and intensify the inflammatory process even before wall rupture.[8]

Clinical Presentation and Assessment

The differential diagnosis of acneiform eruptions includes (a) acne vulgaris; (b) rosacea; (c) folliculitis caused by gram-negative bacteria, *Pityrosporum*, or mechanical irritation; (d) drug-induced acne (acne medicamentosa) such as that caused by topical or systemic corticosteroids, or by anabolic steroids; and (e) perioral dermatitis. Detailed discussions of severe acne variants, such as acne conglobata and acne fulminans, are beyond the scope of this chapter.[8,15] In addition, acne may be secondary to systemic diseases such as SAPHO (synovitis, acne, pustulosis, hyperostosis, osteitis) and Apert syndromes.[17,18]

Table 40-3 lists factors potentially contributing to acne. The effects of sunlight and diet are controversial. Studies of sunlight exposure have found contradictory results; ultraviolet light may make sebum more comedogenic, but some of the visible wavelengths may reduce the follicular bacterial population.[19] As for diet, studies have investigated lower milk intake and lower glycemic load diets for potential benefit in acne,[23] but research on dietary modifications is not yet sufficiently robust to alter routine patient care.

Although no single severity scale has emerged as a standard, clinicians must use some acne grading scale consistently to evaluate treatment options and clinical response. Often, clinicians describe acne as mild (few lesions, little or no inflammation), moderate (many lesions, significant inflammation), or severe (numerous lesions, extreme inflammation, significant scarring; see Table 40-4).[24] Lesion counts per se are not practical for clinicians, but are used by researchers.

The major long-term complication of acne is scarring, often exacerbated by tissue excoriation caused by picking at or squeezing the lesions. Acne can also cause psychological distress, low self-esteem, and social withdrawal, affecting quality of life as much as more physically disabling diseases such as asthma and diabetes.[25]

TABLE 40-3
Potential Contributing Factors to Acne Vulgaris

Stress (in predisposed patients)[20]
Late luteal phase of menstrual cycle (premenstrual exacerbations)[8]
Hyperandrogenic states (e.g., polycystic ovary syndrome)[1]
Oil-based cosmetics, pomades, and moisturizers (acne cosmetica)[13]
Hot or humid conditions[11]
Ultraviolet light[19]
Environmental exposure to halogenated compounds, animal fats, dioxin, or petroleum derivatives[21]
Mechanical irritation from hats, chin straps, backpacks, or shoulder pads (acne mechanica)[13,22]

Overview of Therapy

No known cure exists for acne, but treatment can reduce its severity and minimize scarring. In most cases, especially in severe forms, treatment is individualized, depending on the particular clinical presentation of the patient. The goals of treatment are to relieve discomfort, improve skin appearance, prevent scarring, and minimize the psychosocial impact of the condition.

Treatment is largely preventive because little can be done for existing lesions. Slow improvement over the course of weeks to months is the rule for all treatments. Patients can generally expect 20%, 60%, and 80% resolution of lesions within 2, 6, and 8 months, respectively, after starting effective therapy (slower resolution with hormonal therapies, faster resolution with oral isotretinoin).[8] Therefore, treatment regimens should not be modified more often than every 6 to 8 weeks. Patients should be counseled on the basic pathophysiology of acne, proper drug administration or application technique, delay in onset of therapeutic effect, potential adverse effects, and steps to take if adverse effects occur. Clinical practice guidelines are available.[1,20,26]

TABLE 40-4
Acne Severity

Mild	Comedones with or without a few or several pustules or papules
Moderate	Comedones, several pustules or papules, with or without a few or several nodules
Severe	Numerous or extensive pustules or papules and many nodules; can include cases with persistent nodules, extensive scarring, drainage, or formation of sinus tracts
Very severe	Acne variants such as acne conglobata or acne fulminans

Source: Rigopoulos D et al. The role of isotretinoin in acne therapy: why not as first-line therapy? Facts and controversies. *Clin Dermatol.* 2010;28:24.

NONDRUG THERAPY

Nondrug therapy plays a minimal role in the management of acne. In general, patient education regarding nondrug therapy amounts to "first, do no harm." Twice-daily washing with warm water and a mild facial cleanser suffices; poor hygiene does not cause acne, and aggressive skin washing and abrasive cleansers needlessly traumatize the skin.[8] To minimize scarring, patients must resist squeezing or picking at acne lesions. Drugs known to cause acne, oil-based cosmetics, and other known precipitants should also obviously be avoided. Oil-free, noncomedogenic moisturizers formulated for facial skin can improve the penetration and tolerability of many topical acne drugs by improving the skin's hydration, especially in patients with sensitive skin. Many such moisturizers also contain sunscreen, which is recommended for use with many of the available acne therapies.[4]

Dermatologists may use procedures such as surgical comedo extraction, chemical peels, and microdermabrasion as adjunct therapy to improve cosmetic appearance. Current guidelines recommend drug therapy over light and laser therapies because of less stringent clinical testing for devices versus drugs, concern about long-term effects of therapies aimed at sebaceous gland function, and the inadequate research done on light and laser therapies to date.[20] Acne scarring is treated with various microsurgical techniques, dermabrasion, laser therapy, chemical peels, and tissue augmentation.[27]

DRUG THERAPY

Available drug therapies exhibit one or more of the following mechanisms: (a) normalizing follicular keratinization (e.g., retinoids, benzoyl peroxide to some degree, azelaic acid); (b) decreasing sebum production (e.g., isotretinoin, hormonal therapies); (c) suppressing *P. acnes* (e.g., antibiotics, benzoyl peroxide, azelaic acid, systemic isotretinoin); and (d) reducing inflammation (e.g., antibiotics, retinoids).

Topical therapy is generally preferable for mild to moderate acne. Guidelines emphasize using a retinoid as monotherapy for mild acne, initially augmented in moderate acne with a course of topical antibiotics.[26]

ONLINE CONTENT

For an evidence-based treatment algorithm, go to http://thepoint.lww.com/AT10e.

Treatments are applied to the entire acne-prone area, not just to existing lesions, as the available therapies are more effective at preventing future lesions than resolving existing lesions. With topical therapy, choice of vehicle is as important to treatment success as choice of drug. Gels and solutions are highly drying and suitable for oily skin, whereas less drying creams and moderately drying lotions are more suitable for dry or sensitive skin; ointments are generally too comedogenic owing to their occlusive effects to be useful in acne.

Moderate to severe acne often requires combination therapy using agents with different mechanisms of action, such as a topical retinoid plus a systemic antibiotic. Hormonal therapies (e.g., oral contraceptives) are an option in female patients who are not pregnant and not planning to become pregnant. Acne can be controlled but not cured, and patients should generally continue using maintenance therapy of a retinoid and possibly benzoyl peroxide after control is achieved. The most effective option for severe acne is oral isotretinoin. Because oral isotretinoin addresses every known pathophysiologic mechanism of acne, combining it with other medications is unnecessary.

CLINICAL ASSESSMENT

Mild Acne

CASE 40-1

QUESTION 1: L.Y., a fair-skinned, 15-year-old, Caucasian girl asks a pharmacist the best way to treat "zits." The problem began when she was 13 and has progressively worsened. At first, lesions occasionally appeared on her chin and forehead; now she consistently has about two to four lesions, which have spread to her cheeks and nose. She is increasingly frustrated that "zits are now the rule and not the exception" and wants to see a dermatologist, but her mother insists acne "is just part of being a teen."

L.Y. uses a nonprescription 10% benzoyl peroxide gel as needed on lesions when her acne "gets really bad," but doesn't think it works very well. She tried a "medicated" soap in the past, but stopped because it dried out her skin. She would like to know whether any other nonprescription products work better than the ones she has tried.

L.Y. has no other medical problems and no known drug allergies and takes no chronic prescription medications. She has had normal menstrual periods since menarche at age 12. Both her older brothers have acne, one mild and one severe. L.Y. denies alcohol, tobacco, or illicit drug use. She has a boyfriend, but denies sexual intercourse. After school, she works part time at a fast-food restaurant, plays varsity tennis, and practices violin. She wears a sweatband around her head while playing tennis and uses a hair-styling gel.

Examination reveals one pustule on L.Y.'s forehead, three papules on her cheeks and chin (which are covered with makeup), a well-healing area on her nose, and no open comedones or nodules. Her skin is slightly oily. Her chest, back, and arms are clear. She has no facial hair, and her voice is normal in pitch.

What subjective and objective data support a diagnosis of acne vulgaris? What potentially contributing factors are present? What is your assessment of L.Y.'s acne?

The patient interview is an important component in gathering the necessary information to develop a treatment plan. Table 40-5 lists several historical components that should be addressed.

Through discussion with L.Y., the pharmacist was able to identify subjective evidence consistent with acne. L.Y.'s age puts her in the highest acne prevalence category. In addition, she first

TABLE 40-5
Pertinent Historical Components To Be Obtained from a Patient with Acne

- Duration, including onset and peak severity
- Location and distribution
- Seasonal variation
- For female patients, relation to menstrual periods, pregnancy status, scalp hair thinning, contraceptive method (if used)
- Present and past treatments, topical and systemic, prescription and over-the-counter
- Family history, including severity
- Other skin disorders or medical problems
- Medications and drug allergies
- Occupational exposure to chemicals or oils
- Skin care routine; use of cosmetics, moisturizers, hairstyling products (pomades)
- Areas of skin friction or irritation

experienced acne with the onset of puberty, as is usually the case. Her positive family history and the fact that her condition has waxed and waned, but progressively worsened, are also consistent with acne. The types of lesions and the facial distribution of lesions, while sparing most other areas, provide objective evidence.

Several potentially contributing factors are present. L.Y. may be experiencing mechanical irritation caused by sweatband use and the violin chin rest. Sweating while playing tennis may create humid conditions promoting follicular occlusion. In addition, her occupational exposure to oils may be comedogenic. The pharmacist also noted that L.Y. covers lesions using makeup that may be oil-based and thereby comedogenic. Finally, L.Y.'s use of hair gel may be contributory.

As noted in the pathophysiology discussion, androgens play an important role in acne development. Clinicians should be cognizant of signs and symptoms that may indicate that a patient has a hyperandrogenic state. Potential signs in prepubertal individuals include genital or axillary hair growth, early onset body odor, and accelerated growth. Signs in individuals after puberty include male or female pattern baldness, hirsutism, irregular menses, infertility, and polycystic ovaries.[1] L.Y. did not report any past medical history or signs that indicate a hyperandrogenic state. If the pharmacist had identified a potential sign of elevated androgens, L.Y. would require referral to a physician.

The psychosocial impact of acne on L.Y.'s quality of life is finally significant enough to spur her to discuss her problem with a health care provider, although her mother does not appreciate how much acne bothers L.Y. Such dismissal is, sadly, common. Assessment must draw on the patient's perception rather than the clinician's perception of the severity of the problem, because considerable psychological morbidity can result from even mild to moderate acne.[28] Although not necessary for L.Y., questionnaires are available to measure the psychosocial impact of acne.[29]

L.Y.'s acne should be classified as mild because she has relatively few lesions, which are limited to her face.

DRUG THERAPY

CASE 40-1, QUESTION 2: What are the treatment options for L.Y.'s mild acne?

Topical therapy is considered first-line treatment for mild acne. Topical options appropriate for mild acne include retinoids, benzoyl peroxide, azelaic acid, salicylic acid, and sulfur.

TOPICAL RETINOIDS

Retinoids, analogs of vitamin A, normalize keratinization by decreasing horny cell cohesiveness and stimulating epidermal cell turnover. These actions combine to unplug follicles and prevent microcomedo formation. Retinoids also reduce inflammation by inhibiting the production of inflammatory mediators. Topical retinoids have no antibacterial properties.[14]

As the most potent comedolytic agents, topical retinoids are preferred therapy in mild acne cases with mostly noninflammatory lesions.[26] They are also a core component of combination therapies for moderate to severe acne, and first-line treatment to maintain remission of acne once it is controlled. They are usually applied once daily; bedtime administration is standard because older formulations rapidly degrade in ultraviolet light.[30] Common adverse effects include skin irritation, peeling, erythema, and dryness.[31] Patients must use a sunscreen because the newly exfoliated skin burns easily.[30] Concomitant use of a gentle moisturizing cream with sunscreen may increase patient adherence by relieving skin irritation secondary to retinoid use and providing photosensitivity protection. Patients should recognize that acne may initially worsen during therapy,[30] although this rarely occurs if topical antibiotics are also being used.[32]

Tretinoin (e.g., Retin-A), or all-*trans*-retinoic acid, is the naturally occurring form of vitamin A acid. Creams are available in concentrations ranging from 0.02% to 0.1% and gels in concentrations ranging from 0.01% to 0.1%. Newer dosage forms, delayed-release cream and gel (0.03%; Avita) and microsphere gel (0.04%, 0.1%; Retin-A Micro), are less irritating but more expensive. Another topical retinoid, adapalene (0.1% cream, lotion, gel; 0.3% gel; Differin), is a well-tolerated alternative that binds to different receptors than tretinoin and has more anti-inflammatory activity.[33] Adapalene 0.1% gel seems as effective as, yet better tolerated than, tretinoin 0.025% gel or 0.05% cream; tretinoin 0.05% gel may be more effective but also less well tolerated.[31] Irritation from topical tretinoin can darken skin if used too aggressively in dark-skinned patients, but adapalene may reduce hyperpigmentation in such patients.[34] Tazarotene (0.05% or 0.1%; cream or gel; Tazorac), meanwhile, is an effective, but perhaps less well tolerated, agent in this class.[31]

Among the topical retinoids, adapalene and the older dosage forms of tretinoin are available generically. Topical isotretinoin is not yet available in the United States. Benzoyl peroxide inactivates some formulations of tretinoin, so they should not be used together, or should at least be applied at different times (morning and evening, respectively).[30] However, benzoyl peroxide can be used in combination with either adapalene or tazarotene to provide additive benefit. Two fixed-dose combination products (0.1% adapalene/2.5% benzoyl peroxide gel, Epiduo, and 0.025% tretinoin/1.2% clindamycin gel, Ziana) are available to boost adherence when combination therapy is appropriate. Although some data suggest percutaneous absorption of tretinoin and adapalene is inconsequential,[31] tazarotene is pregnancy category X (contraindicated in pregnancy), and all topical retinoids should be avoided during pregnancy because systemic agents are so notoriously teratogenic and alternative acne therapies have better-characterized pregnancy risk potential.

BENZOYL PEROXIDE

Topical benzoyl peroxide primarily works as an antibacterial, but can also relieve comedones by exfoliating and opening pores through keratolytic activity. The lipophilic nature of benzoyl peroxide allows it to penetrate to the site of *P. acnes* growth and release oxygen free radicals that damage bacterial cell walls.[35] Because resistance cannot develop to this bactericidal mechanism, benzoyl peroxide is often paired with antibiotics to prevent the development of antibiotic resistance. The irritant effects of benzoyl peroxide also cause vasodilation and increase blood flow, which may hasten resolution of inflammatory lesions.

Benzoyl peroxide is available over the counter and by prescription in a variety of dosage forms (cleansers, lotions, creams, gels, foams, pledgets) and concentrations (2.5%–10%). Combination products exist with adapalene, erythromycin, clindamycin, salicylic acid, and sulfur. It is usually applied to the affected area once or twice daily. Cleansers allow less contact time compared with other dosage forms, but they can enhance adherence to therapy when patients must apply medication to the trunk, because cleansers are easy to apply and leave on for a few minutes in the shower.

The possibility that benzoyl peroxide may be a carcinogen has been widely debated in previous years. A Food and Drug Administration (FDA) review of new benzoyl peroxide animal studies concluded that benzoyl peroxide is not a carcinogen.[36]

AZELAIC ACID

Azelaic acid 20% cream (Azelex) carries an indication for acne vulgaris, whereas the 15% gel (Finacea) formulation is indicated for rosacea. This dicarboxylic acid normalizes keratinization and also reduces inflammation by suppressing *P. acnes*.[37] *P. acnes* resistance has not been reported.[38]

Azelaic acid causes less skin irritation than other topical therapies (except for antibiotics), but may not be as effective.[1,3] In addition to being less irritating than other comedolytic therapies, azelaic acid inhibits tyrosinase and thereby melanin production, giving it a useful niche in treating patients of color with postinflammatory hyperpigmentation.[39] A small amount of azelaic acid cream is applied twice daily. Because of its cost and possibly lower efficacy, it is usually reserved for patients who cannot tolerate benzoyl peroxide or topical retinoids.

MISCELLANEOUS TOPICAL AGENTS

Salicylic acid, sulfur, and resorcinol have been used for decades in the treatment of acne, but are not well studied. Topical salicylic acid, a concentration-dependent keratolytic, is more effective than placebo, but less effective than topical benzoyl peroxide or tretinoin.[1] It may be useful in patients with mild acne who cannot tolerate other comedolytics and may augment the effectiveness of other agents when used in combination. It is available in nonprescription creams, lotions, and gels in strengths ranging from 0.5% to 2% (higher strength products are intended for other uses, such as wart removal). Chronic use over large body surfaces increases the risk of percutaneous absorption that could lead to systemic salicylate toxicity.[40] Sulfur preparations have mild comedolytic properties, but can produce skin discoloration and odor, and may be comedogenic with continued use.[11] Anecdotally, however, sulfur products succeed for some patients who have failed first-line therapies. They are available in strengths of 2% to 10%, in a variety of vehicles, often in combination products with resorcinol or benzoyl peroxide. Resorcinol alone is ineffective,[8] but is combined in a 2% concentration with sulfur preparations to enhance the keratolytic effect. It can cause dark scaling on some patients.[11] Topical nicotinamide, a form of vitamin B_3, appears to be as effective as 1% clindamycin gel monotherapy in treating inflammatory acne, but is often unavailable in the United States.[8]

CASE 40-1, QUESTION 3: Is L.Y.'s current acne medication appropriate?

L.Y.'s current antiacne regimen is suboptimal, which explains her progressively worsening course. Benzoyl peroxide is excellent for mild to moderate inflammatory acne, but the product is failing to control L.Y.'s acne because she applies it infrequently to existing lesions only. Routine use over the entire susceptible area is required for long-term acne control.

CASE 40-1, QUESTION 4: What factors may impact the choice of therapy for L.Y.?

Guidelines favor initiating therapy with topical retinoids, because they best attack comedogenesis, the core pathology of acne. However, as a practical matter, L.Y. faces difficulty obtaining a prescriber visit for her acne, and a retinoid prescription is likely to be relatively expensive and possibly not covered by her health care insurance. Benzoyl peroxide, readily and cheaply available, is an adequate alternative for mild acne because it has modest keratolytic properties and reduces bacterial inflammation. Azelaic acid is more expensive and should be reserved for patients who cannot tolerate other comedolytic topical therapies. Antibiotics and oral isotretinoin are not warranted in mild acne. Combination oral contraceptives would have been a reasonable alternative choice if L.Y. were sexually active or had menstrual abnormalities, and she were willing to wait longer for onset of effect.

CASE 40-1, QUESTION 5: Provide L.Y. with a treatment recommendation for benzoyl peroxide. How can L.Y. reduce the risk of developing skin irritation and dryness? What other counseling is appropriate for this product?

Topical application of benzoyl peroxide may cause transient warmth or stinging, significant drying, or skin irritation. Factors that worsen skin irritation include increased benzoyl peroxide concentration and contact time, gels or nonhydrophilic vehicles, thin and sensitive skin, low environmental humidity, use of irritating adjunctive therapies, and increased application frequency.[41] Ideally, patients begin with benzoyl peroxide products in a less drying vehicle (cream) and at lower strength (2.5%) to minimize the risk of intolerable skin irritation while still achieving the desired therapeutic effect. The 2.5% and 5% concentrations are less irritating than the 10% concentration and equally effective overall.[41] Unfortunately, 2.5% concentrations are less frequently stocked in community pharmacies. L.Y. tolerated the 10% gel when she was using it sporadically, so she may be able to use nonprescription products successfully.

Recommend L.Y. apply a 2.5% to 5% cream or gel product every other day for the first week or two, and then advance to daily application as tolerated. L.Y. should use the product regularly over her entire face (avoiding eyes and mucous membranes), and wait several weeks before judging its effectiveness. She should apply the product at bedtime, ideally 30 minutes after washing her face with a mild cleanser, and wash it off in the morning (or after several hours, if excessive skin dryness or peeling occurs). She should be reminded of the product's potential to bleach fabrics.

To minimize skin irritation, L.Y. should avoid medicated cleansers. Oil-free moisturizer increases skin hydration and comfort, and can perform double duty if it also contains sunscreen. Patients using benzoyl peroxide should use a sunscreen every day that blocks ultraviolet (UV) light in both A and B wavelengths and that provides a sun protection factor (SPF) of at least 15. (See Chapter 42, Ultraviolet Radiation Exposure, Photoaging, and Burn Injuries, for a more detailed discussion of sunscreens.) If L.Y. is applying benzoyl peroxide in the morning, she should apply it before applying the moisturizer with sunscreen.

CASE 40-1, QUESTION 6: Two months later, L.Y. returns to the pharmacy. She has been using a benzoyl peroxide 5% gel daily. It has helped some, but she still has frequent breakouts. About a week ago, she began noticing significant redness and itching on her face. She denies any changes in sun exposure or skin care routine. She stopped using the medication until last night, when the irritation had almost resolved. Last night, she attempted to resume benzoyl peroxide therapy. Within 10 minutes after applying a small amount of gel, her skin reddened, and began to burn and itch. She immediately washed the area well with cool, soapy water, but the skin irritation prevented her from getting a good night's sleep. The area is better this morning, but remains red and itchy. Is this a typical adverse reaction to benzoyl peroxide?

In L.Y.'s case, sun exposure or dryness from a change in skin cleanser did not appear to provoke the skin reaction, so it is unlikely caused by benzoyl peroxide's direct irritating effects. The intense itching and burning after rechallenge is more consistent with an allergic-type contact dermatitis, which occurs in up to 2.5% of patients.[40] Those who develop such contact dermatitis should discontinue benzoyl peroxide use.

CASE 40-1, QUESTION 7: L.Y. discontinued treatment with benzoyl peroxide. What therapy is indicated now?

At this point, effective therapy requires prescription agents. If her mother still does not want to take her to a dermatologist, L.Y. could see her primary-care provider. After the allergic reaction resolves, L.Y. should begin using a more tolerable formulation of tretinoin, or adapalene. Because benzoyl peroxide monotherapy did not achieve optimal results, therapy should be intensified by adding a course of topical clindamycin to retinoid therapy. Compared with clindamycin, erythromycin is associated more with the development of resistance.[42] In addition, benzoyl peroxide cannot be used concomitantly to prevent resistance. Ziana is an appropriate treatment recommendation for L.Y. at this time as it offers clindamycin and tretinoin as a combination product to facilitate adherence. It is usually applied at bedtime. Case 40-2 includes additional details about antibiotic therapy.

L.Y. should be counseled to treat the entire face (avoiding eyes and lips), not just the lesions, for optimal results. She should continue protecting her skin with sunscreen and moisturizer. An oral antibiotic is not indicated at this time because only a small area is affected. If a 3-month course of Ziana achieves good results, the antibiotic should be discontinued, and L.Y. should be switched to a tretinoin-only product for maintenance therapy.

Moderate Acne

DRUG THERAPY

CASE 40-2

QUESTION 1: R.P., a fair-skinned, 18-year-old Hispanic man, has had acne since his early teens. He "mostly put up with it," occasionally using nonprescription benzoyl peroxide products. Now, however, his acne is getting noticeably worse. He has increasing numbers of lesions on his face, and the problem has spread to his chest and back. Currently, he has many closed comedones and about 12 papules and pustules on his face, primarily in the T-zone (forehead and nose). He has one painful nodule on his cheek and another on his back. R.P. is embarrassed by the appearance of his skin, especially on his trunk, which is exposed when he wears his basketball jersey while playing on the school team. A freshman in college, he wants his acne to be controlled quickly so that "it doesn't become the permanent part of my image it was in high school." He denies taking any medications or using any drugs, including anabolic steroids. He has no other significant medical conditions and no known drug allergies. What is your assessment of R.P.'s acne severity and contributing factors? What drug therapy options should be considered?

The quantity, location (on face and trunk), and types of lesions (including nodules) indicate that R.P. has moderate acne. R.P. has tried benzoyl peroxide in the past with unknown success, but his adherence is unclear. It is clear that acne has had a psychosocial impact on R.P.'s quality of life as he is concerned about his image.

The treatment of moderate acne should include reduction of contributing factors if possible. Playing basketball exposes R.P.'s skin to a hot, humid environment that may promote comedogenesis, but it also helps control another potential exacerbating factor: the stress of starting college. R.P. should be educated regarding the pathogenesis of acne, proper skin care, and common contributing factors.

Guidelines state that moderate acne should be treated with a topical retinoid coupled with a topical or oral antibiotic. Additionally, benzoyl peroxide may be used for nodular involvement or to reduce development of antibiotic resistance.

ANTIBIOTICS

Although *P. acnes* is part of the skin's normal flora, under the conditions leading to acne it helps transform comedones into inflammatory pustules or papules. Antibiotics do not resolve existing lesions, but they can prevent future lesions by decreasing *P. acnes* colonization and decreasing inflammation. Antibiotic courses used in acne are months long for two reasons. First, *P. acnes* colonies encase themselves within polysaccharide biofilms that shield them from antibiotics.[16] Second, antibiotics exert anti-inflammatory effects independent of their antibacterial activity. Tetracyclines and macrolides can reduce neutrophil chemotaxis and inhibit cytokines, even at subminimal inhibitory concentrations.[43,44] The antibiotics that are most effective in acne have antioxidant properties. In addition, antibiotics inhibit the release of reactive oxygen species by *P. acnes*, which in turn reduces leukocyte recruitment.[20] As a result of this multifactorial mechanism of action, clinical efficacy does not correlate perfectly with reductions in bacterial load; successful antibiotic courses do not necessarily eradicate *P. acnes*.[45] Investigators are beginning to research the use of sub-antimicrobial doses of systemic antibiotics. Pilot studies have found that just 20 mg of doxycycline orally twice daily reduced acne lesion counts similarly to 100 mg orally daily,[46] despite causing no changes in the numbers or resistance patterns of bacteria on the skin surface.[47]

Topical Antibiotics

Topically applied antibiotics avoid systemic exposure and achieve high follicular concentrations. They can augment topical retinoids when initiating therapy in mild to moderate acne cases involving inflammatory lesions, or they can be added to regimens for patients failing monotherapy. Topical antibiotic monotherapies are more effective than placebo, but not superior to benzoyl peroxide monotherapy, and are avoided because of bacterial resistance concerns.[40,48] Topical antibiotic and benzoyl peroxide combinations outperform either ingredient alone.[40,49]

Clindamycin and erythromycin are commonly used agents. Clindamycin (e.g., Cleocin T) is available as a 1% gel, lotion, solution, and foam; 1% gel in combination with 5% benzoyl peroxide (BenzaClin, Duac CS, generic); and 1.2% gel in combination with 2.5% benzoyl peroxide (Acanya) or 0.025% tretinoin (Ziana). Erythromycin (e.g., Erygel) is available as 2% solution, gel, ointment, and pledgets, and as 3% gel in combination with 5% benzoyl peroxide (Benzamycin, generic). Sodium sulfacetamide is not as well studied, but offers an option in patients who have failed first-line agents.[50] It is available at 10% strength, often with 1% to 5% sulfur, in a variety of vehicles. Dapsone 5% gel (Aczone) is a new alternative that has been recently reviewed.[51] Topical tetracycline is no longer used because it is cosmetically unacceptable.

Topical antibiotics are usually applied once or twice daily for 3 months. Although rare reports of systemic adverse effects exist, topical effects such as stinging and tingling are the most common adverse effects, and even these occur more rarely with topical antibiotics than with other topical therapies. Of interest, however, one British study found that acne patients using antibiotics—even topical ones—experienced twice the rate of upper respiratory infections, presumably as a result of changes in the normal flora of the oropharynx affecting vulnerability to infection.[52]

Oral Antibiotics

Oral antibiotics should be paired with topical retinoids and potentially also benzoyl peroxide in patients with moderate to severe

TABLE 40-6
Frequently Used Oral Antibiotics

Drug	Dose
Doxycycline	100 mg orally twice daily
Tetracycline	500 mg orally twice daily
Minocycline	50–100 mg orally twice daily (or 1 mg/kg/d)
Erythromycin	250–500 mg orally twice daily
Trimethoprim/ sulfamethoxazole	160/800 mg orally twice daily

Source: Tan HH. Antibacterial therapy for acne: a guide to selection and use of systemic agents. *Am J Clin Dermatol*. 2003;4:307.

acne; they should not be used as monotherapy. Oral administration is preferred over topical if lesions are widespread or in difficult-to-reach areas, as in R.P.'s case. Oral antibiotics can also replace topical antibiotics when topical combination regimens fail.

Doxycycline is most convenient and effective; tetracycline is an alternative.[53] Minocycline is sometimes tried if other antibiotics fail, but is significantly more expensive and not clearly better in efficacy, even in resistant acne.[54] It is also associated with a higher rate of serious adverse effects than other tetracycline antibiotics, including autoimmune disorders (such as lupus-like syndrome), intracranial hypertension, pseudotumor cerebri, eosinophilic pneumonitis, and hepatotoxicity. Tetracyclines cannot be prescribed for children younger than 9 years of age because of potential impairment of bone growth and discoloration of forming teeth. Pregnant women must avoid tetracyclines because of bone growth effects on the fetus. Trimethoprim/sulfamethoxazole is effective, but has a less favorable adverse effect profile than tetracyclines.[55,56] Erythromycin is associated with higher rates of resistance, but can be useful in patients who cannot use the drugs previously mentioned, such as pregnant women. Azithromycin has also been studied.[57] Clindamycin is not used systemically to treat acne owing to high rates of diarrhea and the risk of pseudomembranous colitis.

Most oral antibiotics are given twice daily for a 3-month course (Table 40-6). Many prescribers still then reduce dose frequency to daily for a maintenance course, but guidelines no longer support this practice, instead recommending topical retinoids for maintenance therapy.[20]

If gram-negative folliculitis is suspected, oral trimethoprim/sulfamethoxazole should be considered (this is probably not the case for R.P.). Rather than continued gradual deterioration, gram-negative folliculitis usually presents as worsening of acne in long-term antibiotic patients whose control had improved. Gram-negative organisms overgrow in the anterior nares and cause pustules on the central and lower face, often in the nasolabial folds.[3]

Antibiotic Resistance

Resistance of *P. acnes* to antibiotics frequently used for acne is increasing and correlates to prescribing patterns. Erythromycin resistance is highest; clindamycin resistance follows similar patterns, and cross-resistance between these two agents is high.[42] More than half of acne patients in Europe harbor resistant bacteria.[58] At one British site, resistance rates almost doubled during a span of 6 years.[42] Resistance to tetracyclines is less common, and is increasing at a slower rate than resistance to other antibiotics. Nonetheless, up to 20% of European patients and nearly one-third of patients in the United States are colonized with tetracycline-resistant strains, reflecting higher historical use of tetracyclines to treat acne in the United States than in Europe.[42,45] One reason tetracycline resistance may lag behind erythromycin and clindamycin resistance is that in environments free of tetracycline, tetracycline-resistant bacteria do not grow as well as susceptible bacteria. Because the genetic material that allows survival in tetracycline-containing environments is a liability in normal environments, selection pressure reduces resistance levels once tetracycline use is discontinued.[42] Erythromycin- or clindamycin-resistant bacteria grow reasonably well (though not as well as susceptible strains) in antibiotic-free environments, so resistance to these antibiotics fades less quickly after antibiotic use stops.[42] Tetracycline resistance is often accompanied by erythromycin and clindamycin resistance.[45]

The increasing rates of antibiotic resistance have had limited impact on prescribing patterns because resistance is not consistently linked to treatment failure in prescribers' everyday clinical experience, and research on the significance of resistance has been conflicting and sparse. Notwithstanding the extra-antimicrobial mechanisms of action of antibiotics, bacterial resistance to antibiotics does appear related to higher rates of treatment failure.[20,45,48] Increasing bacterial resistance is also postulated to explain why recent clinical trials of erythromycin obtain far lower efficacy rates than trials from earlier decades.[59] Although acne treatment failure may not be clearly linked to antibiotic resistance, it is also not the only possible consequence. Acne patients are more likely to carry not only resistant *P. acnes*, but also resistant strains of more clinically significant pathogens such as *Streptococci* and *Staphylococci*.[45,49] Topical antibiotic use is correlated with resistant bacteria at the application site, but systemic antibiotics foster resistant bacteria at all body sites.[20]

Because of growing concerns about antibiotic resistance, guidelines increasingly emphasize that antibiotics should be reserved for acne of at least moderate severity. They should be teamed with drugs exerting additional mechanisms of action, ideally topical retinoids, rather than used as monotherapy, and should be used for the shortest effective duration to obtain acne control (trials to stop antibiotics every 3 months). Antibiotics should not be used for maintenance of control (rather, the retinoid should be continued for maintenance). Including benzoyl peroxide in regimens containing antibiotics reduces the development of resistance, and is particularly recommended if antibiotic therapy needs to be continued beyond 3 months to maintain control.[20] If adherence to therapy with an antibiotic and both topical retinoid and leave-on benzoyl peroxide formulations is challenging, even a benzoyl peroxide wash product can be helpful.[60,61] Dual antibiotic use is inappropriate because it increases the risk of bacterial resistance without offering therapeutic gain, as bacterial eradication is not a therapeutic goal.

HORMONAL THERAPIES

Although hormonal therapies are not appropriate for R.P., they may be used for the treatment of moderate acne in female patients. Hormonal therapies with antiandrogenic effects, such as androgen receptor antagonists and combination oral contraceptives, are the only treatments besides oral isotretinoin to attack acne by reducing sebum production. Hormonal therapies may be helpful in patients with normal serum androgen levels, as well as in patients with elevated serum androgen levels, because hypersensitivity to androgens sometimes occurs at the follicular level despite normal circulating androgen levels.[62] Well-conducted comparative studies are needed to clarify the place of these therapies relative to other treatments suitable for moderate to severe acne, such as antibiotics, but they are good options for women with acne who are not pregnant and not planning to get pregnant, for those who desire contraception, and for women with polycystic ovary syndrome or other hyperandrogenic conditions or symptoms.[63] However, their systemic effects limit the use of hormonal therapies to female patients. Because their mechanism of action, reducing sebum production, is an early step in the cascade of acne pathology, response to hormonal therapies can require 3 to 6 months.[3]

Androgen Receptor Antagonists

Spironolactone at doses of 50 to 200 mg/day reduces acne because it is an androgen receptor antagonist and inhibits 5-α-reductase.[64] Flutamide (Eulexin), an antiandrogen licensed for metastatic prostate cancer, is effective, but potentially hepatotoxic.[65] Cyproterone is an antiandrogen that has orphan drug status in the United States but is used for acne abroad, often in combination with ethinyl estradiol. Gynecomastia precludes the use of antiandrogens in males. Female patients may exhibit menstrual irregularities and should use contraception because of the potential for antiandrogen exposure to impair the sexual development of male fetuses.[66]

Combination Oral Contraceptives

Estrogen, usually administered as ethinyl estradiol in a combination oral contraceptive, improves acne in females by reducing ovarian androgen production and by increasing sex hormone binding globulin concentrations in the serum, thereby lowering free testosterone levels. The manufacturers of Ortho Tri-Cyclen (ethinyl estradiol, norgestimate), Estrostep (ethinyl estradiol, norethindrone acetate), and Yaz (ethinyl estradiol, drospirenone) specifically sought and obtained FDA approval for acne indications. Studies of ethinyl estradiol in combination with levonorgestrel, desogestrel, or gestodene (not available in the United States) demonstrate efficacy in acne for those products as well.[63] Comparative trials have not yet clearly established clinically significant superiority of one product over another.[63] In individual patients, products containing progestins with androgenic effects (e.g., norgestrel, levonorgestrel) may override the effect of ethinyl estradiol and worsen acne. Conversely, patients already on a combination oral contraceptive may improve when switched to a formulation with a less androgenic progestin (norgestimate, desogestrel).[67] Other estrogen-containing contraceptives (transdermal patches, vaginal rings) may have similar beneficial effects to combination oral contraceptives, but studies have not been conducted.

CASE 40-2, QUESTION 2: Please provide a specific drug therapy recommendation for R.P.'s moderate acne treatment. What are the appropriate counseling points?

One appropriate regimen includes a well-tolerated topical retinoid such as adapalene 0.1% gel, applied every night at bedtime; doxycycline 100 mg by mouth twice daily with food; and benzoyl peroxide 5% wash used daily in the shower. Doxycycline may cause gastrointestinal effects such as heartburn, nausea, and diarrhea, and dermatologic effects such as rash and photosensitivity. R.P. should take the drug with a full glass of water to avoid esophageal erosions from prolonged esophageal contact, and wear protective clothing and use UVA/UVB sunscreen with an SPF of at least 15 on a daily basis. Because tetracycline may cause less photosensitivity, it may be an alternative to doxycycline if R.P. spends a lot of time outdoors (although he should still use sunscreen).[53] Tetracycline must be taken at least 1 hour before or 2 hours after eating because food, particularly dairy, impairs its absorption.

CASE 40-2, QUESTION 3: How should R.P.'s doxycycline regimen be monitored?

Assuming R.P. tolerates it, he should continue doxycycline for 6 to 8 weeks, at which point changes can be made if there is no improvement.[55,68] Routine laboratory monitoring is not necessary for most young, healthy patients receiving long-term oral tetracyclines or erythromycin because the incidence of serious adverse effects is low.[53,56] If the response is adequate, R.P. should try to stop doxycycline after 3 months. Topical retinoid therapy and any benzoyl peroxide product should continue during doxycycline therapy and then after the antibiotic course to maintain treatment benefit. If R.P. relapses again in the future after successful use of an oral antibiotic, another course of the same antibiotic should be used; switching offers no therapeutic benefit and can promote multidrug resistance.[56]

Severe Acne

DRUG THERAPY

CASE 40-3

QUESTION 1: K.S., an olive-skinned, 24-year-old Hispanic woman, first noticed acne when she was 10 years old. As a teen, she used topical benzoyl peroxide and systemic erythromycin with limited success. Two years ago, she was diagnosed with polycystic ovary syndrome and began taking Ortho Tri-Cyclen, after which her acne improved, but remained inadequately treated despite the addition of tazarotene gel. Ten months ago, she also began taking minocycline 100 mg orally twice daily. After a few months, she experienced significant improvement, but she has not been able to stop antibiotics because of predictable flare-ups. She now has at least a dozen nodules widely distributed among multiple papules and pustules on her face and back.

K.S. is 5′6″ and weighs 180 pounds (81.8 kg). She has no other health problems and no known drug allergies. She does not smoke, but she occasionally drinks three to four alcoholic beverages on weekends. She is sexually active with one partner, her husband. A month ago, a comprehensive metabolic panel, thyroid-stimulating hormone level, complete blood count with platelets, and lipid panel were normal. How would you assess K.S.'s acne severity? What drug therapy options should be considered?

K.S. has severe acne based on the large number of lesions, wide distribution to multiple body sites, and presence of multiple inflammatory lesions, including nodules. Oral isotretinoin monotherapy should be used to treat severe acne unless contraindicated.

ORAL ISOTRETINOIN

Isotretinoin (Amnesteem, Claravis, Sotret), a synthetic 13-*cis*-isomer of tretinoin, has greater pharmacologic activity than tretinoin. It is administered orally as 10-, 20-, 30-, and 40-mg capsules and is the only effective agent for severe nodular acne. In addition to exhibiting the comedolytic and anti-inflammatory properties of topical retinoids, systemic (oral) isotretinoin indirectly reduces *P. acnes* colonization by reducing the production of sebum, which *P. acnes* requires for survival.[14] Systemic isotretinoin therefore exhibits all four of the mechanisms of action currently used to attack acne, making it a uniquely effective monotherapy. Essentially all patients will respond to systemic isotretinoin; in most cases, one or two 5-month-long courses of therapy induce a remission lasting for several months or even years after the drug is stopped. Use of oral isotretinoin is perhaps more cost effective than use of long-term oral antibiotics in patients with severe acne, owing to its superior efficacy and the long-term cost savings realized by a shorter total duration of therapy.[69] Because of its risk and adverse effect profile, however, it is reserved for patients with severe acne and severe variants such as acne conglobata or acne fulminans, or moderate acne resistant to treatment or prone to scarring. Studies are investigating the role of lower-dose or intermittent courses of isotretinoin to increase tolerability in patients with moderate acne.[70,71]

CASE 40-3, QUESTION 2: Suggest a drug therapy plan for K.S.'s acne.

The most effective medication for K.S. will be oral isotretinoin at an initial dose of 20 mg twice daily (targeting 0.5 mg/kg/day). The dosage should be increased to 40 mg twice daily (1 mg/kg/day) as tolerated after 1 month. The dose is divided twice daily and given with food. For best results and minimal risk of relapse, treatment should continue until a cumulative dose of approximately 120 mg/kg is reached, usually about 5 months.[71] Higher dosages are associated with an increased risk of adverse effects. K.S. should stop taking minocycline when isotretinoin therapy begins because isotretinoin is effective monotherapy, and co-administration of isotretinoin and tetracyclines increases the risk of intracranial hypertension.[55] Tazarotene is also unnecessary once isotretinoin begins. Her acne should significantly improve within the first month of therapy and gradually resolve by the third or fourth month. A second course of therapy is usually not necessary.

CORTICOSTEROIDS

CASE 40-3, QUESTION 3: Should K.S. be pre-medicated with corticosteroids before isotretinoin therapy?

Although corticosteroids sometimes cause acne, under some circumstances they are used in treatment protocols for severe acne. If severe acne flaring is a concern, patients may pretreat 1 to 2 weeks with prednisone 40 to 60 mg/day before isotretinoin therapy begins and continue concomitant prednisone for the first 2 weeks of isotretinoin therapy.[15] Corticosteroids are co-administered with isotretinoin when treating acne fulminans to decrease the inflammatory response.[8] Acne patients with diagnosed adrenal hyperplasia may take prednisone 2.5 to 5 mg/day in the evening to suppress diurnal corticotropin release and thus adrenal hypersecretion of endogenous steroids.[67] Intralesional triamcinolone injections markedly improve severe nodules, but repeated or careless use of the technique can lead to atrophic scarring. Topical application of corticosteroids is ineffective.

K.S.'s acne is severe but stable enough that premedication with prednisone is unnecessary.

CASE 40-3, QUESTION 4: K.S.'s prescriber discusses enrolling her in iPLEDGE. What is the iPLEDGE program? What should K.S. know about avoiding pregnancy while taking isotretinoin?

Isotretinoin is severely teratogenic. A strict risk-management program called iPLEDGE regulates the prescription and distribution of isotretinoin in the United States.[72] The program requires all patients, prescribers, pharmacies, and even drug wholesalers involved in distribution and use of the drug to register with a national database. Proper patient monitoring and education, including negative pregnancy tests in female patients of child-bearing potential, must be documented in the database each month before initial or refill medication can be dispensed to a patient.

Female patients of child-bearing potential must use two forms of contraception for at least a month before, during, and for at least a month after isotretinoin therapy. At least one contraception method must be a "primary" method. K.S. is already using an approved primary method with Ortho Tri-Cyclen; approved primary methods also include bilateral tubal ligation, partner's vasectomy, some intrauterine devices, or hormonal methods (other than progestin-only minipills). However, she must also begin using a backup method, such as condoms. The program requires that all female patients of child-bearing potential must have two negative pregnancy tests before beginning isotretinoin therapy, one at the time of screening and then another, from an appropriately certified laboratory, after a month on their chosen contraception regimen. The program also requires a negative pregnancy test before each monthly refill is prescribed, immediately after therapy, and a month after therapy. K.S. and her prescriber will both have to verify with the program on a monthly basis that she has been counseled again regarding contraception.

Like all isotretinoin patients, male and female, K.S. must also be reminded not to donate blood during therapy and for a month after therapy, to ensure no pregnant woman receives isotretinoin-contaminated blood products.

CASE 40-3, QUESTION 5: In addition to the pregnancy testing discussed, which baseline and periodic laboratory monitoring parameters should be followed in this patient?

Before beginning isotretinoin therapy, all patients, male and female, should have the following baseline laboratory tests: a fractionated lipid panel; a liver function panel, including both serum transaminases and bilirubin; and a complete blood count, including platelets.[1,15] If a particular patient's other medical history suggests potential risk, providers might order baseline serum glucose levels, erythrocyte sedimentation rate, and creatine phosphokinase. For accurate triglyceride results, the blood sample should be collected at least 36 hours after alcohol consumption and 10 hours after eating food. The laboratory results measured a month ago will suffice for K.S. because they likely would not be significantly different now.

A lipid panel should be redrawn 4 and 8 weeks into isotretinoin therapy to document the effect of the drug.[15] About 20% of patients develop significant triglyceride elevations.[73] Triglyceride levels greater than 400 mg/dL should be treated with diet and reduced alcohol intake; monthly monitoring should continue throughout isotretinoin therapy. In the unusual event that triglyceride levels exceed 700 to 800 mg/dL, isotretinoin should be discontinued, or continued at a reduced dosage with concomitant gemfibrozil therapy to reduce the risk of pancreatitis.[15] If pancreatitis develops, isotretinoin must be discontinued. High-density lipoprotein concentrations may decrease slightly, and low-density lipoprotein concentrations may increase, during isotretinoin therapy; however, the clinical significance of these changes is unknown. These lipid abnormalities usually resolve within several weeks of completion of therapy.[73]

Liver function tests and blood counts only need to be redrawn during therapy if symptoms suggestive of hepatitis or blood dyscrasias appear,[15] although some guidelines suggest periodic monitoring.[1] Many practitioners draw liver function tests 4 and 8 weeks into therapy.[74] Mild elevations in serum transaminases may simply be monitored if they occur; however, isotretinoin dosage reduction or drug discontinuation should be considered in asymptomatic patients with persistent enzyme elevations greater than twice the upper limit of normal. Clinical hepatitis occurs rarely, but requires drug discontinuation if suspected.

Adverse effects on bone such as hyperostosis, premature epiphyseal closure, and reduced bone mineral density have not been observed when isotretinoin is used at the doses and durations typical in acne treatment, so monitoring for this toxicity is

TABLE 40-7
Adverse Effects of Systemic Retinoids

Body System	Adverse Effect	Management
Common, Pharmacologic		
Reproductive	Teratogenicity (birth defects, premature birth, neonatal death)	Avoid pregnancy; patients should not donate blood during therapy
Skin	Dryness, erythema, peeling, pruritus, photosensitivity	Use moisturizers, sunscreens, protective clothing; avoid skin waxing, dermabrasion, and other dermatologic procedures during and 6 months after therapy
Hair, nails	Hair dryness, hair thinning, nail fragility	None; discontinue drug if severe
Mucous membranes	Cheilitis, dry mouth, dry nose, nosebleeds, dry eyes, blepharoconjunctivitis	Use lip balms, sugarless gum or candy, saline nasal spray, artificial tears or ophthalmic ointment; avoid contact lenses; lower dosage if severe or bothersome
Metabolic	Elevated triglycerides, LDL; lowered HDL (rare reports of pancreatitis)	Reduce/eliminate alcohol; consume low-fat diet; consider drug discontinuation if changes are extreme
Liver	Elevated transaminases	Monitor if elevation is mild; usually transient despite continued therapy; avoid drug in patients with previous liver dysfunction
Uncommon, Toxic		
CNS	Pseudotumor cerebri, hearing loss, tinnitus	Discontinue drug if patient develops severe headache, nausea, vomiting, papilledema, visual changes (suggest pseudotumor cerebri), or hearing changes
Bones	Pain	Monitor at each visit
	Bone mineral density loss (osteopenia), premature epiphyseal closure, hyperostosis	Routine monitoring is not recommended for usual durations of therapy
Muscle, ligaments	Pain, calcifications	Monitor; more likely in physically active patients; discontinue if severe
Eyes	Impaired night vision, corneal opacities	Patients should use caution when driving
Liver	Hepatitis	Discontinue drug
Hematologic	Anemia, neutropenia, thrombocytopenia	Monitor CBC for changes necessitating drug discontinuation
Psychiatric	Depression, suicide	Monitor for depressed mood and suicidal thoughts

CBC, complete blood count; CNS, central nervous system; HDL, high-density lipoprotein; LDL, low-density lipoprotein.
Source: Goldsmith LA et al. American Academy of Dermatology Consensus Conference on the safe and optimal use of isotretinoin: summary and recommendations. *J Am Acad Dermatol.* 2004;50:900; Marqueling AL, Zane LT. Depression and suicidal behavior in acne patients treated with isotretinoin: a systematic review. *Semin Cutan Med Surg.* 2007;26:210.

not required unless a patient is undergoing multiple isotretinoin courses or has pertinent medical history.[1,75]

CASE 40-3, QUESTION 6: How should K.S. be counseled with regard to adverse effects of isotretinoin?

K.S. should expect significant skin and mucous membrane dryness, which is reported by virtually all patients taking isotretinoin. Severe photosensitivity can occur in any patient taking isotretinoin; K.S. should be advised to wear protective clothing and to use a UVA- and UVB-blocking, high-SPF sunscreen daily, even if she does not anticipate sun exposure. She should also limit alcohol consumption, which can enhance isotretinoin-induced hypertriglyceridemia and hepatotoxicity. Another possible adverse effect is muscle or joint pain, especially if she exercises more than usual. She should avoid waxing, dermabrasion, and other skin procedures during and for 6 months after therapy because her skin would be likelier than usual to scar. She should drive with caution, paying attention to any potential vision changes, particularly at night. Bone growth is not impaired when isotretinoin is used in recommended dosages. Table 40-7 summarizes common and significant adverse effects of isotretinoin. Patients should also be warned that acne may worsen initially because flares occur in up to about half of patients.[73]

CASE 40-3, QUESTION 7: K.S. has never had problems with depression, but her prescriber asked her psychiatric history and current symptoms, and her iPLEDGE patient education materials warn against possible drug-induced depression. The thought of suddenly becoming violent or suicidal concerns her. How significant is this risk?

Isotretinoin product labeling includes a warning that isotretinoin may cause depression, including suicide attempts, psychosis, and violent behavior. Case reports suggest that isotretinoin causes psychiatric symptoms in some patients. Severe acne is itself associated with depression, however, and prospective trials and literature reviews have not established a causal relationship between isotretinoin and depressive symptoms.[76] Although the absolute risk is low, drug-induced depression is a possible idiosyncratic reaction to isotretinoin in individual patients. In any case, all patients with severe acne, whether receiving isotretinoin or not, should be monitored for the development or worsening of depression.[1] K.S. should be reassured that the risk of drug-induced psychiatric symptoms is low. If she does notice any of the psychiatric symptoms listed in her medication guide, she should contact her prescriber immediately about stopping isotretinoin.

CASE 40-3, QUESTION 8: After 3 weeks of therapy, K.S. complains of dry eyes, dry skin, and cracks with bleeding at the corners of her mouth. How might these bothersome mucocutaneous adverse effects be managed?

K.S. should use artificial tears to relieve the discomfort of her dry eyes; if she is still uncomfortable after several days, she can also apply lubricating ophthalmic ointment at bedtime. She should liberally apply moisturizer to dry skin, particularly after bathing (see Chapter 39, Dermatotherapy and Drug-Induced

Skin Disorders). Frequent application of a lip balm or emollient, ideally one containing sunscreen, will treat cheilitis. If the symptoms become intolerable, a small reduction in the isotretinoin dose (e.g., reduction of 10–20 mg/day) usually decreases the intensity of skin and mucous membrane reactions. Drug discontinuation is rarely necessary.[73]

Postinflammatory Hyperpigmentation

DRUG THERAPY

CASE 40-4

QUESTION 1: J.H., a 23-year-old African American woman with medium brown skin tone, has had acne vulgaris for the past 10 years. During this time, she has tried several medications. Benzoyl peroxide was somewhat helpful, but even low concentrations caused excessive irritation. She also tried extended courses of topical erythromycin and clindamycin, with little clinical improvement. Oral tetracycline was moderately effective, but caused her to get frequent yeast infections. A year ago, she began using Yaz for contraception. During that time, she has also noticed improvement in her acne; however, she still has about 20 open and closed comedones on her forehead, cheeks, and chin. She has two papules on her nose and one papule along the jawline. J.H.'s biggest concern about her skin is that lesions "take forever to clear completely." She indicates eight hyperpigmented macules on her cheeks and forehead at the sites of lesions that healed during the past 6 months. She has no other pertinent medical history and no known drug allergies. Recommend a new treatment strategy for J.H.

Because J.H.'s acne is mostly comedonal, a topical retinoid would be an effective addition to the hormonal therapy provided by her contraceptive. Given her history of sensitive skin and propensity toward postinflammatory hyperpigmentation, it is important that therapy not be so irritating as to prompt severe inflammation. Adapalene would be a good option because it has less irritation potential than tretinoin and can reduce postinflammatory hyperpigmentation as well.[9]

For a photo of postinflammatory hyperpigmentation, go to http://thepoint.lww.com/AT10e.

Cream is a less irritating vehicle than gel. J.H. should apply the cream to her entire face every night. Some acne might appear worsened within the first 1 to 2 weeks as preclinical lesions may become visible. Sun exposure significantly intensifies skin irritation, so all patients regardless of skin color (and especially those prone to postinflammatory hyperpigmentation) should be instructed to apply sunscreen to sun-exposed areas when using comedolytic therapies. It is also important to ask J.H. about her skin care regimen and use of hair products to identify the use of any counterproductive cleansing strategies or comedogenic hair pomades.

Like many patients with postinflammatory hyperpigmentation, J.H. is more distressed by the splotchy aftermath of her acne than by the acne itself.[10] She should be assured that the adapalene cream will likely aid the resolution of her current hyperpigmentation in addition to interrupting the comedogenic process behind future lesions. If the hyperpigmentation shows no signs of improvement when J.H. returns for follow-up in 6 weeks, once- or twice-daily application of nonprescription skin-lightening hydroquinone 2% cream can be added to speed resolution.[9] Hydroquinone is applied only to the areas of hyperpigmentation and only until they fade, typically 1 to 3 months. If it is applied at the same time of day as acne medication, it should be applied after the acne medication.

ACKNOWLEDGMENT

The authors wish to thank Terry L. Seaton. This is a revision of his chapter in an earlier edition.

KEY REFERENCES AND WEBSITES

A full list of references for this chapter can be found at http://thepoint.lww.com/AT10e. Below are the key references and websites for this chapter, with the corresponding reference number in this chapter found in parentheses after the reference.

Key References

Gollnick H et al. Management of acne: a report from a Global Alliance to Improve Outcomes in Acne. *J Am Acad Dermatol.* 2003;49(1 Suppl):S1. (26)

Strauss JS et al. Guidelines of care for acne vulgaris management. *J Am Acad Dermatol.* 2007;56:651. (1)

Thiboutot D et al. New insights into the management of acne: an update from the Global Alliance to Improve Outcomes in Acne group. *J Am Acad Dermatol.* 2009;60(5 Suppl):S1. (20)

Webster GF, Graber EM. Antibiotic treatment for acne vulgaris. *Semin Cutan Med Surg.* 2008;27:183. (53)

Key Websites

iPLEDGE: Committed to Pregnancy Prevention. https://www.ipledgeprogram.com/. Accessed December 1, 2010. (73)

Mayo Clinic Acne. http://www.mayoclinic.com/health/acne/DS00169.

Medline Plus Acne. http://www.nlm.nih.gov/medlineplus/acne.html.

Nemours Foundation Acne. http://kidshealth.org/kid/grow/body_stuff/acne.html.

U.S. Food and Drug Administration. Facing Facts About Acne. http://www.fda.gov/ForConsumers/ConsumerUpdates/ucm174521.htm.

41 Psoriasis

Katie L. Kiser and Timothy J. Ives

CORE PRINCIPLES

	CHAPTER CASES
1 Psoriasis is a chronic, proliferative skin disease that is characterized by well-delineated, thickened erythematous skin plaques and is both topical and systemic in nature. It is immune mediated with both vascular and inflammatory changes, which precede epidermal changes.	Case 41-1 (Question 1)
2 Precipitating factors for psoriasis include cold weather, anxiety and stress, viral or bacterial infections, epidermal trauma, or drugs.	Case 41-1 (Question 2)
3 Topical corticosteroids are first-line treatment for mild psoriasis because of their prompt relief, convenience, and anti-inflammatory, immunosuppressant, and antipruritic properties.	Case 41-1 (Question 5)
4 Alternative topical treatments for mild psoriasis—coal tar, anthralin, calcipotriene, and tazarotene—and phototherapy are not as convenient as topical corticosteroids, but have well-established efficacy for initial management.	Case 41-1 (Question 6)
5 Treatment goals for severe psoriasis include both safe and effective resolution of the disease and long-term maintenance using agents to induce immunosuppressive or remittive cellular changes.	Case 41-2 (Question 1)
6 Psoriatic arthritis can occur in up to 40% of patients with psoriasis, and mild disease is treated first with nonsteroidal anti-inflammatory drugs and second with an immunosuppressive agent, methotrexate.	Case 41-3 (Question 1)
7 Use of immunosuppressive agents can be limited as a result of adverse effects, monitoring requirements, or toxicity. There is also a lack of evidence to support that they modify the long-term disease process. Immunomodulatory therapy, including T-cell agents and TNF-α inhibitors, are thought to target the immune-mediated mechanism of psoriasis.	Case 41-3 (Question 2)

EPIDEMIOLOGY

Psoriasis, a term derived from the Greek word *psora* (meaning itch), a chronic, proliferative skin disease, is one of the most common immune-mediated disorders occurring in 1.5% to 3% of the population worldwide, with northern Europeans and Scandinavians affected most.[1,2] It is characterized by well-delineated, thickened erythematous epidermis or dermal plaques covered with a distinctive silvery scale. Of patients, 75% present with symptoms of psoriasis before the age of 46 years.[2] A family history of psoriasis is found in nearly half of patients. At least nine chromosomal loci have been identified that increase psoriasis susceptibility.[3,4] The primary genetic determinant is *PSORS1*, a region of the major histocompatibility complex on chromosome 6p2, which accounts for 35% to 50% of the heritability of the disease.[2,3] Environmental triggers also play a major role in disease expression.

Pathogenesis

Innate and adaptive immunity are both involved in the initiation and maintenance of psoriatic plaques. As the epidermis is the body's main barrier to environmental insult, epidermal hyperplasia forms a key component of the innate immune response. Natural killer cells and natural killer T cells are part of the cutaneous inflammation in psoriasis.[5]

As CD4$^+$ and CD8$^+$ T-lymphocytic cells constitute most of the leukocyte infiltrate found in plaques early in the development of lesions, current evidence supports an autoimmune mechanism for psoriasis. Cytokines such as interferon-α_2 or interleukin-2 are also found in psoriatic plaques.[6] T cells in the cutaneous infiltrate are positive for cutaneous lymphocyte-associated antigen, a marker for skin-homing leukocytes. Pathogenesis also involves vascular and inflammatory changes, which precede epidermal changes.[7] Alterations in the dermal vasculature also appear to be a result of angiogenesis, the development of new blood vessels, similar to a number of other disease processes, including tumor growth. Many commonly used therapeutic agents for psoriasis have antiangiogenic activity.[1]

The epidermal changes of psoriasis are based on the time required for affected epidermal cells to travel to the surface and be cast off, which is markedly reduced (3–4 days, vs. 26–28 days in normal cells).[8] This sixfold to ninefold transit time decrease does not allow the normal events of cell maturation and keratinization to take place and is reflected clinically as diffuse scaling. T cells contribute to this keratinocyte hyperproliferation through the secretion of various growth factors.[9,10] Memory T lymphocytes marked with cutaneous lymphocyte-associated antigen, to remember the anatomic site where they first encountered antigen, migrate to the (epi)dermis by a number of immunologic and inflammatory triggering mechanisms released from keratinocytes after minor trauma. On entry into the skin, these T cells complex with epidermal self-antigens presented by major histocompatibility complex molecules that confer the risk of psoriasis. The subsequent release of T-cell cytokines results in further inflammation, the recruitment of additional marked (i.e., with cutaneous lymphocyte-associated antigen) T cells, and ultimately the development of psoriatic lesions in susceptible persons.[9,10]

Prognosis

Similar to those with diabetes, cancer, and heart disease, patients with psoriasis experience a reduced quality of life related to an impairment of social, psychological, and physical functioning.[11,12] Although psoriasis is a treatable disease, there is no known cure. Optimism and encouragement are justified and make it easier for patients to conscientiously apply sometimes awkward and messy topical treatments or take medications that have significant adverse effects. The goal of therapy should be to achieve complete clearing of psoriatic lesions, particularly during emotionally critical times, such as the commencement of school, puberty, and the summer months.

Clinical Presentation of Psoriasis

CASE 41-1

QUESTION 1: M.M., a 35-year-old man, presents with complaints of several thick, well-defined erythematous areas on both his elbows and knees that have silvery scales on them. He complains of itching in these areas and that the areas bleed when he removes the scales. M.M. states that he has had these lesions for some time; however, he has used over-the-counter hydrocortisone and some of his friend's triamcinolone 0.025% cream on them for the itching. He feels that the lesions have gotten worse since he went on vacation in the Dominican Republic and got "a pretty bad sunburn." His medical history is noncontributory. His only medications, besides topical corticosteroids, include a recent course of chloroquine for malaria prophylaxis during his recent travel. On physical examination, M.M. also has a few scattered, circumscribed, erythematous, scaly plaques on the flexural surfaces of both arms and legs and a dense scale on his forehead and scalp. Approximately 4% of his body surface area (BSA) is estimated to be affected with psoriasis. The rest of M.M.'s physical examination and laboratory results are within normal limits.

Laboratory values and vital signs include the following:

BP, 132/78 mm Hg
HR, 64 beats/minute
Sodium, 140 mEq/L
Potassium, 4.3 mEq/L
BUN, 13 mg/dL
Creatinine, 0.9 mg/dL

What classic signs and symptoms suggestive of psoriasis are demonstrated by M.M.?

Most psoriatic lesions are asymptomatic, but not always. Pruritus, for example, is noted in 50% of patients, and it can be severe.[13] The primary psoriatic lesion is a relapsing eruption of scaling papules that rapidly coalesce or enlarge to form circumscribed, erythematous, scaly, plaques. The scale is adherent and silvery white, and may reveal bleeding points when removed, called the *Auspitz sign*. Scales can become extremely dense on the scalp or macerated and dispersed in intertriginous areas.

ONLINE CONTENT

For an image of psoriatic lesions, go to http://thepoint.lww.com/AT10e.

The development of lesions of active psoriasis at the site of epidermal trauma is known as the *Koebner phenomenon*. Scratch marks, sunburn, or surgical wounds may heal, leaving psoriatic lesions in their place. The elbows, knees, scalp, gluteal cleft, fingernails, and toenails are favored areas of involvement. Extensor surfaces are affected more than the flexor surfaces, but the disease usually spares the palms, soles, and face. Nail beds may show punctate pitting, profuse collections of keratotic material, yellow-brown discoloration ("oil spot"), or onycholysis (nail plate separation) in approximately 50% of patients.[14] Psoriatic arthritis is a seronegative inflammatory arthritis that occurs in approximately 25% of all patients with psoriasis, with combined features of both rheumatoid arthritis and the seronegative spondyloarthropathies.[2,13]

Most patients (90%) have chronic localized disease (plaque-type or *psoriasis vulgaris*), but several other presentations exist. The most severe form of the disease is *erythrodermic psoriasis*, a condition of acute inflammatory erythema and scales involving greater than 90% of the BSA. *Pustular psoriasis* is generally localized to palms and soles, but there is also a generalized version. Both generalized pustular psoriasis and erythrodermic psoriasis can be accompanied by systemic symptoms (i.e., hyperthermia, tachycardia, edema, dehydration, shortness of breath) and can have life-threatening consequences (i.e., hypovolemia, electrolyte imbalance, septicemia) if not promptly treated.[15] Lesions of *Guttate psoriasis* are small, fine, erythematous scales, usually found on the trunk, arms, or legs, classically after β-hemolytic streptococcal pharyngitis. *Flexural* or *inverse psoriasis* is shiny and red, and typically lacks scales and looks more like intertrigo.[2] Of interest, psoriatic skin is rarely secondarily infected, because of the overexpression of the endogenous peptides cathelicidins and beta-defensins.[14]

Systemic disorders that can have a causative association with psoriasis include type 2 diabetes mellitus, Crohn disease, metabolic syndrome, depression, and cardiovascular disease.[2,11,12] This increased risk is thought to be caused by the presence of endothelial activation, proinflammatory cytokines, and hyperlipidemia.[2,15] Disease severity is also thought to be a factor, as psoriatic patients with more severe conditions have an increased risk of metabolic or coronary heart disease or stroke compared with those with milder forms of psoriasis.[11]

M.M. presents with many classic signs of psoriasis including symmetric, distinctive, chronic, erythematous plaques covered with silvery scales on the extensor surfaces of the elbows and knees as well as the flexural surface of his arms and legs. He also shows scalp involvement, but does not appear to have plaques on his trunk or nail or systemic involvement. He exhibits the Auspitz sign and evidence of the Koebner phenomenon because his lesions worsened after skin trauma from the sunburn. His notation of pruritus is consistent with presentation in 50% of patients.

CASE 41-1, QUESTION 2: What are factors that can precipitate or aggravate psoriasis? What are the potential causes of M.M.'s psoriatic exacerbation?

A thorough medical history may reveal a cause for exacerbations of psoriatic lesions. Most patients report that hot weather, sunlight, and humidity help clear psoriasis, whereas cold weather has an adverse effect on its course. Anxiety or psychological stress is believed to contribute adversely. Viral or bacterial infections, especially streptococcal pharyngitis, may precipitate the onset or flare-up of psoriasis. Cuts, burns, abrasions, injections, and other trauma can also elicit the development of lesions. Any drug that causes a skin eruption to develop can exacerbate psoriasis via this response.

Drug-Induced Psoriasis

A number of drugs have been reported to exacerbate pre-existing psoriasis, induce psoriatic lesions on apparently normal skin in patients with psoriasis, or precipitate psoriasis in persons with or without a family history of psoriasis (Table 41-1).[16] Antimalarial agents, such as chloroquine (taken by M.M.), may have an adverse effect on the course of psoriasis and can cause exfoliative erythroderma.[17] Hydroxychloroquine, however, has not shared this association (except for one case report) and usually induces a beneficial response in 75% of patients with psoriatic arthritis.[17] It is preferred over chloroquine in patients with psoriasis who need prophylactic treatment for malaria when both are effective against the particular plasmodium species in the area (see Chapter 78, Parasitic Infections).[17]

Lithium also can precipitate psoriasis and contribute to resistance to treatment through its effects on cell kinetics (increase in circulating neutrophils, accelerated neutrophil turnover, increased epidermal cell proliferation).[16] Psoriasis is not a general contraindication, however, to lithium therapy. More intensive psoriasis treatment can be used if these reactions occur and lithium must be continued.[16]

β-Blockers and some nonsteroidal anti-inflammatory drugs (NSAIDs) also can precipitate a psoriasiform state.[16] As both lithium and propranolol inhibit cyclic adenosine monophosphate (cAMP), cyclic nucleosides may play a role in the onset and clinical course of psoriasis. Chemotactic substances, including 12-hydroxyeicosatetraenoic acid and leukotrienes, may accumulate in the epidermis of some patients taking indomethacin, thereby precipitating psoriasis.

When compared with other NSAIDs, indomethacin may selectively inhibit cyclooxygenase more than lipoxygenase pathways of arachidonic acid metabolism. As a result, indomethacin may have a more significant adverse psoriatic effect than other NSAIDs that have been reported to ameliorate psoriasis.[16]

TABLE 41-1
Drugs Reported to Induce Psoriasis

Anesthetics	Procaine
Antimicrobial agents	Amoxicillin, ampicillin, imiquimod, penicillins, sulfonamides, terbinafine, tetracyclines, vancomycin
Anti-inflammatory drugs	Corticosteroids (after withdrawal), NSAIDs (indomethacin, salicylates)
Antimalarial agents	Chloroquine, hydroxychloroquine
Cardiovascular drugs	Acetazolamide, amiodarone, angiotensin-converting enzyme inhibitors (captopril, enalapril), β-blockers (atenolol, metoprolol, propranolol, timolol), calcium-channel blockers (dihydropyridines, diltiazem, verapamil), clonidine, digoxin, gemfibrozil, quinidine
H_2-antagonists	Cimetidine, ranitidine
Hormones	Oxandrolone, progesterone
Opioid analgesics	Morphine
Psychotropics	Lithium carbonate, valproic acid, fluoxetine, carbamazepine, olanzapine
Miscellaneous	Potassium iodide, mercury, α-interferon, β-interferons, granulocyte-macrophage colony-stimulating factor (GM-CSF)

NSAIDs, nonsteroidal anti-inflammatory drugs.
Source: Dika E et al. Drug-induced psoriasis: an evidence-based overview and the introduction of psoriatic drug eruption probability score. *Cutan Ocul Toxicol.* 2006;25:1; Basavaraj KH et al. The role of drugs in the induction and/or exacerbation of psoriasis. *Int J Dermatol.* 2010;49:1351; Facts & Comparisons eAnswers, accessed January 12, 2011, with permission.

Flare-ups of pustular psoriasis also can be precipitated by withdrawal from systemic corticosteroids or withdrawal from high-potency topical corticosteroids that are applied under occlusion to large areas.[18] Systemic corticosteroids are not routinely used to treat psoriasis because of this problem, and because fatalities have been associated with systemic corticosteroid use and withdrawal.

Chloroquine prophylaxis, a Caribbean sunburn, and triamcinolone tachyphylaxis probably all contributed to the exacerbation of M.M.'s psoriasis.[17,18]

Categorization of Psoriasis

CASE 41-1, QUESTION 3: How would you categorize M.M.'s psoriasis?

The Self-Administered Psoriasis Area and Severity Index (SAPASI) is a validated, structured instrument that can be used for patient assessment of psoriasis severity and the response to therapy. It closely correlates with the standard clinician assessment instrument, Psoriasis Area and Severity Index (PASI), which includes quantification of the percentage of body involvement and severity of lesions.[19] A PASI of 75 (a $\geq$75% decrease in PASI score) at 3 months from baseline has become the most prominent marker to assess systemic agent efficacy (see **http://dermatology-s10.cblib.org/102/original/pasi/feldman.html**, which is *Dermatol Online J.* 2004 Oct 15;10(2):7, for a good reference to teach someone the PASI and SPASI).[19]

The National Psoriasis Foundation has released a clinical consensus statement on the classification of severity of disease. Rather than using a mild (less than 5% BSA affected) to moderate (5% to 10%) to severe (greater than 10% BSA affected) classification system, the statement recommends two categories for patients, those who are candidates for topical therapy (less than

TABLE 41-2
Topical Agents for the Treatment of Psoriasis (Mild to Moderate; < 5% Body Surface Area Involvement)

Treatment Modality	Advantages	Disadvantages
Emollients	Basic adjunct for all treatments; safe, inexpensive, reduces scaling, itching, and related discomfort	Provide minimal relief alone
Keratolytics (salicylic acid, urea, α-hydroxy acids [i.e., glycolic and lactic acids])	Reduce hyperkeratosis; enable other topical modalities to better penetrate; inexpensive	Provide minimal relief individually; nonspecific; salicylism (tinnitus, nausea, vomiting) with salicylic acid if applied extensively
Topical corticosteroids	Rapid response; control inflammation and itching; best for intertriginous areas and face; convenient, not messy; mainstay topical treatment modality for psoriasis	Temporary relief; less effective with continued use (tachyphylaxis occurs); withdrawal can produce flare-ups; atrophy, telangiectasia, and striae with continued use after skin returns to normalized state; expensive; adrenal suppression possible
Coal tar	Particularly effective for "flaky" scalp lesions; newer preparations are more cosmetically appealing; efficacy enhanced in combination with UVB (i.e., Goeckerman regimen)	Effective only for mild psoriasis or scalp psoriasis; inconvenient with difficult application; stains clothing and bedding, not skin; strong smelling; folliculitis and contact allergy (bronchospasm in atopic patient with asthma after inhalation of vapor); carcinogenicity in animals
Anthralin	Effective for widespread, refractory plaques; produces long remissions; short, concentrated programs preferred; enhanced efficacy in combination with UVB (i.e., Ingram regimen)	Purple-brown staining (skin, clothing, and bath fixtures); irritating to normal skin and flexures; careful application is required; can precipitate generalized psoriasis
Calcipotriene	As effective as topical corticosteroids, although slower onset, without long-term corticosteroid adverse effects; convenient, well tolerated	Slow onset; expensive; potential effects on bone metabolism (hypercalcemia); irritant dermatitis on face and intertriginous areas; contraindicated during pregnancy
Tazarotene	Extended response; convenient (applied once daily, in gel formulation); maintenance therapy; effective on scalp and face; used in combination with topical corticosteroids	Slow onset; local irritation and pruritus; teratogenic (adequate contraception is required)
Ultraviolet B (UVB)	Effective as maintenance therapy; eliminates problems of topical corticosteroids	Expensive; office-based therapy; sunburn (exacerbates psoriasis); photoaging; skin cancers

5% of BSA affected), and those who are candidates for systemic or phototherapy (more than 5% of BSA affected).[20]

M.M. would be categorized as having mild psoriasis and is a candidate for topical therapy because less than 5% of his BSA is currently affected by psoriasis.

TREATMENT OF MILD PSORIASIS

Many topical and systemic therapeutic agents are available, varying from simple topical emollients to systemic, highly potent immunosuppressant drugs for more recalcitrant conditions. Often, treatment modalities are chosen on the basis of disease severity, cost, convenience, and patient response. Patients with mild disease can generally be treated with topical therapy (Table 41-2). Patients with psoriasis covering more than 5% of the body require more specialized systemic or phototherapy treatment programs (Table 41-3). Nonpharmacologic treatment is also very important and can range from spa therapy to support groups.

Initial Therapy

NONPHARMACOLOGIC MODALITIES

CASE 41-1, QUESTION 4: What role can emotional support play in the comprehensive management of M.M.'s psoriasis?

Psoriasis is often more emotionally or psychologically disturbing than is recognized, and it may cause a reluctance of patients to participate in sports and other outdoor activities that may expose their skin to sunlight. Although exposure to sunlight helps most patients with psoriasis, there is an unwillingness to sunbathe if the lesions can be seen. Furthermore, if the psoriatic lesions become pruritic and are scratched, there can be further deterioration at the site. Many patients alter their lifestyles or use nontraditional medications and modalities, often in desperation.

Emotional support should begin with explanation of the psoriatic condition. M.M. needs to be reassured that many other people have the same affliction, that the disorder is not contagious or fatal, and that it can be controlled although, as yet, no cure exists.[21] Patients usually are comforted in the knowledge that a wide range of treatments is available. Clinical optimism and psychological encouragement and support are justified and make it easier for the patient to conscientiously apply sometimes awkward and messy topical treatments or to take toxic medications.

TOPICAL CORTICOSTEROIDS

CASE 41-1, QUESTION 5: What topical corticosteroid therapy is appropriate for M.M.?

Topical corticosteroids, the most widely prescribed treatment for psoriasis, are effective in the treatment of psoriasis because of their anti-inflammatory, antimitotic, immunosuppressant, and antipruritic properties.[18,22] These properties are explained by a reduction in phospholipase A_2, DNA synthesis, and epidermal mitotic activity, as well as their vasoconstrictive actions. They provide prompt relief, and patients find them convenient and acceptable. As an added advantage, mild-strength topical products or intermediate-strength products, for limited periods, can be used on facial lesions or intertriginous areas, or for maintenance therapy.[23] However, topical corticosteroids also can become less effective with continued use, called tachyphylaxis,[24] and long-term use after the skin has returned to a normalized state leads to typical corticosteroid adverse effects (atrophy, telangiectasia,

TABLE 41-3
Agents for the Treatment of Severe Psoriasis (>5% Body Surface Area Involvement)

Treatment Modality	Advantages	Disadvantages
UVA and psoralen (PUVA)	80% efficacy; "suntan" effect is cosmetically desirable	Time-consuming; expensive, office-based therapy (restrictive); sunburn (exacerbates psoriasis); photoaging; both nonmelanoma skin cancer and melanoma; contraindicated during pregnancy and lactation
Acitretin	Not as effective as other systemic agents; efficacy enhanced if given with PUVA or UVB (i.e., RePUVA or ReUVB); less hepatotoxic than methotrexate	Teratogenic (contraception required); contraindicated with liver or renal dysfunction, drug or alcohol abuse, hypertriglyceridemia, hypervitaminosis A
Methotrexate	Effective for both skin lesions and arthritis, as well as psoriatic nail disease	Hepatotoxicity (liver biopsy may be indicated); bone marrow toxicity; folic acid protects against stomatitis (but not against hepatic or pulmonary toxicity); drug interactions; contraindicated during pregnancy and lactation, drug or alcohol abuse; use with caution during acute infections
Cyclosporine	Toxicities and short-lived remissions; used in patients with extensive disease who are unresponsive to other agents; however, given changing pathophysiology and increasing experience at lower dosages, increasing role in rotational therapy to induce remissions	Renal impairment; suppressive therapy (relapse occurs when discontinued); increased risk of skin cancer, lymphomas, and solid tumors; phototoxic; contraindicated during pregnancy and lactation, and with hypertension, hyperuricemia, hyperkalemia, acute infections
Immunomodulators (alefacept, efalizumab, etanercept, infliximab, adalimumab, golimumab)	Specific, targeted therapy; effective for both moderate to severe skin lesions and arthritis; maintains remission	Expensive; parenteral therapy (often administered in an office-based practice) therapy; long-term safety unknown; increased risk of serious infections

PUVA, psoralens plus ultraviolet A light; RePUVA, retinoid-PUVA; UVA, ultraviolet A; UVB, ultraviolet B.

and striae). Thin-skinned areas (i.e., facial and intertriginous) are particularly susceptible.

Psoriasis is generally a relatively corticosteroid-resistant disease; therefore, the more potent corticosteroids are frequently necessary, often with occlusion (e.g., plastic food wrap on top of the topical steroid-treated area), for best results (see Table 39-8 in Chapter 39, Dermatotherapy and Drug-Induced Skin Disorders, for a listing of topical corticosteroids by potency). Less-potent agents are more appropriate in intertriginous areas, on the face, and for maintenance. Potent fluorinated corticosteroid preparations should be used cautiously and only for short periods on the face and flexures, if at all. Potent topical corticosteroids may clear psoriasis in 25% of patients in 3 to 4 weeks, with 75% clearing in 50% of treated patients.[25]

Intermittent dosing or "pulse therapy" with several weeks between successive courses appears to yield the best long-term results and minimizes tachyphylaxis and adverse effects. An additional drawback of chronic corticosteroid therapy is an associated acute flare-up of psoriasis when corticosteroid therapy is terminated.[26] Continuous application for more than 3 to 4 weeks should be discouraged in patients with psoriasis, and systemic corticosteroids have no place in therapy.[24,25] Topical corticosteroids occasionally can cause a reversible suppression of the hypothalamic-pituitary-adrenal (HPA) axis, as indicated by a decrease in the morning plasma cortisol level.[24] For anything more extensive than mild disease and short duration of therapy, topical corticosteroids are best used in an adjunctive role. During a flare-up, corticosteroids help reduce inflammation, redness, and irritation and prepare the involved area for initiation of other potentially irritating, but more appropriate, maintenance topical treatments (e.g., coal tar, anthralin, calcipotriene, or tazarotene).

A short course of a potent topical corticosteroid is appropriate for this flare-up of erythematous plaque psoriasis in M.M. This will help reduce inflammation, redness, and irritation before possible initiation of more appropriate chronic topical treatments, such as calcipotriene, coal tar, or anthralin with UVB. Topical corticosteroids also may continue to be useful for M.M. on the face and flexures, where the alternative topical agents are poorly tolerated. His scalp psoriasis can be treated with corticosteroid preparations in gels, lotions, or aerosol sprays. This will allow for a more effective treatment of scaling and pruritus using an agent like coal tar shampoo lathered into the scalp for 5 to 10 minutes, then rinsed out.

The response to once- or twice-daily corticosteroid application is as effective or better than that observed with more frequent regimens (owing to a corticosteroid reservoir effect) and is much less expensive. M.M. should apply a topical corticosteroid preparation after a bath, at bedtime with occlusion (which is covered in Chapter 39, Dermatotherapy and Drug-Induced Skin Disorders), and possibly again during the day without occlusion. As the lesions subside, occlusion should be decreased or omitted, emollient use should increase, and the corticosteroid potency should decrease. After lesions have flattened, the topical corticosteroid products can be continued intermittently (e.g., 1–2 weeks on, 1–2 weeks off; or on alternate days [e.g., days 1, 3, 5, 7]).

ALTERNATIVE TOPICAL TREATMENTS

CASE 41-1, QUESTION 6: M.M.'s acute psoriasis flare-up has responded well to a short course of topical corticosteroid. What alternative topical therapeutic regimens are available for patients such as M.M. who have localized or mild disease?

Four effective alternative topical therapies are available for patients with localized, mild psoriasis. Older, well-known agents are crude coal tar and anthralin, with more recent additions of calcipotriene and tazarotene. Although anthralin has irritating properties and both coal tar and anthralin generally stain clothing and skin and are somewhat inconvenient to apply, their efficacy is well established, and may be an option to consider for initial management. Tachyphylaxis does not occur with chronic use of any of these alternative agents. Once the inflammation and erythema have lessened with corticosteroid use or when a twice-daily, high-potency corticosteroid regimen along with bedtime application of coal tar is ineffective, calcipotriene ointment applied twice daily or tazarotene gel applied once daily is effective in treating flare-ups and maintaining remission. Ointment vehicles are favored because they help moisturize the plaques (in contrast to creams, which dry the plaques further). Also, moisturizers or emollients are often helpful for psoriasis.

COAL TAR

Crude coal tar is a complex mixture of thousands of hydrocarbon compounds.[27] It is a time-honored modality for treating psoriasis. It affects psoriasis by enzyme inhibition and antimitotic action (antiproliferative and anti-inflammatory).[27] The efficacy of the combination of tar and ultraviolet B (UVB) light (i.e., Goeckerman regimen) led to its increased popularity beginning in the 1920s. Tar preparations of 2% to 10% are processed as creams, ointments, lotions, gels, oils, shampoos, and coal tar solution. Newer purified preparations, using refined coal tar, are less messy and more cosmetically acceptable, but perhaps not as effective.[27] Tar may be helpful for patients with mild to moderate disease, and tar shampoos are useful for psoriasis of the scalp. The potential severity of adverse drug effects from topical tar products is less than that from anthralin, and much less than that from topical corticosteroids. Because tar, in every form, is messy, stains the skin, has an odor, and is low potency compared with anthralin, it has been relegated to second-line therapy for most patients, despite its moderate price and newer, more cosmetically appealing formulations.[24,28]

Tar preparations generally are used once or twice daily, and a bedtime application (as a shampoo or cream overnight) is particularly useful in psoriasis of the scalp. Patients should be warned about the staining properties of tar on clothing and bedding. Other adverse effects include photosensitivity, acneiform eruptions, folliculitis, and irritation dermatitis. Care should be taken to avoid use of tar on the face, flexures, and genitalia and with inflammatory psoriasis because of tar's irritant properties.

The polyaromatic hydrocarbons contained in coal tar may be metabolized to active carcinogens by epidermal microsomal enzymes. The incidence of hyperkeratotic lesions, including squamous cell carcinoma, is increased after prolonged industrial exposure to tar; however, extensive reviews of patients who have used tar preparations in psoriasis have not revealed an increased risk of carcinoma.[29]

ANTHRALIN

Anthralin (dithranol in the United Kingdom) is a hydroxyanthrone derivative that inhibits DNA synthesis, mitotic activity, and a variety of enzymes crucial to reducing cell proliferation.[25] It is effective for treatment of widespread, discrete psoriatic plaques, but its use has declined in recent years with the availability of more cosmetically appealing preparations. Traditionally, it was applied as a stiff paste overnight and used in conjunction with coal tar baths and UVB light (i.e., Ingram regimen). Most cases of chronic plaque psoriasis clear in 3 weeks. The primary disadvantages of anthralin are its irritant nature and staining properties to skin and clothing. Anthralin also can precipitate generalized psoriasis if applied to unstable psoriasis (i.e., plaque transformation to pustular form).

When used, the most current anthralin regimen is a once-daily application of a 1 or 1.2% cream (Psoriatec, and Zithranol-RR, respectively) for a short-contact anthralin therapy (SCAT; apply for 20 to 30 minutes, then wash off). One factor that limits its use is the brown to purple staining of the skin, hair, clothing, furniture, and bedding that occurs immediately with use. Plastic gloves should be used, as well as old bed linens and clothing for sleep. If possible, contact with the face, eyes, mucous membranes, and nonpsoriatic skin should be avoided because of irritant properties. According to tolerance or for resistant plaques, potency can be increased (up to 1%) and the contact time shortened. Irritation can be more of a problem with the higher concentrations, and irritation should be checked for at least every 48 hours. Both methods are used daily for clearing of psoriasis, then once or twice weekly for maintenance therapy, which is instituted after a response is seen at 2 to 3 weeks. Short-course regimens clear 32% of lesions and produce greater than 75% improvement in half of patients after 5 weeks. These regimens are comparable in effectiveness to the Ingram regimen, and topical corticosteroids are associated with fewer adverse drug events.[24,30] Application of petrolatum ointment around the psoriatic lesion may help to prevent perilesional irritation. The duration of the petrolatum application is determined by the ongoing severity of the lesions. A topical corticosteroid cream may be used during the remainder of the day.

CALCIPOTRIENE

Calcipotriene (calcipotriol in Europe) is a topical vitamin D_3 analog that suppresses keratinocyte proliferation and has anti-inflammatory effects.[31] It can be applied twice daily as a cream, ointment, or solution. Although systemic absorption is slight and the vitamin D effects of calcipotriene on calcium and bone metabolism are about 100 to 200 times less than that of 1,25-dihydroxyvitamin D_3, serum calcium levels and urinary calcium excretion should be monitored to prevent serious adverse effects. A 100-g/week limit should be enforced; exceeding this limit results in negative effects on calcium and bone metabolism. Other adverse effects of calcipotriene include lesional and perilesional irritation, burning, stinging, pruritus, erythema, and scaling, which occurs in about 30% of patients, and precludes use on the face or in intertriginous areas.[32] When used concurrently with topical salicylic acid, calcipotriene will be chemically inactivated.

Calcipotriene may be the topical maintenance treatment of choice in patients with generalized mild to moderate psoriasis. The drug is usually effective, relatively easy to apply, odorless, and nonstaining (cream, ointment, or scalp solution). Most patients see improvement, although not clearing, of psoriatic plaques at 2 weeks when treated with calcipotriene, often in combination with potent topical corticosteroids.[33] A maximal response is usually seen at 6 to 8 weeks. Of treated patients, 57% experience greater than 75% clearance of psoriatic plaques, which is comparable to that achieved with corticosteroids, albeit slower in onset and associated with more skin irritation.[22,30] Tachyphylaxis has not been a problem.[33]

TAZAROTENE

Tazarotene is a topical synthetic retinoid that is rapidly converted to its biologically active metabolite, tazarotenic acid.[34] By interacting with the predominant retinoid receptors on the skin surface regulating gene transcription, retinoic acids normalize abnormal keratinocyte differentiation, reduce hyperproliferation, and decrease inflammation associated with psoriasis.[34] Treatment success rates compare favorably with corticosteroids (52% clearing of all lesions; 70% clearing of trunk and limb lesions). The antipsoriatic effects of tazarotene are sustained for a longer period after treatment compared with corticosteroids.[25,35] Because local skin irritation and pruritus are common adverse effects of tazarotene use, combination therapy with corticosteroids not only provides additive antipsoriatic effects, but also reduces retinoid-induced irritation.[36] Because oral retinoids are known teratogens, tazarotene is a Category X drug and is contraindicated during pregnancy. Women should be warned of the potential risk and the need to use adequate contraception while using these preparations.[34,35]

Similar to calcipotriene, tazarotene works slowly. It is formulated as a gel, which many patients find more cosmetically appealing than an ointment. It is also effective in a once-daily regimen, which might help to improve compliance.

PHOTOTHERAPY

If available locally, UV light can be used as an outpatient modality; it produces comparatively long-lasting remissions, is pleasant to use, and is relatively nontoxic. Different protocols require exposure daily or multiple times per week for varied lengths of time, depending on patient variables. The optimal effect of UVB on psoriasis is a dose that produces minimal erythema at 24 hours. The usual time to induce clearing of psoriasis is approximately 4 to 6 weeks.

ULTRAVIOLET B

Ultraviolet B light, sunburn spectrum 290 to 320 nm, induces pyrimidine dimers, inhibits DNA synthesis, and depletes intraepidermal T cells found in psoriatic epidermis (i.e., UVB has antiproliferative and local immunologic effects).[18] UVB light, unlike ultraviolet A (UVA) light, is effective without additional sensitizers (i.e., psoralens). UVB therapy is generally considered pleasant to use and relatively nontoxic. Typically, 60% of patients with chronic plaque psoriasis experience clearing, and an additional 34% achieve a 75% clearance with UVB treatment for 7 to 8 weeks.[26] Humidity and heat from sunlight provide additional positive effects. Narrow-band UVB (NB-UVB) phototherapy, sunburn spectrum 311 nm, has been found to be more effective than broad-band UVB (BB-UVB)[35,37]; however, it has not demonstrated superiority to psoralens plus ultraviolet A light (PUVA) therapy in terms of clearing psoriatic lesions.[38] The greater efficacy of PUVA, however, may be offset by the short-term adverse effects of psoralens (e.g., nausea, headaches), the greater incidence of phototoxic reactions (erythema), and the inconvenience of wearing photoprotective eyewear after treatments. At present, NB-UVB may be preferred as the available data suggest no or minimal risk of carcinogenesis compared with PUVA, it is safer to use in children and pregnant patients, it is devoid of drug-related (psoralen) adverse drug events, and there is no requirement for use of posttreatment photoprotective eyewear. Although not definitively proven, it is hypothesized that NB-UVB will produce less long-term photodamage and fewer skin cancers (i.e., squamous cell carcinoma) than PUVA.

Ultraviolet B treatments are administered three times weekly. The use of pretreatment emollients (e.g., petrolatum, mineral or "baby" oil, Eucerin) applied before UVB exposure, long thought to improve results, actually inhibits the penetration of UVB and should not be used.[39] After the skin clears, therapy is discontinued gradually over the course of 2 to 4 months to prolong remissions. The risks of UVB radiation and sunlight are similar: sunburn, photoaging, and skin cancer.

Regimens combining UVB with anthralin (Ingram regimen) or tar (Goeckerman regimen) have been used for years, theoretically taking advantage of the photosensitizing properties of tar and anthralin. The Goeckerman regimen involves daily application of coal tar for at least 4 hours along with exposure to UVB light. The Ingram regimen combines daily application of anthralin plus tar baths with exposure to UVB light, with combination results superior to UVB monotherapy. These two regimens are reported to clear plaques in 75% of patients treated for 6 weeks for chronic plaque psoriasis (vs. 56% with UVB alone). The total number of treatments and the total UVB dose required for clearing are less in the combination groups.[40] Both the Goeckerman and Ingram regimens can clear widespread psoriasis in 3 to 4 weeks, induce remissions that last for weeks to months, and may reduce the long-term adverse effects of UVB exposure.[40]

In summary, the first step in the treatment of M.M. would be a high-potency corticosteroid ointment twice daily, along with a coal tar ointment at night. If this is ineffective, either calcipotriene ointment can be added twice daily or tazarotene gel can be used once a day for 8 weeks. Once control is achieved, M.M. may use calcipotriene or tazarotene without topical corticosteroids; these products do not cause corticosteroid atrophy and they do not have the potential for systemic adverse effects associated with topical corticosteroids. Topical anthralin, with or without UVB, can be used for resistant cases.

TREATMENT OF SEVERE PSORIASIS

CASE 41-2

QUESTION 1: G.L., a 42-year-old man with a several-year history of psoriasis (fairly localized), presents with diffuse, erythematous plaquelike lesions now extending over 80% of his body. The areas have become inflamed, and application of his maintenance topical medication (anthralin) causes pain and irritation. He expresses frustration with the messiness of the current topical regimen. He has reinstituted topical steroids, which helped the redness and itching but are too expensive to use long term. He is free of cardiovascular, renal, or hepatic disease and takes no systemic medications. He is self-employed as a business consultant. Which "systemic" therapy would be most appropriate for G.L.'s psoriasis at this point?

Systemic therapies for psoriasis include PUVA; the systemic retinoid, acitretin; methotrexate; and cyclosporine. Newer biologics, including the tumor necrosis factor (TNF)-α inhibitors (infliximab, etanercept, adalimumab, golimumab, ustekinumab) and the immunosuppressants (alefacept, efalizumab), have also been used for skin lesions.

Although PUVA and methotrexate are used most often, cyclosporine and the newer immunomodulatory agents are being used increasingly as more experience is gained with them for treatment of severe psoriasis.[18,41] The choice of agents depends on patient and drug characteristics. Because patients with psoriasis generally have the disease for the rest of their lives, the goal of treatment is not just safe and effective resolution of lesions at a specific point in time, but also maintenance therapy. Long-term maintenance therapy for psoriasis can generally be achieved even with a weaning or discontinuation of UVB, PUVA, and methotrexate. From a histologic perspective, these drugs have been shown to induce remittive cellular changes. In contrast, partial to full doses of acitretin or cyclosporine are necessary to maintain therapeutic effects, because they induce suppressive rather than remittive histopathologic changes. For example, relapse will occur in most patients in a predictable manner 2 to 4 months after cyclosporine is discontinued.[42]

Photochemotherapy

Photochemotherapy combines psoralens with UVA light in the 320 to 400 nm spectrum. The psoralens (methoxsalen, 8-methoxypsoralen, and trioxsalen) are a group of photoactive compounds that, on absorption of UV light, are both antiproliferative and immunomodulatory. When photoactivated by UVA, psoralens form monofunctional adducts and cross-links with pyrimidine bases. PUVA also inhibits cytokine release and depletes both epidermal and dermal T cells. As measured by extent of T-cell depletion and decreases in delayed hypersensitivity, PUVA has greater immunomodulatory effects in the skin than UVB. Use of PUVA for scalp or nail involvement is limited, however, because of lower exposure.[18,43] Remissions are longer in duration than with UVB. Psoralens are not active without UVA.

Photochemotherapy is used to control severe, recalcitrant, disabling plaque psoriasis. After 10 to 20 treatments over the course of 4 to 8 weeks, more than 80% of patients experience clearing of symptoms, which can be maintained with periodic (twice monthly) treatments.[43] UVA penetrates the skin more deeply than UVB and may have marked effects on the dermis. The use of PUVA requires careful consideration and adherence to strict photoprotective measures. Patients unwilling to adhere to PUVA-related precautions may prefer UVB treatment because it is much less restrictive.

The peak range for UVA light's therapeutic action is between 320 and 335 nm. The most widely used agent, 8-methoxypsoralen, at an oral dosage of 0.6 to 0.8 mg/kg of body weight rounded to the nearest 10 mg, is taken approximately 1.5 hours before exposure to UVA light.[38] The initial dose is selected based on the patient's skin type (i.e., ease of sunburn and inherent skin color). Other options for combination therapy with UVA include calcipotriol-PUVA (D-PUVA) and retinoid-PUVA (RePUVA). Both of these modalities have been shown to have greater efficacy as compared with PUVA alone.[37]

Acute adverse phototoxic effects, such as erythema and blistering, are dose related and, therefore, controllable. Other acute adverse drug effects include nausea, lethargy, headaches, pruritus, and hyperpigmentation. Topical corticosteroid therapy should be continued until the psoriasis is brought under control. If topical corticosteroids are discontinued at the start of PUVA, an exacerbation of psoriasis usually occurs. Patients should wear protective clothing (with long sleeves and high necklines), use sunscreens that filter out both UVA and UVB, and wear sunglasses that block UVA after PUVA (see Chapter 42, Photosensitivity, Photoaging, and Burns). Because methoxsalen has a short half-life and 80% is eliminated within 6 to 8 hours, physical barriers are most important during the 8 hours immediately after PUVA therapy.

Of greater concern are the potential long-term adverse effects: mutagenicity, carcinogenicity, and cataract formation. Squamous cell carcinoma has been associated with cumulative PUVA treatments (11-fold increase in patients who receive more than 260 treatments compared with patients who received fewer than 160 treatments).[44] Male patients have an increased risk of having genital squamous cell carcinoma. A relationship exists between the exposure to PUVA and the risk of malignant melanoma. At present, there appears to be a dose-dependent increase in the risk of melanoma associated with high-dose exposure to PUVA. The risk is first manifested at least 15 years after initial exposure to PUVA.[44–46] Long-term maintenance and high cumulative dosages should be avoided. Shielding the face and genitalia during treatment and performing annual examinations to detect skin cancer at an early stage may lessen the risk of long-term adverse effects of photochemotherapy.

Topical psoralens are extremely photosensitizing, hence difficult to administer. Application of methoxsalen 0.1% followed by small UVA doses (i.e., ≤20% of the level of usual doses for oral PUVA) has been used, however, to treat localized areas and to prevent adverse gastrointestinal effects.[43]

SYSTEMIC PHARMACOTHERAPY

Acitretin

Second-generation systemic retinoids are effective for treatment of recalcitrant psoriatic disease. Antipsoriatic effects stem from the drug's ability to modulate epidermal differentiation and immunologic function in addition to an anti-inflammatory action.[47] This latter effect may alleviate the arthritis that accompanies psoriasis.[18,43] Acitretin, a systemic second-line therapy for severe psoriasis, is the principal metabolite of etretinate. It is 50 times less lipophilic than etretinate, and has a considerably shorter elimination half-life; however, patients taking any retinoid product should still be monitored closely. It is indicated for patients who have received extensive radiation with PUVA, as a pretreatment for PUVA (1–3 weeks) to accelerate the response rate, for patients who fail to respond to UVB with anthralin or tar, or for patients who are not candidates for methotrexate.[48] Most patients require maintenance or intermittent therapy to prevent relapses.[49]

Numerous other adverse effects are associated with acitretin use, including hypervitaminosis A syndrome (i.e., dry skin, skin thinning and fragility, chapped lips, dry nasal mucosa, skin peeling, alopecia, and nail dystrophy), retinoid rash, extraspinal tendon and ligament calcification and bone changes in children, hyperlipidemia with elevated levels of serum triglycerides and cholesterol, and liver enzyme alteration and hepatitis.[50] Many patients find the adverse effects of the retinoids intolerable and discontinue treatment. Topical corticosteroids can reduce some of the cutaneous retinoid adverse effects.

Acitretin is teratogenic and accumulates in fatty tissues, where it is slowly released into the bloodstream for up to 1 year after final administration.[47] Therefore, strict contraception during treatment and for 2 to 3 years afterward is recommended in women of childbearing age.[46,51] Patients also need to be advised not to donate blood while taking acitretin and up to 1 year after the end of treatment.[47]

Immunosuppressive Agents

METHOTREXATE

Methotrexate, a folic acid analog, inhibits dihydrofolate reductase needed for synthesis of several amino acids, pyrimidines, purines, and subsequently DNA, RNA, and protein synthesis. Methotrexate therapy greatly suppresses rapidly proliferating cells, such as those in psoriatic skin. Antipsoriatic mechanisms of methotrexate action include inhibition of keratinocyte differentiation and immunomodulation by destruction of lymphoid cells.[18,52]

Unlike other cytotoxic drugs, methotrexate produces antipsoriatic effects at dosages that are much lower than those used in cancer chemotherapy. Methotrexate is relatively safe and well tolerated, yet the long-term concerns for myelosuppression and hepatotoxicity (fibrosis and cirrhosis) and the need for periodic liver biopsies can discourage many patients and physicians from using it.[53,54] Alcohol and methotrexate are a particularly potent hepatotoxic combination. Patients with psoriasis receiving methotrexate have a 2.5- to 5-fold higher incidence of advanced liver changes than patients with rheumatoid arthritis receiving comparable regimens.[55] Methotrexate hepatotoxicity may be related to both cumulative doses and constant blood levels. Daily administration has been replaced by weekly dosage schedules for this reason. Liver chemistry tests (i.e., serum alanine aminotransferase, serum aspartate aminotransferase, serum albumin, bilirubin) can be within normal limits, even in the presence of methotrexate-induced liver disease.[52] Therefore, consensus guidelines call for risk stratification for liver biopsies in all patients with psoriasis at baseline, and at intervals of approximately 1 to 1.5 g of cumulative methotrexate dose. Liver function tests, bilirubin, and albumin should be monitored monthly for the first 6 months, and then every 1 to 2 months thereafter.[52]

Bone marrow depression, nausea, diarrhea, and stomatitis are other adverse effects associated with methotrexate. Pneumonitis can occur early in the course of treatment, particularly when methotrexate is given at higher dosages similar to those used in cancer chemotherapy regimens. Folic acid, at 1 mg daily, may prevent some of these adverse events, but not hepatitis or pulmonary toxicities. Teratogenesis and miscarriage have occurred, and methotrexate may cause reversible oligospermia. A number of clinically significant drug interactions may enhance the toxicity of methotrexate. Drug interactions are most likely to be clinically relevant problems in patients with decreased renal function.[52]

Relative contraindications to treatment with methotrexate include decreased renal function, significant abnormalities in liver function (i.e., fibrosis, cirrhosis, hepatitis), pregnancy or breastfeeding, anemia, leukopenia, thrombocytopenia, active peptic ulcer disease or infectious disease (tuberculosis, pyelonephritis), alcohol abuse, and patient unreliability.[52] Conception must be avoided during methotrexate therapy and for at least 3 months after cessation of methotrexate in men or one full ovulatory cycle in women.[52] Monthly monitoring of complete blood count with differential and a platelet count should be performed 7 to 14 days after starting therapy, and every 2 to 4 weeks for the first few months, then every 1 to 3 months. Renal function tests (i.e., serum creatinine, BUN) should be obtained at 2- to 3-month intervals.

CYCLOSPORINE

The positive dermatologic effects of cyclosporine, an immunosuppressive agent, highlight the importance of immune alterations in the pathogenesis of psoriasis. The toxicity and the short duration of remissions induced by cyclosporine and tacrolimus limit their usefulness. Cyclosporine is generally reserved for patients with extensive psoriasis who have not responded adequately to topical agents, UVB, PUVA, and other systemic agents.

In psoriasis, cyclosporine primarily acts by inhibition of calcineurin, which is necessary for interleukin-2 (IL-2) production. Interleukin-2 amplifies helper T cells and cytotoxic lymphocytes. Decreased IL-2 production leads to a decline in activated CD4 and CD8 cells in the epidermis. Cyclosporine also inhibits TNF-α and interferon-α_2, both of which are involved in the chemotaxis of inflammatory cells; it inhibits release of cytokines and the growth of keratinocytes.[56]

Cyclosporine is used at relatively low dosages for the treatment of psoriasis. In general, 2.5 to 6 mg/kg of cyclosporine, in one or two divided doses, is recommended for the initiation of psoriasis treatment. Rapid improvement of plaque psoriasis is expected, with 30% of patients experiencing clearing of psoriatic plaques and 50% achieving greater than 75% clearing of lesions within 10 weeks at a dose of 2 to 3 mg/kg/day. Many people relapse 2 to 4 months after the discontinuation of cyclosporine therapy.[57] Cyclosporine showed comparable efficacy to methotrexate in patients with psoriasis with average doses of 4.5 mg/kg/day and 20.6 mg/week, respectively.[53]

Drug-induced renal impairment is common with cyclosporine use, but usually reversible. Hypertension, secondary to vasoconstrictive effects on the smooth muscle of renal blood vessels or drug-induced arteriolar hyalinosis, is dose dependent and gradual in onset. Blood pressure and serum creatinine should be monitored closely in patients receiving cyclosporine.[54] Hypokalemia, hypomagnesemia, hyperuricemia, gingival hyperplasia, hypercholesterolemia, hypertriglyceridemia, adverse gastrointestinal effects, hypertrichosis, fatigue, myalgia, and arthralgia also have been attributed to cyclosporine therapy.[55] The risk of skin cancer, lymphomas, and solid tumors also can increase.[56,57] Patients should be cautioned about excessive sun exposure and should not receive concurrent UVB or PUVA treatment during cyclosporine therapy because of an increased risk of nonmelanoma skin cancers.[58]

PUVA is effective in 80% to 90% of patients, and G.L.'s severe, extensive, plaque psoriasis should be expected to respond accordingly. The systemic drugs (e.g., methotrexate, cyclosporine) may be preferred if G.L. had systemic symptoms (e.g., psoriatic arthritis). Although three times weekly PUVA treatments can be disruptive to work schedules, G.L. is self-employed and presumably has some flexibility in his working hours, and this would be a good option for him.

Rotational Therapy

CASE 41-2, QUESTION 2: Does G.L. have options to decrease adverse effects and cost of his PUVA therapy?

No form of therapy used in psoriasis today is without toxicity. Rotational therapy involves the use of alternating monotherapies, which allows the patient to experience extended intervals off a particular treatment.[59] When used in long-term maintenance, rotational therapy limits adverse effects associated with either long-term use of one specific agent or the additive or synergistic interactions when multiple therapies are used concurrently. As discussed, the relative risk of skin cancer associated with PUVA increases after 160 treatments. If a patient in remission is rotated off PUVA to another treatment after 100 exposures, the skin has time to recuperate from the light therapy, and PUVA can eventually be reinstated presumably with lesser risk. Rotational therapy assumes that the patient can tolerate three to four alternative treatments with unrelated toxicity profiles.[42] By rotating each treatment after 12 to 18 months of cumulative use, the potential for long-term toxicity associated with any single treatment is minimized. With this theoretic rationale, cyclosporine could be used for a limit of possibly 3 to 6 months, thus inducing a remission. The patient could then be rotated to another treatment (e.g., methotrexate or PUVA) for maintenance.

Psoralens and UVA irradiation become noticeably effective in 80% to 90% of patients in 6 to 8 weeks.[18] The regimen is time-consuming because UV radiation treatments must be administered at least three times a week. Methoxypsoralen (8-MOP) is administered (0.6–0.8 mg/kg of body weight), followed by UVA (dose selected based on skin type, ease of sunburn, and inherent skin color) about 75 to 90 minutes later when psoralen blood levels peak. PUVA-induced erythema generally appears later than with UVB therapy, reaching a peak by 48 hours. Consequently, treatment should not be administered more frequently than every second day. The time to produce clearing of psoriatic plaques with PUVA takes longer than with UVB therapy (average 10 weeks compared with $\leq$3 weeks for UVB).[43] PUVA treatment must be decreased slowly once plaques have been cleared (frequency of treatment is reduced during 2 to 3 months) to prevent recurrence of psoriatic plaques. In contrast, UVB therapy can be ceased abruptly.

Taking time off from work three times weekly for photochemotherapy can be disruptive to some patients' work or school schedules. Technological advances in home phototherapy equipment have provided patients with choices for therapy in settings that are familiar and comfortable, in addition to continued improvements in efficacy and safety.[60] Advantages of home phototherapy include improved quality of life, greater convenience, lower cost, and less time lost from work and social activities.

Psoralens and UVA should be avoided in patients with a history of skin cancer, in children, during pregnancy, in patients who are immunosuppressed, and in those who have light-colored skin that burns rather than tans. Absolute contraindications to treatment with PUVA include a history of photosensitivity diseases (i.e., lupus erythematosus, porphyria), idiosyncratic or allergic reactions to psoralens, arsenic intake, exposure to ionizing radiation, skin cancer (relative contraindication), pregnancy, and lactation. Techniques to minimize cumulative dosage of radiation and reduce the risk of long-term adverse effects of photochemotherapy include use of sunscreen, protective clothing, and sunglasses and use of combination therapy (RePUVA). Other photosensitizing drugs (e.g., fluoroquinolones, phenothiazines, sulfonamides, sulfonylureas, tetracyclines, thiazides) should be avoided in patients receiving PUVA.

Rotational therapy could be considered at a later time depending on G.L.'s response and tolerance of PUVA.

Alternative Therapy

CASE 41-2, QUESTION 3: What alternative therapies are available for G.L.?

Balneology (bathing in the sea) and spa therapy are not accepted as mainline dermatologic treatment modalities for psoriasis; however, these approaches are used throughout the world. The antipsoriatic properties of the Dead Sea area may be attributed to its unique climatic characteristics and natural resources. Mechanisms may involve mechanical, thermal, and chemical effects.[61] Available data suggest that balneotherapy may be associated with improvement in several rheumatologic diseases; however, skin improvement is transient, with most benefits lost after 4 months.[62] Short-term balneotherapy and photobalneotherapy could be a temporary option for patients who need to temporarily discontinue pharmacotherapy; however, existing research is not strong enough to draw firm conclusions or to recommend.

Climatotherapy is the combination of bathing in the sea (thalassotherapy or balneotherapy) and exposure to sunlight (heliotherapy).[63] A major aspect of climatotherapy, in addition to daily sunbathing, is bathing in salt (sea) water. Relaxation, rest, and simple topical remedies (e.g., petrolatum) are also important. When rigorously studied, little difference is found in therapeutic outcomes of bathing in salt water or tap water, or the application of various topical ointments (e.g., 2% salicylic acid in white petrolatum, Eucerin, or mineral oil) when used in the current UVB phototherapy protocols. Psychological factors (especially relaxation), however, may contribute substantially to the favorable results of natural heliobaleotherapy. If UV phototherapy is administered via artificial UV sources on an outpatient basis, the psychological effect will certainly be much less than when the patient receives this treatment far from home, when cares and social problems are left behind.

Hydroxyurea, thioguanine, and azathioprine are nonstandard antineoplastic agents that have antipsoriatic activity. The therapeutic effects of these agents are not as potent as methotrexate, but they cause less hepatotoxicity with continuous use.[64]

Traditional Chinese medicine provides an alternative method of therapy that emphasizes the importance of using many herbs that are combined in different formulations for each patient.[65,66] This has become popular among some segments of the population. Both topical and systemic use of herbs has been administered to treat psoriasis, as well as a combination of herbal medications used with UVA; however, studies have not demonstrated the overall efficacy of these modalities.

PSORIATIC ARTHRITIS

CASE 41-3

QUESTION 1: R.T. is a 46-year-old male aerospace machinist with psoriasis and increasing joint complaints. He describes a flare-up during the last month involving predominantly the middle finger of his right hand. He also has arthralgias of the shoulders, knees, and the rest of his hands. Concomitantly, his skin disease has once again become active, despite nightly betamethasone dipropionate administration. He has a history of chronic depression and alcoholism, although he is currently sober and not being treated with antidepressant medications. Physical examination reveals a significant amount of tenderness of the right third metacarpophalangeal joint, without a great deal of active synovitis. He also has a moderate effusion of his right knee, but the rest of the joint examination is otherwise benign. Active psoriatic lesions are noted on his feet, knees, and elbows, and he has characteristic psoriatic nail changes. An erythrocyte sedimentation rate is mildly elevated. Which systemic therapy would be most appropriate to treat both R.T.'s skin and joint complaints?

Psoriatic arthritis (PsA) is a distinct form of inflammatory arthritis that is usually seronegative for rheumatoid factor. In various reports, 6% to 39% of patients with psoriasis experience PsA, and the prevalence is increased among patients with severe cutaneous disease.[13] Nail involvement occurs in greater than 80% of patients with PsA, as compared with 30% of patients with only cutaneous psoriasis.[13,67] Five clinical subsets of PsA have been identified: distal interphalangeal arthritis (classic; 5% to 10%, often accompanied by nail changes), arthritis mutilans (5%, starts in early age, accompanied by osteolysis with severe deformities of fingers and toes), symmetric polyarthritis (rheumatoid-like; <25% incidence, milder course), asymmetric oligoarthritis (most prevalent; 70%, proximal and distal interphalangeal joints, metacarpophalangeal joints, knee, and hip), and spondylitis (5% to 40%, often asymptomatic).

The presentation of R.T. is representative of asymmetric oligoarthritis. Traditionally, treatment of this form of PsA consists of an NSAID, local corticosteroid injections, and immunosuppressive agents, including TNF inhibitors. Despite scant clinical evidence of efficacy, NSAIDs are commonly used to suppress the musculoskeletal symptoms of PsA, but do not induce remissions.[67] Systemic corticosteroids are avoided because they destabilize psoriasis (transformation to pustular forms), induce resistance to other effective therapies, and re-exacerbate the skin disease during withdrawal.[68] PUVA and acitretin have negligible antiarthritic efficacy.

Methotrexate

Methotrexate is one of the most common agents used to produce symptomatic benefits (approximately 30%) in patients with PsA, but data on its efficacy to inhibit articular damage are limited.[68] TNF-α inhibitors have also been demonstrated to slow down or halt radiographic progression.[69] For mild joint disease, NSAIDs and intra-articular glucocorticoid injections may be adequate, whereas moderate to severe joint disease optimally will be treated with systemic oral disease-modifying antirheumatic drugs or biologics. After a sufficient trial of an NSAID, initiation of a second-line agent such as methotrexate before progression to a biologic intervention is a reasonable approach to manage R.T.'s arthralgias in his shoulders, knees, and hands, as well as his active skin disease.

After obtaining the history and physical examination, baseline laboratory tests should be obtained, which include a complete blood count, platelets, renal function tests (serum creatinine, BUN), liver function tests (LFTs: alanine aminotransferase, aspartate aminotransferase, alkaline phosphatase, bilirubin), HIV antibody determination, and a PPD. Although standard in the past for all patients about to receive methotrexate therapy, a baseline aspiration needle biopsy of the liver, not an innocuous procedure, is obtained currently only in those patients with pre-existing severe liver disease.[52] Patients with one or more risk factors for hepatic fibrosis (e.g., persistent abnormal liver chemistries, previous exposure to hepatotoxic agents, obesity, hyperlipidemia, diabetes mellitus, family history of inheritable liver disease, etc.) should receive a baseline liver biopsy and every 2 to 6 months until the drug's efficacy and lack of toxicity have been established. A repeat liver biopsy after 1.0 to 1.5 g of methotrexate have been received is appropriate as it is rare for life-threatening liver disease to develop at this lower cumulative dose.[70]

Therapy with methotrexate usually is initiated with a 2.5- to 5-mg test dose.[52] If no idiosyncratic reaction occurs, doses are gradually increased to a maintenance dose of 10 to 25 mg/week. Methotrexate is best given in a single weekly oral dose or in three 2.5- to 7.5-mg doses at 12-hour intervals during a 24-hour period (e.g., 8 AM, 8 PM, and again at 8 AM). With the introduction of biologic agents in the management of psoriasis and its associated conditions, an increased level of monitoring has developed. Hepatotoxicity, however, may not be apparent on routine laboratory evaluation. Every 4 to 12 weeks, LFTs should be obtained, preferably at least 1 week after the last methotrexate dose because these values are often elevated 1 to 2 days after therapy. If a significant abnormality in the LFTs is noted, therapy should be withheld for 1 to 2 weeks, and the LFT testing should be repeated. LFT values should return to normal in 1 to 2 weeks. If significantly abnormal LFTs persist for 2 to 3 months, a liver biopsy should be considered. As noted previously, a liver biopsy is recommended when the cumulative dosage level reaches 1.0 to 1.5 g, as well as after each subsequent 1.5-g increase in the cumulative dose. Liver function abnormalities may improve after cessation of methotrexate therapy for 6 months.

Immunomodulatory Therapy

CASE 41-3, QUESTION 2: During a follow-up visit to his family physician several months later, R.T. had several somatic complaints that led to a diagnosis of recurrent depression. Subsequent history reveals that he also has resumed use of alcohol. He tends to drink four to five beers a night on weekends or when he is feeling low, although he does admit that his level of alcohol use is sometimes higher. His skin lesions are relatively well controlled, but joint complaints have persisted. What additional options now exist for R.T.?

Methotrexate should be discontinued because the risks probably now exceed the benefits, particularly because rheumatic complaints have not been controlled and alcohol consumption has resumed. Agents such as methotrexate and cyclosporine may reduce inflammatory joint activity in the short-term, but evidence of their ability to modify the long-term disease process remains elusive. Close monitoring of the effects of these agents is also required because the toxicities often limit long-term use. R.T. should be referred for physical and occupational therapy, encouraged to exercise regularly, and if needed, referred for orthotics. An NSAID can be given for symptomatic relief. Sulfasalazine and hydroxychloroquine might be beneficial for mild joint symptoms alone, but the cutaneous manifestations may be controlled with topical agents. Other alternative second-line agents include immunomodulatory agents, anticytokines, TNF-α inhibitors, infliximab, and etanercept. In the case of R.T., it is clear that better therapies for PsA are necessary.

Immunomodulatory Agents

With advances in biotechnology immunomodulatory therapy, specifically the use of anticytokines, important treatment alternatives are becoming available for moderate to severe plaque psoriasis and PsA that is resistant to other systemic therapies. These agents are thought to target the immune-mediated and elevated levels of TNF found in psoriasis.

T-CELL AGENTS: ALEFACEPT AND EFALIZUMAB

Alefacept and efalizumab act as immunosuppressants mainly by inhibiting activation of T lymphocytes in plaques on the skin. The mechanism is by binding to CD2 on memory effector T lymphocytes (alefacept) or binding to a subunit of leukocyte function antigen-1 (efalizumab). Both agents are US Food and Drug Administration (FDA)-approved for the treatment of plaque psoriasis. Administered subcutaneously or intramuscularly on a weekly regimen, benefits include approximately 25% obtaining a PASI of 75 after 12 weeks of alefacept and 30% obtaining a PASI of 75 after 12 weeks of efalizumab when compared with placebo. Some patients have sustained clinical response even after cessation of therapy.[71] The most frequent short-term adverse effect of efalizumab is a flulike syndrome that occurs during the first 2 weeks of therapy. Alefacept is also effective in combination with NB-UVB phototherapy.[72] Because of immunosuppression, these agents are contraindicated in pregnancy or in patients already immunocompromised because of malignancy, infection, or medications. Monitoring includes complete blood counts monthly for the first 9 months and liver function tests at baseline and at 3 months.[73]

TNF-α INHIBITORS: INFLIXIMAB, ETANERCEPT, ADALIMUMAB, GOLIMUMAB, USTEKINUMAB

As a potent cytokine, TNF-α is involved in inflammation and joint damage. Inhibition of TNF-α reduces direct actions as well as the action of other proinflammatory cytokines. The TNF-α inhibitors, infliximab, etanercept, and adalimumab, are FDA-approved for the treatment of both plaque and PsA. Adalimumab and golimumab are approved only for PsA. Ustekinumab is approved only for moderate to severe plaque psoriasis. The mechanism of action of these agents is through blocking the interaction of TNF-α with cell-surface TNF receptors, and ustekinumab is a specific inhibitor of interleukin-12 (IL-12) and anti-interleukin-23 (IL-23).[74] Dosing is either subcutaneous injection (etanercept, adalimumab, golimumab, ustekinumab) or intravenous infusion (infliximab), on a biweekly, weekly, every other week, or monthly schedule during the initiation phase.

In a 24-week trial to assess the efficacy and safety of etanercept 50 mg administered once weekly in patients with moderate-to-severe plaque psoriasis, at week 12, 37.5% of patients achieved a PASI 75 response, with 71.1% achieving PASI 75 at week 24. No deaths, serious infections, opportunistic infections, demyelinating disorders, or malignancies were reported.[75]

Infliximab is a human/mouse chimeric anti-TNF-α antibody. One hundred eighty-six patients were given infliximab for moderate-to-severe plaque and nail psoriasis for 46 weeks. A PASI of 75% was demonstrated in 74.6% of patients and a PASI of 90% was demonstrated in 54.1% at week 50.[76] In spite of clinically significant improvements, induction of antinuclear antibodies and antidouble-stranded DNA antibodies is frequently observed in patients receiving infliximab. To investigate the development of autoimmunity in patients receiving infliximab for severe, recalcitrant forms of psoriasis, 28 patients with psoriasis refractory to three or more systemic treatments were given infliximab 5 mg/kg for 22 weeks.[77] Detection of antinuclear antibodies and of IgM and IgG antidouble-stranded DNA antibodies was performed at baseline and at week 22. The prevalence of positive detection of antinuclear antibodies increased from 12% at baseline to 72% at week 22, and was also observed for IgM antidouble-stranded DNA antibodies. Three patients exhibited nonerosive polyarthritis, without any other criteria for systemic lupus. This study suggests that the incidence of biological autoimmunity is high in patients with refractory psoriasis receiving infliximab.[77]

Pharmacotherapy with TNF-α inhibitors has the best number-needed-to-treat-to-benefit (NNTB) to number-needed-to-harm (NNTH) ratio of all disease-modifying antirheumatic drugs (DMARDs) in psoriatic arthritis, and is able to induce clinical remission in at least 30% of patients. Of interest, however, is that in many of these clinical studies, the NNTB presented comparisons with placebo. Many studies of TNF-α inhibitor therapies have allowed inclusion of patients who had not received other systemic therapies beyond topical therapies alone.[78] When interpreting the NNTB for TNF-α inhibitors, it is important to compare them with the NNTB for other systemic therapies. Also, having a comparable outcome measure (e.g., PASI 75) is necessary, especially because most established treatments have not been compared with placebo.[79]

For a patient like R.T., whose disease cannot be treated successfully or safely with methotrexate, proceeding with a TNF-α inhibitor remains an option. These agents produce rapid, well-tolerated, beneficial responses compared with placebo. Benefit is seen anywhere from 2 to 12 weeks with a PASI 75 being obtained in at least 80% of patients after 10 weeks of infliximab, at least 50% after 12 weeks of etanercept, and at least 50% after 48 weeks of adalimumab treatment.[80,81] R.T. does not have any contraindications to therapy, such as active infection or New York Heart Association (NYHA) class III or IV heart failure. If available, etanercept (25–50 mg subcutaneously twice weekly [3 or 4 days apart] for the first 3 months, followed by 50 mg once a week) may be preferred for convenience; however, in a recent comparative trial of ustekinumab (administered at weeks 0 and 4) and etanercept (administered twice weekly for 12 weeks), ustekinumab patients experienced a superior improvement in PASI 75 scores.[82]

Screening for tuberculosis before beginning therapy with anti-TNF agents is prudent, and those with evidence of prior tuberculous chest infection or with a positive skin test for tuberculosis should be offered prophylactic antitubercular therapy. If further studies continue to confirm long-term effectiveness and safety of the anti-TNF-α inhibitor therapies, then these may become the preferred treatments for patients with moderate to severe disease.

KEY REFERENCES AND WEBSITES

A full list of references for this chapter can be found at http://thepoint.lww.com/AT10e. Below are the key references and websites for this chapter, with the corresponding reference number in this chapter found in parentheses after the reference.

Key References

Gladman DD et al. Psoriatic arthritis: epidemiology, clinical features, course, and outcome. *Ann Rheum Dis*. 2005;64(Suppl 2):ii-14. (13)

Griffiths CEM, Barker JNWN. Pathogenesis and clinical features of psoriasis. *Lancet*. 2007;370:263. (2)

Laws PM, Young HS. Topical treatment of psoriasis. *Expert Opin Pharmacother*. 2010;11:1999. (24)

Leon A et al. An attempt to formulate an evidence-based strategy in the management of moderate to severe psoriasis: a review of the efficacy and safety of biologics and prebiologic options. *Expert Opin Pharmacother*. 2007;8:617. (37)

Mease PJ. Psoriatic arthritis: pharmacotherapy update. *Curr Rheumatol Rep*. 2010;12:272. (68)

Menter A et al. Guidelines of care for the management of psoriasis and psoriatic arthritis: section 5. Guidelines of care for the treatment of psoriasis with phototherapy and photochemotherapy. *J Am Acad Dermatol*. 2010;62:114. (40)

Naldi L. Scoring and monitoring the severity of psoriasis. What is the preferred method? What is the ideal method? Is PASI passé? Facts and controversies. *Clin Dermatol*. 2010;28:67. (19)

Pariser DM et al. National Psoriasis Foundation clinical consensus on disease severity. *Arch Dermatol*. 2007;143:239. (20)

Key Websites

American Academy of Dermatology Current Psoriasis Guidelines: http://www.aad.org/education-and-quality-care/clinical-guidelines/current-and-upcoming-guidelines

American Academy of Dermatology Current Psoriasis Pharmacotherapy Reviews: http://www.aad.org/skin-conditions/dermatology-a-to-z/psoriasis

Arthritis Foundation (psoriatic arthritis): http://www.arthritis.org/disease-center.php?disease_id = 21&df = definition

National Psoriasis Foundation: http://www.psoriasis.org

42 Photosensitivity, Photoaging, and Burn Injuries

Katherine R. Gerrald and Timothy J. Ives

CORE PRINCIPLES

	CHAPTER CASES
PHOTOSENSITIVITY	
1 Ultraviolet radiation (UVR) exposure has been linked to many adverse effects, including malignant melanoma.	**Case 42-1 (Questions 1, 2)**
2 Photoprotection encompasses all methods of UVR blocking, including sunscreens, protective clothing, and sunglasses. Sunscreens are widely used to prevent sunburn and reduce the incidence of premature aging and carcinogenesis, although clothing and avoiding direct sunlight offer greater protection.	**Case 42-1 (Questions 3–9)**
3 The use of tanning beds that use artificial ultraviolet A (UVA) has not been shown to reduce long-term damage to the skin or to provide protection from natural UVR. The use of tanning beds should be minimized, and adherence to Food and Drug Administration (FDA) recommendations on length of exposure should be encouraged.	**Case 42-2 (Questions 1, 2)**
4 Sunburn is a self-limiting condition, which is generally managed with symptomatic treatment including oral analgesics, topical analgesics, and topical anesthetics. Treatment beyond self-management is necessary if the sunburn is accompanied by constitutional symptoms, involves second- or third-degree burns, or is infected.	**Case 42-3 (Question 1)**
5 Phototoxicity and photoallergy are often drug- or chemical-induced reactions to UVR exposure and account for up to 8% of adverse drug reactions.	**Case 42-4 (Questions 1–3)**
PHOTOAGING	
1 Photodamaged skin is characterized as being wrinkled, yellowed, and sagging.	**Case 42-5 (Question 1)**
2 Topical retinoid therapy is most effective for patients 50 to 70 years of age with moderate to severe photoaging and for prophylactic use in patients undergoing the initial changes of photoaging.	**Case 42-5 (Questions 2–5)**
BURN INJURIES	
1 Most burn injuries are minor, and can be managed in ambulatory settings.	**Case 42-6 (Question 1)**
2 Major second- or third-degree burns should be immediately triaged to a health system with a multidisciplinary team that can adequately manage all of the potential complications.	**Case 42-6 (Question 1)**
3 Synthetic dressings and skin substitutes have expanded the options and the desired outcomes for recovery.	**Case 42-6 (Question 2)**

ULTRAVIOLET RADIATION (UVR) EXPOSURE

Incidence, Prevalence, and Epidemiology

Changing lifestyles have considerably increased human exposure to sunlight: more outdoor recreational activities, more emphasis on tanning, longer life spans, seasonal population shifts to the Sunbelt, and most recently, a nationwide emphasis on vitamin D deficiency. Epidemiologic evidence clearly implicates sunlight as a causative factor in many skin diseases, and public attitudes toward tanning and sun exposure have slowly begun to change. Squamous cell carcinoma (SCC) and basal cell carcinoma (BCC), which together account for more than half of all malignancies in the United States, are linked closely to exposure to ultraviolet radiation (UVR).[1] Malignant melanoma, the incidence of which has increased more than 100% in the last decade, most likely is linked to UVR exposure.[2] The American Cancer Society estimated that greater than 1 million of all skin cancers that were diagnosed in 2008 were preventable.[3] Sunburn, photoaging, immunologic changes in the skin, cataracts, photodermatoses, phototoxicity, and photoallergy are other commonly encountered photosensitivity reactions that occur after UVR exposure. Phototoxicity and photoallergy are often drug- or chemical-induced reactions to UVR exposure and account for up to 8% of adverse drug reactions.[4] The appropriate use of sunscreens or other photoprotective behaviors can help mitigate the incidence of the adverse effects of UVR.

Etiology

ULTRAVIOLET RADIATION SPECTRUM

Ultraviolet radiation, the primary inducer of photosensitivity reactions in humans, is divided into ranges according to the effects of the four primary wavelengths: UVA1 (340–400 nm), UVA2 (320–340 nm), UVB (290–320 nm), and UVC (200 to 290 nm) (Fig. 42-1, Table 42-1). UVA, with a wavelength of 320 to 400 nm, is closest in wavelength to visible light.[5] UVA radiation levels have small fluctuations during the day, and are present from sunrise to sunset every day, all year round, even in the winter and on cloudy days. UVA is considerably less likely than a comparable dose of UVB to cause a similar degree of erythema.[6,7] In contrast to UVB, UVA penetrates to the dermal layer and may cause harmful effects not caused by UVB.[5] About 10 to 100 times more UVA reaches the earth's surface than UVB. Consequently, UVA may contribute up to 15% of the erythemal response at midday.[5,8] UVB is the most erythemogenic and melanogenic of the three UVR bands.[5,9] Up to 90% of UVB is blocked by the earth's stratospheric ozone layer, and it is absorbed completely by the epidermal layer of the skin.[10,11] In addition, UVB radiation can alter the immune system,[11] thereby increasing the incidence of certain cancers, including skin cancers. The only known beneficial effect of UVR in humans is exposure to small amounts of UVB, most commonly through sunlight, which converts 7-dehydrocholesterol to cholecalciferol (vitamin D_3). Vitamin D enhances calcium homeostasis and has direct and indirect effects

TABLE 42-1
Types of Ultraviolet Radiation and Characteristics

Radiation	Wavelength (nm)	Characteristics
UVA1 (long UVA; long-wave radiation)	340–400	Not absorbed by the ozone layer Passes through glass Produces some tanning, photoaging, and skin cancers Lower carcinogenic potential than UVA2, but harmful over long-term exposure Levels remain relatively constant throughout the day
UVA2 (short UVA)	320–340	Similar characteristics to UVA1, but greater carcinogenic potential with erythema production similar to UVB
UVB (sunburn range of radiation)	290–320	Partially absorbed by the ozone layer before reaching earth Does not pass through glass Causes erythema, sunburn, tanning, wrinkling, photoaging, skin cancers Daily and seasonal variation, with highest intensity at noon

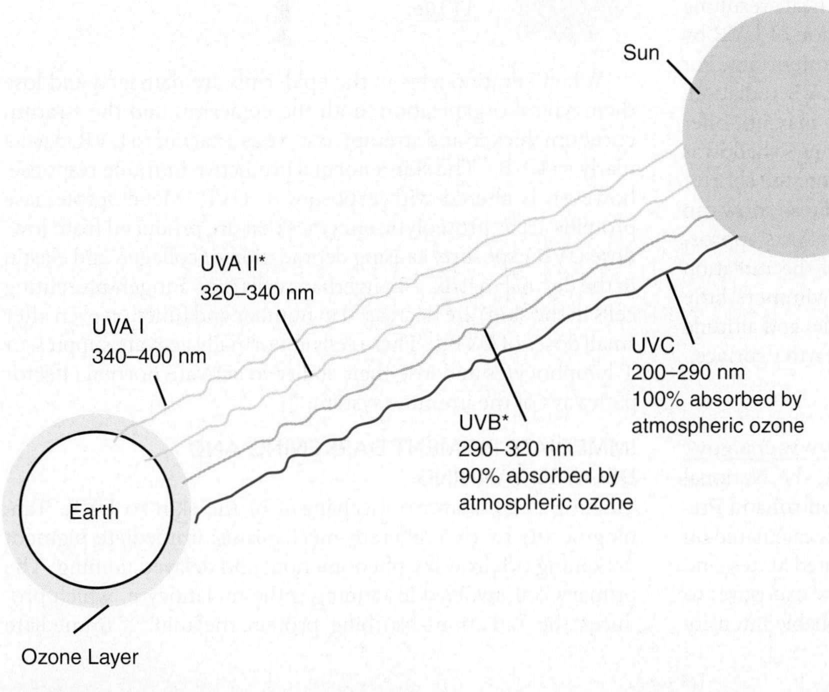

FIGURE 42-1 Ultraviolet radiation (UVR) spectrum. *Erythrogenic and melanogenic bands of UVR.

on cells involved with bone remodeling. As a result, vitamin D can decrease the risk of rickets in childhood and fractures and osteomalacia in adults.[12]

The UVC wavelengths are absorbed completely by the earth's stratospheric ozone layer. Artificial sources of UVC have been used in the sterilization and preservation of food and in minimizing bacterial growth in laboratories and hospital operating rooms by germicidal lamps, which can cause erythema or cataracts if mishandled.[5,9]

ENVIRONMENTAL EFFECTS ON UVR

OZONE AND CHLOROFLUOROCARBONS

The amount of UVR that reaches the earth's surface is influenced by many factors. Concern has been focused on the implications of depletion of the ozone layer.[8,13] In the decade after this effect was first detected in 1983, ozone levels above the Antarctic had fallen to 50% of normal.[13] In the early 1990s, worldwide estimates from the Environmental Protection Agency (EPA) predicted that for every 1% decrease in ozone, UVB radiation reaching the earth's surface would increase by 2% per year, possibly resulting in a 1% to 3% increase per year in nonmelanoma skin cancer.[14] These losses in the ozone layer are thought to be caused by man-made pollutants, e.g., nitrous oxides from jet airliners in stratospheric aviation and chlorofluorocarbons (CFCs) as propellants and refrigerants. The effect of the ban on the commercial use of CFCs by many of the industrialized nations is being seen, as evidenced by a slow decline in these ozone-depleting compounds.[14] Further, all the major emitters of greenhouse gases (GHGs) have agreed under the Copenhagen Accord that global average temperature increase should be kept below 2°C.[15] As GHGs contribute to ozone depletion, and because UVA is only slightly filtered by the ozone layer, any decrease in the ozone layer would result in a disproportionate increase in UVB reaching the earth.

TIME OF DAY, CLOUD COVER, AND SURFACE REFLECTION

The time of day influences the amount of UVR reaching the earth's surface; 20% to 30% of the total daily UVR is received from 11 AM to 1 PM, with 75% between 9 AM and 3 PM. Cloud cover can decrease UV intensity by 10% to 80% and decreases infrared radiation to an even greater extent. This greater attenuation of infrared radiation by cloud cover can lead to an increased risk of UVR overexposure because less infrared radiation will be absorbed by the body and transformed into heat, resulting in less warning of overexposure to UVR. Reflection of UVR by substances (e.g., sand, water, snow) also may be important. For example, sand reflects about 25% of incident UVB radiation; therefore, sitting under an umbrella at the beach may not offer adequate protection. In general, whenever someone's shadow is shorter than his or her height, care should be taken; the shorter the shadow, the more likely a sunburn will occur. Fresh snow can reflect 50% to 95% of incident sunlight. Water reflects approximately 5% of erythemal UVR, whereas 75% of the radiation is transmitted through 2 m of water, offering swimmers little protection.[5] Seasonal changes, geographic latitude, and altitude also influence the amount of UVR reaching the earth's surface.

UV INDEX

The UV Index/Global UV Index (**http://www.epa.gov/sunwise/uvindex.html**), developed by the EPA, the National Weather Service, and the Centers for Disease Control and Prevention, is a public health education service that is calculated on a next-day basis for every ZIP code across the United States, and worldwide.[16] This index, with a scale from 1 (low exposure) to 11+ (extremely high exposure), forecasts the probable intensity of skin-damaging UVR expected to reach the surface during the noon hour when the sun is highest in the sky. Theoretically, the UV Index can range from 0 (e.g., during the night) to 15 or 16 (in the tropics at high elevations under clear skies). The higher the UV Index, the greater the dose received of skin- and eye-damaging UVR, and the less time it takes before skin damage occurs.

The amount of UVR exposure needed to damage an individual's skin is affected by the elevation of the sun in the sky, the amount of ozone in the stratosphere, and the amount of clouds present. Clear skies transmit 100% of UVR to the earth's surface, with scattered clouds transmitting 89%, broken clouds, 73%, and overcast clouds, 32%. The darker an individual's skin tone, the longer (or the more UVR) it takes to cause erythema.

Pathophysiology

ERYTHEMA, SUNBURN, AND TANNING

ERYTHEMA AND OXYGEN FREE RADICALS

Excessive exposure of the epidermal and dermal layers of the skin to UVR can result in an inflammatory erythematous reaction. Excess UVA and UVB causes the release of vasodilatory mediators (e.g., histamine, prostaglandins, cytokines), resulting in increased blood flow, erythema, tissue exudates, swelling, increased sensation of warmth, and a characteristic sunburn.[5,9] Severe UVR exposure, primarily UVB, can cause blister formation, desquamation, fever, chills, weakness, and shock. Erythema caused by UVB begins within 3 to 5 hours after exposure, is maximal after 12 to 24 hours, and usually resolves during the ensuing 3 days.[9] In contrast, erythema caused by UVA begins immediately, plateaus between 6 and 12 hours, and remains for 24 hours. UVA-induced changes in the dermis are characterized by greater damage to the vasculature and dense cellular infiltrates that penetrate to deeper levels of the skin.[9] The dermis also may be damaged when endogenous components of the skin absorb UVR energy and subsequently interact with oxygen to form tissue-damaging oxygen free radicals.[11]

HISTOLOGY OF SUNBURN

The skin undergoes adaptive changes in response to UVR exposure.

ONLINE CONTENT

For a visual of skin response to ultraviolet radiation, go to http://thepoint.lww.com/AT10e.

When keratinocytes in the epidermis are damaged and lose their typical organization, both the epidermis and the stratum corneum thicken and attempt to serve as a barrier to UVR, particularly to UVB.[8] The skin's normal protective immune response, however, is altered with exposure to UVR. Metalloproteinase proteins act as proteolytic enzymes that are produced from low-dose UVR exposure, causing degradation of collagen and elastin in the dermal matrix.[17] Langerhans cells (i.e., antigen-presenting cells in the skin) are decreased in number and function even after small doses of UVB.[17] These cells abnormally activate suppressor T lymphocytes and lose their ability to activate normal effector pathways of the immune system.[18]

IMMEDIATE PIGMENT DARKENING AND DELAYED TANNING

Tanning is an adaptive mechanism of the skin to UVR. Tanning occurs by two different mechanisms: immediate pigment darkening (Meirowsky phenomenon) and delayed tanning. The primary cell involved in tanning is the melanocyte, which produces the radiation-absorbing protein melanin.[5,8] Immediate pigment darkening begins during the actual exposure to UVA and certain bands of visible light,[5,8] and the oxidation of existing melanin in the epidermis transiently turns the skin grayish brown. The degree of immediate pigment darkening depends on the duration and intensity of exposure, the extent of previous tanning (or amount of pre-existing melanin), and the skin type of the individual.[5] Immediate pigment darkening is not protective against UVB erythema.[8]

Delayed tanning occurs 48 to 72 hours after exposure to either UVA or UVB. It is most intense 7 to 10 days after UV exposure and can last for weeks to months.[5] Delayed tanning is the result of increased production of melanin, an increase in the size of dendritic processes, increased melanization of melanosomes, and an increase in the rate of transfer of melanosomes (particulate bodies of melanin) to keratinocytes.[5,8] The keratinocyte, now pigmented with melanosomes, migrates to the epidermis, producing the characteristic suntan. Delayed tanning caused by UVA is less protective against sunburn than delayed tanning caused by UVB, as epidermal thickening is not induced by UVA.[5]

PHOTOCARCINOGENESIS

SQUAMOUS CELL AND BASAL CELL CARCINOMA

The association of skin cancer in humans to UVR exposure is based primarily on clinical and epidemiologic evidence. Nonmelanoma skin cancers, such as SCC and BCC, occur most commonly on areas that are maximally exposed to sunlight (e.g., the face, neck, arms, back of the forearms, and hands).[5] The prevalence of nonmelanoma skin cancers is inversely related to geographic distance from the equator and to the melanin content of the skin, with SCC more strongly linked than BCC to UVR.[5,19] Persons of skin types most sensitive to sunlight, as well as persons working outdoors, have higher incidences of nonmelanoma skin cancers.[5] A family history of SCC and BCC increases the risk at least twofold, depending on the histology, number of lesions, and degree of invasiveness.[20] Albinism, a genetic disease characterized by partial or total absence of pigment in the skin, hair, and eyes, is associated with increased and premature development of skin cancers.[5]

ONLINE CONTENT

For visuals showing squamous cell carcinoma of the lip, nodular basal cell carcinoma, and malignant melanoma, go to <u>http://thepoint.lww.com/AT10e.</u>

CUTANEOUS MALIGNANT MELANOMA

The development of cutaneous malignant melanoma (CMM) also may be linked to UVR exposure, specifically exposures that induce sunburn. A history of five or more severe sunburns during adolescence more than doubles the risk of CMM.[19] Similarly to nonmelanoma skin cancers, CMM demonstrates an inverse relationship to geographic distance from the equator and melanin content of the skin.[5] Unlike nonmelanoma skin cancers, however, CMM does not demonstrate a clear relationship to the cumulative dose of UVR, and it occurs on areas of the body exposed to the sun intermittently (e.g., on the back in men and the lower legs in women). In addition, it occurs most commonly in the middle-aged population and in individuals who work indoors, as well as in those whose sun exposure is limited to weekends and vacations.[19] A family history of melanoma is a strong risk factor for melanoma as 8% to 12% of melanoma patients display a familial propensity for the disease.[21]

ONLINE CONTENT

For a visual showing types of skin cancer, go to <u>http://thepoint.lww.com/AT10e.</u>

MECHANISMS OF CARCINOGENESIS

Mechanisms of carcinogenesis may include damage to DNA and alterations in immunologic status. Epidermal and dermal DNA can absorb UVR, which can contribute to abnormal formation of pyrimidine dimers. Under normal circumstances, these dimers are excised and repaired; however, if left uncorrected, these DNA lesions, as well as an inactivity of p53 tumor suppressor gene activity, can lead to interruption of transcription, with possible mutagenesis and malignancy.[22]

PHOTOEFFECTS ON THE EYE

Age-related opacification of the ocular lens, or senescent cataracts, has been attributed to a lifetime of exposure to sunlight. The incidence of cataracts increases steadily after age 50, reaching nearly 30% in individuals older than 74.[23] UVB is absorbed by the cornea and lens, which slowly results in protein oxidation and precipitation within the lens. UVA penetrates the ocular lens and can cause cumulative damage to deeper structures of the eye. Decreased transmittance and increased scattering of light by the opacified lens eventually result in blurred vision, rings or halos around lights, changes in color perception, and blindness.[24] In advanced cases, the only treatment is surgical removal of the cataract.

High exposure of the eye to UVR (which can range from a few seconds of exposure to arc welding, a few minutes of exposure to a UVC-emitting germicidal lamp, commercial tanning, or UVR reflection by snow or sand) can cause conjunctivitis or photokeratitis, a painful inflammation of the cornea. Photokeratitis usually begins 30 minutes to 24 hours after the exposure, and time to onset depends on the intensity of the exposure.[25] Conjunctivitis commonly accompanies photokeratitis and is characterized by the sensation of a foreign body or grit in the eyes. Varying degrees of photophobia, lacrimation, and blepharospasm also may accompany photokeratitis.[25] Because the corneal epithelium has a great regenerative capacity, photokeratitis tends to be transient, with regression in 24 to 48 hours. Treatment consists of cool, wet compresses and mild anti-inflammatory analgesics, such as ibuprofen, aspirin, or naproxen sodium.

PHOTOTOXICITY AND PHOTOALLERGY

The most common type of drug-induced photosensitivity reaction is phototoxicity, which is an immediate or delayed inflammatory reaction that occurs when a compound with photosensitizing ability absorbs a sufficient concentration of UVR in or on the skin, and when the skin is exposed simultaneously to a specific wavelength of light.[26] When the offending agent is deposited on the skin surface, it is thought to act as a chromophore, absorbing UVR. When the chromophore reaches a sufficient concentration in or on the skin and when the skin is exposed to the appropriate wavelength of UVR, energy is emitted and transferred to the surrounding molecules, which damages the adjacent tissue to cause a phototoxic reaction. The wavelength of radiation necessary to produce such a reaction depends on the absorption spectrum of the offending agent.[27]

Photoallergy results from a similar mechanism to phototoxicity, except that the immune system is involved. Most commonly, it is caused by polycyclic photosensitizers that react with UVA to form antigenic macromolecules, evoking a delayed hypersensitivity response. In photoallergic photosensitivity reactions, the suspected medication or chemical agent is altered in the presence of UVR to become antigenic or to become a hapten (i.e., an incomplete antigen), which can combine with a tissue antigen. These antigen-antibody or immune-mediated processes differentiate photoallergic from phototoxic reactions. Photoallergic reactions do not occur on first exposure to the medication, but as with other allergic reactions, they require prior or prolonged exposure (sensitization period) to the offending agent.[26] Once sensitization has occurred, subsequent exposure to even small amounts of the offending product will produce a photoallergic reaction.

Photoprotection

Photoprotection encompasses all methods of UVR blocking, including sunscreens, protective clothing, and sunglasses. Sunscreens are widely used to prevent sunburn and reduce the incidence of premature aging and carcinogenesis,[28–30] although clothing and avoiding direct sunlight offer greater protection. Sunburn preventive agents are those active ingredients that absorb greater than 95% of UVB radiation, and have the potential to prevent sunburn. Suntanning agents are those with active ingredients that absorb 85% to 95% of UVB radiation, thereby allowing suntanning without significant sunburn in the average individual. Chemical sunscreens include both of the aforementioned designations. Opaque sunblocks, or physical sunscreens, are those active ingredients that reflect or scatter all UVA, UVB, and visible light, thereby preventing or minimizing sunburn and suntanning.[31] The original formulations were developed to protect against the effects of UVB radiation before adverse effects of UVA were recognized. Because UVA plays a significant role in many of the adverse effects associated with UVR exposure, broad-spectrum sunscreen products with absorption spectra in the UVA range have become commercially available, in combination with UVB absorbers. These broad-spectrum products provide additional benefit for patients with photosensitivity reactions caused by wavelengths not covered by single-ingredient sunscreens. Table 42-2 lists the available sunscreen chemicals that have been judged to be both safe and effective.

There is a clear association between UV exposure and the development of BCC and SCC,[32] and limiting UV exposure by starting sunscreen use during childhood is key to reducing the lifetime risk of nonmelanoma skin cancers; however, some investigators have suggested that sunscreen use, through increased UV exposure, may actually cause melanoma, perhaps because its use allows for a longer exposure to the sun,[33,34] and because historically there was a lack of UVA protection in most products.[35] Sunscreen use has been thought to be associated with the occurrence of nevi (pigmented moles), an important risk factor for melanoma development[36]; however, epidemiologic analyses have refuted this proposed association, largely on the basis of a longer exposure to UVR and less protective clothing in individuals who developed nevi.[37,38]

TABLE 42-2
Sunscreens and UVR Absorption

Sunscreen	Absorption
Anthranilates	
Meradimate (menthyl anthranilate)	260–380
Benzophenones	
Dioxybenzone	250–390
Oxybenzone (benzophenone-3)	270–350
Sulisobenzone (Eusolex 4360)	260–375
Cinnamates	
Cinoxate (diethanolamine *p*-methoxycinnamate)	280–310
Octocrylene	250–360
Octinoxate (octyl methoxycinnamate, Parsol MCX)	290–320
Dibenzoylmethanes	
Avobenzone (butyl methoxydibenzoylmethane, Parsol 1789)	320–400
Aminobenzoic Acid and Ester Derivatives	
Para-aminobenzoic acid (PABA)	260–313
Padimate O (octyl dimethyl PABA)	290–315
Salicylates	
Homosalate	295–315
Octisalate (octyl salicylate)	280–320
Trolamine salicylate	260–320
Camphor Derivatives	
Ecamsule (terephthalylidene dicamphor sulfonic acid; Mexoryl)	290–400
Others	
Ensulizole (phenylbenzimidazole sulfonic acid)	290–340
Physical Sunscreens	
Titanium dioxide	290–700
Zinc oxide	290–700

UVR, ultraviolet radiation.

Clinical Application of Photosensitivity

SKIN TYPES

CASE 42-1

QUESTION 1: R.J., a 26-year-old woman, and her husband J.J., 28 years old, are spending a week in August vacationing on the Outer Banks of North Carolina with their two children, P.J., a 6-month-old girl, and L.J., an 18-month-old boy. They have plans for time at the beach, bicycling, and sailing. They come to your pharmacy to inquire about sunscreens for the trip. R.J. has a light brown complexion with brown hair and brown eyes, and J.J. has fair complexion with blond hair and blue eyes. On first exposure to the sun with about an hour of intense midday sunlight, J.J. almost always develops a deep red, painful sunburn, with only minimal subsequent tanning. He freckles easily when exposed to sunlight and remembers being severely sunburned on several occasions as a child. When R.J. is first exposed to the sun in the summer, she usually develops mild erythema, followed by moderate tanning. She cannot recall being severely sunburned as a child, but does recall becoming moderately tanned each summer as a child and adolescent. R.J. is employed as a receptionist for an accounting firm, and J.J. is a lawyer for a local law firm. Both spend considerable amounts of time participating in outdoor activities. Using subjective and objective data in this history, determine the skin types of R.J. and J.J. to guide you to a recommendation of a sunscreen product.

One of the most important pieces of information to include in the patient history is the patient's skin type.[39] Patients can be classified into six sun-reactive skin types based on their response to initial sun exposure, skin color, tendency to sunburn, ability to tan, and personal history of sunburn (Table 42-3). This skin typing system is used by the US Food and Drug Administration (FDA) in its guidelines for sunscreen agents. J.J.'s fair complexion, propensity to sunburn, and minimal tanning classify him as skin type II. R.J.'s light brown complexion, minimal sunburn reaction, and moderate tanning classify her as skin type IV.

Hair and eye colors also provide an indication to skin reactiveness to sunlight. People who have blond, red, or light brown hair or blue or green eyes tend to have greater skin reactivity to sunlight than people with darker-colored hair or eyes. A history of severe sunburn also can be associated with skin reactivity to sunlight, although self-reported patient histories of sunburn or

TABLE 42-3
Suggested SPF for Various Skin Types

Complexion	Skin Type	Skin Characteristics	Suggested Product SPF
Very fair	I	Always burns easily; never tans	20–30
Fair	II	Always burns easily; tans minimally	15–20
Light	III	Burns moderately; tans gradually	10–15
Medium	IV	Burns minimally; always tans well	8–10
Dark	V	Rarely burns; tans profusely	8
Very dark	VI	Never burns; deeply pigmented	8

SPF, sun protection factor.

tanning may not be consistently reliable and personal interviews may be a better indicator. J.J.'s propensity to freckle and his history of severe sunburns as a child may give an indication as to his skin's sun reactiveness. Other important information to consider in the patient before recommending a certain product is medication history, history of sun-reactive dermatoses, history of allergies (particularly contact hypersensitivities to cosmetics or other topical agents), and the intended activities during sunscreen use.

RISK FACTORS

CASE 42-1, QUESTION 2: R.J. and J.J. exhibit several risk factors that place them at risk for the long-term adverse effects of UVR. What are the risk factors for these long-term adverse effects of UVR?

The long-term effects of UVR include photocarcinogenesis and premature aging of the skin (photoaging). The associated risks for development of these long-term effects are directly related to the congenital pigmentation of an individual (which includes skin type and hair and eye color) and intensity, duration, and frequency of exposure to UVR. With skin type II, J.J. is at high risk for carcinogenesis and photoaging, whereas R.J., with skin type IV, may be at a lower risk. Excessive sun exposure, especially during early childhood, increases the risk of nonmelanoma and melanoma skin cancers. During the first 18 years of life, the average child receives three times the dose of UVB of the average adult; consequently, most sun exposure occurs during childhood.[22,40,41] A history of frequent sunburn or intermittent high-intensity exposures to UVR may be associated with the occurrence of malignant melanoma, whereas large cumulative doses of UVR during a lifetime may contribute to the incidence of nonmelanoma skin cancers. J.J.'s history of several severe sunburns as a child may more than double his risk of CMM.[40,41] Cumulative doses of UVR received unintentionally from working outdoors or from participating in outdoor recreational activities also can contribute significantly to the risk of photocarcinogenesis and photoaging.[6] A large number of moles, congenital moles more than 1.5 cm wide, and abnormal moles also appear to be a risk factor for malignant melanoma.[19] Risk for skin cancer is increased among first-degree relatives of patients with skin cancer[42] because frequent sunburns, suboptimal sunscreen use, and high rates of tanning bed use are common among children with a personal or family history of skin cancer.[43]

PHOTOPROTECTION

Sun Protection Factor

CASE 42-1, QUESTION 3: Before deciding on the exact product for R.J., J.J., and their children, R.J. and J.J. want to know how to differentiate among products and how to interpret the SPF of a product. How will you explain this to them?

The effectiveness of a sunscreen formulation is based on its SPF and its substantivity.[44] SPF is a measure of how much solar energy (UV radiation) is required to produce sunburn on protected skin (i.e., in the presence of sunscreen) relative to the amount of solar energy required to produce sunburn on unprotected skin. As the SPF value increases, sunburn protection increases. It is defined as the ratio of the minimal dose of UVR required to produce an erythemal response in sunscreen-protected skin compared with unprotected skin.[28] The SPF is based on tests of volunteers with skin types I through III, using either natural sunlight or a solar simulator that generates both UVB and UVA.[28,44] Because the SPF can be influenced by the composition, chemical properties, emollient properties, and pH of the vehicle, sunscreen formulations must be evaluated on an individual basis.[44] SPF also is influenced by the amount applied to the skin, the time of initial application before UVR exposure, the frequency of application, and environmental factors, such as photodegradation during UVR exposure; therefore, the SPF achieved during actual use can be significantly less than indicated on the label.[45–49] Consumers have been shown to routinely apply only one-fourth to one-half thickness of the layer of sunscreen used to determine the SPF before marketing.[50]

A popular misconception is that SPF relates to time of solar exposure. For example, many people believe that if they normally get sunburn in 1 hour, then an SPF 15 sunscreen allows them to stay in the sun for 15 hours (i.e., 15 times longer) without getting sunburn. This is untrue because SPF is not directly related to time of solar exposure, but to the amount of solar exposure. Although solar energy amount is related to solar exposure time, other factors have an impact on the amount of solar energy. For example, the intensity of the solar energy has an impact on the amount. Generally, it takes less time to be exposed to the same amount of solar energy at midday compared with early morning or late evening because the sun is more intense at midday relative to other times. The following exposures may result in the same amount of solar energy: 1 hour at 9 AM versus 15 minutes at 1 PM. Solar intensity is also related to geographic location, with greater solar intensity occurring at lower latitudes. Also, as clouds absorb solar energy, solar intensity is generally greater on clear days than on cloudy days.

In 1978, the FDA Over-the-Counter (OTC) Review Panel on sunscreens reclassified sunscreens from cosmetics to drugs intended to protect the structure and function of the human integument against actinic damage. In 1999, the FDA finalized its original regulations for OTC sunscreens (available at **http://www.fda.gov/downloads/Drugs/DevelopmentApprovalProcess/DevelopmentResources/Over-the-CounterOTCDrugs/Statusof-OTCRulemakings/ucm090244.pdf**). The 1999 regulations list the active ingredients that can be used in sunscreens and labeling and testing requirements, and also provide for uniform, streamlined labeling for all OTC products intended for use as sunscreens to assist consumers in making decisions on sun protection. These regulations include the following:

- Similar labeling requirements for all OTC products intended for use as sunscreens (including sunscreen–cosmetic combinations, such as makeup products carrying sun protection claims) to provide good, useful information to consumers.

- Uniform, streamlined labeling for all sunscreens. Accommodations in labeling must be made for sunscreens that are labeled for use only on specific small areas of the face (e.g., lips, nose, ears, or around eyes).
- Both required and optional label claims, warnings, and directions.
- Required SPF testing for all agents.
- A "Sun Alert" statement that reflects the important role that sunscreens play in a total program to reduce the harmful effects of the sun (i.e., "Sun alert: Limiting sun exposure, wearing protective clothing, and using sunscreens may reduce the risks of skin aging, skin cancer, and other harmful effects of the sun").
- Cessation of unsupported, absolute, or misleading and confusing terms such as *sun block, waterproof, all-day protection, deep tanning,* and *visible and/or infrared light protection.*

In addition to the aforementioned changes, cosmetic regulations require tanning preparations that do not contain a sunscreen ingredient to display the following warning: "Warning—this product does not contain a sunscreen and does not protect against sunburn. Repeated exposure of unprotected skin while tanning may increase the risk of skin aging, skin cancer, and other harmful effects to the skin even if you do not burn."

In 2006, the FDA introduced further regulations on sunscreen labeling. The term *sunscreen* was redefined: "A product with active ingredients to affect the structure or function of the body by absorbing, reflecting, or scattering the harmful, burning rays of the sun, thereby altering the normal physiological response to solar radiation." These ingredients also help to prevent diseases such as sunburn and may reduce the chance of premature skin aging, skin cancer, and other harmful effects attributable to the sun when used in conjunction with limiting sun exposure and wearing protective clothing. Sunscreen ingredients may also be used in some products for nontherapeutic, nonphysiologic uses (e.g., as a color additive or to protect the color of the product). Further, for sunscreen products that retain SPF after 40 minutes of activity in the water, sweating, or perspiring, the term *water resistant* is used. For products that retain SPF activity after 80 minutes, the term *very water resistant* is allowed. Further, the following phrases may be used for sunscreen products: *reapply as needed or after towel drying, swimming, or sweating* (or *perspiring*).

In 2007, the FDA proposed a new amendment to its original regulations that sets standards for formulating, testing, and labeling sunscreen products.[51] The goal of this proposed rule is to improve the current rating system for sunscreens and to improve consumer understanding of the rating system. In this amendment, the FDA recommends changing "SPF" to "UVB SPF" and to add a UVA rating system for products. This UVA rating system uses one to four stars (one star indicating low UVA protection and four stars indicating high UVA protection). If the product does not rate at least one star, then it would have to bear a "no UVA protection" marking on the front label. This star rating system would appear next to the currently used SPF rating. Similar tests to what are currently used to determine SPF ratings would be conducted to determine UVA ratings. One would measure the product's ability to reduce UVA radiation that passes through it, and the second would measure the product's ability to prevent tanning. Under the new rule, the FDA would now validate SPF ratings up to 50 and require manufacturers to label products with SPF over 50 as 50+ to avoid misleading assurance of protection. Currently, the FDA only validates SPF ratings up to 30; however, several products currently marketed have SPFs of greater than 30 and up to 100+. Additionally, this amendment would include a new warning statement on all products, saying "UV exposure from the sun increases the risk of skin cancer, premature skin aging, and other skin damage. It is important to decrease UV exposure by limiting time in the sun, wearing protective clothing, and using a sunscreen." As of late 2010, this proposed amendment has not yet been finalized.

Evaluation of Sunscreens

Substantivity is a measure of the sunscreen formulation's effectiveness. The substantivity of a sunscreen formulation is its ability to be absorbed by, or adhere to, the skin while swimming or perspiring. In the past, labeling of a product as "waterproof" or "water-resistant" indicated that the SPF of the product was maintained after 80 minutes of moderate activity or 40 minutes while swimming, respectively. Because testing is performed indoors under close to ideal conditions (e.g., lower humidity), the effects of the actual environment where it is used and the evaporation of the vehicle may reduce considerably the overall effectiveness of the sunscreen. The substantivity of a product largely depends on the vehicle, as well as the active ingredient (Table 42-4).[52] The affinity of a sunscreen to the keratinaceous layer of the stratum corneum is directly related to the keratin or vehicle partition coefficient. The saturation of the active agent in keratin depends on the drug's lipophilicity, whereas its substantivity is independent of its lipophilicity. Sunscreen compounds with a high solubility in the product's vehicle penetrate the skin most easily. Classically, vehicles such as water-in-oil emulsions or ointments tend to have a higher degree of substantivity. Some of the newer products have improved substantivity with the addition of a polymer, such as polyacrylamide, to the formulation.

Molar Absorptivity, Absorption Spectrum, and Photostability

The molar absorptivity and absorption spectrum determine the effectiveness of an individual sunscreen agent, mostly by its chemical structure. *Molar absorptivity* is a measure of the amount of UVR absorbed by a particular sunscreen, and it depends on the concentration of the sunscreen in the product and the amount applied to the skin. Sunscreens with an absorption spectrum in the UVB range, with a maximal absorption between 310 and 320 nm, are the most effective at preventing a sunburn.[44] Sunscreens with absorption spectra in the UVB range are para-aminobenzoic acid (PABA) and its esters, cinnamates, and the salicylates. Sunscreens with absorption spectra that extend into the UVA range are the anthranilates (e.g., meradimate), dibenzoylmethanes (e.g., azobenzene), and benzophenones (e.g., oxybenzone). *Photostability* means the ability to stabilize under sunlight. The process of photostability is a key factor in sunscreen protection efficacy. High photostability means the sunscreen will maintain a higher UVA protective barrier longer, and not degrade as quickly as other UVA filters when exposed to the sun.

Table 42-2 shows the 17 ingredients that act as sunscreens currently approved in the United States, along with their FDA-allowable maximal concentration and absorption spectrum.

CHEMICAL ORGANIC SUNSCREENS

Chemical organic sunscreens are compounds capable of absorbing UVR, thereby protecting the skin structures from the adverse effects of the selective wavelengths absorbed.[28] After application to the skin, these aromatic compounds convert the high UVR energy into harmless longer-wave radiation, which may or may

TABLE 42-4
Examples of Commercially Available Sunscreen Products

Name (Active Ingredients)	Formulation	SPF
Anthelios SX (avobenzone, ecamsule, octocrylene)	Cream	15
Banana Boat Baby Sunblock (octinoxate, octisalate, homosalate, titanium dioxide)	Lotion	50
Banana Boat Sport Sun Gear Sunblock (avobenzone, homosalate, octocrylene, oxybenzone, octisalate)	Lotion	50
Banana Boat Kids Quik Blok (octinoxate, homosalate, octisalate, oxybenzone, avobenzone)	Lotion	25+
Banana Boat Sport Sunblock (octinoxate, octisalate, oxybenzone, octocrylene)	Lotion	50
Blistex Ultra Protection (homosalate, meradimate, octinoxate, octisalate, oxybenzone)	Lip balm	30
Blue Lizard Australian Suncream (octinoxate, octocrylene, oxybenzone, zinc oxide)	Lotion	30+
Bullfrog Superblock (octocrylene, octinoxate, oxybenzone)	Lotion	45
Bullfrog for Kids (octocrylene, octinoxate, oxybenzone, octisalate, titanium dioxide, meradimate)	Gel	36
Bullfrog Extreme Sport (octocrylene, octinoxate, octisalate, oxybenzone)	Lotion	30
Bullfrog Sunblock (octinoxate, oxybenzone, octisalate, octocrylene)	Gel	36
ChapStick (padimate O)	Lip balm	15
ChapStick Ultra (octocrylene, octinoxate, oxybenzone, octisalate)	Lip balm	30
ChapStick Sunblock (oxybenzone, padimate O)	Lip balm, or ointment	15
Coppertone BUG & SUN for Adults (with DEET; octocrylene, octinoxate, oxybenzone)	Lotion	30
Coppertone KIDS Quick Cover Sunblock (avobenzone, octocrylene, octisalate, oxybenzone, homosalate)	Lotion/Spray	50
Coppertone Sport (octinoxate, oxybenzone, octisalate)	Lotion	15/30/50
Coppertone Ultra Sheer Faces (avobenzone, homosalate, octisalate, octocrylene, oxybenzone)	Lotion	30
DuraScreen (octinoxate, octisalate, oxybenzone, ensulizole, titanium dioxide)	Lotion/Stick	15, 30
Eau Thermale Avene (titanium dioxide, zinc oxide)	Cream	25, 50
Hawaiian Tropic Ozone (octocrylene, oxybenzone, avobenzone)	Lotion	70
Hawaiian Tropic Kids (avobenzone, octocrylene, oxybenzone)	Lotion	60+
Hawaiian Tropic 45 Plus Sunblock (octinoxate, octisalate, titanium dioxide)	Lotion	45
Neutrogena MoistureShine Lip Soother (octinoxate, oxybenzone)	Lip balm	20
Neutrogena Healthy Defense Oil-Free Sunblock (avobenzone, homosalate, octinoxate, octisalate)	Lotion/Spray/Stick	30, 45
Neutrogena Age Shield Sunblock (avobenzone, homosalate, octocrylene, octisalate, oxybenzone)	Lotion	30, 45
Neutrogena Ultra Sheer Dry-Touch Sunblock (octinoxate, octocrylene, homosalate, octisalate, oxybenzone, avobenzone)	Lotion	30, 45 55, 70
Off! Skintastic with Sunscreen (with DEET; octinoxate, octocrylene, oxybenzone)	Lotion	30

SPF, sun protective factor.

not be perceived as warmth.[28] Chemical organic sunscreens usually are nonopaque because they do not absorb the wavelengths of visible light.

UVB FILTERS

Aminobenzoates

Commonly used in the past and the first widely used UV filter, PABA absorbs UVR in the UVB range from 260 to 313 nm, with maximal absorption around 290 nm; its molar absorptivity is considered to be high.[44] PABA readily penetrates and binds to the stratum corneum and, after several days of application, may remain in the skin and provide protection even after swimming, perspiration, and bathing, making it an ideal candidate for water-resistant sunscreens.[44] It is commonly formulated as an alcoholic mixture, which can cause stinging, dryness, or tightness, particularly when applied to the face. Its major disadvantage is the potential to cause contact or photocontact dermatitis, which has been reported to happen in approximately 4% of the population.[53] Responsible for more sensitivity reactions than any other sunscreen,[47] PABA can also cause cross-sensitivity reactions with benzocaine, thiazides, sulfonamides, paraphenylenediamine (a common ingredient in hair dyes), and other PABA derivatives. It can cause discoloration of clothes as well. The use of PABA in commercial sunscreens has decreased to the point where many of the newer sunscreens are promoted as being PABA-free.

The PABA esters include octyldimethyl PABA (Padimate O) and glyceryl PABA. These esters are incorporated easily into formulations, demonstrate good substantivity, and do not discolor clothing. Their absorption spectra are similar to that of PABA (Table 42-2). With a maximal absorption of 311 nm, Padimate O has the lowest likelihood of any PABA ester to cause cross-sensitivity reactions or contact and photocontact dermatitis.[54]

Cinnamates

Octinoxate (octyl methoxycinnamate, Parsol MCX), which has high molar absorptivity and a maximal absorption of 305 nm, is the most commonly used cinnamate and most potent UVB filter.[55] Cinnamates are related chemically to balsam of Peru, balsam of Tolu, coca leaves, cinnamic acid, cinnamic aldehyde, and cinnamic oil, ingredients that are used in perfumes, topical medications, cosmetics, and flavorings.[56] These agents do not bind well to the stratum corneum, leading to poor substantivity. Cinnamate-based sunscreens tend to be comedogenic because the vehicle may contain other occlusive ingredients that are added to improve the substantivity. Cinnamates are often used in combination with benzophenones, appear to be nonstaining, and rarely cause contact dermatitis.[55]

Salicylates

Salicylates are weak UVB absorbers often found in PABA-free products. Topical salicylates are considered among the safest sunscreens, even though they must be used in high concentrations to meet the SPF requirement.[57] Salicylates have low molar absorptivities, are incorporated easily into formulations, and are used to boost the SPF of combination products, particularly oxybenzone and avobenzone.[58] Octisalate and homosalate are water insoluble, which leads to high substantivity. Sensitization to the salicylates is rare[57]; however, it has been reported with the use of octisalate.[59]

Octocrylene

Octocrylene has a similar absorption profile to the salicylates and cinnamates, with a peak absorption at 307 nm. It has low irritation potential and low substantivity; however, it has become increasingly popular because of its ability to photostabilize avobenzone.[60]

UVA FILTERS

Benzophenones

Benzophenones, such as oxybenzone and dioxybenzone, are UVB-absorbing sunscreens that have absorption spectra extending into the UVA range.[61] Benzophenones are also found in shampoos, soaps, hair sprays and dyes, paints, varnishes, and lacquers. The maximal absorption for each is about 290 nm, but both are limited because of poor substantivity and sensitization.[61] Photocontact dermatitis with oxybenzone and contact dermatitis with dioxybenzone occur commonly, with the latter usually occurring as a contact urticaria.[62] Systemic absorption has also been noted with oxybenzone, and it can be detected in the urine and bloodstream.[63]

Anthranilates

Anthranilates, such as meradimate (menthyl anthranilate), are weak UVB-absorbing sunscreens with an absorption spectrum extending into the UVA range. As with the salicylates, they have low molar absorptivity, with a maximal absorption of approximately 336 nm.[44] Meradimate has a low risk of sensitization and a desirable absorption spectrum, especially when it is used in combination with other sunscreens to give broad-spectrum protection.

Dibenzoylmethanes

As a prototype of the dibenzoylmethanes class, avobenzone (butyl methoxydibenzoylmethane, Parsol 1789) has high molar absorptivity and absorption spectra exclusively in the UVA range, with maximal absorption at approximately 360 nm.[64] It is commonly formulated with UVB sunscreens to broaden UVR coverage. Avobenzone loses approximately 35% of its absorption capacity about 15 minutes after UVR exposure, because of the photoinstability of the compound, thereby reducing its UVA protection efficacy.[2] One molecule of avobenzone can absorb UVA radiation only once, making it inactive from that time forward as opposed to zinc oxide or titanium dioxide, which can reflect UVA radiation over and over again with minimal decay. All of the avobenzone applied to the skin is virtually rendered inactive after 5 hours of UVA exposure. Avobenzone is also not compatible with octinoxate, the most powerful UVB filter.[65] Photostability of avobenzone can be increased with the use of UV absorbers, as well as non-UV filters. One such combination is marketed under the trade name of Helioplex (Neutrogena; avobenzone, octocrylene, oxybenzone, and diethylhexyl 2,6-napthalate [Corapan TQ]).

Ecamsule

Ecamsule is a camphor derivative that protects against short UVA rays and is photostable and water resistant, and has low systemic absorption.[66] The FDA has only approved ecamsule for use in certain formulations such as the combination of 2% ecamsule/2% avobenzone/10% octocrylene cream (Anthelios SX, L'Oreal USA). This OTC product is only available in the United States as a moisturizing cream with an SPF rating of 15, although it is available in Europe up to SPF 50. This combination provides continuous protection across most of the UV spectrum (290–400 nm range), with ecamsule providing protection within the short UVA range (320–340 nm), filling the gap between octocrylene and avobenzone capabilities (210–290 nm, and 340–400 nm, respectively). The photostability of the ecamsule and octocrylene–avobenzone combination provides residual protection at 1 and 5 hours (1 hour, 100% UVB protection and 97% UVA protection; 5 hours, 90% UVB protection and 80% UVA protection). Adverse events associated with its use are infrequent and include acne, dermatitis, dry skin, eczema, erythema, pruritus, skin discomfort, and sunburn.

There are two additional formulations of ecamsule. Mexoryl SX is a water-soluble form suitable for daytime sunscreens, including sunscreen-containing moisturizers and facial foundations. Mexoryl XL, an oil-soluble formulation, is suitable for water-resistant sunscreen formulations, including those worn on the beach and during vigorous physical exercise.

INORGANIC SUNSCREENS

Inorganic sunscreens are opaque formulations made of particulate insoluble compounds, incorporated into a vehicle, which scatter and absorb UV rays. Both size of the particles and thickness of the film determine the degree of protection.[67] Currently, there are only two inorganic sunscreens approved by the FDA, titanium dioxide and zinc oxide.[67,68] Other inorganic sunscreens include magnesium oxide, red veterinarian petrolatum, iron oxides, kaolin, ichthammol, and talc.

These compounds are often used in conjunction with chemical sunscreens to formulate products of higher SPF and as single-ingredient sunblocks. When used alone, they are usually placed in an ointment base designed specifically for vulnerable parts of the body, such as the nose, cheeks, lips, ears, and shoulders.[31] Inorganic sunscreens are important in individuals who are unusually sensitive to UVA and visible light, such as those with vitiligo, a skin condition with amelanotic lesions (white patches) surrounded by areas of normally pigmented skin. Appropriately colored formulations can be used to camouflage and protect these vulnerable amelanotic lesions.[31] Inorganic sunscreen agents are preferred for persons who need absolute UVR and visible light protection (e.g., young children; persons with skin types I through IV who receive constant exposure; and persons with drug photosensitivity reactions, xeroderma pigmentosa, lupus erythematosus, and other photosensitive skin reactions).[31]

Despite some advantages, inorganic sunscreens are not widely accepted because they are visible to others, messy, and occlusive when applied to the skin. They have a higher substantivity, but may melt in the heat of the sun, limiting their protection to a few hours. Physical sunscreen products tend to be so occlusive that they may cause or worsen acne or obstruct sweat glands.[31] Substantial effort has been made to improve the shortcomings of these products by reducing the particle size to improve the cosmetic appearance. This has created a growing trend toward incorporating nanoparticles of titanium dioxide and zinc oxide, which have been shown to have superior UV protection while maintaining cosmetic elegance. Concern about toxicity of these agents has been raised because of the potential for increased skin penetration and interaction with lower portions of the epidermis; however, this has been disproved in both in vivo and in vitro studies.[69–73] There is no current regulation in the United States regarding the testing and labeling of nano-sized titanium or zinc oxides.

ANTIOXIDANTS

The addition of botanical antioxidants and vitamins C and E to a broad-spectrum sunscreen may further decrease UV-induced damage compared with sunscreen alone.[68] Antioxidants have received increased attention for use as photoprotective agents, particularly because of the observation that vitamin C levels in the skin can be severely depleted after UVR exposure.[74]

Vitamins C and E, either taken orally or applied topically (incorporated into a commercially available sunscreen product), may provide additive protection against both UVA- and UVB-induced photodamage.[74,75] Topically applied antioxidants do not have adequate diffusion into the epidermal layer, however, and are susceptible to chemical instability.[58] If recommended, they should only be used in conjunction with adequate sunscreen.

Given their plans for the week of vacation and amount of UV exposure likely, R.J. and J.J. should consider a broad-spectrum product with high substantivity and a high degree of water resistance to offer the best protection.

CROSS-SENSITIVITY

CASE 42-1, QUESTION 4: According to your assessment of R.J. and J.J., you determine that they have type IV skin and type II skin, respectively. On further inquiry you learn that R.J. has no medication allergies; however, she has a history of contact dermatitis on her scalp and around her hairline on several occasions after dyeing her hair and using certain shampoos. As a teenager, J.J. suffered from frequent sinus infections and often was treated with trimethoprim-sulfamethoxazole (TMP-SMX) because of an allergy to penicillin. He remembers developing a severe sunburn after minimal exposure to the sun while taking the sulfa-containing antibiotic. He recently has been started on hydrochlorothiazide (HCTZ), 12.5 mg PO daily, for hypertension. What considerations are important in recommending sunscreens for R.J. and J.J.?

The first consideration for recommending an appropriate sunscreen for R.J. and J.J. is their skin type. R.J. has skin type IV, suggesting that a sunscreen with an SPF of at least 15 would provide adequate protection for her (Table 42-3). J.J. has skin type II, suggesting that a sunscreen with an SPF of 30 to 50 would be required to provide adequate protection for him. Furthermore, the history of contact dermatitis and photosensitivity reaction exhibited by R.J. and J.J., respectively, is important when recommending use of a sunscreen.[76] The contact dermatitis that R.J. experienced from hair dyes and shampoos may have been caused by para-phenylenediamine, an ingredient of hair dyes,[77] or a benzophenone, which sometimes is included in products such as hair dyes and shampoos.[61]

Because cross-reactivity between para-phenylenediamine and PABA or its derivatives is possible, a sunscreen for R.J. that does not contain PABA or a benzophenone should be recommended. Cinnamates and anthralates rarely cause contact dermatoses, which would be ideal for R.J.

Because both contain sulfa moieties, the photosensitivity reaction that J.J. experienced while taking TMP-SMX may indicate that he might be susceptible to a cross-sensitivity reaction with PABA or its derivatives. This reaction to TMP-SMX also indicates that J.J. may be susceptible to a photosensitivity reaction with HCTZ. If a photosensitivity reaction is likely, it is advisable to recommend an SPF of 30 or more. Because drug-induced photosensitivity reactions are caused by UVA, a PABA-free, broad-spectrum sunscreen that absorbs UVA as well as UVB would be necessary to provide J.J. with adequate protection. Broad-spectrum chemical sunscreens commonly contain a benzophenone and a cinnamate. A broad-spectrum sunscreen containing both of these chemical classes (e.g., Coppertone Sport, with octinoxate, oxybenzone, and octisalate; Table 42-4) would be an acceptable broad-spectrum product. Alternatively, because Padimate O is the least likely of the PABA ester derivatives to cause photocontact dermatitis,[77] a broad-spectrum combination product that contains Padimate O could be recommended for J.J. If the photosensitivity reaction is caused by visible light, it would also be necessary to recommend an inorganic physical sunscreen to block all sunlight or complete avoidance of the sun.[48] With all of these issues considered, it may be preferable to recommend an alternative antihypertensive medication for J.J. that would not place him at risk for a photosensitivity reaction.

PHOTOPROTECTION FOR CHILDREN

CASE 42-1, QUESTION 5: What photoprotective measures should be provided for P.J. and L.J.?

Sun protection during childhood is very important, considering that most of a person's lifetime of sun exposure occurs in childhood and that the harmful effects of UVR are cumulative.[36] The FDA has recommended that sunscreen agents not be used for children younger than 6 months of age because of the possible chemical absorption through the skin and lowered ability of children of this age to metabolize the absorbed drug.[78] P.J. needs to be kept out of direct sunlight and, when outside, must be protected with proper clothing and shading.[79–82] The FDA has recommended that children younger than 2 years of age be treated with an SPF greater than 4 because of inadequate UVR protection with lower SPF products for most individuals.[78]

L.J. should be protected with a PABA-free sunscreen with an SPF of at least 15. Regular use of a sunscreen with an SPF of at least 15 for the first 18 years of life can reduce the lifetime incidence of nonmelanoma skin cancers by about three-fourths.[82] If L.J. is in the sun during 6 hours of maximal exposure (i.e., 10 AM–4 PM), or otherwise for an extended period, he should wear protective clothing, covering as much of his body as possible.[81] Tightly woven clothing, long sleeves, and pants protect the skin from almost all UVR, whereas loosely woven clothing or wet T-shirts can allow up to 30% of UVR to pass through to the skin. Although not complete, water is thought to reduce UVR scattering, thus decreasing its transmission. An average-weight cotton T-shirt provides only an SPF of 7 or 8.[81]

The transmission of UVR through a fabric is measured using a spectrophotometer or spectroradiometer. The ultraviolet protection factor (UPF), rather than SPF, has been recommended as a measure of the sun-protective properties of fabrics.[83,84] It is calculated using a formula based on UV transmission through the fabric and the erythema response for human skin. For example, if a fabric has a UPF of 20, then only one-twentieth of the UVR at the surface of the fabric actually passes through it. Certain synthetic fabrics have UPF values that exceed 500, making them vastly superior to sunscreens.[81] Table 42-5 compares the UPF with the amount of effective UVR transmitted and absorbed.

No woven fabric provides complete coverage because the holes between the threads permit UVR transmission. A baseball cap shields little more than the upper central forehead. Broad-rimmed hats can protect the ears, neck, nose, and cheeks, but may provide inadequate protection against SCC of the head or neck.[85] The use of an ultraviolet-absorbing ingredient for fabric softeners

TABLE 42-5
Relative Ultraviolet Protection Factor (UPF) by Ultraviolet Ray (UVR) Transmission and Absorption

UVR Transmitted (%)	UVR Absorbed (%)	UPF	Protection Category
10	90.0	10	Moderate protection
5	95.0	20	High protection
3.3	96.7	30	Very high protection
2.5	97.5	40	Extremely high protection
<2.0	>98.0	50	Maximal protection

(e.g., Tinosorb-M, Ciba) are promoted to reduce transmission of excessive UVA and UVB radiation through fabrics to the skin, through absorption of UV radiation without impairing whiteness. This chemical absorption process has a high affinity for cotton fibers at various washing temperatures. Available as a laundry additive (e.g., SunGuard, Phoenix Brands), it works by binding to laundered fibers, and through accumulation, it increases the UV protection up to UPF 30 through up to 20 wash and rinse cycles.[86,87] Studies are in progress to assess the role of these agents as sunscreens, or as additives to sunscreen products.[87]

PRODUCT SELECTION

Two types of sunscreens are appropriate for use in children. A lotion is preferred for total body application versus an alcoholic lotion or gel because alcoholic preparations can cause stinging, burning, and irritation of the skin and eyes. Physical sunscreens (e.g., zinc oxide) are available in bright colors and are recommended for selected body areas, such as the nose, cheeks, and shoulders. PABA and its derivatives are considered potentially harmful to a child's tender skin. For adolescents with acne vulgaris, the use of an oil-free, noncomedogenic sunscreen formulation (e.g., Neutrogena Healthy Defense Oil-Free Sunblock) and a lip balm that contains a sunscreen of at least SPF 15 (e.g., ChapStick or Blistex Regular [SPF 15], Blistex Ultra [SPF 30], or ChapStick Ultra [SPF 30]) would be appropriate.

APPLICATION

CASE 42-1, QUESTION 6: What instructions should you provide R.J. and J.J. on how to apply the sunscreen that you have chosen for each of their family members?

Because R.J. and J.J. are planning to be active on the beach, sunscreens that are water-resistant or waterproof are recommended (Table 42-4). Before complete application of the sunscreen to the body, because of the risk of cross-sensitivity reactions, patients can perform a patch test by applying a small quantity of the sunscreen to the inner aspect of the forearm and covering with a small bandage overnight.

Most persons apply 20% to 60% of the required amount of sunscreen needed to achieve the SPF of their product.[46,50] Because of this, a method has been developed to determine an approximate volume of sunscreen product needed for adequate protection.[88] This rule states that you should use more than half a teaspoon on each of your head and neck area and arms, and more than a teaspoonful on each of your anterior and posterior torso and your legs. This application size was determined based on the dose used in FDA sunscreen testing (2 mg/m^2). One study of sunscreen application techniques at the beach demonstrated inadequate application at all body sites.[89] The worst protected areas were the ears and top of the feet, and the back was poorly protected if sunscreen was self-applied. Patients should be reminded to apply sunscreen on those often forgotten areas, such as the hands, cheeks, neck, ears, and dorsum of the feet. It is best to reapply the sunscreen every 1 to 2 hours or after sweating, swimming, or toweling off.

CASE 42-1, QUESTION 7: How long might J.J. expect to be protected with the sunscreen properly applied?

If J.J. (skin type II) normally burns after 30 minutes of exposure to the sun, a sunscreen with an SPF of 15 to 30 may provide up to 7.5 hours (0.5 hours × 15 [SPF 15]) of photoprotection from UVB. However, a high SPF product may provide only partial protection against UVA, with little or no protection from infrared radiation.[44] Because of this, sun exposure should be limited to 90 to 120 minutes for each outing after appropriate sunscreen application. Further, environmental factors, such as elevated atmospheric humidity, and inadequate application techniques may reduce photoprotection by as much as half.

Sunscreen formulations with SPF as high as 50 can be made using combinations of chemical and physical sunscreen agents (e.g., Hawaiian Tropic Baby Faces Sunblock Lotion, with octinoxate, octocrylene, oxybenzone, octisalate, and titanium dioxide; Table 42-4).[5] Individuals who are extremely sensitive to the sun may benefit from formulations with higher SPF, but the average fair-skinned person gains adequate protection for sunbathing or for average daily exposure from a product with an SPF of 30.[46]

CASE 42-1, QUESTION 8: Would J.J. gain additional benefit from a product with an SPF greater than 50?

Protection from sunburn increases with higher SPF; however, it is important to remind J.J. that this protection does not correlate to the extent of skin damage from UVA rays. One study reported less sunburn in patients who applied SPF 85 compared with those who applied SPF 50 and spent a similar amount of time in direct sunlight.[90] In the proposed FDA amendment there is specific discussion about the validity of SPF testing over 50. There is concern that the SPF testing is only accurate and reproducible up to SPFs of 50. J.J. should also be reminded that the SPF is only accurate if he correctly applies the sunscreen in the adequate amount.

PROTECTIVE EYEWEAR

CASE 42-1, QUESTION 9: Recommend appropriate protective eyewear for R.J. and J.J.'s family while they are on vacation.

R.J. and J.J. should wear sunglasses when outdoors to decrease their lifelong exposure to solar radiation and while at the beach to prevent high exposure of UVR and possible photokeratitis or conjunctivitis. Many manufacturers of sunglasses label their products according to three categories: cosmetic, general purpose, and special purpose. Cosmetic sunglasses block at least 70% of UVB, at least 20% of UVA, and less than 60% of visible light and are appropriate for casual wear when high exposure to UVR is unlikely. General-purpose sunglasses block at least 95% of UVB, at least 60% of UVA, and 60% to 92% of visible light and are appropriate for most activities in sunny environments.[91] Special-purpose sunglasses block at least 99% of UVB, at least 60% of UVA, and at least 97% of visible light and are appropriate for very bright environments, such as ski slopes or tropical beaches.[91] Special- or general-purpose sunglasses are appropriate recommendations for R.J., J.J, and their children to wear while on vacation.

TANNING BOOTHS

CASE 42-2

QUESTION 1: B.P., a 32-year-old woman, is preparing for a business trip to Cancun. She is seeking advice about the use of a tanning bed to stimulate melanin for the prevention of sunburn while on her trip. B.P. has skin type III and light brown hair and green eyes. She recently heard, however, that a tan produced by artificial sunlight may not protect against sunburn and may even cause skin cancer. What advice will you offer her?

Most tanning beds, booths, or salons use an artificial light source that emits about 95% UVA with minimal (i.e., 1% to 5%) UVB.[92,93] It was originally thought that UVA is much less likely to produce photoaging and photocarcinogenic changes of the skin than UVB; however, UVA has now been found to cause many of the same effects on the skin as UVB, including immunologic, degenerative, and neoplastic changes, as well as damage to DNA and the formation of reactive oxygen species.[94] UVA also contributes to cataract formation and the activation of herpetic lesions.[23] The high doses of UVA received during a tanning session, as well as increasing cumulative UVA doses over time, raise great concern about the long-term effects of UVA.[95] In addition, UVA may augment the photocarcinogenic effect of UVB,[2] and extensive evidence indicates a relationship between indoor tanning and melanoma.[96] Tanning bed use has dramatically increased during the past 20 years from less than 1% of Americans in 1988 to 27% of Americans in 2007, and this growth is particularly alarming in the adolescent population.[97] This issue is compounded by recent evidence that suggests that excessive UV exposure, particularly tanning beds, may have a behavioral component similar to other substance-related disorders. As many as 12% to 53% of young adults meet the criteria for having an addictive component to indoor tanning behavior.[98–100]

With a skin type III, B.P. may be able gradually to achieve a moderate tan with minimal burning, thus providing some protection from UVR because of increased melanization of the skin. This UVA-induced tan, however, may not be as protective as a tan achieved under normal sunlight conditions because UVA does not thicken the stratum corneum.[99] An artificially produced tan plus subsequent sun exposure has not been found to provide any net reduction in long-term damage to the skin when compared with the same amount of tan obtained by sunbathing alone.[99] For these reasons, B.P. should not use the tanning booth to obtain a protective tan, and she should use appropriate photoprotective measures during her trip.

CASE 42-2, QUESTION 2: What precautions would you recommend if she decides to visit a tanning salon?

If B.P. decides to artificially tan despite your recommendation, she should undertake some precautions. The FDA has recommended exposure schedules for first-time users based on skin type, which determines a person's minimal erythemal dose (MED) of UV radiation. MED is determined by the amount of UV exposure necessary to produce any visible reddening of the skin 24 hours after exposure. This policy suggests that exposure be limited to no more than 0.75 MED three times the first week, followed by a gradual increase to maintenance doses of a maximum of 4.0 MED delivered weekly or biweekly.[101] It is important to remember that MED is specific to an individual, and therefore will be different depending on his or her skin type. Correlating the FDA's policy into time limits for an individual is therefore dependent on skin type as well as the amount of UV exposure provided by the tanning apparatus the individual will use. To minimize cataract development, B.P. should always wear protective eye wear that absorbs all UVA, UVB, and visible light up to 500 nm; simply closing her eyes or wearing regular sunglasses provides no protective effect against eye damage.

SUNLESS TANNING PRODUCTS

CASE 42-2, QUESTION 3: B.P. decides to accept your recommendations to avoid tanning beds; however, she would still like to have a tan before going to Cancun. Will the use of sunless tanning agents confer any photoprotection for B.P. against sunburn?

Sunless tanner is a commercial term that denotes a product that provides a tanned appearance without exposure to the sun or other sources of UVR. One commonly used ingredient in these products is dihydroxyacetone (DHA), a color additive that darkens the skin to orange-brown by reacting with amino acids in the stratum corneum. The term *bronzer* is used to describe a variety of products intended to achieve a temporary tanned appearance. For example, among the products marketed as bronzers are tinted moisturizers and brush-on powders. These produce a temporary effect, similar to other types of makeup, and wash off over time. Some products are marketed with other ingredients in addition to DHA to provide a tanned appearance. Neither sunless tanners nor bronzers provide any protective activity to UV exposure by themselves.[77] As previously described, the FDA now requires that all suntanning preparations that do not contain sunscreen ingredients are required to carry a warning statement on the label that they do not protect against sunburn.

Tanning pills are promoted for tinting the skin by ingesting massive doses of color additives, usually canthaxanthin. At large doses, canthaxanthin is deposited in various organs, including skin, imparting an orange-bronze color. This color varies from individual to individual. This colorization is not the result of an increase in the skin's supply of melanin. Although canthaxanthin is approved by the FDA for use as a color additive in foods, in which it is used in small amounts, its use in these so-called tanning pills is not approved. Reported adverse events include drug-induced retinopathy, nausea, gastrointestinal cramping, diarrhea, pruritus, and urticaria. None of the above noted unapproved agents should be recommended for use.

TREATMENT OF SUNBURN

CASE 42-3

QUESTION 1: G.B., a 31-year-old man with skin type IV, returned a few hours ago from an afternoon of activity in the sun. His shoulders, back, neck, and arms are bright red and are beginning to feel hot, stretched, and painful. G.B. has been otherwise healthy, has no significant medical history, and has no known allergies to medications. What treatment recommendations would you give G.B. for his sunburn?

Sunburn is a self-limiting condition, and treatment is usually symptomatic.[102] Suggested treatments that G.B. can try for his first-degree burn are oral (e.g., ibuprofen, aspirin) or topical (e.g., camphor, menthol) analgesics, topical anti-inflammatory agents (e.g., hydrocortisone cream or aloe vera gel), cooling compresses (tap water, saline, or aluminum acetate solution [Burow's solution]) applied to the skin, or cool protectant baths (e.g., colloidal oatmeal). Nonsteroidal anti-inflammatory drugs (NSAIDs), such as aspirin or ibuprofen, may be preferred over acetaminophen because of blockade of the inflammatory prostaglandin-mediated sunburn process; however, although offering symptomatic relief, corticosteroids, NSAIDs, antioxidants, antihistamines, or emollients offer only mild improvement at decreasing the time to recovery.[102]

Topical anesthetics, such as benzocaine or lidocaine, provide only transient analgesia for up to 15 to 45 minutes. These topical agents should not be used in large quantities or applied more than three or four times a day. In addition, they should not be used on raw, blistered, or abraded skin. Benzocaine has minimal systemic toxicities, but is commonly associated with contact sensitization.[103] In contrast, lidocaine is associated with a low incidence of contact sensitization.[104] Topical corticosteroids have been shown to provide minimal clinical benefit when applied after UV exposure.[105] If G.B. wants to try a topical agent, application or administration is recommended when the pain is particularly bothersome, such as at bedtime. Oral antihistamines may help control pruritus associated with sunburn, as well as aid with sleep, if taken at bedtime; however, no definitive studies have shown benefit in reducing symptoms or benefit of one agent over another.

Treatment beyond self-management is generally unnecessary unless the sunburn is extensive with constitutional symptoms (i.e., fever, chills, nausea, vomiting), involves second- or third-degree burns (particularly if on the eyes or genitalia), or becomes infected. In such cases, referral of the patient to his or her health care provider is indicated as a short course (i.e., up to 3 days) of an oral corticosteroid may need to be given (e.g., 1 mg/kg of prednisone or equivalent, given once daily).

Clinical Application of Phototoxicity or Photoallergy

Phototoxic photosensitivity reactions are dose dependent and occur in almost any person who takes or applies an adequate amount of the offending agent. The dose necessary to produce such a reaction varies from person to person and depends on such factors as complexion, hair and eye color, usual ability to tan, and type and amount of UVR exposure. Phototoxic photosensitivity reactions are not immunologically mediated or true allergic reactions; they can occur on first exposure to the agent, and generally show no cross-sensitivity to chemically related agents.

A phototoxic reaction usually has a rapid onset, often within several hours after UVR exposure, and presents as an exaggerated or intensified sunburn with erythema, pain, and prickling or burning. Blistering, desquamation, and hyperpigmentation can occur in severe cases.[26] Symptoms generally peak 24 to 48 hours after the initial exposure and are usually limited to the areas of UVR-exposed skin. Because phototoxicity reactions do not involve the immune system, prior exposure to the photosensitizer is unnecessary for this reaction to occur.

Clinically, photoallergy differs from phototoxicity in that it produces an intensely pruritic, eczematous form of dermatitis.[26] The rash is preceded by pruritus and may subside within an hour. In 5% to 10% of cases, persistent hypersensitivity to light occurs, even after the offending chemical has been eliminated.[26] Photoallergic reactions are not dose related, and eruptions can also be caused by chemically related agents via cross-sensitivity or cross-allergenicity. As a type of delayed hypersensitivity reaction, time is required to develop an immune response, and the onset of a photoallergic reaction is often delayed for 1 to 3 days. These reactions can present as macular, bullous, or purpuric lesions. Acute urticaria can occur within minutes after UVR exposure. Recovery is slower than from a phototoxic reaction, and it can persist after the offending product has been removed. These reactions may present with erythema and possible edema secondary to the inflammation, but are most commonly found to be eczematous, characterized by erythema; pruritus (possible severe); and papules, vesicles, or both, with weeping, oozing, and crusting. Scaling, lichenification, and pigmentation may occur later.

CASE 42-4

QUESTION 1: D.L., a 16-year-old, blond-haired, blue-eyed teenager with skin type II, presents with a severe sunburn. He states that he started a new summer job 2 days ago with typical sun exposure. He is surprised at the severity of this sunburn, which is worse than normal for the same amount of sun exposure. What further information do you need to know before making treatment recommendations?

Because D.L. is reporting symptoms that differ from previous sun exposures, further questions should be asked regarding the history of the current scenario. Information that may be important in the history of the condition include the temporal relationship between sun exposure and onset of symptoms; the nature and duration of symptoms; recent ingestion or topical application of medications; possible exposure to photosensitizers, chemical irritants, or plants that can cause allergic contact dermatitis (e.g., poison ivy); and the potential for arthropod bites. Information that may be important from the physical examination includes the distribution and morphology of the reaction, as well as areas of the body spared of the reaction.

A drug-induced photosensitivity reaction most commonly appears as a sunburn of greater severity than would normally be expected or as a rash in areas exposed to the sun or tanning apparatus. These reactions can be secondary to oral medications; however, it is important to remember that chemicals with photosensitization potential are found in cosmetics, shampoos, moisturizing lotions, hair dyes or tints, soaps, and other topically applied medications and agents.

Drug-induced photosensitivity reactions can be subdivided into phototoxic and photoallergic reactions. The same medication or agent may produce both phototoxic and photoallergic reactions, and it may at times be difficult to differentiate clinically between the two types of reactions.

CASE 42-4, QUESTION 2: On further questioning, you discover that D.L. first experienced painful erythema of the extensor surface of his hands and forearms, the anterior aspect of his neck, and parts of his face within hours of starting his new job at an outdoor garden and greenhouse. Besides painful erythema, the symptoms also included an immediate prickling and burning sensation. The symptoms continued to worsen until the following morning, about 24 hours after initial exposure to the sun. D.L. does not recall orally ingesting or topically applying any medication or other preparation to his skin, nor does he recall exposure to any chemical irritants, or poison ivy or oak. The morphology of the skin lesions is that of an exaggerated sunburn. The skin lesions are patchy in distribution with greater density on his forearms and hands than on his neck and face. The posterior aspect of his neck and covered areas of his body were spared completely. What are some possible causes of his exaggerated sunburn reaction?

The most likely explanation for D.L.'s exaggerated sunburn reaction is *phototoxicity,* secondary to contact with psoralenlike chemicals from the plants at his job at the outdoor garden and greenhouse. Photoallergy is another possible cause of D.L.'s symptoms. Although much less common than phototoxicity, photoallergy requires prior or prolonged exposure to the photosensitizing compound.

Presumably, D.L. came into contact with psoralen-containing plants and simultaneous exposure to sunlight. With an unusual distribution of lesions on his hands, forearms, neck, and face and the lack of lesions on areas not contacted by the plants or sunlight, the temporal relationship between the exposure and onset of symptoms place phototoxicity higher in the differential diagnosis. D.L. is unlikely to have a photoallergic reaction because of the lack of a delayed temporal relationship between the onset of symptoms and combined exposure to a psoralen-containing plant and sunlight. Unlike phototoxicity reactions, photoallergic reactions can spread to areas that have not been exposed to sunlight; however, D.L.'s lesions were limited to areas of skin exposed to sunlight.

CASE 42-4, QUESTION 3: What nonprescription remedies might you recommend for D.L. at this time?

General recommendations for the management of phototoxicity and photoallergy reactions are focused on the removal of exposure to the potential photosensitizer and reduced exposure to the sun. Patients should be counseled not to take any medications, orally or topically, without first consulting with their health care provider to minimize exposure to other photosensitizers. D.L. should try wearing long-sleeved shirts, pants, and gloves when working to limit exposure to plant photosensitizers. He also may try applying a broad-spectrum sunscreen to protect his skin from UVB and UVA radiation. If these measures do not prevent further photosensitivity reactions, D.L. should consider a different type of employment. His presenting symptoms should be managed in a manner similar to that for an exaggerated sunburn.

PHOTOAGING

Incidence, Prevalence, and Epidemiology

Photoaging, or premature aging of the skin, involves skin changes that differ from those associated with normal chronologic aging.[106,107] Aside from advancing age, risk factors that have been associated with photoaging include fair skin, difficulty tanning, ease of sunburning, and sunburns before the age of 20 years.[108] Attempting to correct aged skin and photodamage has become a large financial market in the United States. The antiaging cosmeceutical market was estimated at $12.4 billion in 2004, and is predicted to soar to more than $16.5 billion in 2010.[109] Because recognizing photoaging and photodamage may prevent the progression or development of skin cancer, it is important that they are recognized as real medical problems, not just cosmetic or aesthetic concerns.

Etiology

Normal aging of the skin involves fine wrinkling of the skin, atrophy of the dermis, and a decrease in the amount of subcutaneous adipose tissue, all of which lead to a state of hypocellularity of the skin.[106] Photoaging involves a chronic inflammatory state induced by long-term exposure to UVA radiation from reactive oxygen species (ROS), leading to a hypermetabolic state of the skin.[110] Photodamaged skin is characterized histologically by an accumulation of excessive quantities of thickened, degenerated elastic connective tissue fibers (elastosis).[106] Type I collagen predominates in normal skin, but in photodamaged skin, type III collagen increases about fourfold, and the mature matrix of type I collagen slightly decreases.[94] These degenerative changes in connective tissue may be caused by hyperactive fibroblasts or by enzymatic degradation via cellular infiltrates in inflamed skin.[5] The elastic connective tissue then replaces the collagen in the upper parts of the dermis.[110] The ground substance, composed of proteoglycans and glycosaminoglycans, also is increased considerably in photoaged skin.[5] Capillaries in the dermis become dilated and tortuous, resulting in telangiectasias, ecchymosis, and purpura.[107] The epidermis thickens, and epidermal cells become hyperplastic and possibly neoplastic. Actinic keratosis, a premalignant lesion found mostly in the older population, is a risk factor for the development of SCC because a low percentage of these lesions transform into SCC.[28,107] Large cumulative doses of UVA, UVB, and possibly infrared radiation during the course of a lifetime are strongly implicated as the cause of these changes in photoaged skin.[5]

Photodamaged skin is characterized as being wrinkled, yellowed, and sagging. Mildly affected skin becomes irregularly pigmented, rough, and dry, with mild wrinkles. Moderately affected skin becomes deeply wrinkled, sagging, thickened, and leathery, with vascular lesions.[107] Largely irreversible, severely affected skin can become deeply furrowed and permanently (and irregularly) pigmented, and may manifest premalignant and malignant lesions.[107] Areas of the body most commonly affected are the face, back of the neck, back of the arms and hands, the V-line of the neck of women, and balding areas of the head of men.

For a visual showing photoaging, go to http://thepoint.lww.com/AT10e.

Clinical Application of Photoaging

CASE 42-5

QUESTION 1: P.B. is a 38-year-old woman who has enjoyed many outdoor activities over the years. She lives in a moderate climate, with hot, sunny summers and cold winters. She feels that she appears older than other women her age because of wrinkling and color changes of her skin. Her facial color is somewhat yellowish in appearance, and the fine wrinkles at the corners of her eyes and mouth have become more obvious. She has noticed the formation of small brown spots mottling parts of her face, hands, and forearms. P.B. has skin type III, a clear complexion, and skin that is sensitive to soaps, heavy cosmetics, and perfumes. What nonprescription recommendations can you provide P.B. for treatment of her photoaged skin?

Many nonprescription agents known as cosmeceuticals, products marketed as cosmetic products that contain biologically active ingredients, are targeted at reducing visible signs of aged skin. These products range from peptides to topical antioxidants. One particular product class widely used is alpha-hydroxy acids and polyhydroxy acids. In normal concentrations (4%–12%), they are included in many products to lessen the appearance of damage; however, in high concentrations they are used as peels because of their keratolytic properties. They have been shown in studies to reduce skin roughness and sallowness; however, minimal impact was seen on wrinkles or actinic keratoses.[107,111] In patients who choose to use these products, it should be strongly recommended that they wear at least SPF 15 to 30 because they allow for greater absorption of UVR.

It is important to remember that these agents are not regulated by the FDA and therefore do not have substantial evidence supporting their effectiveness and can be very costly. Emphasis should be placed on protection from the sun, using photoprotective strategies previously discussed.

CASE 42-5, QUESTION 2: Are there any prescription products that you would recommend to P.B. to discuss with her physician?

There are several topical retinoids currently available that are derivatives of vitamin A and are effective for the signs of photoaging (see Chapter 41, Psoriasis). Tretinoin (all-trans-retinoic acid) is available as a cream (0.025%, 0.05%, and 0.1%), gel (0.01%, 0.025%, 0.04% [in microspheres], 0.1% [in microspheres]), or liquid (0.05%). Tazarotene, another retinoic acid, is available as a 0.05% or 0.1% cream. Adapalene is available as a 0.1% cream, and a 0.1% or 0.3% gel. These agents are effective in partially reversing some of the clinical and histologic changes of photoaging by lessening fine wrinkles, mottled pigmentation, and the tactile roughness associated with photoaged skin through mechanisms such as inhibition of metalloproteinase expression.[112–115] Additional benefits of retinoid therapy include the formation of new dermal collagen and vessels, reduction in the number and melanization of freckles, resorption of degenerated connective tissue fibers, and treatment of premalignant and malignant skin lesions.[116] In one of the initial trials, all subjects treated (100%) demonstrated global improvement in the signs of photoaging, with 53% showing moderate changes and the remainder having at least slight improvement. Of the clinical parameters assessed, the most impressive improvements were found with facial skin sallowness, with respondents developing a healthy, rosy glow.[113]

CASE 42-5, QUESTION 3: Would P.B. be an appropriate candidate for therapy with a topical retinoid product (e.g., tretinoin)?

Topical retinoid therapy is most effective for patients 50 to 70 years of age with moderate to severe photoaging and for prophylactic use in patients undergoing the initial changes of photoaging.[112] Recently, P.B. has noticed some of the skin changes consistent with early photoaging and would be a good candidate for prophylactic therapy with topical tretinoin. Treatment may improve her sallow skin color and lessen the mottling on her face and forearms and fine wrinkles at the corners of her eyes and mouth, as well as prevent worsening of the photoaging process that she is experiencing.

CASE 42-5, QUESTION 4: P.B.'s physician calls you asking for dosing recommendations for tretinoin. What advice do you provide?

Because both the beneficial and adverse effects of topical retinoid therapy are dose-dependent, the underlying goal is to provide the maximal benefit by using the highest concentration that causes minimal skin irritation. Considering P.B.'s skin sensitivity to soaps, cosmetics, and perfumes, her skin is likely to be irritated easily by tretinoin; therefore, it would be best to initiate therapy with the lowest strength (e.g., tretinoin 0.025% cream). An alternative retinoid is tazarotene 0.1% cream. These agents are usually applied every night at bedtime, but in some instances, they are applied initially on an every-other-night basis until the skin accommodates to the irritant effects. The likelihood of irritation depends on the type of vehicle more than the concentration of the agent.[116] The cream or the microsphere gel formulations cause the least skin irritation and would be preferred for initiating therapy for P.B. The microsphere gel formulation is preferred for patients with persistent acne or for those with focal actinic lesions. Younger patients often prefer the gel because it leaves no residue and is compatible with most cosmetics. The solution and gel may be better tolerated in older patients with oily, thick, pigmented skin.

CASE 42-5, QUESTION 5: You are now dispensing tretinoin cream 0.025% to P.B. What patient counseling should P.B. be given?

Before applying the cream to her face at bedtime, P.B. should wash her face gently, using her fingertips and mild soap, then pat her skin dry with a towel. If gentle washing with her fingers does not remove the dry, peeling skin, a washcloth can be used gently on the face. The treated stratum corneum is fragile, and erosions could occur if P.B. is not careful when washing. After waiting about 15 minutes, she should apply a pea-sized amount of cream to her forehead and spread the cream evenly over her entire face. Care should be exercised while applying the cream to the areas adjacent to the eyes and mouth because tretinoin can cause irritation and burning of mucous membranes.

Skin irritation can be expected to start in the first 3 to 5 days of therapy and, hopefully, will subside in 1 to 3 months. Irritation can manifest as erythema, peeling, burning, and stinging. If P.B. experiences excessive irritation, she can reinitiate the regimen on a slower timeline by applying the cream on an every-other-night or every-third-night basis for the first 2 weeks to reduce skin irritation, or she can also apply a topical corticosteroid product such as hydrocortisone 1% cream. As she begins to tolerate the therapy, her frequency of applications and strength of cream should be titrated to cause mild scaling with only occasional mild erythema. A thicker film of cream can be applied to photodamaged areas. After 9 to 12 months of therapy, she can begin maintenance therapy, which consists of application 2 or 3 nights a week indefinitely.

Because these agents can dry the skin, P.B. should be counseled to use moisturizers during the day to help decrease the dryness and irritation of the skin. Nighttime application of moisturizers should be discouraged when topical tretinoin is being used because the moisturizers can cause a pH incompatibility with the cream and possibly dilute the concentration of tretinoin. With a thinning of the stratum corneum, P.B.'s skin may be more susceptible to the effects of UVR. For this reason, as well as to prevent further actinic damage, P.B. should begin prophylactic daytime application of a sunscreen. Considering her skin type (III) and early photoaging changes, a sunscreen with an SPF of at least 30 would be appropriate. P.B. should be counseled not to become discouraged by any apparent lack of response; her skin damage is mild, her response to therapy will be gradual, and part of the goal of therapy is to prevent further damage. Her wrinkles may actually appear to worsen early in therapy owing to an initial buildup of the stratum corneum. P.B. should avoid facial saunas and irritating soaps and cosmetics.

BURN INJURIES

Incidence, Prevalence, and Epidemiology

More than 700,000 Americans are treated for burns yearly.[117] Although admission for and mortality from burn injuries are declining, the total number of emergency department visits continue to increase, with 45,000 individuals requiring hospitalization; burns cause an overall yearly mortality of approximately 6,500.[117,118] Complications such as fluid and electrolyte imbalances, metabolic derangements, respiratory failure, sepsis, scarring, and functional impairment are the primary causes of hospitalization for these cases. Most burns, however, are minor and can be managed in an ambulatory environment, provided the burned patient is evaluated carefully, the severity of the burn is assessed accurately, and proper and continuous follow-up care is ensured. Most partial-thickness burns in this country are managed by practitioners in hospital and community settings who do not treat burns on a regular basis.[119]

Burn injuries range from relatively minor, superficial injuries to severe, extensive skin loss resulting from contact with hot solids and liquids, steam, chemical agents, electricity, or other physical agents, such as UVR or infrared radiation. House fires, commonly caused by cigarettes or malfunctioning heating or electrical equipment, are responsible for the majority of fire- and burn-related deaths.[117] The peak incidence of burn injuries occurs in up to 10% of preschool-aged children, who are often scalded by or immersed into hot liquids, frequently as a result of child abuse and neglect that crosses all socioeconomic classes.[120,121] School-aged children and adolescents often are injured when experimenting with matches or gasoline or in association with cars, motorcycles, fireworks, or flammables.[117,122] Teenagers and adults between 17 and 30 years of age most commonly are involved in accidents with flammable liquids, but the mortality associated with clothing ignition continues to decrease as a result of the use of flame-retardant forms of fabric in clothing. Categories of individuals who have a higher reported incidence of burn injuries are the very young, elderly, males, blacks, economically disadvantaged, individuals who have ingested alcohol, handicapped children, and children with previous history of burn.[123]

With the development of multidisciplinary burn centers and a better understanding of the pathophysiology of the burn wound, survival of patients with second- and third-degree burns has improved by five to six times during the last three decades.[124] The number of serious burns is decreasing in the United States because of better prevention (smoke detectors, water temperature regulations, and decreased smoking), but approximately 3,200 deaths from residential fires still occur yearly.[123] The techniques of improved burn wound management have contributed to this decline as well, including topical antimicrobial therapy, early excision or enzymatic débridement of devitalized tissue, and skin grafting or substitutes.[125–127]

Etiology

ZONES OF INJURY

The skin functions as a protective barrier of the underlying organ systems from trauma, temperature variations, harmful penetrations, moisture, humidity, radiation, and invasion by microorganisms (see Fig. 39-1 in Chapter 39, Dermatology and Drug-Induced Skin Disorders). It also is involved with carbohydrate, protein, fat, and vitamin D metabolism, produces secretions that lubricate the skin, is involved with the immune response, and provides the body with the sense of touch.

Burn wounds caused by thermal injury can be described by varying zones of injury.[126] The most peripheral area of injury is the *zone of hyperemia*. The tissue in this area is characterized by inflammatory changes with minimal tissue damage. The *zone of stasis* is the next area of injury, extending inward from the zone of hyperemia. This area involves ischemic, damaged tissue, with blood vessels only partially thrombosed. The damaged endothelial linings of blood vessels within this zone of injury may trigger further thrombosis, resulting in further ischemia, cell death, and deepening of the burn wound. This process of further injury can occur 24 to 48 hours after the initial injury. Drying of the burn wound or infection can cause deepening of the burn wound by preventing re-establishment of circulation to injured tissue. The central-most area, or the *zone of coagulation*, is characterized by thrombotic vessels and necrotic tissue. This area absorbs the most thermal energy, resulting in the greatest tissue damage. Minor burns may involve only the most peripheral zones of injury, whereas severe burns encompass all three zones of injury.

EXTENT OF INJURY

RULE OF NINES

Burn severity is proportional to the percent of body surface area (BSA) involvement and wound depth. The percent of BSA for adults can be estimated by using the "rule of nines," in which each arm constitutes 9% of the BSA, the head 9%, each leg 18%, the front and back of the torso 18% each, and the genitalia 1%.[128] For children younger than 10 years of age, the percent BSA must be adjusted because their bodies have different proportions. Variations of the Lund and Browder chart have been used for this purpose.[128] At birth, the infant's head constitutes about 19% of the BSA. For each additional year of age, the head decreases by about 1%, and the BSA of the legs increases by about 1% of the patient's total body surface area (TBSA), so a quick estimation of the percent BSA of a burn can be made.[120]

ONLINE CONTENT

For a visual showing how to estimate the extent of burns, go to http://thepoint.lww.com/AT10e.

CLASSIFICATION OF WOUNDS

Burn wounds also are classified according to the depth of tissue damage. Determining the depth of the burn wound can be difficult during the first 24 to 48 hours because of the presence of edema and continued tissue ischemia and infection, both of which can cause deepening of the wound. In addition, the depth of destruction can vary within the same burn, and skin surface characteristics may not match underlying tissue damage, making assessment of the burn wound difficult.[127]

ONLINE CONTENT

For a visual showing classification of burns by depth of injury, go to http://thepoint.lww.com/AT10e.

First-Degree Burns (Superficial-Thickness Burn)

First-degree burns result from injury to the superficial cells of the epidermis; a common example is a mild sunburn. The burned skin does not form blisters, but it does become erythematous and mildly painful. This partial-thickness burn heals within 3 to 4 days without scarring.

Second-Degree Burns (Partial-Thickness to Superficial Burn)

Second-degree burns may be superficial or deep, depending on the depth of dermal involvement. Superficial second-degree burns involve the epidermis and the upper layer of the dermis. The burn surface often is erythematous, blistered, weeping, painful, and very sensitive to stimuli. The erythema blanches with pressure, and the hair follicles, sweat, and sebaceous glands are spared. Superficial second-degree burns heal spontaneously within 3 weeks with little, if any, scarring. Deep second-degree burns involve the deeper elements of the dermis and may be difficult to distinguish from third-degree burns. The burn surface is pale, feels indurated or boggy, and does not blanch with pressure. This wound is less painful than more superficial wounds; some areas may be insensitive to stimuli. Healing occurs slowly over the course of about 35 days with eschar formation and possible severe scarring and permanent loss of hair follicles and sweat and sebaceous glands.

Third-Degree Burns (Partial-Thickness to Deep Burn)

Third-degree burns entail complete destruction of the full thickness of the skin, including all skin elements. The wound may appear pearly white, gray, or brown and is dry and inelastic. Pain is sensed only when deep pressure is applied. If the wound is small, healing over the course of several months can occur by epithelial migration from the margins of the injury, with scar and contracture formation. Third-degree burns are repaired most often by excision and grafting of the wound to prevent contractures of the skin.[129]

Fourth-Degree Burns (Full-Thickness Burn)

Fourth-degree burns are similar to third-degree burns except that devitalized tissue extends into the subcutaneous tissue, fascia, and bone. These burns are blackened in appearance; they are dry and generally painless because of destruction of nerve endings, and are at great risk for infection.

COMPLICATIONS OF SEVERE BURN WOUNDS

FLUID LOSS

In severe burns, release of vasoactive mediators and capillary injury cause sequestration of large amounts of body fluid, plasma, and electrolytes in extravascular compartments, resulting in edema both locally and throughout the entire body. This redistribution of fluid is compounded by the loss of large amounts of fluid, electrolytes, and protein into the open wound. The cumulative effect is a marked decrease in blood volume, a fall in cardiac output, and decreased tissue and organ perfusion. During the first 24 to 48 hours after a severe burn injury, adequate fluid must be given to replace fluid lost from the vascular space to prevent shock and, possibly, multiple-organ failure and death.[129]

INFECTION

The most important threat to survival of the fully resuscitated patient is infection, with burn wound sepsis and pneumonia being the leading causes of death.[129] The local mechanical defenses of the skin and respiratory tract often are damaged in burn victims, making these common foci for fatal infections. Loss of circulation to the burn wound margins does not allow proper functioning of cellular and humoral defense mechanisms, which increases susceptibility to infection. Devitalized tissue and tissue exudates provide an ideal environment for the proliferation of bacteria. Colonization of gram-positive bacteria occurs if topical antimicrobial therapy is not initiated promptly, and gram-negative bacteria may predominate by the fifth day after injury.[129] Systemic antibiotics are of limited benefit in full-thickness burns and are used only to treat infections documented by wound biopsy, which reveal in excess of 10^5 bacteria per gram of burn tissue.[130] Topical antimicrobials, local wound care, and strict infection control practices are the mainstays of controlling burn wound infections. Devitalized tissue initiates and perpetuates a sepsislike state in the absence of an identifiable focus of infection.[129] For this reason, as well as for infection control, early excision of devitalized tissue and closure of the burn wound by skin grafting or substitutes have been adopted by many burn centers.

INHALATION INJURY

Burn injuries complicated by inhalation injury are associated with greatly increased mortality rates. Injury to the tracheobronchial mucosa is caused by inhalation of smoke or flames and may result in bronchospasm, ulceration of the mucous membranes, damage to cell membranes, edema, and impairment of bacterial ciliary clearance. Even patients with minor burns can have inhalation injury and require hospital admission. The early symptoms of pulmonary injury (hoarseness, dyspnea, tachypnea, and wheezing) may not be evident for 24 to 48 hours, so patients with suspected inhalation injury (i.e., facial burns or entrapment in a closed space) must be examined carefully. Singed nasal hair, a soot-coated tongue or oropharynx, and upper airway edema are indications of inhalation injury. The diagnosis is established by bronchoscopy, and management may include endotracheal intubation and mechanical ventilation. Maintenance of the patient's fluid status is essential. Corticosteroids do not influence survival rates and should not be routinely administered to patients with inhalation injury. They can also increase morbidity and mortality associated with burns and inhalation injury by increasing the risk of infection.[129]

Clinical Management of Minor Burns

TRIAGE

CASE 42-6

QUESTION 1: S.T., a 17-year-old, nonobese boy, has just burned the calf of his right leg on the muffler of his motorcycle. Immediately after being burned, S.T. was able to rinse his leg with cool water from a garden hose. The burn on his leg is about twice the size of the palm of his hand and appears erythematous and weeping. He sustained no other injury, but now he is in considerable pain. S.T. has no significant medical history. Should S.T. be referred to a health care provider or can he safely self-treat his burn? What patient information is necessary to consider in making this decision?

Before recommending treatment for a patient with a minor burn, it is important to accurately assess the patient to determine whether he or she can self-treat safely or whether referral or hospitalization is necessary. The location and severity of the burn, the patient's age and state of health, and the cause of the burn injury all must be considered.

AMERICAN BURN ASSOCIATION TREATMENT CATEGORIES

Three treatment categories for burn injuries are recommended by the American Burn Association: major burn injuries; moderate, uncomplicated burn injuries; and minor burn injuries.[131]

- *Major burn injuries* are second-degree burns with greater than 25% BSA involvement in adults (20% in children); all third-degree burns with 10% BSA involvement; all burns involving the hands, face, eyes, ears, feet, and perineum that may result in functional or cosmetic impairment; high-voltage electrical injury; and burns complicated by inhalation injury, major trauma, or poor-risk patients (elderly patients and those with debilitating disease).
- *Moderate, uncomplicated burns* are second-degree burns with 15% to 25% BSA involvement in adults (10%–20% in children); third-degree burns with 2% to 10% BSA involvement; and burns not involving risk to areas of specialized function, such as the eyes, ears, face, hands, feet, or perineum.
- *Minor burn injuries* include second-degree burns with less than 15% BSA involvement in adults (10% in children), third-degree burns with less than 2% BSA, and burns not involving functional or cosmetic risk to areas of specialized function.

Patients with minor burn injuries may be treated on an outpatient basis if no other trauma is present; if circumferential burns of the neck, trunk, arms, or legs are not present; and if the patient is able to comply with therapy. After initial evaluation by a health care provider, patients may self-treat a second- or third-degree burn only if less than 1% BSA is involved.

Major or moderate, uncomplicated burns necessitate hospital admission, and surgical referral is recommended for patients of all ages who have deep second- or third-degree burns covering 3% of the TBSA.

Both the American Burn Association and the American College of Surgeons recommend transfer to a burn center for all acutely burned patients who meet any of the following criteria[131]:

- Partial-thickness burns of at least 20% TBSA in patients aged 10 to 50 years
- Partial-thickness burns of at least 10% TBSA in children younger than 10 or adults older than 50 years
- Full-thickness burns of at least 5% TBSA in patients of any age
- Patients with partial- or full-thickness burns of the hands, feet, face, eyes, ears, perineum, or major joints
- Patients with high-voltage electrical injuries, including lightning injuries
- Patients with significant burns from caustic chemicals
- Patients with burns complicated by multiple trauma in which the burn injury poses the greatest risk of morbidity or mortality (in such cases, if the trauma poses the greater immediate risk, the patient may be treated initially in a trauma center until stable before being transferred to a burn center)
- Patients with burns who suffer an inhalation injury
- Patients with significant ongoing medical disorders that could complicate management, prolong recovery, or affect mortality
- Patients who were taken to hospitals without qualified personnel or equipment for the care of children
- Burn injury in patients who will require special social, emotional, or long-term rehabilitative support, including cases involving suspected child abuse or substance abuse

AGE-RELATED RECOMMENDATIONS

Children younger than 2 years of age and elderly patients with a burn injury should be referred for evaluation because these patients may not tolerate any trauma associated with the burn. In addition to medical issues, children with burns that result from suspected child abuse should be hospitalized for legal, psychosocial, and protective reasons. Burns in varying stages of healing, demarcated patterns of burns (e.g., stocking or glove distribution), or more than two burn sites may be clues in identifying an abused child.[122]

DISEASE-RELATED RECOMMENDATIONS

Burn patients with any other medical condition, such as diabetes mellitus, cardiovascular disease, immunodeficiency disorders (e.g., human immunodeficiency virus [HIV]-associated disease, patients receiving cancer chemotherapy), renal disease, obesity, or alcoholism, may be more susceptible to complications from the burn and may have compromised wound healing.

ETIOLOGY

The etiology of a burn should always be considered because this may provide some insight into the burn presentation and its management. Electrical burns can appear to be superficial because external injury may occur at only the entrance and exit sites of the current. These burns, however, can cause extensive damage to underlying nerve and muscle tissue that is not initially evident. Except for very minor electrical burns, these patients should be referred for further evaluation. S.T. has sustained a superficial second-degree burn over about 2% of his BSA. Even though the burn wound on his leg was caused by thermal injury and is relatively minor, S.T. should be referred for further evaluation and treatment.

TREATMENT

CASE 42-6, QUESTION 2: How should S.T.'s burn be treated? What treatment alternatives may be used for S.T.? What immunization should S.T. be questioned about?

GOALS OF TREATMENT AND IMMEDIATE CARE

Treatment goals for first- and second-degree burns are to relieve the pain associated with the burn; to prevent desiccation and deepening of the wound and infection; and to provide a protective environment for healing. Immediate care of the wound should be application of cold, wet compresses or immersion in cool water.

S.T. may have prevented extension of the burn to deeper layers of tissue and alleviated some of his pain from the burn by immediately irrigating the wound with cool water. Next, the area should be cleansed with a mild hypoallergenic soap (e.g., Basis, Purpose) and water. A sterile, nonadherent, fine-mesh gauze dressing that is impregnated with hydrophilic petrolatum (Xeroflo, Adaptic) should be placed over the wound. This type of dressing prevents the gauze from adhering to the wound and allows the burn exudate to flow freely through the dressing, thus preventing maceration.

A second layer of absorbent gauze should be placed over the petrolatum gauze, and a supportive layer of rolled gauze can be used to keep the dressing in place. The outer layer must not be too constricting, and the dressing should be replaced every 48 hours after recleaning the area and inspecting for signs of infection. If S.T.'s wound continues to weep, it may be beneficial to soak his wound or apply a towel saturated with water, normal saline, or Burow's solution (diluted 1:20 or 1:40) for 15 to 30 minutes at least four times daily (see Chapter 39, Dermatotherapy and Drug-Induced Skin Disorders). The use of butter, grease, or similar home remedies should be avoided in the treatment of burns because these measures tend to retain the thermal energy sustained in the burn and may increase the area of thermal injury. Because burn patients are susceptible to secondary tetanus infections, S.T. should receive a tetanus toxoid booster if he has not been immunized within the previous 10 years.

SKIN SUBSTITUTES AND SYNTHETIC DRESSINGS

Advances in the development of skin substitutes are being used to achieve the elusive goal of finding a skin replacement to mimic completely the interaction and functions of dermis and epidermis. Although this goal has yet to be achieved, a growing number of synthetic and biologic products are available that can serve important roles in caring for burn patients.[132] Some of the current modalities are as follows.

Human Cadaver Skin

Fresh human cadaver skin (allograft) is considered the sine qua non for temporary closure of burn wounds. It adheres well to a healthy wound bed, resulting in reduced contamination and reduced protein, heat, and water loss. With improved stabilization techniques, rejection and disease transmission (e.g., hepatitis) can be delayed for 3 to 5 weeks, and the risk of infection transmission (e.g., hepatitis) is minimized.

Epidermal Substitute: Cultured Epithelial Allografts

Deep injuries lead to dermal damage that impairs the ability of the skin to heal and regenerate on its own. Skin autografting after burn excision is considered the current gold standard of care, but lack of patient's own donor skin or unsuitability of the wound for autografting may require the temporary use of dressings or skin substitutes to promote wound healing, reduce pain, and prevent infection and abnormal scarring. These alternatives include deceased donor skin allograft, xenograft, cultured epithelial cells, and biosynthetic skin substitutes. Allotransplantation is the transplantation of cells, tissues, or organs, sourced from a genetically nonidentical member of the same species as the recipient. Human deceased donor skin allografts represent a suitable and much used temporizing option for skin cover after burn injury. The main advantages for their use include dermoprotection and promotion of re-epithelialization of the wound and their ability to act as a skin cover until autografting is possible or reharvesting of donor sites becomes available. Disadvantages of its use include the limited abundance and availability of donors, possible transmission of disease, the eventual rejection by the host, and its handling, storing, transporting, and associated costs of provision. The technique of culturing autologous human epidermal cells grown from a single full-thickness skin biopsy into confluent keratinizing sheets suitable for grafting has been available for more than two decades and is especially useful for patients with large wounds.[133] A lack of mechanical stability of cultured epithelium, causing an imperfect cover, remains a major concern; therefore, the development of a dermal substitute (or a vascularized remnant of allogeneic dermis), in combination with cultured epithelial allografts to increase mechanical stability and decrease wound contracture, or a laboratory-derived autologous composite continues to receive scientific investigation.[134]

Animal Substitute: Porcine Skin

Porcine skin (xenograft; Permacol, Oasis, EZ-Derm) has gained acceptance as a temporary dressing alternative to allograft because of its lower cost and greater availability.[132] At 0°C, frozen porcine skin has a storage life of 6 to 18 months from the date of manufacture. As with an allograft, it has the desirable properties of being able to adhere initially to a clean wound; to cover nerve endings to decrease pain; to function as an autograft test graft; and to diminish heat, protein, and electrolyte loss. A porcine-derived xenograft in a premeshed, de-epithelialized, collagen matrix that can be stored at room temperature (EZ-Derm, Brennen Medical) is thought to be more resistant to bacterial degradation.

Dermal Substitutes: Allodermal Grafts

Unlike the epidermis, the dermis can be rendered acellular and still perform its basic protective and supportive functions. With removal of the dermal cells, the antigenic elements are also eliminated; therefore, an alloplastic transplantation can occur without rejection. The principle of allodermal grafting is that an ultrathin (0.01 cm) meshed autograft laid on top of the allodermis provides skin quality that is comparable to that obtained from thick partial-thickness skin grafts. As one example, AlloDerm (LifeCell) is a shelf-stored, freeze-dried, acellular human cadaveric dermal matrix. Integra (Integra LifeSciences) is used in life-threatening burns. The inner layer of this material is a 2-mm-thick combination of collagen fibers isolated from bovine tissue and the glycosaminoglycan chondroitin-6-sulfate that has a 70- to 200-μm pore size to facilitate host fibrovascular ingrowth. The outer layer is a 0.009-inch polysiloxane polymer with vapor transmission characteristics that simulate normal epithelium.[84]

Hyaluronic Acid

Produced by fibroblasts, this group of dermal matrices has a demonstrated positive impact on scar-free fetal wound healing, and is also used commercially as a dermal filler. It can be obtained from *Streptococcus* fermentation or extracted from rooster combs. It is available as a scaffold for keratinocytes (Laserskin), an acellular dermal matrix (Hyalomatrix), and as a cellular dermal matrix (Hyalograft-3D).[135]

Semisynthetic or Synthetic Dressings

Biobrane (Smith & Nephew), a nylon-collagen mesh, is used commonly for partial-thickness burns.[129,132] It is a bilaminar, semisynthetic, temporary skin substitute made of a silicone film that is bonded to nylon mesh. Once applied to the burn site, blood or sera clot in the nylon matrix to adhere the mesh to the wound until epithelialization occurs. Its adherence is facilitated by collagen peptides bonded to the nylon underlayer. This substitute has been shown to be as effective as frozen human allograft for the temporary coverage of freshly excised full-thickness burn wounds before autografting.[133] Duoderm (ConvaTec) is a hydrocolloid dressing, whereas OpSite (Smith & Nephew) and Tegaderm (3M) are elastomeric polyurethane films. Comfeel (Coloplast) is a semipermeable polyurethane film coated with a flexible, cross-linked adhesive mass containing sodium carboxymethylcellulose (NaCMC) as the principal absorbent and gel-forming agent. This product is permeable to water vapor, but impermeable to exudates and microorganisms. In the presence of an exudate, NaCMC absorbs fluids and swells to form a cohesive gel that does not disintegrate or leave residues in the wound bed.

Alternatives in treating S.T.'s second-degree burn include the use of synthetic dressings and topical antimicrobial agents. Synthetic dressings serve as skin substitutes that are applied to fresh, clean, and moist burns. They are trimmed to about the size of the burn and left in place until the burn is healed or the dressing separates from the wound spontaneously. Indicated for superficial second-degree burns, synthetic dressings keep the wound warm and moist, allowing for a faster rate of healing. These dressings offer a significantly lower rate of infection, less frequent dressing changes, with less pain and electrolyte and albumin loss. The rate of healing in the amniotic membrane group was significantly faster than in the polyurethane group.[136]

Tissue-Engineered Biological Dressings

Tissue-engineered biological dressings have promise in the treatment of burns, chronic ulcers, surgical wounds, and other desquamating dermatologic conditions.[137,138] Although expensive, repeated applications of skin cells, whether keratinocytes or fibroblasts, autologous (the patient's own) or allogeneic (from human donors), can all offer some benefit to chronic nonhealing wounds in prompting them to restart healing. In this setting, cultured cells assist the body's own wound repair mechanisms. Products include Dermagraft, Apligraf, and Oasis. As an example, Apligraf is a bilayer approximating the structure of normal skin. The product is applied in a polyethylene bag containing a 10% CO_2 to air ratio and agarose nutrient medium and must be stored at 20°C to 23°C until use. The first intended indication for Apligraf was full-thickness burns. In a multicenter trial, the use of meshed Apligraf in conjunction with meshed autograft resulted in better scores on the Vancouver Scar Assessment Scale than the use of meshed autograft alone. In most patients, Apligraf-treated burns were judged to have healed better than those treated with meshed autograft alone. Investigators rated Apligraf-treated sites superior to control in 58% of patients, equivalent in 16%, and worse in 16%.[138] The principle of using an appropriate biologically active matrix is now well established for accelerating wound healing and achieving skin reconstruction. Cellular components migrate to the wound from preexisting cell populations in adjacent tissue. Increasing evidence suggests that both circulating marrow-derived stem cells and preexisting organ-specific stem cells can contribute to tissue regeneration.[137] Although important issues concerning wound pretreatment, choice of matrix support for cell growth, and the use of allogeneic cells remain to be fully resolved, tissue-engineered approaches to wound repair still offer significant therapeutic possibilities. Such benefits may include the following:

- Reduced donor site morbidity in burn wounds
- Increased potential for healing of recalcitrant lesions
- Reduced rates of lesion recurrence (as a result of improved dermal quality)
- Reduced wound contracture and scarring
- More rapid closure (epithelialization) of large acute excisional wounds
- Delivery of exogenous growth factors (autologous, allogeneic, or genetically engineered)
- Reduced overall treatment costs and hospital stay

TOPICAL ANTIMICROBIAL AGENTS

Silver Sulfadiazine

Silver sulfadiazine (Silvadene) is the usual agent of choice because it has broad-spectrum gram-positive and gram-negative antibacterial activity, provides reasonable eschar penetration, and is easy and painless to apply and wash off. The cream is a 1% suspension of silver sulfadiazine in a water-miscible base. As a consequence of poor water solubility, the active agent shows only limited diffusion into the eschar. Silver sulfadiazine cream is most effective when applied to burn wounds immediately after thermal injury to prevent bacterial colonization of the burn wound surface as a prelude to intraeschar proliferation. This agent has the advantages of being painless when applied to the wound and being free from acid–base and electrolyte disturbances. The limitations of silver sulfadiazine cream include the potential for allergic reactions owing to its sulfadiazine moiety, silver staining of the treated burn wound, hyperosmolality, methemoglobinemia, and hemolysis as a result of a congenital lack of glucose-6-phospate dehydrogenase.[139] Leukopenia, previously considered to be an adverse drug event associated with use of silver sulfadiazine, occurs when using other topical agents during burn care.[139] An evidence-based review of use of silver sulfadiazine in burns suggested that whereas there is evidence of antibacterial activity, no direct evidence is seen of improved healing or reduced infection compared with normal dressings.[140] This agent should not be applied around the eyes or mouth in patients with hypersensitivity to sulfonamides or in pregnant or breast-feeding women.

Mafenide Acetate

Mafenide acetate (Sulfamylon) is an 11.1% cream formulation of mafenide acetate in a water-dispersible base, or a 5% powder for topical solution. As a water-soluble agent, mafenide diffuses freely to establish an effective antibacterial concentration throughout the eschar and at the interface of viable–nonviable tissue, where bacteria characteristically proliferate before invasion. Because of this characteristic, mafenide is the best agent for use if the patient to be treated has heavily contaminated burn wounds, if treatment is delayed for several days after the burn occurred, or if a dense bacterial population already exists on and within the eschar. Adverse effects include hypersensitivity reactions in 7% of patients (usually responsive to antihistamines), pain or discomfort of 20 to 30 minutes' duration when applied to partial-thickness burns (seldom a cause for discontinuation), and inhibition of carbonic anhydrase. The inhibition of carbonic anhydrase can produce both an early bicarbonate diuresis and an accentuation of postburn hyperventilation. The resulting overall reduction of serum bicarbonate levels renders such patients liable to a rapid shift from an alkalotic to an acidotic state. If acidosis should develop during use of mafenide, the frequency of application should be reduced to once daily, or it should be omitted for 24 to 48 hours, with buffering used as necessary and with efforts made to improve pulmonary function.

Either topical silver sulfadiazine or mafenide should be applied in a one-eighth-inch-thick layer to the entire burn wound with a sterile gloved hand immediately after initial débridement and wound care. Twelve hours later, to ensure continuous topical treatment, a one-eighth-inch coat of cream should be reapplied to those areas of the burn wound from which it has been abraded by clothing. The topical cream should be cleansed gently once each day from all of the burn wound, and the wound should be inspected. Daily débridement should be carried out to a point of bleeding or pain without the use of general anesthesia. After débridement, the wound should be covered again by the topical cream.

Silver Nitrate

If topical antimicrobial creams are unavailable, multilayered occlusive gauze dressings, saturated with a 0.5% solution of silver nitrate, can be used. These soaks are changed two or three times each day and moistened every 2 hours. Evaporation should be avoided to prevent raising the silver nitrate concentration to cytotoxic levels within the soaks. Transeschar losses of sodium, potassium, chloride, and calcium should be anticipated and appropriately replaced. Similar to therapy with silver sulfadiazine cream, silver nitrate soak therapy is best for bacterial control in burn patients who are received immediately after injury before significant microbial proliferation has occurred. Silver nitrate is immediately precipitated on contact with proteinaceous material; it does not penetrate the eschar and, consequently, is ineffective in the treatment of established burn wound infection. For these reasons, it is not routinely recommended.

In S.T.'s case, silver sulfadiazine cream could be chosen to treat his burn on an outpatient basis if an assessment determines that he is at particular risk for infection. The cream would be applied in a thin layer over the wound and covered with absorbent gauze and wrapped with rolled gauze. The dressing must be changed twice daily to maintain an application of cream that is biologically active. Topical bacitracin and the combination of polymyxin B and bacitracin are transparent formulations that also can be used, but because of limited efficacy, may be desirable for use only on small, second-degree burns on the face.

ORAL ANALGESICS AND TOPICAL PROTECTANTS

S.T.'s burn pain can be treated with oral OTC analgesics, aspirin, acetaminophen, or ibuprofen. If these analgesics do not provide adequate relief, oxycodone or acetaminophen (or equivalent) may be of additional benefit. Topical protectants, such as allantoin, calamine, white petrolatum, or zinc oxide, are safe and effective in treating first-degree and minor second-degree burns. These agents protect the burn from mechanical irritation caused by friction and rubbing and prevent drying of the stratum corneum.

POSTWOUND CARE

Postwound care is an essential part of total burn management to ensure adequate follow-up subsequent to wound healing, including psychological support. Good burn care that helps to alleviate physical discomfort, pain, and scarring and that promotes good wound healing will also provide psychological benefits for the patient. Healed wounds should be moisturized on a regular basis. Pruritus can be a major problem after burn injury. To reduce itching, moisturizers can be applied, and oral antihistamines may be necessary.[141] Protection from the sun will help to prevent further thermal damage or pigmentation changes to the affected area. Patients in this population should avoid the sun after a burn injury whenever possible, with use of a sunscreen with an SPF of at least 50 recommended.[129] If surface changes occur (e.g., skin becomes hypertrophic, or blisters or new wounds appear), the patient should be advised to return for evaluation.

KEY REFERENCES AND WEBSITES

A full list of references for this chapter can be found at http://thepoint.lww.com/AT10e. Below are the key references and websites for this chapter, with the corresponding reference number in this chapter found in parentheses after the reference.

Key References

Brusselaers N et al. Skin replacement in burn wounds. *J Trauma*. 2010;68(2):490. (132)

Bylaite M et al. Photodermatoses: classification, evaluation and management. *Br J Dermatol*. 2009;161(Suppl 3):61. (4)

Hexsel CL et al. Current sunscreen issues: 2007 Food and Drug Administration sunscreen labelling recommendations and combination sunscreen/insect repellent products. *J Am Acad Dermatol*. 2008;59(2):316. (78)

Moyal DD, Fourtanier AM. Broad-spectrum sunscreens provide better protection from solar ultraviolet-simulated radiation and natural sunlight-induced immunosuppression in human beings. *J Am Acad Dermatol*. 2008;58(5 Suppl 2):S149. (28)

Rigel DS. Cutaneous ultraviolet exposure and its relationship to the development of skin cancers. *J Am Acad Dermatol*. 2008; 58(5 Suppl 2):S129. (1)

Spanholtz TA et al. Severe burn injuries: acute and long-term treatment. *Dtsch Arztebl Int*. 2009;106(38):607. (129)

Wang SQ et al. U. Photoprotection: a review of the current and future technologies. *Dermatol Ther*. 2010;23(1):31. (7)

Key Websites

American Academy of Dermatology, Sun Safety: http://www.aad.org/public/sun/smart.html

Centers for Disease Control and Prevention, Skin Cancer Prevention: http://www.cdc.gov/cancer/skin/basic_info/prevention.htm

Skin Cancer Organization: http://www.skincancer.org/

SECTION EDITOR: TRICIA M. RUSSELL

43 Osteoarthritis

Dominick P. Trombetta

CORE PRINCIPLES

		CHAPTER CASES
1	Osteoarthritis (OA) is a chronic, progressive condition, primarily affecting women, that causes loss of articular cartilage in the hands, knees, hips, and cervical and lumbar spine. OA causes significant pain and functional disability, and increases costs to our health care systems.	**Case 43-1 (Question 1), Figure 43-2**
2	The evolving role of cytokines and the resultant imbalance between cartilage maintenance and destruction contribute to the pathophysiology of OA. There are no current disease-mitigating therapies.	**Case 43-1 (Questions 2, 3), Figure 43-1**
3	The typical presentation includes stiffness and pain unilaterally in one or more joints lasting less than 30 minutes after a period of immobility. This causes significant limitations in activities of daily living as well as overall quality of life.	**Case 43-1 (Questions 1, 2)**
4	Conservative treatment strategies include weight loss, self-management, aerobic exercise, strength training, and physical and occupational therapies to best maintain optimal functional status.	**Case 43-1 (Question 4)**
5	Initial trials of routine dosing of acetaminophen, topical agents, nonsteroidal anti-inflammatory drugs (NSAIDs) or cyclo-oxygenase-2 (COX-2) inhibitors, tramadol, opioid analgesics, and intra-articular injections into the knee are all attempted before surgical interventions are offered.	**Case 43-1 (Questions 5, 6), Case 43-2 (Questions 1–4), Tables 43-1 through 43-5, Figure 43-3**
6	The decision to use an oral NSAID or COX-2 inhibitor rests in the clinical judgment and the balancing of the risks for gastrointestinal bleeding versus cardiovascular risks in addition to other patient comorbidities. Older patients tend to be more sensitive to the adverse effects and are unable to tolerate these medications because of their effects on blood pressure, kidney, or liver.	**Case 43-2 (Questions 1–3), Table 43-1, Table 43-2, Figure 43-3**
7	A consistent and systematic approach to the management of chronic pain caused by OA can help identify patients with limitations in activities of daily living (ADLs) and prevent further disability. Then, the effectiveness of current therapies can be more appropriately evaluated and the treatment plan updated.	**Case 43-1 (Questions 5, 7), Case 43-2 (Questions 1–6) Case 43-3 (Question 2)**
8	The general recommendation to consider the use of alternative therapies or supplements cannot be justified at this time based on lack of consistent clinical evidence.	**Case 43-3 (Question 3)**

INCIDENCE, PREVALENCE, AND EPIDEMIOLOGY

Osteoarthritis (OA) is a chronic, progressive disorder characterized by the loss of articular cartilage primarily in the hands, knees, hips, and spine. Incidence rates for OA of the hand have been estimated to be 100 per 100,000 person-years, hip OA, 88 per 100,000 person-years, and knee OA, 240 per 100,000 person-years. Incidence rates increase with advancing age until the octogenarian status. The Centers for Disease Control and Prevention (CDC) reported in 2005 that approximately 26.9 million people older than 65 years of age are affected, particularly after the age of 50. Women seem to be affected by more severe OA of the knees than men, particularly after the age of 50. Men have a lower incidence of knee and hip OA than women. However, there are clear dis-associations with the prevalence of radiologic and symptomatic OA. Radiologic OA is more prevalent than symptomatic OA. The reason for the dissociation is unclear at this time. The prevalence of knee OA is estimated to be 0.9% (1.2%, female; 0.4%, male) per 100, whereas the prevalence of symptomatic OA is reported as 12.1% (13.6%, female; 10%, male) per 100 for adults older than 60 years of age as reported by the CDC.[1]

OA accounts for about 0.2 to 0.3 deaths per 100,000 (1979–1988). This could be considered an underestimation because those deaths associated with medication-related toxicities (e.g., renal disease or gastrointestinal [GI] bleeding) are not factored in.[1] However, the associated disability, pain, ambulatory dysfunction, and costs are quite staggering. OA is ranked tenth, slightly below diabetes, among causes of disability-adjusted life-years (DALYs).[2] Pain is more likely to cause disability when the weight-bearing joints are affected. The clinical consequences of knee OA have a significant clinical impact, affecting approximately 20% of community-dwelling adults. Many affected adults describe their health quality of life as fair or poor. Productivity and work absence can be directly impacted by clinically significant knee OA. Limitations in walking can impact activities of daily living (ADLs), with 11% of patients requiring assistance with personal care. Nearly 20% of all ambulatory care visits to primary care providers are secondary to pain and disability associated with OA. There are 7.1 million (4.9 million women and 2.2 million men) total provider visits for the primary diagnosis of OA. However, large percentages (39%) of patients with OA have reported their inability to gain access to rehabilitation providers. The costs of knee and hip replacements have been estimated at $7.9 billion in 1997. As last reported, the total cost of the disease in the year 2000 was $5,700 with consumers paying $2,600 yearly.[1]

ETIOLOGY

The exact etiology of OA is not completely understood. The morphology and clinical complications are the result of a convergence of risk factors. In primary OA, the cause or causes elude determination of any particular identifiable factors. In secondary OA, metabolic conditions such as hemochromatosis, acromegaly, and deposition of crystalline calcium can be identified. Inflammatory diseases such as septic or rheumatoid arthritis and ankylosing spondylitis have been implicated. Structural anomalies such as leg length discrepancies and joint or hip dislocation can contribute to the development of secondary OA. Chronic repetitive joint injury by either occupational, recreational, or major joint trauma will result in cartilage deterioration.[3]

Various risk factors have been identified and can be classified as modifiable and nonmodifiable (Fig. 43-1). Modifiable risk factors of OA include obesity and joint trauma. Increased body weight has been correlated with increased risk of OA of the knee, but not the hip. Intuitively, weight contributes to the biomechanical forces and stresses on the knee joints. The cascade of increased pain leading to decreased function and further worsening of obesity can be a difficult cycle to break. Weight loss and moderate amounts of activity improve symptoms of OA of the knee and improve overall health. Nonmodifiable risk factors are advancing age, sex, genetics, and joint location. Typically, the development of symptomatic OA occurs with increased age predominantly in the weight-bearing joints, although many women are affected by localized inflammation of the proximal and distal interphalangeal joints known as Bouchard's and Heberden's nodes, respectively. Approximately 80% of patients older than 75 years are affected by OA.

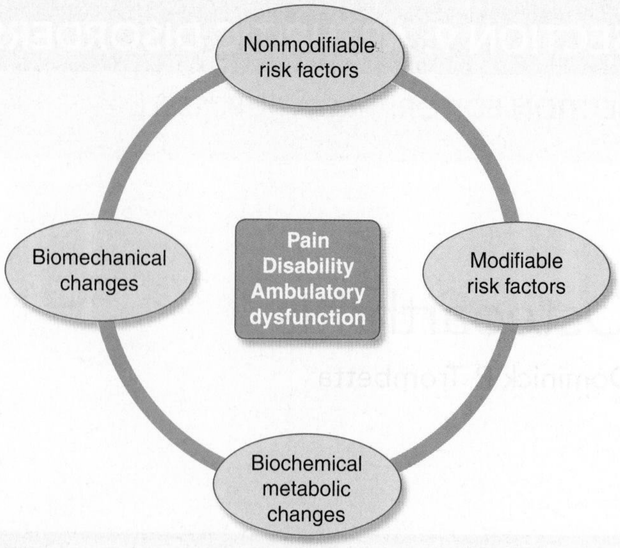

FIGURE 43-1 Schematic representation of the convergence of modifiable, nonmodifiable risk factors, and morphologic changes associated with osteoarthritis. (Source: Sellam J, Berenbaum F. Clinical features of osteoarthritis. In: Firestein GS et al, eds. *Kelley's Textbook of Rheumatology.* 8th ed. Philadelphia, PA: Saunders/Elsevier; 2010:1547; Di Cesare PE et al. Pathogenesis of osteoarthritis. In: Gary S. Firestein et al, eds. *Kelley's Textbook of Rheumatology.* 8th ed. Philadelphia, PA: Saunders/Elsevier; 2010:1525; Dieppe PA, Lohmander LS. Pathogenesis and management of pain in osteoarthritis. *Lancet.* 2005;365:965.)

Epidemiological studies provide support for a genetic component to the development of OA as well as the characteristic Heberden's and Bouchard's nodes. Studies in twins have also supported the influence of genetics and the development of OA. Multiple genes have been identified that are associated with increased risk for OA as well as some genetic mutations associated with OA of early onset. With the increasing development of isolating specific genotypes and pharmacogenomics, more targeted interventions could be implemented to arrest disease progression. OA is particularly more common in the hips and knees than in the ankle joint. Increased interleukin-1 (IL-1) concentrations have been associated with destruction of articular cartilage. It is unknown whether this is the result of disease progression or part of the pathophysiology.[3,4]

Joint trauma can result in the evolution of OA. Biochemical and mechanical changes can occur, resulting in the characteristic joint pain and stiffness. The consequences are articular cartilage with less functionality and resultant characteristics of cartilage, joint capsule, and subchondral bone that are distinctively different from those of normal bone. Regular exercise and physical activity do not increase the risk of OA in normal joints and are necessary to maintain cartilage.[3,4]

The development of radiologic evidence of OA precedes the clinical symptoms; thus the initial presentation may not always correlate with disease prognosis. Diminished ability of chondrocytes to maintain and repair articular cartilage has been correlated with resultant cartilage degradation. These age-related changes in chondrocyte function are associated with a decreased response to anabolic stimuli such as insulinlike growth factor-1 (IGF-1). Thus, the biochemical signal to spur production of proteoglycans and collagen that maintain the strength of cartilage decreases and results in an imbalance between breakdown and repair. The effect of age on chondrocyte apoptosis seems to be strongly related. Perhaps, because of occupational or recreational injury, men tend to have more OA before the age of 50. One theory that tries to explain the sex-based disparity in the prevalence of OA is the effect of menopause and decreasing levels of circulating estrogen. Basic science in humans and animals suggests upregulation of chondrocytes as a direct effect of estrogen. Observational data confirm a reduction in knee OA in patients receiving estrogen replacement therapy (ERT). However, in the absence of randomized controlled trials examining the efficacy and safety of ERT in the treatment of OA, it cannot be recommended.[3,4]

PATHOGENESIS

Osteoarthritis has been known as a "wear and tear" disease of cartilage. The dynamic interactions between biochemical, morphologic, and mechanical processes that affect articular cartilage are relatively new developments. Subchondral bone, ligaments, and the entire joint are clearly affected by the disease. Once the disease process has progressed clinically to the point of requiring surgical intervention, the journey backward to clearly elucidate the mechanisms, etiologies, and pathogenesis becomes very difficult. The observations may reflect the end product of disease progression rather than true disease pathogenesis. Insult to the articular cartilage can result from repetitive damage with time. Alternatively, another theory has been proposed that examines articular damage after superficial or deep penetration injury. Either repetitive or traumatic injury to articular surfaces initiates the cascade leading to release of inflammatory cytokines (tumor necrosis factor [TNF], IL-1), nitric oxide, and enzymes that break down the extracellular matrix. The breakdown of extracellular matrix results in cartilage that is less elastic and less able to support joint loads, and stiffening of subchondral bone. The cartilage is less able to support forces, with diminished efficacy for providing joint lubrication and weight distribution across the joint. Cartilage is avascular, however, and contains chondrocytes that under normal conditions are responsible for cartilage breakdown and repair. In early osteoarthritis, chondrocytes attempt to repair joint damage by forming osteophytes, which try to stabilize the joint or alter the biochemical properties of cartilage. The formation of osteophytes may provide an increased surface area over which to distribute the forces across the joint.[5]

Osteophytes or bony outgrowths may be responsible for the patient reports of pain and limited mobility. It is unclear whether osteophytes are formed as a result of abnormal stress fracture healing of the subchondral bone proximal to the joint margins. Alternatively, osteophyte formation may occur secondary to vascularization of the cartilage that has been altered through etiologies and risk factors mentioned previously. Cyst formation is thought to be created by synovial fluid pressure exerted on the fissures or other structural defects in subchondral bone.[5]

Early in the disease process, the water content of the cartilage is increased. However, this less viscous cartilage is structurally weaker than normal cartilage. There are many structural alterations that contribute to the weakened collagen network. One of the early changes is a smaller diameter of type II collagen, in comparison to that in the more structurally intact disease-free joint. With disease progression, the proteoglycan concentrations diminish with shorter glycosaminoglycan side chains resulting in decreases of net aggregate proteins. Type I collagen within the extracellular matrix increases, and keratin sulfate concentrations decrease. Some of the biochemical changes are reflective of those produced in culture by immature tissue. The deposition of calcium crystals represents a curious finding. It is unknown whether calcium deposition has a direct involvement or is reflective of increased chondrocyte activity. Eventually, the initial water swelling of the cartilage is replaced by cartilage with reduced propensity to allow bone to distribute the force and slide on bone.[5]

Chondrocytes are unable to maintain production of essential macromolecules necessary for healthy cartilage. However, the syntheses of those enzymes that break down the matrix are increased by the same chondrocytes. The enzymes that degrade proteoglycans and collagen are called aggrecanases and collagenases, respectively. The control of these enzymes is complicated by enzymatic activation of latent proteins and inactivation by proteinase inhibitors. In OA, the expression and production of proteinases is increased. Collagen is typically cleaved by matrix metalloproteinases (MMP), MMP-1, MMP-8, and MMP-13. Of the three, MMP-13 may be the most important in OA because it preferentially degrades type II collagen. Bench science has substantiated the increased expression of MMP-13 in cartilage cultures. Upregulated by IL-1 and TNF, MMPs cleave collagen and break down other important elements of the extracellular matrix. Ultimately, the imbalance between cartilage maintenance and degradation leads to erosion and eventual cartilage destruction.[5]

OVERVIEW OF DRUG THERAPY

The current treatment of OA is to provide analgesia to support ADL, engage or facilitate participation in physical or occupational therapies, and recommend appropriate self-managed exercise programs. There are no disease-mitigating strategies that have demonstrated acceptable safety and efficacy in the treatment of OA. The initial treatment for OA pain and stiffness is acetaminophen given on a routine basis for a 2- to 3-week trial in doses typically less than 4 g/day or less than 3 g/day in patients older than 65 years, unless clinically contraindicated. Acetaminophen offers a considerable degree of safety over nonsteroidal anti-inflammatory drugs (NSAIDs) for mild to moderate OA disease.[6] However, many clinical trials have demonstrated significantly better efficacy of NSAIDs as compared with acetaminophen in selected patients, such as those who present with both pain and inflammation, because acetaminophen lacks significant anti-inflammatory effects.[7–9] These patients are more likely to have more moderate to severe disease.[10] Many nonprescription medications contain acetaminophen, as do many prescription analgesic products, especially opioid/acetaminophen combinations. Most recently, the use of acetaminophen and related products has gained the attention of the US Food and Drug Administration (FDA), prompting consumer and health professional awareness to potential liver injury as a result of unintentional misuse. A trial of an NSAID or cyclooxygenase-2 (COX-2) inhibitor would be a reasonable consideration in selected individuals. A careful risk and benefit analysis must be individualized for each patient starting an NSAID or COX-2 inhibitor. Adverse events of GI bleeding, diminishing renal function, liver toxicity, and cardiovascular risk of the specific medication considered need to be carefully assessed and a plan for therapeutic monitoring implemented. Additionally, consideration of drug–drug interactions or drug–disease interactions is also warranted. Topical therapies may be therapeutic for selected patients unable to tolerate oral NSAIDs. Tramadol may represent a useful option for many patients unless precluded because of history of seizures or drug–drug interactions. There are currently no recommendations for the use of oral glucocorticoids in the treatment of OA. In patients presenting with effusions of the knee, aspiration of the affected joint and intra-articular injections of corticosteroids may be therapeutic. Intra-articular injections of hyaluronic acid derivatives are the last of the conservative strategies before surgical interventions are considered. Currently, the use of over-the-counter (OTC) supplements such as glucosamine and chondroitin or cat's claw maybe considered for selected patients, but the cost may be prohibitive for those elderly patients on limited incomes. A trial time limit of 6 months can be discussed with those patients interested in pursuing this type of therapy. The use of oral or transdermal opioids or opioid/acetaminophen combinations for pain management could be entertained cautiously owing to the risks of adverse consequences exceeding the benefits.[11]

CLINICAL MANIFESTATIONS

Clinical Presentation of Osteoarthritis

CASE 43-1

QUESTION 1: R.T., a 60-year-old nonsmoking woman, presents to her primary-care physician reporting pain and stiffness in her right knee. The pain is usually worse in the morning and lasts for about 15 to 20 minutes and then subsides throughout the day. She reports some increased difficulty taking care of her grandchildren while her daughter is working. Her medical history is significant for hypertension, dyslipidemia, and a history of peptic ulcer disease. R.T. currently takes hydrochlorothiazide 12.5 mg daily and simvastatin 40 mg daily. On physical examination, there is a varus misalignment of the knees. The right knee has no swelling or synovial effusions, and crepitus is noted on examination of passive motion. A radiograph shows right knee joint space narrowing with osteophyte formation at the joint margins.

Laboratory values and vital signs obtained at this visit include the following:

Blood pressure (BP), 135/78 mm Hg
Heart rate (HR), 80 beats/minute
Height, 64 inches
Weight, 175 pounds
Sodium, 140 mEq/L
Potassium, 4.5 mEq/L
Blood urea nitrogen (BUN), 10 mg/dL
Creatinine, 0.9 mg/dL
Estimated glomerular filtration rate (eGFR), 70 mL/minute
Thyrotropin (TSH), 3.08 mIU/mL
White blood cells (WBC), 5 × $10^3/\mu L$
Red blood cells (RBC), 4.7 × $10^6/\mu L$
Hemoglobin, 12.7 g/dL
Hematocrit, 38.2%
Uric acid, 5 mg/dL
C-reactive protein (CRP), 0.9 mg/dL
Erythrocyte sedimentation rate (ESR), 18 mm/hour
Total cholesterol, 160 mg/dL
High-density lipoprotein (HDL), 45 mg/dL

What signs and symptoms suggestive of OA are present in R.T.?

R.T. presents with unilateral right knee pain that is worse in the morning and subsides throughout the day. The OA diagnosis can be made by a good history and physical examination. Laboratory studies are not needed to confirm the diagnosis of OA, but a normal ESR rules out inflammatory conditions such as gout or septic arthritis. Radiographs demonstrate joint space narrowing that is consistent with OA. However, radiographs do not reliably assess disease severity.

CASE 43-1, QUESTION 2: How do the subjective and objective findings of OA correlate with disease pathogenesis in R.T.?

The characteristic joint space narrowing as seen on radiograph without joint destruction is characteristic for OA. Osteophyte formation and bone rubbing against bone are most likely responsible for the pain, stiffness, and crepitus demonstrated on physical examination. Crepitus is an audible "crackling" sound that can be heard with passive or active movement of the joint. Instead of the opposing joint surfaces gliding past each other, the movement of the joint now creates the characteristic crunching or crackling sounds. Additionally, the varus misalignment contributes to the stress on the knee joint and some of the functional impairments R.T. reported to her primary-care physician. A varus misalignment is described as the patient in a standing position with his or her knees appearing further apart (bow-legged), and valgus is when the knees are closer together. Both of these deformities can affect a patient's function and quality of life.

The clinical presentation of OA is usually unilateral pain and stiffness of the knee, hip, or cervical or lumbar spine; the distal interphalangeal joints generally are not painful. More often than not, OA tends to affect more than one joint. There are some distribution associations described between knee and hand OA and knee and hip OA. Elbows, wrists, and shoulders tend not to be affected by OA. Diagnostic criteria from the American College of Rheumatology (ACR) hip criteria have a sensitivity and specificity of 91% and 89%, respectively, and a sensitivity of 91% and specificity of 86% for knee OA.[3] These criteria usually are not used in clinical practice outside of research studies. Clinical trials typically provide outcome data based on assessment tools such as the Western Ontario and McMaster Universities (WOMAC), predominantly used for knee OA. A WOMAC functional subscale exists to assess for functional disability.[12] The knee OA outcome score (KOOS) has gained popularity and is readily available for use at http://www.koos.nu/.[13]

Patients usually present to their primary-care provider with complaints of increased pain or stiffness lasting less than 30 minutes, usually in the morning or after periods of prolonged immobility. They usually will report decreases in their ADL, functional status, and overall health-related quality of life. Typically, household activities such as kneeling, stair climbing, and walking tend to be limited. The associated decrease in activities, range of motion and overall physical activity contribute to muscle weakness and unsteadiness. Problems with sleep and depression can occur, compromising attempts to lose weight, increase activity, and participate in physical or occupational therapy or in Tai Chi.

The diagnosis usually can be made by the primary-care provider based on a careful history, brief physical examination, and observation of the patient's gait in the cases of knee or hip OA. More detailed information on physical examination of the hip and knee, including videos that demonstrate techniques used for eliciting an effusion, can be found at **http://meded.ucsd.edu/clinicalmed/joints.htm** (physical knee examination) and **http://meded.ucsd.edu/clinicalmed/joints5.htm** (physical hip examination).

Joint involvement can be characterized with swelling, easily recognized in the fingers and knees. Joints usually are tender when examined during active motion or application of pressure. Bursitis, tendonitis, muscle spasms, and torn meniscus can cause limitations in range of motion and need to be ruled out. Synovial effusions can be chronic but can also present during times of disease exacerbations. The patellar tap test or the wave test can elucidate joint effusions (see above web pages). Patients with advanced disease may present with the expected loss of cartilage, but also deformities in surrounding bone and soft tissue affecting the ligaments. Joint misalignment is common and contributes to joint unsteadiness (Fig. 43-2). Fingers of patients with the characteristic Bouchard's and Heberden's nodes are misaligned. Muscle atrophy is demonstrated by simply measuring the circumference of the quadriceps muscles. The use of radiographs is usually not necessary for the diagnosis of OA, but rather is used to rule out conditions such as avascular necrosis, Paget disease of the bone, rheumatoid arthritis, or gouty arthropathies. However, radiographs can be useful to establish disease severity or monitor for disease progression; otherwise a radiograph is not completely satisfying for providing additional information. The clinical features described on radiographs that are characteristic of OA are joint space narrowing, osteophytes at the joint margins, and sclerosis of subchondral bone. As demonstrated in the above case study, R.T.'s knee radiograph revealed joint space narrowing with osteophyte formation.

An ultrasound can be useful for detecting or confirming joint effusion, popliteal cysts, or other erosive inflammatory conditions. Laboratory assessments are usually unnecessary, as the ESR and CRP are typically within reference ranges. Serum uric acid can help differentiate between similar inflammatory presentations. Synovial fluid aspiration is appropriate if septic or inflammatory arthritis is suspected. In the patient with OA, the WBC count is less than 2,000 μL, synovial fluid is clear, and crystals are absent. There are no relevant biomarkers of bone or cartilage remodeling that are used in the routine care of patients with OA. Magnetic resonance imaging (MRI) scans represent an exciting area of research for assessing cartilage, synovium, and bone, but are not routinely used in the diagnosis of OA.

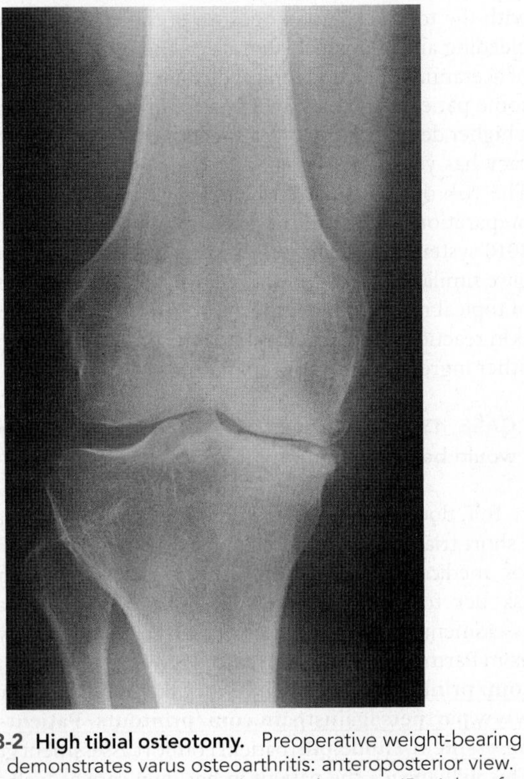

FIGURE 43-2 High tibial osteotomy. Preoperative weight-bearing radiograph demonstrates varus osteoarthritis: anteroposterior view. Reprinted with permission from Koval KJ, Zuckerman, JD. *Atlas of Orthopaedic Surgery: A Multimedia Reference*. Philadelphia, PA: Lippincott Williams & Wilkins; 2004.

CASE 43-1, QUESTION 3: Cytokines are involved in the pathophysiology of OA. Is it possible to modulate these cytokines and thereby slow or delay the disease process to benefit R.T. before her condition worsens?

The role of IL-1 and TNF in rheumatoid arthritis pathogenesis represented exciting discoveries that have led to highly effective disease remissions. The IL-1 receptor antagonist, anakinra, has been used in the treatment of rheumatoid arthritis to prevent joint erosion and destruction. In a trial of 170 patients with OA of the knee, subjects were given varied doses of anakinra as a one-time injection. This randomized, multicenter trial did not find any symptomatic improvements in the treatment versus the placebo-controlled populations studied.[14] However, in OA, the role of these cytokines in upregulating MMP and the exact mechanism that they play in the disease process have not been clearly elucidated. There have been attempts to arrest or slow disease progress with doxycycline without demonstrating any clinically significant benefits.[15]

TREATMENT OF OSTEOARTHRITIS

Nonpharmacologic Management of OA

Nonpharmacologic modalities are a primary strategy for OA treatment. As previously discussed, there are no interventions that effectively attenuate the disease process. Pharmacologic strategies have significant untoward effects and modest efficacy in the management of OA pain and disability. Patients typically have difficulty adhering to self-management, aerobic, or strength-training programs. Many times, nonpharmacologic strategies are not even attempted until pharmacologic interventions have failed or side effects necessitate discontinuation of the offending agent.

The ACR outlines a variety of patient education, self-management, weight-loss, aerobic, and physical and occupational therapies.[12] A study in middle-aged patients with knee OA has demonstrated equivocal efficacy in comparing self-management with strength training and the combination of both programs. Outcomes assessed were pain, disability, and physical conditioning during the 2 years of the trial.[16] One clinical trial examined the comparison of NSAID therapy with quadriceps home exercise. Quality-of-life surveys and pain scores were not different between the groups reviewed in this small trial.[17] In older patients, Tai Chi has established efficacy through randomized controlled trials in the treatment of knee OA. Wang et al. demonstrated the beneficial effects of Tai Chi not only in improving physical function and lessening pain in patients with OA, but also in having a positive effect on their mental health and overall quality of life. Trial limitations included a small sample size (40 patients) and 3-month study duration. It is unknown whether those demonstrated benefits were sustained.[18] Patients can be referred to the Arthritis Foundation website (**http://www.arthritis.org/osteoarthritis.php**) for further information on various programs or activities in their areas.[19] The Osteoarthritis Research Society International

(OARSI) reiterates the effectiveness of nonpharmacologic interventions of self-management, weight loss, exercise, referral to physical therapy, and effective use of bracing for varus or valgus misalignments.[20] Nonpharmacologic interventions remain the most effective, but yet underutilized, interventions for the treatment of OA.[6]

CASE 43-1, QUESTION 4: What nonpharmacologic therapies should be recommended in R.T.?

R.T. should be encouraged to lose weight and participate in either self-management or a structured exercise program that includes aerobic and strength-training exercises. Additionally, R.T. should be encouraged to participate in local Tai Chi classes. Weight loss can be very helpful in patients with OA of the knee. Exercise improves muscle strength and helps prevent falls. The use of knee bracing may offer some degree of support in patients with misalignments of the knee joints.

Pharmacologic Management of Osteoarthritis

CASE 43-1, QUESTION 5: What is the initial pharmacologic treatment recommendation for R.T.?

A trial of acetaminophen 1,000 mg PO three to four times a day should be attempted for 2 to 3 weeks. More aggressive medications are usually reserved for those patients who have failed acetaminophen. Medications such as NSAIDs and COX-2 inhibitors can increase blood pressure, cause GI ulceration, inhibit renal prostaglandins that are vasodilatory and, therefore, diminish renal function, and potentially increase cardiovascular risks. Given R.T.'s past medical history of peptic ulcer disease and lack of knee inflammation on physical examination, the initial trial of acetaminophen is warranted.

ACETAMINOPHEN

Acetaminophen remains the first choice for the treatment of mild to moderate OA of the hands and knees. A more recent update on the management of OA of the hip, knee, and hand from the ACR is expected and pending publication. Clinical practice guidelines from the ACR can be found at http://www.rheumatology.org/practice/clinical/guidelines/index.asp. Treatment recommendations from the ACR, the OARSI, Agency for Healthcare Research and Quality (AHRQ), the National Institute for Clinical Excellence (NICE), and the European League Against Rheumatism (EULAR) have consistently suggested a reasonable trial of acetaminophen in divided doses of less than 4 g per 24 hours.[11,20–24] Chronic acetaminophen use in patients with alcoholism (more than three drinks per day) can increase risk of GI bleeding and elevations of liver enzymes.[25] A 12-week randomized, controlled trial reported in 2007 that extended-release acetaminophen 3,900 mg/day was safe, well tolerated, and more effective than 1,950 mg/day in patients with hip and knee OA.[26] More recently, it has been suggested that those selected patients presenting with both pain and inflammation without contraindications begin an initial trial with an NSAID instead of acetaminophen.[21]

TOPICAL THERAPY

CASE 43-1, QUESTION 6: What is the role of topical agents in the treatment plan for R.T.?

There are three topical products available, capsaicin, diclofenac gel, and diclofenac topical solution, that can be used alone or in combination with other pharmacologic therapies for OA. Topical capsaicin cream is applied to the hands or knees three to four times daily. If used, R.T. should be counseled regarding proper application, initial burning and sensitivity reactions, and expectations of benefits that may take up to a few weeks. There are no systemic effects or drug interactions with topical capsaicin cream.[27]

Topical diclofenac gel alone or in combination with oral acetaminophen represents another therapeutic option. Topical diclofenac gel is indicated in the treatment of OA of the upper extremities such as the hands, elbows, and wrists, and the lower extremities (ankles, feet, and knees). The gel is applied according to "dosing cards" in either 2-g or 4-g measurements. The dose for the upper extremities is 2 g four times a day, and 4 g four times daily to the lower extremities.[28]

Diclofenac topical solution 1.5% w/w in dimethyl sulfoxide, USP (DMSO) 45.5% w/w has recently been approved for treatment of signs and symptoms of OA of the knee.[29] In a 12-week, randomized, placebo-controlled trial, oral and topical diclofenac solution were equivocal for the outcome measures of pain and physical function. Patients receiving the topical solution reported minor skin irritation, but fewer GI symptoms and abnormal liver function tests than those patients receiving oral diclofenac.[30] Similarly, in another comparison trial, diclofenac topical solution was found to be better than placebo and dimethyl sulfoxide alone, but similar in efficacy to oral diclofenac with better tolerability.[31]

Topical agents may be the next step in the planned care of the patient with progressing OA, or those unable to tolerate oral NSAIDs because of GI, liver, renal, or cardiac side effects. However, the warnings about these potential untoward effects for topical NSAIDs and oral NSAIDs are the same.[28,29] There are limited data with regard to topical diclofenac and comparative efficacy with other oral NSAIDs or topical capsaicin than previously mentioned. Outside of short-term efficacy trials, the risk for systemic complications with chronic therapy has not been investigated. Oral NSAIDs should not be used concomitantly with the topical solution because of the increased risk of rectal bleeding and abnormal laboratory findings.[29] The combination of acetaminophen and topical diclofenac may be therapeutic for some patients and may avoid use of other combinations having a higher degree of untoward effects; however, the safety and efficacy has yet to be evaluated in the rigor of randomized trials. The risk of significant GI bleeding would be less with topical preparations as a result of less systemic absorption.[21,30–32] In a 2010 systematic review, oral and topical NSAIDs were noted to have similar rates for discontinuation because of a high incidence of topical reactions with the latter.[33] It is unclear whether these skin reactions are caused by the type of formulation, vehicle, or other ingredients in the preparation.

CASE 43-1, QUESTION 7: What monitoring parameters would be appropriate for R.T.?

R.T. does not have a history of liver disease or hepatitis C, so a short trial of acetaminophen does not require any monitoring for medication safety. However, it would be important to ask her to keep a daily pain log and complete a comfort assessment on her next visit. These tools are readily available from Partners Against Pain (http://www.partnersagainstpain.com/printouts/Daily_Pain_Diary.pdf [pain diary] and http://www.partnersagainstpain.com/printouts/Patient-Comfort-Assessment-Guide.pdf[patient comfort assessment guide]).[34,35] This will engage the patient in her own care as well as provide the clinician with information regarding baseline data, medication efficacy, and the impact of medication on functional impairments. Additionally, limitations or improvements in ADLs and instrumental activities of daily living (IADLs) can provide useful information in helping the clinician determine whether any changes in the plan of care need to occur.

NSAIDS AND OTHER PHARMACOLOGIC TREATMENT

CASE 43-2

QUESTION 1: S.L., a 67-year-old woman, presents to her primary-care physician with increased pain and stiffness in her left knee. S.L. reports her left knee as "weak," and she has difficulty getting out of bed in the morning and after sitting on the recliner for some time. She has tried acetaminophen 1,000 mg four times daily for 1 month without adequate relief. She also takes metoprolol succinate 50 mg daily, lisinopril 20 mg daily, ranitidine 150 mg twice daily, and citalopram 20 mg daily. Her medical history includes hypertension, osteopenia, depression, gastroesophageal reflux disease, osteoarthritis, and a right knee replacement 2 years ago. Her recent laboratory values and vital signs include the following:

BP, 145/78 mm Hg
HR, 76 beats/minute
Height, 66 inches
Weight, 190 pounds
Sodium, 145 mEq/L
Potassium, 4.8 mEq/L
BUN, 16 mg/dL
Creatinine, 1.2 mg/dL
eGFR, 48 mL/minute
WBC, 4.5 × $10^3/\mu L$
RBC, 4.2 × $10^6/\mu L$
Hemoglobin, 12.1 g/dL
Hematocrit, 36.6%

Select and recommend a medication to provide adequate pain relief for S.L.

In this patient who has failed an adequate trial of acetaminophen, therapeutic options include celecoxib, a nonselective NSAID, tramadol, or an opioid analgesic (Fig. 43-3). There are no data to suggest any particular NSAID is more effective than another.[6] S.L. does not have any known history of coronary heart disease or peptic ulcer disease. On the basis of the risk factors identified in Tables 43-1 and 43-2, S.L. has one risk factor of age, placing her at moderate risk for GI ulceration. Data suggest appropriate treatment of *Helicobacter pylori*, if present, reduces the risk of GI ulceration in patients taking NSAIDs chronically.[36] Therefore, if the decision is made to recommend a nonselective NSAID, then ranitidine would need to be discontinued because of a lack of protection against gastric ulcers, and a proton-pump inhibitor (PPI) such as omeprazole or misoprostol should be initiated to prevent GI bleeding.[37] Either option would represent a reasonable therapeutic recommendation.

For those patients with insufficient pain relief from acetaminophen or topical agents, an oral NSAID should be considered. As with any decision regarding pharmacotherapy, the safety and efficacy of the chosen therapy needs to be evaluated in the context of a patient's specific case. The historical perspective and the knowledge of increased cardiovascular risk versus GI safety with COX-2 agents have had a tremendous impact on the use of these agents in clinical practice.

TABLE 43-1
Risk Factors for GI Complications With NSAIDs[36]

Age >65
NSAID dose
Concurrent steroid use
Previous GI adverse event
Oral antiplatelet agents (aspirin, clopidogrel)
Oral anticoagulant therapy
History of
PUD
Upper GI bleeding
GI hospitalization
Dyspepsia
Cardiovascular disease

GI, gastrointestinal; NSAID, nonsteroidal anti-inflammatory drug; PUD, peptic ulcer disease.

ONLINE CONTENT

For a multimedia slide set describing the cardiovascular risks of COX-2 agents, go to http://thepoint.lww.com/AT10e.

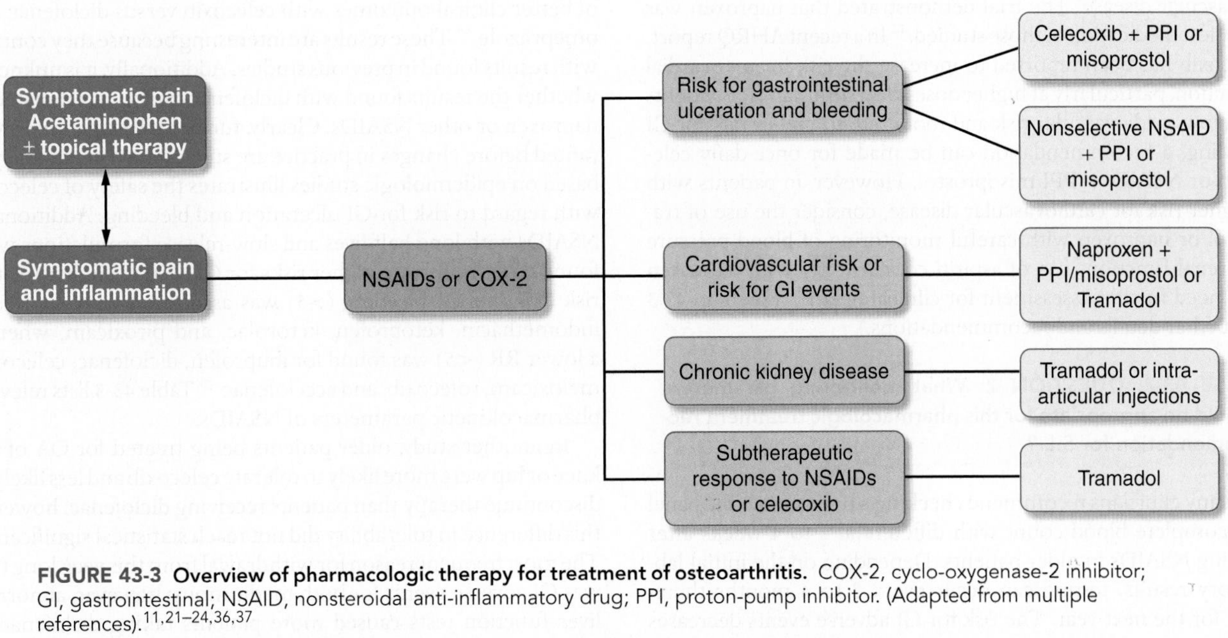

FIGURE 43-3 Overview of pharmacologic therapy for treatment of osteoarthritis. COX-2, cyclo-oxygenase-2 inhibitor; GI, gastrointestinal; NSAID, nonsteroidal anti-inflammatory drug; PPI, proton-pump inhibitor. (Adapted from multiple references).[11,21–24,36,37]

TABLE 43-2
Recommendations for NSAID Selection Based on Gastrointestinal and Cardiovascular Risks[36]

Risk Category	Low GI Risk	Moderate GI Risk	High GI Risk
	0 risk factors	1–2 risk factors	Multiple risk factors, history of previous ulcer events, or continued use of corticosteroids or anticoagulants
Low CV risk	NSAID alone	NSAID + PPI/misoprostol	Alternative therapy or COX-2 + PPI/misoprostol
High CV risk (low-dose aspirin required)	Naproxen + PPI/misoprostol	Naproxen + PPI/misoprostol	Alternative therapy recommended

COX-2, cyclo-oxygenase-2 inhibitor; CV, cardiovascular; NSAID, nonsteroidal anti-inflammatory drug; PPI, proton-pump inhibitor.

Patients at increased risk for cardiovascular disease include those with unstable angina, a history of myocardial infarction, coronary artery bypass surgery, or ischemic stroke, or a high Framingham risk score.[38] Some clinicians have recommended the addition of low-dose aspirin 81 mg to attenuate the increased risk of cardiovascular disease; however, this practice has not been the primary focus of vigorous clinical trials. The addition of aspirin can potentially increase the risk of GI ulceration and compromise cardioprotection.[39] Additionally, randomized controlled studies have not clearly demonstrated the efficacy and safety of this approach.[39,40] In a 52-week double-blind study comparing the cardiovascular outcomes of ibuprofen, naproxen, or lumiracoxib in patients with OA, there were three interesting findings. Ibuprofen users taking aspirin had the highest risk of cardiovascular outcomes and heart failure in comparison with lumiracoxib. This suggests that ibuprofen can interfere with the ability of aspirin to acetylate platelets, thereby inhibiting platelet aggregation. Patients taking naproxen without aspirin had the best safety profile with regard to cardiovascular outcomes. Whether or not naproxen has the lowest risk for cardiovascular side effects has not been clearly elucidated. Conflicting data regarding dose, duration of therapy, and methodological differences in trials have not yet produced clear and concise evidence. Lastly, heart failure was observed more frequently in patients taking ibuprofen than in those patients receiving lumiracoxib or naproxen.[41] The question of how these agents affect morbidity and mortality in healthy patients has been the topic of speculation for a number of years. Most recently, a trial was designed to assess and evaluate the cardiovascular risk of the NSAIDs rofecoxib, diclofenac, celecoxib, ibuprofen, and naproxen in healthy patients without known cardiovascular disease. The trial demonstrated that naproxen was the safest medication of those studied.[42] In a recent AHRQ report, celecoxib has been reported to increase the risk for myocardial infarction, particularly at higher doses.[32] In summary, for patients with low cardiovascular risk and moderate to higher risk for GI bleeding, a recommendation can be made for once-daily celecoxib or NSAID + PPI/misoprostol. However, in patients with a higher risk for cardiovascular disease, consider the use of tramadol or naproxen with careful monitoring of blood pressure and renal function (use of aspirin concurrently with naproxen may need further assessment for clinical need).[11] (See Fig. 43-3 for further details and recommendations.)

CASE 43-2, QUESTION 2: What monitoring parameters would be appropriate for this pharmacologic treatment recommendation for S.L.?

Many clinicians recommend checking a basic metabolic panel and complete blood count with differential 2 to 4 weeks after starting NSAIDs in older patients. Depending on the initial laboratory results, testing can occur every 3 to 4 months thereafter for the next year. The risk for GI adverse events decreases after 1 month, but is always present. Liver function should be checked regularly during the first year of treatment and periodically thereafter. Patients with significant comorbidities may need more stringent follow-up and monitoring. Analgesic efficacy is best evaluated using a consistent systematic assessment approach.[34,35] If S.L. is to remain on chronic NSAID therapy, then monitoring her liver function every 3 months for the first year would be reasonable.

Gastrointestinal ulceration and bleeding remain a cardinal concern when evaluating patients for treatment of chronic pain in OA. The addition of a PPI to a nonselective NSAID has been proposed as a less expensive alternative to the more expensive COX-2 inhibitor agent, celecoxib. In a 2002 trial, 287 patients with a history of GI ulceration and bleeding were randomly assigned to receive diclofenac and omeprazole or celecoxib for 6 months. The results indicated there were no differences in the rates of bleeding between the populations studied.[43] Older patients with OA have comorbidities requiring aspirin in addition to a COX-2 or NSAID. Goldstein et al. compared celecoxib and aspirin with naproxen, lansoprazole, and aspirin with endoscopically diagnosed ulcers after 12 weeks of therapy. Gastrointestinal ulceration rates were found to be statistically insignificant among groups.[44] In contrast, another randomized controlled trial compared celecoxib with diclofenac and omeprazole in patients with OA and rheumatoid arthritis for 6 months. The risk for GI bleeding was evaluated across the small bowel.[45] Consideration of clinically significant anemia not responsive to acid-suppressive interventions (PPIs) distal to the duodenum may provide the clinician with more evidence in patients at increased risk for GI ulceration and bleeding. The results are suggestive of better clinical outcomes with celecoxib versus diclofenac and omeprazole.[45] These results are interesting because they contrast with results found in previous studies. Additionally, it is unknown whether the results found with diclofenac can be extrapolated to naproxen or other NSAIDs. Clearly, further investigation is warranted before changes in practice are suggested. A meta-analysis based on epidemiologic studies illustrates the safety of celecoxib with regard to risk for GI ulceration and bleeding. Additionally, NSAIDs with long half-lives and slow-release formulations were found to demonstrate higher risks for GI events. Higher relative risk (RR) for GI bleeding (>5) was associated with naproxen, indomethacin, ketoprofen, ketorolac, and piroxicam, whereas a lower RR (<5) was found for ibuprofen, diclofenac, celecoxib, meloxicam, rofecoxib, and aceclofenac.[46] Table 43-3 lists relevant pharmacokinetic parameters of NSAIDs.

In another study, older patients being treated for OA of the knee or hip were more likely to tolerate celecoxib and less likely to discontinue therapy than patients receiving diclofenac; however, this difference in tolerability did not reach statistical significance. The most frequent reason for withdrawal from this year-long trial was GI adverse events for both medications; however, abnormal liver function tests caused more patients taking diclofenac to

TABLE 43-3
Pharmacokinetic Parameters of NSAIDs

NSAID	Bioavailability (%)	Half-Life (hours)	Volume of Distribution	Clearance	Peak (hours)	Protein Binding (%)	Renal Elimination (%)	Fecal Elimination (%)
Acetic Acids								
Diclofenac	50 to 60	2	0.1–0.2 L/kg	350 mL/min	2	>99	65	—
Indomethacin	98	4.5	0.29 L/kg	0.084 L/h/kg	2	90	60	33
Sulindac	90	7.8	NS	≈2.71 L/h	2–4	>93	50	25
Tolmetin	NS	2–7	NS	NS	0.5–1	NS	≈100	—
COX-2 Inhibitor								
Celecoxib	NS	11	400 L	27.7 L/h	3	97	27	57
Fenamates								
Meclofenamate	≈100	1.3	23 L	206 mL/min	0.5–2	>99	70	30
Mefenamic acid	NS	2	1.06 L/kg	21.23 L/h	2–4	>90	52	20
Naphthylalkanones								
Nambumetone	>80	22.5	0.1–0.2 L/kg	26.1 mL/min	9–12	>99	80	9
Oxicams								
Piroxicam	NS	50	0.15 L/kg	0.002–0.003 L/kg/h	3–5	98.5	NS	NS
Meloxicam	89	15–20	10 L	7–9 mL/min	4–5	99.4	50	50
Propionic Acids								
Fenoprofen	NS	3	NS	NS	2	99	90	
Flurbiprofen	NS	5.7	0.1–0.2 L/kg	1.13 L/h	≈1.5	>99	>70	
Ibuprofen	>80	1.8–2	0.15 L/kg	≈3–3.5 L/h	1–2	99	45–79	
Ketoprofen	90	2.1	0.1 L/kg	6.9 L/h	0.5–2	>99	80	
Ketoprofen ER	90	5.4	0.1 L/kg	6.8 L/h	6–7	>99	80	
Naproxen	95	12–17	0.16 L/kg	0.13 mL/min/kg	2–4	>99	95	
Oxaprozin	95	42–50	10–12.5 L	0.25–0.34 L/h	3–5	>99	65	35
Pyranocarboxylic Acid								
Etodolac	≥80	7.3	0.362 L/kg	47 mL/h/kg	≈1.5	>99	72	16
Pyrrolizine Carboxylic Acid								
Ketorolac	100	5–6	≈0.2 L/kg	≈0.025 L/h/kg	2–3	99	91	6

COX-2, cyclo-oxygenase-2; NS, not studied; NSAID, nonsteroidal anti-inflammatory drug.
Adapted with permission from Facts & Comparisons eAnswers. Accessed August 17, 2010, from http://online.factsandcomparisons.com/MonoDisp.aspx?monoID=fandc-hcp11516 (select Actions to see information).

withdraw from the study.[47] Diclofenac is associated with elevations in alanine aminotransferase and aspartate aminotransferase levels; however, increases in aminotransferase levels alone are not predictive of liver injury. The FDA recognizes increases in both bilirubin and aminotransferase levels as surrogate markers for drug-induced liver disease. In a study completed by Laine et al., the risk of hospitalization associated with diclofenac therapy is described as relatively rare (0.023% per 100,000 patient-years). The low rate of hospitalization may be secondary to clinical vigilance. This study also found elevations in liver function test concentrations to occur in the initial 4 to 6 months of therapy and do not necessarily parallel clinical significant liver injury.[48]

TRAMADOL AND OPIOIDS

CASE 43-2, QUESTION 3: One week later after starting naproxen 500 mg twice daily, S.L. has been adherent with therapy, and had a basic metabolic panel completed before this office visit. S.L. reported a decrease in pain since she had been started on naproxen. Laboratory values and vital signs obtained at this visit include the following:

BP, 155/78 mm Hg
HR, 88 beats/minute
Height, 66 inches
Weight, 194 pounds
Sodium, 135 mEq/L
Potassium, 5.5 mEq/L
BUN, 40 mg/dL
Creatinine, 2.2 mg/dL
RBC, 4.7 × 10^6/μL
Hemoglobin, 11.4 g/dL
Hematocrit, 33.8%

What changes, if any, need to be made with her OA therapy?

TABLE 43-4
Tramadol Drug Interactions

Precipitant Drug	Object Drug[a]		Description
Carbamazepine	Tramadol	↓	Coadministration may significantly reduce the analgesic effect of tramadol. Because carbamazepine increases the metabolism and because of the seizure risk associated with tramadol, coadministration is not recommended.[1]
CNS depressants (e.g., alcohol, other opioids)	Tramadol	↑	Coadministration may increase the risk of CNS and respiratory depression. Use tramadol with caution and in reduced dosages.[1]
CYP2D6 inhibitors (e.g., fluoxetine, paroxetine, amitriptyline)	Tramadol	↑	Coadministration may inhibit some of the metabolism of tramadol to various degrees. The full pharmacological impact of these alterations is unknown.[1]
CYP3A4 inducers (e.g., rifampin, phenytoin)	Tramadol	↓	May produce increased clearance of tramadol; use with caution.[1]
CYP3A4 inhibitors (e.g., ketoconazole, erythromycin)	Tramadol	↑	Coadministration may produce increased tramadol concentrations.[1]
TCAs and other tricyclic compounds (e.g., cyclobenzaprine, promethazine)	Tramadol	↑	Concomitant use increases the risk of seizures.[1]
Tramadol	Digoxin	↑	Postmarketing surveillance revealed rare reports of digoxin toxicity.[1]
Tramadol	MAOIs	↑	Tramadol inhibits norepinephrine and serotonin reuptake.
MAOIs	Tramadol		Concomitant use increases the risk of adverse reactions, including seizures and serotonin syndrome.[1]
Tramadol	SSRIs	↑	The serotonergic effects of these agents may be addictive.
SSRIs	Tramadol		The risk of seizures is also increased with coadministration.[1,2]
Tramadol	Warfarin	↑↓	Postmarketing reports revealed alteration of warfarin effects, including elevation of prothrombin times. Use with caution and monitor international normalized ratio.[1,2]

[a]↑ = object drug increased; ↓ = object drug decreased.

1. Ultram ER [package insert]. Raritan, NJ: Ortho-McNeil Pharmaceutical Inc; 2006.
2. Tramadol. *Drug Interaction Facts*. Facts & Comparisons [database online]. 2003. St. Louis, MO: Wolters Kluwer Health Inc. Accessed August 21, 2006.

In the week that has passed, there has been an increase in potassium, serum creatinine, and BUN. Naproxen and COX-2 inhibitors have the same potential to cause adverse renal effects. Naproxen should be discontinued, and additional monitoring should be ordered to ensure laboratory values return to baseline.

In many patients with contraindications or subtherapeutic response to acetaminophen, NSAIDs, or COX-2 inhibitors, a trial of tramadol should be considered. Therapeutic alternatives for analgesia are now limited to opioids or tramadol for S.L. Tramadol is a centrally acting analgesic that binds to the mu opioid receptor and also inhibits the uptake of norepinephrine and serotonin.[49] The ACR recommends tramadol in those patients who have failed or have contraindications to NSAIDs.[20] Tramadol should not be used in patients with a history of seizures or receiving medications with serotonergic activity and requires dose adjustment with diminished renal function.[49] Tramadol can be used with acetaminophen, and the combination can be therapeutic. However, she is taking citalopram for depression, and there is a drug interaction with tramadol; therefore, this option should be avoided.[49] (Refer to Table 43-4 for a complete description of drug–drug interactions with tramadol.) Opioid/acetaminophen combinations may be a short-term option in the interim while S.L. is being evaluated for intra-articular injection of either corticosteroid or viscosupplementation (hyaluronic acid injection) by her physician.

In patients in whom the use of tramadol is ineffective or contraindicated, the use of an opioid or opioid/acetaminophen combination can be considered.[20] Side effects from opioids include constipation, confusion, hallucinations, respiratory depression, tolerance, and addiction. A recent Cochrane review evaluated the use of oral and transdermal opioids in the treatment of OA of the hip and knee. Although the findings did conclude opioids are effective, their benefits are mild to moderate; however, the benefits are outweighed by their side effect profiles.[50] The American Pain Society recommends chronic opioid therapy for selected patients with close monitoring. Clinicians need to monitor for medication safety and efficacy, functional status, and progress toward therapeutic goals, and reassess for continued need of chronic opioid therapy.[51] As with any medication, the smallest effective dose for the shortest possible duration is a strategy that is important in the treatment of osteoarthritis with opioids.

DULOXETINE

Recently, duloxetine has been approved for the treatment of chronic musculoskeletal pain. Duloxetine is a selective serotonin and norepinephrine reuptake inhibitor that also is indicated for major depressive disorder, generalized anxiety disorder, fibromyalgia, and diabetic peripheral neuropathic pain.[52] In a 13-week randomized, double-blind, placebo-controlled trial involving 231 patients, duloxetine demonstrated statistically significant reductions in osteoarthritic pain of the knee. The magnitude of difference in average pain between duloxetine and placebo in the reported mean end points and the mean change from baseline was modest. The number of adverse effects between placebo and the treatment groups was low and statistically not significantly different. However, this can only be fully evaluated in the context of larger randomized, placebo-controlled trials. The average age of the patients in this trial was 62 years.[53] Despite the statistical significance demonstrated, the clinical benefit of long-term duloxetine in older and more symptomatic patients is unknown. Until more trial data become available, duloxetine may be an option for selected patients who can tolerate it and have no contraindications. S.L. is currently receiving citalopram for

TABLE 43-5
Hyaluronic Acid Products

Euflexxa (Ferring Pharmaceuticals, Inc.)	**Injection**: sodium hyaluronate 10 mg/mL	In 2-mL prefilled syringes.[a]
Hyalgan (Sanofi-Synthelabo, Inc.)		In 2-mL vials and prefilled syringes.[b]
Supartz (Smith & Nephew)		In 2.5-mL prefilled syringes.[c]
Orthovisc (Anika Therapeutics[d])	**Injection**: hyaluronan 15 mg[e]	Sodium chloride 9 mg/mL. In 2-mL prefilled syringes.
Synvisc (Genzyme Corp)	**Injection**: hylan polymers 8 mg/mL[f]	In 2-mL prefilled syringes.
Synvisc-One (Genzyme Corp)	**Injection**: hylan polymers 8 mg/mL[f]	Sodium chloride 8.5 mg/mL. In 6-mL prefilled syringes.

[a]Molecular weight is 2,400,000–3,600,000 Da.
[b]Molecular weight is 500,000–730,000 Da.
[c]Molecular weight is 620,000–1,170,000 Da.
[d]Anika Therapeutics; 160 New Boston St, Woburn, MA 01801; 1-781-932-6616; http://www.anikatherapeutics.com.
[e]Molecular weight is 1,000,000–2,900,000 Da.
[f]Molecular weight is 6,000,000 Da on average.
Adapted with permission from Facts & Comparisons eAnswers. Accessed August 18, 2010, from http://online.factsandcomparisons.com/MonoDisp.aspx?monoid=fandc-hcp12890&book=DFC&search=423991|21&isStemmed=True&asbooks=.

the treatment of major depressive disorder. The risk-to-benefit analysis of switching citalopram to duloxetine has many considerations. The treatment of the depression and the significant medical history of the patient need to be carefully assessed. S.L. has a past medical history of recurrent depression resistant to several different medications and has been stable for the last year on citalopram. Next, tolerability and cost need to be evaluated as duloxetine may have a higher copay than the generic citalopram. Higher copays have been associated with poor medication adherence. In this case, the mild to modest improvements that could possibly be achieved with duloxetine do not warrant changing therapy in S.L.

Intra-Articular Therapy

CASE 43-2, QUESTION 4: S.L. has seen commercials on television advertising "knee injections." Describe the available therapeutic options.

Ultimately, many patients fail oral or topical therapies, and intra-articular injections represent the last conservative efforts before surgical intervention for OA of the knee. Aspiration of synovial fluid and injections of glucocorticoids or viscosupplementation of hyaluronic acid are strategies that have been offered to patients with severe knee OA. Injections of triamcinolone or methylprednisolone with lidocaine 1% have been shown to be effective for approximately 4 to 8 weeks. Typically, intra-articular glucocorticoids are given no more frequently than every 3 months. Side effects include a paradoxical localized inflammatory reaction.[54,55]

ONLINE CONTENT

For a video that shows knee joint aspiration and injection with steroid, go to http://thepoint.lww.com/AT10e.

In a small multicenter, randomized trial, the safety and efficacy of intra-articular treatment with hyaluronic acid in OA of the knee was demonstrated. However, there was a rather large placebo response and a small effect size with treatment in this trial.[56] In a 2005 meta-analysis, intra-articular hyaluronic acid supplementation did not demonstrate clinical efficacy in OA of the knee.[55,57] In contrast, a more recent Cochrane review found intra-articular injection of hyaluronic acid products to be effective and provide more sustained clinical effects than intra-articular injections of glucocorticoids. The authors acknowledged considerable product variability and corresponding times to clinical response.[58] A 2009 multicenter, randomized, placebo-controlled trial did not find any efficacy of hyaluronic acid in hip OA.[59] Table 43-5 illustrates the various hyaluronic acid products available.

CASE 43-2, QUESTION 5: Two years have passed, and S.L. has now failed all conservative strategies including intra-articular injections into her knee. After discussing all of her options with her physician, S.L. is referred to an orthopedic surgeon for elective left total knee replacement. She is awaiting discharge from the acute care hospital, pending transfer to a short-term rehabilitation facility to facilitate her return home and resumption of her previous level of function. S.L.'s current medications are metoprolol succinate 50 mg daily, lisinopril 20 mg daily, citalopram 20 mg daily, enoxaparin 30 mg subcutaneously twice daily, oxycodone CR 10 mg every 12 hours, senna/docusate one tablet twice daily, and oxycodone/acetaminophen 5 mg/325 mg one tablet every 4 hours as needed for moderate pain and two tablets every 4 hours as needed for severe pain. S.L. asks you, as the counseling pharmacist, why she still needs "shots in the belly"?

The American College of Chest Physicians' (ACCP) highest level of evidence for elective knee arthroplasty recommends low-molecular-weight heparin, fondaparinux, or warfarin (international normalized ratio [INR] goal of 2.5) for patients in whom a risk for significant bleeding does not exist. A minimal duration of therapy is for 10 days after surgery and up to 35 days for some patients.[60] It is important to educate S.L. with this information, providing her with the reason for enoxaparin is to prevent blood clots in her legs or lungs. In cases in which the creatinine clearance is less than 30 mL/minute, the appropriate dosage of enoxaparin would be 30 mg subcutaneously once daily.[61]

CASE 43-2, QUESTION 6: How long will S.L. need oxycodone CR and oxycodone/acetaminophen therapy?

Patients typically need the sustained-release dosing of their opioid analgesic given on a routine schedule only while undergoing aggressive physical and occupational therapy immediately after orthopedic surgery. By the time most patients return to their home environments, the use of as-needed dosing of opioid/acetaminophen combinations may be necessary for the completion of the short-term rehabilitation process. However, the long-term use of opioids in the treatment of chronic pain should be discouraged.

Falls and the Elderly

CASE 43-3

QUESTION 1: L.P. is an 80-year-old woman who was recently admitted to the emergency department (ED) after sustaining a fall at home. L.P. was seen by her physician 1 week ago and was given a prescription for oxycodone/acetaminophen 5 mg/325 mg every 4 hours as needed for left knee pain. Her medical history is significant for type 2 diabetes, diabetic peripheral neuropathy, hypertension, dyslipidemia, OA left knee, a right knee replacement, and Bouchard's nodes on the left upper extremity. Medications include glipizide 10 mg daily in the morning before breakfast, metformin 850 mg twice daily, amitriptyline 100 mg at bedtime, lisinopril 20 mg daily, atorvastatin 40 mg daily, gabapentin 600 mg three times daily, and oxycodone/acetaminophen 5 mg/325 mg one tablet every 4 hours as needed for left knee pain. The physical examination revealed a confused elderly woman, and her hip radiographs were negative for fractures.

Select and recommend the most appropriate therapy for treating L.P.'s OA left knee pain.

The benefits and risks of all medications need to be carefully assessed. L.P. is currently receiving several medications that possess sedating properties, amitriptyline, gabapentin, and oxycodone/acetaminophen. Sedating medications can contribute to an increased risk for falls. Efforts to taper and discontinue amitriptyline, decrease the gabapentin dose to the smallest effective dose, and discontinue oxycodone/acetaminophen should occur. A trial of acetaminophen 500 mg four times daily could be attempted to manage her pain.

Managing Complicated Care

CASE 43-3, QUESTION 2: In the ED, L.P. is diagnosed with new-onset atrial fibrillation. Warfarin 5 mg daily is prescribed. Are there any drug interactions that need consideration in L.P.?

The addition of warfarin to an already complex medical regimen is always challenging. The primary concern with the addition of warfarin is the increased prothrombin time (PT) and increased INR. Acetaminophen in doses of 2 to 4 g/day have been shown to increase the PT and subsequently the INR.[62–64] In many situations, as-needed dosing of acetaminophen along with many common acetaminophen combination products available by prescription and OTC are the underrecognized causes of overanticoagulation and bleeding with warfarin. Often, the dose of acetaminophen can be reduced to 500 mg three times daily and hence the effects of the interaction minimized, with continued monitoring of INR and signs and symptoms of bleeding.

Dietary Supplements

Dietary supplements offer patients an alternative to prescription medications. Some patients often either fail multiple prescription drugs or have intolerable side effects. Others confuse dietary supplements with natural products and consider them safer than traditional medications. In the case of OA, the role of glucosamine, chondroitin, and the combination products have represented such an alternative to many patients. As with any OTC dietary supplement, the vigor of product consistency and standardization are not the same as FDA requires for legend drugs. Researchers have found in evaluating the use of glucosamine, chondroitin, and the combinations in OA of the knee that they were all ineffective in reducing pain. However, it is worth noting that treatment effects were more pronounced in the subgroup of patients with moderate to severe reports of pain. Also, this trial included a celecoxib treatment group that also did not reach statistical significance with regard to primary outcomes measured.[65] Similar findings were published, concluding the lack of efficacy with glucosamine in treatment of OA of the hip as well as degenerative lumbar OA.[66–68]

Another natural product, *S*-adenosylmethionine (SAMe), was a focus of the Cochrane Collaboration in 2009. The authors concluded, based on the outcomes of pain and function, that SAMe lacked demonstrated efficacy and cannot be recommended for the pain and disability associated with OA at this time.[69] In a recent review by Rosenbaum et al., cat's claw (*Uncaria guianensis*) use was supported by an 8-week trial in OA patients to reduce the pain and stiffness and to increase overall functional status with decreased use of analgesics for breakthrough pain. Vitamin E, ginger, combination ginger/galanga, and omega-3 fatty acids were not found to have any effects in patients suffering from OA.[70]

Nontraditional alternatives for the pain, stiffness, and discomfort of OA are few and certainly lack the vigor of large scale, long-term, clinical trials. However, in selected patients who wish to try either cat's claw or glucosamine/chondroitin, a time-limited trial can be considered in patients who fail or refuse more traditional approaches to pharmacologic management. However, a general recommendation cannot be made for all patients.

CASE 43-3, QUESTION 3: Can any glucosamine and chondroitin product be recommended for L.P.?

The data on the use of glucosamine and chondroitin, either separately or in combination, have not conclusively demonstrated efficacy in patients with OA. At this time, no general recommendations can be made for these products for L.P. In addition, these products are expensive and contribute to L.P.'s daily pill burden and thereby may lead to reduced adherence to more proven therapies.

KEY REFERENCES AND WEBSITES

A full list of references for this chapter can be found at **http://thepoint.lww.com/AT10e**. Below are the key references and websites for this chapter, with the corresponding reference number in this chapter found in parentheses after the reference.

Key References

Jordan KM et al. EULAR Recommendations 2003: an evidence based approach to the management of knee osteoarthritis: Report of a Task Force of the Standing Committee for International Clinical Studies Including Therapeutic Trials (ESCISIT). *Ann Rheum Dis.* 2003;62:1145. (23)

Lanza FL et al. Guidelines for prevention of NSAID-related ulcer complications. *Am J Gastroenterol.* 2009;104:728. (36)

Zhang W et al. EULAR evidence based recommendations for the management of hip osteoarthritis: report of a task force of the EULAR Standing Committee for International Clinical Studies Including Therapeutics (ESCISIT). *Ann Rheum Dis.* 2005;64:669. (24)

Zhang W et al. OARSI recommendations for the management of hip and knee osteoarthritis, Part II: OARSI evidence-based, expert consensus guidelines. *Osteoarthritis Cartilage.* 2008;16:137. (21)

Key Websites

Arthritis Foundation. Osteoarthritis. **http://www.arthritis.org/osteoarthritis.php.** (19)

Chou R et al. Comparative effectiveness and safety of analgesics for osteoarthritis. Comparative effectiveness review no. 4. (Prepared by the Oregon Evidence-based Practice Center under Contract No. 290-02-0024.) Rockville, MD. Agency for Healthcare Research and Quality. September 2006. **http://effectivehealthcare.ahrq.gov/reports/final.cfm.** Accessed December 3, 2010. (32)

Hickman D et al. Choosing Non-Opioid Analgesics for Osteoarthritis. Clinician's Guide. Agency for Healthcare Research and Quality. **http://www.effectivehealthcare.ahrq.gov/ehc/products/2/5/Osteoarthritis_Clinician_Guide.pdf.** Accessed December 3, 2010. (11)

National Institute for Health and Clinical Excellence. Osteoarthritis: The Care and Management of Osteoarthritis in Adults. **http://www.nice.org.uk/nicemedia/live/11926/39557/39557.pdf.** Accessed August 18, 2010. (22)

Partners Against Pain. **http://www.partnersagainstpain.com.** (34,35)

44 Rheumatoid Arthritis

Steven W. Chen, Rory E. O'Callaghan, and Alison M. Reta

CORE PRINCIPLES

RHEUMATOID ARTHRITIS	CHAPTER CASES
1 Rheumatoid arthritis (RA) is a chronic systemic inflammatory disorder characterized by potentially deforming polyarthritis and a wide spectrum of extra-articular manifestations. Diagnosis of RA is based on joint involvement, serology, acute-phase reactants, and symptom duration.	**Case 44-1 (Questions 1, 2)**
2 Treatments for RA include nonpharmacologic (heat or cold therapy, range-of-motion exercises, physical therapy, occupational therapy) and pharmacologic options (nonsteroidal anti-inflammatory drugs [NSAIDs], traditional and biologic disease-modifying antirheumatic drugs [DMARDs], corticosteroids). NSAIDs are for symptom management only and must be used cautiously, if at all, because of serious health risks, including gastrointestinal complications and thromboembolic cardiovascular events.	**Case 44-1 (Questions 3–5), Case 44-2 (Question 1), Case 44-3 (Questions 1, 2), Case 44-4 (Question 1), Case 44-5 (Questions 1–3)**
3 Owing to the destructive nature of the disease, DMARDs should be initiated shortly after a diagnosis has been established. Methotrexate is the most common selection because of efficacy, safety, rapid onset, and cost-effectiveness. Other traditional DMARDs and combinations of traditional DMARDs are selected based on disease severity, disease duration, and the presence of poor prognostic indicators. Several traditional DMARDs are no longer used as a result of poor efficacy or intolerable adverse effects. Regardless of the DMARD chosen, all require diligent monitoring.	**Case 44-5 (Questions 4–7), Case 44-6 (Questions 1–9), Case 44-7 (Questions 1–8)**
4 Patients with RA who experience an inadequate response to traditional DMARDs, either alone or in combination, or intolerable adverse effects should consider the addition of or switching to a biologic DMARD. Diligent monitoring is also critical with biologic agents owing to the risk of serious adverse effects such as infections and lymphoma.	**Case 44-7 (Questions 9–13), Case 44-8 (Question 1)**
5 Corticosteroids, when used judiciously at the lowest effective doses and for limited durations, are very effective at quickly controlling inflammation while awaiting onset of DMARD therapy. In rare instances when long-term corticosteroid therapy is prescribed, appropriate therapy must be used to help prevent steroid-induced osteoporosis.	**Case 44-9 (Questions 1–4)**
6 Although systemic corticosteroids can be prescribed for short-term flares of RA disease activity, intra-articular corticosteroid injections are very effective at managing flares that are limited to a few joints and are not associated with the adverse effects of systemic therapy.	**Case 44-9 (Question 5)**

continued

JUVENILE IDIOPATHIC ARTHRITIS

1	Juvenile idiopathic arthritis (JIA) describes an assortment of arthritis conditions affecting adolescents. Symptoms of JIA such as joint inflammation and range-of-motion limitation present before 16 years of age. As in RA, the diagnosis of JIA is based on clinical manifestations, and all infectious, traumatic, and other etiologies must be ruled out.	**Case 44-10 (Questions 1, 2)**
2	Pharmacologic treatment options for JIA include NSAIDs, traditional and biologic DMARDs, and corticosteroids.	**Case 44-10 (Questions 3, 4), Case 44-11 (Questions 1, 2), Case 44-12 (Question 1), Case 44-13 (Questions 1, 2), Case 44-14 (Question 1)**
3	Many nonpharmacologic treatment options are also available to supplement JIA pharmacologic therapy, including exercise, massage, and physical and occupational therapy.	**Case 44-14 (Question 2)**

Epidemiology

The term *arthritis* refers to more than 100 diseases causing pain, swelling, and damage to joints and connective tissue.[1] Rheumatoid arthritis (RA) is a chronic systemic inflammatory disorder characterized by potentially deforming polyarthritis and a wide spectrum of extra-articular manifestations. The diagnosis of RA is based primarily on clinical criteria (Table 44-1) because no single chemical or laboratory finding is specific for this disease.[2] The prevalence of RA is estimated to be 1% worldwide, but varies greatly between geographic regions.[3,4] In the United States, RA afflicts approximately 1.5 million individuals, occurring nearly twice as often in women as in men.[4] The onset of RA typically occurs between the third and fourth decades of life, and prevalence increases with advancing age up to the seventh decade.[1,3] The prevalence of RA increased from 0.62% to 0.72% between 1995 and 2005, and the average age of RA prevalence increased from 63.3 years in 1965 to 66.8 years in 1995.[5] RA-related morbidity, mortality, and disability are expected to increase substantially in future years as the US boomer population ages.[5]

TABLE 44-1
Criteria for Diagnosis of Rheumatoid Arthritis

Criteria	Score[a]
Joint Involvement	
1 large joint	0
2–10 large joints	1
1–3 small joints	2
4–10 small joints	3
>10 small joints	5
Serology	
Negative RF and negative anti-CCP	0
Low-positive RF or low-positive anti-CCP	2
High-positive RF or high-positive anti-CCP	3
Acute-Phase Reactants	
Normal CRP and normal ESR	0
Abnormal CRP or abnormal ESR	1
Duration of Symptoms	
<6 weeks	0
≥6 weeks	1

[a] Score-based algorithm: add score of all categories; score of ≥6/10 needed to classify patient as having definite RA.
anti-CCP, anti–cyclic citrullinated peptide; CRP, C-reactive protein; ESR, erythrocyte sedimentation rate; RA, rheumatoid arthritis; RF, rheumatoid factor.
Source: Aletaha D et al. 2010 rheumatoid arthritis classification criteria: an American College of Rheumatology/European League Against Rheumatism collaborative initiative [published correction appears in *Ann Rheum Dis.* 2010;69:1892]. *Ann Rheum Dis.* 2010;69:1580.

The cause of RA seems to be an interplay among multiple factors (e.g., genetic susceptibility, environmental influences, the effects of advancing age on somatic changes in the musculoskeletal and immune systems).[3] It is suspected that genetics contribute to 50% or 60% of the risk of developing RA.[6] The genes with the strongest implication include the *HLA-DRB1* gene of the major histocompatibility complex (MHC), and chromosome 1's *PTPN22* gene. Epidemiologic associations between cigarette smoking and RA have now been clearly established; cigarette smoking increases the production of rheumatoid factor (RF) and anti-cyclic citrullinated peptide antibody (anti-CCP, another clinical marker for RA).[6] It appears that female sex hormones may play a role in RA development. In women, peak incidence occurs at the fifth decade, a time when many enter menopause or perimenopause. Estrogen is known to stimulate the immune system; pregnant patients often experience a remission of RA symptoms, and women who take oral contraceptives appear to be protected somewhat against the development of RA.[4,6] Diets rich in fish, olive oil, and other omega-3 fatty acid sources are associated with a lower risk of developing RA.[6] A deficiency of vitamin D is also associated with RA.[4]

The course of RA is variable and can be categorized as *polycyclic, monocyclic,* or *progressive.*[7] The polycyclic course occurs in approximately 70% of patients, who initially experience mild intermittent symptoms that resolve over the course of several weeks to months. The patient can be symptomfree for several weeks to months and then experience symptoms that can be more severe than those experienced initially. Monocyclic patients (~20% of patients) experience a relatively sudden onset of symptoms followed by a prolonged clinical remission of disease activity. Patients with the progressive form (~10% of patients) experience advancing disease that usually evolves uninterrupted over the course of a few months, but the rate of disease progression in this group can be rapid or slow. Patients within this group can be subdivided further into those who respond to "aggressive" therapy and those who do not. Patients with more aggressive disease (multiple joint involvement, positive RF) have a greater than 70% probability of developing joint damage or erosions within 2 years of disease onset.[8]

The rate of RA disease remission was low before medications capable of halting or slowing disease progression became more available and commonly used in clinical practice. American College of Rheumatology (ACR) criteria for RA remission were established in 1981[9]; however, the criteria did not incorporate some common RA symptoms and were so stringent that very few patients were able to meet remission criteria. As a result, the majority of RA clinical trials use modified remission criteria, often removing one or more of the ACR criteria and making meaningful comparisons between trials very difficult. This variance in remission criteria is highlighted in a systematic review of literature that evaluated RA remission rates.[10] Among 17 observational trials involving RA patients treated with traditional and biologic disease-modifying antirheumatic drugs (DMARDs), 27% of patients were reported to experience disease remission; however, rates differed when using ACR criteria (17%) versus Disease Activity Score (DAS) criteria (33%). Importantly, many patients deemed to be in remission continued to experience radiological progression of disease, although less progression was noted with combination DMARD therapy versus monotherapy. In response to the need for stringent yet achievable criteria for RA remission that would be more uniformly accepted, updated criteria were recently released jointly by the ACR and the European League Against Rheumatism (EULAR) (Table 44-2).[11] These criteria state that patients with RA in clinical trials will be considered "in remission" if either of the following occurs: (1) tender joint count, swollen joint count (of 28 joints), C-reactive protein in mg/dL, and patient global assessment scores (scale of 0 to 10) are all 1 or less, or (2) Simplified Disease Activity Index is 3.3 or less.

TABLE 44-2

Provisional Criteria for Rheumatoid Arthritis Remission in Clinical Trials From the American College of Rheumatology/European League Against Rheumatism

A patient with rheumatoid arthritis is considered to be "in remission" if either of the following applies:

1. **Boolean-based definition:**
   At any time, patient must satisfy ALL of the following:
   - Tender joint count ≤1[a]
   - Swollen joint count ≤1[a]
   - C-reactive protein ≤1 mg/dL
   - Patient global assessment ≤1 (on a 0–10 scale)[b]
2. **Index-based definition:**
   At any time, patient must have a Simplified Disease Activity Index score of ≤3.3[c]

[a] For tender and swollen joint counts, use of a 28-joint count may miss actively involved joints, especially in the feet and ankles, and it is preferable to include feet and ankles also when evaluating remission.

[b] For the assessment of remission, the following format and wording is suggested for the global assessment questions. *Format:* a horizontal 10-cm visual analog or Likert scale with the best anchor and lowest score on the left side and the worst anchor and highest score on the right side. *Wording of question and anchors:* For patient global assessment, "Considering all of the ways your arthritis has affected you, how do you feel your arthritis is today?" (anchors: very well–very poor). For physician or assessor global assessment, "What is your assessment of the patient's current disease activity?" (anchors: none–extremely active).

[c] Defined as the simple sum of the tender joint count (using 28 joints), swollen joint count (using 28 joints), patient global assessment (0–10 scale), physician global assessment (0–10 scale), and C-reactive protein level (mg/dL).

Source: Felson DT et al. American College of Rheumatology/European League Against Rheumatism provisional definition of remission in rheumatoid arthritis for clinical trials. *Arthritis Rheum.* 2011;63:573.

During the first 10 years of the disease, survival rates of patients with RA appear to be no different from those of the general population.[12,13] However, more recent data indicate that patients with RA have an overall lower life expectancy (median age at death is 3 to 10 years less than non-RA populations),[6] with lower life expectancy associated with more severe disease.[14] The excess mortality has been attributed primarily to accelerated cardiovascular disease, which in turn might be related to RA-induced vascular inflammation, hyperhomocysteinemia, dyslipidemia, or elevations in tumor necrosis factor-alpha (TNF-α).[15] About one-third to one-half of deaths among adults with RA are attributable to cardiovascular disease, compared with one-fourth to one-fifth of deaths among adults without RA. RA is associated with a twofold to threefold increased rate of myocardial infarction (MI), as well as lower MI survival. An evidence-rated guideline for reducing cardiovascular disease risk in patients with RA was recently published by EULAR (Table 44-3).[16] Core recommendations from the guideline include annual cardiovascular risk evaluations for all patients, multiplying risk scores by 1.5 for patients with more than one marker of severe disease activity, use of statins and cardiovascular medications known to reduce cardiovascular risk, caution when prescribing nonsteroidal anti-inflammatory drugs (NSAIDs) owing to associated cardiovascular risk, and smoking cessation.[16]

Pathophysiology

RA-induced joint destruction begins with inflammation of the synovial lining that surrounds the joint space.[17] This normally thin membrane proliferates and transforms into the synovial pannus. The pannus, a highly erosive enzyme-laden inflammatory exudate, invades articular cartilage (leading to narrowing of joint spaces), erodes bone (resulting in osteoporosis), and destroys periarticular structures (ligaments, tendons), resulting in joint deformities (Fig. 44-1).

Familiarity with the basic cellular processes involved in tissue destruction and sustained inflammation in rheumatoid synovium is essential to understanding pharmacologic therapies for RA.[17,18] Under normal circumstances, the body can distinguish between self (i.e., proteins found within the body) and nonself (i.e., foreign substances such as bacteria and viruses). On occasion, immune cells (T or B lymphocytes) can react to a self-protein while developing in the thymus or bone marrow. These developing cells are usually killed or inactivated before release from their place of formation; sometimes, however, a self-targeted immune cell can escape destruction and become activated years later to initiate an autoimmune response. Some experts believe the activation of RA is initiated by bacteria (possibly *Streptococcus*) or a virus containing a protein with an amino acid sequence similar to tissue protein, but this assertion remains disputable.[6] When the activation source (i.e., the self-targeted immune cell) reaches the joint, complex cell–cell interactions take place, leading to the pathology associated with RA.

The initiating interaction for an autoimmune response takes place between antigen-presenting cells (APC), which display complexes of class II MHC molecules, and CD4-lineage T-cell lymphocytes (Fig. 44-2). In addition, B cells (previously thought to have little to do with the inflammatory response) can become activated, leading to antibody formation (including RF and anti-CCP), proinflammatory cytokine production, and accumulation

TABLE 44-3
Recommendations for Reducing Cardiovascular Risk[a] in Patients With Rheumatoid Arthritis (Evidence/Strength Rating)[b]

1. Rheumatoid arthritis should be considered as a disease in which cardiovascular risk is elevated, because of both an increased prevalence of traditional cardiovascular risk factors and the inflammatory burden. Although the evidence base is less, this may also apply to ankylosing spondylitis and psoriatic arthritis (2b–3/B).
2. To lower cardiovascular risk, adequate control of arthritis disease activity is necessary (2b–3/B).
3. All patients with rheumatoid arthritis should undergo annual cardiovascular risk evaluation with use of national guidelines. This should also be considered for all patients with ankylosing spondylitis and psoriatic arthritis. When antirheumatic treatment has been changed, risk assessments should be repeated (3–4/C).
4. For patients with rheumatoid arthritis, risk score models should be adapted by introducing a 1.5 multiplication factor when the patient meets two of the following three criteria: disease duration of more than 10 years, rheumatoid factor or anti–cyclic citrullinated peptide positivity, and the presence of certain extra-articular manifestations (3–4/C).
5. When using the Systematic Coronary Risk Evaluation model for determination of cardiovascular risk, triglyceride to high-density lipoprotein cholesterol ratio should be used (3/C).
6. Intervention for cardiovascular risk factor management should be performed according to national guidelines (3/C).
7. Preferred treatment options are statins, angiotensin-converting enzyme inhibitors, or angiotensin II blockers (2a–3/C–D).
8. The effect of cyclo-oxygenase-2 inhibitors and most nonsteroidal anti-inflammatory drugs on cardiovascular risk is not completely determined and should be studied further. Clinicians should therefore be very cautious in prescribing these drugs, especially to patients with cardiovascular risk factors or with documented cardiovascular disease (2a–3/C).
9. When corticosteroids are prescribed, this should be at the lowest possible dose (3/C).
10. Patients should be actively encouraged to stop smoking (3/C).

[a] Cardioprotective treatment is recommended when 10-year cardiovascular risk is above the threshold of "moderate" that is established for each country (i.e., either 10% or 20%).

[b] Level of Evidence: Category 1A, from meta-analysis of randomized, controlled trials; 1B, from at least one randomized, controlled trial; 2A, from at least one controlled study without randomization; 2B, from at least one type of quasi-experimental study; 3, from descriptive studies, such as comparative studies, correlation studies, or case-control studies; 4, from expert committee reports or opinions or from clinical experience of respected authorities; strength of recommendation directly based on: A, category 1 evidence; B, category 2 evidence or extrapolated recommendations from category 1 evidence; C, category 3 evidence or extrapolated recommendations from category 1 or 2 evidence; D, category 4 evidence or extrapolated recommendations from category 2 or 3 evidence.

Source: Peters MJ et al. EULAR evidence-based recommendations for cardiovascular risk management in patients with rheumatoid arthritis and other forms of inflammatory arthritis. *Ann Rheum Dis.* 2010;69:325.

of polymorphonuclear leukocytes that release cytotoxins and other substances destructive to the synovium and joint structures. B cells also act as APCs, leading to T-cell activation and acceleration of the inflammatory process.[18] T-cell activation requires two signals: (a) an antigen-specific signal occurring when a class II MHC antigen molecule on an APC binds to a T-cell receptor; and (b) binding of CD39 on the T cell to either CD80 or CD86 on the APC. T-cell activation leads to activation of macrophages and secretion of cytokines, polypeptides that serve as important mediators of inflammation, and cytotoxins, which can directly destroy cells and tissues. Proinflammatory cytokines such as interleukin (IL)-1 and TNF-α stimulate both synovial fibroblasts and chondrocytes in neighboring articular cartilage to secrete enzymes that cause degradation of proteoglycan and collagen tissues. In healthy individuals, the inflammatory process is regulated by balancing the ratios of proinflammatory cytokines (e.g., IL-1, IL-6, TNF-α) with anti-inflammatory cytokines—for example, IL-1 receptor antagonist (IL-1Ra), IL-4, IL-10, and IL-11. In the synovium of patients with RA, however, this balance is heavily weighted toward the proinflammatory cytokines, which results in sustained inflammation and tissue destruction.

Treatment

The treatment of RA involves a combination of interventions, which include rest, exercise (physical therapy), emotional support, occupational therapy, and drugs.[8] Specific treatment should be individualized based on joint function, degree of disease activity, patient age, sex, occupation, family responsibilities, drug costs, and results of previous therapy. The ultimate goal of RA treatment is disease remission; however, because sustained remission is uncommon, minimizing disease activity to provide pain

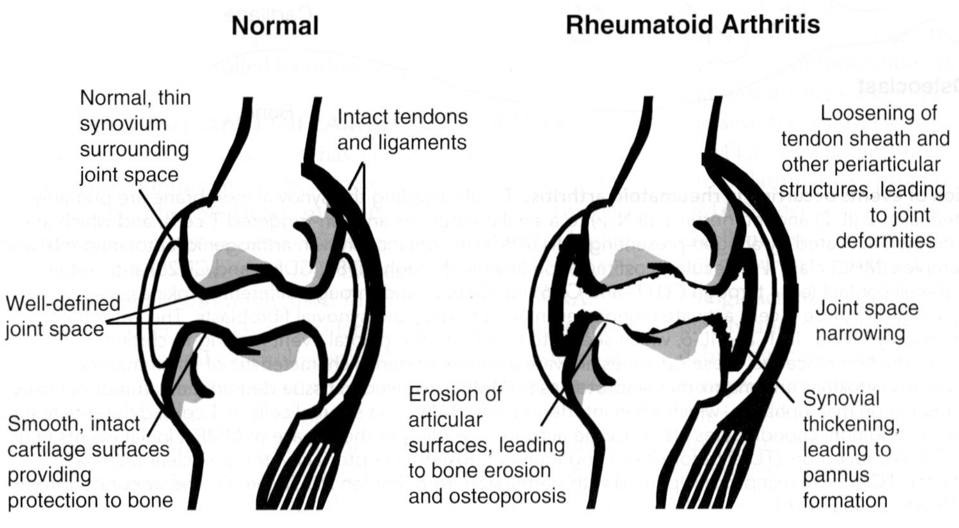

FIGURE 44-1 Overview of joint changes in rheumatoid arthritis.

CASE 44-5

QUESTION 1: T.Z., a 68-year-old man with heart failure previously managed with furosemide 40 mg/day, digoxin 0.125 mg/day, metoprolol 50 mg twice daily, and lisinopril 40 mg/day, returns for a prescription refill of ibuprofen 600 mg three times daily, which he takes for his RA. During the past 2 weeks, he has noted increased leg swelling, a weight gain of several pounds, exacerbated shortness of breath, and easy fatigability. Why might these signs and symptoms be associated with ibuprofen use?

Mild fluid retention occurs in approximately 5% of NSAID users, and NSAID-induced kidney disease occurs in less than 1% of patients.[105,106] NSAID therapy should be avoided, if possible, in patients with pre-existing heart failure, kidney disease, or cirrhosis.[104] If a patient with these conditions requires NSAID therapy, or patients are taking angiotensin-converting enzyme inhibitors and angiotensin receptor blockers, serum creatinine should be checked soon after NSAID initiation. Inhibition of COX by NSAIDs within the kidney reduces prostaglandin concentrations and unopposed vasoconstriction. Consequently, urine output declines, serum blood urea nitrogen and serum creatinine levels rise, and fluid is retained. This potential complication is associated with all of the currently marketed NSAIDs.[106] In addition, ibuprofen and all other NSAIDS besides naproxen are associated with an increased risk of MI, which is a concern for T.Z. because of his risk of thrombotic cardiovascular events.[24]

The provider of T.Z.'s cardiovascular care should be informed of his symptoms of fluid overload, and an alternative to NSAID therapy should be pursued.

CASE 44-5, QUESTION 2: If NSAID therapy is discontinued, what analgesic or anti-inflammatory alternatives are available for T.Z.? What other renal syndromes are associated with NSAID use?

In several studies, sulindac has been associated with fewer adverse effects on the kidney than other NSAIDs.[24] The reasons for this are unclear, but one explanation is that the active sulfide metabolite undergoes renal metabolism and, therefore, might not achieve tissue concentrations within the kidney sufficient to reduce prostaglandin production.[107] Unfortunately, patients do not seem to benefit from sulindac as much as from other NSAIDs, and the evidence overall supporting the safety of sulindac in renal impairment is weak. COX-2 inhibitors do not appear to offer an advantage for renally impaired patients.[24] Although celecoxib has been associated with a slightly lower risk of death and heart failure exacerbation when compared with traditional NSAIDs,[108] it is not a reasonable initial option for T.Z. because celecoxib is also associated with an increased risk of MI and it may contribute to worsening of heart failure.

NSAIDs should be used at their lowest effective doses for minimal periods for T.Z. High-dose NSAIDs should be avoided owing to increased MI risk. Although acetaminophen is not an anti-inflammatory agent, it can provide analgesic relief. Intra-articular corticosteroid injections can be useful if inflamed joints are limited in number, or a short course of oral corticosteroids can provide rapid control of inflammation while reducing the need for longer courses of anti-inflammatory therapy. If T.Z. is not yet being treated with a DMARD, it should be seriously considered because all patients with RA are candidates for DMARDs, and DMARD use could preclude T.Z.'s need for an NSAID. If an NSAID or short course of systemic corticosteroid is selected, close monitoring of renal function and fluid retention status is warranted.

In addition to acute renal failure, NSAIDs can induce various adverse renal effects (e.g., nephrotic syndrome, interstitial nephritis, hyponatremia, abnormalities of water metabolism, hyperkalemia).[109] The nephrotic syndrome, unlike NSAID-induced acute renal failure, can appear anytime (i.e., from days to years) after initiation of therapy, and can resolve as quickly as 1 month, or as long as 1 year, after discontinuation of the NSAID. Hematuria, pyuria, and proteinuria without prior renal disease differentiates nephrotic syndrome from other NSAID-induced renal problems. Histologically, NSAID-induced nephrotic syndrome is characterized by interstitial lymphocytic infiltrates, vacuolar degeneration of proximal and distal tubules, and fusion of epithelial foot processes of glomeruli.

Prostaglandin-mediated inhibition of active chloride transport, regulation of medullary blood flow within the kidney, and antagonism of antidiuretic hormone can be suppressed by NSAIDs. As a result, urine is maximally concentrated, free water clearance is limited, and water retention that is disproportionate to sodium retention can occur. The resulting hyponatremia can be severe and could be potentiated by thiazide diuretics.[109,110] Local prostaglandin synthesis can also stimulate renin production within the kidney. NSAID therapy can critically attenuate this regulatory mechanism in some situations, resulting in reduced aldosterone-mediated potassium excretion and hyperkalemia.

Although the mechanism is poorly understood, some NSAIDs have been associated with sustained mean arterial pressure increases of 5 to 6 mm Hg,[24,111] presumably the result of COX-2 inhibition and sodium and water retention. Several studies suggest that only patients taking antihypertensive medications experienced NSAID-induced mean arterial pressure elevations, whereas those who controlled their hypertension without medications were unaffected by NSAID therapy.

CASE 44-5, QUESTION 3: How frequently should T.Z.'s renal and liver function be tested during his NSAID therapy?

Patients at high risk for NSAID-induced renal disease, like T.Z. (see Case 44-5, Questions 1 and 2), should have their serum creatinine levels checked regularly (e.g., weekly) for several weeks after initiation of NSAID therapy because renal insufficiency more commonly occurs early in the course of therapy rather than later.[110] NSAID-induced nephrotic syndrome and allergic interstitial nephritis occur, on average, about 6.6 months and 15 days after NSAID initiation, respectively.[109]

In most cases, liver function testing (LFT) is unnecessary.[110] Although NSAIDs can elevate liver enzymes, severe hepatotoxicity is rare. Abnormal LFTs without clinical symptoms have no impact on patient outcome and have not been associated with severe hepatotoxicity. Patients who seem to be at greatest risk for hepatotoxicity are those with established or suspected intrinsic liver disease and those taking diclofenac. These patients should have LFTs performed no later than 8 weeks after initiation of therapy because liver toxicity manifests early in therapy, if at all.

TRADITIONAL DISEASE-MODIFYING ANTIRHEUMATIC DRUGS

CASE 44-5, QUESTION 4: T.Z. was diagnosed with RA 18 months ago. He exhibits no features of a poor prognosis, and has low disease activity. Which traditional DMARD therapies are most appropriate for him?

Every RA patient should receive DMARD therapy, unless a contraindication exists.[19] As previously discussed, initial DMARD selection is based on three factors: (a) disease activity (low vs. moderate-high), (b) whether poor prognostic findings

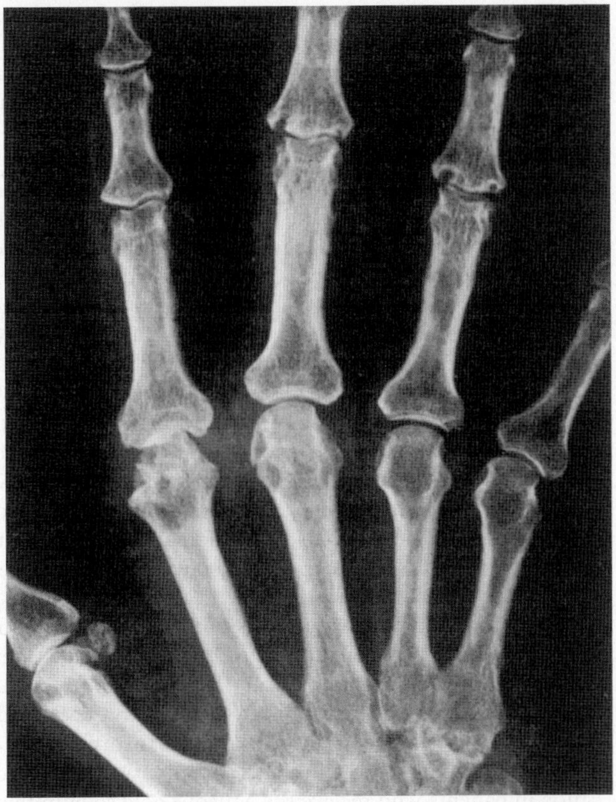

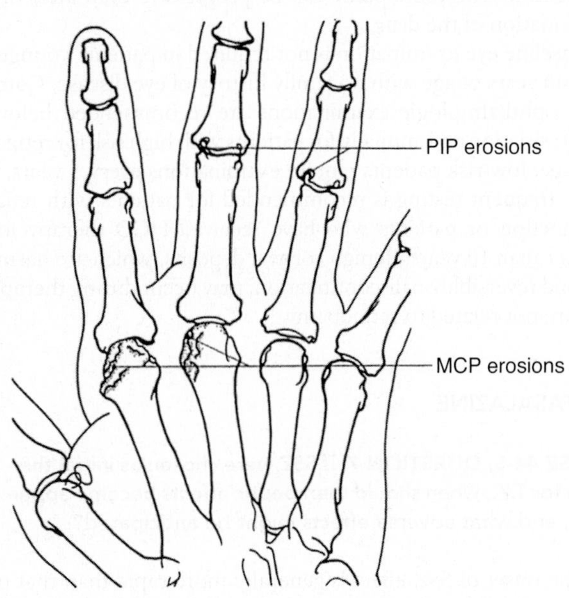

FIGURE 44-7 Radiograph of the hand in rheumatoid arthritis showing both active erosions at the metacarpophalangeal joints (MCPs) and old well-demarcated erosions at the proximal interphalangeal joints (PIPs).

are present, and (c) disease duration. For most patients, MTX or LEF are chosen initially because of high rates of clinical response for all levels of RA severity and radiographic evidence of slowing joint erosion, which is most rapid during the first several years of active disease[19] (Fig. 44-7). Although most DMARDs are associated with potentially serious adverse effects, these generally are reversible and seldom lead to serious complications if the patient has been monitored appropriately.

Most patients with RA are treated with at least one DMARD along with an NSAID.[20] In addition, low-dose oral corticosteroids are often prescribed on an as-needed basis for brief periods of severe disease activity or while awaiting the onset of DMARD action. During periods of disease remission, NSAID therapy can be discontinued; however, attempts to discontinue traditional DMARDs have resulted in disease reactivation or "rebound flare," and resumption of the discontinued agent is not always successful in re-establishing control. Therefore, successful traditional DMARD therapy should be continued indefinitely. Safety and efficacy data, which reflect several years of DMARD therapy combined with biologic agents, have been excellent, and the combination is now commonly prescribed for patients who fail MTX monotherapy (see Case 44-7, Questions 9–11). Guidelines for DMARD selection were discussed previously (see Treatment section). Combination DMARD therapy is indicated for more severe or more advanced RA patients (see Case 44-7, Question 8).

ANTIMALARIAL DRUG DOSING

CASE 44-5, QUESTION 5: Although T.Z.'s presentation could warrant an alternative DMARD, treatment was initiated with HCQ. What dosages would be appropriate, and when should clinical improvement be expected?

Although the manufacturer's literature recommends an initial HCQ adult dose of 400 to 600 mg/day (310 to 465 mg of base), dosages for HCQ generally range from 2 to 6.5 mg/kg/day.[20] If the patient responds well, the maintenance dose can be reduced by 50% and the medication continued at a dose of 200 to 400 mg/day (155 to 310 mg of base). About two-thirds of patients who tolerate HCQ respond favorably. Benefits usually are apparent within 2 to 4 months of therapy, but can vary between 1 and 6 months.[8] About 37% of patients discontinued HCQ within a year and 54% within 2 years, primarily owing to lack of efficacy.[110]

Risk of Retinopathy

CASE 44-5, QUESTION 6: When being counseled regarding HCQ, T.Z. was told that the drug can cause vision problems. How great is the risk of retinopathy from antimalarials when used for the treatment of RA? What monitoring parameters are appropriate?

HCQ is usually well tolerated. The most serious toxicity, retinal damage and subsequent visual impairment, is rare.[20,110] Risk of retinopathy is increased with high cumulative doses (>800 g), increased age (>60 years), liver disease, and retinal disease. The increased risk of retinopathy in the elderly seems to be related to the increased prevalence of macular disease in this age group. HCQ doses exceeding 6.5 mg/kg are associated with increased risk of retinal damage, particularly in patients with renal or hepatic dysfunction. HCQ should not be used for patients with significant renal impairment.

Patients should be instructed to stop therapy immediately and undergo an ophthalmologic evaluation if they are experiencing symptoms of antimalarial-associated retinopathy (e.g., difficulty seeing faces or entire words, glare intolerance, poor night vision, loss of peripheral vision).[111] The fully developed lesion of antimalarial retinopathy is seen on ophthalmoscopy as a pigmentary disturbance with a characteristic bull's-eye appearance in the macular region. The 4-amino-quinolines bind to melanin, and as a result, concentrate in the uveal tract and retinal pigment epithelium. The retinopathy can be progressive even after discontinuation of the drug.

Baseline eye examination is not required in patients younger than 40 years of age with no family history of eye disease. Complete ophthalmologic examinations are recommended before HCQ initiation and annually for patients with high risk for retinal damage; low-risk patients require examinations every 5 years.[20] More frequent testing is recommended for patients with renal dysfunction or patients who have received HCQ therapy for greater than 10 years. Benign corneal deposits, which are harmless and reversible on discontinuation, may occur during therapy and are not related to retinopathy.[76]

SULFASALAZINE

CASE 44-5, QUESTION 7: If SSZ were chosen as initial therapy for T.Z., when should therapeutic effects become apparent, and what adverse effects might be anticipated?

The onset of SSZ effect is generally more rapid than that of HCQ and can become apparent within a month[8,20]; however, a clinical response might be delayed for up to 3 to 4 months, and doses should be adjusted only after this period has elapsed.

Overall, SSZ adverse effects are relatively mild, but SSZ is considered to be more toxic than HCQ.[20] Adverse effects include nausea, abdominal discomfort, heartburn, dizziness, headaches, skin rashes, and, rarely, hematologic effects such as leukopenia (1% to 3%) or thrombocytopenia (rare). A complete blood count (CBC) is recommended every 2 to 4 weeks for the first 3 months of therapy, then every 3 months thereafter. Leukopenia, agranulocytosis, or hepatitis are rare but serious side effects of SSZ, and usually manifest within the first 2 to 3 months of therapy. To minimize GI-related adverse effects, SSZ is initiated at 500 mg/day or 1 g/day, and the dosage is increased at weekly intervals by 500 mg until 1,000 mg two or three times daily is reached.

GOLD PREPARATIONS AND ADVERSE REACTIONS

CASE 44-6

QUESTION 1: S.S., a 41-year-old Asian woman diagnosed with RA, presents with inflammation in both hands (MCP and PIP joints), wrists, elbows, shoulders, knees, hips, ankles, and MTP joints. Objective test results include radiographic evidence of joint erosion in both hands and elbows, positive RF (dilution of 1:1,280), positive anti-CCP at 102 units, and ESR of 78 mm/hour. Her SDAI score is 30. Her symptoms were managed during the past year with ibuprofen 800 mg three times daily; however, pain and inflammation have progressively worsened over the course of several months. ROM testing reveals deficits in wrist flexion and extension (20 degrees bilaterally for both motions; normal, 90 and 70 degrees, respectively), elbow flexion (90 degrees bilaterally with flexion contracture; normal, 160 degrees), shoulder abduction (70 degrees right, 90 degrees left; normal, 180 degrees), and plantar flexion of both ankles (20 degrees bilaterally; normal, 45 degrees). Three firm, pea-sized, nontender moveable subcutaneous nodules are found on both elbows at the ulnar border, two on the right and one on the left. In your discussion about considering DMARD therapy, S.S. states that she does not want gold therapy "because I've heard that it has terrible side effects." What gold preparations are available, and is S.S.'s concern about adverse effects warranted?

Two parenteral gold preparations are available: gold sodium thiomalate, an aqueous solution, and aurothioglucose, an oil suspension. Although an oral gold formulation, AUR, is also available, it is slow in onset (4 to 6 months) and is less efficacious.[8,20] The parenteral formulations, containing approximately 50% gold by weight expressed as milligrams of complex, are equally effective.[20] Aurothioglucose must be shaken thoroughly before withdrawal from its vial, and a large-bore needle is necessary to draw up this viscous suspension. Lumps at the intramuscular injection site sometimes can be troublesome to the patient.

Toxicities with both injectable gold preparations are numerous and largely responsible for their high rate of discontinuation. In a 6-year prospective trial, nearly half of patients receiving gold sodium thiomalate discontinued therapy, with 95% of those discontinuing because of toxicity.[27] The toxicity profiles of the parenteral gold preparations differ. A vasomotor reaction (also termed *nitritoid reaction*), which manifests as nausea, weakness, flushing, tachycardia, or syncope, can occur in up to 5% of patients receiving gold sodium thiomalate. These reactions generally are mild, are transient, and often can be alleviated by having the patient lie down.

Nonvasomotor reactions, consisting of transient stiffness, arthralgias, and myalgias, developed in 15% of patients after initiation of gold sodium thiomalate therapy,[112] and substituting aurothioglucose for the thiomalate formulation decreased the severity of this adverse reaction in 40% of patients.

Skin eruptions, stomatitis, and albuminuria are more common in patients who receive the aqueous gold sodium thiomalate preparation than in patients who receive the oil suspension of aurothioglucose.[113] Aurothioglucose also is more commonly associated with renal toxicity than gold sodium thiomalate, although the overall incidence is rare.[76] Membranous nephropathy (most common), nephrotic syndrome, and interstitial nephritis have been reported. Hematuria and proteinuria may be early indicators of membranous nephropathy; however, proteinuria can occur transiently in up to 50% of patients receiving aurothioglucose. Patients who experience proteinuria should undergo a renal evaluation and a urinalysis. Gold therapy should be discontinued if protein excretion is greater than 500 mg/24 hours.

Parenteral gold preparations have been associated with sudden occurrence of idiosyncratic thrombocytopenia (1%–3%) or aplastic anemia (<1%).[76] Screening for urine protein and a CBC should be performed before each weekly injection for the first 20 to 22 weeks, then before every other injection. In addition, patients should be asked about the occurrence of pruritus, skin eruptions, purpura, sore throat, and stomatitis before each dose of gold is administered.

Dermatologic reactions to gold occur in 15% to 30% of patients.[76] Pruritus, erythema, or a fine morbilliform rash on the neck or extremities can develop after the first few injections of gold. These cutaneous reactions are common, usually subside within several days, and do not seem to be affected by subsequent injections. Although a highly pruritic localized eruption resembling pityriasis rosea is common, gold dermatitis may assume many different forms, including exfoliative dermatitis.[76] Therapy should be discontinued if a pruritic dermatitis develops. Mild dermal reactions may be managed with topical corticosteroids. Because of fears of subsequent exfoliative dermatitis and the belief that dermatologic reactions recur on rechallenge, there is a natural reluctance to continue gold treatment after the appearance of dermatitis or stomatitis. However, in one series of patients, gold treatments were reinstituted successfully in 28 of 30 patients in whom dermatologic reactions developed.[114]

AUR capsules, containing 3 mg of gold, are 25% bioavailable.[115] The recommended AUR daily dose of 6 mg can be given either as single or divided doses. AUR is better tolerated than parenteral gold formulations, but is significantly less effective.[8,19] Like parenteral chrysotherapy, benefit can occur as early as 6 to 8 weeks after starting AUR, but objective benefits might not be apparent for several months. AUR must be monitored in a manner similar to parenteral therapy. The incidence of rashes necessitating AUR withdrawal is lower than with parenteral gold therapy, but loose stools and diarrhea are encountered more commonly (47%).

S.S.'s concerns have merit. Although gold is an effective DMARD and can induce complete RA remission, none of the gold formulations are ideal. Gold sodium thiomalate is easier to administer, but is associated with more frequent side effects compared with aurothioglucose. Aurothioglucose carries a low but serious risk of nephrotoxicity. Both parenteral forms of gold are commonly discontinued because of side effects. AUR is the best-tolerated gold preparation, but the least effective, and is associated with significant diarrhea.

Dosing

CASE 44-6, QUESTION 2: How should gold be administered to S.S., if she agrees to therapy? Is serum drug monitoring of value in gold therapy?

The standard treatment schedule for parenteral gold consists of an initial intramuscular (IM) test dose of 10 mg followed by a 25-mg IM dose 1 week later. The third and subsequent weekly IM injections of 25 to 50 mg should be continued until the cumulative dose reaches 1 g, toxicity occurs, or major benefit is derived.[76] If a satisfactory response is achieved, maintenance doses of 25 to 50 mg every other week are recommended. If the disease remains stable, doses can be administered every third and subsequently every fourth week for an indefinite period. The dose of AUR is 3 mg twice daily or 6 mg once daily.

Attempts to correlate serum gold concentrations with clinical outcomes generally have been unsuccessful. Furthermore, toxicity has not been correlated with serum gold concentrations.[116]

METHOTREXATE

CASE 44-6, QUESTION 3: S.S. will be treated with MTX. Why is MTX a good selection for her?

MTX or LEF are recommended as initial DMARD therapy for all patients with RA.[19] S.S. has many indicators of severe disease (e.g., an SDAI score indicating high disease activity [see Table 44-7], multiple joint involvement, extra-articular manifestations [i.e., subcutaneous nodules], radiographic evidence of erosions, elevated ESR, positive anti-CCP, positive RF with a high titer of 1:1,280 [positive RF is generally a titer less than or equal to 1:20 and titers correlate with disease severity]).

The disease prognosis for S.S. is clearly poor, and a relatively potent DMARD should be initiated to maximize the preservation of joint function and minimize the risk of RA-related cardiovascular disease. MTX has a rapid onset (usually 1 to 2 months before a plateau of effectiveness), a high efficacy rate, and a long history of successful use.[19] In one study, the probability of continuing MTX therapy for at least 5 years was 62%.[117] It is an excellent choice for treating S.S.'s very active RA.

Dosing

CASE 44-6, QUESTION 4: How should MTX be dosed and administered to S.S.?

In general, MTX is administered orally at an initial dose of 7.5 mg once a week, usually in a single weekly dose.[20] The dose can also be divided into three equal parts (e.g., starting dose of 2.5 mg every 12 hours for a total of three doses) for patients who are unable to tolerate adverse effects, particularly hepatotoxicity. If S.S.'s RA shows no objective response in 1 to 2 months, the dose is increased to 15 mg/week (or 5 mg every 12 hours for three doses) for at least 12 additional weeks.[25] If no response is seen at this time, then (a) the dose can be increased to the maximum of 25 mg/week, (b) the dose can be administered as a subcutaneous or IM injection to address bioavailability concerns, (c) the same dose can be continued for a longer time, or (d) another DMARD can be added to MTX or MTX can be substituted.[19] When subcutaneous MTX was compared with oral MTX in a 6-month randomized, controlled trial of 384 MTX-naïve patients with active RA,[118] 78% of patients treated with subcutaneous MTX achieved an ACR-20 response, and only 70% of those treated with oral MTX achieved a similar response. At week 16 of this study, patients treated with oral MTX, who failed to attain an ACR-20 response, were switched to subcutaneous MTX; patients treated with subcutaneous MTX who failed to attain an ACR-20 response were given a larger MTX dose (20 mg) subcutaneously. The patients who were converted from oral dosing to subcutaneous dosing and the patients who were given a larger subcutaneous dose had a 30% and 23% ACR response rate at week 24, respectively. As a result, subcutaneous MTX seems to be more effective than oral MTX and not associated with a higher incidence of adverse effects.

In a 6-month clinical trial, RA patients with a short disease duration (i.e., <3 years) who achieve disease remission with weekly MTX therapy remained in remission when the same MTX dose was administered every other week (i.e., monthly dose reduced by 50%).[119] It is unknown, however, whether every-other-week dosing of MTX prevents joint destruction as effectively as weekly dosing.

Adverse Effects

CASE 44-6, QUESTION 5: What subjective and objective data should be evaluated for evidence of MTX adverse effects in S.S.?

S.S. should be monitored for nausea and other GI distress, malaise, dizziness, mucositis, and mild alopecia, which are commonly encountered adverse effects associated with low-dose MTX therapy.[110] More serious, but less common, adverse effects include myelosuppression, pneumonitis, and hepatic fibrosis and cirrhosis. A CBC, LFTs, and a serum creatinine concentration should be obtained for her at baseline, monthly for the first 6 months of therapy, and then every 4 to 8 weeks during MTX therapy. Renal dysfunction can result in accumulation of MTX and higher risk of myelosuppression. Hypersensitivity pneumonitis, occurring in 1% to 2% of patients, has no known risk factors for development, although it may be more common in patients with a history of lung disease.[20] In addition, hypersensitivity pneumonitis can occur at any time during therapy and at any MTX dosage. A baseline chest radiograph is recommended within the year before MTX initiation. If the patient is found to have pre-existing lung disease, MTX treatment should be reconsidered because further pulmonary damage could be devastating to the patient. S.S. also should be monitored carefully for cough, dyspnea on exertion, and shortness of breath at each clinic visit.

MTX-induced liver disease is rare, but increased age, long duration of therapy, obesity, diabetes mellitus, ethanol consumption, and a history of hepatitis B or C increase the risk of hepatotoxicity.[110] MTX should be prescribed with great caution, if at all, in patients with pre-existing liver disease. The serum

TABLE 44-10
Recommended Monitoring Intervals for Complete Blood Count, Liver Function Tests, and Serum Creatinine Levels for Rheumatoid Arthritis Patients Receiving Traditional (Nonbiologic) Disease-Modifying Antirheumatic Drugs

DMARD	Frequency of Monitoring Based on Duration of Therapy		
	<3 Months	3–6 Months	>6 Months
Hydroxychloroquine (HCQ)	None after baseline	None	None
Minocycline (MIN)			
Leflunomide (LEF)			
Methotrexate (MTX)	2–4 weeks	8–12 weeks	12 weeks
Sulfasalazine (SSZ)			

DMARD, disease-modifying antirheumatic drug.
Source: Saag KG et al. American College of Rheumatology 2008 recommendations for the use of nonbiologic and biologic disease-modifying antirheumatic drugs in rheumatoid arthritis. *Arthritis Rheum.* 2008;59:762.

concentrations of liver enzymes commonly are modestly increased after administration for 1 to 2 days. However, MTX should be withheld if liver enzymes increase to three times the baseline value or if the liver enzyme serum concentrations remain elevated for sustained periods during therapy. Patients taking MTX should avoid alcohol and be instructed to report symptoms of jaundice or dark urine to their primary-care provider. Routine liver biopsies to monitor for MTX-induced hepatotoxicity are unnecessary (see Case 44-6, Question 6). Monitoring recommendations for MTX and other commonly used traditional DMARDs are listed in Table 44-10.

Liver Biopsy and Methotrexate

CASE 44-6, QUESTION 6: The following laboratory test results were obtained for S.S. before starting MTX:

ALT, 28 international units/L
Aspartate aminotransferase (AST), 30 international units/L
Alkaline phosphatase, 100 international units/L
Albumin, 4.5 g/dL
Total bilirubin, 0.8 mg/dL

Should a baseline liver biopsy be performed before S.S. starts MTX?

At one time, routine liver biopsies were recommended for RA patients receiving MTX because cirrhosis developed in up to 26% of MTX-treated psoriasis patients.[120] In patients with RA, however, serial liver biopsies are neither recommended nor cost-effective. Nevertheless, the liver should be biopsied before treatment in patients with suspected liver disease and in patients with persistent LFT abnormalities (defined as elevations above the upper limit of normal [ULN] in AST for 5 of 9 tests within a 12-month period [or 6 of 12 if tests are performed every month] or a reduction in serum albumin below normal range) during, or after discontinuation of, MTX therapy.[121] Because S.S.'s LFTs are normal and there is not a history of liver disease noted, there is no reason to consider a baseline liver biopsy.

Methotrexate and Folate or Folinic Acid

CASE 44-6, QUESTION 7: When should folate (or folinic acid) be administered to reduce the risk of MTX-related toxicity in S.S.?

Folate supplementation appears to reduce the incidence of several MTX-related adverse effects including GI disturbances, mucositis (mouth or GI ulcerations), and LFT elevations.[122–126] When folic acid (1 mg/day), folinic acid (2.5 mg/week), or placebo was added to MTX therapy (7.5 mg/week, titrated up to 25 mg/week) in more than 400 RA patients, hepatotoxicity developed in 26% in the placebo group, but in only 4% of patients in the folic acid and folinic acid groups ($p < 0.001$ for treatment groups vs. placebo). Because hepatotoxicity is one of the most common reasons for MTX discontinuation, the benefit of folate supplementation is clearly important.

A slightly higher dose of MTX might be needed in folate users to produce clinical benefits similar to that achieved by patients without folate supplementation, perhaps because MTX is a folate antagonist.[127] Clinically, however, there does not seem to be a significant attenuation of MTX efficacy associated with concomitant folate supplementation, and, very importantly, folate supplementation reduces the incidence of MTX discontinuation secondary to ALT elevation.

Folic acid 1 to 4 mg daily or folinic acid 2.5 to 10 mg weekly 24 hours after MTX dose can be initiated in S.S.[20] Both regimens are effective, although folic acid may be simpler for patients to self-administer and is inexpensive. Although either folic acid or folinic acid is effective, folic acid 1 mg/day or 7 mg once a week is preferred over folinic acid because of cost and ease of administration.[110]

Methotrexate-Related Pulmonary Disorders

CASE 44-6, QUESTION 8: S.S. is treated with MTX 7.5 mg and with folic acid 7 mg orally once a week. Nine weeks later, she returns to the clinic with subjective and objective improvement in morning stiffness, fatigability, and joint tenderness and swelling. However, she has noted increased shortness of breath and dyspnea in the past week. Why might these symptoms be related to MTX?

Pneumonitis, a rare complication of MTX therapy, is characterized by a nonproductive cough, malaise, and fever, progressing to severe dyspnea.[128] Recognition of this unusual reaction is important to ensure that MTX is discontinued before the pneumonitis progresses to respiratory failure (see Case 44-6, Question 5). After discontinuation of MTX, pulmonary function improves. Corticosteroids can accelerate improvement in pulmonary symptoms associated with pneumonitis. S.S.'s dyspnea and shortness of breath might be related to MTX. If appropriate tests rule out other causes for her pulmonary complaints, MTX-induced pulmonary toxicity should be considered and MTX treatment discontinued.

Methotrexate Interactions

CASE 44-6, QUESTION 9: What major MTX food and drug interactions need to be discussed with S.S. by her providers?

NSAIDs increase MTX serum concentrations and increase the risk of toxicity.[20] MTX doses should be adjusted cautiously if S.S. is taking NSAIDs concurrently to manage her RA pain. Trimethoprim, frequently used as part of the treatment for urinary tract infections, can increase the risk of MTX-induced bone marrow suppression. The concurrent use of MTX and LEF has been associated with major liver damage, requiring diligent monitoring for liver toxicity if used in combination. When 39 MTX-treated RA patients consumed low doses of caffeine (less than 120 mg/day), morning stiffness and joint pain were improved by more than 30% compared with high caffeine consumption (greater than 180 mg/day).[129] Caffeine may interfere with the anti-inflammatory effects of MTX. Because MTX is protein bound and renally excreted, other drugs (e.g., salicylates, probenecid, penicillin, ciprofloxacin) also might interact with MTX.

LEFLUNOMIDE: PLACE IN THERAPY

CASE 44-7

QUESTION 1: B.W., a 36-year-old woman, has severe, progressive RA and is not responding sufficiently to MTX therapy. Would LEF be a reasonable consideration for her?

LEF, an oral traditional DMARD, seems to be similar in efficacy to MTX with regard to ACR-20, radiographic response, and work productivity.[19,63] The onset of benefit (as early as 4 weeks) and the percentage of patients who discontinue LEF therapy because of either lack of efficacy or toxicity are similar for LEF, MTX, and SSZ. It can be used in place of MTX for initial drug therapy, combined with MTX therapy (see Case 44-7, Question 8), or serve as a replacement for MTX-intolerant patients.

Dosing and Monitoring

CASE 44-7, QUESTION 2: How should therapy with LEF be initiated in B.W.? How would you monitor B.W. for adverse effects?

The active metabolite of LEF, A77 1726 or M1, is responsible for virtually all the pharmacologic activity of LEF.[25] The serum half-life of the M1 metabolite is approximately 2 weeks. As a result, LEF should be initiated with a loading dose of 100 mg orally once daily for 3 days to reduce time to steady state, followed by 20 mg once daily. If this dose is not tolerated, the dose should be reduced to 10 mg once daily.

Monitoring for Adverse Effects

Diarrhea (20%–30%), rash (10%), alopecia (10%–17%), and reversible liver enzyme elevations more than three times the ULN (2%–4%) are common adverse effects of LEF.[25] Routine laboratory testing includes a baseline ALT followed by monthly ALT testing for several months. When it is evident that ALT results are stable and within normal limits, testing can be performed less often according to the clinician's judgment. Because of the risk of liver toxicity and the need for activation by the liver to the M1 active metabolite, LEF is not recommended in patients with pre-existing liver disease, including hepatitis B or C.

Potential hepatotoxicity is the greatest concern with LEF; however, the rate of LEF-induced liver enzyme elevation is not significantly different than MTX. Guidelines for managing potential hepatotoxicity include dosage reduction from 20 to 10 mg/day if ALT increases more than two times the ULN.[25] If ALT elevations remain steady between two and three times the ULN and treatment continuation is desired, a liver biopsy is recommended. If ALT elevations are persistently more than three times the ULN despite dosage reduction and cholestyramine administration to enhance elimination (see Case 44-7, Question 3), then the drug should be discontinued and another course of cholestyramine elimination therapy should be given.

Enhancement of Elimination With Cholestyramine

CASE 44-7, QUESTION 3: After 2 months of therapy, B.W. does not respond to LEF and the treatment was discontinued, especially because she is beginning to consider starting a family. What precautions must be taken when discontinuing LEF?

LEF (pregnancy category X) has not been tested in pregnant women, but greatly increases the risk of fetal death or teratogenicity in animals receiving as little as 1% of human equivalent doses.[20,25] After discontinuation of therapy, however, up to 2 years may need to elapse before plasma M1 metabolite levels of LEF are undetectable. As a result, cholestyramine is recommended for all women who discontinue LEF and who are hoping to become pregnant. After stopping the medication, cholestyramine 8 g three times daily is administered for 11 days (which need not be consecutive). Plasma levels of the M1 metabolite are reduced by 40% to 65% in 24 to 48 hours and should become undetectable (<0.02 mg/L) at the end of therapy. B.W.'s blood should be tested at least 14 days apart to verify the absence of the metabolite. If plasma M1 levels remain greater than 0.02 mg/L, more cholestyramine should be administered. Cholestyramine also can be used to enhance elimination of LEF in patients who experience hepatotoxicity or who overdose with this drug. Activated charcoal also can reduce plasma M1 levels by 50% after 48 hours, and can be an effective alternative to cholestyramine when LEF overdosages need to be managed.

HYDROXYCHLOROQUINE AND SULFASALAZINE

CASE 44-7, QUESTION 4: Would it have been reasonable to switch B.W. from MTX to either HCQ or SSZ?

Although both HCQ and SSZ are recommended first-line DMARDs for patients with mild to moderate RA, it is more common to add either or both of these to the regimen of patients who are not achieving adequate RA control from MTX.[19] HCQ, usually dosed at 200 to 400 mg daily, is a very well-tolerated DMARD. The greatest adverse effect of concern, retinal damage, is rare and easily prevented with diligent monitoring and dose limitations (see Case 44-5, Question 6). SSZ, dosed at 2 to 3 g per day divided into two or three doses, is also well tolerated, although toxicity in general is greater than that with HCQ. GI distress (nausea, anorexia) and rash are common. Although leukopenia, agranulocytosis, and hepatitis are serious side effects, they are rare and, if they do occur, normally manifest in the first 2 to 3 months of therapy. As a result, CBC, LFTs, and renal function testing is recommended more frequently early in the course of therapy (see Table 44-10). Both HCQ and SSZ appear to be safe in pregnancy.[20]

MINOCYCLINE

CASE 44-7, QUESTION 5: What evidence is there supporting the use of MIN, a tetracycline antibiotic, as a DMARD? How does it compare with HCQ?

MIN appears to be a useful adjunctive agent in the treatment of RA, and its successful use supports a speculation that RA might have an infectious etiology. It is the immunomodulatory and anti-inflammatory effects of MIN, however, that more likely contribute to its efficacy in RA than its antibiotic properties. A double-blind, placebo-controlled trial involving 46 patients with recent-onset RA evaluated the benefit of adding MIN 100 mg twice daily to conventional therapy with NSAIDs, DMARDs, and corticosteroids.[130] At 4-year follow-up, eight MIN-treated patients without DMARD or steroid therapy were in remission compared with one patient in the placebo group ($p = 0.02$).

Perhaps even more impressive are the results of a randomized trial comparing MIN 100 mg twice daily with HCQ

200 mg/day in patients with early-onset RA.[131] At 2 years, significantly more MIN-treated patients experienced relief of RA signs and symptoms, required less prednisone, and were more likely to be completely tapered off prednisone.

AZATHIOPRINE INDICATIONS AND ADVERSE EFFECTS

CASE 44-7, QUESTION 6: In considering options for B.W., AZA is mentioned. B.W. knows someone who is using AZA for prevention of kidney transplant rejection and thinks AZA is a highly toxic drug. How can adverse effects to AZA be minimized?

AZA is FDA approved for transplant rejection prophylaxis and for treatment of severe RA. The starting dose of AZA for RA is 1 mg/kg/day in single or divided doses.[20] If the patient does not respond, the dose can be increased by 0.5 mg/kg/day after 6 to 8 weeks, and subsequently increased by the same magnitude every 4 weeks if needed until a maximal dose of 2.5 mg/kg/day is reached.

The most common adverse effect of AZA is GI intolerance, and about 10% of patients discontinue therapy because of this problem.[110] Myelosuppression can occur, but is reversible on discontinuation of therapy. Patients with renal insufficiency are at increased risk for myelosuppression, and doses should be adjusted accordingly. Allopurinol decreases metabolism and elimination of AZA via inhibition of xanthine oxidase, thereby increasing the risk of toxicity of AZA because of increased serum concentrations. If concomitant allopurinol therapy cannot be avoided, the dose of AZA must be reduced by 75%. Monitoring for AZA adverse effects should include a baseline CBC, renal function, and LFTs. When AZA doses are increased, a CBC should be monitored every 1 to 2 weeks; thereafter, a CBC should be monitored every 1 to 3 months. Although serious adverse effects have limited the use of AZA for RA, diligent laboratory and clinical monitoring can minimize risk to patients.

D-PENICILLAMINE

CASE 44-7, QUESTION 7: When should D-penicillamine be considered as therapy for B.W.?

D-Penicillamine is no longer considered for the treatment of RA because of a lengthy dose titration schedule and serious toxicities (e.g., myelosuppression, autoimmune diseases).[19] Because D-penicillamine must be given in a "go low, go slow" approach (initial dose usually is 250 mg daily), dose increases cannot be made sooner than every 4 to 8 weeks. As a result, up to 6 months of therapy may be necessary before therapeutic benefits become apparent.

Rash, stomatitis, and dysgeusia are the most common adverse effects associated with D-penicillamine.[20,110] Myelosuppression (particularly thrombocytopenia), proteinuria, renal toxicity, and autoimmune syndromes (e.g., systemic lupus erythematosus, myasthenia gravis, polymyositis, Goodpasture syndrome) are rare but potentially serious adverse effects.[8] Baseline laboratory monitoring includes a renal function test, CBC, and urine protein assay. A CBC and urine protein testing should be monitored every 2 weeks until dosing is stabilized, then every 1 to 3 months thereafter.

Although B.W. has failed to respond to MTX and LEF, DMARDs other than D-penicillamine (including biologics) have a more rapid onset of action, greater efficacy, and less toxicity, and are therefore preferable.

TRADITIONAL DISEASE-MODIFYING ANTIRHEUMATIC DRUG COMBINATION THERAPY

CASE 44-7, QUESTION 8: Is there evidence to support the early and safe use of DMARDs in combination for B.W.?

Because most RA patients develop joint erosions within the first 2 years of disease, the initiation of disease-modifying agents early in the course of therapy, and using them in combination, has been associated with improved patient outcomes. The rationale for combination therapy is based on the premise that a combination of drugs might improve outcomes because of different pharmacological mechanisms of action or different sites of actions. A combination of drugs also may allow the use of lower doses of individual drugs, thereby reducing the risk of toxicity while maintaining or possibly increasing efficacy. The early use of combinations of potent disease-modifying agents also can expose the patient to increased risks of drug adverse effects.

Several DMARD combinations are currently recommended based on literature supporting their efficacy and safety.[19] The combination of MTX and HCQ is recommended for patients with moderate to high disease activity regardless of prognosis or disease duration, as well as for patients with low disease activity and disease duration greater than 24 months. MTX plus LEF is recommended for patients with high disease activity regardless of prognosis, but disease duration should be 6 months or longer. MTX plus SSZ is recommended for patients with poor prognosis and all disease durations. The combination of HCQ plus SSZ is recommended for only one circumstance: patients with high disease activity, no features of poor prognosis, and disease duration between 6 and 24 months. The triple combination of MTZ, HCQ, and SSZ is recommended for all patients with moderate to high disease activity levels and poor prognosis, regardless of disease duration. In one study, a 2-year disease remission rate of 37% was associated with this three-drug combination versus 21% in patients treated with SSZ or MTX monotherapy, with no significant differences in adverse effects.[132] Another trial compared the triple-drug regimen with MTX alone and with the combination of HCQ and SSZ.[133] At 2-year follow-up, 77% of the triple-drug–treated patients responded significantly as compared with 33% of the patients treated with MTX monotherapy ($p < 0.001$) and 40% of the patients treated with SSZ plus HCQ ($p = 0.003$). Toxicity did not differ among the treatment groups. At 5-year follow-up, the triple-drug therapy combination remained efficacious and safe in 36 of 58 patients (62%).

A randomized, controlled trial of 263 MTX-treated patients with active persistent RA found that the addition of LEF resulted in significant clinical improvement without an increase in adverse event and treatment discontinuation rates.[134] Similarly, studies evaluating concurrent use of MTX and HCQ or MTX and SSZ have demonstrated clinical improvement without significantly greater adverse events.[135,136]

As described in the Quantifying Response to Drug Therapy section, clinical assessment tools (e.g., DAS, CDAI, SDAI, Global Arthritis Scale, Routine Assessment of Patient Index Data, Easy Rheumatoid Activity Measure) integrate measures of RA activity (e.g., swollen joint count, tender joint count, pain, questionnaire-derived patient- and clinician-evaluated global disease activity) into a simple summary score.[19,71] These scores can be used to categorize disease severity and modify DMARD or biologic agent therapy accordingly. The BeSt Study used the DAS44 (44 joints) to compare four different treatment approaches for patients with early-onset RA (<2 years). Three of these treatments included exclusively traditional DMARDs.[62] Group 1 patients initially received MTX monotherapy, with dose escalation and sequential addition of SSZ and LEF if DAS44 was greater than 2.4.

Group 2 patients also began therapy with MTX, followed by additions of SSZ, HCQ, and then prednisone if DAS44 was greater than 2.4. In contrast, group 3 patients started with a prednisone taper (60 mg/day tapered down to 7.5 mg/day after 7 weeks), MTX, and SSZ. Group 4 started with infliximab and MTX. DAS44 was evaluated every 3 months. After 1 year of treatment, all groups had similar remission rates (defined by DAS44 <1.6), average DAS44 scores, and adverse events. The BeSt Study demonstrated that an aggressive, DAS-based titration regimen, using a variety of traditional-based DMARDs, is a successful method of using combination DMARD therapy for early RA.

In summary, every RA patient, including B.W., should receive DMARD therapy at or shortly after diagnosis, either as monotherapy or as combination therapy depending on disease duration, disease activity, and prognosis. Although significant attention and resources have most recently been invested in biologic DMARDs, recent evaluations indicate that traditional DMARDs are equally effective at managing symptoms and preventing bone and joint destruction. Patients who experience loss of efficacy or intolerable adverse effects from traditional DMARDs will need to add another DMARD or substitute with an alternative DMARD. Various combinations of traditional DMARDs, when titrated aggressively, have proven to be very effective in RA management. Results from studies of biologic DMARDs have demonstrated a reduction in joint erosions along with symptom improvement, which is why they must also be considered as therapeutic alternatives to traditional DMARDs.

BIOLOGIC AGENTS

Etanercept: Place in Therapy

CASE 44-7, QUESTION 9: After 6 months of treatment with nonbiologic DMARDs (MTX with LEF, then MTX with HCQ), B.W.'s response is inadequate and her RA remains highly active. She is prescribed etanercept. Why is etanercept a reasonable therapeutic option?

Etanercept is the first biologic response modifier to be approved by the FDA for reducing the signs and symptoms of moderate to severe active RA, either alone or in combination with MTX.[137] Etanercept is also approved for use in juvenile RA, ankylosing spondylitis, psoriatic arthritis, and plaque psoriasis. Etanercept is a soluble TNF receptor that competitively binds two TNF molecules, rendering both molecules inactive. Etanercept consists of two extracellular portions of the TNF receptor, and TNF primarily exists as a trimer in the human body. The dimeric structure of etanercept is believed to have a higher binding affinity for the trimeric TNF than the naturally occurring monomeric receptor.

In a randomized, placebo-controlled trial of 234 patients with active RA, significantly more patients met ACR-20 criteria after 6 months of treatment with etanercept 10 mg (51% of patients) and 25 mg (59% of patients) than with placebo (11%).[30] Etanercept was administered subcutaneously twice weekly for 26 weeks. All patients who were enrolled in this study had experienced an inadequate response to at least one of several DMARDs, similar to patient B.W. Furthermore, 24% and 40% of the patients taking etanercept 10 mg and 25 mg, respectively, met ACR-50 response criteria compared with 5% of the placebo group (p <0.001 for both doses compared with placebo, no significant difference between doses). Significant ACR-20, ACR-50, and ACR-70 responses to either etanercept dose were seen after only 2 weeks of therapy.

Another randomized, placebo-controlled trial evaluated the use of combination MTX and etanercept therapy in 89 patients with active RA refractory to at least 6 months of MTX therapy.[138] A dose of 25 mg etanercept or placebo was given subcutaneously twice weekly, and a stable dose of MTX (between 15 and 25 mg/week) was provided to all patients. At 24 weeks of follow-up, an ACR-20 response was found in 71% of the MTX plus etanercept group and 27% of the MTX plus placebo group (p <0.001). Similarly, 39% of the MTX plus etanercept group met ACR-50 response criteria compared with 3% of the MTX plus placebo group (p <0.001). Etanercept was also associated with significantly greater improvement in ESR or CRP test results. The addition of etanercept to MTX provided greater clinical efficacy when compared with MTX monotherapy. Etanercept provides rapid and significant improvement in subjective and objective measures of RA, either alone or in combination with MTX. In other studies, etanercept has demonstrated decreased radiographic progression and long-term safety and efficacy.[139–141] Although cost is a significant consideration, etanercept is a reasonable choice for B.W.

Dosing and Monitoring

CASE 44-7, QUESTION 10: How should etanercept therapy be initiated in B.W., and what are the most common and serious potential adverse effects about which she should be counseled?

The FDA-approved dose of etanercept for the treatment of active RA is 50 mg once weekly with or without MTX.[137] This medication may be self-injected subcutaneously by the patient after proper training. Etanercept is available in a prefilled syringe or a multiple-use vial. If the multiple-use vial is used, it must be reconstituted using only the diluent supplied; the contents should be swirled, not shaken, to avoid excessive foaming. Injection sites (e.g., thigh, abdomen, upper arm) should be rotated. Clinical response usually appears within 1 to 2 weeks of treatment, and nearly all patients respond within 3 months. In fact, patients who fail to respond to DMARD or biologic agent therapy within 3 months should receive consideration for an alternative treatment. When reviewing pooled data from early RA trials, which evaluated MTX, anti-TNF, and the combination of MTX with anti-TNF, a significant response at 3 months correlated with response 1 year after start of therapy based on SDAI, CDAI, and DAS28 scores.[142]

Injection site reactions (37% vs. 10% with placebo), upper respiratory infections (29% vs. 10% with placebo), and the development of autoantibodies are encountered with etanercept treatments. Injection site reactions generally are mild to moderate in severity and usually occurred within the first month of treatment with decreased frequency with time. Upper respiratory infections (e.g., sinusitis) occur at a rate of 0.82 events per patient-year in patients treated with etanercept versus 0.68 events per patient-year in the placebo group. Autoantibodies that developed during etanercept treatment included ANA (11% vs. 5% in placebo group) and new positive anti–double-stranded DNA antibodies (15% vs. 4% in placebo group). Patients with severe heart failure (e.g., NYHA class III or IV) may be at increased risk for heart failure exacerbation and mortality when taking any anti-TNF agent.[19,20,141] Although not a contraindication, caution is advised if etanercept is prescribed for patients with heart failure. An increased incidence of lymphoma has been observed among patients with RA receiving any of the available anti-TNF agents; however, causation has not been established because both RA and MTX are associated with an increased rate of lymphoma.[137] Additionally, the FDA has recently received reports of hepatosplenic T-cell lymphoma, a rare cancer of the white blood cells, in patients being treated with TNF blockers, AZA, or mercaptopurine. The majority of these cases were found in adolescents and young adults with Crohn's disease or ulcerative colitis. Incidence was also more common in patients on a combination of immunosuppressant agents. Although it is difficult to measure the added risk associated with anti-TNF agents, caution and monitoring is advised.[143] Other adverse effects, in order of decreasing frequency, include headache, rhinitis, dizziness, pharyngitis, cough, asthenia, abdominal pain, and rash.

The greatest concern with etanercept therapy is the risk of immunosuppression and subsequent serious infections, including sepsis. TNF-α is a key mediator of inflammation and plays a major role in immune system regulation. Approximately 6 months after FDA approval of etanercept, 30 patients receiving etanercept experienced serious infections.[137] Although the number of reports was not more than what was expected from clinical trials, six of these patients died within 2 to 16 weeks of starting therapy. Postmarketing reports of other infections such as TB (a black-box warning for all anti-TNF agents), mycobacterial infections, and fungal infections further reinforces the strong recommendation against the initiation of etanercept therapy in patients with sepsis or any chronic or localized active infection.[8,19,20] *Mycobacterium tuberculosis* skin testing and a baseline chest radiograph should be undertaken before initiation of anti-TNF therapy. Therapy should be postponed for patients identified as having latent TB until appropriate antituberculosis therapy has been completed. Clinicians also must be cautious when prescribing etanercept to patients with a history of recurring infection or with underlying illnesses that predispose them to infection (e.g., diabetes). B.W. should receive a TB skin test, undergo a chest radiograph, and be warned of the potential adverse effects of etanercept, particularly the risk of immunosuppression and subsequent infection. Any sign of infection must be reported immediately to her health care provider.

INFLIXIMAB AND ADALIMUMAB: DOSING AND PLACE IN THERAPY

CASE 44-7, QUESTION 11: After 3 weeks of etanercept therapy, B.W. seems to respond well. However, she dislikes the subcutaneous administration of etanercept once weekly and wants another medication that can be administered on a more convenient basis. How do the other TNF inhibitors differ from etanercept? Is B.W. a candidate for one of these alternatives?

Four anti-TNF monoclonal antibodies are FDA approved for the treatment of RA. Infliximab and adalimumab have been available since 1998 and 2002, respectively. CZP and GLM have been available since 2008 and 2009, respectively, and will be discussed in the next section.

Infliximab is a chimeric (mouse–human) IgG antibody directed against TNF that is approved for the treatment of a variety of conditions including Crohn's disease, ulcerative colitis, ankylosing spondylitis, psoriatic arthritis, plaque psoriasis, and RA. Specifically, infliximab is approved in combination with MTX for the treatment of moderately to severely active RA.[144] The usual dose of infliximab is 3 mg/kg IV at 0, 2, and 6 weeks, then every 8 weeks thereafter; thus, the convenience of infrequent dosing is tempered by the need for supervised IV administration. Infliximab should be given with MTX therapy to prevent the formation of antibodies to infliximab.

In a randomized, placebo-controlled trial of 101 patients with active RA who responded suboptimally to MTX therapy, 60% of patients receiving 3 or 10 mg/kg of infliximab with or without MTX (7.5 mg/week) responded to treatment after 26 weeks.[145] In another randomized, double-blind, multicenter, placebo-controlled trial of 428 active RA patients who failed to respond adequately to at least 12.5 mg/week of MTX, infliximab 3 or 10 mg/kg or placebo was administered every 4 or 8 weeks along with MTX therapy. This study was unblinded after 1 year because of radiographic evidence of disease modification in patients receiving infliximab. Analysis of radiographic results after 2 years demonstrated that infliximab significantly protected against joint erosion.[146]

Adalimumab is a genetically engineered, fully humanized IgG1 monoclonal antibody, as opposed to the chimeric infliximab. Adalimumab is self-administered subcutaneously by the patient as a 40-mg injection every other week, either as monotherapy or in combination with traditional DMARDs (e.g., MTX).[147] When administered weekly or every other week, monotherapy with adalimumab 40 mg significantly improved ACR-20 response rates in a randomized, controlled trial of 544 RA patients refractory to traditional DMARDs.[148] Patients receiving 40 mg/week had a higher response rate than patients who received the drug every other week. When adalimumab 40 mg every other week was added to the treatment regimen of RA patients receiving stable MTX doses, significantly more adalimumab-treated patients (67%) achieved an ACR-20 response than those receiving only MTX (14.5%, $p < 0.001$) after 24 weeks.[149] In radiographic data reflecting 1 or 2 years of treatment, adalimumab slowed the progression of joint damage.[150] Data are available supporting the efficacy and safety of adalimumab for more than 8 years.[151]

Adverse Effects of Anti-Tumor Necrosis Factor Antibodies

Infliximab and adalimumab have treatment risks and side effect profiles very similar to etanercept (e.g., injection site pain, local reactions, upper respiratory tract infections, nausea, flulike symptoms, rash).[147] Serious adverse effects (e.g., serious infections, increased incidence of lymphoma) are similar as well. As with all anti-TNF agents, a TB skin test result and chest radiograph must be obtained before initiating treatment. The development of antibodies against infliximab occurs frequently with monotherapy owing to the chimeric nature of the medication, and concurrent use with MTX decreases the formation of these HACA antibodies. Although adalimumab is a fully humanized product, approximately 5% of patients develop antibodies against it at least once during therapy when used as a single agent.[148] This reaction is attenuated with weekly dosing of adalimumab or concurrent use of MTX. Patients who switch from one anti-TNF agent to another owing to loss of efficacy of the initial agent are able to attain a good response from the second.[152,153] After the switch, many patients respond even better to the second drug as demonstrated by HAQ score improvement.[154]

B.W. seems to be a reasonable candidate for either infliximab or adalimumab therapy. Her interest in a biologic agent with less frequent dosing is understandable. Although clinical trials have not directly compared the biologic agents, key differentiating variables among these drugs need to be considered. No evidence suggests that there are any significant efficacy differences among etanercept, infliximab, and adalimumab. Although infliximab is ultimately administered every 2 months, it must be administered IV and in combination with MTX (or possibly at a higher dose) to minimize HACA formation. Adalimumab's ease of administration (self-injected subcutaneous injection) and infrequent dosing interval compares favorably with etanercept (once-weekly injections) and anakinra (daily injections), but it is administered more frequently than infliximab (Table 44-6). Although it is difficult to estimate exact costs of these agents, the ACR lists approximate annual costs to be similar among etanercept, infliximab, and adalimumab ($15,436, $13,940, and $14,522, respectively).[155] These costs are subject to change based on patient weight for infliximab, and optional adjusted intervals for adalimumab and infliximab. Additional therapeutic benefit might be achieved from weekly dosing of adalimumab or monthly dosing of infliximab.[144,147]

If the dosing interval is decreased, the costs of therapy would increase considerably.

Anti-TNF Agents: Dosing, Administration, Efficacy, and Safety

CASE 44-7, QUESTION 12: B.W.'s physician has little experience with the two newest anti-TNF-α agents CZP and GLM. He would like to know how these newer agents compare with the older TNF-α inhibitors in regard to efficacy, safety, and administration.

CZP and GLM have demonstrated similar efficacy and safety data when compared with the other approved TNF-*α* inhibitors. CZP is a novel pegylated anti-TNF agent approved for the treatment of adult patients with moderately to severely active RA and Crohn's disease.[31] CZP consists of a Fab attached to a 40-kDa PEG moiety. The attachment to the PEG moiety increases the half-life of CZP to approximately 2 weeks, which allows dosing every 2 to 4 weeks.[156] Additionally, CZP's unique structure lacks an Fc region, so it may not induce complement- or antibody-dependent cell-mediated cytotoxicity, which has been observed in vitro with adalimumab, etanercept, and infliximab.[157]

The efficacy of CZP has been demonstrated in patients with moderate to severe active RA in combination with MTX and as monotherapy.[158–161] In a randomized, double-blind, placebo-controlled study in 619 patients with active RA, significantly more patients met ACR-20 response rates at week 24 with CZP 200 mg and 400 mg plus MTX (57.3% and 57.6%, respectively) than patients treated with placebo plus MTX (8.7%, $p < 0.001$).[160] Additionally, ACR-50 and ACR-70 response rates were significantly improved in the CZP treatment groups versus the placebo group ($p < 0.001$). Physical function, as evidenced by the mean change in the HAQ disability index (DI) score, as well as DAS28 remission were improved in patients who received combination treatment compared with MTX monotherapy. CZP 200 mg and 400 mg also significantly inhibited radiographic progression of RA.[160] An open-label extension of this trial demonstrated that ACR responses and improvements in DAS28, HAQ-DI, and pain from baseline were sustained for patients remaining on CZP for up to 3 years. The progression of structural damage was sustained until the final radiograph evaluation at 2.5 years.[161]

GLM is a human IgG1 monoclonal antibody specific for human TNF-*α*. It was created using genetically engineered mice immunized with human TNF. GLM binds to both the soluble and transmembrane bioactive forms of human TNF. This binding prevents the binding of TNF-*α* to its receptors, thus inhibiting the biologic activity of TNF-*α*.[32] GLM shares common characteristics with both adalimumab and infliximab. Similar to adalimumab, GLM is a fully humanized bivalent immunoglobulin monoclonal antibody.[162] GLM is made up of light and heavy chains, which are identical to infliximab, but whereas infliximab is derived from both mice and humans, GLM is completely humanized. GLM is approved for the treatment of moderate to severe active RA in combination with MTX, as well as active psoriatic arthritis and active ankylosing spondylitis.[32]

Clinical trials have demonstrated GLM efficacy in patients with no previous MTX use and in patients with an inadequate response to MTX or a TNF-*α* inhibitor.[163,164] A randomized, placebo-controlled trial conducted in 444 patients examined the efficacy of GLM in patients with active RA despite concomitant MTX use.[165] In this double-blind, four-arm, dose-ranging, 52-week trial, patients were allowed stable doses of NSAIDs and corticosteroids, but no history of prior biologic use. Significantly more patients in the combined GLM plus MTX groups achieved an ACR-20 response compared with the MTX plus placebo group (55.6% vs. 33.1%, respectively, $p < 0.001$). These results were sustained at 52 weeks.

A Cochrane review of the efficacy and safety data available for GLM showed that patients treated with GLM plus MTX were 2.6 times more likely to reach ACR-50 and were no more likely to have any adverse event when compared with patients treated with placebo plus MTX. Additionally, patients treated with GLM were significantly more likely to achieve remission, low disease activity, and improvement in functional ability compared with patients treated with placebo.[166]

Adverse Effects and Safety

CZP and GLM have been found to be generally well tolerated, with similar safety profiles to the other anti-TNF agents.[31,32] As with all of the anti-TNF agents, the labeling for these agents contains black-box warnings for increased risk of serious infections, and lymphoma and other malignancies. The manufacturer recommends that all patients be screened for latent TB before treatment. Patients found to be TB positive should initiate TB treatment before therapy (see Case 44-7, Questions 10 and 11).

For CZP, the most commonly reported infectious adverse effects included urinary tract infections, nasopharyngitis, and upper respiratory tract infections.[31] Serious infections were observed more frequently in the CZP groups than in the placebo group (5.3 and 7.3 per 100 patient-years in the 200-mg and 400-mg CZP groups, respectively, versus 2.2 per 100 patient-years in the placebo group).[167] The incidence of injection site pain was low across all randomized, controlled trials. A 2-year open-label extension of one randomized, controlled trial showed no evidence of increased incidence of adverse effects after longer-term exposure to CZP.[168] The overall percentage of patients with antibodies to CZP detectable on at least one occasion was 7% (105 of 1,509 patients). Patients treated with concomitant immunosuppressants (MTX) had a lower rate of antibody development than patients not taking immunosuppressants at baseline.[31]

GLM has also produced relatively consistent data across available clinical trials. In one randomized, controlled clinical trial injection site reactions occurred most commonly in patients receiving GLM 100 mg (8.8%–10.8%), followed by GLM 50 mg plus MTX (4.4%), and placebo plus MTX (1.9%).[169] Incidence of injection site reactions were similar across clinical trials, and in all studies none of the injection site reactions were considered severe or resulted in discontinuation of the study drug.[110,169,170] Based on the summarized data from four randomized, controlled trials, GLM 50 mg was associated with no significantly higher risk of infections, serious infections, lung infections, TB, cancer, or death than placebo.[166] The presence of MTX treatment has been shown to decrease anti-GLM antibody incidence.[32]

Dose and Administration

For the treatment of moderately to severely active RA, CZP is initiated with a dose of 400 mg injected subcutaneously at weeks 0, 2, and 4, and maintained with 200 mg per week every other week thereafter.[31] A more convenient dosing regimen of 400 mg every 4 weeks can be considered. CZP is self-administered subcutaneously in 200 mg/mL prefilled syringes or as a lyophilized powder for reconstitution. The lyophilized powder solution should be reconstituted and administered by a health care professional.[171] For a video demonstration on how to use the prefilled syringe, please go to **http://www.cimzia.com/rheumatoidarthritis/hcp/dosing-administration/cimziaprefilled-syringe.aspx.**

The usual dose of GLM is 50 mg/0.5 mL administered subcutaneously every 4 weeks. GLM is administered every 4 weeks, but has similar pharmacokinetics to adalimumab, which is dosed every 2 weeks; thus, dosing may be adjusted for each drug based on patient response to therapy. The dosing regimen for GLM does not require adjustment for patient weight, age, sex, or ethnicity.[32] It is available as a single-dose prefilled SmartJect autoinjector or as a single-dose prefilled syringe. GLM may be self-injected by patients. For an instructional video on how to use the GLM SmartJect autoinjector, go to https://www.simponi.com/about-simponi/smartject-autoinjector. For a video demonstration on how to use the prefilled syringe, please go to https://www.simponi.com/about-simponi/prefilled-syringe.

ANAKINRA

CASE 44-7, QUESTION 13: B.W. would prefer to avoid anakinra because it requires daily subcutaneous injection dosing. Apart from this inconvenience, how does anakinra compare with the anti-TNF agents?

Anakinra is currently the only available IL-1Ra that is almost identical in composition to human IL-1Ra (see Biologic Agents in the Treatment section). Anakinra is approved for the treatment of moderate to severe active RA in patients who have failed one or more DMARDs. It may be used alone or in combination with MTX or other DMARDs.[172] The recommended dose of anakinra is 100 mg daily by self-administered subcutaneous injection.[20] Anakinra significantly, but modestly, improves signs and symptoms and radiographic evidence of joint erosion in RA patients.[20,173] In a study of 472 patients with serious active RA, three different doses of anakinra monotherapy (30, 75, and 150 mg/day) were compared with placebo.[174] At 24-week follow-up, 34% of patients receiving anakinra 75 mg demonstrated an ACR-20 response; however, 27% of placebo patients achieved the same response. Although modest, this difference is statistically significant. Although the higher dose of 150 mg produced improvement in 43% of patients, this dose exceeds the manufacturer's recommended dose. The most commonly reported adverse event with anakinra is local injection site reaction. Injection site reactions have been reported in up to 71% of clinical trial patients, usually occurring within the first month of treatment.[172] Although neutropenia and severe infections are more common with anakinra than placebo, there have been no reports of patients experiencing TB reactivation. Combining anakinra with an anti-TNF agent seems to be logical based on their different mechanisms of action; however, the combination is not recommended because of a significantly increased incidence of serious infections and leukopenia.[172] Unlike anti-TNF agents, anakinra is not associated with decompensation of heart failure.

Although the anti-TNF agents have not been compared directly, anakinra seems to be relatively less effective. In a Cochrane review of biologic agents for RA, anakinra was found to be less effective when trial data were compared with data for TNF-α inhibitors, RXB, and abatacept.[65] In addition, the advantage of being able to self-administer anakinra is offset by the need for daily injections. Anakinra is a therapeutic alternative for RA patients in whom traditional DMARD treatment fails; however, it seems to offer no advantages and some real and potential disadvantages when compared with the other available biologic agents.

MANAGEMENT OF METHOTREXATE NONRESPONDERS

CASE 44-8

QUESTION 1: S.K., a 71-year-old woman, was diagnosed with RA approximately 15 years ago. Her initial drug therapy included MTX, followed by the addition of SSZ and HCQ, which seemed to keep her RA in near-remission until 2002. She began etanercept along with MTX (without SSZ and HCQ) with good results until 2005. In response to declining disease control, infliximab was substituted for MTX with excellent results. Then last month, she experienced a flare in RA activity. At that time, her CRP was 5.1 mg/dL, ESR was 90 mm/hour, and anti-CCP was positive at 112 units. She also experienced morning stiffness lasting several hours and multiple joints with swelling (n = 26) and tenderness (n = 38). What are reasonable treatment options for S.K. at this stage of her disease?

Clinical studies have consistently demonstrated that TNF-α inhibitors improve the signs and symptoms of RA, as well as slow the progression of structural damage. However, TNF-α inhibitors fail to produce an ACR-20 response in approximately 30% of patients (primary failure). Even more patients experience acquired resistance to treatment, known as secondary failure, which is defined as a loss of response with time and is illustrated by S.K.[175] Most patients who lose responsiveness to an initial trial of anti-TNF therapy can often be successfully treated with an alternative anti-TNF agent (see Case 44-7, Questions 11 and 12). However, no evidence supports switching to a third anti-TNF agent if the first two agents fail. Abatacept (inhibitor of T-cell activation), RXB (selective depletor of $CD20^+$ B cells), and TZB (anti-IL-6 receptor antibody) have demonstrated great potential to fill this void. These agents have demonstrated excellent efficacy in patients with inadequate response to traditional DMARDs (e.g., MTX) as well as to anti-TNF therapy (see discussion in Treatment section, Biologic Agents).[19,155] Although there is a lack of head-to-head comparisons of these agents, there is a strong body of evidence detailing efficacy and safety data for each agent, which will be considered for S.K.

Abatacept

Abatacept is a selective costimulation inhibitor of T-cell activation indicated for the treatment of moderately to severely active RA.[41] Abatacept may be prescribed as monotherapy or in combination with other DMARDs other than TNF antagonists. The Abatacept in Inadequate Responders to Methotrexate (AIM) study compared abatacept 10 mg/kg plus MTX versus placebo plus MTX.[44] At 12-month follow-up, significantly more patients in the abatacept group attained ACR-20 response when compared with the placebo group (73.1% vs. 39.7%, respectively, $p < 0.001$). Patients in the abatacept group also achieved better quality-of-life survey scores. After 1 year of abatacept therapy, patients demonstrated statistically significant slowing of structural damage progression compared with patients receiving placebo. Abatacept efficacy was maintained in the 5-year open-label extension of this trial. At year 5, 83.6% of patients had achieved ACR-20 and 33.7% had achieved DAS28 remission.[176] Structural damage progression was reduced by 50% in the second year relative to the first year, with approximately half (45.1%) of the 120 patients who completed all 5 years of abatacept treatment exhibiting no structural damage progression.

Abatacept has also demonstrated efficacy in patients such as S.K. with an inadequate response to one or more TNF-α inhibitors. In the Abatacept Trial in Treatment of Anti-TNF Inadequate Responders study, patients in the abatacept arm achieved an ACR-20 response of 50.4% compared with 19.5% in the placebo arm.[177] The ACR-50 and ACR-70 responses were also significantly improved in the abatacept arm versus the placebo arm. Efficacy and safety data from 7 years of abatacept therapy indicate that abatacept maintains sustained improvements in disease activity and ACR-70 scores during this period, with no change in safety profile.[46]

The side effects of greatest concern include infections such as pneumonia, cellulitis, urinary tract infection, bronchitis, diverticulitis, and acute pyelonephritis (see Treatment section,

Biologic Agents). Infections are significantly more common when abatacept is combined with anti-TNF therapy; thus this combination is not recommended.[41] A few case reports of malignancy have been associated with abatacept, and patients with chronic obstructive pulmonary disease are noted to suffer from more respiratory-related and nonrespiratory-related adverse effects than patients with chronic obstructive pulmonary disease treated with placebo.[41]

Rituximab

RXB is a chimeric monoclonal antibody that binds to the antigen CD20 on B cells. It is approved in combination with MTX for the treatment of moderately to severely active RA in patients who have had an inadequate response to one or more TNF antagonist medications. In a placebo-controlled trial of 161 RA patients who responded inadequately to MTX therapy (≥10 mg/week), the ACR-50 response was significantly higher among treatment groups receiving RXB (33%, 41%, and 43% in the RXB only, RXB plus cyclophosphamide, and RXB plus MTX groups, respectively) versus the MTX only group (13%). At week 48, however, significantly more patients in the RXB plus MTX group (35%) maintained an ACR-50 response than patients in the RXB plus cyclophosphamide group (27%). Although cyclophosphamide is reserved for severe cases of RA (usually involving rheumatoid vasculitis), the combination of RXB plus cyclophosphamide does not seem to be as effective as RXB plus MTX.[178]

The REFLEX (Randomized Evaluation of Long-Term Efficacy of Rituximab in RA) trial evaluated the use of RXB (two IV infusions 2 weeks apart, 1,000 mg/infusion) plus MTX versus placebo plus MTX in 499 patients with active, long-standing RA who responded inadequately to one or more anti-TNF medications, such as S.K.[179] At 24-week follow-up, significantly more patients in the RXB group demonstrated an ACR-20 response than those in the placebo group (51% vs. 18%, respectively). Peripheral CD20$^+$ B cells were depleted among RXB-treated patients at about 4 to 5 months after treatment. The incidence of all side effects was similar in the two treatment groups (85% of RXB patients, 88% of placebo patients), as were side effects identified as being related to any of the study drugs, including placebo (39% and 47%, respectively). Infusion reactions were common during or soon after the first dose among RXB-treated patients (23% vs. 18% of placebo patients). In another randomized, controlled trial, it was found that premedication with IV methylprednisolone reduced the frequency and intensity of first infusion adverse drug reactions, but the addition of oral prednisone did not provide additional benefit.[179] The rate of infections was slightly higher among RXB patients (41%) than placebo patients (38%). Similarly, the rate of serious infections was higher among RXB than placebo-treated patients (5.2 versus 3.7 per 100 patient-years). No cases of TB or opportunistic infections were reported. In a 56-week follow-up report of the REFLEX trial, RXB significantly inhibited radiographic progression of joint damage.[180] In the 2-year extension of this trial, MTX showed significant and sustained inhibition of joint damage. Patients were eligible for repeat courses of RXB every 6 months. Within the RXB group, 87% who had no progression of joint damage at 1 year remained nonprogressive at year 2. These findings support the efficacy and appropriateness of RXB for RA patients such as S.K. who are refractory to anti-TNF therapy.

The safety and efficacy of repeated courses of RXB was reported in an open-label extension analysis of three randomized, controlled trials. Patients were eligible for retreatment with RXB if they demonstrated a greater than or equal to 20% reduction in both the swollen joint count and the tender joint count at any visit 16 weeks after initial treatment or later and had active disease, defined as a swollen joint count of 8 (in 66 joints) or a tender joint count of 8 (in 68 joints). Patients were eligible for additional courses after the second course if they had active disease as described above.[181] A minimum interval of 16 weeks between courses was required. Retreatment courses were administered as 1,000 mg on days 1 and 15. The ACR (20, 50, and 70) response rates at week 24 were comparable after courses 1 and 2 of RXB. Additionally, EULAR good and moderate response rates were comparable after course 2 compared with course 1, and EULAR remission was doubled after course 2 compared with course 1. Safety data were consistent with previous trials and retreatment demonstrated no additional safety issues.

Although repeated treatment with RXB has demonstrated efficacy and raised no additional safety concerns, it is still unclear what dosage regimen is optimal for retreatment. Another randomized trial studied the safety and efficacy of various repeat treatment regimens for RXB.[182] The results of this trial showed no statistically significant difference between retreatment with RXB 500 mg on days 1 and 15, 500 mg on day 1 and 1,000 mg on day 15, or 1,000 mg on days 1 and 15. The 1,000 mg × 2 group produced consistently improved ACR and EULAR response rates; however, statistical significance was not reached. It was found that retreatment at week 24 produced sustained benefits through week 48.

Tocilizumab

TZB is a humanized anti-IL-6 receptor antibody indicated for the treatment of adult patients with moderately to severely active RA who have had an inadequate response to one or more TNF antagonist therapies, such as S.K.[43] It may be prescribed as monotherapy or in combination with MTX or other DMARDs other than TNF antagonists. In a double-blind, placebo-controlled, multicenter study of 1,216 patients with moderately to severely active RA despite treatment with DMARDs, the ACR-20 response was significantly higher in the TZB 8 mg/kg than in the placebo group (61% and 25% respectively, $p < 0.0001$) at week 24.[183] The superiority of TZB plus DMARD therapy versus placebo plus DMARD therapy was also demonstrated with improved results for all of the secondary end points (ACR-50, ACR-70, DAS28, DAS28 remission [<2.6], and CRP and hemoglobin levels).

In another 24-week double-blind, placebo-controlled, multicenter trial (RADIATE), 499 patients with an inadequate response to one or more TNF-α inhibitors were randomly assigned to receive 8 mg/kg or 4 mg/kg of TZB or placebo every 4 weeks for 24 weeks.[184] An ACR-20 response was achieved at 24 weeks by 50.0%, 30.4%, and 10.1% of patients in the TZB 8 mg/kg, 4 mg/kg, and placebo arms, respectively ($p < 0.001$). The impact of TZB on radiographic progression of RA compared with conventional DMARD therapy was studied in 302 Japanese patients with active RA.[185] At week 52, patients in the TZB group showed significantly less radiographic progression compared with the traditional DMARD group. However, it remains unclear how these changes translate to patient quality of life or disability.

The most serious side effects associated with TZB therapy include severe infections, GI perforation, and laboratory abnormalities (see Treatment section, Biologic Agents). As with the TNF-α inhibitors, TZB has a black-box warning for increased risk of developing serious infections, especially those caused by opportunistic pathogens. The risk for infection is increased when TZB is taken in combination with other immunosuppressant agents (e.g., MTX, corticosteroids). As with the anti-TNF agents, a TB skin test result and chest radiograph must be obtained before initiating treatment. In clinical studies the rates of serious infections in the 4-mg/kg and 8-mg/kg TZB plus DMARD groups were 4.4 and 5.3 events per 100 patient-years, respectively, compared with 3.9 events per 100 patient-years in the placebo plus DMARD group. The most common serious infections included pneumonia, urinary tract infection, cellulitis, herpes zoster, gastroenteritis, diverticulitis, sepsis, and bacterial arthritis. The overall rate of fatal serious infections was low at 0.13 per 100 patient-years.[43]

The risk of GI perforation is also connected with TZB use, with a rate of 0.26 per 100 patient-years in the 6-month controlled clinical trial population. The reports of GI perforation in these trials were primarily found to be complications of diverticulitis; thus patients with a history of diverticulitis should be monitored closely.[20,43]

TZB has also been associated with a number of blood chemistry changes including neutropenia, thrombocytopenia, elevated LFTs, and lipid changes. In the 6-month, controlled clinical studies, decreases in neutrophil counts to less than 1,000 cells/μL occurred in 1.8% and 3.4% of patients in the 4-mg/kg and 8-mg/kg TZB plus DMARD groups, respectively, compared with 0.1% of patients in the placebo plus DMARD group. A relationship between decreases in neutrophils less than 1,000 cells/μL and the occurrence of serious infections was not established. Platelet counts less than 100,000 platelets/μL occurred in 1.3% and 1.7% of patients on 4 mg/kg and 8 mg/kg TZB plus DMARD, respectively, compared with 0.5% of patients on placebo plus DMARD, without associated bleeding events. In the 6-month, controlled clinical studies, increases in ALT to 3 times the ULN occurred in 45% and 48% of patients in the 4-mg/kg and 8-mg/kg TZB plus DMARD group, respectively, compared with 23% of patients in the placebo plus DMARD group. In patients experiencing liver enzyme elevations, modifications of the treatment (dosage adjustment of TZB or concomitant DMARD or interruption of TZB therapy) regimen resulted in decrease or normalization of liver enzymes. Liver enzyme elevations were not associated with clinical evidence of hepatitis or hepatic insufficiency. Increases in lipids (total cholesterol, low-density lipoprotein, high-density lipoprotein, and triglycerides) have been shown in clinical trials. This increase in lipids may be caused in part by the decrease in inflammatory activity with TZB use. Lipid elevations respond to lipid-lowering agents, and further studies are necessary to assess the effects of TZB on cardiovascular risk factors. The most common adverse reactions with TZB include upper respiratory tract infections, nasopharyngitis, headache, hypertension, and increased ALT.[43]

In addition to the role of IL-6 on the joint inflammation associated with RA, IL-6 also participates in osteoclast maturation and activation and may alter osteoblast differentiation and function.[49] Systemic and periarticular bone loss, which is associated with severe RA, is correlated with increased IL-6 levels in the bone marrow. In patients with RA, increased levels of IL-6 are present in the serum and synovial fluid. The impact of IL-6 inhibition with TZB on bone health has been examined in one randomized, controlled trial. This study included 416 of the 623 patients included in the OPTION study. In this study, TZB treatment resulted in dose-dependent decreases in markers of bone resorption and cartilage turnover and increased bone formation markers.[186] More data are needed to assess the impact of TZB on bone health and fracture risk.

Dosing and Administration for Abatacept, Rituximab, and Tocilizumab

Abatacept is supplied as a lyophilized powder in preservative-free, single-use vials containing 250 mg of abatacept.[41] Abatacept must be reconstituted with 10 mL of sterile water for injection, using only the silicone-free syringe provided, along with an 18- to 21-gauge needle. Reconstitution using a siliconized syringe can result in the development of translucent particles in the medication solution; solutions prepared using siliconized syringes must be discarded. The reconstituted solution must be diluted to 100 mL using 0.9% sodium chloride, with a final concentration of no more than 10 mg/mL. Abatacept dosing is based on body weight (500 mg for patients <60 kg, 750 mg for patients 60–100 kg, and 1,000 mg for patients >100 kg) and should be infused IV for 30 minutes. The abatacept dose should be repeated at 2 and 4 weeks after the first dose, then every 4 weeks thereafter. Abatacept can be given as monotherapy or in combination with nonbiologic (traditional) DMARDs.[20]

RXB, provided in 100-mg and 500-mg single-use vials at a concentration of 10 mg/mL, is administered as two 1,000-mg IV infusions separated by 2 weeks.[42] RXB must be diluted to a final concentration of 1 to 4 mg/mL with either 0.9% sodium chloride or 5% dextrose in water. To reduce the incidence and severity of infusion-related adverse effects, premedication with IV methylprednisolone 100 mg, or its equivalent, 30 minutes before each infusion is strongly recommended; other premedications (e.g., acetaminophen, antihistamine) may also be beneficial. Antihypertensive medications should be discontinued 12 hours before RXB administration to avoid transient hypotension, which has been reported during RXB infusions. RXB must be given with MTX for maximal efficacy based on clinical trials and to help reduce the risk of developing HACA, which occurs in approximately 9% of patients receiving RXB.

The first IV infusion of RXB solution should be initiated at a rate of 50 mg/hour. In the absence of infusion reactions, the infusion rate can be increased in 50-mg/hour increments every 30 minutes to a maximal rate of 400 mg/hour. In the event of an infusion reaction, the infusion should be halted or slowed until symptoms improve, at which time the infusion can continue at one-half the previous rate. In patients who tolerated the first infusion well, subsequent infusions of RXB can be initiated at a higher rate (100 mg/hour) and increased by 100-mg/hour increments every 30 minutes to a maximal rate of 400 mg/hour. Patients poorly tolerant to the first infusion should receive subsequent RXB infusions at 50 mg/hour.[42] It is recommended that subsequent courses of RXB be given every 24 weeks. The dosing interval may be decreased on the basis of clinical evaluation, but must be no less than every 16 weeks.

TZB is provided in 80-mg, 200-mg, and 400-mg single-use vials with a concentration of 20 mg/mL.[43] The recommended initial dose of TZB is 4 mg/kg, infused IV every 4 weeks. Doses can be increased to 8 mg/kg as needed based on clinical response. The maximal dose must not exceed 800 mg per infusion. The indicated dose should be diluted to 100 mL in 0.9% sodium chloride using aseptic technique. This infusion should be administered by a health care professional through an IV drip for 1 hour. Dose adjustments are recommended for certain dose-related laboratory changes including elevated liver enzymes, neutropenia, and thrombocytopenia. TZB should not be initiated in patients with an absolute neutrophil count less than 2,000 cells/μL, platelet count less than 100,000 platelets/μL, or in patients who have an ALT or AST value greater than 1.5 times the ULN.[43] TZB treatment should be interrupted if a patient experiences a serious infection; therapy may be resumed once the infection is controlled. The half-life of TZB is concentration-dependent. For the 4-mg/kg dose, the half-life is up to 11 days, whereas the half-life for the 8-mg/kg dose is up to 13 days.

Abatacept, RXB, and TZB are all appropriate agents for S.K. Efficacy has been demonstrated in patients with inadequate response to DMARDs, including anti-TNF agents. All three of these agents are generally well tolerated, and unlike the anti-TNF agents, they have not been associated with cardiovascular events or worsening heart failure. However, both RXB and TZB have a black-box warning as described in the Treatment section, Biologic Agents, and the risk of infection in S.K., an older patient, must be taken into consideration when selecting a treatment option. Experience with these agents remains relatively limited compared with experience with etanercept, adalimumab, and infliximab; therefore, the full range of adverse effects from these agents may not be fully manifested. In summary, abatacept, RXB, and TZB are potent treatment options with novel mechanisms of action and proven efficacy at improving RA symptoms and slowing joint erosion. However, based on a combination of current research findings, lack of long-term safety data, and cost, these agents should generally not be used before a trial with anti-TNF agents, except for patients with relative contraindications to anti-TNF agents (e.g., multiple sclerosis, moderate to severe heart failure).

CORTICOSTEROIDS

CASE 44-9

QUESTION 1: W.M., a 57-year-old man, has progressive RA that has not been responsive to SSZ. He is having difficulty working a full day and is seeking an alternative medication. After a discussion of therapeutic options, W.M. declines MTX therapy and asks to start HCQ. Would it be appropriate to initiate corticosteroids concurrently?

Despite the potential for serious adverse effects with long-term therapy, the judicious use of low-dose corticosteroids represents an important component of treatment during the course of unremitting disease. In addition, low-dose corticosteroids may offer some disease-modifying properties, although this is controversial because of the long-term negative effects of corticosteroid use.[20] Considering that W.M.'s RA is sufficiently active to compromise his ability to earn an income, MTX is a much better DMARD selection. Regardless, concurrent initiation of a DMARD and an intermediate-acting corticosteroid (e.g., prednisone in a daily or divided dose of 5 to 10 mg) is justified.[70] In large cohort studies, prednisone doses greater than 7.5 mg/day have been associated with a greater than twofold increased risk of cardiovascular events (MI, stroke, heart failure), as well as the risk of developing hypertension with long-term use (at least 6–12 months).[39,187] Therefore, the lowest effective corticosteroid dose is preferred for the shortest duration of time possible. The onset of action of corticosteroids is relatively rapid, and their immediate benefits will allow W.M. to maintain his current employment and continue taking care of home responsibilities. The corticosteroid dose can be decreased gradually and eventually discontinued as W.M. begins to respond to HCQ therapy. An important goal of low-dose corticosteroid treatment is to provide bridge therapy until the DMARD therapy becomes effective, in hopes of then being able to taper and discontinue the corticosteroid.

DOSING

CASE 44-9, QUESTION 2: How should corticosteroids be dosed for W.M.? What are the considerations regarding divided daily doses rather than as single daily doses or an every-other-day regimen when used to treat RA?

Administering intermediate- or short-acting corticosteroids as a single daily dose each morning most closely mimics the early morning physiological secretion of cortisol, and, thereby, minimizes hypothalamic-pituitary-adrenal axis suppression. Administering corticosteroids on alternate mornings further reduces the risk of hypothalamic-pituitary-adrenal axis suppression by allowing the adrenal glands to respond to hypothalamic and pituitary mediators during the "off" day.[188] Once-a-day and alternate-day steroid therapies are most advantageous when used to prevent reactivation of some diseases (e.g., asthma, ulcerative colitis, chronic active hepatitis, sarcoidosis).[76] In contrast, when corticosteroids are used to provide symptomatic relief in RA during periods of active, ongoing inflammation, switching patients to single daily doses or every-other-day regimens frequently results in increased symptoms during the latter part of each day and during the "off" day. The anti-inflammatory effect of prednisone or prednisolone is attenuated after 12 hours, and is either diminished or absent after 24 hours. As a result, daily prednisone doses may need to be divided in half and administered twice daily to ensure 24-hour anti-inflammatory activity. Although a larger single daily dose may provide comparable therapeutic benefits, dividing the daily dose of prednisone is preferable because larger doses are associated with more frequent and severe adverse effects. To minimize adverse effects and maximize 24-hour symptom relief, an initial prednisone dose of 2.5 mg administered twice daily should be recommended for W.M.

CASE 44-9, QUESTION 3: Why are corticosteroids given in the evening in RA as opposed to the usual morning dosing?

It has been well studied that RA patients experience diurnal variations in symptoms such as joint pain, stiffness, and functional disability, with the worst symptoms occurring in the early morning.[189] Nocturnal surges in proinflammatory cytokines (IL-6, cortisol) have been implicated in the occurrence of these typical early morning symptoms. Corticosteroids have been shown to promote increased reduction in morning stiffness if administered in the evening or during the night as opposed to usual morning dosing.[51] Recently a modified-release prednisone has been developed, which releases active drug approximately 4 hours after ingestion. This is designed to deliver the drug during nighttime hours and prevent nocturnal surges in inflammatory cytokines. Two large phase III clinical trials have been conducted to assess the efficacy and safety of modified-release prednisone. The CAPRA-1 trial randomly assigned patients to receive 3 to 10 mg/day of either the immediate-release or modified-release prednisone for 12 weeks. A statistically significant decrease in duration of morning stiffness was demonstrated in the modified-release prednisone group (reduction of 29 minutes in the modified-release group vs. the immediate-release group).[190] The safety profile did not differ between the treatment groups. These effects were sustained in the 9-month open-label extension of this trial.[191] The use of modified-release prednisone may provide decreased morning stiffness for W.M.; however, this agent has not yet been approved in the United States.

STEROID-INDUCED OSTEOPOROSIS

CASE 44-9, QUESTION 4: Is W.M. at risk for developing glucocorticoid osteoporosis? What therapeutic interventions are available to prevent it?

Chronic corticosteroid therapy induces osteoporosis by inhibiting bone formation and enhancing bone resorption. Steroids impair bone formation by inhibiting the production of bone-forming osteoblasts and enhance bone resorption by reducing GI calcium absorption and increasing the renal excretion of calcium.[76] In addition, corticosteroids reduce the secretion of luteinizing hormone from the pituitary, resulting in a reduction in estrogen production in women and testosterone production in men.[192] This leads to deficiencies in circulating levels of anabolic hormones (e.g., estradiol, estrone, androstenedione, progesterone), which contribute to the development of osteoporosis. Trabecular bone of the spine and ribs seems to be affected primarily by corticosteroid therapy, with most rapid skeletal wasting occurring during the first 6 months (see Chapter 105, Osteoporosis).

allopurinol, although some have been able to be desensitized and tolerate low doses.[109]

Febuxostat

Febuxostat, a nonpurine XO inhibitor, was approved by the FDA in February 2009 for chronic management of hyperuricemia in patients with gout.[110] Febuxostat is more selective than allopurinol for XO and does not inhibit other enzymes involved in purine and pyrimidine metabolism. Several studies during the past few years (FACT,[111] APEX,[112] EXCEL,[113] CONFIRMS,[114] FOCUS[115]) have compared febuxostat to allopurinol for clinical SUA-lowering effect, and all have found febuxostat superior or equivalent to allopurinol 300 mg in achieving SUA less than 6 mg/dL. An important consideration in evaluating these trials is that although the studies allowed upward titration of febuxostat to achieve maximal SUA lowering, the allopurinol dosage was not titrated to greater than 300 mg daily. Because the urate-lowering effect with allopurinol is known to be dose-related,[105] and some patients have required up to 900 mg/day to achieve a SUA less than 6 mg/dL, this study design may not have allowed for an adequate comparison of efficacy between the two drugs. Interestingly, the efficacy of febuxostat in reducing gout flares and decreasing the size of tophi was similar to that of allopurinol in the two trials that included these as secondary end points.[111,116] In addition, adverse effects were shown to be minor and similar between both drugs in all of the comparative studies with increases in liver function tests, nausea, diarrhea, arthralgias, and rash being the most common adverse effects with greater than 1% incidence.[110–114] As febuxostat is more widely used, the clinician should watch postmarketing surveillance reports for further adverse effects such as liver dysfunction or cardiovascular events. The starting dose of febuxostat is 40 mg once daily with a recommended dose increase to 80 mg once daily if SUA concentration is not less than 6 mg/dL by 2 weeks of therapy. It does not require dose adjustments for CrCl greater than 30 mL/minute, and the labeling provides no recommendations for use in patients with more severe renal impairment.[110]

CHOICE OF AGENT

CASE 45-3, QUESTION 4: Because an XO inhibitor is first-line therapy to lower SUA concentration, which product should be chosen for V.D.?

Although febuxostat is clearly efficacious in lowering SUA concentrations and preventing gout flares, allopurinol is also effective when the dose is appropriately titrated to response and goal SUA concentration. The clinician should keep in mind the significantly higher cost for febuxostat and consider patient affordability when choosing drug therapy. National Institute for Health and Clinical Excellence (NICE), an organization that provides medical guidance to health care practitioners of the public health system in the United Kingdom, has recently issued a document that recommends febuxostat be used only in patients who are intolerant of or have contraindications to allopurinol therapy or for those who cannot achieve adequate SUA concentration lowering on allopurinol therapy.[117] V.D. does not have any contraindications to allopurinol therapy. She is on chronic warfarin, which may interact with allopurinol[118] (Table 45-6), but this just warrants monitoring her international normalized ratio 5 to 7 days after allopurinol therapy is initiated and with any allopurinol dosage adjustments.

CASE 45-3, QUESTION 5: V.D. is started on allopurinol 100 mg orally once daily for initial ULT. Her SUA concentration will be checked, and her allopurinol will be increased by 50 to 100 mg/day in 2 to 4 weeks if needed until she reaches the goal of less than or equal to 6 mg/dL. What other drug therapy should also be considered when starting ULT?

TABLE 45-6
Allopurinol and Febuxostat Drug Interactions[118,119]

Precipitant Drug	Object Drug	Management
Allopurinol	Xanthine oxidase substrate drugs (azathioprine, mercaptopurine, theophylline)	Monitor theophylline levels and adjust as necessary; decrease azathioprine/mercaptopurine by 1/3 to 1/4.[120]
Febuxostat		Concurrent use is contraindicated.[113]
ACE inhibitors Ampicillin and amoxicillin Theophylline	Allopurinol	May increase risk for allopurinol hypersensitivity reactions; monitor.
Allopurinol	Vitamin K antagonists	Allopurinol may prolong half-life of dicumarol and warfarin; monitor INR.
Allopurinol	Cyclophosphamide	Allopurinol may increase bone-marrow suppression; monitor.
Febuxostat	Desipramine	Febuxostat may modestly increase desipramine levels; no dose adjustment necessary.

ACE, angiotensin-converting enzyme; INR, international normalized ratio.
Adapted with permission from Facts & Comparisons eAnswers. http://online.factsandcomparisons.com/MonoDisp.aspx?monoID=fandc-hcp15339&quick=364112%7c5&search=364112%7c5&isstemmed=True; http://online.factsandcomparisons.com/MonoDisp.aspx?monoID=fandc-hcp13090&quick=176221%7c5&search=176221%7c5&isstemmed=True. Accessed November 14, 2010.

Paradoxically, initiation of ULT can precipitate acute gout attacks, so both guidelines[38,39] recommend prophylaxis for up to 6 months with either colchicine or NSAIDs. The FACT[111] and EXCEL[113] febuxostat trials used colchicine 0.6 mg daily or naproxen 250 mg twice daily for 8 weeks as gout prophylaxis and found an increase of gout attacks beyond 8 weeks after prophylaxis ceased. This led to a modification in design in the CONFIRMS[115] trial, in which one of these regimens was administered for 6 months to each group. With the long duration of NSAID therapy, patients in this group were also given GI protection with lansoprazole 15 mg daily. This led to an overall decrease in acute gouty flares with time. So, in addition to allopurinol, V.D. will also be started on colchicine 0.6 mg orally once daily (to minimize drug interaction with diltiazem) for 6 months.

URICOSURIC AGENTS

The uricosuric agent probenecid is an alternative to XO inhibitors for patients who are underexcretors, unable to tolerate XO inhibitors, or have significant drug interactions[118] (Table 45-6). Uricosurics should not be administered to patients with impaired renal function or urolithiasis.

Probenecid

Probenecid is well absorbed orally, and plasma concentrations peak within 2 to 4 hours. Its biological half-life is 6 to 12 hours,

Section 9 Arthritic Disorders

and its active metabolites extend the duration of action. The usual initial dose of probenecid (250 mg twice daily for the first week of therapy) can be increased to 500 mg twice a day. If necessary, the dose can be increased further to 2 g/day. Uricosuric therapy should begin with small doses because the excretion of large amounts of uric acid increases the risk of urate stone formation in the kidney. High fluid intake to maintain urine flow of at least 2 L/day also minimizes renal stone formation. This gradual approach to the initiation of ULT also decreases the likelihood of precipitating an acute attack of gout.

Drug Interactions

Probenecid inhibits secretion of penicillins into the renal tubule, and thereby prolongs the serum half-life of penicillin and increases penicillin serum concentrations. Probenecid can also compete with salicylates for renal tubular transport, but its interactions with salicylates involve several mechanisms.[121] Two 300-mg tablets of aspirin every 6 hours can completely antagonize the uricosuric effects of 2 g of probenecid. Doses of salicylate that do not produce serum salicylate levels of greater than 5 mg/dL do not significantly affect probenecid uricosuria.[48] Therefore, low-dose aspirin for cardioprotection is unlikely to interfere with probenecid therapy. Interestingly, high-dose aspirin (e.g., greater than 1 g) has uricosuric activity of its own.[91] Acetaminophen and NSAIDs do not interfere with probenecid, and are reliable alternatives for antipyresis and mild analgesia in patients taking uricosuric agents.

Sulfinpyrazone and Benzbromarone

Sulfinpyrazone, with only limited availability in the United States, and benzbromarone, which is not available in the United States, are other effective uricosuric agents. Sulfinpyrazone should only be used in patients with normal renal function and should be initiated slowly, as with probenecid, and the dose increased gradually. Benzbromarone is safe in patients with CrCl 30 to 60 mL/minute, but should be used with caution because of its association with hepatotoxicity.

RECOMBINANT URATE OXIDASE DRUGS (URICASE)

Uricase, an enzyme endogenous in many animal species other than humans, converts uric acid to allantoin, which is much more soluble than uric acid and, therefore, more readily excreted into urine. Recently, two recombinant urate oxidase drugs have been developed for the treatment of hyperuricemia and gout.

Rasburicase

Rasburicase was initially approved by the FDA for the management of hyperuricemia in children who are receiving cytotoxic chemotherapy likely to result in tumor lysis syndrome, and later received approval for the same indication in adults. Rasburicase is administered as a short IV infusion of 0.2 mg/kg daily for up to 5 days (see Chapter 90, Adverse Effects of Chemotherapy and Targeted Agents).[120] It is not indicated for the treatment of hyperuricemia in patients with gout, but there are a few case reports in which rasburicase has been successfully used in patients refractory to or with contraindications for allopurinol treatment.[122,123] There is also one comparative short-term study in patients with renal impairment that found rasburicase was significantly more effective than allopurinol in lowering SUA concentrations at the end of 7 days of therapy.[124] Until further studies confirm safety and longer term efficacy in nonchemotherapy-related hyperuricemia, rasburicase should be reserved for patients with hyperuricemia who are at risk for tumor lysis syndrome.

Pegloticase

Pegloticase, the other available recombinant uricase drug available, was approved by the FDA in 2010 for the treatment of chronic gout in adult patients who are refractory to or unable to tolerate conventional therapy.[125] It has been shown to be effective in reducing SUA concentrations in patients who were refractory to conventional treatment in one published phase II trial[126] that compared a variety of dosing schemes, as well as in two unpublished manufacturer studies[125] that were placebo controlled. In the latter, there was also a decrease in the number and size of tophi at 6 months in 44% of patients.[127] Of note, pegloticase is administered IV for 2 hours as a dose of 8 mg every 2 weeks. It has a significant risk of anaphylaxis and infusion site reactions, so each dose must be preceded by prophylaxis with an antihistamine and corticosteroid (80% of withdrawals in the published trial[126] were attributable to these effects). It is contraindicated in patients with glucose-6-phosphate dehydrogenase deficiency, and the usual gout flare prophylaxis is recommended for the first 6 months after initiation. Finally, antipegloticase antibodies occurred in the majority of patients studied, and this can ameliorate the SUA lowering effects by decreasing the half-life of pegloticase. This effect occurred less in the every 2-week as compared with the every 4-week dosing regimen.[126] The full implication of this is unknown.

ASCORBIC ACID

Vitamin C has a urate-lowering effect that is believed to be mediated by competition with urate for renal tubular reabsorption.[128] In a study of 184 healthy, nonsmoking adults, ascorbic acid 500 mg daily for 2 months significantly decreased SUA concentrations.[129] Overall, ascorbic acid reduced the SUA concentration a mean of 0.5 mg/dL (range, 0.3–0.7 mg/dL), but the decrease in subjects with baseline SUA concentrations of greater than 7 mg/dL was a mean of 1.5 mg/dL. This would have brought those patients' SUA concentration below goal if they required treatment for their hyperuricemia. A newer trial using data from the men's Health Professional Follow-Up Study achieved similar results. As compared with men taking less than 90 mg of ascorbic acid per day, up to 500 mg per day resulted in average decreases in SUA of 0.6 to 0.7 mg/dL.[130] More important than decreasing SUA would be an actual decrease in gout attacks. Another study using the same Health Professional Follow-Up data in men without gout at baseline found that the risk of developing gout decreased with doses of vitamin C greater than or equal to 500 mg daily, in which the greater the dose, the lower the risk of gout.[131] Vitamin C may be considered as an option for adjunct therapy for patients requiring additional urate lowering to reach goal although further evaluation through randomized controlled trials should done before its use is widely recommended.

Comorbid Conditions

DYSLIPIDEMIA

CASE 45-4

QUESTION 1: L.M. is a 57-year-old man who presents to his family physician for a regular checkup. He is currently controlled on allopurinol 300 mg/day for the management of hyperuricemia. For his dyslipidemia, L.M. takes simvastatin 40 mg/day. Although his low-density lipoprotein is at goal of less than 130 mg/dL, he requires further lowering of his non–high-density lipoprotein cholesterol (goal of less than 160 mg/dL). What would be the best option to consider in this patient?

In addition to therapeutic lifestyle changes, fibrates (i.e., gemfibrozil, fenofibrate) or niacin are effective in lowering total cholesterol, low-density lipoprotein, and triglycerides, and increasing the beneficial high-density lipoprotein. A fibrate or niacin can also be used in combination with this patient's current simvastatin. However, with a history of gout and hyperuricemia, a fibrate would be preferred over niacin because niacin can induce hyperuricemia (Table 45-5). Specifically, fenofibrate has been shown to decrease SUA concentrations and could be beneficial in this dyslipidemic patient with a history of gout; however, the selection of a medication to manage dyslipidemia or other comorbid condition also involves other clinical variables that might be equally applicable.[39,132,133] Fenofibrate modestly increases renal urate excretion.[128]

HYPERTENSION

CASE 45-5

QUESTION 1: Because one of the first-line agents for the treatment of HTN, thiazide diuretics, is known to increase SUA concentrations, what other antihypertensives might be particularly beneficial for hyperuricemic patients?

Both amlodipine and losartan have positive effects on SUA concentrations. Amlodipine, a calcium-channel blocker, decreased SUA concentrations by increasing glomerular filtration rate in a study of renal transplant patients taking cyclosporine.[134] Losartan, an angiotensin II receptor blocker, appears to increase renal excretion of uric acid by interacting with the URAT-1 protein in the proximal tubule of the nephron.[2] When used with diuretics, it appears to alleviate the hyperuricemic effect of the diuretic.[128] This does not seem to be a class effect of angiotensin II receptor blockers because, in one study, patients on losartan achieved significantly lower SUA concentrations than an irbesartan-treated group.[135] Some advocate losartan for patients with hyperuricemia.[39]

Both fenofibrate and losartan have urate-lowering effects and often patients with hyperuricemia have HTN and dyslipidemia as comorbid conditions; therefore, the use of these two drugs in combination is of potential benefit under appropriate circumstances. In a small study of healthy male patients, concurrent daily losartan 100 mg and fenofibrate 300 mg decreased SUA concentrations by a mean of about 1 mg/dL compared with the decrease during treatment alone with these drugs.[133] If further studies show promise, some patients with hyperuricemia might be managed better by selecting drugs to manage comorbid conditions rather than requiring the use of the more traditional ULT.

Asymptomatic Hyperuricemia

CASE 45-6

QUESTION 1: T.M., a 50-year-old man, is seen by his physician for a routine evaluation. His physical examination is unremarkable, and his laboratory evaluations are all within normal limits except for a SUA concentration of 9.5 mg/dL. Should his hyperuricemia be treated?

Individuals with high SUA concentrations are more likely to develop acute gouty arthritis than normouricemic individuals, and the magnitude of the risk increases with increasing degrees of hyperuricemia. Nevertheless, it would be excessive to treat all hyperuricemic individuals with uric acid–lowering medications for a lifetime solely to prevent acute attacks of gouty arthritis. A large percentage of hyperuricemic patients may never experience an acute attack of gout.[136] If an attack should occur, it can be treated easily within 48 to 72 hours, and if the patient has at least two attacks in a year, ULT can then be considered.

The key issue in the treatment of hyperuricemia concerns the effect of uric acid on renal function. Renal disease was commonly associated with gout, and renal failure was believed to be the eventual cause of death in as many as 25% of gouty patients. Thus, treatment of asymptomatic hyperuricemia is justifiable if renal disease is prevented. However, this renal damage was noted to occur in a setting that included HTN, diabetes, renal vascular disease, glomerulonephritis, pyelonephritis, renal calculi, or some other cause of primary nephropathy independent of gout.[137] In fact, the coexistence of gout and renal insufficiency without HTN is so rare that its presence should raise the suspicion of chronic lead toxicity.[24,138] Therefore, the consensus now seems to be that hyperuricemia by itself has no deleterious effect on renal function.[139,140] Considering the financial costs, risks of adverse drug reactions, and practical considerations such as patient compliance, drug treatment of asymptomatic hyperuricemia is difficult to justify.[136] Although hyperuricemia may represent an important risk factor for the development of CHD,[18] the evidence is not sufficiently compelling to justify the treatment of asymptomatic hyperuricemia at this time.

KEY REFERENCES AND WEBSITES

A full list of references for this chapter can be found at **http://thepoint.lww.com/AT10e**. Below are the key references and websites for this chapter, with the corresponding reference number in this chapter found in parentheses after the reference.

Key References

Becker MA et al. Clinical efficacy and safety of successful longterm urate lowering with febuxostat or allopurinol in subjects with gout. *J Rheumatol.* 2009;36:1273. (113)

Becker MA et al. The urate-lowering efficacy and safety of febuxostat in the treatment of the hyperuricemia of gout: the CONFIRMS trial. *Arthritis Res Ther.* 2010;12:R63. (114)

Choi HK et al. Intake of purine-rich foods, protein, and dairy products and relationship to serum levels of uric acid: the Third National Health and Nutrition Examination Survey. *Arthritis Rheum.* 2005;52:283. (66)

Choi HK et al. Obesity, weight change, hypertension, diuretic use, and risk of gout in men: the health professionals follow-up study. *Arch Int Med.* 2005;165:742. (65)

Cronstein BN, Terkeltaub R. The inflammatory process of gout and its treatment. *Arthritis Res Ther.* 2006;8(Suppl 1):S3. (58)

Dalbeth N et al. Dose adjustment of allopurinol according to creatinine clearance does not provide adequate control of hyperuricemia in patients with gout. *J Rheumatol.* 2006;33:1646. (107)

Jordan KM et al. British Society for Rheumatology and British Health Professionals in Rheumatology guideline for the management of gout. *Rheumatology (Oxford).* 2007;46:1372. (38)

Rundles RW et al. Allopurinol in the treatment of gout. *Ann Intern Med.* 1966;64:229. (105)

Sundy JS et al. Reduction of plasma urate levels following treatment with multiple doses of pegloticase (polyethylene glycol-conjugated uricase) in patients with treatment-failure gout: results of a phase II randomized study. *Arthritis Rheum.* 2008;58:2882. (126)

Terkeltaub RA et al. High versus low dosing of oral colchicine for early acute gout flare: twenty-four-hour outcome of the first multicenter, randomized, double-blind, placebo-controlled, parallel-group, dose-comparison colchicine study. *Arthritis Rheum.* 2010;62:1060. (40)

Zhang W et al. EULAR evidence based recommendations for gout. Part 1: Diagnosis. Report of a task force of the standing committee for international clinical studies including therapeutics (ESCISIT). *Ann Rheum Dis.* 2006;65:1301. (11)

Zhang W et al. EULAR evidence based recommendations for gout. Part II: Management. Report of a task force of the EULAR standing committee for international clinical studies including therapeutics (ESCISIT). *Ann Rheum Dis.* 2006;65:1312. (39)

Key Websites

American College of Rheumatology. **http://www.rheumatology.org/.** Accessed March 29, 2011.

Gout and Uric Acid Education Society. **http://gouteducation.org/.** Accessed March 29, 2011.

MedlinePlus. **http://www.nlm.nih.gov/medlineplus/gout.html.** Accessed March 29, 2011.

National Health Service. National Institute for Health and Clinical Excellence. Febuxostat for the management of hyperuricaemia in people with gout. 2008. **http://www.nice.org.uk/nicemedia/live/12101/42738/42738.pdf.** Accessed October 30, 2010. (117)

46 Connective Tissue Disorders

Julie L. Olenak and Jonathan D. Ference

CORE PRINCIPLES

	Core Principle	CHAPTER CASES
1	Systemic lupus erythematosus (SLE) is an autoimmune disease that involves multiple organ systems and possible organ damage (i.e., musculoskeletal, skin, renal, pulmonary, cardiac, gastrointestinal, central nervous system, hematological).	**Case 46-1 (Question 1)**
2	Diagnosing SLE can be difficult because of early generalized symptoms and overlap with other connective tissue diseases. The diagnosis should be based on a combination of physical findings and serology testing.	**Case 46-1 (Question 1)**
3	SLE is commonly treated with antimalarials, nonsteroidal anti-inflammatory drugs, corticosteroids, and immunosuppressant medications. Pharmacotherapy should be selected based on individual cases considering the severity of symptoms, response to previous therapies, and extent of organ involvement.	**Case 46-1 (Question 2)**
4	Patients with SLE should have inactive disease for approximately 6 months before pregnancy. Disease flares are possible during pregnancy and can be treated with corticosteroids. Certain immunosuppressant medications (mycophenolate mofetil, cyclophosphamide, and methotrexate) are not recommended in pregnancy.	**Case 46-1 (Question 3)**
5	Drug-induced lupus is associated with several medications. The typical presentation involves musculoskeletal and constitutional symptoms. The patient will have a positive antinuclear antibody serology test.	**Case 46-2 (Question 1)**
6	Symptoms occurring with drug-induced lupus resolve after discontinuation of the offending drug and rarely require pharmacologic interventions to treat symptoms.	**Case 46-2 (Question 2)**
7	Ninety percent of patients who are affected by systemic sclerosis also have signs and symptoms consistent with Raynaud phenomenon.	**Case 46-3 (Questions 1, 2)**
8	Nifedipine, prazosin, and losartan may decrease severity and frequency of symptoms of Raynaud syndrome.	**Case 46-3 (Question 3)**
9	Many authorities believe polymyalgia rheumatica and temporal arteritis are manifestations of the same underlying process occurring at different times during the clinical course. However, they each have characteristic symptoms and are treated differently.	**Case 46-4 (Questions 1–3)**
10	Empiric antibiotic therapy does not reduce the risk of recurrence of Reiter syndrome and is not routinely recommended. Patients with documented *Chlamydia trachomatis* infection and their partners should be offered antibiotics.	**Case 46-5 (Question 1)**
11	Polymyositis and dermatomyositis should initially be treated with high-dose corticosteroids for several months. Methotrexate or azathioprine are recommended first-line immunosuppressive agents if the disease is not controlled with corticosteroids alone.	**Case 46-6 (Questions 1, 2)**

INTRODUCTION

Despite new knowledge in the immunology and the pathogenesis of the different connective tissue diseases (CTDs), the etiology of these conditions remains unclear.[1] Diagnosing CTDs can be difficult because of the complexity of the diseases and the varying presentation of symptoms. The patient's reported history of symptoms, results of the physical examination, and laboratory testing help guide the diagnosis of a CTD.[1] Diffuse CTDs include systemic lupus erythematosus (SLE), scleroderma, polymyositis, dermatomyositis, rheumatoid arthritis, and Sjögren syndrome. Patients may present with findings consistent with more than one CTD, and symptoms generally do not all appear simultaneously. Mixed CTD is an overlap of autoimmune disease features that can include myositis, scleroderma, and lupus.[1,2]

GENERAL SIGNS AND SYMPTOMS

Many patients can have arthralgias and arthritis as part of the inflammatory disease associated with their CTD, such as those patients with SLE. Inflammatory disease is suggested by morning stiffness of greater than 1 hour (a similar problem occurs with sitting or resting), swelling, fever, weakness, and systemic fatigue. In some patients, activities of daily living and function may be excellent despite pain and deformity; in others, because of psychologic and systemic disease, there may be poor function with minimal articular involvement. Other psychosocial aspects of their life, including sexuality, may be affected by many of the inflammatory disorders.

Dermatologic changes are often associated with a particular rheumatic disease. Examples include alopecia with SLE, onycholysis and keratoderma blennorrhagica with Reiter syndrome, buccal or genital ulcers with SLE or Reiter syndrome, Raynaud phenomenon with SLE or systemic sclerosis, calcinosis and rash over the knuckles (Gottron papule) with dermatomyositis, and sun sensitivity malar rash with SLE. The presence of nodules, tophi, telangiectasia, or vasculitic changes also may be detected, helping the clinician differentiate which inflammatory disease is present and what management is necessary.

The CTDs are commonly associated with musculoskeletal changes. Joints may display warmth, redness and effusion, synovial thickening, deformities, decreased range of motion, pain on motion, tenderness on palpation, and decreased function. Often, a patient's hand and arm function, as well as gait, may be altered. In addition to the signs and symptoms used to differentiate various rheumatic diseases, laboratory evaluation of patients with rheumatic complaints can often define the extent of disease or detect other organ systems that may be involved.

SELECTED CONNECTIVE TISSUE DISEASES

CTDs and rheumatic diseases encompass a wide range of disorders that are inflammatory in nature and related to the immune system. The following are some of the conditions that are encountered in clinical practice and will be discussed in this chapter: SLE, scleroderma, polymyalgia rheumatica, temporal arteritis, Reiter syndrome, polymyositis, and dermatomyositis.

LUPUS ERYTHEMATOSUS

SLE is a complex autoimmune disease that affects multiple organ systems. The word lupus was used as early as the tenth century but only to recognize the cutaneous lesions. Discoid lupus erythematosus is a form of lupus in which cutaneous lesions appear primarily on the face, ears, and scalp; it affects the skin only and spares the systemic organ involvement associated with SLE. These lesions are generally red, inflamed, raised, and round, and have an appearance of scaling. They can lead to permanent scarring and hair loss. Approximately 10% of patients with discoid lupus will develop SLE. It was not until 1954 that the term SLE was used to define this disease that had unique skin rashes but also internal systemic organ involvement. SLE can affect the cardiovascular, gastrointestinal, musculoskeletal, renal, pulmonary, vascular, and hematologic systems.[3,4]

ONLINE CONTENT

For an illustration of the organs affected by SLE, go to http://thepoint.lww.com/AT10e.

Epidemiology

The Lupus Foundation of America estimates that there are 1.5 million people in the United States with lupus. SLE occurs primarily in women ages 15 to 45,[5] and the female to male ratio is 9:1.[6] Fifteen to twenty percent of cases are diagnosed in childhood,[7] and half of all people are diagnosed by age 30. Lupus is two to three times more common in African American and Hispanic populations; those with Asian and Native American backgrounds are also at higher risk. The disease tends to be more severe in African American and Hispanic patients.[5] In the 1950s, SLE was considered a fatal disease with a 5-year survival rate of 50%; currently it has a 15-year survival rate of 80%.[8] Lupus patients are still at a fivefold increased risk of death.[7] The improved survival rates can be attributed to increased frequency of diagnosis detecting mild forms of the disease, earlier diagnosis, and treatment.[6] Although survival rates have improved, quality-of-life issues related to chronic disease symptoms and disease flares remain.

Pathophysiology

The complexity of the immune dysfunction that occurs in a patient with SLE continues to be studied to develop targeted therapies. It has been hypothesized that a combination of genetic and environmental factors leads to a scenario that allows the disease to spontaneously become active. The basis of the disease is autoantibody formation related to immunoglobulin G, which results in immune complexes and tissue damage. A dysfunction of the T cell, B cell, and signaling pathways contribute to autoimmunity and trigger an inflammatory reaction.

ONLINE CONTENT

For an animation that demonstrates the immune response, go to http://thepoint.lww.com/AT10e.

An increase in programmed cell death and decreased clearance of apoptotic cells are problematic.

Various factors have been associated with the development of lupus. Recent genome analysis identified genes that contribute to lupus, but they only explain 15% of the heritability. Studies of twins do reveal a certain extent of genetic susceptibility. In identical twins there is a 25% chance of developing SLE, whereas in fraternal twins, there is only a 2% chance of developing SLE.[8] It is reported that 4% to 5% of SLE patients have a family member with lupus, although it is more common (10%) to have a family member with a different autoimmune disease.[9] Additional factors have been identified that may contribute to the environment triggering autoimmunity. Ultraviolet (UV) light is known to exacerbate lupus, with 70% of patients experiencing a disease flare after significant exposure to UV light.[5] Some patients report the start of symptoms and the clinical presentation of their disease after a significant exposure to UV light, which may be caused by changes to the DNA in the dermal cells as well as increased cell death.[10] More recent information has shown that patients with lupus have an increased number of cells infected with the Epstein-Barr virus. The Epstein-Barr virus lives in and interacts with B cells, which may be a trigger for autoimmunity in patients with genetic predisposition.[5,6] Exposure to silica and pesticides as an occupational hazard, tobacco use, severe stress, and hormones have been shown to contribute to the development of SLE.[6,10]

Clinical Presentation

CASE 46-1

QUESTION 1: K.H. is a 22-year-old African American college student who presents to her primary-care physician, stating that "I'm just not feeling well." On further questioning she explains that she feels very tired, has significant pain in her body, has been running a fever, and has swollen lymph nodes that will not go down. She also reports that her face gets a red rash after she studies outside in the sun. K.H. has been experiencing these symptoms for 2 months, and they are only getting worse. She has not been able to maintain her normal activities. On physical examination, it is noted that there are several ulcers in her nose and mouth, and three of her joints are tender and inflamed. The examination is otherwise normal. The primary-care physician refers her to a rheumatologist whom K.H. sees 3 weeks later after having some blood work. The following are laboratory values from that visit:

Antinuclear antibodies (ANA), positive 1:640
Anti-Smith antibodies, positive
Anti–double-stranded DNA (dsDNA) antibodies, negative
Rheumatoid factor, negative
C3, 40 mg/dL (normal 72–156 mg/dL)
C4, 10 mg/dL (normal 20–50 mg/dL)
Anti-Ro/Sjögren syndrome A antibodies (anti-Ro/SSA), negative
Anti-La/Sjögren syndrome SSB antibodies (anti-La/SSB), negative
Anti-cardiolipin antibodies, negative
Lupus anticoagulant, negative
Erythrocyte sedimentation rate (ESR), 40 mm/hour
White blood cell (WBC) count, 3 × $10^3/\mu L$
Red blood cells (RBCs), 4 × $10^6/\mu L$
Platelets, 300 × $10^3/\mu L$
Serum creatinine (SCr), 0.8 mg/dL
Aspartate aminotransferase (AST), 20 units/L
Alanine aminotransferase (ALT), 15 units/L
Urinalysis, negative for WBC, RBC, and protein

What signs and symptoms are present in K.H. that support a diagnosis of SLE?

The multiple organ system involvement and generalized symptoms can make it difficult to diagnosis lupus. Many of the individual symptoms and components of SLE mimic other autoimmune diseases. It has been reported that patients on average see three physicians and go 4 years before being diagnosed.[11] Table 46-1 describes the signs and symptoms of SLE. The American College of Rheumatology (ACR) recommends consideration of SLE if a patient is experiencing symptoms in two or more organ systems.[3] Patients often present initially with symptoms such as fatigue, fever, lymphadenopathy, and arthralgia that may mimic the body's response to a virus. Although a classic sign of lupus is the malar butterfly rash, not all patients initially present with this rash or may develop cutaneous lesions later in the course of the disease.

TABLE 46-1
Signs and Symptoms of Systemic Lupus Erythematosus

Organ System	Sign
Cutaneous	Malar rash, discoid rash, mouth/nasal sores, Raynaud phenomenon, cutaneous vasculitis, alopecia
Musculoskeletal	Arthritis, arthralgia, myositis
Renal	Proteinuria, hematuria, red blood cell casts, nephrotic syndrome, elevated creatinine
Cardiopulmonary	Pericarditis, pleurisy, pleural effusions, pneumonitis, pulmonary emboli, pulmonary hypertension, myocardial infarction
Hematologic	Anemia, leukopenia, thrombocytopenia, antiphospholipid syndrome
Neurologic	Seizure, psychosis, stroke, transverse myelitis, peripheral neuropathy
Gastrointestinal	Esophageal dysmotility, intestinal vasculitis, nausea, abdominal pain
Constitutional	Fever, weight loss, lymphadenopathy

Source: [No authors listed]. Guidelines for referral and management of systemic lupus erythematosus in adults. American College of Rheumatology Ad Hoc Committee on Systemic Lupus Erythematosus Guidelines. *Arthritis Rheum*. 1999;42:1785.

For a photo of malar butterfly rash characteristic of SLE, go to http://thepoint.lww.com/AT10e.

The rash may last for a short time (a few days) or persist for weeks. The cutaneous manifestations are typically in response to UV light exposure. Musculoskeletal symptoms are present in 53% to 95% of patients with SLE.[12] The inflammatory arthritis present in SLE usually does not damage the joint as rheumatoid arthritis does. The ulcers or sores that can develop on mucous membranes are generally painless and are observed by the practitioner on physical examination. Renal involvement occurs in up to 70% of all patients and is a serious complication of SLE. Pleuritis is a common complication in SLE, with approximately half of all patients experiencing pleuritic pain.[12] Hematologic manifestations are common, with many patients experiencing anemia. Leukopenia usually does not become severe, but during a flare half of patients have a decreased WBC count as well as reduced platelets. Antiphospholipid syndrome may also occur in patients with SLE, leading to a hypercoagulable state. Nervous system involvement can range from cerebrovascular disease to altered cognitive function. The ACR has defined various symptoms and conditions that affect both the central and peripheral nervous systems as neuropsychiatric systemic lupus erythematosus. Gastrointestinal symptoms are generally limited to dyspepsia, abdominal pain, ulcers, nausea, and vomiting, which can also be linked to the pharmacologic treatment of lupus (i.e., nonsteroidal anti-inflammatory drugs [NSAIDs]). Gastrointestinal

TABLE 46-2
1997 Revised Criteria for Classification of Systemic Lupus Erythematosus

Criteria	Explanation[a]
Malar rash	Fixed erythema, flat or raised
Discoid rash	Erythematosus raised patches with adherent keratotic scaling and follicular plugging; atrophic scarring may occur in older lesions
Photosensitivity	Skin rash resulting from an unusual reaction to sunlight by patient history or observed by physician
Oral ulcers	Painless oral or nasopharyngeal ulcers observed by physician
Arthritis	Nonerosive arthritis involving two or more peripheral joints; characterized by tenderness, swelling, or effusion
Serositis	Evidence of pleuritis or pericarditis documented by ECG or rub heard by physician or evidence of pericardial effusion
Renal disorder	As manifested by persistent proteinuria (>0.5 g/d or >3+) or cellular casts
Neurologic disorder	Seizures or psychosis occurring without any other explanation
Hematologic disorder	Leukopenia (<4,000/μL), or hemolytic anemia, or lymphopenia (<1,500/μL), or thrombocytopenia (<100,000/μL)
Immunologic disorder	Anti-double stranded DNA antibody, or anti-Smith antibody, or antiphospholipid antibodies
Antinuclear antibody	An abnormal ANA titer in the absence of drugs known to be associated with drug-induced lupus

[a] The diagnosis of systemic lupus erythematosus is made when a patient has 4 or more of the 11 criteria at any time during the course of the disease with 95% specificity and 85% sensitivity.
ANA, antinuclear antibody; ECG, electrocardiogram.
Adapted with permission from Tan EM et al. The 1982 revised criteria for the classification of systemic lupus erythematosus. *Arthritis Rheum.* 1982;25:1271; Hochberg MC. Updating the American College of Rheumatology revised criteria for the classification of systemic lupus erythematosus [letter]. *Arthritis Rheum.* 1997;40:1725; [No authors listed]. Guidelines for Referral and Management of Systemic Lupus Erythematosus in Adults. American College of Rheumatology Ad Hoc Committee on Systemic Lupus Erythematosus Guidelines. *Arthritis Rheum.* 1999;42:1785.

symptoms should be evaluated to determine whether a more serious problem, such as abdominal vasculitis or peritonitis, is occurring.[12]

With multiple presenting symptoms and varied chronological onset, making a diagnosis of SLE can be difficult. The ACR created criteria for classification of SLE in 1971 and revised the criteria in 1982, with the most recent update published in 1997 specifically addressing the immunologic disorder section. The original intent of the criteria was to ensure that patients in clinical trials actually had lupus. The criteria are currently used to help in the evaluation of patients. The diagnosis of SLE is made when 4 of the 11 criteria presented in Table 46-2 are met.[13,14] The diagnosis is based on a combination of physical findings and serology testing. The ANAs indicate that an autoimmune process is occurring, but are not specific to lupus. Autoantibodies to dsDNA are 95% specific for lupus and are useful not only for diagnosis, but also to monitor disease activity. Anti-Smith antibodies are unique to lupus, but only 10% to 30% of SLE patients present with this serologic finding. They are most useful for diagnosis.[15] Additional antibodies (i.e., to U1 ribonucleoprotein [U1-RNP], Ro/SSA, and La/SSB) may be present, but are not included in the classification criteria owing to overlap with other conditions such as Raynaud phenomenon, neonatal lupus, and Sjögren syndrome.[3] Some patients may present with fewer than four of the required symptoms as listed in the criteria; they should be monitored closely and may be classified as having undifferentiated CTD.[2] A small percentage (10%–20%) of patients referred for evaluation of SLE are diagnosed with undifferentiated CTD; 10% to 15% will meet lupus diagnostic criteria 5 years later.[16]

K.H. meets the criteria for diagnosis of SLE, as she has 5 of the 11 criteria. Her physical symptoms include photoreactive rash, fatigue, and joint pain and swelling, and her examination revealed mucosal ulcers. The supporting laboratory findings are a high ANA, positive anti-Smith, and low WBC count. Other relevant laboratory findings include an elevated ESR showing increased inflammation in the body and low complement levels. Both markers indicate a current flare. The negative anti-dsDNA, normal SCr, and negative urinalysis for RBC and protein indicate she is not currently experiencing renal complications. K.H. also tested negative for antibodies (lupus anticoagulant and anticardiolipin) associated with antiphospholipid syndrome.

Overview of Treatment

Because there is no cure for SLE, therapy generally involves (a) controlling the acute symptoms of SLE and (b) providing maintenance therapy to prevent exacerbations and to keep clinical manifestations of SLE at acceptable levels. Appropriate therapy includes both nonpharmacologic and pharmacologic strategies. Nonpharmacologic treatment should be instituted when the diagnosis is made. Appropriate treatment includes the use of sunscreen, protective clothing (with sun protection factor [SPF]), avoiding UV light (including tanning beds), stress management strategies, and exercise.[17] Ice therapy can be used to relieve pain and swelling of joints. Patients with SLE are at high risk for cardiovascular disease; there is a 7- to 10-fold higher risk of nonfatal coronary heart disease, and the risk of fatal coronary heart disease is 17 times higher.[11] Smoking cessation, exercise, and weight loss should be recommended when appropriate. In addition, patients chronically using steroids should be encouraged to reach adequate intake of vitamin D and calcium through diet or supplements.

Pharmacological treatment of SLE can be selected based on mild, moderate, or severe disease activity. Current treatments include NSAIDs, antimalarials, corticosteroids, and immunosuppressant medications. Table 46-3 lists common dose ranges for these medications in the treatment of SLE. The mechanism of actions, side effects, and monitoring of these medications are covered extensively in other chapters (see Chapter 31, Chronic Kidney Diseases, Chapter 43, Osteoarthritis, and Chapter 44, Rheumatoid Arthritis), with the exception of belimumab. NSAIDs are used to help relieve pain and swelling associated with SLE (see Chapter 43, Osteoarthritis). Cardiovascular risk, renal toxicity, and gastrointestinal effects should be taken into consideration when recommending an NSAID.[7] Hydroxychloroquine is the primary antimalarial drug used and is preferred over chloroquine in the treatment of SLE owing to a safer side effect profile. Hydroxychloroquine can be used to help treat skin manifestations as well as constitutional symptoms.[7,17–19]

Corticosteroids can be used in oral, intravenous (IV), or topical formulations. When used orally, they primarily decrease disease activity and symptoms during initial diagnosis and exacerbation (i.e., flare). Steroids should generally be used for a short period considering the long-term side effects (i.e., decreased bone mineral density, decreased glucose tolerance, negative effects on the lipid profile, weight gain, hypertension, and cataracts). IV pulse therapy with methylprednisolone, given for 3 days, is used

TABLE 46-3
Common Doses of Medications in Treatment of Systemic Lupus Erythematosus

Medication	Dose
Hydroxychloroquine[a,b]	200–400 mg orally divided twice daily
Prednisone (or equivalent)[c,d]	0.125–2 mg/kg orally once daily or divided twice daily if high dose
Mycophenolate mofetil[a,b,d]	1–3 g orally divided twice daily
Azathioprine[d]	1–3 mg/kg once or twice daily
Cyclophosphamide[b,d]	IV: 0.5–1 g/m^2 monthly for initial dose plus 6 months then quarterly for 1 year once remission achieved Oral: 1–2 mg/kg/d
Belimumab[a]	10 mg/kg IV every 2 weeks for the first three doses and then monthly
Methotrexate[a,d]	5–15 mg orally as a single weekly dose or as three divided doses per week every 12 hours (i.e., 2.5 mg × three doses 12 hours apart)

IV, intravenous.
[a] Facts and Comparison database online. **http://online.factsandcomparisons.com/.** Accessed June 15, 2011
[b] Lexi-comp database online. **http://www.crlonline.com/crlsql/servlet/crlonline.** Accessed June 15, 2011.
[c] Kirou K et al. Systemic Glucocorticoid Thaerapy in Systemic Lupus Erythematosus. In: Wallace D, Hahn BH, eds. *Dubois' Lupus Erythematosus.* 7th ed. Philadelphia, PA: Lippincott Williams & Wilkins; 2007:1181.
[d] Tassiulas I, Boumpas D. Clinical features and treatment of systemic lupus erythematosus. In: Firestein G et al, eds. *Kelley's Textbook of Rheumatology.* 8th ed. Philadelphia, PA: Saunders Elsevier; 2009:1263.

in lupus nephritis and other severe disease flares not responding to oral steroids. Pulse therapy is generally not given more frequently than monthly. Topical steroid creams or steroids used intralesionally are used primarily in discoid lupus to help treat dermatological lesions.

Several immunosuppressants are available including mycophenolate mofetil, cyclosporine, belimumab, methotrexate, azathioprine, and cyclophosphamide. Immunosuppressants are indicated if disease symptoms are severe, organ damage is occurring, or symptoms are not responding to other therapies.[7,12] Mycophenolate mofetil has gained popularity in recent years as a treatment for renal disease related to lupus because of positive study results in efficacy and side effect profile. It has also been used in patients with nonrenal disease including refractory cases, patients unable to decrease high-dose steroids, and those with severe hematological manifestations.[7,12,17] Cyclosporine is not commonly used, and methotrexate is generally used for resistant arthritis. Azathioprine has been used for moderate disease activity and is thought to be steroid sparing. Some patients are poor metabolizers, owing to thiopurine methyltransferase enzyme deficiency, and are at risk for increased toxicities (i.e., myelosuppression and hematologic). Cyclophosphamide can be used in oral or IV formulation, most commonly in combination with steroids for induction therapy for lupus nephritis.

The newest medication, belimumab, was approved in 2011 and is the first medication in a half a century to be US Food and Drug Administration approved for the treatment of lupus. Belimumab is a human monoclonal antibody and has a unique mechanism of action. It is a B-lymphocyte stimulator (BLyS) specific inhibitor. Belimumab binds to B-lymphocyte stimulator (BLyS), a protein that is responsible for binding to B cells to cause proliferation and differentiation of B lymphocytes, thus decreasing the survival of B cells including those making autoantibodies.[20–22] In clinical trials, belimumab was not studied in patients with severe lupus nephritis, active central nervous system disease, or in combination with cyclophosphamide or other biologicals. It is indicated to treat patients with active disease, who are auto-antibody positive, and already receiving treatment for SLE. Concomitant medications during clinical trials, including mycophenolate, azathioprine, methotrexate, antimalarials, NSAIDs, aspirin, and steroids, did not demonstrate clinically significant interactions with belimumab. There are several warnings associated with the use of belimumab, including increased mortality, risk of serious infections, hypersensitivity reactions, and depression and suicide.[22]

Patients on immunosuppressive drug therapy should receive both the influenza and pneumococcal vaccines if no contraindications are present. Infections account for 20% to 40% of deaths in SLE patients.[16] The influenza vaccine is now recommended in all people 6 months of age and older. It should be offered to patients with SLE in the injectable form and not the intranasal formulation, which is a live vaccine. The pneumococcal polysaccharide vaccine is administered twice in a lifetime. It should be readministered 5 years after the initial vaccination if a patient is immunocompromised and received the vaccine before 65 years of age. Patients should keep up to date with other routine vaccinations (i.e., tetanus and diphtheria, or tetanus, diphtheria, and pertussis); having lupus is not a contraindication to any vaccine.[23] However, live vaccines (i.e., herpes zoster, intranasal influenza, varicella) should be avoided in patients who are on immunosuppressant drug therapy or are taking greater than 20 mg of prednisone or equivalent for more than 2 weeks.[24,25]

CASE 46-1, QUESTION 2: What treatment options are appropriate for K.H. to control her current symptoms associated with SLE?

Because K.H. is experiencing primarily musculoskeletal, dermatological, and constitutional symptoms it would be appropriate to start an antimalarial and an NSAID and to consider steroids to help provide initial control over her SLE. Hydroxychloroquine 200 mg twice daily should be initiated. It will take several weeks to see improvement and months to see full efficacy. An ophthalmologic examination is recommended at baseline and periodically thereafter. The risk of retinopathy is low, but patients who are taking more than 6.5 mg/kg and receiving treatment for more than 5 years are at increased risk.[25] Various recommendations exist for follow-up screening intervals. The American Academy of Ophthalmology recommends patients at low risk for retinopathy who have a normal baseline examination be checked again in 5 years. The high-risk group (long-term treatment for more than 5 years, high doses, altered liver or kidney function, existing retinal disease, and older than 60 years of age) should have a yearly examination.[26] The manufacturer recommends that with long-term treatment an ophthalmologic examination should be performed every 3 months.[27] With varying recommendations, patients should work with their ophthalmologist to determine the appropriate screening interval based on patient-specific factors. Any NSAID would be appropriate to treat the musculoskeletal complaints.

Because K.H. is experiencing difficulty maintaining daily activities and her laboratory results indicate active disease, a short burst of corticosteroids should be recommended. A low-dose steroid such as prednisone 10 mg once daily in the morning can help control her disease activity. There is an increased risk of infection when corticosteroids are combined with immunosuppressive drugs; therefore, typically lower doses are used. Long-term intermittent use of steroids is sometimes required for patients experiencing organ damage or severe disease; however, the goal is to use corticosteroids for short periods. Corticosteroids are discussed further in Chapter 44, Rheumatoid Arthritis. Immunosuppressants would not be indicated for K.H. at this time. If her disease were to progress or be refractory, azathioprine or mycophenolate mofetil would likely be the next choice.

The follow-up period for patients with SLE is determined by severity of the disease and medications used. Patients with mild or controlled SLE typically should be followed every 3 to 6 months. The following laboratory measurements are recommended: complete blood count, platelet count, SCr, urinalysis, complement levels, ESR, and anti-dsDNA. Patients with renal damage should have additional tests, including 24-hour urine collection specimen for protein, cholesterol, calcium, phosphorus, alkaline phosphatase, sodium, and potassium. Patients with organ-threatening, severe, or refractory disease should be seen more often as determined by their rheumatologist. Use of immunosuppressants would also require more frequent laboratory monitoring.[3]

Additional education to be provided to K.H. would include avoidance of UV light, use of sunscreen, stress-management strategies, and appropriate intake of calcium and vitamin D.

CASE 46-1, QUESTION 3: K.H. returns for her follow-up visit 1 month later. She completed her 2 weeks of steroid therapy and is on celecoxib 200 mg daily and hydroxychloroquine 200 mg twice daily. She shares with you that she is getting married and is concerned because she heard that some of the medications used for lupus can affect fertility. What information can be provided to K.H. regarding fertility, pregnancy, and oral contraceptives?

K.H. is currently not receiving any medication that would affect her fertility. The primary medication associated with premature ovarian failure is cyclophosphamide. This treatment is primarily used in lupus nephritis and severe refractory disease. SLE does not alter fertility although it is associated with a higher miscarriage rate and low-birth-weight infants. Pregnancy may also induce mild to moderate disease flares.[12] Because K.H. has been recently diagnosed and is not in remission, it is recommended that her disease be inactive for 6 months before trying to conceive. Some medications have been used in pregnancy, such as hydroxychloroquine and steroids. Mycophenolate, cyclophosphamide, and methotrexate are not recommended in pregnancy.[7,11,17,28] Barrier (i.e., condoms) or hormonal (oral contraceptives) methods can be used to prevent pregnancy. Some practitioners have avoided estrogen-based contraceptives in patients with SLE. It has been shown that patients with stable SLE who took oral contraceptives for 1 year had similar disease activity to those who did not.[29,30] Hormone-replacement therapy has been associated with an increase in mild to moderate disease activity.[31] Caution should be used in patients who have previously had a clot or have antiphospholipid antibodies as they are at increased risk of thrombotic events. Oral contraceptives can be considered in K.H. because she does not have antiphospholipid antibody syndrome and has mild disease activity.

Drug-Induced Lupus

CASE 46-2

QUESTION 1: S.O. is a 60-year-old white man who has a past medical history of hypertension and diabetes. His current medications include lisinopril 20 mg once daily, metoprolol succinate 100 mg once daily, metformin 1,000 mg twice daily, aspirin 81 mg once daily, and hydralazine 50 mg four times daily, which was added 3 months ago. He presents to his primary-care provider with complaints of new onset of fatigue and joint pain, stating that he has not been feeling like himself. He reports that these symptoms are bothersome, but are not interfering with his normal activities. His laboratory results are normal with the exception of his ANA, which is positive 1:320. He tested negative for all other rheumatology tests, including anti-dsDNA, anti-Smith, and rheumatoid factor. What is the likely cause of S.O.'s elevated ANA and symptoms?

TABLE 46-4
Medications Associated With Drug-Induced Lupus

Risk	Medications
High	Procainamide, hydralazine, and tumor necrosis factor-α blockers
Moderate	Quinidine
Low	Methyldopa, captopril, enalapril, acebutolol, chlorpromazine, isoniazid, minocycline, carbamazepine, propylthiouracil, interferon-α, D-penicillamine, and sulfasalazine

Source: Tassiulas I, Boumpas D. Clinical features and treatment of systemic lupus erythematosus. In: Firestein G et al, eds. *Kelley's Textbook of Rheumatology*. 8th ed. Philadelphia, PA: Saunders Elsevier; 2009:1263; Rubin R. Drug-induced lupus. In: Wallace D, Hahn BH, eds. *Dubois' Lupus Erythematosus*. 7th ed. Philadelphia, PA: Lippincott Williams & Wilkins; 2007:870.

Many medications have been associated with drug-induced lupus. Table 46-4 highlights the drugs with the greatest propensity to cause drug-induced lupus. Hydralazine (as with S.O.) and procainamide have been most commonly implicated, with an incidence of 5% to 8% and 20%, respectively. Drug-induced lupus occurs when a patient develops autoantibodies and presents with symptoms similar to lupus. This is different than drug-induced autoimmunity, which occurs if antibodies are present but the patient does not clinically exhibit symptoms. The symptoms of drug-induced lupus are usually musculoskeletal (i.e., arthralgias and myalgias) and constitutional (i.e., fatigue and fever). Pleuropericarditis has been reported with procainamide. Symptoms generally do not include multiorgan systems, and the kidneys, skin, and central nervous system are spared. The symptom onset is slow with patients being on treatment for a least a month. The risk of developing drug-induced lupus increases with longer treatment durations and higher doses. The patient may have a positive ANA, but will rarely test positive for the lupus-specific antibodies. Unlike in SLE, with drug-induced lupus there is more of a balance in sex and less occurrence in certain ethnic groups (i.e., African American patients).[15,32]

CASE 46-2, QUESTION 2: What pharmacological treatments could be recommended for S.O.?

Hydralazine should be discontinued in S.O. and alternative therapy instituted for his hypertension, if needed. The symptoms associated with drug-induced lupus usually resolve within days to weeks after stopping the offending drug, but he may continue to test positive for autoantibodies for months. NSAIDs can be used to help if severe symptoms or manifestations are present. Because S.O. has hypertension, his blood pressure should be closely monitored with NSAID treatment. However, if S.O. is not experiencing bothersome symptoms, treatment is not needed. More rigorous treatment with medications used for moderate to severe lupus is not indicated in drug-induced lupus. It is not advisable to rechallenge with the drug, especially when alternatives are available.[15]

SYSTEMIC SCLEROSIS (SCLERODERMA)

Systemic sclerosis, or systemic scleroderma, is a CTD associated with autoimmunity characterized by excessive extracellular matrix deposition and vascular injury to the skin and other visceral organs.[33] Systemic sclerosis can be classified into distinct clinical subsets based on the patterns of skin and internal organ involvement, autoantibody production, and patient survival.[33] The most common subsets include limited cutaneous (approximately 60% of patients) and diffuse cutaneous (approximately 35% of patients).[33] The term overlap syndrome may be applied to patients when features common in one or more of the other CTDs are present. The limited cutaneous subset is diagnosed when skin thickening is limited to the areas distal to the elbows and knees. A constellation of dysfunctions known as CREST (calcinosis cutis, Raynaud phenomenon, esophageal dysfunction, sclerodactyly, telangiectasia) syndrome is a subtype of limited cutaneous systemic sclerosis.[33]

For a photo of sclerodactyly in CREST syndrome, go to http://thepoint.lww.com/AT10e.

More women than men suffer from systemic sclerosis (female to male ratio 4.6:1), although the mean age at diagnosis does not differ between men and women.[34] Onset of systemic sclerosis generally begins in adults between 30 and 50 years of age and is rare in children and seniors older than 80 years of age.[35] The prevalence is estimated at 276 cases per million adults in the United States.[34] African American patients are twice as likely as non–African American patients to have diffuse disease.[34] Likely and possible risk factors for the disease include environmental exposure to silica dust (e.g., coal miners) and the presence of a connective-tissue growth factor polymorphism, respectively.[36] At this time there is no conclusive evidence to support an association between silicone breast implants and systemic sclerosis, or any other CTD.[36]

The underlying pathophysiologic changes that lead to systemic scleroderma remain unknown, but many believe that it results from a lymphocyte-mediated autoimmune reaction with endothelial cells, activated immune cells, and fibroblasts playing a key role in the process. It is hypothesized that the process is initiated by an immune attack on the endothelium leading to endothelial cell activation or injury. This is followed by activation of the fibroblasts, resulting in subendothelial connective tissue proliferation, narrowing of the vascular lumen, and Raynaud phenomenon. T cells are then selectively activated and populate the affected areas such as the dermis and lung tissue. These cells produce cytokines that stimulate resident fibroblasts to produce excessive amounts of procollagen, which is then converted extracellularly to mature collagen. Later, when the inflammatory process subsides, the fibroblasts revert back to normal. Complications of systemic scleroderma include, but are not limited to, poor wound healing, arrhythmia, heart failure, renal failure, lung tissue destruction, and esophageal strictures.[36]

CASE 46-3

QUESTION 1: T.P., a 48-year-old African American woman with known limited cutaneous scleroderma, presents to your outpatient clinic complaining of pain and discoloration of the fingers on both hands. She describes discoloration as an intermittent loss of color from normal to a pale appearance, and the pain as intermittent numbness and tingling accompanying the loss of color. T.P. states the symptoms only appear when she is exposed to a cold environment. These symptoms are interfering with her quality of life and activities of daily living. In terms of other symptoms, T.P. also experiences intermittent development of thickened, pitted, rough skin patches located distal to her elbows bilaterally. She has no other significant past medical history, nor takes any medications on a regular basis. The physical examination findings revealed patches of skin thickening and nonpitting induration on upper torso. Telangiectasias are also noted in this area. Laboratory samples drawn last week show her ANA is negative and the basic metabolic panel, complete blood count, and liver function tests are all normal. What subjective and objective data present in T.P.'s case are consistent with limited cutaneous scleroderma?

T.P. is complaining of classic symptoms of Raynaud syndrome, which is a common clinical feature of limited cutaneous scleroderma. In addition, skin fibrosis that is present distal to the elbow or knees and telangiectasias are suggestive of limited cutaneous scleroderma as opposed to diffuse cutaneous scleroderma. Because ANAs may be present in unaffected patients and absent in afflicted patients, ANA test results must be interpreted within the clinical context and should not be relied on as a sole diagnostic marker.[37]

CASE 46-3, QUESTION 2: Based on these signs and symptoms, which variant(s) of limited cutaneous scleroderma is likely present?

Ninety percent of patients who are affected by systemic sclerosis also have signs and symptoms consistent with Raynaud phenomenon, as is seen with T.P. Patients will typically complain of recurrent, intermittent vasospastic episodes resulting in a color change in the fingers or toes after being exposed to

TABLE 46-5
Common Clinical Features of Systemic Sclerosis

Subset	Skin Fibrosis	Lung Involvement	Visceral Organ Involvement	Physical Examination Findings
Limited cutaneous	Areas distal to the elbows and knees[a]	Pulmonary arterial hypertension	Severe GERD and Raynaud phenomenon	Telangiectasia, calcinosis cutis, sclerodactyly, digital ischemic complications
Diffuse cutaneous	Areas proximal or distal to the elbows and knees[a]	Interstitial lung disease	Scleroderma renal crisis	Tendon friction rubs, pigment changes

[a] May affect the face.
GERD, gastroesophageal reflux disease.
Adapted with permission from Hinchcliff M, Varga J. Systemic sclerosis/scleroderma: a treatable multisystem disease. *Am Fam Physician*. 2008;78:961.

cold temperatures. Vasoconstriction may lead to local cyanosis and accompanying pain and numbness, with flushing noted on rewarming. Other parts of the body may also be affected, such as the nose, ears, tongue, and nipples.

Common clinical features can be used to distinguish between limited and diffuse cutaneous systemic sclerosis subsets (Table 46-5).[33] In addition, variants of the condition may exist within each subset based on the presence of other symptoms. Manifestations of systemic sclerosis differ based on the organ system(s) involved (Table 46-6).[33] Other disorders that may have similar clinical characteristics, such as amyloidosis and mixed CTD, should be considered and ruled out before the diagnosis of systemic sclerosis. The ACR preliminary criteria for the diagnosis of systemic sclerosis requires the presence of one lone major criterion (proximal scleroderma) or two minor criteria (sclerodactyly, digital pitting scars or a loss of substance from finger pads, or bibasilar pulmonary fibrosis).[38] Skin biopsy is recommended to confirm scleroderma if the clinical picture is unclear. The overall course of systemic sclerosis is highly variable and unpredictable. However, after a remission occurs, relapse is uncommon.

CASE 46-3, QUESTION 3: At this time, which therapeutic agent(s) is recommended to treat T.P.'s manifestations and symptoms of systemic sclerosis?

There is not a specific therapy for systemic sclerosis. Rather treatment is mainly supportive and symptomatic in nature, targeting the specific organ(s) affected (Table 46-7).[39] Therefore, the primary goals of therapy are to improve quality of life and minimize the risk of complications. Based on T.P.'s current symptoms, initiating therapy with the dihydropyridine calcium-channel blocker nifedipine is an appropriate option to achieve symptom control. Compared with placebo, nifedipine and prazosin modestly reduced the severity and frequency of Raynaud ischemic attacks.[40,41] However, when losartan was compared with low-dose nifedipine in a nonblinded, randomized, controlled trial (RCT), losartan users experienced a decrease in severity and frequency of Raynaud symptoms in a 12-week period.[42] This should not be considered as definitive evidence that losartan is superior as the lack of blinding may have resulted in an overestimation of losartan's benefit. Bosentan (which is restricted in the United States and approved for the treatment of symptomatic pulmonary hypertension) has been shown to decrease the occurrence of digital ulcers caused by Raynaud phenomenon.[43] Early treatment with an angiotensin-converting enzyme inhibitor may improve prognosis in scleroderma renal crisis.[44,45] The effects of cyclophosphamide, an antineoplastic agent, demonstrated in clinical trials are conflicting. In an RCT comparing cyclophosphamide with placebo in patients with scleroderma lung disease, use of this agent modestly reduced dyspnea and disability while improving lung function.[46] However, a meta-analysis of three RCTs and six cohort studies concluded that cyclophosphamide does not result in significant clinical improvement of pulmonary function.[47] Because this is a potentially toxic drug, patients who take it require close monitoring.

TABLE 46-6
Manifestations of Systemic Sclerosis

Organ System	Manifestations
Cardiovascular	Abnormal cardiac conduction, congestive heart failure, pericardial effusion, digital ischemic changes, Raynaud phenomenon
Gastrointestinal	Barrett esophagitis or strictures, gastroesophageal reflux disease, dysphagia, halitosis, chronic cough, dental erosions
Genitourinary	Sexual dysfunction, dyspareunia, impotence
Musculoskeletal	Flexion contractures, muscle atrophy, puffy hands, inability to make a tight fist, weakness
Pulmonary	Interstitial lung disease, pulmonary arterial hypertension, basilar and course crackles, dyspnea on exertion
Renal	Renal crisis
Skin	Calcinosis, pruritus, thickened skin, tight skin, excoriations, scabbing, loss of pigmentation

Adapted with permission from Hinchcliff M, Varga J. Systemic sclerosis/scleroderma: a treatable multisystem disease. *Am Fam Physician*. 2008;78:961.

TABLE 46-7
Treatment Options for Manifestations of Systemic Sclerosis

Manifestation	Treatment Options
Raynaud phenomenon	Nifedipine, verapamil, losartan, prazosin, iloprost
Pulmonary hypertension	Bosentan, sildenafil, enalapril, iloprost
Interstitial lung disease	Cyclophosphamide, prednisone
Renal crisis	Angiotensin converting enzyme inhibitors, dialysis or kidney transplant
Skin fibrosis	Methotrexate, cyclosporine, D-penicillamine
Arthralgias	Acetaminophen and NSAIDs
GERD	Proton pump inhibitors, H2 antagonists, prokinetic agents
Pruritus	Antihistamines, low-dose topical steroids

GERD, gastroesophageal reflux disease; NSAID, nonsteroidal anti-inflammatory drug; H2, Type 2 histamine receptor.
Adapted with permission from Usatine RP, Diaz L. Scleroderma (progressive systemic sclerosis). Ebell MH et al. database online. October 15, 2009. John Wiley & Sons. Accessed March 18, 2011.

POLYMYALGIA RHEUMATICA AND TEMPORAL ARTERITIS (GIANT CELL ARTERITIS)

Polymyalgia rheumatica (PMR) and temporal arteritis, also known as giant cell arteritis (GCA), are closely related clinical syndromes that usually affect the elderly and frequently occur together. Many authorities believe them to be different phases of the same underlying disease process. About 50% of persons with GCA also have PMR, and 10% of those with PMR also have GCA.[48] PMR is characterized by aching and morning stiffness in the cervical region and shoulder and pelvic girdles.[49] Inflammation as a result of GCA most commonly involves the temporal artery, but arteries in other parts of the body can also be affected.[48]

The incidence of PMR and GCA increases in patients after the age of 50 and peaks in those 70 to 80 years of age.[49] GCA is the most common vasculitis among the elderly and can lead to blindness if not diagnosed and treated in a timely manner. Likewise, without treatment PMR can lead to significant morbidity and disability. Patients with PMR are also at an increased risk of peripheral arterial disease. The primary risk factor for both conditions is age, and both occur more frequently in women than in men. PMR is seen mainly in people of north European ancestry and generally affects whites more commonly than African Americans, Hispanics, Asians, and Native Americans.[50] The incidence of PMR is 5.9/10,000 patients/year in the United States, with an overall prevalence in the United States of about 740 per 100,000: 532 for men and 925 for women.[51] The incidence of GCA is 0.17

new cases annually per 1,000 persons older than 50 years of age with a prevalence of 2 per 1,000 persons.[52]

Although the exact pathogeneses of PMR and GCA are yet to be determined, they are both thought to arise from an autoimmune or inflammatory dysfunction involving similar cellular immune responses from T cells, antigen-presenting cells, macrophage-derived inflammatory cytokines, genetic human leukocyte antigen molecules, and macrophages. A viral cause has been suspected but not confirmed for both PMR and GCA, and some studies demonstrate a cyclical pattern in PMR incidence pointing to environmental infectious triggers (e.g., parvovirus B19, *Mycoplasma pneumoniae,* and *Chlamydia pneumoniae*) as potential causes.[49,53] Branches of the internal and external carotid arteries are most commonly affected in those with GCA, and biopsies often reveal inflammatory changes that lead to a narrowing or occlusion of the vessel and ischemia distal to the lesion.[48] Systemic inflammation is the most prominent feature in PMR, but inflammation of the blood vessels is often clinically undetectable.[48]

TABLE 46-8

Common Findings Associated With Polymyalgia Rheumatica and Giant Cell Arteritis

Polymyalgia Rheumatica	Giant Cell Arteritis
Age ≥50 years	Age ≥50 years
ESR >50 mm/h	ESR >50 mm/h
Anemia (mild, normochromic, normocytic)	Anemia
Aching, pain, and morning stiffness in the shoulders and upper arms, hips and thighs, or neck and torso	Headache: temporal with temporal artery involvement, or occipital with occipital artery involvement
Symptoms of systemic inflammation	Visual symptoms or jaw claudication
	Fever, weight loss, depression, fatigue
	Arthralgias

ESR, erythrocyte sedimentation rate.
Adapted with permission from Unwin B et al. Polymyalgia rheumatica and giant cell arteritis. *Am Fam Physician*. 2006;74:1547.

CASE 46-4

QUESTION 1: D.C. is an 80-year old white man presenting to the emergency department complaining of new-onset morning aching pain and stiffness in his shoulders and upper arms. He states his symptoms developed 3 weeks ago and have progressed to the point where his pain and limited range of motion are keeping him from performing activities of daily living. D.C. denies headaches or vision disturbances, but is complaining of overall malaise, fatigue, and anorexia. He has a past medical history significant for hyperlipidemia, type 2 diabetes mellitus, and hypertension. He has been taking his current medications for the past 2 years, which are adequately controlling his hyperlipidemia, diabetes, and hypertension. His current medications include simvastatin 40 mg daily, metformin 1,000 mg twice daily, lisinopril/hydrochlorothiazide 40/25 mg daily, and aspirin 81 mg daily. His physical examination was negative for decreased muscle strength. Limited range of shoulder and upper arm motion is noted along with tenderness of these areas on palpation. Routine baseline laboratory values are within normal limits, with an ESR of 75 mm/hour. D.C. was admitted to a general medical ward with a diagnosis of PMR and was started on prednisone. What signs and symptoms present in this case differentiate PMR from GCA?

No conclusive laboratory test for PMR or GCA exists, and nonspecific clinical features and the absence of physical signs often complicate diagnosis. Distinguishing between the two disorders is of importance, as GCA can lead to blindness and requires higher doses of treatment medications. The typical onset of PMR is acute in nature. However, as is the case with D.C., most who present for a medical evaluation describe their symptoms as occurring for 1 month or longer.[48] D.C. is also exhibiting common complaints associated with PMR, which include aching pain and morning stiffness in the shoulders and upper arms, hips and thighs, or neck and torso. New-onset GCA often manifests as a new headache or a headache that is described as different from previous headaches and has been occurring for 2 to 3 months. The absence of headache in D.C. further supports the diagnosis of PMR. Common findings associated with both conditions are presented in Table 46-8.[48] The most useful laboratory test for diagnosing PMR is the ESR. Patients with GCA usually have an ESR greater than 40 to 50 mm/hour; rates of greater than 100 mm/hour are common.[48] A normal ESR is very helpful in ruling out GCA in corticosteroid-naïve patients; however, an elevated ESR (>100 mm/hour) is only minimally helpful in ruling in GCA.[54] The presence of three or more of the following criteria are 93% sensitive and 91% specific for GCA: age of onset of disease greater than or equal to 50 years, new headache, temporal artery abnormality, ESR greater than or equal to 50 mm/hour, or abnormal findings on biopsy of the temporal artery.[55]

CASE 46-4, QUESTION 2: What other inflammatory conditions should be considered and excluded before making the diagnosis of PMR or GCA in D.C.?

Other inflammatory or autoimmune disorders, such as fibromyalgia, myalgias from statin therapy, osteoarthritis, polymyositis, and rheumatoid arthritis, should be considered and excluded before the diagnosis of PMR or GCA.[48]

CASE 46-4, QUESTION 3: What is the preferred initial treatment approach for PMR in D.C.? Explain the difference(s) in this approach as compared with those for GCA.

Owing to its anti-inflammatory properties, prednisone is considered first-line therapy for either PMR or GCA. Initiation of treatment should not be delayed pending temporal artery biopsy results if CGA is suspected. Beginning low-dose prednisone (10 to 20 mg/day) may improve D.C.'s PMR symptoms within days, but some optimal results could take several weeks to achieve.[56] Attempts to taper the dose to avoid long-term adverse drug events (e.g., osteoporosis, hypothalamus-pituitary-adrenal axis suppression) should be made once acute relief has been achieved. Tapering the dose (e.g., 1 mg/day per week) should be individualized and based on symptom response as it may take years owing to symptom flares. The Polymyalgia Rheumatica Activity Scale, a disease activity assessment, may be used to monitor and adjust therapy and patient response.[48]

As opposed to PMR, treatment for GCA should begin with high-dose prednisone (40 to 60 mg/day); IV treatment (e.g., methylprednisolone) for 3 days should be considered in patients exhibiting visual symptoms.[48] Oral therapy should be continued until symptoms resolve and ESR returns to normal (usually 2–6 weeks), then begin a slow taper (reduction of 2.5 to 5 mg/day every 2 weeks until 25 mg/day is reached, then even more slowly afterward). Most will achieve a dose of 7.5 to 10 mg/day after 6 months of therapy, but relapses are common and are managed by restarting steroid therapy or increasing the dose to previous beneficial amounts.[49] The use of low-dose aspirin may reduce the incidence of cranial ischemic complications.

The use of methotrexate as adjuvant therapy for PMR and GCA is not routinely recommended, and its evidence of symptom relief benefit is conflicting.[48] However, a single RCT demonstrated that the use of methotrexate 10 mg once weekly in addition to prednisone in those with GCA resulted in an overall decrease in the amount of prednisone required and in relapse rates.[57] All patients on long-term corticosteroids should be offered calcium (1,200 mg/day) and vitamin D (800 international units/day) for prevention of osteoporosis and be monitored for other complications of steroid therapy.

REITER SYNDROME

Reiter syndrome is a form of reactive arthritis defined as peripheral arthritis often accompanied by one or more extra-articular manifestations that appear after certain infections of the genitourinary or gastrointestinal tracts. The "classic Reiter triad" consists of arthritis, urethritis, and conjunctivitis. The clinical course of Reiter syndrome is variable and usually runs a self-limited course of 3 to 12 months.[58] Mortality from reactive arthritis is not common and results from cardiac complications such as aortitis. Approximately 10% to 20% of patients may continue to have chronic, destructive and disabling arthritis or enthesitis (inflammation of the sites where tendons or ligaments insert into bone) 2 years after the onset of symptoms. Ten to fifteen percent may progress to ankylosing spondylitis.[59]

The annual incidence is 4.6/100,000/year for *Chlamydia*-induced arthritis and 5/100,000/year for *Enterobacteriaceae*-induced reactive arthritis.[60,61] Reiter syndrome most frequently occurs in patients in their fourth or fifth decade of life, but it can occur at any age.[62,63] In general, Reiter syndrome occurs more frequently in men than in women. Reiter syndrome that occurs as a result of exposure to a venereal disease is seen in more men than women.[61] The form that develops after bowel infection (dysentery) occurs in equal frequency in men and women.[64]

Reiter syndrome is considered a sterile inflammatory response to a remote infection. Reactive arthritis usually occurs after an infection in a genetically susceptible person. Genetics may play a role in pathogenesis; more than two-thirds of patients are surface antigen HLA-B27 positive, which presents antigenic peptides to T cells.[59] Reiter syndrome is strongly associated with ankylosing spondylitis.

Onset of symptoms typically occurs 1 to 3 weeks later and may present in an insidious or acute manner. Patients usually present with a chief complaint of mucocutaneous lesions, joint stiffness, myalgia, and low back pain that is worse with rest.[65] Table 46-9 describes the clinical manifestations of Reiter syndrome.[59] It may present as arthritic in nature or as dysfunctions of the ocular, skin, genitourinary, or cardiac systems.[59] Urethritis, mild dysuria, and a mucopurulent urethra are the most common symptoms that occur in men. Women may have dysuria, vaginal discharge, and purulent cervicitis or vaginitis. Arthritic complaints are usually asymmetrical, involving the lower extremities, and are associated with the appearance of a "sausage finger" digit.[59]

TABLE 46-9
Clinical Manifestations of Reiter Syndrome

Manifestation Type	Manifestations
Arthritic	Asymmetric, lower extremities, enthesitis, sacroiliitis
Cardiac	Aortitis, aortic insufficiency, heart block
Genitourinary	Nonspecific urethritis, cervicitis, cystitis
Ocular	Conjunctivitis, acute anterior uveitis
Skin	Keratoderma, balanitis circinata, tongue ulcerations

Adapted with permission from Barth WF, Segal K. Reactive arthritis (Reiter's syndrome). *Am Fam Physician*. 1999;60:499.

CASE 46-5

QUESTION 1: C.T. is a 47-year-old man who presented to the outpatient primary-care clinic 2 weeks after the onset of a low-grade fever associated with pain and stiffness in his left knee, pain on urination, and a thick yellow discharge from both eyes. The patient is not married and frequently has unprotected sex with multiple partners; the last time he engaged in unprotected sex was 3 weeks ago. C.T. denies experiencing chest pain, skin rash, photosensitivity, genital lesions, or urethral discharge and hematuria. Swelling, erythema, and tenderness of the left knee joint, as well as signs of conjunctivitis, were the only findings noted on physical examination. A urine *Chlamydia* rapid test with first void was positive.

Based on the history of symptoms present in this case, what is an appropriate initial treatment strategy for C.T.?

Empiric antibiotic therapy does not reduce the risk of recurrence of Reiter syndrome, and antibiotics are therefore not routinely recommended for uncomplicated cases. As is the case with C.T., those with documented *Chlamydia trachomatis* infection and their partners should be offered antibiotics (azithromycin 1 g orally as a single dose or doxycycline 100 mg twice per day for 7 days).[66] Oral NSAIDs may be useful for pain control, but there is no evidence they affect arthritis itself or shorten the clinical course.[67] Intra-articular corticosteroid injections do not have as dramatic or as sustained a response as in those with rheumatoid arthritis. However, they may be helpful for the treatment of pain and swelling. If C.T. does not respond to initial antibiotic therapy, additional therapy may be required. For those who suffer from a persistence of Reiter syndrome, a disease-modifying antirheumatic drug such as sulfasalazine is well tolerated and effective at a dose of 1 g two or three times daily.[68,69] Aggressive and unremitting Reiter syndrome may be treated with immunosuppressants. Physical therapy modalities may be an integral part of management to improve mobility and strength and to prevent stiffness and deformities if needed.[67]

POLYMYOSITIS AND DERMATOMYOSITIS

Polymyositis (PM) and dermatomyositis (DM) are idiopathic autoimmune and inflammatory disorders of unknown etiology involving a number of voluntary skeletal muscles simultaneously. PM and DM are characterized by the presence of inflammatory myopathies. In addition, DM involves specific skin manifestations, whereas PM does not.[70] Therapy is aimed at reducing the risk of respiratory failure, renal failure, and cardiomyopathy as potential complications of either disorder.

PM typically presents between the ages of 40 and 60 and is rarely seen in children.[71] DM exhibits a bimodal distribution, and affects adults between the ages of 40 years and 70 years, as well as children. African Americans are at an increased risk for these disorders, and both women and men (2:1) are affected.[72] The exact frequencies of either condition as a stand-alone disorder or in combination are not known. It is estimated that annual incidence rates range from 2.5 cases per million in patients younger than 15 years to 10.5 cases per million in those older than 65 years.[72] The prevalence is thought to lie between 25 and 35.3 cases per million.

There is no clear cause of either disorder, and both are thought to involve immune-mediated processes triggered by environmental factors (autoimmune or viral) in genetically susceptible individuals.[73] DM is thought to be a complement-mediated microangiopathy in which inflammatory infiltrates arise owing to ischemic phenomena. In patients with PM, muscle fibers may be damaged by cytotoxic CD8 T lymphocytes. Infectious agents implicated as causative factors include Coxsackie virus, influenza virus, retroviruses, cytomegalovirus, and Epstein-Barr virus. Various autoantibodies are found in up to 60% of patients. Expression of a genetic-specific HLA subtype (HLA DRB1-03 in whites and HLA DRB1-14 in Koreans) places individuals from certain ethnic groups at an increased risk.[74] Exposure to UV radiation also increases the risk of developing DM.

Symptom onset for both PM and DM is insidious, and patients initially complain of muscle weakness of the trunk, shoulders, hip girdles, upper arms, thighs, neck, and pharynx. These patients usually report increasing difficulties in everyday tasks requiring the use of proximal muscles such as getting up from a chair, climbing stairs, stepping onto a curb, lifting objects, and combing hair. Frequent falls, fatigue, malaise, weight loss, shortness of breath, and low-grade fever are also often present.[75] Classification of PM and DM can be accomplished by assessing the presence or absence of certain characteristics presented in Table 46-10.[70] Systemic and cutaneous signs or symptoms may manifest as complications of either disorder. Specific manifestations seen in DM are described in Table 46-11.[70] A proportion of patients (approximately 11% to 40% of those with DM) will meet the diagnostic criteria for other CTDs. This overlap syndrome is thought to occur more frequently in men than women (9:1 ratio).[70] At present, no diagnostic criteria for PM and DM have been clearly defined and validated. After other conditions (e.g., human immunodeficiency virus infection, lichen planus, SLE, psoriasis, or drug-induced causes) have been considered and ruled out, diagnosis may be confirmed by generally accepted criteria including the presence of proximal muscle weakness, elevated serum concentrations of skeletal muscle enzymes (e.g., creatine kinase, lactate dehydrogenase), myopathic changes on electromyography, evidence of inflammation on muscle biopsy, and skin rash (for DM only).[73]

TABLE 46-10
Classification of Polymyositis and Dermatomyositis

Polymyositis	Dermatomyositis

• Adult
• Pediatric
• Inclusion-body myositis
• Overlap (myositis associated with another CTD)
	• Without muscle weakness:
	  • Amyopathic dermatomyositis or dermatomyositis sine myositis
	• With muscle weakness:
	  • Adult: associated with cancer or not associated with cancer
	  • Pediatric

CTD, connective tissue disorder.
Adapted with permission from Drake LA et al. Guidelines of care of dermatomyositis. *J Am Acad Dermatol.* 1996:34(5 Pt 1):824.

CASE 46-6

QUESTION 1: J.A. is a 55-year-old African American man with a history of PM. He was initially diagnosed 3 years ago and was treated with high-dose oral prednisone for 5 months, at which time an attempt to taper the corticosteroid to the lowest effective dose was initiated. Since that time, J.A. has not been able to completely stop corticosteroid therapy without the recurrence of muscle weakness, which affects his ability to perform activities of daily living. In the past 3 months his symptoms have progressed to the point where he was titrated back to his initial high-dose prednisone regimen in an attempt to gain adequate relief. At this point J.A. and his primary-care physician are considering alternative options for symptom control. What is a reasonable pharmacotherapeutic option to recommend that may provide J.A. with symptom relief?

The initial and long-term goals of therapy are to improve muscle weakness, thereby improving the activities of daily living. The clinical course of both PM and DM varies in severity from mild to more severe progressive disease. Those with mild forms of the disease usually have a rapid response to therapy, whereas those with more severe or slowly progressive forms of the disease are more likely to not respond to treatment; this is a marker for a poor prognosis.[75] As demonstrated in J.A.'s case, initial therapy with high-dose corticosteroids is usually recommended for several months, followed by slow tapering to the

TABLE 46-11
Manifestations and Complications of Dermatomyositis

Cutaneous (Type of Manifestation)	Systemic
Gottron papules (pathognomic)	Proximal muscle weakness, dysphonia, dysphagia (common)
Gottron sign (pathognomic)	Respiratory muscle weakness, visual changes, abdominal pain (less common)
Shawl sign/V-sign (characteristic)	Cardiomyopathy, cardiac conduction defects
Heliotrope (characteristic)	Aspiration pneumonia (secondary to respiratory muscle weakness)
Periungual telangiectasias (characteristic)	Diffuse interstitial pneumonitis or fibrosis
Mechanic's hand (characteristic)	Large-bowel infarction (secondary to vasculopathy occurring in pediatric patients with myositis)
	Muscle atrophy and calcification
	Ocular complications (iritis, nystagmus, cotton-wool spots, optic atrophy, conjunctival edema, and conjunctival pseudopolyposis)

Adapted with permission from Koler RA, Montemarano A. Dermatomyositis. *Am Fam Physician.* 2001;64:1565.

ONLINE CONTENT

For photos of the types of manifestations listed in Table 46-11, go to http://thepoint.lww.com/AT10e.

lowest effective dose, depending on response to therapy.[76] Patients who respond early to high-dose corticosteroids typically respond better to corticosteroid-sparing agents (e.g., methotrexate, azathioprine) in the future. J.A.'s failure to respond to corticosteroids should prompt further investigation for possible other pathologic processes including muscular dystrophy, hypothyroidism, or malignancy-associated myopathy. Should those investigations yield no conclusive results, J.A. may be offered methotrexate or azathioprine as recommended first-line immunosuppressive agents if the disease is not controlled with corticosteroids alone or if the disease is rapidly progressive.[77] If patients do not respond to typical therapeutic modalities, IV gamma globulin, rituximab, cyclophosphamide, cyclosporin A, chlorambucil, tacrolimus, and mycophenolate mofetil may be considered and have all been suggested as alternatives.[78]

CASE 46-6, QUESTION 2: What preventive health measures may be offered to J.A. to augment his pharmacotherapeutic treatment regimen?

Supportive therapy such as bed rest, physiotherapy, warm baths, and moist heat applications to the affected areas can improve muscle stiffness. If oral lesions are present, irrigation of these lesions with warm saline solution is helpful. Preventive health measures for those experiencing either disorder include application of sunscreen, osteoporosis prevention, minimizing aspiration risk in patients with esophageal dysmotility, and physical therapy in patients with muscle weakness.[76]

KEY REFERENCES AND WEBSITES

A full list of references for this chapter can be found at **http://thepoint.lww.com/AT10e.** Below are the key references and websites for this chapter, with the corresponding reference number in this chapter found in parentheses after the reference.

Key References

Amato AA, Griggs RC. Treatment of idiopathic inflammatory myopathies. *Curr Opin Neurol*. 2003;16:569. (76)

Barth WF, Segal K. Reactive arthritis (Reiter's syndrome). *Am Fam Physican*. 1999;60:499. (59)

Bertsias GK et al. Therapeutic opportunities in systemic lupus erythematosus: state of the art and prospects for the new decade. *Ann Rheum Dis*. 2010;69:1603. (16)

Dasgupta B et al. BSR and BHPR guidelines for the management of polymyalgia rheumatica. *Rheumatology (Oxford)*. 2010;49:186. (53)

Hinchcliff M, Varga J. Systemic sclerosis/scleroderma: a treatable multisystem disease. *Am Fam Physician*. 2008;78:961. (33)

Kowal-Bielecka O et al. EULAR recommendations for the treatment of systemic sclerosis: a report from the EULAR Scleroderma Trials and Research group (EUSTAR). *Ann Rheum Dis*. 2009;68(5):620. (45)

Mosca M et al. European League Against Rheumatism recommendations for monitoring patients with systemic lupus erythematosus in clinical practice and in observational studies. *Ann Rheum Dis*. 2010;69:1269. (25)

[No authors listed]. Guidelines for referral and management of systemic lupus erythematosus in adults. American College of Rheumatology Ad Hoc Committee on Systemic Lupus Erythematosus Guidelines. *Arthritis Rheum*. 1999;42:1785. (3)

Sontheimer R, McCauliffe D. Lupus-specific skin disease (cutaneous LE). In: Wallace D, Hahn BH, eds. *Dubois' Lupus Erythematosus*. 7th ed. Philadelphia, PA: Lippincott Williams & Wilkins; 2007:576. (4)

Tassiulas I, Boumpas D. Clinical features and treatment of systemic lupus erythematosus. In: Firestein G et al, eds. *Kelley's Textbook of Rheumatology*. 8th ed. Philadelphia, PA: Saunders Elsevier; 2009:1263. (12)

Yildirim-Toruner C, Diamond B. Current and novel therapeutics in the treatment of systemic lupus erythematosus. *J Allergy Clin Immunol*. 2011;127:303. (18)

Key Websites

Bertsias GK et al. EULAR recommendations for the management of Systemic Lupus Erythematosus (SLE) Report of a task force of the European Standing Committee for International Clinical Studies Including Therapeutics (ESCISIT). **http://ard.bmj.com/content/early/2007/07/05/ard.2007.070367#related-urls.** Accessed January 24, 2011.

Lupus Foundation of America. **http://www.lupus.org/newsite/index.html.** Accessed March 17, 2011.

SECTION EDITOR: SHAREEN Y. EL-IBIARY

47 Contraception

Shareen Y. El-Ibiary and Jennifer L. Hardman

CORE PRINCIPLES

		CHAPTER CASES
1	Contraceptive choice is based on several factors that include formulation, hormone content, effectiveness, side effect profile, cost, accessibility, past medical history, medication use, privacy of use, prevention of sexually transmitted infections (STIs), and return to fertility time.	**Case 47-1 (Question 1)**
2	Combined hormonal contraceptive (CHCs) agents are a combination of estrogen and progestin. They are available in a variety of formulations that include a combination of estrogen and progestin (oral tablet, vaginal ring, and transdermal patch). CHCs may be classified by estrogen content into high dose (50 mcg of ethinyl estradiol), low dose (30 to 35 mcg of ethinyl estradiol), and very low dose (10–25 mcg of ethinyl estradiol) and can vary in cycle length (e.g., 21, 24, or 84 days of active hormone). Combined oral contraceptives (COCs) can be further classified by hormone content into monophasic, biphasic, triphasic, and quadriphasic.	**Case 47-1 (Questions 3–5, 7)**
3	CHCs have benefits aside from pregnancy prevention that include treatment of acne, hirsutism, premenstrual syndrome (PMS) and premenstrual dysphoric disorder (PMDD), and endometrial cancer; menstrual cycle regulation; and prevention of ovarian cancer and functional ovarian cysts.	**Case 47-2 (Questions 1–3)**
4	Breakthrough bleeding, nausea, acne, and weight gain are among the most commonly reported side effects in women taking hormonal contraceptives. Risks and side effects may be linked to estrogenic, progestogenic, or androgenic properties of hormonal contraceptives.	**Case 47-2 (Questions 4–8), Case 47-3 (Question 1)**
5	There are risks associated with CHCs and contraindications for use in some women. Estrogen-containing contraceptives should be avoided in women who are 35 years or older and smoke more than 15 cigarettes per day, have uncontrolled hypertension, history of gallbladder disease, stroke, migraines with aura, cardiovascular disease, and history of thromboembolic events.	**Case 47-1 (Question 2)**
6	Progestin-only contraceptives are alternative agents for women with contraindications to CHCs. Progestin-only contraceptives vary in formulations that include oral tablet, depot and subcutaneous injection, and subdermal implant. Common side effects include weight gain, acne, mood changes, and irregular menses.	**Case 47-3 (Questions 2–6)**
7	Effectiveness of hormonal contraceptives is in part based on proper use and counseling. Patients need to understand how to use the contraceptive, what to do for mishaps (e.g., missed dose, vaginal ring falls out, transdermal patch falls off), and when to use a backup method. Directions for missed doses of progestin-only contraceptives vary from those for COCs.	**Case 47-1 (Question 6, 7), Case 47-3 (Questions 2–6)**

continued

	CHAPTER CASES
8 Concomitant use of certain drugs may increase or decrease the levels of hormonal contraceptive agents. In particular, antibiotics and hepatic inducers may decrease the effectiveness of CHCs. Progestin-only contraceptives or nonhormonal contraceptives including backup methods may be alternatives in these cases.	**Case 47-1 (Question 8)**
9 Intrauterine devices (IUDs) or intrauterine systems (IUSs) are available in two formulations (copper IUD and levonorgestrel IUS) and are best for long-term pregnancy prevention. To avoid the risk of pelvic inflammatory disease, the products should be used in women involved in a monogamous relationship.	**Case 47-3 (Question 7)**
10 Some nonhormonal contraceptives include diaphragms, condoms, and spermicides. Male and female condoms are the only contraceptive products that also provide protection against STIs.	**Case 47-4 (Questions 1, 2)**
11 Timing is key for emergency contraception (EC) to be effective. It is best taken as soon as possible after unprotected sexual intercourse but may be effective up to 120 hours after coitus. Emergency contraception can be in the form of high-dose progestin pills, high-dose estrogen and progestin pills (known as Yuzpe method), selective progesterone receptor modulator (SPRM), or copper IUD.	**Case 47-4 (Question 3)**
12 Medical abortion generally consists of mifepristone or methotrexate (to stop development of the pregnancy), or both, in combination with misoprostol (to induce uterine contractions and expel the pregnancy.	**Case 47-4 (Question 4)**

EPIDEMIOLOGY

The world population is greater than 6.8 billion people. At the predicted rate of growth, the population is projected to reach 7.5 billion by 2020 and more than 9 billion by 2050.[1] In the United States, there are approximately 300 million people, and there is one birth every 7 seconds and 1 death every 13 seconds. This results in an increase in one person every 11 seconds.[2]

Contraception is currently an issue worldwide. Preventing unintended pregnancy is an important goal of contraceptive use, particularly in countries where population control is a goal. Economic implications play a role as well. In 2005, an estimated 49% of pregnancies in the United States were unintended, and of these, nearly half resulted in abortions (22% of all pregnancies).[3–5] Proper use and understanding of contraceptives is important for preventing unintended pregnancies.

HORMONAL CONTRACEPTION BACKGROUND AND PHARMACOLOGY

Hormonal contraceptives include combinations of estrogens and progestins known as combination hormonal contraceptives (CHCs) or progestin-only contraceptives. Estrogens prevent the development of the dominant follicle by suppressing follicle-stimulating hormone (FSH) secretion and stabilize the endometrial lining to minimize breakthrough bleeding (see Chapter 50, Disorders Related to the Menstrual Cycle, for more information about the menstrual cycle).[6] Progestins prevent ovulation by suppressing luteinizing hormone (LH) secretion. They may work in combination with estrogen in CHCs such as combination oral contraceptives (COCs), the contraceptive patch, and the contraceptive ring, or alone in formulations such as the progestin-only pill (POP), depot intramuscular or subcutaneous injection, subdermal implant, and as part of intrauterine systems. Progestin-only contraceptives hamper the transport of sperm through the cervical canal by thickening cervical mucus and causing alterations in the endometrial lining (so that it is not favorable for implantation) and in the fallopian tubes (affecting ovum transport).

COMBINATION HORMONAL CONTRACEPTIVES

Patient Evaluation

CASE 47-1

QUESTION 1: S.F., a healthy 33-year-old woman, presents to clinic stating she is getting married soon and would like birth control pills as a method of contraception. She does not have children but would like to start a family in a year or two. Her past medical history is noncontributory other than occasional headaches for which she takes ibuprofen 200 mg by mouth (PO) as needed.

Vital signs: Weight, 128 pounds
Height, 5′4″
Blood pressure, 122/72 mm Hg
Heart rate, 85 beats/minute
Temperature, 98.6°F
Social history: Smokes 1 pack per day, denies alcohol
Family history: Sister gestational diabetes, mother hypertension, father unknown

Which factors are important in the selection of a contraceptive agent for S.F.?

There are several factors that affect selection of a contraceptive. Among them is effectiveness in preventing pregnancy. It is important to determine the importance of pregnancy prevention for S.F. and choose a method based on this information. For example, patients taking teratogenic medications or those with underlying medical conditions in which pregnancy may not be desired will require a highly effective birth control method or multiple methods. Others may not desire a pregnancy, but for a variety of reasons an unintended pregnancy may be more acceptable.

The effectiveness of contraceptive methods depends on the mechanism of action, availability (e.g., prescription required), patients' concurrent medications, past medical history, and acceptability (e.g., side effects, ease of use, adherence, cost, and religious and social beliefs). Any or all of these factors can account for the discrepancy between the lowest failure rate observed for 1 year in clinical trials (perfect-use failure rate) and the actual failure rate in users (typical-use failure rate) and should be taken into account when selecting a method of contraception (Table 47-1).[6] Return to fertility time is also an important factor to consider. Some contraceptive methods allow a woman to conceive shortly after discontinuation, whereas others may delay fertility longer. S.F. indicated she would like to have children in the near future. Given her age of 33 (fertility decreases more rapidly after age 30) and desire for future pregnancy, it would be best to select a product with a faster return to fertility.[7] However, other factors to consider when selecting a contraceptive agent for S.F. include contraindications and risks for her that may indicate one method over another. A combined hormonal contraceptive (CHC) is used commonly in women and may be appropriate for S.F. once all factors are considered.

Contraindications to Combined Hormonal Contraceptive Use

CASE 47-1, QUESTION 2: Are CHCs an appropriate form of contraception for S.F.? What contraindications to CHC therapy must be considered?

To determine whether any contraindications or precautions exist, the clinician should first obtain baseline health information from S.F. such as past medical history, social history, and family history (Fig. 47-1).[8] The World Health Organization has developed medical eligibility criteria to identify appropriate contraception for patients with specific conditions. In 2010, the Centers for Disease Control and Prevention adopted those guidelines for recommendations in the United States (see **http://www.who.int/reproductivehealth/publications/family_planning/9789241563888/en/index.html** for the WHO Medical Eligibility Criteria).[9] Most data regarding contraindications are based on COCs, but the conclusions are applied to all CHCs (e.g., vaginal ring and transdermal patch).

CIGARETTE SMOKING AND USE OF CHCs

S.F. should be strongly encouraged to stop smoking (see Chapter 88, Tobacco Use and Dependence). Women who are 35 years of age or older and smoke 15 or more cigarettes per day should not use CHCs as a method of contraception. Although S.F. is not yet 35, she is smoking one pack per day (20 cigarettes). In her case, many clinicians would not prescribe CHCs. Although S.F. currently does not have any medical problems that would preclude her from using CHCs, she should be informed that CHCs should not be prescribed for her in 2 years if she continues to smoke. In addition, S.F. should be informed that smoking may decrease fertility and has adverse effects on birth outcomes, which is important given her plans to start a family in the near future.

CARDIOVASCULAR DISEASE

An increased risk of cardiovascular death in women who use COCs has been reported in several studies.[10–13] One study reported that in women who do not smoke or use COCs, the risk of cardiovascular death is 0.59 per 100,000 women younger than 35 years and 3.18 per 100,000 women at least 35 years of age. Among nonsmokers, using COCs increased the risk to 0.65 per 100,000 and 6.21 per 100,000 women younger than 35 years or at least 35 years of age, respectively. For COC users who smoke, the risk is 3.3 per 100,000 women younger than 35 years and 29.4 per 100,000 women at least 35 years of age.[14] The increase in mortality is concentrated in smokers 35 years and older.

Several studies have focused on the effect of COCs on serum lipoprotein concentrations because of the association between lipoproteins and atherosclerotic cardiovascular disease.[15–17] High levels of total cholesterol (TC), triglycerides (TG), low-density lipoprotein (LDL) cholesterol, and very low-density lipoprotein (VLDL) cholesterol serum concentrations are associated with the risk of developing atherosclerotic circulatory diseases, whereas high-density lipoprotein (HDL) cholesterol has an inverse relationship. Apolipoprotein levels also affect atherosclerotic risk (e.g., elevations in apolipoprotein increase risk).

Patients taking COCs may be more likely to experience a myocardial infarction (MI) than nonusers.[18] The risk is higher with higher doses of estrogen and especially if the patient is a smoker or has hypertension. It is not clear whether certain types of progestin are more likely to cause MI than others.[12,19] Combined oral contraceptive users may also be at a slightly higher risk of stroke, but some data are conflicting.[18] Those at highest risk of stroke are smokers, patients with hypertension, and patients older than 35 years.

S.F. and her fiancé should understand that the risk of adverse cardiovascular effects may be increased with CHC use, but the absolute risk is still very low no matter which product is used. S.F.'s cigarette smoking, however, is a much more significant risk factor for MI in combination with a CHC product.

MIGRAINES AND STROKE

Ischemic stroke is more likely to occur in CHC users with a history of migraines and is thought to be caused by the estrogen component. The risk is further elevated in women who have migraines with aura or among those who smoke.[6,20] Women experiencing migraines without aura should use CHCs with caution or avoid use if they smoke or are at least 35 years of age.[21] Clinical experience indicates that women who have increasing migraine attacks with CHCs are not likely to improve when the product is changed to one with a different hormone balance. Headaches or migraines may start with initiation of CHCs (see Case 47-2, Question 6); however, if a patient experiences a migraine with aura while taking CHCs, she should discontinue the product and switch to a nonestrogen method.[20,21] Evidence does not show an increased stroke risk with progestin-only contraceptives, and these agents may be used in women with risk factors for stroke.[21]

S.F. does have a history of occasional headaches but does not have a history of migraines or migraines with aura. Therefore, she is still a candidate for CHCs but should be informed of the increased risk of stroke from cigarette smoking.

THROMBOEMBOLIC EVENTS

Combined hormonal contraceptives contribute to thromboembolic events by several mechanisms. Estrogens increase coagulability and thereby increase the possibility of clot formation. Although they have been shown to significantly increase some clotting factors, other studies have shown no changes or decreases in prothrombotic factors.[15,17] Long-term COC use is

TABLE 47-1

Percentage of Women Experiencing an Unintended Pregnancy During the First Year of Typical Use and the First Year of Perfect Use of Contraception and the Percentage Continuing Use at the End of the First Year: United States

Method	% of Women Experiencing an Unintended Pregnancy Within the First Year of Use: Typical Use[a]	Perfect Use[b]	% of Women Continuing Use at 1 Year[c]	Relative Cost[k]
Chance[d]	85	85	—	
Periodic abstinence	25	—	51	None
Calendar	—	9	—	
Ovulation method	—	3	—	
Symptothermal[e]	—	2	—	
Postovulation	—	1	—	
Withdrawal	19	4	—	
Spermicides[f]	29	18	42	\$–\$\$
Barrier methods				
Cap[g]				\$\$\$
Parous women	32	20	46	
Nulliparous women	16	9	57	
Sponge				\$\$
Parous women	40	20	42	
Nulliparous women	20	9	57	
Diaphragm[g]	16	6	57	\$\$\$
Condom[h]				\$
Female (Reality)	21	5	49	
Male	15	2	53	
Hormonal contraceptives				
Injectable MPA (Depo-Provera)	3	0.3	56	\$\$\$[l]
Pill				
Progestin-only	8	0.3	68	\$\$
Combined	8	0.3	68	\$\$
Transdermal patch	8	0.3	68	\$\$
Vaginal ring	8	0.3	68	\$\$
IUD/IUS	—	—	—	\$\$\$\$[l]
Copper (ParaGard T 380 A)	0.8	0.6	78	
Levonorgestrel (Mirena)	0.2	0.2	80	
Female sterilization	0.5	0.5	100	\$\$\$\$[m]
Male sterilization	0.15	0.10	100	\$\$\$\$[m]
Emergency contraceptive pills				\$\$\$
Treatment initiated within 72 hours after unprotected intercourse reduces the risk of pregnancy by at least 75%.[i]				
Lactational amenorrhea method				None
LAM is a highly effective, temporary method of contraception.[j]				

[a]Among *typical* couples who initiate use of a method (not necessarily for the first time), the percentage who experience an accidental pregnancy during the first year if they do not stop use for any other reason.

[b]Among couples who initiate use of a method (not necessarily for the first time) and who use it *perfectly* (both consistently and correctly), the percentage who experience an accidental pregnancy during the first year if they do not stop use for any other reason. For patch and ring, the percentage comes from the package insert.

[c]Among couples attempting to avoid pregnancy, the percentage who continue to use a method for 1 year.

[d]The percentages becoming pregnant in first year are based on data from populations in which contraception is not used and from women who cease using contraception to become pregnant. Among such populations, about 89% become pregnant within 1 year. This estimate was lowered slightly (to 85%) to represent the percentages who would become pregnant within 1 year among women now relying on reversible methods of contraception if they abandoned contraception altogether.

[e]Cervical mucus (ovulation) method supplemented by calendar in the preovulatory and basal body temperature in the postovulatory phases.

[f]Foams, creams, gels, vaginal suppositories, and vaginal film.

[g]With spermicidal cream or jelly.

[h]Without spermicides.

[i]The treatment schedule is one dose within 72 hours after unprotected intercourse, and a second dose 12 hours after the first dose. The US Food and Drug Administration has declared the following brands of oral contraceptives to be safe and effective for emergency contraception: Ovral or Ogestrel (1 dose is 2 white pills); Alesse, Lessina, or Levlite (1 dose is 5 pink pills); Nordette or Levlen (1 dose is 4 light-orange pills); Lo/Ovral, Lo/Ogestrel, Cryselle, Levora, or Quasence (1 dose is 4 white pills); Triphasil or Tri-Levlen (1 dose is 4 yellow pills); Jolessa, Portia, Seasonale, or Trivora (1 dose is 4 pink pills); Seasonique (1 dose is 4 light blue-green pills); Lutera (1 dose is 5 white pills); Aviane (1 dose is 5 orange pills); Enpresse (1 dose is 4 orange pills).

[j]However, to maintain effective protection against pregnancy, another method of contraception must be used as soon as menstruation resumes, the frequency or duration of breast-feeding is reduced, bottle feeds are introduced, or the baby reaches 6 months of age.

[k]\$ up to \$10 per item, \$\$ up to \$50 per unit, \$\$\$ up to \$80 per unit, \$\$\$\$ more than \$80 per unit *(These are approximate costs and may vary based on location of purchase and patient insurance.)*

[l]Administration or clinic costs not included. Initial cost of product reported but over time similar to \$\$ cost (e.g., injectable MPA 150 mg/mL suspension one syringe approximately \$95, but works for 3 months making its monthly cost similar to COCs or POPs which range from \$20 to \$45 per pack, copper IUD and levonorgestrel IUS may cost more initially but will work for up to 10 years and 5 years, respectively).

[m]Initial cost for procedure but over time may be more cost-effective than other products used frequently (e.g., monthly contraceptives, condoms, or spermicides).

IUD, intrauterine device; IUS, intrauterine system; LAM, lactational amenorrhea method; MPA, medroxyprogesterone acetate.

(Adapted with permission from Hatcher RA et al. *Contraceptive Technology.* 19th ed. New York, NY: Ardent Media Inc; 2007:24, Table 3-2; includes additional information from www.drugstore.com (accessed May 13, 2011), http://www.americanpregnancy.org/preventingpregnancy/diaphragm.html (accessed May 13, 2011), and http://www.plannedparenthood.org/health-topics/birth-control/cervical-cap-20487.htm (accessed May 13, 2011).)

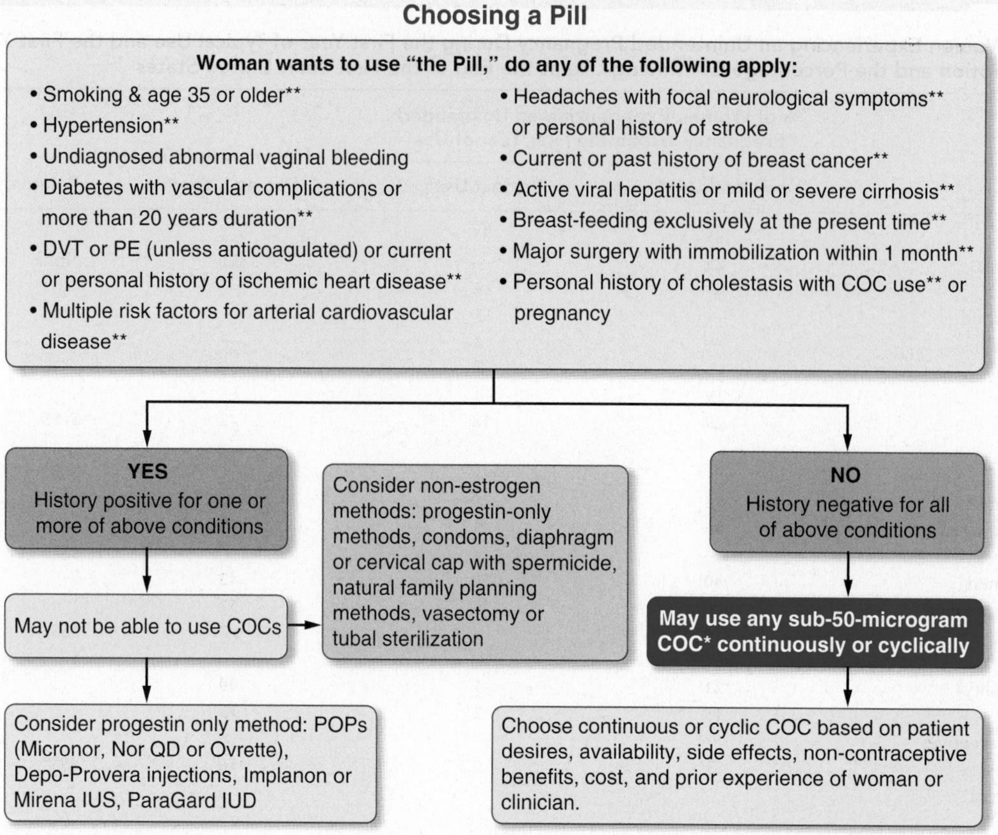

- The World Health Organization and the Food and Drug Administration both recommend using the lowest dose pill that is effective. All combined pills with less than 50 mcg of estrogen are considered "low-dose" and are effective and safe.
- There are no studies demonstrating a decreased risk for deep vein thrombosis (DVT) in women on 20-mcg pills. Data on higher dose pills have demonstrated that the less the estrogen dose, the lower the risk for DVT.
- All COCs lower free testosterone. Class labeling in Canada for all combined pills states that use of pills may improve acne.
- To minimize discontinuation due to spotting and breakthrough bleeding, warn women in advance, reassure that spotting and breakthrough bleeding become better over time.

*The package insert for women on Yasmin and Yaz states [Berlex-2001]: "Yasmin is different from other birth control pills because it contains the progestin drospirenone. Drospirenone may increase potassium. Therefore, you should not take Yasmin if you have kidney, liver or adrenal disease, because this could cause serious heart and health problems. Other drugs may also increase potassium. If you are currently on daily, long-term treatment for a chronic condition with any of the medications below, you should consult your healthcare provider about whether Yasmin is right for you, and during the first month that you take Yasmin, you should have a blood test to check your potassium level: NSAIDs (ibuprofen [Motrin®, Advil®], naproxen [Naprosyn®, Aleve®, and others] when taken long-term and daily for treatment of arthritis or other problems]; potassium-sparing diuretics (sprironolactone and others); potassium supplementation; ACE inhibitors (Capoten®, Vasotec®, Zestril® and others); Angiotensin-II receptor antagonists (Cozaar®, Diovan®, Avapro® and others); heparin."

**These are conditions that receive a WHO:3 or a WHO:4 (based on WHO Medical Eligibility Criteria for Contraceptive Use, 4th ed. 2009, Category 3—A condition in which theoretical or proven risks usually outweigh the benefit of contraceptive method use, Category 4—A condition that represents an unacceptable health risk if contraceptive method is used).

FIGURE 47-1 Choosing a pill. ACE, angiotensin-converting enzyme; COC, combined oral contraceptive; DVT, deep venous thrombosis; IUD, intrauterine device; IUS, intrauterine system; NSAIDs, nonsteroidal anti-inflammatory drugs; PE, pulmonary embolism; POP, progestin-only pill. (Adapted with permission from Zieman M et al. *Managing Contraception for Your Pocket 2010–2012*. Tiger, GA: Bridging the Gap Communications; 2010:108, Figure 26.2.)

associated with an increased platelet count and increased platelet aggregation similar to that seen late in pregnancy; this is generally thought to be caused by the estrogen component. More recent data showing increased thrombosis rates in users of third-generation progestins (desogestrel and gestodene [not available in the United States]) suggest that progestin may also have a role in thromboembolism risk.[22]

The baseline risk of venous thromboembolism (VTE) in women is low, at 1 case per 10,000 person-years, but increases to 3 to 4 cases with COC use.[23] The best studies looking at thromboembolism in COC users found that most users have a twofold to sixfold increased risk of having superficial or deep venous thrombosis or pulmonary embolism (PE).[22] Patients requiring emergency major surgery while taking COCs are more prone to VTE than nonusers. The risk of venous thrombosis does not seem to be associated with duration of COC use or past COC use. A greater risk is associated with ethinyl estradiol (EE) doses greater than 35 mcg.[22]

TABLE 47-2
Pill Early Danger Signs (ACHES)[8]

Signals	Possible Problem
Abdominal pain (severe)	Gallbladder disease, hepatic adenoma, blood clot, pancreatitis
Chest pain (severe), shortness of breath, or coughing up blood	Blood clot in lungs or myocardial infarction
Headaches (severe)	Stroke, hypertension, or migraine headache
Eye problems: blurred vision, flashing lights, or blindness	Stroke, hypertension, or temporary vascular problem
Severe leg pain (calf or thigh)	Blood clot in legs

Women with a mutation in clotting factor V (also called factor V Leiden) or a deficiency in protein C, protein S, or antithrombin are more likely to experience a VTE with COCs than women without a hereditary prothrombotic defect.[24] Women with factor V Leiden using COCs have a 30-fold increase in VTE compared with women without the mutation.[24]

The minimal risk of thrombosis associated with CHCs in the general population does not justify the cost of routine screening for deficiencies and mutations in the coagulation system; however, if a patient has a family history of thrombosis then measurement of antithrombin III, protein C, activated protein C resistance ratio, protein S, anticardiolipin antibodies, prothrombin G mutation, factor V Leiden, and homocysteine levels should be considered.[8]

Whether third-generation progestins (desogestrel, gestodene) are associated with a higher risk of VTE relative to other progestins is controversial.[22] It was believed that the risk of thrombosis with third-generation progestins would be lower than with other progestins because they have more beneficial effects on HDL. However, most studies that compared the risk of thrombosis with third-generation progestins to second-generation progestins found that desogestrel and gestodene are associated with a greater VTE risk. Although the risk may be increased, the overall rate of thrombosis is still low. All patients using CHCs should be counseled about the VTE warning signs (Table 47-2).[8]

S.F. does not have a history of clotting disorders or previous clots. Therefore, she is still a candidate for CHCs. Her smoking status, however, puts her at higher risk for VTE. If she experiences a VTE while taking CHCs, a progestin-only method or nonhormonal contraceptive method should be recommended and the CHC discontinued.

HYPERTENSION

Combined hormonal contraceptives appear to increase blood pressure. Small studies have found systolic blood pressure to increase by 7 to 8 mm Hg and diastolic blood pressure to increase by 6 mm Hg in normotensive or mildly hypertensive women, and these women may have poorer blood pressure control.[25,26] Other studies have shown differing results on whether women with hypertension who use COCs are more likely to suffer an MI than nonusers.[6,27] A small study of adolescent women showed similar systolic and diastolic blood pressures in users versus nonusers.[28]

The underlying mechanisms for CHC-induced hypertension may be sodium and water retention and increased renin activity.[29,30] Hypertension secondary to COCs may develop slowly during 3 to 36 months and may not decline for 3 to 6 months after COC discontinuation.[31] Women with controlled hypertension may attempt a trial of CHCs with blood pressure monitoring; however, progestin-only contraceptives have not been shown to increase blood pressure and may be preferable for women with uncontrolled hypertension.[25]

S.F.'s blood pressure is not elevated at 122/72 mm Hg. Therefore, she is still a candidate for CHCs. If her blood pressure were greater than 140/90 mm Hg, a nonhormonal method or a progestin-only contraceptive would be a preferred form of contraception.

HEPATOTOXICITY

Combined oral contraceptives have been associated with benign liver tumors, hepatic adenomas, and liver cancer.[6,32] The risk of liver cancer is low, and COCs are thought to cause only a modest increase in risk.[32,33] A European study found a small, statistically significant increase in the risk of liver cancer in women without cirrhosis and without hepatitis B or C, which are the types of women that usually use COCs. In this study, COC use in these women increased the risk of liver cancer by 1 case per 1.5 million woman-years.[33] S.F. should be reassured that it is very unlikely for her to develop benign or malignant liver tumors associated with COC use.

DIABETES

Generally, low-dose COCs do not alter glucose tolerance.[17,34] Women with a history of gestational diabetes like S.F.'s sister and those with a strong family history of diabetes in parents or siblings are at greater risk for COC-induced glucose intolerance.[25] Combined oral contraceptives have complex effects on carbohydrate metabolism. Progestins decrease and estrogens increase the number of insulin receptors on the cell membrane. Progestins also may alter insulin receptor affinity. The different progestins in CHCs have different propensities to induce glucose intolerance. Desogestrel seems to have the best glucose values compared with other progestins, but insulin results are not consistent.[34]

Results of one controlled, randomized, prospective study showed no adverse effect on carbohydrate or lipid metabolism in women with a history of gestational diabetes after 6 to 13 months of low-dose CHC use.[35] Both the users and nonusers showed a significant and similar deterioration in glucose tolerance with an overall prevalence of 14% impaired glucose tolerance and 17% diabetes mellitus. The authors concluded that low-dose COCs could be prescribed safely and that serum lipids and glucose tolerance should be monitored closely, regardless of contraceptive choice.

For women with diabetes, the World Health Organization recommends avoiding COCs if they have been diabetic for more than 20 years or they have end-organ damage such as retinopathy, neuropathy, or nephropathy.[9] For women without diabetes, CHC use may protect against developing diabetes. One large prospective, observational study found that women who used COCs had lower fasting glucose levels and lower odds of developing diabetes.[36]

S.F.'s sister having a history of gestational diabetes does not preclude S.F. from using a CHC at this time. Preferably S.F. should start on a low-dose CHC.

GALLBLADDER DISEASE

The incidence of gallstones has been reported to increase with COC use; however, conflicting data exist. Estrogens and progestins may contribute to bile stasis and gallstones by reducing cholesterol clearance and altering bile acid composition.[37] The incidence of gallbladder disease has been reported to increase during the first year of use but then to decline steadily to a rate lower than that of control women.[38] Conversely, in another large study, long-term COC users experienced slightly lower rates of gallbladder disease than nonusers.[39] In addition, another study found that women who had ever used COCs were not more likely to have symptomatic gallstones, but current and long-term users were. An analysis of 482 women with benign gallbladder disease from the Oxford/Family Planning Association contraception study concluded that it is unlikely that COCs cause gallbladder disease.[40]

The newer COCs with lower progestin and estrogen concentrations should have little effect, if any, on gallstone formation in normal patients. Women who are obese, young, or long-term users of COCs may be the most likely to develop gallstones. At this time, this is not a concern of S.F. in starting COCs.

Combined Oral Contraceptives

CASE 47-1, QUESTION 3: S.F. has decided to quit smoking. Based on her past medical history, she is a candidate for CHCs and indicates she wants to start a COC. Which COC should be selected for her?

Selecting a CHC for S.F. can be confusing because of the multitude of products available, the lack of studies directly comparing products, and health insurance medication formulary restrictions. The failure rate of COCs ranges from 0.3% with perfect use to 8% with typical use (Table 47-1).[6]

The COCs are available in varying strengths of estrogens and progestins. Table 47-3[41–53] lists the brand-name and generic COCs in the United States. Almost all COCs available in the United States contain the synthetic estrogen, EE. Doses of EE generally range from 10 to 50 mcg with 10- to 25-mcg formulations considered very low dose, 30- to 35-mcg formulations, low dose, and 50-mcg formulations, high dose. Mestranol, another estrogen available in the United States and used internationally, is an inactive prodrug that is hepatically metabolized to EE. Mestranol 50 mcg has approximately the same activity as EE 35 mcg.[6] Estradiol valerate is a third estrogen available in one oral formulation. The formulation of estradiol valerate 2 to 3 mg with 2 to 3 mg of dienogest was compared against EE 20 mcg with levonorgestrel 100 mcg in clinical trials.[49,54]

The COCs also contain one of the following progestins: ethynodiol diacetate, desogestrel, dienogest, drospirenone, levonorgestrel, norethindrone, norethindrone acetate, norgestimate, and norgestrel (a mixture of dextronorgestrel and levonorgestrel; dextronorgestrel appears to be progestationally inert compared with levonorgestrel).[6] Progestins differ significantly in their progestational potency and in the extent of their metabolism to estrogenic substances. Progestins have both estrogenic and antiestrogenic effects. Because the progestins have a chemical structure similar to that of testosterone, they also have varying degrees of androgenic activity (Table 47-3).[55] Minor structural changes in all of the progestins may lead to significant changes in their progestational, estrogenic, antiestrogenic, and androgenic activities, which may affect patients differently (Table 47-4).[6] Drospirenone is a unique progestin because it has antiandrogenic and antimineralocorticoid properties. Drospirenone is chemically similar to the potassium-sparing diuretic spironolactone, and therefore may increase potassium levels. Drospirenone should be used with caution in patients using medications that can increase potassium levels (e.g., high-dose nonsteroidal anti-inflammatory drugs [NSAIDs], angiotensin-converting enzyme [ACE] inhibitors, heparin, potassium-sparing diuretics, aldosterone antagonists, and angiotensin II blockers).[42]

Because no COC has been shown to be superior to the others, any COC with less than 50 mcg of EE can be used for patients who are COC candidates.[56] The information in Figure 47-1 may be used to select an initial COC for most patients and to change formulations when side effects necessitate an alternative choice.[9] Increased body weight (>70.5 kg) has been associated with increased COC failure.[57] If S.F. were heavier, a COC with a higher dose of EE (e.g., 35 mcg) would be a better option. Any pill containing less than 50 mcg EE can be used for S.F. because she is a healthy woman without medical complications or active medications.

LENGTH OF ACTIVE HORMONE: 21-DAY, 24-DAY, OR 28-DAY

The COCs are available in a variety of cycle lengths. The most common is the 28-day pack that contains 21 days of active pills (pills that contain estrogen and progestin) followed by 7 days of placebo pills. Some newer products contain 24 days of active pills followed by 4 days of placebo. Combined hormonal contraceptives with 4 days of placebo may shorten menses and minimize the hormonal withdrawal side effects (e.g., headaches, mood changes) that some women experience during the placebo week.[58] It is also possible that efficacy is improved; however, this has not been proven in clinical trials.

The 21-day pill packs contain only the active pills. Most patients are instructed to take one pill daily for 21 days and then take nothing for 1 week. Many clinicians prefer the use of 28-day pill packs to minimize confusion; the patient takes one pill daily regardless of whether it is an active or placebo pill. After taking the last pill of a 28-day pack, the patient should begin a new pack the next day. However, when continuous ovarian suppression is indicated to treat estrogen-dependent disorders such as endometriosis, the 21-day cycle products are preferred to facilitate taking active pills continuously. Alternatively, the placebo pills could be removed from 28-day cycle packs. S.F. will not be taking COCs continuously, so a 24-day or 28-day pack is recommended.

MULTIPHASIC ORAL CONTRACEPTIVES

CASE 47-1, QUESTION 4: Should S.F. start a monophasic or multiphasic COC? What are the advantages and disadvantages of the monophasic versus multiphasic COC?

COCs have varying amounts of hormones in the active pills, which can be divided in phases that include monophasic, biphasic, triphasic, or quadriphasic (Table 47-3).

Monophasic COCs contain the same dose of estrogen and progestin in each active pill throughout the pill pack, whereas multiphasic COCs have varying amounts of hormones. Because of metabolic and physiologic effects related to the progestin component of COCs, multiphasic products were initially formulated to contain less progestin overall. Some products, however, are now marketed with varying amounts of estrogen to reduce the overall exposure to estrogen or to minimize estrogen withdrawal side effects (e.g., norethindrone/EE [Estrostep, Estrostep Fe]).

A biphasic formulation usually contains a certain amount of progestin and estrogen for the first half of the cycle, then a different amount for the second half, and then a week of placebos. Triphasic formulations have a different amount of hormones for each of the 3 weeks of active pills. These products attempt to provide adequate endometrial support while also providing adequate contraception.[59] No studies, however, show a superiority of one triphasic over another or compared with monophasics. The reduced progestin content is desirable for women with complaints of progestin-associated side effects (e.g., increased appetite, acne, weight gain) or in women with cardiovascular disease or metabolic abnormalities.[6] Women with side effects related to progestin deficiency (e.g., late-cycle bleeding) or conditions necessitating progestin dominance (e.g., benign breast disease) may do better with monophasics. Recently, a quadriphasic

TABLE 47-3
Oral Contraceptives and Relative Progestin, Estrogen, and Androgen Activities[41–53]

Ingredients	Brand Name Examples	Progestin Activity	Estrogen Activity	Androgen Activity	Unique Properties
Monophasic Formulations					
Levonorgestrel 0.1 mg/EE 20 mcg	Alesse, Aviane, Lessina, Levlite, LoSeasonique, Lutera, Sronyx	Low	Low	Low	LoSeasonique contains 84 active pills, contains 7 pills of EE 10 mcg instead of placebos
Levonorgestrel 0.09 mg/EE 20 mcg	Lybrel	Low	Low	Low	Lybrel is a 1-year continuous formulation available in packs of 28 active pills
Norgestimate 0.25 mg/EE 35 mcg	MonoNessa, Ortho-Cyclen, Previfem, Sprintec	Low	Intermediate	Low	
Norethindrone 0.5 mg/EE 35 mcg	Brevicon, Modicon, Necon 0.5/35, Nortrel 0.5/35	Low	High	Low	
Norethindrone 0.4 mg/EE 35 mcg	Blaziva, Femcon Fe, Ovcon-35, Ovcon-35 Chewable, Zenchent	Low	High	Low	Femcon Fe and Ovcon-35 Chewable are chewable pills
Levonorgestrel 0.15 mg/EE 30 mcg	Levlen, Levora, Introvale, Jolessa, Nordette-28, Portia, Quasence, Seasonale, Seasonique	Intermediate	Low	Intermediate	Introvale and Seasonale contain 84 active pills, 7 placebo pills. Seasonique contains 84 active pills, 7 pills of EE 10 mcg instead of placebos
Norgestrel 0.3 mg/EE 30 mcg	Cryselle, Lo-Ovral, Low-Ogestrel	Intermediate	Low	Intermediate	
Norethindrone 1 mg/ mestranol 50 mcg	Necon 1/50, Norinyl 1+50, Ortho-Novum 1/50	Intermediate	Intermediate	Intermediate	
Norethindrone 1 mg/EE 35 mcg	Genora 1/35, Cyclafem 1/35, Necon 1/35, Norethin 1/35, Norinyl 1+35, Nortrel 1/35, Ortho-Novum 1/35	Intermediate	High	Intermediate	
Norethindrone 1 mg/EE 50 mcg	Ovcon-50	Intermediate	High	Intermediate	
Norethindrone acetate 1 mg/EE 20 mcg	Junel Fe 1/20, Junel 21 Day 1/20, Loestrin 21 1/20, Loestrin Fe 1/20, Loestrin 24 Fe, Microgestin Fe 1/20	High	Low	Intermediate	"Fe" contains 75 mg ferrous fumarate instead of placebos, Loestrin 24 Fe contains 24 active pills and 4 pills of ferrous fumarate
Norethindrone acetate 1.5 mg/EE 30 mcg	Junel 1/35, Loestrin 21 1.5/30, Loestrin Fe 1.5/30, Microgestin Fe 1.5/30	High	Low	High	"Fe" contains 75 mg ferrous fumarate instead of placebos
Ethynodiol diacetate 1 mg/35 mcg EE	Demulen 1/35, Kelnor 1/35, Zovia 1/35E	High	Low	Low	
Desogestrel 0.15 mg/EE 20 mcg	Kariva, Mircette	High	Low	Low	Only 2 days of placebos, other 5 days contain EE 10 mcg
Desogestrel 0.15 mg/EE 30 mcg	Apri, Desogen, Ortho-Cept, Reclipsen, Solia	High	Intermediate	Low	
Ethynodiol diacetate 1 mg/EE 50 mcg	Demulen 1/50, Zovia 1/50 E	High	Intermediate	Low	
Norgestrel 0.5 mg/EE 50 mcg	Ovral, Ogestrel	High	High	High	

(continued)

TABLE 47-3
Oral Contraceptives and Relative Progestin, Estrogen, and Androgen Activities[41–53] (Continued)

Ingredients	Brand Name Examples	Progestin Activity	Estrogen Activity	Androgen Activity	Unique Properties
Norethindrone 0.8 mg/EE 25 mcg	Generess Fe	No data	No data	No data	"Fe" contains 75 mg ferrous fumarate instead of placebos, Generess Fe contains 24 active pills and 4 pills of ferrous fumarate, chewable formulation
Norethindrone 1 mg/EE 10 mcg	Lo Loestrin Fe	No data	No data	No data	Lo Loestrin Fe contains 24 active pills and 2 pills of 10 mcg EE, 2 pills of 75 mg ferrous fumarate
Drospirenone 3 mg/EE 20 mcg levomefolate calcium 0.451 mg	Beyaz	No data	No data	None[a]	Provides folate supplementation, FDA-approved use for treatment of acne and PMDD, 24 active pills and 4 days of 0.451 mg of levomefolate calcium instead of placebos
Drospirenone 3 mg/EE 20 mcg	Gianvi, YAZ, Loryna	No data	No data	None[a]	Antimineralocorticoid properties, FDA-approved use for treatment of acne and PMDD, only 4 days of placebos
Drospirenone 3 mg/EE 30 mcg/levomefolate calcium 0.451 mg	Safyral	No data	Intermediate	None[a]	Provides folate supplementation, 21 active pills and 7 days of 0.451 mg of levomefolate calcium instead of placebos
Drospirenone 3 mg/EE 30 mcg	Ocella, Yasmin, Zarah, Syeda	No data	Intermediate	None[a]	Antimineralocorticoid properties
Biphasic Formulations					
Norethindrone 0.5, 1 mg/EE 35 mcg	Necon 10/11, Ortho-Novum 10/11	Intermediate	High	Low	
Triphasic Formulations					
Norgestimate 0.18, 0.215, 0.25 mg/EE 25 mcg	Ortho Tri-Cyclen Lo	Low	Low	Low	
Norgestimate 0.18, 0.215, 0.25 mg/EE 35 mcg	Ortho Tri-Cyclen, Tri-Previfem, Tri-Sprintec	Low	Intermediate	Low	FDA-approved use for treatment of acne
Levonorgestrel 0.05, 0.075, 0.125 mg/EE 30, 40, 30 mcg	Enpresse, Levonest, Tri-Levlen, Triphasil, Trivora	Low	Intermediate	Low	
Norethindrone 0.5, 1, 0.5 mg/EE 35 mcg	Aranelle, Leena, Tri-Norinyl	Low	High	Low	
Norethindrone 0.5, 0.75, 1 mg/EE 35 mcg	Cyclafem 7/7/7, Necon 7/7/7, Ortho-Novum 7/7/7	Intermediate	High	Low	
Norethindrone 1 mg/EE 20, 30, 35 mcg	Estrostep 21, Estrostep Fe	High	Low	Intermediate	Estrophasic (estrogen content changes), FDA-approved use for treatment of acne, "Fe" contains 75 mg ferrous fumarate instead of placebos
Desogestrel 0.1, 0.125, 0.15 mg/EE 25 mcg	Cyclessa, Velivet	High	Low	Low	

(continued)

TABLE 47-3
Oral Contraceptives and Relative Progestin, Estrogen, and Androgen Activities[41–53] (*Continued*)

Ingredients	Brand Name Examples	Progestin Activity	Estrogen Activity	Androgen Activity	Unique Properties
Quadriphasic Formulation					
Dienogest 0, 2, 3, 0 mg/ estradiol valerate 3, 2, 2, 1 mg	Natazia	No data	Low	No data	Has 2 placebo pills, has 2 pills with 3 mg of estradiol valerate only, 5 pills with 2 mg of dienogest and 2 mg of estradiol valerate, 17 pills with 3 mg of dienogest and 2 mg of estradiol valerate and 2 pills of 1 mg estradiol valerate
Progestin-Only					
Norethindrone 0.35 mg	Camila, Errin, Jolivette, Micronor, Nor-QD, Nora-BE	Low	None	Low	No placebos, 28 days of active pills
dl-Norgestrel	Ovrette	No data	None	No data	No placebos, 28 days of active pills

[a]Preclinical studies have shown that drospirenone has no androgenic, estrogenic, glucocorticoid, antiglucocorticoid, or antiandrogenic activity.
EE, ethinyl estradiol; FDA, US Food and Drug Administration; PMDD, premenstrual dysphoric disorder.
Source: Facts and Comparisons eAnswers. http://online.factsandcomparisons.com/index.aspx.

COC (Natazia) became available, and it contains four different amounts of hormones throughout the pill pack.[48] Advantages of the product remain to be seen, but it may help decrease hormone-withdrawal side effects and intermenstrual bleeding.

One drawback associated with triphasic and quadriphasic COC use is the confusion caused by the different-colored pills in each of the three different phases, making the missed-dose instructions more complicated. Monophasics are preferred for women who will be taking COCs continuously (i.e., skipping the placebo pills) because of the same weekly hormone content.

Other unique formulations include Mircette, which is classified more appropriately as monophasic because the hormone content is consistent throughout the 21-day cycle like other monophasic formulations, but is sometimes referred to as biphasic because it does not contain 7 days of placebos. It provides a unique regimen containing 21 days of 0.15 mg of desogestrel plus 20 mcg of EE, then only 2 days of placebo, followed by 5 days of 10 mcg of EE alone.[51] The patient does not need to take missed 10-mcg EE doses or use a backup method when those specific pills are missed. Adding low-dose estrogen for 5 days during the typical placebo week helps minimize breakthrough bleeding with this product and may be useful for patients who have estrogen-deficiency symptoms such as headaches during the hormone-free week. Because S.F. has not been on a CHC before and does not have a history of side effects associated with COCs, she may be started on any of the COC formulations.

EXTENDED CYCLE

CASE 47-1, QUESTION 5: S.F. has heard that she can skip the placebos from her pill pack to have fewer menses each year. She is interested in this approach. Is this a reasonable option for S.F.?

TABLE 47-4
Estrogenic, Progestogenic, and Combined Effects of Oral Contraceptive Pills

Achieving Proper Hormonal Balance in an Oral Contraceptive			
Estrogen		**Progestin**	
Excess	**Deficiency**	**Excess**	**Deficiency**
Nausea, bloating	Early or mid-cycle breakthrough bleeding	Increased appetite	Late break-through bleeding
Cervical mucorrhea, polyposis	Increased spotting	Weight gain	Amenorrhea
Melasma	Hypomenorrhea	Tiredness, fatigue	Hypermenorrhea
Hypertension		Hypomenorrhea	
Migraine headache		Acne, oily scalp[a]	
Breast fullness or tenderness		Hair loss, hirsutism[a]	
Edema		Depression	
		Monilial vaginitis	
		Breast regression	

[a]Result of androgenic activity of progestins.
Reprinted with permission from Facts and Comparisons eAnswers. http://online.factsandcomparisons.com/index.aspx.

Continuous- or extended-cycle COC regimens (i.e., skipping the placebo pills and taking no break between pill packs, thus having no menses) are often prescribed in women with underlying conditions including anemia, dysmenorrhea (less cramps with fewer menstrual cycles), menorrhagia (heavy menstrual bleeding), and endometriosis (to decrease hormone fluctuations that affect endometrial tissues).[8] In addition, for convenience and lifestyle reasons many women prefer to take COCs continuously to minimize the number of menstrual periods. Regardless of the reason, any woman who is a candidate for CHCs can use them continuously.

Any CHC (e.g., pill, patch, vaginal ring) may be used continuously; however, from the COCs, monophasic pills are recommended because of the consistent hormone content throughout the cycle. Any duration of continuous pill use is acceptable, but many providers recommend that patients take the active pills for 3 to 4 months (3 to 4 pill packs) and then stop COCs for 2 to 7 days. Alternatively, providers may prescribe COCs that are specifically packaged for continuous use (e.g., Seasonale, Seasonique, Lo Seasonique, Lybrel). Patients should be informed that continuous COC use usually results in more breakthrough bleeding or spotting than traditional COC dosing regimens, with up to 41% of women experiencing some form of irregular bleeding in the first few months of the 1-year regimen.[52]

Concerns raised with extended-use regimens include harmful effects on the endometrium; however, one study showed no harmful changes to the endometrium with extended cycles.[60] Long-term side effects of the extended regimens are still being studied. If breakthrough bleeding continues beyond 6 months of continuous COC use, a pelvic examination may be considered. If S.F. is willing to tolerate more irregular bleeding during the first 6 months of continuous COC use, then the extended-cycle regimen may work for her.

Patient Instructions

CASE 47-1, QUESTION 6: What instructions should be given to S.F. about her COC?

WHEN TO START ORAL CONTRACEPTIVES

S.F. should start the first cycle of COCs according to the manufacturer's package instructions or according to one of the following recommendations[6]:

1. Quick start: Take the first COC tablet as soon as possible regardless of cycle day.[61]
2. Day 1 start: Take the first tablet in the COC pack on the first day of menses.
3. Sunday start: Take the first tablet in the COC pack on the first Sunday after the beginning of menstruation. If menses begins on Sunday, start that day.

The quick start method is not described in COC package inserts; however, this method is used by family-planning providers.[61,62] The quick start method can minimize the confusion that many patients have about when to start their first pack and can increase adherence. Also, the quick start method provides contraceptive protection sooner and would, therefore, likely lower the risk of unintended pregnancy. More research on and awareness about this method are needed for it to be used routinely by all health care providers.

WHEN TO USE A BACKUP METHOD OF CONTRACEPTION

Some clinicians recommend that a woman use an alternative method of contraception for the entire first COC cycle. Others believe that alternative methods of contraception are unnecessary if the COC is started on or before the fifth day of the menstrual cycle. Most COC package inserts with the exception of Natazia (estradiol valerate/dienogest) state that a backup method of contraception (e.g., male or female condoms, spermicides, diaphragms) is not necessary if patients use the day 1 start method.[6] If patients use the Sunday or quick start methods, backup contraception should be used for the first week of the COC cycle. A backup method is also recommended when doses are missed, as described in the following section. S.F. has decided to use the quick start method, so she will need to use another method of contraception for her first week of COC use.

COC ADMINISTRATION AND MISSED DOSE INSTRUCTIONS

S.F. should take her COC at the same time each day. Nausea may be prevented or alleviated by taking the dose at bedtime or with food. The best time to take COCs depends on the patient. The optimal time for S.F. is the time when she will have the fewest problems remembering to take her pill each day.

If a woman forgets to take one pill, she must take it as soon as she remembers and refer to the patient instructions in the package insert for further information.[6] Some unique formulations such as estradiol valerate/dienogest (Natazia) have more specific recommendations based on the cycle day missed. If she is taking Natazia, she should be referred to the package insert for information (see http://www.natazia.com), as the advice varies from that listed below.

For the majority of COCs, most manufacturers recommend that if she forgets to take one pill, she should take two pills on the day she remembers (e.g., if she forgets her pill on Monday, she should take two pills on Tuesday). Then she should take the remaining pills as usual. A backup method of contraception is not necessary. If she misses two pills in a row in week 1 or 2 of her pack, she must take two pills on the day she remembers and two pills the next day. She should use an alternative method of contraception for 7 days after missing the pills and may consider emergency contraception.

If a woman misses two pills in a row during the third week (for day 1 starters), she must discard the rest of the pack, start a new pack on that same day, and use an alternative contraceptive method for 7 days. For Sunday starters, she should keep taking one pill every day until Sunday, then start a new pack on Sunday. She must use an alternative method of contraception for 7 days after missing the pills and may consider emergency contraception. She may miss her menstrual period this month.

If a woman misses three or more pills in a row during the first 3 weeks (for day 1 starters), she must discard the rest of her pack, start a new pack that same day, and use an alternative method of contraception for 7 days; Sunday starters should keep taking one pill every day until Sunday, start a new pack on Sunday, and use an alternative method of contraception for 7 days after missing the pills, and they may consider emergency contraception. She may not have a menstrual period this month. If two pills are missed from a low-dose COC (less than EE 30 mcg), some references suggest following the instructions as if three pills were missed.[6] Other references and organizations may cite different recommendations. The recommendations described here are recommended by manufacturers.

CONTRACEPTIVE PATCH AND RING

CASE 47-1, QUESTION 7: S.F. returns to the clinic 3 months later and is very concerned about getting pregnant because

she has trouble remembering to take her pill each day. She wants an effective contraceptive method but is wondering whether other dosage formulations are available. She also indicates concern about high doses of estrogen because she has heard high doses of estrogen can lead to blood clots. She wants the lowest possible dose. What do you tell her?

Contraceptive Patch

The contraceptive patch has an estimated failure rate of 0.3% with perfect use and 8% with typical use (Table 47-1). The contraceptive patch (Ortho Evra) contains 6 mg of norelgestromin and 750 mcg of EE. It was originally formulated to transdermally deliver 150 mcg of norelgestromin and 20 mcg of EE daily into the systemic circulation; however, higher doses of ethinyl estradiol are now thought to be delivered (see below).[63] The patch is a 1.75-inch square with rounded corners and is beige and thin. One patch is applied each week for 3 consecutive weeks for a total of 3 patches used, followed by 1 week with no patch. The day of the week the patch is applied is called the patch change day. Then this cycle is repeated. Menses should begin during the patch-free week. If a woman wants to avoid menses, the patch-free week may be skipped by applying a new patch on week 4 for an extended-use regimen.

ONLINE CONTENT **For photos that show a contraceptive transdermal patch applied to different areas, see the PowerPoint presentation at http://thepoint.lww.com/AT10e.**

The contraceptive patch may be worn on the buttock, abdomen, upper torso, or upper outer arm.[63] The patch should not be applied to the breasts to prevent direct administration of estradiol to the breast tissue. To minimize irritation from the adhesive, S.F. should rotate the patch application sites and not apply the patch to the same location within each month. When applying the patch, S.F. should select the application site and be sure it is clean and dry. She should press firmly on the patch for 10 seconds and trace her finger around the edge of the patch to be sure it adheres securely to the skin. The patch should stay attached during usual activities, including exercising, swimming, and bathing. If the patch falls off and is off less than 24 hours, she should reapply it or apply a new one as soon as possible, and her patch change day will stay the same. No backup contraception is needed. If the patch is off for more than 24 hours, she should start a new cycle of patches, and she will have a new patch change day. She should use backup contraception for 1 week (http://www.orthoevra.com/).

The patch may be started using the quick, Sunday, or day 1 start method, and the recommendations for backup contraception are the same as described earlier with CHCs.[63] If S.F. forgets to start the first patch of a new cycle, she should apply it as soon as she remembers. This day will become her new patch change day, and she should use backup contraception for 1 week. If she forgets to change the patch for 1 or 2 days during week 2 or 3, she should apply a new patch as soon as she remembers. This becomes her new patch change day. No backup contraception is needed. If she forgets to wear the patch for more than 2 days, she should start a new cycle as soon as she remembers. She will need to use backup contraception for 1 week and will have a new patch change day.

The effectiveness of the patch is reduced in patients weighing more than 90 kg and should not be used alone for prevention of pregnancy is these women.[63] S.F. does not weigh more than 90 kg, which does not preclude her from using this method.

The most common side effects reported with the patch are breast tenderness, headache, application site reaction, and nausea. Most risks and benefits with the contraceptive patch are thought to be similar to COCs. One notable difference is the rate of VTE. A small pharmacokinetics trial found that overall monthly serum levels of EE are significantly higher in patch users compared with ring or COC users.[64] With the patch, the peak levels of estrogen are lower, but the steady-state concentrations are higher. It has been noted that the patch provides 60% more ethinyl estradiol than an oral 35-mcg tablet.[63] This raised concern that the patch may have a higher incidence of VTE than the other methods; however, it is controversial. One study found no difference in the rate of nonfatal VTE in patch versus COC users, whereas another study found a doubling of VTE risk in patch users compared with COC users.[65–68] The package insert for Ortho Evra (see http://www.orthoevra.com/) was modified to include this new information.[63] Future studies may find that there are other differences in certain risks or benefits between the patch and pill. Given the higher amounts of EE and controversy surrounding VTE with the transdermal patch, this may not be the most appropriate method for S.F. based on her concerns of VTE associated with COC use.

Contraceptive Ring

The failure rate for the contraceptive ring is also 0.3% with perfect use and 8% with typical use (Table 47-1).[6] The contraceptive ring (NuvaRing) delivers 120 mcg of etonogestrel and 15 mcg of EE daily through the vaginal mucosa.[69] The ring is flexible, and transparent, and has a diameter of just over 2 inches. The ring is inserted vaginally and kept in place for 3 weeks in a row. After 3 weeks, the ring is removed for 1 week, and then a new ring is inserted (see http://www.spfiles.com/pinuvaring.pdf). For extended use, the ring-free week may be skipped by inserting a new ring on week 4.

The ring may be placed anywhere in the vagina, so S.F. does not need to worry about its exact position.[69] To insert the ring, she should compress it so the opposite sides of the ring are touching, and gently insert it into the vagina.

If she feels discomfort with the ring, it has probably not been inserted into the vagina far enough. Most women do not feel the ring once it is in place. To remove the ring, S.F. should grasp the ring between two fingers or hook one finger inside the ring and pull it out. Menses will usually begin within 3 days of removing the ring. If the ring slips out, it should be rinsed with lukewarm water and reinserted. If the ring is out for less than 3 hours, backup contraception is not needed. If the ring is out for more than 3 hours, backup contraception should be used for 1 week. If the ring has been left in the vagina for longer than 3 weeks but no more than 4 weeks, S.F. should remove it, wait 1 week, then reinsert a new ring. The ring is formulated to contain approximately 35 days of medication but should not be promoted for use beyond 21 days.[69] If it has been in place for more than 4 weeks, she should remove it, confirm that she is not pregnant, reinsert a new one, and use backup contraception for 1 week.

The contraceptive ring should be inserted anytime during the first 5 days of the menstrual cycle or inserted using the quick start method.[6,69] Backup contraception should be used for the first week. When changing from the COC, S.F. should insert the ring within 7 days of the last active pill and no backup contraception is needed.

The ring is believed to have the same contraindications and precautions as COCs. The most common side effects with the ring are vaginal infections, irritation, and discharge; headache;

weight gain; and nausea. Unlike the patch, the ring has not been shown to increase VTE risk or have reduced efficacy in obese women.[69] A study of 1,950 women using the contraceptive ring for 13 months found a high degree of patient satisfaction and adherence to the contraceptive method.[70] The ring provides the least amount of EE exposure when compared with other CHCs.[64] Given the good adherence rates and lower EE levels, the vaginal ring would be appropriate for S.F. if she is comfortable with the dosage form.

Drug Interactions

CASE 47-1, QUESTION 8: S.F. returns to the clinic 2 months later for a sore throat. She indicates that she is using the contraceptive vaginal ring.

Current vitals at clinic: Weight, 132 pounds
Height, 5′4″
Blood pressure, 125/78 mm Hg
Heart rate, 97 beats/minute
Respiratory rate, 16 breaths/minute
Temperature 101.1°F
Physical examination: Head, eyes, ear, nose, and throat: tonsils 2+, bright red, soft palate erythematous

Laboratory test results: Rapid streptococcal antigen test, positive

S.F.'s primary-care physician prescribes Augmentin 875 mg/125 mg (amoxicillin/clavulanate) twice daily by mouth for 10 days. Could this medication affect her contraception? What advice should be provided to S.F.? What other drug interactions are of concern with CHCs?

A variety of drugs may alter the levels of CHCs and in turn affect their efficacy (Table 47-5).[71–74] Currently, most data available regarding drug interactions are with COCs. However, as a precaution the potential drug–drug interactions observed with COCs are also applied to the other CHC dosage formulations (e.g., vaginal ring and transdermal patch).

ANTIBACTERIALS

The antibacterials rifampin and griseofulvin are known to cause contraceptive failure, as these products increase the metabolism of estrogen. For other antibacterials, the possible interaction is more complicated.

EE is conjugated in the liver, excreted in the bile, hydrolyzed by intestinal bacteria, and reabsorbed as active drug.[74] Antibacterials, by reducing the population of intestinal bacteria, interrupt the enterohepatic circulation of the estrogen, resulting

TABLE 47-5
Common Combined Oral Contraceptive Drug[a] Interactions[41,71–73]

Drugs That Increase Effect of CHCs or Side Effects of CHCs	Drugs/Herbals That Decrease the Effect of CHCs	Drugs That *May* Decrease the Effect of CHCs (controversial)	Metabolism or Clearance Altered by CHCs (levels of drug listed may either increase or decrease depending on patient)
Acetaminophen	Amprenavir	Amoxicillin	Acetaminophen
Ascorbic acid	Aprepitant	Ampicillin	Amprenavir
Atazanavir	Barbiturates	Ciprofloxacin	Antidepressants, tricyclic
Atorvastatin	Bexarotene	Clarithromycin	Benzodiazepines
Ginseng	Bosentan	Colesevelam	Beta blockers
Indinavir	Carbamazepine	Doxycycline	Caffeine
Red clover[b]	Darunavir	Erythromycin	Clofibric acid
Rosuvastatin	Efavirez	Fluconazole	Corticosteroids
Tranexamic acid	Felbamate	Itraconazole	Cyclosporine
Voriconazole	Griseofulvin	Ketoconazole	Lamotrigine
	Isotretinoin	Metronidazole	Levothyroxine
	Lopinavir	Minocycline	Morphine
	Modafinil	Penicillins	Paclitaxel
	Mycophenolate mofetil	Phenylbutazone	Salicylic acid
	Nelfinavir	Ofloxacin	Selegiline
	Nevirapine	Tetracyclines	Tacrine
	Oxcarbazepine	Topiramate	Tacrolimus
	Phenobarbital		Theophyllines
	Phenytoin/Fosphenytoin		Tizanidine
	Pioglitazone		Valproic acid
	Primidone		Voriconazole
	Red clover[b]		Warfarin[c]
	Rifamycins		
	Ritonavir		
	Rufinamide		
	Saquinavir		
	St. John's wort		
	Tipranavir		

[a] Drug list is not all inclusive. Some drug interactions may exist that are not cited in this table.
[b] Indicates drug may have variable effect on CHC either increasing or decreasing effect.
[c] May decrease anticoagulant effect of warfarin, not warfarin drug levels.
CHC, combined hormonal contraceptive.
Source: Borgelt L et al., eds. *Women's Health Across the Lifespan: A Pharmacotherapeutic Approach.* Washington DC: American Society of Health Systems Pharmacists; 2010.

in a decreased concentration of circulating estrogen. Theoretically, any antimicrobial with significant effects on intestinal bacterial flora could affect COC efficacy. Numerous reports of changes in bleeding patterns and contraceptive failure have been documented.[74] Cases of pregnancy in COC users taking antibiotics have been reported.[74–76] About 30 case reports of contraceptive failure with concomitant COC and antibiotic use have been published.[74] The antibacterials in the case reports include rifampin, ampicillin, penicillin G, tetracycline, and minocycline. In addition, surveys conducted on patients in clinics have revealed about 20 other cases of COC failure.[74] A major limitation of survey data is that it relies on patient reporting, which is often unreliable.

Some believe that the probability of a clinically significant drug interaction between COCs and antibacterials is low.[9,76,77] Numerous factors also effect the likelihood of an interaction: the hormonal content of the COC relative to the patient's requirements, the dosage and duration of use of the interacting drug, variation in the patient's response to bacterial flora alteration, and the fertility of the couple.[74] The number and complexity of these variables make prediction of outcome in a specific patient exceedingly difficult. Even if a drug produces a several-fold increase in unintended pregnancies in women taking COCs, the likelihood of pregnancy in a given patient still will be low. For patients who require long-term, low-dose tetracycline use for acne therapy (e.g., tetracycline 250 mg by mouth daily), it is unlikely to interfere with COC efficacy.[76] Alternatively, topical antibacterials often can control acne and are viable alternatives to oral medications.

A practical approach to managing patients taking COCs and antibacterials is to educate patients about the available data. To be conservative, S.F. should be advised to use backup contraception while taking the amoxicillin/clavulanate and to continue the backup method until her next menses occurs. For other antibiotics such as rifampin and griseofulvin, backup contraception should be used while taking the medication and for 4 weeks after discontinuation of the antibiotics.[6]

HEPATIC ENZYME INDUCTION

Ethinyl estradiol is a substrate of cytochrome P-450 3A4 (CYP3A4), so drugs that induce CYP3A4 activity may decrease COC efficacy. In earlier years, COC efficacy was not decreased significantly by other drugs because of their high hormone content. Because the estrogen and progestin concentrations of COCs have gradually been decreasing, reports of menstrual irregularities (e.g., spotting) and unintended pregnancies attributable to drug interactions have been increasing.

Anticonvulsants such as carbamazepine, oxcarbazepine, phenytoin, phenobarbital, primidone, and topiramate are CYP3A4 inducers and are known to cause increased metabolism of COCs (see Chapter 58, Seizure Disorders).[78] Some studies have shown that another inducer of COC metabolism is St. John's wort.[79,80] Although drugs can influence COC efficacy, COCs also can affect the activity of other drugs. For example, COCs have been reported to increase or decrease serum levels of lamotrigine and can affect seizure control.[81] Other drugs may increase the hormone levels of COCs (Table 47-5), increasing the risk of COC side effects (Table 47-4).

Unlike many drug classes that are carefully dosed to maintain a therapeutic range of monitored blood levels, contraceptive estrogen and progestin blood levels are obtained only in clinical drug studies. Therefore, patients are managed by monitoring side effects and by changes in menstrual patterns. Some prescribers suggest using a 50-mcg EE COC in patients on interacting drugs, although others might recommend using an alternative method of contraception if drug interactions are an issue.

Noncontraceptive Benefits of Combined Hormonal Contraceptives

ACNE

CASE 47-2

QUESTION 1: D.S., a 20-year-old woman, presents to her primary-care physician for a yearly pelvic examination and also complains of moderate acne flares. She has tried a variety of treatments without resolution and is currently using only topical medications. She heard birth control pills can help acne, especially if it occurs right before her period. She also complains of fatigue most days of the month and mood changes, cravings, cramps, and bloating near the time of her period.

Vitals: Weight, 118 pounds
Height, 5′3″
Blood pressure, 118/75 mm Hg
Heart rate, 86 beats/minute
Respiratory rate, 13 breaths/minute
Temperature, 98.6°F
Past medical history: Acne (since age 16)
Social history: Denies tobacco and alcohol use, not sexually active
Family history: Older sister cervical dysplasia grade 2 (age 26), maternal grandmother breast (age 61) and ovarian cancer (age 68)
Allergies: No known drug allergies
Current medications: Benzoyl peroxide 5% cream, apply topically twice daily
Benzoyl peroxide 2.5% wash, wash affected area twice daily
Retin-A micro 0.1%, apply topically twice a week as tolerated
Multivitamin with iron by mouth daily
Past medications: Doxycycline 100 mg by mouth twice daily for acne, stopped because of vaginal yeast infections
Physical examination: Unremarkable with the exception of moderate facial acne
Laboratory test results: White blood cells, 6.0 × $10^3/\mu L$
Red blood cells, 3.9 × $10^6/\mu L$
Hemoglobin, 10.8 g/dL
Hematocrit, 32%
Mean cell volume, 79 μL
Mean corpuscular hemoglobin concentration, 31 g/dL
Red blood cell diameter width, 15%

What effect, if any, would CHCs have on her acne? Does D.S. qualify for CHC treatment of acne, and if so, which COC would you recommend for D.S.?

Depending on the patient, a CHC may cause acne to appear, disappear, or significantly improve.[6] D.S. is interested in COCs. Four COC products (norethindrone acetate/EE [Estrostep, Estrostep Fe], norgestimate/EE [Ortho Tri-Cyclen], and drospirenone/EE [YAZ, Beyaz]) are US Food and Drug Administration (FDA)-approved for the treatment of moderate acne vulgaris in women at least 15 years old (at least 14 years old for Beyaz and YAZ), who have no known contraindications to CHCs, reached menarche, desire contraception, and have failed topical acne treatments (Estrostep, Estrostep Fe, and Ortho Tri-Cyclen). Most CHCs, however, improve acne mainly as a result of the estrogen component. Higher doses of estrogen may decrease acne by suppressing the activity of sebaceous glands, decreasing the production of androgens, and increasing the synthesis of sex hormone–binding globulin (SHBG). The SHBG binds androgens and thereby diminishes their effects.[82] Progestins with higher androgenic activity may be more likely to increase acne because they stimulate sebaceous glands to produce more sebum. Both desogestrel- and norgestimate-containing oral contraceptives are less androgenic, whereas drospirenone has antiandrogenic properties, thereby decreasing acne associated with androgenic activity.[83,84] D.S. is 20 years old, has reached menarche, and has not responded to different acne treatments, and she therefore is a candidate for COC therapy. Her acne appears to be hormonally mediated, particularly because it appears around the time of her menses. It is likely that D.S.'s acne should improve with COC use, particularly if she uses a formulation with higher estrogenic activity and low androgenic activity (e.g., Beyaz, Safyral YAZ, Yasmin, Ortho Tri-Cyclen, Ortho Tri-Cyclen Lo, Mircette, Estrostep; see Table 47-3).

MENSTRUAL CYCLE BENEFITS

CASE 47-2, QUESTION 2: D.S. has iron-deficiency anemia, likely attributed to heavy menses. Will a COC help reduce her menstrual bleeding or menstrual cramps?

COCs help regulate menstrual cycles and reduce monthly blood loss.[27] This may reflect the progressive thinning of the endometrium of COC users and the lack of irregular bleeding. Bleeding may be decreased the most by COCs that have a high ratio of progestin to estrogen because endometrial thinning is maximized.[55] Some COCs have iron pills instead of placebos, often denoted with "Fe" in the name (e.g., Estrostep Fe, Femcon Fe, Loestrin Fe, Lo Loestrin Fe). Others have folic acid (e.g., Beyaz, Safyral) but D.S. would likely benefit more from the formulations with iron. Another option would be to have D.S. take COCs continuously so she has fewer menses.

Dysmenorrhea, or painful menstruation, may be of unknown origin or may be attributable to endometriosis or uterine fibroids. Data suggest menstrual pain might decrease by 60% after the initiation of a COC.[6] A COC with decreased estrogenic and increased progestational activity may be the best at relieving dysmenorrhea (see Chapter 50, Disorders Related to the Menstrual Cycle).

PREMENSTRUAL SYNDROME AND PREMENSTRUAL DYSPHORIC DISORDER

CASE 47-2, QUESTION 3: D.S. also complains of PMS symptoms such as bloating and mood changes. What treatment approaches are appropriate? What other noncontraceptive benefits do CHCs have?

Premenstrual syndrome (PMS) is a cyclic occurrence of one or more symptoms before the onset of menses. Most women complain of at least one PMS symptom, which include irritability, bloating, and depressed mood.[85] Premenstrual dysphoric disorder (PMDD) is a more severe form of PMS and has diagnostic criteria by the American Psychiatric Association. Premenstrual tension has been reported to be reduced in COC users, and other premenstrual symptoms seem to improve as well. Nevertheless, the effect of COCs on PMS symptoms is inconsistent and unpredictable, probably because PMS symptoms are neither consistent nor predictable.[86]

There may be augmentation of depression and mood swings by the progestational component, although the probability of this effect is low with a low-dose product (see Chapter 50, Disorders Related to the Menstrual Cycle, for further discussion of PMS). Some patients may also notice depressed mood during the hormone-free period, in which case a continuous-use COC may be helpful.

Two products, drospirenone/EE (YAZ, Beyaz), have the FDA-approved indication for treatment of symptoms of PMDD. Drospirenone/EE has been studied most extensively in patients with PMDD.[41] D.S. may try any CHC to help with her PMS symptoms; however, because YAZ and Beyaz have more data to show that they are effective for PMDD and acne, one of them may be the preferred initial product for her. In addition, both products are 24-day formulations, which may help minimize her menstrual bleeding and help her iron-deficiency anemia.

ENDOMETRIAL CANCER

Clinical data suggest that COCs protect against endometrial cancer. This effect continues for 20 years after the last pill.[86] The protection is directly related to duration of use and may persist for many years after discontinuation of the COC.[6] A meta-analysis of 11 studies showed a 56%, 67%, and 72% reduction in endometrial cancer risk after 4, 8, and 12 years of COC use, respectively.[87]

OVARIAN CANCER AND FUNCTIONAL OVARIAN CYSTS

The risk of developing functional ovarian cysts is decreased, preexisting cysts are more rapidly resolved, and surgery rates for ovarian masses are reduced in women taking COCs.[88,89] This is likely attributable to reducing ovulation, suppressing androgen production, or increasing progesterone levels.

Each year of COC use decreases the relative risk of developing ovarian cancer by 7% to 9%.[89] The risk reduction continues to be seen in women using COCs for more than 15 years and persists after discontinuation.[86] D.S. should be reassured that COC use may decrease her risk of ovarian cancer given that she has a positive family history.

Combined Hormonal Contraceptive Risks and Adverse Effects

Some patients may not be candidates for CHCs because of the risks and adverse effects associated with their use. Other patients may experience minor side effects with CHCs that may be managed by changing to a CHC with different types or doses of estrogen or progestin. All patients should be counseled on the most serious side effects, which include pulmonary embolism or VTE, hepatotoxicity, or visual disturbances (could be a sign of retinal and corneal changes in the eye) and stroke. A helpful acronym to remember when counseling is "ACHES" (Table 47-2),[6] which can be used to increase a patient's awareness of serious potential adverse effects that warrant immediate medical attention.

Other less severe adverse effects are listed (Table 47-4).[55] Most side effects resolve within 3 months of use. If a patient experiences adverse effects other than those described in "ACHES," (Table 47-2) she should be encouraged to continue the CHC for at least 3 months before switching to a different contraceptive.

BREAKTHROUGH BLEEDING, SPOTTING, AND AMENORRHEA

CASE 47-2, QUESTION 4: D.S. comes to the family planning clinic after taking EE 20 mcg/drospirenone 3 mg (YAZ) for 2 months. She had been started on YAZ to help with her acne. She feels her acne has improved but reports irregular menstrual bleeding during her last two menstrual cycles that occurs around the third week of the pill pack and requires a

pad. What action should be taken to correct D.S.'s bleeding pattern?

Intermenstrual bleeding is bleeding that occurs at times other than the regular menses timing. Intermenstrual bleeding that requires a pad or tampon is designated breakthrough bleeding, whereas a lesser amount of intermenstrual bleeding is called spotting. Intermenstrual bleeding is the most frequent reason for the discontinuation of COCs.[90] Intermenstrual bleeding may also occur if a patient is not adherent to her COCs or taking medications that decrease COC effectiveness (Table 47-5).

Most clinicians will recommend that patients continue the same COC for at least 3 months if breakthrough bleeding or spotting is the only complaint, because this complication usually resolves within 3 months.[6] Early-cycle intermenstrual bleeding, which usually starts before the 14th day of the menstrual cycle (or never ceases completely after menses), is usually caused by insufficient estrogen. Late-cycle intermenstrual bleeding, occurring after day 14, is usually attributable to insufficient progestational support of the endometrium. Another cause of intermenstrual bleeding is drug interactions (see Case 47-1, Question 8, for more information about drug interactions).

The balance between estrogen and progestin components in COCs determines its endometrial activity and, therefore, the likelihood of intermenstrual bleeding problems. It may be helpful to envision the estrogen component as the basic building blocks or "bricks" of the endometrium and the progestational component providing the mortar that holds the bricks together. The estrogenic activity of the progestin component increases the number of bricks, whereas its antiestrogenic activity decreases their numbers. If there are not enough bricks or mortar or if they are present in the wrong proportions, the wall will crumble and bleeding will occur (Table 47-3).

If D.S.'s intermenstrual bleeding continues late in her cycle after 3 months, another COC with the same estrogen activity, more progestin activity, and low androgen activity should be prescribed. Desogestrel 0.15 mg/EE 30 mcg (Desogen, Ortho-Cept, Apri, Reclipsen) would be a good choice because progestational activity would be increased and estrogenic activity would be maintained with minimal androgenic liability (Table 47-3). If D.S. had experienced intermenstrual bleeding early in the cycle after several months of use, she should be changed to a formulation with a higher ratio of estrogen to progestin such as norethindrone 0.4 mg/EE 35 mcg (Ovcon-35, Femcon Fe, Balziva, Zenchent). For D.S., products with low androgenic activity should be selected because of her acne.

Intermenstrual bleeding may also be the sign of other health conditions such as cervical or uterine cancer. If a patient presents with intermenstrual bleeding and has not had a recent pelvic examination, a health care provider may perform an examination to rule out other possible causes of intermenstrual bleeding. D.S. recently had a normal pelvic examination 2 months ago. Given the timing of when she began her COCs, it is likely her intermenstrual bleeding is caused by her COCs.

Some patients experience amenorrhea (no menstrual bleeding) with CHCs. If this occurs, pregnancy should first be ruled out. If the patient is not pregnant and amenorrhea is acceptable to the patient, then the CHC need not be changed. But this does make it difficult for the patient to recognize if she may become pregnant in the future.

NAUSEA

CASE 47-2, QUESTION 5: D.S. continues to have intermenstrual bleeding late in her cycle after 3 months of use and is placed on a new COC. Five days after starting norethindrone 0.4 mg/EE 35 mcg (Ovcon-35), D.S. calls with complaints of nausea. What counseling should the clinician provide to D.S.?

Nausea from COCs can generally be attributed to the estrogen component. About 38% of women in one study reported nausea as the reason for discontinuing using COCs.[91] To help alleviate nausea, D.S. can take her pill at bedtime rather than in the morning. Another alternative may be to take it with food or to try another COC with a lower estrogen strength or property. Ovcon-35 has a higher amount of EE as compared with YAZ (35 mcg of EE vs. 20 mcg of EE), which may be causing D.S.'s nausea. D.S. should be advised that nausea generally resolves within 3 months of use.

HEADACHE

CASE 47-2, QUESTION 6: Three months later, D.S. returns to the clinic for follow-up and states that she has daily headaches during her placebo week but not when she is taking active pills. How should she be managed?

Headache is a common complaint in women taking CHCs or COCs, as is the case with D.S. Women may notice headaches while taking active pills, which may be related to sensitivity of estrogen. Others may experience headaches during the placebo week as a result of the withdrawal of estrogen.[90] Women with migraines may find that their headaches either improve or worsen when CHCs are initiated.

Mild headaches may improve with time or if the woman is changed to a pill with less estrogen or progestin. Headaches that occur during the placebo week can be managed by trying desogestrel 0.15 mg/EE 10 to 20 mcg (Mircette, Kariva), which minimizes the estrogen withdrawal by having only 2 days of placebos, or by taking CHCs continuously (i.e., skipping placebo pills or the hormone-free week). Patients with severe headaches should discontinue CHCs and should be evaluated by their health care provider (see Contraindications above). D.S. is experiencing headaches during the placebo week, indicating withdrawal of estrogen as the cause. Skipping the placebo pills and using an extended-cycle regimen may help decrease D.S.'s headaches.

WEIGHT GAIN

CASE 47-2, QUESTION 7: During the same visit D.S. states she is gaining weight and feels "bloated on and off" since starting the new birth control pill. What might be happening, and how should the clinician respond?

Weight gain associated with CHC use is another common concern for women. A few studies concluded that women using low-dose CHCs did not experience weight gain.[92,93] A Cochrane review of three trials concluded that available evidence was insufficient to determine an association between COCs and weight gain and also stated no large effect was seen.[94] If weight gain is a concern, a low-dose estrogen and low-dose progestin product should be considered. Cyclic weight gain is generally caused by the mineralocorticoid effects of EE stimulating aldosterone receptors to retain sodium, causing water retention and bloating. Too much progestin may cause an increased appetite and noncyclic weight gain. Drospirenone with antimineralocorticoid properties opposes EE effects, resulting in less water retention and weight gain, and increases in appetite may not be as apparent. D.S. recently increased her estrogen dose, which may be causing the "on and off" bloated feeling and weight gain. She also stopped taking a drospirenone-containing product, which may be why she did not experience the effects of bloating and weight gain with the previous product. The clinician should explain that weight gain is a potential side effect associated with COC use and is likely related to the estrogen component. It is reasonable to consider an alternative COC because she is having estrogen withdrawal headaches and weight gain. Desogestrel/EE 10 to 20 mcg (Mircette) has lower estrogen activity than norethindrone 0.4 mg/EE 35 mcg (Ovcon-35; Table 47-3), which may help to decrease the cyclic weight gain and headaches while still helping to control her acne. In addition, Mircette retains high progestational activity to address D.S.'s previous breakthrough bleeding and has low androgenic activity that will likely help her acne.

BREAST CANCER, CERVICAL DYSPLASIA, AND CERVICAL CANCER

CASE 47-2, QUESTION 8: The medical history and physical examination of D.S. are negative for breast and cervical diseases, except for a history of breast cancer in her maternal grandmother and a history of cervical dysplasia in her sister. D.S. asks how COC use will affect her risk of breast cancer and cervical cancer.

There are conflicting data regarding the association of COC use and breast cancer. The reported overall lifetime risk of breast cancer in American women is 12% to 13%.[95] Older studies have indicated a possible link between COC use and breast cancer.[96–99] More recent studies suggest that COC use does not increase breast cancer risk even with long-term use (e.g., 10 years).[100–102] In addition, other studies concluded breast cancer rates in high-risk women with BRCA 1 and 2 mutations or strong family history of breast cancer did not increase with COC use.[103,104] The American Congress of Obstetricians and Gynecologists (ACOG) does not consider a family history of breast cancer (including BRCA 1 and 2) or benign breast disease a contraindication to COC use.[25]

COCs would not be expected to increase the risk of breast cancer in D.S. She should be instructed to perform monthly breast self-examinations and to return annually for a physical examination by her primary-care physician.

With regard to D.S.'s concern of cervical cancer, it is important to educate D.S. about the incidence of cervical cancer and its relation to COC use. The American Cancer Society estimates that more than 12,000 cases of invasive cervical cancer will be diagnosed in 2010 and more than 4,000 women will die of it.[105] Behavior, not genetics, is the usual cause of cervical cancer. Women at highest risk for cancer are those who are positive for certain subtypes of human papillomavirus (HPV), who have certain sexual behaviors, who are immunosuppressed, or who smoke.[6] Sexual behaviors associated with cervical cancer include beginning sexual activity at a young age, having multiple male sexual partners, and having a male sexual partner who has had multiple partners. Women at low risk for cancer are those who have two or fewer partners, whose partners use condoms, and who do not smoke.

Pooled data on cervical cancer risk from eight case-control studies found that oral contraceptive users positive for HPV were more likely to develop cervical cancer.[106] Women who had ever used oral contraceptives and those who had used oral contraceptives for more than 5 years were 1.5 and 3.4 times, respectively, more likely to develop cervical cancer. This is consistent with older studies that suggest that oral contraceptive users have an increased risk of developing or dying of cervical cancer. In contrast, a large cohort study conducted in England found no significant increase in deaths attributable to cervical cancer in women who had ever used COCs.[107]

Epidemiologic comparisons of the prevalence of cervical cancer in oral contraceptive users versus nonusers often are difficult to interpret because yearly medical examinations and regular Pap smears of COC users result in early detection and treatment of precancerous lesions. Two vaccines for HPV are available for women ages 9 to 27 years old. Because D.S. is 20 years old, she may be a candidate for the HPV vaccine (see Chapter 11, Vaccinations). D.S. may use COCs, should be encouraged to have regular Pap smears, and should be counseled on the behaviors that put her at risk for cervical cancer and the risks and benefits of the HPV vaccine.

USE DURING PREGNANCY AND BREAST-FEEDING

CASE 47-3

QUESTION 1: P.K., a 35-year-old woman, comes to clinic stating that she recently took a home pregnancy test that reported a positive result. Her last menstrual period (LMP) was 9 weeks ago. She would like to confirm the results and discuss the effects of her current medications on her unborn baby.

Vitals: Weight, 143 pounds
Height, 5′6″
Blood pressure, 128/82 mm Hg
Heart rate, 97 beats/minute
Respiratory rate, 16 breaths/minute
Temperature, 98.6°F
Past medical history: History of abnormal menses, initiated on COC therapy to help regulate
Medications: Desogestrel 0.15 mg/EE 30 mcg (Ortho-Cept)
Laboratory test results: Blood test, qualitative human chorionic gonadotropin > 25 mIU/mL

P.K. was started on Desogestrel 0.15 mg/EE 30 mcg (Ortho-Cept) extended regimen 3 months ago because of a history of abnormal menstrual periods. Unknowingly, she became pregnant in the first month and continued her COC for two cycles and is now 8 weeks' pregnant. What can you tell P.K. about the possible effects of CHC use on her unborn child?

The fact that CHCs are classified as pregnancy category X (contraindicated, fetal risks clearly outweigh maternal benefit) is very misleading.[108] Although older, poorly designed studies found an association between COC use and cardiac or limb anomalies, newer data suggest that CHC use does not substantially increase the risk of anomalies over that expected in other uneventful pregnancies.[6]

Although a CHC should not be started in a woman who might possibly be pregnant, P.K. should be instructed to stop using her COC and be reassured that the risks to her fetus from the use of a low-dose CHC during the first trimester are likely minimal, while also informing her no drug is without risk and she should follow up with her obstetrician.

CASE 47-3, QUESTION 2: P.K. plans to breast-feed her infant and begin some type of contraception after her discharge from the hospital. Her past experience with condoms and concurrent spermicidal foams or gels resulted in itching and burning. She indicates she would like a contraceptive that would be suitable for long-term use while

breast-feeding. What contraceptives are best for her while she is breast-feeding?

P.K. may use CHCs 6 weeks after she has her baby even if she is breast-feeding, although it is preferable for her to use a progestin-only method.[25] The ACOG recommends waiting at least 6 weeks before starting any estrogen-containing contraceptive regardless of breast-feeding status. By this time, the increased risk of thrombosis that occurs during pregnancy should be reduced to baseline. For non–breast-feeding women, a progestin-only contraceptive may be used immediately postpartum and 6 weeks postpartum if solely breast-feeding and in some cases 3 weeks postpartum if partially breast-feeding.[25] However, COCs have been reported to decrease milk quantity and quality.[25] Therefore, many providers suggest avoiding CHCs in women who are exclusively breast-feeding. If P.K. is planning to breast-feed, a progestin-only contraceptive is probably best and may be started 6 weeks postpartum to ensure the newborn is able to metabolize and clear the medication because progestins enter breast milk.

PROGESTIN-ONLY CONTRACEPTIVES

Progestin-Only Pill (Minipill)

CASE 47-3, QUESTION 3: What advantages and disadvantages of the minipill should you discuss with P.K.?

ADVANTAGES

The minipill is devoid of some of the nuisance side effects (Table 47-4) caused by estrogen (e.g., headaches, chloasma).[6] More importantly, estrogen-mediated hypertension and clotting factor changes will be avoided. Confusion with pill taking is minimized because there is no placebo week and all 28 pills in each pack are the same. Therefore, the missed-dose directions are the same whenever any pill is missed. Minipills also have noncontraceptive benefits, including decreased dysmenorrhea and bleeding and possible protection against pelvic inflammatory disease (PID) and endometrial cancer.[6] Women may also choose them because they are not estrogen containing and fertility returns rapidly after discontinuation.[6]

Theoretically, progestin use in the early postpartum period may decrease milk production because milk production is triggered by the decline in progesterone that occurs after delivery. However, no data have consistently shown this to be a problem in postpartum women.[25] Once breast-feeding has been established, progestins have not been shown to interfere with the quantity or quality of milk produced by a nursing mother. Thus, a contraceptive method that is nonhormonal or only contains progestin is preferred for a patient who plans to breast-feed her infant.

DISADVANTAGES

The minipill, with a failure rate of 0.3% to 8%, is similarly effective as COCs in preventing pregnancies (Table 47-1).[6] Minipills however, must be taken even more regularly than COCs, and therefore are not used often in women who are not breast-feeding (see Patient Instructions below). Some women on minipills ovulate regularly, and some shift back and forth between ovulatory and anovulatory (no ovulation occurring) menstrual cycles. Women who consistently have menses on the minipill may be ovulating and should consider using a backup contraception or changing to a different method.

Irregular menses, decreased duration and amount of menstrual flow, spotting, or amenorrhea commonly occurs in women taking the minipill.[6] Because of this, patients often are concerned that they may be pregnant. Women who are exclusively breast-feeding will usually have amenorrhea. The high incidence of irregular menses associated with the minipill may mask underlying disease such as uterine fibroids or uterine cancer causing irregular bleeding. Other side effects reported with minipills include headaches, breast tenderness, mood changes, and nausea.

Minipills should be avoided if there is a personal history of breast cancer or unexplained vaginal bleeding. Caution should be exercised when using minipills in women with hepatic disease, multiple risk factors for cardiovascular diseases, ischemic heart disease, a current deep venous thrombosis or PE, or complicated diabetes (e.g., diabetes with nephropathy, neuropathy, retinopathy), or those taking medications that may interact with COCs such as hepatic inducers, St. John's wort, and Bosentan (Table 47-5).[109,110]

PATIENT INSTRUCTIONS FOR THE PROGESTIN-ONLY PILL

CASE 47-3, QUESTION 4: What instructions should P.K. receive regarding the use of a minipill?

P.K. may begin taking the minipill on the first day of her menses.[6] Because she is breast-feeding and recently postpartum, she is less likely to have a menses. She could begin taking minipills immediately postpartum if she were not breast-feeding. Because she is breast-feeding, it is recommended that she wait until 3 weeks postpartum if partially breast-feeding and 6 weeks postpartum to begin minipills if solely breast-feeding. If at 6 weeks postpartum, P.K. started her minipills on the first day of her menses, a backup contraception is not needed with the day 1 start. Alternatively, P.K. can use the quick start method; starting any day of her cycle and using a backup method for 48 hours.[6]

P.K. should be instructed to take the pill at the exact same time each day. If she is more than 3 hours late taking a pill, she should take the pill as soon as she remembers and should use backup contraception for 48 hours. This is quite different from the directions for COCs, so this point should be stressed with patients.

Injectable Medroxyprogesterone Acetate

Progestin-only contraceptives are available in two different injectable formulations of medroxyprogesterone acetate (MPA). Depo-Provera is given as a 150-mg intramuscular injection in the deltoid or gluteus maximus every 11 to 13 weeks.[6,111] Since its development in the early 1960s, Depo-Provera has been approved for use in more than 90 countries and has been used by more than 30 million women worldwide.[112] More recently, depo-subQ provera 104 was approved. This product also contains MPA; however, it is given subcutaneously as a 104-mg dose every 12 to 14 weeks.[113] Injectable MPA inhibits ovulation, thickens the cervical mucus, and suppresses endometrial growth, making it a very effective contraceptive. Package inserts instruct the patient to begin the injectable MPA methods in the first 5 days of her menses and then no backup is required; however, P.K. may also begin any other time and use backup for 1 week.[6,111]

CASE 47-3, QUESTION 5: P.K. is now lactating and returns to the gynecology clinic for her second IM injection of

MPA. She was given her first injection 3 months ago, immediately postpartum. She is experiencing prolonged intermenstrual bleeding and a 3- to 5-pound weight gain. Is this to be expected? What are the advantages and disadvantages of injectable MPA? How are the side effects managed?

ADVANTAGES

Injectable MPA is a reasonable contraceptive choice for P.K. because she is breast-feeding and indicated she needed a long-term contraceptive. Among its benefits are a low failure rate of 0.3% to 3% (Table 47-1), ease of use, lack of estrogenic side effects, decreased dysmenorrhea and monthly blood loss, and a reduced risk of endometrial cancer.[6,25] Other noncontraceptive benefits may include a reduction in seizure frequency in epileptic patients and a possible reduction in ovarian cancer.[6,25] Furthermore, contraceptive efficacy is not reduced by the concurrent use of anticonvulsants or certain antibacterials as is seen with COCs.[9] Depo-subQ provera 104 is also indicated for pain caused by endometriosis.[113]

DISADVANTAGES

Patients with breast cancer should not use injectable MPA owing to concerns that breast cancers are hormonally sensitive and the prognosis may worsen for some women.[9] Injectable MPA should be used with caution in women with unexplained vaginal bleeding (MPA may cause irregular bleeding and may mask conditions resulting in vaginal bleeding such as cervical or uterine cancer), multiple risk factors for cardiovascular diseases, ischemic heart disease or multiple risk factors for cerebrovascular disease, or a current VTE or PE (for medical eligibility, see **http://who.int/reproductivehealth/publications/family_planning/9789241563888/en/index.html**).[9] Because clotting factors have not been shown to be clinically affected by injectable MPA, some experts disagree with the manufacturer's labeling for the injectable MPA products, which lists a history of prior thromboembolism as a contraindication.[8,9,111,113] Some clinicians also begin injectable MPA immediately postpartum rather than waiting 6 weeks postpartum, as directed by the package insert.[24] Patients given injectable MPA immediately postpartum are more likely to report frequent episodes of bleeding or spotting, however.[114,115]

Estrogen production declines in women using injectable MPA, so P.K. should be told that injectable MPA may decrease bone mineral density (BMD).[111] Loss of BMD may be of particular concern in adolescent patients. Numerous studies have found that women receiving injectable MPA have lower BMD compared with nonusers.[116] Although there have been reports of stress fractures in injectable MPA users, no studies to date have documented an increased rate of hip or vertebral fractures in injectable MPA users.[117] Also, BMD has been shown to recover after discontinuation of the injections.[118,119] The manufacturer of both products recommends that patients do not use injectable MPA longer than 2 years unless they are unwilling or unable to use other methods.[111]

P.K. must understand that injectable MPA frequently causes irregular bleeding or spotting during the first few months or more of use because estrogen is insufficient to maintain the endometrium. After 1 and 2 years of Depo Provera use, 55% and 68% of women experience amenorrhea, respectively.[111] With depo-subQ provera 104, 56.5% of patients experienced amenorrhea after 1 year.[113] In addition, during the postpartum period irregular bleeding may occur as well. Although not harmful, amenorrhea leads to discontinuation of injectable MPA in 13% of patients.[111] All patients beginning injectable MPA should be informed that during the first year of use they might have menstrual changes. If unusually heavy or continuous bleeding occurs, P.K. should be evaluated. P.K. should be counseled and reassured that her intermenstrual bleeding probably will resolve in the next few months. If the bleeding is bothersome, a 4- to 21-day course of oral estrogen (e.g., conjugated estrogen 0.625 to 2.5 mg/day) or a COC with 20 mcg of EE will minimize or eliminate the bleeding.[8] However, the bleeding may recur after discontinuation of the estrogen. Low-dose estrogen may be continued if bleeding recurs.

Weight gain is another concern with injectable MPA. The mean weight gain after 1 year of therapy with injectable MPA was about 5 pounds in two-thirds of users.[111] Depo-Provera users typically gain a total of about 8 pounds in 2 years, nearly 14 pounds in 4 years, and 16.5 pounds in 6 years. Depo-subQ provera users gain a little less weight, 3.5 pounds in the first year of use and 7.5 pounds after 2 years.[113] Other side effects include mood changes, hair loss, and headaches. P.K. should be counseled on the weight gain associated with injectable MPA. P.K. has already reported an increase in weight since she gave birth 3 months ago, which may be caused by injectable MPA, or possibly her weight is fluctuating because of her recent delivery.

The long return to fertility time is another disadvantage of injectable MPA. After the last injection of 150 mg of MPA, conception was delayed approximately 10 months in half of users.[104] The remaining users took longer to become pregnant, with nearly all users becoming pregnant by 18 months. There are less data on return of fertility with the 104-mg dose of MPA. A small study showed that the median time to ovulation was 10 months, with most women ovulating within 1 year of their last injection.[113] Because P.K. is 35 years old, she should be counseled on the return to fertility time with injectable MPA use in case she desired to have children in the near future. She has indicated that she is not interested in having any more children; however, the long return to fertility time with injectable MPA should be explained to all women, especially those older than 35 years of age.

Subdermal Implant

CASE 47-3, QUESTION 6: P.K. returns to the clinic 7 months postpartum for her third MPA injection. She started menstruating today after missing two appointments; she is now 1 month late for her MPA dose. She states her busy family life and work schedule make it difficult to attend appointments. She also does not like the weight gain and prolonged intermenstrual bleeding that has occurred during the past few months. She read that an implant is available and she would like to know whether this might be a better option for her. What information should you give P.K.?

The contraceptive implant (Implanon) contains 68 mg of etonogestrel in a single, thin rod.[120] The rod is inserted subdermally in the upper inner arm using a needle and a local anesthetic. Once inserted, the implant is effective for up to 3 years. A small incision is required to remove the implant. The etonogestrel implant has the same mechanism of action as injectable MPA. Implanon should be inserted during the first 5 days of menses and no backup contraception is required.

ADVANTAGES

The contraceptive implant is a relatively new product, so information on its protection against cancers or effects on other diseases such as cardiovascular disease is limited. Women using the implant reported amenorrhea, decreased menstrual cramping, and less anemia than nonusers.[6] Also, decreases in BMD have not been shown with this product. Fertility returns quickly after the removal of the implant, and this will be a benefit to P.K. if she decides to have another child, given her age.

DISADVANTAGES

As with the injectables, irregular bleeding is likely and is the most common cause of discontinuation. Side effects reported with the implant are headaches, mood changes, and acne. Implanon is not recommended for patients on medications that induce hepatic enzymes (e.g., anticonvulsants) as they may decrease contraceptive efficacy.[120] Weight gain is also common, with users gaining 2.8 pounds after 1 year and 3.7 pounds after 2 years.[121] So P.K. may still experience weight gain with this product. The implant is not recommended for patients with a current VTE; however, it may be used in patients with a personal or family history of VTE.[9]

INTRAUTERINE DEVICE AND INTRAUTERINE SYSTEM

CASE 47-3, QUESTION 7: P.K. is concerned about weight gain and is not interested in a subdermal implant. What other long-term, reversible contraceptive methods might work for her? Is P.K. a candidate for an intrauterine device (IUD) or intrauterine system (IUS), and if so, what information would you provide her?

Background and Mechanism of Action

Despite concerns (increased risk of PID, tubal scarring, and infertility) with early IUDs, also known as intrauterine contraceptives (IUCs), the current devices offer a safe and effective method of contraception.[121] The ParaGard T 380A (copper) IUD was introduced in 1988 and the Mirena (levonorgestrel) IUS in 2000. Although the IUDs and IUSs available today are a safe and effective method of contraception, they are still not as popular in the United States (1%–6% of women are users) as they are worldwide (12% of married women of reproductive age are users).[122–124]

The copper IUD has a polyethylene body that is wound with copper wire. Once inserted, the copper IUD may be left in place for 10 years.[125] The levonorgestrel IUS also has a polyethylene body, with a levonorgestrel reservoir in the vertical stem of the T that provides 20 mcg of levonorgestrel daily and is effective for 5 years.[126]

ONLINE CONTENT

For a visual of a copper IUC, see the PowerPoint presentation at http://thepoint.lww.com/AT10e.

Failure rate of the copper IUD is 0.6% to 0.8% for the first year compared with 0.2% for the levonorgestrel IUS (Table 47-1). Both IUDs and IUSs are inserted by a health care provider in the office. The procedure usually takes only a few minutes and does not require sedation. Many providers will recommend that patients take a dose of an NSAID before the insertion visit.

Possible mechanisms of action for copper IUDs include prevention of fertilization and implantation and the copper interfering with sperm transport, viability, or number.[126] The levonorgestrel IUS is believed to work by thickening the cervical mucus, preventing sperm from entering the uterus, altering the endometrial lining, preventing ovulation, and altering sperm activity.[126]

Advantages

Both the copper IUD and the levonorgestrel IUS are very effective, reversible, long-term methods that are easy to comply with.[6] The copper IUD is a particularly beneficial option for women who desire a nonhormonal method of contraception. The levonorgestrel IUS has the advantages of reducing menstrual bleeding and cramping as a result of the progestin.

Although the initial cost of inserting an IUD or IUS is high (around $500 for the device plus insertion costs), there are no ongoing monthly costs to P.K. as there are with other methods. Therefore, the IUD or IUS becomes more cost effective when used for more than 1 year.

Disadvantages

Menstrual changes are the most common side effect of IUDs and IUSs.[6] Copper IUD users are more likely to have heavier menstrual bleeding and cramping. Levonorgestrel users should expect to have irregular bleeding and spotting during the first 3 months after insertion. After 3 months, however, levonorgestrel IUS users report lighter menses and reduced cramping.

Both IUDs and IUSs are contraindicated in women with certain anatomic abnormalities of the uterus (e.g., distortion of the uterus, cervical stenosis, or cervical lacerations), unexplained vaginal bleeding, cervical cancer, and PID or other active genital infection. They should be used with caution in women who are HIV positive or are immunosuppressed (for medical eligibility, see http://www.who.int/reproductivehealth/publications/family_planning/9789241563888/en/index.html).[9] The levonorgestrel IUS should be used with caution in women with a current VTE or PE. Although the serum levels of levonorgestrel are low, the manufacturer currently does not recommend that women with active or past breast cancer use the device.

Both IUDs and IUSs are preferred for women in monogamous relationships or who are able to have strict use of condoms as IUD users are more likely to experience PID than nonusers. For all patients, the greatest risk of PID occurs shortly after insertion.[127] To prevent this from occurring, all patients should be tested for gonorrhea and chlamydia before IUD or IUS insertion and evaluated for risk factors of contracting STIs (e.g., multiple partners, unprotected intercourse). Women who are positive for an STI should consider an alternative form of contraception. Alternatively, once treatment is provided, an IUD or IUS may be initiated and the woman counseled on ways to prevent STIs.[9]

If an IUD or IUS user becomes pregnant, the likelihood that the pregnancy is ectopic is higher (i.e., the ratio of ectopic to uterine pregnancies is higher in IUD or IUS users).[125,126] Common complaints of IUD use include excessive uterine bleeding, spotting, or pain. The device may be removed as a result of these issues. Spontaneous expulsion of the IUD occurs in about 2% to 6% of women within the first year.[6] Rarely, IUDs or IUSs may become embedded in the endometrium or partially or totally perforate the uterine wall. P.K. should be instructed to look for the warning signs of a possible complication with IUD or IUS use, such as abdominal pain or abnormal vaginal discharge.

OTHER NONHORMONAL CONTRACEPTION

CASE 47-4

QUESTION 1: C.J. is a 22-year-old HIV+ woman presenting to the clinic for routine checkup and depot medroxyprogesterone acetate injection. She is currently using

a new dose of spermicide should be applied before each act of intercourse.

Spermicides may cause genital irritation and in some patients lead to ulceration. Likely for this reason, spermicides have been shown to increase the transmission of STIs, including HIV, gonorrhea, and chlamydia. Spermicides may not be the best choice for C.J. and her partner to prevent the risk of STI transmission.

EMERGENCY CONTRACEPTION

CASE 47-4, QUESTION 3: C.J. presents to a pharmacy 4 months later and says she missed her MPA injection last month. She had intercourse 4 nights ago with a condom and is worried she might become pregnant. She wants to know whether she should use the "morning-after pill." What do you tell C.J. about emergency contraception options? Is C.J. a candidate for emergency contraception?

Emergency contraception (EC), also referred to as the morning-after pill, is postcoital contraception useful for women who did not use a contraceptive (e.g., forgot, were assaulted) or whose method failed (e.g., broken condom, missed pill). Emergency contraception is available in a few methods, which include oral pills or an IUD.

Emergency Contraception Pills

Emergency contraceptive pills (ECPs) are available in a variety of formulations known as progestin-only, Yuzpe, and progesterone receptor modulators.

Next Choice and Plan B–One Step are the currently marketed progestin-only ECPs.[131] Next Choice is a generic product of the brand formerly known as Plan B and consists of two white levonorgestrel 0.75-mg pills. According to the packaging, one tablet is taken as soon as possible within 72 hours of unprotected intercourse, and the second is taken 12 hours later. Studies, however, have shown that progestin-only ECPs are still effective if taken up to 120 hours (5 days) after unprotected sex and if both pills are taken together in a single dose.[131,132] Most women's health providers give patients these instructions to increase adherence. Plan B–One Step is formulated into one tablet consisting of levonorgestrel 1.5 mg that can be taken at one time within the same time frame as Next Choice.

Progestin-only ECPs reduce the risk of pregnancy by a few potential mechanisms: preventing ovulation, preventing fertilization, or preventing implantation.[6] They reduce the average risk of pregnancy by 89% after a single act of intercourse when taken within 72 hours. ECPs are most effective when taken as soon as possible after intercourse; therefore, treatment should not be delayed. The most common side effects with ECPs are nausea and vomiting.[6] C.J. should be instructed that if she vomits within 1 hour of taking ECPs, the dose should be repeated. C.J.'s menses may come early or late, but she should take a pregnancy test if her menses does not come within 3 weeks of taking ECPs. This may further be complicated if C.J. gets her next scheduled dose of injectable MPA.

Progestin-only ECPs are currently over-the-counter to those older than 17 years old, sold at pharmacies, and stored behind the pharmacy counter. Purchasers must show an ID for proof of age. Both products are also still available by prescription for women younger than 17.

As an alternative to progestin-only ECPs, regular COCs may be used as long as they contain levonorgestrel or norgestrel as the progestin. This is known as the Yuzpe method, which consists of high-dose progestin and high-dose estrogen. There are no marketed formulations of this method. Depending on the brand of COCs used, a differing number of pills are taken within 120 hours of unprotected intercourse as two separate doses 12 hours apart (see Table 47-1 footnote).[6] Compared with progestin-only ECPs, the Yuzpe method is associated with higher incidence of nausea and vomiting, and patients may wish to take an antiemetic before each dose.[131] Because progestin-only ECPs are widely available, easy to use, and more effective and have limited side effects, COCs are being used less often for EC.

A newer ECP classified as an oral selective progesterone receptor modulator (SPRM), ulipristal acetate (Ella), was recently approved for use in the United States.[133] The 30-mg oral tablet should be taken within 120 hours of unprotected intercourse.[134] It is available by prescription only. Its mechanism of action is somewhat different from that of progestin-only ECPs. It has progesterone receptor antagonist and agonist effects; however, its main mechanism is through receptor antagonism at the uterus, cervix, hypothalamus, and ovaries, thus preventing ovulation even after the LH surge, which progestin-only ECPs may not do.[135] The only other SPRM on the market is mifepristone (RU-486), known for medical abortion use. Concerns were raised about the mechanism of ulipristal disrupting an existing pregnancy and leading to abortion. Current pregnancy exposure data do not suggest an increase in miscarriage. Headache, dysmenorrhea, nausea, and abdominal pain were the most reported side effects in clinical trials.[133–135] If nausea occurs within 3 hours of taking the dose, a repeat dose is recommended.[132]

In C.J.'s case, progestin-only ECPs are the better choice because she is taking medications that interact with COCs. She is within the window of 120 hours postcoitus and older than 17 years of age, therefore making over-the-counter progestin-only ECPs an option. If approved, ulipristal would require a prescription and may delay C.J. from receiving timely emergency contraception.

Intrauterine Devices for Emergency Contraception

The copper-T IUD is also an effective method of emergency contraception when inserted within 5 days of unprotected sex.[6,131] There is no evidence that the progestin IUD is effective. Because some women are not good candidates for IUDs (see discussion above) and IUDs must be inserted by a health care provider, they are not used as regularly for emergency contraception. The biggest advantage of using an IUD for emergency contraception is that it provides continued contraception for the patient. Because C.J. is HIV positive, an IUD may not be the best choice for her due to infection risk. Also, having to see a provider for an IUD is less convenient and makes ECPs the better choice for accessibility and timing.

MEDICAL ABORTION

CASE 47-4, QUESTION 4: C.J. presents to the clinic 4 weeks later stating that she missed her period and is concerned she may be pregnant. Her human chorionic gonadotropin test is positive, confirming pregnancy. C.J. considers terminating the pregnancy, stating she is not ready to have a child and is concerned about the antiretroviral medication effects on the baby. What options are there for medical abortion?

It is estimated that about one-half of pregnancies are unintended, so it is important for these women to have safe options.[3] C.J. should be counseled extensively about her options, including keeping the baby, adoption, and medical or surgical abortion. Compared with surgical abortion, medical abortion does not require a surgical procedure, so it is less likely to cause infection and is less costly.[6] Thus, some women feel more in control when choosing this option. However, some patients may not prefer medical abortion because it usually requires more medical visits and follow-up, has a slightly lower success rate (94%–97%; failures will need a surgical procedure), and involves more bleeding and cramping that usually lasts for 2 weeks.

There are many variations in how medical abortions are carried out, but the general treatment remains the same.[6] C.J. would first obtain baseline laboratory tests, including blood type and hemoglobin. She would be given either methotrexate, mifepristone, or both that same day to stop development of the pregnancy. In the United States, mifepristone, a progesterone receptor blocker, is more commonly used. Misoprostol is given to induce uterine contractions and expel the pregnancy.

Typically for a gestational age of 63 days or less, C.J. would be given mifepristone 200 mg orally on day 1, then misoprostol 800 mcg vaginally on day 2 or 3 (6 to 72 hours after the mifepristone dose).[6] Misoprostol may also be given as 400 or 600 mcg orally or buccally with higher doses of mifepristone (600 mg orally).[6,136–138] If using methotrexate, 50 mg/m^2 is given IM on day 1 followed by misoprostol 800 mcg vaginally 3 to 7 days later.[6] Side effects may include nausea, vomiting, diarrhea, cramping, and vaginal bleeding (heavier than a menses). With either method, patients should follow up with their health care provider on about day 15 to make sure the abortion is complete. If complete miscarriage has not occurred, another method may be used, such as aspiration, to remove all pregnancy tissue.

KEY REFERENCES AND WEBSITES

A full list of references for this chapter can be found at http://thepoint.lww.com/AT10e. Below are the key references and websites for this chapter, with the corresponding reference number in this chapter found in parentheses after the reference.

Key References

ACOG Committee on Practice Bulletins-Gynecology. ACOG practice bulletin. No. 73: Use of hormonal contraception in women with coexisting medical conditions. *Obstet Gynecol.* 2006; 107:1453–1472. (25)

ACOG practice bulletin No. 110: Noncontraceptive uses of hormonal contraceptives. *Obstet Gynecol.* 2010;115:206–218. (86)

American College of Obstetricians and Gynecologists. ACOG Practice Bulletin No. 112: Emergency contraception. *Obstet Gynecol.* 2010;115:1100–1109. (131)

Dickey RP. *Managing Contraceptive Pill Patients.* 14th ed. Dallas, TX: Essential Medical Information Systems; 2010. (55)

Hatcher RA et al. *Contraceptive Technology.* 19th ed. New York, NY: Ardent Media Inc; 2008. (6)

Zieman M et al. *Managing Contraception for Your Pocket 2010–2012.* Tiger, GA: Bridging the Gap Communications; 2010. (8)

Key Websites

Association of Reproductive Health Professionals. http://www.arhp.org/.

The Emergency Contraception Website. http://ec.princeton.edu.

Guttmacher Institute. http://www.guttmacher.org. (123)

International Consortium for Emergency Contraception. http://www.cecinfo.org/.

Planned Parenthood Federation of America. http://www.plannedparenthood.org/. (121)

US Medical Eligibility Criteria for Contraceptive Use, 2010. Adapted from the World Health Organization Medical Eligibility Criteria for Contraceptive Use, 4th ed. http://www.cdc.gov/Mmwr/preview/mmwrhtml/rr59e0528a1.htm.

A WHO Family Planning Cornerstone. Medical Eligibility Criteria for Contraceptive Use. 4th ed. 2009. Geneva: World Health Organization; 2010. http://www.who.int/reproductivehealth/publications/family_planning/9789241563888/en/index.html. (9)

48 Infertility

Erin C. Raney

CORE PRINCIPLES

		CHAPTER CASES
1	Infertility is the inability to conceive after twelve months of unprotected intercourse. A major predictor of infertility is the age of the woman. Additional risk factors for both men and women include lifestyle factors, such as tobacco use and obesity, as well as primary and secondary causes of hypogonadism.	**Case 48-1 (Questions 1–3, 6), Case 48-2 (Questions 1, 2)**
2	The evaluation of infertility in women incorporates data from physical examination and laboratory assessments of pituitary and ovarian function. In men, the semen analysis and laboratory assessments of hormone levels provide key information related to gonadal function.	**Case 48-1 (Questions 3–5, 7), Case 48-2 (Questions 1, 2)**
3	Unexplained infertility is diagnosed after a thorough evaluation of both the man and woman reveals no identifiable cause. Treatment is empiric and often combines controlled ovarian stimulation with intrauterine insemination or in vitro fertilization.	**Case 48-1 (Questions 8–12)**
4	Clomiphene citrate is a selective estrogen receptor modulator that is considered a first-line agent for controlled ovarian stimulation in patients with unexplained fertility. Aromatase inhibitors are under investigation as alternative oral agents.	**Case 48-1 (Questions 9–12)**
5	In vitro fertilization is the most commonly used assisted reproductive technology, or procedure that involves manipulation of oocytes and sperm. Medications are used to stimulate multiple follicles for oocyte retrieval and to optimize implantation after embryo transfer.	**Case 48-2 (Questions 3–9)**
6	Controlled ovarian stimulation with gonadotropins is accomplished with follicle stimulating hormone alone or in combination with luteinizing hormone. A gonadotropin-releasing hormone agonist or antagonist is administered to prevent interruption of the cycle by endogenous hormones. Human chorionic gonadotropin is injected in a single dose to finalize follicular development for oocyte retrieval.	**Case 48-2 (Questions 4–8)**
7	A rare but serious complication of controlled ovarian stimulation is ovarian hyperstimulation syndrome. The risk is minimized by monitoring the development of follicles carefully with sequential transvaginal ultrasounds and serum estradiol levels.	**Case 48-2 (Questions 6, 8)**
8	Multiple gestation pregnancies are associated with maternal and neonatal risks, including preterm birth and extended neonatal intensive care. These risks are considered when determining embryo transfer and cryopreservation plans.	**Case 48-2 (Questions 3, 10, 11)**
9	The diagnosis and treatment of infertility affects the couple emotionally, financially, and socially. Psychosocial support is an important aspect of care from the early phases of evaluation and diagnosis through all stages of treatment.	**Case 48-2 (Questions 3, 11)**

INTRODUCTION

Infertility is defined as the inability to conceive after one year of unprotected intercourse.[1] The definition is based upon the observation that roughly 85% of couples with normal fertility will achieve pregnancy within one year.[2] Data from the 2002 National Survey of Family Growth revealed that 7.4% of married women 15 to 44 years old, or 2.1 million, were infertile and approximately 12% of women in this age group had used infertility services.[3] Many factors affect infertility rates, but advancing maternal age appears to be a prominent influence. In 2002, the incidence of infertility in women 15 to 29 years old was 11%, whereas in women 40 to 44 years old it was 27%.[3] Fecundity, or the probability of achieving a live birth in one menstrual cycle, is approximately 20% for couples without infertility. There is a downward trend after age 30, with average fecundity rates of 5% or less between ages 30 and 40.[4] This is accompanied by an age-related increase in chromosomal abnormalities and spontaneous abortion rates.[5] The physiologic factors of reproductive aging are amplified by a trend toward delayed childbearing in the United States. In 1970, 1 out of 100 women had their first child at age 35 or older. In 2006, this increased to 1 out of 12 women.[6] Male fertility is impacted by age as well, with a documented decline after age 35. However, determining the exact contribution of male age to infertility is complicated by the influence of female age.[7]

The complex physical, psychological, and social implications have led to a national focus on infertility as a public health priority.[8] Treatment plans vary widely depending on the contributions of both female and male factors. An individualized approach is necessary to balance the risks and benefits of the various therapeutic options and maximize clinical outcomes.

PATHOPHYSIOLOGY AND DIAGNOSIS

CASE 48-1

QUESTION 1: T.R. is a 32-year-old woman who presents to her gynecologist with concerns that she and her husband, age 37, have not conceived despite having unprotected intercourse on average 2 to 3 times per week for the past 14 months. Her prior contraceptive method was a combined oral contraceptive which she used for 12 years and discontinued 2 years ago. At that time, the couple used male condoms until 14 months ago when they stopped using contraception altogether. What is the recommended initial approach to this couple's concern?

Evaluation of infertility generally begins after a couple has attempted to conceive for at least 12 months without success. Evaluation after just 6 months of unsuccessful conception is recommended in women older than age 35 or in those with a history of conditions associated with infertility, such as amenorrhea, endometriosis, or pelvic inflammatory disease.[2]

This couple has failed to conceive after 14 months of regular, unprotected intercourse, which supports an evaluation of both partners at this time. The diagnostic process first involves a thorough assessment of medical conditions, lifestyle parameters, and medication exposures. This is followed by complete physical examinations and laboratory assessments with other diagnostic procedures as warranted.

General Risk Factors

CASE 48-1, QUESTION 2: Additional information is obtained about the couple's social history. T.R. works as a bank teller and her husband is a financial planner. Neither T.R. nor her husband smoke tobacco or use illicit substances. Both drink one to two cups of caffeinated coffee each day and drink alcohol socially, an average of one to three drinks each on weekends. What lifestyle factors may contribute to infertility in this couple?

Lifestyle factors such as tobacco or illicit drug use and caffeine intake are known contributors to infertility. Tobacco use can be linked to 13% of infertility cases.[9] In addition to the negative effects on fetal development during pregnancy, tobacco use can worsen ovulatory function. It also induces chromosomal changes that alter sperm production and function.[9,10] Caffeine is associated with decreased fertility with higher levels of intake, but moderate use of one to two cups of coffee or equivalent appears to have minimal impact. Although a link between alcohol use and infertility is not definitive, it is recommended that women limit their use to no more than one drink per day. Complete abstinence from alcohol is recommended once pregnancy is confirmed.[11] Use of illicit substances such as marijuana impairs fertility and decreases the success of fertility treatments.[11,12] Occupational and environmental exposures to pesticides, heavy metals, and toxins such as organic solvents used in dry cleaning and printing are additional contributors.[11]

The couple's lack of tobacco or illicit drug use eliminates these as potential contributors and their occupations do not fit known high-risk exposure profiles. Their pattern of caffeine and alcohol use is not greater than the amount currently documented to affect fertility. Assessment of other causes of infertility is warranted.

Female Factor Infertility

OVULATORY DYSFUNCTION

CASE 48-1, QUESTION 3: T.R.'s medical history is significant for exercise-induced asthma diagnosed at age 10. Her medications include an albuterol inhaler used as needed for shortness of breath. She is 5 feet 5 inches tall and weighs 140 pounds. Her reproductive history reveals menarche at age 13, no prior pregnancies, and regular menstrual cycles approximately 25 to 26 days in length since discontinuing the oral contraceptive. She reports the menstrual bleeding phase to be 4 to 5 days in length and does not complain of excessive bleeding. A physical exam is performed along with a pelvic exam with no notable abnormalities. What information does this provide about possible female factors associated with infertility?

An important focus when evaluating causes of infertility is ovulatory function, which is associated with up to 40% of female factor infertility.[2] A thorough reproductive history should document age of menarche, menstrual cycle patterns, premenstrual symptoms, and previous pregnancies. A history of regular menstrual cycles of 22 to 35 days with premenstrual symptoms or dysmenorrhea is considered consistent with ovulatory cycles.[2,13]

Ovarian function is regulated through complex feedback mechanisms within the hypothalamic-pituitary-ovarian axis (see Chapter 50, Disorders Related to the Menstrual Cycle, Fig. 50-1). This involves release of gonadotropin-releasing hormone (GnRH) from the hypothalamus, follicle-stimulating hormone (FSH) and luteinizing hormone (LH) from the pituitary, and estrogen and progesterone from the ovaries.[4] Anovulation results from the disruption of communication at any of these levels and is associated with a variety of causes.[13] Table 48-1 provides an overview of abbreviations commonly associated with diagnosis and management of infertility for use throughout the chapter.

TABLE 48-1
Common Abbreviations Associated with Infertility Diagnosis and Treatment

ART	Assisted reproductive technology
CC	Clomiphene citrate
COS	Controlled ovarian stimulation
FSH	Follicle stimulating hormone
GnRH	Gonadotropin releasing hormone
hCG	Human chorionic gonadotropin
HSG	Hysterosalpingogram
hMG	Human menopausal gonadotropin
IUI	Intrauterine insemination
ICSI	Intracytoplasmic sperm injection
IVF	In vitro fertilization
LH	Luteinizing hormone
OHSS	Ovarian hyperstimulation syndrome
OI	Ovulation induction

Conditions such as thyroid dysfunction, hyperprolactinemia, and polycystic ovary syndrome (PCOS) can induce anovulation. Signs may be evident upon physical examination, including an enlarged thyroid (thyroid dysfunction), abnormal discharge from the breast (hyperprolactinemia), or signs of hyperandrogenism (PCOS). Obesity is another feature associated with PCOS. Conversely, extremely low body weight and excessive exercise may negatively impact ovulatory function at the hypothalamic level. Weight gain improves menstrual regulation in women with anovulation associated with low body fat. Primary ovarian failure can result from exposure to chemotherapy agents or radiation treatments as well as ovarian surgery. As previously discussed, the aging process itself is characterized by diminished ovarian follicular reserve.[13,14]

T.R.'s reproductive history is consistent with regular menstrual cycles which are likely ovulatory. It would be helpful to identify if she reports any symptoms of premenstrual syndrome or dysmenorrhea which are associated with ovulatory cycles. Her physical examination is unremarkable and her medical history does not reveal any conditions associated with anovulation. Her weight is not likely a factor because her body mass index of approximately 23 kg/m^2 is in the normal range. She has no known history of exposure to chemotherapy or ovarian surgery which could directly impact ovarian function. The only parameter consistent with female factor infertility is T.R's age. At 32 years old, she may be experiencing an initial age-related decline in ovarian function consistent with infertility.

CASE 48-1, QUESTION 4: T.R. reports using a home ovulation test kit for the last two menstrual cycles which both yielded positive results. She is referred for a series of laboratory tests with the following findings:

Thyroid stimulating hormone, 3.2 milli-international units/L
Prolactin, 8.4 ng/mL
Cycle day 3 FSH, 4 milli-international units/mL
Cycle day 3 estradiol, 38 pg/mL

What additional information about her ovulatory function can be determined from these results?

Several methods are available to further define ovulatory function. Basal body temperature monitoring is accomplished through the measurement of body temperature every morning upon waking with a basal or digital thermometer. Temperature fluctuations typically follow a biphasic pattern during the menstrual cycle, with a sustained rise in basal body temperature of approximately 0.5°F to 1.0°F after ovulation. If this pattern is apparent through daily documentation in a temperature diary, it can be assumed that ovulation occurred during that cycle. The accuracy of this method is complicated by daily temperature fluctuations, inconsistent measurement technique, and illness. It has largely been replaced by the use of home ovulation test kits that detect urinary LH. The patient initiates daily urine tests during the follicular phase, with the initial testing day determined by the length and regularity of her menstrual cycle (Fig. 48-1). A positive test documents the LH surge, signaling that ovulation will occur in an average of 24 hours.[2,15] Home ovulation test kits that detect changes in cervical mucus or saliva samples are not typically used for diagnostic purposes. They are useful, however, for patients who are timing intercourse during their most fertile period around ovulation.[11,15]

Indirect measurements of ovulation are available, but not widely performed. A serum progesterone concentration measured in the mid-luteal phase greater than 3 ng/mL is considered consistent with an ovulatory cycle. Alternatively, an endometrial biopsy performed just prior to menses measures the degree of progesterone-stimulated growth, signifying whether ovulation likely occurred. The invasive nature of this test limits its feasibility in most diagnostic evaluations.[2]

In patients who are anovulatory, additional laboratory assessments of thyroid function and prolactin levels document potential secondary causes. Anovulation associated with hyperprolactinemia is treated with oral dopamine agonists such as bromocriptine. Prolactin levels should normalize after 4 weeks of treatment in most patients, with 80% reporting successful ovulation once this occurs.[13,16] Elevated testosterone levels may correspond with physical signs of hyperandrogenism and PCOS. The treatment of PCOS is discussed elsewhere (See Chapter 50, Disorders Related to the Menstrual Cycle).

Assessment of ovarian reserve is often recommended for women older than age 35 to help guide fertility treatment choices. There are multiple methods that can be used. One involves the measurement of basal levels of serum FSH and/or estradiol on day 3 of the menstrual cycle, with day 1 being the first day of menses.[2,17] As the number of ovarian follicles declines with age, pituitary release of FSH increases. Therefore, elevated levels of basal FSH suggest diminished ovarian function. Unfortunately, the interpretation is complicated by individual variability in FSH levels from cycle to cycle as well as varying laboratory-specific reference ranges. A serum estradiol level of 80 pg/mL or above during this testing is associated with a poor prognosis for success with infertility treatments.[17] Measurement of inhibin B, which is secreted from the ovarian granulosa cells during the follicular phase of the menstrual cycle, is an additional marker. Low levels of inhibin B correlate with elevated FSH levels and a possible decline in ovarian function.[4,17]

The clomiphene citrate challenge test provides another option for assessing ovarian reserve. This involves the administration of clomiphene citrate (CC), a selective estrogen receptor modulator, at a dose of 100 mg once daily on days 5 through 9 of the menstrual cycle. In addition to the estradiol and FSH measurements measured on day 3 as described previously, FSH is also measured on day 10. The expected response is suppression of FSH by the developing ovarian follicles. Elevated levels at either day 3 or 10 suggest diminished ovarian reserve. The value of this test as a predictor of response to ovarian stimulation is not clearly supported in the literature.[4,18]

Direct visualization of the ovaries through a transvaginal ultrasound may be used in conjunction with the hormone testing described previously. An assessment of ovarian volume and the antral follicle count can be made. The antral follicles, or those at least 2 mm in diameter, are responsive to FSH in the early follicular phase and decline in number with age. This

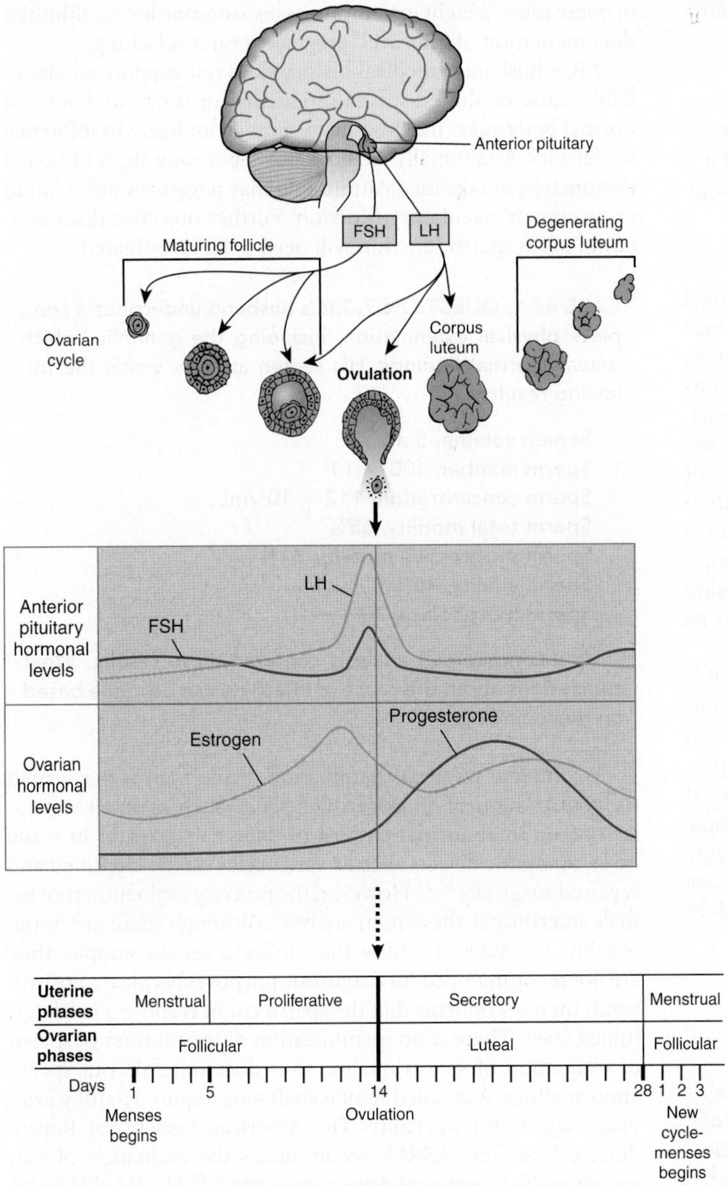

FIGURE 48-1 The menstrual cycle.

measurement may predict ovarian response to various infertility treatments.[4,19]

The laboratory assessment of T.R. provides additional data regarding her ovarian function. Ovulatory cycles are supported by the positive urinary LH surge with the home test kit as well as the normal (non-elevated) day 3 FSH and estradiol levels. Her normal thyroid stimulating hormone and prolactin levels indicate a low probability of secondary causes of anovulation. Because T.R. is younger than 35 and there are no other indicators of ovulatory dysfunction, additional testing of ovarian reserve may not be necessary. The initial findings of T.R.'s infertility assessment show that ovulatory dysfunction is not likely to be a contributor.

STRUCTURAL FACTORS

CASE 48-1, QUESTION 5: Because T.R. has normal ovulatory function, further causes of female factor infertility will be investigated. What testing is recommended to rule out structural causes of infertility?

Structural abnormalities in the uterine cavity or fallopian tubes are additional causes of female factor infertility. These may develop in utero or result from scar tissue or lesions secondary to conditions such as endometriosis. In some cases of endometriosis surgical interventions improve fertility outcomes, but this is highly dependent on the severity and location of the lesions.[20] Further discussion of the diagnosis and treatment of endometriosis is provided elsewhere (see Chapter 50, Disorders Related to the Menstrual Cycle). Pelvic inflammatory disease from sexually transmitted infections such as chlamydia or gonorrhea is a risk factor for tubal infertility. The risk increases with each subsequent infection and is more pronounced in older women. The incidence of infertility in a woman older than age 25 with a history of 3 or more episodes of pelvic inflammatory disease is 75%.[21]

The use of invasive procedures to explore structural causes of female infertility is dictated by the reproductive history and findings of the physical examination and laboratory tests. Abnormalities of the ovaries, uterus, and fallopian tubes are evaluated through various procedures. Transvaginal ultrasonography utilizes vaginal insertion of an ultrasound probe to visualize ovarian structure and developing follicles. A hysterosalpingogram (HSG) is performed to confirm normal fallopian tube structure. During this process, dye is injected into the uterus through a catheter and visualized on x-ray to determine any blockages or malformations. Hysteroscopy and laparoscopy are more invasive procedures that allow for direct visualization of the uterus or pelvic anatomy. These are typically reserved for further examination of abnormalities detected by initial testing.[2]

For visuals of a transvaginal ultrasound, a hysterosalpingogram, a hysteroscopy, and a laparoscopy, see PowerPoint slides 2 through 6 at http://thepoint.lww.com/AT10e.

Impaired cervical mucus production or quality is an additional structural factor that can impact sperm motility and the fertilization process. Cervical mucus increases in volume and becomes thinner as the follicular phase progresses to facilitate sperm transport at ovulation. The "postcoital test" or microscopic examination of cervical mucus within hours of intercourse can be performed to confirm the presence of motile sperm. The validity of the test is debated due to the high variability in the interpretation of results.[2,22] The use of the oral mucolytic guaifenesin in doses of 600 mg twice daily or 200 mg three times daily is a popular recommendation within patient forums to improve the quality of cervical mucus.[23] However, there are few data to support its impact on pregnancy rates.[23,24]

In the evaluation of this couple, it is important to verify T.R.'s sexual history and any possible exposures to sexually transmitted infections, such as chlamydia. An HSG should be ordered to determine whether she has patent fallopian tubes and to provide basic information about the shape of her uterine cavity. If there are abnormal findings from this test, further hysteroscopic or laparoscopic procedures can be performed. A laparoscopy would be necessary to fully evaluate any peritoneal adhesions from undetected endometriosis, but her medical history does not warrant this invasive procedure at this time.

Male Factor Infertility

CASE 48-1, QUESTION 6: The results of the HSG are normal, so the infertility assessment turns now to the evaluation of T.R.'s husband. He is healthy with no chronic medical conditions or medication use. His body mass index is 24.6 kg/m^2. He denies symptoms of low libido or signs of erectile or ejaculatory dysfunction during intercourse. What causes of male factor infertility does he display?

Female factors account for the majority of cases of infertility, but male factors are present in up to 40%.[22] Male factor infertility is often an outcome of impaired sperm production or function, which can originate from a variety of causes. Impaired sperm production may be associated with hypogonadism resulting from testicular trauma, cryptorchidism, radiation, or antiandrogen medications.[25] Varicoceles, or dilated scrotal veins, affect testicular function in up to 40% of men with infertility. It appears that the resulting abnormal venous perfusion and elevated testicular temperature impair spermatogenesis.[26] Genetic conditions may disrupt androgen synthesis or cause defects in the LH or FSH receptor. Azoospermia, or no presence of sperm in the ejaculate, is also apparent in the genetic disorder Klinefelter syndrome. Pituitary tumors can reduce FSH and LH secretion and impair sperm production. Sperm transport defects result from erectile dysfunction, retrograde ejaculation, or obstruction of the vas deferens or epididymis. Medications such as antidepressants or antihypertensives can worsen libido and ejaculatory function. A dosage reduction or switching to an alternative medication can improve sexual function.[25] Weight may play a role in male fertility due to elevated estrogen and lower testosterone levels observed in obese men. Weight loss improves testosterone levels, although documentation of improved pregnancy rates is lacking.[27]

T.R.'s husband's medical history does not support an identifiable cause of altered sperm production or function. He has a normal body mass index so his weight is not likely to influence his fertility. Additionally, he does not report any signs of sexual dysfunction or take medications that may negatively affect libido or erectile or ejaculatory function. Further objective documentation of his sperm function will need to be investigated.

CASE 48-1, QUESTION 7: T.R.'s husband undergoes a complete physical examination, including the genitalia, which reveals normal findings. His semen analysis yields the following results:

Semen volume, 5 mL
Sperm number, 400 × 10^6
Sperm concentration, 112 × 10^6/mL
Sperm total motility, 65%
Sperm progressive motility, 61%
Sperm vitality, 80%
Sperm morphology 30%

A second semen analysis confirms these results. What conclusions about the cause of infertility can be made based on these findings?

A complete physical examination of the man is performed to identify signs of androgen deficiency such as small testicular size or an abnormal pattern of male hair growth. In some cases, anatomic defects such as varicoceles can be identified and repaired surgically.[22,26] However, the primary evaluation tool for male infertility is the semen analysis. Although there are home test kits for male infertility that utilize a semen sample, they are not recommended for diagnostic purposes because a positive result merely confirms that the sperm count is above a predetermined level. There is no quantification of the number of sperm or evaluation of sperm quality, so it does not rule out sperm abnormalities. A detailed semen analysis is required to fully evaluate male factor infertility. The American Society for Reproductive Medicine (ASRM) recommends the evaluation of two semen analyses performed one month apart.[22] The World Health Organization publishes reference values for semen characteristics (Table 48-2).[28] The reference range is based upon semen analyses of a study population of men who successfully conceived within

TABLE 48-2
Semen Analysis: Lower Reference Limits for Selected Parameters

Parameter	Lower Reference Limit (5th percentile with 95% confidence interval)
Semen volume (mL)	1.5 (1.4–1.7)
Total sperm number (10^6 per ejaculate)	39 (33–46)
Sperm concentration (10^6 per mL)	15 (12–16)
Total motility (progressive + nonprogressive, %)	40 (38–42)
Progressive motility (%)	32 (31–34)
Vitality (live spermatozoa, %)	58 (55–63)
Sperm morphology (normal forms, %)	4 (3–4)

Reprinted with permission from World Health Organization, Department of Reproductive Health and Research. *WHO Laboratory Manual for the Examination and Processing of Human Semen.* 5th ed. Geneva, Switzerland: World Health Organization Press; 2010:224.

12 months of discontinuing use of contraceptives. The lower reference limit for each characteristic reflects the fifth percentile value from this cohort of men. Results lower than these cut-off values are not definitive for male factor infertility, but do suggest the need to confirm the findings with a second semen analysis.[28]

Abnormal findings on the semen analysis may be suggestive of the underlying cause of infertility. Low semen volume suggests structural causes of ejaculatory dysfunction. Additional hormone testing, including FSH, testosterone, and prolactin levels, may be necessary to distinguish factors associated with a low sperm count or motility. Low FSH and testosterone are consistent with hypogonadotropic hypogonadism.[22] If hyperprolactinemia is evident, any secondary causes such as medications are investigated. Certain antipsychotics, antihypertensives, or antidepressants can increase prolactin levels and should be discontinued and replaced with agents that do not increase prolactin. If the underlying cause cannot be addressed, a dopamine agonist such as bromocriptine may restore testicular function and sperm production.[16]

All components of the semen analysis for T.R.'s husband are above the lower limit defined by the World Health Organization. His normal physical examination and medical history also support a lack of identifiable male causes of infertility. In this case, the extensive testing of both T.R. and her husband has revealed no obvious contributor to infertility.

TREATMENT APPROACHES

CASE 48-1, QUESTION 8: The couple completes their evaluation and is diagnosed with unexplained infertility. What is the initial approach to treatment?

The diagnosis of unexplained infertility, or no identifiable cause after evaluation, accounts for up to 30% of cases.[29] The treatment approach is empiric but typically incorporates medications to stimulate ovulation. This may or may not be combined with intrauterine insemination or other infertility procedures which are discussed later in the chapter. If untreated, the fecundity rates are low, ranging from approximately 2% to 4%.[29]

Regardless of the treatment approach, all couples pursuing pregnancy are encouraged to avoid tobacco, alcohol, and illicit substances, and limit caffeine intake.[11] The female partner should take a daily supplement containing 400 to 800 mcg of folic acid to reduce the risk of neural tube defects once pregnancy occurs.[30] Any chronic medications must be evaluated for potential safety issues during pregnancy and discontinued or switched to a safer alternative. Patients are encouraged to achieve and maintain a normal weight, which is associated with a lower risk for failed treatment cycles and pregnancy loss.[31] Recommendations pertinent to T.R. include discontinuation of alcohol use, limited caffeine intake, and initiation of a daily multivitamin with 400 to 800 mcg of folic acid. T.R. should also confirm plans for monitoring her asthma symptoms during pregnancy. Albuterol use during pregnancy will be continued, but the frequency of use will be monitored carefully.[32]

Ovulation Induction/Controlled Ovarian Stimulation

There are two general treatment strategies that focus on ovulation: "ovulation induction" (OI) and "controlled ovarian stimulation" (COS). The approach depends on a patient's underlying ovulatory function. Ovulation induction is pursued in patients who are not ovulating to promote an ovulatory cycle. This method may be accompanied by timed natural intercourse or the use of insemination procedures to achieve pregnancy. Controlled ovarian stimulation incorporates many of the same medications, but is appropriate for women who are already having ovulatory cycles but are still experiencing infertility. Additionally, COS is appropriate for infertility procedures where the development of multiple ovarian follicles is desirable (Case 48-2). The general approach to medication use with both strategies is described subsequently.

OVULATION INDUCTION

Anovulatory women with adequate ovarian reserve and no other treatable cause are candidates for OI. This process is designed to mimic the hormonal patterns of the normal menstrual cycle. Follicle-stimulating hormone guides the initial recruitment and development of ovarian follicles early in the menstrual cycle. This is followed by development of a dominant follicle and increased estradiol levels. The elevated estrogen triggers the LH surge and the release of the ovum mid-cycle for fertilization (Figure 48-1). The goal of OI is the development of a single dominant follicle.[13,14]

The choice of medications for OI is dictated by hypothalamic-pituitary-ovarian function. With adequate hypothalamic function, an oral regimen of CC, which exhibits estrogen agonist and antagonist activity, is often utilized first line. Clomiphene citrate inhibits estrogen binding in the hypothalamus to stimulate release of GnRH and pituitary gonadotropins and induce ovarian follicular development. Ovulation is successful in 80% of patients using CC.[33] Oral aromatase inhibitors are not approved by the US Food and Drug Administration (FDA) for OI, but also increase release of GnRH and pituitary gonadotropins through an estrogen antagonist effect.[14,34] An alternative method of stimulating gonadotropin release is through direct administration of gonadorelin, a synthetic version of GnRH. When administered in a pulsatile manner every 1 to 2 hours, it induces pituitary release of FSH and LH and resulting follicular development. The inconvenience of the portable pump device required for this administration schedule has led to a phase-out of this method.[13,14]

If hypothalamic or pituitary dysfunction is detected or if oral regimens are not successful, injectable gonadotropins are administered. The most common gonadotropin regimens use FSH administered alone or in combination with LH (Table 48-3).[35] A "step-up" protocol represents the natural progression of gonadotropin release during the menstrual cycle. Initial daily injections of 50 to 75 international units are increased in increments of 37.5 international units as necessary for a follicular response. A "step-down" protocol uses higher initial daily doses of 150 international units until a dominant follicle is apparent on ultrasound. The daily dose is then decreased incrementally until ovulation is triggered.[36]

An injection of human chorionic gonadotropin (hCG) is administered during the OI process to simulate the LH surge that naturally occurs midcycle. The timing is based on the growth of ovarian follicles monitored with intravaginal ultrasound. As one follicle matures to 16 to 18 mm in diameter, a single dose of hCG is injected and ovulation is expected to occur within 24 to 48 hours. This is timed with natural intercourse or other infertility procedures to achieve pregnancy.[14]

CONTROLLED OVARIAN STIMULATION

The oral and injectable medications used for OI are also incorporated into regimens for COS. They are administered in doses and schedules intended to develop multiple ovarian follicles, rather than one dominant follicle. This results in a greater number of oocytes available for fertilization. Because T.R. has ovulatory

TABLE 48-3
Gonadotropins for Ovulation Induction/Controlled Ovarian Hyperstimulation

Ingredient	Product Name	Strength/Dosage Form	Route of Administration
hMG (menotropin)	Repronex	Powder for reconstitution: 75 international units FSH activity and 75 international units LH activity/vial	IM or SC
hMG (menotropin)	Menopur	Powder for reconstitution: 75 international units FSH activity and 75 international units LH activity/vial	SC
Urinary FSH (urofollitropin)	Bravelle	Powder for reconstitution: 75 international units FSH activity/vial	IM or SC
Recombinant FSH (follitropin alfa)	Gonal-f Multi-Dose	Powder for reconstitution: 450 or 1,050 international units FSH activity/vial	SC
	Gonal-f RFF 75 international units	Powder for reconstitution: 75 international units FSH activity/vial	SC
	Gonal-f RFF pen	Solution: 300, 450, or 900 international units FSH/pen	SC
Recombinant FSH (follitropin beta)	Follistim AQ Vial	Solution: 75 or 150 international units FSH/vial	IM or SC
	Follistim AQ Cartridge for Follistim Pen	Solution: 175, 350, 650, or 975 international units/cartridge (delivers 150, 300, 600, or 900 international units FSH)	SC
Recombinant LH (lutropin alfa)	Luveris	Powder for reconstitution: 75 international units LH/vial	SC
Urinary hCG	Chorionic gonadotropin (generic)	Powder for reconstitution: 10,000 international units LH activity/vial	IM
	Pregnyl	Powder for reconstitution: 10,000 international units LH activity/vial	IM
	Novarel	Powder for reconstitution: 10,000 international units LH activity/vial	IM
Recombinant chorionic gonadotropin alfa	Ovidrel	Prefilled syringe: 250 mcg r-hCG	SC

FSH, follicle stimulating hormone; hCG, human chorionic gonadotropin; hMG, human menopausal gonadotropin; IM, intramuscular; LH, luteinizing hormone; r-hCG, recombinant human chorionic gonadotropin; SC, subcutaneous.
Adapted with permission from Facts & Comparisons eAnswers. http://online.factsandcomparisons.com/MonoDisp.aspx?monoID=fandc-hcp10484; http://online.factsandcomparisons.com/MonoDisp.aspx?monoID=fandc-hcp11267; http://online.factsandcomparisons.com/MonoDisp.aspx?monoID=fandc-hcp11305; http://online.factsandcomparisons.com/MonoDisp.aspx?monoID=fandc-hcp10483; http://online.factsandcomparisons.com/MonoDisp.aspx?monoID=fandc-hcp10893; http://online.factsandcomparisons.com/MonoDisp.aspx?monoID=fandc-hcp10894; http://online.factsandcomparisons.com/MonoDisp.aspx?monoID=fandc-hcp12150. Accessed November 4, 2011.

cycles, but has unexplained infertility, COS will be the medication approach considered most appropriate.

CASE 48-1, QUESTION 9: What medication regimen is recommended for controlled ovarian stimulation for T.R.?

There are multiple approaches to ovulation stimulation that utilize oral or injectable medications. Clomiphene citrate is the most common initial choice because of the convenience and low cost of an oral regimen and the widespread experience with its use.

CLOMIPHENE CITRATE

The competitive binding of CC to estrogen receptors in the hypothalamus stimulates release of GnRH. This promotes gonadotropin release from the anterior pituitary, leading to follicular development, increased estradiol production, and ovulation. As previously described, the mechanism of action of CC requires an intact hypothalamic-pituitary-ovarian axis.[33]

The typical initial dosing regimen for CC is 50 mg once daily for 5 days starting on day 5 of the menstrual cycle. Some clinicians prefer initiating therapy on day 3, although there is no clinical advantage.[33] Ovulation typically occurs 5 to 12 days after the fifth dose is taken. If ovulation is documented but pregnancy does not occur, the same dose of CC is used in future cycles. If ovulation does not occur, then the dose is increased by 50 mg with each subsequent cycle. Although the product labeling does not recommend doses above 100 mg per day, CC doses as high as 250 mg have been described in the literature.[33,37] Alternative medication approaches are typically recommended if daily doses of 150 mg are not successful.[13]

T.R.'s evaluation shows no evidence of hypothalamic or pituitary dysfunction, so she is an appropriate candidate for CC. Once her next cycle begins, she should initiate a 5-day regimen of CC 50 mg once daily starting on the fifth day of menstrual bleeding.

CASE 48-1, QUESTION 10: T.R. begins a regimen of CC and experiences hot flashes and nausea, but chooses to complete the 5-day course. What is the likely cause of her symptoms?

Vasomotor symptoms are a common complaint during a short treatment course of CC, occurring in 10% to 20% of patients. Additional side effects include headache, irritability, mood swings, and nausea.[13,33,38] The peripheral antiestrogenic effects of CC are associated with altered cervical mucus and impaired endometrial proliferation, although this is inconsistently demonstrated in clinical studies. It remains controversial whether this affects pregnancy rates.[33] Although visual disturbances are reported in less than 2% of patients, symptoms such as blurred vision or light sensitivity should be reported and evaluated to prevent serious complications.[39] Ovarian cysts occur in 5% to 10% of users. Subsequent cycles of CC are delayed if cysts are documented on transvaginal ultrasound.[13,29]

Long-term concerns related to CC are linked to pregnancy outcomes. All medications for COS can result in multiple gestation pregnancies. Clomiphene citrate is associated with a risk of multiple gestation in 8% to 10% of cases, primarily resulting in twins.[29] Early concerns about increased rates of ovarian cancer in women exposed to more than 12 cycles of CC have been minimized based on data from more recent studies.[33,40,41] The risk of birth defects with CC and other ovulation inducers is debated and inconclusive. A recent case-control study documented an association between CC and several defects, however conclusions are limited by small case numbers and varying reporting mechanisms.[42] A more detailed discussion of cancer and birth defects related to infertility procedures is provided in Case 48-2.

In this case, T.R. is experiencing side effects commonly associated with CC. They are not treatment limiting, and she is not reporting a change in vision that would require further evaluation. She can safely proceed with treatment by monitoring for an LH surge using a home ovulation test kit.

CASE 48-1, QUESTION 11: T.R. receives a positive test with her urinary LH test kit on day 13 of her cycle. She is scheduled for intrauterine insemination. What is the role of this procedure in the treatment of unexplained infertility?

Controlled ovarian stimulation for unexplained infertility with CC alone is associated with per-cycle pregnancy rates ranging from 3% to 8%.[29] It is frequently combined with intrauterine insemination (IUI) as an additional empiric method. Intrauterine insemination introduces a processed semen sample directly to the uterus via a catheter placed through the cervix. The procedure is timed with ovulation to maximize sperm exposure for fertilization. This is accomplished by using a urinary ovulation home test kit to identify the natural LH surge or injecting hCG to trigger ovulation and planning the IUI 24 to 36 hours later.[43] In general studies of IUI, the use of an hCG trigger does not appear to improve pregnancy outcomes.[44] Due to the nature of the procedure, patients with bilateral obstruction of the fallopian tubes are not candidates for IUI.

Despite the expectation that the combined methodologies of CC plus IUI would increase pregnancy rates, results from clinical trials have been conflicting, with per-cycle pregnancy rates often similar to those of CC alone.[29,43] There are no identifiable contraindications for IUI in this couple, although the use of the procedure may not greatly improve chances of success.

CASE 48-1, QUESTION 12: The pregnancy test after the first cycle of CC and IUI is negative. What other options are available for this couple?

Multiple treatment cycles with the combination of CC and IUI are commonly pursued, but there is little evidence for effectiveness beyond six attempts.[13] In some cases, alternatives to CC for COS may be desirable because of poor tolerability or treatment failure. Aromatase inhibitors or gonadotropins are suitable alternatives to combine with IUI.

AROMATASE INHIBITORS

The aromatase inhibitors letrozole and anastrazole are emerging as oral alternatives to CC, although they are not FDA-labeled for ovulation induction or COS. Aromatase is an enzyme that converts androstenedione to estrone and testosterone to estradiol. Aromatase inhibitors reduce systemic estrogen levels by blocking this conversion in the ovary, resulting in increased gonadotropin secretion and follicular development. The higher concentration of androgens that remains in the ovary increases follicular sensitivity to FSH and further facilitates development.[34]

The recommended administration schedule is similar to clomiphene: once daily for 5 days beginning on cycle days 3 to 5. Although daily doses of letrozole 2.5 or 5 mg or anastrozole 1 mg have been studied for this purpose, there is more evidence available for letrozole. The selection of agent is most commonly determined by physician preference and experience. Ongoing studies are investigating optimal dosing and the possibility of single doses versus 5-day regimens.[45] Pregnancy rates with letrozole appear to be similar to that of CC.[34,46] A prospective comparative trial of CC with IUI versus letrozole with IUI in more than 400 women resulted in statistically similar overall rates of pregnancy (approximately 38% and 36%, respectively).[47]

Adverse effects experienced with aromatase inhibitors during the short treatment course for COS resemble those of CC. Studies of letrozole identify vasomotor symptoms in 11% of patients, with nausea and fatigue occurring in less than 10%.[48] The aromatase inhibitors do not affect cervical mucus or endometrial development, but this finding has not translated into improved pregnancy outcomes in clinical studies. There is a reduced incidence of multiple gestation pregnancy compared with CC because of the development of fewer follicles.[48] Initial concerns of the teratogenic potential of aromatase inhibition during fetal development prompted a warning against use in premenopausal women who are or may become pregnant to be included in the product labeling.[49,50] Recent surveillance studies of letrozole cycles do not demonstrate higher rates of congenital malformations as compared to CC.[51] The early timing of administration in the cycle reduces the risk of fetal exposure. Continued monitoring of pregnancy outcomes is needed to confirm safety.

GONADOTROPINS

If oral agents are unsuccessful, COS can be attempted with injectable gonadotropins including FSH alone or in combination with LH (Table 48-3). The per-cycle conception rates are higher than that of CC or aromatase inhibitors in most studies.[29] However, a recent meta-analysis of COS for IUI documented an overall pregnancy rate of 21% with gonadotropins and 16% for CC, a difference that was not statistically significant.[43] More direct comparative trials are needed to confirm the advantage of parenteral gonadotropins over oral formulations.

A standard protocol involves daily injections of FSH or a combination of FSH and LH to stimulate follicular development. Human chorionic gonadotropin is administered as a single injection to finalize follicular development and induce ovulation. There are many variations, with some protocols combining initial doses of CC or aromatase inhibitors with later doses of gonadotropins to reduce the total gonadotropin dose and duration of injections.[52] Dosing recommendations, key differences between formulations and risks associated with gonadotropin use are reviewed in more detail in Case 48-2.

T.R.'s complaints of vasomotor symptoms are well documented with CC. Although the aromatase inhibitors are another oral option for COS, the likelihood of hot flashes is similar. However, if the couple continues to be unsuccessful with future cycles of CC plus IUI, letrozole could be considered as an alternative to the injectable gonadotropins. In a study of couples with three unsuccessful cycles of CC with IUI, switching to letrozole resulted in pregnancy rates similar to gonadotropins without the inconvenience and added cost of injections.[53]

The conventional treatment approach for unexplained infertility is to delay the use of more complex procedures such as in vitro fertilization (IVF) until multiple CC plus IUI or gonadotropin plus IUI cycles are attempted. However, a recent clinical trial challenged this by accelerating directly to IVF after only three unsuccessful cycles of CC plus IUI. The pregnancy rate was 25% higher in the group that utilized IVF and avoided the interim trial of gonadotropins with IUI. The authors concluded that the extra time and cost associated with trying both oral and injectable COS regimens with IUI can be avoided with earlier progression to IVF.[54] This may be an alternative consideration

TABLE 48-4
Description of Select Infertility Procedures

Classification	Procedure	Description
Insemination	Intrauterine, intracervical, intravaginal	Delivery of a prepared semen sample to the intended site (vagina, cervix, uterus) during ovulation
Assisted reproductive technology	Assisted hatching	Mechanical or chemical separation of the blastocyst from the zona pellucida (membrane surrounding the oocyte) during embryonic development in vitro
	Embryo cryopreservation	Freezing and storage of embryos for future ART cycles
	Gamete intrafallopian transfer	Laparoscopic transfer of the unfertilized oocytes and sperm to the fallopian tube for fertilization
	In vitro fertilization—embryo transfer	Transfer of one or more embryos resulting from in vitro fertilization into the uterus through the cervix
	Intracytoplasmic sperm injection	In vitro injection of the sperm into the oocyte
	Preimplantation genetic diagnosis/screening	Examination of oocytes, zygotes, or embryos for specific genetic conditions (diagnosis) or for general genetic alterations (screening)
	Zygote intrafallopian transfer	Laparoscopic transfer of the fertilized oocyte (zygote) into the fallopian tube

ART, assisted reproductive technology.
Source: Zegers-Hochschild F et al. The International Committee for Monitoring Assisted Reproductive Technology (ICMART) and the World Health Organization (WHO) revised glossary on ART terminology, 2009. *Hum Reprod.* 2009;24:2683.

for this couple if the IUI procedures continue to be unsuccessful. In vitro fertilization is discussed in more detail in Case 48-2.

Assisted Reproductive Technology

OVERVIEW

There are a variety of procedures to address the infertility factors specific to each couple. Insemination processes (intrauterine, intracervical, and intravaginal) are categorized separately from those using assisted reproductive technology (ART), or the manipulation of oocytes and embryos (Table 48-4).[55] The Centers for Disease Control and Prevention monitors ART in the United States through the National ART Surveillance System. The use of ART is trending upward, with the number of cycles increasing from just below 88,000 in 1999 to more than 148,000 in 2008. This represents an estimated 1% of live births.[56]

Procedures using ART provide a valuable treatment option for many couples who are not candidates for OI/COS alone or IUI. Of the 104,673 fresh, non-donor ART cycles in 2008, 37% resulted in a pregnancy and 30% in a live birth.[56] The evaluation of outcomes from these births is complex and controversial. Most pregnancies result in healthy offspring without long-term complications. However, infants born from multiple gestation pregnancies, which make up approximately 30% of pregnancies from ART, may experience health complications as a result of preterm birth and low birth weight.[56,57] The data regarding birth defects remain conflicting. Whereas some studies document no increased risk with ART, others report an elevated risk of 30% or higher.[58,59] The National Birth Defects Prevention Study, an ongoing investigation of major birth defects in the United States, revealed associations between ART and septal heart defects, cleft lip, and certain gastrointestinal malformations, predominantly in the singleton births. Because infertility itself has been linked to an increased risk for birth defects, it is difficult to determine whether the underlying condition or the treatment is the cause.[59,60] Additionally, the relatively small incidence of congenital malformations (less than 5%) and ill-defined patient histories complicate the comparisons of data between studies.[57] Birth outcomes will continue to be an area of focus as data accumulate from the rising numbers of ART procedures.

INDICATIONS

Assisted reproductive technology procedures are utilized to address both female and male factor infertility. For women with adequate ovarian reserve, COS can be combined with ART procedures that facilitate fertilization if there are additional male factors and/or implantation if there are female structural factors. Each couple undergoes a thorough infertility evaluation to determine an individualized approach.

CASE 48-2

QUESTION 1: F.J., a 39-year-old woman, and her 42-year-old husband are a recently married couple undergoing a comprehensive infertility evaluation after 6 months without conceiving. F.J.'s medical history is positive for seasonal allergic rhinitis, dysmenorrhea, and a history of chlamydia at age 21. Her current screen for sexually transmitted infections is negative. F.J.'s reproductive history reveals menarche at age 11, no prior pregnancies, and regular menstrual cycles approximately 30 days in length. Her body mass index is 21 kg/m^2. There are no abnormal findings on her physical exam. She undergoes a CC challenge test and her FSH and estradiol levels on cycle day 3 are 7 milli-international units/mL and 46 pg/mL, respectively. The day 10 FSH is 6 milli-international units/mL. Her HSG shows complete occlusion of the left fallopian tube and partial occlusion of the right fallopian tube. What findings support female factor infertility?

This couple is undergoing evaluation of infertility after only 6 months without conceiving because of F.J.'s advanced age (older than 35) and history of chlamydia, which places her at increased risk of complications from pelvic inflammatory disease. The occlusion of her fallopian tubes is most likely from the chlamydial infection at age 21, which may or may not have been detected at that time. Laparoscopy would be necessary to rule out any additional causes such as endometriosis. Further hysteroscopic procedures are warranted to define the location and type of obstruction and to determine whether surgical repair is feasible.[61] Her regular menstrual cycle length and history of dysmenorrhea is supportive of an ovulatory menstrual cycle and her CC challenge test shows adequate ovarian reserve, with normal levels of FSH and estradiol. She is within the normal weight range and has normal findings upon physical examination. However, further laboratory testing may be warranted to confirm normal thyroid and pituitary function and rule out of findings associated with PCOS.

CASE 48-2, QUESTION 2: F.J.'s husband has normal findings upon physical exam. His semen analysis yields the following results:

Semen volume, 3 mL
Sperm number, 41 × 10^6
Sperm concentration, 18 × 10^6/mL
Sperm total motility, 35%
Sperm progressive motility, 30%
Sperm vitality, 60%
Sperm morphology, 2%

A repeat analysis produces similar results. Additional laboratory findings include:

Testosterone, 650 ng/dL
FSH, 4 milli-international units/mL
Prolactin, 14.2 ng/mL

What is the significance of these findings for male factor infertility?

The semen analysis is significant for sperm motility and morphology values below the lower reference limit defined by the World Health Organization. The semen volume, sperm number, and vitality measurements are just above the lower reference limit (Table 48-2).[28] Interventions to improve sperm parameters typically target the underlying cause if possible, such as treatment of hyperprolactinemia or supplementation with testosterone. In some cases, sperm production can be stimulated through the use of medications that influence the hypothalamic-pituitary-testicular axis. For example, CC improves sperm concentrations in men with hypogonadotropic hypogonadism by stimulating hypothalamic release of GnRH. There is no consensus regarding the optimal dosage regimen, which is FDA-labeled for use in women only. Small clinical studies have examined CC 50 mg once daily and alternate-day dosing for treatment periods of several months with positive results.[62] Administration of various regimens of injectable gonadotropins (FSH, LH, or hCG) also improves pregnancy rates.[63] Given the patient's normal serum testosterone and FSH, CC or gonadotropins are not recommended therapies. His prolactin is normal as well, ruling out this potential secondary cause. In this case, there is no identifiable cause of the abnormal parameters so it is deemed idiopathic, without a known etiology.[22]

Antioxidants such as vitamin C, vitamin E, folic acid, zinc, selenium, and L-carnitine are reported to counteract negative effects from oxidative stress on sperm. Initial studies have demonstrated improvement in sperm motility, concentration, and morphology.[64] A systematic review documented a fourfold increase in pregnancy rates with the use of zinc, magnesium, vitamin E, and L-carnitine.[65] F.J.'s husband may choose to take a daily antioxidant supplement as they move forward with other treatment decisions.

Insemination procedures are one approach to address abnormal findings on semen analysis. Bypassing the cervix and placing the sperm closer to the fallopian tubes near the time of ovulation can overcome lower sperm counts and motility issues. In regards to this couple, however, F.J. does not have patent fallopian tubes and would not be a candidate for IUI.[38] An ART procedure will be necessary to address both female and male infertility factors.

PROCEDURES

CASE 48-2, QUESTION 3: The couple is eager to become pregnant and inquires about procedures using ART. They have saved in anticipation of paying out of pocket for subsequent expenses because their medical insurance provides minimal coverage. Which procedure is recommended for this couple based upon their female and male factors?

The primary ART is IVF, which involves retrieval of oocytes after COS, fertilization in vitro, and transfer of the embryo directly to the uterus through the cervix, bypassing the fallopian tubes (Fig. 48-2; Table 48-4).[55] Intracytoplasmic sperm injection (ICSI), or the injection of sperm directly into the oocyte during the fertilization process, accompanies IVF if severe sperm dysfunction is evident. This procedure has been linked to a risk of transferring certain chromosomal abnormalities called imprinting disorders (Beckwith-Wiedemann syndrome, Angelman syndrome) in less than 1% of births. For most couples it is generally regarded as a safe and effective procedure and was performed

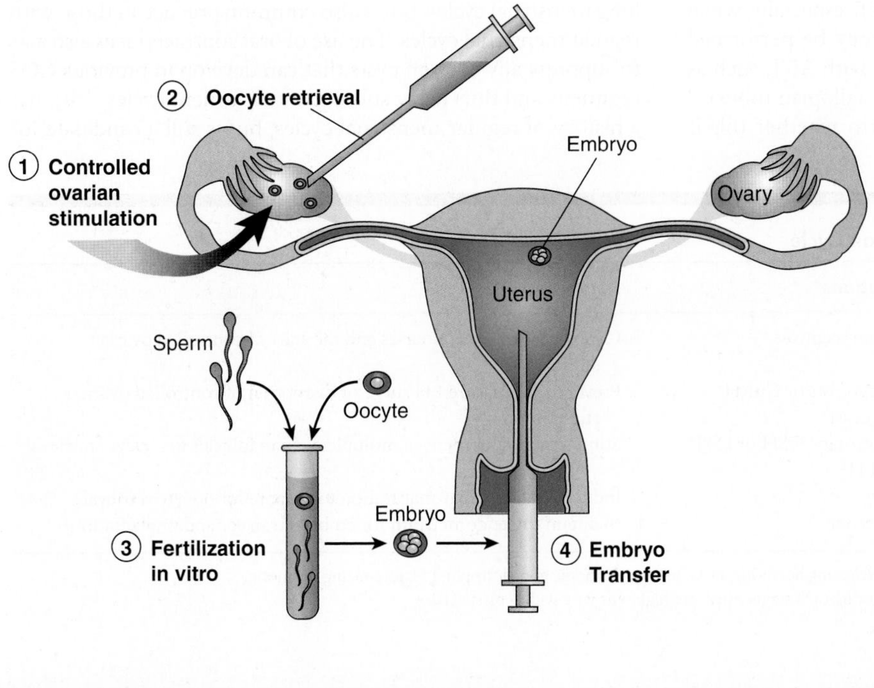

FIGURE 48-2 In vitro fertilization process.

in more than 67,000 fresh nondonor ART cycles in the United States in 2008.[56,66,67]

For a visual of ICSI, see PowerPoint slide 7 at http://thepoint.lww.com/AT10e.

Alternate procedures include gamete intrafallopian transfer and zygote intrafallopian transfer, which alter the timing of fertilization and location of transplantation. In gamete transfer, the retrieved oocytes are transferred with the sperm to the fallopian tube to allow for natural fertilization. In zygote transfer, the oocytes are fertilized in vitro, but are transferred at an earlier stage of development to the fallopian tubes, rather than the uterus.[55] The gamete and zygote transfer procedures are associated with slightly lower live birth rates than IVF (21% and 18% vs. 34%).[56] A variety of ancillary procedures can be used based upon each couple's history and clinical presentation. These include genetic screening and cryopreservation of embryos.[55]

Assisted reproductive technology also allows couples to use donor sperm and/or oocytes to overcome severe sperm or ovarian dysfunction that cannot be addressed through other methods. The option of using donor oocytes uniquely targets infertility due to diminished ovarian reserve. Recent data documented the use of donor oocytes in only 3% of ART procedures in women younger than age 35, but this rate increased to 71% of procedures in women older than age 44.[56]

The financial impact of ART is substantial. A 2006 survey by RESOLVE: The National Infertility Association identified the median cost of an IVF cycle to be $7,500 plus an additional $3,000 to $5,000 for medications. Procedures such as ICSI added an additional $1,500 to the per-cycle cost. This is compared to a median cost of $350 for an IUI cycle.[68] A recent study documented the costs associated with the treatment of infertility in approximately 300 women during an 18-month period. For the 186 women who experienced IVF, the median per-person cost during this time was $24,373 due to multiple procedures.[69] Costs vary widely between clinics and many offer financial counseling and payment packages to facilitate treatment.

In regards to this couple, IVF is more appropriate than gamete intrafallopian transfer and zygote intrafallopian transfer due to F.J.'s tubal findings. Although surgical repair of the obstructed fallopian tubes may be possible in some cases, many couples choose to bypass this option and pursue ART, especially when there are additional male factors. Surgery may be performed in select candidates to improve success rates with ART, such as with hydrosalpinx (fluid accumulation in the fallopian tubes).[70] F.J. will need a surgical evaluation to confirm whether this is recommended prior to proceeding to ART. F.J. is ovulatory with adequate ovarian reserve, so the use of donor oocytes is not required. Her husband's abnormal sperm parameters can be addressed through ICSI, with the option of using donor sperm in the future, if necessary. The couple has already anticipated the financial considerations of the procedures, which will be finalized prior to initiating the treatment plan.

IN VITRO FERTILIZATION

CASE 48-2, QUESTION 4: After the completed evaluation, the couple chooses to undergo IVF with intracytoplasmic sperm injection. Although F.J. is very excited to begin the process, she is anxious about administering the multiple injectable medications associated with the procedure. What medication regimen is recommended to initiate the IVF protocol?

The basic steps in an IVF protocol include COS, oocyte retrieval, fertilization, embryo culture and embryo transfer. Medications are primarily used during three main stages of IVF: COS, oocyte retrieval, and luteal phase support (Table 48-5). (For a step-by-step guide to all the steps in this complex process, go to http://www.sart.org/detail.aspx?id=1903) Treatment protocols vary widely in the medications used, dosing regimens, and timing of administration. A sample in vitro fertilization protocol representing F.J.'s experience is provided in Figure 48-3.

STAGE ONE: CONTROLLED OVARIAN STIMULATION

The purpose of COS for IVF is the development of multiple follicles for oocyte retrieval. Although oocyte retrieval and fertilization can be performed during a normal ovulatory cycle without stimulation, it is more common and many times necessary to use this process.

Oral Contraceptives

Controlled ovarian stimulation for IVF is designed to manipulate follicular development for oocyte retrieval at the most optimal stage of maturation. Many protocols start with the administration of oral contraceptives for up to 28 days in the preceding menstrual cycle. This serves to control the timing of the onset of the next menses in order to plan for initiating the COS regimen. This is particularly pertinent in women who have irregular or long menstrual cycles, but is also common practice in those with regular menstrual cycles. The use of oral contraceptives also acts to suppress any ovarian cysts that can develop in previous COS regimens and thus delay subsequent treatment cycles.[71] F.J. has a history of regular menstrual cycles, but is still a candidate for

TABLE 48-5
Role of Medications in an In Vitro Fertilization Cycle

IVF Stage	Medications[a]	Role
Stage One: Controlled ovarian stimulation	Oral contraceptives	Control the onset of menses and the start of controlled ovarian stimulation
	GnRH agonists or GnRH antagonists	Prevent a premature LH surge or disruption of controlled ovarian stimulation
	Gonadotropins (FSH or FSH plus LH)	Stimulate development of multiple ovarian follicles for oocyte retrieval
Stage Two: Oocyte retrieval	hCG	Induce final follicular maturation to prepare for oocyte retrieval
Stage Three: Luteal phase support	Progesterone	Maintain the endometrium for embryo transfer and implantation

FSH, follicle stimulating hormone; GnRH, gonadotropin releasing hormone; hCG, human chorionic gonadotropin; LH, luteinizing hormone.
[a] This list reflects the medications most commonly used during each stage. Alternate regimens vary widely by specialist.

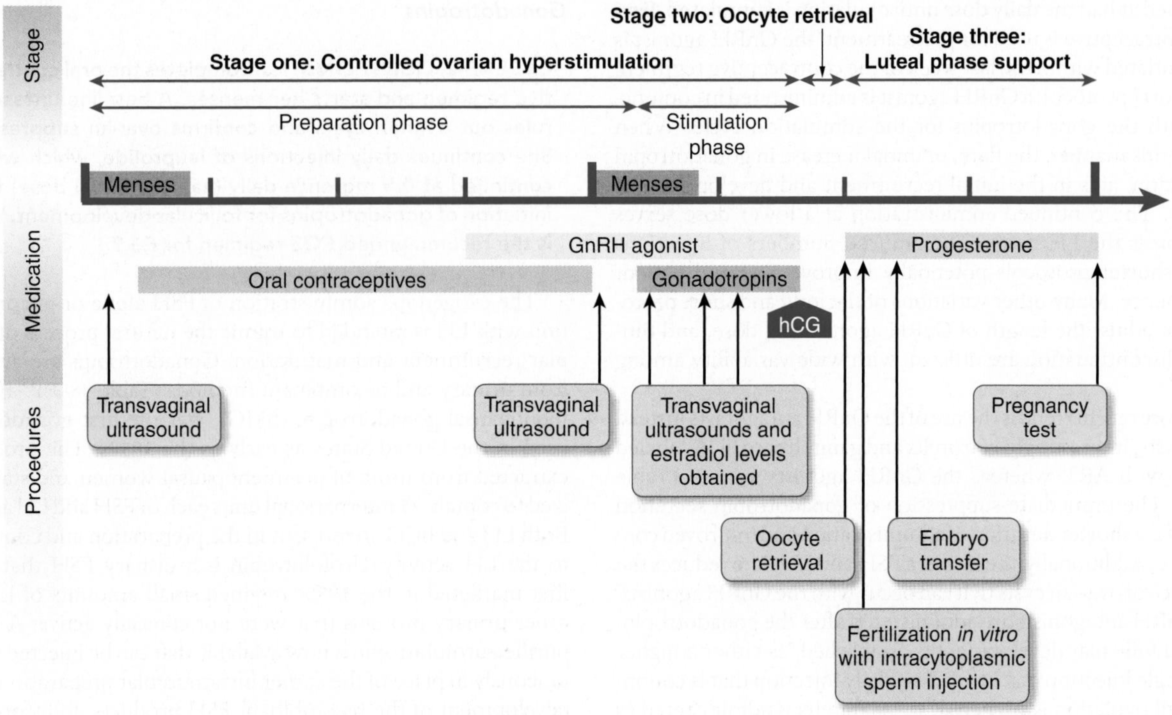

FIGURE 48-3 Sample in vitro fertilization protocol (Case 48-2).

oral contraceptive therapy to conveniently time the remainder of the treatment course.

Gonadotropin-Releasing Hormone Analogs

Once the COS process begins it can be interrupted by an endogenous surge of LH that triggers ovulation prematurely and threatens the success of the cycle. Most protocols use medications to limit the influence of any endogenous hormone levels as the cycle progresses. Gonadotropin-releasing hormone agonists have been used for this purpose for several decades. Administration of a GnRH agonist initially increases pituitary gonadotropin release, often referred to as a "flare." Continued daily administration leads to receptor downregulation and reduced pituitary secretion of LH and FSH, allowing for direct administration of the gonadotropins by injection.[71]

The most common IVF regimens in the United States use either subcutaneous leuprolide or intranasal nafarelin (Table 48-6).[35] The leuprolide formulation is often dosed in "units" using an insulin syringe to permit measurement of small volumes. Daily doses of 10 to 20 "units" correspond with 0.5 to 1 mg using the 1 mg /0.2 mL product. The depot formulations used for endometriosis or hormone-dependent cancers are not ideal for IVF. The prolonged pituitary suppression is associated with a need for higher doses and longer duration of gonadotropin administration for COS.[72] Intranasal nafarelin has been studied in doses of 200 to 400 mcg twice daily.[73] Intranasal absorption can be variable depending on the administration technique, dosage interval, sneezing, or use of nasal decongestants.[71,74] However, studies indicate that pregnancy rates between the GnRH agonists are similar.[73]

Treatment protocols are identified by the timing of GnRH agonist administration.

ONLINE CONTENT

For a comparison of IVF protocols, see PowerPoint slide 8 at <u>http://thepoint.lww.com/AT10e.</u>

In a traditional "long" protocol, a GnRH agonist is initiated during the follicular or luteal phase of the preceding menstrual cycle. Once gonadotropins are initiated, the GnRH agonist is

TABLE 48-6
Gonadotropin Releasing Hormone Analogs for In Vitro Fertilization

Analog	Product Name	Strength/Dosage Form	Route of Administration
GnRH agonist	Nafarelin acetate (Synarel)	2 mg/mL solution (200 mcg/spray)	Intranasal
	Leuprolide acetate	1 mg/0.2 mL solution	SC
GnRH antagonist	Cetrorelix acetate[a] (Cetrotide)	0.25 mg, 3 mg kit	SC
	Ganirelix acetate[a]	250 mcg/0.5 ml solution	SC

GnRH, gonadotropin releasing hormone; SC, subcutaneous.
[a] FDA-labeled for use with assisted reproductive technology procedures.
Adapted with permission from Facts & Comparisons eAnswers. http://online.factsandcomparisons.com/MonoDisp.aspx?monoID=fandc-hcp10444; http://online.factsandcomparisons.com/MonoDisp.aspx?monoID=fandc-hcp10921; http://online.factsandcomparisons.com/MonoDisp.aspx?monoID=fandc-hcp11447; http://online.factsandcomparisons.com/MonoDisp.aspx?monoID=fandc-hcp11213. Accessed November 4, 2011.

continued at half the daily dose until ovulation is stimulated. If an oral contraceptive is used for pretreatment, the GnRH agonist is often initiated within the last week of the contraceptive regimen. In a "short" protocol, a GnRH agonist is administered in conjunction with the gonadotropins for the stimulation cycle. When used in this manner, the flare, or initial increase in gonadotropin production, aids in the initial recruitment and development of follicles. The continued administration at a lower dose serves to suppress the LH surge. The reduced numbers of injections in the shorter protocols potentially improve cost and patient convenience. Many other variations of the long and short protocols that adjust the length of GnRH agonist use, dose, and timing of discontinuation are utilized, with wide variability among clinics.[71]

A more recent trend is the use of the GnRH antagonists instead of agonists. Interestingly, cetrorelix and ganirelix are FDA-labeled for use with ART, whereas the GnRH agonists are not (Table 48-6).[35] The immediate suppression of gonadotropin secretion allows for a shorter duration of administration and improved convenience. Additionally, the lack of a FSH and LH flare reduces the incidence of ovarian cysts that can occur with the GnRH agonists. The GnRH antagonists are administered after the gonadotropin-induced follicular development is established, as either a higher dose single injection or a lower dose daily injection that is continued until ovulation is triggered.[75,76] Ganirelix is administered as a daily 250-mcg subcutaneous injection and cetrorelix is either a daily subcutaneous injection of 0.25 mg or a single 3-mg dose.[35] The timing of initiation is either "fixed" on a particular day of stimulation or "flexible" based on follicular development.[75,76] Protocols that avoid oral contraceptive pretreatment may be advantageous as they appear to require a shorter duration and lower dose of gonadotropins.[76,77]

Available trials comparing GnRH agonist long protocols versus GnRH antagonists show up to 16% lower per-cycle pregnancy rates with the antagonists.[75,76,78] As GnRH antagonist protocols continue to be studied, additional data will help determine the best candidates for this alternative approach.

The administration of GnRH analogs in the long protocol is associated with hot flashes, headaches, and sleep disturbances due to hypoestrogenic effects. Concurrent administration of oral contraceptives may help lessen these responses.[79] The prolonged ovarian suppression with the longer protocols using GnRH agonists has been associated with symptoms of depression and anxiety in some studies, but this has not been replicated in all trials.[80,81] Currently, there is disagreement on whether the symptoms are associated with the low estrogen levels during pituitary downregulation or the fluctuating estrogen levels seen during the COS phase that follows.[80] Local reactions at the injection site and nasal and throat irritation are adverse effects expected with the subcutaneous and intranasal routes of administration.[79]

In this case, a protocol using a GnRH agonist would reflect the most traditional first-line approach. For the preparation phase, an injectable (leuprolide) or intranasal (nafarelin) product can be used. An intranasal product may appear preferable given F.J.'s concerns about injections. However, the symptoms and duration of her seasonal allergic rhinitis should be clarified because the absorption of the intranasal product can be affected by sneezing, congestion, and use of other intranasal medications. Thorough discussion and demonstration of the subcutaneous injection technique can also reduce a patient's fears regarding this route of administration. After discussion, F.J. agrees to administer leuprolide injections. Once she experiences her next menses, she will begin 21 days of an oral contraceptive. On day 16 of this regimen she will initiate leuprolide 1 mg once daily as a subcutaneous injection in conjunction with the oral contraceptives. A calendar will be provided to help her track the daily doses.

Gonadotropins

CASE 48-2, QUESTION 5: F.J. completes the oral contraceptive regimen and starts her menses. A baseline ultrasound rules out ovarian cysts and confirms ovarian suppression. She continues daily injections of leuprolide, which will be continued at 0.5 mg once daily (half the initial dose) upon initiation of gonadotropins for follicular development. What is the recommended COS regimen for F.J.?

The exogenous administration of FSH alone or in combination with LH is intended to mimic the natural process of follicular recruitment and maturation. Gonadotropins are available from urinary and recombinant methods (Table 48-3).[35] Human menopausal gonadotropin, (hMG), was the first gonadotropin used in the United States as early as the 1950s. The product is extracted from urine of postmenopausal women and standardized to contain 75 international units each of FSH and LH activity. Both LH and hCG are present in the preparation and contribute to the LH activity. Urofollitropin is a urinary FSH that when first marketed in the 1980s retained small amounts of LH and other urinary proteins that were not clinically active. A highly purified urofollitropin is now available that can be injected subcutaneously in place of the earlier intramuscular preparations. The development of the recombinant FSH products (follitropin alfa and follitropin beta) further expanded treatment options in the late 1990s. Although they have unique chemical structures they result in clinically similar effects. A recombinant LH product is also available for use in combination with urinary or recombinant FSH.[82]

Women with hypogonadic hypogonadism require administration of both FSH and LH for COS because their low endogenous LH levels do not support follicular development. This is achieved through the administration of hMG or a combination of recombinant FSH plus recombinant LH. Women with normal pituitary function can receive injections of FSH alone, either as urofollitropin or a recombinant product. Although it is generally demonstrated that urinary hMG and recombinant FSH result in similar pregnancy rates, recent meta-analyses documented a relative increase in live birth rate of approximately 20% with the urinary hMG. At this time there is no consensus recommendation for the preferred formulation among experts.[83–86]

Dosage regimens for the gonadotropins are intended to promote multiple follicles for oocyte retrieval and vary widely among clinics. A common starting dose in fixed-dose protocols is 150 to 225 international units daily, with further dose adjustments made based on the status of the developing follicles. Treatment may continue for 7 to 12 days, although longer courses may be necessary depending on follicular response. If subsequent cycles are needed, the initial treatment doses are chosen based on the stimulation achieved in the first cycle.[36]

F.J. is undergoing her first cycle of IVF, so there are no data regarding prior gonadotropin response to guide the dose selection. She has no signs of hypothalamic or pituitary dysfunction so she can receive FSH alone or in combination with LH. All of the available highly purified or recombinant products require daily subcutaneous injections. Although this may be a concern for F.J., this is an advantage over earlier formulations that required intramuscular injection. All products require reconstitution of one or more vials of lyophilized powder just prior to injection except certain formulations of the recombinant follitropin alfa and beta. The two recombinant FSH formulations are available in pen injection devices that avoid the need for reconstitution and reduce the complexity of the dose preparation and injection procedure (Table 48-3).[35] Medication costs vary widely among pharmacies, but the common initial daily doses of any of the formulations can average up to $350 per day.[87] Patient education should focus on product-specific instructions for storage, preparation for injection, and the correct subcutaneous injection technique. All products have patient-friendly video demonstrations or handouts available on the Internet to facilitate this process. (For helpful training videos and patient handouts that walk through the dose preparation and injection technique, see http://www.ferringfertility.com/medications/trainingguide.asp, http://www.fertilitylifelines.com/resources/medicationguide.jsp, and http://www.follistim.com/Consumer/FollistimAQCartridge/FollistimPen/index.asp.) The patient should be instructed to anticipate possible injection-site reactions as well as psychological symptoms of irritability, mood swings, and depression which may increase during the COS phase.[38]

After consideration of these issues, a recombinant FSH product is chosen for F.J. because of the convenience of the pen device. She will begin a dose of 225 IU of recombinant follitropin alfa injected subcutaneously once daily.

CASE 48-2, QUESTION 6: F.J. begins daily subcutaneous injections of follitropin alfa in addition to her leuprolide injections. What medication monitoring should be provided at this time?

The goal of gonadotropin therapy is to guide the development of multiple follicles for oocyte retrieval without increasing the risk for ovarian hyperstimulation syndrome (OHSS), a rare but serious complication of COS. In its most severe form, this syndrome is characterized by increased systemic vascular permeability that can result in ovarian rupture, thromboembolism, renal failure, and adult respiratory distress syndrome. The risk for this condition correlates most directly with the development of multiple ovarian follicles during COS. Additional risk factors include younger age, low body weight, and history of PCOS. Routine monitoring of ovarian follicular development allows the clinician to maximize efficacy and reduce the risk for overstimulation.[88]

The recommended monitoring includes vaginal ultrasounds and serum estradiol measurements performed every 1 to 3 days during the COS phase. The monitoring frequency increases as the follicular development advances, and the gonadotropin doses may be reduced or increased depending on the number and size of the follicles. If hyperresponse is evident, the cycle may be cancelled prior to oocyte retrieval.[88] An alternative to cycle cancellation is "coasting," or discontinuation of gonadotropins until serial estradiol measurements show a plateau or declining trend.[89] One protocol recommends cycle cancellation or coasting if estradiol levels are greater than 3,500 pg/mL and/or there are more than 20 follicles at least 16 mm in diameter.[90] According to the most recent ART data, approximately 5% of cycle cancellations are due to exaggerated medication response. Most result from inadequate oocyte development.[56]

As F.J. initiates therapy, she is scheduled for serum estradiol and vaginal ultrasound measurements every other day. This increases to daily monitoring on day 7 of the combination of leuprolide and follitropin alfa as the number and size of the follicles continues to increase.

STAGE TWO: OOCYTE RETRIEVAL

Chorionic Gonadotropin

CASE 48-2, QUESTION 7: F.J. presents for her daily monitoring on day 10 and it is determined that she is ready for oocyte retrieval. What medication regimen is recommended at this time?

Chorionic gonadotropin is administered in preparation for oocyte retrieval to simulate the effect of the physiologic LH surge on final oocyte maturation. The oocyte retrieval must be carefully timed to coincide with the completion of the oocyte maturation process, just prior to ovulation. Many centers schedule oocyte retrieval between 34 and 36 hours after chorionic gonadotropin is injected.

Chorionic gonadotropin is available from urinary or recombinant sources. The urinary hCG product is administered as a single intramuscular injection of 5,000 to 10,000 international units.[81] Doses of 5,000 international units may be administered to patients who are deemed to be high risk for OHSS.[88] The dose of the recombinant product is 250 mcg injected subcutaneously.[81]

The recombinant LH product is not routinely administered for oocyte maturation because the required dose equivalent of 25,000 to 30,000 international units in a single injection is not feasible with the 75 international-unit vial. A single dose of a GnRH agonist is an alternate method of triggering LH release in IVF protocols that incorporate a GnRH antagonist for COS. A recent review documented a reduced risk for OHSS with the GnRH antagonist, but the live birth rate was 56% lower.[91] F.J. received the GnRH agonist leuprolide in her prestimulation period so she would not be eligible for this approach.

Given F.J.'s concerns regarding injections and the fact that she has been administering the follitropin alfa subcutaneously, it is prudent to continue with this route of administration. F.J. is instructed to inject a single 250 mcg dose of recombinant chorionic gonadotropin subcutaneously. She will discontinue leuprolide and the follitropin alfa at this time.

Ovarian Hyperstimulation Syndrome

CASE 48-2, QUESTION 8: F.J. undergoes a transvaginal oocyte retrieval procedure 36 hours after the administration of recombinant chorionic gonadotropin and there are 9 oocytes available for fertilization. What additional counseling is recommended for F.J. after the oocyte retrieval?

As previously described, OHSS is a rare complication associated with COS. Careful monitoring of estradiol levels and follicular development on ultrasound limits the incidence. However, if symptoms develop, it is typically within 1 to 2 weeks after oocyte retrieval. OHSS is generally categorized as mild, moderate, or severe, and can occur early (within 9 days after oocyte retrieval) or late (after 10 days, often associated with a pregnancy).[79,89] The clinical signs of OHSS are thought to result from increased capillary permeability due to high levels of vascular endothelial growth factor. However, the specific underlying pathology is poorly understood. A mild presentation of OHSS consists primarily of gastrointestinal symptoms (abdominal pain, nausea, diarrhea, bloating) or weight gain, especially abdominal distension. A patient experiencing these symptoms will be instructed to avoid physical activity, maintain oral fluid intake of at least 1 liter per day, and monitor daily weights and urine output. The patient should report any weight gain of 2 pounds or more to allow for more intensive outpatient monitoring of liver and renal function, electrolytes, and hematologic parameters. If the condition progresses, the patient may require hospitalization for monitoring and treatment of severe outcomes such as thromboembolism, renal failure, pulmonary distress, or ovarian rupture.[79,88]

There were no initial indications of hyperstimulation during F.J.'s COS regimen, so she will be instructed to monitor for signs of OHSS during the 2 weeks after oocyte retrieval. She should notify her physician if she experiences gastrointestinal symptoms or weight gain, even if the symptoms are mild. This will facilitate early monitoring to maximize safety during the remainder of the IVF process.

STAGE THREE: LUTEAL PHASE SUPPORT

Progesterone

CASE 48-2, QUESTION 9: After the oocyte retrieval, F.J. is in need of a regimen for luteal phase support. Which agent should be selected?

Supplemental progesterone is administered immediately after oocyte retrieval to provide additional "luteal phase support" during IVF. The luteal phase of the menstrual cycle (Fig. 48-1) is dominated by progesterone released by the corpus luteum that prepares the endometrium for implantation of the fertilized ovum. The disruption of follicles during the oocyte retrieval process delays production of progesterone, necessitating supplementation. Additionally, cycles that utilize a GnRH agonist may be complicated by residual inhibition of pituitary LH secretion and progesterone production into the luteal phase.[92]

Progesterone is available in oral, vaginal, or injectable formulations (Table 48-7).[35] The intramuscular injection of progesterone in oil in a daily dose of 50 mg was the first method used for supplementation and continues to be widely used. However, alternatives to progesterone in oil have been sought due to frequent reports of rash and discomfort at the injection site.[92] Intramuscular injection of a progesterone derivative, 17-α-hydroxyprogesterone caproate, was viewed as a potential alternative requiring less frequent administration (every 3 days) with fewer injection site reactions. Although several studies have indicated benefit for luteal phase support, its primary use in the United States has focused on the prevention of preterm birth when initiated in the second trimester of pregnancy.[35,93–95]

Vaginal progesterone preparations have gained popularity for luteal phase support due to ease of administration and the avoidance of injection-site reactions. The 8% progesterone vaginal gel and the 100 mg vaginal insert are the only commercially available FDA-labeled preparations for use in ART procedures. The gel is administered as one 90 mg applicator once or twice daily. The dose of the vaginal insert is 100 mg either twice a day (every 12 hours) or three times a day (every 8 hours).[35,92,96] Patient education should focus on the correct technique for intravaginal administration. Both products utilize a disposable applicator to facilitate correct placement. Detailed patient instructions are provided by both manufacturers. **http://www.ferringfertility.com/medications/endometrin/admin_instructions.pdf** and **http://www.crinoneusa.com/patients/Patient_Information.pdf.** The vaginal preparations are associated with local irritation and vaginal discharge, although the vaginal gel is generally associated with less discharge than the inserts or suppositories.[97] Clinical studies suggest no difference in pregnancy rates between vaginal and intramuscular formulations, so clinician and patient preferences often dictate the selection .[92,96,97]

Oral formulations range from 100 to 400 mg per day and are associated with nausea, sedation, and dizziness. They are less commonly used due to initial reports of lower pregnancy rates with this route of administration.[92] Compounded formulations are widely available, including oral micronized progesterone and progesterone vaginal suppositories, gels, and creams. In some cases, patients are instructed to insert oral progesterone formulations intravaginally.

Progesterone is administered daily until a pregnancy test is performed and continued until at least 7 to 9 weeks gestation. In terms of safety, data suggest that there are no significant risks to the mother or fetus from supplemental progesterone during this time period.[92] An association between first-trimester exposure to progesterone and the development of hypospadias, or a malformed urethral opening, in male fetuses has been proposed.[98] It is not clear whether the type of progestogen, either natural progesterone or a synthetic progestin, is important due to varying androgenicity profiles. At this time, all products recommended for luteal phase support are progesterone-based. The FDA does not require product labeling for progesterone products used for luteal phase support to contain a warning regarding fetal exposure risk.[92]

Luteal phase support after oocyte retrieval is especially important for F.J. because she received a GnRH agonist in her long cycle protocol. Because the efficacy of the parenteral and vaginal formulations is similar, the patient chooses the vaginal route to avoid further injections. She determines that she is most comfortable with 8% progesterone vaginal gel applied once daily and is given instructions regarding the appropriate administration technique.

TABLE 48-7
Commercially Available Progesterone Products Used in Assisted Reproductive Technology

Product Name	Strength/Dosage Form	Route of Administration
Crinone	8% vaginal gel[a]	Vaginal
Endometrin	100 mg vaginal insert[a]	Vaginal
FIRST-Progesterone VGS	25, 50, 100, 200, 400 mg vaginal suppository (compounding kit)	Vaginal
Progesterone	50 mg/mL (oil)	Intramuscular
Prometrium	100, 200 mg capsule	Oral

[a] FDA-labeled for luteal phase support.
Adapted with permission from Facts & Comparisons eAnswers. **http://online.factsandcomparisons.com/MonoDisp.aspx?monoID=fandc-hcp11740.** Accessed November 4, 2011.

Embryo Transfer

CASE 48-2, QUESTION 10: The in vitro fertilization process using intracytoplasmic sperm injection yields four cleavage-stage embryos. What considerations are necessary for embryo transfer?

After fertilization, timing of the embryo transfer into the uterus depends on the stage of development. Cleavage-stage embryos are transferred 2 to 3 days postfertilization, whereas embryos in the blastocyst stage are transferred at day 5 or 6.[99] (To reference a tool that gives a representation of the embryo at different stages, see **http://visembryo.com/baby/pregnancy1.html.**) The number of embryos placed during this process must balance the risks of a multiple gestation pregnancy with the likelihood of successful implantation.

Multiple gestation pregnancies are associated with increased maternal and neonatal morbidity. The mother is at risk for complications such as premature labor, pregnancy-induced hypertension, and gestational diabetes.[100] Preterm labor occurs in approximately 15% of single gestation pregnancies compared with 75% of triplet pregnancies. The neonates are more likely to experience fetal growth restriction and require intensive care for pulmonary, gastrointestinal, and neurologic complications.[101] Additional stressors include the financial and psychosocial implications of raising children with complex medical needs that may persist beyond infancy.[100,101]

The transfer of a single embryo has the lowest risk for multiple gestation, but is associated with lower pregnancy rates each cycle than the placement of two or more embryos.[102,103] However, the cumulative live birth rate of a single embryo transfer followed by a frozen thawed embryo transfer is similar to that of one cycle of double embryo transfer.[102] The cryopreservation of embryos for use in subsequent cycles circumvents the need for additional oocyte retrieval procedures.

The 2008 ART data indicate that half of the cycles using fresh, nondonor oocytes involved transfer of two embryos.[56] The ASRM has developed embryo transfer recommendations to limit high-order multiple pregnancies (3 or more implanted embryos). The guidelines define the most favorable prognostic criteria to be the first cycle of IVF, embryos of high quality morphology, and excess embryos available for cryopreservation. The transfer of a single embryo is recommended in women under the age of 35 who meet these favorable criteria due to the high rates of success. The guidelines then recommend limits for the number of embryos transferred for additional age groups: 35 to 37 years, 38 to 40 years and 41 to 42 years. Higher numbers of embryos are recommended for those who do not meet the most favorable prognostic criteria.[99]

F.J. is 39 years old experiencing her first cycle of IVF. If the embryos are judged to have good quality morphology, no more than three cleavage-stage or two blastocysts should be transferred according to ASRM guidelines.[99] A pregnancy test will be performed 9 to 12 days after the embryo transfer to determine the outcome of the cycle.

LONG-TERM CONSIDERATIONS

Alternate Protocols

CASE 48-2, QUESTION 11: After careful consideration, the couple decides to transfer two cleavage-stage embryos and reserve two for cryopreservation. Unfortunately, the embryo transfer procedure is unsuccessful and the couple plans to pursue a second procedure. What considerations are necessary for future cycles?

Determining an action plan for subsequent procedures requires a thorough evaluation of the response to therapy during the first cycle. If COS is repeated for oocyte retrieval, hormone levels, follicular development, fertilization rates, and numbers of viable embryos are all considered to determine if dosage adjustments are necessary. Patients considered poor responders to COS with a GnRH agonist may have an improved response to a shorter flare protocol or a GnRH antagonist protocol due to less prolonged pituitary and ovarian suppression.[104]

In this case, F.J. experienced adequate follicular development for oocyte retrieval without signs of OHSS. The fertilization procedure was successful and two embryos were cryopreserved for future procedures. The couple can choose to avoid another stimulation process for oocyte removal and move to frozen embryo transfer. The benefit of a shorter process is countered by lower live birth rates with transfer of frozen embryos (30%) versus fresh embryos (37%). Implantation rates of frozen embryos are highest in women under age 35 (24%). For a 39-year-old like F.J., the rate decreases to 17%.[56] Medications remain important for the frozen embryo transfer process, which may begin as soon as the next cycle, although some clinicians recommend waiting one menstrual cycle. Ovulation may be induced through the use of injectable gonadotropins. Supplementation with estradiol and/or progesterone may also be necessary to prepare the endometrium for implantation.[105,106]

Beyond planning the actual protocol, the long-term safety of any repeated medication exposure as well as the psychosocial effects of continuing therapy must be considered. The time needed to gather available information and weigh all considerations will be specific to each couple.

Cancer

Studies of infertility treatments published in the early 1990s suggested a link with ovarian cancer.[40,107] However, data accumulated since that time fail to document an increased risk with medications for COS.[41,108–111] Interpretation of the data is complicated by the observation that infertility itself is associated with a higher risk for ovarian cancer and women who are infertile are more likely to be of increased age and nulliparous, both characteristics associated with ovarian cancer risk.[41,112] The association between infertility medications and other cancers such as breast and endometrial is limited and inconclusive.[109,113,114] This is largely due to small study populations, lack of standard infertility treatment protocols, and limited reporting of full medical histories. At this time, there is no recommendation for modifying COS protocols based on cancer risk. This will continue to be a subject of interest.

Based on the current data, F.J.'s risk for various cancers should be based on standard criteria, such as family history and lifestyle risk factors. She should participate in the recommended routine screening procedures for cancer as she ages.

Psychosocial Issues

The psychological stress of the diagnosis and treatment of infertility must be considered at all stages. There is an observed fluctuation of mood during the course of an IVF cycle, with higher stress points identified at oocyte retrieval and pregnancy testing. This is complicated by potential side effects of medications as well as the baseline mental health of the couple. It is generally observed that women who are infertile have higher rates of depression and anxiety.[115,116] For couples who undergo successive ART procedures, repeated failures are commonly accompanied by feelings of grief and frustration, and psychological distress is often the reason for discontinuing treatments. Levels of emotional distress, including symptoms of depression and anxiety increase with each unsuccessful cycle.[117] This response appears to remit immediately with a successful pregnancy, but in those who continue to be unsuccessful, symptoms can still be significant even 6 months posttreatment.[117,118]

This couple should be offered individual counseling and social support that extends beyond the initial pretreatment

TABLE 48-8
Patient-Focused Infertility Resources

Sponsor	Website
American Infertility Association	http://www.theafa.org/
American Society of Reproductive Medicine	http://www.reproductivefacts.org/
Centers for Disease Control and Prevention	http://www.cdc.gov/art/PreparingForART/index.htm
Resolve: The National Infertility Association	http://www.resolve.org/
Society for Assisted Reproductive Technology	http://www.sart.org/

consultation to promote positive outcomes.[119] There are several patient-focused resources for informational fact sheets and videos highlighting the financial, medical, and psychosocial issues of infertility (Table 48-8).

KEY REFERENCES AND WEBSITES

A full list of references for this chapter can be found at **http://thepoint.lww.com/AT10e.** Below are the key references and websites for this chapter, with the corresponding reference number in this chapter found in parentheses after the reference.

Key References

American College of Obstetricians and Gynecologists. ACOG Practice Bulletin No. 34. Management of infertility caused by ovulatory dysfunction. *Obstet Gynecol.* 2002;99:347. (13)

Centers for Disease Control and Prevention, American Society for Reproductive Medicine, Society for Assisted Reproductive Technology. 2008 Assisted Reproductive Technology Success Rates: National Summary and Fertility Clinic Reports. Atlanta, GA: US Department of Health and Human Services; 2010. (56)

Humaidan P et al. Preventing ovarian hyperstimulation syndrome. *Fertil Steril.* 2010;94:389. (89)

The Male Infertility Best Practice Policy Committee of the American Urological Association and the Practice Committee of the American Society for Reproductive Medicine. Report on optimal evaluation of the infertile male. *Fertil Steril.* 2006;86(Suppl 4):S202. (22)

Practice Committee of the American Society for Reproductive Medicine. Effectiveness and treatment for unexplained infertility. *Fertil Steril.* 2006;86(Suppl 4):S111. (29)

Practice Committee of the American Society for Reproductive Medicine. Optimal evaluation of the infertile female. *Fertil Steril.* 2006;86(Suppl 4):S264. (2)

Practice Committee of the American Society for Reproductive Medicine. Use of clomiphene citrate in women. *Fertil Steril.* 2006;86(Suppl 4):S187. (33)

Practice Committee of the American Society for Reproductive Medicine. Use of exogenous gonadotropins in anovulatory women. *Fertil Steril.* 2008;90(Suppl 3):S7. (14)

Practice Committee of the American Society for Reproductive Medicine in collaboration with the Society for Reproductive Endocrinology and Infertility. Optimizing natural fertility. *Fertil Steril.* 2008;90(Suppl 3):S1. (11)

Practice Committee of the American Society for Reproductive Medicine in collaboration with the Society for Reproductive Endocrinology and Infertility. Progesterone supplementation during the luteal phase and in early pregnancy in the treatment of infertility: an educational bulletin. *Fertil Steril.* 2008;90(Suppl 3): S150. (92)

World Health Organization, Department of Reproductive Health and Research. *WHO Laboratory Manual for the Examination and Processing of Human Semen.* 5th ed. Geneva, Switzerland: World Health Organization Press; 2010:224. (28)

Zegers-Hochschild F, Adamson GD, de Mouzon J et al. The International Committee for Monitoring Assisted Reproductive Technology (ICMART) and the World Health Organization (WHO) revised glossary on ART terminology, 2009. *Hum Reprod.* 2009;24:2683. (55)

Key Websites

American Society for Reproductive Medicine **http://www.asrm.org/.**

Society for Assisted Reproductive Technology **http://www.sart.org/.**

49

Obstetric Drug Therapy

Kimey D. Ung and Jennifer McNulty

CORE PRINCIPLES

PREGNANCY	CHAPTER CASES
1 The timing and quality of prenatal care can influence an infant's health and survival. Early comprehensive care can promote healthier pregnancies through early detection of risk factors, disease state management, and encouragement of healthy behaviors.	**Case 49-1 (Questions 1, 2)**
2 Determining pregnancy and predicting date of delivery are important to ensure proper prenatal care.	**Case 49-1 (Questions 3, 4)**
3 Important physiologic changes occur in almost all maternal organs during pregnancy to support the growth and development of the fetus.	**Case 49-1 (Question 5)**
4 Drug use during pregnancy presents a great challenge to clinicians because of the potential adverse effect on the embryo, fetus, and newborn. A thorough assessment, including knowledge of the teratogenic potential of the drug, the critical period of exposure, and magnitude of risk, must be compared with the background risk.	**Case 49-1 (Question 6)**
5 Gastrointestinal disturbances such as nausea and vomiting and gastric reflux that occur during pregnancy are common. Treatments include intravenous hydration, pyridoxine (vitamin B_6), antihistamines, and antiemetics for nausea and vomiting. Calcium carbonate, H_2 receptor antagonists, and proton-pump inhibitors may be used for common complaints from reflux.	**Case 49-1 (Questions 7–11)**
6 Urinary tract infections can frequently occur during pregnancy and can easily be treated with nitrofurantoin, cephalexin, or penicillin if cultures are sensitive. If left untreated or treated inadequately, pyelonephritis can develop, which may put the mother at risk for acute respiratory distress syndrome. Intravenous antibiotics such as aminoglycosides, penicillins, and cephalosporins are usually used.	**Case 49-1 (Questions 12, 13)**
7 Diabetes mellitus is the most common maternal medical complication during pregnancy. Tight glycemic control can minimize neonatal and fetal morbidity and mortality associated with diabetic embryopathy.	**Case 49-2 (Questions 1–4), Case 49-3 (Questions 1, 2), Case 49-4 (Questions 1–4)**
8 Women with pregnancy-associated hypertension can be grouped into the following categories: chronic hypertension, pre-eclampsia–eclampsia, pre-eclampsia superimposed on chronic hypertension, and gestational hypertension.	**Case 49-5 (Questions 1–13)**
9 The induction of labor involves the artificial stimulation of uterine contractions that lead to labor and delivery.	**Case 49-6 (Questions 1–5)**
10 Premature birth is the leading cause of neonatal mortality (infant death <1 month of age). Tocolytic therapy to stop contractions, corticosteroids for fetal lung maturity, and antibiotics for preterm premature rupture of membranes can help to prolong the pregnancy.	**Case 49-7 (Questions 1–7)**

continued

PREGNANCY *CONTINUED*

11	Infectious complications including bacterial vaginosis and urinary tract infections can lead to preterm labor. Chorioamnionitis, an infection of the chorion and amnion usually diagnosed during labor with elevations in temperature, should be treated with intravenous antibiotics until delivery. Human immunodeficiency virus–infected mothers should receive intravenous zidovudine during labor and continue their antiretroviral regimens during labor also.	**Case 49-7 (Questions 8–11), Case 49-8 (Questions 1, 2)**
12	Obstetrical postpartum hemorrhage is one of the top three causes of maternal mortality in the United States. Pharmacological therapy for uterine atony includes oxytocin, methylergonovine, carboprost, misoprostol, and dinoprostone.	**Case 49-8 (Questions 3, 4)**
13	Alloimmunization occurs when an Rh D-negative mother becomes immunized after exposure to fetal erythrocytes that carry the D antigen. Rh_o(D) immune globulin should be given to all mothers who are Rh D negative at 28 weeks' gestation.	**Case 49-9 (Questions 1–5)**

LACTATION AND DRUGS IN BREAST MILK

1	Breast milk is recognized as the optimal source of nutrition for infants, with documented benefits not only to infants but also to mothers, families, and societies, and breast-feeding should be encouraged if possible.	**Case 49-10 (Questions 1, 2), Case 49-11 (Question 1)**
2	Most drugs are excreted in the breast milk. The pharmacologic and adverse effects on the infant will be determined by the extent of oral bioavailability, distribution, metabolism, and rate of elimination. A milk to plasma ratio can be used to estimate the drug concentration in milk. The relative infant dose can be calculated to estimate the infant's exposure based on volume of milk ingested.	**Case 49-8 (Question 2), Case 49-12 (Question 1), Case 49-13 (Question 1)**

Placental Physiology

Conception begins with the fertilization of an ovum. The time after conception is the conceptional or developmental age. The gestational age is the time from the start of the last menstrual period (LMP) and generally exceeds the developmental age by 2 weeks.[1] The fertilized ovum, or zygote, undergoes mitotic divisions that lead to the formation of the blastocyst, a hollow fluid-filled sphere. The outer cell mass of the blastocyst differentiates into trophoblasts, whereas the internal cell mass gives rise to the embryo. About 5 to 6 days after fertilization, the blastocyst adheres to the endometrial epithelium, where it undergoes implantation between postconception days 7 and 12.[2] The outer cell mass, or trophoblast, invades the endometrium, and the blastocyst becomes completely buried within the endometrium. Once trophoblastic invasion of the endometrium occurs, the endometrium is transformed into the decidua, the functional layer of the pregnant endometrium, and is referred to by this term throughout pregnancy.[3]

ONLINE CONTENT **For an illustration of a blastocyst, go to http://thepoint.lww.com/AT10e.**

The trophoblast secretes human chorionic gonadotropin (hCG), which maintains the corpus luteum so that menstruation is prevented and pregnancy can continue.[4] (See Chapter 50, Disorders Related to the Menstrual Cycle, for a detailed discussion of the menstrual cycle). As more of the decidua is invaded, the walls of the decidual capillaries are eroded, thereby leaking maternal blood into spaces called lacunae.[2] This initial contact with the maternal blood allows hCG to enter the maternal circulation by 8 to 10 days after conception, at which time it can be measured to aid in the diagnosis of pregnancy.[4]

The placenta has both fetal and maternal components. The placenta is made up of the amnion, chorion, chorionic villi and intervillous spaces, decidual plate, and the myometrium.[1] The fetal surface of the placenta is covered by the amnion, beneath which the fetal chorionic vessels cross. Figure 49-1 describes the structure of the placenta and its maternal–fetal circulation. Maternal–fetal circulation to the intervillous space is not fully established until the second trimester.[1] Maternal uteroplacental arteries perfuse the intervillous spaces, and as the maternal blood flows around the villi, exchanges of oxygen and nutrients occur with fetal blood contained within capillaries found inside these villi.[1] Although the placenta serves as a strong barrier between the fetal and maternal circulations, a few cells are able to cross between the two circulations.[1] Placental blood flow reaches the fetus through a single umbilical vein. At the juncture of the placenta and umbilicus, the umbilical vein and arteries repeatedly branch and traverse the fetal surface of the placenta (between the amnion and the chorionic plate), forming capillary networks that terminate within the villi. These vessels are termed the *chorionic veins and arteries.* Fetal blood flow reaches the placenta through two umbilical arteries; carbon dioxide and waste products diffuse into the intervillous spaces and are carried away by the maternal decidual veins.[1]

Definitions

PARITY AND GRAVIDA

Parity and *gravida* are terms used to describe a pregnant woman. Parity is the number of deliveries after 20 weeks' gestation. Parity is independent of the number of fetuses delivered (live or

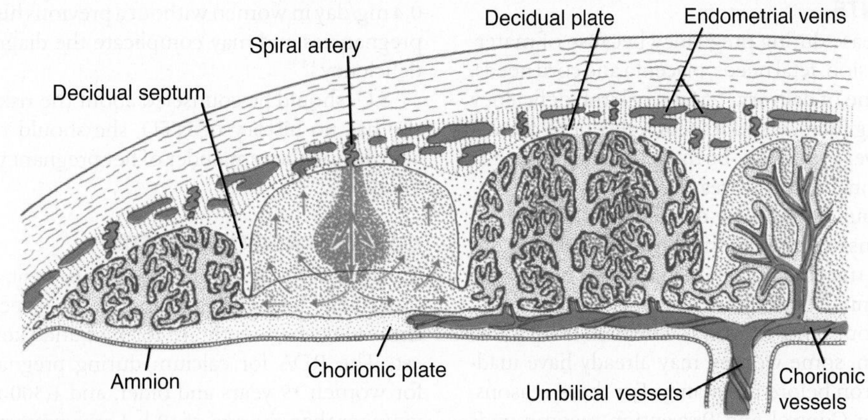

FIGURE 49-1 Term placenta 1. The relation of the villous chorion (C) to the decidua basalis (D) and fetal placental circulation. 2. The maternal placental circulation. Maternal blood flows into the intervillous spaces in funnel-shaped spurts, and exchanges occur with the fetal blood as the maternal blood flows around the villi. 3. The inflowing arterial blood pushes venous blood into the endometrial veins, which are scattered over the entire surface of the decidua basalis. Note also that the umbilical arteries carry deoxygenated fetal blood to the placenta and that the umbilical vein carries oxygenated blood to the fetus. (Adapted with permission from Sadler T. *Langman's Medical Embryology,* Ninth Edition Image Bank. Baltimore: Lippincott Williams & Wilkins, 2003.)

stillborn, single fetus, or twins) or the method of delivery. *Gravida* refers to the number of pregnancies a woman has had regardless of the outcome. For example, a woman who is currently pregnant and has previously delivered one set of twins and had two spontaneous abortions is described as a gravida 4, para 1 (G4, P1).

TRIMESTERS OF PREGNANCY

ONLINE CONTENT

For an illustration showing the fetal development that occurs during each trimester of pregnancy, go to http://thepoint.lww.com/AT10e.

The average pregnancy is approximately 40 weeks when calculated from the first day of the LMP. Pregnancy is typically divided into three trimesters, approximately 13 to 14 weeks each.[5] The first trimester includes the critical period of organogenesis, the time in which most of the vital organs are developing, which occurs between weeks 5 and 10. The time between the end of the 20th week of gestation and the end of the 28th day after birth is considered the perinatal period.

DELIVERY

Depending on the gestational age at the time of delivery, the result can be an abortion, preterm, term, or postterm birth. An abortion is a delivery before 20 weeks' gestation. A term infant is a fetus delivered between 37 and 42 weeks' gestation. A preterm birth is one occurring between 20 and 37 weeks' gestation, and a postterm (postmaturity) birth occurs after the beginning of 42 weeks' gestation. Parturition refers to labor, and the puerperium is the 6 to 8 weeks after delivery.

Preconceptional Care

CASE 49-1

QUESTION 1: S.C. is a 29-year-old, G1, P1 woman who is interested in becoming pregnant. Her past medical history is significant for hypothyroidism. She currently is taking levothyroxine 88 mcg by mouth daily. What advice should be given to S.C. in regards to preconceptional care?

More than 4.2 million live births were registered in the United States in 2008, with an estimated 70.8% of women beginning prenatal care in the first trimester.[6,7] Although much improved, prenatal care is still not easily accessible to all women. Early comprehensive care can promote healthier pregnancies through early detection of risk factors, disease state management, and encouragement of healthy behaviors and will help to ensure normal fetal organogenesis. Appropriate preconception counseling and treatment of women with pre-existing high-risk medical conditions, such as diabetes, hypertension, and epilepsy, can greatly improve pregnancy outcomes. In 2006, the mortality rate in the United States (from birth through the first year of life) for infants of mothers beginning prenatal care in the first trimester was 5.49 per 1,000 live births. However, the infant mortality rate increased to 6.47 per 1,000 live births for women with late care, and was 26.67 per 1,000 live births for women with no prenatal care.[8] S.C. should see her primary-care provider for regular physical examinations and evaluation of her thyroid function before becoming pregnant. Her first prenatal visit should generally occur by 8 weeks' gestational age when she becomes pregnant.[9]

Vitamins and Minerals Supplementation

CASE 49-1, QUESTION 2: What vitamin and mineral supplementation would you recommend for S.C.? When should she begin taking these vitamins and minerals?

A balanced diet that provides S.C. with multiple B vitamins, oil-soluble vitamins (A, E, D, and K), folic acid, and minerals (iron, calcium, phosphorus, magnesium, iodine, zinc) should be encouraged. S.C. should be started on a prenatal multivitamin if she has not yet started taking one. Prenatal vitamins should be taken months before conception to ensure that proper nutritional requirements are met during critical periods of organogenesis and fetal growth.

IRON REQUIREMENTS

Iron requirements increase during pregnancy because of maternal blood volume expansion, fetal needs, placenta and cord needs, and blood loss at the time of delivery.[10] Maternal iron deficiency can cause anemia during infancy, spontaneous abortion, premature delivery, and delivery of a low-birth-weight infant and is associated with low neonatal iron stores.[10,11]

A woman needs about 18 to 21 mg of iron/day during pregnancy; the body compensates by increasing iron absorption from the gastrointestinal (GI) tract by about 15% to 50%.[10] The average diet of women in the United States does not meet these requirements because only about 6 mg of iron is absorbed from 1,000 kcal of food. In addition, some women may already have inadequate body stores of iron before pregnancy. For these reasons, the Centers for Disease Control and Prevention recommends screening for iron deficiency in pregnancy in addition to universal iron supplementation except when genetic conditions such as hemochromatosis are present.[12] Prenatal vitamins usually contain 30 to 60 mg of elemental iron. Women with iron deficiency anemia should be given 60 to 120 mg of elemental iron daily. Iron deficiency anemia during pregnancy generally is associated with a hemoglobin and hematocrit less than 11 mg/dL and less than 33%, respectively, during the first and third trimesters or less than 10.5 mg/dL and less than 32%, respectively, during the second trimester. The classic morphologic changes observed in the erythrocytes in iron deficiency outside of pregnancy, hypochromia and microcytosis, are not prominent in pregnant women. Serum ferritin, however, is low, which has the highest sensitivity and specificity for diagnosing iron deficiency.[11] S.C.'s hemoglobin and hematocrit should be assessed now and again at 26 to 28 weeks' gestation. If her hemoglobin and hematocrit are normal, the amount of iron in her prenatal vitamin should be sufficient.

FOLATE REQUIREMENTS

Folic acid is essential in the synthesis of DNA and RNA. Pregnant women who take 0.4 to 0.8 mg of folic acid daily during the first trimester of pregnancy are significantly less likely to have a child with neural tube defects (NTD), such as spina bifida and anencephaly.[13,14] NTD can lead to stillbirth, neonatal death, or serious disabilities. Approximately 4,000 pregnancies in the United States are affected by NTD each year.[15]

NTDs develop within the first month of pregnancy at a time when many women are unaware of their pregnancy.[14,15] In 1992, the US Public Health Service recommended that all women with child-bearing potential should consume 0.4 mg/day of folic acid to reduce the risk of an NTD-affected pregnancy.[14]

It may be difficult to meet the recommended daily allowance (RDA) for folic acid because foods contain only a small amount of this vitamin; overcooking and high-fiber diets also can reduce the amount of available folic acid from food. Most prenatal vitamins contain 0.8 to 1 mg of folic acid.

Folic acid supplementation is especially important in women with a history of infants born with NTD. Women who have had an NTD-affected pregnancy should receive genetic counseling because they have a 2% to 3% risk of having another such outcome. Women with previous NTD-affected pregnancies who plan another pregnancy should take 4 mg/day of folic acid at least 1 month before conception and through the first 3 months of pregnancy.[16]

Women who require 4 mg/day of folic acid should be prescribed folic acid tablets as an addition to combination prenatal multivitamins (which contain folic acid), rather than just increasing the number of multivitamin tablets. When several fixed-combination multivitamin tablets are taken daily, the mother could be exposed to a potentially teratogenic dose of vitamin A. High doses of folic acid do not prevent NTD better than 0.4 mg/day in women without a previous history of NTD-affected pregnancies and may complicate the diagnosis of a vitamin B_{12} deficiency.[14]

S.C. should be counseled about the risks for NTD, and given she has no history of NTD, she should receive adequate folic acid during the remainder of her pregnancy from a daily prenatal vitamin.

CALCIUM REQUIREMENTS

Calcium is needed during pregnancy for adequate mineralization of the fetal skeleton and teeth, especially during the third trimester when teeth are formed and skeletal growth is greatest. The RDA for calcium during pregnancy is 1,000 mg/day for women 19 years and older, and 1,300 mg/day for teenagers younger than the age of 19.[17] Large maternal stores can provide calcium if dietary intake is inadequate; however, depleting maternal stores may put S.C. at risk for osteoporosis later in life. Foods rich in calcium (e.g., milk, cheese, yogurt, legumes, nuts, dried fruits) or calcium supplements can be used to meet the calcium RDA.

CASE 49-1, QUESTION 3: S.C. starts her prenatal vitamins that contain iron and folic acid immediately. Two months have passed, and now S.C. believes that she may be pregnant because her period is 2 weeks late. She requests help in selecting an over-the-counter commercially available home pregnancy test. How do these home pregnancy tests work, and how should S.C. be counseled?

Commercially available home pregnancy tests are enzyme immunoassays with monoclonal or polyclonal antibodies that bind to hCG in the urine.[18] hCG is detected in the maternal circulation and urine approximately 8 to 10 days after conception.[4] Concentrations in the urine closely parallel those in the maternal blood. The hCG serum concentrations increase rapidly, doubling every 2 days. Peak concentrations are achieved at 60 to 70 days of pregnancy. Thereafter, hCG concentrations decline and reach a low by approximately 120 days, at which point concentrations are maintained for the remainder of the pregnancy.[4]

hCG is composed of an α- and a β-subunit. The α-subunit is identical to the α-subunit of other pituitary hormones (e.g., follicle-stimulating hormone, luteinizing hormone, thyroid-stimulating hormone); however, the β-subunit is specific to hCG. Pregnancy tests specific for this β-subunit are useful diagnostic tests for confirming pregnancy.[5] They can provide accurate results within 1 to 2 weeks after ovulation.[5,18] Several kits are available. The tests can be performed privately and quickly, and are easily interpreted. The results are obtained rapidly—within 1 and 5 minutes—and are highly accurate when performed at the start of the first missed menstrual period. Although home pregnancy tests are reportedly 98% to 100% accurate when used correctly, consumer studies have documented accuracy rates as low as 50% to 75% if product directions are not precisely followed.[18] Many home pregnancy tests include a second test, which should be repeated at a specified time after the first negative test result.

S.C. should purchase a product containing two tests and follow the instructions carefully. If the first test result is negative, S.C. should repeat the test in 1 week if she has not started menstruating. False-negative results occur when testing is done before the first day of a missed period or if the urine is not at room temperature.[18] False-negative results can also occur with an ectopic (outside the uterus) pregnancy or in women with ovarian cysts and in those receiving menotropins or chorionic gonadotropin.[18] False-positive pregnancy test results are rare, but can occur with serum testing if the woman has circulating heterophilic antibodies directed against the animal-derived antigens use in pregnancy tests. These antibodies will not interfere with urine assays, however, as they are not present in urine.[19] If the test is positive, S.C. should be counseled on the possible fetal effects of any medications or herbal products she may be taking and advised to see her primary-care provider as soon as possible.

Date of Confinement (Due Date)

CASE 49-1, QUESTION 4: What is S.C.'s "due date" based on her LMP?

The assessment of gestational age is important to determine the expected date of confinement (EDC), schedule a cesarean section, or determine when it is safe to end a pregnancy prematurely. Gestational age can be determined by several methods, including the date of the LMP, pelvic examination, uterine size, and measurement of fetal parameters by ultrasound. The onset date of the LMP is most commonly used to estimate the gestational age of the fetus.

Because the day of conception rarely is known, it is more practical to measure the duration of pregnancy from the first day of the LMP. The EDC is generally determined by adding 7 days to the first day of the LMP, counting back 3 months, and adding 1 year (Naegele rule).[5] This method assumes that ovulation occurs on day 14 of a 28-day menstrual cycle. The problems with this method are that many pregnant women do not know the date of their LMP, and it is inaccurate in women with irregular or prolonged menstrual cycles. S.C.'s first day of her LMP was estimated to be 6 weeks ago on August 6. It is now September 17; therefore, her EDC or "due date" is May 13. Although this may not be an accurate date, a more exact date will be estimated using first-trimester sonography.

Pregnancy-Induced Pharmacokinetic Changes

CASE 49-1, QUESTION 5: S.C. is concerned about any possible changes that might occur with her medications (levothyroxine 88 mcg orally [PO] daily, prenatal vitamins) now that she is 6 weeks pregnant. Are there any pregnancy-induced pharmacokinetic changes that might occur that will affect her medication use?

Important physiologic changes occur in almost all maternal organs during pregnancy to support the growth and development of the fetus. These physiologic changes affect the cardiovascular, respiratory, and GI systems; plasma volume, renal function, and hepatic enzymes, which can alter the absorption, distribution, metabolism, and elimination of drugs.[20] Alterations in the pharmacokinetics of drugs are influenced by mainly by two factors: (a) maternal physiologic changes and (b) the effects of the placental–fetal compartment.[21]

ABSORPTION

Pregnancy-induced changes affecting drug absorption are (a) a decrease in intestinal motility owing to smooth muscle relaxation by progesterone, resulting in a 30% to 50% increase of gastric and intestinal emptying times; (b) a 40% decrease in gastric acidity, which increases gastric pH; and (c) altered bioavailability or absorption attributable to increased incidence of nausea and vomiting. Bioavailability may be increased for acid-labile drugs and decreased for drugs that require acid medium for stability. Prolonged gastric and intestinal emptying times may decrease the maximum concentration (C_{max}) of a drug and the time to reach C_{max}, whereas the increased intestinal transit time may increase the area under the curve (AUC) and bioavailability of a drug. In contrast, pregnancy-induced vomiting may decrease the amount of drug ingested; it is therefore better to schedule medications during the evening when the incidence of nausea and vomiting is lower, or to use the rectal route for drug administration. In summary, the effect of pregnancy on drug absorption is variable and depends greatly on the physicochemical properties of the drug.[21] Increased blood flow to the maternal skin, which helps dissipate fetal heat production, may also increase the absorption of a topically (transdermal) administered medication.[20]

DISTRIBUTION

Changes in protein binding and increased plasma volume can theoretically increase the apparent volume of distribution (Vd) of drugs during pregnancy. Plasma volume increases by 6 to 8 weeks' gestation and continues to expand to 40% to 50% above pregnancy volumes by 32 to 34 weeks' gestation.[20,21] Plasma volume expands even more with multiple gestations. The total body water (TBW) increases by 8 L; 40% of this increase can be attributable to the mother and 60% to the fetal–placental unit. This increase in TBW necessitates larger loading doses of water-soluble drugs (e.g., aminoglycosides) because of the increase in Vd. A decrease in the C_{max} would be expected.

Plasma albumin concentrations decrease during pregnancy, mostly because of dilution by the increased plasma volume.[20,21] Albumin concentrations may also be decreased as a result of decreased synthesis or increased catabolism.[20] In addition, increased concentrations of steroid and placental hormones may decrease protein-binding sites for drugs.[22] These changes in protein binding generally result in decreased protein binding, increased free fraction (f_u) of drugs, and increased clearance of drugs when clearance is dependent on f_u (e.g., valproic acid, carbamazepine).[23] When both f_u and intrinsic clearance are increased as is the case with increased cytochrome P-450 enzyme activity, both the total and free concentrations are decreased (e.g., phenytoin, phenobarbital).[23] Total protein and α_1-acid glycoprotein concentrations remain fairly unchanged.

METABOLISM

Protein binding, activity of hepatic enzymes, and liver blood flow determine the hepatic clearance of drugs. Increases in estrogen and progesterone during pregnancy affect the hepatic metabolism by stimulating or decreasing different hepatic enzymes of the cytochrome P-450 (CYP) system.[24] CYP3A4 and CYP2D6 activities are increased during pregnancy, which results in increased metabolism of certain drugs such as phenytoin.[21,24] On the other hand, CYP1A2, xanthine oxidase, and *N*-acetyltransferase activity are decreased, resulting in reduced hepatic elimination of drugs such as theophylline and caffeine.[22,23,25] The clearance of caffeine can be decreased by 70%.[25] Hepatic blood flow as a percentage of the cardiac output is decreased; however, the absolute rate (in liters per minute) remains unchanged.[20] The activity of nonhepatic enzymes (e.g., plasma cholinesterase) is also decreased.[23] The extent of the effect on drug therapy of these hepatic physiologic changes during pregnancy is difficult to quantify.

ELIMINATION

The glomerular filtration rate (GFR) begins to rise in the first half of the first trimester and increases by 50% by the beginning of the second trimester.[22] Renal blood flow also increases by 25% to 50% early during gestation. As a result, renal drug excretion (e.g., β-lactams, enoxaparin, digoxin) can increase.[21,25] This increase in GFR necessitates dosage adjustments up to 20% to

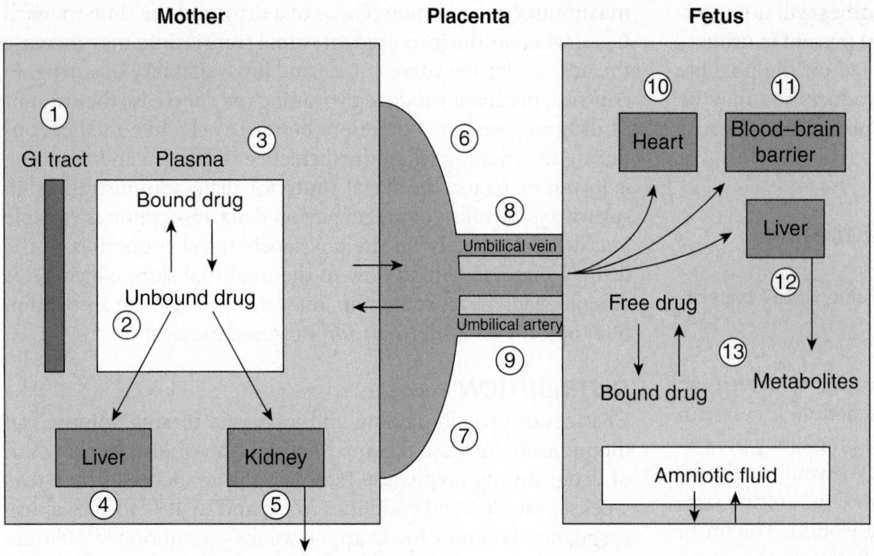

FIGURE 49-2 Drug disposition in the maternal–fetal placental system. The factors affecting the pharmacokinetics and drug effects on mother and fetus are **(1)** altered maternal absorption; **(2)** increased maternal unbound drug fraction; **(3)** increased maternal plasma volume; **(4)** altered hepatic clearance; **(5)** increased maternal renal blood flow and glomerular filtration rate; **(6)** placental transfer; **(7)** possible placental metabolism; **(8)** placental blood flow; **(9)** maternal–fetal blood pH difference; **(10)** preferential fetal circulation to the heart and brain; **(11)** undeveloped fetal blood–brain barrier; **(12)** immature fetal liver enzyme activity; and **(13)** increased fetal unbound drug fraction. GI, gastrointestinal. (Adapted with permission from Loebstein R et al. Pharmacokinetic changes during pregnancy and their clinical relevance. *Clin Pharmacokinet.* 1997;33:328.)

65% for renally excreted drugs throughout pregnancy to maintain therapeutic concentrations.[24] The increased cardiac output and regional blood flow (e.g., renal blood flow) primarily are caused by increased stroke volume and increased heart rate, which can increase drug distribution and drug excretion.

During pregnancy, the serum creatinine concentration is lower because of the increased GFR, resulting in normal serum creatinine values of 0.3 to 0.7 mg/dL in the first and second trimesters.[26] A normal value for serum creatinine in nonpregnant adults is 0.6 to 1.2 mg/dL.[26] Similar changes occur with serum urea nitrogen and uric acid concentrations. These differences have important implications when assessing renal function during pregnancy. A serum creatinine indicative of normal renal function in a nonpregnant woman may be indicative of renal insufficiency in a woman who is pregnant in her third trimester.

PLACENTAL–FETAL COMPARTMENT EFFECT

Maternal and fetal drug concentrations are dependent on the amount of drug that crosses the placenta, the extent of metabolism by the placenta, and fetal distribution and elimination of drug (Fig. 49-2).[21,26] Diffusion across the placenta is the main mechanism of drug transfer; nonionized lipophilic substances are more readily transferred, whereas less lipid-soluble (e.g., ionized) substances less readily cross the placenta.[21] Highly protein-bound or large molecular weight drugs (e.g., heparin and insulin) do not cross the placenta. Both the immature fetal liver and placenta can metabolize drugs. Fetal drug accumulation can be problematic secondary to limited metabolic enzymatic activity along with the concern that approximately half of the blood flow from the umbilical vein bypasses the fetal liver and goes to the cardiac and cerebral circulations.[21] Another mechanism that can also lead to prolonged effects of drugs in the fetal compartment is ion trapping. This phenomenon occurs because the fetal plasma pH is more acidic than the maternal plasma, causing weak bases (e.g., usually nonionized and lipophilic substances) to diffuse across the placental barrier and become ionized in the more acidic fetal blood. The net effect is movement of drugs from the maternal to fetal compartment. This equilibrium between the maternal and fetal compartments becomes important when therapeutic fetal drug concentrations are desired (e.g., digoxin therapy for intrauterine fetal arrhythmias). Drugs are eliminated by the fetus primarily through diffusion back to the maternal compartment. As the fetal kidney matures, metabolites of drugs are excreted into the amniotic fluid.[21]

S.C.'s thyroid function should be checked regularly to assess the need for an increase in her levothyroxine dosage. During S.C.'s pregnancy, an increase in the Vd of thyroid hormones in the vascular, hepatic, and fetal–placental units, an increase in thyroxine-binding globulin resulting from a rise an estrogen, and an increase in placental transport and maternal metabolism of thyroxine will occur.[27] Most women with hypothyroidism who are taking oral thyroid hormones before pregnancy, similar to S.C., will require an increase in their dosage by about 30% to 50% throughout their pregnancy, and then will need decreased dose adjustments post partum.[27]

TERATOGENICITY

CASE 49-1, QUESTION 6: S.C. is currently 8 weeks pregnant and now is concerned about her medication use during pregnancy and the risk of birth defects. How should S.C. be counseled about the teratogenicity potential of levothyroxine use during pregnancy?

Prevalence of Congenital Malformations

The largest concern with medication use during pregnancy is the risk of congenital malformations, defined as "structural abnormalities of prenatal origin that are present at birth and that seriously interfere with viability or physical well-being."[28] Congenital anomalies or birth defects are the leading cause of infant mortality in the United States, accounting for 20% of all infant deaths.[8] Some drug-induced defects relate to changes in functions or conditions that are not structural abnormalities (e.g., mental retardation, central nervous system [CNS] depression, deafness, tumors, or biochemical changes). The broader term *congenital anomalies* include the four major manifestations of abnormal fetal development, which include growth alterations, functional deficits, structural malformations, and fetal death.[29]

The background incidence of birth defects in the general population must be taken into consideration when interpreting the risk of drug-induced birth defects. The prevalence of major congenital malformations discovered at or shortly after birth in the general population is approximately 3%.[29] This number has been derived from large epidemiologic studies completed during the past several decades and depends on how terms are defined (e.g., major versus minor congenital malformations), the thoroughness with which the infant is examined, and how long the exposed person is followed after birth.[29] The collection of malformations data is a complicated task subject to numerous errors and biases. Some studies examined only "significant anomalies," others "major malformations," whereas still others reported only "live births" or "single births" or "birth weights greater than 500 g." Stillbirths and spontaneous abortions, both often associated with congenital malformations, often were excluded from epidemiologic data. Neurodevelopmental delays and growth retardation also are potential long-term effects that will not be diagnosed in the immediate postpartum period. The prevalence of congenital anomalies is likely greater than 3% if minor anomalies and long-term adverse effects are considered.

Despite the significant impact of drug-induced birth defects, it is difficult and unethical to conduct randomized, controlled trials to assess the risk of fetal exposure to drugs in humans. Much of the data available is derived from epidemiologic studies, anecdotal experiences in humans, and animal studies. Because birth defects are species specific and influenced by many factors including genetic predisposition, the data must be carefully interpreted and the results not overgeneralized.

Causes of Malformations

CLASSIFICATION

Causes of congenital malformations are generally classified into one of five categories: (a) monogenic origin, (b) chromosomal abnormalities, (c) multifactorial inheritance, (d) environmental factors, and (e) unknown.[29] Single gene– and chromosomal-related defects account for approximately 25% of all congenital malformations in live-born infants (monogenetic, 7.5%–20%; chromosomal, 5%–6%).[28–30] *Multifactorial inheritance* refers to defects that are polygenic in origin; it has an environmental component. One surveillance program estimated that this interaction between genetic and environmental factors causes 23% of defects.[30] Congenital dislocation of the hip is an example of a defect in this category: the depth of the acetabular socket and joint laxity are genetically determined, and a frank breech malposition is one of the environmental factors.[31] In most cases, however, the environmental factors in multifactorial inheritance are unknown.

Environmental factors account for approximately 10% of malformations.[32] These include maternal conditions, mechanical effects, chemicals and drugs, and certain infectious agents. Maternal diseases associated with malformations include diabetes, phenylketonuria, virilizing tumors, and maternal hyperthermia. About 9% (range, 6.6%–13.0%) of infants of diabetic mothers develop major congenital defects, primarily consisting of cardiovascular, neural tube, and skeletal malformations.[33] Mechanical effects, such as intrauterine compression and abnormal cord constriction, may result in fetal deformations.[32,33]

Probably the best known of the teratogenic viruses is rubella, which can cause a fetal rubella syndrome consisting of cataracts, heart disease, and deafness.[34] In utero exposure to rubella in the first trimester can cause defects in up to 85% of fetuses. Cytomegalovirus infection occurs in 0.5% to 1.5% of newborns in the United States, resulting in deafness and mental retardation in 5% to 10% of these infants.[28] Characteristics of cytomegalic inclusion disease, the syndrome produced by cytomegalovirus, include intrauterine growth restriction (IUGR), microcephaly, and at times chorioretinitis, seizures, blindness, and optic atrophy. Herpes simplex 1 and 2 and varicella are also associated with malformations.[32]

The protozoan generally accepted as a teratogen is *Toxoplasma gondii* which may be present in cat litter.[28] Most infants infected with *T. gondii* show no symptoms and develop normally. When toxicity does occur, the anomalies may consist of hepatosplenomegaly, icterus, maculopapular rash, chorioretinitis, cerebral calcifications, and hydrocephalus or microcephalous.[35] Because of the possible presence of *T. gondii* in cat litter, women should avoid cleaning or touching cat litter while pregnant. *Treponema pallidum* (syphilis) can cross the placenta and cause congenital syphilis as well as other defects, such as hydrocephaly, chorioretinitis, and optic atrophy.[34] In utero exposure to syphilis after the fourth month of pregnancy is associated with higher risk.

ONLINE CONTENT

For a photograph of chorioretinal scars, go to http://thepoint.lww.com/AT10e.

The final category, defects of unknown cause, comprises the greatest percentage of congenital malformations, accounting for about 60% to 65% of the total.[30]

Medication Use in Pregnancy and Teratogenicity

The term *teratogen* is used to denote an agent that has the potential under certain exposure conditions to produce abnormal development in the fetus.[29] Many women have the general perception that use of any medication during a pregnancy can harm the developing fetus.[36] This thought may lead to consideration of terminating wanted pregnancies or withholding necessary drug therapy during the course of the pregnancy. The extent to which a drug will affect the development of the fetus depends on the physical and chemical properties of the drug as well as the dose, duration, route, and timing of exposure and the genetic composition and biological susceptibility of the mother and fetus.[37] Numerous drugs have been associated with congenital anomalies, but only in a few cases has a consensus been reached that a specific agent is teratogenic. Table 49-1[38–40] lists those agents generally considered or suspected to be proven human teratogens. Not all these teratogens will cause developmental toxicity with every exposure, however.

Because every pregnancy has the risk of an abnormal outcome regardless of drug exposure, the objective of evaluating data on drug exposure during pregnancy is to ascertain whether a particular drug increases the risk of developmental toxicity in the fetus beyond the background rate. The following basic principles of teratogenicity should be applied when assessing the potential for teratogenicity of drugs.

CRITICAL STAGE OF EXPOSURE

After fertilization, the development of the embryo and fetus is divided into three main stages: pre-embryonic period, embryonic period, and fetal period.[32] In the first 2 weeks after fertilization or the pre-embryonic period (0–14 days), little is known about the effects of drugs on human development. Exposure to a teratogenic agent during this period usually produces an "all or none" effect on the ovum[35]: the ovum either dies from exposure to a lethal dose of a teratogenic drug or it regenerates completely after exposure to a sublethal dose. Some animal studies have suggested, however, that exposure to some drugs during the preimplantation stage can halt growth and development before implantation.[41] Although the damage can be repaired, intrauterine growth may be retarded in the offspring.

During the embryonic period (14–56 days after fertilization), when organogenesis occurs, the embryo is most susceptible to

TABLE 49-1
Drugs With Suspected or Proven Teratogenic Effects in Humans[a,b]

Alcohol	Growth restriction, mental retardation, midfacial hypoplasia, renal and cardiac defects
Androgens (testosterone)	Masculinization of female fetus
Angiotensin-converting enzyme inhibitors and angiotensin receptor blockers	Pulmonary hypoplasia, hypocalvaria, oligohydramnios, fetal kidney anuria, and neonatal renal failure
Antithyroid drugs	Fetal and neonatal goiter with iodine use; small risk of aplasia cutis with methimazole
β-Blockers	IUGR and decrease in placental weight in β-blockers with intrinsic sympathomimetic activity if used in second and third trimesters
Carbamazepine	Neural tube defects, minor craniofacial defects, fingernail hypoplasia
Cigarette smoking	IUGR, functional and behavioral deficits
Cocaine	Bowel atresias; heart, limbs, face, and genitourinary tract malformations; microcephaly; cerebral infarctions; growth restriction
Corticosteroids (systemic)	Oral cleft lip and palates if used during organogenesis
Cyclophosphamide	Craniofacial, eye, and limb defects; IUGR; neurobehavioral deficits
Diethylstilbestrol	Vaginal carcinoma and other genitourinary defects
Lamotrigine	Oral cleft lip and cleft palate[38]
Lithium	Ebstein anomaly
Methotrexate	CNS and limb malformations
Misoprostol	Möbius sequence (high doses) and spontaneous abortions
Nonsteroidal anti-inflammatory drugs	Constriction of the ductus arteriosus, oral clefts, cardiac defects, and possible spontaneous abortion
Paroxetine	Cardiovascular defects[39]
Phenytoin	Fetal hydantoin syndrome, growth retardation, CNS deficits
Streptomycin and kanamycin	Hearing loss, eighth cranial damage; no ototoxicity reported with gentamicin, tobramycin, amikacin
Systemic retinoids (isotretinoin and etretinate)	CNS, craniofacial, cardiovascular defects
Tetracycline	Permanent discoloration of deciduous teeth
Thalidomide	Limb and skeletal shortening defects, internal organ defects
Topiramate	Cleft lip and cleft palate[40]
Trimethoprim	Neural tube defects and cardiac defects
Vaccines (live)	Live attenuated vaccines can potentially cause fetal infection
Valproic acid	Neural tube defects, developmental delay and deficits
Vitamin A	Microtia, anotia, thymic aplasia, cardiovascular defects (high dose)
Warfarin	Fetal warfarin syndrome with nasal hypoplasia, stippled epiphyses, and skeletal and CNS defects

[a] Teratogenic effects include the four major manifestations of abnormal fetal development which include growth alterations, functional deficits, structural malformations, and fetal death.
[b] Only drugs that are teratogenic when used at clinically recommended doses are listed. List is not all inclusive.
CNS, central nervous system; IUGR, intrauterine growth restriction
Source: Briggs G et al. *Drugs in Pregnancy and Lactation: A Reference Guide to Fetal and Neonatal Risk.* 9th ed. Philadelphia, PA: Lippincott Williams & Wilkins; 2011; Koren G et al. Drugs in pregnancy. *N Engl J Med.* 1998;338:1128.

the effects of teratogens or other chemicals.[29,35] Exposure during this sensitive period may produce major morphologic changes (Fig. 49-3). These stages of development differ significantly from other species, and knowledge of these stages is essential for the interpretation of the relationship between congenital malformations and drugs. For example, if a specific drug exposure occurs after the time of organ development, then a structural defect in that organ is less likely to be caused by that specific drug.

The fetal period (57 days to term) includes most of the stages of histogenesis and functional maturation, although the latter continues for some time after birth.[32] Minor structural changes are still possible during histogenesis, but anomalies are more likely to involve growth and functional aspects such as mental development and reproduction.

DOSE–RESPONSE CURVE

All teratogens follow a toxicologic dose–response curve.[29] All teratogens have a threshold dose below which adverse effects will not occur. The threshold dose is the dosage in which the incidence of structural malformations, rate of fetal death, growth restriction, and functional deficits does not exceed the background rate in the general population.[29] Conversely, developmental toxicity may occur when the fetus is exposed to doses above the maximum or threshold dose. There may be an increase in the severity and incidence of malformations when the fetus is exposed to increasingly higher dosages. For example, the risk for major congenital malformations, including NTD and minor anomalies, are increased statistically in patients taking valproic acid dosages greater than 1,000 mg/day during the first trimester.[42]

EXTRAPOLATION FROM ANIMAL STUDIES

In the absence of human trials, data derived from animal studies are used to assess the level of risk of developmental toxicity in humans. Most newly marketed drugs often have to rely on preclinical data to develop an estimation of teratogenic risk based on animal studies until human data become available. The dose used in experimental animal data is expressed as multiples of the human dose using plasma or serum AUC or dose per unit based on body surface area.[43] The drug appears to have a low risk for teratogenicity if the toxic dose in animals (based on AUC or mg/m^2 comparison) is greater than ten times the anticipated human dose.[44] Risk assessment using animal data is more complicated than just considering the dosage alone. Other major factors, including the effects of metabolism and active metabolites, species differentiation, route of administration, and type of defects, must be considered.[29]

GENETIC VARIABILITY

The most potent teratogenic agent will not produce malformations with every exposure.[29] The teratogenic potential of some drugs is influenced by the genotype of both the mother and fetus. Although the effects of known teratogens can be predictable

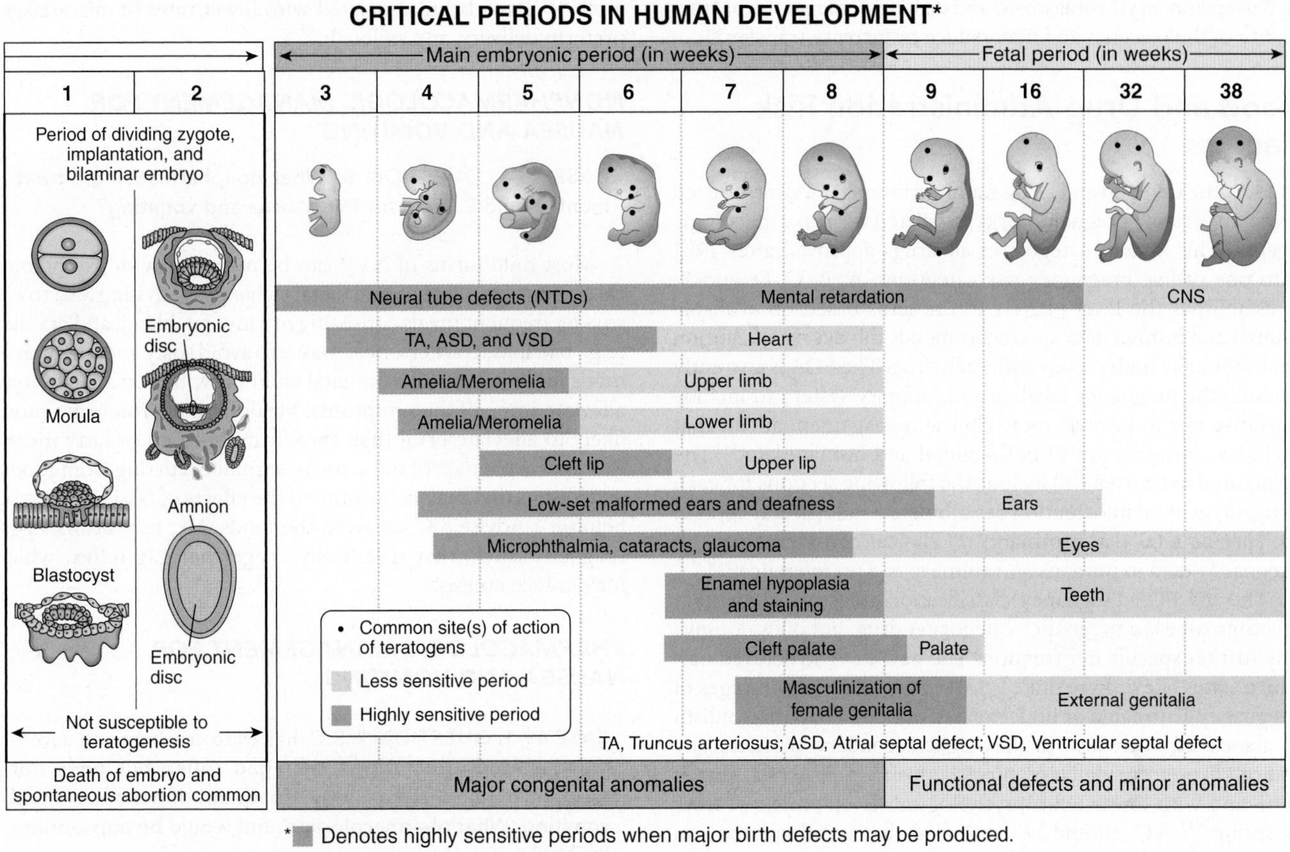

FIGURE 49-3 Critical stages of human development. (Adapted with permission from Moore KL, Persaud TVN. *The Developing Human: Clinically Oriented Embryology.* 7th ed. Philadelphia, PA: Saunders; 2003.)

in the general population, the possibility of individual assessment is difficult. The same dose of a teratogenic agent exposed at the same gestational window will produce variable outcomes in different people. Genetic variability can confer differences in cell sensitivities, placental transport, drug metabolism, enzyme composition, and receptor binding, which may affect how much active drug will reach fetal tissues.[45] One study showed an increased susceptibility to the teratogenic effect of phenytoin, most likely caused by elevated levels of oxidative metabolites (epoxides). These epoxides are normally eliminated from the systemic circulation by enzymes called microsomal epoxide hydrolase. Women who are homozygous for the recessive allele produce low levels of epoxide hydrolase, which may expose the fetus to higher levels of epoxides. These fetuses may be at a higher risk for fetal hydantoin syndrome.[46]

PLACENTAL TRANSFER OF DRUGS

At one time, the placenta was thought to present a barrier to the passage of drugs and noxious chemicals to the fetus. It is now known, however, that most medications cross the placenta to the fetus and, in general, what the mother consumes also is consumed by the fetus. Although the placenta acts as a biologic membrane, it initially is composed of four layers effectively separating two distinct individuals.[47] These layers are (a) the endothelial lining of the fetal vessels, (b) the connective tissue in the core of the villus, (c) the cytotrophoblast layer, and (d) the covering syncytium. During gestation, the placenta's surface area increases while its thickness decreases from approximately 25 μm during the first trimester to 2 to 6 μm at term. Both processes tend to favor the transfer of chemicals to the fetus.

Drugs, nutrients, and other substances cross the placenta by five mechanisms: (a) simple diffusion (e.g., most drugs), (b) facilitated diffusion (e.g., glucose), (c) active transport (e.g., some vitamins, amino acids), (d) pinocytosis (e.g., immune antibodies), and (e) breaks between cells (e.g., erythrocytes).[47,48] The latter two mechanisms are of no practical importance in the transfer of drugs.

Several factors influence the rate of drug transfer across the placenta, including molecular weight, lipid solubility, ionization, protein binding, uterine and umbilical blood flow, and maternal diseases.[48] Drugs with molecular weights of less than 600 cross easily, whereas those of greater than 1,000 (e.g., heparin) cross with difficulty or not at all. Because most drugs have molecular weights of less than 600, it is safe to assume that most drugs reaching the mother's circulatory system also will reach the fetus. As with other biologic membranes, lipid-soluble substances are transferred rapidly, with the rate of entry primarily governed by the lipid solubility of the nonionized molecule. Conversely, those molecules that are ionized at physiologic pH (e.g., the cholinergic quaternary amines) cross slowly, whereas weak acids and bases with dissociation constant (pK_a) values between 4.3 and 8.5 are transferred rapidly to the fetus. The penetration of highly protein-bound drugs also is inhibited; only the free, unbound drugs cross the placenta.[47]

Uterine blood flow, a major factor in determining the rate of drug transfer, increases throughout gestation. Several variables can affect uterine blood flow and the rate of drug transfer, including maternal blood pressure, cord compression, and drug therapy. Maternal hypotension reduces uterine blood flow and the rate at which substances are delivered to the membrane. Cord compression reduces the blood flow on the fetal side of the membrane. The use of drugs with α-adrenergic property (e.g., epinephrine) may constrict uterine vessels and thereby reduce blood flow.[43] Maternal diseases, such as pregnancy-induced hypertension, erythroblastosis, and diabetes, change the permeability of the placenta and may reduce or increase transfer.[48]

Food and Drug Administration Risk Factors

In 1979, the US Food and Drug Administration (FDA) introduced a system of rating pregnancy risks associated with pharmacologic agents. This system categorizes all drugs approved after 1983 into one of five pregnancy risk categories, A, B, C, D, and X. It establishes the level of risks to the fetus based on available animal and human data and recommends the degree of caution that should be undertaken with each drug. The FDA is currently revising the pregnancy labeling and category system to include narrative text to provide more clinical management advice that includes consideration of both animal and human data.[44] The structured narratives will include the following sections for each drug: (a) general information describing overall risk and benefit; (b) specific fetal risk summary; (c) clinical considerations; (d) pregnancy data in humans and animals; and (e) references.[49]

The old FDA pregnancy classification structure states that levothyroxine is a pregnancy category A drug, but does not give any further specific information. The new FDA structured narrative states "Levothyroxine (T_4) is compatible with all stages of pregnancy. Untreated or undertreated maternal hypothyroidism is associated with low birth weight secondary to medically indicated preterm delivery, pre-eclampsia or placental abruption, and with lower neuropsychological development of their offspring."[43] S.C. should be counseled that levothyroxine can safely be used during all trimesters of pregnancy including the period of organogenesis, which she is currently in at 8 weeks' gestation. She should not discontinue her levothyroxine. Thyroxine insufficiency has been shown to impair fetal and neonatal development. Levothyroxine therapy has not been observed to increase the risk of congenital malformations beyond the reported background risk of 3%.[43]

MANAGEMENT OF CONDITIONS IN PREGNANCY

Nausea and Vomiting

CASE 49-1, QUESTION 7: S.C. is now 10 weeks pregnant and complaining of nausea throughout the day with occasional emesis occurring two to three times daily. She is able to tolerate at least two meals a day and oral liquids. She reports very little weight gain since she became pregnant. Her current weight is 72 kg. S.C. states that certain smells such as fish, eggs, spaghetti sauce, and beans cause her to gag. How long is her nausea and vomiting likely to last?

Nausea and vomiting during pregnancy (NVP) is a common condition occurring in approximately 50% to 80% of pregnancies, during weeks 5 to 12 of gestation.[50] For most women, NVP is a self-limiting condition that usually resolves after the first trimester with no long-term detrimental effect on the fetus.[51] About 91% of cases will resolve by 20 weeks of gestation.[52] The effects of NVP can have an impact on a woman's daily activities, work productivity, and quality of life. Studies estimate $130 million per year is spent on the hospitalization for severe NVP.[51] The cause of NVP is unknown, but is most likely multifactorial including hormonal, psychological, and neurologic factors. Changes in hormonal levels of estrogen, progesterone, and hCG have been implicated as a possible cause of NVP. Mild to moderate NVP has been associated with lower rates of miscarriage, preterm delivery, and stillbirth.[53]

NONPHARMACOLOGIC MANAGEMENT FOR NAUSEA AND VOMITING

CASE 49-1, QUESTION 8: What nonpharmacologic treatment should S.C. try for her nausea and vomiting?

Most mild forms of NVP can be managed with psychological support and lifestyle and dietary changes. Advising S.C. to eat smaller frequent meals consisting of a low-fat, bland, and dry diet (e.g., bananas, crackers, rice, toast), to avoid spicy and highly aromatic foods, and to take prenatal vitamins with iron at night may alleviate some of the symptoms. Meals high in protein are more likely to alleviate NVP than carbohydrate-laden or fatty meals. Rest and avoidance of the sensory stimuli occurring from foods, and lotions that may contribute to the effects of NVP can also be helpful.[51] Advise S.C. to avoid the foods (i.e., fish, beans, eggs, spaghetti sauce) that specifically trigger her gag reflex, which may induce emesis.

PHARMACOLOGIC MANAGEMENT FOR NAUSEA AND VOMITING

CASE 49-1, QUESTION 9: S.C. has tried crackers and avoiding the foods that trigger her gag reflex but does not respond to nonpharmacologic treatment of her nausea and vomiting. What pharmacologic agent would be appropriate for her?

Antiemetics are indicated for the treatment of moderate to severe nausea and vomiting that fails to respond to nonpharmacologic interventions or when the nausea or vomiting threatens the mother's metabolic or nutritional status (e.g., hyperemesis gravidarum). Traditionally, medications for NVP have been avoided during the first trimester because of fear of the possible teratogenic effects. Most antiemetic therapies (e.g., antihistamines, multivitamins, phenothiazines) can be taken during pregnancy safely. Table 49-2[43,52,54–56] shows the most common antiemetics used during pregnancy. The goal of antiemetic therapy is to choose an effective medication to improve a woman's quality of life by maintaining her nutrition and hydration needs, while ensuring fetal safety.

Doxylamine with pyridoxine (vitamin B_6) can be considered first-line therapy for the treatment of NVP. This combination, formerly known as Bendectin, was commercially available from 1958 to 1983, but was withdrawn from the market owing to claims of teratogenicity.[52] Subsequently, a meta-analysis including 17,427 first-trimester exposures failed to find an association between the medication and an increased risk of malformations.[54] Several randomized, controlled trials have demonstrated its effectiveness in reducing NVP. Because of its safety and efficacy profile, doxylamine and pyridoxine are still considered a first-line therapy and are available separately as over-the-counter products.[52]

Other antihistamine H_1 receptor blockers (e.g., diphenhydramine, hydroxyzine, meclizine, dimenhydrinate) have been studied for NVP. The safety of antihistamines was supported in a meta-analysis including more than 200,000 first-trimester exposures, which did not find an increase in teratogenic risk.[55] Sedation is the main side effect that limits the use of this class of antiemetics.

Phenothiazines or metoclopramide are usually prescribed if antihistamines fail.[52] Phenothiazines (e.g., promethazine, prochlorperazine) are generally considered safe for both the

TABLE 49-2

Common Antiemetics Used for Nausea and Vomiting During Pregnancy

Drug	Dose	Comments
Vitamin B_6 (pyridoxine)	10–25 mg PO TID	First-line therapy[52]; Documented safety in pregnancy.
Vitamin B_6 (pyridoxine)–doxylamine combination	Pyridoxine 10–25 mg PO TID–QID; Doxylamine 12.5 mg PO TID–QID	First-line therapy; Available OTC; Well-documented safety in pregnancy through large meta-analysis.[54]
Antihistamines		
Diphenhydramine	25–50 mg PO every 8 hours	First-line therapy;
Meclizine	25 mg PO every 6 hours	Antihistamines have not been shown to be teratogenic.[43,55]
Hydroxyzine	25–50 mg PO every 4–6 hours	
Dimenhydrinate	50–100 mg PO every 4–6 hours	
Phenothiazines		
Promethazine	12.5–25 mg PO, PR every 6 hours	Second line of therapy;
Prochlorperazine	5–10 mg PO every 6–8 hours	Available as suppositories; Also suppositories and buccal tablets; Usually add phenothiazine or metoclopramide to therapy if antihistamines fail[52]; Can cause EPS.
Dopamine Antagonists		
Metoclopramide	10 mg PO every 6 hours	Usually add phenothiazine or metoclopramide to therapy if antihistamines fail[52]; Avoid treatment greater than 12 weeks' duration, risk of tardive dyskinesia; Can cause EPS;
Droperidol	1.25–2.5 mg IV/IM or Continuous infusion 1 mg/h for treatment of hyperemesis gravidarum[56]	Boxed warning regarding torsades de pointes, may need ECG during administration. Continuous infusion of droperidol requires concomitant diphenhydramine 50 mg IV every 6 hours.
5-HT_3 Receptor Antagonists		
Ondansetron	4–8 mg IV/PO every 6–8 hours	Available as ODT tablets; Does not cause sedation; Studies suggest low risk in pregnancy.[43]
Glucocorticoids		
Methylprednisolone	16 mg PO every 8 hours × 3 days, then taper over 2 weeks	For refractory cases, last line of therapy; Avoid use before 10th week of gestation, associated with oral cleft and palate.[43,52]
Ginger extract	125–250 mg PO every 6 hours	Available OTC as food supplement.

ECG, electrocardiogram; EPS, extrapyramidal symptoms; IM, intramuscular; IV, intravenous; ODT, oral disintegrating tablet; OTC, over the counter; PO, by mouth; QID, four times a day; TID, three times a day.

Source: Briggs G et al. *Drugs in Pregnancy and Lactation: A Reference Guide to Fetal and Neonatal Risk.* 9th ed. Philadelphia, PA: Lippincott Williams & Wilkins; 2011; Niebyl JR. Clinical practice. Nausea and vomiting in pregnancy. *N Engl J Med.* 2010;363:1544; McKeigue PM et al. Bendectin and birth defects: I. A meta-analysis of the epidemiologic studies. *Teratology.* 1994;50:27; Seto A et al. Pregnancy outcome following first trimester exposure to antihistamines: meta-analysis. *Am J Perinatol.* 1997;14:119.

mother and fetus if used occasionally in low doses. A recent randomized trial compared intravenous (IV) metoclopramide versus IV promethazine in the treatment of hyperemesis gravidarum and found both agents have similar efficacy. However, metoclopramide caused less drowsiness and dizziness.[57] Metoclopramide, a dopaminergic antagonist with prokinetic abilities, can control vomiting and gastric reflux associated with pregnancy. Oral metoclopramide can be added to an antihistamine (e.g., hydroxyzine) or a regimen of doxylamine and pyridoxine.[52] A large cohort study of 3,458 women exposed to metoclopramide in the first trimester failed to show an increase in congenital malformations. The FDA recently issued a black-box warning concerning the risk of rare incidences of tardive dyskinesia.[52] Risk of tardive dyskinesia increases with longer duration of treatment and total cumulative doses, thus length of therapy beyond 12 weeks should be avoided.[52]

Data supporting the use of ondansetron, a 5-hydroxytryptamine type 3 antagonist, during pregnancy are limited, including only a small randomized trial and a few case reports with no malformations reported with first-trimester use. It is increasingly used for NVP and hyperemesis owing to ease of administration with oral disintegrating tablets and tolerability with minimal sedating side effects.[52] Methylprednisolone is an option for refractory cases; however, its use during the first trimester is associated with a small but significant risk of fetal oral clefts.

Alternative therapies (e.g., vitamin B_6, ginger root, acupuncture, acupressure) have improved NVP in a small number of patients.[43,52] S.C. may be started on doxylamine 12.5 mg and pyridoxine 25 mg by mouth four times daily 30 minutes before meals and at bedtime because of its safety and efficacy profile. Drug selection for S.C. mostly depends on the tolerability of adverse effects. If S.C. continues to have significant nausea and emesis on these antiemetics and fails to tolerate any oral liquids or solids, she should be advised to return to the clinic for evaluation and possibly be admitted for IV hydration and IV antiemetic therapy.

CASE 49-1, QUESTION 10: S.C. returns to the clinic a few weeks later at 12 weeks' gestation stating that she has lost about 4 kg in the past 3 weeks, has been unable to tolerate any liquids or medication for 2 weeks, and feels dehydrated and dizzy. S.C. is referred for admission to the hospital. What recommendations should be given to S.C. to help control her nausea and vomiting?

Severe NVP can persist in less than 1% of pregnancies, leading to a condition called *hyperemesis gravidarum,* which can lead to detrimental effects on the mother and fetus. Weight loss of more than 5% of prepregnancy weight, ketonuria, and electrolyte abnormalities are associated with this condition. Treatment of hyperemesis gravidarum often requires hospitalization for parental fluid administration, electrolyte replacement, vitamin supplementation, and antiemetic therapy.[51] Metabolic acidosis, ketosis, hypovolemia, electrolyte disturbances, and weight loss may ensue if patients are not treated.[51] Reductions in lower esophageal pressure, gastric peristalsis, and gastric emptying may worsen nausea and vomiting.

In addition to ondansetron as mentioned above used for NVP, droperidol, an IV dopamine antagonist, has been used extensively for many years in the treatment of hyperemesis and the prevention and treatment of postoperative nausea and vomiting.[43] Although the FDA has mandated electrocardiographic monitoring for concern about the risk of prolonged QTc interval, large meta-analysis studies have failed to show an increased risk of arrhythmias when using droperidol at the low doses used for nausea and vomiting.[52] Limited experience with droperidol use in hyperemesis gravidarum has been documented in a small controlled trial.[56] Human and animal data suggest droperidol carries a low risk of teratogenicity to the fetus.[43]

S.C. should be hydrated with IV fluids with electrolyte replacement therapy and multivitamins including pyridoxine. If hydration with multivitamins does not quell her nausea, IV ondansetron 4 to 8 mg every 4 to 6 hours should be given. IV droperidol therapy should be considered if ondansetron does not work. She should also be evaluated for other causes of nausea and vomiting if her symptoms persist (e.g., gastroenteritis, cholecystitis, pancreatitis, hepatitis, peptic ulcer disease, pyelonephritis, and fatty liver of pregnancy).[51] Enteral nutrition may be needed in the treatment of hyperemesis gravidarum if S.C. cannot tolerate oral liquid and solid intake despite continuous IV antiemetics and hydration. Total parental nutrition should be reserved after multiple antiemetic regimens and enteral therapies have failed because of the substantial risks of catheter sepsis (25%) and thromboembolic clots.[52]

REFLUX ESOPHAGITIS

CASE 49-1, QUESTION 11: S.C. is now 30 weeks pregnant and no longer complains of nausea or vomiting. However, now she has heartburn that worsens when she lies down. What causes reflux esophagitis in pregnancy, and how should S.C. manage this problem?

Reflux esophagitis or heartburn is a normal occurrence in pregnancy affecting approximately two-thirds of women. The enlarging uterus increases intra-abdominal pressure, and estrogen and progesterone relax the esophageal sphincter. These two factors cause the reflux of stomach acid into the lower esophagus, producing symptoms of substernal burning worsened by eating, lying down, or bending over. Lifestyle and dietary modifications, such as eating smaller meals, avoiding late meals close to bedtime, and elevation of the head of the bed, should be tried first. Avoidance of salicylates, caffeine, alcohol, and nicotine are encouraged to reduce the symptoms of reflux and fetal exposure to these harmful substances.

If these modifications are not successful, S.C. should try a calcium carbonate antacid. Animal studies have not shown antacids to have teratogenic effects.[43] Sodium bicarbonate can cause metabolic alkalosis and fluid overload and should be avoided. Despite evidence of fetal toxicity with aluminum, available data suggest that usual doses of aluminum-containing medications are not harmful to the fetus of a pregnant woman with normal renal function. Sucralfate, which contains aluminum, appears to be safe in pregnancy. The American College of Gastroenterology has classified sucralfate as a medication with benefits that outweigh the risks when used in pregnant women.[43]

H_2-receptor antagonists can be used safely during pregnancy because most studies in animals and humans have not found fetal harm with cimetidine, ranitidine, famotidine, or nizatidine.[43] If H_2-receptor antagonists fail to control symptoms, proton-pump inhibitors (PPIs) should be used as the next treatment option. Recent studies have shown that PPI use during the first trimester and throughout pregnancy is not associated with a significant increase in the risk of congenital anomalies. These studies suggest that PPIs can be safely used at any gestational age.[58,59]

URINARY TRACT INFECTIONS

CASE 49-1, QUESTION 12: S.C. is now 31 weeks pregnant, and a routine urine dip was positive for leukocyte esterase and nitrates. Her urine was sent for urinalysis at her most recent prenatal visit and was positive for 10^5 colony-forming units (CFU) of *Escherichia coli.* She does not complain of any frequency and urgency when urinating and denies any fevers. Her temperature is currently 98.9°F. She denies any allergies to medications. What are the risks of having a urinary tract infection during pregnancy, and how should S.C. be treated?

Pathogenesis

Urinary tract infections are one of the most common complications of pregnancy owing to hormonal and mechanical changes that increase the likelihood of bacteriuria. During pregnancy, increases in progesterone cause relaxation of ureteral smooth muscle, promoting urinary stasis. The enlarging gravid uterus can also mechanically compress the ureters, which may lead to urinary retention. Approximately 90% of pregnant women may exhibit ureteral dilation or hydronephrosis, which can decrease bladder tone and ureteral tone. These physiological changes along with increases in the GFR, urine alkalization, and glucosuria help to promote bacterial growth.

Asymptomatic Bacteriuria and Acute Cystitis

Urinary tract infections during pregnancy can present as either asymptomatic bacteriuria (ASB) or acute cystitis. ASB is defined as the presence of significant bacteria, greater than 10^5 CFU of bacteria, obtained by two consecutive clean-catch samples in the absence of any urinary symptoms.[60] In contrast, acute cystitis involves an infection of the bladder and manifests with signs and symptoms of frequency, urgency, dysuria, and hematuria without fever or evidence of systemic illness along with significant presence of bacteria of at least 10^5 CFU. Counts of less than 10^5 CFU with two or more organisms likely represents contamination and not true bacteriuria.

ASB is estimated to occur in 2.5% to 15% of pregnant women with about 80,000 to 400,000 cases occurring each year in the United States.[61–63] If ASBs are left untreated, they can lead to complications such as pyelonephritis, low-birth-weight infants, and premature delivery.[64,65] During pregnancy, treatment of ASB reduces the risk of developing pyelonephritis dramatically down from 20% to 35% to only 1% to 4%.[65] The US Preventive Services

Task Force recommends screening for ASB with a urine culture for all pregnant women between 12 and 16 weeks of gestation or at the first prenatal visit if it occurs later.[66] The American College of Obstetrics and Gynecology (ACOG) further recommends repeating a urine culture during the third trimester.[67]

Risk factors for ASB during pregnancy include diabetes, sickle cell disease, immunosuppression, human immunodeficiency virus (HIV) or acquired immunodeficiency syndrome, urinary tract anatomic anomalies, and spinal cord injuries.[63] The primary sources of organisms that cause bacteriuria originate from existing vaginal and perineal flora and migrate up the urethra to cause ASB and cystitis; they include *E. coli* (most common pathogen isolated), *Klebsiella pneumoniae, Proteus mirabilis, Enterobacter* species, *Enterococcus, Staphylococcus saprophyticus,* and group B β-hemolytic *Streptococcus.*[60] Commonly used antibiotics include penicillins, cephalosporins, and nitrofurantoin. Antibiotic selection should be guided by antimicrobial susceptibility testing. For coverage of the most common organism, *E. coli,* oral nitrofurantoin or cephalexin is often used. *E. coli* resistance has been increasing to amoxicillin and trimethoprim-sulfamethoxazole.[60] The antibiotic chosen should produce adequate concentration in the urine, have a low resistance rate, and be safe to use during pregnancy. Table 49-3 lists common antibiotics used for urinary tract infections during pregnancy. A 7-day regimen of antibiotics should be used whenever possible.[60] A recent WHO multicenter, randomized, noninferiority trial found a 7-day regimen with nitrofurantoin was more effective than a 1-day regimen in treating pregnant women with ASB, with bacteriological cure rates of 86.2% and 75.7%, respectively.[62] Optimal antibiotics and duration of therapy have not been clearly identified and must be individualized for each patient based on cultures and sensitivity results.[64] For S.C., who likely has ASB, a 7-day course of nitrofurantoin is reasonable. At this gestation age of 31 weeks, nitrofurantoin can still be used safely. There is a small risk of hemolytic anemia in newborns when nitrofurantoin is used close to delivery.[43]

Pyelonephritis in Pregnancy

CASE 49-1, QUESTION 13: S.C. returns to the obstetric clinic 2 weeks later stating that she has finished her course of antibiotics of nitrofurantoin 100 mg PO twice daily for 7 days. She reports subjective fevers, right flank pain, shaking chills, and nausea and vomiting. On examination, she was found to have costovertebral angle tenderness, an area on the back overlying the kidney that when gently tapped elicits pain in patients with a kidney infection. She is admitted to the hospital for acute pyelonephritis during pregnancy. What are the risks of having pyelonephritis during pregnancy, and how should S.C. be treated?

Acute pyelonephritis occurs in about 1% to 2% of all pregnancies, usually resulting in antepartum hospitalization. Pyelonephritis is an infection of the upper urinary tracts involving

TABLE 49-3
Fetal Risk Assessment of Common Antibiotics Used During Pregnancy

Drug	Fetal Risk	Comments
Aminoglycosides (gentamicin)	Low risk	Gentamicin used for many indications during pregnancy (i.e., chorioamnionitis, pyelonephritis). Dose to target peak of 8 mcg/mL and trough of less than 1 mcg/mL. Ototoxicity reported with older aminoglycosides (kanamycin, streptomycin). No reports with gentamicin.
Cephalosporins	Compatible	First-line therapy for UTI.
Clindamycin	Compatible	Used for many indications during pregnancy.
Erythromycin	Compatible	Excludes estolate salt, can cause maternal hepatotoxicity.
Fluoroquinolones	Animal data suggest risk; Human data suggest low risk	Reports of fetal cartilage damage and arthropathies in animal studies, not confirmed in human data. Avoid use in first trimester. Reserve use only if needed for drug-resistant organisms (not susceptible to first-line agents).
Metronidazole	Animal data suggest risk; Human data suggest low risk	Mutagenic in bacteria and carcinogenic in rodents. Avoid use in first trimester. Acceptable to use in second and third trimesters.
Nitrofurantoin	Low risk	First-line therapy for UTI. Avoid use close to term in third trimester if possible. May induce hemolytic anemia in G6PD-deficient women and neonates who are deficient in glutathione.
Penicillins	Compatible	Resistance to *E. coli* is high. Can use if GBS is cultured in urine.
Trimethoprim-sulfamethoxazole	Contraindicated in first trimester Caution use in third trimester	Avoid use in first trimester because folate antagonism of trimethoprim can cause NTDs. Avoid use close to term in third trimester owing to theoretical risk of kernicterus in newborns from competitive binding between bilirubin and sulfonamides, to plasma albumin.
Tetracyclines	Contraindicated in all trimesters	Permanent discoloration of deciduous teeth.
Vancomycin	Compatible	Reserve use for drug-resistant gram-positive organisms not sensitive to first-line agents.

GBS, group B Streptococcus; G6PD, glucose-6-phosphate dehydrogenase; NTDs, neural tube defects; UTI, urinary tract infection.
Source: Briggs G et al. *Drugs in Pregnancy and Lactation: A Reference Guide to Fetal and Neonatal Risk.* 9th ed. Philadelphia, PA: Lippincott Williams & Wilkins; 2011.

the kidneys as a result of bacterial ascent through the urethra and bladder.[68] Signs and symptoms of pyelonephritis can include fever, shaking chills, flank pain, nausea and vomiting, and costovertebral angle tenderness on examination.[68] Symptoms of cystitis such as dysuria, urgency, and frequency of voids can occur but are less common.[69] In most cases, urine samples should be obtained by a midstream clean-catch and can be obtained through urethral catheterization if necessary.[68] Blood cultures are usually not obtained unless a systemic infection is suspected with signs and symptoms of sepsis, acute respiratory distress syndrome (ARDS), or temperature elevations above 102.2°F.[69]

Pyelonephritis during pregnancy can be detrimental to both the mother and fetus if not treated appropriately. In the mother, endotoxins produced from gram-negative bacteria can trigger the release of cytokines, histamine, and bradykinin, which can attack capillary endothelial function. Complications such as septic shock, disseminated intravascular coagulation, or ARDS can occur. Approximately 1% to 8% of women with antepartum pyelonephritis can exhibit ARDS, which usually is managed with supplemental oxygen and diuretics, but can progressively worsen to need ventilation support.[70] Risk factors for ARDS include maternal heart rate greater than 110 beats/minute, fever greater than 103°F in the first 24 hours, greater than 20 weeks of gestation, use of β-sympathomimetic tocolytics such as terbutaline, and excessive fluid overload greater than 3 L.[71]

S.C. should be treated with IV hydration, parenteral antibiotics, and antipyretics such as acetaminophen.[69] Her urine output should be closely monitored to avoid fluid overload.[71] IV cephalosporins or penicillin derivatives are commonly used to treat pyelonephritis because of their safety during pregnancy, coverage of uropathogens, and ability to penetrate into tissues and concentrate in the urine.[43,69] Ampicillin is used less frequently owing to increasing resistance to *E. coli* of up to 60% in some areas.[69] Gentamicin, an aminoglycoside, has widely been used during pregnancy because of its ability to reach effective concentrations in the tissues with low resistance rates, and broad coverage of gram-negative organisms. No reports of congenital anomalies have been reported with gentamicin use; however, ototoxicity has been reported with older aminoglycosides such as kanamycin and streptomycin.[43] Optimal antibiotic regimens have not been established universally. Antimicrobial resistance and cost must be taken into account.

S.C. should be started on cefazolin 2 g IV every 8 hours in addition to gentamicin (targeted peak of 8 mcg/mL and trough less than 1 mcg/mL) and continued for at least 48 hours after becoming afebrile. An alternative treatment regimen would be ceftriaxone 2 g IV every 24 hours. Afterward, S.C. should be transitioned to oral antibiotics based on culture and susceptibility results such as cephalexin 500 mg PO four times daily for a total of 10 to 14 days of antibiotic therapy (both PO and IV).[68,69] Antibiotic suppression is recommended after treatment because the rate of recurrence is about 6% to 8%.[69] S.C. should receive antibiotic prophylaxis after treatment with nitrofurantoin 100 mg PO each night during the pregnancy until 4 to 6 weeks post partum. Nitrofurantoin should be discontinued close to term because it can cause hemolytic anemia in infants with G6PD deficiency.[43] Nitrofurantoin should never be used for the treatment of pyelonephritis, a deep tissue infection, because it only concentrates in urine and does not penetrate tissue.

DIABETES MELLITUS

Diabetes mellitus is the most common maternal medical complications during pregnancy. Diabetes during pregnancy can be detected before or during pregnancy and can be separated into two groups: (a) *pregestational diabetes,* which includes women who have been diagnosed before pregnancy with either diabetes type 1 or diabetes type 2, or (b) *gestational diabetes mellitus* (GDM), defined as carbohydrate intolerance first detected during pregnancy.[72]

More prevalent than pregestational diabetes, GDM accounts for more than 90% of diabetes cases during pregnancy and affects approximately 5% to 9% of live births each year.[73] More than half of women with GDM will go on to develop type 2 diabetes later in life.[74] Some believe that GDM is a diagnosis of type 2 diabetes that has been discovered during pregnancy.[74]

Pregestational diabetes accounts for the remaining 10% of cases. In the United States, more than 8 million women have pregestational diabetes, affecting about 1% of live births each year.[73] Most women with pregestational diabetes have type 2 diabetes characterized by peripheral insulin resistance and relative insulin deficiency.[72] The incidence of type 2 pregestational diabetes has been rapidly rising in the past decade, most likely because of the increasing prevalence of obesity. In contrast to type 2 diabetes, type 1 diabetes is characterized by complete insulin deficiency resulting from autoimmune destruction of pancreatic β cells.[72] Less than 0.5% of all pregnancies in the United States are complicated by type 1 diabetes.[75]

Fluctuating glucose levels during the first trimester may be the first signs of pregnancy for women with pregestational diabetes owing to increased insulin resistance and reduced sensitivity to insulin action. Placental hormones (e.g., human placental lactogen, progesterone, prolactin, placental growth hormone, and cortisol) are thought to be responsible for the increase in insulin resistance during pregnancy. The ACOG classifies diabetes in pregnancy according to the White classification, modified to include gestational diabetes according to glycemic control. The White classification relies on age at onset, duration of diabetes, and presence of vascular complications for patient classification (Table 49-4).

Pre-existing Diabetes Mellitus

FETAL AND INFANT RISKS

CASE 49-2

QUESTION 1: K.H., a 27-year-old, 60-kg woman known to have type 1 diabetes since age 12, has married recently and wishes to have children. She has been conscientious in her diabetes care and self-monitors her blood glucose concentrations two to three times a day (fasting and before meals). During the past month, her fasting blood glucose concentrations have ranged from 90 to 140 mg/dL. Today, her fasting blood glucose and glycosylated hemoglobin (Hgb A_{1c}) laboratory results are 134 mg/dL and 7.8%, respectively. Her blood pressure (BP) is 145/94 mm Hg, renal function is normal, serum creatinine is 0.8 mg/dL, and she does not have proteinuria. K.H. reports tingling and pain in her toes. Her current medications include lisinopril 5 mg PO daily, insulin glargine (Lantus) 16 units subcutaneously (SC) every day at bedtime with an insulin lispro (Humalog) sliding-scale of 2 to 10 units before each meal. She reports eating only two meals a day and no snacks in between. How will diabetes affect the health of a child she would like to conceive?

Perinatal mortality for infants of diabetic mothers has declined dramatically with strict maternal metabolic control, improved fetal surveillance, and neonatal intensive care.[76] Fetal and neonatal mortality rates are approximately 2% to 4%, and the risk of spontaneous abortion in patients with well-controlled type 1 diabetes is equal to that of women without diabetes.[77] The

TABLE 49-4
Modified White's Classification of Diabetes During Pregnancy

Class of Diabetes	Age of Onset	Duration	Vascular Complications	Treatment of Choice During Pregnancy
Class A1	First diagnosed during pregnancy	During pregnancy	None	Diet, exercise
Class A2	First diagnosed during pregnancy	During pregnancy	None	Diet, exercise plus oral hypoglycemics or insulin
Class B	Older than 20 years	Less than 10 years	None	Insulin therapy
Class C	Between 10 and 19 years	More than 10 years, less than 19	None	Insulin therapy
Class D	Younger than 10 years	More than 20 years	Background retinopathy Hypertension Microalbuminuria	Insulin therapy
Class F	At any age	Any duration	Nephropathy Macroalbuminuria (>500 mg/d)	Insulin therapy
Class H	At any age	Any duration	Arteriosclerotic heart disease	Insulin therapy
Class R	At any age	Any duration	Proliferative retinopathy Vitreous hemorrhage	Insulin therapy
Class T	At any age	Any duration	Renal transplantation	Insulin therapy

Source: Cunningham FG et al. Diabetes. In: *Williams Obstetrics.* 23rd ed. New York, NY: McGraw-Hill; 2010:1104; White P. Classification of obstetric diabetes. *Am J Obstet Gynecol.* 1978;130:228.

incidence of stillbirth is greatest after 36 weeks' gestation in women with poor glycemic control, fetal macrosomia (see subsequent discussion), maternal vascular disease, ketoacidosis, or pre-eclampsia.[72]

The leading cause of perinatal mortality is major congenital anomalies that occur in 9% to 14% of infants born to mothers with diabetes. The major malformations observed include NTDs and other anomalies involving the cardiac, renal, and GI systems, and rarely caudal regression syndrome.[73] Many congenital anomalies occur during organogenesis, before the seventh week of gestation, when women are often unaware that they are pregnant.[78] A direct correlation exists between higher Hgb A_{1c} levels and increased frequency of anomalies.[78] Women with elevated Hgb A_{1c} values during the time of conception have a significantly higher incidence of infants with anomalies compared with women with Hgb A_{1c} closer to the normal range of 4.0% to 5.6%.[77] The risk of fetal anomalies increases dramatically to approximately 20% to 25% when Hgb A_{1c} levels are near 10%.[78] Hgb A_{1c} levels greater than 12% are associated with the same risk of anomalies as infants exposed to known teratogens such as thalidomide, isotretinoin, or alcohol during organogenesis.

Macrosomia, defined as birth weight greater than 4 kg, is thought to be caused in part by fetal hyperglycemia and hyperinsulinemia.[72] Fetal hyperglycemia occurs when glucose crosses the placenta and subsequently stimulates fetal pancreatic β cells to release excessive insulin. Hyperinsulinemia promotes excessive fetal growth in adipose tissue, causing disproportional fat concentration around the shoulders and chest and doubling the risks of trauma (e.g., shoulder dystocia) during vaginal delivery.

Infants of diabetic mothers also are at increased risk for prolonged hypoglycemia after delivery, respiratory distress syndrome (RDS), hypocalcemia, polycythemia, and hyperbilirubinemia during the neonatal period.[73]

K.H. should be informed that stringent preconception glycemic control is essential for preventing early pregnancy loss and congenital malformations in the infant.[76] Tight glucose control, especially in the months before pregnancy and early in the first trimester, will maximize her chance of having a healthy baby. She should be educated before pregnancy about healthy practices she can institute now to improve a successful pregnancy outcome.

MATERNAL RISKS

CASE 49-2, QUESTION 2: K.H. wants to know what health risks she might incur from becoming pregnant and what measures could minimize these risks?

A prepregnancy assessment, including a history and physical examination, is necessary to determine the risks of or contraindications to pregnancy for K.H. She should be evaluated for ischemic heart disease, neuropathies, or retinopathy, and her renal status must be assessed.[76] Pregnancy can exacerbate the vascular complications of diabetes. For instance, diabetic retinopathy can worsen if strict glycemic control is implemented quickly in pregnant women with proliferative retinopathy; progression to end-stage renal disease can occur in women with mild to moderate renal insufficiency (e.g., serum creatinine >1.5 mg/dL or proteinuria >3 g/24 hours).[73] The presence of gastroparesis should be noted because it will make controlling her glucose more difficult.[75]

Controlling K.H.'s diabetes before she becomes pregnant may benefit her hypertension and neuropathies and will minimize maternal and fetal problems. Good metabolic control of her diabetes can minimize progression of her diabetes.[76]

PRECONCEPTION MANAGEMENT

CASE 49-2, QUESTION 3: What prepregnancy interventions relative to her general health and diabetes should K.H. undertake before she attempts to become pregnant?

Pregestational care for K.H. should ideally begin 6 months before conception.[76] Recommendations for women with diabetes who want to conceive include suggesting birth control methods until stringent glycemic control can be achieved, consulting a dietitian to develop a patient-specific nutritional diet to attain healthy weight targets, and implementing a self-monitoring blood glucose regimen.[76] Good glycemic control (Hgb A_{1c} levels close to normal) should be achieved months before conception to minimize risks of major congenital anomalies. K.H.'s current regimen may not achieve euglycemia (see Chapter 53, Diabetes Mellitus). Her insulin therapy should be titrated to reduce her average blood glucose range from 90 to

120 mg/dL, targeting an Hgb A_{1c} of less than 6% without frequent episodes of hypoglycemia.[76] Additionally, K.H. should be started on prenatal vitamins containing at least 400 mcg of folic acid.

Her BP of 145/94 mm Hg is high and should be decreased to a diastolic BP of about 80 mm Hg to minimize risks for preeclampsia (see Case 49-5, Question 6) or exacerbation of her disorder. Many women with pregestational diabetes, such as K.H., are likely on an angiotensin-converting enzyme inhibitor (ACEI) or angiotensin receptor blocker for hypertension treatment or for renal protective effects. Before pregnancy and during preconception planning, K.H. should be switched to another antihypertensive (e.g., methyldopa, labetalol, or calcium-channel blockers) such as methyldopa or labetalol because recent studies have observed possible increased rates of congenital cardiac malformation associated with the use of ACEIs in the first trimester.[79] Further confirmatory studies are needed to define the risk of using ACEIs during the first trimester. However, use of ACEIs is absolutely contraindicated during the second and third trimesters of pregnancy.[43,79]

TYPE 1 DIABETES TREATMENT IN PREGNANCY

CASE 49-2, QUESTION 4: After lowering her BP to 125/80 mm Hg with labetalol 200 mg PO twice daily and her Hgb A_{1c} to 7.3%, K.H. discontinues her oral contraceptive and returns to the clinic 5 months later and is noted to be about 4 weeks pregnant. How should her diabetes be managed at this time?

GOALS OF THERAPY

The overall goals of treatment of K.H.'s diabetes are to reduce the maternal and fetal morbidity and mortality associated with diabetes. Treatment of diabetes (see Chapter 53, Diabetes Mellitus) should include dietary management, appropriate maternal weight gain, insulin therapy to normalize glycemic control, and exercise.

DIETARY MANAGEMENT

The goals of dietary management for diabetes during pregnancy are directed at ensuring fetal growth and development, appropriate maternal weight gain, and normalizing maternal glucose concentrations. Patients often benefit from individualized diets developed by a dietitian. Neonatal macrosomia has been associated with high postprandial glucose levels; therefore, a reduction in postprandial hyperglycemia is an important goal.

BLOOD GLUCOSE AND GLYCOSYLATED HEMOGLOBIN MONITORING

K.H. should be begin to self-monitor her blood sugars more intensively at fasting, before meals, 1 hour postprandially, at bedtime, when she feels symptomatic hypoglycemia, and at 3:00 AM to rule out dawn phenomenon versus Somogyi effect.[80] The goal of therapy is to maintain fasting glucose levels less than 90 mg/dL, premeal values of less than 100 mg/dL, and 1-hour postprandial levels of 100 to 120 mg/dL.[73] Tight glycemic control without incidence of hypoglycemic episodes, targeting Hgb A_{1c} levels in the normal range, is the goal. Adjusting therapy based on postprandial glucose levels (as opposed to preprandial levels) can lower Hgb A_{1c} levels and decrease the risk of macrosomia, neonatal hypoglycemia, and cesarean delivery. Hgb A_{1c} levels can be drawn at each trimester to reveal the glycemic control during the previous 3 months.[73]

INSULIN THERAPY

Insulin analogs (e.g., lispro, aspart, glargine) are genetically engineered by recombinant DNA technology and usually differ by a few amino acids from human insulin. Concerns about insulin analog use during pregnancy include placental drug transfer and antibody formation.[81] The use of lispro (Humalog) and aspart (Novolog) insulin during pregnancy is supported by several studies that found minimal passage across the placenta, an absence of antibody formation, and no adverse maternal or fetal effects. Although the rapid onset of insulin lispro and aspart can increase adherence and patient satisfaction, it also may increase the incidence of hypoglycemia. Insulin glargine (Lantus), a long-acting insulin analog, allows for once-daily dosing and produces a peakless basal level of insulin. Only case reports have examined the safety and efficacy of insulin glargine during pregnancy.[43] Glargine is usually reserved for very brittle and sensitive insulin-dependent type 1 diabetes patients. Neutral protamine Hagedorn (NPH) insulin is usually used twice daily during pregnancy in lieu of insulin glargine as a basal insulin because it helps to control fasting blood sugars better than a peakless basal insulin. Newer insulin analogs such as insulin detemir (Levemir) and insulin glulisine (Apidra) have not yet been adequately studied during pregnancy and should not be used until further studies clarify their teratogenicity risk.[43]

Glycemic control is most difficult to establish during the first trimester of pregnancy because of the effect on blood sugars of maternal fluctuating hormones.[73] K.H.'s insulin regimen should be optimized by changing from insulin glargine to NPH insulin (with a 1 : 1 ratio) to help better control her fasting blood sugars and instituting a standard insulin lispro dosage before meals based on her carbohydrate intake. Sliding-scale insulin therapy is rarely used during pregnancy.[73] Insulin dosages commonly need to be monitored more strictly (every 2–4 days until glycemic control is achieved) during the first trimester and adjusted usually upward every 2 to 3 weeks during pregnancy.

TYPE 2 DIABETES TREATMENT IN PREGNANCY

CASE 49-3

QUESTION 1: V.W. is a 36-year-old G3, P0 with class B diabetes at 15 weeks' gestation with a history of two spontaneous miscarriages occurring last year. She was diagnosed with diabetes 5 years ago during a routine physical examination. She is morbidly obese with a body mass index (BMI) of 49 kg/m^2, height of 5 feet 5 inches, and weight of 295 pounds. She recently found out that she was pregnant and has not had any prenatal care. Her current medications include metformin 1,000 mg PO twice daily and glipizide 5 mg PO daily. She states she has been noncompliant with checking her blood sugars, maintaining a diabetic diet, and taking her medication. Her last Hgb A_{1c}, which was 8.3%, was 2 months ago. Which medication and treatments should V.W. be started on?

INSULIN THERAPY

Insulin is the hypoglycemic agent of choice during pregnancy because it does not cross the placenta and has an established safety record for both mother and fetus. The goal with insulin therapy is to imitate the glucose levels of a healthy pregnant woman. Rapid glycemic control is of utmost importance during this critical period of organogenesis when vital organs are developing.[78]

Insulin requirements may vary, depending on the trimester. The first trimester is characterized by unstable diabetes, followed by a stable period.[72] During the first trimester, glucose and gluconeogenic substances in the blood are taken up by the fetus, which can lead to a decrease in maternal insulin requirements and increased episodes of hypoglycemia. On average, insulin dosages range from 0.7 to 0.8 units/kg/day in the first trimester.[73] If nausea and vomiting occurs during this time, glycemic control may be unstable and should be monitored closely. At about 24 weeks' gestation, insulin requirements begin to increase to 0.8 to 1 units/kg/day, and insulin doses may need to be adjusted every 5 to 10 days.[73] These needs continue to increase during the third trimester to 0.9 to 1.2 units/kg/day, which may be twice as much as the prepregnancy dose, in part because of the placental hormones (i.e., lactogen, prolactin, estrogen, and progesterone), which antagonize the action of insulin. Weight-based dosing may not accurately assess the insulin requirements in all pregnant women, especially in the obese population. Insulin regimens must be individualized for each patient, taking into consideration their educational level, compliance, and schedule constraints. Dosage adjustments must take into account the level of activity, meal plan, and other factors (e.g., steroid use, stress, infections) that may affect glucose control. Some women may be admitted into the hospital in the first trimester to (a) rapidly gain glucose control, (b) accurately assess their insulin requirements, and (c) institute an individualized insulin regimen under careful monitoring of blood sugars.[72]

An insulin regimen with three to four daily injections is most successful at maintaining adequate glucose control. Biosynthetic human insulin (e.g., regular and NPH insulin) is the usual treatment of choice in pregestational diabetes mellitus because of its chemical, biological, and immunological equivalency to pancreatic human insulin.[43] These insulins have the most established safety profile during pregnancy, but they require more stringent timing of meals during the day.[43]

V.W. should be switched from her oral hypoglycemic agents to insulin therapy with biosynthetic human regular insulin and NPH insulin. Metformin and glipizide should be discontinued. The total daily insulin dosage can be calculated by taking into account V.W.'s gestational age and actual body weight. Her total daily dose equals 0.8 units/kg × 134 kg, or 107 units daily. Using three injections per day, her dosage would be 47 units of NPH insulin plus 24 units of regular insulin SC 30 minutes before breakfast, 18 units of regular insulin SC 30 minutes before dinner, and 18 units SC of NPH insulin at bedtime. V.W.'s treatment plan needs to include dietary management; appropriate counseling on maternal weight gain during pregnancy given her morbid obesity; instructions on how to draw up, mix, and inject her insulin therapy to normalize glycemic control; and moderate exercise and walking 20 to 30 minutes after each meal. She should be taught to inject only in the subcutaneous abdomen area where insulin is best absorbed during pregnancy. V.W. should also be given a glucometer and taught how to self-monitor her blood sugars four times daily, at fasting and 1-hour postprandially (after the last bite of food from each meal) to target fasting blood glucose levels below 90 mg/dL and 1-hour postprandial levels less than 120 mg/dL.

ORAL HYPOGLYCEMIC USE IN TYPE 2 DIABETES DURING PREGNANCY

Although oral hypoglycemic agents are used commonly to treat type 2 diabetes in nonpregnant women, they are rarely used as monotherapy during pregnancy. A switch to insulin therapy is recommended before conception, if possible, or at the time the pregnancy is confirmed because many patients have inadequate control with oral hypoglycemic agents.[73] If insulin is not started before conception, women should be strongly counseled to stay on oral hypoglycemics to adequately control blood glucose until insulin therapy can be implemented. Often, patients will discontinue oral hypoglycemics from fear of taking any medication in pregnancy, resulting in hyperglycemia during the critical period of organogenesis.

The ACOG recommends that the use of oral hypoglycemics for the treatment of type 2 diabetes during pregnancy be individualized until more safety and efficacy data become available.[73] There is limited experience with oral hypoglycemic use in type 2 diabetes during pregnancy. Metformin, a biguanide, has been used during pregnancy for hyperinsulinemic insulin resistance or in the treatment of infertility in women with polycystic ovarian syndrome (see Chapter 50, Disorders Related to the Menstrual Cycle). Women taking metformin should be switched to insulin therapy unless specific circumstances (e.g., high insulin requirements during the second or third trimester) warrant its use.[81]

CASE 49-3, QUESTION 2: Should an oral hypoglycemic be added to V.W.'s insulin regimen?

V.W. should remain on insulin therapy with three injections daily. Her insulin regimen should be adjusted every 2 to 3 days until glycemic control is achieved and targeted blood glucose levels are reached without significant hypoglycemia episodes. Metformin should only be added if V.W.'s total daily insulin requirement exceeds 250 to 300 units. If metformin is added, insulin dosages should be decreased to at least half the amount in anticipation of increased insulin sensitivity.

Gestational Diabetes Mellitus

DIAGNOSTIC CRITERIA

CASE 49-4

QUESTION 1: J.B. is a 22-year-old, Asian woman in the 24th week of her first pregnancy. She is 5 feet 2 inches, 75 kg (prepregnancy weight), and her BMI is 30 kg/m^2. At her regular prenatal visit, her obstetrician recommends an oral glucose-screening test for GDM. Her Hgb A_{1c} was 5.8%. Although her mother has diabetes, J.B. has had no glucosuria during pregnancy. Why is J.B. at risk for GDM?

GDM is defined as carbohydrate intolerance that develops or is recognized during pregnancy regardless of severity, necessity for treatment, time of onset, or persistence after pregnancy.[82] GDM occurs in about 7% (range, 1%–14%), and the prevalence varies with the population and methods of detection.[82] Complications noted in the offspring of affected women include macrosomia, hypocalcemia, hypoglycemia, polycythemia, and jaundice. Women with GDM are more likely to experience pregnancy-induced hypertensive disorders or require a cesarean delivery. They also are at risk for type 2 diabetes later, and their children have an increased risk for obesity and diabetes later in life.

Risk factors for GDM include age older than 25 years, obesity (BMI $\geq$25 kg/m^2), family history of diabetes, previous delivery of an infant weighing more than 4 kg, a history of a stillbirth, a history of glucose intolerance, or current glycosuria.[82] Blacks, Hispanic, Asian, and Native American women also are at increased risk for GDM.[82]

J.B. is at risk for GDM because she is Asian and obese, and she has a family history of diabetes. Her Hgb A_{1c} at 26 weeks' gestation was normal and ruled her out for overt diabetes. J.B. should undergo the standard screening for gestational diabetes with a 50-g 1-hour glucose challenge. It is not essential for J.B. to fast before this test. The diagnosis of GDM is important to the mother and the fetus because of the increased risks of fetal hyperinsulinemia and macrosomia.

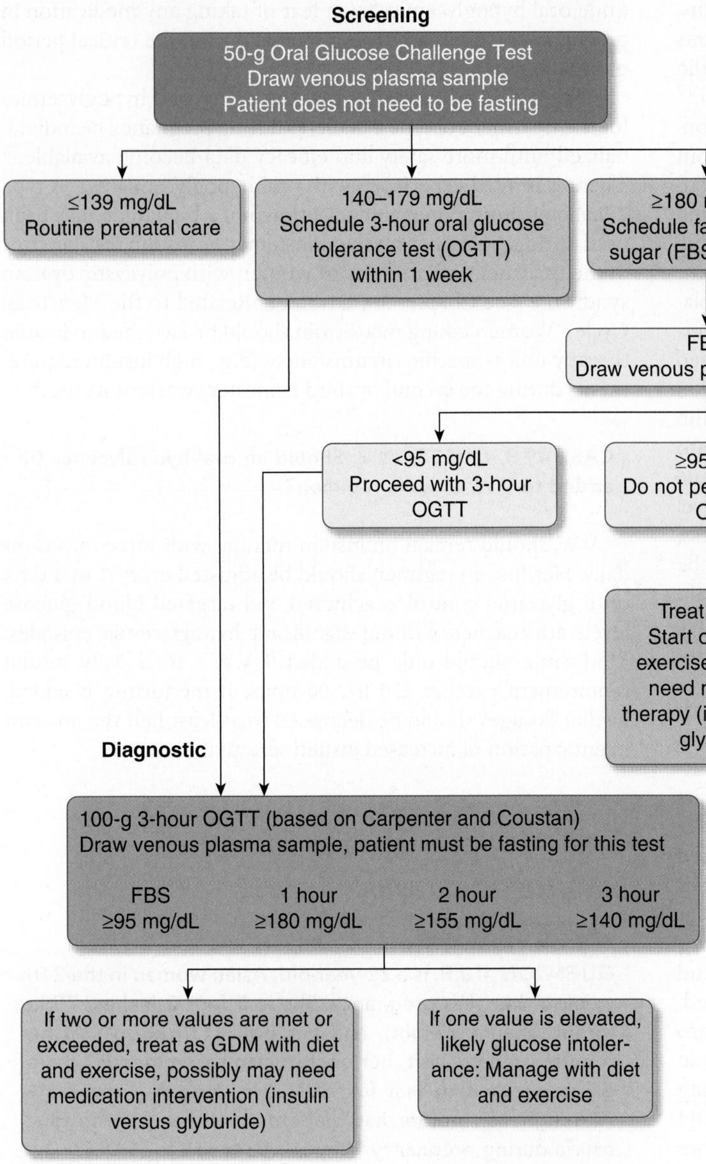

50-g Oral Glucose Challenge Test
Draw venous plasma sample
Patient does not need to be fasting

100-g 3-hour OGTT (based on Carpenter and Coustan)
Draw venous plasma sample, patient must be fasting for this test
FBS ≥95 mg/dL
1 hour ≥180 mg/dL
2 hour ≥155 mg/dL
3 hour ≥140 mg/dL
If two or more values are met or exceeded, treat as GDM with diet and exercise, possibly may need medication intervention (insulin versus glyburide)
If one value is elevated, likely glucose intolerance: Manage with diet and exercise

FIGURE 49-4 Recommendations for screening and diagnosis of gestational diabetes. A1C, hemoglobin A1C; FBG, fasting blood glucose; GDM, gestational diabetes mellitus; OGTT, oral glucose tolerance test. (Adapted with permission from Screening and diagnosis of gestational diabetes mellitus. Committee Opinion No. 504. American College of Obstetricians and Gynecologists. *Obstet Gynecol.* 2011;118: 751–753.)

GESTATIONAL DIABETES MELLITUS TREATMENT

CASE 49-4, QUESTION 2: J.B. is screened with a 50-g 1-hour glucose challenge resulting at 161 mg/dL. Because her screening test was elevated, a diagnostic 3-hour oral glucose tolerance test (OGTT) was given to her the next day, which required her to be fasting. The results of the 3-hour OGTT showed a fasting plasma glucose of 96 mg/dL, a 1-hour glucose of 183 mg/dL, 2-hour glucose of 140 mg/dL, and 3-hour glucose of 126 mg/dL. These results confirm that J.B. has GDM. How should she be managed?

J.B. requires extensive education about a gestational diabetes diet, use of a glucometer, the signs and symptoms of hyperglycemia and hypoglycemia, and treatment of low blood glucose. She should start to monitor her blood glucose four times daily, at fasting and 1 hour after the end of each meal. She should return to the clinic in 1 week for an assessment of her blood sugars to evaluate the need for medication therapy (insulin versus glyburide treatment).

Most women with GDM can control their glucose with dietary modifications and regular exercise; however, management with medications (insulin versus oral hypoglycemics) should be initiated if dietary management fails to maintain fasting plasma blood glucose concentrations at 90 mg/dL or less or to achieve a 1-hour postprandial plasma concentration of less than 130 mg/dL.

CASE 49-4, QUESTION 3: J.B. returns to clinic at 30 weeks' gestation with glucometer and logbook for a blood glucose assessment. She has been compliant with her diabetic diet and blood sugar monitoring for the past 4 weeks. She has been able to control her blood sugars with diet and moderate walking after meals. However, she has noticed that her fasting blood glucose has risen in the past week to an average of 98 mg/dL and her dinner postprandial values are averaging 139 mg/dL. How should J.B. be managed at this time?

Treatment of GDM with insulin therapy is implemented similarly to the treatment for pregestational diabetes. An optimal insulin regimen for GDM has not been determined. Similar dosing with a weight-based, split-mixed multidose regimen is used. The insulin regimen must be tailored specifically to the needs of the woman to successfully achieve target blood glucose levels.

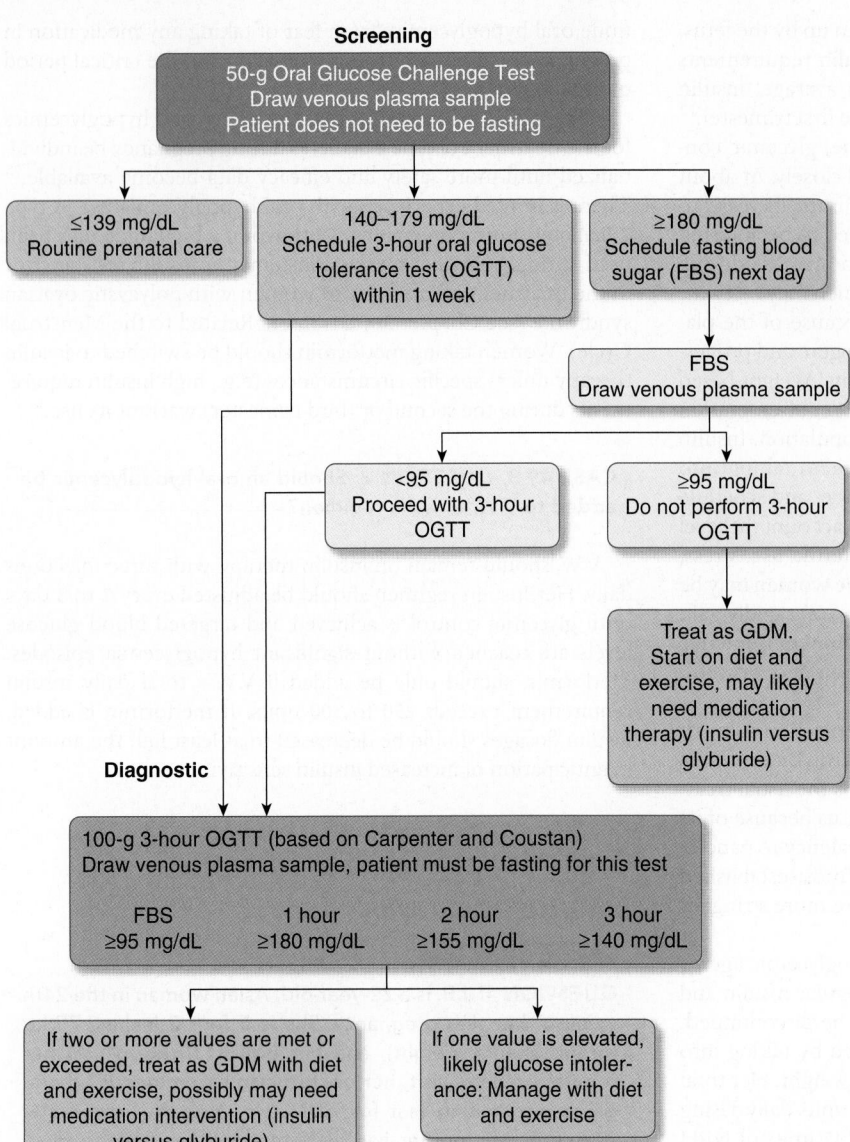

Routine prenatal care
140–179 mg/dL
Schedule 3-hour oral glucose tolerance test (OGTT) within 1 week
≥180 mg/dL
Schedule fasting blood sugar (FBS) next day
FBS
Draw venous plasma sample
<95 mg/dL
Proceed with 3-hour OGTT
≥95 mg/dL
Do not perform 3-hour OGTT
Treat as GDM. Start on diet and exercise, may likely need medication therapy (insulin versus glyburide)

More recently in the past 10 years, the role of oral hypoglycemic agents for the treatment of GDM has increased. Traditionally, oral hypoglycemics have not been used during pregnancy because early animal studies implicated some agents as teratogens. The studies failed to show whether the primary teratogen was the drug itself or the effect of hyperglycemia and altered maternal metabolism.[84] Glyburide, a second-generation sulfonylurea, has been used in several studies as an alternative treatment modality in women with GDM who have relatively mild hyperglycemia.[85] A gestational age of more than 30 weeks, fasting blood glucose level of less than 110 mg/dL, and 1-hour postprandial values of less than 140 mg/dL are parameters that have been shown in one study to predict glyburide success in women with GDM who have failed diet therapy.[86] In a randomized trial, glyburide therapy was compared with an intensive insulin protocol in women between 11 and 33 weeks of gestation with GDM who failed to achieve target blood glucose goals with diet alone.[85] Equivalent glycemic control was achieved with treatment of glyburide or insulin therapy. In addition, both groups had similar pregnancy outcomes, including rates for cesarean delivery, pre-eclampsia, macrosomia, and neonatal hypoglycemia.[85] Although the analysis of the cord serum of the infant did not detect any glyburide in this randomly selected small sample, the drug has been shown to cross the placenta.[85]

More recently, the Metformin in Gestational Diabetes trial examined whether metformin treatment could provide equivalent outcomes to insulin treatment. Women with GDM at 20 to 33 weeks' gestation were randomly assigned to open-label treatment with metformin (titrated up to 2,500 mg with the option to add supplemental insulin if glycemic control was not achieved) or to insulin treatment alone.[87] The two groups achieved similar primary outcomes (composite score of neonatal morbidities), but 46% of the group allocated to metformin required supplemental insulin therapy. Those requiring supplemental insulin were more obese and had higher elevations of glycemic values at presentation. The results indicate that metformin can be used during pregnancy for GDM, but will less likely be successful as monotherapy in women with higher glucose levels.[87] Metformin is usually reserved for patients with high insulin requirements (>300 units daily) in the second and third trimesters.[43] More randomized trials are needed to further determine and to better understand the role of oral hypoglycemic agents in pregnancy.

J.B. is a good candidate for glyburide therapy because she is greater than 30 weeks' gestation and has a fasting blood sugar level less than 110 mg/dL. Glyburide 2.5 mg PO daily 30 minutes before dinner should be started. Doses should be increased or decreased to achieve glycemic control. If maximal dosages of glyburide are reached and glycemic control is not achieved, J.B. should be transitioned to SC insulin therapy.

RISK OF DEVELOPING DIABETES MELLITUS

CASE 49-4, QUESTION 4: Why is J.B. at risk for developing diabetes mellitus after delivery?

Glucose tolerance normalizes after delivery for most women. Women with GDM, however, have a 15% to 50% chance of developing nongestational diabetes within 5 to 16 years.[74] The highest risk is in women who are obese or were diagnosed before 24 weeks' gestation or who had marked hyperglycemia during or soon after pregnancy. The risk of developing GDM in a future pregnancy is estimated to be 50% to 70%.[82]

J.B. should try to minimize the potential for development of insulin resistance by exercising and maintaining a normal weight. She should also have her glucose checked with a 2-hour OGTT at her postpartum appointment 6 weeks after delivery and then at least every 1 to 3 years with screening of either fasting blood sugar or HgbA1c. In addition, J.B. should be instructed about the importance of using an effective birth control method to prevent unplanned pregnancies. She also needs to schedule regular appointments with her primary-care clinician.

HYPERTENSION AND PRE-ECLAMPSIA

Chronic Hypertension

CLINICAL PRESENTATION

CASE 49-5

QUESTION 1: T.D., a 37-year-old G1, P0, obese black woman was diagnosed with stage 1 hypertension several months before her pregnancy (BP, 135 to 145 mm Hg systolic and 90 to 95 mm Hg diastolic). She had no cardiovascular risk factors (i.e., smoking, diabetes mellitus, dyslipidemias) and was prescribed a trial of lifestyle modification (i.e., weight loss and exercise). When she initiated prenatal care at 16 weeks' gestation, her BP ranged from 130 to 135 mm Hg systolic pressure and 82 to 85 mm Hg diastolic pressure. Her BP today at 28 weeks is 142/90 mm Hg. Her serum chemistry values are creatinine (SCr), 0.6 mg/dL, and uric acid (UA), 4 mg/dL. A random urinalysis did not demonstrate proteinuria. Ultrasound confirms an adequately growing fetus at 28 weeks' gestation. What type of hypertension does T.D. have? What is the likelihood T.D. has pre-eclampsia?

Hypertensive disease occurs in 5% to 8% of all pregnancies and is a major cause of maternal and perinatal morbidity and mortality.[88] From 15% to 24% of maternal deaths in developed countries are attributed to hypertensive disorders in pregnancy.[89,90] *Hypertension in pregnancy* is defined as a systolic BP of at least 140 mm Hg or a diastolic BP of at least 90 mm Hg on two separate occasions at least 6 hours apart.

Women with pregnancy-associated hypertension can be grouped into the following categories: chronic hypertension, pre-eclampsia–eclampsia, pre-eclampsia superimposed on chronic hypertension, and gestational hypertension.[88] After delivery, *gestational hypertension* is ultimately delineated as either (a) transient hypertension of pregnancy if pre-eclampsia is absent during delivery and BP normalizes by 12 weeks post partum or (b) chronic hypertension if BP remains elevated.[88]

Chronic hypertension is defined as hypertension diagnosed before conception or before the 20th week of gestation, or hypertension persisting beyond 12 weeks post partum.[88] Hypertension noted after the 20th week of gestation might be difficult to classify, particularly if a woman has had inadequate prenatal care without appropriate BP monitoring.

Women with chronic hypertension, similarly to T.D., commonly have a normal BP during the first half of pregnancy because of the physiologic decline of BP during the second trimester.[91] BP usually returns to the prepregnancy level by the third trimester. T.D.'s diastolic pressure decreased from the prepregnancy levels of 90 to 95 mm Hg to 86 to 90 mm Hg during the second trimester. It is normal for T.D.'s BP to increase during the third trimester. These changes in BP make it difficult to differentiate chronic hypertension from pre-eclampsia during the second half of pregnancy in women with late prenatal care or inadequate BP monitoring. It is also difficult to diagnose pre-eclampsia superimposed on existing hypertension using BP measurements alone. A sharp increase in T.D.'s pressure of more than 30 mm Hg systolic or more than 15 mm Hg diastolic could be consistent with pre-eclampsia. Without coexisting proteinuria (≥0.3 g/24 hours or ≥1+ in a random urine sample) or evidence of renal dysfunction, a diagnosis of pre-eclampsia would be a reach.[88] T.D. has no proteinuria, and a normal SCr and serum uric acid. T.D has chronic hypertension, but it is unlikely that T.D. has pre-eclampsia at this time.

RISK FACTORS FOR PRE-ECLAMPSIA

CASE 49-5, QUESTION 2: What risk factors does T.D. have for developing pre-eclampsia?

Pre-eclampsia is a pregnancy-specific condition usually occurring after 20 weeks' gestation and consisting of hypertension with proteinuria.[88] Pre-eclampsia can affect multiple organ systems (e.g., kidney, liver, hematologic, CNS). The signs and symptoms are often unpredictable and can be mistaken for other disorders. Because edema is so common in normal pregnancy and is not specific, it is no longer used as a criterion for the diagnosis of pre-eclampsia. Pre-eclampsia is a consequence of progressive placental and maternal endothelial cell dysfunction, increased platelet aggregation, and loss of arterial vasoregulation. A variant of pre-eclampsia is HELLP syndrome, which consists of hemolysis (H), elevated liver enzymes (EL), and low platelet count (LP). HELLP can be also be life threatening and may not always present with proteinuria and increases in BP.[92]

When women with pre-eclampsia exhibit seizures, the term *eclampsia* is used. Women with pre-eclampsia may unpredictably progress rapidly from mild to severe pre-eclampsia and to eclampsia within days or even hours. Eclampsia is a potentially preventable complication of pre-eclampsia. About 20% of women who experience eclampsia have a diastolic BP less than 90 mm Hg or no proteinuria.[93]

The term *gestational hypertension* is used when BP is increased during pregnancy or is increased in the first 24 hours post partum in a woman without signs or symptoms of pre-eclampsia and without pre-existing hypertension.[88] Women with gestational hypertension are at high risk of recurrence during subsequent pregnancies.

Pre-eclampsia occurs most commonly during the first pregnancy (two-thirds of cases). Obesity and increasing maternal age are risk factors.[94] Chronic diseases that increase the risk for pre-eclampsia include diabetes mellitus or insulin resistance and renal disease. Pregnancy-associated risk factors include multifetal gestations, urinary tract infection, certain fetal chromosomal anomalies, and hydatiform moles. A family history of a sister or mother with pre-eclampsia significantly increases the risk of developing pre-eclampsia. Women with previous pre-eclampsia are at high risk for recurrence in subsequent pregnancies, particularly if it developed before 30 weeks' gestation.[94,95] In addition to her age and obesity, chronic hypertension is the most significant aspect of T.D.'s medical history, which confers a 25% risk of developing superimposed pre-eclampsia.[95]

MONITORING

CASE 49-5, QUESTION 3: What subjective and objective data should be monitored in T.D. for the development of pre-eclampsia?

T.D. should have her BP monitored frequently. If protein is detected in a random urinalysis, then a 24-hour urine collection for protein and creatinine can be repeated to determine accurately the degree of proteinuria and severity of disease.[88] Periodic ultrasounds should be obtained to assess fetal growth because IUGR is common in pregnant women with chronic hypertension. T.D. should be taught to recognize and immediately report all signs and symptoms of pre-eclampsia, such as nondependent edema (i.e., swelling of face or hands), headaches, and visual disturbances. The latter two are signs of severe pre-eclampsia and may indicate impending eclampsia. Upper abdominal pain also can be a sign of severe pre-eclampsia, indicating hepatic subcapsular hemorrhage.[94] Because T.D. has chronic hypertension, worsening of hypertension alone may not be a reliable sign of superimposed pre-eclampsia. Proteinuria is the best indicator of superimposed pre-eclampsia in a pregnant woman with chronic hypertension and no renal disease.[93]

ANTIHYPERTENSIVE DRUG THERAPY

CASE 49-5, QUESTION 4: Should T.D.'s chronic hypertension be treated with antihypertensive drugs to prevent pre-eclampsia?

The goal of antihypertensive therapy for women with chronic hypertension during pregnancy is to minimize the risks to the mother of an elevated BP without compromising placental perfusion.[88] The value of treating pregnant women with chronic antihypertension drugs remains an area of ongoing debate. A sustained diastolic BP of more than 100 mm Hg may cause maternal vascular damage, especially if the diastolic pressure is more than 105 to 110 mm Hg.[94] Morbidity is unlikely with a diastolic BP of less than 100 mm Hg. Therefore, many clinicians recommend treatment with antihypertensive drugs to lower diastolic pressures of more than 100 to 110 mm Hg.[88] Treatment of a diastolic BP of less than 100 mm Hg should be reserved for women with chronic hypertension and target organ damage (e.g., left ventricular hypertrophy) or underlying renal disease because antihypertensive drugs can decrease placental blood flow, which might increase fetal growth restriction.[97,98] Treatment of mild to moderate hypertension is associated with a decrease in the risk of developing severe hypertension by approximately 50%, but the overall risk of developing pre-eclampsia is unchanged.[99] Furthermore, there is no evidence of a reduction in the risk of stillbirth, fetal growth restriction, or preterm birth if women with chronic hypertension with systolic BP of 140 to 169 mm Hg or diastolic BP of 90 to 109 mm Hg are given antihypertensive therapy.[99] Moreover, women treated with antihypertensive therapy were more likely to experience adverse drug effects compared with those who received placebo or were untreated. Antihypertensive therapy, however, is required to reduce the risk of cardiovascular morbidity such as heart or renal failure and acute risk of stroke in pregnant women with severe hypertension (diastolic >110 mm Hg).

T.D. has normal renal function and her BP is less than 100 mm Hg; she does not need antihypertensive drug treatment at this time. If T.D. had been on drug therapy before conception, some experts would have her continue during the pregnancy.[88,93,97] In such cases, however, the doses of the antihypertensive agents often need to be lowered or discontinued altogether to prevent hypotension because the maternal BP naturally decreases during the second trimester. Perinatal outcomes in women with untreated chronic hypertension who do not progress to pre-eclampsia are similar to those of the general obstetric population.[93] Although chronic hypertension is a major risk factor for pre-eclampsia, treating T.D.'s uncomplicated mild chronic hypertension is unlikely to prevent the development of pre-eclampsia.

METHYLDOPA

CASE 49-5, QUESTION 5: When T.D. returns to the clinic 2 weeks later at 30 weeks' gestation, her BP ranged from

160 to 165 mm Hg systolic pressure and 85 to 92 mm Hg diastolic pressure. Which medication should T.D. be started on?

Methyldopa, a centrally acting α-agonist that decreases sympathetic outflow to decrease BP, is the most commonly used antihypertensive agent for chronic treatment of hypertension in pregnancy in the United States. The usual starting dose of 750 to 1,000 mg/day, to be administered in three to four daily divided doses, can be increased to 2 or 3 g/day if needed. Higher doses may be needed to control BP in pregnancy.[100]

Methyldopa, classified as category B for fetal risk, has the longest and best safety record of all antihypertensive agents during pregnancy. Despite its common use, few adverse effects have been reported in neonates exposed to methyldopa in utero. In addition, no congenital anomalies are associated with methyldopa.[43]

Dizziness and sedation, accompanied by a loss of energy, are among the most common adverse effects reported by pregnant women.[100] Generally, these adverse effects occur early in therapy and tend to subside, but may recur with an increased dosage. Problems with postural hypotension usually do not occur in pregnant women.[100] Patients should be monitored for methyldopa-induced liver damage.[93] Other drugs used to treat hypertension in pregnancy include labetalol and calcium-channel blockers. A review of drug therapies for the treatment of chronic hypertension in pregnancy is listed in Table 49-5.[101–106]

T.D. should be started on methyldopa 500 mg PO three times daily. If T.D. cannot tolerate the side effects, she can be switched to labetalol 200 mg PO twice daily. The only antihypertensive drugs absolutely contraindicated during pregnancy are ACEI and angiotensin II receptor blockers because of the association with fetal and newborn morbidity and mortality.[97]

Mild Pre-Eclampsia

CASE 49-5, QUESTION 6: T.D. returns to her obstetrician 1 week later at 31 weeks' gestation complaining of mild hand and leg edema. She has 1+ proteinuria by dipstick, and her BP is 155/102 mm Hg. An ultrasound demonstrates fetal growth restriction. Laboratory results are as follows:

SCr, 0.9 mg/dL
Serum UA, 6.0 mg/dL
Aspartate aminotransferase (AST), 25 units/L
Alanine aminotransferase (ALT), 16 units/L
Platelets, 230,000/μL

She is currently on labetalol 200 mg PO twice daily and has been compliant with her medications. What signs and laboratory evidence are consistent with pre-eclampsia in T.D.? Does she have mild or severe pre-eclampsia?

ETIOLOGY AND PATHOGENESIS

The causes of pre-eclampsia currently remain unknown. Although the pathogenesis begins early in pregnancy, the disease is not clinically evident until the latter half of the pregnancy and persists until the fetus is delivered.[107] Incomplete physiologic placental vascular bed changes and endothelial cell dysfunction are integral to the pathogenesis of pre-eclampsia (see Placental Physiology section).

PLACENTAL ISCHEMIA

Early in a normal pregnancy, the trophoblastic migration and invasion of the uterine spiral arteries result in physiologic changes within the placental vascular bed that facilitate maximal intervillous blood flow. The physiologic changes within these spiral

TABLE 49-5
Drugs for Treatment of Chronic Hypertension in Pregnancy and Lactation

Drug	Dose	Comments
Methyldopa	750–1,000 mg/d start twice a day, increase up to 2–3 g/d, divided in three to four doses if needed[99]	Longest safety record in pregnancy. Considered a first-line drug.[91] Dizziness, sedation, and lack of energy are common symptoms, which tend to resolve. Can cause liver toxicity. Low breast milk concentrations, so considered safe in breast-feeding.
Labetalol	200–400 mg/d start, increase to up to 2,400 mg/d, divided in two or sometimes three doses	Combined α- and β-receptor antagonist properties. Considered a first-line drug.[91] Increasingly preferred to methyldopa owing to fewer side effects. Neonatal effects could include bradycardia and hypotension. Low concentration in breast milk and generally considered safe in breast-feeding.[101]
Other β-blockers	Various	Atenolol in particular associated with decreased placental weight and IUGR.[102,103] IUGR thought to be related to β-blocker–induced increased vascular resistance in mother and fetus. Atenolol, acebutolol, metoprolol, nadolol, and sotalol can have high milk to plasma ratios and accumulate in breast milk, creating potential risk for neonatal blockade.[104,105] Propanolol found in only small amounts in breast milk and generally considered safe, but infants should be monitored for hypotension, bradycardia, and blood glucose changes.
Nifedipine, long-acting	30 mg/d start, increase to up to 120 mg/d, once daily	Limited pregnancy data on nifedipine or other calcium-channel blockers such as verapamil, diltiazem, and amlodipine. Concentrations of nifedipine in breast milk are low and considered compatible with breast-feeding.[101,106]
Diuretics	Various	Not first-line agents, although probably safe.[88] Concern regarding potential interference with normal blood volume expansion in pregnancy. Avoid if pre-eclampsia or IUGR already present. Concentration low in breast milk, but may decrease milk production.
ACEI or ARB	Contraindicated	Contraindicated in pregnancy in all trimesters. Fetal renal failure when used after first trimester, resulting in oligohydramnios, limb contractures, pulmonary hypoplasia, skull hypoplasia, and irreversible neonatal renal failure.[43] Increased risk major birth defects with first-trimester ACEI exposure.[79] Minimal amounts of captopril and enalapril in breast milk and both considered compatible with breast-feeding.[101] Minimal amounts of benazepril in breast milk.

ACEI, angiotensin-converting enzyme inhibitor; ARB, angiotensin II receptor blocker; IUGR, intrauterine growth restriction.

arteries are responsible for creating a fixed low-resistance arteriolar circuit, which increases blood supply to the growing fetus. In pre-eclampsia, these physiologic changes do not occur completely, resulting in decreased perfusion and, consequently, placental ischemia.[107,108]

ENDOTHELIAL DAMAGE

An intact vascular endothelium assists in preserving the integrity of vasculature, mediating immune and inflammatory responses, preventing intravascular coagulation, and modulating the contractility of the underlying smooth muscle cells.[108]

In normal pregnancy, prostacyclin is increased eight to ten times, creating an increased ratio of prostacyclin to thromboxane A_2.[107] The biologic dominance of prostacyclin along with nitric oxide plays an important role in maintaining vasodilation throughout pregnancy. Prostacyclin may be responsible for vascular refractoriness to angiotensin II in normal pregnancy. In pre-eclampsia, the ratio of prostacyclin to thromboxane A_2 is reversed. Thromboxane A_2 is biologically dominant during pre-eclampsia, leading to increased vascular sensitivity to angiotensin II and norepinephrine.[107] The increased release of thromboxane A_2 is believed to be caused by endothelial cell dysfunction. The end result is vasospasm, which further increases endothelial cell dysfunction and increases BP.[107] Reduced activity of nitric oxide synthase and decreased nitric oxide–dependent or nitric oxide–independent endothelium-derived relaxing factor are believed to increase the vasoconstrictive potential of pressors such as angiotensin II.[88]

Endothelial cell dysfunction in pregnancy is thought to be caused by oxidative stress. Intermittent hypoxic and reperfusion injury that occurs as a consequence of decreased placental perfusion may increase oxidative stress.[107,108] Endothelial damage eventually leads to disruption of the vascular lining, which causes leaking capillary membranes, allowing fluid to leak into the interstitium.[108] In severe pre-eclampsia, this results in hypovolemia, hemoconcentration, and consequently an increase in hematocrit. The loss of plasma volume, vasospasm, and microthrombi decrease perfusion of the kidney, CNS, liver, and other organs. The loss of intravascular proteins in the urine secondary to renal damage, and through damaged epithelia, decreases plasma oncotic pressure and leads to a rapid onset of nondependent edema. The imbalance of endogenous procoagulants and anticoagulants produces platelet consumption and results in thrombocytopenia and coagulation defects.[108]

T.D.'s diastolic BP is now higher than it was before her pregnancy and has increased by 12 mm Hg in the last 3 weeks. Although an increase in BP by itself is not diagnostic of pre-eclampsia, the new finding of proteinuria confirms the diagnosis. Other evidence for pre-eclampsia includes the elevated serum UA concentration, which is a sensitive marker for pre-eclampsia, and elevated SCr.[94] T.D. denies headaches, visual disturbances, and abdominal pain, which are symptoms of severe pre-eclampsia. The transaminases and platelet count are normal; therefore she does not have HELLP syndrome at this time. T.D.'s clinical presentation is consistent with mild pre-eclampsia; however, a 24-hour urine collection should be obtained to measure protein excretion, quantify the urine output, and further rule out severe pre-eclampsia.

TREATMENT OF PRE-ECLAMPSIA

GENERAL PRINCIPLES

CASE 49-5, QUESTION 7: T.D. is admitted to the hospital. The 24-hour urine protein is 500 mg/24 hours. Although fetal growth is restricted, all other fetal testing is reassuring. After 24 hours, her BP decreased to 140/95 mm Hg. Her platelet counts remained stable and greater than 200/μL, and transaminases were normal. No other signs and symptoms of pre-eclampsia were noted. How should T.D.'s mild pre-eclampsia be managed?

The delivery of the fetus is the only cure for pre-eclampsia and would be the best treatment option for T.D. if she were at more than 37 weeks' gestation. T.D. has mild disease, however, and is not close to term. Her delivery should be postponed because premature delivery increases neonatal morbidity and mortality. T.D.'s fetus is somewhat growth restricted, which is common in women with chronic hypertension, with or without superimposed pre-eclampsia. If T.D.'s fetus is severely growth restricted or if subsequent fetal biophysical testing is abnormal, premature delivery would be indicated.[88] Because neither of these is evident in the present circumstances, T.D. should continue her pregnancy under very close medical supervision. It has been suggested that continued hospitalization is appropriate for women with preterm onset of mild pre-eclampsia, such as T.D.[88] This would allow for rapid intervention in case of rapid progression of disease or associated complications. Probably a role exists for outpatient monitoring of some select women with very frequent maternal and fetal monitoring, and rehospitalization for worsening disease.[88]

T.D. is also a candidate for administration of glucocorticoids for fetal lung maturation (see Case 49-7, Question 7). Bed rest in the lateral decubitus position is usually suggested and may help reduce BP and promote diuresis by decreasing vasoconstriction and improving renal and uteroplacental perfusion.

ONLINE CONTENT

For an illustration showing the lateral decubitus position, go to http://thepoint.lww.com/AT10e.

T.D. should have her BP measured regularly each day. Liver transaminases, platelets, and creatinine should be measured periodically and whenever her clinical status changes. She also should be assessed for symptoms of severe pre-eclampsia (e.g., headaches, visual disturbances, epigastric or right upper quadrant pain). Fetal surveillance is indicated.[88] One approach is to perform a modified biophysical profile, a test performed to ensure fetal well-being using ultrasonography measuring fetal breathing, tone, movement, and amniotic fluid volume with an assessment in fetal heart rate, twice a week and whenever maternal clinical status changes, and an ultrasound for fetal growth every 3 to 4 weeks.

Severe Pre-Eclampsia

CLINICAL PRESENTATION

CASE 49-5, QUESTION 8: T.D.'s BP for about 2 weeks ranged from 140 to 150 mm Hg systolic and 90 to 100 mm Hg diastolic with bed rest. Her proteinuria remained stable at 1+ to 2+ by dipstick. During the past 2 days T.D.'s BP started to increase again, and today her BP is 160/112 mm Hg and her urine dipstick is 3+. She complains of headaches, dizziness, and visual disturbances and has significant edema in her face, hands, legs, and ankles. T.D. is transferred to the Labor and Delivery Unit for delivery. Pertinent laboratory results are as follows:

SCr, 1.3 mg/dL
UA, 6.7 mg/dL
AST, 30 U/L

ALT, 16 U/L
Total bilirubin, 1 mg/dL
Platelets, 95,000/μL
Hematocrit, 38%
Hemoglobin, 13 g/dL
Random urine protein, 4+

Estimated fetal weight by ultrasound is 1,700 g, which is between the 10th and 25th percentile for a gestational age of 34 weeks. What signs, symptoms, and laboratory evidence of severe pre-eclampsia support this diagnosis in T.D., and what complications may occur?

T.D. has developed severe pre-eclampsia.[92] Her systolic and diastolic BP are greater than 160 and 112 mm Hg, respectively. She has greater than 3+ protein in a random urine sample, and her SCr is elevated. She complains of headaches and visual disturbances. T.D. is also thrombocytopenic as her platelet count is 95,000/μL. Although her liver transaminases are currently normal, she may be developing HELLP syndrome, a variant of severe pre-eclampsia associated with a high incidence of maternal and perinatal morbidity and mortality. Therefore, her laboratory values should continue to be monitored even as delivery is being planned.

COMPLICATIONS

T.D. is at risk for cerebral hemorrhage, cerebral edema, encephalopathy, coagulopathies, pulmonary edema, liver failure, renal failure, and eclamptic seizures.[93,94] Severe pre-eclampsia is dangerous not only to T.D. but also to her fetus because uteroplacental perfusion is compromised. T.D. requires drug treatments to both lower her BP and prevent eclampsia, as well as delivery.

ACUTE TREATMENT OF SEVERE HYPERTENSION

CASE 49-5, QUESTION 9: How should T.D.'s severe hypertension be treated?

The goal of antihypertensive therapy in T.D. is to prevent cerebral complications (e.g., encephalopathy, hemorrhage).[93] Although it is important to reduce the maternal BP, it must be accomplished gradually while the fetus is in utero because a sudden large drop in maternal BP could result in the reduction of uteroplacental perfusion.[94] Because of the potential for fetal bradycardia during or after acute treatment of maternal hypertension, continuous fetal heart rate monitoring should be considered.

HYDRALAZINE

Hydralazine, a direct arterial smooth muscle dilator, has in the past been the drug of choice for the acute treatment of severe hypertension in pregnancy.[93,100] This drug induces a baroreceptor-mediated tachycardia and increases cardiac output, which increases uterine blood flow as the BP is lowered.[94]

The onset of antihypertensive effect for hydralazine ranges from 10 to 20 minutes, and duration of action ranges from 3 to 6 hours after an IV dose.[94,109] Therefore, doses of hydralazine should not be repeated more frequently than every 20 to 30 minutes to prevent drug accumulation.[100] Nausea, vomiting, tachycardia, flushing, headache, and tremors could occur. Some of these hydralazine-induced adverse effects mimic symptoms associated with severe pre-eclampsia and imminent eclampsia, making it difficult for a clinician to differentiate between drug-associated and disease-related problems.[100] Fetal hydralazine serum concentrations are reportedly the same as or higher than maternal serum concentrations, but drug-associated fetal abnormalities have not been reported.[43]

LABETALOL

Labetalol is also a commonly used drug to treat severe hypertension during pregnancy. It should be administered IV in increasing doses of 20, 40, and 80 mg every 10 minutes to a cumulative dose of 300 mg or until the diastolic pressure is less than 100 mm Hg.[110] The onset of action is within 5 minutes, and its effect peaks in 10 to 20 minutes with a duration of action ranging from 45 minutes to 6 hours.

IV labetalol is as effective as IV hydralazine in lowering BP in patients with hypertension during pregnancy, but has fewer reported adverse effects.[100,111] In a meta-analysis of β-blocker trials for the treatment of hypertension in pregnancy, labetalol was associated with less maternal hypotension, fewer cesarean deliveries, and no increase in perinatal mortality.[111] Labetalol also does not appear to decrease uteroplacental blood flow even with a decrease in maternal BP.[100] Labetalol reduces cerebral perfusion pressure, which occurs in up to 43% of women with severe pre-eclampsia, without negatively affecting cerebral blood flow.[112] Decreased cerebral perfusion pressure may prevent progression to eclampsia. However, it should be avoided in women with asthma and decompensated heart failure.[88,109] Labetalol has also been associated with higher rates of neonatal bradycardia and hypotension than hydralazine, but not higher rates of neonatal intensive care admission.[113,114]

NIFEDIPINE

Nifedipine has been used in doses of 10 mg for acute treatment of severe hypertension during pregnancy because it can be given orally.[100] Nifedipine is effective in decreasing BP without reducing uteroplacental blood flow or decreasing fetal heart rate. Short-acting nifedipine capsules are no longer recommended for the treatment of acute hypertensive urgency, however, because of the risk of stroke or myocardial infarction, and it was never FDA approved for this indication. Immediate-release nifedipine continues to be used to treat hypertension in pregnancy, however, because this unique patient population may not be at high risk for ischemic events secondary to atherosclerotic disease.[97] Calcium gluconate or calcium chloride should be available for IV administration in the event of sudden hypotension. Caution should be used when giving nifedipine to women concomitantly treated with magnesium sulfate because these drugs have synergistic effects, causing hypotension and neuromuscular blockade.[115]

Several studies comparing immediate-release oral nifedipine with IV labetalol in hypertensive emergencies of pregnancy have found them to be equally effective in lowering BP.[116,117] Nifedipine lowers BP to less than 160 mm Hg systolic and less than 100 mm Hg diastolic earlier than labetalol,[116] but it increases cardiac index[117] (see Chapter 21, Hypertensive Crises). The use of sustained-release nifedipine capsules as an alternative is associated with a delay in BP control to 45 to 90 minutes, which is probably not acceptable.[109]

Hydralazine 5 mg IV for 1 to 2 minutes should be administered to T.D. and repeated in doses of 5 to 10 mg every 20 to 30 minutes to a cumulative dose of 20 mg.[93] T.D. should have repeated measurements of her BP at 15-minute intervals. Because intervillous blood flow depends on maternal perfusion pressure, the goal is to decrease the diastolic pressure to not less than 90 mm Hg.[93,109] Lowering the maternal BP excessively may decrease uteroplacental perfusion and compromise the fetus. A hypotensive overshoot can be observed with hydralazine, particularly in the setting of volume depletion, which is typical of pre-eclampsia.[109] If one or two doses of hydralazine are not effective in lowering T.D.'s diastolic to less than 100 mm Hg, labetalol 20 mg IV every 10 to 15 minutes can be given.

Eclampsia

MAGNESIUM SULFATE PROPHYLAXIS

CASE 49-5, QUESTION 10: T.D. will undergo an induction of labor for her severe pre-eclampsia. Which medication should be given to T.D. to prevent seizures?

The precise mechanism of anticonvulsant action of magnesium for the prevention and treatment of eclamptic seizures is unknown. The anticonvulsant activity may be partly mediated through blockade of an excitatory amino acid receptor, *N*-methyl-D-aspartate.[115] Seizures are thought to be caused by decreased cerebral blood flow because of vasospasm. Magnesium sulfate is a potent cerebral vasodilator and increases the synthesis of prostacyclin, an endothelial vasodilator. It also causes a dose-dependent decrease in systemic vascular resistance, which may explain its transient hypotensive effect. Magnesium may also protect against oxidative injury to endothelial cells.[115]

Although termination of the pregnancy is the definitive treatment for severe pre-eclampsia, the intrapartum and immediate postpartum periods are also the periods of greatest risk for eclampsia.[94] Although the incidence of eclampsia is extremely low, maternal morbidity and mortality are high.[118] In the United States, it has been usual practice to treat all pre-eclamptic women with magnesium sulfate during labor and for 12 to 24 hours postpartum.[88,93] In the United Kingdom, however, it is common to reserve magnesium sulfate therapy for severe pre-eclampsia.[119] The evidence for magnesium sulfate prevention of the progression of disease in mildly pre-eclamptic women had been largely anecdotal in the past. In a large international study of more than 10,000 women, published in 2002, magnesium sulfate clearly decreased the risk of eclampsia in pre-eclamptic women by 58% compared with placebo.[119] An observational study of nearly 2,500 women with mild pre-eclampsia (BP of 140/90 mm Hg and 1+ protein) found an incidence of eclampsia of about 1% without the use of seizure prophylaxis.[120]

In a prospective, randomized study, magnesium sulfate was superior to phenytoin for the prevention of eclampsia in hypertensive pregnant women.[118] In addition, magnesium sulfate was more effective than nimodipine for seizure prophylaxis in severely pre-eclamptic women.[121]

A regimen of magnesium sulfate 4 to 6 g IV as a loading dose followed by a continuous infusion of 2 g/hour is the most commonly used regimen in the United States.[122] Lower dosages (e.g., 1 g/hour) have been associated with treatment failures.[123] IV loading doses of 6 g followed by continuous infusions of 2 g/hour maintain therapeutically effective magnesium serum concentrations between 4 and 8 mg/dL.[123] Because magnesium is excreted by the kidneys and will accumulate in cases of renal dysfunction, the continuous infusion rate must be lowered with oliguria or an elevated SCr.

Because of the potential for infusion errors and significant patient morbidity and even mortality with accidental overdoses of magnesium sulfate, the Institute of Medicine has identified magnesium sulfate as a high-risk medication.[124] All infusions of magnesium sulfate must be given through a controlled pump designed to protect against free flow. If such an infusion pump is not available, the intramuscular (IM) route of administration should be used. Dispensing premixed IV bags from the central pharmacy with a standardized concentration of magnesium sulfate and limiting the total grams of magnesium sulfate in each dispensed IV bag also can help guard against inadvertent overdose. Dispensing the loading dose in a separate small bag (e.g., 4 g in 100 mL) from the maintenance bag (e.g., 20 g in 200 mL) also may be helpful.[125]

Magnesium sulfate should be given to T.D. to prevent eclamptic seizures during labor.[88] T.D. should be loaded with magnesium sulfate 4 g IV given for 30 minutes and then started on a continuous infusion of 2 g/hour.

MONITORING MAGNESIUM SULFATE THERAPY

CASE 49-5, QUESTION 11: T.D. has been given magnesium sulfate 4 g IV for 30 minutes and was then started on a continuous infusion of 2 g/hour. What subjective and objective data should be monitored during treatment of T.D. with magnesium?

Deep tendon reflexes (patellar reflex), respiratory rate, and urine output should be monitored periodically during treatment with magnesium sulfate.[118] The loss of patellar reflexes, the first sign of magnesium toxicity, generally occurs at serum concentrations of 8 to 12 mg/dL. The respiratory rate should be monitored hourly and should be greater than 12 breaths/minute. Respiratory arrest can occur with serum concentrations of greater than 13 mg/dL. Urine output should be carefully monitored and should be at least 100 mL every 4 hours (or 25 mL/hour).[118] Magnesium serum concentrations are not routinely measured unless renal dysfunction is evident with oliguria or elevated SCr because magnesium is almost entirely excreted by the kidney.[115,118] Hypocalcemia and hypocalcemic tetany also can occur secondary to elevated magnesium and can be reversed by calcium gluconate 1 g (10 mL of a 10% solution) slow IV push for 3 minutes. Neuromuscular depression can occur in infants whose mothers received magnesium sulfate.[43] Parenteral magnesium sulfate is safe and rarely causes maternal or neonatal toxicity when administered properly but requires stringent, built-in system safeguards to avoid unintended dosing errors.[125]

CASE 49-5, QUESTION 12: How long should magnesium sulfate be continued in T.D.?

Depending on the severity of pre-eclampsia, magnesium sulfate therapy usually is continued for 24 hours after delivery, which should be the same for T.D.[126] Women with severe pre-eclampsia or pre-eclampsia superimposed on chronic hypertension are at greater risk for disease exacerbation when magnesium sulfate is discontinued too soon.

TREATMENT OF ECLAMPSIA

CASE 49-5, QUESTION 13: T.D. delivers vaginally and her magnesium infusion was discontinued by mistake 3 hours postpartum. T.D. experiences an eclamptic seizure 4 hours later when her nurses discover that the magnesium is disconnected. What is appropriate drug therapy for eclampsia?

Lorazepam, diazepam, phenytoin, and magnesium sulfate have all been used to treat eclampsia. The use of magnesium sulfate to treat these seizures results in less maternal morbidity and mortality and less neonatal morbidity.[118,127] Generally, higher serum concentrations of magnesium sulfate are needed to treat than to prevent eclamptic seizures. The same therapeutic range guides both prophylaxis and treatment, however.[122] Seizures unresponsive to magnesium sulfate treatment should prompt an evaluation for other cerebrovascular events (e.g., cerebral hemorrhage or infarction).[122] Lorazepam 2 to 4 mg slow IV push stat should be given for seizure cessation. T.D. should be reloaded with magnesium sulfate and continued on a magnesium infusion for 24 to 48 hours.

DRUG THERAPY MANAGEMENT IN LABOR AND DELIVERY

Induction of Labor

MECHANISMS OF TERM LABOR

In pregnancy, many hormones and peptides, including progesterone, prostacyclin, relaxin, nitric oxide, and parathyroid hormone-related peptide, inhibit uterine smooth muscle contractility. Labor at term occurs because the myometrium is released from its quiescent state.[128] For example, as progesterone concentrations decrease near term gestation, estrogen may stimulate uterine contractility.

Uterine activity is divided into four phases: quiescence (phase 0), activation (phase 1), stimulation (phase 2), and involution (phase 3). Each of these phases is stimulated or inhibited by several factors.[128] During activation, uterotropins such as estrogen, and possibly others, stimulate a complex series of uterine changes (e.g., increased myometrial prostaglandin and oxytocin receptors and myometrial gap junctions), which are important for the coordination of contractions. These changes help prime the myometrium and cervix for stimulation by the uterotonins oxytocin and prostaglandins E_2 and $F_{2\alpha}$. The cervix softens, shortens, and dilates, a process referred to as *cervical ripening*. Uterine stimulation is responsible for the change in myometrial activity from irregular to regular contractions. During phase 3, involution of the uterus occurs after delivery and is mediated mostly by oxytocin.[128]

The exact stimulus of the biochemical scheme leading to labor in humans is unknown. The fetus may help facilitate this process by affecting placental steroid production through mechanical distension of the uterus and by activating the fetal hypothalamic-pituitary-adrenal axis. Ultimately, these lead to increased production of oxytocin and prostaglandins by the fetoplacental unit.

Labor is divided into three stages. Weak, irregular, rhythmic contractions (Braxton-Hicks contractions or "false labor") may happen for weeks before the onset of true labor. The first stage begins with the start of regular uterine contractions and ends with complete cervical dilation. Stage 1 is divided further into the latent phase, active phase, and deceleration phase. During the latent phase, the cervix effaces (thins) but dilates minimally. The contractions become progressively stronger and longer, better coordinated, and more frequent. The duration of the latent phase is the most varied and unpredictable of all aspects of labor and can continue intermittently for days. During the active phase, contractions are strong and regular, occurring every 2 to 3 minutes. The cervix dilates from 3 to 4 cm to full dilation, usually 10 cm. The second stage starts with complete cervical dilation and ends with the delivery of the fetus. The third stage of labor is the time between the delivery of the fetus and the delivery of the placenta.

INDICATIONS, CONTRAINDICATIONS, AND REQUIREMENTS

CASE 49-6

QUESTION 1: J.T., a 28-year-old primigravida, is admitted to the labor and delivery suite for labor induction. She is at 42 weeks' gestation by dates and ultrasound and has a normal obstetric examination. Cervical examination reveals an unfavorable cervix for labor induction; Bishop score is 4. What are the indications and contraindications for labor induction in J.T.?

The induction of labor involves the artificial stimulation of uterine contractions that lead to labor and delivery. Induction of labor is indicated when the benefits to either the mother or fetus outweigh those of continuing the pregnancy. Examples may include pre-eclampsia, chorioamnionitis (infection of the fetal membranes, see Case 49-7, Question 11), fetal demise, significant fetal growth restriction, maternal medical problems, and postterm pregnancy.[129] Postterm pregnancy (≥42 weeks' gestation), as in J.T.'s case, is one of the most common indications for induction of labor.[129] Contraindications to labor induction are similar to those for spontaneous labor and vaginal delivery and include, but are not limited to, active genital herpes infection, placenta previa (placenta implanted over the internal cervical opening), prior classic uterine incision, transverse fetal lie (laying longitudinally across the uterus), and prolapsed umbilical cord. Maternal complications that are associated with induction include increased rates of chorioamnionitis and uterine atony (loss of tone in uterine musculature) (see Case 49-8, Question 4) resulting in hemorrhage, as well as a twofold to threefold increased risk of cesarean delivery, particularly in primigravida women.[130]

A complete assessment of both mother and fetus should be performed before inducing labor.[129,130] Gestational age must be assessed accurately before the induction of labor to avoid the inadvertent delivery of a preterm fetus.[129,130] When delivery is necessary before 34 weeks' gestation with intact membranes or before 32 weeks' gestation with ruptured membranes, antenatal corticosteroids should be administered (see Case 49-7, Question 7).[131,132]

The degree of cervical ripeness and readiness for induction of labor should be assessed.[129,133] Success of labor induction is directly related to the favorability of the cervix.[134,135] The Bishop method of evaluating cervical ripeness assigns a score based on the station of the fetal head relative to the maternal ischial spines and the extent of cervical dilation, effacement (thinning of the cervix), consistency, and position.[130,133] Bishop scores of greater than 8 are associated with rates of vaginal delivery similar to those after spontaneous labor.[129] Conversely, Bishop scores of 4 or less, as documented in J.T., are associated with a high likelihood of failed induction and cesarean delivery. As a result, significant research has been directed toward methods of improving the Bishop score and cervix ripeness before stimulation of uterine contractions. However, women with low Bishop scores who undergo cervical ripening before induction of labor still have higher rates of cesarean delivery compared with spontaneous labor.[133] Nevertheless, cervical ripening appears to have some benefit in decreasing time to delivery, shortening labor, and successfully improving Bishop score.[129]

Cervical ripening can be accomplished pharmacologically or mechanically. Pharmacologic methods include the administration of prostaglandins (E_2 and E_1) or low-dose oxytocin. Mechanical methods include membrane sweeping (or membrane stripping), and intracervical balloons.[129,130,133] Osmotic or hygroscopic dilators (e.g., Dilapan, Lamicel) work by absorbing cervical mucus and gradually swelling, thereby dilating the cervical canal.[130,133] In the setting of a favorable Bishop score, labor induction is accomplished most commonly by amniotomy (artificial rupture of the fetal membranes) and oxytocin administration.[129,130]

Although labor induction is medically indicated in J.T. to decrease the risk of an adverse fetal outcome with continuing a postterm pregnancy, such as macrosomia, asphyxia, meconium aspiration, and intrauterine infection, her cervix is unfavorable for induction and she is a candidate for cervix ripening.

CERVICAL RIPENING

CASE 49-6, QUESTION 2: What pharmacological agents can be used for cervical ripening in J.T.?

which stimulate uterine activity, induce cervix softening and dilation, and weaken the chorioamniotic membranes.[160] Variations in maternal and fetal genes coding for cytokines have been implicated in the apparent genetic predisposition to preterm birth found in some families and racial groups.[161] Thrombin is another uterotonic agent, which can cause uterine contractions, and has been implicated in causing preterm labor associated with vaginal bleeding caused by placental abruption.[162] Studies have shown a relationship between increasing maternal corticotropin-releasing hormone (CRH) and delivery timing.[163] Maternal and fetal stress can activate the hypothalamic-pituitary system and result in the rapid increase of maternal CRH before premature birth. Infection can also activate the fetal hypothalamic-pituitary system, increasing CRH, cortisol, and, ultimately, prostaglandins.[160,162] Despite some progress in recent years, much remains unknown about the etiology of preterm birth, and little is known about how preterm birth can be prevented.

CLINICAL PRESENTATION AND EVALUATION

CASE 49-7

QUESTION 1: B.B., a 17-year-old white woman, G2, P1, and 29 weeks' gestation, is admitted to the obstetrical unit with complaints of backache, cramps, and uterine contractions. She has no symptoms of preterm premature rupture of the membranes (PPROM). She had a previous preterm birth at 32 weeks' gestation. Cervicovaginal secretions are positive for fetal fibronectin. A pelvic examination reveals that her cervix is 2 cm dilated and 80% effaced, which is increased from 1 cm at her prenatal visit last week. Cervical cultures for *Chlamydia trachomatis* and *Neisseria gonorrhoeae* from her previous visit are negative. Vaginal wet-mount preparations are also negative for bacterial vaginosis and *Trichomonas vaginalis*. Vital signs, urinalysis, and complete blood count with differential are normal. Uterine contractions and fetal heart rate are being monitored. Ultrasound reveals a fetus of 30 weeks' gestation size with an estimated weight of 1,200 g. What signs, symptoms, and laboratory evidence support a diagnosis of preterm labor?

B.B. has backache and uterine contractions, which are symptoms of preterm labor. Most women with preterm contractions are not in labor, however, which results in frequent overdiagnosis. In addition, contractions during preterm labor are frequently not painful, are not detected by the woman and, thus, are not a sensitive marker for preterm labor. Fibronectin, a protein that serves as an adhesive between the fetal membranes and decidua, normally disappears from the cervical secretions after the first half of pregnancy, reappearing only at term as labor approaches.[164] A negative fibronectin test can exclude imminent preterm delivery in a woman at risk for preterm delivery, between 24 and 34 weeks' gestation with intact amniotic membranes, and with cervical dilatation of less than 3 cm.[165] Because of fibronectin's high negative predictive value of greater than 95% for delivery in the next 1 to 2 weeks, it can be used to avoid overdiagnosis of preterm labor. Although fibronectin testing will yield false-positive results in the presence of blood, vaginal bleeding itself is independently associated with preterm birth. B.B. has the criteria necessary to establish a firm diagnosis of preterm labor. Not only is her fibronectin test positive, but she has persistent contractions with a documented change in cervix dilatation.

RISK FACTORS

CASE 49-7, QUESTION 2: What risk factors does B.B. have for spontaneous preterm labor?

B.B. has several risk factors for preterm delivery. The strongest predictor of preterm birth is prior preterm birth. She has a twofold or higher increased risk of preterm delivery because of one previous preterm delivery.[164] If this pregnancy also ends prematurely, her risk for a third preterm birth in her next pregnancy will be sixfold higher than that in the normal population.[164] Recurrence risk rises as the gestational age of the prior preterm birth decreases, especially for deliveries at less than 32 weeks. Her young age may also be a risk factor. A maternal age younger than 18 or older than 35 years is associated with spontaneous preterm birth, although it is difficult to separate age from the confounding factors associated with age.[164] Her race likely does not contribute to her risk. Black race is an independent risk factor for both preterm labor and lower neonatal birth weight. Other risk factors include low maternal weight before pregnancy, smoking, second- or third-trimester bleeding, multiple gestation, and uterine anomalies, which B.B. does not have.[128,164] Studies of cervix length by transvaginal ultrasound imaging have demonstrated that shorter lengths are associated with greater risk for preterm delivery; however, the positive predictive value varies widely.[164,165] Maternal infections, such as untreated urinary tract infections and pneumonia, are associated with preterm delivery. In addition, genital organisms such as *Gardnerella vaginalis, C. trachomatis, N. gonorrhoeae, Ureaplasma urealyticum,* and *T. vaginalis,* are also associated with preterm births.[150] Although it is important to identify women at risk for spontaneous preterm delivery, only half of all preterm deliveries occur in women with known risk factors.[164]

TOCOLYSIS

GOALS OF THERAPY

CASE 49-7, QUESTION 3: What are the goals of tocolysis for B.B.?

Treatment of spontaneous preterm labor primarily has been directed at slowing or stopping contractions (tocolysis), which are the obvious, although likely late, sign of impending preterm birth. It has been presumed that if successful, this should prevent or delay preterm birth. Few placebo-controlled trials have been conducted of agents used to diminish contractions (tocolytics), and most data suggest delay of delivery by at most 1 to 2 days.[166] This might be because of the heterogeneous causes of spontaneous preterm birth and because tocolytic agents may not arrest the underlying process that led to contractions. Most studies have been unable to demonstrate a clear benefit of tocolysis on neonatal morbidity and mortality. Instead, they have evaluated surrogate end points, such as pregnancy prolongation or number of preterm births before various cutoff points.[167] The value of prolonging pregnancy will vary by gestational age, and might be substantial if time is gained to administer glucocorticoids to improve fetal lung maturation and decrease the risk of intraventricular hemorrhage (see Case 49-7, Question 7). All women at risk for preterm birth within 7 days and between 24 and 34 weeks' gestation should be considered for glucocorticoid therapy.[132,168] Delay of delivery can also allow transport to a facility best equipped to care for both mother and premature newborn.

Numerous factors affect the decision to treat preterm labor with a tocolytic agent. Fetal factors precluding tocolysis include nonreassuring fetal monitoring, significant IUGR, and lethal congenital anomalies. Maternal factors include evidence of chorioamnionitis, other significant maternal infections or illness, pre-eclampsia, and advanced labor.[164] Tocolysis is less likely to be effective in women with cervical dilation of greater than 3 cm and is usually unsuccessful if the patient is in advanced labor (cervical dilation >5 cm).[164] Because the etiology of preterm labor is multifactorial, B.B. should be evaluated thoroughly and periodically for potential causes of preterm labor and treated appropriately when diagnosed. For example, urinary tract infections are associated with preterm labor, and they should be diagnosed and treated if present.[164] Additionally, some would also perform amniocentesis to exclude subclinical chorioamnionitis as a cause of preterm labor before initiating or continuing tocolysis, and to evaluate lung maturity at later gestational ages.[168] B.B. has no evidence of overt infection or other complications and has no contraindications to tocolysis. Prolonging gestation, even for a few days, would be beneficial because B.B. is only at 29 weeks' gestation.

TOCOLYTIC AGENTS

CASE 49-7, QUESTION 4: How should B.B.'s preterm labor be managed? Which tocolytic agent should be used?

MAGNESIUM SULFATE

Magnesium sulfate is the most frequently used parenteral tocolytic agent in the United States and is also prescribed for the prevention and treatment of eclampsia. Magnesium sulfate relaxes uterine smooth muscle at maternal serum levels of 5 to 8 mg/dL.[164] The mechanism by which it exerts this effect is not understood completely, but involves inhibition of myosin light-chain kinase activity by competition with intracellular calcium, reducing myometrial contractility.[167]

Despite its widespread use, the evidence for magnesium's efficacy in prolonging gestation is inadequate. In two published randomized, placebo-controlled trials, no benefit in mean prolongation of pregnancy or mean neonatal birth weight was demonstrated. In meta-analyses of both placebo-controlled trials of magnesium for tocolysis compared with other active drugs, no prolongation of pregnancy was seen with magnesium.[166,169] Several small randomized, controlled studies have directly compared magnesium with parenteral β-adrenergic agonists, mostly ritodrine.[166] Three of the four showed no differences in birth outcomes. One of the four suggested prolonged pregnancy with magnesium added to ritodrine compared with ritodrine alone. Studies on the efficacy of β-adrenergic agonists (mostly ritodrine) versus placebo have been mixed but on balance suggest delay of delivery for 48 hours, but not for 7 days. Therefore, because most trials comparing magnesium with β-adrenergic agonists did not show differences, it has been presumed that magnesium is equally effective. Magnesium is better tolerated than the β-adrenergic agonists, with fewer maternal side effects.[166] Magnesium is contraindicated in patients with myasthenia gravis, and must be used with caution in renal failure.

β-ADRENERGIC AGONISTS

β-Adrenergic agonists are not the first-line choice for preterm labor because of high costs and the significant potential for maternal adverse effects described subseequently.[164,166] Both ritodrine, the only medication approved by the FDA for the treatment of preterm labor, and terbutaline bind to β_2-adrenergic receptors in uterine smooth muscle and ultimately inhibit smooth muscle cell contractility. Results of randomized, controlled trials of ritodrine have been mixed; however, a meta-analysis that included 1,320 women treated with β-agonists demonstrated fewer births at 48 hours but no change in number of births at 7 days. No benefit on neonatal morbidity or mortality was seen; however, the studies are limited by sample size.[170,171] The continued use of β-agonists can result in the development of tachyphylaxis to its effects on the myometrium and may in part explain treatment failures with these drugs.[164,170]

Terbutaline is available for IV, SC, and oral administration. One dose of terbutaline 0.25 mg SC is often administered to women with mild contractions and cervical dilation less than 2 cm. Intravenous β-sympathomimetics are used in cases with more severe and frequent contractions and cervical dilation greater than 2 cm. However, because of potential adverse maternal side effects such as increased heart rate, transient hyperglycemia, hypokalemia, cardiac arrhythmias, pulmonary edema, and myocardial ischemia, the FDA issued a black-box warning in 2011 against the use of injectable terbutaline beyond 48 to 72 hours. The FDA also recommended against any use of oral terbutaline for preterm labor owing to both lack of efficacy and the potential for significant maternal side effects.

β-Adrenergic Adverse Effects

β-Adrenergic agonists are not selective for myometrial β_2-adrenergic receptors at pharmacologic doses, and this accounts for their high incidence of adverse effects.[172] Maternal adverse effects such as pulmonary edema, palpitations, tachycardia, myocardial ischemia, hyperglycemia, hypokalemia, and hepatotoxicity result in discontinuation of therapy in up to 10% of patients.[164] Pulmonary edema can occur and, if not recognized promptly, can lead to ARDS and death.[164,172] β-Sympathomimetics should not be used in women with underlying cardiac disease or arrhythmias, hypertension, diabetes mellitus, severe anemia, or thyrotoxicosis.[164] In addition, these drugs should be avoided if there are signs of chorioamnionitis such as maternal leukocytosis, fetal tachycardia, or maternal fever.[164]

The most commonly reported fetal or neonatal adverse effects associated with β-agonist therapy include tachycardia, hypotension, hypoglycemia, and hypocalcemia, especially if the drug is being administered within hours of delivery.[164,172] Maternal hyperglycemia causing fetal hyperglycemia and hyperinsulinemia can lead to neonatal hypoglycemia if not properly monitored postnatally. Fetal tachycardia rarely leads to fetal myocardial ischemia or hypertrophy.[172] In summary, although β-sympathomimetic drugs have been used commonly in the past, they are now used much less frequently because of side effect profiles and safety concerns.[164]

INDOMETHACIN

Prostaglandins $F_{2\alpha}$ and especially E_2 are important regulators of myometrial contractility and cervical ripening.[128] Prostaglandin synthesis requires cyclo-oxygenase (COX), also known as prostaglandin synthetase, to convert arachidonic acid to prostaglandin G_2. COX inhibitors such as indomethacin decrease prostaglandin production, which decreases contractions and inhibits cervical change. As with other tocolytics, these drugs have not been adequately studied in multiple randomized controlled trials. A review of available randomized trials of indomethacin compared with placebo found significant reductions in women delivering at less than 37 weeks' gestation, an increase in gestational age at delivery, and a trend toward fewer deliveries at 48 hours and 7 days.[173] In three of eight trials comparing COX inhibitors with other tocolytics, a reduction in both delivery before 37 weeks' gestation and maternal drug reactions was noted. Also, seen in these studies was a trend toward a reduction in delivery within 48 hours.[173] Indomethacin is well tolerated, and GI upset can be mitigated by antacids when it occurs. The available studies are inadequately powered to evaluate neonatal safety and outcomes, however.[173,174]

Although well tolerated by the mother, concerns exist about the fetal and neonatal effects of prostaglandin synthetase inhibition. Indomethacin crosses the placenta rapidly, and fetal levels rapidly approach maternal levels.[172,174] Because indomethacin can decrease fetal urine output leading to oligohydramnios, the amniotic fluid index should be followed and indomethacin discontinued if it falls below 5 cm (normal range, 5–25 cm). Oligohydramnios generally resolves within 48 to 72 hours of the discontinuation of indomethacin. The fetal ductus arteriosus, which is critical to allow blood from the right ventricle to bypass the fluid-filled lungs, constricts in 25% to 50% of fetuses exposed to indomethacin in utero, but generally is reversible.[164] Permanent closure of the ductus arteriosus, however, can lead to fetal right heart failure and even intrauterine demise. The risk for neonatal adverse effects is increased with drug exposure of longer than 48 hours, as well as use after 32 weeks' gestation when premature closure of the ductus occurs more frequently.[164] An increased risk for maternal postpartum hemorrhage has also been reported with indomethacin use but did not reach significance in a meta-analysis.[173] Indomethacin should not be used in the presence of oligohydramnios or suspected fetal renal or cardiac anomaly (see Chapter 100, Neonatal Therapy).

More serious fetal and neonatal effects have been reported in some retrospective and observational studies, including neonatal necrotizing enterocolitis, intraventricular hemorrhage, and renal failure.[174–176] It is difficult, however, to discern whether these complications are causally related to indomethacin or to the use of the drug in cases of refractory preterm labor caused by subclinical intra-amniotic infection.[174,177] An analysis of the risks and benefits of indomethacin suggested its continued use as second-line treatment for preterm labor between 24 and 32 weeks' gestation in women with contraindications to other tocolytics.[174] Typical dosing regimens include a loading dose of 50 to 100 mg either rectally or orally followed by a maintenance dose of 25 mg orally every 4 to 6 hours for 24 to 48 hours.[175]

CALCIUM-CHANNEL BLOCKERS

The calcium-channel blockers nifedipine and nicardipine inhibit preterm contractions by decreasing calcium influx into uterine smooth muscle and inhibiting myometrial contractions. No placebo-controlled trials have been performed with nifedipine, the most commonly used calcium-channel blocker. A meta-analysis of 12 randomized trials including a total of 1,029 women found that calcium-channel blockers were superior to other tocolytics (mostly β-mimetics) in reducing preterm births within 7 days and before 34 weeks' gestation.[178] A more recent study of 192 women comparing nifedipine with magnesium sulfate for preterm labor found no differences in delivery in 48 hours, gestational age at delivery, or deliveries before 32 or 37 weeks' gestation.[179] Maternal side effects were significantly fewer in patients receiving calcium-channel blockers compared with other tocolytics.[178,179]

Maternal side effects can include tachycardia, headache, flushing, dizziness, nausea, and hypotension in the hypovolemic patient.[172] Nifedipine does not adversely affect uteroplacental blood flow or fetal circulation. Concurrent use with magnesium should be avoided because the combination may potentiate neuromuscular blockade.[115,168,172,180] The starting dose is usually 10 mg PO with repeated doses of 10 mg every 15 to 20 minutes for persistent contractions, up to a maximum of 40 mg in the first hour.[181,182] Depending on the tocolytic effect, nifedipine is then maintained at 10 to 20 mg PO every 4 to 6 hours.[181] Overall, nifedipine appears to be an attractive alternative for short-term tocolysis because the drug is usually well tolerated.[181]

B.B. should be started on a magnesium sulfate 6-g IV loading dose for 30 minutes followed by 2 g/hour continuous IV infusion through a controlled infusion pump. The hourly rate of magnesium administration for B.B. may be increased until she has one or fewer contractions per 10 minutes or a maximum of 4 g/hour is attained. B.B.'s deep tendon reflexes, respiratory rate, and urine output should be monitored regularly. Close monitoring of fluid balance is important because fluid overload has been associated with pulmonary edema and the drug is renally excreted.[183]

Magnesium serum concentrations are commonly evaluated every 6 to 12 hours in an effort to minimize adverse effects.[184] The patellar reflex disappears with magnesium serum concentrations between 9 and 10 mg/dL, and as long as deep tendon reflexes are present, many practitioners will not measure concentrations. To prevent inadvertent overdoses, a controlled infusion device should always be used to deliver magnesium as a continuous infusion. Hypocalcemia and tetany can occur with hypermagnesemia. Neuromuscular blockade and respiratory arrest develop with magnesium serum concentrations of 15 to 17 mg/dL, and cardiac arrest develops with greater concentrations. The toxic effects of magnesium can be rapidly reversed with 1 g of parenteral calcium gluconate, which should be readily available when patients are receiving magnesium infusion.[172]

The most common side effects of magnesium loading doses are transient hypotension, flushing, a sense of warmth, headache, dizziness, lethargy, nystagmus, and dry mouth.[164,183] Other adverse effects reported with magnesium are hypothermia, paralytic ileus, and pulmonary edema, which may occur in 1% to 2% of patients treated with magnesium sulfate.[183] Pulmonary edema occurs less frequently with magnesium sulfate than with parenteral β-sympathomimetics but is more commonly encountered with prolonged infusions, multifetal pregnancy, and the use of multiple tocolytics.[172,183] Treatment consists of discontinuing magnesium sulfate and administration of the diuretic furosemide.

Fetal magnesium serum concentrations are similar to maternal concentrations.[183] The most common neonatal adverse effects are hypotonia and sleepiness. Hypotonia may continue for 3 or 4 days in the neonate because of decreased renal elimination of magnesium. Rarely, assisted mechanical ventilation for neuromuscular depression may be needed.[183]

OTHER BENEFITS OF MAGNSIUM SULFATE

Magnesium sulfate is chosen as a tocolytic over nifedipine in B.B. because it offers other benefits at the current gestational age of 29 weeks. A possible role for magnesium sulfate in the prevention of cerebral palsy has been an area of significant recent investigation.[185] Historically, a number of observational retrospective studies suggested that antenatal maternal treatment with magnesium sulfate might be associated with reduced rates of cerebral palsy in the premature neonate.[186] Subsequently, several large randomized controlled trials have been performed to evaluate this possibility. In the largest study, a total of 2,241 women at risk of imminent delivery at less than 32 weeks' gestation received either placebo or magnesium sulfate specifically for neuroprotection. There was no difference in the primary outcome (a composite of total numbers of stillbirths, infant deaths at younger than 1 year, or moderate to severe cerebral palsy at older than 2 years of age). However, in secondary analyses there was a reduction in moderate to severe cerebral palsy as well as total overall cerebral palsy in the group that received magnesium sulfate.[187] In addition, meta-analysis of all clinical trials of magnesium sulfate for neuroprotective purposes demonstrated reduced occurrence of cerebral palsy.[188,189] Of note, the reduction in cerebral palsy was not associated with pregnancy prolongation associated with magnesium sulfate use. The mechanism by which magnesium sulfate may provide neuroprotection is not precisely known. However, in adults, magnesium minimizes fluctuations in cerebral blood flow, reduces reperfusion injuries, and blocks intracellular damage. Magnesium may also reduce cytokine production and minimize the inflammatory effects associated with an infection associated with bacterial endotoxin production.[180] In 2010, the ACOG recommended that physicians could consider using magnesium sulfate for fetal neuroprotection based on the currently available evidence. The duration of therapy associated with neuroprotection has ranged from a loading dose only just before delivery to up to 12 to 24 hours before anticipated delivery.[190] As the several studies have thus far used a variety of doses and duration of therapy, it was also suggested that each hospital choosing to use magnesium for neuroprotection develop specific local guidelines for treatment and monitoring.[190]

DURATION OF TOCOLYSIS

ACUTE THERAPY

CASE 49-7, QUESTION 5: B.B. has been maintained on magnesium sulfate continuous IV infusion for approximately 48 hours. The dose was increased to 3 g/hour shortly after the start of the infusion. B.B. has had no contractions for the past 24 hours. How long does she need to be treated? Should she be weaned off magnesium sulfate?

B.B.'s contractions have completely stopped for 24 hours. Some protocols maintain magnesium sulfate for 12 to 24 hours after successful tocolysis, or for the time it takes to complete the course of corticosteroids. The weaning of magnesium sulfate is unnecessary and simple discontinuation of the magnesium infusion is an easier and less costly option.[184]

CHRONIC MAINTENANCE THERAPY

CASE 49-7, QUESTION 6: B.B. heard that preterm labor can return once stopped and asks whether she should stay on medication. Should B.B. be started on chronic maintenance tocolytic therapy?

Maintenance tocolysis has been used in an attempt to prevent recurrence of preterm labor and prolong gestation in women in whom preterm labor was terminated successfully with parenteral tocolytics. β-Adrenergics and oral calcium-channel blockers have been evaluated for maintenance therapy. Results of meta-analysis of trials comparing placebo or no treatment with oral β-adrenergics for maintenance therapy after acute preterm labor showed no benefit in delay of delivery, births at less than 34 or 37 weeks' gestation, or neonatal complications.[191] Moreover, increases in maternal adverse effects occurred, primarily tachycardia, hypotension, and palpitations. Lastly, inadequate data exist to support the use of calcium-channel blockers as maintenance therapy.[168,192–194] B.B. should not be started on chronic maintenance tocolysis, as there is not compelling evidence that continued suppression of contractions after acute tocolysis reduces the rate of preterm birth or neonatal morbidities.[164,168]

ANTENATAL GLUCOCORTICOID ADMINISTRATION

CASE 49-7, QUESTION 7: Given B.B. is in preterm labor at 29 weeks' gestation, what medication can be given to help facilitate fetal lung maturation?

B.B. should be given betamethasone 12 mg intramuscularly now and a second dose 24 hours later to facilitate fetal lung maturation by increasing production of fetal lung surfactant, thereby reducing the incidence and severity of RDS.[131] Antenatal corticosteroid administration (betamethasone and dexamethasone) also decreases the incidence of intraventricular hemorrhage, necrotizing enterocolitis, and neonatal death.[131] The greatest reduction in RDS occurs when delivery can be delayed 24 hours up to 7 days after starting treatment. Repeated weekly corticosteroid courses should not be given because of the association with decreased birth weight and head circumference, hypothalamic-pituitary-adrenal axis suppression, deleterious effects on cerebral myelination and lung growth, and neonatal death (particularly in neonates born to mothers who received three or more courses).[132,195] However, a randomized clinical trial has now demonstrated a significant reduction in neonatal respiratory morbidity and composite neonatal morbidity when women with preterm labor and intact membranes who had received an initial course of steroids at less than 30 weeks' gestation were treated again with a single rescue course of steroids (betamethansone 12 mg IM × 2 doses, 24 hours apart) if more than 2 weeks had passed and the gestational age was less than 33 weeks.[196] This rescue course was administered if there was judged to be a recurrent risk of preterm birth. Although long-term outcome data are not yet available, the ACOG now recommends consideration of a single rescue course of steroids under these specific circumstances.[132]

The National Institutes of Health (NIH) Consensus Panel and the ACOG recommends a course of antenatal betamethasone or dexamethasone (dexamethansone 4 mg IM × every 12 hours, for 4 doses) for all women in preterm labor between 24 and 34 weeks' gestation.[131,132] Betamethasone, however, might be the preferred agent because fewer IM injections are needed and because in meta-analysis it was associated with a greater reduction in RDS compared with dexamethasone.[195] That conclusion, however, is not based on direct comparison of betamethasone with dexamethasone and should be interpreted with caution. One study, although limited by its retrospective nature, also suggested an advantage of betamethasone over dexamethasone in the reduction of periventricular leukomalacia, a finding associated with later risks for cerebral palsy.[197] In cases of PPROM, the NIH Consensus Panel recommends that corticosteroids may be given up to 32 weeks' gestation in the absence of chorioamnionitis.[131,132] Recent meta-analysis supports the efficacy of corticosteroids in the reduction of neonatal death, RDS, duration of ventilator use, and intraventricular hemorrhage in infants born after ruptured membranes.[195] Women at more than 32 weeks' gestation can be considered for amniotic fluid testing for the presence of phosphatidylglycerol or a lecithin to sphingomyelin ratio of greater than 2 because these are indicators of fetal lung maturation.[198] Corticosteroids are not recommended for use in pregnant women who are at more than 34 weeks' gestation unless there is an indication of fetal lung immaturity (see Chapter 100, Neonatal Therapy).

Infectious Complications During Pregnancy and Labor

CASE 49-7, QUESTION 8: Preterm labor is often associated with an infectious etiology or source. Does B.B. need to be started on any antibiotic therapy because she is in preterm labor?

PRETERM PREMATURE RUPTURE OF MEMBRANES

Increasing evidence associates preterm labor with intra-amniotic infections.[160,199] Of preterm births, 20% to 40% may be caused by an infectious or inflammatory process.[162] Intrauterine infection is associated with approximately 80% of early preterm deliveries.[160] Most of the bacteria found in amniotic fluid and the placenta are believed to have ascended from the vagina.[162] It has been suggested that the microbes responsible for preterm birth are already present in the endometrium before conception or early in the pregnancy, causing a chronic, subclinical infection weeks to months before eventually causing PPROM or labor.[160,162]

When PPROM has occurred, spontaneous labor and delivery occurs on average within 7 days, although longer intervals from PPROM to delivery occur with earlier gestational ages.[200] The use of a short course of antibiotics has been shown to prolong the period between PPROM and delivery (the latency period) and decrease neonatal morbidity.[200] In the largest and best-designed trial of antibiotic treatment of PPROM, women between 24 and 32 weeks' gestation treated with ampicillin and erythromycin had both prolonged pregnancies and lower rates of chorioamnionitis.[201] Their newborns experienced decreased mortality, as well as decreased morbidity including RDS and necrotizing enterocolitis. These effects were not owing to tocolytics or corticosteroids because these were exclusionary factors. These results were confirmed by the results of a large meta-analysis including more than 6,000 women, although information on the best choice of antibiotics was less clear.[202] Therefore, women with PPROM benefit from antibiotic therapy with a broad-spectrum regimen, and IV ampicillin plus erythromycin for 48 hours followed by 5 days of oral amoxicillin plus erythromycin for a total of 7 days treatment is a reasonable choice.[203]

B.B. should not be started on any PPROM antibiotic regimens because her membranes are not ruptured. Antibiotics have not been proved to prevent premature births in the setting of acute preterm labor.[164,168] There is currently no role for antibiotic use to prolong pregnancy or reduce neonatal morbidity in preterm labor with intact membranes, and it may be associated with long-term harm.[164,203] There may be a role for treatment of bacterial vaginosis antenatally to reduce the risk of preterm birth in women with a past history of spontaneous preterm birth.

BACTERIAL VAGINOSIS

Some, but not all, studies have demonstrated that screening and treating asymptomatic women who are at high risk for preterm delivery for bacterial vaginosis (BV) may reduce the risk of preterm birth.[165,167] A polymicrobial overgrowth of mostly anaerobic bacteria, BV is one of the most common genital infections in pregnancy, and it is associated with an increased risk of preterm delivery.[200] Treatment of women with BV who had a prior preterm delivery with oral metronidazole in combination with erythromycin decreased the risk of recurrent preterm delivery in one randomized clinical trial, but there was no difference for women without a history of recurrent preterm birth.[204,205] In addition, a meta-analysis including 622 women with prior preterm birth found no reduction in the risk of preterm birth before 37 weeks' gestation after treatment of BV with antibiotics, but did find a reduction in PPROM. In addition, in women with BV who were treated with oral antibiotics before 20 weeks' gestation, there was a reduction in preterm birth at less than 37 weeks.[205] B.B. does not have BV; therefore, treatment with metronidazole is unnecessary.

GROUP B STREPTOCOCCUS INTRAPARTUM PROPHYLAXIS

Antibiotics should be given to women if delivery is anticipated resulting either from preterm labor with intact membranes or after PPROM to prevent group B streptococcal (GBS) infection in the newborn. Other broad-spectrum antibiotic therapy to prevent preterm delivery should not be given routinely to women in preterm labor with intact membranes.

Approximately 10% to 30% of pregnant women are colonized with GBS or *Streptococcus agalactiae* in the vagina or rectum, and 1% to 2% of neonates born to colonized women experience early-onset invasive GBS disease in the absence of IV intrapartum antibiotic prophylaxis.[206] One-fourth of all cases of neonatal GBS infections occur in preterm newborns. B.B.'s fetus, therefore, is at risk for invasive GBS infection from vertical transmission (mother to infant) of bacteria during labor or delivery. The mortality rate for GBS is reported to be between 5% and 20%. Fortunately, the incidence of GBS has declined to a rate of 0.34 to 0.37 cases per 1,000 live births in recent years owing to prevention efforts.[206] During pregnancy, GBS infection can cause maternal urinary tract infection, amnionitis, endometritis, and wound infection. Antibiotics given to the mother during preterm labor and delivery help to prevent neonatal GBS disease, which may lead to sepsis, pneumonia, and meningitis. In the past decade, the routine administration of intrapartum antibiotic prophylaxis to certain subsets of pregnant women has led to a 70% reduction in the overall incidence of GBS disease.[206] The decision to treat women with intrapartum antibiotics has been based on either a positive vaginal and rectal GBS culture routinely obtained at 35 to 37 weeks' gestation or one or more of the following risk factors without culture screening: (a) previous infant with invasive GBS disease; (b) GBS bacteriuria during any trimester of the current pregnancy; (c) unknown GBS status at onset of labor and any of the following: delivery at less than 37 weeks' gestation, amniotic membrane rupture at 18 hours or more, intrapartum temperature of 38°C (100.4°F) or greater.[206] This treatment algorithm prevents an estimated 85% of all early-onset GBS disease (Fig. 49-5).

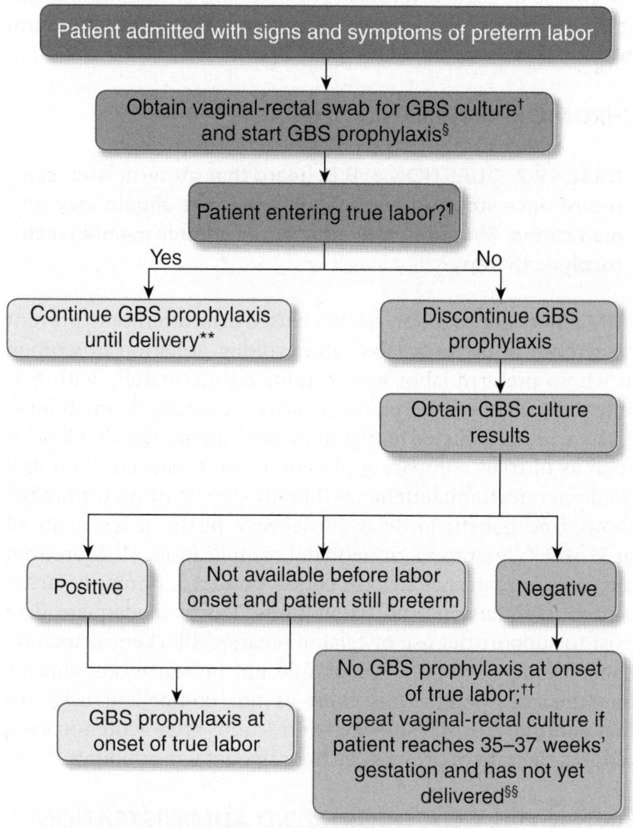

FIGURE 49-5 Sample algorithm for group B streptococcus (GBS) prophylaxis for women with threatened preterm delivery. *At <37 weeks and 0 days' gestation. †If patient has undergone vaginal-rectal GBS culture within the preceding 5 weeks, the results of that culture should guide management. GBS-colonized women should receive intrapartum antibiotic prophylaxis. No antibiotics are indicated for GBS prophylaxis if a vaginal-rectal screen within 5 weeks was negative. §See Figure 49-6 for recommended antibiotic regimens. ¶Patient should be regularly assessed for progression to true labor; if the patient is considered not to be in true labor, discontinue GBS prophylaxis. **If GBS culture results become available prior to delivery and are negative, then discontinue GBS prophylaxis. ††Unless subsequent GBS culture prior to delivery is positive. §§A negative GBS screen is considered valid for 5 weeks. If a patient with a history of PTL is readmitted with signs and symptoms of PTL and had a negative GBS screen >5 weeks prior, she should be rescreened and managed according to this algorithm at that time. (Reprinted from Verani JR et al. Prevention of perinatal group B streptococcal disease—revised guidelines from CDC, 2010. *MMWR Recomm Rep.* 2010;59(RR-10):1.)

Vaginal and rectal GBS cultures should be obtained from B.B., and she should be given a loading dose of penicillin G injection 5 million units, followed by 2.5 to 3.0 million units IV every 4 hours until delivery, while awaiting success of tocolysis and culture results. The Centers for Disease Control and Prevention guidelines recommend that the benchmark for optimal prophylaxis should be antibiotics given at least 4 or more hours before delivery. Penicillin G is preferred over ampicillin because it has a narrower spectrum of antimicrobial activity. If B.B. had a severe allergy to penicillin, sensitivities to clindamycin and erythromycin should be requested at the time of culture in the event GBS is found because of increasing resistance to these drugs. If the isolate is susceptible to both clindamycin and erythromycin, then clindamycin 900 mg IV every 8 hours should be used until delivery. Erythromycin is no longer recommended as an option for treatment because it is often associated with inducible resistance to clindamycin. If the isolate is not susceptible to both clindamycin and erythromycin or if sensitivities are not available, penicillin-allergic women at high risk for anaphylaxis should receive vancomycin 1 g IV every 12 hours until delivery. Penicillin-allergic women at low risk for anaphylaxis should receive cefazolin 2 g IV initially, then 1 g IV every 8 hours until delivery.[206] Antibiotic regimens for intrapartum antimicrobial prophylaxis are listed in Figure 49-6. Because B.B is only at 29 weeks' gestation and is in preterm labor, she has not yet had her GBS culture obtained, which normally occurs at 35 to 37 weeks. Until the results of her rapid testing for GBS culture returns, she should receive penicillin G, 3 million units IV every 4 hours until delivery to prevent perinatal GBS infection (Fig. 49-4).

CASE 49-7, QUESTION 9: B.B.'s culture results are negative for GBS growth. She is still at high risk for imminent delivery. Should penicillin G administration be discontinued?

Penicillin should be discontinued at this time. Vaginal and rectal cultures need not be repeated if B.B. delivers within the next 4 weeks. If tocolysis is successful and delivery is delayed for more than 4 weeks, obtaining cultures and starting penicillin G pre-emptively should be repeated at that time. Intrapartum prophylaxis is effective only if antibiotics can be given immediately before and during delivery.

CASE 49-7, QUESTION 10: B.B.'s contractions are gone, and her cervical examination remains unchanged for 48 hours. She is able to be discharged home undelivered, but is counseled to stay on bed rest for the duration of the pregnancy.

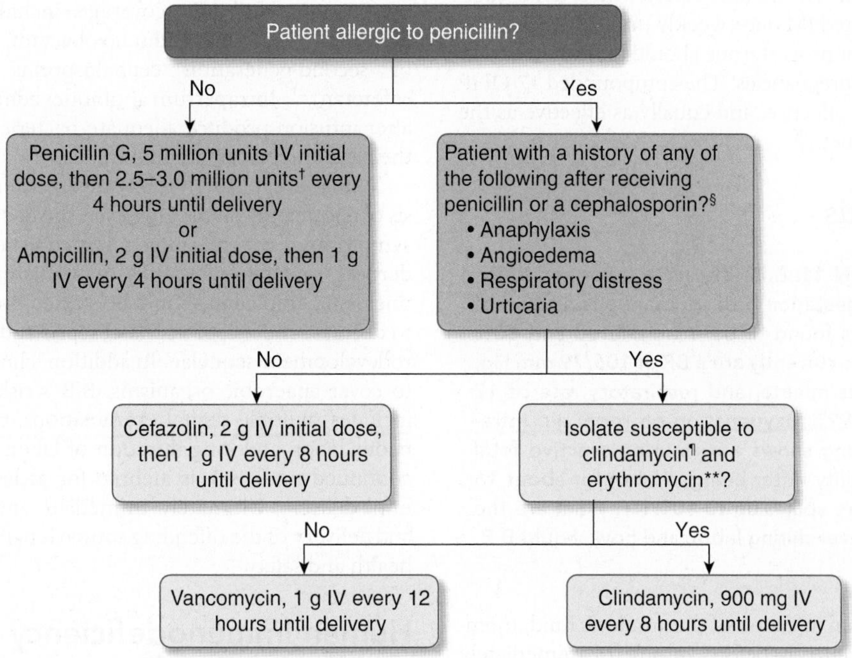

FIGURE 49-6 Intrapartum antibiotic prophylaxis to prevent perinatal group B streptococcus (GBS) disease. Indications for intrapartum antibiotic prophylaxis to prevent perinatal group B streptococcus (GBS) disease under a universal prenatal screening strategy based on combined vaginal and rectal cultures collected at 35–37 weeks' gestation from all pregnant women. IV, intravenously. *Broader-spectrum agents, including an agent active against GBS, might be necessary for treatment of chorioamnionitis. †Doses ranging from 2.5 to 3.0 million units are acceptable for the doses administered every 4 hours following the initial dose. The choice of dose within that range should be guided by which formulations of penicillin G are readily available to reduce the need for pharmacies to specially prepare doses. §Penicillin-allergic patients with a history of anaphylaxis, angioedema, respiratory distress, or urticaria following administration of penicillin or a cephalosporin are considered to be at high risk for anaphylaxis and should not receive penicillin, ampicillin, or cefazolin for GBS intrapartum prophylaxis. For penicillin-allergic patients who do not have a history of those reactions, cefazolin is the preferred agent because pharmacologic data suggest it achieves effective intraamniotic concentrations. Vancomycin and clindamycin should be reserved for penicillin-allergic women at high risk for anaphylaxis. ¶If laboratory facilities are adequate, clindamycin and erythromycin susceptibility testing should be performed on prenatal GBS isolates from penicillin-allergic women at high risk for anaphylaxis. If no susceptibility testing is performed, or the results are not available at the time of labor, vancomycin is the preferred agent for GBS intrapartum prophylaxis for penicillin-allergic women at high risk for anaphylaxis. **Resistance to erythromycin is often but not always associated with clindamycin resistance. If an isolate is resistant to erythromycin, it might have inducible resistance to clindamycin, even if it appears susceptible to clindamycin. If a GBS isolate is susceptible to clindamycin, resistant to erythromycin, and testing for inducible clindamycin resistance has been performed and is negative (no inducible resistance), then clindamycin can be used for GBS intrapartum prophylaxis instead of vancomycin. (Reprinted from Verani JR et al. Prevention of perinatal group B streptococcal disease—revised guidelines from CDC, 2010. *MMWR Recomm Rep.* 2010;59(RR-10):1.)

B.B. has a significant history of a prior preterm delivery at 32 weeks' gestation. What medication should be recommended to B.B. now and in her next pregnancy, to decrease her risk and prevent another preterm delivery from occurring?

Recent studies have shown that progesterone supplementation can help to reduce preterm births, but should only be used in women who have had a prior documented history of a spontaneous preterm birth before 37 weeks' gestation.[207] The optimal progesterone product is not known (vaginal suppositories, oral capsules, or IM injectables). Progesterone should be offered to women like B.B. who have had a prior history of spontaneous preterm delivery.[207] A recent randomized, double-blinded, placebo-controlled trial found a significant reduction in the rate of preterm deliveries in these high-risk women with a prior documented history of preterm delivery with the use of 17-α hydroxyprogesterone (17-OHP).[208] The rate of preterm delivery in the treatment group was 6.3% versus 54.9% in the placebo group.[208] 17-OHP is given as an IM injection prepared as 250 mg/mL once weekly. Therapy should be initiated at 16 to 20 weeks' gestation and continued until 37 weeks' gestation.[207] 17-OHP is widely available from compounding pharmacies, and most recently, a commercially marketed FDA-approved drug called Makena has been released into the market.[209] Although B.B. is already 29 weeks pregnant, she should be started on 17-OHP therapy at 250 mg/mL injected IM once weekly until 37 weeks. She should be counseled that progesterone should be started earlier at 16 weeks in her next pregnancies. The compounded 17-OHP is more affordable, cost-effective, and equally as effective as the marketed Makena product.[209]

Chorioamnionitis

CASE 49-7, QUESTION 11: B.B. returns to labor and delivery at 36 5/7 weeks' gestation with spontaneous rupture of the membranes and is found to be 4 cm dilated and 80% effaced. Her vital signs currently are a BP of 106/79 mm Hg, heart rate of 80 beats/minute, and respiratory rate of 12 breaths/minute with 99% oxygenation on room air. Intrapartum fetal monitoring shows a reassuring reactive fetal heart rate with variability. After being in labor for about 16 hours, her temperature spikes up to 101.1°F. What are the risks of an elevated fever during labor, and how should B.B. be treated?

Chorioamnionitis is an infection of the amniotic fluid, membranes, and placenta occurring before, during, or immediately after birth.[210] Intra-amniotic infections occur in approximately 1% to 5% of term pregnancies and may complicate up to 15% of cases of preterm labor.[211] Maternal fevers are usually the most common clinical presentation in many patients. Diagnosis is based on the presence of fever, defined as 100.4°F (38°C) or greater measured twice at least 4 hours apart, or a temperature of 101°F (38.3°C) measured once. Patients may also present with maternal tachycardia (>100 beats/minute), fetal tachycardia (160 beats/minute), uterine tenderness, foul odor from amniotic fluid, and maternal leukocytosis.[210,211] The exclusion of other sources of infection such as urinary tract infection, viral illness, abscesses, and drug-induced fever (i.e., epidural, misoprostol) must be made. Common organisms ascending from vaginal flora causing polymicrobial intra-amniotic infections include genital mycoplasmas such as *U. urealyticum* and *Mycoplasma hominis,* anaerobes including *G. vaginalis,* enteric gram-negative bacilli, and GBS.[211,212] The two most prominent risk factors of intra-amniotic infections are the number of digital examinations and duration of labor.[210]

Maternal complications from intra-amniotic infections include bacteremia, suboptimal uterine contractility, and risk for postpartum hemorrhage.[211] Increases in rates of neonatal sepsis, pneumonia, meningitis, and mortality have been shown in infants whose mothers had chorioamnionitis.[213] Furthermore, inflammation, intrapartum fever, and infection increases the risk of long-term neurodevelopmental delay and cerebral palsy in these neonates.[214] The risk of cerebral palsy is at least twofold to fourfold higher in infants who were exposed to intra-amniotic infection in utero.[214]

Early administration of broad-spectrum antibiotics immediately after the diagnosis of chorioamnionitis has been shown to have both maternal and neonatal benefit versus postpartum antibiotic administration. A common regimen implemented is ampicillin 2 g IV every 6 hours in addition to gentamicin dosed to a target peak of 8 mcg/mL and trough of 1 mcg/mL.[211] Standard dosing of gentamicin dosed every 8 hours is preferred over once-daily dosing to prevent elevated fetal serum peak levels, although no adverse effects of high-dose therapy were noted.[215] Clindamycin 900 mg IV every 8 hours may be added to the regimen to cover anaerobic organisms. If fevers persist for longer than 24 hours on triple antibiotics with ampicillin, gentamicin, and clindamycin, metronidazole can be substituted for clindamycin to help broaden anaerobic coverage.[211] Other options for antibiotic coverage include extended-spectrum penicillins (i.e., piperacillin-tazobactam, ampicillin-sulbactam) or second-generation cephalosporins (i.e., cefoxitin and cefotetan).[211] Intrapartum antibiotics administered about 1 hour after infusion produce adequate bactericidal concentrations in the fetus and placental membranes.

With a fever of 101.1°F, B.B. meets criteria for a clinical diagnosis of chorioamnionitis. However, she does not exhibit any other symptoms of systemic infection such as tachycardia, uterine tenderness, or fetal tachycardia, which is quite common. Gentamicin and ampicillin should be started promptly after diagnosis to decrease the risk of neonatal sepsis and to avoid possible neurodevelopment sequelae. In addition, clindamycin can be added to cover anaerobic organisms. B.B.'s risk for chorioamnionitis includes multiple digital examinations, preterm labor, spontaneous labor, and long duration of labor. Antibiotics should be continued until B.B. is afebrile for at least 24 to 48 hours or until delivery. Ultimately, immediate antibiotic administration and delivery of the offending source is paramount to ensure fetal health and safety.

Human Immunodeficiency Virus in Labor and Breast-Feeding

CASE 49-8

QUESTION 1: S.L. is a 23-year-old G1, P0 at 38 weeks' gestation and is positive for human immunodeficiency virus (HIV). She is presenting to labor and delivery with spontaneous rupture of membranes and is having regular contractions every 5 minutes. Her last HIV RNA levels were undetectable, and her CD4 count was 400 cells/μL. Her current antiretroviral therapy (ART) consists of zidovudine (AZT), lamivudine, and lopinavir/ritonavir, which was started 2 years ago. What are the risks of HIV perinatal transmission in S.L., and what medications must be started while she is in labor?

Current recommendations state that all HIV-infected pregnant women should receive intrapartum AZT, and their infants should receive neonatal AZT immediately after delivery for

TABLE 49-6

Intrapartum Maternal and Neonatal Zidovudine Dosing for Prevention of Perinatal Human Immunodeficiency Virus Transmission

Drug	Dose	Duration
Maternal zidovudine (intravenous)	**Load:** 2 mg/kg (actual body weight) intravenously for 1 hour **Maintenance:** Continuous infusion of 1 mg/kg/h	Onset of labor until delivery of infant
Neonatal zidovudine (oral syrup)[a]	Greater than 35 weeks' gestation: 4 mg/kg per dose orally every 12 hours	Start within 6–12 hours of birth and continue for 6 weeks
	Greater than 30 weeks' but less than 35 weeks' gestation: 2 mg/kg per dose orally every 12 hours, then after 2 weeks, advanced to every 8 hours	Start within 6–12 hours of birth and continue for 6 weeks
	Less than 30 weeks' gestation: 2 mg/kg per dose orally every 12 hours, then after 4 weeks, advanced to every 8 hours	Start within 6–12 hours of birth and continue for 6 weeks
Neonatal combination therapy (zidovudine + nevirapine)[b]	Zidovudine 4 mg/kg per dose orally every 12 hours Nevirapine (total of 3 doses given orally in first week of life: at birth, at 48 hours, and 96 hours after second dose) Birthweight 1.5–2 kg: 8 mg per dose Birthweight: Greater than 2 kg: 12 mg per dose	Start within 6–12 hours of birth and continue AZT for 6 weeks. Nevirapine given only during first week of life.

[a] Intravenous neonatal zidovudine dose of 1.5 mg/kg/dose every 6 hours if oral zidovudine cannot be given.

[b] In mothers who have not received antepartum ARV medication, infants will need combination ARV therapy.

Source: Panel on Treatment of HIV-Infected Pregnant Women and Prevention of Perinatal Transmission. Recommendations for Use of Antiretroviral Drugs in Pregnant HIV-1-Infected Women for Maternal Health *and* Interventions to Reduce Perinatal HIV Transmission in the United States. Sep. 14, 2011; pp. 1–207. **http://aidsinfo.nih.gov/ContentFiles/PerinatalGL.pdf.** Accessed November 7, 2011.

6 weeks regardless of the ART regimen taken during the pregnancy (Table 49-6).[216] Many factors must be taken into consideration, including cost, ease of administration for compliance, individual ART resistance patterns, and risks of side effects with the possibility of teratogenicity.[217] Generally, if a woman on ART becomes pregnant, she should continue on therapy throughout the pregnancy, including the first trimester.[216] Women who did not require ART before becoming pregnant should start ART prophylaxis after the first trimester but not later than 28 weeks of gestation.[216] ART is more effective in preventing perinatal HIV transmission if it is started earlier, before 28 weeks' gestation versus 36 weeks' gestation.[216] All HIV-infected women should be counseled and offered ART during pregnancy to prevent perinatal transmission regardless of HIV RNA levels.[216] Avoiding the use of efavirenz or combination of stavudine and didanosine in women of childbearing age and during the first trimester, if possible, may be prudent owing to possible teratogenicity reported with these agents.[216] Three ART regimens, in particular, have been shown to decrease mother-to-child HIV transmission, including (a) zidovudine/lamivudine/nevirapine, (b) zidovudine/lamivudine/lopinavir-ritonavir, and (c) zidovudine/lamivudine/abacavir.[217] Further studies are needed to help identify the effectiveness and safety of other ART regimens.

Antepartum ART provides maternal virologic suppression, reducing HIV RNA levels in blood and genital secretions and limiting the potential for exposure. These medications cross the placenta and produce systemic levels in the fetus, which are vital during labor and delivery when the infant is at the highest risk of virus exposure through genital secretions, maternal-fetal transfusion, or accidental ingestion.[216]

S.L. should continue on her ART (AZT, lamivudine, and lopinavir-ritonavir) during labor without missing any doses. She should also be started on intrapartum IV AZT therapy. A loading dose of AZT 2 mg/kg (actual body weight) should be administered IV for 1 hour, followed by a continuous infusion of 1 mg/kg (actual body weight) per hour. If S.L. were having a cesarean section, the infusion must be started 3 hours before surgery to ensure adequate systemic levels. After S.L. delivers, the infusion should be discontinued. Prophylactic neonatal AZT should be administered to the infant at a dose of 4 mg/kg (actual weight) PO every 12 hours, within 6 to 12 hours of birth, for a total duration of 6 weeks.[216] In the event that S.L. failed to receive any antepartum ARV medications, her infant would be started on a combination ARV therapy including neonatal AZT and nevirapine immediately after delivery.

CASE 49-8, QUESTION 2: Should S.L. breast-feed her infant if her HIV RNA levels are undetectable and her CD4 counts are 400 cells/μL?

Although S.L. is currently on effective ART to suppress her HIV RNA levels and maintain her CD4 levels, she should not breast-feed. Breast-feeding is not recommended for HIV-infected women in the United States because of safer and affordable alternatives such as formula. Prophylactic ART in the infant and mother does not entirely eliminate the risk of perinatal transmission through breast milk.[216]

POSTPARTUM HEMORRHAGE

Prevention

CASE 49-8, QUESTION 3: S.L. successfully has a normal spontaneous vaginal delivery with an estimated blood loss of 400 mL. Which medications should be given to S.L. routinely after delivery?

Oxytocin is administered routinely after the delivery of the placenta to promote uterine contraction and vasoconstriction. Meta-analysis of randomized clinical trials demonstrates that the use of oxytocin preventatively in the third stage of labor reduces the risk of hemorrhage and need for medical therapy for uterine atony.[218] Uterine atony, the condition in which the uterus fails to contract after delivery of the placenta, is the most common cause of postpartum hemorrhage.[219] Risks for uterine atony include induction and augmentation of labor, prolonged labor, an overdistended uterus such as with twins or polyhydramnios, and previous postpartum hemorrhage.[219] Oxytocin 10 to 20 units IM or diluted in 0.5 to 1 L of parenteral fluid and given as an IV infusion of 200 milli-units/minute until the uterus is firmly contracted reduces the risk for postpartum hemorrhage secondary to uterine atony.[220] Oxytocin should never be administered undiluted as a bolus dose because it can cause severe hypotension and cardiac dysrhythmias.[220]

MISOPROSTOL

Misoprostol 400 to 600 mcg can be administered orally in the third stage of labor to prevent postpartum hemorrhage.[221,222] In a comparison of 600 mcg of oral misoprostol with parenteral oxytocin for prevention of postpartum hemorrhage, oxytocin was marginally but statistically more effective and had fewer side effects.[223] Misoprostol also can be administered rectally. Rectal administration is associated with a lower incidence of fever and shivering, which is common with orally administered misoprostol during the third stage of labor.[223] The rectal route of administration also is associated with lower maximal serum concentrations and lower time to maximal concentrations than when the drug is administered orally. Although not as effective as oxytocin in preventing postpartum hemorrhage, misoprostol, which is inexpensive, stable at room temperature, and not administered parenterally, may be preferred in settings of meager resources for management of the third stage of labor.

S.L. should receive an infusion of oxytocin 20 units in 1 L of lactated Ringer solution at 125 mL/hour.

Treatment

CASE 49-8, QUESTION 4: Within a few hours of delivering her baby, S.L. has visible vaginal bleeding. She has a distended uterus, and the hemorrhage is attributed to uterine atony. Uterine massage, which is standard treatment, does not control the bleeding. What other pharmacologic options are available to treat her postpartum hemorrhage in addition to the infusion of more oxytocin at this time?

ERGOT ALKALOIDS

If the postpartum hemorrhaging does not respond to oxytocin administration, ergonovine maleate (Ergotrate) and its semisynthetic derivative, methylergonovine maleate (Methergine), can be used because of their potent uterotonic effects. IM administration is associated with less frequent adverse effects (nausea, vomiting, hypertension, headache, chest pain, dizziness, tinnitus, diaphoresis) than the IV route.[220] Ergot alkaloids should be avoided in hypertensive and eclamptic patients because of the potential for arrhythmias, seizures, cerebrovascular accidents, and rarely myocardial infarction. The dose of both drugs is 0.2 mg administered IM every 2 hours as needed. This may be followed by 0.2 to 0.4 mg administered PO two to four times daily for 2 to 7 days to promote involution of the uterus (Table 49-7).[220]

15-METHYL PROSTAGLANDIN $F_{2\alpha}$ (CARBOPROST TROMETHAMINE)

Bleeding caused by uterine atony that is unresponsive to oxytocin can be treated with 15-methyl prostaglandin $F_{2\alpha}$-tromethamine, also known as carboprost tromethamine (Hemabate).[219] Carboprost tromethamine, as with naturally occurring prostaglandins, stimulates uterine contraction and decreases postpartum hemorrhage; it is more potent and has a longer duration of effect than its parent compound, prostaglandin $F_{2\alpha}$.

Carboprost tromethamine is approved for IM use, but also has been also administered through direct myometrial injection.[220,224] Intramyometrial administration has been associated with severe hypotension and pulmonary edema.[225] An initial dose of 0.25 mg IM is given followed by 0.25 mg every 15 to 90 minutes.[220,224] The total cumulative dose should not exceed 2 mg (eight doses maximum).[224] Carboprost tromethamine is effective in treating 60% to 85% of women with uterine atony who have failed standard treatment.[220] Improvement in bleeding typically occurs after one to two injections.

The most common adverse effects of carboprost tromethamine are GI, including nausea, vomiting, and diarrhea. Flushing and fever also occur frequently. Many of the adverse effects are related to the contractile effect of this drug on smooth muscle.[224] Hypertension, although rare, typically occurs in women with pre-existing hypertension or pre-eclampsia. The potent vasoconstricting and bronchoconstricting properties of carboprost can cause uterine rupture, as well as pulmonary and cardiac problems. Carboprost must be used with caution in women with asthma, and is relatively contraindicated in the presence of pulmonary, cardiac, renal, or hepatic disease.[219,224]

MISOPROSTOL

Several case series and small randomized trials have reported that misoprostol might be useful in the treatment of postpartum hemorrhage caused by uterine atony. The available data are very limited, however, and large randomized trials are needed to clarify the efficacy of misoprostol compared with standard therapies, as well as the optimal dose and route of administration.[226] A recent double-blind, randomized, placebo-controlled clinical trial was performed to clarify the role of misoprostol for the treatment of postpartum hemorrhage.[227] Treatment was either 800 mcg of sublingual misoprostol or 40 international units of oxytocin in 1 L of IV fluid given for 15 minutes. Resolution of active bleeding occurred within 20 minutes in 89% to 90% of women in each study arm, demonstrating no advantage to misoprostol over standard IV therapy with oxytocin. Furthermore, women who received misoprostol had significantly more shivering and fever greater than 40°C. In areas with meager resources, misoprostol may offer advantages (low cost, prolonged stability,

TABLE 49-7
Uterotonic Medications Used for Postpartum Obstetric Hemorrhage

Drug	Dose	Comments
Oxytocin (Pitocin)	40 international units in 1 L NS or lactated Ringer solution 10 international units IM if no IV site available	Do not give as undiluted IV bolus, can cause hypotension.
Methylergonovine maleate (Methergine)	0.2 mg IM every 2–4 hours	Contraindicated in hypertensive patients.
Carboprost tromethamine (Hemabate)	0.25 mg IM every 15–90 minutes, not to exceed eight doses	Caution in use with patients with asthma, can cause bronchoconstriction.
Misoprostol	1,000 mcg rectally given once	Can be also be given orally or sublingually, but PR is preferred route.

IM, intramuscular; IV, intravenous; NS, normal saline; PR, per rectum.
Source: Cunningham FG et al. Obstetrical hemorrhage. In: *Williams Obstetrics.* 23rd ed. New York, NY: McGraw-Hill; 2010:757.

and oral formulation), but the role for misoprostol as an adjunctive therapy when oxytocin is already available remains uncertain.[220]

S.L. does not have any contraindications (i.e., asthma or hypertension) to any of the postpartum hemorrhage medications. She should be given oxytocin 40 international units in 1 L of lactated Ringer solution given for 15 minutes. Methylergonovine maleate 0.2 mg IM and misoprostol 1,000 mcg rectally can be given in succession after oxytocin if bleeding does not subside. Lastly, carboprost tromethamine 0.25 mg IM is an option if those medications fail to control bleeding.

PREVENTION OF RH D ALLOIMMUNIZATION

Maternal–Fetal Rh Incompatibility

CASE 49-9

QUESTION 1: G.G., a 34-year-old primigravida, had her ABO blood group and Rh status determined during her initial prenatal visit. She is found to be type O, Rh negative. Her husband is type O, Rh positive. What are the risks associated with Rh incompatibility that could affect G.G.'s unborn?

Blood group incompatibility between a pregnant woman and her fetus can result in alloimmunization of the mother and hemolytic anemia in the fetus. When a woman is exposed during pregnancy, labor, or delivery to an antigen found on the fetus's red blood cells (i.e., AB, Rh complex) that is not found on her own red blood cells (RBCs), she forms antibodies against fetus's antigen. This is referred to as *alloimmunization*. These antibodies, particularly immunoglobulin (Ig) G antibodies, cross the placenta and can interact with the fetal RBC antigens. The pregnancy in which the alloimmunization has occurred usually results in an unaffected child. The risk is carried on in subsequent pregnancies when maternal antibodies from a tiny amount of blood (less than 0.1 mL) can cross from the mother to child, which can result in the destruction of RBCs and lead to hemolytic disease of the newborn (HDN). Most serious cases of HDN are caused by Rh alloimmunization involving the D antigen. The other four alleles of the Rh gene complex code for the antigens C, c, E, and e. They are also serious, but less common, causes of alloimmunization.[228]

An Rh D-negative mother becomes immunized after exposure to fetal erythrocytes that carry the D antigen. The likelihood of having an Rh D-positive offspring is determined by whether an Rh D-positive father is homozygous or heterozygous for the D antigen. If the father is homozygous for the D antigen, all of his offspring will be D positive (Rh positive). If he is heterozygous for the D antigen, then there is a 50% chance that his offspring will be Rh positive.

Pregnant women can produce detectable IgG antibodies to Rh antigens within 6 weeks to 6 months.[229] These antibodies can cross the placenta during subsequent pregnancies and destroy fetal Rh D-positive RBCs. Of Rh D-negative women who do not receive Rh_o(D) immune globulin during pregnancy, 17% will become alloimmunized during a term pregnancy, with most cases occurring at the time of delivery.[230]

The severity of Rh-associated HDN or erythroblastosis fetalis depends on the concentration of maternal antibodies. The placental transfer of large amounts of antibody can cause substantial RBC destruction. This initially results in anemia and hyperbilirubinemia with compensatory extramedullary erythropoiesis (e.g., liver, spleen). In severe hemolytic diseases, the fetus might develop hepatosplenomegaly, portal hypertension, edema, ascites, and hepatic and cardiac failure. The clinical presentation of profound anemia, anasarca, hepatosplenomegaly, cardiac failure, and circulatory collapse is termed *hydrops fetalis*.[229]

The severity of Rh-associated HDN generally worsens with each pregnancy in the alloimmunized mother if her fetus is Rh positive. Thus, it is important to discuss the consequences of alloimmunization with any woman who is known to be alloimmunized and wishes to have more children in the future.[230]

Rh_o(D) Immunoglobulin

CASE 49-9, QUESTION 2: What interventions should be undertaken to prevent G.G. from becoming alloimmunized?

ANTEPARTUM PROPHYLAXIS

G.G. should have antibody screens at the beginning of each pregnancy and postpartum. Although the American Association of Blood Banks recommends that an antepartum screen should also be obtained at 28 weeks' gestation, the cost-effectiveness of such screening has not been studied, and it is estimated that sensitization before 28 weeks occurs at a rate of less than 0.18%. Therefore, the ACOG has suggested that the decision to obtain a third-trimester antibody screen should be dictated by individual circumstances.[230] As pregnancy progresses, both the incidence and the degree of fetomaternal hemorrhage increase. Administrating Rh_o(D) immune globulin to G.G. before or shortly after exposure to fetal Rh D-positive RBCs will prevent her from becoming alloimmunized. Giving Rh_o(D) immune globulin at 28 weeks' gestation has been shown to decrease the antepartum sensitization rate from approximately 2% to 0.1%.[230] One mechanism by which Rh_o(D) immune globulin might prevent sensitization is by suppression of the primary immune response to the D antigen.[229] The anti-D immune globulin binds the D antigen, and this complex is filtered by the spleen and lymph nodes whereby it inhibits D antigen–specific B cells from proliferating.

POSTPARTUM PROPHYLAXIS

A second dose of Rh_o(D) immune globulin should be repeated within 72 hours of delivery. A larger dose is needed if a large transplacental bleed occurs at the time of delivery (0.4% of cases). Therefore, all Rh_o(D)-negative women who deliver an Rh_o(D)-positive newborn should be tested to detect fetal RBCs in maternal blood (e.g., Kleihauer-Betke test) to calculate the correct dose of Rh_o(D) immune globulin. If a woman at risk for sensitization has not been given Rh_o(D) immune globulin within 72 hours, she should still be treated as soon as possible because it has been demonstrated that protection can be seen in some individuals up to 13 days after exposure to Rh-positive RBCs.[230]

ADVERSE EFFECTS OF RH_o(D) IMMUNE GLOBULIN

The plasma from which immune globulin is obtained is tested for viral infections, and the manufacturing process used to produce Rh_o(D) immune globulin inactivates viruses such as HIV, hepatitis B virus, and hepatitis C virus.[231] Adverse reactions associated with the use of anti-D immune globulin are rare. Pain and swelling at the injection site and rash are the most common adverse reactions. Hypersensitivity reactions such as anaphylaxis, although rare, can occur owing to a small amount of IgA in the product. Rh_o(D) immune globulin (RhoGAM) is latexfree and thimerosalfree (contains no mercury).[231]

Prophylaxis for First- and Second-Trimester Events and Procedures

CASE 49-9, QUESTION 3: G.G. will undergo amniocentesis at 16 weeks' gestation. Will she need a dose of Rh_0(D) at that time?

Rh_0(D) immune globulin should be given after all clinical events (e.g., spontaneous abortion) or procedures (e.g., abortion, amniocentesis, fetal blood sampling, or chorionic villus sampling) in which fetomaternal hemorrhage is a risk in an Rh-incompatible pregnancy.[231] Although little evidence supports the need for prophylaxis in the early first trimester, adverse effects are rare and potential benefits are thought by most experts to outweigh the risks.[230,231] Although a 50-mcg dose (MICRhoGAM) is available for first-trimester use (e.g., chorionic villus sampling or abortion), many hospitals do not stock this dose and so a 300-mcg standard dose is often given.

LENGTH OF PROTECTION

CASE 49-9, QUESTION 4: G.G. had an amniocentesis at 16 weeks for which she received Rh_0(D) immune globulin 300 mcg IM. Will she need another dose at 28 weeks' gestation? How long will this dose protect G.G. against alloimmunization?

G.G. will still need a dose of 300 mcg repeated at 28 weeks' gestation and within 72 hours postpartum if her infant is Rh_0(D)-positive. The half-life of Rh_0(D) immune globulin is approximately 23 to 26 days.[231] Without a large fetomaternal hemorrhage, a standard dose of 300 mcg will protect against alloimmunization for up to 12 weeks. If more than 12 weeks have lapsed between receipt of anti-D immune globulin and delivery, many practitioners recommend administering another antepartum dose.[230,231]

Failure of Immunoprophylaxis

CASE 49-9, QUESTION 5: What are the most common reasons for Rh D alloimmunization during pregnancy?

The most common reasons for Rh D alloimmunization are (a) failure to give a dose of anti-D immune globulin at 28 weeks' gestation, (b) failure to give Rh_0(D) immune globulin in a timely manner postpartum to women who have delivered an Rh_0(D)-positive or untyped fetus, and (c) failure to recognize clinical procedures and situations that increase maternal risk for alloimmunization (i.e., amniocentesis, abortions).[229,230]

Thus, G.G. should be told that with proper prophylaxis with anti-D immune globulin, there is little chance for her to become alloimmunized. She need not worry about her present pregnancy or future pregnancies.

LACTATION

Lactation is controlled primarily by prolactin (PRL), but the entire process is under the intricate control of several hormones. Breast tissue maturation during pregnancy is influenced by many factors, including estrogen, progesterone, PRL, insulin, growth hormone, cortisol, thyroxine, and human placental lactogen.[232] PRL concentrations gradually increase during pregnancy, but high estrogen and progesterone concentrations inhibit milk secretion by blocking PRL's effect on the breast epithelium.[232,233] It is the dramatic decrease in progesterone that triggers lactogenesis or milk secretion for the first 3 days after delivery. Infant suckling at the breast is necessary to maintain an adequate milk supply beyond postpartum day 3 or 4. Nipple stimulation transmits sensory impulses to the hypothalamus to initiate PRL release from the anterior pituitary and oxytocin from the posterior pituitary. PRL stimulates the production and secretion of breast milk, and oxytocin stimulates the contraction of the myoepithelial cells in the breast alveoli and ducts so that milk can be ejected from the breast (milk letdown). Oxytocin also can be secreted through other sensory pathways, which is why women can release milk on hearing, smelling, or even thinking about their infants. PRL, however, is released only in response to nipple stimulation.

PRL synthesis and release depend on the inhibition of hypothalamic prolactin inhibitory factor (PIF) secretion. PRL secretion is regulated primarily by dopamine-releasing neurons. Activating the dopamine receptors on the PRL-secreting cells of the anterior pituitary inhibits the release of PRL. PIF is believed to be closely associated with dopamine.[232,233]

Although PRL controls the volume of milk produced, once lactation is established, milk production is regulated by infant demand. Lactation eventually ceases if milk is not removed from the breast. Absence of suckling stops milk letdown and restores the normal production of PIF. Decreased blood flow to the breast reduces oxytocin delivery to the myoepithelium. Consequently, milk secretion stops within a few days.[232,233]

Stimulation

NONPHARMACOLOGIC MEASURES

CASE 49-10

QUESTION 1: C.C., a 22-year-old woman, vaginally delivered her first child, a healthy term infant. C.C. plans to breast-feed and was educated about breast-feeding during obstetric visits and prenatal classes. After giving birth, C.C. tried to breast-feed in the delivery room with great difficulty. Afterward, she became extremely apprehensive and continued to have trouble breast-feeding. What can be done to encourage C.C. and help her with lactation?

The most effective stimulus for lactation is suckling. Many women nurse in the delivery room after uncomplicated vaginal deliveries because nursing increases maternal–infant bonding and helps establish good milk production. If a mother does not nurse immediately after delivery, she should be encouraged to do so as soon as she is physically able. C.C. did try to nurse after delivery, but experienced problems that may have been related to her emotional or physical state, or to the physical state of her infant. The nursing staff should encourage and support C.C. emotionally to help her relax, be comfortable, and relieve her anxiety about breast-feeding. Health care personnel also should emphasize appropriate feeding techniques and proper positioning for breast-feeding. Allowing C.C.'s infant to sleep in her room, rather than the nursery, may help C.C. develop a breast-feeding routine.

Most new mothers who have difficulty breast-feeding initially respond to the emotional and educational support of a good obstetric nursing staff. Few require pharmaceutical intervention.

ENHANCEMENT OF MILK PRODUCTION

CASE 49-10, QUESTION 2: C.C. was successful in establishing breast-feeding. Despite good technique and adequate nutrition, however, she had trouble maintaining adequate milk production after about 2 to 3 weeks and was forced to supplement her infant with formula. How can C.C.'s milk production be enhanced?

Although not an FDA-approved indication, metoclopramide can be used to stimulate lactation in women with decreased or inadequate milk production.[43,234–237] Metoclopramide, a dopamine-antagonist, increases PRL secretion. This is particularly useful in women whose infants do not breast-feed effectively (e.g., preterm infants).[234] Metoclopramide 10 mg PO three times daily for 1 to 2 weeks has been shown to help restore milk production.[43,234–236] Improvement in lactation occurs within 2 to 5 days of starting therapy and persists after discontinuing metoclopramide.

The estimated total daily dose of metoclopramide ingested by the nursing infant of a woman on 30 mg/day is 1 to 45 mcg/kg/day.[43] This is below the maximal recommended infant daily dose of 0.5 mg/kg/day. Maternal doses of 30 mg/day do not alter PRL, thyroid-stimulating hormone, or free thyroxin serum concentrations in breast-fed infants.[237] The only adverse effect reported in nursing infants has been intestinal gas.[43,236] The short-term use of metoclopramide for re-establishing lactation appears to be safe, even in preterm infants.[43,234]

Recent randomized control trials have examined the effects of metoclopramide on breast milk volume and duration in women with recent preterm deliveries and found that breast-feeding outcomes were poor despite medication treatment and lactation support.[238,239] In this special population, women likely need lactation support through various resources addressing nutritional, medical, and psychosocial interventions.

Suppression

CASE 49-11

QUESTION 1: After delivery of a nonviable fetus at 24 weeks' gestation, J.G., a 26-year-old G2, P2, informs her obstetrician that she wishes to suppress her lactation. What methods are available to suppress lactation?

Suppression of lactation is indicated for women who do not want to breast-feed, women who have delivered a stillborn infant, and those who have had an abortion. Both drugs and nonpharmacologic methods have been used. In 1988, the FDA, however, recommended against drug-induced suppression of lactation.[240] The only drug therapy that the FDA recommends in women who are not breast-feeding are analgesics for the relief of breast pain. Bromocriptine was approved for the postpartum suppression of lactation; however, the FDA rescinded its approval for that indication because of cardiovascular complications (e.g., stroke, myocardial infarction) associated with its use.[233]

If breast stimulation is avoided (with or without the use of a breast binder), breast milk production will continue, leading to engorgement and distension of breast alveoli. This leads to the termination of lactation after several days. Approximately 40% of women using this method experience breast discomfort and pain; 30% experience milk leakage from their nipples.[240,241] Ice packs may be applied to the breasts for comfort, and a mild analgesic may be used if necessary.

DRUG EXCRETION IN HUMAN MILK

Breast milk is recognized as the optimal source of nutrition for infants, with documented benefits not only to infants, but also to mothers, families, and societies.[242] Evidence indicates that breast-feeding decreases the incidence or severity of many infectious processes (e.g., otitis media, respiratory infections, urinary tract infections) in infants. In children and adults who were breast-fed, the risk of developing certain medical illnesses also may decrease (e.g., obesity, inflammatory bowel disease, celiac disease, childhood leukemia).[243] Breast-feeding may also positively influence cognitive and intellectual development in children and young adults.[244] Numerous benefits to the mother also have been identified, such as decreased postpartum blood loss, more rapid uterine involution, earlier return to prepregnancy weight, and decreased risks of breast cancer, ovarian cancer, and osteoporosis.[242]

The perception that nursing should be discontinued while the mother is medicated persists, although only a finite number of drugs are absolutely contraindicated during lactation.[104] Unlike the use of drugs during pregnancy, drug excretion in breast milk can be approximated to a certain extent. Actual measurements of drug concentrations in milk and clinical observations in breast-fed infants have been published for selected drugs.

Pharmacokinetics

Different pharmacokinetic models of drug excretion in milk have been described.[245] A two-compartment open model presents the maternal fluids as one compartment and breast milk as the other. After ingestion, the drug gets absorbed into the maternal compartment, with a proportion of drug passing into breast milk and the remaining portion distributed in, and eliminated from, the maternal system. Drugs reaching breast milk will ultimately leave this compartment either by diffusing back into maternal fluids or through milk production and nursing.[246] A more popular model describes drug excretion in milk using a three-compartment model that incorporates the pharmacokinetics of the mother, mammary tissues, and infant.[245] The overall risk to the infant depends on the amount of drug bioavailable to the mother, the amount reaching breast milk, and the actual amount of drug ingested and bioavailable to the nursing infant.

Transfer of Drugs From Plasma to Milk

Transfer of drugs from maternal plasma to milk is generally through passive diffusion.[247] Low-molecular-weight, water-soluble substances diffuse through small, water-filled pores, whereas lipid-soluble compounds pass through lipid membranes.[246] Many factors affect the excretion of drugs in breast milk, and they should be carefully assessed before making a recommendation. The extent of drug passage into breast milk is often expressed quantitatively as the milk to plasma (M/P) ratio. This ratio should not be used as the sole determinant of whether a drug is safe for use during breast-feeding (see Estimating Infant Exposure section).

Several parameters affect drug excretion into breast milk (Table 49-8). The pK_a of a drug partially determines how much drug can reach the milk, because only the nonionized portion of free drug is transferred. Human milk, with an average pH of 7.1, is slightly more acidic than plasma. In general, drugs that are weak acids (e.g., penicillin) tend to have a higher concentration in plasma than milk (M/P <1). Conversely, the concentration of weak bases (e.g., erythromycin) in milk are more likely to be higher or to reach an equilibrium with that measured in plasma (M/P ≥ 1).[246] Once in the milk, the proportion of ionized weak base rises in the relatively acidic solution, and thus drug trapping occurs. Drug reabsorption has been found for some agents, and the prevention of passage back into the plasma by trapping may be clinically important. Lipid solubility also is determined to a large extent by the degree of ionization because drugs with relatively high lipid solubility exist in the nonionized form. Diffusion through lipid membranes is probably the most important pathway for drug transfer. Although pH, pK_a, and lipid solubility are important elements, other factors may significantly modify predictions based solely on these chemical characteristics. Two of these other factors are protein binding and molecular weight.[246,247] Drugs with high molecular weights such as insulin (MW $>6{,}000$) are less likely to transfer into breast milk, whereas those less than 300 transfer more readily.[43] Highly protein-bound

TABLE 49-8

Factors Affecting the Fate of Drugs in Milk and the Nursing Infant

Maternal Parameters	• Drug dosage and duration of therapy • Route and frequency of administration • Metabolism • Renal clearance • Blood flow to the breasts • Milk pH • Milk composition
Drug Parameters	• Oral bioavailability (to mother and infant) • Molecular weight • pK_a • Lipid solubility • Protein binding
Infant Parameters	• Age of the infant • Feeding pattern • Amount of breast milk consumed • Drug absorption, distribution, metabolism, elimination

pK_a, dissociation constant.
Source: Anderson PO. Drugs and breast milk [letter]. *Pediatrics.* 1995;95:957; Dillon AE et al. Drug therapy in the nursing mother. *Obstet Gynecol Clin North Am.* 1997;24:675; Begg EJ et al. Studying drugs in human milk: time to unify the approach. *J Hum Lact.* 2002;18:323; Bennett PN, ed. *Drugs and Human Lactation.* 2nd ed. New York, NY: Elsevier; 1996; Hale TW. *Medications and Mothers' Milk.* 13th ed. Amarillo, TX: Pharmasoft Medical Publishing; 2008.

drugs such as glyburide (99% protein bound) are less likely to be transferred into breast milk, although infants should still be monitored for signs of hypoglycemia.

Drug transfer also is influenced by the yield of milk, which is related to blood flow and PRL secretion.[246] Lactation is associated with a high blood flow to the breasts, but little is known about this flow during or between feedings. The milk yield (volume) differs slightly depending on the duration of lactation and the time of day. A diurnal pattern has been observed, with highest yields at 6 AM and lowest yields at 6 PM or 10 PM. The mean composition of mature human milk is approximately 87% aqueous solution, 3.5% lipids, 8% carbohydrate (83% of which is lactose), 0.9% protein, and 0.2% nitrogen.[248] The proportions of these components may vary widely from woman to woman and even within the same woman. For example, hind milk (breast milk that is expressed last and contains more fat) contains fourfold to fivefold the fat content of foremilk (breast milk that is expressed first and is high in water content, water-soluble vitamins, carbohydrates, and protein), whereas colostrum (first milk, secreted late in pregnancy and in the first few days after delivery) contains little fat. Fat content also has exhibited a diurnal variation.

After a drug reaches the milk, it equilibrates between the aqueous and lipid phases. The nature of this equilibration can modify how much drug actually reaches the infant. Infant feeding patterns differ significantly from one baby to another. The time spent suckling at each breast, and the volume of milk taken in, also determine the amount of drug ingested, especially if the drug has partitioned into one phase more so than the other. Once the infant ingests the drug via breast milk, the pharmacologic and adverse effects on the infant will be determined by the extent of oral bioavailability, distribution, metabolism, and rate of elimination. These pharmacokinetic parameters differ, depending on the infant's age and whether he or she was born prematurely or at term.

CASE 49-12

QUESTION 1: H.P. is 25-year-old woman G3, P3 who recently was diagnosed with a distal deep vein thrombosis (DVT) in her lower left extremity confirmed by a Doppler ultrasound at 5 weeks' gestation. She has a significant history of having multiple DVTs in her prior pregnancies, and her thrombophilia workup was negative. During her pregnancy, she was on therapeutic low-molecular-weight heparin (LMWH) 80 mg (weight, 76 kg) SC every 12 hours. Her dosage was increased to 100 mg SC every 12 hours after subsequent anti-factor Xa levels were subtherapeutic. Her LMWH was discontinued 24 hours before she received an epidural for labor pain. After delivery, H.P. is restarted on LMWH and then changed to warfarin on day 5. H.P. also is breast-feeding. Do either of these drugs present a risk to the nursing infant?

Heparin does not cross into breast milk (see Drug Excretion in Human Milk section) because of its high molecular weight (~12,000) and is therefore safe in breast-feeding. Warfarin is a weakly acidic drug (pK_a 5.05) that is highly ionized at physiologic pH (>99%) in maternal serum.[246] It also is highly protein bound (97%).[43] These pharmacokinetic parameters make warfarin very unlikely to transfer into breast milk. Case reports in lactating mothers confirm that warfarin is not detected in breast milk or infant plasma.[43] The American Academy of Pediatrics (AAP) considers warfarin compatible with breast-feeding,[101] and it is widely considered to be safe in breast-feeding.[249] There are no studies to guide duration of anticoagulation in women who have had a DVT associated with pregnancy. However, most recommend anticoagulation for at least 6 weeks post partum, with total duration of anticoagulation of a minimum of 6 months after the thromboembolic event.[249] H.P. can safely breast-feed her infant while she is on LMWH and warfarin.

Estimating Infant Exposure

The actual amount an infant will ingest is difficult to determine owing to varying maternal, drug, and infant parameters. Available data generally are from single or small numbers of case reports or pharmacokinetic studies involving few mother–infant pairs. An M/P ratio is sometimes used alone as the basis for a recommendation, but this should be avoided because its accuracy can be affected by many factors such as the time of sampling after maternal ingestion (peak versus steady state), dose, length of therapy, route of administration, and milk composition.[250] A relative infant dose (RID) is sometimes reported in resources or literature, which is expressed as a percentage of the maternal dose.[251] Generally, an RID of less than 10% is interpreted as an acceptable level. This must be interpreted with caution, however, taking into account other variables such as the age and health of the infant and the safety profile of the drug. It is also important to note that these are estimated values, often based on data collected from one or only a few individuals. Applying these equations using measurements specific to a woman and her infant is not clinically practical, however. Compared with the M/P ratio, experts believe that the RID is a better estimate of infant exposure.

Sampling during maternal peak drug concentration attempts to approximate the highest amount of drug that can reach the infant. This assumption is inherently flawed because peak drug concentration in the mother does not necessarily equate with peak drug concentration in milk at that same point in time.[245,250] The amount of drug an infant actually receives also depends on the volume of milk ingested. Even if a drug has a high M/P ratio, the actual amount received by the infant could be low if only a small volume of milk was consumed. Therefore, an M/P ratio describes the likelihood of drug excretion into breast milk, but it does not indicate the level of infant exposure. In general, drugs with lower M/P ratios (<1) are preferred over those with higher M/P ratios (>1) during breast-feeding, but other parameters such as maternal condition and therapeutic efficacy should be considered.

Infant exposure to a drug via ingestion of breast milk can be estimated for some drugs. The M/P ratio is used to estimate the drug concentration in milk (Eq. 49-1) and the dose the infant may ingest (Eq. 49-2).[245,252] The variables required to calculate Equation 49-1 can be located in the published literature, but only for some drugs. The actual volume of milk ingested by the infant is difficult to estimate, but the average consumption is approximately 150 mL/kg/day.[252] The estimated infant dose can then be used to calculate an RID, which is expressed as a percentage of the maternal dose.[251]

$$\text{Drug concentration in milk} = \text{Maternal plasma drug concentration} \times \text{M/P} \qquad \textit{(Eq. 49-1)}$$

$$\text{Infant dose (mg/kg/day)} = \text{Drug concentration in milk} \times \text{milk volume (mL/kg/day)} \qquad \textit{(Eq. 49-2)}$$

$$\text{RID \%} = \text{Infant dose (mg/kg/day)/maternal dose (mg/kg/day)} \times 100 \qquad \textit{(Eq. 49-3)}$$

CASE 49-13

QUESTION 1: K.J., a breast-feeding, 91-kg woman, is taking hydrochlorothiazide 50 mg PO daily. The drug has a long elimination half-life of about 12 hours. Peak milk levels of the drug occur 5 to 10 hours after a dose. In a recent study, the drug was excreted into milk with a mean concentration of 80 ng/mL. Based only on dose, does this drug represent a significant risk to K.J.'s nursing infant?

The maternal dose is 50 mg/91 kg = 0.55 mg/kg/day. The infant dose is calculated to be 80 ng/mL (1 mcg/1,000 ng) (1 mg/1,000 mcg) (150 mL/kg/day), which equals 0.012 mg/kg/day. The RID equals the actual infant dose (0.012 mg/kg/day) divided by the actual maternal dose (0.55 mg/kg/day) × 100, which equals 2.18%. Therefore, the exposure likely does not represent a risk. K.J. can continue to take hydrochlorothiazide while breast-feeding. The AAP classifies hydrochlorothiazide as compatible with breast-feeding.[43,101]

Reducing Risk of Exposure

If pharmacologic treatment is medically necessary for a nursing mother, every attempt should be made to minimize infant exposure to the drug. Methods of reducing risks have been proposed.[245,250,253] Table 49-9 summarizes critical factors that should be considered. Except for drugs that are contraindicated during lactation, the decision to continue or discontinue nursing while receiving medication is ultimately the mother's. Therefore, patient education is an integral component in this decision-making process. The mother should be informed of the potential risks, or lack thereof, associated with a drug. She also should be made aware that certain risks may be minimized by altering feeding pattern and drug administration time and by carefully monitoring the infant for early signs of adverse effects.

Resources for Drugs and Lactation

Comprehensive sources reviewing drug use in lactation are available to assist clinicians in weighing the potential risks versus benefits of mothers using medications while breast-feeding.

TABLE 49-9
Reducing Risk of Infant Exposure to Drugs in Breast Milk

A drug should be used only if medically necessary and treatment cannot be delayed until the infant is ready to be weaned.
Drug Selection
Consider whether the drug can be safely given directly to the infant.
Select a drug that passes poorly into breast milk with the lowest predicted M/P ratio, and an RID <10%.
Avoid long-acting formulations (e.g., sustained-release).
Consider possible routes of administration that can reduce drug excretion into milk.
Determine length of therapy and if possible avoid long-term use.
Feeding Pattern
Avoid nursing during times of peak drug concentration.
If possible, plan breast-feeding before administration of the next dose.
Other Considerations
Always observe the infant for unusual signs (e.g., sedation, irritability, rash, decreased appetite, failure to thrive).
Discontinue breast-feeding during the course of therapy if the risks to the fetus outweigh the benefits of nursing.
Provide adequate patient education to increase understanding of risk factors.

M/P, milk to plasma ratio; RID, relative infant dose.
Source: Anderson PO. Drugs and breast milk [letter]. *Pediatrics.* 1995;95:957; Begg EJ et al. Studying drugs in human milk: time to unify the approach. *J Hum Lact.* 2002;18:323; Howard CR, Lawrence RA. Drugs and breastfeeding. *Clin Perinatol.* 1999;26:447.

Table 49-10 lists some medications that are contraindicated during lactation. The AAP Committee on Drugs periodically reviews the transfer of drugs and other chemicals into human milk and publishes their findings.[101] The Committee identifies drugs that should be avoided during breast-feeding, drugs that should be used with caution, drugs whose effects on infants are unknown but of concern, and those considered usually compatible with breast-feeding. This rigorous review is an ongoing process, and new guidelines are published every few years; therefore, the reader should locate the latest AAP recommendations available. In addition to the AAP guidelines, several other references also offer comprehensive information and recommendations on drug use in lactation.[43,252]

Most drugs are excreted into breast milk to some extent; the reader is referred to specialty sources for an in-depth review of the drug in question. The best sources for information regarding drugs in lactation are (a) *Drugs in Pregnancy and Lactation: A Reference Guide to Fetal and Neonatal Risk* by Briggs, Freeman, and Yaffe[43] and (b) TOXNET, an online lactation database (LactMed) sponsored by the NIH, accessible at http://toxnet.nlm.nih.gov and click on LactMed. These two databases are peer-reviewed and contain referenced sources. Categories assigned to these drugs may change as new data become available for specific drugs.

ACKNOWLEDGMENT

The authors acknowledge Gerald G. Briggs, BPharm, for his contributions to this chapter in earlier editions.

KEY REFERENCES AND WEBSITES

A full list of references for this chapter can be found at http://thepoint.lww.com/AT10e. Below are the key references

TABLE 49-10
Drugs Considered Contraindicated During Lactation[a]

Drug or Drug Class	Effects on Nursing Infants
Amphetamines[b]	Accumulate in breast milk and may cause irritability and poor sleep patterns
Antineoplastics	Potential for immune suppression; cytotoxic effects of drugs on dividing cells in infants unknown[2]
Cocaine[b]	Excreted in milk; contraindicated because of CNS stimulation and intoxication
Ergotamine	Potential for suppressing lactation; vomiting, diarrhea, and convulsions have been reported.[217] Considered contraindicated by some clinicians. AAP recommends using with caution
Heroin[b]	Possible addiction if sufficient amounts ingested
Immunosuppressants	Potential for immune suppression
Lithium	Milk and serum concentrations average 40% of maternal serum levels. Potential for toxicity exists. Considered contraindicated by some clinicians. AAP recommends using with caution.
Lysergic acid diethylamide (LSD)[b]	Probably excreted in milk
Marijuana[b]	Excreted in milk
Misoprostol	Excretion in milk has not been studied but contraindicated because of potential for severe diarrhea in infant
Phencyclidine[b]	Potent hallucinogenic properties
Phenidone	Massive scrotal hematoma and wound oozing after herniotomy in one infant; contraindicated
Requiring Temporary Cessation of Breast-Feeding	
Radiopharmaceuticals	Halt breast-feeding temporarily to allow clearance of radioactivity from milk. Suggested times for individual agents are[244]: copper-64 (^{64}Cu) 50 hours; gallium-67 (^{67}Ga) 2 weeks; indium-111 (^{111}In) 20 hours; iodine-123 (^{123}I) 36 hours; iodine-125 (^{125}I) 12 days; iodine-131 (^{131}I) 2–14 days; radioactive sodium 96 hours; technetium-99m (^{99m}Tc) 15 hours–3 days; ($^{99m}TcO_4$) (^{99m}Tc macroaggregates) 15 hours–3 days

[a] This list is not all-inclusive. Selected drugs are listed by drug class and not by individual names.
[b] All drugs of abuse are contraindicated during lactation.
Source: Briggs G et al. *Drugs in Pregnancy and Lactation: A Reference Guide to Fetal and Neonatal Risk*. 9th ed. Philadelphia, PA: Lippincott Williams & Wilkins; 2011; American Academy of Pediatrics Committee on Drugs. Transfer of drugs and other chemicals into human milk. *Pediatrics*. 2001;108:776; Hale TW. *Medications and Mothers' Milk*. 13th ed. Amarillo, TX: Pharmasoft Medical Publishing; 2008.

and websites for this chapter, with the corresponding reference number in this chapter found in parentheses after the reference.

MEDICATION USE IN PREGNANCY AND LACTATION

Key References

Briggs G et al. *Drugs in Pregnancy and Lactation: A Reference Guide to Fetal and Neonatal Risk*. 9th ed. Philadelphia, PA: Lippincott Williams & Wilkins; 2011. (43)

Hale TW. *Medications and Mothers' Milk*. 13th ed. Amarillo, TX: Pharmasoft Medical Publishing; 2008.

Ito S. Drug therapy for breast-feeding women [published correction appears in *N Engl J Med*. 2000;343:1348]. *N Engl J Med*. 2000;343:118. (104)

Key Websites

American Congress of Obstetrics and Gynecology. www.acog.org.

Motherisk. www.motherisk.org.

National Library of Medicine: Drugs and Lactation Database (LACTMED). http://toxnet.nlm.nih.gov.

Organization of Teratology Specialists (OTIS). www.otispregnancy.com.

Perinatology. www.perinatalogy.com/index.html.

REPROTOX (Reproductive Toxicology). www.reprotox.org.

GENERAL INFORMATION

Key References

ACOG Committee on Obstetric Practice. ACOG Committee Opinion No. 475: antenatal corticosteroid therapy for fetal maturation. *Obstet Gynecol*. 2011;117(2 Pt 1):422. (132)

ACOG Committee on Practice Bulletins. ACOG Practice Bulletin. Chronic hypertension in pregnancy. ACOG Committee on Practice Bulletins. *Obstet Gynecol*. 2001;98(1):suppl 177. (91)

American College of Obstetricians and Gynecologists. ACOG Practice Bulletin: Clinical Management Guidelines for Obstetrician-Gynecologists Number 76, October 2006: postpartum hemorrhage. *Obstet Gynecol*. 2006;108:1039. (219)

Bates SM et al. Venous thromboembolism, thrombophilia, antithrombotic therapy, and pregnancy: American College of Chest Physicians Evidence-Based Clinical Practice Guidelines (8th Edition). *Chest*. 2008;133(Suppl):844S. (249)

Coustan DR et al. The Hyperglycemia and Adverse Pregnancy Outcome (HAPO) study: paving the way for new diagnostic criteria for gestational diabetes mellitus. *Am J Obstet Gynecol*. 2010;202:654.e1.

Loebstein R, Koren G. Clinical relevance of therapeutic drug monitoring during pregnancy. *Ther Drug Monit*. 2002;24:15. (21)

Niebyl JR. Clinical practice. Nausea and vomiting in pregnancy. *N Engl J Med*. 2010;363:1544. (52)

[No authors listed]. Use of progesterone to prevent preterm births. ACOG Committee Opinion No. 419 (Replaces No. 291, November 2003). American College of Obstetricians and Gynecologists. *Obstet Gynecol*. 2008;112:963. (207)

Disorders Related to the Menstrual Cycle

50

Laura M. Borgelt and Karen M. Gunning

CORE PRINCIPLES

		CHAPTER CASES
1	A normal menstrual cycle involves the hypothalamus, anterior pituitary gland, ovaries, and endometrial lining of the uterus to create hormonal release. This process results in follicle development, ovulation, and either pregnancy or menstruation every 28 days (average) during reproductive life.	
2	Polycystic ovary syndrome (PCOS) is a heterogenous disorder that presents with signs and symptoms of hyperandrogenism (e.g., acne, hirsutism) or ovulatory dysfunction.	Case 50-1 (Question 1)
3	Long-term complications of PCOS may include impaired glucose tolerance, diabetes, metabolic syndrome, infertility, endometrial cancer, and obstructive sleep apnea.	Case 50-1 (Question 2)
4	Treatment for PCOS involves nonpharmacologic and pharmacologic management. Pharmacologic management targets the pathophysiologic aspects of the syndrome and individual goals of treatment. Oral contraceptives are preferred when contraception is desired; clomiphene citrate alone or in combination with metformin is warranted when pregnancy is desired.	Case 50-1 (Questions 3–7)
5	Dysmenorrhea, or painful cramping that occurs with the onset and first days of menstruation, can be categorized as either primary (without underlying uterine pathology) or secondary as a result of uterine conditions, including endometriosis, uterine polyps, or fibroids; complications of intrauterine contraceptive device use; or pelvic inflammatory disease. A careful history can distinguish most cases of primary dysmenorrhea that can be effectively treated with over-the-counter medications from secondary dysmenorrhea, which should always be investigated further for its underlying etiology.	Case 50-2 (Questions 1, 2)
6	Dysmenorrhea is the single largest cause of lost productivity and school absence among adolescent girls. Health care providers can play a significant role in patient education and development of rational evidence-based drug therapy plans that include nonsteroidal anti-inflammatory drugs (NSAIDs) or hormonal contraceptives to decrease symptoms and improve functionality.	Case 50-2 (Questions 4–8)
7	Nonpharmacologic agents, particularly the use of heat, have been shown to provide benefit in patients with primary dysmenorrhea. Vitamin B_1 and magnesium have also demonstrated benefit with few significant adverse effects.	Case 50-2 (Questions 3, 8)
8	Endometriosis is defined as the presence of functional endometrial tissue occurring outside the uterine cavity. It is the most common cause of secondary dysmenorrhea in young women, and can result in chronic pelvic pain, infertility, and dyspareunia. A significant delay in diagnosis of endometriosis is common and can result in negative effects on fertility and pain control. Recognition of the potential for a diagnosis of endometriosis, through a careful history and physical, is key for clinicians to provide appropriate care.	Case 50-3 (Question 1)

continued

	CHAPTER CASES
9 Pain control in endometriosis is directed at suppression of endometrial implants that respond to estrogen with bleeding, resulting in subsequent inflammation and pain. Pharmacologic therapy is directed at reducing inflammation (via use of NSAIDs) and reduction in estrogen (through use of hormonal contraception), or the use of gonadotropin-releasing hormone (GnRH) analogs to induce a pseudomenopausal state. A treatment plan should take into account cost, ease of use of therapy, and the patient's desire for future fertility.	**Case 50-3 (Questions 2–5), Case 50-4 (Question 1), Case 50-5 (Question 1)**
10 Endometriosis treatment plans that include GnRH analogs or aromatase inhibitors may also require the use of "add-back" therapy. Add-back therapy is the addition of progestins or estrogens that may be used with GnRH analogs and aromatase inhibitors to decrease menopausal side effects including hot flashes, vaginal dryness, and decreases in bone density.	**Case 50-4 (Question 1)**
11 More than 200 premenstrual symptoms (such as increased energy, libido, ability to relax, abdominal distension, fatigue, headaches, and crying spells) have been described as occurring during the days before menstruation. It is not until the symptoms have a decidedly negative influence on the physical, psychological, or social function of a woman that premenstrual syndrome (PMS) or premenstrual disphoric disorder (PMDD) exists. Both PMS and PMDD have symptoms that occur in the luteal phase with resolution within a few days of menstruation, lasting across at least two menstrual cycles, and disrupt normal activities.	**Case 50-6 (Questions 1, 3)**
12 Nonprescription options that have been studied and have shown at least minimal benefit in PMS and PMDD include calcium, magnesium, pyridoxine, chastetree or chasteberry, and some mind–body approaches.	**Case 50-6 (Question 2)**
13 Treatment for PMS and PMDD includes lifestyle modifications, psychological interventions, selective serotonin reuptake inhibitors (SSRIs), other psychotropic medications, oral contraceptives, GnRH agonists, and danazol. Because serotonin is critical in the pathogenesis of these disorders, SSRIs have become the treatment of choice for PMDD and severe PMS.	**Case 50-6 (Question 4)**

MENSTRUAL CYCLE PHYSIOLOGY

Feedback biologic mechanisms involving the hypothalamus, anterior pituitary gland, ovaries, and endometrial lining of the uterus control the average 28-day menstrual cycle.[1–3] The hypothalamus synthesizes gonadotropin-releasing hormone (GnRH) and secretes the hormone in a pulselike manner with varying frequencies throughout the menstrual cycle (typically every 60–90 minutes). GnRH stimulates the anterior pituitary to produce and release follicle-stimulating hormone (FSH) and luteinizing hormone (LH). FSH is important for stimulating growth of ovarian follicles and LH is critical for ovulation and sex steroid production. FSH and LH act on the ovaries to produce estrogen and progesterone. Estrogen in turn acts on the hypothalamus and anterior pituitary, in a negative feedback manner, to stop FSH and LH secretion (Fig. 50-1).

The menstrual cycle can be divided into three phases: the follicular phase, ovulation, and the luteal phase (Fig. 50-2).[1–3] The day bleeding begins is referred to as the first day (or day 1) of the menstrual cycle. Bleeding usually occurs from days 1 to 5 of the cycle, although may be longer in some women. The follicular phase begins at the onset of menstruation and lasts approximately 10 to 14 days (see Fig. 50-2). At the beginning of this phase, several follicles begin to develop within the ovary. In the second half of the follicular phase most of the developing follicles atrophy, while the dominant follicle develops further and produces estrogen in increasing amounts. Elevated estradiol levels during the ovulatory phase leads to a surge in LH and FSH. The LH surge is responsible for final-stage growth and maturation of the follicle, ovulation, and the formation of the corpus luteum. Ovulation usually occurs 14 days before the last day of the cycle, and is followed by the luteal phase. The luteal phase is 13 to 15 days in duration and is the least variable part of the human reproductive cycle.[1] During this progesterone-dominant phase, the corpus luteum produces progesterone and estrogen. Progesterone prepares the endometrium for implantation of a fertilized ovum. If implantation does not occur, corpus luteum regression causes a decrease in the levels of estrogen and progesterone. When these hormone levels decrease, the endometrium cannot be maintained and is sloughed off (menstrual phase). Using the average 28-day cycle as an example, day 28 is the last day of the cycle and is the day before bleeding begins again for the next menstrual cycle.

POLYCYSTIC OVARY SYNDROME

Polycystic ovary syndrome (PCOS) affects approximately 6% to 8%, or 1 in 15, women of reproductive age, making it the leading cause of anovulatory infertility and the most common endocrine abnormality for this age group.[4] This syndrome, or constellation of symptoms, was first described in 1935 by Stein and Leventhal when they reported infertility and amenorrhea in seven women with enlarged cystic ovaries.[5] Excessive male-patterned hair growth and obesity were added later to the description of this syndrome.[6] PCOS also has been referred to as Stein-Leventhal

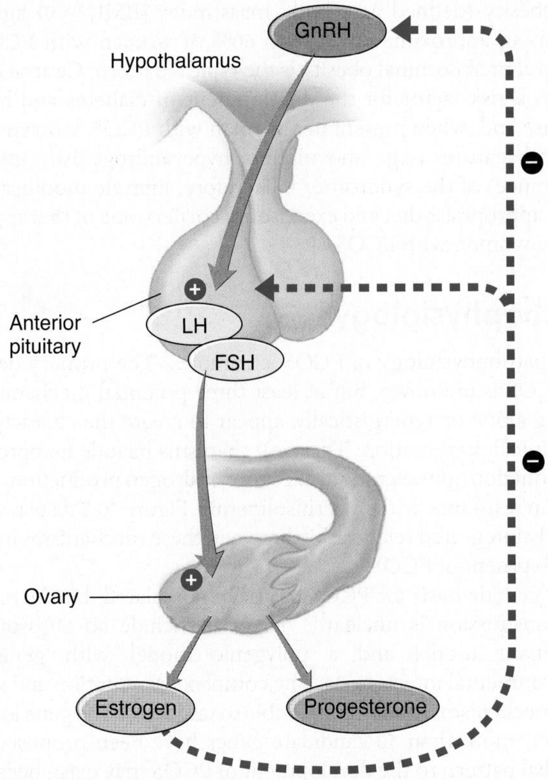

FIGURE 50-1 Menstrual cycle physiology. FSH, follicle-stimulating hormone; GnRH, gonadotropin-releasing hormone; LH, luteinizing hormone. (Adapted with permission from Premkumar K. *The Massage Connection: Anatomy and Physiology*. Baltimore, MD: Lippincott Williams & Wilkins; 2004.)

syndrome, polycystic ovary, polycystic ovarian disease, hyperandrogenic chronic anovulatory syndrome, and functional ovarian hyperandrogenism. The name *polycystic ovary syndrome* has been most widely accepted because it best describes the heterogeneous nature of this disorder.

Diagnostic Criteria

The diagnosis of PCOS is complicated by variations among women presenting signs and symptoms of PCOS and because precise and uniform criteria for diagnosis have not been firmly established. Three major diagnostic criteria for PCOS have been proposed by different organizations.

The initial diagnostic criteria were developed in 1990 during an expert conference sponsored by the US National Institutes of Health and US National Institute of Child Health and Human Development. The panel concluded that the major criteria for PCOS should include (in order of importance): (a) hyperandrogenism (clinical signs of hyperandrogenism such as hirsutism) or hyperandrogenemia (biochemical signs of hyperandrogenism such as elevated testosterone levels), (b) oligo-ovulation (infrequent or irregular ovulation with fewer than nine menses per year), and (c) exclusion of other known disorders such as hyperprolactinemia, thyroid abnormalities, and congenital adrenal hyperplasia.[7] The second set of criteria was proposed at an expert conference in Rotterdam sponsored by the European Society for Human Reproduction and Embryology and the American Society for Reproductive Medicine in 2003.[8] They concluded that the presence of two of these three features, after exclusion of related disorders, confirmed diagnosis of PCOS: (a) oligo-ovulation or anovulation, (b) clinical or biochemical signs of hyperandrogenism, or (c) polycystic ovaries. The third set of criteria was developed by a task force of the Androgen Excess Society in

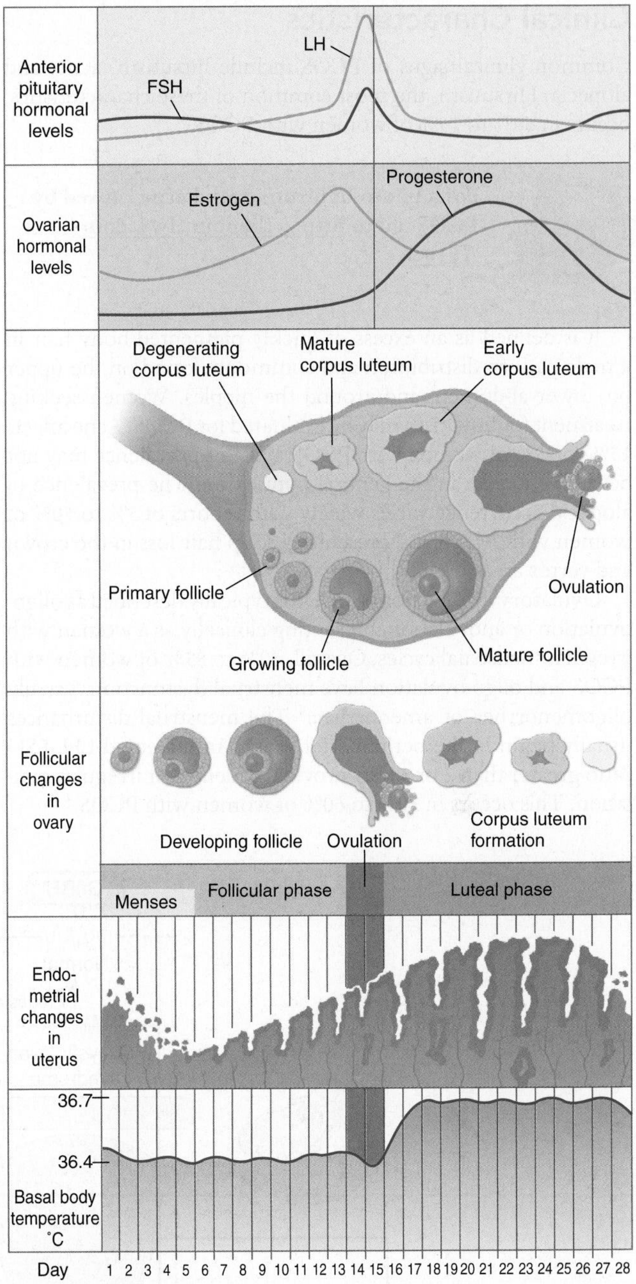

FIGURE 50-2 The menstrual cycle. FSH, follicle-stimulating hormone; LH, luteinizing hormone. (Adapted with permission from Premkumar K. *The Massage Connection: Anatomy and Physiology*. Baltimore, MD: Lippincott Williams & Wilkins; 2004.)

For a full-color version of Figure 50-2, go to http://thepoint.lww.com/AT10e.

2006 with a complete report including phenotyping in 2009.[9,10] Their criteria include hyperandrogenism (hirsutism or hyperandrogenemia), ovarian dysfunction (oligo-ovulation or polycystic ovaries), and exclusion of other androgen excess or related disorders. Strengths and weaknesses exist in each of the criteria proposed, but it is clear that the definition of and diagnostic criteria for PCOS will continue to evolve as new information is released.

For a visual of polycystic ovaries, go to http://thepoint.lww.com/AT10e.

Clinical Characteristics

Common clinical signs of PCOS include hirsutism, acne, and alopecia. Hirsutism, the most common of these characteristics, occurs in 60% to 75% of women with PCOS.[9–10]

ONLINE CONTENT **For a photo of hirutism and acne caused by PCOS, go to http://thepoint.lww.com/AT10e.**

It is defined as an excess of thickly pigmented body hair in a male pattern distribution and commonly found on the upper lip, lower abdomen, and around the nipples. Women seeking treatment for hirsutism may be evaluated for PCOS. Acne affects 15% to 25% of women with PCOS, but this prevalence may not be different than in the general population. The prevalence of alopecia occurrence varies widely with reports of 5% to 50% of women with PCOS and presents as scalp hair loss in the crown and vertex areas.[9,11]

Ovulatory dysfunction in PCOS is typically described as oligo-ovulation or anovulation, presenting clinically as a woman with irregular menstrual cycles. Overall, 60% to 85% of women with PCOS and oligo-ovulation have menstrual dysfunction, usually oligomenorrhea or amenorrhea.[4] The menstrual disturbances usually begin in the peripubertal years. An increased LH–FSH ratio greater than 2 or 3 may provide evidence for irregular ovulation. This occurs in 20% to 60% of women with PCOS.[4]

Obesity (defined as a body mass index [BMI] ≥ 30 kg/m^2) occurs in approximately 30% to 60% of women with PCOS.[4] Central or abdominal obesity is the typical pattern. Central obesity is a risk factor for the development of diabetes and heart disease and, when present in a woman with PCOS, worsens the clinical features (e.g., anovulation, hyperandrogenism, insulin resistance) of the syndrome.[12] Therefore, lifestyle modification with appropriate diet and exercise is a cornerstone of therapy for many women with PCOS.

Pathophysiology

The pathophysiology of PCOS is complex. The primary defect in PCOS is unknown, but at least three potential mechanisms, acting alone or synergistically, appear to create the characteristic clinical presentation. These mechanisms include inappropriate gonadotropin secretion, excessive androgen production, and insulin resistance with hyperinsulinemia. Figure 50-3 displays the closely integrated relationship between these mechanisms in the development of PCOS.

A genetic basis for PCOS has been postulated, but its mode of transmission is unclear.[13] Theories include an autosomal-dominant model and a polygenic model with genetic–environmental interactions. The complex presentation and various mechanisms make it impossible to target just one gene locus; in fact, more than 50 candidate genes have been proposed. A familial pattern to the development of PCOS may exist, because the incidence is higher in women with relatives with the disorder.

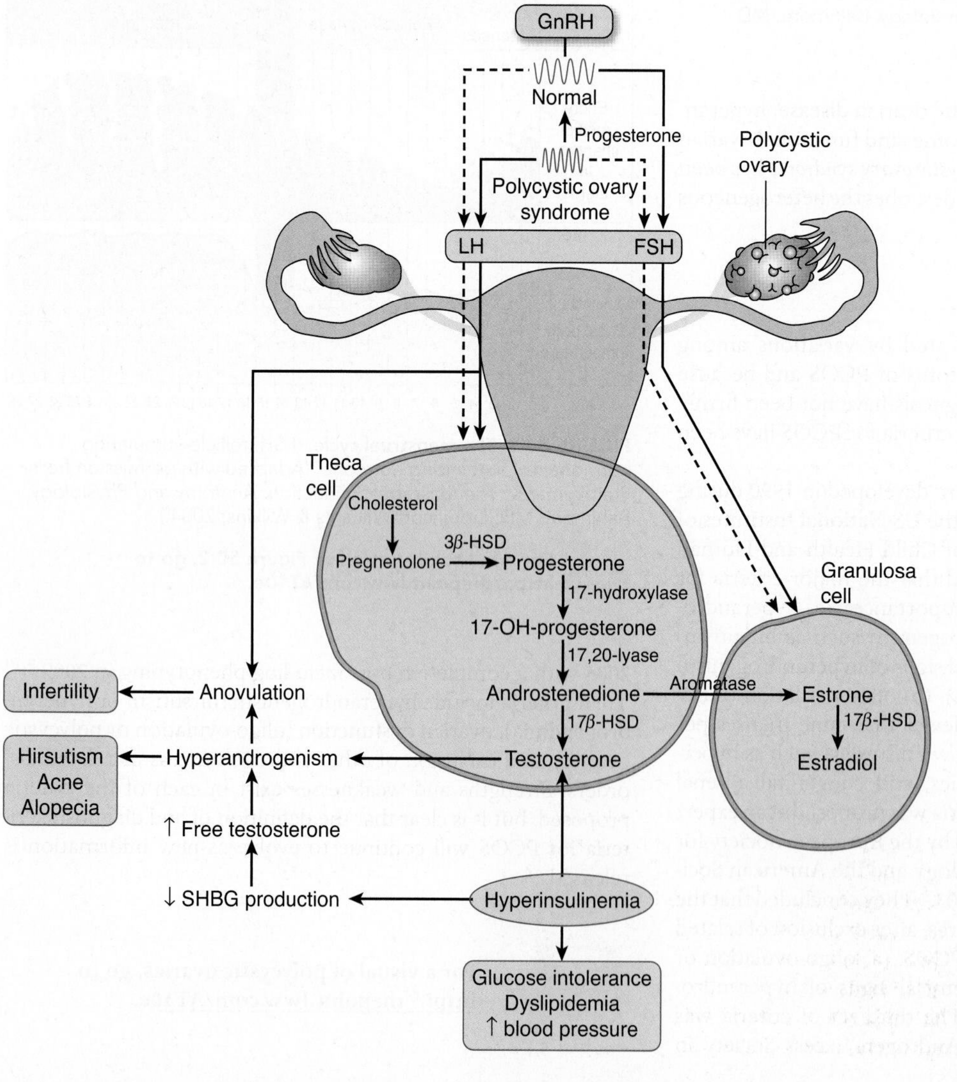

FIGURE 50-3 Relationship of gonadotropin secretion, androgen production, and insulin in polycystic ovary syndrome (PCOS). Inappropriate gonadotropin secretion and hyperinsulinemia in PCOS lead to excess androgen production and potential anovulation. Long term consequences, such as glucose intolerance, dyslipidemia, and increased blood pressure, also can occur as a result of these abnormal processes. (Adapted with permission from Borgelt LM, Cheang KI. Polycystic ovary syndrome. In: Borgelt LM et al, eds. *Women's Health Across the Lifespan: A Pharmacotherapeutic Approach.* Bethesda, MD: American Society of Health-System Pharmacists; 2010:237.)

GONADOTROPIN SECRETION

In PCOS, there is an increased frequency of GnRH stimulation, leading to an increase in LH pulse frequency and amplitude, while FSH secretion remains normal. The development of a dominant follicle does not occur because LH secretion occurs too early in the menstrual cycle. Therefore, a woman is left with several immature follicles and usually will not ovulate. It is not clear whether the abnormal pulse frequency of GnRH is an intrinsic problem in the GnRH pulse generator in the hypothalamus or a result of relatively low progesterone concentrations from infrequent ovulation.[14] A woman with this abnormality does not enter the luteal phase of her menstrual cycle, leaving estrogen unopposed. Unopposed estrogen leads to endometrial hyperplasia and increases the risk for endometrial cancer. Increased LH stimulation also leads to increased steroidogenesis in the ovary, leading to excess androgen production.

EXCESS ANDROGEN PRODUCTION

Androgen production occurs in the theca cell of the ovary to facilitate follicular growth and estradiol synthesis in the granulosa cell. In women with PCOS, hypersecretion of LH and insulin increase the production of androgens, causing abnormal sex steroid synthesis, hyperandrogenism, and hyperandrogenemia. The dysregulation in steroid synthesis and metabolism is believed to result primarily from a dysfunction of the cytochrome P-450 (CYP) C17 enzyme in the ovaries, an enzyme with 17-hydroxylase and 17,20-lyase activities that are required to form androstenedione.[14,15] Androstenedione is then converted to testosterone or is aromatized by the aromatase enzyme to form estrone. Theca cells in women with PCOS are more efficient at the conversion to testosterone than normal theca cells.[16] Also, a similar steroid pathway occurs in the adrenal cortex and, when hyperandrogenism or hyperinsulinemic states exist, androgen production is further enhanced.

Elevated androgen levels are seen in approximately 60% to 80% of women with PCOS, mostly as increased free testosterone concentrations.[9,10] Assays for testosterone tend, however, to be highly variable and inaccurate, so measurement of androgen concentrations should be used only as an adjuvant test and never as the sole criterion for diagnosis. Clinical assessment is the primary tool for assessment of excess androgen.

INSULIN

Women with PCOS generally exhibit an increased risk of insulin resistance with compensatory hyperinsulinemia.[4] Insulin resistance is associated with reproductive and metabolic abnormalities in women with PCOS and can occur in both obese and nonobese women. There are several mechanisms by which this occurs. One proposed mechanism is a postbinding defect in insulin-receptor signaling.[17] Specifically, abnormal receptor autophosphorylation increases serine phosphorylation in targeted cells, which contributes to insulin resistance.[18,19] The insulin resistance in PCOS has been shown to be a selective, tissue-specific process where insulin sensitivity is increased in the ovarian androgenic pathway (causing hyperandrogenism), but insulin resistance is seen in other tissues involved with carbohydrate metabolism, specifically in the fat and muscle. Hyperinsulinemia results because of the compensatory increase in insulin secretion secondary to insulin resistance.

Insulin has both direct and indirect roles in PCOS. In the ovary, insulin acts alone or synergistically with LH to increase androgen production in theca cells. In the liver, insulin inhibits synthesis of sex hormone–binding globulin (SHBG), a key protein that binds to testosterone, and thus increases the free fraction of androgens available for biologic activity. Therefore, hyperinsulinemia is a major contributor to both hyperandrogenism and hyperandrogenemia in PCOS. Treatments targeted to improve insulin resistance in women with PCOS have shown improvements in ovulatory function, hirsutism, androgen levels, and metabolic profiles.[20,21] Indirectly, insulin may enhance the amplitude of LH pulses, further exacerbating the gonadotropin secretion defect in PCOS.[22]

CASE 50-1

QUESTION 1: E.F. is a 27-year-old woman with mild hair growth above her upper lip, mild acne, and a history of irregular menstrual periods. Since age 12, she has had six to nine periods per year at intervals that vary from 30 to 90 days. When she does have a period, she considers them to be "normal" without pain or excessive bleeding. Her irregular periods were not bothersome until recently when she became sexually active and worries about becoming pregnant. She uses condoms for birth control. She reports no other medical conditions. E.F. is 5 feet 7 inches tall and weighs 180 pounds (BMI 28.2 kg/m^2). Her vital signs today are blood pressure (BP) 118/84 mm Hg, heart rate (HR) 70 beats/minute, temperature 98.6°F, and respiratory rate (RR) 18 breaths/minute. Her physical examination is normal, with the exception of noted excessive facial hair and mild acne. She takes a multivitamin daily and acetaminophen as needed for headaches. She has no known medication allergies. What signs and symptoms does E.F. have that are consistent with PCOS?

E.F. exhibits several signs and symptoms that would indicate the presence of PCOS. According to the criteria of all organizations, her history of abnormal menstrual periods (oligomenorrhea) and clinical signs of hyperandrogenism, including hirsutism and acne, would indicate PCOS. E.F. is overweight, which is common in women with PCOS but is not considered a criterion for diagnosis. Before a diagnosis of PCOS is made, laboratory testing to exclude other related causes of her symptoms would have to be performed. Studies may include prolactin, thyroid-stimulating hormone, testosterone, and 17-hydroxyprogesterone concentrations to rule out hyperprolactinemia, hypothyroidism, virilizing tumor, and congenital adrenal hyperplasia, respectively. PCOS is primarily diagnosed by clinical assessment; therefore, these tests assist only in confirming or excluding a diagnosis. To determine the presence of polycystic ovaries, defined as more than eight follicles per ovary that are less than 10 mm (usually 2–8 mm) in diameter, a transvaginal ultrasound should be performed.

Long-Term Complications

CASE 50-1, QUESTION 2: E.F has a mother with diabetes and hypertension and a father with diabetes, hypertension, and dyslipidemia. Her significant laboratory values include the following:

Fasting glucose, 102 mg/dL
Low-density lipoprotein (LDL), 150 mg/dL
High-density lipoprotein (HDL), 52 mg/dL
Triglycerides, 130 mg/dL
Total cholesterol, 228 mg/dL

What risk does E.F. have for experiencing long-term complications from PCOS?

E.F. has an increased risk for experiencing impaired glucose tolerance, diabetes, and metabolic syndrome, especially considering her family history. Furthermore, the diagnosis of PCOS places her at possible increased risk for sleep apnea and endometrial cancer.

IMPAIRED GLUCOSE TOLERANCE AND DIABETES

Studies have shown that women with PCOS have a higher prevalence of impaired glucose tolerance, diabetes, and insulin resistance compared with women without the syndrome.[23] A family history increases the risk of these conditions further. In a study of 254 women with PCOS, 38.6% were found to have either impaired glucose tolerance (IGT) or undiagnosed diabetes.[24] Compared with those without PCOS, the prevalence of IGT and diabetes was significantly higher in both obese and nonobese (BMI <27 kg/m^2) women. Waist–hip ratio and BMI appeared to be the most clinically important predictors of glucose intolerance. Women with PCOS who have IGT appear to exhibit type 2 diabetes at higher rates than the general population.[23] Therefore, screening and diagnosis of these conditions is important for women with PCOS. E.F. is overweight and her mildly elevated fasting glucose and overweight suggest that she may be at increased risk for impaired glucose tolerance.

Glucose tolerance should be assessed in all women with PCOS using a fasting and 2-hour oral (75 g) glucose tolerance test.[23,25] Routine screening for diabetes with an oral glucose tolerance test should be performed for all women with PCOS by the age of 30 years.[26] The American Diabetes Association or World Health Organization criteria should be used for the appropriate diagnosis of IGT or diabetes. Insulin concentrations are typically not obtained in clinical settings because they are inaccurate.

METABOLIC SYNDROME AND CARDIOVASCULAR RISK

Approximately one-third to one-half of women with PCOS have metabolic syndrome. Using the National Cholesterol Education Panel-Adult Treatment Panel III criteria,[27–30] metabolic syndrome is present when the patient exhibits any three of these symptoms: abdominal obesity (>40 inches in men and >35 inches in women), triglycerides greater than or equal to 150 mg/dL, low HDL cholesterol (<40 mg/dL in men and <50 mg/dL in women), blood pressure greater than or equal to 130/85 mm Hg, and fasting glucose greater than or equal to 110 mg/dL. The incidence of a metabolic syndrome in women with PCOS is significantly higher than the rate for the general US population (45% vs. 6%, ages 20–29 years; 53% vs. 14%, ages 30–39 years) and independent of body weight.[30] It is believed that insulin resistance is the primary contributing factor to metabolic syndrome in women with PCOS.[31] Insulin resistance in the metabolic syndrome has been associated with a twofold increased risk of cardiovascular disease and a fivefold increased risk of type 2 diabetes.[32] Low HDL cholesterol (HDL-C) is seen most frequently in women with PCOS (68%), followed by increased BMI and waist circumference (67%), high blood pressure (45%), hypertriglyceridemia (35%), and elevated fasting glucose (4%).[28] Another group found that elevated fasting insulin concentrations, obesity, and a family history of diabetes conferred higher risk of having the metabolic syndrome in women with PCOS.[29]

Compared with women without PCOS, women with PCOS are reported to have a higher prevalence of cardiovascular risk factors, including hypertension, dyslipidemia, and surrogate markers for early atherosclerosis (e.g., increased C-reactive protein concentrations).[31] With increasing age, and especially as women with PCOS become postmenopausal, the risk of hypertension increases twofold.[33] Dyslipidemia in women with PCOS typically presents as decreased HDL-C (which is a strong predictor of cardiovascular disease in women), elevated triglycerides, elevated LDL cholesterol (LDL-C), and higher LDL–HDL ratios.[34] Women with PCOS are noted to have more atherogenic, small, dense LDL-C compared with controls and this substantially increases cardiovascular risk.[35] Women with PCOS may have other surrogate markers for early atherosclerosis and cardiovascular disease, impaired endothelial dysfunction, and other markers of cardiovascular risk such as coronary artery calcifications and increased carotid intima-media thickness.[31] Women with PCOS are considered to be at risk when any of these risk factors are present: obesity, cigarette smoking, hypertension, dyslipidemia, subclinical vascular disease, IGT, or family history of premature cardiovascular disease.[36] They are considered to be high risk when they have metabolic syndrome, type 2 diabetes mellitus, or overt vascular or renal disease. Although cardiovascular risk exists, data are inconclusive about whether women with PCOS have increased rates of morbidity and mortality from cardiovascular disease.

OBSTRUCTIVE SLEEP APNEA

Obstructive sleep apnea is cessation of breathing that occurs during sleep. It can disrupt sleep and cause daytime fatigue. Patients may not be aware that they are having the symptoms of sleep apnea, which include snoring and a gasping or snorting when breathing resumes. Studies indicate that the prevalence of obstructive sleep apnea in the PCOS is higher than expected and cannot be explained by obesity alone.[37–39] Insulin resistance appears to be a strong predictor of sleep apnea—more so than age, BMI, or the circulating testosterone concentration.[39]

ENDOMETRIAL HYPERPLASIA AND CANCER

Chronic anovulation in women with PCOS results in an endometrium that is exposed to the prolonged effects of estrogen unopposed by progesterone. Therefore, PCOS is a risk factor for endometrial hyperplasia. It is unknown if this translates into an increased risk for endometrial cancer because it is a rare occurrence in young women (4% of all cases occur in women younger than 40 years).[40] It is considered prudent management to induce artificial withdrawal bleeding by administering a course of progestin at least every 3 months to prevent endometrial hyperplasia in women with PCOS who experience either amenorrhea or oligomenorrhea. Alternatively, ultrasound scans can also be used to measure endometrial thickness and morphology every 6 to 12 months.

Treatment Goals

CASE 50-1, QUESTION 3: E.F. worries about becoming pregnant when she does not have regular periods. She also has mild hair growth above her upper lip which is somewhat bothersome. Given these concerns, what are the treatment goals for E.F.?

The primary goals for E.F. are to prevent pregnancy and address her hirsutism. Additionally, treatment goals in E.F. would include maintaining a normal endometrium, blocking the actions of androgens at target tissues, reducing insulin resistance and hyperinsulinemia, reducing weight, and preventing long-term complications. Other goals of treatment in patients with PCOS may include correcting anovulation or oligo-ovulation and improve fertility.

Therapy goals should encompass both long-term and short-term objectives because response to nonpharmacologic and pharmacologic therapy is slow, often requiring 3 to 9 months. Addressing long-term goals can minimize the risk for future complications and specifying short-term goals can improve motivation and adherence to therapy.

NONPHARMACOLOGIC TREATMENT

CASE 50-1, QUESTION 4: E.F. has indicated that she would like to lose weight. E.F. does not smoke, drinks one to two beers on weekends, and exercises by walking 20 minutes twice weekly. What nonpharmacologic method(s) would be most effective?

Weight reduction programs designed for a modest weight loss (5%–10%) with the incorporation of fitness are effective in reducing metabolic disease, cardiovascular risk, and improving ovulatory potential.[36] A 5% to 10% weight loss in E.F. would be 9 to 18 pounds. Diet modification and exercise are the most efficient, cost-effective, and safe ways to produce weight loss and improve the endocrine and metabolic parameters of PCOS.[36] Weight reduction should be considered first-line therapy in all overweight or obese women with PCOS and this should be recommended for E.F.

IMPACT OF WEIGHT LOSS IN POLYCYSTIC OVARY SYNDROME

A minimum 5% weight loss has consistently demonstrated restoration of regular menstrual cycling and ovulation in overweight and obese women with PCOS.[12,41,42] When lifestyle modification is implemented, free testosterone concentrations decrease, but clinical outcomes of acne and hirsutism are not often reported.[12] Obesity in PCOS is associated with a higher risk of developing endometrial cancer, but very limited evidence exists to determine the impact of weight loss on the incidence of endometrial cancer.[12] Studies of weight loss in women without PCOS indicate a 25% to 50% reduced risk of endometrial cancer, so it is logical that addressing weight reduction may lower that risk as well.[43,44] The Diabetes Prevention Program trial demonstrated a 53% prevalence of metabolic syndrome; the incidence of this was reduced 41% in the lifestyle modification group.[45,46] This was significantly better than treatment with metformin. Studies specifically evaluating cardiovascular improvements with weight loss in women with PCOS are limited, but improvements in dyslipidemia and insulin sensitivity have been noted.

DIET COMPOSITION

No single diet has been proven to be ideal for women with PCOS. A diet low in saturated fat and high in fiber from mostly low-glycemic-index–carbohydrate foods may, however, be suitable and is recommended.[12,47] Glycemic index is a classification of carbohydrates based on the blood glucose response during 2 hours. Low–glycemic index foods include bran cereals, mixed grain breads, broccoli, peppers, lentils, and soy. High–glycemic index foods, or those that should be minimized, include white rice and bread, potatoes, chips, and foods containing simple sugars (e.g., juice). It has been shown that in women with PCOS, oral glucose intake causes larger fluctuations in plasma glucose, increased hyperinsulinemia, and stimulated adrenal steroid secretion; protein was found to be a preferred nutrient over glucose.[48] The composition of a diet should be individualized to promote adherence and achieve specific goals.

EXERCISE

Exercise is a key component in the attainment and maintenance of weight loss. Exercise with muscle strengthening improves insulin sensitivity.[12] The American Heart Association recommends 150 minutes per week of moderate exercise or 75 minutes per week of vigorous exercise.[49] E.F. should continue to eat a healthy diet. A diet consisting of low saturated fats, high fiber, and foods with a low glycemic index should be encouraged. E.F. should increase her exercise to at least 75 minutes per week for at least 3 days of the week. If she is going to continue walking as her exercise, she should walk at a brisk pace. Titrating her time to a goal of exercising 60 minutes daily will help her lose weight.

Pharmacologic Treatment

CASE 50-1, QUESTION 5: E.F. would like to improve her menstrual irregularity, and be sure that she will not get pregnant. If possible, she would also like to minimize her hirsutism and acne. What options would be appropriate to recommend for E.F.?

Several different pharmacologic options could be recommended to E.F (Table 50-1). A combined oral contraceptive (COC) will address her concerns about irregular menstruation, hyperandrogenism, and pregnancy prevention. An insulin sensitizer would improve her menstrual irregularity and possibly reduce her hirsutism and acne, but it does not address her desire to prevent pregnancy. An antiandrogen, such as spironolactone, would address only hyperandrogenism and other agents would have to be used concurrently to address pregnancy prevention and the other hormonal and metabolic alterations in PCOS.

COMBINED ORAL CONTRACEPTIVES

Estrogen–progestin combination therapy with a COC is the treatment of choice for women seeking regularity in menstrual cycles and relief from hyperandrogenic symptoms (see Chapter 47, Contraception, for a list of possible therapies). The estrogen component suppresses LH, resulting in a reduction of androgen production, and increases hepatic production of SHBG, thereby reducing free testosterone. The progestins in various COCs possess variable androgenic effects, so the choice of the COC is important to minimize androgenic exposure. The potential effects of COCs on insulin resistance, glucose tolerance, and lipids have been debated and should be considered when choosing a progestin component.[50,51] Caution should be used in those who have insulin resistance, a high propensity to develop type 2 diabetes, or abnormal lipid profiles.

Combined oral contraceptive therapy in PCOS should be initiated with a formulation that contains a low dose or very low dose of estrogen (≤35 mcg of ethinyl estradiol) and a progestin with low androgenic or antiandrogen properties. Most COCs manufactured today have low or very low estrogen doses. Desogestrel and norgestimate are progestins with low androgen potential and drospirenone is an antiandrogen. A COC containing ethinyl estradiol and drospirenone would prevent pregnancy, improve menstrual cycle regularity, and reduce E.F.'s signs of hyperandrogenism (hirsutism and acne). If E.F. desired monthly cycles, she could take the typical 21/7 regimen (21 days active pill, 7 days inactive pill) or a 24/4 regimen (24 days active pill, 4 days inactive pill). Although not specifically evaluated in women with PCOS, a monophasic regimen may also be prescribed using extended cycles of 84 or even 365 days. Extended regimens reduce the number of cycles per year while providing contraception. Regardless of the COC selected, one of the long-term benefits is that her risk for endometrial cancer would be reduced by 50%, even up to two decades after discontinuation.[52–54] Ideal initial contraceptive options for E.F. include 30 to 35 mcg of ethinyl estradiol and a low-androgenic or nonandrogenic progestin such as drosperinone or desogestrel. If she would like to have her menstrual cycle monthly, she should take 21 active pills followed by 7 inactive pills. If she does not desire to have her menstrual cycle, then taking continuous active pills in an extended (daily) manner is most appropriate. This therapy would address her concerns of menstrual irregularity, contraception, hirsutism, and acne. She

TABLE 50-1
Selected Treatment Options for Polycystic Ovary Syndrome

Drug Class (Example)	Purpose of Therapy	Mechanism of Action	Effective Dose	Side Effects
Combined oral contraceptive (estrogen and progestin)	Menstrual cyclicity, hirsutism, acne	Suppresses LH (and FSH) and thus ovarian androgen production; increases sex hormone–binding globulin, which decreases free testosterone	One tablet orally daily for 21 (or 24) days, then 7-day (or 4-day) pill-free interval	Breast tenderness, breakthrough bleeding, mood swings, libido changes
Progestins (medroxy-progesterone)	Menstrual cyclicity	Creates withdrawal bleeding by transforming proliferative endometrium into secretory endometrium	5–10 mg orally daily for 10–14 days every 1–2 months	Breakthrough bleeding, spotting, mood swings
Biguanide (metformin)	Menstrual cyclicity, ovulation induction, hirsutism, acne, insulin lowering	Decreases hepatic glucose production, secondarily reducing insulin levels; may have direct effects on steroidogenesis	1,500 mg orally daily in divided doses (up to 2,550 mg/d)	Gastrointestinal problems, diarrhea, abdominal pain
Thiazolidinediones (pioglitazone)	Menstrual cyclicity, ovulation induction, hirsutism, acne, insulin lowering	Improves insulin sensitivity at target-tissue level (muscle, adipocyte); may have direct effects on steroidogenesis	Pioglitazone: 15–30 mg orally daily; maximum 45 mg orally daily	Edema, headache, fatigue, weight gain
Antiandrogen (spironolactone)	Hirsutism, acne	Inhibits androgens from binding to androgen receptor	50–100 mg orally twice daily	Hyperkalemia, polymenorrhea, headache, fatigue
Antiestrogen (clomiphene citrate)	Ovulation induction	Increases GnRH secretion, which induces rise in FSH and LH	50 mg orally daily for 5 days; may increase to 100 mg	Vasomotor symptoms, gastrointestinal problems

FSH, follicle-stimulating hormone; GnRH, gonadotropin-releasing hormone; LH, luteinizing hormone.

should continue therapy for as long as she desires contraception and minimization of the androgenic effects of PCOS.

CASE 50-1, QUESTION 6: Two months later, E.F. reports she is experiencing mood swings and weight gain on her ethinyl estradiol/drospirenone oral contraceptive. She is debating if she wants to continue with the COC and would like to explore other treatment possibilities. What other therapy options may be beneficial for E.F. if she considers her COC to be intolerable?

INSULIN SENSITIZERS

A reduction in insulin levels by using insulin sensitizers can ameliorate the sequelae of hyperinsulinemia and hyperandrogenemia. Currently viable insulin sensitizers include metformin and pioglitazone. More efficacy data are available regarding the use of metformin compared with the thiazolidinediones. Metformin was statistically significantly better in women with PCOS for ovulation induction when compared with rosiglitazone.[55] For these reasons, metformin tends to be the preferred insulin sensitizer for women with PCOS.

METFORMIN

Metformin inhibits hepatic glucose output, providing lower insulin concentrations and reducing androgen production in the ovary. Metformin also appears to influence ovarian steroidogenesis directly.[56] Most studies demonstrate that metformin improves menstrual cycle regulation, ovulation, and fertility in both obese and lean patients with PCOS.[57] Metformin has been used in ovulation induction protocols and has been shown to be very effective when used alone or with clomiphene citrate for inducing ovulation.[58,59] Data also indicate that insulin and free testosterone concentrations may be decreased 20% to 50% with metformin when used in women with PCOS.[60,61] Although few studies have been published on other clinical outcomes in PCOS, results suggest that metformin will produce reductions in hirsutism, acne, and BMI (especially in obese patients).[57] In a Cochrane systematic review comparing COCs and metformin, metformin demonstrated a reduction in fasting insulin and triglyceride levels compared to oral contraceptives, but greater improvement in menstrual pattern and serum androgen levels was observed with COCs.[62]

The most commonly used and most effective dose of metformin in PCOS is 500 mg orally three times daily (TID). It should be titrated slowly to this effective dose; doses up to 2,000 mg daily or 2,550 mg daily may be necessary for individual circumstances. The gastrointestinal (GI) side effects of diarrhea, nausea, vomiting, and abdominal bloating are usually transient and dose-related, and can be minimized by taking with food instead. Serum creatinine should be evaluated at least annually in women using metformin because it is contraindicated in women who have a serum creatinine greater than 1.4 mg/dL.

THIAZOLIDINEDIONES

Rosiglitazone and pioglitazone have been evaluated in women with PCOS, but studies have been small in number. These agents improve insulin action in the liver, skeletal muscle, and adipose tissue. They also are reported to directly affect ovarian steroid synthesis.[63] Rosiglitazone and pioglitazone are extremely effective at reducing insulin and androgen concentrations and have modest effects on hirsutism.[14] Rosiglitazone has demonstrated significantly better ovulation rates in women with PCOS compared with placebo, but it is less effective than metformin.[55] Other abstracts have indicated rosiglitazone may be beneficial for menstrual regularity, hyperandrogenism, and insulin sensitivity. It should be noted that the use of rosiglitazone has been significantly restricted by the US Food and Drug Administration (FDA) and will most likely not be used by women with PCOS.[64] Furthermore, rosiglitazone also appears to have a negative effect on the lipid profile, an unwanted outcome considering the potential long-term consequences of PCOS. Pioglitazone has proved to be as effective as metformin in small studies of women with PCOS and may be especially beneficial when used in combination with metformin for clinical and biochemical improvements.[65,66]

The starting recommended dose for pioglitazone is 15 or 30 mg orally daily. Adverse effects include edema, headache, fatigue, and potential liver enzyme elevations. Liver enzymes should be measured before initiation of treatment and periodically thereafter.

AGENTS FOR HIRSUTISM

Although frequently used, antiandrogens do not have FDA-approved uses for the treatment of female hirsutism or acne in the United States. Spironolactone is commonly prescribed to women for hirsutism. Drospirenone (a derivative of spironolactone), found in COCs has antiandrogenic properties and has also been evaluated in the long-term treatment of hirsutism.[67] Finasteride has been used for female hirsutism, but its lack of specificity for type I 5α-reductase in the pilosebaceous unit and toxicity may make this a suboptimal treatment choice. Flutamide is effective for hirsutism, but it is not used because of hepatoxicity. Eflornithine hydrochloride has been approved for topical use in treating facial hirsutism, but has not been well studied in women with PCOS.

SPIRONOLACTONE

Spironolactone acts by competitively inhibiting dihydrotestosterone (DHT) from interacting with its androgen receptor. This causes a decrease in activity of ovarian-produced testosterone. Spironolactone reduces hair growth by 40% to 88%; however, it takes 6 to 9 months for improvement.[68] Spironolactone may be associated with possible teratogenicity (feminization of the male fetus), so it is prudent to advise women to avoid pregnancy for at least 4 months after the discontinuation of spironolactone. It is recommended that spironolactone be used with a COC to avoid teratogenicity, as well as the side effect of polymenorrhea (more frequent menses) when used as monotherapy. Spironolactone in combination with a COC would also improve hormonal and metabolic manifestations of PCOS as well. The usual effective spironolactone dose is 50 to 100 mg orally twice daily for 6 to 12 months. Serum potassium and renal function should be monitored because this aldosterone antagonist can cause hyperkalemia. Furthermore, spironolactone should not be used with a COC containing drospirenone because of a potential risk for hyperkalemia.

FINASTERIDE

Finasteride is a type II 5α-reductase inhibitor, which decreases the conversion of testosterone to DHT. It provides an approximate 30% reduction from baseline for hirsutism. Compared with spironolactone, finasteride is as or less effective in women with hirsutism.[69] The dose of 5 mg to 7.5 mg orally daily typically takes 6 months for clinical improvement. It is critical to avoid pregnancy while taking this drug owing to the potential teratogenic effect of abnormal genitalia in the male fetus. Finasteride should not be touched or handled by women who are or may be pregnant. This danger limits the usefulness of finasteride in women with PCOS because most are of childbearing age or desire pregnancy.

E.F. should be encouraged to continue her COC for at least 3 months as most COC side effects resolve within 3 months of use. If E.F. decides that the side effects from the COC are intolerable, an appropriate recommendation for E.F. would be metformin orally titrated slowly to 1,500 mg daily (or 850 twice daily). She should continue this therapy for as long as she desires the benefits of this therapy, but it will not provide contraception. If E.F. gets pregnant, metformin should be discontinued.

CASE 50-1, QUESTION 7: E.F. successfully used oral contraceptives for 7 years. After getting married 3 years ago, E.F. and her husband have decided to have children. She lost 30 pounds with diet and exercise when she got married and has been able to maintain that weight loss. They have been trying to get pregnant for the last 18 months. The reason for infertility has been identified as oligo-ovulation associated with PCOS. What treatments for ovulation induction should be used in E.F. and why?

Anovulation or oligo-ovulation in women with PCOS is usually first treated with diet, exercise, and weight reduction. Weight loss improves pregnancy rates and reduces miscarriage rates in women with PCOS.[70] E.F. has been successful at losing weight and now must consider agents for ovulation induction.

AGENTS FOR OVULATION INDUCTION

CLOMIPHENE CITRATE

Clomiphene citrate induces ovulation via an antiestrogenic effect on the hypothalamus. GnRH secretion is increased, which increases LH and FSH production. The increase in FSH concentrations causes appropriate follicle development and estrogen secretion, which produces a positive feedback on the hypothalamic-pituitary system to create a LH surge for ovulation.

The usual initial dose of clomiphene citrate is 50 mg orally daily for 5 days, started on day 5 after a spontaneous or progestin-induced menses. The clinician must determine if ovulation occurs with each cycle through laboratory testing, ultrasound monitoring, or both. If ovulation does not occur, the dose can be increased by 50 mg orally daily up to 150 mg orally daily; however, doses greater than 100 mg orally daily for 5 days are not recommended by the manufacturers.[71] A repeat cycle can be administered as early as 30 days after the previous cycle as long as pregnancy has not occurred. If conception does not occur, women can use clomiphene for three to four cycles before considering another regimen. Long-term cyclic therapy is not recommended beyond a total of six cycles because of potential ovarian cancer risk. Most women respond to clomiphene citrate within three to four ovulatory cycles, but 5% to 10% have demonstrated clomiphene resistance and need to consider other options.[70,71] For women who are clomiphene-citrate–resistant, dexamethasone can be used in conjunction with clomiphene or an aromatase inhibitor can be used (e.g., letrozole, anastrozole) as an alternative for infertility in PCOS.[72–75]

The combination of clomiphene citrate plus metformin initially produced higher ovulation rates than either agent alone.[58] The most clinically relevant outcome for infertility, live birth, however, had not been fully investigated.[59] Investigators performed a randomized, controlled study to determine the live-birth rates in 626 women with PCOS taking extended-release metformin (1,000 mg twice daily), clomiphene citrate (50 mg orally daily and titrated to 150 mg orally daily if needed for ovulation), or both.[76] The live-birth rate was 22.5% in the clomiphene citrate group, 7.2% in the metformin group, and 26.8% in the combination group ($p < 0.001$ for metformin vs. clomiphene citrate and combination therapy). They concluded that clomiphene citrate was superior to metformin in achieving live-birth rates, although multiple births occurred in 6% (3 of 50) of live births. A Cochrane review indicated that metformin may not improve live-birth rates when combined with clomiphene; however, clinical pregnancy and ovulation rates are improved when the combination is used compared to clomiphene alone.[77]

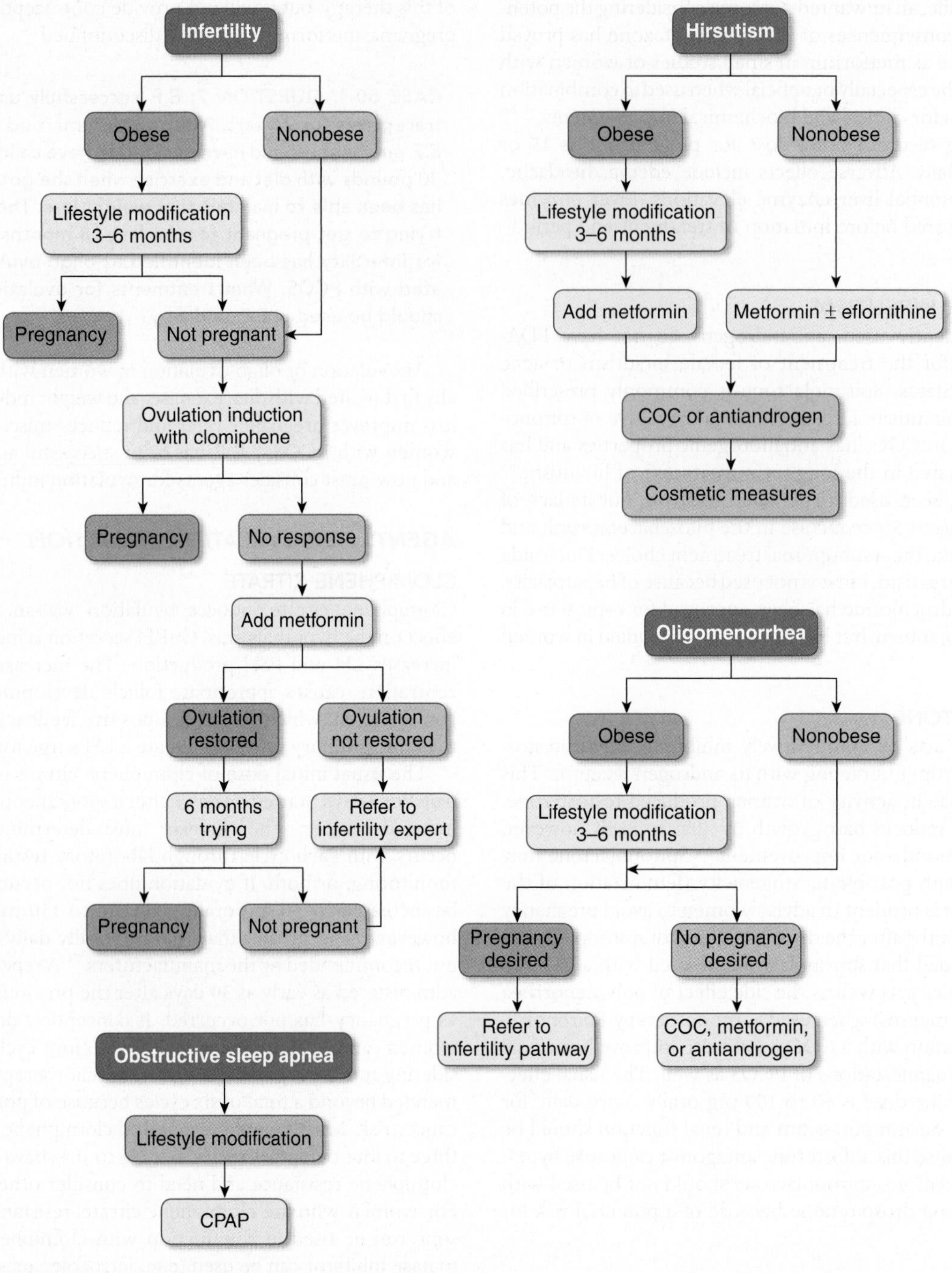

FIGURE 50-4 Treatment algorithm for polycystic ovary syndrome (PCOS). (Adapted with permission from Borgelt LM, Cheang KI. Polycystic ovary syndrome. In: Borgelt LM et al, eds. *Women's Health Across the Lifespan: A Pharmacotherapeutic Approach*. Bethesda, MD: American Society of Health-System Pharmacists; 2010:247.)

OTHER AGENTS

Although clomiphene citrate is the pharmacologic agent of choice in women with PCOS for infertility, it can only be used for a limited number of cycles and resistance can occur (see Chapter 48, Infertility). If clomiphene citrate alone is no longer an option, other regimens, including metformin (alone or in combination with clomiphene citrate), dexamethasone (in combination with clomiphene citrate), aromatase inhibitors, ovarian drilling, or controlled ovarian stimulation with gonadotropins can be recommended (Fig. 50-4).[78] Based on the evidence available, combination clomiphene citrate 50 mg orally daily and metformin 500 mg orally twice daily increasing to a minimum of 1,500 mg total daily dose is recommended in women not responding to clomiphene monotherapy.[71] If the combination of clomiphene and metformin is not successful, dexamethasone 0.25 mg at bedtime can be used in combination with clomiphene. Aromatase inhibitors and ovarian drilling are the next alternatives, followed by administration of gonadotropins or in vitro fertilization. Ovarian drilling is a laproscopic procedure by which a small portion of the ovary is removed via electric current to reduce hyperandrogenemia and improve ovulation. Its effects may only last a few months and it will not help with clinical signs of hyperandrogenism (e.g., hirsutism, acne). Gonadotropins are effective, but are generally reserved as one of the last options because of ovarian hyperstimulation syndrome. Egg retrieval and in vitro fertilization may be used in conjunction with gonadotropins to increase pregnancy rate and minimize the likelihood of multiple pregnancies by limiting the number of transferred embryos.[71]

Women with PCOS exhibit unique clinical features and have individual concerns that should be addressed when making treatment recommendations. Assessment should include gathering relevant medical information, such as menstrual history, signs and symptoms of hyperandrogenism, time course of symptoms, weight history, previous agents tried, and family history. If PCOS is suspected, laboratory assessments should be performed to rule out any other related disorders. Once a diagnosis has been made, a recommendation about treatment must consider the patient's priorities and motivation (Fig. 50-4). For E.F., clomiphene citrate is the pharmacologic agent of choice. Ovulation induction and conception occur in about 50% to 80% and 35% to 40% of women with PCOS, respectively, using clomiphene citrate. The initial dose should be 50 mg orally once daily for 5 days, started on day 5 after a spontaneous or progestin-induced menses. If ovulation does not occur, the dose can be increased by 50 mg orally daily up to 150 mg orally daily; however, doses greater than 100 mg orally daily for 5 days are not recommended. Although side effects (e.g., bloating, nausea, vomiting, and multiple gestation) can occur, the benefit of this therapy outweighs the risk for E.F. Appropriate follow-up for E.F. should include quality-of-life measures, laboratory monitoring when necessary, and medication adherence monitoring. Providers should be educators, facilitators, and empathetic listeners to help women with PCOS become informed and actively engaged in their therapy plan.

DYSMENORRHEA

Dysmenorrhea, or painful cramping that occurs with the onset and first days of menstruation, can be categorized as either primary (without underlying uterine pathology) or secondary (owing to underlying uterine pathology). Secondary dysmenorrhea can result from uterine conditions, including endometriosis, uterine polyps, or fibroids; complications of intrauterine device (IUD) use; or pelvic inflammatory disease.

Up to 93% of adolescents report some pain with menstruation, and up to 15% experience pain that is sufficiently severe and disabling to interfere with activities of daily life.[79] Dysmenorrhea is the single largest cause of lost productivity and school absence among adolescent girls. It most commonly begins within 1 to 2 years after the onset of menses.[80] The prevalence of primary dysmenorrhea decreases with age,[81] although menstrual cramps can occur in up to 50% of menstruating women regardless of age.[82]

Clinical Characteristics

CASE 50-2

QUESTION 1: A.B., a 17-year-old girl, presents at the pharmacy with complaints of severe cramping pain associated with her menstrual cycles. The pain predictably begins with the onset of menses and has been occurring for the past 5 years, but is now limiting A.B.'s ability to play sports in high school. A.B. states that she experienced her first menstrual period at age 11. The pain usually is "like a fist, clenching and relaxing," and it starts in the pelvic area, and radiates to her lower back. She reports no headache, but usually has diarrhea and some nausea, without vomiting. Her symptoms are most severe during the first 12 to 24 hours of her menses, then subside during the next few days. She usually takes two acetaminophen 325-mg tablets when her pain begins and then one tablet every 4 to 6 hours, as needed, with little relief. She has taken no other medications for her symptoms, has no known allergies to medications, and is not taking any other medications. She has no other medical problems. Her social history is significant for occasional social use of less than ten cigarettes and two to three alcoholic beverages per weekend. A recent physical examination was within normal limits. What clinical manifestations in A.B. are consistent with primary dysmenorrhea?

No specific diagnostic criteria exist for primary dysmenorrhea. Typically, the diagnosis is one of exclusion, and is based on response to known effective therapy. Thus, if patients do not respond to therapy, an investigation of pelvic pathology and secondary dysmenorrhea should occur.[82] A.B.'s symptoms that are typical of primary dysmenorrhea include cramping pain in the suprapubic area, which may radiate into the back and thighs, nausea, and diarrhea. Some women also experience vomiting, fatigue, headache, lightheadedness, flushing, loss of appetite, irritability, nervousness, and insomnia.[81] Symptom severity seems to correlate with women who have early menarche (onset of menses before age 8), and those with increased duration and quantity of menstrual flow.[83] Risk factors for dysmenorrhea include age younger than 20 years, depression or anxiety, nulliparity, menorrhagia, and smoking.[84]

Primary dysmenorrhea occurs only with ovulatory cycles, which typically begin after the first year following menarche. Dysmenorrhea occurring several years after menarche is most likely secondary dysmenorrhea, and should be investigated as such. Because A.B.'s pain began within 1 year of menarche and her physical examination is normal, a trial of an effective therapy can be initiated without further investigation into secondary causes of dysmenorrhea. The typical pattern of dysmenorrhea is to have pain beginning up to 12 hours before menses, increasing in severity for up to 24 hours, and continuing with reduced intensity for 24 to 72 hours.[81] A.B.'s description of pain, as a cramping–relaxing cycle, is typical for dysmenorrhea. Likely, her symptoms will decrease with age, after the onset of sexual activity, as well as after childbirth.[83]

Pathophysiology

CASE 50-2, QUESTION 2: What underlying pathophysiology explains A.B.'s symptoms?

In the normal menstrual cycle, prostaglandins are released by the endometrium in the late luteal phase inducing contraction of the uterine smooth muscle and subsequent sloughing of the endometrium, leading to menstrual flow and the beginning of the follicular phase of the next cycle. Women with primary dysmenorrhea appear to have increased prostaglandin secretion, inducing more intense uterine contractions, leading to decreased uterine blood flow and uterine hypoxia, which results in the cramping and pain that are the hallmarks of dysmenorrhea.[82] The decreasing levels of progesterone in the late luteal phase trigger the release of arachidonic acid from cell membranes, ultimately resulting in the production of prostaglandins and leukotrienes.[82]

The importance of prostaglandin secretion in the pathology of primary dysmenorrhea is confirmed by studies of the exogenous administration of prostaglandin $F_{2\alpha}$ ($PGF_{2\alpha}$), and PGE_2, each of which produce pain and uterine contractions similar to those observed in women with primary dysmenorrhea.[85] These prostaglandins, with potent platelet disaggregation and vasodilatory properties, also induce nausea, vomiting, and diarrhea. Thus, A.B.'s pain, nausea, and diarrhea may be caused by elevated prostaglandin levels. This also explains the rationale for the effectiveness of the two main treatments for primary dysmenorrhea: nonsteroidal anti-inflammatory drugs (NSAIDs), which inhibit prostaglandin synthesis, and hormonal contraceptives, which minimize the progesterone increase typically seen in the luteal phase (see Case 50-2, Questions 3–6, for more information).

Nearly 85% to 90% of women initially thought to have primary dysmenorrhea respond to NSAIDs with or without oral contraceptive therapy. The remaining women deserve further investigation into potential causes of secondary dysmenorrhea.[86]

Treatment

NONPHARMACOLOGIC TREATMENT

CASE 50-2, QUESTION 3: What nonpharmacologic therapies may be effective for the treatment of A.B.'s symptoms of primary dysmenorrhea?

A.B. should be educated about the causes of primary dysmenorrhea, its associated symptoms, and the rationale behind nonpharmacologic and pharmacologic treatment options. Nonpharmacologic therapies that may have benefit in the relief of A.B.'s symptoms include aerobic exercise, heat therapy, tobacco cessation, omega-3 polyunsaturated fatty acids, and high frequency transcutaneous electrical nerve stimulation.

Exercise, particularly aerobic exercise, has been correlated with decreased menstrual symptoms in observational studies, and is, in all patients, associated with positive general health benefits.[87] The benefit may be due to improved pelvic blood flow and decreased ischemia, or increased release of β-endorphins. Application of local heat to the lower abdomen has been studied in two clinical trials.[88,89] Heat plus ibuprofen (400 mg orally TID) demonstrated a reduction in the time to pain relief compared with an unheated patch plus ibuprofen.[88] Heat provided better relief than acetaminophen (1,000 mg orally as a single dose).[87] With few adverse effects, heat, in the form of a heating pad or heated patch or wrap device, represents a reasonable suggestion for women with dysmenorrhea.

Women should be advised and assisted in efforts to stop tobacco use. Although no direct evidence links smoking cessation with improvement in dysmenorrhea, an association exists with increased risk and severity of dysmenorrhea in women who smoke.[83] Increased intake of omega-3 polyunsaturated fatty acids, a low-fat vegetarian diet, or both may decrease the intensity and duration of symptoms.[90–92]

Transcutaneous electrical nerve stimulation has been evaluated in seven small trials, and when high frequency stimulation was used, it was more effective than placebo in achieving pain relief.[93] Acupuncture may also be effective, although few trials, using heterogeneous techniques and study designs, have been conducted, which makes interpretation difficult.[91] In extreme cases, surgical interruption of pelvic nerve pathways has been used as a last resort, with continued pain control up to 12 months in clinical trials.[94] Acupuncture has been evaluated as a treatment for primary dysmenorrhea in 27 randomized controlled trials, with positive results in pain reduction seen in several, but this result was diminished in trials that used the gold standard for acupuncture trials—sham acupuncture sites.[95]

A.B.'s therapy should be based on her specific symptoms, response to previous therapy, and any adverse effects of therapy. The regimen of acetaminophen that A.B. is currently using is not providing relief owing to its relative lack of effect on prostaglandin activity. For A.B., discussion of the nonpharmacologic therapies, particularly continuous low level heat applied at onset of symptoms, exercise, and smoking cessation, provide low-risk, potentially beneficial, and low-cost suggestions for pain relief, in addition to drug therapy. A.B should be informed that continuous heat therapy via heat "wraps" or hot water bottle or heating pad should be used cautiously in patients with diabetes, and should not be used while sleeping.

CASE 50-2, QUESTION 4: A.B states that her pain is decreased about 50% with the use of a heating pad, but she would rather not be sedentary for hours at a time. She finds the heat wraps uncomfortable and expensive and asks about Pamprin. What are some over-the-counter pharmacologic options for A.B.?

Although nonpharmacologic therapy with heat, exercise, and smoking cessation may have benefit, often the use of pharmacologic therapies is required to significantly improve functionality.

OVER-THE-COUNTER PHARMACOLOGIC THERAPY

Over-the-counter (OTC) pharmacologic therapy for primary dysmenorrhea is focused on reducing prostaglandin activity. Anti-inflammatory drugs act by directly inhibiting prostaglandin synthesis. NSAIDs provide relief from the symptoms of primary dysmenorrhea for most women (see Case 50-2, Question 5, for further information). Naproxen (as the sodium salt), ibuprofen, and ketoprofen are approved without a prescription for the treatment of primary dysmenorrhea. Acetaminophen is of limited efficacy in the treatment of dysmenorrhea when compared with NSAIDs or hormonal contraception.[96]

Other therapies, including OTC products marketed for dysmenorrhea and other menstrual disorders (e.g., Pamprin, Midol) (particularly combination products including diuretics), weak muscle relaxants (such as pyrilamine, pamabrom), diuretics (caffeine), and acetaminophen have limited efficacy for the specific treatment of dysmenorrhea. Because they do not address the underlying pathophysiology of primary dysmnenorrhea, combination products, narcotic analgesics, and acetaminophen do not have a role in the treatment of primary dysmenorrhea, and may have excessive adverse effects with this minimal benefit.

In adolescents, 91% reported using OTC medications to treat primary dysmenorrhea, usually without consultation from a health care professional.[80] This lack of professional advice resulted, however, in nearly 70% of women using less than 50% of the maximal dose of medication on day 1 of pain. Only 66% of patients choose to use ibuprofen, whereas 44% selected acetaminophen, 30% selected acetaminophen–pyrilamine combinations, and 10% acetaminophen, magnesium salicylate, and pamabrom combination products—which indicates that patients may benefit from professional advice regarding OTC treatments of dysmenorrhea. Other products include Vitamin B_1 100 mg orally daily, magnesium, vitamin B_6, and omega-3 fatty acids, which have all shown some benefit in pain relief compared with placebo, with Vitamin B_1 and magnesium showing the most promise.[92] Other dietary supplements, including fennel, vitamin E, neptune krill oil, and toki-shakuyaju-san, have been evaluated in small trials and need further study.[86] At this point, given the limited efficacy of nonNSAID, nonhormonal methods of treatment, they are not an appropriate alternative for A.B. Ibuprofen 200 mg to 400 mg orally up to three times daily could be a good consideration for A.B.'s menstrual cramps.

PRESCRIPTION PHARMACOLOGIC AGENTS: NONSTEROIDAL ANTI-INFLAMMATORY DRUGS

CASE 50-2, QUESTION 5: A.B has tried OTC ibuprofen 400 mg three times daily starting at onset of her cramping symptoms, but has not had optimal relief. A.B. presents to her family physician for an evaluation. What prescription medications could be recommended for A.B's dysmenorrhea?

The NSAIDs are effective for treatment of dysmenorrhea, but in some cases, OTC doses are not enough and prescription-strength NSAIDs or hormonal contraceptives may be required for adequate relief. Hormonal contraceptives reduce the amount of endometrial proliferation and, as a result, decrease the amount of prostaglandins secreted. By inhibiting ovulation, hormonal contraceptives eliminate the cyclic changes in progesterone that induce prostaglandin release. Choice of therapy depends on the need for contraception, concomitant medical conditions, and patient preference. Treatment efficacy can be monitored by evaluating pain relief, improved functionality, reduced absenteeism, and relief of other symptoms (e.g., diarrhea, nausea) associated with dysmenorrhea. Because A.B. is not sexually active, prescription-strength NSAIDs should be tried for two to three cycles before switching to other agents.

Initial selection of NSAID therapy should be based on effectiveness, incidence of adverse effects, cost, patient history of previous benefit, and availability. In a Cochrane review, 73 trials of NSAIDs for treatment of primary dysmenorrhea were reviewed to assess for any differences in efficacy or safety among the different NSAIDs.[97] When compared with placebo, NSAIDs were significantly more effective (odds ratio [OR], 4.50; 95% confidence interval [CI], 3.85–5.27). When compared with acetaminophen, NSAIDs were, as expected, significantly better at reducing symptoms (OR, 1.90; 95% CI, 1.05–3.44). In limited head-to-head trials comparing NSAIDs, no significant differences in efficacy were seen, with the exception of aspirin being slightly less effective than other NSAIDs when directly compared. Adverse effects seen in these trials were generally mild GI (nausea, upset stomach) and neurologic (sleepiness, dizziness, headache) complaints. When directly compared with each other, no NSAID was found to be better tolerated than another. Naproxen and ketoprofen offer the advantage of less frequent dosing compared with ibuprofen.

Some data suggest that an oral loading dose of naproxen sodium (550 mg) might improve pain control in dysmenorrhea. A randomized trial demonstrated increased relief from dysmenorrhea symptoms in adolescents treated with an NSAID regimen that started with a loading dose, versus those who used a flat dosing regimen.[98] Loading doses generally are twice the regular dose. Although all NSAIDs that have been studied for the treatment of dysmenorrhea appear to be equally effective at reducing pain, there may be theoretic advantages to those that achieve peak serum concentrations 30 to 60 minutes after administration (ibuprofen, naproxen, naproxen sodium, and meclofenamate). Some claim that meclofenamate is more beneficial for the treatment of dysmenorrhea because of its ability to block both the cyclo-oxygenase and the lipoxygenase pathway in the formation of prostaglandins, but this pharmacologic difference does not appear to confer a clinically significant advantage.[81] If A.B. experienced adverse effects with the higher loading dose, an alternative strategy is to initiate dosing 24 hours before menses is expected to start, based on the calendar if the patient has predictable cycles, or based on the start of premenstrual-syndrome–type symptoms. This prophylactic dosing may be helpful especially for patients who have severe dysmenorrhea with absenteeism and decreased work or school productivity.[82,97] Although no specific evidence supports the use of scheduled NSAID dosing regimens, avoiding as needed (PRN) dosing may provide consistent serum levels to maintain reduced prostaglandin levels. As the duration of therapy is typically limited to 2 or 3 days, risk of adverse effects tends to be outweighed by the potential benefit of loading doses, prophylactic dosing, and scheduled versus PRN therapy.

Although the cyclo-oxygenase-2 selective inhibitor, celecoxib, is approved for the treatment of primary dysmenorrhea, it has not been directly compared with conventional NSAIDs for effectiveness for pain control. The FDA-approved dosing of celecoxib is a 400-mg loading dose, followed by 200 mg that same day if needed, then 200 mg twice daily thereafter. Increased cost, lack of increased benefit, and limited data regarding differences in GI safety make celecoxib a second-line therapy for primary dysmenorrhea. A good recommendation for A.B. could include initiating naproxen sodium 550 mg orally at the beginning of menses, followed by 275 mg every 8 hours thereafter for the 2 to 3 days she experiences dysmenorrhea.

Adverse Effects

CASE 50-2, QUESTION 6: What adverse effects might A.B. experience from her NSAID?

All NSAIDs have a similar adverse effect profile. Nausea, vomiting, indigestion, anorexia, diarrhea, constipation, abdominal pain, melena, and bloating are common GI complaints.

Careful attention should be given to previous trials of NSAIDs for dysmenorrhea and other conditions, because women may respond favorably to one NSAID over another. If a 2-month or 3-month trial at appropriate doses of one NSAID is unsuccessful for A.B., another agent from a different class may be tried. Because dysmenorrhea is most prevalent in younger women who tend to be healthy, the risk of adverse events may be lower than would be expected in an older population.

Contraindications

CASE 50-2, QUESTION 7: What medical history information is important to avoid serious adverse effects?

A.B should be questioned about medication allergies and any prior history of ulceration or GI bleeding; a history of cardiovascular and renal disease, although uncommon in young women, should be elicited before prescribing therapy. A thorough medication history, including OTC agents and dietary supplements, should be conducted. Particular attention should be paid to any potential therapeutic duplications (e.g., prescription and OTC NSAIDs), drug–drug (e.g., warfarin), and drug–disease (hypertension) interactions.

Women who are allergic to aspirin or have a history of allergic reaction to any NSAID should not use NSAIDs or celecoxib. Celecoxib should also be avoided in women who are allergic to sulfa drugs. A.B. has not had a previous allergic reaction to NSAID or aspirin; she is not taking any medications that may interact and does not have any history of medical problems that would prevent her from a trial of NSAID therapy.

HORMONAL CONTRACEPTION

Oral Contraceptives

CASE 50-2, QUESTION 8: After 6 months of treatment, A.B. has some relief of her pain, nausea, and diarrhea with the naproxen sodium, but is unhappy with the amount of time that she is spending at home due to menstrual cramps. She is asking about other treatment options for further pain relief. What other options are available for A.B.?

As mentioned previously, hormonal contraceptives may be an option in A.B. if prescription NSAIDs are not adequate for her symptoms. Oral contraceptives (OCs) suppress ovulation, decrease menstrual fluid volume, and subsequently decrease prostaglandin production and uterine cramping.[79,81] OCs alone, or in combination with an NSAID, are appropriate as first-line treatment in women with or without a need for contraception.[99] OCs relieve dysmenorrhea symptoms in 50% to 80% of women within 3 to 6 months after beginning hormone therapy.[100] A study of healthy adolescent women with primary dysmenorrhea evaluated the effects of a 20 mcg ethinyl estradiol/100 mcg levonorgestrel oral contraceptive pill as compared with placebo during a 3-month period.[101] With OC use, women reported decreased severity of pain, and used less pain medication. A Cochrane review of oral contraceptives and primary dysmenorrhea found oral contraceptives containing less than 35 mcg of ethinyl estradiol to be effective at reducing pain, but failed to demonstrate a significant difference between various 35-mcg ethinyl estradiol OC formulations.[100] Selection of an OC should be based on factors presented in Chapter 47, Contraception. Although many providers prescribe extended cycles of oral contraceptives to treat primary dysmenorrhea, no evidence suggests that this practice is more effective than the customary 21-day active pills, 7-day placebo pills regimen.[86,102] A change from this traditional dosing to continuous dosing may be considered if symptoms occur during the placebo week.

Adverse effects and contraindications associated with OC use must be considered (see Chapter 47, Contraception). Although serious complications from OC use are uncommon in young, healthy women, breakthrough bleeding and spotting, nausea, and breast tenderness may occur, especially early in treatment. A.B. may choose to add an OC to her naproxen sodium, with potentially improved pain relief compared with either agent alone. If pain does not respond to either course of therapy, investigation via laparoscopy for causes of secondary dysmenorrhea may be necessary.

Other Hormonal Contraceptive Agents

Other hormonal contraceptive agents that suppress ovulation have also been used in the treatment of primary dysmenorrhea, although none have undergone rigorous trials for this indication.[86] The levonorgestrel intrauterine system (IUS) is associated with amenorrhea and a reduction in dysmenorrhea over time, unlike the copper IUD, which may result in increased pain, cramping, and blood loss. Three years after insertion, fewer women with a levonorgestrel IUS reported menstrual pain (60% baseline, 29% after 3 years), with 47% of women with amenorrhea.[103] In women with primary dysmenorrhea at low risk of sexually transmitted infections, and desiring long term contraception, the levonorgestrel IUS would be an option.

Medroxyprogesterone depot injection is another hormonal contraceptive agent that has been used to treat primary dysmenorrhea. Nearly two-thirds of adolescents reported fewer symptoms of dysmenorrhea with injections every 3 months.[81] Negative effects of medroxyprogesterone injections on bone density should be weighed with potential benefit when considering this option (see Chapter 47, Contraception). Given that A.B.'s past history does not include any absolute contraindications to combined oral contraceptives and her dysmenorrhea symptoms have not been well-controlled with prescription NSAIDs, she is a candidate for combined hormonal contraception. A trial of combined oral contraceptives used in a continuous manner for 3 months (3 months of active pills, then 7 days of placebo pills) would be an appropriate plan for better control of her dysmenorrhea. In addition to smoking cessation, she should be counseled that hormonal contraceptives may require 3 or more months to provide maximal relief of symptoms. The goals of therapy, namely, reduction in pain and associated symptoms, as well as improvement in functionality, should be explained to A.B. and reviewed at each contact.

ENDOMETRIOSIS

Endometriosis is defined as the presence of functional endometrial tissue occurring outside the uterine cavity. It is the most common cause of secondary dysmenorrhea in young women, and can result in chronic pelvic pain, infertility, and dyspareunia.[81] The ovaries are commonly the site of endometriosis, which can also be found in the pelvic peritoneum, cervix, vagina, vulva, rectosigmoid colon, and appendix.

For an illustration that shows common sites of endometriosis, go to http://thepoint.lww.com/AT10e.

Less common sites of implantation of endometrial tissue include the umbilicus, scar tissue resulting from surgery, kidneys, lungs, and even arms and legs.[104] Endometriosis is present in up to 45% of women with infertility. Overall, it is difficult to determine the prevalence of endometriosis, because many women do not experience symptoms or seek treatment, and formal diagnostic criteria currently require visual identification of endometrial tissue during surgery. In women who have laparotomies for any reason, endometriosis is identified in 5% to 15%. This increases to 33% in women with chronic pelvic pain.[104] In contrast to primary dysmenorrhea, endometriosis usually occurs in women who have been menstruating for some time; it can provoke pain that is not limited to the time of the menses, but can occur anytime throughout the cycle. Endometriosis is rarely seen in women near the menarche, after menopause, or in amenorrheic women. Given the many women with endometriosis, the expense of diagnosis and treatment, and the infertility associated with it, endometriosis represents a significant area of cost in the health care system.[105]

Diagnostic Criteria

Diagnosis of endometriosis is difficult, with a delay in diagnosis in the range of 8 to 12 years from initial symptom presentation.[106] Endometriosis, interstitial cystitis, irritable bowel syndrome, and pelvic adhesions represent the four most common causes of chronic pelvic pain (defined as pain not associated with the menses, severe in nature, resulting in functional disability, and lasting at least 6 months).[107] The delay in diagnosis is the unfortunate consequence of the lack of diagnostic laboratory markers, and its similarities to these other conditions. The physical examination is often normal, although the most common physical finding is a fixed retroverted uterus, with scarring and tenderness. A definitive diagnosis is only possible with visualization of endometriosis on laparoscopy, although this is not considered as absolutely necessary today as it has been in the past.[108] Although no diagnostic criteria currently exist, endometriosis can be staged at the time of laparoscopy according to the Revised American Fertility Society Classification of Endometriosis.[109] The stages are classified as minimal (stage I), mild (stage II), moderate (stage III), and severe (stage IV), as determined by an accumulated point total, with points based on the location of the endometrial lesions, the size of the lesions, the presence and extent of the adhesions, and the degree of obliteration of the posterior cul-de-sac. The classification system is designed to document the location and extent of endometriosis and does not predict infertility, aid in treatment selection or outcomes, or predict recurrence of disease. Making diagnosis and prognosis more difficult is that the reported severity of pelvic pain and level of functional disability do not seem to be correlated to the stage of endometriosis.[104]

Pathophysiology

Although the first description of endometriosis was made in the 1860s, the precise etiology of endometriosis remains a mystery. Several theories exist regarding the origins of endometriosis, and the exact etiology is probably a complex interplay between physical and individual patient-specific immunologic factors.[104]

The most commonly cited theory is that of retrograde menstruation or the flow of menstrual fluid, endometrial cells, and other debris backward through the fallopian tubes resulting in implantation in the peritoneal cavity. Once endometrial cells reach the peritoneum, stimulated angiogenesis (potentially by estrogen, among other factors) appears to be a determinant of the development and growth of lesions.[110,111] Also at this point, the lesion stimulates an immune response, triggering the activation of macrophages, as well as cytokine and growth factor release. Peritoneal lesions may contribute to more distant disease by spread via hematogenous or lymphatic routes, or even by movement owing to iatrogenic causes, such as cesarean sections and other forms of gynecologic surgery. Outflow obstruction of the genital tract may also contribute to retrograde menstruation and endometriosis, particularly in adolescents with primary amenorrhea. Investigation and removal of obstruction(s) may impede the course of the disease in those patients.[104,111,112] Although the retrograde menstruation theory makes scientific sense, it has been discovered that retrograde menstruation occurs in nearly all menstruating women (90%), and not all women have endometriosis. This suggests that an additional factor, such as genetic susceptibility or altered immunity, or altered hormone receptor functioning such as progesterone resistance, must be present for the pathogenesis of endometriosis in certain patients.[113]

Another theory for the etiology of endometriosis is the coelomic metaplasia theory. This theory rests on the belief that the coelomic epithelium, the fetal originator tissue for the reproductive tract, retains its ability to differentiate into multiple cell types.[104,112,113] The trigger for differentiation is thought to be, in part, estrogen or environmental factors. This theory would explain the presence of endometriosis in prepubertal girls, in women born without a uterus, and in the rare cases of endometriosis seen in men. Genetics also play a role in the development of endometriosis. For first-degree relatives of women with severe endometriosis, there is a six times higher rate of developing endometriosis when compared with women who do not have affected relatives. These woman also have more severe disease and disease that appears earlier in life.[106,114] More than 15 different gene and gene-product abnormalities have been documented in women with endometriosis. Environmental factors, as discussed, are intriguing in their role as potential causative factors, but are not definitive.[113,114]

Once endometrial tissue becomes implanted, hormones are necessary for their continued growth. As with intrauterine endometrium, the implants of endometriosis possess estrogen, progesterone, and androgen receptors. The endometrial implants may, however, respond differently to hormonal stimulation than normal endometrium. In general, estrogens stimulate the implants, whereas androgens or lack of estrogen results in implant atrophy. Because of their complex hormonal effects, progestins have variable effects on the implants.[109,113,115] In addition, lesions also show high levels of estrogen biosynthesis, owing to abnormally increased aromatase activity, with a concomitant decrease in the inactivation of estrogen, resulting in high intralesional estrogen concentrations.[113,116] The responsiveness of endometrial implants to ovarian hormones plays a role in the pathology of endometriosis. Withdrawal of estrogen and progesterone causes the endometrial implants to bleed, leading to an inflammatory response in the adjacent tissues. Repetitive cycles of bleeding and inflammation lead to the development of scar tissue and adhesions between adjacent peritoneal tissues. On laparoscopy, these areas of involvement appear as multiple hemorrhagic foci composed of endometrial epithelium, stroma, and glands. Ovarian endometriosis usually involves the formation of endometriomas, blood-filled cysts ("chocolate cysts") ranging in size from microscopic to 10 cm. Nodules may form on uterosacral ligaments. Fibrosis usually is present with the endometrial implants, and extensive adhesions may form between pelvic structures.[117]

Clinical Characteristics

CASE 50-3

QUESTION 1: N.H. is a 32-year-old woman who has been married for 6 years, and is currently using the vaginal contraceptive ring to prevent pregnancy. She and her spouse have been contemplating the timing of a pregnancy, but have not yet attempted to become pregnant. She presents to her gynecologist to discuss preconceptual planning, and reports that she has been having severe lower abdominal cramps, associated with her menses, occurring on day 1 and lasting until day 4 or 5. This has been occurring for the past 4 years after many years of pain-free cycles, and has recently been increasing in severity. The pain is slightly relieved by ibuprofen 400 mg orally TID, and during the past 6 months she has had to work from home at least 1 to 2 days per month owing to pain that has been increasing in frequency. On further questioning, she also reports mild to moderate pain that occurs randomly in her cycle, associated with low-back pain, constipation with painful defecation, and pain with intercourse. Her menstrual history reveals menarche at age 10 with regular cycles every 26 to 27 days and heavy menses for 6 to 7 days. She reports discussing her symptoms with her mother, who described similar symptoms during her childbearing years.

N.H. is 5 feet 7 inches and weighs 145 pounds. She smokes one-half pack of cigarettes per day, and does not drink alcohol. She plays recreation league basketball and softball, but does not have a regular exercise regimen. She usually eats five servings of fruits or vegetables per day, but does not like to drink milk. She is concerned about her heart because her father had a cardiac stent placed at age 40, and she has been told she has high cholesterol.

Her physical examination is normal, with the exception of tenderness on palpation of the posterior fornix, and a fixed retroverted uterus. A pregnancy test, and tests for gonorrhea and chlamydia, are negative, and a Pap smear is within normal limits. What subjective and objective data in N.H.'s presentation is compatible with a diagnosis of endometriosis?

A woman presenting with endometriosis may have signs and symptoms that are difficult, initially, to distinguish from primary dysmenorrhea[118] (Table 50-2). N.H.'s symptoms of lower abdominal cramps accompanying her menses are often mistaken for primary dysmenorrhea when other history details are not evaluated in total. N.H.'s age and her nulliparity are consistent with the characteristics of women with endometriosis. Although endometriosis has been diagnosed in women of all ages, it most commonly occurs in women in their late 20s and early 30s who have delayed pregnancy or who have infrequent pregnancies.

N.H.'s menstrual pattern of short cycle length with prolonged flow is characteristic of women with endometriosis. Risk factors for endometriosis are related to exposure to estrogen (i.e.,

TABLE 50-2
Primary Versus Secondary Dysmenorrhea

Characteristic	Primary Dysmenorrhea	Secondary Dysmenorrhea
Onset	Around menarche	Any age (while menstruating)
Timing in menstrual cycle	Worse on day 1, lasts 24–48 hours	Increases in severity, may last days
Change over time	Stable, predictable	Increasing pain with increasing age
Symptoms	Low back pain, premenstrual syndrome, nausea, bloating	Low back pain, dyspareunia, diarrhea or constipation, dysuria, infertility
Signs	Normal pelvic examination	Fixed retroverted uterus, tenderness, but may be completely normal

Source: Reddish S. Dysmenorrhea. *Aust Fam Physician.* 2006;35:82.

early menarche and late menopause), and shorter menstrual cycle length (<28 days) with longer duration of menstrual flow (≥6 days), as well as having a mother or sister with endometriosis, as may be true with N.H.'s mother.[119] Women who have four or more pregnancies lasting greater than 6 months have a 50% lower risk of being diagnosed with endometriosis, and there is a decrease in risk of endometriosis that is parallel to duration of time spent breastfeeding.[119] Higher BMI and shorter stature are associated with a lower risk of endometriosis, with a 12% to 14% decreased likelihood of diagnosis for every unit (kg/m^2) increase in BMI.[119] Potential, but not yet confirmed, risk factors that have been identified include higher social class, exposure to dioxins, and intake of caffeine and alcohol.[119] Cigarette smoking appears to reduce the risk for endometriosis, although studies are not conclusive.[112,114] Women with several immune-mediated conditions, including rheumatoid arthritis, systemic lupus erythematosus, hypothyroidism and hyperthyroidism, and multiple sclerosis, also have a higher rate of endometriosis than women without these immune medicated conditions.[119]

N.H.'s chief complaints center on her progressive pelvic pain occurring throughout the cycle, with worsening during menses, constipation, and pain with intercourse (dyspareunia). Women who report pain during intercourse may have a fixed, retroverted uterus (as N.H. does) or endometriosis located in the posterior fornix of the vagina or along the uterosacral ligaments.[104] This pain may persist for several hours after intercourse. Other symptoms such as the constipation and painful defecation N.H. is experiencing are associated with endometriosis and may (but not always) depend on the organs affected by the location of the endometrial tissue[120,121] (Table 50-3). Depression also is a common symptom in patients with endometriosis, particularly those with chronic pelvic pain, and may express as sadness, somatic complaints, and inability to work or carry on activities of normal living.[122]

Although it is unclear yet whether infertility will be a problem in N.H., endometriosis occurs in up to 45% of women with infertility.[104] The cause of endometriosis-associated infertility is not clear, but is probably caused by a combination of factors, which may include physical distortion of the pelvic architecture, inflammatory factors (including prostanoids, cytokines, and growth factors that may interfere with normal reproductive processes), impaired folliculogenesis (follicle development), or defects in fertilization or implantation.[123,124] Treatment for endometriosis, in inducing a "pseudomenopause," results in impaired fertility while the disease is actively being treated.

N.H.'s limited physical findings are not uncommon in women with endometriosis; physical findings, other than visualization of endometrial tissue during exploratory surgery, may not be present, and outward physical findings may have no correlation with the stage of endometriosis determined with surgery. Many symptoms and physical findings of endometriosis can be associated with other gynecologic conditions or diseases (particularly irritable bowel syndrome), and, if the patient is not responsive to empiric therapy, laparoscopy is indicated to confirm the diagnosis. N.H.'s negative pregnancy, chlamydia, and gonorrhea tests, as well as her normal Pap smear, are reassuring. Other laboratory tests that have been evaluated to diagnose endometriosis have not been sufficiently sensitive or specific in clinical trials to be routinely used. The CA-125 lab test is not sufficiently sensitive or specific enough as a single test to diagnose endometriosis.[125]

Treatment

CASE 50-3, QUESTION 2: N.H.'s pain is uncontrolled after trials of three different NSAIDs (ibuprofen, naproxen, and meloxicam) and she would like relief to improve her functionality at work and home. Given the potential mechanisms behind the pathophysiology of endometriosis, what therapeutic approaches are appropriate for the treatment of endometriosis in N.H.?

Therapy for endometriosis should be individualized and consider N.H.'s desire for future fertility, severity of symptoms, extent

TABLE 50-3
Location of Endometriosis and Associated Symptoms

Sites	Symptoms
Pelvic	
Cervix	Abnormal uterine bleeding
Ovaries	Dysmenorrhea
Peritoneum	Dyspareunia
Rectovaginal septum	Infertility
Uterosacral ligaments	Pelvic pain
Intestinal	
Abdominal scars	Intestinal obstruction
Sigmoid colon	Midabdominal pain
Small intestines	Nausea
	Painful defecation
	Rectal bleeding
Urinary Tract	
Bladder	Cyclic flank pain
Ureter	Hematuria
	Hydronephrosis
	Hydroureter

Source: American College of Obstetricians and Gynecologists. ACDG Practice Bulletin No. 114. Management of endometriosis. *Obstet Gynecol.* 2010;116:223.

of disease, and potential for infertility. This should be done with the knowledge that a high likelihood exists of recurrence and a lack of good prognostic indicators for future severity. The goals of treatment are to relieve symptoms and, if desired, to preserve or improve fertility. Options currently available to treat endometriosis include definitive and conservative surgery, hormonal therapy with estrogen–progestin combinations or progestins alone, danazol, aromatase inhibitors, or the GnRH agonists, and expectant management. Pharmacologic treatment of endometriosis is based on manipulation of this hormonal response: danazol, GnRH agonists, progestins, aromatase inhibitors, and estrogen–progestin combination all result in endometrial tissue atrophy. No treatment has been shown to provide 100% protection against recurrence when discontinued; even surgical removal of the uterus and ovaries is associated with recurrence rates of up to 10%.[111]

PAIN MANAGEMENT: PHARMACOLOGIC THERAPY

NONSTEROIDAL ANTI-INFLAMMATORY DRUGS

NSAIDs, particularly those available as OTC products, are often the first medications that women try for relief of pain from endometriosis, often before they are officially diagnosed. Although typically not thought of as "disease modifying agents," NSAIDs may have a role beyond pain control because of the presence of increased cyclo-oxygenase (both 1 and 2) expression in endometriosis lesions.[116] Although evidence at this point is predominantly in animal models, a potential exists for non–pain-related benefits with NSAIDs in endometriosis. NSAIDs may provide some relief of mild symptoms, particularly in women with endometriosis who have pain associated with the menses (see Dysmenorrhea section), and are an appropriate first choice for women with mild symptoms who do not desire contraception. They should not be the only therapy offered to patients with confirmed endometriosis.[126] Clinicians should be aware of and consider the potential for endometriosis in patients with noncyclic pain, including pain that does not respond to an appropriate trial of an NSAID. N.H. has tried three different NSAIDS with limited relief; a higher dose or trial of another NSAID is not an appropriate strategy at this time. Additional treatment should be considered.

COMBINED HORMONAL CONTRACEPTIVES

For women who do not receive pain relief from a trial of an NSAID, a reasonable next step for those women desiring contraception is the use of oral contraceptives because they are considerably better tolerated over the long term versus other hormonal options. They may be used alone or in combination with NSAIDs. OCs improve symptoms of endometriosis by inhibiting ovulation, decreasing hormone levels, reducing menstrual flow, potentially to the point of amenorrhea. These mechanisms contribute to atrophy of endometrial implants. When used, the most appropriate regimen is continuous OC dosing, so that there is not a "placebo week" that allows for growth of endometrial implants. In a trial of patients who did not respond to cyclic OCs, use of continuous dosing resulted in significant pain reduction.[127] A Cochrane review found that the pain reduction seen with OCs ($\leq$35 mcg of ethinyl estradiol) is similar to a GnRH analog (goserelin).[128] A recent trial directly compared cyclic and continuous administration of a 20 mcg ethinyl estradiol/gestodene 0.075 mg oral contraceptive, and the recurrence rate of endometriomas was improved in both groups, with a nonstatistically significant trend toward an improved response in the continuous group.[129]

Combined contraceptives that are not oral have also been evaluated for their efficacy in the treatment of endometriosis. With the main outcome measure of satisfaction with treatment, a study of 207 women with moderate or severe pelvic pain after conservative surgery found that women who self-selected for the contraceptive ring were more likely to be satisfied with their treatment than those who self-selected the contraceptive patch.[130] Cycle control with continuous use of each regimen was poor, and many patients reverted to cyclic use, with improvement in bleeding rates. Pain and NSAID use rates decreased in both groups.

PROGESTINS

Similarly to oral contraceptives, injectable progestins reduce symptoms of endometriosis by inhibiting ovulation, reducing hormone levels, and inducing endometrial atrophy. They may be particularly useful if estrogen use is contraindicated. Regimens used include oral medroxyprogesterone, depot medroxyprogesterone (see Case 50-3, Question 5), or the levonorgestrel IUS. More recent studies have evaluated the use of the levonorgestrel IUS as a means of providing consistent progestin dosing. The IUS has the advantage of providing longer term contraception. When compared with leuprolide depot (a GnRH agonist), the levonorgestrel IUS provided similar benefits in reducing pelvic pain, with a decreased potential for hypoestrogenic effects, and an increased potential for early breakthrough bleeding, followed by eventual amenorrhea.[131]

A 3-year direct comparison of the levonorgestrel IUS versus depot medroxyprogesterone was conducted in patients with moderate to severe endometriosis for medical control of symptoms after conservative surgery.[132] Although symptoms were improved with both regimens, more IUS patients remained adherent to the regimen, and at 3 years, bone density was increased in the IUS group, and decreased in the depot group.

Progestins, despite being as effective as GnRH agonists in the treatment of pain, have increased side effects when compared with OCs, primarily weight gain (particularly with the depot formulation), initial breakthrough bleeding followed by amenorrhea, and, with depot formulations, decreased bone density with prolonged use, placing them after combined hormonal contraception in choice of therapy.

GONADOTROPIN-RELEASING HORMONE AGONISTS

GnRH agonists induce a pseudomenopausal state, resulting in relief of endometriosis symptoms. Because the GnRH agonists have a longer half-life than endogenous GnRH, their binding to GnRH receptors in the pituitary results in downregulation of the hypothalamic-pituitary-ovarian axis, decreasing release of FSH and LH, leading to low estrogen levels and amenorrhea.[133] GnRH agonists are available in a variety of dosage forms, outlined in Table 50-4. When compared in clinical trials, GnRH agonists have efficacy that is similar to oral contraceptives, progestins, and danazol, but their increased cost and adverse effect profile (including menopausal-type symptoms and decreased bone density) make them second-line agents, after OCs and progestins.[134]

AROMATASE INHIBITORS

The most recently studied therapy for endometriosis, aromatase inhibitors (AIs), were originally developed for use in patients with breast cancer. Aromatase, the enzyme responsible for the synthesis of estrogens, is required for the conversion of androstenedione and testosterone to estrone and estradiol. [135] Although AIs, OCs, progestins, and GnRH agonists all decrease serum levels of estrogen, only AIs decrease secretion and production of estrogen by endometrial tissue itself. Anastrozole and letrozole are type II AIs, binding reversibly to the enzyme to produce a beneficial effect on endometriosis symptoms.[135] Although AIs effectively decrease estrogen conversion in the periphery, addition of an agent to reduce ovarian estrogen levels is also necessary in

TABLE 50-4
Gonadotropin-Releasing Hormone Agonists

GnRH Agonist (Brand Name)	Strength	Dosage Form	Dosage Regimen
Nafarelin (Synarel)	2 mg/mL delivers 200 mcg/spray	Intranasal	200–800 mcg BID
Leuprolide (Lupron)	3.75 mg, 11.25 mg	IM depot	3.75 mg/mo or 11.25 mg every 3 months
Goserelin (Zoladex)	3.6 mg, 10.8 mg	SC implant	3.6 mg implant every month or 10. 8 mg implant every 3 months

BID, twice daily; GnRH, gonadotropin-releasing hormone; IM, intramuscular; SC, subcutaneous.

premenopausal women, hence most of the studies in this population have included double therapy with AIs and oral contraceptives or GnRH analog.

Although the end result of GnRH agonists and AIs is similar, the adverse effects of the AIs are decreased, with fewer hot flashes, and primarily mild headache, nausea, and diarrhea. Although few long-term trials have been conducted, decreased bone density is suspected with the use of AIs and estrogen add-back therapy is appropriate (described later in this section and Case 50-4, Question 1). AIs have been studied alone and in combination with oral contraceptives, progestins, and GnRH agonists. All studies, although small, have demonstrated reduction in pain and reduced lesion size. The largest study to date used a combination of anastrozole with GnRH agonists compared with GnRH agonists alone in patients after surgery.[136] Although effective at controlling pain, the combination resulted in significantly more bone loss than either regimen alone at 6 months, but no difference was seen at the 2-year follow-up.[136] Further research is needed to determine the role of AIs in the treatment of endometriosis, because currently they do not have an FDA indication for the treatment of endometriosis. Their use should be reserved at this time for those patients with severe endometriosis who have failed other therapies.

DANAZOL

Danazol, an androgenic drug derived from 17-ethinyl testosterone, also induces a pseudomenopausal state by increasing androgen levels and decreasing estrogen levels. It inhibits the enzymes involved in ovarian steroidogenesis and increases the metabolic clearance of estradiol. By creating a hypoestrogenic, hypoprogestogenic state, danazol causes anovulation, amenorrhea, and atrophy of endometrial implants. Although effective at decreasing pelvic pain, danazol is poorly tolerated because of its significant side effects, which include weight gain, voice changes, edema, acne, hot flashes, vaginal dryness, hirsutism, liver disease, and increased cholesterol; these occur in up to 85% of treated patients.[111] Because of safety concerns, use should be limited to 6 months at a time, and should only be initiated in women after all other therapy options have failed.[134]

PAIN MANAGEMENT: NONPHARMACOLOGIC THERAPY

DEFINITIVE SURGERY

Definitive surgery, referring to total abdominal hysterectomy, bilateral salpingo-oophorectomy, and removal of all visible endometriosis, theoretically should eliminate the risk of recurrence of the disease. These procedures are not an option for the many women with endometriosis who desire pregnancy in the future. It is invasive surgery, reserved for those patients whose pain is unresponsive to other therapies or to conservative surgery. Furthermore, removal of all endometriosis is difficult, and recurring pain is not uncommon. Sinaii et al. surveyed patients with endometriosis regarding treatments and benefits, and found that, of the 1,160 women surveyed, 12% had had definitive surgery, with 40% reporting the surgery was successful, 33% reporting partial benefit, 5.6% reporting no benefit, and 6% of patients actually reported increased pain and symptoms after surgery.[137]

CONSERVATIVE SURGERY

In contrast to definitive surgery, conservative surgery (involving ablation and removal of implants, and lysis of adhesions) preserves fertility, and is commonly conducted during the initial diagnostic laparoscopy. In the Sinaii et al. survey, 70% of patients had undergone laparoscopy with removal of lesions, with 30% considering the procedure a success, 50% reporting partial benefit, 15% with no difference in symptoms, and 10% reporting increased symptoms.[137] On average, women reported having three surgical procedures.[137] Drug treatment is used after conservative surgery, as it is not possible to remove all lesions, many of which are difficult to visualize. Clinical trials using GnRH agonists for up to 6 months after conservative surgery have provided mixed results, and danazol and medroxyprogesterone trials have shown similar results.[133] Oral contraceptives and progestin intrauterine devices have not been evaluated for prevention of recurrence after surgery.

Clinical trials in endometriosis have not singled out one treatment as the treatment of choice for all women, with most investigations demonstrating equivalence of the studied therapies. An NSAID and combined hormonal contraception (e.g., N.H.'s contraceptive vaginal ring) are the drugs of choice for initial management, owing to their safety profile, and, in this case, the contraceptive agent's dual utility in preventing conception. As a next step, progestins, GnRH agonists, and AIs are options. Because of adverse effects and poor tolerability, danazol should be reserved as an agent of last choice. If N.H. were uninterested in having children in the future, surgical sterilization would be an option. Conservative surgery, including removal of endometriomas and adhesions and ablation of visible lesions is not curative, but may provide pain relief in 50% to 95% of patients at 1 year.[133] A combination of conservative surgery, followed by postoperative progestin, combined hormonal contraceptive, GnRH agonists, or danazol has been shown to prolong the duration of pain relief and decrease recurrence after surgery.[133]

CASE 50-3, QUESTION 3: N.H. has not had a problem in the past tolerating a variety of contraceptive products, but does have some problems with daily medication adherence, and would like to avoid giving herself injections if possible. How does this information assist in the selection of therapy for her endometriosis?

N.H. is a smoker, with poor calcium intake, and some cardiovascular risk factors (family history, high cholesterol), who would rather avoid injectable medication and has trouble with daily medication taking. Danazol, with its ability to increase cardiovascular risk factors, and extensive side effects, is not a good option.

Although some GnRH analogs are available as nasal sprays or injectable implants, the significant risk of decreased bone density and menopauselike adverse effects place it as a second-line option. Progestins, particularly the long-acting progestins, either in the form of the medroxyprogesterone acetate 3-month depot or subcutaneous injection, or the levonorgestrel IUS make these appropriate first-line options for N.H., although the risk of diminished bone density with depot formulations remains an issue.

CASE 50-3, QUESTION 4: N.H. would like to start the levonorgestrel IUS, but her insurance company will not pay for it to be used in the treatment of endometriosis because of its lack of FDA indication. She decides to start depot medroxyprogesterone acetate. What information can you provide her regarding use, and the benefits and risks of treatment?

Depot medroxyprogesterone acetate (DMPA) is available in two dosage forms: 150 mg to be given intramuscularly (IM) every 3 months, and a 104-mg formulation given subcutaneously (SC) every 3 months. Product choice may be based on insurance coverage, or potential for the patient to self-administer (the SC product may be more patient-friendly). Because N.H. does not want to self-inject, either choice, administered by her provider's office, or a pharmacist if law allows, would be an appropriate option. Although the DMPA does provide the contraception N.H. desires, she should be informed that it may take longer than usual (up to 1 year) to become pregnant after its use. More than 80% of patients treated with progestins will experience partial or complete pain relief.[127] Although devoid of the menopauselike adverse effects of other medications used to treat endometriosis, DMPA is associated with weight gain (which may be significant in some patients), bloating, and irregular periods or bleeding for several months, with most users eventually experiencing amenorrhea. To reduce bone density loss, which is significant but less than with GnRH agonists, N.H. should be advised to ensure her daily intake by diet or supplementation of calcium is at least 1,000 mg/day, and at least 400 to 600 international units of vitamin D/day, receive smoking cessation counseling and pharmacotherapy as appropriate, and start a regular weight-bearing exercise regimen.[138] She should be monitored for pain relief, weight gain, amenorrhea or bleeding changes, and adherence to the quarterly injections. When N.H. desires conception, significant planning is required, and she may require a different therapy for her endometriosis as she regains fertility.

GONADOTROPIN-RELEASING HORMONE AGONISTS AND ADD-BACK THERAPY

CASE 50-4

QUESTION 1: M.F., a 24-year-old single woman with a history of moderate to severe endometriosis, has been treated with some benefit with NSAIDs (three different NSAIDs at appropriate doses), combined oral contraceptives, and the levonorgestrel IUS. She has no desire for conception, and is looking for pain relief. She has also had two conservative laparoscopic surgical procedures, each of which was successful, with pain relief lasting 6 months to 1 year. She recently had her "last ever" (by her description) surgical procedure, and is looking to extend the improvement she has seen previously after surgery. She does not mind injections, but has had trouble with adherence in the past. What options are available for the treatment of M.F.'s pain?

M.F. has tried numerous pharmacologic and surgical treatments (NSAIDs, combined oral contraception, and progestin-only contraception) for endometriosis with limited benefit. Given that she does not desire pregnancy at this time, GnRH analogs, aromatase inhibitors, and danazol are other options. Leuprolide, nafarelin, and goserelin are GnRH analogs (agonists) typically used for the treatment of endometriosis (Table 50-4). Although GnRH analogs have not been shown to produce better results than the therapies M.F. has already used, they may provide her with pain relief. Choice of GnRH agonist is driven by patient choice of administration method (nasal twice daily [BID] with nafarelin, monthly SC implant with goserelin, or IM injection either once monthly or once every 3 months with leuprolide). In M.F.'s case, the once every 3 months dosing with leuprolide would be most desirable for her, eliminating the need for daily administration. Efficacy is similar for all the GnRH agonists. Before use of these agents, pregnancy, undiagnosed vaginal bleeding, and breastfeeding should be ruled out. Because M.F. does not desire conception, and use of the GnRH agonists is contraindicated in pregnancy, she should be counseled regarding choices of nonhormonal contraceptive agents.

Onset of response to GnRH therapy depends on the phase in the menstrual cycle during which the agent is initiated. Administration beginning in the luteal phase causes decreased estrogen levels within 2 to 3 weeks, and amenorrhea within 4 to 5 weeks versus the 6 to 8 weeks if started in the follicular phase.[104]

Usual therapy duration is 6 months, although a small pilot study suggested long-term treatment (up to 10 years) with estrogen add-back therapy is without major adverse effects, with continued efficacy.[139] Add-back therapy is based on the concept of an estrogen threshold hypothesis, formulated by Barbieri,[117] which states that there is a critical amount of estrogen that exacerbates endometriosis, and below that level the presence of estrogen serves to decrease adverse effects but does not have an adverse effect on the disease itself. Add-back therapy should be initiated at the beginning of GnRH agonist therapy to try to reduce the occurrence of all hypoestrogenic adverse effects.[139]

Estrogen-containing OCs contain a dose of estrogen that is above the threshold, and they should not be used for add-back therapy. Doses of estrogen equivalent to 0.625 mg of conjugated equine estrogen have been studied in combination with either medroxyprogesterone 2.5 mg daily, or norethindrone 5 mg daily. This dose of norethindrone alone, or a dose of 20 mg of medroxyprogesterone alone, has also demonstrated benefit.[111] To prevent bone loss, a regimen of a progestin plus a bisphosphonate has been studied with positive results. No studies have demonstrated superior efficacy or safety of one regimen over another. Women using add-back therapy should consume in diet or supplements a total of 1,000 mg of calcium daily and have vitamin D levels in the normal range.[116]

Therapy beyond 3 to 6 months requires the use of add-back therapy to reduce the risk of hypoestrogenic complications. Monitoring for efficacy includes monitoring for amenorrhea, decreases in pain and dyspareunia, and quality of life. After discontinuation of GnRH agonists, menses and ovarian function return to normal in 6 to 12 weeks, although benefits may be maintained for another 6 to 12 months.[104]

ADVERSE EFFECTS

Adverse effects should be discussed in detail with M.F. because they differ significantly from the other therapies she has tried. Adverse effects are related to the induction of the pseudomenopausal state (Table 50-5). Nearly all patients experience hot flashes; vaginal dryness and insomnia also are common. GnRH agonists do not affect SHBG or testosterone levels, so the androgenic side effects of danazol, including changes in lipid profiles, are not experienced with these agents.[104] Significant bone loss can occur, necessitating adequate calcium and vitamin D intake, and estrogen add-back therapy to decrease loss.

TABLE 50-5
Adverse Reactions With Danazol and the Gonadotropin-Releasing Hormone Agonists

	Danazol (%)	Nafarelin (%)	Leuprolide (%)	Goserelin (%)
Antiestrogenic Effects				
Hot flashes	67–69	90	84	96
Vaginal dryness or vaginitis	7–43	19	28	75
Abnormal vaginal bleeding[a]	+	+	28	+
Breast atrophy	16–42	10	6	33
Decreased libido	7–44	22	11	61
Androgenic Effects				
Weight gain	23–28	8	13	3
Voice alteration	8	NR	<5	3
Hirsutism	6–7	2	<5	15
Acne	20–42	13	10	55
Central Nervous System Effects				
Sleep disturbances	4	8	<5	11
Headaches	21–63	19	32	75
Depression or emotional lability	18–60	9–15	22	54–56
Other				
Peripheral edema	34	8	7	21
Nausea	14	NR	13	8
Seborrhea	17–52	8	10	26
Nasal irritation	NR	10	NR	NR
Injection site reactions	NR	NR	<5	6
Joint pain	+	<1	8	+

[a] Amenorrhea is an expected consequence of these medications.
+, Reported but percentages not given; NR, not reported.

A reduction in bone density is a significant concern with GnRH agonists, even at 3 months after the onset of therapy, and is particularly concerning because these agents are being used in young women, many of whom have not reached their peak bone mass. Studies have demonstrated a loss of 3.2% in lumbar spine bone mineral density after 6 months, and a 6.3% decrease after 12 months of GnRH agonist treatment.[134] It has also been reported that endometriosis itself is also a risk factor for decreased bone density, although a long-term study did not find any association between endometriosis and fracture risk during a 20-year follow-up period.[140] Interestingly, this same study did not find any association between fracture risk and GnRH agonist therapy, although a significant number of women in the study did take add-back therapy.

Monitoring for decreases in bone density should be accomplished via dual-energy x-ray absorptiometry scan every 24 months if GnRH therapy is continued. M.F. should also be counseled regarding adequate calcium and vitamin D intake, smoking cessation, and a regimen of weight-bearing exercise.

M.F should initate the luprolide 11.25 mg IM once every 3 months, with add-back therapy consisting of conjugated estrogens 0.625 mg daily with 2.5 mg medroxyprogesterone. A 6-month trial followed by an evaluation of symptom control is reasonable.

MANAGEMENT OF ENDOMETRIOSIS-RELATED INFERTILITY

CASE 50-5

QUESTION 1: K.L. is a 32-year-old woman with a history of stage II endometriosis. She currently is using a levonorgestrel IUS for both contraception and control of her pain, with positive results. She also takes ibuprofen 800 mg TID on a regular basis. She and her spouse would like to have a child. About 6 years ago, they attempted to conceive without success after 24 months. K.L is concerned that she will now have even more difficulty becoming pregnant, given her advanced age. What are the recommendations for improving fertility in K.L.?

Of women presenting to the health care system with infertility, 30% to 45% have endometriosis, and 30% to 50% of women with endometriosis are infertile.[141] Proposed mechanisms contributing to infertility include adhesions that impair oocyte transport, changes in the peritoneum not compatible with fertility, changes in hormonal function, endocrine or ovulation dysfunction, and disorders of implantation (see Chapter 48, Infertility). No evidence suggests that hormonal therapy, including therapy with GnRH agonists, improves conception rates for women with stage I/II endometriosis, similar to K.L. On the other hand, surgical ablation or resection of visible endometriosis implants is beneficial in improving pregnancy rates in women with stage I/II endometriosis.

For K.L., removal of her IUS, followed by laparoscopic ablation or resection of visible implants may improve her ability to conceive, barring other factors influencing fertility (e.g., PCOS, male factor infertility, tubal patency).[142] For patients with more advanced disease, or in those patients older than 35 years of age, a more aggressive treatment regimen is appropriate. Options include the use of agents to induce superovulation (clomiphene), and the use of in vitro fertilization techniques with embryo transfer (IVF-ET). In women with endometriosis, the success of IVF-ET is decreased by as much as 20% when compared with women without endometriosis.[104] For women contemplating IVF-ET, three prospective clinical trials have demonstrated a potential benefit in women with stage II–IV endometriosis who were treated for 3 to 6 months or more with GnRH agonists before IVF-ET.[119] The treated subjects had significantly higher pregnancy rates compared with women who did not use GnRH agonists before IVF-ET.[143]

For women who have not yet demonstrated an inability to conceive, a "wait and see" approach, with use of an NSAID for pain, emotional support, and reassurance, for 6 to 12 months is appropriate in women younger than 35 years of age.

PREMENSTRUAL SYNDROME AND PREMENSTRUAL DYSPHORIC DISORDER

Premenstrual symptoms occur in up to 90% of reproductive-age women.[144] Approximately 20% to 40% of these women have more bothersome symptoms of premenstrual syndrome (PMS) and it is estimated that 3% to 8% meet the criteria for premenstrual dysphoric disorder (PMDD), a more severe variant of PMS.[144] More than 200 premenstrual symptoms have been described as occurring during the days before menstruation, including positive symptoms, such as increased energy, libido, and ability to relax, as well as negative symptoms including abdominal distension, fatigue, headaches, and crying spells.[145] It is not until the symptoms have a decidedly negative influence on the physical, psychological, or social function of a woman that PMS or PMDD exists.

Diagnosis

No specific physical findings or laboratory tests can be used to make a diagnosis of PMS. The American College of Obstetricians and Gynecologists (ACOG) published a Practice Bulletin in 2000 that defined diagnostic criteria using cyclical patterns of symptoms in women.[146] PMS can be diagnosed if at least one of the affective and one of the somatic symptoms listed in Table 50-6 is reported 5 days before the onset of menses in the three previous cycles. The symptoms must be prospectively recorded in at least two cycles and must cease within 4 days of onset of menses and not recur until after day 12 of the menstrual cycle. A key factor that separates PMS from "normal" premenstrual symptoms is that work or social activities are adversely affected in PMS. Other diagnoses that may explain premenstrual symptoms should be excluded, including psychological, thyroid, and gynecologic disorders.[147]

TABLE 50-6
ACOG Diagnostic Criteria for Premenstrual Syndrome[a]

Affective Symptoms	Somatic Symptoms
Depression	Breast tenderness
Angry outbursts	Abdominal bloating
Irritability	Headache
Anxiety	Swelling of extremities
Confusion	
Social withdrawal	

[a] Notes: (1) Diagnosis made if at least one affective and one somatic symptom is reported in the three prior menstrual cycles during the 5 days before the onset of menses. (2) The symptoms must resolve within 4 days of onset of menses and do not recur until after day 12 of the cycle. (3) The symptoms must be present in at least two cycles during prospective recording. (4) The symptoms must adversely affect social or work-related activities.

ACOG, American College of Obstetricians and Gynecologists.

Source: American College of Obstetricians and Gynecologists. ACOG Practice Bulletin. Clinical management guidelines for obstetrician-gynecologists. Premenstrual syndrome. April 2000. *Obstet Gynecol.* 2000;95(4); Mishell DR. Premenstrual disorders: epidemiology and disease burden. *Am J Manag Care.* 2005;11:S473.

TABLE 50-7
Diagnostic Criteria for Premenstrual Dysphoric Disorder

- In most menstrual cycles during the past year, at least five of the subsequent symptoms (including one core symptom) were present for most of the time 1 week before menses (luteal phase), began to remit within a few days after the onset of menses, and were absent the week after menses (follicular phase).
  - Core symptoms
    - Markedly depressed mood, feelings of hopelessness or self-deprecating thoughts
    - Persistent and marked anger or irritability or increased interpersonal conflicts
    - Marked anxiety, tension
    - Marked affective lability (i.e., feeling suddenly sad or tearful)
  - Other symptoms
    - Decreased interest in usual activities (e.g., friends, hobbies)
    - Subjective sense of difficulty in concentrating
    - Lethargy, easy fatigability, or marked lack of energy
    - Marked change in appetite, overeating, or specific food cravings
    - Hypersomnia or insomnia
    - A subjective sense of being overwhelmed or out of control
    - Other physical symptoms (e.g., breast tenderness, bloating, weight gain, headache, joint or muscle pain)
- The symptoms seriously interfere with work or school, usual activities, or relationships with others.
- Symptoms are not merely an exacerbation of another disorder, such as major depression, panic disorder, dysthymia, or a personality disorder (although it may be superimposed on any of these disorders).
- Three of these major criteria are confirmed by prospective daily self-ratings for at least two consecutive symptomatic cycles.

Adapted with permission from American Psychiatric Association. *Diagnostic and Statistical Manual of Mental Disorders, DSM-IV-TR.* 4th ed. Washington, DC: APA; 2000.

The American Psychiatric Association has developed criteria for PMDD (Table 50-7).[148] The criteria for PMDD focus on the mood and mental health symptoms, leading to a higher level of dysfunction compared with PMS. Criteria for PMS and PMDD, however, share three essential characteristics: (a) symptoms must occur in the luteal phase and resolve within a few days of menstruation, (b) symptoms are documented for at least two menstrual cycles and are not better explained by other physical or psychological conditions, and (c) symptoms are sufficiently severe to disrupt normal activities.[147]

The symptoms of PMS and PMDD experienced by women can vary widely. Risk factors for PMS include advancing age (older than 30 years) and genetic factors.[147] Symptoms, however, can begin in adolescents around age 14, or 2 years postmenarche, and persist until menopause.[149] Some studies suggest that women with mothers reporting PMS are more likely to develop PMS than those with unaffected mothers (70% vs. 37%, respectively).[150,151] One article found that traumatic events, such as physical threat, childhood sexual abuse, and severe accidents, increased the risk of developing PMDD.[152]

Pathophysiology

The wide range of symptoms exhibited in patients with PMS or PMDD can be explained by multiple possible mechanisms, probably a result of interactions between sex steroids and central neurotransmitters.[153] Alterations in neurotransmitters, primarily reductions in serotonin, triggered by normal hormonal fluctuations of the menstrual cycle appear to be the most probable factors for the development of PMS or PMDD. Other neurotransmitters, including endorphins and γ-aminobutyric acid (GABA), have also been implicated.[154,155] The levels of estrogen, progesterone, and testosterone are normal in women with PMS, but they may be more vulnerable to normal fluctuations.[155] These potential mechanisms provide a rational basis for the symptoms that appear in PMS and PMDD, but also support the therapeutic benefits of treatments that increase serotonin or GABA levels. Many treatments have limited and variable efficacy, which reinforces the argument that PMS or PMDD is a result of multiple factors. Furthermore, placebo responses in trials can be as high as 50% to 80%, which points to an important psychosomatic component and the consideration that PMS or PMDD has relevant biological, psychological, and social factors.[145]

CASE 50-6

QUESTION 1: C.P., a 27-year-old woman, presents complaining of significant mood changes that occur the week before her menstrual cycle. She experiences increased irritability and anxiety as well as breast tenderness and abdominal bloating. These symptoms usually subside the first or second day after her menses begin. For 2 to 3 weeks after her menstrual period, C.P. is her "normal, usual self" until the symptoms begin again just before her next menstruation. She has had these symptoms every month for the past several years. She states that she is very uncomfortable when these symptoms occur. Although she is able to work most of the time, she typically avoids going out with her friends when she has these symptoms. Her menstrual cycles are regular, occurring every 28 to 30 days with a light flow lasting 3 to 4 days.

Pelvic, cardiovascular, and neurologic examinations are normal and all laboratory assessments are within normal limits. Her serum pregnancy test was negative. She is sexually active and uses condoms for contraception. She has no significant past medical history and she does not take any medications. What symptoms does C.P. have that are consistent with a diagnosis of PMS?

C.P. has symptoms that meet the ACOG criteria for PMS. Her affective symptoms include irritability and anxiety and somatic symptoms include breast tenderness and abdominal bloating. These symptoms occur during the luteal phase of the menstrual cycle, resolve within 4 days of menses, and do not recur until after day 12 of her cycle. C.P.'s symptoms appear to be affecting her social activities. She states that these symptoms have been present for years and that they occur every month, although she has not prospectively recorded this information. C.P. does not meet the criteria for PMDD because her symptoms are not severe or markedly impairing her ability to participate in daily activities.

Treatment: Premenstrual Syndrome

CASE 50-6, QUESTION 2: C.P. asks about nonprescription therapy. Which agents, if any, are appropriate for C.P.?

Nonprescription options that have been studied and have demonstrated at least minimal benefit include calcium, magnesium, pyridoxine, chaste tree or chasteberry, and some mind–body approaches. Acetaminophen and NSAIDs may be beneficial for the physical symptoms of PMS, but diuretics found in various OTC products (e.g., ammonium chloride, caffeine, pamabrom) have limited data and unproven efficacy. Given the high placebo response rate in PMS, only agents with clinically proven efficacy should be used.

CALCIUM

Increased estrogen during the middle of a normal menstrual cycle decreases calcium. In women with PMS, intact parathyroid hormone (PTH) increases in response to this change compared with no PTH change in women without PMS.[156] Therefore, women with PMS have midcycle elevations of intact PTH with transient, secondary hyperparathyroidism that increases calcium demands. Calcium supplementation may help to normalize these processes and explains why calcium has demonstrated some benefit in women with PMS.

Three calcium trials have shown efficacy of PMS symptoms. A randomized, double-blind crossover trial of 33 women receiving 1,000 mg elemental calcium daily or placebo for 3 months reported a significant overall 50% reduction in PMS symptoms for women taking calcium compared with placebo.[157] In a double-blind study of 10 women assigned to dietary calcium intake, 1,336 mg daily was found to benefit mood, behavior, pain, and water retention symptoms significantly during the menstrual cycle.[158] Perhaps the most convincing evidence comes from a prospective, multicenter, randomized, double-blind, placebo-controlled, parallel-group trial conducted in 466 women with PMS.[159] Elemental calcium 1,200 mg daily (given as 600 mg BID) for three menstrual cycles significantly decreased negative affect, water retention, food cravings, and pain compared with placebo. Overall, the calcium-treated group had a 48% reduction in luteal symptoms compared with a 30% reduction in the placebo group. Because calcium is well tolerated and may provide other benefits (e.g., osteoporosis prevention) calcium supplementation should be recommended to women with symptoms of PMS if inadequate through diet or other supplementation.

MAGNESIUM

Low levels of red cell magnesium have been correlated with women experiencing PMS, therefore magnesium supplementation has been evaluated for PMS symptoms.[160] A Cochrane review of three small trials comparing magnesium and placebo in women with dysmenorrhea concluded that magnesium was more effective for pain associated with PMS and the need for additional medication was less for those taking magnesium.[92] Magnesium doses that have been studied for PMS vary from 200 to 360 mg orally daily. Trials have reported improvements in fluid retention and negative affect, but findings have not been consistent.[161] The most common side effects affect the gastrointestinal system (e.g., nausea, diarrhea). The conflicting results may be caused by differences in the dosing regimens of the magnesium and differing levels of magnesium stores in the study subjects. Available data support the use of magnesium in PMS, but more research is needed.

PYRIDOXINE (VITAMIN B_6)

Vitamin B_6 has been noted to have positive effects on neurotransmitters, such as serotonin.[162] The most comprehensive information for this nutrient comes from a systematic review of nine trials representing 940 patients with PMS.[163] The overall assessment of the review was that women with PMS are likely to benefit from vitamin B_6 supplementation at a dose of 50 to 100 mg daily. An analysis of four of the trials, which specifically examined depressive symptoms, showed that pyridoxine was more effective than placebo in reducing depressive symptoms (OR, 1.69; 95% CI, 1.39–2.06). Although the conclusions of this review were positive, the authors felt there was insufficient evidence of high quality to recommend vitamin B_6 for PMS. Because neuropathy has been reported with pyridoxine dosages as low as 200 mg/day, patients should be advised to monitor for symptoms and to discontinue therapy and seek medical attention if they occur.[163]

CHASTETREE OR CHASTEBERRY

Chasteberry (Vitex agnus-castus or VAC) is the fruit of the chaste tree, a small shrublike tree native to Central Asia and the Mediterranean region. Liquid or solid extracts from the dried ripe chasteberry are used to make chasteberry capsules and tablets. The mechanism of action of chasteberry relative to PMS is unclear, but several trials have reported its beneficial effects. In a study of 1,542 women with PMS taking chasteberry extract, 33% of subjects reported total relief of symptoms and an additional 57% reported partial relief after 4 months.[164] Of patients, 2% complained of adverse events including nausea, allergy, diarrhea, weight gain, heartburn, hypermenorrhea, and gastric complaints. A randomized, double-blind, placebo-controlled trial of 170 women taking chasteberry extract 20 mg daily for three menstrual cycles showed a treatment response rate of 52% compared with 24% for placebo ($p < 0.001$).[165] Individual symptoms of irritability, mood alteration, anger, headache, and breast fullness were reduced. Bloating was not significantly altered compared with placebo. The incidence of side effects was low, but long-term safety is unknown. A prospective, randomized, placebo-controlled study in 67 Chinese women showed that one VAC tablet daily containing 40 mg of herbal drug produced an 85% efficacy rate compared with a 56% efficacy rate for placebo on symptom scores after three treatment cycles.[166] In general, data indicate that chasteberry may be effective for PMS, but should probably not be used as routine treatment for PMS.[161]

MIND–BODY APPROACHES

Evidence regarding mind–body approaches for PMS is somewhat limited. Because these modalities are risk-free and they are generally accepted as components of a healthy lifestyle, they are favored in the treatment of PMS. Mind–body approaches that have demonstrated benefit in PMS include relaxation response, cognitive-behavioral therapy, yoga, aerobic exercise, and light therapy.[167] Trials that have evaluated acupuncture have demonstrated benefit to patients with PMS, but there are significant flaws in study designs that prevent it from being recommended as a treatment modality.[168]

NONSTEROIDAL ANTI-INFLAMMATORY DRUGS AND DIURETICS

NSAIDs have been used to relieve the physical symptoms (e.g., headache, joint pain) of PMS, but do not improve the mood symptoms.[147] Regimens have included taking naproxen or mefenamic acid during the luteal phase and stopping therapy after menses begin. Diuretics commonly found in OTC products, such as ammonium chloride, caffeine, and pamabrom, are not effective.

Several OTC options are available to C.P. Trials including calcium, magnesium, pyridoxine, and chasteberry have shown some positive findings, but the evidence is not compelling due to methodological limitations. These treatments should not be recommended for the treatment of PMS, but may already be included in a healthy diet or vitamin regimen. Mind–body approaches, such as yoga and relaxation, are part of a healthy lifestyle and could be recommended to C.P. Because C.P. is having mood symptoms (i.e., anxiety), NSAIDs would not be an effective recommendation.

CASE 50-6, QUESTION 3: C.P. has been taking a multivitamin daily for 3 months with adequate amounts of calcium, magnesium, and vitamin B_6 for PMS relief. She also has been taking naproxen sodium 220 mg orally BID without significant reduction of her symptoms. Her physician requests that she keep a daily dairy for two consecutive cycles to document her symptoms. What information should be included in this tool?

C.P. should keep a daily diary for two consecutive menstrual cycles to demonstrate a temporal relationship between her symptoms during the luteal phase and to document the severity of these symptoms (Table 50-8). In addition, she should indicate the presence of menstrual flow, weight, and daily basal body temperature readings to help determine when ovulation occurs. The diary establishes a baseline for each patient and documents the most troublesome symptoms. Once therapy is selected for these symptoms, the diary can aid in assessing patient response.

Treatment: Premenstrual Dysphoric Disorder

CASE 50-6, QUESTION 4: C.P. returns to clinic with the diary presented in Table 50-8. The physician determines that C.P. actually has PMDD. What evidence supports this diagnosis and what should be recommended to C.P. for treatment?

C.P. meets the criteria for PMDD as evidenced by her symptoms during the one week before her menstrual cycle (luteal phase). Specifically, she has at least five symptoms required for the diagnosis of PMDD: sadness or depression (core symptom), fatigue, irritability, inability to concentrate, breast tenderness, and bloating. She rated several of those symptoms as severe, which indicates the symptoms are disabling and she is unable to meet her daily obligations. There is no reason to suspect any other disorder based on her history. PMDD seems to be the most likely diagnosis for C.P.

Therapy options at this time include lifestyle modifications, psychosocial interventions, and pharmacologic therapy. Psychotropic drugs targeted to her most severe symptoms may include selective serotonin reuptake inhibitors (SSRIs), serotonergic tricyclic antidepressants, and anxiolytics. An oral contraceptive has also been approved for PMDD and could be considered.

SELECTIVE SEROTONIN REUPTAKE INHIBITORS

Serotonin is critical in the pathogenesis of PMDD and for that reason, SSRIs have become the treatment of choice for PMDD and severe PMS (Table 50-9).[169] SSRIs have demonstrated efficacy in reducing irritability, depressed mood, dysphoria, psychosocial function, and the physical symptoms of PMDD, including bloating, breast tenderness, and appetite changes. Fluoxetine, sertraline, and paroxetine controlled release each have an approved indication for PMDD.

The onset of SSRI effect in women with PMDD or severe PMS is much more rapid than when these agents are used for treatment of major depression or anxiety disorders.[169] Women may experience symptom relief or resolution within the first menstrual cycle versus the 4 to 8 weeks for other psychological disorders. Several different dosing strategies have been studied, including continuous dosing (once daily), intermittent dosing (last 2 weeks of menstrual cycle or luteal phase), and semi-intermittent dosing (continuous administration throughout the cycle with increased doses during luteal phase).[169] Continuous dosing would be reasonable for women with concurrent mood or anxiety disorders or those who may have difficulty remembering the timing of the intermittent dosing. Intermittent dosing should be considered

TABLE 50-8
Menstrual Cycle Daily Diary Chart

Month 1

Grading Severity of Symptoms:
- 1 = Mild; general awareness of discomfort but does not interfere with daily activities
- 2 = Moderate; interferes with activities but not disabling
- 3 = Severe; symptoms disabling, unable to meet daily social, family, or work obligations
- * = Menstrual bleeding
- Blank = no symptoms

Each Day
1. List the major symptoms (mood, physical, emotional, behavioral) that you experience during your menstrual cycle
2. Grade the severity of the symptom if present (1 to 3)
3. Record daily weight
4. Record basal body temperature, which helps determine ovulation date
5. Check the days of the cycle when menstrual flow occurs

Day of month	1	2	3	4	5	6	7	8	9	10	11	12	13	14	15	16	17	18	19	20	21	22	23	24	25	26	27	28	29	30	31
Day of menstrual cycle	18	19	20	21	22	23	24	25	26	27	28	1	2	3	4	5	6	7	8	9	10	11	12	13	14	15	16	17	18	19	20
Menses												*	*	*	*																
Breast tenderness and pain				1	1	1	1	1	1	1	1																				
Sadness or depression				1	2	3	3	3	3	3	3	2	1																		
Fatigue				3	3	3	3	3	3	3	3	2	1																		
Irritability					2	2	3	3	3	3	3																				
Inability to concentrate							2	2	3	3	3																				
Daily weight (lbs.)	130	130	130	130	130	130	130	130	130	130	130	131	131	131	130	130	130	130	130	130	129	129	129	128	128	129	128	128	128	128	128
Basal body temperature (degrees F)	98.0	98.2	98.0	98.2	98.0	98.0	98.2	97.8	98.0	97.8	97.6					97.8	97.8	97.6	97.8	97.6	97.8	97.8	97.6	97.4	98.4	98.0	98.4	98.6	98.0	98.2	98.0

Month 2

Day of month	1	2	3	4	5	6	7	8	9	10	11	12	13	14	15	16	17	18	19	20	21	22	23	24	25	26	27	28	29	30
Day of menstrual cycle	21	22	23	24	25	26	27	28	1	2	3	4	5	6	7	8	9	10	11	12	13	14	15	16	17	18	19	20	21	22
Menses									*	*	*	*																		
Breast tenderness and pain				1	1	1	1	1	1		1																			
Sadness/depression		1	2	3	3	3	3	3	2	2	1																			
Fatigue		2	2	3	3	3	3	3	2	1																				
Irritability	1	2	2	2	3	3	3	3	3	2	2	1																		
Inability to concentrate			1	1	2	2	3	3																						
Daily weight (lbs.)	128	128	128	128	128	128	128	129	129	129	128	128	128	128	128	128	128	128	128	128	128	128	128	128	128	129	128	128	128	128
Basal body temperature (degrees F)	98.0	98.2	98.4	98.0	98.2	97.8	98.0	97.4					97.6	97.6	97.8	97.8	97.6	97.8	97.6	97.6	97.6	97.2	97.2	97.0	98.4	98.6	98.0	98.2	98.2	98.0

TABLE 50-9

Psychotropic Drugs for the Management of Premenstrual Syndrome or Premenstrual Dysphoric Disorder

Drug (Brand Name)	Daily Dosing Regimen (mg)	Intermittent Dosing Regimen (mg)[a]
SSRI		
Citalopram (Celexa)	5–30	10–30
Escitalopram (Lexapro)	10–20	10–20
Fluoxetine (Prozac or Sarafem[b])	20–60	20 or 90 weekly
Fluvoxamine (Luvox)	50–150	NS
Paroxetine (Paxil)	10–30	NS
Paroxetine controlled release (Paxil CR)[b]	12.5–25	12.5–25
Sertraline (Zoloft)[b]	50–150	100
Other Serotonergic Antidepressants		
Nefazodone (Serzone)	200–600	NS
Venlafaxine (Effexor)	50	NS
Anxiolytics		
Alprazolam (Xanax)	NS	1–2[c]
Buspirone (BuSpar)	NS	25–60

[a] Day 14 until onset of menses.
[b] Medication has FDA-approved indication for premenstrual dysphoric disorder.
[c] Dose to be tapered during 2 days after onset of menses to prevent withdrawal symptoms.
NS, not studied; SSRI, selective serotonin reuptake inhibitors.

for patients with regular menstrual cycles who are able to adhere to the regimen, an absence of symptoms during the follicular phase, concerns about long-term effects (e.g., sexual dysfunction) or cost of daily therapy, and few side effects at treatment initiation.[169] Studies evaluating these dosing strategies have reported conflicting results regarding the most effective method; treatment should be individualized based on patient history, willingness to adhere to therapy, and drug response.

In a meta-analysis of 15 randomized, placebo-controlled trials including 904 women, SSRI treatment demonstrated a significant reduction in overall PMS symptoms (OR, 6.91; 95% CI, 3.9–12.2).[170] SSRIs were effective in treating both physical and behavioral symptoms of PMS. No detectable difference was found in PMS symptoms when comparing continuous or intermittent dosing. SSRIs are generally well tolerated; however, in this analysis, the discontinuation rate in women taking SSRI was 2.5 times higher than in those taking placebo.[170] Common side effects reported with SSRI use were insomnia, fatigue, decreased libido, nausea, and dry mouth.

OTHER PSYCHOTROPIC AGENTS

Non-SSRI antidepressants that affect serotonin are also beneficial in treating PMS and PMDD (Table 50-9). Venlafaxine, dosed daily, is significantly better than placebo at relieving psychological and physical symptoms of PMDD.[171] Alprazolam is a short-acting benzodiazepine that has been assessed for the treatment of PMS in several studies with differing results.[172] With conflicting data and concerns about dependence, alprazolam should be reserved for women who are unresponsive to other PMS treatments. Luteal-phase dosing may limit the risk of drug dependence of this benzodiazepine, but the dose should be tapered during several days to minimize mild withdrawal symptoms. Buspirone, a partial 5-hydroxytryptamine receptor agonist, demonstrated significant reduction in irritability when given daily, but does not seem to affect the physical symptoms of PMS.[173]

COMBINATION ORAL CONTRACEPTIVES

A low-dose Combination Oral Contraceptives (COC) formulation containing 20 mcg ethinyl estradiol and 3 mg drospirenone (an antimineralocorticoid spironolactone analog) with a 4-day hormone-free interval is approved for the treatment of emotional and physical symptoms of PMDD.[174] Studies using this agent have shown efficacy for reduced mood, physical, and behavioral symptoms of PMDD, including a 48% improved response with this agent compared with a 36% response using placebo ($p = 0.015$).[175] Side effects occurring in at least 10% of women treated with this medication included intermenstrual bleeding, headache, nausea, breast pain, and upper respiratory infection. Another COC approved for PMDD contains as well a formulation containing 20 mcg of ethinyl estradiol, 3 mg of drospirenone, and 0.451 mg of levomefolate calcium.[176] For women desiring contraception, these particular agents are approved and have data supporting their use in PMDD. The effects of other contraceptive agents for PMDD symptoms are currently under investigation.

OTHER AGENTS

Treatment with GnRH agonists has been used for the physical and psychological symptoms of PMS.[177] These agents are not typically used for long periods of time, however, because of vasomotor symptoms and the potential for negative long-term effects on bone. They also have to be administered by injection or nasal spray which may affect adherence. This treatment is reserved for women with very severe PMDD who do not respond to other treatments.

Danazol has been investigated for the treatment of PMS with moderate results. Danazol 200 mg orally BID provides greater symptom relief than placebo for symptoms of severe PMS; however, luteal phase treatment does not appear effective for PMS symptoms.[178] Potential side effects are also a concern with this agent, and therefore its use in women should be limited to those who have failed other therapies.

C.P. has PMDD and does not need contraception since she uses condoms. Mood symptoms predominate and are impairing her functionality. An SSRI should be started in either a continuous or intermittent manner. C.P. appears to be a good candidate for intermittent therapy because she can adhere to the regimen and does not have a concurrent depression or anxiety disorder. An appropriate initial treatment regimen is fluoxetine 20 mg orally daily for the last two weeks of the menstrual cycle. Her response rate should be assessed after three cycles of treatment. An anxiolytic could be tried for symptoms not relieved by the SSRI.

KEY REFERENCES AND WEBSITES

A full list of references for this chapter can be found at http://thepoint.lww.com/AT10e. Below are the key references and websites for this chapter, with the corresponding reference number in this chapter found in parentheses after the reference.

Key References

American College of Obstericians and Gynecologists. ACOG Practice Bulletin. Clinical management guidelines for obstetrician-gynecologists. Premenstrual syndrome. April 2000 *Obstet Gynecol.* 2000;95(4). (146)

Azziz R et al. The Androgen Excess and PCOS Society criteria for the polycystic ovary syndrome: the complete task force report. *Fertil Steril.* 2009;91:456. (9)

American College of Obstetricians and Gynecologists. ACOG Practice Bulletin No. 114. Management of endometriosis. *Obstet Gynecol.* 2010;116:223. (116)

Braverman PK. Premenstrual syndrome and premenstrual dysphoric disorder. *J Pediatr Adolesc Gynecol.* 2007;20:3. (147)

Steiner M et al. Expert guidelines for the treatment of severe PMS, PMDD, and comorbidities: the role of SSRIs. *J Womens Health (Larchmt).* 2006;15:57. (169)

Zahradnik HP et al. Nonsteroidal anti-inflammatory drugs and hormonal contraceptives for pain relief from dysmenorrhea: a review. *Contraception.* 2010;81:185. (99)

Key Websites

Androgen Excess Society: **http://www.ae-society.org.** Accessed April 28, 2011.

Polycystic Ovarian Support Association: **http://www.pcosupport.org.** Accessed April 28, 2011.

51

The Transition Through Menopause

Louise Parent-Stevens

CORE PRINCIPLES

	CHAPTER CASES
1 Menopause is a natural progression of reproductive aging in women. It is characterized by declining ovarian function and decreased synthesis of sex hormones.	**Case 51-1 (Question 1)**
2 Many women experience distressing symptoms associated with menopause, including hot flushes and genitourinary atrophy. Management of these women is targeted at relieving symptoms while minimizing risks.	**Case 51-1 (Questions 1–6), Case 51-2 (Questions 1–3)**
3 Estrogen therapy (ET), the most effective treatment for menopausal symptoms, is associated with significant risks, including thromboembolic disease and breast and endometrial cancer. Progestogens are added to systemic estrogen therapy (EPT) to provide protection against endometrial hyperplasia and cancer in women with an intact uterus. Women must be adequately counseled so that they can make educated decisions about treatment.	**Case 51-1 (Questions 3, 5)**
4 Hormone therapy (HT), including ET and EPT, can be achieved through a wide variety of dosage formulations and dosing regimens. Based on the current understanding of the risks and benefits of systemic HT, its use should be limited to the management of menopausal symptoms using the lowest effective dose for the shortest time possible.	**Case 51-1 (Question 4)**
5 The optimal time for the use of HT is controversial; some studies suggest decreased cardiovascular risk when HT is initiated soon after menopause, whereas other studies show an increased risk of breast cancer when HT is started shortly after menopause.	**Case 51-1 (Question 3)**
6 Nonhormonal drugs, including serotonergic antidepressants and antiepileptic drugs, are useful alternatives in women who are unable or unwilling to take HT. Although use of herbal medicines for menopausal symptoms is common, efficacy and safety data on these products are limited.	**Case 51-1 (Questions 2, 6), Case 51-2 (Question 2)**
7 As vaginal atrophy does not wane with time after menopause, long-term use of low-dose vaginal estrogen can be recommended.	**Case 51-2 (Questions 1, 2)**
8 Androgen therapy can be used for women experiencing sexual dysfunction that is unrelated to vaginal atrophy.	**Case 51-2 (Question 3)**

INCIDENCE, PREVALENCE, AND EPIDEMIOLOGY

The perimenopausal or climacteric phase in the female aging process (i.e., the time between the reproductive and nonreproductive years) is distinguished by waning ovarian function and irregular menstrual cycles. Menopause, the last spontaneous episode of physiologic uterine bleeding, is usually identified retrospectively after 12 months of amenorrhea, and typically occurs 4 to 5 years after the onset of the perimenopause. If needed, menopause can be confirmed by measurement of follicle-stimulating hormone (FSH) levels greater than 40 international units/mL. Postmenopause is characterized by significantly decreased hormone levels that may contribute to an increased risk of disease, including osteoporosis and cardiovascular disease.[1,2]

The average age of women at menopause has remained relatively constant at 51 years despite a significant increase in life expectancy.[3] Women today may spend one-third of their lives in the postmenopausal state. There are an estimated 40 million women aged 45 to 65 years in the United States who are at risk for menopause-related health issues.[4] Age at menopause appears to be genetically determined and is not influenced by race, physical characteristics, age at menarche, age at last pregnancy, socioeconomic status, or oral contraceptive use. Cigarette smoking decreases age at menopause by 1 to 2 years.[3] Cytotoxic drugs and radiotherapy may induce ovarian failure, and bilateral oophorectomy results in surgically induced menopause. Onset of menopause before age 40 is termed premature ovarian failure.

TABLE 51-1
Plasma Levels of Hormones in Premenopausal and Postmenopausal Women[5–7]

Hormones	Premenopausal	Postmenopausal
Estradiol	50–350 pg/mL	5–25 pg/mL
Estrone	30–110 pg/mL	20–70 pg/mL
Progesterone		0.17 ng/mL
Follicular	0.2–0.7 ng/mL	
Luteal	3–21 ng/mL	
Testosterone	0.3 ng/mL	0.25 ng/mL
Androstenedione	1.5 ng/mL	0.6 ng/mL

PATHOPHYSIOLOGY

Perimenopause results from an age-related acceleration in oocyte (immature female egg) degeneration and resistance to gonadotropins. The aging follicles produce less inhibin, which triggers increased production of FSH (Fig. 51-1).[3] Despite this increase in FSH levels, the declining ovary is unable to consistently produce mature follicles, resulting in frequent anovulatory cycles during the years approaching menopause. However, spontaneous ovulation can still occur, and contraception should be used if pregnancy is not desired. When all ovarian follicles have been depleted, menopause occurs. This corresponds with a 10- to 20-fold increase in FSH levels and a threefold increase in luteinizing hormone levels, which peak 1 to 3 years after menopause.[3]

As the declining ovary no longer produces estrogen, postmenopausal estrogen production is approximately 10% of premenopausal levels.[3,5] After menopause, the primary circulating estrogen is estrone, rather than the more potent estradiol. Estradiol is the primary estrogen during the reproductive years.[3,6] Estrogen concentrations do not vary in a cyclic fashion as they do during the reproductive years (Table 51-1). The source of postmenopausal estrogen is androstenedione, an androgen that is converted to estrogen by an aromatase enzyme found predominantly in fat, liver, and skin. Enzyme levels increase with age and body weight, resulting in higher estrogen levels in women with greater body fat.[3,6] Progesterone levels after menopause are generally undetectable in the absence of corpus luteum formation by the failed ovary. Despite a 25% to 50% decrease in androgen production after menopause,[3] the androgen to estrogen ratio increases markedly owing to the greater drop in estrogen levels, often resulting in mild symptoms of androgenism, such as hirsutism.[3]

CLINICAL PRESENTATION

Although menopause is a natural progression of aging, the decrease in estrogen production can result in clinical symptoms, such as hot flushes and genitourinary atrophy. The risk for

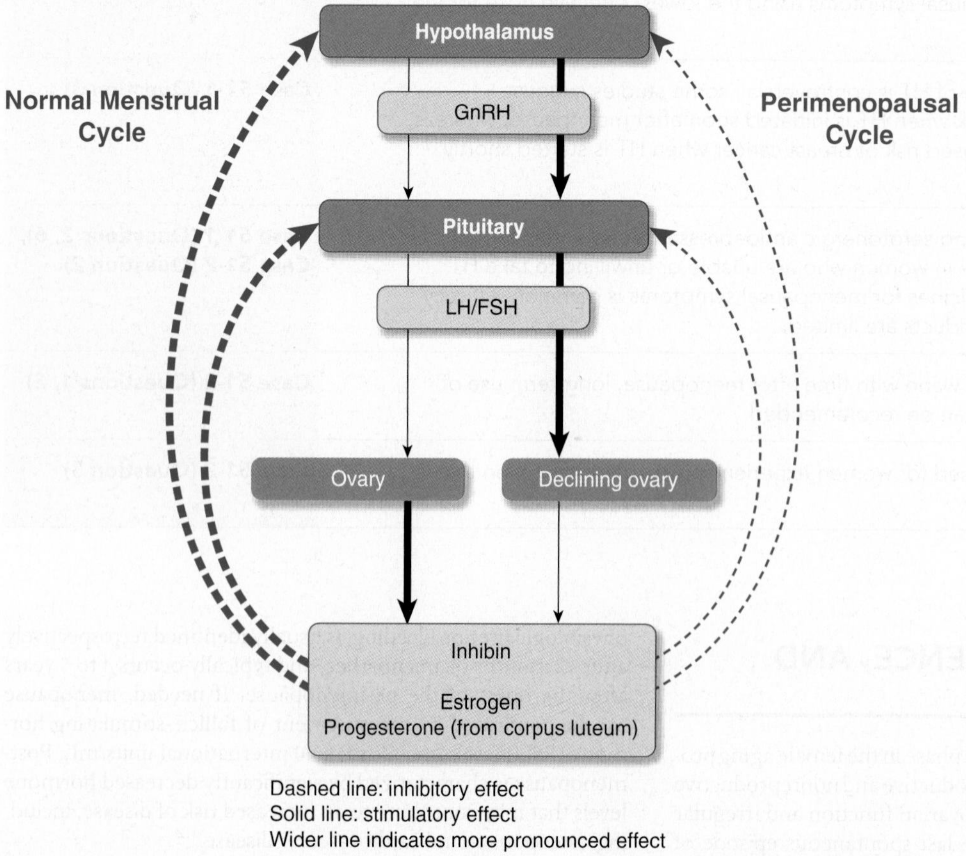

FIGURE 51-1 Perimenopausal changes in hypothalamus–pituitary–ovary axis. FSH, follicle-stimulating hormone; GnRH, gonadotropin-releasing hormone; LH, luteinizing hormone.

cardiovascular disease, the leading cause of death in postmenopausal women, appears to be amplified by estrogen deficiency.[1,2] Postmenopausal osteoporosis may result from estrogen deficiency (see Chapter 105, Osteoporosis). Loss of estrogen has also been associated with adverse effects on cognition and neurologic functioning, wellbeing, and sexual health.[2] Other manifestations of menopause may not yet be elucidated.

ONLINE CONTENT

For a visual of the organs changed by menopause, go to http://thepoint.lww.com?AT10e.

Signs and Symptoms

HOT FLUSHES

CASE 51-1

QUESTION 1: L.K., a 50-year-old woman, has been having sudden feelings of warmth over her chest accompanied by a patchy flushing of her skin and increased sweating for the past month, especially after drinking coffee or wine or if she is upset. She presents to clinic because she has been waking up shivering from a perspiration-drenched gown nightly for the past week. She had a menstrual period 3 weeks ago but recently her menses have been irregular (5 menses in the past 12 months.) Her physical examination is normal for a 50-year-old woman. Her last mammogram 6 months ago was normal. She does not smoke and her body mass index is 24 kg/m^2. She has hypertension that is controlled with hydrochlorothiazide 12.5 mg daily and migraine headaches without aura that she treats with sumatriptan 50 mg orally (PO) as needed. Her family history is positive for osteoporosis but negative for cardiovascular disease and breast cancer. Which of L.K.'s current symptoms are consistent with menopause?

It appears that L.K. is having hot flushes, a vasomotor symptom experienced by 50% to 85% of women during the menopause transition.[3,8] The onset of vasomotor symptoms may precede the last menstrual period, but the prevalence is highest during the 2 years after menopause and declines with time since menopause.[3] Symptoms persist for longer than 1 year in 80% and longer than 5 years in 25% of women.[3,9] Women with surgically induced menopause are more likely to experience moderate to severe hot flushes compared with women with natural menopause.[10] Symptoms include a feeling of warmth in the chest, neck, and facial areas that may be accompanied by visible flushing and increased sweating. Nocturnal hot flushes (night sweats) cause nighttime awakening and may lead to insomnia and sleep deprivation. Hot flushes average approximately 4 minutes in duration and are characteristically episodic rather than continuous, but may occur hourly in women with severe symptoms.[7,9] Increased environmental temperature, ingestion of hot liquids or alcohol, and mental stress also may provoke hot flushes.[3]

The specific trigger for hot flushes is unknown, but they are clearly associated with the declining estrogen concentrations that occur during menopause. It is postulated that the drop in estrogen leads to a decrease in serotonin levels and an increase in the levels of norepinephrine and its metabolite, 3-methoxy-4-hydroxyphenylglycol. These hormones are involved in temperature regulation, and their fluctuations trigger an inappropriate activation of the body's heat-release mechanisms, leading to the cutaneous vasodilation and sweating seen with hot flushes.[3,8,9]

Other symptoms associated with the perimenopause may include irritability, inability to concentrate, forgetfulness, headaches, dizziness, joint stiffness, and fatigue.[7,11] Mood changes, including depression, are not uniformly associated with menopause, but are reported more frequently in women during the perimenopausal period.[12] Vaginal atrophy is also a common manifestation of menopause (see Case 51-2).[7,13]

Overview of Therapy

CASE 51-1, QUESTION 2: L.K. is seeking relief for her hot flushes but is not sure that she wants to use medications for this problem. What nonmedication therapies are appropriate for the management of L.K.'s hot flushes?

Menopausal symptoms may be distressing to women, but they are not associated with increased mortality. Therefore, the goal of drug therapy in a symptomatic postmenopausal woman is to relieve symptoms and improve quality of life without increasing the risk of serious adverse outcomes related to the agents used.

TREATMENT

LIFESTYLE MODIFICATIONS

First-line treatment for hot flushes is lifestyle modification, including avoidance of known triggers (e.g., hot beverages, alcohol, warm environments), wearing layered clothing, and use of personal cooling devices. Data on the effectiveness of regular exercise, biofeedback, and relaxation techniques on hot flush frequency and severity are limited.[14–16] If the patient continues to experience bothersome symptoms, drug therapy should be considered. It is important to note that placebo responses ranging up to 50% have been seen in clinical trials evaluating interventions for hot flushes.[17]

BLACK COHOSH

Black cohosh (*Cimicifuga racemosa*), an herbal product derived from a plant in the buttercup family, has a long tradition of use for the management of menopausal symptoms. Though controversial, it does not appear to have estrogenic effects, but may exert a serotonergic effect.[18,19] Clinical studies of black cohosh for hot flushes have shown mixed results,[19–22] but a beneficial effect on mood symptoms associated with menopause has been reported in some trials.[18] Black cohosh, at a dose of 20 mg orally twice a day is generally well tolerated, but use beyond 12 months has not been evaluated.[19] The most common adverse effects are gastrointestinal in nature though there have been questionable case reports of hepatotoxicity, muscle damage, and pseudolymphoma.[19]

PHYTOESTROGENS

Phytoestrogens, including isoflavones and lignans, are plant-based substances that exert mild estrogenic effects. Epidemiologic studies have found an association between higher dietary soy intake and fewer menopausal symptoms. However, several meta-analyses of clinical trials of phytoestrogens concluded that they have minor, if any, benefits on menopausal symptoms.[23–28] This apparent lack of benefit may be related to the source and dose of isoflavones being evaluated; studies of high doses of the soy-derived isoflavone, genistein, reported significant improvement in hot flushes.[26] In general, isoflavones are well tolerated, the most commonly reported side effect being gastrointestinal intolerance.[29] A 5-year study documented an increased risk of endometrial hyperplasia with phytoestrogen use.[30] Because of their estrogenic effects, phytoestrogens should be avoided or used cautiously in women with a history of estrogen-dependent disease.

TABLE 51-2
Risks and Benefits of Postmenopausal Hormone Therapy

	Evidence	Absolute or Relative Contraindications and Patient Considerations	References
Established Benefits[a]			
Vasomotor symptoms	Systemic ET (in women without a uterus) or EPT (in women with a uterus) is considered the most effective therapy for hot flushes. There may be a dose–response relationship. Oral and TD estrogen are equally effective.	This is the primary indication for the use of systemic hormone therapy.	34,35
Osteoporosis	Numerous clinical trials support reduced risk of vertebral and hip fractures with use of estrogen.	Not a primary indication for use but will provide bone protection during use of HT for menopausal symptoms.	32,36
Vaginal atrophy	Numerous studies show both local and systemic estrogen reverse the atrophy induced by menopause.	Localized therapy should be used for patients with symptoms related solely to vaginal atrophy.	37,38
Established Risks[a]			
Thromboembolic disease	Increased risk of DVT and PE, greatest within the first year of use, risk with EPT possibly greater then with ET. Transdermal estrogen appears to have lower risk than oral estrogen.	**Absolute contraindication:** current tobacco use, history of thrombosis. **Relative contraindication:** obesity, women 65 years and older. Therapy should be discontinued before surgery or anticipated period of immobilization.	33,39,50,52,55
Breast cancer	Numerous clinical trials indicate risk increased ~25% after 5 years of use, increases with continued use. Greater risk with shorter exposure gap, seen with both EPT and ET.	**Absolute contraindication:** personal history of breast cancer. **Relative contraindication:** strong family history of breast cancer.	32,47–49
Cardiovascular disease	Increased risk of MI, especially when started >10 years after menopause or in women ≥60 years old (see also unconfirmed benefit).	**Relative contraindication:** age 60 years or older, >10 years postmenopause.	39,40
Endometrial cancer	Risk related to dose and duration of use. Addition of progestogen reduces or eliminates risk.	Rationale for use of concomitant progestogen in women with uterus. **Absolute contraindication:** undiagnosed postmenopausal vaginal bleeding, prior history of endometrial cancer.	43,44
Ischemic stroke	~30%–40% increased risk for ischemic stroke seen. Risk seen with both ET and EPT and may be dose related. Risk increased with increasing age (because of underlying age-related risk of stroke). HT does not appear to affect risk of hemorrhagic stroke.	**Absolute contraindication:** history of stroke or transient ischemic attacks, current tobacco use. **Relative contraindication:** obesity, uncontrolled hypertension, uncontrolled diabetes.	32,45,46,51,56
Gallbladder disease	~60% increased risk of cholecystitis and cholelithiasis (gallstones) seen with ET and EPT, also increased risk for gallbladder surgery.	**Relative contraindication:** history of gallbladder disease.	33,53
Hypertriglyceridemia	Oral estrogen increases triglycerides. Transdermal estrogen has a less pronounced effect, and EPT may have less effect than ET alone owing to attenuating effect of progestogen.	**Relative contraindication:** hypertriglyceridemia. If estrogen is to be used in woman with elevated TG, select transdermal route, monitor TG levels.	44,54,57

(continued)

TABLE 51-2
Risks and Benefits of Postmenopausal Hormone Therapy (*Continued*)

	Evidence	Absolute or Relative Contraindications and Patient Considerations	References
Unconfirmed Benefits[b]			
Cardiovascular disease	No increased risk or possible decreased risk when initiated soon after menopause (see also established risk).	Prevention of CVD is not a primary indication for use; this information can reassure patient needing HT for menopause symptoms or replacement for women with premature ovarian failure.	41,42
Colorectal cancer	Decreased risk is seen with EPT but not ET.	May be secondary benefit in women using for hot flushes.	39,58
Recurrent UTIs	Low-dose localized estrogen treatment can decrease risk for recurrent UTIs.	May be secondary benefit in women using localized therapy for vaginal atrophy.	59
Diabetes mellitus	Decreased incidence of new-onset diabetes in women taking EPT or ET.	This suggests that DM is not a contraindication for women who wish to use EPT/ET.	56
Unconfirmed Risks[b]			
Ovarian cancer	Increased risk seen with ET and EPT and increased duration is associated with greater risk.	**Relative contraindication:** strong family history of ovarian cancer.	60–63
Lung cancer	Studies showed increased risk of lung cancer diagnosis and mortality with EPT but not ET. Risk seen primarily in current smokers and older women.	**Absolute contraindication:** current tobacco use (owing to increased risk of TED).	64–66
Urinary incontinence	Systemic estrogen caused or worsened urinary incontinence.	Avoid systemic estrogen in women with urinary incontinence, monitor for new onset in women taking HT.	59,67,68
Cognitive effects	Studies report worsening of dementia in women with pre-existing dementia and no improvement or protection in older women taking HT.	**Absolute contraindication:** patients with evidence of dementia. Avoid use in women ≥65 years.	69–71
Migraine headaches	HT may cause worsening of migraine headaches.	**Absolute contraindication:** migraine with aura (increased risk of stroke). **Relative contraindication:** migraine without aura—monitor for changes in HA frequency.	72

[a] Well-documented risk or benefit supported by multiple clinical studies.
[b] Possible risk or benefit shown in limited clinical trials, additional data needed to confirm.
CVD, cardiovascular disease; DM, diabetes mellitus; DVT, deep venous thrombosis; EPT, estrogen and progestogen therapy; ET, estrogen only therapy; HA, headache; HT, hormone therapy; MI, myocardial infarction; PE, pulmonary embolism; TD, transdermal; TED, thromboembolic disease; TG, triglycerides; UTI, urinary tract infection.

OTHER THERAPY

Studies of wild yam extract, ginseng, gingko, evening primrose oil, and St. John's wort do not support a beneficial effect of these agents in the management of hot flushes.[22,31]

L.K. does not have any estrogen-dependent diseases and therefore could try either black cohosh or phytoestrogens for her hot flushes if lifestyle modifications do not provide adequate benefit. She should be counseled that these products have mixed data supporting their benefits and phytoestrogens could potentially have side effects similar to hormone therapy.

HORMONE THERAPY

CASE 51-1, QUESTION 3: L.K. returns to clinic after 2 months. She initiated lifestyle modifications and tried black cohosh but has noted worsening of her flushes, awakening multiple times nightly from night sweats, which is causing daytime fatigue and irritability. She asks about hormone therapy to control her hot flushes. Is L.K. a candidate for hormone therapy?

Hormone therapy (HT) has received a great deal of scientific and media attention during the past decade. The Women's Health Initiative (WHI), a large, prospective study of estrogen therapy (ET) and estrogen/progestogen (EPT) therapy in postmenopausal women, and other large cohort studies have provided a great deal of data, some of it conflicting, on the risks and benefits of hormone use after menopause.[32,33] Before selecting a treatment option, women should be evaluated for contraindications to HT and counseled about its possible risks and benefits (Table 51-2).

ESTABLISHED BENEFITS OF HORMONE THERAPY

Vasomotor Symptoms

The efficacy of estrogen in reducing the frequency and severity of hot flushes is well established. Some studies report a

TABLE 51-3

Agents Labeled for Use in ET and EPT Therapy

Drug (Brand Name)	Route Initial Dosage
Estrogens, Systemic[b]	
Conjugated equine estrogens (Premarin)[a]	PO 0.3 mg
Synthetic conjugated estrogens (A: Cenestin, B: Enjuvia)	PO 0.3 mg
Estropipate (piperazine estrone sulfate) (Ogen, Ortho-Est)[a,c]	PO 0.625 mg
Micronized estradiol (Estrace, Gynodiol)[a,c]	PO 0.5 mg
Estradiol transdermal system (various brand name products)[a]	TD 0.014–0.025 mg/24 h patch applied weekly or twice weekly
Esterified estrogen (Menest)[a]	PO 0.3 mg
Estradiol acetate tablet (Femtrace)[c]	PO 0.45 mg
Estradiol acetate vaginal ring (Femring)[c]	HDV 0.05 mg/24 h ring inserted vaginally every 90 days
Estradiol topical emulsion/gel/solution (Divigel, Elestrin, Estrogel, Estrasorb, Evamist)[c]	TD 0.0125 mg to 0.75 mg (product dependent)
Progestogens	
Medroxyprogesterone acetate (Provera generic and combo products)	PO 5 mg for cyclic regimens; 2.5 mg for continuous regimens
Norethindrone acetate (Aygestin generic and combo products)	PO 2.5 mg for cyclic regimens; 0.5 mg for continuous regimens
Micronized progesterone (Prometrium)[c]	PO 200 mg for cyclic regimens; 100 mg for continuous regimens
Progesterone vaginal gel (Prochieve, Crinone)[c]	V 1 full applicator of 4% gel every other day
Progesterone vaginal suppository (First Progesterone VGS)	V 200 mg/d for 12 days
Levonorgestrel-releasing IUD (Mirena)	IU 0.02 mg/d
Estrogen and Progestogen Combinations	
Prempro[a]	PO 0.3 mg CEE and 1.5 mg MPA
Premphase[a]	PO 0.625 mg CEE for 28 days with 5 mg MPA for last 14 days
CombiPatch	TD 0.05 mg estradiol with 0.14 mg norethindrone
Femhrt[a]	PO 0.0025 mg ethinyl estradiol and 0.1 mg norethindrone acetate
Activella[a]	PO 0.5 mg estradiol and 0.1 mg norethindrone acetate
Prefest[a]	PO 1 mg estradiol and 0.09 mg norgestimate (3 days of ET alternating with 3 days of EPT)
Climara Pro[a]	TD 0.045 mg estradiol/0.015 mg levonorgestrel/24 h patch once weekly
Angeliq	PO 1 mg estradiol and 0.5 mg drospirenone
Estrogen and Androgen Combinations[b]	
Esterified estradiol and Methyltestosterone (Estratest, Covaryx)	PO 0.625 mg esterified estrogens and 1.25 mg MT
Low-dose Vaginal Estrogens (localized effect only)	
Conjugated Equine Estrogen cream (Premarin)	LDV Initial: 0.5–2 g cream (0.3125–1.25 mg CEE) daily Maintenance: 0.5–2 g cream (0.3125–1.25 mg CEE) once/twice weekly based on severity
Estradiol cream (Estrace)[c]	LDV Initial: 2–4 g cream (0.2–0.4 mg estradiol) daily Maintenance: 1 g cream (0.1 mg estradiol) twice weekly
Estradiol ring (Estring)[c]	LDV 2-mg ring (0.0075 mg/d) every 90 days
Estradiol hemihydrate tablets (Vagifem and Vagifem LD)	LDV one tablet (0.01 mg) daily for 2 weeks, then one tablet twice weekly

[a] Approved by the US Food and Drug Administration for prevention of osteoporosis.
[b] Requires addition of progestogen in women with a uterus.
[c] FDA-approved bioidentical hormone.
CEE, conjugated equine estrogens; HDV, high-dose vaginal estrogen, sufficient absorption to produce systemic estrogenic effect (i.e., for treatment of hot flushes); IU, intrauterine; IUD, intrauterine device; LDV, low-dose vaginal estrogen, provides localized estrogenic effect (i.e., for vaginal atrophy), owing to low dose, minimal systemic absorption; MPA, medroxyprogesterone acetate; MT, methyltestosterone; PO, oral; TD, transdermal; V, vaginal.
Adapted with permission from Facts & Comparisons eAnswers. http://online.factsandcomparisons.com/index.aspx?. Accessed November 28, 2011.

dose–response relationship.[34] Oral and transdermal estrogen are equally efficacious, and the addition of a progestogen does not appear to alter this benefit. Estrogen absorption through the vaginal mucosa is efficient—use of higher dose vaginal products can produce levels adequate to relieve systemic symptoms such as hot flushes (Table 51-3). In women with hot flushes, EPT has been shown to improve quality of life and depressive symptoms.[35] During perimenopause, combination hormonal contraceptives are effective in reducing vasomotor symptoms and preventing pregnancy.

Osteoporosis

There are strong clinical data on the efficacy of estrogen, with or without a progestogen, in preventing the bone loss associated with menopause. Estrogen has been shown to decrease the risk of osteoporotic hip and vertebral fractures by approximately 25%.[32,36] Multiple estrogen products are US Food and Drug Administration (FDA)-approved for the prevention of osteoporosis (Table 51-3); however, because of its risks and the availability of effective alternative treatments, ET or EPT should not be used solely for the prevention of osteoporosis. During systemic estrogen therapy, bone density is maintained but bone loss resumes with estrogen discontinuation, so alternative protective therapies should be considered in women at risk who stop ET or avoid its use altogether (see Chapter 105, Osteoporosis).[36]

Other Possible Benefits

There are other less established benefits of HT (Table 51-2), including possible effects on urinary tract infections, cardiovascular disease, diabetes mellitus, and colon cancer.[32]

ESTABLISHED RISKS OF HORMONE THERAPY

Cardiovascular Disease

Estrogens have beneficial effects on lipids (increased high-density lipoprotein and decreased low-density lipoprotein) and endothelial function, suggesting a pharmacologic basis for a heart-protective effect.[73] However, the cardiovascular effects of ET remain controversial. Older case-control and cohort studies found that compared with never users, postmenopausal women who used ET or EPT had a lower risk of coronary heart disease–related death.[74] In the WHI, which was specifically designed to answer questions about ET or EPT and primary prevention of cardiovascular disease, increased cardiovascular events in the EPT group led to early termination of that arm of the study. The estrogen-only arm was also stopped early owing to an increased risk of stroke without evidence of cardiovascular protection.[39,40] Further analysis of data from the WHI and another study found no increased risk of coronary heart disease in women aged 50 to 59 years who began therapy within 10 years of menopause, suggesting that the increased risk of cardiovascular disease occurs primarily in women aged 60 years and older who initiate HT more than 10 years after menopause.[41,42]

Although there are still unanswered questions regarding the cardiovascular effects of ET or EPT, it appears that in younger patients such as L.K. who initiate HT for vasomotor symptoms soon after the onset of menopause, the risk of cardiovascular disease may not be significantly increased.

Endometrial Cancer

Stimulation by exogenous estrogen causes endometrial proliferation leading to hyperplasia rates of 8% to 62% after 1 to 3 years of use.[43] In a woman with a uterus, use of ET alone increases the risk of endometrial cancer by 2-fold to 10-fold, with higher estrogen dose and duration associated with greater risk. The elevated risk persists for at least 5 years after discontinuation of ET.[44] Addition of a progestogen significantly attenuates or eliminates the increased risk of endometrial cancer; therefore, a progestogen should be recommended in addition to ET in a woman with an intact uterus.[43,44,75,76]

Breast Cancer

Numerous studies demonstrate a 25% overall increased risk of breast cancer with EPT use, becoming significant 5 years after initiation, increasing with continued use, and returning to baseline approximately 5 years after EPT is stopped.[32,47] Risk appears to be similar between oral and transdermal estrogen, and no dose–response relationship has been established. Limited data suggest that ET increases the risk of breast cancer less than EPT.[32,48] A short exposure gap (the time from menopause until the start of HT) appears to significantly increase the risk for breast cancer compared with a longer interval.[32,49]

Thromboembolic Disease

ET use increases the overall risk for venous thromboembolic disease (TED), including deep venous thrombosis and pulmonary embolism, twofold.[39,50] The greatest risk is within the first year of treatment. Women who are older or have a higher body mass index are at additional increased risk.[77] The increased risk may be mediated by inhibition of hepatic synthesis of anticoagulant factors, including antithrombin, protein S, and protein C.[52] EPT may incur a greater risk than ET, but transdermal estrogen has a significantly lower risk than oral estrogen as it avoids the first-pass metabolic effects of oral therapy.[32,52,55,78,79] HT should be avoided in women with a history of or at high risk for TED.

Other Possible Risks

Other risks with HT are not as clearly defined (Table 51-2). These include potential adverse effects on cognition and urinary tract function, and the development of ovarian and lung cancer and gallbladder disease.[32]

Recommendations

Current guidelines on systemic HT recommend its use only in women with moderate to severe hot flushes (Fig. 51-2).[56] For women with premature ovarian failure, it is recommended that HT be given until the typical age of natural menopause to avoid early manifestations of estrogen deficiency.[80]

As L.K. continues to experience severe hot flushes that are affecting her quality of life, she is recently postmenopausal, and she has no absolute contraindications to estrogen (such as TED, history of breast or endometrial cancer, uncontrolled hypertension, migraine with aura, tobacco use, obesity), a trial of HT is appropriate.

SELECTION OF THERAPY

CASE 51-1, QUESTION 4: What is an appropriate HT regimen for the management of L.K.'s hot flushes?

ESTROGENS

There are a number of hormonal products (e.g. oral, transdermal patches, transdermal gels, and vaginal rings) currently available for the management of vasomotor symptoms (Table 51-3). Oral and transdermal estrogen appear to be equally efficacious in treating hot flushes.[34] Because it avoids first-pass metabolism, transdermal estrogen is associated with a decreased risk for TED and hypertension but has less of a beneficial effect on the lipid profile compared with oral estrogen. The effect of transdermal estrogen on breast cancer and cardiovascular and gallbladder disease has not been well studied.[81]

BIOIDENTICAL HORMONES

There is strong consumer interest in natural (bioidentical) HT as a potentially safer alternative to synthetic estrogens. Bioidentical hormones are defined as having the same chemical structure as the hormones produced by the human reproductive system and include estradiol, estrone, progesterone, and testosterone. Studies of commercially available bioidentical hormone products demonstrate a similar efficacy to synthetic estrogens; however, clinical evidence to support claims of greater safety is lacking.[82,83] Women desiring to use bioidentical products should be advised of commercially available products (Table 51-3); extemporaneously compounded bioidentical hormones do not carry FDA-approved warnings and may be of inadequate quality.[83]

Current recommendations are to initiate estrogen at a low dose (e.g., 0.3 mg of conjugated equine estrogens or 0.025 mg of transdermal estradiol). If symptoms persist after 2 to 3 weeks of therapy, the dose of estrogen can be increased to the next available dosage strength for the product being used (Table 51-3).

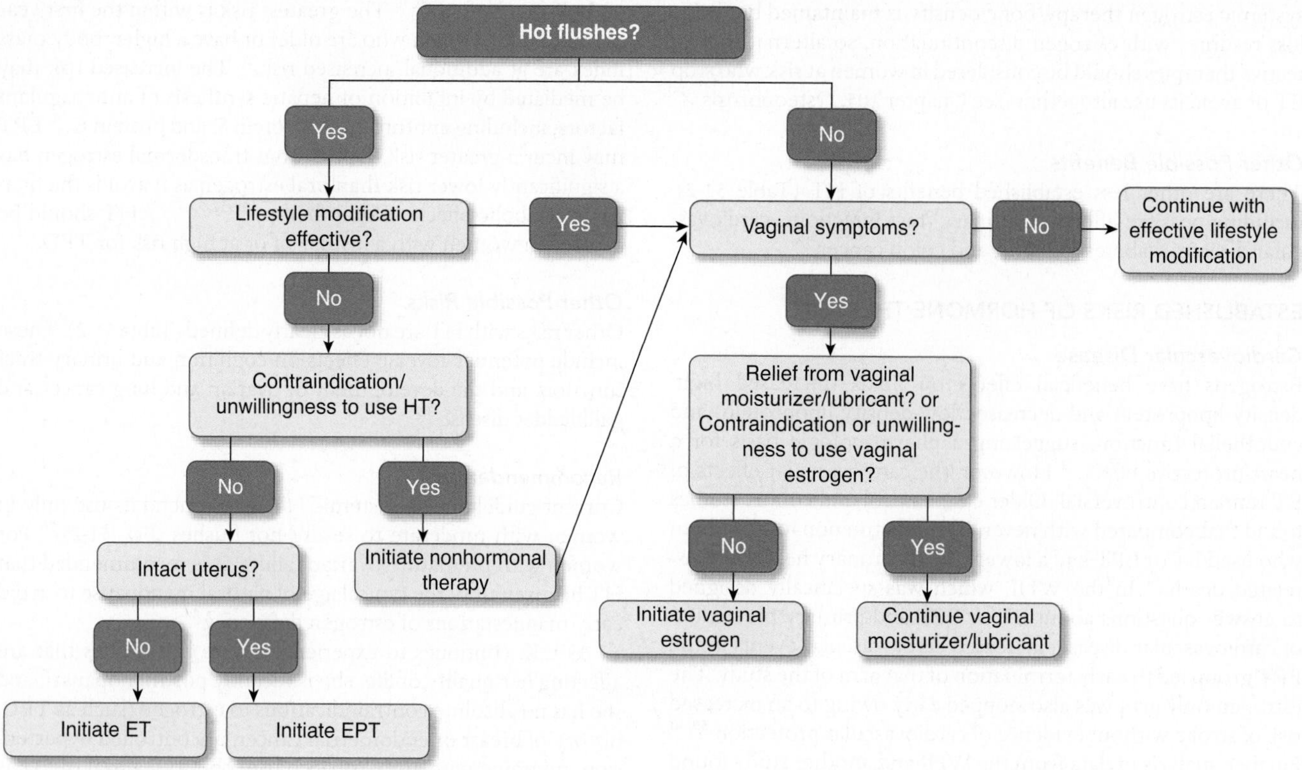

FIGURE 51-2 Algorithm for the management of symptomatic menopausal women. EPT, estrogen/progestogen therapy; ET, estrogen therapy; HT, hormone therapy.

PROGESTOGENS

In women with an intact uterus, such as L.K., a progestogen must also be added to the regimen to minimize the risk of endometrial cancer (Table 51-3).[44,56] Currently, there is no indication for adding a progestogen to ET in women without a uterus. For medroxyprogesterone acetate, the most commonly used EPT progestogen, 5 mg/day for at least 12 days/month is needed to prevent endometrial hyperplasia when used in cyclic regimens (Table 51-4). For continuous regimens, 2.5 mg/day may be adequate. Oral micronized progesterone 100 to 300 mg/day for 12 days/month or the progestogen-releasing intrauterine device also appear to protect against endometrial hyperplasia from ET.[44,85,86]

EPT may result in resumption of uterine withdrawal bleeding. The pattern and frequency of bleeding is dependent on the EPT regimen used (Table 51-4).[84] Patient preference regarding bleeding patterns should be considered when selecting an EPT regimen.

Progestogen monotherapy appears to be similar to estrogen in relieving the symptoms of hot flushes. Effective regimens include megestrol acetate, 40 mg/day orally, and medroxyprogesterone acetate, 10 mg/day orally or 150 mg intramuscularly every 3 months or 400 mg intramuscularly one time.[87,88] Adverse effects of progestogens include vaginal bleeding, fluid retention, increased appetite, breast tenderness, acne, hirsutism, headaches, mood swings, fatigue, and depression. In the absence of ET, progestogens do not appear to increase the risk of TED.[44] However, data on long-term safety, especially in regard to breast cancer, are lacking.[88] Progestogen monotherapy for the treatment of hot flushes is generally reserved for women with contraindications to estrogen use.

DURATION OF HORMONE THERAPY

Because hot flushes are self-limiting, it can be difficult to assess whether symptom relief is related to the treatment or natural resolution of symptoms. Six to 12 months after L.K.'s hot flushes are fully treated, she should attempt discontinuation of EPT. Abrupt discontinuation of ET or EPT may trigger rapid recurrence of hot flushes; therefore, tapering is recommended.[89] There are no specific guidelines for withdrawing therapy; typical taper regimens involve decreasing the daily estrogen dose to the next available dosage strength or increasing the dosing interval. If symptoms recur during the taper, therapy can be resumed at the lowest effective dose and another taper attempted in 6 months.[90]

ADVERSE EFFECTS

CASE 51-1, QUESTION 5: To minimize the risks of TED, L.K. is prescribed a combination estrogen/progestogen patch. How should she be counseled about possible side effects of EPT?

In addition to being counseled about the serious risks of EPT, L.K. should be advised regarding nuisance side effects from HT. These most commonly include resumption of vaginal bleeding and breast tenderness.[34,84] Nausea, weight gain, edema, headache, premenstrual syndromelike symptoms, and increased vaginal discharge have also been reported. Skin irritation may occur with the use of transdermal products. Frequently, these side effects diminish with time or may respond to a change in dosage or product. Although ET and EPT have not been shown to consistently induce or worsen hypertension, patients with hypertension, such as L.K., should be monitored for increases in blood pressure.[91]

NONHORMONAL AGENTS

CASE 51-1, QUESTION 6: L.K. returns 3 months later. Her hot flushes and night sweats resolved with EPT, but she experienced worsening of her migraine headaches, so she

TABLE 51-4
ET/EPT Regimens and Expected Vaginal Bleeding Patterns[84]

Estrogen/Progestogen Dosing	Hormone-Free Interval	Typical Bleeding Pattern
Combined Regimens (EPT) for Patient with Intact Uterus		
CYCLIC REGIMEN		
Estrogen (PO or TD): days 1–25 of each month Progestogen: days 10–25 or 14–25 of each month	3–6 days	Withdrawal bleeding[c] 1–2 days after progestogen dosing ended[a] 80% experience regular bleeding
CYCLIC COMBINED		
Estrogen (PO or TD) and Progestogen: days 1–25 of each month	3–6 days	Withdrawal bleeding[c] 1–2 days after progestogen dosing ended[a] Lower incidence than cyclic regimen
CONTINUOUS CYCLIC		
Estrogen (PO or TD): daily Progestogen: 10–14 days every month	None	Withdrawal bleeding[c] 1–2 days after progestogen dosing ended[a] 80% experience regular bleeding
LONG-CYCLE CYCLIC		
Estrogen (PO or TD): daily Progestogen: 14 days every third month	None	Withdrawal bleeding[c] 1–2 days after progestogen dosing ended[a] ~70% experience regular bleeding
CONTINUOUS COMBINED		
Estrogen (PO or TD) and Progestogen: daily	None	40% have irregular bleeding for first 6–12 months[b] 75%–89% become amenorrheic within 12 months
CONTINUOUS PULSED		
Estrogen PO × 3 days then Estrogen + Progestogen PO × 3 days Repeat continuously	None	~70% experience spotting[d] early during treatment 80% are amenorrheic at the end of 12 months[b]
Estrogen-only Regimens (ET) for Patients Without Uterus		
CONTINUOUS REGIMEN	None	
Estrogen (PO or TD): daily	None	

[a] Bleeding earlier than 11 days after beginning progestogen suggests need for endometrial evaluation.
[b] Bleeding after 6 months of therapy requires endometrial evaluation.
[c] Withdrawal bleed is vaginal bleeding for multiple days (usually <10 days) that resembles menstrual period and requires use of a tampon or sanitary pad.
[d] Spotting is light bleeding that lasts <1 day.
EPT, estrogen therapy with progestogen added; ET, estrogen-only therapy; PO, orally; TD, transdermally.

discontinued HT. Her hot flushes recurred soon thereafter. What alternative therapies are available for the management of L.K.'s symptoms?

Nonhormonal agents are modestly effective in reducing hot flush frequency and severity. Table 51-5 lists the agents and doses that have been shown to be effective along with adverse effects most commonly seen.[14,15,17,23,92–99]

The therapeutic efficacy of selective serotonin reuptake inhibitors and serotonin and norepinephrine reuptake inhibitors in hot flush treatment is thought to be related to their effect on serotonin and norepinephrine levels. In clinical trials, relief of hot flushes was seen at lower doses and with a more rapid onset than is seen for the antidepressant effects of these agents.[17,95] Dosing should be initiated at the lowest effective dose (Table 51-5); this can be increased after 2 to 3 weeks if the patient has an inadequate response. Patients should be advised not to discontinue therapy abruptly to avoid withdrawal symptoms. Venlafaxine and paroxetine, the most studied agents, are considered the drugs of choice; other selective serotonin reuptake inhibitors and serotonin and norepinephrine reuptake inhibitors are considered second-line agents.[95] Commonly seen side effects are listed in Table 51-5. Of particular concern in postmenopausal women is the risk for anorgasmia and loss of libido; similar sexual dysfunction may also occur as a result of menopause. Patients should be advised to discuss the problem with their care provider if it occurs and is bothersome (see Case 51-2, Question 3). The antiepileptic drug gabapentin has been shown in multiple studies to decrease hot flushes through an unidentified mechanism. The therapeutic effect occurs at a dose of 900 mg/day with an onset within 4 weeks of initiation of treatment. To minimize side effects, dosing should be initiated at 300 mg daily and titrated up in 300-mg/day increments as tolerated. Although one study showed benefit with 2,400 mg/day, the optimal dose of gabapentin for hot flushes is unknown.[17,96]

Paroxetine CR at an initial dose of 12.5 mg daily can be tried in L.K. If her symptoms are not improved after 2 to 3 weeks, the dose can be increased to 25 mg daily.

Genitourinary Atrophy

SIGNS AND SYMPTOMS

CASE 51-2

QUESTION 1: D.M., a 58-year-old woman, presents with a complaint of persistent vaginal dryness and irritation as well as pain associated with intercourse. She has tried vaginal lubricants, which help with intercourse-related pain but do not relieve her daily vaginal symptoms. She experienced menopause at age 51, which was accompanied by moderate hot flushes for 2 to 3 years that have since resolved without intervention. She denies symptoms of urinary incontinence. She does not smoke. On physical examination, her labia minora have a pale, dry appearance, and the labia majora appear flattened. Her vagina is small with a pale, dry epithelium. What is causing D.M.'s condition?

D.M. appears to be experiencing symptoms associated with genitourinary atrophy. Estrogen is the dominant hormone of vaginal physiology. With the postmenopausal loss of estrogen production, the vagina decreases in size and loses its rugal

TABLE 51-5
Nonhormonal Agents for the Management of Vasomotor Symptoms[14,15,17,23,92–99]

Drug	Recommended Dosage	Adverse Reactions Reported
Serotonergic Antidepressants		
Citalopram (Celexa)	10–30 mg	Dry mouth, ↓ libido, rash/hives, insomnia, somnolence, bladder spasm, palpitations, arthralgias
Desvenlafaxine (Pristiq)	50–100 mg	Asthenia, chills, anorexia, nausea, vomiting, constipation, diarrhea, dizziness, nervousness, mydriasis, dry mouth
Escitalopram (Lexapro)	10–20 mg	Dizziness, lightheadedness, nausea, vivid dreams, increased sweating
Fluoxetine (Prozac)	10–20 mg	Nausea, dry mouth
Paroxetine (Paxil, PaxilCR)	10–20 mg 12.5–25 mg (CR)	Headache, nausea, insomnia, drowsiness
Sertraline (Zoloft)	50 mg	Nausea, fatigue/malaise, diarrhea, anxiety/nervousness
Venlafaxine (Effexor, Effexor XR)	37.5–75 mg 37.5–150 mg XR	Dry mouth, ↓ appetite, nausea, constipation, possible increase in blood pressure at higher doses
Antiseizure Agents		
Gabapentin (Neurontin)	900 mg, possibly up to 2,400 mg	Somnolence, fatigue, dizziness, rash, palpitations, peripheral edema
Pregabalin (Lyrica)	150–300 mg	Dizziness, sleepiness, weight gain, cognitive difficulty
Antihypertensive Agents		
Clonidine	PO: 0.05–0.15 mg TD: 0.1 mg/24 h	Headache, dry mouth, drowsiness Skin reaction/itching (patch only), risk of rebound HTN if stopped abruptly

HTN, hypertension; PO, orally; TD, transdermally.

pattern: the mucosa becomes pale, thin, and dry, and vaginal blood flow decreases. A decrease in *Lactobacillus* production of lactic acid leads to an increase in vaginal pH to 5.0 or greater (compared with a premenopausal pH of 3.5–4.5).[13,37,100] These changes make the vagina more susceptible to infection from bacterial colonization and localized trauma secondary to intercourse. Unlike hot flushes, vaginal atrophy does not abate with time since menopause.

Symptoms of atrophic vaginitis include dryness, itching, pain, and dyspareunia (painful coitus). About 10% to 40% of postmenopausal women experience symptoms; however, only 25% of those affected seek medical attention.[37] Postmenopausal women who engage in regular coital activity have less atrophic vaginal changes compared with those of similar age and estrogen levels who do not have regular intercourse.

TREATMENT

CASE 51-2, QUESTION 2: What would be an appropriate regimen for D.M. to decrease her vaginal symptoms?

NONHORMONAL TREATMENT

Vaginal moisturizers (e.g., Replens), which adhere to the vaginal mucosa, can improve vaginal symptoms but do not reverse atrophy.[100,101] Personal lubricants (e.g., KY jelly or liquid) can be used for women experiencing dyspareunia related to vaginal atrophy. Nonhormonal treatments used for vasomotor symptoms do not improve vaginal atrophy symptoms.[13,100]

LOCALIZED ESTROGEN TREATMENT

Estrogen therapy reverses vaginal epithelial thinning, decreases the vaginal pH, and improves the symptoms of vaginal atrophy. If hot flushes are also present, oral, transdermal, or high-dose vaginal estrogen can provide relief of both symptoms. For vaginal symptoms alone, low-dose vaginal estrogen is the preferred treatment.[37] The available products (Table 51-3) appear to be equivalent in restoring vaginal cytology and pH and relieving symptoms of vaginal dryness, pruritus, and dyspareunia; product selection should be based on patient preference.[37,38] Vaginal creams and tablets are initiated with once-daily dosing; after symptoms have resolved, the patient should be switched to maintenance dosing of once or twice weekly administration. The low-dose vaginal ring releases a constant dose of estrogen for 90 days.

The most common adverse effects of vaginal estrogens are vaginal irritation and bleeding and breast tenderness. Based on limited studies, the risk of endometrial hyperplasia from low-dose vaginal estrogen is small, and the addition of a progestogen is generally considered unnecessary.[37,38] Women at high risk for endometrial cancer, using higher than usual doses of vaginal estrogen, or experiencing vaginal bleeding during intravaginal ET should be evaluated for endometrial hyperplasia.[37]

Since D.M. has not had relief with nonhormonal therapy, localized ET such as conjugated estrogen, 1 g of 0.625 mg/g cream, applied vaginally once daily is appropriate. After her symptoms have resolved, the dose can be decreased to a maintenance regimen of twice-weekly administration.

ANDROGENS

CASE 51-2, QUESTION 3: D.M. has noted significant improvement in her vaginal symptoms and dyspareunia since initiating estrogen vaginal cream but complains of decreased sexual desire that is affecting her relationship. She asks whether there is anything she can take to help with this problem?

Decreased sexual desire is a common problem in postmenopausal women. Both aging and menopause are associated with low libido, and decreased levels of testosterone are implicated in its etiology.[102] Clinical trials in postmenopausal women have shown that testosterone, with or without concurrent HT, can significantly improve sexual function.[103,104] Oral methyltestosterone in combination with esterified estrogen is FDA-approved for the management of menopausal symptoms (Table 51-3); however, to avoid first-pass hepatic effects, topical administration is the preferred route. The FDA has deferred approval of a transdermal androgen patch for women because of lack of data on long-term safety[102]; use of a small quantity of a gel approved for use in men may provide adequate therapy. The dose of 300 mcg/day of topical testosterone used in clinical trials was associated with a low level of side effects, such as acne and hirsutism,[104] but data on long-term risks, including cardiovascular disease and breast cancer, are minimal.

Based on current recommendations,[103] D.M. is given a prescription for a compounded testosterone gel 150 mcg/day. After 3 months, the dose can be increased to 300 mcg/day if symptoms persist. If improvement in libido is not seen after several months of treatment at a dose that produces a testosterone level in the upper limit of the normal range for ovulating women, testosterone therapy should be discontinued.

KEY REFERENCES AND WEBSITES

A full list of references for this chapter can be found at **http://thepoint.lww.com/AT10e.** Below are the key references for this chapter, with the corresponding reference number in this chapter found in parentheses after the reference.

Key References

Baber R. Phytoestrogens and post reproductive health. *Maturitas.* 2010;66:344. (26)

Borrelli F, Ernst E. Alternative and complementary therapies for menopause. *Maturitas.* 2010;66:333. (22)

Carroll DG, Kelley KW. Use of antidepressants for management of hot flashes. *Pharmacotherapy.* 2009;29:1357. (95)

Cirigliano M. Bioidentical hormone therapy: a review of the evidence. *J Womens Health (Larchmt).* 2007;16:600. (82)

Krapf JM, Simon JA. The role of testosterone in the management of hypoactive sexual desire disorder in postmenopausal women. *Maturitas.* 2009;63:213. (102)

MacBride MB et al. Vulvovaginal atrophy. *Mayo Clin Proc.* 2010; 85:87. (100)

North American Menopause Society. Estrogen and progestogen use in postmenopausal women: 2010 position statement of the North American Menopause Society. *Menopause* 2010;17(2): 242–55. (56)

Santen RJ et al. Executive summary: postmenopausal hormone therapy: an Endocrine Society Scientific Statement. *J Clin Endocrinol Metab.* 2010;95(7 Suppl 1):S1. (32)

Vuvojic S et al. EMAS position statement: managing women with premature ovarian failure. *Maturitas.* 2010;67:91. (80)

Key Websites

NAMS: The North American Menopause Society. **http://www.menopause.org.**

National Heart Lung and Blood Institute, National Institutes of Health, Department of Health and Human Services. *Women's Health Initiative.* **http://www.nhlbi.nih.gov/whi/.**

SECTION EDITOR: LISA A. KROON

52 Thyroid Disorders

Betty J. Dong and Eric F. Schneider

CORE PRINCIPLES

	CHAPTER CASES
1 Thyroid function tests are essential to confirm the presence of thyroid disorders but can be altered by acute and chronic illness and certain drugs. Thyrotropin (TSH) is the most accurate indicator of euthyroidism.	**Case 52-1 (Questions 1, 2), Case 52-2, Case 52-3, Case 52-4, Case 52-5 (Question 5), Case 52-24, Case 52-25, Case 52-26, Case 52-27, Table 52-1**
2 Thyroid hormone deficiency can cause a goiter and hypothyroid symptoms including myxedema coma, heart failure, and hyperlipidemia. The most common cause of hypothyroidism is Hashimoto's thyroiditis.	**Case 52-5 (Question 1), Case 52-8 (Question 2), Case 52-9 (Question 2), Case 52-10 (Question 1), Case 52-11 (Questions 1, 2), Case 52-12, Case 52-13, Case 52-21, Table 52-2, Table 52-3**
3 Generic or branded levothyroxine (L-thyroxine) is the preparation of choice for optimal correction of hypothyroidism. Triiodothyronine (T_3)-containing preparations are not necessary because thyroxine (T_4) is converted to T_3.	**Case 52-5 (Question 2), Case 52-6, Case 52-10 (Question 2), Table 52-4, Table 52-8**
4 The signs and symptoms of hypothyroidism can be corrected by the administration of L-thyroxine on an empty stomach at average oral replacement dosages of 1.6 to 1.7 mcg/kg/day or intravenously. Dosing is altered by weight, comorbidities, and drug interactions.	**Case 52-5 (Questions 3–5), Case 52-7, Case 52-8 (Question 1), Case 52-9 (Question 1), Case 52-10 (Question 2), Case 52-11 (Question 3), Table 52-4, Table 52-9**
5 The signs and symptoms of hyperthyroidism mimic those of adrenergic excess (e.g., tachycardia, tremors, thyroid storm), but symptoms in the elderly may be absent ("apathetic"). Graves disease, a common cause of hyperthyroidism, can be complicated by ophthalmopathy.	**Case 52-14 (Questions 1, 2), Case 52-15 (Question 1), Case 52-22 (Questions 1, 2), Case 52-23 (Questions 1, 2), Table 52-5, Table 52-6**
6 Management of hyperthyroidism includes thioamides, iodides, radioactive iodine, and surgery. β-Blockers can provide symptomatic relief of hyperthyroid symptoms.	**Case 52-15 (Questions 2–9, 12), Case 52-16, Case 52-17, Case 52-20 (Questions 1, 2), Case 52-21, Case 52-23 (Question 2), Case 52-28, Table 52-10**

continued

		CHAPTER CASES
7	Methimazole is preferable to propylthiouracil (PTU) except during the first trimester of pregnancy and during thyroid storm. Thioamide toxicity includes gastrointestinal symptoms, rash, agranulocytosis, and hepatitis.	**Case 52-15 (Questions 4–8, 10, 11), Case 52-19**
8	Both hypothyroidism and hyperthyroidism can alter metabolism of coadministered medications (e.g., digoxin, warfarin).	**Case 52-14 (Questions 2–4)**
9	The management of subclinical hypothyroidism and hyperthyroidism should be individualized.	**Case 52-12, Case 52-18**
10	Certain drugs (e.g., amiodarone, interferon, lithium, tyrosine kinase inhibitors) can cause thyroid disorders.	**Case 52-24, Case 52-25, Case 52-26, Case 52-27, Table 52-2**
11	Thyroid nodules can present as hot, cold, or multinodular. Malignancy should always be excluded. Thyroid-suppression therapy is not recommended for benign nodules.	**Case 52-28, Case 52-29, Case 52-30, Case 52-31, Case 52-32**

OVERVIEW

Thyroid disease is common, affecting approximately 5% to 15% of the general population. Women are three to four times more likely than men to experience any type of thyroid disease. The typical thyroid disorders are emphasized in this chapter, including hypothyroidism, hyperthyroidism, and nodular disease. Thyroid cancer is discussed briefly. The reader is referred to standard medical textbooks for more detailed medical and diagnostic information.

Triiodothyronine (T_3) and thyroxine (T_4) are the two biologically active thyroid hormones produced by the thyroid gland in response to hormones released by the pituitary and hypothalamus. The hypothalamic thyrotropin-releasing hormone (TRH) stimulates release of thyrotropin (i.e., thyroid-stimulating hormone [TSH]) from the pituitary in response to low circulating levels of thyroid hormone. TSH in turn promotes hormone synthesis and release by increasing thyroid activity. When sufficient synthesis has occurred, high circulating thyroid hormone levels block further production by inhibiting TSH release (negative feedback). The intrapituitary deiodination of T_4 to T_3 also plays a critical role in the inhibition of TSH secretion. As the serum concentrations of thyroid hormone decrease, the hypothalamic-pituitary centers again become responsive by releasing TRH and TSH (Fig. 52-1).

T_3 is four times more potent than T_4, but its serum concentration is lower. T_4 is the major circulating hormone secreted by the thyroid. In contrast, about 80% of the total daily T_3 production results from the peripheral conversion of T_4 to T_3 through deiodination of T_4. T_4 has intrinsic biological activity and does not function solely as a prohormone. Approximately 35% to 40% of secreted T_4 is converted peripherally to T_3; another 45% of secreted T_4 undergoes peripheral conversion to inactive reverse T_3 (rT_3). Certain drugs and diseases can modify the conversion rate of T_4 to T_3 and decrease the serum T_3 levels (Table 52-1[1–38]; see Case 52-1, Question 2).

T_3 and T_4 exist in the circulation in free (active) and protein-bound (inactive) forms. About 99.97% of circulating T_4 is bound: 70% to thyroxine-binding globulin (TBG), 15% to thyroxine-binding prealbumin (TBPA), and the rest to albumin. Only 0.03% exists as the free form. This affinity for plasma proteins accounts for T_4's slow metabolic degradation and long half-life ($t_{1/2}$) of 7 days. In contrast, T_3 is considerably less strongly bound to plasma proteins (99.7%); about 0.3% exists as free hormone. The lower protein-binding affinity of T_3 accounts for its threefold greater metabolic potency and its shorter $t_{1/2}$ of 1.5 days.

Hypothyroidism is a clinical syndrome that results from a deficiency of thyroid hormone. The prevalence of hypothyroidism is 1.4% to 2% in women and 0.1% to 0.2% in men. The incidence increases in persons older than 60 years, to 6% of women and 2.5% of men. Hypothyroidism can be caused by either primary

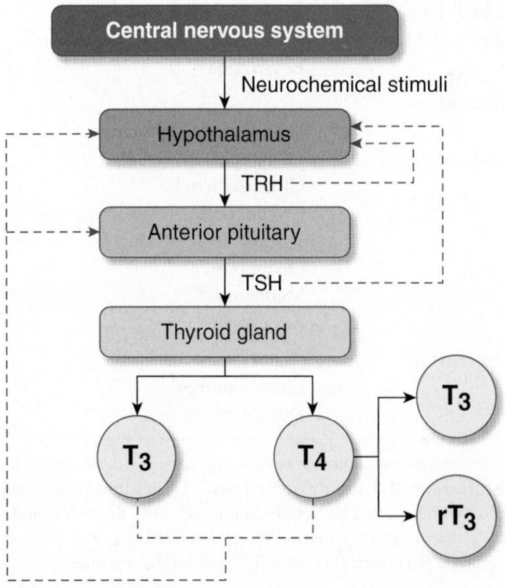

FIGURE 52-1 Regulation of thyroid hormone secretion. Release of thyroid hormones is controlled by the hypothalamic-pituitary-thyroid axis. Dashed lines represent negative feedback.

ONLINE CONTENT **For a narrated PowerPoint that shows regulation of thyroid hormones by the hypothalamic-pituitary-thyroid axis, go to http://thepoint.lww.com/AT10e.**

rT_3, reverse triiodothyronine (inactive); T_4, thyroxine; TRH, thyrotropin-releasing hormone; TSH, thyroid-stimulating hormone or thyrotropin; T_3, triiodothyronine.

TABLE 52-1
Factors That Can Significantly Alter Thyroid Function Tests in Euthyroid Patients

Factors	Drugs/Situations
↑ TBG Binding Capacity	
↑ TT_4	Estrogens,[1,2] tamoxifen,[3] raloxifene[4]
↑ TT_3	Oral contraceptives[5]
Normal TSH	Heroin[6]
Normal FT_4I, FT_4	Methadone maintenance[6]
Normal FT_3I, FT_3	Genetic ↑ in TBG
	Clofibrate
	Active hepatitis[7]
↓ TBG Binding Capacity/Displacement of T_4 From Binding Sites	
↓ TT_4	Androgens[5]
↓ TT_3	Salicylates,[5,8,9] disalcid,[9] salsalate[9]
Normal TSH	High-dose furosemide
Normal FT_4I, FT_4	↓ TBG synthesis-cirrhosis/hepatic failure
Normal FT_3I, FT_3	Nephrotic syndrome[5,7]
	Danazol[5,7]
	Glucocorticoids[5,7,10]
↓ Peripheral $T_4 \rightarrow T_3$ Conversion	
↓ TT_3	PTU
Normal TT_4	Propranolol[11]
Normal FT_4I, FT_4	Glucocorticoids[5,10,12]
Normal TSH	
↓ Pituitary and Peripheral $T_4 \rightarrow T_3$	
↓ TT_3	Iodinated contrast media (e.g., sodium ipodate)[13–17]
↑ TT_4	Amiodarone[18,19,20]
↑ TSH (transient)	Nonthyroidal illness[21–23]
↑ FT_4I	
↑ T_4 Clearance by Enzyme Induction/↑ Fecal Loss[a]	
↓ TT_4	Phenytoin[24,25]
↓ FT_4I	Phenobarbital[24]
Normal or ↓ FT_4	Carbamazepine[24–29]
Normal or ↓ TT_3	Cholestyramine, colestipol[30]
Normal or ↑ TSH	Rifampin[24]
	Bexarotene[31]
↓ TSH Secretion	
	Dopamine,[5,7] dobutamine[32]
	Levodopa,[5] cabergoline[33]
	Glucocorticoids[5,10,12]
	Bromocriptine,[5,12] pramipexole,[10,34] ropinirole[10,34]
	Octreotide[35]
	Metformin[36,37]
	Bexarotene[38]
↑ TSH Secretion	
	Metoclopramide[5,7,12]
	Domperidone[5,7,12]

[a] Can also cause hypothyroidism in patients receiving levothyroxine therapy.
FT_4, free thyroxine; FT_4I, free thyroxine index; FT_3, free triiodothyronine; FT_3I, free triiodothyronine index; PTU, propylthiouracil; TBG, thyroxine-binding globulin; T_4, thyroxine; TSH, thyroid-stimulating hormone; T_3, triiodothyronine; TT_4, total thyroxine; TT_3, total triiodothyronine.

(thyroid gland) or secondary (hypothalamic-pituitary) malfunction. Primary hypothyroidism is more common than secondary causes.

Hashimoto's thyroiditis, an autoimmune disorder, is the most common cause of primary hypothyroidism and appears to have a strong genetic predisposition. The pathogenesis of Hashimoto's thyroiditis results from an impaired immune surveillance, causing dysfunction of normal suppressor T lymphocytes and excessive production of thyroid antibodies by plasma cells (differentiated B lymphocytes). The destruction of thyroid cells by circulating thyroid antibodies produces an underlying defect or block in the intrathyroidal, organobinding of iodide. As a result, inactive prehormones or insufficient amounts of active hormones are synthesized, and this eventually produces hypothyroidism. However, the clinical presentation of Hashimoto's thyroiditis can be variable, depending on the time of diagnosis. Although the typical presentation is hypothyroidism and goiter (thyroid gland enlargement), patients can present with hypothyroidism and no goiter, with euthyroidism and goiter, or rarely (<5%) with hyperthyroidism (Hashitoxicosis).

Other common causes of hypothyroidism are presented in Table 52-2[5,18–20,31,38–54] and include iatrogenic destruction of the gland after radioiodine therapy or surgery and hypothyroidism secondary to nontoxic multinodular goiter. Drug-induced hypothyroidism (e.g., iodides, amiodarone, lithium, tyrosine kinase inhibitors, interferon-α) occurs in susceptible persons (i.e., Hashimoto's thyroiditis) with a pre-existing thyroid abnormality.

TABLE 52-2
Causes of Hypothyroidism

Nongoitrous (No Gland Enlargement)
PRIMARY HYPOTHYROIDISM (DYSFUNCTION OF THE GLAND)
Idiopathic atrophy
Iatrogenic destruction of thyroid
Surgery
Radioactive iodine therapy
X-ray therapy
Postinflammatory thyroiditis
Cretinism (congenital hypothyroidism)
SECONDARY HYPOTHYROIDISM
Deficiency of TSH caused by pituitary dysfunction
Deficiency of TRH caused by hypothalamic dysfunction
Goitrous Hypothyroidism (Enlargement of Thyroid Gland)
Dyshormonogenesis: defect in hormone synthesis, transport, or action
Hashimoto's thyroiditis
Congenital cretinism: maternally induced
Iodide deficiency
Natural goitrogens: rutabagas, turnips, cabbage
Drug-Induced
Aminoglutethimide[5]
Amiodarone[18–20]
Bexarotene[31,38]
Ethionamide[39]
Iodides and iodide-containing preparations[40]
Rifampin[41]
Tyrosine kinase inhibitors (e.g., imatinib, sunitinib, sorafenib)[42–45]
Interleukin[46,47]
Interferon-α[48–51]
Lithium[52–54]
Thiocyanates, phenylbutazone, sulfonylureas[4]

TRH, thyrotropin-releasing hormone; TSH, thyroid-stimulating hormone.

The typical symptoms of hypothyroidism include weight gain, fatigue, sluggishness, cold intolerance, constipation, heavy menstrual periods, and muscle aches. A goiter might or might not be present. Patients with end-stage hypothyroidism, or myxedema coma, can also present with hypothermia, confusion, stupor or coma, carbon dioxide retention, hypoglycemia, hyponatremia, and ileus. Symptoms of "slowing down" would be expected because thyroid hormone is essential for the function and maintenance of all body systems and metabolic processes. In general, hypothyroid symptoms increase with the severity of the

TABLE 52-3
Clinical and Laboratory Findings of Primary Hypothyroidism

Symptoms	Physical Findings	Laboratory
General: weakness, tiredness, lethargy, fatigue	Thin brittle nails	↓ TT_4
Cold intolerance	Thinning of skin	↓ FT_4I
Headache	Pallor	↓ FT_4
Loss of taste/smell	Puffiness of face, eyelids	↓ TT_3
Deafness	Yellowing of skin	↓ FT_3I
Hoarseness	Thinning of outer eyebrows	↑ TSH
No sweating	Thickening of tongue	Positive antibodies (in Hashimoto's)
Modest weight gain	Peripheral edema	↑ Cholesterol
Muscle cramps, aches, pains	Pleural/peritoneal/pericardial effusions	↑ CPK
Dyspnea	↓ DTRs	↓ Na
Slow speech	"Myxedema heart"	↑ LDH
Constipation	Bradycardia (↓ HR)	↑ AST
Menorrhagia	Hypertension	↓ Hct/Hgb
Galactorrhea	Goiter (primary hypothyroidism)	

AST, aspartate aminotransferase; CPK, creatine phosphokinase; DTRs, deep tendon reflexes; FT_4, free thyroxine; FT_4I, free thyroxine index; FT_3I, free triiodothyronine index; Hct, hematocrit; Hgb, hemoglobin; HR, heart rate; LDH, lactate dehydrogenase; Na, sodium; TSH, thyroid-stimulating hormone; TT_3, total triiodothyronine; TT_4, total thyroxine.

hypothyroidism. The exception is the older patient with hypothyroidism, who often presents with minimal or atypical symptoms (e.g., weight loss, deafness, tinnitus, carpal tunnel syndrome). Patients with mild and subclinical hypothyroidism might also have few or no symptoms. Laboratory findings that are diagnostic for overt hypothyroidism include elevated TSH and low free thyroxine (FT_4) levels; for subclinical or early hypothyroidism, the findings are an elevated TSH and normal FT_4 levels. The clinical presentation, physical findings, and laboratory abnormalities of overt hypothyroidism are summarized in Table 52-3.

Levothyroxine (L-thyroxine) is the preferred thyroid replacement preparation. Several brand name and less costly generic preparations are available, and they are interchangeable in most patients. The signs and symptoms of hypothyroidism can be easily corrected in most patients by the administration of L-thyroxine on an empty stomach at an oral replacement dosage of 1.6 to 1.7 mcg/kg/day. Exceptions include older patients, patients with severe and long-standing hypothyroidism, and patients with cardiac disease, in whom administration of full replacement doses might cause cardiac toxicity (Table 52-4). In such patients, minute T_4 doses should be started initially, and the dosage titrated upward as tolerated; complete reversal of hypothyroidism might not be indicated or possible. In myxedema coma, intravenous (IV) therapy with a large initial loading dose of L-thyroxine (e.g., 400 mcg × 1) is necessary to reduce the high mortality rate. In subclinical hypothyroidism, it is controversial whether T_4 replacement therapy is beneficial. There is no justification for treating patients with hypothyroid symptoms and normal TSH findings with T_4.

The goal of therapy is to reverse the signs and symptoms of hypothyroidism and normalize the TSH and FT_4 levels. Some improvement of hypothyroid symptoms is often evident within 2 to 3 weeks of starting T_4 therapy. Overreplacement of L-thyroxine (manifested by below-normal or suppressed serum concentrations of TSH) is associated with osteoporosis and cardiac changes (e.g., atrial fibrillation, heart failure, and tachycardia). The optimal T_4 replacement dosage must be administered for approximately 6 to 8 weeks before steady-state levels are reached. Evaluation of thyroid function tests before this time is misleading. Once a euthyroid state is attained, laboratory tests can be monitored every 3 to 6 months for the first year and then yearly thereafter. Medications that interfere with T_4 absorption (e.g., iron, aluminum-containing products, some calcium preparations [e.g., carbonate], cholesterol resin and phosphate binders, raloxifene) should be separated by at least 4 hours from concomitant T_4 administration.

Hyperthyroidism or thyrotoxicosis is the hypermetabolic syndrome that occurs when the production of thyroid hormone is excessive. Hyperthyroidism affects about 2% of women and about 0.1% of men. The prevalence of hyperthyroidism in older patients varies between 0.5% and 2.3% but accounts for 10% to 15% of all thyrotoxic patients, depending on the population studied.

Graves disease is the most common cause of hyperthyroidism. Toxic autonomous nodular goiters, both multinodular and uninodular, account for a large proportion of the remaining causes. Other causes of hyperthyroidism, including iatrogenic, are outlined in Table 52-5. Graves disease is an autoimmune disorder characterized by one or more of the following features: hyperthyroidism, diffuse goiter, ophthalmopathy (exophthalmos), dermopathy (pretibial myxedema), and acropachy (thickening of fingers or toes). The production of excessive quantities of thyroid hormone is attributed to a circulating immunoglobulin G or thyroid receptor antibody (TRAb), which has a TSH-like ability to stimulate hormone synthesis. The abnormal production of TRAb by plasma cells (differentiated B lymphocytes) results from a deficiency of suppressor T-cell lymphocytes. The peak incidence of Graves disease occurs in the third or fourth decade of life, the duration of the disease is unknown, and its clinical course is characterized by remission and relapse.

Graves disease might be related to Hashimoto's thyroiditis. Both diseases share similar clinical features: positive antibody titers, goiter with lymphocytic infiltration of the gland, familial tendency, and predilection for women. Both diseases can coexist in the same gland. Thyrotoxicosis can precede the onset of Hashimoto's hypothyroidism, and the end result of Graves hyperthyroidism is often hypothyroidism. These common clinical features suggest that Graves disease and Hashimoto's thyroiditis might be the same disease manifesting in different ways.

The classic symptoms of hyperthyroidism, summarized in Table 52-6, mimic a hypermetabolic state and include nervousness, heat intolerance, palpitations, weight loss despite increased

TABLE 52-4
Treatment of Hypothyroidism

Patient Type/Complications	Dose (L-Thyroxine)	Comment
Uncomplicated adult	1.6–1.7 mcg/kg/d; 100–125 mcg/d average replacement dose; usual increment 25 mcg every 6–8 weeks	*Onset of action:* 2–3 weeks; *max effect:* 4–6 weeks. Reversal of skin and hair changes may take several months. An FT_4 and TSH should be checked 6–8 weeks after initiation of therapy because T_4 has a half-life of 7 days and three to four half-lives are needed to achieve steady state. Levels obtained before steady state can be very misleading. Because 80% is bioavailable, adjust IV doses downward. Small changes can be made by varying dose schedule (e.g., 150 mcg daily except Sunday).
Elderly	≤1.6 mcg/kg/d (50–100 mcg/d)	Initiate T_4 cautiously. Elderly may require less than younger patients. Sensitive to small dose changes. A few patients older than 60 years require ≤50 mcg/d.
Cardiovascular disease (angina, CAD)	Start with 12.5–25 mcg/d. ↑ by 12.5–25 mcg/d every 2–6 weeks as tolerated	These patients are very sensitive to cardiovascular effects of T_4. Even subtherapeutic doses can precipitate severe angina, MI, or death. Replace thyroid deficit slowly, cautiously, and sometimes even suboptimally.
Long-standing hypothyroidism (>1 year)	Dose slowly. Start with 25 mcg/d. ↑ by 25 mcg/d every 4–6 weeks as tolerated	Sensitive to cardiovascular effects of T_4. Steady state may be delayed because of ↓ clearance of T_4.[a] Correct replacement dose is a compromise between prevention of myxedema and avoidance of cardiac toxicity.
Pregnancy	Most will require 45% ↑ in dose to ensure euthyroidism	Evaluate TSH, TT_4, and FT_4I. *Goal:* normal TSH and TT_4/FT_4I in upper-normal range to prevent fetal hypothyroidism. TSH should be no higher than 2.5 microunits/mL during the first trimester and 3.0 microunits/mL in the second and third trimesters.
Pediatric (0–3 months)	10–15 mcg/kg/d	Hypothyroid infants can exhibit skin mottling, lethargy, hoarseness, poor feeding, delayed development, constipation, large tongue, neonatal jaundice, piglike facies, choking, respiratory difficulties, and delayed skeletal maturation (epiphyseal dysgenesis). The serum T_4 should be increased rapidly to minimize impaired cognitive function. In the healthy term infant, 37.5–50 mcg/d of T_4 is appropriate. Dose decreases with age (Table 52-9).

[a] In severely myxedematous patients, steady state may require ≥6 months. In patients who are clinically euthyroid but have ↑ TT_4 and FT_4I, use TT_3 and TSH as guide to dose adjustments.

CAD, coronary artery disease; FT_4, free thyroxine; FT_4I, free thyroxine index; IV, intravenous; MI, myocardial infarction; T_4, thyroxine; TSH, thyroid-stimulating hormone; TT_4, total thyroxine.

appetite, insomnia, proximal muscle weakness, frequent bowel movements, amenorrhea, and emotional lability. Hyperthyroid symptoms can be present for 3 to 12 months before the diagnosis is made. The typical symptoms are often absent in the older patient, producing a masked or "apathetic" picture. Because the clinical presentation in the older patient is atypical, occult hyperthyroidism always must be considered, especially in patients with new or worsening cardiac findings (e.g., atrial fibrillation).

TABLE 52-5
Causes of Hyperthyroidism

- Graves disease (toxic diffuse goiter); may be caused by polymorphisms in the TSH receptor[55]
- Toxic uninodular goiter (Plummer disease)
- Toxic multinodular goiter
- Nodular goiter with hyperthyroidism caused by exogenous iodine (Jod-Basedow)
- Exogenous thyroid excess through self-administration (factitious hyperthyroidism)
- Tumors (thyroid adenoma, follicular carcinoma, thyrotropin-secreting tumor of the pituitary, and hydatidiform mole with secretion of a thyroid-stimulating substance)
- Drug-induced (iodides,[56] amiodarone,[18–20] interleukin,[5,46] interferon-α,[48,51] lithium[57,58])

Untreated hyperthyroidism can progress to thyroid storm, a life-threatening form of hyperthyroidism characterized by exaggerated symptoms of thyrotoxicosis and the acute onset of high fever. The diagnosis of hyperthyroidism is confirmed by high serum concentrations of FT_4 and free T_3 (FT_3) or an undetectable TSH level. Positive thyroid antibodies confirm an autoimmune origin for the hyperthyroidism (e.g., Graves disease).

The primary treatment options for hyperthyroidism are antithyroid drugs (thioamides), radioiodine, and surgery. All three modalities are effective, and the treatment of choice is influenced by the etiology of the hyperthyroidism, the size of the goiter, the presence of ophthalmopathy, coexisting conditions (e.g., angina, pregnancy), patient age, patient preference, and physician bias. Older patients and those with coexisting cardiac disease, ophthalmopathy, and hyperthyroidism secondary to a toxic multinodular goiter are treated best with radioactive iodine (RAI). Surgery is preferable if obstructive symptoms are present or concomitant malignancy is suspected. Pregnant patients can be managed with thioamides or surgery in the second trimester; RAI is absolutely contraindicated.

The thioamides are used as primary therapy for hyperthyroidism and as adjunctive short-term therapy to produce euthyroidism before surgery or RAI. The thioamides (e.g., methimazole, propylthiouracil) primarily prevent hormone synthesis but do not affect existing stores of thyroid hormone. Therefore, hyperthyroid symptoms will continue for 4 to 6 weeks after beginning thioamide therapy, and initial treatment with

TABLE 52-6
Clinical and Laboratory Findings of Hyperthyroidism

Symptoms
Heat intolerance
Weight loss common, or weight gain caused by ↑ appetite
Palpitations
Pedal edema
Diarrhea/frequent bowel movements
Amenorrhea/light menses
Tremor
Weakness, fatigue
Nervousness, irritability, insomnia

Physical Findings
Thinning of hair (fine)
Proptosis, lid lag, lid retraction, stare, chemosis, conjunctivitis, periorbital edema, loss of extraocular movements
Diffusely enlarged goiter, bruits, thrills
Wide pulse pressure
Pretibial myxedema
Plummer nails[a]
Flushed, moist skin
Palmar erythema
Brisk DTRs

Laboratory Findings
↑ TT_4
↑ TT_3
↑ FT_4I/FT_4
↑ FT_3I/FT_3
Suppressed TSH
TSI present
TgAb present
TPA present
RAIU >50%
↓ Cholesterol
↑ Alkaline phosphatase
↑ Calcium
↑ AST

[a] The fingernail separates from its matrix, but only one or two nails are generally affected.
AST, aspartate aminotransferase; DTRs, deep tendon reflexes; FT_4, free thyroxine; FT_4I, free thyroxine index; FT_3, free triiodothyronine; FT_3I, free triiodothyronine index; RAIU, radioactive iodine uptake; TgAb, thyroglobulin autoantibodies; TPA, thyroid peroxidase antibody; TSI, thyroid-stimulating immunoglobulin; TSH, thyroid-stimulating hormone; TT_3, total triiodothyronine; TT_4, total thyroxine.

β-blockers or iodides is often required for symptomatic relief. Methimazole is considered the thioamide of choice because propylthiouracil (PTU) has been associated with severe hepatitis that has resulted in fatalities. PTU should be reserved for use during the first trimester of pregnancy, in thyroid storm, and in those experiencing adverse reactions to methimazole (other than agranulocytosis or hepatitis). The onset of action of PTU is more rapid than methimazole in thyroid storm because PTU can also inhibit the peripheral conversion of T_4 to T_3. PTU is also preferred during the first trimester of pregnancy because congenital defects have been reported with methimazole. Although both drugs are secreted in breast milk, no adverse effects have been reported in the exposed infants. Additionally, methimazole can enhance adherence because it can be administered once daily, whereas PTU must be given two or three times daily. The duration of treatment is empiric, and thioamides typically are prescribed for 12 to 18 months in hopes of long-term spontaneous remission once the drug is discontinued. Although thioamides maintain euthyroidism, they do not change the natural course of the disease, and the likelihood of spontaneous remission, once treatment is discontinued, is about 60%. The expectation that the combination of thioamide and T_4 therapy might increase the likelihood of remission has been disappointing and is no longer recommended. The major adverse effects from thioamides include skin rash, gastrointestinal (GI) complaints (e.g., nausea, upset stomach, and metallic taste), agranulocytosis, and hepatitis. Cross-sensitivity between the thioamides is not complete, and the alternative drug can be used if rash or GI complaints do not resolve. This is not true for agranulocytosis and hepatitis, and the alternative agent is not recommended.

Nodular goiters, both multinodular and uninodular, are common thyroid problems. The estimated prevalence is 4% to 5% of the adult population. The origin of thyroid nodules is unknown, although TSH stimulation, iodine deficiency, goitrogens (e.g., iodides, lithium, amiodarone), and radiation exposure are contributory. The nodular goiter is usually found on routine physical examination in asymptomatic and euthyroid patients. However, patients can present with hyperthyroidism caused by autonomous functioning "hot" nodules, overt hypothyroidism, or obstructive symptoms of dysphagia and respiratory difficulty. Thyroid function tests, including TSH and FT_4 levels, and antibodies should be obtained. Additional information can be obtained from radioactive iodine uptake (RAIU), ultrasound, fine-needle aspiration (FNA), or magnetic resonance imaging.

Treatment options include surgery, RAI, or thyroid replacement therapy if necessary to correct hypothyroidism. All goitrogens should be removed if possible. L-Thyroxine suppression therapy is no longer recommended because the dangers from supraphysiologic dosages of T_4 (e.g., osteoporosis and the potential for cardiac arrhythmias) outweigh the benefits.

Malignancy must be considered if there is recent growth in a "cold" single or dominant nodule, a firm nodule clinically suspicious for cancer on a physical examination, a history of thyroid irradiation, or a strong family history of medullary thyroid carcinoma. An FNA of the thyroid nodule can document an underlying malignancy. The risk of malignancy in a toxic multinodular goiter is small, and definitive treatment with RAI is usually required to manage any hyperthyroid symptoms. Surgery is indicated if malignancy is suspected or if any obstructive or respiratory symptoms are present.

After a total thyroidectomy for thyroid cancer, RAI ablation is usually given to remove any remaining thyroid tissue. This dosage is higher than the dosage required for treatment of Graves disease. A yearly evaluation for detection of recurrence of some thyroid cancers requires the patient to be off T_4 for 4 to 6 weeks so that a repeat radioactive uptake and scan can be completed. An elevated TSH level is also necessary to allow thyroglobulin levels, a tumor marker, to rise if any malignant tissue is present. Recurrence of the thyroid cancer is likely if there are positive findings on the scan or an elevation in thyroglobulin levels. The administration of recombinant human TSH may improve quality of life because comparable elevations in TSH occur without stopping L-thyroxine therapy, reducing the duration of hypothyroidism.

THYROID FUNCTION TESTS

The principal laboratory tests recommended in the initial evaluation of thyroid disorders are the TSH and the FT_4 levels.[7,12,35] The relationship between laboratory tests and thyroid disorders is summarized in Figure 52-2. The presence of thyroid antibodies indicates an autoimmune thyroid etiology. Adjuncts to the previous tests include the total T_3 (TT_3), FT_3 or FT_3 index (FT_3I), RAIU and scan, TRAb, ultrasound, and FNA biopsy (Table 52-7).

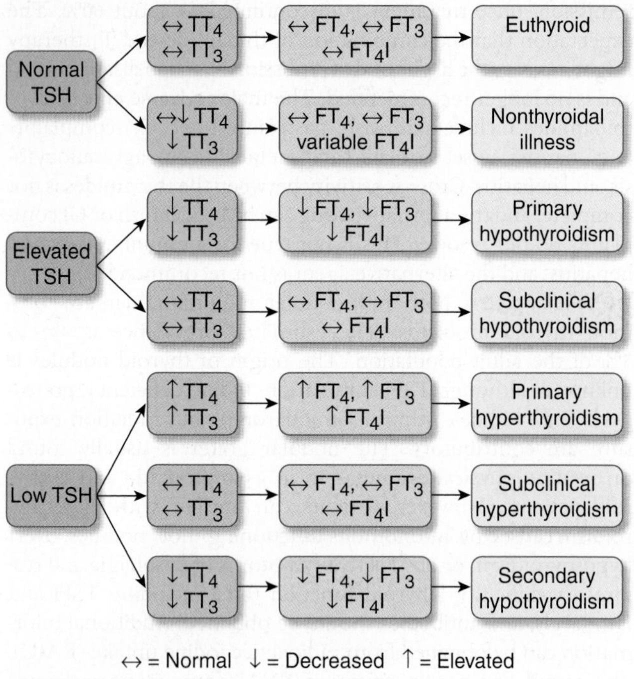

FIGURE 52-2 Evaluation of thyroid function tests. FT_4, free thyroxine; FT_4I, free thyroxine index; FT_3, free triiodothyronine; TSH, thyrotropin; TT_4, total thyroxine; TT_3, total triiodothyronine.

ONLINE CONTENT

For a narrated PowerPoint that shows the evaluation of thyroid status through the interpretation of TFTs, go to http://thepoint.lww.com/AT10e.

Measurements of Free and Total Serum Hormone Levels

FREE THYROXINE, FREE THYROXINE INDEX, FREE TRIIODOTHYRONINE, AND FREE TRIIODOTHYRONINE INDEX

The FT_4 and FT_3 are the most reliable tests for the evaluation of hormone concentrations, especially when thyroid hormone binding abnormalities exist. The FT_3 is most useful in hyperthyroidism but can be normal or low in hypothyroidism. If a direct measure of the free hormone levels is not available, the estimated free hormone indices (FT_4I, FT_3I) can provide comparable information. However, these indices do not correct for changes observed in patients with "euthyroid sick" nonthyroidal illnesses in whom TBG binding affinity is altered. In these circumstances, the FT_4 and FT_3 are preferable.

TOTAL THYROXINE AND TOTAL TRIIODOTHYRONINE

The total thyroxine (TT_4) and TT_3 measure both free and bound (total) serum T_4 and T_3. Because the bound fraction is the major fraction measured, situations that change the hormone's affinity for TBG or the TBG level will influence the results. For example, falsely elevated levels of TT_4 and TT_3 are common in the euthyroid pregnant woman (see Case 52-3). In addition, the TT_3 is often low in older patients and in many acute and chronic nonthyroidal illnesses because the peripheral conversion of T_4 to T_3 is decreased (see Case 52-1, Question 2, and Case 52-2). Therefore, careful interpretation of these tests is necessary in situations that alter thyroid hormone binding, TBG levels, or T_4 to T_3 conversion (Table 52-1). The TT_3 (and FT_3) is particularly helpful in detecting early relapse of Graves disease and in confirming the diagnosis of hyperthyroidism despite normal TT_4 levels. Conversely, TT_3 and FT_3 are not good indicators of hypothyroidism because T_3 levels can be normal. Measurement of only the total hormone levels is less reliable than either the free or estimated free hormone levels when alterations in TBG or nonthyroidal illnesses exist.

Tests of the Hypothalamic-Pituitary-Thyroid Axis

THYROID-STIMULATING HORMONE OR THYROTROPIN

The serum TSH is the most sensitive test to evaluate thyroid function.[7,12,35] TSH, secreted by the pituitary, is elevated in early or subclinical hypothyroidism (when thyroid hormone levels appear normal) and when thyroid hormone replacement therapy is inadequate. TSH can be abnormal even if the FT_4 remains within the normal range because the TSH is specific for each person's physiological set point. Polymorphisms in the TSH receptor contribute to this interindividual variability.[55] Consequently, low-normal free hormone levels can stimulate the pituitary to synthesize increased amounts of TSH. TSH cannot differentiate between primary hypothyroidism (thyroid failure), which is characterized by elevated TSH levels, and secondary (pituitary or hypothalamus failure) hypothyroidism, in which TSH levels may be low or normal. The TSH assay can quantitate the upper and lower limits of normal so that a suppressed TSH level is highly suggestive of hyperthyroidism or exogenous thyroid overreplacement. Of note, TSH is not entirely specific for thyroid disease because abnormal levels are observed in euthyroid patients with nonthyroidal illnesses and in patients receiving drugs that can interfere with TSH secretion. TSH secretion is increased at bedtime and is affected by lack of sleep and exercise.[59] TSH secretion is suppressed physiologically by dopamine, which antagonizes the stimulatory effects of TRH. Therefore, both dopaminergic agonists and antagonists can alter TSH secretion (see Case 52-4). Whether the upper limits of normal for TSH should be lowered to 2.5 microunits/mL is controversial.[55,59]

Tests of Gland Function

RADIOACTIVE IODINE UPTAKE

The radioactive iodine uptake (RAIU), a measure of iodine utilization by the gland, is an indirect measure of hormone synthesis. It is elevated in hyperthyroidism and in early hypothyroidism when the failing gland is trying to increase hormone synthesis. A low or undetectable RAIU occurs in hypothyroidism, thyrotoxicosis factitia, and subacute thyroiditis. Typically, RAIU is used to calculate the dose of RAI therapy for treatment of Graves disease and to determine the activity of one or several nodules in a gland. The RAIU is not necessary to diagnose classic Graves disease or hypothyroidism.

A tracer dose of iodine-131 (^{131}I) is administered, and the radioactivity of the gland is measured at 5 and 24 hours after ingestion. It is necessary to measure both the 5- and 24-hour RAIU so that patients with rapid turnover of iodine will not be missed. In some hyperthyroid patients, the 5-hour uptake is elevated, but the 24-hour uptake can fall to normal or subnormal levels.

The normal range of the RAIU (Table 52-7) is affected by any condition that alters iodine intake. Iodine depletion caused by rigorous diuretic therapy or an iodine-deficient diet increases uptake because of replenishment of depleted total iodide pools.

TABLE 52-7
Common Thyroid Function Tests

Tests	Measures	Normal Values[a]	Assay Interference	Comments
Measurement of Circulating Hormone Levels				
FT_4	Direct measurement of free thyroxine	0.7–1.9 ng/dL (9–24 pmol/L)	No interference by alterations in TBG	Most accurate determination of FT_4 levels; might be higher than normal in patients on thyroxine replacement
FT_4I	Calculated free thyroxine index	*T_4 uptake method:* 6.5–12.5 *$TT_4 \times T_3RU$ method:* 1.3–4.2	Nonthyroidal illness (see Case 52-1, Question 2)	Estimates direct FT_4 measurement; compensates for alterations in TBG
TT_4	Total free and bound T_4	4.8–10.4 mcg/dL (62–134 mmol/L)	Alterations in TBG (Table 52-1)	Specific and sensitive test if no alterations in TBG
TT_3	Total free and bound T_3	79–149 ng/dL (1.2–2.3 nmol/L)	Alterations in TBG levels; T_4 to T_3 (Table 52-1). Nonthyroidal illness (see Case 52-1, Question 2)	Useful in detecting early, relapsing, and T_3 toxicosis. Not useful in evaluation of hypothyroidism
FT_3	Direct measurement of free T_3	145–348 pg/dL (2.2–5.4 pmol/L)	No interference by alterations in TBG	Most accurate determination of FT_4 levels; might be lower than normal in patients on thyroxine replacement
FT_3I	Calculated free T_3 index	17.5–46	Nonthyroidal illness (see Case 52-1, Question 2)	Estimates direct FT_3 measurement; compensates for alterations in TBG
Tests of Thyroid Gland Function				
RAIU	Gland's use of iodine after trace dose of either ^{123}I or ^{131}I	5%–35%	False decrease with excess iodide intake; false elevation with iodide deficiency	Useful in hyperthyroidism to determine RAI dose in Graves disease; does not provide information about hormone synthesis
Scan	Gland size, shape, and tissue activity after ^{123}I or ^{99m}Tc	—	^{123}I scan blocked by antithyroid/thyroid medications	Useful in nodular disease to detect "cold" or "hot" areas
Test of Hypothalamic-Pituitary-Thyroid Axis				
TSH	Pituitary TSH level	0.4–4.0 microunits/mL	Dopamine, glucocorticoids, metoclopramide, thyroid hormone, amiodarone, metformin (Table 52-1)	Most sensitive index for hyperthyroidism, hypothyroidism, and replacement therapy
Tests of Autoimmunity				
TgAb	Thyroglobulin autoantibodies	<20 international units/mL	Nonthyroidal autoimmune disorders	Present in autoimmune thyroid disease; undetectable during remission
TPA	Thyroid peroxidase antibodies	<0.8 international units/mL	Nonthyroidal autoimmune disorders	More sensitive of the two antibodies; titers detectable even after remission
TSI or TRAb	Thyroid receptor or thyroid-stimulating antibody	<125%	—	Confirms Graves disease; detects risk of neonatal Graves disease
Miscellaneous				
Thyroglobulin	Colloid protein of normal thyroid gland	<56 ng/mL	Goiters; inflammatory thyroid disease	Marker for recurrent thyroid cancer or metastases in thyroidectomized patients

[a] At University of California laboratories.

FT_4, free thyroxine; FT_4I, free thyroxine index; FT_3, free triiodothyronine; FT_3I, free triiodothyronine index; RAI, radioactive iodine; RAIU, radioactive iodine uptake; TBG, thyroxine-binding globulin; T_4, thyroxine; TgAb, thyroglobulin auto antibody; TPA, thyroid peroxidase antibody; TRAb, thyroid receptor antibody; TSH, thyroid-stimulating hormone; TSI, thyroid-stimulating antibody; T_3, triiodothyronine; T_3RU, triiodothyronine resin uptake; TT_4, total thyroxine; TT_3, total triiodothyronine.

Conversely, dilution of ^{131}I with exogenous iodide sources (e.g., contrast dyes) decreases RAIU.

IMAGING STUDIES

THYROID SCAN

A scan of the gland is performed simultaneously with the RAIU or after ingestion of technetium-99m (^{99m}Tc) pertechnetate. The scan provides information concerning gland size and shape, and identifies hypermetabolic ("hot") and hypometabolic ("cold") areas. The possibility of carcinoma must be considered if cold areas are present. A scan is often obtained in the evaluation of a patient with nodular thyroid disease.

THYROID ULTRASOUND

A thyroid ultrasound can provide information about gland size and number of clinically palpable or nonpalpable nodules or cysts in the thyroid gland.

Tests of Autoimmunity

THYROID PEROXIDASE AND ANTITHYROGLOBULIN ANTIBODIES

Thyroid peroxidase antibodies (TPA) and thyroglobulin autoantibodies (TgAb) to the thyroid gland indicate an autoimmune process, although the cause of the problem is undetermined.[7,12] About 60% to 70% of patients with Graves disease and 95% of patients with Hashimoto's thyroiditis have positive antibodies to both thyroid antigens. Positive antibodies alone do not indicate thyroid disease because 5% to 10% of asymptomatic patients, as well as patients with other nonthyroidal autoimmune disorders, have positive antibodies.

Clinically, the TPA is more specific than TgAb in assessing disease activity. Although both antibodies are elevated during acute flares of the disease, lower titers of TPA remain positive during quiescent periods of the disease, whereas TgAb levels revert to negative.

THYROID RECEPTOR STIMULATING ANTIBODIES OR THYROID-STIMULATING IMMUNOGLOBULIN

TRAb and thyroid-stimulating immunoglobulin (TSI) are immunoglobulin G immunoglobulins that are present in virtually all patients with Graves disease.[7,12] Like TSH, these immunoglobulins can stimulate the thyroid gland to produce thyroid hormones. High titers of TSI are useful in diagnosing otherwise asymptomatic Graves disease (i.e., ophthalmopathy), in predicting the risk of relapse of Graves disease after discontinuing medication, and in predicting the risk of neonatal hyperthyroidism in utero through transplacental passage of TSI from the pregnant mother. Otherwise, TSI measurement is expensive and offers no additional information in the patient with a typical Graves disease presentation.

Clinical Application and Interpretation

EUTHYROIDISM AND NONTHYROIDAL ILLNESS SYNDROME

CASE 52-1

QUESTION 1: R.K., an obese 42-year-old woman, is admitted to the hospital because of increasing fatigue, sluggishness, shortness of breath (SOB), and pitting edema of the legs during the past 3 weeks. Bilateral pleural effusions found on her chest radiograph indicate a worsening of her congestive heart failure (CHF). Her other medical problems include cirrhosis of the liver, type 2 diabetes, and chronic bronchitis, for which she takes glipizide 10 mg every day and an iodine-containing herbal supplement three times a day (TID).

Pertinent physical findings include a palpable but normal-size thyroid, bibasilar rales, cardiomegaly, hepatomegaly, 4+ pitting edema, and normal deep tendon reflexes (DTRs). A diagnosis of worsening CHF secondary to hypothyroidism is suspected based on the following laboratory findings:

Cholesterol, 385 mg/dL
RAIU at 24 hours, 13% (normal, 5%–35%*)
Scan, normal-size gland with homogenous uptake
TT_4, 1.4 mcg/dL (normal, 4.8–10.4 mcg/dL)
TT_3, 22 ng/dL (normal, 79–149 ng/dL)
TSH, 4 microunits/mL (normal, 0.4–4.0 microunits/mL)
FT_4, 1.0 ng/dL (normal, 0.7–1.9 ng/dL)
TPA, 30 international units/mL (normal, <0.8 international units/mL)
TgAb, 3 international units/mL (normal, <20 international units/mL)

Evaluate and explain R.K.'s thyroid status based on her clinical and laboratory findings.

Although low-output failure can be a presenting sign of hypothyroidism, the normal TSH and FT_4 definitely indicate that R.K. is euthyroid, despite the confusing results of her other thyroid function tests. The depressed RAIU is consistent with her history of iodide ingestion and dilution of the ^{131}I. The low TT_4 and TT_3 may be explained by her cirrhosis and nonthyroidal illness syndrome (see Case 52-1, Question 2). The negative thyroid antibodies, the normal scan, and normal DTRs further substantiate the diagnosis of euthyroidism. In hypothyroidism, a lower rate of cholesterol degradation can produce an elevated serum cholesterol level. However, because many extrathyroidal factors influence the serum concentration of cholesterol, this test is an imprecise reflection of thyroid status. In this case, the elevated cholesterol level is not related to hypothyroidism.

CASE 52-1, QUESTION 2: Assess the results and explain the significance of R.K.'s TT_4, FT_4I, and TT_3 values.

R.K.'s thyroid function test results are consistent with the nonthyroidal illness syndrome. Abnormal thyroid function tests are commonly found in euthyroid patients with various serious systemic diseases, including starvation, infections, sepsis, acute psychiatric disorders, human immunodeficiency virus (HIV) infection, myocardial infarction (MI), bone marrow transplantation, and severe chronic cardiac, pulmonary, renal, hepatic, and neoplastic diseases.[5,7,12,21,22,60–63]

This euthyroid sick syndrome occurs in 37% to 70% of chronically ill or hospitalized patients and must be recognized. In general, the sicker the patient, the greater the degree of abnormal thyroid function findings, even though the patient has no thyroid disease.

The extent of laboratory changes varies with the severity of the illness. The most common finding is a low TT_3 (e.g., 15–20 ng/dL) and high inactive rT_3 levels. Other typical changes include a normal or low TT_4, and suppressed or normal TSH levels. A borderline-high compensatory TSH occurs as patients recover from illness. In more serious illness, the TT_4, FT_4I, and FT_3 are often low. Free hormone levels (e.g., FT_4, FT_3) are often normal or slightly low. However, these inconsistent findings fuel the controversy over whether thyroid hormone therapy is beneficial or detrimental. These findings are believed to be explained by a central hypothyroidism caused by reduction in hypothalamic TRH owing to increased hypothalamic T_3, increased peripheral metabolism of T_3, or a reduction in serum thyroid hormone binding proteins.[60] Impaired protein synthesis of thyroid-binding prealbumin and an increase in the proportion of a lower-binding-capacity form of TBG might account for the lower bound hormone levels, but the concomitant increase in the free hormone concentrations would maintain a euthyroid state. Furthermore, circulating substances that inhibit the binding of T_4 and T_3 to the serum-binding proteins might also be present.

Less common changes include a modestly elevated TT_4 and FT_4I in patients with acute viral hepatitis, psychiatric disorders, renal failure, and advanced HIV infection. The TT_3 is usually normal but can be low in critically ill patients. Modest elevations

*Please note that the normal values used in this chapter are those used at the University of California, San Francisco. Normal values at other locations may differ.

in hormonal binding affinity and increased synthesis of TBG explain these findings.

Several studies have shown a strong inverse correlation between mortality and total serum T_4, T_3, and rT_3 levels.[22,61,62] Of 86 hospitalized, intensive-care patients, 84% of those with a serum T_4 of less than 3 mcg/dL died, whereas 85% of those with a serum T_4 of greater than 5 mcg/dL survived.[61] In 331 patients with acute MI, rT_3 levels greater than 0.41 nmol/L were associated with a significantly greater risk of death at 1 year.[62] During recovery, TSH levels increase and hormone levels start to normalize. Therefore, a favorable outcome is associated with reversal of the hormone indices.

Thyroid experts are divided about whether patients with nonthyroidal illness should be treated, and few randomized studies are available to guide therapeutic decisions.[21,22,60–66] The few available studies found no survival benefits or favorable clinical outcomes after hormone therapy, although cardiac hemodynamics improved. The benefits of hormone replacement are unproven, and might be detrimental. In one trial, the mortality of patients with acute renal failure treated with T_4 was 43% versus 13% in the control group.[63] Opponents argue that T_4 therapy, by inhibiting TSH, may interfere with normal thyroid recovery, whereas proponents argue that there is no clear evidence that therapy is toxic.

In summary, T_4 and T_3 measurements are of limited value in the diagnosis of thyroid dysfunction in patients with significant nonthyroidal illness. A normal or near-normal TSH is necessary to establish euthyroidism in sick patients with nonthyroidal illness. The available data are not supportive of starting thyroid hormone treatment now. The abnormal laboratory findings should reverse when R.K.'s nonthyroid illness is corrected. To confirm euthyroidism, the slightly elevated TSH should be repeated once R.K.'s medical condition improves.

Drug Interference With Thyroid Function Tests

CASE 52-2

QUESTION 1: J.R., a 45-year-old man, complains of fatigue, dry skin, and constipation. His other medical problems include alcoholism for 10 years, cirrhosis, generalized tonic-clonic seizures treated with phenytoin 300 mg/day and phenobarbital 90 mg at night, and rheumatoid arthritis for which he takes aspirin 325 mg, 12 tablets/day. The results of his thyroid function tests are as follows:

TT_4, 4.2 mcg/dL (normal, 4.8–10.4)
FT_4, 0.6 ng/dL (normal, 0.7–1.9)
TSH, 2.5 microunits/mL (normal, 0.4–4.0)

How should these laboratory findings be interpreted? What factors are responsible for the observed changes?

Despite complaints that could be consistent with hypothyroidism (e.g., fatigue, dry skin, constipation) and findings of low serum hormone values, J.R. is euthyroid, as evidenced by the normal TSH level. Secondary hypothyroidism is unlikely at this age without a history of central nervous system (CNS) trauma or tumor. Some nonthyroidal factors could account for J.R.'s low TT_4 and FT_4 values.[5] Anti-inflammatory doses of salicylates greater than 2 g/day and salicylate derivatives can displace T_4 from both TBG and TBPA, causing these abnormal findings.[5,8,9] Elevation in FT_4 levels and suppression of TSH below normal occur transiently (i.e., no longer than first 3 weeks of administration) but normalize with chronic administration. Cirrhosis, stress, severe infections, and hereditary factors can also decrease TBG and TBPA synthesis to produce similar TT_4 findings. A medication history for drugs such as androgens or glucocorticoids that can lower TBG levels, and therefore TT_4 levels, should be elicited (Table 52-1).[5]

Enzyme inducers, such as rifampin and anticonvulsants (phenytoin, phenobarbital, valproic acid, carbamazepine), can alter serum thyroid hormone levels.[5,24–29] A 40% to 60% reduction in TT_4 serum concentrations results from an increase in the metabolism (nondeiodination) of T_4 and from hormone displacement in patients receiving chronic anticonvulsant therapy. Serum T_3 levels are normal or slightly decreased. In addition, therapeutic levels of phenytoin and carbamazepine interfere with the FT_4 assay, causing a 20% to 40% lower FT_4 than would be expected in euthyroid persons.[25] TSH levels remain normal and patients are euthyroid; however, those who previously required T_4 therapy may need a dosage increase to maintain euthyroidism.[28,29] Valproic acid is reported to have similar but less potent effects on thyroid function.[24,26] Phenobarbital can increase T_4 uptake by the liver and increase the fecal excretion of T_4. Serum binding of thyroid hormones is unaffected by phenobarbital.

In summary, J.R. is taking several drugs that can further compromise the already low serum T_4 levels resulting from his liver disease. FT_4 remains subnormal in euthyroid persons receiving phenytoin. For J.R., the normal TSH confirms euthyroidism and no thyroid replacement is necessary.

CASE 52-3

QUESTION 1: S.T., a 23-year-old, sexually active woman whose only medication is birth control pills, comes to the clinic complaining of extreme nervousness, diaphoresis, and scanty menstrual periods. Although she appears healthy, the possibility of hyperthyroidism is considered on the basis of the following laboratory values:

TT_4, 16 mcg/dL (normal, 4.8–10.4)
FT_4, 1.2 ng/dL (normal, 0.7–1.9)
TSH, 1.2 microunits/mL (normal, 0.4–4.0)

Based on this information, what would be a reasonable assessment of S.T.'s thyroid status?

The normal FT_4 and TSH confirm that S.T. is not hyperthyroid. The elevated TT_4 is consistent with increased TBG levels observed in patients with acute hepatitis; in pregnancy; and in persons taking estrogens, estrogen-containing contraceptives, tamoxifen, raloxifene, heroin, or methadone.[1–6] Because TBG and, therefore, bound T_4 levels are increased by estrogens in S.T., serum TT_4 measurements are falsely elevated, but FT_4 levels remain normal. In patients requiring L-thyroxine, the use of estrogens can increase requirements of hormone replacement because the increased pituitary secretion of TSH cannot increase thyroid production needed to offset the increased binding of T_4.[1] Thyroid function tests should return to normal within 4 weeks after estrogen-containing contraceptives are discontinued. A change to progesterone-only contraceptives that do not affect protein binding, do not alter thyroid function tests, and do not increase thyroid requirements can be considered in S.T.

CASE 52-4

QUESTION 1: J.P., a 55-year-old woman, complains of 3 months of progressive tremors, dizziness, and ataxia. Two months ago, she had a silent MI complicated by malignant ventricular ectopy that was responsive only to amiodarone therapy. Her other medical problems include parkinsonism,

type 2 diabetes, and diabetic gastroparesis. Her current medications include amiodarone, insulin, metformin, metoclopramide, pramipexole, and levodopa/carbidopa. Physical examination of the thyroid was unremarkable. Thyroid function tests yielded the following results:

TT_4, 14.5 mcg/dL (normal, 4.8–10.4)
FT_4, 2.3 ng/dL (normal, 0.7–1.9)
TSH, 3.8 microunits/mL (normal, 0.4–4.0)
TT_3, 40 ng/dL (normal, 79–149)
TPA antibodies, 40 international units/L (normal, <0.8)

How should J.P.'s laboratory values be interpreted?

Although the symptoms of tremors, dizziness, and weight loss are suggestive of hyperthyroidism, the low TT_3, negative antibodies, normal TSH, and normal thyroid examination make this diagnosis unlikely. Side effects of amiodarone could be responsible for J.P.'s symptoms. Her drug therapy could also explain her laboratory findings.

Amiodarone produces complex changes in thyroid function tests that are confusing if not properly interpreted.[18,19,67,68] Because amiodarone inhibits both the peripheral and pituitary conversion of T_4 to T_3, FT_4 levels are elevated, and TT_3 levels are subnormal in euthyroid patients. Transient elevations in TSH levels occur (usually <20 microunits/mL) during the first few weeks of therapy but return to normal in approximately 3 months. If TSH levels do not normalize, then amiodarone-induced thyroid disease should be considered. Amiodarone can cause either hypothyroidism or hyperthyroidism in susceptible patients (see Case 52-26, Question 1).

The other drugs J.P. is taking—pramipexole, levodopa, metformin, and metoclopramide—also add to the diagnostic confusion. Although these drugs do not affect the actual circulating hormone levels, they affect the dopaminergic system that controls both TSH and TRH secretion.[5,12,34,35] Infusions of dopamine and dobutamine can decrease both TSH secretion and the TSH response to TRH in euthyroid and hypothyroid patients.[5,10,12,35] Therefore, dopamine agonists such as pramipexole, cabergoline, and levodopa can blunt the normal TSH response.[5,10,34,35] In addition, metformin after 1 year of therapy can cause significant TSH suppression without changes in FT_4 levels by an as yet unknown mechanism of action.[36,37]

Conversely, dopamine antagonists such as metoclopramide or domperidone can elevate TSH levels.[5,35] Fortunately, the alterations in TSH caused by these agents are usually not substantial enough to completely obscure the true thyroid abnormality.

HYPOTHYROIDISM

Clinical Presentation

CASE 52-5

QUESTION 1: M.W., a 70-kg, 23-year-old voice student, thinks that her neck has become "fatter" during the past 3 to 4 months. She has gained 10 kg, feels mentally sluggish, tires easily, and finds that she can no longer hit high notes. Physical examination reveals puffy facies, yellowish skin, delayed DTRs, and a firm, enlarged thyroid gland. Laboratory data include the following results:

FT_4, 0.6 ng/dL (normal, 0.7–1.9)
TSH, 60 microunits/mL (normal, 0.4–4.0)
TPA antibodies, 136 international units/L (normal, <0.8)

Assess M.W.'s thyroid status based on her clinical and laboratory findings.

M.W. presents with many of the clinical features of hypothyroidism as presented in Table 52-3. These include weight gain, mental sluggishness, easy fatigability, lowering of the voice pitch, puffy facies, yellowish tint of the skin, delayed DTRs, and enlarged thyroid.[69] The diagnosis of hypothyroidism is confirmed by her laboratory findings of a low FT_4, an elevated TSH value, and positive TPA antibodies.

A firm goiter, thyroid antibodies, and clinical symptoms of hypothyroidism strongly suggest Hashimoto's thyroiditis. She has no history of prior antithyroid drug use, surgery, or RAI treatment, which are common causes of iatrogenic hypothyroidism. She is also not taking any goitrogens or drugs known to cause hypothyroidism (Table 52-2).[70]

Treatment With Thyroid Hormones

THYROID HORMONE PRODUCTS

CASE 52-5, QUESTION 2: What thyroid preparation should be used to treat M.W.'s hypothyroidism? Are differences, advantages, or disadvantages significant among the various generic and brand name formulations of thyroid hormones?

The principal goals of thyroid hormone therapy are to attain and maintain a euthyroid state. Thyroid preparations (Table 52-8) are synthetic (L-thyroxine, L-triiodothyronine, liotrix) or natural (desiccated thyroid). The latter comes from animal tissues.

DESICCATED THYROID

Desiccated thyroid is derived from pork thyroid glands, although beef and sheep also are used. Today, starting patients on desiccated thyroid is not justified. The US Pharmacopeia requires only that desiccated thyroid contain 0.17% to 0.23% organic iodine by weight. These requirements do not seem stringent enough because potency may vary with changes in the proportion of the two active hormones (T_3 and T_4) or with changes in the amount of organic iodine present.[71,72] This variable potency seems to be particularly true of generic formulations compared with the biologically standardized Armour brand of desiccated thyroid. Inactive desiccated thyroid preparations that contain negligible amounts of T_3 and T_4 or even iodinated casein instead of active hormone have been identified in various brands sold in retail pharmacies and in over-the-counter products found in health-food stores.[72–74] Likewise, preparations with greater-than-expected activity caused by an abnormally high T_3 content have resulted in thyrotoxicosis.

Allergic reactions to the animal protein are another concern. In addition, desiccated thyroid suffers from two problems inherent to all T_3-containing preparations. Because T_3 is absorbed more rapidly than T_4, supraphysiological elevations in plasma T_3 levels occur after oral ingestion, which can produce mild thyrotoxic symptoms in some patients. FT_4 levels are low during T_3 administration and, if misinterpreted, can result in the erroneous administration of more hormone. These problems with T_3 are easily missed unless T_3 levels are routinely monitored. Because significant amounts of T_4 are converted to T_3 peripherally, oral administration of T_3 offers no advantage and is not usually needed (see Triiodothyronine section).

Loss of tablet potency can occur from prolonged storage of desiccated thyroid preparations, but this instability is not as important as once believed. Because the only apparent advantage of desiccated thyroid is its low cost, it should not be

TABLE 52-8
Thyroid Preparations

Drug/Dosage Forms	Composition	Dosage Equivalent	Comments
Thyroid USP (Armour) *Tab:* 0.25, 0.5, 1, 1.5, 2, 3, 4, and 5 grains	Desiccated hog, beef, or sheep thyroid gland Standardized iodine content	1 grain[a] —	Unpredictable T_4:T_3 ratio; supraphysiologic elevations in T_3 levels might produce toxic symptoms; Armour brand preferred
L-Thyroxine (Levoxyl, Levothroid, Synthroid, Unithroid, various) *Tab:* 0.013, 0.025, 0.050, 0.075, 0.088, 0.112, 0.125, 0.137, 0.15, 0.175, 0.2, and 0.3 mg *Inj:* 200 and 500 mcg	Synthetic T_4 — —	60 mcg[a] — —	Stable, predictable potency; well absorbed; more potent than desiccated thyroid. When changing from >2 grains desiccated thyroid to L-T_4, a lower dosage of L-T_4 might be needed to avoid toxicity. Weight should be considered in dosing (1.6–1.7 mcg/kg/d). L-T_4 absorption can be impaired by iron, aluminum-containing products (e.g., antacids, sucralfate), Kayexalate, calcium preparations, proton-pump inhibitors, cholesterol resin and phosphate binders, raloxifene, soy, bran, coffee, fiber-enriched foods. L-T_4 metabolism increased by anticonvulsants, rifampin, imatinib, bexarotene, and pregnancy
L-Triiodothyronine (Cytomel) *Tab:* 5, 25, and 50 mcg *Inj:* 10 mcg/mL (Triostat)	Synthetic T_3 — —	25–37.5 mcg — —	Complete absorption; requires multiple daily dosing; toxicity similar to all T_3-containing products; see desiccated thyroid comments
Liotrix (Thyrolar) *Tab:* 0.25, 0.5, 1, 2, and 3 grains	60 mcg T_4:15 mcg T_3 50 mcg T_4:12.5 mcg T_3	Thyrolar-1 —	No need for liotrix because T_4 is converted to T_3 peripherally; expensive, stable, and predictable content

[a] 60 mg (1 grain) of desiccated thyroid = 60 mcg of T_4.[70]

Inj, injection; L-T_4, levothyroxine; Tab, tablet; T_4, thyroxine; T_3, triiodothyronine; USP, United States Pharmacopeia.

considered the drug of choice for replacement therapy. Patients maintained on desiccated thyroid should be encouraged to change to L-thyroxine (T_4). Although 60 mg (1 grain) of desiccated thyroid is theoretically equal in potency to 75 to 100 mcg of T_4,[70] this equivalency may not hold true if the desiccated thyroid preparation is less active than its labeled content. The patient's weight also should be considered when switching therapy (see Case 52-5, Question 3).

The synthetic thyroid preparations differ from one another in their relative potency, onset of action, and biological half-life.

LEVOTHYROXINE OR L-THYROXINE

L-Thyroxine is the thyroid replacement of choice.[75] Its advantages include stability, uniform potency, relatively low cost, and lack of allergenic foreign protein content. The long half-life of 7 days permits once-a-day dosing and, if necessary, the creation of special convenience schedules, such as the omission of medication on weekends. The mean absorption of a commonly used branded preparation is 81%.[76] Absorption is optimal on an empty stomach, at least 60 minutes before or 2 hours after meals or at bedtime.[77] Several medications can also impair L-thyroxine absorption (see Case 52-9, Question 1).

Concerns about generic and branded L-thyroxine tablet stability and potency, bioavailability, and product interchangeability existed because L-thyroxine preparations were grandfathered in by the 1938 Food, Drug, and Cosmetic Act. To address these concerns, the US Food and Drug Administration (FDA) required that all manufacturers of L-thyroxine products submit a New Drug Application (NDA) by August 2001 or cease production by 2003 if the NDA was not filed.[78] Several FDA-approved brand and generic formulations approved under the NDA received AB or BX ratings, indicating interchangeability for some generic and brand preparations. Raising concerns about the methodology the FDA used to determine bioequivalence, the American Thyroid Association, The Endocrine Society, and the American Association of Clinical Endocrinologists issued joint position statements expressing their displeasure with the FDA's conclusions of interchangeability.[79] Abbot Laboratories, the manufacturer of Synthroid, and others also disagreed with the FDA's findings.[80] Although this issue remains controversial, the preponderance of the evidence supports the FDA ratings and suggests that these preparations are likely to be interchangeable in the majority of patients.[81–84]

TRIIODOTHYRONINE

T_3 (Cytomel) is not recommended for routine thyroid hormone replacement because of the problems identified earlier with T_3 administration (see Desiccated Thyroid section).[75] Numerous randomized studies now conclude that replacement with combination T_4 and small dosages of T_3 offer no advantage to T_4 alone, despite an initial study showing improved cognitive performance and mood changes.[85,86] Furthermore, a prospective study found that T_3 levels after thyroidectomy in 50 patients receiving only levothyroxine were similar to T_3 levels in these euthyroid patients before surgery, confirming that levothyroxine alone is sufficient for replacement.[87] Use of T_3 to enhance contractility in coronary bypass surgery is controversial.[88]

Although T_3 is well absorbed, it has a relatively short half-life (1.5 days), necessitating multiple daily dosing to ensure a uniform response. Other disadvantages include higher expense and a greater potential for cardiotoxicity. Its primary use is for patients who require short-term hormone replacement therapy and rarely in those in whom T_4 conversion to T_3 might be impaired. Proponents favoring thyroid treatment of the euthyroid sick syndrome identify T_3 as the hormone replacement of choice. T_3 therapy should be monitored using the TSH and TT_3 or FT_3 levels.

LIOTRIX

Liotrix is a combination of synthetic T_4 and T_3 in a physiological ratio of 4:1. This preparation is subject to the same disadvantages common to all T_3-containing preparations. It is also stable and potent, but it is more expensive than other thyroid preparations. Because oral administration of T_3 is not needed and there is no advantage of adding T_3 to T_4 therapy, this expensive preparation is not recommended.[85,86] Patients should be changed to an equivalent dosage of L-thyroxine.

THYROXINE

DOSAGE

CASE 52-5, QUESTION 3: What would you recommend as appropriate starting and maintenance dosages of T_4 for M.W.?

The maintenance dosage for M.W. can be estimated from her weight. Average replacement doses of 1.6 to 1.7 mcg/kg/day (e.g., 100–125 mcg) are sufficient in most patients to normalize the TSH.[69,75] L-Thyroxine dosages that suppress TSH levels to below normal or undetectable levels (subclinical hyperthyroidism) should be avoided to prevent osteoporosis and cardiac toxicity.[75,89–93] Excessive l-thyroxine can cause tachycardia, atrial arrhythmias, impaired ventricular relaxation, reduced exercise performance, and increased risk of cardiac mortality.[89] These considerations are especially important in older patients, who might require less T_4 than their younger counterparts and who are particularly sensitive to minute changes in T_4 doses (see Case 52-6). As patients age, the dosage should be evaluated yearly and decreased if necessary to maintain a normal TSH level.

How rapidly T_4 replacement can proceed depends on the likelihood of invoking cardiac toxicity in susceptible patients. Minute doses of T_4 (e.g., <75 mcg) can increase heart rate, stroke volume, oxygen consumption, and cardiac workload before euthyroidism occurs. One double-blind study compared the clinical outcome between starting full replacement doses versus gradual 25-mcg incremental doses in relatively young hypothyroid subjects with asymptomatic cardiac disease and concluded that those receiving full doses normalized thyroid function tests more rapidly (4 weeks) and without any toxicity.[94] Although this strategy may improve symptoms more quickly, further confirmation is needed to eliminate concerns about potential cardiac toxicity. Because M.W. has no identifiable risk factors (see Case 52-11, Question 3) for cardiotoxicity that require careful dosage titration (e.g., old age, cardiac disease, long duration of hypothyroidism), she can be started on an estimated full replacement dose of 125 mcg daily of L-thyroxine (70 kg × 1.7 mcg/kg/day = 120 mcg). An alternative conservative approach would be to start with 100 or 112 mcg/day, check the FT_4 or FT_4I and TSH tests after 6 to 8 weeks of therapy, and if the TSH is still elevated without any symptoms of toxicity, increase the dosage to 125 mcg/day. The appropriate replacement dose will produce a TSH of 1 to 2 microunits/mL, normalize FT_4 or FT_4 I levels, and reverse clinical symptoms of hypothyroidism. Generally, dosing adjustments should not exceed monthly increments of 12.5 to 25 mcg/day.

MONITORING THERAPY

CASE 52-5, QUESTION 4: Ten days after starting L-thyroxine therapy, M.W. continues to complain of tiredness, fatigue, and difficulty singing despite excellent adherence. Thyroid function tests show a TT_4 of 4 mcg/dL, an FT_4 of 0.5 ng/dL, and a TSH of 40 microunits/mL. What therapeutic options are available? How should M.W.'s thyroid function tests be interpreted?

Clinical improvement in the signs and symptoms of hypothyroidism and normalization of laboratory parameters are appropriate therapeutic end points. If the replacement dose is sufficient, some correction of her symptoms should occur after 2 to 3 weeks, but maximal effects will not be evident for 4 to 6 weeks. Typically, improvement of anemia and hair and skin changes is delayed and requires several months of treatment before resolution.[36,70]

In patients with severe myxedema, a transiently elevated T_4 level might occur at 6 weeks because the metabolic clearance of T_4 is decreased by the hypometabolic state associated with hypothyroidism.

FT_4 or FT_4I and TSH should be checked about 6 to 8 weeks after the initiation of therapy because T_4 has a half-life of 7 days, and three to four half-lives are needed to reach steady-state levels. Levels obtained before this time (as in M.W.) may be misleading and should be interpreted cautiously. No change in her L-thyroxine dosage should be attempted at this time.

CASE 52-5, QUESTION 5: Eight weeks later, on a routine follow-up visit, M.W. still feels tired and not back to her normal self. She denies any symptoms of hyperthyroidism. Her thyroid function tests show a TT_4 of 14 mcg/dL, a TT_3 of 100 ng/dL, FT_4 of 1.9 ng/dL, and a TSH of 3.5 microunits/mL. How should M.W.'s thyroid function tests be interpreted? What changes, if any, should be recommended in her therapeutic regimen?

Patients treated with L-thyroxine may develop an elevated TT_4 concentration and FT_4 without overt clinical signs of hyperthyroidism.[87,95] Despite these elevated levels, patients are euthyroid, as evidenced by a normal TSH. Because T_3 is not being released from the nonfunctioning thyroid gland, a higher concentration of T_4 is necessary to increase the amount of T_3 obtained from peripheral conversion. Jonklaas et al. reported that the mean FT_4 was significantly higher (1.34 ng/dL) in patients receiving L-thyroxine postoperatively compared with their euthyroid levels before thyroidectomy (FT_4, 1.06 ng/dL).[87] T_3 levels on L-thyroxine replacement after surgery were also comparable with presurgery levels. However, lower T_3 levels were noted only in those in whom TSH levels were greater than 4.5 microunits/mL, indicating that low T_3 levels are likely a result of suboptimal L-thyroxine replacement. Thus, the TSH appears to be the best indicator of euthyroidism in patients treated with L-thyroxine.

Another possibility is that the elevated thyroid levels may only be an artifact of the laboratory collection time. Before any changes in her dosing regimen are made, M.W. should be asked about the time she takes the drug and its relationship to the time of her blood draw. Random sampling of FT_4 and TSH levels can be significantly different when compared with trough levels.[96,97] In one study, the FT_4 level was 12% higher and the TSH level 19% lower when obtained from random samples compared with trough samples.[97] Transient elevations in FT_4 levels were detected for 9 hours after ingestion of the oral L-thyroxine.

The symptoms of fatigue that M.W. is experiencing are likely not related to her hypothyroidism. Patients may continue to have symptoms of hypothyroidism despite normalization of the TSH value. Although some have suggested that the goal TSH be titrated to 1 to 2 microunits/mL or lower for replacement therapy to improve well-being, this is controversial. One study found that changes in T_4 dosing to achieve TSH concentrations of 2 to 4.8 microunits/mL, 0.3 to 1.9 microunits/mL, or less than 0.3 microunits/mL in hypothyroid patients did not result in improvements in well-being, in psychological or hypothyroid symptoms, or in quality of life.[98] Data justifying the safety of higher T_4 replacement doses found that achievement of a low but detectable TSH level (0.04 to 0.4 microunits/mL) was not associated with an increased risk of cardiovascular disease or fractures compared with those with suppressed (<0.03 microunits/mL) or elevated (>4 microunits/mL) TSH levels.[99]

In conclusion, if an elevated TT_4 and FT_4 are noted without any symptoms of thyrotoxicosis (as in M.W.), the dosage should not be decreased; rather, a trough FT_4 and TSH level should be obtained to eliminate excessive dosing or any laboratory artifacts. Alternatively, obtaining a level at least 9 hours after levothyroxine administration also seems appropriate. Repeat values should be in the normal range if the dosing is correct. An excessively suppressed TSH confirms a dosage that is too high. In M.W., the lack of hyperthyroid symptoms suggests euthyroidism, and no changes in her therapeutic regimen should be attempted until trough levels are available. Evaluation for other causes of fatigue should be explored.

TRIIODOTHYRONINE

CASE 52-6

QUESTION 1: C.B., a 65-year-old woman, complains of fatigue and vague muscle aches and pains, which she attributes to insufficient thyroid medication. On physical examination, the thyroid gland is palpable but not enlarged, and DTRs are 2+ and brisk. Her dose of T_3 was increased from 25 mcg TID to 50 mcg TID about 2 weeks ago based on the results of a recent FT_4 of 0.5 ng/dL. She denies taking any other medications. Is C.B.'s thyroid hormone replacement appropriate?

As noted previously, T_3 is not the drug of choice for thyroid replacement. The use of L-thyroxine would simplify her dosing regimen and facilitate monitoring.

The low FT_4 did not justify increasing C.B.'s T_3 dose. Because she is receiving T_3, the FT_4 will always be low and will never reach normal levels. In fact, her vague complaints may be related to hyperthyroidism because she is receiving the equivalent of 0.2 to 0.3 mg of L-thyroxine daily. TSH and FT_3 levels are most useful in monitoring patients receiving T_3 therapy. A TSH level should be obtained to evaluate her thyroid function. A suppressed TSH and an elevated FT_3 would indicate hyperthyroidism. It is important to remember that in an older patient, hyperthyroidism might not always produce symptoms because of an apathetic sympathetic system.

L-Thyroxine should be initiated cautiously in older patients to avoid exacerbating any pre-existing arteriosclerotic heart disease that might be masked by the hypothyroidism (see Case 52-11, Questions 2 and 3). In general, older patients require smaller replacement dosages (approximately $\leq$1.6 mcg/kg/day of T_4) than their younger counterparts.[100–102] Dosages of less than 50 mcg/day of T_4 are common in patients older than 60 years. However, this lower T_4 dosage is not universal for all older subjects.[102] The reason that older patients need lower dosages is unclear, but it has been suggested that the lower requirements result from an age-related decrease in T_4 degradation rates. Because dosage requirements change with age, patients should be reassessed annually to determine whether the original dosage prescribed is still appropriate.

In C.B., who had been on T_3 without any evidence of cardiac toxicity, a less cautious approach in changing to T_4 can be attempted. An empiric L-thyroxine dosage of 68 mcg/day (40 kg × 1.6 mcg/kg/day) is an approximate dosing end point for C.B. The T_3 should be discontinued and T_4 initiated in a dose of 50 mcg/day; this dosage can be adjusted as needed based on C.B.'s symptoms and thyroid function tests. After T_3 therapy is discontinued, its effects will disappear in 3 to 5 days. In contrast, T_4 levels rise slowly for 4 to 5 days, so no overlap in T_3 administration is necessary to prevent hypothyroidism.

PARENTERAL DOSING

CASE 52-7

QUESTION 1: G.F., a 70-year-old man with long-standing hypothyroidism, has been receiving L-thyroxine 0.2 mg/day. Currently, he is in the hospital with a stroke and paralysis that prohibits him from swallowing oral medications. His last thyroid function tests were normal. What is a reasonable method of administering thyroid hormone to G.F.?

Because L-thyroxine has a half-life of 7 days, administration can be delayed for up to 1 week, assuming G.F. can resume oral intake at that time. However, if parenteral administration is required, L-thyroxine is available as an intramuscular (IM) or IV injection. The IV route is preferred because IM absorption may be slow and unpredictable, particularly if the circulation is compromised. Because the oral absorption of T_4 is approximately 80%,[76] parenteral doses should be decreased. Once IV L-thyroxine replacement is successful, maintenance with a once-weekly IM injection can be continued if oral ingestion is not feasible.[103]

IN PREGNANCY

CASE 52-8

QUESTION 1: P.K. is a 35-year-old woman with Hashimoto's thyroiditis who is 6 weeks pregnant. Laboratory test results showed TT_4 of 5 mcg/dL and FT_4 of 0.7 ng/dL. She takes her medications in the morning, which include L-thyroxine 0.1 mg/day and a prenatal vitamin enriched with iron and calcium. What dosing adjustments are required because of P.K.'s pregnancy?

Inadequately treated or undiagnosed maternal hypothyroidism can be detrimental to the mother and the developing fetus.[104–108] Miscarriage, spontaneous abortion, hypertension, pre-eclampsia, and higher rates of cesarean sections and stillbirths have been reported with maternal hypothyroidism. Congenital defects, congenital hypothyroidism (see Case 52-8, Question 2), abnormal fetal development, and impaired cognitive development in the newborn have been attributed to maternal hypothyroidism. The IQ scores of children born to mothers with undiagnosed hypothyroidism during pregnancy averaged 7 points lower than those of children born to euthyroid mothers.[105] A delay in both mental and motor development was observed in children ages 1 to 2 years old who were born to mothers with hypothyroxinemia but normal TSH levels during the first trimester of pregnancy.[108] Normal maternal thyroid function is essential during early fetal development. Fetal thyroid hormone production begins by the end of the first trimester, with the fetus relying on maternal thyroid hormones until that time. Transfer of maternal thyroid hormones is under the control of the placenta.[109] The risk of congenital hypothyroidism is small if maternal antibodies from Hashimoto's thyroiditis cross the fetal circulation. The infant's cord blood should be assayed at birth to ensure that TSH is normal and that the child is euthyroid.

The majority of women with primary hypothyroidism will require a 30% to 50% increase in the prepregnancy T_4 dosage to maintain euthyroidism during the first trimester of pregnancy.[109–112] The only evidence of increased T_4 demands is an elevated TSH level (e.g., subclinical hypothyroidism) that occurs between weeks 5 (but can be as early as 3) and 16 of gestation. Often, no clinical symptoms of hypothyroidism are evident, and the FT_4 and the FT_4I are normal. Because of the adverse consequences associated with maternal hypothyroidism, some have advocated universal TSH screening of all pregnant women[113] as well as empirically increasing the prepregnancy T_4

dosage by 30% (extra two pills/week) as soon as pregnancy is confirmed.[111] Because there is a physiologic decrease in TSH during pregnancy caused by the TSH-like activity of human chorionic gonadotropin, the upper limit of the normal TSH range should be adjusted for pregnancy.[109] TSH should be no higher than 2.5 microunits/mL during the first trimester and 3.0 microunits/mL in the second and third trimesters.[112]

Physiologic explanations for the increase in thyroid hormone requirements include the twofold increase in TBPA caused by high estrogen levels and increased volume of distribution of thyroid hormones, as well as increased maternal transport of T_4.[109,112] Some authors have challenged the dogma that pregnancy per se increases T_4 demands. Rather, they propose that these increments were recommended before it was recognized that coadministration of iron- and calcium-containing prenatal vitamins reduced T_4 absorption (see Case 52-9, Question 1) and that these drug interactions may be primarily responsible for these increased needs. When prenatal vitamins with iron and calcium were separated by 4 hours from T_4 administration, only 31% of women required an increase in T_4 dose.[114] The increase in thyroid hormone requirements are likely a combination of physiologic and drug interaction causes. Women should be followed closely during the first trimester with monthly monitoring of FT_4 and TSH levels. If necessary, the T_4 dosage should be adjusted to maintain a normal TSH and an FT_4 or FT_4I in the upper limits of normal. Because TBG is elevated, the TT_4 should be kept above the normal range; it is not the best indicator of adequate replacement.

P.K.'s low TT_4 and FT_4 are concerning. The TT_4 should be much higher because of pregnancy-associated increases in TBG. The TSH level should be obtained, and the daily dosage of T_4 should be increased to 125 mcg after eliminating the possibility of patient nonadherence and drug interactions. Ingestion of the prenatal vitamins with iron and calcium should be separated by at least 4 hours from administration of T_4. P.K. could also be instructed to take the T_4 at night for better absorption.[77] The TSH should be repeated in 6 weeks, and the dosage should be adjusted as needed to keep the TSH in the range as above. After delivery, the dosage should be reduced to prepregnancy levels and the FT_4 and TSH rechecked to ensure euthyroidism.

CONGENITAL HYPOTHYROIDISM

CASE 52-8, QUESTION 2: P.K. delivered a healthy baby, T.K., at term without difficulty. T.K.'s postpartum screening serum T_4 level was 5 mcg/dL, and TSH was 35 microunits/mL. At home, T.K. became lethargic, had a weak cry, sucked poorly, and failed to thrive. Assess the situation (including a treatment plan and prognosis). How is mental development affected?

T.K.'s symptoms are suggestive of congenital hypothyroidism, although in most infants the clinical signs and symptoms are so subtle and nonspecific that they are easily missed until the child is several months old. The early clinical findings include prolonged jaundice, skin mottling (cutis marmorata), lethargy, poor feeding, constipation, hypothermia, hoarse cry, large fontanels, distended abdomen, hypotonia, slow reflexes, and piglike facies. Respiratory difficulties, delayed skeletal maturation, and choking (but not palpable goiter) may be present. These infants are also at risk for additional congenital defects or complications.[115] Mass neonatal screening programs have been successful in detecting congenital hypothyroidism within the first few weeks of life before clinical manifestations are apparent and before irreversible changes occur.

The postpartum low serum T_4 concentration and elevated TSH level (>20 microunits/mL) in T.K. are of concern and should be verified. Transient hypothyroidism can result from intrauterine exposure to thioamides or excess iodides, or from transplacental passage of TRAb from the mother. Thyroid function tests often normalize without treatment in 3 to 6 months as the TRAb is cleared by the infant.[115] The diagnosis of hypothyroidism should be confirmed by a low serum T_4, a low FT_4, and an elevated TSH concentration during the next few weeks. Serum T_3 concentrations are often in the normal range and are not helpful. Normal serum T_4 concentrations are higher in the first few weeks of life and gradually return to normal by 2 to 4 months of life. The FT_4I may also be elevated. Because of these confusing changes, thyroid serum levels should be compared with the normal range for the approximate postnatal age.

Thyroid hormones play a critical role in normal growth and development, particularly of the CNS, during the first 3 years of life. If untreated, dwarfism and irreversible mental retardation occur. T.K.'s normal mental (IQ) and physical development will be determined by the age at which treatment is started, the initial dosage of T_4, the serum T_4 level attained during therapy, the adequacy with which treatment is maintained, and the cause and severity of the initial deficiency.[116–122] There is an inverse relationship between the amount of time to reach a euthyroid state and the likelihood of impaired neurologic development.[115]

Sodium L-thyroxine is the preparation of choice for replacement. T_4 tablets can be crushed and mixed with breast milk or formula; suspensions are not stable and should not be used. T_4 tablets should not be mixed with soy-based formulas because decreased absorption and longer time to reach a TSH less than 10 microunits/mL may occur. If a soy-based formula is required, the dosage of T_4 should be administered halfway between feeds.[115] T_3 also can be used, but this form is less desirable because its short half-life causes a greater fluctuation in plasma levels (Table 52-8). The initial replacement dose of T_4 should raise the serum T_4 as rapidly as possible to minimize the consequences of hypothyroidism on cognitive function. A delay in starting therapy of even a few days has resulted in a poorer IQ outcome.[117,118,122] A minimum T_4 dosage of 10 to 15 mcg/kg/day is recommended to raise the serum T_4 to greater than 10 mcg/dL (129 nmol/L) by 7 days.[116] However, some suggest that higher than previously recommended dosages of 12 to 17 mcg/kg/day might be more effective, but concern about negative neurologic outcomes exists.[115,117,118] In the full-term healthy infant, full initial replacement T_4 doses are appropriate unless the infant has underlying heart disease or is extremely sensitive to the effects of thyroid hormones. In these infants, reduced doses of T_4 (approximately 25%–33% of the recommended dose) can be started and increased gradually by similar increments until the therapeutic dose is achieved. The recommended replacement dose decreases with age and is shown in Tables 52-4 and 52-9.

Mental development and attainment of normal growth are not severely impaired if adequate T_4 treatment is initi-

TABLE 52-9
T_4 Recommended Replacement Dose

Age	Daily mcg/kg T_4
3–6 months	10–15
6–12 months	5–7
1–10 years	3–6
>10 years	2–4

T_4, thyroxine.

ated before 3 months of age to achieve a T_4 level greater than 10 mcg/dL.[115–118,120] Children with the most severe congenital hypothyroidism had IQs lower than their siblings.[119] Young adults 20 years after congenital hypothyroidism showed impaired motor and intellectual outcomes after suboptimal T_4 (<7.8 mcg/kg/day) therapy compared with sibling controls.[120] However, those receiving optimal therapy still had some memory, attention, and behavior deficits.[123] Newborns starting L-thyroxine during the first 4 to 6 weeks of life have mean IQs similar to controls. The IQ drops if treatment is delayed until between 6 weeks and 3 months (mean IQ, 95), or until between 3 and 6 months (mean IQ, 75). When treatment is delayed until between 6 months and 1 year of age, normal mental development is impaired despite subsequent treatment. Higher IQs also were found in children who received T_4 dosages greater than 10 mcg/kg/day and achieved a mean T_4 level greater than 14 mcg/dL in the first month of therapy.[115,117,118,122,124] Neurologic deficits were also more likely to occur in infants whose thyroid replacement was delayed or inadequate (T_4 <8 mcg/dL within 30 days of therapy or had delayed TSH normalization [18–24 months]). Additional risk factors for low IQs and poor motor and speech skills despite adequate therapy include clinical signs of hypothyroidism during fetal life, T_4 less than 2 mcg/dL at birth, thyroid aplasia, and retarded bone age.[115,116,118]

The goal of therapy is a T_4 in the upper normal range (e.g., 10–18 mcg/dL or an FT_4 of 2–5 ng/dL) during the first 2 weeks of therapy, and then a lower target thereafter: a T_4 of 10 to 16 mcg/dL (or an FT_4 of 1.6–2.2 ng/dL). IQs are improved if TSH levels are normalized within the first month of therapy, but no later than 3 months.[117,118,122,124] Thyroid function tests should be routinely monitored 2 to 4 weeks after starting therapy, then every 1 to 2 months during the first 6 months of life, every 3 to 4 months until age 3, and finally, every 6 to 12 months until growth is complete.[115] Although TSH suppression is the most reliable index of adequate replacement in older children, normalization of the TSH should not be used as the sole monitoring parameter in infants because the TSH may lag behind correction of the T_4 or FT_4 levels. Overtreatment should be avoided to prevent brain dysfunction, acceleration of bone age, and craniosynostosis (premature closure of the cranial sutures). Normal growth and development should also be a treatment goal. Other clinical end points include an improvement in activity level, skin color, temperature, facial appearance, and reversal of other symptoms and signs of hypothyroidism. The child will require lifelong replacement therapy.

UNRESPONSIVENESS TO LEVOTHYROXINE AND DRUG–DRUG INTERACTIONS

CASE 52-9

QUESTION 1: R.T., a 45-year-old woman, complains of weight gain, heavy menses, sluggishness, and cold intolerance. Her present medical problems include Hashimoto's thyroiditis, treated with L-thyroxine 150 mcg daily; hypercholesterolemia treated with cholestyramine 4 g four times a day (QID); anemia, treated with $FeSO_4$ 325 mg twice a day (BID); dysmenorrhea treated with estrogen-containing birth control pills daily; and a history of peptic ulcer disease, treated with antacids and sucralfate 1 g BID. She was recently started on calcium carbonate 1 g BID and raloxifene 60 mg daily to protect her bones. Her laboratory data include the following findings:

Cholesterol serum concentration, 280 mg/dL
TSH, 21 microunits/mL (normal, 0.4–4.0)
FT_4, 0.6 ng/dL (normal, 0.7–1.9)
Positive TgAb and TPA antibodies

R.T. admits that she self-increased her L-thyroxine dose because she feels better on the higher dose. Why is R.T. apparently unresponsive to thyroid therapy?

R.T.'s complaints and laboratory values confirm inadequate treatment of hypothyroidism despite thyroid therapy. Possible causes of therapeutic failure include nonadherence, error in diagnosis, poor absorption, subpotent medication, rapid metabolism, and tissue resistance.[75,125,126] Thyroid resistance is rare, and nonadherence, error in diagnosis, and rapid metabolism do not appear to be reasonable explanations in R.T.

The most likely explanations are poor bioavailability or a subpotent preparation. The timing of T_4 administration with her meals should be ascertained because its bioavailability is improved when it is taken on an empty stomach and at night.[75,77,127,128] Significantly lower TSH levels are achieved when levothyroxine is taken on an empty stomach than with food or at night.[128] Simultaneous coadministration of T_4 with soy proteins, coffee, or high-fiber diets (e.g., oat bran, soybean) should also be avoided because T_4's absorption can be impaired.[129–131] R.T.'s history does not include surgical bowel resection or GI disorders (e.g., steatorrhea, malabsorption). Evidence for incomplete absorption of the hormone can be obtained by comparing R.T.'s response to oral and parenteral T_4.[125]

L-Thyroxine bioavailability can also be compromised by the numerous medications that R.T. is taking. Estrogen therapy can increase T_4 requirements by increasing TBG to increase T_4 binding.[1] Cholestyramine, colestipol, iron sulfate, antacids, sucralfate, calcium preparations—particularly the carbonate salt—and raloxifene can impair thyroid absorption if these medications are administered at the same time.[30,75,132–138] Cholesterol-lowering agents (e.g., lovastatin) and phosphate binders are also reported to interfere with thyroid hormone absorption.[134,139] R.T. should be questioned about the time she takes her thyroid medication. She should be instructed to take it on an empty stomach or at night,[77] and at least 12 hours apart from the raloxifene and 4 hours apart from the iron, calcium, and cholestyramine.[30,132–138] Aluminum-containing products (i.e., antacids, sucralfate) should be discontinued because separating the concurrent administration of T_4 and her aluminum-containing preparations does not consistently correct this interaction.[135,136] R.T. should be changed to an aluminum- and calciumfree antacid and, if necessary, an H_2-receptor antagonist. Proton-pump inhibitors (e.g., omeprazole) should be avoided because decreased acid secretion may reduce T_4 absorption, although data are conflicting.[140,141] After R.T. has been instructed on the proper times of administration for her medications, the therapeutic response and thyroid function tests should be re-evaluated in 6 to 8 weeks before any changes are made.

CASE 52-9, QUESTION 2: Could R.T.'s hypothyroidism be responsible for her hypercholesterolemia?

Type IIa hypercholesterolemia is the most common lipid abnormality observed in patients with primary hypothyroidism.[142] Although the rate of cholesterol synthesis is normal in hypothyroid patients, the rate of cholesterol clearance is decreased. Similarly, slow removal of triglycerides may result in hypertriglyceridemia. Hypercholesterolemia is frequently observed before the appearance of clinical hypothyroidism. Treatment with T_4 alone should lower the cholesterol levels if no other causes are contributing.

Myxedema Coma

CLINICAL PRESENTATION

CASE 52-10

QUESTION 1: R.B., a 65-year-old, agitated woman arrived at the emergency department complaining of chest pain unrelieved by nitroglycerin (NTG). Her medical problems include alcoholic cardiomyopathy, angina, and hypothyroidism. Although she has been advised repeatedly to take her T_4 regularly, she continues to take it sporadically. An FT_4 drawn 4 months ago was 0.5 ng/dL. Haloperidol 2 mg IM and morphine sulfate 10 mg IM were given for the agitation. After the injection, the nurse noticed mental depression, lethargy, and shallow breathing. R.B.'s oral temperature was 34.5°C, and she exhibited chills and shakes. What is your assessment of R.B.'s subjective and objective data?

R.B. has several symptoms consistent with myxedema coma.[143] Myxedema coma is the end stage of long-standing, uncorrected hypothyroidism. The classic features are hypothermia, delayed DTRs, and an altered sensorium that ranges from stupor to coma. Other predominant features include hypoxia, carbon dioxide retention, severe hypoglycemia, hyponatremia, and paranoid psychosis. Typical physical findings (Table 52-3) include a puffy face and eyelids, a yellowish discoloration of the skin, and loss of the lateral eyebrows. Pleural and pericardial effusions and cardiomegaly may be present. Because myxedema coma frequently occurs in older women, it is often difficult to distinguish the signs and symptoms from dementia or other disease states, as illustrated by R.B. Precipitating factors include cold weather or hypothermia, stress (e.g., surgery, infection, trauma), coexisting disease states such as MI, diabetes, hypoglycemia, or fluid and electrolyte abnormalities (especially hyponatremia), and medications such as sedatives, narcotic analgesics, antidepressants, and other respiratory depressants and diuretics.

Haloperidol and morphine might be responsible for what appears to be impending myxedema coma in R.B. In severely myxedematous patients, respiratory depressants (anesthetics, narcotic analgesics, phenothiazines, sedative-hypnotics) alone or in combination with the hypothermic effects of the phenothiazines can aggravate the pre-existing hypothermia and carbon dioxide retention to precipitate myxedema coma.[143,144] Tranquilizers such as haloperidol should not be given; small doses of less-depressive sedative-hypnotics such as the benzodiazepines should be used only when necessary. Myxedematous patients are also inherently sensitive to the respiratory depressant effects of narcotic analgesics, especially morphine. A dose as small as 10 mg may induce coma in a hypothyroid patient or cause death in a patient who is already comatose. If morphine is required, the dose should be decreased to one-third to one-half the usual analgesic dose, and the respiratory rate should be monitored closely.

TREATMENT

CASE 52-10, QUESTION 2: What would be a reasonable therapeutic plan for the management of R.B.'s myxedema coma?

Emergency treatment, usually in the intensive care unit, of myxedema coma is directed toward thyroid replacement, maintenance of vital functions, and elimination of precipitating factors. Despite immediate and aggressive therapy with large replacement doses of thyroid, mortality rates of 60% to 70% are common.[143]

Whether T_4 or T_3 is the drug of choice in myxedema coma is controversial because no comparative trials have been conducted. Although T_3 is potentially more cardiotoxic, it has been recommended because its more rapid onset might reverse coma faster, and the peripheral conversion from T_4 to the biologically active T_3 might be inhibited in severe systemic disease.[144–148] T_4 alone, T_3 alone, and a combination of the two have all been used successfully to treat myxedema coma. However, L-thyroxine is generally regarded as the hormone of choice because of greater clinical experience with T_4 than with T_3. Also, mortality has occurred despite the higher T_3 levels achieved after T_3 administration.[148] T_3 might be considered after failure of T_4 or if concomitant systemic illness (e.g., heart failure) is likely to impair conversion of T_4 to T_3. Supraphysiological elevations in T_3 levels occur only after oral administration but are not seen after IV T_3 infusion. Factors associated with a higher mortality 1 month after therapy include older age, cardiac complications, and T_4 replacement of at least 500 mcg/day or T_3 replacement of greater than 75 mcg/day.[144,148]

L-Thyroxine 400 to 500 mcg should be given IV initially in patients younger than 55 years of age without cardiac disease to saturate empty TBG sites and raise the serum T_4 level to 6 to 7 mcg/dL.[143,149] This initial dose can be adjusted based on the patient's weight and other restrictive factors (e.g., age, cardiac disease). The initial T_4 dosage for R.B. should be reduced to 300 mcg/day to avoid worsening her angina. If the proper dosage is given, consciousness, restoration of vital signs, and decreased TSH levels should occur within 24 hours. If T_3 is preferred, the usual dose is 10 to 20 mcg IV, followed by 10 mcg every 4 hours for the first 24 hours, and then 10 mcg every 6 hours for a few days until oral therapy can be started.[143]

Maintenance doses should be titrated to the patient's clinical response. Because myxedema can impair oral absorption, the IV route is preferred to ensure adequate drug concentrations. Oral administration is permitted once GI function returns to normal. The smallest dosage (without untoward effects) administered should be 50 to 100 mcg/day of T_4 or 10 to 15 mcg of T_3 every 12 hours.[143,149]

Supportive measures include assisted ventilation, glucose for hypoglycemia, restriction of fluids for hyponatremia, and the use of blood or plasma expanders to prevent circulatory collapse and to maintain blood pressure. The use of blankets to treat R.B.'s hypothermia is not advised because vasodilation will occur and further compromise the cardiovascular components of shock. Although steroids have not been shown to be clearly beneficial in primary myxedema, they may be lifesaving in patients with hypopituitarism masquerading as myxedema coma. Because it is difficult to distinguish between primary and secondary myxedema, hydrocortisone 50 to 100 mg every 6 hours should be given empirically.[143]

Appropriate measures should be taken to relieve R.B.'s chest pain while ruling out the possibility of an MI. The use of a narcotic antagonist such as naloxone may be beneficial in this instance because it can reverse the effects of the morphine. Naloxone can also arouse comatose patients intoxicated with alcohol.

Hypothyroidism With Congestive Heart Failure

CLINICAL PRESENTATION

CASE 52-11

QUESTION 1: E.B., a 45-year-old woman, is admitted with complaints of substernal pressure and chest pain, SOB, dyspnea on exertion, and orthopnea. Other subjective and

objective data suggest CHF complicated by MI. Significant past medical history reveals exertional angina and Graves disease, which was treated with RAI ablation 10 years ago. Symptoms have not recurred. Physical examination reveals cardiomegaly, diastolic hypertension, obesity, facial edema and puffiness, delayed DTRs, and nonpitting pretibial edema. Pertinent laboratory findings include the following results:

FT_4, 0.2 ng/dL (normal, 0.7–1.9)
TSH, 100 microunits/mL (normal, 0.4–4.0)
Creatinine phosphokinase, 300 units/L with negative MB bands
Aspartate aminotransferase (AST), 80 units/L
Lactate dehydrogenase (LDH), 250 units/L
Brain natriuretic protein, 550 pg/mL
Troponin, 0.3 ng/mL (normal, 0.3–1.5)

A chest radiograph reveals cardiomegaly and pericardial effusions, and an electrocardiogram (ECG) shows bradycardia and flattened T waves with ST depression. Diuretics, nitrates, angiotensin-converting enzyme inhibitor, and digitalis are instituted. E.B.'s symptoms improve, but her cardiac abnormalities are not reversed. Why do these clinical findings suggest hypothyroidism?

E.B.'s abnormal thyroid function tests, symptoms, physical findings, and history of RAI therapy are consistent with severe hypothyroidism. "Myxedema heart" can be confused with low-output CHF because the symptoms are similar: cardiomegaly, dyspnea, edema, pericardial effusions, and abnormal ECG.[89,143] Therefore, hypothyroidism should be excluded in all patients with new or worsening symptoms of cardiovascular disease (e.g., angina, arrhythmia). Although hypothyroidism alone rarely causes CHF, it can worsen an underlying cardiac condition. Rarely, ventricular arrhythmia, including torsades de pointes, can occur from a prolonged QT interval.

Although E.B.'s enzyme elevations (i.e., AST, LDH, creatine phosphokinase) are suggestive of an MI, they all may be moderately or significantly increased as a result of chronic skeletal or cardiac muscle damage or decreased enzyme clearance secondary to hypothyroidism. The normal troponin level and negative creatine phosphokinase-MB bands eliminate the possibility of an MI.

TREATMENT

CASE 52-11, QUESTION 2: What might be the effect of hypothyroidism on the cardiac treatment and status of E.B.?

If E.B.'s cardiac abnormalities are caused by hypothyroidism rather than organic disease, adequate doses of T_4 will restore the heart size, normalize the diastolic blood pressure, reverse the ECG findings, and normalize the serum enzyme elevations within 2 to 4 weeks. However, improvement in myocardial function begins only at dosages of 50 to 75 mcg/day of T_4, which may be tolerated poorly by cardiac patients.

The relationship between the altered lipid metabolism of hypothyroidism and increased risk of atherosclerosis is controversial and poorly documented.[142] Interestingly, angina pectoris and MI are rather uncommon among hypothyroid patients. Theoretically, the hypometabolic state associated with hypothyroidism may protect the ischemic myocardium by reducing metabolic demands. However, hypothyroidism actually aggravates subendocardial ischemia during an acute MI by decreasing erythrocyte production of 2,3-diphosphoglycerate, which shifts the oxyhemoglobin dissociation curve to the left. This effect further diminishes oxygen delivery to already ischemic tissues. Angina or premature beats can develop or worsen with the institution of T_4 therapy,[150–152] so doses should be titrated carefully (see Case 52-11, Question 3). Without organic disease, digitalis is ineffective and may even be harmful. Hypothyroid patients show an increased sensitivity to digitalis, and digitalis toxicity is possible unless the maintenance dose is decreased (see Case 52-14, Question 4).[153,154] Nitrates may precipitate hypotension or syncope in hypothyroid patients because these patients have a low circulating blood volume and their response to vasodilation can be exaggerated. Furthermore, if β-blockers are required, the cardioselective β-blockers are preferred. The noncardioselective β-blockers have produced coronary spasm by exacerbating the compensatory increase in norepinephrine levels and α-adrenergic tone found in hypothyroidism.

CASE 52-11, QUESTION 3: How aggressively should thyroid hormone therapy be initiated in a patient like E.B. who has angina? What is the hormone replacement of choice in patients with cardiac disease?

Patients with long-standing hypothyroidism, arteriosclerotic cardiac disease, or advanced age tend to be extremely sensitive to the cardiac effects of thyroid hormone. Initiation of normal or even subtherapeutic doses in these patients might produce severe angina, MI, supraventricular and ventricular premature beats, cardiac failure, or sudden death. These effects underscore the need to replace thyroid cautiously, and sometimes suboptimally, to avoid cardiac toxicity.[150–152,155]

The angina and cardiac status should be controlled before initiating T_4 therapy. In the patient with poorly controlled angina, cardiac catheterization is warranted to assess the coronary artery status before starting hormone therapy. Coronary bypass has been performed safely with minimal complications in the hypothyroid patient to control the angina and may allow institution of full replacement doses without cardiotoxicity.[156]

For E.B., 12.5 to 25 mcg daily of T_4 should be initiated cautiously and increased as tolerated by similar increments of T_4 every 4 to 6 weeks until a therapeutic dosage is reached. The rapidity with which the increments can proceed is determined by how well each increased dose is tolerated. If cardiac toxicity occurs, therapy should be stopped immediately. Once symptoms resolve, therapy can be restarted using smaller dosage increments and longer intervals between dosage adjustments. If cardiac symptoms recur, further T_4 therapy should be stopped pending cardiac evaluation. In some patients with severe cardiac sensitivity, complete euthyroidism might never be achieved. In these patients, the correct replacement dosage is a compromise between prevention of myxedema and avoidance of cardiac toxicity.[152] E.B.'s clinical status and ECG should be monitored closely during the titration period. T_4 should be discontinued or decreased at the first sign of cardiac deterioration. It is not necessary to monitor thyroid function tests (e.g., TSH or FT_4) during the titration period because the results will remain low until adequate replacement is achieved. Thyroid function tests should be obtained once maximally tolerated or estimated euthyroid dosages are achieved.

Some suggest that T_3 is the agent of choice in patients with cardiac abnormalities. The onset of action of T_3 is 1 to 3 days compared with 3 to 5 days for T_4. After therapy is withdrawn, the effects of T_3 dissipate in 3 to 5 days, whereas a period of 7 to 10 days is needed for T_4. Thus, if toxicity occurs, the effects of T_3 will disappear rapidly on cessation of therapy, a theoretical advantage in the cardiac patient. Nevertheless, T_3 is not recommended because its greater potency requires finer and more difficult dosage titration to ensure smooth and uniform blood levels. Furthermore, the high serum T_3 levels that occur after oral administration might cause more cardiac toxicity, especially angina.

Subclinical Hypothyroidism

CASE 52-12

QUESTION 1: M.P., a healthy 53-year-old woman, comes in for her regular checkup. She denies any symptoms of hypothyroidism and feels well. She has no other medical problems, takes no medications, and has no known allergies. Her physical examination is within normal limits. Routine screening laboratory tests are normal except for an FT_4 of 1.2 ng/dL and a TSH of 8 microunits/mL. Does M.P. require thyroid treatment, based on her clinical presentation and laboratory findings?

M.P.'s free thyroid hormone levels are normal, but her TSH level is elevated, indicating subclinical hypothyroidism (SH). The prevalence of SH ranges from 4% to 10% and increases to 26% in the elderly population, particularly women.[91,92] It is unclear whether SH represents the early stages of thyroid failure. The estimated risk of developing overt hypothyroidism after 10 years in untreated patients by Kaplan-Meier curves was 0% for a TSH level of 4 to 6 microunits/mL, 42.8% for a TSH level of 6 to 12 microunits/mL, and 76.9% for a TSH level greater than 12 microunits/mL. This risk is increased in patients with positive thyroid antibodies.[157] Because the most common clinical scenarios involve asymptomatic patients with TSH levels less than 10 microunits/mL, negative thyroid antibodies, and no history of prior thyroid disease, routine thyroid screening has been recommended, particularly in elderly women.[61]

Mild symptoms of hypothyroidism, including psychiatric and cognitive abnormalities, are found in approximately 30% of patients with SH, but the average TSH level usually exceeds 11 microunits/mL. Cardiac dysfunction, including impaired left ventricular diastolic function at rest, systolic dysfunction with exercise, atherosclerosis, CHF, and MI has been reported.[89,92,158–160] Data showing an increased risk of coronary heart disease (CHD) are conflicting and influenced by the severity of SH, study design, and length of follow-up. A meta-analysis noted a 1.6 times increased risk of CHD,[161] a cross-sectional analysis noted an odds ratio of 2.2 only in those with TSH levels of at least 10 microunits/mL, whereas a 20-year longitudinal analysis found a significant risk (hazard ratio [HR], 1.7) regardless of the degree of TSH elevation.[162] However, a large prospective cohort study found no significant association with atherosclerotic disease or cardiac mortality, but observed an increase in all-cause mortality at 10 years of follow-up.[163] Compelling data reported from 11 large prospective cohorts with a median follow-up of 2.5 to 20 years involving 3,450 subjects with subclinical hypothyroidism found an increased risk of CHD (HR, 1.89) and mortality (HR, 1.5) but not total mortality only in those with TSH levels greater than 10 microunits/mLafter adjustment for traditional cardiovascular factors. No increased CHD or CHD mortality was noted with more minimal TSH elevations.[164]

Other atypical and nonspecific signs and symptoms reflecting dysfunction of any part of the body may occur, primarily in the elderly. Failure to thrive, mental confusion, weight loss with poor appetite, incontinence, depression, inability to walk, carpal tunnel syndrome, deafness, ileus, anemia, hypercholesterolemia, and hyponatremia have been reported.[91,92,158–160]

Treatment of subclinical hypothyroidism with T_4 is controversial because study results are conflicting. Potential benefits of treatment include (a) preventing progression to hypothyroidism, (b) improving the lipid profile and reducing cardiac risks, and (c) reversing symptoms of hypothyroidism. Patients with higher TSH levels (e.g., >10 microunits/mL), a history of previously diagnosed thyroid disease, elevated lipid levels, or evidence of positive thyroid antibodies gained the most benefit from L-thyroxine therapy.[89,92,157,160,165] L-Thyroxine significantly reduced total cholesterol by 7.9 to 15.8 mg/dL and low-density cholesterol concentrations by 10 mg/dL; serum high-density lipoprotein cholesterol and triglyceride concentrations remain unchanged.[92,159,160,165] Improvement of elevated intraocular pressures, memory, mood, somatic complaints, and diastolic dysfunction has also been reported after T_4 replacement.[157,159,160,165] However, in patients with mild TSH elevations (e.g., <10 microunits/mL), well-designed studies showed no increased CHD risk or mortality or improvement in clinical symptoms of hypothyroidism with T_4 supplementation.[91,92,159,160]

Treatment of older patients requires an assessment of the risks versus benefits of therapy. Thyroid therapy carries the risk of unmasking underlying cardiac disease in older patients. Nevertheless, thyroid replacement appears reasonable in asymptomatic patients with TSH levels greater than 10 microunits/mLand especially those with symptoms of mild hypothyroidism, dyslipidemia, laboratory abnormalities, or end-organ alterations.[91,92,157,159,165] Patients with asymptomatic subclinical hypothyroidism and a TSH level less than 10 microunits/mL do not warrant immediate therapy, but close follow-up is warranted.

Because M.P. is asymptomatic and has a TSH level less than 10 microunits/mL, it is reasonable to delay therapy and recheck the TSH in a few months.

Hypopituitarism and Thyroxine Replacement With a Normal Thyroid-Stimulating Hormone Level

CASE 52-13

QUESTION 1: K.N. is a 65-year-old woman who complains of fatigue, cold intolerance, dry skin, and weight gain for the past several months. Her thyroid examination and DTRs are within normal limits. A TSH level was 2.5 microunits/mL (normal, 0.4–4.0). She denies taking any other medications. J.P. is started empirically on a 3-month trial of L-thyroxine. How should the TSH level be interpreted? Is T_4 therapy indicated, based on her presenting findings?

Despite complaints that could be consistent with hypothyroidism (e.g., fatigue, cold intolerance, dry skin, weight gain), the normal TSH level indicates that K.N. is euthyroid. However, because a diagnosis of hypopituitarism (i.e., TSH level could be normal or low) cannot be ruled out, an FT_4 level should be obtained; a low level would increase the likelihood of hypopituitarism. Some argue that hypopituitarism is underdiagnosed and would advocate adding FT_4 to the primary screening tests.[166]

If the FT_4 level is normal, indicating euthyroidism, then hypopituitarism is unlikely and L-thyroxine therapy is not indicated. A randomized, double-blind, placebo-controlled crossover trial found that T_4 supplementation in patients with hypothyroid symptoms and normal thyroid function tests was not more effective than placebo in improving cognitive function or psychological well-being despite changes in the TSH and FT_4 levels.[167,168]

In K.N., the T_4 should be discontinued because there is no evidence of its efficacy in euthyroid individuals.

HYPERTHYROIDISM

Clinical Presentation

CASE 52-14

QUESTION 1: S.K., a 48-year-old woman, is admitted to the hospital for a possible MI. Her complaints include chest pain that is unrelieved by NTG, increasing SOB with exercise, nervousness, palpitations, muscle weakness, weight loss despite an increased appetite, and epistaxis; she also bruises easily. She has a history of deep venous thrombosis treated with warfarin 5 mg/day; her last international normalized ratio (INR) was 1.8 (normal, 1; therapeutic, 2–3). She has angina, treated with NTG 0.4 mg, and CHF, treated with digoxin 0.25 mg/day.

Physical examination reveals a thin, flushed, hyperkinetic, nervous woman. Her blood pressure is 180/90 mm Hg, pulse is 130 beats/minute, irregularly irregular, respiratory rate is 30 breaths/minute, and temperature is 37.5°C. Other pertinent findings include a lid lag with stare, proptosis with tearing, decreased visual acuity, a diffusely enlarged thyroid gland without nodules, a bruit in the left lobe of the thyroid, positive jugular venous distension, bibasilar rales, warm moist skin with multiple bruises, new-onset atrial fibrillation (AF), slight diarrhea, hepatomegaly, acropachy, 2+ pitting edema, a fine tremor, proximal muscle weakness, and irregular scant menses.

Laboratory data include the following results:

FT_4, 2.9 ng/dL (normal, 0.7–1.9)
TSH, <0.5 microunits/mL (normal, 0.4–4.0)
RAIU at 24 hours, 80% (normal, 5%–35%)
INR, 4.8 (normal, 1; therapeutic, 2–3)
TPA, 200 international units/mL (normal, <0.8)
Alkaline phosphatase, 200 units/L
Total bilirubin, 1.1 mg/dL
AST, 60 units/L
Alanine aminotransferase, 55 units/L

An RAI scan shows a diffusely enlarged gland, three to four times the normal size. What subjective and objective data are suggestive of hyperthyroidism in S.K.?

S.K. presents with many of the clinical and laboratory features[169] associated with an increased metabolic state resulting from excessive T_4 (Table 52-6). Her ocular symptoms are consistent with Graves disease and include lid lag (lid falls behind the movement of the eye and a narrow white rim of sclera becomes visible between the upper lid and cornea, producing a "staring" appearance), ophthalmopathy (protrusion of the eyeball), and decreased visual acuity. The thyroid bruit, palpitations, exertional dyspnea, worsening CHF (jugular venous distension, bibasilar rales, edema, hepatomegaly), diarrhea, irregular scant menses, nervousness, tremor, muscle weakness, weight loss despite increased appetite, increased perspiration, and flushing of the skin are consistent with a hypermetabolic state. Although sinus tachycardia is the most common arrhythmia in hyperthyroidism, new-onset AF is the presenting symptom in 5% to 20% of patients with hyperthyroidism, particularly in those older than 70 years.[170] Together with S.K.'s symptoms, a diagnosis of Graves disease is confirmed by an elevated FT_4 level, an undetectable TSH level, an increased RAIU, positive TPA antibodies, and a diffusely enlarged goiter. Her cardiac status and other medical problems are aggravated by the hyperthyroidism (see Table 52-5 for causes of hyperthyroidism).

Hypoprothrombinemia

CASE 52-14, QUESTION 2: What factors contribute to S.K.'s hypoprothrombinemia? What effect could this have on her subsequent drug treatment?

The hypoprothrombinemia and bleeding observed in S.K. are most likely related to an exaggerated response to warfarin. This may be related to a decrease in the hepatic metabolism of warfarin (secondary to hepatic congestion), but it is more likely that S.K.'s findings are caused by the combined effects of hyperthyroidism and warfarin on vitamin K–dependent clotting factors.

WARFARIN METABOLISM

Warfarin metabolism and the metabolism of vitamin K–dependent clotting factors can be altered by thyroid status. Net circulating levels of vitamin K–dependent clotting factors are generally not altered in hyperthyroid patients because both the synthesis and catabolism of these clotting factors are increased. However, an enhanced anticoagulant response occurs when the warfarin-induced decrease in clotting factor synthesis is combined with the hyperthyroidism-induced increase in clotting factor catabolism.[19,171] This may explain S.K.'s elevated INR, bruising, and history of epistaxis.

The opposite occurs in hypothyroidism, in which a decrease in both the metabolism and synthesis of clotting factors occurs. In hypothyroid patients, the response to oral anticoagulants is delayed because the clotting factors are eliminated more slowly.[19,171] Therefore, hyperthyroid patients need less warfarin, whereas hypothyroid patients require more warfarin to achieve the same hypoprothrombinemic response. The anticoagulant response to warfarin should be monitored carefully in patients with thyroid abnormalities, and the dosage adjusted as the thyroid status changes.

THIOAMIDE EFFECTS

Because S.K.'s hyperthyroidism will most likely be treated with a thioamide, caution must be exercised. Treatment of hyperthyroid patients with thioamides, especially PTU, has been associated with hypoprothrombinemia, thrombocytopenia, and bleeding, albeit rarely.[172] These drugs can depress the bone marrow and the synthesis of clotting factors II, VII, III, IX, X, and XIII; vitamin K and prothrombin times may remain depressed for up to 2 months after discontinuation of therapy. These effects may be caused by a subclinical hepatic alteration in synthesis or hepatotoxicity (see Case 52-15, Question 10).[173–177] Symptoms occur 2 weeks to 18 months after starting therapy. The bleeding is responsive to vitamin K or blood transfusions. (Also see Case 52-15, Questions 3 and 4, for further discussion of treatment with thioamides.)

Response to Digoxin

CASE 52-14, QUESTION 3: S.K.'s dose of digoxin was increased to 0.5 mg daily because of persistent AF with a rapid ventricular response. Why was such a large dose of digoxin required? What other options can be used to control her ventricular rate?

The AF of hyperthyroidism is often resistant to digitalis. When euthyroid patients with AF were given digitalis before and after exogenous T_3 administration, the daily dose of digoxin required to maintain a ventricular rate of 70 was increased from 0.2 to 0.8 mg after T_3 administration.[178] Higher dosages of digoxin without side effects might be tolerated better by the hyperthyroid patient.[153,154,178] Nevertheless, the goal of digoxin therapy should be a higher target heart rate (i.e., 100 beats/minute) than that achieved with digoxin in the euthyroid patient with AF to minimize cardiac toxicity. If additional rate control is required, β-blockers or calcium-channel blockers (e.g., diltiazem or verapamil) can be added. Unless contraindicated by severe bronchospasm, β-blockers rather than calcium-channel blockers are preferred, because they are more effective in controlling the ventricular rate and are less likely to cause hypotension.

This apparent resistance to digitalis is attributed to intrinsic changes in myocardial function, to an increased volume of distribution for digoxin, and to an increased glomerular filtration of the glycoside.[153,154,178] Conversely, hypothyroid patients are inordinately sensitive to the effects of digitalis and require smaller doses to achieve a therapeutic response. Regardless of the mechanism, one should be aware that higher-than-normal doses might be required in patients with thyrotoxicosis and that the initial dosage should be reduced as the hyperthyroid state resolves.

Cardioversion

CASE 52-14, QUESTION 4: If the AF persists, when should cardioversion be attempted in S.K.? Is other treatment indicated?

Because S.K. received RAI 6 weeks ago, her thyroid function tests should be rechecked to determine her present thyroid status. Cardioversion, either medical or electrical, should not be attempted if she is still toxic because the success rate is low. AF spontaneously reverted to normal sinus rhythm (NSR) in 56% to 62% of patients within the first 3 to 4 months after control of the hyperthyroidism.[170] Spontaneous conversion is highly unlikely if the duration of the hyperthyroidism-induced AF exceeds 13 months or if the AF persists after 4 months of euthyroidism.[170] Older patients with or without underlying heart disorders (except CHF) are also less likely to spontaneously convert to NSR. Patients who meet these criteria are candidates for cardioversion at about the third or fourth month after achieving euthyroidism. Age and the duration of thyrotoxicosis are important determinants of successful cardioversion. Ninety percent of patients achieved NSR after cardioversion; of these, 57% and 48% maintained NSR at 10 and 14 years, respectively, of follow-up.[170]

S.K. should be maintained on warfarin because of a high prevalence of systemic embolization in thyrotoxic patients with AF. Anticoagulation should be started when the AF is first diagnosed and continued until S.K. is euthyroid and in NSR. This is especially true for younger patients at low risk of bleeding with warfarin. The risks versus benefits of anticoagulation should be weighed before therapy (see Chapter 16, Thrombosis). Because an increased sensitivity to warfarin is observed, close monitoring is warranted (see Case 52-14, Question 2.)

Thyrotoxicosis: Clinical Presentation

CASE 52-15

QUESTION 1: C.R., a 27-year-old woman, has a 3-month history of intermittent heat intolerance, sweats, tremor, and severe muscle weakness, which has limited her ability to climb stairs. Her weight has increased because of increased appetite. She is also bothered by the pounding of her heart and some minor difficulty in swallowing. There is a family history of thyroid disease, but she denies taking any thyroid medications or any history of radiation to her neck. C.R. previously received iodide drops with symptomatic improvement, but her disease recurred despite its continued administration. Her other medical problems include type 2 diabetes controlled by diet, and osteoarthritis treated with aspirin 650 mg orally (PO) every 4 hours. She has a history of noncompliance with her clinic visits.

Pertinent physical findings include a blood pressure of 180/90 mm Hg, a pulse of 110 beats/minute, hyperreflexia, lid lag, and a diffusely enlarged thyroid gland that is about four times normal (about 100 g). Laboratory data include the following:

TT_4, 6 mcg/dL (normal, 4.8–10.4)
FT_4, 2 ng/dL (normal, 0.7–1.9)
TSH, <0.01 microunits/mL (normal, 0.4–4.0)
TPA, 350 international units/mL (normal, <0.8)
Fasting blood glucose, 350 mg/dL

Assess these subjective and objective data.

C.R.'s laboratory findings of a positive TPA and elevated thyroid hormone levels verify an autoimmune hyperthyroid state. However, the serum FT_4 is elevated only slightly and is disproportionately low relative to the severity of her symptoms, the undetectable TSH level, and her other laboratory findings. The low-normal TT_4 could be explained by displacement of T_4 from TBG by aspirin (see Case 52-2). The possibility of a variant type of hyperthyroidism known as T_3 toxicosis should be considered. The clinical features include signs and symptoms of thyrotoxicosis, normal or borderline high FT_4, an undetectable TSH level, and elevated T_3 levels. The latter occurs through preferential secretion and peripheral conversion of T_4 to T_3. A T_3 level should be obtained to establish the diagnosis.

Asymptomatic elevations of T_3 levels often precede elevation of T_4 levels and the development of overt hyperthyroidism. T_3 toxicosis probably represents an early stage of classic T_4 toxicosis and is useful for early diagnosis or as an early indicator of relapse after discontinuation of thioamide therapy.

Iodides

CASE 52-15, QUESTION 2: Why were the iodide drops initially effective in improving C.R.'s symptoms and later ineffective? When are iodides indicated? What is their mechanism of action?

Iodides have several effects: They inhibit thyroid hormone release, they block iodotyrosine and iodothyronine synthesis by blocking organification, and they decrease the vascularity of the thyroid gland.[179] However, large doses may accentuate hyperthyroidism because they provide a significant increase in available substrate for hormone synthesis (see Case 52-26).[56,179]

The inhibitory effect of exogenous iodides on the intrathyroidal organification of iodides is known as the Wolff-Chaikoff effect. This is an inherent autoregulatory function of the normal gland to prevent excessive hormone synthesis in the event of a large iodide load. The Wolff-Chaikoff effect occurs when intrathyroidal concentrations of iodides reach a critical level, and this is not overcome by TSH stimulation. However, as illustrated by C.R., the gland can escape from this block even with continued iodide use. The gland escapes by decreasing iodide transport or by leaking iodide. Both mechanisms decrease the critical intrathyroidal iodide level, thereby decreasing the block to organification. This effect is illustrated in C.R. Therefore, iodides should not be used as primary therapy for Graves disease.

Conversely, some patients are responsive to iodide therapy, including (a) patients who already have high intrathyroidal iodine stores (i.e., hot nodules, Graves disease); (b) patients with underlying defects in organic binding mechanisms (i.e., Hashimoto's); (c) patients who develop drug-induced thyroid disorders (see Cases 52-24 to 52-27); and (d) patients with Graves disease made euthyroid with RAI or surgery and who are receiving no thyroid replacement.

These patients are so sensitive that small doses of iodide can elicit the Wolff-Chaikoff effect, resulting in either amelioration of hyperthyroid symptoms or precipitation of hypothyroidism.[40,56,179] For this reason, patients with recurrent hyperthyroidism after surgery or RAI can often be managed with iodides alone.

The most important pharmacologic effect of iodides is their ability to promptly inhibit thyroid hormone release when dosages of 6 mg/day are given.[40,179] The mechanism is unknown, but it is not related to the Wolff-Chaikoff effect, which may take several weeks to manifest. Unlike the Wolff-Chaikoff effect, this effect can be overcome partially by an increase in TSH secretion. Thus, the normal gland can escape in 7 to 14 days because inhibition of thyroid hormone release stimulates a reflex increase in TSH secretion. Because patients with hyperthyroidism experience an improvement in symptoms within 2 to 7 days of initiation of therapy, inhibition of hormone release must be the predominant mechanism of action for the iodides. This rapid onset is the reason iodides are used in the treatment of thyroid storm and as an ameliorative measure while awaiting the onset of the therapeutic effects of thioamides or RAI.

Large doses of iodides are also used 2 weeks before thyroid surgery to increase the firmness of the thyroid gland by decreasing its size, vascularity, and friability. Iodides facilitate a smoother, less complicated surgery and reduce the risk of postoperative complications by inducing a euthyroid state.[179]

Stable iodine can be administered orally either as an unpleasant-tasting Lugol iodine solution (5% iodine and 10% potassium iodide), containing 8 mg/drop of iodide, or as the more palatable saturated solution of potassium iodide, containing 50 mg/drop of iodide. The minimal effective daily dose is 6 mg,[179] although larger doses (e.g., 5–10 drops QID of saturated solution of potassium iodide) are often administered.

The advantages of iodide therapy are that it is simple, inexpensive, and relatively nontoxic and involves no glandular destruction. Disadvantages include escape, accentuation of thyrotoxicosis, allergic reactions, relapse after discontinuation of treatment, and subsequent interference with RAI if used before therapy.

Treatment Modalities

CASE 52-15, QUESTION 3: What are the advantages and disadvantages of the different treatment modalities available for C.R.?

The three major treatment modalities for Graves-related hyperthyroidism are the thioamides, RAI, and surgery (Table 52-10).[180–182] In most cases, any of these three modalities can be used, and there is controversy as to which is the most effective therapy. Often the final decision is empiric, depending on the clinician's available resources and the patient's desires. A review of treatment guidelines published by the major endocrine organizations found that RAI is the most common treatment, and surgery is the least common.[183] Patients who are older and those with cardiac disease, concomitant ophthalmopathy, and hyperthyroidism caused by a toxic multinodular goiter are treated best with RAI. Surgery is the preferred therapy for pregnant women who are drug intolerant, when obstructive symptoms are present, or if malignancy is suspected.

THIOAMIDES

The thioamides are the preferred treatment for children, pregnant women, and young adults with uncomplicated Graves disease.[169,184,185] This is the only treatment that leaves the thyroid gland intact and does not carry the added risk of permanent hypothyroidism often associated with RAI or surgery.

Because the thyrotoxicosis of Graves disease might be self-limiting, thioamides are used to control the symptoms until spontaneous remission occurs. Thioamides should also be given before treatment with RAI or surgery to deplete the gland of stored thyroid hormone, which prevents subsequent thyroid storm. Although hyperthyroidism from toxic nodules will also respond to thioamides, more definitive therapy (surgery or RAI) is needed because these conditions do not undergo spontaneous remission.

Disadvantages of thioamide therapy include the numerous tablets required, patient adherence, possible drug toxicity, the long duration of treatment, and the low remission rates after discontinuation of therapy (see Case 52-17).

The use of thioamides in C.R. has several potential drawbacks. Her relatively large gland and severe disease make the prognosis for spontaneous remission somewhat less favorable. A delay in the onset of thioamide's effect may be expected if intraglandular stores of thyroid have been increased by her prior iodide therapy. Furthermore, her nonadherence and difficulty swallowing may necessitate another means of treatment. Thioamides may also be prepared for administration by the rectal routes.[180–182]

SURGERY

Surgery is considered the treatment of choice[169,186–188] when (a) malignancy is suspected; (b) esophageal obstruction, evidenced by difficulty swallowing, is present; (c) respiratory difficulties are present; (d) contraindications to the use of thioamides (e.g., allergy) or RAI (e.g., pregnancy) exist; (e) a large goiter that regresses poorly on RAI or thioamide therapy is present; or (f) it is the patient's preference. Some argue that surgery is underused in the treatment of Graves disease.[186] In a prospective, randomized trial comparing the three treatment modalities, surgery produced euthyroidism more quickly and was associated with a lower relapse rate than either RAI or thioamides.[187] A meta-analysis of 35 studies encompassing 7,241 patients with Graves disease found that thyroidectomy was successful in 92% of patients with a low recurrence (7.2%) of hyperthyroidism.[189] If C.R.'s minor difficulty in swallowing persists because of poor regression of goiter size with drug therapy, then surgery is a reasonable alternative. If surgery is contemplated, C.R. must be brought to surgery in a euthyroid state to prevent rapid postoperative rises in T_4 levels and subsequent thyroid storm (see Case 52-23, Question 1). A total or near-total rather than a subtotal thyroidectomy is the procedure of choice when performed by an experienced surgeon.[186,188,189] Although subtotal thyroidectomy theoretically avoids the predictable risk of hypothyroidism from total thyroidectomy, the likelihood of recurrent hyperthyroidism increases in proportion to the amount of residual thyroid tissue remaining.[186,187] Recurrent thyrotoxicosis after a subtotal thyroidectomy should be treated with RAI because the incidence of surgical complications increases with a second surgery.

Surgical complication rates are low when the procedure is performed by a competent surgeon and when the patient is adequately prepared for surgery. The disadvantages of surgery are expense, hospitalization, hypothyroidism, the small risk of postoperative complications, and the patient's fear of surgery (see Case 52-15, Question 12).[186,187,189]

TABLE 52-10
Treatment for Hyperthyroidism

Modality	Drug/Dosage	Mechanism of Action	Toxicity	Indication
Primary Treatment				
THIOAMIDES				
Methimazole (Tapazole) 5-, 10-mg tablet; rectal suppositories can be made[180]	Methimazole 30–40 mg PO daily or in two divided doses (*max:* 60 mg/d) for 6–8 weeks or until euthyroid, then maintenance of 5–10 mg/d PO × 12–18 months	Blocks organification of hormone synthesis, does not block conversion of T_4 to T_3	Skin rashes, GI symptoms, arthralgias, cholestatic jaundice, agranulocytosis, aplasia cutis and embryopathy syndrome in pregnancy (methimazole only)	DOC in adults/children except in thyroid storm and first trimester of pregnancy (see PTU). Once-daily dosing can improve adherence
PTU 50-mg tablet; rectal formulation can be made[181,182]	100–200 mg PO every 6–8 hours (*max:* 1,200 mg/d) for 6–8 weeks or until euthyroid; then maintenance of 50–150 mg daily PO × 12–18 months	Similar to methimazole, and blocks peripheral conversion of T_4 to T_3 (PTU only)	Hepatitis, some fatal. Similar to methimazole	DOC in thyroid storm, first trimester of pregnancy
Surgery	Preoperative preparation with iodides, thioamides, or β-blockers before surgery; see specific operative agent	Near-total thyroidectomy	Hypothyroidism, cosmetic scarring, hypoparathyroidism, risks of surgery and anesthesia, vocal cord damage	Obstruction, choking, malignancy, pregnancy in second trimester, contraindication to RAI or thioamides
RAI	^{131}I radioactive isotope; 80–100 μCi/g thyroid tissue. Average dose, ≈10 mCi; pretreatment with corticosteroids indicated in patients with ophthalmopathy	Destruction of the gland	Hypothyroidism; worsening of ophthalmopathy; fear of radiation-induced leukemia; genetic damage; malignancy; rarely, radiation sickness	Adults, older patients who are poor surgical risks or have cardiac disease; patients with a history of prior thyroid surgery; contraindications to thioamide usage; increasingly used in children
Adjuncts to Primary Usage				
IODIDES				
Lugol iodine solution 8 mg/drop (5% iodine, 10% potassium iodide; saturated [SSKI] 50 mg/drop)	5–10 drops TID PO for 10–14 days before surgery; minimal effective dose 6 mg/d	↓ Vascularity of gland and ↑ firmness; blocks release of thyroid hormone	Hypersensitivity reactions, skin rashes, mucous membrane ulcers, anaphylaxis, metallic taste, rhinorrhea, parotid and submaxillary swelling; fetal goiters and death	Preoperative preparation before surgery; thyroid storm, provides symptomatic relief of symptoms. *Do not use before RAI or chronically during pregnancy*
β-BLOCKERS				
Propranolol or equivalent β-blocker. *Avoid* those with ISA	Propranolol 10–40 mg PO every 6 hours or PRN to control HR <100 beats/min; IV 0.5–1 mg slowly	Blocks effects of thyroid hormone peripherally, no effect on underlying disease; blocks T_4 to T_3 conversion	Related to β-blockade; bradycardia, CHF, blocks hyperglycemic response to hypoglycemia, bronchospasm, CNS symptoms at high doses; fetal bradycardia	Symptomatic relief while awaiting onset of thioamides, RAI; preoperative preparation for surgery; thyroid storm
CALCIUM-CHANNEL BLOCKERS				
	Diltiazem 120 mg PO TID–QID or verapamil 80–120 mg PO TID–QID PRN to control HR <100 beats/min	Blocks effects of thyroid hormone peripherally, no effect on underlying disease	Bradycardia, peripheral edema, CHF, headache, flushing, hypotension, dizziness	Alternative for symptomatic relief of hyperthyroid symptoms in patients who cannot tolerate β-blockers
CORTICOSTEROIDS				
	Prednisone or equivalent corticosteroids 50–140 mg PO daily in divided doses; IV hydrocortisone 50–100 mg every 6 hours or equivalent for thyroid storm	↓ TSI, suppression of inflammatory process; blocks T_4 to T_3 conversion	Complications of steroid therapy	Ophthalmopathy, thyroid storm (use IV steroid), pretibial myxedema, pretreatment before RAI therapy in patients with ophthalmopathy

CHF, congestive heart failure; CNS, central nervous system; DOC, drug of choice; GI, gastrointestinal; HR, heart rate; ISA, intrinsic sympathomimetic activity; IV, intravenous; PO, orally (by mouth); PRN, as needed; PTU, propylthiouracil; QID, four times a day; RAI, radioactive iodine; SSKI, saturated solution of potassium iodide; T_3, triiodothyronine; T_4, thyroxine; TID, three times a day; TSI, thyroid stimulating immunoglobulin.[91–93]

RADIOACTIVE IODINE

RAI, the most common treatment modality in the United States, is the preferred treatment for (a) debilitated, cardiac, or older patients who are poor surgical candidates; (b) patients who fail to respond to drug therapy or who experience adverse drug reactions; and (c) patients who experience recurrent hyperthyroidism after surgery.[169,183,187,190]

Pregnancy is an absolute contraindication to RAI therapy. Previously, the use of RAI was restricted to adults older than an arbitrary age of 20 to 35 years because it was feared that RAI could result in genetic damage or neoplasia. However, its use in adolescents is increasing after more than 50 years of clinical experience with RAI showing that it is safe and effective.[190–193] There is no reported evidence of genetic damage after ^{131}I ingestion, and the dose of radiation to the gonads is less than 3 rad, which is comparable to other radiographic diagnostic tests (e.g., barium enemas).[194] The incidence of leukemia or malignancy is no higher in recipients of ^{131}I than in thyrotoxic patients treated with drugs or surgery.[191,195] In a retrospective review of 98 adolescents followed for 36 years after receiving ^{131}I, no cancers of the thyroid or leukemia were reported.[193] One interesting finding is that patients receiving RAI should be warned that they can set off radiation detectors at airport screening terminals for up to 12 weeks after RAI and that they should carry documentation of their treatment.[196,197]

RAI is painless, effective, economical, and quick, but unsubstantiated fears about radiation and malignancy, as well as the high incidence of hypothyroidism, may deter its use. RAI could be used safely in this nonpregnant young patient. However, C.R.'s prior use of iodides will dilute the ^{131}I pool. Thus, it will be impossible to achieve therapeutic thyroid concentrations of RAI for as long as 3 to 6 months.

Treatment With Thioamides

PROPYLTHIOURACIL VERSUS METHIMAZOLE

CASE 52-15, QUESTION 4: C.R. is started on PTU 200 mg every 8 hours after baseline FT_4 and TSH levels have been obtained. Three weeks later, she angrily complains that her symptoms are worse and that the medication is not working; however, she reluctantly admits to missing doses because of difficulty swallowing, nausea, vomiting, diarrhea, fatigue, a cough, and a sore throat. What are the advantages of using either PTU or methimazole in the treatment of hyperthyroidism?

Both thioamides are effective in treating hyperthyroidism. The antithyroid effectiveness of the thioamides primarily depends on their ability to block the organification of iodine, thereby inhibiting thyroid hormone synthesis.[184,185] Thyroid autoantibody synthesis may also be suppressed. In most hyperthyroid adults and children, methimazole should be considered the thioamide of choice because of increasing reports of hepatitis, some fatal, from PTU. PTU should be reserved for use in thyroid storm, during the first trimester of pregnancy because of rare teratogenicity from methimazole, and in those allergic to methimazole (except agranulocytosis and hepatitis) who are not candidates for RAI or surgery.[174,175]

DOSING AND ADMINISTRATION

Methimazole is effective when administered initially as a single dose compared with the multiple-dose regimen required with PTU to achieve a euthyroid state.[184,185] Although a single-dose regimen of PTU has been tried acutely, it is most effective when given in divided doses (see Case 52-16). Compared with PTU, methimazole is also less hepatotoxic and less expensive, requires daily ingestion of fewer numbers of tablets, and is not associated with a bitter tablet taste. However, PTU is preferred in thyroid storm because, unlike methimazole, it also blocks the peripheral conversion of T_4 to T_3.[198] Within 24 to 48 hours after PTU administration, a 25% to 40% reduction in peripheral T_3 production is seen, which contributes to PTU's rapid onset. A significantly greater fall in T_3 concentration and the T_3:T_4 ratio can be demonstrated in hyperthyroid patients treated acutely with PTU and iodine than with methimazole and iodides. Lastly, PTU is preferred over methimazole during the first trimester of pregnancy (see Case 52-19).

CASE 52-15, QUESTION 5: Why was the thioamide therapy ineffective in C.R.? Was the dose of PTU appropriate?

The inadequate response in C.R. suggests poor adherence to the thioamide dosing regimen or a delayed response caused by prior iodide loading of the gland.

The onset of action of the thioamides is slow because they block the synthesis rather than the release of thyroid hormone. Therefore, hormone secretion will continue until the glandular stores of hormone are depleted. If adequate doses were given, some improvement of clinical symptoms should be noted after 2 or 3 weeks.[185]

The dosage of PTU is appropriate. Thioamide dosing consists of two phases: initial therapy to achieve euthyroidism, and maintenance therapy to achieve remission. Initially, high blocking dosages of PTU (400–800 mg/day, depending on the severity of the toxicosis) should be given in three or four divided doses, as in C.R.[169,184,185] Rarely, dosages of 1,200 mg/day of PTU or its equivalent may be required in patients with severe disease or storm.[198] Equipotent doses of methimazole (which is 10 times more potent than PTU on a milligram-per-milligram basis) can also be used. However, it is usually unnecessary to use greater than 40 mg/day of methimazole to restore a euthyroid state.[169,184,185] Toxicity is also less common (see Case 52-15, Questions 10 and 11). True resistance to thioamides is rare; thus, most cases of unresponsiveness are caused by poor patient adherence, as in C.R.

C.R.'s adherence is also hindered by the frequency of PTU administration. The serum half-life of PTU is short (1.5 hours), but it is the intrathyroidal drug concentrations that should determine the dosing intervals because they are most clearly related to the drug's antithyroid effects[185] (see Case 52-16). PTU must be dosed every 6 to 8 hours initially, or as frequently as every 4 hours in cases of severe hyperthyroidism and thyroid storm. In contrast, methimazole has a serum half-life of 6 to 8 hours, remains in the thyroid for 20 hours, and has a duration of activity of up to 40 hours.[185,199]

Poor adherence is often difficult to ascertain and is more likely when multiple daily doses are required. The best option for C.R. is to change to 30 to 40 mg of methimazole, given once daily to improve adherence, or divided into two doses to decrease GI distress. After methimazole is given for 4 to 6 weeks to achieve euthyroidism, the daily dosage can be reduced gradually by 25% to 30% monthly to a dosage that maintains euthyroidism, usually 5 to 10 mg/day of methimazole. If C.R. remains hyperthyroid despite adequate doses of thioamides, then the most likely reason is nonadherence.

MONITORING THERAPY

CASE 52-15, QUESTION 6: What additional objective baseline data should be obtained to monitor both the efficacy and toxicity of thioamides?

advised to contact their physician or pharmacist. If they cannot reach their own physician, patients should inform the emergency physician that they are taking thioamides, and a WBC count with differential should be obtained. Routine monitoring of a WBC and differential is not recommended until further studies justify that it is indicated and cost-effective.

PREOPERATIVE PREPARATION

CASE 52-15, QUESTION 12: C.R.'s PTU is discontinued because she experienced agranulocytosis and hepatitis, and surgery is scheduled for when her granulocyte level returns to normal. What thyroid preparation is needed for C.R. before thyroidectomy? What postoperative complications are associated with thyroidectomy?

C.R. should be in a euthyroid state at the time of surgery to avoid precipitation of thyroid storm and morbidity. Generally, iodides (see Case 52-15, Question 2), thioamides, or propranolol can be used.[11,179,198] The combination of iodides and propranolol is more effective than either used alone. Propranolol used alone has been associated with thyroid crisis postoperatively and may be less effective than iodides in decreasing gland friability and vascularity.[11]

Because C.R. received only 1 week of thioamide therapy, it is likely that her gland still contains large stores of hormone; therefore, pretreatment is necessary.

In addition to the risks of anesthesia and surgery, postoperative complications include hypoparathyroidism, adhesions, laryngeal nerve damage, bleeding, infection, and poor wound healing. However, the surgery can be uneventful if it is performed by experienced surgeons.[186–189,212] Complications are also higher if a total rather than a subtotal thyroidectomy is performed, but there is a lower risk of recurrent hyperthyroidism. Development of hypothyroidism, especially subclinical hypothyroidism, is greatest during the first year after surgery, with an insidious rise in incidence during the next 10 years. The incidence of permanent hypothyroidism varies from 6% to 75% and is related inversely to the amount of remnant tissue left behind.[186–189,212] Thyroid function tests should be monitored annually after surgery.

SINGLE DAILY DOSING

CASE 52-16

QUESTION 1: R.G., a 23-year-old man newly diagnosed with Graves disease, remains hyperthyroid after 6 weeks of PTU 200 mg every 8 hours. He admits he has trouble remembering to take it three times a day and desires a more simplified regimen. Could R.G. be placed on a single daily dose of PTU?

A single daily dose of PTU should not be used as initial therapy because euthyroidism is achieved in only 39% to 68% of hyperthyroid patients using this approach.[185,213] However, once euthyroidism occurs, single daily doses of PTU are effective. In contrast, several clinical studies have documented that a single daily dose of methimazole is as effective as multiple daily doses in greater than 90% of treated patients.[184,185] Although a lower dosage of methimazole (e.g., 10–15 mg daily) can produce euthyroidism with fewer side effects, higher initial dosages of 20 to 40 mg/day are recommended to increase the likelihood of euthyroidism in 6 weeks.[169,184,185]

Methimazole is the preferred agent for once-a-day dosing because of its longer intrathyroidal duration of action (40 hours) and safety profile (see Case 52-15, Questions 4 and 10).[185,199,201,202] However, as previously noted, PTU is preferable in thyroid storm because it acts more rapidly. Despite its short plasma half-life of 4 to 6 hours, a single 30-mg dose of methimazole has a duration of action of 40 hours.[199] The duration of action of PTU is unknown, but it is shorter than methimazole. Apparently, the duration of action of the antithyroid agents correlates best with the size of the dose and the intrathyroidal concentration of the drug.

R.G. should be changed to 20 to 40 mg of methimazole given once daily. Thyroid function tests should be obtained after 4 to 6 weeks and the dosage reduced as necessary to maintain euthyroidism. An effective single daily dose regimen of methimazole should increase patient acceptance and adherence.

REMISSION RATES WITH THIOAMIDES

CASE 52-17

QUESTION 1: B.D., a 30-year-old woman, has been maintained on methimazole 5 mg daily for more than 2 years. Her methimazole has been discontinued twice in the past, and each time her hyperthyroidism recurred. She refuses either surgery or RAI therapy. Although she is clinically euthyroid on methimazole, her gland is larger than her usual size and has never decreased with therapy. Recent laboratory tests showed an FT_4 of 1 ng/dL and a TSH level of 6.5 microunits/mL. What is responsible for the enlarging gland? What subjective or objective data in B.D. would influence her remission rate and justify a longer course of thioamide therapy? Would the addition of T_4 be helpful?

The high TSH level suggests that TSH stimulation caused by excessive suppression of hormone synthesis by methimazole is contributing to the enlarging thyroid gland. The easiest solution to this problem is to decrease the maintenance dose of methimazole to 2.5 mg daily to normalize the TSH value and minimize gland stimulation.

Long-term remission rates achieved with the thioamides are disappointing. Remission rates within 6 years after discontinuing therapy average 50% (range, 14%–75%),[184,185,201–203] although relapse rates are as high as 80%. The rate of permanent remission is usually less than 25% if the follow-up period is long enough.[184,185,214] Why some patients remain in remission while others relapse once thioamides are discontinued is unclear, although patients who remain euthyroid for longer than 10 to 15 years after discontinuing therapy probably do so because of disease progression to Hashimoto's thyroiditis rather than as a direct result of treatment.[169] In other words, the natural course of Graves hyperthyroidism might be eventual hypothyroidism regardless of the treatment modality used. Several factors have a limited role in predicting relapse and remission and have been used to guide therapy.

A longer duration of thioamide treatment (see Case 52-15, Question 7) improves the remission rate by changing the basic underlying abnormality of Graves disease.[184,201–203] Numerous studies show that titers of antithyroid receptor (TSI) and antimicrosomal antibodies fall during therapy with the thioamides but are unchanged during therapy with placebo or β-blockers.[184,185,202,215] Patients with low or undetectable TSI titers at the end of 12 to 24 months of thioamide therapy had a 45% chance of remission compared with a less than 10% chance of remission for those with higher titers within 1 to 5 years after completing therapy.[214–217] The best response was obtained in those with smaller goiters, those with less severe disease, and nonsmokers. A higher thioamide dose did not improve the remission rate but resulted in more toxicity, including agranulocytosis, arthralgias, dermatitis, gastritis, and hepatotoxicity.[184,201,214]

Certain clinical features have been associated with a greater chance of disease remission and might help clinicians identify patients who deserve a longer thioamide trial before changing to RAI or surgery. These clinical features include smaller goiter, mild symptoms of short duration, a reduction in goiter size during treatment, nonsmokers, absence of ophthalmopathy, and undetectable or low TSI levels.[185,214,215] Smokers should be advised to discontinue smoking to increase the chance of remission (see Chapter 88, Tobacco Use and Dependence).[218]

In a preliminary study, the addition of L-thyroxine to maintenance doses of thioamides for 1 year, followed by an additional year of L-thyroxine alone, significantly reduced the risk of relapse after thioamides were discontinued.[217] Those receiving the T_4-methimazole combination experienced significant reductions in TSH receptor antibody titers compared with those receiving methimazole alone. At 3 years, the combination-treated patients had a lower rate of recurrence (1.7%) than those receiving methimazole alone (recurrence rate, 34.7%) after all therapy was discontinued. Unfortunately, several prospective studies evaluating the addition of T_4 to thioamides have not validated these initial favorable results.[214,216,219,220] Support for this therapeutic approach has waned, and the addition of T_4 to existing thioamide therapy is not recommended.

B.D.'s large goiter reduces her chance of remission with longer therapy. Although thioamide therapy can be continued indefinitely if well tolerated, surgery or RAI therapy should seriously be considered for B.D., who already has received methimazole for more than 2 years. Alternative therapy is especially crucial if she plans to become pregnant within the next few years (see Case 52-19).

Subclinical Hyperthyroidism

CASE 52-18

QUESTION 1: J.C. is a 68-year-old man who is found to have a TSH level of 0.25 microunits/mL with normal FT_4 and FT_3 levels on routine blood tests. He is otherwise healthy and denies any symptoms of thyroid dysfunction. On physical examination, his thyroid gland is normal. He denies any family history of thyroid disease and is taking no medications. How should these tests be interpreted? How should J.C. be managed?

J.C.'s laboratory values of a suppressed TSH value below the limits of normal with normal free thyroid hormone levels are consistent with subclinical hyperthyroidism (SHyper)[91–93] Other causes of a suppressed TSH value that are unlikely in J.C. include medications (e.g., metformin, bexarotene, glucocorticoids) (Table 52-1), pituitary hypothyroidism, and nonthyroidal illness (see Case 52-1, Questions 1 and 2).[36,38] A suppressed TSH may also be a normal finding in healthy elderly patients.

The dangers of SHyper are similar to those of overt hyperthyroidism, and include cardiac findings (e.g., atrial and ventricular premature beats, AF, left ventricular hypertrophy, diastolic dysfunction), loss of bone mass, higher fracture rates, especially in postmenopausal women, and, if present, subtle symptoms of hyperthyroidism.[89–93] In elderly patients, hyperthyroid symptoms, even if overtly hyperthyroid, may be apathetic or not be apparent owing to impaired sympathetic nervous system responsiveness. A significant relationship between AF and degree of SHyper is clear, whereas an association with increased atherosclerotic heart disease or mortality is weak.[163] The relative risk of AF in SHyper may be as high as 5.2 and increased by older age, male sex, higher FT_4 levels, and degree of TSH suppression. In two cohorts followed for 10 to 13 years, the relative risk of AF ranged from 1.6 to 3.1, depending on the degree of TSH suppression.[163,221]

The management of SHyper is controversial, especially in asymptomatic patients, because data evaluating treatment outcomes are limited.[91–93] A study of 2,024 patients with a 7-year follow-up of SHyper importantly found that less than 1% progressed to overt hyperthyroidism, whereas 36% reverted back to normal within 7 years, especially those with TSH levels between 0.1 and 0.4 microunits/mL.[222] An expert panel concluded that treatment of SHyper (TSH levels <0.1 microunits/mL) should be considered in elderly patients and in those with cardiac disease and osteoporosis.[91,92] For patients with TSH levels of 0.1 to 0.45 microunits/mL, the evidence was insufficient to recommend therapy. A recent review recommends RAI or thioamide therapy only if the TSH level is less than 0.1 microunits/mL in postmenopausal women, in those 60 years or older, and in patients with a history of heart disease, osteoporosis, or hyperthyroid symptoms.[93] For patients with TSH levels of 0.1 to 0.4 microunits/mL, treatment can be considered if they are in the aforementioned groups; otherwise, therapy is not recommended because TSH normalization may occur.

In J.C., his thyroid function tests should be repeated. An RAIU and scan should be obtained to detect any hyperactive areas or nodules that might be responsible for the suppressed TSH. Because J.C. is generally healthy, treatment can be considered if there are concerns about cardiac disease or bone loss; otherwise, no therapy is also reasonable based on the available evidence. Close monitoring of thyroid function tests is recommended every 6 months to a year. If hyperthyroid symptoms or changes in cardiac or bone function occur, then RAI therapy is recommended.

IN PREGNANCY

CASE 52-19

QUESTION 1: N.N., a 32-year-old woman who is 3 months pregnant, is referred for management of her Graves disease. What are the therapeutic ramifications of managing thyrotoxicosis during pregnancy?

Hyperthyroidism develops in 0.02% to 1.4% of pregnant women and often precedes conception.[223] Symptoms of thyrotoxicosis are typically ameliorated during the second and third trimesters and exacerbated early in the postpartum period. Treatment is crucial to prevent damage to the fetus and to maintain the pregnancy. RAI, chronic iodide therapy, and iodine-containing compounds are contraindicated during pregnancy because they will cross the placenta to produce fetal goiter and athyreosis.[223–225] As little as 12 mg/day of iodide has produced neonatal goiter and death. The long-term use of β-adrenergic blockers should also be avoided because it is associated with fetal respiratory depression, a small placenta, intrauterine growth retardation, impaired response to anoxia, and postnatal bradycardia and hypoglycemia.[223,224] However, if rapid control of hyperthyroidism is required, short-term use (<1–4 weeks) of propranolol is safe.[109,112,223–225] Iodide use in pregnancy should be limited to transient preoperative use before thyroidectomy or in the management of thyroid storm.[112,226]

Either surgery or thioamide is the treatment of choice for hyperthyroidism in the pregnant patient. Surgery is safe during the second trimester with adequate preoperative glycosaminoglycans), and water in all retrobulbar tissue. Ocular symptoms include edema, chemosis, excessive lacrimation, photophobia, corneal protrusion (proptosis), scarring, ulceration, extraocular muscle paralysis with loss of eye movements, and blindness from retinal and optic nerve damage.

The eye involvement can occur at any time and is usually bilateral. The ocular symptoms usually subside or remain stable once the patient is euthyroid; however, some cases will progress during the euthyroid period or after RAI treatment of the hyperthyroidism (see Case 52-22, Question 2). Pioglitazone has been associated with a 1- to 2-mm increase in eye protrusion by stimulating adipogenesis and increasing retrobulbar fat production.[247] Although eye changes were more common in people with a history of thyroid disorders, the overall incidence of eye changes associated with pioglitazone is unknown.[247]

MANAGEMENT OF EYE SYMPTOMS

CASE 52-22, QUESTION 2: Was previous treatment of H.R.'s hyperthyroidism appropriate? How should his current ocular symptoms be managed?

The optimal treatment of hyperthyroidism and its effect on the course of ophthalmopathy remain controversial.[243,244,248] Thioamides might improve eye symptoms through an immunosuppressive mechanism of action and control of the hyperthyroidism or exert a neutral effect.[243] Many clinicians believe that gland ablation with RAI or surgical removal is preferable because it removes the antigen source and prevents progression of the ophthalmopathy.[186,243] However, several studies have confirmed development or worsening of eye symptoms immediately after RAI therapy.[246,248] One randomized study demonstrated that the concomitant use of 0.4 to 0.5 mg/kg of prednisone begun 2 to 3 days after RAI and continued for a total of 3 months after RAI therapy in those with any degree of ocular involvement was well tolerated and prevented further deterioration of eye symptoms.[246,248] Regardless of the treatment used, control of the hyperthyroidism often improves most eye findings, except for proptosis.

In H.R., prednisone 40 to 60 mg/day should have been started after his RAI treatment and continued for 2 to 3 months until the eye symptoms improved. Because the pathophysiology of the ophthalmopathy is unclear, treatment is limited to symptomatic and empiric measures once the patient is euthyroid.[243,244] H.R. should also be encouraged to stop smoking to prevent progression of the ophthalmopathy.[218] His pioglitazone should be discontinued, in case this is contributing to his ophthalmopathy.

Periorbital edema and chemosis are worse in the morning after being in the horizontal position; elevating the head of the bed, taking diuretics, and restricting salt intake may be helpful. Protective glasses can relieve photophobia and external irritation. Topical corticosteroid drops are effective in decreasing local irritation, but they should be used cautiously because they increase the risk of infection. Ocular irritants such as smoke and dust should be avoided. Bothersome symptoms (e.g., dry eye, redness, tearing) caused by eyelid retraction can be ameliorated with artificial tears and lubricants.[243] Incomplete lid closure predisposes the patient to corneal scarring and ulceration, so lubricant eye drops should be applied several times daily and at night to keep the bulbs moist. Taping the eyelids shut at night helps prevent drying and scarring. Lateral surgical closure of the lids (tarsorrhaphy) may be required to improve lid closure.

When the ophthalmopathy is severe and progressive, an aggressive approach is necessary. Systemic corticosteroids can produce either dramatic or marginal results in the emergency treatment of progressive exophthalmos associated with decreasing visual acuity. Prednisone at dosages of 35 to 80 mg/day is often effective, although dosages as high as 100 to 140 mg/day may be necessary.[243,244] Pain, irritation, tearing, and other subjective complaints often respond within 24 hours of administration. Therapy for about 3 months is necessary to improve eye muscle and optic nerve function disturbances. Initial large doses should be tapered rapidly once the desired response is obtained to minimize adverse effects. Subconjunctival and retrobulbar injections of steroids are not as effective.

X-ray therapy to the orbit also relieves congestive and inflammatory symptoms.[243] The combination of orbital irradiation and systemic steroids may be required to achieve maximal benefits. Plasmapheresis and immunosuppressive agents, such as cyclophosphamide, azathioprine, cyclosporine, and methotrexate, have also been used with limited success in combination with steroids. Future investigations are focusing on antitumor necrosis factor and anti-interleukin receptor antibody agents that may neutralize some of the inflammatory reactions in the eye.[243,245]

When the previous measures and thyroid ablation fail to arrest the progression of visual loss and exophthalmos, then surgical orbital decompression should be considered.

Thyroid Storm

CLINICAL PRESENTATION

CASE 52-23

QUESTION 1: H.L., a 48-year-old woman, is admitted to the hospital with a 3-week history of fatigue, weakness, dyspnea on exertion, SOB, palpitations, and inability to keep food and liquids down. One year before admission, she began noticing a preference for cold weather and an increase in nervousness and emotional lability. After her husband died a few days ago, she experienced increased nausea and vomiting, irritability, insomnia, tremor, and a 104°F fever, which she attributed to an upper respiratory tract infection. She denies taking any current medications. Her laboratory data obtained on admission included an FT_4 of 4.65 ng/dL and an undetectable TSH level. Assess H.L.'s subjective and objective data.

The presentation is consistent with thyroid storm, a life-threatening medical emergency that might have been precipitated by the stress associated with the death of her husband. The clinical manifestations of thyroid storm[198] include the acute onset of high fever, tachycardia, and tachypnea, and involvement of the following organ systems: cardiovascular (tachycardia, pulmonary edema, hypertension, shock), CNS (tremor, emotional lability, confusion, psychosis, apathy, stupor, coma), and GI (diarrhea, abdominal pain, nausea and vomiting, liver enlargement, jaundice, nonspecific elevations of bilirubin and prothrombin time). Hyperglycemia is also a common clinical finding in thyroid storm.

Thyroid storm develops in about 2% to 8% of hyperthyroid patients. The pathogenesis of thyroid storm is not well understood, but the condition can be described as an exaggerated or decompensated form of thyrotoxicosis. The term *decompensated* implies failure of body systems to adequately resist the effects of thyrotoxicosis. It is not attributed solely to the release of massive quantities of hormones, which can occur after surgery or RAI therapy. Catecholamines also play an important role; the increased quantities of thyroid hormone in conjunction with increased sympathetic and adrenal output contribute to many of the manifestations of thyroid storm. Although thyroid hormones exert an independent effect, many of the symptoms of hyperthyroidism are ameliorated by catecholamine-blocking agents such as β-blockers and calcium-channel blockers (e.g., diltiazem, verapamil).

TREATMENT

CASE 52-23, QUESTION 2: What treatment plan (including route of administration) should be initiated promptly in H.L.?

Intensive, continuous, and immediate treatment can decrease the mortality of thyroid storm significantly. Mortality rates in thyroid storm are high, ranging between 20% and 30%.[198] Treatment of thyroid storm should be directed against four major areas discussed in the following sections.[198]

DECREASE IN SYNTHESIS AND RELEASE OF HORMONES

High dosages of thioamides, preferably PTU 800 to 1,200 mg/day or methimazole 60 to 100 mg/day, should be given orally in four divided doses. If H.L. cannot take oral doses, a rectal formulation of PTU (better bioavailability with enema than suppository) or methimazole, which is as effective as the oral route, can be administered.[180–182] No commercial parenteral preparation is available for either drug, limiting their use by the IV route. PTU is the thioamide of choice because it acts more rapidly than methimazole by blocking the peripheral conversion of T_4 to T_3, a dominant source of the hormone.

Iodides, which rapidly block further release of intraglandular stores of T_4, should be given at least 1 hour after thioamide administration. Given in this way, the substrate for hormone synthesis is not increased, and the therapeutic effect of thioamide is not blocked. The addition of iodides (e.g., Lugol iodine solution 15 to 30 drops/day orally in divided doses) to the thioamides often ameliorates symptoms within 1 day.

Cholestyramine 4 g PO QID may assist in lowering hormone levels rapidly but should be administered apart from other agents to prevent inhibiting their absorption.[249] Other effective modalities include plasmapheresis, charcoal hemoperfusion, and plasma exchange.

REVERSAL OF THE PERIPHERAL EFFECTS OF HORMONES AND CATECHOLAMINES

β-Adrenergic blocking drugs are the preferred agents to decrease the tachycardia, agitation, tremulousness, and other symptoms of excessive adrenergic stimulation seen in thyroid storm. Propranolol is the β-blocker of choice because its clinical efficacy in storm is well documented and because it inhibits the peripheral conversion of T_4 to T_3.[11,198] If rapid effects are necessary, propranolol 1 mg by slow IV push can be given every 5 minutes to lower the heart rate to approximately 90 beats/minute. A 5- to 10-mg/hour IV infusion can maintain the desired heart rate. IV esmolol 50 to 100 mcg/kg/minute can also be given. If perfusion is maintained, oral β-blockers (e.g., propranolol, 40 mg every 6 hours; atenolol, 50–100 mg BID; metoprolol, 50–100 mg daily; nadolol, 40–80 mg daily), titrated to response, can also be given.

SUPPORTIVE TREATMENT OF VITAL FUNCTIONS

This may include sedation, oxygen, IV glucose, vitamins, treatment of infections with antibiotics, digitalization to maintain the cardiac status, rehydration, and treatment of hyperpyrexia with cooling blankets, sponge baths, and the judicious use of antipyretics. Because hypoadrenalism is often suspected, hydrocortisone 100 to 200 mg should empirically be given IV every 6 hours. Because pharmacologic doses of steroids acutely depress serum T_3 levels, a beneficial effect in storm, their routine use is recommended.

ELIMINATION OF PRECIPITATING CAUSES OF STORM

Factors associated with the induction of thyroid storm include infection (most common), trauma, inadequate preparation before thyroidectomy, surgical operations, stress, diabetic ketoacidosis, pregnancy, emboli, discontinuation or withdrawal of antithyroid medications, drug therapy, and RAI therapy.[198]

DRUG-INDUCED THYROID DISEASE

Lithium and Antidepressants

CASE 52-24

QUESTION 1: D.A., a 56-year-old man, complains of sluggishness, cold intolerance, fatigue, and a "rundown" feeling, which doctors attribute to the depressive phase of his bipolar affective illness. He previously had been well controlled with sertraline 100 mg/day, but lithium carbonate 900 mg/day was added 4 months ago because of unreasonable mirthfulness and uncontrollable gift-buying tendencies. Physical examination reveals a puffy face and a large goiter. What is a reasonable assessment of these subjective and objective data?

Thyroid function tests (i.e., TSH, FT_4) and a thyroid ultrasound should be obtained in D.A. to evaluate the possibility of lithium- and possibly sertraline-induced hypothyroidism and goiter.[52–54,250] If the TSH is elevated, T_4 should be initiated and lithium continued if necessary. Although the incidence of goiter and hypothyroidism in the manic-depressive population is unknown, the 10% incidence of baseline elevated TSH appears higher than in the general population.

The antithyroid effects of lithium were noted first in manic-depressive patients. The exact mechanism of lithium's antithyroid effect on the gland is unclear, although it is highly concentrated by the gland. Similar to the iodides, chronic lithium therapy inhibits the release of thyroid hormone from the gland. The fall in serum T_4 and T_3 hormone levels leads to a compensatory and transient increase in serum TSH levels until a new steady state is achieved.[52–54]

The incidence of SH (i.e., increased TSH level) occurs in approximately 19% of patients on chronic lithium therapy.[54] Typically, the serum thyroid hormone levels decrease and the TSH levels increase during the first few months of treatment, returning to pretreatment levels after 1 year. In one study, TSH levels increased within 10 days after starting therapy. Normalization of the TSH level is less likely to occur in patients with pre-existing positive thyroid antibodies before lithium therapy. Induction of thyroid antibodies and increases in baseline antibody titers also occur after chronic lithium therapy. Because abnormal thyroid function tests can be transient, a longer period of observation is justified before starting thyroid hormone therapy in patients with SH.

Overt hypothyroidism appears in a small percentage of the population after 5 months to 2 years of therapy; one 15-year study found an incidence of 1.5% but an 8.4 relative risk in women with antibody positivity compared with negative subjects.[52–54] Lithium-induced goiter with or without hypothyroidism is common after weeks to months of therapy. Although incidences of less than 6% have been reported, higher rates of 40 to 60% are observed if the goiter is diagnosed using more specific imaging techniques (e.g., ultrasound).[52–54] A direct goitrogenic effect of lithium on inducing cell proliferation might explain the occurrence of euthyroid goiter. The goiters respond to discontinuation of lithium or to suppression with thyroid hormone despite continuation of lithium therapy. Surgical removal of the goiter is required if there are local obstructive symptoms. In D.A.'s case, sertraline could be exerting an additive or synergistic antithyroid effect with lithium because antithyroid effects have also been associated with this drug.[250]

Most patients with lithium-induced thyroid abnormalities are women older than 50 years and those who have a prior history of compromised thyroid function (e.g., Hashimoto's thyroiditis), positive thyroid antibodies before lithium therapy, or a strong family history of thyroid disease.[52–54] Therefore, baseline thyroid function tests (i.e., FT_4, TSH), antibodies, and thyroid ultrasound should be obtained before starting lithium therapy, and levels should be checked annually thereafter or more frequently if clinically indicated. Patients should also be questioned about a positive history or family history for thyroid disease and the concurrent use of other, potentially goitrogenic medications (e.g., tricyclic antidepressants, iodides, iodinated expectorants or herbals).

CASE 52-25

QUESTION 1: A.B., a 66-year-old, otherwise healthy man, is admitted for evaluation of new-onset AF. His only other medical problem is a history of bipolar affective disorder treated with lithium for 1 year. However, A.B. discontinued the lithium 1 month before hospitalization without the knowledge of his physician. His laboratory studies are within normal limits except for a TT_3 of 380 ng/dL. What is the potential cause of A.B.'s AF?

AF may be the only manifestation of thyrotoxicosis in older patients.[221,251] Thyrotoxicosis is reported after lithium withdrawal, and A.B.'s AF most likely is the result of excessive thyroid hormone activity. Lithium's antithyroid action is substantial and is comparable to that of the thioamides; T_4 levels decline by 20% to 35%. Therefore, A.B.'s underlying hyperthyroidism has probably been unmasked by his discontinuation of the lithium. Rarely, lithium-induced thyrotoxicosis occurs.[52,54]

Although lithium is not considered the standard of care for hyperthyroidism, it is recommended as an adjunct to RAI therapy in patients allergic to conventional treatment modalities because it does not interfere with RAI uptake. Furthermore, lithium can increase ^{131}I retention by decreasing its rate of elimination from the gland. The increased thyroidal half-life of ^{131}I by lithium is beneficial in localizing the dose of radiation to the gland and producing faster control of the hyperthyroidism.[57]

Because clinical experience with lithium in the treatment of thyrotoxicosis is limited and because it has such a narrow therapeutic index, its use should be restricted to situations when rapid suppression of thyroid hormone secretion is needed, and when thioamides and iodides are contraindicated.

Iodides and Amiodarone

CASE 52-26

QUESTION 1: C.Y., a 54-year-old man with chronic AF, presents with a 6-month history of weakness, fatigue, tremor, heat intolerance, and increased palpitations, previously controlled for the last 2 years on amiodarone 200 mg/day. Physical examination reveals a 50-g multinodular gland, which C.Y. says has "been there forever." He denies any family history of thyroid disease or ingestion of any thyroid medication. His current complaints began after a magnetic resonance imaging procedure with iodinated radiocontrast media. What might be responsible for C.Y.'s hyperthyroid symptoms?

The iodine load from the magnetic resonance imaging procedure or the amiodarone could be responsible for C.Y.'s hyperthyroid symptoms.[18–20,56,68,179] Iodide-induced hyperthyroidism, known as the Jod-Basedow phenomenon, was first described in the 1800s when patients residing in iodide-deficient areas became toxic when given adequate iodide supplementation. Other reports have appeared since then. Both T_3 toxicosis and classic T_4 toxicosis have occurred after iodide ingestion or injection of roentgenographic contrast media.

Although it is presumed that both iodide deficiency and a multinodular goiter, as in C.Y., are required to invoke the Jod-Basedow phenomenon, iodide-induced disease has been reported in patients residing in iodide-sufficient areas, as well as in euthyroid patients with normal glands and no apparent risk factors (e.g., family history).[56,179]

Amiodarone can cause hypothyroidism or hyperthyroidism in susceptible patients because of its high iodine content.[18–20,40,56,68,179] Twelve milligrams (37%) of free iodine is released per 400-mg dose of amiodarone. Patients with multinodular goiters who lose the ability to turn off organification of iodide with increasing iodide loads (Wolff-Chaikoff effect) are most likely to have iodide-induced thyrotoxicosis. Conversely, patients with positive antibodies or with underlying Hashimoto's thyroiditis who cannot escape from the Wolff-Chaikoff block are most likely to have hypothyroidism.

Amiodarone-induced hypothyroidism may occur at any time during therapy and does not appear to be related to the cumulative dose. A normal FT_4 and a persistently elevated TSH (see Case 52-4) are consistent with amiodarone-induced hypothyroidism, which occurs in 6% to 10% of long-term users. The hypothyroidism responds readily to T_4 therapy, and the amiodarone can often be continued.[18,20,68] Hypothyroidism secondary to amiodarone typically resolves with discontinuation of the drug, but resolution may be delayed owing to amiodarone's long half-life.

In contrast, the development of amiodarone-induced thyrotoxicosis occurs early and suddenly during therapy, so that routine monitoring of thyroid function tests is often not useful. Elevated hormone levels, an undetectable TSH level, and clinical symptoms consistent with hyperthyroidism are the best indicators of amiodarone-induced thyrotoxicosis, which occurs in 1% to 5% of long-term users. Worsening of tachyarrhythmias may be the first clinical clue to amiodarone-induced thyrotoxicosis.

Amiodarone-induced hyperthyroidism can be classified as either type I or type II.[3,18,19,68] Type I occurs in patients with underlying risk factors for thyroid disease (e.g., multinodular goiter) and is related to the iodine load. The formation of large amounts of preformed hormone from the massive iodine load produces a protracted course of hyperthyroidism, which is challenging to manage. Type II amiodarone-induced hyperthyroidism is the result of a destructive thyroiditis, with excessive release of thyroid hormone into the systemic circulation. This occurs most often in patients with normal thyroid glands. Unique laboratory findings include a low RAIU and elevated interleukin 6 levels.

The management of amiodarone-induced thyrotoxicosis is complicated because it is not always possible to identify the type of hyperthyroidism and a mixture of the two types can occur. Stopping amiodarone alone does not immediately improve the hyperthyroidism because of the drug's long half-life (22–55 days) and its sequestration in fat. RAI ablation is never appropriate because the high iodine load from amiodarone will suppress RAI uptake. The combination of methimazole and potassium perchlorate is the treatment of choice for type I hyperthyroidism.[18–20,56,68,179] The addition of corticosteroids to block T_4 to T_3 conversion is less effective because of the already potent inhibitory effects of amiodarone on T_4 to T_3 conversion. However, in patients with type II hyperthyroidism, agents that block T_4 to T_3 conversion (e.g., β-blockers, corticosteroids, and iodinated contrast media if available), rather than the aforementioned agents, are the most appropriate choices.[18,20,56,68,252] A total thyroidectomy can rapidly control the thyrotoxicosis, permitting continued therapy with amiodarone if necessary. Despite underlying cardiac disease in these patients, uneventful surgery and a low complication rate have been observed if patients are treated before surgery with a short course of an oral cholecystographic agent.[252] Changing amiodarone to dronedarone, which is devoid of iodine and lacks the undesirable thyroid effects, should be strongly considered in C.Y.

Large doses of iodides should be avoided in patients with nontoxic multinodular goiters who are predisposed to thyrotoxicosis (see Case 52-4 and Case 52-15, Question 2).

Interferon-α

CASE 52-27

QUESTION 1: P.R., a 56-year-old woman, complains of hoarseness, fatigue, "slow movement," and forgetfulness. She is troubled by these new symptoms, which have worsened during the past few weeks. Her medical history includes persistent hepatitis C, which is responding to the combination of pegylated interferon-α injections and ribavirin. Her mother had a history of Graves disease treated with RAI ablation. Her medications include the hepatitis C virus therapy and an over-the-counter kelp supplement to treat fibrocystic breast disease. On examination, facial edema, coarse skin, an enlarged thyroid gland without nodules, and delayed DTRs are noted. Thyroid function tests, including thyroid antibodies, are pending. What might be responsible for her new complaints?

Although the medications that P.R. is taking for hepatitis C virus could be responsible for her complaints of fatigue and forgetfulness as well as her skin changes, her signs and symptoms are consistent with hypothyroidism. A detailed history of any other dietary and herbal supplements, especially those containing thyroid or iodine, should be obtained. The iodine in kelp tablets could cause thyroid illness in susceptible patients (see Case 52-15, Question 2, and Case 52-26).

Another likely cause of hypothyroidism could be the pegylated interferon-α injections that she has been receiving for hepatitis C treatment.[48–50,253] The prevalence of thyroid abnormalities observed with interferon-α ranges from 15% to 46%. De novo development or aggravation of pre-existing antithyroid antibodies is the most common abnormal finding. The presence of pre-existing antithyroid antibodies (seropositivity) before interferon-α therapy or its persistence at the end of therapy is a significant risk factor for the development of overt thyroid dysfunction. Other risk factors include female sex, older patients, and Asian ethnicity.[49] The incidence of thyroid dysfunction was 46% in a seropositive group compared with 5.4% in the seronegative group.[49] Likewise, in a group of 114 patients with no pre-existing thyroid disease, those who were seropositive at the end of therapy had the highest risk of exhibiting SH 6.2 years later (odds ratio of 38.7).[50]

Hypothyroidism, from Hashimoto's thyroiditis or a nonautoimmune basis, is more common (40%–50% of patients) than hyperthyroidism (10%–30%). Two types of hyperthyroidism can occur: an autoimmune Graves-like disorder with positive antibodies and a hyperthyroid thyroiditis, similar to the type II amiodarone hyperthyroidism (see Case 52-26 Question 1), caused by a direct toxic effect of interferon on the thyroid. Approximately 20% of patients with thyroiditis will first have transient symptoms of hyperthyroidism followed by hypothyroidism (biphasic thyroiditis).[51]

In patients with positive thyroid antibodies, reversal of thyroid dysfunction is less likely. However, thyroid dysfunction appears transient in most patients without positive antibodies, and treatment is not always necessary. L-Thyroxine is required only if hypothyroid symptoms are bothersome; otherwise, therapy can be withheld because symptoms often resolve spontaneously within 2 to 3 months after stopping therapy. If T_4 is begun, it should be stopped after 6 months to re-evaluate the need for continued thyroid replacement. Similarly, transient hyperthyroid laboratory indices do not require therapy with β-blockers unless the patient is symptomatic or laboratory values are dangerously elevated. Rarely, thyroid dysfunction is permanent, but it may take up to 17 months after stopping therapy for symptoms to resolve.

P.R. should be advised to stop taking the kelp supplement and to avoid other iodide-containing herbal or dietary supplements. Once laboratory values confirm hypothyroidism, T_4 should be started concurrently with the interferon-α because of the severity of her symptoms. Once interferon therapy is completed, L-thyroxine should be tapered off to evaluate the need for continued replacement. The presence of thyroid antibodies may increase the risk of permanent hypothyroidism.

Iodide Prophylaxis for Radiation Emergencies

CASE 52-28

QUESTION 1: J.M. is a healthy, 43-year-old Japanese woman who lives with her two young children 50 miles from a nuclear reactor damaged by an earthquake and tsunami. J.M. is concerned about the risks of radiation exposure and would like to protect herself and her children. What prophylaxis and benefits, if any, might be indicated for J.M. in case of a nuclear accident?

The most accurate data for irradiation-induced thyroid abnormalities come from the 1986 Chernobyl incident, in which massive amounts of RAI were released into the environment, contaminating air, food, and water supplies. Significant increases in thyroid cancer were found, primarily in children, who received at least 5 cGy ^{131}I exposures.[254]

The thyroid can be protected against radiation-induced thyroid cancer if potassium iodide (KI) is taken immediately before, coincident with, or possibly 3 to 4 hours after the radiation exposure.[255] Administration of KI 130 mg in adults and 65 mg in school-age children lasts approximately 24 hours and should be continued until the risk of exposure is over. Adolescents close to 70 kg should receive the full 130-mg dose; neonates should receive 16 mg. Repeat dosing is not recommended in pregnant women, neonates, or during lactation unless there is ongoing contamination because the risks of repeated KI administration (e.g., neonatal and fetal hypothyroidism) outweigh their protective benefits. In the aforementioned conditions, when repeated doses of KI are not advisable, and in those intolerant of KI, protective measures (e.g., sheltering, evacuation, control of the food supply) should be implemented. Hypothyroidism can be managed with T_4 supplementation. If repeat dosing is necessary during continued contamination, close monitoring for toxicity is recommended. Short-term administration of KI is safer in children than in adults.

Adverse effects include sialadenitis, GI disturbances, rash, and other allergic reactions, which are increased in patients with dermatitis herpetiformis and hypocomplementemic vasculitides. Hyperthyroidism, goiter, and hypothyroidism can occur, especially in adults with underlying thyroid disorders (see Case 52-26). The decision to treat J.M. and her children prophylactically would be based on the extent of radiation leaked into the environment and the amount of time elapsed since the exposure.

NODULES

"Hot" Nodule

CASE 52-29

QUESTION 1: N.S., a 20-year-old woman, noticed a "lump" in the right side of her neck. There is no history of irradiation and no family history of thyroid disease. She has no local symptoms and no symptoms suggestive of hypothyroidism or hyperthyroidism. The right lobe of the thyroid is occupied by a 3 × 3-cm firm, immovable nodule; the left lobe is barely palpable. All thyroid function tests are within normal limits. A scan shows a large hot nodule occupying the right lobe and a nonexistent left lobe. How should N.S.'s single hot nodule, or Plummer disease, be managed?

Hot nodule is a term used to describe a hyperfunctioning or iodine-concentrating area of the thyroid as shown on scan; it appears as an area of greater density than the rest of the gland. The hyperfunctioning autonomous nodule typically suppresses activity in the remainder of the gland, but it need not produce clinical or chemical evidence of hyperthyroidism and may remain unchanged for years. Some nodules may develop into toxic goiters, causing overt symptoms of toxicosis. Most hot nodules are benign; malignancies are rarely reported.[256]

Treatment of the hot nodule depends on the existing clinical situation. If it is suppressing the other lobe of the thyroid, is not causing toxic symptoms, and is the only source of thyroid production, the patient should be left alone and monitored closely for signs of toxicity. A toxic hot nodule is best treated surgically or with RAI ablation. Because hot nodules do not spontaneously resolve, antithyroid drugs are not the treatment of choice. Because the normal thyroid tissue is suppressed, RAI is concentrated only by the hot nodule, sparing the suppressed tissue. After treatment, the suppressed tissue should begin functioning again. It would be reasonable to just watch N.S. then, since she has no symptoms, but definitive treatment with RAI can be considered if the situation changes.

"Cold" Nodule

CASE 52-30

QUESTION 1: P.L., a 29-year-old woman, is found to have a left thyroid nodule on routine physical examination. She has no history of neck irradiation, no family history of thyroid disease, and no symptoms suggestive of hypothyroidism or hyperthyroidism. A firm, nontender 1-cm nodule occupies the left lobe of the gland. Thyroid function tests are within normal limits. The scan shows a cold nodule, and the ultrasound reveals a solid mass, ruling out the possibility of a cyst. The results of the FNA are pending. TPA antibodies are negative. What is the significance of a cold nodule, and how should it be managed?

A cold nodule is a hypofunctioning area of the thyroid that fails to collect RAI. It is depicted on the scan as a lighter or less dense area. The differential diagnosis includes Hashimoto's thyroiditis, benign adenomas, cysts, and malignant tumors. The absence of thyroid antibodies and identification of a solid mass on ultrasound rules out the possibility of a cyst or Hashimoto's thyroiditis. Most cold nodules turn out to be benign adenomas rather than cancers. The FNA can help distinguish a benign from a malignant nodule. However, a benign biopsy in a suspicious nodule or in a patient with risk factors for malignancy does not eliminate the possibility of malignancy. In these patients, surgery is recommended. The incidence of malignancy in a cold nodule varies between 10% and 20%.[174] A history of irradiation increases the likelihood of cancer in a nodule, and surgery is recommended in these instances. The nature of the nodule is important. Fixation of the nodule to the strap muscles or the trachea, a hard bulging mass, any pain or tenderness, or voice hoarseness can indicate malignancy.

If P.L.'s nodule is benign, then close follow-up every 6 to 18 months is recommended to detect any growth. If the nodule increases in size, a repeat FNA is recommended to rule out any malignancy. Although T_4-suppressive therapy can be considered, only about 10% to 20% of nodules shrink with therapy.[257,258] Furthermore, L-thyroxine may not actually shrink the nodule itself, but rather the surrounding thyroid tissue, making the nodule appear smaller. Spontaneous resolution of the nodule can also occur. The dangers of excessive L-thyroxine therapy (e.g., osteoporosis, cardiac arrhythmias) exceed the benefits of benign nodule suppression.[90,221] Therefore, watchful waiting, with no therapy, is recommended for P.L.[174]

Multinodular Goiter

CASE 52-31

QUESTION 1: G.D., a 35-year-old woman, is referred for a goiter discovered on routine physical examination. She denies any symptoms of hyperthyroidism or hypothyroidism or any history of irradiation. Her grandmother had hypothyroidism and a goiter. A large "lumpy, bumpy" gland is present, but she has no problems with breathing or swallowing. The FNA shows a benign lesion. The assessment is a nontoxic multinodular goiter. How should this be managed?

Nontoxic multinodular goiter is a common finding, occurring in about 5% of the population.[256] In low-risk patients, longstanding asymptomatic nodules that have not exhibited recent growth are likely to be benign and can be followed or excised surgically for cosmetic reasons. If the patient experiences symptoms (swallowing or respiratory difficulty), surgery is the treatment of choice. Observation with close follow-up is the preferred treatment option for most benign multinodular goiters.

T_4 suppression therapy to decrease TSH stimulation and further gland enlargement can be considered if the patient has no cardiac contraindications. Whether T_4 suppression is effective is controversial; studies have noted both reductions in nodular growth and no changes.[256–258] Some gland shrinkage has been reported 3 to 6 months after the initiation of T_4 0.1 to 0.2 mg/day to suppress the TSH to subnormal levels. However, the dangers of long-term thyroid suppression therapy (e.g., osteoporosis, cardiac toxicity) outweigh any potential benefits.[89–93] Levothyroxine therapy is not recommended for the suppression of benign nodules, especially in iodine-sufficient areas such as the United States.[174] Patients should be carefully monitored for the development of hyperthyroidism. Most multinodular goiters contain autonomously functioning nodules that are independent of TSH control and could produce excessive thyroid hormone secretion spontaneously.[256] Toxic multinodular goiters are optimally treated with RAI therapy.[239] If the nodules enlarge, repeat biopsy or surgery is recommended.

Thyrotropin-α and Thyroid Suppression Therapy for Thyroid Cancer

CASE 52-32

QUESTION 1: L.H., a 28-year-old man, had a total thyroidectomy last year for papillary cancer followed by RAI therapy. He is clinically euthyroid on 200 mcg L-thyroxine daily with a TSH level of less than 0.2 microunits/mL. He is hesitant to discontinue his L-thyroxine so that an RAIU scan and thyroglobulin testing can be done to evaluate for tumor recurrence. His doctor is concerned about his suppressed TSH level and is also worried about taking L.H. off his L-thyroxine because the patient says he "feels incapacitated" while carrying out these tests. What can you tell his physician about the TSH level and the need to stop L-thyroxine during these tests?

In patients with thyroid cancers, total thyroidectomy, followed by RAI and L-thyroxine therapy to suppress the TSH to subnormal levels, was associated with improved overall survival.[259] The actual degree of thyroid suppression required is complex and depends on the severity and extent of the thyroid cancer and the likelihood of a diseasefree prognosis. The benefits of prolonged thyrotropin suppression with L-thyroxine to prevent cancer recurrence need to be balanced against the risks and adverse effects (e.g., osteoporosis, cardiac toxicity) of lifelong T_4 excess. Lifelong TSH suppression less than 0.1 microunits/mL is preferred for patients with high to intermediate risk of recurrent cancer or metastastes.[256] A low-normal TSH of 0.3 to 2 microunits/mL can be considered for diseasefree patients.

Annually, it is important to assess recurrence of the malignancy by determining whether any residual cancerous or normal thyroid tissue remains. This is done by elevating the endogenous TSH levels. A rise in thyroglobulin concentrations or a positive RAIU scan is an indication for additional RAI therapy. If no thyroid tissue is detected, patients are considered free of cancer, and an evaluation is repeated in 1 year. Before recombinant human TSH or thyrotropin alfa (Thyrogen) was available, it was necessary to allow recovery of endogenous TSH secretion by discontinuing T_4 for 4 to 6 weeks. The development of hypothyroidism during this withdrawal period is often distressing. Now, thyrotropin-α is indicated as an adjunctive tool for the follow-up assessment of patients with thyroid cancer.[260]

Thyrotropin-α is intended to improve the quality of life in these patients by allowing these procedures to be undertaken without stopping the T_4. Clinical trials show that thyrotropin-α is comparable to the traditional method of T_4 withdrawal to detect distant metastases but that complete thyroid hormone withdrawal is still superior in identifying recurrent thyroid cancers. Thyrotropin-α failed to detect localized tumor recurrence in 7% of patients compared with 100% detection after hormone withdrawal but detected 100% of patients with metastatic disease.[256,260]

Thyrotropin-α is generally well tolerated. Nausea, headaches, and asthenia are the most common adverse effects noted. Recombinant human TSH is available as a 0.9-mg vial and is administered once daily for 2 days IM. Thyrotropin-α costs approximately $1,118 per two-vial kit and is covered under most health insurance plans. Improved quality of life, avoidance of hypothyroidism, and increased patient productivity may offset the direct costs of thyrotropin-α. However, concerns exist about the efficacy of thyrotropin-α to detect tumor recurrence compared with the current standard of practice, which is withdrawal of T_4 therapy. Further studies are needed to identify its role in care.

L.H. should be maintained on his current L-thyroxine suppression dosage because his TSH level is appropriately suppressed without hyperthyroidism.

KEY REFERENCES AND WEBSITES

A full list of references for this chapter can be found at http://thepoint.lww.com/AT10e. Below are the key references and websites for this chapter, with the corresponding reference number in this chapter found in parentheses after the reference.

Key References

American Thyroid Association (ATA) Guidelines Taskforce on Thyroid Nodules and Differentiated Thyroid Cancer et al. Revised American Thyroid Association management guidelines for patients with thyroid nodules and differentiated thyroid cancer [published correction appears in *Thyroid*. 2010;20:674]. *Thyroid*. 2009;19:1167. (174)

Bach-Huynh TG et al. Timing of levothyroxine administration affects serum thyrotropin concentration. *J Clin Endocrinol Metab*. 2009;94:3905. (128)

Biondi B, Cooper DS. Benefits of thyrotropin suppression versus the risks of adverse effects in differentiated thyroid cancer. *Thyroid*. 2010;20:135. (259)

Biondi B, Cooper DS. The clinical significance of subclinical thyroid dysfunction. *Endocr Rev*. 2008;29:76. (92)

Brent GA. Clinical practice: Graves' disease. *N Engl J Med*. 2008;358:2594. (169)

Cohen-Lehman J et al. Effects of amiodarone therapy on thyroid function. *Nat Rev Endocrinol*. 2010;6:34. (68)

Cooper DS. Antithyroid drugs. *N Engl J Med*. 2005;352:905. (185)

Fitzpatrick DL, Russell MA. Diagnosis and management of thyroid disease in pregnancy. *Obstet Gynecol Clin North Am*. 2010;37:173. (226)

Flynn RW et al. Serum thyroid-stimulating hormone concentration and morbidity from cardiovascular disease and fractures in patients on long-term thyroxine therapy. *J Clin Endocrinol Metab*. 2010;95:186. (99)

Grozinsky-Glasberg S et al. Thyroxine-triiodothyronine combination therapy versus thyroxine monotherapy for clinical hypothyroidism: meta-analysis of randomized controlled trials. *J Clin Endocrinol Metab*. 2006;91:2592. (86)

Haugen BR. Drugs that suppress TSH or cause central hypothyroidism. *Best Pract Res Clin Endocrinol Metab*. 2009;23:793. (10)

Jonklaas J et al. Triiodothyronine levels in athyreotic individuals during levothyroxine therapy. *JAMA*. 2008;299:769. (87)

Ross DS. Radioiodine therapy for hyperthyroidism. *N Engl J Med*. 2011;364:542. (190)

Toft A. Which thyroxine? *Thyroid*. 2005;15:124. (81)

Key Websites

American Thyroid Association. ATA Frequently Asked Questions (FAQS). **http://www.thyroid.org/patients/faqs.html.**

American Thyroid Association. ATA Patient Education Web Brochures. **http://www.thyroid.org/patients/brochures.html.**

American Thyroid Association. The Professional Community. **http://www.thyroid.org/professionals/.**

Graves' Disease Foundation. **http://www.ngdf.org/.**

National Cancer Institute. Thyroid Cancer. **http://www.cancer.gov/cancertopics/types/thyroid.**

ThyCa: Thyroid Cancer Survivors' Association. **http://www.thyca.org/.**

53

Diabetes Mellitus

Lisa A. Kroon and Craig Williams

CORE PRINCIPLES

	CHAPTER CASES
1 A glycosylated hemoglobin (A1C) level can be used to diagnose diabetes, in addition to a fasting plasma glucose or oral glucose tolerance test. Each test must be confirmed on a subsequent day.	**Case 53-2 (Question 1), Case 53-14 (Question 1)**
2 The primary metabolic goals for diabetes are an A1C less than 7%, a systolic blood pressure less than 130 mm Hg, and a low-density lipoprotein cholesterol less than 100 mg/dL. Management of cholesterol should include a statin drug, and management of hypertension should include an angiotensin-converting enzyme inhibitor or angiotensin II receptor blocker.	**Case 53-2 (Question 2), Case 53-14 (Question 2)**
3 Glycemic treatment goals should be individualized. For patients with a short duration of diabetes, long life expectancy, and no significant vascular disease, a goal closer to an A1C of 6% can be considered, if it can be achieved without increasing hypoglycemia. For patients with existing vascular disease, other significant macrovascular or microvascular disease, a history of hypoglycemia, or limited life expectancy, or for those with longstanding diabetes who have difficulty lowering their A1C, a less stringent A1C goal should be considered.	**Case 53-2 (Question 2), Case 53-4 (Question 2), Case 53-14 (Question 2), Case 53-22 (Question 3)**
4 Medical nutrition therapy and physical activity are cornerstones to the treatment of diabetes.	**Case 53-2 (Questions 11, 12), Case 53-6 (Question 1), Case 53-14 (Question 3), Case 53-22 (Question 4)**
5 Self-monitoring of blood glucose should be performed by all patients with type 1 diabetes and most patients with type 2 diabetes, particularly those on antidiabetic therapy that can cause hypoglycemia or those engaged in self-management. The key to self-monitoring of blood glucose is to educate patients on how to respond to their blood glucose levels.	**Case 53-2 (Questions 9–11), Case 53-4 (Question 5), Case 53-14 (Question 6)**
6 Basal-bolus insulin regimens should be used for patients with type 1 diabetes. These can be administered by either multiple daily injections or by an insulin pump. Basal-bolus insulin regimens are also effective for patients with type 2 diabetes who no longer are able to achieve A1C goals with noninsulin therapies.	**Case 53-2 (Questions 3–6), Case 53-4 (Question 3), Case 53-17 (Question 6)**
7 Metformin is the first-line therapy for type 2 diabetes unless a patient has a contraindication to its use or is unable to tolerate this agent. It should be added at diagnosis along with lifestyle changes.	**Case 53-14 (Questions 3–5)**
8 After monotherapy, a second antidiabetic agent should be added to the regimen. Factors to consider include the patient's A1C goal, the amount of reduction in A1C required, the patient's kidney and liver function, medication side effects, and cost of therapy.	**Case 53-14 (Question 7), Case 53-15 (Question 1), Case 53-17 (Questions 2–4)**
9 In type 2 diabetes, insulin therapy should be considered any time the patient's A1C is severely uncontrolled (e.g., A1C >10%) and also when the A1C is more than 8.5% to 9% and a patient is already on combination oral therapy.	**Case 53-14 (Question 7), Case 53-15 (Question 1), Case 53-17 (Question 5)**

continued

	CHAPTER CASES
10 Owing to concerns about the effects of hypoglycemia and new trials indicating a lack of benefit of very tight glucose control in acutely ill patients, the current recommended goal blood glucose in hospitalized patients is 140 to 180 mg/dL.	**Case 53-10 (Question 1)**
11 Although acute hyperglycemic crises can occur in patients with diabetes, most morbidity and mortality occurs over the course of years and can be classified as either microvascular (nephropathy, neuropathy, and retinopathy) or macrovascular (coronary heart disease, stroke, and peripheral vascular disease).	**Case 53-24 (Questions 1–5), Case 53-25 (Questions 1–3)**
12 Patients with established vascular disease should remain on lifelong aspirin therapy, whereas patients without established vascular disease need to be carefully considered to determine the appropriateness of antiplatelet therapy.	**Case 53-24 (Question 6)**
13 The incidence and severity of microvascular complications has a strong correlation with long-term glycemic control as measured by A1C. Macrovascular complications are influenced by glycemic control but are more dependent on multiple etiologic factors including dyslipidemia, hypertension, and smoking.	**Case 53-14 (Question 2)**

An estimated 23.6 million people, or 7.8% of the United States population, currently have diabetes.[1] Of these, 5.7 million or about one-third are undiagnosed. In 2007 alone, more than 1.6 million new cases in adults were diagnosed. Globally, the prevalence of diabetes for all ages is estimated to be 2.8% in 2000 and projected to increase to 4.4% by 2030.[2] The incidence of type 2 diabetes is now epidemic, with alarming increases in prevalence in both adults and children. Estimates by the Centers for Disease Control and Prevention indicate that new cases of diabetes annually will increase from 8 per 1,000 people to about 15 per 1,000 in 2050, with as many as 1 in 3 Americans having diabetes in 2050.[3] The dramatic increase in type 2 diabetes in the population is related to obesity and decreased physical activity levels, and also the fact that people with diabetes are living longer. Additional individual factors include a genetic predisposition for increased insulin resistance and progressive β cell failure. Clinical studies have affirmed that type 2 diabetes can be delayed or prevented in high-risk populations and that good glycemic control and other interventions can slow its devastating complications. Therefore, broad implementation of guidelines and goals established by the American Diabetes Association (ADA) and others, as well as progress in processes of care, which could help to eliminate health disparities, should be national priorities.[4]

Definition, Classification, and Epidemiology

Diabetes is a chronic condition caused by an absolute lack of insulin or relative lack of insulin as a result of impaired insulin secretion and action. Its hallmark clinical characteristics are symptomatic glucose intolerance resulting in hyperglycemia and alterations in lipid and protein metabolism. In the long term, these metabolic abnormalities contribute to the development of complications such as cardiovascular disease (CVD), retinopathy, nephropathy, and neuropathy and a higher risk of cancer.[5,6]

Genetically, etiologically, and clinically, diabetes is a heterogeneous group of disorders. Nevertheless, most cases of diabetes mellitus can be assigned to type 1 or type 2 diabetes (Table 53-1). The term gestational diabetes mellitus (GDM) is used to describe glucose intolerance that has its onset during pregnancy. Glucose intolerance that cannot be ascribed to causes consistent with these three classifications include specific genetic defects in β cell function or insulin action (usually genetically defective insulin receptors); diseases of the exocrine pancreas; endocrinopathies; drug- or chemical-induced; infections; and other genetic syndromes.[7] Early glucose intolerance or prediabetes is identified as impaired fasting glucose (IFG) or impaired glucose tolerance (IGT). The pathophysiology of IFG and IGT are somewhat different, and there is not 100% concordance between them.[8] IFG results predominantly from the failure to suppress hepatic gluconeogenesis caused by insulin resistance, whereas IGT results from inadequate insulin secretion and actions in the postprandial state.

Approximately 5% to 10% of the diagnosed diabetic population has type 1 diabetes, which usually results from autoimmune destruction of the pancreatic β cells.[7] At clinical presentation, these patients have little or no pancreatic reserve, have a tendency to develop ketoacidosis, and require exogenous insulin to sustain life. The incidence of autoimmune-mediated type 1 diabetes peaks during childhood and adolescence, but it can occur at any age. A minority of patients diagnosed with type 1 diabetes, mostly of African or Asian ancestry, can have no evidence of autoimmunity; the etiology is, therefore, unknown. In these individuals, the rate of pancreatic destruction seems to occur more slowly, leading to a later onset and less acute presentation.

Most people with diabetes have type 2 diabetes, a heterogeneous disorder that is characterized by obesity, β cell dysfunction, resistance to insulin action, and increased hepatic glucose production. Both the incidence and prevalence of diabetes increase dramatically with age and obesity. The prevalence of self-reported diagnosed diabetes is 2.6% among persons 20 to 39 years of age and 23.1% among persons age 60 and older.[1] One study estimates that the prevalence of diabetes in persons older than 65 years of age increased 62% from 2003 to 2004.[9] Among adults 65 years of age or older, increased adiposity increases the risk for diabetes more than fourfold.[10] The prevalence of type 2 diabetes also differs among ethnic populations. Relative to non-Hispanic whites (6.6%), the prevalence of diagnosed diabetes is higher in Asian Americans (7.5%), Hispanics (10.4%), African Americans (11.8%), and American Indians and Alaskan Natives (14.2%).[1] Although part of the difference in rates of diabetes in different ethnic populations can be explained by obesity and lifestyle, these factors do not explain the entire difference.[11] Patients of Asian ancestry experience diabetes at lower levels of adiposity, possibly because of less reserve for insulin secretion in the pancreatic β cells.[12] Although the role of genetics continues to be explored,

TABLE 53-1
Type 1 and Type 2 Diabetes

Characteristics	Type 1	Type 2
Other names	Previously, type I; insulin-dependent diabetes mellitus (IDDM); juvenile-onset diabetes mellitus	Previously, type II; non–insulin-dependent diabetes mellitus (NIDDM); adult-onset diabetes mellitus
Percentage of diabetic population	5%–10%	90%
Age at onset	Usually <30 years; peaks at 12–14 years; rare before 6 months; some adults develop type 1 during the fifth decade	Usually >40 years, but increasing prevalence among obese children
Pancreatic function	Usually none, although some residual C-peptide can sometimes be detected at diagnosis, especially in adults	Insulin present in low, "normal," or high amounts
Pathogenesis	Associated with certain HLA types; presence of islet cell antibodies suggests autoimmune process	Defect in insulin secretion; tissue resistance to insulin; ↑ hepatic glucose output
Family history	Generally not strong	Strong
Obesity	Uncommon unless "overinsulinized" with exogenous insulin	Common (60%–90%)
History of ketoacidosis	Often present	Rare, except in circumstances of unusual stress (e.g., infection)
Clinical presentation	Moderate to severe symptoms that generally progress relatively rapidly (days to weeks): polyuria, polydipsia, fatigue, weight loss, ketoacidosis	Mild polyuria, fatigue; often diagnosed on routine physical or dental examination
Treatment	MNT Physical activity Insulin Amylin mimetic (pramlintide)	MNT Physical activity Antidiabetic agents (biguanides, glinides, sulfonylureas, thiazolidinediones, α-glucosidase inhibitors, incretin mimetics/analogs, DPP-4 inhibitors) Insulin Amylin mimetic (pramlintide)

DPP-4, dipeptidyl peptidase-4; HLA, human leukocyte antigen; MNT, medical nutrition therapy.

the metabolic consequences of overweight, sedentary lifestyles can clearly vary greatly among individuals.[13]

Diabetes is a serious condition that places people at risk for greater morbidity and mortality relative to the nondiabetic population. Diabetes is the seventh leading cause of death in the United States, although deaths attributed to diabetes and its complications are likely to be underreported.[1] Compared with the general population, the mortality rate for people with diabetes is about twice that for people without diabetes. In addition, disparities in morbidity and mortality attributed to acute and chronic complications associated with diabetes have been documented in certain groups, such as underrepresented minorities and the uninsured.[14]

Medical management of people with diabetes is costly. In 2007, the total cost of diabetes in the United States was estimated to be $174 billion, with 1 of 5 health care dollars being spent on people with diabetes.[15] The average health care expenditures for people with diabetes were approximately 2.3 times higher than those for individuals without diabetes. The majority (56%) of all health care expenditures attributed to diabetes are used by people age 65 years and older. Hospital inpatient costs, nursing facility resources, home care, physician visits, and medications (not just diabetes agents) made up the majority of these expenditures. Because many expenditures are related to treatment of long-term complications, considerable effort has been directed toward early diagnosis and metabolic control of patients with diabetes.

Carbohydrate Metabolism

An understanding of the signs and symptoms associated with diabetes is based on a knowledge of glucose metabolism and the metabolic effects of insulin in nondiabetic and diabetic subjects during the fed (postprandial) and fasting (postabsorptive) states.[16] Homeostatic mechanisms maintain plasma glucose concentrations between 55 and 140 mg/dL. A minimum concentration of 40 to 60 mg/dL is required to provide adequate fuel for the central nervous system, which uses glucose as its primary energy source and is independent of insulin for glucose utilization. When blood glucose (BG) concentrations exceed the reabsorptive capacity of the proximal tubule in the kidneys (~180 mg/dL), glucose spills into the urine (glucosuria), resulting in a loss of calories and water. Muscle and fat, which use glucose as a major source of energy, require insulin for glucose uptake. If glucose is unavailable, these tissues are able to use other substrates such as amino acids and fatty acids for fuel.

POSTPRANDIAL GLUCOSE AND LIPID METABOLISM IN THE NONDIABETIC INDIVIDUAL

After food is ingested, BG concentrations rise and stimulate insulin release. Insulin is the key to efficient glucose utilization. It promotes the uptake of glucose, fatty acids, and amino acids and their conversion to storage forms in most tissues. Insulin also inhibits hepatic glucose production by suppressing glucagon and its effects. In muscle, insulin promotes the uptake of glucose and its storage as glycogen. It also stimulates the uptake of amino acids and their conversion to protein. In adipose tissue, glucose is converted to free fatty acids and stored as triglycerides. Insulin also prevents a breakdown of these triglycerides to free fatty acids, a form that may be transported to other tissues for utilization. The liver does not require insulin for glucose transport, but insulin facilitates the conversion of glucose to glycogen and free fatty acids.

Free fatty acids are esterified to triglycerides, which are transported by very-low-density lipoproteins (VLDLs) to adipose and muscle tissue. Normal insulin signaling suppresses VLDL secretion by reducing the production of fatty acids in the liver.[17] Once secreted by the liver, VLDL is acted on primarily by hepatic lipase in the liver and by lipoprotein lipase on endothelial cells.[17] Acting through apolipoprotein (apo) CII on the surface of the VLDL particle, these lipases remove free fatty acids from the lipoprotein and convert VLDL to IDL (intermediate-density lipoprotein) and then IDL to LDL (low-density lipoprotein). Insulin plays a role in stimulating apoCII expression, which partly explains the hypertriglyceridemia that occurs in type 2 diabetes.

FASTING GLUCOSE METABOLISM IN THE NONDIABETIC INDIVIDUAL

As BG concentrations drop toward normal during the fasting state, insulin release is inhibited. Simultaneously, a number of counter-regulatory hormones that oppose the effect of insulin and promote an increase in blood sugar are released (e.g., glucagon, epinephrine, growth hormone, cortisol). As a result, several processes maintain a minimum BG concentration for the central nervous system. Glycogen in the liver is broken down into glucose (glycogenolysis). Amino acids are transported from muscle to liver, where they are converted to glucose through gluconeogenesis. Uptake of glucose by insulin-dependent tissues is diminished to conserve glucose for the brain. Finally, triglycerides are broken down into free fatty acids, which are used as alternative fuel sources.

Type 1 Diabetes

PATHOGENESIS

The loss of insulin secretion in type 1 diabetes mellitus results from autoimmune destruction of the insulin-producing β cells in the pancreas, which is thought to be triggered by environmental factors, such as viruses or toxins, in genetically susceptible individuals.[18] This form of diabetes is associated closely with histocompatibility antigens (human leukocyte antigen [HLA]-DR3 or HLA-DR4) and the presence of circulating antibodies, including insulin autoantibodies, glutamic acid decarboxylase autoantibodies (GAD65), islet cell autoantibodies (ICA), and autoantibodies to tyrosine phosphatases (e.g., islet cell antibody 512). The capacity of normal pancreatic β cells to secrete insulin far exceeds the normal amounts needed to control carbohydrate, fat, and protein metabolism. As a result, the clinical onset of type 1 diabetes is preceded by an extensive asymptomatic period during which β cells are destroyed (Fig. 53-1). β cell destruction may occur rapidly, but is more likely to take place over a period of weeks, months, or even years. The earliest detectable abnormality in insulin secretion is a progressive reduction of immediate or first-phase plasma insulin response. However, this initial impairment has few detrimental effects on overall glucose homeostasis, and plasma glucose concentrations remain normal. Most affected individuals have circulating antibodies to islet cells or to their own insulin at this stage of the disease. These represent markers of an ongoing autoimmune process that culminates in type 1 diabetes. Fasting hyperglycemia occurs when the β cell mass is reduced by 80% to 90%. One or more of the above autoantibodies is usually present in 85% to 90% of individuals at this point.[7] Initially, only postprandial hyperglycemia occurs, but as insulin secretion becomes further compromised, progressive fasting hyperglycemia is seen. Within 8 to 10 years of clinical presentation, β cell loss is complete and insulin deficiency is absolute.

CLINICAL PRESENTATION

Although the onset of type 1 diabetes seems to be abrupt, evidence now exists for an extended preclinical period that can precede obvious symptoms by several years. As insulin secretion becomes compromised, progressive fasting hyperglycemia

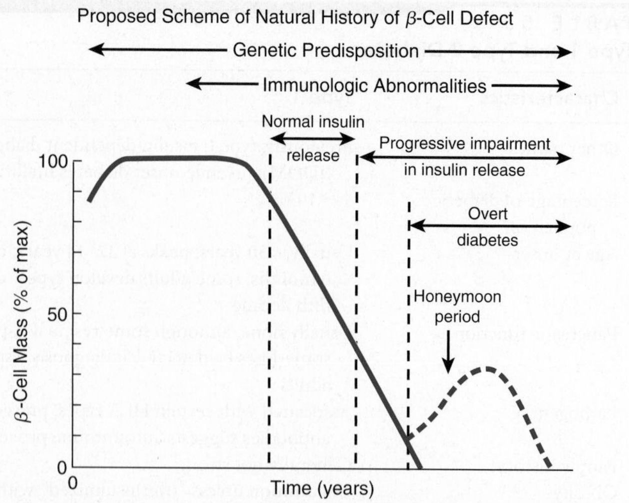

Timing of trigger in relation to immunologic abnormalities is unknown. Note that overt diabetes is not apparent until insulin secretory reserves are <10%–20% of normal.

FIGURE 53-1 Pathogenesis of type 1 diabetes. In an individual with a genetic predisposition, an event (such as a virus or toxin) triggers autoimmune destruction of the pancreatic β cells, probably during a period of several years. When the number of β cells diminishes to approximately 250,000, the pancreas is unable to secrete sufficient insulin and intolerance to glucose ensues. At this point, a stressful event, such as a viral infection, can produce acute symptoms of hyperglycemia and ketoacidosis. Once the acute event has passed, the pancreas temporarily recovers, leading to a remission (honeymoon period). Continued destruction of the β cell ultimately leads to an insulin-dependent state.

occurs. Glucosuria, which occurs when BG levels exceed the renal threshold, results in an osmotic diuresis, producing the classic symptoms of polyuria with compensatory polydipsia. If symptoms are untreated, weight loss occurs as glucose calories are lost in the urine and body fat and protein stores are broken down owing to increased rates of lipolysis and proteolysis. Muscle begins to metabolize its own glycogen stores and fatty acids for fuel, and the liver begins to metabolize free fatty acids that are released in response to epinephrine and low insulin concentrations. An absolute lack of insulin may cause excessive mobilization of free fatty acids to the liver, where they are metabolized to ketones. This can result in ketonemia, ketonuria, and, ultimately, ketoacidosis. Patients present with complaints of fatigue, significant weight loss, polyuria, and polydipsia. A significant elevation in glycosylated hemoglobin (A1C) confirms weeks or months of preceding hyperglycemia.

Because glucose provides an excellent medium for microorganisms, patients may present also with recurrent respiratory, vaginal, and other infections. Patients also may experience blurred vision secondary to osmotically induced changes in the lens of the eye. Treatment with insulin is essential to prevent severe dehydration, ketoacidosis, and death.

HONEYMOON PERIOD

Within days or weeks after the initial diagnosis and implementing treatment, many patients with type 1 diabetes experience an apparent remission, which is reflected by decreased BG concentrations and markedly decreased insulin requirements. This is called the *honeymoon period* because it may last for only a few weeks to months. Once hyperglycemia, metabolic acidosis, and ketosis resolve, endogenous insulin secretion recovers temporarily (Fig. 53-1). Although the honeymoon period may last for up to a year, increasing exogenous insulin requirements are inevitable and should be anticipated. During this time, patients should be maintained on insulin even if the dose is very low, because interrupted treatment is associated with a greater incidence of resistance and allergy to insulin.

Type 2 Diabetes

PATHOGENESIS

Type 2 diabetes is characterized by impaired insulin secretion and resistance to insulin action. In the presence of insulin resistance, glucose utilization by tissues is impaired, hepatic glucose and free fatty acid production is increased, and excess glucose accumulates in the circulation. This hyperglycemia stimulates the pancreas to produce more insulin in an attempt to overcome insulin resistance. The simultaneous elevation of both glucose and insulin levels is strongly suggestive of insulin resistance. Genetic predisposition may play a role in the development of type 2 diabetes. People with type 2 diabetes have a stronger family history of diabetes than those with type 1. There is no association with HLA types, however, and circulating ICAs are absent.[7,19] People with type 2 diabetes also exhibit varying degrees of tissue resistance to insulin, impaired insulin secretion, and increased basal hepatic glucose production. Finally, environmental factors such as obesity and a sedentary lifestyle also contribute to the development of insulin resistance.

Despite being the most common form of diabetes, the exact pathogenesis of type 2 is less well understood. Basal insulin levels are typically normal or elevated at diagnosis. First- or early-phase insulin release in response to glucose often is reduced, and pulsatile insulin secretion is absent, resulting in postprandial hyperglycemia. The effects of other insulinotropic substances such as incretin hormones, which contribute to meal-stimulated insulin release, are also altered.[20] With time, β cells lose their ability to respond to elevated glucose concentrations, leading to increasing loss of glucose control. In patients with severe hyperglycemia, the amount of insulin secreted in response to glucose is diminished and insulin resistance is worsened (glucose toxicity).

Most individuals with type 2 exhibit decreased tissue responsiveness to insulin.[19] Excess weight or hyperglycemia may contribute to hyperinsulinemia, which in time may lead to a decrease in or downregulation of the number of insulin receptors on the surface of target tissues and organs. Evidence suggests that decreased peripheral glucose uptake and utilization in muscle is the primary site of insulin resistance and results in prolonged postprandial hyperglycemia. Resistance may be secondary to decreased numbers of insulin receptors on the cell surface, decreased affinity of receptors for insulin, or defects in insulin signaling and action that follows receptor binding. Defects in insulin signaling and action are referred to as postreceptor or postbinding defects and are likely to be the primary sites of insulin resistance.

Patients with type 2 diabetes also exhibit increased hepatic glucose production (glycogenolysis and gluconeogenesis) reflected by an elevated fasting plasma or BG concentration.[19] As noted, hepatic glucose production is the primary source of glucose in the fasting state. In patients with type 2 diabetes, altered hepatic glucose production may also contribute to or cause postprandial hyperglycemia. Glucagon, produced by the α cells in the pancreatic islets and secreted in response to low BG, stimulates hepatic glucose production.[21] Its production is inhibited by insulin. Glucagon response to carbohydrate ingestion is altered in patients with type 2 diabetes who have a defective or absent early insulin response secondary to β cell dysfunction or failure. For patients with type 2 diabetes, untreated fasting and postprandial hyperglycemia caused by decreased glucose uptake and increased hepatic glucose production, hyperinsulinemia, and insulin resistance lead to a vicious cycle that inflicts ongoing damage to tissues and organs.

Patients with type 2 diabetes are often subclassified based on weight. Obese individuals account for more than 80% of patients with type 2 diabetes.[19] Patients with type 2 diabetes who are not obese often have increased body fat distributed in the abdominal area. Nonobese individuals account for about 10% of the type 2 population. Typically, they develop a mild form of diabetes during childhood, adolescence, or as young adults (usually before age 25), and their insulin levels are low in response to a glucose challenge. Included in this group are patients who have maturity-onset diabetes of the young (MODY).[7,19] MODY is associated with a strong family history that suggests an autosomal-dominant transmission. The underlying defect is heterogeneous, and multiple abnormalities at loci on different chromosomes have been discovered. More common defects include those for hepatic transcription factors and glucokinase (the "glucose sensor" in β cells). Patients with MODY may present with moderate to severe symptoms with or without ketosis. Unlike type 1 diabetes, however, the disease generally is mild and controlled with diet, oral agents, or low doses of insulin. With the increasing prevalence of obesity and type 2 diabetes in children and adolescents, it is important to distinguish between a youth with type 2 diabetes and one who really has autoimmune type 1 diabetes and is also obese.[22]

Type 2 diabetes is associated with a variety of disorders, including dyslipidemia, hypertension, and premature atherosclerosis (Fig. 53-2). Currently termed the metabolic syndrome, this triad

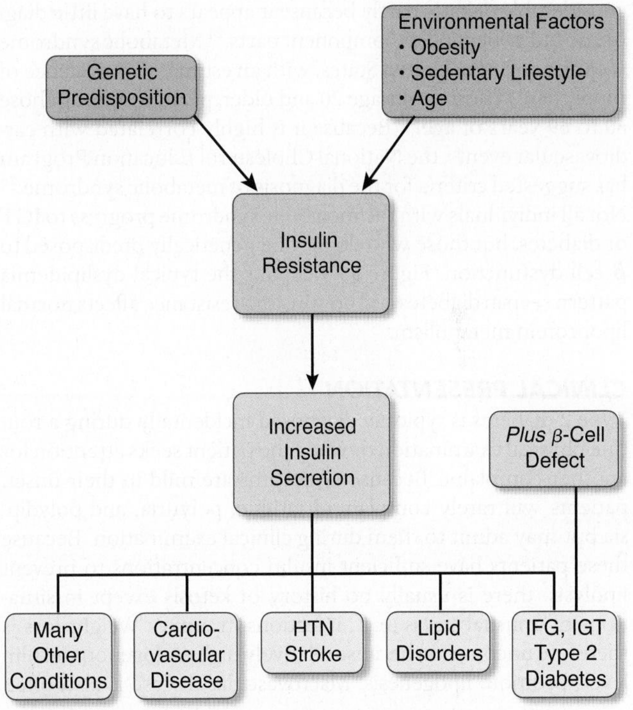

FIGURE 53-2 Metabolic syndrome. Genetic and environmental factors (visceral obesity, sedentary lifestyle, aging) predispose some individuals to insulin resistance. To overcome the resistance, the pancreas secretes more insulin, leading to hyperinsulinemia. People with insulin resistance and hyperinsulinemia commonly develop a cluster of medical problems and biochemical abnormalities: cardiovascular disease, hypertension, dyslipidemia, hyperuricemia, and type 2 diabetes mellitus. Only those individuals who are further genetically predisposed to β cell failure go on to develop impaired glucose tolerance (IGT), impaired fasting glucose (IFG) and type 2 diabetes. Many people with type 2 diabetes already have evidence of cardiovascular disease at the time of diabetes diagnosis. The cause-and-effect relationship between insulin resistance or hyperinsulinemia and these clinical conditions has not been clarified. See text for expanded discussion. DM, diabetes mellitus; HTN, hypertension.

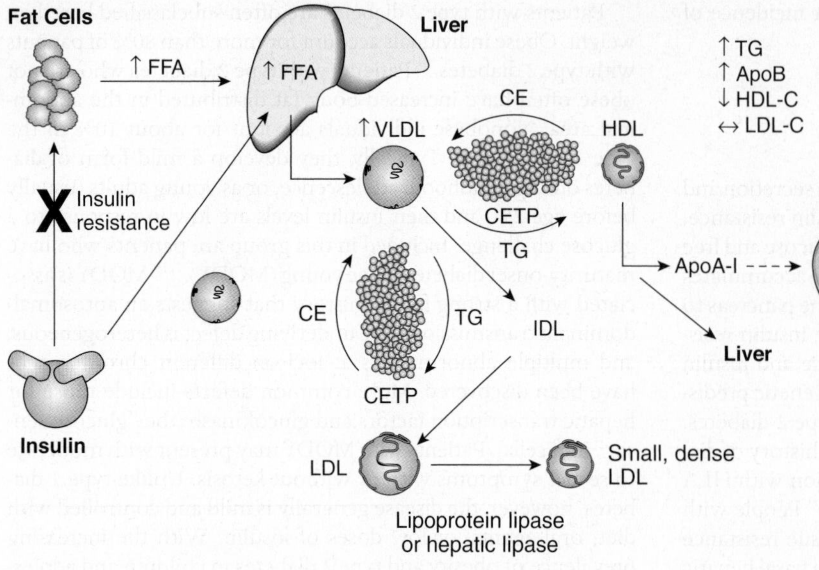

FIGURE 53-3 Changes in lipoprotein metabolism are a direct consequence of insulin resistance and are present before the onset of overt diabetes.

For a narrated PowerPoint on Figure 53-3, go to http://thepoint.lww.com/AT10e.

of clinical findings (hypertension, elevated fasting glucose, and dyslipidemia) is proposed to derive from insulin resistance itself and the resulting compensatory hyperinsulinemia.[23] The labeling of this triad as a separate "syndrome" remains the subject of considerable debate, partly because it appears to have little diagnostic utility beyond its component parts.[24] Metabolic syndrome is common in the United States, with an estimated prevalence of more than 34% in adults age 20 and older, peaking among those 60 to 69 years of age.[25] Because it is highly correlated with cardiovascular events, the National Cholesterol Education Program has suggested criteria for the diagnosis of metabolic syndrome.[26] Not all individuals with the metabolic syndrome progress to IGT or diabetes, but those who do may be genetically predisposed to β cell dysfunction. Figure 53-3 depicts the typical dyslipidemia pattern seen in diabetes and how insulin resistance affects normal lipoprotein metabolism.

CLINICAL PRESENTATION

Type 2 diabetes is typically diagnosed incidentally during a routine physical examination or when the patient seeks attention for another complaint. Because symptoms are mild in their onset, patients will rarely complain of fatigue, polyuria, and polydipsia but may admit to them during clinical examination. Because these patients have sufficient insulin concentrations to prevent lipolysis, there is usually no history of ketosis except in situations of unusual stress (e.g., infections, trauma). Weight loss is therefore uncommon because relatively high endogenous insulin levels promote lipogenesis. Macrovascular disease is also often evident at diagnosis. Microvascular complications at diagnosis suggest the presence of undiagnosed or subclinical diabetes for 7 to 10 years. Because type 2 diabetes patients retain some pancreatic reserve at the time of diagnosis, they generally can be treated with medical nutrition therapy (MNT), physical activity, and noninsulin antidiabetic medications for several years. Nevertheless, many eventually require insulin for control of their symptoms.

Gestational Diabetes Mellitus

GDM affects about 7% of all pregnancies and is defined as "any carbohydrate intolerance with onset or first recognition during pregnancy."[7,27] The onset of diabetes during pregnancy and its duration affect the prognosis for a good obstetric and perinatal outcome (see Chapter 49, Obstetric Drug Therapy).

Diagnosis

DIAGNOSTIC CRITERIA

The categories for normal, increased risk for diabetes, and diabetes for fasting plasma glucose (FPG), A1C, and the oral glucose tolerance test (OGTT) are listed in Table 53-2.[7] The Expert Committee of the ADA has established the diagnostic criteria for diabetes for nonpregnant individuals of any age. For these individuals, a diagnosis of diabetes can be made when one of the following is present[7]:

TABLE 53-2
Normal and Diabetic Plasma[a] Glucose Levels in mg/dL (mmol/L) and Glycosylated Hemoglobin and Normal and Diabetic Plasma Glucose Levels for the Oral Glucose Tolerance Test[7]

	FPG	A1C	OGTT
Normal	<100 (5.6)	≤5.6%	<140 (7.8)
Prediabetes (i.e., impaired fasting glucose, impaired glucose tolerance)	100–125 (5.6–6.9)	≥5.7–6.4%	140–199 (7.8–11.0)
Diabetes (nonpregnant adult)	≥126 (7.0)	≥6.5%	≥200 (11.1)

[a]Equivalent venous whole blood glucose concentrations are approximately 12%–15% lower. Arterial samples are higher than venous samples postprandially because glucose has not yet been removed from peripheral tissues. Capillary whole blood samples contain a mixture of arterial and venous blood. Fasting levels are equivalent to whole blood venous samples.
A1C, glycosylated hemoglobin; FPG, fasting plasma glucose; OGTT, oral glucose tolerance test.

1. An A1C of 6.5% or more. The test must be performed in a laboratory (not with a point-of-care test). It should be performed using a method certified by the National Glycohemoglobin Standardization Program.[28]
2. An FPG of 126 mg/dL or more. *Fasting* means no caloric intake for at least 8 hours.
3. Classic signs and symptoms of diabetes (polyuria, polydipsia, ketonuria, and unexplained weight loss) combined with a random plasma glucose of 200 mg/dL or more.
4. After a standard OGTT (75 g of glucose for an adult or 1.75 g/kg for a child), the venous plasma glucose concentration is 200 mg/dL or more at 2 hours.

The diagnosis must be confirmed by repeating the test, preferably the same test. If two different tests are performed (e.g., FPG and A1C), with only one test's value above the diagnostic cut point, that test should be repeated.[8]

At times, it may be difficult to classify patients as having type 1 or type 2 diabetes mellitus. Type 1 is more likely when a patient is younger than 30 years of age and lean, and has an elevated FPG and signs and symptoms of diabetes. The presence of moderate ketonuria with hyperglycemia in an otherwise unstressed patient also strongly supports a diagnosis of type 1 diabetes. Absence of ketonuria, however, is not of diagnostic value. The presence of autoantibodies to insulin or islet cell components may also indicate the need for eventual insulin therapy.[18] Relatively lean older adults believed to have type 2 diabetes because they are initially responsive to oral agents or low doses of insulin may be subsequently diagnosed with type 1 diabetes. In addition, clinicians are beginning to observe more cases of type 2 diabetes in obese children and adolescents.[29]

Individuals with A1C, FPG, or OGTT values that are intermediate between normal and those considered diagnostic of diabetes are considered to have prediabetes. The terms IFG and IGT should not be used interchangeably because each results from somewhat different physiologic processes. These individuals are not given the diagnosis of diabetes because of broad social, psychological, and economic implications. It is important to interpret the categories listed in Table 53-2 as a continuum of increased risk for diabetes, rather than focus on the absolute cut-off points for prediabetes or diabetes.

Many factors can impair glucose tolerance or increase plasma glucose. These must be excluded before a definitive diagnosis is made. For example, an individual who has not fasted for a minimum of 8 hours may have an elevated FPG. Patients who are tested for glucose tolerance during, or very soon after, an acute illness (e.g., a myocardial infarction [MI]) or who are on corticosteroids (e.g., prednisone, dexamethasone) may be misdiagnosed because of the presence of high concentrations of counter-regulatory hormones that increase glucose concentrations. Glucose tolerance often returns to normal in these individuals.

Screening for Type 2 Diabetes

The ADA advises that adults without risk factors should be screened starting at age 45.[8] Repeat testing should take place every 3 years. Adults may be tested at a younger age and more frequently if they are overweight (body mass index [BMI] ≥25 kg/m²) and have one or more of the risk factors listed in Table 53-3. An FPG or A1C is preferred over the OGTT to test for diabetes, as they are much less cumbersome. Asymptomatic children who are age 10 or who experience the onset of puberty before age 10 should be screened every 2 years for type 2 diabetes if they are overweight (BMI >85th percentile for age and sex; weight for height >85th percentile; or weight >120% of ideal for height) and have two or more of the risk factors listed in Table 53-3.

TABLE 53-3
Risk Factors for Type 2 Diabetes Mellitus[8]

Adults	Children[a]
Overweight (≥25 kg/m²)	Overweight (BMI >85th percentile for age and sex; or weight >120% of ideal for height)
Family history of diabetes (first-degree relative)	Family history of diabetes (first- or second-degree relative)
Physical inactivity	
Ethnic predisposition[b]	Ethnic predisposition[b]
Previous IFG, IGT, or A1C ≥5.7%	
History of PCOS, GDM, or macrosomia	Maternal history of diabetes (including GDM)
Clinical conditions associated with insulin resistance (e.g., severe obesity and acanthosis nigricans)	Signs of insulin resistance (e.g., acanthosis nigricans)
Hypertension (≥140/90 mm Hg or on antihypertensive therapy)	Conditions associated with insulin resistance (e.g., hypertension, dyslipidemia, or PCOS)
Dyslipidemia HDL-C <35 mg/dL (0.90 mmol/L) Triglyceride >250 mg/dL (2.82 mmol/L)	
Cardiovascular disease	

[a]Children are younger than 18 years of age.
[b]Ethnic predisposition includes individuals of African American, Latino, Native American, Asian, or Pacific Islander descent.
A1C, glycosylated hemoglobin; BMI, body mass index; GDM, gestational diabetes mellitus; HDL-C, high-density lipoprotein cholesterol; IFG, impaired fasting glucose; IGT, impaired glucose tolerance; PCOS, polycystic ovarian syndrome.

Long-Term Complications

Although acute hyperglycemic crises can occur in patients with diabetes, the long-term sequelae of diabetes account for most of the morbidity and mortality in the diabetic population. Complications are typically designated as microvascular or macrovascular in nature. Glucose toxicity contributes most to the development and progression of microvascular complications (retinopathy, nephropathy, and neuropathy) owing to the particular susceptibility of these cell systems to elevated glucose.[30] Diabetes is the leading cause of new cases of adult blindness and kidney failure in the United States.[1] About 60% to 70% of people with diabetes also have some manifestation of peripheral or autonomic neuropathy. Severe peripheral neuropathy coupled with abnormalities in immune function likely contribute to the high rate of lower extremity amputations among patients with diabetes.[1,31] Finally, poor glucose control promotes development of dental and oral complications and increases the risk of complications during pregnancy for both mother and fetus.[32–34]

Macrovascular complications are multifactorial in their etiology and less dependent on hyperglycemia. Diabetes mellitus itself is a well-known risk factor for macrovascular disease (peripheral vascular disease, CVD, stroke). Patients with diabetes have a threefold to fourfold elevated risk for MI and cardiovascular death compared with nondiabetic subjects.[35] Insulin resistance and the resultant hyperinsulinemia in type 2 diabetes mellitus contribute to the development of hypertension, dyslipidemia, and platelet hypersensitivity, all of which then contribute to the increased CVD risk in patients with diabetes.[36] Thus, although tight glycemic control (A1C <7.0%) will dramatically reduce the risk for microvascular disease, its relationship to macrovascular disease is still under intense debate.

Relationship of Glycemic Control to Microvascular and Macrovascular Disease

Although epidemiologic studies have shown a general relationship between glucose control and cardiovascular events, recent randomized trials have failed to confirm a benefit of tight glucose control compared with standard control, which highlights the multifactorial nature of macrovascular disease.[37] However, the clear relationship between microvascular events and glycemic control is well established from randomized, clinical trials. The Diabetes Control and Complications Trial (DCCT) and the open-label follow-up trial, DCCT-EDIC (Epidemiology of Diabetes Interventions and Complications) established the benefits of intensive glycemic control on microvascular end points.[38,39] In the DCCT, intensive treatment (A1C 7.1% versus 9.0%) reduced the risk of clinically meaningful retinopathy, nephropathy, and neuropathy by approximately 60%. The EDIC study followed as an open-label extension of the DCCT cohorts. Patients originally assigned to the intensive treatment group were shown to have a persistently lower incidence of microvascular complications even after the glucose control reached parity between the two study groups after the end of the randomized portion of the trial.[39,40] The EDIC study also showed a significant reduction in cardiovascular complications among patients previously assigned to the intensive therapy DCCT arm.[41] See Table 53-4 for the glycemic goals of intensive insulin therapy (herein called physiological or basal-bolus therapy). This persistence of the microvascular benefits of glycemic control has also been demonstrated in patients with type 2 diabetes in the UKPDS (United Kingdom Prospective Diabetes Study) (see Case 53-14, Question 2).[42]

The relationship between glycemic control and macrovascular disease has always been less clear. Evidence of early atherosclerosis in patients with type 1 diabetes in whom dyslipidemia and hypertension are typically absent argues strongly for a role of hyperglycemia itself in the development or progression of macrovascular disease.[43] The UKPDS trial was the first to report the benefit of tight BG control on cardiovascular complications in type 2 diabetes.[44] Although the microvascular benefits were clear, the 21% relative risk reduction for fatal and nonfatal MI and sudden cardiac death failed to reach statistical significance ($p = 0.052$). However, in a planned 10-year follow-up of patients enrolled in the trial, a significant 15% reduction was seen in the risk of MI ($p = 0.01$).[42] A similar finding for macrovascular benefit was reported in a 17-year follow-up of the DCCT-EDIC study.[41] Thus, although glycemic control benefited macrovascular disease, it took more than a decade to see the benefit. Reducing macrovascular risk in patients with diabetes thus takes a more comprehensive approach than just glycemic control. In a trial of multiple risk factor control in type 2 diabetes, the STENO-2 trial found a significant 53% reduction in macrovascular events with modest control of hypertension, dyslipidemia, and glycemia simultaneously.[45] Control of all major CVD risk factors is highlighted by the ADA for its importance in reducing macrovascular disease risk.[8] See Table 53-5 for the metabolic goals for adults with diabetes.

TABLE 53-5

American Diabetes Association Metabolic Goals[a] for Adults With Diabetes Mellitus[8]

Glycemic goals	
• A1C	<7.0% (normal, 4%–6%)[b]
• Preprandial plasma glucose	70–130 mg/dL (3.9–7.2 mmol/L)[c]
• Postprandial plasma glucose	<180 mg/dL (<10.0 mmol/L)[d]
Blood pressure	<130/80 mm Hg
Lipids	
• Low-density lipoprotein cholesterol	<100 mg/dL (<2.6 mmol/L)[e]
• Triglycerides	<150 mg/dL (<1.7 mmol/L)
• High-density lipoprotein cholesterol	
– Men	40 mg/dL (>1.0 mmol/L)
– Women	50 mg/dL (>1.3 mmol/L)

[a]Goals must be individualized to the patient. See Case 53-2, Question 2, Case 53-14, Question 2, and Case 53-24, Questions 1–4, for broader discussion.
[b]More stringent goals (i.e., <6%) can be considered for select individuals. American Association of Clinical Endocrinologists/American College of Endocrinology recommends A1C goal of ≤6.5%.
[c]American Association of Clinical Endocrinologists recommends a fasting blood glucose goal of <110 mg/dL (6.1 mmol/L).[46]
[d]American Association of Clinical Endocrinologists/American College of Endocrinology recommends goal of <140 mg/L (7.8 mmol/L).[46]
[e]More stringent goals (i.e., <70 mg/dL [1.8 mmol/L]) may be considered for individuals with overt cardiovascular disease.
A1C, glycosylated hemoglobin.

TABLE 53-4

Goals of Physiological (Basal-Bolus) Insulin Therapy[a]

Monitoring Parameter	Adults (mg/dL)	School Age (6–12 years) (mg/dL)	Adolescents and Young Adults (13–29 years) (mg/dL)	Pregnancy (mg/dL)
Premeals	70–130	90–180	90–130	60–99
2-hour postprandial plasma glucose	<180	Not routinely recommended	Not routinely recommended	100–129
Bedtime/overnight (2–4 AM) plasma glucose	>70	100–180	90–150	60–99
A1C[b]	<7.0%[c]	<8.0%	<7.5%[d]	<6%
Urine ketones[e]	Absent to rare	Absent to rare	Absent to rare	Rare

[a]See Case 53-2, Question 2, and Case 53-4, Question 2, for discussion. Basal-bolus insulin therapy is a complete therapeutic program of diabetes management and requires a team approach.
[b]A1C, glycosylated hemoglobin, referenced to a nondiabetic range of 4%–6% using a Diabetes Control and Complications Trial (DCCT)-based assay.
[c]Acceptable values should be individualized to levels that are attainable without creating undue risk for hypoglycemia. These results are similar to the results achieved in the DCCT trial. The American Diabetes Association recommends consideration for a lower goal (e.g., <6%) in individuals with a short duration of diabetes, long life expectancy, and no significant cardiovascular disease. Less stringent goals may be appropriate for patients with hypoglycemic unawareness, history of severe hypoglycemia, counterregulatory insufficiency, advanced microvascular or macrovascular complications, or other complicating features (Table 53-12).
[d]A lower goal (<7%) is reasonable if it can be achieved without creating excessive risk for hypoglycemia.
[e]Does not apply to type 2 diabetes patients.
Modified and extrapolated from American Diabetes Association. Standards of medical care in diabetes—2011. *Diabetes Care.* 2011;34(Suppl 1):S11; American Diabetes Association. Preconception care of women with diabetes. *Diabetes Care.* 2004;27(Suppl 1):S76; Kitzmiller JL et al. Managing preexisting diabetes for pregnancy: summary of evidence and consensus recommendations for care. *Diabetes Care.* 2008;31:1060; [No authors listed]. The effect of intensive treatment of diabetes on the development and progression of long-term complications in insulin-dependent diabetes mellitus. The Diabetes Control and Complications Trial Research Group. *N Engl J Med.* 1993;329:977.

Three trials published in 2008 and 2009 have raised new questions about tight glycemic control in patients with type 2 diabetes. In the Action to Control Cardiovascular Risk in Diabetes (ACCORD) trial a higher rate of mortality was seen in the intensive treatment arm, which achieved an A1C of 6.4% compared with the standard arm, which achieved 7.5%.[47] The ACCORD study was a National Heart, Lung, and Blood Institute study of more than 10,000 patients with type 2 diabetes with known heart disease or multiple cardiovascular risk factors. The intensively treated group had an excess of three deaths per 1,000 participants per year compared with the standard group during an average of 4 years on treatment (257 vs. 203 deaths). The higher mortality rate was not attributable to a specific drug therapy or to severe hypoglycemia.[48] A second trial, the Action in Diabetes and Vascular Disease a Controlled Evaluation (ADVANCE) was an even larger study of more than 11,000 patients, which had different findings from ACCORD. In ADVANCE, there was an insignificant trend for reduced cardiovascular mortality and reduced overall mortality with tight glycemic control (A1C of 6.3% compared with 7.0%).[49] Lastly, in the smaller Veterans Affairs Diabetes Trial (VADT), nearly 2,000 patients were studied and found to have an insignificant 12% relative risk reduction in macrovascular end points but a 7% relative increase in overall mortality (95 vs. 102 deaths). Neither finding was statistically significant.[50]

In the face of these new data, the ADA, along with the American Heart Association (AHA) and the American College of Cardiology (ACC) issued a position statement in 2009.[51] Although acknowledging the findings of the ACCORD trial, the persistent trend for reductions in macrovascular events in all three trials was found to be reassuring. The position of the committee (which continues to be the official position of the ADA in the 2011 guidelines) is that although intensive glycemic control did not improve macrovascular outcomes, a goal of less than 7% is still reasonable based on microvascular benefits and a clear lack of harm across the trials of intensive versus standard glycemic control.[8] However, the ADA does acknowledge that there is room to individualize the A1C goal and that achieving an A1C of less than 7% has limited macrovascular benefit compared with A1C values of 7% to 8%. Patients with type 2 diabetes and CVD or multiple risk factors for CVD should discuss their treatment goals with their providers. In these patients, a less intensive goal may be appropriate, particularly for patients who have difficulty achieving the goal of less than 7%.[8]

For a narrated PowerPoint on the ACCORD, ADVANCE and VADT studies and the effect of tight glycemic control in reducing cardiovascular events, go to http://thepoint.lww.com/AT10e.

Prevention of Type 1 and Type 2 Diabetes Mellitus

Because the clinical symptoms of type 1 diabetes mellitus are the overt expression of an insidious pathogenic process that begins years earlier, investigators are focusing attention on strategies that alter the natural history of the disease (Fig. 53-1). First-degree relatives of individuals with type 1 diabetes mellitus have an increased risk for developing the diabetes and can be identified by the presence of immune markers that may herald the disease by many years.[18] This has led to attempts at immune intervention at the prediabetes stage with such drugs as nicotinamide and low doses of insulin, but neither was found to delay or prevent diabetes.[52–54] In contrast, treatment of newly diagnosed diabetes with agents that modify cytotoxic T cells may slow pancreatic destruction and progression of diabetes.[55]

In addition to the 23.6 million people with diabetes in the United States, an estimated additional 57 million Americans aged 20 years and older have prediabetes (IGT, IFG, A1C 5.7% to 6.4%; see Table 53-3 for a list of risk factors associated with prediabetes).[1] The Diabetes Prevention Program Research Group studied a diverse group of 3,234 individuals at high risk for developing diabetes to determine whether lifestyle interventions or metformin (850 mg by mouth [PO] twice a day [BID]) would prevent or delay the onset of type 2 diabetes.[56] After 3 years, the incidence of diabetes was reduced by 58% and 31% in the intensive lifestyle and metformin groups, respectively, compared with the control group. Diabetes incidence during 10 years of follow-up was persistently lower in the groups originally treated with lifestyle (34% reduction) and metformin (18% reduction) interventions compared with the control group.[57] Other studies have confirmed the value of lifestyle intervention and other drugs (acarbose, orlistat, and various thiazolidinediones) in the prevention of type 2 diabetes.[8,58] Lifelong medication therapy, however, is not without its own risks and complications. Current recommendations regarding the treatment for individuals with prediabetes include lifestyle modification (5%–10% weight loss and 150 minutes/week of moderately intense physical activity).[8] For patients at very high risk of diabetes (BMI $\geq$35 kg/m^2, combined IFG and IGT, and at least one diabetes risk factor such as A1C >6.0%, hypertension, low high-density lipoprotein cholesterol [HDL-C], high triglycerides, or family history of diabetes in a first-degree relative) and who are younger than 60 years old, the addition of metformin may be considered.

CASE 53-1

QUESTION 1: R.P. is a 43-year-old woman visiting a primary-care clinic to obtain a routine physical examination for her new job. Her past medical history is significant for GDM. She was told during her two pregnancies (last child born 3 years ago) that she had "borderline diabetes," which resolved each time after giving birth. Her family history is significant for type 2 diabetes (mother, maternal grandmother, older first cousin), hypertension, and CVD. She appears black and when asked identifies herself as African American. She denies tobacco or alcohol use. She states she tries to walk 15 minutes twice a week. Physical examination is significant for moderate central obesity (5 feet 4 inches; 160 pounds; BMI, 30.2 kg/m^2) and blood pressure (BP) 145/85 mm Hg. R.P. denies any symptoms of polyphagia, polyuria, or lethargy. On checking her electronic medical record, she has documented hypertension and an FPG value of 119 mg/dL, measured 2 months prior. What features of R.P.'s history and examination are consistent with an increased risk of developing type 2 diabetes?

The features of R.P.'s history that are consistent with an increased risk of developing type 2 diabetes include her age, ethnicity, weight, family history of diabetes, history of GDM, and a documented IFG. In addition, type 2 diabetes is also often associated with other disorders such as hypertension. The fact that R.P. has hypertension that is not well controlled and has a family history of hypertension and CVD may indicate that she is predisposed to insulin resistance, further putting her at risk for developing type 2 diabetes.

CASE 53-1, QUESTION 2: The physician orders an A1C for R.P., which comes back at 6.1%. How should R.P. be managed at this time?

Both the A1C and FPG values are in the prediabetes range. R.P. should be educated about her risk for developing type 2 diabetes. Working with her physician or other health care providers, R.P. should be encouraged and educated on how to institute lifestyle modifications (MNT, physical activity) that will help her to lose weight, improve her cardiovascular health, and decrease her risk for developing type 2 diabetes. A weight loss goal of 5% to 10% during the next 6 to 12 months should be recommended, and she should increase her level of moderate physical activity to at least 150 minutes/week. Her hypertension should be managed. At this time, the use of pharmacologic agents (i.e., metformin) to prevent the development of type 2 diabetes is not recommended.

Treatment

There are three major components to the treatment of diabetes: diet, drugs (insulin and antidiabetic agents [oral and injectable]), and exercise. Each of these components interacts with the others to the extent that no assessment and modification of one can be made without knowledge of the other two.

BARIATRIC SURGERY FOR TYPE 2 DIABETES

Gastric reduction surgery, with either gastric banding or bypass procedures, has become an option for adult patients with type 2 diabetes who are obese (BMI >35 kg/m^2), unable to lose weight by other methods, and whose diabetes or other comorbidities are difficult to control through lifestyle and drug therapy.[8] Bariatric surgery can lead to complete resolution of diabetes (normalization of BG) in up to 78% of patients.[59] Glycemia can normalize after intestinal bypass procedures (Roux-en-Y gastric bypass) quickly after surgery, independent of weight, possibly owing to increases in incretin hormone levels.[60,61] Although this evidence is exciting, bariatric surgery is not risk-free, and patients may endure long-term problems such as malabsorption.

MEDICAL NUTRITION THERAPY

PRINCIPLES

MNT plays a crucial role in the therapy of all individuals with diabetes.[62] Unfortunately, patient acceptance and adherence to diet and meal planning is often poor, but revised evidence-based recommendations that are more flexible than previous approaches offer new opportunities to increase the effectiveness of nutrition therapy.

Nutrition therapy is designed to help patients achieve appropriate metabolic and physiological goals (e.g., glucose, lipids, BP, proteinuria, weight), select healthy foods, and take into consideration personal and cultural preferences. Appropriate levels and types of physical activity to achieve a healthier status are incorporated into the nutrition plan.

NUTRITION THERAPY AND TYPE 1 DIABETES MELLITUS

For patients with type 1 diabetes taking fixed doses of insulin, a meal plan is designed to provide adequate carbohydrates timed to match the peak action of exogenously administered mealtime insulin. Regularly scheduled meals and snacks should contain consistent carbohydrate amounts, which are required to prevent hypoglycemic reactions. Fortunately, newer insulins and insulin regimens provide much more flexibility in the amount and timing of food intake. Patients who are taught to count carbohydrates can inject rapid- or short-acting insulin doses designed to match their anticipated intake. Integration of food intake, physical activity, and insulin dose is critical and discussed extensively in the cases that follow.

NUTRITION THERAPY AND TYPE 2 DIABETES MELLITUS

For patients with type 2 diabetes, meal plans emphasize normalizing plasma glucose and lipid levels as well as maintaining a normal BP to prevent or mitigate cardiovascular morbidity. Although weight loss reduces insulin resistance and improves glycemic control, traditional dietary strategies incorporating hypocaloric diets have not been effective in achieving long-term weight loss. A sustainable weight loss of 5% to 7% can be achieved within structured programs that emphasize lifestyle changes, physical activity, and food intake that modestly reduces caloric and fat intake. For weight loss, the ADA recommends either low-carbohydrate (<130 g/day) or low-fat, calorie-restricted diets for up to 1 year.[62]

SPECIFIC NUTRITION COMPONENTS

MNT is an integral and critical component of diabetes care. For a more extensive discussion of the principles underlying nutrition therapy, the reader is directed to other sources.[62–64] A few key principles are briefly noted below because they are common sources of misunderstanding.

Carbohydrates and Artificial Sweeteners

Carbohydrates include sugar (sucrose), starch, and fiber and are liberally incorporated into the diet of a person with diabetes. In fact, the amount of dietary carbohydrate is the main determinant of insulin demand and is commonly used to determine the premeal insulin dose. Furthermore, patients using fixed doses of insulin or antihyperglycemic medications (e.g., sulfonylureas) must eat meals containing consistent amounts of carbohydrate to avoid hypoglycemia. Because isocaloric amounts of sucrose and starch produce the same degree of glycemia, sucrose can be substituted for a portion of the total carbohydrate intake and should be incorporated into an otherwise healthful diet.

Whole grains, fruits, and vegetables high in fiber are recommended for people with diabetes, as they are for the general population. There is no evidence that larger amounts produce a differential metabolic benefit with regard to plasma glucose and lipid levels. Nonnutritive sweeteners (saccharin, aspartame, neotame, acesulfame potassium, sucralose) and sugar alcohols have been rigorously tested by the US Food and Drug Administration (FDA) for safety in people with diabetes and are safe at approved daily intakes. Fructose and the reduced-calorie sweeteners called sugar alcohols produce lower postprandial glucose responses than sucrose, glucose, and starch. When sugar alcohols (e.g., sorbitol, mannitol, lactitol, xylitol, and maltitol) are consumed, it is recommended to subtract half of their grams from the total carbohydrate amount because their effect on BG is less. Patients should be advised that when these sweeteners are used in foods labeled "dietetic" or "sugar free," they still add to the carbohydrate content and provide substantial calories (2 cal/g). Furthermore, excessive intake of sorbitol-sweetened foods (e.g., 30–50 g/day) can induce an osmotic diarrhea, and excessive amounts of fructose can increase total and LDL cholesterol (LDL-C).

Counting Carbohydrates

When patients are taught to estimate the grams of carbohydrate in a meal they are given the following guideline: One carbohydrate serving = 1 starch or 1 fruit or 1 cup milk = 15 g carbohydrate. Patients vary with regard to their insulin to carbohydrate ratio throughout time and throughout the day; however, a typical starting point is 1 unit/15 g carbohydrate.

ONLINE CONTENT

For a table with examples of 15-g carbohydrate servings, go to http://thepoint.lww.com/AT10e.

Fat

CVD is a major cause of morbidity and mortality in patients with diabetes. Therefore, saturated fats should be limited to less than 7% of calories. The intake of *trans* fat should also be minimized. The recommended cholesterol intake is less than 200 mg/day for patients with diabetes. Two or more servings per week of fish to provide *n*-3 polyunsaturated fatty acids and omega-3 fatty acids are advised.

Protein

Data are insufficient to support special dietary protein recommendations for persons with diabetes if kidney function is normal. Generally, 15% to 20% of the daily caloric intake comes from animal and vegetable protein sources in the US diet. This amount may be liberalized in pregnant and lactating women or in elderly people. With the onset of nephropathy, a lower protein intake of 0.8 to 1.0 g/kg/day is considered sufficiently restrictive. For patients in later stages of nephropathy, reduction of protein intake to 0.8 g/kg/day is recommended. High-protein diets are not recommended as a long-term method for weight loss, because the effects on kidney function are not known.

Sodium

The ADA recommends a reduced sodium intake of less than 2,300 mg/day in normotensive and hypertensive individuals. For patients with diabetes and symptomatic heart failure, sodium should be further restricted to less than 2,000 mg/day to help reduce symptoms. For all other patients, the ADA has no particular restrictions on sodium intake, but recommends individualizing amounts based on the patient's sensitivity to salt and concurrent conditions such as hypertension or nephropathy.

Alcohol

The ADA's recommendation for alcohol is consistent with general recommendations of no more than two alcoholic drinks per day for men or one drink per day for women. A drink is equivalent to 12 ounces of beer, 5 ounces of wine, or 1.5 ounces of distilled spirits (each contains about 15 g of carbohydrate). Nevertheless, its caloric contribution must be considered (1 alcoholic beverage = 2 fat exchanges), and it should always be taken with food to minimize its hypoglycemic effect. In people with diabetes, light to moderate alcohol intake (one to two drinks per day) is associated with a decreased risk of CVD. A note of caution: Evening consumption of alcohol may increase the risk of nocturnal and fasting hypoglycemia, particularly in people with type 1 diabetes.

Physical Activity

Physical activity is a key factor in the treatment of diabetes, particularly in type 2 diabetes, because obesity and inactivity contribute to the development of glucose intolerance in genetically predisposed individuals.[65,66] Regular exercise reduces cholesterol levels, raises HDL-C, lowers BP, augments weight-reduction diets, reduces the dose requirements or need for insulin or antihyperglycemic agents, enhances insulin sensitivity, and improves psychological well-being by reducing stress. Exercise increases glucose utilization, which is provided initially from the breakdown of muscle glycogen and, subsequently, from hepatic glycogenolysis and gluconeogenesis. These effects are mediated through norepinephrine, epinephrine, growth hormone, cortisol, and glucagon, along with the suppression of insulin secretion. In patients using insulin, hyperglycemia, normoglycemia, or hypoglycemia can occur secondary to exercise depending on the degree of control, recent administration of rapid-acting insulin, and food intake. Exercise in patients taking insulin must be tempered by increased food intake, potential delay in insulin administration, decreased doses of insulin, or a combination of these actions to minimize hypoglycemia (see Case 53-6).

In patients with type 2 diabetes, plasma glucose concentrations usually decrease in response to exercise, but symptomatic hypoglycemia is uncommon. The vascular benefits of exercise are particularly helpful in patients with diabetes given their predisposition to CVD. In general, exercise that produces moderate exertion (increase in heart rate of 20%–40% from resting baseline) is recommended with a starting goal of 150 minutes per week. The eventual goal is for patients to be able to achieve 50% to 70% of their age-adjusted maximal heart rate.[8]

Resistance exercise has been shown to improve insulin sensitivity. Therefore, in the absence of any contraindications, people with type 2 diabetes are encouraged to perform resistance training three times per week. Patients with conditions that may preclude certain types of physical activity (e.g., coronary artery disease, uncontrolled hypertension, severe autonomic neuropathy, severe peripheral neuropathy or history of foot lesions, and advanced retinopathy in which retinal detachment may occur) should be carefully evaluated before starting an exercise regimen.

PHARMACOLOGIC TREATMENT

Insulin, along with diet, is crucial to the survival of individuals with type 1 diabetes and plays a major role in the therapy of people with type 2 diabetes when their symptoms cannot be controlled with diet or noninsulin antidiabetic agents. Insulin also is used for people with type 2 diabetes during periods of intercurrent illness or stress (e.g., surgery, pregnancy). The use of antidiabetic agents is reserved for the treatment of patients with type 2 diabetes whose symptoms cannot be controlled with diet and exercise alone (however, metformin is an exception to this). The clinical use of these agents and the complications associated with their use are discussed later in this chapter.

PANCREAS AND ISLET CELL TRANSPLANTS

Pancreas transplantation, by either whole pancreas or pancreatic islet cells, is the only available treatment for type 1 diabetes that induces an insulin-independent, normoglycemic state. Benefits can include improvement in quality of life, retinopathy, and nephropathy.[67–69] Whole-organ pancreas transplantation continues to be widely used in uremic diabetic patients because it can be performed at the same time as kidney transplantation (simultaneous kidney and pancreas transplant [SPK]) or after (pancreas after kidney transplant [PAK]). SPK graft survival rates are 86% and 71% at years 1 and 5, respectively. For PAK, survival rates are slightly lower, at 78% and 57% at years 1 and 5, respectively.[67,70]

Islet cell transplants (infusions) have received increased attention with the success of the Edmonton protocol, which used a steroid-free immunosuppression regimen as well as other techniques. All patients achieved insulin independence after 1 year in contrast with a previous success rate of 8%.[71] At 5 years, approximately 80% of patients had C-peptide present, but only 10% maintained insulin independence with a median duration of insulin independence of 15 months.[72] Since then, an international trial of the Edmonton protocol, organized by the Immune Tolerance Network, was published demonstrating proof of concept that the protocol could be replicated, although 28% of patients had complete graft loss at 1 year.[73]

Although islet cell transplantation does not achieve sustained insulin independence, it can improve quality of life, mainly from reduced hypoglycemia, and should be considered for patients with hypoglycemic unawareness.[71,73] The Collaborative Islet Transplant Registry reported 408 recipients of islet infusion procedures from 1999 to 2008 in North America. Many issues remain regarding islet cell transplantation, including availability of islet cell transplant material, islet cell preparation, types of immunosuppression, and assessment of long-term outcomes.

OVERALL GOALS OF THERAPY

The overall goal of diabetes management is to prevent acute and chronic complications. Periodic assessments of A1C coupled with regular measurement of fasting, preprandial, and postprandial glucose levels should be used to assess therapy. The following overall goals of therapy are agreed on by most endocrinologists:

1. Strive for glycemic control achieved in DCCT and UKPDS. The landmark randomized, prospective trials of various interventional therapies in patients with both types 1 and 2 diabetes have clearly demonstrated that reductions in hyperglycemia significantly decrease microvascular complications. In both the UKPDS and the DCCT follow-up studies, significant reductions in macrovascular complications were also observed. Target BG goals may need to be adjusted for patients with frequent, severe hypoglycemia or hypoglycemia unawareness (see Case 53-11, Questions 1–3, and Case 53-12), or with CVD. In addition, established renal insufficiency, proliferative retinopathy, severe neuropathy, and other advanced complications are not likely to be improved by tight glucose control. See Table 53-5 for the ADA glycemic goals. The American Association of Clinical Endocrinologists and the American College of Endocrinology established glycemic goals as well (Table 53-5).[46] We elected to discuss ADA guidelines throughout this chapter.
2. Try to keep patients free of symptoms associated with hyperglycemia (polyuria, polydipsia, weight loss, fatigue, recurrent infection, ketoacidosis) or hypoglycemia (hunger, anxiety, palpitations, sweatiness).
3. Maintain normal growth and development in children. Intensive therapy is not recommended for children younger than 7 years of age and should be used cautiously in children ages 7 to 13 years old (see Case 53-4, Questions 2 and 3).
4. Eliminate or minimize all other cardiovascular risk factors (obesity, hypertension, tobacco use, hyperlipidemia; see Table 53-5 for BP and lipid goals).
5. Try to integrate the patient into the health care team through intensive education. The patient's knowledge and understanding of this disease can favorably influence its outcomes (see Table 53-16 later in this chapter).

Methods of Monitoring Glycemic Control

In addition to monitoring signs and symptoms associated with hyperglycemia, hypoglycemia, and the long-term complications of diabetes, an ongoing assessment of metabolic control is an integral component of diabetes management. Ideally, self-monitoring of blood glucose (SMBG) results combined with laboratory measures of acute and chronic glycemia can be used to evaluate and adjust therapy.[74] SMBG and A1C levels continue to be the two primary methods used to access glycemic control. Continuous glucose monitoring (CGM) of interstitial fluid is also available for people with diabetes. CGM is discussed somewhat briefly here because this method is currently recommended for consideration, along with SMBG, for patients with type 1 diabetes only, especially those with hypoglycemic unawareness.[8]

KETONE TESTING

Ketone testing is recommended for patients with gestational and type 1 diabetes. Urine ketones (acetoacetic acid) should be evaluated when glucose concentrations consistently exceed 300 mg/dL or during acute illness.[74] In addition, a glucose monitor that is able measure blood β-ketones (e.g., the Precision Xtra has a specific test strip to measure β-hydroxybutyric acid), can be used. Persistently high glucose concentrations of this magnitude signal insulin deficiency that can, in turn, lead to lipolysis and ketoacidosis. A positive test may indicate impending or established ketoacidosis and demands a more extensive diagnostic workup. Testing also is recommended during pregnancy and if the patient has symptoms of ketoacidosis. Although there are generally no ketones in the urine, they may be present in people who are on extremely low-caloric diets and in the first morning sample of women who are pregnant. Also, see discussions of sick day management and ketoacidosis in other sections of this chapter (Cases 53-7 and 53-13).

PLASMA GLUCOSE

FPG concentrations are commonly used to assess glycemic control in the fasting state because this is when glucose concentrations are most reproducible. FPG concentrations generally reflect glucose derived from hepatic glucose production because this is the primary source of glucose in the postabsorptive state. The FPG is the most frequent test performed by patients when self-monitoring. Postprandial glucose concentrations (1–2 hours after the start of the meal) also are used to assess glycemic control when fasting glucose concentrations are within normal limits or when there is a need to assess the effects of food or drugs (e.g., rapid-acting insulins, glinides) on meal-related glycemia. In nondiabetic individuals, glucose concentrations generally return to less than 140 mg/dL within 2 hours after a meal. One- to 2-hour postprandial concentrations primarily reflect the efficiency of insulin-mediated glucose uptake by peripheral tissue.

Because glucose concentrations are affected by various factors (e.g., meals, medications, stress), single-time point measurements cannot be used to assess a patient's overall control. Most laboratories measure plasma glucose concentrations rather than whole blood because these values are not subject to changes in the hematocrit. The majority of glucose monitors report plasma-referenced glucose concentrations. Whole BG concentrations are approximately 10% to 15% lower than plasma glucose concentrations because glucose is not distributed into red blood cells. To convert plasma glucose concentrations (mg/dL) to whole BG values (and vice versa), the following equation can be used:

$$\text{Whole blood glucose (mg/dL)} = \text{plasma glucose (mg/dL)} \div 1.12 \quad \textbf{(Eq. 53-1)}$$

To convert a glucose concentration in mg/dL to mmol/L, a factor of 18 is used:

$$\text{Plasma glucose (mmol/L)} = \text{plasma glucose (mg/dL)} \div 18 \quad \textbf{(Eq. 53-2)}$$

SELF-MONITORING OF BLOOD GLUCOSE

SMBG has made euglycemia, both preprandially and postprandially, an achievable goal (70–130 mg/dL). Patients and their health care providers can use SMBG to assess directly the effects of drug dose changes, meals, exercise, and illness on BG concentrations. With improved technology, decreasing costs, and increased coverage by health plans, SMBG is the day-to-day monitoring test of choice for all patients with diabetes. However, SMBG remains expensive for patients without health insurance, is invasive, and can be difficult for some patients to perform depending on their technical ability. Furthermore, to achieve maximal benefit from SMBG, both the clinician and patient must be motivated and willing to spend the time required to interpret the data and modify therapy to improve glycemic control. According to the results of the DCCT and UKPDS, most people with diabetes should attempt to achieve and maintain BG levels as close to normal as is safely possible. This goal can realistically be achieved only by using SMBG. The frequency and timing of performing SMBG should be dictated by the individual's needs and goals. Selection and use of SMBG testing materials are discussed in Case 53-2, Questions 9 and 10. Patients in whom SMBG is particularly valuable include the following:

- *Patients with type 1 diabetes:* Frequent BG measurements help the patient to correlate meals, exercise, and insulin dose with BG concentrations. This instant feedback gives the patient an increased sense of control and motivation, leading to improved glucose control.
- *Pregnant patients:* Infant morbidity and mortality are associated with the mother's overall glucose control. Using SMBG, the mother with diabetes who achieves normoglycemia before conception and throughout pregnancy improves her chances of delivering a live, healthy infant.
- *Patients having difficulty recognizing hypoglycemia:* With time, patients with diabetes can develop a sluggish counterregulatory response to hypoglycemia whereby hypoglycemic symptoms are blunted or even absent. This is often referred to as hypoglycemic unawareness. Routine SMBG to detect asymptomatic hypoglycemia is essential in these individuals (see Case 53-12). In addition, acute anxiety attacks or signs and symptoms associated with a rapidly falling BG concentration may mimic a true hypoglycemic reaction. This can be evaluated easily by measuring a fingerstick BG concentration.
- *Patients who are using physiological (e.g., basal-bolus) insulin therapy:* Individuals who are on multiple daily doses of insulin or those using an insulin pump should perform SMBG to evaluate the effectiveness of their insulin regimens and meal plans and to check for hypoglycemic or hyperglycemic reactions (see Case 53-2, Question 10). Knowledge of preprandial, postprandial, bedtime, and nocturnal (e.g., 2 AM) BG concentrations is essential in determining basal and preprandial insulin requirements.
- *Patients with type 2 diabetes who are on therapy that can cause hypoglycemia:* Individuals taking glinides, a sulfonylurea, or insulin therapy should know how to perform SMBG to detect hypoglycemia when experiencing symptoms consistent with hypoglycemia.
- *Patients with type 2 diabetes who are engaged in self-management of their diabetes:* Even individuals using noninsulin therapies can benefit from SMBG to evaluate the impact of food, exercise, and antidiabetic medications on their BG.

CONTINUOUS GLUCOSE MONITORING

Like SMBG, CGM provides real-time information on glucose concentrations. However, the difference is that the CMG system automatically detects glucose concentrations (subcutaneous interstitial fluid glucose concentrations) on a continual basis. The three main CGM systems in the United States are DexCom Seven Plus, Medtronic Diabetes Guardian Real-Time, and Abbott Diabetes Care FreeStyle Navigator. The CGM systems use electrochemical sensors that are inserted into the skin. Sensor probe length varies as does the duration that the sensor can remain in the skin (3–7 days). The sensors transmit a signal to a receiver (wired or wireless), which records and displays the data every 1 to 5 minutes. The sensors require a warm-up or initialization period and have very specific calibration requirements. Calibration is performed by using a BG monitor. Interstitial glucose levels lag behind plasma or BG levels by 8 to 18 minutes, depending on the glucose rate of change.[75] Therefore, if a person's glucose is low, or trending downward, SMBG is required. CGM systems have alarms that can go off at certain high and low glucose thresholds. The ability to detect hypoglycemia during the night with these alarms has been a very attractive reason for using CGM. Another key feature is the ability to follow trends and rates of change in BG levels. Small, short-term studies have demonstrated modest improvements in A1C (0.3%–0.6% reductions) in adults and children with type 1 diabetes.[76–79] However, just as for SMBG with a glucose meter, use of CGM requires a person to actively assess and react to their readings for this self-management tool to have an impact on A1C.[80]

GLYCOSYLATED HEMOGLOBIN

The glycosylated hemoglobin, or A1C, has become the gold standard for measuring chronic glycemia and is the clinical marker for predicting long-term complications, particularly microvascular complications. A1C is most commonly measured because it comprises the majority of glycosylated hemoglobin and is the least affected by recent fluctuations in BG. A1C measures the percentage of hemoglobin A that has been irreversibly glycosylated at the *N*-terminal amino group of the β-chain; the plasma glucose level and the life span of a red blood cell (RBC; ~120 days) determine its value. Thus, A1C is an indicator of glycemic control during the preceding 2 to 3 months. In patients without diabetes, A1C comprises approximately 4% to 6% of the total hemoglobin. Values may be three times this level in patients with diabetes.

The current A1C assay actually measures several different molecules of hemoglobin A ($HgbA_{1c}$, $HgbA_{1a}$, $HgbA_{1b}$, $HgbA_0$), not just A1C. Each laboratory establishes its own normal values for the A1C test (most are referenced to the normal range of 4%–6%). The International Federation of Clinical Chemistry has developed a new reference method that only measures glycated A1C (with a new unit of millimoles of A1C per mole of total hemoglobin).[81] The downside of this method is that the A1C values are 1.3% to 2.0% lower than the current values, which would cause great confusion among practitioners. The international A1C-derived Average Glucose (ADAG) trial provided correlations of A1C with mean plasma glucose by measuring both SMBG and CGM glucose values for a 3-month period, resulting in ~2,800 readings per A1C.[82] The following formula was developed to convert an A1C into an average glucose: $28.7 \times \text{A1C} - 46.7 = \text{eAG}$ (estimated average glucose). A formula that approximates this very closely and is much easier to use in practice is $(\text{A1C} - 2) \times 30$. The ADA now recommends reporting an eAG (units, mg/dL, or mmol/L) along with the A1C. An eAG calculator is available on their website to do this conversion (**http://diabetes.org/professional/eAG**). The correlation between A1C and eAG is shown in the following table.

A1C (%)	Estimated Average Plasma Glucose (mg/dL)
6	126
7	154
8	183
9	212
10	240
11	269
12	298

Hemoglobinopathies, such as sickle cell trait or chemically modified derivatives of hemoglobin as seen in uremia, in which hemoglobin becomes carbamylated, or acetylated hemoglobin with high-dose aspirin, can affect A1C values (increase or decrease depending on the assay), resulting in inaccurate indications of glycemic control. Alterations in red blood cell survival or turnover, seen in hemolytic anemia and acute blood loss, can falsely lower the A1C. Also a recent blood transfusion or use of intravenous (IV) iron therapy or erythropoietin-stimulating

TABLE 53-6
Factors Affecting A1C

Cause	Effect on A1C
Hemoglobinopathies (sickle cell trait, acetylated or carbamylated[a] hemoglobin)	Decreased or increased
Anemias	
Hemolytic	Decreased
Iron deficiency	Increased
Blood loss	Decreased
Blood transfusion	Decreased
Erythropoietin-stimulating agents	Decreased
Antioxidants	Decreased[b]

[a]Carbamylated hemoglobin equaling 0.063% of total hemoglobin is formed for every 1 mmol/L of serum urea.
[b]Reported with vitamins C (1 g/d) and E (1,200 mg/d). Possible mechanism is competitive inhibition of hemoglobin glycosylation.
A1C, glycosylated hemoglobin; RBC, red blood cell.
A detailed listing of factors that interfere with A1C test results is available at http://www.ngsp.org/factors.asp.

agents in patients with chronic kidney disease[83] can falsely lower A1C values. A glycated serum protein (fructosamine) should be considered for these patients. Antioxidants such as vitamins C and E also may interfere with the glycosylation process[84,85] (see Table 53-6 for details).

A1C can be measured without any special patient preparation (e.g., fasting) and generally is not subject to acute changes in insulin dosing, exercise, or diet. A1C values can be used as an adjunct to assessing overall glycemic control in patients with diabetes or to diagnose diabetes and prediabetes.[28] Normalization can indicate whether euglycemia has been achieved. However, A1C does not replace the day-to-day monitoring of BG concentrations, which is essential for evaluating acute changes in BG concentrations. These values are needed to adjust the meal plan or medication doses. Sometimes, an A1C is used to verify clinical impressions related to glucose control and patient adherence. It should be measured quarterly in patients who do not meet treatment goals, and at least semiannually in stable patients who are meeting treatment goals.

GLYCATED SERUM PROTEIN, GLYCATED SERUM ALBUMIN, AND FRUCTOSAMINE

Assays for glycated serum proteins reflect the extent of glycosylation of a variety of serum proteins, including glycated serum albumin.[74] The fructosamine assay is one of the most widely used methods to measure glycated proteins (normal, 2–2.8 mmol/L). Because the half-life of albumin is approximately 14 to 20 days, fructosamine provides an indication of glycemic control during a shorter time frame (1–2 weeks) than does the A1C. The ADA does not consider measurement of fructosamine equivalent to that of A1C, although it correlates well with this value. Fructosamine levels may be useful as an adjunct to A1C in determining whether a patient is improving or worsening in the short term (e.g., a patient on insulin therapy undergoing multiple dosage adjustments; for women with type 2 diabetes during pregnancy or gestational diabetes) or in patients with conditions such as hemolytic anemia in whom the A1C test is inaccurate (Table 53-6).

INSULIN

Insulin is a hormone secreted from the pancreatic β cell in response to glucose and other stimulants (e.g., amino acids, free fatty acids, gastric hormones, parasympathetic stimulation, β-adrenergic stimulation).[86,87] The hormone is made up of two polypeptide chains (a 21-amino acid A chain and a 30-amino acid B chain), which are connected by two disulfide bonds. Proinsulin, the precursor of insulin, is a single-chain, 86-amino acid polypeptide that is processed in the Golgi apparatus of β cells and then packaged into granules.[86] In the storage granule, the connecting or C-peptide is cleaved from proinsulin to produce equimolar amounts of insulin and C-peptide. Insulin and C-peptide are cosecreted, thus, measurable C-peptide levels indicate the presence of endogenously produced insulin and functioning β cells. Insulin is crucial to the survival of individuals with type 1 diabetes, whose β cells have been destroyed. It also plays a major role in the therapy of individuals with type 2 diabetes when their symptoms cannot be controlled with diet and exercise alone or a combination of antidiabetic agents. Insulin also is used in patients with type 2 diabetes during pregnancy or periods of intercurrent illness or stress (e.g., surgery).

ONLINE CONTENT

For a visual of the structure of the insulin molecule, go to http://thepoint.lww.com/AT10e.

Commercially available insulin products differ in their physical and chemical properties as well as in the pharmacokinetics of their action. Prior issues with immunogenicity have been eliminated through modern manufacturing processes and the cessation of use of animal-derived insulin products. Consequently, immunologically mediated sequelae, such as lipodystrophy, hypersensitivity, and insulin resistance caused by "blocking" antibodies, are extremely rare.

Pharmacokinetics: Absorption, Distribution, and Elimination

Regular insulin, a solution, is the only insulin that can be administered by any parenteral route: IV, intramuscularly (IM), or subcutaneously (SC). All other insulins are only to be used SC.

After SC injection, insulin is absorbed directly into the bloodstream, bypassing the lymphatic system. The rate-limiting step of insulin activity after SC administration is absorption of insulin from the injection site, which depends on the type of insulin administered, as well as a multitude of other factors. Variations in SC absorption can occur, primarily related to changes in blood flow around the injection site.

Endogenous insulin is secreted directly into the portal circulation and thus is primarily cleared by the liver in nondiabetic individuals (60%), with the kidneys removing only 35% to 40% of it.[86] Exogenous insulin is degraded at both renal and extrarenal (liver and muscle) sites. Degradation also takes place at the cellular level after internalization of the insulin–receptor complex. In contrast to endogenously secreted insulin, up to 60% of exogenous insulin is cleared from the systemic circulation by the kidneys, with the liver accounting for only 30% to 40% of its clearance. Insulin is filtered by glomerular capillaries, but more than 99% is reabsorbed by the proximal tubules. The insulin is then degraded in glomerular capillary cells and postglomerular peritubular cells.[88] See Case 53-8 for changes in insulin requirement in renal dysfunction.

When insulin is given IV, the half-lives for the three compartments are 2.3 to 2.4 minutes, 14 minutes, and 133 minutes. Insulin action most closely corresponds to the last compartment.[89] Therefore, it is unnecessary to adjust the dose more frequently than every 2 hours.

TABLE 53-7
Insulins Available in the United States[a]

Type/Duration of Action	Brand Name	Manufacturer
Rapid-Acting		
Insulin lispro	Humalog	Lilly
Insulin aspart	NovoLog	Novo Nordisk
Insulin glulisine	Apidra	sanofi-aventis
Short-Acting		
Regular	Humulin R[b] Novolin R	Lilly Novo Nordisk
Intermediate-Acting		
NPH (isophane insulin suspension)	Humulin N Novolin N	Lilly Novo Nordisk
Long-Acting		
Insulin glargine	Lantus	sanofi-aventis
Insulin detemir	Levemir	Novo Nordisk
Premixed Insulins		
NPH/regular (70%/30%)	Humulin 70/30 Novolin 70/30	Lilly Novo Nordisk
Insulin aspart protamine suspension/insulin aspart (70%/30%)	NovoLog Mix 70/30	Novo Nordisk
Insulin lispro protamine suspension/insulin lispro (75%/25%)	Humalog Mix 75/25	Lilly
Insulin lispro protamine suspension/insulin lispro (50%/50%)	Humalog Mix 50/50	Lilly

[a]Insulin is made through recombinant DNA technology. Only regular and NPH are human insulin. All other insulins are human insulin analogs. All insulins available in the United States have a concentration of 100 units/mL (U-100), except as noted.
[b]A U-500 concentration is available for use in rare circumstances in patients with severe insulin resistance requiring very large insulin doses.
NPH, neutral protamine Hagedorn, or isophane insulin suspension.

Pharmacodynamics

Clinically, the most important differences among insulin products relate to their onset, peak, and duration of action (not the actual insulin levels, which is pharmacokinetics). Current insulin products can be categorized as rapid-acting, short-acting, intermediate-acting, and long-acting insulin. Products available in the United States are listed in Table 53-7, and the onset of action, peak effect, and durations of action of each insulin category are listed in Table 53-8. However, these data are derived primarily from studies in normal, healthy volunteers in the fasting state or in well-controlled patients with diabetes stabilized in a metabolic ward. In actuality, intersubject and intrasubject variations in response to insulin can be substantial because an individual pattern of response to insulin can be affected by numerous factors (e.g., the formation of insulin hexamers, the presence of insulin-binding antibodies, dose, exercise, site of injection, massage of the injection site, ambient temperature, and interactions between insulins that have been mixed together; see Table 53-10 later in this chapter and Case 53-2, Question 14).[89,90] Nevertheless, knowledge of when one might expect the various insulins to exert their effects is absolutely essential to the rational adjustment of insulin dosages.

RAPID-ACTING INSULIN

INSULIN LISPRO

Insulin lispro (Humalog) was the first available rapid-acting insulin analog. The natural amino acid sequence of the insulin B chain at positions 28 (proline) and 29 (lysine) is inverted to form lispro. This change results in an insulin molecule that more loosely self-associates into hexamers than does regular human insulin. Consequently, the active monomeric form is more readily available, resulting in an onset of activity (15 minutes), peak action (60–90 minutes), and duration (3–4 hours) that more closely simulates physiological insulin secretion relative to meals. Because it can be injected shortly before eating (0–15 minutes), lispro, and all rapid-acting insulins, provide patients greater flexibility in lifestyle. These insulins lower 2-hour postprandial BG levels, and can decrease the risk of late postprandial and nocturnal hypoglycemia compared with regular insulin formulations.[91] Patients who use an insulin pump most often use a rapid-acting insulin instead of regular insulin. One randomized, two-way, crossover, open-label study compared lispro with regular insulin administered for 3 months by continuous SC insulin infusion.[92] Lispro resulted in A1C values that were significantly lower than those produced by regular insulin (7.41% vs. 7.65%). There were no differences in adverse events. Because lispro has a shorter duration of action than regular insulin, hyperglycemia and ketosis may occur more rapidly in patients with type 1 diabetes if insulin pump delivery is inadvertently interrupted or if the basal insulin dose is missed. Insulin lispro is approved for use in pediatrics (studies included children age 3 and older), and it is pregnancy category B.[93]

INSULIN ASPART

Insulin aspart (NovoLog) is a rapid-acting insulin analog that differs from human insulin by substitution of aspartic acid at B28. Insulin aspart is approved for use in pediatric patients,

TABLE 53-8
Insulin Pharmacodynamics[a]

Insulin	Onset (hours)	Peak (hours)	Duration (hours)	Appearance
Rapid-acting (insulin aspart, glulisine, and lispro)	5–15 minutes	30–90 minutes	<5	Clear
Regular	0.5–1	2–4	5–7	Clear
NPH	2–4	4–12	12–18	Cloudy
Insulin glargine	1.5	No pronounced peak	20–24	Clear[b]
Insulin detemir	0.8–2	Relatively flat	5.7–23.2	Clear[b]

[a]The onset, peak, and duration of insulin activity may vary considerably from times listed in this table. See text and Table 53-12.
[b]Should not be mixed with other insulins. Some patients require twice-daily dosing.
Source: Levemir [package insert]. Bagsværd, Denmark: Novo Nordisk Inc; July 2009; DeWitt DE, Hirsch IB. Outpatient insulin therapy in type 1 and type 2 diabetes mellitus: scientific review. *JAMA*. 2003;289:2254.

age 2 and older.[94] It is pregnancy category B. Insulin aspart controls postprandial glucose excursions similarly to insulin lispro.

INSULIN GLULISINE

Insulin glulisine (Apidra) is a rapid-acting insulin analog that differs from human insulin by substitution of lysine for asparagine at position B3 and glutamic acid for lysine at position B23. Insulin glulisine has been studied in pediatric patients age 4 and older.[95] It is pregnancy category C. Insulin glulisine lowers postprandial glucose excursions similarly to insulin lispro and insulin aspart.

Other routes for insulin have been studied, including dermal, nasal, buccal, oral, and pulmonary inhalation. Previously, an inhaled human insulin powder was available, but has since been discontinued owing to infrequent use. Another inhaled insulin, Technosphere human insulin inhalation powder (Afrezza, MannKind Corp.), a mealtime insulin, is under review by the FDA.[96] Oral-lyn (Generex Biotechnology Corp.), an oral insulin spray in which insulin is absorbed across the lining of the mouth, is available for restricted use through the FDA's Treatment Investigational New Drug Program.

SHORT-ACTING INSULIN

Regular insulin has an onset of action of 30 to 60 minutes, a peak effect at 2 to 4 hours, and a duration of action of 5 to 7 hours. The broad range in peak effect and duration reflects the many variables that affect insulin action (Table 53-8). The 30- to 60-minute onset of action requires proper timing of premeal regular insulin, which is difficult for most patients. Use of regular insulin in patients with type 1 diabetes is much less common with the advent of the rapid-acting insulins.

INTERMEDIATE-ACTING INSULIN

NPH

NPH (neutral protamine Hagedorn or isophane) is an intermediate-acting insulin. Its onset of action is approximately 2 hours (range, 1–3 hours), peak effects occur at approximately 6 to 14 hours, and the duration of action of NPH is approximately 16 to 24 hours. Again, it must be emphasized that this pattern of response is at best a generalization. Patients may have a variable pattern of response to NPH insulin with time, and those on higher doses are likely to have a later peak and a longer duration of action. Up to 80% of these day-to-day fluctuations in BG responses can be accounted for by variation in the absorption of this intermediate-acting insulin.[89]

LONG-ACTING INSULIN

INSULIN GLARGINE

Insulin glargine (Lantus) is a long-acting insulin that serves to provide a basal level of insulin. It is pregnancy category C.[97] It is approved for once a day SC administration for the treatment of adult and pediatric patients (age $\geq$6 year) with type 1 diabetes or adult patients with type 2 diabetes. It can be administered any time during the day, but it is important to take it at the same time each day. It is usually administered at bedtime or, less commonly, in the morning.

Insulin glargine is an insulin analog in which asparagine in position A21 is substituted with glycine and two arginines are added to the *C*-terminus of the B chain. This change in the amino acid sequence causes a shift in the isoelectric point from pH 5.4 to 6.7, making it more soluble at an acidic pH.[98] Once injected, insulin glargine (which is a clear solution with a pH of 4.0) precipitates at physiological pH, forming a depot that releases insulin slowly for 24 hours. This results in delayed absorption and a less pronounced peak compared with NPH insulin.[99] Zinc is added to further prolong the duration of insulin glargine. In clinical trials of patients with types 1 and 2 diabetes, once-daily injections of insulin glargine were as effective as NPH in lowering A1C values, with less nocturnal hypoglycemia.[100] Insulin glargine is associated with more injection site pain compared with NPH (6.1% vs. 0.3% in one study and 2.7% vs. 0.7% in another), which is likely related to its acidity.[97,101] Some patients report that they feel the insulin glargine injection more than they do other insulins.

Recently, several epidemiologic studies have assessed the risk of cancer from insulin use. Three studies have reported an increased risk of cancer with insulin glargine; one found a dose-dependent increased risk of cancer for insulin glargine compared with human insulin (e.g., hazard ratio of 1.09, 1.19, and 1.31 for total daily doses of 10 units, 30 units, and 50 units, respectively).[102] A second found a significantly increased risk of breast cancer in women who used insulin glargine alone (relative risk, 1.99) but not in those on insulin glargine plus other insulins.[103] A third trial reported an increased risk of cancer (hazard ratio, 1.55) in patients on insulin glargine alone, whereas those on insulin glargine plus other insulins had a slight, insignificantly lower incidence of cancer (hazard ratio, 0.81).[104] These findings contrast with those of a UK study[105] and an analysis of 31 randomized controlled trials from the sanofi-aventis safety database (phase 2, 3, and 4 studies),[106] in which no link between insulin glargine and cancer was identified. Given the significant limitations of these studies (potential for different pretreatment characteristics of the groups, selection bias, the small numbers of cancer cases found, and short duration of follow-up) and that type 2 diabetes itself is associated with an increased risk of cancer (e.g., colon, pancreas, and breast), we feel these studies do not provide conclusive evidence of an increased risk of cancer associated with insulin glargine.

INSULIN DETEMIR

Insulin detemir (Levemir) is the other basal insulin available in the United States and is approved for once- or twice-daily SC administration for the treatment of adult and pediatric patients (age $\geq$6 years) with type 1 diabetes or adult patients with type 2 diabetes. It is pregnancy category C.[107] Unlike other insulin analogs, in which the amino acid sequence is modified, for insulin detemir a fatty acid moiety is added to the last amino acid on the end of the B chain. Insulin detemir is a neutral, soluble insulin preparation in which the B30 threonine has been removed and the B29 lysine residue has been covalently bound to a 14-carbon fatty acid. The result is an insulin that is more slowly absorbed in the SC tissue because the fatty acid moiety binds to albumin, creating a long-acting insulin.[108] Insulin determir's kinetics and dynamics are dose dependent.[109] When used in type 1 diabetes, two injections daily are usually required to provide adequate basal coverage. Insulin detemir demonstrates less intrasubject variability than NPH or insulin glargine.[110] The clinical significance and impact of this observation is unclear.

ONLINE CONTENT

For a summary table of the amino acid changes for the insulin analogs compared with human insulin, go to http://thepoint.lww.com/AT10e.

PREMIXED INSULIN

Products that contain premixed NPH and regular insulin in a fixed ratio of 70:30 are available from Lilly as Humulin 70/30 and from Novo Nordisk as Novolin 70/30. Additional premixed formulations are available in which both insulin lispro and insulin aspart have been cocrystallized with protamine to create an intermediate-acting insulin similar to NPH. Humalog Mix 75/25 and Humalog Mix 50/50 (Lilly) are products with lispro protamine and insulin lispro in a fixed ratio of 75:25 and 50:50, respectively. NovoLog Mix 70/30 (Novo Nordisk) is aspart protamine and insulin aspart in a fixed ratio of 70:30. These premixed insulins are useful for patients who have difficulty measuring and mixing insulins and are dosed twice daily. These insulins are compatible when mixed together and retain their individual pharmacodynamic profiles (see Table 53-20 later in this chapter and Case 53-2, Question 15).

TREATMENT OF TYPE 1 DIABETES: CLINICAL USE OF INSULIN

Clinical Presentation of Type 1 Diabetes

CASE 53-2

QUESTION 1: A.H., a slender, 18-year-old woman who was recently discharged from the hospital for severe dehydration and mild ketoacidosis, is referred to the Diabetes Clinic from the University Student Health Service (no records available). A fasting and a random plasma glucose ordered subsequently were 190 mg/dL and 250 mg/dL. Approximately 4 weeks before she was hospitalized, A.H. had moved across the country to attend college—her first time away from home. In retrospect, she remembers that she had symptoms of polydipsia, nocturia (six times a night), fatigue, and a 12-pound weight loss during this period, which she attributed to the anxiety associated with her move away from home and adjustment to her new environment. Her medical history is remarkable for recurrent upper respiratory infections and three cases of vaginal moniliasis in the past 6 months. Her family history is negative for diabetes, and she takes no medications.

Physical examination is within normal limits. She weighs 50 kg and is 5 feet 4 inches tall. Laboratory results are as follows: FPG, 280 mg/dL; A1C, 14%; and trace urine ketones as measured by Keto-Diastix. On the basis of her history and laboratory findings, the presumptive diagnosis is type 1 diabetes. Which findings are consistent with this diagnosis in A.H.?

A.H. meets several of the diagnostic criteria for diabetes. She has classic symptoms of the disease (polyuria, polydipsia, weight loss, glucosuria, fatigue, recurrent infections), a random plasma glucose greater than 200 mg/dL, an FPG of 126 mg/dL or more on at least two occasions, and an A1C of 6.5% or more[7] (Tables 53-1 and 53-2). Features of A.H.'s history that are consistent with type 1 diabetes, in particular, include the relatively acute onset of symptoms in association with a major life event (moving away from home), ketones in the urine, negative family history, and a relatively young age at onset.

Treatment Goals

CASE 53-2, QUESTION 2: A.H. will be started on insulin therapy on this visit. What are the goals of therapy? Will normoglycemia prevent the development or progression of long-term complications?

The goal of diabetes management is the prevention of acute and chronic complications. The results of the DCCT and DCCT-EDIC studies convincingly demonstrated that lowering BG concentrations through intensive insulin therapy in persons with type 1 diabetes slows or prevents the development of microvascular complications.[38,39] The ADA recommends an A1C goal of less than 7% for patients in general and an individual goal as close to normal as possible (<6%) without significant hypoglycemia.

It is important to understand that physiological or basal-bolus insulin therapy involves a *complete* program of diabetes management that includes a balanced meal plan, physical activity, frequent SMBG, and insulin adjustments based on these factors (Tables 53-4 and 53-9). Because the patient is the key member of the team, A.H. must be highly motivated and able to learn about the complex metabolic interplay between insulin therapy and lifestyle.

In summary, A.H. is a patient newly diagnosed with type 1 diabetes who has not yet developed any signs or symptoms of long-term complications. Therefore, she is an ideal candidate for basal-bolus insulin therapy, and if she is willing and motivated, normoglycemia with rare hypoglycemic reactions is a reasonable long-term goal. This goal should be achieved gradually over the course of several months with insulin therapy, diet, education, and strong clinical support. A desirable goal is an A1C value as close to the normal range as possible with rare hypoglycemic reactions.

TABLE 53-9
Components of Physiological Insulin Therapy

Multicomponent insulin regimen of basal plus preprandial insulin doses
Balance of carbohydrate intake, exercise, and insulin dosage
Daily, multiple self-monitoring of blood glucose levels
Patient self-adjustment of carbohydrate intake and insulin dosage with use of correction or supplemental rapid- or short-acting insulin according to a predetermined plan
Individualized target blood glucose and A1C levels
Frequent contact between patient and diabetes team
Intensive patient education
Psychological support
Regular objective assessment (as measured by A1C)

A1C, glycosylated hemoglobin.
Source: Skyler JS. Tactics for type I diabetes. *Endocrinol Metab Clin North Am.* 1997;26:647.

Basal-Bolus (Physiological) Insulin Therapy

CASE 53-2, QUESTION 3: What methods of insulin administration are available to achieve optimal glucose control?

A physiological insulin regimen is designed to mimic normal insulin secretion as closely as possible. Problems with insulin delivery include factors that affect the SC absorption of insulin (Table 53-10). Before the development of the rapid-acting insulin analogs and basal insulins, previous insulins lacked pharmacodynamic profiles that allowed one to closely simulate normal pancreatic release of the hormone. In the nondiabetic individual, the pancreas secretes boluses of insulin in response to snacks and meals. Between meals and throughout the night, the pancreas secretes small amounts of insulin that are sufficient to suppress lipolysis and hepatic glucose output (basal insulin). Clinicians now have more tools to mimic this basal-bolus model. Two methods have been used to achieve this pattern of insulin release: (a) insulin pump therapy (previously referred to as continuous subcutaneous infusion of insulin) and (b) basal-bolus insulin regimens consisting of once- or twice-daily doses of basal insulin

TABLE 53-10
Factors Altering Onset and Duration of Insulin Action

Factor	Comments
Route of administration	Onset of action more rapid and duration of action shorter for IV > IM > SC.[111,112] Intrapulmonary insulin has onset and duration comparable to SC rapid-acting insulins.[113]
Factors altering clearance	
Renal function	Renal failure lowers insulin clearance; may prolong and intensify action of exogenous and endogenous insulin.[86]
Insulin antibodies	IgG antibodies bind insulin as it is absorbed and release it slowly, thereby delaying or prolonging its effect.[114]
Thyroid function	Hyperthyroidism increases clearance, but also increases insulin action, making control difficult; patients stabilize as they become euthyroid.[115]
Factors altering SC absorption	Factors that raise SC blood flow ↑ absorption rates of regular insulin; effect on intermediate- and long-acting insulins is minimal.
Site of injection	Rate of absorption is fastest from the abdomen, intermediate from the arm, and slowest from the thigh.[112] Less variation is observed in type 2 diabetes patients; less variation is observed with current rapid-acting and long-acting insulins.
	Site — *Half-life absorption (minutes)*
	Abdomen — 87 ± 12
	Arm — 141 ± 23
	Hip — 153 ± 28
	Thigh — 164 ± 15
Exercise of injected area	Strenuous exercise of an injected area within 1 hour of injection can increase absorption rate; rate of absorption of regular insulin is increased, but little effect on intermediate-acting insulin.[116,117]
Ambient temperature	Heat (e.g., hot weather, hot bath, sauna) increases absorption rate; cold has opposite effect.[117–119]
Local massage	Massaging injected area for 30 minutes substantially increases absorption rate of regular insulin as well as longer-acting insulins.[115]
Smoking	Controversial; vasoconstriction may decrease absorption rate.[89]
Jet injectors	Insulin absorption is more rapid, probably secondary to increases in surface area for absorption.[120,121]
Lipohypertrophy	Insulin absorption is delayed from lipohypertrophic sites.[122]
Insulin preparation	More soluble forms of insulin are absorbed more rapidly and have shorter durations of action (see Table 53-8 and text); human insulin may have shorter action than animal insulin.
Insulin mixtures	The short-acting properties of rapid-acting insulins may be blunted if mixed with NPH insulin (see Case 53-2, Question 15).
Insulin concentration	More dilute solutions (e.g., U-40, U-10) are absorbed more rapidly than more concentrated forms (U-100, U-500).
Insulin dose	Lower doses are absorbed more rapidly and have a shorter duration of action than larger doses.

IgG, immunoglobulin G; IM, intramuscular; IV, intravenous; NPH, neutral protamine Hagedorn; SC, subcutaneous.

coupled with premeal doses of rapid- or short-acting insulin (see Case 53-2, Questions 3–5).

INSULIN PUMP THERAPY

The use of an insulin pump is currently the most precise way to mimic normal insulin secretion. This consists of a battery-operated pump and a computer that can program the pump to deliver predetermined amounts of insulin (i.e., regular, lispro, aspart, or glulisine) from a reservoir to a subcutaneously inserted catheter or needle.[123,124] These systems are portable and designed to deliver various basal amounts of insulin over the course of 24 hours as well as meal-related boluses. Most patients using an insulin pump use a rapid-acting insulin, rather than regular insulin. For meal coverage, the rapid-acting insulin can be given 0 to 15 minutes before eating. The delivery of the bolus can be adjusted depending on the type of food eaten (e.g., piece of cake versus slice of pizza). Caveat: If SC delivery is discontinued, check for rise in glucose and urine ketones after 2 or 3 hours. Because there is no SC pool, effects dissipate quickly.

The preferred meal-planning approach for patients using an insulin pump is carbohydrate counting. The insulin to carbohydrate ratio, or how much carbohydrate is covered by 1 unit of insulin, must be determined. One method is to use the "500 Rule." The number 500 (or 450 for regular insulin) is divided by the total daily dose of insulin the patient is using to determine the insulin to carbohydrate ratio (see Case 53-2, Question 11). Insulin pumps are capable of delivering many basal insulin rates. The basal insulin infusion rate may be adjusted depending on the situation. Many patients find it advantageous to decrease the basal rate during the middle of the night when nocturnal hypoglycemia is most likely to occur. The basal rate also may be increased before awakening to avoid hyperglycemia secondary to the "dawn phenomenon"—adjustments that are not possible using SC basal insulin injections.

ONLINE CONTENT

For a narrated PowerPoint presentation on an example of an insulin pump basal rate and bolus (insulin:carbohydrate) ratios go to http://thepoint.lww.com/AT10e.

Features of the current pump models include the "bolus wizard," which calculates bolus doses based on preset carbohydrate to insulin ratios and correction factors, carbohydrate counts for selected foods, and an "insulin-on-board" feature, which helps avoid excessive dosing of insulin by indicating how much insulin from a previously administered dose should still be acting. Most insurance plans provide coverage for insulin pumps for patients with type 1 diabetes and for some patients with type 2 diabetes. Factors to consider when choosing a pump include safety features, durability, ability of the manufacturer to provide service, availability of training, clinically desirable features, and cosmetic attractiveness for the user.[124,125] The ADA website (www.diabetes.org) contains helpful information about insulin pumps for patients under the Living with Diabetes section.

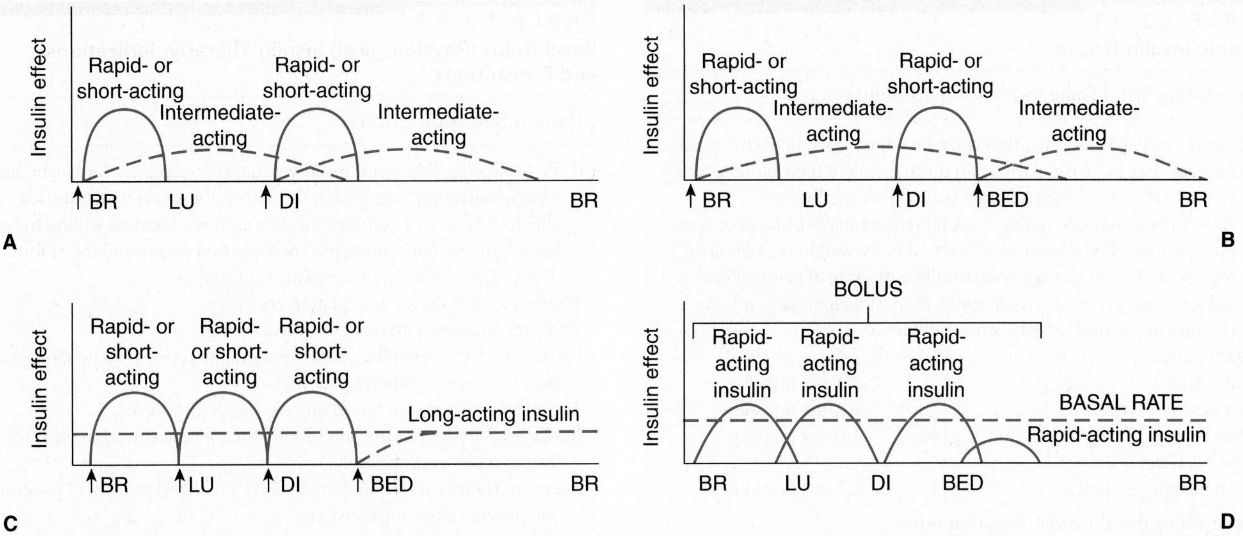

FIGURE 53-4 Theoretical insulin effect provided by various insulin regimens. A: Two daily injections of rapid-acting (insulin aspart, glulisine, or lispro) or short-acting (regular) and intermediate-acting insulin (NPH). **B:** Morning injection of rapid-acting or short-acting insulin and intermediate-acting insulin, a predinner injection of rapid-acting or short-acting insulin, and a bedtime injection of intermediate-acting insulin. Suggested for patients with early-morning hypoglycemia, and also those who have early-morning hyperglycemia (owing to rebound phenomenon from hypoglycemia). **C:** Premeal injections of rapid-acting or short-acting insulin and long-acting (e.g., insulin glargine or detemir) or intermediate-acting insulin (NPH) at bedtime. **D:** Continuous subcutaneous insulin infusion, showing an example with bolus given for a bedtime snack. BR, breakfast; Bed, bedtime; LU, lunch; DI, dinner. Arrows indicate time of insulin injection (<15 minutes before meals for rapid-acting insulin and 30 minutes before meals for short-acting insulin).

MULTIPLE DAILY INJECTIONS

CASE 53-2, QUESTION 4: How can insulin injections be administered to A.H. in a way that mimics the physiological release of insulin from the pancreas?

Endocrinologists have developed a variety of insulin regimens that are intended to mimic the release of insulin from the pancreas.[126,127] Examples of these are displayed in and illustrated in Figure 53-4. A total daily dose of insulin is estimated empirically (e.g., 0.5 units/kg/day) or according to guidelines listed in Table 53-11. The total daily dose of insulin then is split into several doses. In general, the basal dose comprises approximately 50% of the total daily dose.

A regimen much less commonly used in patients with type 1 diabetes involves injecting a mixture of intermediate-acting and regular or rapid-acting insulin twice daily, before breakfast and before dinner (Fig. 53-4A). The morning dose of regular or rapid-acting insulin is intended to take care of the breakfast meal; the morning dose of NPH takes care of the noon meal and provides basal insulin throughout the day; the evening dose of regular or rapid-acting insulin takes care of the evening meal; and the evening dose of NPH provides basal insulin levels during the night and takes care of any evening snack that is ingested. Because NPH is an intermediate-acting insulin and has a peak effect, it does not provide true basal insulin coverage. Also, when NPH is injected in the morning, the patient must eat lunch on time because of this peak effect; otherwise he or she will experience hypoglycemia. Also, when NPH is taken with mealtime insulin before dinner, the patient is at risk for nocturnal hypoglycemia from the peak effect of the evening dose of NPH. The advantage of using a rapid-acting insulin (e.g., insulin lispro, insulin aspart, or insulin glulisine) instead of regular insulin in this regimen is to facilitate the patient being able to take insulin doses immediately before a meal. However, the peak effect of the NPH component in this combined dose still presents the same problems. This type of insulin regimen does not mimic physiological insulin release.

Figure 53-4B depicts a variation of this method. It is the same except that the evening dose of NPH is given as a third injection at bedtime. This shifts the time of peak effect from approximately 2 to 3 AM to approximately 7 AM. By administering NPH at bedtime, nocturnal hypoglycemia is reduced, and peak insulin activity occurs when the patient is more likely to be awake and ingesting food. This method may be useful for patients in whom nocturnal hypoglycemia and fasting hyperglycemia are particularly troublesome; however, this regimen also does not mimic physiological insulin release.

The regimen that most closely mimics physiological insulin release besides the use of an insulin pump is the use of a once-daily basal insulin such as insulin glargine or insulin detemir to provide basal insulin levels throughout the day, along with doses of a rapid-acting insulin (preferred) or regular insulin before meals (Fig. 53-4C depicts the long-acting insulin given at bedtime, but it can be given alternatively in the morning). When smaller doses are used, twice-daily insulin detemir and possibly insulin glargine will be required for 24-hour coverage.[128–130] This method theoretically provides insulin similar to the insulin pump: constant basal levels plus small boluses for meals and snacks. In doing so, it offers some of the same advantages of the pump in that it permits some degree of flexibility in the patient's lifestyle. For example, if a patient with diabetes chooses to skip a meal, he or she omits a premeal bolus; if the patient chooses to eat a larger meal than usual, he or she increases the premeal bolus. Similar dose adjustments can be made to accommodate snacks, exercise patterns, and acute illnesses. Caveat: Insulin glargine and insulin detemir must be injected separately; that is, they may not be mixed in the same syringe with other insulins.

CASE 53-2, QUESTION 5: Should A.H. use an insulin pump or multiple insulin injections?

Indications for basal-bolus insulin therapy are listed in Table 53-12. Patients with type 1 diabetes should be placed on a basal-bolus insulin regimen. A.H. is an ideal candidate to strive for an A1C close to 6%. She is newly diagnosed, has not yet developed the long-term complications of diabetes, and should derive the benefits of normoglycemia. Assuming A.H. will be able to manage a basal-bolus insulin regimen, individualized target BG levels

TABLE 53-11
Empiric Insulin Doses

Estimating Total Daily Insulin Requirements

These are initial doses only; they must be adjusted using SMBG results. Patients may be particularly resistant to insulin if their blood glucose concentrations are high (glucose toxicity); once glucose concentrations begin to drop, insulin requirements often decrease precipitously. The weight used is actual body weight. Insulin dose requirements can change dramatically with time depending on circumstances (e.g., a growth spurt, modest weight gain or loss, changes in physical activity, stress or illness).

Type 1 diabetes	
Initial dose	0.3–0.5 units/kg
Honeymoon phase	0.2–0.5 units/kg
With ketosis, during illness, during growth	1.0–1.5 units/kg
Type 2 diabetes	
With insulin resistance	0.7–1.5 units/kg

Estimating Basal Insulin Requirements

These are empiric doses only and should be adjusted using appropriate SMBG results (fasting or premeal). Basal requirements vary throughout the day, often increasing during the early morning hours. The basal requirement also is influenced by the presence of endogenous insulin, the degree of insulin resistance, and body weight. Basal requirements are approximately 50% of total daily insulin needs. Thus, basal insulin dose is approximately 50% of TDD. A conservative approach is to reduce the calculated 50% basal dose by 20% to avoid hypoglycemia.[127]

Estimating Premeal Insulin Requirements

The premeal insulin requirements are approximately 50% of the TDD, usually divided equally into three doses initially, taken with each meal (i.e., breakfast, lunch, and dinner), and then each premeal dose is individually adjusted based on BG readings.

The "500 rule" estimates the number of grams of carbohydrate that will be covered by 1 unit of rapid-acting insulin. The rule is modified to the "450 rule" if using regular insulin.

500/TDD of insulin = number of grams covered

Example: For a patient using 50 units/d, 500/50 = 10. Therefore, 10 g of carbohydrate would be covered by 1 unit of insulin lispro, glulisine, or aspart. This equation works very well for type 1 diabetes patients in estimating their premeal insulin requirements. Because patients with type 2 diabetes have insulin resistance, the rule may underestimate their insulin requirements.

Determining the "Correction Factor"

Supplemental doses of rapid-acting insulin are administered to acutely lower glucose concentrations that exceed the target glucose concentration. These doses must be individualized for each patient and again are based on the degree of sensitivity to insulin action. For example, if the premeal blood glucose target is 120 mg/dL and the patient's value is 190 mg/dL, additional units of rapid-acting insulin could be added to the premeal dose. The correction factor determines how far the blood glucose drops per unit of insulin given and is known as the "1,700 rule." For regular insulin, the rule is modified to the "1,500 rule." The equation is as follows:

1,700/TDD = point drop in blood glucose per unit of insulin

Example: If a patient uses 28 units/d of insulin, their correction factor (or insulin sensitivity) would be 1,700/28 = 60 mg/dL. Therefore, the patient can expect a 60-mg/dL drop for every unit of rapid-acting insulin administered. Patients with a higher sensitivity factor have lower insulin requirements. Individuals with a lower sensitivity factor (higher insulin requirements) typically achieve a smaller reduction in blood glucose per unit of insulin.

SMBG, self-monitored blood glucose; TDD, total daily dose.
Source: DeWitt DE, Hirsch IB. Outpatient insulin therapy in type 1 and type 2 diabetes mellitus: scientific review. *JAMA*. 2003;289:2254; Walsh J, Roberts R. *Pumping Insulin: Everything You Need For Success On A Smart Insulin Pump*. 4th ed. San Diego, CA: Torrey Pines Press; 2006; Walsh J et al. *Using Insulin: Everything You Need for Success With Insulin*. San Diego, CA: Torrey Pine Press; 2003.

TABLE 53-12
Basal-Bolus (Physiological) Insulin Therapy: Indications and Precautions

Patient Selection Criteria

Type 1 diabetes, otherwise healthy patients (>7 years of age) who are highly motivated, engaged in diabetes self-management, and are able to adhere to a complex insulin regimen. Must be willing to test blood glucose concentrations multiple times daily and inject four doses of insulin daily, on average.
Women with diabetes who plan to conceive.
Pregnant patients with diabetes (pre-existing).
Patients poorly controlled on conventional therapy, 2–3 injections daily (includes type 2 diabetes patients).
Technical ability to test blood glucose concentrations.
Intellectual ability to interpret blood glucose concentrations and adjust insulin doses appropriately.
Access to trained and skilled medical staff to direct treatment program and provide close supervision.

Avoid or Use Cautiously in Patients Who Are Predisposed to Severe Hypoglycemic Reactions or in Whom Such Reactions Could Be Fatal

Patients with counterregulatory insufficiency.
β-Adrenergic blocker therapy.
Autonomic insufficiency.
Adrenal or pituitary insufficiency.
Patients with coronary or cerebral vascular disease.
(*Note:* Counterregulatory hormones released in response to hypoglycemia may have adverse effects in these individuals.)
Unreliable, nonadherent individuals, including those who abuse alcohol or drugs and those with psychiatric disorders.

that strive for the best level of glucose control possible without placing her at undue risk for hypoglycemia should be prescribed. She must be willing to test her BG concentrations four or more times daily and inject herself four times daily or learn about the use and care of an insulin pump. She also must be willing to keep detailed BG and food records and participate in an extensive education program that enables her to adjust her insulin doses based on BG concentrations, physical activity, and the carbohydrate content of her snacks and meals.

Transition to an insulin pump is facilitated by patients being able to attain these skills using multiple daily SC insulin injections before insulin pump initiation. The ADA recommends that the use of insulin pumps be limited to highly motivated individuals under the guidance of a health care team trained and knowledgeable in their use. Pumps offer the patient the ability to use multiple basal rates during the 24-hour period and assist with the calculation of bolus and correction insulin doses. Most studies have shown that pump therapy provides equivalent and sometimes better glycemic control than does intensive management with multiple injections.[131,132]

Insulin pumps are particularly useful in patients with frequent, unpredictable hypoglycemia or marked dawn phenomena (see Case 53-3). Others have described the methods by which insulin doses are established and altered in patients using the insulin pump.[125,133] Because A.H. has just been diagnosed, she should be initiated on a basal-bolus SC insulin therapy. Once she has acquired these skills, she may be considered for pump therapy.

Clinical Use of Insulin

INITIATING INSULIN THERAPY

CASE 53-2, QUESTION 6: How should multiple-dose insulin therapy be initiated in A.H.?

TABLE 53-13
Self-Monitored Blood Glucose Testing: Areas of Patient Education

When and How Often To Test

Technique

How and when to calibrate the glucose monitor.
Review all "buttons" and their purposes. Identify battery type. Review cleaning procedures, if applicable.
Preparation
1. Calibrate monitor/set code for batch of test strips, if required.
2. Insert test strip to turn machine on (some meters require user to turn machine on).
3. Prepare all materials: tissue, strip, lancet.
4. Remember to close the lid of the strip container immediately. Strips exposed to air and moisture deteriorate rapidly.
5. Wash hands with warm water. *Dry thoroughly.* A wet finger causes blood to spread rather than form a drop. Milk the finger from the base to ensure an adequate flow of blood.
6. Lance the tip of the finger. Avoid the pads of the finger where nerve endings are concentrated.
7. Hold the finger *below* the heart with the lanced area pointing toward the floor.
8. Once a sufficient amount of blood is available, *quickly* apply blood to designated area of the test strip. Depending on the strip type, the blood sample is placed in an area on the surface of the strip or it is applied to the side of the strip where it is taken up by capillary action.

Record Results in a Log Book and Bring to All Clinician Visits. Include relevant information regarding diet or exercise.

How To Use Results To Achieve Glycemic Targets; Educate Patients on What To Do With Their Blood Glucose Readings (e.g., adjust their insulin dose; modify their carbohydrate content).

A conservative total daily dose of insulin is estimated empirically or according to guidelines similar to those listed in Table 53-11 in newly diagnosed patients. For a basal-bolus insulin regimen, insulin glargine or insulin detemir is used as the basal insulin with bolus doses of a rapid- or short-acting insulin (insulin lispro, insulin aspart, insulin glulisine, or regular) given at mealtime. During the initial visit, A.H. needs to learn how to inject her insulin (see Case 53-2, Question 8), how to test her BG (Table 53-13), how and when to test her urine for ketones, and how to recognize and treat hypoglycemia (Table 53-14). She also needs to understand the importance of meal planning and the relationship between carbohydrate intake and insulin action (Table 53-15). It is very important not to overwhelm A.H. with information on the first visit. One should be particularly sensitive to the psychological impact of this diagnosis on A.H., address her major concerns, and provide only the information that is absolutely essential before the next visit. Between visits, she should be assessed and provided information on an as-needed basis by phone. Table 53-16 lists important areas of patient education.

A reasonable first approach for A.H. is to provide a total daily dose of insulin of 24 units (~0.5 units/kg). Because 50% of the daily dose should be given as basal insulin with the remainder given as rapid-acting insulin divided into three doses, A.H. would take the following: 12 units of insulin glargine once daily (morning or bedtime) with 4 units of insulin aspart given approximately 15 minutes before each meal.[134] Alternatively, if insulin detemir is used, the dose would generally be split twice daily, or 6 units BID. An alternative regimen using NPH would be 8 units of NPH in the morning with 8 units of aspart, 4 units of aspart with dinner, and 4 units of NPH at bedtime. Caveat: As A.H.'s glucose concentration returns to normal, glucose toxicity will recede and she may require less insulin.

TABLE 53-14
Hypoglycemia

Definition

Blood glucose concentration <60 mg/dL: Patient may or may not be symptomatic.
Blood glucose <40 mg/dL: Patient is generally symptomatic.
Blood glucose <20 mg/dL: Can be associated with seizures and coma.

Signs and Symptoms

Blurred vision, sweaty palms, generalized sweating, tremulousness, hunger, confusion, anxiety, circumoral tingling, and numbness. Patients vary with regard to their symptoms. Behavior can be confused with alcohol inebriation. Patients become combative and use poor judgment.
Nocturnal hypoglycemia: nightmares, restless sleep, profuse sweating, morning headache, morning "hangover." Not all patients have symptoms during nocturnal hypoglycemia.

Clinical Considerations

Irregular eating patterns
↑ Physical exercise
Gastroparesis (delayed gastric emptying)
Defective counterregulatory responses
Excessive dose of insulin or insulin secretagogues (sulfonylureas, glinides)
Alcohol ingestion
Drugs

Treatment

Ingest 10–20 g of rapidly absorbed carbohydrate. Repeat in 15–20 minutes if glucose concentration remains less than 60 mg/dL or if patient is symptomatic. Follow with complex carbohydrate/protein snack if mealtime is not imminent.
The following are examples of food sources that provide 15 g of carbohydrate:

Orange, grapefruit, or apple juice; regular, nondiet soda	1/2 cup
Fat-free milk	1 cup
Grape juice, cranberry juice cocktail	1/3 cup
Sugar	1 Tbsp or 3 cubes
Lifesavers	5–6 pieces
Glucose tablets	3–4 tablets

If patient is unconscious the following measures should be initiated:
Glucagon 1 mg SC, IM, or IV (generally administered IM in outpatient setting; mean response time, 6.5 minutes)
Glucose 25 g IV (dextrose 50%, 50 mL; mean response time, 4 minutes)

IM, intramuscular; IV, intravenous; SC, subcutaneous.

SELECTING AN INSULIN DELIVERY DEVICE

CASE 53-2, QUESTION 7: What kind of insulin delivery device should be prescribed for A.H.?

Delivery of insulin with a syringe is still the most common method of insulin administration in the United States. Insulin syringes are plastic, disposable syringes with needles that are very fine (28–31 gauge), sharp, and well lubricated to ease insertion. Needles and syringes have been improved so that insulin injections are relatively painless if proper technique is used. Less pain is associated with the smaller 30- or 31-gauge needles. The dead space (air space at the hub of the needle) has been virtually eliminated so that mixing and measuring problems previously associated with its presence are no longer a concern. The lengths of needles are 5/16 inch (8 mm), 3/8 inch (9.5 mm), or 1/2 inch (12.7 mm).[134] The shortest needle can be used for children or patients with little SC fat. A longer needle length (1/2 inch) may

TABLE 53-15
Interpreting Self-Monitored Blood Glucose Concentrations[a]

Test Time	Target Insulin Dose	Target Meal/Snack
Prebreakfast (fasting)	Predinner/bedtime intermediate-acting or basal insulin	Dinner or bedtime snack
Prelunch	Prebreakfast regular or rapid-acting insulin	Breakfast or midmorning snack
Predinner	Prebreakfast intermediate-acting insulin or prelunch regular or rapid-acting insulin	Lunch or midafternoon snack
Bedtime	Predinner regular or rapid-acting insulin	Dinner
2-hour postprandial	Premeal regular or rapid-acting insulin	Preceding meal or snack
2–3 AM or later	Predinner intermediate-acting insulin or basal insulin if given in AM	Dinner or bedtime snack

[a]Considerations: (a) Assumes a regular meal pattern. For patients who travel, have odd working or sleeping hours, or have irregular meal patterns, these guidelines may not apply. (b) Assumes administration of regular insulin 30–60 minutes before meals or rapid-acting insulin 0–15 minutes before meals and a normal pattern of insulin response (see Table 53-10 for factors that can alter insulin absorption and response). (c) If prebreakfast concentrations are high, rule out reactive hyperglycemia (Somogyi reaction or posthypoglycemic hyperglycemia). Consider contribution of dawn phenomenon as well. Whenever blood glucose concentrations are high, consider reactive hyperglycemia (excessive insulin doses). (d) Consider accuracy of reported test results: (i) Do they correlate with the glycosylated hemoglobin and patient's signs and symptoms? (ii) What is the patient's medication adherence? Could results be fabricated? (iii) Is the patient's technique appropriate? Check timing, adequate blood sample, machine, strips, and calibration (Table 53-13). (iv) Are insulin kinetics altered? (v) What is the carbohydrate content, quality, and regularity of meals?

be required in patients with excess abdominal fat; use of a short needle may result in insulin leakage.

Manufacturers produce 1-, 0.5-, and 0.3-mL syringes for U-100 insulin. For patients such as A.H., using fewer than 30 units of insulin per injection, the 0.3-mL syringe is preferred for ease of reading the dose markings on the syringe. This allows the patient to measure insulin more easily. Insulin syringes are available in 1-unit increments or 0.5-unit increments. One-half-unit increments are useful for pediatric patients and for patients who count carbohydrates, because mealtime insulin doses can be rounded to the 0.5 unit.

Insulin pen devices are also available for injecting insulin. Pen devices are often preferred as they make insulin administration much easier, especially for patients who need to take their insulin doses away from home. They also can increase dosing accuracy. The pens are particularly useful for patients with (a) regimens consisting of multiple daily doses of rapid- or short-acting insulin before meals and snacks (such as A.H.), (b) a fear of needles, (c) impaired visual or dexterity problems, (d) hectic work schedules or lifestyle, or (e) a need to train alternative individuals who administer insulin (e.g., school nurses, siblings).

Pens eliminate the need to withdraw insulin, and the insulin dose is dialed up on the device. Pen devices are available as a disposable prefilled pen or a durable pen in which an insulin cartridge is replaced. A prefilled pen contains a built-in, single-use insulin cartridge designed to deliver 300 units of insulin. These are helpful for patients who have difficulty handling the cartridges in reusable pens or for patients with busy schedules who prefer not to have to change cartridges. Pen devices are available to dose insulin in 2-unit, 1-unit (most), and 0.5-unit increments (NovoPen Junior and HumaPen Luxura HD). Pen needles are available in 29-, 30-, 31-, and 32-gauge needles and 4-mm, 3/16-inch (5-mm), 1/4-inch (6-mm), 5/16-inch (8-mm), or 1/2-inch (12.7-mm) lengths.[134] Patients are advised to use a new disposable needle for each injection. Unfortunately, limited health insurance coverage and higher copays can deter pen use. A detailed review of pen devices was published in 2009.[135]

For insulin delivery using an insulin pump, see Case 53-2, Questions 3 and 5.

If she elected to use a syringe, a 0.3-mL U-100 insulin syringe with a 5/16-inch (8-mm), 30- or 31-gauge needle should be prescribed for A.H. Subjectively, patients can "feel" the difference between different brands, or they may prefer the "ease of bubble removal," physical characteristics, or packaging of one syringe over another. If she elected to use an insulin pen, a prefilled pen for insulin glargine and insulin aspart are available. An 8-mm, 30- or 31-gauge pen needle should be prescribed for A.H. as well. Needle length can be adjusted depending on patient comfort.

TABLE 53-16
Areas of Patient Education

Diabetes: Pathogenesis and the complications
Hyperglycemia: Signs and symptoms
Ketoacidosis: Signs and symptoms (Table 53-23)
Hypoglycemia: Signs, symptoms, and appropriate treatment (Table 53-14)
Exercise: Effect on blood glucose concentrations and insulin dose (Table 53-21)
Diet: See text. Emphasis placed on carbohydrate counting because the carbohydrate is responsible for 90% of the rise in blood glucose after a meal.
Insulins:
- Injection technique
- Types of insulin
- Time action profiles (onset, peak and duration)
- Storage
- Stability (look for crystallization and precipitation with NPH insulin)

Therapeutic goals: A1C, fasting, preprandial and postprandial blood glucose levels, cholesterol, triglyceride, blood pressure
SMBG testing: Table 53-15
Interpretation of SMBG testing results
Foot care: Inspect feet daily; wear well-fitted shoes; avoid self-care of ingrown toenails, corns, or athlete's foot; see a podiatrist
Sick day management: Table 53-22
Cardiovascular risk factors: Tobacco use, high blood pressure, obesity, elevated cholesterol
Importance of annual ophthalmologic examinations; tests for microalbuminuria; keeping up-to-date with immunizations

A1C, glycosylated hemoglobin; NPH, neutral protamine Hagedorn; SMBG, self-monitored blood glucose.

MEASURING AND INJECTING INSULIN

CASE 53-2, QUESTION 8: How should A.H. be instructed to administer her insulin injections?

INJECTION

A.H. should prepare an area for injection. Alcohol swabs may be used to clean the rubber stopper of the insulin vial (or pen device). To inject the insulin subcutaneously, A.H. should be instructed to firmly pinch up the area to be injected (this creates a firm surface for the injection) and to quickly insert the needle perpendicularly (90-degree angle) into the center of this area. The syringe should be held toward the middle or back of the barrel, like a pencil. Anxious patients have a tendency to "choke" the hub of the syringe, and this prevents proper needle insertion. A 45-degree angle of injection may be used for infants and very thin individuals who have little SC fat, especially in the thigh area. The skin pinch should be released and the insulin injected.[136] Gentle pressure should be applied at the site of injection for 5 to 8 seconds to prevent back leakage of the insulin as the needle is removed. The site should not be massaged, because this may accelerate the absorption and onset of action of insulin (Table 53-10). When using an insulin pen, the needle should be embedded within the skin for about 5 to 10 seconds after depressing the dosing knob to ensure full delivery of the insulin dose. For a video of a SC insulin injection demonstration, see http://www.youtube.com/watch?v=0PX4R14N68Y&feature=related.

ROTATING INJECTION SITES

The primary sites used for injecting insulin are the lateral thigh, abdomen (avoid 2-inch radius around the navel), and upper arm (Fig. 53-5). The ADA recommends that insulin injections be rotated within the same anatomic region to decrease chances of variability in insulin absorption.[136] Many practitioners recommend using the abdominal area because absorption from this site is least affected by exercise and is the most predictable. Alternatively, A.H. can be instructed to rotate her morning injection within one region (e.g., the abdomen) and her evening injection in another anatomic region. This minimizes the variables that can alter her response to insulin.

Rotating injection sites also was recommended at one time to avoid the lipodystrophic effect of insulin (lipohypertrophy and lipoatrophy); however, because insulin has been purified, these complications are less common and the importance of rotation is less critical. Nevertheless, repetitive use of the same site of injection may still result in lipohypertrophy, and it does toughen the skin, making needle penetration more difficult. Furthermore, insulin absorption from lipohypertrophic sites can be slowed.[136]

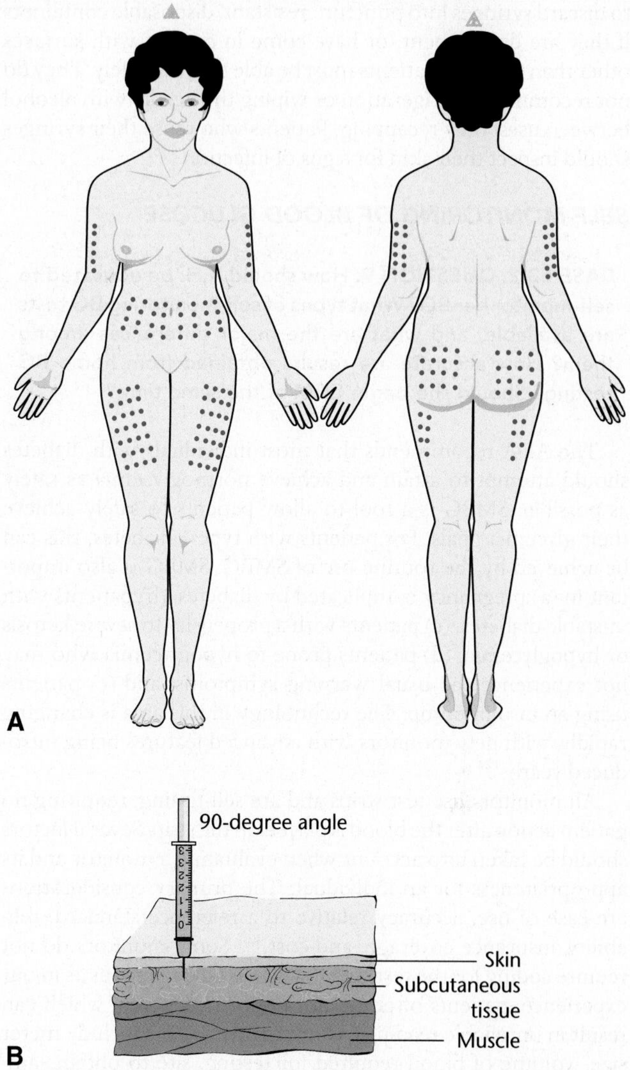

FIGURE 53-5 Selecting insulin injection sites. A: Areas of the body most suitable for insulin injections. The actual point of injection should be varied each time within a chosen body area. Give injections at least one inch apart. Patients should consult with their provider or diabetes educator about which area is most appropriate for use. LifeART image © 2011. Lippincott Williams & Wilkins. All rights reserved. **B:** The site where insulin should be injected. Insulin is injected in the subcutaneous tissue (between the skin and the muscle layer). If the skin is pinched up and the needle is pushed all the way in, the need will reach the proper space under the skin. Adapted with permission from Springhouse. Lippincott's Visual Encyclopedia of Clinical Skills. Philadelphia: Wolters Kluwer Health, 2009.

AGITATION

A.H. does not need to agitate insulin glargine or aspart because these are clear insulins. For NPH insulin, which is a suspension, the vial or pen must be agitated before use. A new, unused vial of NPH insulin may require vigorous agitation to loosen the sediment, which may have become packed down with storage. The vial should be rolled between the palms of the hands to minimize foaming. A pen device is inverted back and forth to mix the insulin. Agitation is only required for insulin suspensions (i.e., insulin mixtures).

MEASUREMENT

First, A.H. should make sure her hands and the injection site are clean (it is not necessary to use alcohol to clean the site). She should withdraw the plunger to the level of insulin she intends to inject (e.g., 12 units for her insulin glargine dose), then she should insert the needle into the vial and inject the air to prevent creation of a vacuum within the vial. The vial then should be inverted with the syringe inserted, and 12 units of insulin glargine should be withdrawn. The bevel of the needle should be well below the surface of the insulin to avoid withdrawing air or bubbles into the syringe. Insulin glargine must not be mixed in the same syringe with her insulin aspart, and it should be injected into a different site if it is injected at the same time as her aspart dose.

The barrel of the syringe should be held at eye level to check for air bubbles and to allow accurate placement of the plunger tip at the 12-unit mark. If bubbles are present, they should be removed by tapping the syringe gently to coax the bubbles to the top of the barrel, where they can be injected back into the insulin vial. To remove air bubbles in an insulin pen, prime the pen with 2 units of insulin before each use (repeat until insulin drop appears at tip of pen needle). Also, remove the needle from the pen device in between uses to prevent air bubbles from accumulating.

REUSING INSULIN SYRINGES AND PEN NEEDLES

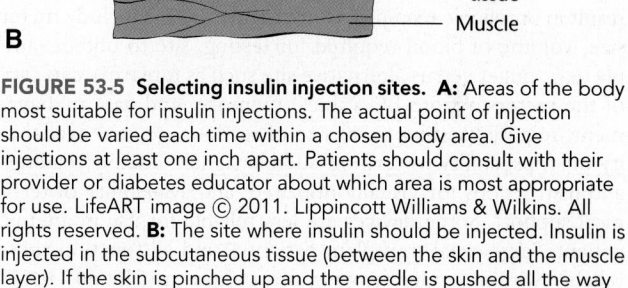

A frequently encountered practice is the reuse of disposable syringes. In a small survey of 56 patients with diabetes who reused syringes, even with poor adherence to aseptic technique, no adverse effects were noted in the patients.[137] The ADA does not encourage the reuse of syringes or pen needles. Smaller gauge needles (e.g., 30–32) seem particularly susceptible to bending and can form hooks. The ADA recommends that patients who do reuse syringes inspect injection sites for redness or swelling and to discard syringes into puncture-resistant, disposable containers if they are dull or bent, or have come in contact with surfaces other than the skin. Patients must be able to recap safely. They do not recommend refrigeration or wiping the needle with alcohol between uses, only recapping. Patients who reuse their syringes should inspect their skin for signs of infection.[136]

SELF-MONITORING OF BLOOD GLUCOSE

CASE 53-2, QUESTION 9: How should A.H. be educated to self-monitor her BG? What types of self-monitoring BG tests are available, and what are the major differences among them? How accurate are results obtained from home BG testing? Should she begin CGM at the same time?

The ADA recommends that most individuals with diabetes should attempt to attain and achieve normoglycemia as safely as possible. SMBG is a tool to allow patients to safely achieve their glycemia goals. For patients with type 1 diabetes, this can be achieved by the routine use of SMBG. SMBG is also important in (a) pregnancy complicated by diabetes, (b) patients with unstable diabetes, (c) patients with a propensity to severe ketosis or hypoglycemia, (d) patients prone to hypoglycemia who may not experience the usual warning symptoms, and (e) patients using an insulin pump. The technology in this area is changing rapidly, with new monitors with advanced features being introduced yearly.[124]

All monitors use test strips and are self-timing, requiring no patient action after the blood is placed on the strip. Several factors should be taken into account when evaluating a monitor and its appropriateness for an individual. The primary considerations are ease of use, accuracy relative to a reference standard, reliability, insurance coverage, and cost.[124] Some monitors do not require coding for the test strips, which is advantageous as in our experience, patients often do not perform this step, which can result in unreliable readings. Convenience factors include meter size, volume of blood required for testing, site to obtain sample (e.g., finger versus alternative site such as forearm), capacity of the meter to store BG values (memory) and data management, required testing time, size of readout, general availability of strips, ability to turn off audible signals, audible readings and instructions for visually impaired, and availability of technical support. Some devices are less reliable for use in anemic patients (e.g., renal transplant patients), and all function most reliably within certain temperature ranges (usually 60°–95°F) and humidity (generally <90%) conditions. Strips are sensitive to light, moisture, and temperature extremes and must be stored and handled with care.

Periodically, patients should compare the results they get on their monitor with the laboratory BG test for accuracy. The majority of monitors are calibrated to plasma levels (i.e., plasma referenced). Only a few monitors report whole BG; in these monitors, capillary values measured are likely to be 10% to 15% lower than values measured by the laboratory.

Patient education regarding any coding procedures, testing procedures, the importance of logging results in a diary, and test times are critical. Ultimately, A.H. should be taught how to adjust her insulin dose based on her glucose values, dietary intake, and exercise pattern (Table 53-17).

Used properly, available monitors provide reasonably accurate results that can be used by patients to manage their diabetes. However, several factors can affect the accuracy of monitor results—most commonly, equipment malfunction and human error (e.g., not coding). Problems with a monitor can be detected by performing a quality-control test once weekly and with each

TABLE 53-17
Guidelines for Dosing Insulin

Basic Insulin Doses
First, adjust the basic insulin dose (i.e., the dose that the patient will be instructed to take daily).
Only adjust insulin doses if a *pattern* of response is observed under stable diet and exercise circumstances. That is, the same response to insulin is observed for ≥3 days, particularly for the basal insulin dose. It is important to verify the stability of diet and exercise. Consider adjusting these variables as well.
Unless all levels are >200 mg/dL, try to adjust one component of insulin therapy at a time.
Start with the insulin component affecting the FBG concentration. This glucose level often is the most difficult to control and often affects all other glucose concentrations measured throughout the day. The basal insulin dose is often what is adjusted to control the FBG. However, if the dinner insulin dose (of rapid-acting or short-acting insulin) is not adequate, this can result in hyperglycemia that can persist into the morning. The basal dose is typically adjusted by 2–4 units, no sooner than every 3 days.[138]
Prandial/mealtime insulin dose:
• For patients eating a set amount of carbohydrate at meals: typically adjust the basic insulin dose by 1–2 units at a time. The amount given is based on the individual patient's response to insulin. This can be determined by looking at the patient's total daily dose using the "500 rule" (see the following, and Table 53-11).
• For patients using the insulin to carbohydrate method (i.e., 1 unit rapid-acting or short-acting insulin for every *x* g of carbohydrate), adjust the "ratio" based in the patient's response to insulin (e.g., 1:8, 1:10, 1:12, 1:15, 1:18, 1:20).
General Principles
Assumes that diet and physical activity are stable. Set a reasonable goal initially. This may mean the upper limits of the acceptable concentrations may be high initially (e.g., <200 mg/dL). Move toward a more ideal goal slowly.
Supplementary Insulin Doses (with rapid-acting or short-acting insulin)
Once the basic dose of prandial insulin has been established, supplemental doses of rapid- or short-acting insulin can be prescribed to correct *preprandial* hyperglycemia. For example, if the goal is 140 mg/dL and the glucose value is 190 mg/dL, administer one additional unit. Supplemental doses also can be used when the patient is ill (Table 53-22).
Algorithms for correction doses are based on the patient's sensitivity to insulin using the "1,500 or 1,700 rule" (Table 53-11).
If premeal glucose concentrations are <60–70 mg/dL, the dose of aspart, glulisine, lispro, or regular insulin administered before the meal is ↓ by 1–2 units; insulin administration is delayed until just before the meal; the meal should include an extra 15 g of glucose if the value is <50 mg/dL.
If supplemental doses before a given meal are required for ≥3 days, the basic insulin dose should be adjusted appropriately. For example, if a patient taking lispro before meals requires an extra 2 units before lunch for ≥3 days, 2 units should be added to the prebreakfast dose, or the insulin to carbohydrate ratio at breakfast should be adjusted (e.g., if patient was using a 1:15 ratio, a 1:12 ratio could be used).
Anticipatory Insulin Doses (with rapid-acting or short-acting insulin)
The basic insulin dose is ↑ or ↓ based on the anticipated effects of diet or physical activity.
↑ Aspart/glulisine/lispro or regular insulin by 1 unit for each additional 15 g of carbohydrate ingested (e.g., holiday meal) or ↓ the usual dose by 1–2 units if the meal is smaller than usual (Table 53-11).
See Table 53-21 for recommended insulin adjustments for exercise.

FBG, fasting blood glucose.

TABLE 53-18
Factors That Can Alter Self-Monitored Blood Glucose Test Results: Troubleshooting

Glucose monitor not coded for batch of test strips[a]
An inadequate amount of blood applied to test strip[b]
Improper storage of test strips (temperature and humidity)[a]
Dirty glucose monitor[a]
Low battery[a]
Test performed outside of altitude, temperature, and humidity operating conditions[a]
Low[c] or high[b] hematocrit
Dehydration[b]
Hyperosmolar, nonketotic state[b]
Lipemia[a]
Interfering substances
Nonglucose sugars (e.g., maltose, xylose, galactose) in meters using GDH-PQQ test strips[139]
Large amounts of acetaminophen[c]
Large amounts of ascorbic acid or salicylates (rare)[b]

[a]Effect unpredictable.
[b]Values tend to be lower.
[c]Values tend to be higher.
GDH-PQQ, glucose dehydrogenase pyrroloquinolinequinone.
Source: Heinemann L. Quality of glucose measurement with blood glucose meters at the point-of-care: relevance of interfering factors. *Diabetes Technol Ther.* 2010;12:847.

new vial of strips; human error can be minimized with adequate training. Table 53-18 lists factors that can affect results of SMBG test results. Any time SMBG values are inconsistent with the patient's symptoms or A1C values, sources of error should be evaluated. A.H.'s technique should be reviewed periodically, because clinical decisions are based on the patient's BG testing record.

Because A.H. is just starting insulin therapy and SMBG, it would be reasonable to hold off on considering CGM until she becomes comfortable with these skills. Then, she and her practitioner could assess whether CGM would be useful.

TESTING FREQUENCY

CASE 53-2, QUESTION 10: How often should A.H. test her BG concentrations?

Although the exact frequency and timing of BG tests should be dictated by individualized patient goals, most patients with type 1 diabetes using basal-bolus insulin regimens should perform SMBG at least three times daily or more according to the ADA.[8] Glucose monitoring should also be performed more frequently whenever therapy is modified. Because A.H. is being initiated on insulin therapy with the goal of normoglycemia, she should ideally self-monitor her BG four times per day (before meals and at bedtime) for 2 weeks until the pattern of blood sugar fluctuation can be assessed and adjustments can be made. Motivated patients may continue this degree of monitoring, but it may be reduced to twice daily for patients on long-term insulin. Varying the time of day in which testing is performed will allow the clinician and patient to make informed decisions on how to make adjustments.

The objective of ongoing, frequent BG testing is to determine whether normoglycemia is being achieved and to assess the action of specific insulin doses as well as the impact of meals, food, illness, or exercise on BG levels. Ideally, patients should test their BG before meals, 60 to 120 minutes after the start of meals to assess postprandial glycemic control and to determine their insulin to carbohydrate ratio, at bedtime, and occasionally at 2 or 3 AM (i.e., eight times daily). However, it can be challenging for patients to adhere to such a rigorous regimen. A.H. should set her alarm for 3 AM two or three times per week and test her BG. BG concentrations measured before meals allow patients and clinicians to determine whether the rapid-acting insulin dose is appropriate for the amount of carbohydrate consumed; FPG levels are used to determine whether the basal insulin dose is adequate; and the 2 to 3 AM BG level is used to identify nocturnal hypoglycemia. For example, the BG measured before dinner reflects the action of A.H.'s prelunch aspart dose on food she has eaten for lunch, as well as hepatic glucose production between meals. Increasingly, patients who use carbohydrate counting with rapid-acting insulins test 2-hour postprandial levels when initiating therapy to enhance proper dosage adjustment (Table 53-15).

The importance of frequent BG testing cannot be overemphasized. When BG is tested less frequently than four times daily, it becomes difficult to adjust insulin doses based on infrequent readings or to assess patterns in glucose levels (i.e., pattern management). If patients refuse to test four times daily, they should be encouraged to test four times daily on representative days of the week or to test at different times of the day each day so that a weekly profile can be developed. A.H. also should be encouraged to test her BG concentration any time she is feeling unusual, if she is experiencing hypoglycemic symptoms, or to evaluate the effect of unusual circumstances on her BG concentration (e.g., increased physical exercise, a large holiday meal, final examinations, a family crisis).

USING BLOOD GLUCOSE TEST RESULTS TO EVALUATE INSULIN DOSES

CASE 53-2, QUESTION 11: A.H. was instructed to inject herself with 12 units of insulin glargine each evening and to give 4 units of insulin aspart just before each meal. She was asked to test her BG four times daily (before meals and at bedtime), to record her results and other unusual events or symptoms during the day, and to bring her BG logbook to the clinic. A.H. was also instructed to track her food and record the number of carbohydrates she ingested at each meal. The initial goal of therapy is to lower her BG to eliminate symptoms of hyperglycemia. The ultimate goal is to achieve fasting glucoses of 70 to 130 mg/dL and postprandial values of less than 180 mg/dL. One week later, trends in her BG concentrations were as follows:

Time	Glucose Concentration (mg/dL)
7 AM	160–200
Noon	220–260
5 PM	130–180
11 PM	140–180

Occasional 3 AM tests averaged 160 mg/dL, and A.H.'s urine is negative for ketones. She eats approximately four carbohydrate servings for breakfast (60 g) and two to four carbohydrate servings for lunch and dinner (30–45 g). Subjectively, A.H. feels a bit better, and her weight has stabilized, but she still urinates two to three times nightly. How would you interpret these results, and how should A.H.'s insulin doses be altered?

TABLE 53-19
Factors That Can Alter Blood Glucose Control

Diet
Insufficient calories (e.g., alcoholism, eating disorders, anorexia, nausea, and vomiting)
Overeating (e.g., during the holidays)
Irregularly spaced, skipped, or delayed meals
Dietary content (e.g., fiber, carbohydrate content)
Physical Activity
See Table 53-21 and Case 53-6
Stress
Infection
Surgery/trauma
Psychological
Drugs
Certain medications can increase or decrease blood glucose levels. It is important to assess for potential effects on the blood glucose when starting new medications.
Hormonal Changes
Menstruation: Glucose concentrations may increase premenstrually and return to normal after menses.
Pregnancy
Puberty: hyperglycemia probably related to high growth hormone levels
Gastroparesis
Delays gastric emptying time. Peak insulin action and meal-related glucose excursions may become mismatched.
Altered Insulin Pharmacokinetics
See Table 53-10
Insulin Injection Technique
Measuring
Timing
Technique
Inactive Insulin
Outdated insulin
Improperly stored insulin (heat or cold)
Crystallized insulin

Values from SMBG appropriately form the basis for insulin adjustments. Ultimately, the goal is to move motivated patients toward being able to recognize their own glucose trends and make insulin adjustments accordingly.[74] Before using A.H.'s BG results to adjust her insulin dose, it is important to observe and reassess her testing technique. One also should determine whether there were any unusual circumstances in her life, illness, diet changes, or exercise patterns during the past week that might have affected her response to insulin. Once these have been ruled out as confounding factors, one can begin making gross adjustments in A.H.'s insulin dose, realizing that fine-tuning will be impossible until a consistent diet and exercise pattern have been instituted.

Several principles must be kept in mind whenever BG tests are used to adjust a patient's basic insulin dose (Table 53-19). Because many factors can alter a patient's response to insulin, it is important to review BG concentration *trends* measured for a minimum of 3 days to adjust the basic insulin dose (i.e., the dose the patient will use every day). The only exception to this rule is the use of supplemental insulin doses to correct exceptionally high glucose concentrations after A.H. has acquired sophisticated insulin adjustment skills (see Case 53-2, Question 16). SMBG results should be evaluated in conjunction with the A1C.

The daily dose of insulin glargine is inadequately controlling A.H.'s fasting blood glucose (FBG) and should be increased by 2 to 4 units, although published algorithms would recommend increasing her dose by 4 to 6 units. A more conservative approach would be to increase the dose to 14 units each evening (or a designated time of day that she will be able to do consistently) and further titrate as needed.[126,140] She is achieving some response from her lunchtime dose of insulin aspart, but there is room for improvement in her meal insulin coverage overall. The BG concentration of 160 mg/dL at 3 AM indicates that rebound hyperglycemia is an unlikely cause of her high fasting levels (see Case 53-2, Question 13, and Case 53-3). As an initial step toward control, A.H.'s daily dose of insulin glargine should be increased in an attempt to control her fasting hyperglycemia. However, this approach does not address A.H.'s elevated prelunch values. Her intake of carbohydrates also varies from meal to meal. Thus, a more appropriate method would be to calculate the insulin to carbohydrate ratio for A.H. and allow her to determine her premeal aspart dose based on the amounts of carbohydrates she will ingest at each meal. A typical starting point for the insulin to carbohydrate ratio is 1 unit to every 15 g of carbohydrate. To calculate her insulin to carbohydrate ratio, the "500 rule" is used: Divide the number 500 by her total daily dose of insulin (14 units of insulin glargine plus 12 units of insulin aspart for meal coverage = 26 units):

$$500/26 = 19 \text{ g of carbohydrate covered by 1 unit of insulin}$$

Because most single servings of carbohydrate contain 15 g, A.H. decides to start with a ratio of 1 unit for every 15 g or single serving of carbohydrates she consumes at each meal. If A.H. were using regular insulin for meal coverage, she could use the "450 rule": 450 divided by the total daily insulin dose yields grams of carbohydrate covered by 1 unit of insulin.

To evaluate the accuracy of her insulin to carbohydrate ratio, A.H. will need to check her BG values 2 hours after each meal (postprandial) to assess the appropriateness of her ratio. She agrees to test her BG level eight times per day and return in 2 weeks.

CASE 53-2, QUESTION 12: A.H. is getting more comfortable with carbohydrate counting and adjusting her insulin doses accordingly. A review of her food diary reveals that for the most part, she is able to determine the appropriate serving sizes for 15 g of carbohydrate. She admits to difficulty determining carbohydrate amounts when eating out. As a result, A.H. notices that her preprandial BG concentrations exceed her goal of 80 to 120 mg/dL on occasion. Sometimes they are as high as 200 mg/dL. Evaluate A.H.'s BG trends. How should occasional preprandial glucose concentrations that exceed the desired goal of 80 to 120 mg/dL be managed?

ONLINE CONTENT

For a PowerPoint presentation that shows A.H.'s food diary and the units of premeal insulin she injected, go to http://thepoint.lww.com/AT10e.

Once the basal insulin dose and insulin to carbohydrate insulin dose have been established, one can begin to teach A.H. how to use a correction factor to adjust her dose of insulin when preprandial BG concentrations fall above or below the range of BG concentrations that have been established as her goal of therapy (70–130 mg/dL per the ADA; Table 53-17).

A correction insulin dose is used to compensate for unusually high BG concentrations (high-sugar correction). To reemphasize, this assumes there are no unusual changes in the patient's overall diet or exercise patterns. Many clinicians favor rapid-acting insulin versus regular insulin because its action is brief and patients do not have to worry about residual effects 3 to 4 hours after its injection. This is particularly valuable when correctional doses of insulin are needed at bedtime.

The patient's sensitivity to insulin, as reflected by his or her total daily dose on a unit per kilogram basis, is a major determinant of any algorithm developed. A general approach is to give an additional 1 to 2 units of supplemental rapid-acting insulin for each 30- to 50-mg/dL elevation above the target level.[127] An alternative method of estimating the drop in a person's BG per unit of regular insulin is the "1,500 rule."[133] The derived value is referred to as the "sensitivity factor": The rule was modified to the "1,800 rule" for use with rapid-acting insulin (insulin lispro, aspart, or glulisine). Because these insulins tend to drop the BG level faster and farther, 1,500 turns out to be too aggressive. Others have recommended other numerators such as 1,600, 1,700, 2,000, and 2,200.[141] For this case, the "1,700 rule" will be used. The calculation for A.H. would be as follows:

$$1{,}700/24 = 70 \text{ mg/dL}$$

Thus, 1 unit of insulin aspart for A.H. will drop her BG level by about 70 mg/dL. People with a lower sensitivity factor (higher insulin requirements) typically achieve a smaller reduction in BG per unit of insulin compared with those with a higher sensitivity factor (lower insulin requirement). Thus, an algorithm of 1 unit of insulin aspart for every 70-mg/dL excursion above her goal of 120 mg/dL is a reasonable place to begin. If this dose of insulin is insufficient, one can decrease the BG excursion required per unit of insulin dose (e.g., 50 mg/dL). Correctional insulin doses also are used for sick day management (see Case 53-7). The following is an example of a high-sugar correction algorithm for A.H.

Glucose Concentrations (mg/dL)	Insulin Aspart
<80	1 unit less
80–120	Usual dose
120–190	1 unit extra
191–260	2 units extra
261–330[a]	3 units extra
331–400[a]	4 units extra

[a] Check urine ketones. If urine ketones are positive and BG concentrations remain >300 mg/dL for ≥12 hours, call the physician for directions.

EVALUATING FASTING HYPERGLYCEMIA

CASE 53-2, QUESTION 13: A.H. returns after 1 month. She is currently using 14 units of insulin glargine each evening, 1 unit of insulin aspart for each 15 g of carbohydrate ingested at mealtime, and a high-sugar correction factor of 1 unit of insulin aspart for every 70 mg/dL above 120 mg/dL. Her SMBG results are as follows:

Time	Glucose Concentration mg/dL
7 AM	140–180
Noon	120–150
5 PM	90–130
11 PM	90–120
3 AM	60–90

Overall, A.H. feels her diabetes is in good control. Her energy level has returned to normal, and her nocturia has diminished, but she occasionally gets up one or two times nightly to urinate. A.H. has also noticed that nightmares or "sweats" sometimes awaken her. When this occurs, she generally has something to eat because she is "famished." She is able to get back to sleep, but wakes up the next morning with a "splitting headache" and a "hungover" feeling. A.H.'s weight remains the same, and she has begun to develop some consistency in her dietary patterns with the help of a dietitian. She has been consistently correcting her prelunch and predinner insulin doses by adding or subtracting 2 units from her premeal insulin doses based on her premeal BG values. The A1C from her last visit is 7.3%. Evaluate A.H.'s BG values. What are possible causes of A.H.'s fasting hyperglycemia?

When evaluating morning hyperglycemia, several causes must be considered:

- An insufficient basal dose of insulin. If the basal dose is insufficient, hepatic glucose output during the fasting state will be excessive, thereby producing hyperglycemia.
- Insufficient dinner coverage with insulin aspart, resulting in hyperglycemia that persists into the morning. This can be distinguished from an insufficient basal insulin by assessing glucose control at bedtime.
- Reactive hyperglycemia in response to a nocturnal hypoglycemic episode (Somogyi effect or rebound hyperglycemia).
- An excessive bedtime snack.
- The dawn phenomenon (see Case 53-3).

The presence of normoglycemia at bedtime, low BG concentrations at 3 AM, and symptoms of nocturnal hypoglycemia (nightmares, sweating, hunger, morning headache) in A.H. are consistent with a rebound hyperglycemic reaction in the morning (i.e., posthypoglycemic hyperglycemia, also referred to as the Somogyi effect).[142]

Theoretically, this effect occurs after any episode of severe hypoglycemia and is secondary to an excessive increase in glucose production by the liver that is activated by insulin counterregulatory hormones such as cortisol, glucagon, epinephrine, and growth hormone. The waning effects of the basal insulin dose can also be a cause of fasting hyperglycemia because insulin is needed to suppress hepatic glucose output during the fasting state; however, this is not likely in A.H.'s case.[128] Asymptomatic nocturnal hypoglycemia can occur in patients taking evening doses of insulin and may account for morning hyperglycemia. By correcting the nocturnal hypoglycemia, normalization of A.H.'s fasting hyperglycemia also may be achieved. Thus, a decrease in the daily dose of insulin glargine by 2 units is warranted. A.H. should continue to monitor her BG concentrations at 3 AM.

Caveat: If A.H. were using NPH BID to supply her basal insulin, one option would be to shift the evening injection of NPH from before dinner to bedtime. This preferred method effectively shifts the peak action of NPH to the early morning, when she is awake, and decreases the risk of nocturnal hypoglycemia.[127,143] This peak action also corresponds to the dawn phenomenon (see Case 53-3) and the breakfast meal.

Another option if a patient is using NPH and experiencing nocturnal hypoglycemia is to change from NPH to either insulin glargine or insulin detemir because these insulins are associated with less nocturnal hypoglycemia.[144,145] In this case, the daily dose of NPH should be decreased by 20% to determine the insulin glargine dose to err on the conservative side. When switching from NPH to insulin detemir, a one-to-one dose conversion may be used, although higher doses of detemir may be required. In one crossover study of type 1 diabetes patients, the average detemir basal dose was approximately double that of the NPH basal dose.[146]

Although A.H.'s prelunch BG values are above her goal, this may be attributable to the fasting BG being elevated and then continuing to be elevated midmorning, like a domino effect. It is important to first correct the fasting hyperglycemia, and generally correct one BG concentration at a time.

MIXING INSULINS

CASE 53-2, QUESTION 14: If A.H. were to use NPH as basal insulin, how should she be instructed to measure and withdraw this insulin mixture?

Although mixing two insulins in the same syringe has become less common with use of basal-bolus therapy (because insulin glargine and detemir cannot be mixed) and the use of rapid-acting insulin pen devices, the procedure used to mix and withdraw NPH and mealtime insulin (regular or rapid-acting insulin) is basically the same as that described in Case 53-2, Question 8. The major difference is that an adequate volume of air must be injected into the NPH vial before the regular or insulin aspart is measured and withdrawn. Also, the mealtime clear insulin is measured and withdrawn into the insulin syringe *first* to avoid contamination of the vial of regular, aspart, lispro, or glulisine insulin with NPH. For example, contamination with NPH ultimately alters the NPH to regular insulin ratio that is administered. When patients withdraw NPH insulin first, the vial of regular insulin eventually becomes cloudy. In contrast, contamination of the NPH insulin with regular insulin probably is insignificant because the protamine contained in NPH can bind the regular insulin (see Case 53-2, Question 15). The procedure A.H. should use to mix her insulins is described in the following section, using her morning dose as an example.

- After dispersing the NPH insulin suspension, inject 14 units of air into the NPH vial and withdraw the needle.
- Inject 7 units of air into the insulin aspart vial, and withdraw the 7 units of insulin as described in Case 53-2, Question 8.
- Insert the needle into the NPH vial, and pull the plunger down to the 21-unit mark (14 units of NPH plus 7 units of insulin aspart).

STABILITY OF MIXED INSULINS

CASE 53-2, QUESTION 15: Will mixing NPH with a rapid-acting or regular insulin blunt the rapid action of the mealtime insulins? How stable are other insulin mixtures?

Regular insulin and all of the rapid-acting insulin analogs (aspart, lispro, and glulisine) may be mixed with NPH. In general, it is recommended to mix the insulins just before administration. See Table 53-20 for details on compatibility and stability of insulin mixtures. Although the manufacturer advises against mixing insulin glargine, small studies with pediatric patients have demonstrated that insulin glargine, when mixed with a rapid-acting analog, is effective for glycemic control.[148,149] The reason for doing this would be to reduce the number of injections for a pediatric patient. However, with the increased use of insulin pen devices, mixing of insulins in the same syringe has become a less common practice.

TABLE 53-20
Compatibility of Insulin Mixtures[136]

Mixture	Proportion	Comments
Regular + NPH[147]	Any proportion	The pharmacodynamic profiles of regular and NPH insulin are unchanged when premixed and stored in vials or syringes for up to 3 months.
Regular + normal saline	Any proportion	Use within 2–3 hours of preparation.
Regular + insulin diluting solution	Any proportion	Stable indefinitely.
Rapid-acting + NPH[93–95]	Any proportion	The absorption rate and peak action of the rapid-acting insulins are blunted; total bioavailability is unaltered. Rapid-acting insulin and NPH should be mixed just before use (within 15 minutes).
Insulin glargine and detemir[97,107]	Do not mix with other insulins	Pharmacodynamics could be modified.

NPH, neutral protamine Hagedorn.

PREMEAL HYPERGLYCEMIA

CASE 53-2, QUESTION 16: After reducing the dose of insulin glargine to 14 units each evening, A.H.'s FBG is now 110 to 125 mg/dL. However, her noon BG concentrations remain in the 120- to 150-mg/dL range.

When evaluating midmorning hyperglycemia, it is important to remember that the FPG concentration can contribute up to 50% of this plasma glucose excursion. Therefore, a key to the control of midmorning hyperglycemia may be to normalize the fasting glucose concentration. However, for A.H., the reduction in the insulin glargine has now corrected the reactive fasting hyperglycemia.

Hyperglycemia before a meal can be a result of several factors. The following are possible explanations for A.H.'s midmorning hyperglycemia:

- An insufficient dose of insulin aspart before breakfast. For A.H., this means that her insulin to carbohydrate ratio needs to be adjusted.
- Excessive carbohydrate ingestion at breakfast or inaccurate (under) counting of the carbohydrates ingested. Patients having difficulty accurately counting their carbohydrates should meet with a dietitian or diabetes educator for education; this is often necessary periodically throughout their lives as a refresher, just like many other skills require.

- Poor synchrony between meal intake and insulin action. This could be caused by administration of rapid-acting insulin too long before or after the meal (e.g., ≥30 minutes). If regular insulin is used, this could be caused by administering regular insulin just before or after meals.
- An insufficient dose of evening insulin glargine to suppress hepatic glucose production (glycogenolysis and gluconeogenesis) during the fasting state or the dawn phenomenon (see Case 53-3). However, in A.H.'s case, her FBG values are in target, so this is not likely.

The following interventions may be considered:

- Adjust her insulin to carbohydrate ratio to increase her insulin aspart dose at breakfast. The ratio should be changed to 1 unit of aspart for every 10 or 12 g (which are typical ratios used) of carbohydrate for the breakfast meal. This assumes a patient is technically able to use a different "ratio" at different mealtimes.
- Alter the carbohydrate content of the meals. This may include decreasing the amount of carbohydrate in the breakfast meal, changing the type of carbohydrate ingested, or adding fiber to that meal to minimize glucose excursions.
- Adjust the high-sugar correction factor if the glucose excursions appear to be caused by reduced insulin sensitivity in the morning. For example, the high-sugar correction can be adjusted to give 1 unit of aspart for every 50 mg/dL above 120 mg/dL.

PREPRANDIAL HYPOGLYCEMIA

CASE 53-2, QUESTION 17: A.H. is now taking insulin glargine 12 units each night and using an insulin to carbohydrate ratio of 1:15 (1 unit of insulin aspart for every 15 g of carbohydrate) at lunch and dinner and 1:12 at breakfast. She is continuing with the same high-sugar premeal correction of 1 unit of insulin aspart for every 70 mg/dL more than her premeal BG target of 120 mg/dL. Two weeks later, she brings in her BG records.

Time	Glucose Concentration (mg/dL)
7 AM	110–120
Noon	90–115
5 PM	60–110
11 PM	80–110
3 AM	110–120

A.H. feels that she is now "back to normal." She has no signs or symptoms of hyperglycemia, and her weight has remained stable. Occasionally, she becomes hypoglycemic before dinner, but this most often occurs when her dinner is delayed because of a hectic work schedule. Evaluate A.H.'s BG trends. What could be the cause of her predinner hypoglycemia, and how could she be managed?

A.H.'s BG concentrations indicate that her basic insulin regimen is generally adequate to achieve the overall goal of preprandial BG concentrations of less than 120 mg/dL.

The hypoglycemia A.H. is experiencing before dinner could be caused by insufficient carbohydrate intake at lunch (inaccurate carbohydrate counting), increased activity during the day, or an excessive dose of insulin aspart (insulin to carbohydrate ratio too high). Thus, the problem could be resolved by augmenting A.H.'s lunch meal, adjusting the lunch insulin to carbohydrate ratio to 1 unit of insulin aspart for every 18 (or 20) g of carbohydrate, or adding a midafternoon snack.

DAWN PHENOMENON

CASE 53-3

QUESTION 1: R.D., a 37-year-old man, has had type 1 diabetes since age 14. During the past 2 years, he has been very well controlled on the following insulin regimen: insulin glargine 20 units each morning with insulin lispro 3 to 4 units depending on carbohydrate intake before meals. On this regimen, his BG concentrations for the past 2 weeks have been as follows:

Time	Glucose Concentration (mg/dL)
7 AM	140–170
Noon	100–120
5 PM	100–130
11 PM	115–140
3 AM	100–120

What are the likely causes of R.D.'s fasting hyperglycemia?

As discussed in Case 53-2, Question 13, fasting hyperglycemia may be the result of insufficient doses of insulin in the evening and, possibly, reactive hyperglycemia. In R.D.'s case, the dawn phenomenon also must be considered.[150] The *dawn phenomenon* is a rise in the BG concentration that occurs between 4 and 8 AM after a physiological nadir in the BG concentration that occurs between midnight and 3 AM. This 30- to 40-mg/dL increase in the morning BG concentration cannot be attributed to increases in counterregulatory hormones secondary to an antecedent hypoglycemic event, but it may be secondary to rising growth hormone levels. This phenomenon is inconsistently observed in individuals with type 1 and type 2 diabetes as well as nondiabetic individuals; furthermore, it is inconsistently present from one day to the next.[151]

R.D.'s normal 3 AM BG concentration indicates that posthypoglycemic hyperglycemia is an unlikely cause of his fasting hyperglycemia. Thus, the modest increase in his BG concentration between 3 and 8 AM may be attributed to the waning effects of insulin or the dawn phenomenon. In both cases, an increase in R.D.'s daily dose of insulin glargine would be indicated. If hypoglycemia begins occurring 4 to 8 hours after the glargine dose, then twice-daily dosing can be tried. Somewhat more rapid absorption and clearance of glargine has been noted in nonobese patients, and splitting the total daily dose into two injections can help create smoother 24-hour plasma levels in these patients. Another option would be to switch R.D. to an insulin pump. He has demonstrated a desire and the ability for intensive management with multiple daily injections, frequent SMBG, recordkeeping skills, the ability to make appropriate insulin dose adjustments, and accurate carbohydrate counting. The advantage to using a pump is the ability to program an increase in the basal infusion rate in the early morning hours (e.g., beginning around 2 to 3 AM and continuing until 7 to 9 AM).

ONLINE CONTENT

For an example of basal rate and bolus (insulin:carbohydrate) ratios for a patient using an insulin pump, go to http://thepoint.lww.com/AT10e.

Type 1 Diabetes in Children

DIAGNOSIS AND CLINICAL PRESENTATION

CASE 53-4

QUESTION 1: J.C., a 7-year-old, 30-kg (95th percentile), 50 inches tall (90th percentile) girl, was brought to the emergency department by her parents because of nausea, vomiting, and a persistent stomachache secondary to the flu. For the past week, J.C. had flulike symptoms, resulting in a 6-pound weight loss. Initial laboratory values revealed a BG of 600 mg/dL, serum pH of 6.8 with bicarbonate level of 13 mEq/L, plasma ketone level of 5.2 mmol/L, and positive ketonuria. J.C. was diagnosed with diabetic ketoacidosis (DKA) secondary to new-onset type 1 diabetes. In retrospect and on further questioning, J.C.'s parents realized that she probably had symptoms as early as 4 weeks before her hospitalization. While on a driving vacation, she drank large quantities of juice and had to stop hourly to urinate. She began experiencing enuresis, which her parents attributed to her increased fluid intake. What signs and symptoms are consistent with the diagnosis of type 1 diabetes in a child?

The diagnosis of type 1 diabetes in children is generally straightforward. Presenting symptoms include a several-week history of polyuria, polydipsia, polyphagia, and weight loss, with hyperglycemia, glucosuria, ketonemia, and ketonuria. J.C.'s presentation is typical for a child newly diagnosed with diabetes who is brought in for medical attention because of severe symptoms related to the flu. An acute viral illness can trigger autoimmune destruction of the pancreas and abdominal pain, which may masquerade as gastroenteritis. Abdominal pain is a common presenting symptom of DKA.[152] J.C.'s weight loss probably represents fluid and caloric loss secondary to uncontrolled diabetes as well as decreased caloric intake from the flu. The symptoms of polyuria are less obvious in an infant and are frequently missed until metabolic derangement has occurred. Unlike J.C., infants frequently present with severe dehydration and metabolic acidosis despite a negative history of diarrhea or significant vomiting.

GOALS OF THERAPY

CASE 53-4, QUESTION 2: What are the goals of therapy for J.C.? Do the results of the DCCT apply to children such as J.C.? Are there age-specific goals?

The glycemic goals of therapy for children such as J.C. and adolescents with diabetes mellitus are technically not different than those for adults, but age should be considered and goals individiualized.[8] Additional targets should also be kept in mind, including (a) to achieve normal growth and development, (b) to facilitate positive psychosocial adjustment to diabetes, and (c) to prevent acute and chronic complications. Attainment of these goals requires a tremendous amount of support and education for the parents and can best be provided by a multidisciplinary team of professionals, including a pediatric endocrinologist, nurse educator, pharmacist, dietitian, and mental health professional.[153]

Growth serves as an important clinical indication of overall general health and well-being in children with diabetes. Height and weight should be measured at each visit and plotted on standard growth grids. If, at the time of diagnosis, a child has fallen behind in height or weight, prompt and appropriate treatment should quickly return the child to the appropriate percentile and pattern of growth. An overweight child should be encouraged to achieve a more appropriate percentile of weight gradually, over the course of several months.

Although recommendations for glycemic control are based on data from studies in adult patients with diabetes, achieving the same near-normalization of BG levels in children and adolescents is recommended. However, special consideration must be given to the unique risks and consequences of hypoglycemia in young children. A cohort of adolescents included in the DCCT was analyzed separately. The intensive group achieved an A1C about 1% higher than the current ADA recommendations for patients in general.[154] Similar to the adults in the DCCT, adolescents had sustained benefits from intensive management with little further progression to proliferative retinopathy 4 years after the DCCT was terminated.[155] Thus, J.C.'s pediatrician must strive for the best glucose control that she, her family circumstances, and currently available treatment regimens will permit.

The risk of hypoglycemia and potential neuropsychological impairment is of great concern in young children. Children younger than 6 to 7 years of age can have a form of hypoglycemic unawareness that results partly from their reduced capacity to communicate symptoms of hypoglycemia, but may be contributed to by less-developed counterregulatory mechanisms.[8] In addition, food intake and physical activity are unpredictable in this age group. To minimize the risk of hypoglycemia and hyperglycemia, an A1C value between 7.5% and 8.5% is recommended.[153]

The management of diabetes in children 6 to 12 years of age, such as J.C., is particularly challenging because many children require insulin with lunch or at other times when they are away from home. Administration of insulin at school demands flexibility and close communications between the parents, the health care team, and school personnel. An A1C goal of 8% or lower is recommended (Table 53-4).[8,153]

The greatest amount of evidence-based data exists for adolescents with diabetes (13–19 years). As mentioned, teenagers included in the DCCT achieved a mean A1C level of 8.06% in an era before the availability of rapid-acting or basal insulins. An A1C goal of less than 7.5% is recommended in this age group.[8,153]

INSULIN THERAPY

CASE 53-4, QUESTION 3: How should J.C. be started on insulin? Is the use of an insulin pump appropriate in children such as J.C.?

Generally, rapid-acting or short-acting insulin, intermediate-acting insulin (i.e., NPH), and basal insulin analogs are used in children. Insulin requirements are generally based on body weight, age, and pubertal status. Newly diagnosed children with type 1 diabetes usually require an initial total daily dose of approximately 0.5 to 1.0 unit/kg.[153] The small insulin requirements of infants and toddlers may be delivered by using diluted insulin (e.g., 10 units/mL, U-10; or 50 units/mL, U-50)[93,94] to measure doses in less than 1-unit increments. Diluents are available for insulin aspart and lispro. Insulin syringes and pens that deliver insulin in 0.5-unit increments are also very useful. Most children are now treated with basal-bolus regimens. These regimens have demonstrated lower FBG levels with less nocturnal hypoglycemia versus regimens using NPH in children and adolescents.[156] In newly diagnosed children with type 1 diabetes, lower A1C levels can be achieved with basal-bolus therapy compared with a more conventional regimen with NPH twice daily (breakfast and bedtime) and rapid-acting insulin at breakfast and dinner only.[157] However, if the lunchtime dose at school is too difficult, a small dose of NPH can be given with the morning rapid-acting insulin dose to cover the lunch meal.[158] Basal-bolus insulin regimens combined with carbohydrate counting are attractive regimens for middle and high school students. Because children often have erratic eating habits, rapid-acting insulins are advantageous over regular insulin because they can even be injected immediately after a meal, accounting for the portion of the meal a child actually consumed. J.C. should be started on approximately a total daily dose of 15 units (i.e., 0.5 units/kg/day), such as 3 units of rapid-acting insulin before meals and 7 units of insulin glargine at bedtime.[153,159] In some patients, insulin glargine may not last a full 24 hours; in this case, the dose of insulin glargine should be divided and given twice daily, and then each adjusted based on the BG patterns.[153]

When J.C. and her caregivers become skilled with carbohydrate counting, insulin kinetics, dosing insulin based on her carbohydrate intake, and diabetes management, the use of an insulin pump can be considered. The insulin pump therapy in the pediatric population is increasing rapidly as it provides increased flexibility with meal timing and has been shown to improve glycemic control and quality of life.[160,161] Young children (not just adolescents) are now recommended for consideration of insulin pump therapy.[160] Family and adult support both at home and school is critical for successful pump use until the child is able to manage his or her diabetes independently.

INJECTION SITES

CASE 53-4, QUESTION 4: Where should J.C. administer her insulin? Are the recommended sites of injection different for children? Does the age of the child play a factor?

For infants with abundant SC tissue, injection sites are usually plentiful. For some toddlers who have lost their "baby fat," locating an appropriate site for injection can be difficult. Injecting insulin into the abdomen of children with minimal SC abdominal fat or in very young children may not be advisable. Rotation of injection sites among arms, thighs, and the upper-outer quadrant of the buttock or hip area, as well as the abdominal area in older children, is recommended. To achieve consistent absorption, insulin injections can be patterned; for example, using the arms for the morning injection and the thighs for the evening injection. Children and teens should be cautioned to not consistently inject their insulin into a single area, which may be more convenient for them.[162] Fatty deposits and scar tissue can develop secondary to insulin action at the local tissue level. Insulin absorption from these hypertrophied areas is generally poor and unpredictable, resulting in variability in glycemic control. Insulin pen devices are very helpful for use in children because they are less intimidating (see Case 53-2, Question 7). Also, spring-loaded injection devices may be helpful in reducing the child's fear of needles and easing access to difficult-to-reach injection sites such as the back of the arms or buttocks.

BLOOD GLUCOSE MONITORING

CASE 53-4, QUESTION 5: How often should J.C. monitor her BG?

The eventual goal for children with diabetes is self-management, with insulin dosing decisions based on interpretation of BG results. Self-management skills and basal-bolus insulin regimens rely on frequent SMBG. For children with type 1 diabetes, four or more BG tests per day are generally necessary. Most newer meters allow for alternative site testing (arm or thigh), which decreases the discomfort of fingersticks. For infants, the earlobes and heels provide alternative blood sources to fingersticks. Enthusiasm for frequent BG testing tends to wane with duration of diabetes. However, families who are instructed on managing diabetes on the basis of test results are better motivated to persevere with SMBG. CGM may also be considered at some point for improved assessment of her metabolic control, particularly to detect nocturnal hypoglycemia. J.C. should test her BG before each meal and at bedtime, at a minimum. Additional tests should be performed whenever J.C. experiences hypoglycemia or ketonuria or when she becomes acutely ill.

HONEYMOON PERIOD

CASE 53-4, QUESTION 6: During the next 2 months, J.C.'s insulin requirements decreased to a total daily dose of 10 units (~0.3 unit/kg). Has her diabetes gone into remission?

Approximately 20% to 30% of individuals with type 1 diabetes go into a remission phase (honeymoon period) within days to weeks of their diagnosis.[153] During this phase, which can last for weeks to months, insulin requirements can fall well below the usual initial dose of 0.5 to 1.0 units/kg/day, and C-peptide can be detected, indicating a return of pancreatic function. A child may require minimal to no basal insulin replacement, and mealtime replacement requirements may need to be reduced. As illustrated by J.C., this presents clinically as markedly decreased insulin requirements to maintain normoglycemia. J.C. should continue to perform SMBG and closely monitor for rising BG concentrations, as β cell destruction continues during the honeymoon phase and she will eventually return to higher insulin requirements.

HYPOGLYCEMIA

CASE 53-4, QUESTION 7: J.C.'s parents contacted the clinic to report that J.C. is having nightmares and is awakening in the middle of the night complaining of a headache and stomach pain. However, these symptoms resolve by noon the following day. Her current insulin regimen is insulin aspart 2 units before meals and 3 units of insulin glargine twice daily (at breakfast and bedtime). Could J.C. be experiencing nocturnal hypoglycemia? How do the symptoms of hypoglycemia differ in a child compared with an adult? How can the risk of hypoglycemia be minimized for J.C.?

J.C.'s parents are appropriately worried. Hypoglycemia is a serious and often life-threatening complication of diabetes management in children, and the risk of hypoglycemia increases with attempts to maintain meticulous control of BG levels. Cognitive dysfunction may be increased in children and adolescents who continually experience severe hypoglycemia, and this can persist.[153,163] Common causes of hypoglycemia include changes in carbohydrate intake, late or skipped meals or snacks, exercise or unusual activity, and administration of excessive insulin. Because very young children may not be able to identify or express symptoms of hypoglycemia, caretakers must observe the child closely and identify symptoms or behaviors associated with a falling BG. Symptoms of hypoglycemia may include crankiness, sudden crying, restless sleep, or nightmares as seen in J.C.

Hypoglycemia is more frequent in children with lower A1C values, a prior history of severe hypoglycemia, larger insulin doses, and younger children.[164] Nocturnal hypoglycemia is reported in 14% to 47% of children with type 1 diabetes and is thought to be related to impaired counterregulatory response to hypoglycemia during sleep.[165] Bedtime BG levels are poor predictors of nocturnal hypoglycemia. J.C.'s parents should be instructed to test her BG at 2 AM closely for the next few nights, and then continue to check at least twice weekly. In children, insulin glargine can exhibit a small peak effect during the initial 3 to 5 hours after administration, increasing the risk for nocturnal hypoglycemia.[153] The insulin glargine dose should be moved to dinnertime. If this does not correct the nocturnal hypoglycemia, then the dose should be reduced. Use of insulin glargine is associated with less nocturnal hypoglycemia (and asymptomatic nocturnal hypoglycemia) compared with NPH insulin in children and adolescents.[156,159,166] A bedtime snack may also be needed. Treatment of hypoglycemia is addressed in Case 53-11, Question 3.

Using Insulin in Special Situations

INSULIN STABILITY: FACTORS ALTERING CONTROL

CASE 53-5

QUESTION 1: T.M., a 31-year-old farmer, has had type 1 diabetes for 20 years. He has been relatively well controlled on his current regimen of premeal insulin lispro and insulin glargine each evening for some time. During the winter and spring seasons, his BG concentrations have ranged from 90 to 140 mg/dL, and the A1C measured at his last clinic visit 3 months ago was 7.5%. It is now August. For the past 2 months, T.M. has noticed that his diabetes is not very well controlled. His BG concentrations vary widely from concentrations as low as 60 mg/dL to as high as 240 mg/dL. He has no explanation for this. On inspection, his vials of insulin lispro and glargine are cloudy. Both vials are approximately one-third full. What factors may be contributing to T.M.'s poor glycemic control?

Many factors may be contributing to T.M.'s poor control. Both of T.M.'s insulin vials have changed in appearance. T.M. should be instructed to immediately use new vials of insulin lispro and glargine. He should be educated to inspect his insulin before use, and to discard it if it has discoloration, clumping, frosting, or precipitation, which can result in loss of potency.[167]

TEMPERATURE

Insulin is a fragile molecule that can be damaged by temperature extremes. All commercially available insulins are stable for at least 28 days (e.g., ~1 month) at room temperature (68°–86°F), and the ADA recommends avoiding temperature extremes (<36°F or >86°F).[136,167] Some insulins are recommended to only be stored up to 77°F (insulin aspart, Novolin N, and Novolin 70/30). In practice, most patients store vials currently in use at room temperature because injection of cold insulin is uncomfortable. All unopened, extra vials or pen devices should be stored in the refrigerator (36°–46°F or 2°–8°C). For most insulins, patients should discard vials that have not been completely used in 28 days if they have been kept at room temperature (exceptions are insulin detemir, Novolin N, and Novolin 70/30, which can be kept for up to 42 days at room temperature). As a practical method, we recommend patients to obtain a new vial or pen, for basal and rapid-acting insulins, every month.

Insulin should not be used if it has been frozen or exposed to temperatures >98.6°F (37°C).[167] If T.M. lives in an area where temperatures frequently exceed 100°F during the summer months, he should be instructed to avoid storing his insulin in an automobile or in the sun, where it may be subject to deterioration. An insulated container or cooling packet (such as the FRIO Wallet) is recommended for T.M. It also is of interest that many wholesale drug distributors and some mail-order pharmacies do not take special packaging precautions when delivering insulins to pharmacies or homes during the summer months. Thus, inadvertent exposure to high temperatures during these months may alter the potency and actions of insulins. If T.M. were using an insulin suspension (e.g., NPH), freezing may cause aggregation of the precipitate and improper resuspension.[167]

PHYSICAL CHANGES

T.M.'s insulin appears cloudy or opaque. His insulin (insulin glargine and lispro) should always be completely clear.

Although not pertinent to T.M., in patients using NPH, a common cause of cloudiness is from contamination of the mealtime insulin (e.g., regular or rapid-acting insulin) with NPH (see Case 53-2, Question 15). NPH can sometimes flocculate or crystallize onto the insulin bottle, where a white precipitate clings to the vial, giving it a frosted appearance.[168]

OTHER FACTORS ALTERING INSULIN RESPONSE

Many other factors may be altering T.M.'s response to insulin. The heat in the summer months may increase circulation to the injected site, thus speeding the onset and shortening the duration of action of his insulin. Exercise of the injected limb may affect insulin action similarly. During the summer months, farmers typically are more physically active and, as a consequence, require less insulin than usual. Other factors that can alter insulin action are listed in Tables 53-10 and 53-19.

When patients like T.M. observe that their insulin seems to work less well even when the product is well within the expiration date and there are no obvious physical changes, they should inject insulin from a fresh vial to assess whether insulin from the original vial has deteriorated. If the response remains the same, they should work with a clinician to identify other reasons for their decreased responsiveness to insulin.

EXERCISE AND INSULIN REQUIREMENTS

CASE 53-6

QUESTION 1: J.S. is a 17-year-old, nonobese, patient with type 1 diabetes who was diagnosed at age 12. He currently is moderately well controlled on a single daily dose of insulin glargine 18 units at bedtime with 4 to 6 units of insulin aspart with meals (depending on carbohydrate intake). His A1C is 7.8%, and his BG levels before meals range from 150 to 190 mg/dL. FBG concentrations in the clinic range from 130 to 170 mg/dL. He has rare hypoglycemic reactions that are associated with skipped meals, and he generally adheres to his prescribed meal plan. J.S. would like to start running as his exercise program. What effect is running likely to have on his glycemic control? What precautions, if any, should he take?

Exercise has varying effects on plasma glucose levels in patients, such as J.S., who are taking insulin (Table 53-21). In the resting state, muscle derives approximately 10% of its metabolic requirement from glucose. In contrast, almost all of the muscle's metabolic requirements are derived from glucose during moderate to heavy exercise. Muscle glycogen stores are depleted quite rapidly, after which glucose is derived from the peripheral circulation. To meet the increased glucose demands, hepatic glycogenolysis and gluconeogenesis increase. This is mediated primarily through suppression of insulin secretion and increased secretion of counterregulatory hormones such as glucagon. Low, permissive levels of insulin are required for glucose utilization by the muscle. In nondiabetic individuals, hepatic glucose output and peripheral utilization are balanced such that euglycemia is maintained during exercise.[169,170]

In a patient like J.S., exercise may cause hyperglycemia or hypoglycemia if he does not take proper precautions. If he

TABLE 53-21
Exercise in Patients With Diabetes

1. Test blood glucose before, during, and after exercise.
2. For moderate exercise (e.g., bicycling or jogging for 30–45 minutes), ↓ the preceding dose of regular or rapid-acting insulin by approximately 30%–50%. If glucose concentration is normal or low before exercise, supplement the diet with a snack containing 10–15 g of carbohydrate.
3. To avoid ↑ absorption of regular insulin by exercise, inject into the abdomen or exercise 30–60 minutes after injection. Avoid exercise when rapid-acting insulin is peaking.
4. Individuals with low glycogen stores may be predisposed to the hypoglycemic effects of exercise. Examples include alcoholics, fasted individuals, or patients on extremely hypocaloric (<800 calories), low-carbohydrate (<10 g/d) diets.
5. Patients taking insulin are more susceptible to hypoglycemia than those taking oral insulin secretagogues (sulfonylureas, glinides). Patients with type 2 diabetes treated with diet are unlikely to develop hypoglycemia.
6. Watch for postexercise hypoglycemia. Individuals who have been exercising during the day will likely need to ↑ their carbohydrate intake and should test their blood glucose during the night to detect nocturnal hypoglycemia. Hypoglycemia can occur 8–15 hours after exercise.
7. If the glucose concentration is >240–300 mg/dL, the patient should not exercise. This indicates severe insulin deficiency. These patients are predisposed to hyperglycemia secondary to exercise.
8. Patients with severe proliferative retinopathy or retinal hemorrhage should avoid jarring exercise or exercise that involves moving the head below the waist.

is insulin deficient when he commences exercise, hepatic glucose output will be increased, but peripheral utilization will be decreased and hyperglycemia will ensue. Thus, patients like J.S. with type 1 diabetes should not exercise if their BG concentrations exceed 250 mg/dL and they have ketosis or if levels exceed 300 mg/dL (with or without ketosis), because these levels usually indicate insulin deficiency.[170]

Conversely, excess insulin enhances peripheral utilization of glucose by muscle and suppresses hepatic glucose output. Both can contribute to hypoglycemia. Hypoglycemia is more likely to occur in patients whose BG concentrations are normal or low just before exercise. Thus, if J.S.'s BG concentration is normal or low (<100 mg/dL) before he begins exercise, he should eat a carbohydrate snack (10–20 g) and have additional carbohydrates readily available during and after exercise.[170] He should delay his dose of insulin lispro until after exercising and adjust the amount according to his postexercise BG level. Consistent exercise may increase tissue sensitivity to insulin and eventually lower J.S.'s insulin requirements.

It is less well appreciated that peripheral glucose utilization remains high after exercise has been discontinued. This is thought to be related to the replenishment of glycogen stores in the liver and muscle. Thus, J.S. may need to use a lower dose of insulin aspart at the meal after his exercise, as hypoglycemia can occur 10 to 12 hours after exercise.[171] To err on the safe side, insulin should be injected at a site that is not exercised, for example, the abdomen in the case of J.S., to minimize the potential for exercise to enhance insulin's absorption (e.g., if injected into the thigh before running or jogging).

In overweight or obese individuals with type 2 diabetes who are treated with diet, exercise is unlikely to cause hypoglycemia. Patients with type 2 diabetes who are treated with insulin secretagogues or insulin may become hypoglycemic; thus, patients with type 2 diabetes who are normoglycemic before exercise also should consider increasing their carbohydrate intake.[172] Because patients with type 2 diabetes do not have an absolute lack of insulin, they are less likely to become hyperglycemic in response to exercise.

SICK DAY MANAGEMENT

CASE 53-7

QUESTION 1: G.M. a 32-year-old woman with type 1 diabetes, has been well controlled on a basal-bolus regimen (four injections daily) for the past 6 months. However, 2 days ago, she began to exhibit signs and symptoms consistent with the flu. This has made her nauseated, and now she has begun to vomit; consequently, her food intake has been minimal. Because R.D. is not eating at this time, should she discontinue her insulin?

Insulin requirements always increase in the presence of an infection or acute illness, even if food intake is diminished. Patients with type 1 diabetes, such as G.M., commonly decrease or eliminate insulin doses under these circumstances, and it is in just this setting that ketoacidosis occurs.

Therefore, G.M. should be instructed to maintain her usual dose of insulin and test her BG and urine ketones every 3 to 4 hours. If BG concentrations are above the usual range, extra doses of her rapid-acting insulin should be administered according to a prescribed algorithm based on her body's sensitivity to insulin (e.g., 1 unit for each 50 mg/dL above her BG target). People with type 1 diabetes should be instructed to test for ketones if their BG concentration is 300 mg/dL or higher. G.M. should call her physician if her BG concentration remains more than 240 mg/dL after three corrective insulin doses; if she has moderate to large amounts of ketones in her urine or blood (if using a meter that can measure these); if she has been vomiting or having diarrhea for longer than 6 hours; or if she begins to experience signs and symptoms related to ketoacidosis (polyuria, polydipsia, dehydration, ketonuria, and a fruity breath [see Case 53-13]). G.M. also should attempt to maintain her fluid, mineral, and carbohydrate intake with easily digested food and fluids (Table 53-22).[173]

TABLE 53-22
Sick Day Management[173]

1. Continue taking your basic dose of insulin *even* if you are not eating well or have nausea or vomiting.
2. Test your blood glucose more frequently: every 3–4 hours.
3. If indicated, give yourself extra doses (high-sugar correction) of lispro, aspart, glulisine, or regular insulin: for example, 1–2 units for every 30–50 mg/dL over an agreed-on target glucose concentration (e.g., 150 mg/dL). Correction doses must be individualized based on the patient's sensitivity to insulin (Table 53-11).
4. Begin testing your ketones (urine or blood) if you have type 1 diabetes. If you have type 2 diabetes, begin testing especially when glucose readings exceed 300 mg/dL.
5. Try to drink plenty of fluids (1/2 cup/h for adults) and maintain your caloric intake (50 g carbohydrate every 4 hours). Foods such as gelatin, noncarbonated soft drinks, crackers, soup, and soda may be used.
6. Call a physician if your blood glucose concentration remains >300 mg/dL, or your urine ketones remain high after two or three supplemental doses of insulin, or your blood glucose level remains >240 mg/dL for more than 24 hours.

INSULIN REQUIREMENTS IN RENAL FAILURE

CASE 53-8

QUESTION 1: M.B., a 32-year-old woman, has had type 1 diabetes for 15 years. During the past 2 years, a gradual deterioration of her renal function—as reflected by increased proteinuria, serum creatinine (SCr), and blood urea nitrogen (BUN) values, and reduced glomerular filtration rate (GFR)—has been observed. What are the anticipated effects of decreased renal function on M.B.'s insulin requirements?

The effects of renal failure on insulin requirements are complex, and under various circumstances, insulin requirements may increase or decrease. The kidney is the most important site of extrahepatic insulin metabolism and excretion. In nondiabetic individuals, the liver extracts approximately 60% of insulin secreted endogenously before it reaches the peripheral circulation.[86] Because exogenous insulin is delivered directly to the periphery, the kidneys play a more important role in its elimination. Insulin is filtered by the glomerulus and reabsorbed in the proximal tubules, where it is destroyed enzymatically. The kidney also clears insulin from the peritubular circulation.[88,174] At that site, insulin can enhance the reabsorption of sodium, which may account for the edema occasionally observed after the initiation of insulin therapy in some individuals.

Diminished renal function can be accompanied by decreased clearance of endogenous and exogenous insulin, resulting in increased plasma concentrations of insulin. Therefore, M.B.'s insulin requirements may diminish as her renal disease progresses. Patients with moderate degrees of renal failure (GFR >22.5 mL/minute) remove 39% of insulin from arterial plasma, similar to normal subjects. In contrast, patients with severe renal insufficiency (GFR <6 mL/minute) have a marked reduction in insulin removal from arterial plasma (9%).[175] Decreased insulin clearance in conjunction with the nausea and decreased food intake associated with uremia can lead to hypoglycemia in such individuals. In some patients with diabetes, particularly those with residual endogenous insulin secretion (e.g., type 2 diabetes), glucose tolerance may normalize as renal function diminishes, eliminating the need for insulin. In contrast, severe uremia is associated with glucose intolerance. This seems to be related to tissue resistance to insulin secondary to an unknown factor that can be removed by dialysis.

As M.B.'s renal function worsens, a reduction in her insulin requirements should be anticipated.

TRAVELING WITH DIABETES

CASE 53-9

QUESTION 1: J.R. is a 42-year-old woman with type 1 diabetes mellitus who has just taken a position that requires extensive overseas air travel. She is concerned about potential problems she may encounter managing her diabetes under these circumstances. What are some basic travel tips J.R. should consider?

The following sections discuss basic considerations for people with diabetes when traveling.[176] Before a trip, she should obtain a letter from her health care provider indicating her diagnosis (type 1 diabetes), diabetes therapy, and the supplies she requires (e.g., pens, pen needles). She should also obtain a prescription for all of her insulin therapy in case of an emergency.

When going through airport security, J.R. should alert the security officer that she has diabetes and is carrying her supplies with her. All diabetes medications, supplies, and equipment are allowed through the checkpoint once they have been screened. She should carry a plentiful backup supply (e.g., twice as much as she anticipates needing) of insulin, syringes, blood-testing supplies (including an extra battery for her meter), and glucose tablets.[176] J.R.'s insulin supply should be insulated (e.g., using a FRIO Wallet) and separated in various bags she will carry with her (i.e., not placed in checked luggage). J.R. should take with her a brief medical history and a prescription for insulin for emergency situations.

J.R. should carry some identification that alerts medical personnel or others to her diagnosis in emergency situations. This can take the form of a wallet card or a medical alert bracelet.

J.R. should try to maintain some regularity in her diet (time and amounts). When flying, she can request a low-carbohydrate, low-fat meal. She should inject her rapid-acting insulin only when her meal has been served to her (or sees the food coming down the aisle) to prevent hypoglycemia. To avoid unforeseen events (e.g., travel delays), J.R. should carry sufficient food and snacks with her on the plane.

J.R. needs to adjust her basal insulin doses when she flies across several time zones to account for time lost or gained.[176] When traveling east, the insulin dose should be decreased proportionately for the time lost and a shorter day. Conversely, when traveling west, the basal insulin dose should be increased for the time gained and a longer day.[177] The principle is to provide the same amount of basal insulin per hour. For example, if J.R. is using 10 units of insulin glargine and is traveling from New York to London (a 5-hour difference), her dose would be reduced to 8 units. This is because she is receiving about 0.4 units/hour and she will be losing 5 hours as she crosses the time zones ($0.4 \times 5 = 2$ units). When she arrives in London and changes her watch, she may resume her insulin glargine 10 units at the usual time of administration.

MANAGEMENT OF THE HOSPITALIZED PATIENT

CASE 53-10

QUESTION 1: A.G., a 55-year-old, 60-kg woman with a 35-year history of type 1 diabetes, was admitted to the critical care unit for an abdominal hysterectomy. Before admission, she was well controlled on 24 units of insulin glargine at bedtime and premeal doses of insulin aspart. How should A.G.'s diabetes be managed while in the critical care unit?

Patients with diabetes account for more than 1 in 5 hospital days in the United States. Of the nearly $174 billion that is spent annually on diabetes, nearly half is spent on inpatient care.[15] A clear, linear relationship exists between hyperglycemia and adverse clinical outcomes in the hospitalized patient.[178] However, this relationship exists regardless of a baseline diagnosis of diabetes at the time of admission, and iatrogenic hyperglycemia in the hospital does not have the same relationship morbidity that spontaneous hyperglycemia does.[178–180] These observations have raised important questions about the relationship between hyperglycemia and morbidity in the hospitalized patient.

Complex responses to acute illness including excess secretion of catecholamines and cortisol result in peripheral insulin resistance and so-called stress hyperglycemia. This makes it difficult to discern whether glycemia is a marker or a mediator of adverse outcomes in the acutely ill patient. Accordingly, historic practice had been to only aim for BG concentrations that prevent glucosuria (<200 mg/dL) and the subsequent risk for dehydration in the hospitalized patient. However, beginning in 2001, a series of randomized trials tested glycemic control in the critically ill patient. Significant changes have subsequently been made to practice recommendations for both the critically and the noncritically ill hospitalized patient.

Although several trials beginning in the 1990s tested intensive insulin regimens in patients with acute MI, they were small, placebo-controlled studies and reached different conclusions that proved difficult to rectify.[181–184] In 2001, the first of the van den Berghe trials tested two different levels of glycemic control in a relatively large number of surgical intensive care unit (ICU) patients with hyperglycemia with or without known diabetes.[185] A liberal glucose control strategy (reduction only if BG rose above 215 mg/dL) was compared with normalization of BG (80–110 mg/dL). Overall, normalization of BG significantly reduced ICU mortality from 8.0% to 4.5%.[185] However, the same researchers were unable to replicate their findings in a subsequent, similarly designed study in medical ICU patients with substantially higher baseline mortality rates.[186] Although a substudy showed that an ICU stay of 3 days or longer was predictive of benefit from tight control, a subsequent and much larger trial not only failed to confirm that finding but found increased mortality from a blood sugar of 80 to 110 mg/dL compared with 140 to 180 mg/dL (27.5%, 829 of 3,010 vs. 24.9%, 751 of 3,012).[187] The incidence of severe hypoglycemia (<40 mg/dL) in the different study groups assigned to tight control was between 7% and 18% and did not explain the different findings between studies. However, several important differences between these trials, which helped to inform current guidelines, should be noted.

The 2001 van den Berghe trial used parenteral nutrition in all patients and allowed for higher glucose values (insulin started if blood sugar exceeded 215 mg/dL) to occur in the conventional glycemia arm.[185] It is therefore possible that the aggressive insulin therapy in the tight control group helped to blunt the excessive glucotoxicity that may have been occurring from the parenteral nutrition. In the second van den Berghe trial as in the NICE-SUGAR study, parenteral nutrition was rarely used and initiation of insulin therapy in the conventional arms began at blood sugar values greater than 180 mg/dL.[186] Additionally, in NICE-SUGAR, a more aggressive target of 140 to 180 mg/dL was used rather than 180 to 200 mg/dL as in the two van den Berghe studies.[185–187] Table 53-23 summarizes these three trials assessing level of glucose control in critically ill patients.

Overall, numerous individual studies as well as meta-analyses have reached different conclusions regarding whether or not tight control of BG is superior to conventional control in the hospitalized, acutely ill patient.[188,189]

In 2009, the ADA made substantial changes to its 2005 guideline on management of inpatient hyperglycemia.[190] Although existing randomized trials of glycemic control have been performed in critical care settings, the ADA guideline included non-ICU settings. To make recommendations for non-ICU patients, ADA relied on case series and retrospective analyses, which will ultimately need to be subjected to randomized, prospective trials.[191–193] In the meantime, recommendations for both critically ill and noncritically ill hospitalized patients are the same: a premeal or fasting BG target less than 140 mg/dL and random values of less than 180 mg/dL.[190]

For perioperative insulin needs, A.G. should receive her usual basal insulin dose (insulin glargine 24 units) on the night before surgery. If the basal insulin is normally administered in the morning, the usual dose can still be given for patients with type 1 diabetes; for those with type 2 diabetes, 50% to 100% of the basal insulin is administered the morning of surgery. Correction doses of rapid-acting insulin can be administered the morning of surgery if the BG is more than 180 mg/dL.[194] If a current A1C is not available, it can be measured to assess the patient's glycemic control before admission.

Most insulin infusion protocols include the use of IV regular insulin and maintenance IV fluids, either 5% dextrose in water (D5W) or D5W with 0.45% normal saline (0.45% NaCl). For a patient requiring fluid restriction, 10% dextrose in water (D10W) may be used.[194] The adjustment algorithms are used by nursing to change the rate of infusion (in units/hour) depending on the BG level. Most often, the insulin infusion is prepared in a solution of 1 unit/1 mL normal saline (e.g., 100 units of regular insulin in 100 mL of 0.9% NaCl). A dedicated IV line is used for the insulin infusion to avoid iatrogenic hypoglycemia. The insulin infusion is connected to the maintenance IV containing dextrose (can be Y-connected). Because insulin binds to plastic, the insulin solution should be flushed (e.g., with 20 mL) through the IV tubing before the line is connected to the patient. An IV dextrose infusion is maintained while a patient is on an insulin infusion. Most patients need 5 to 10 g of glucose per hour (or D5W or D5W/0.45% NaCl at 100–200 mL/hour). Additional maintenance fluids (and electrolytes) can be administered via a different port or line. Some protocols include an initial bolus dose of insulin. The initial insulin infusion rate is primarily based on current BG level and BMI; other factors such as body weight, current daily insulin requirements, and renal function should be taken into consideration. An initial rate of 1 unit/hour is common (can range from 0.5 units/hour to ≥2 units/hour). The choice of initial infusion rate is not critical but should be based on patient history. A rate of 0.5 units/hour is appropriate for a patient who has never previously received insulin, whereas 2 units/hour would be appropriate for a patient with known insulin-dependent diabetes. Adjustments in the insulin infusion rate are determined by BG levels every 60 minutes until the BG is stable and close to target. Then the frequency of BG testing may be reduced to every 2 to 3 hours. Algorithms should consider both the current and previous BG level, the rate of change of the BG level, and the current infusion rate.[8]

Insulin infusion should be started at least 2 to 3 hours before the surgery to titrate to the desired level of glucose control. Examples of protocols are available on the Institute for Healthcare Improvement's website (available at http://www.ihi.org/IHI/Topics/PatientSafety/MedicationSystems/Tools/), and many are published in the medical literature.[195,196]

TABLE 53-23
Summary Data of Three Major Trials of Intensive vs. Conventional Glycemic Control With Insulin in Critically Ill Patients

		Glucose Target (mg/dL)		Glucose Achieved (mg/dL)				
Trial	N	Intensive	Conventional	Intensive	Conventional	Primary Outcome	End Point	OR (95% CI)
van den Berghe et al.[185]	1,548	80–110	180–200	103	153	ICU mortality	4.6% vs. 8%	0.58 (0.38–0.78)
van den Berghe et al.[186]	1,200	80–110	180–200	111	153	Hospital mortality	37.3% vs. 40.0%	0.94 (0.84–1.06)
NICE-SUGAR[187]	6,104	81–108	<180	115	145	90-day mortality	27.5% vs. 24.9%	1.14 (1.02–1.28)

CI, confidence interval; OR, odds ratio.

Thus, A.G.'s usual SC insulin regimen should be discontinued, and she should be initiated on an insulin infusion that is adjusted according to an algorithm. Throughout the perioperative period, she should receive a minimum of 100 g of glucose daily to prevent starvation ketosis.

Assessment of interfering substances with point-of-care BG testing is particularly important for hospitalized patients. Some immunoglobulins and dialysates contain nonglucose sugars (including maltose, xylose, and galactose), which can interfere with glucose measurements with glucose dehydrogenase pyrroloquinolinequinone test strips (will falsely elevate the reading, Table 53-18). BG concentrations should only be performed by the laboratory in these patients.[139]

Adverse Effects of Insulin

HYPOGLYCEMIA

CASE 53-11

QUESTION 1: G.O., a 42-year-old, slightly overweight (5 feet 11 inches, 200 pounds, BMI 27.9 kg/m^2) man, has had a history of type 1 diabetes mellitus for 17 years. G.O.'s medical care was sporadic until 1 year ago when he referred himself to a diabetes clinic because he was beginning to experience pain and numbness in his feet. At that time, he was poorly controlled on a single daily dose of a premixed NPH and regular insulin mixture (Humulin 70/30), 45 units. He had not been testing his BG concentrations, and his A1C was 13%.

On physical examination, G.O. was found to have an elevated BP (160/94 mm Hg), background retinopathy, and decreased pedal pulses bilaterally. He had decreased sensation to vibration and monofilament testing in both feet. G.O. also complained of impotence and "shooting pains" in both legs. A spot collection for microalbuminuria was 450 mg of albumin/g creatinine (normal, 30–299 mg/g creatinine).

G.O. was transitioned to a basal-bolus insulin regimen. His physician gave him a premeal BG target of 70 to 130 mg/dL.[8] For the past several months, he has been treated with the following regimen: 14 to 18 units of insulin glulisine before breakfast; 14 to 18 units of insulin glulisine before lunch; 16 to 18 units of insulin glulisine before dinner; and 40 units of insulin glargine at bedtime. If his BG level is high after lunch, he takes additional glulisine (~2 hours after eating). If his BG is high at bedtime (e.g., > 150 mg/dL), he takes additional insulin glulisine (7–10 units) because his physician told him his BG level needed to be lowered significantly. BG concentrations have been as follows:

Time	Glucose Concentration (mg/dL)
7 AM	60–320
Noon	140–280
5 PM	40–300

In the past year, G.O.'s A1C has decreased to 7.1%. Currently, he has approximately five hypoglycemic episodes per week, primarily in the late afternoon and early morning hours. These are characterized by intense hunger, sweating, palpitations, and (according to his wife) a short temper. He has found that he can avoid nocturnal hypoglycemia (night sweats, nightmares, and headaches) by eating a large bedtime snack. During the past 3 months, he has gained 15 pounds. Are G.O.'s signs and symptoms consistent with mild, moderate, or severe hypoglycemia? What are the causes?

G.O.'s case illustrates one of the major hazards of aggressive BG targets and intensive insulin therapy: hypoglycemia. Hypoglycemia is a fact of life for patients with type 1 diabetes, virtually all of whom experience a hypoglycemic episode at one time or another. Nocturnal hypoglycemia is of particular concern. A syndrome called "dead-in-bed" has been described for patients with type 1 diabetes, who experience repeated hypoglycemia and have an underlying cardiovascular pathology, and die in their sleep.[197]

Hypoglycemia is a BG concentration less than 60 mg/dL, and its occurrence is potentially fatal if not promptly recognized and treated. However, the exact level at which a patient experiences symptoms is difficult to define. Clinical hypoglycemia is associated with typical autonomic (neurogenic) and neuroglycopenic symptoms relieved by the administration of a quickly absorbed carbohydrate.

PATHOPHYSIOLOGY

Normal brain function depends on glucose, the exclusive fuel for cerebral metabolism. Because the brain is unable to synthesize or store glucose, it must be provided with a constant exogenous quantity via the brain's blood supply. As BG concentrations fall, a series of physiological responses occur to restore glucose levels. These responses create symptoms warning a patient to take corrective action by consuming carbohydrates. If these counterregulatory responses fail to alert the patient and BG concentrations fall below a critical level, cognitive function becomes impaired, and confusion and coma may ensue.

In people without diabetes, the peripheral responses to hypoglycemia are so efficient that clinically important hypoglycemia probably never occurs. As glucose levels fall to between 50 and 60 mg/dL, a series of neuroendocrine events occur, raising the plasma glucose concentration back toward normal by increasing hepatic glucose output. The major hormone responsible for producing acute recovery from insulin-induced hypoglycemia is glucagon; however, epinephrine alone also can produce near-normal recovery. Rising levels of adrenergic and cholinergic hormones generate warning symptoms of hypoglycemia. When hypoglycemia is prolonged, growth hormone and cortisone play a greater role in producing recovery.

Patients with type 1 diabetes who maintain insulin depots throughout the day are predisposed to severe hypoglycemic reactions because deficiencies in the normal feedback system occur with time. Glucagon secretion becomes deficient within the first 2 to 5 years after diagnosis, and by 10 years or longer, epinephrine secretion may become impaired. The latter defect leads to asymptomatic hypoglycemia or hypoglycemic unawareness (see Case 53-12).

Certain circumstances predispose patients with type 1 diabetes to severe hypoglycemia. These include (a) a defective counterregulatory hormonal response to hypoglycemia (see Case 53-12), which may be further diminished with frequent hypoglycemia, (b) medications such as β-blockers that diminish early warning signs of impending hypoglycemia, (c) intensive insulin therapy that can alter secretion of counterregulatory hormones, (d) skipped meals or inadequate carbohydrate intake relative to the insulin dose, (e) physical activity, and (e) excessive alcohol intake (Table 53-14).

SYMPTOMS

The signs and symptoms associated with hypoglycemia vary in intensity according to the presence of cognitive deficits and the patient's ability to self-treat the reaction. They vary substantially from one patient to another. Symptoms are conventionally divided into two categories: neurogenic (or autonomic) and neuroglycopenic.[198]

Autonomic symptoms include sweating, intense hunger, palpitations, tremor, tingling, and anxiety. Epinephrine is thought to mediate many of the neurogenic responses to hypoglycemia.

Neuroglycopenic symptoms resulting from neuronal fuel deprivation (glucose) include difficulty concentrating, lethargy, confusion, agitation, weakness, and possibly, slurred speech, dizziness, and fainting. Profound behavioral changes, seizures, and coma are more severe manifestations of neuroglycopenia. Prolonged, severe neuroglycopenia ultimately results in death. Symptoms of mild, moderate, severe, and nocturnal hypoglycemia are as follows:

- *Mild hypoglycemia:* Symptoms include tremor, palpitations, sweating, and intense hunger. Diminished cerebral function is not present, and patients are capable of self-treating.
- *Moderate hypoglycemia:* Moderate hypoglycemic reactions include neuroglycopenic as well as autonomic symptoms: headache, mood changes, irritability, decreased attention, and drowsiness. Patients may require assistance in treating themselves because of the presence of impaired judgment or weakness. Symptoms are more severe, usually last longer, and often require a second dose of a simple carbohydrate.
- *Severe hypoglycemia:* Symptoms of severe hypoglycemia include unresponsiveness, unconsciousness, or convulsions. These reactions require assistance from another individual for appropriate treatment. Approximately 10% of patients treated with insulin experience at least one severe, disabling episode of hypoglycemia per year that requires emergency treatment with parenteral glucagon or IV glucose.[198]
- *Nocturnal hypoglycemia:* Tingling of the lips and tongue are common complaints of patients who experience nocturnal hypoglycemia. These patients also may complain of headache and difficulty arising in the morning, nightmares, or nocturnal diaphoresis.[198] Family members should be conscious of any unusual sounds or activity while the patient is sleeping.

G.O. has mild to moderate hypoglycemic reactions, which he is able to self-treat. These are likely caused by overinsulinization and insulin "stacking" (giving rapid or short-acting insulin injections too close together, so that the doses "stack" on top of the other) with his rapid-acting insulin.

OVERINSULINIZATION

CASE 53-11, QUESTION 2: Evaluate G.O.'s overall control. What signs and symptoms in G.O. are consistent with overinsulinization and insulin stacking? How should he be managed?

The following is a list of signs and symptoms of overinsulinization in G.O.:

- A total daily insulin dose of more than 1.0 unit/kg. This dose is unusually high for a patient with type 1 diabetes, who should not be resistant to the action of insulin.
- Weight gain in the past several months. This is secondary to the anabolic effects of insulin as well as G.O.'s increased carbohydrate intake to match his high insulin doses for treatment of hypoglycemia.
- Frequent hypoglycemic reactions.
- High glycemic variability (i.e., BG concentrations that fluctuate wildly between hypoglycemia and hyperglycemia). In G.O.'s case, high BG concentrations may represent reactive hyperglycemia or overtreatment of hypoglycemic episodes. His low BG level may represent excessive rapid-acting insulin at bedtime and insulin stacking of his rapid-acting insulin after lunch. At lunchtime, he is administering a high-sugar correction dose of insulin glulisine too soon; his mealtime glulisine is still likely at a peak action and working to lower his prandial BG. By administering additional glulisine soon after the meal, the two insulin doses are adding up, or stacking, causing hypoglycemia.
- Near-normal A1C levels indicate mean BG concentrations that must be within the normal range even though the patient has recorded numerous high BG concentrations. Patients treated with intensive insulin therapy in the DCCT experienced hypoglycemic episodes three times more often than patients treated with standard insulin therapy.[38] A1C levels were approximately 7.2%.

G.O. should be managed by discontinuing his high-sugar corrections at bedtime and after lunch. He should SMBG premeal, 1 to 2 hours after meals, and at bedtime to obtain a better picture of his glucose patterns and insulin requirements. He should avoid the large bedtime snack because one should not have to add food just to avoid hypoglycemia (i.e., the insulin regimen should be adjusted). He should also begin testing his BG at 2 or 3 AM to assess whether he is still experiencing nocturnal hypoglycemia after stopping the bedtime insulin glulisine. It will be important that he record the actual dose he administers before each meal and bring the record to clinic so that his insulin doses can be fine-tuned. Next, if he is capable, an algorithm for adjusting his preprandial insulin glulisine doses should be provided to minimize hypoglycemic and hyperglycemic reactions (see Case 53-2, Question 12), eventually he can transition to counting carbohydrates (see Case 53-2, Questions 11 and 12).

TREATMENT OF HYPOGLYCEMIA

CASE 53-11, QUESTION 3: How should G.O.'s hypoglycemic episodes be managed?

As G.O. illustrates, many patients with diabetes are frightened of hypoglycemia and have a tendency to overtreat their reactions with, for example, large quantities of juice or regular soda. This should be discouraged because overcorrection together with glucose generated by counterregulatory hormones ultimately results in hyperglycemia.

The key to successful management of hypoglycemia is recognition and prevention. Because early warning symptoms of hypoglycemia vary from person to person, it is important that G.O. learn to recognize and pay attention to his earliest warning symptoms and treat early. Patients generally can recall prodromal symptoms after recovery from a severe hypoglycemic reaction if they have not developed hypoglycemic unawareness (see Case 53-12). As a caveat, we occasionally have seen patients who "feel" hypoglycemic after their BG concentrations have been normalized from very high levels with intensive insulin therapy, owing to the amount of BG change. We encourage patients to test their BG level any time they "feel unusual" to verify a low BG concentration before treatment. G.O. should treat his symptoms only if he is truly hypoglycemic.

A second component of prevention is determining its cause and taking preventive or corrective action. This entails assessment of his diet (did he skip or delay a meal or change its content?), exercise pattern, time of insulin administration, insulin dose, and accuracy of carbohydrate counting and dose administered. If hypoglycemic reactions consistently occur at a certain time of day, he should determine whether this corresponds with a mealtime dose of his rapid-acting insulin and reduce that insulin dose by 1 to 2 units. If his FBG is running low, his insulin glargine dose can be reduced.

If a reaction occurs, G.O. should be instructed to treat it as follows (Table 53-14).

MILD HYPOGLYCEMIA

Most hypoglycemic reactions are managed readily with the equivalent of 10 to 20 g of glucose (see Table 53-14 for examples of carbohydrate sources containing 15 g of glucose). If the blood concentration remains low after 15 minutes, the patient should ingest another 10 to 20 g of carbohydrate. This quick-acting source of glucose should be followed by a small complex carbohydrate or protein snack (e.g., milk, peanut butter sandwich) to provide a continual source of glucose if a meal is not scheduled within the next 1 to 2 hours. An easy rule of thumb that can be used by patients is "15-15-15": 15 g of glucose followed by a second 15 g if the patient is still symptomatic after 15 minutes.

Glucose tablets are available and have the added benefit of being premeasured to prevent overtreatment of hypoglycemia. Glucose gels or small tubes of cake frosting are useful for children or patients who become uncooperative and combative when hypoglycemic.

MODERATE TO SEVERE HYPOGLYCEMIA

Glucagon can be injected by the SC or IM (preferred) route into the deltoid or anterior thigh region. Glucagon is used when a patient is unable to self-treat their hypoglycemia caused by exogenous insulin. The dose of glucagon recommended to treat moderate or severe hypoglycemia for a child younger than 5 years of age is 0.25 to 0.5 mg; for children 5 to 10 years of age, 0.5 to 1 mg; and for patients older than 10 years, 1 mg. Parents, spouses, or other close contacts should be taught how to mix, draw up, and administer glucagon during emergency situations. Kits with prefilled syringes containing 1 mg glucagon are available. Patients who are given glucagon should be positioned so that their face is turned toward the floor to prevent aspiration in the event of vomiting. As soon as the patient awakens (10–25 minutes), he or she should be fed.

Intravenous Glucose

If glucagon is unavailable, the patient should be taken to the hospital's emergency department, where he or she can be treated with IV glucose (~10–25 g administered as 20–50 mL of 50% dextrose for 1–3 minutes) in preference to glucagon. After the bolus injection of glucose, IV glucose (5–10 g/hour) should be continued until the patient has gained consciousness and is able to eat.

HYPOGLYCEMIC UNAWARENESS

CASE 53-12

QUESTION 1: M.M., a 35-year-old, 75-kg, unemployed man, has had type 1 diabetes since the age of 3. As a consequence of the diabetes, he has developed proliferative retinopathy and progressive diabetic nephropathy (current SCr, 2.2 mg/dL). M.M. has an erratic lifestyle. Because he does not work, he often stays out late at night and sleeps late into the morning. His insulin is injected whenever he awakens, and his meals are irregularly spaced. Each time he comes to the clinic, he brings with him a complete log of glucose concentrations that range from 80 to 140 mg/dL. He has two to three severe hypoglycemic reactions a month that require trips to the emergency department for treatment with IV glucose. On several occasions, his BG concentration has been 30 mg/dL, and he states he may feel a little weak, but otherwise feels "not too bad." M.M.'s last A1C was 10%. He says that he adheres to the following insulin regimen: 18 units NPH/11 units regular insulin before breakfast, 10 units regular insulin before lunch and dinner, and 14 units NPH at bedtime.

At this visit, M.M. comes with his girlfriend. He has a large gash on his nose that occurred 3 days ago when he lost consciousness at approximately 1:30 PM while pushing his stalled car. He was unable to eat lunch at the usual hour because he had problems with his car. Assess M.M.'s hypoglycemic reactions and BG control. Should his current insulin regimen be continued? How should he be managed?

M.M. illustrates a patient with type 1 diabetes who has defective glucose counterregulation and, as a result, is unable to counteract a hypoglycemic reaction effectively. He also is an example of a patient who should not have aggressive BG targets because he does not feel the symptoms of a low blood sugar and has already developed end-stage organ damage (proliferative retinopathy and nephropathy). Neither is likely to be reversed with improved glycemic control. In fact, proliferative retinopathy may actually worsen with intensive insulin therapy initially.[38] In the DCCT study, severe hypoglycemic reactions were three times more common among patients treated with intensive insulin therapy, and nocturnal hypoglycemia accounted for 41% of the total hypoglycemic episodes.[38] In patients with defective counterregulation, the risk of severe hypoglycemia may be 25 times higher than in patients with adequate counterregulatory mechanisms treated with intensive insulin therapy.[198] M.M. is at great risk for death secondary to hypoglycemia.

M.M.'s lifestyle is erratic, he eats irregularly, and his reported BG concentrations (80–140 mg/dL) do not correspond to his elevated A1C value. This may indicate that M.M.'s technique is incorrect or that he simply fills in the log with fictitious numbers before he comes to the clinic. Irregular entries in different colored inks and bloodstains usually indicate authentic records.

As noted, the primary hormones that are secreted in response to a low BG concentration are glucagon and epinephrine. In patients who have had type 1 diabetes for longer than 2 to 5 years, a deficiency in glucagon secretion is a relatively consistent finding, and these patients must rely on epinephrine to reverse low BG concentrations.[199] Unfortunately, approximately 40% of patients with long-standing type 1 diabetes (8–15 years) have defective epinephrine secretion as well, and this may be related to the development of autonomic neuropathy. Patients whose diabetes is tightly controlled also have reduced counterregulatory hormone responses to hypoglycemia. As illustrated by M.M., patients with defective epinephrine secretory responses also lose the warning signs and symptoms of hypoglycemia. These patients are said to have hypoglycemia unawareness because they have no awareness of BG concentrations less than 50 mg/dL. In these individuals, loss of consciousness, seizures, or irrational behavior may be the first objective signs of exceedingly low BG concentrations. The glycemic threshold for symptoms also is lowered in patients on intensive insulin therapy whose glucose concentrations have been lowered to normal or near-normal levels.[198] Consequently, their hypoglycemic reactions may go unnoticed and untreated until they lose consciousness. M.M. should be managed as follows:

- Because his waking, sleeping, and eating patterns are highly irregular, M.M. should be treated with an insulin regimen that addresses his lifestyle. For example, he could be switched to a basal-bolus insulin regimen, in which he can give himself a rapid-acting insulin just before he actually intends to eat. A dose of insulin glargine or detemir could be given before his first meal to supply a basal level of insulin between meals.

- Because M.M. has no warning symptoms for hypoglycemia, the importance of regular SMBG should be emphasized. When BG testing was reviewed with M.M., it was discovered that his eyesight was so poor that he was unable to distinguish between the right and wrong side of the glucose test strip. Furthermore, because he had lost his depth of field, he was unable to apply the drop of blood into the test strip. To address this situation, M.M.'s girlfriend was taught how to perform BG testing. Also, a glucose monitor that requires a very small blood sample and beeps with an adequate blood sample (e.g., Abbott Freestyle Freedom Lite) was provided to him.
- M.M.'s girlfriend also was taught how to recognize and treat symptoms of hypoglycemia and how to administer glucagon. Often, patients ignore early warning symptoms and progress to a point that they lose the judgment needed to treat the condition. If M.M. has not yet become combative, a quick-acting carbohydrate source should be offered. If he has lost consciousness, glucagon should be injected.

All of these maneuvers diminished the frequency of M.M.'s severe hypoglycemic reactions. On the whole, his BG concentrations were maintained below 180 mg/dL, and he remained relatively free of hyperglycemic symptoms. M.M.'s A1C using a basal-bolus insulin regimen was 8.0%.

DIABETIC KETOACIDOSIS

CASE 53-13

QUESTION 1: J.L., a 40-year-old, 60-kg woman with an 8-year history of type 1 diabetes, is moderately well controlled on 24 units of insulin glargine plus premeal doses of insulin lispro. Her family brings her to the emergency department, where she complains of abdominal tenderness, nausea, and vomiting. According to her family, J.L. was well until 2 days ago when she awoke with nausea, vomiting, diarrhea, and chills. Because she has been unable to eat, she has omitted her usual morning dose of insulin for the past 2 days. Her gastrointestinal (GI) symptoms progressed, and she was brought to the emergency department when she became lethargic.

Physical examination reveals an ill-appearing woman who is lethargic but responsive. Her temperature is 37°C. Skin turgor is poor, mucous membranes are dry, and her eyeballs are shrunken and soft. J.L.'s lungs are clear, but respirations are deep and her breath has a fruity odor. Cardiac examination is within normal limits.

In the supine position, J.L.'s pulse rate is 115 beats/minute and her BP is 105/60 mm Hg. In the upright position, her pulse increased to 140 beats/minute, and her BP dropped to 85/40 mm Hg. There is mild, diffuse tenderness over her abdomen.

Laboratory results on admission disclosed the following:

BG, 450 mg/dL
Sodium (Na), 150 mEq/L
Potassium (K), 5.4 mEq/L
Chloride (Cl), 106 mEq/L
HCO_3, 10 mEq/L
SCr, 2.0 mg/dL
Hemoglobin, 15.7 g/dL
Hematocrit, 49%
White blood cell count, 15,000/μL with 3% bands (normal, 3%–5%), 70% polymorphonuclear neutrophils (normal, 54%–62%), and 27% lymphocytes (normal, 25%–33%)
Serum ketones, moderate at 1:10 dilution (normal, negative)

The urinalysis showed the following:

Glucose, 2+ (normal, 0)
Moderate ketones (normal, 0)
pH, 5.5 (normal, 4.6–8)
Specific gravity, 1.029 (normal, 1.020–1.025)
No white blood cells, red blood cells, bacteria, or casts

Arterial blood gas results were as follows:

pH, 7.05 (normal, 7.36–7.44)
P_{CO_2}, 20 mm Hg (normal, 35–45)
P_{O_2}, 120 mm Hg (normal, 90–100)

What supports the diagnosis of DKA in J.L.?

The fact that J.L. has type 1 diabetes puts her at risk for developing ketoacidosis. About 80% of DKA cases occur in patients older than 18 years of age with about one-third of those occurring in patients older than 45 years of age.[200] In DKA, an absolute or relative insulin deficiency promotes lipolysis and metabolism of free fatty acids to β-hydroxybutyrate, acetoacetic acid, and acetone in the liver. Excess glucagon enhances gluconeogenesis and impairs peripheral ketone utilization. Physiologic stress contributes to the development of DKA by stimulating release of insulin counterregulatory hormones including glucagon, catecholamines, glucocorticoids, and growth hormone. Common stress factors include infection, pregnancy, pancreatitis, trauma, hyperthyroidism, and acute MI.

J.L. presented with symptoms of nausea, vomiting, diarrhea, and chills, and these are suggestive of an acute viral gastroenteritis. Patients such as J.L. commonly discontinue their insulin in this setting, which can rapidly precipitate the development of DKA (see Case 53-7). Table 53-24 lists patient education points with regard to DKA.

As illustrated by J.L., patients with DKA present with moderate to high serum glucose concentrations secondary to decreased peripheral utilization and increased hepatic production (Table 53-25). This increases serum osmolality, which initially shifts fluid from the intracellular to the extracellular space. When serum glucose concentrations exceed the renal threshold for reabsorption of about 200 mg/dL, glucose "spills" over into the urine and causes an osmotic diuresis that depletes the total body water and electrolytes. J.L. also has lost fluid and electrolytes from vomiting and diarrhea. Eventually, as losses exceed input, the patient becomes dehydrated (dry mucous membranes; dry skin; soft, shrunken eyeballs; increased hematocrit), and intravascular volume becomes depleted (orthostatic BP and pulse changes).

The finding of hyperkalemia in J.L. is also common in DKA because insulin contributes to the intracellular shift of potassium.[200] The relative deficiency of insulin in DKA results in an extracellular shift of potassium that is worsened by the acidosis that often develops.[200] A finding of hypokalemia in DKA (<3.3 mg/dL) is uncommon and is a marker of more severe disease. In the hypokalemic patient, the combination of the extracellular shift of potassium and polyuria has led to excessive depletion of total body potassium. Care must be used in these patients to replace potassium intravenously before beginning insulin therapy, which will cause further hypokalemia as potassium shifts back into cells.[200]

TABLE 53-24
Diabetic Ketoacidosis: Patient Education

Definition: DKA occurs when the body has insufficient insulin.

Questions to Ask

1. Has insulin use been discontinued or a dose skipped for any reason?
2. If an insulin pump is being used, is the tubing clogged or twisted? Has the catheter become dislodged?
3. Has the insulin being used lost its activity? Is the bottle of rapid-acting/regular or basal insulin cloudy? Does the bottle of NPH look frosty?
4. Have insulin requirements increased owing to illness or other forms of stress (infection, pregnancy, pancreatitis, trauma, hyperthyroidism, or MI)?

What to Look For

1. Signs and symptoms of hyperglycemia: thirst, excessive urination, fatigue, blurred vision, consistently elevated blood glucose concentrations (>300 mg/dL)
2. Signs of acidosis: fruity breath odor, deep and difficult breathing
3. Signs of dehydration: dry mouth; warm, dry skin; fatigue
4. Others: stomach pain, nausea, vomiting, loss of appetite

What to Do

1. Review "sick day management" (Table 53-22)
2. Test blood glucose ≥4 times daily
3. Test urine for ketones when blood glucose concentration is >300 mg/dL
4. Drink plenty of fluids (water, clear soups)
5. Continue taking insulin dose
6. Contact physician immediately

DKA, diabetic ketoacidosis; MI, myocardial infarction; NPH, neutral protamine Hagedorn.

Evidence of excessive ketone production in J.L. includes ketonuria, ketonemia, and the characteristic fruity odor of acetone on the breath. Elevated levels of these organic acids increase the anion gap and decrease the pH and carbonate levels. The respiratory rate is increased to compensate for the metabolic acidosis leading to hypercapnia.[200,201]

Treatment

CASE 53-13, QUESTION 2: How should J.L. be treated?

Treatment of patients with DKA is aimed at expansion of intravascular and extravascular volume, replacement of electrolyte losses, and cessation of ketone production (Table 53-26).

FLUIDS

Rapid correction of fluid loss is most crucial. The usual fluid deficit is difficult to estimate in the absence of overt hypernatremia but approximates 5% to 10% of body weight in most patients depending on the severity of the DKA. In the absence of cardiac compromise, hypernatremia, or significant renal dysfunction, isotonic saline (0.9% NaCl) should be used.[200]

J.L. has evidence of significant dehydration and intravascular volume depletion. Based on body weight, if the patient has

TABLE 53-25
Common Laboratory Abnormalities in Diabetic Ketoacidosis

Glucose	250 mg/dL
Serum osmolarity	Variable, can be >320 mOsm/kg in presence of coma
Sodium	Low, normal, or high[a]
Potassium	Normal or high
Ketones	Present in urine and blood
pH	Mild: 7.25–7.30 Moderate: 7.00–7.24 Severe: <7.00
Bicarbonate	Mild: 15–18 mEq/L Moderate: 10 to <15 mEq/L Severe: <10 mEq/L
WBC count	15,000–40,000 cells/μL even without evidence of infection

[a]Total body sodium is always low.
WBC, white blood cell.

TABLE 53-26
Management of Diabetic Ketoacidosis[200]

Fluid Administration

Start IV fluids using normal saline (0.9% NaCl) unless patient has cardiac compromise.

Rate is 15–20 mL/kg body weight or 1–1.5 L during first hour.

Then, if corrected sodium is normal or elevated, use 0.45% NaCl at a rate of 4–14 mL/kg/h (250–500 mL/h). Use 0.9% NaCl if corrected sodium is low.

Once serum glucose reaches 200 mg/dL, change to 5% dextrose with 0.45% NaCl at 150–250 mL/h.

Insulin

Continuous IV infusion of regular insulin is preferred. Use IM route only if infusion is not available.

Bolus dose: 0.1 units/kg IV

Maintenance dose: 0.1 units/kg/h IV

If blood glucose level has not decreased by 50–75 mg/dL after 1 hour, double infusion rate.

Once blood glucose reaches 200 mg/dL, reduce infusion rate to 0.05–0.1 units/kg/h and change fluid to 5% dextrose with 0.45% NaCl (do not stop insulin infusion).

When SC insulin can be initiated, administer dose 1–2 hours before discontinuing IV infusion.

For uncomplicated DKA, SC rapid-acting insulin can be considered. A bolus dose of 0.2 units/kg followed by 0.1 units/kg every hour *or* an initial dose of 0.3 units/kg followed by 0.2 units/kg every 2 hours until the blood glucose reaches <250 mg/dL; then the SC insulin dose is decreased by half (to either 0.05 or 0.1 units/kg every 1–2 hours).

Potassium

Establish adequate renal function (urine output ~50 mL/h). If K is <3.3 mEq/L, hold insulin and give 20–40 mEq/h until K >3.3 mEq/L. If K is >5.5mEq/L, do not give K and check serum K every 2 hours. If K is >3.3 but <5.3 mEq/L, give 20–30 mEq in each liter of IV fluid to maintain K between 4 and 5 mEq/L.

Phosphate

Initiate if level <1 mg/dL, or in patients with cardiac dysfunction, anemia, or respiratory depression. Use potassium phosphate salt, 20–30 mEq added to replacement fluid. Rarely needed.

Bicarbonate

Replacement is controversial and may be dangerous.

For adults with pH <6.9, 100 mmol of sodium bicarbonate may be added to 400 mL of sterile water with 20 mEq of KCl; infuse for 2 hours (200 mL/h). For adults with pH of 6. 9–7.0, 50 mmol of sodium bicarbonate diluted in 200 mL of sterile water with 10 mEq of KCL; infuse for 1 hour (200 mL/h). No bicarbonate is necessary if pH >7.0.

DKA, diabetic ketoacidosis; IM, intramuscular; IV, intravenous; SC, subcutaneous.

the typical 5% to 10% weight loss, that would indicate approximately 3 to 6 L of fluid will be needed to fully replete (10% of 60 kg = 6-kg loss and 1 L = 1 kg). It is recommended that fluids be replaced at the rate of 15 to 20 mL/kg/hour during the first hour (~1 to 1.5 L in the average adult). The subsequent choice for fluid replacement depends on the patient's state of hydration, serum electrolyte levels, and urinary output. If the corrected sodium is normal or elevated, 0.45% NaCl infused at a rate of 4 to 14 mL/kg/hour is appropriate. If the corrected serum sodium is low, 0.9% NaCl is preferred.[200] When serum glucose concentrations approach 200 mg/dL, solutions should be changed to D5W/0.45% NaCl. Glucose is added to allow the continuation of insulin therapy without causing hypoglycemia (see Case 53-13, Question 5).[200]

SODIUM

Total body sodium usually is depleted by 7 to 10 mEq/kg of body weight in patients with DKA. In assessing serum sodium in these patients, it is important to remember that falsely low values (i.e., pseudohyponatremia) may be the result of hyperglycemia and hypertriglyceridemia. A corrected sodium value can be estimated by adding 1.6 mEq/L to the observed sodium value for every 100 mg/dL glucose in excess of 100 mg/dL. Sodium is replaced adequately with normal saline, which has a sodium concentration of 154 mEq/L.[200]

POTASSIUM

Potassium balance is altered markedly in patients with DKA because of combined urinary and GI losses. Invariably, total body potassium is at least partly depleted; however, the serum potassium concentration may be high, normal, or low, depending on the degree of acidosis and volume contraction and severity of insulin deficiency. Usual potassium deficits in this situation average 3 to 5 mEq/kg of body weight, although they may be as high as 10 mEq/kg.[200,201]

Thus, J.L. needs approximately 200 to 350 mEq of potassium to replenish her body stores, assuming her normal weight is 70 kg. To prevent hypokalemia, potassium replacement should be started after her serum potassium concentrations decreases to less than 5.3 mEq/L (assuming an adequate urine output of 50 mL/hour). The addition of 20 to 30 mEq/L is usually sufficient to maintain the serum potassium at greater than 4 mEq/L. In cases when serum potassium is low at presentation (<3.3 mEq/L), potassium replacement should be initiated with fluid therapy, and insulin therapy delayed until the potassium level is greater than 3.3 mEq/L to avoid severe hypokalemia and the risk of cardiac arrhythmias and diaphragmatic weakness. In these cases, initial IV solutions should contain 20 to 30 mEq/L of potassium chloride.

PHOSPHATE

Phosphate is lost as the result of increased tissue catabolism, impaired cellular uptake, and enhanced renal excretion. Like other electrolytes, serum levels initially may seem normal, even though body stores are depleted. However, replacement can result in hypocalcemia, and the use of phosphate in DKA has resulted in no clinical benefit to patients.[200] Severe hypophosphatemia (<1.0 mg/dL) can cause cardiac and skeletal muscle weakness as well as respiratory depression. To avoid this, phosphate can be carefully replaced in patients with cardiac dysfunction or respiratory depression when phosphate concentrations are less than 1.0 mg/dL. Potassium phosphate can be added to the replacement fluids in the amount of 20 to 30 mEq/L.

INSULIN

CASE 53-13, QUESTION 3: What is an appropriate insulin dose and route of administration for J.L.?

Insulin therapy is the key to DKA management because it is what stops the production of ketones. As insulin allows glucose metabolism to resume, the counterregulatory signals for ketone production are turned off. Unless the episode of DKA is mild (pH 7.25–7.30) and uncomplicated, regular insulin by continuous infusion is the treatment of choice. Once hypokalemia (K^+ <3.3 mEq/L) is excluded or treated, an IV bolus of regular insulin at 0.1 units/kg followed by a continuous infusion at a dose of 0.1 units/kg/hour should be administered. This should decrease the plasma glucose by at least 10% in the first hour. If there is not at least a 10% reduction in the first hour, then a second bolus of 0.15 units/kg should be administered. Once the plasma glucose reaches 200 mg/dL, the insulin infusion can be decreased to 0.05 units/kg/hour. Alternatively, insulin can be switched to SC at a dose of 0.1 units/kg every 2 hours. Regardless of the route of insulin therapy, serum glucose should be maintained at less than 200 mg/dL.[200] At this point, the fluid should be changed to D5W with 0.45% NaCl. Thereafter, the rate of insulin administration and the rate of infusion of D5W with 0.45% NaCl are adjusted to maintain the glucose value at around 200 mg/dL until the ketosis is resolved.[200] Resolution of ketosis is marked by a serum bicarbonate level of at least 15 mEq/L, a venous pH greater than 7.3, and a calculated anion gap of 12 mEq/L or less. Once any two of those three findings are present, the patient can be converted to a longer-acting SC regimen.

For mild DKA (serum bicarbonate ≥15 mEq/L, anion gap <15), SC rapid-acting insulin has been used with no differences in patient outcomes. The advantage is that patients can be treated in a non-ICU setting, thus reducing hospital costs. The dosing for rapid-acting insulin is included in Table 53-26.

SODIUM BICARBONATE

CASE 53-13, QUESTION 4: J.L. was treated with fluids, electrolytes, and insulin as discussed in previous questions. Laboratory and clinical data 4 hours after therapy are as follows:

pH, 7.1
BG, 400 mg/dL
K, 3.8 mEq/L
SCr, 3.1 mg/dL
Serum ketones, strongly positive at a 1:40 dilution

Her BP was 120/70 mm Hg with no orthostatic changes. Urine output for the past 3 hours has been 500 mL. Because serum ketones have increased, should J.L. receive more insulin? Should she receive bicarbonate therapy?

The assumption that ketosis is worse in J.L. is incorrect. In DKA, low levels of insulin and elevated glucagon levels promote the metabolism of free fatty acids in the liver to acetoacetate and β-hydroxybutyrate. The standard nitroprusside reaction test for ketones measures only acetoacetate, even though β-hydroxybutyrate is the more important ketone. The conversion of acetoacetic acid to β-hydroxybutyrate is coupled closely with the reduced NADH:NAD ratio. If this ratio is high (as in the presence of alcohol), so much β-hydroxybutyrate may be formed that acetoacetate is virtually undetectable; thus, the absence of ketones in the serum does not rule out ketoacidosis.

Conversely, treatment with insulin begins to suppress lipolysis and fatty acid oxidation; nicotinamide adenine dinucleotide is regenerated, shifting the reaction back in favor of acetoacetate.[200] Thus, even though there seem to be higher concentrations of ketones in the serum, J.L.'s declining BG concentration, improved bicarbonate concentrations, and improved acid–base and cardiovascular responses indicate that she is responding appropriately. Therefore, no change in the insulin dose is indicated. It is important to emphasize that the glucose concentrations normalize before ketones (4–6 hours vs. 6–12 hours) because the latter are metabolized more slowly. For this reason, it is important to continue insulin to maintain suppression of lipolysis until plasma and urine ketones have cleared.

The use of bicarbonate in patients with DKA has been controversial.[200] Most investigators discourage its routine use, reserving it for patients with severe acidemia (pH <6.9) or those in clinical shock. Coma is correlated most closely with BG concentrations (>700 mg/dL) and hyperosmolality (calculated osmolality >340 mOsm/kg).[200] In a small randomized, prospective study, bicarbonate did not affect recovery in patients with severe DKA (arterial pH, 6.9–7.14).[202] Thus, even though J.L.'s acidosis seemed severe on admission (pH, 7.05; bicarbonate, 10 mEq/L; Kussmaul respirations [deep, frequent respirations resulting in blowing off of CO_2]), bicarbonate was not administered. It is apparent that with fluid and insulin therapy alone, her acidosis is beginning to improve.

CASE 53-13, QUESTION 5: What is the expected course of DKA in J.L.?

After 3 L of fluid and a constant insulin infusion of 6 units/hour for 3 hours, J.L.'s glucose concentration had dropped to 400 mg/dL and she had no orthostatic BP changes, reflecting recovery from her volume-depleted status. Potassium (40 mEq/L) was added to her fluids, which were administered at a reduced rate of 300 mL/hour.

Three hours later, the glucose concentration had dropped to 350 mg/dL and her pH had increased to 7.21 with an anion gap of 24 mEq/L. The serum potassium remained low-normal at 3.4 mEq/L, and serum sodium increased to 151 mEq/L. In view of these changes, the IV infusion fluid was changed to half-normal saline with 5% dextrose to which 40 mEq/L of potassium was added. The rate was slowed to 250 mL/hour, and the insulin infusion was continued at 6 units/hour.

Four hours later (10 hours after admission), the BG was 205 mg/dL and the serum potassium was 3.5 mEq/dL. The IV fluids were changed to 5% dextrose with 40 mEq/L of potassium chloride, administered at a rate of 250 mL/hour, and the regular insulin infusion was decreased from 6 to 3 units/hour. J.L. continued to improve during the next 12 hours, and she began taking full oral liquids by the second hospital day. At that time, her IV infusion rate was decreased to 200 mL/hour, but her insulin infusion was continued.

Approximately 24 hours after admission, J.L.'s BG concentration was 175 mg/dL, potassium was 4.6 mEq/L, sodium was 144 mEq/L, and the anion gap had closed down to 16 mEq/L. There were no ketones in the plasma. The urine contained 1% glucose and moderate amounts of ketones. IV fluids were discontinued, and a rapid-acting insulin was administered SC 1 hour before the insulin infusion was discontinued. J.L. continued to receive rapid-acting insulin SC every 4 hours according to a sliding scale (see Case 53-2, Question 12). Thirty-six hours after admission, J.L. was given her usual dose of insulin glargine and insulin lispro and was sent home for follow-up in the clinic.

TREATMENT OF TYPE 2 DIABETES: ANTIDIABETIC AGENTS

Type 2 diabetes must be managed in the context of the metabolic syndrome. At the time of diagnosis, many people with type 2 diabetes already have evidence of macrovascular and microvascular disease. Every effort to lower glucose concentrations toward normal values and to control BP and lipids is important to delay the onset or slow the progression of these complications, improve the overall quality of the patient's life, and save the health care system millions of dollars in hospitalization costs to treat these complications. MNT, physical activity, and SMBG are cornerstones in treating of people with type 2 diabetes. Unfortunately, these measures alone are usually not successful in achieving control for the majority of patients, and drug therapy is eventually required. Because these patients also often require a number of medications to treat related conditions (e.g., hypertension, dyslipidemia, CVD, and depression) and may also be medicating themselves with over-the-counter drugs, herbal products, and nutritional supplements, the aim of therapy for type 2 diabetes should be the simplest and safest regimen that provides the best glycemic control possible.

Figure 53-6 depicts the sources of hyperglycemia in people with type 2 diabetes and the primary site of action for each class of agents. Tables 53-27 and 53-28 summarize the comparative pharmacology, pharmacokinetics, and dosing of the noninsulin antidiabetic drugs. The clinical use of these agents in specific situations is illustrated in cases presented later in this chapter.

Biguanides

Metformin belongs to the biguanide class of oral antidiabetic agents. It has been available in the United States since 1995 and became generically available in 2002. The clinical pharmacology of metformin has been extensively reviewed.[203]

MECHANISM OF ACTION

The biguanides are described more accurately as antihyperglycemic agents. Although they lower BG concentrations in people with type 2 diabetes, they do not cause hypoglycemia in nondiabetic individuals or individuals with diabetes when used as monotherapy. Partly because of this lack of hypoglycemia, metformin is the only agent recommended by the ADA for consideration of use to reduce the risk for developing diabetes in patients at high risk (IGT and IFG).[8] Metformin primarily lowers FPG concentrations by decreasing hepatic gluconeogenesis, but it also increases insulin-stimulated glucose uptake by skeletal muscle and adipose tissue.[203]

Metformin has been shown to activate 5′ adenosine monophosphate–activated protein kinase (AMPK), a major regulator of glucose and lipid metabolism.[204] The primary cellular site of metformin is thought to be complex I in the mitochondria, whose inhibition by metformin leads to the activation of AMPK.[205] Through AMPK activation, acetyl-CoA carboxylase is inactivated, resulting in decreased lipid synthesis and increased fatty acid oxidation. Sterol regulatory element–binding protein-1, a key lipogenic transcription factor, is also suppressed, leading to a reduction in hepatic lipid production. AMPK activation is also thought to play a role in metformin's inhibition of hepatocyte glucose production and induction of muscle glucose uptake.[204,206]

Metformin modestly lowers total cholesterol (5%–10%) and triglycerides (10%–20%) and may maintain or improve HDL-C levels.[207] The observed effects on lipid metabolism as well as others on clotting factors, platelet function, and vascular

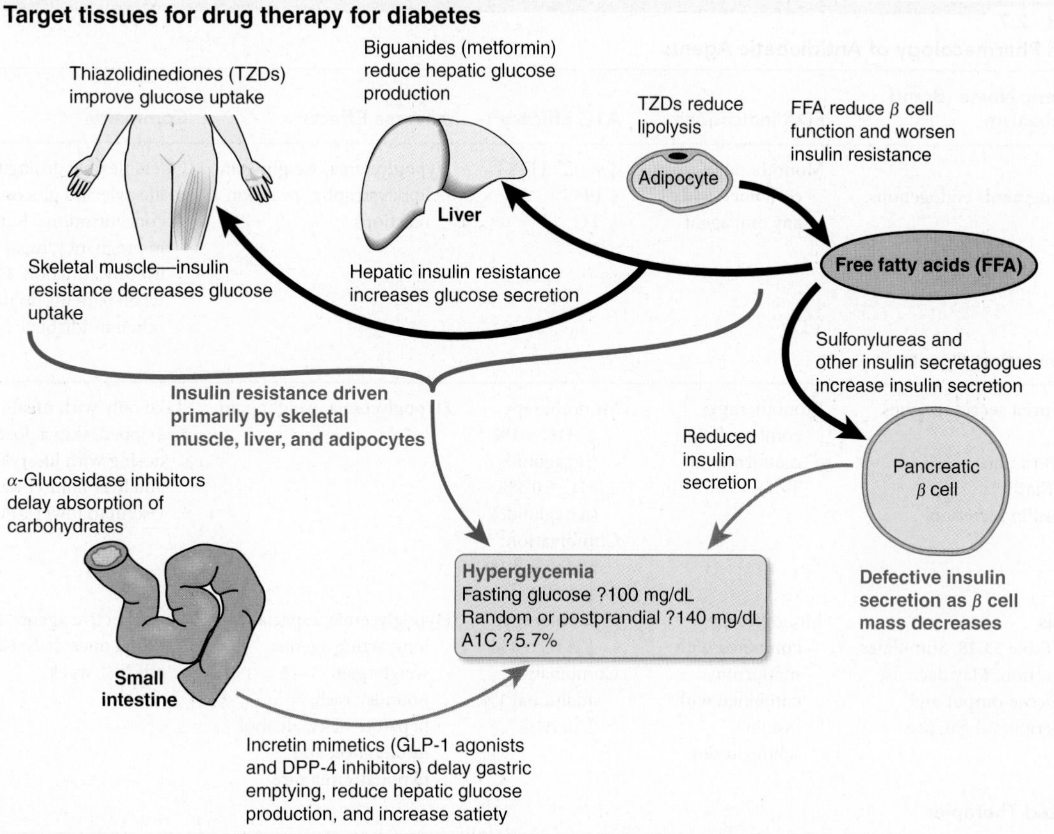

FIGURE 53-6 Sources of hyperglycemia in type 2 diabetes and site of action of antidiabetic agents. [a]Glucagonlike peptide-1 (GLP-1) agonists and dipeptidyl peptidase-4 (DPP-4) inhibitors have been added to the original figure. TZDs, thiazolidinediones.

function may impart some of metformin's favorable effects on CVD and outcomes (see Case 53-14, Question 3). A key advantage with metformin is that weight loss rather than weight gain is more likely to occur with its use (mean weight loss of 1.2 kg compared with 1.7 kg increase with sulfonylurea or insulin therapy).[208]

PHARMACOKINETICS

Approximately 50% to 60% of metformin is absorbed from the small intestine.[209] It is eliminated entirely by the kidney unchanged (primarily by tubular secretion) and has a plasma half-life of 6.2 hours and a whole blood half-life of 17.6 hours.[207] It is not bound to plasma proteins.

ADVERSE EFFECTS

GASTROINTESTINAL EFFECTS

Transient side effects include diarrhea and other GI disturbances such as nausea, abdominal discomfort, metallic taste, and anorexia.[207] Relative to placebo, diarrhea is the most common GI complaint (53.2% metformin vs. 11.7% placebo-treated patients). Symptoms can be minimized by taking metformin with food and slowly titrating the dose. To enhance adherence to therapy, patients should be informed of the possibility of GI side effects that will likely subside with time and instructed to discuss any suspected side effects with their provider before discontinuing therapy (see Case 53-14, Question 4).

LACTIC ACIDOSIS

Much of the perceived risk of lactic acidosis secondary to metformin use is based on historical data for phenformin, a biguanide that was withdrawn from the market in 1977.[210] The risk of lactic acidosis secondary to metformin is 10 to 20 times lower than with phenformin.[203] Unlike phenformin, metformin is not metabolized, does not inhibit peripheral glucose oxidation, and does not enhance peripheral lactate production.[211] However, it may decrease conversion of lactate to glucose (decreased gluconeogenesis) and increase lactate production in the gut and liver.[203,212] Metformin has rarely been associated with lactic acidosis. The few patients in whom this event has been reported had renal, liver, or cardiorespiratory contraindications to the use of biguanides. Patients should be warned to bring the following symptoms of lactic acidosis to the attention of their physician: weakness, malaise, myalgias, abdominal distress, and heavy, labored breathing (see Case 53-20, Question 2).

CONTRAINDICATIONS AND PRECAUTIONS

Patients with renal impairment, liver disease, or other states predisposing them to hypoxia, acute or chronic metabolic acidosis, or a history of lactic acidosis should be excluded from therapy.[207] Metformin can accumulate in patients whose renal function is impaired, thereby increasing their risk for lactic acidosis. Its use is not recommended in patients with decreased GFR (see Case 53-20, Question 2, for detailed discussion) or elevated creatinine levels (≥1.4 mg/dL for women or ≥1.5 mg/dL for men[207]). Because even a temporary reduction in renal function could cause lactic acidosis in patients taking metformin, the manufacturer recommends withholding it after some radiologic procedures (see Drug Interactions section). Other predisposing factors for lactic acidosis include the following: excessive alcohol ingestion, dehydration, surgery, decompensated congestive heart failure (HF), hepatic failure, shock, or sepsis. Because aging is associated with reduced renal function, metformin should be titrated to the minimal effective dose and renal function should be monitored regularly. An estimated GFR (eGFR) or creatinine clearance (ClCr) should be measured in patients older than

TABLE 53-27
Comparative Pharmacology of Antidiabetic Agents

Agent/Generic Name (Brand Name)/Mechanism	FDA Indications	A1C Efficacy[a]	Adverse Effects	Comments
Insulin Replaces or augments endogenous insulin	Monotherapy; combined with any oral agent	↓ A1C[b] ↓FPG[b] ↓ PPG[b] ↓ TG	Hypoglycemia, weight gain, lipodystrophy, local skin reactions	Offers flexible dosing to match lifestyle and glucose concentrations. Rapid onset. Safe in pregnancy, renal failure, and liver dysfunction. Drug of choice when patients do not respond to other antidiabetic agents.
Insulin-Augmenting Agents				
Nonsulfonylurea secretagogues (glinides) Repaglinide (Prandin) Nateglinide (Starlix) Stimulates insulin secretion	Monotherapy; combined with metformin or TZD	Monotherapy: ↓ A1C ~1% (repaglinide) ↓ A1C ~0.5% (nateglinide) Combination: additional 1% ↓ A1C	Hypoglycemia, weight gain	Take only with meals. If a meal is skipped, skip a dose. Flexible dosing with lifestyle. Safe in renal and liver failure. Rapid onset. Useful to lower PPG.
Sulfonylureas Various; see Table 53-28. Stimulates insulin secretion. May decrease hepatic glucose output and enhance peripheral glucose utilization.	Monotherapy; combined with metformin; combined with insulin (glimepiride)	Monotherapy: ↓ A1C ~1% Combination: additional 1% ↓ in A1C	Hypoglycemia, especially long-acting agents; weight gain (5–10 pounds); rash, hepatotoxicity, alcohol intolerance, and hyponatremia rare	Very effective agents. Some can be dosed once daily. Rapid onset of effect (1 week).
Incretin-Based Therapies				
Glucagonlike peptide-1 receptor agonists/incretin mimetic Exenatide (Byetta) Liraglutide (Victoza) Stimulates insulin secretion, delays gastric emptying, reduces postprandial glucagon levels, improved satiety	Monotherapy (exenatide only) Combined with metformin, SFU, or TZD, combined with metformin + SFU; combined with metformin + TZD	Monotherapy: ↓ A1C 0.8%–0.9% Combination: additional 1% ↓ in A1C	GI: nausea, vomiting, diarrhea; hypoglycemia (with SFUs); weight loss; reports of acute pancreatitis	Weight loss. Exenatide: take within 60 minutes before morning and evening meals or before two main meals of the day (≥6 hours apart). Liraglutide: Do not use if personal or family history of medullary thyroid carcinoma or in patients with multiple endocrine neoplasia syndrome type 2. Do not use in patients with gastroparesis or severe GI disease. Administered by SC injection; pen device in use does not need to be refrigerated. Rare cases of pancreatitis with both drugs.
DPP-4 inhibitors Sitagliptin (Januvia) Saxagliptin (Onglyza) Linagliptin (Tradjenta) Stimulates insulin secretion and reduces postprandial glucagon levels	Monotherapy; combined with metformin, SFU, or TZD; insulin (sitagliptin only)	Monotherapy: ↓ A1C 0.5%–0.8% Combination: ↓ A1C 0.5%–0.9%	Headache, nasopharyngitis, hypoglycemia (with SFU), rash (rare)	Dosed once daily. Taken with or without food. No weight gain or nausea. Need to adjust sitagliptin and sazagliptin dose in renal dysfunction. Reduce dose of SFU when combined. Rare reports of pancreatitis.
Amylin Receptor Agonists				
Amylin mimetic Pramlintide (Symlin)	Type 1: Adjunct to mealtime insulin	T1: ↓ A1C 0.33% T2: ↓ A1C 0.40%	GI: nausea, decreased appetite	Take only immediately before meals; administered by SC injection. Do not use in patients with gastroparesis.
Stimulates insulin secretion, delays gastric emptying, reduces postprandial glucagon levels, improved satiety	Type 2: Adjunct to mealtime insulin; ± SFU and metformin		Headache; hypoglycemia; weight loss (mild)	
Insulin Sensitizers				
Biguanides Metformin (Glucophage) ↓ Hepatic glucose output; ↑ peripheral glucose uptake	Monotherapy; combined with SFU or TZD; or with insulin	Monotherapy: ↓ A1C ~1% Combination: additional 1% ↓ in A1C	GI: nausea, cramping, diarrhea; lactic acidosis (rare)	Titrate dose slowly to minimize GI effects. No hypoglycemia or weight gain; weight loss possible. Mild reduction in cholesterol. Do not use in patients with renal or severe hepatic dysfunction.

(*continued*)

TABLE 53-27
Comparative Pharmacology of Antidiabetic Agents (*Continued*)

Agent/Generic Name (Brand Name)/Mechanism	FDA Indications	A1C Efficacy[a]	Adverse Effects	Comments
Thiazolidinediones Rosiglitazone (Avandia) Pioglitazone (Actos) Enhances insulin action in periphery; increases glucose utilization by muscle and fat tissue; decreases hepatic glucose output	Monotherapy; combined with SFU, TZD, or insulin; combined with SFU + TZD	Monotherapy: ↓ A1C ~1% Combination: additional 1% ↓ in A1C	Mild anemia; fluid retention and edema, weight gain, macular edema, fractures (in women)	Can cause or exacerbate HF; do not use in patients with symptomatic HF or class III or IV HF. Rosiglitazone may increase risk of MI. Increased risk of distal fractures in older women. Pioglitazone may increase risk of bladder cancer when used for >1 year. Slight reduction in TG with pioglitazone; slight increase in LDL-C with rosiglitazone. LFTs must be measured at baseline and periodically thereafter. Slow onset (2–4 weeks).
Delayers of Carbohydrate Absorption				
α-Glucosidase inhibitors Acarbose (Precose) Miglitol (Glyset) Slow absorption of complex carbohydrates	Monotherapy; combined with SFUs, metformin, or insulin	Monotherapy: ↓ A1C ~0.5% Combination: additional ~0.5% ↓ A1C	GI: flatulence, diarrhea. Elevations in LFTs seen in doses >50 mg TID of acarbose	Useful for PPG control (↓ PPG 25–50 mg/dL). LFTs should be monitored every 3 months during the first year of therapy and periodically thereafter. Because miglitol is not metabolized, monitoring of LFTs is not required. Titrate dose slowly to minimize GI effects. No hypoglycemia or weight gain. If used in combination with hypoglycemic agents, advise patients to treat hypoglycemia with glucose tablets because absorption is not inhibited as with sucrose.
Bile acid sequestrant Colesevelam (Welchol)	Combined with metformin, SFU, or insulin	↓ A1C 0.3%–0.4%	Constipation, dyspepsia, and nausea; ↑ TG	Added benefit of ↓ LDL-C (by 12%–16%). Administer certain drugs 4 hours before. Take with a meal and liquid.

[a]Comparative effectiveness data provided for SFUs, glinides, TZDs, and α-glucosidase inhibitors.[307]
[b]Theoretically, unlimited glucose lowering with insulin therapy.
A1C, glycosylated hemoglobin; DPP-4, dipeptidyl peptidase-4; FDA, Food and Drug Administration; FPG, fasting plasma glucose; GI, gastrointestinal; HF, heart failure; LDL-C, low-density lipoprotein cholesterol; LFTs, liver function tests; MI, myocardial infarction; PPG, postprandial glucose; SC, subcutaneously; SFU, sulfonylureas; TG, triglycerides; TID, three times a day; T1, type 1 diabetes; T2, type 2 diabetes; TZD, thiazolidinediones.

80 years of age to ensure adequate renal function because these patients are more susceptible to experiencing lactic acidosis.[207]

DRUG INTERACTIONS

- Alcohol potentiates the effect of metformin on lactate metabolism. Patients should be warned against excessive alcohol intake while taking metformin.
- Cimetidine increases peak metformin plasma concentrations by 60%; use of an alternative H_2 blocker or a reduction in metformin dose is recommended.
- Parenteral contrast studies (e.g., pyelography or angiography) that use iodinated materials can result in acute renal failure and increases the risk of metformin-induced lactic acidosis. For patients requiring such a study, metformin should be withheld at the time of or before and for 48 hours after the procedure. Metformin should be reinstituted only after renal function has been re-evaluated and determined to be normal.

EFFICACY

As monotherapy, metformin can be expected to reduce the A1C by 1.5% to 1.7% and the FPG by 50 to 70 mg/dL.[203] Research suggests that certain genetic variations may impact patient response to metformin therapy. Patients exhibiting reduced function polymorphisms of organic cation transporter 1, which is involved in the hepatic uptake of metformin, may be less responsive to metformin therapy.[213]

DOSAGE AND CLINICAL USE

Metformin is the first line of therapy for type 2 diabetes.[8] The ADA recommends its initiation as monotherapy in combination with lifestyle interventions (e.g., MNT, physical activity) on diagnosis. To minimize GI side effects, metformin should be initiated at 500 mg once or twice daily, to be taken with food, followed by weekly or biweekly increases in increments of 500 mg daily (see Case 53-14, Question 4). Metformin is dosed two to three times daily (500–1,000 mg/dose; maximal dose, 2,550 mg/day or 850 mg PO three times a day [TID]), unless an extended-release preparation is prescribed. Clinicians should obtain an SCr/eGFR (using the Modification of Diet in Renal Disease equation) and hepatic function tests at baseline and then annually. Metformin should not be used in patients older than 80 years unless a ClCr/eGFR demonstrates normal renal function. Patients are good candidates for treatment if the ClCr

TABLE 53-28
Antidiabetic Pharmacokinetic Data

Drug (Brand Name), Available Tablet Strengths (mg)	Typical Dosing Regimen (mg)	Usual Minimum and Maximum Total Daily Dose/How Divided	Mean Half-Life	Approximate Duration of Activity	Bioavailability, Metabolism, and Excretion	Comments
α-Glucosidase Inhibitors						
Acarbose (Precose) 25, 50, 100 mg	25–100 mg with first bite of each meal Begin with 25 mg; ↑ by 25 mg/meal every 4–8 weeks	Minimum: 25 mg TID Maximum dose is 50 mg TID if ≤60 kg; 100 mg TID if >60 kg	2.8 hours	Affects absorption of complex carbohydrates in a single meal	F = 0.5%–1.7%; extensively metabolized by GI amylases to inactive products; 50% excreted unchanged in the feces	Titrate doses slowly to avoid GI effects
Miglitol (Glyset) 25, 50, 100 mg	25–100 mg with first bite of each meal Begin with 25 mg; ↑ by 25 mg/meal every 4–8 weeks	Minimum: 25 mg TID Maximum: 100 mg TID	2 hours	Affects absorption of complex carbohydrates in a single meal	Dose of 25 mg is completely absorbed; dose of 100 mg 50%–70% absorbed; elimination by renal excretion as unchanged drug	
Biguanides						
Metformin (Glucophage) 500, 850, 1000 mg; 500 mg/mL liquid	Begin with 500 mg daily or BID; ↑ by 500 mg daily every 1–2 weeks	0.5–2.5 g BID or TID	Plasma, 6.2 hours. Whole blood, 17.6 hours	6–12 hours	F = 50%–60%; excreted unchanged in urine	Take with food. Avoid in patients with renal dysfunction or those who could be predisposed to lactic acidosis (e.g., alcoholism, severe HF, severe respiratory disorders, liver failure)
Metformin extended-release (Glucophage XR) 500, 750, 1000 mg	500–1,000 mg daily with evening meal; ↑ by 500 mg every 1–2 weeks	1,500–2,000 mg daily	As for metformin, but active drug is released slowly	24 hours	As for metformin	As for metformin
Nonsulfonylurea Insulin Secretagogues (Glinides)						
Repaglinide (Prandin) 0.5, 1, 2 mg	If A1C is <8% or if this is first drug, begin with 0.5 mg with each meal. For others, begin with 1–2 mg/meal	0.5–4 mg with each meal (16 mg/d) TID or QID	1 hour	C_{max} is at 1 hour; duration is approximately 2–3 hours	F = 56%; 92% metabolized to inactive products by the liver; 8% excreted as metabolites unchanged in the urine	Take only with meals. Skip dose if meal is skipped. Maximum dose per meal is 4 mg
Nateglinide (Starlix) 60, 120 mg	120 mg TID 1–30 minutes before meals; 60 mg TID for patients with near-normal A1C at initiation	60 or 120 mg TID	1.5 hours	Onset, 20 minutes; peak, 1 hours; duration, 2–4 hours	F = 73%; metabolized to inactive products (predominantly) that are excreted in the urine (83%) and feces (10%)	Skip dose if meal is skipped
First-Generation Sulfonylureas						
Acetohexamide (Dymelor) 250, 500 mg	250 or 500 mg daily; ↑ by 250 mg daily every 1–2 weeks	0. 25–1.5 g daily or BID	5 hours (active metabolite)	12–18 hours	Activity of metabolite greater then parent drug. Metabolite excreted, in part, by kidney	Caution in elderly and patients with renal disease. Significant uricosuric effects
Chlorpropamide (Diabinese) 100, 250 mg	100 or 250 mg daily; ↑ by 100 or 250 mg every 1–2 weeks	0.1–0.5 g daily	≥35 hours	24–72 hours	Inactive and weakly active metabolites; 20% excreted unchanged; varies widely	Caution in elderly and patients with renal impairment. Highest frequency of side effects relative to other sulfonylureas

First-Generation Sulfonylureas (*continued*)						
Tolazamide (Tolinase) 100, 250, 500 mg	100–250 mg daily; ↑ by 100 or 250 mg every 1–2 weeks	0.2–1 g daily or BID	7 hours (4–25)	12–24 hours	Some metabolites with moderate activity excreted via kidney	Active metabolites may accumulate in renal failure
Tolbutamide (Orinase) 250, 500 mg	250 mg BID before meals; ↑ by 250 mg daily every 1–2 weeks	0.5–3 g BID or TID	7 hours	6–12 hours	Metabolized to compounds with negligible activity	No special precautions Shortest-acting sulfonylurea
Second-Generation Sulfonylureas						
Glimepiride (Amaryl) 1, 2, 4 mg	1–2 mg daily initially; usual maintenance dose is 1–4 mg	1–8 mg daily	9 hours	24 hours	F = 100% completely metabolized by liver. Principal metabolite is slightly active (30% of parent compound). Excreted by the urine (60%) and feces (40%).	Probably safe in patients with renal failure, but low initial doses recommended for older patients and those with renal insufficiency. Incidence of hypoglycemia may be lower than other long-acting sulfonylureas.
Glipizide (Glucotrol) 5, 10 mg	2.5 mg daily in elderly, 5 mg daily in others; ↑ by 2.5 or 5 mg every 1–2 weeks	2.5–40 mg daily or BID[a]	2–4 hours	12–24 hours	Metabolized to inactive compounds	No special precautions daily dose >15 mg should be divided. Dose 30 minutes before meals.
Glipizide extended-release (Glucotrol XL) 5 mg	5 mg daily; ↑ by 5 mg every 1–2 weeks	5–20 mg daily	4–13 hours	24 hours	Same as glipizide	Use with caution in patients with pre-existing GI narrowing owing to possible obstruction.
Glyburide (Diabeta, Micronase) 1.25, 2.5, 5 mg	1.25 mg daily in elderly, 2.5 mg daily in others; ↑ by 1.25 or 2.5 mg every 1–2 weeks	1.25–20 mg daily or BID	4–13 hours	12–24 hours	Metabolized to inactive or weakly inactive compounds; 50% excreted in urine and 50% in feces.	Caution in elderly patients with renal failure and others predisposed to hypoglycemia. Daily doses >10 mg should be divided.
Micronized glyburide (Glynase presTab) 1.5, 3 mg	1.5 mg daily; ↑ by 1.5 mg every 1–2 weeks	1.0–12 mg daily	4 hours	24 hours	Metabolized to inactive or weakly inactive compounds; 50% excreted in urine and 50% in feces.	Daily doses >6 mg should be divided. ↑ Bioavailability relative to original formulation. Resulted in reduced dose.
Thiazolidinediones						
Rosiglitazone (Avandia) 2, 4, 8 mg	4 mg daily; ↑ to 8 mg daily (or 4 mg BID)	4–8 mg daily in single or divided doses	3–4 hours	Onset and duration poorly correlated with half-life because of mechanism of action. Onset at 3 weeks; max at ≥4 weeks. Offset likely to be similar.	F = 99%; extensively metabolized in liver into inactive metabolites; excreted 2/3 in urine and 1/3 in feces.	Food has no effect on absorption. BID dosing may have greater A1C lowering effect. No dose adjustments required in renal failure. Avoid in patients with liver disease and heart failure.
Pioglitazone (Actos) 15, 30, 45 mg	15–30 mg daily; ↑ to 45 mg daily. If used with insulin, ↓ insulin dose by 10%–25% once FPG <120 mg/dL	15–45 mg daily	3–7 hours (16–24 hours for all metabolites)	Same as previous	Extensively metabolized in liver; 15%–30% excreted in urine, remainder eliminated in the feces.	Food delays absorption but is not clinically significant. No dose adjustments required in renal disease. Avoid in patients with liver disease and heart failure.

(continued)

TABLE 53-28
Antidiabetic Pharmacokinetic Data (*Continued*)

Drug (Brand Name), Available Tablet Strengths (mg)	Typical Dosing Regimen (mg)	Usual Minimum and Maximum Total Daily Dose/How Divided	Mean Half-Life	Approximate Duration of Activity	Bioavailability, Metabolism, and Excretion	Comments
GLP-1 Receptor Agonists/Incretin Mimetics						
Exenatide (Byetta)	5 mcg SC BID; ↑ to 10 mcg SC BID after 1 month	5–10 mcg BID	2.4 hours	C_{max} is at 2.1 hours; duration 10 hours	Glomerular filtration	Take within 60 minutes before morning and evening meal. Nausea usually subsides with time.
Liraglutide (Victoza)	0.6 mg daily for 1 week; ↑ to 1.2 mg daily	0.6–1.8 mg daily	13 hours	24 hours; C_{max} is 8–12 hours after dosing	Metabolized as other large proteins	Take daily without regard to meals. Nausea usually subsides with time.
DPP-4 Inhibitors						
Sitagliptin (Januvia)	100 mg daily CrCl ≥30 to <50 mL/min: 50 mg daily CrCl <30 mL/min: 25 mg daily	100 mg daily	12.4 hours	24 hours	F = 87%; ~79% excreted unchanged in urine	Requires dose adjustment in renal insufficiency
Saxagliptin (Onglyza)	5 mg daily CrCl ≤50 mL/min: 2.5 mg daily	2.5–5 mg daily	2.5 hours (3.1 hours for active metabolite)	24 hours	Metabolized by CYP 3A4/5 Excreted by renal and hepatic pathways	Active metabolite is 1/2 as potent Reduce dose to 2.5 mg with strong CYP 3A4/5 inhibitors
Linagliptin (Tradjenta)	5 mg daily	5 mg daily	12 hours	24 hours	F = 30%; ~90% excreted unchanged (80% enterohepatic system, 5% urine). Small fraction metabolized to inactive metabolite	No dose adjustment needed in liver or renal disease
Amylin Mimetics						
Pramlintide (Symlin)	Type 1 DM: 15 mcg SC before major meals; ↑ by 15-mcg increments after minimum of 3 days Type 2 DM: 60 mcg SC before major meals; ↑ to 120 mcg after 3–7 days	Type 1: 15–60 mcg before major meals Type 2: 60 or 120 mcg before major meals	48 minutes	C_{max} is 20 minutes	F = 30%–40%; metabolized by kidneys	Reduce mealtime insulin dose by 50%. Titrate dose if no significant nausea.
Bile Acid Sequestrants						
Colesevelam (Welchol)	6 tablets once daily or 3 tablets BID [625 mg tablets]	3.75 g	N/A	N/A	Drug is not absorbed systemically and not metabolized	Take with food and liquid. Do not use if history of bowel obstruction, TG >500 mg/dL, or history of pancreatitis from ↑ TG.

A1C, glycosylated hemoglobin; BID, twice a day; C_{max}, maximal concentration; CrCl, creatinine clearance; CYP, cytochrome P-450; DM, diabetes mellitus; DPP-4, dipeptidyl peptidase-4; F, bioavailability; FPG, fasting plasma glucose; GI, gastrointestinal; GLP-1, glucagonlike peptide-1; HF, heart failure; N/A, not available; QID, four times a day; SC, subcutaneously; TG, triglycerides; TID, three times a day.

ONLINE CONTENT

For a table of the oral combination medications, go to http://thepoint.lww.com/AT10e.

is more than 60 mL/minute (or eGFR >60 mL/minute/1.73 m^2). Although many articles discuss the issue of use of metformin in patients with renal dysfunction,[214–216] we use metformin cautiously in these patients and avoid it if the eGFR is less than 40 mL/minute/1.73 m^2. Although a reduced dose can be tried in patients with an eGFR of 20 to 40 mL/minute/1.73 m^2, we generally do not recommend it.[217] For patients unable to achieve goals of therapy with metformin alone within 3 to 6 months of initiating therapy, addition of insulin or another agent should be considered (also see Case 53-17).

Nonsulfonylurea Insulin Secretagogues (Glinides)

Repaglinide (Prandin) and nateglinide (Starlix) are nonsulfonylurea insulin secretagogues (i.e., they stimulate insulin secretion). They belong to a class of agents referred to as meglitinides and amino acid (D-phenylalanine) derivatives, respectively, and collectively often called "glinides."[138] Repaglinide was approved by the FDA in December 1997, and nateglinide was approved in December 2000 (Table 53-27).

MECHANISM OF ACTION

These agents close the adenosine triphosphate (ATP)-sensitive potassium channels in the β cell, which leads to cell membrane depolarization, an influx of calcium, and secretion of insulin.[86] Unlike the sulfonylureas, they have a rapid onset and shorter duration of action, so they are given with meals to enhance postprandial glucose utilization.

PHARMACOKINETICS

Repaglinide has a bioavailability of 56% and is rapidly absorbed and excreted.[218] Its maximal serum concentration (C_{max}) occurs at approximately 1 hour, and its half-life is 1 hour. Repaglinide is highly (>98%) protein bound (volume of distribution, 31 L). It is completely metabolized (via cytochrome P-450 [CYP] 3A4) by the liver to inactive products, with 90% excreted in the feces and 8% excreted in urine. Nateglinide has a bioavailability of 73%.[219] It is rapidly absorbed, with a C_{max} occurring within 1 hour after dosing and a half-life of 1.5 hours. Nateglinide is metabolized (CYP 2C9, 70%; CYP 3A4, 30%) to less potent compounds, which are 75% excreted in the urine and 10% in the feces. Sixteen percent is excreted unchanged in the urine. It is highly (98%) protein bound, primarily to albumin, and, to a lesser extent, to α_1-acid glycoprotein.

ADVERSE EFFECTS

Mild hypoglycemia may occur, particularly if patients delay or forget to eat after the dose. A weight gain of 0.9 to 3 kg compared with baseline has been observed.[218,219] Rare side effects include elevated hepatic enzymes and hypersensitivity reactions. There has been at least one case report of repaglinide-induced hepatic toxicity.[220]

CONTRAINDICATIONS AND PRECAUTIONS

Because a functioning pancreas is required, these agents should not be used in people with type 1 diabetes. They should be used with caution in patients with liver dysfunction. Repaglinide clearance is reduced in patients with severe renal insufficiency, but may still be used safely at a reduced dose.[218] The clearance of nateglinide is not affected in patients with moderate to severe renal insufficiency.[219]

DRUG INTERACTIONS

Clinically relevant drug interactions include those that occur when these drugs are taken in combination with other glucose-lowering agents or drugs known to induce or inhibit their metabolism.[221] Therefore, BG levels should be closely monitored when either drug is taken in combination with other agents known to lower BG or affect their metabolism. Repaglinide is metabolized by CYP 2C8 and 3A4.[218] Studies have shown that repaglinide has no pharmacokinetic effects on digoxin or warfarin. Cimetidine does not affect its absorption or efficacy. Gemfibrozil should be avoided in combination with repaglinide owing to the risk of hypoglycemia. The combination of gemfibrozil and itraconazole synergistically inhibits repaglinide metabolism and should be avoided. Nateglinide is metabolized largely by CYP 2C9 (70%) and to a lesser extent by 3A4 (30%).[219] When evaluated in clinical studies, there were no clinically relevant interactions with nateglinide and glyburide, metformin, digoxin, diclofenac, or warfarin. Concomitant use of either repaglinide or nateglinide with rifampin may lower their efficacy.[221]

EFFICACY

The efficacy of repaglinide is comparable to metformin and the sulfonylureas.[222] When used as monotherapy, the mean decrease in FPG, postprandial glucose, and the A1C values were 61 mg/dL, 104 mg/dL, and 1.7%, respectively, compared with placebo (–31.0 mg/dL, –47.6 mg/dL, and –0.6% compared with baseline). Nateglinide as monotherapy results in a mean decrease in FPG and A1C of 13.6 mg/dL and 0.7%, respectively, compared with placebo (–4.5 mg/dL and –0.5% compared with baseline). In comparison with metformin monotherapy, both drugs produce a similar or slightly smaller reduction in A1C.

DOSAGE AND CLINICAL USE

Repaglinide and nateglinide are approved to treat people with type 2 diabetes as monotherapy or in combination with metformin or a thiazolidinedione (TZD). Because they have the same mechanism of action as the sulfonylureas, combining these agents does not produce any additional benefit. The agents are usually added to therapy for patients with postprandial hyperglycemia, particularly nateglinide. When repaglinide is used as the initial treatment in patients who are naïve to oral antidiabetic therapy or in patients with A1C values less than 8%, the recommended starting dose is 0.5 mg with each meal. When used in patients who have failed sulfonylureas or in those with A1C values greater than 8%, the initial dose is 1 to 2 mg with each meal. Doses can be titrated weekly at a rate of 1 mg/meal to a maximum of 4 mg/dose or 16 mg/day. The recommended starting dose of nateglinide is 120 mg TID 0 to 30 minutes before meals. For patients close to their A1C goal, a dose of 60 mg TID may be used. Doses should be omitted if a meal is skipped and added if an extra meal is ingested (repaglinide only). Repaglinide should be initiated at a 0.5-mg dose in patients with severe renal dysfunction and should be titrated cautiously in patients with liver dysfunction.

Sulfonylureas

Until metformin and other antidiabetic agents became available in the United States, sulfonylureas were the first-line pharmacologic treatment for people with type 2 diabetes who had failed diet and exercise therapy. Six sulfonylureas are available in the United States. The three first-generation sulfonylureas (chlorpropamide, tolazamide, and tolbutamide) are considered equally effective despite differences in their pharmacokinetic properties and adverse effect profiles (see the following discussion and Table 53-26).

American Diabetes Association. Standards of medical care in diabetes—2011. *Diabetes Care*. 2011;34(Suppl 1):S11. (8)

Duckworth W et al. Glucose control and vascular complications in veterans with type 2 diabetes [published corrections appear in *N Engl J Med*. 2009;361:1028; *N Engl J Med*. 2009;361:1024]. *N Engl J Med*. 2009;360:129. (50)

Holman RR et al. Long-term follow-up after tight control of blood pressure in type 2 diabetes. *N Engl J Med*. 2008;359:1565. (296)

Holman RR et al. 10-year follow-up of intensive glucose control in type 2 diabetes. *N Engl J Med*. 2008;359:1577. (42)

Knowler WC et al. Reduction in the incidence of type 2 diabetes with lifestyle intervention or metformin. *N Engl J Med*. 2002; 346:393. (56)

Nathan DM et al. Intensive diabetes treatment and cardiovascular disease in patients with type 1 diabetes. *N Engl J Med*. 2005; 353:2643. (41)

Nathan DM et al. Medical management of hyperglycemia in type 2 diabetes: a consensus algorithm for the initiation and adjustment of therapy: a consensus statement of the American Diabetes Association and the European Association for the Study of Diabetes. *Diabetes Care*. 2009;32:193. (138)

NICE-SUGAR Study Investigators et al. Intensive versus conventional glucose control in critically ill patients. *N Engl J Med*. 2009;360:1283. (187)

[No authors listed]. Effect of intensive blood-glucose control with metformin on complications in overweight patients with type 2 diabetes (UKPDS 34). UK Prospective Diabetes Study (UKPDS) Group [published correction appears in *Lancet*. 1998;352:1558]. *Lancet*. 1998;352:854. (293)

[No authors listed]. Intensive blood-glucose control with sulphonylureas or insulin compared with conventional treatment and risk of complications in patients with type 2 diabetes (UKPDS 33). UK Prospective Diabetes Study (UKPDS) Group [published correction appears in *Lancet*. 1999;354:602]. *Lancet*. 1998;352:837. (44)

[No authors listed]. Retinopathy and nephropathy in patients with type 1 diabetes four years after a trial of intensive therapy. The Diabetes Control and Complications Trial/Epidemiology of Diabetes Interventions and Complications Research Group [published correction appears in *N Engl J Med*. 2000;342:1376]. *N Engl J Med*. 2000;342:381. (39)

[No authors listed]. The effect of intensive treatment of diabetes on the development and progression of long-term complications in insulin-dependent diabetes mellitus. The Diabetes Control and Complications Trial Research Group. *N Engl J Med*. 1993;329:977. (38)

[No authors listed]. Tight blood pressure control and risk of macrovascular and microvascular complications in type 2 diabetes: UKPDS 38. UK Prospective Diabetes Study Group [published correction appears in *BMJ*. 1999;318:29]. *BMJ*. 1998; 317:703. (295)

Key Websites

American Diabetes Association. http://www.diabetes.org.

54 Eye Disorders

Steven R. Abel and Suellyn J. Sorensen

CORE PRINCIPLES

	CHAPTER CASES
GLAUCOMA	
1 There are different types of glaucoma, including open-angle and angle-closure. Angle-closure glaucoma is a medical emergency requiring immediate intervention. Open-angle glaucoma is a chronic condition, which can result in progressive loss of vision leading to blindness if left untreated.	**Case 54-1 (Question 1)**
2 Treatment for open-angle glaucoma is targeted toward reducing intraocular pressure, a clinical measure of drug efficacy. β-Adrenergic blockers, prostaglandin analogs, and α-adrenergic agonists are the mainstay of treatment. Treatment is not curative.	**Case 54-1 (Question 2)**
OCULAR AND SYSTEMIC SIDE EFFECTS OF DRUGS	
1 Many widely used medications for various conditions cause ocular side effects. The true incidence is frequently not known, making the reporting of ocular side effects of drugs an important function for any health care practitioner.	**Case 54-3 (Question 1)**
2 Conversely, many topically administered ocular medications may cause systemic symptoms.	**Case 54-10 (Question 1)**
COMMON OCULAR DISORDERS	
1 Stye (hordeolum) is a common ocular disorder for which no viable over-the-counter treatment exists.	
2 Conjunctivitis (pinkeye) is frequently related to bacterial or viral infection, or allergy. Viral conjunctivitis is generally self-limiting. Bacterial conjunctivitis should be treated with an appropriate antimicrobial, recognizing that gram-positive organisms are frequently the cause. A number of agents are available for the treatment of allergic conjunctivitis. Among those, decongestants (e.g., tetrahydrozoline) should be used for no more than 72 hours, as they may mask a more serious condition or result in rebound redness.	**Case 54-5 (Question 1)**
CORTICOSTEROIDS	
1 Topical corticosteroids are used for a variety of ocular inflammatory conditions. The most potent topical corticosteroid is prednisolone acetate 1%.	**Case 54-8 (Question 1)**
2 Topical and oral corticosteroids may be associated with serious side effects such as increases in intraocular pressure and cataracts (with long-term use).	**Case 54-8 (Question 1)**

continued

AGE-RELATED MACULAR DEGENERATION

1	There are two forms, dry (affecting 85% of patients) and the more serious form, wet (affecting 15% of patients).	**Case 54-13 (Question 1)**
2	Wet macular degeneration is associated with abnormal growth of blood vessels behind the retina (choroidal neovascularization) and may be treated by vascular endothelial growth factor (VEGF) inhibitors.	**Case 54-13 (Question 1)**

The eye is a highly complex organ composed of various parts, all of which must function in integration to permit vision. A brief overview of the anatomy and physiology of the eye prefaces the presentation of specific eye disorders. Readers should consult an ophthalmology textbook for an understanding of ocular anatomy, physiology, and general ophthalmology (e.g., *Vaughan and Asbury's General Ophthalmology*).[1]

OCULAR ANATOMY AND PHYSIOLOGY

The eyeball is approximately 1 inch wide and is housed in a cavity (i.e., eye socket) formed by two bony orbits that are lined with fat, which serves to protect the eyeball. Six ocular muscles facilitate movement of the eyeball (Fig. 54-1).

The outer coat of the eye is made up of the sclera, conjunctiva, and cornea. The *sclera* is the white, dense, fibrous protective coating. The episclera, a thin layer of loose connective tissue, contains blood vessels that cover and nourish the sclera. The *conjunctiva* is a mucous membrane that covers the anterior portion of the eye and lines the eyelids. The *cornea* is the transparent, avascular tissue that functions as a refractive and protective window membrane through which light rays pass en route to the retina.

ONLINE CONTENT **For a visual of a corneal cross section, go to http://thepoint.lww.com/AT10e.**

The corneal epithelium and endothelium are lipophilic, and the centrally located stroma is hydrophilic. These three corneal layers are particularly important because they affect drug penetration through the cornea. Ophthalmic medications, which are both fat- and water-soluble, are best able to penetrate through the intact cornea.

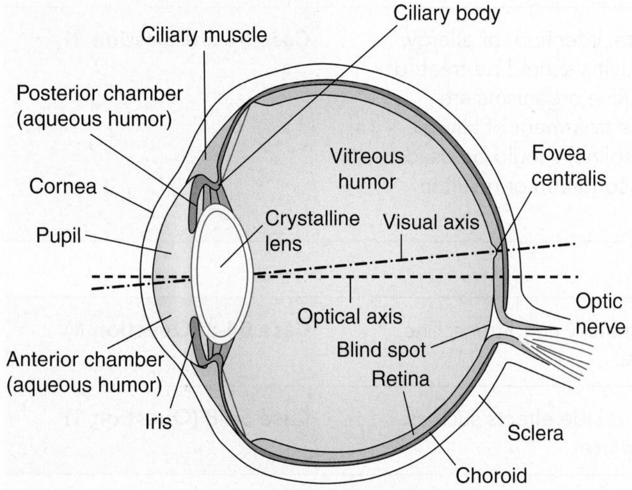

FIGURE 54-1 Anatomy of the human eye. (Adapted from http://commons.wikimedia.org/wiki/File:Eyesection.svg)

The iris, choroid, and ciliary body are known collectively as the uveal tract. The *iris* is a colored, circular membrane suspended between the cornea and the crystalline lens. It controls the amount of light that enters the eye. The *choroid*, located between the sclera and retina, is largely made up of blood vessels, which nourish the retina. The *ciliary body* is adherent to the sclera and contains the ciliary muscle and ciliary processes. The ciliary muscle contracts and relaxes the zonular fibers, which hold the crystalline lens in place. The ciliary processes are responsible for the secretion of aqueous humor, a clear liquid that occupies the anterior chamber. The anterior chamber is bounded anteriorly by the cornea and posteriorly by the iris. The posterior chamber lies between the iris and the crystalline lens.

The inner segment of the eye contains the retina with the optic nerve. The *retina*, the light-sensitive tissue at the back of the eye, contains all of the sensory receptors for light transmission. The *optic nerve*, a bundle of more than a million nerve fibers, transmits visual impulses from the retina to the brain.

The crystalline lens, aqueous humor, and vitreous humor assist the cornea with the refraction of light. The *lens*, located behind the iris, functions to focus light onto the retina by changing its shape to accommodate near or distant vision. The innermost part of the lens (i.e., the nucleus) is surrounded by the softer material of the cortex. The *aqueous humor*, the thin watery fluid that fills the anterior chamber (i.e., the space between the cornea and the iris) and posterior chamber of the eye, functions to provide nourishment to the cornea and lens. Disorders involving the aqueous humor are presented in the section on glaucoma. The primary function of the *vitreous humor* (i.e., the jellylike substance between the lens and the retina) is to maintain the shape of the eye and allow the transmission of light to the retina.

The eyelids and eyelashes are the outermost means of protection for the eye. The eyelids contain various sebaceous and sweat glands, which may become infected or inflamed, contributing to many ocular disorders.

The eye is innervated by both the sympathetic and parasympathetic nervous systems. Parasympathetic fibers, originating from the oculomotor nerve in the brain, innervate the ciliary muscle and sphincter pupillae muscle that constrict the pupil. As a result, parasympathomimetic (cholinergic) medications generally are associated with *miosis* (pupillary contraction), and parasympatholytic (anticholinergic) agents with *mydriasis* (pupillary dilation) and *cycloplegia*. The term *cycloplegia* refers to a paralysis of the ciliary muscle and zonules (fibrous strands connecting the ciliary body to the lens) that results in decreased accommodation (adjustment of the lens curvature for various distances) and blurred vision. Tear secretion by the lacrimal glands also is a parasympathetic function.

Sympathetic fibers from the superior cervical ganglion in the spinal cord innervate the dilator pupillae muscle, the blood vessels of the ciliary body, the episclera, and the extraocular muscles. Sympathomimetics cause mydriasis without affecting accommodation.

In this chapter we will discuss glaucoma, ocular and systemic side effects of drugs, common ocular disorders, ocular inflammatory conditions, and age-related macular degeneration. These are all common conditions that the pharmacist may encounter in all practices of pharmacy. It is important for the pharmacist to be educated on these disorders and their associated treatment so that the pharmacist can evaluate the appropriateness of pharmacotherapy, screen for adverse effects and drug interactions, and counsel patients on their ocular medications.

GLAUCOMA

Glaucoma, a leading cause of blindness worldwide, is a nonspecific term used for a group of diseases that can irreversibly damage the optic nerve, resulting in visual field loss. Increased intraocular pressure (IOP) is the most common risk factor for the development of glaucoma; however, even people with "normal" IOPs can experience vision loss from glaucoma. Generally, the higher the IOP is, the greater the risk for developing glaucoma. Increasing age, African American race, family history, thinner central corneas, and larger vertical cup–disc ratios are other risk factors for glaucoma.[1,2]

Intraocular Pressure

The inner pressure of the eye (i.e., IOP) is influenced by the production of aqueous humor by the ciliary processes and the outflow of aqueous humor through the trabecular meshwork. The tonometry test to measure the IOP is based on the pressure required to flatten a small area of the central cornea. Generally, an IOP of 10 to 20 mm Hg is considered normal. An IOP of 22 mm Hg or greater should arouse suspicion of glaucoma, although a more rare form of glaucoma is associated with a low IOP.

Ocular Hypertension

Ocular hypertension has been defined as an IOP exceeding 21 mm Hg, normal visual fields, normal optic discs, open angles, and the absence of any ocular disease contributing to the elevation of IOP. Only a small percentage of patients with ocular hypertension have open-angle glaucoma. An ophthalmoscope can examine the inside of the eye, especially the optic nerve, and a diagnosis of glaucoma can be applied when pathologic cupping of the optic nerve is observed.

ONLINE CONTENT **For a visual of a normal optic disc and an optic disc showing changes caused by glaucoma, go to http://thepoint.lww.com/AT10e.**

Open-Angle Glaucoma

Primary open-angle glaucoma occurs in about 1.8% of people older than 40 years of age in the United States; however, glaucoma can affect other age groups, including children.[1–3] About 2.2 million people in the United States have glaucoma, and this number likely will increase to about 3.3 million by the year 2020 as the population ages.[3] In patients with primary open-angle glaucoma (POAG), aqueous humor outflow from the anterior chamber is continuously subnormal primarily because of a degenerative process in the trabecular meshwork. The IOP can vary in the course of a day from normal to significantly high pressures.[1] The decreased outflow appears to be caused by degenerative changes in outflow channels (i.e., the trabecular meshwork and Schlemm canal) and tends to worsen with the passage of time.[1] In rare cases, the outflow is normal even during a phase of elevated IOP, and the elevation appears to be to the result of hypersecretion of aqueous humor.[1]

ONLINE CONTENT **For an illustration of how aqueous humor flows through the eye, go to http://thepoint.lww.com/AT10e.**

The onset of POAG usually is gradual and asymptomatic. A defect in the visual field examination may be present in early glaucoma, but loss of peripheral vision usually is not seen until late in the course of the disease. Visual field defects correlate well with changes in the optic disc and help differentiate glaucoma from ocular hypertension in patients with increased IOP. Patients with normal visual fields and an IOP of 24 mm Hg or greater have a 10% likelihood of developing glaucoma in 5 years.[3]

Angle-Closure Glaucoma

Examination of the anterior chamber angle by gonioscopy, using a corneal contact lens, a magnifying device (e.g., a slit-lamp microscope), and a light source, assists in differentiating between open-angle glaucoma and angle-closure glaucoma. Angle-closure glaucoma accounts for approximately 5% to 10% of all primary glaucoma cases. The sole cause of the elevated IOP in angle-closure glaucoma is closure of the anterior chamber angle.[1,4]

Angle-closure glaucoma, which is a medical emergency, usually presents as an acute attack with a rapid increase in IOP, blurring or sudden loss of vision, appearance of haloes around lights, and pain that is often severe. When patients are predisposed to angle-closure glaucoma, their pupils should not be dilated (e.g., during an ophthalmic examination) and they should be taught the signs and symptoms of angle closure. Acute attacks can terminate without treatment, but if the IOP remains high, the optic nerve can be irreparably damaged.[1] Patients with chronic angle-closure generally experience a gradual closure of aqueous humor outflow channels, and patients can be asymptomatic until the glaucoma is in an advanced stage.[1] Permanent medical management of acute or chronic angle-closure glaucoma is difficult: surgical procedures (e.g., peripheral iridectomies) often are needed.

PRIMARY OPEN-ANGLE GLAUCOMA

Therapeutic Agents for Treatment of Primary Open-Angle Glaucoma

INITIAL THERAPY

Historically, β-adrenergic blockers have been the most commonly prescribed first-line agents for the treatment of POAG. In recent years, prostaglandin analog use has reached, if not exceeded, β-adrenergic blocker use. All of the ophthalmic β-blockers currently on the market are available in generic formulation, allowing for cost-effective treatment. Unlike β-blockers, generic versions of prostaglandin analogs are not yet available; hence the cost of this class of medications can be prohibitive for some patients, depending on their insurance plans.

β-ADRENERGIC BLOCKERS

Ophthalmic β-adrenergic antagonists block the β-adrenergic receptors in the ciliary epithelium of the eye and lower IOP primarily by decreasing aqueous humor production. On average, β-blockers decrease IOP by 20% to 35% depending on the strength used and the frequency of administration.[5–13]

Timolol (Timoptic)

Timolol, a nonselective β_1- and β_2-adrenergic antagonist, is one of the most commonly prescribed glaucoma medications. Because timolol was the first ocular β-adrenergic blocker marketed, subsequently marketed ophthalmic β-blockers usually are compared with timolol for safety and effectiveness. Concentrations or dosages exceeding one drop of timolol 0.5% twice daily (BID) do not produce further significant decreases in IOP.[14] Therapy usually is initiated with a 0.25% solution administered as one drop BID. Monocular administration of timolol has resulted in equal bilateral IOP reduction and can reduce the cost of therapy and side effects for some patients.[15] An escape phenomenon, or tachyphylaxis, can occur with timolol.

Timolol has been associated with a modest reduction of resting pulse rate (5–8 beats/minute),[16,17] worsening of heart failure, and adverse pulmonary effects (e.g., dyspnea, airway obstruction, pulmonary failure).[18,19] After chronic administration in susceptible individuals, timolol can cause corneal anesthesia.[20,21] Although uveitis has been reported in patients receiving ophthalmic timolol, a cause-and-effect relationship has not been established.[22,23]

Systemic absorption after topical administration does occur, but it may not be significant in the majority of patients. Care should be taken when timolol is used in patients with sinus bradycardia, heart failure (see Chapter 19, Heart Failure), or pulmonary disease. Systemic side effects could be exaggerated in elderly patients secondary to inadvertent overdosing associated with poor administration technique (see Case 54-1, Question 3).

Timoptic XE

Timoptic XE, a timolol ophthalmic gel-forming solution, is administered once daily. The ophthalmic vehicle, gellan gum (Gelrite), is a solution that forms a clear gel in the presence of monovalent or divalent cations.[24] This ion-activated gelation prolongs precorneal residence time and increases ocular bioavailability, allowing timolol to be administered once daily.[24] Timoptic XE is comparable to timoptic solution in lowering IOP.[25]

Levobunolol (Betagan)

Levobunolol, a nonselective β-adrenergic antagonist, is approved for either once daily or BID administration. Levobunolol 0.5% and 1% are comparable to timolol in lowering IOP. The incidence of adverse reactions, including decreases in heart rate, are also comparable to that for timolol.[6,26]

Metipranolol (OptiPranolol)

Another nonselective β-adrenergic blocking agent, metipranolol 0.1% to 0.6%, is comparable to timolol 0.25% to 0.5% in reducing IOP.[7,8] Like timolol, metipranolol produces corneal anesthesia, which occurs within 1 minute of instillation and returns to baseline after 10 minutes.[21] Metipranolol is associated with a greater incidence of stinging or burning on administration and has been associated with granulomatous anterior uveitis.[27,28] As a result of these side effects, the use of metipranolol is limited.

Carteolol (Ocupress)

Carteolol, a nonselective β-adrenergic blocking agent with partial β-adrenergic agonist activity, theoretically should minimize the bronchospastic, bradycardic, and hypotensive effects associated with other ocular β-adrenergic blockers.[29] However, no clinical differences were seen when the cardiovascular and pulmonary function effects of carteolol were compared with those of timolol. Carteolol 1% and timolol 0.25% administered BID are equally effective in reducing IOP.[10–12]

Betaxolol (Betoptic)

In contrast to other β-adrenergic blocking ophthalmic agents, betaxolol is a selective β_1-adrenergic blocker. This cardioselective property may result in less adverse effects on pulmonary function than nonselective β-adrenergic blockers in patients with reactive airway disorders. Betaxolol is slightly less effective than timolol in IOP reduction, and more patients tend to need adjunctive therapy with betaxolol.[13,30–32]

PROSTAGLANDIN ANALOGS

Latanoprost (Xalatan), travoprost (Travatan), and bimatoprost (Lumigan), are all prostaglandin analogs. Latanoprost and travoprost are analogs of prostaglandin $F_{2\alpha}$, and they lower IOP by serving as selective prostaglandin $F_{2\alpha}$-receptor agonists. Bimatoprost is a synthetic prostamide analog. The prostaglandin analogs (PGAs) increase uveoscleral outflow of aqueous humor and, thereby, decrease IOP.[33] These agents often are prescribed as first-line agents for the treatment of POAG because they are at least as effective as the β-blockers, can be administered once a day, and are associated with minimal systemic adverse effects.

Latanoprost

Latanoprost (Xalatan) is approved for the initial treatment of POAG or ocular hypertension.[34] When administered once daily in the evening, latanoprost is at least as effective as timolol in decreasing IOP. When the effectiveness of latanoprost 0.005% once daily was compared with timolol 0.5% BID, the IOP-lowering effects of latanoprost were superior to those of timolol.[35,36] In addition, the nocturnal control of IOP with latanoprost was superior to that with timolol. Latanoprost 0.005% should be dosed once daily in the evening because the IOP-lowering effects of latanoprost might actually be inferior when administered more frequently.

Systemic side effects are minimal with latanoprost, but local reactions (e.g., iris pigmentation; eyelid skin darkening; eyelash lengthening, thickening, pigmentation, and misdirected growth; conjunctival hyperemia; ocular irritation; superficial punctate keratitis) are relatively common. Latanoprost can gradually increase the amount of brown pigment in the iris by increasing the melanin content in the stromal melanocytes of the iris. This pigment change occurs in 7% to 22% of patients and is most noticeable in those with green-brown, blue/gray-brown, or yellow-brown eyes.[34,35] The onset of increased iris pigmentation usually is noticeable within the first year of treatment and can be permanent. The nature and severity of adverse events are not affected by the increased pigmentation of the iris.

Latanoprost has additive effects when administered with β-blockers (e.g., timolol), carbonic-anhydrase inhibitors (e.g., dorzolamide), and α_2-adrenergic agonists (e.g., brimonidine, apraclonidine). When added to existing therapy, latanoprost decreases IOP an additional 2.9 to 6.1 mm Hg. As a result, latanoprost is a good adjunctive ophthalmic agent for patients who are unable to adequately lower their IOP with single-agent therapy. Although the complementary IOP-lowering effects of latanoprost are comparable with those of brimonidine (at least a 15% reduction in IOP) in patients inadequately controlled on β-adrenergic blocking agents, brimonidine (an α_2-adrenergic agonist) in a comparative study was associated with fewer adverse effects on the quality of life. For example, watery or teary eyes and cold hands and feet were reported more frequently in latanoprost-treated patients.[37] The effectiveness of latanoprost when used once a day alone or as an adjunct to other IOP-lowering drugs and its relative tolerability make it one of the most common if not the most common treatment option for POAG and ocular hypertension.[36,38–40]

Travoprost

Travoprost (Travatan Z) is US Food and Drug Administration (FDA)–approved for the reduction of elevated IOP and ocular hypertension in patients who are intolerant or who fail to respond to other agents. Travoprost is used as a first-line agent in clinical practice because it is more effective than timolol and at least as effective as latanoprost. The mean IOP reduction with travoprost in African American patients was 1.8 mm Hg greater than in non–African American patients. Travoprost, as adjunctive therapy to timolol in patients not responding adequately to timolol alone, reduced IOP an additional 6 to 7 mm Hg. The side-effect profile of travoprost is similar to that for latanoprost, including increased iris pigmentation and eyelash changes.[41–43] Local irritation may be less because it is free of the preservative benzalkonium chloride.

Bimatoprost

Like travoprost, bimatoprost (Lumigan) once daily or BID achieved lower target IOPs than did timolol BID. Bimatoprost BID, however, was less effective than bimatoprost once a day. Iris pigmentation changed in 1.1% of bimatoprost-treated patients. In a 6-month randomized multicenter study, bimatoprost once a day lowered IOP more effectively than latanoprost once a day. Side effects were similar between treatment groups; however, conjunctiva hyperemia was more common ($p < 0.001$) in bimatoprost-treated patients. Overall, the side effect profile of bimatoprost appears to be similar to that for latanoprost and travoprost.[44–46] The local side effects seen with other PGAs also appear to be relatively common with bimatoprost. As a result, the FDA approved the cosmetic use of bimatoprost solution under the trade name Latisse. Latisse solution is applied with an applicator to the base of the upper eyelashes for the treatment of hypotrichosis (inadequate eyelashes). Eyelash lengthening, thickening, and darkening or pigmentation is seen after 8 to 16 weeks of use.[47]

α_2-ADRENERGIC AGONISTS

Apraclonidine (Iopidine) and brimonidine (Alphagan) are selective α_2-adrenergic agonists similar to clonidine. Apraclonidine is less lipophilic than clonidine and brimonidine, does not cross the blood–brain barrier as readily, and theoretically has fewer systemic side effects (e.g., hypotension, decreased pulse, dry mouth). Brimonidine is more highly selective for α_2-adrenergic receptors than clonidine or apraclonidine and, theoretically, should be associated with fewer ocular side effects. α_2-Adrenergic agonists appear to lower IOP by decreasing the production of aqueous humor and by increasing uveoscleral outflow.[48]

Brimonidine is an alternative first-line agent in the treatment of POAG. It may also be used as adjunctive therapy in patients not responding to other agents. Apraclonidine 1% is indicated to control or prevent postsurgical elevations in IOP after argon laser trabeculoplasty or iridotomy. The 0.5% apraclonidine solution is indicated for short-term adjunctive therapy in patients on maximally tolerated medical therapy. Long-term IOP control should be monitored closely in patients taking α_2-adrenergic agonists because tachyphylaxis can occur. Common ocular side effects include burning, stinging, blurring, conjunctival follicles, and an allergiclike reaction consisting of hyperemia, pruritus, edema of the lid and conjunctiva, and foreign body sensation. Although ocular side effects are less common with brimonidine than with apraclonidine, systemic side effects (e.g., dry nose and mouth, mild hypotension, decreased pulse, and lethargy) are more common with brimonidine. α_2-Adrenergic agonists should be used with caution in patients with cardiovascular disease, orthostatic hypotension, depression, and renal or hepatic dysfunction.[48,49] Brimonidine (Alphagan P) is available with Purite as a preservative, which facilitates drug delivery into the eye, allowing use of a lower drug concentration.[49]

The IOP-reduction effects (peak and trough) of brimonidine 0.2% BID are 14% to 28%. Although the approved dosing schedule of brimonidine is three times a day (TID), brimonidine 0.2% BID lowers IOP comparably to timolol 0.5% BID, and both are slightly better than betaxolol 0.25% BID.[49–51] The IOP-lowering effect of brimonidine also may be comparable with that of latanoprost; however, conflicting efficacy and tolerability results in clinical studies may be related to differences in study design.[52] The combination of brimonidine and timolol is as equally tolerable and effective as the combination of dorzolamide and timolol.[53] The FDA-approved Combigan ophthalmic solution combines an α_2-adrenergic agonist (brimonidine tartrate 0.2%) with a β-adrenergic blocker (timolol maleate 0.5%).

TOPICAL CARBONIC ANHYDRASE INHIBITORS

Carbonic anhydrase occurs in high concentrations in the ciliary processes and retina of the eye. Carbonic anhydrase inhibitors (CAIs) lower IOP by decreasing bicarbonate production and, therefore, the flow of bicarbonate, sodium, and water into the posterior chamber of the eye, resulting in a 40% to 60% decrease in aqueous humor secretion.

Although CAIs have been used orally for many years in the treatment of elevated IOPs, they have been replaced by the topical ophthalmic CAIs, dorzolamide (Trusopt) and brinzolamide (Azopt), which are safer and better tolerated. Topical CAIs are excellent alternatives to β-blockers in the initial management of elevated IOPs, and are effective as adjunctive agents. Brinzolamide 1% TID reduces IOP comparably to that achieved with dorzolamide 2% TID and to betaxolol 0.5% BID, but slightly less than timolol 0.5% BID. The IOP-reduction effects (peak and trough) of dorzolamide 2% TID are 16% to 25%. Brinzolamide and dorzolamide are approved for TID dosing; however, BID dosing may be adequate. Dorzolamide provides additional IOP-lowering effects when added to existing β-blocker therapy.[54,55] An ophthalmic solution of dorzolamide hydrochloride and timolol maleate is marketed as Cosopt. The combined use of topical dorzolamide and oral acetazolamide does not result in additive effects and might increase the risk of toxicity. Therefore, the concomitant use of topical and oral CAIs is not advised.[56–58]

The topical CAIs are well tolerated with few systemic side effects. The most common adverse effects reported with dorzolamide are ocular burning, stinging, discomfort and allergic reactions, bitter taste, and superficial punctate keratitis. Brinzolamide causes less burning and stinging of the eyes than dorzolamide, because its pH more closely resembles that of human tears. Dorzolamide and brinzolamide are sulfonamides and may cause the same types of adverse reactions attributable to sulfonamides. These drugs should not be used in patients with renal or hepatic impairment.

PILOCARPINE

Pilocarpine (Isopto Carpine) historically was an initial treatment of choice, but with the introduction and widespread use of newer agents, pilocarpine has fallen out of favor. Therapy usually is begun using lower concentrations (1%), one drop four times a day (QID). Pilocarpine is a direct-acting cholinergic (parasympathomimetic) that causes contraction of ciliary muscle fibers attached to the trabecular meshwork and scleral spur. This opens the trabecular meshwork to enhance aqueous humor outflow. There also may be a direct effect on the trabecular meshwork. Pilocarpine causes miosis by contraction of the iris sphincter muscle, but the miosis is not related to the decrease in IOP.

CARBACHOL

Carbachol (Isopto Carbachol) is reserved as a third-line agent in patients who are unresponsive or intolerant to initial medications. In addition to having direct cholinergic effects, carbachol is more resistant to cholinesterase than pilocarpine. Added benefits include increased release of acetylcholine from parasympathetic nerve terminals and a weak anticholinesterase effect. Carbachol is administered TID.

ANTICHOLINESTERASE AGENTS

If control of IOP is not achieved with optimal use of other topical monotherapy and combination therapy agents, then anticholinesterase agents may be prescribed as a last topical therapy option. Anticholinesterase agents inhibit the enzyme cholinesterase, thereby increasing the amount of acetylcholine and its naturally occurring cholinergic effects.

ECHOTHIOPHATE IODIDE

Echothiophate iodide (Phospholine Iodide), an irreversible cholinesterase inhibitor, primarily inactivates pseudocholinesterase and secondarily inhibits true cholinesterase. Echothiophate iodide may be used if maximal doses of other agents and combination therapy are ineffective. Echothiophate iodide has a long duration of action that affords good control of IOP; however, miosis and myopia are significant side effects. Concentrations higher than 0.06% are associated with a significant increase in subjective complaints (e.g., brow ache).[59]

COMBINATION THERAPY

In general, drugs with different pharmacologic actions have at least partially additive effects in lowering IOP in the treatment of glaucoma. Drugs with similar pharmacologic actions (i.e., from the same pharmacologic class) should not be combined because dose-related adverse effects are more likely and the incremental increase in benefits is likely to be more modest.

Timolol and other β-adrenergic blocking drugs have additive IOP-lowering effects when used in combination with miotic agents, prostaglandin analogs,[37,60] α_2-agonists,[61] and CAIs.[62,63] For example, the IOP-lowering effect is greater when timolol is used in combination with pilocarpine,[36,64] dorzolamide,[64] brimonidine,[37,61,65] and travoprost.[36,39] Likewise, for example, latanoprost has additive effects when administered with timolol,[36,41] dorzolamide,[38,39] and α_2-adrenergic agonists.[37,38,65] The trend toward the development of fixed-combination products offers many advantages in the treatment of POAG. These advantages include improved adherence because of a reduction in the number of dosages and bottles, eliminating the need to instill two separate drugs 5 to 10 minutes apart to prevent a washout effect from the second medication, improving safety and tolerability by limiting the exposure to the benzalkonium chloride preservative, and a cost savings for the patient by potentially eliminating a copay for one of the medications. There are two β-adrenergic blocker combination products currently on the market, timolol/dorzolamide (Cosopt) and brimonidine/timolol (Combigan). The IOP-lowering effects of timolol/dorzolamide (Cosopt) are comparable to or greater than those of latanoprost monotherapy.[66] Several other combination products are under investigation for POAG, which will offer a wide range of options for patients. These investigational agents include timolol/latanoprost (Xalacom), timolol/travoprost (DuoTrav, Extravan), and timolol/bimatoprost.[67,68]

Predisposing Factors

CASE 54-1

QUESTION 1: M.H., a 52-year-old African American woman with brown eyes, presented for routine ophthalmic examination. Visual acuity without correction was 20/40 right eye and 20/80 left eye. Tonometry measured an IOP of 36 mm Hg in both eyes. Ophthalmoscopy revealed physiologic cupping of the optic discs in both eyes, and visual field examination revealed a nerve fiber bundle defect consistent with glaucoma. Pupils were normal in both eyes, and gonioscopy indicated that anterior chamber angles were open in both eyes. There were no signs of cataract formation. M.H. related a positive family history for glaucoma and presently is being treated for hypertension, chronic heart failure (CHF), chronic obstructive pulmonary disease, and asthma. Her medications include the following:

Amitriptyline, 75 mg at bedtime
Chlorpheniramine, 4 mg every 6 hours as needed (PRN)
Lisinopril, 10 mg once daily
Furosemide, 40 mg BID
Nitroglycerin, 0.3 mg sublingual PRN
Fluticasone/salmeterol 250 mcg/50 mcg dry powder inhaler, one inhalation twice daily
Albuterol 90 mcg metered-dose inhaler, 1-2 puffs QID PRN
Tiotropium bromide inhaler, 18 mcg inhaled once daily

Findings on examination indicate that M.H. has POAG. What other factors may predispose M.H. to an increased IOP?

POAG is thought to be determined genetically, and M.H. has a positive family history. The disease is more prevalent and aggressive in African Americans.[1] In addition, she is taking several medications that have been associated with increases in IOP.

ANTICHOLINERGIC DRUGS

Most reports dealing with drug-induced increases in IOP center around precipitation of angle-closure glaucoma by ophthalmic mydriatic or cycloplegic agents (anticholinergics). In patients with open-angle glaucoma, topical anticholinergics can significantly increase resistance to aqueous humor outflow and elevate IOP while the anterior chamber remains grossly open.[2] As part of any routine ophthalmic examination, the pupils are dilated with a mydriatic or cycloplegic agent (unless otherwise contraindicated). The IOP is always measured before this procedure, so the use of these agents would not have influenced the IOP readings in M.H.

If systemic anticholinergic agents are administered in doses sufficient to cause pupillary dilation, the risk of precipitating angle-closure increases. However, it is unlikely that these agents will aggravate open-angle glaucoma unless the amount reaching the eye is sufficient to cause cycloplegia.[2] Although literature documentation of POAG exacerbation by these agents is scarce, medications with anticholinergic side effects (e.g., antihistamines, benzodiazepines, disopyramide, phenothiazines, tricyclic antidepressants, tiotropium) should be considered. M.H. is receiving chlorpheniramine as needed, amitriptyline at bedtime, and tiotropium bromide once daily, but her pupil examination is normal with no evidence of mydriasis or cycloplegia. Therefore, it is highly unlikely that these medications contributed to her increased IOP.

ADRENERGIC DRUGS

Adrenergic agents, such as central nervous system stimulants, vasoconstrictors, appetite suppressants, and bronchodilators, may produce minimal pupillary dilation. These have no proven adverse influences on IOP in patients with either normal eyes or eyes with open-angle glaucoma. Consequently, the use of salmeterol and albuterol in M.H. is also an unlikely source of the increased IOP.

OTHER DRUGS

Conclusive evidence for the production of angle-closure glaucoma by vasodilators is lacking, although slight increases in IOP have been reported. Use of nitroglycerin as needed in M.H. is not a cause for concern. There have been isolated reports of other medications causing mydriasis in glaucoma patients. These include muscle relaxants (carisoprodol), monoamine oxidase inhibitors, fenfluramine, ganglionic blocking agents, salicylates, and oral contraceptives. Succinylcholine, ketamine, and caffeine have been associated with increases in IOP. Corticosteroid-induced IOP elevation will be addressed in Case 54-8, Question 2. If M.H. requires administration of any other medications associated with increases in IOP, the risk of potential adverse effects can be minimized by routine follow-up.

Initial Therapy

CASE 54-1, QUESTION 2: What is the best initial therapeutic treatment in M.H.?

Topical β-blockers or PGAs are the initial agents of choice in the treatment of POAG (Fig. 54-2). Their efficacy is well documented in numerous studies, and side effects are well characterized. Brimonidine (Alphagan) and topical CAIs are alternative first-line agents. Table 54-1 lists the common topical agents used in the treatment of primary open-angle glaucoma.

Timolol or other nonselective β-adrenergic blockers should not be initiated for M.H. because of her history of asthma (the indications and use of β-blockers for patients with heart failure are described in Chapter 19, Heart Failure). Betaxolol, a β_1-adrenergic blocker, is better tolerated than the nonselective β-adrenergic blocker, timolol, in patients with reactive airway disease and should be considered when topical β-blocker therapy is indicated in patients such as M.H.[13,30,31,69] Betaxolol 0.25% suspension BID would be reasonable for the initial treatment of M.H.'s glaucoma. Nevertheless, adverse pulmonary and cardiac side effects can occur with betaxolol: M.H. should be followed up closely for these adverse effects. Although ocular burning and stinging have been associated more frequently with betaxolol and metipranolol than with other topical β-blockers, the 0.25% suspension is better tolerated than the 0.5% solution and is as effective.[32] Brimonidine, a topical CAI, or a PGA (e.g., latanoprost) are acceptable alternatives to betaxolol as initial therapy. Although brimonidine, topical CAIs, and latanoprost may not exacerbate her asthma or CHF, they can cause localized side effects and brimonidine can cause systemic hypotension and lethargy.

Patient Education

CASE 54-1, QUESTION 3: Betaxolol 0.25% suspension, one drop in both eyes BID, is ordered for M.H. How should M.H. be instructed regarding the proper use of her betaxolol and expected therapeutic side effects?

M.H. should be instructed to hold the inverted betaxolol bottle between her thumb and middle finger and to rest that hand on her forehead to minimize the risk of inadvertent eye injury caused by sudden unexpected movement of the hand. The index finger is left free to depress the bottom of the container, releasing one drop for the dose. With a little practice, this technique is easy to master. The lower eyelid should be drawn downward with the index finger of the opposite hand or pinched between the thumb and index finger to form a pouch. The patient should look up and administer the drug into the pouch of the eye.

Patients must be encouraged to continue regular use of their medications for effective treatment of glaucoma. Chronic glaucoma is a silent disease and often not associated with symptoms; therefore, the continuation of therapy should be encouraged continuously in patients, especially when side effects to drug therapy can be encountered. Betaxolol is best administered every 12 hours because this schedule of administration is consistent with its duration of action (see Table 54-1).

Systemic side effects (e.g., bradycardia, heart block, CHF, pulmonary distress, central nervous system) are rare with betaxolol, but M.H. should be instructed to report any of these effects to her primary-care provider.

NASOLACRIMAL OCCLUSION

CASE 54-1, QUESTION 4: How much would occlusion of the nasolacrimal ducts (punctal occlusion) by M.H. influence systemic absorption or alter the therapeutic effects of betaxolol?

Nasolacrimal, or punctal, occlusion is a technique that can decrease the amount of drug absorbed systemically.[70] Occlusion of the puncta (through the application of slight pressure with the finger to the inner corner of the eye closest to the nose for 3 to 5 minutes during and after drug instillation) can minimize systemic absorption of ophthalmic medications (e.g., betaxolol), decrease the incidence of side effects, and improve medication effectiveness.[70–72] When a single drop of ophthalmic timolol 0.5% was instilled into the eyes of patients at various times before cataract surgery and the nasolacrimal duct was occluded for 5 minutes, drug levels in the aqueous humor were significantly greater in patients who had their nasolacrimal ducts occluded than those who did not.[71] The average measured maximal aqueous humor timolol concentration of 1.66 mcg/mL in the occlusion group was significantly greater than 0.85 mcg/mL in the nonocclusion group. The area under the curve was 1.7 times greater in patients who used the technique of nasolacrimal occlusion, and the duration of action was prolonged.[71]

ONLINE CONTENT

For a video demonstrating nasolacrimal occlusion, go to http://thepoint.lww.com/AT10e.

Nasolacrimal occlusion is effective and can maximize drug benefits because a lower concentration of an ophthalmic formulation can be used and the dose can be administered less

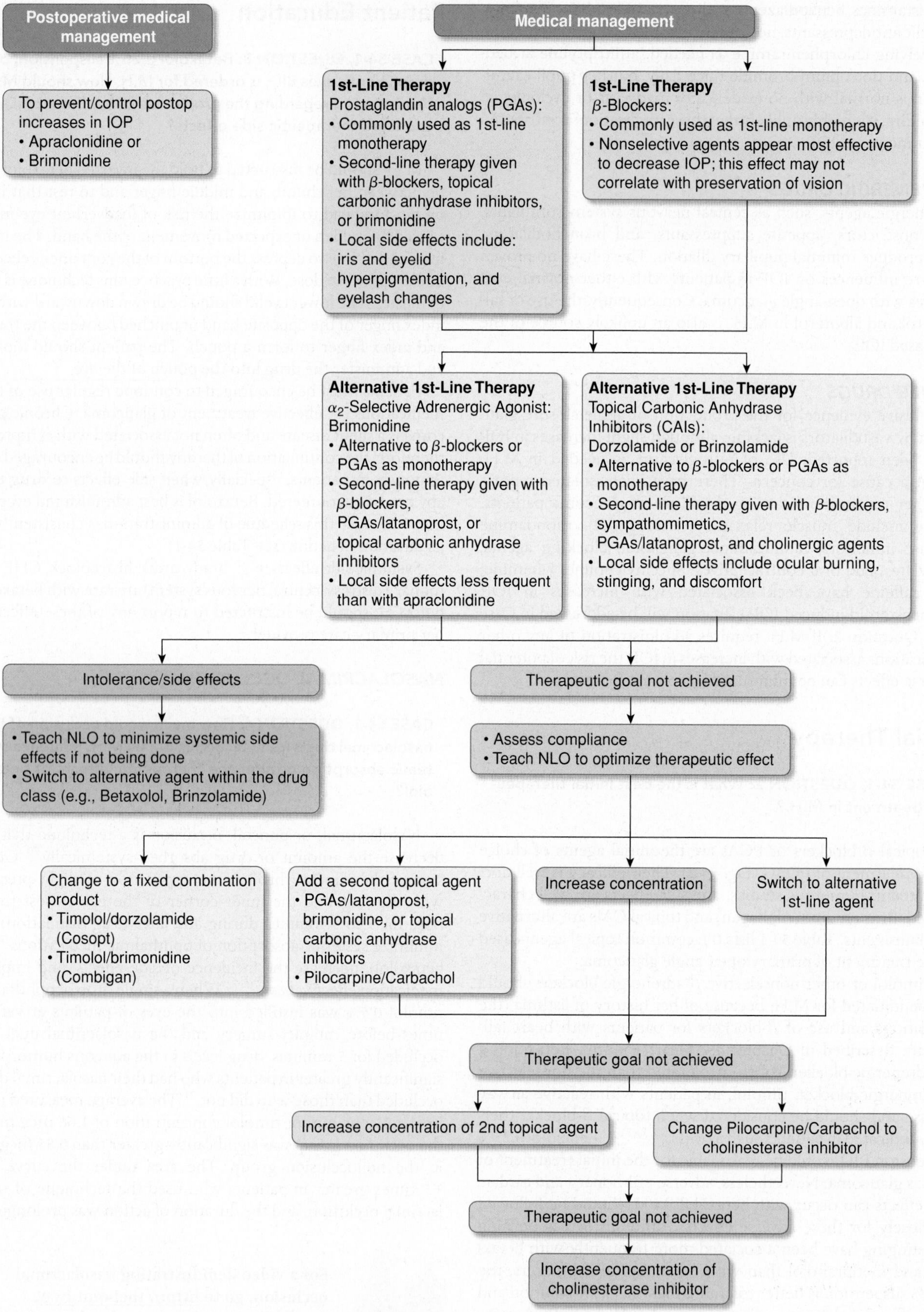

FIGURE 54-2 Medical management of glaucoma. IOP, intraocular pressure; NLO, nasolacrimal occlusion.

TABLE 54-1
Common Topical Agents Used in the Treatment of Open-Angle Glaucoma

Generic	Mechanism	Strength	Usual Dosage	Comments
β-Blockers				
Betaxolol (Betoptic [solution], Betoptic S [suspension])	Sympatholytic Sympatholytic	0.25% (suspension) 0.5% (solution)	1 drop BID 1 drop BID	Effective with few associated ocular side effects. BID dosage enhances compliance. Considered β-blocker of choice in patients with pre-existing HF or pulmonary disease because of β_1-adrenergic specificity. Patient response may be less than that seen with timolol.
Carteolol (Ocupress)	Sympatholytic	1%	1 drop BID	Effective with few associated side effects. BID dosage enhances compliance. Use with caution in patients with pre-existing HF or pulmonary disease.
Levobunolol (Betagan)	Sympatholytic	0.25%, 0.5%	1 drop daily or BID	Effective with few associated ocular side effects. Daily and BID dosage enhances compliance. Use with caution in patients with pre-existing HF or pulmonary disease.
Metipranolol (OptiPranolol)	Sympatholytic	0.3%	1 drop BID	Effective with few associated side effects. BID dosage enhances compliance. Use with caution in patients with pre-existing HF or pulmonary disease.
Timolol (Timoptic)	Sympatholytic	0.25%, 0.5%	1 drop BID	Effective with few associated ocular side effects. BID dosage enhances compliance. Use with caution in patients with pre-existing HF or pulmonary disease. Proven long-term effectiveness, with well-defined side effect profile.
Timolol Gel Forming Solution (Timoptic XE)	Sympatholytic	0.25%, 0.5%	1 drop daily	Once-daily timolol formulation. The ophthalmic vehicle, gellan gum (Gelrite), prolongs precorneal residence time and ↑ ocular bioavailability, allowing once daily administration.
α_2-Selective Adrenergic Agonists				
Apraclonidine (Iopidine)	Sympathomimetic	0.5%, 1%	1 drop preoperatively and postoperatively or 1 drop BID to TID	May be used preoperatively and postoperatively for the prevention of ↑ IOP after anterior-segment laser procedures. Use of NLO minimizes systemic side effects and allows for BID dosing. Does not penetrate the blood–brain barrier; therefore, negligible systemic hypotension. Local adverse effects fairly common. Tachyphylaxis may be observed.
Brimonidine (Alphagan)	Sympathomimetic	0.15%, 0.2%	1 drop BID to TID	Effective long-term monotherapy or adjunctive therapy. Use of NLO minimizes systemic side effects and allows for BID dosing. Penetrates the blood–brain barrier; therefore, may cause mild systemic hypotension and lethargy. Local adverse effects less common than with apraclonidine.
Brimonidine (Alphagan P)	Sympathomimetic	0.1%, 0.15%	1 drop BID to TID	Contains PURITE preservative. PURITE preservative and lower concentrations may improve tolerability.
Topical Carbonic Anhydrase Inhibitors				
Brinzolamide (Azopt)	Decreased aqueous humor production	1%	1 drop TID	Effective long-term monotherapy or adjunctive therapy. Well tolerated with few systemic side effects. Less burning and stinging compared with dorzolamide.
Dorzolamide (Trusopt)	Decreased aqueous humor production	2%	1 drop TID	Effective long-term monotherapy or adjunctive therapy. Well tolerated with few systemic side effects.

(continued)

TABLE 54-1

Common Topical Agents Used in the Treatment of Open-Angle Glaucoma (*Continued*)

Generic	Mechanism	Strength	Usual Dosage	Comments
Prostaglandin Analogs				
Latanoprost (Xalatan)	Prostaglandin $F_{2\alpha}$ agonist	0.005%	1 drop once a day at bedtime	BID dosing may be less effective than once a day at bedtime dosing. May cause increased pigmentation of the iris and eyelid. Systemic side effects are rare, but may cause muscle, joint, back pain, headaches, migraines, and skin rash. Effective monotherapy or adjunctive therapy. Store unopened bottles in refrigerator. Opened bottles may be stored at room temperature up to 6 weeks.
Travoprost (Travatan Z)	Prostaglandin $F_{2\alpha}$ agonist	0.004%	1 drop once a day at bedtime	BID dosing may be less effective than once a day at bedtime dosing. May cause increased pigmentation of the iris and eyelid. Systemic side effects are rare, but may include colds and upper respiratory tract infections. Effective monotherapy or adjunctive therapy with timolol. May be more effective than timolol and latanoprost and more effective in African Americans. Benzalkonium chloride preservative free. Contains a preservative that may be better tolerated.
Bimatoprost (Lumigan)	Prostamide	0.01%, 0.03%	1 drop once a day at bedtime	BID dosing may be less effective than QHS dosing. May cause increased pigmentation of the iris and eyelid. Systemic side effects are rare but include colds and upper respiratory tract infections and headache. May be more effective than timolol and latanoprost.
Miotics				
Pilocarpine (Isopto Carpine)	Parasympathomimetic	1%, 2%, 4% 4% (ointment)	1–2 drops TID or QID ½ inch in cul-de-sac daily at bedtime	Long-term proven effectiveness. Little rationale for administration more frequently than every 4 hours. Side effects of miosis with decreased vision and brow ache are common sources of patient complaints. Once-daily administration of ointment may increase compliance. Effectiveness for 24 hours should be assessed in patients receiving the ointment. Ointment may cause a visual haze and blurred vision.
Carbachol (Isopto Carbachol)	Parasympathomimetic	1.5%, 3%	1–2 drops TID or QID	Used in patients allergic to or intolerant of other miotics. May be used as frequently as every 4 hours. Corneal penetration is enhanced by benzalkonium chloride in commercial preparations. Side effects are similar to those of pilocarpine.
Echothiophate iodide (Phospholine iodide)	Anticholinesterase	0.125%	1 drop BID	Long duration, although usually dosed BID, which enhances compliance. Available as powder + diluent; after reconstitution, stable 30 days at room temperature, 6 months refrigerated. Side effects similar to those of pilocarpine. Increased cataract formation has been associated with its use.
Combination Products				
Brimonidine tartrate 0.2%/timolol 0.5% (Combigan)	Sympathomimetic/ sympatholytic	0.2%/0.5%	1 drop BID	Combination products may improve adherence. Eliminates the 5- to 10-minute wait between instillation of drops.
Dorzolamide 2%/timolol 0.5% (Cosopt)	Decreased aqueous humor production/ sympathomimetic	2%/0.5%	1 drop BID	Combination products may improve adherence. Eliminates the 5- to 10-minute wait between instillation of drops.

BID, twice daily; HF, heart failure; IOP, intraocular pressure; NLO, nasolacrimal occlusion; QHS, every day at bedtime; QID, four times a day; TID, three times a day.

frequently. Pilocarpine 1% and 2% significantly decreased IOP at 6, 8, and 12 hours after instillation when the technique of nasolacrimal occlusion was applied.[70] Similarly, carbachol 1.5% and 3%, and the combination of carbachol 1.5% with timolol 0.25% every 12 hours also were maximally beneficial with nasolacrimal occlusion.[70] Timolol reduced IOP by 15% and maintained this reduction of IOP at 24 hours in 92% of patients when nasolacrimal occlusion was used; in comparison, only 55% achieved comparable IOP reductions when nasolacrimal ducts were not occluded.[70] When nasolacrimal occlusion is used, pilocarpine 2% and carbachol 1.5% can be administered every 12 hours rather than the usual TID or QID regimens needed when the technique of nasolacrimal occlusion is not applied.[70] The every 12-hour regimen of treatment then can be adjusted according to the patient's response. Timolol can be administered every 24 hours if the nasolacrimal occlusion technique is used.[64] If nasolacrimal occlusion is used consistently and properly, maximal drug effect can be achieved with a reduced frequency of administration and at about half of the drug concentrations typically used. Nasolacrimal occlusion should be incorporated into patient counseling for instillation of all eye drops.[70]

Alternative Therapy

CASE 54-1, QUESTION 5: Two weeks after initiation of therapy, M.H. returns to clinic for a follow-up evaluation. Her IOP measures 32 mm Hg in the right eye and 30 mm Hg in the left eye. She denies nonadherence and has no complaints of intolerable side effects. How should therapy be altered? Are there alternative dosage forms or drugs that can be used?

Betaxolol may not be as effective as other ocular β-blockers. Therefore, adjunctive therapy may be required. However, M.H. should be evaluated to determine whether she has been using the technique of nasolacrimal occlusion. If not, M.H. should be again instructed on the technique of nasolacrimal occlusion and the importance of this technique in achieving the maximal therapeutic effect of her therapy (see Case 54-1, Question 4).

After the initiation of therapy, patients should be seen for a follow-up evaluation within about 2 weeks. If M.H. has been adherent to therapy and has been occluding her nasolacrimal ducts, a new course of action is needed because her IOP still is elevated. When the goal of therapy has not been achieved, the drug concentration of the ophthalmic formulation can be increased, adjunctive therapy (e.g., brimonidine, a topical CAI, a PGA) can be initiated, or an alternative first-line agent can be selected. Patients who are experiencing unstable reductions of IOP should be followed up within 4 months.[3] Stable patients usually are evaluated every 6 to 12 months.[3]

Adverse Effects

CASE 54-1, QUESTION 6: Several weeks later, dorzolamide 2% solution, one drop both eyes BID, is added to M.H.'s betaxolol therapy. Two weeks later, M.H. returns for a follow-up evaluation and complains of bilateral stinging and foreign body sensation. Her IOP measures 30 mm Hg in the right eye and 29 mm Hg in the left eye. What are the possible causes of her side effects and poor response to therapy?

The exposure of dorzolamide to the outside environment may result in the aggregation of dry white granules on the tip of the dorzolamide bottle. These granules can drop into a patient's eyes when instilling the medication, leading to local side effects, such as stinging and foreign body sensation. Such foreign bodies may cause enough discomfort to induce nonadherence, resulting in a poor response to therapy. These granules may be rinsed off of the tip with sterile water. M.H. should be questioned about the presence of dry white granules on the tip of her dorzolamide bottle.[73]

These complaints may also be a side effect from the medications, regardless of the granule presence. Ocular burning, stinging, and discomfort were reported in one-third of patients in dorzolamide clinical trials. M.H.'s administration technique should also be assessed to determine whether she is administering the two drugs at least 5 to 10 minutes apart so that the first drug is not washed away by the second drug. This should be a consideration when assessing her response to therapy.[14]

CASE 54-1, QUESTION 7: After further discussions with M.H., it is determined that she has not been adherent to her dorzolamide therapy because of intolerable side effects. The dorzolamide is discontinued and replaced with travoprost 0.004% one drop both eyes once a day at bedtime. Why might this drug selection be especially appropriate for M.H.? What patient education information should be provided to M.H. about travoprost side effects?

Prostaglandin analogs are first-line agents and are appropriate in patients who are not responding to or are having intolerable side effects from other medications. Travoprost is an ideal choice for M.H., because African Americans respond especially well to travoprost.[41] M.H. still needs to be informed about the PGA-induced potential for hyperpigmentation of the iris, which may be permanent. She also needs to be educated on the possibility of eyelid skin darkening and increased thickness, length, and pigmentation of her eyelashes, which all may or may not be reversible. These side effects might not be as cosmetically concerning to M.H., because she has brown eyes and will be instilling travoprost eye drops into both eyes.

ANGLE-CLOSURE GLAUCOMA

Treatment

CASE 54-2

QUESTION 1: D.H., a 72-year-old man, presents to the emergency department with an intensely red right eye, a "steamy" appearing cornea, complaints of haloes around lights, and extreme pain. A diagnosis of acute angle-closure glaucoma is made. How should D.H. be managed?

D.H. should be seen by an ophthalmologist because acute angle-closure glaucoma is a medical emergency. Medical treatment usually consists of pilocarpine 2% to 4%, one drop every 5 minutes for four to six administrations. It is recommended that the puncta be covered during administration to decrease the possibility of systemic absorption. Stronger miotic agents are contraindicated because they may potentiate angle closure. Topical timolol also has been used in acute angle-closure glaucoma, commonly in combination with pilocarpine. However, drugs that decrease aqueous humor production may be ineffective in this situation because they have a decreased ability to reduce aqueous production if the ciliary body is ischemic.[4]

TABLE 54-2
Hyperosmotic Agents

Generic	Mode of Administration	Strength	Onset	Peak	Duration	Dose	Ocular Penetration	Distribution
Mannitol	IV	5%, 10%, 15%, 20%	30–60 minutes	1 hour	6–8 hours	1–2 g/kg	Very poor	E
Glycerin	PO	50%	10–30 minutes	30 minutes	4–5 hours	1–1.5 g/kg	Poor	E
Isosorbide	PO	45%	10–30 minutes	1 hour	5 hours	1.5–2 g/kg	Good	TBW

E, Extracellular water; IV, intravenous; PO, orally; TBW, total body water.

HYPEROSMOTIC AGENTS

Hyperosmotic agents (Table 54-2) act by creating an osmotic gradient between the plasma and ocular fluids.[74] Agents that are confined to the extracellular fluid space (e.g., mannitol) provide a greater effect on blood osmolality at the same dosage than do agents distributed in total body water.[74] Intravenously administered drugs provide a faster, somewhat greater effect than oral agents. Palatability may be a problem with oral agents and can be improved by serving these agents over crushed ice or with lemon juice or cola flavoring.

Orally, 50% glycerin is the usual drug of choice and is administered in dosages of 1 to 1.5 g/kg.[75] Isosorbide is an alternative, especially in diabetic patients because it is not metabolized to provide calories.[76] Parenterally, mannitol is the drug of choice. It is administered in doses of 1 to 2 g/kg, is not metabolized to provide calories, and may be used in patients with renal failure.[77,78]

Primary side effects of hyperosmotic agents include headache, nausea, vomiting, diuresis, and dehydration. It is important that the patient not be allowed to drink because this will counteract the osmotic effects of these agents.

Precipitation of pulmonary edema and CHF has been reported with hyperosmotic agents, and an allergic reaction has been reported with mannitol.[79]

Acetazolamide (Diamox) 500 mg intravenously may be administered in addition to hyperosmotic agents.

OCULAR SIDE EFFECTS OF DRUGS

CASE 54-3

QUESTION 1: B.C., a 64-year-old man, has a history of hypertension managed with hydrochlorothiazide 25 mg/day. He takes amiodarone 800 mg/day for cardiac arrhythmia, and chlorpheniramine 12 mg BID PRN for allergies. Four weeks ago, risperidone 1 mg BID was added to his medication regimen. He also takes sildenafil 100 mg an average of twice weekly. He complains of occasional blurred vision. Could these symptoms be related to his medications?

All the drugs that B.C. is taking have been associated with ocular side effects. Thiazide diuretics have been associated with acute myopia that may last from 24 to 48 hours.[80,81] However, hydrochlorothiazide is an unlikely cause of B.C.'s blurred vision considering its recent onset.

Amiodarone can cause keratopathy, but it is asymptomatic.[82,83] A high percentage of patients who receive this drug exhibit microdeposits within the corneal epithelium that resemble the verticillate keratopathy induced by chloroquine.[80] These corneal deposits are bilateral, dose and duration related, reversible, and unassociated with visual symptoms.

Risperidone has been associated with disturbances of accommodation and blurred vision.[84]

B.C. may be in the approximately 1% of the population who experiences blurred vision with chlorpheniramine. This effect has been seen in patients receiving 12 to 14 mg/day.[80] If an antihistamine is indicated, an agent such as cetirizine would be less likely to cause such an effect. Sildenafil has been associated with change in color and light perception as well as blurred vision.[85] These effects generally subside within 4 hours of the dose.

Table 54-3[86–109] outlines some of the more common ocular side effects associated with systemic medications. Each case should be evaluated individually and alternative therapy considered in intolerant patients.

OCULAR EMERGENCIES

Chemical Burns

CASE 54-4

QUESTION 1: S.J., a 24-year-old construction worker, has splashed an unidentified chemical in his eyes and runs into a nearby pharmacy complaining of burning in both eyes. Should the pharmacist attempt to treat S.J. or refer him to the emergency department?

Chemical burns require immediate attention. The immediate treatment is copious irrigation using the most accessible source of water (e.g., shower, faucet, drinking fountain, hose, bathtub). After at least 5 minutes of initial irrigation, S.J. should be taken immediately to the emergency department. A water-soaked towel or cloth should be kept on his eyes during transport.

Other Ocular Emergencies

When health care professionals are approached by patients with acute ocular emergencies (e.g., chemical burns, corneal trauma, corneal ulcers, acute angle-closure glaucoma), patients require immediate treatment and should be referred to an ophthalmologist if the practitioner has even the slightest doubt about appropriate therapy. It is difficult to effectively evaluate the severity of ocular disorders without the benefit of a thorough ophthalmologic workup and specialized training. In situations of corneal trauma from abrasion or foreign bodies, the patient often complains of a gritty, scratchy feeling and can be aware of a foreign body's presence. The corneal tissue is an excellent culture medium for bacteria (e.g., *Pseudomonas aeruginosa*), and therapy should be initiated as soon as possible to avoid corneal perforation and possible blindness.[1] Signs and symptoms of acute angle-closure glaucoma are reviewed in Case 54-2, Question 1.

Gonococcal conjunctivitis is an ocular emergency, and patients should be referred immediately to an ophthalmologist to minimize the potential of corneal perforation.[1] These patients, who can present with symptoms of red, tender, swollen eyelids with exophthalmos and mild pain, may be suffering from orbital cellulitis or endophthalmitis, which require immediate treatment with systemic antibiotics. Conjunctivitis of other

TABLE 54-3
Ocular Side Effects of Systemic Medications

Drug Class	Effect(s)	Clinical Remarks
Analgesics		
Ibuprofen	Reduced vision	Rare; blurred vision reported in patients taking from four 200-mg tablets/wk to six tablets/d; changes in color vision rarely reported.[86]
Narcotics, including pentazocine	Miosis	Miosis often with morphine in normal doses: slight with other agents; effect secondary to CNS action on the pupilloconstrictor center.[80]
	Tearing Irregular pupils Paresis of accommodation Diplopia	Effects associated with narcotic withdrawal.[80]
Antiarrhythmics		
Amiodarone	Keratopathy	Dose and duration related; resembles chloroquine keratopathy. Corneal deposits are bilateral, reversible, and unassociated with visual symptoms. Patients taking 100–200 mg/d have only minimal deposits. Deposits occur in almost 100% of patients receiving 400 mg/d.[80–83]
	Cataracts	Previously reported as insignificant, anterior subcapsular lens opacities have been associated with amiodarone therapy. Rarely, such opacities may progress, increasing in density and in the diffuse distribution of the deposits, ultimately covering an area somewhat larger than the undilated pupil's aperture. The mechanism for this effect is unclear, but like chlorpromazine, amiodarone is a photosensitizing agent. Given that the lens changes are limited largely to the pupillary aperture, light exposure may result in the lens changes.[80–83]
	Optic neuropathy	Approximately 2% of patients experience optic neuropathy.[85]
Anticholinergics		
Atropine Dicyclomine Glycopyrrolate Propantheline Scopolamine Trihexyphenidyl	Mydriasis Cycloplegia with ↓ accommodation Photophobia	Systemic and transdermal anticholinergic agents may cause mydriasis and, less frequently, cycloplegia. Mydriasis may precipitate angle-closure glaucoma. Photophobia is related to the mydriasis. Accommodation for near objects.[80,87]
Anticonvulsants		
Carbamazepine	Diplopia Blurred vision	Ocular adverse reactions when dosage >1–2 g/d; disappear when dosage is reduced.[80]
Phenytoin	Nystagmus Cataracts	Nystagmus in patients with high blood levels (>20 mcg/mL); rarely occurs with other hydantoins. Cataracts may occur rarely with prolonged therapy.[80,88]
Topiramate	Acute myopia Secondary angle-closure glaucoma	Topiramate has been associated with angle-closure glaucoma. Symptoms including ocular pain, headache, nausea, vomiting, hyperemia, visual field defects, and blindness have been reported. This process is usually bilateral, but if symptoms are recognized and the drug is stopped in a timely manner, adverse outcomes may be minimized.[85]
Trimethadione	Visual glares	A prolonged glare or dazzle occurs when eyes are exposed to light. The glare is reversible, occurs at the retinal level, and is more common in adolescents and adults; rarely in young children.[80]
Vigabatrin	Visual field abnormalities	Visual field abnormalities including bilateral, symmetrical, and irreversible peripheral constriction occur in up to 30% of patients. Most patients are asymptomatic and <0.1% of patients are clinically affected.[85]
Anesthetics		
Propofol	Inability to open eyes	6 of 50 patients undergoing ENT procedures using standardized anesthesia with propofol were unable to open their eyes either spontaneously or in response to verbal commands. This effect lasted from 3 to 20 minutes after the end of anesthetic administration. Two patients showed complete loss of ocular motility. This was a transient, myasthenialike weakness.[89]
Antidepressants		
Tricyclic antidepressants (TCAs)		Mydriasis is the most common ocular side effect of TCAs. Cycloplegia is rare. Reports of precipitation of angle-closure glaucoma.[80]
Fluoxetine	Mydriasis Cycloplegia Eye tics	Administration of fluoxetine 20–40 mg/d has been associated with paroxysmal contractions of the muscles around the lateral aspect of the eye. This effect occurred 3–4 weeks after initiation of fluoxetine therapy and resolved within 2 weeks of discontinuation.[90]
Antihistamines		
Chlorpheniramine	Blurred vision	Blurred vision occurs rarely (about 1% of patients taking 12–14 mg/d).[80]
	Mydriasis, decreased lacrimal secretions	Rare.[80]

(continued)

TABLE 54-3
Ocular Side Effects of Systemic Medications (*Continued*)

Drug Class	Effect(s)	Clinical Remarks
Antihypertensives		
Clonidine	Miosis	Miosis is seen in overdose.[80]
	Dry itchy eyes	Rare.[80]
Diazoxide	Lacrimation	About 20% experience lacrimation, which may continue after drug is discontinued.[80]
Guanethidine	Miosis Ptosis Conjunctivitis Blurred vision	Sporadically documented. One study reported a 17% incidence of blurred vision in patients taking guanethidine 70 mg/d.[80]
Reserpine	Miosis	Miosis is slight, but can last up to 1 week after a single dose.[80]
	Conjunctivitis	Common, secondary to dilation of conjunctival blood vessels.[80]
Anti-Infectives		
Amantadine	Corneal lesions	Diffuse, white punctate subepithelial corneal opacities have been reported, occasionally associated with superficial punctate keratitis. Onset has been 1–2 weeks after initiation of therapy with dosages of 200–400 mg/d. Resolves with drug discontinuation.[91]
Chloramphenicol	Optic neuritis	Rare unless a total dose of 100 g and duration >6 weeks are exceeded. Vision usually improves after the drug is discontinued.[80]
Chloroquine	Corneal deposits	Some patients using ordinary doses may develop corneal deposits in a few months. The deposits are visible with use of a biomicroscope and appear as white-yellow in color, but are of no consequence.[80]
	Retinopathy (macular degeneration)	Serious retinopathy when total dose >100 g. Usually develops after 1–3 years; can occur in 6 months. Visual loss may be peripheral, with progression to central vision loss and disturbance of color vision. Rarely, effects such as blurred vision are seen earlier when larger doses (500–700 mg/d) are used. Macular changes may progress after drug is discontinued. These agents concentrate in pigmented tissue.[80]
Ethambutol	Retrobulbar neuritis	At dosages of 15 mg/kg/d, virtually void of ocular side effects. Such effects are rare at dosages of 25 mg/kg/d for a duration of a few months. Patients treated for prolonged periods should have routine visual examinations including visual fields. Most effects are reversible after the drug is discontinued, but optic neuritis may continue to progress for 1–2 months after the drug has been discontinued.[80,85]
Gentamicin	Pseudotumor cerebri	Rare, but has been well documented with secondary papilledema and visual loss.[8]
Isoniazid	Optic neuritis	Prevalence not well defined, but appears to be significantly less than peripheral neuritis. Evaluation difficult because most patients are malnourished, chronic alcoholics, or receiving multiple medications. Pre-existing eye disease does not appear to be a predisposing factor.[80]
Nalidixic acid	Visual sensations	Most common ocular side effect. Main feature is a brightly colored appearance of objects; occurs soon after the drug is taken. Although quinolone antibiotics are nalidixic acid derivatives, they have rarely been associated with these ocular side effects.[80]
	Visual loss	Temporary effect (30 minutes–3 days).
	Papilledema	Primarily in infants and young children and secondary to intracranial pressure; reversible on withdrawal of the drug.
Sulfonamides	Myopia	Acute and reversible; most common ocular side effect.[80]
	Conjunctivitis	Primarily with topical sulfathiazole, 4% incidence between 5 and 9 days of therapy.[80]
	Optic neuritis	Even in low dosages. Usually reversible with complete recovery of vision.[80]
	Photosensitivity	Associated with use of sulfisoxazole lid margin therapy.[92,93]
Tetracyclines	Myopia	Appears to be acute, transient, and rare.[80]
	Papilledema	More common in children and infants than adults; rare.[80]
Voriconazole	Altered visual perception Blurred vision	May be associated with higher doses or plasma concentrations.[94]
Anti-Inflammatory Agents (also see Analgesics; Corticosteroids)		
Cyclo-oxygenase-2 inhibitors	Blurred vision Conjunctivitis	Discontinuation of therapy leads to resolution without long-term effects.[85]
Gold	Corneal Conjunctival deposits	Deposition in the conjunctiva and superficial cornea more common than in the lens or deep cornea. Incidence in cornea of 40%–80% in total doses of 1.5 g; visual acuity is unaffected. One reported case after oral therapy.[80]
Indomethacin	Decreased vision	Rare; also changes in color vision have been rarely reported.[80]
Phenylbutazone	Decreased vision	Most common ocular side effect with this drug may be caused by lens hydration.[80]
	Conjunctivitis Retinal hemorrhage	Occurs less often than vision. The conjunctivitis may be associated with development of Stevens-Johnson syndrome or an allergic reaction.[80]

(continued)

TABLE 54-3
Ocular Side Effects of Systemic Medications (*Continued*)

Drug Class	Effect(s)	Clinical Remarks
Antilipemic Agents		
Lovastatin	Cataracts	The crystalline lenses of hypercholesteremic patients were assessed before and after 48 weeks of treatment with lovastatin 20–80 mg/d. Statistical analyses of the distribution of cortical, nuclear, and subcapsular opacities at 48 weeks showed no significant differences between placebo-treated and lovastatin-treated groups. Visual acuity assessments also were not significantly different among the groups.[95]
Antineoplastic Agents		
Busulfan	Cataracts	Reported with high dosages.[80]
Carmustine	Arterial narrowing Nerve fiber-layer infarcts Intraretinal hemorrhages	These ocular side effects are not well established. Evidence of delayed bilateral ocular toxicity developed in 2 of 50 patients treated with high-dose IV carmustine (800 mg/m^2). Symptoms of ocular toxicity became evident 4 weeks after IV treatment. Evidence of delayed ocular toxicity (mean onset 6 weeks) ipsilateral to the site of infusion developed in 7 of 10 patients treated with intra-arterial carotid doses of carmustine to a cumulative minimum of 450 mg/m^2 in two treatments.[96]
Cytarabine	Keratoconjunctivitis Ocular burning Photophobia Blurred vision	Corneal toxicity and conjunctivitis have been reported with high-dose (3 g/m^2) therapy.[97]
Doxorubicin	Conjunctivitis Excessive tearing	May last for several days after treatment.[80]
Fluorouracil	Ocular irritation Lacrimation	Reversible and seldom interfere with continued therapy.[80]
Tamoxifen	Corneal opacities Decreased vision Retinopathy	Generally occurs in patients receiving more than 1 year of treatment when a total dose exceeding 100 g has been taken.[80]
Vinca alkaloids (especially vincristine)	Extraocular muscle paresis (EMP) Ptosis	The onset of EMP or paralysis may be seen as early as 2 weeks. Dose related. Most recover fully when drug is discontinued.[80]
Barbiturates		
	Miosis Mydriasis Disturbances in ocular movement Ptosis	Most significant ocular side effects occur in chronic users or in toxic states. Pupillary responses are variable; miosis seen most frequently except in toxicity when mydriasis predominates. Nystagmus and weakness in extraocular muscles may be seen. Chronic abusers have a characteristic ptosis.[80]
Bisphosphonates (Alendronate, Etidronate, Pamidronate, Risedronate)		
	Blurred vision, pain, photophobia, conjunctivitis, scleritis, uveitis	Adverse events more common with pamidronate. Scleritis and uveitis are of greatest concern. After persistent reduction in vision of sustained ocular pain, refer patient to an ophthalmologist. Ocular NSAID treatment may be of symptomatic benefit.[85]
Calcium-Channel Blockers		
	Blurred vision Transient blindness	Primarily blurred vision; transient blindness at peak concentrations has been observed in several patients.[98]
Corticosteroids		
	Cataracts	Posterior subcapsular cataracts have been associated with systemic corticosteroids in patients who have received >15 mg/d of prednisone or its equivalent daily for periods >1 year.[99,100] Rare reports of bilateral posterior subcapsular cataracts associated with nasal aerosol or inhalation of beclomethasone dipropionate have been received. Most patients had received therapy for >5 years, often in higher than the recommended dosage. Approximately 40% of patients also were receiving systemic corticosteroids.[101] (Also see Case 54-8, Question 1.)
	↑ Intraocular pressure	More common with topical corticosteroids than with systemic therapy. Of little consequence in patients without pre-existing glaucoma. Glaucoma patients should be monitored routinely if receiving systemic corticosteroids.[80] (See Case 54-8, Question 1.)
	Papilledema	Intracranial hypertension or pseudotumor cerebri from systemic corticosteroids has been well documented. The incidence appears to be greater in children than in adults; primarily associated with chronic therapy.

(continued)

TABLE 54-3
Ocular Side Effects of Systemic Medications (*Continued*)

Drug Class	Effect(s)	Clinical Remarks
Digitalis		
	Altered color vision, visual acuity	Changes in color vision. A glare phenomenon and a snowy appearance in objects have been associated primarily with digitalis intoxication. In a small number of cases, reversible reduction in visual acuity has been noted. Also associated with changes in the visual fields.[80]
	Decreased intraocular pressure	Digitalis derivatives can decrease intraocular pressure, but clinical use for glaucoma is not practical because the therapeutic systemic dose for this effect is very near the toxic dose.[80]
Diuretics		
Carbonic anhydrase inhibitors Thiazides	Myopia	Acute myopia that may last from 24 to 48 hours. Probably caused by an increase in the anteroposterior diameter of the lens, which may be reversible even if drug use is continued.[80]
Estrogens		
Clomiphene	Blurred vision Mydriasis Visual field changes Visual sensations	5%–10% experience ocular side effects. Blurred vision is the most common effect, although visual sensations such as flashing lights, distortion of images, and various colored lights (primarily silver) may occur.[80]
Oral contraceptives (OCs)	Optic neuritis Pseudotumor cerebri Retrobulbar neuritis	Quite rare. In patients with retinal vascular abnormalities, use of OCs is questionable. Numerous other possible ocular side effects are associated with these agents, and further documentation is required.[80]
Hypouricemics		
Allopurinol	Cataracts	Conflicting reports have suggested allopurinol may be associated with anterior and posterior lens capsule changes and with anterior subcapsular vacuoles; 42 cases of cataracts have been reported; these have been observed primarily in age groups in whom normal lens aging changes would not be expected. No cause-and-effect relationship has been proven.[80,102]
Immune Modulators		
Imatinib	Visual deficits	Ocular symptoms include blurred vision, conjunctivitis, dry eyes, epiphora, and periorbital edema. The latter occurs in up to 74% of treated patients.[103]
Interleukin 2	Visual deficits	Interleukin 2 visual complications have occurred during the first or second treatment cycle, usually within 5–6 days of initiation of therapy. Ocular symptoms included diplopia, binocular negative scotomas (isolated areas of varying size and shape in which vision is absent or depressed; these are not perceived ordinarily, but would be apparent on completion of a visual field examination), and palinopsia (abnormal recurring visual imagery). In most cases, treatment was continued for the entire planned duration of therapy. Symptoms resolved after discontinuation.[104]
Phenothiazines		
Chlorpromazine	Deposits on the lens	Rare when total dose $<$0.5 kg. Visible after a total dose of 1 kg in most cases; incidence may increase to 90% after $\geq$2.5 kg. Usually, deposits do not affect vision appreciably. The cornea and conjunctiva may be affected after the lens shows pigment changes.[80]
	Retinal pigment deposits	The number of reported cases is small; further documentation is necessary.[80]
Thioridazine	Pigmentary retinopathy	Primarily associated with maximal daily dosages or average doses $>$1,000 mg. Daily dosages up to 600 mg are relatively safe; 600–800 mg is uncertain, but rarely suspect. If $>$800 mg/d is used, periodic ophthalmoscopic examinations may uncover problems before visual acuity is compromised.[80]
Therapy for Erectile Dysfunction		
Sildenafil Tadalafil Vardenafil α-Blockers	Changes in color or light perception, blurred vision, conjunctival hyperemia, ocular pain, photophobia	Color vision alterations are mild to moderate. Blurred vision does not impair visual acuity. Visual alterations usually subside within 4 hours after the dose.[105–107] Ocular adverse effects are uncommon, dose dependent, and fully reversible to date. Incidence is not related to age, but is related to blood concentration. Peak visual effects usually occur within 60 minutes after ingestion.[85]
Alfuzosin	Visual defects	Amblyopia, blurred vision, and floppy iris have been reported.[108]
Tamsulosin	Floppy iris Floppy iris	Approximately 3% of patients taking tamsulosin for benign prostatic hyperplasia (BPH) experience floppy iris during cataract surgery. Modification of the surgical procedure usually results in successful surgery.[109]

CNS, central nervous system; ENT, ear, nose, and throat; NSAID, nonsteroidal anti-inflammatory drug.

origins (see Acute Bacterial Conjunctivitis [Pinkeye] and Allergic Conjunctivitis sections) generally is not an ocular emergency.

Any loss of vision (whether sudden, complete, or transient), flashes of light, pain, or photophobia can signify potentially damaging ocular disorders (e.g., retinal artery occlusion, optic neuritis, amaurosis fugax, retinal detachment), and an ophthalmologist should evaluate the patient as soon as possible. Referral also is recommended for patients with blurred vision, pupil disorders, diplopia, nystagmus, or ocular hemorrhage.

COMMON OCULAR DISORDERS

Stye (Hordeolum)

Sties are infections of the hair follicles or sebaceous glands of the eyelids. The most common infecting organism is *Staphylococcus aureus*. Treatment consists of hot, moist compresses and topical antibiotics (e.g., sulfacetamide). Over-the-counter products should not be recommended. An ophthalmologist should evaluate sties that do not respond to warm compresses within a few days.

Conjunctivitis

Conjunctivitis, a common external eye problem that involves inflammation of the conjunctiva, usually is associated with symptoms of a diffusely reddened eye with purulent or serous discharge accompanied by itching, smarting, stinging, or a scratching foreign-body sensation. Patients with pain, decreased vision, unequal distribution of redness, irregular pupils, or opacity should be referred immediately to an ophthalmologist because these are signs of more serious eye disease.

Conjunctivitis can be bacterial, fungal, parasitic, viral, or allergic in origin. Most cases of bacterial conjunctivitis are caused by *S. aureus*, *Streptococcus pneumococcus* (in temperate climates), or *Haemophilus aegyptius* (in warm climates), although a number of other organisms may be responsible. The infection usually starts in one eye and is spread to the other by the hands. It also may be spread to other persons. Unlike bacterial conjunctivitis, corneal infections can obliterate vision rapidly; therefore, accurate diagnosis is important.

ACUTE BACTERIAL CONJUNCTIVITIS (PINKEYE)

CASE 54-5

QUESTION 1: L.T. is a 6-year-old boy with diffuse bilateral conjunctival redness that has been present for 2 days. A crusting discharge is deposited on his lashes and the corners of his eyes. His vision is normal, and his pupils are round and equal. The diagnosis of acute bacterial conjunctivitis is made, and sodium sulfacetamide 10% ophthalmic drops, two drops in both eyes every 2 hours while awake, are prescribed. What other measures should be used? What instructions should his caregivers receive?

Although treatment of typical bacterial conjunctivitis such as this is empirical, a culture should be obtained. Other ophthalmic antibiotic drops or ointments, such as neomycin-polymyxin-B-gramicidin combination (Neosporin), also are used in these situations. Although other antimicrobials, such as the ocular quinolones, may be used for bacterial conjunctivitis, these agents should be reserved as second-line therapies because of cost and the potential development of resistance. Proper management of this infection also includes mechanical cleaning of the eyelids and hygienic measures that prevent spreading the infection to other children. The deposits should be removed as often as possible with moist cotton swabs or cotton-tipped applicators. A mild baby shampoo can be used to moisten the applicator. Firm adherent crusts may be softened with warm, moist compresses. Because this material is infectious, it should be disposed of in a sanitary fashion. The common use of washcloths by several individuals will spread bacterial conjunctivitis.

ALLERGIC CONJUNCTIVITIS

CASE 54-6

QUESTION 1: N.V., a 10-year-old girl, has experienced redness in both eyes accompanied by "hay fever" for the past 2 months (June and July). There is no crusting on her eyelids, and her vision is normal; she rubs her eyes often because they itch. What treatment is best for N.V.'s allergic conjunctivitis?

Topical vasoconstrictors (e.g., naphazoline, tetrahydrozoline) with or without antihistamines (e.g., antazoline, pheniramine) may be used to treat hyperemia, but they should not be used excessively because rebound congestion can occur secondary to the vasoconstrictors. Therefore, use of topical vasoconstrictors for longer than 72 hours is not recommended owing to the potential for rebound congestion and masking of more serious ocular inflammatory conditions. Antihistamine tablets or syrup can provide considerable, but temporary, relief. Several ophthalmic histamine H_1-receptor antagonists are effective in the treatment of allergic conjunctivitis. Levocabastine 0.05% is administered BID to QID, olopatadine 0.1% BID (separating doses by 6–8 hours) or 0.2% once daily, emedastine 0.05% QID, and ketotifen 0.025% BID to QID.[110–112] Ketotifen, olopatadine, azelastine, and epinastine exhibit both antihistamine and mast cell stabilizing effects. Olopatadine inhibits the release of other mast cell inflammatory mediators such as tryptase and prostaglandin. Ketotifen and azelastine suppress the release of mediators from cells involved in hypersensitivity reactions and decrease chemotaxis and activation of eosinophils. Azelastine inhibits other mediators involved in allergic reactions such as leukotrienes and platelet activating factor. Epinastine produces antileukotriene, anti–platelet activating factor, and antibradykinin effects. Emedastine was more efficacious than levocabastine when used BID for 6 weeks in adult and pediatric patients with seasonal allergic conjunctivitis.[113] Olopatadine provided superior efficacy and a more rapid resolution of the signs and symptoms of allergic conjunctivitis when compared with ketotifen in a small trial involving adult patients.[114] Azelastine has a slightly quicker onset of therapeutic effect when compared with olopatadine and placebo.[115] Information to date is insufficient to definitively recommend one of these products as superior to the others. The ideal treatment would be removal of the allergen, but this usually is impossible when the conjunctivitis is secondary to seasonal allergies. Topical corticosteroids provide dramatic relief, but their use must be limited because of potential adverse effects (see Ophthalmic Corticosteroids section).

Cromolyn sodium ophthalmic, a drug that inhibits the release of histamine in response to antigen, may be effective as an alternative for patients who fail to respond to more conservative measures. Lodoxamide, pemirolast, and nedocromil have a similar mechanism of action to cromolyn sodium ophthalmic, but these agents also decrease chemotaxis and activation of eosinophils. In comparative studies, lodoxamide

reuptake inhibitors and tricyclic antidepressants. It is contraindicated with drugs that prolong the QT interval and are metabolized by CYP 2D6. Dextromethorphan–quinidine should be used with caution with drugs that inhibit CYP 3A4. Because quinidine inhibits CYP 2D6, dose adjustments for CYP 2D6 substrates are necessary. Quinidine also inhibits P-glycoprotein, requiring caution and perhaps dose adjustments when this treatment is used in combination with digoxin.

KEY REFERENCES AND WEBSITE

A full list of references for this chapter can be found at http://thepoint.lww.com/AT10e. Below are the key references and website for this chapter, with the corresponding reference number in this chapter found in parentheses after the reference.

Key References

Aktas O et al. Neuroprotection, regeneration and immunomodulation: broadening the therapeutic repertoire in multiple sclerosis. *Trends Neurosci.* 2010;33:140. (2)

Petratos S et al. Novel therapeutic targets for axonal degeneration in multiple sclerosis. *J Neuropathol Exp Neurol.* 2010;69:323. (3)

Thompson AJ et al. Pharmacological management of symptoms in multiple sclerosis: current approaches and future directions. *Lancet Neurol.* 2010;9:1182. (43)

Key Website

National Multiple Sclerosis Society. http://www.nationalmssociety.org

56

Headache

Brian K. Alldredge

CORE PRINCIPLES

		CHAPTER CASES
1	Primary headaches (i.e., those that lack an identifiable and treatable underlying cause) include migraine, tension-type, and cluster headaches. These headaches are among the most common presenting complaints in emergency departments and outpatient clinics, and they tend to have their onset in the first several decades of life. Women are more often affected by migraine and tension-type headaches than men.	**Case 56-1 (Question 1), Case 56-5 (Question 1), Case 56-6 (Question 1)**
2	Virtually all patients who suffer from migraine, tension-type, and cluster headaches are candidates to receive abortive (or symptomatic) medications during an acute attack. In a minority of patients, adjunctive medications are also used to treat symptoms associated with acute headaches (e.g., antiemetics, muscle relaxants, sedatives). In all patients with cluster headache, and some patients with migraine and tension-type headache (i.e., those with frequent headaches or those who fail to respond to abortive or symptomatic treatments), prophylactic headache therapies are indicated.	**Case 56-1 (Questions 3, 5–8, 11, 12, 14, 15), Case 56-2 (Question 1), Case 56-5 (Questions 2, 3), Case 56-6 (Questions 1, 2)**
3	Triptans (e.g., sumatriptan and second-generation agents such as zolmitriptan and eletriptan) are the drugs of choice for acute treatment of migraine headaches. These agents are effective when given early or late in a migraine attack, and they relieve the associated symptoms of migraine including nausea, photophobia, and phonophobia. Oral, subcutaneous, and intranasal dosage forms are available.	**Case 56-1 (Question 5)**
4	Common adverse effects of triptans include malaise, dizziness, and chest or throat tightness or pressure. Local injection site pain is common with subcutaneous sumatriptan. Nasal irritation and bad taste is common with intranasal formulations of sumatriptan and zolmitriptan. Because of potential vasoconstrictive effects, triptans are contraindicated in patients with uncontrolled hypertension and those with established or probable coronary artery disease.	**Case 56-1 (Question 5)**
5	Prophylactic drug therapy of migraine is indicated for patients who experience two or more headaches per month, who fail to respond to abortive treatments (e.g., triptans and alternatives), and who experience frequent or bothersome migraine auras. Propranolol, amitriptyline, topiramate, and valproate are the agents of choice for migraine prophylaxis. The choice among agents is often based on adverse effects and comorbidities.	**Case 56-1 (Questions 14, 15), Case 56-2 (Question 1)**
6	Overuse of symptomatic or abortive agents (including triptans and over-the-counter, combination, and narcotic analgesics) can increase the intensity and chronicity of all headache types. To prevent medication overuse headache, use of these agents should be limited to fewer than 10 days per month.	**Case 56-4 (Question 1)**
7	Cluster headaches are severely painful, short-duration attacks that tend to occur nightly during susceptible periods and then enter remission for a period of months or years. Treatments of choice for abortive treatment must be fast acting, and include subcutaneous sumatriptan, intranasal zolmitriptan, and oxygen inhalation. Evidence supports the use of verapamil, lithium, suboccipital steroid injections, and civamide (currently investigational) for cluster headache prophylaxis.	**Case 56-5 (Questions 1–3)**

continued

	CHAPTER CASES
8 Tension-type headaches (previously known as tension or muscle contraction headaches) usually cause mild to moderate discomfort and respond to over-the-counter analgesics. Acetaminophen, aspirin, and various nonsteroidal anti-inflammatory drugs are all equally effective for most patients.	**Case 56-6 (Question 1)**
9 Patients who experience frequent episodic tension-type headaches (and who are therefore at risk for analgesic overuse) should be considered for prophylactic headache treatment. Amitriptyline is the drug of choice for tension-headache prevention. Mirtazapine and venlafaxine are reasonable alternatives.	**Case 56-6 (Question 2)**

Prevalence

In the United States, migraine headache affects approximately 23 million persons, and 11 million experience significant headache-related disability.[1] Headache accounts for 3% of emergency department (ED) visits and 1.3% of outpatient visits,[2,3] and the health care expenses associated with migraine are estimated to be between $1 billion and $17 billion dollars annually.[4] Overall, the prevalence of headache is highest in adolescence and early adulthood and declines with age through the elderly years.[5] Despite numerous potential causes of headaches, the vast majority of patients with a chief complaint of continuous or sporadically recurring headaches are eventually diagnosed as having either tension-type or migraine headache.

Classification

Headache is a symptom that can be caused by many disorders. For example, head pain can result from traction, displacement, or inflammation of pain-sensitive structures within the head, or it can be attributable to disorders of extracranial structures such as the eyes, ears, or sinuses. For diagnostic and therapeutic purposes, it is useful to categorize headache into one of two major types (*primary* and *secondary*) on the basis of the underlying etiology. *Primary headache disorders* are characterized by the lack of an identifiable and treatable underlying cause. Migraine, tension-type, and cluster headaches are examples of primary headache disorders. *Secondary headache disorders* are those associated with a variety of organic causes such as trauma, cerebrovascular malformations, and brain tumors. Depending on the cause, headache may manifest in a variety of ways or may be accompanied by other associated signs or symptoms. A comprehensive classification scheme of the different types of headaches, modified from the International Headache Society, is shown in Table 56-1.[6] Readers are referred to the second edition of the International Headache Society classification report (ICHD-II) for the comprehensive headache classification scheme (including the variety of secondary causes of headache) and a detailed description of the specific diagnostic features of each headache type.[6] This classification scheme is useful for grouping headaches with similar clinical features or etiologies. Headache must be accurately evaluated and classified because this symptom may reflect an ominous problem such as the presence of a brain tumor or a much more benign process such as muscle tension. Moreover, effective intervention depends on a correct diagnosis.

TABLE 56-1
Classification of Primary Headaches[6]

Migraine
Migraine without aura
Migraine with aura
Tension-Type Headache
Episodic tension-type headache
Chronic tension-type headache
Cluster Headache
Episodic cluster headache
Chronic cluster headache
Other Primary Headaches
Cough headache
Exertional headache

PRIMARY HEADACHE DISORDERS

MIGRAINE HEADACHES

Migraine headaches usually develop over a period of minutes to hours, progressing from a dull ache to a more intense pulsating pain that worsens with each pulse. The headache usually begins in the frontotemporal region and may radiate to the occiput and neck; it may occur unilaterally or bilaterally. Migraine headaches often are accompanied by nausea and vomiting and may last for up to 72 hours. These headaches usually are alleviated by relaxation in a dark room and sleep. Migraine is more common in women than men. Migraine headaches are divided into those with and without an aura. The term *aura* refers to the complex of focal neurologic symptoms (e.g., alterations in vision or sensation) that initiate or accompany a migraine attack. Migraine may be precipitated by a variety of dietary, pharmacologic, hormonal, or environmental factors.

CLUSTER HEADACHES

Cluster headaches derive their name from a characteristic pattern of recurrent headaches that are separated by periods of remission that last from months to even years. During those periods when clusters of headaches are experienced, the headaches usually occur at least once daily. The headache generally is unilateral, occurs behind the eye, reaches maximal intensity over several minutes, and lasts for less than 3 hours. Unilateral lacrimation, rhinorrhea, and facial flushing may accompany the cluster headache. During cluster periods, headache is commonly precipitated by alcohol, naps, and vasodilating drugs. In contrast to migraine headaches, cluster headaches are more common in men than women.

TENSION-TYPE HEADACHES

A dull, persistent headache, occurring bilaterally in a hatband distribution around the head is characteristic of tension-type headaches. The headache is usually not debilitating and may fluctuate in intensity throughout the day. Tension-type headaches often occur during or after stress, but chronic tension-type headaches may persist for months even in the absence of recognizable stress. Skeletal muscle overcontraction, depression, and occasionally nausea may accompany the headache. Prodrome neurologic symptoms do not occur in association with tension-type headache. More detailed descriptions of migraine, cluster, and tension-type headaches appear in subsequent sections of this chapter.

SECONDARY HEADACHE DISORDERS

In addition to migraine, cluster, and tension-type headaches, patients may also experience headache associated with head trauma, vascular disorders, central nervous system (CNS) infection (including human immunodeficiency virus), or metabolic disorders. Examples of secondary headache disorders are given in the ICHD-II report.[6]

The length of time that a patient has experienced headaches provides highly useful information for assessing the nature and etiology of the headaches. A new severe headache in a patient without a previous history is the single most useful piece of information for identifying potentially destructive intracranial or extracranial causes of headache. Such headaches may develop suddenly, during a period of hours to days (acute headache), or more gradually for days to months (subacute headache).

ACUTE HEADACHES

Acute headaches can be symptomatic of subarachnoid hemorrhage, stroke, meningitis, or intracranial mass lesion (e.g., brain tumor, hematoma, abscess). The headache that accompanies subarachnoid hemorrhage is typically severe (often described by the patient as the "worst headache of my life") and may occur in conjunction with alteration of mental status and focal neurologic signs. The headache of meningitis is usually bilateral and develops gradually over hours to days; symptoms such as fever, photophobia, and positive meningeal (Kernig and Brudzinski) signs often accompany the meningeal headache. Although the acute onset of headache associated with coughing, sneezing, straining, or change in head position is commonly thought to indicate a cranial mass lesion with cerebrospinal fluid pathway obstruction, several varieties of exertional headache are benign.

SUBACUTE HEADACHES

Subacute headaches may be a sign of increased intracranial pressure, intracranial mass lesion, temporal arteritis, sinusitis, or trigeminal neuralgia. Trigeminal neuralgia usually occurs after the age of 40 and is more common in women than men. The pain usually occurs along the second or third divisions of the trigeminal (facial) nerve and lasts only moments. Trigeminal neuralgia is characterized by sudden, intense pain that recurs paroxysmally, often in response to triggers such as talking, chewing, or shaving.

The clinical manifestations of headache, as described previously, focus on the onset, frequency, duration, site, sex of the patient, distribution, and other unique characteristics of the head pain. A comprehensive medical history and physical examination of the patient often provide sufficient information to make an adequate assessment of a patient's headache complaint, and may enable the practitioner to rule out headache as a manifestation of more serious illness. Physical examination of the patient suffering from the common, benign forms of headache (e.g., migraine, cluster, and tension-type headaches) is usually normal. When the medical history of the patient is suggestive of a secondary cause of headache, a more extensive evaluation with referral to or consultation by a neurologist is necessary.

Pathophysiology

Intracranially, only a limited number of structures are sensitive to pain. The most important pain-sensitive structures within the cranium are the proximal portions of the cerebral arteries, large veins, and the venous sinuses.[7] Headache may result from dilation, distension, or traction of the large intracranial vessels.

ONLINE CONTENT

For an illustration of vascular changes in headache, go to http://thepoint.lww.com/AT10e.

The brain itself is insensitive to pain. Referred pain from inflammation of frontal or maxillary sinuses or refractive errors of the eye are also potential causes of headache. Scalp arteries and muscles are also capable of registering pain and have been implicated in the pathophysiology of migraine and tension-type headache. Extracranially, most of the structures outside the skull (e.g., periosteum, eye, ear, teeth, skin, deeper tissues) have pain afferents. In general, pain can be produced by activation of peripheral pain receptors (nociceptors), injury to the CNS or peripheral nervous system, or displacement of the pain-sensitive structures mentioned earlier.

Historically, the primary headache disorders have been thought to be related either to vascular disturbances (migraine and cluster headache) or muscular tension (tension-type headache). However, clinical and experimental evidence now suggests that these headaches have their origin in an underlying disturbance in brain function.[8] Evidence in this regard is particularly strong for migraine and cluster headache. Many authors now hold the opinion that these clinically dissimilar primary headache syndromes represent variable manifestations of a common pathogenetic phenomenon that involves neural innervation of the cranial circulation. The specific mechanisms that lead to primary headaches have not been identified. However, a *neurovascular hypothesis* has been proposed in which headache is triggered by disturbances in central pain processing pathways (the trigeminocervical complex), leading to the release of potent neuropeptides (calcitonin gene-related peptide [CGRP], substance P, and neurokinin A) and subsequent vasodilation.[9] Serotonin, a vasoactive neurotransmitter released by brainstem nuclei of the trigeminovascular system, has for decades been suspected of playing a significant role in migraine pathogenesis.[10] Furthermore, drugs that alter serotonergic function are highly effective for the symptomatic treatment of migraine and cluster headache.

Drug Therapy

Drug therapy for headache is divided into two major categories: (a) abortive therapy to provide relief during an acute headache attack and (b) prophylactic therapy to prevent or reduce the severity of recurrent headaches. Most people with infrequent tension-type headaches self-medicate with over-the-counter (OTC) analgesics to abort the acute event and do not require prophylactic therapy. By contrast, migraine and cluster headache sufferers who experience frequent headaches and who respond poorly to abortive measures are good candidates for preventive therapy.

Although analgesics are often useful for the treatment of episodic tension-type headaches, most patients with migraine and all patients with cluster headaches require other abortive measures. Until recently, ergot alkaloids (e.g., ergotamine and dihydroergotamine) were the most commonly prescribed agents for relief of migraine and cluster headaches. Now, the triptan class of agents (e.g., sumatriptan, zolmitriptan, naratriptan, rizatriptan, almotriptan, frovatriptan, and eletriptan) is preferred because of their favorable efficacy and tolerable adverse effect profiles.[5] However, the greater expense of the triptans limits the availability of these drugs for some patients.

Antidepressant agents (e.g., amitriptyline) are useful for prophylactic treatment of migraine and tension-type headaches. Because many patients suffer from mixed headache types, these agents can be useful for patients who might otherwise require preventive polytherapy. Other agents useful for migraine headache prophylaxis include β-blocking agents (e.g., propranolol), valproate, calcium-channel blocking agents (particularly verapamil), nonsteroidal anti-inflammatory drugs (NSAIDs), and select antiepileptic drugs (valproate, topiramate). Among the agents effective for prophylaxis against cluster headaches, verapamil, suboccipital steroid injections, and lithium are usually preferred.

MIGRAINE HEADACHE

The word *migraine* comes from the Greek *hemicrania* and historically was used to describe unilateral headaches with associated symptoms. More recently, migraine is described as "paroxysmal attacks of moderate-to-severe, throbbing headache with associated symptoms that may include nausea, vomiting, and photophobia or phonophobia."[5] Migraine headaches are subclassified according to the presence or absence of aura symptoms. Most persons who suffer from migraine do not experience aura symptoms. In patients with aura, visual symptoms are most common.

Pathophysiology

Past theories of pathogenesis have focused on alterations in cranial vessel diameter and blood flow as the primary cause of migraine. In this "vascular hypothesis," it was thought that focal neurologic symptoms preceding or accompanying the headache were caused by vasoconstriction and reduction in cerebral blood flow. The headache was thought to be caused by a compensatory vasodilation with displacement of pain-sensitive intracranial structures. Although blood flow is decreased during the aura of migraine,[11] there are conflicting observations regarding blood flow alterations during migraine headache. Olesen et al. found that the headache phase of migraine with aura began while blood flow is reduced,[11] and that migraine without aura was not associated with alterations in regional cerebral blood flow.[12] Furthermore, Limmroth et al. found that the therapeutic effect of sumatriptan, a drug highly specific for neurovascular headaches, was not temporally related to its vasoconstrictive effect.[13] More recently, however, Asghar et al. used a novel high-resolution magnetic resonance angiography imaging technique to show significant dilatation in select cerebral arteries during a migraine attack; this dilatation was ipsilateral to the headache in those with unilateral headache pain. Furthermore, sumatriptan caused significant contraction in the middle meningeal artery—one of the vessels found to dilate during migraine.[14]

Although vasodilation may be a feature of migraine, recent evidence also suggests that the pain of migraine is generated centrally and involves episodic dysfunction of neural structures that control the cranial circulation (the *trigeminovascular system*). The availability of functional brain imaging has had a dramatic effect on the ability to visualize the pathophysiologic events of a migraine attack.[9] The trigeminovascular system consists of neurons originating in the trigeminal ganglion, which innervate the cerebral circulation. Several potent vasodilator neuropeptides are contained within these trigeminal neurons, including CGRP, substance P, and neurokinin A. In animals, stimulation of the trigeminal ganglion significantly alters regional brain blood flow.[9] Stimulation of the trigeminal ganglion in humans causes facial flushing, an increase in facial temperature,[15] and increases in extracerebral venous concentrations of CGRP and substance P.[16]

The specific events leading to trigeminovascular dysfunction in migraine are unknown. However, evidence from positron emission tomography scanning (a technique to measure regional cerebral blood flow as an index of neuronal activity) suggests that episodic dysfunction of the brainstem, with corresponding effects on the trigeminal system, are involved. Using this technique, Weiller et al.[17] found activation of the brainstem (periaqueductal gray, dorsal raphe nucleus, and locus ceruleus) at the onset of migraine headaches in nine patients. This area may represent an endogenous "migraine generator." Sporadic dysfunction of the nociceptive system (periaqueductal gray and dorsal raphe nucleus) and the neural control of cerebral blood flow (dorsal raphe nucleus and locus ceruleus) is hypothesized to trigger migraine headache via effects of these brain structures on the trigeminovascular system. Further support for a trigeminovascular mechanism for migraine comes from studies that demonstrate inhibition of trigeminal neurons and associated nociceptive responses by various antimigraine drugs such as dihydroergotamine,[18] rizatriptan,[19] and zolmitriptan.[20]

Abnormalities in serotonin (5-HT) activity are also thought to play a role in migraine headache. Plasma 5-HT levels decrease by nearly half during a migraine attack,[21] with a corresponding rise in the urinary excretion of 5-hydroxyindoleacetic acid,[22] the primary metabolite of 5-HT. Also, reserpine, a drug that depletes 5-HT from body stores, has been found to induce a stereotypical headache in migraineurs and a dull discomfort in patients not prone to migraine.[21,23] An intravenous (IV) injection of 5-HT effectively relieved both reserpine-induced and spontaneous migraine headache.[21,23] The therapeutic effects of drugs that stimulate 5-HT_1 receptors (e.g., dihydroergotamine, sumatriptan), antagonize 5-HT_2 receptors (e.g., methysergide, cyproheptadine), prevent 5-HT reuptake (e.g., amitriptyline) or release (e.g., calcium-channel blockers), or inhibit brainstem serotonergic raphe neurons (e.g., valproate) all lend support to the hypothesis that 5-HT is an important mediator of migraine. Furthermore, brainstem nuclei activated during migraine have high densities of serotonergic neurons. Specific 5-HT receptor subtypes, 5-HT_{1B} and 5-HT_{1D}, are largely distributed in blood[24] and nerves,[25] respectively. These same 5-HT receptor subtypes are the targets of antimigraine drugs such as the triptans and ergot alkaloids.

GENETICS

A familial predisposition for migraine has been well recognized, although not until recent advances in gene mapping techniques has the genetic basis of a specific migraine disorder been discovered. The first identified migraine gene was found among several unrelated families with familial hemiplegic migraine. The mutations involved a gene encoding the α_1 subunit of a voltage-gated P/Q-type neuronal calcium channel.[26] The relevance of this discovery to other migrainous disorders is unknown, but it suggests that some forms of migraine may be fundamentally related to other episodic disorders of neurologic dysfunction known as "channelopathies."[8] More recently, genomewide linkage analysis in families with migraine (both with and without aura) have identified susceptibility loci on chromosomes 4 and 14.[27,28] An improved understanding of the genetics of migraine is likely to improve our understanding of the pathophysiology of the disorder as well as to hold promise for the identification of homogenous subgroups of patients in whom targeted drug (or other) interventions are likely to be highly effective.

In summary, the pathophysiology of migraine probably involves dysfunction of the trigeminal neurons that provide sensory innervation and modulate blood flow for intracranial blood vessels. The endogenous stimulus causing this dysfunction may arise from a migraine generator in the brainstem. Disturbances in 5-HT activity are also probably involved, and it is this feature that serves as the target for many migraine-specific therapies. (For an animation that depicts migraine pathophysiology, go to http://www.youtube.com/watch?v=cnath-Oe5Ds.)

Signs and Symptoms

MIGRAINE WITH AND WITHOUT AURA

CASE 56-1

QUESTION 1: H.R., a 29-year-old woman, presents to the clinic with a 5-month history of left-sided pulsatile head pain recurring on a weekly basis. Her headaches are usually preceded by unformed flashes of light bilaterally and a sensation of light-headedness. The ensuing pain is always unilateral and is commonly associated with nausea, vomiting, and photophobia. The headache is not relieved by two tablets of either aspirin 325 mg or ibuprofen 200 mg and generally lasts all day unless she is able to lie in a dark room and sleep. The headaches usually interfere with her ability to continue work. H.R. is unable to identify any external factors that precipitate a migraine attack. Both H.R.'s mother and grandmother also were affected by migraine headaches. Medical history is unremarkable, and H.R. denies any other medical problems. Current medications include only the OTC analgesics for headache and the contraceptive, Ortho-Novum 7/7/7. General physical and neurologic examinations are within normal limits. What subjective and objective data from the above description are consistent with a diagnosis of migraine with aura?

Given H.R.'s headache description, normal physical examination, and age of onset, she is most likely suffering from migraine with aura, a benign, though often disabling, disorder.

Approximately 17% of women and 6% of men in the United States experience migraine headaches.[1] The lifetime cumulative incidence of migraine is 43% in women and 18% in men.[5] The typical age of onset of migraine headaches is 15 to 35 years; after the age of 50, the onset of new migraine headaches is less common and is suggestive of a secondary cause. Although influenced by physiologic and environmental factors, migraine headaches occur more frequently among first-degree relatives, suggesting a genetic basis for this disorder. H.R.'s sex (female), age (29 years), and positive family history are compatible with these aspects of migraine.

In the assessment of headache, the site or location of the pain, the quality of the pain, the duration and time course of the pain, and the conditions that provoke or palliate the pain should be considered.

The site or location of head pain can provide the clinician with clues as to the potential for secondary causes (e.g., lesions in the frontal sinuses, eyes, ears, teeth, or cerebral arteries). However, pain often is referred from other regions and the location of pain can provide misleading information. Thus, the site of head pain need not be related to the apparent site of the focal neurologic symptoms that accompany migraine with aura. Head pain may be either unilateral or bilateral, and the pain need not recur on the same side if unilateral. In fact, 50% of patients with unilateral headache report that either side of the head may be affected during any individual migraine attack.[29]

The quality of migraine head pain usually begins as a dull ache that intensifies over a period of minutes or hours to a throbbing headache, which worsens with each arterial pulse. If left untreated, the headache often lasts from several hours to as long as 3 days or until the patient goes to sleep. The pain usually is intense enough to interfere with daily activities. Although migraine headaches seldom occur more often than once every few weeks, there is great interpatient variability in the frequency of occurrence. A patient may experience only several migraines in a lifetime, whereas others may suffer several headaches weekly on a chronic basis. H.R., like half of all patients with migraine, describes headaches that recur between one to four times monthly.[29] In this patient, the quality of the pain (i.e., interferes with H.R.'s ability to continue work), the duration and the time course of the pain (i.e., usually lasts all day), and the conditions that palliate the pain (i.e., lie in a dark room and sleep) are all compatible with the description of migraine headaches.

Aura symptoms are focal neurologic features that precede or accompany the headache in up to 30% of migraine sufferers.[30] When they precede the headache, aura symptoms usually begin 10 minutes to 1 hour before the onset of head pain. Light-headedness and photopsia (unformed flashes of light) are frequently reported and were described by H.R. before the onset of her head pain. Visual disturbances, such as scotoma (an isolated area within the visual field where vision is absent), occur in 30% of migraine patients.[30] At times, the scotoma is preceded only by a sensation that something is wrong with vision that cannot be more specifically characterized. At other times, the scotoma may be preceded by other visual distortions (e.g., the "halves of peoples' faces were vertically displaced in such a way that one eye appeared to be 1 or 2 cm lower than the other").[31] When scotomata are surrounded by a shiny pattern, they are termed *scintillating scotomata*. (For an animated example of a migraine aura with scotomata, go to http://www.migraine-aura.org/content/e27891/index_en.html.) These scintillating scotomata can have "the visual quality of images in the kaleidoscopes we looked into as children, with the difference that the scotoma are silvery instead of multicolored as in the toy."[31] Other neurologic symptoms of cortical origin (e.g., paresthesias, temporal lobe symptoms) occur less commonly in patients who suffer from migraine with aura. H.R.'s physical and neurologic examinations were within normal limits. The nausea and vomiting that were experienced by H.R. accompany migraine headaches (with or without aura) in 90% of patients. Vomiting is occasionally followed by a gradual resolution of migraine symptoms. Diarrhea may also occur.

In summary, H.R.'s history and relative lack of important physical findings are compatible with a diagnosis of migraine with aura.

Diagnostic Tests

CASE 56-1, QUESTION 2: What further laboratory or diagnostic tests should be ordered for H.R.?

Headaches are common medical complaints, and evaluation of these headaches with sophisticated diagnostic procedures (e.g., computed tomography [CT], magnetic resonance imaging [MRI] scans) is generally unnecessary in the uncomplicated migraine patient. Because H.R.'s headaches are not of recent origin, not progressive, and unassociated with traumatic injury or persistent neurologic deficits, CT or MRI imaging should be unnecessary. Her headaches are unaccompanied by fever or nuchal rigidity, and she does not present with headache described as being "the worst headache of my life." Therefore, a lumbar puncture would not likely be of diagnostic value because meningitis or subarachnoid hemorrhage is unlikely. The signs and symptoms experienced

results, and these agents are not recommended for migraine prophylaxis.

On the basis of efficacy, either NSAIDs (i.e., naproxen, naproxen sodium, flurbiprofen, ketoprofen, or mefenamic acid) or verapamil could be considered for prophylactic therapy to reduce the frequency of S.A.'s migraine headaches. However, NSAIDs are likely to interact with her lithium therapy, resulting in an increase in serum concentration and risk for adverse effects. For this reason, NSAIDs are best avoided at this time. S.A. should be started on verapamil 80 mg three times a day with gradual dosage titration to side effects, cessation of migraine attacks, or a maximal dose of 480 mg/day. She should be counseled regarding the possible occurrence of constipation and the appropriate management of this common side effect of verapamil. A 2-month trial may be necessary to demonstrate optimal therapeutic effect. Prophylactic therapy for migraine should be continued for 3 to 6 months. If a satisfactory response is achieved, the prophylactic agent should be gradually discontinued for several weeks to assess the continued need for this mode of therapy.

Medication Overuse

CASE 56-4

QUESTION 1: L.D. is a 39-year-old woman with a 7-year history of migraine (without aura) and tension-type headache who comes to the clinic requesting a refill of her Fiorinal (aspirin, butalbital, and caffeine) and acetaminophen with codeine (30 mg). She reports an increase in the frequency of both her "throbbing" and "dull, pressure-sensation" headaches during the past year, and lately she has had difficulty distinguishing the two types. In the past 2 months, she has had only 5 days with no headache, and she has been much less productive in her work as a magazine editor. A review of her medication refill records indicates that she has had four refills of Fiorinal (30 tablets) and three refills of acetaminophen with codeine (20 tablets) in the past 2 months and that her use of these drugs has increased in the past year. During the visit, she also indicates that she uses OTC acetaminophen and naproxen sodium on an as-needed basis. Although L.D. had experienced relief of mild headaches in the past with the use of OTC analgesics, these medications no longer reduce the intensity of her pain. What is the potential role of analgesic overuse in the worsening of L.D.'s headaches? How should her condition be managed?

Medication overuse is defined as the use of triptans, ergot alkaloids, narcotic analgesics, or combination analgesics on 10 or more days per month (the criterion for use of simple OTC analgesics is 15 or more days per month).[129] Medication overuse can increase the frequency and intensity of migraine and other headache types. In severe circumstances, a pattern of chronic daily headache can emerge. These chronic daily headaches often have features of both migraine and tension-type headaches.[160] L.D. displays many of the features of medication overuse headache. She reports an increase in the frequency of headaches to a near-daily pattern, and she is no longer able to distinguish between migrainous and tension-type headaches. Furthermore, the exacerbation of her headaches appears to coincide with the escalating use of combination analgesics. L.D. should be questioned carefully to determine the total amount of acetaminophen, naproxen sodium, and aspirin that she consumes daily and weekly. Daily users of analgesics are at increased risk for chronic renal disease, chronic liver disease, and acute GI bleeding.[161–163] Laboratory tests should be ordered to assess L.D.'s renal and hepatic function, and she should be questioned regarding the occurrence of GI discomfort, acute bleeding, or a change in her stool color.

In general, patients who receive abortive agents for headache treatment should be counseled to restrict their use of these agents to no more than twice per week.[106] However, in patients with medication overuse headache, a reduction in the use of these drugs will likely worsen their headache condition. The management of medication overuse headache is a challenge to clinicians and the patients who suffer from them. These headaches are often unresponsive to the usual abortive and prophylactic therapy measures discussed in earlier sections of this chapter. Successful management requires gradual withdrawal from the overused drugs. This process can be protracted and made even more difficult when barbiturate, codeine, or ergotamine-containing drugs are involved.[160] Withdrawal can usually be accomplished on an outpatient basis, although in some patients, inpatient detoxification is preferred. Once the frequency and quantity of analgesic use by L.D. have been adequately quantified, a process of gradual drug removal should be initiated. Medications taken on an infrequent basis (e.g., fewer than two times per week) can be abruptly stopped. For medications currently taken on a daily basis, L.D. should be counseled to reduce the dose of medication by approximately 10% every 1 to 2 weeks.[129] She should be informed that her headaches may worsen during this period but that symptoms will gradually improve as she proceeds through the detoxification process.

L.D.'s use of acetaminophen with codeine does not appear to be frequent enough to place her at risk for the development of opiate withdrawal symptoms. However, she should be counseled to report symptoms such as anxiety, tremulousness, insomnia, or diarrhea. If these symptoms occur, the rate of drug withdrawal should be reduced.

When use of analgesics has been substantially reduced, L.D. may benefit from a preventive headache medication if her headaches persist. The range of agents discussed earlier can be considered (Table 56-5). Recent evidence suggests that topiramate may be particularly effective for headache prevention in patients who are withdrawing from overused medication.[164] After medication withdrawal has been achieved, treatments other than the withdrawn drugs should be considered for treatment of her acute attacks. For example, a triptan agent may be useful for abortive treatment of her migraine headaches. An NSAID may be considered for acute treatment of her tension-type headaches. L.D. must clearly understand that these agents should not be used more than twice per week, and her use of all abortive or symptomatic therapies should be monitored closely.

CLUSTER HEADACHE

Cluster headache is an uncommon headache disorder (estimated prevalence 0.07%–0.4%) that derives its name from the characteristic pattern of headache recurrence—headaches tend to occur nightly during a relatively short time (i.e., several weeks or months), followed by a long period of complete remission.[165] Cluster headaches occur more commonly in men than women. There may be a seasonal predilection to cluster attacks, with the spring and fall being common times for headache recurrence. Headaches are usually of short duration (15 to 180 minutes) and present as severe, unrelenting, unilateral pain occurring behind the eye with radiation to the territory of the ipsilateral trigeminal nerve (temple, cheek, or gum).

The different clinical characteristics between cluster and migraine headaches (e.g., sex ratio, periodicity of attacks, duration of headaches, aura symptoms) suggest that these two types of vascular headaches are different clinical entities.

Pathophysiology

The pathophysiology of cluster headache is undetermined. As in migraine headaches, vascular, neurogenic, metabolic, and humoral factors have been proposed to play a role in cluster headache pathogenesis. Precipitation of headaches during a cluster period by vasodilators and response to vasoconstrictors suggests an underlying vascular component. During a cluster headache, thermography shows increased periorbital heat emission ipsilateral to the head pain.[166] Also, patients commonly report flushing in the same area, and these observations suggest that extracranial vasodilation occurs in cluster headache. However, intracranial blood flow studies fail to show consistent changes during a cluster attack,[167–169] and the alterations in extracranial blood flow follow the onset of head pain,[170] suggesting that vasodilation occurs in response to some other initiating stimulus. Abnormal plasma levels of melatonin, growth hormone, testosterone, and prolactin have been reported in patients with cluster headache. These findings, along with the cyclic recurrence pattern of the disorder, suggest a disturbance in hypothalamic function.[171]

In recent years, the role of heredity in cluster headache has been appreciated.[172] Cluster headache has been reported in monozygotic twins,[173] and first-degree relatives of individuals with cluster headache have a 14-fold higher risk of also having cluster headaches.[174] However, the mode of heritability is not clear, and a specific genetic basis for the disorder remains elusive.[172]

Signs and Symptoms

CASE 56-5

QUESTION 1: R.H. is a 31-year-old man with a 3-year history of episodic cluster headache. He has been headachefree for the past year, but today states that the headaches are returning in their characteristic fashion. He reports abrupt onset of right-sided retro-orbital pain with occasional superimposed knifelike "jabs" that increase in intensity for several minutes to a severe, unrelenting pain lasting about 90 minutes. The headache then gradually subsides. Associated symptoms include right-sided lacrimation, conjunctival injection, and rhinorrhea. He denies any premonition of ensuing headache or GI upset during the attacks. Physical examination during a cluster headache shows right eyelid droop and pupillary miosis. R.H.'s cluster periods characteristically last about 2 months and usually recur once or twice yearly. The first headache of the current bout awoke him from a short nap. R.H. expects to suffer one or two such headaches daily because this has been the usual pattern during each cluster period. Previous cluster headaches have been symptomatically treated with aspirin and codeine 30 mg. However, R.H. reports only modest relief with this treatment approach.

R.H.'s medical history is unremarkable. He does not use tobacco but admits to occasional social drinking. What subjective and objective evidence in this case is consistent with a diagnosis of cluster headaches?

R.H.'s sex, age of onset, quality and intensity of headache pain, periodicity of headache attacks, and associated symptoms all support the diagnosis of cluster headaches.

Cluster headaches affect men more commonly than women by a ratio of 5:1,[166] and have their usual onset between the second and fourth decades of life.[175] R.H.'s sex (male) and age of onset (28 years) are compatible with these aspects of cluster headaches.

Recurrent cluster headaches are usually severe and throbbing and affect the same side of the head. Occasionally, cluster headaches may involve the entire hemicranium. The pain starts abruptly, often waking the patient from sleep, reaches maximal intensity in 5 to 15 minutes, and usually lasts 45 to 60 minutes.[166] Unlike migraine, cluster headache is not preceded by an aura. Thus, patients have no warning before onset of head pain. Cluster periods often last from 2 to 3 months and recur once or twice yearly.[166] Patients suffering from *chronic cluster headaches* have bouts that last 12 months or longer. R.H.'s headache quality (severe, unrelenting pain), site (unilateral), evolution and resolution pattern (worsens over several minutes and resolves within 90 minutes), and periodicity of attacks (one or two headaches occurring daily for about 2 months followed by a period of remission that lasts about 1 year) are all compatible with the usual character of cluster headaches.

Associated features may include ipsilateral lacrimation, injected conjunctiva, and rhinorrhea or blocked nasal passage. A partial Horner syndrome (ptosis with miosis) occurs in one-third of patients and is often the only abnormal physical finding during a cluster headache.

ONLINE CONTENT

For a photo of a woman with Horner syndrome, go to http://thepoint.lww.com/AT10e.

Nausea, vomiting, and focal neurologic symptoms are often absent. Associated symptoms reported by R.H. during headache attacks (e.g., lacrimation, rhinorrhea, conjunctival injection) and the absence of GI or neurologic disturbances are also compatible with the diagnosis of cluster headaches.

During a cluster period, headaches may be precipitated by alcohol (even in small amounts), vasodilators, stress, warm weather, missed meals, and excessive sleep. Therefore, during the current cluster period, R.H. should be counseled to avoid all alcohol and daytime naps.

Abortive Therapy

CASE 56-5, QUESTION 2: What abortive measures are available for symptomatic treatment of individual headaches during R.H.'s current cluster period?

The treatments of choice for abortive treatment of cluster headaches are sumatriptan by subcutaneous injection, zolmitriptan nasal spray, and oxygen inhalation.[176] Among these agents, subcutaneous sumatriptan is often preferred.[177] The expense and inconvenience of having oxygen inhalation apparatus close at hand limit the usefulness of this treatment for many patients. A community-based study found that most patients suffering from cluster headaches do not receive optimal treatment for their condition.[178] Table 56-6 is a summary of drugs commonly used for the acute treatment of cluster headache.

SUMATRIPTAN

Sumatriptan 6 mg subcutaneously has been shown to effectively relieve cluster headache in randomized, double-blind, placebo-controlled trials. Cluster headaches are reduced in severity in 74% of attacks within 15 minutes, compared with 26% of attacks treated with placebo.[177] An additional injection of 6 mg does not appear to give additional headache relief.[177] However, in patients who experience a recurrent headache after initial relief with sumatriptan, a second injection is often useful.[171] Sumatriptan

TABLE 56-6
Drugs Recommended for Acute Treatment of Cluster Headache[a]

Drug	Route	Dose	Contraindications	Adverse Effects	Comments
Sumatriptan (Imitrex)	SC	6 mg at HA onset	Ischemic heart disease, within 24 hours of ergot alkaloids	Heavy sensation in head or chest, tingling, pain at injection site	Not an FDA-approved indication; costly but well tolerated
Zolmitriptan (Zomig)	IN	5–10 mg at HA onset	Ischemic heart disease, within 24 hours of ergot alkaloids	Bad taste, nasal irritation, somnolence	Not an FDA-approved indication; onset likely slower than SC sumatriptan although no direct comparisons performed
Oxygen	Inhalation	6–12 L/min for 15 minutes			Fast onset of effect

[a] Class 1 randomized controlled trials document the effectiveness of these therapies. See text for references and additional details.
FDA, Food and Drug Administration; HA, headache; IN, intranasal; SC, subcutaneous.

should not be used more often than twice daily during cluster bouts. For patients who experience more than two attacks per day, adjunctive therapy with oxygen inhalation should be considered.

Intranasal and oral sumatriptan have also been evaluated in patients with cluster headache. A randomized, open-label comparison of sumatriptan by intranasal (20 mg) and subcutaneous (6 mg) routes found a much higher response with the injectable form of the drug at 15 minutes after treatment (13% versus 94%, respectively). Patients included in this study indicated a clear preference for the subcutaneous dosage form.[179] Oral sumatriptan (100 mg three times a day) was studied as a prophylactic agent during cluster headache bouts and found to be ineffective.[180]

OXYGEN

Oxygen inhalation is often preferred not only for in-hospital treatment of cluster headache but also for use by some patients at home or at work. Two randomized, controlled trials have documented the effectiveness of 100% oxygen for treatment of acute cluster headache attacks.[181,182] Response rates of 56% to 78% were reported in these trials with the administration of 6 L/minute and 12 L/minute, respectively.[181,182] Oxygen is also useful for patients with frequent cluster headaches who would otherwise exceed maximal dosing restrictions of sumatriptan.[165] Most patients experience headache relief within 15 minutes of beginning inhalation. The mechanism of oxygen's effect is unknown but may be related to a direct vasoconstrictive action.[165]

ZOLMITRIPTAN

Two controlled trials have established the effectiveness of intranasal zolmitriptan for the acute treatment of cluster headache attacks. Cluster headache relief rates were 40% and 50% with 5 mg of zolmitriptan, and 62% and 63% with 10 mg of intranasal zolmitriptan in these two studies, respectively.[183,184] The onset of action of zolmitriptan nasal spray appears to be slower than that of subcutaneous sumatriptan; however, no direct comparative studies have been performed. The most common adverse effects of zolmitriptan nasal spray are bad taste, nasal irritation, and somnolence. Oral zolmitriptan (5 mg and 10 mg at headache onset) has been shown to be superior to placebo for relief of acute cluster headache (episodic type) at 30 minutes, and this treatment can be considered when other therapies discussed earlier are either ineffective or unavailable.

OTHER THERAPEUTIC INTERVENTIONS

Cluster headaches also can be relieved by less commonly used therapeutic interventions such as intranasal capsaicin,[185] dexamethasone 8 mg orally,[171] methoxyflurane inhalation (10–15 drops applied to a handkerchief and inhaled for several seconds),[72] somatostatin IV infusion (25 mcg/minute for 20 minutes),[186] octreotide (100 mcg self-administered subcutaneously),[187] and local anesthesia with either intranasal application of 1 mL of 4% lidocaine hydrochloride[188] or 0.3 mL of a 5% to 10% solution of cocaine hydrochloride[189] to the ipsilateral sphenopalatine fossa. In general there is insufficient evidence to recommend these therapies for the acute relief of cluster headache attacks.[176]

Orally administered narcotic analgesics are usually ineffective in cluster headache,[166] and R.H. has suffered several cluster periods with inadequate therapy. Improved response can be expected with the use of a more effective agent that has a faster onset of action. Reasonable options for the acute treatment of R.H.'s acute cluster headaches include subcutaneous sumatriptan, oxygen inhalation, and intranasal zolmitriptan. The success rate with each of these therapies is high. For many patients, oxygen is a less convenient therapy because the equipment is not easily portable and the patient must sit still during the treatment. The choice can be made on the basis of patient preference or cost.

Prophylactic Therapy

CASE 56-5, QUESTION 3: What therapeutic agents are available for headache prophylaxis during an active cluster period?

Pharmacotherapy aimed at preventing cluster headaches during an active period should be considered if symptomatic therapy is ineffective or intolerable, or if headaches occur more frequently than twice daily. Table 56-7 contains a list of available drugs for cluster headache prophylaxis.

VERAPAMIL

Verapamil is effective for the prevention of cluster headaches,[154,189,190] and many authors now consider this agent to be the prophylactic agent of choice.[166,177] The usual effective daily dose is 360 mg/day, and approximately two-thirds of patients have a 50% or greater reduction in headache frequency. In one randomized comparative trial, verapamil was more effective than lithium for cluster headache prophylaxis.[190]

LITHIUM CARBONATE

Lithium carbonate is effective in preventing episodic and chronic cluster headache, but it is sometimes considered a second-line agent because of its adverse effect profile, need for blood level monitoring, and propensity for drug interactions.[176,190,191] Benefits from lithium prophylaxis are observable 1 to 2 weeks after

TABLE 56-7
Drugs for Prophylaxis of Cluster Headache[a]

Drug	Dose	Route	Comments
Suboccipital steroid injection	12.46 mg betamethasone dipropionate and 5.26 mg betamethasone disodium phosphate with 0.5 mL 2% lidocaine	Suboccipital injection (near periosteum)	RCT demonstrated efficacy compared with placebo. Response evident within 72 hours
Civamide	100 μL of 0.025% civamide into each nostril daily × 7 days	IN	Civamide is investigational agent that may become available soon. RCT demonstrated efficacy compared with placebo. Response lasts for 20 days after treatment
Verapamil	360 mg/d divided TID–QID	PO	Two RCTs support efficacy for reduction in cluster headache. Verapamil may be more effective than lithium
Lithium carbonate	800–900 mg daily	PO	RCTs support some efficacy
Melatonin	10 mg daily × 2 weeks	PO	Efficacy demonstrated in 1 randomized controlled trial; patients with chronic cluster headache did not respond
Prednisone	20 mg every other day	PO	Supportive evidence is limited. May be considered for short bouts of cluster HA owing to long-term adverse effects

[a] See text for references and additional details.
IN, intranasal; HA, headache; PO, oral; QID, four times a day; RCT, randomized controlled trial; TID, three times a day.

initiation of therapy[72,192] and are maintained with long-term use.[193] Lithium serum levels associated with efficacy in cluster headache prophylaxis are usually between 0.4 and 0.8 mEq/L.[177] Adverse effects from long-term lithium use (e.g., renal toxicity) are discussed in Chapter 84, Mood Disorders II: Bipolar Disorders.

SUBOCCIPITAL STEROID INJECTION

One high-quality randomized, controlled trial demonstrated the efficacy of suboccipital steroid injection for the prophylaxis of cluster headache in 26 patients.[194] Injections included 12.46 mg of betamethasone dipropionate and 5.26 mg of betamethasone disodium phosphate mixed with 0.5 mL of 2% lidocaine. Eighty-five percent of patients had relief of headache attacks within 72 hours of injection (compared with none in the placebo group). Transient pain at the injection site may occur.

CIVAMIDE

Civamide is an investigational agent, used for pain conditions, which may be approved for use in the near future. One high-quality randomized, controlled trial demonstrated the efficacy of intranasal civamide for cluster headache prophylaxis in 28 patients.[195] Treatment consisted of 100 μL of 0.025% civamide into each nostril daily for 7 days. There was a significant reduction in headache attacks throughout the 20-day observation period. Thus, the effectiveness of civamide persists beyond the administration period. The most common adverse effects of civamide were nasal burning, lacrimation, and pharyngitis.

OTHER THERAPIES

Melatonin was shown to be superior to placebo for prophylaxis of cluster headache in a randomized, controlled trial of 20 patients.[196] Prednisone has long been used for the prophylaxis of cluster headache, but the strength of the evidence supporting its use is not strong.[177] One randomized, controlled trial found that prednisone 20 mg PO every other day reduced the frequency of attacks.[197]

R.H. should be evaluated at his next clinic visit for response to abortive sumatriptan or oxygen therapy. Prompt consideration should be given to the aforementioned additional treatments if suppression of headaches during the cluster period is warranted. In general, after response to prophylactic agents such as verapamil and lithium has been established and maintained for at least 2 weeks, attempts can be made to discontinue the drug. Treatment should be reinstituted if headaches recur. Other treatments (e.g., suboccipital steroid injection, intranasal civamide) are administered on a more limited basis, with benefits persisting beyond the direct treatment period.

TENSION-TYPE HEADACHE

Tension-type headache is the most common headache type with a lifetime prevalence of 88% in women and 69% in men.[198] Women are slightly more affected by tension-type headaches than men, with a ratio of 5:4.[199] Highest prevalence rates are found in women between 30 and 39 years of age and, in both sexes, those with higher education levels.[200] Tension-type headaches (previously known as *tension* or *muscle contraction* headaches) are usually characterized by a dull aching sensation bilaterally that occurs in a hatband distribution around the head. The pain is usually mild to moderate in severity and has a nonpulsating quality.[201]

Tension-type headaches are classified into three subtypes based on the frequency of headache attacks: infrequent episodic tension-type headache (<1 day of headache per month); frequent, episodic tension-type headache (1 to 14 days of headache per month); and chronic tension-type headache (≥15 days of headache per month).[6,202] Chronic tension-type headache occurs in approximately 2% of the population (1-year prevalence rate), and sufferers may have headache continuously for months or even years.[200] Tension-type headaches are not associated with aura symptoms, nor are they accompanied by nausea, vomiting, or photophobia. The headache is usually not of sufficient intensity to interfere with daily activities but may be a nuisance by virtue of its persistent nature.

Pathophysiology

For many years, excessive muscle contraction with constriction of pain-sensitive extracranial structures was thought to be the cause of tension-type headache.[203] More recent evidence shows no correlation between muscle contraction and the presence of tension-type headache.[195,204] Abnormal vascular reactivity was also thought to play a role in tension-type headache, but temporal muscle blood flow is unaltered compared with control subjects.[204] Platelet 5-HT content is lower in patients with chronic tension-type headache, suggesting that migraine and tension-type headaches share some pathophysiologic features.[201]

Tension-type headaches also may be associated with depression,[205] repressed hostility, or resentment.[206] However, these psychological associations may be the result of the chronic pain syndrome rather than a cause or feature of the headache disorder.[195] Patients with recurrent tension-type headaches probably do not experience more frequent stressful events, but may use less effective coping strategies in stressful situations.[207]

There is some evidence to suggest that the different subtypes of tension-type headache have distinct pathophysiological mechanisms.[202] Patients with infrequent episodic tension-type headache have an increased sensitivity to myofascial pain, and peripheral mechanisms are thought to play a role.[202] Central pain mechanisms appear to be involved in patients with chronic tension-type headache.[195,202]

General Management and Abortive Therapy

CASE 56-6

QUESTION 1: K.B., a 27-year-old female financial analyst, presents to her general practitioner with a complaint of recurring headaches that worsened when she started her current job. Before this time, she had experienced infrequent headaches, which she associated with periods of stress. The headaches would occur three to four times yearly, were of a constant, dull, or "pressing" character and were present around the entire head. Recently, headaches of similar character have been occurring about one to two times weekly, usually toward the end of her workday. The pain usually lasts the rest of the day but varies in intensity. Occasionally, a headache is present when she wakes up in the morning as well. K.B. denies GI and aura symptoms associated with her headaches. She has noticed that relaxation and alcohol ingestion seem to relieve these headaches, but aspirin and acetaminophen have been ineffective. Her blood pressure is 120/74 mm Hg; her physical and neurologic examinations are completely normal. What measures should be taken to relieve K.B.'s headaches? What is an appropriate goal for treatment?

K.B. appears to be suffering from frequent episodic tension-type headaches. She reports approximately four to eight headache episodes per month, and these headaches have features that are stereotypical for tension-type headache. As in the treatment of other chronic headache disorders, a cure for recurrent tension-type headache is unlikely. K.B. should clearly understand that the goal of treatment is a reduction in the frequency and severity of headache. Drug therapy and relaxation techniques are the primary means by which tension-type headaches are treated.

ANALGESICS

Analgesics are the drugs of choice for treatment of acute tension-type headache attacks.[195] The initial choice of an analgesic should be based on the severity of the pain. Acetaminophen, aspirin, and NSAIDs are often effective, although their benefits may be short lived. Acetaminophen 1,000 mg provides equal relief from moderately severe tension-type headache when compared with 650 mg of aspirin; both are superior to placebo.[208] Ibuprofen is as effective as aspirin for relief from tension-type headache discomfort, and side effects with both 400 and 800 mg of ibuprofen are less common than with aspirin.[209] Ibuprofen 400 mg is superior to acetaminophen 1,000 mg for relief of tension-type headache pain.[210] Naproxen sodium 550 mg is more effective than placebo and acetaminophen 650 mg for relieving the pain of tension-type headache.[211] The potency of some analgesics may be enhanced by combination with an antihistamine (e.g., doxylamine).[212] Because the relative potencies of nonnarcotic analgesics are equivalent, the choice among agents should be guided by cost and patient preference.

Sedatives (e.g., butalbital),[72] anxiolytics (e.g., meprobamate,[211] diazepam[213]), and skeletal muscle relaxants (e.g., orphenadrine) have also been used to treat tension-type headache, and occasionally patients respond to their concomitant use when an analgesic alone affords insufficient relief. However, combination analgesic products are best avoided because of an increased risk of dependence, and their association with the transformation of episodic tension-type headache into chronic tension-type headache.[195,202]

NONDRUG TECHNIQUES

Nondrug techniques such as massage, physical therapy, hot baths, acupuncture, and various relaxation methods can provide relief from tension-type headache and are often effective adjuncts to drug therapy.[214] However, the evidence basis to support their use is sparse.[202,215] The literature both supports and refutes the effectiveness of acupuncture,[216] electromyography biofeedback,[217–219] and other relaxation techniques in the therapy of tension-type headache.[215] The utility of biofeedback and other relaxation techniques is based on the premise that voluntary control of muscle contraction could benefit the headache sufferer. These techniques are most successful in young, episodic headache sufferers who are motivated to apply the techniques as instructed.[220] A randomized, controlled trial of spinal manipulation for the treatment of tension-type headache failed to demonstrate a benefit of this approach.[221]

An NSAID (e.g., ibuprofen or naproxen) would be an appropriate recommendation for therapy of K.B.'s tension-type headaches because of her previous inadequate responses to aspirin and acetaminophen. Drug use should be carefully monitored because analgesic abuse in patients with frequently recurring tension-type headache is a primary factor in the perpetuation of chronic pain syndromes.[195]

Prophylactic Therapy

CASE 56-6, QUESTION 2: Ibuprofen 400 mg every 4 to 6 hours as needed for headache was prescribed for acute relief of K.B.'s recurrent tension-type headaches. At her next scheduled follow-up visit, K.B. reported moderate relief with ibuprofen but complained of GI upset with each dose, even when taken with food. Because headaches have been occurring more frequently, her use of ibuprofen has also increased. What prophylactic agents are available for continuous suppression of K.B.'s tension-type headaches?

Antidepressants are the most useful group of agents in the prophylaxis of tension-type and mixed-type headaches. Amitriptyline is considered the drug of choice because it is most effective[202,222]; 65% of patients improved by more than 50%, and 25% became headache-free in an early report.[205] The effective daily dose of amitriptyline for most patients is 30 to 75 mg.[202] Response to amitriptyline does not require a history of depressive symptoms, and benefit to the tension-type headache sufferer is usually evident within 2 to 10 days.[72] Amitriptyline should be initiated at a dose of 10 to 25 mg/day at bedtime and increased gradually as needed to allow for the development of tolerance to the sedative and anticholinergic side effects of this drug. Mirtazapine (Remeron; 30 mg/day) and venlafaxine (Effexor; 150 mg/day) are reasonable alternative prophylactic agents for patients who fail or are intolerant to amitriptyline.[202] The efficacy of both agents has been demonstrated in randomized, controlled trials. These agents appear to be effective for prevention of both episodic and chronic tension-type headache. As a class, SSRIs are less effective than amitriptyline for prophylaxis of tension-type headache.[223] Randomized, placebo-controlled trials of citalopram[224] and sertraline failed to find a benefit with these agents.[225]

Given K.B.'s increasing frequency of tension-type headache and her intolerance to moderate doses of ibuprofen, prophylactic treatment with amitriptyline would be appropriate. A starting dose of amitriptyline 10 mg nightly, increasing by 10 to 25 mg at 1-week intervals to a maintenance dose of 50 mg/day, should be prescribed, at which time headache response can be assessed and the dose increased or decreased as necessary. If effective, amitriptyline should be continued for 3 to 4 months before gradually decreasing the dose until the drug is completely discontinued. Therapy should be reinstituted if headaches return.

KEY REFERENCES AND WEBSITES

A full list of references for this chapter can be found at http://thepoint.lww.com/AT10e. Below are the key references and websites for this chapter, with the corresponding reference number in this chapter found in parentheses after the reference.

Key References

Bendtsen L et al. EFNS guideline on the treatment of tension-type headache—report of an EFNS task force. *Eur J Neurol* 2010;17:1318. (202)

Fenstermacher N et al. Pharmacological prevention of migraine. *BMJ*. 2011;342:1583. (106)

Francis GJ et al. Acute and preventive pharmacologic treatment of cluster headache. *Neurology*. 2010;75:463. (176)

Goadsby PJ, Sprenger T. Current practice and future directions in the prevention and acute management of migraine. *Lancet Neurol*. 2010;9:285. (129)

Headache Classification Subcommittee of the International Headache Society. The International Classification of Headache Disorders. 2nd edition. *Cephalalgia*. 2004;24(Suppl 1):9. (6)

Key Websites

American Headache Society. http://www.americanheadachesociety.org

International Headache Society. http://www.ihs-headache.org

Migraine Action Association. http://www.migraine.org.uk

57 Parkinson Disease and Other Movement Disorders

Michael E. Ernst and Mildred D. Gottwald

CORE PRINCIPLES

	CHAPTER CASES
PARKINSON DISEASE	
1 Parkinson disease (PD) is a chronic, progressive movement disorder resulting from loss of dopamine from the nigrostriatal tracts in the brain, and is characterized by rigidity, bradykinesia, postural disturbances, and tremor.	**Case 57-1 (Questions 1, 2)**
2 Treatment for PD is aimed at restoring dopamine supply through one, or a combination, of the following methods: exogenous dopamine in the form of a precursor, levodopa; direct stimulation of dopamine receptors via dopamine agonists; and inhibition of metabolic pathways responsible for degradation of levodopa.	**Case 57-1 (Questions 3–18), Case 57-2 (Questions 1, 2)**
3 Therapy for PD is usually delayed until there is a significant effect on quality of life; generally younger patients start with dopamine agonists, whereas older patients may start with levodopa.	**Case 57-1 (Questions 4, 10)**
4 Initial therapy with dopamine agonists is associated with a lower risk of developing motor complications than with levodopa, but all patients will eventually require levodopa.	**Case 57-1 (Questions 4, 10–15)**
5 Advanced PD is characterized by motor fluctuations including a gradual decline in on time, and the development of troubling dopaminergic-induced dyskinesias. Dopamine agonists, monoamine oxidase type B (MAO-B) inhibitors, and catechol-*O*-methyltransferase (COMT) inhibitors can reduce motor fluctuations; amantadine can improve dyskinesias. Deep brain stimulation of the globus pallidus interna or subthalamic nucleus may benefit patients with advanced PD.	**Case 57-1 (Questions 15–18), Case 57-2 (Question 1), Case 57-3 (Questions 1, 2)**
6 It is controversial whether any therapies for PD are truly disease-modifying or neuroprotective.	**Case 57-2 (Question 1)**
7 Comprehensive therapy for patients should include attention to the many progressive complications of PD, including neuropsychiatric disturbances and autonomic dysfunction.	**Case 57-4 (Questions 1, 2)**
RESTLESS LEG SYNDROME	
1 Dopamine agonists are first-line treatments for restless leg syndrome (RLS). They are preferred because they are longer acting than levodopa, and reduce symptoms throughout the entire night. Other effective therapies include carbidopa/levodopa, gabapentin, benzodiazepines, and opiates.	**Case 57-5 (Question 3)**
2 A common problem with long-term use of dopaminergic agents in RLS, particularly levodopa, is an augmentation effect. This refers to a gradual dosage intensification that occurs in response to a progressive worsening of symptoms after an initial period of improvement. Gradual withdrawal of therapy and substitution with other agents should be performed, rather than continued dopaminergic dose escalation.	**Case 57-5 (Question 4)**

continued

ESSENTIAL TREMOR

1	Essential tremor should be distinguished clinically from tremor associated with PD or other causes.	**Case 57-6 (Question 1)**
2	Treatments of choice for essential tremor include propranolol or primidone. In refractory cases, targeted botulinum toxin A injections can be useful.	**Case 57-6 (Question 2)**

PARKINSON DISEASE

Incidence, Prevalence, and Epidemiology

Parkinson disease (PD) is a chronic, progressive movement disorder in which drug therapy plays a central role. Since its original description in 1817 by Dr. James Parkinson, the term *parkinsonism* has come to refer to any disorder associated with two or more features of tremor, rigidity, bradykinesia, or postural instability.[1] Most cases of PD are of unknown cause, and referred to as *idiopathic parkinsonism;* however, viral encephalitis, cerebrovascular disease, and hydrocephalus have symptoms similar to PD as part of their clinical presentation.[1] Unless otherwise stated, all references to PD in this chapter refer to the idiopathic type.

The age at onset of PD is variable, usually between 50 and 80 years, with a mean onset of 55 years.[2] Both the incidence and prevalence of PD are age-dependent, with annual incidence estimates ranging from 10 cases per 100,000 (age 50–59 years) to 100 cases per 100,000 (age 80–89 years), and an estimated prevalence of 1% of the population older than 65 years of age.[3,4] Men are affected slightly more frequently than women.[5] Despite the availability of effective symptomatic treatments to improve both quality of life and life expectancy, no cure exists. The symptoms of PD are progressive, and within 10 to 20 years, significant immobility results for most patients.[6] More rapid rates of symptom progression and motor disability have been observed in patients who are older at the onset of clinically recognizable disease.[7] PD itself does not cause death; however, patients often succumb to complications related to impaired mobility and function (e.g., aspiration pneumonia, thromboembolism) and overall frailty.[6]

For a supplemental table listing contact information for organizations that can serve as a resource to persons with PD (as well as other movement disorders) and their families, go to http://thepoint.lww.com/AT10e.

Etiology

The etiology of PD is poorly understood. Most evidence suggests it is multifactorial, and attributable to a complex interplay between age-related changes in the nigrostriatal tract, underlying genetic risks, and environmental triggers. Support for this hypothesis can be found in several historic observations, most notably the postviral parkinsonian symptoms occurring after epidemics of encephalitis in the early 1900s, and the discovery that ingestion of a meperidine analog, 1-methyl-4-phenyl-1,2,3,6-tetrahydropyridine (MPTP), by heroin addicts in northern California during the early 1980s caused a rapid and irreversible parkinsonism.[8] (For an excellent in-depth discussion of the importance of the MPTP discovery and its influence on PD research, please view the episode "My Father, My Brother, and Me" from the Public Broadcasting System program *Frontline* at http://www.pbs.org/wgbh/pages/frontline/parkinsons/).

The relative contributions of environment and genetics to the occurrence of PD remains controversial; rural living, pesticide exposure, and consumption of well water have consistently been associated with increased lifetime risk of PD, whereas cigarette smoking and caffeine ingestion appear protective.[9] Mutations in several genes, including α-synuclein (*SNCA*), leucine-rich repeat kinase-2 (*LRRK2*), *parkin,* PTEN-induced kinase-1 (*PINK1*), and *DJ-1,* have been observed in rare familial inherited cases of PD, but these genes lack typical Mendelian patterns of inheritance, and do not account for the threefold increased risk of developing PD for individuals who have a first-degree relative affected with sporadic PD.[10] Recent advances in molecular genetics and genome-wide association studies have revealed other novel risk genes; however, the exact linkage between genetics, environment, and clinical expression of disease remains uncertain.[11]

Pathophysiology

PD affects the portion of the extrapyramidal system of the brain involving the basal ganglia, an area composed of the substantia nigra, neostriatum, and globus pallidus. Together, they are involved with maintaining posture and muscle tone and regulating voluntary smooth motor activity. The pigmented neurons within the substantia nigra have dopaminergic fibers that project into the neostriatum and globus pallidus, and in PD, these dopamine-producing neurons are progressively depigmented.

For an image of the areas of the brain affected by PD, go to http://thepoint.lww.com/AT10e.

Postmortem pathologic examination of the basal ganglia reveals the presence of Lewy bodies within the remaining dopaminergic cells of the substantia nigra.[12] These abnormal intraneuronal protein aggregates are considered pathognomonic for the disease. Lewy body pathology appears to ascend the brain in a predictable manner in PD, beginning in the medulla oblongata in preclinical stages (which may explain observations of anxiety, depression, and olfactory disturbance), ascending to the midbrain (motor dysfunction), and spreading eventually to the cortex (cognitive and behavioral changes).[13]

The exact pathological sequence leading to neurodegeneration is unclear, but free radicals formed as by-products of dopamine auto-oxidation have been implicated. The oxidative stress imparted by these events may provide the stimulus for inflammation and cellular apoptosis, thereby initiating the cascade of neurodegeneration. The finding that a critical threshold of neuronal loss (at least 70%–80%) occurs before PD becomes clinically apparent suggests that adaptive mechanisms (e.g., upregulation of dopamine synthesis or downregulation of synaptic dopamine reuptake) may somehow influence disease progression during the preclinical stages.

Overview of Drug Therapy

Because the salient pathophysiologic feature of PD is the progressive loss of dopamine from the nigrostriatal tracts in the brain, drug therapy for the disease is aimed primarily at replenishing the supply of dopamine (Table 57-1). This is accomplished through one, or a combination, of the following methods: (a) administering exogenous dopamine in the form of a precursor, levodopa; (b) stimulating dopamine receptors within the corpus striatum through the use of dopamine agonists (e.g., pramipexole, ropinirole); or (c) inhibiting the major metabolic pathways within the brain that are responsible for the degradation of levodopa and its metabolites. This latter effect is achieved through the use of aromatic L-amino acid decarboxylase (AAD) inhibitors (e.g., carbidopa), catechol-*O*-methyltransferase (COMT) inhibitors (e.g., entacapone), or monoamine oxidase type B (MAO-B) inhibitors (e.g., selegiline, rasagiline). Additional therapies such as anticholinergics may be used to improve tremor thought to be attributable to the relative increase in cholinergic activity that occurs as a consequence of loss of dopamine-mediated inhibition of acetylcholine neurons. Their routine use, however, is limited by central nervous system adverse effects, particularly in older patients. Amantadine is also used occasionally, and may provide modest benefits via both dopaminergic and nondopaminergic (inhibition of glutamate) mechanisms.

Despite optimization of both pharmacologic and nonpharmacologic therapies in PD, physical disability is progressive and unavoidable. In many instances, adverse effects of the medications themselves can lead to additional problems. Supportive drug treatment of the associated comorbidities of PD is also necessary. These include neuropsychiatric problems (cognitive impairment and dementia, hallucinations and delirium, depression, agitation, anxiety), autonomic dysfunction (constipation, urinary problems, sexual problems, orthostasis, thermoregulatory imbalances), falls, and sleep disorders (insomnia or sleep fragmentation, nightmares, restless leg syndrome).

CLINICAL PRESENTATION OF PARKINSON DISEASE

CASE 57-1

QUESTION 1: L.M., a 55-year-old, right-handed male artist, presents to the neurology clinic complaining of difficulty painting because of unsteadiness in his right hand. On questioning, he notes that it is becoming increasingly difficult to get out of chairs after sitting for a long period because of tightness in his arms and legs. He also reports having a loss in sense of smell and has noticed excessive drooling, especially at night. His wife claims that he has become more "forgetful" lately, and L.M. admits that his memory does not seem to be as sharp as it once was. His medical history is significant for depression for the past year, gout (currently requiring no treatment), constipation, benign prostatic hypertrophy, and aortic stenosis. He does not smoke, but usually drinks one alcoholic beverage in the evenings. His only prescription medication is citalopram 10 mg/day. On physical examination, L.M. is noted to be a well-developed, well-nourished man who displays a notable lack of normal changes in facial expression and speaks in a soft, monotone voice. A strong body odor is noted. Examination of his extremities reveals a slight ratchetlike rigidity in both arms and legs, and a mild resting tremor is present in his right hand. His gait is slow but otherwise normal, with a slightly bent posture. His balance is determined to be normal, with no retropulsion or loss of righting reflexes after physical threat. His genitourinary examination is remarkable only for prostatic enlargement. The remainder of L.M.'s physical examination is within normal limits. Laboratory values and vital signs obtained at this visit include the following:

Blood pressure, 119/66 mm Hg
Heart rate, 71 beats/minute
Sodium, 132 mEq/L
Potassium, 4.4 mEq/L
Blood urea nitrogen, 19 mg/dL
Creatinine, 1.1 mg/dL
Thyroid stimulating hormone, 3.65 microunits/L
Vitamin B_{12}, 612 pg/mL
Folate, 5.2 ng/mL
White blood cells, 4,400 cells/μL
Red blood cells, 5.9 $\times$ 10^6/μL
Hemoglobin, 13.8 g/dL
Hematocrit, 41%
Uric acid, 6.3 mg/dL

How is PD diagnosed? What signs and symptoms suggestive of PD are present in L.M.? Which of these symptoms are among the classic symptoms for diagnosing PD, and which are considered associated symptoms? Is neuroimaging or any other testing helpful in establishing the diagnosis of PD?

The foundation for establishing the diagnosis of PD remains firmly grounded in obtaining a careful history and physical examination.[12] The neurologic examination to assess motor function, along with a positive response to levodopa, is highly diagnostic. The search for biomarkers of premotor PD in blood, cerebrospinal fluid, and urine has not uncovered any useful candidates.[10] Likewise, although positron emission tomography and single photon emission computed tomography imaging can visualize nigrostriatal nerve terminals of dopamine synthesis and identify presymptomatic pathology, their use remains investigational and largely confined to enriched populations of asymptomatic first-degree relatives of patients with PD.[10] Although these methods are highly sensitive and specific, the application of such imaging techniques into routine practice in asymptomatic at-risk individuals is not yet justified. Other associated premotor symptoms, such as hyposmia (a reduced ability to smell and detect odors) and rapid eye movement sleep disorder, are among the earliest symptoms to appear; screening for these findings may prove more economically practical and identify a population at higher risk and worthy of further study.[14] An example of such a strategy can be found in the longitudinal Parkinson Associated Risk Study (http://www.parsinfosource.com), which uses an inexpensive but sensitive screening test of olfactory disturbances to select asymptomatic individuals at risk for PD to undergo further neuroimaging.[10] Those with pathology identified from neuroimaging are then observed longitudinally for the development of motor symptoms. By the time patients present with symptoms such as L.M., a substantial burden of neuropathologic evidence has accumulated, and the diagnosis can be made clinically. Therefore, further laboratory or radiological testing is unnecessary.

TABLE 57-1
Medications Used for the Treatment of Parkinson Disease

Generic (Trade) Name	Dosage Unit	Titration Schedule	Usual Daily Dose	Adverse Effects
Amantadine (Symmetrel)	100-mg capsule Liquid: 50 mg/5 mL	100 mg every day; increased by 100 mg 1–2 weeks	100–300 mg	Orthostatic hypotension, insomnia, depression, hallucinations, livedo reticularis, xerostomia
Anticholinergic Agents				
Benztropine (Cogentin)	0.5-, 1-, and 2-mg tablets Injection: 2 mL (1 mg/mL)	0.5 mg/d increased by 0.5 mg every 3–5 days	1–3 mg given every day to BID	Constipation, xerostomia, dry skin, dysphagia, confusion, memory impairment
Trihexyphenidyl (Artane)	2- and 5-mg tablets Liquid: 2 mg/5 mL	1–2 mg/d increased by 1–2 mg every 3–5 days	6–15 mg divided TID to BID	Constipation, xerostomia, dry skin, dysphagia, confusion, memory impairment
Combination Agents				
Carbidopa-Levodopa (immediate-release)/ entacapone (Stalevo)	12.5/50/200, 25/100/200, and 37.5/150/200 mg tablets	Titrate with individual dosage forms (carbidopa/levodopa and entacapone) first, then switch to combination tablet	Varies (see listings for individual drugs)	See listing for individual drugs
Dopamine Replacement				
Carbidopa-Levodopa (Regular) (Sinemet)	10/100, 25/100, and 25/250 tablets	25/100 mg BID, increased by 25/100 weekly to effect and as tolerated	30/300 to 150/1,500 divided TID to QID	Nausea, orthostatic hypotension, confusion, dizziness, hallucinations, dyskinesias, blepharospasm
Carbidopa-Levodopa (CR) (Sinemet CR)	25/100 and 50/200 tablets	25/100 mg BID (spaced at least 6 hours apart), increased every 3–7 days	50/200 to 500/2,000 divided QID	Same as regular Sinemet
Carbidopa-Levodopa ODT (Parcopa)	10/100, 25/100, and 25/250 mg tablets	25/100 BID, increased every 1–2 days; if transferring from regular levodopa <1,500 mg/d) start 25/100 mg TID to QID (start 25/250 mg TID to QID if already on >1,500 mg/d of regular levodopa)	25/100 to 200/2,000 divided TID to QID	Same as regular Sinemet; may occur more rapidly than with regular Sinemet
Dopamine Agonists				
Bromocriptine (Parlodel)	2.5-mg tablet, 5-mg capsule	1.25 HS, titrate slowly as tolerated for 4–6 weeks	10–40 mg divided TID	Orthostatic hypotension, confusion, dizziness, hallucinations, nausea, leg cramps; retroperitoneal, pleural, pericardial fibrosis; cardiac valve thickening
Pramipexole (Mirapex, Mirapex ER)	0.125-, 0.25-, 0.50-, 1-, 1.5-mg tablets 0.375-, 0.75-, 1.5-, 3-, 4.5-mg tablets (ER)	0.375 divided TID; titrate weekly by 0.125–0.25 mg/dose	1.5–4.5 mg divided TID	Orthostatic hypotension, confusion, dizziness, hallucinations, nausea, somnolence
Ropinirole (Requip, Requip XL)	0.25-, 0.5-, 1-, 2-, 4-, 5-mg tablet 2-, 4-, 6-, 8-, 12-mg tablets (XL)	Titrate weekly by 0.25 mg/dose	3–12 mg divided TID	Orthostatic hypotension, confusion, dizziness, hallucinations, nausea, somnolence
Apomorphine (Apokyn)	10 mg/mL injection	Initial 2-mg test dose, then begin 1 mg less than tolerated test dose; increase by 1 mg every few days; approved for "rescue" during periods of hypomobility	2–6 mg TID	Nausea, vomiting; administer with trimethobenzamide (not 5-hydroxytryptamine-3 [5-HT_3] antagonists)
Rotigotine (Neupro)[a]	2-, 4-, 6-mg/24 h transdermal delivery system	2 mg/24 h; titrate weekly by 2 mg/24 h until response noted or maximal dose of 6 mg/24 h reached. Application site should be rotated daily between abdomen, thigh, hip, flank, shoulder, or upper arm	4–6 mg/24 h	Hallucinations, abnormal dreaming, insomnia, somnolence, nausea, vomiting, application site reactions; avoid in patients with known sulfite sensitivity

(continued)

TABLE 57-1
Medications Used for the Treatment of Parkinson Disease (*Continued*)

Generic (Trade) Name	Dosage Unit	Titration Schedule	Usual Daily Dose	Adverse Effects
COMT Inhibitors				
Entacapone (Comtan)	200-mg tablet	One tablet with each administration of levodopa/carbidopa, up to 8 tablets daily	3–8 tablets daily	Diarrhea, dyskinesias, abdominal pain, urine discoloration
Tolcapone (Tasmar)	100-, 200-mg tablet	100–200 mg TID	300–600 mg divided TID	Diarrhea, dyskinesias, abdominal pain, urine discoloration, hepatotoxicity
MAO-B Inhibitors				
Selegiline (Eldepryl)[b]	5-mg tablet, capsule	5 mg AM; may increase to 5 mg BID	5–10 mg (take 5 mg with breakfast and 5 mg with lunch)	Insomnia, dizziness, nausea, vomiting, xerostomia, dyskinesias, mood changes; use caution when coadministered with sympathomimetics or serotoninergic agents (increased risk of serotonin syndrome); avoid tyramine-containing foods
Selegiline ODT (Zelapar)	1.25-mg tablet	1.25 mg every day; may increase to 2.5 mg every day after 6 weeks	1.25–2.5 mg every day	Insomnia, dizziness, nausea, vomiting, xerostomia, dyskinesias, mood changes; use caution when coadministered with sympathomimetics or serotoninergic agents (increased risk of serotonin syndrome); avoid ingestion large amounts of tyramine-containing foods
Rasagiline (Azilect)	0.5-mg tablet	0.5 mg every day; may increase to 1 mg every day	0.5–1 mg/d	Similar to selegiline

[a]Not currently available in the United States.
[b]A transdermal formulation is also available, but not approved for use in PD.
BID, twice daily; COMT, catechol-*O*-methyltransferase; HS, bedtime; MAO-B, monoamine oxidase type B; ODT, orally disintegrating tablet; QID, four times daily; TID, three times daily.

The classic features of PD—tremor, limb rigidity, and bradykinesia—are easily recognized, particularly in advanced stages of disease. However, it is important to note that not all are required to be present to make the diagnosis of PD. The presence of two or more features indicates clinically probable PD.[15] Tremor, which is most often the first symptom observed in younger patients, is usually unilateral on initial presentation. Frequently, the tremor is of a pill-rolling type involving the thumb and index finger (3–6 Hz); it is present at rest, worsens under fatigue or stress, and is absent with purposeful movement or when asleep.[1] These features help distinguish it from essential tremor, which usually manifests as a symmetric tremor in the hands, often accompanied by head and voice tremor.[12] Approximately 30% of patients with idiopathic PD do not present with tremor.[16] Muscular rigidity resulting from increased muscle tone often manifests as a cogwheel or ratchet (catch-release) type of motion when an extremity is moved passively.[1] Rigidity may also be experienced as stiffness or vague aching or limb discomfort.[12] Bradykinesia refers to an overall slowness in initiating movement. Early in the disease, patients may describe this as weakness or clumsiness of a hand or leg.[12] As the disease progresses, difficulty initiating and terminating steps results in a hurried or festinating gait; the posture becomes stooped (simian posture), and postural reflexes are impaired.[1] Symptoms that were unilateral on initial presentation progress asymmetrically and often become bilateral and more severe with disease progression.[1] Patients with PD develop masked facies, or a blank stare with reduced eye blinking (Fig. 57-1).

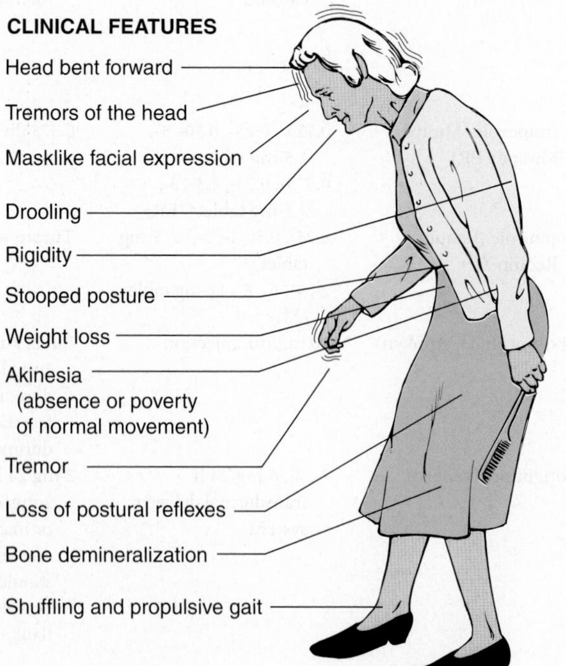

FIGURE 57-1 Clinical features of Parkinson disease. (Reprinted with permission from Rosdahl CB. *Book of Basic Nursing*. 7th ed. Philadelphia, PA: Lippincott-Raven; 1999:1063.)

For a visual of the features of Parkinson Disease, and for a video overview of motor function testing in an individual with PD (titled Impairments), go to http://thepoint.lww.com/AT10e.

Because the diagnosis of PD is clinical, misdiagnosis can occur, leading to inappropriate, ineffective, or delayed treatment. Patients with PD may have an insidious onset of nonspecific symptoms such as generalized malaise and fatigue.[1] Several conditions can be mistaken for PD, and include multiple system atrophy (formerly known as Shy-Drager syndrome), progressive supranuclear palsy, and normal pressure hydrocephalus. These atypical parkinsonian conditions (also referred to as "parkinson-plus" syndromes) are important to distinguish from PD because they respond poorly to dopaminergic medications and are associated with worse prognosis.[12] Magnetic resonance imaging can be useful in some situations to exclude these conditions, particularly when clinical signs suggest an alternate diagnosis. Falls or dementia early in the disease, symmetric parkinsonism, wide-based gait, abnormal eye movements, marked orthostatic hypotension, urinary retention, and marked disability within 5 years after the onset of symptoms suggest alternative diagnoses other than PD.[16] Drugs that act as antagonists at dopaminergic D_2 receptors (e.g., neuroleptics, prochlorperazine, and metoclopramide), and others such as valproate, amiodarone, phenytoin, and lithium may cause a state of drug-induced parkinsonism that mimics idiopathic PD. Drug-induced parkinsonism should be excluded before the diagnosis of PD is established. Although reversible, symptoms may persist for weeks or months after discontinuation of the offending agent.[16]

L.M. presents with many of the classic symptoms of PD. A noticeable unilateral resting tremor is present along with decreased manual dexterity, as evidenced by his difficulty handling a paintbrush. Rigidity (ratcheting of the arms), bradykinesia (slowness of movement), and a masklike facial expression also are present. Although he has a partially stooped posture, it is difficult to attribute this entirely to the disease because postural changes commonly occur with advancing age and, on physical examination, his balance was normal. To confirm the diagnosis of PD, a therapeutic trial of levodopa may be considered. A positive response to levodopa, as evidenced by an improvement in motor or cognitive function, suggests the diagnosis of PD. Patients with the tremor-predominant form of the disease may, however, not respond to levodopa, especially in the early stages of the disease.[16]

Numerous nonmotor clinical features are associated with PD. Handwriting abnormalities occur frequently, particularly micrographia, a symptom of bradykinesia.

For a video that shows how Parkinson disease can affect the upper extremities, go to http://thepoint.lww.com/AT10e.

Because L.M. is an artist, this abnormality would be particularly troublesome. He also is showing signs of autonomic nervous system dysfunction, such as drooling (sialorrhea), seborrhea, and constipation, all of which can be particularly embarrassing to the patient. Drooling may be a consequence of impaired swallowing. The strong body odor exhibited by L.M. could be ascribed to excess sebum production. L.M.'s seborrhea can be treated with coal tar– or selenium-based shampoos, or topical ketoconazole. His constipation should be managed first by evaluating his diet and exercise level, discontinuing anticholinergic medications (including over-the-counter cold and sleep medications) that may exacerbate constipation, and using a stool softener such as sodium or calcium docusate. In more severe cases, polyethylene glycol, lactulose, milk of magnesia, or enemas may be required.

L.M. should be evaluated for other manifestations of autonomic dysfunction, including urinary problems, increased sweating, orthostatic hypotension, erectile dysfunction, pain or dysesthesias, and problems swallowing.

For a video that shows the postural control challenges posed by Parkinson disease, go to http://thepoint.lww.com/AT10e.

L.M. has benign prostatic hypertrophy and may benefit from further evaluation. He should be counseled to avoid anticholinergic agents that may exacerbate this problem. He should be referred to a speech and swallowing expert because dysphagia can result in impaired swallowing and lead to aspiration; a soft diet may be indicated. The soft, mumbled, monotone voice noted in L.M. is frequently observed in PD and often one of the early symptoms noted. Speech therapy can be of benefit.[17]

Psychiatric disturbances, such as nervousness, anxiety, and depression, occur commonly in patients with PD, and regular screening for these symptoms should occur.[16,18] L.M. has a history of depression treated with citalopram that could be attributable to PD, and his therapy should be periodically evaluated. Finally, the prevalence of cognitive decline and dementia among patients with PD ranges from 10% to 30% and may be associated with a more rapid progression of disease-related disability.[7] The development of hallucinations in patients with PD with dementia is a poor prognostic sign.[19] The forgetfulness and decreased memory described by L.M. could be early signs of cognitive decline and warrant close observation.

Staging of Parkinson Disease

CASE 57-1, QUESTION 2: What are the stages of PD? In what stage of the disease is L.M.?

To assess the degree of disability and determine the rate of disease progression relative to treatment, various scales have been developed. The most common of these is the Hoehn and Yahr scale (Table 57-2).[2] In general, patients in Hoehn and Yahr stage 1 or 2 of PD have mild disease that does not interfere with activities of daily living or work and usually requires minimal or no treatment. In stage 3 disease, daily activities are restricted and employment may be significantly affected unless effective treatment is initiated. L.M. appears to be in late stage 2, early stage 3 of the disease according to the scale.

TABLE 57-2
Staging of Disability in Parkinson Disease

Stage 1	Unilateral involvement only; minimal or no functional impairment
Stage 2	Bilateral involvement, without impairment of balance
Stage 3	Evidence of postural imbalance; some restriction in activities; capable of leading independent life; mild to moderate disability
Stage 4	Severely disabled, cannot walk and stand unassisted; significantly incapacitated
Stage 5	Restricted to bed or wheelchair unless aided

With advanced-stage disease (3 to 4), most patients require levodopa therapy (with a peripheral decarboxylase inhibitor such as carbidopa) and often in combination with a COMT inhibitor such as entacapone or a dopamine agonist such as pramipexole or ropinirole. In some cases, selegiline, rasagiline, or amantadine may provide further symptomatic relief. Patients with end-stage disease (stage 5) are severely incapacitated and, because of advanced disease progression, often do not respond well to drug therapy.

TREATMENT OF PARKINSON DISEASE

CASE 57-1, QUESTION 3: When should L.M. begin treatment for his PD?

In choosing when to treat the symptoms of PD and which therapy to use, care must be taken to approach each patient individually. Although no consensus has been reached about when to initiate symptomatic treatment, most health care professionals agree that treatment should begin when the patient begins to experience functional impairment as defined by (a) threat to employment status, (b) symptoms affecting the dominant side of the body, or (c) bradykinesia or rigidity. Individual patient preferences also should be considered. Judging by the symptoms L.M. is displaying, he would likely benefit from immediate treatment. His symptoms are unilateral but are occurring on his dominant side and are interfering with his ability to paint, thus affecting his livelihood. He is also showing signs of rigidity and bradykinesia but can otherwise live independently.

An algorithm for the management of patients with PD is presented in Figure 57-2. The long-term, individualized treatment

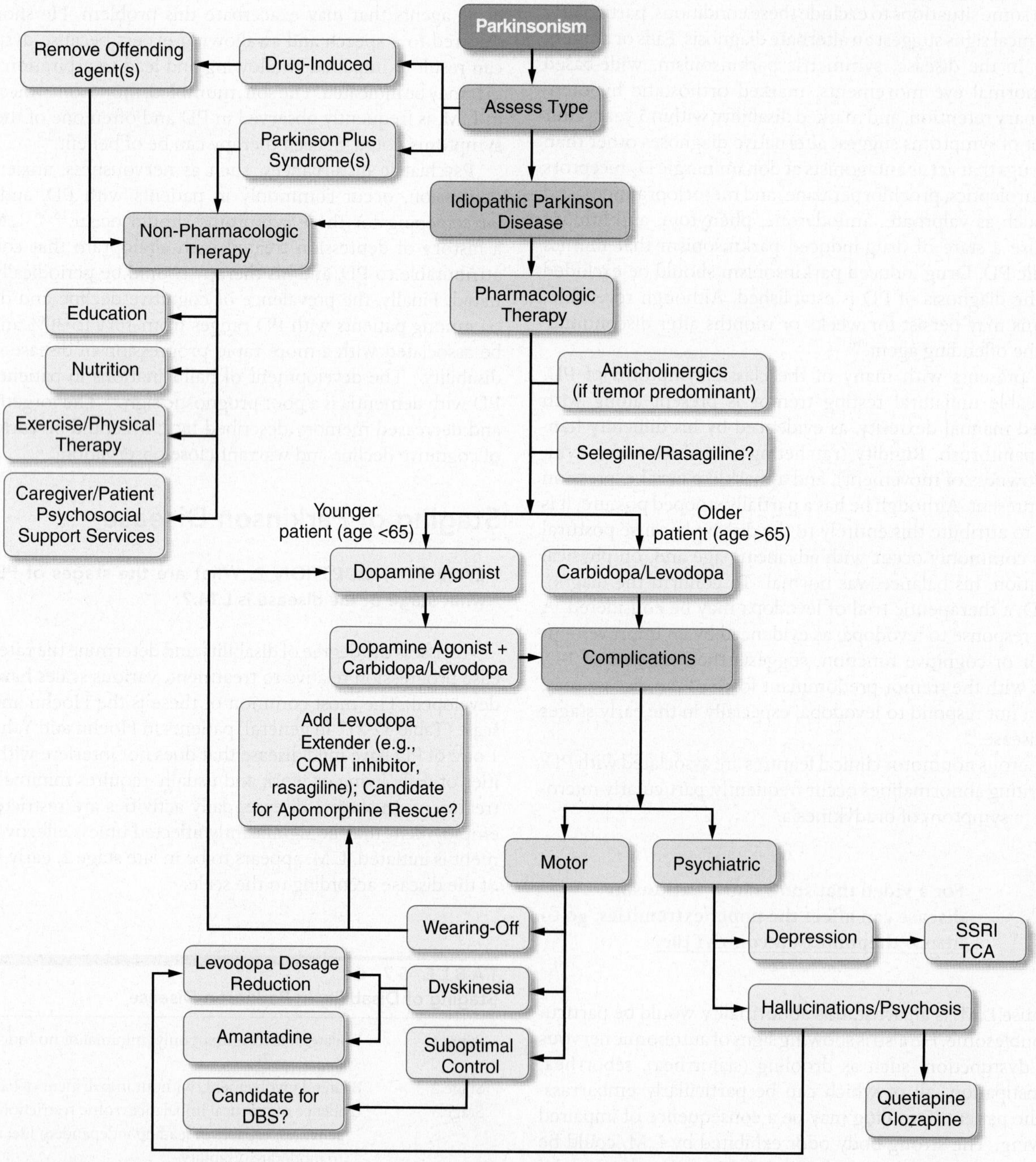

FIGURE 57-2 Suggested treatment algorithm for the management of Parkinson disease. DBS, deep brain stimulation. (Modified with permission from the American College of Clinical Pharmacy. Ernst ME. Parkinson's disease. In: Dunsworth T et al, eds. *Pharmacotherapy Self-Assessment Program*. 6th ed. Neurology and Psychiatry module. Lenexa, KS: American College of Clinical Pharmacy; 2007:22.)

plan is usually characterized by frequent dosage adjustments with time because of the chronic and progressive nature of the disease. Although most of this chapter is devoted to the drug therapy of PD, the importance of supportive care cannot be overemphasized. Exercise, physiotherapy, and good nutritional support can be beneficial at the earlier stages to improve mobility, increase strength, and enhance well-being and mood.[16] Psychological support is often necessary in dealing with depression and other related problems. Newly diagnosed patients and their family members need to be educated about what to expect from the disease and the various forms of treatment available. The support of family members is vital in establishing an overall effective therapeutic plan.

Dopamine Agonists

INITIAL THERAPY

CASE 57-1, QUESTION 4: The decision is made to begin drug therapy for L.M. Should therapy be initiated with a dopamine agonist or levodopa?

Levodopa remains the most effective antiparkinsonian agent.[12] However, monotherapy with levodopa throughout the entire course of the disease is limited by response fluctuations and declining efficacy as PD progresses. Escalating doses of levodopa are accompanied by a high frequency of undesirable side effects; thus, other methods of enriching dopamine supply have been developed. Dopamine agonists, which directly bind to dopamine receptors, are one such group of agents. In clinical trials comparing dopamine agonists with levodopa, activities of daily living (ADLs) and motor features are improved 40% to 50% with levodopa compared with 30% with dopamine agonists.[20] Although they are not as effective as levodopa, the dopamine agonists have a number of potential advantages. Because they act directly on dopamine receptors, they do not require metabolic conversion to an active product and therefore act independently of degenerating dopaminergic neurons. Unlike levodopa, circulating plasma amino acids do not compete with dopamine agonists for absorption and transport into the brain. Dopamine agonists have a longer half-life than levodopa formulations, reducing the need for multiple daily dosing. Initial therapy with dopamine agonists is associated with fewer motor complications such as dyskinesias, and can delay the need for initiation of dopaminergic therapy.[21–23] As a class, dopamine agonists provide adequate control of symptoms when given as monotherapy in up to 80% of patients with early-stage disease. These benefits are sustained for 3 years or more in most patients. However, with disease progression, levodopa therapy will eventually be required.

Guidelines from the American Academy of Neurology support either dopamine agonists or levodopa as initial therapy for PD.[24] In younger patients (e.g., age <65 years) with milder disease, such as L.M., the initiation of a dopamine agonist as a first-line agent is a strategy used to delay the introduction of levodopa. Delaying levodopa allows patients to have a longer period of time before experiencing motor complications, particularly troubling peak-dose levodopa-induced dyskinesias, which eventually develop with advancing PD. In older patients (e.g., age >65 years) with PD, it may be more appropriate to initiate treatment with levodopa instead of a dopamine agonist because these patients are more likely to experience intolerable central nervous system side effects from dopamine agonists.[16]

In the case of L.M., his relatively young age (<65 years) and mild disease make him a good candidate for initial therapy with a dopamine agonist. L.M. will require levodopa therapy at a later time, when he reaches more advanced stages of the disease. By initiating therapy first with a dopamine agonist, rescue levodopa therapy can likely be started at smaller doses, and the onset of motor complications that often occur with escalating doses and extended therapy with levodopa may be delayed.

SELECTION OF AGENTS

CASE 57-1, QUESTION 5: L.M. is to be started on a dopamine agonist. Which agent should be selected?

Two generations of dopamine agonists have been used for the treatment of idiopathic, early-stage PD as monotherapy, or as an adjunct to levodopa in patients with advanced disease. The comparative pharmacologic and pharmacokinetic properties of these agents are shown in Table 57-3. The first-generation dopamine agonists, which are derived from ergot alkaloids, include bromocriptine, pergolide, and cabergoline. These older agents are now rarely used because of increased risk of retroperitoneal, pleural, and pericardial fibrosis, as well as a twofold to fourfold increased risk for cardiac valve fibrosis, when compared with nonergoline dopamine agonists and controls.[25,26] Pergolide was voluntarily withdrawn in the United States in 2007 for this reason, and although cabergoline continues to be used in Europe, it is only indicated in the United States for treating hyperprolactinemia. Pramipexole, ropinirole, apomorphine, and rotigotine are second-generation nonergoline dopamine agonists. Of

TABLE 57-3
Pharmacologic and Pharmacokinetic Properties of Dopamine Agonists

	Bromocriptine	Pramipexole	Ropinirole	Apomorphine	Rotigotine[a]
Type of compound	Ergot derivative	Nonergoline	Nonergoline	Nonergoline	Nonergoline
Receptor specificity	D_2, D_1,[b] α_1, α_2, 5-HT	D_2, D_3, D_4, α_2	D_2, D_3, D_4	D_1, D_2, D_3, D_4, D_5, α_1, α_2, 5-HT_1, 5-HT_2	D_1, D_2, D_3, 5-HT_1
Bioavailability	8%	>90%	55% (first-pass metabolism)	<5% orally; 100% subcutaneous	<1% orally
T_{max} (minutes)	70–100	60–180	90	10–60	15–18 (hours); no characteristic peak observed
Protein binding	90–96%	15%	40%	>99.9%	89.5%
Elimination route	Hepatic	Renal	Hepatic	Hepatic and extrahepatic	Hepatic
Half-life (hours)	3–8	8–12	6	0.5–1	3

[a]Not currently available in the United States.
[b]Antagonist.
5-HT, serotonin.

these agents, pramipexole and ropinirole are primarily used. Apomorphine is available only in injectable form, for use as a rescue agent in the treatment of hypomobility or off episodes in patients with PD. A once-daily transdermal formulation of rotigotine was briefly available in the United States, but withdrawn in March 2008 owing to manufacturing problems with crystal formation in the patches. It remains available in several European countries, but no timeline has been given for its reintroduction in the United States.

Dopamine agonists work by directly stimulating postsynaptic dopamine receptors within the corpus striatum. The two families of dopamine receptors are D_1 and D_2. The D_1 family includes the D_1 and D_5 dopamine subtype receptors and the D_2 family includes D_2, D_3, and D_4 dopamine subtype receptors. Stimulation of D_2 receptors is largely responsible for reducing rigidity and bradykinesia, whereas the precise role of the D_1 receptors remains uncertain.[27] Although the dopamine agonists differ slightly from each other in terms of their affinities for dopamine receptor subtypes, these agents produce similar clinical effects when used to treat PD, and no compelling evidence favors one agent over another strictly on efficacy measures. Instead, experience with the nonergoline dopamine agonists, pramipexole or ropinirole, makes them currently preferred as initial dopamine agonists. No studies have directly compared these two agents, and individual studies of efficacy appear to demonstrate similar benefits. Thus, either agent would be acceptable as initial therapy in L.M.

CASE 57-1, QUESTION 6: The decision is made to begin pramipexole in L.M. How effective is pramipexole in the initial treatment of PD? How does ropinirole compare?

PRAMIPEXOLE

Pramipexole has been well studied as monotherapy in patients with early-stage PD,[28–30] and as an adjunct to levodopa therapy in advanced-stage disease.[31,32] These trials were multicenter, placebo-controlled, parallel-group studies, and the primary outcome measures included improvement in ADLs (part II) and motor function scores (part III) as measured by the Unified Parkinson Disease Rating Scale (UPDRS). (Go to http://www.mdvu.org/library/ratingscales/pd/ to download this document.) Each evaluation on the UPDRS is rated on a scale of 0 (normal) to 4 (can barely perform). Lower scores on the UPDRS after treatment indicate an improvement in overall performance.

The evidence for pramipexole's efficacy in early PD comes from two large-scale, double-blind, placebo-controlled studies that included a total of 599 patients with early-stage PD (mean disease duration of 2 years).[28,29] In the first study, 264 patients were randomly assigned to receive one of four fixed doses (1.5, 3.0, 4.5, or 6.0 mg/day) or placebo.[28] The pramipexole-treated patients had a 20% reduction in their total UPDRS scores compared with baseline values, whereas no significant improvement was observed in the placebo-treated patients. A trend toward decreased tolerability was noted as the pramipexole dosage was escalated, especially in the 6.0-mg/day group. A second study of 335 patients titrated doses up to the maximal tolerated dose (not to exceed 4.5 mg/day) and then followed patients for a 6-month maintenance phase.[29] The mean pramipexole maintenance dosage was 3.8 mg/day. Those treated with pramipexole experienced significant improvements in both the ADL scores (22%–29%) and motor scores (25%–31%), whereas there were no significant changes in the placebo group ($p < 0.0001$).

Against levodopa as initial therapy, pramipexole appears to delay the onset of dyskinesias. In a randomized, controlled trial evaluating the development of motor complications with the two therapies, 301 untreated patients with early PD were randomly assigned to receive either pramipexole 0.5 mg three times daily or carbidopa/levodopa 25/100 mg three times daily.[23] Doses could be escalated during the first 10 weeks of the study, after which open-label levodopa was permitted if necessary. The primary end point was the time to the first occurrence of wearing off, dyskinesias, or on-off motor fluctuations. After a mean follow-up of 24 months, patients in the pramipexole group were receiving a mean daily dose of 2.78 mg pramipexole and 264 mg of supplemental levodopa, whereas patients in the levodopa group were receiving a mean total of 509 mg/day levodopa. Fewer pramipexole-treated patients reached the primary end point (28% vs. 51%; $p < 0.001$) than the patients initially randomly assigned to levodopa therapy. Dyskinesias were noted in only 10% of pramipexole-treated patients compared with 31% of levodopa-treated patients ($p < 0.001$), and fewer patients experienced wearing-off effects with pramipexole (24% vs. 38%; $p = 0.01$). Long-term follow-up of this cohort (mean = 6.0 years) has revealed a persistently lower rate of dopaminergic motor complications in the pramipexole-treated patients compared with those receiving levodopa (50.0% vs. 68.4%, respectively; $p = 0.002$).[33]

ROPINIROLE

Ropinirole is a synthetic nonergoline dopamine agonist with selectivity for D_2 receptors; as with pramipexole, however, it has no significant affinity for D_1 receptors.[34] Although the drug is pharmacologically similar to pramipexole, it has some distinct pharmacokinetic properties, as shown in Table 57-3. Unlike pramipexole, which is primarily eliminated by renal excretion, ropinirole is metabolized by the cytochrome P-450 (primarily CYP1A2) oxidative pathway and undergoes significant first-pass hepatic metabolism.[35] Similar to pramipexole, ropinirole is approved for use as monotherapy in early-stage idiopathic PD and as an adjunct to levodopa therapy in patients with advanced-stage disease.

Ropinirole has not been directly compared with pramipexole in a randomized, double-blind trial, but it appears to have comparable efficacy as inferred from indirect comparison. In several randomized, double-blind, multicenter, parallel group studies comparing it with placebo, bromocriptine, or levodopa, 6 months of monotherapy with ropinirole in patients with early PD significantly improves UPDRS motor scores (approximately 20%–30%) compared with baseline values.[36–38] In a long-term study, patients treated initially with ropinirole were less likely to experience dyskinesias compared with those treated initially with levodopa.[21] At the end of 5 years, the mean daily dose of ropinirole was 16.5 mg plus 427 mg of open-label levodopa, compared with a mean daily dose of 753 mg of levodopa for the levodopa group. Of patients in the ropinirole group, 66% required open-label levodopa supplementation compared with 36% in the levodopa group. Dyskinesias developed in 20% of the ropinirole-treated patients compared with 45% of the levodopa-treated patients (hazard ratio for remaining free of dyskinesia in the ropinirole group, compared with the levodopa group, 2.82; $p < 0.001$). For ropinirole-treated patients who were able to remain on monotherapy without open-label levodopa supplementation, only 5% experienced dyskinesia, compared with 36% of those receiving levodopa monotherapy. The lower incidence of dyskinesia in ropinirole-treated patients was shown to persist in long-term open-label follow-up of this study cohort.[39]

DOSING

CASE 57-1, QUESTION 7: How are pramipexole and ropinirole dosed?

Pramipexole and ropinirole should always be initiated at a low dosage and gradually titrated to the maximal effective dose, as tolerated. This approach minimizes adverse effects that may result in nonadherence or discontinuation of the drug. In clinical trials, the maximal effective doses are variable and correlate with disease severity and tolerability. One fixed-dose study of pramipexole in early PD showed that most patients responded maximally at a dosage of 0.5 mg three times daily.[29] In patients with advanced-stage disease, an average of 3.4 mg/day is usually required to reach the maximal effect of pramipexole.[32]

L.M. has normal renal function and his pramipexole should be started at an initial dosage of 0.125 mg three times daily for 5 to 7 days. At week 2, the dosage should be increased to 0.25 mg three times daily. Thereafter, his dosage may be increased weekly by 0.25 mg/dose (0.75 mg/day) as tolerated and up to the maximal effective dose, not to exceed 1.5 mg three times daily.[40] The titration period usually takes about 4 to 7 weeks, depending on the optimal maintenance dose. Patients with a creatinine clearance of less than 60 mL/minute should be dosed less frequently than those with normal renal function.[40] Patients with a creatinine clearance of 35 to 59 mL/minute should receive a starting dose of 0.125 mg twice daily up to a maximal dose of 1.5 mg twice daily; patients with a creatinine clearance of 15 to 34 mL/minute should receive a starting dose of 0.125 mg daily up to a maximal dose of 1.5 mg daily. Pramipexole has not been studied in patients with a creatinine clearance of less than 15 mL/minute or those receiving hemodialysis. A once-daily extended-release formulation of pramipexole is also available; patients can be switched overnight from immediate-release pramipexole at the same daily dose.

Ropinirole should be initiated at a dosage of 0.25 mg three times daily with gradual titration in weekly increments of 0.25 mg/dose over the course of 4 to 6 weeks.[41] Clinical response to ropinirole is usually observed at a daily dose of 9 to 12 mg given in three divided doses. Doses may be increased to a maximal daily dose of 24 mg/day. Patients wishing to take the drug less frequently can be switched directly to an extended-release once-daily formulation, selecting the dose that most closely matches the total daily dose of the immediate-release formulation. No dose adjustments for ropinirole are necessary in patients with renal dysfunction.

ADVERSE EFFECTS

CASE 57-1, QUESTION 8: What are the adverse effects of pramipexole and ropinirole? How can these be managed?

Because pramipexole and ropinirole are both approved for use as monotherapy in early-stage disease and as adjunctive therapy in advanced-stage disease, the adverse events of these agents have been evaluated as a function of disease stage. In studies of patients with early-stage disease, the most common adverse effects were nausea (~28%–44%), dizziness (~25%–40%), somnolence (~22%–40%), insomnia (~17%), constipation (~14%), asthenia (~14%), hallucinations (~9%), and leg edema (~5%).[28–30,36–38,40,41] Nausea, with or without vomiting, can be a significant problem, particularly with higher doses. Administering these drugs with food may partially alleviate this problem. With continued use, many patients exhibit tolerance to the gastrointestinal side effects. Central nervous system side effects were the most common reason for discontinuation of these agents. Older patients are particularly more likely to experience hallucinations and other central nervous system adverse effects with dopamine agonists. The incidence of orthostatic hypotension was relatively low (1%–9%) and may in part reflect the exclusion of patients with underlying cardiovascular disease in several of the studies.

In advanced-stage disease, the most common adverse events of dopamine agonists were nausea (25%), orthostatic hypotension (10%–54%), dyskinesias (26%–47%), insomnia (27%), somnolence (11%), confusion (10%), and hallucinations (11%–17%).[32,40–42] As expected, in patients with advanced-stage disease, the most common reasons for discontinuing these agents are mental disturbances (nightmares, confusion, hallucinations, insomnia) and orthostatic hypotension. Dyskinesias experienced when dopamine agonists are used in combination with levodopa in advanced-stage disease may require lowering the dose of levodopa or, in some cases, the dopamine agonist.

Sudden, excessive daytime somnolence, including while driving, has been reported with dopamine agonists and has resulted in accidents.[40,41,43] Affected patients have not always reported warning signs before falling asleep and believed they were alert immediately before the event. Labeling for these drugs includes a warning that patients should be alerted to the possibility of falling asleep while engaged in daily activities. Patients should be advised to refrain from driving or other potentially dangerous activities until they have gained sufficient experience with the dopamine agonist to determine whether it will hinder their mental and motor performance. Caution should be advised when patients are taking other sedating medications or alcohol in combination with pramipexole and ropinirole. If excessive daytime somnolence does occur, patients should be advised to contact their physician.

Dopamine agonist therapy in patients with PD is associated with a 2- to 3.5-fold increased odds of developing an impulse control disorder.[44] The frequency appears similar for both pramipexole and ropinirole. In one study, a prevalence of 6.1% was noted for pathologic gambling in patients with PD compared with 0.25% for age- and sex-matched controls.[45] These cases may represent variations of a behavioral syndrome termed *hedonistic homeostatic dysregulation* or *dopamine dysregulation syndrome.*[46] Other features of the syndrome have been reported, including punding (carrying out repetitive, purposeless motor acts), hypersexuality, walkabout (having the urge to walk great distances during on times, often with no purpose or destination and abnormalities in time perception), compulsive buying, binge eating, drug hoarding, and social independence or isolation.[46] The syndrome appears to be more common among younger, male patients with early-onset PD, as well as those having novelty-seeking personality traits, depressive symptoms, and current use of alcohol or tobacco.[44,47]

Management of impulse control disorders can be challenging, as it often requires modification of dopaminergic therapies, which must be carefully balanced with the accompanying risk of worsening motor function. Underlying depression, if present, should be treated and may improve impulse control. Nonpharmacologic measures (such as limiting access to money or the Internet) may be helpful; in some cases, antipsychotic drugs may be considered, but must also be used carefully to avoid precipitating motor disability.[48]

Although L.M. is younger than 65 years of age, he is experiencing memory difficulty and may be at increased risk for visual hallucinations and cognitive problems from dopamine agonist therapy. He should be monitored closely for occurrence or exacerbation of these problems. He should also be evaluated for lightheadedness before initiation of pramipexole and counseled to report dizziness or unsteadiness, because this may lead to falls. He should also be reassured that if these effects are caused by pramipexole, they should subside with time and that he should not drive or operate complex machinery until he can assess the drug's effect on his mental status. L.M. should be counseled about the possibility of excessive, and potentially unpredictable, daytime somnolence as pramipexole is introduced. L.M. does not appear to have a problem with excessive alcohol use; however, he and his family should be educated about his increased risk for impulse control disorders and advised to report any new, unusual or uncharacteristic behaviors or increased use of alcohol.

ROTIGOTINE

CASE 57-1, QUESTION 9: What type of dopamine agonist is rotigotine? How is it used?

Rotigotine is a nonergoline dopamine receptor agonist that was briefly available in the United States for the treatment of early-stage idiopathic PD. It remains available in Europe. Rotigotine is formulated in a transdermal patch delivery system designed for once a day application. Transdermal delivery may provide a more continuous stimulation of dopamine receptors than traditional oral formulations, which in theory may translate into improved efficacy. Rotigotine has demonstrated efficacy as monotherapy in early-stage PD,[49–51] and as adjunctive therapy to levodopa in patients with advanced stages of PD.[52] Adverse events with rotigotine were similar to those observed with other dopamine agonists (nausea, vomiting, somnolence, dizziness).

Rotigotine was voluntarily withdrawn from the US market in 2008 because of problems with crystal formation in the patches, and faces an uncertain future. Although it continues to be available in Europe, no timeline has been given for its reintroduction into the United States.

Levodopa

TIMING OF INITIATION OF THERAPY

CASE 57-1, QUESTION 10: L.M. has responded well to pramipexole 1.0 mg three times daily (TID) for the past 18 months, with an increased ability to paint and carry out ADLs. During the past few weeks, however, he has noticed a gradual worsening in his symptoms and once again is having difficulty holding a paintbrush. He currently complains of feeling more "tied up," he has more difficulty getting out of a chair, and his posture is slightly more stooped. He also notes that he feels tired throughout much of the day. He remains able to carry out most of his ADLs without assistance. Should levodopa be considered for the treatment of L.M.'s PD at this time?

Dopamine itself does not cross the blood–brain barrier. Levodopa, a dopamine precursor with no known pharmacologic action of its own, crosses the blood–brain barrier, where it is converted by aromatic amino acid (dopa) decarboxylase to dopamine. For patients with advancing PD, levodopa has been a mainstay of treatment since the 1960s.[53] Nearly all patients will eventually require treatment with the drug, regardless of their initial therapy. Although it is the most effective therapy for treating the rigidity and bradykinesia of PD, as with other dopaminergic agents, levodopa does not effectively improve postural instability, or reduce dementia, autonomic dysfunction, or freezing, an extreme type of akinesia that often occurs in advanced-stage disease.

The question of when to begin levodopa in the treatment of PD has been historically debated. With long-term use, the efficacy of levodopa decreases (as measured by the total on time), and the development of motor fluctuations and dyskinesias occurs. These observations led to the belief that chronic levodopa therapy may actually accelerate the neurodegenerative process through formation of free radicals generated by dopamine metabolism.[54] The Earlier versus Later Levodopa Therapy in Parkinson's Disease (ELLDOPA) study was designed to determine whether long-term use of levodopa accelerates neurodegeneration and paradoxically worsens PD.[55] The investigators of this study randomly assigned 361 patients with early PD to either carbidopa/levodopa 37.5/150 mg/day, 75/300 mg/day, or 150/600 mg/day or placebo for 40 weeks followed by a 2-week withdrawal of treatment. After 42 weeks, the severity of symptoms as measured by changes in the total UPDRS increased more in the placebo group than in all of the groups receiving levodopa. The findings of this study provide assurance that levodopa use does not result in accelerated progression of the disease based on clinical evaluations.

The optimal time to initiate levodopa therapy must be individualized. In untreated individuals, there is little reason to start levodopa until the patient reports worsening of function (socially, vocationally, or otherwise). As discussed previously, the need for levodopa therapy may be delayed by initiating therapy first with a dopamine agonist. This approach is a particular advantage in younger patients who will likely live many years with PD. In the case of L.M., he is now experiencing bothersome symptoms despite near-maximal dopamine agonist therapy, and it has progressed sufficiently to threaten his job performance. Although the dose of pramipexole could be increased, he may experience more daytime somnolence; thus, levodopa should be added to his regimen.

LEVODOPA: ADVANTAGES AND DISADVANTAGES

CASE 57-1, QUESTION 11: What are the advantages and disadvantages of carbidopa/levodopa versus levodopa alone?

Although levodopa is the most effective agent for PD, it is associated with many undesirable side effects, such as nausea, vomiting, and anorexia (50% of patients); postural hypotension (30% of patients); and cardiac arrhythmias (10% of patients).[12] In addition, mental disturbances (see Case 57-1, Question 13) are encountered in 15% of patients, and abnormal involuntary movements (dyskinesias) can be seen in up to 55% of patients during the first 6 months of levodopa treatment.[56] Because significant amounts of levodopa are peripherally (extracerebrally) metabolized to dopamine by the enzyme aromatic amino acid (dopa) decarboxylase, extremely high doses are necessary if administered alone. For this reason, levodopa is always coadministered with a dopa decarboxylase inhibitor.

By combining levodopa with a dopa decarboxylase inhibitor that does not penetrate the blood–brain barrier, a decrease in the peripheral conversion of levodopa to dopamine can be achieved, while the desired conversion within the basal ganglia remains unaffected (Fig. 57-3).[57] The two peripheral decarboxylase inhibitors in clinical use are benserazide (unavailable in the United States) and carbidopa. A fixed combination of carbidopa and levodopa is available in ratios of 1:4 (carbidopa/levodopa 25/100) and 1:10 (carbidopa/levodopa 10/100 and 25/250). A controlled-release product is available in a ratio of 25/100 and 50/200. In addition, carbidopa/levodopa is also available as an orally disintegrating tablet.

Combining carbidopa with levodopa enhances the amount of dopamine available to the brain and thereby allows the dose of levodopa to be decreased by 80%.[58] This combination also shortens the time needed to achieve optimal effects by several weeks, because carbidopa substantially decreases the often dose-limiting levodopa-induced nausea and vomiting.

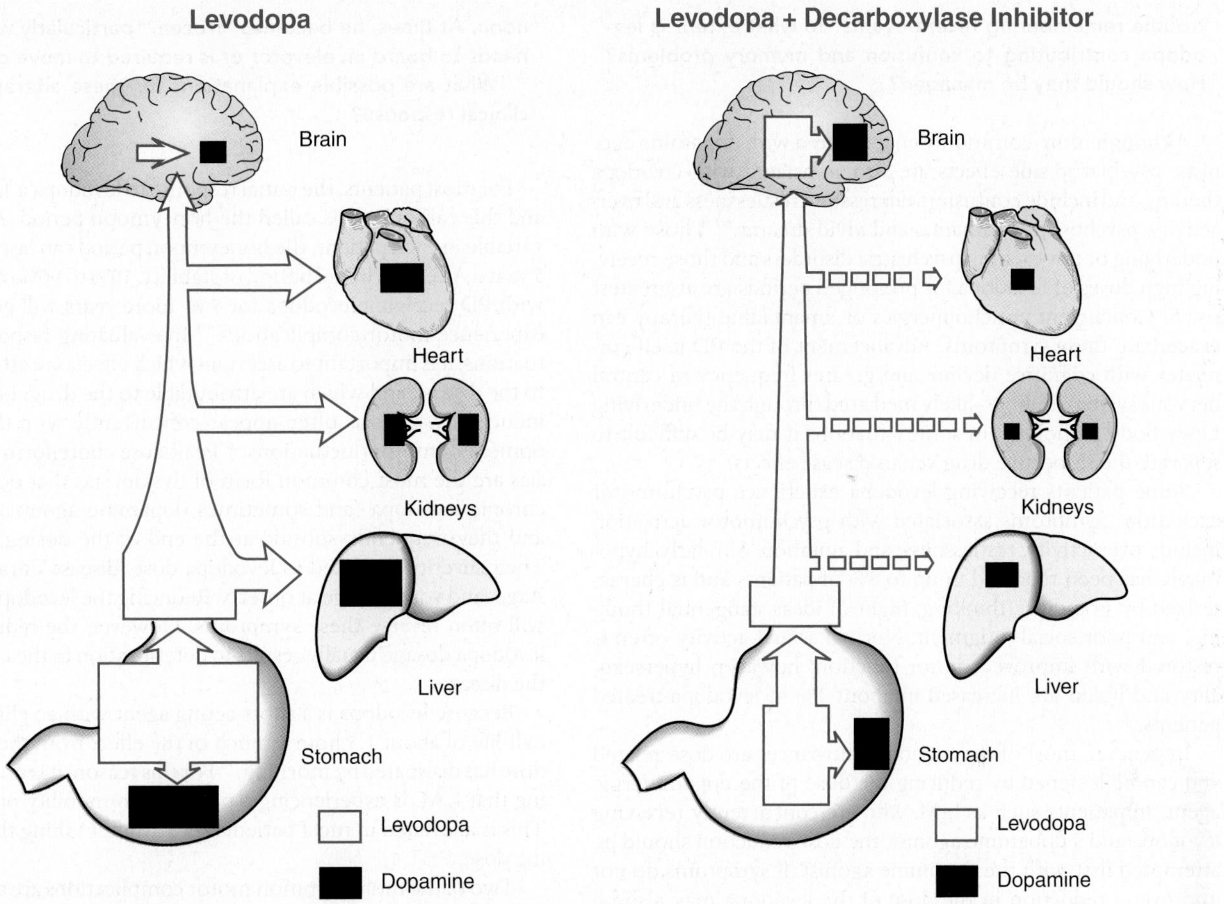

FIGURE 57-3 Peripheral decarboxylation of levodopa when given alone (*left*) and with a peripheral decarboxylase inhibitor (*right*). When combined with a decarboxylase inhibitor, less drug is required and more levodopa reaches the brain. (Reproduced with permission from Pinder RM et al. Levodopa and decarboxylase inhibitors: a review of their clinical pharmacology and use in the treatment of parkinsonism. *Drugs*. 1976;11:329.)

CARBIDOPA/LEVODOPA DOSING

CASE 57-1, QUESTION 12: The decision is made to begin L.M. on carbidopa/levodopa. How should it be dosed?

About 75 to 100 mg/day of carbidopa is necessary to saturate peripheral dopa decarboxylase.[16] It is usually unnecessary and more costly to give higher amounts of carbidopa than this. Therapy should be initiated with immediate-release carbidopa/levodopa 25/100 at a dose of one tablet three times a day. The immediate-release formulation is preferred because it allows for much easier adjustment of the levodopa dose. In L.M.'s case, the dose can then be increased by 100 mg of levodopa every day or every other day up to eight tablets (800 mg) or to the maximal effective dose, to individual requirements, or as tolerated.

If troublesome peak-dose dyskinesias occur, the following strategies should be considered: the levodopa dose can be lowered but given more frequently; consideration can be given to switching patients to immediate-release if taking controlled-release carbidopa/levodopa (for ease in refining dose adjustments); agents that prolong the half-life of levodopa but do not provide stable levodopa plasma concentrations (e.g., COMT inhibitor, MAO-B inhibitor) can be added; or an antidyskinetic agent such as amantadine can be used. The goal of optimizing therapy lies in balancing the most useful dose (i.e., maximizing the patient's on time) with that which does not produce unacceptable side effects (i.e., troublesome dyskinesias). Because L.M. is currently being treated with a dopamine agonist, he must be monitored closely for the development of motor complications with the addition of levodopa.

Most patients respond to levodopa doses of 750 to 1,000 mg/day when given with carbidopa.[16] When levodopa doses exceed 750 mg/day, patients such as L.M. can be switched from the 1:4 ratio of carbidopa/levodopa to the 1:10 ratio to prevent providing excessive amounts of decarboxylase inhibitor. For example, if L.M. needed 800 mg/day of levodopa, two carbidopa/levodopa 10/100 tablets four times daily could be given. If L.M. had not been initially treated with a dopamine agonist, some clinicians would consider adding a dopamine agonist after the daily levodopa dose has been increased to more than 600 mg because dopamine agonists directly stimulate dopamine receptors, have longer half-lives, and result in a lower incidence of dyskinesias, thus providing a smoother dopaminergic response.[16]

L.M.'s clinical response to levodopa therapy may be improved by modifying dietary amino acid ingestion.[16,59] Levodopa is actively transported across the blood–brain barrier by a large neutral amino acid transport system. This transport system also facilitates the blood-to-brain transport of amino acids such as L-leucine, L-isoleucine, L-valine, and L-phenylalanine. Levodopa and these neutral amino acids compete for transport mechanisms, and high plasma concentrations of these amino acids can decrease brain concentrations of levodopa.[59] Patients should be instructed to take immediate-release carbidopa/levodopa 30 minutes before or 60 minutes after meals for optimal efficacy.

ADVERSE EFFECTS: MENTAL CHANGES

CASE 57-1, QUESTION 13: Since initiating carbidopa/levodopa, L.M. reports he feels confused at times and has

trouble remembering recent events. To what extent is levodopa contributing to confusion and memory problems? How should they be managed?

Although more commonly encountered with dopamine agonists, psychiatric side effects are also associated with levodopa therapy, and include confusion, depression, restlessness and overactivity, psychosis, hypomania, and vivid dreams.[60] Those with underlying or pre-existing psychiatric disorders and those receiving high doses of levodopa for prolonged periods are at greatest risk.[60] Concurrent anticholinergics or amantadine therapy can exacerbate these symptoms. Advancement of the PD itself correlates with cognitive decline and greater frequency of central nervous system findings, likely mediated through the underlying Lewy body pathology. In some situations it may be difficult to separate the respective drug versus disease effects.

Some patients receiving levodopa experience psychomotor excitation. Symptoms associated with psychomotor activation include overactivity, restlessness, and agitation. Similarly, hypomania has been reported in up to 8% of patients and is characterized by grandiose thinking, flight of ideas, tangential thinking, and poor social judgment. Normal sexual activity often is restored with improved motor function; however, hypersexuality and libido are increased in about 1% of levodopa-treated patients.[60]

In general, most of the mental disturbances are dose-related and can be lessened by reducing the dose of the dopaminergic agent. In patients such as L.M. who are concurrently receiving levodopa and a dopamine agonist, the dose reduction should be attempted first with the dopamine agonist. If symptoms do not improve, a reduction in the dose of the levodopa may also be warranted. These dose reductions may, however, be impractical for L.M. because a return of parkinsonian symptoms is likely, and the benefits of levodopa therapy may outweigh the risk for mental disturbances.

Motor Complications

CASE 57-1, QUESTION 14: L.M. had a dramatic improvement in all of his parkinsonian symptoms with the initiation of levodopa therapy after being maintained on 25/250 regular carbidopa/levodopa four times a day.

For a video showing an example of the effects of dopaminergic medication on the mobility of a Parkinson patient, go to http://thepoint.lww.com/AT10e.

After 6 months of treatment, he began to experience dyskinesias. These usually occurred 1 to 2 hours after a dose and were manifested by facial grimacing, lip smacking, tongue protrusion, and rocking of the trunk. These dyskinetic effects were lessened by decreasing his pramipexole dose to 0.5 mg TID and gradually decreasing his dosage of carbidopa/levodopa to 25/250 TID.

After 3 years of levodopa therapy, more serious problems have begun to emerge. In the mornings, L.M. often experiences immobility. Nearly every day, he has periods (lasting for a few minutes) in which he cannot move, followed by a sudden switch to a fluidlike state, often associated with dyskinetic activity. He continues to take carbidopa/levodopa (25/250 TID), but gains symptomatic relief only for about 3 to 4 hours after a dose. Also, the response to a given dose varies and is often less in the afternoon. At times, he becomes "frozen," particularly when he needs to board an elevator or is required to move quickly.

What are possible explanations for these alterations in clinical response?

For most patients, the initial response to levodopa is favorable, and this early phase is called the honeymoon period. Although variable in each patient, the honeymoon period can last for up to 5 years. After this initial period of stability, 50% to 90% of patients with PD receiving levodopa for 5 or more years will eventually experience motor complications.[16] In evaluating response fluctuations, it is important to ascertain which effects are attributable to the disease and which are attributable to the drug. Levodopa-induced dyskinesias often appear concurrently with the development of motor fluctuations.[16] Peak-dose choreiform dyskinesias are the most common form of dyskinesias that occur with chronic levodopa (and sometimes dopamine agonist) therapy and they frequently subside at the end of the dosing interval. Their severity is related to levodopa dose, disease duration and stage, and younger age at onset.[61] Reducing the levodopa dosage will often reverse these symptoms. However, the reduction in levodopa dosage usually results in deterioration in the control of the disease.

Because levodopa is a short-acting agent with an elimination half-life of about 1.5 hours, much of the effect from the evening dose has dissipated by morning.[58] For this reason, it is not surprising that L.M. is experiencing a period of immobility on arising. This is alleviated in most patients shortly after taking the morning dose.

Two of the more common motor complications are the *on–off* effect and the *wearing off*, or *end-of-dose deterioration* effect. The on–off effect is described as random fluctuations from mobility (often associated with dyskinesias) to the parkinsonian state, which appear suddenly as if a switch has been turned on or off. These fluctuations can last from minutes to hours and increase in frequency and intensity with time. Although most patients prefer to be on despite accompanying dyskinesias, rather than in an off or akinetic state, dyskinesias in some patients can be more disabling than the parkinsonism.[16] Early in the course of disease, it is usually possible to adjust the amount and timing of the doses of levodopa to control parkinsonian symptoms without inducing dyskinesias; however, as the disease advances and the therapeutic window narrows, cycling between on periods complicated by dyskinesia and off periods with resulting immobility is common.[16] Eventually, despite adjustments in levodopa dose, many patients with advanced PD experience either mobility with severe dyskinesias or complete immobility. In most patients, this effect bears no clear relationship to the timing of the dose or levodopa serum levels.[62] The wearing off or end-of-dose effect is a more predictable effect that occurs at the latter part of the dosing interval after a period of relief; it can be improved by various means such as shortening the dosing interval or by adjunctive therapy with a dopamine agonist (if not already present) or levodopa extender such as a COMT inhibitor.

The pathophysiologic basis for motor complications and dyskinesias is not entirely clear, but incomplete delivery of dopamine to central receptors is likely responsible.[61] As the disease progresses, dopamine terminals are lost and the capacity to store dopamine presynaptically is diminished.[61] This dopaminergic denervation impairs the ability to maintain striatal dopamine concentrations at a relatively constant level. As a consequence, dopamine receptors are subject to intermittent or pulsatile stimulation rather than by a more natural physiologic tonic stimulation. Overactivity of excitatory pathways mediated by neurotransmitters such as glutamate may also be involved.[61] Variations in the rate and extent of levodopa absorption, dietary substrates

TABLE 57-4
Levodopa Drug Interactions

Drug	Interaction	Mechanism	Comments
Anticholinergics	↓ Levodopa effect	↓ Gastric emptying, thus ↑ degradation of levodopa in gut, and ↓ amount absorbed	Watch for ↓ levodopa effect when anticholinergics used in doses sufficient to ↓ GI motility. When anticholinergic therapy discontinued in a patient on levodopa, watch for signs of levodopa toxicity. Anticholinergics can relieve symptoms of parkinsonism and might offset the reduction of levodopa bioavailability. Overall, interaction of minor significance.
Benzodiazepines	↓ Levodopa effect	Mechanism unknown	Use together with caution; discontinue if interaction observed.
Ferrous sulfate	↓ Levodopa oral absorption by 50%	Formation of chelation complex	Avoid concomitant administration.
Food	↓ Levodopa effect	Large, neutral amino acids compete with levodopa for intestinal absorption	Although levodopa usually taken with meals to slow absorption and ↓ central emetic effect, high-protein diets should be avoided.
MAOI (e.g., phenelzine, tranylcypromine)	Hypertensive crisis	Peripheral dopamine and norepinephrine	Avoid using together; selegiline and levodopa used successfully together. Carbidopa might minimize hypertensive reaction to levodopa in patients receiving an MAOI.
Methyldopa	↑ or ↓ levodopa effect	Acts as central and peripheral decarboxylase inhibitor	Observe for response; may need to switch to another antihypertensive.
Metoclopramide	↓ Levodopa effect	Central dopamine blockade	Avoid using together.
Neuroleptics (e.g., butyrophenones, phenothiazines)	↓ Levodopa effect	Central blockade of dopamine neurotransmission	Important interaction; avoid using these drugs together.
Phenytoin	↓ Levodopa effect	Mechanism unknown	Avoid using together if possible.
Pyridoxine	↓ Levodopa effect	Peripheral decarboxylation of levodopa	Not observed when levodopa given with carbidopa.
TCA	↓ Levodopa effect	Levodopa degradation in gut because of delayed emptying	TCA and levodopa have been used successfully together; use with caution.

GI, gastrointestinal; MAOI, monoamine oxidase inhibitor; TCA, tricyclic antidepressants.

(e.g., large neutral amino acids) that compete with cerebral transport mechanisms, levodopa drug–drug interactions (Table 57-4), and competition for receptor binding by levodopa metabolites can further explain the variable responses observed to levodopa.

CASE 57-1, QUESTION 15: What options are available to reduce L.M.'s motor fluctuations?

CONTROLLED-RELEASE CARBIDOPA/LEVODOPA

A more sustained delivery of levodopa than that achieved with routine oral dosing has been suggested to reduce motor complications, because it would more effectively replicate normal physiology. Several studies have documented the efficacy of continuous infusions of levodopa in patients with advanced PD,[63,64] but this strategy is not widely used outside of research protocols. A controlled-release formulation of carbidopa/levodopa is available, containing 25 mg carbidopa and 100 mg levodopa or 50 mg carbidopa and 200 mg levodopa in an erodible polymer matrix that retards dissolution in gastric fluids. Although off time should theoretically be reduced by the slower rate of plasma levodopa decline, clinical study has generally not found a difference in off time, or a reduction in dyskinesias, with the controlled-release preparation compared with the immediate-release preparation.[65] As a result, the American Academy of Neurology Practice Parameter for treatment of motor fluctuations and dyskinesias does not recommend switching to controlled-release carbidopa/levodopa as a primary strategy to reduce off time or lessen dyskinesias.[66]

A likely reason for the lack of superior effect with controlled-release carbidopa/levodopa as compared with the regular release formulation is its variable absorption. Controlled-release carbidopa/levodopa is about 30% less bioavailable than the immediate-release formulation. Patients converted from standard carbidopa/levodopa to the controlled-release formulation should receive a dose that will provide 10% more levodopa, and then the dose should be titrated upward to clinical reponse.[16] Given that there is no obvious advantage to controlled-release carbidopa/levodopa, L.M.'s levodopa formulation should not be switched. Rather, L.M.'s condition may be improved by taking his immediate-release carbidopa/levodopa more frequently and avoiding substantial increases in the total daily dose, which could worsen his dyskinesias. Taking his morning dose before arising from bed may help with his early morning problems and prevent other response fluctuations. If L.M.'s symptoms are not improved with adjustment of his carbidopa/levodopa dose, a number of adjunctive agents such as dopamine agonists, apomorphine rescue, COMT inhibitors, and MAO-B inhibitors can be considered.

DOPAMINE AGONISTS

The effectiveness of pramipexole added to levodopa therapy in advanced PD was evaluated in a multicenter, placebo-controlled study of 360 patients with a mean disease duration of 9 years.[32] Pramipexole was titrated gradually to the maximal effective dose as tolerated, and doses did not exceed 4.5 mg/day in three divided doses. At the end of a 6-month maintenance period, patients treated with pramipexole had a 22% improvement in their ADLs ($p < 0.0001$) and a 25% improvement in their motor scores ($p < 0.01$) compared with baseline values. Patients treated with pramipexole also had a 31% improvement in the mean off time, compared with a 7% improvement in the placebo-treated group ($p < 0.0006$). Dyskinesias and hallucinations were more common in pramipexole-treated patients, and necessitated levodopa dose reduction in 76% of the pramipexole group compared with 54% in the placebo group. The total daily levodopa dose was decreased by 27% in those treated with pramipexole compared with 5% in the placebo group.

Ropinirole has also shown efficacy in improving motor scores when added to levodopa therapy in patients with advanced-stage disease.[42] In a multicenter, double-blind, randomized parallel-group study, patients treated with ropinirole experienced an average off time that was decreased by 1.9 hours daily. In those treated with ropinirole, the total daily levodopa dose was decreased by an average of 19%. At least a 35% reduction in off time and a reduction in levodopa dose were observed for 28% of ropinirole-treated patients, compared with 13% of those in the placebo group. In a study of 208 PD patients not optimally controlled with levodopa after up to 3 years of therapy with less than 600 mg/day of levodopa, a prolonged-release, once-daily formulation of ropinirole was found to improve motor scores in a similar fashion to increasing the levodopa dose; however, only 3% of ropinirole-treated subjects experienced dyskinesias compared with 17% of levodopa-treated patients ($p < 0.001$).[67] In moderate-to-advanced PD, treatment benefits were observed within 2 weeks of initiation.[68]

Because L.M. has advanced disease and is experiencing motor fluctuations despite a treatment regimen that includes a dopamine agonist, further dose adjustments of the dopamine agonist may provide little additional benefit. Any adjustments must be made with consideration of worsening his dyskinesias, and the possibility of exacerbating central nervous system adverse effects.

APOMORPHINE

Apomorphine is a dopamine agonist that is approved as rescue therapy for treatment of hypomobility or off episodes in patients with PD. It is available only in injectable form. In a randomized, double-blind, parallel-group study of 29 patients, rescue treatment with apomorphine resulted in a 34% reduction (~2 hours) in off time compared with 0% in the placebo group ($p = 0.02$).[69] Mean UPDRS motor scores were reduced by 23.9 points (62%) in those treated with apomorphine, compared with 0.1 (1%) in those receiving placebo ($p < 0.001$). Adverse events in the apomorphine group included yawning (40%), dyskinesias (35%), drowsiness or somnolence (35%), nausea or vomiting (30%), and dizziness (20%), although only yawning was statistically different from placebo (40% vs. 0%; $p = 0.03$).

Because nausea and vomiting frequently occur with apomorphine treatment, it should be administered with an antiemetic such as trimethobenzamide. The antiemetic should be started 3 days before initiating apomorphine and continued for the first 2 months of treatment.[70] Apomorphine should not be used with ondansetron and other serotonin antagonists used to treat nausea because the combination may cause severe hypotension. In addition, other antiemetics, such as prochlorperazine and metoclopramide, should not be given concurrently with apomorphine because they are dopamine antagonists and can decrease the effectiveness of apomorphine.

Doses of apomorphine range from 2 to 6 mg per subcutaneous injection. A 2-mg test dose is recommended while monitoring blood pressure. If tolerated, the recommendation is to start with a dose of 1 mg less than the tolerated test dose, and increase the dose by 1 mg every few days if needed. Peak plasma levels are observed within 10 to 60 minutes after dosing, so the onset of therapeutic effect is rapid. Two main disadvantages of apomorphine are that the test dose and titration are time-consuming and must be done under physician supervision, and that patients may require someone else to inject the drug once hypomobility has occurred. For these reasons, apomorphine is not widely used. Given that L.M. is experiencing motor fluctuations almost daily, long-term frequent apomorphine use would not be a viable solution in his situation.

AMANTADINE

The antiviral agent, amantadine, was serendipitously found to improve PD symptoms when a patient given the drug for influenza experienced a remission in her parkinsonism.[71] Amantadine reduces all the symptoms of parkinsonian disability in about 50% of patients, usually within days after starting therapy; however, long-term use is limited in many patients by the development of tachyphylaxis within 1 to 3 months.[72]

The pathophysiologic basis for amantadine's benefit in PD is not entirely understood, but it probably augments dopamine release from presynaptic nerve terminals and possibly inhibits dopamine reuptake into storage granules.[73] Anticholinergic action has also been suggested. More recently, amantadine has been found to be an antagonist at *N*-methyl-D-aspartate (NMDA) receptors and to block glutamate transmission.[74] Because excess glutamatergic activity has been implicated in the pathophysiology of dopaminergic dyskinesias, the finding of NMDA antagonism by amantadine has shifted its emphasis from use as monotherapy in early disease to that of an adjunctive agent in managing levodopa-induced dyskinesias. In several studies, amantadine has consistently shown approximately 50% reductions in dyskinesia severity and duration, without adversely impacting motor performance.[75–78] The long-term efficacy of this approach has been questioned; however, a recent study indicates benefit can persist beyond 1 year.[79]

The decision to use amantadine in L.M. should be based on whether his dyskinesias are deemed more problematic than his duration of off time. If so, amantadine should be started 100 mg/day taken at breakfast; an additional 100-mg can be taken with lunch 5 to 7 days after initiation. The dose can be increased to a maximum of 300 mg/day; however, doses in excess of 200 mg/day are associated with increased adverse effects and should be used cautiously. Amantadine is renally excreted, and the dose should be reduced in patients with renal impairment.[80] If L.M.'s dyskinesias are tolerable but the duration of off time is more problematic, then selection of another agent such as a COMT inhibitor (discussed subsequently) may be more appropriate than instituting amantadine at this time.

Side effects of amantadine mainly involve the gastrointestinal (nausea, vomiting) and central nervous systems (dizziness, confusion, insomnia, nightmares, and hallucinations). Amantadine possesses anticholinergic properties, and patients receiving concomitant anticholinergic therapy may experience more prominent central nervous system side effects.[80] Livedo reticularis, a rose-colored mottling of the skin usually involving the lower extremities, can occur with amantadine as early as 2 weeks after initiating therapy. It is believed to be caused by local release of catecholamines, which lead to vasoconstriction and alter the permeability of cutaneous blood vessels. The consequences of livedo reticularis are entirely cosmetic and discontinuation of therapy is unnecessary. Ankle edema may be seen in association with livedo reticularis. Elevation of the legs, diuretic therapy, and dosage reduction often alleviate the edema.

CATECHOL-O-METHYLTRANSFERASE INHIBITORS

COMT is an enzyme widely distributed throughout the body, and it is responsible for the biotransformation of many catechols and hydroxylated metabolites, including levodopa. When carbidopa, an inhibitor of aromatic AAD, is coadministered with levodopa, the peripheral conversion of levodopa to dopamine via this pathway is inhibited; as a consequence, the conversion of levodopa to 3-*O*-methyldopa (3-OMD) by COMT is amplified and becomes the major metabolic pathway for levodopa degradation. The metabolite 3-OMD lacks antiparkinsonian activity and may compete with levodopa for transport into the circulation and brain. The therapeutic effect of levodopa can be extended

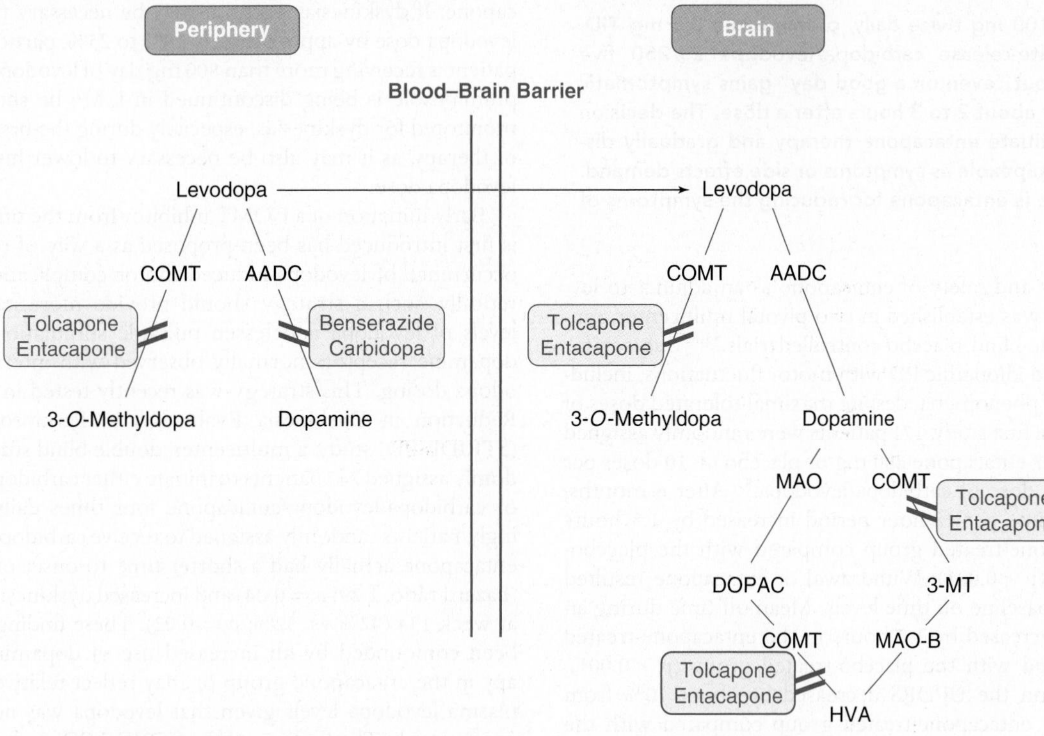

FIGURE 57-4 Levodopa metabolism in the human body. AADC, aromatic amino acid decarboxylase; COMT, catechol-*O*-methyltransferase; DOPAC, 3,4-dihydroxyphenylacetic acid; MAO, monoamine oxidase; 3-MT, 3-methoxytyramine.

by preventing its peripheral degradation though inhibition of COMT.

Entacapone and tolcapone are selective, reversible, and potent COMT inhibitors that increase the amount of levodopa available for transport across the blood–brain barrier (Fig. 57-4). This effect prolongs the response to levodopa as measured by an increase in the amount of on time and a decrease in the daily levodopa dose.[81] The pharmacologic and pharmacokinetic effects of entacapone and tolcapone are compared in Table 57-5. Tolcapone is slightly more potent and has a longer duration of action than entacapone.[82,83] Entacapone is usually given with every administration of carbidopa/levodopa (up to eight tablets per day), whereas tolcapone is dosed three times daily. Tolcapone is associated with cases of fatal, acute fulminant liver failure, which has led to stringent liver function monitoring requirements and limited clinical use. If initiated, liver function monitoring should be performed at baseline and every 2 to 4 weeks for the first 6 months, followed periodically thereafter as clinically necessary.[84] Because of the risks for hepatotoxicity associated with tolcapone, entacapone is the preferred COMT inhibitor and would be a good choice for L.M. if he desires an increase in his on time. Entacapone has a Level A evidence recommendation to reduce off time in the American Academy of Neurology Practice Parameter addressing the treatment of motor fluctuations and dyskinesias.[66]

ENTACAPONE

CASE 57-1, QUESTION 16: Six months after adjusting the frequency of his carbidopa/levodopa and adding amantadine, L.M. reports that his dyskinesias are not too bothersome, but he is having increased periods (lasting a few minutes) in which he cannot move. He is currently taking

TABLE 57-5

Pharmacologic and Pharmacokinetic Properties of Catechol-*O*-Methyltransferase Inhibitors

	Tolcapone	Entacapone
Bioavailability	65%	30%–46%
T_{max} (hours)	2.0	0.7–1.2
Protein binding	99.9%	98%
Metabolism	Glucuronidation; CYP3A4, 2CYPA6 Acetylation; methylated by COMT	Glucuronidation
Half-life (hours)	2–3	1.6–3.4
Time to reverse COMT inhibition (hours)	16–24	4–8
Maximal COMT inhibition at 200-mg dose	80%–90%	60%
Increase in levodopa AUC	100%	30%–45%
Increase in levodopa half-life	75%	60%–75%
Dosing method	TID, spaced 6 hours apart	With every administration of levodopa

AUC, area under the curve; COMT, catechol-O-methyltransferase; CYP, cytochrome P-450; TID, three times daily.

amantadine 100 mg twice daily, pramipexole 0.5 mg TID, and immediate-release carbidopa/levodopa 25/250 five times a day, but "even on a good day" gains symptomatic relief for only about 2 to 3 hours after a dose. The decision is made to initiate entacapone therapy and gradually discontinue pramipexole as symptoms or side effects demand. How effective is entacapone for reducing the symptoms of PD?

The efficacy and safety of entacapone as an adjunct to levodopa therapy was established in two pivotal multicenter, randomized, double-blind, placebo-controlled trials.[85,86] Subjects for both studies had idiopathic PD with motor fluctuations, including wearing off phenomena, despite maximal tolerated doses of levodopa. In the first study, 171 patients were randomly assigned to receive either entacapone 200 mg or placebo (4–10 doses per day) with each dose of carbidopa/levodopa.[85] After 6 months, the mean on time per 18-hour period increased by 1.5 hours in the entacapone-treated group compared with the placebo-treated group ($p < 0.001$). Withdrawal of entacapone resulted in a return to baseline on time levels. Mean off time during an 18-hour day decreased by 1.2 hours in the entacapone-treated group compared with the placebo-treated group ($p < 0.001$). Motor scores on the UPDRS decreased by about 10% from baseline in the entacapone-treated group compared with the placebo group ($p < 0.01$). Improvements of approximately 10% to 20% in these motor scores usually produce clinically significant improvements as indicated by increased functional capacity and decreased parkinsonian symptoms (bradykinesia and rigidity). Patients who received entacapone could also lower their levodopa daily dose by an average of 79 mg, whereas placebo-treated subjects required an increase of 12 mg in their average daily levodopa dose ($p < 0.001$). A 3-year open-label extension of this trial demonstrated continued efficacy and tolerability of entacapone.[87]

In the second study, 205 patients were randomly assigned to receive either entacapone 200 mg or placebo (up to 10 doses per day) with each dose of carbidopa/levodopa.[86] At baseline, patients had experienced about 4 years of motor fluctuations and had been taking levodopa for about 9 years. Approximately 80% of the study subjects continued to take other antiparkinsonian therapies, including anticholinergic agents, selegiline, dopamine agonists, and amantadine. Compared with placebo over the course of 8 to 24 weeks, daily on time increased by about 1 hour ($p < 0.05$) in patients treated with entacapone, with the greatest improvements observed in those who had a smaller percentage of on time at baseline. Those treated with entacapone also had about a 10% reduction in their total UPDRS scores, and they decreased their daily levodopa dose by about 100 mg (13%).

Dosing

CASE 57-1, QUESTION 17: When should entacapone be initiated, and what is the most effective method for dosing the drug? If initiated at the same time as levodopa, can it prevent the onset of levodopa-induced dyskinesias?

Entacapone is approved for use as adjunctive therapy to levodopa for the treatment of PD in patients experiencing wearing-off or end-of-dose deterioration. It is not necessary to titrate the dose; rather, it is given as one 200-mg tablet with each carbidopa/levodopa administration, up to eight tablets per day. It is available in a combination tablet with a 1 : 4 ratio of immediate-release carbidopa/levodopa that patients can be switched to once they are stabilized individually on carbidopa/levodopa and entacapone. If dyskinesias occur, it may be necessary to lower the levodopa dose by approximately 10% to 25%, particularly if the patient is receiving more than 800 mg/day of levodopa. Although pramipexole is being discontinued in L.M., he should still be monitored for dyskinesias, especially during the first few weeks of therapy, as it may also be necessary to lower his carbidopa/levodopa dose.

Early initiation of a COMT inhibitor from the time levodopa is first introduced has been proposed as a way of reducing the occurrence of levodopa-induced motor complications[88]; theoretically, such a strategy should provide more-stable plasma levels of levodopa and lessen pulsatile stimulation of striatal dopamine receptors normally observed with intermittent levodopa dosing. This strategy was recently tested in the Stalevo Reduction in Dyskinesia Evaluation in Parkinson's Disease (STRIDE-PD) study, a multicenter, double-blind study that randomly assigned 747 patients to initiate either carbidopa/levodopa or carbidopa/levodopa/entacapone four times daily.[88] Surprisingly, patients randomly assigned to receive carbidopa/levodopa/entacapone actually had a shorter time to onset of dyskinesia (hazard ratio, 1.29; $p = 0.04$) and increased dyskinesia frequency at week 134 (42% vs. 32%; $p = 0.02$). These findings may have been confounded by an increased use of dopaminergic therapy in the entacapone group or may reflect relatively unstable plasma levodopa levels given that levodopa was not delivered continuously. The findings of the STRIDE-PD study do not support the early administration of entacapone in combination with levodopa to reduce the occurrence of motor complications.

Adverse Effects

CASE 57-1, QUESTION 18: What are the adverse effects of entacapone, and how should they be managed?

Most entacapone-induced adverse effects are consistent with increased levodopa exposure. They include dyskinesias (50%–60%), nausea (15%–20%), dizziness (10%–25%), and hallucinations (1%–14%).[85,86] Reducing the levodopa dosage by 10% to 15% as a strategy for circumventing these effects was successful in about one-third of patients experiencing dyskinesias. Other adverse effects related to entacapone include urine discoloration (11%–40%), abdominal pain (6%), and diarrhea (10%).[85,86] Urine discoloration (brownish-orange) is attributed to entacapone and its metabolites and is considered benign, but patients should be counseled regarding this effect to avoid undue concern. The most common reason for withdrawal from clinical studies and discontinuation of therapy was severe diarrhea (2.5%). No monitoring of liver function tests is required during entacapone therapy.

Recently, the Food and Drug Administration notified health care professionals that it is undertaking a meta-analysis to examine the cardiovascular risks associated with entacapone.[89] This action was prompted by an evaluation of data from the STRIDE-PD study, which indicated that patients taking the combination carbidopa/levodopa/entacapone may be at an increased risk for cardiovascular events (heart attack, stroke, and cardiovascular death) compared with those taking carbidopa/levodopa.

Monoamine Oxidase-B Inhibitors

SELEGILINE AND RASAGILINE

CASE 57-2

QUESTION 1: K.B. is a 61-year-old woman who presents to the movement disorders clinic after referral from her family doctor for a presumptive diagnosis of PD. She is Hoehn

and Yahr stage 1, with slightly decreased arm swing on the left side and unilateral resting hand tremor. Her past medical history is significant for hypertension and mild renal insufficiency (serum creatinine of 1.4 mg/dL), likely owing to the fact that she was born with only one functioning kidney. Since her initial visit with her family physician, she has been researching information about different PD treatments from several PD-related websites. She is particularly interested today in learning more about possible neuroprotective effects of medications for PD. What role do MAO-B inhibitors have in the treatment of PD, and is there any evidence for neuroprotection?

The development of effective disease-modifying therapies for PD is largely precluded by the inability to readily identify individuals in the presymptomatic state. By the time patients present with clinical symptoms, substantial neuropathology has accumulated during the long preclinical evolution of the disease; an ability to recognize PD at an earlier stage would be a major breakthrough. A number of agents have exhibited neuroprotective effects in animal models, but none have had a clear impact on clinical outcomes in human studies.[90]

SELEGILINE

Selegiline (also referred to as deprenyl) is an irreversible inhibitor of MAO type B, a major enzymatic pathway responsible for the metabolism of dopamine in the brain.[91] The discovery of MPTP fostered the development of animal models in which it was found that the neurotoxicity associated with MPTP is not directly caused by MPTP itself, but rather the oxidized product, L-methyl-4-phenylpyridinium (MPP).[92] The conversion to MPP is a two-step process mediated in part by MAO-B. Inhibition of MAO-B can inhibit the oxidative conversion of dopamine to potentially reactive peroxides. In animals, pretreatment with selegiline protects against neuronal damage after the administration of MPTP.[93]

The Deprenyl and Tocopherol Antioxidative Therapy of Parkinsonism (DATATOP) study was designed to test the hypothesis that the combined use of selegiline and an antioxidant (α-tocopherol) early in the course of the disease may slow disease progression.[94] The primary outcome was the length of time that patients could be sustained without levodopa therapy (an indication of disease progression). Early treatment with selegiline 10 mg/day delayed the need to start levodopa therapy by approximately 9 months compared with patients given placebo; however, long-term observation showed that the benefits of selegiline were not sustained and diminished with time. During an additional year of observation, patients originally randomly assigned to selegiline tended to reach the end point of disability even more quickly than did those not assigned to receive selegiline. Initial selegiline treatment did not alter the development of levodopa's adverse effects such as dyskinesias and wearing-off and on–off phenomena.

Although selegiline does not appear to have neuroprotective effects in humans, it may have a role as a symptomatic adjunct to levodopa in more advanced disease. Studies have found improvement in the wearing off effect of levodopa in 50% to 70% of patients treated with selegiline and a reduction in as much as 30% in the total daily dose of levodopa.[95,96] The on–off effect is less responsive to the addition of selegiline.

Selegiline is available in a 5-mg capsule or tablet, and as a 1.25-mg orally disintegrating tablet. It is also available in a transdermal patch, but this formulation is not approved for use in PD (approved for treatment of depression). The bioavailability of conventional selegiline is low, and it undergoes extensive hepatic first-pass metabolism into amphetamine-based metabolites, which have been hypothesized to be neurotoxic.[91] The usual dosage of conventional selegiline is 10 mg/day given in 5-mg doses in the morning and early afternoon. It is not given in the evening because excess stimulation from metabolites (L-methamphetamine and L-amphetamine) can cause insomnia and other psychiatric side effects.[91] The orally disintegrating tablet formulation dissolves in the mouth on contact with saliva and undergoes pregastric absorption. This is an improvement over conventional selegiline because it minimizes the effect of first-pass metabolism and results in higher plasma concentrations of selegiline and reductions in the amphetamine-based metabolites.[97] Indeed, this formulation was shown to reduce off time by 32% (2.2 hours) compared with 9% (0.6 hours) for placebo in a 12-week, randomized, multicenter, parallel group, double-blind study.[98] Because selegiline selectively binds to MAO-B in usual doses ($\leq$10 mg/day), it does not produce a hypertensive reaction ("cheese effect") with dietary tyramine or other catecholamines. It is still recommended, however, that patients be counseled regarding this potential risk.

RASAGILINE

Rasagiline is a second-generation, propargylamine-type irreversible selective inhibitor of MAO-B. It is indicated as monotherapy in early disease or as adjunct therapy to levodopa in advanced disease. Rasagiline is differentiated from selegiline primarily in that it is a more potent inhibitor of MAO-B, and it is not metabolized into amphetamine-based metabolites.[99] Like selegiline, rasagiline has also been found to protect from MPTP-induced parkinsonism in animal models.[100]

Rasagiline was studied as monotherapy in early PD in a randomized, double-blind, placebo-controlled trial comparing rasagiline 1 mg ($n = 134$) or 2 mg ($n = 132$) daily with placebo ($n = 138$). After 6 months of therapy, the mean adjusted change in UPDRS scores compared with placebo were –4.2 and –3.56 in the 1- and 2-mg groups, respectively ($p < 0.001$ for both).[101] These changes are quantitatively similar to those observed with levodopa therapy. This study used a delayed-start design, wherein at the end of the initial 6 months of treatment, patients who received placebo were then switched over to receive active treatment with rasagiline, and the rasagiline-treated patients continued on therapy. After an additional 6 months of study, it was found that patients receiving rasagiline for all 12 months had less functional decline than patients in whom rasagiline was delayed.[102] The mean adjusted difference at 12 months for patients receiving rasagiline 2 mg/day for all 12 months was –2.29 compared with the delayed-start rasagiline 2-mg group ($p = 0.01$). These encouraging findings suggested that neuroprotection might be afforded by rasagiline, and prompted a larger, more definitive study.

The Attenuation of Disease Progression with Azilect Given Once-daily (ADIAGO) study was conducted in follow-up to the earlier findings that suggested the possibility of neuroprotection with rasagiline. This was also a randomized, placebo-controlled trial using the delayed-start methodology, but with a much larger sample size ($n = 1{,}176$).[103] Patients were randomly assigned to receive rasagiline (either 1 or 2 mg/day) or placebo for 36 weeks. At 36 weeks, rasagiline-treated subjects continued therapy, and the placebo group was switched to either 1 or 2 mg/day of rasagiline; all patients were then followed for an additional 36 weeks. To prove disease modification attributable to rasagiline with either dose, the early-start treatment group had to meet each of three hierarchical end points, based on magnitude and rate of change of UPDRS scores during different periods of the study. At the end of the study, the early-start group receiving rasagiline 1 mg/day met all end points, suggesting a possible disease-modifying effect, but the 2-mg dose failed to meet all three of the required end points. The inconsistency between doses led the authors to state that they could not definitively conclude that rasagiline 1 mg/day has disease-modifying effects.[103]

Rasagiline has also been studied as an adjunct to levodopa in advanced disease. When added to levodopa therapy, rasagiline can improve motor fluctuations, reducing off time by 1.4 hours and 1.8 hours compared with 0.9 hours for placebo ($p = 0.02$ and $p < 0.0001$ for 0.5- and 1-mg/day groups, respectively).[104] Significant improvements were reported in the UPDRS subscores for ADLs in the off state and motor performance in the on state, as well as clinician global assessments. Dyskinesias were slightly worsened in the 1-mg/day group. As adjunctive therapy to levodopa, rasagiline appears to provide similar benefit to entacapone, and is also given a Level A evidence rating for reducing off time in the Practice Parameter addressing motor fluctuations and dyskinesias.[66] When compared with entacapone 200 mg administered with each levodopa dose, rasagiline 1 mg/day reduced total daily off time in a similar manner (decrease of 21% or 1.18 hours for rasagiline and 21% or 1.2 hours for entacapone).[105]

Rasagiline is available in 0.5- and 1-mg tablets. When used as monotherapy, it is initiated at 1 mg daily. When combined with levodopa, the initial dose is lowered to 0.5 mg daily, and can be increased to 1 mg daily based on response. Although tyramine-challenge studies have not demonstrated any clinically significant reactions, the product labeling still contains a warning that patients should be advised to restrict tyramine intake.[106,107] Rasagiline is well-tolerated; headache, dizziness, and nausea appear to be the most common adverse effects when rasagiline is given as monotherapy.[107] Reduction of levodopa dose may be necessary if dyskinesias occur when rasagiline is added in combination to levodopa. Similar precautions regarding drug interactions exist with rasagiline as selegiline; that is, sympathomimetics, meperidine, dextromethorphan, other MAO inhibitors, and selective serotonin reuptake inhibitors (SSRI) should be avoided or used with caution. Because rasagiline is metabolized by CYP1A2, inhibitors such as ciprofloxacin may increase plasma concentrations of rasagiline.

The search for agents capable of clinically apparent neuroprotection remains a primary focus in the management of PD. The disappointing legacy of selegiline and the ambiguity of the ADIAGO study results with rasagiline underscore the fact that overt and tangible neuroprotective effects of PD therapies remain elusive. Nevertheless, given the efficacy of rasagiline in early disease, it would be a reasonable agent to try in a patient such as K.B. who presents very early in her disease course and seeks a possible neuroprotective agent. Depending on her degree of functional impairment caused by the tremor, additional therapy may be necessary.

Anticholinergics

CASE 57-2, QUESTION 2: Should K.B. receive an anticholinergic agent? What role do anticholinergic drugs play in the treatment of P.D.?

Anticholinergic drugs have been used to treat PD since the mid-1800s, when it was discovered that symptoms were reduced by the belladonna derivative hyoscyamine sulfate (scopolamine).[16] These drugs work by blocking the excitatory neurotransmitter acetylcholine in the striatum, which minimizes the effect of the relative increase in cholinergic sensitivity. Until the late 1960s, when amantadine and levodopa were introduced, anticholinergics were a mainstay of treatment; however, because of their undesirable side effect profile and poor efficacy relative to levodopa in treating bradykinesia and rigidity, anticholinergic agents are no longer used as first-line agents. Instead, they are usually reserved for the treatment of resting tremor early in the disease, particularly in younger patients with preserved cognitive function. Given her history and clinical presentation, K.B. would probably benefit from an anticholinergic drug such as trihexyphenidyl 1 mg/day.

K.B. should be observed carefully for adverse effects on initiation of an anticholinergic. These drugs produce both peripherally and centrally mediated adverse effects. Peripheral effects, such as dry mouth, blurred vision, constipation, and urinary retention, are common and bothersome.[16] Anticholinergic agents can increase intraocular pressure and should be avoided in patients with angle-closure glaucoma. Central nervous system effects can include confusion, impairment of recent memory, hallucinations, and delusions.[16] Patients with PD are more susceptible to these central effects because of advanced age, intercurrent illnesses, and impaired cognition.[16] As K.B.'s disease eventually progresses and she develops other nonmotor complications, the benefit versus risk of anticholinergic therapy should be periodically re-evaluated.

Investigational Pharmacotherapy

CASE 57-2, QUESTION 3: Are there any antioxidants, dietary supplements, or other investigational therapies that may benefit K.B.?

ANTIOXIDANTS

Antioxidants have been hypothesized to benefit patients with PD through their ability to act as free radical scavengers. The most comprehensive evaluation of antioxidant therapy for PD comes again from the DATATOP study.[95,108,109] In this study, patients were assigned to one of four treatment regimens: α-tocopherol (2,000 international units/day) and selegiline placebo; selegiline 10 mg/day and α-tocopherol placebo; selegiline and α-tocopherol active treatments; or dual placebos. The primary end point was time to requirement of levodopa therapy. After approximately 14 months of follow-up, no difference was seen between the α-tocopherol group and placebo group in time to require levodopa.[109] Thus, despite the theoretic benefit, clinical data are lacking to support the routine use of α-tocopherol, and it would not be recommended in K.B.[17]

COENZYME Q10

Coenzyme Q10 (CoQ_{10}) is an antioxidant involved in the mitochondrial electron transport chain, and has been shown to have reduced levels in patients with PD.[110] The finding that MPTP can induce parkinsonism through inhibition of complex I in the mitochondrial electron transport chain led to the hypothesis that supplementation with CoQ_{10} may help restore dysfunctional mitochondria.[111] Early results in a trial of 80 patients with untreated PD, randomly assigned to placebo or CoQ_{10} at dosages of 300, 600, or 1,200 mg/day in four divided doses, were promising.[112] Subjects were followed for up to 16 months or until therapy with levodopa was required. The primary outcome was a change in total score on the UPDRS from baseline to the last visit. Total UPDRS scores increased (indicating worsening of symptoms) to a greater extent in placebo-treated patients than in those treated with CoQ_{10} (+11.99 for placebo, +8.81 for 300 mg/day, +10.82 for 600 mg/day, and +6.69 for 1,200 mg/day).

A larger study was undertaken in follow-up, using a futility design, randomly assigning 213 untreated PD patients to CoQ_{10} 600 mg four times daily or placebo.[113] The primary outcome measure was the mean change in total UPDRS score from baseline to either the time required for symptomatic therapy or 12 months, whichever came first. The threshold value for futility of CoQ_{10} was defined as 30% less progression on the total UPDRS than the 10.65-unit change observed historically in the placebo arm of the DATATOP trial, or 7.46. After 12 months of therapy, the mean change in the CoQ_{10} group was 7.52 compared with 6.31 in the placebo group. Based on the prespecified criteria, although CoQ_{10} did not meet the prespecified end point of a change of 7.46 or less, it could not be rejected as futile and met criteria for further clinical testing. Further testing of CoQ_{10} in phase 3 trials is currently being conducted. In the meantime, given the small likelihood of harm from CoQ_{10}, K.B. can be counseled about the possibility for modest benefits and advised to make an informed decision about using it.

CREATINE AND MINOCYCLINE

Similar to the theory for efficacy of CoQ_{10}, creatine plays a role in mitochondrial energy production and has been shown to protect from MPTP-induced dopamine depletion in animal models.[114] Minocycline is an anti-infective agent that also displays anti-inflammatory effects, and is hypothesized to alter the neuroinflammatory response that occurs as dopaminergic neurons are lost in PD. Minocycline has been shown to be protective in MPTP animal models of PD.[115]

The use of both creatine and minocycline in PD was examined in a futility-design study, in which 200 patients with early PD not requiring therapy were randomly assigned to receive creatine ($n = 67$) 10 g/day, minocycline 200 mg/day ($n = 66$), or placebo ($n = 67$).[116] The study was identically designed to the CoQ_{10} study discussed previously and used the same primary end points. After 12 months, the mean change in the total UPDRS was 5.6 units in the creatine group, 7.09 in the minocycline group, and 8.39 in the placebo group. Based on the prespecified criteria, neither creatine nor minocycline could be rejected as futile and met criteria for further clinical testing. Additional studies of these agents are currently ongoing. Given the unresolved issues surrounding the induction of antibiotic resistance with long-term use of an agent such as minocycline, it should be avoided in K.B. Likewise, given her mild renal insufficiency, she should also be advised to avoid creatine.

Surgical Therapies for PD

CASE 57-3

QUESTION 1: S.L. is a 68-year-old man with a 10-year history of PD, now considered to be in Hoehn and Yahr late stage 3. His current regimen includes sustained-release carbidopa/levodopa 50/200 mg twice daily, immediate-release carbidopa/levodopa 25/100 mg TID, ropinirole 2 mg TID, and amantadine 100 mg twice daily. S.L.'s overall control of his PD has diminished greatly in the last couple of months. His on time averages around 6 hours/day, with the majority of it accompanied by troublesome dyskinesias. Most days he needs some assistance with ADLs. His cognitive function remains well preserved, and he is not depressed. He has heard about surgical procedures that might benefit patients with PD. Is surgical therapy superior to medical therapy in patients with advanced PD?

Two types of surgical therapies have been used in patients with advanced PD who cannot be adequately controlled with medications. The first involves making an irreversible surgical lesion in a specific location in the brain (e.g., posteroventral pallidotomy or stereotaxic thalamotomy); the second involves surgical implan-

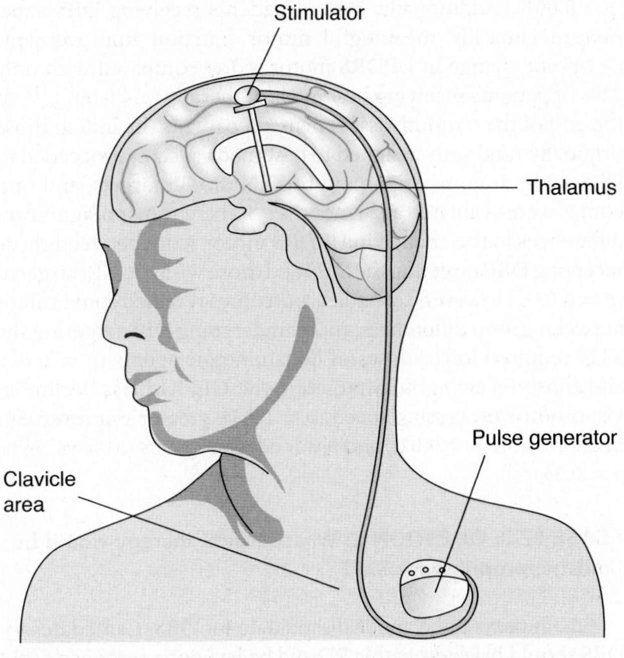

FIGURE 57-5 Deep brain stimulation. A pulse generator, surgically implanted in a pouch beneath the clavicle, sends high-frequency electrical impulses to the thalamus, thereby blocking the nerve pathways associated with tremors in Parkinson disease. (Adapted with permission from Smeltzer SC, Bare BG. *Textbook of Medical-Surgical Nursing*. 9th ed. Philadelphia, PA: Lippincott Williams & Wilkins; 2000.)

tation of a device that sends electrical impulses to specific parts of the brain (e.g., deep brain stimulation [DBS]) (Fig. 57-5). Posteroventral pallidotomy has been shown to reduce dyskinesias on the contralateral side and may permit the use of higher dosages of levodopa for managing rigidity and bradykinesia.[117] However, a significant disadvantage is the need to make a lesion near the optic tract, which may risk visual loss. Other possible risks of pallidotomy include weakness, paralysis, and hemorrhage that can cause stroke and speech difficulty. Stereotaxic thalamotomy has been shown to reduce symptoms of debilitating tremor and improve rigidity in patients with PD.[118] This intervention has eliminated contralateral tremor in 80% of patients, and improvement has been sustained for up to 10 years. However, as with pallidotomy, a disadvantage of thalamotomy is the need to make an irreversible lesion in the basal ganglia that may limit the effectiveness of newer procedures as they become available. Thus, DBS is now the preferred surgical method for treating advanced PD that cannot be adequately controlled with medications. DBS uses an implanted electrode in the brain, in either the subthalamic nucleus (STN) or the globus pallidus interna (GPi), that is connected to a subcutaneously implanted pacemaker. This permits delivery of a high-frequency stimulation to the desired target. Advantages of DBS include no need for an irreversible brain lesion, and it provides flexibility for altering the target site and program stimulation parameters.

The efficacy of DBS in advanced PD was shown in a two-part study of 255 patients with idiopathic PD responsive to levodopa but with persistent and disabling motor symptoms.[119] Patients were randomly assigned to DBS (further randomly assigned to either STN or GPi targets) or best medical therapy (management by movement disorders specialists) and followed for 6 months for the primary outcome of time spent in the on state without troubling dyskinesias. Patients receiving DBS gained a mean of 4.6 hours/day of on time without troubling dyskinesias compared with 0 hours/day for best medical therapy

($p < 0.001$). Additionally, 71% of patients receiving DBS experienced clinically meaningful motor function improvements (≥5-point change in UPDRS motor score) compared with only 32% of patients receiving best medical therapy ($p < 0.001$).[119] At the end of the 6 month assessment, all patients (including those originally randomly assigned to best medical care) proceeded to DBS with random assignment to STN or GPi targets, and outcomes were evaluated at 24 months.[120] There were no significant differences in the change in UPDRS motor score between those receiving DBP targeting the STN and those with the GPi targeted ($p = 0.05$). However, secondary outcomes revealed some minor between-group differences; those undergoing DBS targeting the STN required lower doses of dopaminergic agents ($p = 0.02$), and those receiving DBS targeting the GPi had less decline in visuomotor processing speed ($p = 0.03$), greater improvement in depression ($p = 0.02$), and fewer adverse events (51% vs. 56%; $p = 0.35$).[120]

CASE 57-3, QUESTION 2: What surgical therapy would be most appropriate for S.L.?

S.L. appears to be an ideal candidate for DBS. Candidates for DBS should have idiopathic PD and be levodopa-responsive, but continue to experience motor complications or tremor despite optimal pharmacotherapeutic regimens. Ideally, DBS should be avoided in patients with pre-existing cognitive or psychiatric problems owing to a slight risk of decline in cognition. No strict age limitation for DBS exists, but patients younger than 70 years of age, such as S.L., appear to recover from surgery more quickly and show greater motor improvements. Although both the GPi and STN would be acceptable targets of therapy in S.L., nonmotor factors may be considered when selecting the surgical target for DBS. DBS of the STN consistently demonstrates marked reduction in the need for escalating levodopa dosages compared with DBS of the GPi,[120–123] but the results of the most recent comparative trial suggest other nonmotor symptoms may be affected more favorably when targeting the GPi.[120]

Treatment of Nonmotor Symptoms of Parkinson Disease

Although PD is mostly recognized for its cardinal features of motor dysfunction, nonmotor symptoms are an important part of the disease throughout all stages and a key determinant of quality of life.[124] More than 98% of patients with PD have at least one nonmotor symptom; the average per patient is nearly eight, with the number and impact increasing in parallel with disease duration and severity.[125] Common nonmotor symptoms include autonomic dysfunction (gastrointestinal disorders, orthostatic hypotension, sexual dysfunction, urinary incontinence), sleep disorders (restless leg syndrome, periodic limb movements of sleep, excessive daytime somnolence, insomnia, rapid eye movement [REM] sleep behavior disorder), fatigue, and anxiety.[125] In one longitudinal study of patients with PD, the most common nonmotor symptoms were psychiatric symptoms (68%, most commonly anxiety), fatigue (58%), leg pain (38%), insomnia (37%), urinary symptoms (35%), drooling (31%), and difficulty concentrating (31%).[125] The management of several commonly encountered nonmotor symptoms are reviewed below. Table 57-6 summarizes pharmacological treatments for several nonmotor symptoms of PD.

DEMENTIA

CASE 57-4

QUESTION 1: J.D. is a 74-year-old man with advanced PD, Hoehn and Yahr stage 4. During the last year, his family has noticed that he is increasingly forgetful and anxious. Twice recently, he left home alone for brief periods, and called

TABLE 57-6

Summary of Pharmacological Treatments for Common Nonmotor Symptoms of Parkinson Disease[10,18,124,126]

Domain	Symptom	Possible Treatments	Adverse Effect Considerations
Cognitive	Dementia	Rivastigmine, donepezil	Deterioration of motor function (tremor), sialorrhea, excessive lacrimation, incontinence, nausea, vomiting, and orthostasis
Psychiatric	Depression	Dopamine agonists (pramipexole), TCAs (amitriptyline, desipramine, nortriptyline), SSRIs (citalopram, paroxetine)	Impulse control disorders (dopamine agonists); anticholinergic adverse effects (TCAs) on cognition, urinary symptoms, autonomic nervous system (orthostasis, falls); tremorogenic (SSRIs)
	Anxiety	Benzodiazepines	Decreased attention, cognition; increased risk of falls
	Psychosis	Clozapine, quetiapine	White cell count monitoring for clozapine (agranulocytosis)
Autonomic	Falls	If possible, avoid using medications that increase risk of falls	N/A
	Erectile dysfunction	Sildenafil	N/A
	Constipation	Polyethylene glycol, fiber, stool softeners	N/A
	Drooling	Botulinum toxin, glycopyrrolate	Focal weakness
	Orthostatic hypotension	Midodrine, fludrocortisone	Hypertension, piloerection (midodrine)
Sleep	Excessive daytime sleepiness	Modafinil	Dizziness, insomnia, anxiety
	Insomnia	Melatonin, benzodiazepines	Sedation, dizziness, falls, ataxia, cognitive dysfunction (benzodiazepines)
	Periodic limb movements of sleep	Carbidopa/levodopa, dopamine agonists	Impulse control disorders, psychosis
Miscellaneous	Fatigue	Methylphenidate	Tachycardia, weight loss, nausea

N/A, not applicable; SSRI, selective serotonin reuptake inhibitor; TCA, tricyclic antidepressant.

9-1-1 because he thought someone was trying to break into the house. He also calls his daughter two or three times each day, often repeating the same questions and forgetting that he called her earlier. His wife is his primary caregiver, and he is nearly entirely reliant on her for help in performing ADLs. He scored 20 (below normal) on his most recent Mini-Mental Status Examination, and his family reports that he is no longer interested in social activities or hobbies. Neuropsychiatric testing is performed and demonstrates a significant depressive component to his dementia. Subsequent recommendations from the neuropsychiatrist are that he receive 24-hour supervision, along with participation in structured leisure activities, such as adult day-care, several hours per week to help relieve his wife's caregiver burden. How should J.D.'s progressive cognitive decline be treated?

The prevalence of dementia in patients with PD increases with age and duration of disease and is approximately 6- to 12-fold greater than in age-matched control subjects.[16] One longitudinal study of 136 incident cases of PD followed for 20 years found that nearly 100% eventually exhibited dementia.[127] Successful management of cognitive impairment in patients with PD first requires that all potentially reversible causes and underlying contributing factors be addressed. These include treating infections, dehydration, and metabolic abnormalities, as well as eliminating unnecessary medications (particularly anticholinergics, sedatives, anxiolytics) that can exacerbate dementia or delirium.

Experience with cholinesterase inhibitors such as donepezil and rivastigmine for treating cognitive impairment in PD indicates marginal improvements with their use.[128–130] Outcomes of these studies are measured using a variety of scales, such as the Mini Mental Status Examination, the Alzheimer's Disease Assessment Scale—Cognitive Subscale, the Alzheimer's Disease Assessment Scale—Clinician's Global Impression of Change, and the Clinician's Interview-Based Impression of Change Plus Caregiver Input. Compared with placebo, the cholinesterase inhibitors often result in a statistically significant change of a couple of points in these scales. It is unclear, however, to what extent the changes in the scores of these outcome measures are clinically relevant in such areas as ability to perform ADLs without assistance and delay in nursing home placement.

Although the American Academy of Neurology Practice Parameter addressing depression, psychosis, and dementia in PD suggests that either donepezil or rivastigmine can be considered for patients such as J.D.,[18] he must be monitored closely for signs of deterioration of motor function such as worsening of tremor. Cholinesterase inhibitors are associated with other adverse events that may be overlooked and attributed to the PD itself, including sialorrhea, excessive lacrimation, incontinence, nausea, vomiting, and orthostasis. Perhaps more important than any medication therapy, adequate social support for J.D. should be ensured. As he becomes further dependent on family members for assistance with ADLs, the increased needs of the caregiver(s) should also be considered. In J.D.'s case, attending adult day-care several times weekly, if available, would provide a structured, supervised environment for interaction with others, as well as providing a rest period for his caregiver. Dementia is a leading cause of nursing home placement for patients with PD.[18]

DEPRESSION/ANXIETY

CASE 57-4, QUESTION 2: How should J.D.'s anxiety and depression be treated?

Despite being one of the strongest predictors of quality of life in PD patients, depression is often poorly recognized and inadequately treated.[131,132] This is likely because of the fact that depression and PD share overlapping features that often confound the identification of depression. Such features may include withdrawal, lack of motivation, flattened affect, decreased physical activity, or bradyphrenia.[18]

Treatment of depression in PD should first focus on providing adequate treatment of the symptoms of PD by attempting to restore mobility and independence, particularly in patients whose depression can be attributed to lengthy off periods. Antiparkinson drugs, such as pramipexole, can be associated with mood-enhancing effects independent of their ability to reduce time in the off state.[133,134] Small trials and case reports have shown that depression in patients with PD can be successfully treated with antidepressant drugs, including tricyclic agents such as amitriptyline, desipramine, nortriptyline, bupropion, and SSRIs such as citalopram and paroxetine.[18,135,136] Given the overall lack of controlled trials, it is difficult to know whether expected benefits reflect class responses or are unique to the individual agents studied. Importantly, the potential for adverse effects should always be considered when selecting an antidepressant in PD. For example, some SSRIs, such as fluoxetine, can be activating. Although this may be beneficial in patients who are apathetic or withdrawn, it may worsen symptoms in patients with PD who are agitated.[16,137] With tricyclic antidepressants, care must be taken to observe for anticholinergic side effects that may worsen PD symptoms, such as impaired cognition, delayed gastric emptying (which may reduce levodopa effectiveness by increasing levodopa degradation in the gut), urinary problems, orthostatic hypotension, and increased risk of falls. Electroconvulsive therapy may be considered in refractory cases, but may adversely affect cognition.

Based on J.D.'s symptoms, it is reasonable to start him on an antidepressant. Clinical experience suggests a good initial choice for balancing efficacy and safety is probably an SSRI, such as citalopram. As with other patients with depression, the choice of agent should be individualized based on other pragmatic factors such as cost, potential for adverse effects, and personal or family history of response to prior agents. Regardless of which agent or class of antidepressant is selected, therapy should be started at the lowest dose and gradually titrated to effect. He should be monitored closely for side effects, particularly anticholinergic symptoms with tricyclic antidepressants, and for any adverse effects on mobility. He should be observed carefully for changes in parkinsonian symptoms, including development of extrapyramidal symptoms, as well as any signs of psychomotor agitation. Short-term use of benzodiazepines, such as lorazepam or alprazolam, may also provide relief of anxiety symptoms,[124] but must be used cautiously owing to adverse effects on cognition and risk of falling. Generally, anxiety symptoms should improve with treatment of the underlying depression.

PSYCHOSIS

The incidence of psychotic symptoms increases with age and cognitive impairment in patients with PD. Other risk factors include higher age at PD onset, high doses of dopaminergic drugs, and REM sleep behavior disorder.[138] Symptoms are often more pronounced at night (the "sundowning" effect), and hallucinations are typically visual. As with the management of cognitive impairment, it is important to eliminate or minimize any potential causative factors, particularly anticholinergic medications that could be contributing to the hallucinations or delirium. In some patients, reducing the dose of levodopa improves mental function and also provides satisfactory control of motor features. If it is not possible to achieve a balance between preserving motor control and decreasing neuropsychiatric symptoms through reduction in levodopa dosage, antipsychotics may be considered.

Older antipsychotic medications, such as haloperidol, perphenazine, and chlorpromazine, block striatal dopamine D_2 receptors and may exacerbate parkinsonian symptoms. Therefore, these agents are not recommended.[16] Newer atypical antipsychotics are more selective for limbic and cortical D_3, D_4, D_5 receptors; they have minimal activity at D_2 receptors and may control symptoms without worsening parkinsonism. Of these agents, clozapine has the best evidence of efficacy in patients with PD without adversely affecting motor function, and should be preferentially considered.[18,139] However, its use is complicated by the need for frequent monitoring of white blood cell counts because of the risk of agranulocytosis. Other newer agents, particularly quetiapine, appear promising and have controlled psychosis without worsening parkinsonism.[140,141] Risperidone and olanzapine have also been studied, but both worsened parkinsonism and were inferior to clozapine in patients with PD.[142,143] Aripiprazole, also a newer atypical antipsychotic, has been associated with worsening motor function in patients with PD, whereas experience with ziprasidone has yielded mixed results.[144]

AUTONOMIC DYSFUNCTION

Patients with PD frequently experience dysautonomia, including orthostasis, erectile dysfunction, constipation, nocturia, sensory disturbances, dysphagia, seborrhea, and thermoregulatory imbalances. Management of these symptoms is generally supportive, and appropriate medical interventions similar to those used in other geriatric patients can be used to treat these symptoms whenever encountered. In some cases, fludrocortisone or midodrine can be considered if orthostatic hypotension is severe, although they have been subject to little study in PD patients specifically.[124] Other possibly effective treatments for symptoms of autonomic dysfunction outlined in the American Academy of Neurology Practice Parameter include sildenafil for erectile dysfunction and polyethylene glycol for constipation.[124]

FALLS

Patients with PD and their caregivers should be counseled on the prevention of falls because they can result in serious morbidity and mortality. Falls generally result from one of several factors, including postural instability, freezing and festination, levodopa-induced dyskinesia, symptomatic orthostatic hypotension, coexisting neurologic or other medical disorders, and environmental factors.[16] Prevention remains the best strategy and includes environmental precautions, such as proper lighting, use of handrails, removing tripping hazards, and incorporating physical and occupational therapy. Reversible causes of postural or gait instability should be addressed whenever suspected.

SLEEP DISORDERS

Parasomnias often experienced by elderly persons are accentuated in PD patients.[16] Insomnia, sleep fragmentation owing to PD symptoms, restless leg syndrome, and REM sleep disorder (characterized by vivid dreams that are often acted out, especially if frightening) are common and a source of decreased quality of life. When sleep dysfunction can be directly attributed to PD symptoms, such as akinesia, tremor, dyskinesia, or nightmares, dosage adjustment of dopaminergic medications is indicated. Proper sleep hygiene should be encouraged. Short-acting benzodiazepines can be used if insomnia occurs; however, a longer-acting agent or controlled-release formulation may be preferred if the patient wakes early and is unable to return to sleep. If excessive daytime drowsiness occurs, modafinil may be considered.[124] Similar to dysautonomia, management of sleep disorders that are not directly attributable to PD symptoms can be managed supportively, as in other geriatric patients.

ONLINE CONTENT

For a brief video summarizing the clinical features of a patient with PD, go to http://thepoint.lww.com/AT10e.

RESTLESS LEG SYNDROME AND PERIODIC LIMB MOVEMENTS OF SLEEP

Clinical Presentation

CASE 57-5

QUESTION 1: J.J., a 47-year-old woman, presents to her family physician complaining of daytime fatigue and difficulty sleeping at night because of "jumpy legs." She reports being able to sleep only 4 to 5 hours per night because of the leg restlessness, and feels unrefreshed after sleep. On further questioning, she describes the sensation in her legs as being like "bugs crawling under the skin." The sensation is not painful. She explains that the symptoms worsen in the evening and at night, and are partially relieved with walking. She recalls that her mother had similar symptoms. J.J.'s spouse notes that she often "kicks" him in her sleep. Review of her medical history shows an otherwise healthy postmenopausal woman. What signs and symptoms are suggestive of restless legs syndrome (RLS) in J.J.? What laboratory tests or diagnostic procedures should be performed in J.J. to evaluate her condition?

Restless legs syndrome, also known as Ekbom disease, is a disabling sensorimotor disorder estimated to affect approximately 2% of the adult population.[145] Although most patients with mild symptoms will not require treatment, RLS can be associated with adverse health outcomes, including sleep-onset insomnia, missed or late work, anxiety, depression, marital discord, and even suicide in severe cases.

Four essential criteria have been established by the International Restless Legs Syndrome Study Group to diagnose RLS (Table 57-7).[146] The pathognomonic trait of RLS is an almost irresistible urge to move the legs (akathisia), often associated

TABLE 57-7
Clinical Features of Restless Legs Syndrome

Essential Criteria
Urge to move legs, associated with paresthesias or dysesthesias
Relief of symptoms with movement
Onset or exacerbation of symptoms at rest
Onset or worsening of symptoms during nighttime
Supportive Clinical Features
Accompanying sleep disturbance (sleep-onset insomnia)
Periodic leg movements
Positive response to dopaminergic therapy
Positive family history of RLS
Otherwise normal physical examination

RLS, restless legs syndrome.

with uncomfortable paresthesias or dysesthesias felt deep inside the limbs. Patients describe the sensation as "creepy-crawly" or "like soda water in the veins."[147] The symptoms may occur unilaterally or bilaterally, affecting the ankle, knee, or entire lower limb. With progressive disease, symptoms can begin earlier in the day, and progressive involvement of the arms or trunk may occur. Temporary or partial relief of symptoms can be achieved with movement. If patients attempt to ignore the urge to move the legs, akathisia will progressively intensify until they either move their legs or the legs jerk involuntarily.[147] Symptoms usually manifest in a circadian pattern with onset or worsening during nighttime hours (usually between 6 PM and 4 AM, with peak symptoms between midnight and 4 AM). The circadian pattern persists even in patients with inverted sleep–wake cycles. As a result of their symptoms, patients with RLS become "nightwalkers," spending significant time walking, stretching, or bending the legs in an effort to relieve symptoms.

J.J.'s case is an example of a classic presentation of RLS. The prevalence of RLS increases with age and appears to be slightly more common in women.[148] She describes "creepy-crawly" sensations that are relieved partially with walking, a core feature of RLS. Her symptoms are worse during the evening hours. J.J. reports her mother suffered from similar symptoms. The observation of a familial tendency suggests a genetic component, and several chromosomal loci have been linked to the disease.[149] A strong family history of RLS appears to correlate with an early age of onset (<45 years), whereas presentation at a later age is associated with more neuropathy and accelerated disease progression.[147]

Most cases of RLS are considered primary or idiopathic; therefore, the diagnosis does not require elaborate laboratory tests or diagnostic procedures. Several conditions are associated with RLS, and include iron deficiency, pregnancy, and end-stage renal disease. A thorough medical history should be taken in J.J. to rule out reversible causes of RLS or other conditions with similar characteristics. Several medications and substances are known aggravators of RLS, including medications with antidopaminergic properties, such as metoclopramide and prochlorperazine. Nicotine, caffeine, and alcohol can aggravate RLS through their own ability to interfere with quality of sleep. Additionally, SSRIs, tricyclic antidepressants, and commonly used over-the-counter antihistamines, such as diphenhydramine, can trigger or worsen RLS symptoms.[149] Hypotensive akathisia, leg cramps, and other conditions such as arthritis, which can cause positional discomfort with extended periods of sitting in one position, can mimic RLS. These conditions are easily distinguished from RLS because they are usually localized to certain joints or muscles, do not have a circadian pattern, and are not associated with an uncontrollable urge to move.

With an otherwise unremarkable physical examination and medical history, specific laboratory tests that should be performed in J.J. are limited to serum ferritin and percent transferrin saturation (total iron-binding capacity) to rule out iron deficiency anemia. It is important to note that ferritin is an acute-phase reactant and may be artificially elevated if there is an underlying inflammatory or infectious condition. Therefore, the ferritin level should always be accompanied by the percent transferrin saturation. Several studies have documented a relationship between low ferritin concentrations and increased symptom severity.[150,151] J.J. is postmenopausal, so a pregnancy test is not necessary. Polysomnography is not usually indicated unless there is clinical suspicion for sleep apnea or if sleep remains disrupted despite treatment of RLS. When clinical suspicion from the physical examination or medical history suggests a possible peripheral nerve or radiculopathy cause, a routine neurologic panel, including thyroid function tests, fasting glucose, vitamins B_6 and B_{12}, and folate, should be obtained.[149] Renal function tests (serum creatinine and blood urea nitrogen) can be obtained to screen for uremia, although RLS does not usually occur in this situation until the patient has reached end-stage renal failure.

CASE 57-5, QUESTION 2: What is the difference between RLS and periodic limb movements of sleep (PLMS)?

In addition to the presence of RLS, J.J.'s spouse has noticed what are likely PLMS. PLMS, also known as nocturnal myoclonus, are best described as involuntary clonic-type movements of the lower extremities while sleeping that usually involve bilateral ankle dorsiflexion, knee flexion and hip flexion. Approximately 80% of patients with RLS will also have PLMS, but PLMS can occur by itself and is also associated with significant sleep dysfunction. The diagnosis of PLMS usually requires a polysomnogram; the universally accepted criteria for diagnosis are that there should be at least four periodic leg movements (PLMs) in a 90-second period, with contractions typically lasting 0.5 to 5 seconds and recurring every 5 to 90 seconds.[152] A PLM index (PLMI) is calculated by dividing the total number of PLMs by sleep time in hours; an index of more than 5 but less than 25 is considered mild, a PMLI of more than 25 and less than 50 is moderate, and a PLMI of more than 50 is severe. The diagnosis of PLM disorder can be made when patients present with insomnia, tiredness, and daytime sleepiness in the presence of a high PLMI.[153] There is considerable overlap in the treatments of PLMS and RLS. Because J.J. clearly has RLS there is no need to perform a polysomnogram. The diagnosis of PLMS in her case is incidental and would not alter the clinical management. An exception to this would be if J.J.'s medical history revealed the possibility of sleep apnea, as there is a high association between PLMS and upper airway resistance[154]; a polysomnogram would then be indicated.

Treatment

CASE 57-5, QUESTION 3: The decision is made to treat J.J.'s symptoms with medication. What pharmacologic therapy should be selected? What nonpharmacologic therapies should be recommended?

Figure 57-6 presents an approach to the treatment of RLS. Iron supplements can potentially cure RLS symptoms in patients found to be iron deficient.[155] If J.J. is iron deficient, she should be prescribed 50 to 65 mg of elemental iron one to three times daily on an empty stomach with 200 mg of vitamin C to enhance absorption. After ruling out possible reversible causes of RLS, it is important to establish the frequency of J.J.'s symptoms and whether or not they are associated with pain. This information will help determine appropriate therapy.

Several classes of medications are effective for treating RLS.[156] Dopaminergic therapies are most consistently effective in relieving RLS symptoms, improving sleep, and reducing leg movements. The available dopaminergic therapies that have been evaluated in RLS include carbidopa/levodopa, pramipexole, ropinirole, bromocriptine, and rotigotine (not currently available in the United States).[156,157] Dopamine agonists are now the preferred dopaminergic class to treat RLS because they are longer acting than levodopa, which allows for more sustained efficacy and control of symptoms throughout the entire night. J.J. should be started on either ropinirole (0.25 mg initially, up to 0.5–8.0 mg/day) or pramipexole (0.125 mg initially, up to 0.5–1.5 mg/day), as both are both Food and Drug Administration–approved for treating RLS. Several randomized, controlled clinical trials have

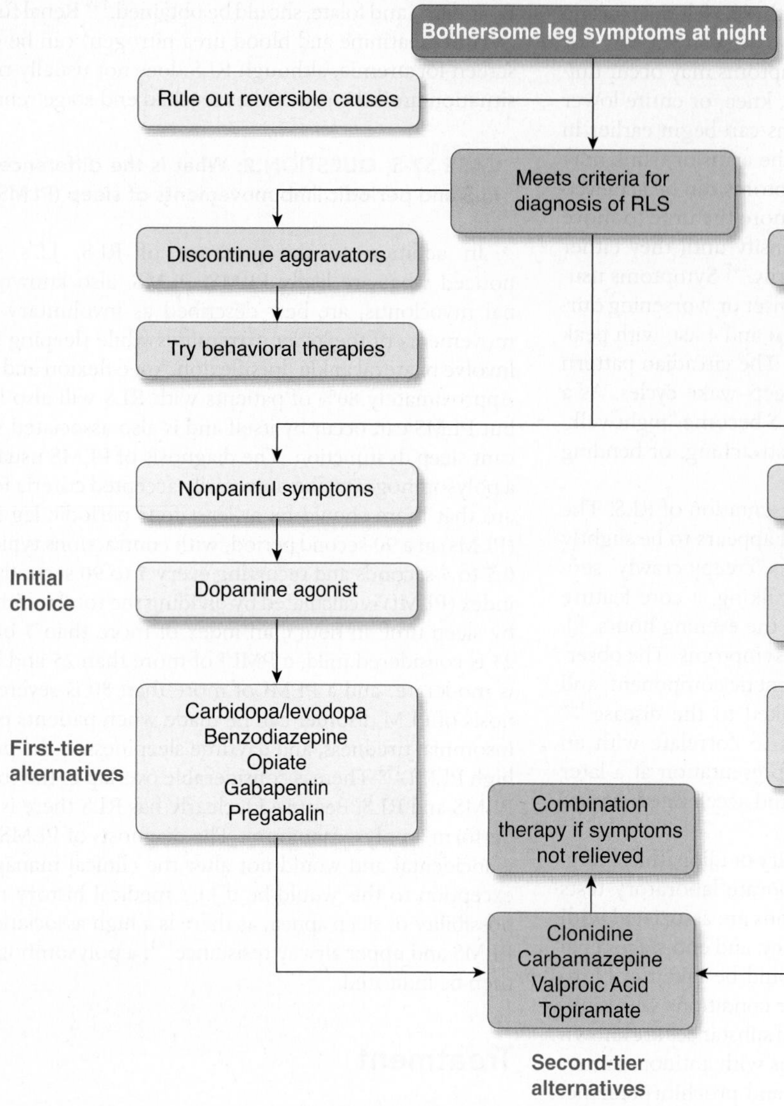

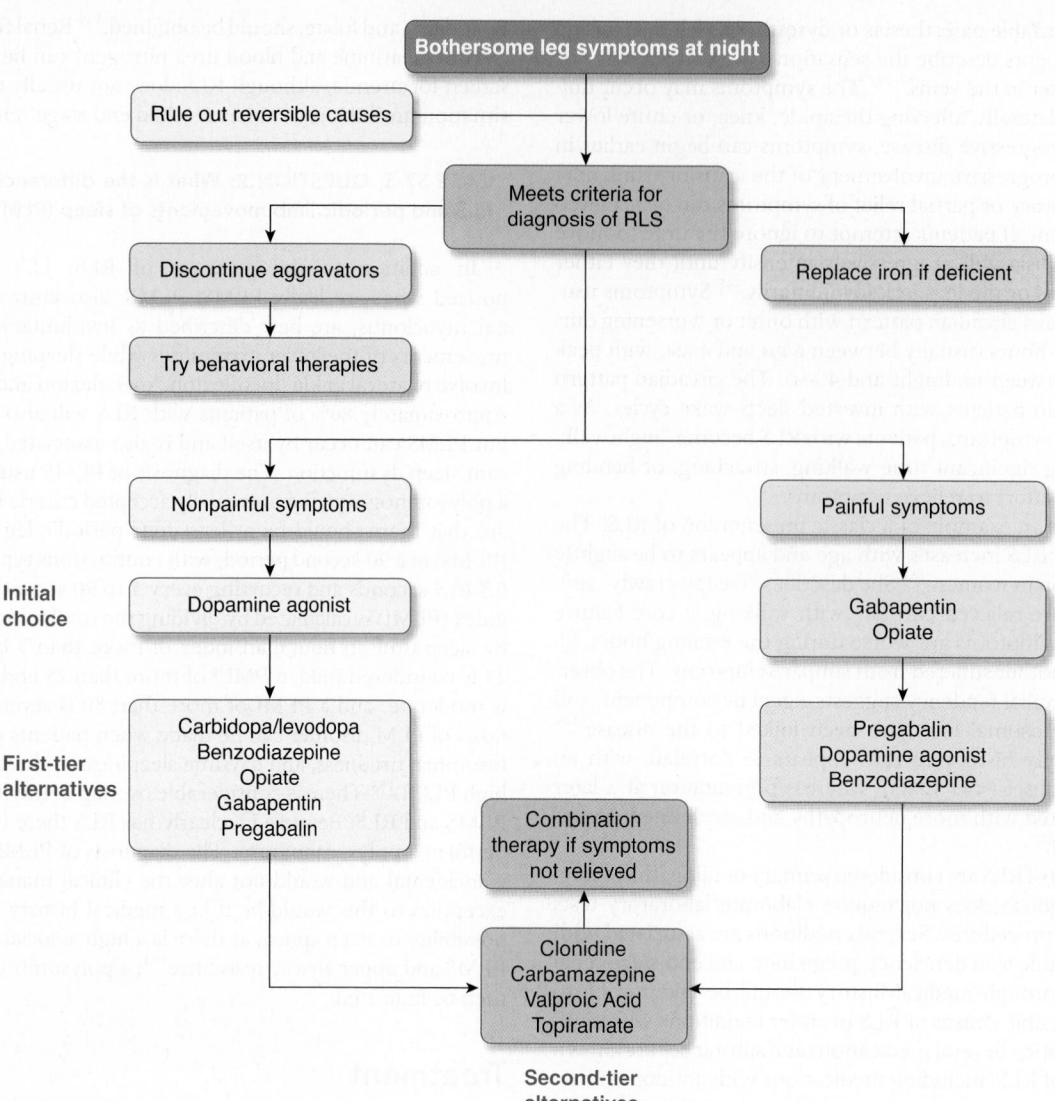

FIGURE 57-6 Approach to the treatment of restless legs syndrome.

documented efficacy of these agents in both objective and subjective ratings of improvement by patients and clinicians with either short- or long-term use.[158–162] Ropinirole and pramipexole do not appear to differ with regard to efficacy or adverse effects. When used for RLS, ropinirole and pramipexole should be administered 2 hours before bedtime. Adverse effects are similar to those seen with the use of these agents in PD, and patients should be counseled accordingly.

Other medications may also provide modest benefit in RLS, including benzodiazepines, opiates, anticonvulsants, and clonidine.[156] With the exception of gabapentin or opiates,[163,164] which could be considered initially if J.J.'s discomfort was primarily caused by pain, all are considered to be alternatives to the dopaminergics. The dosing and adverse effects of the benzodiazepines used in RLS are similar to their use in the general population. No evidence suggests that one benzodiazepine is more effective than another for RLS, and selection should be based on the patient's primary sleep disorder complaint. For example, a newer short-acting benzodiazepine with quick onset of action may be preferred in a patient whose primary problem is getting to sleep. Older anticonvulsants such as carbamazepine and valproic acid may be efficacious, but lack substantial study in RLS patients.[156] Newer agents such as pregabalin and topiramate have also been studied with favorable preliminary results.[156,165]

In addition to a dopamine agonist, nonpharmacologic therapies and behavioral techniques should also be recommended for J.J. Most important among these include discontinuing all RLS aggravators and practicing good sleep hygiene. Physical and mental activity (e.g., reading, playing card games, or working on the computer) if patients are unable to sleep can reduce symptoms.[149] Counter stimuli such as massage or hot baths may be helpful.[149]

CASE 57-5, QUESTION 4: After carefully considering the costs of therapy, J.J. and her physician choose levodopa to treat her RLS. She initially responds well to the therapy. One year later, J.J. returns for follow-up. Her dose of carbidopa/levodopa has progressively increased to three 25/100 mg tablets at bedtime. She describes continued worsening of her symptoms, and they do not seem to be relieved with increasing doses of carbidopa/levodopa. Her symptoms are now starting earlier in the evening, occur almost every night, and are now painful. How should J.J.'s therapy be further adjusted?

J.J. is likely experiencing augmentation, a common problem with long-term use of dopaminergic drugs, particularly levodopa.[166] Augmentation is described as a progressive worsening of RLS symptoms after an initial improvement, and is manifested by gradually intensified symptoms that occur earlier in the evening and spread to other parts of the body.[167] It is the most common side effect occurring with long-term use (>3 months) of dopaminergic agents, and usually occurs 6 to 18 months after therapy is initiated.[149] Doses of dopaminergic agents are often increased in response; however, with each incremental dose increase symptoms progress more rapidly until they may occur continuously throughout the day.[149] Although augmentation has been clinically recognized for many years, it has not been systematically studied. The exact etiology is uncertain, but it likely relates to the finding that RLS, unlike PD, is actually a hyperdopaminergic condition with an apparent postsynaptic desensitization that overcompensates during the circadian low point of dopaminergic activity in the evening and night. Adding dopamine in the evening initially corrects the symptoms, but ultimately leads to increasing postsynaptic desensitization.

The highest risk for augmentation is with levodopa. An estimated 50% to 85% of patients on levodopa will develop augmentation, compared with only 20% to 30% with dopamine agonists.[156] The primary treatment strategy in dealing with augmentation is to withdraw the dopaminergic agent and substitute other nondopaminergic agents. Given her presentation, J.J. should have her carbidopa/levodopa discontinued. She should be counseled that her symptoms will likely rebound severely for 48 to 72 hours, but approximately 4 to 7 days later her symptoms should gradually return to baseline or pretreatment state.[149]

With the discontinuation of carbidopa/levodopa in J.J., an alternative therapy should be selected. The selection of an alternative agent in cases in which the initial therapy failed or augmentation occurs must be approached on an individual basis. Although a number of agents are available to choose from, clinical experience generally guides the decision as lack of comparative trials precludes development of any formal recommendations. Because J.J. describes increasing pain with her RLS, it would be appropriate to initiate a trial of gabapentin. If gabapentin is ineffective or not tolerated, J.J. could be prescribed an opiate, which is also an acceptable choice in patients with RLS who have neuropathy or painful dysesthesias. Hydrocodone, oxycodone, methadone, codeine, and tramadol have all demonstrated efficacy in RLS.[149] Augmentation does not prevent a future reintroduction of dopaminergic therapy; in J.J.'s case, a dopamine agonist could be added after an extended dopaminergic-free period if her symptoms are not completely controlled on gabapentin.

ESSENTIAL TREMOR

Clinical Presentation

CASE 57-6

QUESTION 1: K.H. is a 52-year-old white female office manager who was referred to a neurologist for evaluation of bilateral tremor. She is otherwise healthy and reports not taking any regularly prescribed medications. She describes her tremor as being present mainly when she performs voluntary movements. The tremor is not noticeable during rest. She also notices the tremor seems to disappear in the evening after drinking a couple of glasses of wine. The tremor interferes with several of her ADLs, including writing, eating, drinking from a cup, and inserting her keys into the ignition. She reports mild interference with her job function and some social embarrassment. No bradykinesia or rigidity is elicited on physical examination. A handwriting sample reveals large characters that are difficult to decipher. Family history reveals that her maternal grandmother and mother both had similar symptoms. What signs and symptoms are consistent with essential tremor in K.H.?

Beginning in the mid-20th century, the term *essential tremor* (ET) has been consistently used to describe a kinetic tremor for which no definite cause has been established. ET is a common neurologic disorder with an estimated incidence of 616 cases per 100,000 person-years, and a prevalence of about 0.9% to 4.6%.[168,169] Despite its commonness, it is underrecognized and undertreated, likely because it has been traditionally viewed as a monosymptomatic disorder of little consequence; more recently, it is recognized to be complex and progressive, resulting in significant disability in ADLs and job performance, and social embarrassment.[170] Both the incidence and prevalence of ET increase with age. In addition, ethnicity and family history of ET are consistently identified risk factors; it is approximately five times more common in whites than blacks, and approximately 50% of patients report a positive family history. The latter finding suggests that genetic predisposition may play a role in ET; however, differences in intrafamilial onset and severity suggest environmental factors may also influence underlying susceptibility to the disease. Several environmental toxins have been proposed as causes of ET, including β-carboline alkaloids (e.g., harmane and harmine) and lead, both of which have been found in elevated concentrations in patients with ET compared with normal control subjects.[171,172]

Because parkinsonian tremor and ET are the most common forms of tremor observed in practice, it is important to distinguish between the two because the treatments differ substantially. Diagnostic criteria for ET developed by the Movement Disorder Society are summarized in Table 57-8.[173] Tremor should first be identified as either an action or resting tremor. Action tremors include kinetic, postural, and isometric tremors. The defining feature of ET is a bilateral, largely symmetrical, 5- to 10-Hz kinetic and postural tremor of the arms. The tremor can also affect head or voice. Kinetic tremor can be elicited in patients during voluntary movement, such as finger-to-nose test, signing their name, drawing spirals, or drinking water from a cup. Postural tremor occurs during sustained arm extension. Although both types of action tremors (kinetic or postural) can be present in ET and PD,

TABLE 57-8
Diagnostic Criteria for Essential Tremor

Inclusion Criteria
Bilateral postural tremor with or without kinetic tremor, involving hands and forearms, that is visible and persistent
Duration >5 years
Exclusion Criteria
Other abnormal neurological signs (except Froment sign)
Presence of known causes of increased physiological tremor
Concurrent or recent exposure to tremorogenic drugs or the presence of a drug withdrawal state
Direct or indirect trauma to the nervous system within 3 months before the onset of tremor
Historical or clinical evidence of psychogenic origins
Convincing evidence of sudden onset or evidence of stepwise deterioration

TABLE 57-9
Differentiation of Essential Tremor and Parkinson Disease

Characteristic	Essential Tremor	Parkinson Disease
Kinetic tremor in arms, hands, or head	++	++
Hemibody (arm and leg) tremor	0	++
Kinetic tremor > resting tremor	++	+
Resting tremor > kinetic tremor	0	++
Rigidity or bradykinesia	0	++
Postural instability	0	++
Usual age of onset (years)	15–25, 45–55	55–65
Symmetry	Bilateral	Unilateral > Bilateral
Family history of tremor	+++	+
Response to alcohol	+++	0
Response to anticholinergics	0	++
Response to levodopa	0	+++
Response to primidone	+++	0
Response to propranolol	+++	+
Handwriting analysis	Large, tremulous script	Micrographia

0, not observed; +, rarely observed; ++, sometimes observed; +++, often observed.

the presence of resting tremor is much more common in PD. Lack of resting tremor and absence of bradykinesia or rigidity in K.H. suggest the tremor is not parkinsonian. She describes interference of her tremor occurring with voluntary movement, such as in her ADLs and drinking from a cup. Other signs and symptoms that support a diagnosis of ET include her age, family history, large and tremulous handwriting (as opposed to micrographia in PD), and improvement in tremor with alcohol consumption. Table 57-9 summarizes the similarities and differences of ET and parkinsonian tremor.

Several medications and substances are known to cause tremors. All patients with tremor should have thorough medication history to rule out these possible causes. Medications commonly implicated include corticosteroids, metoclopramide, valproate, sympathomimetics (e.g., albuterol, amphetamines, pseudoephedrine), SSRIs, tricyclic antidepressants, theophylline, and thyroid preparations.[174] In addition, caffeine, tobacco, and chronic alcohol use can cause tremor that resembles ET. K.H. does not report taking any regularly prescribed medications; however, she should be questioned regarding any over-the-counter medication use as well as her caffeine and smoking habits, and alcohol use if applicable.

The diagnosis of ET is based solely on clinical examination and neurological history. Neuroimaging is not useful, and there are no available biological markers or diagnostic tests that are specific to ET. The evaluation of K.H.'s tremor should include laboratory analysis to rule out possible medical conditions associated with tremor. If clinical signs suggest the possibility of hyperthyroidism, thyroid function tests should be performed. In patients younger than 40 years of age who present with action tremor, serum ceruloplasmin can be tested to evaluate for possible Wilson disease.[174]

Treatment

CASE 57-6, QUESTION 2: What therapies are effective in treating ET? How should K.H. be treated?

Patients with ET who have mild disability that does not cause functional disability or social embarrassment can go without treatment. Because K.H. is experiencing tremor that is interfering with her occupation and causing social embarrassment, she should be considered for pharmacotherapy (Table 57-10). It is important to note that although effective treatments exist, tremor is rarely eliminated completely. Factors predicting lack of response have not been readily identified.

Propranolol, a nonselective β-adrenergic receptor blocker, or primidone, an anticonvulsant, are recommended as first-line agents to treat ET.[175,176] Propranolol is typically effective in doses of at least 120 mg/day, with about 50% of patients having long-lasting benefit.[175] Long-acting propranolol is as effective as the regular-release formulation. Other β_1-selective blockers such as atenolol and metoprolol have also been studied, but with mixed findings.[177] Propranolol has demonstrated greater efficacy than these β_1 selective agents, suggesting that blockade of β_2 receptors is of importance. β-Adrenergic receptor blockers with intrinsic sympathomimetic activity, such as pindolol, appear ineffective in ET.[175] Caution should be exercised with propranolol in patients with asthma, congestive heart failure, diabetes mellitus, and atrioventricular block.

Several studies have compared propranolol and primidone in ET,[178,179] and they are considered to have similar efficacy.[175,176] Primidone is metabolized to a phenobarbital-based metabolite; however, phenobarbital is inferior to primidone in treating ET.[180] Acute adverse effects of primidone include nausea, vomiting, and ataxia, which can occur in up to one-fourth of patients, often limiting its use.[175] The long-term tolerability of primidone is very good, however, and may actually be superior to propranolol.[179] Primidone should be initiated at 12.5 mg/day and administered at bedtime to reduce the occurrence of acute side effects. It can be titrated gradually as tolerated up to 750 mg/day in divided doses, although side effects become more common at doses greater than 500 mg/day.[175]

Other agents that have demonstrated variable efficacy in ET include gabapentin, pregabalin, topiramate, zonisamide, levetiracetam, and benzodiazepines (specifically, alprazolam and clonazepam).[175,177] They are generally considered to be less-proven, second-line therapies, however. Adverse effects and potential for abuse (specifically with benzodiazepines) should be considered when an agent is selected.

If oral pharmacotherapy options for ET are not beneficial, intramuscular injections of botulinum toxin A or surgical treatments can be used in selected patients.[181] Targeted botulinum toxin A injections can reduce hand, head, and voice tremor; however, they are associated with focal weakness of the adjacent

TABLE 57-10
Pharmacotherapy for Essential Tremor

Drug	Initial Dose	Usual Therapeutic Dose	Adverse Effects
β-Blockers			
Propranolol	10 mg every day to BID	160–320 mg divided every day to BID	Bradycardia, fatigue, hypotension, depression, exercise intolerance
Atenolol	12.5–25 mg every day	50–150 mg every day	Bradycardia, fatigue, hypotension, exercise intolerance
Nadolol	40 mg every day	120–240 mg every day	Bradycardia, fatigue, hypotension, exercise intolerance
Anticonvulsants			
Primidone	12.5 mg every day	50–750 mg divided every day to TID	Sedation, fatigue, nausea, vomiting, ataxia, dizziness, confusion, vertigo
Gabapentin	300 mg every day	1,200–3,600 mg divided TID	Nausea, drowsiness, dizziness, unsteadiness
Topiramate	25 mg every day	200–400 mg divided BID	Appetite suppression, weight loss, paresthesias, concentration difficulties
Pregabalin	75 mg BID	75–300 mg divided BID	Weight gain, dizziness, drowsiness
Benzodiazepines			
Alprazolam	0.125 mg every day	0.75–3 mg divided TID	Sedation, fatigue, potential for abuse
Clonazepam	0.25 mg every day	0.5–6 mg divided every day to BID	Sedation, fatigue, ataxia, dizziness, impaired cognition
Miscellaneous			
Botulinum toxin A	Varies by injection site: 50–100 units/arm for hand tremor; 40–400 units/neck for head tremor; 0.6–15 units/vocal cords for voice tremor; retreat no sooner than every 3 months (extend as long as possible)		Hand weakness (with wrist injection); dysphagia, hoarseness, breathiness (with neck or vocal cord injection)

BID, two times daily; TID, three times daily.

areas.[175] Injections in the wrist can cause hand weakness, and dysphagia, hoarseness, and breathiness can occur with injections into the neck or vocal cords. The use of botulinum toxin injections in the United States is also limited by cost. Treatment should occur with the lowest dose, and the interval should be as long as possible between injections. DBS of the ventral intermediate nucleus of the thalamus or unilateral thalamotomy is highly efficacious in reducing ET.[176] Greater improvement in self-reported measures of function and fewer adverse events make DBS the preferred surgical option of the two.[176,182]

Because K.H. is otherwise healthy, she is a good candidate for propranolol therapy. Propranolol can be initiated as needed or on a scheduled basis depending on the degree of impairment and desire of the patient. If the decision is made with K.H. to use propranolol on an as-needed basis, she should begin with one-half of a 20-mg tablet administered 30 minutes to 1 hour before the desired effect. The dose can be increased from one-half to two tablets. An example of a situation in which this may occur is if she wants to avoid embarrassment with attending a social activity or before certain tasks requiring manual dexterity at work. Given the degree of her impairment, she is probably a better candidate for chronic suppressive therapy with propranolol. In this situation, she can be prescribed 10 mg twice daily and titrated every few days up to 120 to 360 mg/day in divided doses.

KEY REFERENCES

A full list of references for this chapter can be found at http://thepoint.lww.com/AT10e. Below are the key references for this chapter, with the corresponding reference number in this chapter found in parentheses after the reference.

Key References

Parkinson Disease

Miyasaki JM et al. Practice parameter: evaluation and treatment of depression, psychosis, and dementia in Parkinson disease (an evidence-based review). Report of the Quality Standards Subcommittee of the American Academy of Neurology. *Neurology.* 2006;66:996. (18)

Miyasaki JM et al. Practice parameter: initiation of treatment for Parkinson's disease: an evidence-based review. Report of the Quality Standards Subcommittee of the American Academy of Neurology. *Neurology.* 2002;58:11. (24)

Morley JF, Hurtig HI. Current understanding and management of Parkinson disease: five new things. *Neurology.* 2010; 75(18 Suppl 1):S9. (10)

Nutt JG, Wooten GF. Clinical practice. Diagnosis and initial management of Parkinson's disease. *N Engl J Med.* 2005;353:1021. (12)

Pahwa R et al. Practice parameter: treatment of Parkinson disease with motor fluctuations and dyskinesia (an evidence-based review): report of the Quality Standards Subcommittee of the American Academy of Neurology. *Neurology.* 2006;66:983. (66)

Suchowersky O et al. Practice parameter: diagnosis and prognosis of new onset Parkinson disease (an evidence-based review): report of the Quality Standards Subcommittee of the American Academy of Neurology. *Neurology.* 2006;66:968. (7)

Suchowersky O et al. Practice parameter: neuroprotective strategies and alternative therapies for Parkinson disease (an evidence-based overview): report of the Quality Standards Subcommittee of the American Academy of Neurology. *Neurology.* 2006;66:976. (17)

Zesiewicz TA et al. Practice parameter: treatment of nonmotor symptoms of Parkinson disease: report of the Quality Standards Subcommittee of the American Academy of Neurology. *Neurology.* 2010;74:924. (124)

Restless Leg Syndrome

Gamaldo CE, Earley CJ. Restless legs syndrome: a clinical update. *Chest.* 2006;130:1596. (149)

Trenkwalder C et al. Treatment of restless legs syndrome: an evidence-based review and implications for clinical practice. *Mov Disord.* 2008;23:2267. (156)

Essential Tremor

Deuschl G et al. Treatment of patients with essential tremor. *Lancet Neurol.* 2011;10:148. (175)

Zesiewicz TA et al. Practice parameter: therapies for essential tremor. Report of the Quality Standards Subcommittee of the American Academy of Neurology. *Neurology.* 2005;64:2008. (176)

58

Seizure Disorders

James W. McAuley, Rex S. Lott, and Brian K. Alldredge

CORE PRINCIPLES

		CHAPTER CASES
1	Epilepsy is a disorder characterized by spontaneously recurring seizures. Seizures can arise from a focal area of the brain (focal or partial seizures) or arise diffusely from both brain hemispheres (primary generalized seizures).	**Case 58-1 (Questions 1, 2)**
2	The optimal choice of antiepileptic drug (AED) treatment is based on patient-specific considerations including seizure type (or epilepsy syndrome, if defined), age, sex, concomitant medical conditions and therapies, and AED adverse effects. Monotherapy is preferred; polytherapy should be considered for patients with multiple seizure types and/or when monotherapy (with 2 or 3 agents) fails at maximal tolerated doses.	**Case 58-1 (Question 3), Case 58-7 (Question 1), Case 58-8 (Questions 1, 4), Case 58-14 (Question 2)**
3	Standard AEDs, such as carbamazepine, phenytoin, and valproate, are used commonly for patients with newly diagnosed epilepsy. Newer AEDs (e.g., lacosamide, lamotrigine, levetiracetam, oxcarbazepine, pregabalin, topiramate, zonisamide) are often initially approved for add-on therapy in patients with partial-onset seizures who do not respond to other AEDs. Lamotrigine, oxcarbazepine, topiramate, and felbamate are indicated for monotherapy.	**Case 58-1 (Question 3), Case 58-2 (Question 1), Case 58-7 (Question 1)**
4	Enzyme-inducing AEDs (carbamazepine, phenobarbital, phenytoin) increase the metabolism of many other drugs (e.g., warfarin, contraceptive hormones) and can influence the concentrations of other AEDs and other AED metabolites (e.g., valproate effect on carbamazepine epoxide). In addition, carbamazepine induces its own metabolism and levels may decline during the first month of therapy despite excellent adherence.	**Case 58-1 (Question 5), Case 58-11 (Question 1), Case 58-12 (Questions 1, 2), Case 58-14 (Question 1)**
5	Serious idiosyncratic adverse effects have been associated with most standard and new AED and include carbamazepine-associated hematologic abnormalities; lamotrigine-associated skin rash; valproate-induced hepatotoxicity; and hypersensitivity syndrome seen with carbamazepine, phenobarbital, and phenytoin. The role of routine laboratory monitoring for detection of these adverse effects is controversial. Patients should know the signs or symptoms that should prompt them to seek medical attention.	**Case 58-1 (Question 4), Case 58-2 (Question 1), Case 58-8 (Questions 8, 9), Case 58-13 (Questions 1, 2)**
6	Unlike other AEDs, phenytoin displays capacity-limited pharmacokinetics at serum concentrations that are clinically useful for epilepsy treatment. As a consequence, phenytoin blood levels often change disproportionately to changes in dosage, and time to steady-state varies significantly in individual patients based on the phenytoin concentration.	**Case 58-3 (Questions 2, 3)**
7	Serum concentration monitoring can be useful for selected AEDs when there is a good correlation between concentration and therapeutic or toxic responses. However, clinical criteria (seizure control, medication tolerability) are the primary determinants of the need for dosage adjustments.	**Case 58-8 (Question 7)**
8	The occurrence of seizure clusters (acute repetitive seizures) and status epilepticus (prolonged or repeated seizures without recovery of consciousness) warrant emergent AED therapy. Acute repetitive seizures are often treated by parents or caregivers with rectal diazepam. Status epilepticus is a life-threatening emergency and should be treated with intravenous lorazepam as initial therapy.	**Case 58-9 (Question 1, Case 58-15 (Questions 1–5)**

Incidence, Prevalence, and Epidemiology

Approximately 10% of the population will experience a seizure at some time in their life. Up to 30% of all seizures are provoked by central nervous system (CNS) disorders or insults (e.g., meningitis, trauma, tumors, and exposure to toxins); these seizures may become recurrent and require chronic treatment with antiepileptic drugs (AEDs). Reversible conditions such as alcohol withdrawal, fever, and metabolic disturbances may provoke acute, isolated seizures. These seizures are not considered to be epilepsy and usually do not require long-term AED therapy. Approximately 1% of the general population has epilepsy.[1]

Terminology, Classification, and Diagnosis of Epilepsies

CLASSIFICATION OF SEIZURES AND EPILEPSIES

A seizure is the "transient occurrence of signs and/or symptoms due to abnormal excessive or synchronous neuronal activity in the brain" (p. 471).[2] These signs or symptoms "may include alterations of consciousness, motor, sensory, autonomic, or psychic events" (p. 593).[1] Epilepsy is a "disorder of the brain characterized by an enduring predisposition to generate epileptic seizures and by the neurobiologic, cognitive, psychological and social consequence of this condition" (p. 471).[2] By definition, epilepsy requires the occurrence of two or more seizures that are not acutely provoked by other illnesses or conditions.[3] A commonly used classification scheme for epileptic seizures is shown in Table 58-1.[4] Older terms such as "grand mal" and "petit mal" should not be used, because their use may create confusion in the clinical setting. For example, it is common for patients or caregivers to identify any seizure other than a generalized tonic-clonic seizure as a "petit mal" seizure. This labeling may result in the selection of an inappropriate medication.

Generalized tonic-clonic seizures are common. The patient loses consciousness and falls at the onset. Simultaneously, tonic muscle spasms begin and may be accompanied by a cry that results from air being forced through the larynx. Bilateral, repetitive clonic movements follow. After the clonic phase, patients return to consciousness but remain lethargic and may be confused for varying periods of time (postictal state). Urinary incontinence and tongue biting is common. Primary generalized tonic-clonic seizures affect both cerebral hemispheres from the outset. Secondarily generalized tonic-clonic seizures begin as either simple or complex partial seizures. The aura described by some patients before a generalized tonic-clonic seizure represents an initial partial seizure that spreads to become a secondarily generalized seizure. Identification of secondarily generalized tonic-clonic seizures is important because some AEDs are more effective at controlling primary generalized seizures than secondarily generalized seizures. In general, partial seizures are often more difficult to control with AEDs as compared to primary generalized seizures.[3,5,6]

Absence seizures occur primarily in children and often remit during puberty; affected patients may exhibit a second type of seizure. Absence seizures consist of a brief loss of consciousness, usually lasting several seconds. Simple (typical) absence seizures are not accompanied by motor symptoms; automatisms, muscle twitching, myoclonic jerking, or autonomic manifestations may accompany atypical (complex) absence seizures. Although consciousness is lost, muscle tone is maintained and patients do not fall during absence seizures. Patients are unaware of their surroundings and will have no recall of events during the seizure. Consciousness returns immediately when the seizure ends, and postictal confusion does not occur. Differentiation of atypical absence seizures from complex partial seizures may be difficult if only a second-hand account of the episodes is available; identification of a focal abnormality by an electroencephalogram (EEG) often is necessary to identify complex partial seizures. This distinction is important for the proper selection of AED.

Simple partial (focal motor or sensory) seizures are localized in a single cerebral hemisphere or portion of a hemisphere. Consciousness is not impaired during these events. Various motor, sensory, or psychic manifestations may occur depending on the area of the brain that is affected. A single part of the body may twitch, or the patient may experience only an unusual sensory experience.

Complex partial seizures result from the spread of focal discharges to involve a larger area. Consciousness is impaired and patients may exhibit complex but inappropriate behavior (automatisms) such as lip smacking, picking at clothing, or aimless wandering. A period of brief postictal lethargy or confusion is common.

In 2010, the International League Against Epilepsy recommended modifications to the traditional seizure classification scheme and terminology. While some of the terminology remained unchanged, seizures limited to one hemisphere are now termed "focal seizures" (instead of partial seizures) and the formal distinction between complex partial and simple partial seizures is eliminated.[7] Since most of the existing literature on

TABLE 58-1
Classification of Epileptic Seizures

Partial Seizure (Focal)
Simple Partial Seizures (Without Impairment of Consciousness)
Motor symptoms
Special sensory or somatosensory symptoms
Autonomic symptoms
Psychic symptoms
Complex Partial Seizures (With Impairment of Consciousness)
Progressing to impairment of consciousness
With no other features
With features as in simple partial seizures
With automatisms
With impaired consciousness at onset
With no other features
With features as in simple partial seizures
With automatisms
Partial Seizures That Evolve to Generalized Seizures
Simple partial seizures evolving to generalized seizures
Complex partial seizures evolving to generalized seizures
Simple partial seizures evolving to complex partial seizures to generalized seizures
Generalized Seizures (Convulsive or Nonconvulsive)
Absence Seizures
Typical seizures (impaired consciousness only)
Atypical absence seizures
Myoclonic Seizures
Clonic Seizures
Tonic Seizures
Tonic-Clonic Seizures
Atonic (Astatic or Akinetic) Seizures
Unclassified Epileptic Seizures
All seizures that cannot be classified because of inadequate or incomplete data and some that cannot be classified in previously described categories

epilepsy makes use of the traditional seizure terminology, we have retained the use of "partial," "complex partial" and "simple partial" for this chapter.

EPILEPSY SYNDROMES

Epilepsy can be classified based on seizure type as shown in Table 58-1. Epilepsy syndromes can be defined on the basis of seizure type as well as cause (if known), precipitating factors, age of onset, characteristic EEG patterns, severity, chronicity, family history, and prognosis. Accurate diagnosis of epilepsy syndromes may better guide clinicians regarding the need for drug therapy, the choice of appropriate medication, and the likelihood of successful treatment.[1,5,6] Many epilepsy syndromes have been defined; a complete listing is beyond the scope of this chapter. Several are of interest with respect to pharmacotherapy and are described in Table 58-2.[6]

Diagnosis

Optimal treatment of seizure disorders requires accurate classification (diagnosis) of seizure type and appropriate choice and use of medications. Seizure classification may be straightforward if an adequate history and description of the clinical seizure are available. Physicians often do not observe patients' seizures; thus, family members, teachers, nurses, and others who have frequent direct contact with patients should learn to observe accurately and objectively describe and record these events. The onset, duration, and characteristics of a seizure should be described as completely as possible. Several aspects of the events surrounding a seizure may be especially significant: the patient's behavior before the seizure (e.g., did the patient complain of feeling ill or describe an unusual sensation?), deviation of the eyes or head to one side or localization of convulsive activity to one portion of the body, impaired consciousness, loss of continence, and the

TABLE 58-2
Selected Epilepsy Syndromes

Syndrome	Seizure Patterns and Characteristics	Preferred AED Therapy	Comments
Juvenile myoclonic epilepsy	Myoclonic seizures often precede generalized tonic-clonic seizures. Myoclonic and generalized tonic-clonic episodes on awakening. Absence seizures also common. ↓ sleep, fatigue, and alcohol commonly precipitate seizures.	Valproate. Levetiracetam FDA-approved as adjunct for myoclonic seizures. Phenytoin possibly an adjunct to valproate in resistant cases. Carbamazepine reported to exacerbate seizures in some patients.	5%–10% of all epilepsies; 85%–90% response to valproate. Lifelong therapy usually needed. High relapse rate with attempts to discontinue AED therapy.
Lennox-Gastaut syndrome	Generalized seizures: atypical absence, atonic/akinetic, myoclonic, and tonic most common. Abnormal interictal EEG with slow spike-wave pattern. Cognitive dysfunction and mental retardation. Status epilepticus common.	Valproate and benzodiazepines may be effective. Lamotrigine, rufinamide and topiramate FDA-approved. Felbamate also may be effective, but potential hematologic toxicity limits use. Poorly responsive to AED.	Oversedation with aggressive AED trials may ↑ seizure frequency. Tolerance to benzodiazepines limits their usefulness.
Childhood absence epilepsy	Typical absences often in clusters of multiple seizures. Tonic-clonic seizures in ~40%. Onset usually between ages 4 and 8 years. Significant genetic component. EEG shows classic 3-Hz spike-and-wave pattern.	Ethosuximide or valproate. Lamotrigine probably effective.	80%–90% response rate to AED therapy. Good prognosis for remission. Tonic-clonic seizures may persist.
Reflex epilepsy	Tonic-clonic seizures most common. Induced by flicker or patterns (photosensitivity) most commonly. Reading also may precipitate partial seizures affecting the jaw, which may generalize. Some cases involve precipitation of underlying seizures; some seem primary.	AED specific to underlying seizures. Avoidance of precipitating stimuli when possible. Valproate usually effective for cases of spontaneous seizures precipitated by photosensitivity.	Relatively rare; seizures may be precipitated by television or video games.
Temporal lobe epilepsy	Complex partial seizures with automatisms. Simple partial seizures (auras) common; secondary generalized seizures occur in 50%.	Carbamazepine, phenytoin, valproate, gabapentin, lamotrigine, topiramate, tiagabine, levetiracetam, oxcarbazepine, zonisamide, pregabalin, lacosamide.	Often incompletely controlled with current AEDs. Emotional stress may precipitate seizures; psychiatric disorders seen with temporal lobe epilepsy; surgical resection can be effective when patient is identified as a good surgical candidate.

AED, antiepileptic drug; EEG, electroencephalogram; FDA, US Food and Drug Administration.
Source: Dreifuss FE. The epilepsies: clinical implications of the international classification. *Epilepsia.* 1990;31(Suppl 3):S3; Serratosa JM. Juvenile myoclonic epilepsy. In: Wyllie E et al, eds. *The Treatment of Epilepsy: Principles and Practice.* 3rd ed. Philadelphia, PA: Lippincott Williams & Wilkins; 2001:491; Farrell K. Secondary generalized epilepsy and Lennox-Gastaut syndrome. In: Wyllie E et al, eds. *The Treatment of Epilepsy: Principles and Practice.* 3rd ed. Philadelphia, PA: Lippincott Williams & Wilkins; 2001:525; Kotagal P. Complex partial seizures. In: Wyllie E et al, eds. *The Treatment of Epilepsy: Principles and Practice.* 3rd ed. Philadelphia, PA: Lippincott Williams & Wilkins; 2001:309; Berkovic SF et al. Absence seizures. In: Wyllie E et al, eds. *The Treatment of Epilepsy: Principles and Practice.* 3rd ed. Philadelphia, PA: Lippincott Williams & Wilkins; 2001:357; Zifkin BG et al. Epilepsy with reflex seizures. In: Wyllie E et al, eds. *The Treatment of Epilepsy: Principles and Practice.* 3rd ed. Philadelphia, PA: Lippincott Williams & Wilkins; 2001:537.

patient's behavior after the seizure (e.g., was there any postictal confusion?). In addition, it is helpful if the observer can record the length of the event and how long it took for the patient to return to baseline. The patient and caregivers should have a seizure calendar or diary to record events. Those who observe a seizure should not try to label the seizure but should be encouraged to describe the event fully and objectively.

Accurate seizure diagnosis and identification of the type of epilepsy or epilepsy syndrome also depend on neurologic examination, medical history, and diagnostic techniques, such as EEG, computed tomography (CT), and magnetic resonance imaging (MRI). The EEG often is critical for identifying specific seizure types. CT scanning may help assess newly diagnosed patients, but MRI is preferred. MRI may locate brain lesions or anatomic defects that are missed by conventional radiographs or CT scans.[8]

Treatment

Early control of epileptic seizures is important because it allows normalization of patients' lives and prevents acute physical harm and long-term morbidity associated with recurrent seizures. In addition, early control of tonic-clonic seizures is associated with a reduced likelihood of seizure recurrence. Early control of epileptic seizures also correlates with successful discontinuation of AED treatment after long-term seizure control.[9–11]

NONPHARMACOLOGIC TREATMENT OF EPILEPSY

Alternatives or adjuncts to pharmacotherapy may be helpful in some patients. Surgery is an extremely effective treatment in selected patients. Depending on the epilepsy syndrome and procedure performed, up to 90% of patients treated surgically may improve or become seizurefree. A study of 80 patients with medically refractory temporal lobe epilepsy randomly assigned to either surgery or continued medical treatment showed that after 1 year patients were more likely to be seizurefree after surgery.[12] Surgery is advocated as early therapy for some patients with specific epilepsy syndromes, such as mesial temporal sclerosis. Early surgical intervention may prevent or lessen neurologic deterioration and developmental delay.

Dietary modification may be used for patients who cannot tolerate AEDs or to treat seizures that are not completely responsive to AEDs. In most circumstances, dietary modification consists of a ketogenic diet. This low-carbohydrate, high-fat diet results in persistent ketosis, which is believed to play a major role in the therapeutic effect. Ketogenic diets seem to be most beneficial in children; they are also used as adjuncts to ongoing AED treatment.[13,14]

The vagus nerve stimulator is an implantable device approved for treatment of intractable partial seizures. This device uses electrodes attached around the left branch of the vagus nerve. The electrodes are attached to a programmable stimulator that delivers stimuli on a regular cycling basis; patients can also use "on demand" stimulation at the onset of seizures by swiping the magnet over the subcutaneously implanted stimulator. Approximately 30% to 40% of patients who are so treated have a positive response (50% reduction in seizures).[15] The primary side effect of this device is hoarseness during stimulation; infrequently, this is accompanied by left vocal cord paralysis.

AVOIDANCE OF POTENTIAL SEIZURE PRECIPITANTS

It is impossible to generalize about environmental and lifestyle precipitants of seizure activity in persons with epilepsy. Individual patients or caregivers may identify specific circumstances such as stress, sleep deprivation, acute illness, or ingestion of excessive amounts of caffeine or alcohol, which may increase the likelihood of a recurrent seizure event. Some women experience an increase in the frequency and/or severity of seizures around the time of menstruation or ovulation. Patients with epilepsy should avoid activities that seem to precipitate seizures; as always, the goal is complete seizure control with as little alteration in quality of life as possible.

ANTIEPILEPTIC DRUG THERAPY

Pharmacotherapy is the mainstay of treatment for epilepsy. Therefore, patient education regarding medications and consultation among health care professionals regarding the optimal use of AEDs are essential to quality patient care. Optimal AED therapy completely controls seizures in approximately two-thirds of patients.[16,17] Optimization of drug therapy depends on several factors, with the choice of appropriate AED, individualization of dosing, and adherence being the most important.

For a narrated PowerPoint presentation of mini case studies addressing multiple aspects of AED therapy, go to http://thepoint.lww.com/AT10e.

CHOICE OF ANTIEPILEPTIC DRUG

Many AEDs have a relatively narrow spectrum of efficacy against selected seizure types; therefore, choice of appropriate drug therapy for a specific patient depends on an accurate diagnosis of epilepsy. In addition, toxicity must be considered when selecting an AED. Preferred drugs for specific types of seizures and common epileptic syndromes are listed in Tables 58-2 and 58-3. Although certain drugs are preferred, the identification of the most effective drug for a particular patient may be a process of trial and error; several medication trials may be necessary before success is achieved. The consensus method was used to analyze expert opinion on treatment of three epilepsy syndromes and status epilepticus.[18] The experts recommended monotherapy first, followed by a second monotherapy agent if the first failed. If the second monotherapy failed, the experts were not in agreement on whether to try a third monotherapy agent or to combine two therapies. The experts recommended epilepsy surgery evaluation after the third failed AED for patients with symptomatic localization-related epilepsies.

To assess the evidence on efficacy, tolerability, and safety of many of the new AEDs in treating children and adults with new-onset and refractory partial and generalized epilepsies, a panel evaluated the available evidence.[19,20] They concluded that AED choice depends on seizure and syndrome type; patient age; concomitant medications; and AED tolerability, safety, and efficacy. The results of these two evidence-based assessments provide guidelines for the use of newer AEDs in patients with new-onset and refractory epilepsy.

THERAPEUTIC END POINTS

The individual patient's response to AED treatment (i.e., seizure frequency and severity, and symptoms of toxicity) must be the major focus for therapy assessment. In general, the goal of AED treatment is administration of sufficient medication to completely prevent seizures without producing significant toxicity.[21] Realistically, this goal may be compromised for many patients; it may not be possible to completely prevent seizures without producing intolerable adverse effects. Thus, the therapeutic end points achieved can vary among patients; optimization of AED therapy for a specific person depends on tailoring therapy to the patient's needs and lifestyle. It is rarely optimal to administer "standard" or "usual" doses of an AED to a patient or to adjust doses to achieve a "therapeutic blood level" without considering the effect of the dose or serum concentration on the patient's

TABLE 58-3
Antiepileptic Drugs Useful for Various Seizure Types[a]

Primary Generalized Tonic-Clonic	Secondarily Generalized Tonic-Clonic	Simple or Complex Partial	Absence	Myoclonic, Atonic/Akinetic
Most Effective With Least Toxicity				
Valproate	Carbamazepine	Carbamazepine	Ethosuximide	Valproate
Carbamazepine	Oxcarbazepine	Oxcarbazepine	Valproate	Clonazepam
Lamotrigine	Levetiracetam	Levetiracetam	Lamotrigine[b]	Rufinamide (Lennox-Gastaut Syndrome)
	Valproate	Valproate	(Topiramate)[b]	Levetiracetam (Juvenile Myoclonic Epilepsy)
(Levetiracetam)[b]	(Gabapentin)[b]	Lamotrigine		Lamotrigine[b]
(Oxcarbazepine)[b]	Lamotrigine	(Gabapentin)[b]		(Topiramate)[b]
(Topiramate)[b]	(Topiramate)[b]	(Levetiracetam)[b]		
(Zonisamide)[b]	(Tiagabine)[b]	(Topiramate)[b]		
	(Zonisamide)[b]	(Tiagabine)[b]		
	(Levetiracetam)[b]	(Pregabalin)[b]		
	(Pregabalin)[b]	(Zonisamide)[b]		
	(Lacosamide)[b]	(Lacosamide)[b]		
Effective, but Often Poorly Tolerated or Cause Unacceptable Toxicity				
Phenobarbital	Phenobarbital	Clorazepate	Clonazepam	(Felbamate)[c]
Primidone	Primidone	Phenobarbital		
(Felbamate)[c]	(Felbamate)[c]	Primidone		
Phenytoin	Phenytoin	(Felbamate)[c]		
		Phenytoin		
Of Little Value				
Ethosuximide	Ethosuximide	Ethosuximide	Phenytoin	
			Carbamazepine	
			Phenobarbital	
			Primidone	
			Oxcarbazepine	
			Levetiracetam	
			Lacosamide	
			Rufinamide	
			Tiagabine	

[a] Drugs are listed in general order of preference within each category. Recommendations by various authorities may differ, especially regarding the relative place of valproate and the role of phenytoin as a first-line AED. The use of phenobarbital and primidone is now discouraged.

[b] The place of gabapentin, lacosamide, rufinamide, lamotrigine, oxcarbazepine, levetiracetam, topiramate, tiagabine, pregabalin, and zonisamide is yet to be determined. They are placed on this table only to indicate the types of seizures for which they appear to be effective. More clinical experience is needed before their roles as possible primary AEDs are clarified.

[c] The place of felbamate is yet to be determined. It is placed on this table only to indicate the types of seizures for which it appears to be effective. Felbamate has been associated with aplastic anemia and hepatic failure; until a possible causative role is clarified, felbamate cannot be recommended for treatment of epilepsy unless all other, potentially less toxic, treatment options have been exhausted.

Source: French JA et al. Efficacy and tolerability of the new antiepileptic drugs I: treatment of new onset epilepsy: report of the Therapeutics and Technology Assessment Subcommittee and Quality Standards Subcommittee of the American Academy of Neurology and the American Epilepsy Society. *Neurology.* 2004;62:1252; French JA et al. Efficacy and tolerability of the new antiepileptic drugs II: treatment of refractory epilepsy: report of the Therapeutics and Technology Assessment Subcommittee and Quality Standards Subcommittee of the American Academy of Neurology and the American Epilepsy Society. *Neurology.* 2004;62:1261; Pellock JM. Efficacy and adverse effects of antiepileptic drugs. *Pediatr Clin North Am.* 1989;36:435; Mattson RH et al. Comparison of carbamazepine, phenobarbital, phenytoin, and primidone in partial and secondarily generalized tonic-clonic seizures. *N Engl J Med.* 1985;313:145; Mattson RH et al. A comparison of valproate with carbamazepine for the treatment of complex partial seizures and secondarily generalized tonic-clonic seizures in adults. The Department of Veterans Affairs Epilepsy Cooperative Study No. 264 Group. *N Engl J Med.* 1992;327:765; Fisch BJ et al. Generalized tonic-clonic seizures. In: Wyllie E et al, eds. *The Treatment of Epilepsy: Principles and Practice.* 3rd ed. Philadelphia, PA: Lippincott Williams & Wilkins; 2001:369.

condition and quality of life. As with many conditions requiring chronic drug therapy, patient participation in developing and evaluating a therapeutic plan is extremely important. Patients should be educated regarding the expected positive and negative effects of their AED therapy, and they must be encouraged to communicate with their health care provider regarding their responses to prescribed AED.

SERUM DRUG CONCENTRATIONS

Relation to Dosage

For some AEDs, a good correlation exists between serum concentrations and both therapeutic response and toxicity. For these agents, the wide availability of AED serum concentration determinations has had a significant impact on the treatment of seizure disorders. The correlation between the administered maintenance dose of an AED and the resulting steady-state serum concentration is poor. Administration of "usual therapeutic doses," even when calculated on the basis of body weight, is equally likely to produce subtherapeutic, therapeutic, or potentially intoxicating serum concentrations. Interindividual variation in hepatic metabolic capacity probably accounts for most of this variability.

Relation to Clinical Response

For selected AEDs, proper use and interpretation of serum concentrations are important for optimizing treatment regimens in epilepsy.[22,23] An individual patient's clinical response to AED treatment must be the major focus for therapy assessment.

Neither therapeutic effects nor toxic symptoms are "all or none"; in most situations, there are gradations of efficacy and toxicity. Dosage increases and titration to AED serum concentrations within and occasionally above the "therapeutic range" may significantly improve therapeutic responses without producing significant toxicity.[23] Individual patients often differ dramatically in their response to a particular serum drug concentration; therefore, therapeutic serum concentrations should be considered only as guidelines for treatment. Many patients' condition may be controlled with serum drug concentrations below the usual therapeutic range.[24] In these patients, dosage adjustment to increase the serum drug concentration is not warranted. In this case, it is better to "treat the patient, not the level."

Interestingly, a recent Cochrane Review found no evidence that measuring AED concentrations routinely to inform dose adjustments is superior to dose adjustments based on clinical information.[25] However, the authors do state that their review does not exclude the possibility that AED serum concentration might be useful in special situations or in selected patients.

Indications for Use

Measurement of serum drug concentrations may provide clinically useful information in the following situations:

- Uncontrolled seizures despite administration of greater-than-average doses: Serum concentrations of AED may help distinguish drug resistance from subtherapeutic drug concentrations caused by malabsorption, nonadherence, or rapid metabolism.
- Seizure recurrence in a patient whose seizures were previously controlled: This is often owing to nonadherence with the prescribed medication regimen.
- Documentation of intoxication: In patients who exhibit signs or symptoms of dose-related AED toxicity, documentation of the dose and serum concentration of the responsible drug is helpful.
- Assessment of patient adherence: Although monitoring AED serum concentrations can be used to assess patient adherence with therapy, conclusions must be based on comparisons with previous steady-state serum concentrations that reflected reliable intake of a given dose of AED.
- Documentation of desired results from a dose change or other therapeutic maneuver (e.g., administration of a loading dose): When patients are receiving multiple AEDs, it is often appropriate to measure serum concentrations of all drugs after a change in the dose of one agent because changes to one drug frequently affect the pharmacokinetic disposition of other drugs.
- When precise dosage changes are required: On occasion, small changes in the dose of a drug (e.g., phenytoin) can result in large changes in both the serum concentration and clinical response. In addition, cautious titration of dosage and serum concentration may be necessary to avoid intoxication. Knowledge of the serum drug concentration before the dosage change may allow the clinician to select a more appropriate new maintenance dose.
- During pregnancy, AED serum concentrations often decline and dosage adjustments may be warranted to maintain adequate seizure protection. Free (unbound) concentrations should be monitored for highly protein-bound AEDs. AED serum concentrations should be monitored after delivery, particularly when dosage escalations have been made during pregnancy.

Frequent, "routine" determinations of serum AED concentrations are costly and not warranted for patients whose clinical status is stable. Clinicians may tend to focus attention on normal variability in serum concentrations rather than on the patient's clinical status; as a result, unnecessary dosage adjustments may be made to make serum concentrations fit the "normal range." A plan of action for what the clinician is going to do with the information once it is obtained should be in place before obtaining the sample. Therefore, the results of individual serum concentration determinations must be evaluated carefully to decide whether a significant, clinically meaningful change has occurred.[26]

Interpretation of Serum Concentrations

Several factors can alter the relationship between AED serum concentration and the patient's response to the drug. Whenever a change in serum concentration is apparent, pharmacokinetic factors (Table 58-4) should be considered (along with the patient's clinical status) before a decision is made to adjust the AED dosage. Laboratory variability can cause minor fluctuations in reported AED serum concentrations. Under the best conditions, reported values for serum concentrations may be within plus or minus 10% of "true" values.[27,28] Therefore, the magnitude of any apparent change must be considered. Therapeutic ranges are not well established for some drugs (e.g., valproate and the newer AEDs such as lamotrigine, topiramate, and tiagabine). Published therapeutic ranges may have been determined in small numbers of patients or may more accurately represent average serum concentrations at usual doses. As an example, many clinicians agree that "pushing" valproate serum concentrations up to 150 to 200 mcg/mL may be beneficial for some patients; these higher concentrations are not consistently associated with specific toxicity symptoms.[29–32] Nevertheless, most laboratories report 50 to 100 mcg/mL as a therapeutic range for valproate. Inappropriate sample timing can result in inconsistent and clinically meaningless changes in AED serum concentrations.[22] Generally, serum concentrations of AED should not be measured until a minimum of four to five half-lives have elapsed since initiation of therapy or a dosage change. Blood samples should be obtained in the morning, before any doses of the AED have been taken; this practice provides reproducible, postabsorptive (i.e., "trough") serum concentrations. Interindividual variability in response to a given serum concentration of medication is common. Excellent therapeutic response or even symptoms of intoxication may be associated with AED serum concentrations that are classified as "subtherapeutic."[33] Active metabolites of AEDs usually are not measured when serum concentrations are determined.[28,34] Alterations in the relative proportion of parent drug and active metabolite may result in an apparent alteration in the relationship between the serum concentration of the parent drug and the patient's response. Binding to serum proteins is significant for some AEDs (e.g., phenytoin, valproate, tiagabine). Changes in protein binding can result from drug interaction, renal failure, pregnancy, or changes in nutritional status. These changes can alter the usual relationship between the measured total drug concentration (bound and unbound to plasma proteins) and the unbound (pharmacologically active) drug concentration. This change may not be apparent when only total serum concentrations are measured. Determination of serum concentrations of free (i.e., unbound) AEDs is available from many commercial laboratories; these determinations are expensive and results may not be available for several days. If significant changes in protein binding are suspected, measurement of free concentrations of AED may provide additional information useful for adjustment of doses or interpretation of the patient's symptoms.[27,28,34]

MONOTHERAPY VERSUS POLYTHERAPY

Decades ago, epilepsy was often treated initially with multiple AEDs (polytherapy). A second, third, or even fourth drug was added when seizures were incompletely controlled with a single

TABLE 58-4
Pharmacokinetic Properties of Antiepileptic Drugs

Drug	Oral Absorption (%)	Half-Life (hours)	Time to Steady State	Dosage Schedule	Usual Therapeutic Serum Concentration	Plasma Protein Binding (%)	Volume of Distribution (L/kg)
Carbamazepine	90–100	*Chronic:* 5–25	2–4 days	BID to TID	5–12 mcg/mL	75 (50–90)	0.8–1.6
Ethosuximide	90–100	*Pediatric:* 30 *Adult:* 60	5–10 days	Daily (BID)	40–100 mcg/mL	0	0.7
Felbamate	90	12–20	3–4 days	BID to TID	50–110 mcg/mL	24	0.7–0.8
Gabapentin	40–60; ↓ with ↑ dose	*Normal renal function:* 5–9; ↑ with ↓ renal function	*Normal renal function:* 1–1.5 days	TID to QID (every 6–8 hours)	2 mcg/mL (proposed)	0	≈0.8
Lacosamide	100	13 ↑ slightly with renal impairment	2–3 days	BID	Not determined	<15	0.6
Lamotrigine	90–100	*Monotherapy:* 24–29 *Enzyme inducers:* 15 *Enzyme inhibitor (VPA):* 59	4–9 days	BID	4–18 mcg/mL (proposed)	55	0.9–1.2
Levetiracetam	100	*Normal renal function:* 6–8; ↑ with ↓ renal function	*Normal renal function:* 1–1.5 days	BID	Not determined	<10	≈0.7
Oxcarbazepine	100	8–13	2–3 days	BID to TID	Not determined	40	
Phenobarbital	90–100	2–4 days	8–16 days	Daily	15–40 mcg/mL	50	0.5–0.6
Phenytoin	90–100	Varies with dose	5–30 days	Daily to BID	10–20 mcg/mL	95	0.5–0.7
Pregabalin	≥90	*Normal renal function:* 6; ↑ with ↓ renal function	24 hours	BID to TID	Not determined	0	0.5
Rufinamide	>85	9	1–2 days	BID	Not determined	<35	Dose dependent
Tiagabine	90	*Monotherapy:* 7–9 *Enzyme inducers:* 4–7	1–2 days	BID to QID	Not determined	96	1.1
Topiramate	≥80	12–24	3–4 days	BID	Not determined	10–15	0.7
Valproate	100 (≈ 80% with divalproex ER)	10–16	2–3 days	BID to QID (daily with divalproe × ER)	50–150 mcg/mL	90+	0.09–0.17
Vigabatrin	80–90	8–12 (not clinically important. Irreversible enzyme inhibitor)	NA	Daily to BID	NA	NA	NA
Zonisamide	≈80	*Monotherapy:* ≈60 *Enzyme inducers:* 27–36	2 weeks	Daily to BID	Not determined	50–60	1.3

[a] Based on four half-lives. This lag time should allow determination of steady-state serum concentrations within limits of most assay sensitivities.
BID, twice daily; NA, not applicable; QID, four times daily; VPA, valproic acid.

AED. Evaluation of the effectiveness of polytherapy in subsequent years has shown little advantage for most patients. Use of a single drug at optimal tolerated serum concentrations produces excellent therapeutic results and minimal side effects in most patients. Addition of a second AED significantly improves seizure control in only 10% to 20% of patients.[35,36] Reduction or elimination of existing polytherapy in patients with longstanding seizure disorders often lessens or eliminates cognitive impairment and other side effects; seizure control actually may improve.[35,37–40]

Most experts advocate the use of a single AED (monotherapy) whenever possible. Successful monotherapy may require higher-than-usual AED doses or serum concentrations greater than the upper limit of the usual therapeutic range.[41,42] Addition of a second drug may be necessary in some patients; however, polytherapy should be reserved for patients with multiple seizure types or for patients in whom first-line AEDs have failed to control seizures when titrated to maximal tolerated doses.[18,38,41] When a new AED is added to a patient's regimen with the goal of improving seizure control, the existing AED regimen should be scrutinized for continued value. In some cases, a patient's AED regimen can accumulate drugs that may be unnecessary because they were started and never re-evaluated. Continued vigilance and critical assessment of every drug in a patient's regimen is important.

Use of polytherapy creates several disadvantages that must be weighed against possible benefits. Seizure control may not significantly improve; in fact, our experience and information from studies in which patients were converted from polytherapy to monotherapy indicate that even with use of an optimal AED, seizure control may be worsened in some patients by polytherapy regimens.[40] Health care costs, for medications and for increased laboratory monitoring, may increase significantly with polytherapy. In addition, drug interactions among AEDs can complicate assessment of the patient's response and serum concentrations. Patient adherence often is worsened when multiple medications are prescribed, and adverse effects often increase.

Although AED monotherapy is preferred whenever feasible, the recent introduction of several new AEDs has increased the use of polytherapy.[42] Owing to limitations on the patient populations used for clinical trials of new drugs (i.e., patients with seizure disorders not completely controlled by previous medications), most new AEDs are labeled only for use as add-on therapy. Although reports exist on the efficacy of the new AEDs as monotherapy,[43–46] only lamotrigine, topiramate, oxcarbazepine, and felbamate are US Food and Drug Administration (FDA) approved for monotherapy. Lamotrigine is indicated for conversion to monotherapy in adults with partial seizures who are receiving treatment with carbamazepine, phenytoin, phenobarbital, primidone, or valproate as the single AED.[47] Topiramate is approved as initial monotherapy in patients 10 years of age and older with partial-onset or primary generalized tonic-clonic seizures.[48] Oxcarbazepine is approved for monotherapy of partial seizures in adults and children.[49] Felbamate should be considered (as monotherapy or polytherapy) only when other AEDs have failed. More AEDs will undoubtedly follow with monotherapy indications.

DURATION OF THERAPY AND DISCONTINUATION OF ANTIEPILEPTIC DRUGS

A diagnosis of epilepsy may not necessitate lifelong drug therapy. Several long-term studies have shown that AED therapy may be successfully withdrawn from some patients after a seizure-free period of 2 to 5 years.[9–11] Seizures recurred in only 12% to 36% of patients who were followed for up to 23 years after AED withdrawal. Therefore, many patients whose epilepsy is completely controlled with medication can stop therapy after a seizurefree period of at least 2 years.

Discontinuation of medications is advantageous for economic, medical, and psychosocial reasons. Costs associated with health care visits, serum concentration determinations, and the medications themselves are eliminated or reduced. The risk of adverse effects from long-term medication use is eliminated, and patients can expect fewer lifestyle restrictions. Attempts to withdraw AED therapy are associated with risks, however. Primary among them is the reappearance of seizure activity which can result in status epilepticus, loss of driving privileges, employment difficulties, and/or physical injury.

Risk factors for seizure recurrence after discontinuation of AED have been identified in observational studies; complete agreement, however, is not found among studies regarding the nature and importance of specific risk factors. Opinions and data also differ regarding the optimal duration of the seizurefree period before discontinuation of AED is attempted. Nevertheless, at least some consensus has been reached regarding certain factors that may predict a higher risk of seizure recurrence (Table 58-5).[9–11,50,51]

In nonemergency situations, AED should be withdrawn slowly; if a patient receives multiple drugs, each drug should be withdrawn separately. Too-rapid withdrawal can result in status epilepticus. Clinical studies of AED discontinuation usually used a 2-month to 3-month withdrawal schedule for each drug. The optimal rate of withdrawal of AED has not been identified. One study compared withdrawal of individual drugs for a 6-week and a 9-month period and found no difference in seizure recurrence between the groups.[52] Another study compared seizure frequencies in patients withdrawn from carbamazepine rapidly (for 4 days) and in patients withdrawn more slowly (for 10 days).[53] Significantly more generalized tonic-clonic seizures occurred when carbamazepine was withdrawn rapidly; complex partial seizures, however, did not occur at a higher rate with rapid withdrawal. Therefore, withdrawal of each AED for at least 6 weeks would seem to be a safe approach. Gradual withdrawal is recommended even for medications such as phenobarbital that have long half-lives and should theoretically be "self-tapering." In our experience, gradual reduction of medications such as phenobarbital is associated with a significantly higher success rate. If AEDs are withdrawn at an appropriate rate and seizures recur, drug treatment is usually reinstituted. In most patients, good seizure control is regained by restarting therapy. However, in approximately 1% of patients, seizure control is not easily

TABLE 58-5

Risk Factors Possibly Predicting Seizure Recurrence After Antiepileptic Drug Withdrawal[9–11,50,51]

- <2 years seizure-free before withdrawal
- Onset of seizures after age 12
- History of atypical febrile seizures
- Family history of seizures
- 2–6 years before seizures controlled
- Large number of seizures (>30) before control or total of >100 seizures
- Partial seizures (simple or complex)
- History of absence seizures
- Abnormal EEG persisting throughout treatment
- Slowing on EEG before medication withdrawal
- Organic neurologic disorder
- Moderate to severe mental retardation
- Withdrawal of valproate or phenytoin (higher rate of recurrence than withdrawal of other AED)

AED, antiepileptic drug; EEG, electroencephalogram.

regained.[54] This uncommon, but potentially serious, outcome should be considered when therapy withdrawal is considered.

CLINICAL ASSESSMENT AND TREATMENT OF EPILEPSY

Complex Partial Seizures with Secondary Generalization

DIAGNOSIS

CASE 58-1

QUESTION 1: A.R. is a 14-year-old, 40-kg female high school student. A.R. had three febrile seizures when she was 3 years old. She received phenobarbital prophylaxis "off and on," according to her parents, for about 6 months after her second febrile seizure. Since then, she had no reported seizures until 24 hours before admission. At that time she had a "convulsion" shortly after arriving at school in the morning. A teacher who witnessed the episode describes her as behaving "oddly" before the seizure. She abruptly got up from her desk and began to walk clumsily toward the door; she bumped into several desks and did not respond to the teacher's attempts to redirect her back to her seat. After approximately 1 minute of this behavior, she fell to the floor and experienced an apparent generalized tonic-clonic seizure that lasted approximately 90 seconds. During the episode, she was incontinent of urine and was described as "turning kind of blue." After this episode, A.R. was transported to the hospital.

On arrival at the hospital, A.R. appeared drowsy and confused. Laboratory studies—a complete blood count (CBC), serum glucose, electrolytes, drug and alcohol screen, and lumbar puncture—were normal. Physical examination and a complete neurologic evaluation were normal. An EEG showed diffuse slowing with focal epileptiform discharges in the left temporal area; it was interpreted as abnormal. There was no history of recent illness or injury, although A.R. had stayed up late several nights recently studying for an examination.

A second seizure occurred in the hospital. The nursing staff described an episode similar to the one that occurred at school. After recovery from each episode, A.R. had no memory of events during the seizures; she only remembered a "funny feeling" in her stomach and a "buzzing" in her head before she lost consciousness. She described having these feelings "a couple of times" in the past; she attributed them to "just getting dizzy" and had not reported them to her parents. After these previous episodes, A.R. described feeling "mixed up" and groggy for a few minutes. What subjective and objective features of A.R.'s seizures are consistent with a diagnosis of complex partial seizures with secondary generalization?

A.R.'s clinical pattern of observed seizure activity (an apparent aura preceding her loss of consciousness), her history of apparent complex partial seizures not accompanied by generalized seizures, and the findings of focal abnormal activity on EEG are all concordant with this diagnosis. Postictal confusion and grogginess are common after both generalized tonic-clonic and complex partial seizures. Her unusual or inappropriate behavior represents a complex partial seizure that subsequently generalized. The clinical features, accompanied by her EEG findings, also help rule out possible atypical absence seizures, which can be confused with complex partial epilepsy syndromes based on only clinical presentation. In both syndromes, patients may briefly appear to lose contact with their surroundings and display automatisms and mild clonic movements during seizure activity. In A.R.'s case, the EEG and the generalized tonic-clonic seizures during her episodes would rule out atypical absence as a likely possibility.

DECISION TO USE ANTIEPILEPTIC DRUG THERAPY

CASE 58-1, QUESTION 2: What factors should be considered in a decision to treat A.R.'s seizures with AED therapy?

Once a diagnosis of epilepsy is established, the decision to treat the patient with medication is based on the likelihood of recurrence. The need for AED therapy after a single seizure is controversial; however, recurrence of generalized tonic-clonic seizures is less likely if AED therapy is initiated after the first generalized tonic-clonic seizure.[55] Therefore, at least for this one specific seizure type, early use of AED is supported. Whether this information applies to other types of seizures is not known. Clinical wisdom, however, holds that "seizures beget seizures," and most experts advocate early treatment of epilepsy (i.e., after a first or second unprovoked seizure).

In A.R.'s case, the potential benefits of immediate introduction of AED therapy appear to outweigh potential risks. She experienced complex partial seizures and some were followed by secondarily generalized tonic-clonic seizures. Recurrence of seizure activity is likely to result in physical injury, social embarrassment, and interference with her participation in activities typical of a person her age. If her seizures are not controlled, she faces future limitation of her driving privileges and may face barriers to employment. Although AED therapy is associated with risks, they probably are outweighed by the potential benefits.

CHOICE OF ANTIEPILEPTIC DRUG

CASE 58-1, QUESTION 3: Which AED are commonly used for A.R.'s seizure type? Based on the subjective and objective data available, recommend a first-choice AED for A.R. and a plan for initial dosing of this medication.

Many AEDs would be appropriate choices for A.R.'s complex partial seizures that can secondarily generalize (Table 58-3).[36,56,57] Some AEDs are not FDA-approved as initial monotherapy. Although valproate is effective for treating both generalized and complex partial seizures,[58] it would not be a good initial choice for this patient owing to the increased risks in a woman of childbearing age (see Women's Issues in Epilepsy section).

Felbamate, gabapentin, lacosamide, lamotrigine, levetiracetam, oxcarbazepine, pregabalin, tiagabine, topiramate, and zonisamide are effective for control of partial seizures with or without secondary generalization. Most experience with these drugs was obtained when they were used as adjunctive agents when previous AED therapies were unsuccessful. Initial clinical trials with these medications indicate that several of them may be useful as single agents. Felbamate, lamotrigine, oxcarbazepine, and topiramate have monotherapy indications. Most of the more recently approved medications appear to be safe and are usually well tolerated. The usefulness of felbamate is limited, however, owing to its potential for serious hematologic and hepatic toxicity.

Carbamazepine has several advantages that make it a preferred first-choice agent in the opinion of many clinicians. In comparison with phenytoin, carbamazepine is less sedating and is not associated with dysmorphic effects, such as hirsutism, acne, gingival hyperplasia, and coarsening of facial features. Carbamazepine's pharmacokinetic profile also makes dosage adjustment easier. In A.R.'s case, the lack of cosmetic side effects may be especially significant because she may be taking medication for many years. In addition, reduced sedation may be important with respect to her school performance.

CARBAMAZEPINE THERAPY

INITIATION AND DOSAGE

Initiation of treatment with full therapeutic maintenance doses of carbamazepine often causes excessive side effects such as nausea, vomiting, diplopia, and significant sedation. Therefore, carbamazepine therapy should be initiated gradually and patients should be allowed time to acclimate to the effects of the drug. Final dosing requirements are difficult to anticipate in individual patients. A reasonable starting dosage of carbamazepine for A.R. would be 100 mg twice a day; her dosage could be increased by 100 to 200 mg/day every 7 to 14 days. The rapidity of increases will depend on A.R.'s tolerance for the drug and the frequency of her seizures.

HEMATOLOGIC TOXICITY

CASE 58-1, QUESTION 4: Carbamazepine has been associated with hematologic and hepatic toxicities. What is the incidence and significance of these toxicities? How should A.R. be monitored for them?

Aplastic anemia and agranulocytosis have occurred in association with carbamazepine therapy.[59] Several cases have been fatal; however, most cases occurred in older patients treated for trigeminal neuralgia. Many patients were receiving other medications, and occasionally the reports were incomplete; thus, assessment of a causal role for carbamazepine is difficult.[60] Severe blood dyscrasias from carbamazepine seem rare (estimated prevalence <1/50,000) and have predominantly occurred in nonepileptic patients. The lack of severe hematologic toxicity in various published series and clinical trials in patients with epilepsy has been notable.[61,62]

Leukopenia is relatively common in patients taking carbamazepine. It is usually mild and often reverses despite continued administration of the drug.[61] Total leukocyte counts may fall to less than 4,000 cells/μL in some patients, but differentials and platelet and erythrocyte counts remain normal. Symptoms (e.g., fever, sore throat) that might suggest early stages of agranulocytosis do not occur. Carbamazepine-associated hematologic disorders are unrelated to drug dosage; thus, these reactions appear to be idiosyncratic.

Routine Hematologic Testing

Laboratory monitoring of A.R.'s hematologic status is recommended during carbamazepine therapy. The likelihood of early detection of aplastic anemia or agranulocytosis through frequent blood counts is low, however, and such monitoring is costly.[61,63] Because hematologic toxicity from carbamazepine primarily occurs early in therapy, a CBC should be obtained before therapy and at monthly intervals during the first 2 to 3 months of therapy; thereafter, a yearly or every-other-year CBC, white blood cell count with differential, and platelet count should be sufficient.

HEPATOTOXICITY

Carbamazepine-related liver damage is extremely rare despite its being frequently mentioned as a potential problem and strong warnings in the package insert.[64,65] Hepatic adverse reactions are believed to be idiosyncratic or immunologically based. Aggressive laboratory monitoring of liver function tests (LFTs) probably is unnecessary.[63] Alkaline phosphatase and γ-glutamyltransferase concentrations often are elevated in patients taking carbamazepine (and other AEDs). This is believed to result from hepatic enzyme induction and is not necessarily evidence for hepatic disease.[66]

In summary, hepatic and hematologic toxicities of carbamazepine are rare. Although potentially serious, they are best monitored on clinical grounds rather than by ongoing, intensive laboratory testing. Patients, families, or caregivers should be aware that the appearance of unusual symptoms (e.g., jaundice, abdominal pain, excessive bruising and bleeding, or sudden onset of severe sore throat with fever) should be reported to a health care professional. Baseline (pretreatment) determination of A.R.'s hepatic and hematologic status, possibly with monthly follow-up testing for 2 to 3 months, probably will be sufficient.[62,63] Thereafter, a CBC and a liver function battery should probably be evaluated only every 1 to 2 years, unless signs or symptoms of hepatic or hematologic disorders are observed.

PHARMACOKINETICS AND AUTOINDUCTION OF METABOLISM

CASE 58-1, QUESTION 5: For the subsequent 6 weeks, A.R.'s carbamazepine dosage was gradually increased to 400 mg twice daily (BID) (20 mg/kg/day). Until the last dose increase, she had been experiencing one or two complex partial seizures weekly; she had experienced only one generalized tonic-clonic seizure since her hospitalization. One week after the increase to 20 mg/kg/day, her serum carbamazepine concentration was 9 mcg/mL just before her first dose of the day. No seizures occurred for 4 weeks, and she tolerated the medication well. Subsequent to the 4-week seizurefree period, she again began experiencing one seizure weekly. What factor(s) might be responsible for this reversal of seizure control?

Several factors may account for this change. It is important always to consider the possibility of poor medication adherence when clinical response changes unexpectedly. This should be investigated, and A.R. and her family should be educated regarding the importance of regular medication intake.

The observed changes in A.R.'s seizure control may also be due to unique features of carbamazepine pharmacokinetics. Carbamazepine is a potent inducer of hepatic cytochrome P-450 (CYP3A4). The drug is also a substrate for this enzyme. As a result, carbamazepine not only stimulates the metabolism of other CYP3A4 substrates but also induces its own metabolism by autoinduction. Carbamazepine's half-life after single acute doses is approximately 35 hours; with chronic dosing, its half-life decreases to 15 to 25 hours. This induction of metabolism may be enhanced by combined administration of carbamazepine and other enzyme-inducing AEDs; with polytherapy, carbamazepine's half-life may be as short as 6 to 10 hours.[28] This increase in clearance necessitates increased carbamazepine doses, increased frequency of administration, or both. Autoinduction of carbamazepine metabolism appears to be related to dose and serum concentration. Approximately 1 month may be required for the autoinduction process to reach completion after each increase in carbamazepine dose.[67]

Assuming that adherence was not the main problem, A.R.'s carbamazepine dose should be increased. The drug's pharmacokinetics are generally linear with respect to acute dosage changes.[68] A 50% increase in dosage to 1,200 mg/day should re-establish seizure control. Depending on A.R.'s clinical status, further increases in dosage may be necessary.

BIOEQUIVALENCE OF GENERIC DOSAGE

CASE 58-1, QUESTION 6: A.R.'s dosage was increased to 600 mg BID. Four weeks later, she was still experiencing approximately one complex partial seizure weekly. A repeat trough serum carbamazepine concentration was 6.5 mcg/mL. On questioning, A.R. denied missing doses of medication, and a tablet count confirmed apparently accurate drug intake. A.R. relates that she experiences some mild nausea after her doses, but she has not vomited. It is noted that her pharmacist has begun substituting a generic carbamazepine tablets for the Tegretol that was previously dispensed. What role, if any, might this change in carbamazepine formulation have played in the failure of A.R.'s serum concentrations to increase as expected? What other factors might be considered in explaining this situation?

Several manufacturers market generic carbamazepine tablets. Bioavailability data supplied by the manufacturers are based on single-dose or short multiple-dose studies in healthy subjects. Therefore, it is impossible to completely predict the results of a change from Tegretol to generic carbamazepine for maintenance therapy in an individual patient.[69] Because of variations in amount of drug available from different products, some patients with epilepsy cannot tolerate changes in formulations between brand and generic, generic and generic, or generic and brand.[70] Changes in seizure control from too little drug or toxicity from too much drug have been reported with changes between formulations for several AEDs. Additionally, increased costs to the health care system which offset savings achieved by the use of generic drugs have been identified in some studies.[71–75] Bioavailability data and one author's (R.S.L.) experience with institutionalized patients with severe seizure disorders suggest that the generic carbamazepine preparations currently on the market may be substituted for Tegretol with little need for dosage adjustment. Nonetheless, in A.R.'s case, substitution of generic carbamazepine may be a possible cause for the loss of seizure control. Readjustment of her dose to gain seizure control and consistent use of one manufacturer's product (either brand or generic) might alleviate this problem.

Three extended-release forms of carbamazepine (Tegretol XR, Carbatrol, and Equetro) are available and may provide an alternative for A.R. These formulations allow more reliable absorption of drug when administered on a twice-daily dosing schedule. Many patients can better tolerate carbamazepine when these forms are used because large fluctuations in plasma concentrations are avoided. Use of Tegretol XR to avoid three-times-daily or four-times-daily dosing schedules has been shown to increase adherence for many patients.[76] It is important to counsel patients on the fact that the empty Oros tablet shell from the Tegretol XR dose does not dissolve as it passes through the gastrointestinal (GI) tract, and it may be visible in the stool. Patients need to understand that the carbamazepine has been absorbed, and that this is an empty shell. Tegretol XR tablets lose their extended-release properties when broken or crushed; Carbatrol beads may be emptied onto food or administered via feeding tube.[77] Equetro is not FDA-approved for epilepsy, it is indicated for the treatment of acute manic and mixed episodes associated with bipolar I disorder.

In conclusion, it may be impossible to identify a single cause for the unexpected change in A.R.'s seizure control. Common reasons for loss of seizure control include sleep deprivation, increased stress, acute illness, and/or medication nonadherence.

TREATMENT FAILURE AND ALTERNATIVE ANTIEPILEPTIC DRUGS

CASE 58-2

QUESTION 1: R.H., a 19-year-old, 64-kg young woman, has experienced simple partial seizures, complex partial seizures, and secondarily generalized tonic-clonic seizures for the past 2 years. She could not tolerate treatment with phenytoin (severe gingival hyperplasia and mental "dullness") or valproate (hair loss, tremor, and a weight gain of 8 kg). In addition, neither phenytoin nor valproate was dramatically effective in reducing her seizures. She currently receives carbamazepine 600 mg three times daily (TID). For the past 3 months, while being treated with carbamazepine, she has had approximately five simple partial seizures, three complex partial seizures, and one generalized tonic-clonic seizure. This represents an approximate 30% reduction in her frequency of seizures. She tolerates her present dose of carbamazepine but has experienced significant drowsiness, incoordination, and mental confusion at higher doses. What are possible therapeutic options for R.H.? Evaluate the newer AEDs and their possible usefulness for R.H.

R.H. is exhibiting a partial response to maximally tolerated doses of carbamazepine. An alteration in her current AED regimen is indicated. She has not tolerated other AEDs because of side effects. Although valproate is effective for control of partial seizures, it is not considered an alternative in a woman of child-bearing age. R.H.'s CNS side effects (e.g., persistent drowsiness) with other AEDs would make many clinicians reluctant to consider medications such as phenobarbital or primidone as either alternatives or adjunctive agents to her current carbamazepine regimen. Use of one of the newer AEDs as adjunctive medication may be of value for R.H.

New AEDs marketed in the United States since 1993 for maintenance treatment of epilepsy include the following: felbamate, gabapentin, lacosamide, lamotrigine, levetiracetam, oxcarbazepine, pregabalin, tiagabine, topiramate and zonisamide (Table 58-6).[78–91] Clinical trials for new AEDs are most often carried out in patients with partial seizures refractory to standard AEDs. Most of these newer or "second-generation" AEDs were initially FDA-approved as "add-on" or adjunctive treatment in patients with partial seizures with or without secondary generalization. Also, consensus is that some of these AEDs may be effective as broad-spectrum agents; for example, lamotrigine appears to be a useful treatment in absence seizures.

SIDE EFFECTS

Common side effects for the newer AEDs are described in Table 58-6. Most of them are less sedating than older medications such as phenobarbital or phenytoin. Felbamate causes insomnia and irritability in a significant proportion of treated patients. Other side effects that may be prominent during felbamate therapy include headaches, weight loss, and GI effects. Felbamate's usefulness is seriously limited by its association with aplastic anemia and hepatic failure. A conservative estimate of the occurrence rate is 1 case per 2,000 to 5,000 patients treated.[92] Some cases of felbamate-associated aplastic anemia and hepatotoxicity were fatal. Routine hematologic studies and LFTs should be performed and patients and their families should be fully informed of the potential risks. Because of the relationship between felbamate therapy and aplastic anemia and hepatic failure, felbamate is much lower on the list of options for patients with epilepsy.

Gabapentin and tiagabine have not been associated with serious side effects; gabapentin can cause weight gain[93] and tiagabine can cause nonspecific dizziness relatively frequently.[94]

TABLE 58-6

Drugs Used for the Treatment of Partial and Generalized Tonic-Clonic Seizures

AED	Regimen	Adverse Effects	Comments
Carbamazepine (Tegretol, Tegretol XR, Carbatrol, Equetro)	Initial 200 mg BID (adults) or 100 mg BID (children) and weekly until therapeutic response or target serum concentrations. Usual maintenance doses 7–15 mg/kg/d in adults; 10–40 mg/kg/d in children.	Sedation, visual disturbance may limit dosage. Severe blood dyscrasias extremely rare. Mild leukopenia more common. Laboratory monitoring of little value. Asian patients positive for HLA-B*1502 are at 10-fold higher risk for Stevens-Johnson syndrome/toxic epidermal necrolysis. Hepatotoxicity rare. May cause hyponatremia. Long-term use may cause osteomalacia.	Usually little sedation and minimal interference with cognitive function or behavior. Preferred by most for partial or secondarily generalized seizures. Extended-release products may allow less frequent dosing with fewer peak serum concentration-related side effects. These products may also facilitate adherence.
Phenytoin (Dilantin, Phenytek)	Initiate at maintenance dose of 4–5 mg/kg/d (300–400 mg/d). Titrate on basis of clinical response and target serum concentration. 3–4 weeks between dose ↑ recommended because of potentially slow accumulation.	Nystagmus, ataxia, sedation may limit dosage. Gum hyperplasia, hirsutism common. Long-term use may cause osteomalacia. Peripheral neuropathy, hypersensitivity with liver damage rare. Possible increased risk of Stevens-Johnson syndrome/toxic epidermal necrolysis in Asian patients positive for HLA-B*1502.	Clearance and half-life change with dose. Small ↑ in dose (30 mg capsule) recommended as plasma concentrations exceed 7–10 mcg/mL. Cautious use of suspension; dose measurement and potential mixing difficulties. IM administration not recommended. Potential precipitation in IV solutions. Fosphenytoin (Cerebyx) recommended for IM and IV use due to faster administration rate, admixture compatibility and lower rate of injection site complications.
Valproate (Depakene, Depakote, Depakote-ER)	See Table 58-7.	–	–
Phenobarbital	Initial 1 mg/kg/d; titrate to therapeutic response. 2–3 weeks between dose ↑	Sedation (chronic), behavior disturbances common, especially in children. Possibly impairs learning and intellectual performance. Long-term use may cause osteomalacia.	Considered outmoded for AED therapy in most patients; adverse effects outweigh benefits. IV use for refractory status epilepticus.
Pregabalin (Lyrica)	Initial 50 mg BID then titrate to therapeutic response with maximal daily dose at 600 mg/d in divided doses (BID or TID)	Potential side effects include dizziness, blurred vision and weight gain.	No significant interactions with other AEDs. Can be useful for patients with concomitant pain disorders.
Gabapentin (Neurontin)	Initial 300 mg/d with titration to 900–1,800 mg/d for 1–2 weeks. Doses of 2,400 mg/d and higher have been well tolerated. Owing to short half-life, TID or QID dosing recommended.	Sedation, dizziness, and ataxia relatively common with initiation of therapy. Gabapentin therapy usually not associated with prominent side effects. Commonly associated with weight gain.	Excreted unchanged by kidneys. No significant drug–drug interactions. Absorption dose dependent; fraction absorbed ↓ as size of individual dose ↑
Lamotrigine (Lamictal)	*When added to enzyme inducers alone:* Initiate at 50 mg daily HS or 50 mg BID. Daily dose can be ↑ by 50–100 mg every 7–14 days. Usual maintenance doses of 400–500 mg/d. BID dosing may be necessary with enzyme inducer cotherapy.		
	When added to valproate alone: Initiate at 25 mg QOD HS. Daily dose can be ↑ by 25 mg every 14 days. Usual maintenance doses of 100–200 mg/d. *When added to valproate and enzyme inducers:* Initiate at 25 mg QOD HS. Daily dose can be ↑ by 25 mg every 14 days. Usual daily doses of 100–200 mg/d.	Dizziness, diplopia, sedation, ataxia, and blurred vision can be common with initiation of therapy; limit speed of titration. Incidence of serious rash ranges from 0.8–8.0 per 1,000.	Significant ↑ in clearance of lamotrigine when coadministered with enzyme inducers. Significant ↓ in clearance when coadministered with valproate. Slow, gradual titration of dose may reduce risk of skin rash. Estrogen increases clearance.

(continued)

TABLE 58-6
Drugs Used for the Treatment of Partial and Generalized Tonic-Clonic Seizures *(continued)*

AED	Regimen	Adverse Effects	Comments
Tiagabine (Gabitril)	Initial 4 mg/d. ↑ by 4 mg/d at 7 days. Then ↑ daily dose by 4–8 mg every week. Maximal recommended dose of 32 mg/d in adolescents or 56 mg/d in adults. BID to QID dosing recommended.	Drowsiness, nervousness, difficulty with concentration or attention, tremor. Nonspecific dizziness described by some patients.	Increased clearance when given with enzyme inducers. TID or QID doses probably needed. Potential for protein-binding displacement interactions with other highly protein bound drugs (e.g., valproate). Significance of protein-binding displacement not known. Substrate for CYP3A4.
Topiramate (Topamax)	Initial 50 mg HS. ↑ daily dose by 50 mg every 7 days. 200–400 mg/d recommended as target dosage range. Larger daily doses associated with increased CNS side effects. BID dosing recommended.	Sedation, dizziness, difficulty concentrating, confusion. May be dose related. Possible weight loss. Weak CA inhibitor; may cause or predispose to kidney stones; CA inhibition also possibly related to paresthesias in up to 15%. Risk of hypohidrosis and hyperthermia especially in children. Rarely associated with angle closure glaucoma.	Approximately 70% renal elimination. Phenytoin and carbamazepine may reduce topiramate plasma concentrations and potentially increase dosage requirements. Topiramate may cause small ↑ in phenytoin plasma concentration. Advise patients to drink plenty of fluids. May affect oral contraceptives above 200 mg/d.
Levetiracetam (Keppra)	Initial 250–500 mg BID. ↑ by 500–1,000 mg/d every 2 weeks. Usual maximal dose is 3,000 mg/d. Doses up to 4,000 mg/d have been used. BID dosing recommended.	Somnolence, dizziness, asthenia are commonly reported. Behavioral symptoms (agitation, emotional lability, hostility, depression, and depersonalization) reported.	No hepatic (CYP450 or UGT) metabolism. 66% excreted unchanged in urine. Less than 10% protein bound. No significant drug interactions reported.
Rufinamide	Initial: In adults 400–800 mg/d given BID. ↑ by 400–800 mg/d every 2 days. Target dose of 3,200 mg/d. In children, initiate at 10 mg/kg/d given BID. ↑ by 10 mg/kg/d every other day. Target dose of 45 mg/kg/d or 3,200 mg/d.	Sedation, dizziness, vomiting and headache. Shortens QT interval.	Presently only approved for treatment of seizures in Lennox-Gastaut syndrome in patients older than 4 years of age. Extensively metabolized through enzymes other than CYP. Weakly induces CYP3A; may decrease effectiveness of hormonal contraceptives. VPA significantly decreases rufinamide clearance; potentially significant increases in rufinamide clearance caused by carbamazepine, phenytoin, and phenobarbital.
Lacosamide	Initiate at 50 mg BID. Increase weekly by 100 mg/d. Target doses of 200–400 mg/d. Maximum recommended dose is 400 mg/d.	Dizziness, ataxia, diplopia, headache, nausea. May slow cardiac conduction. Caution is advised in patients with second-degree AV block. Syncope has been reported.	Currently only indicated for treatment of partial seizures in adults. IV form available; currently only approved for short-term replacement of oral therapy. Little evidence of significant risk of drug–drug interactions. Some hepatic metabolism by CYP2C19; significant renal elimination.
Oxcarbazepine (Trileptal)	*Monotherapy:* Initial 300 mg BID. ↑ weekly up to 1,200 mg/d. Can increase to 2,400 mg/d. *Adjunctive therapy:* Initial 300 mg BID. ↑ weekly up to 1,200 mg/d.	Dizziness, somnolence, diplopia, nausea, and ataxia are commonly reported. May cause hyponatremia; most cases asymptomatic, more common in elderly. A 25% cross-sensitivity reported between oxcarbazepine and carbamazepine.	Parent is a prodrug; the MHD is the active component. Readily converted to MHD via omnipresent cytosolic enzymes. Lacks autoinduction properties. In doses >1,200 mg/d, may affect oral contraceptives.
Zonisamide (Zonegran)	Initial 100 mg daily. ↑ by 100 mg/d every 2 weeks. Usual maintenance doses of 200–400 mg/d; maximum 600 mg/d.	Somnolence, nausea, ataxia, dizziness, headache, and anorexia are common. Weight loss and nephrolithiasis reported. Serious skin eruptions, oligohidrosis, and hyperthermia have also occurred.	Broad spectrum, long half-life. 35% of dose is excreted unchanged in the urine. Also a substrate of CYP3A4; enzyme induction may increase clearance. Advise patients to drink plenty of fluids.

AED, antiepileptic drugs; AV, atrioventricular; BID, twice daily; CA, carbonic anhydrase; CNS, central nervous system; CYP, cytochrome P-450; GI, gastrointestinal; HS, at bedtime; IM, intramuscular; IV, intravenous; MHD, monohydroxy derivative; PE, phenytoin sodium equivalent; QID, four times daily; QOD, every other day; SIADH, syndrome of inappropriate antidiuretic hormone secretion; TID, three times daily; UGT, uridine diphosphate glucuronosyltransferase; VPA, valproic acid.

Common adverse effects associated with lacosamide include dizziness, headache, diplopia, and nausea. Gradual escalation to the desired dose reduces the adverse event risk.

The most serious adverse effect associated with lamotrigine is skin rash. Rashes occur in approximately 10% of treated patients, usually in the first 8 weeks.[95] Rashes leading to hospitalization occurred in 1 of 300 adults and 1 of 100 children. Widespread, maculopapular rashes usually appear and may progress to erythema multiforme or toxic epidermal necrolysis. Lamotrigine-related rashes may resolve rapidly when lamotrigine is discontinued. Coadministration of valproate with lamotrigine may increase the likelihood of dermatologic reactions; it is partly for this reason that more conservative dosage titration and lower maintenance doses of lamotrigine are recommended for patients receiving concomitant valproate. Higher starting doses and more rapid dose escalation than those recommended by the manufacturer also increase the risk of skin rash.

Levetiracetam is generally well tolerated, with the most common adverse events in clinical trials being asthenia, vertigo, flu syndrome, headache, rhinitis, and somnolence. The most serious adverse effects are behavioral and are more common in patients with a history of behavioral problems.[96] Levetiracetam should be used with caution in patients with a history of suicidal ideations.

Oxcarbazepine, a keto derivative of carbamazepine, is essentially a prodrug for the monohydroxy active metabolite.[97] Oxcarbazepine probably causes less frequent, less severe adverse effects compared with carbamazepine, with the exception of hyponatremia. Hyponatremia is more common with oxcarbazepine than with carbamazepine. Baseline and periodic serum sodium monitoring is indicated during oxcarbazepine therapy. The most commonly reported side effects of oxcarbazepine in clinical trials include ataxia, dizziness, fatigue, nausea, somnolence, and diplopia.

Adverse effects of pregabalin are dose-dependent and usually occur within the first 2 weeks of treatment.[90] Somnolence, dizziness, and ataxia are most common. Pregabalin also appears to be associated with a dose-related weight gain.

Topiramate can cause cognitive disturbances, lethargy, and impaired mental concentration when given in large daily doses (especially in combination with other AEDs) or when the dosage is titrated too aggressively.[97] Topiramate has caused nephrolithiasis in approximately 1.5% of treated patients. This adverse effect is believed to be related to inhibition of carbonic anhydrase by topiramate, with resulting increased urinary pH and decreased citrate excretion. Topiramate can also cause acute, secondary angle-closure glaucoma which presents within the first month of therapy. Topiramate is associated with weight loss.

Zonisamide is a sulfonamide derivative and thus is contraindicated in patients allergic to sulfonamides.[98] The most commonly reported adverse events include ataxia, somnolence, agitation, and anorexia. Kidney stones have developed in 3% to 4% of patients, some of whom had a family history of nephrolithiasis.

PHARMACOKINETICS

The newer AEDs have somewhat different pharmacokinetic profiles from those of older agents. They also differ in their tendency to interact with other AEDs. Gabapentin is excreted entirely by the kidneys as unchanged drug and is not significantly bound to plasma protein. Gabapentin has a relatively short half-life and should be administered three times daily.[99]

Lacosamide is excreted mostly by the kidneys. Dosage reductions are warranted for patients with renal impairment (creatinine clearance <30 mL/minute). It is less than 15% bound to plasma protein, has a 12 to 13 hour half-life and is administered twice daily.[91]

Lamotrigine is primarily eliminated by hepatic glucuronidation and excretion of metabolites in the urine. Other AEDs, such as carbamazepine and phenytoin, induce the hepatic metabolism of lamotrigine. When lamotrigine is coadministered with enzyme-inducing drugs, its half-life decreases from approximately 24 hours to 15 hours. Valproate inhibits lamotrigine metabolism, causing increases in half-life and serum concentrations.[100,101] Patients treated with both lamotrigine and carbamazepine may experience more nausea, drowsiness, and ataxia. Although this interaction has been attributed to lamotrigine-induced increases in serum concentrations of carbamazepine's active metabolite, carbmazepine-10,11-epoxide (CBZ-E) in some patients,[102] lamotrigine does not consistently produce increases in this metabolite. It appears more likely that this interaction represents a pharmacodynamic interaction between lamotrigine and carbamazepine.[103]

Levetiracetam has a short half-life and is eliminated primarily by renal mechanisms. Dosage reductions are warranted for patients with renal impairment (creatinine clearance <80 mL/minute). The drug has a low potential for interactions with other drugs.[104]

Oxcarbazepine is a prodrug that is converted to the monohydroxy derivative, its primary active metabolite. It may cause less hepatic enzyme induction than carbamazepine and may therefore be less likely to interact with other medications. Oxcarbazepine, however, does increase the metabolism of oral contraceptive hormones.[105] Because oxcarbazepine probably has a similar mechanism of action to that of carbamazepine, it is unlikely that it would offer significant benefits to R.H. because she has not responded to maximal tolerated doses of carbamazepine.[97]

Pregabalin is excreted entirely by the kidneys as unchanged drug and is not significantly bound to serum proteins. Unlike gabapentin, which requires more frequent dosing, pregabalin can be administered two or three times daily.[90]

Tiagabine has a relatively short half-life (4–7 hours). It should be administered at least twice daily.[85] Concurrently administered enzyme-inducing AEDs may reduce the half-life of tiagabine to 2 to 3 hours and necessitate use of larger daily doses and, possibly, shorter dosing intervals. Tiagabine is highly protein-bound (96%), and it is displaced from protein-binding sites by valproate, salicylate, and naproxen. The clinical significance of these protein-binding interactions is unknown.

Topiramate has a half-life of approximately 20 hours, which allows twice-daily administration. It is only partially excreted by hepatic metabolism; approximately 70% of the drug is excreted unchanged by the kidneys. Topiramate is minimally protein-bound (~10%–15%). When topiramate is coadministered with enzyme-inducing agents, such as carbamazepine, hepatic metabolism is increased and topiramate clearance is increased. This interaction may necessitate titration to somewhat higher doses when topiramate is used with enzyme-inducing drugs. Inconsistently, topiramate can cause a small and often insignificant decrease in phenytoin plasma concentrations.

Zonisamide has a long half-life and low protein binding. It is eliminated by both hepatic metabolism and renal excretion. The average half-life of zonisamide is 63 hours, but there is wide interpatient variation. Serum levels of zonisamide are reduced by enzyme-inducing AEDs but clinical consequences of pharmacokinetic interactions with zonisamide are rare.[98]

On the basis of efficacy and side effect characteristics, gabapentin, lacosamide, lamotrigine, levetiracetam, pregabalin, tiagabine, topiramate or zonisamide could be considered for use as adjunctive therapy for R.H. In young, active patients such as R.H., sedation might prove to be a problem; however, it is not clear that any of these drugs predictably causes more initial or long-term sedation. The short half-lives of gabapentin and tiagabine and the associated need for R.H. to take several doses during the day might decrease her adherence. Therefore, lamotrigine, levetiracetam, pregabalin, topiramate or zonisamide would be reasonable choices on the basis of convenience. As the patient is not tolerating carbamazepine, it does not make sense to switch to oxcarbazepine. Additionally, as lacosamide is the newest AED at the time of this writing, it would make sense to try other more established agents first.

POTENTIAL THERAPIES

Other AEDs that may become available in the near future include brivaracetam, eslicarbazepine, perampanel, and retigabine.[106] These drugs may become useful as alternatives or adjuncts to established and newer medications in the future.

With advancing technology and knowledge about genes and brain networks, future treatment strategies should move from controlling symptoms of epilepsy with AEDs to prevention and cure.[107] For AED-resistant epilepsy, much research is examining the role of multidrug transporters (e.g., P-glycoprotein) at the blood–brain barrier. These proteins may act as a defense mechanism by limiting the accumulation of AED in the brain.[108] Although it has not yet had much of an impact on the clinical care of patients with epilepsy, pharmacogenetics of AED therapy is continually advancing.[109]

LAMOTRIGINE THERAPY

INITIATION AND DOSAGE TITRATION

CASE 58-2, QUESTION 2: R.H. is to be started on lamotrigine as adjunctive therapy to her carbamazepine. Outline a treatment plan for initiating and monitoring therapy for R.H. What should R.H. and her family be told about this medication and how to use it?

Lamotrigine therapy should be initiated in R.H. with a slow upward dosage titration to minimize early sedative effects and reduce the likelihood of skin rash. An initial dosage of 50 mg/day given at bedtime is recommended; the daily dose can be increased by 50 mg every 1 to 2 weeks. Because R.H. is currently receiving carbamazepine, induction of liver enzymes is likely to increase her dosage requirements for lamotrigine and allow a less conservative dosage titration. A twice-daily schedule is recommended for maintenance therapy. Usual maintenance dosages of lamotrigine are approximately 300 to 500 mg/day, although there is some experience with dosages of up to 700 mg/day. A patient's ability to tolerate this medication ultimately determines dosage limitations. Onset of side effects (e.g., nausea, diplopia, ataxia, and dizziness) may prevent further dosage increases.

R.H. should be told that she may feel drowsy and possibly experience headache and upset stomach, but that these side effects usually disappear with ongoing therapy. She should contact her physician or other health care professional if severe side effects occur that make it difficult to take the medication; this is especially important if she exhibits a rash.

SIDE EFFECTS AND POSSIBLE INTERACTION WITH CARBAMAZEPINE

CASE 58-2, QUESTION 3: Two days after her dosage of lamotrigine was increased to 300 mg/day (12 weeks after beginning therapy), R.H. noticed that her vision was blurring; she also complained of feeling dizzy and having difficulty maintaining her balance. Previously, she had experienced only mild, occasional nausea. She had continued to experience seizures at approximately the same frequency she had before the initiation of lamotrigine. Her physician had encouraged her to continue taking the medication and explained that it would take time to increase the dose to possibly effective levels. Her current carbamazepine serum concentration is essentially unchanged when compared with when she was taking it in monotherapy. Do these new side effects represent treatment failure with lamotrigine? If not, how might these new side effects be managed?

R.H.'s seizure disorder may be unresponsive to lamotrigine therapy, and her side effects may limit further dosage increases. Her current side effects might represent carbamazepine intoxication, lamotrigine side effects, or an interaction between these two medications. Because R.H. tolerated the same carbamazepine dose previously, carbamazepine "intoxication" seems a less likely cause. Assessing the role of lamotrigine as the only cause is difficult. Obtaining a lamotrigine serum concentration to aid in assessing her adverse effects is not likely to be helpful. A usual "therapeutic range" for lamotrigine serum concentrations has not been established. Clinical studies have failed to demonstrate a significant correlation between lamotrigine serum concentrations and either therapeutic or adverse responses.[110,111] Her symptoms may also be related to an apparent pharmacodynamic interaction between lamotrigine and carbamazepine.[103] The effects experienced by some patients taking both drugs may be relieved by reducing the carbamazepine dosage.

LEVETIRACETAM THERAPY

INITIATION AND DOSAGE TITRATION

CASE 58-2, QUESTION 4: R.H.'s carbamazepine dosage was reduced from 1,800 mg/day to 1,400 mg/day. After 5 days, her symptoms persisted and her seizure frequency appeared to be increasing. The clinician decides to abandon lamotrigine therapy and institute treatment with levetiracetam. Recommend a plan for initiating R.H.'s levetiracetam treatment.

R.H. previously tolerated and had a better therapeutic response to a higher carbamazepine dose. Therefore, the dosage of carbamazepine should be returned to 1,800 mg/day before levetiracetam therapy is initiated. Little specific information is available to help determine how lamotrigine can be safely discontinued. As a general rule, rapid discontinuation of AEDs is not recommended in other than emergency situations. Therefore, immediate reduction of R.H.'s lamotrigine dosage to 200 mg/day would seem reasonable. This dosage could then be reduced by 50 to 100 mg every week until lamotrigine is discontinued.

Levetiracetam treatment should be instituted immediately for R.H. because of her continuing seizures. Levetiracetam does not interact with other AEDs. Therefore, discontinuing lamotrigine during initiation of levetiracetam should not create difficulties in assessing R.H.'s response. Levetiracetam should be initiated at a dosage of 250 to 500 mg two times daily.[89,104] Although the manufacturer recommends initiating treatment at 500 mg twice daily, patients may better tolerate lower initial doses and more gradual titration.[104] R.H.'s daily levetiracetam dose can be increased by 500 to 1,000 mg every 2 or 3 weeks, according to her tolerance of side effects and her change in seizure frequency. Although the drug reaches steady state quickly, allowing at least 2 weeks for observation before dosage increases may improve patient tolerability and allow for a more thorough evaluation of therapeutic response. At present, the relationship between serum concentrations of levetiracetam and therapeutic response or symptoms of intoxication is not well defined. Therefore, R.H.'s dose should be titrated to the maximal tolerated amount required to control her seizures. There is limited published experience with levetiracetam dosages as high as 4,000 mg/day. However, in controlled trials, no clear benefits were apparent at doses greater than 3,000 mg/day.

PATIENT EDUCATION

R.H. should be informed that with levetiracetam she may experience side effects similar to those she had with lamotrigine. R.H.'s mood should be assessed at each visit. Much reassurance and encouragement may need to be given along with this information to help ensure that R.H. adheres to her treatment regimen. Many patients become discouraged when multiple trials of medication are necessary and side effects are prominent. They may express feelings of being "guinea pigs" and may become uncooperative with the therapeutic plan.

PHENYTOIN THERAPY

INITIATION AND DOSAGE

CASE 58-3

QUESTION 1: J.N., an 18-year-old, 88-kg male college student, was diagnosed with epilepsy. He experiences generalized tonic-clonic seizures that last 2 minutes approximately three times monthly. J.N. describes a "churning" feeling in his abdomen before his seizures; this is followed by involuntary right-sided jerking of his upper extremities. An EEG showed diffuse slowing with focal epileptiform discharges in the left temporal area; it was interpreted as abnormal. No correctable cause for his seizure disorder was identified despite a thorough workup. He has no other medical conditions and takes no routine medications. He was treated initially with carbamazepine up to 600 mg/day. He could not tolerate the medication because of nausea and diplopia despite relatively low doses. J.N.'s physician has elected to implement a therapeutic trial of phenytoin. Recommend an initial dosage. What information should be provided to J.N. about his new medication?

Selecting a nontoxic, therapeutic dose of any AED is difficult without having information about the drug's disposition in the individual patient (i.e., prior dosages and clinical response). Although "average" dosages and resulting serum concentrations for phenytoin often are quoted, interpatient variability is significant. An initial phenytoin dosage of 400 mg/day (approximately 4.5 mg/kg/day) would be appropriate for J.N. To avoid patient nonadherence because of transient side effects, J.N. could be instructed to take 100 mg every 12 hours for 1 week. The following week he could take 100 mg in the morning and 200 mg 12 hours later. If he can tolerate this regimen, he could then take 200 mg every 12 hours.

PATIENT EDUCATION

In addition to the name and strength of the medication and instructions for when and how it should be taken, J.N. should be informed that he may experience initial mild sedation from phenytoin. He should be cautioned that symptoms such as blurred or double vision, dysarthria, dizziness, or staggering may indicate that his dosage is too high; he should be instructed to notify his physician, pharmacist, or other health care professional of these symptoms. It is also a good idea to inform patients, at the beginning of therapy, that adjustments of medication dosage may be necessary before the regimen is stabilized.

ACCUMULATION PHARMACOKINETICS

CASE 58-3, QUESTION 2: What are the characteristics of phenytoin accumulation pharmacokinetics?

Phenytoin exhibits dose-dependent (Michaelis-Menten or capacity-limited) pharmacokinetics; therefore, the usual pharmacokinetic concepts of "clearance" and "half-life" are meaningless. The apparent half-life of phenytoin changes with the dose and serum concentration. Thus, the time required to reach a new steady state after dose alteration is difficult to predict because it depends on the dose itself and the patient's pharmacokinetic parameters, V_{max} and K_m.[112] V_{max} is a kinetic constant representing the maximal rate of phenytoin elimination from the body. K_m is the Michaelis constant, the serum concentration at which the rate of elimination is 50% of V_{max}. Values for these parameters vary widely among patients; as a result, patterns of phenytoin accumulation and the time required to achieve steady state also are variable.

Many clinicians assume that phenytoin's apparent half-life is approximately 24 hours, and they wait 5 to 7 days before assessing the patient's clinical response and measuring serum phenytoin concentrations. Both clinical studies[113] and model simulations[114] using observed values for K_m and V_{max} have been used to estimate time required for serum concentrations of phenytoin to reach steady state. Up to 30 days may be needed for this to occur either with doses sufficient to produce steady-state serum concentrations of 10 to 15 mcg/mL or with doses of 4 mg/kg/day.[112,115] Occasionally, such a dose may exceed a patient's V_{max}; the result is extremely high serum phenytoin concentrations, with probable intoxication. It is important not to assume that steady state has been reached unless widely spaced, serial serum concentrations indicate that accumulation has ceased. Alterations in phenytoin dosage before steady state has been reached can result in significant fluctuations in serum concentrations and the patient's clinical status. Such situations occur frequently and result in unnecessary confusion and expense. As always, serum concentrations in J.N. must be interpreted in the context of his clinical response.

PHENYTOIN INTOXICATION

CASE 58-3, QUESTION 3: J.N. was started on phenytoin and is now taking 200 mg every 12 hours. One week after achieving this dose, mild lateral gaze nystagmus was noted, but J.N. had no subjective complaints and was seizure-free. After 3 weeks, J.N. complained of double vision and feeling "drunk" and "unsteady." Significant nystagmus was present. How should J.N.'s phenytoin dosage be altered?

J.N.'s signs and symptoms indicate phenytoin intoxication. Dosage reduction is indicated. Reducing J.N.'s dosage to 360 mg/day (accomplished using both 100-mg and 30-mg phenytoin capsules) would be reasonable. A larger reduction may result in a loss of seizure control. Many clinicians also would have J.N. omit one day's dose of phenytoin before beginning the new maintenance dosage. This would accelerate the decline in phenytoin serum levels. After this dosage change, clinical response should be monitored closely. The new maintenance dose may still be excessive, if J.N.'s V_{max} for phenytoin is low. If this were the case, continued accumulation of drug would occur despite the dosage reduction.[112]

INTRAMUSCULAR PHENYTOIN AND FOSPHENYTOIN (PHENYTOIN PRODRUG)

CASE 58-4

QUESTION 1: S.D. is a 24-year-old, male state hospital patient with a history of complex partial and secondarily generalized tonic-clonic seizures. Within the past year, his phenytoin formulation was switched from phenytoin sodium capsules to phenytoin suspension because S.D. was suspected of "cheeking" his medicines and not swallowing the capsules properly. He has had no seizures in the past 3 months on 275 mg/day of phenytoin suspension. S.D. has now been transferred to the acute medical unit after a 2-day history of anorexia, nausea, occasional vomiting, and abdominal pain accompanied by diarrhea. His chart now states "nothing by mouth." Intramuscular (IM) fosphenytoin, 275 mg (phenytoin sodium equivalents [PE]) per day, has been ordered. Discuss the use of IM fosphenytoin, and devise a dosage regimen for S.D.

S.D. is a candidate for parenteral administration of his AED. If placement of an intravenous (IV) line for fluid administration is not planned, then IM administration is probably an acceptable approach to treatment. Previously, sodium phenytoin injection was the only parenteral preparation available for replacement of oral phenytoin. Fosphenytoin sodium injection is now available. Although preparations of sodium phenytoin injection are still available, their IM administration is not recommended. Injectable phenytoin is highly alkaline (pH 12) and extremely irritating to tissue. After IM injection, the drug may precipitate at the injection site because of the change in pH. As a result, phenytoin crystals form a repository or depot from which the drug is slowly absorbed.[116–118] Often injection site discomfort is noted, although severe muscle damage does not seem to occur.[118]

Fosphenytoin, a phosphate ester prodrug of phenytoin, is highly water-soluble. Its solubility allows this preparation to be administered parenterally without the need for solubilization using propylene glycol or the adjustment of pH to nonphysiologic levels. Therefore, fosphenytoin may be administered either IM or IV with less risk of tissue damage and venous irritation than with parenteral administration of phenytoin.[119–121] (See also subsequent discussion of IV administration of phenytoin and fosphenytoin.) After administration, fosphenytoin is rapidly absorbed and converted to phenytoin by phosphatase enzymes. Ultimately, the bioavailability of phenytoin from IM fosphenytoin administration is 100%.

Fosphenytoin is available as a solution containing 50 mg PE/mL. By labeling fosphenytoin this way, no dosing adjustments are necessary when converting from phenytoin sodium to fosphenytoin or vice versa. Although the prescriber ordered 275 mg PE, S.D. may be underdosed. His oral dosage of phenytoin suspension is providing the equivalent of 300 mg/day of sodium phenytoin. Phenytoin suspension and chewable tablets contain free acid, whereas capsules contain sodium phenytoin. Therefore, phenytoin capsule products contain only 92% of the labeled content as phenytoin acid (i.e., a 100-mg sodium phenytoin capsule contains only 92 mg of phenytoin acid). He should receive a 300-mg dose of fosphenytoin daily to fully replace his current dosage of phenytoin suspension.[121]

Assuming that S.D. will be given 300 mg PE of fosphenytoin daily, he will require a total of 6 mL of this injection given IM. This medication is well tolerated when given IM, and S.D.'s full daily dose can probably be given in a single injection without causing excessive discomfort. Some clinicians report administering IM injections of fosphenytoin as large as 20 mL in a single site without adverse consequences or serious discomfort.[122] It is also possible to divide his daily dosage into two injections given in two different sites, although many patients prefer to receive fewer injections.

ADVERSE EFFECTS

CASE 58-5

QUESTION 1: M.N., a 10-year-old boy receiving 150 mg/day of phenytoin as chewable tablets, is to be fitted with orthodontic braces. He exhibits moderate gingival hyperplasia resulting in poor oral hygiene and halitosis. Discuss phenytoin-related gingival hyperplasia and management techniques that may be helpful for M.N.

Gingival Hyperplasia

Gum hyperplasia related to phenytoin is common and troublesome. Prevalence is estimated at up to 90%,[123] depending on the rating system used and the degree of gum change rated as hyperplastic. A realistic prevalence estimate is probably 40% to 50% of treated patients.[124] Prevalence and incidence rates, however, are misleading because the occurrence and severity of hyperplasia are related to the dose and serum concentration of phenytoin.[124,125] Gingival hyperplasia is of obvious cosmetic importance. Also, as in M.N., formation of pockets of tissue leads to difficulties with oral hygiene, and severe halitosis may result.

The mechanism of phenytoin-induced gingival hyperplasia is not well understood. The drug is excreted in saliva and saliva phenytoin concentrations and hyperplasia are correlated; however, this correlation may simply reflect higher serum concentrations producing a greater pharmacologic effect. Phenytoin may stimulate gingival mast cells to release heparin and other mediators that may encourage synthesis of excessive amounts of new connective tissue by fibroblasts. Local irritation caused by dental plaque and food particles may further stimulate this process.[124,125]

Three approaches to the treatment of existing hyperplasia[125] are (a) dosage reduction or replacement of phenytoin with an alternative AED, if possible, which will permit partial or complete reversal of hyperplasia; (b) surgical gingivectomy, which will correct the problem temporarily, but hyperplasia eventually recurs; and (c) periodontal treatment, which will eliminate local irritants and maintains oral hygiene. Because M.N. is to be fitted with braces, oral hygiene will be further complicated. Treatment for existing hyperplasia and prevention of further tissue enlargement is important. Assuming that phenytoin is producing adequate seizure control, a combination of gingivectomy and follow-up periodontal treatment may be the best approach.

Theoretically, the use of chewable phenytoin tablets in M.N. may aggravate hyperplasia. Exposure of the gingiva to high localized concentrations of phenytoin may result from braces holding tablet fragments in close physical contact with gum tissue. The significance of this relationship is questionable, but if M.N. can swallow capsules, a change to this dosage form may be beneficial. The most appropriate dosage of phenytoin sodium capsules for M.N. would be 160 mg/day. If chewable tablets are to be continued, having M.N. rinse and swallow after each dose may minimize problems.

Oral hygiene programs appear to reduce the degree and severity of gingival hyperplasia when they are initiated before phenytoin therapy is started.[125] Patients who are beginning phenytoin therapy should be educated about the role of oral hygiene in diminishing this side effect. The use of dental floss, gum stimulators, and water-flossing appliances may be beneficial adjuncts to other oral hygiene techniques.

CASE 58-6

QUESTION 1: G.R. is a 53-year-old man with epilepsy characterized by occasional tonic-clonic seizures. He has taken phenytoin since he was 25 years of age. His dosage of phenytoin was recently reduced from 400 mg/day to 360 mg/day because of symptoms of AED intoxication (mild confusion, occasional diplopia, ataxia, and lateral gaze nystagmus). After the dose reduction, his confusion and diplopia decreased significantly. The neurologic evaluation at the lower dose was within normal limits. No seizures occurred during the subsequent 8 weeks. He continued to complain of being mildly "unsteady" on his feet. Because G.R.'s seizures are apparently under complete control, is there any problem maintaining him on this dose of phenytoin?

Neurotoxicity

Patients chronically maintained on intoxicating doses of phenytoin appear to be at risk for developing irreversible cerebellar damage and/or peripheral neuropathy. Cerebellar degeneration, resulting in symptoms such as dysarthria, ataxic gait, intention tremor, and muscular hypotonia, is of particular concern; this complication has been observed after episodes of acute phenytoin intoxication.[126,127] Generalized seizures also can cause cerebellar degeneration secondary to hypoxia. For this reason, the relative importance of phenytoin in the development of this condition is controversial. Nevertheless, cerebellar degeneration has been reported in several patients without hypoxic seizures.[127,128]

Symptomatic phenytoin-related peripheral neuropathy is rare, although electrophysiologic evidence of impaired neuronal conduction may be found in many patients.[126,129] Symptomatic patients may complain of paresthesias, muscle weakness, and occasional muscle wasting. Knee and ankle tendon reflexes are absent in 18% of patients on long-term phenytoin therapy; the upper limbs are rarely affected. Although areflexia may be irreversible,[130] electrophysiologic abnormalities may be closely related to excessive serum phenytoin concentrations and are reversible after dosage reduction or discontinuation.[128]

In G.R., the general discomfort of mild phenytoin intoxication and the potential for producing cerebellar degeneration necessitates a therapy alteration. The phenytoin dose should be reduced to 330 mg/day because it may produce adequate seizure control without toxic symptoms. Should seizures recur at this lower dosage, it may be advisable to consider an alternative AED.

ANTIEPILEPTIC DRUG IMPACT ON BONE

Some AEDs have a negative impact on bone density. People with epilepsy treated with these drugs are at increased risk for bone disorders and fractures.[131] Although bone disorders are more common in women, the negative impact of AEDs on bone is not sex-specific. Longer duration of AED therapy and exposure to multiple AEDs are thought to predict bone loss. Enzyme-inducing AEDs (carbamazepine, phenytoin, and phenobarbital) have been associated with bone loss and an increased risk for fracture. Valproate, although not an enzyme inducer, is associated with decreased bone mineral density in children.[132] Less is known about the impact of newer AEDs on bone mineral metabolism, although a report suggests lamotrigine has no effect.[133] Because of the length of phenytoin use, G.R. is at risk. His bone health should be further evaluated. Oral calcium and vitamin D supplementation should be implemented. Depending on the outcome of evaluation, a change from phenytoin to an AED with less or no effect on bone should be considered.

NEW-ONSET SEIZURES IN THE ELDERLY

CASE 58-7

QUESTION 1: J.R., a 74-year-old man with newly diagnosed partial seizures, is referred to the neurology clinic for evaluation and treatment. The etiology of his new-onset seizures is presumed to be a recent cerebral infarct. His seizures are complex partial seizures (he "blacks out" and loses track of time). He has no history of secondarily generalized tonic-clonic convulsions. He has had three seizures in the last 4 weeks. His last seizure resulted in a fall down a flight of stairs. His wife reports that he is more likely to have a seizure if he gets "overtired" or "stressed-out." He is also being treated for hypertension and diabetes. What options are available for the treatment of J.R.'s epilepsy?

There are relatively few head-to-head comparative studies of AEDs in patients with epilepsy. Even fewer studies address the comparative efficacy of AEDs in elderly patients. Two studies, in particular, are important when discussing AED treatment in elderly persons with epilepsy.

Brodie et al.[134] compared lamotrigine ($n = 102$) with carbamazepine ($n = 48$) in elderly patients with newly diagnosed epilepsy via a double-blind, randomized, parallel study. Discontinuation rates because of adverse effects (the primary outcome parameter) were higher for carbamazepine (42%) than for lamotrigine (18%). Using time to first seizure as a measure of efficacy, no differences were found between the two AEDs, and the authors suggested that lamotrigine is "acceptable" as initial treatment in elderly patients with newly diagnosed epilepsy.

Carbamazepine (600 mg/day), gabapentin (1,500 mg/day), and lamotrigine (150 mg/day) were compared for efficacy and tolerability in 593 patients older than 55 years of age (mean age, 72 years) with newly diagnosed epilepsy.[135] Although efficacy was similar in all three groups, study termination for adverse events varied between treatment groups. Carbamazepine had the highest termination rate (31%), followed by gabapentin (21.6%), and then lamotrigine (12.1%) ($p = 0.001$). The authors concluded that lamotrigine and gabapentin should be considered as initial therapy for new-onset seizures in older patients with epilepsy.

These two studies in elderly patients with epilepsy suggest that either gabapentin or lamotrigine would be good choices for initial treatment of J.R.'s epilepsy. It is noteworthy that neither AED is FDA-approved for newly diagnosed epilepsy.

It is also important to consider drug-interaction profile, dosing frequency, and drug costs when selecting AED therapy. Generally, elderly persons take more medicines than younger individuals. For example, the average number of concomitant medications in the study by Rowan et al.[135] was seven. J.R. is likely to be taking other medicines for diabetes and hypertension. Neither gabapentin nor lamotrigine cause drug–drug interactions, although lamotrigine is influenced more so than gabapentin by other medicines. Gabapentin may need to be dosed more frequently than lamotrigine; this may negatively impact adherence.

ADVERSE EFFECTS

Both comparative studies identified minimal differences in efficacy. Newer AEDs, however, showed better tolerability than the older AEDs. In general, elderly patients not only respond to AEDs at lower doses and concentrations but they also exhibit toxicity symptoms at lower doses than do younger patients. Age-related declines in renal and hepatic function may account for those observations. The pharmacokinetics of many AEDs have been studied in the elderly and a decrease in clearance is noted as compared with the young.[136] Decreased clearance of AEDs in the elderly has often been cited as a reason for their increased responsiveness to these drugs. Newer pharmacokinetic studies, however, appear to indicate that the alterations in pharmacokinetics for at least some AEDs may not be as significant as previously thought.[137,138]

The impact of AEDs on cognition is an important issue for all patients with epilepsy and perhaps it is an even greater issue in elderly patients. Martin et al. evaluated cognitive functioning using several standardized measures in 25 older (>60 years of age) adults with epilepsy and compared them with healthy older adults ($n = 27$).[139] Patients with epilepsy fared worse than their healthy counterparts, especially if they were receiving AED polytherapy. Piazzini et al. found similar results in 40 patients older than 60 years of age compared with 40 controls.[140] Additionally, Bambara et al. reported that 20 older adults (age >60 years) with epilepsy demonstrated deficits in their ability to provide informed consent for medical treatment.[141] These authors expressed concern for their patients' medical decision-making abilities.

As evidenced from the study by Rowan et al.,[135] CNS toxicities such as dizziness, unsteady gait, and ataxia are common adverse effects of AEDs in elderly patients. These symptoms may increase the risk of falls, which are of particular concern in light of the potential negative effects of AEDs on bone mineral density. Fife et al.[142] prospectively examined the effects of carbamazepine, gabapentin, or lamotrigine monotherapy on balance in patients with epilepsy who were older than 50 years of age. Ten patients on each drug were extensively evaluated. Patients receiving lamotrigine exhibited significantly better scores on select measures of balance than did patients receiving carbamazepine. Although not statistically significant (perhaps owing to a small sample size), gabapentin showed a trend toward better balance scores than carbamazepine.

J.R. and his family should be informed about the benefits and risks associated with each AED and they should also be incorporated into the decision-making process. AED therapy in the elderly should follow the "start low and go slow" adage, and elderly patients should be monitored for both efficacy (via a seizure calendar) and toxicity (reporting any intolerable side effects).

Absence Seizures

CHOICE OF MEDICATION AND INITIATION OF ETHOSUXIMIDE THERAPY

CASE 58-8

QUESTION 1: T.D., a 7-year-old, 25-kg girl, is reported by her teacher to have three or four episodes of "staring" daily. Each spell lasts 5 to 10 seconds. Although no convulsive movements occur, her eyelids appear to flutter during the episodes. She is fully alert afterward. T.D.'s school performance is somewhat below average, despite an intelligence quotient (IQ) of 125. An EEG shows 3 Hertz (Hz) spike-and-wave activity. Typical absence epilepsy is diagnosed. Physical examination and laboratory evaluation findings are normal, and no other positive findings are evident on the neurologic examination. What drug should be prescribed for T.D., and how should therapy with this drug be initiated?

Ethosuximide and valproate are commonly used to treat absence epilepsy in the United States. Both drugs are equally effective. Lamotrigine also has been recommended as an initial monotherapy agent for treatment of absence epilepsy, although it is not FDA-approved for this indication[143–145] (Tables 58-2 and 58-6). Valproate, ethosuximide, and lamotrigine were compared for treatment of newly diagnosed childhood absence epilepsy.[146] Efficacy rates for valproate and ethosuximide (based on freedom from treatment failure) were not significantly different, but were significantly higher than for lamotrigine. Attentional dysfunction

TABLE 58-7
Common Drugs for the Treatment of Absence Seizures

AED	Regimen	Adverse Effects	Comments
Valproate (Depakene, Depakote, Depakote ER)	Initial 5–10 mg/kg/d (sprinkle caps or syrup); then ↑ by 5–10 mg/kg/d weekly to therapeutic effect or target serum concentration. Manufacturer's recommended usual maximal dose of 60 mg/kg/d often must be exceeded clinically (especially for patients receiving enzyme-inducing AED) to achieve optimal clinical results. Daily dosing recommended for ER product; doses should be 8%–20% higher than non-ER products.	GI upset, hair loss, appetite stimulation, and weight gain common. Tremor may occur. Serious hepatotoxicity extremely rare with monotherapy and in patients younger than 2 years of age.	Enteric-coated tablets or capsules or ER tablets may ↓ GI toxicity. Time to peak serum concentrations delayed for 3–8 hours with enteric coating; longer delay if given with food; serum concentrations must be interpreted carefully. Also effective against primarily generalized tonic-clonic seizures.
Lamotrigine (Lamictal)	See Table 58-6.		
Ethosuximide (Zarontin)	Initial 20 mg/kg/d or 250 mg daily or BID; then ↑ by 250 mg/d every 2 weeks to therapeutic effect or target serum concentration.	GI upset and sedation common with large single dose, especially on initiation. Daily divided doses may be necessary despite long half-life. Leukopenia (mild, transient) in up to 7%; serious hematologic toxicity extremely rare.	Parents/patient should be informed that GI effects and sedation may occur but tolerance usually develops. No good evidence it precipitates tonic-clonic seizures. Up to 50% of patients with absence may exhibit tonic-clonic seizures independent of ethosuximide.

AED, antiepileptic drug; BID, twice daily; ER, extended release; GI, gastrointestinal.

was significantly more common with valproate than with ethosuximide. Valproate was also more efficacious than lamotrigine for treatment of idiopathic generalized seizures (including absence) in the SANAD (Standard and New Antiepileptic Drugs) trial.[147] Most authorities now consider ethosuximide the drug of first choice for treatment of absence seizures. Valproate is more likely to cause significant nausea and initial drowsiness and it is more likely to interact with other drugs, including AEDs. Valproate usually is reserved for patients whose absence seizures do not respond to ethosuximide.[148] Clonazepam, a benzodiazepine, often is effective for control of absence seizures. Therapy with this drug is limited by prominent CNS side effects (sedation, ataxia, and mood changes) and development of tolerance to its antiepileptic effect after long-term use.[149] Most authorities consider clonazepam a fourth-choice drug for treatment of absence seizures.

T.D. should be started on ethosuximide at a dosage of 15 to 20 mg/kg/day or 250 mg twice daily. The daily dose can be increased by 250 mg every 10 to 14 days as necessary to control seizures. Because the average half-life of ethosuximide in children is ~30 hours, a delay of 10 to 14 days between dosage increments allows ~7 days for achievement of steady state and 7 days for assessment of response.[28]

PATIENT OR CAREGIVER EDUCATION

Educating T.D. and her parents regarding the importance of regular drug administration is extremely helpful in ensuring successful therapy. Nonadherence is common in patients taking AEDs, and rapid discontinuation of these drugs (often secondary to nonadherence) may precipitate status epilepticus. The concept that medication controls rather than cures the seizure disorder should be strongly reinforced. It is also critical to inform both the parents and T.D. that a therapeutic response may not occur immediately and that dosage adjustments may be necessary.

THERAPEUTIC MONITORING

CASE 58-8, QUESTION 2: What subjective or objective clinical data should be monitored in T.D. for evidence of ethosuximide's therapeutic and adverse effects?

T.D.'s seizure frequency and any side effects she experiences are the primary monitoring parameters. If ethosuximide serum concentrations are used to assist in dosing, 40 to 100 mcg/mL is the usual target range; however, a clearly defined toxicity syndrome does not reliably develop when ethosuximide serum concentrations exceed 100 mcg/mL. Gradual and cautious increases in ethosuximide dosage when serum concentrations are beyond the upper limits of the "usual therapeutic range" may improve response in resistant patients. Although ethosuximide traditionally is administered in divided doses, its long half-life allows successful use of single daily doses for many patients. Clinicians should be alert to acute side effects of nausea and vomiting that are associated with large single doses of ethosuximide; should these occur, divided daily doses may be necessary.[28]

Laboratory monitoring for idiosyncratic hematologic toxicity from ethosuximide often is recommended. Ethosuximide causes neutropenia in approximately 7% of patients. Although this reaction often is transient, even if the drug is continued, rare patients may exhibit fatal pancytopenia. Presumably, early detection of neutropenia by means of periodic CBC will allow discontinuation of the drug and potential reversal of this adverse effect.[150] These hematologic reactions, however, can occur unpredictably at any time during therapy and often are missed by routine laboratory monitoring. Patient or caregiver education regarding signs and symptoms associated with leukopenia and pancytopenia (e.g., sudden onset of severe sore throat with oral lesions, easy bruisability, increased bleeding tendency) and instructions to consult the physician if these symptoms occur may be more important than laboratory monitoring.[63]

T.D.'s parents should be informed that nausea or sedation may occur with initiation of ethosuximide. Tolerance to these effects usually develops, although temporary dose reductions may be necessary. Subtle degrees of sedation may persist throughout therapy and may not be recognized until the drug has been discontinued and alertness improves.

Generalized Tonic-Clonic Seizures Accompanying Absence Seizures

CASE 58-8, QUESTION 3: Three months later, T.D.'s absence seizures have been reduced to a frequency of one every 2 weeks with an ethosuximide dosage of 750 mg/day. Her initial drowsiness has almost disappeared, and nausea was alleviated by administering doses with food. She has, however, experienced two tonic-clonic convulsions in the past month. Both seizures were witnessed by her parents and were well described. No auras or signs of focal seizure activity were apparent, and each episode consisted of typical tonic-clonic activity lasting 3 to 4 minutes. T.D. was incontinent of urine on both occasions, and postictal confusion and drowsiness were significant. Physical examination and laboratory testing showed no abnormalities. A repeat EEG continued to show infrequent 3-Hz spike-and-wave discharges; no abnormal focal discharges were noted. What is the relationship between T.D.'s tonic-clonic seizures and ethosuximide therapy?

It is commonly believed, and often stated in the literature, that ethosuximide may precipitate or worsen tonic-clonic seizures; however, this effect has not been clearly demonstrated. As many as 50% of patients who initially present with absence seizures also experience tonic-clonic seizures.[151] It had been common practice to add phenobarbital or phenytoin to ethosuximide therapy to prevent this. Livingston et al. found that 80.5% of their patients treated with a drug specific for absence seizures experienced "grand mal" seizures, whereas only 36% did so while receiving combined therapy.[152] On the other hand, Browne et al. pointed out that a child with absence seizures who has not yet had a tonic-clonic seizure has only a 25% chance of doing so in the future.[151] In addition, routine use of drugs for prophylaxis of tonic-clonic seizures may increase the risk of toxicity and potentially reduce adherence with medication regimens. Sedative drugs, especially phenobarbital, actually may aggravate absence seizures in some patients.[153]

In summary, subsequent generalized tonic-clonic seizures are common in patients who initially experience absence spells. It is not possible to assess the causative role of ethosuximide for this development in T.D.

ASSESSMENT REGARDING NEED FOR ALTERATION IN ANTIEPILEPTIC DRUG THERAPY AND CHOICE OF ALTERNATIVE ANTIEPILEPTIC DRUG

CASE 58-8, QUESTION 4: What alterations are indicated in T.D.'s drug therapy because of the appearance of generalized tonic-clonic seizures?

Drug therapy for prevention of further tonic-clonic seizures is indicated. Phenytoin, carbamazepine, or valproate might be considered for use in T.D. Owing to her age and sex, many clinicians would avoid using phenytoin because of its dysmorphic and cosmetic side effects. Carbamazepine is widely used for secondarily generalized tonic-clonic seizures and some cases of tonic-clonic seizures in children. It lacks many of the troublesome, common side effects associated with phenytoin. Carbamazepine, however, is not effective for control of absence seizures. Therefore, it is likely that both ethosuximide and carbamazepine would be needed by T.D. Carbamazepine also has been associated with exacerbation of seizures (including atonic, myoclonic, and absence seizures) in children with mixed seizure disorders who exhibit bilaterally synchronous 2.5- to 3-Hz discharges on the EEG.[154,155] The need for polytherapy and the possible risk of seizure exacerbation make carbamazepine a less attractive treatment option for T.D.

Valproate is effective for controlling both absence and primary generalized tonic-clonic seizures.[41,57] T.D. appears to have primary generalized tonic-clonic convulsions; focal signs (e.g., unilateral or single limb involvement) were not observed, and focal discharges (e.g., isolated abnormal electrical activity localized to one portion of the brain) were not found on the EEG. Although neither observation completely rules out secondarily generalized tonic-clonic seizures, the likelihood seems low. Therefore, valproate may offer advantages over carbamazepine in terms of efficacy. In addition, both of T.D.'s seizure types potentially could be controlled with a single medication.

VALPROATE THERAPY

INITIATION AND DOSAGE

CASE 58-8, QUESTION 5: T.D.'s physician elects to use valproate. The therapeutic goal is control of her seizures with valproate alone. What procedure should be followed regarding discontinuation of ethosuximide and initiation of valproate?

Techniques used by clinicians to substitute one AED for another depend largely on experience and judgment. Generally, it is best to attain a potentially therapeutic dose of a new medication before attempting to discontinue the previous drug. Serum concentration monitoring may be helpful for some AEDs. Ethosuximide has a relatively long half-life, whereas valproate's half-life is short. Therefore, if necessary, steady-state serum concentrations of valproate can be established and evaluated rapidly; evaluation of the effect of decreases in the ethosuximide dosage must await the prolonged elimination of this drug. Once a desired valproate dose or serum concentration has been achieved, the ethosuximide dosage can be reduced gradually by 250 mg/day every 2 to 4 weeks.

Valproate should be initiated at 125 to 250 mg twice daily. Valproic acid syrup or capsules or divalproex sodium can be used. Divalproex often is preferred because it may cause fewer GI side effects than valproic acid. Syrup forms of valproate probably should be avoided unless extremely small doses are required (e.g., infants) or patients cannot swallow. Valproate syrup has an unpleasant taste, and its rapid absorption increases the likelihood of acute, dose-related side effects such as nausea. Lower initial valproate doses are less likely to cause acute side effects (e.g., drowsiness and GI upset). Weekly dosage increases of 5 to 10 mg/kg/day usually are well tolerated and would be appropriate for T.D. More rapid increases may be desirable if tonic-clonic seizures occur frequently. The maximal recommended dosage of valproate is 60 mg/kg/day. Many patients, especially those receiving enzyme-inducing drugs, require higher-than-recommended doses to achieve adequate clinical effect; other patients may respond at much lower doses. Valproate can be titrated in T.D. to produce a "target" serum concentration of approximately 75 mcg/mL. As ethosuximide is withdrawn, the valproate dose can be further adjusted on the basis of seizure frequency and side effects.

DOSAGE FORMS

CASE 58-8, QUESTION 6: T.D. has been taking valproic acid capsules, 250 mg TID, for 3 weeks. Ethosuximide was discontinued 2 weeks ago; at that time, a valproate serum level just before her morning dose was 68 mcg/mL. She has not experienced generalized tonic-clonic seizures for 6 weeks but continues to have an absence seizure every 2 to 3 weeks. T.D. complains of nausea, epigastric burning pain, and occasional vomiting lasting approximately 1 hour after her doses of valproate. All recent laboratory tests were within normal limits. Administration of the drug with meals is only partially helpful. What alterations can be made in T.D.'s dosing regimen to relieve these symptoms and possibly improve seizure control?

T.D. appears to be a candidate for the use of an enteric-coated valproate preparation or extended-release divalproex. Enteric-coated valproic acid capsules are available, but are expensive and are not commonly used. Divalproex tablets are available as an enteric-coated delayed-release preparation which causes delayed rather than extended absorption of valproate; therefore, these tablets are not a sustained-release product formulation. When patients are switched from nonenteric-coated formulations to divalproex tablets, the frequency of administration should not be decreased. Valproic acid and enteric-coated dosage forms of valproic acid or divalproex are completely absorbed; these can be interconverted at the same total daily dose of medication.[156,157] An extended release formulation of divalproex sodium is also available that can be administered as a single daily dose. Extended release divalproex (divalproex ER), however, is not bioequivalent to other dosage forms of valproate.[158] When equal doses are administered, the ER formulation produces serum concentrations that are approximately 89% of those produced by other valproate dosage forms. Accordingly, when patients are converted to divalproex ER from other forms of valproate, the manufacturer recommends an increase of 8% to 20% in the administered dose. T.D.'s valproic acid capsules can be replaced with an equal daily dose of divalproex tablets. Divalproex should be administered on a three-times-daily dosing schedule. Alternatively, T.D. could be given 1,000 mg of divalproex ER once daily. The results of this change should be apparent within approximately 1 week. By that time, significant relief from GI side effects should have occurred. It may then be possible to increase the dose of divalproex in an effort to improve seizure control.

Capsules containing enteric-coated beads of divalproex also are available; the capsule contents can be dispersed in food for administration to children or others who have difficulty swallowing tablets or capsules. In addition, use of the "cap" end of the capsule to measure half of the contents can approximate doses of 62.5 mg. Patients with feeding tubes in place may be given these opened divalproex capsules through their feeding tubes; however, patients with certain types of feeding gastrostomies should be assessed frequently for possible leakage at the insertion point. This complication may occur because of adherence of undissolved medication beads to the exterior of the feeding tube. The beads may also clog the lumen of smaller-bore feeding tubes.

PHARMACOKINETICS AND SERUM CONCENTRATION MONITORING

CASE 58-8, QUESTION 7: Two weeks later, T.D. returns for follow-up. Her GI symptoms have almost completely disappeared. She has been taking divalproex tablets 250 mg with breakfast and lunch and 375 mg with a bedtime snack for the past week. She has had no seizures in the past 2 weeks and complains of no side effects. A valproate serum level before her morning dose today was 117 mcg/mL (considerably higher than her previous valproate level of 68 mcg/mL). The laboratory reports that duplicate determinations of this level agreed within 5 mcg/mL. T.D. denies taking her medication incorrectly; her parents support this, and the tablet count in her prescription bottle is correct. She has taken no other drugs except a multivitamin. How can this disproportionate increase in her valproate serum concentration be explained, and what is its clinical significance? Does valproate exhibit dose-dependent pharmacokinetics?

Changes in valproate serum concentrations of this nature are, in one author's experience (R.S.L.), relatively common with use of enteric-coated, delayed release divalproex. They are probably not the result of saturable, dose-dependent metabolism as is seen with phenytoin; instead, these changes are more readily explained by the absorption characteristics of divalproex tablets. Peak serum concentrations of valproate after administration of divalproex may be delayed for 3 to 8 hours, and administration of food may further delay absorption.[159] In addition, diurnal fluctuation in both the rate and extent of absorption of divalproex may be significant. Absorption may be reduced by approximately one-third and peak plasma concentrations may be delayed for up to 12 hours for divalproex doses administered in the evening.[34] Twelve to 15 hours probably elapsed between the administration of T.D.'s last dose and blood sampling; therefore, the currently reported blood level may more closely approximate a peak concentration. Previous blood levels, determined while she was receiving rapidly absorbed valproic acid capsules, are more likely to have been trough concentrations. T.D.'s adherence to her prescribed dosage regimen also may have increased because of the change in dosage form and reduced side effects; her previous serum concentrations may not have reflected administration of the prescribed dose.

Other pharmacokinetic factors may have actually moderated this unusual increase in valproate concentrations. Valproate concentrations may fluctuate throughout the day in a pattern that does not reflect the timing of doses.[160] This fluctuation may be partially related to changes in serum concentrations of endogenous fatty acids that displace valproate from protein-binding sites.[29] Valproate's hepatic clearance is restrictive (i.e., valproate has a low extraction ratio and its clearance is limited by the free fraction of drug in plasma); therefore, when protein-binding displacement occurs, free fraction of drug in plasma and clearance increase. As a result, free serum concentrations of valproate increase only transiently, whereas total serum concentrations decrease persistently. Valproate also exhibits dose dependency in its binding to serum proteins. As concentrations approach 70 to 80 mcg/mL, binding sites on albumin molecules become saturated, and the free fraction of drug in plasma increases.[28,156] This effect also increases valproate clearance and reduces total serum concentrations. Both of these effects may actually "dampen" the apparent increase in plasma concentrations seen in T.D. When also considering the poorly established "therapeutic range" for this drug, it becomes apparent that monitoring serum concentrations is a less useful tool in valproate therapy than with some other AEDs.[29,156]

The clinical significance of T.D.'s elevated valproate serum concentrations is minimal. She is not experiencing symptoms suggestive of valproate toxicity, and it is too soon after the dosage increase to assess the effect of this change on her seizure frequency. Therefore, alteration in her drug therapy is unnecessary at present and might only confuse evaluation of her response to this drug. She should be observed for an additional 4 to 6 weeks to evaluate seizure frequency before further alterations in her dosing regimen are considered. Further increases in her dosage are not contraindicated as long as she is tolerating the medication and such increases are justified on the basis of seizure frequency.

HEPATOTOXICITY

CASE 58-8, QUESTION 8: Two months later, T.D. is taking 375 mg of divalproex TID with meals. She has had no absence seizures for 5 weeks and no generalized tonic-clonic seizures for 10 weeks. Yesterday, her valproate plasma concentration was 132 mcg/mL. In addition, her alanine aminotransferase (ALT) was 32 international units/mL and her aspartate aminotransferase (AST) was 41 international units/mL. All other laboratory tests (bilirubin, alkaline phosphatase, lactate dehydrogenase, prothrombin time, and serum albumin) were normal. T.D.'s LFTs have been monitored monthly since she began taking valproate, and they were previously normal. Physical examination was negative for scleral icterus, abdominal pain, or other signs of liver disease. Discuss these laboratory abnormalities and physical findings in relation to possible valproate-induced hepatotoxicity in T.D.

Liver damage related to valproate therapy appears to be caused by accumulation of hepatotoxic metabolites of valproate (probably 4-en-valproate) in certain patients.[161,162] These metabolites may be formed in larger quantities in patients who also receive enzyme-inducing drugs such as phenobarbital. Most cases of fatal hepatotoxicity have occurred in young (<2 years of age) patients with neurologic and metabolic abnormalities who also had severe, difficult-to-control seizures and who were taking multiple AEDs.[161–166] It is important to recognize, however, that severe hepatotoxicity is not limited to this population.[167] Liver damage occurs early in therapy and symptomatically resembles fulminant hepatitis with hepatic failure. Patients may experience vomiting, drowsiness, lethargy, anorexia, edema, and jaundice; these symptoms often precede laboratory evidence of hepatic damage. Liver biopsies in affected patients show evidence of hepatic necrosis and steatosis. Laboratory findings consist of dramatic elevations of AST, total bilirubin, and serum ammonia; coagulation disturbances accompanied by prolonged prothrombin times, low fibrinogen concentrations, and thrombocytopenia also may be observed. Death results from hepatic failure or a Reyelike syndrome.[162,164,168]

Asymptomatic elevations in liver enzymes (such as those found in T.D.) occur commonly during the first 6 months of treatment with valproate and usually are not associated with severe or potentially fatal valproate-induced hepatotoxicity. These changes in aminotransferase usually disappear without alteration in therapy; in some cases, temporary dosage reduction is followed by normalization of laboratory tests within 4 to 6 weeks.[162,164] Without systemic symptoms or other signs of significant liver damage, it is unlikely that the laboratory abnormalities observed in T.D. represent severe liver toxicity from valproate. Because T.D. is responding well to valproate therapy, no change in therapy is warranted at this time. Laboratory testing probably can be repeated in 4 to 6 weeks. T.D. and her family should be educated regarding the possible signs and symptoms of valproate-induced liver damage and instructed to consult their physician if these symptoms are noted.

Routine Liver Function Tests

CASE 58-8, QUESTION 9: What is the usefulness of routinely monitoring LFTs in patients receiving valproate?

Serious hepatotoxicity related to valproate therapy is extremely rare. Historically, the rate of fatal hepatotoxicity decreased significantly (despite substantial increases in the use of valproate) after the use of the drug in high-risk patients (e.g., the very young) decreased and its use as monotherapy increased. Hepatotoxicity is estimated to occur in less than 0.002% of patients treated with valproate.[162,163,165] In children younger than 2 years of age who receive AED polytherapy, the incidence of this complication is 1 in 500 to 1 in 800. Because asymptomatic, apparently benign elevations in liver enzymes are common early in therapy with valproate and symptoms of liver damage often precede laboratory changes, frequent LFTs during early valproate therapy are unlikely to detect serious hepatotoxicity.[63,162–164,169] In addition, this type of laboratory monitoring adds significant cost while providing little benefit for patients. Education of caregivers or patients regarding potential symptoms of hepatotoxicity, with careful observation and follow-up by health care professionals, is recommended as the most effective method to monitor for this drug-induced illness.

Especially careful monitoring should be provided for predisposed patients (i.e., very young children with associated neurologic abnormalities and those receiving polytherapy). In predisposed patients, significant increases in LFT values that are noted early in therapy may be clinically significant. At the onset of symptoms suggesting this condition, laboratory testing may help confirm its presence. Practitioners who feel compelled to perform frequent laboratory testing for liver dysfunction on the basis of manufacturer's package insert recommendations should be cautious not to overinterpret common, transient, and apparently benign elevations in aminotransferases or ammonia levels.

Acute Repetitive ("Cluster") Seizures

RECTAL DIAZEPAM GEL

CASE 58-9

QUESTION 1: B.N., a 7-year-old, 28-kg boy, has had seizures since age 3 months. He suffered anoxia at birth. His seizures usually involve initial confusion and disorientation, shortly followed by generalized tonic-clonic convulsive activity. Despite treatment with carbamazepine at maximal tolerated doses and serum concentrations (300 mg TID; 9–11 mcg/mL), he continues to have approximately two seizures monthly. Recent trials of topiramate and tiagabine as additions to his carbamazepine were unsuccessful and caused intolerable sedation and lethargy. During the past year, he has been admitted to the emergency department (ED) five times because of seizure "flurries" consisting of three to six seizures occurring during a period of 12 or fewer hours. Although he regains consciousness between these "flurry" seizures, he remains lethargic. During ED admissions, IV diazepam was administered. This was rapidly successful in terminating seizure activity. B.N.'s mother relates that she usually can identify the onset of seizure flurries; B.N.'s behavior changes and he becomes "clinging" and "whiny" and hyperactive. She also indicates that the initial seizure in a flurry differs from B.N.'s typical episodes. Before the onset of generalized seizure activity, he experiences much briefer periods of confusion. In addition, the generalized seizures are longer and more severe (often with dramatic cyanosis) at the beginning of a "flurry." Why is prophylactic or abortive therapy for B.N.'s seizure flurries indicated? What factors about B.N. predict successful use of such treatment, and how can it be administered?

B.N.'s relatively frequent flurries or clusters of seizures are causing him and his family significant difficulty. Frequent ED visits are expensive and frightening for many patients and their families. B.N. continues to experience seizure flurries despite carbamazepine therapy. He responds well to IV diazepam and has a caregiver who can identify the onset of seizure clusters. His seizure clusters appear to be distinct from the other seizures that he experiences. All of these factors indicate that a trial of caregiver-administered treatment to abort these cluster episodes is likely to be helpful and should be initiated.

Rectal diazepam gel is available for home administration to patients with acute episodes of repetitive seizure activity.[170] When diazepam gel is administered rectally, it is absorbed relatively rapidly (peak plasma concentrations occur in approximately 1.5 hours[171]), and is often effective in terminating cluster seizures within 15 or fewer minutes. Use of diazepam rectal gel is recommended only when caregivers can recognize the onset of cluster seizures, which are different from a patient's usual seizure activity, and when the caregivers can be trained to administer the preparation safely and to monitor the patient's response (e.g., respiratory status) after administration. Caregivers should be informed that this preparation is not for as needed use with every seizure; it should be used only for identifiable cluster seizures or prolonged seizures. Home use of rectal diazepam may result in significant reduction in the costs of treating these events and may decrease ED visits.[172]

B.N.'s mother should administer rectal diazepam gel at the onset of identifiable cluster seizure activity. A dose of approximately 0.3 mg/kg (10 mg) should be given and repeated, if necessary, within 4 to 12 hours of the first dose. B.N.'s mother should be counseled on the administration of this product and given the patient package insert, which gives complete instructions for the administration of rectal diazepam. After administration, B.N. should be monitored for at least 4 hours to ensure that no respiratory depression or other adverse side effects are occurring and to assess the effect of the medication on his seizures. The most common adverse effect seen with rectal diazepam is somnolence, occasionally accompanied by dizziness and ataxia. Respiratory depression is very uncommon.

Febrile Seizures

INCIDENCE AND CLASSIFICATION

CASE 58-10

QUESTION 1: J.J., a 14-month-old girl, is brought to the ED after having a generalized tonic-clonic convulsion lasting approximately 5 minutes. The episode occurred in association with an upper respiratory infection. On arrival in the ED, her temperature was 39.5°C rectally. She was alert at that time; all laboratory and neurologic findings, including lumbar puncture, were normal. J.J. has no history of neurologic

abnormality. Her 7-year-old brother suffers from both absence and generalized tonic-clonic seizures. What is the relationship between febrile seizures and epilepsy? How may J.J.'s convulsion be classified on the basis of the data available?

Up to 8% of children have a febrile seizure between 6 months and 6 years of age.[173,174] Simple febrile seizures occur with a fever of greater than or equal to 38°C in previously normal children younger than 5 years of age. They last less than 15 minutes and have no focal features. The associated seizure does not arise from CNS pathology. Complex febrile seizures show focal characteristics or are prolonged longer than 15 minutes. The child may or may not have previous neurologic abnormalities. The risk of occurrence of unprovoked afebrile seizures after a febrile seizure is four times greater than in the general population. A family history of afebrile seizures, complex febrile seizures, and pre-existing neurologic abnormality are risk factors associated with the later development of chronic epilepsy.[173,174]

J.J.'s seizure appears to be a typical simple febrile seizure that developed in association with her upper respiratory tract infection. The lack of previous neurologic abnormality and normal findings on lumbar puncture and laboratory evaluation help confirm this assessment.

TREATMENT OF ACUTE SEIZURE

CASE 58-10, QUESTION 2: How should J.J.'s febrile seizures be treated?

Because J.J. is not having a seizure at present, AED therapy is not required. Measures to reduce her elevated temperature should be initiated; however, these measures may not reduce the risk of further seizures. Acetaminophen and tepid sponge baths usually are helpful.

If patients experience prolonged or repeated febrile seizures, either diazepam or, less commonly, midazolam may be administered.[174,175] Rectal diazepam gel can be used for this purpose.

PROPHYLAXIS AND CHOICE OF ANTIEPILEPTIC DRUG

CASE 58-10, QUESTION 3: On the basis of the subjective and objective data available for J.J., is AED therapy indicated on a long-term basis? What are the benefits and risks of AED prophylaxis for febrile seizures?

Long-term treatment or prophylaxis with AED for simple febrile seizures is not recommended. Up to 54% of affected patients will have recurrent febrile seizures, and the risk of recurrence is even greater when the first episode occurs before 13 months of age. Nonetheless, recurrent febrile seizures are not associated with brain damage or development of epilepsy.[173] The efficacy of prophylactic AED for prevention of chronic epilepsy after febrile seizures has not been evaluated.[176] The primary potential benefit of long-term AED therapy would be prevention of recurrent febrile seizures.

Phenobarbital and, occasionally, valproate were historically used as prophylaxis in patients with febrile seizures.[177] A reanalysis of published British trials of both valproate and phenobarbital for febrile seizure prophylaxis found that neither drug was reliably effective.[178] Although phenobarbital had been considered at least partially effective, the high rate of side effects (40%) preclude recommending its use. When the effects on intelligence of phenobarbital versus placebo prophylaxis for febrile seizures in young children were evaluated, IQ scores were significantly lower in children treated with phenobarbital.[179] This effect persisted for at least 6 months after discontinuation of drug therapy. In addition, reduction in the recurrence rate of febrile seizures in children treated with phenobarbital was not statistically significant compared to placebo. Therefore, phenobarbital has no beneficial effect on preventing febrile seizure recurrence and may adversely affect cognitive function.[180]

Antiepileptic drug prophylaxis for febrile seizures is probably not warranted for J.J., even though she is at risk for both development of epilepsy and recurrence of febrile seizures. No evidence supports that medication will significantly affect her later development of epilepsy. Phenobarbital's use for this purpose is difficult to justify when considering the risk of learning impairment. In addition, phenobarbital therapy is associated with hyperactivity and behavioral disturbance in up to 75% of children receiving the drug.[181–184] J.J.'s age places her at higher risk of valproate-related hepatotoxicity, and this risk probably outweighs any potential benefit from treatment with this drug. Close medical follow-up of J.J. is warranted. In addition, her parents should be instructed to institute antipyretic measures (i.e., acetaminophen and tepid sponge baths) at the onset of any febrile illness. Many febrile seizures occur early in the course of an illness before fever is detected[174]; nevertheless, vigilance by her parents and early antipyretic therapy may help prevent further febrile seizures. The intermittent administration of oral diazepam 0.33 mg/kg orally given every 8 hours at the onset of a febrile illness may be of value. In one large randomized trial, 22% of diazepam-treated patients had seizure recurrence by 36 months compared with 31% of placebo-treated patients; a modest reduction.[184] Diazepam, initiated at the onset of fever and continued for 24 hours after fever has resolved, can be considered for J.J., but the modest benefits should be weighed against sedating her with each febrile episode. Furthermore, sedation and other CNS side effects of diazepam, such as dysarthria and insomnia, may confuse assessment of the condition of children with febrile illnesses.[173]

ANTIEPILEPTIC DRUG INTERACTIONS AND ADVERSE EFFECTS

AED–Warfarin Interaction

CASE 58-11

QUESTION 1: T.C. is a 50-year-old woman with a history of complex partial seizures and a mechanical valve replacement. She had been concomitantly treated for many years with carbamazepine 600 mg/day and warfarin 7.5 mg/day. Her international normalized ratio (INR) values during the past 18 months were within the desired range (2.0–3.0). She recently experienced an increase in seizures. Upon questioning, they were unprovoked by common precipitating factors like increased stress, sleep deprivation, and so forth. She states very good adherence. The decision is made to convert her from carbamazepine to levetiracetam, thinking that the latter AED will not have an adverse effect on her bone density compared to carbamazepine. Though not routinely done, this AED changeover was accomplished during a nonrelated hospital stay and she was discharged only on levetiracetam 500 mg BID and warfarin 7.5 mg/day. Twelve days after hospital discharge and before she could be seen in the anticoagulation clinic, she presented to the ED with abdominal pain, rhinorrhagia, ecchymosis, and petechiae on

her back and legs. Her INR is 10.4. Could the "supraphysiologic" INR and signs of excessive bleeding be related to the recent change in her AED regimen?

This scenario depicts a drug interaction between carbamazepine and warfarin. When T.C. was originally put on warfarin, her dose probably had to be increased to attain the goal INR due to the enzyme-inducing effect of carbamazepine increasing the clearance of warfarin. Once that was accomplished, she was maintained on the combination for many years and the drug interaction was managed successfully. Though the details of the original warfarin dosing are not known, the problem arose when the warfarin dose was not adjusted accordingly when the enzyme-inducer was removed from TC's drug regimen.[185] Levetiracetam has no impact on the metabolism of warfarin and is not known to cause problems with excessive bleeding.[186] T.C. wound up being "over-anticoagulated" when her enzyme-inducing AED (carbamazepine) was switched to a non-enzyme-inducing AED (levetiracetam). It is prudent to think about drug interactions not only when drugs are added to a regimen but also when drugs are removed. In this case, it would have been preferable if T.C.'s INR were monitored more frequently during and after the removal of carbamazepine, with appropriate adjustments to her warfarin dosage as needed.

Valproate–Carbamazepine Interaction

CASE 58-12

QUESTION 1: D.H., a 21-year-old, 84-kg man, was taking carbamazepine 1,400 mg/day (600 mg every morning and 800 mg at bedtime) for treatment of generalized tonic-clonic seizures. Despite carbamazepine serum concentrations of 14 mcg/mL, he continued to have a seizure every 6 to 8 weeks. Higher serum levels were associated with toxicity symptoms. Valproate (divalproex) was recently added and gradually increased to a dosage of 1,000 mg TID; the therapeutic goal is replacement of carbamazepine with valproate. At this dose, D.H. experienced symptoms of carbamazepine intoxication (double vision, unsteady gait, and drowsiness), although his carbamazepine serum concentration was 12 mcg/mL. Valproate serum levels were 40 mcg/mL and 43 mcg/mL on two occasions. D.H. has continued to experience seizures at his previous rate. He appears to be adherent with his prescribed medication regimen. How can D.H.'s symptoms and low valproate levels be explained on the basis of an interaction between his two AEDs?

Difficulty in achieving serum valproate concentrations adequate for improvement in seizure control frequently is encountered in patients who receive concomitant therapy with potent enzyme inducers such as carbamazepine. Clinicians frequently note that it is difficult to administer doses of valproate sufficiently large to achieve desired serum levels under these circumstances.[28,187] Serum concentrations of valproate in patients receiving carbamazepine may be only approximately 50% of those expected on the basis of single-dose valproate pharmacokinetic studies.

D.H.'s symptoms of carbamazepine intoxication at plasma levels that were previously tolerated suggest possible accumulation of CBZ-E. This compound is an active metabolite of carbamazepine. Valproate may inhibit epoxide hydrolase and cause accumulation of CBZ-E sufficient to exert significant pharmacologic effects, including intoxication. One author (R.S.L.) has observed a patient receiving both valproate and carbamazepine who developed serum concentrations of CBZ-E equal to the concentration of carbamazepine itself (both compounds were measured at ~12 mcg/mL) and experienced significant intoxication. Determination of the serum concentration of carbamazepine and CBZ-E could help confirm the clinical impression. Unfortunately, the assay for CBZ-E is not readily available in many clinical laboratories.

CASE 58-12, QUESTION 2: What recommendations can be made for alteration in D.H.'s drug therapy regimen to alleviate the effects of this drug interaction and enhance his therapeutic response to the medication?

On clinical and empiric grounds, D.H.'s dosage of carbamazepine should be reduced; this would seem especially appropriate because the therapeutic goal was replacement of carbamazepine with valproate. Dosage reduction will result in a decrease in serum concentrations of both carbamazepine and CBZ-E and a reduction in symptoms of intoxication. An initial decrease of 10% to 20% (200 mg) of D.H.'s daily carbamazepine dose would be reasonable. Subsequently, his carbamazepine dose can be tapered using reductions of 200 mg every 1 to 2 weeks. During tapering of carbamazepine, D.H. should be monitored carefully for increased seizure activity.

Valproate-Related Thrombocytopenia

CASE 58-12, QUESTION 3: D.H.'s symptoms abated significantly within 3 days of reduction of his carbamazepine dosage to 1,200 mg/day. A CBZ-E serum concentration was not determined. His carbamazepine dosage was reduced by 200 mg/day in weekly steps, with no increase in seizure activity. A serum valproate concentration after his carbamazepine dosage reached 600 mg/day was 53 mcg/mL. At that time, he had not had a seizure in approximately 6 weeks. A serum valproate concentration was repeated when his carbamazepine dosage reached 200 mg/day and it was 58 mcg/mL. Three weeks after discontinuation of carbamazepine, D.H. noted the onset of tremor affecting his hands and a "fuzzy sensation in my head" accompanied by difficulty concentrating on tasks. His serum valproate concentration was 126 mcg/mL on a dose of 3,000 mg/day. In addition, a CBC showed a platelet count of 60,000 cells/μL; no other abnormalities were seen. No bleeding tendencies were noted, and D.H. denied easy bruisability or unusual bleeding. Previous CBC had been normal. Is this pattern of increase in valproate serum concentrations consistent with the loss of carbamazepine-related enzyme induction? What is the relationship between D.H.'s new symptoms, his reduced platelet count, and the elevation in his valproate serum concentration?

D.H.'s valproate serum concentrations were expected to increase with "deinduction" of hepatic microsomal enzymes while carbamazepine was being discontinued. The pattern and timing of deinduction are not consistently predictable. Although a somewhat linear increase in valproate concentrations might be anticipated as enzyme-inducers such as carbamazepine are gradually reduced, it is not unusual for valproate levels to remain relatively constant until 1 to 2 weeks after discontinuation of enzyme inducers.[187] Therefore, patients should be monitored for signs or symptoms of possible valproate intoxication during and for several weeks after such a discontinuation process; clinicians and patients should be aware that dosage adjustment may not be required until the enzyme-inducing drug has been completely discontinued.

D.H.'s new symptoms appear to be consistent with mild to moderate intoxication with valproate. Tremor is a relatively common side effect of valproate that is likely to appear as serum concentrations exceed approximately 80 mcg/mL.[28] This side effect may be troublesome for some patients because the tremor is usually an intention tremor, which worsens with physical activity. In most patients, dose reduction will improve or eliminate tremor.[188] The neurologic symptoms exhibited by D.H. also are typically seen with valproate intoxication. All of these symptoms are reversible with dosage reduction.

Reductions in platelet counts are not rare in patients treated with valproate. Significant thrombocytopenia with bleeding manifestations is extremely uncommon, although measurable changes in platelet function may occur.[189,190] The mechanism underlying thrombocytopenia is not known; evidence exists for both a dose-related or serum-concentration–related effect[190] and an immunologic mechanism.[191] Affected patients usually can be continued on valproate therapy at reduced doses without adverse effects. One author (R.S.L.) has observed two patients who experienced significant valproate-related thrombocytopenia without bleeding complications; both cases were associated with dramatic increases in valproate serum concentrations after discontinuation of enzyme-inducing drugs.

Both the neurologic symptoms and thrombocytopenia exhibited by D.H. probably can be corrected by reducing his dose of divalproex. The magnitude of dose reduction should be determined by titration using symptom remission and normalization of his platelet count as endpoints. Periodically rechecking valproate serum concentrations may help establish a safe upper limit dose and serum levels for D.H. Ongoing monitoring also will be important for several weeks because the process of deinduction of hepatic enzymes may not yet be complete. Further dose reductions may be necessary as this process reaches completion and D.H.'s valproate clearance gradually decreases. Reduction of D.H.'s dosage to 2,000 mg/day should approximate serum concentrations between those that were previously subtherapeutic and those that are causing his current adverse effects.

Skin Rash: Hypersensitivity Reactions to Antiepileptic Drugs

CASE 58-13

QUESTION 1: R.S., a 34-year-old man, has been taking phenytoin 200 mg BID for the past 7 weeks to control complex partial and secondarily generalized tonic-clonic seizures. Seizures began approximately 4 months ago after surgical evacuation of a subdural hematoma. Today he appears at the walk-in clinic and complains of an "itchy rash" that began 2 days ago. He describes "feeling lousy" for the past week. On examination he is febrile (38.5°C orally). A maculopapular, scaly, erythematous rash covers his upper extremities and torso, and the mucous membranes of his mouth appear to be mildly inflamed. Cervical lymphadenopathy is noted, and the liver is found to be enlarged and tender. R.S. also relates that his urine has become very dark in the past 2 days and that his stools are light colored. What is the significance of R.S.'s skin rash and other signs and symptoms? Are these likely to be related to his phenytoin therapy?

Skin rash is a relatively common (2%–3% of patients) side effect related to AED therapy. It is most commonly associated with phenytoin, lamotrigine, carbamazepine, and phenobarbital. Most cases are relatively mild, but severely affected patients may exhibit Stevens-Johnson syndrome or a systemic hypersensitivity syndrome accompanied by severe hepatic damage. In R.S.'s case, signs and symptoms suggesting hepatic involvement accompany the skin rash. Fever, lymphadenopathy, and apparent inflammation of mucous membranes also suggest a hypersensitivity reaction to phenytoin with multisystem involvement and the potential for progression to Stevens-Johnson syndrome. Viral infection (e.g., hepatitis, influenza, infectious mononucleosis) should be considered and ruled out as a possible cause of R.S.'s symptoms before they are attributed to phenytoin therapy.[123,192–195]

Phenytoin hypersensitivity syndrome is most commonly seen in adults. Typically, patients with this syndrome present with complaints of fever, skin rash, and lymphadenopathy during the first 2 months of phenytoin therapy. Hepatomegaly, splenomegaly, jaundice, and bleeding manifestations such as petechial hemorrhage also are relatively common. Laboratory manifestations usually include leukocytosis with eosinophilia, elevated serum bilirubin, and elevated AST and ALT. When a phenytoin hypersensitivity reaction includes significant hepatotoxicity, fatality may occur in as many as 38% of affected patients.[192]

A high likelihood exists that R.S. has developed a severe reaction to phenytoin; the clinical manifestations and the timing of their appearance are typical of this reaction. Phenytoin should be discontinued immediately pending diagnostic clarification (i.e., evaluation for other possible causes of his symptoms such as viral illness). R.S. should be hospitalized for further diagnostic evaluation and treatment. Treatment of phenytoin-related hypersensitivity and hepatotoxicity is symptomatic and supportive. Intensive therapy with corticosteroids has commonly been used, although little objective evidence exists for beneficial effects of this treatment. Potential complications of this reaction include sepsis and hepatic failure; these conditions should be treated specifically.

CASE 58-13, QUESTION 2: R.S. was hospitalized and treated with oral prednisone and topical corticosteroids. Other potential causes for his condition were ruled out, and his signs and symptoms were attributed to phenytoin hypersensitivity. His fever resolved within 5 days; the skin rash became exfoliative but resolved without infectious complications. Laboratory parameters began to normalize after 10 days. While he was hospitalized, R.S. experienced three episodes of generalized seizure activity that were treated with acute administration of IV lorazepam. R.S. was afebrile at the time these episodes occurred. What information regarding the pathogenesis of phenytoin hypersensitivity and hepatotoxicity can be used to guide selection of an alternative AED for R.S.?

Further administration of phenytoin to R.S. is contraindicated on the basis of his history of a severe hypersensitivity reaction to this drug. Readministration of phenytoin is likely to result in rapid recurrence of severe symptoms of this syndrome. Although the mechanism of this reaction is not fully understood, research implicates reactive arene oxide metabolites of phenytoin (and other chemically similar AEDs) as possible causative agents for hypersensitivity reactions. Affected patients purportedly are predisposed genetically to the development of hypersensitivity, possibly because a relative deficiency of epoxide hydrolase enzymes allows the accumulation of toxic concentrations of reactive epoxide metabolites. These metabolites are believed to exert a direct cytotoxic effect and to interact with cellular macromolecules, thereby functioning as haptens that stimulate an immunologic reaction.[196,197] Carbamazepine, phenytoin, and phenobarbital all are metabolized by similar pathways and converted to reactive arene oxides. It is hypothesized that carbamazepine-induced liver damage also may result from the effects of accumulation of reactive epoxide metabolites; these reactive metabolites differ from the 10,11-epoxide metabolite that accumulates during carbamazepine therapy. For this reason, these drugs potentially cross-react in susceptible patients. Cases of apparent cross-reactivity between phenytoin and phenobarbital or carbamazepine have been documented.[198–200] In addition, both carbamazepine and phenobarbital can produce hypersensitivity reactions similar to those seen with phenytoin. This potential for cross-reactivity should be considered when an alternative AED is selected for R.S. An analysis of cases of AED-related skin rashes found that the most significant nondrug predictor of skin rash was the occurrence of a rash with another AED.[201]

Valproate has been suggested as the preferred alternative AED for patients who have exhibited hypersensitivity reactions to phenytoin.[199] Valproate is not metabolized to arene oxides and also is chemically dissimilar to all other AEDs. Because valproate often shows good efficacy for complex partial seizures with secondary generalization, it would seem to be a safe and potentially effective alternative AED for R.S. Of the newer AEDs, lamotrigine should probably be avoided in R.S. because of its likelihood of causing skin rash and apparent hypersensitivity reactions. Oxcarbazepine is potentially an alternative AED for R.S. because it is not metabolized through the arene oxide pathway. Nevertheless, 25% to 30% of patients who experience a rash in response to carbamazepine will also experience a rash with oxcarbazepine.[202] Therefore, many clinicians would avoid oxcarbazepine. Gabapentin, lacosamide, levetiracetam, pregabalin, tiagabine, topiramate, or zonisamide could be considered as alternative medications for R.S. These medications appear less likely to cause skin rash or hypersensitivity reactions.[201,203]

It is suggested that R.S. be advised to add phenytoin to his list of medication allergies.

WOMEN'S ISSUES IN EPILEPSY

Although epilepsy affects men and women equally, many health issues are of specific importance to women, such as contraceptive interactions with AEDs, teratogenicity, pharmacokinetic changes during pregnancy, breast-feeding, menstrual cycle influences on seizure activity (catamenial epilepsy), AED impact on bone, and sexual dysfunction.[204] It is noteworthy that the latter two issues can also occur in men. A great need exists to educate both health care professionals and patients about the many complex issues facing women with epilepsy.

For women of childbearing potential, prepregnancy planning and counseling are important, because significant AED exposure of the fetus often occurs by the time pregnancy is confirmed. This is especially important because of the potential for unplanned pregnancies from the AED–contraceptive drug interactions. Prepregnancy counseling also should include the importance of folic acid supplementation and medication adherence. Patients should be informed about the risk of teratogenicity and the importance of prenatal care.

Although complete seizure control is desirable for all patients with epilepsy, it is especially favorable for a woman's seizures to be well controlled before conception. Monotherapy is preferred whenever possible, because the relative risk of birth defects dramatically increases with AED polytherapy.[205,206] Monotherapy also improves patient adherence. The AED should be given at the lowest effective dose to reduce the possibility of birth defects.[207] Gradual discontinuation of AED before pregnancy may be considered if a woman has been seizurefree for 2 years or longer.

Antiepileptic Drug–Oral Contraceptive Interaction

CASE 58-14

QUESTION 1: P.Z., a 26-year-old woman, experiences complex partial and secondarily generalized tonic-clonic seizures. She is taking phenytoin 400 mg/day and divalproex 2,000 mg/day. She reports having two or three partial seizures and one generalized seizure every 3 to 4 months. Despite taking Lo/Ovral (norgestrel 0.3 mg with ethinyl estradiol 30 mcg), she has just learned she is pregnant. Her last menstrual period was 6 weeks ago. What is the relationship between P.Z.'s apparent contraceptive failure and her antiepileptic drug therapy?

There have been several reports of reduced efficacy of oral contraceptives in patients receiving various AEDs.[208,209] These reports describe both breakthrough bleeding and pregnancy. Phenobarbital, phenytoin, carbamazepine, oxcarbazepine, and felbamate have been shown to increase the metabolism of ethinylestradiol and progestogens.[210] This effect is not associated with valproate, lamotrigine, gabapentin, tiagabine, zonisamide, levetiracetam, lacosamide or pregabalin.[90,91,204,211] Topiramate in polytherapy and at high dosages (200–800 mg/day) appears to have a mild though measurable effect on oral contraceptive pharmacokinetics; apparent clearance of the estrogen component of combined oral contraceptives is increased in patients taking topiramate.[212] In contrast, topiramate monotherapy in lower dosages (50–200 mg/day) has a lesser impact on the pharmacokinetics of the oral contraceptive.[213]

A lack of contraceptive efficacy may present as irregular or breakthrough menstrual bleeding. Decreased efficacy is not always associated with breakthrough bleeding, however. Oral contraceptive doses can be increased to compensate for the effect of an AED.[214] However, estrogens also may exacerbate seizures in some women.[215] Women older than 35 years of age and those who smoke must consider the risk of thromboembolic complications associated with higher doses of contraceptives. A second contraceptive method (e.g., condoms, intrauterine devices, or spermicide) is recommended to avoid contraceptive failure.[203] Tubal ligation is also an alternative. An additional alternative that could be considered is injectable depot medroxyprogesterone acetate. Although there is a lack of clinical studies substantiating its effectiveness in patients on enzyme-inducing AED, the pharmacokinetic characteristics of this agent suggest that its effect is not reduced by enzyme induction. Medroxyprogesterone is a high-clearance drug; its clearance is directly dependent on hepatic blood flow. Thus, enzyme induction would have little effect on the metabolism of this drug when it is administered by injection. Depot medroxyprogesterone acetate may, however, have other negative effects that would limit its choice as an alternative contraceptive in this situation.[216]

Assuming P.Z. was taking her contraceptive pills on a regular basis, it is possible that her enzyme-inducing AED (phenytoin) is responsible for their failure. Patients receiving enzyme-inducing AED should be prospectively informed that this interaction can occur and advised concerning the use of alternative contraceptives (see Chapter 47, Contraception).

Interestingly, a different drug interaction exists between oral contraceptives and lamotrigine. It is currently thought that the estrogen component in oral contraceptives increases the clearance of lamotrigine. Lamotrigine clearance may increase twofold when contraceptive steroids are begun and fall by 50% when contraceptive steroids are discontinued. Changes in lamotrigine levels associated with initiation and discontinuation of contraceptive steroids can result in increased seizure activity in some patients and toxicity in others.[217]

Teratogenicity

CASE 58-14, QUESTION 2: What are the risks of teratogenic effects from P.Z.'s medications? What steps might be taken to minimize these risks?

P.Z.'s child is at risk of congenital malformations because of exposure to several potentially teratogenic drugs: estrogen–progestin combination oral contraceptives, valproate, and phenytoin (also see Chapter 49, Obstetric Drug Therapy).

Many AEDs have teratogenic effects.[218] Animal data regarding the teratogenic potential of felbamate, gabapentin, lacosamide, levetiracetam, oxcarbazepine, pregabalin, tiagabine, and zonisamide are encouraging, but conclusions regarding the teratogenic potential of these AEDs cannot be made because of limited experience in pregnant women. Controversy has been significantly reduced regarding the relative contributions of parental epilepsy itself, genetic influences, and drug therapy since data have shown that the infants of AED-untreated women with epilepsy had fewer abnormalities compared with those born to women with epilepsy who were taking AED.[219] The risk of major congenital malformations (e.g., facial clefts, cardiac septal defects) in children exposed to AED in utero may be as high as two to three times the baseline risk in the general population.[220] In addition, maternal epilepsy increases the risk of complications of pregnancy, prenatal or postnatal infant mortality, premature birth, and low infant birth weight.

The American Epilepsy Society and the American Academy of Neurology have published a series of three Practice Parameter updates on management issues for women with epilepsy focused on pregnancy. They deal with obstetrical complications and change in seizure frequency; teratogenesis and perinatal outcomes; and vitamin K, folic acid, blood levels, and breast-feeding.[221–223] The authors evaluated the available evidence based on a structured literature review and provide recommendations.

Most AEDs are believed to exert their teratogenic effects (and possibly other adverse effects such as hepatotoxicity) partly via reactive epoxide metabolites.[220] Enhancement of the formation of these metabolites via hepatic enzyme induction (e.g., by carbamazepine or phenobarbital) or inhibition of their breakdown (e.g., through inhibition of epoxide hydrolase by valproate) would increase the risk of teratogenicity. Combined administration of enzyme inducers and valproate (specifically the combination of carbamazepine, phenobarbital, and valproate with or without phenytoin) is associated with an especially high risk of teratogenicity.[224] In addition, each of the present major AEDs has been associated with congenital malformations when administered alone. Meador et al. provide data from 333 pregnancies in women with epilepsy taking an AED in monotherapy and enrolled in the Neurodevelopmental Effects of Antiepileptic Drugs (NEAD) study.[225] Serious adverse outcomes (major malformations and fetal death) were significantly more likely to occur with exposure to valproate (20.3%) than with carbamazepine (8.2%), phenytoin (10.7%), or lamotrigine (1%).

The NEAD study included one newer AED, lamotrigine. The North American AED Pregnancy Registry reported that the risk for a major malformation after first trimester monotherapy exposure to lamotrigine was not increased compared to the risk for the nonexposed control population. The risk for nonsyndromic cleft lip or palate was increased in the babies exposed to lamotrigine, although this has not been identified in other registries.[226] The reason for this incongruence is not known.

In March 2011, the FDA changed the Pregnancy Category of topiramate from "C" to "D" due to an increased risk of development of cleft lip and/or cleft palate (oral clefts) in infants born to women treated with it during pregnancy.[227]

In addition to physical malformations, AED exposure in utero may have an effect on neurodevelopment. An interim analysis of the NEAD study raised concerns about the effects of in utero exposure to valproate on neurodevelopment.[228] It was found that valproate-exposed children have low scores (mean, 85) on the children's mental development index (MDI), even after controlling for the mother's IQ and seizure type. The MDI scores were significantly lower for children exposed in utero to valproate compared with scores of children exposed to carbamazepine (mean, 94), phenytoin (mean, 90), and lamotrigine (mean, 97) monotherapy.

Several strategies can be used to reduce the potential adverse effects of AEDs on pregnancy outcomes. If feasible, before conception, seizure control should be optimized using the AED of first choice for the prospective mother's seizure type or epilepsy syndrome. Monotherapy at the lowest effective dose is the goal. Maintenance of adequate folic acid stores before conception and during fetal organogenesis is also important. Folic acid supplementation can reduce the risk of congenital neural tube malformations in infants at risk who are born to women without epilepsy, but folate supplementation does not reliably reduce the teratogenic effects of AED. Nevertheless, supplementation of folic acid (and ensuring adequate folate levels) is recommended. Because about half of pregnancies are unplanned and not evident until weeks after conception, folate supplementation should be given routinely to women of childbearing age with epilepsy. No study has been conducted to determine the optimal dose of folic acid supplementation in patients taking AEDs. Clinicians engage in much discussion of this topic, but the current practices are not evidence-based. Even though this is the case, P.Z. should start taking 4 mg of folic acid supplementation each day.

Physiologic changes in pregnant women may affect the pharmacokinetics of AEDs.[204] Absorption can be influenced by nausea and vomiting. Hepatic metabolism and renal function both increase during pregnancy. The binding capacity of albumin is decreased during pregnancy, resulting in decreased protein binding for highly bound drugs. Unbound fractions of phenobarbital, phenytoin, and valproate increase with decreased concentrations of albumin.[229–231] For drugs predominately metabolized by the liver with a restrictive clearance (e.g., carbamazepine and valproate), decreased protein binding without changes in intrinsic clearance should result in a decrease in total drug concentrations; unbound drug concentrations usually remain unchanged. For drugs with both increased hepatic metabolism and decreased protein binding (e.g., phenytoin and phenobarbital), both total and unbound plasma concentrations decrease, but not necessarily proportionately.

The clearance of lamotrigine increases as pregnancy progresses, presumably related to the impact of estrogen on lamotrigine metabolism as mentioned here.[232] This alteration in clearance changes immediately postpartum. Preliminary data suggest that oxcarbazepine concentrations may also decrease as pregnancy progresses.[233]

The effects of changes in renal function during pregnancy on AED concentrations are not well known.[233] Renal blood flow and glomerular filtration rate increase during pregnancy. Thus, the renal clearance of drugs that are predominately excreted through the kidneys, such as gabapentin, levetiracetam, and pregabalin, may increase during pregnancy.

During pregnancy, serum levels of AEDs (including free serum levels for highly protein-bound drugs) can be monitored. In this case, a prepregnancy level would be optimal for comparison. Dosage adjustments may help to prevent the increase in seizure frequency that is seen in approximately 25% of pregnant women with epilepsy. Because falls and anoxia associated with uncontrolled generalized tonic-clonic seizures may increase the risk to the unborn baby, P.Z. should be educated on the value of adherence to her AED regimen.

For P.Z., it can be presumed that significant exposure of the fetus to any teratogenic influence of AED has already occurred. Optimization of seizure control is a primary concern for this woman. Any major alterations in P.Z.'s AED regimen should be made cautiously to avoid precipitating seizures. In addition, she should be instructed to contact the AED pregnancy registry at Massachusetts General Hospital (1-888-233-2334 or www.aedpregnancyregistry.org). Information provided to the registry will aid in the ongoing monitoring of outcomes of babies born to mothers taking AEDs. Reports from this registry have provided risk information on two of the older AEDs (phenobarbital and valproate). In utero exposure to either of these AEDs in monotherapy caused a significantly increased incidence of major birth defects compared with controls.

VITAMIN K SUPPLEMENTATION

Babies born to women with epilepsy who are taking enzyme-inducing AED are at risk of hemorrhage owing to decreased vitamin-K–dependent clotting factors. Although some question the evidence, women taking carbamazepine, phenobarbital, primidone, or phenytoin should receive vitamin K 10 mg orally every day from 36 weeks of gestation until delivery, and babies should also receive vitamin K 1 mg IM at birth.[234]

BREAST-FEEDING

In a lactating woman who is taking medications, the risk of drug exposure to the infant needs to be weighed against the benefits of breast-feeding.[235] All drugs transfer into milk to some extent. The extent of protein binding of the drug is the most important predictor of drug passage into milk.[236,237] For the AED, a large intersubject variability in the milk/plasma (M/P) ratio is seen, presumably owing to a difference in volume and composition of the milk. Thus, the M/P ratio is not useful for predicting infant AED exposure. Reviews on AED and breast-feeding are available.[238,239] For most first-generation AEDs (carbamazepine, phenytoin, valproic acid), breast-feeding results in negligible AED plasma concentrations in the infants. For the second-generation AEDs, breast-feeding should be done cautiously and the infant should be monitored for excess AED plasma concentrations and toxicity, if possible. This information should be presented to P.Z. in an appropriate manner. Once she delivers her baby, re-evaluation and optimization of P.Z.'s AED therapy should occur.

STATUS EPILEPTICUS

Characteristics and Pathophysiology

CASE 58-15

QUESTION 1: V.S., a 22-year-old, 85-kg man, was recently diagnosed as having idiopathic epilepsy with generalized tonic-clonic seizures. For the past 3 months, he has been treated with 600 mg/day of carbamazepine, which completely eliminated his seizures. His steady-state carbamazepine serum concentration was 10 mcg/mL. While at his parents' home, he had two tonic-clonic seizures, each lasting 3 to 4 minutes. On arrival at the hospital (~30 minutes after the first seizure began), he was noted to be only semiconscious. His blood pressure was 197/104 mm Hg, his pulse was 124 beats/minute, respirations were 23 breaths/minute, and his body temperature was 38°C rectally. Shortly after his arrival, another generalized tonic-clonic seizure began. How does V.S.'s current condition meet accepted diagnostic criteria for status epilepticus? What risks are associated with status epilepticus?

Status epilepticus (SE) is operationally defined as "either continuous seizures lasting at least five minutes or two or more discrete seizures between which there is incomplete recovery of consciousness."[240] Because V.S. has had three seizures within slightly more than 30 minutes and remains unconscious, his present condition meets this definition. V.S. is experiencing generalized convulsive SE; this is the most common type and it is associated with the greatest risk of physical and neurologic damage. SE also may be characterized by nonconvulsive seizures that produce a persistent state of impaired consciousness, or by partial seizures (with or without impaired consciousness). These forms of SE are associated with much lower morbidity and mortality than generalized convulsive SE.

Uncontrolled, convulsive SE can cause severe metabolic and hemodynamic alterations. V.S.'s vital signs (tachycardia, elevated blood pressure, increased respiratory rate, and elevated body temperature) are typical for a patient in SE. Prolonged, severe muscle contractions and CNS dysfunction from uncontrolled seizure discharges result in hyperthermia, cardiorespiratory collapse, myoglobinuria, renal failure, and neurologic damage. Even in the absence of convulsive muscle movements, neurologic damage can occur from excessive electrical activity and the resultant alterations in brain metabolism. When seizure activity persists longer than approximately 30 minutes, failure of mechanisms that regulate cerebral blood flow is more likely; this failure accompanies dramatic increases in brain metabolism and demand for glucose and oxygen. Failure to meet the metabolic demands of brain tissue results in accumulation of lactate and cell death. Peripherally, lactate accumulates and serum glucose and electrolytes are altered. After 30 minutes of seizure activity, the body often fails to compensate for increased metabolic demands, and cardiovascular collapse can occur.[241,242] For these reasons, SE is considered a medical emergency that requires immediate treatment to prevent or lessen both physical and neurologic damage. Mortality in adults with SE is approximately 20%[240]; fatal outcome is often the result of the condition that precipitated SE (e.g., cardiopulmonary arrest, stroke). Long-term neurologic consequences of severe SE may include cognitive impairment, memory loss, and worsening of seizure disorders. The effect of SE on cognitive function is not clearly established, however; cognitive impairment may result from the neurologic disorder underlying SE rather than from SE itself.[243]

General Treatment Measures and Antiepileptic Drug Therapy

CASE 58-15, QUESTION 2: Describe a general treatment plan for V.S.'s episode of status epilepticus.

The immediate therapeutic concern in V.S. is to ensure ventilation and terminate current seizure activity. If possible, an airway should be placed for airway protection and if ventilatory support is needed; however, this may not be possible while he is convulsing. Objects (e.g., spoons, tongue blades) should never be placed into the mouth of a patient during a seizure. If airway placement is impossible, V.S. should be positioned on his side to allow drainage of saliva and mucus from the mouth and prevent aspiration. An IV line should be established using normal saline, and blood should be obtained for serum chemistries (especially glucose and electrolytes), AED serum concentrations, and toxicology screens. Glucose, 25 g (50 mL of 50% dextrose solution) by IV push should be administered to correct any hypoglycemia, which may be responsible for SE. Glucose administration should be preceded by IV thiamine 100 mg or vitamin B complex to prevent Wernicke encephalopathy.[244]

Intravenous administration of rapidly effective anticonvulsant medication should begin as soon as possible to terminate V.S.'s seizure activity. Treatment is more likely to be effective in stopping seizures the sooner it is administered.[240] IM or rectal administration of medication is not recommended as initial treatment unless IV access is impossible. IM medications are unlikely to be absorbed sufficiently rapidly to achieve the CNS concentrations needed to terminate status seizures.

CASE 58-15, QUESTION 3: Which anticonvulsants are available for IV administration? Evaluate the available drugs and recommend a drug, dosage, and regimen for initial treatment of status epilepticus in V.S.

Lorazepam, diazepam, phenytoin, and fosphenytoin are the agents most commonly used as IV therapy in the initial treatment of SE.[240,245] Phenytoin and fosphenytoin are indicated for treatment of SE, but owing to limitations on their rates of infusion, the onset of their peak effect may be delayed. Therefore, phenytoin or fosphenytoin are usually used after initial treatment with a benzodiazepine.

Intravenous sodium valproate (Depacon) is available, but it is not indicated for the treatment of SE. Although the manufacturer recommends that Depacon be administered slowly (<20 mg/minute), it has been administered safely at high doses and faster infusion rates.[244] Currently, IV valproate is indicated only for use in patients who cannot take oral dosage forms of valproate. However, there is growing experience with the use of IV valproate for SE who fail to respond to benzodiazepines and phenytoin, and for patients in whom phenytoin is contraindicated (e.g., phenytoin allergy).[245] An IV form of levetiracetam is available. This drug also is indicated only for patients who cannot receive oral dosage forms of levetiracetam. Rapid IV administration of levetiracetam has been used; however, experience with this agent is limited.[246] Lacosamide is also available in an IV formulation and there are several case reports of its successful use for refractory nonconvulsive SE.[247,248] IV phenobarbital is usually reserved for SE that does not respond to benzodiazepines and phenytoin.[240]

Four IV regimens for generalized convulsive SE were directly compared in one randomized controlled trial.[249] The study evaluated diazepam (0.15 mg/kg) followed by phenytoin (18 mg/kg), lorazepam (0.1 mg/kg) alone, phenobarbital (15 mg/kg) alone, and phenytoin (18 mg/kg) alone. For initial IV treatment of overt generalized SE, lorazepam was more effective than phenytoin alone. Lorazepam was as effective as the other two regimens, and it was easier to use.

Intravenous administration of either diazepam or lorazepam is usually effective for rapid termination of seizure activity in SE.[250] Owing to diazepam's higher lipid solubility, it redistributes from the CNS to peripheral tissues rapidly after administration; this results in a short duration of action (<60 minutes).[251] Lorazepam's lower lipid solubility prevents rapid redistribution and accounts for its longer duration of action.[251] Lorazepam may be effective for up to 72 hours.[252,253] Owing to this longer duration, lorazepam is now the preferred benzodiazepine for immediate treatment of SE in most centers.[244,245] At adequate doses, the onset of antiepileptic activity and efficacy of lorazepam and diazepam are equal.[250]

Lorazepam 0.1 mg/kg given intravenously at 2 mg/minute would be appropriate initial therapy for V.S.[244] Lorazepam may cause significant venous irritation, and the manufacturer recommends dilution with an equal volume of normal saline solution or water for injection before IV administration. Lorazepam may be repeated after 5 minutes if seizure activity has not stopped. The efficacy of lorazepam (and diazepam) depends on rapid achievement of high serum and CNS concentrations. Although lorazepam can be administered IM, this route should not be used for treatment of SE because it is unlikely that it would achieve serum concentrations necessary for termination of seizure activity. Diazepam should not be given by the IM route because it is absorbed slowly and erratically from gluteal IM injection sites.[251] The most common adverse effects after IV administration of benzodiazepines are sedation, hypotension, and respiratory arrest.[251] These side effects are usually short-lived and, when adequate facilities are available for assisted ventilation and administration of fluids, they usually can be managed without major risk to the patient. Respiratory depression occurs most commonly in patients who receive multiple IV medications for control of SE.

INTRAVENOUS PHENYTOIN AND FOSPHENYTOIN

CASE 58-15, QUESTION 4: V.S. was given lorazepam 8 mg IV. Seizure activity ceased 2 minutes after the injection was completed. What drug should be administered to V.S. for prolonged control of seizures? Recommend a dose, route, and method of administration.

Continued effective seizure control is important for patients who experience SE. Previously, when diazepam was the benzodiazepine predominantly used for immediate control of SE, a long-acting AED such as phenytoin was routinely administered at the same time to ensure continued suppression of seizure activity. Routine use of phenytoin has been somewhat de-emphasized with increased use of lorazepam[244]; lorazepam's apparent longer duration of effect may make routine use of IV phenytoin less necessary. Nevertheless, many centers still use phenytoin in conjunction with lorazepam.

The availability of fosphenytoin for IV administration has provided an additional option for administration of phenytoin in the treatment of SE. Use of this phenytoin prodrug allows more rapid administration of large IV loading doses of phenytoin with less risk of injection site complications and potentially fewer cardiovascular adverse effects. Fosphenytoin itself is inactive; the therapeutic effect results from its conversion to phenytoin.[120,121] Because fosphenytoin is more expensive in both brand and generic formulations as compared with phenytoin, many facilities have been reluctant to place this product on their formularies. Pharmacoeconomic studies, however, seem to indicate that, although it is initially more expensive, fosphenytoin may be more economical because it causes fewer adverse effects than phenytoin.[254]

Phenytoin (administered as either sodium phenytoin injection or as sodium fosphenytoin injection) is presently considered the long-acting anticonvulsant of choice for most patients with generalized convulsive SE.[240] Extensive clinical experience with the use of IV loading doses of phenytoin has established its efficacy and general safety. Phenytoin causes much less sedation and respiratory depression than drugs such as phenobarbital when it is used in conjunction with IV benzodiazepines.[244] V.S.'s maintenance carbamazepine therapy was previously effective. Without obvious precipitating factors such as head trauma, CNS infection, and drug or alcohol abuse, SE, in a patient with a history of epilepsy, most commonly results from poor adherence with maintenance AED medication. Therefore, IV use of either phenytoin or fosphenytoin is a good choice for re-establishing effective AED therapy for V.S.

LOADING DOSE

Whether or not V.S. has a detectable serum concentration of carbamazepine, he should be given an IV loading dose of either phenytoin (20 mg/kg IV at 50 mg/minute) or fosphenytoin (20 mg/kg PE IV at 150 mg/minute). After administration of either of these loading doses, serum phenytoin concentrations should remain greater than 10 mcg/mL for approximately 24 hours; this will allow time for determination of V.S.'s serum carbamazepine concentration and estimation of an appropriate maintenance dose of oral carbamazepine once oral therapy can be restarted. In this setting, the use of IV phenytoin or fosphenytoin is a temporary measure. V.S.'s previous positive response to carbamazepine indicates that he should likely continue to receive this drug as his oral maintenance medication.

Intravenous phenytoin can be administered by direct injection into a running IV line. The rate of administration should be no faster than 50 mg/minute to minimize the risk of hypotension and acute cardiac arrhythmias. Cardiovascular status (blood pressure, electrocardiogram) should be monitored closely during administration. Hypotension or electrocardiographic abnormalities usually reverse if the administration of phenytoin is slowed or stopped temporarily. If fosphenytoin is administered, it can be given by either direct IV injection or, after dilution in any suitable IV solution, by infusion at up to 150 mg PE/minute.[120] Absence of propylene glycol as a diluent renders fosphenytoin potentially less likely than phenytoin to cause cardiovascular adverse effects. Nonetheless, adverse cardiac events have been associated with fosphenytoin administration.[255] Electrocardiographic and blood pressure monitoring is recommended when this drug is given IV. Pruritus and paresthesias, usually localized to the face and groin, are relatively common side effects during IV fosphenytoin administration. These sensations are not allergic reactions to the medication. Their occurrence is related to the administration rate, and they are reversible with temporary discontinuation or slowing of the injection.[120] These side effects are thought to be related to the phosphate component of fosphenytoin.

INTRAVENOUS INFUSION

CASE 58-15, QUESTION 5: V.S.'s physician is reluctant to administer this dose of either phenytoin or fosphenytoin by direct IV injection. What are the guidelines for administration of phenytoin and fosphenytoin by IV infusion?

Practical difficulties associated with administration of phenytoin by direct IV push undoubtedly have contributed to its low usage rate. In many hospitals or other facilities, direct IV injections must be administered by a physician, and many physicians would be unwilling to commit the 30 to 45 minutes necessary to administer V.S.'s loading dose at a safe rate. In addition, the rate of direct IV administration is difficult to control, and too-rapid administration resulting in cardiac toxicity is a risk. Although fosphenytoin can be given at a faster injection rate with a lower risk of complications, direct IV administration of this drug still presents practical difficulties.

The compatibility of phenytoin injection with IV solutions has been controversial. Phenytoin's chemical properties (weakly acidic with a pK_a of 8 and low water solubility) require that the commercial injectable dosage form of sodium phenytoin be dissolved in a mixture of 40% propylene glycol and 10% alcohol; the pH of the final product is adjusted to approximately 12 with sodium hydroxide. Addition of the preparation to IV fluids dilutes the drug's solvent system and reduces pH. A possible result would be precipitation of phenytoin. Several studies indicate, however, that phenytoin can be diluted, preferably in small total volumes, with saline solution.[256,257] Despite the formation of crystals in many solutions, measured phenytoin concentrations are essentially identical to those predicted. Thus, dilution of the required volume of phenytoin injection in approximately 100 to 500 mL of 0.45% or 0.9% saline should provide an appropriate solution for IV administration. An in-line filter of 0.45 to 0.22 micron pore size may be used to prevent the infusion of crystals. The administration rate should be no faster than 50 mg/minute. This method of administration is both safe and effective when the infusion rate is monitored carefully. Burning pain at the IV infusion site, hypotension, and cardiac arrhythmias can occur during the infusion and appear to be related to the infusion rate. Either slowing or temporarily stopping the infusion may relieve these side effects.[258,259] IV administration of phenytoin is also associated with phlebitis; extravasation has resulted in chemical cellulitis and tissue necrosis.[260]

Intravenous infusion of fosphenytoin is less troublesome. Fosphenytoin is compatible with virtually all IV fluids because of its high water solubility and the lower pH required to maintain the drug in solution. Hypotension can occur during fosphenytoin infusion, and cardiovascular status should still be monitored closely.[255] Fosphenytoin should not be infused at a rate greater than 150 mg PE/minute. Injection site complications and phlebitis are significantly less likely with administration of fosphenytoin.[119]

Maintenance Therapy

CASE 58-15, QUESTION 6: After administration of IV phenytoin, no further seizures occurred. The laboratory reported that serum chemistries were all normal. The carbamazepine serum concentration was less then 1.0 mcg/mL on admission. A serum phenytoin concentration determined 1 hour after administration of the IV loading dose was 24 mcg/mL. How should V.S.'s maintenance AED therapy be altered?

The undetectable serum carbamazepine concentration appears to confirm the role of nonadherence in this episode of SE. As V.S. was previously well controlled on 600 mg/day, this would be a reasonable target dose. As carbamazepine cannot be restarted at this dose, due to autoinduction (see earlier), gradually escalating up to this dose should be initiated as soon as V.S. can take oral medication. V.S. should be counseled regarding the importance of taking his medication according to directions.

Alternative Therapies for Refractory Status Epilepticus

CASE 58-15, QUESTION 7: What other medications are options for treatment of SE that does not respond to benzodiazepines or phenytoin?

Phenobarbital may be useful for treatment of SE if the patient cannot tolerate phenytoin or when seizures continue after administration of appropriate loading doses of phenytoin. Patients who receive phenobarbital after being treated with IV benzodiazepines should be monitored closely for respiratory depression because this effect may be additive. Equipment and personnel to provide ventilatory assistance should be available.[244] Administration of IV phenobarbital can cause hypotension, which may necessitate discontinuation of the drug or the use of pressor agents. An initial dose of 20 mg/kg given IV at a rate no faster than 100 mg/minute is recommended.[244] IM administration of phenobarbital results in slow absorption, and this route of administration is not recommended for treatment of SE.

Pentobarbital or other anesthetic barbiturates are administered for treatment of SE that has not responded to more conservative measures, including phenobarbital. Significant respiratory depression is expected with this therapy; patients require intubation and mechanical ventilation. In addition, vasopressors, such as dopamine or dobutamine, may be required to control hypotension. Constant EEG monitoring also is required to assess the effect of the drug.

Pentobarbital is given as a loading dose of 5 mg/kg IV and is followed by an IV infusion of 0.5 to 3 mg/kg/hour.[244] The dose and infusion rate are adjusted to produce either a flat or a burst-suppression EEG pattern.[261] Most protocols for pentobarbital coma recommend attempts at gradually reducing the dose of medication after 12 to 24 hours of treatment. If clinical or EEG seizure activity recurs, the dose is increased again to produce continued EEG suppression. Pentobarbital coma may need to be continued for several days in some patients.

Continuous intravenous infusions of propofol or midazolam are also useful for refractory SE. These therapies appear to be less likely than pentobarbital to cause severe hypotension that is refractory to vasopressors.[262–265] Because no direct comparative trials of pentobarbital, propofol, and midazolam have been performed, physician familiarity and preference often guides the choice between these agents for the treatment of refractory SE.

Several other drugs have been used for treatment of refractory SE, but experience with these agents is limited. Valproate has been used for treatment of refractory SE and as an alternative to phenytoin in early SE therapy.[266] Other drugs that have been used for refractory SE include IV levetiracetam, IV lacosamide, topiramate (via nasogastric tube), intravenous lidocaine, and general anesthetics (halothane or isoflurane).[240,246,247,267]

KEY REFERENCES AND WEBSITES

A full list of references for this chapter can be found at http://thepoint.lww.com/AT10e. Below are the key references and websites for this chapter, with the corresponding reference number in this chapter found in parentheses after the reference.

Key References

Asconapé JJ. The selection of antiepileptic drugs for the treatment of epilepsy in children and adults. *Neurol Clin.* 2010;28(4):843.

Berg AT et al. Revised terminology and concepts for organization of seizures and epilepsies: Report of the ILAE Commission on Classification and Terminology, 2005–2009. *Epilepsia.* 2010;51:676. (7)

Bialer M et al. Progress report on new antiepileptic drugs: a summary of the Tenth Eilat Conference (EILAT X). *Epilepsy Res.* 2010;92:89. (106)

Brodie MJ et al. Epilepsy in later life. *Lancet Neurol.* 2009; 8(11):1019.

French JA, Pedley TA. Clinical practice. Initial management of epilepsy. *N Engl J Med.* 2008;359:166. (3)

Glauser TA et al. Ethosuximide, valproic acid, and lamotrigine in childhood absence epilepsy. *N Engl J Med.* 2010;362:790. (146)

Harden CL et al. Management issues for women with epilepsy-Focus on pregnancy (an evidence-based review): I. Obstetrical complications and change in seizure frequency, II. Teratogenesis and perinatal outcomes, III. Vitamin K, folic acid, blood levels, and breast-feeding. Report of the Quality Standards Subcommittee and Therapeutics and Technology Subcommittee of the American Academy of Neurology and the American Epilepsy Society. *Epilepsia.* 2009;50:1229. (221–223)

Marson AG et al. The SANAD study of effectiveness of carbamazepine, gabapentin, lamotrigine, oxcarbazepine, or topiramate for treatment of partial epilepsy: an unblended randomised controlled trial. *Lancet.* 2007;369(9566):1000.

Marson AG et al. The SANAD study of effectiveness of valproate, lamotrigine, or topiramate for generalised and unclassifiable epilepsy: an unblinded randomised controlled trial. *Lancet.* 2007;369:1016. (147)

Meador KJ et al. Cognitive function at 3 years of age after fetal exposure to antiepileptic drugs. *N Engl J Med.* 2009;360:1597. (228)

Potschka H. Transporter hypothesis of drug-resistant epilepsy: challenges for pharmacogenetic approaches. *Pharmacogenomics.* 2010;11:1427. (108)

Shorvon S. The treatment of status epilepticus. *Curr Opin Neurol.* 2011;24:165. (245)

Key Websites

American Epilepsy Society. http://www.aesnet.org.

Epilepsy and Seizure Information for Patients and Health Professionals. http://www.epilepsy.com.

Epilepsy Foundation. http://www.epilepsyfoundation.org.

Cerebrovascular Disorders

59

Timothy E. Welty

CORE PRINCIPLES

		CHAPTER CASES
1	Cerebrovascular disease includes a broad range of disorders involving the vascular system of the brain. In the United States, approximately 85% of cerebrovascular events are ischemic in nature and 15% are hemorrhagic.	**Case 59-1 (Question 1)**
2	Important modifiable risk factors for ischemic stroke include cardiovascular disease, hypertension, smoking, diabetes, atrial fibrillation, dyslipidemia, obesity, and physical inactivity. Nonmodifiable risk factors include older age, family history of stroke, race, and sex.	**Case 59-1 (Question 1), Case 59-2 (Question 2)**
3	Ischemic and hemorrhagic stroke are medical emergencies, requiring prompt medical attention at the first sign of symptoms. Signs and symptoms of cerebrovascular disease usually occur acutely, and vary depending on the area of the brain involved. Ischemic and hemorrhagic events have similar symptoms and must be distinguished before initiating treatment.	**Case 59-3 (Questions 1, 2, 8)**
4	Primary prevention is vital to reducing the risk of a stroke. However, antiplatelet agents or other pharmacotherapies are recommended only for women older than 65 years with some exceptions (see Core Principle 5). Lifestyle modification is the mainstay of primary prevention.	**Case 59-1 (Question 2)**
5	Atrial fibrillation and patent foramen ovale are exceptions to the guidelines for primary prevention pharmacotherapy. Antiplatelet agents or anticoagulants should be used in patients with these conditions, with selection of an agent dependent on patient characteristics.	**Case 59-1 (Question 2)**
6	Secondary prevention of cerebral infarction involves the use of antiplatelet agents. Selection of an agent is dependent on patient characteristics.	**Case 59-2 (Questions 5, 7)**
7	Acute treatment of ischemic events includes the use of alteplase given intravenously. Alteplase should be started after confirming an event is ischemic and not hemorrhagic. The treatment window for use of alteplase is limited to 4.5 hours after the onset of neurologic symptoms. Strict criteria for administration of alteplase must be followed, and hemorrhagic complications should be carefully monitored.	**Case 59-3 (Question 6)**
8	Subarachnoid hemorrhage is the second most common type of cerebrovascular hemorrhagic event. Complications of subarachnoid hemorrhage include rebleeding, cerebral vasospasm, and hydrocephalus. Surgical clipping of the aneurysm is preferred to control the risk of rebleeding. Nimodipine is used to reduce the risk of cerebral vasospasm.	**Case 59-4 (Questions 1–4)**
9	Rehabilitation after a cerebrovascular event is essential to patient recovery. Common complications encountered in rehabilitation included spasticity, depression, and neurogenic bowel or bladder. Pharmacotherapy interventions should be directed at each of these complications with the goal of improving the patient's quality of life and ability to function independently.	**Case 59-3 (Questions 10, 11)**

TRANSIENT ISCHEMIC ATTACKS

Cerebrovascular disease is a broad term encompassing many disorders of the blood vessels of the central nervous system (CNS). These disorders result from either inadequate blood flow to the brain (i.e., cerebral ischemia) with subsequent infarction of the involved portion of the CNS or hemorrhages into the parenchyma or subarachnoid space of the CNS and subsequent neurologic dysfunction. This group of disorders is the third leading cause of deaths among adults in the United States.[1]

Definitions

TRANSIENT ISCHEMIC ATTACK

A transient ischemic attack (TIA) describes the clinical condition in which a patient experiences a temporary focal neurologic deficit such as slurred speech, aphasia, weakness or paralysis of a limb, or blindness. These symptoms appear rapidly and are temporary, lasting less than 24 hours (usually only 2–15 minutes). The clinical presentation depends on the portion of the cerebrovascular tree (e.g., carotid artery, vertebrobasilar artery, or both) affected by diminished or absent blood flow. TIAs frequently result from small clots breaking away from larger, distant blood clots. These emboli are then dissolved by the fibrinolytic system, allowing re-establishment of blood flow and return of neurologic function.

CEREBRAL INFARCTION

A cerebral infarction is a permanent neurologic disorder characterized by symptoms similar to a TIA. The patient with a cerebral infarction presents with neurological deficits caused by the death of neurons in a focal area of the brain. The two primary causes of infarction and persistent ischemia are atherosclerosis of cerebral blood vessels and an embolus to cerebral arteries from a distant clot. Cerebral infarctions can present in three forms: stable, improving, or progressing. A *stable infarction* describes the condition in which the neurologic deficit is permanent, will not improve, and will not deteriorate. An *improving infarction* is marked by return of previously lost neurologic function over the course of several days or weeks. A *progressing infarction* is one in which the patient's neurologic status continues to deteriorate after the initial onset of focal deficits.

CEREBRAL HEMORRHAGE

Cerebral hemorrhage involves escape of blood from blood vessels into the brain and its surrounding structures. The leakage of blood causes clinical symptoms similar to those associated with a TIA or cerebral infarction. The neurologic dysfunction that is associated with TIAs or cerebral infarction results from the lack of blood flow to a given portion of the brain. In a cerebral hemorrhage, the initial neurologic deficits are attributable to the direct irritant effects of blood that is in direct contact with brain tissue. Primary causes of a cerebral hemorrhage include cerebral artery aneurysm, arteriovenous malformation, hypertensive hemorrhage, and trauma.

The terms *apoplexy, stroke,* and *paralytic stroke* are commonly used by laypersons to describe a sudden neurologic affliction that usually is related to the cerebral blood supply. The term *stroke* is used to describe a cerebral vascular event when neurologic deficits persist for at least 24 hours.

Epidemiology

Annually, approximately 700,000 individuals in the United States experience a cerebral infarction, and approximately 160,000 will die as a result of the stroke.[2] Of the 700,000 strokes annually, 500,000 are first-ever strokes and 200,000 are recurrent events.[3] Cerebrovascular disease is the third most common cause of death in adults and is one of the more commonly encountered causes of neurologic dysfunction. Nevertheless, this represents a dramatic decrease in the mortality rate of ischemic stroke from 88.8 per 100,000 population in 1950 to 54.3 per 100,000 in 2003. There are important racial and ethnic differences in incidence and mortality rates for ischemic stroke as shown in Table 59-1. The precise reasons for these differences are unclear, but genetic, geographic, dietary, and cultural factors have been considered.[4] In addition, the incidence of risk factors for stroke such as hypertension, diabetes, and hypercholesterolemia differ among racial groups.[4]

In the United States, ischemic stroke is the most common type of infarction (Fig. 59-1). Atherothrombotic disease of the large

TABLE 59-1
Epidemiology of Stroke by Race or Ethnic Group[1–4]

Ethnic/Racial Group	First-Ever Age-Adjusted Stroke Incidence (per 100,000 people)	Death Rate (per 100,000 people)
Overall	208	54.3
Black men	323	78.8
Black women	260	69.1
White men	167	51.9
White women	138	50.5
Hispanic men		44.3
Hispanic women		38.6
Asian men		50.8
Asian women		45.4
Native American men		37.1
Native American women		38

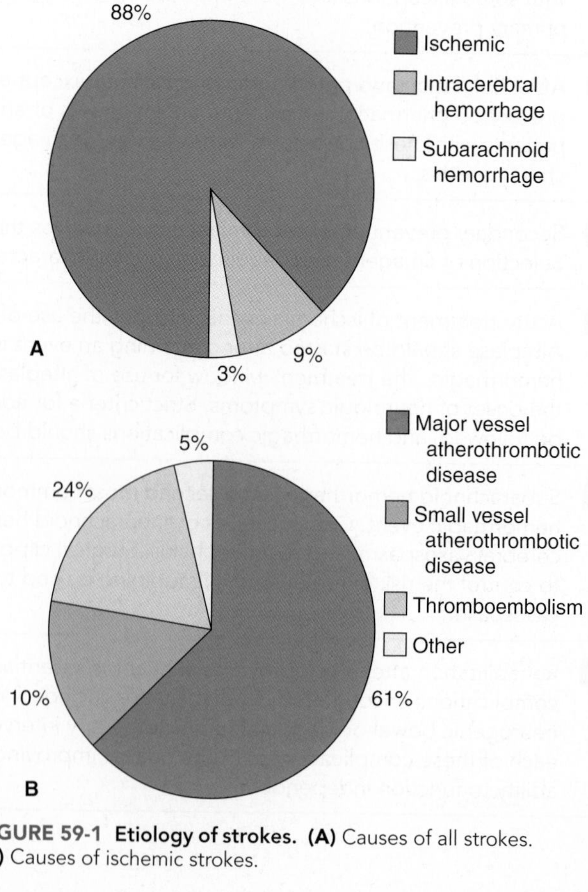

FIGURE 59-1 Etiology of strokes. (A) Causes of all strokes. **(B)** Causes of ischemic strokes.

TABLE 59-2
Risk Factors for Ischemic Stroke

Modifiable	Potentially Modifiable	Nonmodifiable
Cardiovascular disease (coronary heart disease, heart failure, peripheral arterial disease) Hypertension Cigarette smoking Diabetes Asymptomatic carotid stenosis Atrial fibrillation Sickle cell disease Dyslipidemia (high total cholesterol, low HDL) Dietary factors (sodium intake <2,300 mg/d; potassium intake <4,700 mg/d) Obesity Physical inactivity Postmenopausal hormone therapy (women 50–74 years old)	Metabolic syndrome Alcohol abuse (≥5 drinks daily) Hyperhomocysteinemia Drug abuse (e.g., cocaine, amphetamine, methamphetamine) Hypercoagulability (e.g., anticardiolipin, factor V Leiden, protein C deficiency, protein S deficiency, antithrombin III deficiency) Oral contraceptive use (women 25–44 years old) Inflammatory processes (e.g., periodontal disease, cytomegalovirus, *Helicobacter pylori* seropositive) Acute infection (e.g., respiratory infection, urinary tract infection) CD40 ligand >3.71 ng/mL in women free of cardiovascular disease IL-18 upper tertile hs-CRP >3 mg/L in women 45 years or older Migraine headaches High Lp(a) High Lp-PLA$_2$ Sleep-disordered breathing	Age (doubling each 10 years after age 55) Race (blacks > Hispanics > whites) Sex (men > women) Low birth weight (<2,500 g) Family history of stroke (paternal > maternal)

HDL, high-density lipoprotein; hs-CRP, high sensitivity C-reactive protein; IL, interleukin; Lp(a), lipoprotein(a); Lp-LPA$_2$, lipoprotein associated phospholipase A$_2$.
Source: Goldstein LB et al. Primary prevention of ischemic stroke: a guideline from the American Heart Association/American Stroke Council: cosponsored by the Atherosclerotic Peripheral Vascular Disease Interdisciplinary Working Group; Cardiovascular Nursing Council; Clinical Cardiology Council; Nutrition Physical Activity, and Metabolism Council; and the Quality of Care and Outcomes Research Interdisciplinary Working Group: The American Academy of Neurology affirms the value of this guideline [published correction appears in *Stroke.* 2007;38:207]. *Stroke.* 2006;37:1583.

cerebral blood vessels is responsible for the majority of cerebral ischemic events and infarctions. Disease of penetrating arteries that are responsible for oxygenation and nutrition of the CNS, thromboembolic causes (e.g., atrial fibrillation), and other causes such as infection or inflammation of arteries are also responsible for ischemic stroke.[1,2]

There is a strong relationship between the occurrence of TIA and an increased risk for subsequent cerebral infarction.[1] The risk of an ischemic stroke is highest in the first 30 days after a TIA, and the risk within 90 days of a TIA is 3% to 17.3%. Additionally, nearly 25% of patients who experience a TIA will die within a year.[1]

Risk factors for cerebral infarction are listed in Table 59-2. A key element in the prevention of stroke is the elimination or modification of risk factors.[5,6] The control of risk factors is of primary importance in managing a patient with a TIA or cerebral infarction.

Hemorrhage into the brain accounts for 12% of all strokes in North America. Hypertensive hemorrhage is the most common cause of intracerebral hemorrhages (ICHs), with 46% of ICHs resulting from hypertension.[7] Subarachnoid hemorrhage is the second most common cause of hemorrhagic stroke and has a mortality rate of approximately 50%. Patients with subarachnoid hemorrhage are usually 20 to 70 years old, and the majority of survivors have permanent neurologic deficits. A less common cause of ICH is an arteriovenous malformation (AVM), which is a clump of arteries and veins that are intertwined, resulting in weakened blood vessel walls. AVMs usually result from a congenital defect or trauma.

Pathophysiology

THROMBOTIC EVENTS

The neurologic sequelae of cerebral ischemia or infarction directly result from an embolic or thrombotic source. A clot may form in the heart, along the wall of a major blood vessel (e.g., aorta, carotid, or basilar artery), or in small arteries penetrating deep into the brain. If the clot is located near the infarction, it is considered to be a thrombus; however, when the clot has migrated to the brain from a distant source, it is considered an embolus. Either can diminish or block blood flow to the affected area of the brain.

Clots, both embolic and thrombotic, affecting the cerebral vasculature are typically arterial in origin and are formed primarily by fibrin. Tissue injury or turbulent blood flow causes the release of adenosine diphosphate (ADP), thrombin, epinephrine, and a variety of other substances to stimulate platelet migration. Exposure of collagen and other subendothelial surfaces of the blood vessel wall causes adhesion of platelets to the damaged vessel wall. As platelets adhere and aggregate, phospholipase is activated, leading to the splitting of arachidonic acid from platelet membrane phospholipids. This begins a cascade of events ultimately ending in the formation of thromboxane A$_2$ (TXA$_2$) and prostacyclin. Prostacyclin inhibits platelet aggregation and is a powerful vasodilator, whereas TXA$_2$ is a potent inducer of platelet release and aggregation. Prostacyclin is formed in and released from arterial and venous walls. TXA$_2$ is formed in and released from platelets. The delicate balance between the actions of these two compounds controls thrombogenesis. When a clot is formed, it can either embolize to the cerebral vasculature or occlude a cerebral artery.

Inflammatory mechanisms also contribute to the development of ischemia, especially thrombotic lesions. Substances like C-reactive protein, a mediator of inflammation, are elevated in patients with an acute stroke. Inflammation is thought to enhance the development of thrombotic lesions and result in sudden, intermittent occlusion of blood vessels.

Cerebral blood flow in the normal adult brain is 30 to 70 mL/100 g/minute. When a thrombotic or embolic clot partially occludes a cerebral artery, causing a reduction in blood flow

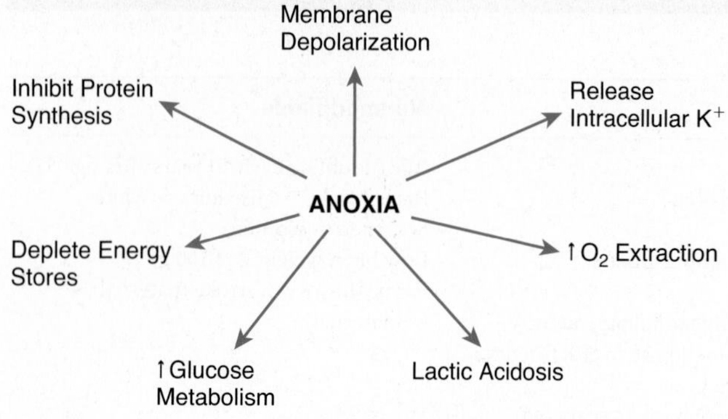

FIGURE 59-2 Physiologic effects of cerebral anoxia.

to less than 20 mL/100 g/minute, various compensatory mechanisms are activated. These include vasodilation and increased oxygen extraction. If the artery is further occluded and cerebral blood flow is reduced to less than 12 mL/100 g/minute, the affected neurons become sufficiently anoxic to die within minutes (Fig. 59-2).[8] Rapid re-establishment of blood flow to the ischemic area can delay, prevent, or limit the onset of infarction, improving the outcome of the acute stroke.

Ischemia in the brain usually involves a core or focal region of profound ischemia that results in neuronal death. The extent of this region is dependent on the amount of brain that is perfused directly by the blood vessel that becomes occluded. There is a surrounding area of brain that becomes marginally ischemic with normal function being disrupted. This region of marginal ischemia is frequently called the *ischemic penumbra.* If ischemia continues, neurons in this region will die. However, if normal blood flow is restored quickly, neurons in this area will survive.

When neurons become ischemic, excitatory neurotransmitters are released, causing neurons to rapidly and repeatedly discharge. Increased neuronal activity results in extreme metabolic demands, disrupts neuronal homeostasis, depletes stores of adenosine triphosphate (ATP), and synergistically increases the effects of hypoxia. Especially vulnerable to ischemic effects are neurons in the middle layers of the cerebral cortex; portions of the hippocampus (CA1 and subiculum regions), a structure running parallel to the parahippocampal gyrus; and Purkinje cells in the cerebellum.[9] There is also a rapid intracellular influx of calcium. Both voltage-dependent and chemical-dependent calcium channels are unable to act as a gate to prevent the movement of calcium, owing to depletion of cellular energy sources. Intracellular stores of calcium ions also are disrupted, causing release of calcium into the cytoplasm. Increased concentration of calcium ions enhances phospholipase and protease activity and increases reactive metabolites, such as superoxide and hydroxide ions, and nitric oxide (Fig. 59-3). This eventually causes neuronal death.[8,9] In addition, lipolysis of cell membranes occurs in the presence of an accumulation of neurotoxic free radicals.

Immediate therapeutic intervention is needed to limit and prevent permanent neurologic damage from these rapidly occurring events.

EMBOLIC EVENTS

The pathophysiology of infarction of brain tissue and neuronal death is similar for both embolic and thrombotic events. However, rather than forming locally in the vasculature of the brain, embolic events result from clots that are formed in distant parts of the body. Portions of these clots may break away and travel through the blood to the brain. When they become lodged in the cerebral vasculature, blood flow is partially or totally occluded. This occlusion initiates the cascade of ischemic events in the brain and neurons. Disorders like atrial fibrillation, mitral or aortic valve disease, patent foramen ovale, or coagulopathies are associated with formation of clots that may embolize to the brain.

INTRACEREBRAL HEMORRHAGE

Cerebral aneurysms, AVMs, hypertension, and adverse drug reactions are the primary causes of ICH. One type of ICH, subarachnoid hemorrhage, can result from weakened blood vessel walls (i.e., aneurysms) caused by congenital defects, trauma, infection, and hypertension. Blood slowly leaks from the involved vessel, or the aneurysm may rupture suddenly. In this type of hemorrhage, blood typically is released into the subarachnoid space and, depending on the severity of the hemorrhage, into the ventricles of the brain. Direct contact of blood with brain tissue irritates and damages brain cells. Rebleeding, hydrocephalus, and delayed cerebral ischemia frequently occur after the aneurysm ruptures, further worsening the patient's neurologic function.

AVMs attributable to congenital causes or traumatic injury, and uncontrolled hypertension also can cause devastating intracerebral bleeding. In these patients, blood is usually released directly into the brain parenchyma. In more severe cases, blood is released into the surrounding brain structures. ICHs can be the result of adverse reactions to drugs, such as anticoagulants, thrombolytics, and sympathomimetics.

General Treatment Principles

Rapid recognition of stroke symptoms and immediate initiation of treatment are essential to the management of ischemic or

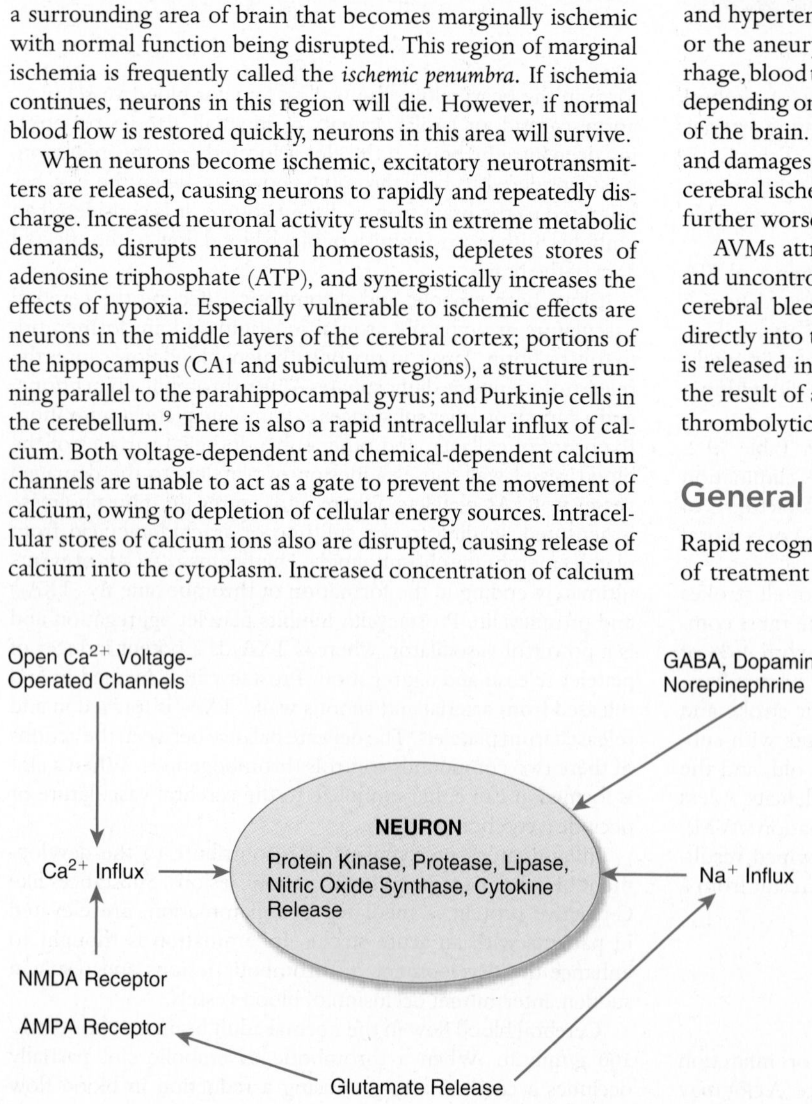

FIGURE 59-3 The effects of membrane depolarization. AMPA, α-amino-3-hydroxy-5-methyl-4-isoxazoleproprionate; GABA, γ-aminobutyric acid; NMDA, N-methyl-D-aspartate.

hemorrhagic stroke. Appropriate pharmacotherapy of cerebrovascular disease requires a precise diagnosis. It is vital to differentiate between an ischemic stroke and a hemorrhagic stroke, because an inaccurate diagnosis can lead to the use of drugs that may cause severe morbidity or mortality. Interventions to prevent and treat ischemic strokes are directed at reducing risk factors, eliminating or modifying the underlying pathologic process, reducing secondary brain damage, and rehabilitation.

Treatments for ischemic stroke and hemorrhagic stroke vary. In ischemic stroke, treatment involves acute management, chronic management of the effects of the stroke, and prevention of further events. In hemorrhagic stroke, the emphasis of treatment is on supportive therapy to maximize neurological function, prevention of further hemorrhagic events, and management of complications. This involves wise management of blood pressure, pulmonary function, fluid and electrolytes, and elimination of drugs that inhibit coagulation. There are no proven direct therapies for hemorrhagic events.

PRIMARY PREVENTION

Lifestyle Modification

CASE 59-1

QUESTION 1: R.B. is a 60-year-old, 5 feet 6 inches tall, 85-kg woman who is concerned about having a stroke. Her father died of a stroke, and her 85-year-old mother has had several episodes diagnosed as TIAs. R.B.'s blood pressure is 140 to 150/90 to 100 mm Hg, and she was recently diagnosed with diabetes mellitus. She does not have a history of TIA or stroke. Additionally, she smoked for 25 years, but has not used tobacco for the past 10 years. Her current medications include lisinopril, metformin, conjugated estrogen/medroxyprogesterone, and acetaminophen. She approaches her pharmacist because of concerns about having a stroke and being "like her parents." What can R.B. do to reduce her risk of stroke?

Any plan for *primary prevention* (i.e., prevention of a first event) of TIA or stroke must address the control or reduction of risk factors (Table 59-3).

For R.B., hypertension is a risk factor that requires immediate attention. Nearly 70% of strokes result from hypertension, and blood pressure control is vital for stroke prevention. Both systolic and diastolic hypertension increase the risk of stroke.[10,11] Adequate control of her blood pressure should reduce R.B.'s risk of stroke by 35% to 44%.[12] On the basis of the Seventh Report of the Joint National Committee on Prevention, Detection, Evaluation, and Treatment of High Blood Pressure (JNC-7) guidelines, R.B.'s blood pressure goal should be less than 130/80 mm Hg because of the additional risk factor of diabetes.[13] Because she is already receiving lisinopril and her blood pressure is poorly controlled, it is likely that combination therapy is needed. Addition of hydrochlorothiazide 25 mg/day is advisable.[5]

Diabetes is another important risk factor for stroke. In older women, diabetes is a more significant risk factor for stroke than it is for men.[14] There is controversy regarding the intensity of glucose control that optimally reduces stroke risk. Clearly, good control of diabetes results in better control of hypertension and other risk factors for stroke.[15] Additionally, use of oral hypoglycemics may reduce the risk of stroke through mechanisms other than glycemic control. However, strict control of blood glucose did not reduce the risk of stroke over the course of 9 years in one study.[15] There is evidence that angiotensin-converting enzyme inhibitors (ACEIs) and angiotensin receptor blockers (ARBs) reduce the risk of stroke in diabetics, with or without

TABLE 59-3
Primary Prevention of Ischemic Stroke

Factor	Goal	Recommendation
Hypertension	Blood pressure <140/90 mm Hg; with diabetes <130/80 mm Hg	Follow JNC-7 guidelines; after lifestyle modification thiazide-type diuretic, angiotensin-converting enzyme inhibitor, or angiotensin receptor blocker
Atrial fibrillation	When warfarin is used, INR 2–3	Aspirin 75–325 mg/day or warfarin as determined by the use of the $CHADS_2$ score
Dyslipidemia	National Cholesterol Education Program III goals	Lifestyle modification, HMG-CoA reductase inhibitor
Women (>65 years, history of hypertension, hyperlipidemia, diabetes, or 10-year cardiovascular risk ≥10%)	Reduce risk without bleeding complications	Aspirin 75–325 mg/d; use the lowest possible dose
Cigarette smoke	Elimination of cigarette smoke	Smoking cessation; avoidance of environmental tobacco smoke
Physical inactivity	≥30 minutes daily of moderate-intensity activity	Establish exercise program of aerobic activity
Excessive alcohol intake	Moderation	≤2 drinks/d for men or ≤1 drink/d for nonpregnant women
Diet and nutrition	≤2.3 g/d of sodium; ≥4.7 g/d of potassium	Institute a diet that is high in fruits and vegetables and low in saturated fats
Elevated lipoprotein(a)	Reduction of lipoprotein(a) by ≥25%	Niacin 2,000 mg/d as tolerated

HMG-CoA, β-hydroxy-β-methylglutaryl-CoA; INR, international normalized ratio; JNC-7, Seventh Report of the Joint National Committee on Prevention, Detection, Evaluation, and Treatment of High Blood Pressure.
Source: Goldstein LB et al. Primary prevention of ischemic stroke: a guideline from the American Heart Association/American Stroke Council: cosponsored by the Atherosclerotic Peripheral Vascular Disease Interdisciplinary Working Group; Cardiovascular Nursing Council; Clinical Cardiology Council; Nutrition Physical Activity, and Metabolism Council; and the Quality of Care and Outcomes Research Interdisciplinary Working Group: The American Academy of Neurology affirms the value of this guideline [published correction appears in *Stroke.* 2007;38:207]. *Stroke.* 2006;37:1583.

hypertension.[16,17] For diabetic patients with at least one additional risk factor for cardiovascular disease, taking a β-hydroxy-β-methylglutaryl-CoA (HMG-CoA) reductase inhibitor appears to reduce the risk of stroke by approximately 24% even in the absence of hypercholesterolemia.[18,19] For R.B., she should maintain tight control of her diabetes, continue her lisinopril, and start an HMG-CoA reductase inhibitor, such as simvastatin or atorvastatin.

The body mass index for R.B. is 30.2 kg/m^2, placing her in the obese category. Multiple large studies have demonstrated a direct relationship between increased body weight and an increased risk of stroke.[20,21] There are no data available to establish the precise effect of weight reduction on reducing the risk of stroke. Data are available to show that an average weight reduction of 5.1 kg results in a reduction in systolic blood pressure of 4.4 mm Hg and a reduction in diastolic pressure of 3.6 mm Hg.[22] In addition to weight loss, a proper diet and exercise are important for controlling risk factors. A diet high in sodium is associated with an increased risk in stroke, whereas a diet high in potassium appears to reduce the risk of stroke.[23,24] Current recommendations for diet are for sodium intake of 2.3 g/day or less and potassium intake of at least 4.7 g/day.[5] Several studies have shown an inverse relationship between physical activity and risk of stroke.[25,26] At least 30 minutes of moderate-intensity exercise daily is recommended.[5] On the basis of these data, R.B. should initiate a weight-reduction program that includes a low-sodium and high-potassium diet with an exercise program.

Cigarette smoking is an independent risk factor for stroke and potentiates other risk factors. In addition to active smoking, passive inhalation of cigarette smoke also appears to be a risk factor for stroke.[27] Smoking cessation does result in a rapid reduction in the risk of stroke, but the risk never returns to levels seen in individuals who have never smoked.[28] R.B. should be encouraged to avoid passive smoke and to continue avoiding the use of tobacco.

Three studies have specifically investigated the effect of hormone replacement on stroke risk. The Women's Estrogen for Stroke Trial (WEST) investigated the effect of hormonal therapy on the secondary prevention of stroke.[29] In the first 6 months of the study, those randomly assigned to receive estradiol had a significantly higher risk of recurrent stroke and were less likely to recover if they had a stroke. A second study, the Heart and Estrogen/Progesterone Replacement Study (HERS) evaluated the effect of hormone therapy on the secondary prevention of myocardial infarction in postmenopausal women.[30] In a post hoc analysis, hormone-replacement therapy had no effect on stroke risk.[31] The Women's Health Initiative (WHI) study specifically evaluated the effect of conjugated estrogens and medroxyprogesterone on primary prevention of cardiovascular events, including stroke, in women who were postmenopausal.[32] The study was terminated early because of a significant increase in stroke rates and other cardiovascular events in women receiving hormone-replacement therapy. Similar findings were seen in a parallel group of women who were surgically postmenopausal.[33] On the basis of results from these studies, R.B. should discontinue her conjugated estrogen/medroxyprogesterone product unless she is taking this medication for a specific reason other than control of menopausal symptoms or prevention of cardiovascular events.

Pharmacotherapy Primary Prevention

CASE 59-1, QUESTION 2: Are there specific pharmacotherapeutic treatments to reduce the risk of stroke for R.B.?

Aspirin has been carefully investigated for primary prophylaxis of stroke. Although aspirin is recommended in the primary prevention of coronary heart disease, it is not generally recommended for the primary prevention of stroke. In a study of 22,071 male physicians who took 325 mg of aspirin or placebo every other day for 5 years, there was not a reduced incidence of stroke.[34] This group of individuals who had no previous history of cerebrovascular disease experienced 217 strokes, 119 in the aspirin group and 98 in the placebo group. In addition, there was an increased risk of cerebrovascular events caused by hemorrhage in the aspirin group. Chen et al. reported a meta-analysis of 40,000 patients randomly assigned to aspirin and found a reduction from 47% to 45.8% in death and disability attributable to stroke.[35] Another study considered the role of aspirin for primary stroke prevention in women.[36] Women who took one to six aspirins per week had a slightly reduced risk of stroke and a lower risk of large-artery occlusive disease (relative risk, 59%; 95% confidence level, 0.29–0.85; $p = 0.01$). An increased risk of stroke was seen in women who took more than 7 aspirin weekly, and an excess risk of subarachnoid hemorrhage was seen in those taking more than 15 aspirin a week. The Women's Health Study also investigated the use of 100 mg/day in asymptomatic women and followed them for 10 years, monitoring for nonfatal cardiovascular events including stroke.[37] In this study there was a 17% reduction in the risk for all strokes and a 24% reduction in the risk for ischemic stroke, whereas there was a not significant increase in the risk for hemorrhage. Women 65 years of age and older at entry into the trial showed the most consistent risk reduction, but hemorrhagic strokes negated some of the benefit. Additionally, women with a history of hypertension, hyperlipidemia, or diabetes, or a 10-year cardiovascular risk of at least 10% had the most benefit. There are very limited data currently available regarding the use of other antiplatelet drugs for primary prevention of stroke. Aspirin should only be considered in women who are 65 years or older or have other important risk factors for stroke.

Although oral anticoagulants are not generally considered safe for primary prevention of stroke, a major exception is patients with atrial fibrillation. These individuals are at risk for an embolic event arising from clot formation in the atrium of the heart. Numerous studies have clearly shown that warfarin prevents embolic cerebrovascular events for patients with nonvalvular atrial fibrillation.[38–42] In these studies, the warfarin dose was adjusted to maintain an international normalized ratio (INR) of 1.5 to 4.5, with most recommendations to adjust the dose for an INR of 2 to 3. The Stroke Prevention in Atrial Fibrillation (SPAF) trial included aspirin combined with warfarin in one study arm and indicated that some benefit may be derived by combining antiplatelet agents with anticoagulants.[38] A follow-up study was performed and showed no difference between warfarin and aspirin in preventing stroke in atrial fibrillation.[42] Aspirin can be used as an alternative to warfarin in patients with atrial fibrillation, based on the $CHADS_2$ score (Table 59-4).[5,43,44] Additionally,

TABLE 59-4
$CHADS_2$ Score: Primary Stroke Prevention in Atrial Fibrillation

Add points for the following items. If score is <2, aspirin can be considered. If score is ≥2, then warfarin is recommended.
Congestive heart failure = 1 point
Hypertension = 1 point
Age >75 years = 1 point
Diabetes mellitus = 1 point
Prior stroke or TIA = 2 points

TIA, transient ischemic attack.
Source: Gage BF et al. Validation of clinical classification schemes for predicting stroke: results from the National Registry of Atrial Fibrillation. *JAMA.* 2001;285:2864; Gage BF et al. Selecting patients with atrial fibrillation for anticoagulation: stroke risk stratification in patients taking aspirin. *Circulation.* 2004;110:2287.

warfarin may be used in primary prevention of embolic stroke due to a patent foramen ovale.

For R.B., primary prevention of stroke with aspirin 81 mg/day can be considered because of her history of hypertension and diabetes.

SECONDARY PREVENTION AND TRANSIENT ISCHEMIC ATTACKS

Clinical Presentation

CASE 59-2

QUESTION 1: J.S., a 55-year-old, 5 feet 11 inches tall, 120-kg man, experienced a rapidly progressive paralysis of his right arm and slurred speech yesterday. These symptoms lasted for 15 to 20 minutes and resolved rapidly. His neurologic examination is entirely normal, and he denies any feeling of weakness. He smokes two packs of cigarettes daily and drinks three to six cans of beer each evening. His physical examination is entirely normal except for a left carotid bruit, which was first noted 2 years ago. His blood pressure is 165/100 mm Hg, and he has a long history of hypertension. His hemoglobin is 16.5 g/dL (normal, 12–16 g/dL), his hematocrit is 51% (normal, 42%–52%), and his total serum cholesterol concentration is 275 mg/dL (normal, < 200 mg/dL). A Doppler examination of his carotid arteries shows a 90% stenosis on the left and a 40% stenosis on the right. What subjective and objective data in J.S.'s history are consistent with a TIA?

A TIA can present with any type of neurologic symptoms. The presentation is determined by the location of the involved arteries and the portion of the brain that they supply. For example, if the affected artery provides circulation to the motor area in the left hemisphere of the brain, the expected result would be impairment of muscle strength on the right side of the body. Symptoms of TIA may include paresis or paralysis of one or more limbs, paresthesia, slurred speech, blurred vision, blindness (amaurosis fugax), facial droop, dizziness, or difficulty in swallowing (Table 59-5). Patients rarely lose consciousness. Symptoms of TIA always resolve within 24 hours, and there is no residual clinical focal neurologic deficit. Most often, the neurologic deficits last for only 2 to 15 minutes, and neurologic function rapidly returns to normal.

J.S.'s rapid onset of right arm paralysis and slurred speech suggest involvement of the left cerebral cortex. The 15- to 20-minute duration of these symptoms and the entirely normal neurologic examination on the day after these symptoms also are compatible with a TIA. The left carotid bruit heard on physical examination suggests a left-sided process.

Right-sided neurologic deficits generally suggest left-sided cerebral dysfunction because motor and sensory neuronal tracts cross over in the midbrain. Thus, the left hemisphere of the cerebral cortex controls the right or contralateral side of the body. CNS lesions occurring below the midbrain will cause ipsilateral neurologic deficits. Therefore, J.S.'s right arm paralysis suggests a left-sided cerebral lesion above the midbrain.

TABLE 59-5
Symptoms Associated With Transient Ischemic Attacks

Symptom	Right Carotid	Left Carotid	Vertebrobasilar
Aphasia	Possible	Yes	No
Ataxia	No	No	Yes
Blindness	Right	Left	Right or left side
Clumsiness	Yes	Yes	Yes
Diplopia	No	No	Yes
Dysarthria	Yes	Yes	No
Paralysis	Left side	Right side	Any limb
Paresthesia	Left side	Right side	Any limb
Vertigo	No	No	Yes

Risk Factors

CASE 59-2, QUESTION 2: How can another TIA be prevented in J.S.?

As with primary prevention, the initial interventions for secondary prevention of stroke are reduction of the risk factors. J.S. has several risk factors for TIA and ischemic stroke (Table 59-2): a smoking history, excessive alcohol consumption, obesity, older age, male sex, hypercholesterolemia, and hypertension. He should be instructed and counseled to change his lifestyle by discontinuing his smoking, limiting his alcohol consumption, reducing his weight, and increasing his physical exercise. Hypoxia and hypercarbia induced by cigarette smoking may have caused his increased hematocrit, and his high serum cholesterol and obesity suggest the need for dietary changes. The goal of a weight control program should be for his body mass index to be 18.5 to 24.9 kg/m^2, and a waist circumference of less than 40 inches.[6] A smoking cessation program, substance abuse program, and consultation with a dietitian should be useful in reducing his risk factors. Additionally, steps should be taken to ensure at least 30 minutes of moderate-intensity physical activity for 5 to 7 days of the week.[6]

The goals of antihypertensive therapy should be individualized. A mean blood pressure reduction of approximately 10/5 mm Hg has been associated with risk reduction for stroke.[6] Further reductions may be useful, but in managing his blood pressure all reductions should be gradual. A sudden or dramatic decrease in blood pressure could compromise cerebral perfusion and result in a decreased level of consciousness or cerebral infarction. The degree of his carotid artery stenosis will contribute to the problem of decreased perfusion if the blood pressure is decreased rapidly. A mild degree of hypertension may be temporarily acceptable because of the extent of carotid stenosis. Data are lacking to indicate an optimal treatment regimen, and pharmacotherapy plans should be individualized to the patient. The use of a diuretic or a diuretic combined with an ACEI is supported by available literature.[6] Initiation of hydrochlorothiazide at a dosage of 12.5 mg/day or a combination of hydrochlorothiazide with an ACEI should be considered.

Reduction of serum cholesterol is important for J.S. The first step in managing his cholesterol is to institute lifestyle and dietary modifications. In addition, HMG-CoA reductase inhibitors significantly reduce the risk of stroke and TIA.[45–49] For example, individuals with coronary disease who received pravastatin had a 20% to 40% reduction in the risk of stroke. A study of atorvastatin showed similar risk reductions.[50] These findings are reinforced by two meta-analyses that reported a 25% to 32% reduction in the risk of stroke.[51,52] It is known that HMG-CoA reductase inhibitors have anti-inflammatory activity that may influence the development of atherosclerotic plaques and cerebral ischemic processes.[53–55] Because of these effects of HMG-CoA reductase inhibitors, these drugs should be started after a TIA or stroke even in patients who do not have dyslipidemia.[56] Targets for managing cholesterol in patients with atherosclerotic disease are a low-density lipoprotein cholesterol of less than

100 mg/dL or, in extremely high-risk patients, a low-density lipoprotein cholesterol of less than 70 mg/dL.[6] Niacin or gemfibrozil can be considered for patients who do not tolerate HMG-CoA reductase inhibitors or have low high-density lipoprotein cholesterol concentrations. On the basis of these data, J.S. should receive an HMG-CoA reductase inhibitor. The benefits of HMG-CoA reductase inhibitors appear to be a class effect, so selection of a specific agent should be based on the individual characteristics of the patient.

Treatment

GOALS OF THERAPY

CASE 59-2, QUESTION 3: What are the initial and long-term goals in treating J.S.?

The immediate goal is to re-establish adequate blood flow in his diseased cerebral vessels. Longer-range objectives are to prevent reocclusion, decrease the risk of future symptomatic TIAs, and ultimately, prevent a cerebral infarction.[57]

SURGICAL INTERVENTIONS

CASE 59-2, QUESTION 4: What nonpharmacologic interventions might be available to prevent another TIA? What would be the best choice for J.S.?

Various surgical interventions are available to prevent TIA or infarction. These are designed to either remove the source for an embolism or improve circulation to ischemic areas of the brain.

CAROTID ENDARTERECTOMY

Carotid endarterectomy (CEA) is a common surgical procedure for correcting atheromatous lesions responsible for causing a TIA. In this procedure, the carotid artery is surgically exposed, and the atheromatous plaque is excised.

To see a visual of the surgical removal of plaque from the carotid artery, go to http://thepoint.lww.com/AT10e.

Balloon angioplasty and placement of stents also can improve blood flow through a stenosed artery. During this procedure, a catheter with a small, deflated balloon is placed in the stenosed artery and the atherosclerotic lesion is pressed into the arterial wall when the balloon is inflated. A small, plastic tube stent is placed in the artery to prevent the vessel from collapsing at the site of the lesion.

CEA is most effective for patients with an ulcerated lesion or stenotic clot that occludes greater than 70% of blood flow in the ipsilateral carotid artery and who experience symptoms of a TIA or stroke. Use of CEA in these patients may result in a 60% reduction in stroke risk during the subsequent 2 years.[58] Of six to eight patients treated with CEA, one stroke will be prevented within 2 years.[59] The use of CEA in other patient groups must be balanced with the risk of the procedure and life expectancy.[60] CEA is beneficial in patients with 50% to 69% stenosis of the carotid artery.[6] Surgery should be done within 2 weeks of a TIA or stroke. Generally, CEA is not indicated in patients who have permanent neurologic deficits or total occlusion of the carotid artery.[58] CEA should be done by a surgeon with less than 6% morbidity and mortality rates.[6]

Carotid artery angioplasty and stenting (CAS) is another alternative. The initial study of this procedure was halted because of poor outcomes.[61] Subsequently, two studies have shown that CAS is not inferior to CEA, but further study is underway to determine whether CAS is more beneficial than CEA.[62,63] CAS can be used in patients who are not candidates for CEA.

J.S. should undergo CEA for his left carotid lesion as soon as possible. The lesion on the right should be monitored closely for continued progression. If further TIAs occur or the right carotid stenosis is greater than 60%, he should have a CEA performed on the right carotid artery.

DRUG THERAPY

CASE 59-2, QUESTION 5: Which antiplatelet agents should be considered for J.S., and which one is best to prevent stroke?

Because platelets play a key role in the formation of atheromatous clots (Fig. 59-4), various antiplatelet drugs, such as aspirin, sulfinpyrazone, dipyridamole, ticlopidine, and clopidogrel, have been tried to prevent ischemic strokes. These agents generally work by either preventing the formation of TXA_2 or increasing the concentration of prostacyclin. These actions seek to re-establish the proper balance between these two substances, thus preventing the adhesion and aggregation of platelets (Table 59-6).

ASPIRIN

Aspirin acts primarily by irreversibly inactivating platelet cyclo-oxygenase.[64] Inactivation of cyclo-oxygenase decreases platelet aggregation, prevents release of vasoactive substances, and prolongs the bleeding time. Because binding of cyclo-oxygenase by the acetyl component of acetylsalicylic acid (aspirin) is irreversible and the platelet cannot synthesize new protein, platelet function is altered for the duration of the platelet's life, usually 5 to 7 days. Aspirin's ability to prevent clot formation and subsequent embolic or thrombotic events also can be attributed to an inhibition of TXA_2-mediated vasoconstriction, activation of fibrinolysis, inhibition of synthesis of vitamin K–dependent clotting factors, and inhibition of lipoxygenase pathways.

TABLE 59-6
Drugs for Preventing Transient Ischemic Attacks and Ischemic Stroke

Drug	Action	Dose	Adverse Effects
Aspirin	Antiplatelet	50–1,300 mg/d	Diarrhea, gastric ulcer, GI upset
Dipyridamole	Antiplatelet (use in combination with aspirin)	200 mg sustained-release twice daily	GI upset
Ticlopidine	Antiplatelet	500 mg/d	Diarrhea, neutropenia, rash
Clopidogrel	Antiplatelet	75 mg/d	Thrombocytopenia, neutropenia
Warfarin	Anticoagulant	Titrate to INR 2–3	Bleeding, bruising, petechiae

GI, gastrointestinal; INR, international normalized ratio.

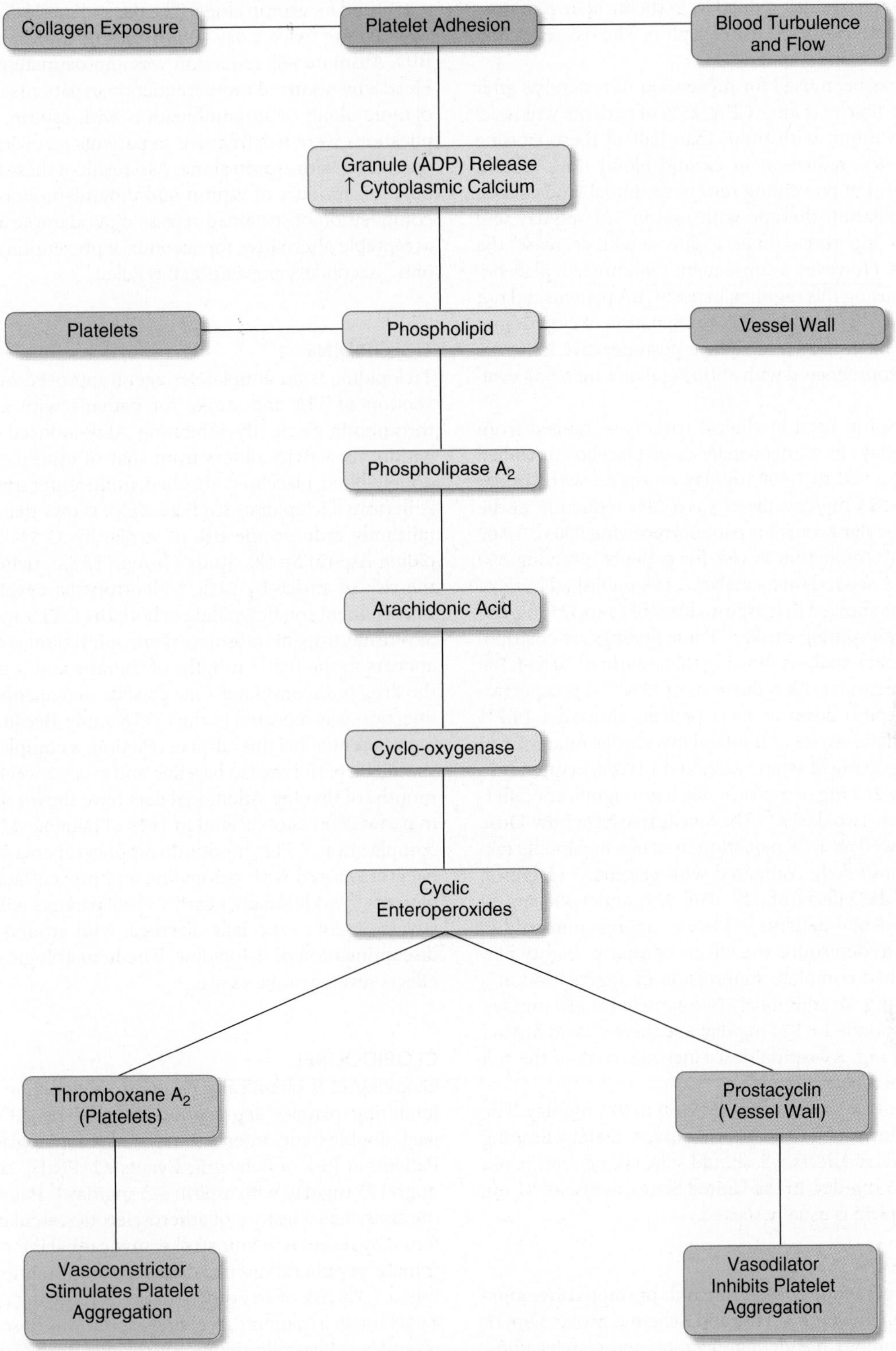

FIGURE 59-4 Arachidonic acid cascade and platelet plug formation. ADP, adenosine diphosphate.

In addition to its action on platelet cyclo-oxygenase, high concentrations of aspirin also inhibit prostacyclin synthesis in the walls of blood vessels. Because prostacyclin inhibits platelet aggregation, depletion of prostacyclin could result in an undesirable increase in aggregation of platelets. However, depletion of prostacyclin is not prolonged because the vascular endothelium is able to synthesize new enzymes. Higher dosages of aspirin (1.3 g/day) also may decrease vascular plasminogen activator, thereby enhancing thrombus formation.[65] Therefore, aspirin should be dosed carefully.

At least 15 randomized trials, with 7 being placebo-controlled, have studied aspirin alone or in combination with other antiplatelet drugs in the prevention of vascular events.[36,66–70] Patients were enrolled in these studies for as long as 5 years after experiencing a vascular event (i.e., TIA, stroke, unstable angina, or myocardial infarction). Follow-up periods lasted from 1 to 6 years. The incidence of ischemic stroke or TIA ranged from 7% to 23%: the aspirin-treated patients experienced an average 22% decrease in relative risk of a stroke compared with those receiving placebo. In 10 trials that considered only TIA or stroke patients, there was a 24% relative risk reduction in the incidence of nonfatal stroke associated with the use of aspirin. The risk reduction rate is equal for men and women.[66,71]

Aspirin also has been used for prevention of restenosis after CEA. During the first year after CEA, 25% of patients will redevelop a stenotic lesion, with more than half of these causing a greater than 50% reduction in carotid blood flow.[72] Stent placement is useful in preventing restenosis. Initial studies indicated that combination therapy with aspirin 325 mg/day and dipyridamole 75 mg three times a day would decrease the rate of restenosis. However, a subsequent randomized, placebo-controlled study using this regimen in post-CEA patients did not substantiate the earlier findings.[73] A combination of clopidogrel with aspirin has been shown to reduce postoperative ischemic events.[74] Stents impregnated with anticoagulants are being evaluated.

Dosages of aspirin used in clinical trials have ranged from 30 to 1,500 mg/day. In a meta-analysis of placebo-controlled studies comparing 900 to 1,500 mg/day of aspirin with similar studies of 300 to 325 mg/day, there was a 23% reduction in the risk of cerebrovascular events for patients receiving 900 to 1,500 mg/day and a 24% reduction in risk for patients receiving 300 to 325 mg/day.[68] A second meta-analysis of all published trials of antiplatelet agents showed that aspirin doses of 75 to 325 mg/day were effective in preventing stroke.[75] These findings are corroborated by a third meta-analysis showing that aspirin of 50 to 1,500 mg/day produced similar risk reductions of 15%.[76] A prospective comparison of aspirin doses in 3,131 patients showed a 14.7% frequency of nonfatal stroke or nonfatal myocardial infarction in patients receiving 30 mg of aspirin a day and a 15.2% frequency in patients receiving 283 mg of aspirin a day, a not significant difference between these two doses.[77] The Swedish Aspirin Low-Dose Trial (SALT) showed an 18% reduction in stroke in patients taking 75 mg of aspirin daily compared with placebo.[78] Helgason et al. compared the effects of 325, 650, 975, and 1,300 mg of aspirin a day in stroke patients.[79] Platelet aggregation studies were performed to determine the effects of aspirin. Eighty percent of patients had complete suppression of aggregation at a daily dose of 325 mg, an additional 5% responded at 650 mg/day, only 1% more responded at 975 mg/day, and there was no further response at 1,300 mg. As aspirin doses increase, so does the risk of gastrointestinal (GI) bleeding.[80]

The recommended dose for aspirin is 50 to 975 mg/day. The goal is to use the lowest effective aspirin dosage, thereby limiting the risk of GI adverse effects. J.S. should start taking aspirin at a dosage of 50 to 75 mg/day. In the United States, a dose of 81 mg enteric-coated aspirin is usually started.

DIPYRIDAMOLE

Two pharmacologic actions of dipyridamole prompted investigations into its use in preventing TIAs and ischemic stroke. Dipyridamole weakly inhibits platelet aggregation and platelet phosphodiesterase and has potential vasodilating properties through its inhibition of adenosine uptake in vascular smooth muscle.[64]

Two European studies have shown benefit with a combination of aspirin and dipyridamole. In the first study, a combination of aspirin 975 mg/day and dipyridamole 225 mg/day was compared with placebo.[81] Results from this study showed that the combination reduced the combined risk of stroke and death by 33% and the risk of stroke by 38%. The Second European Stroke Prevention Study enrolled patients who had experienced a previous stroke or TIA and found that aspirin combined with dipyridamole was more effective than placebo, dipyridamole alone, and aspirin alone.[82] A sustained-release formulation of dipyridamole was used for this study. A 37% relative risk reduction was found for the combination treatment, and a 23% relative risk reduction was found for aspirin alone. The dipyridamole dose for this study was 200 mg twice a day (BID), and the aspirin dose was 25 mg BID. Absolute risk reduction was approximately 1.5% annually. Headache occurred more frequently in patients receiving dipyridamole alone or in combination with aspirin. Bleeding complications were less frequent in patients receiving dipyridamole compared with aspirin alone. As a result of these findings, a combination product of aspirin and dipyridamole is available. The combination of sustained-release dipyridamole and aspirin is an acceptable alternative for secondary prevention of stroke when initial secondary prevention has failed.

TICLOPIDINE

Ticlopidine is an antiplatelet agent approved only for the prevention of TIA and stroke for patients with a prior cerebral thrombotic event. By inhibiting ADP-induced platelet aggregation, its activity differs from that of aspirin. A randomized, double-blind, placebo-controlled, multicenter trial, the Canadian American Ticlopidine Study (CATS), shows that ticlopidine significantly reduced the risk of stroke by 33.5%.[83] In the Ticlopidine Aspirin Stroke Study Group (TASS), ticlopidine reduced the risk of stroke by 21%.[84] Neutropenia developed in 1% to 2% of patients on ticlopidine in both the CATS and TASS studies. Severe neutropenia (absolute neutrophil count $<450/\mu L$) usually appears in the first 3 months of therapy and is reversible when the drug is discontinued. One episode of neutropenia-associated infection was reported in the CATS study. Because of the rather high potential for this adverse reaction, a complete blood count should be performed at baseline and every 2 weeks for the first 3 months of therapy. Additional data have shown that severe bone marrow depression is fatal in 16% of patients who develop this complication.[85] Thrombotic thrombocytopenia purpura has also been associated with ticlopidine and proved fatal in 33% of 60 patients.[86] Additionally, nearly 25% of patients will experience GI adverse events, especially diarrhea, with around 10% requiring discontinuation of ticlopidine. The hematologic and GI adverse effects severely limit its use.

CLOPIDOGREL

Clopidogrel is chemically related to ticlopidine and works by inhibiting platelet aggregation induced by ADP. A randomized, double-blind, international trial (Clopidogrel vs. Aspirin in Patients at Risk of Ischaemic Events [CAPRIE]) compared clopidogrel 75 mg/day with aspirin 325 mg/day.[87] Patients enrolled in the study had a history of atherosclerotic vascular disease manifested by recent ischemic stroke, myocardial infarction, or symptomatic peripheral vascular disease. Using intention-to-treat analysis, a 5.3% risk of an event in patients receiving clopidogrel and a 5.83% risk in patients receiving aspirin was observed. This represents a statistically significant relative risk reduction of 8.7%, favoring clopidogrel. On-treatment analysis showed a relative risk reduction of 9.4%, again in favor of clopidogrel. For patients whose primary condition for entry into CAPRIE was stroke, the relative risk reduction was 7.3%; however, this difference was not statistically significant. Patients receiving clopidogrel more frequently experienced rash and diarrhea compared with those receiving aspirin. Patients receiving aspirin were more frequently affected by upper GI distress, intracranial hemorrhage, and GI hemorrhage. Significant reductions in neutrophils occurred in 0.10% of patients on clopidogrel and in 0.17% of patients on aspirin. Some cases of thrombocytopenia purpura are reported in the literature.[88]

Clopidogrel is as effective and safe as aspirin. Clopidogrel is an alternative to aspirin in secondary prevention of stroke.

WARFARIN AND ANTICOAGULANTS

Large randomized trials have compared oral anticoagulants with aspirin in the secondary prevention of stroke and TIA. In one study, aspirin 30 mg/day was compared with oral anticoagulants in doses adjusted to maintain an INR between 3.0 and 4.5.[89] This study was terminated early when the mortality rate attributable to major bleeding events in the anticoagulant group was double the rate in the aspirin group. In this study, there was no difference between anticoagulants and aspirin in the frequency of stroke. A second study compared warfarin, dosed to maintain the INR between 1.4 and 2.8, and aspirin 325 mg/day.[90] Results from this study did not demonstrate a significant difference between aspirin and warfarin with regard to the prevention of stroke or major hemorrhagic events. However, minor hemorrhages were significantly more frequent among patients receiving warfarin. A third study was terminated early because of safety concerns in the warfarin arm of the study.[91] The target INR for this study was 2 to 3 in the warfarin arm compared with aspirin. The study was stopped owing to significantly higher rates of adverse events in individuals receiving warfarin and no difference in the risk of stroke. Events including major hemorrhage, myocardial infarction, or sudden death, and overall death were increased in those receiving warfarin. Warfarin is not generally recommended for secondary prevention of stroke.

J.S. is clearly at risk for additional TIAs or an ischemic stroke. Because J.S. has experienced a TIA, he also should be placed on an antiplatelet agent. Aspirin, dipyridamole combined with aspirin, or clopidogrel are acceptable alternatives for J.S. Warfarin is not an acceptable alternative in J.S. for initial, secondary prevention of TIA or stroke. Considering the overall costs of therapy and that he does not have any definite contraindications to aspirin, J.S. should be started on aspirin 81 mg/day. Clopidogrel or a combination of aspirin and dipyridamole can be used if J.S. is unable to tolerate aspirin or he experiences a recurrent TIA or a stroke while taking aspirin (Table 59-6).

Aspirin: Patient Education

CASE 59-2, QUESTION 6: The physician decides to begin J.S. on aspirin 81 mg/day. How should he be counseled on the use of aspirin? Should J.S. be advised to discontinue aspirin before surgical and dental procedures?

Even low dosages of aspirin may cause gastric erosions and gastric ulcers. J.S. should be instructed to take aspirin with the largest meal of the day, inform his physician of any epigastric pain, and seek medical attention at the first sign of any gastric bleeding (e.g., dark stools). Enteric-coated aspirin may cause less gastric upset than uncoated aspirin formulations.

J.S. should inform all of his health care providers, especially his physicians, pharmacist, and dentist, that he is taking aspirin daily. The decision to discontinue aspirin is at the discretion of his physician or dentist. This decision is based on the possibility of bleeding complications from the procedure and the risk of J.S. having a TIA while off aspirin. If aspirin is to be temporarily discontinued, it should be stopped at least 5 to 7 days before the procedure and restarted several days after the procedure.

Combination Antiplatelet Pharmacotherapy

CASE 59-2, QUESTION 7: Six months later, J.S. has another TIA, despite taking aspirin. What is an appropriate intervention to prevent further TIA or stroke?

Possible interventions at this point are to switch to a different antiplatelet therapeutic regimen, to add clopidogrel to aspirin, or to increase the aspirin dose. A major study has compared clopidogrel 75 mg/day with the combination of clopidogrel 75 mg/day and aspirin 75 mg/day.[92] There was no difference in the risk of recurrent stroke or other cardiovascular outcomes between the groups, but the combination therapy group had a significant increase in life-threatening bleeding. Some individuals may be resistant to aspirin's effects on platelets.[64] Although poorly understood and studied, aspirin resistance may be related to the presence of extraplatelet sources of TXA_2 and an interaction with over-the-counter nonsteroidal anti-inflammatory drugs or high levels of circulating 11-dehydro-thromboxane B_2.[93–95] There are no data to suggest that increasing the aspirin dose will overcome possible resistance to the antiplatelet effects of aspirin, but it is clear that an increased dose of aspirin increases his risk of major bleeding.

On the basis of the available data, the antiplatelet therapy for J.S. should be switched to clopidogrel monotherapy or the combination product of aspirin with dipyridamole.

CEREBRAL INFARCTION AND ISCHEMIC STROKE

Clinical Presentation and Diagnostic Tests

CASE 59-3

QUESTION 1: P.C., a 65-year-old man, is admitted through the emergency department (ED) after collapsing to the ground and experiencing a brief loss of consciousness. He regained consciousness by the time he arrived in the ED, one hour after the initial event. Both right extremities are flaccid. He is unable to speak but is capable of understanding instructions (i.e., expressive aphasia). Gross ophthalmologic examination indicates right-sided neglect (inability of his eyes to track to the right or acknowledge the right side of his body). His blood pressure is 175/105 mm Hg; other vital signs are normal. Laboratory studies are all within normal limits. By the next day, his neurologic status is unchanged, and he is diagnosed as having an ischemic stroke. What interventions should have been initiated before arrival in the ED?

Immediate recognition of, and response to, stroke symptoms are essential to an optimal outcome. As soon as stroke symptoms are recognized, the emergency medical system should be activated. Emergency medical personnel should be trained to gather important historical information, especially when the symptoms started. Use of a standardized evaluation tool like the Cincinnati Prehospital Stroke Scale or Los Angeles Prehospital Stroke Screen are useful in distinguishing stroke symptoms from other disorders like conversion disorder, hypertensive encephalopathy, hypoglycemia, complicated migraine, or seizures.[96] General supportive care for respiratory and cardiovascular function should be initiated before transporting the patient to the ED. An important key to effectively managing acute stroke patients is to have a well-designed evaluation and treatment algorithm that addresses assessment and care of the patient from initial onset of symptoms through rehabilitation (Fig. 59-5).[96]

CASE 59-3, QUESTION 2: What diagnostic tests and evaluations will be helpful in guiding P.C.'s therapy?

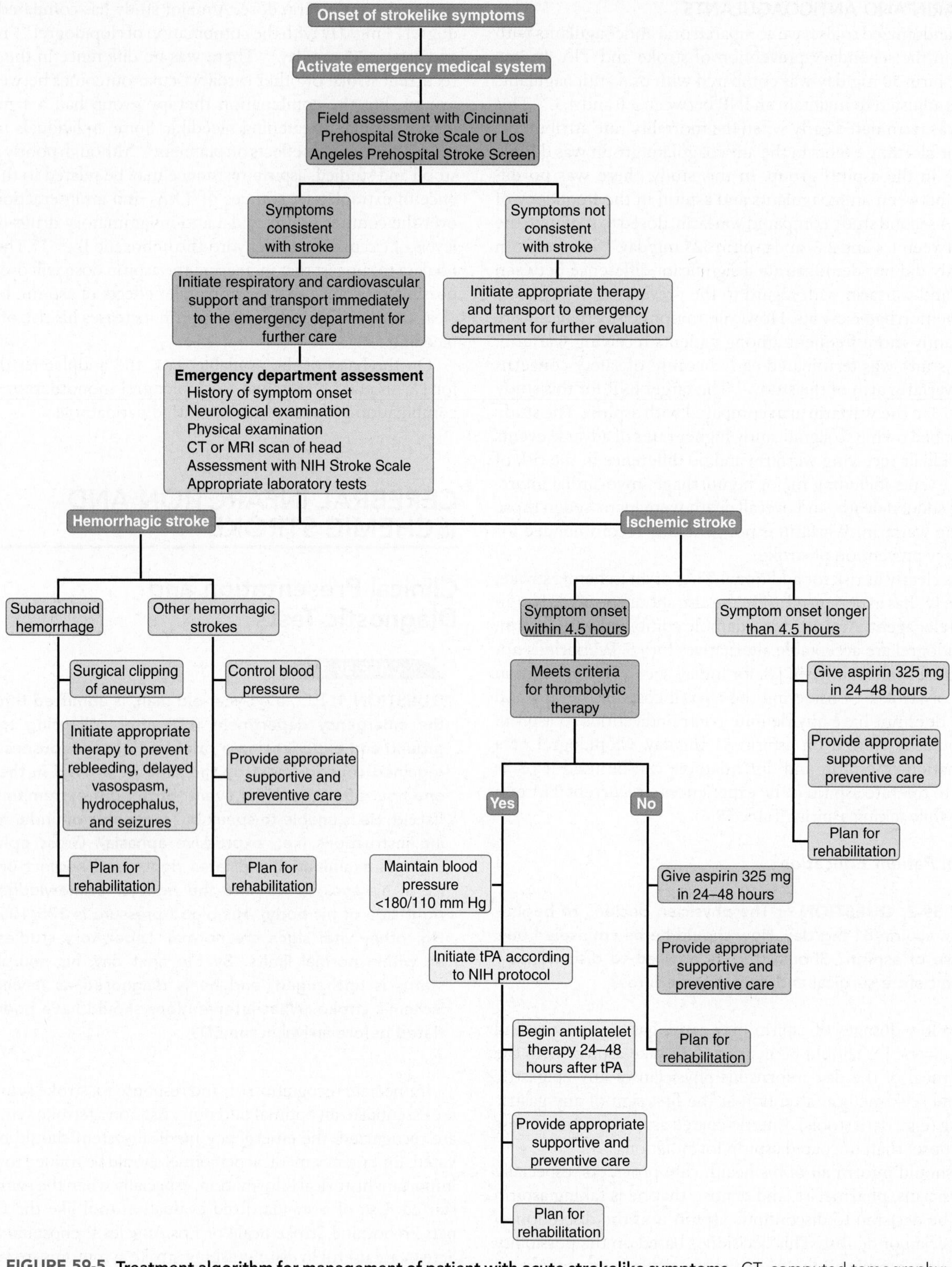

FIGURE 59-5 Treatment algorithm for management of patient with acute strokelike symptoms. CT, computed tomography; MRI, magnetic resonance imaging; NIH, National Institutes of Health; t-PA, alteplase. (Source: Adams HP et al. Antifibrinolytic therapy in patients with aneurysmal subarachnoid hemorrhage: a report of the cooperative aneurysmal study. *Arch Neurol.* 1981;38:25.)

Basic laboratory and diagnostic tests should be quickly performed to exclude noncerebrovascular causes of P.C.'s symptoms, such as metabolic or toxicologic derangement or infections. These tests include a routine serum chemistry profile (electrolytes, blood urea nitrogen, serum creatinine, hepatic enzymes, calcium, phosphorus, magnesium, albumin), complete blood count, and toxicology screen. Coagulation studies, including a prothrombin time with INR and partial thromboplastin time, should be performed to provide baseline values for potential anticoagulation or thrombolytic therapy. In addition, a thorough physical, neurologic, cardiovascular, and mental status examination should be performed. The neurologic examination will assist in localization of the lesion in the CNS. The physical examination should include use of the National Institutes of Health Stroke Scale.[97] In addition to providing important information for diagnosis of his neurologic compromise, these tests will provide baseline data for ongoing assessment of P.C.'s progress and recovery.

The etiology of a stroke is difficult to discern based solely on a physical and neurologic examination. As a result, computed tomography (CT) or magnetic resonance imaging (MRI) is valuable in the evaluation of these patients. An MRI is preferred to a CT because of its superior tissue contrast, ability to obtain images in multiple planes, absence of artifacts caused by bone, vascular imaging capabilities, absence of ionizing radiation, and safer contrast media. MRI also allows for a magnetic resonance angiogram to be performed, allowing visualization of the cerebrovasculature and possible identification of the precise location of the thrombus or embolus. Within the first 24 hours of an ischemic stroke, an MRI is clearly more sensitive than a CT. After 48 hours, the MRI and CT are equally effective in detecting ischemic infarcts. The primary disadvantages of the MRI are that it is more sensitive to artifacts, more difficult to perform in unstable patients, and not always available in smaller hospitals or communities.

ONLINE CONTENT

To see a CT scan of a person who has experienced an ischemic stroke, go to http://thepoint.lww.com/AT10e.

P.C. must have either a CT or an MRI before initiation of anticoagulation, thrombolytic agents, or other therapies for stroke. A follow-up CT or MRI in 5 to 7 days is useful to determine the extent of neurologic damage resulting from the ischemic stroke.

Angiographic, Doppler, or sonographic examination of the cerebral vasculature may be helpful in identifying the location of the vascular lesion. These tests usually are performed after the patient has been stabilized, unless angioplasty with stents or use of intra-arterial fibrinolytics is anticipated. A lumbar puncture with collection of cerebrospinal fluid (CSF) for evaluation may be helpful in identifying the presence of blood in the CNS. In the presence of suspected increased intracranial pressure, a lumbar puncture must be avoided because of the potential for tentorial herniation. Tentorial herniation occurs when the ventral half of the midbrain (i.e., the cerebral peduncles) pass through the tentorial notch (i.e., a portion of the dura mater that provides support for the occipital lobe and covers the cerebellum). This causes pressure on blood vessels that supply the cerebral cortex, resulting in restricted blood flow.

Treatment

CASE 59-3, QUESTION 3: What general treatment interventions should be made for P.C.?

In addition to the general supportive therapy needed for a hospitalized patient, several issues are important to the proper management of a stroke patient. Careful attention should be given to fluid and electrolyte control. Excessive hydration or inadequate sodium supplementation may result in hyponatremia, thereby forcing fluid into neurons to further increase the damage from ischemia. In addition, hyponatremia can produce seizures, which increases the metabolic demand on compromised neurons. Thus, it is advisable to initiate fluid therapy with a solution containing at least 0.45% saline and preferably 0.9% saline.

Attention to body temperature needs to be given. Studies have shown that even small increases in temperature are associated with worse outcomes after acute stroke.[98,99] Hypothermia is neuroprotective, and a reduction in body temperature of 0.26°F can be beneficial in stroke patients.[96,100] Use of antipyretics, such as acetaminophen, are advised to maintain normal or slightly subnormal body temperatures.

Another metabolic parameter that must be followed carefully is the serum glucose concentration, because hyperglycemia may adversely affect ischemic infarction outcomes. A review of multiple studies on the effects of hyperglycemia in acute stroke concluded that hyperglycemia results in poor outcomes and increased mortality.[101] If hyperglycemia is detected, appropriate insulin therapy should be initiated to keep the serum glucose concentration less than 140 mg/dL without causing hypoglycemia.[96]

Caution should be exercised in the acute management of P.C.'s blood pressure. Decreasing the blood pressure too rapidly will compromise cerebral blood flow and expand the region of ischemia and infarction, whereas hypertension will place him at a greater risk for cerebral hemorrhage, especially if a thrombolytic agent is used. However, a study comparing treated and untreated patients who were hypertensive in association with an acute stroke failed to demonstrate any difference in outcomes between the groups.[102] For patients with a systolic blood pressure greater than 185 mm Hg or diastolic blood pressure greater than 110 mm Hg, who are otherwise candidates for intravenous fibrinolytic treatment, labetalol, nitroglycerin paste, or intravenous nicardipine should be used to reduce the blood pressure to these goals before starting alteplase.[96] After administration with alteplase, blood pressure should be kept less than 180/105 mm Hg. In other patients, the only consensus on blood pressure control is that treatment is required when pressures exceed 220/120 mm Hg.[96] If there is a clinical deterioration of neurologic function associated with the reduction of blood pressure, the infusion rate of the antihypertensive agent should be slowed or the drug discontinued. Maintenance antihypertensive therapy can then be initiated using an oral agent, such as a calcium-channel antagonist or ACEI.

The general daily needs of the patient should be assessed and provided on an as-needed basis. These include nutrition, urination, defecation, and prevention of decubitus ulcers. Neurologic deficits will compromise the ability of many patients to adequately meet these needs, increasing the necessity for medical assistance.

Two interventions that have been shown to improve outcomes of ischemic stroke are reducing the time to treatment of stroke and admitting patients to specialized stroke care units. Reduction of the time to treatment permits the use of interventions shown only to work within the first 2 hours of a stroke.[103] In addition, Indredavik et al. have shown that stroke care units significantly improve long-term survival and functionality of patients after a stroke.[104]

CASE 59-3, QUESTION 4: Should anticoagulation or antiplatelet agents be used acutely in P.C.?

Several studies have evaluated the use of anticoagulants and antiplatelet agents in the treatment of acute strokes. However, most of these studies are poorly designed or underpowered to determine the efficacy of these agents. Despite these problems with published studies, many physicians prefer to use anticoagulants or antiplatelet agents in the management of patients with acute stroke.

HEPARIN AND HEPARINOIDS

Three studies have evaluated the use of heparin in acute stroke.[105–107] In one double-blind study, heparin doses were adjusted to maintain the partial thromboplastin time at 1.5 to 2 times control and continued for 7 days.[105] There were no significant differences in death at 7 days, no differences in functional ability 1 year after the stroke, and a greater mortality rate at 1 year for heparin-treated patients. Another study compared aspirin, subcutaneous heparin (5,000 international units or 12,500 international units BID), both, and neither treatments for patients with acute ischemic stroke.[106] There was no reduction of mortality or morbidity for patients receiving either dose of heparin. Heparin use has also been studied in progressing stroke (stroke with evolving neurologic symptoms), and no benefit was demonstrated with its use.[107] No studies have demonstrated that heparin is useful in mitigating the neurological effects of a stroke.

Low-molecular-weight heparins and heparinoids have been evaluated in several studies for acute stroke. Two doses of nadroparin were compared with placebo in one randomized, double-blind, placebo-controlled trial.[108] There were no differences in death rates or functional ability at 3 months among the three treatment arms. However, at 6 months, patients receiving high-dose nadroparin (i.e., 4,100 anti-Xa international units BID) had improved function. A large randomized, placebo-controlled trial of dose-adjusted danaparoid, a low-molecular-weight heparinoid, did not demonstrate improvement in danaparoid-treated patients.[109] In addition, no improvements were observed in studies of dalteparin and certoparin.[110,111] Similar to heparin, low-molecular-weight heparins and heparinoids are not indicated in the acute treatment of stroke.

ASPIRIN

One study evaluated early administration of aspirin in acute stroke. The Chinese Acute Stroke Trial (CAST) compared 160 mg/day of aspirin administered within 48 hours of the onset of stroke symptoms with placebo.[112] Patients who received aspirin had reduced early mortality rates, but there was no difference in the primary end point of death or dependency at discharge from the hospital. Two other studies did not demonstrate benefit with aspirin.[106,113] When data from these studies are combined, a slight beneficial effect of aspirin is seen with regard to reducing the risk of early stroke recurrence. Current recommendations are for aspirin 325 mg to be administered within 24 to 48 hours of the onset of stroke symptoms, except when alteplase is administered.[96] If alteplase is used, aspirin should not be given until 24 to 48 hours after the alteplase infusion.

GLYCOPROTEIN IIB/IIIA INHIBITORS

Platelet glycoprotein IIb/IIIa inhibitors have also been studied in acute stroke. A placebo-controlled phase II trial of abciximab given within 24 hours of acute stroke showed a trend toward improved functionality in abciximab-treated patients, but the study was not powered to show significance for this outcome.[114] In another placebo-controlled, phase II study of patients with acute stroke, the direct thrombin inhibitor, argatroban, was associated with statistically significant improvements in neurologic symptoms and daily living activities.[115] The number of patients enrolled in this study was small, but the results show promise. Currently, the use of these agents is limited to clinical trials.

CASE 59-3, QUESTION 5: When might antiplatelet agents or anticoagulants be used in the treatment of acute stroke?

Deep vein thrombosis and pulmonary embolism are common complications in patients following a stroke. The incidences of deep vein thrombosis and pulmonary embolus were reduced in most studies in which patients received heparin, low-molecular-weight heparins, or heparinoids.[116]

Two systematic reviews of the literature in this area resulted in the following recommendations and guidelines[96,116]:

1. Aspirin 325 mg/day should be initiated within 48 hours of the onset of stroke symptoms, unless alteplase is used. If alteplase is used, aspirin should not be started until 24 to 48 hours after alteplase administration.
2. Heparin, low-molecular-weight heparins, and heparinoids may be considered for prevention of deep vein thrombosis and pulmonary embolus. Use of these agents must be weighed against the risk of hemorrhagic complications.
3. Fixed-dose heparin may have some early benefit in the treatment of acute stroke, but this benefit is negated by an increased risk of hemorrhage and is not recommended.
4. Dose-adjusted heparin is associated with increased bleeding complications and is not recommended.
5. Low-molecular-weight heparins and heparinoids at high doses are not recommended in patients with acute stroke.
6. Intravenous heparin, high-dose low-molecular-weight heparins, or heparinoids are not recommended for any subgroup or specific type of stroke.

On the basis of these recommendations, P.C. should receive 325 mg/day of aspirin to be started within 24 to 48 hours of onset of his stroke symptoms, unless alteplase is administered. If alteplase is used, then aspirin should be started 24 to 48 hours after the alteplase infusion. Use of other anticoagulants is not recommended.

THROMBOLYTICS

CASE 59-3, QUESTION 6: Would thrombolytic agents be useful to treat P.C.'s acute ischemic stroke?

The critical primary event in a thromboembolic stroke is the development of an acute thrombus. Prospective cerebral angiography has demonstrated an arterial occlusion corresponding to the area of acute neurologic deficit in greater than 90% of cases.[117] Occlusion of cerebral arteries does not cause complete ischemia because collateral circulation from other arterial sources provides unstable and incomplete circulation to the ischemic region of the brain.[118] When blood flow is sustained in the range of 10 to 18 mL/100 g/minute, irreversible cellular damage may occur. Blood flow must be restored quickly after the event. Experimental studies in dogs and cats have shown that when blood flow is restored within 2 to 3 hours, neurologic deficits are prevented.[119,120] Thrombolytic agents can re-establish blood flow to ischemic regions of the brain.

A total of five large, placebo-controlled trials using either alteplase or streptokinase for acute stroke have been published. In three studies, streptokinase was used as the thrombolytic, and all of these studies were terminated early owing to high rates of mortality and intracranial hemorrhage associated with streptokinase.[113,121,122] These trials clearly demonstrate that streptokinase is associated with increased mortality and disability. The rates of intracranial hemorrhage ranged from 6% to 17% for patients receiving streptokinase compared with 0.6% to 3% for patients receiving placebo. In all three trials the mortality rates were significantly greater for patients receiving streptokinase. Streptokinase should not be used for P.C.

Studies with alteplase demonstrate some benefit associated with its use.[123,124] The National Institute of Neurological Disorders and Stroke (NINDS) alteplase trial and the European Cooperative Acute Stroke Study (ECASS) used different doses, inclusion criteria, and treatment protocols. Both trials showed the benefit of alteplase in at least some outcome parameters. In the NINDS alteplase study, patients were enrolled within 3 hours of symptom onset using strict inclusion and exclusion criteria (Table 59-7). When enrolled, patients received either alteplase 0.9 mg/kg (maximal dose, 90 mg), with 10% of the dose given as a bolus for 1 minute and the remainder infused for 60 minutes,

TABLE 59-7
Criteria for Alteplase Use in Treatment of Acute Stroke

Inclusion Criteria	Exclusion Criteria
18 years of age or older	Minor or rapidly improving symptoms
Clinical diagnosis of stroke with clinically meaningful neurologic deficit	CT signs of intracranial hemorrhage
	History of intracranial hemorrhage
Clearly defined onset within 180 minutes before treatment	Seizure at onset of stroke
	Stroke or serious head injury within 3 months
Baseline CT with no evidence of intracranial hemorrhage	Major surgery or serious trauma within 2 weeks
	GI or urinary tract hemorrhage within 3 weeks
	Systolic BP >185 mm Hg, diastolic BP >110 mm Hg
	Aggressive treatment to lower BP
	Glucose 400 mg/dL
	Symptoms of subarachnoid hemorrhage
	Additional Exclusion Criteria for Alteplase Use 3–4.5 hours After Onset of Symptoms
	Age >80 years
	NIHSS score >22
	Major ischemic infarction with 30% of the middle cerebral artery involved

BP, blood pressure; CT, computed tomography; GI, gastrointestinal; NIHSS, National Institutes of Health Stroke Scale.

or placebo. In this study, there were no differences at 24 hours in responses between the placebo group and those who received alteplase. However, at 3 months, patients who received alteplase were 30% more likely to have minimal or no disability. There was an 11% to 13% absolute increase in the number of patients with excellent outcomes and a corresponding decrease in the number of patients with severe neurologic impairment or death at 3 months. Intracranial hemorrhage occurred more frequently among patients receiving alteplase (6.4%) than in patients receiving placebo (0.6%). Despite the increased incidence of intracranial hemorrhage, outcomes remained better for patients receiving alteplase.

Three ECASS studies have been completed. For the ECASS I trial, patients were enrolled within 6 hours of the onset of symptoms.[124] The treatment protocol consisted of intravenous alteplase 1.1 mg/kg (maximal, 100 mg) or placebo. There was no difference in the primary outcome measures of functionality at 3 months. However, with target population analysis, there was a significant difference favoring alteplase. Of alteplase-treated patients, 41% had minimal or no disability compared with 29% of placebo-treated patients. A variety of secondary outcome measures favored alteplase. There was no difference in 30-day mortality rates, but 19.8% of alteplase-treated patients had major parenchymal hemorrhages compared with 6.5% of placebo-treated patients. The ECASS II study used an alteplase dose of 0.9 mg/kg and replicated the NINDS trial.[125] However, patients were enrolled up to 6 hours after the onset of stroke symptoms. This study found no difference between alteplase and placebo. Too few patients were enrolled with stroke symptoms within 3 hours to reliably evaluate the influence of this variable on outcome. Finally, the ECASS III study used the NINDS alteplase dose, but focused on the efficacy and safety of alteplase administered 3 to 4.5 hours after the onset of symptoms.[126] There were differences in exclusion between the ECASS III study and the NINDS trial. A significantly greater number of patients receiving alteplase had favorable outcomes compared with placebo (odds ratio, 1.34; 95% confidence interval, 1.02–1.76). Although the rate of intracranial hemorrhage was greater with alteplase, mortality and reports of adverse events were similar between the two groups. When considering the use of alteplase in the 3- to 4.5-hour window, the ECASS III criteria should be followed (Table 59-7).

Several studies have reported the use of intra-arterial thrombolytic therapy, primarily with prourokinase.[127,128] Both studies of prourokinase found significantly improved outcomes with this treatment. Other investigators have attempted to combine intra-arterial thrombolytic therapy with systemic alteplase or with mechanical manipulation of the clot to increase penetration of the thrombolytic agent into the clot. Although useful in major medical centers, various approaches to the use of intra-arterial thrombolytics present technical obstacles that limit their use in small hospitals.

Because P.C. presented to the ED within 1 hour of the onset of his stroke symptoms, he is a candidate for alteplase therapy in accordance with the NINDS study protocol. A thorough history and CT scan must be performed before initiation of alteplase to ensure compliance with inclusion and exclusion criteria.

MECHANICAL THROMBECTOMY

CASE 59-3, QUESTION 7: What other interventions might be also considered for P.C.?

Response to alteplase is less likely with a large vessel (e.g., carotid artery, middle cerebral artery) stroke, as a result of the large size clots that occlude these arteries. Several devices for intra-arterial removal of a clot have been developed, but the Merci Retriever has been most studied. Mechanical removal of the clot has been done with and without alteplase. In one study, 68% of patients had successful recanalization with the Merci Retriever, and response rates were not different between patients who received concomitant thrombolytics and those who did not receive thrombolytics.[129] Use of this device is limited to major medical centers with an interventional radiologist skilled in its use.

Stroke Education

CASE 59-3, QUESTION 8: What information and instruction should be given to P.C. regarding future stroke symptoms?

Early treatment of acute stroke with available or investigational drugs appears to be the most important factor in determining optimal outcome. Nearly every clinical trial demonstrating some benefit of pharmacotherapy for acute stroke has shown the greatest effect for patients who are treated within a few hours of the onset of stroke symptoms. Immediate detection of stroke symptoms and initiation of treatment are imperative. The primary rate-limiting step in diagnosis and provision of medical care is recognition by the patient of stroke symptoms. Every patient who is at increased risk of stroke should be carefully instructed to seek emergent medical attention if they experience any weakness or paralysis, speech impairment, numbness, blurred vision or sudden loss of vision, or altered level of consciousness. These symptoms should be handled with the same urgency as the symptoms of a myocardial infarction. The pharmacist should ensure that P.C. and his caregivers know the symptoms of stroke and understand what to do if they occur.

Complications

CASE 59-3, QUESTION 9: What complications associated with stroke might P.C. experience?

Agitation, delirium, stupor, coma, cerebral edema, and increased intracranial pressure are other symptoms that can be associated with ischemic stroke. These symptoms correlate with the specific blood vessels that are affected, and the development of these complications in P.C. would depend on the progression of his stroke.

Seizures may occur in up to 20% of stroke patients. Pneumonia, pulmonary edema, cardiac arrest, deep vein thrombosis, and arrhythmias commonly are associated with ischemic stroke and should be managed as they occur. In P.C., these may occur soon after his stroke, or be related to a rapidly developing neurologic event such as further infarction, hemorrhage, or severe cerebral edema. Pneumonia or deep venous thromboses are related primarily to inactivity, and the risk of these events will increase the longer P.C. remains immobile.

Stroke patients frequently experience psychologic reactions. The most common psychiatric complication is depression, occurring in 30% to 50% of patients.[130] The severity of depression varies from mild to major depressive episodes. If the depression interferes with recovery and the rehabilitative process, it should be managed with the use of a selective serotonin reuptake inhibitor or other appropriate agent. Severe psychomotor depression may respond to CNS stimulants, such as methylphenidate or dextroamphetamine. Because of P.C.'s hypertension, stimulants should be used only with careful blood pressure monitoring.

Prognosis

CASE 59-3, QUESTION 10: After 4 days in the hospital, P.C.'s neurologic status is stabilized. Will further neurologic improvements be realized?

Neurologic deficits in stroke patients are not considered stable or fixed until at least 8 to 12 months have elapsed. During this time, neurologic function may return, but rarely to normal. The prognosis after ischemic stroke depends on a variety of factors including age, hypertension, coma, cardiopulmonary complications, hypoxia, and neurogenic hyperventilation. However, infarction of the middle cerebral artery is associated with a poor chance for recovery. Recently, physical and occupational therapy techniques involving restriction of activity in the unaffected limb or limbs has proven to be effective in patients regaining lost function. Therefore, it is possible that P.C. will experience further neurologic improvement.

Rehabilitation

CASE 59-3, QUESTION 11: As P.C. enters rehabilitation, what interventions will aid his recovery?

Rehabilitation for P.C. is directed at managing daily functions, enhancing existing neurologic function, and attempting to regain lost function. Considerations for daily functions include activities of daily living and bowel and bladder management through balanced pharmacologic interventions. Efforts should be made to allow P.C. to function independently with activities of daily living and manage the psychologic effects of stroke. Enhancement of current neurologic function and minimizing depression includes elimination of drugs that may compromise P.C.'s memory and mental function. These include benzodiazepines, major tranquilizers, and sedating antiepileptic drugs.

Spasticity of the affected limb may present a problem for P.C. Because spasticity often is localized to a single limb after ischemic stroke, it frequently responds to regional motor nerve blocks with botulinum toxin. Aggressive physical therapy also is essential to the management of spasticity. Systemic antispasticity agents such as diazepam, baclofen, or dantrolene sodium are not used routinely because of the risk for toxicity. They are used only when spasticity involves multiple parts of the body or is unresponsive to other therapies.

Other less common impediments to P.C.'s recovery include decubitus ulcers, hypercalcemia, and heterotopic ossification (e.g., the laying down and calcification of a bone matrix in muscle surrounding major joints). Prevention through meticulous skin care is the key to the management of pressure ulcers. Mobilizing P.C. as soon as possible after the stroke can prevent hypercalcemia and heterotopic ossification. If necessary, these complications may be treated with etidronate.

SUBARACHNOID HEMORRHAGE

Clinical Presentation and Treatment

CASE 59-4

QUESTION 1: R.A., a 65-year-old woman, suddenly collapsed in the bathroom of her home. An ambulance was immediately called, and on arrival at the ED she had regained consciousness. She complained of a severe headache and kept dropping off to sleep during the examination. Nuchal rigidity (i.e., a stiff and painful neck when flexed) and mild mental confusion with regard to place also were observed. A CT scan demonstrated blood in the subarachnoid space and in her ventricles. A cerebral angiogram demonstrated a posterior communicating artery aneurysm. Electrolytes, coagulation studies, and blood counts were within normal limits. What pharmacotherapy is used for subarachnoid hemorrhage?

R.A.'s neurologic symptoms and the appearance of blood on her CT scan are consistent with a diagnosis of subarachnoid hemorrhage.

ONLINE CONTENT

To see an illustration of a subarachnoid hemorrhage and a cranial computed tomographic scan showing diffuse subarachnoid hemorrhage, go to http://thepoint.lww.com/AT10e.

Unfortunately, there are no direct pharmacotherapeutic interventions that are effective for subarachnoid hemorrhage. Surgical repair and clipping of the aneurysm is the definitive intervention. Pharmacotherapy is directed at preventing or managing complications of subarachnoid hemorrhage (Fig. 59-5).

Complications

CASE 59-4, QUESTION 2: R.A.'s neurologic status deteriorated approximately 3 days after admission. What complications may be responsible for these changes?

After the initial hemorrhagic event, there are three major complications that usually are responsible for neurologic changes

TABLE 59-8
Therapy for Subarachnoid Hemorrhage Complications

Rebleeding	Hydrocephalus	Delayed Ischemia
Surgical clip	Ventricular drain	Nimodipine 60 mg every 4 hours for 21 days
Aminocaproic acid 5 g loading dose and 1–2 g/h	Ventricular-peritoneal shunt	Hypervolemia PCWP 12–15 mm Hg Hypertension Systolic BP 170–220 mm Hg

BP, blood pressure; PCWP, pulmonary capillary wedge pressure.

(Table 59-8). *Rebleeding* from an aneurysm occurs in 20% of patients, usually within the first 48 hours after the initial event. In some cases, rebleeding can happen as long as 14 days later. From 24 hours to weeks after the hemorrhage, *hydrocephalus* (i.e., accumulation of excessive CSF within the ventricular system of the brain) may be caused by blood interrupting CSF flow through the ventricles and reabsorption of CSF through the arachnoid villa. Another 20% to 40% of patients will experience *delayed cerebral ischemia,* usually within 5 to 12 days after the initial hemorrhage. Delayed ischemia caused by vasospasm of the cerebral vessels is evidenced by development of new neurologic deficits and confirmed by a cerebral angiogram. At least half of these individuals will die or experience permanent neurologic damage. Approximately 5% to 15% of patients have seizures.

CASE 59-4, QUESTION 3: How should each of these complications (rebleeding, hydrocephalus, vasospasm, seizures) be managed in R.A.?

REBLEEDING

Surgical clipping of the aneurysm is the best method to prevent rebleeding. If early surgery is contraindicated or unavailable, antifibrinolytic therapy with epsilon aminocaproic acid (EACA) may be instituted. EACA blocks the activation of plasminogen and inhibits the action of plasmin on the fibrin clot. EACA enhances hemostasis when fibrinolysis contributes to bleeding and stabilizes the clot that has formed around the ruptured aneurysm. The incidence of rebleeding is decreased from 20% to 30% to 10% to 15% by EACA.[131,132] However, delayed cerebral ischemia occurs more frequently in patients receiving EACA.[131] It is unclear whether this is a direct effect of EACA or whether more individuals survive to experience delayed cerebral ischemia. EACA usually is given as a 5-g intravenous bolus followed by a continuous infusion of 1 to 2 g/hour. Dosages can be adjusted to maintain serum concentrations of 200 to 400 mg/mL. R.A. may benefit from receiving EACA as soon as a subarachnoid hemorrhage is diagnosed, and it should be continued until surgical clipping can be performed or for at least 2 weeks after the initial hemorrhage. It is preferable to surgically repair the aneurysm as soon as possible after R.A. is admitted to the hospital.

HYDROCEPHALUS

The only effective treatment for hydrocephalus is surgical intervention. If a CT scan demonstrates hydrocephalus, a ventricular drain should be surgically placed after the aneurysm has been clipped. When hydrocephalus becomes a chronic problem, the drain can be replaced with a permanent ventriculoperitoneal shunt.

Ventriculitis is a common complication of a ventricular drain and is most likely caused by staphylococci or Gram-negative bacteria. Antibiotic therapy for this complication should consist of an intravenous agent (e.g., chloramphenicol, ceftriaxone, ampicillin, penicillin, vancomycin, ceftazidime, cefuroxime, nafcillin, rifampin) that readily crosses the blood–brain barrier with inflamed meninges. Alternatively, gentamicin and vancomycin can be instilled through the ventricular drains directly to the site of infection. The antibiotic solution is prepared using a preservativefree sterile powder for injection. Gentamicin 4 to 8 mg or vancomycin 5 to 20 mg is instilled once a day. Systemic and intraventricular antibiotics should be continued until three consecutive CSF cultures are free of bacterial growth.

DELAYED CEREBRAL ISCHEMIA (VASOSPASM)

The occurrence of delayed cerebral ischemia probably is attributable to vasospasm of the cerebral blood vessels. Current therapy for delayed ischemia is not optimal and is rather confusing. Volume expansion with normal saline or plasma protein fraction usually is initiated when focal neurologic changes develop, with the goal of maintaining a pulmonary capillary wedge pressure of 15 to 20 mm Hg.[133–135] Some clinicians may institute hypervolemia therapy in anticipation of delayed cerebral ischemia. If the neurologic deficits are not reversed with hypervolemia, systolic blood pressure can be increased to as high as 200 to 220 mm Hg using dopamine or norepinephrine. A high systolic pressure allows the brain to redirect flow to ischemic areas, and such therapy is often continued for 7 to 14 days.

Nimodipine also is indicated for the prevention of delayed cerebral ischemia for patients with a subarachnoid hemorrhage. Its mechanisms of action may include preventing cerebral vasospasm that is responsible for delayed ischemia, inhibiting calcium influx into ischemic neurons, or re-establishing cerebrovascular autoregulation (i.e., the ability of the brain to control blood flow in accordance with metabolic needs). Nimodipine has been administered in clinical studies intravenously, orally, or topically (i.e., direct application to the brain's surface and the cerebral vasculature during surgery). Several studies of nimodipine in subarachnoid hemorrhage have used oral formulations.[134–139] In these studies, angiographic improvement was not significantly different in patients treated with nimodipine or placebo, but neurologic outcomes improved significantly in nimodipine-treated patients who presented with a mild to moderately severe subarachnoid hemorrhage. Nimodipine 60 to 90 mg every 4 hours for 21 days was initiated within the first 96 hours after the original subarachnoid hemorrhage in these studies. The recommended dose of nimodipine is 60 mg orally every 6 hours.

Recently, the use of magnesium infusions to prevent vasospasm has been incorporated into many treatment regimens. However, one study failed to demonstrate a relationship between magnesium serum concentrations and reduced cerebral vasospasm.[140] Another study failed to show any benefit with the use of a magnesium sulfate infusion titrated to maintain serum magnesium concentrations twice the baseline concentration.[141]

R.A. should receive nimodipine 60 mg orally every 4 hours for 21 days because she was diagnosed within several hours of her subarachnoid hemorrhage.

CASE 59-4, QUESTION 4: Should seizure prophylaxis be initiated for R.A.?

Seizures occur in approximately 9% of patients experiencing a subarachnoid hemorrhage. Only two factors associated with subarachnoid hemorrhage have been identified as predictive of seizures: rebleeding or large amounts of cisternal blood on CT scan.

Phenytoin often is used for seizure prophylaxis. However, no trials have investigated the efficacy of phenytoin in preventing seizure in patients with subarachnoid hemorrhage. The usual dose of phenytoin is 15 to 20 mg/kg administered as an intravenous bolus at a rate less than 50 mg/minute. A maintenance dose of 5 to 7 mg/kg/day either orally or intravenously is titrated to maintain steady-state serum concentrations of 10 to 20 mcg/mL. Alternatively, fosphenytoin, a phenytoin prodrug, can be administered intravenously or intramuscularly at a loading dose of 15 to 20 mg phenytoin equivalents/kg and a maintenance dose of 5 to 7 mg phenytoin equivalents/kg/day. Infusion rates of fosphenytoin should be less than 150 mg phenytoin equivalents/minute. Maintenance phenytoin usually is continued for 1 to 2 years or longer if the patient experiences seizures. Valproic acid and levetiracetam are available in intravenous formulations. However, there is little experience with the use of these agents for seizures in the setting of subarachnoid hemorrhage. Because there is a 5% to 20% risk of seizures for R.A., she should receive an antiepileptic drug such as phenytoin to prevent seizures.

KEY REFERENCES AND WEBSITES

A full list of references for this chapter can be found at http://thepoint.lww.com/AT10e. Below are the key references and websites for this chapter, with the corresponding reference number in this chapter found in parentheses after the reference.

Key References

Adams HP Jr et al. Guidelines for the early management of adults with ischemic stroke: a guideline from the American Heart Association/American Stroke Association Stroke Council, Clinical Cardiology Council, Cardiovascular Radiology and Intervention Council, and the Atherosclerotic Peripheral Vascular Disease and Quality of Care Outcomes in Research Interdisciplinary Working Groups: the American Academy of Neurology affirms the value of this guideline as an educational tool for neurologists [published corrections appear in *Stroke.* 2007;38:e38; *Stroke.* 2007;38:e96]. *Stroke.* 2007;38:1655 (96).

Coull BM et al. Anticoagulants and antiplatelet agents in acute ischemic stroke report of the Joint Stroke Guideline Development Committee of the American Academy of Neurology and the American Stroke Association (a division of the American Heart Association). *Neurology.* 2002;59:13. (116)

Goldstein LB et al. Primary prevention of ischemic stroke: a guideline from the American Heart Association/American Stroke Council: cosponsored by the Atherosclerotic Peripheral Vascular Disease Interdisciplinary Working Group; Cardiovascular Nursing Council; Clinical Cardiology Council; Nutrition Physical Activity, and Metabolism Council; and the Quality of Care and Outcomes Research Interdisciplinary Working Group: The American Academy of Neurology affirms the value of this guideline [published correction appears in *Stroke.* 2007;38:207]. *Stroke.* 2006;37:1583. (5)

Hacke W et al. Thrombolysis with alteplase 3 to 4.5 hours after acute ischemic stroke. *N Engl J Med.* 2008;359:1317. (126)

Rosamond W et al. Heart disease and stroke statistics—2007 update: a report from the American Heart Association Statistics Committee and Stroke Statistics Subcommittee [published correction appears in *Circulation.* 2007;115:e172]. *Circulation.* 2007;115:e69. (1)

Sacco RL et al. Guidelines for the prevention of stroke in patients with ischemic stroke or transient ischemic attack: a statement for healthcare professionals from the American Heart Association/American Stroke Association Council on Stroke: cosponsored by the Council on Cardiovascular Radiology and Intervention: The American Academy of Neurology affirms the value of this guideline. *Stroke.* 2006;37:577. (6)

Key Websites

American Heart Association. http://www.americanheart.org/presenter.jhtml?identifier=4755.

American Stroke Association. http://www.strokeassociation.org/STROKEORG/.

Center for Disease Control and Prevention. http://www.cdc.gov/stroke/.

National Institute of Neurological Disorders and Stroke. http://www.ninds.nih.gov/disorders/stroke/stroke.htm.

Principles of Infectious Diseases

60

B. Joseph Guglielmo

CORE PRINCIPLES

		CHAPTER CASES
1	Although acute infection generally is associated with an increased white blood cell count, fever, and localizing signs, these symptoms may be absent in less severe disease. More severe infection, including sepsis, may be associated with hypotension, disseminated intravascular coagulation, and end-organ dysfunction.	**Case 60-1 (Questions 1, 2)**
2	Other disease states, particularly autoimmune disease and malignancy, may mimic infectious diseases. Although it should be considered a diagnosis of exclusion, drug-induced fever should be ruled out, particularly in patients without other classic signs and symptoms of infection.	**Case 60-1 (Question 3)**
3	Site-specific signs and symptoms and host factors generally predict the most likely pathogens, and empirical antimicrobial therapy should be directed against these organisms.	**Case 60-1 (Questions 4, 5, Tables 60-1, 60-2)**
4	Isolation of an organism may reflect infection; however, colonization and contamination must be ruled out to avoid unnecessary antimicrobial exposure. Once a pathogen is identified, susceptibility tests, particularly disk diffusion or broth dilution, can demonstrate the most active antimicrobial agents.	**Case 60-1 (Questions 6, 7, Tables 60-3 through 60-7)**
5	Once the site of infection is confirmed and the likely pathogens are identified, antimicrobial toxicity and side effects, costs, site of infection, drug distribution, and route of admistration must be considered before selection of therapy.	**Case 60-1 (Questions 8–10, Table 60-8)**
6	Antimicrobial dosing should reflect site of infection, route of elimination, and pharmacokinetics and pharmacodynamics.	**Case 60-1 (Questions 11–13, Table 60-9)**
7	Antimicrobial failure may be related to pharmacologic factors (inadeqate dosing, insufficient penetration to the site of infection, and inadequate duration) and host factors (presence of prosthetic material, undrained focus of infection, and immune status).	**Case 60-1 (Questions 14–16)**

APPROACHING THE PROBLEM

The proper choice, dose, and duration of antimicrobial therapy are based on several factors. Before initiating therapy, it is important first to confirm an infectious versus noninfectious process. Once infection has been documented, the most likely site must be identified, and signs and symptoms (e.g., erythema associated with cellulitis) generally direct the clinician to the likely source. Because certain pathogens are known to be associated with a specific site of infection, empirical therapy often can be directed against these organisms. Additional laboratory tests, including the Gram stain, serologic analysis, and antimicrobial susceptibility testing, generally identify the primary pathogen and active agents. Spectrum of activity, established clinical efficacy, adverse effect profile, pharmacokinetic disposition, and cost considerations ultimately guide the choice of therapy. Once an agent has been selected, the dosage and duration should be based on the size of the patient, site of infection, route of elimination, and other factors.

ESTABLISHING THE PRESENCE OF AN INFECTION

CASE 60-1

QUESTION 1: R.G., a 63-year-old, 70-kg man in the intensive care unit, underwent emergency resection of his large bowel. He has been mechanically ventilated throughout his postoperative course. On day 20 of his hospital stay, R.G. suddenly becomes confused; his blood pressure (BP) drops to 70/30 mm Hg, with a heart rate of 130 beats/minute. His extremities are cold to the touch, and he presents with circumoral pallor. His temperature increases to 40°C (axillary), and his respiratory rate is 24 breaths/minute. Copious amounts of yellow-green secretions are suctioned from his endotracheal tube.

Physical examination reveals sinus tachycardia with no rubs or murmurs. Rhonchi with decreased breath sounds are observed on auscultation. The abdomen is distended, and R.G. complains of new abdominal pain. No bowel sounds can be heard, and the stool is guaiac positive. Urine output from the Foley catheter has been 10 mL/hour for the past 2 hours. Erythema is noted around the central venous catheter.

A chest radiograph demonstrates bilateral lower lobe infiltrates, and urinalysis reveals >50 white blood cells/high-power field (WBC/HPF), few casts, and a specific gravity of 1.015. Blood, endotracheal aspirate, and urine cultures are pending. Other laboratory values include the following:

Sodium (Na), 131 mEq/L (normal, 135 to 147)
Potassium (K), 4.1 mEq/L (normal, 3.5 to 5)
Chloride (Cl), 110 mEq/L (normal, 95–105)
CO_2, 16 mEq/L (normal, 20–29 mEq/L)
Blood urea nitrogen (BUN), 58 mg/dL (normal, 8–18)
Serum creatinine (SCr), 3.8 mg/dL (increased from 0.9 mg/dL at admission; normal, 0.6–1.2)
Glucose, 320 mg/dL (normal, 70–110)
Serum albumin, 2.1 g/dL (normal, 4–6)
Hemoglobin (Hgb), 10.3 g/dL
Hematocrit (Hct), 33% (normal, 39%–49% [male patients])
WBC count, 15,600/μL with bands present (normal, 4,500–10,000 μL)
Platelets, 40,000/μL (normal, 130,000–400,000)
Prothrombin time (PT), 18 seconds (normal, 10–12)
Erythrocyte sedimentation rate (ESR), 65 mm/hour (normal, 0–20)
Procalcitonin, 1 mcg/L (normal <0.25mcg/L)

Which of R.G.'s signs and symptoms are consistent with infection?

R.G. has numerous signs and symptoms consistent with an infectious process. His WBC count (15,600/μL) is increased, and a "shift to the left" (bands, i.e., premature neutrophils) is observed on the differential. An increased WBC count commonly is observed with infection, particularly with bacterial pathogens. The WBC differential in patients with a bacterial infection often demonstrates a shift to the left (i.e., presence of immature neutrophils) owing to the bone marrow response to infection. Although infection is usually associated with an increased WBC, overwhelming sepsis can also be associated with a markedly decreased WBC count. In less acute infection (e.g., uncomplicated urinary tract infection, abscess), the WBC count may remain within the normal range. In the case of a localized abscess, less of a bone marrow response would be anticipated; thus, the WBC count may or may not be increased.

R.G.'s temperature is 40°C by axillary measurement. Fever is a common manifestation of infection, with oral temperatures generally greater than 38°C. Oral and axillary temperatures tend to be approximately 0.4°C lower compared with rectal measurement. As a result, R.G.'s temperature would be expected to be 40.4°C if his temperature had been taken rectally. In general, rectal measurement of temperature is a more reliable determination of fever. Some patients with overwhelming infection, however, may present with hypothermia with temperatures less than 36°C. Furthermore, patients with localized infections (e.g., uncomplicated urinary tract infection, chronic abscesses) may be afebrile.

The bilateral lower lobe infiltrates on R.G.'s chest radiograph, the presence of copious amounts of yellow-green secretions from his endotracheal tube, and the erythema surrounding his central venous catheter also are compatible with one or more infectious processes. Furthermore, R.G. has signs and symptoms consistent with sepsis, which are discussed next.

ESTABLISHING THE SEVERITY OF AN INFECTION

CASE 60-1, QUESTION 2: What signs and symptoms manifested by R.G. are consistent with a serious systemic infection?

The term *sepsis* is used to describe a poorly defined syndrome; however, sepsis generally suggests a more systemic infection with the presence of pathogenic microorganisms or their toxins in the blood. A uniform system for defining the spectrum of disorders associated with sepsis has been established, but it remains difficult to precisely define.[1]

The pathogenesis of sepsis is complex (Fig. 60-1) and only partially understood.[2,3] Gram-negative aerobes produce endotoxin that results in a cascade of endogenous mediator release, including tumor necrosis factor (TNF), interleukin 1 (IL-1) and interleukin 6 (IL-6), platelet-activating factor (PAF), and various other substances from mononuclear phagocytes and other cells. Although this initial stimulus commonly is associated with gram-negative endotoxin, other substances, including gram-positive exotoxin and fungal cell wall constituents, also may be associated with cytokine release. After release of TNF, IL-1, and PAF, arachidonic acid is metabolized to form leukotrienes, thromboxane A_2, and prostaglandins, particularly prostaglandin E_2 and prostaglandin I_2. IL-1 and IL-6 activate the T cells to produce interferon, IL-2, IL-4, and granulocyte-macrophage colony-stimulating factor (GM-CSF). Increased endothelial permeability ensues. Subsequently, the endothelium releases two hemodynamically active substances: endothelium-derived relaxing factor (EDRF) and endothelin-l. Activation of the complement cascade (fragments C3a and C5a) follows, with additional vascular abnormalities and neutrophil activation. Other potentially important agents in this cascade include adhesion molecules, kinins, thrombin, myocardial depressant substance, endorphins, and heat shock protein. The net result of this cascade involves several hemodynamic, renal, acid-base, and other disorders. Uncontrolled inflammation and coagulation have a particularly important role in this sepsis cascade.[3]

Hemodynamic Changes

Critically ill patients often have central intravenous (IV) lines in place for measuring cardiac output and systemic vascular resistance (SVR). In other words, these lines are placed in the pulmonary artery and allow for more precise measurement

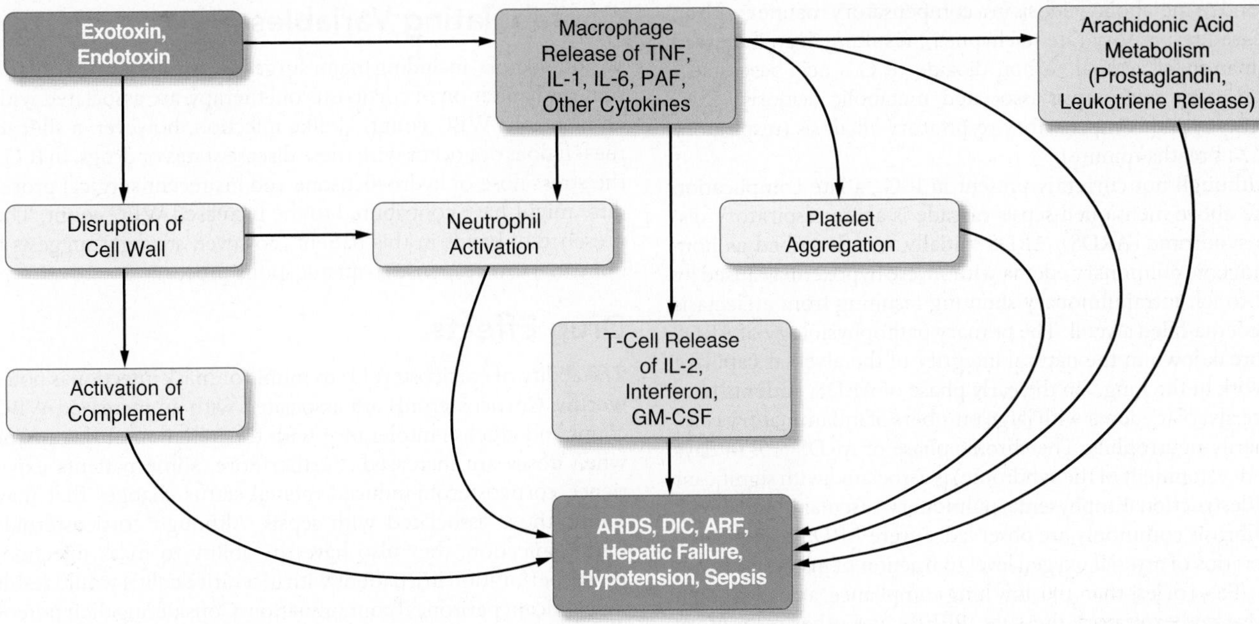

FIGURE 60-1 The sepsis cascade. ARDS, acute respiratory distress syndrome; ARF, acute renal failure; DIC, disseminated intravascular coagulation; GM-CSF, granulocyte-macrophage colony-stimulating factor; IL-1, interleukin-1; IL-2, interleukin-2; IL-6, interleukin-6; PAF, platelet-activating factor; TNF, tumor necrosis factor.

of critical hemodynamics. A normal SVR of 800 to 1,200 dyne · s · cm^{-5} may fall to 500 to 600 dyne · s · cm^{-5} in septic shock as a result of extensive vasodilation. In response to vasodilation, the heart reflexively increases cardiac output from a normal 4 to 6 L/minute to up to 11 to 12 L/minute in septic patients. This reflex increase in cardiac output is caused by an increased heart rate; stroke volume remains unchanged or decreased. Although the heart rate increases because of reflex tachycardia, stress-induced catecholamine release (norepinephrine, epinephrine) also is a source for the increased heart rate. Although cardiac output initially increases in response to arterial vasodilation, this increase generally is insufficient to overcome the vasodilatory state, and hypotension ensues. In overwhelming septic shock, myocardial depression may result, resulting in a decreased cardiac output. The combination of decreased cardiac output and decreased SVR results in hypotension often unresponsive to pressors and IV fluids. R.G. has hemodynamic evidence of septic shock. He is hypotensive (BP, 70/30 mm Hg) and tachycardic (130 beats/minute), presumably in response to vasodilation and catecholamine release.

Although vasodilation commonly occurs in sepsis, this dilation is unequal and chaotic. Some vascular beds constrict and others dilate, resulting in maldistribution of blood flow. In sepsis, blood generally is shunted away from the kidneys, mesentery, and extremities.

Normal urine output of approximately 0.5 to 1.0 mL/kg/hour (30–70 mL/hour for a 70-kg patient) can decrease to less than 20 mL/hour in sepsis. The urine output for R.G. has decreased to 10 mL/hour, consistent with sepsis-induced perfusion abnormalities. Decreased blood flow to the kidney as well as mediator-induced microvascular failure can cause acute-tubular necrosis (ATN). R.G.'s uremia (BUN, 58 mg/dL) and increased serum creatinine concentration (3.8 mg/dL) are consistent with decreased renal perfusion secondary to sepsis. When sepsis has progressed to septic shock, blood flow to most major organs is decreased. Decreased blood flow to the liver may result in "shock liver," in which liver function tests, including alanine aminotransferase (ALT), aspartate aminotransferase (AST), and alkaline phosphatase, become elevated. The liver function tests for R.G. are not available; however, his serum albumin concentration is low (2.1 g/dL) and his PT of 18 seconds is prolonged. Decreased blood flow to the musculature classically is characterized by cool extremities, and decreased blood flow to the brain can result in decreased mentation. R.G. is confused, his extremities are cold, and the area around his mouth appears pale. All these signs and symptoms provide strong evidence that he is in septic shock.

Cellular Changes

The sepsis syndrome is associated with significant abnormalities in cellular metabolism. Glucose intolerance commonly is observed in sepsis, and patients with previously normal blood glucose levels may experience sudden increases in blood sugar. In some cases, an increase in glucose is one of the first signs of an infectious process. R.G.'s increased blood glucose concentration (320 mg/dL) is, therefore, consistent with infection. Other sensitive indicators of sepsis-associated inflammation include the ESR, C-reactive protein, and procalcitonin, nonspecific tests that are commonly elevated in various inflammatory states, including infection. The ESR, C-reactive protein, or procalcitonin can be used to follow the progression of infection; currently, R.G.'s ESR is elevated at 65 mm/hour. With appropriate management of infection, the ESR would be expected to decrease; inadequate treatment would be associated with persistent elevation of the ESR and C-reactive protein. Procalcitonin is a marker that is a more specific indicator for infection than ESR or C-reactive protein and has been used as a tool to discontinue antibiotics in patients with noninfectious inflammation.[4] At the present, R.G.'s procalcitonin is 1.0 mcg/L, which is consistent with infection-associated inflammation.

Respiratory Changes

Production of organic acids, such as lactate, increased glycolysis, decreased fractional extraction of oxygen, and abnormal delivery-dependent oxygen consumption are observed in sepsis.[3] This process results in metabolic acidosis, with accompanying decreased serum bicarbonate levels. The lungs normally respond to metabolic acidosis in a compensatory manner with an increased respiratory rate (tachypnea), resulting in an increased elimination of arterial carbon dioxide. R.G.'s acid-base status is consistent with sepsis-associated metabolic acidosis (CO_2, 16 mEq/L) and compensatory respiratory alkalosis (respiratory rate, 24 breaths/minute).

Although not currently present in R.G., a late complication of the above-mentioned sepsis cascade is acute respiratory distress syndrome (ARDS). ARDS initially was described as noncardiogenic pulmonary edema with severe hypoxemia caused by right-to-left intrapulmonary shunting resulting from atelectasis and edema-filled alveoli. The primary pathophysiology of ARDS is a breakdown in the natural integrity of the alveolar capillary network in the lung.[5] In the early phase of ARDS, patients have severe alveolar edema with large numbers of inflammatory cells, primarily neutrophils. The chronic phase of ARDS (10–14 days after development of the syndrome) is associated with significant lung destruction. Emphysema, pulmonary vascular obliteration, and fibrosis commonly are observed. Severe ARDS is associated with ratios of arterial oxygen level to fraction of inspired oxygen (PaO_2/FIO_2) of less than 100, low lung compliance, a need for high positive end-expiratory pressure (PEEP), and other respiratory maneuvers. At present, the treatment for this syndrome primarily is supportive, including mechanical ventilation, high inspired oxygen, and PEEP. If patients fail to show improved gas exchange by day 7, the mortality associated with ARDS is high (>80%).[6] Although R.G. currently does not have ARDS, the severity of his sepsis strongly suggests he may develop this complication.

Hematologic Changes

Disseminated intravascular coagulation (DIC) is a well-recognized sequel of sepsis. Huge quantities of clotting factors and platelets are consumed in DIC as widespread coagulation and inflammation take place throughout the circulatory system. As a result, the ratio of PT to international normalized ratio (INR) and the activated partial thromboplastin time (aPTT) are prolonged, and the platelet count commonly is decreased in sepsis. Decreased fibrinogen levels and increased fibrin split products generally are diagnostic for DIC. The PT of 18 seconds and the decreased platelet count of 40,000/μL in R.G. are consistent with sepsis-induced DIC.

Neurologic Changes

Central nervous system (CNS) changes, including lethargy, disorientation, confusion, and psychosis, are commonly observed in septic patients. Altered mental status is a well-recognized symptom associated with CNS infections, such as meningitis and brain abscess. These changes, however, also are commonly observed with other sites of infection as well. R.G.'s confused state is consistent with that expected with septic shock.

PROBLEMS IN THE DIAGNOSIS OF AN INFECTION

CASE 60-1, QUESTION 3: R.G.'s medical history includes temporal arteritis and seizures chronically treated with corticosteroids and phenytoin. Perioperative "stress doses" of hydrocortisone recently were administered because of his surgical procedure. What medications or disease states confuse the diagnosis of infection?

Confabulating Variables

Various factors, including major surgery, acute myocardial infarction, and initiation of corticosteroid therapy, are associated with an increased WBC count. Unlike infection, however, a shift to the left does not occur with these disease states or drugs. In R.G., the stress dose of hydrocortisone and his recent surgical procedure might have contributed to the increased WBC count. The presence of bands in this patient, however, strongly suggests a bone marrow response to an infectious process.

Drug Effects

The ability of corticosteroids to mimic or mask infection is noteworthy. Corticosteroids are associated with an increased WBC count and glucose intolerance with the initiation of therapy or when doses are increased. Furthermore, some patients experience corticosteroid-induced mental status changes that may mimic those associated with sepsis. Although corticosteroids mimic infection, they also have the ability to mask infection. Bowel perforation in a patient with ulcerative colitis would result in significant peritoneal contamination. Considering their potent anti-inflammatory effects, concomitant receipt of glucocorticoids may, however, reduce the classic findings of peritonitis. Furthermore, corticosteroids can reduce and sometimes ablate the febrile response. Thus, these corticosteroid-treated patients may be asymptomatic but at great risk for gram-negative septic shock.

Another example of the influence of corticosteroids on the diagnosis of infection relates to neurosurgical procedures. Dexamethasone is a corticosteroid commonly used to reduce the inflammation and swelling associated with neurosurgical procedures. Certain neurosurgical procedures are associated with significant trauma to the meninges; however, the patient often is asymptomatic while receiving high-dose dexamethasone. When the dexamethasone dose is decreased, the patient subsequently may experience classic meningismus, including stiff neck, photophobia, and headache. The lumbar puncture may demonstrate cloudy cerebrospinal fluid (CSF), an elevated WBC count, high CSF protein, and low CSF glucose. Although the signs and symptoms are consistent with infectious meningitis, if no bacteria grow from the CSF sample, this disease state represents an aseptic meningitis (i.e., inflammation of the meninges without an infectious origin).[7] Certain drugs may cause aseptic meningitis, including OKT3, nonsteroidal anti-inflammatory agents, sulfonamides, and certain antiepileptics.[8]

Fever

Fever also is a common finding with autoimmune diseases, such as systemic lupus erythematosus and temporal arteritis.[9,10] Cancers, such as leukemia and lymphoma, also may present with low-grade fevers, similar to those observed in an infectious process. One evaluation of fever of unknown origin (FUO) in community hospitals demonstrated a 25% incidence of FUO caused by cancer.[10] Other diseases associated with fever include sarcoidosis, chronic liver disease, and familial Mediterranean fever. Acute myocardial infarction, pulmonary embolism, and postoperative pulmonary atelectasis also are commonly associated with fever. Factitious fever or self-induced disease must be considered in certain patients. After infection, autoimmune disease, and malignancy have been ruled out, drug fever should be considered. Drugs, including certain antimicrobials, have been associated with drug fever. Drug fever generally occurs after 7 to 10 days of therapy and resolves within 48 hours of the drug's discontinuation.[11] Some clinicians claim that patients with drug fever generally feel "well" and are unaware of their fever. A rechallenge with the offending agent usually results in recurrence of fever within hours of administration. Drug fever should be considered a diagnosis of exclusion, however, and should be considered only after eliminating the presence of other disease states.

Neoplasms may be radiographically indistinguishable from an abscess. An example of this dilemma is the differential diagnosis of toxoplasmosis versus lymphoma in patients with human immunodeficiency virus (HIV) with brain lesions documented by a computed axial tomography scan. One method for diagnosis is to use empirical therapy against *Toxoplasma gondii*. If the lesions are unresponsive to therapy, a presumptive diagnosis of malignancy can be made.

In summary, R.G. has an autoimmune disease, temporal arteritis, which is known to be associated with fever. Similarly, his corticosteroid administration and phenytoin use may confound the diagnosis of infection. His other signs and symptoms, however, strongly suggest that R.G.'s problems are of an infectious origin.

ESTABLISHING THE SITE OF THE INFECTION

CASE 60-1, QUESTION 4: What are the most likely sources of R.G.'s infection?

Independent of the presumed site of infection, in septic patients a series of blood samples for culture tests must be drawn to demonstrate the presence of bacteremia. After blood culture sampling, a thorough physical examination often documents the source of infection. Urosepsis, the most common cause of nosocomial infection, may be associated with dysuria, flank pain, and abnormal urinalysis.[12] Tachypnea, increased sputum production, altered chest radiograph, and hypoxemia may direct the clinician toward a pulmonary source. Evidence for an infected IV line might include pain, erythema, and purulent discharge around the IV catheter. Other potential sites of infection include the peritoneum, pelvis, bone, and CNS.

R.G. has several possible sites of infection. The copious production of yellow-green sputum, tachypnea, and the altered chest radiograph suggest the presence of pneumonia. The abdominal pain, absent bowel sounds, and recent surgical procedure, however, suggest an intra-abdominal source.[13] Lastly, the abnormal urinalysis (>50 WBC/HPF) and the erythema around the central venous catheter suggest urinary tract and catheter infections, respectively.

DETERMINING LIKELY PATHOGENS

CASE 60-1, QUESTION 5: What are the most likely pathogens associated with R.G.'s infection(s)?

R.G. has several possible sources of infection with probable associated pathogens. Table 60-1 provides a classification of infectious organisms (e.g., gram-positive, gram-negative, aerobic,

TABLE 60-1
Classification of Infectious Organisms

1. Bacteria

Aerobic

Gram-positive

Cocci

- Streptococci: pneumococcus, viridans streptococci; group A streptococci
- *Enterococcus*
- Staphylococci: *Staphylococcus aureus, Staphylococcus epidermidis*

Rods (bacilli)

- *Corynebacterium*
- *Listeria*

Gram-negative

Cocci

- *Moraxella*
- *Neisseria (Neisseria meningitidis, Neisseria gonorrhoeae)*

Rods (bacilli)

- Enterobacteriaceae (*Escherichia coli, Klebsiella, Enterobacter, Citrobacter, Proteus, Serratia, Salmonella, Shigella, Morganella, Providencia*)
- *Campylobacter*
- *Pseudomonas*
- *Helicobacter*
- *Haemophilus* (coccobacilli morphology)
- *Legionella*

Anaerobic

Gram-positive

Cocci

- *Peptococcus*
- *Peptostreptococcus*

Rods (bacilli)

- Clostridia (*Clostridium perfringens, Clostridium tetani, Clostridium difficile*)
- *Propionibacterium acnes*

Gram-negative

Cocci

- None

Rods (bacilli)

- Bacteroides (*Bacteroides fragilis, Bacteroides melaninogenicus*)
- Fusobacterium
- Prevotella

2. Fungi

Aspergillus, Candida, Coccidioides, Cryptococcus, Histoplasma, Mucor, Tinea, Trichophyton

3. Viruses

Influenza; hepatitis A, B, C, D, E; human immunodeficiency virus; rubella; herpes; influenza; cytomegalovirus; respiratory syncytial virus; Epstein-Barr virus; severe acute respiratory syndrome (SARS) virus

4. Chlamydiae

Chlamydia trachomatis
Chlamydia psittaci
Chlamydia pneumoniae
Lymphogranuloma venereum (LGV)

5. Rickettsiae

Rocky Mountain spotted fever, Q fever
Ureaplasma

6. Mycoplasmas

Mycoplasma pneumoniae, Mycoplasma hominis

7. Spirochetes

Treponema pallidum, Borrelia burgdorferi (Lyme disease)

8. Mycobacteria

Mycobacterium tuberculosis
Mycobacterium avium intracellulare

TABLE 60-2
Site of Infection: Suspected Organisms

Site/Type of Infection	Suspected Organisms
1. Respiratory	
Pharyngitis	Viral, group A streptococci
Bronchitis, otitis	Viral, *Haemophilus influenzae, Streptococcus pneumoniae, Moraxella catarrhalis*
Acute sinusitis	Viral, *Streptococcus pneumoniae, Haemophilus influenzae, Moraxella catarrhalis*
Chronic sinusitis	Anaerobes, *Staphylococcus aureus* (as well as suspected organisms associated with acute sinusitis)
Epiglottitis	Viral, *Haemophilus influenzae*
Pneumonia	
Community -acquired	
Normal host	*Streptococcus pneumoniae*, viral, mycoplasma
Aspiration	Normal aerobic and anaerobic mouth flora
Pediatrics	*Streptococcus pneumoniae, Haemophilus influenzae*
COPD	*Streptococcus pneumoniae, Haemophilus influenzae, Legionella, Chlamydia, Mycoplasma*
Alcoholic	*Streptococcus pneumoniae, Klebsiella*
Hospital-acquired	
Aspiration	Mouth anaerobes, aerobic gram-negative rods, *Staphylococcus aureus*
Neutropenic	Fungi, aerobic gram-negative rods, *Staphylococcus aureus*
HIV	Fungi, *Pneumocystis, Legionella, Nocardia, Streptococcus pneumoniae, Pseudomonas*
2. Urinary Tract	
Community-acquired	*Escherichia coli*, other gram-negative rods, *Staphylococcus aureus, Staphylococcus epidermidis*, enterococci
Hospital-acquired	Resistant aerobic gram-negative rods, enterococci
3. Skin and Soft Tissue	
Cellulitis	Group A streptococci, *Staphylococcus aureus*
IV catheter infection	*Staphylococcus aureus, Staphylococcus epidermidis*
Surgical wound	*Staphylococcus aureus*, gram-negative rods
Diabetic ulcer	*Staphylococcus aureus*, gram-negative aerobic rods, anaerobes
Furuncle	*Staphylococcus aureus*
4. Intra-Abdominal	*Bacteroides fragilis, Escherichia coli*, other aerobic gram-negative rods, enterococci
5. Gastroenteritis	*Salmonella, Shigella, Helicobacter, Campylobacter, Clostridium difficile*, amoeba, *Giardia*, viral, enterotoxigenic-hemorrhagic *Escherichia coli*
6. Endocarditis	
Pre-existing valvular disease	*Viridans streptococci*
IV drug user	*Staphylococcus aureus*, aerobic gram-negative rods, enterococci, fungi
Prosthetic valve	*Staphylococcus epidermidis, Staphylocccus aureus*
7. Osteomyelitis and Septic Arthritis	*Staphylococcus aureus*, aerobic gram-negative rods
8. Meningitis	
<2 months	*Escherichia coli*, group B streptococci, *Listeria*
2 months–12 years	*Streptococcus pneumoniae, Neisseria meningitidis, Haemophilus influenzae*
Adults	*Streptococcus pneumoniae, Neisseria meningitidis*
Hospital-acquired	*Streptococcus pneumoniae, Neisseria meningitidis*, aerobic gram-negative rods
Postneurosurgery	*Staphylococcus aureus*, aerobic gram-negative rods

COPD, chronic obstructive pulmonary disease; IV, intravenous.

anaerobic), and Table 60-2 lists the most likely organisms associated with sites of infection. Bacterial pneumonia is caused by various pathogens, including *Streptococcus pneumoniae, Enterobacteriacae*, and atypical pathogens (e.g., *Legionella pneumophila*).[14] However, empirical antimicrobial therapy directed against all the above organisms is not necessary in all patients. Community-acquired pneumonia in normal hosts is generally associated with *S. pneumoniae, Haemophilus influenza*, and "atypical" bacterial pathogens.[15] In contrast, nosocomial (hospital, nursing home) pneumonia is associated with gram-negative bacilli (e.g., *Escherichia coli, Klebsiella* species, *Enterobacter* species, and *Pseudomonas aeruginosa*) and *Staphylococcus aureus*. If the pneumonia is a result of a gastric aspiration, empirical antibacterial treatment of mouth anaerobes generally takes place; however, their true pathogenicity in aspiration pneumonia is not clear. For the empirical treatment of hospital-associated pneumonia or ventilator-associated pneumonia, knowledge of a hospital epidemiology is useful. If *P. aeruginosa* or *Enterobacter cloacae* predominate in an institution, then broad-spectrum agents should be used directed against these pathogens. Similarly, prior or concurrent receipt of antimicrobial therapy significantly impacts on the choice of empirical therapy. Age is an important determinant in the epidemiology of infection. For example, meningitis in a neonate is commonly caused by group B streptococci, *E. coli*, and *Listeria monocytogenes*, whereas these bacteria are uncommon meningitis pathogens in normal adults. The presence of concomitant diseases, such as chronic obstructive pulmonary disease (COPD) or alcohol and IV drug use, also influences the specific pathogen.

As an example, patients with COPD-associated pneumonia are more likely to be infected by *S. pneumoniae* and *H. influenzae*, whereas chronic alchoholics are more likely to have *Klebsiella* species as a source of pneumonia.

Immune status is an important predictor of likely pathogens. HIV/AIDS patients or those receiving Atgam, cyclosporine (or tacrolimus), and corticosteroids have lymphocyte deficiency or dysfunction-associated infections, including those caused by cytomegalovirus, *Pneumocystis jiroveci*, atypical mycobacteria, and *Cryptococcus neoformans*. Patients with leukemia and neutropenia are at risk for infection caused by aerobic gram-negative bacilli, including *P. aeruginosa*, *Candida* species, and *Aspergillus* species, as well as the above-mentioned pathogens.

In R.G., the abdomen, respiratory tract, urinary tract, and IV catheter are all potential sites of infection. Intra-abdominal infection is likely caused by aerobic gram-negative enteric bacteria, *Bacteroides fragilis*, and possibly enterococcus; nosocomial urinary tract infection is usually caused by aerobic gram-negative bacteria. Consequently, R.G.'s pneumonia could be attributable to gram-negative bacilli and staphylococci, as well as other organisms. Furthermore, his long-term use of corticosteroids may predispose him to infection caused by more opportunistic organisms, including *Legionella*, *P. jiroveci*, and fungi. Lastly, his IV catheter infection suggests infection caused by staphylococci, including *Staphylococcus epidermidis* and *S. aureus*.

MICROBIOLOGIC TESTS AND SUSCEPTIBILITY OF ORGANISMS

CASE 60-1, QUESTION 6: A Gram stain of R.G.'s tracheal aspirate shows gram-negative bacilli. What tests may assist with the identification of the pathogen(s)?

TABLE 60-3
Classification of Antibacterials

β-Lactam Antibiotics
Cephalosporins
- *First-generation*
  - Cefadroxil (Duricef)
  - Cefazolin (Ancef)
  - Cephalexin (Keflex)
- *Second-generation*
  - Cefaclor (Ceclor)
  - Cefamandole (Mandol)
  - Cefonicid (Monocid)
  - Ceforanide (Precef)
  - Cefotetan (Cefotan)
  - Cefoxitin (Mefoxin)
  - Cefprozil (Cefzil)
  - Cefuroxime (Zinacef)
  - Cefuroxime axetil (Ceftin)
- *Third-generation*
  - Cefdinir (Omnicef)
  - Cefditoren (Spectracef)
  - Cefixime (Suprax)
  - Cefotaxime (Claforan)
  - Cefpodoxime proxetil (Vantin)
  - Ceftazidime (Fortaz)
  - Ceftibuten (Cedax)
  - Ceftizoxime (Cefizox)
  - Ceftriaxone (Rocephin)
- *Fourth-generation*
  - Cefepime (Maxipime)
- *Fifth-generation*
  - Ceftaroline (Teflaro)

Carbacephems
- Loracarbef (Lorabid)

Monobactams
- Aztreonam (Azactam)

Penems
- Doripenem (Doribax)
- Ertapenem (Invanz)
- Imipenem (Primaxin)
- Meropenem (Merem)

Penicillins
- *Natural penicillins*
  - Penicillin G
  - Penicillin V
- *Aminopenicillins*
  - Ampicillin (Omnipen)
  - Amoxicillin (Amoxil)
  - Bacampicillin (Spectrobid)

β-Lactam Antibiotics
- *Penicillinase-resistant penicillins*
  - Isoxazolyl penicillins (dicloxacillin, oxacillin, cloxacillin)
  - Nafcillin (Unipen)
- *Combination with β-lactamase inhibitors*
  - Augmentin (amoxicillin plus clavulanic acid)
  - Timentin (ticarcillin plus clavulanic acid)
  - Unasyn (ampicillin plus sulbactam)
  - Zosyn (piperacillin plus tazobactam)

Aminoglycosides
- Amikacin (Amikin)
- Gentamicin (Garamycin)
- Neomycin (Mycifradin)
- Netilmicin (Netromycin)
- Streptomycin
- Tobramycin (Nebcin)

Protein synthesis inhibitors
- Azithromycin (Zithromax)
- Clarithromycin (Biaxin)
- Clindamycin (Cleocin)
- Chloramphenicol (Chloromycetin)
- Dalfopristin/Quinupristin (Synercid)
- Dirithromycin (Dynabac)
- Erythromycin (Erythrocin)
- Linezolid (Zyvox)
- Telithromycin (Ketek)
- Tetracyclines (doxycycline, minocycline, tetracycline, tigecycline)

Folate inhibitors
- Sulfadiazine
- Sulfadoxine (Fansidar)
- Trimethoprim (Trimpex)
- Trimethoprim-sulfamethoxazole (Bactrim, Septra)

Quinolones
- Ciprofloxacin (Cipro)
- Gemifloxacin (Factive)
- Levofloxacin (Levoquin)
- Moxifloxacin (Avelox)
- Norfloxacin (Noroxin)
- Ofloxacin (Floxin)

Daptomycin (Cubicin)
Televancin (Vibativ)
Vancomycin (Vancocin)
Metronidazole (Flagyl)

Once the site of infection has been determined and host defense and other epidemiologic factors have been evaluated, additional tests can be performed to identify the pathogen. The Gram stain uses crystal violet solution and iodine, which results in bacteria staining gram positive or gram negative; some organisms are gram variable. In addition, the shape of the organism (cocci, bacilli) is readily apparent with the use of the Gram stain. Streptococci and staphylococci are gram-positive cocci, whereas *E. coli, E. cloacae,* and *P. aeruginosa* appear as gram-negative bacilli (Table 55-1).[16] If the Gram stain of the tracheal aspirate demonstrates gram-positive cocci in clusters, empirical antistaphylococcal therapy is indicated. In contrast, if the Gram stain shows gram-negative rods, antimicrobials with activity against these pathogens should be used.

Similar to the Gram stain in bacterial infection, the India ink and potassium hydroxide (KOH) stains are helpful in the identification of certain fungi. The acid-fast bacilli (AFB) stain is critical in the diagnosis of infection caused by *Mycobacterium tuberculosis* or atypical mycobacteria.

In R.G.'s case, the Gram stain suggests that antimicrobials active against gram-negative bacilli should be used. Table 60-3 provides a classification of antibacterials (e.g., different generations of cephalosporins). Tables 60-4, 60-5, and 60-6 list in vitro susceptibilities of aerobic gram-positive organisms, gram-negative aerobes, and anaerobic organisms, respectively.

Culture and Susceptibility Testing

Culture and susceptibility testing provides final identification of the pathogen, as well as information regarding the likely effectiveness of various antimicrobials. Although these tests provide more information than the Gram stain, they generally require 18 to 24 hours to complete. After the pathogen has been identified, Table 60-7 can be used in conjunction with institution-specific susceptibility studies to select the most appropriate antimicrobial.

DISK DIFFUSION

The most widely used tests for bacterial susceptibility are the disk diffusion and the broth dilution methods. The disk diffusion (Kirby-Bauer) technique uses an agar plate on which an inoculum of the organism is placed. After inoculation, several antimicrobial-laden disks are placed on the plate, and evidence of bacterial growth is observed after 18 to 24 hours. If the antimicrobial is active against the pathogen, a zone of growth inhibition is observed around the disk. Based on guidelines provided by the Clinical and Laboratory Standards Institute (CLSI), the diameter of inhibition is reported as susceptible, intermediate, or resistant.

BROTH DILUTION

The broth dilution method involves placing a bacterial inoculum into several tubes or wells filled with broth. Serial dilutions

TABLE 60-4
In Vitro Antimicrobial Susceptibility: Aerobic Gram-Positive Cocci

Drugs	Staphylococcus Aureus	Staphylococcus Aureus (MR)	Staphylococcus Epidermidis	Staphylococcus Epidermidis (MR)	Streptococci[a]	Enterococci[b]	Pneumococci
Ampicillin	+		+		++++	++	+++
Augmentin	++++	+	++++		++++	++	++++
Aztreonam							
Cefazolin	++++		++++		++++		++
Cefepime	++++		++++		++++		+++
Cefoxitin/Cefotetan	++		++		++		+
Cefuroxime	++++		++++		++++		+++
Ciprofloxacin[c]	+++	++	+++	++	+	+	++
Clindamycin	++++	+	++++	+	+++		+++
Cotrimoxazole	++++	+++	++	+	++	+	+
Daptomycin[f]	++++	++++	++++	++++	++++	++++	++++
Erythromycin (azithromycin/ clarithromycin)	++		+		+++		++
Imipenem	++++		++++		++++	++	+++
Levofloxacin (gemifloxacin, moxifloxacin)	++++	++	+++	++	+++	++	++++
Linezolid[f]	++++	++++	++++	++++	++++	++++	++++
Nafcillin	++++		++++		++++		++
Penicillin	+		+		++++	++	+++
Quinupristin/ dalfopristin[d,f]	++++	++++	++++	++++	++++	++++	++++
TGC[e]	+++		++		++++		+++
Televancin	++++	++++	++++	++++	++++	++++	++++
Tigecycline[f]	++++	++++	++++	++++	++++	++++	++++
Timentin	++++		++++		++++	+	+
Unasyn	++++		++++		++++	++	+++
Vancomycin	++++	++++	++++	++++	++++	+++	++++
Zosyn	++++		++++		++++	++	+++

[a]Nonpneumococcal streptococci.
[b]Usually requires combination therapy (e.g., ampicillin and an aminoglycoside) for serious infection.
[c]Levofloxacin (gatifloxacin, gemifloxacin, moxifloxacin) is more active than ciprofloxacin against staphylococci and streptococci.
[d]Active against *E. faecium* but unpredictable against *E. faecalis.*
[e]Cefotaxime, ceftizoxime, ceftriaxone, cefoperazone. Ceftazidime has comparatively inferior antistaphylococcal and antipneumococcal activity. Cefotaxime and ceftriaxone are the most reliable cephalosporins versus *S. pneumoniae.*
[f]Active versus vancomycin-resistant *Enterococcus faecium.*
MR, methicillin resistant; TGC, third-generation cephalosporin.

TABLE 60-5
In Vitro Antimicrobial Susceptibility: Gram-Negative Aerobes

Drugs	Escherichia Coli	Klebsiella Pneumoniae	Enterobacter Cloacae	Proteus Mirabilis	Serratia Marcescens	Pseudomonas Aeruginosa	Haemophilus Influenzae	Haemophilus Influenzae[a]
Ampicillin	++			+++			++++	
Augmentin	+++	++		++++			++++	++++
Aztreonam	++++	++++	+	++++	++++	++++	++++	++++
Cefazolin	+++	+++		++++			+	
Cefepime	++++	++++	+++	++++	++++	++++	++++	++++
Ceftazidime	++++	++++	+	++++	++++	++++	++++	++++
Cefuroxime	+++	+++		++++	+		++++	++++
Cotrimoxazole	++	+++	+++	++++	+++		++++	++++
Ertepenem	++++	++++	++++	++++	++++	+	++++	++++
Gentamicin	++++	++++	++++	++++	++++	+++	++	++
Imipenem/ meropenem/ doripenem	++++	++++	++++	+++	++++	++++	++++	++++
Quinolones	+++	++++	+++	++++	++++	++	++++	++++
TGC[b]	++++	++++	+	++++	++++	+	++++	++++
Tigecycline	++++	++++	++++	++	++++	–	++++	++++
Timentin	+++	++	+	++++	+++	+++	++++	++++
Tobramycin	++++	++++	++++	++++	+++	++++	++	++
Unasyn	+++	+++		++++	++		++++	++++
Zosyn	++++	++++	++	++++	++++	++++	++++	++++

[a]β-Lactamase-producing strains.
[b]Cefataxime, ceftizoxime, ceftriaxone.
TGC, third-generation cephalosporin.

of antimicrobials (e.g., nafcillin 0.5, 1.0, and 2.0 mcg/mL) are placed in the respective wells. After bacteria are allowed to incubate for 18 to 24 hours, the wells are examined for bacterial growth. If the well is cloudy, bacterial growth has occurred, suggesting resistance to the specific antimicrobial at that concentration. As an example, if bacterial growth is observed with *S. aureus* at 0.5 mcg/mL of nafcillin but not at 1.0 mcg/mL, then 1.0 mcg/mL would be considered the minimum inhibitory concentration (MIC) for nafcillin against *S. aureus*.

Similar to the disk diffusion method, the CLSI provides guidelines[17] that also take into account the pharmacokinetic characteristics of an antimicrobial to determine whether the MIC should be reported as susceptible, intermediately susceptible, or resistant. MIC interpretations are both pathogen- and antimicrobial-specific. For example, ciprofloxacin achieves serum concentrations of only 1 to 4 mcg/mL, whereas the fourth-generation cephalosporin, cefepime, achieves peak serum concentrations of 75 to mcg/mL; consequently an MIC of 4.0 mcg/mL for *E. coli* would be interpreted by CLSI as resistant to ciprofloxacin, but susceptible to cefepime.

Although these tests provide an accurate assessment of in vitro susceptibility, the time delay (18–24 hours) can hinder

TABLE 60-6
Antimicrobial Susceptibility: Anaerobes

Drugs	Bacteroides Fragilis	Peptococcus	Peptostreptococcus	Clostridia
Ampicillin	+	++++	++++	+++
Aztreonam				
Cefazolin		+++	+++	
Cefepime	+	+++	+++	+
Cefotaxime	++	+++	+++	+
Cefoxitin	+++	+++	++++	+
Ceftazidime		+	+	+
Ceftizoxime	+++	+++	+++	+
Ciprofloxacin	+	+	+	+
Clindamycin	+++	++++	++++	++
Moxifloxacin	+++	+++	+++	++
Imipenem (doripenem/ ertapenem/meropenem)	++++	++++	++++	++
Metronidazole	++++	+++	++	+++
Penicillin	+	++++	++++	++++
Timentin	++++	+++	+++	+++
Unasyn	++++	++++	++++	++++
Vancomycin		+++	+++	+++
Zosyn	++++	++++	+++	+++

TABLE 60-7
Antimicrobials of Choice in the Treatment of Bacterial Infection

Organism	Drug of Choice	Alternatives	Comments
Aerobes			
Gram-positive cocci			
Streptococcus pyogenes (group A streptococci)	Penicillin	Clindamycin, macrolide, cephalosporin	Clindamycin is the most reliable alternative for penicillin-allergic patients.
Streptococcus pneumoniae	Ceftriaxone, ampicillin, oral amoxicillin	Macrolide, cephalosporin, doxycycline	Although the incidence of penicillin-nonsusceptible pneumococci is 20%–30%, high-dose penicillin or amoxicillin is active against most of these isolates. Penicillin-resistant pneumococci commonly demonstrate resistance to other agents, including erythromycin, tetracyclines, and cephalosporins. Antipneumococcal quinolones (gemifloxacin, levofloxacin, moxifloxacin), ceftriaxone, and cefotaxime are options for treatment of high-level penicillin-resistant isolates.
Enterococcus faecalis	Ampicillin ± gentamicin	Piperacillin-tazobactam; vancomycin ± gentamicin; daptomycin, linezolid, tigecycline	Most commonly isolated enterococcus (80%–85%). Most reliable antienterococcal agents are ampicillin (penicillin, piperacillin-tazobactam), vancomycin, and linezolid. Monotherapy generally inhibits but does not kill the enterococcus. Daptomycin is unique in its bactericidal activity against enterococci. Aminoglycosides must be added to ampicillin or vancomycin to provide bactericidal activity. High-level aminoglycoside resistance should be determined for endocarditis.
Enterococcus faecium	Vancomycin ± gentamicin	Linezolid, daptomycin, dalfopristin/quinupristin (D/Q), tigecycline	Second most common enterococcal organism (10%–20%) and is more likely than *E. faecalis* to be resistant to multiple antimicrobials. Most reliable agents are daptomycin, D/Q, and linezolid. Monotherapy generally inhibits but does not kill the enterococcus. Aminoglycosides must be added to cell wall–active agents to provide bactericidal activity. Ampicillin and vancomycin resistance is common. Daptomycin, D/Q, and linezolid are drugs of choice for vancomycin-resistant isolates.
Staphylococcus aureus (nafcillin-resistant)	Nafcillin	Cefazolin, vancomycin, clindamycin, trimethoprim-sulfamethoxazole linezolid,	10%–15% of isolates inhibited by penicillin. Most isolates susceptible to nafcillin, cephalosporins, trimethoprim-sulfamethoxazole, and clindamycin. First-generation cephalosporins are equal to nafcillin. Most second- and third-generation cephalosporins adequate in the treatment of infection (exceptions include ceftazidime and cefonicid). Methicillin-resistant *S. aureus* must be treated with vancomycin; however, trimethoprim-sulfamethoxazole, daptomycin, D/Q, linezolid, or minocycline can be used.
	Vancomycin	Trimethoprim-sulfamethoxazole, minocycline, daptomycin, tigecycline, televancin	
Staphylococcus epidermidis (nafcillin-resistant)	Nafcillin	Cefazolin, vancomycin, clindamycin	Most isolates are β-lactam-, clindamycin-, and trimethoprim-sulfamethoxazole–resistant. Most reliable agents are vancomycin, daptomycin, D/Q, and linezolid. Rifampin is active and can be used in conjunction with other agents; however, monotherapy with rifampin is associated with development of resistance.
	Vancomycin	Daptomycin, linezolid, D/Q	
Gram-positive Bacilli			
Diphtheroids	Penicillin	Cephalosporin	
Corynebacterium jeikeium	Vancomycin	Erythromycin, quinolone	
Listeria monocytogenes	Ampicillin (± gentamicin)	Trimethoprim-sulfamethoxazole	
Gram-negative Cocci			
Moraxella catarrhalis	Trimethoprim-sulfamethoxazole	Amoxicillin-clavulanic acid, erythromycin, doxycycline, second- or third-generation cephalosporin	
Neisseria gonorrhoeae	Cefixime	Ceftriaxone	
Neisseria meningitidis	Penicillin	Third-generation cephalosporin	

Gram-negative bacilli			
Campylobacter fetus	Imipenem	Gentamicin	
Campylobacter jejuni	Quinolone, erythromycin	A tetracycline, amoxicillin-clavulanic acid	
Enterobacter	Trimethoprim-sulfamethoxazole	Quinolone, carbapenem, aminoglycoside	Not predictably inhibited by third-generation cephalosporins. Carbapenems, quinolones, trimethoprim-sulfamethoxazole, cefepime, and aminoglycosides are most active agents.
Escherichia coli	Third-generation cephalosporin	First- or second-generation cephalosporin, gentamicin	Extended-spectrum β-lactamase (ESBL) –producers should be treated with a carbapenem.
Haemophilus influenzae	Third-generation cephalosporin	β-Lactamase inhibitor combinations, second-generation cephalosporin, trimethoprim-sulfamethoxazole	
Helicobacter pylori	Amoxicillin + clarithromycin + omeprazole	Tetracycline + metronidazole + bismuth subsalicylate	
Klebsiella pneumoniae	Third-generation cephalosporin	First- or second-generation cephalosporin, gentamicin, trimethoprim-sulfamethoxazole	Extended-spectrum β-lactamase (ESBL) –producers should be treated with a carbapenem.
Legionella	Fluoroquinolone	Erythromycin ± rifampin, doxycycline	
Proteus mirabilis	Ampicillin	First-generation cephalosporin, trimethoprim-sulfamethoxazole	
Other *Proteus*	Third-generation cephalosporin	β-Lactamase inhibitor combination, aminoglycoside, trimethoprim-sulfamethoxazole	
Pseudomonas aeruginosa	Antipseudomonal penicillin (or ceftazidime) ± aminoglycoside (or quinolone)	Quinolone or imipenem ± aminoglycoside	Most active agents include aminoglycosides, doripenem, imipenem, meropenem, ceftazidime, cefepime, aztreonam and the extended-spectrum penicillins. Monotherapy is adequate for most pseudomonal infections.
Salmonella typhi	Quinolone	Ceftriaxone	
Serratia marcescens	Third-generation cephalosporin	Trimethoprim-sulfamethoxazole, aminoglycoside	
Shigella	Quinolone	Trimethoprim-sulfamethoxazole, ampicillin	
Stenotrophomonas maltophilia	Trimethoprim-sulfamethoxazole	Ceftazidime, minocycline, β-lactamase inhibitor combination (Timentin)	
Anaerobes			
Bacteroides fragilis	Metronidazole	β-Lactamase inhibitor combinations, penems	Most active agents (95%–100%) include metronidazole, the β-lactamase inhibitor combinations (ampicillin-sulbactam, piperacillin-tazobactam, ticarcillin-clavulanic acid), and penems. Clindamycin, cefoxitin, cefotetan, cefmetazole, ceftizoxime have good activity but not to the degree of metronidazole. Aminoglycosides and aztreonam are inactive.
Clostridia difficile	Metronidazole	Vancomycin	Oral vancomycin is the drug of choice for severe infection.
Fusobacterium	Penicillin	Metronidazole, clindamycin	
Other Oropharyngeal			
Prevotella	β-Lactamase inhibitor combination	Metronidazole, clindamycin	
Peptostreptococcus	Penicillin	Clindamycin, cephalosporin	Most β-lactams active (exceptions include aztreonam, nafcillin, ceftazidime).
Other			
Actinomyces israelii	Penicillin	Tetracyclines	
Nocardia	Trimethoprim-sulfamethoxazole	Amikacin, minocycline, imipenem	
Chlamydia trachomatis	Doxycycline	Azithromycin	
Chlamydia pneumoniae		Azithromycin, clarithromycin	
Mycoplasma pneumoniae	Doxycycline	Azithromycin, clarithromycin	
Borrelia burgdorferi	Doxycycline	Ampicillin, second- or third-generation cephalosporin	
Treponema pallidum	Penicillin	Doxycycline	

streamlining of therapy. An alternative efficient, but more expensive, MIC test is the E test, which uses an antibiotic-laden plastic strip with increasing concentrations of a specific antimicrobial from one end to the other. The strip is placed on an agar plate with the actively growing pathogen. Inhibition of growth observed at specific marks on the strip coincides with the MIC of the organism. Numerous studies have confirmed that the E test is as effective as traditional susceptibility testing. Several automated antimicrobial susceptibility systems are available in the United States, including Phoenix (Becton Dickinson, Franklin Lakes, NJ), Vitek (bioMérieux, Durham, NC), MicroScan WalkAway (Siemens Healthcare Diagnostics, Tarrytown, NY), and Sensititre (Trek Diagnostics, Cleveland, OH). These systems generally use a computerized algorithm for interpreting results and determine the antibiotic MIC for the organism by using specialized decision technology. Two major advantages of automated susceptibility methodologies include a reduction in labor and faster reporting of susceptibility results, potentially leading to the earlier initiation of appropriate antibiotic therapy. Although these represent advantages, disadvantages exist, particularly with cystic fibrosis isolates. Most clinical microbiology laboratories use automated susceptibility testing systems.

Although susceptibility testing is relatively well standardized for aerobic gram-negative and gram-positive organisms, its utility is not as established for anaerobes[18] and fungi.[19] In general, despite improvements in the standardization of testing in anaerobes, institutions do not routinely perform susceptibility testing for these bacteria. In contrast, susceptibility testing is now available for *Candida* species, and these in vitro data have been demonstrated to predict clinical success in the patient care setting.

The consensus of the CLSI and other experts is that anaerobic isolates from blood, bone and joint sources, brain abscesses, empyemic fluid, and other body fluids that are normally sterile should be considered for susceptibility testing. However, in general, these susceptibilities are rarely performed.[18] Although progress has been made in developing a standardized test for determining fungal susceptibility, the primary emphasis has been on the susceptibility of *Candida* species to azoles in the treatment of candidiasis.[19] Although standardized susceptibility testing for molds is established by the CLSI, this testing is rarely performed in the clinical setting.[20]

The MIC is the minimum concentration at which an antimicrobial inhibits the growth of the organism; the test does not provide information regarding whether the organism is actually killed. In some disease states (e.g., endocarditis), bactericidal therapy is necessary. The minimum bactericidal concentration (MBC) is the test that can be used to determine the killing activity associated with an antimicrobial. The MBC is determined by taking an aliquot from each clear MIC tube for subculture onto agar plates. The concentration at which no significant bacterial growth (i.e., 99.9% of the original inoclum) is observed on these plates is considered the MBC.

DETERMINATION OF ISOLATE PATHOGENICITY

CASE 60-1, QUESTION 7: *Serratia marcescens* grows from a culture of R.G.'s endotracheal aspirate. How can it be determined whether an isolate represents a true bacterial infection versus colonization or contamination?

A positive culture may represent colonization, contamination, or infection. Colonization indicates that bacteria are present at the site; however, they are not actively causing infection. Poor sampling techniques or inappropriate handling of specimens can result in contamination. Contamination differs from colonization in that these isolates are not truly at the site in question. The *S. marcescens* growing from this sample could represent infection, colonization, or contamination. If a suction catheter was used to sample R.G.'s endotracheal aspirate, the infecting organism likely would be cultured; however, other nonpathogenic flora would also appear in the culture medium (colonization). Furthermore, if the sample is not handled aseptically by the clinician or the microbiology laboratory, bacterial contamination is possible.

In summary, culture results do not solely identify true pathogens. In R.G., the *Serratia* may be a pathogen, contaminant, or colonizer. Nevertheless, considering the severity of R.G.'s illness and his associated respiratory symptoms, treatment directed against this pathogen is necessary.

ANTIMICROBIAL TOXICITIES

CASE 60-1, QUESTION 8: In light of the positive culture for *Serratia*, his increased respiratory secretions, and a worsening chest radiograph, ventilator-associated pneumonia (VAP) is likely. Pending susceptibility results, R.G. is empirically started on imipenem and gentamicin. In review of his patient records, R.G. has no known allergies. Are there equally effective, less toxic options for this patient?

Adverse Effects and Toxicities

Before antimicrobial therapy is started, it is important to elicit an accurate drug and allergy history. When "allergy" has been reported by the patient, it is necessary to determine whether the reaction was intolerance, toxicity, or true allergy. Table 60-8 lists the most common adverse effects and toxicities associated with antimicrobial therapy. For example, gastric intolerance caused by oral erythromycin or doxycycline is common; however, this adverse effect does not represent an allergic manifestation. Although R.G. has no known allergies, neither imipenem nor gentamicin are optimal choices. Imipenem is associated with seizures, particularly in patients with renal failure and in doses in excess of 50 mg/kg/day. Considering R.G.'s acute onset of renal failure and his history of seizures, other carbapenems, such as meropenem or doripenem, or alternative classes of antibacterials would be preferable. Gentamicin similarly may not be a good choice in R.G. His increased age and declining renal function predispose him to aminoglycoside nephrotoxicity and ototoxicity (cochlear and vestibular).[21] A reasonable recommendation pending susceptibility results would be to discontinue imipenem and gentamicin and treat with meropenem or doripenem with or without a fluoroquinolone.

Concomitant Disease States

Concomitant disease states also should be considered in the selection of therapy. As discussed above, older patients with hearing deficits are poor candidates for potentially ototoxic aminoglycoside therapy. Diabetic or kidney transplant patients with candidemia may be better treated with fluconazole or an echinocandin rather than nephrotoxic amphotericin B products. Patients with a pre-existing seizure history should not receive imipenem if less toxic therapy can be used. In summary, the toxicologic profile of a drug must be taken into account in the selection of antimicrobial therapy.

TABLE 60-8

Antibiotic Adverse Effects and Toxicities

Antibiotic	Side Effects	Comments
β-Lactams, (penicillin, cephalosporins, monobactams, penems)	*Allergic:* anaphylaxis, urticaria, serum sickness, rash, fever	Many patients will have "ampicillin rash" or "β-lactam rash" with no cross-reactivity with any other penicillins/β-lactams. Most commonly observed in patients with concomitant EBV disease. Likelihood of IgE-mediated cross-reactivity between penicillins and cephalosporins approximately 5%–10%. Most recent data strongly suggest minimal IgE cross-reactivity between penicillins and imipenem/meropenem. No IgE cross-reactivity between aztreonam and penicillins.
	Diarrhea	Particularly common with ampicillin, augmentin, ceftriaxone, and cefoperazone. Antibiotic-associated colitis can occur with most antimicrobials.
	Hematologic: anemia, thrombocytopenia, antiplatelet activity, hypothrombinemia	Hemolytic anemia more common with higher doses. Antiplatelet activity (inhibition of platelet aggregation) most common with the antipseudomonal penicillins and high serum levels of other β-lactams. Hypothrombinemia more often associated with those cephalosporins with the methyltetrazolethiol side chain (cefamandole, cefotetan). Reaction preventable and reversible with vitamin K.
	Hepatitis or biliary sludging	Hepatitis most common with oxacillin. Biliary sludging and stones reported with ceftriaxone.
	Phlebitis	
	Seizure activity	Associated with high levels of β-lactams, particularly penicillins and imipenem.
	Potassium load	Penicillin G (K^+).
	Nephritis	Most common with methicillin; however, occasionally reported for most other β-lactams.
	Neutropenia	Nafcillin.
	Disulfiram reaction	Associated with cephalosporins with methyltetrazolethiol side chain (cefamandole, cefotetan).
	Hypotension, nausea	Associated with fast infusion of imipenem.
Aminoglycosides (gentamicin, tobramycin, amikacin, netilmicin)	Nephrotoxicity	Averages 10%–15% incidence. Generally reversible, usually occurs after 5–7 days of therapy. *Risk factors:* dehydration, age, dose, duration, concurrent nephrotoxins, liver disease.
	Ototoxicity	1%–5% incidence, often irreversible. Both cochlear and vestibular toxicity occur.
	Neuromuscular paralysis	Rare, most common with large doses administered via intraperitoneal instillation or in patients with myasthenia gravis.
Macrolides (erythromycin, azithromycin, clarithromycin)	Nausea, vomiting, "burning" stomach	Oral administration. Azithromycin and clarithromycin associated with less nausea than erythromycin.
	Cholestatic jaundice	Reported for all erythromycin salts, most common with estolate.
	Ototoxicity	Most common with high doses in patients with renal or hepatic failure.
Telithromycin	Hepatoxicity; upper GI	Severe, sometime fatal hepatoxicity associated with telithromycin.
Clindamycin	Diarrhea	Most common adverse effect. High association with antibiotic-associated colitis.
Tetracyclines (including tigecycline)	Allergic	
	Photosensitivity	
	Teeth and bone deposition and discoloration	Avoid in pediatrics (<8 years old), pregnancy, and breast-feeding.
	GI	Upper GI predominates.
	Hepatitis	Primarily in pregnancy or the elderly.
	Renal (azotemia)	Tetracyclines have antianabolic effect and should be avoided in patients with ↓ renal function. Less problematic with doxycycline.
	Vestibular	Associated with minocycline, particularly high doses.

(continued)

TABLE 60-8
Antibiotic Adverse Effects and Toxicities (*Continued*)

Antibiotic	Side Effects	Comments
Vancomycin	Ototoxicity	Only with receipt of concomitant ototoxins such as aminoglycosides or macrolides.
	Nephrotoxicity	Nephrotoxic only with high doses or in combination with other nephrotoxins.
	Hypotension, flushing	Associated with rapid infusion of vancomycin. More common with increased doses.
	Phlebitis	Needs large volume dilution.
Dalfopristin/quinupristin	Phlebitis	Generally requires central line administration.
	Myalgia	Moderate to severe in many patients.
	Increased bilirubin	
Daptomycin	Myalgia	Primarily at high doses and reversible.
Linezolid	Thrombocytopenia, neutropenia, anemia, MAO inhibition, tongue discoloration	
Televancin	Renal toxicity, prolonged QT	
Sulfonamides	GI	Nausea, diarrhea.
	Hepatic	Cholestatic hepatitis, ↑ incidence in HIV.
	Rash	Exfoliative dermatitis, Stevens-Johnson syndrome. More common in HIV.
	Hyperkalemia	Only with trimethoprim (as a component of trimethoprim-sulfamethoxazole).
	Bone marrow	Neutropenia, thrombocytopenia. More common in HIV.
	Kernicterus	Caused by unbound drug in the neonate. Premature liver cannot conjugate bilirubin. Sulfonamide displaces bilirubin from protein, resulting in excessive free bilirubin and kernicterus.
Chloramphenicol	Anemia	Idiosyncratic irreversible aplastic anemia (rare). Reversible dose-related anemia.
	Gray syndrome	Caused by inability of neonates to conjugate chloramphenicol.
Quinolones	GI	Nausea, vomiting, diarrhea.
	Prolonged QT	Moxifloxacin; possibly all quinolones as a class.
	Drug interactions	↓ Oral bioavailability with multivalent cations.
	CNS	Altered mental status, confusion, seizures.
	Cartilage toxicity	Toxic in animal model. Despite this toxicity, appears safe in children including patients with cystic fibrosis.
	Tendonitis or tendon rupture	Common in elderly, renal failure, concomitant glucocorticoids.

Antifungals		
Amphotericin B products	Nephrotoxicity	Common. May depend on patient sodium load. Caution with concomitant nephrotoxins (e.g., aminoglycosides, cyclosporine).
	Hypokalemia	Predictable. Probably caused by renal tubular excretion of potassium. More common in patients receiving concomitant piperacillin-tazobactam.
	Hypomagnesemia	Less commonly observed than hypokalemia.
	Anemia	Long-term adverse effect. Similar to anemia of chronic disease.
Caspofungin, micafungin, anidulofungin	Mild LFT increase with concomitant cyclosporine; anidulofungin is reconstituted with alcohol (about the equivalent of a beer).	
Flucytosine	Neutropenia, thrombocytopenia	Secondary to metabolism of flucytosine to fluorouracil. More commonly observed with flucytosine levels >100 mg/mL. More common in patients with HIV.
	Hepatitis	Usually moderate ↑ in LFT. Rarely clinical hepatitis.
Ketoconazole (fluconazole, itraconazole, posaconazole, voriconazole)	Drug interactions	↓ Oral bioavailability of ketoconazole tablet, and itraconazole capsules with ↑ gastric pH. Azoles are CYP450 substrates and also inhibitors of CYP450 3A4 and other CYP isoenzymes.
	Hepatitis	Ranges from mild ↑ in LFT to occasional fatal hepatitis.
	Gynecomastia, ↓ libido	More common with high-dose ketoconazole (>400 mg/d). Less common with other azoles.
	Visual disturbance	Unique to voriconazole, particularly first week of therapy.
Antivirals (excluding antiretrovirals)		
Acyclovir	Phlebitis	Caused by poor solubility of IV preparation. Reported in 1%–20% of cases.
	Renal failure	Low solubility of acyclovir associated with renal failure. Dehydrated patients, as well as rapid infusions, predispose to toxicity.
	CNS	1% incidence in AIDS. ↑ Incidence with dose in >10 mg/kg/d.
Foscarnet	Nephrotoxicity	Occurs in up to 60% of patients. May be prevented with normal saline bolus before dose. Frequent monitoring of renal function imperative.
	Mineral and electrolyte abnormalities	↑ and ↓ calcium or phosphate may be observed. Hypocalcemia, hypo- and hyperphosphatemia, hypomagnesemia, hypokalemia. ↑ Risk of cardiomyopathy and seizures.
	Anemia	Anemia in 33%; usually manageable with transfusions and discontinuation of foscarnet.
	Nausea, vomiting	
Ganciclovir	Neutropenia, thrombocytopenia	↑ Incidence in AIDS. ↑ Incidence with doses in excess of 10 mg/kg/d.
	Hepatitis	Usually mild to moderate in LFT.
Oseltamavir	Nausea	

AIDS, acquired immunodeficiency syndrome; CNS, central nervous system; EBV, Epstein-Barr virus; GI, gastrointestinal; HIV, human immunodeficiency virus; IV, intravenous; LFT, liver function tests; MAO, monoamine oxidase.

ANTIMICROBIAL COSTS OF THERAPY

CASE 60-1, QUESTION 9: What factors should be included in calculating the cost of R.G.'s antimicrobial therapy?

The true cost of antimicrobial therapy is difficult to quantify.[22] Although acquisition cost traditionally has been the primary factor in the overall cost of therapy, drug administration labor costs (i.e., nursing and pharmacy) and the use of IV sets, piggyback bags, and infusion control devices must be included in the analysis. As a result, a drug that must be administered several times daily, such as intravenous penicillin, will incur increased administration costs compared with one, such as ceftriaxone, that requires once-a-day dosing.

Some drugs, such as aminoglycosides, are associated with increased laboratory costs (e.g., aminoglycoside serum concentrations, serum creatinine, audiometry) that are not required for other agents,[23] such as the third-generation cephalosporins and quinolones. Similarly, drugs with a high potential for misuse or toxicity can be associated with increased costs because of monitoring (e.g., medication use evaluation, pharmacokinetic monitoring). If meropenem with or without ciprofloxacin had been selected for R.G., this therapy would be expected to be associated with relatively few laboratory costs. However, the broad spectrum of activity[24] of these agents, potential for misuse, and development of resistance might, however, result in increased monitoring costs and overall cost to society.

Costs that are difficult to quantitate include those associated with failure of antimicrobial therapy and antimicrobial toxicity. Ineffective or toxic therapy can prolong hospitalization and may require expensive interventions, such as hemodialysis,[23] mechanical ventilation, and intensive care unit admission. The net effect of these latter costs can be significantly greater than the acquisition and administration costs of antimicrobial therapy.

In summary, determining the true cost of antimicrobial therapy is complex. Acquisition cost, IV bags, infusion controllers, and labor must be incorporated into the analysis. Although they are difficult to estimate, other costs, including antibiotic toxicity and failure of therapy, also should be included.

ROUTE OF ADMINISTRATION

CASE 60-1, QUESTION 10: The *Serratia* was determined to be susceptible to ciprofloxacin. Oral ciprofloxacin was considered for the treatment of R.G.'s presumed *Serratia* pneumonia, but the IV route was prescribed. Why is the oral administration of ciprofloxacin reasonable (or unreasonable) in R.G.?

The proper route of antibiotic administration depends on many factors, including the severity of infection, antimicrobial oral bioavailability, and other patient factors. In patients who appear "septic," blood flow often is shunted away from the mesentery and extremities, resulting in unreliable bioavailability from the gastrointestinal (GI) tract or muscles. Consequently, hemodynamically unstable patients should always receive antimicrobials by the IV route to ensure therapeutic antimicrobial levels. Furthermore, some drug interactions with oral agents can result in subtherapeutic serum concentrations (e.g., reduced bioavailability associated with concomitant quinolone and antacid administration and the decreased absorption of itraconazole with concurrent proton-pump inhibitor [PPI] therapy).

R.G. is clinically septic with a possible *Serratia* pneumonia. Considering his unstable state, the bioavailability of oral ciprofloxacin cannot be guaranteed; thus, he should be treated with IV antimicrobials.

ANTIMICROBIAL DOSING

CASE 60-1, QUESTION 11: What dose of IV ciprofloxacin should be given to R.G.? What factors must be taken into account in determining a proper antimicrobial dose?

The choice of dosing regimen is based on many factors. Table 60-9 provides a guide for the dosing of more commonly administered antimicrobials. Selection of the appropriate dosage should be based on evidence confirming the efficacy of the dosage in the treatment of a specific infection. Patient-specific factors, including weight, site of infection, and route of elimination, also must be considered in dosage selection. The patient's weight is important, particularly for agents with a low therapeutic index (e.g., aminoglycosides, imipenem, flucytosine); these drugs should be dosed on a milligram per kilogram per day basis. Other agents with a more favorable adverse effect profile, such as cephalosporins, are less likely to require weight-specific dosing in most disease states.

Site of Infection

Site of infection results in different dosage requirements. An uncomplicated urinary tract infection requires lower doses considering the high urinary drug concentrations that are achieved with most renally cleared agents. In contrast, a more serious upper urinary tract infection, such as pyelonephritis, requires increased doses to ensure therapeutic drug levels in tissue and in serum.

Anatomic and Physiologic Barriers

Anatomic and physiologic barriers also must be considered in evaluating a dosing regimen. For example, penetration into cerebrospinal fluid requires high doses to ensure adequate antimicrobial concentrations.[25] Vitreous humor[26] and the prostate gland[27] are additional sites in which therapeutic antimicrobial concentrations are more difficult to achieve.

Route of Elimination

Route of elimination must also be considered in the dosage calculation. In general, antimicrobials are eliminated renally or nonrenally (metabolic or biliary). Renal function can be estimated via 24-hour urine collection or with equations, such as the Cockcroft and Gault equation[28]:

$$\text{Creatinine clearance} = ([140 - \text{age}] \times [\text{weight in kg}])/(72 \times \text{SCr})$$

Several anti-infectives are eliminated renally (Table 60-9). Most β-lactams are eliminated by the kidney. In contrast, ceftriaxone and most antistaphylococcal penicillins (e.g., nafcillin, oxacillin, dicloxacillin) are eliminated both renally and nonrenally. Aminoglycosides, vancomycin, acyclovir, and ganciclovir are cleared primarily by the kidney. Thus, dosage adjustment is recommended for these drugs in patients with renal failure (Table 60-9). Because azithromycin, clindamycin, and metronidazole are primarily eliminated by the liver, no dose reduction is required in

TABLE 60-9

UCSF/Mt. Zion Medical Center Adult Antimicrobial Dosing Guidelines[a]

Approved by the Antibiotic Advisory Subcommittee and the Pharmacy and Therapeutics Committee 7/10
Department of Pharmaceutical Services

Drug	CrCl > 50 mL/min	CrCl 10–50 mL/min	CrCl < 10 mL/min (ESRD not on HD)	Dialysis (HD or CRRT)
Acyclovir	*Herpes simplex infections* 5 mg/kg/dose IV every 8 hours *HSV encephalitis/Herpes zoster* 10 mg/kg/dose IV every 8 hours	5 mg/kg/dose IV every 12–24 hours 10 mg/kg/dose IV every 12–24 hours	2.5 mg/kg IV every 24 hours 5 mg/kg IV every 24 hours	HD: 2.5 mg/kg IV ×1 now then 2.5 mg/kg every evening (give after HD on HD days) CRRT: 5 mg/kg every 24 hours HD: 5 mg/kg IV ×1 now then 5 mg/kg every evening (give after HD on HD days) CRRT: 5–10 mg/kg every 12–24 hours
Amphotericin B	0.6–1.0 mg/kg IV every 24 hours	No Change	No Change	No Change
Dosage reductions in renal disease unnecessary; however, due to the drug's nephrotoxicity, consider reducing the dose or holding the drug in the setting of a rising SCr.				
AmBisome	*Invasive mold infections* 3–5 mg/kg IV every 24 hours Doses up to 10mg/kg have been used for invasive mucormycosis *Invasive yeast infections* 3 mg/kg IV every 24 hours *Prophylaxis (heme-onc)* 1 mg/kg IV every 24 hours	No Change	No Change	No Change
Amikacin	≥60 mL/min 15–20 mg/kg/dose IV every 24 hours	See Below	See Below	
Consultation with ID/ID pharmacy recommended before use. Dose is based on ideal body weight (IBW) except in obese patients or those under their ideal body weight. Use actual body weight if patient weight is less than IBW. Use adjusted body weight (ABW) in patients who are obese. Amikacin is generally used as a second-line aminoglycoside because of its increased cost and need to send out levels. The total daily dose of amikacin can be administered as a single daily dose in patients with normal renal function (CrCl ≥60 mL/min). Patients with decreased renal function or abnormal body composition should have doses adjusted according to the recommendations below. Turnaround time on amikacin levels is usually 2–4 days. Peak levels are not useful with this dosing regimen; trough levels are recommended and should be <5 mg/L.				
	40–60 mL/min 5–7.5 mg/kg IV every 12 hours	20–40 mL/min 5 mg/kg IV every 12–24 hours	<20 mL/min 5 mg/kg loading dose *(Consult pharmacy for maintenance dose)*	HD: 5 mg/kg ×1, then 3 mg/kg IV after HD CRRT: 5 mg/kg ×1, then 3 mg/kg IV every 24 hours
With traditional dosing of amikacin, peak (20–30 mg/L) and trough (<8mg/L) levels are recommended in patients anticipated to receive aminoglycosides for severe gram-negative infection. Those patients with CrCl <60 mL/min, obesity, or increased fluid volume should be monitored with serum amikacin levels.				
Ampicillin	1–2 g IV every 4–6 hours	1–1.5 g IV every 6 hours	1 g IV every 8–12 hours	HD: 1–2 g IV every 12 hours CRRT: 1–2 g IV every 6 hours
Ampicillin/ sulbactam	1.5–3 g IV every 6 hours	1.5 g IV every 6–8 hours	1.5 g IV every 12 hours	HD: 1.5 g IV every 12 hours CRRT: 1.5 g IV every 6 hours
Aztreonam	2 g IV every 8 hours	2 g IV every 12 hours	1 g IV every 12 hours	HD: 1 g IV ×1 now then 1 g every evening (give after HD on HD days) CRRT: 2 g IV every 12 hours

(continued)

TABLE 60-9

UCSF/Mt. Zion Medical Center Adult Antimicrobial Dosing Guidelines[a] (*Continued*)

Drug	CrCl > 50 mL/min	CrCl 10–50 mL/min	CrCl <10 mL/min (ESRD not on HD)	Dialysis (HD or CRRT)
Cefazolin	1–2 g IV every 8 hours	1–2 g IV every 12 hours	1 g IV every 24 hours	HD: 2 g after HD only CRRT: 2 g IV every 12 hours
Caspofungin Severe hepatic dysfunction: 70 mg LD, then 35 mg IV daily	LD: 70 mg × 1, then 50 mg every 24 hours Increase maintenance dose to 70 mg when given with phenytoin, rifampin, carbamazapine, dexamethasone, nevirapine, efavirenz	No Change	No Change	No Change
Cefepime Febrile neutropenia, meningitis, pseudomonas infections, critically ill patients	>60 mL/min 2 g IV every 12 hours 2 g IV every 8 hours	30–60 mL/min: 2 g IV every 24 hours; 2 g IV every 12 hours 10–30 mL/min: 1 g IV every 24 hours; 2 g IV every 24 hours	<10 mL/min 500 mg IV every 24 hours 1 g IV every 24 hours	HD: 2 g after HD only CRRT: 2 g IV every 12 hours
Ceftazidime	2 g IV every 8 hours	2 g IV every 12–24 hours	0.5 g IV every 24 hours	HD: 1 g after HD only CRRT: 2 g IV every 12 hours
Ceftriaxone Meningitis: 2 g every 12 hours Endocarditis and osteomyelitis: 2 g every 24 hours	1 g IV every 24 hours	No Change	No Change	No Change
Ciprofloxacin[IV-PO] Pseudomonas infections	400 mg IV every 12 hours 500–750 mg PO every 12 hours 400 mg IV every 8 hours 750 mg PO every 12 hours	30–50 mL/min: No Change; No Change 10–30 mL/min: 200–400 mg IV every 12 hours; 250–500 mg PO every 12 hours	200 IV every 12 hours 250 mg PO every 12 hours	HD: 400 mg IV every 24 hours or 500 mg PO every 24 hours CRRT: 400 mg IV every 12 hours
Clindamycin	600–900 mg IV every 8 hours	No Change	No Change	No Change
Colistin Consultation with ID pharmacy recommended	2.5 mg/kg IV every 12 hours	2.5 mg/kg IV every 12–24 hours	1.5 mg/kg IV every 24 hours	HD: 1.5 mg/kg every 24 hours CRRT: 1.5 mg/kg every 24 hours
Daptomycin Dose on total body weight	4–10 mg/kg IV every 24 hours Dose depends on indication	<30 mL/min 4–10 mg/kg IV every 48 hours		HD: 4–10 mg/kg IV every 48 hours CRRT: 4–10 mg/kg IV every 48 hours
Doxycycline[IV-PO]	100 mg IV/PO every 12 hours	No Change	No Change	No Change
Ertapenem	1 g IV every 24 hours	<30 mL/min 500 mg IV every 24 hours		HD: 500 mg every 24 hours CRRT: 500 mg every 24 hours
Ethambutol	15–20 mg/kg PO every 24 hours	<30 mL/min 15–25 mg/kg three times per week		HD: 15–25 mg/kg three times per week (after HD) CRRT: 15–25 mg/kg three times per week

(continued)

TABLE 60-9
UCSF/Mt. Zion Medical Center Adult Antimicrobial Dosing Guidelines[a] *(Continued)*

Drug	CrCl > 50 mL/min	CrCl 10–50 mL/min	CrCl < 10 mL/min (ESRD not on HD)	Dialysis (HD or CRRT)
Fluconazole[IV-PO]	100–400 mg IV/PO every 24 hours	50–200 mg IV/PO every 24 hours	50–100 mg IV/PO every 24 hours	HD: 400 mg after HD only CRRT: 400–800 mg every 24 hours
Flucytosine (5FC)	25 mg/kg/dose PO every 6 hours	<u>25–50 mL/min</u> 25 mg/kg/dose PO every 12 hours <u>10–25 mL/min</u> 25 mg/kg/dose PO every 24 hours	12.5 mg/kg/dose PO every 24 hours	HD: 12.5–25 mg/kg PO every 24 hours CRRT: 12.5–37.5 mg/kg/dose PO every 12–24 hours
Ganciclovir	<u>>70 mL/min</u> 5 mg/kg/dose IV every 12 hours <u>50–69 mL/min</u> 2.5 mg/kg/dose IV every 12 hours	<u>25–49 mL/min</u> 2.5 mg/kg IV every 24 hours	<u>10–24 mL/min</u> 1.25 mg/kg IV every 24 hours	HD: 1.25 mg/kg after HD only CRRT: 2.5–5 mg/kg every 24 hours
Gentamicin	<u>≥60 mL/min</u> 5 mg/kg/dose IV every 24 hours	See Below See Below		
Dose is based on ideal body weight (IBW) except in obese patients or those under their ideal body weight. Use actual body weight if patient weight is less than IBW. Use adjusted body weight (ABW) in patients who are obese. The total daily dose of gentamicin can be administered as a single daily dose in patients with normal renal function (CrCl ≥60 mL/min). Peak levels are not useful in this regimen; however, trough levels are recommended and in most cases will be undetectable. Patients with decreased renal function or abnormal body composition should have doses adjusted according to the recommendations below.				
	Alternative: 1.6 mg/kg iv every 8 hours (total 5 mg/kg/day) for clinically tenuous patients or patients with changing volume status	<u>40–60 mL/min</u> 1.2–1.5 mg/kg IV every 12 hours <u>20–40 mL/min</u> 1.2–1.5 mg/kg IV every 12–24 hours	<u><20 mL/min</u> 2 mg/kg loading dose *(Consult pharmacy for maintenance dose)*	HD: 2 mg/kg ×1, then 1 mg/kg IV after HD CRRT: 2 mg/kg ×1, then 1.5 mg/kg IV every 24 hours
With traditional dosing of gentamicin, peak (5–8 mg/L) and trough (<2 mg/L) levels are recommended for patients receiving aminoglycosides for severe gram-negative infection. Lower doses (1 mg/kg/dose every 8 hours) are suggested when aminoglycosides are used synergistically in gram-positive infections. Those patients with CrCl <60 mL/min, obesity, or increased fluid volume should be monitored with serum gentamicin levels. Goals for gram-positive synergy dosing peak (3–4 mg/L) and trough (<1 mg/L)				
Imipenem	500 mg IV every 6–8 hours *max 50 mg/kg/d*	500 mg IV every 8 hours	<u><20 mL/min</u> 250–500 mg IV every 12 hours	HD: 250 mg IV every 12 hours CRRT: 500 mg IV every 8 hours
Isoniazid	300 mg PO every 24 hours	No Change	No Change	No Change
Levofloxacin[IV-PO] Nosocomial pneumonia/ Pseudomonas infections	250–500 mg IV/PO every 24 hours 750 mg IV/PO every 24 hours	500 mg ×1, then 250 mg IV/PO every 24 hours 750 mg ×1; then 750 IV/PO every 48 hours	500 mg ×1, then 250 mg IV/PO every 48 hours 750 mg ×1, then 500 mg IV/PO every 48 hours	HD: 500 mg ×1, then 250 mg every 48 hours CRRT: 500 mg ×1, then 250–500 mg every 24 hours
Linezolid[IV-PO]	600 mg IV/PO every 12 hours	No Change	No Change	No Change
Meropenem Meningitis/documented or suspected *Pseudomonas* infections or critically ill	0.5–1 g IV every 8 hours 2 g IV every 8 hours	<u>25–50 mL/min</u> 0.5–1 g IV every 12 hours 2 g IV every 12 hours <u>10–25 mL/min</u> 0.5 g IV every 12 hours 1 g IV every 12 hours	0.5 g IV every 24 hours 1 g IV every 24 hours	HD: 500 mg IV ×1 now then 500 mg every evening (give after HD on HD days) CRRT: 1 g IV every 12 hours
Metronidazole[IV-PO]	500 mg IV/PO every 8 hours	500 mg IV/PO every 8 hours	500 mg IV/PO every 12 hours ESRD not on HD	500 mg IV/PO every 8 hours
Moxifloxacin[IV-PO]	400 mg IV/PO every 24 hours	No Change	No Change	No Change
Nafcillin	1–2 g IV every 4–6 hours	No Change	No Change	No Change
Penicillin G	2–3 MU IV every 4–6 hours	1–2 MU IV every 4–6 hours	1 MU IV every 6 hours	HD: 1 MU IV every 6 hours CRRT: 2 MU IV every 4–6 hours

(continued)

TABLE 60-9
UCSF/Mt. Zion Medical Center Adult Antimicrobial Dosing Guidelines[a] (*Continued*)

Drug	CrCl > 50 mL/min	CrCl 10–50 mL/min	CrCl < 10 mL/min (ESRD not on HD)	Dialysis (HD or CRRT)
Pip/Tazo (Zosyn®) Documented/suspected *Pseudomonas* infections	3.375–4.5 g IV every 6–8 hours 4.5 g every 6 hours for ClCr >20 mL/min	3.375–4.5 g every 6–8 hours	2.25–3.375 g every 8 hours	HD: 2.25 g IV every 8 hours CRRT: 4.5 g IV every 8 hours or 3.375 g IV every 6 hours
Posaconazole Must be administered with high-fat meal or nutritional shake, i.e., Ensure	400 mg PO every 12 hours or 200 mg PO every 6 hours	No Change	No Change	No Change
Pyrazinamide	20–25 mg/kg/day PO every 24 hours	<30 mL/min 25–35 mg/kg three times per week		HD: 25–35 mg/kg three times per week after HD CRRT: 25–35 mg/kg three times per week
Rifampin Endocarditis Prosthetic infection	600 mg PO every 24 hours 300 mg PO every 8 hours 450 mg PO every 12 hours	No Change	No Change	No Change
Tigecycline Severe hepatic disease: 100 mg IV × 1, then 25 mg IV every 12 hours	100 mg IV × 1, then 50 mg IV every 12 hours	No Change	No Change	No Change
Tobramycin	See Gentamicin	See Gentamicin	See Gentamicin	See Gentamicin
TMP/SMX[IV-PO] When switching to oral therapy, consider that a single-strength tablet has 80 mg of TMP, a double-strength tablet 160 mg of TMP.	*Systemic GNR infections* 10 mg TMP/kg/d IV divided every 6–12 hours *Pneumocystis pneumonia* 15–20 mg TMP/kg/d IV divided every 6–12 hours	5–7.5 mg TMP/kg/d IV divided every 12–24 hours 10–15 mg TMP/kg/d IV divided every 12–24 hours	2.5–5.0 mg TMP/kg IV every 24 hours 5–10 mg TMP/kg IV every 24 hours	HD: 2.5–5 mg TMP/kg/d every 24 hours CRRT: 5–7.5mg TMP/kg/d divided every 12–24 hours
Voriconazole[IV-PO]	LD = 400 mg every 12 hours × 1 day, then 200 mg every 12 hours (PO)	No Change	No Change*	No Change*

PO should be used when possible, as oral bioavailability >95%. IV dose: LD = 6 mg/kg/dose every 12 hours × 1 day, then 4 mg/kg/dose every 12 hours. *The use of the IV formulation should be avoided in patients with CrCl <50 mL/min owing to accumulation of IV vehicle and is contraindicated in ESRD and hemodialysis. May require dose adjustment in hepatic dysfunction. ID approval required except for heme-onc and lung transplant services.

Drug	>60 mL/min	40–60 mL/min	20–40 mL/min	10–20 mL/min	<10 mL/min	Dialysis (HD or CRRT)
Vancomycin Uncomplicated infections Serious infections	10–15 mg/kg IV every 12 hours[1] 15–20 mg/kg IV every 8–12 hours[2]	10–15 mg/kg IV every 12–24 hours	5–10 mg/kg IV every 24 hours	5 –10 mg/kg IV every 24–48 hours	10–15 mg/kg IV loading dose ×1; redose according to serum levels	HD: 15–20 mg/kg load, then 500 mg IV after HD only CRRT: 10–15 mg/kg IV every 24 hours

Round dose to 250 mg, 500 mg, 750 mg, 1 g, 1.25 g, 1.5 g, 1.75 g, or 2 g (maximum 2 g/dose). Trough levels should be obtained within 30 minutes before fourth dose of a new regimen or dosage change. Vancomycin troughs are not recommended in patients in whom anticipated duration of therapy is ≤3 days.

[1]For patients with uncomplicated infections requiring vancomycin, trough levels of 10–15 mcg/mL are recommended.

[2]For patients with serious infections caused by MRSA (central nervous system infections, endocarditis, ventilator-associated pneumonia, bacteremia, or osteomyelitis), trough levels of 15–20 mcg/mL are recommended. ID CONSULT IS RECOMMENDED.

[a] Doses are those recommended for systemic infections commonly treated with these agents.

CrCl, creatinine clearance; CRRT, continuous renal replacement therapy (assumes an ultrafiltration rate of 2 L/h with continuous venovenous hemofiltration and an ultrafiltration rate of 1 L/h and dialysate flow rate of 1 L/h with continuous venovenous hemodiafiltration and residual native glomerular filtration rate <10 mL/min); ESRD, end-stage renal disease; HD, intermittent (high-flux) hemodialysis (when administering a daily dose with HD, the drug should be administered after the HD session); HSV, herpes simplex virus; IV, intravenous; IV-PO, high oral bioavailability (consider initiating with or switching to PO therapy when patient tolerating orals); LD, loading dose; MRSA, methicillin-resistant *Staphylococcus aureus*; PO, by mouth; SCr, serum creatinine.

Estimate of renal function using Cockcroft and Gault equation: $\text{CrCl (mL/min)} = \dfrac{(140 - \text{age}) \times \text{Wt (kg)}}{72 \times \text{SCr (mg/dL)}}$ (for females multiply by 0.85)

Ideal body weight equation: Males : IBW = 50 kg + 2.3 kg for each inch over 5 feet.
Females : IBW = 45.5 kg + 2.3 kg for each inch over 5 feet.

Adjusted body weight: ABW = IBW + 0.4 (actual weight − IBW).

renal failure for these agents. Using the Cockcroft and Gault equation, R.G.'s age (63 years), weight (70 kg) and current serum creatinine (3.8 mg/dL) results in a calculated creatinine clearance of 14 mL/minute. R.G. normally would be given an IV dosage of ciprofloxacin at 400 mg every 12 hours. His increasing creatinine, however, suggests that his dosage should be decreased to 200 to 300 mg every 12 hours.

Although renal function can be approximated with the use of the Cockcroft and Gault equation (or a similar equation), hepatic function is more difficult to evaluate. No standard liver function test (AST, ALT, alkaline phosphatase) has been demonstrated to correlate well with hepatic drug clearance. Some tests, such as PT, INR, and albumin, are markers of hepatic function, but even these tests do not clearly predict drug clearance. Patients receiving hemodialysis or continuous hemofiltration provide additional dosing challenges. Table 60-9 provides dosing recommendations in patients receiving hemodialysis or continuous hemofiltration.

Patient Age

It is important to note that most dosing information is derived from a younger, relatively healthy patient population. It is clear that the very young and the elderly have a decreased ability to clear drugs; thus, dosage requirements for many agents are likely to be decreased in neonatal and geriatric patients.

Fever and Inoculum Effect

The impact of other factors on the selection of an antimicrobial dose is less clear. Fever increases and decreases blood flow to mesenteric, hepatic, and renal organ systems[29] and can either increase or decrease drug clearance. Inoculum effect has taken place when higher concentrations of a bacterial inoculum result in an increase in the MIC.[30] As an example, piperacillin may demonstrate an MIC of 8.0 mcg/mL against *P. aeruginosa* at a concentration of 10^5 colony-forming units/mL (CFU/mL); however, at 10^9 CFU/mL, the MIC may increase to 32 to 64 mcg/mL. This phenomenon is well recognized, particularly with β-lactamase–producing bacteria treated with β-lactam antimicrobials. The more stable the antimicrobial is to β-lactamase, the less the influence of the inoculum effect. Aminoglycosides, quinolones, and imipenem appear to be less affected by the inoculum effect than β-lactams. The inoculum effect probably is most relevant in the treatment of a bacterial abscess, in which extremely high concentrations of bacteria would be expected. As a result, antimicrobials that are more susceptible to the inoculum effect may require increased drug dosages for optimal outcome in the treatment of abscesses.

PHARMACOKINETICS AND PHARMACODYNAMICS

CASE 60-1, QUESTION 12: R.G.'s respiratory status remains unchanged; thus, the ciprofloxacin is discontinued and cefotaxime and gentamicin are started empirically. The use of a constant IV infusion of cefotaxime is being considered in R.G. In addition, the use of single daily dosing of gentamicin is being discussed. What is the rationale for these approaches, and would either be advantageous for R.G.?

β-Lactams, such as cefotaxime, are not associated with increased bacterial killing with increasing drug concentrations. Pharmacodynamic activity with β-lactams best correlates with the duration of time that antimicrobial levels are maintained above the MIC.[31] The animal model suggests that β-lactam antimicrobials should be dosed such that their serum levels exceed the MIC of the pathogen as long as possible.[31] This observation appears to be most important in the neutropenic model, in which the use of a constant infusion more reliably inhibits bacterial growth compared with traditional intermittent dosing. An additional benefit of the use of constant infusions of β-lactams is that smaller daily doses appear to be as effective as higher doses administered intermittently. Other than this latter outcome, it is unclear, however, whether constant infusions have any distinct advantages or disadvantages compared with usual dosing of β-lactams. The efficacy of quinolone antimicrobials appears to correlate with the peak plasma concentration to MIC ratio or area under the curve (AUC) to MIC ratio.[31] In light of this pharmacodynamic principle, it is possible that ciprofloxacin was underdosed in this patient, contributing to the therapeutic failure, particularly if the MIC was in the upper range of susceptibility for this agent.

Aminoglycosides traditionally have been administered every 8 to 12 hours to achieve peak serum gentamicin levels of 5 to 8 g/mL to ensure efficacy in the treatment of serious gram-negative infection.[32,33] Gentamicin troughs of greater than 2 mcg/mL have been associated with an increased risk for nephrotoxicity.[33,34] These studies attempting to correlate efficacy and toxicity with serum levels and the association of peaks or troughs with clinical outcomes have been questioned.[21] Vancomycin troughs of 5 to 10 mcg/mL have been traditionally recommended[35,36]; however, more recent recommendations suggest higher troughs (10 to 20 mcg/mL) depending on the site of infection and severity of illness.[37]

Several antimicrobials (e.g., aminoglycosides) have been associated with a pharmacodynamic phenomenon known as a postantibiotic effect (PAE). PAE is delayed regrowth of bacteria after exposure to an antibiotic[31,38] (i.e., continued suppression of normal growth in the absence of antibiotic levels above the MIC of the organism). As an example, if *P. aeruginosa* is cultured in broth, it will multiply to a concentration of 10^9 CFU/mL. If piperacillin is added in a concentration above the MIC for the organism, a reduction in the bacterial concentration is observed. When piperacillin is removed from the broth, immediate bacterial growth takes place. As described, a β-lactam antibiotic should be present in concentrations above the MIC to optimize its time-dependent killing. If the above experiment is repeated with gentamicin, a reduction in bacterial CFU is observed. In contrast to that observed with β-lactam antibiotics, if the gentamicin is removed from the system, a lag period of 2 to 6 hours takes place before characteristic bacterial growth occurs. This lag period is defined as the PAE. A PAE also has been observed with quinolones and imipenem against gram-negative organisms. Although most β-lactam antibiotics, such as antipseudomonal penicillins or cephalosporins, do not exhibit PAE with gram-negative organisms, PAE has been demonstrated with β-lactam with gram-positive pathogens such as *S. aureus*.

Once-Daily Dosing of Aminoglycosides

As a result of PAE and other pharmacodynamic factors, certain antimicrobials may be dosed less frequently. The greatest clinical experience has been with the aminoglycosides in the treatment of gram-negative infection.[39,40] Earlier data suggested that the maximal aminoglycoside peak level to MIC ratio correlates well with clinical response. Thus, the higher the achievable peak, the greater likelihood of a favorable outcome. Consequently, greater, less frequent doses of aminoglycosides should work at least as well as the more traditional lower, more frequent doses. Once-daily dosing of aminoglycosides in the treatment of gram-negative infection is as efficacious as traditional multiple daily dosing.[21]

Single daily dosing of aminoglycosides has been investigated primarily in patients with normal renal function, and few critically ill patients have been treated with this nontraditional regimen. Thus, patients in septic shock are less clear candidates for once-daily dosing. The utility and proper timing of serum aminoglycoside concentrations and association with clinical outcomes are debatable with nontraditional once-daily aminoglycosides.

In summary, the use of a constant IV infusion of cefotaxime is possible in R.G., but the benefit of this mode of administration is not clear. Considering the severity of R.G.'s infection and his elevated serum creatinine level, he is not a candidate for single daily dosing of aminoglycosides (i.e., 5 to 6 mg/kg every 24 hours). Independent of the aminoglycoside-associated PAE, his current renal function requires a reduced gentamicin dose to treat his infection.

Antimicrobial Protein Binding

CASE 60-1, QUESTION 13: Ceftriaxone (Rocephin), rather than cefotaxime (Claforan), is being considered for the treatment of R.G.'s infection. Ceftriaxone is more highly protein bound than cefotaxime. Why is protein binding important in the selection of therapy?

Free (i.e., unbound) rather than total drug levels are best correlated with antimicrobial activity,[41] and the degree of protein binding may have important clinical consequences in some patients. Chambers et al.[42] reported treatment failures with the highly protein-bound cefonicid (98% protein bound) in patients with endocarditis caused by *S. aureus.* Despite achievable serum drug concentrations well above the MIC of the organism, breakthrough bacteremia occurred in three of four patients. Although total drug concentrations greatly exceeded the MIC of the pathogen, free concentrations were consistently below the level necessary to inhibit bacterial growth. Similar experiences have been reported with daptomycin (90% to 93% protein bound).[43] Thus, clinical cure appears to be more likely if unbound antibiotic concentrations exceed the MIC of the infecting organism. Although ceftriaxone is 85% to 90% protein bound, the free concentrations probably remain far above the MIC of the *Serratia*. Therefore, protein-binding considerations are unlikely to be important in the treatment of R.G.'s infection.

ANTIMICROBIAL FAILURE

ONLINE CONTENT

For a narrated PowerPoint presentation on antimicrobial failure, go to http://thepoint.lww.com/AT10e.

Antibiotic-Specific Factors

CASE 60-1, QUESTION 14: Despite "appropriate" treatment, R.G. is unresponsive to antimicrobial therapy. What antibiotic-specific factors may contribute to "antimicrobial failure"?

Antimicrobials may fail for various reasons, including patient-specific host factors, drug or dosage selection, and concomitant disease states. One of the most common reasons for antimicrobial failure is drug resistance.[44–46] Several clinically important pathogens have been associated with emergence of resistance during the past decade, including *M. tuberculosis,*[47] enterococci,[48] gram-negative rods,[44] *S. aureus,*[49] *S. pneumoniae,*[50] and others. Of particular concern is the isolation of glycopeptide-resistant *S. aureus*[49] and multiresistant *Acinetobacter* and *Pseudomonas.*[51] Development of resistance during therapy, although less common than initial intrinsic resistance, may also account for failure to respond to therapy. Organisms that produce extended-spectrum (ESBL) or amp C β-lactamases may be unresponsive to β-lactam therapy despite associated in vitro susceptibility.[52]

Superinfection also may play a role in the unsuccessful treatment of infection. Superinfection has taken place when a new pathogen resistant to the current antimicrobial regimen is isolated. If R.G.'s ceftriaxone-treated *Serratia* pneumonia subsequently worsens and a tracheal aspirate returns positive for *P. aeruginosa,* then supercolonization and, perhaps, superinfection have occurred.

Combination Therapy

Most infections can be treated with monotherapy (e.g., an *E. coli* wound infection is treatable with a cephalosporin). Some infections, however, require two-drug therapy, including most cases of enterococcal endocarditis and perhaps certain *P. aeruginosa* infections. Hilf et al.[53] studied 200 consecutive patients with *P. aeruginosa* bacteremia and demonstrated a 47% mortality in those receiving monotherapy (antipseudomonal β-lactam or aminoglycoside) versus 27% in those in whom two-drug therapy was used. Thus, monotherapy appeared to contribute to antimicrobial failure in this specific study.

In contrast to the findings of the previous trial, more current investigations do not support the use of two drugs over monotherapy in the treatment of serious gram-negative infection, including *P. aeruginosa.*[54–56] An exception to this rule is bacteremia caused by *P. aeruginosa* in neutropenic patients.

If two antimicrobials are used in the treatment of infection, one of three sequelae will result: indifference, synergism, or antagonism.[57] Indifference occurs when the antimicrobial effect of drug A plus that of drug B equals the anticipated sum activity of the two drugs. Although numerous definitions exist, synergism generally occurs when the addition of drug A to drug B results in a total antibiotic activity greater than the expected sum of the two agents. Antagonism occurs if the addition of drug A to drug B results in a combined activity less than the sum of drug A plus drug B. An example of antagonism is the combination of imipenem with a less β-lactamase–stable β-lactam, such as piperacillin.[58] If *P. aeruginosa* is exposed to imipenem and piperacillin, the imipenem induces the organism to produce increased β-lactamase. Imipenem is remarkably β-lactamase stable, and is not degraded by this β-lactamase. In direct contrast, piperacillin is easily degraded by the β-lactamase. Thus, imipenem antagonized the effectiveness of piperacillin. Antagonism is not unique to antibacterials; itraconazole may antagonize amphotericin B in the treatment of certain fungal infections.[59]

Pharmacologic Factors

CASE 60-1, QUESTION 15: What pharmacologic or pharmaceutic factors may be implicated in failure of therapy?

Subtherapeutic dosing regimens are commonplace, particularly for agents with a low therapeutic index, such as the aminoglycosides. For example, a serious gram-negative pneumonia may not respond to aminoglycoside therapy if the achievable peak gentamicin serum levels are only 3 to 4 mcg/mL.[21,32] Considering that only 20% to 30% of the aminoglycoside penetrates from serum into bronchial secretions, only 0.5 to 1.0 mcg/mL may exist at the site of infection,[60] a level that may be inadequate to treat pneumonia. Another example of dosing contributing to antimicrobial failure centers on the use of loading doses. Aminoglycosides or vancomycin should be intiated with a loading dose, particulary in patients with renal failure. If the clinician neglects to use a loading dose, it may take several days before a therapeutic level is achieved. As described previously, yet another reason for subtherapeutic antimicrobial levels and potential drug failure is reduced oral absorption secondary to drug interactions (e.g., concomitant oral ciprofloxacin with antacids or iron).

An emerging problem relates to the use of vancomycin in the treatment of serious methicillin-resistant *S. aureus* infection (MRSA). By CLSI standards, an isolate of MRSA with an MIC of 2 mcg/mL is considered susceptible. Retrospective analyses have, however, demonstrated a high failure rate associated with vancomycin in the treatment of MRSA isolates with an MIC of 2 mcg/mL.[37,61,62] Hidayat et al.[61] observed that an MIC of 2 mcg/mL was associated with a decreased likelihood of vancomycin response. Unfortunately, achievement of therapeutic to supratherapeutic vancomycin trough levels did not improve efficacy. Similarly, in another retrospective analysis of MRSA bacteremia, investigators noted that a vancomycin MIC of 2 mcg/mL was an independent risk factor for increased mortality.[62] The pharmacodynamic parameter that serves as the best predictor of vancomycin activity against *S. aureus* is the AUC to MIC ratio, with a value greater than 350 independently associated with success. The probability of attaining this value with isolates with an MIC of 2 mcg/mL is 0%, even when achieving vancomycin trough concentrations of 15 mcg/mL.[63]

The infection site also potentially contributes to antimicrobial failure. Most antimicrobials concentrate in the urine, resulting in therapeutic levels even with low doses. In some infections, such as meningitis, prostatitis, and endophthalmitis, antimicrobial penetration to the site of infection may be inadequate. Agents that penetrate well into these sites are associated with a more favorable outcome.

Another potential reason for antimicrobial failure is inadequate therapy duration. A woman with a first-time uncomplicated cystitis may respond adequately to a 3-day course of an antibiotic. In contrast, patients with recurrent urinary tract infections are not candidates for this short course of therapy, however, and failure would be expected with only 3 days of therapy.

Host Factors

CASE 60-1, QUESTION 16: What host factors may contribute to the failure of antimicrobial therapy?

Several host factors may limit the ability of an antibiotic to cure infection. Infection of prosthetic material (e.g., IV catheters, orthopaedic prostheses, mechanical cardiac valves, and vascular grafts) is difficult to eradicate without removal of the hardware. In most cases, surgical intervention is necessary. To treat R.G.'s IV catheter infection adequately, removal of his central intravenous catheter would be optimal. Similar to removal of prostheses, large undrained abscesses are difficult, if not impossible, to treat with antimicrobial therapy. These infections generally require surgical drainage for successful outcome.

Diabetic foot ulcer cellulitis may not respond adequately to antimicrobial therapy. Reasons for antimicrobial failure in patients with diabetes include poor wound healing and reduced delivery of antibiotics to the infection site.

Immune status, particularly neutropenia or lymphocytopenia, also affects the outcome in the treatment of infection. Profoundly neutropenic patients with disseminated *Aspergillus* infections are unlikely to respond to even the most appropriate antifungal therapy. Similarly, patients with AIDS who have low CD4 lymphocyte counts cannot eradicate various infections, including those caused by cytomegalovirus, atypical mycobacteria, and cryptococci.

Once these factors have been eliminated as causes for antimicrobial failure, noninfectious sources must be ruled out. As discussed, malignancy, autoimmune disease, drug fever, and other diseases must be evaluated.

CASE 60-1, QUESTION 17: Other than initiation of adequate antimicrobial therapy, what adjunct measures can be considered in this patient with septic shock?

The 2008 Surviving Sepsis Campaign: International Guidelines for Management of Severe Sepsis and Septic Shock consultants developed key recommendations toward the early goal-directed resuscitation of the septic patient.[64] Key recommended adjuncts include administration of broad-spectrum antibiotics within 1 hour of diagnosis of septic shock, administration of either crystalloid or colloid fluid resuscitation, and norepinephrine or dopamine to maintain mean arterial pressure of at least 65 mm Hg. In addition, stress-dose steroid therapy can be given to those patients whose blood pressure is poorly responsive to fluid resuscitation and vasopressors. Recombinant activated protein C (rhAPC) is controversial, but may be considered in those patients at high risk of death as documented by Acute Physiology and Chronic Health Evaluation (APACHE) II scores of 25 or greater or with multiple-organ failure; however, those patients with severe sepsis and low risk of death, as measured by APACHE II scores of less than 25 or single-organ failure should not receive rhAPC.[65] Contraindications, including recent major surgery and other bleeding disorders, must also be evaluated before administering rhAPC. Other adjuncts include targeting lower blood glucose levels, stress ulcer prophylaxis, and prevention of deep vein thrombosis in septic patients.[64]

KEY REFERENCES AND WEBSITES

A full list of references for this chapter can be found at http://thepoint.lww.com/AT10e. Below are the key references and websites for this chapter, with the corresponding reference number in this chapter found in parentheses after the reference.

Key References

Boucher HW, Talbot GH, Bradley JS et al. Bad bugs, no drugs: No ESKAPE! An update from the Infectious Diseases Society of America. *Clin Infect Dis.* 2009;48(1):1. (44)

Cantón E et al. Trends in antifungal susceptibility testing using CLSI reference and commercial methods. *Expert Rev Anti Infect Ther.* 2009;7(1):107. (19)

Czock D et al. Pharmacokinetics and pharmacodynamics of antimicrobial drugs. *Expert Opin Drug Metab Toxicol.* 2009;5(5):475. (31)

Dellinger RP et al. Surviving sepsis campaign: international guidelines for management of severe sepsis and septic shock [published correction appears in *Crit Care Med.* 2008;36(4):1394–1396]. *Crit Care Med.* 2008;36(1):296. (64)

Drusano GL et al. Back to the future: using aminoglycosides again and how to dose them optimally. *Clin Infect Dis.* 2007;45(6):753. (21)

Giamarellou H, Poulakou G. Multidrug-resistant gram-negative infections: what are the treatment options? *Drugs.* 2009; 69(14):1879. (45)

Hooton TM et al. Diagnosis, prevention, and treatment of catheter-associated urinary tract infection in adults: 2009 International Clinical Practice Guidelines from the Infectious Diseases Society of America. *Clin Infect Dis.* 2010;50(5):625. (12)

López-Cabezas C et al. Antibiotics in endophthalmitis: microbiological and pharmacokinetic considerations. *Curr Clin Pharmacol.* 2010;5(1):47. (26)

Mandell LA et al. Infectious Diseases Society of America/American Thoracic Society consensus guidelines on the management of community-acquired pneumonia in adults. *Clin Infect Dis.* 2007;44(Suppl 2):S27. (15)

Rybak MJ et al. Vancomycin therapeutic guidelines: a summary of consensus recommendations from the infectious diseases Society of America, the American Society of Health-System Pharmacists, and the Society of Infectious Diseases Pharmacists. *Clin Infect Dis.* 2009;49(3):325. (37)

Solomkin JS et al. Diagnosis and management of complicated intra-abdominal infection in adults and children: guidelines by the Surgical Infection Society and the Infectious Diseases Society of America [published correction appears in *Clin Infect Dis.* 2010;50(12):1695]. *Clin Infect Dis.* 2010;50(2):133. (13)

Vincent JL, Martinez EO, Silva E. Evolving concepts in sepsis definitions. *Crit Care Clin.* 2009;25(4):665, vii. (1)

Weisfelt M et al. Bacterial meningitis: a review of effective pharmacotherapy. *Expert Opin Pharmacother.* 2007;8(10):1493. (25)

Yang K, Guglielmo BJ. Diagnosis and treatment of extended-spectrum and AmpC ß-lactamase-producing organisms. *Ann Pharmacother.* 2007;41(9):1427. (52)

61

Antimicrobial Prophylaxis for Surgical Procedures

Daniel J. G. Thirion

CORE PRINCIPLES

		CHAPTER CASES
1	Surgical antibiotic prophylaxis is indicated for patients at high risk of infection or in those at high risk of complications from postoperative infection.	**Case 61-1 (Question 1), Case 61-3 (Question 1)**
2	The choice of agent is based on the most likely pathogen associated with the surgical site infection that may occur.	**Case 61-1 (Question 2), Case 61-5 (Questions 1, 2), Case 61-7 (Question 1)**
3	To maximize the benefit of prophylaxis, antibiotics should be given within 1 hour before incision to achieve adequate drug levels at the surgical site.	**Case 61-1 (Question 3), Case 61-4 (Question 1)**
4	Antimicrobials with shorter half-lives may require administration of an additional intraoperative dose in prolonged surgical cases.	**Case 61-1 (Question 4)**
5	Single-dose preoperative prophylaxis is sufficient for most surgical procedures.	**Case 61-2 (Questions 1, 2), Case 61-4 (Question 1)**
6	Continuation of postoperative prophylaxis for up to 48 hours in cardiac surgery has been recommended by some professional organizations.	**Case 61-3 (Question 1)**
7	Continuation of prophylaxis beyond these time frames is not associated with improved outcomes and increases the risk of superinfections, emergence of resistance, adverse effects, and cost.	**Case 61-7 (Question 2)**
8	Surgical site infections are classified as superficial or deep incisional and usually occur within 30 days after the surgical procedure. Deep organ or space infections can occur up to several months after surgery and up to a year after implantation of prosthetic material.	**Case 61-4 (Question 2)**
9	Continuous quality improvement is critical in the prevention of surgical infection and should be overseen by a multidisciplinary team.	

Surgical site infection occurs when a pathogenic organism multiplies in a surgical wound leading to local and sometimes systemic signs and symptoms. Infections complicate surgical procedures in about 1% to 5% of cases, depending on the surgical procedure and the patient.[1,2] Surgical site infections increase morbidity, extend the duration of hospitalization,[3] and are associated with an annual cost of up to $1.6 billion for the estimated 26.6 million inpatient surgical procedures performed annually in the United States.[2,4]

Prophylactic antibiotics are widely used in surgical procedures and account for substantial antibiotic use in many hospitals.[5] The purpose of surgical antibiotic prophylaxis is to reduce the prevalence of postoperative wound infection at or around the surgical site.[6] Appropriate use of prophylactic antimicrobial agents results in decreased patient morbidity and hospitalization costs for many surgical procedures. However, the benefits of prophylaxis are controversial and not justified for some surgical procedures (e.g., urologic operations in patients with sterile urine).[7] Consequently, inappropriate or indiscriminate use of prophylactic antibiotics increases the risk of drug toxicity, the risk of superinfections, the selection of resistant organisms, and costs.[8,9]

RISK FACTORS FOR INFECTION

The likelihood for development of postoperative site infection is related to the degree of bacterial contamination during surgery, the virulence of the infecting organism, and host defenses. Risk factors for postoperative site infection can be classified according to procedure-specific factors and patient characteristics.[10–13]

TABLE 61-1
National Research Council Wound Classification

Classification	Criteria	Infection Rate (%)
Clean	No acute inflammation or entry into GI, respiratory, GU, or biliary tracts; no break in aseptic technique occurs; wounds primarily closed	>5
Clean-contaminated	Elective, controlled opening of GI, respiratory, biliary, or GU tracts without significant spillage; clean wounds with major break in sterile technique	>10
Contaminated	Penetrating trauma (>4 hours old); major technique break or major spillage from GI tract; acute, nonpurulent inflammation	15–20
Dirty	Penetrating trauma (<4 hours old); purulence or abscess (active infectious process); preoperative perforation of viscera	30–40

GI, gastrointestinal; GU, genitourinary.
Adapted with permission from Berard F, Gandon J. Postoperative wound infections: the influence of ultraviolet irradiation of the operating room and of various other factors. *Ann Surg.* 1964;160(Suppl 2):1.

Bacterial contamination can occur from exogenous sources (e.g., the operative team, instruments, airborne organisms) or from endogenous sources (e.g., the patient's microflora of the skin, respiratory, genitourinary, or gastrointestinal [GI] tract).[10] Infection control procedures to minimize all sources of bacterial contamination, including patient and surgical team preparation, operative technique, and incision care, are compiled in Centers for Disease Control and Prevention guidelines for surgical site infection.[14]

The risk of postoperative wound infection is influenced by host factors, such as extremes of age, obesity, tobacco use, malnutrition, and comorbid states, including diabetes mellitus, glycemic control in diabetic patients, remote infection, ischemia, oxygenation and body temperature during the procedure, colonization with microorganisms, and immunosuppressive therapy.[7,15] In addition, the longer the surgical procedure, the greater the likelihood of developing a postoperative wound infection, presumably because of the greater amount of bacterial contamination occurring as a function of time.[7]

Measuring and predicting risk of infection determines which patients benefit from antibiotic prophylaxis. The Centers for Disease Control and Prevention Study on the Efficacy of Nosocomial Infection Control (SENIC) developed an index that included the level of wound contamination and three other criteria based on procedure-related and patient-related factors.[12] Modification of this tool has led to the National Nosocomial Infection Surveillance system (NNIS) risk index that takes into account the patient's preoperative assessment (American Anesthesiology Assessment)[16], the level of contamination of the procedure, the duration of the procedure, and the use of a laparoscope.[17] This last criterion was added because of the associated decreased incidence of infection with the introduction of laparoscopic procedures. Indexes like these are particularly useful for comparison of performance among institutions and public reporting.

Based on these risk factors for infection, the decision whether a given patient should receive antimicrobial prophylaxis depends on a number of factors. Antimicrobial prophylaxis should be given for surgical procedures (a) with a high rate of infection, (b) involving the implantation of prosthetic materials, or (c) in which an infection would have catastrophic consequences.[7] A widely used surgical wound classification system to assist in this decision-making process follows.

CLASSIFICATION OF SURGICAL SITE INFECTIONS

From 1960 to 1964, the National Academy of Sciences National Research Council conducted a landmark study of surgical site infections and formulated a widely used standard classification based on the risk of intraoperative bacterial contamination (Table 61-1).[18] Current recommendations for surgical prophylaxis pertain to clean surgeries involving implantation of prosthetic material, clean-contaminated surgeries, and select contaminated wounds. Antimicrobial therapy for most contaminated and all dirty surgeries in which infection already is established is considered treatment instead of prophylaxis and is not discussed further in this chapter. Table 61-2 lists suspected pathogens and recommendations for site-specific prophylactic antimicrobial regimens; a detailed examination of clinical trials supporting these recommendations is presented elsewhere.[19,20]

PRINCIPLES OF SURGICAL ANTIMICROBIAL PROPHYLAXIS

ONLINE CONTENT

For a PowerPoint presentation on evaluating an antibiotic prophylaxis regimen, go to http://thepoint.lww.com/AT10e.

Decision to Use Antimicrobial Prophylaxis

CASE 61-1

QUESTION 1: M.R., a 72-year-old woman, is admitted to the hospital with severe abdominal pain, nausea and vomiting, and temperature of 39.3°C. A diagnosis of acute cholecystitis is made, and M.R. is scheduled for biliary tract surgery (cholecystectomy). Why is antimicrobial prophylaxis warranted for M.R.?

Biliary tract surgery is considered a clean-contaminated procedure and, therefore, carries a risk of surgical wound infection approaching 10% (Tables 61-1, 61-2). Prophylaxis for biliary tract surgery is limited to high-risk procedures, which include obesity, age older than 70 years, diabetes mellitus, acute cholecystitis, obstructive jaundice, or common duct stones.[7,20] Prophylaxis is not recommended for low-risk procedures such as elective laparoscopic cholecystectomy. Thus, prophylaxis is warranted in M.R., who falls into at least two high-risk categories (age older than 70 years and acute cholecystitis).

TABLE 61-2
Suggested Prophylactic Antimicrobial Regimens for Surgical Procedures

Procedure	Predominant Organism(s)	Antibiotic Regimen (Alternative)	Adult Preoperative IV Dose (Alternative)
Clean			
Neurosurgery	*Staphylococcus aureus, Staphylococcus epidermidis*	Cefazolin (vancomycin[b])	1–2[a] g (1 g)
Cardiac (all with sternotomy, cardiopulmonary bypass, pacemaker and automated defibrillator placement)	*S. aureus, S. epidermidis*	Cefazolin (vancomycin[b])	1–2[a] g (1 g)
Thoracic	*S. aureus, S. epidermidis,* gram-negative enterics	Cefazolin (vancomycin[b])	1–2[a] g (1 g)
Vascular (aortic resection, groin incision, prosthesis)	*S. aureus, S. epidermidis,* gram-negative enterics	Cefazolin (vancomycin[b])	1–2[a] g (1 g)
Orthopedic (total joint replacement, internal fixation of fractures)	*S. aureus, S. epidermidis*	Cefazolin (vancomycin[b])	1–2[a] g (1 g)
Clean-Contaminated			
Head and neck (involving incisions through mucosa)	*S. aureus,* oral anaerobes, streptococci	Cefazolin (clindamycin-gentamicin)	2 g (600 mg clindamycin-1.5 mg/kg gentamicin)
Gastroduodenal (only for procedures entering the stomach)	Gram-negative enterics, *S. aureus,* mouth flora	Cefazolin	1–2[a] g
Appendectomy (uncomplicated)	Gram-negative enterics, anaerobes (*B. fragilis*), enterococci	Cefoxitin	1–2 g
Biliary tract (only for high-risk procedures)	Gram-negative enterics, *Enterococcus faecalis, Clostridia*	Cefazolin	1–2[a] g
Colorectal	Gram-negative enterics, anaerobes (*Bacteroides fragilis*), enterococci	Oral neomycin-erythromycin base (IV cefoxitin)	1 g each at 1 PM, 2 PM, and 11 PM day before surgery (1 g)
Cesarean section	Group B streptococci, enterococci, anaerobes, gram-negative enterics	Cefazolin	2 g before umbilical cord clamped
Hysterectomy	Group B streptococci, enterococci, anaerobes, gram-negative enterics	Cefazolin or cefoxitin	1–2[a] g
Abortion (only for high-risk in first trimester)	Group B streptococci, enterococci, anaerobes, gram-negative enterics	Aqueous penicillin G (doxycycline) (first trimester)	2 million units (100 mg PO before and 200 mg PO after)
		Cefazolin (second trimester)	1–2[a] g
Genitourinary (only for high-risk procedures)	Gram-negative enterics, enterococci	Ciprofloxacin[b]	400 mg

[a] Cefazolin should be dosed at 2 g in patients weighing more than 80 kg.
[b] Vancomycin and ciprofloxacin require longer infusion times and should be administered within 2 hours before surgery.

CASE 61-1, QUESTION 2: An order for intravenous (IV) cefazolin 1 g on call to the operating room (OR) is written for M.R. Why is this an appropriate (or inappropriate) antibiotic selection?

The selected prophylactic agent should be directed against likely infecting organisms (Table 61-2), but need not eradicate every potential pathogen. Cefazolin has been proved effective for most surgical procedures, including biliary tract surgery, given that the goal of prophylaxis is to decrease bacterial counts below critical levels necessary to cause infection. Broad-spectrum agents, such as third-generation cephalosporins, should be avoided for prophylaxis because they are no more effective than cefazolin and may alter microbial flora, increasing the emergence of microbial resistance to these otherwise valuable agents.

Timing of Antimicrobial Administration

CASE 61-1, QUESTION 3: Why is the administration time for this antimicrobial appropriate (or inappropriate) for M.R.?

Classic animal studies conducted by Burke[21] and others[22] clearly demonstrated the need for therapeutic antibiotic concentrations in the bloodstream and in vulnerable tissue at the time of wound contamination. Bacteria were most likely to enter the tissue beginning with the initial surgical incision and continuing until the wound was closed; antibiotics administered more than 3 hours after bacterial contamination were ineffective in decreasing the rate of wound infection.[21,22] This 2- to 3-hour period after the surgical incision was deemed the "effective" or "decisive" period for prophylaxis, when the animal's wound was most susceptible to the beneficial effects of the antibiotic. This decisive period for administration of prophylactic antibiotics has been confirmed in humans.[23–25]

For maximal efficacy, an antibiotic should be present in therapeutic concentrations at the incision site as early as possible during the decisive period and continuing until the wound is closed. Because an antibiotic administered postoperatively cannot achieve therapeutic concentrations during the decisive period, postoperative administration does not prevent postoperative wound infections, and infection rates are similar to those in patients who receive no antibiotics.[24]

Consequently, prophylactic antibiotics should be administered before the surgical procedure in the operative suite.[19]

Prophylactic antibiotics are most effective when given within the 1-hour window before surgical incision; rates of infection increase significantly if antibiotics are administered more than 1 hour before incision or postoperatively.[26,27] If a tourniquet is required to control blood flow to a limb during surgery, then the entire antibiotic dose should be administered before inflation of the tourniquet.

The "on-call" prescribing practice for surgical prophylaxis, as with M.R., has fallen into disfavor because the time between antibiotic administration and the actual incision may exceed 1 hour. This delay may result in subtherapeutic antibiotic concentrations during the decisive period.[19,28] M.R.'s cefazolin should be ordered preoperatively and should be administered in the OR within 1 hour of the surgical incision.

CASE 61-1, QUESTION 4: Will M.R. require a second dose of cefazolin during the surgical procedure?

The duration of the surgical procedure and the half-life of the administered antibiotic should be considered when determining the need for an additional intraoperative dose. The longer the duration of the surgical procedure, particularly with short half-life antibacterials, the greater the incidence of postoperative infection.[29] Cefazolin, with a half-life of approximately 1.8 hours, is effective in a single preoperative dose for most surgical procedures. For procedures lasting longer than 3 hours, or those with major blood loss, additional intraoperative doses should be administered every one to two times the half-life of the drug.[19,29] M.R. should require an additional intraoperative cefazolin dose only if the surgical procedure is prolonged (>3 hours).[29]

Route of Administration

CASE 61-2

QUESTION 1: G.B., a 55-year-old woman recently diagnosed with carcinoma of the large bowel, is admitted to the hospital for an elective colorectal surgical resection; the surgery is expected to last 5 hours. Physical examination reveals a cachectic woman with a 9-kg weight loss during the previous 3 months (current weight, 60 kg). Increased frequency of bowel movements and chronic fatigue are noted; all other systems are normal. Laboratory data include the following:

Hemoglobin (Hgb), 10.4 g/dL (normal, 12.1–15.3 g/dL; SI units, 104 g/L)
Hematocrit (Hct), 29.7% (normal, 36%–45%; SI units, 0.297)
Prothrombin time (PT), 15 seconds (normal, 10–13 seconds)

Stool guaiac is positive. Vital signs are within normal limits. G.B. is taking no medications and has no history of drug allergies. The following orders are written to begin at home on the day before surgery: (a) clear liquid diet; (b) mechanical bowel cleansing with polyethylene glycol-electrolyte lavage solution (CoLYTE, GoLYTELY); and (c) neomycin sulfate 1 g and erythromycin 1 g orally (PO) at 1 PM, 2 PM, and 11 PM. Comment on the appropriateness of the oral route of administration of antibiotic prophylaxis for G.B.

In general, oral administration of surgical antimicrobial prophylaxis is not recommended because of unreliable or poor absorption of oral agents in the anesthetized bowel. Oral nonabsorbable agents, however, function effectively as GI decontaminants because high intraluminal drug concentrations are sufficient to decrease bacterial counts.[30] The concentration of bacteria in the colon may approach 10^{16} bacteria/μL, and colorectal procedures, such as the one G.B. will undergo, carry a relatively high risk of postoperative infection. Antimicrobial regimens with activity against aerobic and anaerobic bacterial fecal flora (*Escherichia coli* and other Enterobacteriaceae and *Bacteroides fragilis*) are effective in preventing postoperative wound infections.[31]

A widely used oral antimicrobial regimen is 1 g each of the nonabsorbable antibiotics neomycin sulfate (for gram-negative aerobes) and erythromycin base (for anaerobes), given 1 day before surgery at the times indicated for G.B.[24,31] Mechanical bowel cleansing, such as with polyethylene glycol-electrolyte or sodium phosphate lavage solution, precede administration of this regimen; the purpose of bowel purging is to evacuate the colonic contents as completely as possible to decrease colonic bacterial counts. Effective oral alternatives to neomycin plus erythromycin include metronidazole with or without neomycin or with kanamycin, or kanamycin plus erythromycin[32]; however, clinical situations warranting the use of such alternatives over the well-established neomycin-erythromycin regimen are practically nonexistent. Thus, the regimen selected for G.B. is highly appropriate.

CASE 61-2, QUESTION 2: The surgical resident has canceled the oral neomycin-erythromycin bowel regimen for G.B. Instead, he orders cefoxitin (Mefoxin) 1 g IV preoperatively. Why is (or is not) this change in therapy an effective and rational choice for G.B.?

Numerous parenteral regimens, specifically with agents that possess both aerobic and anaerobic activity, are effective as surgical prophylaxis in colorectal procedures. The second-generation cephalosporins with significant anaerobic activity (e.g., cefoxitin) are superior to first-generation cephalosporins, which lack sufficient anaerobic activity.[33] At present, it is not clear whether oral antimicrobial prophylaxis is superior to parenteral therapy in preventing infection after colorectal surgery.[34]

However, the cefoxitin order for G.B. would be unacceptable if the surgery lasts longer than 3.5 hours (the relatively short half-life of cefoxitin could be associated with inadequate antibacterial levels and predispose her to infection).[35] For prolonged procedures (>3 hours) such as anticipated for G.B., an alternative agent with a longer half-life, such as ertapenem, or a second dose of cefoxitin should be considered. Ertapenem has been found to be superior to cefotetan in preventing infection after colorectal surgery.[36] This improved efficacy may be because of the long half-life or broader antibacterial activity.[37,38] Whereas ertapenem may offer certain advantages as a prophylactic antibiotic, its use in this indication is discouraged by most clinicians. Although unproven, the potential impact of widespread ertapenem utilization on subsequent carbapenem resistance is of hypothetical concern. The increased acquisition cost of ertapenem also needs to be considered. Thus, for G.B., the importance of duration for intravenous regimens in prolonged surgery should be stressed to the resident.

CASE 61-2, QUESTION 3: The surgical resident has reconsidered the cefoxitin order and decided to prescribe both the oral and parenteral prophylactic regimens for G.B. Will the combination significantly reduce the rate of postoperative wound infection compared with either regimen administered singly?

Although the coadministration of both oral and parenteral prophylactic regimens occurs commonly in practice (75% of one survey's respondents),[39] data in support of this practice are conflicting.[32,41] Oral plus parenteral antimicrobial prophylaxis combination is equivalent or superior to either regimen administered alone in reducing infection rates.[32,41] As a result, a combination of oral and parenteral antimicrobial prophylaxis is recommended for colorectal surgery.[7,20]

Duration of Administration

CASE 61-3

QUESTION 1: L.G., a 28-year-old man with a history of rheumatic heart disease, has a 12-year history of a heart murmur consistent with mild mitral stenosis and mitral regurgitation. During the past 4 months his murmur has become much more prominent. In addition, he has experienced severe dyspnea with light physical activity and 3+ pitting edema over both lower legs. Physical examination is notable for coarse rales and an S_3 gallop. For the past 6 weeks he has been maintained on digoxin and diuretics without significant relief of his shortness of breath (SOB). The cardiothoracic surgeon recommends mitral valve replacement and orders the following surgical antibiotic prophylaxis regimen: cefazolin 1 g IV preoperatively, then every 8 hours for 48 hours. Why is cefazolin the most appropriate antimicrobial for L.G.? Why was prophylaxis ordered for only 48 hours?

Although the incidence of postoperative wound infection for cardiothoracic procedures is low (<5%), the devastating consequences of a postoperative endocarditis (after valve replacement) and mediastinitis or sternal osteomyelitis (after sternotomy) warrant antimicrobial prophylaxis.[42–44] Common pathogens associated with cardiothoracic surgery include *Staphylococcus aureus* and *Staphylococcus epidermidis* (particularly with hardware placement) (Table 61-2); based on these potential pathogens, successful prophylactic regimens include cefazolin and cefuroxime. When cefazolin has been compared with cefuroxime or cefamandole, a statistical trend in favor of the second-generation cephalosporins has been noted, and collective wound infection rates were slightly higher in the cefazolin group.[45–47] In contrast, a comparison of prophylactic cefazolin and cefuroxime in patients having open heart surgery noted a significantly greater incidence of sternal wound infection and mediastinitis in the cefuroxime group.[48] Other studies similarly have not observed improved efficacy with cefuroxime compared with cefazolin.[49,50] In conclusion, cefazolin probably is at least as effective as second-generation cephalosporins; therefore, the choice of agent should be based on an institution's antimicrobial susceptibility and cost data. Hospital-specific antimicrobial resistance patterns are especially important in determining the incidence of methicillin-resistant *S. aureus* (MRSA) or methicillin-resistant *S. epidermidis* (MRSE) surgical site infection rates. Although vancomycin has not been determined to be superior to cefazolin, vancomycin is the drug of choice for prophylaxis in patients colonized with MRSA or in institutions with high rates of MRSA or MRSE surgical site infections.[19,51] Patients at high risk of MRSA carriage should be screened on hospital admission.[52]

Meta-analyses reveal no differences between first- and second-generation cephalosporins or between β-lactams and glycopeptides in the prevention of surgical wound infection.[53,54] Thus, the cefazolin prophylaxis selected for L.G. is acceptable, provided the patient is not colonized with MRSA or MRSE.

With regard to duration, the shortest effective prophylactic course of antibiotics should be used (i.e., single dose preoperatively or not more than 24 hours postoperatively for most procedures).[55] Postoperative doses after wound closure are usually not required and may increase the risk of resistance. Single-dose prophylaxis, a viable option for many surgical procedures (see Case 61-4, Question 1), is controversial for cardiac procedures.[56] In practice, cardiothoracic antimicrobial prophylaxis often is continued up to 48 hours after surgery, as in L.G. No benefit is seen to prolonging prophylaxis to more than 48 hours, and such use should be discouraged. The duration of antimicrobial prophylaxis ordered for L.G. is appropriate.

CASE 61-4

QUESTION 1: G.J., a 27-year-old woman, is admitted to the obstetrics unit at term with her first pregnancy. She is scheduled for a cesarean section because the baby is in a breech presentation. Cefazolin 1 g IV to be administered after the cord is clamped and every 8 hours for 24 hours is ordered. Why is this surgical prophylaxis inappropriate?

As noted previously, the shortest effective duration of prophylaxis should be used. In the past, 5- or 6-day antimicrobial regimens were commonly used for cesarean section, but 24-hour regimens have been proven to be as effective as these longer regimens.[57] Faro et al.[57] demonstrated that a single 2-g dose of cefazolin was superior to either a single 1-g dose or to a three-dose, 1-g prophylactic regimen. Others have noted similar results (i.e., a single cefazolin dose administered after the umbilical cord is clamped is sufficient in preventing postoperative wound infections in cesarean section).[58–60] Single-dose prophylaxis is less costly[61] and minimizes the development of bacterial resistance.[9] Antibiotic prophylaxis has traditionally been administered after clamping of the umbilical cord to minimize infant drug exposure. This early exposure could theoretically mask the signs of neonatal sepsis and favor the acquisition of resistant organisms. However, administration before initial incision and cord clamping decreases the incidence of maternal infections without adverse consequences to the child.[62–64] Thus, G.J. should receive a single 2-g dose of cefazolin before the cord has been clamped, without the three additional doses.

Single-dose prophylaxis has been found to be effective in a variety of GI tract, orthopaedic, and gynecologic procedures.[29] A single dose of an antibiotic with a short half-life, however, may provide insufficient antimicrobial coverage during a prolonged surgical procedure. Repeated intraoperative dosing or selection of an agent with a longer half-life is recommended when the duration of surgery is long to maintain adequate tissue concentrations throughout the procedure.[19,65]

Signs of Surgical Site Infection

CASE 61-4, QUESTION 2: G.J. is discharged on the fifth hospital day and instructed to observe her incision site carefully for signs of infection. What are the typical signs of site infection? What is the typical time course for signs of site infection to manifest?

Most surgical site infections involve the incision site and are defined as either *superficial* (involving the skin and subcutaneous fat) or *deep incisional* (involving fascia and muscle). Typically, an infected incision site wound is red, warm, and purulent and sometimes swollen, tender, or painful. Poor wound healing or dehiscence (premature opening of the incision) is highly suggestive of infection. The purulent drainage should be cultured to identify the causative pathogen and to direct antimicrobial therapy. Empiric therapy directed against the most likely pathogens should be instituted while awaiting culture and sensitivity test results. Although most incision site infections are diagnosed shortly after surgery (within 30 days), some deep-seated infections present indolently during weeks to months, e.g., abscess formation.[10,18] Infection of surgically implanted prosthetic hardware may take place up to a year after the surgical procedure.[66]

ONLINE CONTENT

For a PowerPoint presentation on classification and assessment of surgical site infections, go to http://thepoint.lww.com/AT10e.

Selection of an Antimicrobial Agent

CASE 61-5

QUESTION 1: L.T., a 46-year-old woman, has a recent history of abnormal uterine bleeding and vaginal discharge. Endometrial biopsy is positive for squamous cell carcinoma; however, there does not appear to be invasive disease. The diagnosis is carcinoma in situ, and a vaginal hysterectomy is scheduled. What would be an appropriate surgical prophylaxis antimicrobial regimen for L.T.?

The selection of a prophylactic regimen should be based on the spectrum of activity of the agents and the most likely pathogens associated with the given surgical procedure (Table 61-2), pharmacokinetic characteristics (e.g., half-life), adverse event profile, impact on bacterial resistance selection, and cost.

The usefulness of antimicrobial prophylaxis in vaginal hysterectomies is well established and should be directed against vaginal microflora, including gram-positive and gram-negative aerobes and anaerobes (Table 61-2). The most-effective, yet most narrow-spectrum agent should be selected considering that the goal of prophylaxis is not to eradicate every potential pathogen but to reduce bacterial counts below a critical level necessary to cause infection. Cefazolin has been proven to be as effective a prophylactic agent as ceftriaxone for vaginal hysterectomy.[67] This finding reinforces the fact that a more broad-spectrum agent (e.g., a third-generation cephalosporin) is unwarranted.

Similar to vaginal hysterectomy, cefazolin and numerous agents decrease the incidence of postoperative surgical infection when the abdominal approach is used.[68,69] As with vaginal hysterectomy, most trials have not revealed significant differences between first- and second-generation cephalosporins.[69] In contrast, Hemsell et al.[70] observed a significantly higher incidence of major postoperative surgical infections in patients receiving the first-generation agent cefazolin when compared with the second-generation cephalosporin cefotetan. Cefazolin exhibits a favorable toxicity profile and has a relatively long half-life (~1.8 hours), and a single dose has proven prophylactic efficacy.[67] Cefazolin also is considerably less expensive than broader-spectrum agents and is currently recommended by the American College of Obstetricians and Gynecologists.[71] Although it has a broader spectrum of coverage, a single dose of cefoxitin would also be an appropriate choice for this patient.

CASE 61-5, QUESTION 2: Because cefoxitin has an increased spectrum of activity against the anaerobe *B. fragilis*, it is being considered as an alternative to cefazolin prophylaxis for L.T. Comment on the appropriateness of this proposed change in prophylaxis.

The second- and third-generation cephalosporins and ampicillin-sulbactam generally are not more effective than the first-generation cephalosporins for surgical prophylaxis in vaginal hysterectomy or in gastroduodenal, biliary, and clean surgical procedures.[20] One exception to these findings is in the prevention of infection after colorectal procedures and perhaps hysterectomy. Several investigations have documented the failure of first-generation agents when used as prophylaxis in colorectal procedures, probably a consequence of their weak anaerobic coverage.[33] As stated previously, second- and third-generation agents and ampicillin-sulbactam generally are no more efficacious than cefazolin and should not be used for surgical prophylaxis in most procedures. Cefoxitin, however, would be a reasonable choice in colorectal surgery or hysterectomy. Considering that this patient is having a hysterectomy, either cefazolin or cefoxitin is appropriate.

CASE 61-6

QUESTION 1: S.N., a 57-year-old woman with rheumatoid arthritis and degenerative joint disease, has been admitted for total hip arthroplasty. She states that she had an anaphylactic reaction to penicillin in the past. How does this allergy history impact on the selection of surgical prophylaxis for S.N.?

Cefazolin is the preferred prophylactic agent for most clean procedures, including cardiac, vascular, and orthopedic procedures[20] (Table 61-2). Although the risk of cefazolin cross-allergenicity to penicillin is relatively low, S.N. experienced a serious, accelerated reaction (hives, shortness of breath) with penicillin; consequently, she should not receive cefazolin. The organisms most likely to cause postoperative infection after total hip replacement are *S. aureus* and *S. epidermidis* (Table 61-2). Nafcillin, cefazolin, and vancomycin possess excellent activity against *S. aureus;* however, the β-lactams have only marginal activity against *S. epidermidis*. Regardless, nafcillin (and cefazolin) should be avoided because of the penicillin allergy, and the preferred agent for S.N. is vancomycin.

Preoperative vancomycin 1 g should be administered IV slowly, during at least 60 minutes. This slow rate of infusion is necessary to reduce the risk of infusion-related hypotension.[72,73]

CASE 61-7

QUESTION 1: B.K., an 18-year-old woman, complains of severe acute abdominal pain and nausea; the pain is localized to the periumbilical region. B.K. has a temperature of 39.5°C. After initial examination by her pediatrician, she is admitted to the hospital with presumed appendicitis, and an exploratory laparotomy is scheduled. What surgical antimicrobial prophylaxis should be ordered for B.K.?

As with colorectal surgery, the most likely infecting organisms in appendectomy are *Bacteroides* species and gram-negative enterics (Table 61-2). On surgical inspection, if the appendix appears normal (not inflamed, without perforation), then antimicrobial prophylaxis is unnecessary.[74] If the appendix is inflamed without perforation, a single preoperative antibiotic dose is necessary. If the appendix is perforated or gangrenous (complicated), infection is already established and postoperative treatment is warranted. The status of the appendix, however, cannot be determined before surgery; therefore, all patients should receive at least one preoperative dose of an appropriate antibiotic.[75] After surgical inspection of the appendix, the need for postoperative antibiotic therapy can be determined.

Based on the pathogens likely to be encountered, an antimicrobial agent with both aerobic and anaerobic activity should be used. Consequently, cefoxitin is an acceptable choice for prophylaxis.[76]

Risks of Indiscriminate Antimicrobial Use

CASE 61-7, QUESTION 2: On surgical exploration, B.K. was found to have uncomplicated (nonperforated, nongangrenous) appendicitis; however, cefoxitin therapy was continued for 3 days. What are the risks of indiscriminate use of antimicrobials for surgical prophylaxis?

The risks of indiscriminate use of antimicrobials include the potential for adverse effects and superinfection. The administration of any β-lactam agent poses the risk of a hypersensitivity reaction, and many antibiotics, including cefoxitin, as is being used in B.K., predispose patients to *Clostridium difficile*–associated disease. The risk of developing this superinfection increases with duration of antibiotic exposure.[8] Avoiding unnecessary initial and prolonged exposure reduce the risk of this superinfection and its associated complications.[77] In addition, prolonged use of antimicrobials increases the selection of resistant organisms in a given patient that could be nosocomially spread to other hospitalized patients.[78]

OPTIMIZING SURGICAL ANTIMICROBIAL PROPHYLAXIS

Antibiotic control strategies have improved the appropriate use of antimicrobial agents for surgical prophylaxis. Numerous factors including individual knowledge, attitudes, beliefs, and practice; team communication and allocation of responsibilities; and institutional support for promoting and monitoring practice influence antibiotic prophylaxis measures.[79] Interventions for improvement are focused on education of practitioners, standardization of the ordering, the delivery and the administration processes, and providing feedback on performance as measured by infection rates and compliance with improvements. The Surgical Care Improvement Project (SCIP), a national multidisciplinary initiative developed by the Centers for Medicare and Medicaid Services, aims at improving surgical care. Reducing surgical site infections is among one of the targeted goals of this initiative.[80] Prophylactic antimicrobial received within 1 hour before surgical incision, prophylactic antimicrobial consistent with published guidelines, and prophylactic antimicrobial discontinued within 24 hours of surgery end time are three performances measures included in this quality improvement process. This approach achieved a decrease in the surgical infection rate from 2.3% to 1.7% during a 1-year period.[81]

Smaller scale projects have also been successful at improving antibiotic use and decreasing infection rates. A multidisciplinary team generated electronic quick orders allowing for a computer-enhanced decision-making process and developed an antibiotic administration protocol. Appropriate selection of antibiotics increased from 78% to 94%, timely administration improved from 51% to 98%, and clean wound infection rate decreased from 2.7% to 1.4%.[82]

In collaboration with other health care providers, pharmacists should be responsible for optimizing the timing, choice, and duration of antimicrobial surgical prophylaxis.[83] Education of surgical, anesthesia, and nursing staff, supported by hospital policy changes initiated by pharmacists, improved appropriate timing from 68% to 97% and resulted in significant cost avoidance.[83] Postdischarge surveillance is also critical in reducing surgical site infections.[84]

KEY REFERENCES AND WEBSITES

A full list of references for this chapter can be found at http://thepoint.lww.com/AT10e. Below are the key references and websites for this chapter, with the corresponding reference number in this chapter found in parentheses after the reference.

Key References

Anderson DJ, et al. Strategies to prevent surgical site infections in acute care hospitals. *Infect Control Hosp Epidemiol.* 2008; 29(Suppl 1):S51. (14)

Bratzler DW, Houck PM. Antimicrobial prophylaxis for surgery: an advisory statement from the National Surgical Infection Prevention Project. *Clin Infect Dis.* 2004;38:1706. (19)

Bratzler DW, Hunt DR. The surgical infection prevention and surgical care improvement projects: national initiatives to improve outcomes for patients having surgery. *Clin Infect Dis.* 2006;43:322. (80)

Classen DC, et al. The timing of prophylactic administration of antibiotics and the risk of surgical-wound infection. *N Engl J Med.* 1992;326:281. (26)

Edwards FH, et al. The Society of Thoracic Surgeons Practice Guideline Series: antibiotic prophylaxis in cardiac surgery, part I: duration. *Ann Thorac Surg.* 2006;81:397. (56)

[No authors listed]. ASHP Therapeutic Guidelines on Antimicrobial Prophylaxis in Surgery. American Society of Health-System Pharmacists. *Am J Health Syst Pharm.* 1999;56:1839. (7)

Key Websites

Centers for Diseases Control and Prevention (CDC). Healthcare Associated Infections. Surgical Site Infection (SSI). http://www.cdc.gov/HAI/ssi/ssi.html.

Centers for Diseases Control and Prevention (CDC). Healthcare Infection Control Practices Advisory Committee (HICPAC). General Guidelines. http://www. cdc.gov/hicpac/pubs.html.

Centers for Diseases Control and Prevention (CDC). National Healthcare Safety Network. Data and Statistics. http://www.cdc.gov/nhsn/dataStat.html.

Safer Healthcare Now! Surgical Site Infection (SSI). http://www.saferhealthcarenow. ca/EN/Interventions/SSI/Pages/default.aspx.

National Institute for Health and Clinical Excellence. Surgical Site Infection. http://www.nice.org.uk/CG74.

62 Central Nervous System Infections

Gregory A. Eschenauer, Brian A. Potoski, and Victoria J. Dudas

	CHAPTER CASES
1 The most common symptoms of meningitis include the triad of fever, stiff neck, and altered mental status. In neonates and infants, irritability and poor feeding may be reported along with fever. In the elderly, signs may be absent or more subtle.	**Case 62-1 (Question 1)**
2 All children should be vaccinated against *Haemophilus influenzae* and *Streptococcus pneumoniae*. In addition, all persons aged 21 years or younger should receive a dose of the *Neisseria meningitidis* conjugate vaccine within 5 years of enrollment to college. Adults with certain risk factors and those older than 65 years of age should be vaccinated against *S. pneumoniae*.	**Case 62-1 (Questions 11, 12), Case 62-2 (Question 5)**
3 Adjunctive dexamethasone should be initiated in all patients with suspected bacterial meningitis either before or concomitant with the first dose of antibiotic.	**Case 62-1 (Question 4)**
4 Intraventricular antibiotics should be considered for patients with meningitis who have an external drainage device in place. Such therapy should be used in combination with systemically administered therapy.	**Case 62-4 (Question 4)**
5 Cerebrospinal fluid (CSF) is essential in confirming the diagnosis of meningitis. The CSF typically contains many white blood cells with a predominance of neutrophils. Additionally, CSF protein is typically elevated to greater than 100 mg/dL with a low CSF glucose concentration.	**Case 62-1 (Question 2)**
6 Response to therapy should be monitored by fever, altered mental status, and stiff neck. A baseline level of mental status should be evaluated for this reason. Delays in response to therapy may require a repeat lumbar puncture to re-examine CSF cultures, which are usually sterile after 18 to 24 hours of therapy. Clinical response should be seen between 24 and 48 hours of initiation of therapy.	**Case 62-1 (Question 6)**
7 The combination of ceftriaxone or cefotaxime (in patients without severe penicillin allergy) with vancomycin represents the most reasonable approach to empiric therapy for potential penicillin-resistant pneumococcal meningitis.	**Case 62-2 (Question 2)**
8 Brain abscess is associated with a different spectrum of pathogens, including oral anaerobes, staphylococci, and aerobic gram-negative bacilli, depending on the patient. The barrier from the blood to brain parenchyma differs from that between blood and CSF. Consequently, the choice of antimicrobial for brain abscess may differ from that associated with meningitis.	**Case 62-5 (Questions 1–3)**

The pharmacotherapy of central nervous system (CNS) infections presents numerous challenges. Antibiotic penetration often is limited, and host defenses are absent or inadequate. Thus, morbidity and mortality from infections of the CNS remain high despite the availability of highly potent, bactericidal antibiotics. In a review of 696 episodes of adult patients treated for community-acquired bacterial meningitis between October 1998 and April 2002, the mortality rate was 21%.[1] Although eradication of bacteria is essential, it is only one of the variables that affect mortality from CNS infections. In an attempt to decrease morbidity and mortality, the pathophysiologic mechanisms of CNS infections continue to be studied.[2–4]

A number of infectious processes can occur within the CNS (e.g., meningitis, encephalitis, meningoencephalitis, brain abscess, subdural empyema, and epidural abscess).[5,6] In addition, prosthetic devices placed into the CNS (e.g., cerebrospinal fluid [CSF] shunts for management of hydrocephalus) often are complicated by infection.[7] Many etiologic agents are capable of inducing CNS infections, including bacteria, viruses, fungi, and certain parasites. This chapter focuses primarily on bacterial infections of the CNS, with an emphasis on the pharmacotherapy of bacterial meningitis and brain abscess. (Also see Chapter 73, Pharmacotherapy of Human Immunodeficiency Virus Infection, and Chapter 74, Opportunistic Infection in HIV-Infected Patients, for presentations pertaining to CNS infections in these populations.)

REVIEW OF CENTRAL NERVOUS SYSTEM

Anatomy and Physiology

MENINGES

Proper therapy of CNS infections requires an understanding of the anatomic and physiologic characteristics. The brain and spinal cord are ensheathed by a protective covering known as the meninges and suspended in CSF, which acts as a shock absorber to outside trauma.[8,9] The meninges consist of three layers of fibrous tissue: the *pia mater, arachnoid,* and *dura mater.* The pia mater, the innermost layer of the meninges, is a thin, delicate membrane that closely adheres to the contours of the brain. Separating the pia mater from the more loosely enclosed arachnoid membrane is the subarachnoid space, in which the CSF resides. The pia mater and arachnoid, known collectively as the *leptomeninges,* lie interior to the dura mater, a tough outer membrane that adheres to the periosteum and vertebral column.[8,10] *Meningitis* is a term describing inflammation (often the result of infection) of the subarachnoid space.[8] Abscesses also can form outside the dural space (epidural abscess), often with devastating consequences.[6]

CEREBROSPINAL FLUID

The CSF is produced and secreted by the choroid plexus in the lateral ventricles and, to a lesser extent, by the choroid plexuses within the third and fourth ventricles.[9,11] CSF flows unidirectionally from the lateral ventricles through the foramina of the third and fourth ventricles into the subarachnoid space, then over the cerebral hemispheres and downward into the spinal canal. CSF is absorbed through villous projections (arachnoid villi) into veins, primarily the cerebral venous sinuses.[9,11] About 550 mL/day of CSF is produced, with complete exchange occurring every 3 to 4 hours.[9,11] The flow of CSF is unidirectional from the ventricles to the intralumbar space. Therefore, intrathecal injection of antibiotics results in little, if any, antibiotic reaching the cerebral ventricles.[12,13] This unidirectional flow of CSF presents a problem because ventriculitis commonly occurs in conjunction with bacterial meningitis. Direct intraventricular instillation of antibiotics, usually by means of a reservoir, is preferable in the setting of ventriculitis (see Case 62-4, Question 4).[12,13]

In adults, children, and infants the volume of CSF is approximately 150 mL, 60 to 100 mL, and 40 to 60 mL, respectively.[9,11] Knowledge of approximate CSF volume facilitates estimation of the CSF concentration of a drug subsequent to intrathecal administration. For example, administration of gentamicin 5 mg (5,000 mcg) intrathecally should result in a CSF concentration of approximately 33 mcg/mL in an adult shortly after administration.

The composition of CSF differs from other physiologic fluids. The pH of CSF is slightly acidic (normal pH, 7.3) and, with the exception of chloride ion, electrolyte concentrations are slightly less than those in serum.[9,11] Under normal conditions, the protein concentration in CSF is less than 50 mg/dL, CSF glucose values are approximately 60% those of plasma, and few if any white blood cells (WBCs) are present (<5 cells/μL).[9,11] When the meninges become inflamed (i.e., in meningitis), the composition of the CSF is altered. In particular, the protein concentration in the CSF increases, and the glucose concentration in the CSF usually declines with meningitis. Therefore, careful evaluation of CSF chemistries is useful when establishing a diagnosis of meningitis.

BLOOD–BRAIN BARRIER

The blood–brain barrier plays a crucial role in protecting the brain and maintaining homeostasis within the CNS.[9,14,15] Actually, two distinct barriers exist within the brain: the blood–CSF barrier and the blood–brain barrier.[14,15] The blood–CSF barrier is located in the choroid plexus and circumventricular organs (e.g., area postrema) and is characterized morphologically by fenestrated (porous) capillaries (Fig. 62-1).[14] This arrangement allows proteins and other molecules (including antibiotics) to pass freely into the immediate interstitial space. Diffusion of substances into the CSF is restricted by tightly fused ependymal cells lining the ventricular side of the choroid plexus (Fig. 62-1).[14] Cerebral capillary endothelial cells make up the blood–brain barrier, which separates blood from the interstitial fluid of the brain. Unlike capillaries in other areas of the body, the capillary endothelia of the brain are packed closely together, forming tight junctions that in effect produce a barrier physiologically similar to a continuous lipid bilayer.[14] The surface area of the blood–brain barrier is more than 5,000 times greater than that of the blood–CSF barrier; thus, the blood–brain barrier plays a more important role in protecting the brain and regulating its chemical composition.[11,14] Many antimicrobials traverse the blood–brain barrier with difficulty, particularly agents having low lipid solubility (see section on Antimicrobial Penetration Into the Cerebrospinal Fluid below).[15]

ONLINE CONTENT

For an illustration of the blood–brain barrier, go to http://thepoint.lww.com/AT10e.

MENINGITIS

Meningitis is the most common type of CNS infection. The signs and symptoms associated with bacterial meningitis usually are acute in onset, evolving over the course of a few hours.[5] Prompt recognition and early institution of therapy are essential to ensuring beneficial outcomes. In contrast, a diverse group of infectious (e.g., viruses, fungi, and mycobacteria) and noninfectious (e.g., chemical irritants) agents produce a meningitic picture often of a less acute or chronic nature.[16] On occasion, such "aseptic" causes can produce signs and symptoms nearly indistinguishable from those of acute bacterial meningitis.[5,16] Drugs that can induce aseptic meningitis include trimethoprim-sulfamethoxazole (TMP-SMX), the antirejection monoclonal antibody muromonab-CD3, azathioprine, and nonsteroidal anti-inflammatory drugs such as ibuprofen, naproxen, and sulindac.[17]

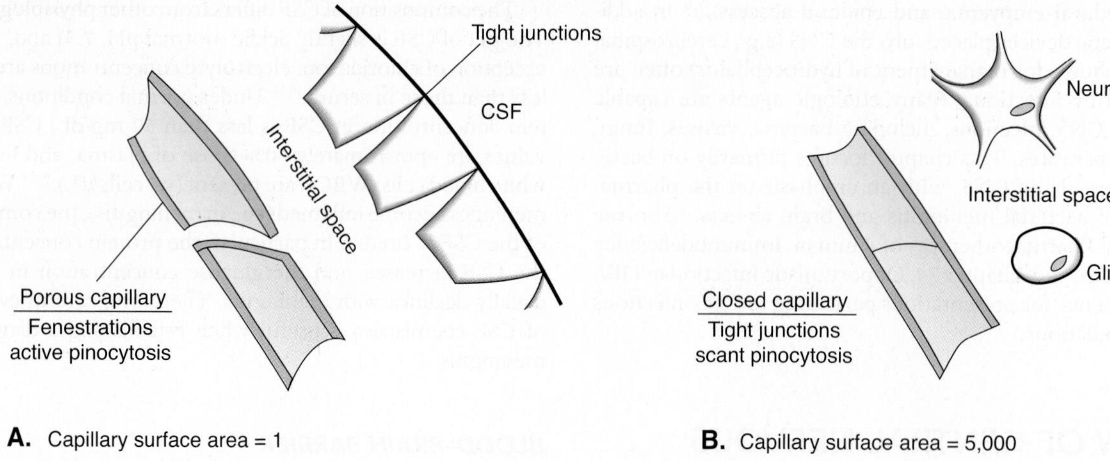

FIGURE 62-1 The two membrane barrier systems in the central nervous system: the blood–cerebrospinal fluid (CSF) barrier (left) and the blood–brain barrier. (Reprinted with permission from Pardridge WM et al. Blood–brain barrier: interface between internal medicine and the brain. *Ann Intern Med.* 1986;105:82.)

Microbiology

The bacterial causes of meningitis correlate well with age and underlying conditions, such as head trauma or recent neurosurgery (Table 62-1).[18–21] Generally, meningitis is a disease of the very young and very old: most cases occur in children younger than 2 years of age and in elderly adults.[18,19]

TABLE 62-1
Microbiology of Bacterial Meningitis

Age Group or Predisposing Condition	Most Likely Organisms[a]
Neonates (<1 month)	Group B streptococcus *(Streptococcus agalactiae), E. coli, (Klebsiella species, Listeria monocytogenes)*
Infants and children (1–23 months)	*Streptococcus pneumoniae, Neisseria meningitidis, S. agalactiae, Haemophilus influenzae,*[b] *E. coli*
Children and adults (2–50 years)	*N. meningitidis, S. pneumoniae*
Adults (>50 years)	*S. pneumoniae, N. meningitidis, L. monocytogenes, E. coli, Klebsiella* species, and other aerobic gram-negative bacilli
Postneurosurgical	*Staphylococcus aureus,* aerobic gram-negative bacilli (e.g., *E. coli, Klebsiella* species, *Pseudomonas aeruginosa), Staphylococcus epidermidis*[c]
Closed head trauma	*S. pneumoniae, H. influenzae,* group A β-hemolytic streptococci
Penetrating trauma	*S. aureus, S. epidermidis,* aerobic gram-negative bacilli (e.g., *E. coli, Klebsiella* species, *P. aeruginosa)*
CSF shunt	Coagulase-negative staphylococci (particularly *S. epidermidis*), *S. aureus,* aerobic gram-negative bacilli (including *P. aeruginosa*), *Propionibacterium acnes*
Presence of risk factor (alcoholism and altered immune status)	*S. pneumoniae, L. monocytogenes, H. influenzae, N. meningitidis*

[a]Organisms listed in descending order of frequency.
[b]Need to consider this pathogen only in children not vaccinated with Hib.
[c]Most commonly seen in association with prosthetic devices (e.g., cerebrospinal fluid shunts).
CSF, cerebrospinal fluid.

Neonates (infants <1 month) are at an especially high risk of experiencing meningitis. Meningitis in neonates most often is caused by group B streptococci (*Streptococcus agalactiae*) or coliform organisms such as *Escherichia coli*.[18,19,22] These highly virulent pathogens usually are acquired during passage through the birth canal or from the hospital environment and are associated with significant morbidity and mortality, particularly in premature infants.[18,19,22] Case fatality rates of greater than 20% and 30% have been reported for meningitis caused by group B streptococci and gram-negative bacilli, respectively.[18] *Listeria monocytogenes* is another important and often overlooked pathogen in neonates.[18,19,23] Because *L. monocytogenes* is resistant to many antimicrobial agents, including third-generation cephalosporins, selection of initial (empiric) therapy in neonates must be approached with this pathogen in mind.[23]

Infants older than 1 month of age and children younger than 4 years of age are at the highest risk for meningitis. Historically, in this age group, the disease was caused predominantly by three pathogens: *Haemophilus influenzae, Streptococcus pneumoniae,* and *Neisseria meningitidis*.[18,19]

Up to 45% of all cases of meningitis in the United States before 1985 were caused by *H. influenzae* type b (Hib).[19] From 1987 through 1997, however, Hib meningitis cases in children younger than 5 years of age decreased by 97%.[24,25] This reduction in *H. influenzae*–induced meningitis correlates with the widespread vaccination of children against invasive *H. influenzae* disease with the Hib polysaccharide–protein conjugate vaccines. Invasive *H. influenzae* infection now is considered a vaccine-preventable disease in the United States as well as in other countries, highlighting the importance of vaccinating children against Hib invasive disease.[26] Further follow-up from 1998 to 2000 indicates that the incidence of Hib has remained extremely low. One of the national health objectives in *Healthy People 2010* was to reduce the incidence of Hib to zero.[25] In addition, widespread vaccination has caused a shift in the age distribution of bacterial meningitis. Before the Hib vaccine was available, more than two-thirds of cases occurred in children younger than 5 years of age. With the dramatic reduction of Hib cases in this age group, most cases now are observed in adults.[26,27]

In adults and children who have received the conjugated Hib vaccine, community-acquired meningitis most often is caused by *S. pneumoniae* (the pneumococcus) and *N. meningitidis* (the meningococcus).[4,18,19] Meningococci more commonly are implicated in individuals ages 5 to 30 years, whereas pneumococci are the predominant pathogens in adults older than 30 years of age.[18] In the past several years, meningococcal meningitis has been occurring in clusters within the general population with increased frequency. The observed clusters, defined as two or more cases of the same serogroup that are closer in time or space than expected, usually occur in secondary schools or university settings.[27]

Traditionally, pneumococci and meningococci have been highly susceptible to penicillin G (minimum inhibitory concentration [MIC] $\leq$0.06 mcg/mL). Pneumococcal strains showing resistance (MIC $\geq$0.12 mcg/mL), however, are a problem in many areas of the world, including the United States. Penicillin-resistant pneumococci are of particular concern in relation to meningitis because there is the additional challenge of delivering adequate levels to the site of infection, the CSF.[1,28] Optimal therapy for resistant pneumococci is controversial and is discussed in greater detail in Case 62-2, Question 2.

The elderly also are susceptible to experiencing meningitis, and the infection-related mortality in this population often is higher than in other age groups.[18,19,29] For example, the case-fatality rate for pneumococcal meningitis is 5% in children younger than 5 years of age but 19% to 37% in adults.[19,30] Patients of advanced age are most susceptible to meningitis from pneumococci and meningococci. Enteric gram-negative bacilli (e.g., *E. coli, Klebsiella pneumoniae*) also are occasionally isolated.[18,19,29] Furthermore, *L. monocytogenes* is a problem pathogen in the elderly, especially in immunocompromised patients.[18,19,23,29,31]

Meningitis after neurosurgical procedures or open trauma to the head most often is caused by enteric gram-negative bacilli (predominantly *E. coli* and *K. pneumoniae*) and, to a lesser extent, staphylococci, particularly *Staphylococcus aureus.*[1,20,31] Meningitis that occurs after neurosurgery is occasionally caused by resistant pathogens, such as *Enterobacter* species and *Pseudomonas aeruginosa,* often with devastating consequences.[20,32–34] In addition, patients requiring ventriculostomy or placement of CSF shunts can exhibit infections of these prosthetic devices by coagulase-negative staphylococci (e.g., *Staphylococcus epidermidis*) or diphtheroids.[7,20] Closed head trauma, particularly when associated with CSF rhinorrhea or otorrhea, can lead to pneumococcal meningitis or, to a lesser extent, *H. influenzae* meningitis.[20]

Pathogenesis and Pathophysiology

The steps leading to the development of meningitis and the underlying pathophysiologic processes involved have become more clearly understood in the past few years.[2,4] In general, meningitis can develop from *hematogenous* spread of organisms (the most common mechanism), by *contiguous* spread from a parameningeal focus (e.g., sinusitis or otitis media), or by direct bacterial *inoculation,* as occurs with head trauma or neurosurgery.

The list of pathogens causing bacterial meningitis is relatively short because only bacteria possessing certain virulence factors are capable of invading the meninges. Specifically, the presence of a polysaccharide capsule and other cell surface structures (e.g., pili) are necessary for bacteria to evade host defenses and gain entry into the subarachnoid space.[2–4] Once in the CSF, virulence factors contained within the cell wall (e.g., lipopolysaccharide or endotoxin in the case of *H. influenzae*) initiate a complex cascade of events culminating in neurologic damage.[2,3] These cell wall substances trigger the release of various cytokines, which act as mediators of the inflammatory response.[2–4]

Colonization of mucosal surfaces is a necessary first step in the pathogenesis of meningitis (Fig. 62-2).[3,4] The polysaccharide capsule and pili or fimbriae on the bacterial cell surface allow attachment to oropharyngeal or nasopharyngeal mucosa.[2–4] Secretion of protease enzymes that neutralize the protective activity of mucosal immunoglobulin A (IgA) and intrinsic resistance to ciliary clearance mechanisms allow meningeal pathogens to adhere to, and penetrate through, the epithelial surface and enter the intravascular space.[3] The presence of a capsule prevents binding by the alternative complement pathway and prolongs survival within the bloodstream.[3,4] Eventually, organisms multiply to sufficient numbers that allow invasion of the blood–brain barrier. The exact mechanism by which bacteria invade the blood–brain barrier is not well understood. Bacteria, however, probably adhere to cerebral capillary endothelia or perhaps the epithelium of the choroid plexus.[3,4]

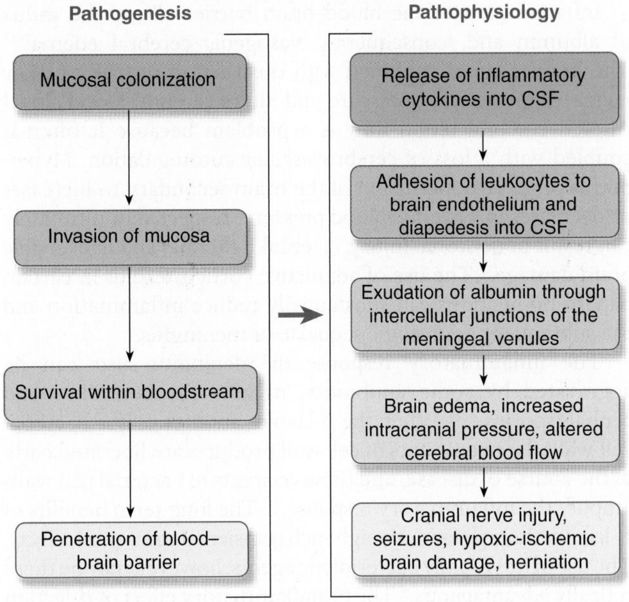

FIGURE 62-2 Summary of the pathogenesis and pathophysiology of bacterial meningitis. (Adapted with permission from Quagliarello VJ, Scheld WM. New perspectives on bacterial meningitis. *Clin Infect Dis.* 1993;17:603; Quagliarello VJ, Scheld WM. Bacterial meningitis: pathogenesis, pathophysiology, and progress. *N Engl J Med.* 1992; 327:864.)

Once bacteria gain entry into the CSF, host defenses are inadequate to contain the infection, and bacteria replicate rapidly. Humoral immunity (both complement and immunoglobulin) essentially is absent within the CSF.[2–4] In addition, opsonic activity in CSF is negligible, and although leukocytosis ensues shortly after bacterial invasion, phagocytosis also is inefficient.[3,4] Therefore, this relative immunodeficiency state necessitates the initiation of bactericidal therapy.[2]

Inflammation of the meninges is initiated by contents within the bacterial cell wall.[2–4] Specifically, gram-negative bacteria possess lipopolysaccharide, or endotoxin, and gram-positive bacteria contain teichoic acid in their cell walls. Release of lipopolysaccharide (or teichoic acid) induces the production and secretion of inflammatory cytokines such as interleukin 1, interleukin 6, prostaglandin E_2, and tumor necrosis factor from astrocytes, endothelial cells, and circulating monocytes.[3,4] These cytokines play an essential role in promoting the adherence of leukocytes to cerebral capillary endothelial cells, and they also facilitate the migration of leukocytes into the CSF.[2,3] On attachment to brain endothelium, leukocytes release toxic oxygen products that damage endothelial cells. This increases pinocytotic activity, widens tight junctions, and eventually increases blood–brain barrier permeability (Fig. 62-2).[2–4]

Inflammation of the blood–brain barrier allows the influx of albumin and, consequently, vasogenic cerebral edema.[2,3] The brain edema combined with obstruction of CSF outflow increases intracranial pressure and alters cerebral blood flow.[3] Altered cerebral blood flow is a problem because it often is coupled with a loss of cerebrovascular autoregulation. Hyperperfusion or hypoperfusion of the brain secondary to increases or decreases in systemic blood pressure, respectively, ultimately can result in neuronal injury, cerebral ischemia, and irreversible brain damage.[3] The use of adjunctive corticosteroids in certain patient populations can substantially reduce inflammation and the subsequent neurologic sequelae of meningitis.[2]

The inflammatory response in meningitis also can be aggravated by some antibiotics, notably the penicillins and cephalosporins.[2,34] When the β-lactam antibiotics lyse bacterial cell walls, large amounts of cell wall products are liberated early in the course of disease, and these contents of bacterial cell walls amplify the inflammatory response.[34] The long-term benefits of β-lactam therapy far outweigh such transient detrimental effects. The use of less rapidly bacteriolytic agents, however, may be theoretically advantageous.[2] The proinflammatory effect of β-lactam antibiotics is attenuated by concomitant corticosteroid therapy.[2]

In a systemic review of approximately three decades of data surrounding neurologic sequelae, the median risk of developing at least one major or minor sequela was 19.9% (12.3%–35.3%).[35] The type and severity of neurologic complications vary with the specific infecting organism, the severity of the infection, and the susceptibility of the host. In children, pneumococcal meningitis carries the highest risk of permanent neurologic sequelae, particularly sensorineural hearing loss.[5] In a long-term prospective study of 185 children with acute bacterial meningitis, permanent hearing loss occurred in 6%, 10.5%, and 31% of children with meningitis caused by *H. influenzae, N. meningitidis,* and *S. pneumoniae,* respectively.[36] Although seizures are fairly common on initial presentation, long-term epilepsy occurs in approximately 7% of patients.[36] Other important long-term complications include spastic paraparesis, behavioral disorders, and learning deficits.[36]

Diagnosis and Clinical Features

CLINICAL AND LABORATORY FEATURES OF BACTERIAL MENINGITIS

CASE 62-1

QUESTION 1: S.C., a 5-year-old boy, is brought to the emergency department (ED) by his mother, who says her son has a temperature of 39°C, is irritable and lethargic, and has a rash. S.C. was in his usual state of good health until last night, when he awoke crying. When she went to investigate, her son began to stiffen up and rock back and forth in his bed. Because he was not arousable, S.C.'s mother rushed him to the hospital. S.C.'s medical history is noncontributory except for an allergy to amoxicillin described as a skin rash. S.C., his mother and father, and his 7-year-old brother recently moved to the United States. S.C.'s vaccination history currently is unknown. S.C. and his brother currently attend a community day-care center.

On physical examination, S.C. was in marked distress, with a temperature of 40°C, blood pressure of 90/60 mm Hg, and a respiratory rate of 32 breaths/minute. His weight on admission was 20 kg. Neurologic examination showed evidence of nuchal rigidity; he was lethargic and difficult to arouse. Brudzinski and Kernig signs were positive. On head, eyes, ears, nose, and throat examination, S.C. demonstrated photophobia (he squinted severely when the examiner shone a light in his eyes), but no evidence was noted of papilledema. A petechial rash was visible on his extremities. The remainder of S.C.'s examination was essentially normal.

Blood drawn for laboratory tests revealed the following results:

Sodium (Na), 128 mEq/L
Potassium (K), 3.2 mEq/L
Chloride (Cl), 100 mEq/L
Bicarbonate (HCO_3), 25 mEq/L
Blood urea nitrogen (BUN), 16 mg/dL
Serum creatinine (SCr), 0.6 mg/dL
Serum glucose, 80 mg/dL

The WBC count was 18,000 cells/μL with 95% polymorphonuclear (PMN) cells; the hemoglobin (Hgb), hematocrit (Hct), and platelet count all were within normal limits. What clinical and laboratory features does S.C. display that are suggestive of meningitis?

S.C.'s presentation contains many features typical of acute bacterial meningitis. For example, the boy was in good health until he awoke at night confused and disoriented. When symptoms present abruptly and evolve quickly during a period of several hours, an acute bacterial process is a strong possibility.[37,38] S.C. has several predisposing factors for the development of meningitis: young age, an unknown vaccination history, and day-care exposure.[1,36]

The clinical features of bacterial meningitis are summarized in Table 62-2.[1,5,20,37,38] The most common symptoms include the triad of fever, stiff neck (nuchal rigidity), and altered mental status.[1,5,37] When all three of these features are present, as is S.C.'s case, meningitis should be strongly suspected. Other less common signs and symptoms include headache, photophobia (unusual intolerance to light), and focal neurologic deficits, including cranial nerve palsies.[1,5,37,38] A positive Brudzinski sign (reflex flexion of the hips and knees produced on flexion of the neck when lying in the recumbent position) and Kernig sign (pain on extension of the hamstrings when lying supine with the thighs perpendicular to the trunk) provide physical evidence of meningeal irritation.[39] Brudzinski and Kernig signs both were positive in S.C. Seizures occur on initial presentation in 15% to 30% of patients and may be focal or generalized.[1,5,35] The presence of seizures or a severely depressed mental status (i.e., obtundation or coma) generally is associated with a poorer prognosis.[1,5,35,37,38,40] According to the most recent practice guidelines for the management of bacterial meningitis, a computed tomographic (CT) scan should be obtained before lumbar puncture in patients with specific criteria. These include immunocompromised state, history of CNS disease, new-onset seizure, papilledema, abnormal level of consciousness, and focal neurologic defect.[21] Although controversial, brain herniation

TABLE 62-2
Signs and Symptoms of Acute Bacterial Meningitis

Fever	Anorexia
Nuchal rigidity (stiff neck)	Headache
Altered mental status	Photophobia
Seizures	Nausea and vomiting
Brudzinski sign[a]	Focal neurologic deficits
Kernig sign[a]	Septic shock
Irritability[b]	

[a]See text for description of sign.
[b]Symptoms seen in infants with meningitis.

can occur when lumbar puncture is performed in such patients because of the pressure changes induced within the cranial vault.[21]

S.C. has many of the clinical features associated with acute bacterial meningitis. High fever, stiff neck, altered mentation, photophobia, and positive Kernig and Brudzinski signs all are consistent with bacterial meningitis. Furthermore, the low blood pressure (hypotension) and increased respiratory rate are characteristic findings in severe, life-threatening types of bacterial infection (e.g., septic shock, meningitis) and are likely the result of endotoxin release.

The signs and symptoms of meningitis in the very young and very old differ from those in older children and adults.[5,22,29,40] In neonates, signs of meningeal irritation may be absent; fever, irritability, and poor feeding are often the only symptoms manifested.[5,22] Fullness of the fontanel in infants also may reflect the increased intracranial pressure that occurs with meningitis.[5,36] Because S.C. is 5 years of age, accurate assessment of his mental status is challenging. Irritability (crying), as was manifested by S.C., is an important finding that suggests an altered mental status.

In elderly patients, many of the classic signs of meningeal irritation are absent as well, and the disease presentation can be subtler.[5,29,37] Therefore, given the grave consequences of a misdiagnosis, clinicians caring for infants and elderly patients must have a particularly high index of suspicion for meningitis.

Laboratory evaluation of meningitis should include serum chemistries and a hemogram as well as a detailed examination of the CSF.[5,11,37] The peripheral WBC count often is markedly elevated in acute bacterial meningitis, usually with a left shift evident on the differential. This finding, however, is nonspecific and occurs in many acute inflammatory and infectious diseases. S.C. has a marked leukocytosis with a predominance of PMN cells on the differential. A low serum sodium value, which is present in S.C., reflects the syndrome of inappropriate secretion of antidiuretic hormone (SIADH), a frequent complication of acute bacterial meningitis.[4,5] SIADH is an important finding in meningitis because it worsens cerebral edema.[4,5]

The abrupt onset of S.C.'s clinical symptoms is consistent with an acute bacterial process rather than a fungal or viral etiology. Given his age (5 years) and the community-acquired nature of the infection, the most likely pathogens for his meningitis are *H. influenzae, N. meningitidis,* and *S. pneumoniae.* The presence of maculopapular lesions argues for *N. meningitidis* as the causative pathogen because this is a common finding in cases of meningococcemia or meningococcal meningitis.[3] To make an accurate clinical and microbiologic diagnosis in S.C., it is necessary to obtain CSF for analysis. Thus, a lumbar puncture is required as soon as possible.

CEREBROSPINAL FLUID EXAMINATION

CASE 62-1, QUESTION 2: The resident in the ED performs a lumbar puncture, which yielded the following:

Opening pressure, 300 mm CSF (normal, < 20)
CSF glucose, 20 mg/dL (normal, 60% of plasma glucose)
Protein, 250 mg/dL (normal, < 50 mg/dL)
WBC count, 1,200 cells/μL, with 90% PMN, 4% monohistiocytes, and 6% lymphocytes

The CSF red blood cell (RBC) count was 50/μL. A stat Gram stain of CSF revealed numerous WBCs but no organisms. CSF, blood, and urine cultures are pending. What CSF findings in S.C. are consistent with a diagnosis of bacterial meningitis?

TABLE 62-3
Cerebrospinal Fluid Findings in Various Types of Meningitis

Microbial Etiology	WBC Count (cells/μL)	Predominant Cell Type	Protein	Glucose
Bacterial	>500	PMN	Elevated	Decreased
Fungal	10–500	MN	Elevated	Variable
Viral	10–200	PMN or MN	Variable	Normal

MN, mononuclear cells; PMN, polymorphonuclear neutrophils; WBC, white blood cell.

Careful examination of the CSF is essential to confirm the diagnosis of meningitis.[9] Table 62-3 compares the typical findings in CSF obtained from patients with acute bacterial meningitis with those seen with fungal or viral causes.[5,16,37] In acute bacterial meningitis, the CSF is purulent, containing numerous WBCs (usually >500 cells/μL) with a predominance of PMNs, and often is turbid.[11,37] CSF protein nearly always is elevated, usually greater than 100 mg/dL, and the CSF glucose concentration is low, either less than 50 mg/dL or less than 50% of a simultaneously obtained serum glucose value.[9,12] In contrast, CSF obtained in viral and fungal cases of meningitis usually is clear and characterized by a much lower WBC count (<100 cells/μL), with a mononuclear or lymphocyte predominance.[16,37] Although the CSF protein concentration often is elevated, it may be normal.[16] A variable effect is observed with CSF glucose.[16]

MICROBIOLOGIC EVALUATION

Microbiologic evaluation should include examination of CSF by Gram stain and culture as well as cultures obtained from other potential sites of infection (e.g., blood, sputum, urine).[5,37] Gram stain of the CSF is positive in more than 50% of acute bacterial meningitis cases and directs initial (empiric) antimicrobial therapy.[5,9,37] The presence of organisms on smear is indicative of a high bacterial inoculum (i.e., inoculum $>10^5$ colony-forming units/mL) and is associated with more fulminant disease.[2] The absence of organisms on Gram stain by no means rules out infection but does make selection of empiric therapy more difficult.

S.C. has a negative Gram stain, which may be the result of previous antibiotic therapy or the early detection of disease. Given the negative CSF Gram stain result, S.C. must receive antibacterial therapy sufficiently broad to cover all pathogens associated with meningitis in his age group until the results from his CSF culture are available (usually within 24 to 48 hours). The CSF culture nearly always is positive in purulent meningitis, and the presence of any organism in this normally sterile fluid is concerning.[5,37,41] In a few instances, particularly with antecedent receipt of antibiotic therapy, CSF cultures can be negative in a patient who clearly has meningitis.[9,36,41] In this setting, newer diagnostic tests, such as latex particle agglutination, which reliably detect antigens of *H. influenzae, S. pneumoniae, N. meningitidis, E. coli* (K-1 capsular antigen), and group B streptococci in CSF, are available. Latex particle agglutination should be considered for S.C., especially if his cultures fail to yield any growth. Finally, results from cultures of other sites, such as the blood, urine, and sputum (when appropriate), can yield very useful microbiologic information.[37,41]

The CSF findings in S.C. also strongly support the diagnosis of bacterial meningitis. He has a markedly elevated opening CSF pressure, CSF leukocytosis (with a predominance of PMNs), an elevated CSF protein concentration, and a depressed CSF glucose value. A few RBCs are present in the CSF, which suggests contamination with peripheral blood caused by the traumatic nature of the lumbar puncture. Precise identification of the offending organism is not possible until CSF culture results are available.

Treatment Principles

Prompt institution of appropriate antimicrobial therapy is essential when treating meningitis.[37] Delay in antibiotic administration is associated with increased morbidity and mortality.[42] When choosing antimicrobial therapy, a number of factors must be considered. First, the antibiotics selected must penetrate adequately into the CSF.[12,15,43] In addition, the regimen chosen must have potent activity against known or suspected pathogens and exert a bactericidal effect.[15]

ANTIMICROBIAL PENETRATION INTO THE CEREBROSPINAL FLUID

In cases of purulent meningitis, the concentration of bacteria in the CSF can be greater than the standard inoculum (~10^5 colony-forming units/mL) used in routine antimicrobial susceptibility testing.[15,44] As a result, extrapolation of in vitro sensitivity results to clinical efficacy is difficult, particularly for antimicrobials susceptible to an inoculum effect (i.e., an increase in the MIC with an increase in inoculum size). Cefuroxime, for example, is affected by an inoculum effect against *H. influenzae,* and piperacillin-tazobactam is similarly affected by enteric gram-negative bacilli.[15,45] In addition, some antimicrobials (e.g., aminoglycosides, fluoroquinolones) have reduced bactericidal activity in the acidic milieu of purulent CSF.[15,43,46,47] For example, gentamicin has a minimum bactericidal concentration (MBC) of 1 mcg/mL against *E. coli* at a pH of 7.35, and a decrease in the pH to 7.0 results in an eightfold increase in MBC.[48] This may partially explain why aminoglycoside therapy for gram-negative bacillary meningitis is suboptimal, even when direct intrathecal therapy is given.[31,34] The ability of antimicrobials to penetrate into the CSF is affected by lipid solubility, degree of ionization, molecular weight, protein binding, and susceptibility to active transport systems operative within the choroid plexus.[12,15,44,49] In general, the penetration of most antibiotics into the CSF is increased when the meninges are inflamed. The rabbit meningitis model suggests that bactericidal effects are maximal when CSF antibiotic concentrations exceed the MBC of the infecting pathogen by 10- to 30-fold.[15,43,48] Antimicrobial penetration into the CSF is most commonly reported as a ratio of CSF to serum antimicrobial levels. Table 62-4 summarizes the CSF penetration characteristics of various antimicrobials during acute bacterial meningitis.[12,13,43,48,50] Chloramphenicol, metronidazole, and trimethoprim are highly lipophilic compounds and penetrate into the CSF extremely well, achieving high concentrations even when meningeal inflammation is absent.[12,43,51] Rifampin has satisfactory CSF penetration and may be combined with vancomycin to treat coagulase-negative staphylococcal infections in the CNS.[7,43,51] Because β-lactams and aminoglycosides usually are ionized at physiologic pH, they are more polar and do not penetrate into the CSF as well. β-Lactams penetrate poorly when the meninges are intact, but when the meninges are inflamed, most penicillins and the third-generation cephalosporins achieve CSF concentrations sufficient to treat meningitis (~10%–30% of simultaneously obtained serum concentrations).[12,43,49–51] An additional factor working against maintenance of therapeutic concentrations of β-lactams in the CSF is the active transport system of the choroid plexus, which pumps these organic acids out of the CSF.[15] Meropenem achieves CSF levels 10% to 40% of serum levels.[48]

TABLE 62-4
Cerebrospinal Fluid Penetration Characteristics of Various Antimicrobials

Very Good[a]
Chloramphenicol, metronidazole, TMP-SMX, linezolid
Good[a]
Penicillins: Penicillin G, ampicillin, nafcillin *Other β-lactams:* Aztreonam, clavulanic acid, imipenem, meropenem, sulbactam *Cephalosporins:* Cefepime, cefotaxime, ceftazidime, ceftizoxime, ceftriaxone *Other agents:* Rifampin
Fair to Poor[c]
Aminoglycosides: Amikacin, gentamicin, tobramycin *Other agents:* Azithromycin, clarithromycin, clindamycin, erythromycin, vancomycin, daptomycin

[a]Penetrates CSF well regardless of meningeal inflammation.
[b]Adequate CSF penetration achieved when the meninges are inflamed.
[c]Penetration often inadequate even when the meninges are inflamed.
CSF, cerebrospinal fluid; TMP-SMX, trimethoprim-sulfamethoxazole.

The aminoglycosides have a low therapeutic index, and adequate CSF concentrations are difficult to achieve with intravenous (IV) dosing alone without risking significant toxicity.[13,43] Furthermore, the acidic nature of purulent CSF reduces the antimicrobial activity of the aminoglycosides.[47] Thus, when aminoglycoside therapy is initiated for adults with CNS infections, concomitant intrathecal therapy is required.[13,52] Direct instillation of aminoglycosides into the ventricles is preferred, but this approach requires the surgical insertion of a reservoir (e.g., Ommaya reservoir), which often is not possible, particularly in the early stages of bacterial meningitis.[15,43] The degree of serum protein binding correlates well with the extent of CSF penetration.[15,49] Ceftriaxone is highly bound to serum proteins and, thus, is more confined to the intravascular space and not as readily available for CSF penetration as cefotaxime and ceftazidime, which are less protein bound. Ceftriaxone achieves sustained, reliable bactericidal activity within the CSF despite its high protein binding[43,50] and has been used successfully to treat meningitis in both children and adults.[4,50,53]

Vancomycin and polymyxin B do not diffuse well across the blood–CSF barrier, primarily because of their large molecular size.[11,15,43,51] Therapeutic concentrations in the CSF (up to 22% of serum concentrations) are attained with systemic vancomycin therapy when the meninges are inflamed. In selected circumstances, however, concomitant intraventricular therapy also may be necessary.[7,43] Clindamycin and erythromycin penetrate the CSF poorly[12,43,51] and should not be used in the treatment of meningitis.

Although fluoroquinolones penetrate reasonably well into the CSF on a percentage basis (~20%–30%), CSF concentrations attained are inadequate (≤1 mcg/mL) when standard doses are administered.[43,46]

EMPIRIC THERAPY FOR CHILDHOOD MENINGITIS

CASE 62-1, QUESTION 3: A detailed medication and vaccination history reveals that S.C. and his brother appropriately received vaccination for Hib when they were 2 months of age. What constitutes appropriate empiric therapy for childhood meningitis? Which antibiotic would be appropriate for S.C.? What dose and route of administration should be used?

Because results from culture and sensitivity testing of CSF will not be available for more than 24 hours, empiric therapy must be instituted promptly. The regimen should take into consideration the patient's age, any predisposing conditions,

TABLE 62-5
Empiric Therapy for Bacterial Meningitis

Age Group or Predisposing Condition	Recommended Therapy	Alternative Therapy
Neonates (<1 month)	Ampicillin + cefotaxime	Ampicillin + gentamicin
Infants and children (1–23 months)	Cefotaxime or ceftriaxone + vancomycin	Vancomycin + rifampin + aztreonam
Older children and adults (2–50 years)	Cefotaxime or ceftriaxone + vancomycin	Vancomycin + rifampin + aztreonam
Elderly (>50 years)	Ampicillin, cefotaxime, or ceftriaxone + vancomycin	Vancomycin + TMP-SMX + aztreonam
Postneurosurgical	Vancomycin + ceftazidime	Vancomycin + cefepime or meropenem
Closed head trauma	Cefotaxime or ceftriaxone + vancomycin	Vancomycin + rifampin + aztreonam
Penetrating head trauma	Vancomycin + ceftazidime	Vancomycin + cefepime or meropenem
Presence of risk factor (alcoholism and altered immune status)	Vancomycin + ceftriaxone or cefotaxime + ampicillin	Vancomycin + TMP-SMX + aztreonam

TMP-SMX, trimethoprim-sulfamethoxazole.

results from the CSF Gram stain, history of allergy, and the presence of organ dysfunction. Table 62-5 gives recommendations for empiric antimicrobial therapy for acute bacterial meningitis.[4,5,19,21,38,39,52–54]

S.C. is 5 years of age and has a negative CSF Gram stain. Therefore, therapy with a third-generation cephalosporin, such as ceftriaxone or cefotaxime (Claforan), is preferred. Either of these two agents will provide excellent coverage of the most likely pathogens in this age group (*S. pneumoniae* and *N. meningitidis*).[18,19,54] Of these two pathogens, S.C.'s rash suggests that *N. meningitidis* is likely.[38] *H. influenzae* is not very likely because he was vaccinated against Hib. Thus, initiation of ceftriaxone plus vancomycin would be appropriate for S.C. at this time.

Use of a cephalosporin in this case is appropriate despite the allergic history with amoxicillin (history of skin rash). Patients with penicillin allergy carry a 5% to 12% risk of cross-reactivity when cephalosporins are prescribed, depending on the agent.[55] In this setting, the type of reaction to penicillin is important to consider.[55] Patients with a history of accelerated hypersensitivity reactions (e.g., hives, shortness of breath [SOB], or anaphylaxis) to penicillins should not be given cephalosporins in most instances. Conversely, a benign skin rash would not contraindicate use of a cephalosporin. If S.C. had experienced an accelerated reaction to penicillin, vancomycin plus aztreonam would be the best alternative choice (Table 62-5).[4,5,21]

DOSING CONSIDERATIONS

In general, therapy of meningitis requires the use of high dosages of antimicrobials administered by the IV route. Table 62-6 lists the recommended dosing regimens for the treatment of CNS infections.[4,5,7,13,52,54,56]

TABLE 62-6
Suggested Antibiotic Dosing Regimens for Treatment of Central Nervous System Infections

	Daily Dose (interval in hours)[a]			
	Neonates			
Antibiotic	0–7 days Old	8–28 days Old	Infants and Children	Adults
Ampicillin	150 mg/kg (8)	200 mg/kg (6–8)	300 mg/kg (6)	12 g (4)
Aztreonam				8 g (6)
Nafcillin	75 mg/kg (8–12)	100–150 mg/kg (6–8)	200 mg/kg (6)	12 g (4)
Penicillin G	0.15 million units/kg (8–12)	0.2 million units/kg (6–8)	0.3 million units/kg (4–6)	24 million units (4)
Meropenem			120 mg/kg (8)	6 g (8)
Cephalosporins				
Cefotaxime	100–150 mg/kg (8–12)	150- 200 mg/kg (6–8)	225–300 mg/kg (6–8)	12 g (4)
Ceftriaxone			80–100 mg/kg (12–24)	4 g (12)
Cefazidime	100–150 mg/kg (8–12)	150 mg/kg (8)	150 mg/kg (8)	6 g (8)
Cefepime			150 mg/kg (8)	6 g (8)
Aminoglycoside[b,c]				
Gentamicin	5 mg/kg (12)	7.5 mg/kg (8)	7.5 mg/kg (8)	5–7 mg/kg (24)
Tobramycin	5 mg/kg (12)	7.5 mg/kg (8)	7.5 mg/kg (8)	5–7 mg/kg (24)
Amikacin	15–20 mg/kg (12)	30 mg/kg (8)	20–30 mg/kg (8)	15 mg/kg (24)
Linezolid				1,200 mg (12)
Rifampin		10–20 mg/kg (12)	10–20 mg/kg (12–24)	600 mg (24)
TMP-SMX[d]			10–20 mg/kg (6–12)	10–20 mg/kg (6–12)
Vancomycin[c,e]	20–30 mg/kg (8–12)	30–45 mg/kg (6–8)	60 mg/kg (6)	30–45 mg/kg (8–12)

[a]Recommended daily dose when renal and hepatic functions are normal.
[b]Concurrent intraventricular doses of 5–10 mg (gentamicin, tobramycin) or 20 mg (amikacin) often required when treating gram-negative bacillary meningitis.
[c]Dose should be individualized based on serum level monitoring.
[d]Dose is based on the trimethoprim component.
[e]Concurrent intraventricular doses of 5–20 mg recommended if response to intravenous therapy is inadequate.
TMP-SMX, trimethoprim-sulfamethoxazole.
Source: Tunkel AR et al. Practice guidelines for the management of bacterial meningitis. *Clin Infect Dis.* 2004;39:1267.

S.C. should receive ceftriaxone in a dosage of 100 mg/kg/day given in one or two doses.[5,53,54] A ceftriaxone regimen of 1,000 mg IV every 12 hours is reasonable for S.C. The elimination half-life of ceftriaxone is long (usually 6–8 hours), and once-daily dosing is feasible. Many clinicians, however, prefer to administer ceftriaxone on a twice-daily schedule[4,54] because most published trials used the twice-daily regimen and such a schedule reduces the potential for prolonged periods of subtherapeutic CSF concentrations if a dose is delayed or missed.[4] Nevertheless, the US Food and Drug Administration (FDA) has approved the use of the once-daily dosing regimen of ceftriaxone for treatment of pediatric meningitis.[57]

ADJUNCTIVE CORTICOSTEROID THERAPY

CASE 62-1, QUESTION 4: What is the rationale for adjunctive corticosteroid therapy in acute bacterial meningitis, and would it be appropriate for S.C.? How should dexamethasone be dosed and monitored for S.C.?

Corticosteroids, particularly dexamethasone, can reduce cerebral edema and lower intracranial pressure.[58] In addition, corticosteroids reduce the synthesis and release of the proinflammatory cytokines tumor necrosis factor-α and interleukin 1β from monocytes and astrocytes.[3,4] These two cytokines play a central role in initiating the cascade of events that lead to neuronal tissue damage and neurologic sequelae. Theoretically, then, inhibition of cytokine synthesis by corticosteroids in meningitis should lead to a decreased risk of hearing loss and other neurologic sequelae. Indeed, a prospective, randomized, double-blind multicenter trial evaluating the use of dexamethasone in adults with acute bacterial meningitis supported this theory.[59] A total of 301 patients were randomly assigned to receive dexamethasone or placebo 15 to 20 minutes before or with the first dose of antibiotic every 6 hours for 4 days. Dexamethasone reduced the risk of unfavorable outcome, defined as a Glasgow Coma Scale score of 1 to 4 at 8 weeks (relative risk, 0.59; $p = 0.03$), and of death (relative risk, 0.48; $p = 0.04$). Among the patients with pneumococcal meningitis, 26% in the dexamethasone group and 52% in the placebo group had unfavorable outcomes (relative risk, 0.5; $p = 0.06$). Although this was not statistically significant, patients with pneumococcal meningitis appeared to receive the most benefit from steroids. Dexamethasone did not significantly decrease the risk of neurologic sequelae, including hearing loss. Neither gastrointestinal (GI) bleeding nor other adverse effects were increased in the dexamethasone group. Based largely on the results of this study, the 2004 Infectious Diseases Society of America meningitis guidelines recommend that dexamethasone be initiated before (or concomitant with the first dose of) antimicrobial therapy in all adult patients with suspected or proven pneumococcal meningitis.[21] Controversy remains about whether dexamethasone should be continued in adults if the causative agent is found not to be pneumococcus, but many experts recommend continuing regardless of pathogen.[60]

The use of adjunctive dexamethasone in the treatment of bacterial meningitis for children, however, has been more controversial. Several prospective placebo-controlled, randomized trials have demonstrated that adjunctive dexamethasone therapy significantly reduces audiologic and neurologic sequelae in children older than 2 months of age. *H. influenzae,* however, was the causative pathogen in most of these meningitis cases, whereas the number of children with streptococcal and meningococcal meningitis in these trials was small.[4,61–65] As previously mentioned, the number of Hib cases has decreased dramatically, making the data from these trials difficult to apply to the present day. More recently, of the 166 patients enrolled in a trial comparing dexamethasone with placebo, 35 and 26 cases were caused by *S. pneumoniae* and *N. meningitides,* respectively, in the treatment arm. Few audiologic and neurologic sequelae were observed in the dexamethasone-treated group compared with the placebo group, but the difference did not reach statistical significance.[66]

In 2010, a Cochrane meta-analysis was conducted to ascertain whether an overall effect could be noted when the available studies were combined.[67] Although no significant effect on mortality was noted, use of adjunctive corticosteroids in children with bacterial meningitis was shown to significantly reduce the outcomes of any hearing loss, severe hearing loss, and short-term neurologic sequelae in children in high-income countries. When analyzed separately, the difference in severe hearing loss was significant for children infected with *H. influenzae,* but not for other pathogens.

Although controversy remains, these data provide convincing evidence for the beneficial effects of adjunctive dexamethasone therapy. The risks associated with short-term steroid therapy are low and are outweighed by the benefit of a reduction in neurologic complications. Therefore, children with bacterial meningitis should receive adjunctive dexamethasone therapy. At this time, there can be no firm recommendation as to whether steroids should be continued in children if the pathogen is found not to be *H. influenzae.*[2,4]

Thus, S.C. should receive dexamethasone therapy, 0.15 mg/kg/dose given IV every 6 hours for 2 to 4 days. For S.C., who is 20 kg, this would be 3 mg every 6 hours, with the first dexamethasone dose given 15 minutes before initiating ceftriaxone therapy.

Potential adverse effects associated with dexamethasone include GI bleeding, mental status changes (e.g., euphoria or encephalopathy), increases in blood glucose, and possibly elevations in blood pressure.[4,58,68,69] For S.C., the complete blood count, serum chemistries, and stool guaiac should be monitored daily while he is receiving dexamethasone. He also should be questioned about possible GI upset and assessed for changes in mental status (e.g., confusion, combativeness). Given the short duration of corticosteroid therapy, dexamethasone can be discontinued abruptly without tapering.

EFFECT ON CENTRAL NERVOUS SYSTEM PENETRATION OF ANTIBIOTICS

Another important issue to consider is whether dexamethasone, a potent anti-inflammatory agent, reduces the ability of antimicrobials to penetrate across the blood–brain barrier into the CSF. Because CSF penetration of the penicillins, cephalosporins, and vancomycin is greatest when the meninges are inflamed, a hypothetical concern is that concomitant dexamethasone may reduce CSF concentrations of these agents, resulting in reduced efficacy. Current data suggest that CSF penetration of ceftriaxone is not diminished with concomitant administration of dexamethasone.[70–73] Animal models, however, suggest that vancomycin penetration into the CSF is reduced in dexamethasone-treated animals compared with animals not treated with steroids.[70–72] As such, a concern is that adjunctive dexamethasone may delay CSF sterilization in patients with pneumococcal meningitis attributable to penicillin- or cephalosporin-resistant strains. In a rabbit meningitis model, the coadministration of dexamethasone and vancomycin resulted in 29% less penetration of vancomycin into the CSF. By increasing the daily dose of vancomycin in these rabbits, however, therapeutic CSF levels were achieved, suggesting that giving larger daily doses of vancomycin circumvents the steroid effect on CNS penetration.[74] A study in children receiving concomitant dexamethasone found that vancomycin at a dose of 60 mg/kg/day penetrated reliably into the CSF.[75] Finally, a study evaluated vancomycin levels in the CSF in 14 adult patients receiving adjunctive corticosteroids to treat pneumococcal meningitis.[76] Vancomycin was administered by continuous infusion at 60 mg/kg/day. In this small observational study, vancomycin concentrations in the CSF were therapeutic even in the setting of dexamethasone.[76] Based on these encouraging findings, it is recommended that dexamethasone be used in all patients, regardless of the concern for penicillin- or cephalosporin-resistant pneumococcus.[21]

Neisseria meningitidis Meningitis

DEFINITIVE THERAPY

CASE 62-1, QUESTION 5: Twenty-four hours after admission, S.C.'s culture results from his blood and CSF samples are available. The CSF culture is growing *N. meningitidis* (penicillin MIC, 0.06 mg/L), and *N. meningitidis* is also growing in both of the two collected blood cultures. What modification in S.C.'s antimicrobial therapy is necessary at this time?

Once culture and sensitivity results become available, definitive therapy can be instituted, often with a single agent (Table 62-7).[4,5,32–35,54] As suspected, S.C.'s CSF culture is positive for *N. meningitidis.* Cefuroxime, a second-generation cephalosporin, has activity against *N. meningitides;* however, it is less effective for meningitis than third-generation cephalosporins and should not be used.[77,78] In a prospective, randomized trial involving 106 children with acute bacterial meningitis, 12% of the patients receiving cefuroxime had positive CSF cultures after 18 to 24 hours versus 2% of those who received ceftriaxone ($p = 0.11$), and 17% of cefuroxime-treated patients experienced moderate to severe hearing loss compared with only 4% of those receiving ceftriaxone ($p = 0.05$).[77] Nearly identical findings to these also were noted in a retrospective analysis of four comparative trials of children treated with cefuroxime (159 patients) and ceftriaxone (174 patients) for bacterial meningitis.[78] The reason for the inferiority of cefuroxime relative to ceftriaxone most likely is related to reduced potency and the presence of an inoculum effect (described earlier).[45]

Because *N. meningitidis* is susceptible to penicillin and ampicillin currently, penicillin is the drug of choice. However, S.C.'s questionable history of amoxicillin rash makes the use of ceftriaxone a reasonable choice.

MONITORING THERAPY

CASE 62-1, QUESTION 6: What subjective and objective data should be monitored to evaluate the efficacy and toxicity of treatment of patients with meningitis, and what specifically should be monitored in S.C.?

Clinical signs and symptoms attributable to the disease, such as fever, altered mental status, and stiff neck, should be checked periodically throughout the day and monitored for resolution. S.C.'s temperature and mental status should be assessed often. Accurate assessment of S.C.'s mental status can be difficult because of his young age. Thus, his baseline level of mental status should be evaluated (e.g., whether he is awake and alert, or lethargic and difficult to arouse). If awake and alert, S.C. should be observed for irritability, because this often is the only sign of altered mentation. Questions can be used to assess his orientation: Does he know where he is? Does he know his name? Can he recognize his mother or other family members? In general, signs of clinical improvement should be evident within 24 to 48 hours for most uncomplicated cases of acute bacterial meningitis,[4,5,37,77] and the corticosteroid therapy that S.C. is receiving may accelerate the clinical response.[4]

Laboratory tests should be monitored as well. A complete blood count with differential, serum electrolytes (e.g., Na, K, Cl, HCO_3), blood glucose, and renal function tests (e.g., BUN, SCr) should be performed daily. Abnormal electrolyte results may require more frequent monitoring. Laboratory abnormalities, such as leukocytosis and hyponatremia, may take longer to normalize than clinical symptoms. If S.C. exhibits severe SIADH,

TABLE 62-7
Definitive Therapy for Bacterial Meningitis

Pathogen	Recommended Treatment	Alternative Agents
Haemophilus influenzae		
β-Lactamase-negative	Ampicillin	Cefotaxime or ceftriaxone; aztreonam;
β-Lactamase-positive	Cefotaxime or ceftriaxone	Aztreonam
Neisseria meningitidis	Penicillin MIC <0.1 mcg/mL: Penicillin G or ampicillin	Cefotaxime or ceftriaxone
	Penicillin MIC 0.1–1.0 mcg/mL: Cefotaxime or ceftriaxone	Meropenem
Streptococcus pneumoniae	Penicillin MIC ≤0.06 mcg/mL: Penicillin G or ampicillin	Cefotaxime or ceftriaxone
	Penicillin MIC ≥0.12 mcg/mL: Cefotaxime or ceftriaxone if susceptible	Vancomycin
	Penicillin and cefotaxime/ceftriaxone nonsusceptible: Vancomycin + cefotaxime/ceftriaxone ± rifampin	Vancomycin + meropenem
Streptococcus agalactiae	Penicillin G or ampicillin + gentamicin	Cefotaxime or ceftriaxone
Listeria monocytogenes	Penicillin G or ampicillin ± gentamicin	TMP-SMX
Enterobacteriaceae[a]		
E. coli, Klebsiella species	Cefotaxime or ceftriaxone	Cefepime; aztreonam; meropenem
Enterobacter, Serratia species	Cefepime; meropenem	TMP-SMX; aztreonam
Pseudomonas aeruginosa	Cefepime or ceftazidime; meropenem	Aztreonam
Staphylococcus aureus[a]		
Methicillin-susceptible (MSSA)	Nafcillin or oxacillin	Vancomycin ± rifampin; meropenem; linezolid
Methicillin-resistant (MRSA)	Vancomycin ± rifampin	TMP-SMX; linezolid
Staphylococcus epidermidis[a]	Vancomycin ± rifampin	TMP-SMX; linezolid

[a] Concomitant intrathecal therapy may be required for optimal response (most commonly an intrathecal aminoglycoside for gram-negative or intrathecal vancomycin for gram-positive infections).
MIC, minimum inhibitory concentration; TMP-SMX, trimethoprim-sulfamethoxazole.

as manifested by serum sodium values up to 120 mEq/L with altered mental status or seizures, fluid restriction and short-term (i.e., 6–12 hours) IV administration of 3% sodium chloride may be necessary.

CSF chemistries usually normalize after several days, although CSF protein may remain elevated for a week or more.[5,37] With effective therapy, the CSF culture usually is sterile after about 18 to 24 hours of therapy.[4,77] Delays in CSF sterilization are associated with a higher propensity for neurologic complications.[4,35] If S.C. responds to therapy in a straightforward manner, he need not have a repeat lumbar puncture. If the response is inadequate, as evidenced by persistent fever or deteriorating mental status, S.C. will require a repeat lumbar puncture to re-examine the CSF parameters.[5,37]

In addition to monitoring the therapeutic response, side effects of the antimicrobial regimen also need to be assessed frequently. Meningitis requires high-dose therapy, making the likelihood of adverse effects much greater. Currently, S.C. is being treated with ceftriaxone, a cephalosporin antibiotic. The adverse effects most often associated with ceftriaxone include hypersensitivity reactions, mild pain and phlebitis at the injection site, and GI complaints.[79] S.C. should be observed for the formation of an antibiotic-related skin rash or evidence of an accelerated allergic reaction (e.g., hives, wheezing). The IV catheter site should be observed daily for redness, tenderness, or pain on palpation of the vein. S.C. should be watched closely for loose stools or diarrhea. Although diarrhea is a common side effect of most antimicrobials, this adverse effect is more likely to occur with ceftriaxone because approximately 40% to 50% of the dose is excreted unchanged into the bile. Mild diarrhea, which usually does not require discontinuation of therapy, occurs in 23% to 41% of children receiving ceftriaxone for meningitis therapy.[53,77] Less common, but of concern, is the potential for antibiotic-associated colitis.[79,80] If S.C. experiences diarrhea that is persistent, accompanied by fever and abdominal cramping, a stool sample should be tested for *Clostridium difficile* toxin. (see Chapter 66, Infectious Diarrhea).

CEFTRIAXONE-INDUCED BILIARY PSEUDOLITHIASIS

CASE 62-1, QUESTION 7: After 5 days of treatment, the nurse caring for S.C. notes that his appetite is markedly diminished, and he complains of an upset stomach. S.C. was afebrile and alert and oriented, but abdominal examination revealed "guarding," with pain localized in the right upper quadrant area. Laboratory data at this time are as follows:

WBC count, 6,000 cells/μL
Hgb, 12.5 g/dL
Hct, 34%
Platelets, 120,000/μL
Na, 135 mEq/L
K, 3.6 mEq/L
Cl, 98 mEq/L
Aspartate aminotransferase (AST), 35 units/L
Alanine aminotransferase (ALT), 33 units/L
Alkaline phosphatase, 110 units/L
Total bilirubin, 1.2 mg/dL
Amylase 70 units/L

A stool guaiac is negative. What are possible causes of S.C.'s abdominal discomfort?

A number of possible causes exist for S.C.'s abdominal discomfort. His corticosteroid therapy may have caused acute GI bleeding, however, the dexamethasone was discontinued 3 days ago, and S.C.'s hemoglobin and hematocrit values are in the low-normal range. The negative stool guaiac result also argues strongly against a GI bleed. Acute pancreatitis is unlikely given the normal amylase result. Viral or drug-induced hepatitis is another possibility but also is unlikely given his normal AST, ALT, and bilirubin results. An intra-abdominal infection also is possible, but this is improbable because he is afebrile and has a normal WBC count. Other causes, such as acute cholecystitis or appendicitis, require further diagnostic evaluation.

CASE 62-1, QUESTION 8: An abdominal ultrasound reveals sludge in the gallbladder. What is the significance of this finding in S.C., and how should this abnormality be managed?

The abnormality on S.C.'s abdominal ultrasound explains his right upper quadrant pain. S.C. has what appears to be a condition known as biliary pseudolithiasis (i.e., biliary "sludging"). Biliary sludging can occur in conditions of gallbladder hypomotility (e.g., recent surgery, burns, total parenteral nutrition) and, in some instances, can be drug-induced. S.C. has been receiving ceftriaxone for treatment of his meningitis, and this drug can cause biliary pseudolithiasis.[81–84]

Antibiotic-associated biliary pseudolithiasis is seen almost exclusively with ceftriaxone.[79] The biliary excretion associated with ceftriaxone results in very high concentrations of the drug in gallbladder bile.[81] In selected circumstances, the biliary concentration of ceftriaxone may exceed solubility limits, resulting in formation of a fine, granular precipitate (i.e., sludge),[81] which differs in composition and ultrasound features from true gallstones.[77,82] The precipitate is composed of a ceftriaxone–calcium complex, the formation of which is dose dependent.[81,83] Given the high dosages required for meningitis therapy, it is not surprising that this adverse effect has occurred in S.C.[77,82] In the comparative randomized trial between ceftriaxone and cefuroxime cited previously, evidence of biliary pseudolithiasis on abdominal ultrasonography was observed in 16 of 35 (46%) patients who received ceftriaxone and in none of 35 patients receiving cefuroxime.[77] Pseudolithiasis usually appears 3 to 10 days after the start of therapy, and in most instances, it is clinically asymptomatic. Symptoms similar to acute cholecystitis are evident in some individuals and include nausea with or without vomiting and abdominal right upper quadrant pain. Approximately 10% to 20% of patients with evidence of biliary sludging on ultrasound are symptomatic.[82,84]

Prompt recognition of this adverse effect and discontinuation of ceftriaxone therapy are required to effectively manage biliary pseudolithiasis. Before this complication was recognized, a few patients underwent cholecystectomies, but this intervention is rarely necessary because the condition nearly always is reversible. Once S.C.'s ceftriaxone is discontinued, the condition should resolve gradually during a period of weeks to months; the clinical symptoms should disappear within a few days.[82,84] Cefotaxime can be substituted for ceftriaxone; cefotaxime is not associated with biliary complications, and the efficacy of these two agents is equivalent.[79] For S.C., the cefotaxime dosage would be 1,000 mg IV every 6 hours (Table 62-6).

DURATION OF THERAPY

CASE 62-1, QUESTION 9: What is the recommended duration of antimicrobial therapy for S.C.?

The optimal duration of therapy for meningitis is difficult to ascertain because few trials have been designed to address this issue.[85] Although general guidelines exist, the duration should

TABLE 62-8
Duration of Therapy for Bacterial Meningitis

Etiology	Duration of Therapy (days)
Haemophilus influenzae	7
Neisseria meningitidis	7
Streptococcus pneumoniae	10–14
Group B streptococci *(Streptococcus agalactiae)*	14–21
Listeria monocytogenes	≥21
Gram-negative bacilli	21

be individualized based on the response to therapy, the presence of complicating factors (e.g., immunosuppression), and the specific causative pathogen. Table 62-8 lists the recommended treatment durations for uncomplicated cases of bacterial meningitis according to the specific pathogen.[5,21] Patients such as S.C. with meningitis caused by *N. meningitidis* should be treated for 7 days.[21] Complicated cases, such as those with delayed CSF sterilization, require therapy for longer periods (up to 2 weeks or more).

S.C. had been responding well to therapy, and there is no need for additional oral antibiotics when he is discharged from the hospital. An oral second- or third-generation cephalosporin cannot be recommended in the treatment of meningitis because insufficient concentrations are achieved in the CSF. S.C. should be watched carefully for a possible relapse (e.g., the reappearance of signs and symptoms of meningitis), which would require readmission to the hospital for further evaluation and IV antibiotic therapy.

PREVENTION OF NEISSERIA MENINGITIDIS MENINGITIS

CASE 62-1, QUESTION 10: S.C. is ready to be discharged home. How can the potential spread of meningococcal disease be prevented in persons with whom S.C. has contact?

CHEMOPROPHYLAXIS OF CLOSE CONTACTS

Despite an excellent response to therapy, S.C. still may harbor *N. meningitidis* in his nasopharynx and could transmit this organism to individuals with whom he has close contact.[86–88] Therefore, chemoprophylaxis to reduce nasopharyngeal carriage of *N. meningitidis* is indicated for S.C. and his close contacts.[86,88] In this context, close contacts are defined as individuals who frequently sleep and eat in the same dwelling with an index case: a household member, day-care center contacts, and any person directly exposed to the patient's oral secretions (e.g., boyfriend or girlfriend, mouth-to-mouth resuscitation, or endotracheal intubation).[86,88] The potential for a close contact to become infected with *N. meningitidis* is 500 to 800 times greater than for the total population.[86] S.C.'s 7-year-old brother is at risk for invasive *N. meningitidis* disease and should receive chemoprophylaxis. The children at the day-care center or close contacts at the hospital who have been caring for S.C. should also receive chemoprophylaxis. Because the risk of secondary disease is greatest within 2 to 5 days after exposure to the index case, chemoprophylaxis should be instituted as soon as possible and ideally within 24 hours.[86] Administering chemoprophylaxis 14 days or more after identification of the index case is of little value. The most frequently used regimen to reduce nasopharyngeal carriage of *N. meningitidis* for children older than 1 month is rifampin, given twice daily in a dosage of 10 mg/kg/dose for 2 days.[88] The index patient should also receive prophylaxis if he or she was treated with penicillin as soon as he or she is able to tolerate oral medications. Because S.C. is receiving ceftriaxone, he does not need chemoprophylaxis. For adult close contacts, rifampin 600 mg twice a day for 2 days should be administered. Thus, S.C.'s brother, parents, and day-care contacts should be treated with appropriate doses of rifampin as soon as he is diagnosed. Alternative chemoprophylactic regimens shown to be effective for reducing nasopharyngeal carriage of *N. meningitidis* are ceftriaxone 250 mg or 125 mg intramuscularly in adults and children, respectively, and ciprofloxacin 500 mg orally as a single dose in adults. Because rifampin is not recommended for pregnant women, ceftriaxone would be a viable alternative.[86,88]

PREVENTION OF HAEMOPHILUS INFLUENZAE TYPE B MENINGITIS

CASE 62-1, QUESTION 11: S.C. and his brother were vaccinated for Hib. Are these vaccinations now routinely recommended by the Centers for Disease Control and Prevention Advisory Committee on Immunization Practices (ACIP)?

S.C. appropriately received one of the Hib protein conjugate vaccines when he was 2 months of age.[89] Given the tremendous success that conjugated Hib vaccines have had on reducing the incidence of Hib meningitis in the United States, all children older than 2 months of age should receive the vaccination series with one of the three commercially available products.[89] PRP-OMP (PedvaxHIB or Comvax) links PRP with the outer membrane complex protein of *N. meningitidis*. PRP-T (Hiberix) is a PRP–tetanus toxoid conjugate. In 1990, PRP-OMP received FDA approval for use in infants 2 months of age or older. PRP-T should not be used for doses at ages 2, 4, or 6 months for the primary series, but can be used as the final dose in children aged 12 months through 4 years. Table 62-9 outlines the

TABLE 62-9
Recommended Vaccination Schedule for *Haemophilus influenzae* Protein Conjugated Vaccines

	Schedule				
Vaccine (Trade Name)	2 Months	4 Months	6 Months	12–15 Months	15–18 Months
PRP-T (ActHIB)[a,b]	Dose 1	Dose 2	Dose 3	Booster	
PRP-T/DTaP/IPV (Pentacel)[c]	Dose 1	Dose 2	Dose 3		Booster
PRP-OMP (PedvaxHIB)[d]	Dose 1	Dose 2	—	Booster	

[a]Also approved for reconstitution with diphtheria-tetanus-acellular pertussis vaccine (DTaP/PRP-T, TriHIBit), but only for administration as a booster dose in children 15 months and older (i.e., not as initial doses in vaccination series).
[b]Also available as PRP-T (Hiberix), but only for administration as a booster dose in children 15 months to 4 years (i.e., not as initial doses in vaccination series).
[c]Combination vaccine with diphtheria-tetanus-acellular pertussis vaccine (DTaP) and inactivated poliovirus (IPV) vaccine.
[d]Also available in combination with hepatitis B vaccine (PRP-OMP/hepatitis B, Comvax).

vaccination schedule for PRP-OMP and PRP-T as recommended by the ACIP.[90] In general, the vaccines are well tolerated; fever, redness, and swelling at the injection site are the most common adverse effects and occur in less than 4% of patients.[91]

NEISSERIA MENINGITIDIS VACCINATION RECOMMENDATIONS

CASE 62-1, QUESTION 12: What are the current recommendations for the use of meningococcal vaccine in college students?

Neisseria meningitidis is responsible for causing both outbreaks (clusters of cases) as well as epidemics. Currently, three meningococcal vaccines are available in the United States. MPSV4 or Menomune, a quadrivalent (Men A,C,Y,W-135) polysaccharide vaccine, has been available for more than 25 years and is approved for all age groups. Meningococcal conjugate vaccine (MCV4 or Menactra) was approved in January 2005 for use in persons 11 to 55 years of age. Another quadrivalent conjugate vaccine (MenACWY or Menveo) was approved in 2010. Unlike MPSV4, the conjugate vaccines elicit a more durable initial antibody response and also reduce nasopharyngeal carriage. Meningococci serogroups A, B, and C are responsible for causing more than 90% of cases. After vaccination, protective levels of antibody are usually achieved within 7 to 10 days. No vaccine has activity against meningococci serogroup B.[86–88,92]

In 2005, the ACIP recommended routine vaccination of young adolescents with a conjugate vaccine at age 11 or 12 years. The goal at that time was to protect persons aged 16 to 21 years, when meningococcal disease rates peak. It was believed that vaccinating at this time (rather than at 14 or 15 years of age) would be more effective because more persons have preventive care visits at age 11 or 12, and that conjugate vaccines would protect adolescents through the period of risk. Newer data, however, have shown that adolescents vaccinated at age 11 or 12 years may have decreased protective immunity by ages 16 to 21. As such, the ACIP has recently revised its recommendations, and now recommends a booster dose at age 16 years. Corresponding to this recommendation, all persons aged 21 years or younger should have received a dose of conjugate vaccine within 5 years of enrollment to college.[92]

Streptococcus pneumoniae Meningitis

CLINICAL FEATURES, PREDISPOSING FACTORS, AND DIAGNOSIS

CASE 62-2

QUESTION 1: A.L., a 58-year-old man with a long history of alcohol abuse, is admitted to the ED febrile and unresponsive. During the past several days, A.L. has experienced intermittent episodes of fever, chills, SOB, and a worsening productive cough. A friend visiting A.L. called 9–1-1 when he could not arouse him. A.L.'s medical records indicate that he has hypertension, adult-onset diabetes mellitus, peptic ulcer disease (PUD), and chronic obstructive pulmonary disease (COPD). A splenectomy was performed 10 years ago after trauma to the abdomen. A.L. is divorced and lives alone in a low-income apartment. He has no known drug allergies. His records show him to be a smoker for more than 30 years. Current medications include hydrochlorothiazide 50 mg every other day, glipizide 5 mg orally (PO) twice daily, famotidine 20 mg PO every bedtime, and doxycycline PO twice daily as needed for cough and increased sputum production.

On admission to the ED, A.L. had a temperature of 40°C, blood pressure of 90/50 mm Hg, and pulse and respiratory rates of 115 beats/minute and 25 breaths/minute, respectively. His weight is 59 kg. A.L. was unresponsive but withdrew all extremities to painful stimuli. His pupils were equal and sluggishly reactive to light; papilledema and evidence of meningismus were present. Wheezes and crackles were heard throughout both lung fields, with dense consolidation noted in the left lower lobe. The remainder of his physical examination was noncontributory.

Stat laboratory tests revealed the following:

WBC count, 18,000 cells/μL, with 80% PMN, 15% bands, 3% lymphocytes, and 2% basophils
Hgb, 10.5 g/dL
Hct, 34%
Platelet count, 250,000/μL
K, 3.0 mEq/L
Glucose, 250 mg/dL
AST, 190 mg/dL
ALT, 140 mg/dL
BUN, 35 mg/dL
SCr, 2.4 mg/dL

The prothrombin time was high-normal, and albumin was 3.1 mg/dL. A stat blood alcohol level of 100 mg/dL was reported, and a urine toxicology screen was negative. A.L.'s serum theophylline concentration was 18 mg/dL. Stool guaiac was positive.

A CT scan showed no evidence of mass lesions or cerebral hematoma. Lumbar puncture yielded the following results:

CSF opening pressure, 200 mm Hg
Protein, 120 mg/dL
Glucose, 100 mg/dL
WBC count, 8,500 cells/μL, with 92% PMN, 4% monohistiocytes, and 4% lymphocytes
RBC count, 400/μL

Gram-positive, lancet-shaped diplococci were visible on CSF Gram stain. In addition, a sputum Gram stain revealed numerous WBCs, few epithelial cells, and numerous gram-positive cocci in pairs and in short chains. Blood, CSF, urine, and sputum cultures are pending. What are the clinical and laboratory features of pneumococcal meningitis? What features of pneumococcal meningitis are present in A.L.?

A.L. presents to the ED with many signs and symptoms suggestive of pneumococcal meningitis. He is 58 years of age, and *S. pneumoniae* is the most common bacterial etiology for meningitis in adults older than 30 years of age (Table 62-1).[18,19] As is evidenced by A.L.'s presentation, invasive pneumococcal disease often is associated with significant morbidity, and mortality rates remain high.[19] The incidence of *S. pneumoniae* meningitis in the United States has consistently ranged between 1.2 and 2.8 cases per 100,000 population per year.[18,19] Predisposing factors to invasive pneumococcal disease include advanced age, alcoholism, chronic pulmonary disease, and sickle cell disease.[5,38,86] In addition, individuals infected with the human immunodeficiency virus (HIV), those with Hodgkin disease, and patients who have undergone kidney, liver, or bone marrow transplantation are at higher risk.[5,93,94] Patients with CSF otorrhea or rhinorrhea induced by closed head trauma or neurosurgical procedures are more susceptible to have pneumococcal meningitis as well.[19,86,94]

A.L. has many predisposing factors for pneumococcal meningitis. He has a low socioeconomic status, smokes, has a long history of alcohol abuse, has had a splenectomy, and has diabetes and COPD. Underlying COPD is an important predisposing factor in that chronic colonization with pneumococci occurs in such patients. A diagnosis of pneumococcal meningitis in A.L. is supported by the high fever, stiff neck (meningismus), and altered mental status. He is unresponsive, which is a definite negative prognostic factor.[1,5] Results from CSF chemistries and microbiologic analysis are highly suggestive of pneumococcal meningitis. A.L. has an elevated opening CSF pressure and a markedly elevated CSF protein and WBC count with a predominance of neutrophils on differential examination. The normal CSF glucose level (100 g/dL) is misleading because A.L. is diabetic. The calculated ratio of CSF-to-serum glucose for A.L. is less than 50%, which is consistent with acute bacterial meningitis (Table 62-3). The presence of gram-positive, lancet-shaped diplococci in pairs on the CSF Gram stain strongly supports the diagnosis of pneumococcal disease. The signs and symptoms of pneumococcal pneumonia (cough, SOB, increased sputum production, and pulmonary consolidation) as well as the sputum Gram stain result also lend support to a diagnosis of invasive pneumococcal infection.

EMPIRIC THERAPY IN ADULTS

CASE 62-2, QUESTION 2: What empiric therapy is appropriate for A.L. at this time?

Resistance among pneumococci to penicillin G is a significant concern worldwide and in the United States.[2,28] For this reason, susceptibility testing is required for all pneumococcal isolates obtained from sterile sites (e.g., blood, CSF).[2] For treatment of meningitis caused by strains intermediately resistant to penicillin, ceftriaxone and cefotaxime are the most useful agents because many of these isolates retain cephalosporin sensitivity.[2,7,95] Management of invasive pneumococcal infections in sites other than CSF (e.g., lungs, bloodstream) usually can be accomplished by increasing the dose of penicillin G to 20 to 24 million units/day. This approach is not possible with meningitis caused by intermediately resistant strains because further increases in the penicillin dose are likely to produce unacceptable neurotoxicity. *S. pneumoniae* strains in CSF with MIC greater than 0.5 mcg/mL to cefotaxime or ceftriaxone are resistant.[95] Reduced activity of ceftriaxone and cefotaxime against penicillin-resistant pneumococci affects the therapeutic ratio achieved in CSF and has been associated with clinical failure.[95] Optimal therapy for fully penicillin-resistant pneumococcal meningitis should include vancomycin.[2,95] The combination of vancomycin and ceftriaxone was superior to either agent given alone in a rabbit model of penicillin-resistant pneumococcal meningitis.[96] Ceftriaxone or vancomycin combined with rifampin also may be superior to either drug given alone.[95] Animal data suggest that the use of rifampin reduces early mortality in pneumococcal meningitis by reducing the release of proinflammatory bacterial cell components.[97] Thus, until more information is available, the combination of ceftriaxone or cefotaxime with vancomycin represents the most reasonable approach to empiric therapy for potential penicillin-resistant pneumococcal meningitis.

Until culture and susceptibility results are available, the recommended antibiotic in this situation is ceftriaxone 2 g given IV every 12 hours and vancomycin 30 to 45 mg/kg/day IV divided every 8 to 12 hours. A.L. weighs 59 kg, and because his renal function is not normal (SCr, 2.4 mg/dL; creatinine clearance, 30 mL/minute), a dosage adjustment was made. (See Case 62-5, Question 2, for vancomycin dosing in CNS infections.)

CORTICOSTEROID THERAPY FOR ADULT MENINGITIS

CASE 62-2, QUESTION 3: Should A.L. receive corticosteroid therapy in addition to his antibiotic therapy?

The issue of adjunctive corticosteroid therapy for A.L. needs to be addressed. As previously stated, the efficacy of dexamethasone in adults with meningitis has recently been studied.[67] Clearly, A.L. presents with profoundly altered mental status, and his signs and symptoms are consistent with a fulminant course of disease. Given that he is unarousable, hypotensive, and tachycardic, A.L. likely will be admitted to the intensive care unit. Thus, his age, underlying medical problems, likely streptococcal meningitis, and deteriorating clinical status all point to a poor prognosis and argue for the use of adjunctive dexamethasone. On the other hand, A.L. is diabetic and has an elevated glucose concentration. He also has PUD, which may be active given that he is anemic and has a positive stool guaiac result. High-dose dexamethasone therapy may impact his mental status, making assessment even more difficult. Although each of these issues is a concern, none is so critical as to preclude the use of corticosteroids.[69] Therefore, dexamethasone given in a dosage of 10 mg IV every 6 hours could be instituted before starting ceftriaxone therapy and continued for up to 4 days, provided that the diagnosis of bacterial meningitis is confirmed. To control blood glucose, a sliding-scale dosing schedule of regular insulin is recommended. A.L.'s PUD should be properly worked up and treated if necessary.

TREATMENT OF PENICILLIN-SUSCEPTIBLE PNEUMOCOCCAL MENINGITIS

CASE 62-2, QUESTION 4: Results from A.L.'s CSF, blood, and sputum cultures are available and are positive for *S. pneumoniae* at each site. Sensitivity testing in CSF revealed an MIC of 0.06 mcg/mL to penicillin, 0.25 mcg/mL to cefotaxime and ceftriaxone, and 0.25 mcg/mL to vancomycin. What therapy is indicated for A.L.?

A.L. is infected with a strain of *S. pneumoniae* that is susceptible to penicillin G (Table 62-5).[4,5,37] The dosage usually is 20 to 24 million units/day in adults with normal renal function (Table 62-6). A.L. has renal impairment, however, which means he should receive a reduced penicillin dosage. For A.L., who has a calculated creatinine clearance of 30 mL/minute (according to the method of Cockcroft and Gault), the daily dose would be approximately 8 million units, or 2 million units every 6 hours. This revised regimen should provide penicillin serum concentrations similar to those achieved with high-dose therapy when kidney function is normal. Failure to adjust the dosage appropriately is equivalent to providing massive doses of penicillin, and seizures.[98]

In patients unable to tolerate penicillin G, the best alternatives are ceftriaxone or cefotaxime (Table 62-5).[4,5] First-generation cephalosporins (e.g., cefazolin) have good activity against pneumococci, but their limited CSF penetration makes these agents poor choices for therapy.[43,50] Conversely, the third-generation agent, ceftazidime, penetrates well into CSF, but its usefulness is limited by reduced activity against pneumococci in comparison to other third-generation agents.[49,50] Cefuroxime also has good pneumococcal activity but, as previously mentioned, is inferior to ceftriaxone and cefotaxime.[77] Vancomycin has more limited and variable CSF penetration.[43] Therefore, vancomycin should be reserved for situations in which there is bacterial resistance or penicillin intolerance. TMP-SMX has excellent CSF penetration characteristics but is not active against many strains of *S. pneumoniae.* Limited experience exists with TMP-SMX for the treatment of pneumococcal meningitis.[43,99]

PREVENTION OF MENINGITIS

CASE 62-2, QUESTION 5: Should A.L. have received pneumococcal vaccine? How effective is vaccination in preventing invasive pneumococcal disease?

The pneumococcal vaccine (Pneumovax 23, Pnu-Immune 23) provides protection against invasive pneumococcal disease.[94] The vaccine is composed of purified capsular polysaccharide antigens of 23 serotypes of *S. pneumoniae,* which are responsible for causing approximately 88% of the bacteremic pneumococcal disease in the United States.[86] Individuals such as A.L. who are at high risk for pneumococcal infection should be given the vaccine. Persons with chronic heart disease (except hypertension), chronic lung disease (including asthma and COPD), diabetes, alcoholism, cigarette smokers, chronic liver disease (including cirrhosis), CSF leaks, cochlear implants and asplenia (or splenic dysfunction), hemoglobinopathies (including sickle cell disease), and those older than 65 years of age should be vaccinated with the pneumococcal vaccine.[94] Immunocompromised patients, such as those with Hodgkin disease, lymphoma, multiple myeloma, or chronic renal failure, or patients who have undergone organ transplantation, and HIV-infected individuals also are at high risk for pneumococcal disease and should receive the vaccine.[94] Immunocompromised patients, however, often fail to mount a sufficient immune response to the vaccine to fully protect them against infection.[86] Patients with asymptomatic HIV disease respond more favorably to the vaccine than those with advanced acquired immunodeficiency syndrome.[100]

Thus, given his underlying medical condition (splenectomy) and history of alcoholism, A.L. should receive the pneumococcal vaccine. Revaccination (only once) after 5 years is recommended for persons with chronic renal failure or nephrotic syndrome, functional or anatomic asplenia, and for persons with immunocompromising conditions. For persons older than 65 years of age, one-time revaccination is recommended if they were vaccinated more than 5 years previously and were younger than 65 years of age at the time of primary vaccination.[94]

The antibody response in children younger than 2 years of age to polysaccharide vaccines is poor or absent, and the vaccine is not recommended for these young children.[86] Conjugate vaccines, however, are effective and have resulted in significant decreases in the incidence of invasive pneumococcal disease in children aged younger than 18 years. Routine vaccination with a 7-valent conjugate vaccine (PCV7, Prevnar) began in 2000. In 2010, a 13-valent conjugate vaccine (PCV13, Prevnar-13) was introduced to extend coverage to serotypes not covered by PCV7 (which now constitute the majority of cases of disease). As such, the ACIP now recommends routine vaccination for all children with PCV13.[101]

Gram-Negative Bacillary Meningitis

CASE 62-3

QUESTION 1: R.R., a 40-year-old, 80-kg man, is admitted to the hospital for a cervical laminectomy with vertebral fusion. His surgical procedure was complicated by a dural tear. On the third postoperative day, drainage at his surgical excision site was noted, and R.R. was febrile to 38.2°C. A Gram stain of the drainage revealed few gram-positive cocci and moderate gram-negative bacilli. Therapy with IV cefazolin 1 g every 8 hours was begun. The following morning, R.R. was oriented to person, place, and time, but he was slightly obtunded and had a temperature of 40°C. Neck stiffness could not be assessed because of his recent surgery. A magnetic resonance imaging (MRI) scan of the head and neck was negative, and lumbar puncture yielded the following CSF results:

WBC count, 3,000 cells/μL, with 95% PMN
Glucose, 20 mg/dL
Protein, 280 mg/dL

CSF Gram stain showed numerous gram-negative rods. What important clinical and laboratory features of gram-negative bacillary meningitis are manifested in R.R.?

EPIDEMIOLOGY

R.R. has gram-negative meningitis as a complication of his recent neurosurgical procedure. Although gram-negative bacilli do not cause meningitis nearly as often as *H. influenzae, S. pneumoniae,* and *N. meningitidis,* they are important pathogens, particularly after neurosurgical procedures.[1,18,19,31,34,56] Of 493 episodes of meningitis occurring during a 27-year period (1962–1988) at the Massachusetts General Hospital, enteric gram-negative bacilli accounted for 33% of all nosocomial episodes and 3% of community-acquired cases.[1] Historically, mortality rates from gram-negative bacillary meningitis have been extremely high, ranging from 40% to 70%. With the availability of third-generation cephalosporins, fatalities have declined to less than 40%.[18,31,34,56] Increasing resistance among certain gram-negative bacilli, such as *Enterobacter* species and *P. aeruginosa,* presents a therapeutic dilemma in that mortality associated with these pathogens is high and therapeutic options are fewer.[32,33]

PREDISPOSING FACTORS

Individuals at greatest risk for gram-negative bacillary meningitis include neonates, the elderly, debilitated individuals, patients with open trauma to the head, and individuals such as R.R. undergoing neurosurgical procedures.[18–20,31,56] Although meningitis is a rare complication of clean neurosurgical procedures (e.g., craniotomy, laminectomy), the consequences can be devastating when it does happen.[1,20,102]

MICROBIOLOGY

E. coli and *K. pneumoniae* are the most common gram-negative bacteria causing meningitis, and they represent about two-thirds of all cases.[34,56,102] *E. coli* is the most common gram-negative cause of neonatal meningitis, whereas *K. pneumoniae* is isolated more often in the adult population.[22,34,56,102] The remaining one-third of cases are divided evenly among *Proteus, Serratia, Enterobacter,* and *Salmonella* species, *P. aeruginosa,* and other less common bacilli.[34,56,102]

CLINICAL FEATURES

In general, clinical laboratory features of gram-negative bacillary meningitis are similar to other types of bacterial meningitis.[22,37,56] Because of high virulence, gram-negative bacillary meningitis often is a fulminant, rapidly progressive disease. An exception to this rule is meningitis after neurosurgery.[20] As is evidenced by R.R.'s clinical presentation, postneurosurgical gram-negative bacillary meningitis can present in a more subtle fashion. In such patients, many of the symptoms of meningitis (e.g., altered mental status, stiff neck) are masked by underlying neurologic disease. Thus, a high index of suspicion is warranted in the postsurgical setting. In addition to gram-negative bacilli, staphylococci also are associated with postneurosurgical meningitis.[20] The presence of what looks like staphylococci on R.R.'s wound drainage fluid is of concern, but the abundance of gram-negative rods on his CSF Gram stain supports the latter as being the most likely causative pathogen.

TREATMENT OF GRAM-NEGATIVE BACILLARY MENINGITIS

CASE 62-3, QUESTION 2: What would be appropriate therapy for gram-negative bacillary meningitis in R.R.?

Fewer choices are available for treatment of gram-negative bacillary meningitis than for other meningitides. Ampicillin is active against only *E. coli, Proteus mirabilis,* and *Salmonella* species, but resistance has essentially eliminated its use.[34,56,102] Aminoglycosides are limited by their inability to achieve therapeutic CSF concentrations, as well as reduced activity in the acidic milieu of purulent CSF.[13,15,34,52] Intraventricular administration results in therapeutic CSF concentrations, but repeated administration often is complicated by painful arachnoiditis. Even with this approach, mortality rates are high (>40%).[13,56] Unlike intraventricular administration, intralumbar injections will not result in therapeutic CSF concentrations in the ventricle. The third-generation cephalosporins represent by far the most useful group of agents for treating gram-negative bacillary meningitis, given their high potency against many enteric gram-negative bacilli and good CSF penetration. [4,34,103]

Empiric therapy for R.R. should include an antipseudomonal such as cefepime or meropenem (Table 62-5).[4,20,54] Cefepime has excellent activity against *E. coli* and *K. pneumoniae* and is active against other enteric gram-negative bacilli as well (Table 62-7).[34,103] Resistance to third-generation cephalosporins among *Enterobacter, Citrobacter,* and *Serratia* is so prevalent that these agents cannot be relied on for the treatment of meningitis caused by these pathogens.[33,103] With this in mind, therapy of gram-negative meningitis in situations in which third-generation cephalosporin resistance is likely (e.g., nosocomial or postneurosurgical meningitis) should result in the use of cefepime or meropenem. Of the third-generation cephalosporins currently available, the most experience has been accumulated with cefotaxime and ceftriaxone; success rates are greater than 80% for treatment of gram-negative bacillary meningitis caused by *E. coli* or *K. pneumoniae.*[34,104] For R.R., cefazolin should be discontinued, and treatment with cefepime (2 g IV every 8 hours) should be instituted. The choice of cefepime for empiric therapy is appropriate while waiting for results from culture and sensitivity testing.

TREATMENT OF ENTEROBACTER MENINGITIS

CASE 62-3, QUESTION 3: Culture results from R.R.'s wound drainage and CSF both are positive for *Enterobacter cloacae.* Sensitivity data reveal resistance to ceftriaxone, cefepime, ceftazidime, piperacillin-tazobactam, and aztreonam. Drugs to which the isolate is sensitive include imipenem, meropenem, TMP-SMX, gentamicin, tobramycin, and ciprofloxacin. What alteration in antimicrobial therapy is most appropriate for R.R. at this time?

Treatment of meningitis caused by *Enterobacter* and related species (e.g., *Serratia, Citrobacter* species) presents a particular challenge.[32,34] Furthermore, some isolates that are sensitive to third-generation cephalosporins can become resistant during therapy by virtue of selecting for derepressed mutants.[32] Thus, in contrast to gram-negative bacillary meningitis caused by *E. coli* and *Klebsiella* species, alternative therapies are needed when treating meningitis caused by *Enterobacter, Serratia, Citrobacter,* and *Pseudomonas* species. Based on the sensitivity profile of R.R.'s infecting strain, piperacillin-tazobactam would not be appropriate. Aztreonam, a monobactam antibiotic with good CSF penetration and gram-negative activity comparable to ceftazidime, also is inactive against R.R.'s infecting strain.[105] The isolate is sensitive to imipenem, but the higher propensity for seizures compared with other β-lactams (including penicillin G) argues against its use in R.R.[106–108] Meropenem is not considered to be epileptogenic and should be used preferentially to imipenem for meningitis.[109] Clinical trials have evaluated the efficacy and safety of meropenem versus cefotaxime in the treatment of meningitis in children. Clinical outcomes were similar among the patients randomly assigned to either group, and the incidence of seizures was similar in the treatment groups.[110,111] Thus, after consideration of the aforementioned options, meropenem appears to be the best choice of therapy for R.R, and carries FDA approval for this indication; however, TMP-SMX, although not FDA-approved, may be an option as well.[32] Cefepime should be discontinued and therapy started with meropenem 2 g IV every 8 hours adjusted for renal insufficiency.

DURATION OF THERAPY

The optimal duration of therapy for gram-negative bacillary meningitis has not been clearly established. Because of the high mortality and morbidity associated with these pathogens and the reduced susceptibility of enteric pathogens to antimicrobial agents, 21 days has been suggested (Table 62-8).[21,44,54,56] Although R.R. does not appear to have a fulminant case of gram-negative meningitis, a 21-day course of therapy is recommended with close follow-up.

Staphylococcus epidermidis Meningitis or Ventriculitis

CLINICAL PRESENTATION OF CEREBROSPINAL FLUID SHUNT INFECTIONS

CASE 62-4

QUESTION 1: T.A., a 21-year-old woman with a history of congenital hydrocephalus, is admitted to the neurosurgery unit for worsening mental status and fever. T.A. has a history of multiple revisions and placements of intraventricular shunts for control of hydrocephalus. Currently, she has a ventriculoperitoneal (VP) shunt, which was placed 1 month ago and previously had been functioning normally. During the past few days, T.A. has exhibited worsening obtundation, stiff neck, and a temperature of 39.5°C. A CT scan performed today reveals enlarged ventricles consistent with acute hydrocephalus.

T.A.'s medical history is noncontributory except for a seizure disorder for which she takes phenytoin 400 mg PO at bedtime. She also takes ethinyl estradiol and norgestrel for birth control. T.A. is allergic to sulfa drugs (severe skin rash). Her weight on admission is 60 kg.

Laboratory analysis was significant for the following:

WBC count, 14,000 cells/μL, with a differential of 85% PMNs and 10% lymphocytes
BUN, 19 mg/dL
SCr, 0.9 mg/dL

A tap of T.A.'s shunt was performed, and the ventricular fluid was notable for the following results:

Total protein, 150 mg/dL
Glucose, 40 mg/dL
WBC count, 200 cells/μL, with 85% PMNs and 10% lymphocytes

Gram stain of the ventricular fluid showed numerous gram-positive cocci in clusters. What are the subjective and objective findings of CSF shunt infections, and what manifestations of this type of infection are present in T.A.?

T.A. likely has meningitis with ventriculitis secondary to infection of her VP shunt. The most important way to manage hydrocephalus involves the use of devices that divert (shunt) CSF from the cerebral ventricles to other areas of the body such as the peritoneum (VP shunts) or atrium (ventriculoatrial shunts).[7,112,113] This approach alleviates increased CSF pressure and substantially reduces morbidity and mortality.[112,113] Infection of these devices, however, is a common cause of shunt malfunction, as seen in T.A. The reported incidence of CSF shunt infections varies from 2% to 39% (usually between 10% and 11%) and depends on patient factors, surgical technique, and the type and duration of the procedure performed (i.e., shunt revision versus placement of a new device).[112,113] T.A., who has been hydrocephalic since birth and has a history of multiple shunt procedures, is at high risk for such an infection.

Clinical symptoms associated with infected CSF shunts vary widely from asymptomatic colonization to fulminant ventriculitis with meningitis.[112,113] Fever is common and, in many instances, is the only presenting symptom.[112] CSF findings also are slightly different in shunt infection compared with acute meningitis: the WBC count usually is not as elevated, the decrease in CSF glucose is less pronounced, and the protein value may be normal or slightly elevated.[112,113] CSF culture is positive in most patients.[114] T.A.'s clinical presentation, CSF findings, and radiographic evidence of hydrocephalus are highly suggestive of a VP shunt infection. She is febrile and has altered mental status. The presence of a stiff neck strongly suggests meningeal involvement. Evaluation of T.A.'s ventricular fluid reveals a slightly elevated WBC count, with a predominance of PMNs, an elevated protein concentration, and a slightly lower than normal glucose concentration.

Skin microflora are the most common causes for CSF shunt infections.[114] Staphylococci account for 75% of all cases, with two-thirds of these caused by coagulase-negative staphylococci (usually *S. epidermidis*) and one-third by *S. aureus*.[112–114] Other less common pathogens include diphtheroids, enterococci, and *Propionibacterium acnes*. Enteric gram-negative bacilli are responsible for a small percentage of cases; these cases usually occur when the distal end of the shunt is inserted improperly into the peritoneal cavity.[112–114] The gram-positive cocci in clusters on Gram stain of T.A.'s CSF strongly suggest a staphylococcal shunt infection. Determining the coagulase status of the isolate will allow differentiation between *S. aureus* and coagulase-negative staphylococci, likely *S. epidermidis*.

TREATMENT OF CEREBROSPINAL FLUID SHUNT INFECTIONS

CASE 62-4, QUESTION 2: Culture and sensitivity tests of T.A.'s ventricular fluid are positive for *S. epidermidis*. The isolate is resistant to nafcillin but sensitive to vancomycin, rifampin, and TMP-SMX. How should T.A.'s CSF shunt infection be treated?

For T.A.'s CSF shunt infection to be optimally treated, a combined medical and surgical approach is required.[21] Antibiotic therapy directed against the causative organism, although essential, is only associated with cure rates of less than 40%. In contrast, antibiotic therapy plus surgical removal of the infected device results in clinical cure rates of greater than 80%.[115] Because many patients cannot tolerate the complete removal of their shunt for long, externalization of the distal end of the shunt, or shunt removal and placement of an external drainage device, often is necessary during systemic antibiotic therapy. The presence of an externalized device permits sequential sampling of ventricular fluid and also provides a convenient way to administer antibiotic intraventricularly (see the *Intraventricular Dosing of Vancomycin* section later in this chapter).

GLYCOCALYX

Although *S. epidermidis* is not as virulent a pathogen as *S. aureus*, it is extremely difficult to eradicate this organism from prosthetic devices such as CSF shunts. This is because many strains of *S. epidermidis* produce a mucous film or slime layer known as *glycocalyx*, which allows the staphylococci to adhere tightly to the shunt material, protecting them against phagocytosis.[116] As expected, antibiotic failures are much more likely with slime-producing strains of *S. epidermidis*.

Vancomycin is the drug of choice for treatment of shunt infections caused by *S. epidermidis* and should be instituted immediately in T.A.[7,112] This is because a high percentage (>60%) of coagulase-negative staphylococci are resistant to methicillin (e.g., methicillin-resistant *S. epidermidis* [MRSE]). Furthermore, methicillin-resistant staphylococci (both methicillin-resistant *S. aureus* [MRSA] and MRSE) also are resistant to cephalosporins. T.A.'s isolate also is sensitive to TMP-SMX, as is the case with many strains of MRSE (and also MRSA),[7] but it must be avoided because T.A. is allergic to this drug combination. Although many staphylococcal isolates (both *S. epidermidis* and *S. aureus*) are susceptible to rifampin, monotherapy with this drug is not recommended because of rapid emergence of resistance.

VANCOMYCIN THERAPY

CASE 62-4, QUESTION 3: What would be an appropriate IV dosage for vancomycin in T.A.? What subjective or objective data should be monitored to evaluate the efficacy and toxicity of the treatment?

Vancomycin therapy for T.A.'s CSF shunt infection requires the use of higher than usual doses.[7,54,117] For adults such as T.A., vancomycin dosages of 30 to 45 mg/kg/day have been endorsed.[22] For children with meningitis or infected shunts, the recommended dosage of vancomycin is 40 to 60 mg/kg/day, given IV in two to four divided doses (Table 62-6).[7,54] Targeted serum trough concentrations of vancomycin should be between 15 and 20 mcg/mL.[118]

T.A., who weighs 60 kg, should be started on a vancomycin regimen of 1 g IV every 12 hours (~30 mg/kg/day) because her renal function is normal. In either case, trough serum concentrations should be obtained at steady state to assess whether the initial dosing regimen is adequate. Another consideration for T.A. is the addition of rifampin to her vancomycin regimen. This is based on the excellent staphylococcal activity of rifampin, its moderate CSF penetration, and the potential for synergy between these two agents.[7] Whether rifampin plus vancomycin is superior to vancomycin alone has not been determined. For T.A., it is best to avoid rifampin because evidence supporting its efficacy is weak, and she currently is taking phenytoin and birth control pills. Rifampin is a potent inducer of hepatic microsomal enzymes, which can lower serum phenytoin concentrations (possibly resulting in seizure activity) and increase the possibility of an unplanned pregnancy (from reduced effectiveness of the birth control pill).

Intraventricular Dosing of Vancomycin

CASE 62-4, QUESTION 4: Should T.A. receive intraventricular vancomycin? If so, what would be an appropriate dosage?

T.A. has a long history of hydrocephalus and will require placement of an external drainage device after removal of her VP shunt. The external drainage device allows for intraventricular administration of vancomycin, and such treatment should be instituted promptly. Although dosage recommendations vary from 5 to 20 mg/day, most use 20 mg/day and this dose should be used for T.A. Also, serial (daily) cultures of CSF are recommended to monitor her response to therapy. To summarize, T.A. should receive combined IV and intraventricular vancomycin therapy as described previously. Therapy should be continued for at least 10 days after sterilization of her ventricular fluid is documented, at which time a new VP shunt can be placed.[21]

In contrast to T.A.'s situation, vancomycin therapy for patients with MRSA meningitis not associated with a CSF shunt or indwelling ventricular catheter is more problematic. The latest MRSA clinical practice guidelines from 2011 endorse a 2-week course of IV vancomycin 15 to 20 mg/kg/dose IV every 8 to 12 hours, with the potential addition of rifampin 600 mg daily, or 300 to 450 mg every 12 hours. In the setting of drug allergy, intolerance, or adverse events, alternatives include linezolid 600 mg PO or IV every 12 hours, or TMP-SMX 5 mg/kg/dose IV every 8 to 12 hours. Additionally, in seriously ill patients, including those with meningitis, a loading dose of 25 to 30 mg/kg of actual body weight may be considered. Trough concentrations between 15 and 20 mcg/mL are recommended.[118]

BRAIN ABSCESS

Epidemiology

Although not nearly as common as meningitis, abscesses of the brain parenchyma (brain abscess) remain an important type of CNS infection. The incidence of brain abscess has not varied since the preantibiotic era and is estimated to account for 1 in 10,000 hospital admissions.[119] On a busy neurosurgical service, 4 to 10 cases a year typically are seen.[119,120] For reasons that are not entirely clear, men are more likely to have abscesses within the brain than women.[119] Brain abscess can occur at any age, but the median age is 30 to 40 years, with approximately 25% of cases occurring in children.[119,121,122]

ONLINE CONTENT

For a picture of a brain abscess, go to http://thepoint.lww.com/AT10e.

Despite advances in antimicrobial therapy in the past several decades, mortality rates from brain abscess have remained above 40% until just recently. Developments in imaging techniques (e.g., CT and MRI scanning), which allow early recognition of abscesses and the ability to serially monitor the radiographic response to antimicrobial therapy, have had the most profound impact on reducing morbidity and mortality from brain abscess.[119,120,123] In a review of 102 cases of bacterial abscesses occurring during a 17-year period, mortality was 41% in the period before 1975 (pre-CT scan era), compared with 6% during 1975 to 1986, when CT scanning became routinely available.[120] With the combined medical and surgical approach currently recommended, mortality rates continue to average less than 10%.[119,120,123]

Predisposing Factors

Brain abscesses most commonly arise from a contiguous suppurative source of infection (e.g., sinusitis, otitis, mastoiditis, or dental infections).[119,124] In the United States, abscesses occurring as a complication of sinusitis are more common than abscesses arising from otitic or dental sources.[119] The formation of a single abscess cavity usually is found when infection develops from a contiguous source. In addition, the abscess nearly always is formed in close proximity to the primary focus of infection (Table 62-10).[119,124] For example, abscesses of sinusitic origin more commonly involve the frontal lobe, whereas otitic infections often lead to temporal lobe abscess formation.[124] Brain abscess also occurs as a consequence of metastatic spread of organisms from a primary site of infection (e.g., lung abscess, endocarditis, osteomyelitis, pelvic, and intra-abdominal infections).[121] In children, cyanotic congenital heart disease is a common predisposing factor for brain abscess.[121,122] Multiple abscesses suggest a metastatic source of infection.[119] As with meningitis, brain abscess occurs as an infrequent complication

TABLE 62-10
Predisposing Conditions, Microbiology, and Recommended Therapy for Bacterial Brain Abscess

Predisposing Condition	Usual Location of Abscess	Most Likely Organisms	Recommended Therapy
Contiguous Site			
Otitic infection	Temporal lobe or cerebellum	Streptococci (anaerobic and aerobic), *Bacteroides fragilis*, gram-negative bacilli	Penicillin G + metronidazole + cefotaxime or ceftriaxone
Sinusitis	Frontal lobe	Streptococci (predominantly), *Bacteroides* species, gram-negative bacilli, *Staphylococcus aureus*, *Haemophilus* species	Penicillin G + metronidazole + cefotaxime or ceftriaxone
Dental infection	Frontal lobe	*Fusobacterium* species, *Bacteroides* species, and streptococci	Penicillin G + metronidazole
Primary Infection			
Head trauma or neurosurgery	Related to site of wound	Gram-negative bacilli, staphylococci, streptococci, diphtheroids	Vancomycin + cefepime

of head trauma or neurosurgery.[11,119,124] No identifiable source (cryptogenic abscess) is detected in as many as 30% of cases.[119,124]

Staging

Once an intracranial focus of infection is established, the evolution of brain abscess involves two distinct stages: cerebritis and capsule formation.[121,123] The cerebritis stage evolves gradually during the first 9 to 10 days of infection and is characterized by an area of marked inflammatory infiltrate that contains a necrotic center surrounded by an area of cerebral edema.[121,123] Capsule formation occurs about 10 to 14 days after the initiation of infection, and once formed, the capsule continues to thicken for a period of weeks.[121,123] The stage of abscess development has important implications for therapy. Although it is best to wait until the capsule is fully formed before attempting any type of surgical intervention, antimicrobial therapy alone may resolve the infection if discovered in the early cerebritis stage.[123]

Microbiology

The microbiology of brain abscess is distinctly different from that of meningitis. Streptococci are implicated in 60% to 70% of cases and include anaerobic as well as microaerophilic streptococci of the *Streptococcus milleri* group.[119,124,125] Other anaerobes, particularly *Bacteroides* species (including *Bacteroides fragilis*) and *Prevotella* species, are found in up to 40% of cases, usually in mixed culture.[119,124] In recent years, staphylococci appear to be decreasing and enteric gram-negative bacteria increasing as etiologic agents of bacterial brain abscess.[123] Although somewhat imprecise, a reasonable correlation exists between the various predisposing conditions and the microbiologic etiology of brain abscess (Table 62-10).[119,122,123]

In the immunocompromised patient, a diverse group of microorganisms can induce abscesses within the brain. In patients with acquired immunodeficiency syndrome, *Toxoplasma gondii* is the most common infectious cause of focal brain lesions.[126] Transplant recipients and those receiving immunosuppressive therapy are susceptible to infection from *Nocardia* species.[127] In Mexico and other Central American countries, cysticercosis remains a common cause of intracerebral infection.[128]

Clinical and Radiologic Features

CASE 62-5

QUESTION 1: L.Y., a 40-year-old man, is brought to the ED by a friend. L.Y. complains of severe headache, fever, weakness in his left arm and leg, and increasing drowsiness. During the past week, L.Y. has suffered from headaches, which have gradually worsened in intensity, and from intermittent episodes of fever. Despite getting plenty of sleep, L.Y. has been feeling increasingly drowsy during the past several days. When he noticed weakness in his left arm and difficulty concentrating this morning, he called a friend and asked to be taken in for evaluation.

L.Y. has a history of chronic sinusitis that has been treated with a variety of oral antibiotics. His last episode of sinusitis, which occurred about 1 month ago, was treated with a 10-day course of cephalexin. He denies any nausea or vomiting and has not experienced any seizures in the recent past. L.Y. was tested for HIV 6 months ago, and the result of his antibody test was negative. He takes no current medications, denies smoking and use of recreational drugs, and drinks alcohol only on social occasions a few times a month. L.Y. has no known drug allergies.

Physical examination reveals L.Y. to be in mild distress, with a temperature of 38.2°C. He is slightly lethargic and is oriented to person and place but not time. The strength in L.Y.'s left arm is 3/5; the strength in his left leg is 4/5. The remainder of his neurologic examination is grossly normal. L.Y. described moderate pain on palpation of his frontal sinuses, and a purulent discharge is noted.

Laboratory evaluation shows the following:

WBC count, 8,000 cells/μL, with 70% PMN, 25% lymphocytes, and 5% monocytes
BUN, 16 mg/dL
SCr, 1.2 mg/dL
Erythrocyte sedimentation rate (ESR), 40 mm/hour

Hgb, Hct, platelets, and serum chemistries are within normal limits.

A CT scan with contrast dye reveals a right frontal ring-enhancing lesion with a small amount of surrounding cerebral edema. L.Y. is admitted to the neurosurgery unit for further evaluation and treatment. What clinical signs and symptoms does L.Y. display that are suggestive of bacterial brain abscess? How can brain abscess be diagnosed in L.Y.?

L.Y. has presented to the ED with many signs and symptoms suggestive of bacterial brain abscess. He is 40 years of age and a man, both of which place him in a group with the highest likelihood of having a brain abscess. In contrast to the diffuse nature of meningitis, brain abscess presents as a focal neurologic process.[119,120] Notable in L.Y.'s presentation is left-sided (arm and leg) weakness. Symptoms of brain abscess range in severity from indolent to fulminant, and in most patients, the duration of symptoms at the time of presentation is 2 weeks or less.[119–121] Headache is the most common symptom of brain abscess, occurring in approximately 70% of cases. L.Y.'s clinical manifestations have become gradually worse during the past week, and his worsening headaches, increasing drowsiness, and difficulty in concentrating all are consistent with bacterial brain abscess.

L.Y. presents with the classic triad of fever, headache, and focal neurologic deficits. Although this triad should always be looked for, fewer than half of patients with confirmed bacterial brain abscess present in this manner.[119,120]

The absence of fever does not rule out infection because fever is found in less than 50% of patients.[119,120] Focal neurologic deficits are present in approximately 50% of patients and vary in nature and severity in relation to the location and size of the abscess and surrounding cerebral edema.[119,120,122] Although L.Y. does not have a history of seizure activity, approximately one-third of patients experience partial seizures that often become generalized.[119,122] Papilledema and nuchal rigidity occur in 25% of cases or less and often are not useful in confirming the diagnosis. Symptoms associated with a contiguous focus of infection should always be sought, and in some situations, they may dominate the clinical picture.[119,120] L.Y. has a history of sinus infection, and the pain on palpation of his sinuses coupled with the purulent sinus drainage suggests active infection at this site.

As can be seen from L.Y.'s test results, laboratory evaluation usually is not very helpful when diagnosing brain abscess. L.Y. does not have a peripheral leukocytosis, but he does have an elevated ESR. A normal peripheral WBC count is not unusual in patients with intracranial suppuration. The ESR often is elevated in brain abscess, but this test is nonspecific and only indirectly supports the diagnosis.

L.Y. did not have a lumbar puncture because this procedure is contraindicated for diagnosing brain abscess.[41,119,120] The diagnostic yield from CSF is low because chemistries (e.g., protein, glucose, WBCs) usually are normal and culture of the CSF in patients with brain abscess is unlikely to yield the causative pathogen. More important, performing a lumbar puncture in patients with space-occupying lesions of the brain can produce cerebral herniation as a consequence of the shifting pressure gradient induced within the cranial vault after insertion of the lumbar puncture needle.[41]

Of paramount importance is the abnormality detected on the CT scan of L.Y.'s brain. When dye is injected before the CT scan, brain abscesses will appear to "ring enhance." Furthermore, cerebral edema can be identified as a variable hypodense region immediately surrounding the abscess cavity. As stated earlier, CT and MRI scanning techniques have revolutionized the diagnosis and treatment of brain abscess.[119,120,123] In general, a good correlation exists between the clinical and radiologic response to therapy of bacterial brain abscess.

Treatment

CASE 62-5, QUESTION 2: How should L.Y.'s brain abscess be treated?

SURGICAL TECHNIQUES

A combined medical and surgical approach is the best form of therapy for L.Y.'s brain abscess.[119,123] Response rates to antimicrobial therapy alone have been disappointing and, with a few exceptions, surgical intervention is necessary to ensure optimal results. Medical therapy is indicated when multiple abscesses are present, when the abscess cavity is inaccessible surgically, for patients who are poor surgical candidates, and when the abscess is small (<4 cm).[119,123,129]

The two types of surgical approaches for brain abscess are stereotactic needle aspiration and craniotomy for abscess excision.[123] Stereotactic aspiration of abscess contents can be performed under local anesthesia and is associated with lower morbidity and mortality than craniotomy.[18] Such an approach is highly effective, except when multiloculated abscesses are present.[123] With craniotomy, the abscess cavity can be excised completely, which often allows a shorter duration of antimicrobial therapy. Both techniques are effective, and the decision regarding which procedure is most appropriate must be individualized.

ANTIMICROBIAL PENETRATION INTO BRAIN ABSCESS

Antimicrobial therapy is an essential component of brain abscess therapy. Penetration of antibiotics into brain abscess fluid has not been studied as carefully as penetration into CSF, and as discussed earlier, the barrier involved is different (Fig. 62-1).[14] Penicillins and cephalosporins penetrate adequately into abscess fluid, but certain agents (e.g., penicillin G) may be susceptible to degradation by enzymes present within the abscess milieu.[119,124,130–132] Third-generation cephalosporins (e.g., cefotaxime, ceftriaxone) penetrate sufficiently into the abscess and thus are appropriate choices when gram-negative bacteria are present.[119,132] Metronidazole achieves abscess fluid concentrations equal to or in excess of serum levels and is bactericidal against strict anaerobes. The unique mechanism of action of metronidazole makes it particularly useful in the necrotic core of the cavity, where the oxidation-reduction potential is low and bacteria replicate slowly or are dormant. For these reasons, metronidazole is the drug of choice for anaerobic gram-negative bacterial brain abscess.[119] Vancomycin and carbapenems also penetrate sufficiently into brain abscess fluid.[119,133] Although specific abscess-penetration data are unavailable, successful treatment of cerebral nocardiosis with TMP-SMX and CNS toxoplasmosis with clindamycin suggests that these compounds also achieve adequate penetration into cerebral abscess cavities.[126,127]

ANTIBIOTIC THERAPY

When antibiotic therapy should be instituted depends on the status of the patient and the stage of abscess development. For patients diagnosed during the cerebritis stage, before formation of a well-circumscribed capsule, surgery should be delayed and antimicrobial therapy begun in patients with significant symptoms.[119,123] If capsule formation already has taken place, it is better to delay initiation of antibiotics until after surgery to increase the microbiologic yield from tissue and fluid samples. If the disease is fulminant, antibiotics must be instituted promptly and surgical intervention performed as quickly as possible.[119,123]

L.Y.'s clinical presentation suggests an advanced brain abscess. The presence of ring enhancement on CT and the onset of symptoms for more than 2 weeks support this conclusion. Because he is not critically ill, antibiotic therapy should be delayed until surgery is performed. Specimens obtained from the surgical procedure should be sent for aerobic and anaerobic culture and a stat Gram stain.

Initial antibiotic therapy for brain abscess needs to be sufficiently broad to cover the most likely pathogens (Table 62-10).[119,122,124] In most cases, a combination of high-dose penicillin G and metronidazole is indicated. Penicillin will cover aerobic, anaerobic, and microaerophilic streptococci, whereas metronidazole will provide coverage for strict anaerobes, including *Bacteroides* and *Prevotella* species. If gram-negative bacilli are suspected or documented, as in abscesses related to otitis, head trauma, or neurosurgery, a third-generation cephalosporin is indicated. Staphylococcal abscesses should be treated with nafcillin or vancomycin.[119]

For L.Y., therapy with penicillin G 4 million units IV every 4 hours and metronidazole 500 mg IV every 8 hours should be started postoperatively (Table 62-6). Because his abscess appears to originate from the sinus, the likelihood of gram-negative infection is reduced. With evidence of gram-negative bacteria on the Gram stain of abscess fluid, therapy with ceftriaxone 2 g IV every 12 hours should be included. Outpatient therapy is appropriate for CNS infections as long as patients are carefully selected and monitored, as described in a recent report.[134] Of interest, of the 24 patients treated on an outpatient basis, 46% received ceftriaxone 2 g IV once daily with similar success as that observed for twice-daily dosing.[134] Antimicrobial therapy for L.Y. should be revised once results from culture and sensitivity testing are available.

ADJUNCTIVE CORTICOSTEROID THERAPY

Adjunctive corticosteroid therapy for bacterial brain abscess is controversial.[119,123] Steroids can interfere with antibiotic penetration into abscesses and obscure the interpretation of serial CT scans when assessing response to therapy.[119,123] Therefore, steroids are indicated only if significant cerebral edema is present, particularly if it is accompanied by rapid neurologic deterioration.[119,123] L.Y. should not receive dexamethasone because his mental status is only mildly depressed and the cerebral edema seen on CT scan is not massive.

ADJUNCTIVE ANTICONVULSANT THERAPY

L.Y. has shown no signs of seizure activity thus far and, therefore, does not require anticonvulsant therapy. Anticonvulsants should be used in the acute setting when seizures are present, however.[119,123] Agents with activity against partial and complex partial seizures are preferred (e.g., phenytoin, carbamazepine, and potentially levetiracetam). The long-term use of anticonvulsants depends on whether seizure activity persists. Insufficient information exists regarding how long to continue anticonvulsants in such cases. Therefore, discontinuation of these agents must be individualized.

No formal guidelines are available regarding the optimal duration of therapy for bacterial brain abscess. Given the serious nature of the infection and the difficulty associated with antibiotic penetration, therapy with high-dose IV therapy should continue for at least 6 to 8 weeks.[119,123] The duration of therapy should be evaluated on a case-by-case basis. In an attempt to ensure complete eradication of infection, some experts recommend long-term (2–6 months) oral antibiotics after the IV course, provided agents with good oral absorption and activity against the offending pathogens are available.[119]

MONITORING THERAPY

CASE 62-5, QUESTION 3: How should L.Y. be monitored for therapeutic response and toxicity?

Although L.Y. is on antibiotic therapy, weekly or biweekly CT scans should be obtained to evaluate abscess resolution. His clinical response to therapy also should be assessed daily. If therapy is effective, L.Y.'s mental status should improve gradually (e.g., he will become more alert and oriented) during a period of several days. L.Y.'s headaches and hemiparesis (weakness in his arm and leg) also should resolve eventually. It may take a week or longer, however, to see a complete resolution of symptoms.[119] In general, radiologic improvement (i.e., reduction in abscess size) correlates reasonably well with clinical response, but not always.[119,123] Persistent symptoms or failure to detect a reduction in abscess size on CT scan or the appearance of new abscesses may indicate improper antimicrobial therapy or the need for more surgery.[119,123] Repeated surgical intervention with appropriate reculturing may be required in some instances to optimize therapy.

Adverse effects associated with the penicillin G therapy that L.Y. is receiving are similar to those of other β-lactam antibiotics. Seizures are a potential complication when high doses of penicillin are used in the presence of a mass lesion in the brain.[5,98,135] L.Y. should be observed closely by those providing care and questioned regularly for any evidence of seizure activity. Metronidazole usually is well tolerated, but may also cause neurotoxicity,[119,136] most commonly peripheral neuropathy.[136] L.Y. should be assessed for the presence of numbness or tingling in his hands or feet. Seizures, although uncommon, occasionally occur with metronidazole.[136] If L.Y. experiences peripheral neuropathy or seizures, a switch to chloramphenicol would be appropriate. Other adverse effects associated with metronidazole include mild nausea, brownish discoloration of the urine, and the potential for a disulfiramlike reaction with concomitant ethanol ingestion.[136] L.Y. should be counseled regarding the possibility of gastric upset and discoloration of the urine, and he should be strongly cautioned to avoid alcoholic beverages while receiving metronidazole. Given his young age, the absence of significant underlying diseases, and the relative early detection of his brain abscess, there is every reason to expect a good response to his treatment and, eventually, a complete resolution of his abscess.

KEY REFERENCES AND WEBSITES

A full list of references for this chapter can be found at http://thepoint.lww.com/AT10e. Below are the key references for this chapter, with the corresponding reference number in this chapter found in parentheses after the reference.

Key References

Brouwer MC et al. Corticosteroids for acute bacterial meningitis. *Cochrane Database Syst Rev.* 2010;(9):CD004405. (67)

de Gans J et al. Dexamethasone in adults with bacterial meningitis. *N Engl J Med.* 2002;347:1549. (59)

Liu C et al. Clinical practice guidelines by the Infectious Diseases Society of America for the treatment of methicillin-resistant *Staphylococcus aureus* infections in adults and children: executive summary. *Clin Infect Dis.* 2011;52:285. (118)

Lutsar I, Friedland IR. Pharmacokinetics and pharmacodynamics of cephalosporins in cerebrospinal fluid. *Clin Pharmacokinet.* 2000:39:335. (50)

Lutsar I et al. Antibiotic pharmacodynamics in cerebrospinal fluid. *Clin Infect Dis.* 1998;27:1117. (43)

National Center for Immunization and Respiratory Diseases. General recommendations on immunization—recommendations of the Advisory Committee on Immunization Practices (ACIP). *MMWR Recomm Rep.* 2011;60:1. (91)

Proulx N et al. Delays in the administration of antibiotics are associated with mortality from adult acute bacterial meningitis. *QJM.* 2005;98:291. (42)

Rybak M et al. Therapeutic monitoring of vancomycin in adult patients: a consensus review of the American Society of Health-System Pharmacists, the Infectious Diseases Society of America, and the Society of Infectious Diseases Pharmacists [published correction appears in *Am J Health Syst Pharm.* 2009;66:887]. *Am J Health Syst Pharm.* 2009;66:82.

Scheld WM et al. Pathophysiology of bacterial meningitis: mechanism(s) of neuronal injury. *J Infect Dis.* 2002;186(Suppl 2):S225. (4)

Tunkel AR. et al. Practice guidelines for the management of bacterial meningitis. *Clin Infect Dis.* 2004;39:1267. (21)

van de Beek D et al. Clinical features and prognostic factors in adults with bacterial meningitis [published correction appears in *N Engl J Med.* 2005;352:950]. *N Engl J Med.* 2004;351:1849. (1)

van de Beek D et al. Community-acquired bacterial meningitis in adults. *N Engl J Med.* 2006;354:44. (30)

63

Endocarditis

Annie Wong-Beringer and Michelle Lee

CORE PRINCIPLES

	CHAPTER CASES
1 Infective endocarditis (IE) is a microbial infection of the heart valves or other endocardial tissue, usually associated with an underlying cardiac defect. Disease incidence has remained stable over time accounting for 15,000 to 20,000 new cases per year. *Streptococcus viridans, Staphylococcus aureus*, and *Enterococcus* species are common causes of IE. Other pathogens affecting special populations include *Staphylococcus epidermidis, Pseudomonas aeruginosa*, and *Candida* species.	**Case 63-1 (Question 1), Case 63-2 (Question 1), Case 63-3 (Question 1), Case 63-4 (Question 1), Case 63-5 (Questions 1, 4, 6), Table 63-1**
2 Clinical presentation may be highly variable and characterized by nonspecific symptoms such as fever, weight loss, fatigue, night sweats, and arthralgias. Peripheral manifestations specific to IE include conjunctival petechiae, Janeway lesions, and splinter hemorrhages. Major embolic episodes and infarction involving other organs can develop in up to one-third of cases. Congestive heart failure is the most common cause of death in IE, and the most common indication for surgery.	**Case 63-1 (Question 1), Figures 63-1–63-5**
3 The American Heart Association (AHA) recommends use of the modified Duke criteria as the primary diagnostic schema to evaluate patients suspected of IE. The most important factor confirming IE is positive blood cultures. Transesophageal echocardiogram (TEE) is a valuable tool to strengthen diagnosis and identify patients at risk for complications and need for surgical interventions.	**Case 63-1 (Question 2), Tables 63-2, 63-3**
4 General treatment approach to organism eradication requires the administration of parenteral bactericidal antibiotics at high doses for a prolonged duration of 4 to 6 weeks. Combination therapy may be needed to achieve synergy for some pathogens. Selection of regimen should be based on organism sensitivity, tissue penetration, and host tolerance of the antibiotic agent(s). The AHA treatment guideline by organisms should be followed.	**Case 63-1 (Questions 3, 4), Case 63-2 (Question 3), Case 63-3 (Questions 2–4), Case 63-4 (Questions 1–6), Case 63-5 (Questions 2, 3, 5, 7), Tables 63-4–63-6**
5 Treatment of IE caused by methicillin-resistant *Staphylococcus aureus* (MRSA) and enterococci present significant challenges owing to emergence of resistance to standard therapy, vancomycin. Higher doses of vancomycin targeting trough concentration of 15 to 20 mcg/mL is advocated for treatment of MRSA IE but may be associated with increased incidence of nephrotoxicity. Alternative agents for treatment of IE caused by vancomycin-resistant enterococci have limited clinical success.	**Case 63-3 (Questions 3, 4), Case 63-4 (Questions 5, 6)**
6 Fungal endocarditis is rare but carries poor prognosis. It occurs primarily in intravenous (IV) drug users, patients with prosthetic heart valves or IV catheters, and those with a compromised immune system. Management generally requires early valve replacement and combination antifungal therapy.	**Case 63-5 (Questions 1–3)**
7 The AHA recommends the use of antibiotic prophylaxis in select patients with specific cardiac conditions (e.g., damaged heart valve) associated with the highest risk of adverse outcomes from endocarditis who are undergoing dental or respiratory procedures known to cause significant bacteremia. Antimicrobial prophylaxis should be directed against the viridans group of streptococci.	**Case 63-6 (Questions 1, 2), Tables 63-1, 63-7**

INFECTIVE ENDOCARDITIS

Infective endocarditis (IE) is a microbial infection of the heart valves or other endocardial tissue, often associated with an underlying cardiac defect. IE used to be classified as either acute bacterial endocarditis or subacute bacterial endocarditis based on the clinical presentation and course of the untreated disease. This classification system is nonspecific, however, and it does not account for many nonbacterial causes of endocarditis such as chlamydiae, rickettsiae, and fungi. Hence, the current system based on the causative organism is preferred because it provides information regarding the probable course of the disease, the likelihood of underlying heart disease, and the appropriate antimicrobial regimens.[1]

Pathogenesis

The pathogenesis of endocarditis involves a complex series of events that ultimately results in the formation of an infected platelet β-fibrin thrombus on the valve surface.[1,2] This thrombus is called a *vegetation*.

The first step in the formation of the vegetation involves modification of the endocardial surface, which is normally nonthrombogenic.

For a visual of tissue changes in endocarditis, go to http://thepoint.lww.com/AT10e.

In patients with rheumatic heart disease, endocardial injury occurs as a result of immune complex deposition or hemodynamic disturbances. Valvular insufficiency caused by aortic stenosis or ventricular septal defects can produce regurgitant blood flow, high-pressure gradients, or narrow orifices, resulting in turbulence and endocardial damage.

Once the endocardial surface of the valve is traumatized, small, sterile thrombi consisting of platelets and fibrin are deposited, forming the lesion called nonbacterial thrombotic endocarditis (NBTE). NBTE occurs most commonly on the atrial surfaces of the mitral and tricuspid valves and on the ventricular surface of the aortic valve.

NBTE serves as a nidus for microbial colonization during periods of bacteremia. Table 63-1 lists procedures associated with bacteremia. Organisms such as *Streptococcus viridans, Enterococcus* species, *Staphylococcus aureus, Staphylococcus epidermidis, Pseudomonas aeruginosa,* and *Candida albicans* possess adherence factors that facilitate their pathogenicity. In particular, platelet aggregation has been shown to be an important virulence factor in experimental streptococcal endocarditis; larger vegetations and multifocal embolic spread have been associated with strains that aggregate platelets.[3] Once the NBTE lesion becomes colonized by microorganisms, the surface is rapidly covered with a sheath of fibrin and platelets. This avascular encasement provides an environment protected from host defenses and is conducive to further bacterial replication and vegetation growth. Progression of the infection can be interrupted at any time by various host defense mechanisms, including blocking antibodies that interfere with bacterial adherence, serum bactericidal complement activity, hemodynamic forces that dislodge poorly adherent bacteria, and circulating prophylactic antibiotics.

The vegetation is thought to propagate by continuous reseeding of the thrombus by circulating organisms. As the vegetation enlarges, it takes on a laminar appearance caused by the alternating layers of bacteria and platelet fibrin deposits. The bacterial colony count can be as high as 10^4 to 10^5 bacteria per gram of valvular vegetation.

Endocarditis can result in life-threatening hemodynamic disturbances and embolic episodes. Without antimicrobial therapy and surgical intervention, IE is virtually 100% fatal. Because of bacterial proliferation to high densities in the fibrin mesh protected from normal host defenses, cure of infection requires prolonged therapy of 4 to 6 weeks with relapse not uncommon.

TABLE 63-1
Cardiac Conditions for Which Prophylaxis is Recommended

Cardiac Conditions
Prophylaxis Recommended
• Prosthetic cardiac valves
• Previous bacterial endocarditis
• Congenital heart disease
– Unrepaired cyanotic CHD, including palliative shunts and conduits
– Completely repaired congenital heart defect with prosthetic material device during the first 6 months after the procedure
– Repaired CHD with residual defects at or adjacent to the site of the prosthetic device or patch
– Mitral valve prolapse with valvular regurgitation and/or thickened leaflets
• Cardiac transplantation recipients who develop cardiac valvulopathy

CHD, congenital heart disease.
Source: Wilson W et al. Prevention of infective endocarditis: guidelines from the American Heart Association: a guideline from the American Heart Association Rheumatic Fever, Endocarditis, and Kawasaki Disease Committee, Council on Cardiovascular Disease in the Young, and the Council on Clinical Cardiology, Council on Cardiovascular Surgery and Anesthesia, and the Quality of Care an Outcomes Research Interdisciplinary Working Group. American Heart Association [published correction appears in *Circulation*. 2007;116:e376]. *Circulation*. 2007;116:1736.

Epidemiology

IE accounts for approximately 15,000 to 20,000 new cases per year in the United States.[4] The overall incidence has been stable; however, health care–associated IE has emerged as a result of increased use of invasive medical devices and procedures (e.g., intravenous [IV] catheters, total parenteral nutrition intravenous [TPN] lines, pacemakers, dialysis shunts).[1] The mean patient age has shifted from younger than 30 years in the 1920s to older than 55 years today.[4,5] This increase in age is likely attributable to (a) a decline in the incidence of acute rheumatic fever and rheumatic heart disease counterbalanced by degenerative valvular disease in an increasing elderly population, (b) the increasing longevity of the general population, and (c) increased exposure to more intense and invasive medical procedures in both the overall and the aging populations. Men are infected more often than women (roughly 2:1), and the disease remains uncommon in children, primarily in association with underlying congenital cardiac defect and nosocomial catheter-related bacteremia.[1]

Predisposing Factors

In general, any structural cardiac defect that leads to the turbulence of blood flow predisposes to the development of IE. Rheumatic heart disease was at one time the most common underlying cardiac defect associated with endocarditis; however, the proportion of cases related to rheumatic heart disease have declined to 25% or less in developed countries while remaining the predominant defect in developing countries. Mitral valve prolapse with thickened leaflets and valvular redundancy is a recognized predisposing risk to IE, with a documented occurrence rate of 10%. Clinical presentation is often subtle with lower associated mortality in these individuals compared with left-sided IE of other types. In the absence of underlying valvular defects, degenerative cardiac lesions, such as calcified mitral annulus secondary to atherosclerotic cardiovascular disease and postmyocardial infarction thrombus, may be a significant risk factor for the elderly. In one series of native valve endocarditis cases, 50% of patients 60 years of age or older had degenerative cardiac lesions; however, the actual contribution of these lesions is unknown.[6] Intravenous drug users constitute a unique population at greatest risk for recurrent and polymicrobial IE. In addition, health care–related IE occurs with increasing frequency among hospitalized critically ill patients and others who are subjected to IV access procedures or invasive medical device placement (hemodialysis shunts or fistulas, intracardiac prosthesis, central venous pressure monitoring lines, TPN lines, defibrillators, permanent cardiac pacemakers).[1]

Hemodialysis dependency (8%), diabetes mellitus (16%), and congenital heart disease (12%) are the most common demographic characteristics associated with IE.[7] Up to 25% of all cases are acquired in health care–related settings. Notably, in the United States, health care–associated IE is more likely compared with community acquisition.

Bacteriology

Streptococci and staphylococci are the cause of 80% to 90% of cases of IE. Historically, viridans streptococci were the predominant causative pathogens in IE, accounting for 60% to 80% of all cases.[1] When comparing epidemiologic studies in the aggregate during the past decades, however, staphylococci are increasingly prevalent as a cause of IE. Viridans streptococci remain the predominant cause of IE in children and in young women with isolated mitral valve involvement.[1]

Staphylococcus aureus is the leading cause of IE.[6,7] Acquisition of IE in nearly half of these cases was likely health care–related, supporting a low threshold to evaluate underlying IE in the setting of health care–related *S. aureus* bacteremia. More importantly, methicillin-resistant strains account for up to 40% of IE cases involving *S. aureus*.[4,5]

Endocarditis in IV drug users often is caused by *S. aureus*, whereas prosthetic valve endocarditis is more commonly caused by coagulase-negative staphylococci, such as *S. epidermidis*. Gram-negative bacilli and fungi together account for less than 10% of all endocarditis cases, which usually are associated with IV drug use, valvular prostheses, and hospital IV access procedures. Endocarditis caused by anaerobes and other organisms is rare. Polymicrobial infective endocarditis (caused by at least two organisms), although uncommon in the typical patient, is being recognized more frequently in IV drug users and certain postoperative patients. *Candida* species, *S. aureus, P. aeruginosa, Serratia marcescens*, and non-β group D streptococci are the organisms involved most frequently in these populations.

Site of Involvement

The site of heart valve involvement is determined by the underlying cardiac defect and the infecting organism.[2,4,5,7] The mitral valve is affected in more than 85% of cases caused by viridans streptococci with underlying rheumatic heart disease. The tricuspid valve is the common site of involvement in staphylococcal endocarditis associated with IV drug use. Overall, the distribution ranges from 28% to 45% for mitral valve, 5% to 36% for aortic valves, and 0% to 6% for tricuspid valves, and the pulmonary valve is rarely affected.[8] Multiple heart valves may be affected simultaneously. Some studies have shown that aortic valve involvement is increasing in frequency and is associated with higher morbidity and mortality.

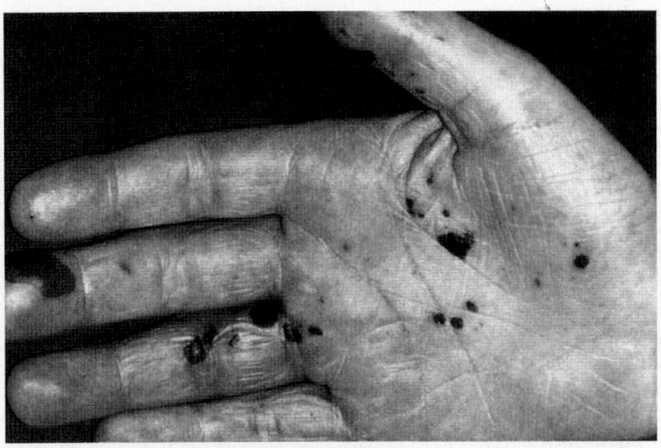

FIGURE 63-1 Janeway lesions. Extensive ecchymotic embolic lesions in a case of acute bacterial endocarditis.

STREPTOCOCCUS VIRIDANS ENDOCARDITIS

Clinical Presentation

CASE 63-1

QUESTION 1: A.G., a 57-year-old, 60-kg man with chief complaints of fatigue, a persistent low-grade fever, night sweats, arthralgias, and a 7-kg unintentional weight loss, is admitted to the hospital for evaluation. Visual inspection reveals a cachectic, ill-appearing man in no acute distress. Physical examination is significant for a grade III/IV diastolic murmur with mitral regurgitation (insufficiency) increased from pre-existing murmur, a temperature of 100.5°F, petechial skin lesions, subungual splinter hemorrhages, and Janeway lesions on the soles of both feet (Figs. 63-1, 63-2, and 63-3). Nail clubbing, Roth spots, or Osler's nodes are not evident (Figs. 63-4 and 63-5).

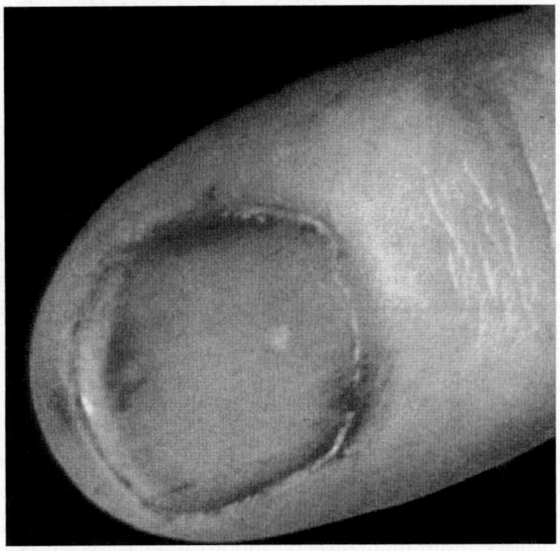

FIGURE 63-2 Splinter hemorrhages in the nailbed.

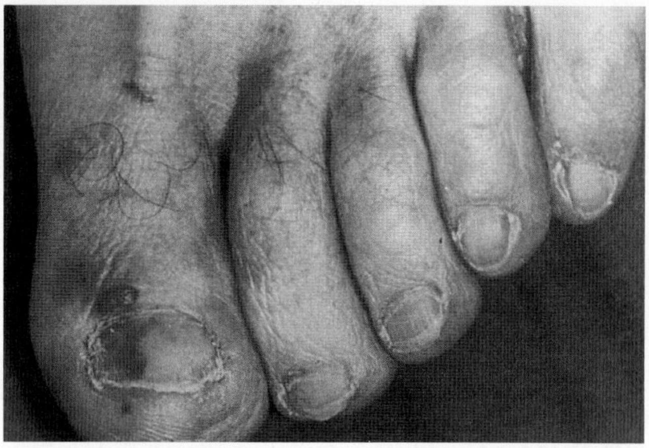

FIGURE 63-3 Petechial skin lesions in a case of acute staphylococcal endocarditis.

The remainder of his physical examination is unremarkable. A.G.'s medical history is significant for mitral valve prolapse and, more recently, a dental procedure involving the extraction of four wisdom teeth. The history of his present illness is noteworthy for the development of symptoms 2 weeks after the dental procedure (about 2 months before admission). His only current medication is ibuprofen 600 mg four times a day (QID).

Relevant laboratory results include the following:

Hemoglobin (Hgb), 11.4 g/dL (SI units, 114 g/L [normal, 140–180])
Hematocrit (Hct), 34% (SI units, 0.34 [normal, 0.39–0.49])
Reticulocyte count, 0.5% (SI units, 0.005 [normal, 0.001–0.024])
White blood cell (WBC) count, 85,000/μL with 65% polys and 1% bands (SI units, 85 × 10/L with 0.65 polys and 0.01 bands [normal, 3.2–9.8 with 0.54–0.62 polys and 0.03–0.05 bands])
Blood urea nitrogen (BUN), 21 mg/dL (SI units, 7.5 mmol/L of urea [normal, 2.9–8.9])
Serum creatinine (SCr), 1.8 mg/dL (SI units, 159 mmol/L [normal, 53–133])

A urinalysis (UA) reveals 2+ proteinuria and 10 to 20 red blood cells (RBCs) per high-power field (HPF). The erythrocyte sedimentation rate (ESR) is elevated at 66 mm/hour, and the rheumatoid factor (RF) is positive. Results from a transthoracic echocardiogram were unrevealing.

Three blood cultures were obtained during 24 hours, and all cultures obtained on day 1 are growing α-hemolytic streptococci. While confirmation and speciation of the organism is being performed, A.G. is started on penicillin G, 2 million units IV every 4 hours (12 million units/day), and gentamicin, 120 mg (loading dose) followed by 60 mg every 12 hours. Antimicrobial susceptibility results are pending. What clinical manifestations and laboratory abnormalities in A.G. are consistent with IE?

The clinical presentation of IE is highly variable and can involve almost any organ system.[1] A.G. appears pale and chronically ill and represents the typical patient with subacute disease (e.g., that caused by viridans streptococci). Nonspecific complaints consistent with endocarditis in A.G. include fatigue, weight loss, fever, night sweats, and arthralgias. Fever alone is present in most (90%) patients with endocarditis. The fever is characteristically low grade and remittent, with peaks in the afternoon and evening. The temperature rarely exceeds 103°F in subacute disease.[1] Fever may be absent or minimal in patients with congestive heart failure (CHF), chronic renal and liver failure, prior use of antimicrobial agents, or IE caused by less virulent organisms.[1] Musculoskeletal complaints (e.g., arthralgias, myalgias, and back pain) are common and may mimic rheumatic disease. Other symptoms can include lethargy, anorexia, malaise, nausea, and vomiting.[1] Because signs and symptoms are nonspecific and subtle, diagnosis is often difficult to make. In addition, the time from bacteremia to diagnosis is often prolonged because of the insidious progression of symptoms.[1] Delayed diagnosis occurs more commonly in the elderly. Fever may be absent in 30% to 40% of patients older than 60 years of age, whereas it can be present in more than 90% of patients younger than 40 years of age. Elderly patients are less likely to have new or changed heart murmurs. The most common presenting complaints in the elderly with endocarditis are confusion, anorexia, fatigue, and weakness, which may be readily attributable to stroke, heart failure, or syncope.

The temporal relationship between A.G.'s dental procedure and the onset of symptoms suggest it was the etiology of bacteremia and subsequent endocarditis. Although it is assumed

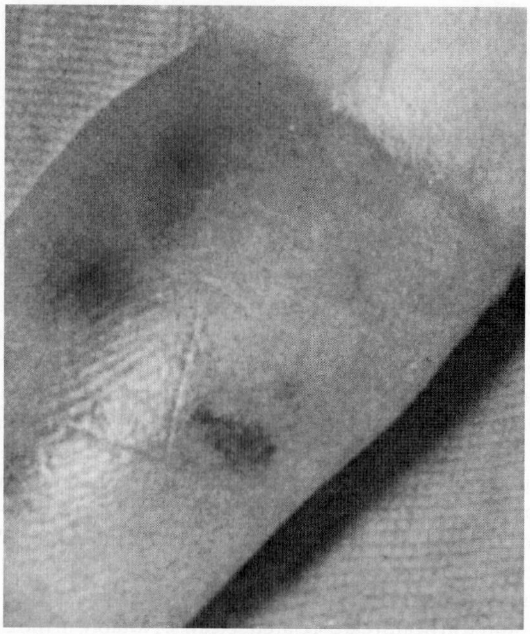

FIGURE 63-4 Osler nodes on the tip of the index finger in a case of endocarditis caused by ***Staphylococcus aureus.***

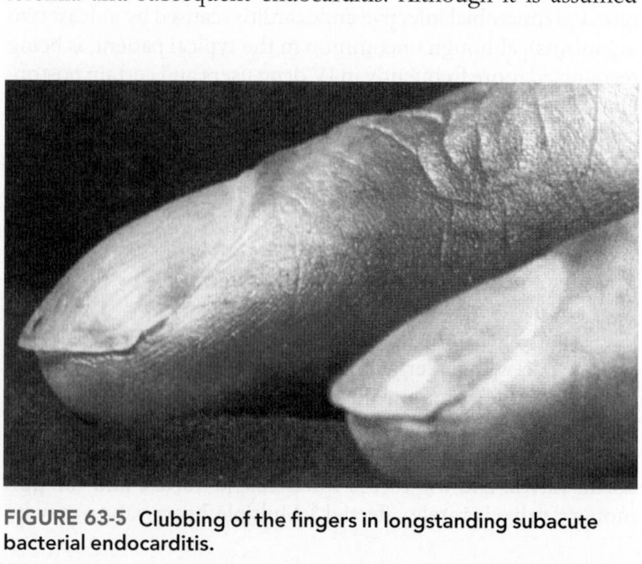

FIGURE 63-5 Clubbing of the fingers in longstanding subacute bacterial endocarditis.

that prophylactic antibiotics were administered before the procedure, endocarditis can develop despite receipt of adequate chemoprophylaxis.[9]

A.G. has an increase in his pre-existing diastolic murmur with mitral insufficiency, a finding consistent with endocarditis. Cardiac murmurs are present in more than 85% of patients with endocarditis. Murmurs frequently are absent in patients with acute disease (e.g., staphylococcal endocarditis), right-sided disease (e.g., endocarditis in IV drug users), or mural infection.[1]

A.G. exhibits several peripheral manifestations of IE, including conjunctival petechiae, Janeway lesions, and splinter hemorrhages. Overall, peripheral manifestations are observed in 10% to 50% of cases, but none of these is pathognomonic for IE. These manifestations are usually a result of septic embolization of vegetations to distal sites or immune complex deposition. Mucocutaneous petechial lesions of the conjunctiva, mouth, or pharynx are present in 20% to 40% of patients, especially those with longstanding disease. These lesions generally are small, nontender, and hemorrhagic in appearance and occur as a result of vasculitis or peripheral embolization. Janeway lesions are painless, hemorrhagic, macular plaques most commonly found on the palms and soles (Fig. 63-1). Splinter hemorrhages are nonspecific findings that appear as red to brown linear streaks in the proximal portion of the fingers or toenails (Fig. 63-2). Other findings can include Roth spots (small, flame-shaped retinal hemorrhages with pale white centers found near the optic nerve) and Osler nodes (purplish, nonhemorrhagic, painful nodules that develop on the subcutaneous pads of the fingers and toes or on palms and soles) (Fig. 63-4). Clubbing (broadening and thickening) of the nails also may be observed in patients with prolonged disease (Fig. 63-5).[1,10] Petechial skin lesions also are seen (Fig. 63-3).

Several laboratory findings are consistent with IE in A.G. A low Hgb and Hct with normal red cell indices suggest anemia of chronic disease. Of patients with subacute disease, 70% to 90% will have a normochromic, normocytic anemia. Leukocytosis with a left shift, although not evident in A.G., commonly is seen in those with acute, fulminant disease such as staphylococcal endocarditis. The ESR nearly always is elevated in IE, but this finding is nonspecific and can be associated with several other disease entities. Rheumatoid factor (an immunoglobulin M antiglobulin) and circulating immune complexes can be detected in most patients with longstanding disease, but both are nonspecific findings.[1]

Major embolic episodes and infarction involving the kidney, spleen, lung, and brain develop as secondary complications in up to one-third of cases.[1] A.G. exhibits some degree of renal damage, as evidenced by moderate hematuria and proteinuria. Erythrocyte and leukocyte cast formation also may be present. Alterations in A.G.'s renal function (increased BUN and creatinine) probably are a result of immune complex deposition (diffuse glomerulonephritis) or secondary to renal embolization (focal glomerulonephritis). Renal impairment usually is reversible with the institution of effective antimicrobial therapy.[1,10]

Cardiac complications occur most frequently. CHF, the most common cause of death in IE, is the most common indication for surgery. Infection-induced valvular damage is responsible for valvular insufficiency causing heart failure.[1,10] As many as two-thirds of patients with endocarditis develop CHF. Aortic valve infection is more frequently associated with CHF than mitral valve infection. Other manifestations include paravalvular abscesses, pulmonary edema, and pericarditis.[10] Mitral valve injury caused by viridans streptococci generally is better tolerated hemodynamically than aortic valve injury caused by staphylococci. Although A.G. has no apparent signs of overt heart failure, he should be monitored closely for the development of hemodynamic instability.

Neurologic complications rank second to cardiac complications in frequency, but they may be the leading cause of death in patients with endocarditis. Stroke is the most common neurologic complication of IE.[10] A stroke syndrome in a patient with underlying valvular abnormalities should prompt the clinician to rule out IE. Other clinical manifestations include headache, mental status change, stroke or transient ischemic attack, seizures, brain abscess, or intracranial mycotic aneurysms.[1,10] Neurologic symptoms take place in up to 35% of with *S. aureus* endocarditis patients who are not drug addicts. Mortality is significantly more likely in those with neurologic manifestations compared with those without.[11]

Splenomegaly, although not part of A.G.'s findings, occurs in 20% to 60% of all cases and is more common in subacute disease. In addition, metastatic abscesses can develop in virtually any organ secondary to systemic septic embolization. The most commonly involved metastatic foci are the spleen, kidney, liver, and iliac and mesenteric arteries.[10]

Diagnosis

CASE 63-1, QUESTION 2: How was the diagnosis of IE established in A.G.?

BLOOD CULTURES

Although A.G.'s medical history (mitral valve prolapse, recent dental procedure) and clinical presentation are highly suggestive of IE, blood culture is the single most important diagnostic workup for IE.[1] Bacteremia secondary to endocarditis is continuous and low grade; more than 50% of the cultures have only 1 to 30 bacteria/mL. Despite the low concentration of organisms, bacteremia (when present) results in at least one of the first two blood cultures being positive in 95% of cases.[1] Administration of antibiotics within the previous 2 weeks may significantly decrease this yield.[12]

At least three sets of blood cultures collected by separate venipunctures should be obtained during the first 24 hours of presentation.[1] In a "stable" patient such as A.G. who has had the disease for several weeks or months, it is important to establish the exact microbiologic cause before initiating antimicrobial therapy. Patients who are acutely ill should have empiric therapy started as soon as the appropriate cultures are obtained to avoid further valvular damage or other complications.[1]

ECHOCARDIOGRAPHY

Echocardiography is a valuable tool in establishing early diagnosis, identifying patients at high risk for complications, and optimizing the timing and mode of surgical intervention by detecting and monitoring associated pathologic changes such as valvular abscess, as well as the presence and size of vegetations.[1,13,14] With echocardiography, high-frequency sound waves are applied, and the reflection by body tissues is processed by a transducer to create images. The transducer may be placed on the chest (transthoracic echocardiogram [TTE]) or in the esophagus (transesophageal echocardiogram [TEE]).[14] TTE is a rapid and noninvasive procedure with 98% specificity for vegetations. Sensitivity for vegetations may be less than 60% to 70%, however, for adult patients with obesity, hyperinflated lungs caused by emphysema, or a prosthetic valve. TEE is more costly and invasive, but is significantly more sensitive in detecting vegetations while maintaining high specificity. All patients with suspected IE should have echocardiography on admission and repeated during their course, as necessary.[14] Two cost-effective analyses support the increased use of TEE to define antibiotic therapy duration for intravascular catheter-related *S. aureus* bacteremia

(2 vs. 4 weeks).[15,16] In particular, compared with TTE, TEE is superior in the diagnosis of pacemaker IE and IE in the elderly, and should be performed in all patients with a complicated course in whom paravalvular extension is suspected unless contraindicated by underlying esophageal disease.[1] A.G. has a negative TTE result on admission. Given the high clinical suspicion for IE in A.G., a follow-up TEE is recommended to rule out a false-negative TTE result. Documentation of valvular morphology, the presence and size of vegetations, ventricular function, and valvular insufficiency is important to establish a baseline and, on completion of therapy, to guide future medical management and appropriate timing of intervention.[7]

In summary, IE should be suspected in any patient who has a documented fever and heart murmur. Prior cardiac disease, peripheral manifestations, splenomegaly, various laboratory abnormalities, and a positive echocardiogram strengthen the diagnosis, but microbiologic documentation is the most important factor in confirming IE. Disease entities with overlapping clinical presentation and laboratory abnormalities should be excluded using the appropriate tests.[1]

Standardized criteria (Duke criteria) for the clinical assessment of patients suspected of having IE were proposed by a group at Duke University in 1994.[17] Limitations of the Duke criteria, such as misclassification of culture-negative endocarditis and the overly broad categorization of "possible" causes as well as the increasing role of TEE and the relative risk of IE with *S. aureus* bacteremia, were addressed in a modified version.[18] Diagnostic criteria for IE are listed in Tables 63-2 and 63-3, which integrate clinical, laboratory, microbiologic, and echocardiographic data.[7,18] Based on published evidence involving nearly 2,000 patients, the 2005 American Heart Association (AHA) guidelines suggest that the modified Duke criteria be used as the primary diagnostic schema to evaluate patients suspected of IE.[7]

A.G. possesses one major criterion (positive blood cultures) and three minor criteria (fever, predisposing heart condition, vascular and immunologic phenomena); therefore, he meets the diagnostic criteria for definite IE.[18]

TABLE 63-2

Definition of Infective Endocarditis (IE) According to the Modified Duke Criteria[a]

Definite Infective Endocarditis
PATHOLOGIC CRITERIA
Microorganisms: Demonstrated by culture or histology examination of a vegetation, a vegetation that has embolized, or an intracardiac abscess specimen, or
Pathologic lesions: Vegetation or intracardiac abscess confirmed by histologic examination showing active endocarditis
CLINICAL CRITERIA
Using specific definitions listed in Table 63-3; two major criteria *or* one major and three minor criteria *or* five minor criteria
Possible Infective Endocarditis
One major criterion and one minor criterion; or three minor criteria
Rejected
Firm alternative diagnosis explaining evidence of IE; *or*
Resolution of IE syndrome with antibiotic therapy for <4 days; *or*
No pathologic evidence of infective endocarditis at surgery or autopsy, with antibiotic therapy for <4 days; or not meet criteria for possible IE as above

[a] Modifications shown in bold.

Reprinted with permission from Li JS et al. Proposed modifications to the Duke criteria for the diagnosis of infective endocarditis. *Clin Infect Dis.* 2000;30:633.

TABLE 63-3

Definitions of Terminology Used in the Modified Duke Criteria for the Diagnosis of Infective Endocarditis (IE)[a]

Major Criteria
BLOOD CULTURE POSITIVE FOR INFECTIVE ENDOCARDITIS
• Typical microorganisms consistent with IE from two separate blood cultures
1. *Viridans streptococci*, *Streptococcus bovis*, HACEK group, *or*
2. ***Staphylococcus aureus*** or community-acquired enterococci in the absence of a primary focus, *or*
• Microorganisms consistent with IE from persistently positive blood cultures defined as follows:
1. At least two positive blood cultures drawn >12 hours apart, *or*
2. All of three or a majority of four separate cultures of blood (with first and last sample drawn at least 1 hour apart)
• **Single positive blood culture for *Coxiella burnetii* or antiphase 1 IgG antibody titer >1:800**
EVIDENCE OF ENDOCARDIAL INVOLVEMENT
• Echocardiogram positive for IE (**TEE recommended for patients with prosthetic valves, rated at least "possible IE" by clinical criteria or complicated IE [paravalvular abscess]; TEE as first test in other patients**) defined as follows:
1. Oscillating intracardiac Masson valve or supporting structures, in the path of regurgitant jets, or on implanted material in the absence of an alternative anatomic explanation; *or*
2. Abscess, *or*
3. New partial dehiscence of prosthetic valve
• New valvular regurgitation (worsening or changing of pre-existing murmur not sufficient)
Minor Criteria
• Predisposition: Predisposing heart condition or intravenous drug use
• Fever >38°C (100.4°F)
• *Vascular Phenomena:* Major arterial emboli, septic pulmonary infarcts, mycotic aneurysm, intracranial hemorrhage, conjunctival hemorrhages, Janeway lesions
• *Immunologic Phenomena:* Glomerulonephritis, Osler nodes, Roth spots, rheumatoid factor
• *Microbiologic Evidence:* Positive blood culture but not meeting major criterion as noted above[b] or serologic evidence of active infection with organism consistent with IE
• **Echocardiographic minor criteria eliminated**

[a] Modifications shown in bold.
[b] Excludes single positive cultures for coagulase-negative staphylococci and organisms that do not cause endocarditis.

HACEK, *Haemophilus* species, *Actinobacillus actinomycetemcomitans*, *Cardiobacterium hominis*, *Eikenella* species, and *Kingella kingae*; TEE, transesophageal echocardiography.

Reprinted with permission from Li JS et al. Proposed modifications to the Duke criteria for the diagnosis of infective endocarditis. *Clin Infect Dis.* 2000;30:633.

Antimicrobial Therapy

GENERAL PRINCIPLES

CASE 63-1, QUESTION 3: What would be a reasonable duration of antibiotic therapy for A.G.? When is determination of minimum bactericidal concentration (MBC) useful in treating bacterial endocarditis?

The avascular nature of the vegetation results in an environment that is devoid of normal host defenses (e.g., phagocytic cells and complement); this permits uninhibited growth of bacteria.[2] Therefore, to eradicate the causative organism, high doses of a parenterally administered, bactericidal antibiotic generally are administered for 4 to 6 weeks.[1,19] For some infections, it may be necessary to use two antibiotics to achieve synergistic activity against the organism.[20] For example, the addition of an aminoglycoside to penicillin results in a more rapid and complete bactericidal effect against enterococci.[21]

Once an organism has been identified, its in vitro susceptibility pattern is determined by the minimum inhibitory concentration (MIC) for various antibiotics. Standard Kirby-Bauer disk diffusion testing is inadequate in the setting of IE to aid in selection of antibiotics without the quantitative information provided by the MIC.[1] In addition, the MBC may be useful in detecting tolerant strains, particularly in the setting of unexplained slow response or treatment failure. Routine MBC determination is not recommended, however.[1] Treatment of endocarditis requires antibiotics with bactericidal activity; therefore, the serum concentration of the antibiotic must greatly exceed the MBC for the particular organism. For endocarditis caused by viridans streptococci acquired from the community, this usually is achieved without much difficulty because most isolates are sensitive to penicillin at an MIC of less than 0.125 mcg/mL; corresponding MBC are, at most, one or two tube dilutions higher.[8] The emergence of strains demonstrating resistance to penicillin and related β-lactams, such as ceftriaxone, is a significant problem, particularly among bloodstream isolates obtained from the nosocomial setting and neutropenic cancer patients.[8,22–24] The increasing prevalence of β-lactam–resistant clinical isolates highlights the importance of determining the MIC and continued close monitoring of the antibiotic susceptibility of viridans streptococci. An increasing number of reports have described suboptimal response to vancomycin therapy for the treatment of invasive infection caused by methicillin-resistant *S. aureus* (MRSA) strains showing borderline susceptibility (MIC 2 mcg/mL).[25] Many such strains demonstrated tolerance to vancomycin as defined by a high MBC-to-MIC ratio ($\geq$32).[26] Thus, these data support the need to determine MBC, especially in the setting in which the treatment option for IE caused by *S. aureus* is limited to vancomycin and suboptimal response is observed.[26]

REGIMEN SELECTION

CASE 63-1, QUESTION 4: What factors must be considered in selecting a regimen for A.G.? Which regimen should be used for A.G.?

Patients with endocarditis caused by penicillin-sensitive strains of viridans streptococci and nonenterococcal group D streptococci (e.g., *Streptococcus bovis;* MIC <0.1 mcg/mL) can be treated with any one of three regimens as outlined in the 1995 AHA treatment guidelines.[19] The suggested regimens (Table 63-4) are associated with cure rates of up to 98% and include (a) high-dose parenteral penicillin for 4 weeks; (b) high-dose parenteral ceftriaxone for 4 weeks; and (c) 2 weeks of combined therapy with high-dose parenteral penicillin and an aminoglycoside.[19,27–33] Ceftriaxone with an aminoglycoside for 2 weeks appears to be equally effective.[34,35]

HIGH-DOSE PENICILLIN FOR 4 WEEKS

Ten to 20 million units/day of IV penicillin G for 4 weeks resulted in a cure rate of 100% for 66 patients with nonenterococcal streptococcal endocarditis.[29] Another study using penicillin monotherapy reported relapse in only 2 of 49 patients; however, both of these patients received less than 4 weeks of therapy.[30] The large range of 12 to 18 million units/day of penicillin is recommended to allow flexibility in dosing based on the patient's renal function and disease severity.

SINGLE DAILY CEFTRIAXONE FOR 4 WEEKS

Ceftriaxone is active against viridans streptococcal strains isolated from patients with endocarditis. In one study, all 49 strains of viridans streptococci and 11 strains of *S. bovis* were inhibited at a concentration of less than 0.125 mcg/mL of ceftriaxone; one strain of *Streptococcus sanguinis* was inhibited at an MIC of 0.25 mcg/mL.[36] Although no direct comparative trials have been performed evaluating ceftriaxone against high-dose penicillin for the treatment of streptococcal endocarditis, it appears to be comparable to high-dose penicillin when treatment is given for 4 weeks.[37,38] Of the 70 assessable patients who received ceftriaxone 2 g as a single daily dose for 4 weeks, all were cured, except for 1 patient who had a probable relapse 3 months after completion of therapy. All strains of viridans streptococci were inhibited by ceftriaxone at an MIC of 0.25 mcg/mL in both studies. Although the simplicity of single daily treatment with ceftriaxone is attractive for outpatient use, careful patient selection based on microbiologic, clinical, and host factors is critical to the success of treatment and the proper and timely management of potential complications. (See Case 63-6, Question 1, for a detailed discussion of outpatient therapy.)

HIGH-DOSE PENICILLIN OR CEFTRIAXONE PLUS AN AMINOGLYCOSIDE FOR 2 WEEKS

The combination of 2 weeks of streptomycin (or gentamicin) with 4 weeks of penicillin is synergistically bactericidal for most streptococci, including enterococci (see Case 63-4, Question 4).[20,33] This in vitro synergy also has been correlated with a more rapid rate of eradication of viridans streptococci from cardiac vegetations in the rabbit model.[31] A shortened combination regimen consisting of high-dose penicillin G and streptomycin for 2 weeks is an effective alternative to the previously described regimens. The reported cure rate in 104 patients treated at the Mayo Clinic with this regimen was 99%.[32,33]

Although clinical experience with combination therapy has been primarily with penicillin and streptomycin, in vitro and animal data support that streptomycin and gentamicin are reasonably interchangeable. Gentamicin is more widely used in clinical practice, and serum concentrations are more readily available to monitor efficacy and toxicities. Administration of gentamicin once daily versus thrice daily when added to penicillin appears equally effective in the treatment of viridans streptococcal endocarditis.[28]

Combination therapy with ceftriaxone and an aminoglycoside for 2 weeks has also been evaluated.[30,34] A 2-week course of ceftriaxone 2 g plus netilmicin (3 mg/kg) (both given once daily) resulted in a clinical cure of 87%.[34] A second open-label study compared ceftriaxone 2 g alone versus the combination of ceftriaxone 2 g plus gentamicin (3 mg/kg), both given once daily, for the treatment of endocarditis caused by penicillin-susceptible streptococci.[35] Patients were randomly assigned to either regimen; 26 monotherapy recipients and 25 combination therapy recipients were evaluable. Clinical cure was observed in 96% of the patients in both groups at completion of therapy and at 3-month follow-up. This study excluded patients with suspected or documented cardiac or extracardiac abscesses and those with prosthetic valve endocarditis. Although the aminoglycoside agent (netilmicin or gentamicin) was administered as a single daily dose in both studies, all of the patients had measurable serum trough levels. Therefore, the efficacy of "extended-interval dosing" of aminoglycoside (whereby trough levels are not detectable, allowing a drug-free interval) in short-course combination therapy remains uncertain.

Based on available data, the 2-week regimen of penicillin or ceftriaxone plus an aminoglycoside appears to be efficacious for uncomplicated cases of penicillin-susceptible viridans streptococci endocarditis. It is not currently recommended for patients with extracardiac complications or intracardiac abscesses. Patients infected with *Abiotrophia* species (formerly

TABLE 63-4

Suggested Regimens for Therapy of Native Valve Endocarditis Caused by *Streptococcus viridans* and *Streptococcus bovis*

Antibiotic	Dose[a,b] and Route	Duration
Penicillin-Susceptible (minimum inhibitory concentration = 0.12 mcg/mL)		
Aqueous crystalline penicillin G[c]	*Adult:* 12–18 million units/24 h IV either continuously or in four to six equally divided doses *Pediatric:* 200,000 units/kg/24 h IV (max: 20 million units/24 h) either continuously or in four to six equally divided doses	4 weeks
Ceftriaxone sodium[c]	*Adult:* 2 g once daily IV or IM *Pediatric:* 100 mg/kg once daily IV or IM	4 weeks
Aqueous crystalline penicillin G	*Adult:* 12–18 million units/24 h IV either continuously or in six equally divided doses *Pediatric:* 200,000 units/kg/24 h IV (max: 20 million units/24 h) either continuously or in six equally divided doses	2 weeks
Ceftriaxone sodium	*Adult:* 2 g once daily IV or IM *Pediatric:* 100 mg/kg once daily IV or IM	
With gentamicin sulfate[d]	*Adult:* 3 mg/kg once daily IV or IM *Pediatric:* 3 mg/kg once daily IV or IM or in three equally divided doses	2 weeks
Relatively Penicillin G Resistant (minimum inhibitory concentration > 0.1 mcg/mL and < 0.5 mcg/mL)		
Aqueous crystalline penicillin G[e]	*Adult:* 24 million units/24 h IV either continuously or in four to six equally divided doses *Pediatric:* 200,000–300,000 units/kg/24 h IV (max: 20 million units/24 h) either continuously or in four to six equally divided doses	4 weeks
Ceftriaxone sodium	*Pediatric:* 100 mg/kg once daily IV or IM	
With gentamicin sulfate[d]	*Adult:* 3 mg/kg once daily IV or IM *Pediatric:* 3 mg/kg once daily IV or IM or in three equally divided doses	2 weeks
β-Lactam Allergic Patients		
Vancomycin hydrochloride[f]	*Adult:* 30 mg/kg/24 h IV in two equally divided doses (max: 2 g/24 h unless serum concentrations are monitored) *Pediatric:* 40 mg/kg/24 h IV in two or three equally divided doses (max: 2 g/24 h unless serum concentrations are monitored)	4 weeks

[a] Pediatric doses should not exceed that of a normal adult.
[b] Antibiotic doses for patients with impaired renal function should be modified appropriately. Vancomycin dosage should be reduced in patients with renal dysfunction; cephalosporin dosage may need to be reduced in patients with moderate to severe renal dysfunction.
[c] Preferred in most patients >65 years of age and in those with impairment of the eighth nerve or renal function.
[d] Two-week regimen not intended for patients with known cardiac or extracardiac abscess or for those with creatinine clearance of <20 mL/min, impaired eighth cranial nerve function or *Abiotrophia, Granullicatella,* or *Gemelia* infection. Gentamicin dosage should be adjusted to achieve peak serum concentrations of 3–4 mcg/mL and trough serum concentrations of <1 mcg/mL when three divided doses are used; nomogram used for single daily dosing. Other potential nephrotoxic drugs should be used with caution in patients receiving gentamicin therapy.
[e] Cefazolin or other first-generation cephalosporins may be substituted for penicillin in patients whose penicillin hypersensitivity is not of the immediate type.
[f] Vancomycin dosage should be reduced in patients with impaired renal function. Vancomycin given on a milligram per kilogram basis produces higher serum concentrations in obese patients than in lean patients. Therefore, in obese patients, dosing should be based on ideal body weight. Each dose of vancomycin should be infused for at least 1 hour to reduce the risk of the histamine-release red man syndrome. Peak serum concentrations of vancomycin should be obtained 1 hour after completion of the infusion and should be in the range of 30–45 mg/mL. Trough concentrations should be obtained within half an hour of the next dose and be in the range of 10–15 mcg/mL.
IM, intramuscular; IV, intravenous.
Source: Baddour LM et al. Infective endocarditis: diagnosis, antimicrobial therapy, and management of complications: a statement for healthcare professionals from the Committee on Rheumatic Fever, Endocarditis, and Kawasaki Disease, Council on Cardiovascular Disease in the Young, and the Councils on Clinical Cardiology, Stroke, and Cardiovascular Surgery and Anesthesia, American Heart Association: endorsed by the Infectious Diseases Society of America. *Circulation.* 2005; 111:e394.

known as nutritionally variant viridans streptococci) or viridans streptococci who have a penicillin MIC greater than 0.1 mcg/mL or patients who have prosthetic valve infections should not receive short-course therapy.[19]

SPECIAL CONSIDERATIONS

The risk of relapse may be higher in patients who have had symptoms for more than 3 months before the initiation of treatment.[1,19,37] These patients should be treated with 4 to 6 weeks of penicillin combined with an aminoglycoside for the first 2 weeks.[1,19,37]

Nutritionally deficient or variant streptococci (NVS) have been reclassified into a new genus, *Abiotrophia,* which includes *Abiotrophia defectiva, Abiotrophia adiacens* (renamed again as *Granulicatella adiacens*), and *Abiotrophia elegans. Abiotrophia* species are slow-growing, fastidious organisms that are responsible for approximately 5% of IE cases. Previously, NVS was the cause of most of the cases of endocarditis diagnosed as "culture-negative" initially owing to its requirement for the addition of vitamin B_6 (pyridoxal HCl) to the culture media for laboratory growth. Laboratory identification is no longer a significant problem, however, because of current culture media and laboratory techniques.[8]

Nutritionally deficient or variant streptococci are less susceptible to penicillin when compared with other streptococci. Many NVS have a relatively high MIC to penicillin (0.2–2.0 mcg/mL), and some show high-level resistance to penicillin (MIC >4 mcg/mL).[8] In addition, tolerance to penicillin has been described in many strains.[8] An animal model of endocarditis indicates that a penicillin–aminoglycoside (streptomycin or gentamicin) combination is significantly better than penicillin alone in reducing bacterial counts.[39] High rates of bacteriologic failure and relapse may be expected in patients despite completion of the treatment course for strains highly susceptible to penicillin.[8] All patients infected with NVS or *Abiotrophia* should receive 4 to 6 weeks of penicillin (or ampicillin) in combination with gentamicin.[19] A 6-week course of combination therapy with penicillin and gentamicin is recommended for patients with symptoms longer than 3 months in duration and those with prosthetic valve endocarditis caused by these strains.[8,19] Patients with endocarditis caused by relatively resistant viridans streptococci with penicillin MIC of greater than 0.5 mcg/mL or enterococci should receive a similar treatment regimen, as described above.[19]

Patients allergic to β-lactams should receive vancomycin 30 mg/kg/day divided into two doses for 4 to 6 weeks. In patients who have had minor reactions to penicillins (e.g., a delayed rash), a first-generation cephalosporin, such as cefazolin (2 g every 8 hours), may be cautiously substituted. Although the addition of an aminoglycoside to a cephalosporin or vancomycin enhances bactericidal activity in vitro, it is unknown whether the addition of an aminoglycoside confers any additional clinical benefit.[19] For most cases of endocarditis caused by penicillin-sensitive viridans streptococci (in patients not allergic to penicillin), all three of the aforementioned regimens are equally acceptable; therefore, the choice should be based on their relative advantages and disadvantages. The 2-week regimen requires the shortest hospital stay, but it has the disadvantage of possible ototoxicity and nephrotoxicity secondary to aminoglycoside administration. Therefore, it may be prudent to consider the use of penicillin or ceftriaxone alone for 4 weeks in older persons (>65 years) and those with impaired renal or vestibular function. For those with uncomplicated viridans streptococci endocarditis who can manage the technical aspects of outpatient therapy, ceftriaxone monotherapy offers the convenience of single daily administration. The combined regimen consisting of penicillin (or ampicillin) and an aminoglycoside for 4 to 6 weeks can be used for patients infected with NVS or relatively penicillin-resistant strains, those with prosthetic valve infections, and those with longstanding disease (symptoms >3 months).[8,19,37]

Assuming the viridans streptococci isolated from A.G. is not resistant to penicillin and he has no other complicating factors, any of the suggested regimens would be appropriate. Because no compelling reason exists to use the 4-week regimens, the 2-week penicillin–aminoglycoside regimen is the optimal choice. Although A.G. has mild renal impairment, this is most likely secondary to the endocarditis and should improve once adequate antimicrobial therapy has been instituted. A.G. was begun on 12 million units/day of penicillin G, which would be reasonable for his age and mild renal impairment. If nephrotoxicity were a major concern in A.G., penicillin or ceftriaxone alone for 4 weeks would be reasonable. If gentamicin is used, A.G.'s dose should be adjusted appropriately and he should be evaluated frequently for signs of toxicity. Periodic peak and trough aminoglycoside concentrations should be monitored.

STAPHYLOCOCCUS EPIDERMIDIS: PROSTHETIC VALVE ENDOCARDITIS

Etiology

CASE 63-2

QUESTION 1: F.T., a 65-year-old man, presents with chief complaints of anorexia, fever, chills, and weight loss. His medical history is significant for replacement of his mitral and aortic heart valves (both porcine) 1 year ago for aortic stenosis, mitral regurgitation, and mitral stenosis secondary to rheumatic heart disease. One month later he was readmitted with fever, a right pleural effusion, a pericardial friction rub, and pericarditis. The impression at that time was either postpericardiotomy or Dressler syndrome. F.T. was sent home on anti-inflammatory agents but failed to improve. After continued complaints of anorexia, nausea, chills, and fever to 101°F, he returned to the hospital. On readmission, his physical examination was noteworthy for a systolic ejection murmur at the left sternal border and 3+ pedal edema. Blood cultures were obtained, and routine laboratory studies were performed. His history and clinical presentation were strongly suggestive of prosthetic valve endocarditis (PVE). What are the most likely organisms responsible for PVE in F.T.?

Prosthetic valve endocarditis is a life-threatening infectious complication of artificial heart valve implantation that accounts for 7% to 25% of cases of IE in developed countries.[40,41] The prevalence of complications resulting in death has been as high as 20% to 40%.[41] The risk of PVE after surgery is approximately 1% at 12 months and 2% to 3% at 60 months. PVE is categorized as early or late, depending on the onset of clinical manifestations after cardiac surgery.[40,41] Early PVE occurs within 2 months after surgery and is thought to represent infection acquired during valve placement. It usually is caused by skin organisms that were implanted into the valve annulus (suture site where the valve is attached to cardiac muscle) at the time of surgery.[40,41] The most common organisms cultured from patients such as F.T. with early PVE are coagulase-negative staphylococci (primarily *S. epidermidis* [>30%], most of which are resistant to methicillin), followed by *S. aureus* (20%), and gram-negative bacilli (10%–15%). Miscellaneous organisms, such as diphtheroids and fungi, account for the remainder.[40,41] In contrast, streptococci are a more common cause of late PVE (>2 months after surgery).[40,41]

Nosocomial bacteremia and fungemia in a patient with prosthetic heart valves contribute to a significant risk for the development of PVE. One study noted that bacteremia caused by staphylococci and gram-negative bacilli resulted in 55% and 33% of subsequent PVE cases, respectively.[42] Another study observed the development of PVE in 25% (11 of 44) of patients after nosocomial candidemia.[43]

Prophylaxis

CASE 63-2, QUESTION 2: What measures can be taken to prevent early PVE?

The overall frequency of early PVE, despite antibiotic prophylaxis, is 1% to 4%.[44] Complications are severe and include valve dehiscence, acute heart failure, arrhythmias, and outflow obstruction. Although antibiotic prophylaxis before valve surgery (a "clean" procedure) has not been proved to reduce the frequency of early PVE, it is indicated nevertheless because the complications of infection are catastrophic. Animal data indicate that antibiotic prophylaxis reduces the infection rate.[44]

CEPHALOSPORINS

The antimicrobial regimen used most commonly for cardiac surgery prophylaxis (see Chapter 61, Antimicrobial Prophylaxis for Surgical Procedures) consists of an antistaphylococcal cephalosporin, such as cefazolin, given in the operating room at the time of induction of anesthesia or within 60 minutes before the procedure. Prophylaxis should only be continued for up to 48 hours because there is no evidence that administration of antibiotics for prolonged duration confers any greater benefit. The Joint Commission has set standards outlining appropriate antibiotic selection and timing based on the type of surgery. These standards are referred to in the focus area, Surgical Care Improvement Project (SCIP).[45] Cephalosporins are the agent of choice because they are active against most strains of *S. aureus*. The prevalence of methicillin- (and cephalosporin-) resistant strains is increasing, with rates exceeding 50% in many centers.

Most strains (87%) of coagulase-negative staphylococci are also methicillin- (and cephalosporin-) resistant.[41,46] Resistance is thought to be caused by an altered penicillin-binding protein (PBP 2a); thus, cross-resistance to all other β-lactams, except ceftaroline, is expected.[47]

VANCOMYCIN

Vancomycin is the prophylactic agent of choice when a first-generation cephalosporin cannot be used. Vancomycin could be considered the prophylactic agent of choice for cardiovascular procedures, including prosthetic valve replacement and implantation of prosthetic grafts, in the presence of any of the following: (a) documented penicillin allergy, (b) prior receipt of broad-spectrum antimicrobial therapy and high likelihood of being colonized with cephalosporin-resistant staphylococci or enterococci, or (c) performance of the procedure in a center experiencing outbreaks or a high endemic rate of surgical infection with methicillin-resistant staphylococci.[48]

Because the frequency of PVE is low, it would be nearly impossible to demonstrate a statistically significant decrease in its incidence after the use of vancomycin compared with conventional agents. Thus, the decision to use vancomycin rests on its superior in vitro activity for methicillin-resistant staphylococci. Arguments against the routine use of vancomycin in this specific setting include the potential for vancomycin-related hypotension.[48] More importantly, the emergence of vancomycin-resistant enterococci (VRE), heterogeneous glycopeptide-intermediate (hGISA) *S. aureus*, glycopeptide-intermediate *S. aureus* (GISA), and glycopeptide-resistant *S. aureus* (VRSA) heightens the need to limit vancomycin use because prior exposure to vancomycin is a recognized predisposing risk for the development of resistance to vancomycin.[49–52]

Of note, ceftaroline, a fifth-generation cephalosporin, is active against methicillin-resistant *S. aureus* and *S. epidermidis*. However, it is not approved for the treatment or prevention of IE.

In summary, selection of the most appropriate prophylactic antibiotic for valve replacement surgery should take into account the SCIP antibiotic recommendations and patient- and institution-specific factors. The choice should be based on drug allergy history, rates of postoperative wound infection, and associated pathogens.

ADVERSE EFFECTS

The most common adverse effect associated with vancomycin administration is the so-called red man or red neck syndrome,[53,54] which most commonly causes erythema of the head and upper torso, pruritus, urticaria, and in some cases hypotension. It is mediated in part by histamine release, and the severity of the reaction is proportional to the quantity released. The total dose of vancomycin administered and the rate of infusion are major determinants of the frequency and severity of this reaction. The reaction can be minimized by administering vancomycin over at least 1 hour. Cutaneous manifestations of the vancomycin-induced red man syndrome still can occur with a 1-hour infusion, but hypotension is uncommon.[53,54]

Several drugs used perioperatively and in anesthesia also cause histamine release; therefore, the possibility of additive toxicity with vancomycin is possible. Most of the serious reactions caused by vancomycin have been associated with perioperative use. Vancomycin-induced hypotension occurred in 7% of patients scheduled for cardiothoracic surgery, despite the 1-hour infusion time.[48]

ADMINISTRATION

Vancomycin is difficult to administer in the operating room because it must be administered by infusion for 1 hour and administration right before the procedure may not provide sufficient time for the vancomycin infusion to achieve adequate serum and tissue levels. Therapeutic serum concentrations of vancomycin can be maintained reliably during surgery if the 15-mg/kg dose is administered within 2 hours before the initial incision.

ANTIBIOTIC-IMPREGNATED HEART VALVES

PVE after heart valve replacement surgery is rare, but early-onset infection is associated with a mortality rate of 23% to 41%.[40] Systemically administered antibiotic prophylaxis before surgery does not confer 100% protection. The infectious process typically begins at the sewing ring and extends to involve the adjacent area between the prosthesis and the annulus of the heart valve. Hence, investigators have evaluated the use of antibiotic-impregnated heart valve sewing rings for the prophylaxis and treatment of bacterial endocarditis. Various antibiotics, including rifampin, gentamicin, and clindamycin, have been studied with respect to their diffusion kinetics and duration of antimicrobial activity both in vitro and in animal experiments.[55–57] It is unknown whether these antibiotic-impregnated heart valve rings decrease the risk of postoperative endocarditis.

Antimicrobial Therapy

CASE 63-2, QUESTION 3: What are the treatment options for F.T.?

As noted earlier, F.T. most likely is infected with coagulase-negative staphylococci. For those rare coagulase-negative staphylococci that remain sensitive to β-lactams (<20%), a penicillinase-resistant penicillin (nafcillin or oxacillin) is the drug of choice (Table 63-5).[46] For the treatment of PVE caused by methicillin-resistant, coagulase-negative staphylococci, vancomycin should be used.[46,58,59] Most staphylococci are sensitive to vancomycin at concentrations of 2 mcg/mL or less; however, strains of staphylococci with intermediate susceptibility to vancomycin have emerged.[58,59]

The AHA currently recommends the use of triple-drug combination therapy for the treatment of PVE caused by methicillin-resistant, coagulase-negative staphylococci.[21] In a retrospective review of 75 episodes of PVE caused by methicillin-resistant *S. epidermidis* (MRSE),[60] 21 of 26 patients treated with vancomycin were cured compared with 10 of 20 patients treated with a β-lactam antibiotic ($p = 0.05$); however, the addition of either rifampin or an aminoglycoside to vancomycin was associated with increased cure (18 of 20 cured) compared with vancomycin alone (3 of 6 cured; $p = 0.06$). A subsequent prospective, multicenter study compared the efficacy of 6 weeks of vancomycin plus rifampin with and without gentamicin for the first 2 weeks for the treatment of PVE caused by MRSE.[41,46] The emergence of rifampin-resistant strains during therapy was reduced by the addition of gentamicin (6 of 15 vs. 0 of 8; $p = 0.04$). Based on current data, a three-drug regimen (vancomycin, gentamicin, and rifampin) should be used for the treatment of PVE caused by MRSE. When isolates of MRSE are resistant to all available aminoglycosides, aminoglycoside treatment should be omitted. A fluoroquinolone active against the isolate may be considered as substitute for the aminoglycoside in the three-drug regimen. In addition to medical therapy, most patients also required valve replacement surgery.[40,41,46]

Although quinupristin/dalfopristin (Synercid), linezolid (Zyvox), daptomycin (Cubicin), telavancin, and ceftaroline have

TABLE 63-5
Treatment of Staphylococcal Endocarditis

Antibiotic	Dosage and Route	Duration
Without Prosthetic Material[a]		
OXACILLIN-SUSCEPTIBLE STAPHYLOCOCCI		
NONPENICILLIN-ALLERGIC PATIENTS		
Nafcillin *or*	*Adult:* 2 g IV every 4 hours *Pediatric:* 150–200 mg/kg/24 h IV (max: 12 g/24 h) in four to six equally divided doses	4–6 weeks
Oxacillin	*Adult:* 2 g IV every 4 hours *Pediatric:* 200 mg/kg/24 h IV (max: 12 g/24 h) in four to six equally divided doses	4–6 weeks
With optional addition of gentamicin[b,c]	*Adult:* 3 mg/kg IV or IM in two or three equally divided doses *Pediatric:* 3 mg/kg IV or IM in three equally divided doses	3–5 days
PENICILLIN-ALLERGIC PATIENTS		
1. Cefazolin[d]	*Adult:* 2 g IV every 8 hours *Pediatric:* 100 mg/kg/24 h IV (max: 6 g/24 h) in equally divided doses every 8 hours	4–6 weeks
With optional addition of gentamicin[b]	*Adult:* See Nonpenicillin-allergic patient *Pediatric:* See Nonpenicillin-allergic patient	
2. Vancomycin[b,e,f]	*Adult:* 30 mg/kg/24 h IV in two or four equally divided doses (max: 2 g/24 h unless serum levels monitored) *Pediatric:* 40 mg/kg/24 h IV in two or four equally divided doses (max: 2 g/24 h unless serum levels monitored)	4–6 weeks
METHICILLIN-RESISTANT STAPHYLOCOCCI		
VANCOMYCIN[b,e,f]	*Adult:* 30 mg/kg/24 h IV in two or four equally divided doses (max: 2 g/24 h unless serum levels monitored) *Pediatric:* 40 mg/kg/24 h IV in two or four equally divided doses (max: 2 g/24 h unless serum levels monitored)	4–6 weeks
With Prosthetic Valve or Other Prosthetic Material[g]		
METHICILLIN-RESISTANT STAPHYLOCOCCI		
VANCOMYCIN[b,c,g]	*Adult:* 30 mg/kg/24 h IV in two or three equally divided doses (max: 2 g/24 h unless serum levels monitored) *Pediatric:* 40 mg/kg/24 h IV in two or four equally divided doses (max: 2 g/24 h unless serum levels monitored)	≥6 weeks
With rifampin[h] *and*	*Adult:* 300 mg IV/PO every 8 hours *Pediatric:* 20 mg/kg/24 h PO (max: 900 mg/24 h) in two equally divided doses	≥6 weeks
With gentamicin[b,g,i,j]	*Adult:* 3 mg/kg IV or IM in two or three equally divided doses *Pediatric:* 3 mg/kg IV or IM in three equally divided doses	2 weeks
METHICILLIN-SUSCEPTIBLE STAPHYLOCOCCI		
Nafcillin or oxacillin[k]	*Adult:* 2 g IV every 4 hours *Pediatric:* 150–200 mg/kg/24 h (max: 12 g/24 h) in four to six equally divided doses	≥6 weeks
With rifampin[h] *and*	*Adult:* 300 mg IV/PO every 8 hours *Pediatric:* 20 mg/kg/24 h PO (max: 900 mg/24 h) in three equally divided doses	≥6 weeks
With gentamicin[b,g,i,j]	*Adult:* 3 mg/kg IV or IM in two or three equally divided doses *Pediatric:* 3 mg/kg IV or IM in three equally divided doses	2 weeks

[a] Antibiotic doses should be modified appropriately for patients with impaired renal function. Shorter antibiotic courses have been effective in some drug addicts with right-sided endocarditis caused by *S. aureus.* (See text for comments on the use of daptomycin and rifampin.)
[b] Dosing of aminoglycosides and vancomycin on a milligram per kilogram basis will give higher serum concentrations in obese than in lean patients.
[c] The benefit of additional aminoglycoside has not been established. The risk of toxic reactions because of these agents is increased in patients >65 years of age or those with renal or eighth nerve impairment.
[d] There is potential cross-allergenicity between penicillins and cephalosporins. Cephalosporins should be avoided in patients with immediate-type hypersensitivity to penicillin.
[e] Peak serum concentrations of vancomycin should be obtained 1 hour after infusion and should be in the range of 30–45 mcg/mL for twice daily dosing and 20–30 mcg/mL for four times a day dosing. Trough serum concentrations should be obtained within half an hour of the next dose and should be in the range of 10–15 mcg/mL. (See text for detailed discussion on the need for high trough target of 15–20 mcg/mL for strains with reduced susceptibility to vancomycin. Each vancomycin dose should be infused for 1 hour.)
[f] See text for consideration of optional addition of gentamicin.
[g] Vancomycin and gentamicin doses must be modified appropriately in patients with renal failure.
[h] Rifampin is recommended therapy for infections caused by coagulase-negative staphylococci. Its use in coagulase-positive staphylococcal infections is controversial. Rifampin increases the amount of warfarin sodium required for antithrombotic therapy.
[i] Serum concentration of gentamicin should be monitored and the dose should be adjusted to obtain a peak level of approximately 3 mcg/mL.
[j] Use during initial 2 weeks. (See text on alternative aminoglycoside therapy for organisms resistant to gentamicin.)
[k] First-generation cephalosporins or vancomycin should be used in penicillin-allergic patients. Cephalosporins should be avoided in patients with immediate-type hypersensitivity to penicillin and those infected with methicillin-resistant staphylococci.
IM, intramuscular; IV, intravenous; PO, orally.
Source: Baddour LM et al. Infective endocarditis: diagnosis, antimicrobial therapy, and management of complications: a statement for healthcare professionals from the Committee on Rheumatic Fever, Endocarditis, and Kawasaki Disease, Council on Cardiovascular Disease in the Young, and the Councils on Clinical Cardiology, Stroke, and Cardiovascular Surgery and Anesthesia, American Heart Association: endorsed by the Infectious Diseases Society of America. *Circulation.* 2005;111:e394.

potent in vitro activity against coagulase-negative staphylococci, clinical experience in the treatment of IE caused by these strains is lacking.[46,61,62]

STAPHYLOCOCCUS AUREUS ENDOCARDITIS

Intravenous Drug User Versus Nonuser

CASE 63-3

QUESTION 1: T.J., a 36-year-old human immunodeficiency virus (HIV)-seropositive man with a long history of IV drug abuse, was admitted to the hospital 4 months after being released from the state prison. His chief complaints included fever, night sweats, pleuritic chest pain, shortness of breath, dyspnea on exertion, and fatigue. Physical examination was remarkable for a temperature of 101.2°F, splenomegaly, and a pansystolic ejection murmur at the left sternal border, best heard during inspiration. The chest radiograph revealed diffuse nodular infiltrates. TTE was positive for a small vegetation on the tricuspid valve leaflet. Significant laboratory results included the following:

WBC count, 14,000/μL with 65% polys and 5% bands (SI units, 14 × 10/L with 0.65 polys and 0.05 bands [normal, 3.2–9.8 with 0.54–0.62 polys and 0.03–0.05 bands])
CD4 cell count, 350/μL
Hgb, 13.1 g/dL (SI units, 131 g/L [normal, 140–180])
Hct, 39% (SI units, 0.39 [normal, 0.39–0.49])
ESR, 55 mm/hour (Westergren)

IE was suspected. Blood cultures were obtained, and all six samples were positive for coagulase-positive, gram-positive cocci, later identified as methicillin-sensitive *S. aureus* (MSSA). How do the clinical presentation and prognosis of endocarditis in the IV drug user differ from that of the nonuser? What impact does HIV infection have on the risk and outcomes of endocarditis in the IV drug user?

The annual incidence of endocarditis among IV drug users is estimated at 1% to 5%; parenteral cocaine addicts have the highest risk.[63] The presentation, pathophysiology, and prognosis of endocarditis in those who acquire the disease secondary to IV drug use differ from those in nonusers.[1,63,64] *S. aureus* is tenfold more likely than other pathogens to cause infection in this population.[7] *S. aureus* is part of the normal skin flora and is introduced when the illicit drug is injected. It is hypothesized that insoluble agents used to "cut" the drug damage the normal heart valve, preparing the surface for bacterial adherence and growth.[1]

The following are differences between addicts and nonaddicts with *S. aureus* endocarditis: addicts are significantly younger; they have fewer underlying diseases and more right-sided (tricuspid) involvement (in contrast to the predominance of left-sided disease in nonaddicts); they are less likely to have heart failure or central nervous system complications; and they exhibit fewer signs of peripheral involvement and have a lower incidence of death.[64] Among patients without history of IV drug use, MRSA was involved in one-third of a cohort of 424 patients with definite *S. aureus* IE. Clinical features that characterized MRSA IE were persistent bacteremia, chronic immunosuppressive therapy, health care–associated infection, a presumed intravascular device source, and diabetes mellitus.[5]

The prevalence of HIV seropositivity is 40% to 90% among IV drug users with IE.[63,65] HIV-related immunosuppression may be an independent risk factor for the development of endocarditis.[66]

Antimicrobial Therapy

METHICILLIN-SENSITIVE STAPHYLOCOCCUS AUREUS

CASE 63-3, QUESTION 2: What are the therapeutic options for treating *S. aureus* endocarditis in T.J.?

The susceptibility of *S. aureus* to methicillin is the major determinant of which antibiotic is selected to treat T.J.'s endocarditis. T.J. is infected with MSSA. Therapy of choice for methicillin-sensitive strains is a penicillinase-resistant penicillin, such as nafcillin or oxacillin[19] (Table 63-5). Penicillin G rarely is appropriate because nearly all isolates of *S. aureus* produce penicillinase. Methicillin is no longer used because it is associated with a high incidence of interstitial nephritis.

A 4- to 6-week course of therapy with high-dose (12 g/day) nafcillin is the therapy of choice.[67,68] Vancomycin may be less efficacious than nafcillin as an antistaphylococcal agent.[19,67] IV drug addicts, for the reasons previously identified, have a higher response rate to appropriate therapy compared with nonaddicts, and 4 weeks of therapy is probably adequate. In one study, 31 addicts were successfully treated with 16 days of parenteral therapy followed by 26 days of oral dicloxacillin.[69]

Addicts with uncomplicated right-sided endocarditis caused by MSSA can be treated successfully with a 2-week course of combination therapy with a penicillinase-resistant penicillin and an aminoglycoside.[70–72] In one study, 47 of 50 patients (94%) were cured after treatment with the combination of IV nafcillin (1.5 g every 4 hours) and tobramycin (1 mg/kg every 8 hours) for a total of 2 weeks. Notably, 2 of 3 patients treated with vancomycin relapsed, resulting in early termination of this arm of study. Thus, vancomycin should not be used to substitute for nafcillin in this regimen. In another study, 71 patients who completed the 2-week course of treatment with cloxacillin (2 g IV every 4 hours) plus amikacin (7.5 mg/kg IV every 12 hours) had a cure rate of 94%.[72] Of the four patients who failed, the 2-week treatment period had to be extended to achieve cure. In contrast to the prior study, most (72%) patients had definite endocarditis with echocardiographic vegetations. Overall, none of the patients who responded promptly to treatment relapsed. In addition, aminoglycoside nephrotoxicity was minimal in this selected patient population. Alternatively, Ribera et al. demonstrated in a study that cloxacillin alone was as effective as combination therapy of cloxacillin plus gentamicin for the treatment of right-sided MSSA endocarditis; the treatment response exceeded 90% in the cloxacillin monotherapy arm.[73] Gentamicin administered at 1 mg/kg every 8 hours for 7 days in the combination group did not improve treatment response.

An abbreviated course of treatment can be used in a defined group of IV drug users with right-sided endocarditis. These patients should have the following characteristics: (a) clinical and bacteriologic response within 96 hours of initiation of therapy; (b) no evidence of hemodynamic compromise, metastatic infection, or neurologic or systemic embolic complications either at the initiation or completion of 2 weeks of therapy; (c) no echocardiographically demonstrable vegetations larger than 2 cm^3; (d) not infected with MRSA; and (e) not receiving antibiotics other than penicillinase-resistant penicillins, such as first-generation cephalosporins and glycopeptides.[19,71] HIV-seropositive patients (CD4 counts >300 × 10^6 cells) with tricuspid involvement included in the above studies also responded favorably to these short-course regimens; thus, a short-course regimen is an option for T.J.[73]

Some studies suggest that the addition of an aminoglycoside to the treatment regimen does not improve overall response for patients who meet the above criteria for short-course therapy. Thus, all patients receiving this regimen should be carefully evaluated for evidence of continuing infection or complications before discontinuing therapy at the end of the 2-week treatment course; extension of therapy with a β-lactam agent to at least 4 weeks' duration is recommended with any evidence of active disease or complications. Although response to antibiotic therapy has been shown to be similar between asymptomatic HIV-seropositive and HIV-seronegative IV drug users, short-course therapy should be avoided in more immunosuppressed individuals (CD4 cell counts <200 μL) until more definitive outcome data are available in this subgroup.[63]

ORAL REGIMEN

An oral treatment regimen consisting of ciprofloxacin (750 mg every 12 hours) plus rifampin (300 mg every 12 hours) has also been evaluated in addicts with uncomplicated right-sided endocarditis. In one small, noncomparative study, 10 addicts were successfully treated with the combination of ciprofloxacin and rifampin for 4 weeks.[74] Ciprofloxacin was given IV (300 mg every 12 hours) for the first 7 days, followed by oral administration (750 mg every 12 hours) for the remaining 21 days of therapy. Another study prospectively compared the oral regimen with standard parenteral therapy for this subgroup.[75] Patients were randomly assigned to receive 28 days of therapy with oral ciprofloxacin plus rifampin or oxacillin (2 g IV every 4 hours) plus gentamicin (2 mg/kg IV every 8 hours). Vancomycin (1 g IV every 12 hours) was substituted for oxacillin in the penicillin-allergic patients. One of 19 patients in the oral group versus 3 of 25 in the IV group failed treatment; however, approximately half of the study patients in either group had possible endocarditis. Given the small number of patients who completed treatment, therapeutic equivalency between the oral and parenteral regimens will need to be confirmed in larger trials. In addition, emerging quinolone resistance in *S. aureus* and the compliance and monitoring required of this regimen when administered in the outpatient setting are of concern. Nonetheless, it appears that a 4-week oral regimen with ciprofloxacin and rifampin may be a useful alternative treatment option in addicts with uncomplicated right-sided endocarditis.

PENICILLIN-ALLERGIC PATIENTS

Treatment of penicillin-allergic patients with *S. aureus* endocarditis is somewhat controversial. First-generation cephalosporins have been used with some success for the treatment of patients with mild penicillin allergy, but treatment failures with cefazolin are difficult to explain.[76] The stability of cefazolin when exposed to staphylococcal β-lactamase has been proposed as a mechanism for these failures.[77] Notably, staphylococci are capable of producing four penicillinase subtypes, to which the stability of cefazolin varies. These susceptibility differences are apparent on MIC testing only if a larger-than-usual inoculum is used (i.e., $>10^6$ organisms).[77] It is possible that treatment failures with cefazolin may be caused by a combination of the recalcitrant nature of the infection and the instability of cefazolin against a particular subtype of penicillinase produced by the staphylococcal strain, which is not readily detectable via routine MIC testing. For patients with endocarditis caused by *S. aureus* who have immediate-type hypersensitivity to penicillin, vancomycin or daptomycin may be used. Other treatment options include linezolid and quinupristin/dalfopristin.[78] Selection of agent depends on organism susceptibility, potential of drug–drug interactions, and host predisposition for development of adverse effects.

COMBINATION THERAPY

An enhanced response to combination therapy in the experimental animal model of MSSA endocarditis has prompted clinical trials to evaluate whether the addition of gentamicin to nafcillin confers any additional benefit. The combination of nafcillin and gentamicin resulted in more rapid clearing of organisms from the blood, but the response rates were similar to patients treated with nafcillin alone.[67] As expected, the group receiving gentamicin had a higher incidence of nephrotoxicity. Thus, for the routine management of endocarditis caused by MSSA, the addition of a second drug does not appear to offer additional benefit when a penicillinase-resistant penicillin is used unless an abbreviated treatment course in a select patient group is desired (see Case 63-3, Question 2, previous discussion). For patients who remain bacteremic or who fail to improve clinically (usually nonaddicts), imaging studies are often performed to identify metastatic sites of infection (i.e., occult abscess) with possible need for surgical intervention.

METHICILLIN-RESISTANT STAPHYLOCOCCUS AUREUS: *VANCOMYCIN*

CASE 63-3, QUESTION 3: How would T.J.'s therapy differ if he were infected with MRSA?

Staphylococcus aureus IE involving methicillin-resistant strains has become increasingly common and accounts for up to 40% of cases.[4,5] MRSA-infected patients have more chronic comorbid conditions (e.g., diabetes mellitus, hemodialysis dependency) and are more likely to have health care–associated infection (76% vs. 37%) and an indwelling intravascular catheter or hemodialysis fistula as the presumed source of infection (60% vs. 31%) when compared with patients infected with MSSA.[4,5] Persistent bacteremia was more common with MRSA IE, occurring in 43% versus 9% of patients infected with MSSA. Of interest, in this study, patients with *S. aureus* IE from the United States were significantly more likely to be infected with MRSA, to receive vancomycin therapy, and to develop persistent bacteremia.[79]

In 20% of patients with MRSA IE, identifiable health care contact was absent. MRSA infection is traditionally associated with health care contact in the nosocomial setting, but is now becoming more prevalent in the community (CA-MRSA).[5] Young and otherwise healthy individuals without the traditional risk factors are infected in the community.[80] CA-MRSA strains are distinct from health care–associated strains in that most possess a distinct virulence gene encoding for the Panton-Valentine leukocidin [PVL]. Expression of this pore-forming toxin that causes severe necrosis in polymorphonuclear neutrophil cells in a rabbit model has been implicated to cause invasive infections, including necrotizing pneumonia and skin abscesses.[81–87] Specifically, CA-MRSA PVL-producing strains causing IE have been reported.[88]

TREATMENT OPTIONS

Vancomycin has been the accepted standard of treatment for MRSA endocarditis. Response to treatment, however, is slower than with semisynthetic penicillins (e.g., nafcillin) for MSSA endocarditis. The mean duration of bacteremia in patients with MSSA endocarditis has been reported to be 3.4 days for nafcillin alone and 2.9 days for the combination of nafcillin and gentamicin.[70] In contrast, the median duration of bacteremia for MRSA endocarditis was 7 days for vancomycin alone. Failure rates of up to 40% have been documented in patients even with right-sided involvement. Of great concern is the emergence of resistant strains of *S. aureus* after repeated and prolonged exposure to vancomycin therapy.[58,89]

Either vancomycin or daptomycin at 6 mg/kg IV once daily (up to 10 mg/kg/day) may be used to treat patients with MRSA endocarditis.[90] Vancomycin 30 mg/kg/day in two divided doses for a total of 4 to 6 weeks is recommended for adults with normal renal function. Ideal body weight should be used to dose vancomycin on a milligram per kilogram basis in obese patients. Dosage adjustment for renal dysfunction is necessary. Vancomycin peak levels are not recommended. Dosage adjustment of vancomycin therapy based on measured trough levels is more reliable. Given the emergence of MRSA strains with reduced susceptibility to vancomycin, published guidelines from the Infectious Diseases Society of America recommend a target trough of 15 to 20 mcg/mL[7,91,92] in an attempt to overcome increasing MIC of clinical strains and limited tissue penetration. Measurement of trough serum vancomycin concentrations is typically within 30 minutes of the fourth dose for patients receiving a dosing interval of every 12 hours. A dosage regimen of vancomycin aimed to achieve an area under the curve-to-MIC ratio of 400 or an unbound trough at four to five times MIC of the infected strain has been proposed as the optimal pharmacodynamic target.[90,93,94]

PERSISTENT BACTEREMIA

CASE 63-3, QUESTION 4: T.J. has been treated with vancomycin 1 g IV every 12 hours for 5 days for his MRSA endocarditis, but does not seem to be clinically improving. His blood cultures are still positive, and his WBC count remains elevated at 12,500/μL with 55% polys and 7% bands. He continues to have a low-grade fever since starting vancomycin. His vancomycin trough level on the second day of therapy was 17 mcg/mL. The infected MRSA strain had a vancomycin MIC of 1.5 mcg/mL as determined by Epsilometer test. What factors may be contributing to T.J.'s poor response to treatment? What other therapeutic options are available for T.J.?

In a large multinational study of nearly 1,800 patients with definite IE, persistent bacteremia, receipt of vancomycin, and health care contact were significantly more common in patients with MRSA IE from the United States compared with those from other geographic regions.[5] The authors speculated that the higher rates of persistent bacteremia in US patients may be attributable in part to the receipt of vancomycin therapy.

Vancomycin MICs against *S. aureus* have been increasing over the years. At one university medical center, vancomycin MICs were determined by broth microdilution for 6,000 nosocomial MRSA isolates collected during a 5-year period. In the year 2000, 80% of the strains had vancomycin MIC of 0.5 mcg/mL; however, by 2004, 70% of isolates had MICs of 2 mcg/mL.[52] In response to increasing reports of vancomycin failures caused by strains that are in the susceptible range, the vancomycin breakpoint for susceptibility was reduced from 4 to 2 mcg/mL for *S. aureus* in 2005 per the Clinical and Laboratory Standards Institute.[95,96]

Widespread use of vancomycin has led to the emergence of GISA or hGISA strains.[58] Reduced susceptibility to glycopeptides results from an increase in the production of peptidoglycan precursors leading to a thickened cell wall and decreased penetration of glycopeptides into the bacterial cell membrane.[97] In the absence of vancomycin, hGISA strains may revert to glycopeptide susceptibility, making it difficult to detect these strains in vitro. As such, several investigators have found that hGISA strains have an MIC range that overlaps with the currently defined susceptible range and that the prevalence among hospitalized patients is increasing.[98–100] Routine susceptibility testing methods performed in the clinical laboratory are unreliable in detecting MRSA strains with hGISA phenotype.[101] MIC determined by Epsilometer test (Etest) best predicts treatment outcome with vancomycin.[26,79,102,103]

Experts have recommended a target vancomycin trough concentration of 15 to 20 mcg/mL to overcome increasing MIC when treating pneumonia or endocarditis caused by MRSA.[79,103] A published study of adult infections with MRSA reported that 54% (51 of 95) of clinical isolates had vancomycin MIC of 2 mcg/mL.[25] Notably, invasive infections, such as bacteremia and pneumonia, were linked to higher MIC. Infections caused by those strains were associated with lower end of treatment responses (62% vs. 85%) and increased mortality (24% vs. 10%) compared with strains with MIC of 1 mcg/mL or less irrespective of attaining a goal trough of 15 to 20 mcg/mL (achieving the goal of four to five times greater than MIC of an infected strain that has an MIC of 2 mcg/mL). Borderline susceptibility (MIC 2 mcg/mL) and severity of underlying disease were independent predictors of poor treatment response. Many strains demonstrated tolerance to vancomycin as defined by the MBC-to-MIC ratio of 32, and up to 10% exhibited heterogeneous vancomycin intermediate resistance phenotype (hVISA).[26,104] Vancomycin monotherapy of hVISA was associated with treatment failure, whereas combination therapy responded favorably. Combination regimens included vancomycin plus rifampin, linezolid, or daptomycin. These findings suggest a role for combination therapy or alternative agents when treating invasive infections caused by MRSA strains with borderline susceptibility. However, the above study was not designed to compare the efficacy of vancomycin monotherapy versus combination therapy for the treatment of MRSA infections, and the sample size of patients infected with hVISA in this study was small. Therefore, the role of vancomycin as the treatment of choice for MRSA IE will need to be re-evaluated against other available treatment options.

Despite attaining a pharmacodynamic goal of unbound vancomycin trough level of at least four times MIC of the infected strain, T.J. fails to clinically improve and has persistent bacteremia. It is possible that T.J. is infected with an hVISA strain; thus, a change in therapy is warranted.

Trimethoprim-sulfamethoxazole has been used successfully in a limited number of patients with right-sided native valve endocarditis caused by susceptible strains of *S. aureus* and may be an alternative to vancomycin.[105] A study of experimental staphylococcal endocarditis, however, found trimethoprim-sulfamethoxazole to be inferior to cloxacillin, vancomycin, and teicoplanin. Alternatively, minocycline has been shown to be a potential treatment alternative to vancomycin in experimental endocarditis caused by MRSA. Although both drugs are equally effective in decreasing the bacterial density of cardiac vegetations, the penetration of minocycline into vegetation was twice that of vancomycin.[106]

Other agents showing promise for the treatment of MRSA IE based on their in vitro activity include quinupristin/dalfopristin, linezolid, daptomycin, telavancin, and ceftaroline. A limited number of patients with MRSA endocarditis have been successfully treated with quinupristin/dalfopristin.[107,108] A cure rate of 56% was reported for patients treated with quinupristin/dalfopristin for MRSA endocarditis in an international open trial in patients intolerant of or failed prior therapy.[107,108] Additional data are needed before quinupristin/dalfopristin can be recommended for therapy.

Linezolid (Zyvox), an oxazolidinone, is not US Food and Drug Administration (FDA)-approved for the treatment of endocarditis, but has been used in cases of treatment failures, intolerability to standard therapy, or in infections with multidrug-resistant gram-positive cocci.[109] In a review article that included 33 case reports of endocarditis treated with linezolid, 63.6% of patients had successful outcomes at the end of the follow-up period.[110] MRSA and vancomycin intermediate *S. aureus* were the most common pathogens, accounting for 24% and 30% of cases, respectively. Failure with linezolid treatment was documented in seven cases, including four deaths attributed to endocarditis and three owing to persistent positive blood cultures. Thrombocytopenia was the most common adverse effect, occurring in eight of nine patients. In a compassionate use program, linezolid achieved 50% clinical and microbiologic cure rates at 6-month follow-up in 32 patients with definite IE; MRSA was the causative agent in 7 of those patients. The most common adverse events reported in this group were gastrointestinal system effects and thrombocytopenia, each occurring in 15% of patients.[111] The degree of thrombocytopenia associated with linezolid correlates with the extent of drug exposure, as measured by area under the concentration curve and duration of treatment.[112] Of note, treatment failure with linezolid for MRSA endocarditis caused by persistent bacteremia has been described in two patients and in one patient with relapse of infection.[109,113] Thus, additional efficacy data are needed before linezolid can be recommended for the treatment of IE caused by MRSA.

Daptomycin (Cubicin) is a cyclic lipopeptide that has been approved for treatment of *S. aureus* bacteremia and right-sided endocarditis. In vivo, it has a wide spectrum of activity against gram-positive bacteria, including *S. aureus* (including MRSA), *Enterococcus faecalis*, *Enterococcus faecium*, streptococci, and most other species of aerobic and anaerobic gram-positive bacteria. It was approved for the treatment of *S. aureus* bacteremia and endocarditis in a noninferiority study in patients receiving daptomycin or standard therapy consisting of an antistaphylococcal penicillin or vancomycin in addition to low-dose gentamicin.[114] Successful outcome was seen in 46% (41 of 90) of patients who had presumed or definite endocarditis at their baseline diagnosis. Of those, MRSA endocarditis was successfully treated in 42% (15 of 36) of cases. In patients with confirmed uncomplicated and complicated right-sided endocarditis, treatment success was similar between the daptomycin group (8 of 18) and the group receiving standard therapy (7 of 16) at 44%. Microbiologic failure occurred in seven patients in the daptomycin group and in five patients receiving standard therapy. Overall, the most common cause of daptomycin failure was persistent or relapsing infections, accounting for 16% of failures. In contrast, failure of standard therapy was more often the result of treatment-limiting adverse events, accounting for 15% of failures. Increase in the MIC of the infected strain was observed more often in the daptomycin group compared with standard treatment (six in the daptomycin group vs. one patient in the standard therapy group). The use of daptomycin for treatment of left-sided endocarditis is not established because only nine patients were treated and only one had treatment success.

Daptomycin at 6 mg/kg/day for a total duration of 6 weeks should be used for the treatment of endocarditis. Considering its concentration-dependent effects, some recommended higher doses of 8 to 10 mg/kg/day, which appear to be safe.[92] Frequency of administration should be increased to every 48 hours for patients with a clearance of creatinine of 30 mL/minute or less. Daptomycin should be dosed based on total body weight because obese patients have a larger volume of distribution as well as increased clearance compared with the nonobese population.[115] Creatinine kinase elevations were more commonly seen in the daptomycin group (6.7%) compared with the standard therapy group (0.9%).[114] Creatinine kinase levels should be obtained at baseline and weekly to monitor for elevations, and more frequently in patients who may be at risk for developing skeletal-muscle dysfunction (e.g., concomitant therapy with hydroxymethylglutaryl-coenzyme A reductase inhibitors). In addition, 9% of patients experienced peripheral nervous system–related adverse events (e.g., paresthesia and peripheral neuropathies), which resolved during continued treatment.[115]

High-dose daptomycin at 10 mg/kg daily[90] should be considered as alternative therapy in T.J. Emergence of cross-resistance to daptomycin after vancomycin exposure has been documented.[51,116] Similar to a thickened cell wall contributing to decreased susceptibility to vancomycin, the same mechanism is thought to contribute to daptomycin resistance in *S. aureus*.[117] Therefore, it is important to confirm MRSA susceptibility to daptomycin when used in a patient who had prior vancomycin exposure. Either gentamicin (at 1 mg/kg every 8 hours or 5 mg/kg daily) or rifampin 300 to 450 mg orally (PO) twice daily or both may be used in combination with daptomycin as in vitro synergy has been demonstrated for the combinations.[79] Alternatively, daptomycin 10 mg/kg/dose IV once daily[118] plus linezolid 600 mg PO twice daily may be used, particularly with concomitant pneumonia. Linezolid is a potential treatment option for T.J. if his infected MRSA strain demonstrates reduced susceptibility to daptomycin; however, clinical experience is limited to case reports and compassionate use.

Once daptomycin therapy is initiated, continued monitoring of clinical response and organism susceptibility to daptomycin is warranted because resistance development has been reported during prolonged therapy.[119–122] Daptomycin MIC increase during therapy for *S. aureus* endocarditis was demonstrated in six patients.[115] Baseline MIC increased from 0.25 to 2 mcg/mL in five isolates and from 0.5 to 4 mcg/mL in one isolate. Five of those six isolates were MRSA.

ENTEROCOCCAL ENDOCARDITIS

Antimicrobial Therapy

ANTIBIOTIC SYNERGY

CASE 63-4

QUESTION 1: G.S., a 35-year-old woman, has been complaining of anorexia, weight loss, and fever for the past 2 months. Her medical history is significant for an aortic aneurysm with insufficiency that resulted in an aortic valve replacement (porcine) 3 years before admission. Approximately 2 months before admission, G.S. had a cesarean section followed by a tubal ligation. She did not receive antibiotic prophylaxis for either procedure. Physical examination revealed a thin woman (5 foot 0 inches, 48 kg) in no acute distress with evidence of a systolic heart murmur, splinter hemorrhages, and petechiae on her soft palate. Her temperature was 100.2°F. Her WBC count was 14,000/μL (SI unit, 14 $\times$ 10/L) with a slight left shift; all other laboratory results were within normal limits. She was not taking any medications, and she has a documented allergy to penicillin (rash, urticaria, and wheezing). The working clinical diagnosis was probable bacterial endocarditis, which was confirmed when four sets of blood cultures grew gram-positive cocci. Biochemical testing subsequently identified the organism as *E. faecalis*, highly resistant to streptomycin (MIC > 2,000 mcg/mL). Antibiotic therapy with gentamicin (50 mg IV every 8 hours) and vancomycin (1,000 mg IV every 12 hours) was begun. Why were two antibiotics prescribed for the treatment of enterococcal endocarditis in G.S.?

Enterococci, unlike streptococci, are inhibited but not killed by penicillin or vancomycin alone.[20,123] The synergistic

TABLE 63-6

Therapy for Endocarditis Caused by Enterococci (or *Streptococci viridans* with an MIC $\geq$0.5 mcg/mL)[a,b]

Antibiotic	Dose and Route	Duration
Nonpenicillin-Allergic Patient		
1. Penicillin G	*Adult:* 18–30 million units/24 h IV given continuously or in six equally divided doses	4–6 weeks
	Pediatric: 300,000 units/kg/24 h IV (max: 30 million units/24 h) given continuously or in four to six equally divided doses	4–6 weeks
With gentamicin[c,d,e]	*Adult:* 1 mg/kg IM or IV every 8 hours	4–6 weeks
or	*Pediatric:* 1 mg/kg IM or IV every 8 hours	4–6 weeks
2. Ampicillin	*Adult:* 12 g/24 h IV given continuously or in six equally divided doses	4–6 weeks
	Pediatric: 300 mg/kg/24 h IV (max: 12 g/24 h) in four to six equally divided doses	4–6 weeks
With gentamicin[c,d,e]	*Adult:* 1 mg/kg IM or IV every 8 hours	4–6 weeks
	Pediatric: 1 mg/kg IM or IV every 8 hours	4–6 weeks
Penicillin-Allergic Patients[f]		
Vancomycin[e]	*Adult:* 30 mg/kg/24 h IV in two equally divided doses (max: 2 g/24 h unless serum levels monitored)	6 weeks
	Pediatric: 40 mg/kg/24 h IV in two to three equally divided doses (max: 2 g/24 h unless serum levels monitored)	6 weeks
With gentamicin[c,d]	*Adult:* 1 mg/kg IM or IV (max: 80 mg) every 8 hours	6 weeks
	Pediatric: 1 mg/kg IM or IV (max: 80 mg) every 8 hours	6 weeks

[a] Antibiotic doses should be modified appropriately in patients with impaired renal function.
[b] Enterococci should be tested for high-level resistance (gentamicin: MIC $\geq$500 mcg/mL).
[c] Serum concentration of gentamicin should be monitored and dosage adjusted to obtain a peak level of approximately 3 mcg/mL. (For shorter course gentamicin therapy for enterococcal endocarditis see comment in text.)
[d] Dosing of aminoglycosides and vancomycin on a mg/kg basis gives higher serum concentrations in obese than in lean patients.
[e] Peak serum concentrations of vancomycin should be obtained 1 hours after infusion and should be in the range of 30–45 mcg/mL for twice daily dosing and 20–30 mcg/mL for four times a day dosing. Trough serum concentrations should be obtained within half an hours of the next dose and should be in the range of 10–15 mcg/mL. Each dose should be infused over 1 hours; 6 weeks of vancomycin therapy recommended because of decreased activity against enterococci.
[f] Desensitization should be considered; cephalosporins are not satisfactory alternatives.
IM, intramuscular; IV, intravenous; MIC, minimum inhibitory concentration.
Source: Baddour LM et al. Infective endocarditis: diagnosis, antimicrobial therapy, and management of complications: a statement for healthcare professionals from the Committee on Rheumatic Fever, Endocarditis, and Kawasaki Disease, Council on Cardiovascular Disease in the Young, and the Councils on Clinical Cardiology, Stroke, and Cardiovascular Surgery and Anesthesia, American Heart Association: endorsed by the Infectious Diseases Society of America. *Circulation.* 2005;111:e394.

combination of penicillin (or ampicillin, piperacillin, or vancomycin) and an aminoglycoside are required to produce the desired bactericidal effect.[20,124] One definition of synergy is when a combination of antibiotics lowers the MIC to at least one-fourth the MIC of either drug alone.[125] The mechanism of synergy against enterococci is caused by an increased cellular uptake of the aminoglycoside with agents that inhibit cell wall synthesis (e.g., β-lactams and vancomycin).[126] Because G.S. is allergic to penicillin, vancomycin was prescribed with an aminoglycoside. Relapse rates are unacceptably high if penicillin is used alone for the treatment of enterococcal endocarditis.[19,21,125,126] The addition of an aminoglycoside to penicillin therapy significantly increases the sterilization rate of vegetations in animal studies.[125,126] Numerous clinical studies have confirmed the in vitro synergy for penicillin in combination with streptomycin or gentamicin for enterococcal endocarditis.[20]

STREPTOMYCIN RESISTANCE

As many as 55% of all enterococcal blood isolates are highly resistant to streptomycin (MIC >2,000 mcg/mL), and the combination of streptomycin with penicillin is not synergistic for those isolates. In contrast, gentamicin in combination with penicillin, ampicillin, or vancomycin is synergistic for most blood isolates of enterococci, regardless of their susceptibility to streptomycin.[1,21,127] In addition, ototoxicity in the form of vestibular dysfunction secondary to streptomycin therapy occurs in nearly 30% of patients in the treatment of enterococcal endocarditis and is most often irreversible. High peak concentrations and prolonged drug therapy have been associated with ototoxicity, but laboratory assays for streptomycin levels are not readily available. For these reasons, gentamicin in combination with penicillin (or ampicillin) or vancomycin is recommended by most authorities for the treatment of aminoglycoside-susceptible and, in particular, streptomycin-resistant enterococcal endocarditis, as it was for G.S.[19] Of note, other aminoglycosides cannot be used to substitute for gentamicin or streptomycin because of the uncertain correlation between in vitro synergy and in vivo efficacy.[19] Table 63-6 lists the suggested regimens for the treatment of enterococcal endocarditis.

GENTAMICIN RESISTANCE

Of the aminoglycosides, gentamicin and streptomycin are often tested with penicillin (or ampicillin) for synergistic bactericidal activity. About 10% to 25% of the clinical isolates of *E. faecalis* and up to 50% of *E. faecium* are resistant to gentamicin.[127,128] Without conclusive data, some groups favor long-term (8–12 weeks) therapy with high-dose penicillin (20–40 million units/day IV in divided doses) or ampicillin (2–3 g IV every 4 hours) for treatment of multiply resistant enterococci. Ampicillin plus the β-lactamase inhibitor sulbactam (Unasyn) would be substituted for β-lactamase–producing, high-level gentamicin-resistant enterococci. In light of the increasing prevalence of enterococci with high-level aminoglycoside resistance, the potential synergistic interaction between ampicillin or amoxicillin and a third-generation cephalosporin was explored in vitro and in experimental models of IE.[129] A bactericidal synergistic effect was shown between amoxicillin and cefotaxime against 50 strains of *E. faecalis*. Amoxicillin MIC decreased from 0.25 to 1 mcg/mL to 0.01 to 0.25 mcg/mL for 48 of 50 strains tested.[130] Additionally, Brandt et al.[131] demonstrated a synergistic bactericidal effect for amoxicillin in combination with imipenem against vancomycin-aminoglycoside–resistant *E. faecium* strains. The authors speculated that saturation of different penicillin-binding proteins by different β-lactam agents may be the underlying mechanism for the synergy observed. Limited clinical data on 13 endocarditis cases caused by high-level aminoglycoside-resistant *E. faecalis* treated with the combination of high-dose ceftriaxone (4 g/day) and ampicillin appear to confirm the above synergistic interaction. All 16 evaluable patients were cured by 1 month of double β-lactam therapy with no evidence of relapse during a 3-month follow-up period. Of note, two patients experienced reversible neutropenia and were withdrawn from the study.[132] Double β-lactam therapy appears promising for infections caused by aminoglycoside-resistant *E. faecalis* strains as well as an aminoglycoside-sparing regimen for patients with renal insufficiency, but the above preliminary results need to be confirmed with a larger number of patients.

GENTAMICIN

DOSING

CASE 63-4, QUESTION 2: What is the optimal dosage of gentamicin for G.S.?

Because patients with enterococcal endocarditis require prolonged therapy with aminoglycosides, the optimal serum concentration should minimize toxicity without jeopardizing clinical cure. Early in vitro data indicated that the bactericidal activity of gentamicin against enterococci was not significantly different between peak concentrations of 5 mcg/mL and 3 mcg/L; however, the differences between 3 mcg/mL and 1 mcg/mL were significant.[129] In the rat model of endocarditis, the bacterial counts in vegetations at 5 and 10 days were compared between those treated with low-dose (1 mg/kg intramuscularly twice daily) and those treated with high-dose (5 mg/kg intramuscularly twice daily) gentamicin with penicillin.[133] Bacterial counts did not differ at 5 days, but at 10 days they were significantly lower in the rats receiving the high-dose regimen. In contrast, results in the rabbit model showed no difference in the amount of bacteria per gram of vegetation in high- and low-dose gentamicin treatment groups.[134] Multiple daily dosing is more effective in reducing bacterial titers in vegetations than single daily dosing in experimental enterococcal endocarditits.[135–137] In contrast, viridans streptococci endocarditis can be managed with single daily dosing[33] (see Case 63-1, Question 4). Thus, extended-interval dosing of aminoglycosides cannot be recommended for the treatment of enterococcal endocarditis at this time.

The only study comparing high-dose (>3 mg/kg/day) and low-dose (<3 mg/kg/day) gentamicin with penicillin in humans with enterococcal endocarditis evaluated 56 patients during a 12-year period (36 with streptomycin-susceptible and 20 with streptomycin-resistant infections).[138] The relapse rate of patients infected with streptomycin-resistant organisms ($n = 20$) was not significantly different between the high- and low-dose treatment groups ($n = 10$ each). Furthermore, patients who received the higher doses of gentamicin experienced a greater prevalence of nephrotoxicity (10 of 10 vs. 2 of 10; $p < 0.001$). Mean peak and trough concentrations of gentamicin in the patients who received the high doses were 5 mcg/mL and 2.1 mcg/mL, respectively; corresponding levels for patients receiving the low-dose regimen were 3.1 mcg/mL and 1 mcg/mL.

Given the available data, it would be reasonable to start G.S. on a gentamicin dosage of 1 mg/kg every 8 hours (assuming her renal function is normal) and to maintain peak concentrations of 3 to 5 mcg/mL and trough concentrations of less than 1 mcg/mL.

IN COMBINATION WITH VANCOMYCIN

CASE 63-4, QUESTION 3: Why was vancomycin used in combination with gentamicin in G.S.? Is this combination effective against enterococci?

G.S. has a history of penicillin allergy. Most clinicians favor a combination of vancomycin and gentamicin for penicillin-allergic patients with enterococcal endocarditis, although vancomycin plus streptomycin is a suitable alternative.[19,21,138] The combination of vancomycin and gentamicin demonstrates bactericidal synergy for about 95% of enterococci strains. In contrast, the vancomycin and streptomycin combination demonstrates bactericidal synergy for about 65% of enterococci. Because G.S. has PVE, she should receive approximately 30 mg/kg/day, or roughly 1.5 g/day (750 mg every 12 hours), of vancomycin in combination with gentamicin (3 mg/kg/day). Serum levels of vancomycin and gentamicin should be monitored as previously discussed.

DURATION OF THERAPY

CASE 63-4, QUESTION 4: How long should G.S. be treated?

Historically, enterococcal endocarditis has been treated with penicillin plus an aminoglycoside for 6 weeks; the overall cure rate with this regimen is about 85%.[19] Four weeks of therapy is probably adequate for most patients with enterococcal endocarditis.[19,138,139] One study evaluated the efficacy of a treatment regimen involving shorter-course aminoglycoside therapy (median of 15 days) in combination with a cell wall–active agent for a median of 42 days in patients with PVE and native valve enterococcal endocarditis.[140] Clinical cure was observed in 75 of 93 (81%) patients overall, 78% of patients with PVE and 82% of patients with native valves. Among those who had a clinical cure, 52% received a β-lactam, 12% received vancomycin, and 36% received a combination of both. Ampicillin was given in 88% of patients receiving a β-lactam. The causative organism was *E. faecalis* in 78 patients and *E. faecium* in 5 patients. Clinical success was also achieved in all eight patients with native valve IE who received either vancomycin (50%), ampicillin (25%), or combination of both (25%) without synergistic aminoglycoside therapy.

Patients with complicated courses should receive 6 weeks of therapy, including patients infected with streptomycin-resistant organisms (such as G.S.), those who have had symptoms for more than 3 months before the initiation of antibiotics, and patients with PVE (such as G.S.).[12,19] Some clinicians recommend 6 weeks of therapy for all patients in whom the duration of illness cannot be firmly established; this accounts for many patients who present with subacute disease.

INCREASED NEPHROTOXICITY WITH VANCOMYCIN COMBINATION THERAPY

CASE 63-4, QUESTION 5: Is the combination of vancomycin and an aminoglycoside more nephrotoxic than either drug alone?

The incidence of nephrotoxicity associated with vancomycin administration in humans is thought to be minimal or nonexistent.[141] In a three-arm study involving more than 200 patients, nephrotoxicity was found in 5% of patients who received vancomycin alone, 22% of those receiving vancomycin with an aminoglycoside, and 11% of those receiving an aminoglycoside alone.[142] The study was well designed in that an aminoglycoside control group was included for comparison of the incidence of nephrotoxicity. Patients in whom increases in the serum creatinine concentration may have been a result of clinical conditions and patients who received drugs known to alter renal function were excluded in the analysis of this study. Serial serum vancomycin and aminoglycoside concentrations, as well as duration of therapy, were reported and analyzed. The authors concluded that vancomycin trough concentrations of more than 10 mcg/mL and concurrent therapy with an aminoglycoside were risk factors associated with an increased incidence of nephrotoxicity.

Another study specifically evaluated the risk of nephrotoxicity in patients receiving high-dose vancomycin therapy achieving trough concentrations of 15 to 20 mcg/mL for MRSA infections.[28] Nephrotoxicity occurred in 12% (11 of 95) of patients, significantly predicted by concomitant therapy with other nephrotoxic agents. An incremental increase in the risk of nephrotoxicity was associated with duration of therapy at high trough levels (15–20 mcg/mL): 6.3% for 7 days or less, 21.1% for 8 to 14 days, and 30% for more than 14 days. In a subanalysis that included only patients without receipt of concomitant nephrotoxic agents, nephrotoxicity occurred in only 1 (2%) of 44 high-trough versus 0 of 24 low-trough (<15 mcg/mL) patients. A review of the published literature confirms that an increased incidence of nephrotoxicity is likely when vancomycin and another nephrotoxic agent (i.e., an aminoglycoside, nonsteroidal anti-inflammatory drug) are given concomitantly, especially when vancomycin is dosed targeting trough concentration of 15 to 20 mcg/mL and administered for prolonged duration (>1 week).[141]

GLYCOPEPTIDE RESISTANCE IN ENTEROCOCCI

CASE 63-4, QUESTION 6: How do enterococci develop resistance to vancomycin? What are the therapeutic implications if G.S. is infected with glycopeptide-resistant enterococci?

VRE, particularly *E. faecium,* have emerged in the United States since 1987.[140,142] The increased use of vancomycin since the mid-1980s has coincided with the increased resistance to this class of compounds. Between 1989 and 1993, the percentage of nosocomial enterococci reported as resistant to vancomycin in the United States rose more than 20-fold, from 0.3% to 7.9%.[143] Enterococcal isolates from intensive care units increased even more dramatically, from 0.4% to 13.6%, during that time. Data from the Centers for Disease Control and Prevention National Nosocomial Infections Surveillance (NNIS) system indicate that the rate of increase has slowed down from 31% in 2000 to 12% in 2003.[144,145] A 12% increase was found in VRE infections in intensive care units between 2003 and the prior 5-year period (1998–2002). Nonetheless, epidemiologic studies conducted by the NNIS system, as well as others, have shown that VRE bacteremia is associated with significantly increased morbidity and mortality.[144,145]

Although *E. faecalis* is responsible for 80% to 90% of infections caused by enterococci, *E. faecium* is more likely to exhibit resistance to glycopeptides compared with *E. faecalis*; more than 95% of VRE recovered in the United States are *E. faecium.* Glycopeptide-resistant enterococci synthesize abnormal peptidoglycan precursors that lower the binding affinity of glycopeptides to peptidoglycans.[140] VRE can be broadly classified into three separate phenotypes (A, B, and C) based on three structurally different genes and gene products (e.g., altered ligases).[140] Most (approximately 70%) of resistant enterococci are of the VanA phenotype, which are resistant to high levels of both vancomycin (MIC >256 mcg/mL) and teicoplanin (MIC >16 mcg/mL). Expression of resistance is inducible, usually plasmid mediated, and transferable to other organisms via conjugation. The VanB strains exhibit moderate vancomycin resistance (MIC 16–64 mcg/mL), but remain susceptible to teicoplanin (MIC ≤2 mcg/mL). Overall, the VanC isolates are the least resistant (vancomycin MIC 8–16 mcg/mL; teicoplanin MIC ≤2 mcg/mL) because of chromosomal-mediated constitutive expression (i.e., not inducible as are VanA and VanB); however, VanC isolates usually are associated with the much less common *Enterococcus gallinarum* and *Enterococcus casseliflavus* infections.

Vancomycin, as well as extended-spectrum cephalosporins and drugs with potent antianaerobic activity, are risk factors for VRE.[140]

Few therapeutic alternatives exist for VRE, and synergistic combinations are required for bactericidal activity and clinical cure in endocarditis. Consequently, the treatment of choice is unknown. As a result, practitioners must make decisions using the available data from in vitro synergy studies, experimental models of endocarditis, and scattered case reports. Of additional concern, glycopeptide-resistant isolates often exhibit concomitant high-level resistance to aminoglycosides and β-lactams (e.g., ampicillin, penicillin) secondary to either β-lactamase production or alteration in the target penicillin-binding proteins.

Several antibiotic combinations appear promising in vitro and in preliminary animal models of endocarditis, but few data are currently available in humans. Those combinations include high-dose ampicillin (20 g/day) or ampicillin/sulbactam plus an aminoglycoside; vancomycin, penicillin or ceftriaxone and gentamicin; ampicillin and imipenem; ciprofloxacin and ampicillin; ciprofloxacin, rifampin, and gentamicin; and teicoplanin and gentamicin (teicoplanin is not available in the United States).[140]

STREPTOGRAMIN AND OXAZOLIDINONE

Quinupristin/dalfopristin (Synercid) and linezolid (Zyvox) are two agents with activity and proven efficacy against some infections caused by VRE approved for use by the FDA in the United States. Quinupristin/dalfopristin, available as a fixed 70:30 combination, is the first drug in the streptogramin class made available in the United States for human use. It belongs to the antibiotic family of macrolides/lincosamides/streptogramins. The agent received accelerated approval by the FDA in late 1999 specifically for the treatment of vancomycin-resistant *E. faecium* bacteremia. The combination is synergistic for glycopeptide-resistant enterococci with an MIC_{90} of 2 mcg/mL. The fixed product is generally bactericidal against susceptible streptococci and staphylococci (including methicillin-resistant strains), but it is bacteriostatic against *E. faecium*. Specifically, *E. faecalis* is not susceptible to the agent because of the presence of an efflux[146] pump conferring resistance to dalfopristin. Emergence of resistance during therapy has been reported on rare occasions.[146] The recommended dosage is 7.5 mg/kg every 8 to 12 hours (depending on the severity of infection).[147,148]

Arthralgias or myalgias were the most frequently reported events (10%) and also most frequently resulted in drug discontinuation.[147,148] A higher incidence of arthralgias or myalgias has been reported by others (up to 50%); those patients had significant comorbidities.[149] All cases were reversible on cessation of therapy. Significant venous irritation occurred (46%) when the drug was administered via a peripheral vein. Each dose can be diluted in 250 to 750 mL of dextrose (lower concentrations may decrease vein irritation) and infused for 1 hour.[62] The drug is not compatible with saline solutions. Laboratory abnormalities most frequently observed were increases in total and conjugated bilirubin in up to 34% of patients. As a result, liver function tests should be obtained once a week during therapy. Because quinupristin/dalfopristin is a potent inhibitor of the cytochrome P-450 3A4 enzyme system, coadministration of drugs (e.g., cyclosporine) metabolized by the same enzyme system should be avoided, if possible, or done only with close monitoring of therapeutic levels.[147]

Linezolid has bacteriostatic activity against enterococci, including vancomycin-resistant *E. faecium* and *E. faecalis*. It is also active against other gram-positive cocci, including *Streptococcus pneumoniae* and methicillin-resistant staphylococci.[147] Vancomycin-resistant *E. faecium* isolates resistant to linezolid have been isolated.[150,151] Treatment experience with linezolid under the compassionate use protocol reported clinical and microbiologic cure rates of 50% at 6-month follow-up for patients with endocarditis. Vancomycin-resistant *E. faecium* was the causative organism for 19 of the 32 patients treated.[111] Common adverse effects associated with linezolid include nausea, headache, diarrhea, rash, and altered taste. Of greater concern is its potential to cause myelosuppression. Thrombocytopenia, leukopenia, anemia, and pancytopenia have all been reported. Up to 30% of patients treated experience thrombocytopenia (platelet counts $<$100,000 platelets/μL).[147] In addition, linezolid is a weak monoamine oxidase inhibitor, which may potentiate the adrenergic effects of sympathomimetic agents (i.e., pseudoephedrine) and precipitate serotonergic syndrome when used concomitantly with selective serotonin reuptake inhibitors. Patients should be advised to avoid tyramine-containing foods (i.e., aged cheese, sausages, sauerkraut, wine) during therapy as well. Linezolid is available both orally and parenterally. Linezolid given orally or via enteral feedings is completely bioavailable.[152] A dosage of 600 mg twice daily is recommended for adults. Persistent MRSA bacteremia caused by suboptimal serum concentrations of linezolid has been described.[109]

DAPTOMYCIN

Daptomycin is active against enterococci in vitro with an MIC range of 0.25 to 4 mcg/mL and MIC_{90} of 4 mcg/mL for 219 vancomycin-resistant *E. faecium* isolates from the United States. For 40 vancomycin-resistant *E. faecalis* isolates, the MIC range is 0.015 to 2 mcg/mL, with a MIC_{90} of 2 mcg/mL.[153] When tested against 20 vancomycin-resistant *E. faecium* strains, daptomycin had MIC_{50} of 2 mcg/mL versus 0.5 mcg/mL and 4 mcg/mL for quinupristin/dalfopristin and linezolid, respectively.[153] Of concern is the emergence of daptomycin resistance during therapy for VRE infections.[154,155] In a case report of a patient with vancomycin-resistant *E. faecium* pyelonephritis, the initial isolate had an MIC of 2 mcg/mL; however, after 17 days of treatment, a blood culture yielded growth of vancomycin-resistant *E. faecium* with an MIC increase to 32 mcg/mL.[156] Clinical experience with daptomycin for vancomycin-resistant *E. faecium* endocarditis is limited, and treatment failure has been reported.[157] Thus, the role of daptomycin in treating VRE endocarditis is uncertain at this point.

FUNGAL ENDOCARDITIS CAUSED BY *CANDIDA ALBICANS*

Prognosis and Treatment

CASE 63-5

QUESTION 1: B.G., a 35-year-old male heroin addict, was admitted to the hospital with chief complaints of pleuritic chest pain and dyspnea on exertion. Physical examination revealed a cachectic man with a temperature of 104°F, a diastolic regurgitant heart murmur heard loudest during inspiration, splenomegaly, and pharyngeal petechiae. Funduscopic examination was noncontributory. On the chest radiograph, several pulmonary infiltrates with cavitation were evident. UA was significant for microscopic hematuria and RBC casts. A transesophageal echocardiogram demonstrated vegetations on both the tricuspid and aortic heart valves. B.G. had evidence of moderate heart failure, although his hemodynamic status at that time was "stable." Six sets of blood cultures were drawn over the course of 2 days, and broad-spectrum empiric coverage consisting of vancomycin, gentamicin, and ceftazidime was initiated. Two days later, two of the cultures grew *Candida albicans*, and a diagnosis of fungal endocarditis was established. What is B.G.'s prognosis, and how should his fungal endocarditis be treated?

Fungal endocarditis is a rare but life-threatening infection that is difficult to diagnose and even more difficult to treat.[1] Most cases are caused by *Candida* and *Aspergillus* species. Fungal endocarditis occurs primarily in IV drug users, patients with prosthetic heart valves, immunocompromised patients, those with IV catheters, or patients receiving broad-spectrum antibiotics.[158–161]

Management of fungal endocarditis generally requires early valve replacement and aggressive fungicidal therapy with amphotericin deoxycholate B 0.6 to 1 mg/kg/day with or without 5-flucytosine (5-FC) 25 mg/kg orally QID. If B.G. had poor renal function, liposomal formulations of amphotericin B 3 to 5 mg/kg daily can be used as an alternative.[162]

These antifungal agents should be prescribed for B.G., and his broad-spectrum antibiotic coverage with vancomycin, gentamicin, and ceftazidime should be discontinued.

B.G.'s clinical presentation and chest radiograph indicate that fragments of vegetation have already embolized to his lungs and possibly to other vital organs (e.g., spleen, kidneys). Because of the morbidity and mortality associated with major emboli and valvular insufficiency, B.G. should undergo surgery within 48 to 72 hours after antifungal therapy has been initiated. The prognosis for B.G. is dismal even with proper medical and surgical treatment. In a series analyzing 270 cases of fungal IE occurring during a 30-year period, mortality for those who received combined medical and surgical management was 45%, compared with 64% for those who received antifungal therapy alone.[158] Despite initial response to treatment, the rate of relapse is high (30%–40%), and relapse can occur up to 9 years after the initial episode of infection.[158–161] Most deaths in IV drug users with endocarditis are secondary to heart failure, a finding already evident in B.G.[1] In addition, replacement of a heart valve for fungal endocarditis in a heroin addict carries a significant risk of late morbidity and mortality.[158]

COMBINATION THERAPY WITH 5-FLUCYTOSINE AND AMPHOTERICIN B

CASE 63-5, QUESTION 2: Why is it important to treat B.G.'s fungal endocarditis with the combination of 5-FC and conventional or lipid-based amphotericin B? What is the optimal duration of therapy?

The importance of adding 5-FC (Ancobon) to amphotericin B (Fungizone) therapy has not been adequately studied; however, the poor prognosis associated with fungal endocarditis warrants the administration of 5-FC, despite its potential for causing bone marrow suppression and hepatotoxicity.[158] The vegetations from his tricuspid or aortic heart valves already have broken off and caused pulmonary cavitation and possibly splenomegaly. His clinical presentation is consistent with a potentially fatal outcome; therefore, his blood isolates should be tested for in vitro susceptibility to amphotericin, 5-FC, and azoles. Fungi resistant to 5-FC alone may still be susceptible to the synergistic effect of the 5-FC–amphotericin B combination.[163] If the organism is resistant to 5-FC, in vitro synergy between these two antifungals should be performed or therapy with an echinocandin should be considered.

The optimal dose and duration of antifungal therapy for fungal endocarditis have not been determined by clinical studies; however, postoperative treatment with amphotericin B and 5-FC (if it has in vitro activity) for a minimum of 6 weeks (total dose, 1.5–3 g of amphotericin B) is recommended and is supported by the poor penetration of amphotericin B into heart valve tissue.[164] In patients with fungal PVE, some experts advocate secondary prophylaxis for a minimum of 2 years or lifelong suppressive treatment with an oral antifungal agent for nonsurgical candidates in light of the high rates of relapse.[1,158,160,163–166]

Nephrotoxicity caused by amphotericin is often a serious dose-limiting factor to completion of therapy, particularly in patients who require a prolonged treatment course. Renal dysfunction secondary to the conventional formulation of amphotericin B may stabilize or improve with the switch to lipid-formulated amphotericin B products (i.e., Abelcet, AmBisome).[167] The efficacy of the new formulations in the treatment of endocarditis has been demonstrated only in anecdotal reports.[158,160,163,164,168] Alternative antifungal agents, including echinocandins and azole, are potential options in patients who experience significant renal toxicities.

ALTERNATIVE ANTIFUNGALS

CASE 63-5, QUESTION 3: If B.G. experiences significant toxicities because of prolonged combination treatment with amphotericin and 5-FC, what alternative antifungal agent(s) can be used to treat his fungal endocarditis?

Fluconazole (Diflucan) is a triazole compound active against *Candida* species, particularly *C. albicans* and *Candida parapsilosis.* It also has a favorable toxicity profile compared with amphotericin and 5-FC.[169] Prolonged combination treatment with amphotericin products and 5-FC often is limited by nephrotoxicity, bone marrow suppression, and hepatic damage. Limited experimental and clinical experience exists using fluconazole in the treatment of candidal endocarditis.

Fluconazole was effective in eradicating cardiac fungal vegetations caused by *C. albicans* and *C. parapsilosis* in a rabbit model.[170] Successful experience with fluconazole treatment of fungal endocarditis in humans has been described in only a few case reports.[171–175] Patients with various *Candida* species (i.e., *C. albicans, C. parapsilosis,* and *Candida tropicalis)* were treated with 200 to 600 mg of fluconazole daily for 45 days to 6 months or until death. Fluconazole therapy reduced or completely removed all cardiac vegetations and resolved clinical symptoms. Because of the lack of adequate clinical experience, however, the use of fluconazole in treating fungal endocarditis cannot be advocated except in patients who require lifelong therapy because of the following situations: (a) the patient is a poor surgical candidate, (b) the patient has relapsed at least once since the initial infection episode, or (c) the patient has PVE.

Another potential alternative is caspofungin, which is a first-line agent in the echinocandin class.[176] Caspofungin is approved for the treatment of invasive candidiasis (primarily bloodstream infections and peritonitis). Caspofungin inhibits fungal cell wall synthesis by inhibiting β-1,3-glucan synthesis. It is fungicidal against most *Candida* species (including *C. albicans),* and with minimal toxicity. Case reports describe successful outcomes with caspofungin in the treatment of IE.[177–179] In a patient with *Candida glabrata* mitral valve endocarditis without surgical intervention, caspofungin was used successfully as induction therapy in combination with amphotericin B and continued as maintenance therapy for 12 weeks.[180] In a second case report of a patient with PVE caused by *C. glabrata* and *Candida krusei*, resolution of vegetation was achieved after 6 weeks of caspofungin therapy alone without valvular replacement. Both patients were deemed to be poor surgical candidates and received medical therapy only.[179] Micafungin and anidulafungin are other potential echinocandin options; however, clinical experience in the treatment of endocarditis is currently lacking.

GRAM-NEGATIVE BACILLARY ENDOCARDITIS CAUSED BY *PSEUDOMONAS AERUGINOSA*

Prevalence

CASE 63-5, QUESTION 4: Fourteen months after completing his course of antifungal therapy, B.G. was readmitted to the hospital with a 48-hour history of fever, shaking chills, rigors, and night sweats. His vital signs at that time were blood pressure, 100/60 mm Hg; pulse, 120 beats/minute; respirations, 24/minute; and temperature, 103.7°F. A new-onset systolic murmur was noted on auscultation. Two-dimensional echocardiography revealed two small vegetations on the prosthetic valve. Empiric therapy consisting of amphotericin B, 5-FC, vancomycin, and gentamicin was initiated. Three blood cultures drawn on the day of admission were positive for *P. aeruginosa* with the following antibiotic susceptibilities[85]: gentamicin (8 mcg/mL), tobramycin (2 mcg/mL), piperacillin-tazobactam (64 mcg/mL), and ceftazidime (2 mcg/mL). A presumptive diagnosis of PVE caused by *P. aeruginosa* was made. Why was the finding of *Pseudomonas* expected in B.G.?

The prevalence of endocarditis caused by gram-negative organisms has increased significantly over the years, especially in IV drug users such as B.G. and patients with prosthetic heart valves. Gram-negative organisms are responsible for about 15% to 20% of endocarditis cases in these populations.[181] Most gram-negative endocarditis cases are caused by *Pseudomonas* species, *S. marcescens,* and *Enterobacter* species, although numerous other gram-negative organisms have been known to cause endocarditis.[181–186] Geographic clustering of certain organisms causing endocarditis in narcotic addicts has been shown in the past, such as the association of *P. aeruginosa* with the Detroit area and *S. marcescens* with San Francisco.[183,187–189] These past epidemiologic findings are not necessarily true today. In narcotic addicts with gram-negative endocarditis, the tricuspid, aortic, and mitral valves are involved in 50%, 45%, and 40% of cases, respectively.[186]

Antimicrobial Therapy

CASE 63-5, QUESTION 5: How should B.G.'s gram-negative endocarditis be treated and monitored?

The previous empirical antimicrobials should be discontinued because *P. aeruginosa* has been cultured from B.G.'s blood. A bactericidal combination of antibiotics usually is required to provide in vivo synergy and to prevent resistant subpopulations from emerging during therapy.[1,190] B.G., therefore, should be treated with ceftazidime (2 g IV every 8 hours) with concurrent high-dose tobramycin (3 mg/kg IV every 8 hours). The duration of therapy is not well defined, but most authorities recommend 4 to 6 weeks.[1,182,187,189] Because B.G. should be receiving both ceftazidime and tobramycin on the same schedule (every 8 hours), the trough titer should be drawn just before dose administration. Finally, the infected valve should be surgically excised for the reasons previously discussed.

Endocarditis caused by *P. aeruginosa* (as in B.G.) should be treated for at least 6 weeks with a combination of an aminoglycoside and an antipseudomonal penicillin (piperacillin-tazobactam) or cephalosporin (ceftazidime).[1,191] The combination of an antipseudomonal penicillin and an aminoglycoside is synergistic in vitro and in the rabbit model of *P. aeruginosa* endocarditis,[191,192] and clinical experience has confirmed this finding in IV drug users. Combination therapy with high dosages of tobramycin or gentamicin (8 mg/kg/day) has been associated with a significantly higher cure rate and lower mortality rate compared with an older, low-dose regimen (2.5–5 mg/kg/day).[181,182,189] Aminoglycosides (tobramycin or gentamicin) should be dosed to produce peak and trough serum concentrations of 15 to 20 mcg/mL and less than 2 mcg/mL, respectively, to ensure maximum efficacy[1]; therefore, high-dose tobramycin should be selected for B.G.

Of note, the use of extended-interval dosing of aminoglycoside has not been evaluated for the treatment of endocarditis caused by gram-negative organisms; therefore, this dosing approach cannot be recommended at this time. The choice of aminoglycoside should be based on the in vitro activity of the organism (i.e., MIC), relative toxicity potential, and cost. In B.G.'s case, tobramycin should be selected over gentamicin because the isolated organism was resistant to gentamicin. Generally, *P. aeruginosa* is more susceptible to tobramycin than to gentamicin. Thus, it is not at all surprising that the *P. aeruginosa* in B.G.'s blood cultures had an MIC of 2 mcg/mL for tobramycin compared with MIC of 8 mcg/mL for gentamicin. Ceftazidime is preferred over piperacillin-tazobactam for B.G. on the basis of its narrower spectrum of activity.[193]

Several compounds such as imipenem (Primaxin), meropenem (Merrem), aztreonam (Azactam), cefepime (Maxipime), and ciprofloxacin (Cipro) are active against many of the gram-negative organisms causing endocarditis. Clinical data regarding their use in the treatment of endocarditis are very limited, however.[194–197]

CULTURE-NEGATIVE ENDOCARDITIS

CASE 63-5, QUESTION 6: B.G.'s history, clinical presentation, and imaging studies are strongly suggestive of infective endocarditis. If his blood cultures had been negative after 48 hours of incubation, the working diagnosis would have been culture-negative endocarditis. What are the possible reasons for culture-negative endocarditis, and what measures should be taken to establish a microbiologic etiology?

The proportion of patients with culture-negative endocarditis has diminished considerably, presumably as a result of improved microbiologic culture techniques. Negative blood cultures are present in only 5% to 7% of patients who meet strict criteria for the diagnosis of IE and have not recently received antibiotics.[198]

The prior administration of antimicrobials is thought to account for most cases of culture-negative endocarditis.[199] B.G.'s blood cultures may remain negative for several days to weeks if he has taken antibiotics recently. The use of antibiotic absorbance resins or the addition of β-lactamases to the blood sample may remove or inactivate some antibiotics.[200]

Slow-growing and fastidious organisms, such as gram-negative bacilli in the *Haemophilus-Actinobacillus-Cardiobacterium-Eikenella-Kingella* group (HACEK), *Brucella, Coxiella,* chlamydiae, strict anaerobes, and fungi, should be pursued in culture-negative patients. This usually is accomplished by the use of special culture media or by obtaining appropriate serologic acute and convalescent titers. Blood cultures should be saved for at least 3 weeks to detect slow-growing organisms.[199] The use of polymerase chain reaction to identify nonculturable organisms in excised valvular specimens or septic emboli has been helpful in some cases.[201] Of note, previously NVS has been the cause of most of the cases of endocarditis diagnosed as culture-negative, initially because of its requirement for the addition of vitamin B_6 (pyridoxal HCl) to the culture media for laboratory growth; however, laboratory identification is no longer a significant problem with current culture media and laboratory techniques.[8]

Empiric Therapy

CASE 63-5, QUESTION 7: The causative organism remains unidentified. Recommend an antimicrobial regimen for the empiric treatment of B.G.'s presumed culture-negative endocarditis.

In the hemodynamically stable patient, antibiotic therapy should be withheld until positive blood cultures are obtained.[1] Based on B.G.'s clinical presentation and echocardiographic findings, empiric antibiotics should be initiated as soon as necessary cultures have been collected. Because staphylococci and gram-negative bacilli account for most cases of endocarditis in the narcotic addict with a prosthetic heart valve, B.G. should be started on a four-drug regimen: vancomycin targeting trough of 15 to 20 mcg/mL, gentamicin targeting peak of 3 to 4 mcg/mL, cefepime 2 g IV every 8 hours, and rifampin 300 mg IV/PO every 8 hours.[7] Because B.G. may be experiencing a relapse caused by *C. albicans,* the addition of amphotericin B and 5-FC would be appropriate. If B.G. is from an area where methicillin-resistant staphylococci are prevalent, vancomycin should be substituted for nafcillin. A third-generation cephalosporin (ceftriaxone or ceftazidime) or piperacillin-tazobactam could be used, depending on the gram-negative pathogens common to the region and their anticipated susceptibilities. This regimen, which contains an aminoglycoside and piperacillin-tazobactam, also will provide coverage for enterococci.

B.G.'s clinical status and the positive echocardiogram indicate that early surgical valve excision and replacement are necessary.[202] Cultures obtained from the excised valve may allow for identification of the causative organism. His antimicrobial regimen may need to be altered if and when subsequent culture information becomes available. Other noninfective conditions, such as atrial myxoma, marasmic endocarditis, and rheumatic fever, can mimic culture-negative endocarditis and should be excluded from the differential diagnosis with the appropriate tests.[1]

PROPHYLACTIC THERAPY

Rationale and Recommendations

CASE 63-6

QUESTION 1: B.B., a 74-year-old man with poor dentition, is scheduled to have all of his remaining teeth extracted for

subsequent fitting of dentures. His medical history is significant for numerous infections of the oral cavity and prosthetic valve replacement 2 years ago. His only current medications are digoxin (Lanoxin) 0.125 mg/day and furosemide (Lasix) 40 mg every morning. What is the rationale for antibiotic prophylaxis?

Because IE is associated with significant mortality and long-term morbidity, prevention in susceptible patients is of paramount importance.[1] Estimates are, however, that less than 10% of all cases are theoretically preventable.[9,203] The incidence of endocarditis in patients undergoing procedures known to cause significant bacteremia, even without antibiotic prophylaxis, is low. In addition, endocarditis may develop after the administration of seemingly appropriate chemoprophylaxis. Therefore, it is not surprising that the efficacy of prophylaxis has never been established through placebo-controlled clinical trials. Approximately 6,000 patients would be necessary to demonstrate a statistical difference (if one exists) between untreated controls and a group receiving prophylaxis.[203,204]

Without conclusive clinical data from prospective trials, recommendations for antibiotic prophylaxis have been based largely on in vitro susceptibility data, evaluation of antibiotic regimens using animal models of endocarditis, and anecdotal experiences.[203,204]

Prophylactic antibiotics are thought to provide protection by decreasing the number of organisms reaching the damaged heart valve from a primary source. Thus, antibiotics theoretically prevent bacterial multiplication on the valve and interfere with bacterial adherence to the cardiac lesion.[203,204]

The 2007 AHA recommendations for antibiotic prophylaxis before common medical procedures are outlined in Table 63-7.[204] Compared with the previous (1997) guideline,[204] the current guidelines only recommend the use of prophylaxis in patients with specific cardiac conditions who are undergoing only dental or respiratory tract procedures. The use of prophylaxis for patients undergoing genitourinary or gastrointestinal procedures is not recommended because of a continuing lack of evidence to support efficacy.

TABLE 63-7

Endocarditis Prophylaxis Regimen Indicated for Patients With Cardiac Conditions[a]

Drug	Dose
Dental or upper respiratory tract procedures	Single dose 30 to 60 minutes before procedure
Standard Regimen	
Amoxicillin	*Adult:* 2 g *Pediatric:* 50 mg/kg
Allergic to penicillin or ampicillin	
Clindamycin	*Adult:* 600 mg
or	*Pediatric:* 20 mg/kg
Cephalexin[b,c]	*Adult:* 2 g
or	*Pediatric:* 50 mg/kg
Azithromycin or clarithromycin	*Adult:* 500 mg *Pediatric:* 15 mg/kg
Unable to Take Oral Medications	
Ampicillin	*Adult:* 2 g IM or IV *Pediatric:* 50 mg/kg IM or IV
Allergic to Penicillin or Ampicillin	
Clindamycin	*Adult:* 600 mg
or	*Pediatric:* 20 mg/kg IV
Cefazolin[b]	*Adult:* 1 g IM or IV *Pediatric:* 50 mg/kg IM or IV

[a] See Table 63-1.

[b] Cephalosporins should not be used in individuals with immediate-type hypersensitivity reaction (e.g., urticaria, angioedema, or anaphylaxis) to penicillins or ampicillin.

[c] Other first- or second-generation oral cephalosporins in equivalent adult or pediatric dose.

IM, intramuscular; IV, intravenous.

Source: Wilson W et al. Prevention of infective endocarditis: guidelines from the American Heart Association: a guideline from the American Heart Association Rheumatic Fever, Endocarditis, and Kawasaki Disease Committee, Council on Cardiovascular Disease in the Young, and the Council on Clinical Cardiology, Council on Cardiovascular Surgery and Anesthesia, and the Quality of Care an Outcomes Research Interdisciplinary Working Group. American Heart Association [published correction appears in *Circulation*. 2007;116:e376]. *Circulation*. 2007;116:1736.

DENTAL AND UPPER RESPIRATORY TRACT PROCEDURES

The current guidelines only recommend prophylaxis in individuals with cardiac conditions associated with the highest risk of adverse outcomes from endocarditis (Table 63-1). Previous 1997 AHA guidelines listed a substantial number of procedures in which prophylaxis is either indicated or not recommended. Analysis of published data shows that viridans streptococci bacteremia can result from any procedure that involves the manipulation of the gingival tissue or the periapical region of the teeth or perforation of the oral mucosa. Placement or removal of prosthodontic or orthodontic appliances, adjustment of orthodontic appliances, taking dental radiographs, bleeding from trauma to the lips or oral mucosa, and instantaneous shedding of deciduous teeth do not require chemoprophylaxis. Endotracheal intubation also does not require prophylactic therapy.

Antimicrobial prophylaxis should be directed against the viridans group of streptococci because these organisms are the most common cause of endocarditis after dental procedures. Invasive surgical procedures involving the upper respiratory tract, such as incision or biopsy of the respiratory mucosa (e.g., tonsillectomy, adenoidectomy), can cause transient bacteremia with organisms that have similar antibiotic susceptibilities to those that occur after dental procedures; therefore, the same regimens are suggested. Prophylaxis is not recommended for bronchoscopies unless the procedure involves incision of the respiratory mucosa. Amoxicillin is currently recommended for oral prophylaxis in susceptible persons having dental or upper respiratory tract surgery. Oral clindamycin, clarithromycin, or azithromycin is recommended for patients with immediate-type hypersensitivity reaction to penicillins. Only patients with outlined cardiac conditions should receive prophylactic antibiotics.

Most cases of endocarditis that are caused by bacterial flora from the mouth do not follow dental procedures but rather are the result of poor oral hygiene. The cumulative exposure to random bacteremias from daily oral activities is estimated to be 5,730 minutes during a 1-month period compared with only 6 to 30 minutes for a dental procedure. Furthermore, it is estimated that the cumulative exposure to bacteremia from routine daily activities may be as high as 5.6 million times greater than a single tooth extraction.[203] Based on the study results, concerns for antimicrobial resistance, and cost, changes to restrict the use of antibiotic prophylaxis to the highest-risk patients before dental procedures may be expected with future guidelines issued by the AHA.

Indications and Choice of Agent

CASE 63-6, QUESTION 2: Is prophylactic antibiotic therapy indicated for B.B.? If so, which antibiotic(s) should be used?

Based on the current recommendations, B.B. is a candidate for antibiotic prophylaxis. Presence of a prosthetic aortic valve while undergoing multiple tooth extractions places him at risk for experiencing endocarditis. He also is scheduled to have all of his remaining teeth extracted, a procedure likely to result in bacteremia. According to Table 63-7, B.B. should receive a single 2-g oral dose of amoxicillin 1 hour before the procedure.

HOME INTRAVENOUS ANTIBIOTIC THERAPY

CASE 63-7

QUESTION 1: T.M., a 48-year-old woman, developed viridans streptococci endocarditis after a dental procedure. Her medical history is significant for rheumatic heart disease and chronic renal insufficiency (measured creatinine clearance, 50 mL/minute). She is hemodynamically stable and has no evidence of vegetation. She is currently on day 7 of therapy with penicillin G, 2 million units IV every 4 hours. The plan is to continue penicillin therapy for a total of 4 weeks. What are the considerations for using home IV therapy for the treatment of infective endocarditis? Is T.M. a candidate for home antibiotic therapy?

The successful use of home IV antibiotic therapy for the patient with endocarditis has been described, although the number of patients treated is relatively small compared with those treated for osteomyelitis.[205–206] The advantages of home therapy include economic benefits to the hospital for early discharge (the diagnosis-related-group allocation for endocarditis is 18.4 days, which is shorter than the usual recommended duration of therapy) and the potential for greater acceptance by the patient.

Home treatment of endocarditis is not without risk, however.[206] Patients must be hemodynamically stable before discharge and free from the risk of sudden valve rupture. The drug abuser is obviously not a candidate for home treatment, nor is the patient receiving frequent doses of medication. The successful management of any infection amenable to home treatment requires careful patient evaluation for suitability and coordination of the health care provided by key personnel.

T.M. represents the typical patient with uncomplicated streptococcal endocarditis. If the sole reason for continued hospitalization is to administer IV antibiotics, she is a potential candidate for home therapy.

Ceftriaxone is an attractive option for outpatient therapy of uncomplicated endocarditis caused by penicillin-susceptible streptococci. The excellent in vitro activity of ceftriaxone and its long half-life of 6 to 9 hours allow once-a-day administration. The feasibility of intramuscular administration of ceftriaxone also obviates the need for IV access, thus avoiding any potential line-related complications when administered in the outpatient setting.

Clinical experience with the use of ceftriaxone in the treatment of patients with penicillin-susceptible streptococcal endocarditis was described in four open-label studies.[38–41] Two of the studies evaluated ceftriaxone monotherapy for 4 weeks; the other two evaluated combination therapy with ceftriaxone and an aminoglycoside for a 2-week duration. All infecting strains of streptococci in the first two studies were inhibited by ceftriaxone at an MIC of less than 0.25 mcg/mL. In one study, ceftriaxone was given at a dosage of 2 g once daily for 4 weeks to most patients, with 15 receiving ceftriaxone for 2 weeks followed by amoxicillin 1 g four times daily for 2 weeks. Most of the patients received therapy predominantly as outpatients. All 30 patients reported in this study responded favorably to treatment with ceftriaxone or ceftriaxone followed by amoxicillin.[38] Patients with cardiovascular risk factors, such as heart failure, severe aortic insufficiency, or evidence of recurrent thromboembolic events, were excluded from the study. Only one probable relapse was noted at 3 months after therapy with presentation of febrile syndrome, elevated sedimentation rate, and negative bacterial blood culture. An uncontrolled study extended the favorable results of the aforementioned study.[34] Treatment was completed in 55 of 59 patients. Patients were followed for 4 months to up to 5 years after the end of treatment with no clinical signs or laboratory evidence of relapse. Of patients, 71% completed therapy without complications; however, 10 required valve replacement secondary to hemodynamic deterioration or recurrent emboli, whereas 4 required a change in therapy because of drug allergy. Adverse side effects were minor, but 3 patients had neutropenia that resolved after cessation of therapy.

Because of the lack of controlled trials comparing the efficacy of ceftriaxone against penicillin with or without an aminoglycoside in the treatment of penicillin-susceptible streptococcal endocarditis, ceftriaxone should be considered primarily in patients such as T.M. for whom home antibiotic therapy is a treatment option and those who are hemodynamically stable with no evidence of vegetation.

The feasibility of home therapy depends on the following additional factors: (a) patient willingness, (b) adequate venous access, (c) psychosocial stability, (d) access to medical care if an emergency occurs, (e) ability to train T.M. (proper aseptic technique, catheter site care, antibiotic preparation, recognition of untoward effects of the antibiotic, and recognition of symptoms associated with worsening infection), and (f) insurance coverage for home IV therapy. These conditions can be accomplished only with the multidisciplinary involvement of the infectious disease physician, a social worker, a pharmacist, a specialty nurse, and the patient. Home care, outpatient care, and other options will be used increasingly because health care reform mandates the decreased use of tertiary care facilities when possible.

KEY REFERENCES

A full list of references for this chapter can be found at http://thepoint.lww.com/AT10e. Below are the key references for this chapter, with the corresponding reference number in this chapter found in parentheses after the reference.

Key References

Archer GL et al. *Staphylococcus epidermidis* and other coagulase-negative staphylococci. In: Mandell GL et al, ed. *Mandell, Douglas, and Bennett's Principles and Practice of Infectious Diseases.* 7th ed. Philadelphia, PA: Elsevier Churchill Livingstone; 2009: Chapter 116;2545. (46)

Baddour LM et al. Infective endocarditis: diagnosis, antimicrobial therapy, and management of complications: a statement for healthcare professionals from the Committee on Rheumatic Fever, Endocarditis, and Kawasaki Disease, Council on Cardiovascular Disease in the Young, and the Councils on Clinical Cardiology, Stroke, and Cardiovascular Surgery and Anesthesia, American Heart Association: endorsed by the Infectious Diseases Society of America. *Circulation.* 2005;111:e394. (7)

Fowler VG Jr et al. Daptomycin versus standard therapy for bacteremia and endocarditis caused by *Staphylococcus aureus. N Engl J Med.* 2006;355:653. (114)

Fowler VJ Jr et al. Endocarditis and intravascular infections. In: Mandell GL et al, eds. *Mandell, Douglas, and Bennett's Principles and Practice of Infectious Diseases.* 7th ed. Philadelphia, PA: Elsevier Churchill Livingston; 2009: Chapter 77. (1)

Fowler VG Jr et al. *Staphylococcus aureus* endocarditis: a consequence of medical progress [published correction appears in *JAMA.* 2005;294:900]. *JAMA.* 2005;293:3012. (5)

Howden BP et al. Reduced vancomycin susceptibility in *Staphylococcus aureus,* including vancomycin-intermediate and heterogeneous vancomycin-intermediate strains: resistance mechanisms, laboratory detection, and clinical implications. *Clin Microbiol Rev.* 2010;23:99. (58)

Karchmer AW. Prosthetic valve endocarditis. In: Mandell GL et al, ed. *Mandell, Douglas, and Bennett's Principles and Practice of Infectious Diseases.* 7th ed. Philadelphia, PA: Elsevier Churchill Livingstone; 2009: Chapter 78;1113. (41)

Le T, Bayer AS. Combination antibiotic therapy for infective endocarditis. *Clin Infect Dis.* 2003;36:615. (20)

Li JS et al. Proposed modifications to the Duke criteria for the diagnosis of infective endocarditis. *Clin Infect Dis.* 2000;30:633. (18)

Liu C et al. Clinical practice guidelines by the Infectious Diseases Society of America for the treatment of methicillin-resistant *Staphylococcus aureus* infections in adults and children. *Clin Infect Dis.* 2011;52:e18. (79)

Pappas PG et al. Clinical practice guidelines for the management of candidiasis: 2009 update by the Infectious Diseases Society of America. *Clin Infect Dis.* 2009;48:503. (162)

Sexton DJ et al. Ceftriaxone once daily for four weeks compared with ceftriaxone plus gentamicin once daily for two weeks for treatment of endocarditis due to penicillin-susceptible streptococci. Endocarditis Treatment Consortium Group. *Clin Infect Dis.* 1998;27:1470. (35)

Wilson W et al. Prevention of infective endocarditis: guidelines from the American Heart Association: a guideline from the American Heart Association Rheumatic Fever, Endocarditis, and Kawasaki Disease Committee, Council on Cardiovascular Disease in the Young, and the Council on Clinical Cardiology, Council on Cardiovascular Surgery and Anesthesia, and the Quality of Care an Outcomes Research Interdisciplinary Working Group. American Heart Association [published correction appears in *Circulation.* 2007;116:e376]. *Circulation.* 2007;116:1736. (204)

Respiratory Tract Infections

Heather M. Arnold, Eli N. Deal, Steven Gelone, and Scott T. Micek

64

CORE PRINCIPLES

	CHAPTER CASES
ACUTE BRONCHITIS	
1 Acute bronchitis is a commonly encountered clinical diagnosis exhibited by cough for more than 5 days and generally does not require treatment with antimicrobial agents.	**Case 64-1 (Questions 1 and 3)**
ACUTE EXACERBATION OF CHRONIC OBSTRUCTIVE PULMONARY DISEASE	
1 Antibiotics should be provided to patients with acute exacerbations of chronic obstructive pulmonary disease (AECOPD) if three primary symptoms (increased dyspnea, increased sputum volume, and increased sputum purulence) are present, if two primary symptoms are present and increased sputum purulence is one of the symptoms, or with required mechanical ventilation.	**Case 64-2 (Question 4)**
2 Corticosteroids should be considered for certain patients with AECOPD, including patients receiving home therapy with severe chronic obstructive pulmonary disease (COPD) and for all patients requiring hospitalization.	**Case 64-2 (Question 6)**
3 Prevention of influenza and *Streptococcus pneumoniae* through vaccinations in patients with COPD or previous pneumonia reduces disease-associated morbidity.	**Case 64-2 (Question 8)**
COMMUNITY-ACQUIRED PNEUMONIA	
1 The first decision after a diagnosis of community-acquired pneumonia (CAP) is to determine need for hospitalization. Several prediction rules including the pneumonia severity index (PSI) and CURB-65 (confusion, uremia, increased respiratory rate, low blood pressure, and age ≥65 years) have been developed to facilitate site-of-care decision making.	**Case 64-3 (Question 2)**
2 The most frequently isolated bacterial pathogen causing CAP, regardless of epidemiological factors and severity of illness, is *S. pneumoniae*.	**Case 64-3 (Question 4)**
3 The most important consideration to be made with selection of empiric therapy is to identify patients at risk for infection with drug-resistant *S. pneumoniae* (DRSP).	**Case 64-3 (Question 5)**
4 Patients who continue to have a positive laboratory test result for influenza more than 48 hours after the onset of illness at high risk or requiring hospitalization who are not improving should also be treated.	**Case 64-4 (Question 2)**

continued

HOSPITAL-ACQUIRED, VENTILATOR-ASSOCIATED, AND HEALTH CARE–ASSOCIATED PNEUMONIA

1	Hospital-acquired pneumonia (HAP) is defined as pneumonia that occurs at least 48 hours after hospitalization not incubating at the time of admission. Ventilator-associated pneumonia (VAP) refers to pneumonia that arises 48 to 72 hours after endotracheal intubation. Health care–associated pneumonia (HCAP) includes any patient who has been hospitalized in an acute-care hospital for 2 or more days within 90 days of infection; resided in a nursing home or long-term care facility; received intravenous antibiotic therapy, chemotherapy, or wound care within the past 30 days of the current infection; lived in close contact with a person with a multidrug-resistant (MDR) pathogen; or attended a hospital or hemodialysis clinic.	**Case 64-5 (Question 1)**
2	The major difference in the bacteriology between CAP and HAP/HCAP/VAP is a shift to gram-negative pathogens, MDR pathogens, and methicillin-resistant *Staphylococcus aureus* (MRSA) in HAP/HCAP/VAP.	**Case 64-5 (Question 2)**
3	Risk factors for pneumonia caused by MDR pathogens include antimicrobial therapy in the previous 90 days, current hospitalization of 5 days or more, immunosuppressive disease or therapy, or any risk factor for HCAP.	**Case 64-5 (Question 2)**
4	Patients with early-onset pneumonia (<5 days) and no MDR risk factors can be treated with a single agent, including nonantipseudomonal third-generation cephalosporins or ertapenem, ampicillin/sulbactam, or an antipneumococcal fluoroquinolone. Empiric therapy in those with late-onset (≥5 days) or MDR risk factors should include a combination of antibiotics active against *Pseudomonas aeruginosa.* This regimen usually includes an antipseudomonal β-lactam, plus either an aminoglycoside or ciprofloxacin/levofloxacin. Vancomycin or linezolid should be added if MRSA risk factors are present or there is a high incidence at the health care facility.	**Case 64-6 (Question 2)**

ACUTE BRONCHITIS

Definition and Incidence

Acute bronchitis (AB) is defined as an acute, self-limiting respiratory illness of the upper bronchi accompanied by cough for more than 5 days that can last up to 3 weeks.[1–3] AB can be associated with or without purulent sputum production, and fever is rare.[1] During the first few days of symptoms, AB is frequently indistinguishable from other upper respiratory illnesses including the "common cold."[1,3] AB is one of the most common conditions encountered in clinical practice as 5% of the adult population are diagnosed annually in the United States, and it ranks as the ninth most common illness among outpatients.[1,4–6] Most cases of AB (>90%) are caused by viruses.[7,8] AB accounts for greater than 10 million office visits per year and is associated with frequent antibiotic overuse.[2,3,8–17]

It is important to delineate the differences between an acute exacerbation of chronic bronchitis associated with chronic obstructive pulmonary disease (COPD) and AB. Chronic bronchitis (CB) is defined as having daily symptoms of sputum production on most days for more than 3 or more consecutive months for greater than 2 successive years.[18] Exacerbations of CB (discussed separately in this chapter) associated with COPD differ from AB in pathogenesis, microbiology, and treatment.

Pathophysiology and Epidemiology

AB is characterized by the inflammatory response to infection in the epithelium of the bronchi. Further progression of this inflammation leads to thickening of the tracheal mucosa.[19] Sloughing of cells from the tracheobronchial epithelium and inflammatory mediators leads to bronchospasm and reduced forced expiratory volume in 1 second (FEV_1) that usually improves after 5 weeks. Spread of pathogen and inflammatory response correlate with patient symptoms. Although bacteria can be isolated from sputum, bacterial invasion of the bronchial tree rarely occurs and the role of bacterial pathogens in AB is limited.[15]

Clinical Presentation

Cough lasting for more than 5 days is the hallmark sign of AB. Although the illness is self-limited, cough can last for up to 3 weeks (typical duration 10–20 days). Sputum production occurs in up to 50% of cases, but does not indicate bacterial infection.[2] Fever is unusual in most cases, but when present should lead to investigation for influenza during appropriate seasons or pneumonia if other clinical signs are present.

Overview of Drug Therapy

Although the available trials are associated with some flaws, antimicrobials do not significantly reduce symptoms of AB. However, antimicrobial use increases adverse drug events and antimicrobial resistence.[8,10,20–22] Expert guidelines in the United States and abroad recommended against the use of antimicrobial agents for the treatment of AB.[2,3,11,17] Despite the evidence refuting use, greater than two-thirds of AB cases are treated with antibiotics in the United States. Furthermore, the agents used for AB are increasingly broad-spectrum drugs, further exacerbating bacterial resistance pressure.[11–14,23] Nonantimicrobial treatment considerations include bronchodilators or antitussives depending on symptoms, even though evidence to support the use of many of these modalities is limited.[1,2,24,25]

Clinical Presentation

CASE 64-1

QUESTION 1: A.R. is a 30-year-old woman presenting with a chief complaint of cough. Her symptoms have persisted for 10 days, and she now produces yellow sputum with each cough. She has had no recent illnesses; however, her 2-year-old daughter in day care has experienced recent colds. She denies nausea, vomiting, or emesis or fever and chills. A review of systems reveals fatigue and difficulty sleeping because of cough. Past medical history includes ulcerative colitis managed with mesalamine and generalized anxiety disorder for which she takes sertraline. Vital signs review indicates a temperature of 37.1°C, heart rate of 70 beats/minute, blood pressure of 130/70 mm Hg, and respiratory rate of 18 breaths/minute with accompanying oxygen saturations of 98% on room air. Her physical examination is positive for coarse breath sounds that clear with coughing, but is otherwise normal. What signs and symptoms in A.R. are consistent with AB?

Persistent cough in the absence of other symptoms including fever or myalgias is typical with AB.[2] Cough can last up to 3 weeks and is usually self-limited. The typical duration of symptoms in AB is 5 to 14 days.[1] Pneumonia must be ruled out; however, normal oxygen saturation and lack of focal signs on pulmonary physical examination makes this diagnosis less likely. Sputum production is common, although not present in all cases of AB. Symptoms can oftentimes be present at night, contributing to A.R.'s symptoms of fatigue.

Microbiology

CASE 64-1, QUESTION 2: What are the most likely causes of A.R.'s case of AB?

The causative agent for AB is identified in a minority of cases (16%–30%); however, when pathogens are isolated, greater than 90% are of viral etiology.[7,8] A limited number of bacterial pathogens are associated with AB and should only be considered in patients with underlying COPD, mechanical ventilation (tracheobronchitis), or in cases of outbreaks and exposures (*Bordetella pertussis*). Common pathogens are listed in Table 64-1.[1] Viral etiologies include influenza A and B, parainfluenza, coronavirus, rhinovirus, adenovirus, respiratory syncytial virus, and human metapneumovirus.[1,26] Atypical bacteria including *Mycoplasma pneumoniae* (1% of cases), *Chlamydophila pneumoniae* (5% of college-aged youths in one series), and *B. pertussis* or *Bordetella parapertussis* have been implicated in cases of outbreaks or previous exposures.[1,27,28]

TABLE 64-1
Causes of Acute Bronchitis

Pathogen	Comments
Virus	
Influenza	Quick onset with fever, chills, headache, and cough. Myalgias are common and may be accompanied by myopathy.
Parainfluenza	Epidemics in autumn. Outbreaks may occur in nursing homes. Croup in child at home suggests presence of the organism.
Respiratory syncytial virus	About 45% of family members exposed to infant with bronchiolitis become infected. Outbreaks prominent in winter or spring. Twenty percent of adults have ear pain.
Coronavirus	Can cause severe respiratory symptoms in elderly. Epidemics present in military recruits.
Adenovirus	Similar presentation as influenza; abrupt onset of fever.
Rhinovirus	Fever is uncommon and infection generally mild.
Atypical Bacteria	
Bordetella pertussis	Incubation period of 1–3 weeks. Whooping occurs in a minority of patients, and fever is uncommon. Marked leukocytosis with lymphocytic predominance can occur.
Mycoplasma pneumoniae	Incubation period is 2–3 weeks. Outbreak cases in military and students have been reported.
Chlamydophila pneumoniae	Incubation period is 3 weeks. Onset of symptoms, which include hoarseness before cough, is gradual. Outbreaks reported in nursing homes, college students, and military personnel.

Source: Wenzel RP, Fowler AA 3rd. Clinical practice. Acute bronchitis. *N Engl J Med*. 2006;355:2125.

Clinical Diagnosis and Treatment

CASE 64-1, QUESTION 3: Should A.R. be provided an antimicrobial agent for her AB?

Antimicrobials are frequently prescribed for AB, despite the lack of clinical data supporting this practice.[12–16,29] Meta-analyses reveal antibiotics reduce AB symptoms, including cough, by only a fraction of a day.[10] A systematic review of double-blind trials revealed limited to no improvement in clinical outcomes with erythromycin, doxycycline, or trimethoprim/sulfamethoxazole compared with placebo; albuterol was determined to be clinically superior to erythromycin.[8] Antibiotics minimally reduce the duration of cough and days with limited activity, but have no impact on sick day reduction. In addition, antibiotic therapy has been associated with an insignificant increase in adverse events.[22] Azithromycin in comparison to vitamin C (both with dextromethorphan and albuterol) has similar effect on quality of life at day 7 and no difference in return to work or school at days 3 and 7.[20] Based on minimal clinical benefit and concerns regarding spread of antimicrobial resistance, guidelines promote antimicrobial abstinence for AB.[3,11,17,24] In A.R.'s case, no antimicrobial agent is warranted.

CASE 64-1, QUESTION 4: Should a sputum culture be obtained from A.R.? What other diagnostics should be considered?

Obtaining a sputum sample for culture to determine the presence of the causative agent or diagnostic screening for atypical pathogens does not routinely take place for AB. The rationale is that most of the identified pathogens have no specific treatment (viral illnesses), and the isolated organisms often are not true pathogens. Diagnostic screening, however, should be performed during influenza season or during outbreaks of *B. pertussis* or other atypical pathogens for infection control purposes. The use of a procalcitonin screen may decrease inappropriate antimicrobial use in AB, but its widespread use cannot be recommended at this time.[30,31]

CASE 64-1, QUESTION 5: Which clinical scenarios including infection associated with influenza or atypical bacteria should result in targeted treatment for A.R.?

Sick contacts, duration of incubation (2–7 days for viruses vs. weeks for atypical bacteria), and previous exposures should be considered when determining the etiological agent responsible for AB. A list of common incubation periods and specific symptoms for particular pathogens is included in Table 64-1. Specific symptoms reveal infection caused by specific pathogens, such as an inspiratory whoop and posttussive emesis (*B. pertussis*), pharyngitis and cough lasting longer than 4 weeks (*M. pneumoniae*), hoarseness with low-grade fever (*C. pneumoniae*), or cough with fever and myalgias (influenza).[1] For *B. pertussis* outbreaks in nursing homes, college dormitories, prisons, or among health care workers, postexposure prophylaxis may be warranted. However, treating *B. pertussis* after the first week in adults does not result in improved clinical outcomes.[32] No specific recommendations can be made after exposure to other atypical infections, and treatment is not warranted. Given A.R.'s lack of sick contacts, time course of present illness, and absence of symptoms suggestive of influenza, a viral etiology (other than influenza) is most likely to be the cause of her symptoms.

CASE 64-1, QUESTION 6: What symptom-guided therapies should be offered to A.R.?

Symptom-guided therapies include the use of inhaled β-agonists (albuterol) for shortness of breath, particularly in patients with underlying reactive airway disease; inhaled or systemic steroids for persistent cough; nonsteroidal anti-inflammatory drugs (NSAIDs), aspirin, or acetaminophen to alleviate myalgias or fever; or antihistamines (brompheniramine), antitussives (codeine or dextromethorphan), or mucolytics (guaifenesin) for cough. However, these potential treatments are not backed with evidence demonstrating a clear benefit.[1,2,24,25,33] As such, each of these treatments should be approached with an appropriate consideration of the balance between perceived benefit and risk of adverse events. Given A.R.'s troublesome cough that has kept her up at night, a trial of an antitussive such as dextromethorphan is a reasonable first option. NSAIDs or aspirin should be avoided given her underlying inflammatory bowel disease and lack of clear indication. An inhaled β-agonist or steroid is also not necessary at this time.

CASE 64-1, QUESTION 7: Should a chest radiograph be ordered for A.R.? What other illnesses may be considered as the cause of her symptoms?

It is important to distinguish AB from pneumonia with chest radiograph or other imaging tests when fever, tachycardia, tachypnea; physical examination findings such as egophony or rales; or hypoxemia or mental status changes (especially in the elderly) are present.[1,2] Clinical differentiation of AB from an acute exacerbation of COPD (AECOPD), postnasal drip, gastroesophageal reflux disorder (GERD), and asthma must also be made (discussed separately in this chapter and in Chapter 27, Upper Gastrointestinal Disorders, and Chapter 23, Asthma, respectively). In A.R.'s case, no sign of pneumonia are seen on physical examination or on reviewing symptomatology; therefore, no chest radiograph is warranted. Frequent symptoms over time or risk factors for COPD would warrant an investigation for CB. Wheezing or frequent AB outbreaks and GERD symptoms would guide evaluations for asthma or gastrointestinal disorders, respectively.

Patient Education

CASE 64-1, QUESTION 8: What education would you provide to A.R. to dissuade her perceived need for an antibiotic?

An evaluation of A.R.'s expectations for therapy is important to alleviate concerns about the decision to not prescribe antimicrobials. Overuse of antibiotics in AB is often driven by either prescriber knowledge or patient request. Communication is key with each patient to provide insight into the causative agents of AB, the natural course of the disease, the role of symptomatic relief, and reasons for avoiding prescriptions for antibiotics.

ACUTE EXACERBATON OF CHRONIC OBSTRUCTIVE PULMONARY DISEASE

Definition, Incidence, and Epidemiology

CB is defined as daily symptoms of sputum production on most days for 3 or more consecutive months for greater than 2 successive years.[18] CB as a component of COPD (discussed separately in Chapter 24, Chronic Obstructive Pulmonary Disease) portends no specific treatment outside of those treatments indicated for the maintenance of COPD. Distinct from COPD, AECOPD is defined by the Global Initiative for Chronic Obstructive Lung Disease (GOLD) as "an event in the natural course of the disease characterized by a change in the patient's baseline dyspnea, cough, and/or sputum that is beyond normal day-to-day variations, is acute in onset, and may warrant a change in regular medication."[34]

In 2000 in the United States, 726,000 hospitalizations were attributable to AECOPD, representing a 10-year increase of 57%.[35] The costs associated with AECOPD hospitalizations in 2002 was estimated to be $18 billion in the United States.[36] The total mortality for each hospitalization reaches 10%, with estimates up to 25% for those requiring intensive care unit (ICU) care.[37,38] Mortality nears 50% 3 years after hospitalization for AECOPD and is worse (40%) at year 1 for those who require mechanical ventilation.[37–43] AECOPD is associated with a decrease in quality-of-life measurements and a decline in lung function, particularly if not treated early.[43–49]

The primary precipitating factors for AECOPD are infection of the bronchial tree and air pollution.[34,50–52] As many as one-third of the cases of AECOPD do not have a cause identified. In some cases, consideration for venous thromboembolism or pulmonary embolism (discussed separately in Chapter 16, Thrombosis) is warranted.[34,53–56]

Pathophysiology

Both bacteria and pollutants lead to inflammatory response.[52] Airway inflammation, associated with increases in interleukin-8, tumor necrosis factor-α, and neutrophils, contributes to pulmonary remodeling as well as decreased ciliary clearance of mucus, worsening airflow obstruction, and the respiratory symptoms associated with AECOPD.

ONLINE CONTENT

For an illustration of chronic bronchitis compared to normal bronchi, go to http://thepoint.lww.com/AT10e.

TABLE 64-2

Micro-organisms Common in Exacerbations of Chronic Obstructive Pulmonary Disease and Recommended Treatment

Group	Micro-organisms	Oral Treatment	Parenteral Treatment
Exacerbation with no risk factors for poor outcomes[a]	*Haemophilus influenzae* *Streptococcus pneumoniae* *Moraxella catarrhalis* *Chlamydophila pneumoniae* Viruses	β-Lactam[b] or β-lactam/β-lactamase inhibitor combination Tetracyclines (doxycycline) Trimethoprim-sulfamethoxazole Macrolides (azithromycin) Cephalosporins from second- or third-generation (cefuroxime or cefpodoxime)	
Exacerbations with risk factors for poor outcomes	Above microorganisms plus: Drug-resistant *S. pneumoniae* *Klebsiella pneumoniae* *Escherichia coli* *Proteus* sp. *Enterobacter* sp.	β-Lactam/β-lactamase inhibitor combination Fluoroquinolone (moxifloxacin)	β-lactam/β-lactamase inhibitor combination (ampicillin/sulbactam) Cephalosporins from third-generation (ceftriaxone) Fluoroquinolone (moxifloxacin)
Exacerbations with risk factors for *Pseudomonas aeruginosa*[c]	Above microorganisms plus: *P. aeruginosa*		β-Lactam with *P. aeruginosa* activity (cefepime) or Ciprofloxacin (added to options above if necessary)

[a] Risk factors for poor outcomes include the following: medical comorbidities (cardiac disease), forced expiratory volume in 1 second of 50% of predicted or less (severe chronic obstructive pulmonary disease), frequent exacerbations (>3 per year), age ≥65 years, and antimicrobial use within last 3 months.

[b] High-dose β-lactams should be used in areas with high incidence of drug-resistant *S. pneumoniae;* β-lactams should not be used without a β-lactamase inhibitor in areas with high rates of *H. influenzae* or *M. catarrhalis* resistant to penicillin owing to β-lactamase production.

[c] Risk factors for *P. aeruginosa* include the following: recent hospitalization, severe chronic obstructive pulmonary disease exacerbations, or isolation of *P. aeruginosa* during previous exacerbation or colonization during a stable period.

Source: Global Initiative for Chronic Obstructive Lung Disease (GOLD). *Global Strategy for the Diagnosis, Management, and Prevention of Chronic Obstructive Lung Disease 2010.* **http://www.goldcopd.org/guidelines-global-strategy-for-diagnosis-management.html.**

Up to 29% of patients with stable COPD have bacteria isolated in the tracheobronchial tree when assessed using protected brush specimens on bronchoscopy. In contrast, 54% of patients with AECOPD will have bacteria identified using the same bronchoscopic technique.[57] In addition to acquisition of a new bacterial species in the development of symptoms associated with AECOPD, acquisition of a new strain of the same colonizing micro-organism has been associated with exacerbating COPD symptoms.[52] Decreases in adaptive immune responses occur as COPD disease progresses, making patients susceptible to more frequent exacerbations caused by bacterial pathogens. Additionally, pathogens associated with exacerbations tend to increase in virulence and antimicrobial resistance as the underlying disease progresses.[34,40,51,52,58] A possible mechanism for prolonged infection and colonization in patients with COPD is suggested by interactions between both viruses and bacteria altering immune respone.[52]

Viruses have been identified as the etiological cause of AECOPD in up to one-third of the cases, and bacteria have been identified in up to one-half.[52] Table 64-2 describes the micro-organisms most commonly associated with AECOPD based on risk factors and presentation severity.

Clinical Presentation and Diagnosis

Common features of AECOPD include the following: breathlessness, increased cough, increased sputum volume, and increased sputum purulence. In contrast to AB, purulent sputum in AECOPD is associated with an acute bacterial infection.[58] Other less specific symptoms include insomnia, fatigue, tachycardia, tachypnea, and a decrease in exercise tolerance. Patients often report a decrease in ability to conduct activities of daily living.[34]

Diagnostic considerations in the evaluation of patients with AECOPD include pulse oximetry and arterial blood gases, electrocardiogram, and complete blood count including white blood cell (WBC) differential. Mechanical ventilation is considered when acidosis (pH <7.36) and hypercapnia ($Paco_2$ >68 mm Hg) are present. Chest radiographs are helpful to rule out pneumonia, pneumothorax, or pleural effusion. Consideration of heart failure based on history, physical signs, and brain natriuretic peptide as well as venous thromboembolism must be made based on patient presentation.[34,50] Collection of sputum samples for Gram stain and culture are not generally recommended, but may be helpful if patients are failing initial therapies.

Overview of Treatment

Pharmacotherapy directed at AECOPD includes bronchodilators and supplemental oxygen, antimicrobial therapy to decrease the burden of microorganisms, and corticosteroids targeting the inflammatory response.[34,50] Methylxanthines (aminophylline or theophylline) are rarely used owing to conflicting and limited evidence of efficacy and concerns about toxicity.[34] Nonpharmacological considerations related to treatment of AECOPD include decisions regarding site-of-care and the level of respiratory support. These nondrug considerations are not discussed in detail in this chapter, but are available in the GOLD Guidelines.[34]

Disease Severity

CASE 64-2

QUESTION 1: T.H. is a 68-year-old white man presenting to the emergency department (ED) because he "cannot catch my breath." At baseline he is on 4 L of oxygen continuously via nasal cannula. However, during the last week he has experienced worsening dyspnea including the need for help with daily activities including bathing and feeding. His wife had contacted T.H.'s primary-care physician who directed the patient to the ED when T.H. seemed "out of it" and was

difficult to arouse. T.H.'s wife indicates that he has been "having a cold" with increased sputum that is more yellow than in the past with frequent coughing spells. Past medical history is significant for very severe COPD, atrial fibrillation, depression, obstructive sleep apnea, morbid obesity, and a left humerus fracture. No medication allergies are noted. Medications at home include aspirin 81 mg daily, citalopram 20 mg daily, diltiazem extended-release capsule 240 mg daily, salmeterol-fluticasone dry powdered inhaler 50/250 one puff twice daily, and albuterol four puffs every 6 hours as needed for shortness of breath. Social history is significant for a greater than 80-pack-year history of cigarette smoking, but he quit 4 to 5 years ago. In the ED he was afebrile, heart rate was 76 beats/minute, respiratory rate was 23 breaths/minute, blood pressure was 135/75 mm Hg, and oxygen saturation was 60% on 4 L of oxygen. T.H. is in some distress, alert and oriented times two, and is using accessory muscles for breathing. Initial physical examination was significant for distant breath sounds and decreased air movement bilaterally, a noted absence of lower extremity edema, and an irregularly irregular heart beat. Laboratory findings are as follows:

pH, 7.34
P_{CO_2}, 60 mm Hg
P_{O_2}, 72 mm Hg
WBC, 9.8 × $10^3/\mu L$ (neutrophils 71%)
Hemoglobin, 12 g/dL
Platelets, 319 × $10^3/\mu L$
Sodium, 135 mmol/L
Potassium, 3.7 mmol/L
Chloride, 91 mmol/L
Bicarbonate, 39 mmol/L
Blood urea nitrogen (BUN), 15 mg/dL
Serum creatinine (SCr), 1.21 mg/dL
Glucose, 104 mg/dL
Brain natriuretic peptide, 66 pg/mL
Troponin, <0.07 ng/mL
Thyrotropin, 1.63 micro-international units/mL

Chest radiograph indicated small pleural effusions, but was otherwise negative for infiltrates or consolidation. An electrocardiogram indicated the presence of atrial fibrillation. Pulmonary function tests obtained 1 year previously indicated an FEV_1 to forced vital capacity ratio of 0.39 and an FEV_1 of 37% predicted. How would you stage the severity of this exacerbation for T.H.?

T.H. has several risk factors for a poor outcome, including the presence of atrial fibrillation and severe COPD defined by his home oxygen requirement and low baseline FEV_1. Additional risk factors for a poor outcome, however, are not present in T.H., including frequent exacerbations (>3/year) and the use of antimicrobials for his respiratory illness in the last 3 months.[34]

Clinical signs and symptoms consistent with a severe exacerbation include the use of accessory respiratory muscles, paradoxical chest wall movements, worsening or new cyanosis, peripheral edema, hemodynamic compromise, signs of right heart failure, and alterations in mental status.[34] T.H. has two of these factors, i.e., reduced alertness and use of accessory muscles.[34,37–41,50,59]

Disease Prevention

CASE 64-2, QUESTION 2: Which therapies should be made available to T.H. to alleviate his shortness of breath?

Supplemental oxygen to alleviate hypoxemia is a foundation of treatment for AECOPD. Controlled provision of oxygen should be implemented to provide an oxygen saturation of greater than 90% or a Pa_{O_2} of greater than 60 mm Hg. Hypoxia that is not easily reversible warrants further examination for venous thromboembolism, pneumonia, or other causes. A repeat arterial blood gas should be obtained within 1 hour of initiation of supplemental oxygen to assess for carbon dioxide retention or acidosis.

The use of short-acting bronchodilators should be initiated promptly in all patients with AECOPD. β-Agonists, such as albuterol, are the preferred agents.[34] If the patient does not respond to β-agonists, an anticholinergic agent such as ipratropium can be considered, although evidence for this class of medication is limited for this indication. Likewise, there is no role for long-acting bronchodilators in AECOPD at this time.

CASE 64-2, QUESTION 3: Which microbiological causes are likely in T.H.?

Table 64-2 outlines the most common pathogens identified in AECOPD along with associated risk factors. *Haemophilus influenzae* (up to 30% of exacerbations) and *Streptococcus pneumoniae* (up to 15% of exacerbations) are the two most common bacterial pathogens, particularly in less severe AECOPD. Less common bacterial etiologies include *Haemophilus haemolyticus, Haemophilus parainfluenzae, Staphylococcus aureus, and Moraxella catarrhalis.* Viral etiologies of AECOPD (about 30% of all cases) include influenza A and B, parainfluenza, coronavirus, rhinovirus, adenovirus, respiratory syncytial virus, and human metapneumovirus.[26,52]

As disease progresses, more frequent exacerbations occur, more antimicrobials are typically administered, and changes in pulmonary anatomy arise including advancing bronchiectasis. These factors promote drug-resistant *S. pneumoniae* (DRSP) and *Pseudomonas aeruginosa*. The GOLD guidelines indicate that recent hospitalization, frequent administration of antibiotics (four courses per year), and isolation of *P. aeruginosa* during a previous exacerbation or colonization during a stable period are risk factors for *P. aeruginosa*.[34]

Atypical bacteria such as *C. pneumoniae* and *M. pneumoniae* are isolated in up to 5% of cases. However, the significance of these bacteria is unknown, and targeting atypical bacteria during AECOPD is often unnecessary.[34,51,52]

Targeting the likely infectious etiologies requires recognition of the risk factors for poor outcomes (see Case 64-2, Question 1, and Table 64-2) as well as local patterns of resistance for *S. pneumoniae* and *H. influenzae*. T.H.'s exacerbation is likely to be associated with one or more of the following (in this order): *H. influenzae, S. pneumoniae* (including drug-resistant types), *M. catarrhalis, C. pneumoniae*, viruses, *Klebsiella pneumoniae, Escherichia coli, Proteus* species, and *Enterobacter* species.

CASE 64-2, QUESTION 4: Does T.H. need to be treated with antimicrobial therapy?

The "cardinal" symptoms of AECOPD include increases in sputum purulence, sputum volume, and dyspnea.[60] "Mild" exacerbation is defined as the presence of one cardinal symptom, "moderate" exacerbation as two cardinal symptoms, and "severe" when all three symptoms are present. The use of cardinal symptoms as a method of staging AECOPD severity has been used in several prospective studies and is recommended in GOLD guidelines.[34,61] Although some studies suggest a benefit in treating severe exacerbations of AECOPD, many of these use flawed methodology, unequal controls, outdated definitions of

AECOPD, and utilization of outdated antimicrobials (penicillins, tetracyclines, and trimethoprim/sulfamethoxazole).[62] Nonetheless, a review of more contemporary trials support the use of antibiotics for AECOPD. Antibiotic administration reduces mortality and treatment failure in patients with moderate and severe exacerbations.[61] Diarrhea was more common in patients treated with antibiotics.[61] Reduced mortality and a decrease in the duration of mechanical ventilation has been associated with antibiotic therapy in those patients requiring mechanical ventilation.[63]

The benefit of antibiotic therapy in combination with corticosteroids is unclear (see Case 64-2, Question 6). The addition of doxycycline in hospitalized, corticosteroid-treated patients was associated with no benefit.[64] In contrast, a retrospective cohort of steroid-treated patients suggested early treatment with antimicrobials was associated with significantly less treatment failure, hospital readmission within 30 days for AECOPD, inpatient mortality, or the need for mechanical ventilation.[65] However, patients receiving antimicrobials had a sevenfold increase in readmissions for *Clostridium difficile* infection.

Experts advocate for the use of antibacterials for AECOPD, particularly when two or three cardinal symptoms are present.[34,50,59] Specifically, the GOLD Guidelines recommend antibiotics for patients with three cardinal symptoms (increased dyspnea, increased sputum volume, and increased sputum purulence), when two cardinal symptoms are present if increased sputum purulence is one of the symptoms, or in all patients requiring mechanical ventilation for their AECOPD.[34]

T.H. is exhibiting all three of the cardinal symptoms and therefore should receive antibiotics. Likely benefits would be increased likelihood of treatment success, prevention of relapse, decreased risk for rehospitalization, improvement in pulmonary function, and reducing the severity of his exacerbation.

CASE 64-2, QUESTION 5: Which antimicrobial agent should be selected for treating T.H.? What duration of treatment would be recommended?

Table 64-2 provides a summary of the GOLD Guideline recommendations for antimicrobial treatment.[34] The choice of agent links with specific underlying risk factors. Macrolides are recommended only in patients with no risk factors for poor outcome. Theoretical benefits of macrolides include anti-inflammatory effects in addition to antibacterial benefit.[66,67] Given T.H.'s history, diminished mental status, and risk factors for poor outcomes, intravenous (IV) administration seems appropriate for the initial antibiotic administration. Evaluation of potential risk factors for *P. aeruginosa* should take place. If T.H. demonstrates risk factors for *P. aeruginosa*, a β-lactam with appropriate coverage, such as cefepime, would be an appropriate initial agent. If no risk factors for *P. aeruginosa* exist, a β-lactam/β-lactamase inhibitor such as ampicillin/sulbactam, a third-generation cephalosporin such as ceftriaxone, or a respiratory fluoroquinolone such as moxifloxacin or levofloxacin should be selected. All these therapies are active against DRSP. If T.H. improves on one of these parenteral agents and is ready for discharge, T.H. could transition to an oral respiratory fluoroquinolone or high doses of amoxicillin/clavulanate.

Another important consideration for initial selection of antimicrobials is an evaluation of antibiotic history. Alternative antimicrobials from another class should be considered if patients have been previously treated in the last 3 months.[34] Additionally, if no improvements in symptoms occur within 72 hours, consider obtaining a sputum sample for directed therapy.[34]

The duration of treatment of antibiotics for AECOPD suffers from lack of solid evidence-based recommendation. Given findings from CB investigations, a duration of 3 to 7 days has been suggested, but this is an area in need of further research.[34]

CASE 64-2, QUESTION 6: Should T.H. be treated with corticosteroids? If so, which dose and duration would be selected?

Corticosteroids are the treatment foundation for patients with AECOPD. A 10% absolute reduction in composite treatment failure, defined by the need for mechanical ventilation, readmission to the hospital for COPD, or intensification of therapy, was observed in patients treated with steroids.[68] Troubling side effects, perhaps owing to the high doses and long tapers used, included a greater than fourfold increase in hyperglycemia requiring intervention and a greater than 3.5-fold increase in hospital stay days.

Reviewing all trials for steroids in AECOPD suggests a relative reduction in treatment failure by 46%, a decrease in hospital length of stay by an average of 1.4 days, and improved FEV_1 by a mean of 0.13 L.[50] These findings have been confirmed in other analyses, along with demonstrated improvement in quality-of-life indices. No mortality benefit has been demonstrated with corticosteroids in AECOPD.[69]

Based on available evidence, the GOLD Guidelines recommend the use of corticosteroids in patients receiving home oxygen therapy at baseline, for patients with FEV_1 of less than 50% predicted, and for all patients hospitalized with AECOPD.[34] As much as 500 mg/day of methylprednisolone tapered over 2 to 6 weeks and as low as 30 mg/day of prednisone for 7 days have been used in clinical trials.[34,50,68–70] The risk of treatment failure, death, or mechanical ventilation has been observed to not be statistically different between high-dose IV and lower-dose oral steroids.[70] Considering that 30 to 40 mg of prednisone has been demonstrated to be effective in most AECOPD, and because high doses are associated with significant side effects, this dose for 7 to 10 days is appropriate for T.H.[34] In those patients receiving more than 3 weeks of steroids or multiple course of steroids in the previous months, tapering the dose should be considered. Inhaled corticosteroids may be an alterative to systemic corticosteroids for some AECOPD to spare some of the complications of systemic steroids, but its use cannot be widely adopted until further research is available.

Enhancing Patient Outcomes

CASE 64-2, QUESTION 7: What factors should be assessed for T.H. during his hospitalization, and what follow-up should be planned to help assure he recovers fully and is not readmitted for COPD?

Hospitalized patients with AECOPD should not only be optimally treated for the exacerbation, but be assessed to decrease the likelihood of readmission. T.H.'s baseline COPD medications should be examined and adjusted based on disease severity (see Chapter 24, Chronic Obstructive Pulmonary Disease, for details). Additionally, an assessment of his understanding of the role of medications (maintenance therapy vs. rescue medications), ability to use inhalers correctly, access to his prescribed medications, and discussions regarding pulmonary rehabilitation should take place.[34,37,44,45,47,49] Consideration for pharmacological venous thromboembolism prophylaxis (see Chapter 16, Thrombosis) should also be made in this high-risk population.[34,55]

PREVENTION OF COMMON RESPIRATORY INFECTIONS BY VACCINATION

CASE 64-2, QUESTION 8: What are the benefits of providing either influenza vaccination or pneumococcal vaccination in T.H.?

Vaccination records for influenza and *S. pneumoniae* should be evaluated in T.H. *S. pneumoniae* is the most common bacterial pathogen associated with community-acquired pneumonia (CAP). Pneumococcal infections cause an estimated 40,000 deaths annually in the United States. The currently available pneumococcal vaccine includes 23 purified capsular polysaccharide antigens. After vaccination, an antigen-specific antibody response develops within 2 to 3 weeks in at least 80% of healthy adults.[71] The levels of antibody to most antigens remains elevated for at least 5 years in healthy adults and decreases to prevaccination levels by 10 years.[72,73]

Pneumococcal vaccine has not been shown to be effective against nonbacteremic pneumococcal disease. Effectiveness against invasive disease is 56% to 81%.[74–77] Pneumococcal polysaccharide vaccine is cost-effective and potentially cost-saving among persons at least 65 years of age for prevention of bacteremia.[78]

The vaccine is both cost-effective and protective against invasive pneumococcal infection when administered to immunocompetent persons at least 2 years of age.[79] Therefore, all persons in the following categories should receive the 23-valent pneumococcal polysaccharide vaccine: patients at least 65 years of age, patients 2 to 64 years of age with chronic illness, patients 2 to 64 years of age with functional or anatomic asplenia, patients 2 to 64 years of age living in special environments or social settings, and immunocompromised patients. If vaccination status is unknown, patients in these categories should be administered pneumococcal vaccine.

The primary option for reducing the effect of influenza is immunoprophylaxis with inactivated vaccine. The effectiveness of influenza vaccination depends primarily on the age and immunocompetence of the recipient and the degree of similarity between viruses in the vaccine and in circulation. Vaccine prevents influenza illness in 70% to 90% of healthy adults younger than 65 years of age. In adults at least 65 years of age, the effectiveness of the vaccine has been reported to be 58%. From 1990 to 1999, there were more than 36,000 deaths, and from 1980 to 2001 there have been an average of 226,000 hospitalizations per year in the United States as a result of influenza. Vaccination has been shown to prevent secondary complications and reduce the risk for influenza-related hospitalization and death. Influenza vaccine is recommended for all persons older than 6 months of age.[80]

COMMUNITY-ACQUIRED PNEUMONIA

Definition, Incidence, and Epidemiology

Pneumonia is an infection of the lung parenchyma. CAP refers to pneumonia acquired outside of the hospital or extended-care facility in patients without recent exposure to the health care system. The diagnosis of CAP requires the presence of clinical features that develop over hours to days in combination with radiological evidence of an infiltrate. These findings can be further supported by characteristic physical examination observations or hypoxemia.

Estimates of the incidence of CAP range from 4 million to 5 million cases per year with an accompanying 10 million physician visits.[81,82] In 2006, there were 1.23 million hospitalizations for pneumonia in the United States, equal to a rate of 41.3 cases per 10,000 discharges. Patients older than 65 years account for one-third of all cases of pneumonia, but are responsible for nearly 60% of the hospitalizations, owing to comorbidities, including cardiac disease, pulmonary disease, and diabetes mellitus.[83,84] In 2006, pneumonia, along with influenza, was the eighth leading cause of death in the United States overall, with 90% of deaths occurring in the population of patients 65 and older. The mortality rate for outpatients is less than 5%, whereas the mortality rate in hospitalized patients averages 12% across all severity levels, and up to 40% in patients requiring intensive care.[81] The cost of care for patients with pneumonia in 2005 was approximately $40 billion, with $34 billion in direct costs.

Pathophysiology

A key pathogenic mechanism in the development of CAP is the inhalation of infectious particles. Aspiration of oropharyngeal or gastric contents with subsequent infection can occur in patients with underlying neuromuscular disease, stroke, or seizure disorder, and in patients with altered states of consciousness resulting in impairments in swallowing and epiglottic closure. Rarely, hematogenous spread of bacteria from distant sources into the lungs may occur, as well as direct extension of infection to the lung from contiguous areas, such as the pleural or subdiaphragmatic spaces.

Once bacteria reach the tracheobronchial tree, defects in local pulmonary defenses facilitate infection. Depressed mucociliary clearance and injured bronchial epithelium triggered by inflammatory mediators contribute to the pathogenic process. In addition, a blunted cellular and humoral response, including reduced granulocyte chemotaxis, leukopenia, dysfunctional alveolar macrophages, and diminished antibody production or function in patients with underlying or acquired immunodeficiencies, compromise the host to invading pathogens.

Clinical Presentation and Diagnosis

In the majority of CAP cases, patients manifest acutely with high fever, chills, tachypnea, tachycardia, and productive cough. Physical examination findings are usually localized to a specific lung zone and can include crackles, rhonchi, bronchial breath sounds, dullness, or egophony. On rare occasion, CAP exhibits a subacute presentation with fever, nonproductive cough, constitutional symptoms, and absent or diffuse findings on lung examination. Both acute and subacute presentations can progress rapidly to respiratory failure with sepsis.

A chest radiograph or other imaging technique is required for the diagnosis of CAP and usually reveals an infiltrate.[85] However, this finding may be absent in the intravascular volume–depleted patient. Importantly, the radiographic manifestations of diseases such as congestive heart failure and malignancy can obscure the infiltrate of pneumonia, reinforcing the need to combine clinical and chest radiographic findings.

Pretreatment blood cultures and a respiratory sample (expectorated or induced sputum or endotracheal aspirate in intubated patients) should be obtained. Although these cultures are often negative, when they are positive, they allow fine-tuning of the empirical antibiotic selection.

Overview of Drug Therapy

Antibiotic therapy for CAP is empirical in the majority of cases and should always be based on the most likely pathogen(s) underlying patient characteristics and the severity of disease. Based on these variables, clinicians can triage patients for risk of infection caused by antibiotic-resistant pathogens and appropriately tailor therapy.

CLINICAL PRESENTATION

CASE 64-3

QUESTION 1: M.R. is a 33-year-old man presenting to the ED with fevers, chills, and chest pain. His symptoms have persisted for 3 days, and he has a productive cough with rusty-colored sputum and dyspnea with exertion. He has had no recent illnesses and no known sick contacts, but he was recently released from a 2-year period of incarceration. He has tried ibuprofen to alleviate his fever and chest pain. Past medical history is positive for asthma, for which he is prescribed fluticasone and albuterol, and depression, for which he takes sertraline. Vital signs reveal a temperature of 40.1°C, heart rate of 128 beats/minute, blood pressure of 130/76 mm Hg, and respiratory rate of 32 breaths/minute with accompanying oxygen saturations of 85% on 5 L of oxygen by nasal cannula. The remainder of the physical examination is notable for orientation to person but not place or time and for diffuse crackles bilaterally, which are most apparent on the right side. Laboratory results include the following:

WBC count, 15,500 cells/μL
Hematocrit, 29.3%
Sodium, 133 mmol/L
Potassium, 3.8 mmol/L
BUN, 23 mg/dL
SCr, 0.8 mg/dL
Glucose 148, mg/dL
pH 7.42
Po_2, 61 mm Hg
Pco_2, 46 mm Hg
HCO_3, 28 mEq/L

A test for human immunodeficiency virus is negative. Chest radiograph reveals a right lower lobe infiltrate. What signs, symptoms, and tests are consistent with CAP in M.R.?

In the majority of cases, patients with CAP present with cough with sputum production, dyspnea, and pleuritic chest pain.[86] Patients also frequently demonstrate signs of the systemic inflammatory response syndrome, including tachycardia, tachypnea, fever, and an abnormal WBC count.[87] In addition, auscultatory examination often reveals decreased breath sounds, more distinctive crackles or rhonchi, or egophony in patients with consolidation. Signs and symptoms associated with severe pneumonia fall under minor and major criteria defined initially in the 1993 American Thoracic Society (ATS) Guidelines for CAP and modified in the 2007 version.[85] Minor criteria include respiratory rate greater than 30 breaths/minute at admission, ratios of the Pao_2 to fraction of inspired oxygen (Fio_2) (Pao_2/Fio_2) less than 250 mm Hg, systolic blood pressure less than 90 mm Hg, or diastolic blood pressure less than 60 mm Hg; confusion; multilobar infiltrates; systolic blood pressure less than 90 mm Hg despite aggressive fluid resuscitation; BUN of at least 20 mg/dL; leukopenia; thrombocytopenia; and hypothermia. Major criteria include requirement of mechanical ventilation and requirement of vasopressors for more than 4 hours.[85]

In addition to the compilation of clinical findings consistent with CAP, a demonstrable infiltrate by chest radiograph or other imaging technique is required for the diagnosis of pneumonia.[85] On occasion, the admission chest radiograph is negative for infiltrate despite a clinical syndrome consistent with pneumonia. For such patients who are hospitalized, imaging should be repeated 24 to 48 hours after admission.

Disease Severity

CASE 64-3, QUESTION 2: Given the clinical condition of M.R. in the ED, where should his care be continued?

The first decision after a diagnosis of CAP is to determine whether the patient should be hospitalized. Several prediction rules have been developed to facilitate site-of-care decision making. The two best studied tools that are endorsed by the Infectious Diseases Society of America (IDSA)/ATS guidelines are the pneumonia severity index (PSI) and the CURB-65 rule, defined subsequently.

The PSI uses demographic characteristics, historical findings, physical examination findings, and laboratory data, each of which are assigned a score that, when cumulated, categorizes patients into one of five classes that are associated with an escalating risk of death (Table 64-3).[88] This tool was developed to define mortality risk, but has been subsequently applied as a method to facilitate disposition of patients. The CURB-65, developed by the British Thoracic Society, is a simple tool that makes five assessments: confusion (owing to pneumonia), uremia (BUN >19 mg/dL), respiratory rate of at least 30 breaths/minute, blood pressure of less than 90 mm Hg systolic or 60 mm Hg or less diastolic, and age of at least 65 years.[89] Each criteria receives one point, and the cumulative score is associated with a rising mortality risk. The recommendation for determining where a patient should receive subsequent care is as follows: score of 0–1 = outpatient, 2 = admission to ward, ≥3 = ICU care. Both scales identify patients at low risk of death, but the CURB-65 has been found to be more discerning of patients who need ICU care (score of 3 or more) and with highest risk of death.[90] There are no specific rules for who should be admitted to the ICU; however, it is recommended that patients with three or more minor criteria or at least one major criteria for severe CAP should be admitted to the ICU.

Using the PSI, the scoring for M.R. is as follows: He is a 33-year-old man (33 points), his respiratory rate is more than 30 breaths/minute (20 points), his heart rate is more than 125 beats/minute (20 points), his temperature is more than 40°C

TABLE 64-3
Predicted Mortality and Recommended Site of Care

System and Score	Predicted 30-Day Mortality (%)	Recommended Site of Care
PSI strata 1–2	0.1–0.7	Outpatient
PSI strata 3	0.9–2.8	Admit to ward
PSI strata 4–5	9.3–27	Admit; consider ICU
CURB-65 score 0–1	0.7–2.1	Outpatient
CURB-65 score 2	9.2	Admit to ward
CURB-65 score ≥3	14.5–57.0	Admit to ICU

CURB-65, confusion, uremia, increased respiratory rate, low blood pressure, and age ≥65 years; ICU, intensive care unit; PSI, pneumonia severity index.

(15 points), his oxygen saturation is less than 60% (10 points), his hematocrit is less than 30% (10 points), and he has an altered mental status (20 points). His score of 118 points places him in risk strata IV, which carries a 30-day mortality risk of 9.3% to 27%. Based on M.R.'s PSI assessment and clinical status, he should be admitted to the hospital. Using the CURB-65, M.R. has a score of "3" (30-day mortality of 9.2%) given that he was confused and had an increased respiratory rate, similarly resulting in the intensive care unit as the preferred site of care.

CASE 64-3, QUESTION 3: What testing should be performed to obtain a microbiological diagnosis in M.R.?

The IDSA/ATS guidelines recommend attempting to make a microbiological diagnosis in patients with CAP who are hospitalized. Microbiological testing is optional for outpatients with CAP.[85] The main reason to test for pathogen etiology is the potential to streamline antimicrobial therapy. Several other reasons for etiologic diagnostic testing include documenting unusual pathogens such as severe acute respiratory syndrome (SARS) or agents of bioterrorism, recognizing cluster cases of pneumonia, and, most importantly, guiding empiric therapy of CAP on the national and local levels.

Culture and Gram stain of a respiratory sample such as expectorated sputum or an endotracheal aspirate in intubated patients is the primary method by which an etiologic diagnosis can be made in hospitalized patients. In addition, pretreatment blood cultures should be obtained in patients with severe CAP. The necessity for drawing blood cultures in less severely ill hospitalized patients is uncertain.

Urine antigen tests for pneumococcus and *Legionella pneumophila* serogroup 1 are available. Both tests are sensitive (>80%) and specific (>90%), but the generalized utility of these studies should be limited to hospitalized patients. One advantage of this methodology compared with respiratory specimen and blood cultures is the ability to detect the pathogen after antibiotic therapy has been given, especially for *S. pneumoniae*. In addition, the turnaround time for the test results is short, often allowing for rapid modification of antibiotic therapy.

The decision to test for influenza should be based on the patient's clinical presentation as well as prevalence of influenza in the community. The recommended test for the detection of influenza is via reverse transcriptase polymerase chain reaction (RT-PCR), which is the most sensitive and specific of all methods, with results available within 4 to 6 hours of collection.[91] Rapid influenza antigen detection tests are widely used and have a prompt turnaround time, but lack the sensitivity and specificity of the RT-PCR, and therefore, RT-PCR should be performed to confirm negative test results reported by the rapid antigen test. Immunofluorescence antibody staining is an option that provides greater sensitivity and specificity than rapid antigen testing, but performance depends on collection of a quality specimen and expert processing. Viral isolation in standard cell culture should be routinely performed with respiratory specimens during the influenza season.

Microbiology

CASE 64-3, QUESTION 4: What pathogens are most likely in M.R.?

The major pathogens for CAP are summarized in Table 64-4. The most frequently isolated bacterial pathogen, regardless of epidemiological factors and severity of illness, is *S. pneumoniae*.[85] This organism is one of many commensal bacteria found on the respiratory epithelium. Two survival strategies are used by *S. pneumoniae*.[92] The first is a noninvasive phenotype that uses surface adhesions, immune evasion strategies, and secretory defenses to promote long-term carriage within the nasopharynx. Deficits in host defense, such as an immunocompromised state, allow colonizing strains of low virulence to cause invasive disease. The second tactic accounting for the infectious success of *S. pneumoniae* depends on efficient person-to-person transmission and associated rapid disease induction by this invasive phenotype. Age younger than 2 or older than 64 years, asplenia, alcoholism, diabetes mellitus, antecedent influenza, defects in humoral immunity, and human immunodeficiency virus infection are risk factors for the invasive pneumococcal phenotype.[93] Other risk factors less likely to cause invasive disease include poverty and crowding, cigarette smoking, chronic lung disease, severe liver disease, recent exposure to antibiotics, and chronic proton-pump inhibitor use. An array of virulence factors must be expressed by *S. pneumoniae* for invasive disease to occur in patients with one or more of these risk factors. The most significant virulence factors include extracellular toxins and enzymes (e.g., pneumolysin), anticomplement invasion factors, metal binding transporters, biofilm formation, and the antiphagocytic and adherence properties of the polysaccharide capsule, which provides the greatest capacity to induce pneumonia and is the antigenic target for vaccine-mediated antibody production.[94]

TABLE 64-4
Microorganisms Common in Community-Acquired Pneumonia

Ambulatory	Hospitalized, Non-ICU	Hospitalized, ICU
Streptococcus pneumoniae *Mycoplasma pneumoniae* *Haemophilus influenzae* *Chlamydophila pneumoniae*	*S. pneumoniae* *M. pneumoniae* *C. pneumoniae* *Staphylococcus aureus*	*S. pneumoniae* *S. aureus* *Legionella* species Gram-negative bacilli
Respiratory viruses[a]	*H. influenzae* *Legionella* species Respiratory viruses[a]	*H. influenzae*

[a] Influenza A and B, adenovirus, respiratory syncytial virus, and parainfluenza.
Source: Mandell LA et al. Infectious Diseases Society of America/American Thoracic Society consensus guidelines on the management of community-acquired pneumonia in adults. *Clin Infect Dis.* 2007;44(Suppl 2):S27.

Although *S. pneumoniae* remains the pathogen most commonly associated with CAP, the overall incidence of invasive disease has decreased by 75% in children older than 5 years from 1999 to 2005.[95] The change was related mainly to reduced rates of infection caused by serotypes contained in the pneumococcal conjugate vaccine. Although the rate of disease caused by these serotypes has decreased, invasive disease attributable to nonvaccine serotypes has greatly increased.[96] The serotype of greatest concern is 19A, which displays significant virulent potential and has the propensity to acquire multiple-drug resistance genes.[97]

The significance of atypical pathogens, including *L. pneumophila, C. pneumoniae,* and *M. pneumoniae,* is perhaps greatest in patients with severe CAP. The frequency of these organisms as CAP pathogens may be as high as 60% of episodes, and these organisms may be copathogens in up to 40% of cases.[98,99] Importantly, when polymicrobial infection occurs with atypical pathogens, a more complicated course with longer lengths of stay are often observed. The significance of the atypical organisms as etiologic agents in CAP has been suggested by studies that use antibiotics with activity against these organisms and demonstrate a survival benefit over regimens without.[100–104] The

TABLE 64-5
Community-Acquired Pneumonia: Underlying Conditions and Commonly Encountered Pathogens

Condition	Commonly Encountered Pathogen(s)
Alcoholism	Oral anaerobes, *Klebsiella pneumoniae, Acinetobacter* sp., *Mycobacterium tuberculosis*
COPD or smoking	*Pseudomonas aeruginosa, Legionella* sp.
Aspiration	Gram-negative enteric pathogens, oral anaerobes
Lung abscess	CA-MRSA, oral anaerobes, endemic fungal pneumonia, *M. tuberculosis*, atypical mycobacteria
Exposure to bat or bird droppings	*Histoplasma capsulatum*
Exposure to birds	*Chlamydophila psittaci* (if poultry; avian influenza)
Exposure to rabbits	*Francisella tularensis*
Exposure to farm animals or parturient cats	*Coxiella burnetii* (Q fever)
HIV infection (early)	*M. tuberculosis*
HIV infection (late)	*M. tuberculosis, Pneumocystis jiroveci, Cryptococcus* sp., *Histoplasma* sp., *Aspergillus* sp., atypical mycobacteria (especially *Mycobacterium kansasii*), *Pseudomonas aeruginosa*
Hotel or cruise ship stay in previous 2 weeks	*Legionella* sp.
Travel to or residence in southwestern United States	*Coccidioides* sp., hantavirus
Travel to or residence in Southeast and East Asia	*Burkholderia pseudomallei*, avian influenza, SARS
Cough >2 weeks with whoop or posttussive vomiting	*Bordetella pertussis*
Structural lung disease (e.g., bronchiectasis)	*P. aeruginosa, Burkholderia cepacia, Staphylococcus aureus*
Injection drug use	*S. aureus*, anaerobes, *M. tuberculosis*
Endobronchial obstruction	Anaerobes, *S. aureus*
In context of bioterrorism	*Bacillus anthracis* (anthrax), *Yersinia pestis* (plague), *F. tularensis* (tularemia)

CA-MRSA, community-acquired methicillin-resistant *Staphylococcus aureus;* COPD, chronic obstructive pulmonary disease; HIV, human immunodeficiency virus; SARS, severe acute respiratory syndrome.

majority of cases of Legionnaires' disease are caused by *L. pneumophila* serogroup 1, but other serogroups are also implicated.[105] A characteristic clinical profile has been described that links *L. pneumophila* as the cause of CAP that includes a high temperature, absence of sputum production, low serum sodium concentration, high concentration of lactate dehydrogenase, and low platelet counts.[106] *L. pneumophila* is more likely to cause CAP that is moderate to severe as demonstrated by an increasing incidence among hospitalized patients and those requiring intensive care compared with outpatients.[107]

Epidemiologic factors may favor the presence of certain bacterial pathogens and are listed in Table 64-5. CAP caused by *Enterobacteriaceae* species and *P. aeruginosa* generally occurs in patients with structural lung diseases and alcoholism.[85,108] In addition, chronic oral steroid use (≥10 mg prednisone/day) or immunosuppression and frequent antibiotic therapy are additional risks for infection caused by these pathogens; however, these characteristics currently place patients into the category of health care–associated pneumonia (HCAP).[109]

S. aureus is recognized as a major cause of nosocomial pneumonia; however, its significance in CAP is less clear. Traditionally, *S. aureus* has not been considered a common cause of CAP, but is most likely to occur in association with influenza or in patients with lung abscess.[85,110,111] However, some studies document *S. aureus* to be second only to *S. pneumoniae* as the etiological pathogen associated with CAP.[112] The proportion of CAP caused by methicillin-resistant strain of *S. aureus* (MRSA) occurs at a significant rate.[113] Community-associated MRSA (CA-MRSA) is significantly different from the typical hospital-acquired strain. These differences include susceptibility to non–β-lactam antibiotics (e.g., clindamycin) and clinical syndrome (necrotizing radiographic presentation, empyema formation, hemoptysis, and profound hypoxemia) associated with toxins including Panton-Valentine leukocidin.[114] Toxin-producing strains are also part of methicillin-sensitive *S. aureus*'s (MSSA) virulence.[115] The outcomes of patients with MRSA and MSSA CAP are similarly poor with prolonged length of hospital stay and a nearly 25% mortality.[116]

Recent epidemics (SARS-associated coronavirus in 2003 and influenza A H1N1 in 2009) have highlighted the contribution of respiratory viruses as an etiology of CAP. Respiratory virus can be the primary cause of CAP, but can also be a major contributing factor that predisposes the patient to infection by another pathogen, often bacterial. Using contemporary nucleic acid amplification tests, the incidence of viral CAP ranges from 19% to 32%.[117–119] Respiratory viruses that cause CAP include influenza A and B, respiratory syncytial virus, rhinovirus, parainfluenza, adenovirus, human metapneumovirus, and coronavirus. Of patients with viral CAP, 11% to 15% have coinfection with a bacterial pathogen, most commonly *S. pneumoniae, S. aureus*, and atypical pathogens.

Possible microbes causing M.R.'s CAP include *S. pneumoniae, M. pneumoniae, C. pneumonia, S. aureus, H. influenzae, Legionella* species, and respiratory viruses.

Antibiotic Therapy

CASE 64-3, QUESTION 5: Which antimicrobial agent(s) should be chosen for the initial management of M.R.?

Delayed antibiotic therapy has been associated with an increased length of stay and decreased survival in CAP; therefore, a rapid and correct diagnosis is imperative.[120,121] The most recent IDSA/ATS CAP treatment guidelines recommend the first dose of antibiotic be given in the ED in effort to avoid treatment delays associated with the hospital admission process.[85]

Initial antimicrobial treatment is empirical because of the limited turnaround time, sensitivity, and specificity of currently available microbiological tests. All patients should be empirically treated for pneumococcus and atypical pathogens. In addition, the choice of the initial regimen should be based on medical comorbidities or epidemiological factors. In addition, an assessment of likelihood for infection caused by an antibiotic-resistant pathogen should take place.

The most important consideration in the selection of empiric therapy is to determine risk for infection with DRSP (Table 64-6).

TABLE 64-6

Risk Factors for β-Lactam-Resistant *Streptococcus Pneumoniae*

Age <2 or >65 years
β-Lactam therapy within the previous 3 months (also at risk for organisms associated with HCAP)
Alcoholism
Medical comorbidities
Immunosuppressive illness or therapy (also at risk for organisms associated with HCAP)
Exposure to a child in a day-care center

HCAP, health care–associated pneumonia.

Combination therapy with a β-lactam plus a macrolide is first-line therapy for all patients at risk as well as all hospitalized patients. Susceptibility to penicillin is the benchmark for evaluating the antibiotic resistance of pneumococcus. For CAP, the current breakpoints (revised in 2008) for IV penicillin G at a dose of 12 million units per day are susceptible at 2 mg/L or less, intermediate at 4 mg/L, and resistant at 8 mg/L or greater. Using these breakpoints, less than 1% of isolates are resistant to penicillin G.[122] β-Lactam resistance occurs through alteration of one or more of the penicillin-binding proteins that mediate the bacterial cell wall production.[123] Penicillin-binding protein alterations in resistant strains decrease the affinity to all β-lactams such that higher concentrations are required for binding and inhibition of the enzyme. Thus, appropriate dosing of β-lactams in the treatment of CAP minimizes development of resistance and promotes optimal clinical outcomes.[124,125]

Macrolides are often a backbone of initial therapy for the treatment of CAP, but rarely should be used as monotherapy with nearly 30% of pneumococcal isolates demonstrating resistance. Several mechanisms are responsible for macrolide resistance, including ribosomal modification mediated by *erm* (B), efflux from the bacterial cell controlled by *mef* (A), or a combination of both.[126]

Respiratory fluoroquinolones including levofloxacin, moxifloxacin, and gemifloxacin are given strong recommendation for use across all sites of care, all severity of illness, in patients at risk for DRSP, and those with comorbid conditions.[85] Fluoroquinolones are the preferred agents for CAP in penicillin-allergic patients. Fluoroquinolone resistance has increased mainly as a result of increased use for a variety of indications; however, overall pneumococcal resistance rates are low.[127] The mechanisms of fluoroquinolone resistance include mutations in the DNA gyrase gene *gyrA* and the topoisomerase IV genes *parC* and *parE*, as well as an efflux pump–mediated mechanism.

An approach to the patient with CAP and recommended antibiotic regimens based on the patient's site of care and severity of illness are provided in Figure 64-1. IDSA/ATS guideline-concordant therapy for hospitalized patients has been associated with improved patient outcomes including decreases in time to achieve clinical stability, total duration of parenteral therapy, and hospital length of stay, as well as improved in-hospital survival.[128,129]

M.R.'s treatment should be started in the ED after obtaining a respiratory specimen and pretreatment blood cultures for Gram stain and culture. A β-lactam (ceftriaxone) plus a macrolide (azithromycin) should be initiated empirically, both initially given parenterally. M.R. does not have risk factors that place him at risk

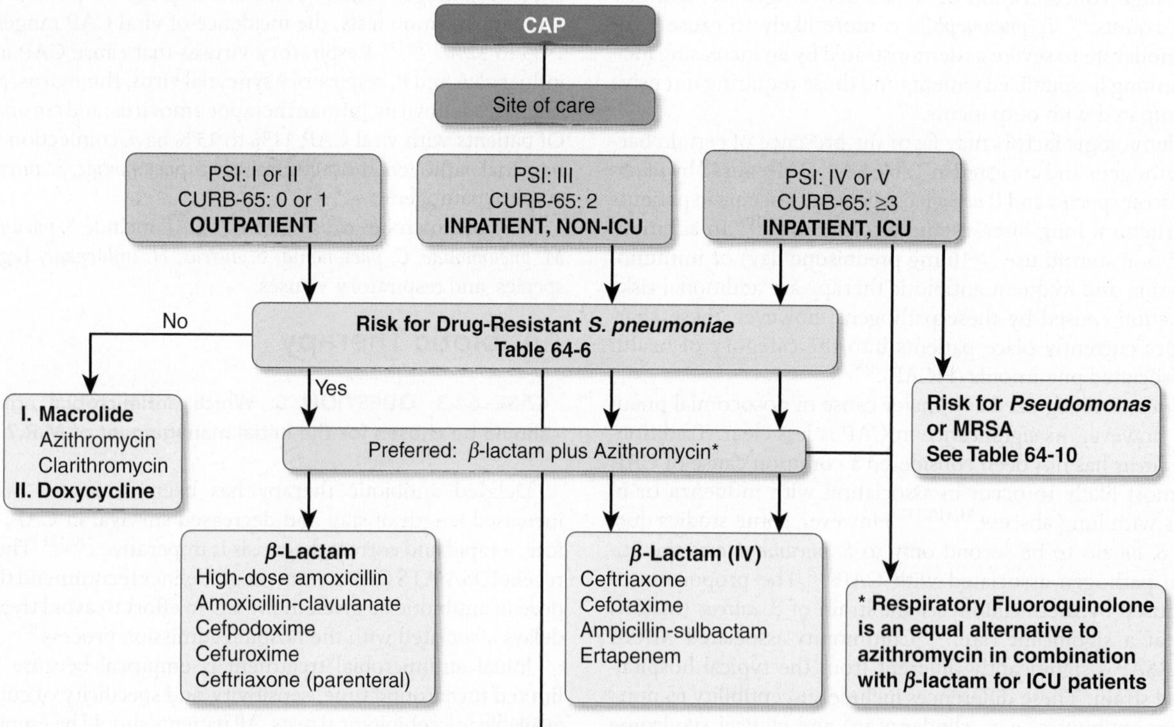

FIGURE 64-1 Approach to empiric antibiotic therapy in patients with community-acquired pneumonia. CAP, community-acquired pneumonia; CURB-65, confusion, uremia, respiratory rate, blood pressure, and age of at least 65 years; IV, intravenous; MRSA, methicillin-resistant *Staphylococcus aureus;* PSI, pneumonia severity index.

for infection caused by *Enterobacteriaceae* or *P. aeruginosa*. Consideration of CA-MRSA infection should be made given M.R.'s recent incarceration and profound hypoxemia, although the rest of his clinical presentation is not compatible with this etiology.

CASE 64-3, QUESTION 6: What is the appropriate length of therapy for M.R.?

A definitive duration of treatment for CAP has not been well established. Significant variation in duration of treatment exists and is independent of severity of CAP.[130] The IDSA/ATS guidelines recommend treatment for a minimum of 5 days, and patients should be afebrile for 48 to 72 hours before therapy is discontinued. In addition, patients should not have therapy discontinued if they meet two or more CAP-associated signs of clinical instability, including temperature of greater than 37.8°C, heart rate of greater than 100 beats/minute, respiratory rate of greater than 24 breaths/minute, systolic blood pressure of less than 90 mm Hg, arterial oxygen saturation of less than 90% or Pao_2 of less than 60 mm Hg on room air, inability to maintain oral intake, or abnormal mental status.[85]

Serial monitoring of biomarkers may guide duration of antibiotic therapy. Procalcitonin (PCT) is a calcitonin precursor that is elevated in infection, trauma, and burns. PCT was initially used as an upfront diagnostic marker for bacterial infection; however, it does not adequately discriminate between bacterial and viral infection. Given this shortcoming, the strongest role for PCT is guiding the duration of antibiotic therapy. Serial measurement of PCT has been associated with a significant reduction in total duration of antibiotic use compared with standard care, suggesting that a fall in PCT level may be a useful indicator of adequate therapy.[31,131]

CASE 64-4

QUESTION 1: R.J. is a 39-year-old man presenting to the ED with the complaints of fever, chills, nausea, and vomiting for the last 7 days, and more recently, shortness of breath with productive cough with white sputum for the past 4 days. He presents to the ED one day after visiting an urgent-care center. Initial assessment reveals the patient to be alert and oriented times three, but falling asleep during assessment, pulses present with brisk capillary refill, decreased lung sounds bilaterally, and no peripheral edema. Past medical history is significant for hypertension and diabetes mellitus. The patient has an allergy to penicillin, with a reported reaction of rash. Medications at home include aspirin 81 mg daily, hydrochlorothiazide 25 mg daily, lisinopril 20 mg daily, and atorvastatin 40 mg daily. Social history is significant for 1 pack of cigarettes per week. In the ED he had a temperature of 38.9°C, heart rate of 112 beats/minute, respiratory rate of 22 breaths/minute, blood pressure of 126/80 mm Hg, and oxygen saturation of 93% on 2 L. Laboratory results include the following:

WBC count, 2,900 cells/μL
Hematocrit, 47.1%
Platelets 129,000 cells/μL
Sodium, 127 mmol/L
Potassium, 4.6 mmol/L
BUN, 7 mg/dL
SCr, 0.73 mg/dL
Glucose 117, mg/dL

Chest radiograph showed bilateral interstitial infiltrates, and RT-PCR was positive for influenza A. What is the most likely reason for R.J.'s influenza infection?

TABLE 64-7
Patients at High Risk of Complications From Influenza

Unvaccinated infants aged 12–24 months
Persons with asthma or other chronic pulmonary diseases (e.g. COPD, cystic fibrosis)
Persons with hemodynamically significant cardiac disease
Persons who have immunosuppressive disorders or who are receiving immunosuppressive therapy
HIV-infected persons
Persons with sickle cell anemia and other hemoglobinopathies
Persons with diseases that require long-term, high-dose aspirin therapy, such as rheumatoid arthritis
Persons with chronic renal dysfunction
Persons with cancer
Persons with chronic metabolic disease, such as diabetes mellitus
Persons with central nervous system disorders that may compromise the handling of secretions such as neuromuscular disorders, cerebral vascular accidents, or seizure disorders
Adults aged ≥65 years
Residents of any age of nursing homes or other long-term care institutions

COPD, chronic obstructive pulmonary disease; HIV, human immunodeficiency virus.

Influenza viruses spread when an infected person coughs or sneezes near a susceptible person.[132] The usual incubation period for influenza is 1 to 4 days, and the time between onset among patients who have come into contact with one another is likely 3 to 4 days.[133] Adults can shed influenza virus from the day before symptoms begin through 5 to 10 days after illness onset[134]; young children shed virus several days before illness onset, and can be infectious for 10 days or more after onset of symptoms. Prolonged viral replication can occur in adults with severe disease, including those with comorbidities or those receiving corticosteroid therapy.[135,136] Severely immunocompromised persons can shed virus for weeks to months.[137,138]

CASE 64-4, QUESTION 2: Should R.J. be treated with antiviral agents?

Patients with laboratory-confirmed influenza virus infection or those suspected of infection who are at high risk of complications (Table 64-7) should receive antiviral therapy within 48 hours of symptom onset whether or not they are hospitalized. Those patients with symptoms greater than 48 hours and requiring hospitalization or those at high risk of complications with illness that is not improving should also be treated. R.J. falls into the latter category and should be treated for influenza A.[91] In addition, antibacterial therapy is recommended for patients with CAP even if influenza is suspected. Antibiotic treatment should be directed at likely bacterial pathogens associated with influenza such as *S. pneumoniae*, *Streptococcus pyogenes*, and *S. aureus*, including MRSA, especially for hospitalized patients.[85]

Antiviral Therapy

CASE 64-4, QUESTION 3: Which antiviral agent(s) should R.J. be treated with?

Influenza susceptibility profiles to antiviral agents evolve rapidly, and treating clinicians should be familiar with updated resistance data found at the Center for Disease Control and Prevention website: www.cdc.gov/flu. Neuraminidase inhibitors including oseltamivir or zanamivir are the primary antiviral

TABLE 64-8
Comparison of Current Neuraminidase Inhibitors for Influenza

	Oseltamivir	Zanamivir
Influenza activity	A and B	A and B
Route of administration	Oral	Oral inhalation
Treatment dosage	Adults: 75 mg PO BID Children ≥12 months: ≤15 kg: 30 mg PO BID 15–23 kg: 45 mg PO BID 24–40 kg: 60 mg PO BID ≥60 kg: 75 mg PO BID	Adults: Two inhalations (5 mg each) PO BID Children ≥7 years: Two inhalations (5 mg each) PO BID
Side effects	Nasal and throat discomfort, headache, bronchospasm	Nausea, vomiting, headache

BID, twice a day; PO, by mouth.

agents recommended for the treatment of influenza (Table 64-8). The inhibition of neuraminidase prevents cleavage of sialic acid residues on the cell surface of the virus, thereby preventing the release of virus from infected cells. Considering the high rate of resistance, adamantines (amantadine and rimantadine) are not currently recommended for treatment of influenza.

The benefits of neuraminidase inhibitor therapy are likely to be greatest if treatment is started as soon as possible after illness onset, ideally within 48 hours of illness onset. However, treatment of any person with confirmed or suspected influenza who requires hospitalization is recommended, even if the patient presents up to 96 hours after illness onset.[139,140] Treatment regimens might need to be altered such that regimens may need to be extended longer than 5 days for patients whose illness is prolonged.

Development of resistance to zanamivir or oseltamivir also has been identified during treatment of seasonal influenza.[141] One elucidated mechanism of oseltamivir resistance is a specific mutation causing a histidine to tyrosine substitution (H275Y) in neuraminidase.[142] Patients receiving oseltamivir who do not respond to treatment might have an infection with an antiviral-resistant influenza virus. Oseltamivir resistance, which can occur within 1 week of treatment initiation, has been reported particularly among immunocompromised patients with the 2009 H1N1 virus infection.[143,144]

HOSPITAL-ACQUIRED PNEUMONIA, HEALTH CARE–ASSOCIATED PNEUMONIA, AND VENTILATOR-ASSOCIATED PNEUMONIA

Definitions and Incidence

Despite advances in therapy and prevention, hospital-acquired pneumonia (HAP), ventilator-associated pneumonia (VAP), and HCAP are associated with significant morbidity and mortality. HAP is defined as pneumonia that occurs at least 48 hours after admission and is not incubating at the time of hospitalization. VAP refers to pneumonia that arises 48 to 72 hours after endotracheal intubation. HCAP occurs within 48 hours of admission in patients with previous risk factors for infection caused by potentially drug-resistant pathogens, including hospitalization in an acute-care hospital for 2 or more days within 90 days of infection; residence in a nursing home or long-term care facility; receipt of recent IV antibiotic therapy, chemotherapy, or wound care within the past 30 days of the current infection; living in close contact with a person with a multidrug-resistant pathogen or attending a hospital or hemodialysis clinic.[109]

Epidemiology

A retrospective cohort study of 4,543 hospitalized patients with culture-positive pneumonia observed that HCAP accounted for 21.7% of cases, HAP, 18.4%, and VAP, 11%. Mortality rates associated with HCAP (19.8%) and HAP (18.8%) groups were comparable, and both were significantly lower than that for VAP (29.3%). Mean lengths of stay differed with pneumonia category with HCAP patients admitted for a mean of 8.8 ± 7.2 days, HAP, 15.2 ± 13.6 days, and VAP, 23 ± 20.2 days.[145]

The onset is an important epidemiologic variable and risk factor for specific pathogens and outcomes in patients with HAP and VAP. Early-onset HAP and VAP are defined as occurring within the first 4 days of hospitalization, usually carry a better prognosis, and are more likely caused by antibiotic-sensitive bacteria. Late-onset HAP and VAP (those cases occurring after ≥5 days of hospitalization) are more likely to be caused by multidrug-resistant (MDR) pathogens and are associated with increased morbidity and mortality.[109]

Pathogenesis

Microorganisms gain access into the lower respiratory tract via aspiration of oropharyngeal pathogens and leakage of secretions around the endotracheal tube cuff in intubated patients.[146,147] Invasive-care devices, contaminated equipment, and transfer of microorganisms among staff and patients serve as the primary pathogen sources,[148] and although more controversial, the gastrointestinal tract may also play a role in bacterial colonization.[149]

Clinical Presentation and Diagnosis

HAP is diagnosed on the basis of radiographic findings and clinical features. Patients must demonstrate new or progressive infiltrates on imaging as well as two of three of the following: fever greater than 38°C, leukopenia or leukocytosis, and purulent sputum. Patients will often experience declines in oxygen saturation, but this finding is less specific for determining the need for empiric antimicrobial agents.[150]

Respiratory cultures may consist of endotracheal aspirates, bronchoalveolar lavage, or protected-specimen brush samples. Blood cultures lack sensitivity, and when positive, consideration should also be given to a potential extrapulmonary source.[151]

TABLE 64-9

Empiric Therapy for Hospital-Acquired Pneumonia, Health Care–Associated Pneumonia, and Ventilator-Associated Pneumonia in Patients With No Known Risk Factors for Multidrug Resistant Pathogens and Onset < 5 Days

Possible Pathogens	Recommended Therapy	Dosage
Streptococcus pneumoniae[a]	Ceftriaxone	1 g IV every 24 hours
Haemophilus influenza	or	
MSSA	Levofloxacin, moxifloxacin, or ciprofloxacin	500–750 mg PO/IV every 24 hours 400 mg PO/IV every 24 hours 500–750 mg PO every 12 hours or 400 mg IV every 8–12 hours
Antibiotic-sensitive enteric GNB		
Escherichia coli	or	
Klebsiella pneumonia	Ampicillin/sulbactam	1.5–3 g IV every 6 hours
Enterobacter sp.	or	
Proteus sp.	Ertapenem	1 g IM/IV every 24 hours
Serratia marcescens		

[a] The frequency of penicillin-resistant *S. pneumoniae and* multidrug-resistant *S. pneumoniae is* increasing; levofloxacin or moxifloxacin are preferred to ciprofloxacin.

GNB, gram-negative bacilli; IM, intramuscular; IV, intravenous; MSSA, methicillin-sensitive *Staphylococcus aureus;* PO, orally.

Overview of Treatment

The IDSA/ATS have published guidelines for the treatment of HAP.[109] The five major principles underlying the management of HAP, HCAP, and VAP include the following: (a) failure to initiate prompt, appropriate therapy is associated with increased mortality; (b) the variability of bacteriology from one institution to another, as well as within specific sites in a hospital, can be significant; (c) the overuse of antibiotics should be avoided by focusing on accurate diagnosis; (d) therapy should be tailored based on lower respiratory tract cultures and the duration of therapy should be shortened; and (e) prevention strategies directed at modifiable risk factors should be applied. The likelihood of an infection with a potential pathogen is based largely on the time to onset of HAP, severity of the condition, and underlying risk factors. In general, patients with early-onset disease who are not severely ill and have no risk factors for MDR organisms can be treated with a single agent, including nonantipseudomonal third-generation cephalosporins or ertapenem, ampicillin/sulbactam, or an antipneumococcal fluoroquinolone (Table 64-9). Empiric therapy in those with late-onset or severe disease should include a combination of antibiotics active against *Pseudomonas.* This regimen usually includes an antipseudomonal β-lactam, such as cefepime, imipenem, meropenem, doripenem, or piperacillin-tazobactam, plus either an aminoglycoside or ciprofloxacin/levofloxacin. Vancomycin or linezolid should be added if MRSA risk factors are present or there is a high institutional incidence (Table 64-10).[109]

CASE 64-5

QUESTION 1: A.S. is a 37-year-old woman with poorly controlled type 1 diabetes and resultant end-stage renal disease who is on intermittent hemodialysis. She completed a course of meropenem for a catheter-associated bloodstream infection 2 weeks ago. A.S. presents to the ED from her home with a 3-day history of dyspnea, cough with purulent sputum production, and intermittent fever.

Examination reveals decreased breath sounds over the right middle and lower lobes consistent with chest radiograph findings of dense consolidation throughout the same areas. Her blood pressure is 159/63 mm Hg, pulse is 88 beats/minute, respiration is 26 breaths/minute, and temperature is 38.3°C. Significant laboratory findings include the following:

WBC, 15,000 cells/μL
Differential polymorphonuclear neutrophil cells, 89%
Bands, 9%
Lymphocytes, 30%

How should A.S.'s pneumonia be classified?

Although A.S. resides in the community, her diagnosis should be considered HCAP as she receives care at a hemodialysis clinic and completed a course of antibiotics within the last 30 days. She is therefore at risk for infection with pathogens distinctly different from those often identified in CAP.

Microbiology

CASE 64-5, QUESTION 2: What pathogens should be suspected in A.S.'s pneumonia?

The major difference in the bacteriology between CAP and HAP, HCAP, or VAP is a shift to gram-negative pathogens, MDR pathogens, and MRSA. Gram-negative bacilli commonly colonize oropharyngeal secretions of patients with moderate to severe acute and chronic illnesses without exposure to broad-spectrum antibiotics.[152] Patients admitted to the hospital with acute illnesses are rapidly colonized with gram-negative organisms. Approximately 20% are colonized on the first hospital day, and this number increases with the duration of hospitalization and severity of illness.[153] Approximately 35% to 45% of hospitalized patients[153] and up to 100% of critically ill patients[152] will be colonized within 3 to 5 days of admission.

In the past, gram-negative bacteria accounted for 50% to 70% of all cases of HAP and VAP[109,154–158]; however, gram-positive organisms have become increasingly common, with *S. aureus* responsible for upward of 40% of cases of HAP, VAP, and HCAP. This is in stark contrast to CAP bacteriology, in which *S. aureus* represents 25% or less of cases. *P. aeruginosa* remains the most prevalent gram-negative organism in HAP, VAP, and HCAP, accounting for approximately 20% to 25% of infections.[145] In patients who are ventilator dependent, *Acinetobacter* species is an increasingly common gram-negative pathogen. Other organisms with special risk factors include *Legionella,* which is associated with high-dose corticosteroid use and outbreaks secondary to water supplies and cooling systems,[152,159] and *Aspergillus,* which is associated with neutropenia or organ transplantation.[160]

TABLE 64-10

Empiric Therapy for Hospital-Acquired Pneumonia, Health Care–Associated Pneumonia, and Ventilator-Associated Pneumonia in Patients With Late-Onset Infection (≥5 days) or Risk Factors for Multidrug Resistant Pathogens

Possible Pathogens	Combination Recommended Therapy	Adult Dosage[a]
Pathogens listed in Table 60-1 and MDR pathogens	Antipseudomonal cephalosporin cefepime	1–2 g IV every 8–12 hours
	Ceftazidime	2 g IV every 8 hours
Pseudomonas aeruginosa	*Or*	
Klebsiella pneumoniae (ESBL$^+$)[b]	Antipseudomonal carbapenem imipenem	500 mg IV every 6 hours or 1 g IV every 8 hours
Acinetobacter sp.[b]	Doripenem	500 mg IV every 6–8 hours[c]
	Meropenem	1 g IV every 8 hours
	Or	
	β-Lactam/β-Lactamase inhibitor piperacillin-tazobactam	4.5 g IV every 6 hours
	Plus	
	Antipseudomonal fluoroquinolone[d]	
	Ciprofloxacin	400 mg IV every 8 hours
	Levofloxacin	750 mg IV every 24 hours
	Or	
	Aminoglycoside	
	Amikacin	15–20 mg/kg IV every 24 hours[e]
	Gentamicin	5–7 mg/kg IV every 24 hours[e]
	Tobramycin	5–7 mg/kg IV every 24 hours[e]
	Plus	
MRSA[d]	Linezolid	600 mg/kg every 12 hours[f]
	Vancomycin	15 mg every 12 hours
Legionella pneumophila[g]	Azithromycin	500 mg IV every 24 hours

[a] Dosages are based on normal renal and hepatic function.
[b] If an ESBL$^+$ strain, such as *K. pneumoniae*, or an *Acinetobacter* sp. is suspected, a carbapenem is a reliable choice.
[c] Studied infusion times range from 30 minutes to 4 hours.
[d] If MRSA risk factors are present, or there is a high incidence locally.
[e] Trough levels for gentamicin and tobramycin should be <1 mcg/mL; for amikacin, they should be <4–5 mcg/mL.
[f] Trough levels for vancomycin should be 15–20 mcg/mL.
[g] If *L. pneumophila* is suspected, a combination antibiotic regimen including a macrolide (e.g., azithromycin) or a fluoroquinolone (e.g., ciprofloxacin or levofloxacin) should be used.
ESBL, extended-spectrum β-lactamase; IV, intravenous; MDR, multidrug-resistant; MRSA, methicillin-resistant *Staphylococcus aureus*.

Risk factors for MDR pathogens include patient-specific factors such as antimicrobial therapy in the previous 90 days, current hospitalization of 5 days or more, and immunosuppressive disease or therapy. Coverage for MDR organisms should also take place with high frequency of community, hospital, or unit antibiotic resistance or if the patient demonstrates any risk factors for HCAP.

A.S. is at risk for MDR pathogens because she attends a hemodialysis clinic and recently completed a course of antibiotics. She should receive therapy targeting MRSA and MDR gram-negative pathogens including *P. aeruginosa*. Some experts would also suggest she receive atypical coverage as she has close contact with others in the community setting.

CASE 64-6

QUESTION 1: M.L. is a 71-year-old man admitted to the hospital for a deep vein thrombosis. His past medical history is significant for chronic kidney disease, diabetes mellitus, COPD, GERD, hypertension, and a recent diagnosis of non–small cell lung cancer for which he is not currently receiving chemotherapy. M.L.'s home medications include lisinopril, famotidine, aspirin, insulin glargine, insulin aspart, tiotropium, fluticasone/salmeterol, and as-needed albuterol. What characteristics does M.L. exhibit that place him at risk for HAP?

Several risk factors for HAP have been identified, including intubation and mechanical ventilation, aspiration, a patient's body position, the administration of enteral feeding, prior use of antibacterial agents, gastrointestinal bleeding prophylaxis (i.e., histamine type 2 antagonists and proton-pump inhibitors), immunosuppressive therapy, and poor nutrition status or glucose control. Other nonmodifiable risk factors associated with developing HAP include age older than 70 years and chronic lung disease.

An important contributing factor in the cause of pneumonia is colonization of the oropharynx common in alcoholism, prolonged hospitalization, and previous antimicrobial exposure.[161] Several factors may contribute to the colonization of M.L.'s oropharynx with gram-negative bacteria. In addition to his pulmonary disease, an altered immune response in diabetics and the elderly can contribute to respiratory infection in M.L. The use of drugs that inhibit the production of gastric acid, such as famotidine, increases the possibility of oropharyngeal colonization and pneumonia.[162–165]

Antibiotic Therapy

CASE 64-6, QUESTION 2: Six days after admission, M.L. exhibits a fever to 39.3°C. He has since been intubated and has increasing secretions coming from his endotracheal tube, an elevated WBC count, and new infiltrate on his daily chest radiograph. Sputum cultures are sent, and the decision is made to start M.L. on antibiotics. How should antimicrobial therapy be managed for M.L.?

Because delays in the administration of appropriate therapy have been associated with increased hospital mortality from HAP, the prompt administration of empiric therapy is essential. Importantly, changing therapy once culture results are available may not reduce the excess risk of hospital mortality if inappropriate initial therapy is selected.[166–168] To this end, local bacteriologic patterns and in vitro susceptibility results should be made available and updated as frequently as possible to allow for more appropriate selection of initial empirical therapy. In addition to the selection of an appropriate agent, the selection of adequate dosing regimens will optimize the pharmacodynamic properties of the antibacterial agent(s) and improve clinical outcomes.

Resolution of HAP can be defined both clinically and microbiologically. Clinical improvement usually is apparent after the first 48 to 72 hours of therapy. During this time, the selected antibacterial regimen should not be changed unless progressive deterioration takes place or microbiologic studies confirm the pathogen.

If culture results are negative or inconclusive (because of known specimen contamination with mouth flora), the patient's response to the initial antibiotic therapy should be used to evaluate modification of the antibiotic regimen. If the patient responds to the initial regimen, consideration should be given to narrowing coverage to the most likely causative pathogens.

If the patient is not responding to the initial antibiotic therapy, one should consider whether (a) the pathogen is not covered in the initial choice of antibiotic therapy, (b) the dose of antibiotic is insufficient, and (c) any other factors are responsible for the failure to respond to therapy. Such factors include poor pulmonary clearance of necrotic tissue and cellular debris, lung abscesses or empyema, and severely altered host defenses with a rapidly fatal underlying disease.

Of note, if one of the following organisms is isolated (*Serratia, Pseudomonas,* indole-positive *Proteus, Citrobacter,* or *Enterobacter* species), in vitro reports indicating susceptibility should be carefully evaluated, as these organisms often possess an inducible β-lactamase gene (also referred to as a type I β-lactamase enzyme).[169] In vitro testing may demonstrate susceptibility to third-generation cephalosporins and extended-spectrum penicillins but may not translate to efficacy in the clinical setting. As a possible scenario of infection with these organisms, after initiation with one of the above agents, the patient may initially respond; however, after approximately 1 week, the patient's condition will begin to worsen. Because treatment with the β-lactam agent induces the expression of the type I enzyme, a subsequent specimen sent after approximately 1 week is now likely to demonstrate resistance to the third-generation cephalosporins and extended-spectrum penicillins.[169] Although cefepime is more likely to be active against these isolates, a large inoculum of organisms (e.g., that present in pneumonia) can result in β-lactamase degradation of this agent as well.[170] Considering that this phenomenon will not be identified by using usual in vitro testing, cefepime should be used cautiously in these patients.[171] The preferred therapy in these patients includes trimethoprim-sulfamethoxazole, a fluoroquinolone, or a carbapenem.[169] *Acinetobacter* species are increasingly resistant to many commonly used antibacterial agents. Treatment of this often multiply-resistant pathogen requires the use of very high doses of ampicillin-sulbactam (up to 24 g/day) or colistin.[172,173]

In summary, M.L. could be started empirically with an anti-MRSA agent (vancomycin), and double coverage for resistant gram-negative pathogens (cefepime and gentamicin or ciprofloxacin). When culture results are known, the antibiotic regimen can be modified and individualized. Seven to 8 days of therapy is recommended for patients with uncomplicated HAP, VAP, or HCAP who have received appropriate empiric antibiotics with a satisfactory subsequent clinical response.[109] However, patients infected with nonfermenting gram-negative bacilli may benefit from longer courses (14 days or greater) to prevent recurrence.[174] M.L.'s clinical response should be monitored to determine whether the selected antibiotics are effective in treating this infection. These parameters include an improvement in Pa_{O_2}/F_{IO_2} and decreases in temperature and WBC count with resolution of the left shift.

CASE 64-6, QUESTION 3: Seventy-two hours after empiric antibiotics were initiated, the microbiology laboratory reports that greater than 100,000 colonies/mL of MRSA have grown on M.L.'s sputum culture. Antibiotics are de-escalated to vancomycin therapy alone, to which the isolate is susceptible. After a loading dose and aggressive maintenance regimen, vancomycin trough concentrations have been 17 to 22 mcg/mL. However, M.L. remains febrile, demonstrates progression of his infiltrates on chest radiograph, and has acute worsening of renal function requiring dialysis. Repeat tracheal cultures again grow only *S. aureus* with susceptibility to vancomycin, sulfamethoxazole-trimethoprim, daptomycin, and linezolid. Should M.L.'s antibiotic therapy be modified?

The first IDSA MRSA infection treatment guidelines[175] were published in 2011 and are discussed subsequently in collaboration with the first vancomycin therapeutic monitoring guidelines jointly developed by the American Society of Health-System Pharmacists, the Society of Infectious Diseases Pharmacists, and the IDSA.[176]

For MRSA pneumonia, IV vancomycin or linezolid 600 mg by mouth (PO) or IV twice daily or clindamycin 600 mg PO or IV three times daily (if the strain is susceptible) is recommended for 7 to 21 days, depending on the extent of infection. Daptomycin should not be used for the treatment of MRSA pneumonia, as its activity is inhibited by pulmonary surfactant, rendering it inactive in the treatment of lung infection.[175]

VANCOMYCIN

The recommended dosing of IV vancomycin is 15 to 20 mg/kg/dose (actual body weight) every 8 to 12 hours, not to exceed 2 g/dose, for patients with normal renal function. A loading dose of 25 to 30 mg/kg (actual body weight) may be considered. Some patients may experience an adverse event during the infusion of vancomycin known as red man syndrome. Extending the infusion time to 2 hours for larger doses or premedicating patients who have experienced this phenomenon with an antihistamine may alleviate this adverse event.[175]

Vancomycin trough concentrations of 15 to 20 mcg/mL are recommended for the treatment of pneumonia[175] as higher trough serum concentrations should increase the likelihood of optimizing the area under the curve (AUC) and minimum inhibitory concentration (MIC) and therefore take into account higher vancomycin MIC values appreciated in some isolates. It has also been postulated that targeting higher trough values may help to overcome vancomycin's inherent impaired penetration into epithelial lining fluid and respiratory secretions.[176] Of note, there are no data confirming that achievement of more aggressive trough levels is associated with improvement in clinical cure. A retrospective trial of patients with MRSA HCAP found no difference in trough serum concentrations or calculated AUCs between survivors and nonsurvivors. Several limitations of this investigation are worth noting. There was considerable variability in both AUCs (range, 119–897 mg · h/L) and trough concentrations (range, 4.2–29.8 mg/L), MICs could not be determined, and time to target achievement was not captured. Furthermore, as no sample size was predetermined, the study may have been underpowered, placing it at risk for type II error.[176,177]

LINEZOLID

Linezolid achieves higher concentrations in lung epithelial fluid than in plasma[178] and serves as an alternative to vancomycin for the treatment of MRSA pneumonia. A retrospective analysis of two prospective trials[179,180] for the treatment of HAP found the subgroup of MRSA cases experienced higher cure rates and lower mortality in patients randomly assigned to linezolid compared with vancomycin.[181] In contrast, a meta-analysis of eight randomized control trials comparing glycopeptide antibiotics to linezolid for suspected MRSA pneumonia found no evidence to support superiority of linezolid.[182] Therefore, it remains uncertain whether linezolid or vancomycin should be considered superior. The ZEPHyR study compared linezolid with vancomycin in patients with proven nosocomial MRSA pneumonia in a randomized, double-blind fashion. This is the largest trial conducted in this population to date and may provide some guidance on the optimal therapy for MRSA pneumonia. [183]

ALTERNATIVE AGENTS

Doxycycline, clindamycin, and sulfamethoxazole-trimethoprim are not reliably active against health care–associated MRSA strains, leading to more research focused on novel agents. Although active against MRSA, tigecycline has been associated with worsened clinical outcomes when used for the treatment of HAP, including MRSA pneumonia.[184] Telavancin has been compared with vancomycin in the treatment of HAP caused by gram-positive pathogens. Treatment with telavancin achieved higher clinical cure rates in patients with monomicrobial *S. aureus* infection and in those with isolates that demonstrated a vancomycin MIC of at least 1 mcg/mL. However, lower cure rates were observed in the telavancin group in those who had mixed infections. Telavancin use was associated with a higher incidence in SCr elevation, and at the time of writing, has not been approved by the US Food and Drug Administration for this indication.

Additional microbiologic testing may reveal M.L.'s isolate has an elevated MIC or demonstrates vancomycin heteroresistance, but in the setting of vancomycin failure, these data would not affect decision making. Despite daptomycin susceptibility, the drug does not penetrate lung surfactant, and therefore it is not appropriate to use in the treatment of pneumonia. Sulfamethoxazole-trimethoprim is a less appealing option owing to the patient's dialysis requirement. M.L. should be switched to linezolid. Linezolid quickly reaches high lung concentrations and is safe to use in the setting of acute renal failure.

CASE 64-7

QUESTION 1: A.T. is a 64-year-old woman discharged from the ICU 8 days ago after a prolonged hospitalization complicated by VAP. At that time, cultures obtained from bronchoalveolar lavage grew *P. aeruginosa,* and she was treated with a 14-day course of cefepime. Today, the patient reports fever up to 39.4°C in addition to increased secretions.

Vital signs on admission are blood pressure of 101/65 mm Hg, pulse rate of 99 beats/minute, and respiration rate of 29 breaths/minute. Significant laboratory findings include a WBC of 18,900 cells/μL and SCr of 0.9 mg/dL. Chest radiography shows progressive bilateral infiltrates. The microbiology laboratory from A.T.'s rehabilitation facility calls to report that oxidase-positive gram-negative bacilli are growing from a sputum sample obtained there 2 days ago. Meropenem and gentamicin are prescribed. How should A.T.'s combination therapy against *P. aeruginosa* be managed?

After return of the susceptibility report, A.T.'s therapy may be de-escalated to monotherapy. A retrospective study evaluating treatment of VAP demonstrated empiric combination therapy significantly decreased the probability of inappropriate therapy, which was an independent variable associated with a higher incidence of mortality. However, there was no difference between combination and monotherapy groups with regard to mortality, length of stay, development of resistance or recurrence, suggesting that switching to monotherapy once susceptibility data are available is safe.[185]

CASE 64-7, QUESTION 2: What pharmacokinetic and pharmacodynamic characteristics must be considered in the dosing of aminoglycosides in A.T.?

Individualization of aminoglycoside dosing is imperative as the efficacy and toxicity of aminoglycosides correlates with plasma concentrations and therapeutic outcome in patients with gram-negative pneumonia.[186–189] In patients receiving multiple daily doses of gentamicin or tobramycin and achieving a 1-hour postinfusion peak plasma concentration of greater than 7 mcg/mL, a successful outcome occurs more often than in those with lower plasma concentrations.

The aminoglycosides are concentration-dependent killing antibiotics. Their rate and extent of killing organisms is maximized by increasing the peak serum concentration relative to the MIC of the pathogen. In addition to maximizing bactericidal activity, in vitro evidence has demonstrated that this concentration goal also minimizes the development of resistance. The use of once-daily dosing strategies to minimize nephrotoxicity of the aminoglycosides has been studied extensively. Single doses of gentamicin and tobramycin (5–7 mg/kg/day) and of amikacin (15–20 mg/kg/day) have been reported to be as effective as standard dosing (smaller single doses provided every 12 or every 8 hours) of these agents in controlled clinical trials. However, none of the trials has enrolled a sufficient number of patients required to demonstrate a lower incidence of nephrotoxicity. There are several advantages of once-daily dose aminoglycoside therapy: (a) it is no more nephrotoxic than traditional dosing, (b) clinicians are ensured that a therapeutic peak serum level will be achieved with the first dose, (c) it is the only safe and effective way to achieve serum peak levels of 10 to 20 times the MIC for difficult-to-treat organisms such as *P. aeruginosa,* and (d) it is a more efficient dosing regimen (fewer doses and administration times per day; fewer serum level measurements are required).

Despite the use of individualized aminoglycoside dosing, morbidity and mortality rates attributable to gram-negative pneumonia remain high. This is because the success of antibiotic therapy depends on the ability of the antibiotic to reach the site of infection and remain biologically active.[189] Concentrations of the aminoglycosides in bronchial secretions range from 1 to 5 mcg/mL (~30%–40% of serum concentrations) 2 to 4 hours after parenteral administration.[190] These concentrations may be insufficient to inhibit the growth of many gram-negative organisms, especially *Pseudomonas.*

The bioactivity of the aminoglycosides is influenced by the local tissue pH. In contrast to the penicillins and cephalosporins, whose activities are little affected over a pH range of 6.0 to 8.0, a 2- to 16-fold increase in the aminoglycoside MIC of most gram-negative bacteria occurs when the pH is decreased from 7.4 to 6.8.[191] The pH of endobronchial fluid in patients with normal lung physiology and pneumonia averages 6.6.

Lastly, aminoglycosides bind to purulent exudates and cellular debris, inactivating these agents.[192–194] In summary, the aminoglycosides penetrate poorly into bronchial secretions and are less active at the site of infection because of local pH effects and binding to cellular debris. These properties may result in the need for increased dosages, placing patients at increased risk for ototoxicity and nephrotoxicity. Therefore, unless no reasonable alternative exists, aminoglycoside monotherapy for the treatment of pneumonia should be avoided.

A.T. is a candidate for once-daily dosing of aminoglycoside therapy as a result of her preserved renal function. This strategy should provide adequate peaks to maximize concentration-dependent killing, while taking advantage of the postantibiotic effect appreciated with aminoglycosides and gram-negative organisms. Random aminoglycoside levels drawn approximately 8 hours or later after dosage administration should be followed and adjustments made as necessary. Serum creatinine, urine output, WBC count, and temperature should be followed frequently to determine safety and efficacy. When possible, audiometric testing should be considered in patients requiring prolonged therapy.

CASE 64-7, QUESTION 3: Susceptibility data show that the *Pseudomonas* isolate is sensitive to meropenem (MIC = 4 mcg/mL), gentamicin, and colistin, and gentamicin is discontinued. A.T. receives an additional 72 hours of appropriately dosed meropenem but remains febrile with an elevated WBC count despite no data to support other infection. Is there a role for inhaled antibiotics in the treatment of A.T.'s VAP?

Because of the growing incidence of pneumonia caused by MDR gram-negative organisms, interest has been renewed in the use of inhaled aminoglycosides and polymyxin products. When given systemically, both classes have been associated with poor pulmonary penetration and nephrotoxicity, with polymyxin carrying the additional risk of neurotoxicity and aminoglycosides, ototoxicity. However, the proposed high drug concentrations at the site of pulmonary infection, minimal systemic exposure after nebulized administration, and data showing benefit in both the prevention and treatment of *Pseudomonas* pulmonary infection in cystic fibrosis patients make aerosolized antibiotic therapy an appealing strategy for the treatment of VAP.

The evidence for use of monotherapy with aerosolized colistin is limited to a single case series describing three patients with VAP and two with HAP. Antimicrobials to which the isolated pathogens were resistant were administered concomitantly with inhaled colistin. Four of the five patients were cured, survived, and were discharged. However, owing to the small sample size, results of this study should be considered hypothesis generating only.[195]

The use of adjunctive inhaled antibiotics has been evaluated in several retrospective studies. A retrospective study with 60 bronchoalveolar lavage–proven episodes of VAP treated with aerosolized tobramycin (300 mg), amikacin (1000 mg), and colistimethate (150 mg) every 12 hours was associated with microbiological (71%) and clinical success (73%) in the majority of cases. Clinical success was also documented in 20 episodes in which patients received inhaled antimicrobials after failure of IV monotherapy.[196] This paper has been criticized for the lack of a control group, but its findings do suggest that the addition of aerosolized antimicrobials may have a role in salvage therapy. A retrospective, matched case-control study compared 43 patients with VAP who received IV colistin alone (9 million units divided into three doses) with 43 patients who received IV and inhaled colistin (2 million units divided into two doses). The majority of subjects were infected with *Acinetobacter*. Investigators found no difference in pathogen eradication, mortality, or reversible renal dysfunction between groups. The combination group demonstrated a numerically better rate of clinical cure, but this finding was not statistically significant.[197]

A single randomized control trial has been published detailing adjunctive nebulized colistimethate sodium in VAP. Investigators enrolled 100 patients, most of whom were infected with *Acinetobacter* or *Pseudomonas;* all received systemic antibiotics according to their responsible physician. Fifty-one patients were randomly assigned to receive 75 mg of colistimethate and 49 patients were to receive sterile normal saline inhalations every 12 hours. All inhaled therapy was continued until systemic therapy was ended. No difference in clinical outcomes was demonstrated between groups, but receipt of aerosolized colistimethate was associated with more favorable microbiological outcomes. Inhaled treatment was also numerically more likely to cause bronchospasm, although this did not reach statistical significance. Duration of treatment was shorter in the inhaled colistimethate group, suggesting that prescription of inhaled adjunctive treatment may result in shorter lengths of antimicrobial therapy.[198]

Aerosolization of antibiotics may cause cough, bronchial irritation, and in some individuals, bronchospasm. These effects most often have been associated with polymyxin B and have resulted in episodes of acute respiratory failure.[199,200] Polymyxin can stimulate the release of histamine, which is believed to be responsible for these adverse effects; it also can decrease ventilatory function.[199] The aminoglycosides have been relatively well tolerated, although minor alterations in ventilatory function have been reported.[201]

The IDSA/ATS guidelines state that aerosolized antimicrobials may be considered in patients with MDR organisms not responding well to IV therapy.[109] A.T. would be a candidate for adjunctive inhaled antimicrobials based on the guideline recommendations and limited evidence suggesting that patients who demonstrate clinical failure while receiving IV monotherapy may experience a higher incidence of clinical success after adjunctive aerosolized antibiotics. Drug selection should be based on susceptibility data and drug availability.

CASE 64-7, QUESTION 4: In light of the decline in new antimicrobial development and increasing rates of antibiotic resistance, are there any proposed β-lactam dosing strategies that could have been used to improve A.T.'s outcome?

Carbapenems, cephalosporins, and extended-spectrum penicillins or β-lactamase inhibitors demonstrate time-dependent killing, and it is known that 30% to 40%, 50% to 60%, and 60% to 70% of the time that free drug concentrations are greater than the MIC optimizes bactericidal killing for these drug classes, respectively. Enhancement of this parameter via prolonged or continuous infusions has been used to increase the time that free drug concentrations are greater than the MIC and may theoretically lead to improved patient outcomes.[202]

Continuous infusions were first used in the late 1970s with suggested improvement in clinical cure rates,[203] but until recently were largely abandoned owing to logistical concerns about medication stability, drug compatibility, and limited IV access. These concerns were lessened by use of contemporary prolonged infusions. This latter strategy is supported primarily by Monte Carlo simulation, a mathematical modeling technique that estimates the probability of pharmacodynamic target attainment at each MIC for a given MIC range.

Patients diagnosed with VAP and treated with cefepime (2 g every 8 hours for 3 hours) have been evaluated using Monte Carlo methodology. Investigators found that at an MIC of 1 mcg/mL, all tested regimens had a probability of target attainment greater than 90%. However, at an MIC of 8 mcg/mL, when compared with 30-minute intermittent infusions of 1 to 2 g every 8 hours and 2 g every 12 hours, only the prolonged infusion (3 hours) of 2 g every 8 hours maintained 90% probability of target attainment. As one might predict, this phenomenon was only demonstrated in patients with preserved renal function as defined as a creatinine clearance of 50 to 120 mL/minute.[204]

Data exist comparing meropenem administered by a continuous versus an intermittent infusion in the setting of VAP caused by gram-negative bacilli. The continuous infusion group (n = 42) received 1 g of meropenem infused over 6 hours and administered every 6 hours and the intermittent infusion group (n = 47) received 1 g of meropenem for 30 minutes every 6 hours. The chosen administration method was at the discretion of the treating physician, but all patients received tobramycin in addition to meropenem for a total of 14 days. The primary causative pathogen was *Pseudomonas,* followed by *E. coli* and *Serratia*. Overall clinical cure rates were greater in the continuous infusion group.[205]

Intermittent and continuous infusion dosing strategies have also been compared when using piperacillin-tazobactam to treat VAP. A retrospective analysis of 83 patients treated for gram-negative VAP compared intermittent dosing (4.5 g IV every 6 hours for 30 minutes) and continuous infusions (4.5 g IV for 30 minutes followed by 4.5 g IV every 6 hours for 6 hours). Mortality, duration of mechanical ventilation, and ICU length of stay were not different between groups. However, clinical cure rates were significantly higher in the continuous infusion group with increasing MICs (MIC = 8, 40% vs. 89%, $p = 0.02$; MIC = 16, 17% vs. 88%, $p = 0.02$). Of note, this study excluded all patients with a creatinine clearance of less than 60 mL/minute and enrolled significantly more patients with higher MICs. However, as this study took place in Spain, MICs of 32 and 64 were considered resistant and therefore not included in the analysis.[206]

Taken together, these limited data suggest it may have been beneficial to use a prolonged or continuous infusion strategy in A.T. as she demonstrates preserved renal function and an elevated MIC (MIC $\leq$4 mcg/mL is considered susceptible for *Pseudomonas.*) However, larger well-designed trials are needed to confirm the proposed favorable effects of alternative dosing of β-lactams in the setting of pneumonia.

Ventilator-Associated Pneumonia Prophylaxis

The substantial risk of pneumonia in the ICU has prompted aggressive methods to prevent this disease.[207] The most important recommendations include the use of the semiupright position to reduce the risk of aspiration,[208] infection control (including hand washing) to prevent the spread of pathogens from one patient to the next, and surveillance for ICU infections.

Several strategies for prevention of VAP are controversial, including selective decontamination of the digestive tract (SDD), selective oral decontamination (SOD), and topical antiseptics applied to the oral mucosa. These three strategies address the concept that VAP occurs after colonization of the upper respiratory tract. Because digestive tract flora may play a role in this colonization, the impact of various decontamination approaches has been studied.

SDD with combination therapy including topical tobramycin, polymixin E, and sometimes amphotericin B is administered to the stomach and oropharynx four times daily in collaboration with IV administration of ciprofloxacin or a second-generation cephalosporin. Three recent prospective, controlled trials collectively enrolling more than 1,500 patients demonstrated significant reduction in mortality in medical/surgical, surgery/trauma, and burn patients.[209–211] Concern exists, however, for the development of resistance with SDD as was demonstrated in a prospective, randomized trial that occurred over the course of 54 months and led to increased rates of colonization with MRSA.[212]

SOD uses a similar antimicrobial strategy to SDD except that the IV agents are omitted. A recent meta-analysis evaluated SOD alone in 1,098 patients, but failed to show a decrease in the incidence of VAP or overall mortality.[213] Since the publication of that trial, a controlled, crossover study has been completed, enrolling 5,939 patients into one of three arms. The SDD arm received 4 days of IV cefotaxime and topical tobramycin, colistin, and amphotericin applied to the stomach and oropharynx until discharge from the ICU; the SOD arm received the same topical regimen applied only to the oropharynx. The final group received three to four washings per day with sterile water. The initial analysis revealed no difference in 28-day mortality among groups, but after adjustment for Acute Physiology and Chronic Health Evaluation II score, intubation status, and study site, among other factors, the odds ratio for mortality was significantly less in the treatment groups as compared with the sterile water group. SDD was associated with an odds ratio of 0.86 (95% confidence interval, 0.74–0.99, $p = 0.045$) and SOD with an odds ratio of 0.83 (95% confidence interval, 0.72–0.97), suggesting that IV and enteral therapy may not be necessary to improve mortality.[214]

Chlorhexidine is the most widely studied agent for oral decontamination as it targets a wide spectrum of pathogens, including *Pseudomonas, Acinetobacter,* and MRSA. However, the literature has been plagued with inconsistencies in study design. A variety of drug concentrations (0.12%, 0.2%, and 2%) and formulations (gel, solution, and paste) have been used with different administration frequencies in a variety of populations. Some studies included patients who were not receiving mechanical ventilation. Although widely used in practice, the data on the use of chlorhexidine in medical/surgical patients undergoing prolonged mechanical ventilation have not shown reductions in VAP. Conversely, cardiothoracic patients have shown consistent improvements in nosocomial infection rates, but the majority of these patients were extubated within 24 hours of study enrollment. Furthermore, the concentration most consistently shown to have an effect is the 2% formulation, which is not available in the United States outside of surgical scrubs.

KEY REFERENCES AND WEBSITES

A full list of references this chapter can be found at **http://thepoint.lww.com/AT10e.** Below are the key references and websites for this chapter, with the corresponding reference number in this chapter found in parentheses after the reference.

Acute Bronchitis

Braman SS. Chronic cough due to acute bronchitis: ACCP evidence-based practice guidelines. *Chest*. 2006;129(1 Suppl): 95S. (2)

Gonzales R et al. Principles of appropriate antibiotic use for treatment of acute respiratory tract infections in adults: background. *Ann Intern Med*. 2001;134:521. (11)

Smucny J et al. Antibiotics for acute bronchitis. *Cochrane Database Syst Rev.* 2004;(4):CD000245. (22)

Chronic Bronchitis/Acute Exacerbation of COPD

Key Reference

Quon BS et al. Contemporary management of acute exacerbations of COPD: a systemic review and meta-analysis. *Chest.* 2008;133:756. (50)

Key Website

Global Initiative for Chronic Obstructive Lung Disease (GOLD). *Global Strategy for the Diagnosis, Management, and Prevention of Chronic Obstructive Lung Disease 2010.* http://www.goldcopd.org/guidelines-global-strategy-for-diagnosis-management.html. Accessed February 16, 2011. (34)

Preventing Common Respiratory Illnesses With Vaccines

Key Reference

[No authors listed]. Prevention of pneumococcal disease: recommendations from the Advisory Committee on Immunization Practices (ACIP). *MMWR Recomm Rep.* 1997;46(RR-8):1. (79)

Key Website

Centers for Disease Control and Prevention. Seasonal Influenza Vaccination Resources for Health Professionals. http://www.cdc.gov/flu/professionals/vaccination/.

Community-Acquired Pneumonia

Harper SA et al. Seasonal influenza in adults and children: diagnosis, treatment, chemoprophylaxis, and institutional outbreak management: clinical practice guidelines of the Infectious Diseases Society of America. *Clin Infect Dis.* 2009;48:1003. (91)

Mandell LA et al. Infectious Diseases Society of America/American Thoracic Society consensus guidelines on the management of community-acquired pneumonia in adults. *Clin Infect Dis.* 2007;44(Suppl 2):S27. (85)

Hospital-Acquired Pneumonia, Health Care–Associated Pneumonia, and Ventilator-Associated Pneumonia

American Thoracic Society; Infectious Diseases Society of America. Guidelines for the management of adults with hospital-acquired, ventilator-associated, and health care-associated pneumonia. *Am J Respir Crit Care Med.* 2005;171:388. (109)

65 Tuberculosis

Michael B. Kays

CORE PRINCIPLES

		CHAPTER CASES
1	Tuberculosis is an infectious disease caused by *Mycobacterium tuberculosis*, and the most common site of infection is the lungs. Active disease is characterized by fever, chills, night sweats, weight loss, and changes on chest radiography. Several risk factors for tuberculosis have been identified, including immune suppression, exposure to close contacts, and smoking.	**Case 65-1 (Questions 1, 2)**
2	Diagnosis of active disease includes tuberculin skin testing, chest radiography, and sputum collection for acid-fast bacilli stain and culture. Nucleic acid amplification tests and interferon-γ release assays may aid in the diagnosis of tuberculosis. Human immunodeficiency virus (HIV) screening is recommended for all patients with tuberculosis.	**Case 65-1 (Questions 3–7)**
3	The goals of therapy include cure and prevention of transmission of *M. tuberculosis.* Treatment of active pulmonary disease requires administration of multiple-drug therapy for a minimum of 26 weeks. Directly observed therapy is a core management strategy for all patients to ensure adherence to therapy.	**Case 65-1 (Questions 8–12)**
4	Patients should be monitored for resolution of symptoms and questioned about the occurrence of adverse events, especially hepatitis. Sputum smears and cultures should be obtained every 2 to 4 weeks initially and then monthly after cultures become negative. If treatment failure occurs, at least two or three new drugs should be added to the treatment regimen.	**Case 65-1 (Questions 13, 14)**
5	Patients with latent tuberculosis infection have a positive tuberculin skin test but no clinical symptoms or radiographic evidence of active disease. Isoniazid for 6 to 9 months is preferred, and rifampin for 4 months is an alternative.	**Case 65-2 (Questions 1, 2)**
6	Adverse events associated with isoniazid include hepatotoxicity and peripheral neuropathy. Rifampin is associated with hepatotoxicity, flulike syndrome, thrombocytopenia, and discoloration of body fluids. Pyrazinamide can cause hepatotoxicity and increased uric acid, whereas ethambutol can cause optic neuritis.	**Case 65-3 (Questions 1–3), Case 65-4 (Question 1)**
7	The case rate for tuberculosis in the elderly is greater than that in all other age groups. Principles of treatment of tuberculosis in the elderly are the same as those for other age groups.	**Case 65-5 (Question 1)**
8	Multidrug-resistant tuberculosis can develop as a result of nonadherence to treatment. Successful treatment of multidrug-resistant tuberculosis is possible depending on the host, adherence to therapy, and the number of drugs to which the organism remains susceptible. Treatment with six to seven drugs may be required in the intensive phase.	**Case 65-6 (Questions 1, 2)**
9	HIV infection is an important risk factor for tuberculosis. The clinical manifestations in HIV-infected persons will vary depending on the severity of immunodeficiency at presentation. Principles and recommendations for treatment of active disease and latent infection in HIV-infected persons are the same as those for HIV-negative persons.	**Case 65-7 (Questions 1–3), Case 65-8 (Question 1)**

continued

10	In antiretroviral-naïve patients, the optimal timing for initiating antiretroviral therapy is unknown. In patients with low CD4+ counts, antiretroviral therapy may be delayed to decrease the potential for immune reconstitution syndrome. If patients are receiving antiretroviral therapy, treatment of tuberculosis should begin immediately with modification of antiviral therapy as needed.	**Case 65-7 (Questions 4, 5)**
11	Treatment of active disease in pregnant women is the same as that for nonpregnant women. Pyrazinamide is not recommended in pregnancy due to insufficient safety data. The minimum duration of therapy is 9 months.	**Case 65-9 (Question 1)**
12	Infants and children have a higher risk of disseminated tuberculosis, and treatment should be initiated promptly. Ethambutol is generally avoided because it is difficult to assess visual acuity in children. Many experts prefer to initiate therapy in children with three drugs, and treat for a minimum duration of 6 months.	**Case 65-10 (Question 1)**
13	Extrapulmonary tuberculosis may require longer durations of therapy. Tuberculous meningitis may require 9 to 12 months of therapy, and corticosteroids reduce sequelae and improve survival.	**Case 65-11 (Question 1)**

History

Tuberculosis (TB) is an ancient disease, dating back to prehistoric times with evidence of spinal TB in pre-Columbian and early Egyptian remains. However, TB did not become a major health problem until the 17th and 18th centuries, when crowded living conditions of the industrial revolution contributed to its epidemic spread throughout Europe and the United States. Early physicians referred to TB as *phthisis,* derived from the Greek term for wasting, because its clinical presentation consisted of weight loss, cough, fevers, and hemoptysis. Although its characteristics were well known, an etiologic agent was not clearly defined until 1882 when Robert Koch isolated and cultured *Mycobacterium tuberculosis* and demonstrated its infectious nature. With this knowledge, early treatment in the mid-1800s to the early 1900s consisted of removing patients with TB from the community and placing them in a sanatorium for bed rest and fresh air. With the advent of radiographic film, pulmonary cavitary lesions were found to be a pivotal component in the evolution of the disease. Therapy would include pneumoperitoneum, thoracoplasty, and plombage to reduce the size of the cavitary lesion, and some of these therapies are still used today for severe and refractory cases.

The modern era of medical therapy for TB began in 1944 with the discovery of streptomycin and, shortly thereafter, *p*-aminosalicylic acid. The addition of isoniazid in 1952 and rifampin in the late 1960s greatly increased treatment success rates and provided hope for the eventual elimination of TB. However, multidrug-resistant TB (MDR-TB) emerged in the 1990s as a threat to the control of TB in the United States and other countries.[1–3] In the subsequent decade, reports were published describing the worldwide emergence of extensively drug-resistant TB (XDR-TB)[4–6] and, more recently, the emergence of new forms of totally drug-resistant (TDR) or super XDR-TB strains in Iran.[7] As TB strains become increasingly resistant to the currently available agents, the likelihood of achieving the goals for global control and elimination of this disease are diminished. Therefore, a high index of suspicion for TB, rapid pathogen identification, susceptibility testing, patient isolation, and appropriate antimicrobial therapy are critical to prevent further development and spread of drug-resistant TB.

Incidence and Epidemiology

Assuming lifelong infection, approximately 2.0 billion people (30% of the world's population) are infected with *M. tuberculosis.*[8] TB is one of the most common causes of death from an infectious disease in the world, second only to human immunodeficiency virus (HIV) and acquired immunodeficiency syndrome (AIDS). Globally, there were an estimated 9.4 million new cases of TB in 2009, which represents an increase of 1.1 million cases compared with 2000.[9] The majority of the new cases in 2009 were identified in the Southeast Asia, African, and Western Pacific regions (35%, 30%, and 20%, respectively).[9] The countries with the largest number of new cases were India (2 million), China (1.3 million), South Africa (0.49 million), Nigeria (0.46 million), Indonesia (0.43 million), and Pakistan (0.42 million).[9] Approximately 12% of the new TB cases in 2009 were identified in patients infected with HIV, with the African region accounting for 80% of these cases.[9] In 2009, approximately 1.3 million deaths were reported among HIV-negative cases of TB and 0.4 million deaths were reported among HIV-positive cases of TB, which represents approximately 4,700 deaths a day.[9]

In the United States, a total of 11,181 cases of TB were reported in 2010, and the incidence rate was 3.6 per 100,000 population, which represents the lowest recorded rate since national reporting began in 1953.[10] However, the incidence rate remained substantially higher than the national goal for elimination of TB (<0.1 case per 100,000 population) that was set for 2010.[10] Thirty-two states had lower rates in 2010 compared with 2009, whereas higher rates were reported in 18 states and the District of Columbia.[10] Four states (California, Texas, New York, and Florida) accounted for 49.2% of all TB cases in 2010.[10] The number of TB cases and the incidence rates declined for both foreign-born and US-born persons, but foreign-born and ethnic and racial minorities continue to be disproportionally affected by TB in the United States (Fig. 65-1). In 2010, 60.5% and 39.5% of all TB cases were reported in foreign-born and US-born persons, respectively, and the TB rate was 11 times greater in foreign-born persons compared with US-born persons (18.1 versus 1.6 per 100,000 population).[10] In 2010, four countries accounted for more than half of TB cases in foreign-born persons: Mexico (23.0%), the Philippines (11.0%), India (8.6%), and Vietnam (7.7%).[10] TB

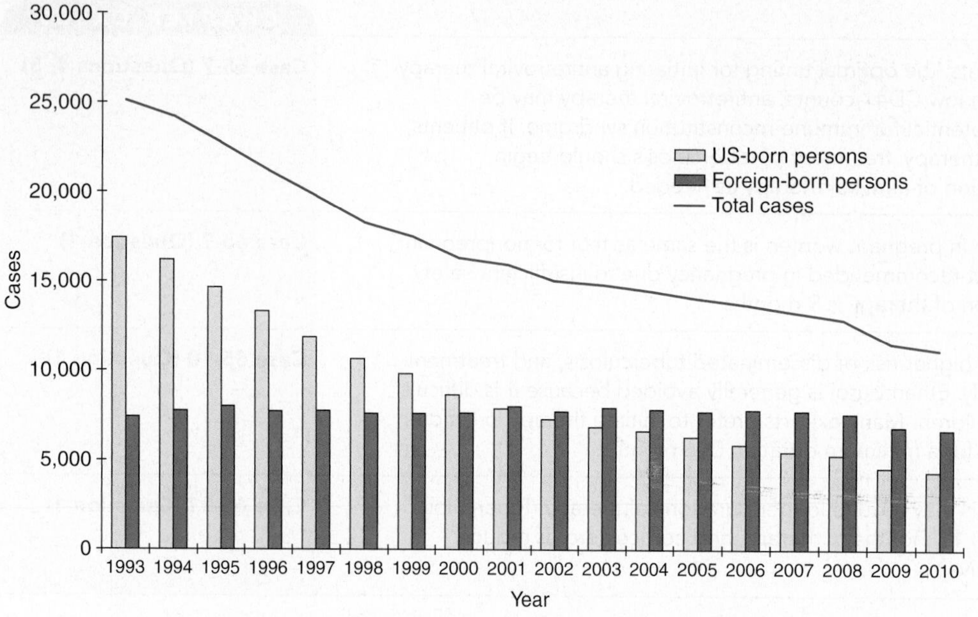

FIGURE 65-1 Reported cases of tuberculosis in the United States, 1993–2010. (Source: Centers for Disease Control and Prevention. Reported tuberculosis in the United States, 2009. Atlanta, GA: U.S. Department of Health and Human Services, CDC, October 2010.)

rates for Hispanics, non-Hispanic blacks, and Asians were 7, 8, and 25 times greater than the rate for non-Hispanic Caucasians.[10] Among US-born persons, the greatest number of TB cases was reported in blacks. Among persons with TB whose HIV status was known, 8.6% of patients with TB were coinfected with HIV.[10]

Globally, there were approximately 440,000 cases of MDR-TB, defined as resistance to both isoniazid and rifampin, in 2008.[9] The largest number of MDR-TB cases were reported in China, India, the Russian Federation, and South Africa.[9] In the United States, a total of 113 cases of MDR-TB were reported in 2009.[10] The overall proportion of MDR-TB cases was similar for 2009 (1.3%) and 2008 (1.1%), and foreign-born persons accounted for 89.4% of the MDR-TB cases.[10] The percentage of MDR-TB is approximately five times greater for persons with a previous history of TB compared with persons without a previous history of TB.[10] Several conditions and risk factors for persons with increased risk of infection with drug-resistant TB are shown in Table 65-1.

In the last few years, XDR-TB has emerged as another major threat to global health.[4–6] The definition of XDR-TB is resistance to isoniazid and rifampin among first-line agents, resistance to any fluoroquinolone, and resistance to at least one second-line injectable drug (amikacin, kanamycin, or capreomycin).[11] According to the World Health Organization, XDR-TB strains have been identified in 58 countries and territories worldwide, including the United States.[9] One of the first reports described 53 patients infected with XDR-TB from South Africa.[12] HIV status was known in 44 patients, and all of these patients were HIV-positive. Fifty-five percent of the patients had no prior history of TB treatment, and 98% died with a median survival period of only 16 days after collection of the first sputum specimen.[12] In the United States, 49 cases of XDR-TB were identified between 1993 and 2006, and mortality was strongly associated with concomitant HIV infection.[13] Four cases of XDR-TB were reported in the United States in 2008, but no cases were reported in 2009 and one case was reported in 2010.[10,14]

Risk factors for XDR-TB include previous treatment for TB, HIV infection, homelessness, and alcohol use.[15] In a retrospective analysis of patients with documented MDR-TB, emergence of XDR-TB was observed in certain patients while receiving treatment for MDR-TB.[16] This study found that the development of XDR-TB was associated with baseline chronic disease and nonadherence to MDR-TB therapy.[16] XDR-TB is significantly less likely to be successfully treated and associated with increased all-cause and TB-related mortality when compared with patients with MDR-TB.[17] However, a recent meta-analysis reported that treatment outcomes were significantly improved when later-generation fluoroquinolones were added to the treatment regimen for XDR-TB, even if fluoroquinolone resistance was demonstrated on susceptibility testing.[18]

The evolution of resistance in TB continued in 2009 with the identification of strains that were reported to be TDR, which was defined as resistance to all first-line and second-line agents.[7] Fifteen (10.3%) strains of 146 MDR-TB strains tested were found to be TDR-TB in Iran, and cultures remained positive in these cases after 18 months of treatment with second-line agents.[7] All of these TDR-TB cases were HIV-negative. This report illustrates the critical need to develop new and effective agents for the treatment of TB caused by MDR, XDR, and TDR strains.

TABLE 65-1

Conditions and Risk Factors for Persons With Increased Risk of Drug-Resistant Tuberculosis

History of treatment for latent tuberculosis infection or active disease
Patients from areas with high prevalence of initial or primary drug resistance (urban population, northeast United States, Florida, California, Texas, United States–Mexico border)
Foreign-born persons from areas with high prevalence of drug-resistant tuberculosis (southeast Asia, Mexico, South America, Africa)
Contact with persons with active infection caused by drug-resistant *Mycobacterium tuberculosis*
Tuberculosis in persons who are homeless, abusers of intravenous drugs, and HIV infected
Patients with positive sputum smears and cultures after 2 months of treatment

HIV, human immunodeficiency virus.

Etiology

TB is caused by *M. tuberculosis*, an aerobic, non–spore-forming bacillus that resists decolorization by acid alcohol after staining with basic fuchsin. For this reason, the organism is often referred to as an acid-fast bacillus (AFB).

For a photo of *M. tuberculosis*, go to http://thepoint.lww.com/AT10e.

It is also different from other organisms in that it replicates slowly—once every 24 hours instead of every 20 to 40 minutes as with some other organisms. *M. tuberculosis* thrives in environments in which the oxygen tension is relatively high, such as the apices of the lung, the renal parenchyma, and the growing ends of bones.

Transmission

M. tuberculosis is transmitted through the air by aerosolized droplet nuclei that are produced when a person with pulmonary or laryngeal TB coughs, sneezes, speaks, or sings. Droplet nuclei may also be produced by other methods, such as aerosol treatments, sputum induction, bronchoscopy, endotracheal intubation, suctioning, autopsy, and through manipulation of lesions or processing of secretions in the hospital or laboratory.[19] These droplet nuclei, which contain one to three *M. tuberculosis* organisms, are small enough (1–5 μm) to remain airborne for long periods and reach the alveoli within the lungs when inhaled. Tubercle bacilli are not transmitted on inanimate objects such as dishes, clothing, or bedding, and organisms deposited on skin or intact mucosa do not invade tissue.

Several factors influence the likelihood of transmission of *M. tuberculosis,* including the number of organisms expelled into the air, the concentration of organisms in the air determined by the volume of the space and its ventilation, the length of time an exposed person breathes the contaminated air, and presumably the immune status of the exposed individual.[19] Family household contacts, especially children, and persons working or living in an enclosed environment (e.g., hospitals, nursing homes, prisons) with an infected person are at a significantly increased risk for becoming infected. Individuals with impaired cell-mediated immunity, such as HIV-infected persons or transplant patients, are more likely to become infected with *M. tuberculosis* after exposure than persons with normal immune function.[19]

Several techniques are effective in limiting airborne transmission of *M. tuberculosis* by reducing the number of droplet nuclei in a given airspace. Adequate room ventilation with fresh air is very important, especially in the health care setting, in which six or more room-air exchanges per hour are desirable.[19,20] New construction or renovation of existing facilities should be designed so that airborne infection isolation rooms achieve 12 or more room-air exchanges per hour.[20] Ultraviolet irradiation of air in the upper part of the room can also reduce the number of viable airborne tubercle bacilli. All healthcare workers and visitors who enter the room of a patient with TB should wear at least N95 disposable respirators, and the mask should be molded to fit tightly around the nose and mouth.[20] Patients with presumed or confirmed infectious TB should wear a protective mask when being transferred to another area of the institution or to another institution.[20] However, the most important means of reducing transmission of *M. tuberculosis* is by treating the infected patient with effective antituberculosis therapy.

Pathogenesis

LATENT INFECTION VERSUS ACTIVE DISEASE

LATENT INFECTION

A clear distinction should be made between latent infection and active disease (tuberculosis). Latent infection occurs when the tubercle bacilli are inhaled into the body. After inhalation, the droplet nuclei containing *M. tuberculosis* settle into the bronchioles and alveoli of the lungs. Development of infection in the lung is dependent on the inoculum of *M. tuberculosis* organisms inhaled, the virulence of the organism, and the innate immune response of the host.[21–23] In the nonimmune (susceptible) host, the bacilli initially multiply unopposed by normal host defense mechanisms. The organisms are then phagocytized by alveolar macrophages and resident dendritic cells, but they may remain viable, multiplying within the cells for extended periods.[23] After 14 to 21 days of replication, the tubercle bacilli spread via the lymphatic system to the hilar lymph nodes and through the bloodstream to many other organs of the body.

For a photo of spread of *M. tuberculosis* from lymph node to the bloodstream, go to http://thepoint.lww.com/AT10e.

Fortunately, certain organs and tissues in the body, such as the bone marrow, liver, and spleen, are resistant to subsequent multiplication of these bacilli. Organs with high blood flow and Pao_2, such as the apices of the lungs, kidneys, bones, and brain, are particularly favorable for growth of the organisms. The organisms replicate for 2 to 12 weeks until they reach a concentration of 10^3 to 10^4, plateauing coincident with T-cell–mediated immune response.[23] $CD4^+$ T cells produce interferon-γ, which is an essential cytokine for activation of macrophages and mycobacterial killing, as well as other cytokines.[23] At this point, the patient has developed cell-mediated immunity, which can be detected by a reaction to the tuberculin skin test, and bacterial replication is halted.[20]

In persons with intact cell-mediated immunity, activated T cells and macrophages may result in formation of a granuloma, a hallmark of TB, that is thought to represent a physical and immunologic barrier to control the infection and limit dissemination of the bacilli to the surrounding environment.[23] Cells found within the granuloma include $CD4^+$ and $CD8^+$ T cells, B cells, neutrophils, macrophages, multinucleated giant cells, and fibroblasts.[23] The organisms tend to localize in the center of the granuloma, which is frequently necrotic, and the tubercle bacilli may remain viable within the granuloma. In addition, maintenance of the integrity of the granuloma allows for control of bacterial replication and depends on the immune status of the patient.[23] Most patients with latent TB infection are asymptomatic with no radiographic evidence of the infection.[21] In some patients, there may be a healed, calcified lesion on chest radiograph, but bacteriologic studies are negative. A positive tuberculin skin test is usually the only indication that the person has been infected with *M. tuberculosis.* Individuals with latent TB infection are not infectious and thus cannot transmit the organism to other individuals.[19]

ACTIVE DISEASE

In the majority of patients, active TB disease results from reactivation of a previously controlled latent infection, termed reactivation TB. It has been estimated that approximately 10% of individuals who acquire TB infection and do not receive therapy for the latent infection will develop active TB disease, and the risk of developing active disease is greatest during the first 2 years after infection.[19] Rates of reactivation among persons with latent TB infection was 0.10 to 0.16 cases per 100 person-years, but these data were derived in the 1950s.[24] In a population-based tuberculin skin test survey conducted in Florida between 1997 and 2001, the rate of reactivation with latent TB infection but without HIV coinfection was 0.040 to 0.058 cases per 100 person-years.[24] The authors suggested that the decline in reactivation rates may have been attributed to the disappearance of old, healed TB in the population.[24]

Reactivation of TB in persons with latent TB infection is primarily a function of the immune status of the host. The ability of the host to respond to *M. tuberculosis* infection is reduced by certain diseases such as diabetes mellitus, silicosis, chronic renal failure, and diseases or drugs associated with immunosuppression (e.g., HIV infection, anti-tumor necrosis factor-α agents, organ transplantation, corticosteroids, and other immunosuppressive agents). The likelihood of developing active TB disease is greater in persons with these conditions.[19,24,25] HIV-infected persons, especially those with low $CD4^+$ T-cell counts, develop active TB disease rapidly after becoming infected with *M. tuberculosis;* up to 50% of these individuals may develop active disease in the first 2 years after infection.[26] In addition, a person with untreated latent TB infection who acquires HIV infection will progress to active TB disease at an approximate rate of 5% to 10% per year.[27,28] Physical or emotional stress, gastrectomy, intestinal bypass surgery, alcohol abuse, hematologic disease, reticuloendothelial disease, and intravenous drug use are risk factors for development of active disease. The elderly, adolescents, and children younger than 5 years of age are at increased risk of developing active disease.[19,29]

ONLINE CONTENT

For a photo of the pathogenesis of tuberculosis infection, go to http://thepoint.lww.com/AT10e.

Overview of Drug Therapy

Drug treatment is the cornerstone for management of patients with TB. In a patient with active TB, the overall treatment goals are to cure the individual patient and to minimize the transmission of *M. tuberculosis.* The primary goals of chemotherapy are rapid bacterial killing, prevention of emergence of drug resistance, and elimination of persistent tubercle bacilli to prevent relapse.[30] To accomplish these goals, treatment must be tailored to each patient's clinical and social circumstances to ensure adherence to and completion of the treatment regimen (patient-centered care). Effective treatment of TB requires a substantial period (minimum 6 months) of intensive drug therapy with at least two active bactericidal drugs. Optimization of this initial phase of treatment prevents emergence of resistance and ensures the success of TB therapy. Current guidelines recommend four drugs for the initial 8-week treatment phase: isoniazid, rifampin, pyrazinamide, and ethambutol.[30] The drug regimen and duration of the continuation phase depends on the susceptibility of the isolate, host factors, the extent of the disease (pulmonary versus extrapulmonary), and drug tolerability.[30] The shortest duration of therapy is 6 months, but longer durations may be required with drug-resistant strains.[30] Because patients must be treated for a long time, directly observed therapy (DOT) is the preferred core management strategy to ensure adherence.[30–32] In patients with latent TB infection, monotherapy with isoniazid for 6 to 9 months is highly effective.

Clinical Presentation of Active Disease

CASE 65-1

QUESTION 1: H.G. is a 35-year-old Hispanic man who presents with a 4-week history of a productive cough. The cough was initially nonproductive but became productive of yellow sputum after 2 weeks. The patient has been self-medicating with over-the-counter antitussives without relief, but he experienced hemoptysis this morning. He also complains of subjective fevers, chills, night sweats, dyspnea on exertion, fatigue, and an unintentional 15-pound weight loss during the last 2 months. He immigrated to the United States from Mexico when he was 12 years old, but he has not traveled outside the United States for more than a decade. He currently works as a laborer on new home construction projects, and several of his coworkers, who moved to the United States from Mexico within the past year, have similar respiratory symptoms. He is currently married with 3 children. The patient has a 20-pack-year smoking history and drinks alcohol on the weekends but denies illicit drug use.

On physical examination, H.G. is a thin-appearing man in mild respiratory distress. His heart rate is 94 beats/minute, his respiratory rate is 24 breaths/minute, and his temperature is 38.9°C. Bronchial breath sounds are noted in the right upper lobe on chest auscultation, and the chest radiograph shows extensive patchy infiltrates in the right upper lobe. Significant laboratory data include the following:

White blood cell count, 13,200/μL (72% polymorphonuclear leukocytes, 3% bands, 12% lymphocytes, 13% monocytes)
Red blood cell count, $3.7 \times 10^6/\mu$L
Hemoglobin, 11.2 g/dL
Hematocrit, 34%
Platelets, $269 \times 10^3/\mu$L

Serum electrolytes, renal function, and hepatic function are within normal limits. He is 69 inches tall, and his weight is 68 kg. The remainder of his physical examination is unremarkable. What signs and symptoms consistent with active TB disease are present in H.G.?

H.G.'s history of cough (which gradually became productive), fever, night sweats, fatigue, and weight loss are consistent with the classic symptoms of active TB.[19] Cough may be nonproductive early in the course of the illness, but with subsequent inflammation and tissue necrosis, sputum is usually produced and is key to most of the diagnostic studies. The sputum may contain blood (hemoptysis) in patients with advanced cavitary disease, which is particularly worrisome because cavitary lesions harbor high concentrations of organisms and the pulmonary location facilitates airborne transmission. Dyspnea is unusual unless there is extensive disease.[19] Other symptoms of TB may include pleuritic chest pain and general malaise.

In pulmonary TB, the chest radiograph usually reveals patchy or nodular infiltrates in the apical or posterior segments of the upper lobes, but changes may be observed in any segment.

ONLINE CONTENT

For a photo of pulmonary lesion due to *M. tuberculosis* on chest radiograph, go to http://thepoint.lww.com/AT10e.

The patchy infiltrates on H.G.'s chest radiograph is consistent with pulmonary TB. Cavitary lesions may be seen; however, these were absent in this patient. Moderate elevation of the white blood cell count, with an increase in monocytes and eosinophils, and anemia are the most common hematologic manifestations of TB.[19] H.G. had an elevated white blood cell count with an increase in monocytes, and he was also anemic.

Many patients with active pulmonary TB have no acute symptoms, and a lack of symptoms may hinder diagnosis. During a 1-year span, approximately 50% of the cases of active TB without classic symptoms are misdiagnosed.[33] More than one-third of the patients with active TB had no sweats, chills, or malaise, and fewer than 50% were febrile. Cough was evident in 80% of these patients, and only 25% had hemoptysis. Although dullness over the apices of the lungs and posttussive rales are expected in TB, less than one-third of these patients had any abnormal pulmonary signs. Similar findings have been reported in other trials.[34] The lack of specific clinical symptoms underscores the importance of skin testing, sputum smears for AFB, and chest radiographs in suspected TB. Lastly, cases of active TB are often found after routine chest radiographs for other illnesses. Because many of the symptoms of TB also occur in persons with pre-existing pulmonary disease or pneumonia, they may be overlooked and not attributed to TB.

CASE 65-1, QUESTION 2: What risk factors for TB are present in H.G.?

The close contact of H.G. with his coworkers who have similar respiratory symptoms, and their geographical origin from Mexico, are risk factors for TB. In addition, studies have now implicated cigarette smoking as a risk factor for TB.[35–37] In a cohort study conducted in Taiwan, smoking was associated with a twofold increase in the risk of active TB. Furthermore, a significant dose–response relationship was identified for number of cigarettes smoked per day, number of years of smoking, and number of pack-years smoked.[37] Smoking impairs mucociliary clearance, decreases phagocytic pulmonary alveolar macrophage function, decreases intracellular production of tumor necrosis factor-α, and causes iron overload in macrophages.[38–41] These defects in host defense mechanisms increase the risk of active disease after exposure to *M. tuberculosis*.

Diagnosis of Active Tuberculosis

CASE 65-1, QUESTION 3: A tuberculin purified protein derivative (PPD) skin test (5 test units [TU]) is ordered and placed on the volar aspect of his left arm. Sputum is collected and sent for AFB stain, culture, and susceptibility testing. His smear is positive for AFB, and the result of the tuberculin skin test, read at 48 hours, was a palpable induration of 14 mm. What is tuberculin PPD skin testing? How should the result be interpreted in H.G.?

The tuberculin skin test (Mantoux method) has been used as a diagnostic tool for infection with *M. tuberculosis* for decades, but a positive skin test is not necessary for the diagnosis of active TB disease. The test is frequently referred to as the PPD (purified protein derivative) test, which contains a protein prepared from a culture of the tubercle bacilli. The skin test is performed by injecting 0.1 mL of solution containing 5 TU of PPD *intracutaneously* into the volar or dorsal surface of the forearm.[19,42] The injection is made using a one-quarter– to one-half–inch, 27-gauge needle and a tuberculin syringe. The solution should be injected just beneath the surface of the skin, avoiding subcutaneous tissue.[19,43] A discrete, pale elevation of the skin (a wheal) 6 to 10 mm in diameter is produced when the injection is performed correctly. If the first injection was administered improperly, another test dose can be given at once, selecting a site several centimeters away from the original injection site.[19]

If the patient has previously been infected with *M. tuberculosis*, sensitized T cells are recruited to the skin site where they release cytokines.[44] These cytokines induce an induration (raised area) through local vasodilatation, edema, fibrin deposition, and recruitment of other inflammatory cells to the area.[19] Typically, the reaction to the tuberculin protein begins 5 to 6 hours after injection with maximal induration observed at 48 to 72 hours. Therefore, the test should be read between 48 and 72 hours after injection because tests read after 72 hours tend to underestimate the actual size of the induration.[19] For standardization, the diameter of the induration should be measured transversely to the long axis of the forearm and recorded in millimeters.[19] The diameter of the induration should be measured and not the erythematous zone surrounding the induration.

ONLINE CONTENT

For a photo of a positive PPD skin test, go to http://thepoint.lww.com/AT10e.

An induration of at least 5 mm in diameter read 48 to 72 hours after injection is a positive reaction in an individual with a recent history of close contact with a person with active TB, a person with fibrotic changes on chest radiograph consistent with previous TB, organ transplant patients and other immunosuppressed patients (receiving the equivalent of $\geq$15 mg/day of prednisone for $>$1 month), or HIV-infected persons.[19,42,45,46]

An induration of at least 10 mm in diameter is a positive reaction with clinical conditions associated with increased risk for TB, such as diabetes mellitus, silicosis, chronic renal failure, malnutrition, leukemia, lymphoma, gastrectomy, jejunoileal bypass, and weight loss of greater than 10% of ideal body weight.[19,42,46] In addition, an induration of at least 10 mm is considered to be positive in recent immigrants ($<$5 years) from countries with a high prevalence of TB, injection drug users, residents and employees of high-risk congregate settings (e.g., prisons, nursing homes, homeless shelters), health care workers, mycobacteriology laboratory personnel, and children younger than 4 years of age or infants, children, and adolescents exposed to adults in high-risk catgories.[19,42,46] The skin test is also considered positive for persons with an increase in induration diameter of at least 10 mm within a 2-year period.[42,46] For individuals with no risk factors for TB, an induration of at least 15 mm is required for a positive reaction.[42,46]

It is very likely that H.G. has been in close contact with persons with active TB, i.e., his coworkers, even though they have not yet been diagnosed with active TB. When all factors are considered, the PPD of 14 mm should be considered to be positive in H.G.

CASE 65-1, QUESTION 4: Because H.G.'s PPD skin test is positive, does this confirm his diagnosis of active TB? What other laboratory tests may be performed to aid in the diagnosis of TB in H.G.?

H.G.'s positive reaction to 5 TU of PPD alone does not imply active TB disease. It only confirms that he has previously been infected with *M. tuberculosis*. To finalize the diagnosis of active TB disease in H.G., *M. tuberculosis* must be detected and isolated from sputum, gastric aspirate, spinal fluid, urine, or tissue biopsy, depending on the site of infection.[19] As was performed in H.G., the detection of AFB in stained smears examined microscopically should be the first test to confirm the presence of mycobacteria in a clinical specimen. It is the easiest and fastest procedure that can be performed, and allows preliminary confirmation of the diagnosis. Sputum samples for AFB stain and culture are best obtained early in the morning on at least 3 separate days.[31] Smears may be prepared directly from clinical specimens or from concentrated preparations by placing the specimen on a glass slide under a microscope with a Ziehl-Neelsen or fluorochrome stain (not a Gram's stain).[19] However, the sensitivity of sputum smear microscopy is low; 5,000 to 10,000 bacilli/mL of specimen must be present to allow for detection of AFB in stained smears.[19,47] In 2009, 43% of pulmonary TB cases had negative sputum smears.[14] Therefore, a negative AFB smear does not rule out active TB disease, and patients with active TB and negative AFB smears may facilitate transmission of *M. tuberculosis*. An additional limitation of the AFB smear is its inability to differentiate among mycobacterial species and between viable and nonviable organisms. In many areas of the United States, *Mycobacterium avium* complex organisms are commonly isolated from the sputum of patients in whom a diagnosis of TB is highly probable, such as the elderly and patients with HIV infection.[48] This finding has resulted in a marked decrease in the specificity and positive-predictive value of the sputum smear, in some cases to as low as 50%.[49]

During the last 20 years, nucleic acid amplification (NAA) techniques have been developed that enhance and expedite the direct identification of *M. tuberculosis* in clinical specimens. These technologies allow for the amplification of specific target sequences of nucleic acids in *M. tuberculosis* that can be detected by a nucleic acid probe within 24 to 48 hours. Two NAA tests have been approved by the US Food and Drug Administration (FDA) for use in the United States. The enhanced amplified *M. tuberculosis* direct test (Gen-Probe, San Diego, CA) is approved for detection of *M. tuberculosis* in AFB smear-positive and smear-negative respiratory specimens from patients suspected of having TB. The sensitivity of this test is greater than 95% for detecting *M. tuberculosis* in respiratory specimens from patients with AFB-positive smears and 75% to 90% for detecting *M. tuberculosis* in respiratory specimens from patients with AFB-negative smears. The Amplicor *M. tuberculosis* test (Amplicor, Roche Diagnostics, Basel, Switzerland) is approved for the detection of *M. tuberculosis* in AFB smear-positive respiratory specimens from patients suspected of having TB. The sensitivity of the Amplicor test is greater than 95% for detecting *M. tuberculosis* in respiratory specimens from patients with AFB-positive smears and 60% to 70% for detecting *M. tuberculosis* in respiratory specimens from patients with AFB-negative smears. The specificity of the NAA tests is greater than 95% for both AFB smear-positive and smear-negative pulmonary specimens.

Compared with AFB smears, the added benefits of NAA testing include the ability to rapidly confirm the presence of *M. tuberculosis* in a majority of patients with AFB-negative smears and the positive-predictive value of greater than 95% for specimens that are AFB positive in settings in which nontuberculous mycobacteria are common.[50] The NAA tests are cost-effective because they prioritize contact investigations, improve decision making regarding respiratory isolation, and decrease unnecessary TB treatment.[51,52] The most recent guidelines recommend NAA testing on at least one respiratory specimen from a patient with signs and symptoms of pulmonary TB for whom a diagnosis has not been established and for whom the test result would alter case management and infection control activities.[50] If the NAA result and the AFB smear result are positive, the patient is presumed to have TB, and drug treatment should be initiated while awaiting culture results.[50] If the NAA result is positive and the AFB smear result is negative, clinical judgment should be exercised regarding initiating drug therapy, and additional diagnostic testing may be needed. If the NAA result is negative and the AFB smear result is positive, a test for inhibitors should be performed and an additional specimen should be tested with NAA. Sputum specimens (3%–7%) might contain inhibitors that prevent or reduce amplification and cause false-negative NAA results.[50] If the NAA result and the AFB smear result are negative, clinical judgment is recommended in the decision to begin drug therapy because NAA tests lack the sensitivity in AFB smear-negative specimens needed to exclude the diagnosis of TB.[50]

The gold standard for laboratory confirmation of TB is culture.[50] Some patients may have a negative AFB smear, but a sufficient number of organisms may be present to produce a positive culture. Only 10 to 100 organisms are needed for a positive culture.[19] As a result of the limitations of the AFB smear, a positive culture for *M. tuberculosis* is necessary to definitively diagnose TB in H.G. and all patients, even if the AFB smear is positive. In addition, the culture is the only widely available technology that allows for genotyping and susceptibility testing of the isolate.[48] Because *M. tuberculosis* grows slowly (i.e., once every 24 hours), it may take several weeks for the cultures to become positive.[19] Broth-based culture systems such as BACTEC, MGIT, MB/BacT, Septi-Check, and ESP, when combined with DNA probes, can result in positive cultures in 2 weeks or less for sputum smear-positive specimens and in 3 weeks or less for smear-negative specimens.[48]

CASE 65-1, QUESTION 5: Would a negative tuberculin skin test have eliminated the possibility of infection with *M. tuberculosis* in H.G.?

A negative response to 5 TU of PPD in H.G. does not exclude active infection with *M. tuberculosis*. The PPD skin test has a reported false-negative rate of 25% during the initial evaluation of persons with active tuberculosis.[19] This high false-negative rate is attributable to poor nutrition and general health, overwhelming acute illness, or immunosuppression. False-negative results usually occur in persons who have only recently been infected or are anergic. Anergy, the decreased ability to respond to antigens, may be caused by severe debility, old age, immaturity in newborns, high fever, sarcoidosis, corticosteroids, immunosuppressive drugs, hematologic disease, HIV infections, overwhelming TB, recent viral infection, live-virus vaccinations, and malnutrition.[19] If anergy is suspected, control skin tests (*Candida*, mumps, or *Trichophyton*) should also be placed in the contralateral arm. If the control test results are positive and the PPD test result is negative, infection with *M. tuberculosis* is less likely. The Centers for Disease Control and Prevention (CDC) changed its recommendations regarding anergy skin testing in HIV-infected patients with a negative PPD. They cite problems with standardization and reproducibility, a low risk for TB associated with a diagnosis of anergy, and the lack of apparent benefit of therapy for latent TB infection in anergic HIV-infected patients. Therefore, the use of anergy testing in conjunction with PPD is no longer routinely recommended in this population or other patients who are immunocompromised.[45,53,54]

CASE 65-1, QUESTION 6: On further questioning, H.G. informs the medical team that he received the BCG vaccine when he was a child in Mexico. What is the BCG vaccine? What effect does the BCG vaccine have on the results of the tuberculin skin test? What other test may be performed in H.G. for detection of *M. tuberculosis* infection?

BCG, or bacille Calmette-Guérin, is a live vaccine derived from an attenuated strain of *Mycobacterium bovis*, and it is used in many foreign countries with a high prevalence of TB to prevent the disease in persons who are tuberculin negative (no immunity to TB infection). Many different BCG vaccines are available worldwide; they differ with respect to immunogenicity, efficacy, and reactogenicity. Additional factors, such as genetic variability in the vaccinated subjects, the nature of the mycobacteria endemic in different parts of the world, and the use of different doses and different immunization schedules, may contribute to the varied degrees of protection afforded by the vaccine. The protective effect derived from BCG vaccines in case-control studies ranges from 0% to 80%.[55] Two meta-analyses regarding the efficacy of BCG vaccination for preventing TB attempted to calculate estimates of the protective efficacy of the vaccines. The results of the first meta-analysis indicated an 86% protective effect against meningeal and miliary TB in children in 10 randomized clinical trials and a 75% protective effect in 8 case-control studies.[56] In the second meta-analysis, the overall protective effect of BCG vaccines was 51% in 14 clinical studies and 50% in 12 case-control studies.[57] Vaccine efficacy rates were higher in studies in which persons were vaccinated during childhood in contrast with those vaccinated at older ages.[57] Unfortunately, neither study could confirm the efficacy of the vaccine for preventing pulmonary TB.

Prior vaccination with BCG usually results in a false-positive tuberculin skin test in patients who are not infected with *M. tuberculosis,* but skin test reactivity does not correlate with protection against TB.[19,55] There is no reliable method of distinguishing tuberculin reactions caused by BCG vaccination from those caused by natural mycobacterial infections.[19,55] Therefore, it is prudent to consider "positive" reactions to 5 TU of PPD in BCG-vaccinated persons as indicating infection with *M. tuberculosis,* especially among persons from countries with a high prevalence of TB.[19] Even though H.G. received the BCG vaccine when he was a child, the results of the PPD skin test should still be considered positive, especially in light of his symptoms.

In general, BCG vaccine is not recommended for use in the routine prophylaxis of TB in the United States because the risk of exposure to TB in this country is relatively low. However, the BCG vaccine should be considered only for very select persons who meet specific criteria and in consultation with a TB expert. BCG vaccination should only be considered for infants or children who are PPD negative and are continually exposed to a highly infectious, untreated patient with active TB or a child who is continually exposed to a person with infectious pulmonary TB caused by *M. tuberculosis* strains resistant to isoniazid and rifampin.[55] BCG vaccination of health care workers should be considered on an individualized basis in settings in which a high prevalence of patients are infected with MDR-TB, transmission of MDR-TB strains to health care workers and subsequent infection are likely, and comprehensive infection control precautions have been unsuccessful.[55] BCG vaccination is contraindicated in pregnancy and in persons who are immunocompromised (e.g., HIV infection) or persons who are likely to become immunocompromised (e.g., organ transplantation).[55] Adverse reactions to the BCG vaccine vary according to the type, dose, and age of the vaccine. Osteitis, prolonged ulceration at the vaccination site, lupoid reactions, regional suppurative lymphadenitis, disseminated BCG infection, and death have been reported.[55]

An interferon-γ release assay (IGRA) is preferred over the tuberculin skin test for testing persons who have received the BCG vaccine.[58] Three IGRAs are currently approved by the FDA as an aid for diagnosing both latent and active *M. tuberculosis* infection: the QuantiFERON-TB Gold test (Cellestis Limited, Carnegie, Victoria, Australia), the QuantiFERON-TB Gold In-Tube test (Cellestis Limited, Carnegie), and the T-SPOT TB test (Oxford Immunotec, Marlborough, MA). These IGRAs assess response to synthetic peptides that represent specific proteins, early secretory antigenic target-6 (ESAT-6) and culture filtrate protein-10 (CFP-10), that are present in all *M. tuberculosis* strains.[58] In sensitized patients, ESAT-6 and CFP-10 are recognized by the T cells and stimulate release of interferon-γ. The QuantiFERON-TB Gold and QuantiFERON-TB Gold In-Tube tests measure the interferon-γ concentrations released using an enzyme-linked immunosorbent assay. The T-SPOT TB test uses an enzyme-linked immunospot assay (ELISpot) to detect increases in the number of cells that secrete interferon-γ. However, ESAT-6 and CFP-10 are not present in BCG vaccine strains and most nontuberculous mycobacteria; therefore, these IGRAs have improved specificity in BCG-vaccinated persons compared with the tuberculin skin test.[58]

CASE 65-1, QUESTION 7: Should H.G. be tested for HIV infection?

The CDC recommends HIV screening for all patients with TB as well as those persons suspected of having TB disease and contacts of patients with TB.[59] Therefore, H.G. should be tested for HIV. HIV infection is the most important risk factor for progression of latent TB infection to active disease, and progression is more rapid in HIV-infected persons. Unlike other AIDS-related opportunistic infections, CD4 count is not a reliable predictor of increased risk of TB disease in HIV-infected persons.[60] TB may be the first manifestation of HIV infection as patients can have a relatively high CD4 count when TB disease develops.[60]

TREATMENT OF ACTIVE DISEASE

Initial Therapy

CASE 65-1, QUESTION 8: H.G.'s HIV test is negative. How should treatment be initiated in H.G., pending the results of sputum culture and susceptibility testing? Can he transmit *M. tuberculosis* to others during treatment?

There are four basic regimens recommended for the treatment of adult patients with TB caused by organisms that are known or presumed to be drug susceptible (Table 65-2).[30] Because H.G. has not been treated previously for TB, he should be started on isoniazid, rifampin, pyrazinamide, and ethambutol. However, he has been in close contact with persons with symptoms resembling TB who are from an area (Mexico) with a high prevalence of drug-resistant TB. Therefore, H.G. must be closely monitored for resolution of symptoms, results of repeated sputum smears, and culture and susceptibility results, regardless of the initial treatment regimen. Previous guidelines recommended the addition of ethambutol only if the local prevalence of isoniazid-resistant *M. tuberculosis* is at least 4%.[31,61] In the United States, 8.6% of *M. tuberculosis* isolates recovered from patients with no previous history of TB in 2009 were resistant to isoniazid.[14] The prevalence of isoniazid resistance was higher in foreign-born persons (10.1%) compared with US-born persons (6.0%).[14] In patients with a history of previous of TB, 15.2% of strains were resistant to isoniazid in 2009, with 20.5% resistance in foreign-born persons versus 4.5% resistance in US-born persons.[14] Because of the relatively high likelihood of TB caused by isoniazid-resistant organisms, four drugs are necessary in the initial 8-week treatment phase.[30]

The initial four-drug regimen may be administered daily throughout the 8-week period (regimen 1), daily for the first 2 weeks and then twice weekly for 6 weeks (regimen 2), or thrice weekly throughout (regimen 3).[30] On the basis of clinical experience, administration of drugs for 5 days/week is considered to be equivalent to 7 days/week administration and either regimen

TABLE 65-2
Treatment Regimens for Pulmonary Tuberculosis Caused by Drug-Susceptible Organisms

Initial Phase			Continuation Phase				Rating (Evidence)[a]	
Regimen	Drugs	Interval and Doses (Minimal Duration)	Regimen	Drugs	Interval and Doses (Minimal Duration)[b]	# Total Doses (Minimal Duration)	HIV–	HIV+
1	INH RIF PZA EMB	7 d/wk for 56 doses (8 weeks) *OR* 5 d/wk for 40 doses (8 weeks)[c]	1a	INH/RIF	7 d/wk for 126 doses (18 weeks) *OR* 5 d/wk for 90 doses (18 weeks)[c]	182–130 (26 weeks)	A (I)	A (II)
			1b	INH/RIF	Twice weekly for 36 doses (18 weeks)	92–76 (26 weeks)	A (I)	A (II)[d]
			1c[e]	INH/RPT	Once weekly for 18 doses (18 weeks)	74–58 (26 weeks)	B (I)	E (I)
2	INH RIF PZA EMB	7 d/wk for 14 doses (2 weeks) *then* twice weekly for 12 doses (6 weeks) *OR* 5 d/wk for 10 doses (2 weeks)[c] *then* twice weekly for 12 doses (6 weeks)	2a	INF/RIF	Twice weekly for 36 doses (18 weeks)	62–58 (26 weeks)	A (II)	B (II)[d]
			2b[e]	INH/RPT	Once weekly for 18 doses (18 weeks)	44–40 (26 weeks)	B (I)	E (I)
3	INH RIF PZA EMB	3 times weekly for 24 doses (8 weeks)	3a	INH/RIF	3 times weekly for 54 doses (18 weeks)	78 (26 weeks)	B (I)	B (II)
4	INH RIF EMB	7 d/wk for 56 doses (8 weeks) *OR* 5 d/wk for 40 doses (8 weeks)[c]	4a	INH/RIF	7 d/wk for 217 doses (31 weeks) *OR* 5 d/wk for 155 doses (31 weeks)[c]	273–195 (39 weeks)	C (I)	C (II)
			4b	INH/RIF	Twice weekly for 62 doses (31 weeks)	118–102 (39 weeks)	C (I)	C (II)

[a]Definitions of evidence ratings: A, preferred; B, acceptable alternative; C, offer when A and B cannot be given; E, should never be given; I, randomized clinical trial; II, data from clinical trials that were not randomized or were conducted in other populations; III, expert opinion.
[b]Patients with cavitation on initial chest radiograph and positive cultures at completion of 2 months of therapy should receive a 7-month continuation phase (31-weeks; either 217 doses [daily] or 62 doses [twice weekly]).
[c]Five-day-a-week administration is always given by directly observed therapy (DOT). Rating for 5 d/wk regimens is A (III).
[d]Not recommended for HIV-infected patients with $CD4^+$ cell counts <100 cells/μL.
[e]Options 1c and 2b should be used only in HIV-negative patients who have negative sputum smears at the time of completion of 2 months of therapy and who do not have cavitation on the initial chest radiograph.
EMB, ethambutol; INH, isoniazid; PZA, pyrazinamide; RIF, rifampin; RPT, rifapentine.

1 or 2 may be considered "daily." However, 5-day-a-week administration should always be given by DOT.[30] Drug dosages for these recommended regimens are listed in Table 65-3. Therefore, H.G. should be started on isoniazid 300 mg daily, rifampin 600 mg daily, pyrazinamide 1,500 mg daily, and ethambutol 1,200 mg daily. He should also receive pyridoxine 25 mg/day to minimize the risk for development of isoniazid-induced peripheral neuropathy. Ethambutol can be discontinued when the results of susceptibility testing demonstrate that the isolate is susceptible to isoniazid and rifampin. The incidence of streptomycin resistance has increased globally; therefore, streptomycin is no longer recommended as being interchangeable with ethambutol unless the organism is known to be susceptible to the drug or the patient is from an area in which streptomycin resistance is unlikely.[30]

Fixed-dose combinations of drugs have been advocated to ensure maximum adherence to the prescribed regimen, especially during the critical initial treatment phase. There are two fixed-dose combination preparations available in the United States: Rifamate, which contains isoniazid 150 mg and rifampin 300 mg per capsule, and Rifater, which contains isoniazid 50 mg, rifampin 120 mg, and pyrazinamide 300 mg per tablet. These formulations are a means of minimizing inadvertent monotherapy, especially when DOT is not possible, and they may decrease the risk of acquired drug resistance while reducing the number of capsules or tablets that must be ingested each day.[30] Recently, the safety and efficacy of a four-drug fixed-dose combination regimen was compared with each drug administered separately in patients with pulmonary TB.[62] The combination tablet contained isoniazid 75 mg, rifampin 150 mg, pyrazinamide 400 mg, and ethambutol 275 mg, and two to five tablets were ingested per day based on body weight. The number of patients who were culture negative at 18 and 24 months was similar between the treatment groups, in addition to the number of treatment failures, relapses, and death, and the four-drug fixed-dose combination was noninferior to each drug administered separately.[62] It should be noted that there was no difference in outcomes based on HIV status, but less than 7% of the study subjects were HIV positive.[62]

The high risk of transmission of *M. tuberculosis* to other persons mandates that hospitalized persons with suspected or confirmed infectious TB be placed in respiratory isolation until they are determined not to have TB, they are discharged from the hospital, or they are confirmed to be noninfectious.[31] Based on H.G.'s subjective and objective findings, he should be placed in respiratory isolation. H.G.'s symptoms of TB should improve within the first 4 weeks. He would be considered to be noninfectious when he is receiving effective drug therapy, is improving clinically, and has had negative results for three consecutive sputum AFB smears collected on different days.[31] Patients who have responded clinically may be discharged to home despite positive smears if their household contacts have already been exposed and these contacts are not at increased risk of TB (e.g., infants,

TABLE 65-3
Drugs Used in the Treatment of Tuberculosis in Adults and Children

Drug	Dosing (Maximum Dose)	Primary Side Effects	Dose Adjustment in Renal Impairment	Comments
First-Line Agents				
Isoniazid	Adults: 5 mg/kg (300 mg) daily; 15 mg/kg (900 mg) once, twice, or thrice weekly Children: 10–15 mg/kg (300 mg) daily; 20–30 mg/kg (900 mg) twice weekly	Increased aminotransferases (asymptomatic), clinical hepatitis, peripheral neuropathy, CNS effects, lupuslike syndrome, hypersensitivity reactions	No	Peripheral neuropathy preventable with pyridoxine 10–25 mg; ↑ serum level of phenytoin. Hepatitis more common in older patients and alcoholics.
Rifampin	Adults: 10 mg/kg (600 mg) once daily, twice weekly, or thrice weekly Children: 10–20 mg/kg (600 mg) once daily or twice weekly	Pruritus, rash, hepatotoxicity, GI (nausea, anorexia, abdominal pain), flulike syndrome, thrombocytopenia, renal failure	No	Orange-red discoloration of body secretions (sweat, saliva, tears, urine). Drug interactions due to induction of hepatic microsomal enzymes (warfarin, antiretroviral agents, corticosteroids, diazepam, lorazepam, triazolam, quinidine, oral contraceptives, methadone, sulfonylureas).
Rifabutin	Adults: 5 mg/kg (300 mg) once daily, twice weekly, or thrice weekly Children: unknown	Neutropenia, uveitis, GI symptoms, polyarthralgias, hepatotoxicity, rash	No	Orange-red discoloration of body secretions (sweat, saliva, tears, urine). Weaker inducer of hepatic microsomal enzymes than rifampin.
Rifapentine	Adults: 10 mg/kg (600 mg) once weekly during continuation phase Children: not approved	Similar to rifampin	Unknown	Drug interactions due to induction of hepatic microsomal enzymes (see rifampin).
Pyrazinamide	Adults: 40–55 kg: 1 g daily, 2 g twice weekly, 1.5 g thrice weekly; 56–75 kg: 1.5 g daily, 3 g twice weekly, 2.5 g thrice weekly; 76–90 kg: 2 g daily, 4 g twice weekly, 3 g thrice weekly Children: 15–30 mg/kg (2 g) daily; 50 mg/kg (2 g) twice weekly	Hepatotoxicity, nausea, anorexia, polyarthralgias, rash, hyperuricemia, dermatitis	Yes	Monitor aminotransferases monthly.
Ethambutol	Adults: 40–55 kg: 800 mg daily, 2 g twice weekly, 1.2 g thrice weekly; 56–75 kg: 1.2 g daily, 2.8 g twice weekly, 2 g thrice weekly; 76–90 kg:1.6 g daily, 4 g twice weekly, 2.4 g thrice weekly Children: 15–20 mg/kg (1 g) daily; 50 mg/kg (2.5 g) twice weekly	Optic neuritis, skin rash, drug fever	Yes	Routine vision tests recommended; 50% excreted unchanged in urine.
Second-Line Agents				
Cycloserine	Adults: 10–15 mg/kg/d (1 g), usually 500–750 mg/d in two divided doses Children: 10–15 mg/kg/d (1 g)	CNS toxicity (psychosis, seizures), headache, tremor, fever, skin rashes	Yes	May exacerbate seizure disorders or mental illness. Some toxicity preventable by pyridoxine (100–200 mg/d). Monitor serum concentrations (peak 20–35 mcg/mL desirable).
Ethionamide	Adults: 15–20 mg/kg/d (1 g), usually 500–750 mg/d in one daily dose or two divided doses Children: 15–20 mg/kg/d (1 g)	GI effects (metallic taste, nausea, vomiting, anorexia, abdominal pain), hepatotoxicity, neurotoxicity, endocrine effects (alopecia, gynecomastia, impotence, hypothyroidism), difficulty in diabetes management	Yes	Must be given with meals and antacids. Monitor aminotransferases and thyroid-stimulating hormone monthly.

(continued)

Chapter 65

Tuberculosis

TABLE 65-3
Drugs Used in the Treatment of Tuberculosis in Adults and Children (*Continued*)

Drug	Dosing (Maximum Dose)	Primary Side Effects	Dose Adjustment in Renal Impairment	Comments
Second-Line Agents (*Continued*)				
Streptomycin	Adults: 15 mg/kg/d (1 g); ≥60 years, 10 mg/kg/d (750 mg) Children: 20–40 mg/kg/d (1 g)	Vestibular or auditory dysfunction of eighth cranial nerve, renal dysfunction, skin rashes, neuromuscular blockade	Yes	Audiometric and neurologic examinations recommended; 60%–80% excreted unchanged in urine. Monitor renal function.
Amikacin	Adults: 15 mg/kg/d (1 g); ≥60 years, 10 mg/kg/d (750 mg) Children: 15–30 mg/kg/d (1 g)	Ototoxicity, nephrotoxicity	Yes	Less vestibular toxicity than streptomycin. Monitoring similar to streptomycin.
Capreomycin	Adults: 15 mg/kg/d (1 g); ≥60 years, 10 mg/kg/d (750 mg) Children: 15–30 mg/kg/d (1 g) as single dose or twice-weekly dose	Nephrotoxicity, ototoxicity	Yes	Monitoring similar to streptomycin.
p-Aminosalicylic acid (PAS)	Adults: 8–12 g/d in two to three doses Children: 200–300 mg/kg/d in two to four divided doses	GI intolerance, hepatotoxicity, malabsorption syndrome, hypothyroidism	Yes	Liver enzymes and thyroid function should be monitored.
Levofloxacin	Adults: 500 to 1,000 mg/d	Nausea, diarrhea, abdominal pain, anorexia, headache, dizziness, QT prolongation, tendon pain or rupture	Yes	Do not give with divalent or trivalent cations (aluminum, magnesium, iron, etc.).
Moxifloxacin	Adults: 400 mg/d	Nausea, diarrhea, abdominal pain, anorexia, headache, dizziness, QT prolongation, tendon pain or rupture	No	See levofloxacin.

CNS, central nervous system; GI, gastrointestinal.

HIV-positive and immunosuppressed persons). In addition, patients discharged to home with positive smears must agree not to have contact with other susceptible persons.[31]

Fluoroquinolones as Initial Therapy

Interest in fluoroquinolones for the treatment of TB dates back more than 25 years with a report describing the use of ofloxacin in 19 patients with chronic, drug-resistant TB disease.[63] In another study from India, 92% to 98% of patients with newly diagnosed pulmonary TB had negative sputum cultures after 2 months of an ofloxacin-containing regimen.[64] However, this study did not have a standard control regimen for comparison. Several fluoroquinolones possess in vitro activity against *M. tuberculosis.* The most potent activity has been reported with moxifloxacin and gatifloxacin; minimum inhibitory concentrations for these agents are fourfold to eightfold lower than for levofloxacin.[65] In murine models of TB, moxifloxacin, in combination with rifampin and pyrazinamide, has been shown to reduce the time to negative lung cultures by up to 2 months and produce stable cure compared with isoniazid, rifampin, and pyrazinamide.[66,67] In mice treated for 4 months, no relapses occurred in the moxifloxacin-containing regimen.[67]

In humans, moxifloxacin was compared with ethambutol in the first 2 months of treatment in adults with smear-positive pulmonary TB.[68] Seventy-four percent of patients had cavitation on chest radiograph, and 22% of patients were infected with HIV. Patients were randomly assigned to receive moxifloxacin 400 mg daily or ethambutol (based on body weight), and all patients received isoniazid, rifampin, and pyrazinamide. Patients receiving moxifloxacin were more likely to have negative sputum cultures at 4 weeks and at 6 weeks, but the 2-month conversion rates were equal in each group.[68] Relapse rates were not evaluated in this study. Nausea was reported more frequently in the moxifloxacin group, but similar proportions of patients in each group completed study treatment.[68] Two additional studies of other fluoroquinolones reported earlier sputum conversion, but there was no difference in the rate of negative cultures at 2 months.[69,70] However, in a recent study conducted in Brazil, sputum culture conversion at 8 weeks was significantly greater in patients treated with moxifloxacin when compared with ethambutol (80% versus 63%).[71] Culture conversion rates were also significantly higher in the moxifloxacin group at weeks 1, 2, 3, and 4, and the median time to consistently negative cultures was 35.0 days in the moxifloxacin group and 48.5 days in the ethambutol group.[71] However, only less than 4% of patients were infected with HIV.[71]

Moxifloxacin has also been compared with isoniazid during the intensive phase of treatment of pulmonary TB.[72] In this study, 76% of patients had cavitation on baseline chest radiographs and 11% were infected with HIV. Patients were randomly assigned to receive moxifloxacin 400 mg or isoniazid 300 mg daily, and all patients received rifampin, pyrazinamide, and ethambutol.[72] After 8 weeks, negative sputum cultures were observed in 60.4% of the patients in the moxifloxacin group and 54.9% of patients in the isoniazid group, but this difference was not statistically significant.[72]

Despite the reported efficacy of the fluoroquinolones in the treatment of TB, clinicians must be cognizant of the potential for development of resistance to this important drug class. Fluoroquinolone resistance in *M. tuberculosis* has been described, occurring more frequently in multidrug-resistant isolates.[73] In addition, fluoroquinolones are the most commonly prescribed antibiotic class in the United States, and outpatient exposure to a fluoroquinolone for infections other than TB could be a potential risk factor for TB resistance in a patient who becomes infected with *M. tuberculosis*. In a recent study evaluating risk factors for fluoroquinolone-resistant *M. tuberculosis*, investigators identified newly diagnosed patients with culture-confirmed TB in a Medicaid population.[74] Of the 640 patients included in the study, 116 (18%) patients had fluoroquinolone exposure within the 12 months before diagnosis with TB, and 16 (2.5%) patients were infected with *M. tuberculosis* strains that were fluoroquinolone-resistant.[74] Fifty-four patients received more than 10 days of fluoroquinolone exposure, and 7 (13%) patients had fluoroquinolone-resistant strains of *M. tuberculosis*.[74] The study found that receipt of a fluoroquinolone for more than 10 days, occurring more than 60 days before diagnosis of TB, was associated with the highest risk for fluoroquinolone resistance.[74] Therefore, judicious use of fluoroquinolones, especially in patients at risk for infection with TB, is mandatory to maintain the utility of fluoroquinolones in the treatment of TB.

Susceptibility Testing

Drug susceptibility testing is essential to ensure proper treatment of patients with active disease and should be performed on the initial isolate of *M. tuberculosis* from all patients.[19] Susceptibility testing should also be performed if cultures remain positive after 3 months of therapy or if negative cultures become positive after some period. Traditionally, susceptibility testing is performed by attempting to grow the organism on solid or in liquid media containing the drug. The agar proportion method allows for quantitation of the proportion of organisms that is resistant to a given drug, which is expressed as a percentage of the total organism population tested.[19] A drug will not be useful for therapy if 1% or more of the total population are resistant to the drug. Unfortunately, susceptibility results may not be available for 6 to 8 weeks using the agar proportion method and for 4 to 5 weeks with liquid culture methods because of the slow growth of the organism and the need to isolate the pathogen before susceptibility testing can be performed.[19]

To expedite reporting of drug susceptibility, molecular drug resistance tests have been developed to detect mutations in the chromosomal sequence encoding for resistance to a specific drug. For example, mutations in the *rpoB* gene block the activity of rifampin by preventing the drug from binding to RNA polymerase, and approximately 95% of rifampin-resistant *M. tuberculosis* carry this mutation.[75] The molecular drug resistance test amplifies the target genetic sequence using polymerase chain reaction, and a second assay, such as DNA sequencing and hybridization assays, is used to determine whether the sequence contains the mutation associated with drug resistance. If a mutation is detected, the organism is considered to be drug-resistant, but the organism is presumed to be drug-susceptible if a mutation is not detected. These molecular tests can reliably detect the presence of mutations within 1 to 2 days, which may result in earlier initiation of effective therapy, shorter durations of infectivity, and reduced spread of TB.

Kits for detecting mutations associated with rifampin resistance include GenoType MTBDR(*plus*) and INNO-LiPA Rif.TB. Compared with culture-based drug resistance tests, the sensitivity and specificity of the MTBDR(*plus*) line-probe assay was 98% and 99%, respectively, for detecting rifampin resistance in isolates or directly from clinical specimens.[76,77] The sensitivity of the INNO-LiPA Rif.TB assay ranged from 80% to 100% and the specificity was 100% for detecting rifampin resistance directly from clinical specimens.[76,77] Molecular beacons are hybridization probes that use fluorescent-labeled, hairpin-shaped DNA probes with a fluorophore adjacent to a molecule that prevents fluorescence.[32] Using a real-time polymerase chain reaction assay, fluorescence occurs if the amplified PCR products have the wild-type gene sequence, but fluorescence is not detected if mutations are present in the target sequence. These tests have high sensitivity (96%–97%) and specificity (99%–100%) for rifampin resistance in clinical specimens.[78] Molecular drug resistance tests for other antitubercular drugs are not fully developed compared with tests for rifampin resistance. For detecting mutations associated with isoniazid resistance, the specificity of the MTBDR(*plus*) assay was 100%, but the sensitivity ranged from 57% to 100% (pooled sensitivity 85%).[78] However, rifampin resistance is a reliable surrogate for MDR-TB in the United States because isolated rifampin resistance is uncommon.

CASE 65-1, QUESTION 9: Is H.G. a risk to the community and does anyone need to know?

Yes! Each case of active TB disease must be reported to the local, state, or both public health departments.[19,31,79] This not only results in optimal therapy by monitoring adherence to therapy, but it also ensures that contact and source-case investigations will be performed. All individuals who have been in close contact to H.G. should be evaluated for latent TB infection or active disease. Considering their close contact to H.G. and his coworkers, his family members should be evaluated. Reporting of cases also permits record-keeping and surveillance to determine whether public health TB control efforts are achieving their goal of preventing the spread of TB.[31,79]

Continuation Therapy

REGIMENS

CASE 65-1, QUESTION 10: Four weeks later, H.G.'s initial sputum cultures were reported to be positive for *M. tuberculosis*. Drug susceptibility testing to isoniazid and rifampin revealed susceptibility to both agents. What drug regimen should be used for continued treatment of H.G.? How long should treatment be continued?

Successful treatment of uncomplicated TB can now be completed in 6 months (26 weeks) if isoniazid, rifampin, pyrazinamide, and ethambutol are used for the first 2 months (8 weeks) and if patient adherence to the regimen and the organism susceptibility can be assured.[30] Therefore, after 8 weeks of DOT with isoniazid, rifampin, pyrazinamide, and ethambutol, H.G.'s regimen may be streamlined to isoniazid and rifampin daily (5 days or 7 days per week) or two to three times per week under continued DOT for an additional 18 weeks (Table 65-2). Because H.G. is HIV-negative and cavitary lesions were not present on his chest radiograph, he may also be a candidate for once-weekly administration of isoniazid and rifapentine, as long as his sputum AFB smear is negative after completing the initial 8 weeks of therapy.[30]

The effectiveness of a primarily twice-weekly treatment regimen has been demonstrated in both pulmonary and extrapulmonary TB.[80] The regimen consisted of isoniazid 300 mg, rifampin 600 mg, pyrazinamide 1.5 to 2.5 g, and streptomycin 750 to 1,000 mg intramuscularly daily for 2 weeks, followed by the same drugs twice weekly at higher doses (except rifampin) for an additional 6 weeks. The regimen was then reduced to isoniazid and rifampin twice weekly for the remaining 16 weeks (4 months). All doses were administered by DOT. Three months after beginning therapy, 75% of all patients studied had negative sputum cultures, and all patients were culture negative at 20 weeks.[80] A 1.6% relapse rate (two patients) and only minor adverse effects were reported. Another important feature of this regimen is that it is highly cost-effective. Among the 6- and 9-month regimens, it is the second lowest in cost, primarily because of the least number of patient–health care worker encounters (62 directly observed doses).

If pyrazinamide cannot be included in the initial regimen, therapy should be initiated with isoniazid, rifampin, and ethambutol for the first 8 weeks. Therapy should be continued with isoniazid and rifampin for 31 weeks given either daily or twice weekly.[30] If drugs other than isoniazid and rifampin are used in the initial phase, treatment must be continued for 18 to 24 months.[61]

Twice-weekly administration of isoniazid (900 mg) and rifampin (600 mg) is recommended for H.G. because this approach requires fewer doses and should result in substantial cost savings.[30,80] In addition, the relapse rates for the twice- and thrice-weekly isoniazid and rifampin continuation regimens are significantly lower than the once-weekly regimen of isoniazid and rifapentine 600 mg.[81,82] Five characteristics were associated with increased relapse risk in the isoniazid and rifapentine group: sputum culture positive at 2 months; cavitation on chest radiograph; underweight; bilateral pulmonary involvement; non-Hispanic Caucasian race.[82] A potential explanation for these results is the high protein binding of rifapentine (97%). A study evaluated the safety and tolerability of rifapentine 600 mg, 900 mg, and 1,200 mg once weekly (with isoniazid 15 mg/kg) in 150 HIV-negative patients.[83] A trend toward more adverse events was observed in the 1,200-mg treatment arm ($p = 0.051$), but the 900-mg dose was well tolerated.[83] However, relapse rates for the higher-dose weekly rifapentine regimens with isoniazid are unknown. A subsequent study demonstrated that low plasma concentrations of isoniazid were associated with failure or relapse with once-weekly isoniazid and rifapentine.[84] Two patients who relapsed with *M. tuberculosis* monoresistant to rifamycin had very low isoniazid concentrations. Rapid acetylation status was a risk factor in those patients who failed or relapsed.[84] Rifamycin pharmacokinetics did not influence patient outcomes, however.[84]

Treatment with isoniazid and rifampin should be continued for a minimum duration of 26 weeks. A full course of therapy can be more accurately determined by the total number of doses ingested, not solely by the duration of therapy.[30] Thus, 26 weeks is the minimum duration of treatment and accurately indicates the amount of time the drugs are given only if there are no interruptions in drug administration.[30] Pyridoxine 10 to 25 mg/day should be continued throughout the treatment period. If H.G. is symptomatic or smear or culture is positive after 3 months of therapy, he should be re-evaluated for possible nonadherence with his therapy or infection with drug-resistant organisms. Evaluation should include a second culture and a second susceptibility test, consideration of DOT (if not already instituted), and consultation with experts in the treatment of TB.[31]

Directly Observed Therapy

CASE 65-1, QUESTION 11: What is directly observed therapy, and why is it important for H.G. to be treated by directly observed therapy?

Directly observed therapy is the practice of a health care provider or other responsible person observing as the patient ingests and swallows the TB medications. DOT is the preferred core management strategy for *all* patients with TB.[30–32] The purpose of DOT is to ensure adherence to TB therapy. DOT not only ensures completion of therapy, but it may also reduce the risk of developing drug resistance. By improving these two factors, it also reduces the risk of transmission of TB to the community. DOT can be administered with daily or two- to three-times-per-week regimens. It can be administered to patients in the office or clinic setting, or it can be given at the patient's home, school, or work.[30,61] Often, enablers or incentives, such as food, clothing, or transportation, are used to improve adherence to DOT. A comprehensive review of DOT-related articles by a consensus panel of public health experts found that the completion rate of TB therapy exceeds 90% when DOT, as recommended by the CDC, is used along with enablers.[32,85] A study from San Francisco, California, found that culture-positive patients treated for active pulmonary TB with DOT had significantly higher cure rates (97.8% vs. 88.6%; $p < 0.002$) and lower TB-related mortality (0% vs. 5.5%; $p = 0.002$) compared with patients treated using self-administered therapy.[86] Rates of treatment failure and relapse were similar between the two groups.[86] Although DOT is recommended for all patients, public health departments may not be able to provide DOT for all patients because of the associated costs. The initial cost of DOT is greater than self-administered therapy; however, when costs of relapse and failure are included in a cost-effectiveness analysis, DOT is significantly less expensive than self-administered therapy.[87] When drug resistance develops (in those instances in which DOT is not used), the cost of salvage therapy increases to $180,000.00 per patient.[88] It is, therefore, widely accepted that patients with TB should receive DOT.[87,89]

Multiple-Drug Therapy

CASE 65-1, QUESTION 12: Why are multiple drugs recommended for the treatment of active TB disease? What is the role of each drug in the treatment of active TB?

The key to treating active TB disease is multiple-drug therapy for a period sufficient to kill the organisms and to prevent development of resistant strains of *M. tuberculosis*. Most cavitary lesions contain a concentration of 10^9 to 10^{12} organisms, and the frequency of mutations that confer resistance to a single drug is approximately 10^{-6} for isoniazid and streptomycin, 10^{-8} for rifampin, and 10^{-5} for ethambutol.[30] Considering the inoculum of organisms involved, patients with active TB disease likely harbor organisms with random mutations that confer drug resistance to a given drug. If a single drug is given, it would reduce the number of drug-susceptible organisms but allow the drug-resistant organisms to replicate. By using multiple-drug therapy, the likelihood of encountering organisms with mutations to multiple drugs is reduced. For example, the frequency of concurrent mutations to isoniazid and rifampin would be 10^{-14} (10^{-6} for isoniazid and 10^{-8} for rifampin), making simultaneous resistance to both drugs an unlikely event in an untreated patient.[30] Therefore, monotherapy should never be used in the treatment of active TB disease.[30,88]

Multiple-drug therapy also serves to sterilize the sputum and lesions as quickly as possible. The drugs available for the treatment of TB vary in their ability to accomplish this task.[30] Drugs effective against tubercle bacilli can be divided into first-line and second-line agents (Table 65-3). The foundation of treatment should be with first-line agents, such as isoniazid, rifampin, pyrazinamide, and ethambutol. Of the various agents, isoniazid has the most bactericidal activity versus rapidly multiplying *M. tuberculosis* during the initial phase of therapy (early bactericidal activity), followed by ethambutol, rifampin, and streptomycin.[90–92] Drugs that have potent early bactericidal activity more rapidly decrease the infectiousness of the patient and reduce the likelihood of developing resistance.[30] Pyrazinamide has weak early bactericidal activity during the first 2 weeks of therapy and is less effective at preventing emergence of drug resistance than isoniazid, rifampin, and ethambutol.[30,90,93] Therefore, pyrazinamide should not be combined with only one other agent when treating active TB disease. Rifampin also has activity against intracellular organisms that are usually dormant but undergo periods of active growth. This ability to penetrate and destroy the persistent intracellular organisms makes rifampin extremely valuable in short-course chemotherapy regimens.[94]

Pyrazinamide is most effective against tubercle bacilli in the acidic environment within the macrophage or areas of tissue necrosis. In addition, it is most effective in sterilizing lesions when used in the first 2 months of treatment, but it does not offer substantial sterilizing activity after 2 months. Pyrazinamide should be considered an essential component of short-course regimens.[30,61]

Ethambutol is bacteriostatic at low doses and bactericidal at higher doses. It is moderately effective against the fast-growing bacilli. It has little sterilizing activity and is primarily used to prevent the emergence of drug-resistant organisms.[61]

Streptomycin is bactericidal against the rapidly multiplying extracellular organisms and is effective when given daily for 2 months followed by twice- or thrice-weekly administration thereafter. In the past, streptomycin was administered by intramuscular injection, but these intramuscular injections were painful. Therefore, although it is not labeled for intravenous use, streptomycin may be given in 50 to 100 mL of 5% dextrose in water or normal saline and infused for 30 to 60 minutes.[95] Also, as with all aminoglycosides, streptomycin can cause ototoxicity and nephrotoxicity.[61,94]

The other drugs used in the treatment of TB (capreomycin, amikacin, cycloserine, ethionamide, *p*-aminosalicylic acid) are usually reserved for cases involving drug-resistant organisms, treatment failures, drug toxicity, or patient intolerance to the other agents. Their use is discussed later in the chapter.

Monitoring Drug Therapy

CASE 65-1, QUESTION 13: What subjective and objective findings should be followed to ensure therapeutic efficacy and to minimize drug toxicity? Should H.G. be followed closely after completion of his treatment regimen?

H.G. should be questioned about the occurrence of adverse reactions associated with his therapy (Table 65-3). Specifically, he should be asked about anorexia, nausea, vomiting, or abdominal pain, which may be an indication of possible hepatitis secondary to isoniazid, rifampin, or pyrazinamide. He should be questioned about numbness and tingling in his extremities; however, isoniazid-induced peripheral neuropathy should not be a problem in H.G. because he is also taking pyridoxine, which should prevent this adverse effect. H.G. also should be examined for, and questioned about, petechiae or bruises, because thrombocytopenia occurs occasionally with intermittent rifampin therapy. This effect purportedly occurs more frequently with intermittent rifampin therapy, but it is rare at the currently recommended intermittent rifampin dose of 10 mg/kg/day (~600 mg).[61]

In a study comparing 6-month versus 9-month antituberculosis therapies of mostly isoniazid and rifampin, the incidence of side effects was similar between the two groups. Adverse effects occurred in 7.7% of patients in the 6-month arm compared with 6.4% in the 9-month arm, a difference that was not statistically significant.[96] Hepatic abnormalities occurred in 1.6% of patients in the 6-month regimen, a nonsignificant difference from patients in the 9-month regimens (1.2%). Hematologic events were rare at 0.2% and 0.0% in the 6-month and 9-month groups, respectively. Other reported effects, gastrointestinal (GI) problems, rash, and arthralgias, were minor and infrequent in both regimens.[96]

OBJECTIVE SIGNS

A pretreatment complete blood count, platelet count, blood urea nitrogen, hepatic enzymes (serum aminotransferases), bilirubin, and serum uric acid should be evaluated. Baseline visual examination should also be considered for patients receiving ethambutol. These tests are performed to detect any abnormality that may complicate or necessitate modification of the prescribed regimen. These tests should be repeated if the patient experiences any evidence of drug toxicity or has abnormalities at baseline.[30,61]

H.G. is 35 years of age and at increased risk for development of drug-induced hepatotoxicity. Isoniazid can cause asymptomatic increases in serum transaminases as well as hepatitis.[30] Pyrazinamide has also been associated with hepatotoxicity, but the incidence is less common at doses of 25 mg/kg/day or less. Transient asymptomatic hyperbilirubinemia and cholestatic hepatitis can occur in patients receiving rifampin.[30] Therefore, it is important that that patient be instructed about possible symptoms of hepatotoxicity, primarily nausea, vomiting, abdominal pain, anorexia, and jaundice. Monthly serum liver function tests (LFTs) are no longer recommended because they are costly; transient, asymptomatic elevations in LFTs may occur, which could result in unnecessary discontinuation of optimal therapy. The CDC recommends that medical personnel question patients about symptoms once monthly.[61]

Sputum cultures and smears for AFB should be ordered every 2 to 4 weeks initially and then monthly after the sputum cultures become negative. With appropriate therapy, sputum cultures should become negative in more than 85% of patients after 2 months. At this point, they will usually need only one more sputum smear and culture at the completion of therapy. Radiologic examination (chest radiographs) is not as important as sputum examination, but it may be useful at the completion of therapy to serve as a comparison for any future films.

Patients who are culture-positive at 2 months need to be carefully re-examined. Drug susceptibility testing should be performed to rule out acquired drug resistance, and special attention should be given to drug adherence (i.e., DOT should be used). If drug resistance is demonstrated, the regimen should be modified as needed. Sputum cultures should also be obtained monthly until negativity is achieved.[61]

As was the case for H.G., weight loss and nutritional depletion are common in patients with active TB disease. In a large TB treatment study, 7.1% of patients experienced relapse, with relapse greatest in patients who were underweight at diagnosis or with a body mass index less than 18.5 kg/m^2.[97] In those patients underweight at diagnosis (defined as $\geq$10% below ideal body weight), weight gain of 5% or less between diagnosis and completion of 2 months of therapy was independently associated with relapse.[97] In addition, the relapse rate was 50.5% in underweight patients with a cavitary lesion on chest radiograph, positive sputum cultures after 2 months of therapy, and a 5% or less weight gain in the first 2 months of therapy.[97] Therefore, it may be prudent to monitor H.G.'s body weight during the initial 2 months of therapy, and he may need to receive more-intensive therapy or a longer duration of therapy.

Routine follow-up usually is not required after the successful completion of chemotherapy with isoniazid and rifampin. It may be prudent, however to re-examine the patient 6 months after completion of therapy or at the first sign of any symptoms suggestive of active TB. This is especially important in patients who were slow to respond to therapy or who have significant radiologic findings at completion of therapy. These recommendations are only for those patients with organisms fully susceptible to the medications being used.[61]

Patients who are culture negative but have radiographic abnormalities consistent with TB should have an induced sputum or bronchoscopy performed to establish a microbiologic diagnosis and monitored radiographically. Patients with extrapulmonary TB should be evaluated according to the site of involvement.[30,61]

Treatment Failure

CASE 65-1, QUESTION 14: If H.G. does not respond to his currently prescribed treatment regimen, should one more drug be added to his regimen?

No! Adding a single drug to a failing regimen is the most common and devastating prescribing error in TB therapy. This practice is essentially monotherapy because the assumption is that the organisms are resistant to the medications currently being used. Resistance to the new drug will eventually develop, further reducing the patient's chance of cure. At least two, and preferably three, new drugs to which susceptibility can be inferred should be added to lessen the probability of further acquired drug resistance. Empiric retreatment regimens may include a fluoroquinolone, an injectable agent (e.g., streptomycin, amikacin, or capreomycin), and an additional oral agent (e.g., *p*-aminosalicylic acid, cycloserine, or ethionamide).[30] New drug susceptibility testing should be performed and treatment adjusted accordingly.[30,88]

TREATMENT OF LATENT TUBERCULOSIS INFECTION

CASE 65-2

QUESTION 1: J.G., the 32-year-old wife of H.G., and her children are tested to determine whether they have been infected with *M. tuberculosis.* For his wife, the induration from 5 TU of PPD was 12 mm, which is reported as positive. J.G. states that she has never received the BCG vaccine. The children were negative. She does not have any clinical symptoms or radiographic findings suggestive of active TB at this time. Is she at risk of developing active disease? What are the current recommendations for drug therapy for persons with latent TB infection? Should his wife receive treatment?

Because J.G. is a household contact of a person with active TB disease and has a positive tuberculin skin test, she is at great risk of becoming infected and developing active disease.[45,46] During the first year after infection from the source case, a household contact's risk of developing active disease is 2% to 4%, and patients with a positive skin test are at the greatest risk.[61] As with active disease, the tuberculin skin test is usually performed to detect the presence of latent TB infection. However, studies have demonstrated that IGRAs are a more accurate indicator of the presence of latent TB infection than tuberculin skin testing.[98,99] Therefore, many health departments in the United States have adopted IGRAs as screening tests for contact investigations.[100] The majority of people with a negative IGRA after exposure to a person with active TB disease do not have TB infection; however, the immune reaction to TB can take several weeks to develop so the IGRA should be repeated 8 weeks after the last exposure to rule out infection.[100]

Treatment of latent TB infection is effective in preventing active TB disease in persons with positive tuberculin skin tests and in those at risk for reactivation of active TB; therefore, it is *strongly* recommended.[31,45,46] Treatment decreases the population of tubercle bacilli and reduces future morbidity from TB in the groups at high risk for developing active disease. Isoniazid prevents active TB in up to 93% of persons who receive the drug, depending on the duration of therapy and patient adherence to the prescribed regimen.[45] Although debate regarding the issue continues, the benefits of treating latent TB infection outweigh the risks of isoniazid-induced hepatitis because all persons infected with TB are at risk for developing active disease throughout their lifetime.[1,61]

J.G. is infected with *M. tuberculosis,* but she does not currently have active TB disease. Studies in HIV-negative patients suggest that 12 months of isoniazid is more effective than 6 months; however, the maximal benefit of isoniazid is likely achieved by 9 months. Daily isoniazid for 6 months and twice-weekly isoniazid for 6 or 9 months are also recommended treatment options for latent TB infection.[45] However, patient adherence to these isoniazid regimens is very poor. In a population of patients beginning isoniazid treatment for latent TB, only 64% of patients completed at least 6 months of therapy.[101] Younger age, Hispanic ethnicity, and non-US country of birth were associated with greater likelihood of completing therapy.[101] Lower completion rates were associated with homelessness, excess alcohol intake, and experiencing an adverse event.[101] In another study conducted in the United States and Canada, 52.7% patients receiving treatment for latent TB infection failed to complete the prescribed course of therapy.[102] More than 93% of these patients were receiving isoniazid. Risk factors for failing to complete therapy included receipt of a 9-month isoniazid regimen, residence in a congregate setting (nursing home, shelter, jail), injection drug use, and employment at a health care facility.[102] In addition, this study reported that employees at health care facilities were more likely to decline treatment for latent TB infection.[102]

Because of concerns about isoniazid toxicity and abysmal adherence secondary to the relatively long duration of therapy, shorter rifampin-based regimens have been recommended. Rifampin monotherapy daily for 4 months and rifampin plus pyrazinamide daily for 2 months or twice weekly for 2 to 3 months were recommended alternatives to isoniazid therapy.[45] In 2001, however, severe and fatal hepatitis was reported in two patients receiving rifampin and pyrazinamide for latent TB infection.[103] Later in the same year, the CDC reported an additional 21 cases of liver injury associated with the 2-month rifampin and pyrazinamide regimen.[104] Of these 21 cases, 16 patients recovered and 5 patients died of liver failure. The onset of liver injury occurred during the second month of the 2-month course in those who died.[104]

The American Thoracic Society and the CDC, with the endorsement of the Infectious Diseases Society of America, published revised recommendations for the treatment of latent TB infection.[104] For persons not infected with HIV, daily isoniazid therapy for 9 months remains the preferred regimen, and 4 months of daily rifampin is an acceptable alternative. The 2-month rifampin and pyrazinamide regimen should be used with caution, if at all, especially in patients receiving medications associated with liver injury or those with alcoholism. No more than a 2-week supply of isoniazid and pyrazinamide should be dispensed at a time to facilitate periodic clinical assessments of the patient. Serum aminotransferases and bilirubin should be measured at baseline, and at 2, 4, and 6 weeks of treatment in patients receiving the rifampin and pyrazinamide regimen.[104]

Daily rifampin for 4 months has been compared with daily isoniazid for 9 months to assess completion of therapy and costs in patients with latent TB infection.[105] For the patients randomly assigned to receive rifampin, 91% took 80% of the doses, and 86% took more than 90% of the doses at 20 weeks.[105] For the patients randomly assigned to receive isoniazid, 76% took 80% of the doses, and only 62% took more than 90% of the doses at 43 weeks.[105] Discontinuation of therapy because of adverse events was more common in the isoniazid group (14%) versus the rifampin group (3%).[105] Another study reported significantly fewer grade 3 to 4 adverse events and hepatitis and significantly higher treatment completion rates with 4 months of rifampin compared with 9 months of isoniazid.[106] Rifampin for 4 months is an effective, safe, and cost-effective strategy to consider when treating latent TB infection in selected populations of patients.[105–109]

In a study of household contacts of patients with newly diagnosed pulmonary TB with a positive PPD, TB rates, adverse events, and adherence to therapy were compared between weekly rifapentine and isoniazid for 12 weeks and daily rifampin and pyrazinamide for 8 weeks.[110] Adherence to therapy was at least 95% in both groups. Four patients experienced active TB disease: three in the rifapentine and isoniazid group and one in the rifampin and pyrazinamide group (not significant).[110] Of the patients in the rifapentine and isoniazid group, 1% experienced hepatotoxicity compared with 10% in the rifampin and pyrazinamide group.[110] Although more data are needed, weekly rifapentine and isoniazid may be an alternative for treatment of latent TB infection.

J.G. should be placed on isoniazid 300 mg/day for at least 6 months and preferably up to 9 months or rifampin for 4 months.[45,104] She should be educated and questioned frequently about the clinical symptoms of hepatitis, such as GI complaints. Pretreatment serum aminotransferases and bilirubin should be assessed to rule out pre-existing liver disease. The American Thoracic Society and the CDC do not recommend routine monitoring of LFTs unless symptoms suggest hepatotoxicity.[61]

ADVERSE DRUG EVENTS

Isoniazid

HEPATOTOXICITY

CASE 65-2, QUESTION 2: After 2 months of isoniazid therapy, J.G. was found to have an aspartate aminotransferase (AST) of 150 international units/L. Discuss the presentation, prognosis, and mechanism of isoniazid-induced hepatitis. What are the risk factors for developing hepatitis? Should isoniazid be discontinued to prevent further liver damage?

Approximately 10% to 20% of patients treated with isoniazid alone for latent TB infection will develop elevated serum aminotransferases, which are generally transient and asymptomatic.[30,111] Most patients with mild, subclinical hepatic damage do not progress to overt hepatitis and recover completely even while continuing isoniazid. In contrast, continuation of isoniazid in patients with symptoms of hepatitis increases the risk of mortality compared with immediate discontinuation.[30] The risk of death from TB, however, is estimated to be 11 times higher than the risk of death from isoniazid hepatotoxicity.[112]

Isoniazid-induced hepatotoxicity generally occurs within weeks to months of initiating therapy; 60% of cases occur in the first 3 months and 80% occur in the first 6 months.[111] Constitutional symptoms may be seen early and may last from days to months. Nausea, vomiting, and abdominal pain are seen in 50% to 75% of patients with severe hepatotoxicity.[111] Jaundice, dark urine, and clay-colored stools may also be seen. Recovery may take weeks after discontinuing isoniazid therapy. The development of isoniazid hepatotoxicity has been linked to several factors, including acetylator phenotype, age, daily alcohol consumption, and concurrent rifampin use. Additionally, women may be at higher risk of death, especially during the postpartum period.[112]

The mechanisms responsible for isoniazid hepatotoxicity remain unclear. Previously, it was thought that rapid acetylators had a greater risk for isoniazid hepatotoxicity than slow acetylators. Rapid acetylators of isoniazid form monoacetylhydrazine, a compound that can cause liver damage, more rapidly than slow acetylators.[113] Rapid acetylators, however, would eliminate monoacetylhydrazine at a faster rate, and this should equalize the risk of toxicity between slow and fast acetylators.[114] One study demonstrated a different incidence of hepatitis between Asian men and women. Because both groups were fast acetylators, this study suggests that hepatitis is associated with factors other than acetylator phenotype.[115] Acetylator status alone does not explain the development of isoniazid hepatotoxicity. Some evidence supports the theory that isoniazid-induced hepatitis is a hypersensitivity reaction; however, many patients tolerate isoniazid on rechallenge, discounting this theory.[116,117]

Age and concurrent daily alcohol ingestion are the most consistent risk factors for isoniazid hepatitis.[61] Progressive liver damage is rare in persons younger than 20 years of age. It occurs in approximately 0.3% of persons between the ages of 20 and 34 years, 1.2% of those between the ages of 35 and 49 years, and 2.3% of persons older than 50 years of age.[61] One prospective cohort study, however, demonstrated a low incidence of isoniazid hepatitis. Of 11,141 patients receiving isoniazid alone for the treatment of latent TB infection, only 11 (0.1% of those starting and 0.15% of those completing therapy) developed clinical hepatitis.[118] Previous studies suggested a higher incidence of clinical hepatitis in patients receiving isoniazid alone, and a meta-analysis of six studies estimated the rate to be 0.6%.[30] However, severe hepatotoxicity may occur with isoniazid treatment of latent TB infection. The CDC reported 17 severe hepatic adverse events with isoniazid in 15 adults and 2 children (ages 11 and 14 years).[119] Five patients, including one child, underwent liver transplantation, and five adults died (including one liver transplant patient).

High-risk patients should be followed with routine monitoring of LFTs. These patients include those who consume alcohol daily, persons older than 35 years of age, those taking other hepatotoxic drugs, those with pre-existing liver disease, intravenous drug users, black and Hispanic women, and all postpartum women. In these high-risk patients, isoniazid should be discontinued if the AST level exceeds three to five times the upper limit of the normal value.[61] Because J.G.'s AST is greater than three times the upper range of the normal value, isoniazid should be discontinued temporarily until the AST returns to normal. At that time, isoniazid should be resumed, and her LFTs rechecked. If the AST increases again, the drug should be discontinued, and J.G. should be followed frequently for development of active TB.

CASE 65-3

QUESTION 1: C.M., a 50-kg, 35-year-old woman, is being treated for active TB disease with isoniazid 1,200 mg and

rifampin 600 mg twice weekly. Is 1,200 mg of isoniazid twice weekly an appropriate dose for a 50-kg patient? What isoniazid side effects, other than hepatotoxicity, should be anticipated?

The usual twice-weekly isoniazid dose is 15 mg/kg, with a maximal dose of 900 mg; therefore, C.M. should be receiving no more than 900 mg rather than 1,200 mg of isoniazid. Although high doses or increased serum concentrations have not been linked with hepatitis, elevated serum isoniazid concentrations have been associated with increased central nervous system (CNS) events, ranging from somnolence to psychosis and seizure. GI complaints are also more commonly observed at doses greater than 20 mg/kg.

PERIPHERAL NEUROPATHY

Although uncommon at the recommended daily and intermittent doses, isoniazid can cause a peripheral neuropathy by interfering with pyridoxine (vitamin B_6) metabolism.[30,45] As many as 20% of patients may experience this problem with isoniazid doses greater than 6 mg/kg/day. Numbness or tingling in the feet or hands are the most common neuropathic symptom. In patients with medical conditions in which neuropathy is common, including diabetes mellitus, alcoholism, HIV infection, malnutrition, and renal failure, supplemental pyridoxine 25 mg/day should be given with isoniazid.[30,45] Women who are pregnant or breastfeeding and persons with seizure disorders should also receive supplemental pyridoxine with isoniazid.[45]

ALLERGIC AND OTHER REACTIONS

Allergic reactions consisting of arthralgias, skin rash, swelling of the tongue, and fever have also been reported. Isoniazid has been associated with arthritic symptoms and systemic lupus erythematosus; approximately 20% of patients receiving isoniazid develop antinuclear antibodies.[30] Other less common reactions reported with isoniazid are dry mouth, epigastric distress, CNS stimulation and depression, psychoses, hemolytic anemia, pyridoxine-responsive anemia, and agranulocytosis.[116]

DRUG INTERACTIONS

Isoniazid is a relatively potent inhibitor of several cytochrome P-450 isoenzymes (CYP2C9, CYP2C19, CYP2E1), but has minimal effects on CYP3A.[30] Isoniazid inhibits the hepatic metabolism of phenytoin and carbamazepine, resulting in increased plasma concentrations of these drugs. Patients receiving either of these two drugs with isoniazid should be observed for signs of phenytoin or carbamazepine toxicity, such as nystagmus, ataxia, headache, nausea, or drowsiness. Plasma phenytoin and carbamazepine concentrations should be monitored periodically so that the doses can be adjusted if necessary. Carbamazepine also may induce isoniazid hepatitis by inducing its metabolism to toxic metabolites.[120] In addition, isoniazid inhibits the metabolism of diazepam and triazolam. It is important to note that rifampin has the exact opposite effect on hepatic metabolism. Rifampin is a stronger inducer than isoniazid and is an inhibitor as documented by the fact that isoniazid–rifampin combination therapy induces the metabolism of diazepam, phenytoin, and other agents metabolized by the cytochrome P-450 system.[121]

Rifampin

FLULIKE SYNDROME

CASE 65-3, QUESTION 2: One month after beginning her twice-weekly DOT regimen, C.M. exhibited symptoms of myalgias, malaise, and anorexia. Laboratory data were normal except for a slightly decreased platelet count. Could C.M.'s symptoms be related to her drug therapy? What adverse reactions other than hepatotoxicity should be anticipated in a patient receiving rifampin?

A flulike syndrome has been reported in about 1% of patients receiving intermittent rifampin administration. This syndrome is rarely seen with usual doses of 600 mg twice weekly, but the incidence increases with twice-weekly doses greater than 900 mg. The incidence also increases if the dosing interval is increased to 1 week or longer.[122,123] Unless the symptoms are severe, discontinuation of the drug is unnecessary. Because C.M. is receiving rifampin 900 mg twice weekly, her dose should be reduced to 600 mg and administered daily until the symptoms subside. The temporary administration of a nonsteroidal anti-inflammatory drug has been used to alleviate the flulike symptoms. Twice-weekly therapy may then be resumed as long as the dose of rifampin dose does not exceed 600 mg.

HEPATOTOXICITY

Rifampin (rifapentine) is associated with a less than 1% rate of hepatotoxicity. Therefore, the risk of drug-induced hepatotoxicity is greater with isoniazid than with rifampin. On occasion, rifampin can cause hepatocellular injury and potentiate hepatotoxicity of other antituberculosis drugs.[111] Although elevations of liver enzymes are seen on occasion, rifampin is more likely to produce cholestasis, as manifested by increases in alkaline phosphatase and hyperbilirubinemia without hepatocellular injury.[111] Elevations of all liver function tests may be seen transiently during the first month of rifampin therapy, but they are usually benign.[30]

THROMBOCYTOPENIA

Thrombocytopenia is more frequently associated with intermittent or interrupted rifampin administration, likely caused by production of immunoglobulin G and immunoglobulin M antibodies to rifampin. These antibodies likely fix complement onto the platelets, resulting in platelet destruction. Hypothetically, intermittent or interrupted rifampin therapy results in increased antibody production, resulting in destruction of platelets. Once thrombocytopenia occurs with rifampin, its subsequent use is contraindicated because the problem will likely recur.[124,125]

MISCELLANEOUS REACTIONS

In addition to the side effects associated with high-dose, intermittent therapy, 3% to 4% of patients taking normal doses of rifampin may experience adverse reactions.[124] The most common of these are nausea, vomiting, fever, and rash. Other reactions to rifampin include the hepatorenal syndrome hemolysis, leukopenia, anemia, and arthralgias as part of a suspected drug-induced lupus syndrome.[30,126] The development of these latter reactions would require discontinuation of the drug.

ACUTE RENAL FAILURE

Acute renal failure has been reported rarely with rifampin.[30] This hypersensitivity reaction may occur with both intermittent and daily administration and may last as long as 12 months.[122] Rifampin should be discontinued, and other drugs (e.g., pyrazinamide and ethambutol) should be given. The dose of ethambutol should be adjusted for renal dysfunction. Both rifampin and isoniazid may, however, be given in normal dosages to patients with pre-existing renal failure.[127,128]

DISCOLORATION OF BODY FLUIDS

Another important characteristic of rifampin relates to its chemical makeup. It is an orange-red crystalline powder that is distributed widely in body fluids. As a result, it can discolor saliva, tears, urine, and sweat.[30] Patients using rifampin should be warned of this effect and cautioned not to use soft contact lenses because of possible discoloration. This effect may also be used to monitor adherence to rifampin therapy.

DRUG INTERACTIONS

Rifampin is a potent inducer of cytochrome P-450 isoenzymes, especially CYP3A4.[30] The rifamycins differ in their ability to induce cytochrome P-450 isoenzymes, in which rifampin is the most potent, rifapentine is intermediate, and rifabutin is the least potent enzyme inducer.[30] Rifampin increases the metabolism of protease inhibitors, non-nucleoside reverse transcriptase inhibitors (NNRTIs), macrolide antibiotics, azole antifungal agents, corticosteroids, oral contraceptives, warfarin, cyclosporine, tacrolimus, theophylline, phenytoin, quinidine, diazepam, propranolol, metoprolol, sulfonylureas, verapamil, nifedipine, diltiazem, enalapril, and simvastatin.[30,121] While the patient is receiving rifampin, it may be necessary to monitor serum concentrations of the aforementioned drugs, when appropriate, or increase their dosages. Also, women who are taking rifampin and oral contraceptives should use an alternative method of birth control. When treating any patient with rifampin, the health care professional should carefully evaluate all concomitant medications for the possibility of drug–drug interactions.

Isoniazid–Rifampin

HEPATOTOXICITY

CASE 65-3, QUESTION 3: Will the combination of isoniazid and rifampin increase the risk of hepatotoxicity in C.M. to a greater extent than either drug alone?

Some initial evidence suggested that the concomitant use of isoniazid and rifampin was associated with a greater incidence of hepatotoxicity. The mechanism was thought to be attributable to rifampin induction of the metabolism of isoniazid to either monoacetylhydrazine or to other hepatotoxic products of hydrolysis. Steele et al.[117] performed a meta-analysis reviewing the incidence of hepatitis using regimens that contained isoniazid without rifampin, rifampin without isoniazid, and regimens containing both drugs. They found the incidence of clinical hepatitis was greater in regimens containing both isoniazid and rifampin (2.7%) versus regimens of isoniazid alone (1.6%), but this effect was additive, not synergistic, and therefore expected.[117] The use of the two drugs together, therefore, is not contraindicated, but caution should be used in high-risk groups such as the elderly, alcoholics, those receiving concomitant hepatotoxic agents, and those with pre-existing liver disease.[111]

Ethambutol

OPTIC NEURITIS

CASE 65-4

QUESTION 1: S.E., a 65-year-old woman, was placed on isoniazid 300 mg/day, rifampin 600 mg/day, pyrazinamide 900 mg/day, and ethambutol 1,200 mg/day for initial treatment of active pulmonary TB. Two months after the initiation of therapy, she began to complain of blurred vision. A routine eye examination and visual field tests yielded a diagnosis of optic neuritis. No evidence was seen of glaucoma, cataracts, or retinal damage. Laboratory tests were within normal limits except for an elevated serum uric acid (9.7 mg/dL) and a slightly elevated serum creatinine (1.6 mg/dL). No symptoms of joint pain were associated with the elevated serum uric acid, and there was no history of gout. Her calculated creatinine clearance based on her weight of 65 kg was 36 mL/minute. Could the visual problem and increased uric acid levels be related to her medications?

S.E.'s decrease in visual acuity is compatible with ethambutol-induced optic neuritis. This condition is characterized by central scotomas, loss of red-green color vision, or less commonly, a peripheral vision defect. The intensity of these ocular effects is related to the duration of continued therapy after decreased visual acuity is first noted. Optic neuritis is related to both dose and duration, and it rarely occurs at doses of 15 mg/kg.[129–131] The incidence is estimated to be 6% for doses of 25 mg/kg and increases to 15% for doses in excess of 35 mg/kg. Recovery, which may take many months, is usually, but not always, complete when the drug is discontinued.

Optic neuritis manifested in S.E. is probably caused by the use of an increased ethambutol dose (18.5 mg/kg) in a patient with impaired renal function. Because ethambutol adds no additional benefit to isoniazid and rifampin after the first 2 months for susceptible organisms, it can be discontinued. Ethambutol is excreted by the kidney (50%–80%), and her ethambutol dosage interval (or dosage) should have been increased based on the decline in creatinine clearance.[127] Her visual acuity should be monitored closely through periodic eye examinations, and she should be instructed to contact her physician immediately if she experiences any further visual changes.

S.E.'s elevated serum uric acid also may be attributed to her ethambutol as well as a decline in her renal function, but it is more likely caused by pyrazinamide, which decreases the tubular secretion of urate.[96] Asymptomatic hyperuricemia secondary to drugs usually does not require treatment.

SPECIAL TREATMENT CONSIDERATIONS

The Elderly

INCIDENCE

CASE 65-5

QUESTION 1: G.H., a 75-year-old, 80-kg man who resides in a nursing home, becomes disoriented, refuses to eat, and has a productive cough. Physical examination reveals a thin man with slight difficulty breathing. Laboratory findings are essentially normal with the exception of a slightly elevated blood urea nitrogen of 25 mg/dL and serum creatinine of 1.3 mg/dL. A chest radiograph reveals infiltrates in the right lower lobe. He has a history of congestive heart failure, which is well controlled. Blood, urine, and sputum samples are sent for culture and susceptibility testing. The initial Gram stain is negative. Because the nursing home has recently had two cases of active TB, a PPD skin test and sputum smear for AFB are ordered. The PPD skin test induration is 16 mm, and the sputum smear is positive for AFB. G.H.'s admission skin test several months ago was negative. Discuss the presentation of TB in the elderly, and the appropriate treatment of active disease in G.H. Is the

incidence of drug side effects higher in the elderly? Should other patients in close contact with G.H. receive isoniazid therapy?

In 2009, the overall case rate of TB in adults 65 years or older was higher than all other age groups (5.8 per 100,000 population).[14] Similar to other age groups, the case rate for persons 65 years or older has declined every year since 1993 when the case rate was 17.7 per 100,000 population.[14] In 2009, 2.2% of TB cases were reported in residents of long-term care facilities,[14] and the case rate for nursing home residents is 1.8 times higher than that for elderly persons living in the community.[132] Active TB disease in the elderly has been attributed to a decrease in the immune system followed by reactivation of an earlier infection, but active disease is a common, endemic infection in nursing home patients with no previous immunity (negative skin test) to *M. tuberculosis*.[132,133] The incidence of positive skin tests increases after patients have been in the nursing home longer than 1 month. Therefore, all patients entering a nursing home should be tested with 5 TU of PPD. If the initial test is negative and a source case is present in the nursing home (as illustrated by this case), this test should be repeated in 1 month. The rate of tuberculin skin test conversion (from negative to positive tests) in this population is approximately 5%. If these recent converters are not treated with isoniazid, approximately 17% will develop progressive pulmonary TB.[134]

DIAGNOSIS

The diagnosis of active TB in elderly patients is difficult because the classic symptoms of TB (cough, fever, night sweats, weight loss) are often absent, and elderly patients may describe their symptoms poorly. The chest radiograph and PPD skin test may be the only signs of TB infection.[132,134] Frequently, the chest radiograph is atypical, resembling pneumonia or worsening heart failure. Chest radiographs in the elderly are less likely to reveal upper lobe infiltration; however, more commonly they will show extensive infiltration of both lungs.[135] If the patient's clinical disease is caused by granuloma breakdown (reactivation), the chest radiograph often shows apical infiltrates or nodules. If the disease is progressing from an initial infection, as in the case of G.H., lower lobe infiltrates may be present.[132] TB in this population may present clinically with changes in activities of daily living, chronic fatigue, cognitive impairment, anorexia, or unexplained low-grade fever. Nonspecific signs and symptoms that range in severity from subacute to chronic and that persist for weeks to months must alert clinicians to the possibility that unrecognized TB is present.[136] Sputum examination for *M. tuberculosis*, and AFB smear and culture should be performed in all patients, including the elderly.

TREATMENT OF ACTIVE DISEASE IN THE ELDERLY

The principles of TB treatment are the same for the elderly as for any other age group.[30,132] Because G.H. has clinical symptoms of a respiratory infection, positive sputum smears for AFB, and a positive tuberculin skin test, he should be treated with a four-drug regimen for active TB disease. Most TB cases in elderly patients are caused by drug-susceptible strains of *M. tuberculosis;* however, notable exceptions would be older patients who are from a country or region where the prevalence of drug-resistant strains is high, persons who have been inadequately treated in the past, or persons who acquired the infection from a recent contact known to be infected with drug-resistant *M. tuberculosis*.[136] G.H.'s drug regimen likely would include isoniazid 300 mg, rifampin 600 mg, pyrazinamide 2,000 mg, and ethambutol 1,600 mg daily for 8 weeks followed by isoniazid and rifampin daily or two to three times a week for 16 weeks (DOT). Another option might be isoniazid, rifampin, pyrazinamide, and ethambutol daily for 2 weeks, followed by twice weekly for 6 weeks, then isoniazid and rifampin twice weekly for 16 weeks.[136] Some clinicians prefer treating the elderly with 9-month regimens of isoniazid and rifampin. G.H. should also receive pyridoxine 10 to 50 mg with each dose.[61]

ADVERSE DRUG EFFECTS

Although isoniazid hepatitis is more common in elderly patients, both isoniazid and rifampin are generally well tolerated within this age group, with major hematologic or hepatic side effects occurring in 3% to 4% of patients.[137] Therefore, serum aminotransferases should be assessed at baseline, and G.H. should be observed monthly for clinical signs of hepatitis. As discussed, routine monitoring of LFTs remains controversial because transient, asymptomatic elevations do occur among the elderly.[137]

Although uncommon at 600 mg, rifampin given twice weekly may cause a greater incidence of flulike symptoms. Because potential drug interactions with isoniazid and rifampin are possible, any medication added to the patient's regimen should be carefully evaluated. Considering that G.H. has age-related decreased renal function, signs of ethambutol-induced visual dysfunction should be monitoring carefully.

TREATMENT OF LATENT INFECTION IN THE ELDERLY

Treatment of elderly patients with positive tuberculin skin tests but no active TB disease with isoniazid 300 mg daily for 6 to 9 months is essential if a source case is present in the nursing home. Stead et al.[134] reported only one case of active disease in patients receiving therapy for latent TB infection compared with 69 cases in untreated patients. In patients with recently converted skin tests, one patient in the group receiving isoniazid therapy had active disease compared with 45 who received no treatment.[134] Rifampin for 4 months is also an acceptable regimen in the elderly.[132]

Multidrug-Resistant Organisms

DEFINITION AND ETIOLOGY

CASE 65-6

QUESTION 1: M.S., an ill-appearing 29-year-old Asian man, is admitted to the hospital with signs and symptoms of pneumonia. He is coughing and his chest radiograph indicates bilateral infiltrates. He is placed in respiratory isolation pending the results of sputum testing for *M. tuberculosis*. He states that he was diagnosed with TB approximately 3 months ago and treatment was initiated with isoniazid, rifampin, pyrazinamide, and ethambutol. However, he stopped taking his medication after 1 month. An HIV test was performed 3 months ago, which was negative. What is the likelihood of acquired drug resistance in *M. tuberculosis*?

Drug-resistant *M. tuberculosis* became increasingly prevalent in the United States in the late 1980s to early 1990s, although this has decreased in more recent years.[2,3,14,138] In 2009, the incidence of isoniazid resistance in the United States was 8.6%, and the incidence of resistance to both isoniazid and rifampin (multidrug resistance) was 1.2%.[14] The prevalence of resistance to isoniazid has increased slightly during the last 10 years, but the prevalence of multidrug resistance has remained stable.[14]

Resistance to *M. tuberculosis* is either primary or acquired. Primary drug resistance occurs when a patient harbors a resistant strain before any drugs have been administered. Acquired drug resistance occurs when resistant subpopulations are selected as a result of treatment errors, such as addition of a single drug to a failing regimen, inadequate primary regimen, failure to recognize resistance, and, most importantly, nonadherence to the prescribed regimen. Sporadic ingestion, inadequate dosages, or malabsorption of medications can cause susceptible *M. tuberculosis* strains to become resistant to multiple drugs within a few months.[139,140] These resistant organisms can then be transmitted to persons who have never received treatment and lead to primary resistance in these patients. Patients with MDR-TB are twice as likely to have cavitary lesions on chest radiography and seven times more likely to have reported prior treatment for TB.[141]

Patterns and prevalence of drug resistance vary throughout the world, and the highest rates of MDR-TB are in countries of the former Soviet Union and China. As mentioned, the incidence of MDR-TB in the United States has declined from 2.5% in 1993 and has remained stable at 1.0% to 1.2% for the past 10 years.[14] Nonetheless, it is important to note that certain populations are at risk for infections caused by MDR-TB. These include HIV-infected persons and those in groups or institutional settings, such as hospitals, prisons, nursing homes, and homeless shelters.

M.S. is a foreign-born person of Asian ethnicity and therefore may have primary resistance from his country of origin, making a detailed exposure history essential for the treatment of his infection. M.S. is also an example of the problem of treatment failure caused by nonadherence and the potential development of drug-resistant organisms. Homelessness and lack of awareness of the severity of TB have been shown to be significantly associated with interruptions in TB therapy.[142] Therefore, educational efforts to improve a patient's understanding of TB disease are critical for appropriate treatment of the disease.

CASE 65-6, QUESTION 2: Can M.S. be cured by drug therapy, and if so, how should he be treated?

Many factors can affect the outcome of therapy for MDR-TB. These include HIV status, treatment adherence, the number of drugs to which the tubercle bacilli remain susceptible, and the time since the first diagnosis of TB.[143–145] In one study, all 11 patients who were HIV-positive died during observation.[144] In another study, 77% of patients with MDR-TB had sputum cultures convert to negative in a median time of 60 days (range, 4–462 days), but 23% of patients never converted to negative cultures.[145] Of the patients who converted, 60% converted after 4 months of therapy.[145] Predictors of a longer time for sputum culture conversion were high initial sputum colony counts, bilateral cavitation on chest radiograph, previous treatment of MDR-TB, and the number of drugs the initial isolate was resistant to at the beginning of therapy.[145]

Because his recent HIV test was negative, M.S. has a high probability of treatment success. In HIV-negative patients, 32 (97%) of 33 patients with MDR-TB were cured, and these patients received an average of five second-line drugs.[144] Only one relapse occurred 5 years after treatment.[144] Therefore, M.S.'s current regimen should be re-evaluated, drug susceptibility testing should be determined, and the patient should be referred to a specialist or consultation at a specialized treatment center.[30] Molecular drug-resistance testing should be performed to evaluate resistance to rifampin, which is a reliable surrogate for MDR-TB. Standard susceptibility testing methods should be performed for the other agents, although results may not be available for several weeks. If the rapid molecular test detects the presence of mutations to rifampin, the patient should then begin therapy for MDR-TB. When initiating or revising therapy, at least three previously unused drugs to which there is in vitro susceptibility should be used, and one of these agents should be injectable.[30] A new regimen should contain at least four drugs, possibly more, depending on the severity of the disease and the resistance pattern. If resistance to isoniazid and rifampin is suspected, M.S. should be started on a regimen of pyrazinamide, ethambutol, a fluoroquinolone (levofloxacin, ciprofloxacin, or moxifloxacin), and an injectable agent (streptomycin, amikacin capreomycin), pending the results of susceptibility testing.[30] Treatment should be given by DOT, and the recommended duration is 18 to 24 months.[30,143]

In a recent study, the efficacy of a standardized treatment regimen for a shorter duration of therapy was evaluated in patients with documented MDR-TB.[146] The study population consisted of 427 patients with a mean age of 34 years, 81.5% had bilateral disease on chest radiograph, and patients had exhibited TB for approximately 30 months on average. The mean body mass index was 16.1 kg/m^2, indicating severe emaciation. The intensive phase consisted of 3 or more months of therapy with six to seven agents, including kanamycin, clofazimine prothionamide, ofloxacin, or gatifloxacin, and doses were based on body weight.[146] Of interest, daily ofloxacin and gatifloxacin doses were 400 mg, 600 mg, and 800 mg for body weights less than 33 kg, 33 to 50 kg, and greater than 50 kg, respectively.[146] The most effective treatment regimen required a minimum of 9 months of therapy with gatifloxacin, clofazimine, ethambutol, and pyrazinamide throughout the treatment period with the addition of high-dose isoniazid, prothionamide, and kanamycin for a minimum of 4 months during the intensive phase. Among 206 patients receiving this regimen, the relapse-free cure rate was 87.9%. The most common adverse events with this regimen were vomiting (21.4%), diminished hearing acuity (6.3%), dysglycemia (3.9%), and ataxia (3.9%).[146] These results suggest that it may be possible to adequately treat patients with MDR-TB with shorter courses of therapy.

The fluoroquinolone antibiotics, ciprofloxacin, levofloxacin, and moxifloxacin, are active against mycobacteria, including *M. tuberculosis*, and they penetrate rapidly into macrophages and exhibit intracellular mycobactericidal activity.[143] Fluoroquinolones inhibit DNA gyrase in *M. tuberculosis*, but the other molecular target of these agents, topoisomerase IV, is absent.[143] Ciprofloxacin, ofloxacin, and levofloxacin have been used long term for the treatment of mycobacterial infections and were well tolerated with few serious adverse effects.[147,148] Of the commercially available fluoroquinolones, moxifloxacin is the most potent agent against *M. tuberculosis*.[65] Limited data suggest that moxifloxacin is an acceptable option in the treatment of MDR-TB.[149] Selection of fluoroquinolone resistance has been observed in vivo, and complete cross-resistance within the class is the accepted rule.[143] Other second-line medications used for MDR-TB include *p*-aminosalicylic acid, cycloserine, ethionamide, and capreomycin. These are all associated with numerous side effects and should not be prescribed without the guidance of an expert in the treatment of MDR-TB.

Human Immunodeficiency Virus Infection

TREATMENT OF ACTIVE DISEASE

CASE 65-7

QUESTION 1: F.R. is a 32-year-old man who presents to the emergency department complaining of mild pleuritic chest pain and a productive cough. He also has experienced weight loss, fatigue, and night sweats for the past 3 weeks. On questioning, F.R. states that he is bisexual and frequently

engages in unprotected sex. A chest radiograph is ordered and reveals bilateral interstitial infiltrates. Sputum samples are ordered, and the workup includes AFB smear and culture. A PPD skin test is placed, and an HIV test is ordered. The results of the AFB smear and HIV test are positive, and the induration from the PPD is 6 mm. A CD4$^+$ count is ordered, which is 150 cells/μL. What are the clinical manifestations of active TB in patients infected with HIV? How effective is skin testing in the diagnosis of TB infection in patients infected with HIV? What diagnostic tests should be performed in F.R.?

HIV infection is an important risk factor for active TB disease because HIV infects and destroys CD4$^+$ cells, leading to decreased cell-mediated immunity. This immunodeficiency allows for the rapid development of active TB disease in a person who is infected with *M. tuberculosis*. TB is a common opportunistic infection in persons infected with HIV, but unlike other opportunistic infections in this population, CD4$^+$ count is not a reliable predictor for risk for TB disease.[60] Patients infected with HIV can have relatively high CD4$^+$ counts when TB disease develops.

The clinical manifestations of TB in persons infected with HIV depend on the severity of the immunodeficiency at the time of presentation. TB in an HIV-infected person will clinically resemble TB in an HIV-uninfected person if the immunodeficiency is less severe (CD4$^+$ count >350 cells/μL).[60] The disease will primarily be limited to the lungs in these patients, and upper lobe involvement with or without cavitation will be seen on chest radiography. However, the findings on chest radiography are markedly different in patients with advanced HIV disease. Lower lobe, middle lobe, and interstitial infiltrates are common, whereas cavitation is seen infrequently.[60] In these patients, TB may be difficult to distinguish from other HIV-related pulmonary opportunistic infections (*Pneumocystis jiroveci*, *M. avium* complex), and TB should be ruled out in any HIV-infected patient with pulmonary symptoms. Patients with advanced HIV disease may also have normal chest radiographs but still have positive sputum smears for AFB and positive cultures for *M. tuberculosis*. Therefore, a normal chest radiograph does not exclude the possibility of active TB disease. Extrapulmonary TB is more common in HIV-infected persons with CD4$^+$ counts less than 200 cells/μL.[60] Because of F.R.'s clinical presentation and positive HIV test, a high index of suspicion and diagnostic workup for active TB are appropriate.

A PPD skin test should be placed on HIV-infected patients with suspected TB infection, but the sensitivity and specificity of skin testing is poor in patients with HIV infection. Only about 30% to 50% of patients with AIDS and TB will respond to a PPD skin test with an induration greater than 10 mm. Therefore, an induration of 5 mm or more is considered to be a positive reaction in this population.[45,61] F.R.'s reaction of 6 mm to the tuberculin skin test should be considered positive. Theoretically, the sensitivity and specificity of IGRAs are also limited in patients with HIV infection because the tests depend on adequately functioning CD4$^+$ cells. In a study of 294 HIV-infected subjects, indeterminate results were more likely to occur in subjects with a CD4$^+$ count less than 100 cells/μL compared with those with a CD4$^+$ count of 100 cells/μL or more.[150] Additional studies found only 64% sensitivity for detection of active TB disease, and false-negative results occurred in approximately 25% of HIV-infected patients with documented pulmonary TB.[151,152] These studies suggest that IGRAs should not be used alone to exclude active TB.

The diagnostic workup for HIV-infected persons is similar to that for HIV-uninfected persons. Chest radiography and sputum samples for AFB smear and culture should be obtained.[60] HIV status does not alter the yield from sputum smears and cultures. NAA tests can be used to assist in evaluation of HIV-infected persons with positive AFB smears, and a positive NAA result in a patient who is AFB smear-positive likely represents active TB.[60] Drug susceptibility testing should be performed for all first-line agents, and testing should be repeated if sputum cultures remain positive after 3 months of treatment or become positive after at least 1 month of negative cultures.[60] Susceptibility of second-line agents should be limited to specimens from patients who have received prior therapy, are contacts of persons with drug-resistant TB disease, have demonstrated resistance to rifampin or other first-line agents, have positive cultures after 3 months of therapy, or are from regions with a high prevalence of MDR-TB or XDR-TB.[153] Molecular drug-resistance tests may also be used to yield faster results. Patients with symptoms of extrapulmonary TB should undergo needle aspiration or tissue biopsy of skin lesions, lymph nodes, or pericardial or pleural fluid, and blood cultures for AFB should be obtained.[60]

CASE 65-7, QUESTION 2: What is the preferred treatment regimen for TB in F.R.?

Given his symptoms and positive AFB smear, F.R. should be started on multiple-drug therapy for treatment of active TB disease. DOT is recommended for all patients with HIV-related TB.[30,60] F.R.'s treatment plan should be based on completion of the total number of doses ingested rather than the duration of therapy. Principles and recommendations for treatment of TB in HIV-infected adults are the same as those for HIV-uninfected adults (Table 65-2). The initial 8-week treatment phase in F.R. should include isoniazid, rifampin or rifabutin, pyrazinamide, and ethambutol administered daily by DOT (7 days/week for 56 doses or 5 days/week for 40 doses) or thrice weekly by DOT for 24 doses.[30,60] He should also receive supplemental pyridoxine. After the initial phase, if no drug resistance is evident on susceptibility testing, F.R. can be treated with isoniazid and rifampin (or rifabutin) daily or two to three times a week by DOT for a minimum of 26 weeks.[60] Although not applicable to F.R. because his CD4$^+$ count is 150 cells/μL, it should be noted that twice-weekly continuation therapy with isoniazid and rifampin or isoniazid and rifabutin is not recommended for HIV-infected patients with a CD4$^+$ count less than 100 cells/μL because of an increased frequency of acquired rifamycin resistance.[30,60,154,155] Twice-weekly administration in the continuation phase may be considered in F.R. because his CD4$^+$ count is greater than 100 cells/μL, but the data supporting this recommendation are limited (Table 65-2).[30,60] In addition, the once-weekly continuation regimen of isoniazid and rifapentine is contraindicated in HIV-infected patients because of a high rate of relapse with organisms that have acquired resistance to the rifamycins.[30,60]

A recent randomized clinical study evaluated the efficacy of 6 months and 9 months of fully intermittent therapy in HIV-infected patients with TB.[156] All patients received 2 months of isoniazid, rifampin, pyrazinamide, and ethambutol, and then patients were randomly assigned to receive either 4 months ($n = 167$) or 7 months ($n = 160$) of isoniazid and rifampin. Throughout the study duration, doses were administered thrice weekly. The median viral load was 155,000 copies/mL, and the median CD4$^+$ count was 160 cells/μL. Favorable clinical response was similar between the two groups; however, bacteriologic recurrence occurred significantly less frequently in the 9-month group compared with the 6-month group (7% vs. 15%; $p < 0.05$).[156] These data may provide support for 9 months of therapy if a fully intermittent regimen is prescribed for TB therapy in HIV-infected patients.

If F.R. had cavitary disease on chest radiograph or if cultures are positive after 2 months of therapy, treatment with isoniazid and rifampin or rifabutin should be continued to complete a total of 9 months of therapy. If F.R. was suspected of having extrapulmonary disease caused by drug-susceptible strains, the recommended treatment is isoniazid, rifampin, pyrazinamide, and ethambutol for 2 months followed by isoniazid and rifampin for 4 to 7 months. However, longer durations of therapy are recommended for extrapulmonary TB involving the CNS (meningitis or tuberculoma) or bone and joints. For these infections, many experts recommend 9 to 12 months of therapy.[60]

CASE 65-7, QUESTION 3: How should TB therapy be monitored in F.R.?

Baseline and monthly evaluations of hepatic function, renal function, complete blood count, and $CD4^+$ cell count are recommended in all HIV-infected patients with active TB disease.[60] For pulmonary TB, at least one sputum specimen should be obtained at least monthly for AFB smear and culture until two consecutive specimens are culture-negative.[60] If the AFB smear is positive at the initiation of treatment, AFB smears may be obtained every 2 weeks to provide an early assessment of bacteriologic response to therapy.[30,60] Results of the sputum sample obtained after the initial 8-week treatment phase are important because determination of the duration of the continuation phase will be based on these results. Susceptibility testing should be performed on all isolates, and susceptibility testing should be repeated on a newly obtained sputum sample if cultures are positive for *M. tuberculosis* after 3 months of therapy.[60] Patients with positive cultures after 4 months of therapy should be considered treatment failures.

At every visit, patients should be questioned about adherence to therapy and possible adverse events to the treatment regimen. If a patient is experiencing adverse events, the first-line drugs should not be discontinued permanently without strong evidence that a specific agent is the cause of the adverse event.[60] Drug concentration monitoring may be useful to help guide therapy in patients who respond slowly to the prescribed treatment regimen.[157] However, routine serum drug concentration monitoring is not recommended.[60]

CASE 65-7, QUESTION 4: When should antiretroviral therapy (ART) be initiated in F.R.?

Because F.R. is ART naïve, the optimal timing for initiating ART is not well defined. One option is to initiate ART at the beginning of TB therapy.[60] In patients with HIV infection, $CD4^+$ cells multiply in response to *M. tuberculosis,* and then HIV replication accelerates within the lymphocytes and macrophages, which leads to progression of HIV disease. Therefore, initiation of ART can possibly prevent the progression of HIV disease and reduce morbidity and mortality associated with TB and other opportunistic infections.[60] However, this approach may be associated with cumulative drug toxicities, significant drug interactions, a higher pill burden, and the potential for development of immune reconstitution inflammatory syndrome (IRIS).[60] Another option is to delay ART for several weeks after initiating TB therapy.

For patients with a $CD4^+$ count less than 100 cells/μL, it is recommended to begin ART after 2 or more weeks of TB therapy.[60,158] In one study, IRIS occurred in almost all HIV-infected patients with TB and a $CD4^+$ count less than 100 cells/μL who began ART within the first month of TB therapy.[159] For patients with a $CD4^+$ count between 100 and 200 cells/μL, like F.R., certain specialists would delay ART until the end of the initial 8-week intensive phase of TB treatment.[60] In patients with sustained $CD4^+$ counts greater than 200 cells/μL, ART could be started during the continuation phase, and ART could be initiated after completion of TB therapy in patients with $CD4^+$ counts greater than 350 cells/μL.[60] In a recently published study in South Africa, HIV-infected patients with TB were randomly assigned to receive ART during TB therapy or after the completion of TB therapy.[160] In patients with $CD4^+$ counts of 200 cells/μL or less and those with $CD4^+$ counts greater than 200 cells/μL, mortality was significantly lower in patients receiving ART during TB therapy compared with patients receiving ART after completion of TB therapy.[160] Consequently, ART should be initiated during treatment for HIV-related TB regardless of $CD4^+$ cell count.

If F.R. was already receiving ART, TB therapy should be started immediately, and ART should be modified to maintain virologic suppression while reducing the risk for drug–drug interactions.[60] ART should not be withheld simply because the patient is being treated for TB, and a rifamycin should not be excluded from the treatment regimen for fear of interactions with certain antiretroviral agents.[30,161] Exclusion of a rifamycin will likely delay sputum conversion, prolong the duration of therapy, and possibly result in a poor outcome.

CASE 65-7, QUESTION 5: Because F.R.'s $CD4^+$ count is 150 cells/μL, the decision is made to begin ART after the initial 8-week intensive phase to decrease the potential for IRIS. What is IRIS? What drug interactions are likely in an HIV-infected patient receiving treatment for TB and HIV?

Immune reconstitution inflammatory syndrome, or IRIS, occurs in approximately 30% of patients who begin therapy for both HIV and TB in close temporal proximity.[161] This syndrome is thought to reflect recovery of immune responses to *M. tuberculosis* and usually occurs in the first 1 to 3 months after initiation of ART.[60,161] The immune response can be an exaggerated inflammatory response during TB therapy in a patient known to have TB infection, or it may unmask a previously undiagnosed TB infection. The risk of IRIS is greater when ART is initiated within the first 2 months of TB therapy and when the $CD4^+$ count is less than 100 cells/μL.[60] Symptoms include high fever, malaise, and local reactions in organs, depending on the location of the mycobacterial infection (e.g., lungs, lymph nodes, CNS). IRIS is usually self-limiting, but supportive therapy may be required if symptoms are severe. Moderate IRIS reactions should be treated with nonsteroidal anti-inflammatory drugs without any changes to TB therapy or ART.[60] No specific treatment recommendations are available for severe IRIS; however, prednisone or methylprednisolone at doses of 1 mg/kg body weight and tapered for 1 to 2 weeks have been beneficial.[60]

The simultaneous treatment of TB and HIV can be complicated by drug interactions with the rifamycins and ART. Rifampin is a potent inducer of cytochrome P-450 isoenzymes (especially CYP3A4), rifapentine is intermediate, and rifabutin is the least potent inducer.[30,32,60] Rifampin should not be used in patients on protease inhibitor–based ART, regardless of boosting with ritonavir.[60] Rifabutin is highly active against *M. tuberculosis,* so it has been recommended in place of rifampin for the treatment of active TB in HIV-infected patients receiving certain protease inhibitors or NNRTIs.[30] Data from clinical trials also suggest that rifabutin- and rifampin-based regimens are equally efficacious.[30] Protease inhibitors and NNRTIs may, however, either induce or inhibit cytochrome P-450 isoenzymes, depending on the specific drug. As a result, these drugs may alter the serum concentrations of rifabutin.[30,154]

For patients receiving treatment for active TB, initiating ART with either an efavirenz- or nevirapine-based regimen is preferred because these NNRTIs have fewer interactions with rifamycins.[60] Delavirdine should not be used with either rifampin or rifabutin.[162] Dose reduction of rifabutin is required with boosted protease inhibitor regimens.[60] Efavirenz decreases rifabutin concentrations, which may necessitate a dosage increase, but nevirapine does not appreciably affect rifabutin concentrations, so dosage adjustment of rifabutin is not required.[60] Underdosing of ART can result in selection of drug-resistant HIV strains, and underdosing of rifabutin can result in acquired rifamycin resistance. Overdosing of rifabutin may result in adverse drug events, which include uveitis, neutropenia, arthralgias, skin discoloration).[60,154] Therapeutic drug monitoring of rifabutin, protease inhibitors, and NNRTIs may be helpful because significant interpatient variability in the degree of enzyme induction or inhibition can occur.[60] HIV nucleotide analogs and the fusion inhibitor enfuvirtide are not affected by CYP enzymes and can be used with the rifamycins.[60] Rifampin appears to decrease the concentrations of maraviroc, raltegravir, and elvitegravir; therefore, these drugs should be used with caution or perhaps avoided until more data are available to guide dose adjustment.[60]

MALABSORPTION IN HUMAN IMMUNODEFICIENCY VIRUS INFECTION

Inadequate treatment of TB is one of the main reasons for treatment failure and development of acquired drug resistance. This can occur in many ways, such as nonadherence to therapy or malabsorption of the TB medications. Malabsorption of TB medications has been documented in HIV-infected patients. In one study, 19 of 20 patients had subtherapeutic serum rifampin concentrations. This phenomenon is particularly common with rifampin and ethambutol and explains, in part, the slow response in HIV-infected patients with TB.[140,163–165] Therefore, serum concentrations of rifampin (or rifabutin) and ethambutol should be monitored in F.R.

TREATMENT OF LATENT TUBERCULOSIS INFECTION IN HUMAN IMMUNODEFICIENCY VIRUS INFECTION

CASE 65-8

QUESTION 1: N.M. is the 32-year-old partner and roommate of F.R. Because of his close contact with F.R., he is evaluated by an infectious diseases specialist for exposure to TB. N.M.'s HIV test is positive, and a tuberculin skin test produces an induration of 8 mm, which is positive. All other studies are negative for active TB. Should N.M. receive treatment for latent TB infection? If so, what therapy should he receive?

The risk of N.M. developing active TB disease is significant; therefore, he should receive treatment for latent TB infection. HIV-infected persons, regardless of age, should be treated for latent TB infection.[60] Pape et al. conducted a randomized, placebo-controlled trial of isoniazid therapy in HIV-infected patients.[166] They found that patients receiving placebo were six times more likely to develop active TB than those receiving isoniazid. The patients receiving isoniazid were also less likely to develop AIDS.[166] Treatment options for latent TB infection in patients with HIV include isoniazid 300 mg daily or twice weekly for 9 months.[60] Therefore, N.M. should be treated with isoniazid. Rifampin or rifabutin for 4 months is an alternative to isoniazid, but the potential for drug interactions should be considered.

Pregnancy

CASE 65-9

QUESTION 1: E.F. is a 25-year-old Hispanic woman who is being treated with isoniazid 900 mg and rifampin 600 mg twice a week for pulmonary TB. She completed 2 months of therapy with isoniazid, rifampin, pyrazinamide, and ethambutol, and began the new regimen 2 months ago. She recently became pregnant, and her obstetrician is concerned about the possible teratogenic effects of her TB regimen. What are the risks of TB and its treatment to the mother and the fetus? Are these drugs teratogenic?

Although concerns about the use of any medication during pregnancy always exist, it is now recognized that untreated TB represents a far greater risk to a pregnant woman and her fetus than the treatment.[30,61] TB is one of the leading nonobstetric causes of maternal mortality.[167] The World Health Organization recommends that treatment of TB in pregnant women should be the same as that for nonpregnant women, with few exceptions.[167] Isoniazid, rifampin, pyrazinamide, and ethambutol are not teratogenic in humans.[168,169] In the United States, pyrazinamide is not recommended for use during pregnancy because of insufficient safety data.[30] If pyrazinamide is not included in the initial treatment regimen, the minimal duration of therapy is 9 months.[30] All pregnant women receiving isoniazid should also receive pyridoxine 25 mg/day because of the possibility of peripheral neuropathy.

Streptomycin should not be used during pregnancy except as a last alternative because it has been associated with mild-to-severe ototoxicity in the fetus.[167] This ototoxicity can occur throughout the gestational period and is not confined to the first trimester. With the exception of streptomycin ototoxicity, the occurrence of birth defects in women being treated for TB with the above agents is no greater than that of healthy pregnant women.[170,171] Therefore, administration of antituberculosis drugs is not an indication for termination of pregnancy.[30] Because E.F. likely became pregnant after completing the first 2 months of therapy, she should continue her current regimen for a total of 6 months because she received pyrazinamide as part of the initial regimen.

MULTIDRUG-RESISTANT TUBERCULOSIS IN PREGNANCY

Little is known about the efficacy and safety of second-line drugs for the treatment of MDR-TB during pregnancy. Two reports with small numbers of patients have suggested that treatment is effective with no adverse effects to mother or child.[172,173] In a study of seven women treated for MDR-TB during pregnancy, no obstetrical complications or perinatal transmission of MDR-TB was observed.[172] Five women were cured, one experienced treatment failure, and one stopped therapy prematurely.[172] No evidence of drug toxicity was seen among their children exposed to second-line drugs in utero, although one child was diagnosed with MDR-TB.[173] Clearly, more data are needed, but pregnancy should not be a limitation to the treatment of MDR-TB.

LACTATION

When the baby is born, E.F. may breast-feed while continuing her medication. Drug concentrations in breast milk are minimal and do not provide sufficient quantities for the treatment or prevention of TB in the nursing infant.[30,61]

Pediatrics

CASE 65-10

QUESTION 1: A.M., a 3-year-old African American boy, is suspected of having TB. His father has been receiving treatment for TB for the last 2 months. A.M. has a productive cough, fever, and general malaise. His sputum is positive for AFB, and his PPD skin test is positive (10 mm). What is the incidence of TB in children? How should A.M. be treated?

The incidence of TB in children younger than 15 years of age has declined from 1,661 cases (2.9 per 100,000 population) in 1993 to 646 cases (1.0 per 100,000 population) in 2009.[14] Children commonly have active TB disease as a complication of the initial infection with *M. tuberculosis,* and the disease is characterized by intrathoracic adenopathy, middle and lower lung lobe infiltrates, and the absence of cavitation on chest radiography.[30,174] Because of the high risk of disseminated TB in infants and children, treatment should be started as soon as the diagnosis of TB is suspected. In general, the regimens recommended for adults are also the regimens of choice for infants, children, and adolescents, with the exception that ethambutol is not used routinely in children.[30] Although it is no more toxic, ethambutol is often avoided because it is difficult to assess visual acuity in children. A.M. should be started on isoniazid 10 to 15 mg/kg/day, rifampin 10 to 20 mg/kg/day, and pyrazinamide 15 to 30 mg/kg/day.[30,61,174] Many experts prefer to treat children with three drugs (rather than four) in the initial phase because the bacillary population is usually lower than in an adult and it may be difficult for an infant or child to ingest four drugs. If resistance is suspected, ethambutol 15 to 20 mg/kg/day or streptomycin 20 to 40 mg/kg/day should be added to the regimen until susceptibility of the organism to isoniazid, rifampin, and pyrazinamide is known. Pyridoxine is recommended for infants, children, and adolescents who are receiving isoniazid.[30]

If resistance is not suspected and drug susceptibility is confirmed, A.M. should receive the isoniazid, rifampin, and pyrazinamide daily for 8 weeks. He can then continue to take the isoniazid and rifampin daily or two to three times a week (DOT) for an additional 4 months. The dosage for isoniazid and rifampin in a two to three times a week regimen would be 20 to 30 mg/kg per dose and 10 to 20 mg/kg per dose, respectively (Table 65-3).

A.M. should be examined routinely for signs and symptoms of hepatitis. Although antituberculosis medications are generally well-tolerated in children, LFTs two to three times normal are common. These are often benign and transient; however, the incidence of hepatitis in children from isoniazid with rifampin may be four to six times more common than in children receiving isoniazid alone. Most hepatitis occurs within the first 3 months of therapy and generally is associated with higher than recommended doses of isoniazid or rifampin.[117,175]

Children and adolescents should be screened for risk factors for TB using a questionnaire, and they should be skin tested with 5 TU of PPD if one or more risk factors are present.[176] Insufficient data are available to recommend use of whole blood interferon-γ assays in children. Isoniazid for 9 months is recommended for treatment of latent TB in this population.[176] Daily rifampin for 6 months is an acceptable alternative, especially in children who cannot tolerate isoniazid or those exposed to a source case whose isolate was isoniazid -resistant.[176]

Extrapulmonary Tuberculosis and Tuberculous Meningitis

CASE 65-11

QUESTION 1: R.U. is a 64-year-old, 82-kg man who is brought to the emergency department after a 4-day period during which he became progressively disoriented, febrile to 40.5°C, and obtunded. He also had severe headaches during this time. Physical examination revealed moderate nuchal rigidity and a positive Brudzinski sign (neck resistant to flexion). An initial diagnosis of possible meningitis was made, and a lumbar puncture ordered. The cerebrospinal fluid (CSF) appeared turbid, and laboratory analysis revealed an elevated protein concentration of 200 mg/dL, a decreased glucose concentration of 30 mg/dL, and a white blood cell count of 500/μL (85% lymphocytes). A Gram stain of the spinal fluid and a sputum smear for AFB were negative; other laboratory tests were within normal limits. A diagnosis of tuberculous meningitis was presumed. Discuss the presentation and prognosis of tuberculous meningitis. How should R.U. be treated?

Tuberculous meningitis is only one of the extrapulmonary complications of infection with *M. tuberculosis.*

For a photo of extrapulmonary TB on computed tomography, go to http://thepoint.lww.com/AT10e.

Successful treatment of extrapulmonary TB can usually be accomplished in 6 to 9 months with an acceptable relapse rate.[30,61,177] Some forms, such as bone or joint TB, miliary TB, or tuberculous meningitis, may require 9 to 12 months of therapy.[30] Because specimens for culture and susceptibility testing may be difficult or impossible to obtain from a site, response to treatment must be based on clinical and radiographic improvement.

Tuberculous meningitis in older persons is usually caused by hematogenous dissemination of the tubercle bacilli from a primary site, usually the lungs. In its early stages, tuberculous meningitis often is confused with aseptic meningitis because the Gram stain is negative. The most common symptoms of tuberculous meningitis are headache, fever, restlessness, irritability, nausea, and vomiting. A positive Brudzinski sign and neck stiffness may be present. As illustrated by R.U., the CSF is usually turbid with increased protein and decreased glucose concentrations. There is an increase in the CSF white blood cell count with a predominance of lymphocytes. Culture of the CSF for *M. tuberculosis* may not be helpful because rates of positivity for clinically diagnosed cases range from 25% to 70%.[178] Early recognition and treatment are essential for a favorable outcome. Thus, empirical treatment before receipt of confirmatory culture and susceptibility results is common in suspected tuberculous meningitis. Multiple-drug therapy should be used because irreversible brain damage or death can occur as soon as 2 weeks after the onset of infection (not clinical symptoms).[178]

TREATMENT

Treatment should be initiated in R.U. with daily administration of isoniazid 300 mg, rifampin 600 mg, pyrazinamide 2,000 mg, and ethambutol 1,600 mg for the first 2 months.[30] After this initial phase of treatment, R.U. should receive daily isoniazid and rifampin for an additional 7 to 10 months, although the optimal duration of therapy is unknown.[30] In addition, because R.U. is older, pyridoxine 10 to 50 mg/day should be given to prevent the occurrence of peripheral neuropathy from isoniazid. It also should be remembered that rifampin may impart a red to orange color to the CSF.

Isoniazid readily penetrates into the CSF, with CSF concentrations reaching up to 100% of those in the serum. Rifampin is often included in tuberculous meningitis regimens and may be associated with reduced morbidity and mortality; however, even with inflammation, CSF concentrations of rifampin are only 6% to 30% of those found in the serum. Ethambutol should be used in the highest dosage to achieve bactericidal concentrations in the CSF because its CSF concentrations are only 10% to 54% of those in the serum. Streptomycin penetrates into the CSF poorly even with inflamed meninges.[179]

CORTICOSTEROIDS

Corticosteroids in moderate to severe tuberculous meningitis appear to reduce sequelae and prolong survival.[180] The mechanism for this benefit is likely owing to reduction of intracranial pressure. Dexamethasone 8 to 12 mg/day (or prednisone equivalent) for 6 to 8 weeks should be used and then tapered slowly after symptoms subside.[180] Corticosteroids are likely indicated for R.U.

KEY REFERENCES AND WEBSITES

A full list of references for this chapter can be found at http://thepoint.lww.com/AT10e. Below are the key references and websites for this chapter, with the corresponding reference number in this chapter found in parentheses after the reference.

Key References

Abdool Karim SS et al. Timing of initiation of antiretroviral drugs during tuberculosis therapy. *N Engl J Med*. 2010;362:697. (160)

Blumberg HM et al. American Thoracic Society/Centers for Disease Control and Prevention/Infectious Diseases Society of America. Treatment of tuberculosis. *Am J Respir Crit Care Med*. 2003;167:603. (30)

Centers for Disease Control and Prevention (CDC). Updated guidelines for the use of nucleic acid amplification tests in the diagnosis of tuberculosis. *MMWR Morb Mortal Wkly Rep*. 2009;58:7. (50)

Centers for Disease Control and Prevention. Reported tuberculosis in the United States, 2009. Atlanta, GA: U.S. Department of Health and Human Services, CDC, October 2010. (14)

Holland DP et al. Costs and cost-effectiveness of four treatment regimens for latent tuberculosis infection. *Am J Respir Crit Care Med*. 2009;179:1055. (109)

Horsburgh CR Jr et al. Latent TB infection treatment acceptance and completion in the United States and Canada. *Chest*. 2010;137:401. (102)

Kaplan JE et al. Guidelines for prevention and treatment of opportunistic infections in HIV-infected adults and adolescents: recommendations from CDC, the National Institutes of Health, and the HIV Medicine Association of the Infectious Diseases Society of America. *MMWR Recomm Rep*. 2009;58(RR-4):1. (60)

Lienhardt C et al. Efficacy and safety of a 4-drug fixed-dose combination regimen compared with separate drugs for treatment of pulmonary tuberculosis. The Study C randomized controlled trial. *JAMA*. 2011;305:1415. (62)

Lin HH et al. Association between tobacco smoking and active tuberculosis in Taiwan: prospective cohort study. *Am J Respir Crit Care Med*. 2009;180:475. (37)

Mazurek GH et al. Updated guidelines for using interferon gamma release assays to detect *Mycobacterium tuberculosis* infection—United States, 2010. *MMWR Recomm Rep*. 2010; 59(RR-5):1. (59)

[No authors listed]. Diagnostic standards and classification of tuberculosis in adults and children. *Am J Respir Crit Care Med*. 2000;161(4 Pt 1):1376. (19)

Schluger NW, Burzynski J. Recent advances in testing for latent TB. *Chest*. 2010;138:1456. (100)

Van Deun A et al. Short, highly effective, and inexpensive standardized treatment of multidrug-resistant tuberculosis. *Am J Respir Crit Care Med*. 2010;182:684. (146)

Key Websites

Centers for Disease Control and Prevention. Tuberculosis (TB). http://www.cdc.gov/tb

World Health Organization. WHO Report 2010. Global tuberculosis control. http://www.who.int/tb/publications/global_report/2010/gtbr10_main.pdf. Accessed April 4, 2011. (9)

66

Infectious Diarrhea

Gail S. Itokazu, David T. Bearden, and Larry H. Danziger

CORE PRINCIPLES

	CHAPTER CASES
1 The most common complication of any diarrheal illness is loss of fluids and electrolytes, which in extreme cases can lead to hypovolemia, shock, and death. Depending on the degree of dehydration, fluid and electrolyte losses are replaced intravenously or orally.	**Case 66-1 (Questions 1, 2)**
2 Classification of infectious diarrheas as either an inflammatory or noninflammatory diarrheal illness provides a basis for preparing a more focused list of suspected pathogens, thus guiding the overall diagnostic and therapeutic plan.	**Case 66-1 (Question 3)**
3 *Vibrio cholerae* 01 and 0139 are toxigenic strains of *Vibrio* species, which cause epidemic cholera; severe dehydration requiring vigorous fluid replacement may be necessary. Noncholera *Vibrio* species do not possess the virulence factors required to cause epidemic cholera. Antimicrobial treatment differs between toxigenic and nontoxigenic *Vibrio* species.	**Case 66-2 (Questions 1–3), Case 66-3 (Questions 1, 2)**
4 *Salmonella* species are classified as nontyphoidal and typhoidal salmonellae. Nontyphoidal salmonellae cause the clinical syndromes of gastroenteritis, bacteremia, and localized infection, whereas typhoidal salmonellae cause typhoid fever. The role of antimicrobials in the management of salmonellosis is based on the clinical syndrome, its severity, and underlying health problems of infected persons.	**Case 66-7 (Questions 1–4, 6, 7)**
5 Patients infected with nalidixic acid–resistant *Salmonella* who are treated with a fluoroquinolone are at greater risk for treatment failure, despite routine susceptibility tests indicating susceptibility to the fluoroquinolone. Measurement of the fluoroquinolone minimum inhibitory concentration will detect isolates with low-level fluoroquinolone-resistance.	**Case 66-7 (Question 5)**
6 Severe dysentery caused by *Shigella* species is most commonly caused by *Shigella dysenteriae*, whereas a milder illness is typically caused by *Shigella sonnei*. Antimicrobials alleviate the symptoms of shigellosis, and decrease the period of time that shigellae can be spread by person-to-person contact.	**Case 66-9 (Questions 1–5)**
7 Fluoroquinolone-resistance in *Campylobacter* species is no longer an unexpected finding in both developed and underdeveloped areas of the world; when indicated, macrolide antimicrobials are recommended.	**Case 66-11 (Questions 1–3)**
8 Travelers departing to destinations with risk for traveler's diarrhea should bring a travel kit including medications (e.g., loperamide and antimicrobials) and instructions for self-treatment at the onset of illness. The selected antimicrobial depends on the area of travel.	**Case 66-12 (Questions 1–7)**
9 *Escherichia coli* O157:H7 is a specific toxin-producing strain of bacteria that can lead to the severe sequelae of hemolytic uremic syndrome.	**Case 66-13 (Questions 3, 4)**

continued

		CHAPTER CASES
10	*Clostridium difficile*–associated diarrhea causes a wide range of severity of illness. Mild to moderate disease is typically treated with metronidazole as first-line therapy, and oral vancomycin is preferred for severe disease.	Case 66-14 (Question 6)
11	Severe *C. difficile*–associated diarrhea can be life-threatening and often necessitates multiple therapeutic interventions.	Case 66-15 (Questions 5, 6)

PREVALENCE AND ETIOLOGY

Worldwide, diarrhea accounts for more than 2 million deaths annually,[1] mainly affecting infants and children living in poverty.[2] Prolonged episodes of diarrhea lead to malnutrition, and in children, contribute to impaired growth and developmental delay.[2] In the United States, more than 5 million cases of bacterial diarrhea occur annually, resulting in an estimated 46,000 hospitalizations and 1,500 deaths.[3]

Infectious diarrhea is caused by the ingestion of food or water contaminated with pathogenic microorganisms (e.g., bacteria, viruses, protozoa, or fungi) or their toxins (Table 66-1).[2] In the United States, viruses account for 30% to 40% of acute diarrheal episodes, and common bacterial pathogens include

TABLE 66-1
Predisposing Factors, Symptoms, and Therapy of Gastrointestinal Infections

Pathogen	Predisposing Factors	Symptoms	Diagnostic Evaluations	Drug of Choice[a,c]	Alternatives[a,c]
Salmonella (nontyphoidal)[b]	Ingestion of contaminated poultry, raw milk, custards, and cream fillings; foreign travel	Nausea, vomiting, diarrhea, cramps, fever, tenesmus Incubation: 6–72 hours	Fecal leukocytes, stool culture	Fluoroquinolone, azithromycin, third-generation cephalosporins	Amoxicillin, TMP-SMX
Salmonella (typhoidal)	Ingestion of contaminated food, foreign travel	High fever, abdominal pain, headache, dry cough	Fecal leukocytes, stool culture, blood culture	Fluoroquinolone, azithromycin, third-generation cephalosporins	TMP-SMX, amoxicillin
Shigella	Ingestion of contaminated food, foreign travel	Fever, dysentery, cramps, tenesmus Incubation: 24–48 hours	Fecal leukocytes, stool culture	Fluoroquinolone, azithromycin, ceftriaxone	TMP-SMX, ampicillin
Campylobacter	Contaminated eggs, raw milk, or poultry; foreign travel	Mild to severe diarrhea; fever, systemic malaise Incubation: 24–72 hours	Fecal leukocytes, stool culture	Erythromycin, azithromycin	—
Clostridium difficile	Antibiotics, antineoplastics	Mild to severe diarrhea, cramps	*C. difficile* toxin, *C. difficile* culture, colonoscopy	Metronidazole	Vancomycin
Staphylococcal food poisoning	Custard-filled bakery products, canned food, processed meat, ice cream	Nausea, vomiting, salivation, cramps, diarrhea; usually resolves in 8 hours Incubation: 2–6 hours	—	Supportive therapy only	—
Travelers' diarrhea (Enterotoxigenic *Escherichia coli*, *Campylobacter*)	Contaminated food (vegetables and cheese), water, foreign travel	Nausea, vomiting, mild to severe diarrhea, cramps	Stool culture	See Table 66-3	—
Shiga toxin–producing *Escherichia coli* (*E. coli* O157:H7)	Beef, raw milk, water	Diarrhea, headache, bloody stools Incubation: 48–96 hours	Stool cultures on MacConkey's sorbitol	Supportive therapy only	—
Cryptosporidiosis	Immunosuppression, day-care centers, contaminated water, animal handlers	Mild to severe diarrhea (chronic or self-limited); large fluid volume	Stool screening for oocytes, PCR, ELISA	See Chapter 74, Opportunistic Infections in HIV-Infected Patients	—
Viral gastroenteritis	Community-wide outbreaks, contaminated food	Nausea, diarrhea (self-limited), cramps Incubation: 16–48 hours	Special viral studies	Supportive therapy only	—

ELISA, enzyme-linked immunosorbent assay; PCR, polymerase chain reaction; TMP-SMX, trimethoprim-sulfamethoxazole.
[a]Source: Navaneethan U, Giannella RA. Mechanisms of infectious diarrhea. *Nat Clin Pract Gastroenterol Hepatol.* 2008;5:637; DuPont HL. Clinical practice. Bacterial diarrhea. *N Engl J Med.* 2009;361:1560. See text for doses and duration of therapy.
[b]Not all cases require antibiotic therapy. See text for details.
[c]If susceptible. See text for details.

Campylobacter, nontyphoidal *Salmonella*, *Shigella*, and Shiga toxin–producing *Escherichia coli*.[3]

This chapter focuses on the diagnosis and management of the common microbial causes of acute infectious diarrhea.

DEFINITIONS

Diarrhea is often defined as three or more episodes of loose stools, or any loose stool with blood during a 24-hour period, which may be accompanied by nausea, vomiting, or abdominal cramping.[1] The duration of illness is considered acute if symptoms are present for less than 2 weeks' duration, persistent if symptoms last for more than 14 days, and chronic if symptoms last beyond 30 days.[1,4]

Diarrheal syndromes should be classified as noninflammatory versus inflammatory illness. This categorization provides a basis for predicting the most likely microbial cause for an intestinal illness.[1]

PATHOGENESIS

The pathogenesis of infectious diarrhea involves an interplay among bacterial virulence factors, host factors, and predisposing factors to infection. Diarrhea is more likely to occur in the setting in which an imbalance among these factors favors the enteropathogen.

Bacterial Virulence Factors

Enteropathogens possess virulence factors that contribute to the organism's pathogenicity.[2] Enterotoxins targeting the small bowel cause net movement of fluid into the gut lumen, leading to voluminous watery stools and potentially life-threatening dehydration. Cytotoxins targeting the colon cause direct mucosal damage, leading to fever and bloody diarrhea. Invasive properties of *Shigella* species and invasive strains of *E. coli* allow these bacteria to invade and destroy epithelial cells, causing bloody or mucoid stools. Some enteropathogens induce a vigorous host response through the release of proinflammatory cytokines from intestinal epithelial cells, leading to diarrhea. Finally, adhesions allow enteropathogens to attach to and colonize the gastrointestinal (GI) mucosa, facilitating toxin delivery, invasion, dissemination, or host cell lysis.[2]

Host Defenses

The human GI tract possesses numerous defense mechanisms to protect against enteric infection.[2] Normal bacterial flora compete for space and nutrients with potentially pathogenic organisms, or produce substances, e.g., short-chain fatty acids, that are inhibitory to enteropathogens.[2] Gastric acidity of the stomach prevents acid-susceptible pathogens from passing from the stomach into the intestinal tract, whereas gastrointestinal mucus and mucosal tissue integrity provide physical barriers against infection. Intestinal immunity includes defensins that are bactericidal to some enteropathogens, the local production of antibodies, and toll-like receptors that recognize enteropathogens and activate the immune response.[2,5] Intestinal peristalsis moves bacteria and their toxins along and out of the GI tract. Finally, specific host genetic factors are protective against enteric infection.[6]

Predisposing Factors

Inadequate sanitation facilities increase the risk that local inhabitants and travelers will be exposed to contaminated food and water. Similarly, outbreaks of foodborne or waterborne illnesses in both industrialized and developing countries facilitate the spread of infectious organisms. Industrialized countries that rely on imported food items risk the possibility of importation of contaminated food products.

TABLE 66-2
Pharmacologic Agents That May Promote Gastrointestinal Infection

Drug	Mechanism
Antacids, H_2-receptor antagonists, proton-pump inhibitors	Increased gastric pH; viable pathogens passed to lower gut
Antibiotics	Eradication of normal (anaerobic) flora
Antidiarrheals	Decreased gut motility; bacterial growth
Immunosuppressives	Inhibition of gut immune defenses

Immunocompromised individuals are more susceptible to intestinal infection, such as various organ transplant recipients and patients receiving immunosuppressive therapies. Institutional settings, such as day-care centers, hospitals, and extended-care facilities, are high-risk settings for dissemination of disease. Poor personal hygiene is also a risk for infectious diarrhea.

The use of pharmacologic agents, e.g., drugs that increase gastric pH (Table 66-2), increases the risk for infection with acid-susceptible pathogens such as *Salmonella* species and *Vibrio cholerae*.[7] Recent data suggest use of proton-pump inhibitors may be a risk factor for *Clostridium difficile*–associated diarrhea (CDAD).[8,9]

MANAGEMENT OVERVIEW

Rehydration Therapy

The most common complication of any diarrheal illness is loss of fluids and electrolytes, which in extreme cases can lead to hypovolemia, shock, and death. Depending on the degree of dehydration, fluid and electrolyte losses are replaced intravenously (IV) or orally.[10] Once replacement of fluid and electrolyte losses have been resolved, additional laboratory tests and drug therapies can be considered.

Laboratory Tests

Inflammatory diarrheal illnesses are characterized by the presence of bloody or mucoid stools. Therefore, stool specimens with red blood cells (RBCs) or occult blood, or those that contain large numbers of white blood cells (WBCs) or markers of fecal leukocytes such as lactoferrin, suggest infection attributable to invasive pathogens.[11] The absence of leukocytes in a stool specimen suggests a noninflammatory diarrheal illness; however, it does not rule out the possibility of an inflammatory diarrheal illness.[11]

Identification of bacterial toxins in stool specimens is a useful diagnostic tool. For example, because only the toxigenic strains of *C. difficile* are pathogenic, the presence or absence of bacterial toxins in stool specimens is more important than a positive culture for the organism.[4]

In clinical practice, routine microbiologic analysis is made using selective media favoring the growth of the pathogen(s) of interest.[4] Stool cultures are recommended for patients with one of the following: severe diarrhea; bloody stools; or stools containing leukocytes, lactoferrin, or occult blood; or an oral temperature of at least 101.3°F; and for patients with persistent diarrhea who have not been given empiric antimicrobials.[12] Culture of specimens from extraintestinal sites of infection may be used to identify the microbial etiology; as an example, *Salmonella* species are well known to cause bloodstream infection.[13]

Molecular assays, which are highly sensitive and specific, are capable of rapidly confirming the microbiologic etiology, although these technologies are generally only available in research settings.[4]

Drug Therapy

Drug therapy for infectious diarrhea includes medications to provide symptomatic relief or to eradicate the causative pathogen.

LOPERAMIDE AND DIPHENOXYLATE/ATROPINE

Loperamide and diphenoxylate/atropine reduce the frequency of diarrheal stools by slowing intestinal transit time; additionally, loperamide possesses antisecretory properties.[14] Loperamide is preferred over diphenoxylate/atropine because of its greater efficacy, decreased adverse effects, and over-the-counter availability. Diphenoxylate/atropine causes drowsiness, dizziness, dry mouth, and urinary retention owing to the atropine component.

Although controversial,[15,16] the use of antimotility drugs in persons with fever or bloody diarrhea or when invasive pathogens are suspected is not recommended. The primary concern is prolongation of clearance of pathogens from the intestinal tract could worsen the severity of illness. Some experts note that as long as effective antimicrobial therapy is administered, there is no definitive evidence that antimotility drugs are harmful.[3,16]

Crofelemer, an investigational antisecretory drug, reduces diarrhea by preventing the secretion of intestinal fluids into the bowel.[17]

BISMUTH SUBSALICYLATE (BSS)

Bismuth subsalicylate's antisecretory effect is attributed to its salicylate moiety.[14] Adverse effects of BSS include darkening of the tongue and stools. Tinnitus, secondary to salicylate absorption, may occur[14]; consequently, BSS is not recommended for persons with chronic intestinal disease in whom absorption may be increased as a result of damaged intestinal mucosa.[14]

PROBIOTICS

Interest in probiotics stems, in part, from their potential to decrease the use of antibiotics. These live microbial mixtures of bacteria and yeasts are used to restore the normal intestinal flora, thereby reducing intestinal colonization with pathogenic organisms.[18] Probiotics also produce pathogen-inhibiting substances, inhibit pathogen adhesion to the GI tract, inhibit the action of microbial toxins, and stimulate immune defense mechanisms.[19]

Disadvantages of probiotics include the lack of both well-controlled trials supporting their efficacy and quality controls on the manufacturing of these products, and the risk for systemic infection, particularly in the immunocompromised host.[19] Some evidence supports the use of probiotics for the treatment of rotavirus diarrhea in children and as an adjunct for the treatment of recurrent *C. difficile* colitis.[19]

ANTIMICROBIALS

In selected cases, antimicrobials are prescribed to decrease the duration and the severity of the diarrheal illness, prevent the progression to invasive infection,[13] and prevent person-to-person transmission of pathogens.[20] Antimicrobials are generally recommended for the severely ill, for patients with conditions compromising normal enteric defenses, or for immunocompromised patients[12] and treatment of extraintestinal infections.

Ongoing surveillance of antimicrobial resistance is important to guide treatment recommendations. Although trimethoprim-sulfamethoxazole (TMP-SMX), the aminopenicillins, tetracyclines, and nalidixic acid have been extensively used in the past, widespread resistance makes them unsuitable options for the empiric treatment of infectious diarrhea.[3] Depending on the circumstances surrounding the diarrheal illness, including the origin of the pathogen (e.g., domestic vs. travel-related), age, and allergy history of the patient, recommended antimicrobials include selected third-generation cephalosporins (e.g., ceftriaxone, cefotaxime), azithromycin, rifaximin, fluoroquinolones, and others.[3]

The fluoroquinolones, although still recommended because of their efficacy against susceptible organisms[12] and their availability as oral formulations, must be used cautiously as common enteropathogens, e.g., *Shigella*,[21] *Salmonella*,[22] and *Campylobacter*[23] species, are commonly fluoroquinolone-resistant. Nalidixic acid–resistant isolates are associated with worse clinical outcomes when compared with susceptible pathogens.[24]

Another consideration with using fluoroquinolones is that they are not U.S. Food and Drug Administration (FDA)–approved for use in children, because lesions on cartilage tissue have been reported in juvenile animals.[17] Nevertheless, because of the emergence of multidrug-resistant enteropathogens in some geographic areas, clinical trials using fluoroquinolones in children have been performed, and the available data suggest that a short course of these agents is safe.[17]

Prevention

Good personal hygiene, along with proper handling, cooking, and storage of foods are essential to prevent the spread of enteropathogens. When visiting areas with inadequate facilities for the disposal of sewage, travelers should follow the rule, "boil it, cook it, peel it, or forget it." In the United States, vaccines to prevent typhoid fever are available.

EVALUATION AND TREATMENT OF PATIENTS WITH INFECTIOUS DIARRHEA

CASE 66-1

QUESTION 1: B.K. is a 78-year-old man presenting to his physician with a diarrheal illness of 1 day's duration. His illness began with vomiting, and was followed by abdominal pain, nausea, and watery, but nonbloody, diarrhea. Despite not feeling well, he is able to drink fruit juices. B.K.'s history of present illness is significant for eating raw oysters at the local seafood restaurant 2 nights ago. He has since learned that other patrons are experiencing a similar illness. B.K. has no significant medical history. He denies recent hospitalization, contact with small children, recent travel, or recent use of antimicrobials. On physical examination, B.K. is alert and oriented, is not "toxic" appearing, is afebrile, and has stable vital signs. The remainder of his examination is significant for decreased skin turgor and dry mucous membranes. What is your general approach to the management of B.K.'s diarrheal illness?

Because infectious diarrhea is typically a self-limiting illness, patients may never seek medical attention, and in many cases, replacement of fluids and electrolytes is all that is required. In general, medical evaluation is warranted for patients with profuse watery diarrhea with dehydration, bloody stools, temperature greater than 101.3°F, or illness of more than 48 hours' duration. Other persons requiring medical evaluation include patients older than 50 years of age with severe abdominal pain, and immunocompromised patients (e.g., acquired immunodeficiency syndrome [AIDS], organ transplant recipients, or patients being treated with cancer chemotherapies.[12] Noninfectious causes for the illness, such as medications, inflammatory bowel disease, radiation colitis, or malabsorption syndromes, should be considered.

CASE 66-1, QUESTION 2: What rehydration plan would you recommend for B.K.?

B.K.'s physical examination is significant for decreased skin turgor and dry mucous membranes, findings consistent with mild to moderate volume depletion.[10] Given that B.K. is not "toxic" appearing, with stable vital signs, and is tolerating oral liquids, oral beverages containing glucose (e.g., lemonades, sweet sodas, or fruit juices) or soups rich in electrolytes are appropriate.[10,25,26] In developing countries, significant reductions in dehydration-related mortality is attributed to oral replacement therapy solutions containing optimal concentrations of sodium, potassium, chloride, bicarbonate and glucose; the glucose content of these solutions is responsible for accelerating the absorption of sodium.[26]

Intravenous replacement therapy is warranted for severe dehydration, which is characterized by lethargy, very sunken and dry eyes, a very dry tongue and mouth, a fast, weak or nonpalpable pulse,[10,26] poor urine output, and low blood pressure, or for persons with intestinal ileus or who are unable to drink on their own.[10]

CLINICAL PRESENTATION

CASE 66-1, QUESTION 3: How does B.K.'s clinical presentation as a noninflammatory versus inflammatory diarrheal illness help to guide further treatment?

Clinical presentation (e.g., the specific symptoms, the severity and duration of symptoms), along with the history of present illness (e.g., predisposing factors for infection), allows for classification of diarrheal syndromes as noninflammatory versus inflammatory illness. Such a classification allows the physician to prepare a more focused list of potential enteropathogen(s); based on the list of suspected organisms, a diagnostic and therapeutic plan can be developed.[1]

B.K.'s history of present illness and clinical presentation are consistent with a noninflammatory diarrheal illness. Voluminous, watery, nonbloody diarrhea is characteristic of pathogens targeting the small bowel, which is responsible for absorption of most fluids entering the GI tract.[4] Specifically, noninflammatory, watery diarrheal illnesses are a consequence of bacterial enterotoxins stimulating the secretion of water and electrolytes into the intestinal lumen or by viruses that infect and damage the absorptive villus tips, resulting in a watery diarrhea.[4] Like B.K., patients with noninflammatory diarrheal illnesses are not severely ill and are afebrile and without significant abdominal pain[2,4]; most patients require only supportive therapies. Noninflammatory diarrheas are typically caused by rotaviruses, noroviruses, *Staphylococcus aureus, Bacillus cereus, Clostridium perfringens, Cryptosporidium parvum,* and *Giardia lamblia.*[12]

In contrast, inflammatory diarrheas are generally a more severe illness characterized by diarrhea with or without dysentery, abdominal pain, and fever.[2] Pathogens targeting the distal small bowel and colon disrupt the epithelial barrier, leading to the bloody or mucoid stools.[2] In addition to supportive therapies, selected persons with inflammatory diarrheal illnesses may benefit from antimicrobial therapy directed at the causative pathogen. Inflammatory diarrheas resulting from the production of cytotoxins are caused by *C. difficile,* Shiga toxin–producing *E. coli* (STEC), and enteroaggregative *E. coli,* whereas disease attributable to the invasion of the intestinal mucosa are caused by *Campylobacter jejuni, Shigella* species, and *Salmonella* species.[27]

VIRAL GASTROENTERITIS

Clinical Presentation and Treatment

CASE 66-1, QUESTION 4: B.K.'s stool is negative for WBCs and RBCs. With B.K.'s history of dining and other patrons having similar illness, the physician calls the Board of Health to find out whether persons with a similar illness have been identified. The physician is informed that an outbreak of norovirus (previously called Norwalk-like virus) gastroenteritis was confirmed at the restaurant where B.K. had dined. Why are B.K.'s history of present illness and clinical presentation consistent with the presumptive diagnosis of a viral gastroenteritis, specifically the norovirus? What supportive therapies are recommended?

Noroviruses are responsible for major outbreaks of foodborne viral illnesses in both adults and children, usually in association with restaurants, schools, and day-care centers.[28] The virus is spread by eating inadequately cooked clams and oysters harvested from contaminated waters, by person-to-person contact, or by exposure to contaminated recreational waters.[28] Like B.K., within 12 to 48 hours after exposure to the virus, patients complain of nausea, vomiting, diarrhea, abdominal cramps, myalgias, headache, and chills; fever occurs in one-third to one-half of cases. Overall, this is generally a mild illness lasting 1 to 3 days. Prevention of illness is aimed at proper food-handling practices.[28]

Rotaviruses and astroviruses are responsible for 30% to 60% of all cases of severe, watery diarrhea in children. After an incubation period of 1 to 3 days, patients experience fever, vomiting, and watery but nonbloody diarrhea; otherwise healthy persons are typically ill for 5 to 7 days.

Supportive therapies to correct fluid and electrolyte losses and to replace ongoing losses are the mainstay of treatment for viral gastroenteritis. Compared with placebo, probiotics administered early (<60 hours) in the course of illness of hospitalized children with acute diarrhea caused by rotaviruses decreased the duration of the diarrheal illness (130 vs. 80 hours).[29]

As rotaviruses are spread by the fecal–oral route, proper hand washing and disposal of contaminated items are essential to limit the spread of infection. In the United States, the FDA-approved vaccine (RotaTeq) is indicated for the prevention of rotavirus gastroenteritis in infants and children. A three-dose series is administered between the ages of 6 and 32 weeks.[30]

VIBRIO SPECIES

Vibrio species are curved gram-negative rods whose natural habitats are the environmental waters throughout the world.

V. cholerae 01 and 0139 are toxigenic (toxin-producing) strains that cause epidemic cholera in humans. Noncholera *Vibrio* species, such as *Vibrio parahaemolyticus,* do not possess the virulence factors required to cause epidemic cholera, but are associated with gastroenteritis, wound infections, and in susceptible hosts, fulminant sepsis.[7]

To view an electron photomicrograph of *Vibrio cholerae,* go to http://thepoint.lww.com/AT10e.

Vibrio cholerae

CLINICAL PRESENTATION

CASE 66-2

QUESTION 1: M.M. is a 50-year-old man hospitalized for severe watery diarrhea, vomiting, and altered mental status. His history of present illness is significant for returning 1 day ago from Latin America, where he visited with relatives, several of whom were recovering from a diarrheal illness caused by *V. cholerae*. Approximately 24 hours before admission, he noted the onset of watery diarrhea, and began drinking the oral rehydrating solution left over from his trip to Latin America. During the past several hours he has been unable to drink on his own, and his family noticed "white flecks" in his stools. His past medical history is significant for peptic ulcer disease for which he takes a proton-pump inhibitor.

In the emergency department, M.M.'s vital signs are as follows: temperature is 101°F, blood pressure is 70/40 mm Hg, and heart rate is 130 beats/minute. His weight is 61 kg, which is 8 kg below his normal weight. Physical examination reveals a critically ill man with sunken eyes, poor skin turgor, and dry mucous membranes. The physician's assessment is severe dehydration, most likely secondary to infection from *V. cholerae*. Why is M.M.'s history of present illness and past medical history consistent with a severe diarrheal illness caused by toxin-producing *V. cholerae*?

In the United States and other developed nations, cholera has been virtually eliminated because of modern sewage and water treatment systems. Sporadic cases of cholera are identified in the United States, particularly in travelers like M.M. returning from areas where epidemics or outbreaks of cholera still occur, such as parts of Latin America (most recently in Haiti),[31] Africa, or Asia; in travelers bringing contaminated seafood (e.g., improperly preserved fish, raw oysters, and shellfish, such as crabs) back to the United States[10]; and from the consumption of undercooked seafood harvested from contaminated waters off the Gulf Coast.[7] M.M.'s additional risk factor for acquiring cholera is his daily use of a proton-pump inhibitor, because the reduced stomach acidity allows the acid-susceptible *V. cholerae* to pass from the stomach into the small intestine.[2]

As was the case with M.M., patients experience a mild to moderate watery diarrheal illness, 12 hours to 5 days after ingestion of contaminated foods. Although disease may progress to life-threatening dehydration,[10] most patients, however, remain asymptomatic carriers of *V. cholerae.* Cholera epidemics are caused by toxin-producing strains of *V. cholerae* 01 or 0139.[7] The voluminous, watery, and colorless stools with "white flecks" of mucus, referred to as rice-water stools, are caused by the cholera toxin, which promotes the intestinal secretion of fluids and electrolytes.[10]

TREATMENT

CASE 66-2, QUESTION 2: What are the signs and symptoms suggestive of severe dehydration, and how should M.M.'s dehydration be treated?

M.M. is one of the 2% to 5% of persons with *V. cholerae* infection who experience severe dehydration and who may, within hours, progress to hypovolemic shock and death. Patients may lose up to 1 L/hour of fluid during the first 24 hours and lose up to 10% of their body weight.

M.M. shows signs of severe dehydration as manifested by his altered mental status, sunken eyes, poor skin turgor, dry mucous membranes, low blood pressure, increased heart rate, and weight loss of more than 10% of his normal body weight.[10] Acidosis may occur as a result of massive bicarbonate losses through the diarrheal stools, and be exacerbated by lactic acidosis from shock and hypovolemic renal failure.[10] M.M. should receive vigorous IV hydration with Ringer's lactate solution to replace the large quantities of sodium, potassium, and bicarbonate being lost through his watery stools. Monitoring of blood pressure and normalization of heart rate are critical interventions. Once M.M. is able to drink fluids, oral hydration can be started, even with ongoing IV hydration. Oral replacement solutions containing less than 75 mEq/L of sodium are inappropriate because of the large amounts of sodium lost through cholera stools.[10]

CASE 66-2, QUESTION 3: Would M.M. benefit from the administration of antibiotics?

Antimicrobials administered to patients with cholera decrease the volume of diarrheal losses, shorten the duration of illness, and reduce the period of carriage.[7] Selection of an antimicrobial should include the susceptibility of the circulating strain,[32] as antimicrobial susceptibility of *V. cholerae* varies and changes with time.[33]

Both single-dose and multiple-dose regimens are effective against susceptible *V. cholerae;* single-dose regimens are preferred because of their ease of administration, and compared with erythromycin, are better tolerated.[32,34] In adults, susceptible *V. cholerae* infections are treated with one of the following single-dose oral regimens: 300 mg of doxycycline,[7] 1 g of ciprofloxacin,[35] or 1 g of azithromycin[32]; multiple-dose regimens include tetracycline (500 mg orally every 6 hours for 48–72 hours),[7] erythromycin (250 mg orally four times daily for 3 days),[10] or TMP-SMX (160 mg TMP/800 mg SMX twice daily for 3 days).[7]

In children, susceptible *V. cholerae* infections are treated with one of the following single-dose oral regimens: ciprofloxacin 20 mg/kg (maximum, 750 mg)[32] or azithromycin 20 mg/kg (maximum, 1 g)[34]; multiple-dose regimens include erythromycin 250 mg orally four times daily for 3 days,[10] erythromycin 12.5 mg/kg/dose (maximum, 500 mg/dose) every 6 hours for 3 days,[32] or TMP-SMX (5 mg/kg/dose TMP, 25 mg/kg/dose SMX twice daily for 3 days).[7]

Vibrio parahaemolyticus

CLINICAL PRESENTATION

CASE 66-3

QUESTION 1: C.T. is a 45-year-old man presenting to his physician with 1 day of nonbloody, watery diarrhea. Two days before this illness, he had dinner at a local restaurant, which included an appetizer of raw oysters. C.T. lives along the coast of Florida, and has no significant medical

history. His physical examination reveals no signs or symptoms of dehydration. Why is C.T.'s history of present illness and clinical presentation consistent with noncholera *Vibrio* gastroenteritis?

A key piece of information from C.T.'s history of present illness consistent with the presumptive diagnosis of noncholera *Vibrio* gastroenteritis is consumption of raw oysters harvested from areas such as the coastal areas of Florida, where *V. parahaemolyticus* species have been identified. Diarrhea, abdominal cramps, nausea, vomiting, and fever begin after a median incubation period of 17 hours (range, 4–90 hours); bloody diarrhea occurs in 9% to 29% of cases. In Japan, *V. parahaemolyticus* is a frequent cause of watery diarrhea because of the popularity of consuming raw fish and shellfish.[7]

TREATMENT

CASE 66-3, QUESTION 2: Should a course of antibiotics be prescribed for C.T.?

In otherwise healthy adults, *V. parahaemolyticus* gastroenteritis is usually a mild, self-limiting illness with a median duration of 2 to 6 days.[7] There are no data to support a benefit of antibiotics in this setting, although patients with diarrhea lasting longer than 5 days may benefit from treatment with tetracycline or a fluoroquinolone; minocycline 100 mg orally every 12 hours and cefotaxime 2 g IV every 8 hours have also been recommended.[7]

Individuals with liver disease or alcoholism are at risk for severe *Vibrio* infections, including septicemia[7]; such individuals should avoid eating raw or undercooked shellfish, and avoid the exposure of wounds to seawater, especially during the warmer months when water temperatures favor the growth of *Vibrio* species.

STAPHYLOCOCCUS AUREUS, BACILLUS CEREUS, AND CLOSTRIDIUM PERFRINGENS

Staphylococcus aureus, B. cereus, and *C. perfringens* are important causes of toxin-mediated foodborne illnesses. Gastrointestinal symptoms typically begin within 24 hours after the ingestion of contaminated foods, which is in contrast to the longer incubation periods for illnesses caused by *Salmonella, Shigella,* and *Campylobacter* species. *B. cereus,* however, causes two different intestinal syndromes: the short-incubation disease characterized by vomiting (emetic syndrome), and a long-incubation disease characterized by a diarrheal illness (diarrheal syndrome).

Clinical Presentation and Treatment

CASE 66-4

QUESTION 1: S.A. is an otherwise healthy 23-year-old college student, who presents to the Student Health Center with an acute gastrointestinal illness after dinner at the school cafeteria. S.A. recalled eating the salad and the cream-filled pastries, and stated that within 3 hours, she felt nauseous and began vomiting. Why is S.A.'s history of present illness and clinical presentation consistent with food poisoning caused by *S. aureus* or *B. cereus* (short-incubation)?

Foodborne illnesses are often grouped by their usual incubation period: less than 6 hours, 8 to 16 hours, and greater than 16 hours.[36] The rapid onset (within 6 hours) of S.A.'s intestinal symptoms after eating suggests the illness is caused by preformed toxins, such as those produced by *S. aureus* or *B. cereus* (short-incubation disease, emetic syndrome). Diarrhea and abdominal cramps may also occur. Although cooking kills the toxin-producing bacteria, it does not destroy toxin that has already been produced. Foods implicated in staphylococcal food poisoning include salads, cream-filled pastries, and meats, whereas foods implicated in *B. cereus* food poisoning include fried rice, dried foods, and dairy products.[36]

CASE 66-5

QUESTION 1: C.P. is also an otherwise healthy 23-year-old college student presenting to the same Student Health Center as S.A., with an acute gastrointestinal illness. C.P. recalled having lunch at the cafeteria, selecting the fish and poultry dishes. Approximately 10 hours after eating, she reported diarrhea and abdominal cramps. Why is C.P.'s history of present illness and clinical presentation consistent with food poisoning caused by *C. perfringens* or *B. cereus* (long-incubation disease)? Should empiric antibiotics be prescribed to either of these students?

In contrast to S.A., the longer incubation period before the onset of symptoms is consistent with illness caused by *C. perfringens* or *B. cereus* (long-incubation disease, diarrheal syndrome). These bacteria are associated with an incubation period of 8 to 16 hours and symptoms of diarrhea and abdominal cramps; vomiting is not a prominent symptom in these illnesses.[36]

C. perfringens or *B. cereus* associated with long-incubation disease produces heat-labile toxins after the ingestion of contaminated foods, resulting in a longer incubation period, compared with illness caused by the ingestion of preformed toxins. Foods implicated in *C. perfringens* food poisoning include improperly stored beef, fish, poultry dishes, pasta salads, and dairy products, whereas foods implicated in long-incubation *B. cereus* food poisoning include meats, vanilla sauce, cream-filled baked goods, and salads.[36]

Foodborne illnesses caused by these toxin-producing bacteria usually resolve within 24 hours, and antibiotic therapy is not indicated.

CRYPTOSPORIDIUM PARVUM

Cryptosporidia parvum is an important cause of human intestinal illness in both healthy and immunocompromised persons. The role of antiprotozoal agents and the clinical response to these agents differs depending on the patient.

Clinical Presentation

CASE 66-6

QUESTION 1: C.K., a 35-year-old, previously healthy man, presented to his physician with complaints of 15 days of watery diarrhea and a 5-pound weight loss. He is concerned that his illness is related to the announcement by the Board of Health, notifying the community of an outbreak of cryptosporidiosis from contaminated water supplies. Why are C.K.'s history of present illness and clinical presentation consistent with cryptosporidiosis? Should antiprotozoal agents be prescribed to treat cryptosporidiosis in otherwise healthy persons such as C.K.?

A key finding from C.K.'s history is his exposure to water supplies known to be contaminated with cryptosporidium oocysts[37]; other modes of spreading cryptosporidiosis include animal contact (cattle and sheep) and person-to-person contact (e.g., health care workers, day-care personnel).[37]

C.K. is presenting with persistent diarrhea, i.e., diarrhea lasting longer than 14 days. Common microbial causes of persistent watery diarrhea include parasites, such as *Isospora belli, Microsporidia, G. lamblia*, and *C. parvum*. The spectrum of infection with *C. parvum* ranges from asymptomatic carriage to a persistent, noninflammatory diarrheal illness[37]; vomiting, abdominal cramps, weight loss, and fever may also occur.[37] Immunocompetent patients like C.K. can generally expect a self-limiting illness lasting approximately 2 weeks.[37]

In contrast, in immunocompromised patients, cryptosporidiosis can be a chronic, debilitating, diarrheal illness associated with malnutrition, increased mortality, and in children, long-term cognitive impairment.[38]

Treatment

For immunocompetent hosts with cryptosporidiosis, other than replacement of fluids and electrolytes, no specific therapy directed at the organism is generally required.[39] Nevertheless, a 3-day course of nitazoxanide taken with food (≥12 years, 500 mg every 12 hours; 4–11 years, 200 mg every 12 hours; and 1–3 years, 100 mg every 12 hours) is approved for the treatment of diarrhea caused by *C. parvum* in persons older than 1 year of age.[40] A randomized, double-blind, placebo-controlled trial in immunocompetent adults and children found that diarrhea resolved in 80% of those treated with nitazoxanide versus 41% of patients given placebo; oocyst shedding was also significantly reduced in the treatment group. Diarrhea generally resolved within 3 to 4 days of starting treatment.[41]

In contrast, for immunocompromised persons, a meta-analysis of treatments for cryptosporidiosis found no evidence to support the role of chemotherapy.[39] These findings are consistent with randomized trials concluding that neither a short, 3-day course of nitazoxanide nor a more intensive regimen of nitazoxanide (200–400 mg twice daily for 28 days) provided any benefit to HIV-positive children. For HIV-infected persons, reconstitution of the immune system is the mainstay of treatment for cryptosporidiosis.

SALMONELLA

Salmonellae are enteric gram-negative bacilli that are important causes of foodborne illness in humans. Nontyphoidal salmonellae (e.g., *Salmonella typhimurium, Salmonella enteritidis, Salmonella choleraesuis*, and many others) cause the clinical syndromes of gastroenteritis, bacteremia, and localized infection,[42] whereas typhoidal salmonellae (*Salmonella typhi* and *Salmonella paratyphi* A, B, and C) cause the syndromes of enteric fever (also referred to as typhoid or paratyphoid fever) and chronic carriage.[43] The role of antimicrobials in the management of salmonellosis depends on the clinical syndrome, its severity, and underlying health problems of infected persons.

ONLINE CONTENT

For a visual of *Salmonella* with flagella., go to http://thepoint.lww.com/AT10e.

Nontyphoidal Salmonellosis

UNCOMPLICATED GASTROENTERITIS IN THE IMMUNOCOMPETENT HOST

CLINICAL PRESENTATION

CASE 66-7

QUESTION 1: B.B., a 35-year-old, otherwise healthy man, presents to his physician with a 1-day history of abdominal pain, nausea, vomiting, and nonbloody stools. One day before the onset of his symptoms, he dined at a local restaurant, ordering the turkey dinner. He later heard news reports of an outbreak of *Salmonella* gastroenteritis attributed to food served at the restaurant. B.B. has no significant medical history. On physical examination, he is not ill appearing, but is febrile. The rest of his examination is normal. B.B. is given the presumptive diagnosis of mild, uncomplicated nontyphoidal *Salmonella* gastroenteritis. Why is B.B.'s history of present illness and clinical presentation consistent with this diagnosis?

A key piece of information from B.B.'s history of present illness that is consistent with the presumptive diagnosis of foodborne *Salmonella* gastroenteritis is his eating of foods associated with an outbreak of *Salmonella* gastroenteritis. Salmonellae are widely found in nature, colonizing animal hosts, including mammals, reptiles, and birds, and consequently are major causes of foodborne illnesses. Frequently contaminated foods include poultry or poultry products (eggs) and dairy products.[13]

Similar to that seen in B.B., patients with *Salmonella* gastroenteritis present with an acute onset of fever, diarrhea, and abdominal cramping within 6 to 72 hours of ingestion of contaminated foods; other manifestations include bloody diarrhea and dehydration.

TREATMENT

CASE 66-7, QUESTION 2: Should B.B. receive a course of antibiotics to treat his presumed diagnosis of uncomplicated nontyphoidal *Salmonella* gastroenteritis?

In otherwise healthy individuals such as B.B., uncomplicated nontyphoidal *Salmonella* salmonellosis is typically self-limiting, lasting for 2 to 5 days, and antibiotics are not routinely recommended. Antimicrobials do not reduce the duration or severity of illness, and may actually prolong asymptomatic carriage of salmonellae, promotes the emergence of antimicrobial-resistant bacteria, and place patients at risk for adverse drug reactions.[44] Most individuals will only require replacement of lost fluids and electrolytes.

Antimicrobials should be reserved for persons who are severely ill or at risk for having extraintestinal *Salmonella* infection; they have also been used when rapid interruption of fecal excretion of organisms is needed to control outbreaks of salmonellosis in institutionalized persons.[13]

CASE 66-7, QUESTION 3: Three weeks after resolution of B.B.'s acute episode of *Salmonella* gastroenteritis, he is found to be still excreting *Salmonella* bacteria from his stool, despite remaining asymptomatic. Should antimicrobials be prescribed to eliminate B.B.'s intestinal carriage of nontyphoidal *Salmonella*?

A randomized, double-blind trial in healthy, asymptomatic adults from areas where nontyphoidal salmonellae are endemic concluded that neither norfloxacin or azithromycin was better than placebo in eradicating intestinal carriage of *Salmonella* species.[27] The median duration of fecal shedding of nontyphoidal *Salmonella* is about 1 month in adults and 7 weeks in children younger than 5 years of age.[13] Thus, antimicrobials should not be prescribed to eliminate intestinal carriage of nontyphoidal *Salmonella* in asymptomatic carriers like B.B.[27]

GASTROENTERITIS IN PATIENTS AT RISK FOR EXTRAINTESTINAL SALMONELLA INFECTION

CLINICAL PRESENTATION

CASE 66-7, QUESTION 4: W.M., a 75-year-old moderately ill-appearing man, presents to his physician with signs and symptoms of *Salmonella* gastroenteritis. His history of present illness is significant for eating the same turkey dinner as B.B. (Case 66-7, Questions 1–3). In contrast to B.B., W.M.'s medical history is significant for recently diagnosed leukemia. Would antimicrobial therapy benefit W.M.?

Overall, less than 5% of patients with nontyphoidal *Salmonella* gastroenteritis become bacteremic, although infection with some serotypes, e.g., *S. choleraesuis* and *Salmonella dublin,* are more likely to be associated with bloodstream infections.[44] Complications of bloodstream infections include osteomyelitis, septic arthritis, meningitis, or infectious endarteritis.[13] Host factors that increase the risk for extraintestinal *Salmonella* infection include a very young age, low gastric pH (e.g., as in infancy, pernicious anemia, or medication-induced), diabetes, malignancy, rheumatologic disorders, HIV infection, and receipt of immunosuppressive therapies.[42] Compared with non–HIV-infected persons, patients with HIV infection and a CD4 count less than 200 cells/μL are significantly more likely to have invasive, nontyphoidal salmonellosis.[45]

Antimicrobial therapy (usually 3–7 days) is recommended for severely ill persons like W.M., and for persons with underlying conditions that increase the risk for extraintestinal infection. Additionally, a short course (duration of 48–72 hours or until the patient is afebrile) of antimicrobials is commonly recommended for persons older than 50 years of age who may have atherosclerotic lesions, which, if bacteremia were to occur, could become hematogenously infected.[13]

TREATMENT

Nalidixic Acid Resistance

CASE 66-7, QUESTION 5: The physician receives from the Board of Health the following susceptibility information for the isolate responsible for the ongoing outbreak of *Salmonella* gastroenteritis.

Microbiology Report:

Salmonella species	
Ampicillin	Resistant
Ceftriaxone	Susceptible
Chloramphenicol	Resistant
Ciprofloxacin	Susceptible
Nalidixic acid	Resistant
TMP-SMX	Resistant

What is the significance of nalidixic acid resistance as it pertains to the use of fluoroquinolones (e.g., ciprofloxacin) for the treatment of salmonellosis?

Patients infected with nalidixic acid–resistant *Salmonella* who are treated with a fluoroquinolone are at greater risk for treatment failure, despite routine susceptibility tests indicating susceptibility to the fluoroquinolone.[46] Nalidixic acid and the fluoroquinolones are related compounds, belonging to the quinolone family of antibiotics.[47] Nalidixic acid is the predecessor of the quinolone family, but is not frequently prescribed because many common enteropathogens are resistant to this agent. In contrast, fluoroquinolones, named so because of the structural modification that added a fluorine atom to the quinolone molecule, are widely prescribed because of their greater antimicrobial activity.[47] Because of the structural similarities between these agents, nalidixic acid resistance is usually, but not always, indicative of low-level fluoroquinolone resistance, and as discussed below, is not readily detected by routine susceptibility testing.[48]

Ciprofloxacin minimum inhibitory concentration (MIC) breakpoints for Enterobacteriace including *Salmonella* are at least 4 mcg/mL (resistant) and 1 mcg/mL or less (susceptible).[48] Comparison of the ciprofloxacin MICs for nalidixic acid–resistant salmonellae cultured from patients failing fluoroquinolone therapy generally reveals these strains have higher ciprofloxacin MICs (0.12–0.5 mcg/mL) compared with nalidixic acid–susceptible strains (MICs <0.03 mcg/mL).[22,48] Because the breakpoint for susceptibility to ciprofloxacin is 1 mcg/mL or less, routine susceptibility testing will not detect isolates with low-level ciprofloxacin resistance. Although nalidixic acid–resistance has been recommended as a surrogate marker for *Salmonella* species with low-level fluoroquinolone resistance, more recent data show that this is not always the case, leading some experts to recommend that the actual fluoroquinolone MIC of isolates be determined.[49]

When fluoroquinolones are used for the treatment of nalidixic acid–resistant infections, treatment failures occur more often compared with infections caused by nalidixic acid–susceptible isolates.[24]

CASE 66-7, QUESTION 6: What antimicrobials are available for the treatment of nontyphoidal *Salmonella* infection?

Fluoroquinolones are widely recommended for the empiric treatment of nontyphoidal salmonellosis,[3] as the prevalence of multidrug-resistant (simultaneous resistance to ampicillin, TMP-SMX, and chloramphenicol) isolates frequently exceeds 50%. During the 1990s, suboptimal clinical responses after treatment with fluoroquinolones raised questions about the effectiveness of this class of antimicrobials for the treatment of salmonellosis.[48] Microbiologic tests revealed these *Salmonella* strains, in addition to being multidrug-resistant, were also resistant to nalidixic acid.[48]

Although nalidixic acid–resistant isolates have been identified in Asia for many years, such isolates are increasingly more common in the United States.[22] A survey of nontyphoidal *Salmonella* species isolated from infected persons revealed an increase in the proportion of nalidixic acid–resistant nontyphi *Salmonella,* from 0.4% in 1996 to 2.3% in 2003.[22] Ninety-one percent of these nalidixic acid–resistant isolates showed decreased susceptibility to ciprofloxacin (MIC ≥0.12 mcg/mL), and 7% were resistant to ciprofloxacin (MIC ≥32 mcg/mL). Among the nalidixic acid–resistant isolates, the most common resistance phenotype was simultaneous resistance to ampicillin, chloramphenicol, streptomycin, sulfamethoxazole, and tetracycline.[22]

If susceptible, antimicrobial options for the empiric treatment of nontyphoidal salmonellosis include azithromycin, ceftriaxone, or a fluoroquinolone.[3] Ceftriaxone resistance, although uncommon, has been identified in many areas of the world; these strains may also exhibit decreased susceptibility to ciprofloxacin.[50] Imipenem has been successfully used for the treatment of invasive infection caused by *Salmonella enterica* serotype choleraesuis, resistant to both ceftriaxone and ciprofloxacin.[51]

INVASIVE NONTYPHOIDAL SALMONELLA INFECTION

CLINICAL PRESENTATION AND TREATMENT

CASE 66-7, QUESTION 7: B.T. is an "ill-appearing," 70-year-old man, hospitalized for severe abdominal pain, bloody diarrhea, new-onset right hip pain, and a temperature of 102°F. His history of present illness is significant for eating the same turkey dinner as B.B. (Case 66-7, Question 1). His past surgical history is significant for a right hip prosthesis. Would B.T. benefit from antibiotic therapy, and if so, what would you recommend?

B.T. is presenting with signs and symptoms of *Salmonella* gastroenteritis, and probable bloodstream infection (i.e., fever) complicated by localized infection of his prosthetic hip (i.e., new-onset right hip pain). Treatment of *Salmonella* bacteremia without localized infection is generally successful after 10 to 14 days of antimicrobial therapy.[3,45] However, if infection of B.T.'s prosthetic hip is confirmed, a longer duration of treatment and surgery may be required to cure the infection.[13] Until susceptibility data are available, empiric antimicrobial treatment with ceftriaxone is a reasonable option. Widespread resistance to ampicillin, TMP-SMX, and fluoroquinolones precludes their empiric use.

Typhoidal Salmonellosis—Typhoid Fever (Enteric Fever)

CLINICAL PRESENTATION

CASE 66-8

QUESTION 1: B.C. is a 49-year-old obese woman, presenting to the emergency department with a 1-week history of fever, confusion and delirium, abdominal pain, headache, anorexia, and diarrhea. One day before admission, she noted a new, red rash on her chest. Her history of present illness is significant for returning 10 days ago from travel to the Indian subcontinent, where she stayed with relatives, some of whom were recovering from typhoid fever. B.C.'s medical history is significant for gallstones. She lives in California with her husband. Admission vital signs are as follows: temperature is 101°F and heart rate is 60 beats/minute; blood pressure is stable. Physical examination is significant for splenomegaly and hepatomegaly. Laboratory tests include the following: WBC is 3.0 × $10^6/\mu L$, liver function tests are mildly elevated, and the results of two sets of blood cultures are pending. B.C. is given the presumptive diagnosis of enteric fever and encephalopathy most likely attributable to *S. typhi*. Why is her history of present illness, clinical presentation, and laboratory results consistent with this diagnosis?

Key pieces of information from B.C.'s history of present illness supporting her diagnosis of typhoid fever (also referred to as enteric fever) are her recent travel history and exposure to relatives recovering from typhoid fever. Typhoid fever is endemic in developing areas of the world such as the Indian subcontinent, Southeast Asia, Africa, and Latin America.[43] In developed countries, enteric fever is a sporadic disease occurring mainly in travelers returning from areas where the disease is endemic. Eighty-five percent of cases of typhoid fever diagnosed in the United States are travel-related, with most persons reporting recent travel to the Indian subcontinent, specifically to India, Pakistan, or Bangladesh.[52]

B.C.'s clinical presentation and laboratory findings are classic for enteric fever. During the 7- to 14-day incubation period,[43] salmonellae multiply within macrophages and monocytes; systemic manifestations of infection appear after the release of bacteria into the bloodstream. Patients present with fever, abdominal pain, anorexia, diarrhea or constipation, headache, dry cough, splenomegaly, and hepatomegaly; severe illness is characterized by concomitant GI bleeding, encephalopathy, and shock.[43] Bacteremia may be followed by localized infection to the liver, spleen, bone marrow, Peyer's patches of the terminal ileum, and gallbladder.[53] Laboratory abnormalities consistent with typhoid fever include B.C.'s low WBC count and mildly elevated liver function tests.[43]

For a visual of the stages of typhoid fever, see http://thepoint.lww.com/AT10e.

TREATMENT

CASE 66-8, QUESTION 2: Would B.C. benefit from a course of antimicrobials to treat her presumptive diagnosis of typhoid fever? If so, what options are available?

Treatment of typhoid fever with effective antimicrobials results in resolution of fever and other symptoms within 3 to 5 days and clearing of all symptoms within 7 to 10 days,[54] decreasing mortality from 5% to 10% to less than 1%,[43] eradicating fecal shedding of *S. typhi*, thereby limiting the spread of infection,[54] and preventing relapse of infection. Relapsing infection occurs in 5% to 10% of patients, typically within 2 to 3 weeks after resolution of fever.[55] Most cases of typhoid fever are treated with oral antimicrobials, with IV therapy reserved for severely ill patients or patients with persistent vomiting and severe diarrhea.[53]

Until the late 1980s, the standard treatments for typhoid fever were 14 to 21 days of chloramphenicol, TMP-SMX, or ampicillin, regimens with cure rates exceeding 90%.[55] By the early 1990s, multidrug-resistant (i.e., simultaneous resistance to chloramphenicol, ampicillin, and TMP-SMX) *S. typhi* caused outbreaks of typhoid fever in India, Pakistan, Bangladesh, Vietnam, the Middle East, and Africa. These isolates, however, remained susceptible to the fluoroquinolones.

Short treatment courses (e.g., 3–5 days) of oral fluoroquinolones were found to be as effective or better than the longer standard treatments.[55] In children and adults, the majority of whom were infected with multidrug-resistant *S. typhi*, ofloxacin (7.5 mg/kg/dose twice daily for 2–3 days[56] or 200 mg every 12 hours for 5 days[42]) cured greater than 89% of patients. In adults, ofloxacin was superior to a 5-day course of ceftriaxone even though all *S. typhi* isolates were susceptible to both study drugs; the six ceftriaxone failures were successfully treated with ofloxacin.[42] Ceftriaxone (3–4 g/day for 3–7 days) is an alternative parenteral agent for seriously ill patients.[57]

By the late 1990s, clinical failures as high as 50% with short courses (less than 5 days) of a fluoroquinolone were reported from parts of Asia,[24] and in the United States, treatment failures in hospitalized patients with invasive *S. typhi* infection were also described. Microbiologic evaluation revealed these isolates were resistant to nalidixic acid, and had higher ciprofloxacin MICs (0.125–1 mcg/mL) compared with *Salmonella* that were fully susceptible to ciprofloxacin (MICs of <0.03 mcg/mL).[49,54] Newer fluoroquinolones (gemifloxacin and moxifloxacin) have lower MICs than the older fluoroquinolones, and may be the best fluoroquinolones for the treatment of multidrug-resistant and nalidixic acid–resistant isolates,[58] although clinical data are lacking.

Cefixime, an oral third-generation cephalosporin, has been used for the treatment of typhoid fever; however, failure rates range from 4% to 27%.[53] In a study from Nepal, in which 83% of isolates were nalidixic acid–resistant compared with gatifloxacin (no longer marketed in the United States), overall treatment failure was higher in the cefixime-treated patients (27% vs. 1%, $p < 0.001$). The lower clinical response to cefixime may be related to the poor intracellular penetration of the β-lactam, which is the primary site of *S. typhi* colonization.[59] In Bangladesh, 10 days of either cefixime (20 mg/kg/day in two divided doses) or cefpodoxime (16 mg/kg/day in two divided doses) cured 95% of infections; however, other than reporting that the MIC of all isolates to both cephalosporins was less than 4 mcg/mL, susceptibilities to other antimicrobials were not reported.[60]

Thus, in the setting of multidrug-resistant *S. typhi*, and increasing clinical failures with fluoroquinolones, treatment options for typhoid fever include ceftriaxone or azithromycin, although resistance and slower treatment responses with these agents have been reported. In a study in which all blood isolates were susceptible to azithromycin, ceftriaxone, and ciprofloxacin (susceptibility to nalidixic acid was not reported),[61] azithromycin (10 mg/kg/day, maximum 500 mg) was as effective as ceftriaxone (75 mg/kg/day for 7 days; maximum, 2.5 g/day), with clinical response rates of 91% and 97%, respectively. However, when infections were primarily caused by multidrug-resistant *S. typhi* or *S. paratyphi* (88% of isolates were resistant to TMP-SMX, chloramphenicol, and ampicillin and 93% were nalidixic acid–resistant), fewer patients were cured with this same 7-day course of azithromycin (51 [82%] patients); the cure rate was 64% with ofloxacin and 76% with azithromycin plus ofloxacin.[62]

Higher doses of azithromycin (20 mg/kg/day for 7 days), however, have been used when nalidixic acid resistance was more prevalent. In a study of children, most of whom were infected with multidrug-resistant *S. typhi* (96% were nalidixic acid–resistant with reduced susceptibility to ofloxacin and ciprofloxacin),[63] clinical cure was greater than 95%, similar to the comparator, gatifloxacin (10 mg/kg/day for 7 days).[63] Fever clearance time was 106 hours for both azithromycin and gatifloxacin, and relapse was uncommon, 0% and 2.9%, respectively.[63] Although gatifloxacin is no longer marketed in the United States, MICs to gatifloxacin are lower (0.19 mcg/mL) compared with ciprofloxacin (0.5 mcg/mL) and ofloxacin (1.5 mcg/mL).[63]

Although ceftriaxone remains very active against *S. typhi*, isolates with decreased susceptibility to ceftriaxone (MIC $\geq$2 mcg/mL) have been identified in the United States and elsewhere.[64] In clinical trials, the median time to defervescence in patients treated with ceftriaxone is in the range of 5 to 7 days, and some patients are febrile for 10 days.[65] Despite in vitro susceptibility, in bacteremic patients, relapse of infection is higher in ceftriaxone- versus azithromycin-treated patients, 14% versus 0%, respectively[66]; however, when a longer course (14 days) of ceftriaxone was used in children with multidrug-resistant *S. typhi*, no child experienced a relapse.[67] Azithromycin resistance in blood isolates of *S. typhi* has been reported to be as high as 95% in Bangladesh.[53]

Future treatment options will rely on ongoing surveillance of resistance patterns in *S. typhi*. The re-emergence of *S. typhi* susceptible to TMP-SMX[68] and chloramphenicol[54] may allow these agents to be useful and inexpensive alternatives for the treatment of *S. typhi* infection.

CASE 66-8, QUESTION 3: What specific empiric antibiotic regimen would you recommend for the treatment of B.C.'s typhoid fever?

B.C.'s clinical presentation, including altered mental status (confusion, delirium) is consistent with severe typhoid fever; thus, empiric therapy with parenteral ceftriaxone is warranted.[55] Uncomplicated typhoid fever can generally be treated with oral antibiotics. For adults, levofloxacin 500 mg once daily for 7 days (other fluoroquinolones can be used) or azithromycin 500 mg daily for 7 days are the primary choices.[3] For children, azithromycin is recommended; parenteral ceftriaxone is an alternative.[3]

Optimal treatment for fluoroquinolone-resistant *S. typhi*, which have been detected in India,[65] is yet to be determined; azithromycin, ceftriaxone, or maximal recommended doses of fluoroquinolones for 10 to 14 days have been recommended.[55] Aztreonam and imipenem are potential third-line alternatives for the treatment of typhoid fever.[53]

ADJUNCTIVE TREATMENT

CASE 66-8, QUESTION 4: Besides the administration of antibiotics, are there adjunctive therapies which could be of benefit to B.C.?

Enteric encephalopathy, i.e., altered mental status, is associated with a mortality rate as high as 56% if prompt treatment is not administered.[69] For persons with enteric encephalopathy, retrospective data have concluded that appropriate antimicrobial therapy combined with high-dose dexamethasone (3 mg/kg IV followed by 1 mg/kg every 6 hours IV for eight doses) improved survival.[69] The mechanism of action of dexamethasone in enteric encephalopathy is not known.[69]

CHRONIC TYPHOID CARRIERS

CLINICAL PRESENTATION

CASE 66-8, QUESTION 5: Fourteen months after discharge from the hospital, B.C.'s stool is still positive for *S. typhi*. During this time, her husband has had two episodes of typhoid fever. Why is B.C.'s clinical syndrome consistent with the chronic carrier state?

Unlike the nontyphoidal salmonellae, humans are the only natural host and reservoir for *S. typhi*.[65] Although most patients excrete *S. typhi* in their stools for 3 to 4 weeks after recovery from their illness, 1% to 3% excrete *Salmonella* from stool or urine for more than 1 year after infection; these individuals are referred to as "chronic carriers." B.C.'s risk factor for becoming a chronic carrier is her history of gallstones, which allows the sequestration of organisms in her diseased biliary tract. Although B.C. remains asymptomatic, she serves as a reservoir for spreading infection to others.

TREATMENT

CASE 66-8, QUESTION 6: What therapeutic options are available to cure B.C.'s chronic carrier state?

Treatment options for chronic *S. typhi* carriers include a prolonged course of antibiotics, cholecystectomy, or suppressive antimicrobial therapy.[55] Fifty-ninety percent of chronic carriers may be cured after prolonged courses of antibiotics,[70–73] although efficacy may be lessened when anatomic abnormalities (e.g., cholelithiasis) are present.[70] Relapse is usually detected within the first several months after completing antimicrobial therapy,[74] but can occur up to 24 months after completing therapy.[70] For susceptible *S. typhi*, antimicrobial regimens proven effective in curing chronic carriers include amoxicillin 2 g three times daily for 28 days,[72] ampicillin 1 g four times daily for 90 days,[71] ampicillin 1.5 g four times daily plus probenecid for 6 weeks,[70] TMP-SMX 160/800 mg twice a day for 3 months,[73] ciprofloxacin 500 to 750 mg twice a day for 3 to 4 weeks,[74–76] or norfloxacin 400 mg twice daily for 4 weeks.[77]

PREVENTION

CASE 66-8, QUESTION 7: B.C.'s sister is planning a trip to the Indian subcontinent and is concerned about acquiring typhoid fever. What can she do to reduce her risk for getting typhoid fever?

The World Health Organization and the U.S. Centers for Disease Control and Prevention recommend vaccination for prolonged (generally more than 1 month) travel to most destinations and for shorter stays in the hyperendemic Indian subcontinent.[65] In the United States, two licensed vaccines are currently available to provide protection against *S. typhi*, but not against *S. paratyphi*. The intramuscular vaccine for persons older than 2 years of age is 51% to 77% effective in preventing typhoid fever; adverse effects include local pain and swelling, fever, headache, and malaise.[55] The oral Ty21a vaccine for persons older than 6 years of age is well tolerated, and affords a protective efficacy rate ranging from 42% to 96%.[55]

As previously noted, neither vaccine is licensed to provide protection against *S. paratyphi*, which is of concern because in some Asian countries, *S. paratyphi* A accounts for up to 50% of blood isolates from patients with enteric fever.[78] Retrospective data indicate the oral Ty21a vaccine may offer some protection against *S. paratyphi* A and B,[65] although the intramuscular vaccine affords no protection against these organisms. Thus, as the available vaccine's protection against *S. typhi* is not 100%, and because neither vaccine is licensed to protect against *S. paratyphi*, it is still necessary to reinforce the importance of good hygiene and the avoidance of foods with a high risk for being contaminated with enteropathogens.

Section 14 Infectious Disease

SHIGELLA SPECIES

Shigella species are the most frequent causes of the dysentery syndrome, an inflammatory diarrheal illness characterized by bloody or mucoid stools with abdominal cramps. Of the four *Shigella* species, severe dysentery is most commonly caused by *Shigella dysenteriae* followed by *Shigella flexneri*, whereas a milder illness characterized by watery diarrhea with or without blood is typically caused by *Shigella sonnei* and *Shigella boydii*.[79]

Shigella dysenteriae

CLINICAL PRESENTATION

CASE 66-9

QUESTION 1: M.T. is a 60-year-old, ill-appearing man hospitalized for worsening bloody diarrhea and fever. Two days before admission, he noted the onset of fever, abdominal cramps, and six to seven nonbloody, watery stools. His diarrhea has since worsened to 10 to 12 small-volume stools with blood and mucus, and he now complains of painful straining while passing his stools. His history of present illness is significant for returning 2 days ago from a business trip to Bangladesh. During the business portion of the trip he remained at the hotel where all his meals were prepared by the hotel staff. However, on the day of his departure, he mingled with the local residents and sampled foods from local street vendors. M.T. lives alone in Florida, has no significant medical history or drug allergies, and takes no medications. On admission, his temperature is 101°F. Physical examination reveals an acutely ill man with severe abdominal tenderness, and with signs and symptoms of mild dehydration. Why are his history of present illness and clinical presentation consistent with the diagnosis of dysentery, most likely caused by *Shigella dysenteriae*?

M.T.'s presumptive diagnosis of dysentery is consistent with his recent travel to Bangladesh, where inadequate systems for disposal of sewage result in endemic shigellosis. Similarly, epidemics or outbreaks of *S. dysenteriae* occur in South Asia, India, and Sri Lanka.[79] Because as few as 10 to 100 *Shigella* organisms may be infectious in healthy hosts,[79] M.T. likely became infected after sampling contaminated foods prepared by local street vendors or through person-to-person contact from symptomatic persons with diarrhea or asymptomatic persons continuing to excrete shigellae from their stool.[80]

As with M.T., symptoms of dysentery begin within 24 to 48 hours after ingestion of *Shigella* bacteria and include fever, fatigue, malaise, and anorexia.[80] Watery diarrhea generally precedes dysentery, and frequently is the only manifestation of mild infection.[80] Progression to dysentery may follow within hours to days, and is characterized by frequent, small-volume, bloody, and mucoid stools, abdominal cramps, and tenesmus (painful straining when passing stools).[80] Acute complications of shigellosis include seizures, hemolytic uremic syndrome (HUS), and toxic megacolon.[80] Longer-term complications that may occur in susceptible hosts with diarrheal illnesses caused by invasive pathogens including *Shigella* species (*Salmonella* and *Campylobacter* species, and others have also been implicated) include a postinfectious irritable bowel syndrome[81] or reactive arthritis.[82]

TREATMENT

CASE 66-9, QUESTION 2: Would M.T. benefit from antimicrobials to treat his presumed diagnosis of shigellosis?

Effective antimicrobial therapy for shigellosis reduces the average duration of illness from 5 to 7 days to about 3 days,[80] and reduces the risk of death and serious infection-related complications. Within 48 hours of starting treatment, M.T. should notice a reduction in stool frequency, volume of bloody stools, and fever. Antimicrobial therapy quickly reduces the carriage and excretion of *Shigella* species, thus limiting the spread of infection.[83]

Despite the aforementioned benefits of antimicrobials, controversy surrounds their use and the risk for developing HUS. A retrospective study reported that early administration of effective antimicrobials is associated with a low risk for developing HUS; the authors speculated that the prior association between HUS and antimicrobial use may have been because effective antibiotics were given later during the course of the illness. Reasons for delay in administration of antimicrobials could have been related to the patient's delay in seeking medical care, or because the *Shigella* species were resistant to the initially prescribed antimicrobials.[84]

CASE 66-9, QUESTION 3: What empiric antimicrobial regimens are available for the treatment of shigellosis?

As *Shigella* species are well known for rapidly developing antimicrobial resistance, empiric antibiotic therapy should be based on the local susceptibility patterns.[80] At one time, effective treatments for shigellosis were TMP-SMX, ampicillin (but not amoxicillin),[85] or nalidixic acid.

During the 1990s, multidrug-resistant (e.g., resistance to ampicillin, TMP-SMX, and chloramphenicol) *Shigella* species were so common that fluoroquinolones, to which isolates remained susceptible, were widely prescribed.[86] In adults, norfloxacin 400 mg twice daily for 5 days[87] or ciprofloxacin 500 mg twice daily for 3 to 5 days[86,88] have been found to be effective against multidrug-resistant *S. dysenteriae* type 1 infection. Even a single dose of ciprofloxacin 1 g[89] or norfloxacin 800 mg[90] was as effective as longer treatment courses in patients with mild to moderate disease, but less effective than the standard 5-day treatment course in patients with more severe illness[89] or in patients infected with *S. dysenteriae* type 1.[89]

Since the introduction of fluoroquinolones as the drugs of choice for the treatment of shigellosis, fluoroquinolone-resistant (MIC 6–24 mcg/mL) *Shigella* species have emerged; however, these isolates remain susceptible to azithromycin and ceftriaxone.[3]

In the setting of epidemic dysentery caused by *S. dysenteriae* type 1, similar clinical outcomes were observed in adults treated with a single 1-g oral dose of azithromycin or multiple doses of ciprofloxacin (500 mg orally twice daily for 3 days). Of note, nearly all of the isolates were resistant to ampicillin and TMP-SMX, but only 17% were nalidixic acid–resistant. In this study, the mean number of days until resolution of symptoms after starting therapy was 2.5 days for azithromycin versus 2.3 days of ciprofloxacin.[91]

In adults with moderate to severe shigellosis caused by multidrug-resistant *Shigella* species, clinical efficacy is similar with oral azithromycin (500 mg on day 1, then 250 mg daily for 4 days) or oral ciprofloxacin (500 mg every 12 hours for 5 days), 89% versus 82%, respectively ($p > 0.2$).[46] Despite in vitro susceptibility to the study antibiotics, a greater proportion of the subset of patients infected with *S. dysenteriae* type 1 failed therapy with either azithromycin (29%) or ciprofloxacin (17%), compared with patients infected with other *Shigella* species (failure rate of 6% for either antibiotic).[46] Nearly all (97%) of the *S. dysenteriae* type 1 isolates were nalidixic acid–resistant, with a median ciprofloxacin MIC of 0.125 mcg/mL, whereas only 6% of the other *Shigella* species were nalidixic acid–resistant, with a median ciprofloxacin MIC of 0.016 mcg/mL. These findings parallel the higher treatment failures observed in patients infected with nalidixic acid–resistant *Salmonella* species who are treated with fluoroquinolones.[24]

Parenteral third-generation cephalosporins have a role in the treatment of multidrug-resistant shigellosis; however, the usefulness of the oral third-generation cephalosporin, cefixime, is less certain. Both ceftriaxone and cefotaxime have excellent in vitro activity against *Shigella* species and have been used alone[39] or with amikacin[46] for patients failing ciprofloxacin therapy. Ceftriaxone resistance in *S. dysenteriae* and other *Shigella* species have emerged in India, Korea, Taiwan, Argentina, and Turkey and is attributed to the production of extended-spectrum β-lactamases.[92]

The oral third-generation cephalosporin, cefixime, is unreliable for the treatment of shigellosis, with failures reported in 11% to 47% of patients.[93] Treatment failure is more common with infection caused by *S. flexneri* and *S. dysenteriae* type 1, the *Shigella* species typically associated with more severe illness.[52]

CASE 66-9, QUESTION 4: Should loperamide be started in patients with dysentery?

The use of loperamide in dysentery is controversial,[15] as prolonging the clearance of pathogens from the intestinal tract could worsen the severity of illness. In non–critically ill adults with bacillary dysentery primarily caused by *Shigella* species, the combination of ciprofloxacin and loperamide did not prolong fever. Rather, the combination decreased the number of unformed stools and shortened the duration of diarrhea.[88]

CASE 66-9, QUESTION 5: What would be an appropriate empiric antimicrobial regimen for patients like M.T. with severe dysentery, likely caused by *S. dysenteriae* type 1?

For severe cases of shigellosis, such as that displayed by M.T., or for the treatment of proven *S. dysenteriae* type 1 infection, 3 to 5 days of therapy is recommended.[3,80] Potential antimicrobials include ceftriaxone[3,21] or azithromycin,[3,21] and if susceptible, fluoroquinolones.[3]

Shigella Species Other Than *S. dysenteriae*

CLINICAL PRESENTATION

CASE 66-10

QUESTION 1: F.F. is a 30-year-old, previously healthy woman, presenting to her physician with nonbloody, watery diarrhea of 3 days' duration. Her history of present illness is significant for the following: 2 days before the onset of her gastrointestinal symptoms, she visited with her 4-year-old nephew who was recovering from *S. sonnei* shigellosis, which he acquired at school. F.F. has no significant medical history. Overall, she feels better compared with the previous day and is afebrile; her physical examination is completely normal. How does F.F.'s clinical presentation of shigellosis differ from that of M.T. (Case 66-9, Question 1)? Should F.F. be treated with antimicrobials for her presumed, mild case of shigellosis?

TREATMENT

F.F.'s diarrheal illness demonstrates the ease with which *Shigella* bacteria are transmitted to others, especially in settings where individuals are in close contact, including day-care centers, institutionalized patients, and military barracks.[80] Secondary attack rates as high as 40% occur within 1 to 4 days after exposure to the primary case.

S. sonnei accounts for 90% of shigellosis in developed countries. Most patients have a mild and self-limiting illness; thus, antimicrobials are not generally required. However, they are often prescribed to shorten the duration of illness and to reduce the infectious period.[21] For adults, a fluoroquinolone or azithromycin can be used. Because fluoroquinolones are not FDA approved for use in children, azithromycin or ceftriaxone are recommended.[3]

Ongoing surveillance to detect changes in antimicrobial susceptibility among *Shigella* species is needed to direct treatment recommendations. In the United States, ciprofloxacin-resistant *Shigella* species has been identified in New York,[21] and *S. sonnei* with reduced susceptibility to azithromycin have been identified.[94] Good hygiene and access to clean water and foods are essential to prevent the spread of shigellosis.

CAMPYLOBACTER JEJUNI

Clinical Presentation

CASE 66-11

QUESTION 1: M.U. is a 20-year-old, previously healthy woman presenting to the Student Health Center with the

following complaints for the past 24 hours: malaise, fever, diarrhea, abdominal pain, and bloody diarrhea. One day before the onset of her symptoms, she dined at a restaurant near campus, noting that the chicken she ate was not thoroughly cooked. She has no significant medical history and no recent travel history. On physical examination, M.U. is not ill appearing. The physician tells her that during the past week, several students with gastrointestinal symptoms similar to hers have been diagnosed with *C. jejuni* gastroenteritis, and all had recently eaten at the same restaurant. Why are M.U.'s history of present illness and clinical presentation consistent with *Campylobacter* gastroenteritis?

M.U.'s presumptive diagnosis of *Campylobacter* gastroenteritis is consistent with her eating undercooked chicken at a restaurant with an ongoing outbreak of *Campylobacter* gastroenteritis. In industrialized nations, the most important risk factor for acquiring *Campylobacter* infection is the consumption of improperly cooked foods, such as unpasteurized foods, and contaminated water. Prevention of *Campylobacter* infection involves careful food preparation and cooking practices.[95] Person-to-person transmission is not a major means of spreading this infection.

Beginning 24 to 72 hours after exposure to contaminated foods, clinical manifestations of *Campylobacter* gastroenteritis include diarrhea and fever (90%), abdominal cramps, and either loose and watery or bloody stools.[96] M.U. does not exhibit signs or symptoms of complicated *Campylobacter* infection, such as meningitis, cholecystitis, pancreatitis, peritonitis, gastrointestinal hemorrhage, and bacteremia; bacteremia occurs in less than 1% of cases, most commonly in immunosuppressed persons, the very young, or the elderly.

Less commonly, complications of *C. jejuni* gastroenteritis[96] include Guillain-Barré syndrome (<1/1,000 cases of infections), postinfectious irritable bowel syndrome, and a reactive arthritis.[82]

For a Gram stain of *Campylobacter jejuni* in stool that shows the curved and S-shaped forms, go to http://thepoint.lww.com/AT10e.

Treatment

CASE 66-11, QUESTION 2: Would M.U. benefit from antimicrobial therapy to treat her *Campylobacter* gastroenteritis?

Because *C. jejuni* gastroenteritis is an acute, self-limiting illness typically resolving within 1 week,[96] antibiotic therapy is usually not necessary.[97] However, antibiotics are recommended for patients with symptoms lasting longer than 1 week, high fevers, bloody stools, pregnant women, or immunocompromised hosts.[96] As M.U.'s clinical presentation includes fever with bloody stools, antimicrobial therapy is warranted.

When administered early in the course of the illness (i.e., before determining the cause of the diarrhea), antimicrobial therapy shortens the duration and the severity of illness and the duration of fecal excretion of pathogens.[95] In contrast, when antimicrobials are initiated later during the course of the illness (i.e., after determining the cause of the diarrhea), antimicrobials do not alter the clinical course of *Campylobacter* gastroenteritis.[98]

CASE 66-11, QUESTION 3: What empiric antimicrobial therapies could be initiated to treat M.U.'s presumed case of *C. jejuni* enteritis?

Although fluoroquinolones were once considered the drugs of choice for *Campylobacter* infection, fluoroquinolone-resistance in *Campylobacter* species is common, ranging from 10% to 29% in Sweden, the United Kingdom, the Netherlands, and United States, and as high as 72% to 84% in Thailand and Spain[96]; resistance to erythromycin remains low (2%).[95] Widespread fluoroquinolone resistance is largely attributed to their use in veterinary medicine and food animals (e.g., poultry); the latter practice has since been banned in the United States.[23]

Infection with fluoroquinolone- or erythromycin-resistant *Campylobacter* species increases the risk for invasive illness or death.[97] In travelers with *Campylobacter* gastroenteritis, a trend is seen toward a longer duration of illness in patients treated with ciprofloxacin versus azithromycin (52 hours vs. 40 hours, respectively), which may be related to the finding that 50% of the *Campylobacter* isolates were resistant to ciprofloxacin, whereas all isolates were susceptible to azithromycin.[99]

Recommended treatments for *C. jejuni* gastroenteritis in adults are 3 days of either azithromycin 500 mg once daily or erythromycin 500 mg four times daily. Children may be treated with azithromycin 10 mg/kg/day once daily for 3 to 5 days or erythromycin 30 mg/kg in two to four divided doses for 3 to 5 days.[3] On the basis of M.U.'s medical history and clinical presentation, empiric therapy with oral erythromycin or azithromycin can be started.

TRAVELERS' DIARRHEA (TD)

Of the nearly one billion people who travel each year, approximately 20% to 60% traveling from industrialized countries to developing areas will experience an acute, self-limiting diarrheal illness; 5% to 10% of these travelers will continue to have enteric symptoms for as long as 5 years after their initial illness, a condition referred to as the postinfectious irritable bowel syndrome (PI-IBS).[14]

Travel to areas with suboptimal sanitation facilities to manage the disposal of sewage is a major risk factor for TD. Antimicrobials with or without antimotility therapy significantly reduce the duration and severity of illness. Many experts now recommend that in addition to pretravel education on the selection of "safe foods" and preventing dehydration, travelers should be bringing with them a travel kit including medications intended for self-treatment of TD at the onset of illness.[14]

Definition, Etiology, and Clinical Presentation

CASE 66-12

QUESTION 1: W.D. and B.D. are otherwise healthy 23-year-olds planning their 2-week vacation through Central America. On the day of their arrival, they both eat fresh fruits and vegetables from street vendors, and drink unbottled water. On the second day of their vacation, W.D. noted the passing of two to three watery stools without blood, and without other GI symptoms. In contrast, B.D. felt "feverish" and passed six to seven loose, bloody stools. Neither traveler felt dizzy or thirsty, and both continued drinking unbottled water and juices to avoid dehydration. Why is their clinical presentation and history of present illness consistent with the diagnosis of TD? What risk factors do they have for acquiring TD? What are the likely enteropathogens causing their illness?

Travelers' diarrhea is defined as three or more loose, unformed stools per day plus at least one symptom of enteric infection, such as abdominal cramps, nausea, vomiting, fever, fecal urgency, tenesmus, or the passage of bloody or mucoid stools. Illness begins within 24 to 48 hours after consuming fecally contaminated foods and, left untreated, is generally a self-limiting illness lasting 5 days.[100]

The major risk factors include destination to an area where the risk for TD is high and eating "unsafe" foods. High-risk destinations (i.e., 40% risk of developing diarrhea) include Africa (excluding South Africa), South and Central America (excluding Chile and Argentina), most of the Middle East, Southern and Southeast Asia, and Oceania; intermediate-risk destinations (e.g., 15% risk of developing diarrhea) include the Caribbean nations, South Africa, Argentina, Chile, Eastern Europe, Russia, and China.[4]

Foods likely to be contaminated with enteropathogens include foods from street vendors, unbottled water, ice cubes, raw milk, unpeeled fruits and vegetables, uncooked foods, moist foods, and foods remaining at room temperature for prolonged periods of time, allowing bacteria to multiply or release their enterotoxins.[100,101]

CASE 66-12, QUESTION 2: What are the likely microbial causes of TD?

Infectious agents are the major cause of TD, with bacteria identified in 80% of cases[4]; less frequently isolated are viruses and parasites. Clues to the likely pathogen include the clinical manifestations of the illness and the travel destination. Enterotoxigenic *E. coli* (ETEC) is suspected in the setting of watery diarrhea in travelers to Latin America, the Caribbean, Africa, and South Asia, but is less likely in travelers to Southeast Asia. Invasive pathogens such as *Campylobacter* species are suspected in the setting of bloody diarrhea and fever (dysentery) in travelers to Southeast Asia (32%), South Asia, North Africa, and Central and South America.[100]

Viral pathogens, e.g., norovirus and rotavirus, identified in 5% to 10% of travelers, are more likely in the setting of watery diarrhea, particularly in groups traveling in close proximity, such as on cruise ships. Parasites such as *G. lamblia* and *Cryptosporidium* species are frequently associated with persistent diarrhea, and *Entamoeba histolytica* is more likely in travelers to Asia.[4]

More recently recognized pathogens include enteroaggregative *E. coli* (EAEC) with or without other pathogens in travelers to Mexico, Jamaica, and India, and enterotoxin-producing *Bacteroides fragilis* has been identified in both high- and low-income areas.[100]

General Management

CASE 66-12, QUESTION 3: What general approach should W.D. and B.D. take to manage their illnesses?

W.D. and B.D. should review the pretravel education information they received from their physician, focusing on preventing dehydration and selecting "safe foods." Neither traveler shows signs and symptoms of dehydration such as thirst, dizziness, or altered mental status, and both are drinking normally. They should continue to drink only bottled or boiled fluids such as tea, broth, carbonated beverages, and fruit juices[101]; electrolytes can be replaced by eating salted crackers or similar sources of sodium chloride. For travelers able to drink fluids ad libitum, a modified World Health Organization oral rehydration solution offers no additional benefit over the administration of loperamide alone.[102]

"Safe foods" include well-cooked foods served steaming hot or foods that have been peeled or adequately washed and prepared by the traveler in their own room.[101] Depending on the severity of their illness, these travelers can consider the use of antimotility agents with or without antimicrobial therapy.

CASE 66-12, QUESTION 4: What drug therapies could W.D. and B.D. consider using to reduce the duration and severity of travelers' diarrhea?

Antimotility agents alone provide rapid relief of symptoms but do not cure the infection, whereas antimicrobials alone will cure the infection but symptoms will persist for a longer time.[101] In combination, antimotility drugs and antibiotics provide the fastest relief of diarrheal symptoms.[14]

Symptomatic Therapy

LOPERAMIDE, DIPHENOXYLATE/ATROPINE, BISMUTH PREPARATIONS

Loperamide relieves diarrheal symptoms more rapidly than bismuth subsalicylate[15] and is better tolerated than diphenoxylate/atropine. Loperamide alone can be considered in patients with a mild diarrheal illness, e.g., two loose stools and mild symptoms. In this setting, an infectious etiology is less likely, and noninfectious causes such as anxiety, diet changes, and stress should be considered. If improvement is not evident within 12 hours, an antimicrobial could be started.[103]

ANTIMICROBIALS

Antimicrobial therapy shortens the duration and severity of TD. Widespread resistance of common enteropathogens to tetracycline and TMP-SMX makes these agents unsuitable choices for the empiric treatment of TD.[101] Depending on the travel destination and clinical manifestations of the diarrheal illness, recommended treatment options include azithromycin, a fluoroquinolone, or rifaximin (Table 66-3).[14]

In travelers to Mexico[104–106] or Kenya,[106] where ETEC is a frequent cause of TD, a single dose of ciprofloxacin 500 mg,[107] azithromycin 1 g,[104] or levofloxacin 500 mg,[104] decreased the median time to passage of the last unformed stool to 22 to 33 hours,[104,106] compared with 54 to 66 hours in travelers given placebo.[104] In travelers to Mexico or India, oral rifaximin 200 mg three times daily or ciprofloxacin 500 mg twice daily for 3 days significantly reduced the median time to passage of the last unformed stool to 32 hours and 29 hours, respectively, versus 66 hours for travelers taking placebo.[108] In this study, rifaximin was as effective as ciprofloxacin against noninvasive bacterial enteropathogens, but less effective than ciprofloxacin when

TABLE 66-3
Therapy for Travelers' Diarrhea in Adults

Drug	Treatment
Ciprofloxacin	500 mg twice daily for 1–3 days[a]
Levofloxacin	500 mg daily for 1–3 days[a]
Azithromycin	1,000 mg in a single dose
Rifaximin	200 mg three times daily for 3 days

[a]Single dose may be effective. If diarrhea improves 12–24 hours after the first dose, the antibiotic can be stopped; otherwise, may continue antibiotic for up to 3 days.

Source: Hill DR, Beeching NJ. Travelers' diarrhea. *Curr Opin Infect Dis.* 2010;23: 481; DuPont HL et al. Expert review of the evidence base for self-therapy of travelers' diarrhea. *J Travel Med.* 2009;16:161.

invasive pathogens were identified. Rifaximin should not be used in patients with diarrhea complicated by fever and bloody stools or diarrhea caused by pathogens other than *E. coli*.[14] Rifaximin is not systemically absorbed; however, it is well tolerated and has a low potential for the development of antibiotic resistance.[109]

Travelers' diarrhea in travelers to Asia is more likely to be associated with invasive pathogens such as *Shigella*, *Campylobacter*, and *Salmonella* species. In a study of military personnel experiencing TD while in Thailand, most were infected with fluoroquinolone-resistant, azithromycin-susceptible *Campylobacter* species. Cure rates were highest with a single dose of azithromycin 1 g (96%), followed by 3 days of azithromycin 500 mg daily (85%) and levofloxacin 500 mg daily (71%).[110] Levofloxacin was inferior to azithromycin with the exception of levofloxacin-susceptible *Campylobacter* species. Nausea during the 30 minutes after receipt of the first antimicrobial dose was more common in persons given 1 g of azithromycin (14% vs. <6%, respectively, for the other regimens).[110]

ANTIMOTILITY DRUGS PLUS ANTIMICROBIALS

Antimotility drugs plus antimicrobials provide the fastest relief of diarrheal symptoms.[111] The antimotility drug quickly acts to reduce the number of stools, whereas the antimicrobial cures the infection.[14] In military personnel stationed in Turkey with TD primarily caused by ETEC, the median time to the passage of the last unformed stool was shortened to as little as 3 hours in recruits taking levofloxacin (single 500-mg dose) plus loperamide (4 mg initially, then 2 mg as needed; maximum 16 mg/day), comparable to that observed in patients treated with azithromycin (single 1-g dose) plus loperamide.[112] In otherwise healthy US students at least 18 years old attending school in Mexico, the combination of rifaximin (200 mg orally three times daily for 3 days) plus loperamide (4 mg initially, then 2 mg after each unformed stool) provided the fastest relief of diarrheal symptoms (27 ± 4.13 hours) compared with rifaximin alone (32.5 ± 4.14 hours) or loperamide alone (69 ± 4.11 hours).[109]

CASE 66-12, QUESTION 5: Based on the severity of their illnesses, what specific drug therapies could W.D. and B.D. consider taking?

Reviewing the contents and instructions for self-treatment of TD, travelers like W.D. with a mild, watery diarrhea of one to two stools per 24 hours and with mild or absent symptoms may choose to forgo specific drug therapy or use bismuth subsalicylate. For a mild to moderate diarrheal illness (more than three stools per 24 hours) with minimal symptoms, the use of loperamide or bismuth subsalicylate can be considered, although patients on a short and critical trip (e.g., business) might also consider the addition of an antibiotic (e.g., azithromycin 1 g for one dose, ciprofloxacin 750 mg once daily for 1 to 3 days, or levofloxacin 500 mg for 1 to 3 days).[14]

Travelers such as B.D., with severe diarrhea or diarrhea with fever or bloody stools, should be treated with a single 1-g dose of azithromycin or azithromycin 500 mg daily for 3 days.[14,113] Rifaximin is not a good choice for B.D., as it is not effective in TD caused by invasive enteropathogens.[14]

POSTINFECTIOUS IRRITABLE BOWEL SYNDROME (PI-IBS)

CASE 66-12, QUESTION 6: Three weeks after returning from their trip, unlike W.D. who is free of intestinal symptoms, B.D. continues to have episodes of loose stools and abdominal discomfort, for which she seeks medical attention. On physical examination, her vital signs are stable and she is afebrile. The physician believes her symptoms are consistent with the postinfectious irritable bowel syndrome (PI-IBS). Why is B.D.'s history and clinical presentation consistent with this diagnosis, and what therapies can be recommended to manage these symptoms?

After an acute episode of infectious gastroenteritis, 10% to 12% of individuals continue to be symptomatic, e.g., bloating, urgency, diarrhea, and increased frequency of passing mucus per rectum, consistent with irritable bowel syndrome (IBS).[114] For these individuals, the diagnosis of PI-IBS is based on an episode of infectious gastroenteritis characterized by the presence of at least two of the following: diarrhea, fever, vomiting, or a positive bacterial stool culture.[115] PI-IBS has been attributed to invasive pathogens including *Campylobacter*, *Salmonella*, and *Shigella* species, and other enteropathogens.[4]

Risk factors for PI-IBS include a prolonged duration of the initial illness (>3 weeks), virulence of the enteropathogen, female sex, and depression.[4] One retrospective study suggested that administration of antimicrobials increased the risk for PI-IBS; however, these findings need to be confirmed with randomized, placebo-controlled trials.[115]

Treatment of PI-IBS is aimed at providing symptomatic relief; antimicrobials have not been proven to be beneficial, and may be harmful.[115] Diarrheal symptoms can be managed with loperamide; if postprandial fecal urgency is problematic, taking loperamide 30 minutes before meals is recommended. Bloating and abdominal discomfort can be managed with simethicone or antispasmodic agents[81]; chronic abdominal symptoms can be managed with low doses of amitriptyline and selective serotonin reuptake inhibitors.[81,115]

The prognosis for patients with PI-IBS suggests that about 50% of patients recover within 6 years, although recovery was less likely in the setting of persistent depression or anxiety.[115] An unproven but likely benefit of chemoprophylaxis of TD is the prevention of PI-IBS; studies are needed to address this issue.[101]

Prophylaxis

CASE 66-12, QUESTION 7: On hearing of the travels of W.D. and B.D., friends J.G. and T.M. begin planning their vacation to Central America, but want to prevent the occurrence of any diarrheal illness that could interfere with their plans. Neither friend has any significant medical history. Besides receiving pretravel education including selection of "safe foods," what drug therapies can be used to minimize their likelihood of experiencing TD?

ANTIMICROBIALS

Chemoprophylaxis could be considered in travelers at greatest risk for infection or its complications, including persons in whom a short-term illness could ruin the purpose of the trip (e.g., athletes, politicians, lecturers, others), persons in whom a diarrheal illness could complicate an underlying medical problem (e.g., insulin-dependent diabetes mellitus, congestive heart failure, reactive arthritis, inflammatory bowel disease, advanced cancer, or HIV infection), persons with conditions that increase the risk for enteric infection (e.g., genetic predisposition, gastric disease or surgery, or use of acid-reducing medications), and persons requesting chemoprophylaxis.[101]

Norfloxacin 400 mg daily or ciprofloxacin 500 mg daily for 7 to 15 days significantly reduces the incidence of diarrheal illness.[116] Rifaximin, although not currently approved for the prophylaxis of TD,[117] is effective in the prevention of TD in students traveling from the United States to Mexico; ETEC was the main enteropathogen identified in this study.[118]

MISCELLANEOUS AGENTS

Bismuth subsalicylate, two tablets (524 mg/dose) four times daily for a maximum of 3 weeks, has a protective efficacy of 65% against TD.[119] Probiotics have been studied on the basis of their ability to prevent enteropathogen colonization. The effectiveness of probiotics has not been determined; more studies are needed before these agents can be routinely recommended.[101]

Despite their efficacy in preventing TD, universal antimicrobial prophylaxis is not uniformly recommended. Most travelers will experience self-limiting TD, and treatment reduces the duration of illness to as little as a few hours.[120] Antimicrobials should be reserved for when the benefit of prophylaxis outweighs the risk for adverse drug reactions, increased bacterial resistance, and expense. If offered, chemoprophylaxis should not extend beyond 2 weeks.[101]

ESCHERICHIA COLI O157:H7

Epidemiology

CASE 66-13

QUESTION 1: P.J., a 3-year-old girl, is brought to the emergency department because of "stomach pains" and nonbloody diarrhea that has progressed to bloody diarrhea during the past 48 hours. Five days before the onset of diarrhea, the family celebrated a birthday at a fast-food restaurant; P.J.'s parents ate fish sandwiches and P.J. ate a hamburger. P.J.'s mother noted that, unlike previous hamburgers eaten at the restaurant, this hamburger was not thoroughly cooked because the juices from the hamburger were still pinkish. P.J. has no significant medical history. During the week, she attends a day-care center.

On physical examination P.J. is afebrile, with signs of mild to moderate dehydration. A stool sample is negative for fecal leukocytes. The physician assesses her illness as bloody diarrhea, possibly caused by STEC. The plan is to admit P.J. to the hospital for hydration, observation, and further workup. What clinical and laboratory findings and epidemiologic history are consistent with the diagnosis of STEC?

Escherichia coli O157:H7 is a strain of *E. coli* that produces Shiga toxins as a primary mechanism of causing GI illness. A second virulence factor of STEC strains is their ability to attach to and damage the intestinal mucosa.[121] These *E. coli* bacteria cause a spectrum of infection, including asymptomatic carriage, mild and nonbloody diarrhea, bloody diarrhea (hemorrhagic colitis), HUS, and thrombotic thrombocytopenia purpura.[122]

Escherichia coli O157:H7 should be suspected in the setting of abdominal cramps with nonbloody diarrhea that progresses to bloody diarrhea during 1 to 2 days.[123] Unlike bloody diarrhea associated with *Shigella* species or *Campylobacter* species, fever is often absent or low grade because this pathogen is not invasive.[124] Patients with severe illness are more likely to have fever.[125]

Shiga toxin–producing *E. coli* is most commonly spread by consumption of undercooked beef products that are contaminated with *E. coli* O157:H7. The incubation period for this infection is usually 3 to 4 days, which is consistent with P.J.'s recent history of eating undercooked hamburger. In most instances, the illness resolves in 5 to 7 days.[123] Fecal leukocytes may or may not be found in stool samples.[126]

Laboratory Diagnosis

CASE 66-13, QUESTION 2: How can P.J.'s diagnosis of *E. coli* O157:H7 infection be confirmed?

In the United States, *E. coli* O157:H7 is the most common STEC serotype identified as causing this infection.[126] Unlike other *E. coli*, O157:H7 does not rapidly ferment sorbitol, thus allowing the use of special culture media (Sorbitol-MacConkey) to identify this organism. P.J.'s stool should be cultured using this media.

Because of sorbitol-fermenting organisms and non-O157 STEC, further testing for Shiga toxins or the genes encoding them is increasingly performed.[122,123,126]

Hemolytic Uremic Syndrome

CASE 66-13, QUESTION 3: Forty-eight hours after admission to the hospital, P.J. is pale and has developed several "bruises" on her extremities. The nurse recorded only a minimal output of darkened urine during the past 24 hours. New laboratory tests reveal the following:

Blood urea nitrogen (BUN), 150 mg/dL
Serum creatinine (SCr), 6 mg/dL
Serum potassium (K), 6.8 mEq/L
WBC count, 20,000 cells/μL
Hemoglobin (Hgb), 7 g/dL
Platelets, 50,000 cells/μL
Urinalysis, positive for blood and protein

The stool specimen sent on admission is positive for *E. coli* O157:H7. What complication of *E. coli* O157:H7 infection does P.J. now display?

The new clinical and laboratory findings support the diagnosis of hemolytic uremic syndrome (HUS), a well-known complication of STEC infection. HUS is characterized by the triad of thrombocytopenia, microangiopathic hemolytic anemia, and acute renal failure with oliguria.[127] On physical examination, P.J.'s "bruises" on her extremities are consistent with thrombocytopenia, which is confirmed by the low platelet count. Her pale appearance is consistent with anemia and is confirmed by the low Hgb. The dark urine is caused by the color imparted from bilirubin because of red cell lysis (hemolytic anemia). Finally, P.J.'s decreased urine output and increased serum creatinine and BUN concentrations are consistent with renal failure.[128] P.J. has several risk factors for HUS: her age (i.e., children aged <5–15 years, median age 4–8 years), fever, increased peripheral WBC count, and the season (i.e., summer).[125,127,129–132] Although not present in this case, another possible risk factor for developing HUS is treatment with antimotility or antidiarrheal agents,[133] although this has not been consistently confirmed.[125,132] In addition to young age, age older than 65 years is a risk factor for HUS.[126] The progression of *E. coli* O157:H7 gastroenteritis to HUS typically takes place 1 week after the onset of diarrhea.[125,127,129] Of children, 3% to 7%[133] may develop HUS, with a mortality rate ranging from 3% to 5%.

In adults, *E. coli* O157:H7 infection progresses to HUS in as many as 27% of patients, with a higher rate in patients older than 65 years of age.[125] HUS-related mortality has been reported to be as high as 42% in patients older than 15 years of age[125]; elderly nursing home patients have a mortality rate of up to 88%.[134]

Treatment

CASE 66-13, QUESTION 4: Would P.J. benefit from drug therapy, including antimicrobial, antimotility, or antidiarrheal agents?

Other than supportive measures to manage the complications associated with illness caused by *E. coli* O157:H7, no specific drug therapy for this infection exists.[123] In retrospective and prospective studies, antibiotics have not influenced the severity of illness, or the duration of diarrhea or other GI symptoms.[135,136] When TMP-SMX was started a mean of 7 days after the onset of diarrhea, the duration of *E. coli* O157:H7 excretion did not change.[135]

The effect of antibiotic administration on the risk of *E. coli* O157:H7 complications (e.g., HUS) remains controversial. A prospective cohort study of 71 children with diarrhea caused by *E. coli* O157:H7 found that antibiotic treatment increased the risk of progression to HUS.[132] Previous publications have supported these findings[133,135,136]; however, others refute these findings.[125,137] A systematic review of these and other studies revealed no association between antibiotic administration and development of HUS.[138] Antibiotic selection, dosing, timing of administration, small sample sizes, and a lack of placebo use in the selected studies complicate the analysis. Thus, the role of antibiotics in the treatment of *E. coli* O157:H7 infection remains controversial. Currently, clinicians do not recommend antibiotic treatment for STEC. P.J. should not receive antibiotic therapy at this time.

Antimotility drugs are not recommended for patients with *E. coli* O157:H7 infection because they have been variably associated with an increased risk of progression to HUS,[133,137] although other studies have not documented this association.[125,132] Although the explanation for the increased risk is unknown, the reduction of bowel motility may decrease the clearance of organisms from the GI tract, thereby increasing the absorption of toxins. Administration of antimotility drugs within the first 3 days of illness has been associated with a longer duration of bloody diarrhea.[139]

Prevention

CASE 66-13, QUESTION 5: P.J.'s family members want to know what they could have done to prevent this infection. On discharge from the hospital, is it safe for P.J. to return to her day-care center?

Shiga toxin–producing *E. coli* is often spread to humans by consumption of contaminated beef products that are not thoroughly cooked.[122] Because thorough cooking kills this organism, meat should be well cooked (i.e., juices from meat should be clear, not pink). In addition, this infection can be acquired by consuming other contaminated foods, including water, unpasteurized milk, apple cider, lettuce, and sprouts.[122,123]

Finally, because contact with infected persons commonly results in transmission of this infection to others,[133,134,136] P.J. should have two consecutive stool cultures that are negative for *E. coli* O157:H7 before returning to day care.[140]

CLOSTRIDIUM DIFFICILE–ASSOCIATED DIARRHEA

Mild to Moderate Infection

CLINICAL PRESENTATION AND DIAGNOSIS

CASE 66-14

QUESTION 1: B.W., a 35-year-old woman, is admitted to a 10-bed medical ward for the treatment of *Streptococcus pneumoniae* meningitis. On arrival, she is started on ceftriaxone (Rocephin) 2 g IV every 12 hours and improves during the next few days. On day 7 of antibiotic therapy, she complained of feeling warm, with cramping abdominal pain and diarrhea. She began passing mucoid, greenish, foul-smelling watery stools, and had a temperature of 101°F. Microscopic examination of a stool sample was positive for fecal leukocytes. The physician's assessment of B.W.'s clinical and laboratory findings is antibiotic-associated diarrhea (AAD), most likely caused by *C. difficile*. What are the primary risk factors for this patient's AAD?

Antibiotic-associated diarrhea is a common complication of antimicrobial therapy.[141] The mechanisms by which antibiotics cause diarrhea include direct allergic and toxic effects on intestinal mucosa and alterations of GI motility (e.g., erythromycin) and of normal intestinal flora. Changes in the normal bowel flora can lead to changes in carbohydrate or bile acid metabolism by intestinal bacteria or to overgrowth of pathogenic bacteria, either of which may be followed by diarrhea.[141] Bacteria known to be associated with AAD include *C. perfringens, S. aureus, Klebsiella oxytoca, Candida* species, and *C. difficile. C. difficile* infection is the most clinically relevant microbial cause and is the focus of this section.

A spore-forming, gram-positive anaerobic bacillus, *C. difficile* can cause a wide spectrum of syndromes, including asymptomatic carriage, diarrhea of varying severity, colitis with or without formation of pseudomembranes, toxic megacolon, colonic perforation, and death.[142]

The pathogenesis of *C. difficile* infection involves disruption of the normal colonic flora, most commonly by antibiotics; however, antineoplastic drugs[143] and tacrolimus[144] have been implicated as well (Table 66-4). An increasing number of

TABLE 66-4
Medications Implicated in *Clostridium difficile*–Associated Diarrhea

Commonly Implicated	Rarely Implicated
Cephalosporins	Aminoglycosides
Clindamycin	Rifampin
Ampicillin	Tetracycline
Fluoroquinolones	Vancomycin
Less Commonly Implicated	Metronidazole
Erythromycin	Antineoplastic agents
Clarithromycin	
Azithromycin	
Other penicillins	
Trimethoprim-sulfamethoxazole	

Source: Owens RC Jr et al. Antimicrobial-associated risk factors for *Clostridium difficile* infection. *Clin Infect Dis.* 2008;46(Suppl 1):S19; Cohen SH et al. Society for Healthcare Epidemiology of America; Infectious Diseases Society of America. Clinical practice guidelines for *Clostridium difficile* infection in adults: 2010 update by the society for healthcare epidemiology of America (SHEA) and the infectious diseases society of America (IDSA). *Infect Control Hosp Epidemiol.* 2010;31:431.

cases in the outpatient setting have been identified without any antibiotic exposure.[145] Recent data suggest use of proton-pump inhibitors may be a risk factor for CDAD.[8,9] Alteration of the colonic microflora is followed by overgrowth of toxin-producing strains of *C. difficile*.[141,142] These toxins are responsible for causing colonic inflammation and the clinical manifestations of this infection.[141,142]

CASE 66-14, QUESTION 2: Why is B.W.'s history and presentation consistent with AAD caused by *C. difficile*?

B.W.'s major risk factor for acquiring CDAD is her receipt of an antibiotic within the last 2 weeks. *C. difficile* is a common cause of nosocomial diarrhea. The clinical and laboratory findings consistent with CDAD include mucoid, greenish, foul-smelling watery stools and crampy abdominal pain. Patients usually present with low-grade fevers, but temperature may be greater than 104°F.[146] Peripheral leukocytosis is common, with CDAD a common cause of WBC greater than 30,000 cells/μL.[146,147] Fecal leukocytes are variably present in CDAD and are not clinically useful for diagnosis.[148]

The onset of symptoms of CDAD varies widely from a few days after the start of antibiotic therapy to 8 weeks after the agent is discontinued.[146] Other risk factors for acquiring CDAD are admission to a hospital in which *C. difficile* is endemic or in which there is an ongoing outbreak of *C. difficile* infection.

CASE 66-14, QUESTION 3: How can B.W.'s diagnosis of CDAD be confirmed?

Several tests are available to make the diagnosis of *C. difficile* infection including culture, cell cytotoxicity studies, and toxin and antigen detection. Although debate continues about the most appropriate test, enzyme immunoassay of toxins A/B is the most frequently performed laboratory test.[149] At a minimum, B.W. should have her stool sent for enzyme immunoassay to look for *C. difficile* toxins. Culture, although helpful, is complicated by the fact that of the *C. difficile* strains isolated from various populations, 5% to 25% do not produce toxins (nontoxigenic) and do not cause colitis or diarrhea.[146,150]

Colonoscopy with biopsy is used to make the diagnosis of *C. difficile* colitis rapidly. The characteristic colonic changes are raised, yellowish nodules or plaquelike pseudomembranes, often with skip areas of normal mucosa.[146] Because the characteristic pseudomembranes may be scattered throughout the colon, the diagnosis of pseudomembranous colitis can be missed with colonoscopy.

CASE 66-14, QUESTION 4: How can B.W.'s CDAD be differentiated from enigmatic AAD?

Only 10% to 20% of cases of AAD are positive for toxigenic *C. difficile*; the remaining cases have an unknown cause and are referred to as simple, benign, or "nuisance" diarrhea.[141] The clinical presentation of benign diarrhea is similar to many cases of CDAD in that it is a self-limited illness that resolves with nonspecific supportive measures and discontinuation of antibiotics. Despite these similarities, these clinical entities can be differentiated from one another by several objective measures. In hospitalized patients, watery diarrhea, low functional capacity, acid suppression, low albumin, and a WBC greater than 13,000 cells/μL were significant predictors of CDAD.[151] Other clinical features that suggest CDAD rather than enigmatic diarrhea are constitutional symptoms, no antibiotic dose relationship to the illness, and hospital-wide epidemics of diarrhea.[152]

TREATMENT

CASE 66-14, QUESTION 5: B.W.'s stool sample is positive for *C. difficile* toxin. What is the general plan for treating B.W.'s CDAD?

After replacement of fluids and electrolytes, there are three options for managing B.W.'s diarrhea. The first is to discontinue the offending drug (if possible), which in B.W.'s case is probably the antibiotic ceftriaxone. In approximately 25% of cases, discontinuation of the offending agent with concomitant fluid and electrolyte replacement leads to resolution of symptoms within 48 to 72 hours.[153] Thus, patients with mild diarrhea may not require any treatment other than discontinuation of the offending agent.[154,155]

Because B.W. is being treated for bacterial meningitis, a life-threatening infection, discontinuing antibiotics is not an option. A second option is to change her antimicrobial therapy to an agent less likely to cause CDAD. B.W. is taking a cephalosporin, which, as with ampicillin, amoxicillin, and clindamycin, is frequently implicated as a cause of *C. difficile* diarrhea (Table 66-4). In contrast, antibiotics such as TMP-SMX and aminoglyclosides are less commonly associated with *C. difficile* infection.[154–156] None of these antimicrobials, however, is a suitable alternative for treating *S. pneumoniae* meningitis.

The third and most reasonable option for B.W. is to receive therapy directed against *C. difficile* while continuing to take ceftriaxone for the treatment of her bacterial meningitis.

METRONIDAZOLE AND VANCOMYCIN

CASE 66-14, QUESTION 6: What antibiotic should be selected to treat B.W.'s CDAD?

The oral agents most commonly used to treat CDAD are metronidazole and vancomycin. The differentiation between these two agents is complex and evolving, but is guided in part by severity of illness.[149,157–160] In patients categorized as having mild to moderate disease severity, metronidazole is generally recommended as the preferred initial agent.[149] In a randomized trial that enrolled patients with CDAD and colitis, no significant difference was found in the efficacy of these drugs after 10 days of treatment.[159] Overall, greater than 95% of patients treated for a first episode of CDAD with either oral metronidazole or vancomycin respond to therapy.[159,160] Recent reports have shown small increases in *C. difficile* resistance to metronidazole and vancomycin, but the clinical significance in treatment selection is unknown.[161] Antibiotic sensitivities, therefore, are not routinely performed on *C. difficile*.

Metronidazole is well absorbed after oral administration and is excreted through the biliary tract before reaching the colon. Common adverse reactions include nausea, vomiting, diarrhea, dizziness, confusion, and an unpleasant metallic taste.[154] A disulfiramlike reaction can occur when alcohol or alcohol-containing medications are taken concurrently with metronidazole.[162] Because metronidazole is a carcinogen and, in some animal species, a mutagen, it should be used in pregnancy only if clearly needed. Similarly, metronidazole's safety in children has not been proved, and many prefer not to use it in this population if other options exist.[154] Further, long-term use of metronidazole has been associated with neurotoxicity.[163]

Oral vancomycin produces fecal concentrations that are several hundred times the concentration needed to inhibit toxin-producing strains of *C. difficile*.[160] A 7- to 10-day course of oral vancomycin (125–500 mg orally four times daily) is recommended for the treatment of CDAD, with all dosing regimens appearing

TABLE 66-5
Costs of Oral Drug Therapy for *Clostridium difficile*–Associated Diarrhea

Drug	Regimen	Cost[a]
Metronidazole tablets (generic)	500 mg TID × 10 days	$8.51/10 days
Vancomycin capsules (Vancocin)	125 mg QID × 10 days	$707.16/10 days
Vancomycin solution (generic)[b]	125 mg QID × 10 days	$45.50/10 days
Nitazoxanide (Alinia)	125 mg BID × 10 days	$345.63/10 days

[a]AWP Red Book 2010.
[b]Prepared from intravenous formulation.

equally effective.[154,160,164,165] Because of equal efficacy and high concentrations in the colon with all doses, 125 mg is the most commonly prescribed dose. Although oral vancomycin is not well absorbed, measurable serum concentrations have been found in patients with both normal and compromised renal function.[166,167]

Because B.W. is not critically ill, metronidazole (500 mg orally three times daily) for 10 to 14 days is recommended as first-line treatment.[149,157,158] Oral metronidazole and oral vancomycin are generally considered equally efficacious in mild to moderate disease,[149] but vancomycin use should be limited to prevent emergence of vancomycin-resistant organisms.[168] In addition, oral vancomycin is significantly more expensive than a course of oral metronidazole (Table 66-5). Some of this cost differential can be offset by using the IV vancomycin preparation to prepare an oral solution.

Once therapy directed against *C. difficile* is initiated, diarrhea or cramping should subside within 2 to 4 days. If B.W.'s symptoms have not resolved, vancomycin can be tried.[152]

ALTERNATIVE THERAPIES

NITAZOXANIDE

Nitazoxanide is an oral nitrothiazolide currently FDA approved for the treatment of *Cryptosporidia* and *Giardia*. Nitazoxanide has in vitro activity against *C. difficile* and has been shown to be as effective as metronidazole in the initial treatment of CDAD in a small comparative trial.[169] An additional small randomized, double-blind trial versus vancomycin showed comparable efficacy in all disease severities.[170] Further studies are needed to determine the appropriate place in therapy.

TOXIN BINDERS

Traditional anion-binding resins (e.g., cholestyramine, colestipol) are not as reliable or as rapidly effective as oral metronidazole or vancomycin, and are not recommended as routine therapy.[171]

An investigational toxin-binding agent, tolevamer is an anionic polymer that binds *C. difficile* toxins A and B. Further studies of variable doses are ongoing. After initially promising clinical trials,[172] larger studies revealed poor efficacy of tolevamer as a single agent for CDAD.[171] However, tolevamer appears to have potential as an adjunct agent for toxin binding, particularly in patients with relapsing infection.

PROBIOTICS

Probiotic microorganisms are introduced into the normal flora to counteract disturbances and reduce the colonization with pathogenic species.[18] Although orally administered *Lactobacillus* species and the yeast *Saccharomyces boulardii* have been used to treat CDAD, no data support the use of probiotics alone to treat CDAD. Adjunctive use has been suggested to prevent CDAD and its recurrences. A hospital trial looking at prevention of all antibiotic-associated diarrhea with *Lactobacillus* suggested probiotics prevented CDAD.[173] However, patients receiving antibiotics, i.e., those at greater risk for CDAD, were excluded from this trial, making generalization to other patient groups difficult. Isolated adverse effects, including fungemia, have been associated with ingestion of viable *S. boulardii*.[149,174]

ANTIDIARRHEALS

CASE 66-14, QUESTION 7: Should B.W. be given any antidiarrheal agent to relieve her symptoms?

Opiates and other antiperistaltic agents should be avoided in patients with CDAD. Although these types of drugs may relieve diarrheal symptoms, they may also delay toxin removal from the GI tract. Although it is not proven that antidiarrheal agents can harm,[16] it is prudent to avoid the use of antimotility agents in B.W.

CASE 66-14, QUESTION 8: After resolution of B.W.'s CDAD, is it necessary to send a follow-up stool sample to determine whether it is negative for *C. difficile* toxin?

There is no need to obtain a follow-up stool sample after resolution of diarrhea. Many patients will continue to be culture positive for *C. difficile* or the toxin, and most patients with positive tests will not experience a recurrence of their diarrhea.[149] In addition, up to 3% of healthy adults carry small numbers of *C. difficile* in their feces, whereas colonization rates are much higher (31%–37%) in hospitalized patients and infants younger than 1 month.[175,176]

Transmission

CASE 66-15

QUESTION 1: H.T., a 76-year-old man with multiple medical conditions, is admitted to the same 10-bed ward as B.W. H.T.'s medical history is significant for a stroke that has left him bedridden in a nursing home. His only medications are those used to manage his hypertension. On day 4 of his hospitalization, H.T. complained of severe abdominal pain and watery, loose stools with blood. Physical examination revealed an ill-appearing man with a temperature of 101°F and hypotension. His WBC is 21,000 cells/μL. A stool specimen is positive for *C. difficile* toxin, and colonoscopy reveals pseudomembranes and colitis. A surgical consultant is considering an emergent colectomy because of possible bowel perforation secondary to the *C. difficile* infection. What are H.T.'s risk factors for acquiring *C. difficile*–associated pseudomembranous colitis during his hospitalization?

H.T.'s risk factors for acquiring *C. difficile* infection include his advanced age, bedridden status,[177] underlying diseases,[178] and admission to the hospital. *C. difficile* infection is spread when hospital personnel or equipment contaminated with *C. difficile* spores come into contact with susceptible patients. Physical proximity to an infected patient has been associated with an increased risk of CDAD.[179] Therefore, measures to prevent the spread of *C. difficile* infection include proper hand washing before and after contact with infected patients, and the use of gloves and enteric isolation precautions when in contact with infected patients with diarrhea. Contaminated equipment should be properly disinfected.[154]

Although *C. difficile* is often thought of as a nosocomial pathogen, it is being increasingly isolated in outpatient settings.[145,180] A European study found that up to 28% of all cases occurred without previous hospitalization.[181]

NEW EPIDEMIC STRAIN

CASE 66-15, QUESTION 2: Could there be a strain difference causing the severe CDAD in H.T.?

A highly pathogenic strain of *C. difficile* has recently been described in outbreaks in the United States and around the world.[142,182] This strain, labeled BI/NAP1 (or ribotype 027), generally causes more severe disease. Among its increased virulence factors are an increased production of both toxins A and B and a binary toxin. These strains are also newly resistant to fluoroquinolones, and these agents may increase the frequency of disease.[156] No currently available clinical tests distinguish BI/NAP1 from other strains, making it unknown whether this strain is causing H.T.'s infection. Although initial reports suggested a possible superiority of vancomycin in treating any infection associated with these strains, these isolates should be treated similar to nonhypervirulent pathogens.[149,158]

CASE 66-15, QUESTION 3: During the next few days, all 10 patients on the ward with B.W. and H.T. are found to have *C. difficile* toxin in their stools. Five patients have diarrhea, and the other five are asymptomatic. What is the role of antibiotic therapy directed at *C. difficile* in controlling this outbreak?

Neither oral metronidazole nor vancomycin is reliably effective in eradicating the carrier state (i.e., asymptomatic fecal excretion), and neither is recommended for use in this situation.[183] The lack of efficacy of these drugs is probably related because, unlike the vegetative forms of *C. difficile,* the spores of *C. difficile* are resistant to the action of antibiotics.[154] Furthermore, compared with placebo, vancomycin administration is associated with a significantly higher rate of *C. difficile* carriage 2 months after treatment.[183]

Controlling overall antibiotic use in the hospital can be a useful strategy. Restricting the use of single agents like clindamycin can be an effective component in efforts to control nosocomial epidemics of CDAD.[177] With the emergence of the BI/NAP1 strain, control of all antibiotic use, including fluoroquinolones, may be important in outbreak control.[184]

CASE 66-15, QUESTION 4: What effect will the current CDAD outbreak have on the outcomes of the infected patients and on health care costs?

In a prospective study, hospitalized patients who experienced CDAD had a 3.6-day increase in length of stay.[185] This increase was accompanied by a doubling of hospital costs. Although 3-month mortality rates were higher in patients with CDAD (48% vs. 22%), no significant differences were observed when adjustments were made for severity of underlying illness. A review of available economic data suggests an incremental hospital cost of $2,800 to $4,800 for each primary case of CDAD.[186] The current outbreak on the hospital ward is likely to increase both hospital costs and individual lengths of stay.

Severe *C. difficile* Infection

CASE 66-15, QUESTION 5: What treatment is recommended for H.T., who is critically ill from a *C. difficile* infection? What criteria should be used to characterize patients as "critically ill"?

Of patients with antibiotic-associated pseudomembranous colitis who require surgical intervention (colectomy), up to 57% die.[187] Although the precise definition of "critically ill" is debated, it generally includes patients with pseudomembranes, age older than 60 years, serum albumin less than 2.5 mg/dL, fever greater than 38.3°C, severe abdominal pain, and marked leukocytosis (>15,000–20,000 cells/μL).[188,189] Recent guidelines from the Society for Healthcare Epidemiology of America and the Infectious Disease Society of America have suggested the definition of severity as the presence of either of the following two parameters: WBC count at least 15,000 cells/μL, or serum creatinine 1.5 times baseline.[149] Growing evidence suggests that vancomycin 125 mg orally four times daily may be more effective than metronidazole in patients with severe disease.[149,189] An additional designation of "severe, complicated" disease has been suggested for patients like H.T. with hypotension, shock, ileus, or megacolon. The recommended therapy for H.T. would be a combination of vancomycin 500 mg orally four times daily and metronidazole 500 mg intravenously every 8 hours.[149] The combination of high-dose therapies is suggested as it may be difficult for either medication to get to the site of action in the colon.

NONORAL TREATMENT

CASE 66-15, QUESTION 6: Three days after oral vancomycin and intravenous metronidazole is initiated, H.T. experiences an ileus and cannot take anything by mouth. What therapeutic options are available to treat H.T.'s pseudomembranous colitis?

Adequate antibiotic levels in the colon are necessary to treat *C. difficile*–associated pseudomembranous colitis. If the oral route is not feasible (e.g., patients with an ileus or bowel obstruction), the clinician must choose an agent that is either secreted or excreted into the GI tract in its active form. IV vancomycin is not a desirable agent in this situation because it is not secreted into the GI tract. In contrast, intravenous metronidazole is eliminated by both renal and hepatic routes; bactericidal concentrations are achieved in both serum and bile.[190]

The literature contains few reports of successful attempts to treat CDAD or pseudomembranous colitis with IV metronidazole (500 mg every 6–8 hours).[191–193] Likewise, unsuccessful attempts to treat CDAD with IV metronidazole have been reported.[191,194] The use of IV vancomycin in the treatment of CDAD cannot be recommended.[160]

In adults, enteral vancomycin 500 mg four times daily can be given through an ileostomy or colostomy (if present). Several reports of successful outcomes using intercolonic vancomycin (as an adjunct to oral or IV antibiotics) in patients with CDAD have been documented. Rectal doses of vancomycin have varied from 500 mg/L every 4 to 8 hours to 1,000 mg/L every 8 hours.[195]

Because patients with CDAD are at risk for colonic perforation, enteral vancomycin should be administered cautiously.

Relapse

CASE 66-16

QUESTION 1: P.V. is a 57-year-old woman who acquired CDAD on the same ward as the other infected patients. P.V. was treated with metronidazole 500 mg orally three times daily for 10 days while in the hospital. One week after discharge from the hospital, P.V. once again had abdominal pain and diarrhea. Her clinic physician assumed these symptoms could not be related to a relapse of her CDAD because she had responded so well to metronidazole. What is the likelihood that CDAD has recurred?

Regardless of the antibiotic regimen prescribed for CDAD, symptomatic relapse occurs in 5% to 30% of patients who respond to their initial treatment regimen.[154,155] Relapses occur 2 weeks to 2 months (median of 7 days) after treatment has been discontinued.[196]

In most instances, relapses are caused by germination of dormant spores that are intrinsically resistant to antibiotics. Reinfection with *C. difficile* from external sources, however, may account for up to half of all second episodes.[197] In rare instances, either vancomycin[198] or metronidazole[199] may have caused CDAD.

Risk factors for recurrent CDAD include increasing age, low quality-of-health score,[196] use of additional antibiotics, onset in the spring, and multiple prior episodes of *C. difficile* infection.[200] Of patients experiencing their first episode of CDAD, 24% experience a relapse, and 65% of patients with a prior history of CDAD have a relapse.[201]

Data suggest that patients with a poor immune response to *C. difficile* toxin A are more likely to have a relapse of CDAD.[202] This finding is not clinically helpful in the case of P.V. because no standard tests are currently available for this immune response. The influence of the immune system, however, has led to the usage of IV immune globulin in refractory or severe cases of CDAD.[203,204] The utility of the usage of immune globulins has been debated in small single-institution reviews. Immune globulins would not be the considered the next line of therapy for B.W.

A recent study of monoclonal antibodies against *C. difficile* toxins has shown promise in preventing recurrent infection[205] but further studies are necessary for this methodology.

CASE 66-16, QUESTION 2: How should P.V.'s CDAD relapse be treated?

Most infections resulting from relapse are not related to bacterial resistance, and they respond to retreatment with the same antibiotic used for initial treatment of the *C. difficile* infection.[155,206] Thus, an appropriate approach for P.V. is to administer another 10- to 14-day course of oral metronidazole.

For patients with multiple recurrences of CDAD, the optimal management plan is unresolved.[154] Different approaches have been tried, including (a) high-dose vancomycin (2,000 mg/day)[207]; (b) a 4- to 6-week course with vancomycin, after which the dose is tapered for a 1- to 2-month period[207,208]; (c) exchange resins[209,210]; (d) "pulse" dosing every 2 to 3 days[207]; or (e) a combination of vancomycin and rifampin (600 mg orally twice daily).[211] Tapered and pulse therapies with vancomycin were shown to be most effective in a clinical trial comparing multiple strategies.[207] When combined with standard antibiotic therapy, a clinical trial with the probiotic *S. boulardii* for cases of relapsing CDAD noted a 65% response rate versus a 36% response rate for combination therapy with placebo.[201] The relapse rate was reduced to 17% when *S. boulardii* was combined with high-dose vancomycin.[212]

Nitazoxanide had a 74% initial response rate in patients who had previously failed metronidazole therapy.[213] Recurrent relapse was successfully treated with a second course of nitazoxanide in a limited number of individuals, representing an overall 66% response rate in a small difficult-to-treat population.

After treatment with vancomycin, a "chaser" course of rifaximin, a poorly absorbed rifamycin derivative, was successful in separate case series for patients with multiple relapses.[214,215] Although obviously a small sample, concern must be raised that the single failure occurred in concert with emerging rifaximin resistance.[214]

KEY REFERENCES AND WEBSITES

A full list of references for this chapter can be found at **http://thepoint.lww.com/AT10e.** Below are the key references for this chapter, with the corresponding reference number in this chapter found in parentheses after the reference.

Key References

Cohen SH et al. Clinical practice guidelines for *Clostridium difficile* infection in adults: 2010 update by the Society for Healthcare Epidemiology of America (SHEA) and the Infectious Diseases Society of America (IDSA). *Infect Control Hosp Epidemiol.* 2010;31:431. (149)

Crump JA et al. Clinical response and outcome of infection with *Salmonella enterica* serotype Typhi with decreased susceptibility to fluoroquinolones: a United States FoodNet multicenter retrospective cohort study. *Antimicrob Agents Chemother.* 2008;52:1278. (49)

DuPont HL. Clinical practice. Bacterial diarrhea. *N Engl J Med.* 2009;361:1560. (3)

DuPont HL et al. Expert review of the evidence base for self-therapy of travelers' diarrhea. *J Travel Med.* 2009;16:161. (14)

Freeman J et al. The changing epidemiology of *Clostridium difficile* infections. *Clin Microbiol Rev.* 2010;23:529. (142)

Lynch MF et al. Typhoid fever in the United States, 1999–2006. *JAMA.* 2009;302:859. (52)

Meltzer E, Schwartz E. Enteric fever: a travel medicine oriented view. *Curr Opin Infect Dis.* 2010;23:432. (65)

Morris JG Jr. Cholera and other types of vibriosis: a story of human pandemics and oysters on the half shell. *Clin Infect Dis.* 2003;37:272. (7)

Navaneethan U, Giannella RA. Mechanisms of infectious diarrhea. *Nat Clin Pract Gastroenterol Hepatol.* 2008;5:637. (2)

Niyogi SK. Shigellosis. *J Microbiol.* 2005;43:133. (80)

Pawlowski SW et al. Diagnosis and treatment of acute or persistent diarrhea. *Gastroenterology.* 2009;136:1874. (4)

Pennington H. *Escherichia coli* O157. *Lancet.* 2010;376:1428. (121)

Zar FA et al. A comparison of vancomycin and metronidazole for the treatment of *Clostridium difficile*-associated diarrhea, stratified by disease severity. *Clin Infect Dis.* 2007;45:302. (189)

67

Intra-Abdominal Infections

Carrie A. Sincak and Sheila K. Wang

CORE PRINCIPLES

		CHAPTER CASES
1	Acute cholecystitis is the acute inflammation of the gallbladder presenting with fever, prolonged abdominal pain, and positive Murphy's sign of the right upper quadrant followed by nausea and vomiting. Acute cholangitis is an acute inflammation of the common bile duct with accompanying classic Charcot's triad: fever, jaundice, and right upper quadrant pain.	**Case 67-1 (Question 1)**
2	Empiric therapy for severe biliary tract infections may include combination therapy with either ciprofloxacin, levofloxacin, or cefepime plus metronidazole or monotherapy with piperacillin/tazobactam or an antipseudomonal carbapenem (imipenem/cilastatin, meropenem, doripenem) if multidrug-resistant gram-negative rods are suspected.	**Case 67-1 (Question 3)**
3	Spontaneous bacterial peritonitis (SBP) is largely a monomicrobial infection commonly caused by aerobic enteric gram-negative rods, such as *Escherichia coli* and *Klebsiella pneumoniae*.	**Case 67-2 (Question 1)**
4	Empiric therapy for SBP may include a third-generation cephalosporin such as ceftriaxone or cefotaxime or parenteral fluoroquinolone with activity versus *Streptococcus pneumoniae*. Length of therapy depends on the reduction of polymorphonuclear leukocyte counts (<250 cells/μL) in peritoneal fluid, generally occurring in 5 days or fewer.	**Case 67-2 (Question 2)**
5	For secondary peritonitis, empiric antimicrobial therapy for community-acquired infections is routinely initiated without obtaining Gram stain and culture. Blood cultures may be useful, however, in health care–associated infections or suspected multidrug-resistant pathogens.	**Case 67-4 (Question 1)**
6	Therapy for secondary peritonitis should include antimicrobial coverage directed at gram-negative bacteria and anaerobes. Therapy may include (a) certain extended-spectrum beta-lactams or beta-lactamase inhibitor combinations, (b) carbapenems, or (c) a fluoroquinolone with metronidazole.	**Case 67-4 (Question 3)**
7	Duration of therapy for intra-abdominal infections typically ranges from 4 to 7 days. Clinical response and source control influence duration of therapy.	**Case 67-4 (Question 4)**
8	Acute penetrating abdominal trauma requires a short course (<24 hours) of antimicrobial therapy. Delay of therapy or development of infection necessitates a 5- to 7-day course of therapy.	**Case 67-7 (Question 2)**

INTRODUCTION

Despite the introduction of new antimicrobial agents and improvements in diagnostic and surgical techniques, the treatment of intra-abdominal infections remains a therapeutic challenge. However, advances in radiographic and interventional techniques with timely source control, improved fluid and nutritional management, and the selection of appropriate antimicrobial agents have decreased mortality in intra-abdominal infections.

Intra-abdominal infections are those contained within the peritoneal cavity, which extends from the undersurface of the diaphragm to the floor of the pelvis or the retroperitoneal space. Intra-abdominal infections can present as a localized infection (appendicitis), a diffuse inflammation throughout the peritoneum (peritonitis), or as abscesses, which can form anywhere within the abdomen, between bowel loops, or in solid organs such as the liver, biliary tract, spleen, pancreas, or female pelvic organs.

Empiric antimicrobial therapy should be initiated as soon as an intra-abdominal infection is suspected. Therapy should be selected on the basis of the suspected pathogens; however, antimicrobial therapy alone is insufficient, especially in the setting of diffuse peritonitis. Source control includes interventional techniques to control and eliminate the infection with efforts to restore normal physiological function. If adequate source control is delayed, bacteremia, multiple organ failure, and mortality are more likely to occur.[1]

Normal Gastrointestinal Flora

The stomach of fasting individuals contains very few bacteria (i.e., <100 colony-forming units [CFU]/mL) as a result of gastric motility and the bactericidal activity of normal acidic gastric fluid.[2] The bacterial population of the stomach can be altered by drugs or diseases that increase gastric pH or decrease gastric motility. Not surprisingly, patients with bleeding or obstructing duodenal ulcers, gastric ulcers, gastric carcinomas, or those receiving proton pump inhibitors or histamine-2 receptor antagonists have an increased number of oral bacteria colonizing the stomach.

The upper small intestine (duodenum and jejunum) usually contains relatively few bacteria and harbors mainly oral flora. The lower small intestine serves as a transitional zone between the sparsely populated stomach and the abundant microbial flora of the colon.[3] The biliary tree is generally sterile, although colonization with aerobic gram-negative bacilli (particularly *Escherichia coli* and *Klebsiella* species) is more likely in patients with gallstones or surgical biliary interventions, and in the elderly.[4]

In the ileum, facultative gram-negative and gram-positive species, as well as obligate anaerobes, are encountered. As the distal ileum is approached, the quantity and variety of bacteria increase. Substantial numbers of anaerobic bacteria are present, including *Bacteroides* species, as well as *E. coli* and *Enterococcus* species, which are the most commonly encountered anaerobic, aerobic gram-negative, and aerobic gram-positive bacteria, respectively.[2,3]

In the large bowel, anaerobic bacteria, particularly *Bacteroides* species, predominate. In the distal colon, bacterial counts average 10^{10} CFU/mL of feces, with anaerobes outnumbering other organisms by a ratio of 1,000 to 10,000:1.[3] Although large numbers of *Clostridium* species, anaerobic gram-positive cocci, and non–spore-forming anaerobic rods are present, the most prevalent anaerobes are *Bacteroides* species. Among the facultative aerobes, *E. coli* is the most frequently isolated species.[2,3] Given these differences in regional microflora populations, it is not surprising that trauma to the colon carries a much higher risk of intra-abdominal infection in comparison with the stomach or jejunum[5] (Fig. 67-1, Table 67-1).

Resistant flora are more common in health care–associated infections, including *Pseudomonas aeruginosa*, *Acinetobacter* species, extended-spectrum β-lactamase (ESBL)–producing *E. coli* and *Klebsiella* species, methicillin-resistant *Staphylococcus aureus* (MRSA), enterococci, and *Candida* species.[6–9]

INFECTIONS OF THE BILIARY TRACT

Cholecystitis and Cholangitis

Cholecystitis and cholangitis originate as inflammatory conditions, usually as a result of obstruction in the gallbladder or common bile duct. The obstruction is typically caused by the presence of stones. The biliary tract is sterile under normal conditions, and the flow of bile, along with its bacteriostatic properties, functions to maintain the sterility. Infection typically occurs as a secondary event to obstruction.[4,5]

Acute cholecystitis is the acute inflammation of the gallbladder. The presence of gallstones in greater than 90% of cases prevents the outflow of gallbladder drainage by obstructing the neck of the gallbladder, Hartmann's pouch, or the cystic duct.[4] The obstruction causes an increase in intraluminal pressure, gallbladder distension, and edema, which triggers an acute inflammatory response. The potential consequences of this obstruction and inflammation include infection, ischemia, perforation, and necrosis.[4,10] The reduction in gallbladder outflow leads to biliary stasis, which provides an ideal environment for bacterial proliferation and subsequent infection (Fig. 67-2).

Acute cholangitis is an acute inflammation of the common bile duct. The most common cause of cholangitis in the United States is common bile duct obstruction as a consequence of choledocholithiasis. Less common causes include neoplastic obstruction, postoperative obstruction after biliary intervention, benign strictures, and primary sclerosing cholangitis.[4] The decrease in biliary outflow results in biliary stasis and bacterial proliferation. Infection results in a rapid rise in biliary pressure, which facilitates the spread of bacteria into lymphatics and the bloodstream via alterations in membrane permeability. In comparison with cholecystitis, acute cholangitis generally carries a poorer prognosis.[4,11]

CLINICAL PRESENTATION AND DIAGNOSIS

CASE 67-1

QUESTION 1: D.S., a 54-year-old man, presents to the hospital with a 1-week history of abdominal pain and tenderness, localized to the right upper quadrant, fever of 38.9°C, and chills. He complains of nausea, with three episodes of emesis occurring in the past 24 hours. D.S. appears jaundiced and reports dark-colored urine. His laboratory values are the following:

White blood cell (WBC) count, 17 × $10^3/\mu L$
Serum creatinine (SCr), 1.1 mg/dL
Total bilirubin, 6 mg/dL
Alkaline phosphatase, 270 U/L

What evidence of cholangitis exists in D.S.? How does the presentation of cholecystitis differ from cholangitis?

The clinical manifestations of acute cholangitis vary, but the classic presentation involves Charcot's triad, which consists of fever, jaundice, and right upper quadrant abdominal pain. Fever is present in 90% of cases, and jaundice and abdominal pain occur in 60% to 70% of cases.[4] A smaller percentage of patients, generally with gram-negative septicemia, may present with changes in mental status and hypotension.[4] Laboratory findings of acute cholangitis include leukocytosis, elevated bilirubin (>2 mg/dL) and alkaline phosphatase, and mildly elevated liver transaminases.[4,12] The clinical signs and symptoms of cholangitis, as exemplified by D.S., include high fevers (38.9°C), chills,

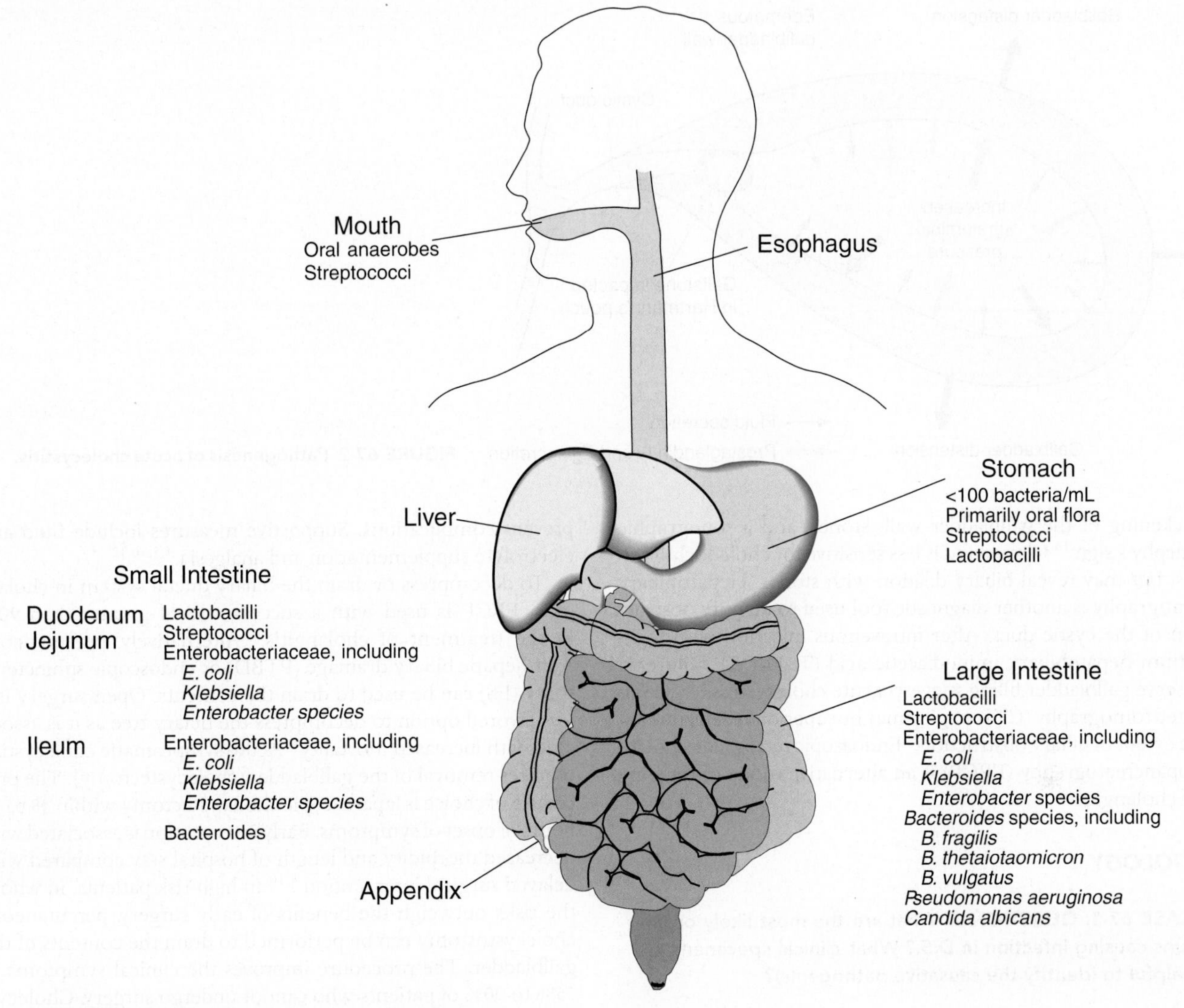

FIGURE 67-1 Microflora of the gastrointestinal tract.

jaundice, and right upper quadrant abdominal pain. Laboratory evidence supportive of cholangitis includes leukocytosis with WBC of $17 \times 10^3/\mu L$, increased bilirubin of 6 mg/dL, and elevated alkaline phosphatase of 270 U/L.

The clinical presentation of acute cholecystitis involves fever and prolonged constant abdominal pain typically localized to the right upper quadrant, followed by nausea and vomiting. On physical examination, tenderness in the right upper quadrant and a positive Murphy's sign (inspiration is inhibited by pain on palpation) are often present.[4,10] Laboratory findings include leukocytosis with increased neutrophils (left shift) and mild elevations in transaminases. Jaundice is less common in patients with cholecystitis (bilirubin <4 mg/dL) compared with cholangitis.[4,10]

Diagnostic imaging for acute cholecystitis and cholangitis involves ultrasonography. Findings for acute cholecystitis may reveal pericholecystic fluid, distension of the gallbladder,

TABLE 67-1
Common Pathogens in Intra-Abdominal Infection

Disease	Pathogens	Comments
Primary peritonitis	*Escherichia coli, Klebsiella pneumoniae, Streptococcus pneumoniae, Streptococcus* species, occasional anaerobes	Predominately in spontaneous bacterial peritonitis in cirrhotic patients. Anaerobes less likely than aerobes.
Secondary peritonitis	*E. coli, Bacteroides fragilis,* other aerobic gram-negative rods and anaerobes, *Enterococcus*	Generally polymicrobial with both aerobic and anaerobic pathogens. *Enterococcus* species are associated with nosocomial infections and chronic surgical infections, particularly in patients receiving broad-spectrum antimicrobials.
Chronic ambulatory peritoneal dialysis	*S. epidermidis, Staphylococcus aureus,* diphtheroids, gram-negative rods	Dwell time of exchange with intraperitoneal antibiotics must be a minimum of 6 hours.
Cholecystitis, cholangitis	*E. coli, K. pneumoniae,* other gram-negative rods, *Enterococcus,* and anaerobes	Unnecessary to use antimicrobials that achieve high biliary concentrations.

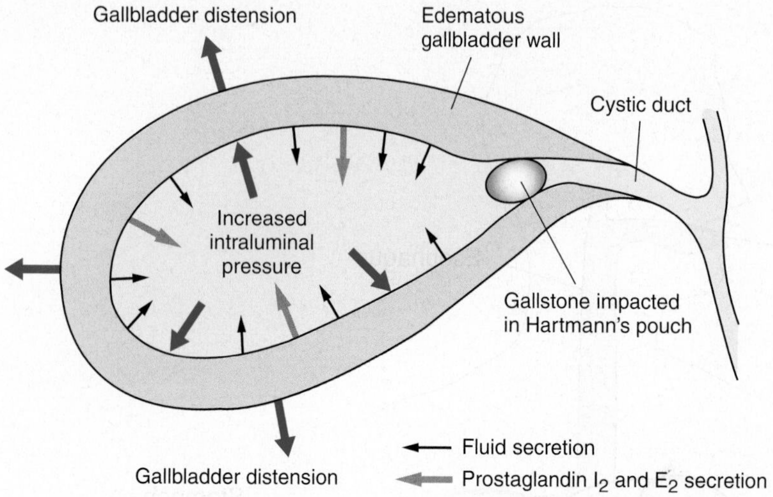

FIGURE 67-2 Pathogenesis of acute cholecystitis.

thickening of the gallbladder wall, stones, and a sonographic Murphy's sign.[13] Ultrasound is less sensitive for choledocholithiasis, but may reveal biliary dilation with stones. Hepatobiliary scintigraphy is another diagnostic tool used to identify obstruction of the cystic duct. After intravenous injection with technetium hepatobiliary iminodiacetic acid (Tc-HIDA), failure to observe gallbladder filling suggests acute cholecystitis.[6,13] Computed tomography (CT) imaging may be superior in determining the extent of biliary obstruction.[4] Endoscopic retrograde cholangiopancreatography (ERCP) is an alternative mode of imaging for cholangitis.[4,12]

ETIOLOGY

CASE 67-1, QUESTION 2: What are the most likely organisms causing infection in D.S.? What clinical specimens are helpful to identify the causative pathogen(s)?

The most common pathogens associated with acute cholangitis include *E. coli*, *Klebsiella* species, *Enterobacter* species, and *Enterococcus* species. However, *Pseudomonas aeruginosa*, skin flora (*Staphylococcus* species, *Streptococcus* species), and oropharynx bacteria may be implicated. Anaerobic organisms, commonly *Bacteroides* species, are associated with approximately 15% of infections, particularly in elderly patients undergoing biliary tract surgery.[4,14] The etiology of cholecystitis typically involves *E. coli*, *Klebsiella* species, and *Enterococcus* species. Anaerobes are less commonly isolated (Table 67-1).[4,10]

As described above, the stasis of bile flow results in proliferation of bacteria within the gallbladder or common bile duct. Acute cholangitis results in increased pressure within the common bile duct with dissemination of bacteria from the biliary tree to the bloodstream. Blood cultures may be positive in up to 40% of patients with symptomatic acute cholangitis.[4] Acute cholecystitis may reveal positive bile cultures in 20% to 75% of patients with symptomatic disease, but the utility of bile cultures has yet to be determined.[3] In contrast to cholangitis, bacteremia is unlikely with cholecystitis. The choice of antibacterial agents is largely empiric covering the aforementioned common causative pathogens.

TREATMENT

Definitive therapy for both cholangitis and cholecystitis must involve source control, using surgery, percutaneous drainage, or endoscopic intervention. Empiric antibacterial therapy should be added owing to the likelihood of secondary infection and to prevent complications. Supportive measures include fluid and electrolyte supplementation and analgesia.[4,5,10,12]

To decompress or drain the biliary ductal system in cholangitis, ERCP is used with a success rate of greater than 90% in the treatment of cholangitis.[4] Alternatively, percutaneous transhepatic biliary drainage (PTBD) or endoscopic sphincterotomy (ES) can be used to drain the contents. Open surgery is a less favored option to decompress the biliary tree as it is associated with increased mortality.[4] Acute symptomatic cholecystitis requires removal of the gallbladder (cholecystectomy). The procedure of choice is laparoscopic cholecystectomy within 48 to 72 hours of onset of symptoms. Early intervention is associated with decreased morbidity and length of hospital stay compared with delayed surgical intervention.[4,10] In high-risk patients, in whom the risks outweigh the benefits of early surgery, percutaneous cholecystostomy can be performed to drain the contents of the gallbladder. The procedure improves the clinical symptoms in 75% to 90% of patients who cannot undergo surgery. Cholecystectomy, however, should take place once the patient is stable enough for surgery.[4]

ANTIMICROBIAL THERAPY

CASE 67-1, QUESTION 3: Based on the most likely causative pathogen(s), what empiric antimicrobial therapy is recommended for D.S., given a diagnosis of cholangitis?

Empiric antimicrobial therapy for acute cholangitis and cholecystitis should be initiated after blood cultures have been collected. The empiric choice of therapy should cover enteric gram-negative pathogens, particularly *E. coli*. In general, the addition of anaerobic coverage is not mandatory for cholecystitis; however, it should be considered in the setting of severe cases such as acute cholangitis, biliary-enteric anastomosis, or health care–associated infections.[6] Empiric coverage for *Enterococcus* species should be considered for patients at risk for health care–associated infections, such as immunocompromised patients, patients who have required long-term hospitalization, patients who have received broad-spectrum antimicrobial therapy, or those with valvular heart disease or prosthetic intravascular materials.[6]

Antimicrobial therapy must be guided by drug pharmacokinetics and pharmacodynamics, local resistance patterns, and patient factors, such as drug allergies, renal or hepatic dysfunction, and cost. Examples of appropriate empiric regimens for biliary infections include combination therapy with either ciprofloxacin, levofloxacin, or cefepime plus metronidazole or monotherapy with piperacillin/tazobactam or an

TABLE 67-2
Empiric Treatment of Biliary Infections[6]

Infection	Regimen
Community-acquired acute cholecystitis (mild-to-moderate)	Cefazolin, cefuroxime, or ceftriaxone
Community-acquired acute cholecystitis with severe physiologic disturbance, advanced age, or immunocompromised state Acute cholangitis associated with biliary-enteric anastomosis	1. Imipenem-cilastatin, meropenem, doripenem, piperacillin-tazobactam monotherapy 2. Ciprofloxacin, levofloxacin, or cefepime PLUS metronidazole[a]
Health care–associated biliary infection	Vancomycin[b] may be added to each regimen in the setting of health care–associated biliary infections.

[a] Selection of fluoroquinolones should be based on local antibiogram or susceptibility reports.
[b] Given for suspected MRSA or ampicillin-resistant enterococcal infection.

antipseudomonal carbapenem (imipenem-cilastatin, meropenem, doripenem) (Table 67-2).[6] The aforementioned regimens are recommended for patients with acute cholecystitis of severe physiologic disturbance, advanced age, or immunocompromised state; acute cholangitis as a result of biliary-enteric anastomosis; or health care–associated biliary infections.[6] Considering their activity versus multidrug-resistant gram-negative bacilli, carbapenems generally should be reserved for infection caused by these pathogens. Vancomycin may be added empirically in health care–associated biliary infections in which ampicillin-resistant enterococci and MRSA are of concern. Empiric broad-spectrum antimicrobial regimens should be narrowed, when possible, based on culture and susceptibility findings. For mild-to-moderate community-acquired acute cholecystitis, monotherapy with cefazolin, cefuroxime, or ceftriaxone is recommended. Ampicillin-sulbactam is the least active agent for Enterobacteriaceae.[15] As a result, empiric coverage with ampicillin-sulbactam for complicated intra-abdominal infections is no longer recommended.[6] Resistance to fluoroquinolones is problematic with unpredictable susceptibility of *E. coli* to ciprofloxacin and levofloxacin.[15] Current guidelines for complicated intra-abdominal infections suggest fluoroquinolones be considered for therapy when institutional antibiograms indicate greater than 90% susceptibility of *E. coli*.[6] Use of aminoglycosides is not routinely recommended because of the need for therapeutic drug monitoring and potential nephrotoxicity and ototoxicity.[6] Furthermore, in comparison with other regimens, aminoglycoside-based regimens are inferior in the treatment of intra-abdominal infections.[16] However, some argue the decreased efficacy of aminoglycosides has been caused by inadequate dosing. An appropriate empiric regimen for D.S. would be piperacillin-tazobactam 3.375 g intravenously (IV) every 6 hours.

BILIARY CONCENTRATIONS

CASE 67-1, QUESTION 4: The physician caring for D.S. questions the need for an antibiotic that concentrates in the bile. Is there a benefit to using an antibiotic that is extensively excreted into bile?

Common bile duct obstruction prevents the entry of antibiotics into the bile, and the need for high biliary concentrations of antibiotics in the treatment of cholangitis has been debated.[17] Nagar and Berger[18] concluded that a number of antibiotics with excellent in vitro susceptibility, but poor biliary excretion, are still clinically effective. Biliary antibacterial concentrations do not correlate with an improved clinical outcome.[4] Highly biliary-excreted versus moderately biliary-excreted antibiotics have been compared.[17] Serum concentrations are more important than biliary levels in reducing the septic complications of biliary tract surgery. Furthermore, biliary excretion of any antibiotic is minimal in the presence of obstruction.[17]

The treatment of D.S.'s biliary tract infection must include biliary drainage. Piperacillin-tazobactam should be continued for 4 to 7 days.

PRIMARY PERITONITIS

Peritonitis is inflammation of the peritoneum as a result of infectious or chemical inflammation within the peritoneal cavity.[3,19] Infectious peritonitis can be classified as primary, secondary, or tertiary. Primary peritonitis involves the development of infection in the peritoneal cavity in the absence of intra-abdominal pathology.[19,20] Secondary peritonitis classically results from contamination of the peritoneum with gastrointestinal (GI) or genitourinary microorganisms as a result of the loss of mucosal barrier integrity. Tertiary peritonitis is clinical peritonitis along with signs of sepsis and multiorgan dysfunction persisting or recurring after the treatment of secondary peritonitis.[3,19]

Primary peritonitis is also known as spontaneous bacterial peritonitis (SBP) and is most frequently identified in adults with cirrhosis and ascites. Nearly 10% to 30% of hospitalized patients with cirrhosis and ascites have SBP.[3,20,21] Primary peritonitis is associated with postnecrotic cirrhosis, chronic acute hepatitis, acute viral hepatitis, congestive heart failure, metastatic malignancy, or systemic lupus erythematosus.[3,19]

Spontaneous Bacterial Peritonitis in Cirrhotic Patients

CLINICAL MANIFESTATIONS AND DIAGNOSIS

Patients with SBP may present with fever; signs of peritonitis, including abdominal pain; altered mental status; changes in GI motility; nausea; vomiting; diarrhea; or ileus.[21] Fever is common, occurring in 50% to 80% of patients.[3] Some patients have an atypical presentation or even lack symptoms.[21] The diagnosis of SBP is made on clinical presentation and examination of the peritoneal fluid via paracentesis. The ascitic fluid is tested for cell counts with WBC differential and the presence of microorganisms based on Gram stain and culture. Ascitic fluid with an elevated polymorphonuclear (PMN) count ($\geq 250/\mu L$) is diagnostic for SBP.[21]

ETIOLOGY AND PATHOGENESIS

CASE 67-2

QUESTION 1: M.W., a 51-year-old man with alcoholic cirrhosis and significant abdominal ascites, presents with a 4-day history of fever of 38.4°C and abdominal pain. Ascitic fluid obtained by paracentesis was cloudy, and culture of the ascitic fluid is pending. Laboratory values include ascitic fluid PMN count, $450/\mu L$; serum WBC count, $12.2 \times 10^3/\mu L$; and total bilirubin, 4.4 mg/dL. What organisms are likely to be cultured from M.W.'s ascitic fluid?

An estimated 70% of cases of SBP are caused by aerobic enteric organisms considered normal flora of the GI tract.[21]

E. coli is the most common pathogen, followed by *K. pneumoniae*.[3] Other common causes of SBP include *S. pneumoniae* and other *Streptococcus* species, accounting for 20% of cases. *Enterococcus* species are isolated in approximately 5% of cases.[21] *Staphylococcus* species, anaerobes, and microaerophilic organisms are rarely reported in community-acquired SBP. SBP is largely a monomicrobial infection.

One of the main mechanisms of pathogenesis associated with the development of SBP is bacterial translocation, which is the migration of microorganisms through the GI wall to mesenteric lymph nodes and other structures outside the intestine, including the bloodstream. Bacteria then infect the ascitic fluid by hematogenous or lymphogenous spread.[21,22] Certain characteristics of cirrhotic patients facilitate the pathogenesis of SBP, including bacterial overgrowth, decreased motility, structural intestinal damage, and decreased host-defense mechanisms that normally function to eliminate microorganisms. Bacterial overgrowth in the face of decreased motility and increased gut wall permeability, secondary to structural damage, facilitates subsequent systemic infection. Reduced opsonic activity and phagocytosis allow the microorganisms to escape the hosts' defenses and subsequently infect the ascitic fluid.[22] Spontaneous bacterial peritonitis with underlying cirrhosis was previously associated with a greater than 90% mortality rate, but with the advances in antibacterial therapy, the rate has been reduced to approximately 20% to 40%.[3,21] Patient characteristics associated with increased mortality include renal insufficiency, hypothermia, hyperbilirubinemia, and hypoalbuminemia. Gram-negative pathogens are associated with increased mortality compared with gram-positive pathogens.[3] Early diagnosis and effective antibacterial treatment of SBP are associated with reduced rates of mortality.[23]

ANTIMICROBIAL THERAPY

CASE 67-2, QUESTION 2: Pending ascitic fluid culture results, what empiric antimicrobial therapy should be recommended for M.W.? What is an appropriate duration of therapy, and how should the response to therapy be monitored?

Although a positive Gram stain and culture guides antibacterial therapy, nearly 60% of patients with signs and symptoms of SBP have negative cultures.[24] Initial antibacterial therapy for patients with a diagnosis of SBP is typically empiric and targeted toward the most likely pathogens as described previously. Ampicillin plus an aminoglycoside was the traditional choice for empiric therapy; however, third-generation cephalosporins (cefotaxime and ceftriaxone) represent safer, more-effective options.[24,25] A fluoroquinolone may be considered an alternative in patients with β-lactam allergies. Levofloxacin and moxifloxacin are preferred over ciprofloxacin, because of their superior activity against *S. pneumoniae*, the most commonly isolated gram-positive bacterial pathogen. Although parenteral therapy is preferred, oral fluoroquinolones may be as effective in patients with uncomplicated SBP.[24] As described earlier, aminoglycosides are not recommended in cirrhotic SBP therapy because of the risk of nephrotoxicity, and the decision whether or not to use fluoroquinolones should be based on institutional antibiogram reports.[21]

Antibiotic therapy is recommended until the PMN count from the ascitic fluid falls below 250 cells/μL, which normally occurs within 5 days.[23] França et al.[26] concluded that a 5-day course of cefotaxime for the treatment of SBP was as effective as a 10-day course.

M.W. should receive empiric therapy with an antimicrobial agent effective against *E. coli* and other common pathogens such as *Klebsiella* species and *S. pneumoniae*. Any of the abovementioned options would be reasonable empiric choices.

PROPHYLAXIS

CASE 67-2, QUESTION 3: After treatment is completed, should prophylactic antimicrobial therapy be initiated in M.W.?

Recurrence rates for primary peritonitis are high. Cirrhotic patients who survive an episode of SBP have a 1-year recurrence rate of nearly 70%. Two other types of cirrhotic patients are also at high risk for the development of SBP: patients with low ascitic protein ($<$1.0 g/dL) or elevated serum bilirubin ($>$2.5 mg/dL) and patients presenting with GI hemorrhage.[21] Prophylactic antimicrobial therapy has been shown to be of some benefit in cirrhotic patients at risk for the development of SBP (primary prophylaxis) and those with a high risk for the recurrence (secondary prophylaxis) of SBP. The risks and benefits must be carefully evaluated.

Secondary prophylaxis in cirrhotic patients is typically initiated with an antibacterial agent to provide selective decontamination of the GI tract. The goal of this therapy is to reduce the burden of bacteria and subsequently prevent bacterial translocation and infection.[21] Prospective, randomized studies in cirrhotic subjects with ascites support the use of oral antibacterial agents to reduce the rate of recurrence. The agents studied include oral norfloxacin,[27] ciprofloxacin,[28] and trimethoprim-sulfamethoxazole.[29] Rifaximin, a nonabsorbable derivative of rifamycin, has also been shown to significantly reduce the occurrence of SBP.[30] Long-term secondary prophylaxis is recommended based on the significant reduction in rates of recurrence in clinical trials. Long-term primary prophylaxis in patients with low ascitic proteins, elevated bilirubin, or both may also be beneficial but has not been associated with decreased overall infection or mortality and, therefore, is not uniformly recommended.[21,22,27–29] Primary prophylaxis is recommended, however, in all cirrhotic patients presenting with a GI hemorrhage.[21] Clinical trials have provided evidence to support the use of short-course therapy (7 days) of norfloxacin or ceftriaxone in patients presenting with GI hemorrhage.[22,31] Prophylactic therapy prevents bacterial infection and reduces the risk of rebleeding.[22] Several cost analyses have been performed demonstrating that prophylactic therapy in high-risk groups of cirrhotic patients is cost-effective.[22]

Concerns have been raised regarding the rapid emergence of bacterial resistance in cirrhotic patients receiving norfloxacin prophylaxis. In one study evaluating the influence of prophylactic norfloxacin (400 mg/day) on fecal flora, fluoroquinolone-resistant isolates developed during treatment. Rates of fluoroquinolone-resistant and trimethoprim-sulfamethoxazole–resistant gram-negative bacilli are more prevalent in patients who receive long-term prophylactic therapy.[32] Because of an increase both in resistance and in gram-positive causative organisms, the use of long-term prophylaxis must be considered when initiating antibacterial therapy for the treatment of new infections in this patient population.[33]

M.W. has cirrhosis, a previous episode of SBP, and a high total bilirubin; thus, he is at high risk for recurrence. Prophylactic antimicrobial therapy should be considered and may be a cost-effective measure. Any of the aforementioned prophylactic regimens would be appropriate for M.W. A specific choice for prophylactic therapy for M.W. would depend on institutional resistance patterns and tolerability.

PENETRATION OF ANTIMICROBIAL AGENTS INTO PERITONEAL FLUID

CASE 67-2, QUESTION 4: The physician asks whether the agents chosen for treatment and prophylaxis of peritonitis in M.W. will penetrate across the peritoneum. What properties determine the penetration of antibiotics into the peritoneal fluid?

The penetration of antimicrobial agents into tissues or abscess cavities depends on the serum-to-tissue fluid concentration gradient; the binding of the antimicrobial to serum and tissue proteins; the diffusibility of the drug, based on its molecular size and acid dissociation constant (pK_a); and lipid solubility.[34] In general, the β-lactam antimicrobials achieve peritoneal fluid concentrations exceeding typical minimum inhibitory concentrations (MIC) for most commonly encountered facultative gram-negative and anaerobic bacteria.[34,35]

Continuous Ambulatory Peritoneal Dialysis–Associated Peritonitis

PATHOGENESIS AND CLINICAL PRESENTATION

CASE 67-3

QUESTION 1: H.M., a 33-year-old woman with HIV and end-stage renal disease, has undergone continuous ambulatory peritoneal dialysis (CAPD) daily for the past year. She presents with abdominal pain and a cloudy dialysate fluid. H.M. has negligible residual urine output. What are the most common causative organisms related to CAPD-associated peritonitis? What empiric antimicrobial therapy should be initiated? How should antimicrobial agents be administered?

Peritonitis continues to remain a major complication of peritoneal dialysis. An estimated 45% of patients undergoing CAPD will experience at least one episode of peritonitis in the first 6 months of dialysis. Approximately 60% to 70% of patients exhibit peritonitis during the first year of dialysis, and recurrent infection occurs in 20% to 30% of patients.[3] CAPD-associated peritonitis is theorized to originate from contamination of the catheter by organisms of the normal skin flora, contamination of the peritoneum from an exit-site or subcutaneous-tunnel infection, contamination of the dialysate fluid, or bacterial translocation.[3] Alterations in host defenses of the peritoneum may also have a role in the development of CAPD-associated peritonitis.[3]

Clinical manifestations of CAPD-associated peritonitis include abdominal pain and tenderness, which is observed in 60% to 80% of patients. Nausea and vomiting occur in approximately 30% of patients, whereas 10% will have diarrhea and 10% to 20% will present with fever. The diagnosis of peritonitis is made on the basis of clinical signs and symptoms along with examination of the dialysate fluid for cell counts, Gram stain, and culture. Characteristically, the dialysate fluid will be cloudy and have a WBC count greater than 100 cells/μL with a neutrophilic predominance (at least 50%).[36] The Gram stain may be negative in 5% to 10% of cases, and blood cultures are typically negative.[3] In most cases, peritonitis is commonly caused by a single organism.[37]

ETIOLOGY

The most common causative organisms are gram-positive bacteria, accounting for 60% to 80% of isolates. Coagulase-negative *Staphylococcus* species (*S. epidermidis*) are the most common causative organisms, followed by *Staphylococcus aureus* and *Streptococcus* species. Gram-negative bacilli are isolated in approximately 15% to 30% of cases, with *E. coli* being the most common. Other common gram-negative organisms include *Klebsiella* species, *Enterobacter* species, *Proteus* species, and *P. aeruginosa*. Anaerobes, fungi, and mycobacteria constitute the less commonly encountered pathogens.[3]

ANTIMICROBIAL THERAPY

In general, empiric antibiotic therapy should be directed against the most common causative organisms, both gram-positive and gram-negative, until cultures of peritoneal fluid are available. Intraperitoneal (IP) delivery of antibacterial agents is the preferred route of administration for the treatment of CAPD-associated peritonitis. The IP route provides very high local concentrations of antibacterial agents as well as the ability to avoid a venipuncture and allow the patient to self-administer therapy at home.[36]

Treatment guidelines for CAPD-associated peritonitis provide a systematic approach for antimicrobial selection, dosing guidelines, and duration of therapy. Initial IP therapy recommendations include vancomycin or a first-generation cephalosporin for gram-positive coverage plus an antibacterial agent with antipseudomonal coverage.[36] Because of the increasing rates of MRSA and methicillin-resistant *S. epidermidis* (MRSE), vancomycin may be the most appropriate initial therapy for gram-positive organisms, although cefazolin remains effective in certain geographical areas.[37–39] Gram-negative therapy options include an aminoglycoside, ceftazidime, cefepime, or a carbapenem.[36,40] For patients who are intolerant of β-lactams or aminoglycosides, aztreonam may be considered as an alternative agent for gram-negative coverage.[36,40] Fluoroquinolones represent an option for CAPD-associated peritonitis given the extent of distribution into the peritoneal cavity; however, oral therapy should not be used in severe cases of peritonitis. The increasing prevalence of fluoroquinolone-resistant gram-negative *E. coli*, however, is decreasing the utility of these agents.[41,42]

When culture and susceptibility results are available, antibacterial therapy should be adjusted as necessary. With appropriate therapy, a clinical response should be expected within the first 48 hours. However, the presence of cloudy effluent after 5 days of therapy suggests refractory peritonitis, requiring removal of the catheter.[36] Antibiotic therapy is recommended for at least 2 weeks; however, 3 weeks of therapy may be required for severe cases such as exit-site and tunnel infections involving *S. aureus* or *P. aeruginosa*. When *S. aureus* is isolated, the infection usually necessitates the removal of the dialysis catheter. Vancomycin is recommended for MRSA (with or without rifampin) for 1 week, although monotherapy with vancomycin is adequate, particularly if the infected catheter is removed. Conversely, cefazolin alone is adequate for MSSA. Coagulase-negative *Staphylococcus* species do not require prompt catheter removal as they typically respond well to antimicrobial therapy. Methicillin resistance is common for *S. epidermidis;* thus, vancomycin is normally used. *Enterococcus* species or *Streptococcus* species should be treated with ampicillin if susceptible. The addition of synergistic gentamicin is not recommended because it does not improve efficacy and is ototoxic in this patient population. Vancomycin should be used for ampicillin-resistant enterococcus; however, vancomycin-resistant *Enterococcus* species (VRE) require treatment with linezolid, quinupristin-dalfopristin, or daptomycin. In the case of culture-negative peritonitis and clinical improvement after 3 days of empiric coverage, a single agent directed toward gram-positive organisms may be continued for a total of 2 weeks.[36]

TABLE 67-3
Intraperitoneal Antibiotic Intermittent Dosing Recommendations for CAPD Patients[a]

	Intermittent Dosing[b]
Amikacin	2 mg/kg
Ampicillin-sulbactam	2 g every 12 hours
Cefazolin	15 mg/kg
Cefepime	1000 mg
Ceftazidime	1000–1500 mg
Ceftizoxime	1000 mg
Fluconazole	200 mg every 24–28 hours
Gentamicin	0.6 mg/kg
Imipenem-cilastatin	1 g twice daily
Levofloxacin	500 mg PO every 48 hours[c]
Linezolid	200–300 mg PO daily
Meropenem	500–1000 mg daily
Polymixin B	150,000 units (IV) every 12 hours
Quinupristin-dalfopristin	25 mg/L in alternate bags[d]
Tobramycin	0.6 mg/kg
Vancomycin	15–30 mg/kg every 5–7 days

[a] Empiric doses for patients with residual renal function (>100 mL/day urine output) should be increased by 25%.
[b] Per exchange, once daily.
[c] Oral levofloxacin is recommended to be given with weekly IP vancomycin in centers with low fluoroquinolone resistance.
[d] Given in conjunction with 500 mg intravenous twice daily.
CAPD, continuous ambulatory peritoneal dialysis; LD, loading dose; MD, maintenance dose; IV, intravenous.
Source: Li PK et al. Peritoneal dialysis-related infections recommendations: 2010 update. *Perit Dial Int.* 2010;30:393.

TABLE 67-4
Intraperitoneal Antibiotic Continuous Dosing Recommendations for CAPD Patients[a]

	Continuous Dosing[b] (mg/L)	
	LD	MD
Amikacin	25	12
Amoxicillin	250–500	50
Amphotericin		1.5
Ampicillin		125
Ampicillin-sulbactam	1000	100
Aztreonam	1000	250
Cefazolin	500	125
Cefepime	500	125
Ceftazidime	500	125
Ceftizoxime	250	125
Ciprofloxacin	50	25
Daptomycin	100	20
Gentamicin	8	4
Imipenem-cilastatin	250	50
Nafcillin		125
Oxacillin		125
Penicillin G	50,000 units	25,000 units
Tobramycin	8	4
Vancomycin	1000	25

[a] Empiric doses for patients with residual renal function (>100 mL/day urine output) should be increased by 25%.
[b] All exchanges.
CAPD, continuous ambulatory peritoneal dialysis; LD, loading dose; MD, maintenance dose.
Source: Li PK et al. Peritoneal dialysis-related infections recommendations: 2010 update. *Perit Dial Int.* 2010;30:393.

When a single gram-negative organism is cultured (e.g., *E. coli, Klebsiella* species, or *Proteus* species), therapy can be narrowed based on susceptibility. Isolation of *P. aeruginosa* most often indicates a severe infection, which may also involve the dialysis catheter. Therapy options include an antipseudomonal β-lactam such as ceftazidime, cefepime, or piperacillin-tazobactam with or without a fluoroquinolone or an aminoglycoside. Aztreonam can be used in the case of severe immunoglobulin E (IgE)-mediated penicillin allergy. Polymicrobial peritonitis is uncommon, and may indicate a more complicated intra-abdominal process. Tables 67-3 and 67-4 list antimicrobial dosing guidelines for the treatment of peritonitis associated with CAPD.[36]

An example of an appropriate regimen for H.M. may include vancomycin plus cefepime or an aminoglycoside given intraperitoneally. The clinician should monitor culture and sensitivity results to adjust therapy based on guidelines, local sensitivity patterns, and therapeutic response.

FUNGAL CAPD-ASSOCIATED PERITONITIS

CASE 67-3, QUESTION 2: Two years later, H.M. presents with abdominal pain and cloudy dialysate fluid. *Candida albicans* is cultured from the dialysate fluid. No other organisms are present. How should H.M. be treated?

Fungal peritonitis is a rare complication of CAPD that is associated with significant morbidity and mortality. The rate of mortality in fungal peritonitis is approximately 25%.[36] Considering the high rate of failure of therapy, CAPD patients with fungal peritonitis should have their catheters removed.[36] Patients who have received prolonged or multiple courses of antibiotics are at increased risk for fungal peritonitis.[43] Most cases are caused by *Candida* species, most commonly *C. albicans;* however, an increase in infection attributable to nonalbicans species has emerged in many areas.[43] Empiric antifungal therapy should be broad and include most *Candida* species; echinocandins are the empiric drugs of choice. Amphotericin B may be administered intravenously (IV) or IP, but when given IP, it is very irritating to the peritoneum.[36] The azole antifungal agents can be administered orally, IV, or IP. Fluconazole is active against *C. albicans* but has decreased activity against certain types of nonalbicans species, such as *Candida glabrata*. In general, fluconazole is the drug of choice for *C. albicans;* however, other options, such as a polyene or echinocandin, would be needed for *C. glabrata*. Therapy should continue for a minimum of 2 weeks after catheter removal, and the total duration may be based on severity and clinical response.[36]

H.M.'s treatment should include temporary catheter removal and administration of antifungal agents. Antifungal therapy with oral fluconazole 200 mg daily should be continued for at least 14 days.

SECONDARY PERITONITIS

Pathogenesis and Epidemiology

Secondary peritonitis usually occurs after fecal or urinary contamination of the peritoneal cavity or its surrounding structures.[2] Infections most often occur after perforation of the GI or genitourinary tract (e.g., appendicitis, diverticulitis, perforated ulcer or uterus, abdominal trauma, bowel neoplasm). Secondary peritonitis most commonly occurs after penetrating or blunt abdominal trauma.

Localization of infection without eradication of bacteria results in intraperitoneal or visceral abscesses. Intraperitoneal abscesses occur most often in the right lower quadrant in association with appendicitis or a perforated peptic ulcer. Other causes can include diverticulitis, pancreatitis, inflammatory bowel disease, trauma, and abdominal surgery. Visceral abscesses generally are found in the pancreas but may also occur in the liver, spleen, or kidney.[3]

Clinical Presentation and Diagnosis

CASE 67-4

QUESTION 1: R.C., a 48-year-old man, presents with severe abdominal pain and nausea. Colonoscopy reveals a perforated peptic ulcer. Vital signs include temperature of 101.6°F and tachycardia (pulse, 105 beats/minute). Bowel sounds are absent. Laboratory values are WBC count, 16.5 × $10^3/\mu L$; and blood urea nitrogen (BUN), 34 mg/dL. What signs and symptoms of secondary peritonitis does R.C. display?

Making the diagnosis of a localized intra-abdominal infection may be difficult, despite the presence of signs and symptoms typical of severe infection. The patient may experience pain and voluntary guarding of the abdomen. Generalized abdominal pain usually is followed by a rigid, "boardlike" tensing of the abdominal muscles.[3] Inflammation around the intestines and peritoneal cavity results in local paralysis and reflex rigidity of the abdominal wall muscles and the diaphragm, causing rapid and shallow respirations.[3] Bowel sounds may be faint or absent with concomitant abdominal distension, nausea, and vomiting. Fever usually is present with tachycardia and decreased urine output secondary to fluid loss into the peritoneum. These signs usually are accompanied by an elevated WBC count with a predominance of neutrophils (left shift). The hematocrit (Hct) and BUN may be elevated as a result of dehydration. Initially, patients are usually alkalotic owing to emesis and hyperventilation, but in the later stages of peritonitis, acidosis usually occurs. Untreated peritonitis can result in generalized sepsis and hypovolemic shock.[2,3]

Gram stain and culture do not need to be routinely obtained in community-acquired intra-abdominal infections before the initiation of antimicrobial therapy. It may be useful in health care–associated infections or with suspected multidrug-resistant pathogens.[3] The presence of pleomorphic gram-negative bacilli, a strong odor, or tissue gas is strongly suggestive of infection with anaerobes, particularly *Bacteroides fragilis*.

ETIOLOGY

CASE 67-4, QUESTION 2: Given these findings, what are the most likely pathogens for R.C.'s secondary peritonitis?

Because secondary peritonitis can result from perforation of the intestinal tract, the normal flora consistent with the perforated segment determine the most likely pathogens. Studies consistently document a mixed culture of aerobes and anaerobes. The presence of anaerobic bacteria in the culture is indicative of a polymicrobial infection with a predictable group of pathogens.[2,3]

The most commonly isolated facultative bacterium is *E. coli*, which is found in approximately 50% of cultures. A variety of other gram-negative bacteria also are isolated, including *Klebsiella* species, *Proteus* species, *Enterobacter* species, and *P. aeruginosa* (Table 67-5).[2,44–47] Highly antibiotic-resistant strains of *P. aeruginosa*, *Serratia* species, *Acinetobacter* species, *Enterobacter* species, and *Enterococcus*, as well as *Candida* species, often are isolated from hospitalized patients who experience secondary peritonitis.[3,6] *B. fragilis* is the most frequently isolated anaerobe after perforation of the colon.[3,48] Anaerobic cocci (*Peptostreptococcus*) and facultative gram-positive cocci, such as streptococci, are also isolated.[3,6,45,48] *Enterococcus* species are isolated less frequently.[3,6,45,48] *B. fragilis* and *E. coli* are the most common pathogens found in blood culture samples after bacteremia related to an intra-abdominal infection.[3]

TABLE 67-5
Bacteriology of Intra-Abdominal Infections[2,44–47]

Bacteria	Patients (%)
Facultative and aerobic gram-negatives	
Escherichia coli[a]	71
Klebsiella species	14
Pseudomonas aeruginosa	14
Proteus mirabilis	5
Enterobacter species	5
Anaerobes	
Bacteroides fragilis[a]	35
Other *Bacteroides* species	71
Clostridium species	29
Prevotella species	12
Peptostreptococcus species	17
Fusobacterium species	9
Aerobic gram-positives	
Streptococcus species	38
Enterococcus faecalis	12
Enterococcus faecium	3
Staphylococcus aureus	4

[a] Most common in community-acquired intra-abdominal infections.

ONLINE CONTENT

For an algorithm on the classification of primary and secondary peritonitis, go to http://thepoint.lww.com/AT10e.

In summary, R.C. is likely to have an intra-abdominal infection caused by mixed flora, containing both aerobic and anaerobic bacteria. His current clinical status, highlighted by an elevated temperature, is probably secondary to the presence of facultative gram-negative bacteria, such as *E. coli*, *Proteus*, *Klebsiella*, or *Enterobacter*. Prolonged hospitalization or receipt of broad-spectrum antimicrobial agents is more likely associated with *P. aeruginosa*, *Candida* species, or other resistant bacteria.

Antimicrobial Therapy

EMPIRIC THERAPY

CASE 67-4, QUESTION 3: How should R.C. be treated? On the basis of clinical studies, what empiric antimicrobial therapy is appropriate for R.C. at this time?

Therapy for secondary peritonitis should include early administration of antimicrobial agents directed at gram-negative bacteria and anaerobes, fluid therapy, and support of vital organ function, as well as source control measures. *Source control* is a term used to involve all physical measures needed to eradicate an infection, such as débridement of necrotic tissue or drainage of an abscess or fluid collection. Surgical débridement and drainage, in conjunction with appropriate antimicrobial therapy, decrease morbidity and mortality.[2,3,49] Although not necessary for R.C., antipseudomonal coverage should be considered if the patient is hospitalized or has received broad-spectrum

TABLE 67-6
Treatment of Intra-Abdominal Infections[6]

Regimen	Dosage
Combination Therapy	
1. Metronidazole	500 mg IV every 8–12 hours
Plus	
Aminoglycoside (gentamicin or tobramycin)	5–7 mg/kg/d (normal renal function)
Amikacin	15–20 mg/kg/d (normal renal function)
2. Metronidazole	500 mg IV every 8–12 hours
Plus	
Aztreonam	1–2 g IV every 6–8 hours
3. Metronidazole	500 mg IV every 8–12 hours
Plus	
Ceftriaxone	1–2 g IV every 12–24 hours
Or	
Cefotaxime	1–2 g IV every 6–8 hours
Or	
Cefepime	2 g IV every 8–12 hours
4. Metronidazole	500 mg IV every 8–12 hours
Plus	
Ciprofloxacin	400 mg IV every 12 hours
Or	
Levofloxacin	750 mg IV every 24 hours
Or	
Moxifloxacin	400 mg IV every 24 hours
Monotherapy	
Cefoxitin	2 g IV every 6 hours
Cefazolin	1–2 g IV every 8 hours
Cefepime	2 g IV every 8–12 hours
Cefotaxime	1–2 g IV every 6–8 hours
Ceftazidime	2 g IV every 8 hours
Ceftriaxone	1 g IV every 24 hours
Cefuroxime	1.5 g IV every 8 hours
Ertapenem	1 g IV every 24 hours
Imipenem-cilastatin	500 mg IV every 6 hours or 1 g every 8 hours
Meropenem	1 g IV every 8 hours
Doripenem	500 mg IV every 8 hours
Piperacillin-tazobactam	3.375 g IV every 4–6 hours or 4.5 g IV every 6 hours
Ticarcillin-clavulanic acid	3.1 g IV every 6 hours
Tigecycline	100 mg initial, then 50 mg IV every 12 hours
Vancomycin	15–20 mg/kg IV every 8–12 hours (normal renal function)

IV, intravenous.

antimicrobials. In general, when an intra-abdominal infection is present, antimicrobial agents should be started immediately after appropriate specimens (e.g., blood, peritoneal fluid, abscess drainage) have been obtained and before any surgical procedures are performed.[2,3,6,50] The parenteral route should be used to ensure adequate systemic and tissue concentrations, especially in patients in whom shock or poor perfusion of the muscles or GI tract precludes the use of oral or intramuscular (IM) routes of administration. Therefore, antimicrobial therapy is generally empiric, based on the expected pathogens at the site of infection. Table 67-6 outlines dosing recommendations for antibiotics commonly used in the treatment of intra-abdominal infections.

Early clinical trials of clindamycin combined with gentamicin demonstrated the efficacy of this regimen.[3] Because of increasing resistance rates and toxicity, aminoglycosides are no longer considered first-line agents. The association of clindamycin with *Clostridium difficile*–associated diarrhea has also resulted in the use of other options.[6,44,51–55] For mild to moderate community-acquired infections, monotherapy with cefoxitin, ertapenem, moxifloxacin, tigecycline, and ticarcillin-clavulanic acid is recommended. Combination therapy with either a cephalosporin or a fluoroquinolone plus metronidazole is also reasonable.[6] For severe community-acquired intra-abdominal infections, meropenem, imipenem-cilastatin, doripenem, and piperacillin-tazobactam are monotherapy options that may be used. A third- or fourth-generation cephalosporin, ciprofloxacin, levofloxacin, aztreonam, or an aminoglycoside in combination with metronidazole represent alternative options for severe infections.[6,51] Meropenem, imipenem-cilastatin, doripenem, or piperacillin-tazobactam[6] should be reserved for presumed or documented multidrug-resistant pathogens or in sepsis. Although meropenem and imipenem should be reserved as last-line agents, ertapenem has a role in mild to moderate intra-abdominal infection. In comparative trials of ertapenem versus piperacillin-tazobactam, the two agents were shown to be similar in efficacy and safety.[51–53] Moxifloxacin with mixed aerobic and anaerobic coverage may be a monotherapy option; however, resistance to *E. coli* and anaerobes may limit its utility.[45] Because monotherapy has been shown to be efficacious in numerous trials, combination therapy is now rarely used.

Meropenem and imipenem-cilastatin, because of their broad spectrum of activity, should be reserved for the treatment of more resistant gram-negative organisms associated with health care–associated infections. Although piperacillin-tazobactam and ticarcillin-clavulanic acid are effective in complicated intra-abdominal infections, ampicillin-sulbactam has inferior activity against health care–associated gram-negative organisms and should not be used in patients with community-acquired or health care–associated intra-abdominal infections.

ONLINE CONTENT

For a narrated PowerPoint presentation on the treatment of intra-abdominal infections, go to http://thepoint.lww.com/AT10e.

R.C. should receive antimicrobial therapy with activity against facultative gram-negative bacteria and anaerobes, including *B. fragilis*. Ertapenem 1 g IV every 24 hours would be an appropriate treatment for R.C.'s mild to moderate infection.

DURATION OF ANTIMICROBIAL THERAPY

CASE 67-4, QUESTION 4: How long should R.C. receive antimicrobial therapy?

Recommendations for the duration of therapy for intra-abdominal infection vary from 4 to 7 days and depend primarily on the patient's clinical response to therapy and need for surgical drainage.[6] In general, antimicrobial therapy should be continued until resolution of signs of infection takes place, including return of WBC count to normal and elimination of fever.

ENTEROCOCCAL INFECTION

CASE 67-5

QUESTION 1: B.B. is a 58-year-old, nonobese woman with gangrene of the bowel from strangulation. One day after undergoing surgical resection of the duodenum, she has a fever of 102°F, shaking chills, and abdominal pain. Laboratory values are a WBC count of 18.4 × 10³/μL and creatinine of 1.1 mg/dL. B.B.'s peritoneal fluid cultures grow *E. coli*,

B. fragilis, C. albicans, and Enterococcus. Blood cultures are negative. Should she receive additional antimicrobial therapy active against Enterococcus?

Although *Enterococcus* is commonly cultured in patients with secondary peritonitis, its pathogenicity has been questioned. *Enterococcus* can cause serious infections (e.g., endocarditis, urinary tract infections), but is less virulent in the setting of polymicrobial infections such as intra-abdominal infections.

An important issue is whether empiric treatment should include antibiotics with activity against *Enterococcus*. Some investigators believe that *Enterococcus* species are commensal organisms that need not be treated in most clinical settings. They point to clinical studies in which antibiotic regimens lacking in vitro activity against *Enterococcus* have been successful. The pathogenicity of *Enterococcus* lies in its ability to enhance the formation of abscesses.[2,3]

In general, coverage is warranted if *Enterococcus* is present in blood cultures, is the sole organism on culture, or is the predominant organism on Gram stain.[3,6] Antienteroccocal therapy may also be recommended in patients with nosocomial or health care–associated infections,[6] particularly those who are immunocompromised, have postoperative infection, or have valvular heart disease or prosthetic intravascular materials.[6] Because B.B.'s blood cultures are negative and ascitic culture has demonstrated mixed pathogens, *Enterococcus* coverage is not necessary. B.B. should be treated with an antimicrobial regimen that has activity against gram-negative pathogens and anaerobes.

ANTIFUNGAL THERAPY: TREATMENT OF CANDIDA

CASE 67-5, QUESTION 2: Should B.B.'s antimicrobial therapy include an agent with antifungal activity?

The need to treat *Candida* species as a solitary isolate or as part of a polymicrobial infection is controversial. Certainly, *Candida* has the potential to cause peritonitis, IP abscesses, and subsequent candidemia. Echinocandins and azoles are options for fungal peritonitis.[6,19] Concerns about the toxicity of conventional amphotericin have limited the use of this agent. To date, no clinical trials have assessed the efficacy and safety of lipid-based amphotericin B, voriconazole, or caspofungin in the treatment of intra-abdominal fungal infections. The use of antifungal agents, such as fluconazole, may offer decreased toxicity in these patients. The potential risk of the development of resistance must, however, be addressed in clinical trials.

Fluconazole is considered an appropriate drug of choice for *C. albicans*.[6] For *C. glabrata* or other fluconazole-resistant species, an echinocandin (caspofungin, micafungin, or anidulafungin) or an amphotericin product is an appropriate option.[6] If critically ill, initial therapy with an echinocandin is recommended.

Therapy with an antifungal agent is not warranted at this time unless positive blood cultures for *Candida* are isolated or B.B. fails to respond to appropriate antimicrobial therapy.

ANTIMICROBIAL IRRIGATIONS

CASE 67-5, QUESTION 3: B.B.'s physician wishes to irrigate the peritoneum with aminoglycosides to achieve high local concentrations. Is irrigation with antimicrobial agents rational or effective in the treatment of intra-abdominal infections?

Hypothetic concerns regarding irrigation of the peritoneal cavity include spread of local infection, damage to the mesothelium, dilution of opsonins, or suspension of bacteria in a fluid medium in which they are less amenable to phagocytosis. Gravity and the movement of the diaphragm during respiration, however, spread bacteria throughout the peritoneal cavity even in the absence of irrigation. In addition, free circulation of fluids within the peritoneal cavity facilitates lymphatic clearance of microorganisms and toxins.[56]

Although data are limited, systemic antibiotic therapy and antibiotic irrigations appear to be efficacious for both the prevention and treatment of postoperative infections.[57,58] However, systemic toxicity resulting from systemic absorption of antimicrobial agents from the peritoneal cavity is possible. Most antimicrobials are readily absorbed from mucosal surfaces, especially when they are inflamed. When large volumes of irrigating solution containing antibiotics are used (especially in combination with IV doses), systemic drug concentrations markedly exceeding the therapeutic range have been observed. Neuromuscular blockade, renal failure, and ototoxicity have been reported after absorption of aminoglycosides from mucosal surfaces. Although a greater margin of safety exists for many of the penicillins and cephalosporins, the potential for toxicity is still of concern.[59]

Few data support the superiority of antibiotic-containing irrigating solutions versus systemic therapy. Given the potential for systemic toxicity secondary to absorption of antimicrobial agents from the peritoneum, the paucity of controlled trials documenting the efficacy of this method of administration, and the proved efficacy of systemic therapy, it seems prudent to use systemic therapy alone for the treatment of intra-abdominal infections.[57,58]

ANAEROBIC BACTERIA

CASE 67-5, QUESTION 4: The surgical resident initiated piperacillin-tazobactam for the treatment of B.B.'s intra-abdominal infection. Should culture and sensitivity results be used to monitor for anaerobic activity?

With the introduction of broad-spectrum antimicrobial agents with in vitro activity against *B. fragilis* and a significant problem of increasing resistance, the choice of a specific antianaerobic agent has become more complex. Multiple mechanisms of resistance are encountered, and resistance rates differ among various geographic areas of the United States. Although *Bacteroides* resistance to metronidazole is rare,[19,60] resistance to clindamycin has increased substantially.[19] Although the carbapenems and the β-lactamase inhibitor combinations are exquisitely active against *Bacteroides*, occasional resistance has been reported.

The Clinical and Laboratory Standards Institute (CLSI) has suggested that susceptibility testing be performed only to determine patterns of anaerobic susceptibility to new antimicrobial agents and to monitor susceptibility patterns periodically on a geographic and local basis.[61]

Because most anaerobes are cultured in the setting of mixed flora, isolation of individual components of a complex mixture can be time-consuming. In addition, most anaerobes are very slow growing, and it may take days to weeks for a definitive culture and sensitivity report. If specimens are not collected and transported in optimal media or in a timely manner, inaccurate or misleading results may be reported. The methods for susceptibility testing of anaerobic bacteria are not well standardized, and many hospital laboratories do not have resources to perform extensive culture and sensitivity testing. Routine cultures rarely impact the choice of antibiotic regimen, and thus the empiric choice of therapy usually determines the outcome.[62] Routine susceptibility testing for patient-specific cases is not recommended because of the prolonged time needed to achieve results but may be useful when resistant organisms are suspected or high-risk patients have been identified.[63]

Intra-Abdominal Abscess

CASE 67-6

QUESTION 1: R.K. is a 28-year-old woman with a history of diverticulitis who presents with abdominal pain and distension, fever, and chills. An intra-abdominal abscess is visualized by CT scan. How did this abscess develop? What considerations should be taken into account in the selection of appropriate antimicrobial agents?

Abscesses are collections of necrotic tissue, bacteria, and WBCs that form during a period of days to years. They generally result from chronic inflammation and the body's attempt to localize organisms and toxic substances by formation of an avascular fibrous wall. This process isolates bacteria and the liquid core from opsonins and antimicrobial agents.

MICROBIOLOGY

Although pathogens encountered in abscesses are similar to those encountered in other intra-abdominal infections, abscesses pose a therapeutic challenge because they typically contain large bacterial inocula that are likely to include subpopulations of resistant bacteria.[49] Furthermore, the rate of penetration of antibiotics into abscesses is hindered by the low surface-to-volume ratio, low pH, and decreased permeability.

Although percutaneous drainage or surgical débridement of R.K.'s abscess is crucial, adjunctive therapy with antimicrobial agents is warranted. The optimal antimicrobial agent should penetrate into the abscess in adequate concentrations and have an adequate spectrum of activity.[19,49] R.K. should be placed on an antimicrobial regimen that covers gram-negative bacteria and anaerobes, such as piperacillin-tazobactam 3.375 g IV every 6 hours.

INFECTIONS AFTER ABDOMINAL TRAUMA AND POSTOPERATIVE COMPLICATIONS

Risk factors for infection after penetrating abdominal trauma include the number, type, and location of injuries; the presence of hypotension; large transfusion requirements; prolonged operation; advanced age; and the mechanism of injury.[64]

Most investigators stress the importance of instituting antimicrobial therapy as close to the time of trauma as possible. Bozorgzadeh et al.[65] demonstrated a significant reduction in the incidence of postoperative infections when antibiotics were administered before surgical repair of the penetrating abdominal trauma.

Antimicrobial Therapy

PENETRATING TRAUMA

CASE 67-7

QUESTION 1: T.I., a 19-year-old man, is admitted to the emergency department within 1 hour after sustaining a gunshot wound to the stomach and colon. He is to undergo emergency laparotomy. What antimicrobial therapy is appropriate at this time?

As with other types of intra-abdominal infections, antibiotics active against both aerobic and anaerobic pathogens should be used.

Anti-infective therapy has been studied in patients who have sustained penetrating trauma to the abdomen (usually from knife or gunshot wounds). In several comparative trials, single-drug therapy with cefoxitin was as effective as the combination of clindamycin or metronidazole plus an aminoglycoside.[66] In evaluating these studies, however, it is important to note that most patients did not sustain injuries to the colon, where the risk of infection is highest. Although the age of this patient suggests he would tolerate aminoglycoside therapy, monotherapy with cefoxitin or one of the β-lactamase inhibitor combinations would be appropriate.

CASE 67-7, QUESTION 2: How long should antibiotic therapy be administered to T.I.?

Consensus guidelines regarding the duration of therapy were published by the Eastern Association for the Surgery of Trauma (EAST) Practice Management Group. These investigators reviewed all literature from 1976 to 1997 regarding the duration of antimicrobial use after penetrating abdominal trauma. They concluded that antimicrobial use should not exceed 24 hours in this patient population.[64]

The shortest duration of therapy that has been shown to be effective has been 12 hours with the possibility that a short course (<48 hours) of antimicrobial therapy is as efficacious as 5- to 7-day courses of therapy if antimicrobial therapy is promptly instituted.[6] Several other trials have confirmed no additional benefit exists in providing a longer treatment duration.[6,62,64,67–69]

Because antimicrobial therapy carries a risk of adverse reactions, the development of resistance, and unnecessary cost, short-term therapy seems warranted as long as it is instituted soon after the injury.[64,70] If the initial dose of antibiotic is administered more than 3 to 4 hours after injury, therapy should be continued for 3 to 7 days because the incidence of infection in this circumstance is high.

Antimicrobial therapy was instituted soon after T.I. sustained the colonic injury; therefore, a short course of antimicrobial therapy is appropriate. Therapy should be continued for 24 hours.

APPENDECTOMY

CASE 67-8

QUESTION 1: S.R. is a 12-year-old girl with a 2-day history of periumbilical pain migrating to the right lower quadrant, abdominal distension, fever of 102.3°F, diarrhea, and decreased bowel sounds. Her WBC count is 15.8 × $10^3/\mu L$. A presumptive diagnosis of acute appendicitis is made. What antimicrobial therapy is indicated, and for how long should it be continued?

Clinical manifestations commonly encountered with acute appendicitis include right lower quadrant abdominal pain, rebound tenderness, and low-grade fever complicated by nausea, vomiting, and anorexia.[3,6,36]

A variety of antimicrobial agents are effective in the treatment of acute appendicitis.[71–75] Most studies, however, have included patients without gangrenous or perforated appendices, which are associated with the highest risk of infection. In several well-designed, randomized, placebo-controlled trials, monotherapy with imipenem-cilastatin, β-lactams, and β-lactamase inhibitor combinations has been found to be as effective as the combination of clindamycin or metronidazole plus an aminoglycoside.[26,72,74] Patients with gangrenous or perforated appendices who were afebrile for 48 hours have been treated for durations ranging from a single dose[75] to 3 or more days.[73]

Overall, the studies justify the use of single-agent therapy with a β-lactam or β-lactamase inhibitor combination active against both gram-negative aerobes and anaerobes. In patients with uncomplicated appendicitis, therapy for less than 24 hours is sufficient; however, patients with gangrenous or perforated appendicitis should be treated for at least 3 days.

S.R. should receive a preoperative dose of any of the aforementioned β-lactam antimicrobials with activity against facultative gram-negative and anaerobic bacteria, such as cefotaxime (1 g IV every 8 hours for 24 hours). Cost, potential side effects, and ease of administration guide selection of a specific agent. If a gangrenous or perforated appendix is found during surgery, antimicrobial therapy should be continued for a minimum of 3 days or until S.R. has been afebrile for 48 hours.

KEY REFERENCES

A full list of references for this chapter can be found at **http://thepoint.lww.com/AT10e.** Below are the key references for this chapter, with the corresponding reference number in this chapter found in parentheses after the reference.

Key References

Garcia-Tsao G. Current management of the complications of cirrhosis and portal hypertension: variceal hemorrhage, ascites, and spontaneous bacterial peritonitis. *Gastroenterology.* 2001;120:726. (21)

Hau T et al. Irrigation of the peritoneal cavity and local antibiotics in the treatment of peritonitis. *Surg Gynecol Obstet.* 1983; 156:25. (56)

Hoban DJ et al. Susceptibility of gram-negative pathogens isolated from patients with complicated intra-abdominal infections in the United States, 2007–2008: results of the Study for Monitoring Antimicrobial Resistance Trends (SMART). *Antimicrob Agents Chemother.* 2010;54:3031. (15)

Horton JD et al. Gallstone disease and its complications. In: Feldman M et al., eds. *Sleisenger and Fordtran's Gastrointestinal and Liver Disease: Pathophysiology/Diagnosis/Management.* 7th ed. Philadelphia, PA: Saunders; 2002:1065. (11)

Levison ME et al. Peritonitis and intraperitoneal abscesses. In: Mandell GL et al., eds. *Mandell, Douglas, and Bennett's Principles and Practices of Infectious Diseases.* 7th ed. Philadelphia, PA: Churchill Livingstone; 2009:1101. (3)

Li PK et al. Peritoneal dialysis-related infections recommendations: 2010 update. *Perit Dial Int.* 2010;30:393. (36)

Luchette FA et al. Practice management guidelines for prophylactic antibiotic use in penetrating abdominal trauma: the EAST Practice Management Guidelines Work Group. *J Trauma.* 2000;48:508. (64)

Sifri CD et al. Infections of the liver and biliary system. In: Mandell GL et al. eds. *Mandell, Douglas, and Bennett's Principles and Practice of Infectious Diseases.* 7th ed. Philadelphia, PA: Churchill Livingstone; 2009:1035. (5)

Sirinek KR. Diagnosis and treatment of intra-abdominal abscesses. *Surg Infect (Larchmt).* 2000;1:31. (49)

Solomkin JS et al. Diagnosis and management of complicated intra-abdominal infection in adults and children: guidelines by Surgical Infection Society and the Infectious Diseases Society of America [published correction appears in *Clin Infect Dis.* 2010;50:1695. Dosage error in article text]. *Clin Infect Dis.* 2010;50:133. (6)

68 Urinary Tract Infections

Douglas N. Fish

CORE PRINCIPLES

		CHAPTER CASES
1	Urinary tract infection (UTI) is usually bacterial in etiology, may be either acute or chronic, and may affect any part of the upper or lower urinary system. UTI is often classified as either uncomplicated or complicated based upon patient characteristics and on the clinical setting in which the infection is acquired (e.g., community-acquired vs. health care–acquired).	**Case 68-1 (Questions 1–6), Case 68-2 (Questions 1–3)**
2	Uncomplicated UTI occurs in women who are otherwise healthy and have normal structure and function of the urinary tract. These infections are primarily caused by *E. coli* (75%–95% of infections) and other gram-negative bacilli, as well as gram-positive organisms such as *Staphylococcus saprophyticus* and *Enterococcus*.	**Case 68-1 (Questions 1–3)**
3	Symptoms commonly associated with lower UTI (e.g., cystitis) include dysuria, frequent urination, suprapubic pain, hematuria, and back pain. Patients with upper tract infection (e.g., acute pyelonephritis) often present with similar findings as well as loin pain, costovertebral angle tenderness, fever, chills, nausea, and vomiting.	**Case 68-1 (Questions 1, 2), Case 68-5 (Questions 1–3)**
4	The cornerstone of effective treatment of UTI is appropriate selection and use of antibiotics. Resistance among *E. coli* and other uropathogens is increasing and is an important consideration in antibiotic selection. Consensus clinical guidelines recommend trimethoprim-sulfamethoxazole (TMP-SMX) for 3 days, nitrofurantoin for 5 days, or a single dose of fosfomycin as preferred first-line antibiotics for treatment of acute uncomplicated cystitis in women.	**Case 68-1 (Questions 1–6), Case 68-2 (Question 1)**
5	Fluoroquinolones are commonly used for treatment of UTI and are highly effective. However, growing concerns regarding increasing resistance and potential adverse effects has limited the recommended use of fluoroquinolones in uncomplicated UTI to patients unable to receive other preferred agents due to drug resistance or other contraindications. Similar recommendations limit the use of β-lactam antibiotics for uncomplicated UTI.	**Case 68-1 (Question 3), Case 68-2 (Questions 1–3)**
6	Complicated UTI is associated with abnormalities of the urinary tract that interfere with normal urine flow or function; men, children, diabetics, pregnant women, and hospitalized patients are examples of commonly affected populations. Complicated infections are more frequently caused by drug-resistant gram-negative bacilli or other pathogens with reduced antibiotic susceptibility. Antibiotic selection for complicated UTI should be guided by culture and susceptibility testing, and patients usually require longer durations of antibiotic therapy (7–14 days).	**Case 68-1 (Questions 1–4), Case 68-2 (Question 1), Case 68-4 (Question 1), Case 68-9 (Questions 1, 2)**
7	Pyelonephritis may be more severe in presentation and is often associated with bacteremia and other complications. However, most cases are uncomplicated and can be treated on an outpatient basis with oral antibiotics such as fluoroquinolones. Patients who cannot take oral antibiotics or who are clinically unstable should be hospitalized for initial treatment with intravenous antibiotics.	**Case 68-5 (Questions 1–5)**

continued

		CHAPTER CASES
8	Recurrent UTI may be caused by either relapse due to treatment failure or reinfection. Relapse usually occurs within two weeks of the original infection and is caused by the same pathogen. Selection of antibiotics for treatment of relapsed UTI should be guided by culture and susceptibility testing, and the duration of antibiotic therapy should be at least 2 weeks in length.	**Case 68-6 (Questions 1–4, 9, 10), Case 68-7 (Questions 1, 2)**
9	Recurrent UTI which occurs more than 2 weeks after the original infection is treated as a new infection with antibiotic considerations similar to those for the initial infection. Women with frequent infections (3 or more/year) may be considered for chronic prophylaxis therapy. Women with identifiable causes of reinfection (e.g., in association with sexual intercourse) may self-administer prophylactic antibiotics.	**Case 68-6 (Questions 6, 7, 9, 10)**
10	Asymptomatic bacteriuria ($\geq 10^5$ bacteria per milliliter of urine in the absence of clinical signs/symptoms of UTI) is particularly common in children, the elderly, pregnant women, and in diabetics. Treatment of asymptomatic bacteriuria for prevention of subsequent infection and associated complications is routinely recommended in children and pregnant women. However, treatment of the elderly and patients with diabetes has not shown clear benefits and is not currently recommended.	**Case 68-7 (Questions 3, 4), Case 68-11 (Questions 1, 2)**
11	Prostatitis is a relatively common infection in men and is caused by bacterial organisms similar to those causing uncomplicated UTI in women. Acute bacterial prostatitis is usually treated with either a fluoroquinolone or TMP-SMX for a period of 2 to 4 weeks. Chronic prostatitis persists in a small percentage of men after acute infection and is usually treated for 4 to 6 weeks, although longer courses may sometimes be required.	**Case 68-12 (Questions 1, 2)**

URINARY TRACT INFECTION

Incidence, Prevalence, and Epidemiology

Urinary tract infection (UTI) is an acute or chronic infection, usually bacterial in origin, that may affect any part of the upper or lower urinary system.

For an illustration showing upper and lower urinary tract infections, see <u>http://thepoint.lww.com/AT10e.</u>

Infections of the bladder are referred to cystitis, and infections involving the parenchyma of the kidneys are known as pyelonephritis. Urinary tract infections occur frequently in both community and hospital environments and are the most common bacterial infections in humans.[1,2] The term UTI encompasses a spectrum of clinical entities ranging in severity from asymptomatic infection to acute pyelonephritis with sepsis.[1–3] Approximately 7 million cases of acute cystitis and 250,000 cases of acute pyelonephritis occur annually in the United States, resulting in more than 100,000 hospitalizations.[4,5] Direct costs associated with the diagnosis and treatment of UTI have been estimated at approximately $3 billion annually in the United States.[2,5,6]

UTI is predominantly a disease of females. The overall likelihood of developing a UTI is approximately 30 times higher in women than in men.[2,6] From ages 5 through 14, the incidence of bacteriuria (bacteria in the urine, either symptomatic or asymptomatic) is 1.2% among girls and only 0.03% among boys (40-fold lower). Of women between the ages of 15 and 24 years, 1% to 5% have bacteriuria; the incidence increases 1% to 2% for each decade of life until approximately 10% to 20% of women are bacteriuric after age 70.[1,7–9] Approximately 25% to 40% of all women will experience at least one UTI during their lifetime.[4] Women have more UTI than men, probably because of anatomic and physiologic differences. The female urethra is relatively short and allows bacteria easy access to the bladder. In contrast, males are partly protected because the urethra is longer and antimicrobial substances are secreted by the prostate.[1,2,6,7]

The incidence of UTI in neonates is about 1% and is more frequent in male neonates, many of whom prove to have congenital structural abnormalities.[10] The mortality rate among newborns with UTI was earlier reported to be as high as 10%[10]; however, this rate is now much lower because of an increased awareness of the high frequency of UTI in children, improved diagnostic techniques, and more effective management.[10] Urinary tract infections in males also occur with increased frequency after age 50, when prostatic obstruction, urethral instrumentation, and surgery influence the infection rate. Infection in younger men is rare and requires careful evaluation for urinary tract pathology.[11,12]

In general, 5% to 20% of the elderly living at home have bacteriuria, increasing to 20% to 50% in extended care facilities and 30% in hospitals.[2,8,13,14] The frequency of infection continues to rise with increasing age for those 65 years or older. Most UTI in these patients are asymptomatic, but often result in symptomatic infection.[8,13,14] Whether bacteriuria in old age is associated with decreased survival is controversial[15,16]; however, the presence of asymptomatic bacteriuria is associated with decreased functional ability of institutionalized persons,[8,13] and symptomatic UTI has been independently associated with a three-fold increased risk of vertebral fractures.[17] Reasons for higher UTI rates in elderly persons include the high prevalence of prostatic hypertrophy in men, incomplete bladder emptying caused by underlying diseases or medications, dementia, and urinary and fecal incontinence.[7,13,14,16]

Etiology

UNCOMPLICATED VERSUS COMPLICATED INFECTIONS

An important distinction in the characterization and treatment of UTI is that of uncomplicated versus complicated infections. Uncomplicated UTI, either cystitis or pyelonephritis, occurs in women who have normal structure and function of the genitourinary tract and who have no other factors which would put them at risk for more severe or complex infections.[2,4,18] By contrast, complicated infections are those which are associated with conditions that increase the risk for acquiring infection, the potential for serious outcomes, or the risk for therapy failure. Such conditions are often associated with abnormalities that may interfere with normal urine flow. Infections in men, children, and pregnant women are automatically considered complicated, as are those which are health care–associated in origin. Other examples of complicated infections include those associated with structural and neurologic abnormalities of the urinary tract, metabolic or hormonal abnormalities, impaired host responses, instrumentation and catheterization of the urinary tract, and those caused by unusual pathogens (e.g., yeasts, *Mycoplasma*).[2,4,18] Uncomplicated infections are invariably community-acquired in etiology and are caused by the organisms typical to that etiology. Complicated UTI may be caused by pathogens usually associated with either community-acquired or health care–associated infections, depending on the source of bacterial acquisition and specific underlying patient risk factors. Complicated infections are also more often polymicrobial in etiology and often associated with more antibiotic-resistant pathogens. Proper drug selection for treatment of complicated UTI is challenging and generally associated with a longer duration of therapy.

COMMUNITY-ACQUIRED INFECTIONS

Most UTI are caused by gram-negative aerobic bacilli from the intestinal tract. *Escherichia coli* cause 75% to 95% of community-acquired, uncomplicated UTIs.[1,2,18] Coagulase-negative staphylococci (i.e., *Staphylococcus saprophyticus*) account for another 5% to 20% of UTIs in younger women.[1,2,4] Other Enterobacteriaceae (*Proteus mirabilis, Klebsiella*) and *Enterococcus faecalis* also are common pathogens.[1,2,18] Uncomplicated infections are nearly always caused by a single pathogen.

HEALTH CARE–ASSOCIATED INFECTIONS

Urinary tract infections occur in up to 10% of hospitalized patients and represent 20% to 30% of all nosocomial infections.[19–21] *E. coli* remains the most common pathogen in hospital-acquired or other complicated UTI, but it is responsible for only 20% to 30% of these infections. Other gram-negative organisms such as *Pseudomonas aeruginosa, Klebsiella, Proteus, Enterobacter,* and *Acinetobacter* cause significantly more infections (up to 25%) than in community-acquired infections.[4,20,21] *Enterococcus* is also a common pathogen in hospital-acquired infections and causes approximately 15% of infections.[20,21] UTIs caused by *Staphylococcus aureus* are usually the result of hematogenous spread, although this pathogen is also associated with urinary catheterization.[1,20–22] Finally, *Candida* is a common pathogen in hospital-acquired infections and may be involved in 20% to 30% of cases.[19–21] In contrast to uncomplicated infections that are usually monomicrobial, UTI associated with structural abnormalities or indwelling urinary catheters are often caused by multiple organisms.[1,19–22]

Pathogenesis and Predisposing Factors

The usual pathway for the spread of bacteria to the urinary tract is the ascending route. A UTI usually begins with heavy and persistent colonization of the introitus (i.e., vaginal vestibule and urethral mucosa) with intestinal bacteria. Once introital colonization has occurred, colonization of the urethra leads to retrograde infection of the bladder and the development of cystitis.[23,24]

The bladder has defense mechanisms that prevent spread of the infection after urethral colonization occurs.[1,2,20] Urination washes bacteria out of the bladder and is effective if urine flows freely and the bladder is emptied completely. Substances in the urine, including organic acids (which contribute to a low pH) and urea (which contributes to a high osmolality), are antibacterial. The bladder mucosa also has antibacterial properties.[1,2,20] Lastly, other substances, including immunoglobulin A and glycoproteins (e.g., Tamm-Horsfall protein), are actively secreted into the urine and act to prevent adherence of bacteria to uroendothelial cells.[20,23,24]

Focal renal involvement leading to pyelonephritis may result from the spread of bacteria via the ureters and may be facilitated by vesicoureteral reflux or decreased ureteral peristalsis. Reflux can be produced by cystitis alone or by anatomic defects.

ONLINE CONTENT

For an illustration of mechanisms of ureterovesical and urethrovesical reflux, go to http://thepoint.lww.com/AT10e.

Ureteral peristalsis is decreased by pregnancy, ureteral obstruction, or gram-negative bacterial endotoxins.[1,23,24]

A variety of factors are associated with the development of UTI. Some of these involve expression of bacterial virulence factors such as specific adhesin molecules, bacterial polysaccharides, and bacterial enzymes. Other factors leading to UTI are dependent on the host. Extremes of age, female sex, sexual activity, use of contraception, pregnancy, urinary tract instrumentation or catheterization, urinary tract obstruction, neurologic dysfunction, renal disease, previous antimicrobial use, and expression of A, B, and H blood group oligosaccharides on the surface of epithelial cells are among the many predisposing factors for the development of UTI.[1,2,16,23,25]

ONLINE CONTENT

For an illustration that shows the pathogenesis of UTI, go to http://thepoint.lww.com/AT10e.

The incidence of bacteriuria in pregnant women is as high as 15%, which is approximately twice that of similarly aged nonpregnant women.[1,8,26,27] The incidence of acute symptomatic pyelonephritis in pregnant women with untreated bacteriuria also is high and may reach 40%.[2] Many factors contribute to the increased susceptibility of the pregnant female to infection; these include hormonal changes, anatomic changes, progressive urinary stasis, and glucose in the urine.[26,27] Hormonal changes have also been linked to a significantly increased risk of UTI in menopausal women.[2] Estrogen promotes an acidic vaginal pH and proliferation of normal flora such as *Lactobacillus,* both factors which reduce pathogenic colonization of the vagina. Reduction of estrogen production at the time of menopause allows significant colonization of the vaginal tract with *E. coli* and other enteric bacilli, thus predisposing to subsequent infection.[2]

Renal disease increases the susceptibility of the kidney to infection.[1] The incidence of UTI among renal transplant recipients ranges from 35% to 80% without prophylactic antibiotic therapy.[28] Patients with spinal cord injuries, stroke, atherosclerosis, or diabetes may have neurologic dysfunction predisposing to UTI. The neurologic dysfunction can cause urinary retention, requiring catheterization. Furthermore, prolonged immobilization facilitates hypercalciuria and stone formation in some of these patients.[1,4,23]

Previous antimicrobial use (within the previous 15–28 days) increases the relative risk for UTI in women by threefold to sixfold.[2] This increased infection risk applies to prior antimicrobial use for treatment of UTI as well as other infections. The proposed mechanism for increased risk is alteration of normal flora of the urogenital tract and predisposition to colonization with pathogenic bacterial strains.[2]

Diabetes mellitus is associated with an increased risk for UTI because of glucose in the urine, which both promotes bacterial growth and impairs leukocyte function. Diabetes is also often associated with anatomic, neurologic, and immunologic abnormalities of the urinary tract that increase risk of infection, often because of increased need for urinary tract instrumentation.[29,30] Several studies have documented a twofold to threefold increase in UTI in diabetic women compared with nondiabetic women; rates of relapses and reinfections, as well as complications such as pyelonephritis, are also increased.[29–31] Autonomic neuropathy also contributes to increased frequency and severity of UTI in diabetic patients.[23,29,30]

Finally, studies have supported an association between sexual intercourse and UTI among otherwise healthy women.[2,23,32,33] Specific contraceptive practices, particularly the use of spermicides, are associated with increased risk for UTI. The use of a diaphragm, cervical cap, or condom in combination with spermicidal jelly increases the risk of UTI compared with the use of the barrier method alone.[25,32,33] Although the greatest risk has been associated with the spermicide nonoxynol-9, the use of other types of spermicidal jellies has also been associated with a significantly higher risk for UTI.[34] Oral contraceptive use has also been associated with increased risk of UTI.[2,32,33] The exact mechanisms of infection related to sexual intercourse and contraceptive methods are unclear but appear to be related to alterations in vaginal flora that allow for bacterial overgrowth and subsequent infection.[2,35]

URINARY CATHETERS

Instrumentation or catheterization of the urinary tract is an important predisposing factor for health care–associated UTI. Catheter-associated UTI, the most common type of hospital-acquired infection, occurs in up to 30% of catheterized patients.[21] Catheterization and other forms of urologic instrumentation take place in 65% to 95% of all hospital-acquired UTI.[20] These UTI also are a major cause of nosocomial gram-negative bacteremia.[19,21] Other urologic procedures, such as cystoscopy, transurethral surgery, prostate biopsy, and upper urinary tract endoscopy, are much less likely to result in infection unless there is pre-existing bacteriuria or other contaminated sites (e.g., prostate, renal stones). Any obstruction to the free flow of urine (e.g., urethral stenosis, stones, tumor) or mechanical difficulty in evacuating the bladder (e.g., prostatic hypertrophy, urethral stricture) also predisposes patients to UTI. Furthermore, infections associated with urethral or renal pelvic obstruction can lead to rapid destruction of the kidney and sepsis.[1]

Catheter infection can occur by bacterial entry from several routes. The urethral meatus and the distal third of the urethra normally are colonized by bacteria; therefore, initial catheter insertion can introduce bacteria into the bladder. Bacteria contaminating catheter junctions and the urine collection bag can migrate through the catheter lumen to the bladder, initiating infection.[21] The extraluminal space in the urethra also has been considered a potential route of contamination. The risk of infection is directly related to catheter insertion technique, care of the catheter, duration of catheterization, and the susceptibility of the patient. A diagnostic or single, short-term catheterization is associated with a much lower risk of infection than indwelling, long-term catheterization.[21] Despite careful technique, the risk of contaminating a sterile bladder with urethral bacteria is always present. The incidence of infection after a single catheterization is 1% in healthy young women and 20% in debilitated patients. Each reinsertion of the catheter introduces a risk of infection.[21]

Infections have been reduced dramatically by the closed, sterile drainage system, the most common type of catheter currently in use. With this system, the drainage tube leads from the catheter directly to a closed plastic collection bag. The overall incidence of infection from the closed system with careful insertion and maintenance is about 20%; the risk increases to 50% after 14 days of catheterization.[21] Condom catheters are associated with a lower incidence of bacteriuria than indwelling urethral catheters. These catheters avoid problems associated with insertion of a tube directly into the urinary tract; nevertheless, urine within the catheters may have high concentrations of organisms so that colonization of the urethra and subsequent cystitis may develop.[21]

Application of antibacterial substances to the collection bag and the catheter–urethral interface do not decrease the incidence of bacteriuria.[21,36,37] The use of antimicrobial-coated catheters (e.g., silver, rifampin plus minocycline) have been shown in some studies to decrease rates of bacteriuria and UTI.[21,36,37] The overall effects of these catheters on infection rates, patient outcomes, and antibiotic resistance are not known, however. The routine use of antibiotic-coated catheters is not currently recommended.[21,36]

Clinical Presentation

Symptoms commonly associated with lower UTI (e.g., cystitis) include burning on urination (dysuria), frequent urination, suprapubic pain, blood in the urine (hematuria), and back pain. Patients with upper tract infection (e.g., acute pyelonephritis) also may present with loin pain, costovertebral angle (CVA) tenderness, fever, chills, nausea, and vomiting.[1–4,38]

Clinical signs and symptoms correlate poorly with either the presence or the extent of the infection. Symptoms common to lower UTI often are the only positive findings in upper UTI (i.e., subclinical pyelonephritis).[1,3] The probability of true infection in women who present with one or more symptoms of UTI is only about 50%.[39] The presence of dysuria, back pain, pyuria, hematuria, bacteriuria, and a history of previous UTI enhance the probability of true infection; the absence of dysuria or back pain, and history of vaginal discharge or irritation significantly decrease the likelihood of infection.[39] The combination of dysuria and frequency in the absence of vaginal discharge or irritation increases the probability of true infection to greater than 90%.[39] Fever, chills, flank pain, nausea and vomiting, or CVA tenderness are highly suggestive of acute pyelonephritis rather than cystitis.[3,4,38] Many elderly patients with UTI are asymptomatic without pyuria. Additionally, because many patients have frequency and dysuria, it is difficult to distinguish between noninfectious and infectious causes based on symptoms.[1] Nonspecific symptoms, such as failure to thrive and fever, may be the only manifestations of UTI in neonates and children younger than 2 years of age.[1]

Diagnosis

Diagnosis of UTI based on clinical findings alone is accurate in only approximately 70% of patients.[40] The urinalysis (UA) is a series of laboratory tests commonly performed in patients suspected of having a UTI; in combination with appropriate clinical findings, the UA effectively improves the overall diagnostic accuracy for UTI.[41] A technician first performs a macroscopic analysis by describing the color of the urine; measuring its specific gravity; and estimating the pH and glucose, protein, ketone, blood, and bilirubin contents using a rapid "dipstick" method. Then the urine sediment, obtained by centrifugation, is examined under a microscope for the presence and quantity of leukocytes, erythrocytes, epithelial cells, crystals, casts, and bacteria.

Microscopic examination of urine sediment in patients with documented UTI reveals many bacteria (usually >20 per high-power field [HPF]). Gram staining of uncentrifuged ("unspun") urine shows at least one organism per immersion oil field and usually correlates with a positive urine culture. Pyuria (i.e., ≥8 white blood cells [WBC] per milliliter (mL) of unspun urine or 2–5 WBC/HPF of centrifuged urine) is frequently seen in patients with UTI. WBC casts in the urine strongly suggest acute pyelonephritis.[1,41]

A rapid diagnostic dipstick test for the detection of bacteriuria, the nitrite test, detects nitrite formation from the reduction of nitrates by bacteria. This test is widely available and easily performed; however, at least 10^5 bacteria/mL are necessary to form sufficient nitrite for the reaction to occur. Although a positive nitrite reading is useful, false-negative results do occur.[40] Dipstick testing can also be used to perform the leukocyte esterase test, which detects the esterase activity of activated leukocytes in the urine. A positive test correlates well with significant pyuria[42]; however, both false-negative and false-positive findings can occur with the leukocyte esterase panel as well.[40] Nitrite and leukocyte esterase tests are useful in ruling out the presence of infection if results of both tests are negative, whereas positive results of both tests in combination are highly suggestive of the presence of infection.[40] Confirmatory tests (e.g., urine culture) should be considered, however, if one or both dipstick test findings is positive owing to the possibility of false-positive test results.[42]

The gold-standard criterion for the diagnosis of UTI is the urine culture with a positive urinanalysis.[1,2,38] Proper interpretation of these cultures depends, however, on appropriate urine collection techniques. Urinating into a sterile collection cup using the midstream clean-catch technique is the most practical method of urine collection. This method of urine specimen collection is especially useful for male patients, but is less useful in female patients because contamination is extremely difficult to avoid.[1] The external urethral area must first be thoroughly cleaned and rinsed, then the urine specimen collected after initiation of the urine stream (hence "midstream").

Urinary catheterization for a urine culture sample yields fairly reliable results if performed carefully. However, infections can result from the procedure itself because organisms might be introduced into the bladder at the time of catheterization. Suprapubic bladder aspiration, although unpleasant from a patient's point of view, generally is not painful and is quite reliable. It is not practical for routine office or clinic practice, but may be useful when voided urine samples repeatedly yield questionable results or when patients have voiding problems. Because contamination is negligible, any number of bacteria found by this method reflects infection.[1,2]

Urine must be plated on culture media within 20 minutes of collection to avoid erroneously high colony counts from bacterial growth in urine at room temperature. Otherwise, urine should be promptly refrigerated until it can be cultured. Colony counts are also affected by the concentration of bladder urine; bacterial counts are higher in first-voided morning urines compared with those obtained from the same patient later in the day.

Greater than 10^5 colonies of bacteria/mL cultured from a midstream urine specimen confirms a UTI. A single, carefully collected urine specimen provides 80% reliability, and two consecutive cultures of the same organism are virtually diagnostic.[1,2] It is important to understand that the classic definition of UTI as greater than or equal to 10^5 bacteria/mL is fairly insensitive in accurately diagnosing patients with UTI. Approximately 30% to 50% of actual cases of acute cystitis have less than 10^5 bacteria/mL.[4,8] Particularly in a symptomatic patient, using a definition of greater than or equal to 10^2 bacteria/mL is much more sensitive and avoids failure to diagnose infection in many patients.[4]

Diagnosis of UTI in men also requires different interpretation of laboratory data. Contamination of urinary specimens is much less likely to occur in men compared with women, and numbers of bacterial colonies in specimens are therefore much lower. Greater than 10^3 bacteria/mL is thus highly suggestive of UTI in men.[11,12,43] In addition, although a positive nitrite test in a symptomatic man is highly indicative of the presence of an acute UTI, a negative nitrite test does not necessarily exclude infection and should be confirmed with a urine culture.[44]

Diagnosis of UTI in children is particularly problematic because of the difficulties and high contamination rates associated with commonly used methods of urine specimen collection. Suprapubic aspiration is the most accurate method in children, followed by urinary bladder catheterization.[2,38] Although clean-catch and bag methods (i.e., collecting urine into a bag placed around the urogenital area) are most susceptible to contamination and inaccurate results, they are also the most preferred methods for parents and health care personnel because they are simple and noninvasive. The choice of diagnostic tests for children will therefore be based on the experience, skill, and preferences of those involved with the child, and no one technique will be ideal in every setting.[38]

Simplified culture methods such as the filter-paper method (e.g., Testuria-R), dip-slide method (e.g., Uricult), and pad-culture method (Microstix) are as reliable as traditional laboratory methods for bacterial identification and quantification. The filter-paper method is relatively inexpensive but does not differentiate between gram-positive and gram-negative organisms. The dip-slide and pad-culture methods are accurate, differentiate between gram-positive and gram-negative organisms, and are similar in cost. The dip-slide method has the added advantages of ease of storage and a nitrite indicator pad.

Overview of Drug Therapy

The cornerstone of the effective treatment of UTI is the appropriate selection and use of antibiotics. Antibiotic treatment of UTI has been well studied and, compared to many infectious diseases, the choice of specific antibiotic and duration of therapy for acute, uncomplicated infections are reasonably clear. Recently published consensus guidelines from the Infectious Diseases Society of America (IDSA) and the European Society for Microbiology and Infectious Diseases (ESMID) recommend a 5-day course of nitrofurantoin, trimethoprim-sulfamethoxazole (TMP-SMX) for 3 days, or a single dose of fosfomycin trometamol as first-line antibiotics for treatment of acute uncomplicated cystitis in women.[18] Whereas nitrofurantoin and TMP-SMX are familiar agents, fosfomycin is a previously little used antibiotic which has been available for many years. However, it has recently made a resurgence in clinical use due to low rates of resistance among common uropathogens. Fosfomycin also has usefulness against multidrug-resistant pathogens which are becoming more common in certain practice settings; these include methicillin-resistant *Staphylococcus aureus*, vancomycin-resistant enterococci, and extended spectrum β-lactamase (ESBL)-producing gram-negative bacteria.[18,45] Fluoroquinolones and β-lactam antibiotics such as amoxicillin-clavulanate or various cephalosporins are recommended by the IDSA/ESMID guidelines as alternative agents for treating acute uncomplicated cystitis.[18] These same guidelines recommend fluoroquinolones, cephalosporins, aminoglycosides, TMP-SMX, extended-spectrum penicillins (i.e., piperacillin-tazobactam), or a carbapenem for the treatment of acute pyelonephritis in women.[18] The choice of a specific agent for pyelonephritis depends primarily on whether or not the patient is hospitalized or treated as an outpatient, local susceptibility patterns, and whether therapy is empiric or based on known susceptibilities. The duration of therapy for acute pyelonephritis ranges from 5 to 14 days and is dependent on which specific antibiotic is being used.[18] The parameters for monitoring response to treatment of either uncomplicated cystitis or pyelonephritis are primarily those indicating resolution of clinical signs and symptoms; repeat urinary cultures are not usually required assuming that signs and symptoms of infection resolve promptly. Patients with complicated UTI or recurrent infections may require additional monitoring and long-term follow-up, and antibiotic selection must be guided by culture and susceptibility testing. Patient monitoring related to the safety and tolerability of antibiotic therapy is required regardless of type of infection, as is effective patient counseling.

LOWER URINARY TRACT INFECTION

Initial Patient Evaluation and Determining Goals of Therapy

CASE 68-1

QUESTION 1: V.Q., a 20-year-old woman with no previous history of UTI, complains of burning on urination, frequent urination of a small amount, and bladder pain. She has no fever or CVA tenderness. A clean-catch midstream urine sample shows gram-negative rods on Gram stain. A urine sample for culture and susceptibility (C&S) testing is ordered, and the results of a urinalysis are as follows:

Appearance, straw-colored (normal, straw)
Specific gravity, 1.015
pH, 8.0
Protein, glucose, ketones, bilirubin, and blood, all negative (normal, all negative)
WBC, 10 to 15 cells/LPF (normal, 0–2 cells/LPF)
Red blood cells (RBC), 0 to 1 cells/LPF (normal, 0–2 cells/LPF)
Bacteria, many (normal, 0 to rare)
Epithelial cells, 3 to 5 cells/LPF (normal, 0 to few cells/LPF)

Based on these findings, V.Q. is presumed to have a lower UTI. What should be the goals of therapy of V.Q.'s infection at this time? What factors should be considered before selecting an antibiotic for V.Q.?

The goals of therapy for treatment of acute cystitis are to effectively eradicate the infection and prevent associated complications, while minimizing adverse effects and costs associated with drug therapy. To accomplish these goals, selection of a specific antimicrobial agent should be made after considering several factors: (a) most likely pathogens, (b) resistance rates within the specific geographic area, (c) desired duration of therapy, (d) clinical efficacy and toxicity profiles of various agents, (e) cost and availability of specific agents, and (f) patient characteristics such as allergies, compliance history, and underlying comorbidities.[18] Because resistance rates among various pathogens vary considerably among geographic areas, clinicians must be familiar with resistance rates prevalent within the specific area within which they practice.[18,46,47]

Drug treatment of a lower UTI often is started before C&S results are known because the most probable infecting organisms and their susceptibility to antibiotics can be predicted reasonably well (Table 68-1). Approximately 75% to 95% of community-acquired infections are caused by Enterobacteriaceae (especially *E. coli*). Although these organisms may be sensitive to ampicillin, amoxicillin, and the sulfonamides (such as TMP-SMX), resistance to these agents is common.[46–50] Ampicillin resistance occurs in 25% to 70% of community-acquired isolates[46–50]; resistance nationwide is currently about 30% to 40%.[1,4,18,46–50] TMP-SMX has been a traditional agent of choice for many years; however, TMP-SMX resistance has significantly increased in recent years and may be as high as 20% to 40% among community-acquired *E. coli* isolates.[18,46–50] Although traditionally associated with hospital-acquired infections, resistance among *E. coli* and

TABLE 68-1
Overview of Treatment of Urinary Tract Infections

Organisms Commonly Found	Antibacterial of Choice
Uncomplicated UTI	
Escherichia coli	TMP-SMX[a]
Proteus mirabilis	TMP-SMX[a]
Klebsiella pneumoniae	TMP-SMX[a]
Enterococcus faecalis	Ampicillin, amoxicillin
Staphylococcus saprophyticus	First-generation cephalosporin or TMP-SMX
Complicated UTI[b,c]	
Escherichia coli	First-, second-, or third-generation cephalosporin; TMP-SMX[c]
Proteus mirabilis	First-, second-, or third-generation cephalosporin
Klebsiella pneumoniae	First-generation cephalosporin; fluoroquinolone
Enterococcus faecalis	Ampicillin or vancomycin ± aminoglycoside
Pseudomonas aeruginosa	Antipseudomonal penicillin ± aminoglycoside; ceftazidime; cefepime; fluoroquinolone; carbapenem
Enterobacter	Fluoroquinolone; TMP-SMX; carbapenem
Indole-positive *Proteus*	Third-generation cephalosporin; fluoroquinolone
Serratia	Third-generation cephalosporin; fluoroquinolone
Acinetobacter	Carbapenem; TMP-SMX
Staphylococcus aureus	Penicillinase-resistant penicillin; vancomycin

[a] Caution in communities with increased resistance (>10%–20%).
[b] Drug selection based on culture and susceptibility testing when possible.
[c] Oral therapy when appropriate.
Nitrofurantoin, fosfomycin, fluoroquinolone, or cephalosporins should be used in areas with increased TMP-SMX resistance.
TMP-SMX, trimethoprim-sulfamethoxazole; UTI, urinary tract infection.

Klebsiella caused by production of ESBL enzymes which confer resistance to penicillins and cephalosporins has also been steadily increasing among community-acquired pathogens.[51,52] Another relatively common organism is *S. saprophyticus.* Most strains are susceptible to sulfonamides, TMP-SMX, penicillins, and cephalosporins. Alternative medications and doses are shown in Table 68-2.

ROLE OF URINE CULTURES

CASE 68-1, QUESTION 2: Is it necessary to order a pretreatment urine C&S test for V.Q.?

Some investigators question the value of pretreatment urine cultures for acute uncomplicated UTI.[1,4] Women with lower UTI usually have pyuria on urinalysis and respond rapidly to appropriate antimicrobial treatment. Pyuria may be a better predictor of treatable infection than the colony count obtained on urine culture. Furthermore, the urine culture accounts for a large portion of the cost of treating a patient with a UTI.[53] Consequently, in patients such as V.Q. with uncomplicated, acute, lower UTI, it is more cost-effective to order a urinalysis and, if pyuria is present, to forego a urine culture. Instead, the patient should be empirically treated with a conventional 3-day to 7-day course of antibiotic therapy. If V.Q. remains symptomatic 48 hours later, a C&S test can then be ordered. Considerations are quite different in patients with complicated infections. In complicated UTI, predisposing factors which lead to infection and frequent history of previous antibiotic use make both causative pathogens and associated antibiotic susceptibilities much less predictable. Use of C&S testing is therefore more necessary and commonly recommended in order to choose appropriate antibiotics for treatment of complicated UTI.[1,2,4,18]

INITIAL ANTIBIOTIC SELECTION

CASE 68-1, QUESTION 3: What antibiotics may be appropriately selected for treatment of V.Q.'s infection?

Updated IDSA/ESMID guidelines for the treatment of acute uncomplicated cystitis and pyelonephritis were published in 2011, and should serve as the basis for selection of antibiotics in V.Q. (Table 68-3).[18] The recommended first-line agents for treatment of this patient's uncomplicated cystitis include TMP-SMX, nitrofurantoin, and fosfomycin trometamol; a fourth recommended antibiotic, pivmecillinam, is not commercially available in the United States.

TMP-SMX is effective for therapy of uncomplicated cystitis.[1,2,18,54,55] Gram-positive and gram-negative organisms, with the notable exceptions of *P. aeruginosa, Enterococcus,* and anaerobes, are generally susceptible to TMP-SMX.[18,56] Although TMP-SMX may appear active against enterococci in vitro, clinical efficacy against this pathogen is variable and does not always correlate well with in vitro susceptibilities. The efficacy of TMP-SMX largely depends on the sensitivity of the organism to the trimethoprim component. Individually, trimethoprim and sulfamethoxazole are bacteriostatic, but in combination they are bactericidal against most urinary pathogens.[56] Furthermore, this combination is almost uniformly successful in the treatment of uncomplicated UTI, even against organisms that originally were resistant to either agent alone. Although rates of trimethoprim resistance have increased over the past several years,[18,46–50,57] resistance rates remain relatively low in many geographic areas and trimethoprim alone would be effective in managing UTI in many patients.

The ratio of trimethoprim to sulfamethoxazole in the available tablet products is 1:5 (e.g., 80 mg trimethoprim and 400 mg sulfamethoxazole). This combination has been chosen to achieve peak serum concentrations of the two drugs that approximate a 1:20 ratio. This ratio is optimal for synergistic activity against most microorganisms, although the drugs remain synergistic and bactericidal in ratios ranging from 1:5 to 1:40 in vitro.[56,58] Urinary concentrations of trimethoprim and sulfamethoxazole far exceed the minimum inhibitory concentrations (MIC) for most susceptible urinary pathogens. Therefore, good in vitro activity, excellent clinical success which is similar to that of the fluoroquinolones and other alternative agents in susceptible strains, relatively low resistance rates among common pathogens in many geographic areas, and low cost make TMP-SMX a reasonable choice in V.Q.[18,54] The 2011 IDSA/ESMID guidelines recommend TMP-SMX as an appropriate initial agent of choice in the treatment of acute, uncomplicated lower UTI in geographic areas where the incidence of TMP-SMX resistance among *E. coli* is less than 20%.[18,54,59]

Nitrofurantoin is also recommended as an appropriate agent for empirical treatment of acute uncomplicated cystitis.[18] Nitrofurantoin is almost completely absorbed after oral administration, but barely reaches detectable levels in the plasma because it is eliminated rapidly (half-life, 20 minutes) into the urine and bile; the resulting high urine levels are 50 to 250 mg/L and are well in excess of the MIC for most common pathogens causing UTI.[60] The Kirby-Bauer disc sensitivity test measures the sensitivity of an organism to the expected serum levels of most antibiotics, whereas in the case of nitrofurantoin, the test measures sensitivity to urinary levels. Food substantially decreases the rate of absorption, but increases the total bioavailability of nitrofurantoin from both the macrocrystalline capsules and the microcrystalline tablets by about 40%. This effect lengthens the duration of therapeutic urine concentrations by about 2 hours.[60]

Nitrofurantoin has a spectrum of activity which includes *E. coli,* some strains of *Pseudomonas, S. saprophyticus,* streptococci, and enterococci; on the other hand, *Proteus, Enterobacter,* and *Klebsiella* are more likely to be resistant (susceptibility <60%).[18,49,61] Nitrofurantoin does not significantly alter the fecal or introital flora, and the development of resistance in previously sensitive strains does not often occur.[18,62,63] In contrast to ampicillin, TMP-SMX, and other drugs with relatively high resistance rates, nitrofurantoin has maintained excellent activity against most uropathogens; resistance rates among *E. coli* currently ranges from 90% to 99% in most geographic areas.[46–50,61,62] Finally, nitrofurantoin has been shown in comparative clinical studies to be as effective as TMP-SMX, fluoroquinolones, or fosfomycin in the treatment of acute uncomplicated cystitis.[18] Nitrofurantoin is thus recommended in the most recent clinical guidelines as an appropriate choice for treatment of uncomplicated UTI in patients such as V.Q. (Table 68-3).[18]

Most practitioners in the United States have little experience with fosfomycin trometamol, but the drug has, nevertheless, been used quite successfully in the treatment of UTI in many other parts of the world.[18,45] Fosfomycin is a phosphonic acid derivative which has been shown to irreversibly block bacterial cell wall synthesis through inhibition of early cytoplasmic stages of peptidoglycan synthesis.[45,64] It has bactericidal activity against a broad range of gram-negative and gram-positive organisms including *E. coli* and other Enterobacteriaceae, *Pseudomonas aeruginosa,* and *Enterococcus* as well as many multidrug-resistant pathogens such as methicillin-resistant *S. aureus,* vancomycin-resistant enterococci, and ESBL-producing gram-negative bacilli.[18,45] Fosfomycin is approximately 40% absorbed after oral administration as granules marketed in a sachet form, is rapidly and almost completely excreted unchanged in the urine,

TABLE 68-2
Commonly Used Oral Antimicrobial Agents for Acute Urinary Tract Infections[1,2,4,27,48,49,96]

Drug	Usual Dose: Adult	Usual Dose: Pediatric	Pregnancy[a]	Breast Milk[a]	Comments[b]
Amoxicillin	250 mg every 8 hours or 3 g single dose	20–40 mg/kg/d in three doses	Crosses placenta (cord) = 30% (maternal)[c]	Small amount present	High resistance rates, not for empiric use.
Amoxicillin + potassium clavulanate	500 + 125 mg every 12 hours	20 mg/kg/d (amoxicillin content) in three doses	Unknown	Unknown	
Ampicillin	250–500 mg every 6 hours	50–100 mg/kg/d in four doses	Crosses placenta	Variable amount (milk) = 1%–30% (serum)[c]	High resistance rates, not for empiric use. Should be taken on an empty stomach.
Cefadroxil	0.5–1 g every 12 hours	15–30 mg/kg/d in four doses	Crosses placenta	Enters breast milk (milk) = 20% (serum)[c]	Alternate choices for patients allergic to penicillins, although cross-hypersensitivity can occur. May be associated with high failure rates.
Cephalexin	250–500 mg every 6 hours	15–30 mg/kg/d in four doses	Crosses placenta		
Cephradine	250–500 mg every 6 hours	15–30 mg/kg/d in four doses	Crosses placenta (cord) = 10% (maternal)[c]		
Norfloxacin[d]	400 mg every 12 hours	Avoid	Arthropathy in immature animals	Unknown	Useful for pseudomonal infection. *Avoid antacids, divalent and trivalent cations, and sucralfate. May cause dizziness.*[e]
Ciprofloxacin[d]	250–500 mg every 12 hours	Avoid	Arthropathy in immature animals	Unknown	Alternate choices for patients allergic to β-lactams
Levofloxacin	250 mg every 24 hours	Avoid	Arthropathy in immature animals	(milk) = 100% (serum)[c]	
Nitrofurantoin	100 mg every 12 hours	5–7 mg/kg/d in two to four doses	Hemolytic anemia in newborn	Variable amounts; not detectable to 30%; may cause hemolysis in G6PD-deficient baby	Alternate choice. *To be taken with food or milk. May cause brown or rust-yellow discoloration of urine.*
Sulfisoxazole	0.5–1 g every 6 hours	50–100 mg/kg/d in four doses	Crosses placenta; hemolysis in newborn with G6PD deficiency; displacement of bilirubin may lead to hyperbilirubinemia and kernicterus; teratogenic in some animal studies	Enters breast milk; displacement of bilirubin may lead to neonatal jaundice; may cause hemolysis in G6PD-deficient baby	Alters bowel flora to favor resistant organisms. *To be taken on an empty stomach with a full glass of water. Photosensitivity may occur.*
Sulfamethoxazole (SMX)	1 g every 12 hours	60 mg/kg/d in two doses			
Trimethoprim (TMP)	100 mg every 12 hours		Crosses placenta (cord) = 60%; (maternal) folate antagonism; teratogenic in rats	(milk) >1 (serum)[c]	Alternate choice.
TMP-SMX	160 + 800 mg every 12 hours or 0.48 + 2.4 g single dose	10 mg/kg/d (TMP component in two doses)	Crosses placenta (cord) = 60%; (maternal) folate antagonism; teratogenic in rats	(milk) >1 (serum)[c]	*To be taken on an empty stomach with a full glass of water. Photosensitivity may occur.* Monitor HIV-infected patients closely for development of adverse hematologic reactions. First-line agent for prostatitis.
Fosfomycin	3 g single dose	No data	Crosses placenta	Unknown	Recommended option for uncomplicated cystitis.

[a] Also see Chapter 49, Obstetric Drug Therapy.
[b] Includes unique patient consultation information in italics.
[c] Denotes drug concentration.
[d] May increase theophylline concentrations when given concurrently. Carefully monitor theophylline serum concentrations during quinolone use.
[e] Same comments apply to all fluoroquinolones.
G6PD, glucose-6-phosphate dehydrogenase; HIV, human immunodeficiency virus; TMP-SMX, trimethoprim-sulfamethoxazole.

TABLE 68-3

Summary of Evidence-Based Recommendations for Treatment of Acute Uncomplicated Cystitis and Pyelonephritis[19]

Recommendations	Recommendation Grades[a]
Cystitis	
Preferred Agents	
Nitrofurantoin monohydrate/macrocrystals 100 mg PO twice daily × 5 days	A-1
TMP-SMX 160/800 mg (1 double-strength tablet) PO twice daily × 3 days	A-1
Trimethoprim 100 mg PO twice daily × 3 days is considered equivalent to TMP-SMX and is the preferred agent in some regions	A-3
Fosfomycin trometamol 3 g PO × one dose	A-1, but appears to have inferior microbiological efficacy compared with standard short-course therapies with agents such as trimethoprim or nitrofurantoin
Pivmecillinam 400 mg PO twice daily × 3–7 days (not commercially available in the United States)	A-1, but may have inferior efficacy compared with other available therapies
RESISTANCE CONSIDERATIONS	
A specific antibiotic is no longer recommended for empirical treatment when the prevalence of resistance is ≥20%	B-3 for TMP-SMX No recommendation for other agents
Alternative agents	
FLUOROQUINOLONES	
Fluoroquinolones (ofloxacin, ciprofloxacin, or levofloxacin) PO × 3 days are highly efficacious for acute cystitis	A-1
Fluoroquinolones should be reserved for other important clinical uses due to propensity for collateral damage	A-3
β-LACTAMS	
β-Lactams (including amoxicillin-clavulanate, cefdinir, cefaclor, and cefpodoxime-proxetil) PO × 3–7 days are appropriate when other recommended agents cannot be used	B-1
Other β-lactams such as cephalexin are less well studied but may also be appropriate in certain settings	B-3
β-Lactams generally have inferior efficacy and more adverse effects compared with other antimicrobials for UTI	B-1
Pyelonephritis	
All Patients	
Urine culture and susceptibility testing should be performed and initial empirical antibiotic therapy tailored appropriately based on results	A-3
Outpatient Treatment	
FLUOROQUINOLONES	
Ciprofloxacin 500 mg PO twice daily × 7 days, ± an initial IV dose of ciprofloxacin 400 mg, a long-acting parenteral cephalosporin (e.g., ceftriaxone 1 g) or a consolidated 24-hour dose of an aminoglycoside (e.g., gentamicin 5–7 mg/kg)	A-1
Ciprofloxacin 1,000 mg extended release tablet PO once daily × 7 days, or levofloxacin 750 mg PO once daily × 5 days	B-2
If the local prevalence of fluoroquinolone resistance among uropathogens is >10%, an initial one-time IV dose of a long-acting parenteral cephalosporin or a consolidated 24-hour dose of an aminoglycoside should be administered	B-3
Alternative agents	
TMP-SMX 160/800 mg (1 double-strength tablet) PO twice daily × 14 days	A-1
If TMP-SMX susceptibility is not known, an initial IV dose of a long-acting parenteral cephalosporin or a consolidated 24-hour dose of an aminoglycoside should be administered	B-2 for a cephalosporin B-3 for an aminoglycoside
Oral β-lactams × 10–14 days are less effective than other available agents	B-3
If an oral β-lactam is used, an initial IV dose of a long-acting parenteral cephalosporin or a consolidated 24-hour dose of an aminoglycoside should be administered	B-2 for a cephalosporin B-3 for an aminoglycoside
Hospitalized Patients	
One of the following antibiotic options may be used initially, based on local resistance data and tailored based on susceptibility results: IV fluoroquinolone; IV aminoglycoside ± IV ampicillin; extended-spectrum IV cephalosporin or extended-spectrum IV penicillin ± aminoglycoside; or IV carbapenem.	B-3

[a] Strength of recommendations: A, B, C = good, moderate, and poor evidence to support recommendation for or against use, respectively.
Quality of evidence: 1 = evidence from ≥1 properly randomized, controlled trial; 2 = evidence from ≥1 well-designed clinical trial without randomization, from cohort or case-control analytic studies, from multiple time series, or from dramatic results from uncontrolled experiments; 3 = evidence from opinions of respected authorities, based on clinical experience, descriptive studies, or reports of expert committees.
IV, intravenous; PO, orally; TMP-SMX, trimethoprim-sulfamethoxazole; UTI, urinary tract infection.

achieves mean urinary concentrations greater than 500 mg/L within 6 to 8 hours after administration, and maintains concentrations greater than 100 mg/L for a duration of more than 26 hours after a single oral dose.[45,64] Single 3-gram oral doses of fosfomycin are clinically as effective as trimethoprim and nitrofurantoin, although microbiological efficacy may be less.[18] Nevertheless, fosfomycin is currently recommended for treatment of acute uncomplicated cystitis in the 2011 IDSA/ESMID guidelines (Table 68-3).[18] It should be noted that although fosfomycin is commercially available in the United States, availability is currently somewhat limited.

Alternative agents for the treatment of UTI in V.Q. include the fluoroquinolones and various oral β-lactam antibiotics.[18] The fluoroquinolones remain highly effective in the treatment of UTI. However, increasing rates of resistance among common uropathogens and the potential for significant collateral affects on normal flora leading to complications such as *Clostridium difficile* infection have led to recent recommendations that the fluoroquinolones not be routinely used as preferred agents in the treatment of uncomplicated UTI such as that present in V.Q.[18] Further details regarding the use of fluoroquinolones for UTI are discussed in Case 68-2.

Amoxicillin-clavulanate and several oral cephalosporins have been studied for the treatment of uncomplicated UTI; these studies have shown the β-lactams to be generally comparable to TMP-SMX, but less clinically or microbiologically effective than the fluoroquinolones.[18,54] β-lactams require longer durations of treatment (see Case 68-1, Question 4), which makes them less attractive from the standpoint of ensuring patient adherence and may also predispose to higher rates of drug-related adverse effects.[18] Finally, these relatively broad-spectrum agents may be associated with more frequent emergence of bacterial resistance, including ESBL-producing gram-negative bacilli.[18,54] Thus, the β-lactam antibiotics (with the exception of pivmecillinam) are currently only recommended for empirical treatment of uncomplicated cystitis when none of the other agents previously discussed are appropriately used (Table 68-3).[18] Of note, ampicillin and amoxicillin are specifically discouraged for empirical treatment of UTI due to the high resistance rates previously noted.[18]

Based on the foregoing discussion, V.Q. could be appropriately treated with either TMP-SMX, nitrofurantoin, or fosfomycin (if available). She has no apparent patient characteristics that would favor the use of one agent over another. In this case, the most important factor to consider would be local antibiotic susceptibilities among community-acquired uropathogens, particularly *E. coli*. Local costs and availability of the different options would also be important to consider in V.Q.

Note that the current IDSA/ESMID guidelines do not apply to the empirical selection of antibiotics for complicated UTI. Complicated infections are often associated with more difficult pathogens (e.g., *P. aeruginosa*) and increased risk of antibiotic resistance; fluoroquinolones are therefore considered preferred agents for initial treatment of complicated UTI with subsequent antibiotic therapy guided by results of C&S testing.[1,2,4,22]

DURATION OF ANTIBIOTIC THERAPY

CASE 68-1, QUESTION 4: V.Q. is started on TMP-SMX for treatment of her infection. What would be the preferred duration of therapy of antibiotic therapy for V.Q.?

Outpatients with acute, uncomplicated UTI can be treated successfully with a traditional 7-day to 14-day course of oral medications, a shorter 3-day to 5-day course of therapy, or with single-dose therapy.[1,4,18,65] The duration of therapy for UTI has been extensively studied and progressively shortened. The traditional 7-day to 14-day course of antibiotic therapy now is considered excessive for most patients with uncomplicated infections and is seldom used.[1,2,4,18,54,65] A 3-day to 5-day antibiotic treatment regimen is just as effective as a 10-day regimen in achieving clinical cures and eradicating urinary tract organisms, although this is somewhat antibiotic-class–specific.[1,2,4,18,54,65] TMP-SMX is recommended as the preferred agent for 3-day treatment regimens; the fluoroquinolones may also be used in this shorter duration (Table 68-3).[18] A recent study has shown that a 5-day course of nitrofurantoin is as effective as a 3-day course of TMP-SMX for acute uncomplicated cystitis, and nitrofurantoin is thus currently recommended as a 5-day regimen.[18,66] β-Lactam antibiotics are more appropriately reserved for longer treatment courses of 3 to 7 days.[4,18,54] Longer treatment courses are also used in cases of treatment failure after regimens of shorter duration, as well as in the treatment of complicated UTI where longer courses of therapy (7 to 14 days) are associated with higher clinical success rates and improved outcomes.[1,2,22]

Even a single dose of an antibiotic may be effective. Bacteria disappear from the urine within hours after antibacterial therapy has been initiated.[54] This, coupled with the urinary bladder's ability to defend itself through micturition, acidification, and inherent antibacterial activity, gives theoretic support to the clinical evidence that a large single dose of an antibiotic can eradicate a UTI. Fosfomycin trometamol is a perfect example of this principle: Very high urinary concentrations (>100 mg/L) of this bactericidal agent are maintained for more than 24 hours after a single 3-gram oral dose and contribute to the favorable clinical efficacy observed in comparative trials.[18,45,64]

Although not recommended in the current guidelines, single doses of antibiotics other than fosfomycin are also occasionally used in treating acute, lower UTI in young women.[4,7,18,54] Commonly used regimens are TMP-SMX (two or three double-strength tablets), trimethoprim 400 mg, amoxicillin-clavulanate 500 mg, amoxicillin 3 g, ampicillin 3.5 g, nitrofurantoin 200 mg, ciprofloxacin 500 mg, and norfloxacin 400 mg.[1,54] Again, choice of a specific agent should be based on local susceptibility patterns, patient allergies, and relative drug costs. Female patients with history or clinical presentation suggestive of complicated infection (e.g., systemic manifestations of infection, renal disease, anatomic abnormalities of the urinary tract, diabetes mellitus, pregnancy), a history of antibiotic resistance, or a history of relapse after single-dose therapy should not receive single-dose regimens. Single-dose therapy is also not appropriate for male patients with UTI. Because V.Q. does not have any of these contraindications, she could theoretically receive single-dose therapy with an appropriate agent.

The advantages of single-dose treatment of UTI include improved compliance, reduced cost, proven efficacy in a defined population of patients (i.e., young women with acute, uncomplicated lower UTI), minimal side effects, and a potentially decreased incidence of bacterial resistance associated with antibiotic overuse. However, several concerns also exist regarding single-dose therapy.[4,7,54] First, sample sizes in most of the comparative studies to date have been relatively small. Consequently, it is difficult to determine whether differences in effectiveness or incidence of side effects between single-dose and multiple-dose therapy are clinically significant. Meta-analysis of studies comparing either single-dose or 3-day regimens with multiple-dose TMP-SMX therapy has demonstrated that single-dose therapy is significantly less effective in eradicating bacteriuria than regimens of either greater than or equal to 5 days (83% vs. 93%, respectively, $p < 0.001$) or greater than or equal to 7 days in duration (87% vs. 94%, respectively; $p = 0.014$).[54,55,65] As discussed in Case 68-1, Question 3, reduced microbiological efficacy was also observed with single-dose fosfomycin.[18] Although fewer studies have directly compared single-dose versus 3-day therapies, numerous studies have shown that 3-day courses are as effective as courses of longer duration.[54,65] A 3-day course of therapy is therefore currently recommended by the IDSA/ESMID for uncomplicated cystitis, with a large single dose of fosfomycin being the sole single-dose regimen endorsed by the guidelines.[18]

A second area of concern relates to recurrences in patients treated with single-dose therapy. Recurrent infections may represent either a relapse caused by incomplete eradication of more deep-seated kidney infection or a true reinfection in a high-risk patient. If it is assumed that patients who receive single-dose therapy are selected properly, then reinfection is a more likely explanation. It has also has been suggested, however, that relapse after single-dose therapy actually suggests subclinical upper urinary tract infection.[4] In either case, single-dose therapies have been associated with higher rates of recurrence compared with therapies of longer duration, and these regimens are not currently recommended.[18]

Based on the preceding information, and according to current guidelines, a 3-day course of TMP-SMX, a 5-day course of nitrofurantoin, or a single dose of fosfomycin would be most appropriate for treatment of V.Q.'s infection (Table 68-3).[18]

When using short-course regimens, it is important to counsel the patient that the clinical signs and symptoms of infection may often not be completely resolved for 2 to 3 days after initiation of therapy. Therefore, symptoms that persist for a short while after beginning therapy (or actually completing therapy, in the case of single-dose regimens) are not necessarily indicative of treatment failure.

PHENAZOPYRIDINE

CASE 68-1, QUESTION 5: Along with TMP-SMX, phenazopyridine is also prescribed because of V.Q.'s complaints of significant dysuria. Is phenazopyridine appropriate for this patient?

Phenazopyridine, a urinary tract analgesic, occasionally is prescribed alone or along with an antibacterial agent for the symptomatic relief of dysuria. Although phenazopyridine at a dose of 200 mg orally three times a day may relieve dysuria, it is ineffective in the actual eradication of true UTI. Phenazopyridine plus an antibiotic is not any better than an antibiotic alone; therefore, the drug is not likely to be of significant value in V.Q. and should not be routinely recommended. However, although most patients have resolution of symptoms within 24 to 48 hours after beginning therapy, certain patients with severe dysuria or delayed response to antibiotic therapy may benefit symptomatically from a short trial (1–2 days) of phenazopyridine.[4] The need for, and duration of, analgesic therapy must be individualized.

Phenazopyridine is an azo dye and may discolor the urine to an orange-red, orange-brown, or red color that can stain clothes. Other adverse effects of phenazopyridine occur after acute overdose, or as a result of accumulation in older patients or in patients with decreased renal function who take the drug chronically. In vivo, about 50% of phenazopyridine is metabolized to aniline, which can cause methemoglobinemia and hemolytic anemia. Hemolytic anemia associated with phenazopyridine occurs primarily in patients with glucose-6-phosphate dehydrogenase (G6PD) deficiency.[67] Cases of reversible acute renal failure and allergic hepatitis have also been rarely reported after brief exposure to phenazopyridine.[67]

INTERPRETATION OF URINE CULTURE AND SUSCEPTIBILITY TEST RESULTS

CASE 68-1, QUESTION 6: Two days after V.Q. begins treatment for her infection with TMP-SMX, results of the C&S studies become available and reveal greater than 10^5 bacteria per milliliter of *P. mirabilis*, which is susceptible to ampicillin, amoxicillin-clavulanate, cephalosporins, and gentamicin. The *Proteus* is intermediately sensitive to nitrofurantoin, and is resistant to TMP-SMX and ciprofloxacin. V.Q. reports that she is symptomatically better since starting antibiotic therapy and that her dysuria and bladder pain are now almost completely resolved. How should these test results be interpreted? Is a change in V.Q.'s antibiotic therapy necessary?

Most women with either lower or upper UTI have greater than 100,000 bacterial colonies/mL of urine. As previously mentioned, a major revision in the diagnostic criteria for symptomatic UTI has been the abandonment of the absolute requirement for growth of at least 10^5 bacterial colonies/mL of urine. The criterion of greater than or equal to 100 bacteria/mL results in excellent sensitivity and specificity in correctly diagnosing and treating women with symptomatic infection.[8] This same criterion should also be applied to lower UTI when *S. saprophyticus* is isolated, because UTI caused by this pathogen often are associated with low urine bacterial colony counts, suboptimal growth on commonly used media, and negative findings on nitrite screening.

Mixed flora (more than two organisms) is unusual except in severely debilitated persons and other complicated infections. Thus, mixed flora in the setting of uncomplicated infection frequently suggests contamination, and a repeat specimen should be obtained.

Bacterial susceptibility to different antimicrobial drugs is usually determined by referencing interpretive criteria which correlate with achievable serum concentrations of those drugs. However, drugs useful in the treatment of UTI are excreted primarily by the kidney, and urine concentrations of these drugs may be 20 to 100 times greater than serum concentrations. Therefore, infections caused by organisms that are only intermediately susceptible, or even "resistant" to the tested concentration of antibacterial drug, might still be effectively treated with the high concentration of drug achieved in the urine.

Although in vitro susceptibility testing is not always predictive of patient response to therapy of UTI, studies clearly show that patients infected with a resistant pathogen are at increased risk of treatment failure.[52,59,68,69] Clinical response to infection occurred in only 24% to 61% of patients with organisms resistant to TMP-SMX compared with 83% to 92% of patients infected with susceptible organisms[52,59,68]; furthermore, patients infected with TMP-SMX-resistant pathogens were 17 times more likely to fail therapy compared with patients with susceptible strains.[70] Patients treated with TMP-SMX who were infected with drug-resistant organisms were also found to have longer median times to symptom resolution (14 vs. 7 days, $p = 0.0002$), more frequent return clinic visits within 1 week (36% vs. 6%, $p < 0.0001$), more frequent need for subsequent antibiotic therapy (36% vs. 4%, $p < 0.0001$), and higher rates of significant bacteriuria after 1 month (42% vs. 20%, $p = 0.04$).[68]

Although 50% to 60% of patients with resistant organisms may experience failure of TMP-SMX therapy, antimicrobial therapy is usually chosen empirically without the benefit of C&S testing results. Appropriateness of antibiotic therapy is thus usually judged according to subsequent clinical response. If the infecting organism is susceptible, the urine will usually be sterile in 24 to 48 hours. If a urine specimen collected 48 hours after initiation of therapy is not sterile and the patient has been taking the medication properly, the antibiotic may be inappropriate or the focus of infection may be deeper (e.g., pyelonephritis, abscess, obstruction). If the urine specimen is sterile and the patient is symptomatically improved, the appropriate antimicrobial is being used (regardless of susceptibility studies) and the full course of therapy should be completed. Because V.Q. reports significant improvement in her subjective symptoms, her 3-day course of TMP-SMX should be completed as originally ordered and V.Q. should be closely monitored for any evidence of relapse. A repeat C&S test should be performed in the event that V.Q. reports any new signs or symptoms which are consistent with antibiotic failure and relapse of her infection, and a different antibiotic should be selected for treatment at that time.

FLUOROQUINOLONE THERAPY

CASE 68-2

QUESTION 1: I.B., a 48-year-old woman, presents with a community-acquired UTI. She has a past medical history significant only for several previous episodes of UTI. A urinalysis is ordered with the following results:

Appearance, straw-colored and turbid (normal, straw-colored and clear)
Specific gravity, 1.028
pH, 6.3
Glucose, ketones, and bilirubin, all negative (normal, all negative)
Blood and protein, both trace positive by dipstick (normal, both negative)
WBC, 10 to 15 cells/LPF (normal, 0–2 cells/LPF)
RBC, 5 to 10 cells/LPF (normal, 0–2 cells/ LPF)
Bacteria, many (normal, 0 to rare)
Epithelial cells, 3 to 5 cells/LPF (normal, 0 to few cells/LPF)
Leukocyte esterase and nitrite tests by dipstick, both positive (normal, both negative)

Of note, I.B. has experienced a rash with TMP-SMX and has a type I hypersensitivity reaction to penicillins in the past. What is the role of fluoroquinolones in the treatment of I.B.'s community-acquired UTI?

Several fluoroquinolones are indicated for the treatment of uncomplicated or complicated UTI; these include norfloxacin, ciprofloxacin, and levofloxacin. The fluoroquinolones are usually administered orally in the treatment of UTI and have excellent in vitro activity against most gram-negative organisms, including *P. aeruginosa*.[71] They are also active in vitro against many gram-positive organisms including *S. saprophyticus*.[71] The activity of many fluoroquinolones in vitro is antagonized by urine (acidic pH, divalent cations); however, this is unlikely to be clinically significant because urine concentrations are several hundred-fold greater than serum levels.[71] A large number of clinical trials have demonstrated the fluoroquinolones to be very effective in the treatment of acute uncomplicated UTI with efficacy rates typically greater than 90%.[18,55]

Although the fluoroquinolones are as effective as TMP-SMX, nitrofurantoin, or β-lactams in treatment of uncomplicated UTI, they are no longer recommended as first-line empirical therapy because they are more expensive and provide no additional treatment benefits.[4,7,54,55,71] Concerns also exist regarding the overuse of fluoroquinolones and the promotion of drug resistance among community-acquired uropathogens. Resistance to fluoroquinolones among organisms causing acute uncomplicated UTI is usually less than 1% to 2%.[19] Fluoroquinolone resistance may, however, be more frequent in some geographic areas and in complicated infections[46–50,57]; recent studies have documented resistance to ciprofloxacin in 2% to 10% of acute uncomplicated infections, but from 8% to 60% in complicated UTI.[18,47–50,72] Furthermore, these quinolone-resistant strains often are resistant to multiple other antimicrobials.[47–50,72] Concerns also exist regarding the potential for fluoroquinolones to produce collateral effects on normal flora, these alterations leading to increased risk of infection due to methicillin-resistant *S. aureus* and hypervirulent *C. difficile*.[18]

Fluoroquinolones are recommended as appropriate alternatives for patients with allergies or other contraindications to the use of other first-line agents, or for patients infected with organisms resistant to multiple antibiotics, such as *P. aeruginosa*. Fluoroquinolones are appropriate initial therapy in geographic areas with greater than 20% resistance of *E. coli* to TMP-SMX[54]; however, many patients in such areas may still often be appropriately treated with nitrofurantoin or some other option (Table 68-3).[18] Finally, the fluoroquinolones are effective in treating patients with structural or functional abnormalities of the urinary tract and other complicated infections.[18,71]

A fluoroquinolone may be considered for I.B. because she has experienced previous adverse reactions to penicillins and sulfonamides. However, nitrofurantoin or fosfomycin should be preferentially considered for I.B. based on current IDSA/ESMID recommendations.[18] If a fluoroquinolone was deemed appropriate for I.B. based on other unspecified factors such as availability, cost, or tolerability issues with other treatment options, the fluoroquinolones are similar in efficacy and the choice would be based on comparative costs and compliance considerations.[18] The duration of fluoroquinolone therapy in I.B. would be 3 days.[18]

DRUG INTERACTIONS

CASE 68-2, QUESTION 2: I.B. also is taking Maalox for a duodenal ulcer. What is the likelihood that this antacid will reduce the efficacy of the fluoroquinolones?

It is imperative that clinicians question patients such as I.B. regarding concomitant medications (both prescription and nonprescription). Products containing multivalent cations (Mg^{2+}, Ca^{2+}, Zn^{2+}, Al^{2+}, Fe^{2+}) significantly decreased fluoroquinolone absorption (20%–70% decrease in the area under the concentration curve [AUC]), and this may result in therapeutic failures. Although this interaction can be avoided by taking the antacids or other products at least 2 hours before or 4 to 6 hours after the fluoroquinolone dose, this practice is complicated and inconvenient for the patient.[73] Patients simply should avoid these products while taking fluoroquinolones. Interactions of the fluoroquinolones with H_2-receptor antagonists and proton pump inhibitors are not clinically significant, and these agents can be used for patients such as I.B. with symptoms of reflux disease or gastrointestinal ulcers.[73] Alternatively, I.B. should be treated with a different antibiotic for her UTI.

Some older fluoroquinolones also interfere with theophylline metabolism, especially ciprofloxacin (20%–90% increase in AUC). Norfloxacin increases the theophylline AUC by approximately 15%.[73] Therefore, theophylline levels should be monitored closely in patients receiving these quinolones and theophylline together. Levofloxacin does not significantly alter methylxanthine metabolism.[73] Whereas ciprofloxacin interferes with the metabolism of caffeine, levofloxacin does not.[73] Although the clinical significance of the interaction between caffeine and most fluoroquinolones is minimal, patients should be monitored carefully for signs and symptoms of caffeine toxicity. This is especially important for patients ingesting large quantities of caffeine and in older patients.

There have been isolated reports of a clinical interaction between certain quinolones (e.g., ciprofloxacin) and warfarin. Although there seems to be no truly relevant pharmacokinetic or pharmacodynamic interactions, patients receiving both warfarin and quinolone therapy should nevertheless be carefully monitored for changes in their anticoagulation.[73] Isolated cases have also been reported of increased toxicity with coadministration of quinolones and nonsteroidal anti-inflammatory drugs, phenytoin, and cyclosporine; whether these interactions truly exist is unknown.[73]

As previously discussed, I.B. should preferentially be treated with a different antibiotic option such as nitrofurantoin or fosfomycin. Use of one of these agents would potentially be more appropriate according to current guidelines and would also avoid the potential drug–drug interaction.[18] If a fluoroquinolone is prescribed for I.B., she should either take the antacid at least 2 hours before or 4 to 6 hours after the fluoroquinolone dose or temporarily switch the antacid to an H_2-receptor antagonist or proton pump inhibitor.[73]

NITROFURANTOIN-INDUCED ADVERSE EFFECTS

CASE 68-2, QUESTION 3: The decision is made to begin I.B. on nitrofurantoin rather than a fluoroquinolone. After beginning nitrofurantoin monohydrate 100 mg twice daily, she complains of nausea and gastrointestinal (GI) upset after the ingestion of each dose. I.B. had her nitrofurantoin prescription filled with nitrofurantoin monohydrate because it was the less expensive product at her local pharmacy. How can these GI effects be minimized in I.B.? What other important adverse effects are associated with nitrofurantoin?

Nausea is a common complication of nitrofurantoin therapy, and the patient's compliance with the prescribed regimen may be affected by this side effect. It is not known whether the mechanism by which nitrofurantoin produces nausea is central or local. Taking nitrofurantoin with food may reduce nausea either through serving as a buffer, or slowing the rate of absorption and reducing peak concentrations of the drug. Food, however, may also increase the bioavailability of nitrofurantoin. Slowing of absorption is particularly beneficial in decreasing the incidence of nausea and vomiting associated with the microcrystalline product.[61] Use of the macrocrystalline preparation may also reduce adverse effects through slowing rates of dissolution and absorption, and producing lower serum levels. A disadvantage of the macrocrystalline form is the cost, which may be 2 to 10 times that of the microcrystalline form, depending on the product source. Finally, because nausea and vomiting appear to be dose related and occur more frequently in small persons, reducing the daily dose of nitrofurantoin may also improve tolerability.[60,61] However, the best-studied dose of nitrofurantoin which has been shown to be clinically effective is 100 mg twice daily,[18] which I.B. is currently receiving. I.B. should remain on her current dose; taking the drug with food and/or switching to a macrocrystalline product should allow her to successfully finish her course of nitrofurantoin at the recommended dose.

Several hundred cases of nitrofurantoin-induced acute, subacute, or chronic pulmonary reactions have been reported.[74] Acute toxicity often manifests within several days of initiating the drug with a sudden flulike syndrome consisting of fever, dyspnea, and cough; eosinophilia may also be present. The subacute form tends to occur after at least a month of exposure; symptoms include fever and dyspnea. The chronic form tends to be more insidious with milder dyspnea and low-grade fever. In all forms, rales are common and pulmonary infiltrates may be present on chest radiograph.[74] Discontinuation of nitrofurantoin results in complete symptomatic recovery after several weeks; however, permanent fibrotic changes may persist with chronic pulmonary reactions. Rechallenge with oral nitrofurantoin results in rapid reappearance of pulmonary symptoms in those who have had an acute reaction; the drug must therefore be avoided in patients with history of nitrofurantoin-induced pulmonary toxicity.[74]

Peripheral neuropathy may also occur during nitrofurantoin therapy and is characterized by symmetric dysesthesia and paresthesia in the distal extremities, which progresses in a central and ascending fashion.[60,75] Neuropathy usually occurs within the first 60 days of chronic nitrofurantoin treatment and is rarely seen during shorter courses of therapy.[60,75] Symptom severity is not dose related and is generally reversible, although more severe cases may require up to several months to resolve completely. Renal failure is a risk factor for both neurotoxicity and pulmonary toxicity, but neuropathy has also been reported in patients with normal renal function.[60,75]

FLUOROQUINOLONE USE IN PEDIATRIC INFECTIONS

CASE 68-3

QUESTION 1: C.S. is a 2-year-old girl with a history of multiple recurrent UTIs caused by congenital urinary tract abnormalities that have not been corrected. She has had at least nine UTIs since birth and has received multiple courses of antibiotics, including ampicillin, amoxicillin, amoxicillin-clavulanate, and TMP-SMX. She has also been on chronic low-dose antibiotic prophylaxis with TMP-SMX. C.S. was brought to her pediatrician 48 hours ago with signs and symptoms consistent with a new UTI. Suprapubital aspiration was performed and urine samples sent for C&S testing at that time, and C.S. was empirically begun on amoxicillin-clavulanate pending laboratory test results. C&S results, however, are now available and show greater than 10^5 colonies/mL of *P. mirabilis*. The organism is susceptible to ciprofloxacin, gentamicin, and ertapenem; and resistant to ampicillin, trimethoprim, TMP-SMX, cephalexin, cefaclor, cefpodoxime, tetracycline, nitrofurantoin, and erythromycin. C.S. has not clinically improved while receiving empiric amoxicillin-clavulanate. What antibiotic therapy would be most appropriate for continued management of this acute infection in C.S.?

This case illustrates the serious dilemmas caused by antibiotic resistance among uropathogens. The pathogen isolated from C.S. is resistant to all commonly used, orally administered antibiotics that have been proved effective in the treatment of UTI in pediatric patients. Although penicillins, cephalosporins, nitrofurantoin, and sulfonamides are frequently recommended for treatment of pediatric UTI, multiple past treatment regimens and chronic antibiotic prophylaxis have led to these agents being unsuitable for treatment of this new infection. Although in vitro susceptibility testing does not accurately predict clinical response to therapy in all cases, the risk of treatment failure and poor patient outcome is significantly increased when agents to which isolates are resistant are administered.[59,68] Alternative treatment is required; however, few desirable options exist for C.S.

The recommended duration of antibiotic therapy in C.S. would be at least 2 weeks for the treatment of this complicated and recurrent infection (refer to subsequent sections of this chapter). Although the organism isolated from C.S. is susceptible to gentamicin and this drug would be effective, parenteral (intramuscular or intravenous) administration would be required and the lengthy required treatment duration makes this far from ideal. Use of aminoglycosides would also be less desirable because of toxicity concerns. Although ertapenem would also likely be effective, there is relatively little clinical experience with this agent in the pediatric population and ertapenem would also require parenteral administration for the duration of the treatment regimen.

Fluoroquinolones are contraindicated in children and adolescents younger than 18 years of age because of concerns regarding potential musculoskeletal toxicities in juvenile populations. Although not approved for pediatric use, fluoroquinolones have been formally studied for febrile neutropenia, infectious gastroenteritis, otitis media, bacterial meningitis, and other uses.[76–78] The use of fluoroquinolones has dramatically increased in children and adolescents, most likely owing to resistance to other antimicrobials; approximately 520,000 prescriptions were written for patients younger than 18 years of age during 2002, of which nearly 3,000 prescriptions were for children younger than 2 years.[76] Several recent reviews have summarized data related to the safety of fluoroquinolones in children. Although tendinopathy or other musculoskeletal toxicities have been recorded, these toxicities have been usually mild in severity, reversible, and occurring at rates comparable to that seen in adults.[76–78] Based on currently available information and in consideration of problems related to antimicrobial resistance, the American Academy of Pediatrics has published recommendations regarding the use of fluoroquinolones in children and adolescents.[76] According to these recommendations, fluoroquinolones may be considered in special circumstances including (a) infections caused by multidrug-resistant pathogens for which there are no other safe and effective alternatives; and (b) times when parenteral therapy is not feasible and no other effective oral agent is available. Treatment of UTI caused by multidrug-resistant, gram-negative pathogens are specifically mentioned as a potentially appropriate use for fluoroquinolones in pediatric patients.[76]

Selection of a specific agent for the treatment of UTI in C.S. should be based on careful consideration of potential risks and benefits of available antibiotic options. The feasibility, risks, expenses, and inconvenience associated with prolonged (≥2 weeks) parenteral administration of an aminoglycoside or carbapenem are problematic; however, the ease of oral fluoroquinolone administration must be carefully balanced against the possible risks of using these agents in this population. Clearly, no antibiotic of choice exists for treatment of C.S. and both the providers and the child's parents must be involved in development of an acceptable and well-informed treatment plan.

TREATMENT OF LOWER-TRACT INFECTION IN RENAL FAILURE

CASE 68-4

QUESTION 1: K.M., a 55-year-old man with a history of hypertension and chronic renal failure, experiences a UTI. His creatinine clearance (CrCl), determined from a recent 24-hour urine collection, is 20 mL/minute. What antimicrobial agent should be prescribed?

The major problem in treating UTI in patients with renal failure is how to achieve adequate urine concentrations of the drug without causing systemic toxicity. The ideal drug would be (a) inherently nontoxic, even at high serum concentrations, making dosage adjustments unnecessary; (b) excreted unchanged in the urine (i.e., not metabolized); and (c) eliminated by renal tubular secretion rather than glomerular filtration. Because renal tubular secretion remains active in all but the most severe cases of renal failure, antibiotics eliminated by this mechanism would reach adequate urinary levels; however, no such ideal drug exists.

Nitrofurantoin, doxycycline, and many sulfonamides are substantially metabolized by the liver and generally produce low urine levels in uremic patients. The aminoglycosides are eliminated almost exclusively by the kidneys, but uremic patients are at high risk of drug-induced toxicities and alternative agents are usually recommended. Penicillins, cephalosporins, and trimethoprim are partially metabolized by the liver but are also eliminated by the kidney to a significant extent. These agents are suitable for use in renal failure according to the criteria described above. Certain fluoroquinolones, specifically ciprofloxacin and levofloxacin, are highly excreted in the urine through a combination of filtration and tubular secretion and reach extremely high urinary concentrations. These agents are also considered safe and effective in the treatment of UTI in patients with renal failure.

Acute Pyelonephritis

SIGNS AND SYMPTOMS

CASE 68-5

QUESTION 1: L.B., a 45-year-old woman with type 1 diabetes mellitus, comes to the emergency department complaining of severe nausea, frequent vomiting, frequent urination, fever, shaking chills, and flank pain. Positive physical findings include a temperature of 103°F, a pulse of 110 beats/minute, blood pressure of 90/60 mm Hg, and CVA tenderness. A Gram stain of L.B.'s urine reveals gram-negative rods, and a urinalysis demonstrates glucosuria, macroscopic hematuria, 20 to 25 WBC/LPF, numerous bacteria, and WBC casts. She also has a blood sugar level of 400 mg/dL. L.B. is admitted to the hospital with a diagnosis of acute bacterial pyelonephritis, and routine laboratory tests including a blood chemistry profile and complete blood count with differential, and specimens of urine and blood for C&S are ordered. L.B. is started on intravenous (IV) normal saline, ampicillin 1 g IV every 6 hours, and a sliding-scale schedule of regular insulin based on every 6-hour blood sugars. Which signs and symptoms in L.B. are consistent with pyelonephritis?

It is not always possible to differentiate clinically between upper and lower urinary tract infections. Symptoms common in lower UTI often are the only positive findings in upper UTI (i.e., subclinical pyelonephritis).[1–4,79] L.B., however, does manifest signs and symptoms of systemic infection consistent with acute bacterial pyelonephritis, including tachycardia, hypotension, fever, nausea and vomiting, shaking chills, flank pain, CVA tenderness, hematuria, and WBC casts. In addition, her diabetes may predispose her to various renal infections, including pyelonephritis, possibly because diabetic patients have altered antibacterial defense mechanisms.[2–4,79]

Treatment

TRIAGE FOR HOSPITALIZATION

CASE 68-5, QUESTION 2: Why was L.B. hospitalized?

Most patients with clinical pyelonephritis have relatively mild infection and usually can be treated as outpatients. The need for hospitalization often is determined by the patient's social situation and ability to maintain an adequate fluid intake and tolerate oral medications.[2–4,7,54] Patients who experience significant nausea and/or vomiting may not be able to maintain adequate hydration and thus may be at higher risk for cardiovascular complications of infection. Such patients may also require parenteral therapy initially in order to guarantee adequate initial antibiotic therapy. Finally, patients such as L.B. with diabetes should be hospitalized because acute pyelonephritis may predispose her to diabetic ketoacidosis.

Although blood cultures are usually obtained in patients with moderate-to-severe pyelonephritis, one study found that blood cultures were of low yield in the setting of acute uncomplicated pyelonephritis; they rarely provided any additional information not already obtained from the urine culture and were not helpful in the clinical management of such cases.[80] Blood cultures may be positive in up to 25% of patients with severe or complicated pyelonephritis, however, and they are still recommended for patients such as L.B.[2–4,79,80]

ANTIMICROBIAL CHOICE FOR PYELONEPHRITIS

CASE 68-5, QUESTION 3: Was ampicillin appropriate treatment for L.B.?

Ampicillin is not an appropriate choice for L.B. because diabetic patients (and patients treated with corticosteroids) are susceptible to colonization with unusual or more resistant organisms. As with lower tract UTI, pyelonephritis is often classified as uncomplicated or complicated. L.B.'s infection would be classified as a complicated infection because of her underlying diabetes.[2–4,7,79]

E. coli remains the predominant pathogen in complicated pyelonephritis, but other gram-negative organisms (e.g., *Klebsiella, Proteus, Pseudomonas*) are found relatively more frequently.[2–4,7] Because L.B. is acutely ill and has gram-negative organisms in her urine, she should be treated with an antibiotic that has a better spectrum of activity against gram-negative organisms. Because of high rates of ampicillin resistance among common uropathogens, ampicillin and amoxicillin are inappropriate for the empirical therapy of UTI, including pyelonephritis.[18] Current IDSA/ESMID recommendations for the initial management of acute pyelonephritis are shown in Table 68-3. Because L.B. is to be hospitalized, broad-spectrum antibiotics appropriate for initial therapy would include parenteral third-generation cephalosporins (e.g., ceftriaxone), IV fluoroquinolones (e.g., ciprofloxacin, levofloxacin), extended-spectrum penicillins such as piperacillin-tazobactam, or carbapenems.[2–4,7,18] Aminoglycosides may initially be used empirically as either monotherapy or in combination with various β-lactams: in combination with ampicillin to provide better activity against enterococci, or together with cephalosporins or piperacillin-tazobactam to provide enhanced gram-negative activity to the β-lactam regimen.[18] The choice of a specific regimen is based on local susceptibility patterns and should be tailored as needed on the basis of C&S test results.[18] It is not always necessary to initially treat patients with antipseudomonal therapy; thus, agents such as ceftriaxone with relatively less activity against *Pseudomonas* are often appropriate as initial therapy in patients such as L.B.[3,7,18] Because most hospital laboratories can report C&S results within 48 hours, these antibiotics can be replaced with more specific ones if appropriate.

SERUM VERSUS URINE CONCENTRATIONS

CASE 68-5, QUESTION 4: Is it necessary to achieve bactericidal concentrations of antimicrobials in the serum, or are high urinary concentrations adequate for L.B.? How long should she be treated? How should therapeutic success be determined?

In patients with pyelonephritis and infection of the renal parenchyma, adequate tissue concentrations of antimicrobial agents are needed. Therefore, antibiotics that achieve bactericidal concentrations in serum and kidney tissues as well as in the urine should be selected.[18,81] Patients requiring hospitalization should be treated with parenteral antibiotics until fluids can be taken orally and the patient is symptomatically improved and afebrile for 24 to 48 hours.[2–4] This should be followed with a course of oral antibiotics for a total duration of antimicrobial therapy of approximately 14 days; less severe infections not requiring hospitalization are usually treated with 7-day to 14-day courses, depending on the specific agent chosen.[18] Although it is customary to observe the patient in the hospital for 24 hours after switching from parenteral to oral antibiotics before discharge, this is probably of limited benefit.[2–4,7] Specimens for C&S testing should be obtained on the second day of therapy (to rule out treatment failure), 2 to 3 weeks after the completion of therapy, and again at 3 months.[1,3]

For patients who have relapsed after 14 days, retreatment for 6 weeks usually is curative. There have been reports of successful therapy with 5 days of treatment[80]; however, longer courses are recommended.[3,7,80]

ORAL THERAPY FOR PYELONEPHRITIS

CASE 68-5, QUESTION 5: Would oral therapy have been appropriate for the initial treatment of acute pyelonephritis in L.B.?

Patients with mild, acute pyelonephritis (no nausea, vomiting, or signs of sepsis) can be treated with oral antibiotics such as fluoroquinolones for 5 to 7 days, or with TMP-SMX for 14 days.[2–4,18] Oral fluoroquinolones are preferred agents for initial empirical therapy of acute pyelonephritis in patients not requiring hospitalization because of lower rates of resistance among common uropathogens compared to TMP-SMX, and higher rates of clinical and microbiological efficacy compared to β-lactams.[18] Fluoroquinolones may be particularly useful for patients potentially infected with resistant organisms because of their excellent in vitro activity against gram-negative organisms and high kidney tissue concentrations (2-fold to 10-fold greater than serum).[71] However, fluoroquinolone resistance and risk of inappropriate initial therapy may be more common in certain geographic areas. If fluoroquinolone resistance among *E. coli* exceeds 10%, treatment for acute pyelonephritis should be initiated with an intravenous dose of extended-spectrum cephalosporin or an aminoglycoside until C&S test results are known (Table 68-3).[18] Oral agents such as amoxicillin-clavulanate, cefixime, or cefuroxime also can be used in this setting, but the most recent guidelines suggest that oral β-lactams are less effective than other available options and their use is somewhat discouraged as first-line treatment options.[18]

Patients such as L.B. with evidence of bacteremia (e.g., fever, shaking chills) or sepsis (e.g., hypotension) should be hospitalized and treated with parenteral antibiotics.[3,7,18] L.B.'s frequent vomiting and potential inability to be successfully treated with oral antibiotics would also make initial therapy with parenteral antibiotics more favorable. Although L.B. will be initially treated with parenteral antibiotics, early switch to oral therapy after as few as 1 to 4 days of treatment is recommended; clinical outcomes with oral are similar to those achieved with continued parenteral therapy (i.e., 5 days or longer).[82]

RECURRENT URINARY TRACT INFECTIONS

Relapse versus Reinfection

CASE 68-6

QUESTION 1: T.W. is a 28-year-old woman with a history of recurrent infections who now exhibits a new *E. coli* UTI. Her last episode occurred 5 months previously. Her current infection is treated with TMP-SMX for 10 days. A repeat UA was scheduled for the completion of antibiotic therapy, but she canceled her appointment because she "felt fine." Twelve weeks later, she returns to the clinic with signs and symptoms of another UTI. The only other medication she has taken is an oral contraceptive. Why would C&S testing of a urine sample be especially useful at this time?

Recurrent infections develop in approximately 20% to 30% of women with acute cystitis.[2,4,33,83,84] Repeat C&S data should help determine whether this infection represents a relapse or a reinfection. Relapse refers to a recurrence of bacteriuria caused by the same microorganism that was present before initial therapy. Most relapses occur within 1 to 2 weeks after the completion of therapy and are caused by persistence of the organism in the urinary tract. Relapses often are associated with an inadequately treated upper UTI, structural abnormalities of the urinary tract, or chronic bacterial prostatitis.[1,33,83,84]

Reinfection implies recurrence of bacteriuria with a different organism than was present before therapy. Reinfections can occur at any time during or after the completion of treatment, but most appear several weeks to several months later. Approximately 80% of recurrences are caused by reinfection.[1,33] Reinfection is generally caused by introital colonization with Enterobacteriaceae from the lower intestinal tract[1]; of these, *E. coli* is the most common. Certain *E. coli* strains have been shown to adhere to vaginal epithelial cells and, in women with recurrent UTI, adherence of these organisms to epithelial cells is increased.[24] Considering T.W. was symptomfree for 8 weeks suggests that this is a reinfection, rather than a relapse.

Oral Contraceptives as a Risk Factor

CASE 68-6, QUESTION 2: Is there an association between T.W.'s use of oral contraceptives and her risk of contracting a UTI?

Information regarding the association between oral contraceptive use and UTI is controversial. As evidence, the two most well-designed studies evaluating this association disagree in their conclusions. A well-designed, prospective study examined 796 women and found the incidence of UTI to be exactly the same between oral contraceptive users and nonusers.[32] A subsequent case-control study in 229 women with recurrent UTI and 253 control subjects, however, found that oral contraceptive users were at significantly higher risk for recurrent infection.[25] The association between oral contraceptive use and risk of UTI remains unclear.

The association between diaphragm use and UTI is much stronger. Diaphragm users are approximately three times more likely to experience a UTI than women using other contraceptive methods, especially when the diaphragm is used in conjunction with spermicidal jelly.[25,32] Possible explanations include urethral obstruction by the diaphragm together with increased vaginal colonization by coliform organisms caused by the spermicide. Use of a spermicide-coated condom also has been shown to increase the risk of UTI.[25,85]

Treatment for Reinfection

CASE 68-6, QUESTION 3: Pending the C&S test results, what therapy should be instituted in T.W.?

T.W. has a history of recurrent infections and now probably has a reinfection. Because reinfection is not caused by failure of previous therapy, TMP-SMX may be a reasonable choice once again. The probability that a resistant organism will be responsible for the infection increases when the interval between infectious episodes is short. If several months elapse between each episode of antimicrobial therapy, normal fecal bacterial flora become re-established and the risk of infection with resistant pathogens is reduced.

The alteration of fecal flora caused by the sulfonamides makes these drugs poor choices for repeated use in cases of frequent reinfection, especially when C&S results are unknown. The development of bacterial resistance also may limit the usefulness of these agents for chronic antimicrobial therapy.[18,33,83,84] However, because her most recent infection was 12 weeks ago and the UTI previous to that was 5 months earlier, TMP-SMX would again be a reasonable choice at this time.

CASE 68-6, QUESTION 4: If T.W. exhibited an adverse reaction to TMP-SMX, what are some other therapeutic alternatives?

Nitrofurantoin is highly effective against *E. coli* with relatively low rates of resistance (<10%) in most geographic areas. It does not significantly alter the fecal or introital flora, and the development of resistance in previously sensitive strains does not often occur.[18,62,63,86] Therefore, it generally is a useful agent for the treatment of recurrent *E. coli*, *S. saprophyticus*, and *Enterococcus* infections.[18]

The fluoroquinolones also are useful in this setting, especially in geographic areas with high rates of TMP-SMX resistance.[33,82] Their widespread use should not be encouraged for reinfections as in T.W. in light of their high cost and concern regarding selection of resistant organisms.[18,33,84] Cephalosporins and trimethoprim also have been recommended as alternative agents in this setting.[2,83,84]

Evaluation Procedures (Localization)

CASE 68-6, QUESTION 5: Greater than 10^5 bacteria per milliliter of *P. mirabilis*, sensitive to ampicillin and TMP-SMX, are cultured from T.W.'s urine. One week after completing her second course of TMP-SMX therapy, signs and symptoms of a UTI again appear. How should T.W. be assessed at this time?

First, an attempt should be made to rule out common causes for relapse in T.W. Inadequate therapy resulting from patient noncompliance with the prescribed treatment, inappropriate antibiotic selection, or bacterial resistance to the prescribed agent should be considered if significant bacteriuria persists despite treatment. Other renal infections (e.g., subclinical pyelonephritis) may predispose to relapse and must be ruled out.[1,2,33,83,84] Finally, if these common causes are not present, radiologic tests (e.g., IV pyelogram) should be performed to rule out surgically correctable structural abnormalities of the urinary tract. Infected kidney stones and unilateral atrophic kidneys are common but correctable abnormalities in females.[1,2,33,83,84]

Radiologic tests are indicated when infections recur in children, in men younger than 50 years of age, and in patients with UTI associated with bacteremia, ureteral colic, or passage of stones. These populations are most likely to have surgically correctable lesions.[1,2,33,83,84] In contrast, these procedures rarely are necessary in adult women and elderly men until the more likely causes of relapse have been eliminated.[4,22,33,84] Chronic bacterial prostatitis should be considered as a frequent cause of recurrent infections in male patients.

Antibiotic Selection for Treatment of Relapse

CASE 68-6, QUESTION 6: Pending C&S results, TMP-SMX is again prescribed. Is this still a reasonable medication for T.W. at this time?

Because the *P. mirabilis* cultured during the last recurrence was still susceptible to TMP-SMX, this agent would again be a reasonable choice until C&S test results are obtained. Alternatively, use of a different agent (e.g., nitrofurantoin, fluoroquinolone) could be considered because the relapse occurred within 1 week of completing the previous treatment and resistance may have developed.[4,33,84]

CASE 68-6, QUESTION 7: How long should antibiotic therapy be continued in T.W. for her relapsed infection?

The duration of therapy for relapsing infections usually is 14 days. In patients who relapse after a second 2-week course of therapy, treatment for 6 weeks should be instituted.[1,2,33] If relapse occurs after a 6-week course, some experts recommend longer courses of 6 months to 1 year.[1,2] These prolonged courses should be reserved for children, adults who have continuous symptoms, or adults who are at high risk for experiencing progressive renal damage. Asymptomatic adults without evidence of obstruction should not receive these longer courses. T.W. should be treated for at least 2 weeks and perhaps as long as 6 weeks.[33,84]

CASE 68-6, QUESTION 8: Although T.W. tolerated TMP-SMX well during her previous treatment, on this occasion she experiences significant nausea and vomiting after taking the medication. Would trimethoprim alone be an appropriate substitute for TMP-SMX in the treatment of T.W.'s infection?

Trimethoprim alone and in combination with sulfamethoxazole is active in vitro against many of the Enterobacteriaceae associated with UTI and is an effective alternative to TMP-SMX in the management of both acute and chronic UTI.[1,2,4] It would be especially appropriate for T.W. because GI intolerance to TMP-SMX is most commonly attributed to the sulfamethoxazole component, and trimethoprim is associated with a lower incidence of side effects. Some concern exists for the potential development of resistant organisms, but studies using trimethoprim alone have failed to demonstrate a significant increase in bacterial resistance.[83,84] Trimethoprim is used for the treatment of acute, uncomplicated UTI in a dosage of 200 mg/day.

Chronic Prophylaxis

CASE 68-6, QUESTION 9: T.W. was treated successfully with trimethoprim for 6 weeks. Is prophylactic antimicrobial therapy indicated? If so, how long should it be continued?

Cases of chronic UTI in adult patients may be managed by treating each recurrent infection with an appropriate antibacterial. Chronic UTI may also be managed by administering chronic, low-dose prophylactic therapy. The frequency of urinary infections probably is the main determinant of whether chronic suppressive therapy should be used, because repeated treatment of recurrent infections eventually will result in a decreased incidence of subsequent infections.[1,33,84,87] Long-term prophylactic therapy clearly reduces the frequency of symptomatic infections in nearly all patients.[13,33,84,87]

From a cost-effectiveness standpoint, women having more than one episode of cystitis per year may benefit from antimicrobial prophylaxis.[83] For women with three or more episodes of cystitis per year, prophylaxis clearly is more cost-effective than treating individual infections. Therefore, chronic antimicrobial prophylaxis should be considered in any adult patient with two or more episodes of UTI per year.[33,84]

The duration of prophylactic therapy is also determined by the frequency of infection. Women with three or more UTIs in the 12 months before a 6-month course of antimicrobial prophylaxis have a significantly higher recurrence rate (75%) in the 6 months after prophylaxis than women who have had only two infections in the 12 months before prophylaxis (26% recurrence rate).[87] Therefore, prophylaxis should be continued for 6 months in patients with fewer than three UTIs per year and for at least 12 months in adult patients with three or more UTIs per year.

Before chronic antimicrobial suppressive therapy is initiated, active infections must be completely eradicated with a full course of appropriate antibiotic therapy. The low doses of antimicrobials used for chronic prophylaxis suppress bacterial growth but do not eliminate active infection. Furthermore, surgically correctable anatomic abnormalities that predispose the patient to recurrent infections (e.g., obstruction, stones) should be ruled out. Patients with urologic abnormalities respond poorly to prophylactic therapy.[33,83,84] Age also should be considered when contemplating chronic antimicrobial therapy. An asymptomatic, elderly patient taking many other medications is usually not an ideal candidate for chronic prophylactic treatment because of problems of noncompliance, cost, and potential drug interactions or toxicities.[83,84] Younger patients, however, are good candidates for long-term suppressive therapy.[84]

Because T.W., a 28-year-old woman, has had at least three UTIs in the past few months, has undergone extensive evaluation, and has just been successfully treated with a standard course of trimethoprim, a 12-month course of antimicrobial prophylaxis would seem reasonable. She also should be evaluated at regular intervals for recurrent UTI and for the development of resistant organisms.

Although the foregoing discussion applies to antimicrobial prophylaxis in adults, the use of long-term prophylaxis of recurrent UTI in children remains controversial. One study examined risk factors for recurrent UTI and associations with antimicrobial prophylaxis in a prospective cohort study involving nearly 75,000 children 6 years of age or younger.[88] Among the children in this study, antimicrobial prophylaxis was not associated with decreased risk of recurrent UTI; however, prophylaxis was associated with a 7.5 times increased risk of infection

TABLE 68-4
Antimicrobial Agents Commonly Used for Chronic Prophylaxis Against Recurrent UTIs[1,2,4,81–83,87]

Agent	Adult Dose	Comments[a]
Nitrofurantoin	50–100 mg nightly	Contraindicated in infant <1 month of age. *To be taken with food or milk. May cause brown or rust-yellow discoloration of urine.*
Trimethoprim	100 mg nightly	Not recommended in children <12 years of age.
Trimethoprim 80 mg + Sulfamethoxazole 400 mg	0.5–1 tablet nightly Or 3/wk	Not recommended for use in infants <2 months. *To be taken on an empty stomach with a full glass of water. Photosensitivity may occur.*
Norfloxacin	200 mg/d	*Avoid antacids;* monitor theophylline levels.
Cephalexin	125–250 mg/d	
Cefaclor	250 mg/d	
Cephradine	250 mg/d	
Sulfamethoxazole	500 mg/d	

[a] Includes unique patient consultation information in italics.

caused by resistant bacteria. A more recent study examined 576 children younger than 18 years of age with a history of one or more microbiologically proven UTIs randomly assigned to receive either placebo or prophylaxis with TMP-SMX for 12 months.[89] Children randomly assigned to receive TMP-SMX experienced a 40% reduction in UTI during the study period; this benefit was independent of underlying risk factors such as history of vesicoureteral reflux. However, other outcomes such as hospitalization, secondary infections, or evidence of parenchymal disease on renal scans were not significantly different between groups; the one exception was that children receiving antibiotics were significantly more likely to experience UTI caused by an organism resistant to TMP-SMX.[89] Finally, a meta-analysis of 11 studies evaluating long-term antibiotic prophylaxis in children found no significant benefits of antibiotic administration overall.[90] Based on the conflicting data in the literature, current recommendations are that long-term antimicrobial prophylaxis should not be routinely recommended for prevention of recurrent UTI in children.[1,2,83,84,90–92]

CASE 68-6, QUESTION 10: What drugs could be appropriately used for long-term suppressive therapy in T.W?

Although numerous drugs are used for prophylaxis, TMP-SMX may be the drug of choice for chronic antimicrobial therapy owing to extensive experience, proven efficacy, infrequent toxicities, and low cost.[33,84] TMP-SMX also has the effect of decreasing vaginal colonization with uropathogens.[33,84] TMP-SMX one-half tablet daily is commonly prescribed for chronic UTI prophylaxis and is an effective, well-tolerated and convenient prophylactic regimen.[33,84]

Successful prophylaxis, however, is significantly decreased in patients with urologic abnormalities or renal dysfunction. Also, infections that are not eradicated by a short-term therapeutic trial of TMP-SMX are not likely to respond to a long-term regimen.[83] Finally, enterococci may colonize introitally in patients taking chronic TMP-SMX.[87]

Fluoroquinolones are effective for chronic suppressive therapy but should be used only when antimicrobial resistance or intolerance to other recommended drugs is present. Cephalosporins also have been recommended, but are best reserved for patients intolerant to or failing prophylaxis with other agents.[83,84]

When selecting a drug for chronic antimicrobial therapy, it is important to consider efficacy, the likelihood that resistant organisms will develop, long-term toxicity, convenience, and cost to the patient. The most commonly used agents are listed in Table 68-4.

Based on the available information, T.W. could be switched to TMP-SMX. Although she has a history of GI distress because of this drug, this may not be a problem with the lower doses used for prophylaxis. If she is intolerant, trimethoprim alone, nitrofurantoin, or a fluoroquinolone also should be effective.

Cranberries and probiotics have long been of interest for their potentially beneficial effects in preventing UTI. Cranberries contain known compounds (i.e., flavonols, anthocyanidins, proanthocyanidin-tannins) that prevent *E. coli* from adhering to uroepithelial cells in the urinary tract.[93] Cranberries have been evaluated in the prophylaxis of UTI, but the results are inconclusive.[93–95] A wide variety of cranberry products (e.g., juice concentrate, juice cocktail, cranberry extracts in capsules and tablets) as well as different dosing regimens have been used.[93,94] Two trials found that cranberry juice may decrease the number of symptomatic UTI during a 12-month period in younger women, whereas another study found cranberry extract to be less effective than daily trimethoprim in preventing recurrent UTI in women older than 45 years of age.[95] Whether cranberry is effective for other groups such as children and elderly men has not been evaluated.[93–95] Probiotics (particularly *Lactobacillus* strains) may prevent colonization with pathogens associated with UTI.[96] Studies of probiotics for prophylaxis, however, are inconclusive at this time. Further research is required to clarify unanswered questions regarding the role of cranberries or probiotics in the prevention of UTI.[93,96]

Rash and Drug Fever

CASE 68-6, QUESTION 11: T.W. is switched to TMP-SMX for chronic suppressive therapy of her UTI. Ten days later she presents to the emergency department with a pruritic maculopapular rash and fever. Are the rash and fever in T.W. typical of that caused by the sulfonamides?

Rash is one of the more common side effects associated with sulfonamide use and occurs in approximately 1% to 2% of patients treated with TMP-SMX. Various hypersensitivity skin and mucous membrane reactions have been reported, including morbilliform, scarlatinal, urticarial, erysipeloid, pemphigoid, purpuric, and petechial rashes. Erythema nodosum, exfoliative dermatitis, photosensitivity reactions, and the Stevens-Johnson syndrome also are associated with sulfonamides. Skin eruptions usually appear after 1 week of treatment, although more rapid onset may occur in a sensitized person.[56] The hypersensitivity reaction that occurred in T.W. signify that an alternate drug should be used for chronic suppressive therapy. The TMP-SMX should be immediately discontinued and a different drug such as nitrofurantoin should be started for continued suppressive therapy.

Urinary Tract Infection and Sexual Intercourse

CASE 68-7

QUESTION 1: On routine screening, asymptomatic bacteriuria is noted in W.W., a 30-year-old pregnant woman in her first trimester. Five years ago, during her first pregnancy, she experienced acute bacterial pyelonephritis, which required hospitalization and treatment with parenteral antibiotics. Since that time, she has had recurrent UTI, apparently related to sexual intercourse. These subsided when she began taking a single dose of nitrofurantoin after coitus, but she discontinued the practice before this pregnancy because she was afraid of the potential effects of this drug on the fetus. What is the association between sexual intercourse and the occurrence of UTI?

Studies strongly support an association between sexual intercourse and UTI.[1,2,25,32] A direct relationship seems to exist between the number of days with intercourse within the previous week and the risk of developing a UTI.[32] One study found the relative risk of infection in women with 1, 4, and 7 days of intercourse within the previous week to be 1.4, 3.5, and 9.0, respectively, compared with women who were sexually inactive within the previous week. Another study found that the risk of UTI was doubled in women having intercourse more than four times per month compared with those women who did not.[25] Studies also indicate that introital colonization by fecal bacteria has a definite role in recurrent infections related to intercourse. The migration of these colonizing bacteria into the bladder appears to be facilitated during intercourse, but the exact mechanism remains unclear.[1,2,32] Because UTI are uncommon in men, transmission of an infection from the man is unlikely. Occasionally, bacteria harbored under the foreskin of an uncircumcised man may be transmitted to his partner through intercourse.[23]

CASE 68-7, QUESTION 2: Was it rational to treat W.W.'s repeated infections with a single dose of an antibiotic after intercourse?

Postcoital antibiotic prophylaxis is useful when recurrent UTI results from sexual intercourse. Theoretically, a single dose of an antimicrobial agent produces bactericidal activity in the urine before bacteria have a chance to multiply, and the infection is averted. Patients should be instructed to empty their bladder just after intercourse and before taking the medication to minimize the number of bacteria present in the bladder and to reduce dilution of the drug in the urine. Because most drugs effective for UTI are rapidly excreted by the kidney and quickly reach high urinary concentrations, this regimen is reasonable and decreases the incidence of postcoital infections.[85,97] However, this practice is not recommended in patients with structural abnormalities of the urinary tract or decreased renal function. Symptomatic infection must be completed before beginning prophylaxis.

Depending on the frequency of intercourse, postcoital prophylaxis may result in less antibiotic use compared with continuous prophylaxis. TMP-SMX or nitrofurantoin is the most commonly recommended agent; however, other agents such as fluoroquinolones and cephalexin may be used.[81,97]

Urinary Tract Infection and Pregnancy

CASE 68-7, QUESTION 3: Because W.W.'s UTI is asymptomatic at this time, should treatment be withheld because of her pregnancy?

W.W. should be treated because acute symptomatic pyelonephritis may develop in pregnant women with untreated bacteriuria. In addition, a UTI during pregnancy has been suggested to be associated with increased rates of preterm labor, premature delivery, and lower birth-weight infants.[25] A cause-and-effect relationship between UTI and maternal or infant risk has not been definitely established; in fact, a recent retrospective cohort study in nearly 86,000 mothers with or without UTI during pregnancy found no adverse pregnancy outcomes.[98] Nevertheless, treatment with an appropriate antimicrobial agent is currently recommended for all pregnant patients with significant bacteriuria.[8,26,27]

Nitrofurantoin is often recommended during pregnancy because teratogenic effects have not been observed clinically.[99,100] In vitro and retrospective investigations, however, suggest a slight mutagenic potential.[101,102] Nitrofurantoin also could cause hemolytic anemia in a G6PD-deficient nursing infant; however, only small amounts have been detected in breast milk.[102] The fluoroquinolones are contraindicated in pregnancy because of the arthropathy observed in immature animals.[71]

The penicillins, cephalosporins, and aminoglycosides are safe for use during pregnancy, although caution with the aminoglycosides is warranted because of possible eighth nerve toxicity in the fetus. These drugs, along with the others listed in Tables 68-3 and 68-4, cross the placental barrier; thus, the risk of toxicity or teratogenicity to the fetus always must be considered before deciding to treat a pregnant patient with a UTI.[102]

In this case, a cephalosporin or sulfisoxazole could be safely prescribed for treatment of W.W.'s UTI. W.W. was correct in discontinuing her nitrofurantoin before pregnancy because of the risk to the fetus, although small, tends to offset the advantage of antimicrobial prophylaxis. W.W. must receive proper follow-up care.

CASE 68-7, QUESTION 4: For how long should W.W. be treated?

Few studies have compared single-dose and 3-day therapy with conventional 7-day therapy in pregnant patients. Available trials suggest, however, that cure rates of single-dose therapy were lower than 7-day to 10-day therapy.[25,99] Although more recent trials have shown that single-dose therapy effectively eradicates bacteriuria in pregnancy, these studies were conducted in a small number of patients. Therefore, similar to other populations, it is recommended that pregnant patients receive either a 3-day regimen or a 7-day to 10-day regimen rather than single-dose therapy.[8,25,99]

Irrespective of the duration of therapy, appropriate follow-up of patients is crucial. Clinicians must document elimination of pathogens 1 to 2 weeks after therapy and follow the patient monthly for the remainder of gestation. If bacteriuria recurs, therapy should be given for relapse or reinfection and the patient evaluated radiologically for structural abnormalities.[1,25]

SYMPTOMATIC ABACTERIURIA

Clinical Presentation

CASE 68-8

QUESTION 1: R.D., a 22-year-old woman, complains of urinary frequency and painful urination, which have developed during the past 4 to 5 days. UA reveals 10 to 15 WBC/LPF, but no bacteria are seen on a Gram stain of the urine. What is a reasonable assessment of R.D.'s clinical presentation?

Acute urethral syndrome is defined as symptoms consistent with lower UTI but with no organisms evident on Gram stain or culture. The lack of detectable pathogens may mean that the urine specimen is sterile or that the concentration of the organism in the urine sample is small. Patients with these findings still may have a UTI even though the voided urine is sterile or contains less than 10^5 microorganisms/mL.[103] The causative organisms and the pathogenesis of infection in these cases are the same as for lower UTI. Other organisms that can cause urethritis in this setting are *Chlamydia trachomatis, N. gonorrhoeae,* and *Trichomonas vaginalis.*[103]

Most cases of UTI with low bacterial counts are associated with bacteriuria or *C. trachomatis* and also demonstrate pyuria (>8 WBC/LPF).[103] Conversely, pathogens are seldom present in patients with the acute urethral syndrome when pyuria is absent. Because R.D. is symptomatic, has 10 to 15 WBC/LPF in her urine, and no bacteria on Gram stain, infection with *C. trachomatis* or some other more atypical pathogen is likely.

Interstitial cystitis is a chronic clinical syndrome characterized by bladder or pelvic pain and urinary frequency or urgency.[104] Although the exact cause of interstitial cystitis is not known, it is apparently not an infection-related disorder and does not respond to antibiotic therapy. The clinical presentation of interstitial cystitis is very similar to that of symptomatic abacteriuria, but absence of pyuria is a key difference. Interstitial cystitis should be suspected in patients with clinical findings suggestive of lower UTI but who do not manifest pyuria and who have not responded to previous empiric antibiotic therapy; no antibiotics should be administered without further diagnostic evaluation.[104]

Antibiotic Treatment

CASE 68-8, QUESTION 2: Should R.D. be treated with antibiotics?

A double-blind, placebo-controlled study evaluated the use of doxycycline 100 mg twice a day (BID) in patients with UTI and low bacterial counts. Clinical cure of bacteriuria and pyuria was significantly greater in the doxycycline-treated group, but doxycycline did not reduce symptoms in patients without pyuria.[103] Because *E. coli,* other gram-negative bacteria, and *C. trachomatis* are the usual causes of acute urethral syndrome, an antibiotic such as doxycycline with activity against *Chlamydia* is reasonable initial treatment for patients such as R.D. presenting with urinary tract symptoms (without bacteriuria) if pyuria also is present. All tetracyclines and sulfonamides, with or without trimethoprim, also are likely to be effective in such patients, but doxycycline has been best studied to date. Of the fluoroquinolones, newer agents, such as levofloxacin, offer promise as alternatives to doxycycline but have not been well studied in this setting.[103] Azithromycin as a single dose also has a major role in treating chlamydial infections (see Chapter 69, Sexually Transmitted Diseases).

Prolonged therapy of 2 to 4 weeks in duration and treatment of sexual partners may be required to prevent reinfection through intercourse. Prolonged therapy is appropriate if the patient has a history consistent with *Chlamydia* urethritis; a sexual partner with recent urethritis; a recent new sexual partner; a gradual, rather than abrupt, onset of symptoms that has occurred during a period of days (as in R.D.); and no hematuria. Patients without such a history can be treated with a short course of antibiotics as any other patient with a lower UTI.

HOSPITAL-ACQUIRED ACUTE URINARY TRACT INFECTION

CASE 68-9

QUESTION 1: P.M., an alert, 70-year-old woman with chest pain, was hospitalized to rule out acute myocardial infarction. This is her third hospitalization for chest pain in the past 6 months. A urinary catheter was temporarily placed as part of her routine medical care. Two days after admission, she complained of burning on urination and bladder pain. TMP-SMX double-strength, one tablet BID was ordered after microscopic examination of the urine indicated a UTI. Why was this empiric therapy appropriate?

Hospital-acquired (or nosocomial) UTI occur in about one-half million patients per year and most are associated with the use of indwelling bladder catheters. Approximately 10% to 30% of catheterized patients exhibit infection.[21] Complications of catheter-associated UTI are significant. Nosocomial UTI are the source of up to 15% of all nosocomial bloodstream infections, occurring in about 4% of all catheterized patients[21]; the associated mortality rate is approximately 15%.[21] Nosocomial UTI also prolongs hospitalization by an average of 2.5 days and cost an additional $600 to $700.[21] Prevention is the best way to manage nosocomial UTI, but antibiotic treatment is usually initiated in hospitalized patients who exhibit UTI symptoms.

The susceptibility of hospital-acquired pathogens to antimicrobial agents differs from community-acquired bacteria, and these susceptibilities frequently vary from one hospital to another. Therefore, the microbiology department of a particular hospital should be consulted to determine current trends in the antibiotic susceptibility of bacteria acquired in that setting. In general, *E. coli* is still the predominant urinary tract pathogen. An increased proportion of infections is caused, however, by other gram-negative bacteria such as *Proteus* and *Pseudomonas,* gram-positive pathogens such as *Staphylococcus* and *Enterococcus,* and yeast (e.g., *Candida*).[19,21]

Repeated courses of antibiotic therapy, anatomic defects of the urinary tract, old age, increased hospital length of stay, and repeated hospital admissions are associated with a higher incidence of infection with antibiotic-resistant organisms.[19,21,105] *Pseudomonas, Proteus, Providencia, Morganella, Klebsiella, Enterobacter, Citrobacter,* and *Serratia* are particularly difficult to eradicate because they usually are less susceptible to commonly used antimicrobial agents.

P.M. is elderly, hospitalized, and has been repeatedly exposed to potentially resistant organisms during her previous hospitalizations. Oral fluoroquinolones are most commonly used as empiric therapy in this setting because of their greater activity against potentially resistant pathogens compared to TMP-SMX.[19,21,106] Cultures of P.M.'s urine should be performed and, once C&S test results are known, therapy promptly changed according to susceptibility reports. To achieve the most cost-effective

TABLE 68-5

Parenteral Antimicrobial Agents Commonly Used in the Treatment of Urinary Tract Infections

Class	Drug	Average Adult Daily Dose: UTI	Average Adult Daily Dose: Sepsis	Usual Dosage Interval[a]	Comments
Penicillins	Ampicillin	2–4 g	8 g	Every 4–6 hours	Use should be based on local susceptibility patterns.
	Ampicillin-sulbactam	6 g	12 g	Every 6 hours	
Extended-spectrum penicillin	Ticarcillin-clavulanate	9–12 g	18 g	Every 4–6 hours	
	Piperacillin-tazobactam	9 g	18 g	Every 4–6 hours	
First-generation cephalosporins	Cefazolin	1.5–3 g	6 g	Every 8–12 hours	More effective than second- or third-generation cephalosporins against gram-positive organisms.
Second-generation cephalosporins	Cefoxitin	3–4 g	8 g	Every 4–8 hours	Intermediate between first- and third-generation cephalosporins against gram-negative organisms.
	Cefuroxime	2.25 g	4.5 g	Every 8 hours	
	Cefotetan	1–4 g	6 g	Every 12 hours	
Third-generation cephalosporins	Cefotaxime	3–4 g	8 g	Every 6–8 hours	Better coverage than first- and second-generation cephalosporins against gram-negative organisms.
	Ceftizoxime	2–3 g	8 g	Every 8–12 hours	
	Ceftriaxone	1 g	2 g	Every 12–24 hours	
	Ceftazidime	1.5–3 g	6 g	Every 8–12 hours	Ceftazidime and cefepime are most effective against *Pseudomonas*. All generations of cephalosporins are ineffective against *Enterococcus faecalis* and methicillin-resistant staphylococci.
Fourth-generation cephalosporins	Cefepime	1–2 g	4 g	Every 12 hours	Has activity against methicillin-resistant staphylococci.
	Ceftaroline	0.6	0.6 g	Every 12 hours	
Carbapenems	Imipenem-cilastatin	1 g	2 g	Every 6 hours	The most broad-spectrum coverage of any antibiotics listed. Ertapenem not active against *Pseudomonas*. Resistance may develop especially with *Pseudomonas*. Toxic in some pregnant animals.
	Meropenem	1.5–3 g	3 g	Every 8 hours	
	Doripenem	0.5 g	0.5g	Every 8 hours	
	Ertapenem	0.5–1 g	1 g	Every 24 hours	
Monobactam	Aztreonam	1–2 g	6–8 g	Every 8–12 hours	Active against gram-negative aerobic pathogens, including *Pseudomonas* sp.
Aminoglycosides	Gentamicin	3 mg/kg	5 mg/kg	Every 8 hours	Potent against gram-negative bacteria including *Pseudomonas*. Associated with possible eighth nerve toxicity in the fetus. Amikacin should be reserved for multiresistant bacteria.
	Tobramycin	3 mg/kg	5 mg/kg	Every 8 hours	
	Amikacin	7.5 mg/kg	15 mg/kg	Every 12 hours	
Quinolones	Ciprofloxacin	400–800 mg	800 mg	Every 12 hours	Use for resistant organisms. Change to oral therapy when indicated.
	Levofloxacin	250–500 mg	500–750 mg	Every 24 hours	

[a] Assuming normal renal function.
UTI, urinary tract infection.

therapy, oral agents should be administered to all patients capable of taking medications by mouth unless the isolated pathogens are resistant to oral medications or underlying GI dysfunction makes adequate absorption of oral antibiotics questionable.[21,79,106] The recommended duration of antibiotic therapy for patients such as P.M. who present with mild to moderate symptoms is 5 to 7 days; patients who do not respond promptly to treatment may be treated for a total of 10 to 14 days.[21]

CASE 68-9, QUESTION 2: If P.M. had additional symptoms of fever, chills, flank pain, and vomiting, how would her treatment differ?

In seriously ill patients with possible sepsis, broad-spectrum parenteral antibiotics with activity against *P. aeruginosa* are usually preferred as initial therapy (Table 68-5). Suitable antibiotic choices include antipseudomonal cephalosporins (e.g., ceftazidime, cefepime), extended-spectrum penicillins (e.g., piperacillin-tazobactam, ticarcillin-clavulanate), carbapenems (imipenem-cilastatin, meropenem, doripenem), IV fluoroquinolones (e.g., ciprofloxacin, levofloxacin), and aztreonam. These antibiotics are at least as effective as the aminoglycosides and lack the ototoxic and nephrotoxic potential. However, these fluoroquinolone and β-lactam agents are more costly and associated with the emergence of resistant organisms and superinfection.

In general, antipseudomonal β-lactam antibiotics remain the drugs of choice for nosocomial urologic sepsis.[106] Although combination therapy may be useful initially in neutropenic patients with urologic sepsis, it should be narrowed to single-agent therapy once culture results are available.[106] The recommended duration of antibiotic therapy in patients with seriously ill patients is 10 to 14 days.[21]

Urinary Catheters

CASE 68-10

QUESTION 1: J.W., an 18-year-old woman, was hospitalized after a diving accident that resulted in a spinal cord injury with paralysis. Included among several initial interventions was insertion of an indwelling catheter with a closed drainage system because of bladder incontinence. Two weeks after admission to the hospital, J.W. has exhibited asymptomatic bacteriuria. Should this be treated?

A systemic antibiotic selected specifically for the infecting organism will temporarily result in sterile urine. Reinfection, often by a resistant organism, occurs in 30% to 50% of these cases if closed drainage catheterization is continued during therapy.[1,21] For this reason, it generally is recommended that systemic antimicrobial therapy be initiated after or just before catheter removal.[1,21] Because long-term catheterization is necessary in many patients and because bacteriuria is an inevitable consequence, it is often recommended that asymptomatic patients (such as J.W.) be left untreated to avoid the complications of recolonization and potential infection with resistant organisms.[1,8,21] Therapy must be started, however, if fever, flank pain, or other symptoms indicative of UTI develop.[1,21]

CASE 68-10, QUESTION 2: Is systemic antimicrobial prophylaxis useful for J.W.?

The benefits of systemic antibiotics in preventing catheter-induced UTI are not clear. Studies using closed drainage systems with diligent catheter care indicate that systemic antibiotics decrease the daily and overall incidence of infection in patients with sterile urines before catheterization.[36,37] The preventive effect of antimicrobials is greatest for short-term catheterizations or during the first 4 to 7 days of long-term catheterization.[36,37] Thereafter, the rate of infection increases. Although the overall infection rate remains lower than in untreated patients, the emergence of resistant organisms is significant. Therefore, in deciding to use systemic antimicrobials, it is important to consider the patient's underlying diseases, risk factors, probable duration of catheterization, and potential complications of drug toxicity or resistant organisms that can result from the chronic use of antimicrobials. Because long-term catheterization is anticipated for J.W., antimicrobial prophylaxis for J.W. is not recommended.[21]

CASE 68-10, QUESTION 3: J.W. eventually recovers urinary continence and the catheter is able to be removed. However, two days after removal of the catheter, she still has asymptomatic bacteriuria. How should she be treated?

Because asymptomatic bacteriuria in patients with urinary catheters is very common (~25% with short-term catheterization and virtually 100% long-term) but is associated with few complications, antibiotic therapy for asymptomatic bacteriuria is not recommended as long as the catheter remains in place.[21] However, antibiotic treatment may be considered in asymptomatic women with catheter-acquired bacteriuria that persists 48 hours after catheter removal.[8,21] Such patients may be treated with either a single large dose or a 3-day regimen of TMP-SMX, even if the patient is asymptomatic.[8,21,107] Older women (>65 years) probably should be treated with a 10-day course; however, the optimal duration in this age group is unknown. Whether these treatment regimens can be used in male patients requires further study.[21]

ASYMPTOMATIC BACTERIURIA

Antibiotic Treatment

CASE 68-11

QUESTION 1: A.K., an asymptomatic 6-year-old girl, is found to have significant bacteriuria on routine screening. Should she be treated with an antimicrobial agent?

The treatment of patients with asymptomatic bacteriuria depends on the clinical setting in which it is found. Asymptomatic bacteriuria occurs in a heterogeneous group of patients with different prognoses and risks. Therefore, recommendations for treatment of asymptomatic patients with significant bacteriuria (two consecutive voided urine specimens showing $\geq 10^5$ bacteria/mL of urine in women, or a single clean-catch voided specimen in men) are based on specific age, sex, and clinical characteristics.[1,8,10,108] These recommendations are based on the risk for development of acute UTI and subsequent long-term complications. Generally, patients who benefit most from antibiotic treatment are those with urinary tract structural abnormalities, immunosuppressive therapy, and procedures requiring urinary tract instrumentation or manipulation.[1,2,8] Short-course regimens (i.e., single-dose or 3-day) are usually recommended when treatment is desired,[2] although longer regimens have also been recommended.[8]

Urinary tract infections in infants and preschool children (predominantly girls) occasionally are associated with renal tissue damage.[109] Asymptomatic bacteriuria of childhood also is important because it may be a manifestation of an anatomic or mechanical defect in the urinary tract. Therefore, it should be evaluated fully. Because most cases of renal scarring as a result of bacteriuria occur within the first 5 years of life, it is controversial whether treatment should be limited to infants and preschool children or whether all children should be treated regardless of age. Screening for bacteriuria in children and treating those with positive cultures, regardless of their clinical presentation, seems reasonable and is frequently recommended.[109] Treatment of A.K., although still controversial, seems prudent because renal damage resulting from asymptomatic bacteriuria generally occurs during childhood. Should the decision be made to treat, principles of therapy are similar to those for symptomatic infections.

Pregnant Patients, the Elderly, and Other Adult Populations

CASE 68-11, QUESTION 2: The decision to treat the asymptomatic bacteriuria of A.K. was based primarily on the increased probability of renal damage during childhood. What other population groups should be treated for asymptomatic bacteriuria?

Without urinary tract obstruction, UTI in adults rarely lead to progressive renal damage.[2,4] Therefore, asymptomatic bacteriuria does not require treatment in most adult patients who have no evidence of mechanical obstruction or renal insufficiency. Aggressive antimicrobial therapy is appropriate during pregnancy, however, because as many as 40% of pregnant women with asymptomatic bacteriuria later develop symptomatic UTI, particularly pyelonephritis.[8] In addition, studies have confirmed associations between acute pyelonephritis during pregnancy with increased rates of preterm labor, premature delivery, and lower birth-weight infants.[25] The treatment of asymptomatic bacteriuria in pregnancy is therefore justified to decrease the risk of associated complications.[8]

Treatment should be based on in vitro susceptibility testing or by selecting the least expensive, least toxic agent. Sulfonamides should be avoided in late pregnancy because they can contribute to kernicterus in the neonate. Fluoroquinolones should be avoided during pregnancy because of the risk of arthropathies to the fetus (see Case 68-7, Question 3).

Bacteriuria in the elderly is common; it is estimated that 20% of all women and 10% of all men age 65 years and older have bacteriuria.[9,13,14] Although bacteriuria in this population often leads to symptomatic infection, clinical studies, however, have consistently documented no beneficial outcomes in treated patients compared with untreated patients.[8,13] Consequently, therapy is not recommended for the asymptomatic older patient because the expense, side effects, and potential complications of drug therapy appear to outweigh the benefits.[8,13] Patients experiencing symptomatic infections should be treated as usual.

The treatment of asymptomatic bacteriuria in women with diabetes does not reduce complications and is not currently recommended.[8,108]

PROSTATITIS

Incidence, Prevalence, and Epidemiology

Prostatitis is an acute or chronic inflammatory condition affecting the prostate, approximately 5% of cases being caused by proven bacterial infections.[11,12] Prostatitis is a common but poorly understood entity, the most prevalent forms include acute and chronic bacterial prostatitis, chronic calculus prostatitis, nonbacterial prostatitis, and prostatodynia.[11,12] Chronic bacterial prostatitis, defined as prostatitis in which symptoms persist for at least 3 months, is one of the most common causes of recurrent UTI in men. The lifetime probability of a man being diagnosed with prostatitis is greater than 25%; recurrence rates reportedly range from 20% to 50%.[11,12] Approximately 5% of men with acute prostatitis will experience chronic infection.[11]

Etiology, Pathogenesis, and Predisposing Factors

ACUTE BACTERIAL PROSTATITIS

Acute bacterial prostatitis in most patients probably begins as an ascending infection of the urethra. A simple UTI then eventually involves reflux of infected urine into the ejaculatory and prostatic ducts through the prostate gland, where bacteria are difficult to eradicate.[12] Acute prostatitis may also result from urethral stricture or after instrumentation of the urinary tract or prostate biopsy, especially in the presence of bacteriuria at the time of the procedure.[12] Bacterial prostatitis is predominantly caused by aerobic gram-negative bacilli, with *E. coli* causing 50% to 90% of cases. Other Enterobacteriaceae such as *Proteus* and *Klebsiella* account for an additional 10% to 30% of cases, followed by *Enterococcus* (5% to 10%) and *Pseudomonas* (<5%); less common causes include staphylococci, streptococci, and atypical organisms such as *Chlamydia trachomatis, Trichomonas vaginalis,* and *Ureaplasma urealyticum*.[11,12]

CHRONIC BACTERIAL PROSTATITIS

Chronic prostatitis is commonly associated with spinal cord injuries, infectious stones, anatomic or physiologic abnormalities of the urinary tract such as obstruction or voiding dysfunction, and immune dysfunction. However, recurrent infections are also commonly caused by relapses of acute prostatitis caused by persistence of bacteria in the prostate.[11,12] Normally, men secrete a prostatic antibacterial factor; however, this substance is often absent or significantly reduced in men with chronic prostatitis. The most common pathogens isolated from chronic bacterial prostatitis are *E. coli* (>80% of cases) and other gram-negative bacilli, although atypical bacteria have also been more commonly reported in chronic prostatitis compared to acute infections.[11,12]

Clinical Presentation and Diagnosis

ACUTE BACTERIAL PROSTATITIS

Acute bacterial prostatitis is characterized by the sudden onset of chills and fever; perineal and low back pain; urinary urgency and frequency; nocturia, dysuria, and generalized malaise; and prostration. Patients also may complain of myalgias, arthralgias, and symptoms of bladder outlet obstruction. Rectal examination usually discloses an exquisitely tender, swollen prostate that is firm and warm to the touch. The pathogens generally can be identified by culture of the voided urine. In patients with acute bacterial prostatitis, prostatic massage (see following discussion) should be avoided because of patient discomfort and the risk of bacteremia.[11,12] The diagnosis of acute prostatitis is therefore usually based on clinical presentation and physical examination.

CHRONIC BACTERIAL PROSTATITIS

The clinical manifestations of chronic bacterial prostatitis are highly variable and, in many patients, are asymptomatic. The disease usually is suspected when a male patient treated for UTI or acute prostatitis relapses. The diagnosis of chronic prostatitis is confirmed by examination of expressed prostatic secretions.[11,12] To ensure accurate localization (i.e., to distinguish prostatic from urethral bacteria), segmented urine samples are taken. The first 10 mL of voided urine represents the urethral sample, the midstream urine collected represents the bladder sample, and the first 10 mL voided immediately after prostatic massage represents the prostate sample. When the bladder sample is sterile or nearly so, bacterial prostatitis is diagnosed if the bacterial count in the prostate sample is at least one logarithm greater than that in the urethral sample.[11,12]

Overview of Treatment

Treatment of bacterial prostatitis is made challenging by poor penetration of many antibiotics across the non-fenestrated prostatic capillaries and through prostatic epithelium into infected tissues and fluids. Fluoroquinolones are often considered the preferred antibiotics for treatment of acute or chronic prostatitis due to good penetration into the prostate (10% to 50% of serum concentrations) and good activity against most causative pathogens, although fluoroquinolone resistance has become a growing problem.[11,12] Trimethoprim alone or TMP-SMX are also commonly used agents. β-Lactams, tetracyclines, macrolides, and clindamycin have also been successfully used in the treatment of both acute and chronic infections, but their penetration into the prostatic tissues and fluids may be somewhat less than the fluoroquinolones and/or the antimicrobial activity of these drugs is not necessarily ideal for covering the most common causative pathogens.[11,12] The duration of antibiotic therapy in acute prostatitis is usually 2 to 4 weeks, depending on the severity of the infection and rate of response to treatment.[11,12] Chronic prostatitis is usually treated for 4 to 6 weeks, although longer courses may be required in the presence of prostate stones or other types of genitourinary pathology and long-term suppressive therapy is sometimes used for patients with a history of rapid and/or multiple recurrences.[11,12] Monitoring parameters consist primarily of clinical signs and symptoms, and the end point of treatment is simply complete resolution of clinical findings.[11,12] Nonpharmacologic treatment consists primarily of drugs such as acetaminophen or non-steroidal anti-inflammatory agents for symptomatic relief; warm compresses to the perineal area are also sometimes recommended, although there are few data to support this practice.[11,12]

CASE 68-12

QUESTION 1: D.G., a 60-year-old man, experienced his first UTI at age 40, with symptoms of frequency, dysuria, nocturia, perineal pain, chills, and fever, but no flank pain. Acute prostatitis was diagnosed. *E. coli* was cultured from the urine, and treatment with a sulfonamide was successful. After 12 asymptomatic years, acute prostatitis caused by *E. coli* recurred and again responded to sulfonamide therapy. Two more *E. coli* infections that responded to sulfonamide therapy occurred during the next 8 years. Why were sulfonamides appropriate treatment for D.G.'s repeated acute episodes of bacterial prostatitis?

Most antibacterial drugs appropriate for UTI, including sulfonamides, can be used to treat acute bacterial prostatitis because the diffuse, intense inflammation of the prostate gland allows many drugs to readily penetrate into the prostatic fluid and tissues. Antimicrobial therapy should be continued for at least 2 to 4 weeks to prevent the development of chronic prostatitis.[11,12,107]

In addition to antibiotics, other supportive measures may provide symptomatic relief to patients with acute bacterial prostatitis. These measures include liberal hydration, nonsteroidal anti-inflammatory drugs for pain relief, sitz baths, and stool softeners.

In retrospect, sulfonamides were appropriate for D.G. because they effectively treated his infections. Other options, particularly the fluoroquinolones, would also have been appropriate in the treatment of D.G.'s episodes of acute prostatitis.

CASE 68-12, QUESTION 2: Taking into account the pathophysiology of prostatitis, what would be a reasonable choice of therapy for D.G. should he have future recurrences of prostatitis?

Most antibiotics that are acidic do not readily cross the prostatic epithelium into the alkaline prostatic fluid except in the presence of acute inflammation. Theoretically, the high alkalinity of prostatic fluids should impair the diffusion of trimethoprim and enhance the diffusion of the tetracyclines, certain sulfonamides, and the macrolide antibiotics, such as erythromycin. Nevertheless, TMP-SMX historically has the best documented cure rates in the treatment of acute and chronic bacterial prostatitis. Long-term therapy of chronic bacterial prostatitis with TMP-SMX for 4 to 16 weeks is associated with a cure rate of 32% to 71%, which significantly exceeds the cure rate associated with short-term therapy of 2 or fewer weeks.[11,12]

The fluoroquinolones have become well-accepted alternatives to TMP-SMX and are now considered by many to be the agents of choice for the treatment of prostatitis.[11,12,107] A number of studies have documented bacteriologic cure in 80% to 90% of patients treated with norfloxacin, ciprofloxacin, or levofloxacin for 4 to 12 weeks, rates comparable to or substantially higher than those achieved with agents such as TMP-SMX.[11,12] The fluoroquinolones have assumed an important role in the treatment of prostatitis owing to their bactericidal activity against common pathogens and excellent penetration into prostatic tissues and fluid. The fluoroquinolones are often used as initial empiric therapy of prostatitis and are also excellent alternatives to other agents in patients who are unresponsive or intolerant to conventional therapy, or in those infected with resistant organisms.[11,12,107] Fluoroquinolones also have been used for chronic suppressive therapy (one-half normal doses) in patients who relapse after conventional treatment.[1]

D.G. should be treated with TMP-SMX for a minimum of 6 weeks; some authorities recommend a 2-month to 3-month total course of therapy. If an adequate trial of TMP-SMX is unsuccessful, fluoroquinolone therapy can be used. Alternatively, a fluoroquinolone could be used as initial therapy for this or future episodes.[11,12,107]

If D.G. continues to experience recurrent infections after a trial of fluoroquinolone therapy, chronic low-dose treatment with TMP-SMX, fluoroquinolones, or nitrofurantoin can alleviate the symptoms of episodic bladder infection associated with chronic bacterial prostatitis. Infections eventually recur with greater frequency in most of these patients, although some become asymptomatic, even with chronic bacteriuria. Chronic, low-dose antibacterial therapy sterilizes the bladder, alleviates symptoms, confines bacteria to the prostate, and prevents infection of and damage to the rest of the urinary tract. Chronic bacterial prostatitis is one of the few indications for continuous antibiotic therapy.

KEY REFERENCES AND WEBSITES

A full list of references for this chapter can be found at **http://thepoint.lww.com/AT10e.** Below are the key references for this chapter, with the corresponding reference number in this chapter found in parentheses after the reference.

Key References

Craig JC et al. Antibiotic prophylaxis and recurrent urinary tract infection in children [published correction appears in *N Engl J Med.* 2010;362:1250]. *N Engl J Med.* 2009;361:1748. (89)

Dielubanza EJ, Schaeffer AJ. Urinary tract infections in women. *Med Clin North Am.* 2011;95:27. (2)

Epp A et al. Recurrent urinary tract infection. *J Obstet Gynaecol Can.*2010;250:1082. (33)

Gupta K et al. International clinical practice guidelines for the treatment of acute uncomplicated cystitis and pyelonephritis in women: a 2010 update by the Infectious Diseases Society of America and the European Society for Microbiology and Infectious Diseases. *Clin Infect Dis.* 2011;52:e103. (18)

Hooton TM et al. Diagnosis, prevention, and treatment of catheter-associated urinary tract infection in adults: 2009 international clinical practice guidelines from the Infectious Diseases Society of America. *Clin Infect Dis.* 2010;50:625. (21)

Karlowsky JA et al. Fluoroquinolone-resistant urinary isolates of *Escherichia coli* from outpatients are frequently multidrug resistant: results from the North American Urinary Tract Infection Collaborative Alliance-Quinolone Resistance Study. *Antimicrob Agents Chemother.* 2006;50:2251. (72)

Katsarolis I et al. Acute uncomplicated cystitis: from surveillance data to a rationale for empirical treatment. *Int J Antimicrob Agents.* 2010;35:62. (50)

Lipsky BA et al. Treatment of bacterial prostatitis. *Clin Infect Dis.* 2010;50:1641. (11)

CHANCROID

1	Uncircumcised men have an increased risk of infection and may not respond to therapy as well as circumcised men. Current treatment options include azithromycin, ceftriaxone, ciprofloxacin, and erythromycin base.	**Case 69-9 (Questions 1, 2)**

VAGINITIS

1	Common causes of vaginitis include bacterial vaginosis, trichomoniasis, and vulvovaginal candidiasis. General symptoms may include itching, burning, irritation, and abnormal discharge, and it can be differentiated based on signs, symptoms, and laboratory testing.	**Case 69-10 (Question 1), Case 69-11 (Questions 2–4), Case 69-12 (Question 1)**
2	Vulvovaginal candidiasis may be effectively treated with nonprescription medications; however, patients must be assessed fully before self-treatment is initiated.	**Case 69-11 (Questions 1–4, 6–9)**

GENITAL HERPES

1	Genital herpes, transmitted either from symptomatic or asymptomatic individuals, often presents with painful vesicles in those with herpes simplex virus type 2 primary infection, and recurrent infections are common, although the frequency decreases with time.	**Case 69-14 (Questions 1–3)**
2	Genital herpes is best treated with oral antivirals, such as acyclovir or valacyclovir, and prevented with either suppressive or standby antivirals.	**Case 69-14 (Question 5)**

GENITAL WARTS

1	Genital human papillomavirus warts are highly contagious and may now be prevented by vaccination, in addition to condoms.	**Case 69-17 (Question 1)**
2	Genital warts often recur even with treatment, which is primarily local, including antimitotics, immune modulators, chemical and surgical ablation, and cryotherapy.	**Case 69-17 (Question 1)**

Sexually transmitted diseases (STDs) are discussed in the earliest written records. However, only in the last several decades have the common STDs been differentiated from each other; unique STD syndromes continue to be described today. For example, of the common STDs, bacterial vaginosis (BV) was not described clearly as a syndrome (initially called *Haemophilus vaginalis* vaginitis) until the 1950s; herpes simplex virus (HSV) type 2 (the cause of genital herpes) was not differentiated from HSV type 1 until the 1960s; the spectrum of genital chlamydial infections was not defined until the 1970s; and the human immunodeficiency virus (HIV) as an STD was not recognized until the 1980s. Since 1980, eight additional sexually transmitted pathogens have been identified. They include the human papillomaviruses (HPV), human T-lymphotropic virus (HTLV-I and -II), *Mycoplasma genitalium, Mobiluncus* species, HIV-1 and -2, and the human herpes virus type 8 (associated with Kaposi sarcoma).[1] More recently, the Centers for Disease Control and Prevention (CDC) reports that 10% of persons with hepatitis C virus (HCV) infection had sexual contact with an HCV-positive partner, many of who were HIV positive and homosexual.[2] See http://www.cdc.gov/std/training/othertraining.htm for general resources from the Centers for Disease Control for various sexually transmitted diseases.

GONORRHEA

Gonorrhea (see http://www.cdc.gov/STD/TRAINING/CLINICALSLIDES/slides-dl.htm for symptoms of this STD) is caused by *Neisseria gonorrhoeae*, a gram-negative diplococcus. In AD 130, Galen coined the term *gonorrhea* (Greek for "flow of seed") for the syndrome associated with this infection because he believed the urethral exudate was semen. Although the role of the gonococcus in causing urethral discharge in men has been known for years, the manifestations of gonorrhea in women were determined much later. In the 1930s, sulfonamides became the first form of effective antimicrobial therapy for gonorrhea until penicillins and tetracyclines became the mainstays of therapy; however, the high levels of resistance to these two antimicrobial agents has eliminated their use in the treatment of this disease state.

In the United States, the incidence of gonorrhea fell 74.3% between 1975 and 1997 after the establishment of national gonorrhea control programs. From 1996 to 2006, the rate fluctuated at around 115 cases per 100,000 individuals, and from 2006 to 2009, it declined from 119.7 cases to 99.1 cases per 100,000 individuals representing a total of 301,174 cases.[3] The current Healthy People 2020 goals for gonorrhea are 257 cases per 100,000 women aged 15 to 44 and 198 cases per 100,000 men aged 15 to 44 (Fig. 69-1).[4] Rates of gonorrhea have remained steady during the past years in most racial and ethnic groups; however, the incidence of infection in African Americans remains higher than in other groups.[3]

The highest incidence of gonorrhea is in men 20 to 24 years of age and in women 15 to 24 years of age.[3] Additional risk factors for women acquiring gonorrhea include a previous gonococcal or other STD infection, new or multiple sex partners, inconsistent condom use, or engaging in commercial sex work or drug use.[2]

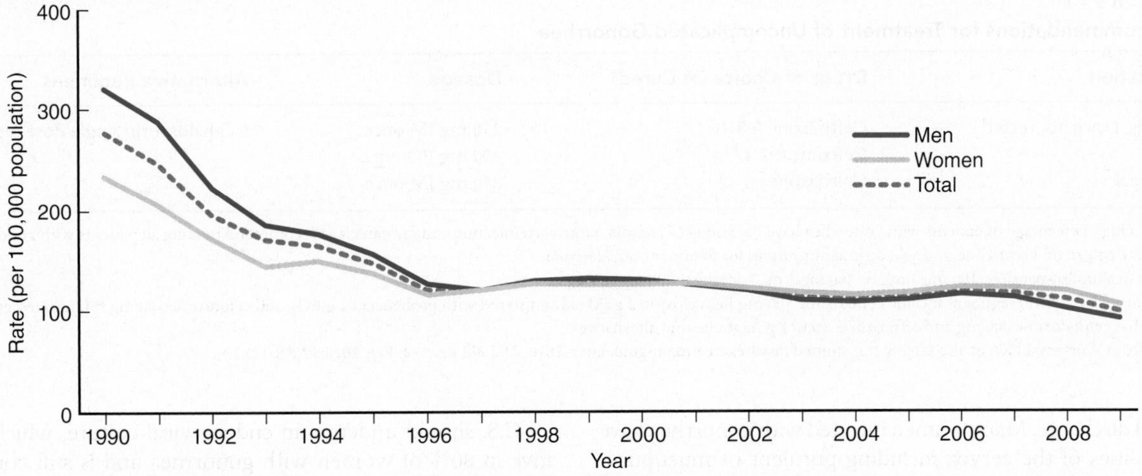

FIGURE 69-1 Gonorrhea rates by sex, United States, 1990–2009. Note: the Healthy People 2020 target for gonorrhea is 257 new cases per 100,000 for women 15 to 44 years of age and 198 new cases per 100,000 for men 15 to 44 years of age. (Reprinted from Centers for Disease Control and Prevention. *2009 Sexually Transmitted Disease Surveillance*. Atlanta, GA: US Dept of Health and Human Services; 2010.)

Although the risk of gonorrhea was greater in homosexual men than in heterosexual men in the past, the incidence dropped in homosexual men during the 1980s AIDS epidemic because of a reduction in risky sexual behaviors. Currently, the incidence of gonorrhea in men who have sex with men (MSM) continues to rise, from 21.5% in 2006 to 25.3% in 2009.[3]

Uncomplicated Gonorrhea

TRANSMISSION

CASE 69-1

QUESTION 1: D.S., a 23-year-old male naval officer recently stationed in the Philippines, complains of dysuria, meatal pain, and a profuse yellow urethral discharge for 2 days. He admits to extramarital sex with a prostitute during the past week. He is accompanied by his pregnant wife, C.S., who is asymptomatic. D.S. engages in vaginal sex, but there is no history of oral or anal sex with either partner. Assuming the prostitute has gonorrhea, what is the likelihood that D.S. and C.S. have been infected?

After one or two episodes of unprotected vaginal intercourse with an infected prostitute, a man has approximately a 50% risk of acquiring a urethral infection; the risk increases with repeated exposures and high prevalence among commercial sex workers.[5] The prevalence of infection in women who are secondary sex contacts of infected men is as high as 80% to 90%.[6] Therefore, the likelihood that D.S. and C.S. are infected is high. Because D.S. had sex with a prostitute, both D.S. and C.S. should also be tested for HIV infection.

SIGNS AND SYMPTOMS: MALES

CASE 69-1, QUESTION 2: What signs and symptoms in D.S. are consistent with the diagnosis of gonorrhea? Describe D.S.'s anticipated clinical course if he remains untreated.

In men, gonorrhea usually becomes clinically apparent 1 to 7 days after contact with an infected source. A purulent discharge associated with dysuria is the first sign of infection; D.S. exhibits both. The discharge, which is presumably caused by chemotactic factors such as C5a released when antigonococcal antibody binds complement, may become more profuse and blood tinged as the infection progresses. Some strains of gonorrhea have a propensity to cause asymptomatic or minimally symptomatic infection with negative Gram stain.

Patients with asymptomatic or minimally symptomatic disease may serve as reservoirs for the infection, evading treatment for prolonged periods.[7] At one time, only women were thought to have asymptomatic gonorrhea, but now it is known that men may be asymptomatic carriers as well.[8]

In the era before antimicrobials, gonococci occasionally spread to the epididymis, causing unilateral epididymitis; the prevalence was 5% or more in patients in some studies. Now epididymitis occurs in less than 1% of men with gonorrhea. Urethral stricture after repeated attacks and sterility after epididymitis are rare complications of gonococcal infection owing to the effectiveness of antibiotics.

DIAGNOSIS: MALES

CASE 69-1, QUESTION 3: Intracellular gram-negative diplococci were seen on the Gram stain of D.S.'s urethral exudate. Is any further diagnostic testing required?

Demonstration of intracellular gram-negative diplococci in the gram-stained exudate confirms the diagnosis in symptomatic men. Until recently, some experts recommended that cultures be reserved for individuals with negative Gram stain of urethral exudate. However, today cultures are recommended for all patients to permit isolation and testing of the bacteria for antibiotic susceptibility. Cultures usually are performed on Thayer–Martin medium, an enriched chocolate agar to which vancomycin, colistimethate, and nystatin have been added. Cultures from the throat should be obtained if D.S. was exposed by cunnilingus to the prostitute. In D.S.'s case, a urethral culture is indicated.

SIGNS AND SYMPTOMS: FEMALES

CASE 69-1, QUESTION 4: C.S., D.S.'s wife, is asymptomatic. What symptoms would be consistent with gonorrhea in C.S.? Do the symptoms differ because she is pregnant? What is the natural course of gonorrhea in women if left untreated?

Because the endocervical canal is the primary site of urogenital gonococcal infection in women, the most common symptom

TABLE 69-1
CDC Recommendations for Treatment of Uncomplicated Gonorrhea

Presentation	Drugs of Choice (% Cured)	Dosage	Alternative Regimens
Urethritis, cervicitis, rectal[a]	Ceftriaxone (98.9)	250 mg IM once	Cephalosporin single-dose regimens[c]
	Cefixime (97.4)[b]	400 mg PO once	
Pharyngeal	Ceftriaxone	250 mg IM once	

[a] Because a high percentage of patients with gonorrhea have coexisting *Chlamydia trachomatis* infections, many clinicians recommend treating all patients with gonorrhea with a 7-day course of doxycycline or single-dose azithromycin for treatment of *Chlamydia*.
[b] Available in a oral suspension (100 mg/5 mL or 200 mg/5 mL) or tablet (400 mg) dosage form.
[c] Additional cephalosporin regimens include ceftizoxime 500 mg IM, cefoxitin 2 g IM (administered with probenecid 1 g PO), and cefotaxime 500 mg IM. Limited evidence suggests that cefpodoxime 400 mg and cefuroxime axetil 1 g might be oral alternatives.
Adapted from Workowski KA et al. Sexually transmitted diseases treatment guidelines, 2010. *MMWR Recomm Rep.* 2010;59(RR-12):1.

is vaginal discharge. Many women infected with gonorrhea have abnormalities of the cervix, including purulent or mucopurulent endocervical discharge, erythema, friability, and edema of the zone of ectopy.[6] The incubation period for urogenital gonorrhea in women is variable.[9] Pelvic inflammatory disease (PID) is a serious complication in 10% to 20% of women with acute gonococcal infection and can lead to infertility and chronic pelvic pain.[2,6] The assessment of signs and symptoms in women with gonorrhea often is confounded by nonspecific signs and symptoms and a high prevalence of coexisting infection, especially with *Chlamydia trachomatis* or *Trichomonas vaginalis*.

Although lower genital tract symptoms in women may disappear, they remain carriers of *N. gonorrhoeae* and should be treated. Complications of urogenital gonorrhea in pregnancy include spontaneous abortion, premature rupture of the fetal membranes, premature delivery, and acute chorioamnionitis.[2,10,11] Other complications include gonococcal arthritis (see Case 69-4, Question 1) conjunctivitis, and ophthalmia neonatorum in the newborn.[12] For these reasons, it is critical that C.S. be worked up thoroughly for gonorrhea.

DIAGNOSIS: FEMALES

CASE 69-1, QUESTION 5: How should gonorrhea be ruled out in C.S.?

C.S. should undergo an endocervical culture, which is positive in 80% of women with gonorrhea and is still considered the "gold standard."[13] This test should be a part of every pelvic examination of sexually active women. Nucleic acid amplification tests (NAATs), such as polymerase chain reaction (PCR), may yield sensitivities and specificities in the 90% to 100% range, but results must be confirmed with endocervical culture in low-prevalence communities (i.e., <4%).[14] In C.S., anal cultures also could be performed because the rectum can serve as a reservoir for gonococci.

TREATMENT

CASE 69-1, QUESTION 6: Compare the various drug regimens used for uncomplicated gonorrhea.

The CDC recommendations are summarized in Table 69-1. Many strains of *N. gonorrhoeae* exhibit plasmid-mediated resistance to penicillin and tetracycline (penicillinase-producing *N. gonorrhoeae* [PPNG] and tetracycline-resistant *N. gonorrhoeae* [TRNG], respectively) (Fig. 69-2). In addition, significant levels of chromosomally mediated resistance to penicillin, tetracycline, and cefoxitin have been reported.[15] In 2009, all isolates in the Gonococcal Isolate Surveillance Project (GISP) were susceptible to ceftriaxone; therefore, a single dose of intramuscular (IM)

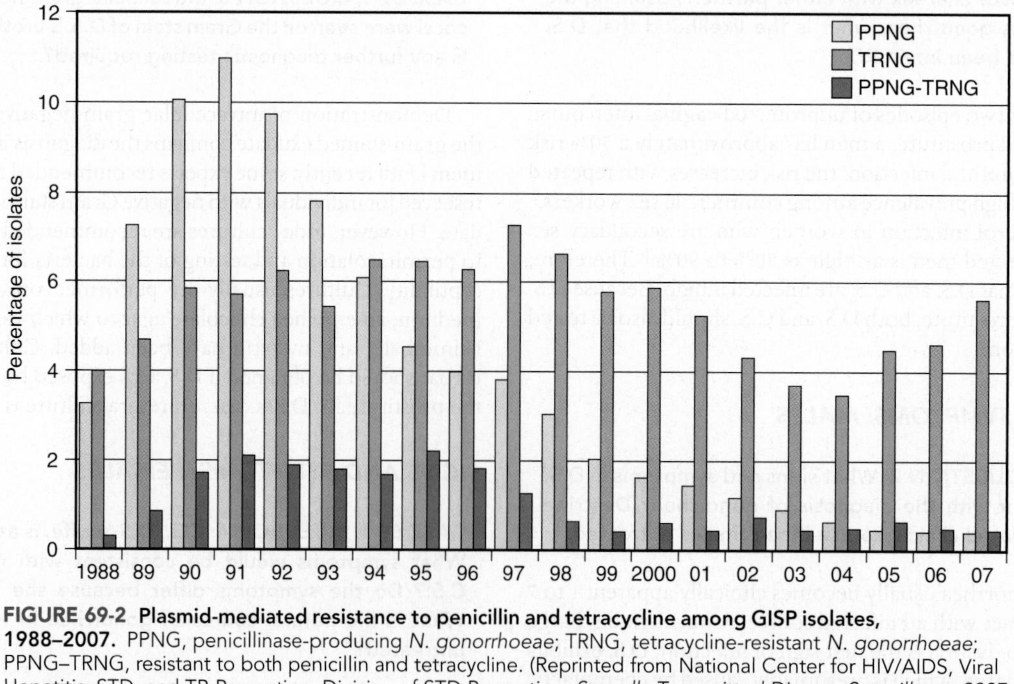

FIGURE 69-2 Plasmid-mediated resistance to penicillin and tetracycline among GISP isolates, 1988–2007. PPNG, penicillinase-producing *N. gonorrhoeae*; TRNG, tetracycline-resistant *N. gonorrhoeae*; PPNG–TRNG, resistant to both penicillin and tetracycline. (Reprinted from National Center for HIV/AIDS, Viral Hepatitis, STD, and TB Prevention, Division of STD Prevention. *Sexually Transmitted Disease Surveillance 2007 Supplement, Gonococcal Isolate Surveillance Project (GISP) Annual Report 2007*. Atlanta, GA: US Dept of Health and Human Services, Centers for Disease Control and Prevention; 2009.)

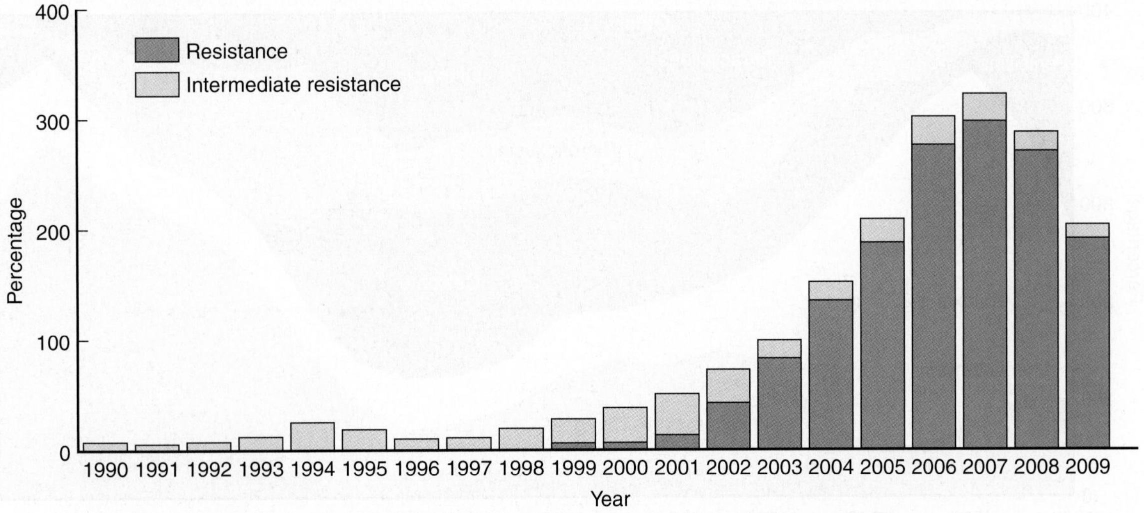

NOTE: Resistant isolates have ciprofloxacin minimum inhibitory concentrations (MICs) ≥1 mcg/mL. Isolates with intermediate resistance have ciprofloxacin MICs of 0.125–0.5 mcg/mL. Susceptibility to ciprofloxacin was first measured in GISP in 1990.

FIGURE 69-3 Gonococcal Isolate Surveillance Project (GISP)—percent of *Neisseria gonorrhoeae* isolates with resistance or intermediate resistance to ciprofloxacin, 1990–2009. (Reprinted from Centers for Disease Control and Prevention. *2009 Sexually Transmitted Disease Surveillance*. Atlanta, GA: US Dept of Health and Human Services; 2010.)

ceftriaxone 250 mg is preferred for the treatment of gonorrhea.[2,3] Cefixime 400 mg orally as a single dose is an alternative option that is also recommended by the CDC. The CDC has withdrawn recommendations for use of fluoroquinolones such as ciprofloxacin and ofloxacin because of unacceptably high levels of quinolone-resistant *N. gonorrhoeae* (QRNG).[2,16] Because a high percentage of patients with gonorrhea are also coinfected with *C. trachomatis*, a single dose of azithromycin or a 7-day course of doxycycline is recommended to be taken concurrently for a presumed infection (see Case 69-5, Question 3).[2]

Intramuscular spectinomycin, which traditionally had been used in individuals who could not tolerate either fluoroquinolones or cephalosporins, is also still unavailable from the manufacturer. Spectinomycin was the recommended treatment option for gonorrhea in those with either penicillin or cephalosporin allergies.[17] Individuals who have either penicillin or cephalosporin allergies should be desensitized to cephalosporins before treatment begins.[18]

CEFTRIAXONE AND OTHER CEPHALOSPORINS

Ceftriaxone, a third-generation cephalosporin, is given as a single, small-volume IM injection that eradicates anal and pharyngeal gonorrhea and is also safe in pregnancy (U.S. Food and Drug Administration [FDA] pregnancy category B). Ceftriaxone is ineffective against *C. trachomatis* and in the prevention of postgonococcal urethritis, whereas ofloxacin and levofloxacin for 7 days have similar efficacy to doxycycline.[2] Other injectable cephalosporins (notably ceftizoxime, cefoxitin, and cefotaxime) have been found to be safe and highly effective, although efficacy in pharyngeal infections is not as well established. Although not meeting the strict CDC definition of success, evidence suggests that cefpodoxime is also effective in the treatment of uncomplicated urogenital gonorrhea; however, it should not be considered a first-line agent.[2]

FLUOROQUINOLONES

Fluoroquinolones have been routinely used since the 1990s for the treatment of gonorrhea; however, the GISP has continuously documented fluoroquinolone resistance in *N. gonorrhoeae* isolates, which has necessitated changes in the CDC Sexually Transmitted Disease treatment guidelines (Fig. 69-3). Because of this increased resistance, the CDC no longer recommends ciprofloxacin, levofloxacin, ofloxacin, or other fluoroquinolones for the treatment of gonorrhea. This recommendation also extends to the treatment of gonorrhea-associated conditions such as PID.[2,16]

PRESCRIBING PATTERNS

The CDC's 2009 Sexually Transmitted Disease Surveillance Program observed that ceftriaxone 125 mg was the most prescribed medication, followed in order by ceftriaxone 250 mg, cefixime, and ciprofloxacin (Fig. 69-4).[3] Cefixime 400-mg tablets were reintroduced on the market in 2008.[19] Their use should increase as they are a CDC-recommended alternative agent for uncomplicated gonorrhea. In addition to tablets, cefixime is also available in a suspension (either 100 or 200 mg/5 mL) dosage form.

CASE 69-1, QUESTION 7: How should D.S.'s urethritis be treated? Because C.S. is totally asymptomatic and the results of her cultures are pending, should she be treated empirically? If so, what drug(s) would you recommend?

Because D.S. has gonococcal infection limited to the urethra (uncomplicated), a few treatment regimens are possible, as outlined in Case 69-1, Question 6. Ceftriaxone is the preferred treatment, but cefixime could also be used. Quinolones should be avoided because of increased resistance in *N. gonorrhoeae* and because D.S.'s infection was likely obtained in the Philippines, where quinolone resistance occurs in more than half of all isolates.[16,20] Both cefpodoxime 400 mg orally (PO) and cefuroxime 1 g PO have limited clinical evidence to support their use and are not as effective as cefixime; however, they are FDA approved to treat uncomplicated *N. gonorrhoeae*.[2] Patients with gonorrhea may also be coinfected with *Chlamydia*, and therefore presumptive cotreatment with either azithromycin 1 g PO as a single dose or doxycycline 100 mg PO twice daily for 7 days could be initiated if coinfection is suspected.[2,21] Although single-dose azithromycin has been used to treat concurrent gonorrhea and *Chlamydia*, it is more expensive and poorly tolerated because of increased gastrointestinal (GI) side effects, and may lead to macrolide-resistant *N. gonorrhoeae* or treatment failure.[2]

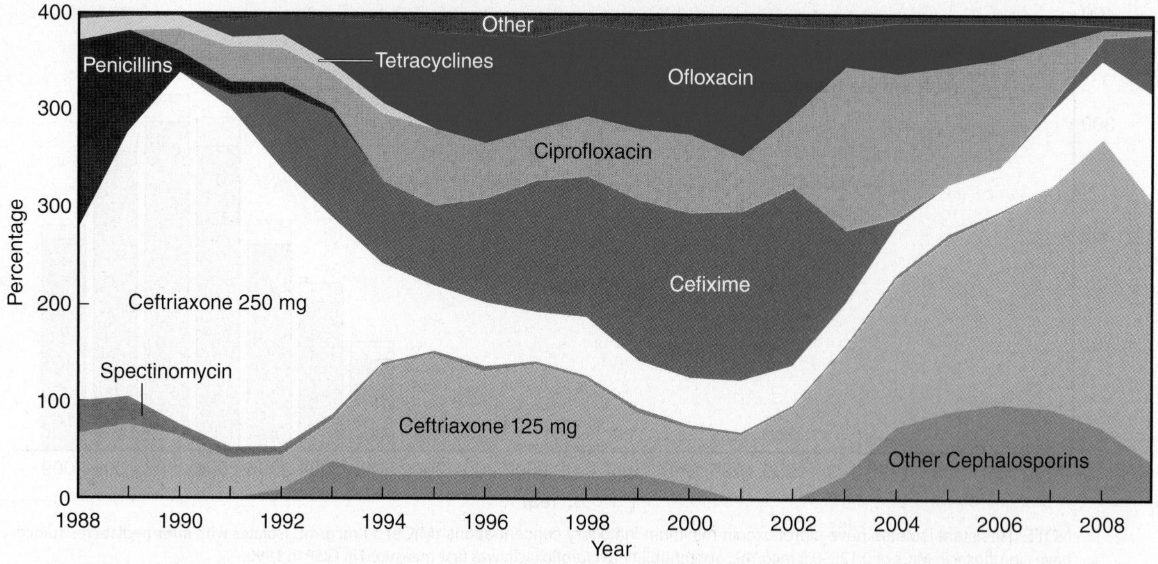

NOTE: For 2009, "Other" includes no therapy (1.5%), azithromycin 2 g (1.7%), and other less frequently used drugs.

FIGURE 69-4 Gonococcal Isolate Surveillance Project (GISP)—drugs used to treat gonorrhea in GISP participants, 1988–2009. (Reprinted from Centers for Disease Control and Prevention. *2009 Sexually Transmitted Disease Surveillance.* Atlanta, GA: US Dept of Health and Human Services; 2010.)

SEXUAL PARTNERS

C.S. also should be treated even though she appears asymptomatic. All partners who have had sexual exposure to patients with gonorrhea within 60 days should be treated. If the patient has not been sexually active for 60 days, the most recent sexual partner should be treated. This is especially true when the partner is pregnant because gonorrhea during pregnancy is associated with chorioamnionitis and prematurity, as well as neonatal infection. Pregnant women can be treated safely with cephalosporins and azithromycin for gonorrhea and *Chlamydia*. Doxycycline should be avoided during pregnancy.

FOLLOW-UP

CASE 69-1, QUESTION 8: How does one determine whether the drug therapy of gonorrhea has been effective in D.S. and C.S.?

If recommended therapies are used for treatment of uncomplicated gonorrhea, a test of cure is not necessary for either C.S. or D.S. because cure rates are close to 100%.[2] If symptoms persist in D.S., who was treated with ceftriaxone, cultures should be done to rule out other causes of urethritis.

ANTIBIOTIC-RESISTANT *NEISSERIA GONORRHOEAE*

CASE 69-1, QUESTION 9: D.S. states that he was treated with penicillin in the past for a gonococcal infection. Why are penicillins not prescribed routinely today?

Failure of penicillin to eradicate the gonococcus can be the result of plasmid (e.g., PPNG) or chromosomally mediated resistant *N. gonorrhoeae* (CMRNG) antibiotic resistance. PPNG contain plasmids, which determine the production of lactamase, an enzyme that hydrolyzes the lactam ring of penicillin G or ampicillin. Chromosomally mediated resistance does not involve β-lactamase production and often is associated with increased resistance to other β-lactams. The clinical significance of CMRNG is questionable because serum levels of approved antibiotics are achieved far above the minimum inhibitory concentration, such that treatment failure is unlikely. However, to date CMRNG remain largely susceptible to ceftriaxone. High-level tetracycline resistance is defined by gonococci that carry plasmid-encoded resistance to 16 g/mL or more of tetracycline. These strains are known as TRNG. Although not of major concern in the United States, development of resistance to alternative therapies is a continuing concern.

The first cases of PPNG infection were reported in the United States in 1976. PPNG are especially prevalent in Southeast Asia, the Far East, and West Africa, where the prevalence often exceeds 50%. In the United States, the percent of PPNG strains reached a peak of about 11% in 1991; since then, cases have steadily declined to 0.4% in 2007, according to the CDC's GISP (Fig. 69-2).[22] Strains of TRNG were first identified in 1985, but fortunately most TRNG isolates still are sensitive to β-lactam antibiotics. The use of tetracycline was officially abandoned by the CDC in 1985, and penicillin was abandoned in 1987. In the late 1990s, the number of TRNG and PPNG plus TRNG cases plateaued at about 5% and 1%, respectively. Therefore, because approximately 21% of gonococcal isolates are resistant to tetracycline or penicillin within the United States, it is not acceptable to use these agents in the initial management of uncomplicated genital gonorrhea; IM ceftriaxone remains the drug of choice. Antibiotic susceptibility testing is recommended in cases of persistent infection after treatment.

Quinolone-resistant *N. gonorrhoeae* was first reported in 1990 and was reported to be 0.2% of isolates in the continental United States.[3,15] In the 2007 GISP report, 28.6% of isolates from Honolulu, Hawaii, were QRNG, whereas among California sites, 18.7% to 36.3% of isolates were QRNG.[15,22] *N. gonorrhoeae* resistance to quinolones has increased almost every year since reporting began in 1990 and has become widespread in the United States, resulting in the CDC recommending against using quinolones for the treatment of gonococcal or related conditions (e.g., PID) acquired in the United States.[2] In 2007, 14.8% of all isolates collected by the GISP demonstrated resistance to ciprofloxacin.[16,22] Resistance to fluoroquinolones is associated with mutations of GyrA and is commonly identified in strains that produce β-lactamase and strains exhibiting chromosomally mediated resistance to penicillin and tetracycline.[23]

N. gonorrhoeae strains may therefore exhibit decreased susceptibility or complete resistance to the recommended dose of quinolones; the clinical importance of strains with decreased susceptibility is unknown.[24]

D.S. was likely infected with *N. gonorrhoeae* in the Philippines, and QRNG is highly likely; thus, an appropriate cephalosporin antibiotic such as IM ceftriaxone should be recommended. If he had been initially treated with ceftriaxone, the expectation would be that he would be free of gonococcal infection within 3 days. To date, ceftriaxone-resistant strains of *N. gonorrhoeae* have not been reported in the United States.

Anorectal and Pharyngeal Gonorrhea

EPIDEMIOLOGY

CASE 69-2

QUESTION 1: M.B. is a 24-year-old, sexually active, homosexual man with a 2-month history of perianal itching, painful defecation, constipation, a bloody mucoid rectal discharge, and a sore throat. Sigmoidoscopy revealed rectal mucosal inflammation but no apparent ulcers or fissures. Stool examination for parasites was negative, and a Venereal Disease Research Laboratory (VDRL) test was nonreactive. Both rectal and pharyngeal cultures revealed *N. gonorrhoeae.* How does gonorrhea in homosexual men compare with gonorrhea in heterosexual men?

Rectal infection occurs rarely in strictly heterosexual men, whereas in the male homosexual population, anorectal (25%) and pharyngeal (10%–25%) gonococcal infections occur more often.[6,25] Because pharyngeal[25,26] and anorectal gonococcal infections are often asymptomatic, a large reservoir of carriers in the homosexual male population may exist, diagnosed only with more sensitive DNA amplification techniques.[27] By comparison, very few urethral gonococcal infections are asymptomatic. In addition, recent data indicate that pharyngeal infections may be an important source of urethral gonorrhea in homosexual men, spread by fellatio.[25]

SIGNS AND SYMPTOMS

CASE 69-2, QUESTION 2: Are M.B.'s signs and symptoms consistent with gonorrhea?

Rectal gonorrhea produces the syndrome of proctitis with anorectal pain, mucopurulent anorectal discharge, constipation, tenesmus, and anorectal bleeding. The differential diagnosis of proctitis in the homosexual male includes rectal infection with *N. gonorrhoeae, C. trachomatis,* HSV, and syphilis. Proctitis, limited to the distal rectum, should be differentiated from proctocolitis, which is often caused by *Shigella* species, *Campylobacter* species, or *Entamoeba histolytica* in homosexual men. The incidence of rectal gonorrhea and *Chlamydia* has risen dramatically since 1996.[28] Rectal *Chlamydia* is often asymptomatic and observed more often than gonorrhea, necessitating testing for both pathogens.[29]

TREATMENT

CASE 69-2, QUESTION 3: How should M.B.'s diagnosis be managed?

The treatment of choice for patients such as M.B. with anorectal or pharyngeal gonorrhea is ceftriaxone 250 mg IM as a single dose (Table 69-1).[2] Azithromycin or doxycycline should also be given to treat possible coexisting rectal chlamydial infection. Patients such as M.B. with either anorectal or pharyngeal gonorrhea should be advised to avoid further unprotected sexual activity and should be counseled and tested for infection with HIV.

CASE 69-2, QUESTION 4: What are alternative regimens for patients with isolated anal or pharyngeal gonorrhea?

Women with anorectal gonorrhea alone can be treated with ceftriaxone or cefixime. Alternative regimens for isolated anorectal infection include a single-dose cephalosporin regimen such as ceftizoxime. Because spectinomycin is unavailable, patients with anorectal gonorrhea who are allergic to penicillin or cephalosporins should be desensitized before treatment is initiated. Patients with gonococcal infections of the pharynx should be treated with ceftriaxone; however, infections of this nature are more difficult to eradicate than infections at anorectal sites. Chlamydial coinfection is uncommon in pharyngeal gonorrhea, but should be treated with either doxycycline or azithromycin.[2]

PREVENTION

CASE 69-2, QUESTION 5: What measures have been used to prevent the sexual transmission of infection?

Condoms, when used properly, seem to provide a high degree of protection against the acquisition and transmission of STDs.[30] Previous studies indicated that the use of the spermicide nonoxynol-9 had activity against gonorrhea and *Chlamydia;* however, in light of recent evidence suggesting that nonoxynol-9 might actually increase the risk of acquiring HIV and other sexually transmitted diseases, the FDA currently requires manufacturers of nonoxynol-9 products to include a warning statement on the product's label that it does not protect against HIV or other STDs.[2,31] Topical antibacterial agents, urinating, and washing after intercourse are of little value in preventing the transmission of STDs. Douching may increase the risk of other STDs such as trichomoniasis.[32]

The prophylactic administration of antibiotics immediately before or soon after sexual intercourse is not recommended owing to increased costs and antimicrobial resistance. Rapid, specific tests and empiric symptomatic management should be used to enhance detection and treatment of gonorrhea.

PELVIC INFLAMMATORY DISEASE

The term pelvic inflammatory disease (PID) refers to a variety of inflammatory disorders of the upper female reproductive tract. This term does not denote the primary infection site (the fallopian tubes) or the causative micro-organisms. PID also has been used to connote an infection that occurs acutely when either vaginal or cervical micro-organisms traverse the sterile endometrium and ascend to the fallopian tubes. Acute salpingitis also may be used to describe an acute infection of the fallopian tubes. Therefore, the terms PID and salpingitis are used interchangeably in this discussion to denote an acute infection involving the fallopian tubes.

PID affects approximately 1 million women annually in the United States.[33] However, since 1985, the rate of hospitalization owing to PID has decreased 68%. Many cases of acute PID occur by sexual transmission, especially in young women 16 to 24 years who are more likely to have multiple sexual partners.[34] Risk factors for the development of PID include unprotected sexual intercourse before age 15, douching, BV, sex while menstruating, and smoking.[35] It is unclear whether an intrauterine device (IUD) increases the risk of PID, but it may be prudent to avoid placement when the patient has chlamydial or gonococcal cervicitis.[36] Two-thirds of PID cases resulting in infertility are asymptomatic, and up to one-third are incorrectly diagnosed owing to low specificity of diagnostic techniques. In the United States, infertility occurs in about 12.1% of women after the first episode of PID.[37] The estimated aggregate cost for PID is $2 billion, with most of this cost associated with treatment of acute PID.[38]

Etiology

Most cases of PID are caused by *C. trachomatis* and *N. gonorrhoeae.* Some micro-organisms that make up the vaginal flora are also associated with PID, including *Gardnerella vaginalis, Haemophilus influenzae*, and *Streptococcus agalactiae. Mycoplasma hominis, Ureaplasma urealyticum, M. genitalium,* and cytomegalovirus (CMV) have also been associated with PID, but a causative role is unclear.[2] Up to 70% of cases may be polymicrobial and include *M. genitalium* and BV.[39] Facultative enteric gram-negative bacilli and a variety of anaerobic bacteria have also been isolated from the upper genital tract of up to 70% of women with acute PID.[39] Women diagnosed with acute PID should be tested for *C. trachomatis* and *N. gonorrhoeae* and screened for HIV.[2]

Signs and Symptoms

The onset of symptoms of abdominal pain attributable to PID caused by either gonococci or chlamydia often occurs soon after the menstrual period. Symptoms of PID, if present, are often nonspecific, which can create a delay in or failure of diagnosis. Vaginal discharge, menorrhagia, dysuria, and dyspareunia are commonly associated with PID. Signs include cervical motion tenderness, uterine tenderness, or adnexal tenderness. Temperatures greater than 101°F, abnormal cervical or vaginal mucopurulent discharge, white blood cells (WBC) on saline microscopy of vaginal secretions, elevated erythrocyte sedimentation rate, an elevated C-reactive protein, or laboratory documentation of cervical infection with *N. gonorrhoeae* or *C. trachomatis* support a diagnosis of PID.[2] Clinical diagnosis has a sensitivity for PID of about 65% to 90%, whereas laparoscopy and a newer technique, transvaginal Doppler ultrasound, are about 100% specific, resulting in the combination of laparoscopy and clinical impression serving as the gold standard.[2,40,41] Unfortunately, laparoscopy and Doppler ultrasound are costly and often not readily available for acute cases, and they are not diagnostic for endometritis; thus, clinical impression is critical. A key to reducing the incidence of PID may be through active screening of *Chlamydia* in young, sexually active women.[42,43]

Clinical Sequelae

An abscess may form in the pelvic or abdominal cavity and in one or both fallopian tubes. Chronic abdominal pain develops in 18% of women with PID and may be the result of pelvic adhesions surrounding the tubes and ovaries. Tubal occlusion and fibrosis secondary to fallopian tube inflammation (salpingitis) result in 12% infertility after a single episode of PID, 25% infertility after two episodes, and 50% infertility after three or more episodes.[37] Other sequelae include ectopic pregnancy (9%) and chronic pelvic pain (18%).[44] The risk of ectopic pregnancy is increased approximately eightfold after one or more episodes of PID.

Diagnosis and Treatment

CASE 69-3

QUESTION 1: H.C., a 19-year-old, sexually active woman, complains of mild dysuria, a purulent vaginal discharge, fever, and moderately severe, bilateral, lower abdominal pain of 3 days' duration. Examination confirms uterine and adnexal tenderness, a purulent cervical exudate, and a temperature of 39°C. Laboratory examinations show a nonreactive VDRL and negative urinalysis. A pregnancy test performed was negative. The peripheral WBC count was mildly elevated (11,000/μL) with 70% polymorphonuclear leukocytes. Does H.C. have PID? How should she be treated?

Although fever and leukocytosis are often absent in mild or subacute PID, these findings in a woman with uterine and adnexal tenderness with cervical exudate increases the likelihood of acute PID. Recommended treatment regimens for PID are listed in Table 69-2 and should be initiated immediately after diagnosis of PID to prevent clinical sequelae; confirmation of the actual pathogen rarely takes place. Patients such as H.C. with mild-to-moderate PID can be hospitalized and treated with parenteral antibiotics; however, clinical efficacy and overall outcomes are equal between parenteral and oral therapy, and H.C. could also be treated on an outpatient basis. For inpatient treatment, the CDC recommends either intravenous (IV) cefotetan 2 g every 12 hours or IV cefoxitin 2 g every 6 hours for at least 24 hours beyond the first signs of clinical improvement along with doxycycline 100 mg every 12 hours. Once clinical improvement is noted, parenteral therapy may be discontinued, and PO doxycycline 100 mg every 12 hours can be continued to complete 14 days of therapy. For outpatient treatment, the CDC guidelines recommend either IM ceftriaxone 250 mg as a single dose or IM cefoxitin 2 g as a single dose (with probenecid 1 g PO for one dose) plus PO doxycycline 100 mg twice a day for 14 days with or without PO metronidazole 500 mg twice daily for 14 days.[2] A tetracycline derivative or an alternative agent that is active against *C. trachomatis* should be included in the treatment of PID; however, monotherapy with a tetracycline is not recommended because of the lack of activity against gram-negative aerobic and anaerobic organisms and *N. gonorrhoeae.* The addition of metronidazole, which covers anaerobic bacteria, should also be considered; anaerobes have been isolated from the upper reproductive tract of women with PID and may cause tubal and epithelial destruction.[2,45] Metronidazole is widely used by clinicians, as BV is frequently associated with PID.[2] Fluoroquinolones such as levofloxacin and ofloxacin are no longer recommended for the treatment of PID because of the increase in prevalence of QRNG in the United States.[16]

Both oral and IV doxycycline have similar bioavailability; therefore, doxycycline should be given PO whenever possible.[2] Substantial clinical improvement is usually seen within 3 days after initiation of therapy. Clindamycin plus gentamicin can be used alternatively in penicillin-allergic and pregnant women.[2] Because H.C. is sexually active, any sexual partners within the previous 60 days (or if >60 days, then the most recent sexual partner) should be empirically treated because of the risk of gonococcal or chlamydial urethritis as well as to reduce the risk of reinfection.[2]

TABLE 69-2

Antimicrobial Regimens Recommended by the CDC for Treatment of Acute Pelvic Inflammatory Disease

Treatment Setting, Drugs, Schedule	Advantage	Disadvantage	Clinical Considerations
Inpatient (Parenteral) Therapy			
Regimen A Cefotetan 2 g IV every 12 hours or cefoxitin 2 g IV every 6 hours plus doxycycline 100 mg IV or PO every 12 hours[a] Continue doxycycline (100 mg PO twice daily) after discharge to complete 14 days of therapy	Optimal coverage of *N. gonorrhoeae* (including resistant strains) and *C. trachomatis*	Possible suboptimal anaerobic coverage	Penicillin-allergic patients also may be allergic to cephalosporins; doxycycline use in pregnant patients may cause reversible inhibition of skeletal growth in the fetus and discoloration of teeth in young children
Regimen B Clindamycin 900 mg IV every 8 hours plus gentamicin loading dose IV or IM (2 mg/kg) followed by a maintenance dose of 1.5 mg/kg every 8 hours[b]	Optimal coverage of anaerobes and gram-negative enteric rods	Possible suboptimal coverage of *N. gonorrhoeae* and *C. trachomatis*	Patients with decreased renal function may not be good candidates for aminoglycoside treatment or may need a dosage adjustment
Alternative regimen Ampicillins/sulbactam 3 g IV every 6 hours plus doxycycline 100 mg PO or IV every 12 hours	Optimal coverage of *N. gonorrhoeae* and *C. trachomatis*	Inadequate coverage of anaerobes necessitates use of metronidazole or ampicillin/sulbactam	Not appropriate in pregnancy or in young children
Outpatient (Oral) Therapy[c]			
Regimen A Ceftriaxone 250 mg IM in a single dose plus doxycycline 100 mg PO twice daily for 14 days with or without metronidazole 500 mg PO twice daily for 14 days OR cefoxitin 2 g IM in a single dose and probenecid 1 g PO administered concurrently in a single dose plus doxycycline 100 mg PO twice daily for 14 days with or without metronidazole 500 mg PO twice daily for 14 days OR other parenteral third-generation cephalosporins (e.g., ceftizoxime or cefotaxime) plus doxycycline 100 mg PO twice daily for 14 days with or without metronidazole 500 mg PO twice daily for 14 days	Good to excellent coverage of *N. gonorrhoeae* and optimal coverage of *C. trachomatis*	Possible suboptimal anaerobic coverage necessitating the addition of metronidazole	Optimal cephalosporin is unclear; more complicated regimen requiring combination of parenteral and oral therapies

[a]Considering the oral bioavailability of doxycycline, PO therapy should be preferentially used over IV.
[b]Single daily dosing may be substituted.
[c]Consider for mild-to-moderate acute PID.
Adapted from Workowski KA et al. Sexually transmitted diseases treatment guidelines, 2010. *MMWR Recomm Rep*. 2010;59(RR-12):1.

COMPLICATED GONORRHEA

Disseminated Gonococcal Infection

SIGNS AND SYMPTOMS

CASE 69-4

QUESTION 1: S.P., a 28-year-old, sexually active woman, was seen for stiffness and pain of the right wrist and left ankle and fever (38°C). On physical examination, the knee and wrist joints were found to be hot, red, and swollen; papules and pustular lesions were observed on S.P.'s legs and forearms. A latex fixation test for rheumatoid factor was negative. A tap of the right knee yielded an effusion with a WBC count of 34,000/μL (80% polymorphonuclear leukocytes). Cultures of the skin lesions were negative, but *N. gonorrhoeae* was isolated from the throat, cervix, blood, and synovial fluid. A chest radiograph, echocardiogram, and electrocardiogram all were normal, and no murmur could be appreciated. Assess S.P.'s clinical presentation.

S.P.'s signs, symptoms, and laboratory findings are consistent with gonococcal bacteremia, which today occurs in less than 1% of women and men with gonorrhea. The most common manifestation of gonococcemia is the gonococcal arthritis–dermatitis syndrome or disseminated gonococcal infection (DGI) exhibited by S.P. Symptoms include fever, occasional chills, a mild tenosynovitis of the small joints, and skin lesions; the latter primarily involving the distal extremities are petechial, papular, pustular, and hemorrhagic in appearance.[2]

TABLE 69-3
Treatment of Disseminated Gonococcal Infection[a]

No Penicillin Allergy
Parenteral
Recommended—Ceftriaxone 1 g IV or IM every 24 hours **Alternative**—Cefotaxime 1 g IV every 8 hours or ceftizoxime 1 g IV every 8 hours
Oral[b]
Cefixime 400 mg PO twice daily

[a] Parenteral treatment should be continued for 24 to 48 hours beyond clinical improvement.
[b] Treat for 7 days after switching from parenteral therapy.
Adapted from Workowski KA et al. Sexually transmitted diseases treatment guidelines, 2010. *MMWR Recomm Rep*. 2010;59(RR-12):1.

Diagnosis of DGI is made by Gram stain and culture. However, blood cultures are positive in only 33% of DGI cases, even when culture samples are obtained early in the course of the infection.[2] The low positive yield from blood cultures may be attributable to the low inoculum or intermittent bacteremic period. Routine culture of the urethra, cervix, pharynx, and rectum should be performed in any patient suspected of having DGI.

TREATMENT

CASE 69-4, QUESTION 2: How should S.P. be managed? How quickly will she respond to therapy?

Patients like S.P. with gonococcal arthritis and bacteremia should be hospitalized for treatment with ceftriaxone 1 g IV or IM daily until clinical improvement, such as decreased fever and pain, is sustained for 24 to 48 hours, at which time therapy may be switched to oral cefixime 400 mg twice daily for 7 days (Table 69-3).[2] Symptoms and signs of tenosynovitis should improve markedly within 48 hours. Septic gonococcal arthritis with purulent synovial fluid may require repeated aspiration and resolves more slowly.

Treatment of Gonococcal Endocarditis and Meningitis

CASE 69-4, QUESTION 3: How should gonococcal endocarditis and meningitis be treated?

Gonococcal endocarditis and meningitis, occurring in only 1% to 3% of DGIs, require high-dose IV therapy such as ceftriaxone (1–2 g IV every 12 hours) for 10 to 14 days in the case of meningitis and for 4 weeks in the case of endocarditis.[2]

Neonatal Disseminated Gonococcal Infection: Treatment

CASE 69-4, QUESTION 4: How should neonatal DGI and meningitis be managed?

Neonatal DGI and meningitis can be treated with either ceftriaxone 25 to 50 mg/kg (IV or IM) daily or cefotaxime 25 mg/kg (IV or IM) every 12 hours. Treatment is for 7 days for DGI; however, meningitis requires 10 to 14 days of treatment.[2] Although ceftriaxone is also effective in the treatment of neonatal DGI and meningitis, cefotaxime is considered a safer choice in the neonatal population.

CHLAMYDIA TRACHOMATIS

Chlamydia trachomatis was first isolated from patients with lymphogranuloma venereum (LGV). However, laboratory diagnoses for this pathogen were not developed until the 1960s and 1970s.[2] The rate of reported *Chlamydia* infections has climbed steadily each year since the 1980s. In 2009, just over 1.2 million cases were reported to the CDC, the most of any reported STD. From 2008 to 2009, there was a 2.8% increase in cases, which corresponds to 409.2 cases per 100,000 individuals.[3] This increase may be attributable to the increased development and use of more sensitive screening tests, improved national reporting efforts, or a true increase in the incidence of disease.[2] Women are three times more likely than men to be infected with *Chlamydia*—592.2 cases versus 219.3 cases per 100,000 individuals, respectively, in 2009. However, from 2005 to 2009, the infection rate among men increased 37.6% compared with 20.3% in women. The highest rate of infection is in women 15 to 19 years of age (3,329.3 cases per 100,000 individuals) and in men 20 to 24 years of age (1,120.6 cases per 100,000 individuals).[3] If left untreated, chlamydial infection in women can lead to serious sequelae such as PID, ectopic pregnancy, and infertility. Asymptomatic infection is also observed in both men and women; however, routine screening is recommended for sexually active women up to 25 years of age and older women with risk factors for infection (e.g., multiple sexual partners or having a new sexual partner). Screening sexually active men for *C. trachomatis* can be considered in settings with a high prevalence of the infection.[2]

C. trachomatis, an intracellular obligate organism, can be diagnosed either by culture, direct immunofluorescence assay (DFA), enzyme immunoassay (EIA), or NAAT of endocervical or male urethral swabs.[2] However, *C. trachomatis* is a difficult organism to demonstrate in clinical specimens because cell culture techniques are not readily available to the practitioner. Because few practitioners have access to facilities for isolation of *C. trachomatis,* most chlamydial infections are diagnosed and treated based on clinical impression and laboratory techniques. Diagnostic tests, such as NAATs, DFAs, and EIAs, are generally sensitive methods for detecting *C. trachomatis.* Ligase chain reaction and PCR are two NAATs with wide commercial availability, are relatively simple to use, can be performed using urine or genital swab specimens, and are more sensitive than non-NAATs.[12] A test of cure is not necessary unless patient compliance is questionable, symptoms persist, or reinfection is suspected. Repeat testing fewer than 3 weeks after initiation of treatment is not recommended because false-negative results may occur as a result of undetectable *C. trachomatis* organisms. Moreover, false positives may occur with repeat NAATs with the continued excretion of dead organisms.

A variety of clinical syndromes are caused by *C. trachomatis,* including cervicitis, urethritis, bartholinitis, endometritis, salpingitis, and perihepatitis in women, and urethritis, epididymitis, prostatitis, proctitis, and Reiter syndrome in men.[2] The spectrum of chlamydial infections closely resembles those caused by the gonococcus, which is why many patients presenting with these syndromes are treated with drugs effective against both organisms.

There is controversy in how *C. trachomatis* is cultured and what the in vitro results mean clinically, especially in the 10% to 15% of cases that fail treatment.[46] The CDC thus uses cure rates instead of microbial susceptibilities to make treatment recommendations. Only azithromycin and doxycycline have 97% and 98%

cure rates, respectively.[2,47] Alternatives include erythromycin, ofloxacin, and levofloxacin. Other agents such as the penicillins, cephalosporins, aminoglycosides, clarithromycin, ciprofloxacin, and metronidazole should not be used because they have not been evaluated adequately or are not reliably effective.[2]

Nongonococcal Urethritis

ETIOLOGY

CASE 69-5

QUESTION 1: T.K., a 26-year-old, sexually active man, complains of mild dysuria and a mucoidlike urethral discharge beginning 15 days after his last intercourse. He has no fever, lymphadenopathy, penile lesions, or hematuria. A Gram stain smear of an anterior urethral specimen showed 20 polymorphonuclear neutrophilic leukocytes (PMNs) per oil immersion (×1,000) field and no gram-negative diplococci. What pathogens are associated with nongonococcal urethritis (NGU)?

In the United States, NGU is the most common STD in men.[48,49] *C. trachomatis* is a frequent cause of NGU, representing 15% to 40% of all cases. Other agents that have been associated with NGU include *M. genitalium*, *T. vaginalis*, HSV, and *adenovirus*; however, the cause for the majority of NGU cases is unknown.[2] The variety of pathogens and disparity among identification techniques require sound clinical judgment and an algorithmic laboratory testing approach to accurately identify and treat the cause. An NAAT, if available, should be performed to rule out the presence of *C. trachomatis*.

SIGNS AND SYMPTOMS

CASE 69-5, QUESTION 2: Describe the clinical presentation of a person with NGU. Is T.K.'s presentation consistent with NGU? How does one differentiate between NGU and gonococcal urethritis?

T.K.'s presentation is typical. Compared with gonococcal urethritis, NGU typically produces less severe and less frequent dysuria and less penile discharge. Chlamydial urethral infection is completely asymptomatic more often than gonococcal urethral infection. The incubation period for gonococcal urethritis is 2 to 7 days, whereas the incubation period for NGU is typically 2 to 3 weeks.

Nonetheless, NGU and gonococcal urethritis cannot be reliably differentiated solely on the basis of symptoms and signs. If there is objective evidence of a urethral discharge (expressed by milking the urethra), a Gram stain with fewer than 5 WBCs per oil immersion field in the urethral secretion, or a positive leukocyte esterase test demonstrating 10 WBCs per high-power field, the diagnosis of NGU is made by excluding the presence of *N. gonorrhoeae* by Gram stain or culture.

Treatment

CASE 69-5, QUESTION 3: How should T.K. be treated?

If *C. trachomatis* cannot be ruled out, therapy with azithromycin 1 g PO for one dose should be ordered to cover both *M. genitalium* and *Chlamydia* as doxycycline does not effectively eradicate *M. genitalium*.[2] Azithromycin also has the advantage of a single-dose regimen, which may aid in patient compliance. However, doxycycline 100 mg PO twice daily for 7 days may be prescribed when chlamydial urethritis is confirmed. Erythromycin base 500 mg PO four times a day or erythromycin ethylsuccinate 800 mg PO four times a day for 7 days are alternative CDC-approved regimens. Additionally, ofloxacin 300 mg PO twice daily or levofloxacin 500 mg PO every day for 7 days are other alternatives, but they offer no significant advantages compared with the previously mentioned agents, may not treat *U. urealyticum* adequately, and are significantly more expensive.[2,50] Ciprofloxacin should be avoided because treatment failures have been reported.[51] Patient counseling should emphasize the need for abstinence from sexual intercourse at least until the prescribed course of therapy has been completed (or 7 days after single-dose therapy) by the patient and his sexual partner(s).[2] There is some indication that the proportion of NGU caused by *C. trachomatis* is declining, potentially being replaced by an increased proportion of *U. urealyticum*, which is variably cured at 2 weeks by azithromycin (73%) and doxycycline (65%).[52]

RECURRENT INFECTION

CASE 69-5, QUESTION 4: T.K. was treated with doxycycline 100 mg twice daily for 7 days. He remained asymptomatic for 14 days after completion of his therapy, when he again noticed similar symptoms of dysuria and a mucoidlike urethral discharge. How should T.K.'s recurrent infection be treated?

The major problem encountered in the treatment of NGU is the high rate of recurrent infections. Approximately 20% to 60% of patients experience recurrent or persistent urethritis within 1 to 2 weeks after treatment.[53] The rate of recurrence is highest in patients with idiopathic urethritis, that is, those not infected with *C. trachomatis* or *U. urealyticum*. Recurrence suggests re-exposure to an untreated partner, whereas persistent urethritis (without improvement during therapy) suggests the presence of other organisms including *M. genitalium*, *U. urealyticum*, or *T. vaginalis*.[2] NGU that persists or recurs should be retreated with the initial regimen if the patient was not compliant or the sexual partner was not treated. For patients with persistent symptoms who were compliant with the initial regimen and were not re-exposed, the CDC recommends using either metronidazole or tinidazole 2 g PO as a single dose plus a single 1-g dose of azithromycin if not used for the initial episode.[2]

Men with acute epididymitis often have chlamydial or gonococcal infection, particularly if they are younger than 35 years of age or have a urethral discharge. *Escherichia coli* and *Pseudomonas* species are common pathogens in homosexual men. In older men, sexually transmitted epididymitis is less common and is more commonly caused by urinary tract instrumentation, surgery, systemic disease, or immune suppression.[2] If testicular tenderness is present with urethritis, and the clinical impression is consistent with epididymitis caused by *Chlamydia* or gonorrhea, the CDC recommend a single dose of ceftriaxone 250 mg IM plus doxycycline 100 mg PO twice for 10 days. For acute epididymitis caused by enteric organisms or with a negative gonococcal culture or NAAT, ofloxacin 300 mg PO twice daily or levofloxacin 500 mg PO once daily for 10 days may be used.[2,45]

SEXUAL PARTNERS

CASE 69-5, QUESTION 5: A.C., T.K.'s girlfriend, comes into the clinic 3 weeks after T.K.'s last visit. She is worried that she may have a similar infection, although she has no signs or symptoms. What clinical manifestations of chlamydial

infections are seen in women? Should A.C. be treated for suspected chlamydial infection?

In the absence of cultures for *Chlamydia,* empirical treatment of women who are sexual partners of men with NGU is recommended. Routine partner referral for presumptive therapy is not indicated for nonchlamydial NGU.[54] Many partners are asymptomatic, but from 30% to 70% are culture positive if tested. A.C. should be examined carefully for mucopurulent cervicitis and salpingitis. Although many women with chlamydial infection of the cervix are asymptomatic, up to one-quarter have evidence of mucopurulent discharge.[55] A Gram stain of appropriately collected mucopurulent endocervical discharge from patients with *Chlamydia* infection shows many PMNs and no gonococci.

Regardless of findings, treatment should be initiated with the same doxycycline regimen used for NGU. However, if A.C. is pregnant, tetracyclines and fluoroquinolones should be avoided. Azithromycin 1 g PO as a single dose or amoxicillin 500 mg PO three times a day for 7 days could be used instead. Alternatively, either erythromycin base 500 mg PO four times a day for 7 days, erythromycin base 250 mg PO four times a day for 14 days, erythromycin ethylsuccinate 800 mg PO four times a day for 7 days, or erythromycin ethylsuccinate 400 mg PO four times a day for 14 days can be used.[2] Erythromycin estolate should be avoided in pregnancy because of the increased risk of hepatotoxicity. Azithromycin is safe and effective during pregnancy.[56,57] High rates of GI side effects limit the use of erythromycin. In pregnant women, a repeat NAAT is recommended 3 weeks after completion of therapy to ensure therapeutic cure.[2] Coinfection with *Chlamydia* is common in heterosexual men and women with gonorrhea. Therefore, drug regimens effective against both organisms are recommended in patients with gonorrhea to prevent postgonococcal chlamydial morbidity (epididymitis, mucopurulent cervicitis, salpingitis) and to reduce the genital reservoir of *C. trachomatis.*

Lymphogranuloma Venereum

ETIOLOGY AND SIGNS AND SYMPTOMS

CASE 69-6

QUESTION 1: S.F., a 32-year-old male student who recently arrived from a trip to Western Europe, presents to the STD clinic with a chief complaint of pain and swelling in the groin. He reports the appearance of a small ulcer on his penis about 2 weeks ago, which resolved rapidly. On examination, he has a bubo (inflammatory swelling of one or more lymph nodes in the groin) with surrounding erythema on his right side. S.F. also has a fever (39°C). Laboratory findings are remarkable for a mild leukocytosis (WBC count, 12,000 cells/μL). What organisms are responsible for LGV? Describe its clinical course. What subjective and objective manifestations in S.F. are consistent with LGV?

LGV (see http://www.cdc.gov/STD/TRAINING/CLINICALSLIDES/slides-dl.htm for symptoms of this STD) or Nicolas-Favre disease has historically been considered a rare disease in the United States and other developed nations; however, outbreaks have been recently reported in the Netherlands and Great Britain as well as in the United States in New York, Texas, and San Francisco.[58,59] The cause of LGV is usually *C. trachomatis* serovars L1, L2, or L3, which are different from those serovars responsible for chlamydia urethritis.[60] Three stages of LGV infection are recognized in heterosexual men.[61]

Stage I is characterized by a small genital papule or vesicle that appears between 3 and 30 days after exposure. The patient usually is asymptomatic; the ulcer heals rapidly and leaves no scar. This primary lesion is consistent with that reported by S.F. Many patients with LGV recall no primary lesion. Stage II is characterized by acute, painful lymphadenitis with bubo formation (the inguinal syndrome); it often is accompanied by pain and fever, as illustrated by S.F. Without treatment, the buboes may rupture, forming numerous sinus tracts that drain chronically. Adenopathy above and below the inguinal ligament results in the "groove sign." Healing occurs slowly, and most patients experience no serious sequelae. Patients in this stage also may present with an anogenitorectal syndrome, which is accompanied by proctocolitis and hyperplasia of intestinal and perirectal lymphatic tissue. Stage III is characterized by perirectal abscesses, rectovaginal fistulae (in women), rectal strictures, and genital elephantiasis.[61] Appropriate treatment of stage II LGV usually prevents these late complications.

An acute anorectal syndrome of LGV occurs in homosexual men who acquire the infection through rectal receptive intercourse. In these cases, a primary anal ulcer may be noted with associated inguinal adenopathy (anal lymphatics drain to inguinal nodes). Subsequently, acute hemorrhagic proctocolitis occurs with tenesmus, rectal pain, constipation, and a mucopurulent, bloody rectal discharge. Rectal biopsy may show granulomatous colitis, mimicking Crohn disease. Perirectal pelvic adenopathy also occurs.

TREATMENT

CASE 69-6, QUESTION 2: How should S.F. be treated?

Current CDC recommendations for LGV include doxycycline 100 mg PO twice daily or erythromycin base 500 mg PO four times a day for 21 days.[2] Surgical intervention may be needed for later forms of the disease. Azithromycin 1 g weekly for 3 weeks may be effective, but clinical data on its use are lacking.[2]

SYPHILIS

Epidemiology

Syphilis (see http://www.cdc.gov/STD/TRAINING/CLINICALSLIDES/slides-dl.htm for symptoms of this STD) is caused by the spirochete, *Treponema pallidum.* The rates of primary and secondary syphilis in the United States increased in the late 1980s secondary to crack cocaine use (and associated unsafe sex practices), but from 1990 to 2000, rates have decreased to those reported in 1941 when reporting began, representing an 87.9% decrease since 1990.[62,63] However, the number of cases of primary and secondary syphilis have steadily risen since 2000, reaching a high of 13,997 cases in 2009.[3] Another concern is that syphilis facilitates the transmission of HIV, and recent outbreaks of syphilis have been associated with HIV-positive men who have sex with men.[64,65] Since 2005, rates of congenital syphilis have increased, and in 2009, 427 cases were reported to the CDC, which represents 10 cases per 100,000 individuals (Fig. 69-5).[3] This increase may be attributable to the increase in primary and secondary syphilis cases in women. The *Healthy People 2020* goals for primary and secondary syphilis among women is 1.4 cases per 100,000 individuals and among men is 6.8 cases per 100,000 individuals (Fig. 69-6).[4]

The clinical manifestations of syphilis have not changed appreciably since their first description. However, early diagnosis, treatment, and greater physician and patient awareness of the disease

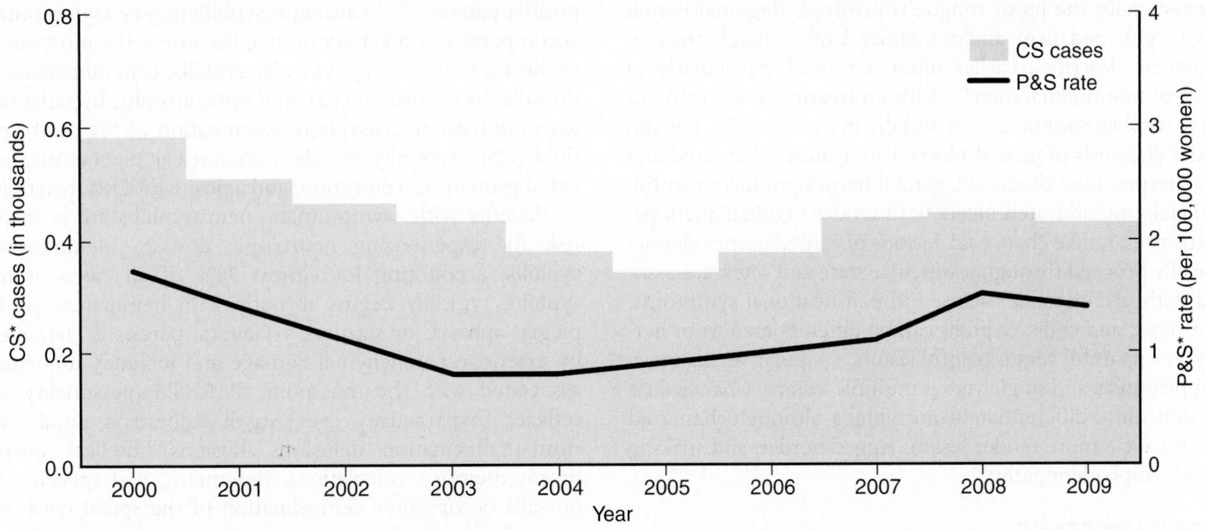

FIGURE 69-5 Congenital syphilis (CS)—reported cases among infants by year of birth and rates of primary and secondary syphilis (P&S) among women, 2000–2009. (Reprinted from Centers for Disease Control and Prevention. *2009 Sexually Transmitted Disease Surveillance*. Atlanta, GA: US Dept of Health and Human Services; 2010.)

have reduced the incidence of its severe forms. Penicillin continues to be the mainstay of therapy.

Clinical Stages

CASE 69-7

QUESTION 1: D.M., a 27-year-old homosexual man, presents to the STD clinic with complaints of malaise, headache, and fever of 4 days' duration. He also reveals that he had a sore on his penis about 8 weeks ago, but it has since resolved. On examination, he is afebrile and has a widespread maculopapular skin rash that involves the soles of his feet; general lymphadenopathy also is appreciated. Medical history is unremarkable except for one episode of gonorrhea 2 years ago that was treated with procaine penicillin. Laboratory findings include a normal peripheral WBC count, a negative serology for HIV antigen, and a positive rapid plasma reagin (RPR) test and fluorescent treponemal antibody absorption (FTA-Abs) test. Describe the clinical course of syphilis. Are D.M.'s symptoms consistent with this infection?

PRIMARY STAGE

The average incubation period for syphilis is 3 weeks and ranges from 10 to 90 days.[66] During this incubation period, *T. pallidum* can be demonstrated in the lymph and blood. The primary chancre develops at the site of inoculation as a painless papule that becomes ulcerated and indurated. The ulcer is nontender and filled with spirochetes. The chancre usually involves the penis in the heterosexual male, the penis or anus in the homosexual male, and the vulva, perineum, or cervix in the female.

ONLINE CONTENT

For a visual of a chancre of syphilis, go to http://thepoint.lww.com/AT10e.

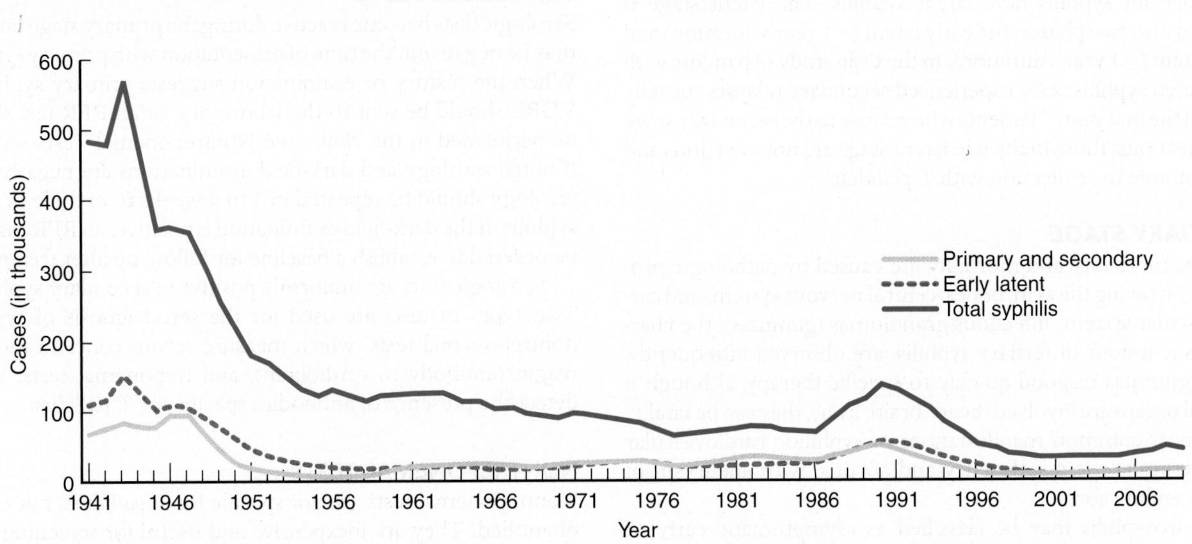

FIGURE 69-6 Syphilis—reported cases by stage of infection, United States, 1941–2009. Note: the Healthy People 2020 target for primary and secondary syphilis is 1.4 new cases per 100,000 for women and 6.8 new cases per 100,000 for men. (Reprinted from Centers for Disease Control and Prevention. *2009 Sexually Transmitted Disease Surveillance*. Atlanta, GA: US Dept of Health and Human Services; 2010.)

Occasionally, the lip or tongue is involved. Regional lymph nodes are enlarged, firm, and nontender. Unfortunately, the typical chancre described earlier often is missed, particularly in women or homosexual men.[67] Without treatment, the primary chancre resolves spontaneously, usually in 2 to 6 weeks. The differential diagnosis of genital ulcers also includes chancroid and genital herpes. Like chancroid, genital herpes produces painful, superficial, nonindurated ulcers with tender inguinal adenopathy. However, unlike chancroid, lesions of genital herpes characteristically proceed through a vesicular state and often are associated with urethritis, cervicitis, and constitutional symptoms, such as fever and chills. Syphilis can be differentiated from herpes by a nonpainful versus painful lesion, a papular versus vesicular appearance, and single versus multiple lesions. Chancroid is more difficult to differentiate from syphilis, although chancroid tends to have a more tender lesion, jagged border, and striking inguinal lymphadenopathy.[66]

SECONDARY STAGE

Approximately 6 weeks after a chancre first appears, the untreated patient manifests signs and symptoms of the secondary stage of syphilis. This stage is currently evidenced by D.M. Skin lesions of secondary syphilis may erupt in a variety of patterns and are usually widespread in distribution. A macular lesion often is the earliest manifestation in this stage. The lesion is round or oval, occurs primarily on the trunk, and is rose or pink in color. As lesions mature, they become papular or nodular with scaling (the so-called papulosquamous rash). The differential diagnosis of diffuse papulosquamous rashes includes psoriasis, pityriasis rosea, and lichen planus. In syphilis, the palms and soles are characteristically involved, and oral lesions (mucous patches) may occur. Generalized lymphadenopathy usually is present, and patchy alopecia may be seen. The most infectious lesion of secondary syphilis is condyloma latum. Condylomata lata are characteristically wet, indurated lesions occurring primarily in the perineum or around the anus as a result of direct spread from the primary lesion. Laboratory studies sometimes reveal anemia, leukocytosis, or an increased erythrocyte sedimentation rate. Other manifestations of secondary syphilis include mild hepatitis, aseptic meningitis, uveitis, neuropathies, and glomerulonephritis.[68]

LATENT STAGE

By definition, untreated, asymptomatic persons with serologic evidence for syphilis have latent syphilis. The latent stage is divided into two phases: the early latent (<1 year's duration) and late latent (>1 year's duration). In the Oslo study of patients with untreated syphilis, 25% experienced secondary relapses, usually within the first year.[69] Patients who relapse to the secondary stage are infectious; those in the late latent stage are not infectious and are immune to reinfection with *T. pallidum.*

TERTIARY STAGE

Serious morbidity and mortality are caused by pathologic processes involving the skin, bones, central nervous system, and cardiovascular system. Infectious granulomas (gummas), the characteristic lesions of tertiary syphilis, are observed infrequently. Most gummas respond quickly to specific therapy, although if critical organs are involved (heart, brain, liver), they can be fatal.[70] The most common manifestations of syphilitic cardiovascular disease are aortic insufficiency and aortitis, with aneurysm of the ascending aorta.

Neurosyphilis may be classified as asymptomatic early or late, meningeal, parenchymatous, or gummatous. Although neurosyphilis has been a rare complication for more than 40 years because of the widespread of use of penicillin, syphilitic meningitis, an early form of neurosyphilis, may be more common in HIV-positive patients.[66,71] Late neurosyphilis may be asymptomatic or accompanied by a variety of manifestations; the most common syndromes are meningovascular syphilis, general paresis, tabes dorsalis (locomotor ataxia), and optic atrophy. In patients with asymptomatic neurosyphilis, examination of the cerebrospinal fluid (CSF) typically reveals mononuclear pleocytosis, an elevated protein concentration, and a positive VDRL reaction.

Patients with asymptomatic neurosyphilis are at increased risk for experiencing neurologic disease. Meningovascular syphilis, accounting for almost 38% of all cases of neurosyphilis, typically begins abruptly with hemiparesis or hemiplegia, aphasia, or seizures.[72] General paresis is characterized by extensive parenchymal damage and includes abnormalities associated with the mnemonic PARESIS (personality, affect, reflexes [hyperactive], eye [Argyll Robertson pupil], sensorium [hallucination, delusions, illusions], intellect [decreased recent memory, calculations, judgment], and speech). Tabes dorsalis occurs after demyelination of the spinal cord. Symptoms observed include an ataxic, wide-based gait and foot slap; paresthesias; bladder irregularities; impotence; areflexia; and loss of position, deep pain, and temperature sensation. The Argyll Robertson pupil, seen in both paresis and tabes dorsalis, is a small, irregular pupil that reacts to accommodation but not to light.

Laboratory Tests

CASE 69-7, QUESTION 2: Evaluate D.M.'s laboratory findings.

DARK-FIELD EXAMINATION

Exudate expressed from the chancre or from condyloma latum is examined with a dark-field microscope. The diagnosis of syphilis is made if spirochetes with characteristic corkscrew morphology and mobility are present. Dark-field examination is the most specific and sensitive method, but only with an experienced microscopist.[73] Three dark-field examinations on consecutive days should be performed before considering the test negative in suspected primary syphilis.

SEROLOGIC TESTS

Serologic tests become reactive during the primary stage but they may be negative at the time of presentation with primary syphilis. When the history or examination suggests primary syphilis, a VDRL should be sent to the laboratory, or an RPR test should be performed in the clinic (see Nontreponemal Tests section). If initial serology and dark-field examinations are negative, the serology should be repeated in 1 to 4 weeks to exclude primary syphilis. If the dark-field examination is positive, an RPR may still be ordered to establish a baseline for follow-up after treatment.

Serologic tests are uniformly positive in secondary syphilis.[66] Two types of tests are used for the serodiagnosis of syphilis: nontreponemal tests, which measure serum concentrations of reagin (antibody to cardiolipin), and treponemal tests, which detect the presence of antibodies specific for *T. pallidum.*

NONTREPONEMAL TESTS

Nontreponemal tests are not specific for *T. pallidum*, but can be quantified. They are inexpensive and useful for screening large numbers of people. The most widely used nontreponemal tests are the VDRL test and the RPR Card Test. The RPR test is the most widely used because it is simpler to perform than the VDRL. Results of the VDRL and RPR are not interchangeable; thus, the

TABLE 69-4
Treatment Guidelines for Syphilis

Stage	Recommended Regimen	Alternative Regimen
Early (primary, secondary, or early latent)[a]	Benzathine penicillin G 2.4 million units single dose IM	Doxycycline 100 mg PO BID for 14 days *or* Tetracycline 500 mg PO QID for 14 days *or* Ceftriaxone 1 g IM/IV every day for 8 to 10 days *or* Azithromycin 2 g PO × 1 dose
Late latent or latent syphilis of unknown duration	Lumbar puncture	Lumbar puncture
	If CSF normal: benzathine penicillin G 2.4 million units/wk × 3 weeks IM If CSF abnormal: treat as neurosyphilis	If CSF normal: doxycycline 100 mg PO BID for 28 days If CSF abnormal: treat as neurosyphilis
Neurosyphilis (asymptomatic or symptomatic)[b]	Aqueous crystalline penicillin G 18–24 million units IV every day × 10–14 days[c]	Procaine penicillin 2.4 million units IM every day plus probenecid 500 mg PO QID, both for 10–14 days
Congenital	Aqueous crystalline penicillin G 100,000–150,000 units/kg/d, administered as 50,000 units/kg/dose IV every 12 hours during the first 7 days of life, and every 8 hours thereafter for a total of 10 days[d] *or* Procaine penicillin G 50,000 units/kg/dose IM a day in a single dose for 10 days	If CSF normal: benzathine penicillin G 50,000 units/kg/dose IM in a single dose
Syphilis in pregnancy	According to stage	According to stage

[a] Some experts recommend repeating this regimen after 7 days for HIV-infected patients.
[b] Because of the shorter duration of therapy as compared with latent syphilis, some experts recommend giving benzathine penicillin G, 2.4 million units/wk for up to 3 weeks, after the completion of these neurosyphilis regimens to provide a comparable total duration of therapy.
[c] Administered as 3–4 million units IV every 4 hours or continuous infusion.
[d] All infants born to women treated during pregnancy with erythromycin must be treated with penicillin at birth.
Adapted from Workowski KA et al. Sexually transmitted diseases treatment guidelines, 2010. *MMWR Recomm Rep.* 2010;59(RR-12):1.

same test should be used throughout the posttreatment monitoring period.[74]

The result reported in the quantitative VDRL test is the most dilute serum concentration with a positive reaction. This test may be used to follow the decline in VDRL titer after effective therapy (see Case 69-7, Question 5). In some individuals, a serofast reaction occurs in which nontreponemal antibodies may remain at a low titer for up to their entire lives. When false-positive tests occur, the titer usually is low (e.g., VDRL or RPR titer of 1:8).[75] In secondary syphilis, sensitivity of the RPR and VDRL approach 100% owing to the high antibody concentrations.[76]

TREPONEMAL TESTS

Specific treponemal tests confirm a positive nontreponemal test. The FTA-Abs test is the most commonly used treponemal test. Because the FTA-Abs test requires fluorescence microscopy, it is relatively difficult and expensive to perform and not appropriate for screening.

Treatment

CASE 69-7, QUESTION 3: How should D.M. be treated?

The CDC recommends penicillin G for the treatment of all stages of syphilis (Table 69-4).[2] Every effort should be made to rule out penicillin allergy before choosing alternative agents. Considering that penicillin-resistant *T. pallidum* has never been observed, treatment regimens for syphilis have changed relatively little during the years.

As shown in Table 69-4, recommended therapy for primary, secondary, or latent syphilis (with negative findings in the CSF) of less than 1 year's duration is a single, IM 2.4-million unit dose of benzathine penicillin G. If penicillin is contraindicated, tetracycline 500 mg PO four times a day or doxycycline 100 mg PO twice a day for 14 days are the main alternatives. If the patient is allergic to penicillin, is not pregnant, and cannot receive tetracycline or doxycycline, a 10- to 14-day regimen of ceftriaxone 1 g IM or IV every day or a single 2-g dose of azithromycin are options.[2] The use of erythromycin as an alternative is no longer recommended by the CDC because of its poor efficacy. The optimal dose, duration, and efficacy of these alternative regimens are not well defined, necessitating close follow-up of patients. Recent studies, however, have shown that azithromycin 2 g PO as a one-time dose is at least equivalent to benzathine penicillin G.[77,78] Skin testing should be performed for individuals who claim allergy to penicillin. If the patient is truly allergic, he or she should be desensitized.[2] Latent syphilis (>1 year's duration) and cardiovascular syphilis are treated with IM benzathine penicillin G (2.4 million units) for a total of 3 weeks.[2]

NEUROSYPHILIS

CASE 69-7, QUESTION 4: Would D.M.'s treatment differ if his CSF had tested positive for syphilis?

Neurosyphilis can present at any stage of syphilis. When conventional IM doses of benzathine penicillin G are administered, measurable levels of penicillin are not obtainable in the CSF. However, this does not mean that penicillin does not concentrate in meningeal tissue.[79] Treatment failures, as well as late clinical progression to neurosyphilis, can occur after treatment with the recommended IM regimen. After one dose, benzathine penicillin reaches peak plasma concentrations slower (13 to 24 hours) but with more prolonged treponemicidal plasma concentrations (7 to 10 days) when compared with procaine penicillin (1 to 4 hours to peak; 12- to 24-hour treponemicidal plasma concentrations).[79] Reports of benzathine penicillin failures in the 1970s has resulted in the CDC recommending treatment with aqueous crystalline penicillin G, 3 to 4 million units IV every 4 hours, or 18 to 24 million units per day continuous infusion, for 10 to 14 days.

Alternatively, neurosyphilis can be treated with procaine penicillin (2.4 million units IM daily) plus probenecid (500 mg PO four times a day) for 10 to 14 days. Some experts add benzathine penicillin G (2.4 million units IM once a week for up to 3 weeks) after the completion of aqueous penicillin G or procaine penicillin.[2] Penicillin-allergic patients should be skin tested to confirm allergy, and if confirmed, the patient should be desensitized and treated with an appropriate penicillin regimen. The World Health Organization also recommends penicillin-allergic nonpregnant patients receive either doxycycline 200 mg PO twice a day or tetracycline 500 mg PO four times a day for 30 days.[80]

FOLLOW-UP

CASE 69-7, QUESTION 5: D.M. was treated with a single IM dose of benzathine penicillin (2.4 million units). How should his response to therapy be monitored?

Physical examination and a quantitative VDRL or RPR test for primary and secondary syphilis should be repeated at least 6 and 12 months after therapy.[2] Retreatment should be considered when the RPR or VDRL titer does not decline fourfold in 6 months. Patients with HIV coinfection should receive periodic serologic testing.[66] Patients with latent syphilis should be retested 6, 12, and 24 months after treatment. Close serologic monitoring is necessary if antibiotics other than penicillin are used; CSF examination should be performed in these patients at their last follow-up visit. Patients with neurosyphilis should be monitored serologically every 6 months; CSF examinations should be repeated at 6-month intervals until normal. If still abnormal at 2 years, retreatment should be considered. Return of lesions, a fourfold increase in titer, or a titer of 1:8 that does not fall at least fourfold within 12 months necessitates retreatment. Suspected treatment failures, especially with abnormal CSF, should be treated as described for neurosyphilis. However, false-positive serologic results should be ruled out.

Within 2 years, most patients with early syphilis become seronegative. However, if the disease is treated during the late stages, complete seroreversion may not occur. Patients treated with oral doxycycline or erythromycin are less likely to become seronegative.[81] Therapy is considered adequate in patients who never become seronegative as long as the titer decreases fourfold. Although the disease process may be halted in patients with tertiary syphilis, existing damage to the cardiovascular or nervous systems cannot be reversed.

PREGNANCY

CASE 69-8

QUESTION 1: N.W., a 27-year-old woman in her 19th week of gestation, has a positive VDRL and FTA-Abs. How should N.W. be managed? How would management be altered in the face of penicillin allergy?

Although pregnancy may be associated with false-positive nontreponemal tests,[68] the presence of both a positive treponemal test (e.g., FTA-Abs) and a nontreponemal test (e.g., RPR) virtually excludes a false-positive reaction.[73] The next step is to determine whether N.W. already has been treated adequately. If she has previously received adequate treatment and follow-up and shows no evidence of persistence or recurrence of syphilis, then she requires no further therapy. Pregnancy has no known effect on the clinical course of syphilis.[82] However, her infant should be observed carefully. If N.W. has not been treated previously for syphilis, then she should be treated with penicillin in the same doses recommended for nonpregnant women; some experts recommend a second dose 1 week later of 2.4 million units of benzathine penicillin.[2]

The goal of therapy should be to treat the mother with syphilis as soon as possible. Syphilis transmission can occur transplacentally as early as 9 to 10 weeks' gestation via direct contact with lesions in the birth canal.[82,83] If the mother is left untreated, 70% to 100% of fetuses born to mothers with primary syphilis or 40% with secondary syphilis may be aborted, stillborn, or born with congenital syphilis (see Case 69-8, Question 3).[84,85]

There is no completely satisfactory alternative for the pregnant woman with an accelerated allergic reaction to penicillin. Tetracycline, as well as doxycycline, should be avoided during pregnancy, especially during the second or third trimester, because of tetracycline's known effects on the fetus (tooth staining and inhibition of bone growth).[86] Erythromycin has been used to treat pregnant patients with syphilis; however, the transplacental transfer rate of erythromycin is inadequate,[87] potentially explaining the increased rate of aborted or stillborn infants in erythromycin-treated patients. Therefore, erythromycin is no longer recommended as therapy for syphilis during pregnancy.[2] A woman with a history of allergy to penicillin should be skin tested; if allergy is confirmed, she should be desensitized and treated with penicillin.[2] It is possible that the newer cephalosporins or azithromycin may ultimately prove to be acceptable alternatives to penicillin G in the pregnant woman with syphilis who is allergic to penicillin, but there is insufficient evidence for the CDC to recommend their use. Adequate treatment with penicillin can prevent up to 98% of fetal infections.[88,89] During pregnancy, the patient should be followed up with monthly quantitative VDRL titers to evaluate the effectiveness of therapy; thereafter, she should be followed up as any other patient with syphilis.

JARISCH-HERXHEIMER REACTION

CASE 69-8, QUESTION 2: N.W. was treated with an IM injection of 2.4 million units of benzathine penicillin G. Six hours later, she complained of diffuse myalgias, chills, headache, and an exacerbation of her rash. She was tachypneic, but normotensive. What is this reaction? How should N.W. be managed?

N.W. has developed the Jarisch-Herxheimer reaction (JHR), a usually benign, self-limited complication of antitreponemal antibiotic therapy that develops within hours after treatment of early syphilis.[2] The cause of JHR is not well understood, but is probably related to release of cytokines.[90] Clinical manifestations include fever, chills, myalgias, headache, tachycardia, and hypotension. The pathogenesis of the syndrome is uncertain, but the reaction should not be interpreted as an allergic reaction to penicillin. It typically begins within the first 1 to 2 hours after antibiotic administration and normally subsides spontaneously, generally subsiding even while antibiotics are continued.[91] Notably, JHR can occur after administration of many antimicrobials and is not exclusive to penicillins, nor is it exclusive to syphilis treatment, occurring in other spirochetal diseases such as Lyme disease and relapsing fever.[92] Usually self-limiting in nonpregnant patients, the primary risk of this reaction in pregnant women is miscarriage, premature labor, or fetal distress.[2,93] Pregnant women should seek medical attention if contractions or a change in fetal movements is noted. Close monitoring of JHR should be observed for patients with ophthalmic or neurologic syphilis. For these patients, prednisolone 10 to 20 mg three times a day for 3 days given 24 hours before syphilis treatment may prevent fever, but will not control local inflammation.[79] Tumor necrosis factor-α has been demonstrated to have some success in the prevention of JHR in spirochete disease.[94] Although there is no proven effective preventive therapy, some experts still recommend antipyretics, hydration, and patient education; antibiotic therapy should not be discontinued.

NEONATAL SYPHILIS

CASE 69-8, QUESTION 3: How should N.W.'s baby be treated if a diagnosis of congenital syphilis is confirmed?

Infants born to mothers who have been treated for syphilis during pregnancy should be carefully examined at birth, at 1 month, every 2 to 3 months for 15 months, and then every 6 months until the VDRL is negative or stable at a low titer. Newborn serology is difficult to interpret because of transplacental transfer of nontreponemal and treponemal immunoglobulin G to the infant. Treatment decisions are largely based on evidence of syphilis in the mother, adequacy of maternal treatment, comparison of maternal and neonatal nontreponemal serology, and presence of clinical or laboratory evidence of syphilis in the neonate. In addition, infants should be treated at birth, even if they are asymptomatic, when maternal treatment is unknown or inadequate, or when infant follow-up cannot be guaranteed. In most cases, a CSF examination should be performed before treatment is begun to rule out neurosyphilis. Although some clinicians recommend a single dose of benzathine penicillin, efficacy data are lacking and this route and form of penicillin cannot be recommended.[2]

CHANCROID

Chancroid (see http://www.cdc.gov/STD/TRAINING/CLINICALSLIDES/slides-dl.htm for symptoms of this STD) or soft chancre is a painful genital ulcer disease that often is associated with tender inguinal adenopathy. It is caused by *Haemophilus ducreyi,* a gram-negative bacillus. Chancroid is endemic in developing countries, but its incidence in the United States has steadily declined from 1987 to 2001 and since has fluctuated. In 2009, 28 cases of chancroid were reported in the United States.[3] Chancroid and other genital ulcers have been implicated in the transmission of HIV. In the United States, up to 18% of people with genital ulcers were also HIV seropositive.[95]

Signs and Symptoms

CASE 69-9

QUESTION 1: T.G., a 31-year-old uncircumcised man, presents to the STD clinic with complaints of tender lesions on the penis and inguinal regions. He noticed the penile lesions on the external surface of the prepuce (foreskin) 2 days before his visit. The lesions were sharply demarcated, but were not indurated; the base of the penile ulcer was covered by a yellow-gray purulent exudate. Right inguinal adenitis was present and extremely painful on palpation. A dark-field examination of the purulent exudate was negative. Gram stain revealed a mixture of gram-positive and gram-negative flora. T.G. claims to have no drug allergies. What is the natural course of chancroid? Does T.G. have signs or symptoms consistent with chancroid? What diagnostic procedures are necessary?

Uncircumcised men may have an increased risk of chancroid infection and may not respond to therapy as well as circumcised men. In fact, evidence suggests circumcision is protective against nearly all STDs, including HIV, as well as protecting women against *Trichomonas vaginalis* and BV.[2] A painful genital ulcer appears 3 to 10 days after exposure and begins as a tender, red papule that becomes pustular and ulcerates within 2 days. As illustrated by T.G., the ulcer may be covered by a grayish or yellow exudate. Multiple ulcers and tender inguinal lymph nodes, which may become fluctuant, are seen in about 50% of cases.[96] Aspiration of fluctuant nodes may be necessary to prevent rupture. A Gram stain can be misleading because of the polymicrobic nature of the ulcer and culture and because isolation of *H. ducreyi* is difficult, requiring specialized specimen collection and growth media.[2]

Treatment

CASE 69-9, QUESTION 2: How should T.G.'s chancroid be treated?

Most strains of *H. ducreyi* produce a TEM-type β-lactamase, and many strains are resistant to the antimicrobials that traditionally were used to treat chancroid, such as sulfonamides and tetracycline.[97,98] Currently recommended treatment regimens include azithromycin 1 g PO for one dose, ceftriaxone 250 mg IM once, ciprofloxacin 500 mg PO twice a day for 3 days, or erythromycin base 500 mg PO three times a day for 7 days.[2] Ciprofloxacin is contraindicated in pregnant and lactating women. Because T.G. does not have a history of penicillin hypersensitivity, ceftriaxone as a single dose is the preferred treatment regimen. Treatment may not be as effective for patients who are coinfected with HIV or who are uncircumcised.[2] Follow-up should occur 3 to 7 days after treatment is initiated. Depending on the size of the ulcer, the time required until complete recovery will vary; larger ulcers may require longer than 2 weeks.[2]

VAGINITIS

Approximately 10 million physician office visits are made annually in the United States for women seeking evaluation and treatment of vaginitis.[99,100] The term *vaginitis* refers to such nonspecific vaginal symptoms as itching, burning, irritation, and abnormal discharge that may be caused by infection or other medical conditions. The most common vaginal infections are BV (22%–50% of cases), vulvovaginal candidiasis (VVC; 17%–39% of cases), and trichomoniasis (4%–35% of cases). However, 7% to 72% of cases of vaginitis may remain undiagnosed.[101]

Bacterial Vaginosis

Bacterial vaginosis (formerly called nonspecific vaginitis, leukorrhea, *G. vaginalis,* or *H. vaginalis*) is associated with an increased, malodorous vaginal discharge. The normal vaginal lactobacillus flora is replaced by *Mobiluncus* species, *Prevotella* species, *Ureaplasma* species, *Mycoplasma* species, and increased numbers of *G. vaginalis.*[2]

The prevalence of BV varies widely owing to differing diagnostic criteria, demographics, and lack of a national reporting system, but a recent estimate places it at 29.2%.[101] Many sexually active women are infected with *G. vaginalis*, yet fewer than 50% are symptomatic or have signs of abnormal vaginal discharge.[102] The evidence for definitive risk factors in BV is inconclusive. Multiple sexual partners, a new sexual partner, douching, lack of condom use, and decreased concentrations of vaginal lactobacilli have been associated with BV. Non–sexually active heterosexual women may also be infected.[2] In addition, studies among lesbians or women who generally have sex with other women show evidence for sexual transmission.[103] The routine treatment of sexual partners is not recommended because a woman's response to therapy or her likelihood of relapse or recurrence is not impacted by treatment of her sexual partner(s).[2]

SIGNS, SYMPTOMS, AND DIAGNOSIS

CASE 69-10

QUESTION 1: H.H. is a 24-year-old, sexually active woman with a 1-week history of moderate vaginal discharge that has a "fishy" odor, most notable after coitus. She has no complaints of vaginal pruritus or burning. On examination, the discharge appears thin, white, homogeneous, and notably malodorous. A wet mount of the vaginal secretion revealed few leukocytes and numerous "clue cells." The vaginal pH was 4.8, and a characteristic fishy odor was noted when the discharge was mixed with 10% potassium hydroxide (KOH). Does H.H. have signs and symptoms consistent with BV? What diagnostic tests are required?

H.H.'s signs and symptoms are typical of BV. The clinical diagnosis can be confirmed by a vaginal Gram stain that shows overgrowth of the vagina with *G. vaginalis* and other organisms as noted earlier. A 10% KOH solution mixed with the vaginal secretions yields a transient fishy odor because of the increased production of biogenic diamines (positive amine test). A wet preparation of the specimen reveals "clue cells" (exfoliated vaginal epithelial cells sometimes with adherent coccobacillary pathogens), pH greater than 4.5, and the characteristic KOH "whiff" test.[104] If there are many white cells, other infections (e.g., *T. vaginalis*) should be suspected. Self-diagnosis is correct only about 3% to 4% of the time because most women attribute symptoms to poor hygiene.[105]

TREATMENT

CASE 69-10, QUESTION 2: How should H.H. be treated?

Nonpregnant women with symptomatic disease require treatment. CDC-recommended regimens include oral metronidazole 500 mg twice a day for 7 days, metronidazole gel 0.75% intravaginally daily for 5 days, or clindamycin cream 2% intravaginally at bedtime for 7 days.[2] The FDA has approved metronidazole extended release 750 mg once daily for 7 days and a single dose of clindamycin intravaginal cream for the treatment of BV; however, limited data have been published comparing these regimens with other established therapies. Patients should be instructed to avoid consuming alcohol during treatment with metronidazole and for 72 hours afterward to avoid disulfiramlike reactions. Additionally, clindamycin cream is oil based and may weaken latex condoms or diaphragms. Alternatively, the CDC recommends either tinidazole 2 g PO every day for 2 days, tinidazole 1 g PO every day for 5 days, clindamycin 300 mg PO two times a day for 7 days, or clindamycin ovules 10 mg intravaginally once at bedtime for 3 days.[2]

BV has been associated with preterm labor and premature delivery. If the decision is made to treat BV during pregnancy, the CDC recommends metronidazole 250 mg PO three times daily for 7 days or 500 mg PO twice a day for 7 days, or clindamycin 300 mg PO twice daily for 7 days. Recent teratogenic data suggest that metronidazole is not harmful to the fetus, but the use of intravaginal clindamycin cream has been associated with preterm delivery.[2]

Vulvovaginal Candidiasis

Candida albicans is the causative organism of VVC in 80% to 92% of cases, with *Candida glabrata* and *Candida tropicalis* accounting for most of the remaining cases.[2,106,107] The latter organisms have been identified increasingly as the causative agents of VVC during the past two decades. Approximately 75% of women will experience at least one episode of VVC, and 40% to 45% will have two or more episodes within their lifetime. Approximately 5% of women who have VVC have recurrent candidal episodes (defined as four or more episodes of VVC in 1 year).[2] Vulvovaginal candidiasis is not usually described as an STD because celibate women can experience VVC; however, the incidence of VVC increases when women become sexually active.[107] Because of this, VVC is often diagnosed during evaluation for a suspected STD when women present with vaginal symptoms.[2]

ASSESSING SELF-TREATMENT

CASE 69-11

QUESTION 1: L.L., a 23-year-old woman, purchases a nonprescription antifungal agent to relieve vaginal symptoms that she believes are caused by a vaginal yeast infection. L.L. asks the pharmacist for assistance in the selection of an antifungal agent. What information should be obtained from L.L. before a medication is recommended?

The pharmacist should ask L.L. whether this is her first episode of vaginitis or whether she has experienced similar symptoms previously that have been diagnosed as a vaginal yeast infection and treated by a physician. The nonprescription antifungal agents are indicated for the treatment of VVC in women who previously were diagnosed and treated by their physician. Additional questions that should be asked by the pharmacist include current symptoms, whether they are pregnant or not, other current medical conditions or medications, and allergies. Patients should be referred to a physician if any of the following are present: first episode of VVC, two episodes of VVC within the past 6 months, pregnancy, younger than 16 years or older than 60 years of age, current abnormal vaginal bleeding or lower abdominal pain, exposure to an STD, or a malodorous vaginal discharge.

SIGNS AND SYMPTOMS

CASE 69-11, QUESTION 2: L.L. has experienced two episodes of vaginal yeast infections, with the most recent case occurring approximately 1 year ago. On both occasions she was diagnosed as having VVC by her physician and responded to antifungal therapy. L.L. currently describes vaginal and vulvar itching, vaginal soreness, and vulvar burning accompanied by a thick, white vaginal discharge that has the consistency of cottage cheese. She has been unable to have sexual intercourse because of pain. These symptoms are similar to those she experienced with her previous vaginal yeast infections. L.L. has no underlying major health problems. Her current medications include oral tetracycline for acne and Ortho Tri-Cyclen for birth control. She has regular menstrual cycles, and her last menstrual period ended 4 days ago. What clinical manifestations does L.L. exhibit that are consistent with VVC? What are other common manifestations?

L.L. exhibits signs and symptoms associated with VVC (i.e., vulvar and vaginal pruritus, vaginal soreness, vulvar burning, dyspareunia, and a thick, white vaginal discharge that appears to be curdlike).[2] Although vulvar pruritus occurs in most

TABLE 69-5
Characteristics of Vaginal Discharge

Characteristics	Normal	Candidiasis	Trichomoniasis	Bacterial Vaginosis
Color	White or clear	White	Yellow-green	White to gray
Odor	Nonodorous	Nonodorous	Malodorous	Fishy smell
Consistency	Floccular	Floccular	Homogeneous	Homogeneous
Viscosity	High	High	Low	Low
pH	<4.5	4–4.5	5–6.0	>4.5
Other characteristics		Thick, curdlike	Frothy	Thin

Source: Ries AJ. Treatment of vaginal infections: candidiasis, bacterial vaginosis, and trichomoniasis. *J Am Pharm Assoc (Wash)*. 1997;NS37:563; Sobel JD. Vaginitis. *N Engl J Med*. 1997;337:1896; Carr PL et al. Evaluation and management of vaginitis. *J Gen Intern Med*. 1998;13:335.

symptomatic patients, many affected women have little or no vaginal discharge.[106] Typically, the vaginal discharge associated with VVC is a nonodorous, highly viscous, white discharge that may vary in consistency from curdlike to watery. Symptoms may be worse before menses and may diminish with the onset of menses.[106]

DIFFERENTIAL DIAGNOSIS

CASE 69-11, QUESTION 3: How can VVC be differentiated from other vaginal infections?

VVC should be differentiated from other vaginal infections because a nonprescription antifungal agent could delay the appropriate treatment of other vaginal infections. The physical appearance of the vaginal discharge may be useful in predicting VVC if it is a viscous, nonodorous, white, curdlike discharge and the patient has a normal vaginal pH (pH <4.5).[2] The quantity of the discharge may be scanty to profuse. Some women with VVC exhibit only vaginal erythema with minimal discharge or an increased amount of normal vaginal secretion. Table 69-5 characterizes the vaginal discharges associated with VVC, BV, and trichomoniasis. The vaginal discharge from a woman with signs and symptoms of VVC should be examined for the microscopic presence of *Candida* using a wet mount preparation with 10% KOH or a Gram stain of the vaginal discharge. The use of KOH improves the visualization of yeast or pseudohyphae that are seen in approximately 70% of women diagnosed with VVC.[2] If the wet mount is negative, the patient's vaginal discharge should be cultured for *Candida* in an appropriate growth medium. Isolation of *Candida* without signs and symptoms should not result in treatment, because *Candida* is part of normal vaginal flora in approximately 10% to 20% of women.[2] It is the proliferation of *C. albicans* or other yeasts that lead to vulvovaginitis symptoms. Several nonprescription home diagnostic tests are available (e.g., Vagisil screening kit and Fem-V), which may allow individuals to identify VVC by measuring pH levels of the vaginal epithelium.

PHYSIOLOGICAL VAGINAL DISCHARGE AND SYMPTOMATIC NORMAL pH VULVOVAGINITIS

CASE 69-11, QUESTION 4: Do women such as L.L., who have an increased vaginal discharge and symptoms consistent with VVC, necessarily have a vaginal infection?

Although the possibility of vaginal infection must be addressed when a woman presents with an increased vaginal discharge with or without symptoms, other conditions are associated with an increased discharge. First, a physiological vaginal discharge must be distinguished from a pathological discharge. Physiological discharges (Table 69-5) characteristically are nonodorous, white or clear, highly viscous or floccular, and acidic (pH ~4.5). Physiological discharge may also become more profuse at midcycle secondary to increased cervical mucus or vaginal epithelial cells. Other conditions resulting in excessive vaginal discharge include retention of foreign bodies (e.g., tampons) and allergic reactions or contact dermatitis secondary to the use of vaginal spermicidal agents, soaps, deodorants, douches, vaginal lubricants, and condoms. Episodes of vulvovaginitislike symptoms can be associated with frequent use of hot tubs, Jacuzzi baths, or swimming pools that contain chemically treated water with high levels of chlorine.[108]

RISK FACTORS FOR VULVOVAGINAL CANDIDIASIS

CASE 69-11, QUESTION 5: What specific groups of women are most susceptible to VVC? Does L.L. fit into any group at high risk for VVC?

Women are most susceptible to VVC during their childbearing years. Approximately 50% of U.S. college women report having an episode of VVC between menarche and age 25.[107] *C. albicans* colonization and symptomatic VVC increases during pregnancy and with use of high-estrogen–containing oral contraceptives. Estrogens increase binding affinity of vaginal epithelial cells to *C. albicans*.[109] Women with high glycogen concentrations (e.g., uncontrolled or poorly controlled diabetes mellitus), women with depressed cell-mediated immunity secondary to disease (e.g., cancer, HIV infection), and women receiving broad-spectrum antibiotics or immunosuppressive drugs (e.g., cytotoxic agents, corticosteroids) are at risk for VVC.[107,109] Individual cases of VVC, although not related to intercourse, may be related to orogenital sex.

L.L. is taking tetracycline, which may increase her risk for VVC. Antibacterials increase the risk for *C. albicans* overgrowth by suppressing the normal vaginal flora (e.g., lactobacilli), which normally protect against *C. albicans*. L.L. is also taking a low-estrogen–containing oral contraceptive; however, low-dose oral contraceptives have not been consistently associated with an increased risk of VVC.[110,111] The use of diaphragms, vaginal sponges, and IUDs also may be risk factors for VVC.[112]

Stress-induced VVC and an increased incidence of VVC before menstruation have been described.[109] The cause of both is currently unknown. Although various dietary factors have been postulated as a cause of vaginal yeast overgrowth, the role of diet in the development of VVC remains inconclusive.[109]

TREATMENT OF VULVOVAGINAL CANDIDIASIS

VAGINALLY ADMINISTERED AZOLES

CASE 69-11, QUESTION 6: What vaginally administered therapy is effective for L.L.'s VVC?

TABLE 69-6

Products Available for the Treatment of *Candida* Vulvovaginitis

Drug	Availability	Trade Names	Dosing Regimens
Nonprescription Products			
Butoconazole	2% vaginal cream[a]	Femstat 3	*Nonpregnant women:* Administer 1 applicatorful intravaginally at bedtime for 3 consecutive days *Pregnant women during second and third trimesters:* Administer 1 applicatorful intravaginally at bedtime for 7 consecutive days
Clotrimazole	1% vaginal cream[a]	Gyne-Lotrimin 7; Mycelex-7; Clotrimazole 7; various generics	Administer 1 applicatorful intravaginally at bedtime for 7 consecutive days
	2% vaginal cream[a]	Gyne-Lotrimin 3; various generics	Administer 1 applicatorful intravaginally at bedtime for 3 consecutive days
	100-mg vaginal suppositories[a]	Mycelex-7; various generics	Insert 1 suppository intravaginally at bedtime for 7 consecutive days
	200-mg vaginal suppositories[a]	Gyne-Lotrimin 3; various generics	Insert 1 suppository intravaginally at bedtime for 3 consecutive days
Miconazole	2% cream[a]	Monistat 7; Femizol-M; various generics	Administer 1 applicatorful intravaginally at bedtime for 7 consecutive days
	4% cream[a]	Monistat 3; various generics	Administer 1 applicatorful intravaginally at bedtime for 3 consecutive days
	100-mg vaginal suppositories[a]	Monistat 7	Insert 1 suppository intravaginally at bedtime for 7 consecutive days
	200-mg vaginal suppositories[a]	Monistat 3	Insert 1 suppository intravaginally at bedtime for 3 consecutive days
	1200-mg vaginal suppositories[a]	Monistat 1 Daytime Ovule	Insert 1 suppository intravaginally at bedtime for 1 dose only
Tioconazole	6.5% vaginal ointment	Vagistat-1, generics	Administer 1 applicatorful intravaginally at bedtime for 1 dose only
Prescription Products			
Butoconazole (sustained release)	2% vaginal cream[a]	Gynazole 1	*Nonpregnant women:* Administer 1 applicatorful at bedtime for 1 dose only
Fluconazole	150-mg oral tablet	Diflucan tablet	Take 1 tablet PO for 1 dose only
Nystatin[b]	100,000 units vaginal tablet	Mycostatin; Nystatin; various generics	Insert 1 tablet intravaginally at bedtime for 14 consecutive days
Terconazole	0.4% vaginal cream[a]	Terazol 7	Administer 1 applicatorful intravaginally at bedtime for 7 consecutive days
	0.8% vaginal cream[a]	Terazol 3	Administer 1 applicatorful intravaginally at bedtime for 3 consecutive days
	80-mg vaginal suppositories[a]	Terazol 3	Insert 1 suppository intravaginally at bedtime for 3 consecutive days

[a] The CDC states that the use of vaginally administered oil-based preparations may weaken latex products such as condoms and diaphragms.

[b] All topically applied azole medications are superior to nystatin.

Adapted from Workowski KA et al. Sexually transmitted diseases treatment guidelines, 2010. *MMWR Recomm Rep.* 2010;59(RR-12):1.

L.L. is an appropriate candidate for nonprescription therapy (Table 69-6) because she had previous vaginal yeast infections with symptoms similar to those she currently is experiencing and her VVC is uncomplicated (defined as sporadic disease with mild to moderate symptoms in a immunocompetent host). When a patient's VVC appears complicated (defined as a recurrent infection, severe symptoms, non–C. *albicans* infection, presence of uncontrolled diabetes, immunosuppression, or pregnancy), she should be referred to her medical practitioner.[2] L.L. should respond well to short-term topical azole therapy. In addition, L.L. should ask her physician whether continuation of antibacterials is truly needed. If L.L. had been evaluated by her physician, a prescription for single-dose oral fluconazole or 3-day intravaginal therapy might have been an option.

The available azole antifungals are equally effective in treating VVC with cure rates between 80% and 90% when a full course of therapy is completed.[2,113] All the azole antifungal products listed in Table 69-6 are superior to nystatin. The medication used to treat L.L.'s VVC should be selected based on response or failure to previous therapy, convenience, ease of use, length of therapy, dosage form, and cost. L.L. should select a non–oil-based product if a latex condom or a diaphragm is used for contraception (Table 69-6).

OTHER TREATMENTS FOR ACUTE VULVOVAGINAL CANDIDIASIS

Oral lactobacillus and lactobacillus-containing yogurt are advocated for the treatment of VVC; however, evidence in support of this treatment is inconclusive.[114] Boric acid 600-mg capsules inserted high in the vagina at bedtime for 14 days are effective for the treatment of VVC, but vaginal burning and irritation occur in approximately 4% of women, and boric acid is poisonous if inadvertently ingested.[2,114] The primary indication for these extemporaneously prepared boric acid capsules primarily has been in the treatment of fluconazole-resistant *Candida* infection, especially that caused by *C. glabrata*. Gentian violet preparations also have limited use in the treatment of candidiasis because they stain clothing and bed linens and cause local irritation and edema. It is important to note that these alternative regimens for the treatment of acute VVC are not currently recommended by the CDC.

ORAL AZOLES

CASE 69-11, QUESTION 7: How effective are orally administered azoles in the treatment of an acute VVC infection such as the one L.L. is experiencing?

Fluconazole is the only oral antifungal agent currently recommended by the CDC for the treatment of acute VVC.[2] A single 150-mg oral dose of fluconazole is as effective as a 3- to 6-day regimen of intravaginal clotrimazole.[115,116] Although some women may prefer an orally administered drug to one that is administered intravaginally, their use for mild-to-moderate VVC is of some concern because of the possibility for systemic adverse effects and drug–drug interactions.

Adverse Effects Associated With Azoles

CASE 69-11, QUESTION 8: What adverse effects might L.L. experience from intravaginally or orally administered azoles?

When used intravaginally, azoles are associated with minimal adverse reactions, similar to symptoms women report from VVC. Thus, it can be difficult to differentiate disease symptoms from adverse drug reactions. If the vaginal symptoms worsen after therapy is started, the patient should contact her health care provider. In addition, if symptoms have not improved within 3 days after initiation of therapy, the patient should contact her physician to rule out more severe disease, treatment of the wrong disease, or drug-related adverse effects. Topical azole therapy has been associated with a variety of adverse drug reactions including headaches; allergic contact dermatitis; vulvovaginal pruritus and irritation; dyspareunia; and general burning, soreness, and genital pain. Oral fluconazole has been associated with headaches, nausea, abdominal pain, diarrhea, dyspepsia, dizziness, taste perversion, angioedema, and rare cases of anaphylactic reactions.[117]

PATIENT COUNSELING

CASE 69-11, QUESTION 9: How should L.L. be counseled about the use of a nonprescription vaginal antifungal product?

The details of intravaginal administration should be reviewed with L.L., including instructions on how to clean the applicator. To minimize leakage and annoyance, L.L. should apply the product at bedtime to increase retention in the vagina. She should be advised that the nonprescription vaginal antifungal creams and suppositories are oil based and thus may weaken condoms or diaphragms, thereby reducing their effectiveness.

L.L. should be informed about the importance of completing a full course of therapy even if her symptoms subside beforehand and to continue her antifungal treatment through her menstrual period should it occur. In addition, L.L. should be instructed to see her physician if her symptoms persist, if she experiences symptoms that signal a more serious problem (e.g., abdominal pain, fever, a foul-smelling or bloody vaginal discharge), or if another yeast infection occurs within 2 months.

L.L. also should be advised to avoid wearing tight-fitting, unventilated underwear (e.g., nylon panties or panty hose) and tight-fitting jeans because a warm, moist environment can facilitate fungal growth. However, a study addressing risk factors for VVC found no relation between type of underwear and the incidence of VVC.[112] L.L. also could be alerted to the possible relation between candidiasis and swimming in a heavily chlorinated pool or frequent use of a Jacuzzi or hot tub.

Complicated Vulvovaginal Candidiasis

CASE 69-11, QUESTION 10: How would management of L.L.'s VVC differ if she had poorly controlled diabetes?

VVC in a woman with uncontrolled diabetes is usually considered to be complicated VVC. A diagnosis of complicated VVC is also warranted when the VVC is severe, recurrent (as defined), caused by non–*C. albicans* species, or when VVC occurs in an immunosuppressed, debilitated, or pregnant woman. Approximately 10% to 20% of VVC cases can be classified as complicated.[2] The treatment of complicated VVC varies depending on the underlying reason for the complication. Severe VVC (e.g., extensive vulvar erythema, edema, excoriation, and fissures) may be treated with either a 7- to 14-day course of topical azoles or two oral doses of fluconazole 150 mg given 72 hours apart.[2] Infection with non–*C. albicans* species should be treated with a 7- to 14-day course of an oral or intravaginal azole; however, the optimal treatment is unknown. Oral fluconazole has poor activity against non–*C. albicans* species and should not be used; however, a 7-day regimen of terconazole 0.4% cream has been shown to eradicate non–*C. albicans* species in 56% of affected patients.[118] Boric acid 600-mg capsules administered intravaginally once daily for 14 days can be used if this regimen is not effective in eradicating the infection in cases unresponsive to azoles.[2]

Recurrent Vulvovaginal Candidiasis

CASE 69-11, QUESTION 11: L.L. experiences another case of VVC 1 month later. Does she have recurrent VVC? How should she be treated?

Most women have only occasional episodes of VVC, but approximately 5% experience recurrent VVC infections defined as four or more episodes per year.[2] To determine whether L.L. has recurrent VVC, a diagnosis of *Candida* needs to be confirmed by vaginal cultures. Then, underlying risk factors for VVC, such as uncontrolled diabetes mellitus, consumption of excess sugars, IUD placement, and use of antibiotics, must be ruled out.[119] Based on the timing of L.L.'s episodes and the absence of risk factors, L.L. does not meet the definition for recurrent VVC. If a patient meets the criteria for recurrent VVC, an underlying cause of the problem may not be determined. In addition, the role of sexual transmission is not currently well understood.[107] In most patients, the pathogenesis of recurrent VVC cannot be determined.

Treatment of recurrent *C. albicans* vulvovaginitis should include a prolonged (7- to 14-day) course of topical therapy or a three-dose regimen of oral fluconazole (100, 150, or 200 mg) administered every 3 days.[2] A 6-month maintenance regimen should be initiated after remission has been achieved (Table 69-7). Despite the efficacy of these regimens, discontinuation of therapy after 6 months can result in relapse in up to 50% of women.[2,119] Azole-resistant strains of *C. albicans* are rare; therefore, culture and sensitivity testing is not usually performed to help guide treatment before initiation.

TABLE 69-7
Maintenance Regimens for Recurrent Vulvovaginal Candidiasis

	Dose	Frequency
Topical agents[a]		
Clotrimazole	200 mg	Intermittently
Clotrimazole vaginal suppositories	500 mg	Intermittently
Oral agents		
Fluconazole tablets	100, 150, or 200 mg	Weekly for 6 months

[a] Given as examples only, CDC does not indicate a preferred regimen.
Adapted from Workowski KA et al. Sexually transmitted diseases treatment guidelines, 2010. *MMWR Recomm Rep.* 2010;59(RR-12):1.

Vulvovaginal Candidiasis During Pregnancy

CASE 69-11, QUESTION 12: What teratogenic risks are associated with the use of azole preparations?

Vaginal colonization with *Candida* and symptomatic VVC are common during pregnancy.[120] Asymptomatic colonization is not associated with increased maternal or fetal risks and need not be treated.[121] However, symptomatic VVC should be treated. Although doses of oral fluconazole used to treat VVC have not been associated with increased fetal defects, higher doses may be teratogenic. Therefore, topical antifungal agents are preferred for treatment of VVC in pregnant women. The CDC currently recommends a 7-day course of topical antifungal therapy for VVC during pregnancy; however, a 3-day regimen with appropriate follow-up to assess efficacy has been shown to be effective in mild-to-moderate cases.[2] Nystatin is classified as a category B drug, is inferior to azoles, and should not be used. Clotrimazole is also classified as a category B drug for fetal risk, and the remaining vaginally administered azoles are designated as category C.[121]

Trichomoniasis

SIGNS AND SYMPTOMS

CASE 69-12

QUESTION 1: N.B. is a 31-year-old woman with a recent history of diffuse vaginal discharge and irritation. A wet mount examination of vaginal secretions revealed numerous trichomonads. Examination confirms the presence of an increased, yellow-green vaginal discharge. What subjective and objective clinical data support a diagnosis of trichomoniasis?

Trichomoniasis is an STD caused by the protozoan *T. vaginalis.* The overall prevalence is estimated at 3.1% with the highest prevalence among African Americans at 13.3%.[3] Trichomoniasis in women is asymptomatic about 20% to 50% of the time.[122] In men, *T. vaginalis* presumably infects the urethra, although the site of infection (urethra versus prostate) is uncertain. Men with *T. vaginalis* infection usually are asymptomatic. Classic symptoms of trichomoniasis in women include a diffuse, yellow-green discharge with pruritus, dysuria, and a "strawberry" cervix (cervical microhemorrhages). The latter are typically only seen in 2% to 25% of cases.[122] In almost all cases of trichomoniasis, a vaginal pH greater than 5 or 6 is observed.[123] The Papanicolaou smear is associated with a 48.4% error in diagnosis when used alone.[122] Direct microscopic observation of trichomoniasis using a wet mount suffers from low sensitivity, but is up to 99% specific.[124] Broth culture is considered to be the gold standard for identification of trichomoniasis, but it requires up to a 7-day incubation period and the culture system is not widely available.[122] The best approach to diagnosis requires clinical and laboratory confirmation.

TREATMENT

METRONIDAZOLE AND TINIDAZOLE

CASE 69-12, QUESTION 2: How should N.B.'s trichomoniasis be treated?

The only class of drugs that are effective for the treatment of trichomoniasis is the nitroimidazoles. In the United States, metronidazole and tinidazole are the only available nitroimidazoles, and both are CDC-recommended first-line agents given as a single 2-g oral dose.[2] In addition, sexual partners should be simultaneously treated. Metronidazole cure rates are reported to be 90% to 95%, whereas tinidazole cure rates are reported to be 86% to 100%; concurrently treating sexual partners might increase these rates.[2] Tinidazole is equivalent or superior to metronidazole in achieving cure and resolution of symptoms.[2] Approximately 2% to 5% of *T. vaginalis* isolates exhibit a low-level resistance to metronidazole therapy; however, higher-level resistance appears to be rare.[2] If metronidazole 2 g PO for one dose fails and reinfection is excluded, either metronidazole 500 mg PO twice daily for 7 days or tinidazole 2 g PO as a single dose can be used. If either of these regimens fails, metronidazole or tinidazole 2 g PO daily for 5 days may be used. Tinidazole has the advantage of a longer half-life and reaching higher genitourinary tissue concentrations than metronidazole. In the case of allergy to nitroimidazole compounds, patients should be desensitized to metronidazole and subsequently treated.[2]

Adverse Effects

CASE 69-12, QUESTION 3: N.B. was treated with metronidazole 500 mg twice a day for 7 days. On the fourth day of therapy while attending a party, N.B. experienced a severe headache, followed by nausea, sweating, and dizziness. Could N.B.'s symptoms be caused by metronidazole?

Minor side effects associated with metronidazole therapy include nausea, vomiting (especially with single-dose therapy), headache, skin rashes, and alcohol intolerance. The alcohol intolerance may be attributable to a metronidazole-induced inhibition of aldehyde dehydrogenase, which results in the buildup of high serum acetaldehyde levels, although the true risk of this interaction has been debated.[125] According to the manufacturer, patients should be warned about the possibility of nausea, vomiting, flushing, and respiratory distress after alcohol consumption, although reliable evidence is lacking.[112] As a general rule, patients should avoid alcohol ingestion during treatment and for 72 hours after metronidazole or tinidazole therapy.

PREGNANCY

CASE 69-13

QUESTION 1: S.G., a 31-year-old woman, is in her first trimester of pregnancy and has a history of recurrent trichomoniasis. She now complains of a diffuse, yellow vaginal discharge. The preliminary diagnosis of trichomoniasis is confirmed by a wet mount examination of vaginal

secretions revealing numerous trichomonads. S.G. has read much of the lay press on metronidazole and is concerned about her own safety as well as that of her fetus. Can metronidazole be used for S.G.?

During pregnancy, trichomoniasis is associated with premature rupture of the membranes, preterm delivery, and low birth weight.[2] In one meta-analysis, an association between metronidazole use and teratogenicity or mutagenicity in infants could not be demonstrated.[126] However, caution should still be exercised if metronidazole must be administered within the first trimester. Metronidazole is mutagenic in facultative bacteria and contains a nitro-reductase enzyme. Long-term, high-dose metronidazole in laboratory mice is associated with the development of pulmonary and hepatic tumors. Midline facial defects have been documented in humans, but two literature reviews indicate that metronidazole is not a teratogen.[127,128] In contrast, the use of metronidazole in asymptomatic women has not been shown to decrease rates of preterm labor despite eliminating the organism from its host.[129]

TREATMENT

CASE 69-13, QUESTION 2: How should S.G. be treated?

All symptomatic women should be treated with metronidazole 2 g PO as a single dose.[2] Metronidazole is classified as pregnancy category B. Tinidazole 2 g PO as a single dose could be suggested as an alternative regimen; however, it is classified as pregnancy category C.

GENITAL HERPES

The word *herpes* is of Greek origin and means "to creep." HSV (see **http://www.cdc.gov/STD/TRAINING/CLINICALSLIDES/slides-dl.htm** for symptoms of this STD) is a DNA-containing virus that consists of two antigenically distinct serotypes: HSV-1 and HSV-2. The primary cause of herpes labialis (cold sores), herpes keratitis, and herpetic encephalitis is HSV-1. Genital herpes and neonatal herpes primarily are the result of HSV-2 infections. However, up to 50% of all reported cases of primary genital herpes are caused by HSV-1 infections acquired through oral sex.[130,131]

Etiology

Most people are exposed to HSV-1 early in life, with more than half being positive for HSV-1 antibodies before 18 years and more than 90% of the population positive by 70 years of age.[132] The infection is often asymptomatic and generally acquired through primary infection of mucocutaneous surfaces. The initial, primary disease is a gingivostomatitis characterized by vesicles in the oral cavity and occasionally an elevated temperature; life-threatening encephalitis or keratitis may appear during this interval. Usually after primary exposure, HSV-1 enters cells of the trigeminal ganglion, where it may remain latent for the lifetime of the host.[133]

Initial HSV-2 infections usually occur after puberty and coincide with the onset of sexual activity, although transfer to a neonate from an infected mother can occur. After primary infection, the virus enters a state of latency in the sacral dorsal root ganglia in many infected individuals; a high percentage of infected persons may never manifest the disease clinically.[133,134]

In both HSV-1 and HSV-2 infections, the latent virus can reactivate. Recurrent disease may occur even when circulating antibody and sensitized lymphocytes are present. Clinically, the lesions periodically erupt usually at the same location, and the interval between episodes varies widely between individuals.

Epidemiology

Although herpes was recognized several thousand years ago, genital herpes was not described until the 18th century. The seroprevalence of genital herpes (HSV-2) has remained the same in the United States since 1999—at approximately 16.2% overall in 19- to 49-year-olds, but 20.9% in women and 39.2% in non-Hispanic blacks—making it still one of the most common STDs in the United States.[135] In 2009, US physicians saw more than 300,000 new patients presenting with genital herpes simplex, and nearly 20% of non-Hispanic whites and more than double that in non-Hispanic blacks are already seropositive in the United States.[3]

Demographic characteristics obtained at the University of Washington indicate that the mean number of lifetime sexual partners before acquisition of the disease was 8.8 in women compared with 32.8 in men, with the overall chance of acquiring HSV-2 of 5 per 1,000 sex contacts.[136] The range of time from the last sexual exposure to the onset of disease is 5 to 14 days.[134] Whether causal or not, HSV-2 infection increases the risk of HIV.[137]

Signs and Symptoms

CASE 69-14

QUESTION 1: B.J., a 28-year-old, sexually active man, complains of painful penile lesions and tender inguinal adenopathy. The lesions are vesicular and limited to the scrotum, glands, and shaft of the penis. The onset of the lesions was preceded by a 1-week period of fever, malaise, headache, and itching. Viral culture of the lesions was positive for HSV infection. Describe the typical course and clinical presentation of herpes genitalis in men and women. What subjective and objective clinical data in B.J. are compatible with herpes genitalis?

Most initial episodes of genital herpes, especially in the male, are symptomatic. As illustrated by B.J., the symptoms usually start about 1 week after the initial exposure with prodromal signs of tingling, itching, paresthesia, or genital burning. The prodromal stage, which can last from a few hours to several days, is followed by the appearance of numerous vesicles. The vesicles eventually erupt, resulting in painful genital ulcers. The pain and edema associated with genital herpetic lesions, especially if they are infected secondarily, can be severe enough to result in dysuria and urinary retention. Bilaterally distributed lesions of the external genitalia are characteristic. The lesions usually are limited to the glans, corona prepuce, and shaft of the penis in men and to the vulva and vagina in women. However, lesions can occur on the buttocks, thighs, and urethra.[134] Asymptomatic or mucopurulent cervicitis occurs in about 15% to 20% of women with primary HSV-2 infections.[138] Rectal and perianal HSV-2 infections are more common in MSM and immunocompromised individuals.[139] Symptoms include anorectal pain and discharge, tenesmus, and constipation.

Prior infection with HSV-1 may ameliorate the severity of the first episode of genital herpes, but does not impact the rate of recurrence.[140] In primary infections, the local symptoms of pain, itching, and urethral or vaginal discharge last from 11 to 14 days, with a complete disappearance of lesions in 3 to 6 weeks.[134,141]

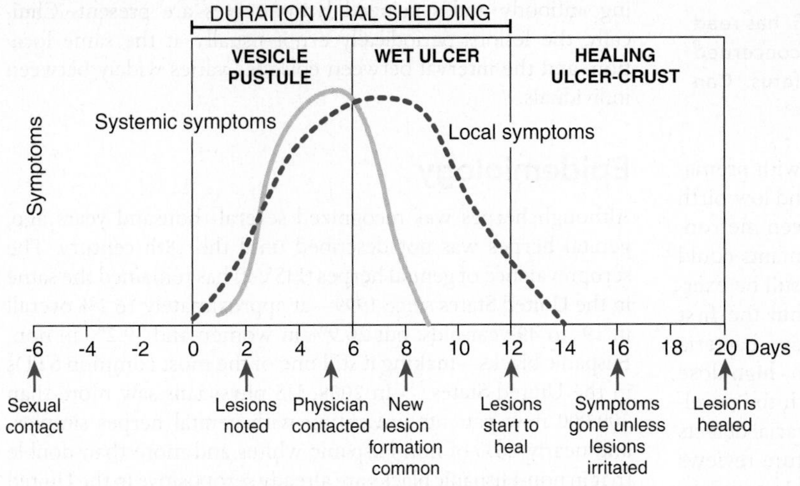

FIGURE 69-7 The clinical time course of primary genital herpes infections. (Adapted with permission from Corey L, Wald A. Genital herpes. In: Holmes K et al., eds. *Sexually Transmitted Diseases*. 4th ed. New York, NY: McGraw-Hill; 2008:399.)

The clinical course of primary herpes is presented in Figure 69-7. Most patients have minor symptoms or are asymptomatic and unaware of their disease; they are most infectious within the first year of acquisition of the virus.[142]

Recurrence

CASE 69-14, QUESTION 2: Is B.J.'s infection likely to recur?

Most patients experience a recurrence of their initial infection. The rate of recurrent infections varies among individual patients. Approximately 38% experience at least six episodes, and 20% have more than ten recurrences.[141] Natural infection with HSV-2 induces type-specific immunity against exogenous reinfection, but does not affect recurrences.[143] The severity of the primary episode and recurrence appear to be influenced by the host's immune status, especially a depressed T-cell response.[134] Recurrent infections usually appear at or near the site of the initial infection, and prodromal symptoms are reported by about 50% of persons with recurrent infection. Men recur more frequently than women. In contrast with primary infections, there are fewer lesions and they are often unilateral.[134] Constitutional symptoms such as lymphadenopathy, fever, and malaise generally are also milder. Recurrent infections are shorter in duration (average, 1 week); local symptoms such as pain and itching last 4 to 5 days and the lesions themselves last 7 to 10 days.[134] Although there is wide variability, patients may have four to five recurrences during the first year, but reactivation frequency can decline by three reactivations per year during the first 2 years.[144,145] By about 5 years after the initial infection, recurrence rates decrease greatly.[146] Genital infections with HSV-1, however, recur infrequently and decrease by 50% between 1 and 2 years after infection.[147]

Transmission

CASE 69-14, QUESTION 3: B.J. states that this is the first time he has had such lesions and that he has had only one sexual partner for the last 14 months. His sexually active female partner has no history of herpes genitalis or any other STD. The couple is very curious as to how B.J. acquired his infection. How is HSV transmitted?

Transmission of HSV occurs by direct contact with active lesions or from a symptomatic or asymptomatic person shedding virus at a peripheral site, mucosal surface, or secretion.[148] Genital HSV-2 infections usually are acquired through sexual (vaginal or anorectal) intercourse, whereas genital HSV-1 infections are acquired through orogenital sexual practices. Because HSV is inactivated readily by drying and exposure to room temperature, aerosol and fomite spread are unusual means of transmission.[149] Condoms may act as an effective barrier to viral transmission in women, but this method does not offer complete protection for men as women often have perigenital lesions.[150] Evidence suggests that the frequency of correct condom use is directly proportional to protection against acquisition of HSV-2 and that condoms are more likely to be worn when lesions are present.[151,152]

A patient with genital herpes is contagious only when shedding the virus. The patient begins to shed virus during the prodromal phase, which may be several hours to days before the actual lesions first appear. Subclinical or asymptomatic viral shedding is the most common means of sexual transmission and, thus, important from a public health standpoint.[153,154] Lesions are most contagious during the ulcerative phase. The median duration of viral shedding as defined from onset to the last positive culture is about 12 days.[134] The mean time from the onset of vesicles to the appearance of the crust stage (~10.5 days) correlates well with the duration of viral shedding. However, there is considerable overlap between the duration of viral shedding and the duration of crusting. Women require a longer healing time than men, 19.5 and 16.5 days, respectively.[134] The mean duration of viral shedding from the cervix is 11.4 days. Therefore, patients should be advised to refrain from sexual activity until the lesions have completely healed; however, asymptomatic viral shedding is just as likely to transmit HSV.

A genital herpes infection may be acquired from an individual who has never had symptomatic genital lesions. States of asymptomatic or subclinical viral shedding occur in the majority of women with recurrent genital herpes as a result of reactivation of latent infection. These recurrent infections can have a primary disease presentation, causing the patient to blame the most proximate sexual partner, when in actuality, the exposure could have occurred in the distant past.[155] Serologic and virologic typing can be used to determine whether this is a true primary infection. Using sensitive detection techniques such as PCR, women with recurrent HSV infections shed virus up to 28% of the time, but the relationship between a PCR-positive HSV test and true communicability has yet to be determined.[156] A recent study of men and women seropositive for HSV-2, but with no previous history of symptomatic genital herpes, demonstrated viral shedding in the genital tract at a rate similar to those who reported symptomatic infection.[157] In addition, asymptomatic spread can occur from multiple anatomic genital sites and in a bilateral fashion, even with previous outbreaks of unilateral lesions.[158]

Seropositive HSV patients also should be counseled to practice safer sex, using male or female condoms, at all times, not just during symptomatic episodes.

Diagnostic Tests

CASE 69-14, QUESTION 4: Viral culture was negative for B.J., but HSV-2 point-of-care (POC) serology was positive for both B.J. and his sexual partner. How should these laboratory tests be interpreted?

The accuracy with which herpes genitalis can be diagnosed without the aid of laboratory tests generally is difficult to achieve, especially if the infection is not symptomatically recurrent in nature. Thus, because of the potentially severe psychological and physiological ramifications of such a diagnosis, either virologic or serologic confirmation of the diagnosis may be obtained.

The laboratory diagnosis of HSV-1 or HSV-2 infection depends on isolation of virus using viral culture, HSV DNA detection by PCR (more expensive than viral culture and not as widely available), or HSV antigen detection using EIA or DFA. Both PCR and EIA can differentiate HSV-1 from HSV-2. Currently, HSV DNA PCR is the most sensitive method for detecting mucocutaneous herpes simplex infection rather than simple viral culture in those with genital ulcers and is the preferred method for CSF samples.[134] Tests that measure serologic response (antibody production) are valuable in documenting primary infection, but they are not very useful in recurrent infections or in determining when the initial infection occurred. It is possible to differentiate between antibodies to HSV-1 and HSV-2 by means of type-specific serologic assay. POC devices using HSV-2–specific antibody testing kits offer ease, reduced time, differentiation between HSV-1 and HSV-2, and high sensitivities and specificities.[2,159,160]

Viral culture is more likely to yield false-negative results than other testing methods.[2] A better antigen detection test could have been used, such as an EIA or DFA. The lack of a positive viral culture does not rule out the diagnosis of a primary infection in B.J., especially because the antibody test was positive. The fact that B.J.'s partner's antibody test was positive without a history of symptomatic disease suggests a distant infection with asymptomatic shedding.

Treatment

CASE 69-14, QUESTION 5: How should B.J.'s lesions be managed? Because the likelihood of recurrence of genital herpes is high, what treatment and prevention measures are recommended currently?

A diagnosis of genital herpes is concerning because there is no cure for the condition. Therapies ranging from antiviral agents and photoinactivation to investigational vaccines have been tried. Currently, only acyclovir (ACV), famciclovir (FCV), and valacyclovir (VCV) are useful in the treatment and prevention of genital herpes.

The ideal anti-HSV agent should (a) prevent infection, (b) shorten the clinical course, (c) prevent the development of latency, (d) prevent recurrence in patients with established latency, (e) decrease transmission of disease, and (f) eradicate established latent infection.[134] To date, no agent has been successful in achieving all of these goals.

All three agents, ACV, FCV, and VCV, are effective for the short-term treatment of some HSV infections. ACV, a nucleoside analog, is a substrate for HSV-specific thymidine kinase. Through a series of phosphorylation steps, ACV is transformed to ACV-triphosphate, a competitive inhibitor of viral DNA polymerase. ACV has potent in vitro activity against both HSV-1 and HSV-2 and is far less active against varicella-zoster and CMV.[161] FCV, a prodrug of penciclovir, has increased oral bioavailability compared with acyclovir. Once converted in the intestine and liver to the active form, penciclovir, it is quickly phosphorylated in HSV in a similar manner as ACV. VCV is the L-valyl ester prodrug of ACV. The oral bioavailability of VCV is also significantly better than ACV, producing plasma levels of ACV comparable to those attained with IV administered ACV, often eliminating the need for parenteral therapy.[162] All three antiviral drugs are equally effective for genital herpes infections.

IV ACV (5 mg/kg/dose every 8 hours) significantly reduced the duration of viral shedding in primary genital herpes, decreasing the duration of signs and symptoms of disease by a mean of 5 days, and the time to healing of lesions by a mean of 6 to 12 days compared with placebo-treated patients.[2,163] Similar findings have been shown in the immunocompromised patient population.[164] IV and oral ACV or VCV also prevent HSV reactivation in seropositive immunocompromised patients who are undergoing bone marrow transplantation.[165] For patients with HIV, ACV 400 mg PO three times daily, FCV 500 mg twice daily, or VCV 500 mg twice daily for 5 to 10 days have been used for recurrent episodes.[2] Currently, IV therapy is recommended only for patients with severe genital or disseminated infections who cannot take oral medication.

Topical therapy with ACV ointment (5% in polyethylene glycol) has minimal effect on the duration of viral shedding, symptoms, and lesion healing in a first episode of primary genital herpes, has no effect on the recurrence rate,[163] and is not recommended for primary genital herpes. Penciclovir 1% cream applied every 2 hours while awake is effective for treatment of herpes simplex labialis,[166] but insufficient data exist to recommend its use for genital herpes infections.

Oral antivirals speed the healing and resolution of symptoms of first and recurrent episodes of genital HSV-2 infections.[167] Treatment of primary infection after the first week of infection does change the natural history of recurrent outbreaks; thus, patients should be educated about risk of sexual transmission, prompt recognition of signs and symptoms, and the early use of antivirals.[168] The frequency of recurrence decreases with time in most patients. Recurrent episodes of genital HSV-2 infection can be treated with any of the three available oral antivirals (Table 69-8). Rather than having to go into clinic, patients with recurrent infection should have a supply of their antiviral drug with them to allow early initiation of therapy, which may abort or reduce symptoms by 1 to 2 days.[169,170]

Daily suppressive therapy with ACV, FCV, or VCV reduces the frequency of recurrent episodes up to 70% to 80% among patients with frequent (five to eight episodes per year) genital herpes.[2,171] Recurrent outbreaks diminish with time; thus, after each year of continuous suppressive therapy, an effort should be made to discuss discontinuing therapy with the patient.[2] The use of suppressive therapy does not completely eliminate viral transmission. However, a randomized, controlled clinical trial of serodiscordant HSV-2–positive couples demonstrated a statistically significant decrease in the rate of transmission to uninfected partners when infected partners took 500 mg/day of VCV.[145] This 8-month study was restricted to heterosexual partners with fewer than ten recurrences per year. The CDC recommends various dosing regimens for VCV, but the 500-mg once-daily dose appears to be less effective than the 1-g once-daily dose in patients with frequent recurrent episodes (i.e., >10 episodes per year).[2] However, one meta-analysis showed a consistent prophylactic benefit whether VCV was dosed at 250 mg twice daily or

TABLE 69-8
Antiviral Chemotherapy of Genital HSV-2 Infections

	Acyclovir	Valacyclovir	Famciclovir	Duration	Comments
First clinical episode	400 mg PO TID *or* 200 mg PO 5 times per day	1 g PO BID	250 mg PO TID	7–10 days	May extend treatment duration if healing is incomplete
Episodic recurrent infection	400 mg PO TID *or* 800 mg PO BID *or* 800 mg PO TID × 2 days	1 g every day *or* 500 mg PO BID × 3 days	125 mg PO BID *or* 1 g PO BID × 1 day *or* 500 mg PO × 1 day, then 250 mg BID × 2 days	5 days	Most effective if initiated within the first 24 hours of onset of lesions or during the prodrome
Daily suppressive therapy	400 mg PO BID[a]	500 mg PO every day[b] *or* 1 g PO every day	250 mg PO BID	Daily	Reduces the frequency of genital herpes recurrences by ≥75% among patients who have frequent recurrences (i.e., ≥6 recurrences per year); use should be reevaluated at 1 year
Severe disseminated	5–10 mg/kg IV every 8 hours	Not indicated	Not indicated	Variable	Hospitalize and treat until clinical resolution of symptoms Follow-up IV therapy with PO acyclovir to complete 10 days
HIV-infected: episodic	400 mg PO TID *or* 200 mg 5 per day	1 g PO BID[c]	500 mg PO BID	5–10 days	Treat until clinical resolution of lesions
HIV-infected: suppressive	400–800 mg PO BID or TID	500 mg PO BID[d]	500 mg PO BID		

[a] Safety and efficacy up to 6 years have been documented with the use of acyclovir.
[b] Valacyclovir 500 mg every day seems less effective in patients with more than 10 episodes per year. Thus, 1 g every day should be used in these patients.
[c] Dosages up to 8 g/d have been used, but an association with a syndrome resembling either hemolytic uremic syndrome or thrombotic thrombocytopenic purpura was observed.
[d] Effective in decreasing both the rate of recurrences and the rate of subclinical shedding among HIV-infected patients.
Note: Regimen recommendations derived from Workowski KA et al. Sexually transmitted diseases treatment guidelines, 2010. *MMWR Recomm Rep.* 2010;59(RR-12):1.

500 mg once daily.[172] Immunocompromised patients may require higher doses or more frequent intervals for suppression.[173] Most cases of ACV-resistant HSV occur in the immunocompromised host; however, the resistance is less than 5%.[174] All ACV-resistant strains are also resistant to VCV, and most are resistant to FCV as well. Foscarnet 40 mg/kg IV every 8 hours may be used for severe ACV-resistant genital HSV infections.[2] Cidofovir 1% gel (not commercially available in the United States, but has been compounded by pharmacists) applied once daily for 5 days may be an alternative to IV foscarnet, but more studies are needed.[2,175]

B.J. is not yet a candidate for daily suppressive ACV therapy. A summary of the indications for ACV, FCV, and VCV is outlined in Table 69-8.

ADVERSE EFFECTS

CASE 69-14, QUESTION 6: What adverse effects associated with ACV, FCV, or VCV should be anticipated?

Overall, all forms of ACV, including VCV and FCV, are associated with relatively few adverse reactions largely because of the drugs' affinity for viral thymidine kinase compared with cellular kinase.

Hematuria and an increase in blood urea nitrogen and serum creatinine may occur, primarily in patients with underlying renal disease or those receiving concomitant nephrotoxic agents. However, this complication is almost entirely associated with the IV route. In addition, severe local reactions are possible with IV administration. In patients with HIV/AIDS, VCV at a dosage of 8 g/day was associated with a hemolytic uremic syndrome or thrombotic thrombocytopenic purpuralike syndrome. However, this complication has not been observed with normal therapeutic doses. As described previously, when given intravenously in high doses or with significant dehydration, ACV crystallizes in the renal collecting tubules of animals, leading to renal insufficiency.[176] ACV should not be rapidly infused or administered at concentrations greater than10 mg/mL. Dose adjustment is necessary for all three antiviral agents in patients with decreased renal function.

Although neurotoxicity is a rare side effect, case reports of coma and delirium have been reported in patients with renal failure.[177,178]

Intravenous ACV occasionally has been associated with cutaneous irritation and phlebitis, reversible leukopenia,[179] and transient elevations of liver transaminases. Oral ACV and VCV are relatively safe and do not produce any serious side effects at normal doses. Patients receiving oral ACV, VCV, or FCV may complain of nausea, dizziness, diarrhea, and headaches.

Patient Education and Counseling

CASE 69-14, QUESTION 7: What are the roles for education and counseling in patients with genital herpes? Are other forms of local or symptomatic care useful?

Most genital herpes infections are benign, and lesions heal spontaneously unless the patient is immunocompromised or the lesions have become infected secondarily. The patient should be instructed to keep the involved areas clean and dry. To prevent autoinoculation, the patient should be told not to touch the lesions and to wash his hands immediately afterward if he comes in contact with the lesion. Local anesthetics provide relief from the pain of genital lesions, but they should be avoided if possible because they counteract efforts to keep the lesions dry.

Local corticosteroid therapy is contraindicated because it may predispose the patient to secondary infections.

Patient counseling should include the source contact and any future partner. Health care practitioners should attempt to relieve patients' feelings of guilt and anxiety; discussion of long-term consequences should take place after the acute symptoms of the infection have resolved.

For individuals with frequent recurrences, efforts should be made to identify and avoid stimulatory factors such as sunlight, trauma, or emotional stress. The limitations of therapy and the decreased severity and frequency of recurrences with time should be explained to the patient. The periods of infectivity and the need to avoid sexual activity even when lesions are not present should be emphasized, indicating the need for continuous barrier protection. Women with herpes genitalis should be scheduled for routine Pap smears and should be instructed to discuss their HSV with their physicians if they become pregnant.

Currently, there is no completely effective way to prevent the transmission of HSV-2 infection. Barrier forms of contraception, in particular condoms, may reduce the transmission of HSV, but this may be limited only to male-to-female transmission owing to the large area that herpes lesions may occupy on the woman.[150] However, greater use of condoms by men can increase protection and is recommended to prevent HSV infections.[151] Nonoxynol-9, a spermicide that has in vitro anti-HSV activity, is ineffective in the prevention of established genital HSV infection and may actually increase the risk of transmission of HSV by causing genital ulceration.[180]

Complications

CASE 69-15

QUESTION 1: M.F. is a 23-year-old, sexually active female student with a history of frequent and severe recurrences of genital herpes since her initial infection 3 years ago. M.F. has tried numerous therapies, including suppressive and episodic antivirals. None of these therapies has provided M.F. with any relief of her symptoms, nor have they decreased the frequency of her recurrences. M.F. has read much in the lay press about herpes and is concerned about the possible complications of the disease, especially cervical cancer. What are the potential complications of herpes genitalis?

Previous research suggested that HSV-2 might be an oncogenic agent responsible for carcinoma of the cervix. However, a large longitudinal nested case-control study using nearly 20 years of seroepidemiologic and epidemiologic data combined with a meta-analysis concluded that it is very unlikely that HSV-2 is associated with the development of invasive cervical carcinoma.[181] Severe complications of herpes genitalis include central nervous system disease, such as meningitis and encephalitis, and disseminated disease.[134]

PREGNANCY

CASE 69-16

QUESTION 1: A.P., a 26-year-old woman in her 32nd week of gestation, was hospitalized with complaints of painful genital lesions, headache, fever, increased vaginal discharge, and dysuria of 1 week's duration. Multiple ulcerative lesions consistent with genital herpes were present on the cervix, vulva, labia minora, and thighs. How should A.P. be treated?

Herpes genitalis seropositivity in pregnant women occurs more frequently than in nonpregnant women, with 20% to 30% of all pregnant women having serologic evidence of HSV-2 infection and 2% acquiring the infection during pregnancy.[182] Unfortunately, a large proportion of those infections occurring during pregnancy are limited to the cervix and are totally asymptomatic, often eluding diagnosis.

Pregnant patients with a history of recurrent genital herpes should be examined carefully when they present in labor for evidence of active disease. The safety of systemic ACV and VCV in pregnant women has not been established in controlled trials and may or may not be indicated for A.P. Some small studies suggest ACV administered for several weeks before delivery may decrease recurrent outbreaks and lessen the need for herpes-related cesarean section,[183] whereas a larger randomized clinical trial did not show a benefit in reducing the need for a cesarean delivery with primary infection.[184] In general, it does seem that patients with symptomatic genital herpes benefit from cesarean section.[185] The manufacturer of Zovirax (ACV) maintains an extensive database of fetal complications related to ACV use. To date, no link between ACV and birth defects has been established.[186] The decision to treat HSV with ACV during pregnancy should depend on the clinical severity of infection. Fetal exposure data to FCV or VCV are limited. If the mother has an active herpes genitalis infection at the time of delivery (either active genital lesions or asymptomatic HSV-2 cervicitis), the baby should be delivered by cesarean section within 4 hours after the membranes have ruptured to prevent exposure of the neonate to the virus.[187] However, if no genital lesions are present at the time of labor, vaginal delivery may be recommended.[2] There is evidence that up to 70% of neonatal herpes cases occur in asymptomatic women, and the use of ACV or VCV after 36 weeks' gestation may decrease clinical disease and viral shedding to the fetus.[188]

Neonatal herpes is a devastating systemic infection of the newborn, associated with high morbidity and mortality, especially when infected with HSV-2 versus HSV-1.[189] HSV is usually transmitted to the newborn during passage through an infected birth canal, approximately 300 times greater than when HSV is not present.[185] The risk of transmission to the newborn is greatest in mothers who acquire an initial infection late in the third trimester and lower in mothers with recurrent infection or those who acquire herpes in the first trimester (25% to 50% vs. $<1\%$ for pre-existing infection).[189]

GENITAL WARTS

CASE 69-17

QUESTION 1: S.L., a 19-year-old woman, presents to the women's health clinic for her annual pelvic examination. One week later, her Pap smear is read as showing koilocytosis. A colposcopy is subsequently performed, revealing changes consistent with cervical flat warts. What is the cause of S.L.'s infection? How should she be managed?

Human papillomavirus (HPV) is the cause of genital warts, or condylomata acuminata. Types 6 and 11 account for more than 90% of genital warts.[190] Other types of HPV, including 16 and 18, account for as much as 70% of cervical cancer.[191,192] They are associated with Pap smear changes, including koilocytosis and cervical dysplasia. In the United States, the seroprevalence of HPV 6, 11, 16, and 18 is 32.5% for women and 12.2% among men 14 to 59 years of age.[193]

Cervical intraepithelial neoplasia (CIN) is a common cervical cancer grading system using histologic changes to classify specimens in three categories, CIN-1, -2, and -3. The higher the number, the greater is the chance of progressing to invasive cervical cancer. Most new cases of HPV infection spontaneously regress, but with progressive histologic changes, the chance of spontaneously regressing diminishes (CIN-1, 60%; CIN-2, 30%; CIN-3, 10%).[194] Types of HPV are also classified as high risk, or those likely to cause cancer, and low risk, those less likely to cause cancer. HPV types 16 and 18 are considered high risk and types 6 and 11 are low risk, the latter mostly resulting in genital warts. In women, visible warts occur on the labia, introitus, and vagina. Subclinical lesions also commonly occur on these sites and on the cervix, as in S.L.'s case. They are visible only by colposcopy after applying acetic acid. Men can sexually transmit HPV infections to women as well as exhibit genital warts, and anal and penile cancer are associated with oncogenic HPV types, especially type 16.[195] The goal of HPV therapy is the removal of symptomatic warts. Several therapeutic options are available and include patient-administered treatments to visible warts such as podofilox 0.5% solution or gel, imiquimod 5% cream and sinecatechins 15% ointment; provider-administered products include topical treatments (podophyllin 10%–25%, trichloroacetic acid 80%–90%, and cryotherapy), surgery (laser or scalpel), and intralesional interferon.[2] In a recent meta-analysis, locally applied interferon showed a 44% lesion clearance compared with 27.4% for systemic interferon.[196] None of these treatments can eradicate HPV infection or alter the natural history of HPV. It is important to individualize therapy, considering location and number of warts, patient preference, cost, and convenience.

Podophyllin, compounded as a 10% to 25% solution in tincture of benzoin, is applied by the health care provider to visible warts. After application, it is washed off 3 to 4 hours later and then reapplied once or twice a week until the warts have disappeared. Podofilox 0.5% solution or gel, the active component of podophyllin resin, may be applied by the patient with a cotton swab, or podofilox gel with a finger, to visible genital warts twice a day for 3 days, followed by 4 days of no therapy. A total of four cycles, 0.5 mL/day, or application of an area larger than 10 cm^2 should not be exceeded. Podofilox solution is not suitable for use with perianal warts; the gel is more practical for this region. Podophyllin is potentially neurotoxic if absorbed in large amounts. Podofilox has the advantage over podophyllin resin in that it has a longer shelf life, does not need to be washed off, and has less systemic toxicity.[197] Therefore, it should be applied in limited doses and should also be avoided in pregnancy. The rate of wart recurrence after podophyllin therapy is extremely high, probably 50%. With the high cost of clinic care and the high recurrence rate, home treatment of HPV with podofilox solution may be more cost effective and equally efficacious.[198]

Imiquimod induces cytokines and activates the cell-mediated immune system. In initial trials, complete clearance of warts took place in 37% to 50% of immunocompetent patients, but up to 20% experienced recurrence.[199] The 5% cream is optimally applied by finger at bedtime three times per week for up to 16 weeks.[200] It is usually left on for 6 to 10 hours before it is washed off with soap and water. Imiquimod may take as long as 8 weeks before warts are cleared. Mild to moderate local irritation occurs in more than half of the patients who use it, especially when used daily instead of three times weekly as directed. The cream may weaken condoms and diaphragms.

Sinecatechins are green-tea extracts that contain active catechins with purported immunostimulatory, antiproliferative, and antitumor properties. In the United States, a 15% topical ointment is available. There are limited data on this product, but literature suggests it may be more effective than imiquimod or podofilox by clearing up to 55% of external genital warts.[201] It is applied by finger directly to the wart three times a day up to 16 weeks, with the most common side effects being local erythema, pruritus or burning, and pain.[2]

Cryotherapy by application of liquid nitrogen can be more effective than podophyllin, but requires special equipment and highly trained personnel. Pain and skin blistering after treatment are common. Cryotherapy is associated with minimal systemic toxicity and is useful against oral, anal, urethral, and vaginal warts.

Trichloroacetic acid (80%–90%) is used topically in the treatment of some genital warts, but its efficacy is uncertain. To date, interferons are not recommended because of expense and toxicity. Cases refractory to topical drug therapy should be considered for surgical treatment.

Prevention

In 2006, the first vaccine to prevent HPV types 6, 11, 16, and 18 was approved in the United States. This quadrivalent vaccine was tested in women from 15 to 26 years of age and demonstrated 98% to 100% protection against HPV types contained in the vaccine.[202,203] In men, the quadrivalent vaccine efficacy was 62.1% to 89.4% against genital warts, depending on previous HPV exposure, leading to its approval for men and boys 9 to 26 years old.[204] This three-dose series can be given as early as 9 years of age, but is CDC recommended at 11 to 12 years as part of a routine adolescent health care visit and ideally before commencement of sexual activity. Because there are more than 30 types of HPV associated with anogenital disease, a previous HPV infection is not a contraindication to vaccination. It is also important to note that receipt of the HPV vaccine does not change the recommendation for Pap smears. Lastly, it should not be considered a therapeutic vaccine as it has no impact on active HPV infection.

VACCINES

Prevention and control of STDs have largely revolved around education and antimicrobials. Immunization, however, holds the promise of protecting large numbers of people before they are at risk for STDs as well as targeting those who already have the infection. Hepatitis B is an example of an STD with a highly effective vaccine that is now mandatory for school-aged children. The quadrivalent HPV vaccine is gaining momentum, and a bivalent (HPV 16 and 18) vaccine is also now approved by the FDA, but the latter is not indicated for prevention of genital warts. Herpes simplex vaccines have been extensively studied, but no candidate vaccine has been submitted for approval.

KEY REFERENCES AND WEBSITES

A full list of references for this chapter can be found at **http://thepoint.lww.com/AT10e.** Below are the key references and websites for this chapter, with the corresponding reference number in this chapter found in parentheses after the reference.

Key References

Centers for Disease Control and Prevention (CDC). Update to CDC's sexually transmitted diseases treatment guidelines,

2006: fluoroquinolones no longer recommended for treatment of gonococcal infections. *MMWR Morb Mortal Wkly Rep*. 2007; 56:332. (16)

National Center for HIV/AIDS, Viral Hepatitis, STD, and TB Prevention, Division of STD Prevention. *Sexually Transmitted Disease Surveillance 2007 Supplement, Gonococcal Isolate Surveillance Project (GISP) Annual Report 2007*. Atlanta, GA: US Dept of Health and Human Services, Centers for Disease Control and Prevention; 2009. (22)

Workowski KA et al. Sexually transmitted diseases treatment guidelines, 2010. *MMWR Recomm Rep*. 2010;59(RR-12):1. (2)

Key Websites

U.S. Department of Health and Human Services. Healthy People 2020 Topics and Objectives: Sexually Transmitted Diseases. **http://www.healthypeople.gov/2020/topicsobjectives2020/objectiveslist.aspx?topicid=37.** Accessed February 3, 2011. (4)

U.S. Food and Drug Administration. New Warning for Nonoxynol 9 OTC Contraceptive Products re: STDs and HIV/AIDS. **http://www.fda.gov/ForConsumers/ByAudience/ForPatientAdvocates/HIVandAIDSActivities/ucm124023.htm.** Accessed August 5, 2010. (31)

70 Osteomyelitis and Septic Arthritis

Bridgette Kram and Ralph H. Raasch

CORE PRINCIPLES

OSTEOMYELITIS	CHAPTER CASES
1 Acute hematogenous osteomyelitis is characterized by the abrupt onset of localized pain and tenderness at a single site, fever, and increased inflammatory markers (erythrocyte sedimentation rate, C-reactive protein). Imaging techniques and blood and bone cultures (if done) may document findings consistent with bone changes in osteomyelitis and the responsible pathogen.	**Case 70-1 (Questions 1, 2), Table 70-1**
2 Initial empiric antibiotic therapy for acute hematogenous osteomyelitis should be directed at gram-positive cocci, including methicillin-resistant *Staphylococcus aureus* (MRSA). Protein binding and bone concentrations of antibiotics are not critical factors in predicting successful treatment, as long as the responsible pathogen is susceptible to the chosen therapy, and treatment is given in high doses for long duration.	**Case 70-1 (Question 3), Table 70-2**
3 If blood or bone cultures grow the likely pathogen, then therapy should be de-escalated when possible based on organism susceptibilities. Assuming no allergies, methicillin-sensitive *Staphylococcus aureus* (MSSA) should be treated with oxacillin or nafcillin. The overall duration of therapy (by intravenous [IV] route and possibly orally) should be at least 4 weeks. Patients should be followed closely for at least 2 years after treatment is completed to detect possible relapse.	**Case 70-1 (Questions 4–7), Tables 70-2, 70-3**
4 Osteomyelitis secondary to a contiguous focus of infection typically occurs after trauma and the consequent orthopedic corrective surgery. Common symptoms are pain, tenderness, erythema and drainage at the site of injury or infection. Imaging studies usually show bone changes consistent with infection.	**Case 70-2 (Questions 1, 2), Table 70-1**
5 Secondary osteomyelitis is often polymicrobial. Surgical efforts should be instituted to reassess the site of bone injury and infection, with deep tissue or bone samples obtained for culture. Treatment is for at least 4 weeks of IV therapy, and the antibiotics chosen should depend on the cultured organisms and their antibiotic susceptibilities.	**Case 70-2 (Questions 3, 4)**
6 Osteomyelitis associated with vascular insufficiency most often occurs in patients with diabetes mellitus. Neuropathy and impaired blood flow leads to the development of chronic lower extremity cellulitis and underlying osteomyelitis. Multiple gram-positive and gram-negative aerobic and anaerobic bacteria may be involved; thus, initial empirical treatment typically includes vancomycin and an antipseudomonal beta-lactam. Definitive therapy should be based on the results of deep surgical cultures. Duration of treatment should be 6 or more weeks, with chronic suppressive therapy considered thereafter.	**Case 70-3 (Questions 1, 2), Case 70-4 (Question 1)**

continued

OSTEOMYELITIS *CONTINUED*

7 Chronic osteomyelitis can present years later at a site of previous bone infection, and is usually characterized by a draining sinus tract from bone to skin. Chronically infected dead bone is involved, and surgery is important in removing necrotic bone when possible. Chronic osteomyelitis is often polymicrobial, and the same organism (especially *S. aureus*) that was causative of a previous bone infection could still be involved in chronic infection. High-dose IV therapy directed at the results of bone cultures for at least 6 weeks is recommended to offer the best chances of preventing the extension of infection to adjacent uninfected bone.	**Case 70-5 (Questions 1–3)**
8 Prosthetic joint infection with adjacent bone osteomyelitis usually requires surgical removal of the infected prosthesis for cure. Antibiotics should be directed at the cultured bacteria from a joint aspirate or from deep surgical specimens. The most common pathogens are *S. aureus* and coagulase-negative staphylococci. In a situation in which the prosthesis cannot be totally removed, lifelong, chronic suppressive oral therapy should be considered.	**Case 70-6 (Questions 1–3)**

SEPTIC ARTHRITIS

1 Nongonococcal septic arthritis is characterized by fever, and the acute onset of joint pain and effusion in a single joint. Infection is typically acquired hematogenously from an originating site that may not always be easily identified. *S. aureus* is the most common pathogen. Duration of treatment should be 4 weeks, with oral therapy for the final 2 weeks.	**Case 70-7 (Questions 1–3)**
2 *Neisseria gonorrhoeae* is the most common cause of polyarticular arthritis in a young, sexually active adult. Skin lesions may also be present in disseminated gonococcal infection (DGI). The diagnosis is frequently based on the clinical syndrome and sexual history, as joint fluid aspirate and blood cultures are frequently negative. Intravenous ceftriaxone is the treatment of choice, and should be continued for 1 to 2 days after improvement begins. Treatment duration is at least 7 days, and therapy can be converted to oral drugs for the last portion of treatment.	**Case 70-8 (Question 1)**

OSTEOMYELITIS

Osteomyelitis is an inflammation of the bone marrow and surrounding bone associated with infection. Any bone can be involved, and substantial morbidity is possible even with early diagnosis and treatment. Despite the continued refinement of diagnostic procedures (e.g., radionuclide imaging, computed tomography, magnetic resonance imaging), advances in antimicrobial therapy, and the use of prophylactic antibiotics before orthopedic procedures, osteomyelitis continues to be difficult to cure.

Osteomyelitis can affect all age groups.[1] The most common causative microorganisms of acute osteomyelitis have historically been streptococci and staphylococci. *Staphylococcus aureus* remains the most common causative organism, although the prevalence of infection caused by methicillin-resistant *S. aureus* (MRSA) is increasing among all age groups. Additionally, osteomyelitis caused by gram-negative and anaerobic bacilli is also becoming more common.[2]

Bone may be infected by three routes: hematogenous spread of bacteria from a distant infection site, direct infection of bone from an adjacent or contiguous source of infection, and infection of bone secondary to vascular insufficiency. Table 70-1 summarizes characteristics associated with osteomyelitis.[1,2] Patients with recurrent osteomyelitis are considered to have chronic osteomyelitis.

Bone Anatomy and Physiology

Understanding the pathophysiology of osteomyelitis requires a basic understanding of bone anatomy and physiology. Figure 70-1 is a graphic representation of a long bone. The bone is divided into three sections: the epiphysis, located at the end of the bone; the metaphysis; and the diaphysis. The epiphysis and metaphysis are separated by the epiphyseal growth plate. This is the rapidly growing area of the bone supported by many blood vessels. Surrounding most of the bone is a fibrous and cellular envelope. The external portion of this envelope is the periosteum, whereas the internal portion is the endosteum.

The blood vessels that supply bone tissue are located predominantly in the bone's epiphysis and metaphysis. The nutrient arteries enter the bone at the metaphyseal side of the epiphyseal growth plate and lead to capillaries that form sharp loops within the growth plate. These capillaries lead to large sinusoidal veins that eventually exit the metaphysis through a nutrient vein. Within the sinusoidal veins, blood flow is slowed considerably, and infection is possible with bacterial colonization.

Differences in the vasculature of bone in different age groups lead to different forms of osteomyelitis. In neonates and adults, vascular communications are present between the epiphysis and metaphysis, which can allow infection to spread from bone to the adjacent joint. During childhood, however, this area often is protected from infection because the epiphyseal plate separates the vascular supply for these two regions.

TABLE 70-1
Features of Osteomyelitis

Feature	Hematogenous	Adjacent Site of Infection	Vascular Insufficiency
Usual age of onset (years)	<20; >50	>40	>40
Sites of infection	Long bones, vertebrae	Femur, tibia, skull, mandible	Feet
Risk factors	Bacteremia	Surgery, trauma, cellulitis, joint prosthesis	Diabetes, peripheral vascular disease
Common bacteria	*S. aureus*, gram-negative bacilli; usually one organism	*S. aureus*, gram-negative bacilli; anaerobic organisms; often polymicrobial	*S. aureus*, coagulase-negative staphylococci, streptococci, gram-negative and anaerobic organisms; usually polymicrobial
Clinical findings			
Initial episode	Fever, chills, local tenderness, swelling; limitation of motion	Fever, warmth, swelling; unstable joint	Pain, swelling, drainage, ulcer formation
Recurrent episode	Drainage	Drainage, sinus tract	As above

For a narrated PowerPoint presentation that emphasizes the different types and pathophysiologies of osteomyelitis, go to http://thepoint.lww.com/AT10e.

Hematogenous Osteomyelitis

Hematogenous osteomyelitis classically has been a disease of children, although the number of cases reported in adults is increasing. Osteomyelitis in children tends to be acute and hematogenous and is often responsive to antibiotic therapy alone. In comparison, osteomyelitis in adults tends to be subacute or chronic, occurs in the fifth or sixth decade of life, and commonly results from trauma, infection of prosthetic devices, or other insult.[1–3] When treating osteomyelitis in adults, surgical débridement is often needed in addition to antimicrobial therapy.

Infection in children develops primarily in the metaphysis of the rapidly growing long bones of the body where the slowed blood flow allows bacteria to colonize and multiply. The acute infectious process (e.g., edema, inflammation, small vessel thrombosis) increases bone pressure, which compromises blood flow and eventually leads to necrosis. Released cytokines alter bone integrity by promoting osteoclast activity. Eventually, the elevated pressure and necrosis cause devitalized bone to fragment from healthy bone (sequestra). With continued spread of the infection into the outer layers of the bone and soft tissue, abscess and draining sinus tracts form.[1,2]

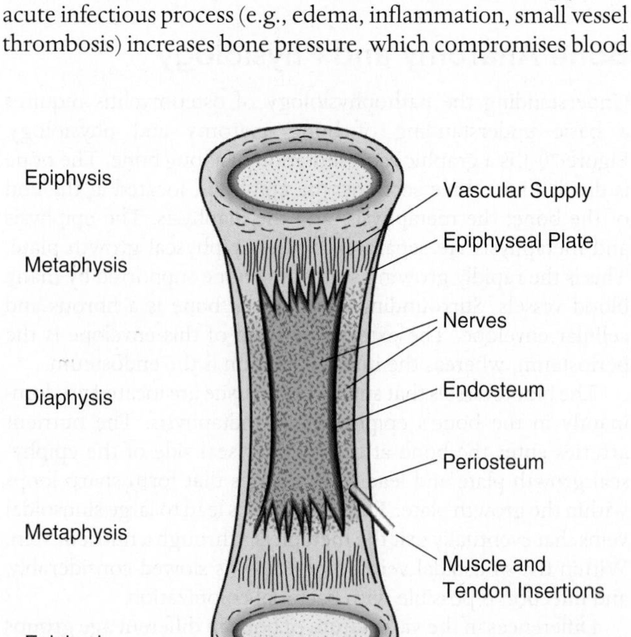

FIGURE 70-1 Long bone anatomy. (Adapted with permission from Triffitt JT. Organic matrix of bone tissue. In: Urist MR, ed. *Fundamental and Clinical Bone Physiology*. Philadelphia, PA: JB Lippincott; 1980:46.)

In children, hematogenous infection most commonly occurs in the long bones as a single focus in the femur and tibia.[1] In neonates, hematogenous osteomyelitis is an especially serious disease that often involves multiple bones, especially the long bones. Rapid spread across the epiphyseal plate can involve the adjacent joint, necessitating immediate, aggressive treatment. In adults, the vertebrae are more commonly involved.[1–3]

The most common organism causing hematogenous osteomyelitis is *S. aureus,* in part because of its proclivity to adhere to bone and cartilage. In recent decades, the rapid emergence of both hospital- and community-acquired strains of MRSA has challenged the management of osteomyelitis. MRSA infections are associated with an increased risk of antibiotic treatment failures and complications, including abscess formation, deep vein thrombosis, and septic emboli.[4,5] Gram-negative bacilli (*Escherichia coli, Klebsiella, Proteus, Salmonella,* and *Pseudomonas*) are responsible for an increasing number of cases of osteomyelitis as well. Intravenous (IV) drug use often leads to infection with *Pseudomonas aeruginosa,* whereas *Salmonella* species is a common cause in patients with sickle cell anemia.[1,2]

The clinical features of hematogenous osteomyelitis vary, depending on the patient's age and the infection site. In children, infection usually is characterized by an abrupt onset of high fever and chills, localized pain, tenderness, and swelling. Systemic symptoms often are absent in neonates, potentially delaying the diagnosis. A diagnosis, therefore, must be made on the basis of localized symptoms such as edema and restricted limb movement. Systemic symptoms are also less common in adults, although patients with vertebral osteomyelitis can present with the insidious onset of localized back pain and tenderness.[1,3]

Acute Osteomyelitis

USUAL CLINICAL PRESENTATION

CASE 70-1

QUESTION 1: L.D., a 7-year-old girl, is unable to go to school today because of fever and worsening leg pain. Her upper left leg started to hurt 3 to 4 days ago, and last night she began limping. Her parents report no history of trauma to the area. Her only past medical history is two episodes of otitis media at ages 2 and 5. In the pediatrician's office,

maximal tenderness is localized over the left distal femur without knee joint effusion. No signs of swelling, warmth, or trauma are seen. Her white blood cell (WBC) count is 8,000 cells/μL with a normal WBC differential. Plain radiographic studies of the left leg are normal, but the erythrocyte sedimentation rate (ESR) is 58 mm/hour. Two blood samples are obtained for culture, and L.D. is sent home with directions for bed rest and use of acetaminophen as needed for fever. Two days later, she is admitted to the hospital with severe pain and tenderness in her left leg and a fever of 38.8°C. The blood cultures obtained 2 days ago are positive for *S. aureus* with susceptibilities still pending. C-reactive protein (CRP) is 14 mg/dL (normal, <2 mg/dL). Another plain radiographic study is normal, but a magnetic resonance imaging (MRI) scan reveals inflammation in her left distal femur. What findings in L.D. are consistent with hematogenous osteomyelitis?

L.D. displays the usual signs and symptoms of acute hematogenous osteomyelitis in children. She is a previously healthy child who experienced acute localized pain and tenderness of the left distal femur, abrupt onset of high fever, and an elevated ESR and CRP. Her plain radiographic studies were normal on two occasions; however, destructive changes to bone often do not appear on plain radiographs for at least 10 to 14 days after onset of infection.[2] Hence, a normal plain film does not rule out acute osteomyelitis if obtained within the first 2 weeks of infection. Although costly, MRI scans can detect bone changes earlier in the course of disease.[2] L.D.'s MRI scan on hospitalization detected inflammation in the left distal femur. Although L.D. did not have a bone biopsy sent for culture, her clinical picture, a positive MRI scan, and blood cultures positive for *S. aureus* establish the diagnosis of osteomyelitis. The specific event that caused bacteremia with dissemination to bone is unknown, as is often the case in children.[2,4]

Laboratory tests that should be routinely obtained in every child suspected of having osteomyelitis include a complete blood count (CBC), ESR, and serum CRP. Although these tests are not specific for the diagnosis of osteomyelitis, they help confirm the clinical diagnosis. An increased WBC count is consistent with osteomyelitis, but leukocytosis is absent in many children with osteomyelitis at the initial examination. Thus, L.D.'s WBC count of 8,000 cells/μL is not unusual. In adults, leukocytosis is more common in an acute infection rather than with recurrent or chronic disease. When leukocytosis is present, the WBC count rarely exceeds 15,000 cells/μL.[2,5] Both ESR and CRP are nonspecific markers of systemic inflammation when elevated. Most patients with osteomyelitis have an ESR greater than 20 mm/hour and a CRP greater than 2.0 mg/dL.[2]

Predisposing factors for hematogenous osteomyelitis include any risk factors for bacteremia (e.g., indwelling catheters such as hemodialysis shunts and chronic central venous catheters). Other risk factors that can potentially lead to bacteremia and subsequently hematogenous osteomyelitis include IV drug use and a distant focus of infection in the gastrointestinal or urinary tract. None of these factors exist in L.D. In children such as L.D. who have no history of fractures or penetrating injury, the most common cause of acute hematogenous osteomyelitis is *S. aureus*, including MRSA.[2,4–6]

PATIENT WORKUP

CASE 70-1, QUESTION 2: What additional patient and diagnostic information should be obtained before L.D. receives her first dose of antibiotics?

Before L.D. receives antibiotic therapy, she should be assessed for drug allergies, especially penicillin allergy. Patient interviews, discussions with her parents, and a comprehensive review of her medical record are necessary, especially with a history of allergy. Details of an allergic reaction, including symptoms, onset of the reaction, probable causative agent, treatment, and exposure to related antibacterials should be evaluated.

Cultures of blood and bone aspirate material optimally identify the pathogen and must be part of the initial workup. Cultures taken after antibiotics are started often are negative, resulting in a prolonged, unnecessary course of empiric broad-spectrum antibiotic therapy.

In L.D.'s case, the positive blood culture and MRI scan establish the diagnosis of osteomyelitis. If the blood cultures had been negative, however, a bone aspirate would be recommended to identify the pathogen.[1,2] Once material has been obtained for culture, empiric therapy should start as soon as possible.

TREATMENT

EMPIRIC ANTIBIOTIC THERAPY

CASE 70-1, QUESTION 3: L.D. has no history of drug allergies. She took amoxicillin for the previous episodes of acute otitis media without incident. What empiric antibiotic(s) should be started? What is the relevance of bone concentrations or protein binding of antibiotics in the selection of therapy for osteomyelitis?

The chosen agent should be administered IV at high dosages to optimize drug concentration in infected bone. Treatment should be initiated as soon as possible to improve the chances for complete eradication of infection and to avoid the need for surgery. Thus, empiric antibiotic therapy is often administered while bacterial cultures are pending or before antibiotic susceptibility results are known.

While cultures are pending or with negative cultures, the age of the child can predict the likely pathogen and empiric antibiotic selection. For example, *S. aureus* and *Streptococcus* species are commonly responsible for osteomyelitis in the neonate.[1] Other organisms that can cause osteomyelitis include *Staphylococcus epidermidis, Streptococcus pyogenes, Streptococcus pneumoniae, Haemophilus influenzae,* and *P. aeruginosa*. Table 70-2 summarizes the common causative organisms of acute hematogenous osteomyelitis in children and recommended drugs and dosages for treatment.[1,6,7]

Considering the epidemiology of L.D.'s infection and the blood cultures, she should be treated for *S. aureus* osteomyelitis. In both children and adults, approximately one-third of cases of acute osteomyelitis are currently caused by MRSA.[6,8,9] Empiric IV vancomycin should be administered pending susceptibility results. There is limited clinical experience treating MRSA osteomyelitis with clindamycin, linezolid, or daptomycin; thus, these agents should be used only in patients who are vancomycin-intolerant. Because there has been an upward drift in vancomycin minimum inhibitory concentrations (MIC) (1–2 mcg/mL) for MRSA, starting doses of vancomycin in children should be 60 mg/kg/day divided into four doses. Daptomycin or linezolid should be considered if the vancomycin MIC is 2 mcg/mL for MRSA.[10]

The importance of antibiotic bone concentration when treating osteomyelitis is unclear, and bone concentrations do not predict outcome of therapy.[1,2,8] Theoretically, protein binding could influence clinical efficacy because free drug is thought to diffuse from plasma into bone tissue; however, protein-bound drug does not. Studies evaluating the penetration of highly protein-bound

TABLE 70-2

Empiric Intravenous Antibiotics for Acute Osteomyelitis in Children

Host	Likely Organisms	Antibiotics	Dosage (mg/kg/d)	Dosage (doses/d)
Neonate	*Staphylococcus aureus*	Oxacillin (or nafcillin) +	100	4
	Group B streptococci	cefotaxime *or*	150	3
	Gram-negative bacilli	Oxacillin (or nafcillin) +	100	4
		gentamicin	5–7.5	3
<3 years	*S. aureus*	Vancomycin *or*	45–60	4
	Haemophilus influenzae type b	Cefuroxime *or*	50	2
		Oxacillin (or nafcillin) +	150	4
		cefotaxime	100	4
≥3 years	*S. aureus*	Vancomycin *or*	45–60	4
		Oxacillin (or nafcillin) *or*	150	4
		Cefazolin *or*	100	3
		Clindamycin	30–40	3
After puncture wound through shoe	*P. aeruginosa*	Ceftazidime	150	3
Child with sickle cell disease	*Salmonella* sp.	Oxacillin (or nafcillin) +	150	4
	S. aureus	cefotaxime *or*	100	4
		Vancomycin +	45–60	4
		cefotaxime	100	4

drugs such as cefazolin (90% protein-bound) show high cefazolin bone levels after a single 1-g IV dose, actually exceeding levels achieved with cephalothin (20% protein-bound). In addition, cefazolin (for sensitive gram-positive cocci) and ceftriaxone (for sensitive gram-negative rods and streptococci), both highly protein-bound drugs, are well established in treating osteomyelitis when appropriate dosages and duration are used. To summarize, antibiotic bone concentrations and protein binding of antibiotics (when appropriate dosages are used) are not significant factors in the selection of appropriate therapy for osteomyelitis.[1,2]

DIRECTED ANTIBIOTIC THERAPY

CASE 70-1, QUESTION 4: The *S. aureus* grown from L.D.'s blood culture is methicillin-sensitive (MSSA). Considering these results, what is the optimal antibiotic regimen? Would other antibiotics given less frequently also be adequate?

L.D. is not allergic to penicillin. Although vancomycin is active against MSSA, it is inferior to β-lactams; thus, β-lactam–based therapy should be used for susceptible organisms.[11,12] De-escalating from vancomycin to oxacillin (or nafcillin) at 150 mg/kg/day every 6 hours is appropriate. Nafcillin and oxacillin are therapeutically equivalent and are given in similar dosages; therefore, selection typically depends on hospital formulary considerations. Her prior exposure to amoxicillin is irrelevant except to establish the absence of a penicillin allergy.

Continuing to treat L.D. with IV oxacillin (or nafcillin) every 6 hours follows treatment recommendations for MSSA osteomyelitis. Antistaphylococcal penicillins are effective therapy with appropriate dose and duration. Changing L.D. to cefazolin would allow slightly less frequent dosing (every 8 hours), a potential advantage for home treatment. Vancomycin use should be discouraged in L.D.'s case because cultures revealed a methicillin-sensitive organism, and vancomycin is more likely to be associated with treatment failure.[11,12] In the absence of susceptibility results or methicillin resistance, IV vancomycin would be required for the duration of therapy. While the logistics of outpatient therapy in L.D. are being investigated, she should remain on oxacillin while in the hospital.

DURATION OF THERAPY

CASE 70-1, QUESTION 5: Both of L.D.'s parents are employed and their work schedules prevent them from leaving their jobs to transport her to an outpatient antibiotic treatment center. Is L.D. a candidate for outpatient IV antibiotic therapy at home, or is oral antibiotic treatment an option? Must L.D. remain in the hospital to receive her oxacillin?

Initially, all patients should receive IV antibiotics because early, aggressive therapy offers the best chance to cure the infection. L.D., however, does not necessarily need to stay in the hospital for the duration of therapy. A peripherally inserted central catheter (PICC) can be placed, and antibiotics can be administered via continuous infusion pump.[1,2,5] The decision to use home IV antibiotic administration must be decided in concert with L.D.'s parents. If L.D.'s parents do not have the resources or are unwilling to oversee IV treatment at home, L.D. should remain hospitalized for a minimum of 1 week to assess the efficacy of IV treatment.

As discussed in Question 6, L.D. can complete most of her treatment with oral antibiotics. Oral antibiotics, however, should not be given until the effectiveness of IV therapy can be assessed. The total duration of antibiotic therapy should be at least 4 weeks or until the ESR has returned to the normal range.[1,2,7] Reports of shorter-course treatment programs exist, but these investigations are not randomized to different durations of treatment.[13] Expert guidelines continue to recommend at least 4 weeks of treatment.[1,2,5]

ORAL ANTIBIOTICS

CASE 70-1, QUESTION 6: After 1 week of IV nafcillin, L.D. is afebrile and reports that the pain and tenderness in her left leg are much better. Her ESR is 40 mm/hour and CRP is 6 mg/dL (normal <2 mg/dL). The plan is to switch L.D. to oral antibiotics to complete at least a 4-week course of therapy at home. What would be an appropriate oral antibiotic regimen for L.D.? How often should she return to the clinic for evaluation?

TABLE 70-3
Oral Antibiotic Doses for the Treatment of Osteomyelitis in Children

Drug	Dosage (mg/kg/d)	Interval Between Doses (hours)
Penicillin V	125	4
Dicloxacillin	100	6
Amoxicillin	100	6
Cephalexin	150	6
Cefaclor	150	6
Clindamycin	40	8

Because IV therapy for several weeks is inconvenient and expensive, even at home, pediatric patients who have responded to IV antibiotics are candidates for oral therapy. Again, oral antibiotics are only appropriate if a clear clinical response has occurred during the first 7 to 10 days of IV therapy, the patient's parents are aware of the vital importance of compliance, and the patient can swallow and tolerate oral therapy.[1,5]

Assuming her parents agree to supervise treatment outside of the hospital, L.D. is a candidate for oral therapy. She has responded promptly to the IV therapy: her symptoms have improved, and the ESR and CRP are trending downward. Oral therapy will be effective only if L.D. consistently takes her medications; therefore, assurances must be in place to facilitate compliance. L.D.'s parents have made arrangements with her teacher to help her take her oral antibiotic during the day.

L.D. can complete her 4-week course of antibiotics with oral cephalexin capsules or suspension, which tastes better (and is usually better tolerated) than dicloxacillin suspension. Cephalexin should begin at 37.5 mg/kg/dose every 6 hours. Weekly follow-up is necessary to monitor compliance and clinical response to therapy. Parenteral therapy should be reinitiated if L.D.'s compliance is not optimal, symptoms recur, or ESR or CRP increase.[5,7,14] Oral therapy with a quinolone is not appropriate for L.D. primarily because of the risk for emergence of quinolone-resistant staphylococci and secondarily because quinolone use is relatively contraindicated in children. Oral antibiotic dosages for children with osteomyelitis are summarized in Table 70-3.[7]

DURATION OF FOLLOW-UP FOR RECURRENT INFECTION

CASE 70-1, QUESTION 7: L.D. has completed 4 weeks of treatment for her acute staphylococcal osteomyelitis. Clinical evidence shows that the osteomyelitis is completely resolved, and the ESR and CRP are normal. How long should L.D. be followed for possible recurrence of her infection?

Relapses of osteomyelitis can occur years after the initial acute episode.[1,2] In L.D.'s case of uncomplicated acute osteomyelitis, she should be evaluated for recurrence at least every 3 months for at least 2 years.

Osteomyelitis Secondary to a Contiguous Source of Infection

CLINICAL PRESENTATION

CASE 70-2

QUESTION 1: M.K., a 30-year-old man, suffered an open left femur fracture 3 weeks ago in a motorcycle accident. His fracture was set by open reduction and internal fixation. M.K. received prophylactic piperacillin/tazobactam pending soft tissue coverage of the open fracture for 72 hours after hospitalization. His postoperative course was unremarkable until yesterday when he experienced left leg pain and spontaneous drainage from the surgical wound. On presentation, his left thigh is tender, warm, swollen, and erythematous, but he is afebrile. Laboratory data, including WBC count, serum creatinine, and blood urea nitrogen (BUN) are normal, but the ESR is 38 mm/hour and CRP is 8 mg/dL (normal <2 mg/dL). Plain bone films and bone MRI show inflammation and nonhealing of the femur fracture. What findings in M.K. are characteristic of secondary osteomyelitis?

Few of the systemic signs and symptoms usually associated with acute osteomyelitis are seen in secondary osteomyelitis. In contrast to hematogenous disease, fever, leukocytosis and an elevated ESR can be absent. The most common subjective complaint in acute contiguous osteomyelitis is pain in the area of infection, localized tenderness, swelling, erythema, and drainage. Considering several weeks might pass before the patient becomes symptomatic, radiographic studies at the time of diagnosis might reveal abnormalities consistent with bone deterioration.[1,2]

M.K.'s case is consistent with osteomyelitis secondary to a contiguous focus of infection. Infection likely is at the site of surgical repair of the left femur fracture. M.K.'s localized symptoms, along with the absence of fever and leukocytosis, are characteristic of secondary osteomyelitis. In these cases, bone becomes infected from an exogenous source or through spread of an infection from adjacent tissue to bone. Infection can result from any trauma with subsequent orthopedic procedure to fix a bone fracture. The bones most commonly involved are the tibia, fibula, femur, and hip.[1,2]

Other conditions potentially associated with secondary osteomyelitis include gunshot wound, nail puncture, or soft tissue infections (e.g., pressure sores, cellulitis involving the fingers and toes).

Unlike hematogenous osteomyelitis, which occurs mostly in children, acute contiguous infection occurs more often in adults. This finding is explained by the higher incidence of precipitating factors within this age group, such as hip fractures, orthopedic procedures, oral cancers, sternotomy incisions for cardiac surgery, craniotomies, and trauma.[1,2]

COMMON PATHOGENS

CASE 70-2, QUESTION 2: What organisms are mostly likely causing infection in M.K.?

Whereas hematogenous osteomyelitis usually involves a single pathogen, polymicrobial infection is common in contiguous-spread osteomyelitis. Although *S. aureus* is the most common pathogen, it is often part of a mixed infection. Other common pathogens include *Pseudomonas, Proteus, Streptococcus,* and *Klebsiella* species, *E. coli,* and *S. epidermidis.* Most cases of osteomyelitis involving the mandible, pelvis, and small bones (e.g., those of the hands and feet) are caused by gram-negative organisms. *Pseudomonas* often is isolated from infections after puncture wounds of the foot.[1,2] Anaerobes also are associated with contiguous-spread osteomyelitis. The anaerobic organisms most commonly isolated are *Bacteroides* species and anaerobic cocci. Possible predisposing factors include previous fractures or injuries resulting from human bites. Adjacent soft tissue infections can also lead to anaerobic bone infections, as in the case of sacral osteomyelitis secondary to severe decubitus ulcers. To identify the true pathogen(s), M.K. should have surgical re-evaluation and a biopsy of involved bone at the probable site of infection.[1,2] Bone films and the MRI scan will help localize the possible infectious process to direct the surgical biopsy.

INITIAL TREATMENT

CASE 70-2, QUESTION 3: M.K. returns to the operating room for surgical exploration, and bone tissue is obtained for culture. He has no drug allergies and weighs 90 kg. The initial postoperative antibiotic order is for vancomycin, 1 g IV every 12 hours. Is this adequate antibiotic treatment for M.K.?

M.K. has had surgery to obtain bone material for culture because cultures of adjacent wound or sinus tract material are not predictive of the bacteria actually infecting the bone.[15] Broad empiric antibiotic coverage is necessary because *S. aureus* and polymicrobial gram-negative aerobic bacilli most likely are causing this infection.[1,2]

M.K. has been started on vancomycin for possible MRSA infection while awaiting results of bone tissue cultures. Although optimal trough concentrations are not defined, aggressive therapy is usually warranted. Many clinicians target goal trough concentrations between 15 and 20 mcg/mL for osteomyelitis.[16–18] Given his normal renal function and weight, M.K.'s vancomycin dosage will likely require at least 1.5 g IV every 12 hours.

To cover possible pathogenic gram-negative aerobic bacilli, a third- or fourth-generation cephalosporin (cefotaxime, ceftriaxone, ceftazidime, or cefepime) or a quinolone (ciprofloxacin, levofloxacin) could be added for gram-negative coverage. Cefepime is suggested in cases involving *P. aeruginosa,* although other antipseudomonal agents (e.g., ciprofloxacin, ceftazidime, aztreonam) would also be appropriate.[2,19] The choice of agent should, in part, be based on local susceptibility patterns. In locations in which quinolone gram-negative resistance approaches 30%, these agents have limited utility. Third-generation cephalosporins or quinolones should not be used alone to treat serious staphylococcal infection; therefore, combination therapy with antistaphylococcal penicillins (if MSSA) or vancomycin is necessary.[1]

Anaerobic coverage is usually not necessary empirically, although it should be initiated if an anaerobe is cultured from bone. Vancomycin has activity against gram-positive anaerobes, but not against an important gram-negative anaerobe, *Bacteroides fragilis.* If *B. fragilis* is cultured from bone, additional therapy with metronidazole is indicated. Alternatively, combined, broad-spectrum aerobic (including *Pseudomonas)* and anaerobic gram-negative coverage could be provided by a β-lactam/β-lactamase inhibitor combination therapy with piperacillin/tazobactam or a carbapenem (e.g., imipenem, meropenem, doripenem).

While cultures are pending, M.K.'s antibiotic regimen is changed to vancomycin 1.5 g IV every 12 hours and cefepime 1 g IV every 6 hours.

DIRECTED THERAPY

CASE 70-2, QUESTION 4: The bone biopsy from M.K. grows *P. aeruginosa,* which is sensitive to ceftazidime, cefepime, imipenem, gentamicin, tobramycin, and ciprofloxacin. His leg pain is no worse than it was 2 days ago, and he remains afebrile. How should M.K. now be treated? Is he a candidate for oral therapy?

Because no gram-positive organisms grew on culture, vancomycin may be discontinued. Therapy should be directed against the *Pseudomonas.* Traditional therapy for M.K. would include gentamicin or tobramycin plus an antipseudomonal β-lactam, such as piperacillin-tazobactam or ceftazidime to complete a 4-week course of therapy.[1] More recently, antipseudomonal therapy with a β-lactam plus ciprofloxacin combination has been used with increasing frequency to avoid the complications associated with aminoglycosides. However, there is no current evidence that combining two antipseudomonal agents to which the responsible bacteria is susceptible is superior to treatment with one agent alone when treating osteomyelitis. Thus, it is justified to treat M.K. with a single agent as long as he is monitored closely, following weekly ESR or CRP levels and his symptoms. Thus, M.K. can continue to receive cefepime in aggressive doses (1 g IV every 6 hours), which can be administered at home with the appropriate home health care. Because there is controversy with respect to the use of monotherapy for pseudomonal infection, some clinicians might add adjunctive gentamicin (or tobramycin) to cefepime. To facilitate antibiotic therapy at home, M.K. is a candidate for once-daily dosing of gentamicin.[1] Because his renal function is normal, a single daily dose of 5 to 7 mg/kg can be administered. Although only a few reports exist of extended-interval aminoglycoside use in osteomyelitis, experience in other gram-negative infections suggests that once-a-day therapy is as effective and possibly less toxic as multiple daily doses.[20,21] At home, M.K. should have weekly serum creatinine and gentamicin levels drawn. He should be followed closely for at least 2 years to detect recurrent infection.

Osteomyelitis Associated with Vascular Insufficiency

CLINICAL PRESENTATION

CASE 70-3

QUESTION 1: M.S., a 55-year-old woman, presents to the diabetes clinic with an ulcer 2 cm wide × 1 cm deep on the left lateral aspect of her foot that she first noted a month ago. Her primary-care physician had prescribed a 2-week course of ciprofloxacin and gave her instructions for regular wound care. A few days before her clinic visit, the callus surrounding the ulcer cracked open and a small piece of bone protruded from the wound. She reports mild swelling and redness but denies any pain, fever, or chills. Her past medical history includes type 2 diabetes mellitus, hypertension, peripheral neuropathy, and chronic kidney disease requiring hemodialysis three times a week. Laboratory findings include a WBC of 5,200 cells/μL with normal differential, BUN of 56 mg/dL, serum creatinine of 5.6 mg/dL, fasting blood glucose of 240 mg/dL, hemoglobin A_{1c} (Hgb A_{1c}) of 12.4%, and ESR of 45 mm/hour. What findings in M.S. are consistent with secondary osteomyelitis?

M.S. has chronic lower extremity vascular insufficiency as a result of type 2 diabetes. Patients with impaired blood flow may develop osteomyelitis in the toes or small bones of the feet. Infection often first presents as cellulitis, as in M.S.'s case, progressing to deep ulcers and finally to the underlying bone.

Similar to contiguous-spread osteomyelitis, systemic signs of infection (e.g., fever and leukocytosis) are often absent in patients who experience bone infection secondary to vascular insufficiency. Local symptoms such as pain, swelling, and erythema usually predominate.[1,2,22]

M.S. may have a bone infection under the chronic, cutaneous ulcer on the bottom of her left big toe. Because of peripheral neuropathy, the skin lesion may not be very painful, and poor blood supply to the site likely contributed to the development of a chronic infection and possibly secondary osteomyelitis. Infection is suggested by her elevated ESR, fasting glucose (consistent with infection), and Hgb A_{1c} (indicating uncontrolled diabetes). In addition, diabetic foot ulcers that are more than 2 cm wide and more than 2 cm deep, or that penetrate to bone, are often predictive for underlying osteomyelitis.[22,23]

ANTIBIOTIC SELECTION

CASE 70-3, QUESTION 2: M.S. is admitted into the hospital for diagnostic workup, wound care, and antibiotics. Plain films show destruction of the distal left fifth metatarsal with bony changes consistent with osteomyelitis. Her wound is débrided, and material obtained from a bone biopsy is sent to the microbiology laboratory for cultures. She has no drug allergies and is started on vancomycin (1 g IV every 12 hours) and oral ciprofloxacin (750 mg every 12 hours). Is this appropriate initial, empiric therapy?

In many cases of osteomyelitis associated with vascular insufficiency, multiple pathogens can be cultured from surgical specimens or the wound. The most commonly isolated pathogens are *S. aureus;* however, gram-negative and anaerobic bacteria are also often recovered. It should be recognized that the bacteria isolated from a wound or soft tissue culture may not correlate with bacteria found in a concomitant bone biopsy.[24] Therefore, empiric antibiotic therapy for osteomyelitis associated with vascular insufficiency should be active against both gram-positive and gram-negative aerobic bacteria. Because anaerobic gram-negative bacteria are cultured from bone in diabetic patients with osteomyelitis up to 15% of the time, empiric anaerobic coverage may not be necessary.[24] Vancomycin plus an antipseudomonal β-lactam (ceftazidime, cefepime) or quinolone (ciprofloxacin, levofloxacin) for gram-negative coverage is frequently used as an empiric regimen. If anaerobic bacteria are believed to be clinically involved (e.g., foul-smelling wound), metronidazole should be added to the regimen; alternatively an antipseudomonal β-lactam/β-lactamase inhibitor combination, such as piperacillin-tazobactam, can be used.

M.S. has risk factors for MRSA and resistant gram-negative bacilli because of her diabetes and recent course of antibiotics. The initial regimen of vancomycin and ciprofloxacin for M.S. is not optimal for several reasons. Because of her recent, prolonged ciprofloxacin exposure, a quinolone-resistant organism may be responsible for infection and a β-lactam–based antibiotic regimen would be more appropriate. Second, IV antibiotics should be used during initial treatment. Lastly, M.S. is dialysis-dependent and the antibiotic regimen selected should be dose-adjusted according to her renal function. A more appropriate empiric regimen for M.S. would be vancomycin intermittently dosed based on serum levels and her dialysis regimen, and cefepime 1 g every 24 hours with the dose administered after dialysis on dialysis days.

Further antibiotic refinement should occur after the results of the deep wound swab culture are available. The optimal duration of IV therapy for diabetic foot osteomyelitis is patient-dependent, and many patients require long-term, oral suppressive therapy. The overall duration of antibiotic treatment can range from 6 weeks to many months depending on the degree of surgical débridement and the healing rate of the ulcer.[25,26] Oral linezolid (600 mg every 12 hours) has been used to treat MRSA osteomyelitis in diabetic patients, although long-term therapy can be associated with hematological and neuropathic adverse effects.[27] Other useful oral drugs for long-term suppressive therapy are clindamycin (300 every 8 hours), trimethoprim-sulfamethoxazole (two double-strength tablets every 12 hours), and amoxicillin/clavulanate (850 mg every 12 hours), depending on susceptibilities and patient tolerance.

M.S. should be made aware that osteomyelitis associated with diabetic foot ulcers is difficult to treat. Despite adequate surgical débridement of the infection followed by appropriate treatment with long-term IV and oral antibiotic therapy, cure rates are low. Even minor amputations (one or two toes) are unsuccessful in eradicating infection. Radical surgical approaches, such as transmetatarsal, below-the-knee, or above-the-knee amputations, often are necessary to cure these infections.[1,2,25]

CASE 70-4

QUESTION 1: H.H., a 58-year-old man, is transferred from an outside hospital with a gangrenous second left toe. He has a foot ulcer that has been present for 6 weeks and has been managed closely by his primary-care provider. In the past week, however, H.H. noted increased pain, redness, and swelling of the toe and surrounding area. He was prescribed doxycycline and clindamycin for his infection, but after 5 days his symptoms worsened, and he now reports odorous drainage from the wound. H.H. has a past medical history of type 1 diabetes mellitus, chronic renal insufficiency, hypertension, and obesity. H.H. is taken for amputation of his toe. Intraoperative deep cultures grow MRSA, *Enterobacter cloacae, Klebsiella oxytoca,* and *Bacteroides fragilis.* What antibiotic regimen options are available for H.H.?

H.H. has polymicrobial osteomyelitis attributable to chronic vascular insufficiency. Diabetic foot infections with multidrug-resistant organisms, such as MRSA, coagulase-negative staphylococci, and resistant gram-negative bacteria, are increasing in prevalence.[28,29] These patients often have repeated health care system exposures and eventually become colonized, and potentially infected, with these organisms. H.H. needs broad-spectrum coverage targeting gram-positive, gram-negative, and anaerobic bacteria. Vancomycin and piperacillin-tazobactam would be an appropriate combination regimen for his polymicrobial infection. Alternative agents to piperacillin-tazobactam that offer both gram-negative and anaerobic coverage would include a carbapenem (ertapenem, meropenem, doripenem), a quinolone plus metronidazole, or a third- or fourth-generation cephalosporin (ceftriaxone, cefepime) plus metronidazole. If combination therapy is not desired or if the patient has drug intolerance or allergy, monotherapy with tigecycline (Tigacyl) may be considered for patients with polymicrobial soft-tissue infections, but probably not osteomyelitis. Tigecycline offers activity against gram-positive organisms, including MRSA; many resistant gram-negative organisms; and anaerobes. Important to note is that tigecycline does not have activity against *Pseudomonas, Proteus, Providencia,* and *Morganella.*

Duration of antimicrobial therapy after amputation varies from several days to several weeks depending on the residual infected soft tissue. If there is suspected residual infection of bone that was not removed during the amputation, then duration of therapy should continue for 4 to 6 weeks.[30]

Chronic Osteomyelitis

CLINICAL PRESENTATION

CASE 70-5

QUESTION 1: J.F., a 52-year-old man, sustained a fracture of the right humerus in a farming accident 6 years ago. That fracture clinically healed without any immediate consequences; however, 1 year ago, a draining sinus tract developed at the site of the previous fracture without any antecedent events. He has taken various oral antibiotics during this last year, including amoxicillin and levofloxacin,

which he stopped taking 2 months ago. Two weeks ago he noted increased sinus drainage, pain, swelling, and erythema of his left upper arm, and levofloxacin was restarted. A swab culture of the sinus drainage grew *S. epidermidis*, *E. coli*, *Peptostreptococcus micros*, and *Bacteroides* species. Surgical débridement of bone and tissue was performed because of increased drainage and poor appearance of the wound. Gentamicin-impregnated polymethylmethacrylate (PMMA) beads were placed in the tissue adjacent to the débrided bone during surgery. Bone cultures grew *Proteus mirabilis* and *B. fragilis*. The *Proteus* was resistant to ampicillin, cefazolin, ticarcillin, levofloxacin, and tigecycline, but sensitive to cefotaxime, ceftriaxone, imipenem, gentamicin, and trimethoprim-sulfamethoxazole. Antibiotic sensitivities for the *Bacteroides* were not tested. What aspects of J.F.'s case are characteristic of chronic osteomyelitis?

Inadequate treatment of an acute episode of osteomyelitis can lead to formation of necrotic, infected bone and recurrent symptoms consistent with chronic disease. Even with appropriate initial therapy, osteomyelitis can reactivate, even with different organisms from the initial episode. Some propose that previously infected bone might be a risk for reinfection. Persistent symptoms or signs lasting longer than 10 days are consistent with chronic osteomyelitis and the development of necrotic bone. Draining sinus tracts often develop from the bone to the skin with chronic osteomyelitis.[1,2]

J.F. probably experienced a chronic bone infection after the farming accident. The reappearance of sinus tract drainage in his left upper arm indicates an indolent infection of bone that was periodically suppressed, but not treated by oral antibiotics. Cultures of sinus drainage now reveal multiple organisms including normal skin flora. These sinus tract cultures usually do not correlate with the organisms actually causing bone infection. J.F.'s recurrent course of bone involvement with drainage and local symptoms, and lack of any remarkable systemic symptoms, is classic for chronic osteomyelitis.[1,2,7]

SURGERY AND ORAL ANTIBIOTICS

CASE 70-5, QUESTION 2: Oral levofloxacin (500 mg daily) was restarted 2 weeks ago when J.F.'s left arm became more painful and drainage increased. Was his poor response to therapy unexpected? How should his case have been managed?

J.F.'s poor response should have been expected for at least two reasons: antibiotic therapy was started before surgical débridement of avascular tissue, and he was given an antibiotic that was inactive against the cultured bone organisms.

Surgery plays an important role in the treatment of chronic osteomyelitis. Bone necrosis will continue to progress if decompression and drainage of the infected area is not carried out as soon as possible. Furthermore, without initial surgical removal of necrotic bone and other poorly vascularized, infected material, even the most optimal IV antibiotics are likely to fail.

After surgery, antibiotic therapy directed against the surgical specimens should be started. As previously discussed, the choice of the regimen should not be selected on the basis of the sinus tract culture results because these isolates generally do not correlate with the actual causative organisms. J.F. should be treated initially with IV antibiotics because of relatively poor blood flow at the infection site. Although the optimal duration of therapy for chronic osteomyelitis is not well established,[1,2,31] parenteral therapy is generally recommended for 6 to 8 weeks, followed by 3 to 12 months of oral antibiotic therapy, depending on the healing rate.[2]

J.F. should continue to be evaluated by an orthopedic surgeon because he may require further surgical treatment to eradicate chronically infected bone.

INTRAVENOUS ANTIBIOTICS

CASE 70-5, QUESTION 3: What would be reasonable antibiotic therapy for J.F.?

On the basis of the bone culture and sensitivity results, J.F. needs high-dose therapy directed at *P. mirabilis* and *B. fragilis*. For convenience and possible future home therapy, ceftriaxone (2 g IV every 24 hours) could be started for coverage of *Proteus* and metronidazole (500 mg IV every 8 hours) also should be started for coverage of *B. fragilis*. Because of excellent oral bioavailability, the metronidazole can be rapidly converted to oral therapy at the same dose before discharge. Ertapenem (Invanz) could be an alternative choice for home IV therapy assuming that the *Proteus* isolate is sensitive. This agent also provides excellent anaerobic activity, and its once-daily dosing (1 g IV every 24 hours) is convenient for home therapy.

After 6 to 8 weeks of home parenteral therapy, J.F. should be evaluated for response. If symptoms have abated, treatment with oral antibiotics (trimethoprim-sulfamethoxazole and metronidazole) may commence and should continue for an additional 6 to 8 weeks or longer depending on resolution of the sinus tract drainage, pain, and tenderness in J.F.'s arm. Under these circumstances, he should be monitored closely for possible long-term adverse effects (hepatitis, cytopenias, neuropathy). If the sinus tract does not heal or if J.F. remains symptomatic, surgical exploration and bone cultures must be repeated.

LOCAL ANTIBIOTICS

CASE 70-5, QUESTION 4: What are the rationale for and effectiveness of local antibiotic administration (the PMMA beads) inserted during J.F.'s orthopedic surgery?

To deliver high concentrations of antibiotics to poorly vascularized bone infection sites, various materials containing antibiotics can be placed at the infection site during surgery. Plaster pellets, fibrin, collagen, hydroxyapatite, and PMMA impregnated with antibiotic, usually an aminoglycoside or vancomycin, have been used. The dosage form is designed for the slow release of antibiotics from the material. The most commonly reported experience with local antibiotic delivery has been with antibiotic-impregnated PMMA cement or beads inserted during joint arthroplasty. Recurrent infection rates have been comparable in patients treated with local antibiotic insertion and those treated with systemic antibiotics. Thus, no evidence suggests that the PMMA beads will improve J.F.'s outcome when added to systemic therapy. Local delivery of antibiotics should never replace systemic antibiotics in the treatment of chronic osteomyelitis.[32]

Osteomyelitis Associated with Prosthetic Material

USUAL CLINICAL PRESENTATION

CASE 70-6

QUESTION 1: A.T., a 47-year-old woman, had a left knee replacement 1 year ago for osteoarthritis. She is seen today

in the orthopedic clinic because of increasing left knee pain for the past 2 months. The knee is painful and warm. She is afebrile, and her peripheral WBC count is 9,800 cells/μL. Aspiration of fluid from the knee reveals a total nucleated cell count of 78,000 cells/μL with 90% neutrophils. A Gram stain of this fluid shows 4+ polymorphonuclear leukocytes (PMN) and 1+ gram-positive cocci. She is started on antibiotic therapy with vancomycin and ciprofloxacin pending culture results, and she is scheduled for operative evaluation and possible removal of her prosthetic joint. Does A.T. have a prosthetic joint infection?

Joint replacement surgery is commonly performed for patients with significant joint destruction as a result of arthritis and other disabling diseases. Prosthetic knee, shoulder, elbow, or hip devices made of metallic alloys are cemented to adjacent bone to re-establish joint function. Infection of these foreign bodies can occur because of hematogenous dissemination of bacteria or by contiguous spread from a topical wound. *Staphylococcus* species are most commonly involved in prosthetic joint infections, followed by *Streptococcus* species, gram-negative bacilli, and anaerobes. Bacteria infect bone adjacent to the joint prosthesis, including the bone–cement interface, resulting in a loosened and less functional prosthesis.[33]

Chronic pain, swelling, erythema, and tenderness over a prosthetic joint are typical findings associated with prosthetic joint infection. A.T. has had a relatively lengthy duration of symptoms associated with her left knee, which could be caused by joint loosening, but the cell count and differential from the joint aspirate suggest joint infection. Also consistent with infected prosthesis is the predominance of neutrophils in her joint fluid and gram-positive cocci on a Gram stain. As is often the case, she has no obvious preceding source of infection from which bacteria may have originated. Occasionally, sources of infection with hematogenous dissemination to the prosthetic joint are identified, such as dental infections, cellulitis, or urinary tract infections. Given the Gram stain result, A.T. should be covered for *Staphylococcus* and *Streptococcus* species with vancomycin while awaiting the results of cultures and sensitivities. *Staphylococcus* species, including coagulase-negative species such as *S. epidermidis,* are the most commonly isolated bacteria responsible for prosthetic infection. Although coagulase-negative staphylococci are usually considered a contaminant in culture, this organism readily adheres to prosthetic material and should be considered pathogenic when cultured from prostheses. Coagulase-negative staphylococci are often methicillin-resistant but susceptible to vancomycin. Because gram-negative bacteria also can infect these joints, gram-negative coverage is reasonable until the results of joint fluid cultures are available.

SURGERY

CASE 70-6, QUESTION 2: Does A.T. need surgery and antibiotics to cure her infection?

Surgical removal of A.T.'s knee prosthesis with antibiotics for 6 weeks are the current recommendations for optimal eradication of prosthetic joint infection.[1,33] A two-stage orthopedic procedure is frequently used that involves removal of the infected prosthesis, placement of an antibiotic-filled spacer or block, joint immobilization, and antibiotics for 6 weeks. If the joint space remains culture-negative, a new joint prosthesis is then reinserted. Because avascular bone cement and prosthetic material can become seeded with bacteria, complete removal of this material is necessary to have the greatest chance of curing the infection. Six weeks of systemic antibiotic therapy in combination with orthopedic surgery results in restoration of joint function in 85% to 95% of cases. High rates of treatment failure (~70%) occur if the joint prosthesis is not removed, if the antibiotic duration is too short, and if chronic suppressive antibiotics are not given.[33,34]

ANTIBIOTICS

CASE 70-6, QUESTION 3: The surgeon is unable to completely remove A.T.'s prosthetic joint. The removed lining material and three swabs of the left knee prosthesis grow MRSA. What antibiotic regimen could be used? How long should A.T. be treated?

To prevent recurrence of infection, A.T. will need a prolonged course of antibiotics, perhaps indefinitely if the original prosthesis remains in place. Lifelong therapy is impractical, expensive, and likely to provoke adverse effects. Initially, A.T. may be treated with IV vancomycin (15 mg/kg/dose IV every 12 hours) for at least 2 weeks, although the optimal duration of this initial parenteral therapy is unknown. Daptomycin (Cubicin) is an appropriate alternative for patients with vancomycin allergy or intolerance, or to facilitate home IV therapy with the convenience of once-daily administration.[35]

After 2 weeks of parenteral therapy, A.T. may be switched to oral antibiotics. Combination therapy with rifampin should be used for prosthetic joint infection caused by staphylococci, particularly if removal of the infected prosthesis is not possible.[36] Rifampin penetrates bacterial membranes and biofilms to enhance bactericidal activity of the antibiotic regimen; however, monotherapy with rifampin should never be used because of rapid development of resistance.[36,37] Limited success has been reported with the use of quinolones with rifampin for patients with retained staphylococcal prosthetic joint infections, although patients presenting with a long duration of symptoms (>1 month) or prosthetic infection with MRSA are more likely to fail treatment. A.T.'s symptoms have lasted 3 months, suggesting that her infection may not respond well to therapy. Nevertheless, a prolonged course of levofloxacin (500 mg PO daily) and rifampin could be tried for at least 3 months.[38] Rifampin increases the metabolism of multiple other agents (e.g., warfarin, anticonvulsants, azole antifungals); therefore, a thorough review of A.T.'s medication profile is critical. A.T.'s baseline liver function should also be evaluated, and rechecked at least monthly while she is taking rifampin.[36]

Another option for oral therapy is linezolid (Zyvox), although limited data exist on its role in treating prosthetic joint infection and chronic use is associated with thrombocytopenia, neutropenia, and neuritis. If linezolid is used for more than 2 weeks, A.T.'s platelet and WBC count should be followed weekly.[39]

SEPTIC ARTHRITIS

Septic arthritis or infectious arthritis is usually acquired hematogenously. The highly vascular synovium of the joint allows easy passage of bacteria from blood into the synovial space. Bacteremia, secondary to *Neisseria gonorrhoeae* or *S. aureus* in particular, often is associated with joint infections. Septic arthritis also can develop secondary to the spread of osteomyelitis into the joint. This is especially a problem in children younger than 1 year of age who still have capillaries penetrating the epiphyseal growth plate.[2,6]

Several factors predispose patients to the development of infectious arthritis. Trauma can directly inoculate the synovium or allow infecting organisms to penetrate it more easily. Patients with certain systemic disorders, such as diabetes mellitus, rheumatoid arthritis (RA), osteoarthritis, chronic granulomatous disease, cancer, or chronic liver disease, are more susceptible to the development of infection. Endocrine factors predispose pregnant or menstruating women to the development of gonococcal arthritis. In the menstruating patient, this can be explained partially by the increased endocervical shedding of *N. gonorrhoeae*.[40]

Clinical Presentation of Nongonococcal Arthritis

CASE 70-7

QUESTION 1: C.H., a 35-year-old man, is referred to the rheumatology clinic for left knee swelling. Two days ago, his left knee became painful and swollen, and he is unable to flex the joint. He also recorded temperatures at home of 100.7°F to 102°F for at least 4 days. In clinic, a joint effusion is noted, and fluid is aspirated for cell count, a Gram stain, and culture. His medical history is unremarkable except for an episode of hives after receiving cephalexin for cellulitis 2 years ago. C.H.'s WBC count is 16,000 cells/μL, and his ESR is 42 mm/hour. The synovial fluid from his right knee contains 30,000 WBCs/μL with 90% neutrophils, and the Gram stain shows gram-positive cocci in clusters. Culture results are pending. His temperature is 38.5°C. What findings in C.H. are consistent with septic arthritis?

C.H. has an acute onset of monoarticular joint pain and swelling, with reduced range of motion and fever. These findings are classic for septic, nongonococcal arthritis. The joint effusion shows a predominance of neutrophils, which confirms the diagnosis. C.H.'s knee has been infected hematogenously from a distant, usually unrecognized, source of infection. The knee is infected most commonly, and *S. aureus* is the usual organism. If C.H. had a urinary tract infection, however, gram-negative bacilli would be more likely to be responsible for joint infection. Occasionally, a predisposing factor is present in the involved joint, such as pre-existing arthritis (i.e., RA) or trauma.

A single joint is infected in 90% of bacterial arthritis cases. Other possible sites of infectious arthritis in adults include the hip, shoulder, sternoclavicular, and sacroiliac joints; the ankle and elbow are common sites of infection in children. The wrist and interphalangeal joints of the hand also may be involved, but in these cases, the infectious pathogens are most often *N. gonorrhoeae* and *Mycobacterium tuberculosis*.[40] The most common systemic symptom in infectious arthritis is fever. Localized symptoms include pain, decreased mobility of the involved joint, and swelling.

As illustrated by C.H., most patients have joint effusion on physical examination. When evaluating a patient with possible septic arthritis, any purulent joint effusion should be considered septic until proven otherwise. Alternatively, noninfectious conditions may be present, such as single joint involvement with synovial effusions (e.g., acute RA, gout, chondrocalcinosis).[40]

Aspirated joint fluid should be cultured because isolation of bacteria is the only definitive diagnostic test for bacterial arthritis. C.H.'s joint fluid picture is typical. The leukocyte count in the synovial fluid usually is significantly elevated, with counts ranging from 50,000 to 200,000 cells/μL. Leukocyte counts of less than 20,000 cells/μL rarely are seen during infection, except in early cases of bacterial arthritis or in patients with disseminated gonococcal infection (DGI).

Another laboratory finding in C.H. consistent with infectious arthritis is the elevated ESR. Viral or fungal arthritis also can increase the ESR. Leukocytosis is common in younger patients, but rare in adults. Anemia also can be associated with infection, especially in patients with chronic involvement or in cases in which predisposing factors such as RA are present.

The patient's age impacts the most common bacterial causes of infection. In adults older than 30 years of age such as C.H., and in children older than 2 years of age, *S. aureus* is the most common cause. In adults younger than 30 years of age, *N. gonorrhoeae* is more likely to be the causative agent. Streptococci, such as group A β-hemolytic streptococci, can cause infection in children and adults. Other organisms, such as group B streptococci, anaerobic streptococci, and gram-negative bacteria, can cause infection. Gram-negative bacilli are responsible for approximately 15% of cases and often infect multiple joints. Infections with gram-negative bacteria usually are associated with predisposing factors, such as RA, osteoarthritis, or heroin use. The organism most commonly isolated from patients with bacterial arthritis who have a history of IV drug use is *P. aeruginosa*.[40,41]

Initial Antimicrobial Therapy

TREATMENT IN β-LACTAM ALLERGIC PATIENTS

CASE 70-7, QUESTION 2: C.H. describes his reaction to cephalexin as intense pruritic skin lesions over his trunk and upper extremities that appeared acutely (several hours) after he had received three doses. He did not experience wheezing or shortness of breath, and his reaction was treated symptomatically with diphenhydramine and discontinuation of the cephalexin. He had received several types of oral antibiotics before this episode of pruritus without difficulty, but has not taken antibiotics since then. How should C.H. be treated?

Treatment of nongonococcal arthritis includes drainage of purulent joint fluid (by needle aspiration or surgery) and appropriate antibiotic therapy. Because *S. aureus* is most likely involved, initial empiric therapy with a penicillinase-resistant penicillin, a cephalosporin, or vancomycin should be initiated. C.H.'s reaction to cephalexin is worrisome because readministration of a penicillin or cephalosporin might result in similar or worse (e.g., anaphylaxis) allergic symptoms. Consequently, because C.H.'s septic arthritis is probably caused by *S. aureus* and, perhaps, streptococci, vancomycin (15 mg/kg/dose IV every 12 hours), which covers both organisms, should be started as soon as possible. In patients who are not allergic to penicillin, oxacillin or nafcillin (2 g IV every 4 hours) is recommended for MSSA infections. Because of the increasing frequency of community-acquired MRSA causing infection,[41] and even in the absence of penicillin allergy, vancomycin would be initially indicated empirically. And in the nonallergic patient, vancomycin then can be changed on the basis of sensitivity testing to oxacillin or nafcillin if *S. aureus* is susceptible.[40,41]

DURATION OF THERAPY

CASE 70-7, QUESTION 3: How long should C.H. be treated? How should the efficacy of treatment be monitored?

No high-quality studies have been performed to determine the optimal duration of therapy for bacterial arthritis.[41] Previous recommendations based on early clinical trials recommended treating for 2 to 3 weeks.[42] However, current recommendations are to initiate therapy with at least 2 weeks of IV antibiotics, followed by oral antibiotics (if possible based on susceptibilities) for at least 4 more weeks.[40,41]

C.H. should be treated for at least 4 to 6 weeks.[40,41] His response to therapy should be monitored clinically (resolution of symptoms, fever, and falling ESR, CRP, or both) as well as by periodic evaluation of joint fluid. Frequent aspirations of joint fluid, initially on a daily basis, should take place, with evaluation of cell count and fluid culture. Effective therapy should result in a decreasing WBC count in the joint fluid and negative cultures, usually within 3 to 4 days of treatment. Worse outcomes (permanent joint dysfunction) are likely if joint fluid cultures remain positive after 6 days of treatment for gram-positive infection. If fluid cultures are persistently positive, more aggressive surgical management is necessary to preserve joint function.[40,41]

Most joint fluid cultures become negative after 7 days of treatment with IV antibiotics. Joint inflammation and other symptoms also should diminish by this time. The duration of articular symptoms before antibiotic therapy is begun correlates with the subsequent time required to sterilize the synovial fluid. Therefore, delay in initiating antibiotic treatment may necessitate a longer course of therapy.

Similar to hematogenous osteomyelitis, oral antibiotics have been used in septic arthritis to complete treatment if the initial response to IV therapy is adequate. Oral therapy should not be considered until the patient is afebrile, joint fluid cultures are negative, the ESR or CRP is normal, and there is decreased joint pain and increased joint mobility.[41] Case series reveal generally positive results, but adequately controlled, randomized clinical trials comparing IV and oral therapy are not available.[42,43] Because of C.H.'s allergy to cephalexin, the choice of adequate oral therapy to complete at least 3 weeks of treatment is difficult. Because of the continuing emergence of resistance among gram-positive organisms to ciprofloxacin, use of this agent is not recommended. Oral clindamycin could be used, but published experience in adults is not substantial, and there would be concern about the possible development of antibiotic-associated colitis. Linezolid (Zyvox) has been used in septic arthritis in a few case series.[27] If the *S. aureus* isolated is sensitive to trimethoprim-sulfamethoxazole, this agent may be an alternative to clindamycin for oral treatment. Published experience with this mode of treatment also is not vast. C.H. should be advised that parenteral treatment with vancomycin, which can be accomplished at home, would be the most effective mode of treatment. Finally, injections of antibiotics into the joint space are of no value. Most systemic antibiotics readily penetrate the joint space and enter the synovial fluid.[40,41]

Gonococcal Arthritis

Polyarticular arthritis in a young, sexually active adult is caused most commonly by *N. gonorrhoeae.* Arthritis in multiple joints is a common feature of DGI. Unlike nongonococcal arthritis, which is almost exclusively monoarticular, gonococcal arthritis involves multiple joints in approximately 50% of cases. Clinically, patients present initially with a migratory polyarthralgia and later with fever, dermatitis, and tenosynovitis. Skin lesions are an important clue to the diagnosis of DGI and often begin as tiny erythematous papules and develop into larger vesicles. Other symptoms, such as purulent and swollen joints, are present in only 30% to 40% of patients. As in hematogenously acquired nongonococcal arthritis, the synovial fluid leukocyte count usually is elevated, but to a lesser degree. *N. gonorrhoeae* is recovered in less than 50% of purulent joint effusions. However, blood cultures often are positive for this organism and, coupled with the patient's clinical presentation, can be used to make a definitive diagnosis.[40,43]

CLINICAL PRESENTATION OF GONOCOCCAL ARTHRITIS

CASE 70-8

QUESTION 1: E.D, a 21-year-old woman, presents to the walk-in clinic with right knee and right shoulder pain, nausea, and vomiting. On physical examination, her right knee is swollen and she has decreased range of motion of her right shoulder. Several erythematous, papular skin lesions are noted on both hands. She also has a vaginal discharge. Her temperature is 38.2°C, and her WBC count is 15,000 cells/μL. She gives a history of having two recent sexual partners. Cultures of blood, joint fluid, and vaginal discharge are obtained; a joint fluid Gram stain shows 4+ PMNs, but no organisms are seen. Why is E.D. considered to have gonococcal arthritis?

E.D. has systemic signs of infection (fever, nausea, vomiting, leukocytosis), skin lesions, and multiple joint involvement, which are classic for DGI. Her history of recent sexual activity and the presence of a vaginal discharge are consistent with gonococcal infection, although evidence of mucosal infection with *N. gonorrhoeae* is not necessary for disseminated infection to occur.[40,43]

PATIENT WORKUP AND TREATMENT IN THE CLINIC

CASE 70-8, QUESTION 2: What additional workup should be done in E.D.? Can she be treated immediately in the clinic?

E.D. should be evaluated for other sexually transmitted diseases, specifically syphilis and HIV infection. Serologic testing for syphilis (rapid plasma reagent [RPR] or venereal disease research laboratory [VDRL] testing) and for antibody to HIV should be obtained. In addition, she should have a pregnancy test because some of the antibiotics that may be used are contraindicated during pregnancy, including doxycycline.

Because of possible penicillinase production by *N. gonorrhoeae,* recommended therapy is with ceftriaxone (1 g intramuscularly or IV every 24 hours) initially. E.D. should receive her first dose of ceftriaxone in the clinic today. Parenteral treatment should continue for 1 to 2 days after improvement begins; at that point, oral cephalosporin therapy (cefixime 400 mg twice daily or cefpodoxime 400 mg twice daily) can be started. Quinolone-resistant *N. gonorrhoeae* are prevalent throughout the United States, so the use of ciprofloxacin or levofloxacin as treatment is no longer recommended by the Centers for Disease Control and Prevention (CDC). The duration of antibiotic treatment is 7 to 14 days.[43,44]

E.D.'s sexual partners should also be evaluated and treated for relevant sexually transmitted diseases.

FULL COURSE OF THERAPY

CASE 70-8, QUESTION 3: Results of RPR and pregnancy testing in E.D. are negative. How should she complete her course of therapy?

E.D.'s DGI should be treated for at least 7 days. E.D. also should begin treatment with azithromycin (1 g orally once) or doxycycline (100 mg orally twice daily for 7 days) for the possibility of concomitant chlamydial infection. E.D. can complete her course of treatment for DGI orally, although parenteral therapy is recommended until signs and symptoms resolve. This course usually takes 2 to 4 days.[43] She will have to return to the clinic for daily ceftriaxone administration unless other arrangements for parenteral therapy can be made. Current recommendations from the CDC are that oral treatment should be with either cefixime (400 mg twice daily) or cefpodoxime (400 mg twice daily).[44] Treatment guidelines for DGI are also included in the gonorrhea section of Chapter 69, Sexually Transmitted Diseases.

KEY REFERENCES AND WEBSITES

A full list of references for this chapter can be found at **http://thepoint.lww.com/AT10e.** Below are the key references and website for this chapter, with the corresponding reference number in this chapter found in parentheses after the reference.

Key References

Berbari EF et al. Osteomyelitis. In: Mandell GL, Bennett JE, Dolin R, eds. *Mandell, Douglas, and Bennett's Principles and Practice of Infectious Diseases*, 7th ed. Philadelphia, PA: Elsevier Churchill Livingstone; 2010:1457. (2)

Brause BD. Infections with prostheses in bones and joints. In: Mandell GL, Bennett JE, Dolin R, eds. *Mandell, Douglas, and Bennett's Principles and Practice of Infectious Diseases*. 7th ed. Philadelphia, PA: Elsevier Churchill Livingstone; 2010:1469. (33)

Byren I et al. Pharmacotherapy of diabetic foot osteomyelitis. *Expert Opin Pharmacother*. 2009;10(18):3033. (23)

Forrest GN, Tamura K. Rifampin combination therapy for nonmycobacterial infections. *Clin Microbiol Rev*. 2010;23(1):14. (36)

Game F. Management of osteomyelitis of the foot in diabetes mellitus. *Nat Rev Endocrinol*. 2010;6(1):43. (25)

Lazzarini L et al. Antibiotic treatment of osteomyelitis: what have we learned from 30 years of clinical trials? *Int J Infect Dis*. 2005;9(3):127. (31)

Lipsky BA et al. Infectious Diseases Society of America. Diagnosis and treatment of diabetic foot infections. *Clin Infect Dis*. 2004;39(7):885. (30)

Ohl CA. Infectious arthritis of native joints. In: Mandell GL, Bennett JE, Dolin R, eds. *Mandell, Douglas, and Bennett's Principles and Practice of Infectious Diseases*. 7th ed. Philadelphia, PA: Elsevier Churchill Livingstone; 2010:1443. (40)

Zimmerli W. Vertebral osteomyelitis. *N Engl J Med*. 2010;362(11):1022. (3)

Key Websites

Center for Disease Control and Prevention, Sexually Transmitted Diseases Treatment Guidelines, 2010. Accessed from **http://cdc.gov/std/treatment/2010/gonococcal-infections.htm** February 4, 2011. (44)

71

Traumatic Skin and Soft Tissue Infections

James P. McCormack and Glen R. Brown

CORE PRINCIPLES

		CHAPTER CASES
CELLULITIS		
1	Cellulitis (an acute inflammation of the skin and subcutaneous fat) is characterized by local tenderness, pain, swelling, warmth, and erythema with or without a definite entry point.	**Case 71-1**
2	Local treatment (i.e., cleaning or irrigation of the site with soap and water) is all that is required for mild cellulitis in patients with no evidence of a systemic infection.	**Case 71-1**
3	Cellulitis most often is caused by group A β-hemolytic streptococci (*Streptococcus pyogenes*) and, less often, *Staphylococcus aureus*.	**Case 71-1 (Question 1)**
4	Community-acquired methicillin-resistant *S. aureus* (CA-MRSA) may be a causative pathogen, especially in high-risk patients (children, competitive athletes, prisoners, soldiers, selected ethnic populations, Native Americans/Alaska Natives, Pacific Islanders, intravenous drug users, men who have sex with men), and empiric treatment should have activity against CA-MRSA.	**Case 71-1 (Question 1)**
5	The value of topical antibiotics in treating skin infections is questionable.	**Case 71-1 (Question 6)**
6	For most cases of cellulitis requiring antibiotics, the least expensive of cloxacillin, dicloxacillin, or cephalexin should be chosen. Although macrolides and quinolones are effective in treating some cellulitis, they do not provide any therapeutic advantage over older and less expensive agents.	**Case 71-1 (Question 1)**
SOFT TISSUE INFECTIONS IN DIABETIC PATIENTS		
1	Skin and soft tissue infections are very common in diabetic patients with approximately 25% of patients reporting a history of skin and soft tissue infection.	**Case 71-4 (Question 1)**
2	No "best" regimens exist to treat diabetic soft tissue infections.	**Case 71-4 (Question 2)**
3	Many diabetic soft tissue infections can be prevented with proper foot care.	**Case 71-4 (Question 4)**
NECROTIZING SOFT TISSUE INFECTIONS		
1	Necrotizing soft tissue infections can progress rapidly to cause local (e.g., necrosis and loss of skin sensation) and severe systemic effects (e.g., hypotension, shock).	**Case 71-5 (Question 1)**
2	Initial treatment of necrotizing soft tissue infections involves extensive débridement to remove all necrotic tissue, fluid resuscitation, and broad-spectrum antibiotics.	**Case 71-5 (Question 1)**

continued

ERYSIPELAS

1 Erysipelas is a superficial skin infection caused by streptococci, predominantly group A, although groups C or G also are associated.	**Case 71-6 (Question 1)**
2 Oral or parenteral penicillins, with activity against group A streptococci, are the drugs of choice for treatment.	**Case 71-6 (Question 1)**

ACUTE TRAUMATIC WOUND

1 Routine antibiotic therapy is not indicated for traumatic wounds unless the patient has risk factors for impaired clearance of bacteria or involvement of high-risk (e.g., joint, tendons) tissues. For all traumatic wounds, aggressive wound care (e.g., irrigation, removal of foreign objects) is required.	**Case 71-7 (Question 1)**

ANIMAL BITES

1 All animal bites should be washed thoroughly with clean water as soon as possible after the bite. Irrigation of the wound may be the only treatment necessary.	**Case 71-9 (Question 1)**
2 Animals have different oral flora, which alters the potential pathogens associated with bites.	**Case 71-9 (Question 2)**

HUMAN BITES

1 Treating a human bite is similar to any other laceration, including cleansing, irrigating, exploring, débriding, draining, excising, and suturing, as required.	**Case 71-10 (Question 1)**
2 Various treatment options are available for preventing or treating human bite infections.	**Case 71-10 (Question 1)**

TETANUS

1 Tetanus is a preventable disease through primary prophylaxis and appropriate wound management. Tetanus can develop in patients who have not been immunized or who have not received a booster dose within the past 10 years.	**Case 71-11 (Question 1)**

Skin and soft tissue infections may involve any or all layers of the skin (epidermis, dermis), subcutaneous fat, fascia, or muscle. Many terms or classifications are used to describe various skin and soft tissue infections, and these often are based on the site of infection and causative organism(s).[1] These terms or classifications add little to the understanding and treatment of these infections. This chapter focuses on skin and soft tissue infections that are primarily the result of a break in the skin after an abrasion, skin puncture, ulceration, surgical wound, intentional or unintentional insertion of a foreign body, or blunt soft tissue contusion. Treatment of traumatic skin and soft tissue infections often is empiric and based on the severity and site of infection, the patient's underlying immunocompetence, and the triggering event (e.g., abrasion, bite, insertion of a foreign object) because attempts to isolate the causative organism often are futile.

CELLULITIS

Cellulitis (an acute inflammation of the skin and subcutaneous fat) is characterized by local tenderness, pain, swelling, warmth, and erythema with or without a definite entry point. Cellulitis is usually secondary to trauma or an underlying skin lesion that allows bacterial penetration into the skin and underlying tissues. Cellulitis most often is caused by group A β-hemolytic streptococci (*Streptococcus pyogenes*) and, less often, *Staphylococcus aureus* (Table 71-1).[2] However, unless there is an abscess or penetrating trauma, *S. aureus* rarely causes cellulitis.[2] Local treatment (i.e., cleaning or irrigation of the site with soap and water) is all that is required for mild cellulitis in patients with no evidence of a systemic infection. An elevated temperature, increasing pain, and lymphadenopathy suggest a more serious infection, and antibiotics, in addition to local wound care, should be prescribed. Wound cultures often are negative and fail to identify the causative organism. Other organisms (*Escherichia coli, Pseudomonas aeruginosa, Klebsiella pneumoniae*) also can cause cellulitis, but should be suspected only in immunocompromised patients or in patients who fail to respond to antibiotics that have activity limited to gram-positive organisms. Recently, the incidence of community-acquired methicillin-resistant *S. aureus* (CA-MRSA) has been increasing.[3]

CASE 71-1

QUESTION 1: N.P., age 25 years, presents to her family doctor with a 2- to 3-day history of worsening pain, redness, and swelling on her left leg after an abrasion that occurred by sliding during a soccer game. The area is warm to the touch with a defined erythematous border. During

TABLE 71-1
Potential Organisms Causing Skin and Soft Tissue Infections

	Gram-Positive		Gram-Negative		Anaerobes			
	Staphylococcal	Streptococcal	*Escherichia coli*, *Klebsiella* species, *Proteus* species	*Pasteurella multocida*	*Eikenella corrodens*	Oral Anaerobes	*Clostridium* species	*Bacteroides fragilis*
Cellulitis	X	X						
Diabetic soft tissue	X	X	X					X
Necrotizing infections	X	X	X			X	X	X
Erysipelas		X						
Animal bites	X	X	X	X		X		
Human bites	X	X	X		X	X		

X, organisms that should be covered empirically with appropriate antibiotic therapy.

the past 24 to 36 hours, the leg has become increasingly painful and "tight." Mild lymphadenopathy is present, and N.P. has a temperature of 38.2°C. The presumptive diagnosis is a moderate cellulitis, and cloxacillin is prescribed. Why is cloxacillin appropriate empiric treatment for N.P.?

Oral cloxacillin is appropriate empiric therapy for cellulitis in an otherwise healthy individual. Cloxacillin has predictable activity against methicillin-sensitive staphylococcal (MSSA) and streptococcal organisms and is better tolerated than erythromycin or clindamycin. Dicloxacillin, another antistaphylococcal penicillin, produces slightly higher total serum concentrations than cloxacillin but is more highly protein bound, resulting in slightly lower free serum concentrations. Flucloxacillin provides similar total serum concentrations to dicloxacillin but is less protein bound and produces higher free concentrations than either cloxacillin or dicloxacillin. These small differences in pharmacokinetics do not affect clinical outcome, and the choice between these agents should be based on cost. If the cellulitis is well demarcated and there are no pockets of pus or evidence of vein thrombosis, penicillin alone can be appropriate because the causative organism is likely to be streptococcal. Many other available antibiotics that have activity against staphylococcal and streptococcal organisms have been evaluated for effectiveness in skin and soft tissue infections. In a surveillance study in the United States, all 405 isolates of *S. pyogenes* isolated from skin and soft tissue infections were sensitive to penicillin. *S. pyogenes* was also 100% susceptible to ceftriaxone, vancomycin, levofloxacin, and moxifloxacin; 6% of the organisms were resistant to azithromycin.[4] Although many antibiotics are effective for the treatment of cellulitis, none is more effective than cloxacillin or dicloxacillin. A recent review concluded that the available evidence does not allow specific recommendations for the best antibiotic regimen for cellulitis.[5] Cephalexin is probably as effective and as well tolerated as cloxacillin or dicloxacillin and is comparable in cost. The gram-negative activity of cephalexin (not present with cloxacillin or dicloxacillin) is not required for most cases of cellulitis in otherwise healthy patients. In many emergency departments (ED), a single dose of a long-acting parenterally administered cephalosporin (e.g., ceftriaxone), followed by oral therapy with one of the agents mentioned above, is often the preferred treatment regimen. However, this regimen is not more effective than oral therapy alone, and ceftriaxone adds to the cost of treatment.

In this case, antibiotic treatment is required, and N.P. should receive the least expensive of cloxacillin, dicloxacillin, or cephalexin. Although some of the macrolides and quinolones are effective in treating cellulitis, they do not provide any therapeutic advantage over older and less expensive agents.[2] In cases in which there is an abscess, drainage is often all that is needed as antibiotic therapy (cephalexin) has been shown to be no better than placebo for uncomplicated skin abscesses in a population at risk for CA-MRSA infection.[6]

In geographical areas where the incidence of CA-MRSA has become clinically important (>10% of isolates), particularly with additional risk factors (children, competitive athletes, prisoners, soldiers, selected ethnic populations, Native Americans/Alaska Natives, Pacific Islanders, intravenous [IV] drug users, men who have sex with men), empiric treatment should include antibiotics with activity against CA-MRSA.[7] At present, most CA-MRSA are still susceptible to trimethoprim-sulfamethoxazole, clindamycin, and doxycycline, but definitive clinical trials of these agents for CA-MRSA infections are lacking.[2,8] In a small randomized, controlled trial ($n = 34$) doxycycline was compared with trimethoprim-sulfamethoxazole, and although no statistical difference in outcome was observed, all three failures occurred in patients receiving trimethoprim-sulfamethoxazole.[9] If these agents are used, a reasonable suggestion would be to re-evaluate (by the patient if they are competent) within 24 to 48 hours to verify that an improvement is occurring. Some clinicians avoid the use of clindamycin because of concerns of inducible resistance. In areas with a clinically important incidence of CA-MRSA, laboratories should test for inducible clindamycin resistance.[2] If N.P. is from an area of high CA-MRSA prevalence and has associated risk factors, the combination of trimethoprim-sulfamethoxazole or doxycycline with amoxicillin would provide therapy for the anticipated pathogens. However, even in areas of high CA-MRSA prevalence, some investigations have found cephalexin to be as effective as therapy specifically targeted for CA-MRSA,[10,11] although this has not been supported in all studies.[12] If CA-MRSA does not require antibacterial coverage, this practice may reduce antibacterial selection pressure and expense.[13]

In addition to systemic therapy, N.P. should be instructed to keep the area clean with soap and water (if an open wound is present) and to protect the area.

CASE 71-1, QUESTION 2: What agents could be chosen if N.P. is allergic to penicillin?

Clindamycin or moxifloxacin could be chosen for patients with a documented history of penicillin or cephalosporin allergy. In certain geographical areas, group A streptococci macrolide resistance approaches 15% to 20%, decreasing the potential value of these agents. Clindamycin is superior to macrolides with respect to group A streptococcal coverage; however, it causes diarrhea in 20% of patients and is one of the main agents responsible for antibiotic-associated colitis. Moxifloxacin is well tolerated and has the convenience of once-daily dosing, but it is more expensive. Although trimethoprim-sulfamethoxazole has good activity against *S. aureus,* its activity against *S. pyogenes,* i.e., group A streptococci, is weak, making this antibiotic undesirable alone as empiric therapy. The decision about which agent to choose should likely come down to cost.

CASE 71-1, QUESTION 3: What dose should be prescribed for N.P.?

The recommended dosages in the literature for cloxacillin and dicloxacillin are 250 to 500 mg orally every 6 hours and 125 to 250 mg orally every 6 hours, respectively. Although lower dosages of dicloxacillin can be used, cloxacillin and dicloxacillin produce relatively similar free serum concentrations and should be prescribed at similar dosages. The dosage for mild to moderate infections should be 250 mg orally every 6 hours; for moderate to severe infections, it should be 500 mg orally every 6 hours. The dosage for mild to moderate infections should be 250 mg orally every 6 hours; for moderate to severe infections, it should be 500 mg orally every 6 hours. For the beta-lactams, dosages up to 1,000 mg orally every 6 hours have been used, but gastrointestinal intolerance (usually diarrhea) can occur. The dosage for penicillin V is 250 to 500 mg orally every 6 hours; for oral clindamycin, the dosage is 150 to 450 mg orally every 6 hours. Because cloxacillin is the drug chosen for N.P., a dosage of 250 mg orally every 6 hours should be sufficient. If she were more severely ill, however, the higher dosage of 500 mg orally every 6 hours could be chosen. The dose for doxycycline is 100 mg orally every 12 hours, and the dose for trimethoprim-sulfamethoxazole is two double-strength tablets orally every 12 hours. The recommended dose for moxifloxacin is 400 mg orally every 24 hours and 500 mg orally every 24 hours for levofloxacin.

CASE 71-1, QUESTION 4: How long should N.P. be treated?

Although the usual recommended duration of therapy for cellulitis is 10 days, 5 days of antibiotics has been shown to be as efficacious as 10 days for uncomplicated cellulitis.[14] A reasonable recommendation to the patient would be to continue oral antibiotics for 2 to 3 days after the patient has become afebrile and has clinically improved. N.P. should be counseled to expect a response within 1 to 2 days after therapy begins (although erythema may persist longer). In addition, she should be instructed to return for re-evaluation if the condition does not improve or worsens during the next few days.

CASE 71-1, QUESTION 5: What further diagnostic evaluation should be undertaken for N.P.?

In otherwise healthy individuals, identification of the causative organism in cases of cellulitis is unnecessary. Needle aspiration, fine-needle aspiration biopsy, and punch biopsy identify the causative organism in only 15% to 25% of patients. Appropriate empiric treatment is effective in most patients, and an attempt to isolate the organism does not improve success of treatment and adds significantly to the cost of care. However, failure of initial empirical therapy, cellulitis in immunocompromised patients, patients with potential joint or tendon damage, and patients with life-threatening infections requiring hospitalization may benefit from additional cultures. In these cases, a swab of the primary wound and a needle aspiration or punch biopsy of the leading edge of the cellulitis should be obtained for Gram stain and culture before initiating antimicrobial therapy. Blood and wound cultures should be drawn in these patients. Anaerobic cultures need to be drawn only when the wound contains necrotic tissue, the wound is foul smelling, or crepitus is present. Even if wound and blood cultures are obtained, many infections will be culture negative (74%). Blood culture results are positive in less than 5% of cellulitis cases. Culture information, in conjunction with clinical course, can be used to modify subsequent treatment. Because N.P. has only a moderate cellulitis, cultures are not required and therapy can be given empirically.

CASE 71-1, QUESTION 6: Could topical antibiotics be used to treat N.P.'s cellulitis?

The value of topical antibiotics in treating skin infections is questionable. Most topical antibiotics have not been evaluated in appropriately designed trials. Although mupirocin is superior to placebo in treating some types of wound infections, its value in more severe disease is uncertain. Mupirocin has been compared favorably with erythromycin and cloxacillin in the treatment of patients with impetigo, minor wound infections, and mild cellulitis; however, most cases of mild cellulitis improve with only local wound care (e.g., cleansing or irrigation of the area) and no additional systemic antibiotics. In patients with moderate to severe infections, mupirocin or any topical antibiotics (neomycin, bacitracin, polymyxin B) should not be used to replace or augment systemic antibiotics. Topical antibiotics likely do little but add to the cost of therapy, and they occasionally cause a contact dermatitis. Therefore, N.P. should not be treated with topical antibiotics because her moderate cellulitis should be managed adequately by her systemic antimicrobial therapy.

CASE 71-2

QUESTION 1: O.A., age 49 years, presents to the ED with a 3- to 4-day history of increasing pain around his left hip, secondary to an injury he received falling on the sidewalk. In addition, he has a fever and feels weak, lethargic, and nauseated. Examination reveals a swollen, warm, and extremely tender hip. O.A. has a temperature of 39.8°C and appears quite ill. A diagnosis of moderate to severe cellulitis is made, and O.A. is hospitalized because of the severity of the infection. O.A. has no other underlying medical problems. What empiric antibiotic regimen would be reasonable for O.A.?

In moderate to severely ill patients, when hospitalization is required, antibiotics should be administered parenterally. The parenteral agent of choice is nafcillin, or cloxacillin (in Canada). Cefazolin (1–2 g IV every 8 hours) would be an appropriate alternative if it is less expensive than nafcillin. Second- and third-generation cephalosporins (cefuroxime, cefoxitin, ceftriaxone, cefotaxime) and some quinolones may be as effective as nafcillin but provide no clinical advantages for most cellulitis and are more expensive. Linezolid is also effective for the treatment of complicated skin and soft tissue infections, but it is no more effective than cloxacillin.[15] In a large study (1,080 subjects) of complicated soft tissue infections, linezolid produced similar cure rates to vancomycin overall (92% vs. 89%), but in a subset analysis of subjects with MRSA, linezolid was associated with a better outcome rate (89% vs. 67%).[16] Linezolid does have a potential for drug interactions with serotonin uptake inhibitors, so concurrent therapies must be considered. Newer agents, like daptomycin and tigecycline, are effective in serious soft tissue infections, but should only be used if other first-line agents are ineffective or are not tolerated.

Therefore, O.A. should receive either nafcillin or cefazolin, whichever is less expensive. Once O.A. has become afebrile and has clinically improved for 2 days, the parenteral antibiotic should be discontinued and appropriate oral therapy (cloxacillin) initiated to complete at least a 10-day course (2 weeks if the patient responds slowly). In settings where 10% to 15% of community isolates of *S. aureus* are methicillin resistant, in severe infections (sepsis, necrotizing fasciitis, etc.), or if the patient has risk factors, empiric treatment with vancomycin, linezolid, or daptomycin should be considered until the results of cultures and sensitivities are known.

CASE 71-2, QUESTION 2: Two days after starting therapy, O.A. develops a maculopapular skin rash. What alternative therapy should be chosen?

Regardless of when during the course of therapy a drug rash occurs (early or late), the precipitant drug should be discontinued because there is a chance, although small, that the reaction could worsen. In patients who have a penicillin allergy and who still require parenteral therapy, clindamycin, vancomycin, linezolid, moxifloxacin, or levofloxacin could be chosen. Because all of these agents are equally effective, the choice should be based on cost and dosing convenience and presence of risk factors for CA-MRSA (clindamycin 600 mg IV every 8 hours, vancomycin 1,000 mg IV every 12 hours, linezolid 600 mg IV every 12 hours, moxifloxacin 400 mg IV every 24 hours, and levofloxacin 500 mg IV every 24 hours).

CASE 71-2, QUESTION 3: After 48 hours of therapy, culture and sensitivity results are available. What changes, if any, should be made in O.A.'s treatment?

If cultures show only streptococcal organisms in a patient who is not allergic to penicillin, therapy should be switched to penicillin because it is effective, well tolerated, and less expensive than nafcillin. If cultures show staphylococcal species (*S. aureus*) that are sensitive to methicillin, the initial empiric therapy should be continued. If the organisms are resistant to methicillin, therapy should be switched to vancomycin 15 mg/kg IV every 12 hours or linezolid 600 mg IV every 12 hours (unless the patient has very much improved on the present therapy). The choice between these two agents should be based on side effect profile, drug interactions, and cost. Although more expensive than vancomycin, linezolid can be used orally. Because O.A. has a presumed penicillin allergy and does not require therapy for CA-MRSA, he should continue with clindamycin or vancomycin.

CASE 71-2, QUESTION 4: After 72 hours of therapy, O.A. has improved considerably and has been afebrile for 24 hours. Can he be switched to oral therapy?

Once O.A. has been afebrile for at least 24 hours and is significantly improved, he can be switched to oral therapy, assuming he can tolerate oral medications. Although clinicians often switch to an oral version of the drug that was given parenterally, this may not always provide the patient with the most convenient and cost-effective therapy. Clinicians should select the oral agent on the basis of culture results (if available), anticipated pathogens (if no culture results), convenience, and cost.

CASE 71-3

QUESTION 1: M.C., age 22 years, presents to the ED with a 3- to 4-day history of pain in her left forearm. On examination, she has a swollen and erythematous area of approximately 8 × 12 cm in the antecubital fossa of the left arm. The area is warm and tender to the touch. M.C. has a temperature of 39.2°C. She admits to injecting heroin daily; track marks are present on both arms. She states that she uses "filtered tap water" as a diluent for her narcotics and that her arm "has only been hurting for the last 3 days." No signs of lymphangitis or thrombophlebitis are seen. What tests are needed to confirm the diagnosis?

M.C. has all the cardinal signs of cellulitis (i.e., induration, edema, erythema, and tenderness to touch). Given her history of an injury (injection), her presentation is compatible with cellulitis. No additional tests are required unless, on clinical examination, there is a suspicion of additional injury beyond the injection site or of a deeper infection (e.g., osteomyelitis). Obtaining a specimen from the infection site (by aspiration) to identify the organism(s) is unnecessary unless the patient has a concurrent condition that could impair her immunologic response. The sensitivity in identifying the infecting organism via needle aspiration at the edge of the wound or at the site of greatest inflammation is only about 10%. Therefore, aspiration of the wound is not warranted. The sensitivity of needle aspiration increases to 25% in patients with underlying immunologic dysfunction (e.g., diabetes, malignancy, poor peripheral circulation) and may be beneficial in identifying the infecting organism(s) in these patients. M.C. has a risk factor (IV drug use) for CA-MRSA.[17] She should be closely examined for any sign of abscess and drained if present. Cultures should be sent of any abscess fluid, but routine cultures for CA-MRSA in pure cellulitis is not required unless this is a repeat presentation or is part of an infection control measure for a community outbreak.[17] For patients such as M.C. with signs and symptoms (e.g., fever) in whom the injury is a significant risk for bacteremia and endocarditis, blood cultures are warranted. Blood cultures should be drawn before antibiotics are started to maximize the ability to isolate the pathogen. If the blood cultures return positive for *S. aureus*, further assessment for potential endocarditis is warranted.

CASE 71-3, QUESTION 2: Are the suspected organisms in this patient population similar to those found in other patients with cellulitis?

A wide range of organisms are associated with cellulitis in an IV drug user. Despite the efforts of an IV drug user to make as sterile an IV product as possible, it is commonplace to inject inadvertently contaminated solution. Although almost any organism can be found, the infecting bacteria causing cellulitis in an IV drug user are similar to those found in normal hosts. β-Hemolytic group A streptococci and staphylococci, particularly *S. aureus*, are the most common infecting organisms. Intravenous drug use is a risk factor for infection with CA-MRSA and should be particularly considered if the patient has had recurrent infections or has failed to respond to MSSA-directed antibiotic therapy.[17] *Staphylococcus epidermidis* and gram-negative organisms, including *P. aeruginosa*, are rarely pathogens unless the IV drug user has taken oral cephalexin concurrent with his or her injections, a common practice in IV drug users. In areas with a high prevalence of methicillin-resistant *S. aureus*, this organism will appear in a similar percentage of IV drug users with cellulitis. Some investigators report a high incidence of mouth anaerobic bacteria in cellulitis of IV drug users and hypothesize that these result from the transfer of oral flora.

CASE 71-3, QUESTION 3: What is the appropriate empiric therapy?

Antibiotic therapy directed at eradicating all possible infecting organisms is not required. Because streptococci and staphylococci account for more than 94% of all infecting organisms in IV drug users with soft tissue infections, therapy need cover only the sensitivity patterns of these organisms in the treatment area. Oral therapy is appropriate for mild cases of cellulitis. Infections that involve a large area or that are associated with lymphangitis should be treated with parenteral antibiotics. Likewise, infections involving the hand should be treated parenterally. Because M.C. may be at risk for CA-MRSA, if this organism is common in her local community, initial therapy with cotrimoxazole (1 double strength tablet twice daily) or doxycycline (if confirmed not pregnant) would be appropriate. If treatment does not result in some resolution of inflammation within 48 hours, antimicrobial coverage should be expanded to cover gram-negative organisms and cotrimoxazole- or doxycycline-resistant streptococci. The anaerobic organisms found in IV drug users with cellulitis usually respond to treatment with penicillins or cephalosporins.

For patients not responding to initial therapy and for patients with signs or symptoms of a systemic response (e.g., rigors, hypotension), parenteral therapy that covers CA-MRSA is required, such as vancomycin, linezolid, daptomycin, or tigecycline.[17] Antibiotic therapy that provides coverage against the other common organisms causing cellulitis (i.e., *E. coli* and *K. pneumoniae*) in the IV drug user population should be added, based on the sensitivity patterns in the local area. This may include the use of a parenteral cephalosporin or quinolone or tigecycline. Tigecycline is unique in providing activity against the potential streptococcal and staphylococcal pathogens, including CA-MRSA, as well as potential gram-negative pathogens. Tigecycline may be as effective used alone as a combination of cephalosporin, carbapenem, or extended penicillin with vancomycin.[18] Treatment of cellulitis in an IV drug user should include rest, immobilization and elevation of the infected arm, antibiotics, and surgical drainage or débridement as required. If any sign of pus collection in the wound is noted, the wound must be surgically explored and drained. If no area of pus collection can be seen or palpated, immobilization and elevation, combined with systemic antibiotic therapy, is appropriate treatment. The wound should be assessed daily for local tenderness, pain, erythema, swelling, ulceration, necrosis, and wound drainage until signs of resolution to ensure that subsequent surgical treatment is not required.

SOFT TISSUE INFECTIONS IN DIABETIC PATIENTS

Skin and soft tissue infections are common in patients with diabetes mellitus. Approximately 25% of diabetic patients report a history of skin and soft tissue infections,[19] and 5% to 15% of diabetic patients may undergo limb amputation. In addition to the cost associated with treating skin and soft tissue infections, functional disability can occur, which can significantly decrease the patient's quality of life. Diabetic patients are at particular risk for foot problems, primarily because of the neuropathies and peripheral vascular diseases associated with longstanding diabetes. The decreased pain sensation allows the patient to continue to bear weight in the presence of skin damage, thereby promoting the formation of an ulcer. In addition, minor trauma (e.g., cuts, foreign body insertion) can go unnoticed and, when left untreated, can become infected and extensive. Although these infections are common, preventive measures should likely reduce the frequency of amputations. Mild infections can be treated empirically with those agents used for soft tissue infections in nondiabetic patients because these are commonly caused by aerobic gram-positive cocci. In moderate to severe infections, antibiotic coverage should be expanded because multiple organisms may be responsible for the infection. Although it is often difficult to determine colonizers from true pathogens, an average of two to six organisms are cultured from foot ulcers in patients with diabetes. The following organisms (in no particular order) have been isolated in more than 20% of wounds in patients with diabetes: *S. aureus, S. epidermidis, Enterococcus faecalis,* other streptococci, *Proteus* species, *E. coli, Klebsiella* species, *Peptococcus* species, *Peptostreptococcus* species, and *Bacteroides* species.[20] These infections are often polymicrobic, but treatment can be effective even if not all cultured pathogens are covered.[20] To determine the pathogens most accurately, a specimen of infected tissue should be obtained that is not directly communicating with an ulcer. If this is not possible, cultures of purulent exudate or curettage should be obtained, versus superficial swab, to determine the true pathogens in the wound.[19] Although antibiotics have an important role, drainage and surgical débridement to remove necrotic tissue are essential and may be the mainstay of treatment.[20]

Cultures of the affected areas may not be that useful unless bone is infected. Although anaerobic organisms often are difficult to culture, anaerobic organisms must be considered if an abscess or devitalized, necrotic, foul-smelling tissue is present or the wound is a result of abdominal surgery. Empiric coverage for *E. faecalis* is required only for severe (necrotizing) infection in which the severity of the infection puts the patient at risk for significant morbidity if this pathogen is not covered. Even if enterococci are found in the wound, enterococcal coverage probably is needed only if it is the predominant organism. Blood cultures should be obtained for patients who have severe infection and systemic signs of infection.[21]

CASE 71-4

QUESTION 1: T.U., a 67-year-old man with diabetes, presents to his general practitioner for a routine checkup and has no specific complaints. T.U. has a 15-year history of poorly controlled type 2 diabetes and a 3-year history of recurrent foot ulcers. On examination, the physician observes that an ulcer on the underside of the foot, which had previously healed over, is open and inflamed; purulent fluid can be expressed from the wound. T.U. reports no pain around the area and was unaware that the ulcer had worsened. He is afebrile and demonstrates no other signs of a systemic infection. Does T.U. have an active infection, and is antibiotic therapy required?

All open wounds, in diabetic and nondiabetic patients, will become colonized with bacteria, but only infected wounds should be treated with antibiotic therapy.[20,21] Often it is difficult to determine whether an open wound is infected, but signs and symptoms (e.g., purulent drainage, erythema, pain, and swelling around the area) are suggestive of infection. Based on his symptoms, T.U. has an infection that requires treatment.

CASE 71-4, QUESTION 2: What treatment should T.U. receive?

Mild diabetic foot infections should not be treated with topical antibiotic preparations as the evidence of efficacy is limited; the preparations do not allow sufficient penetration of antibiotic into the tissues; and many preparations are detrimental to wound healing.[22] Mild infections can be treated empirically in a similar way to other soft tissue infections[20] because these are commonly caused by aerobic gram-positive cocci. A penicillinase-resistant penicillin (e.g., cloxacillin, nafcillin) or cephalexin will be effective in most cases. The choice between these agents should be based on tolerability and cost. If anaerobes are suspected (based on malodorous aroma, if the infection is severe or long-standing or has recently been treated with antibiotics), metronidazole or clindamycin should be added to the regimen.[19] If metronidazole is selected, concurrent use of an antibiotic with good activity against aerobic pathogens is required because metronidazole has no activity against aerobic bacteria. In patients with significant vascular compromise, crepitus, or gangrene, a radiograph should be taken to identify any bone involvement suggestive of osteomyelitis.

No "best" regimens exist to treat diabetic soft tissue infections.[23] Clindamycin 600 mg IV every 8 hours in combination with either ciprofloxacin 400 mg or a third-generation cephalosporin is an effective combination that will provide coverage against most potential pathogens (gram-positive, gram-negative, and anaerobes), with the exception of *E. faecalis.* Clindamycin (and other antibacterials), however, can cause *Clostridium difficile*–associated diarrhea. Aminoglycosides are associated with serious toxicity if used for an extended period and should probably be avoided in diabetic patients. A β-lactam–β-lactamase inhibitor combination, such as piperacillin and tazobactam, ticarcillin and clavulanic acid, or ampicillin and sulbactam, provides similar coverage but also adds coverage against enterococci (piperacillin and ampicillin, but not ticarcillin) and offers the advantage of monotherapy.

Other single-agent therapies could include the use of a carbapenem (ertapenem, imipenem, or meropenem) or tigecycline, but the increased cost and broad spectrum of activity of these agents should limit their use to patients unresponsive to other therapies.[24] Linezolid could be used for patients with low likelihood of gram-negative or anaerobic pathogens.[19] However, if osteomyelitis or severe infection is present, the need for prolonged therapy with the associated risk of linezolid-induced myelosuppression and neuropathies make other agents more desirable.[19]

Because T.U. is an elderly diabetic patient and does not appear to be severely ill, the least expensive of ciprofloxacin–clindamycin or piperacillin–tazobactam, cefoxitin, or ceftizoxime should be chosen as empiric therapy. In addition, ampicillin and sulbactam or ticarcillin and clavulanate could be chosen if either is less expensive than the aforementioned agents or if local sensitivity patterns suggest that organisms typically found in these types of infections are routinely resistant to the other less expensive agents. The broad spectrum of carbapenems (e.g., imipenem, meropenem) may appear desirable, but frequent use in individual patients and patient populations contributes to isolation of more resistant pathogens, such as *Stenotrophomonas* organisms. Their use should be limited when possible.

Treatment should be continued for 3 to 4 days after all signs of infection have resolved. Oral therapy should be considered once the patient has clinically improved; treatment can be stopped even if the underlying ulcer has not completely healed.[19]

CASE 71-4, QUESTION 3: Despite aggressive antibiotic therapy and débridement, T.U.'s infection spreads and an amputation is required. How long should antibiotics be prescribed for T.U. after surgery?

The best option for uncontrollable, life-threatening infections often is amputation to remove the infected area. Once the infected area has been removed, antibiotic therapy is no longer required.

CASE 71-4, QUESTION 4: What measures could have been taken to prevent this complication in P.U.?

Many of the foot problems associated with diabetes can be prevented with proper foot care (Table 71-2), and these preventive measures must be emphasized. Diabetic patients with neuropathies or those who are elderly should carefully examine their feet on a regular basis (every 1–2 days).

TABLE 71-2
Foot Care for the Diabetic Patient

Inspect feet daily for cuts, blisters, or scratches. Pay particular attention to the area between the toes and use a mirror to examine the bottom of the foot.
Wash feet daily in tepid water and dry thoroughly.
Apply lotion to feet to prevent calluses and cracking.
Ensure that shoes fit properly (not too tight or too loose), and inspect them daily.
Trim nails regularly, making sure to cut straight across the nail.
Do not use chemical agents to remove corns or calluses.

Necrotizing Soft Tissue Infections

Skin and soft tissue infections are described as *necrotizing* when the inflammation is rapidly progressing and necrosis of the skin or underlying tissue is present. The following clinical signs suggest necrotizing infections, as opposed to simple cellulitis: edema beyond the area of erythema, skin blisters or bullae, localized pallor or discoloration, gas in the subcutaneous tissues (crepitus), and the absence of lymphangitis and lymphadenitis. Pain out of proportion to the apparent extent of the infection or the hard wood feel of the infected area may be the only clues of necrotizing infection.[2] Necrotizing soft tissue infections can progress rapidly to cause additional local effects (e.g., necrosis and loss of skin sensation) and severe systemic effects (e.g., hypotension, shock).[25] Necrotizing soft tissue infections are rare,[26] with approximately 1000 cases per year in the United States,[27] but they can be lethal. Necrotizing infections can occur in healthy individuals, but are more commonly associated with IV or subcutaneous injections of illicit drugs.[28]

ONLINE CONTENT

For a visual of a necrotizing soft tissue infection, go to http://thepoint.lww.com/AT10e.

Necrotizing cellulitis involves the skin and subcutaneous tissues. Necrotizing fasciitis involves both superficial and deep fascia, and necrotizing infections involving the muscle are termed *myonecrosis.* Group A β-hemolytic streptococci, *S. aureus,* other staphylococci, *Pseudomonas* species, other gram-negative organisms, *Clostridium perfringens,* peptostreptococci, *B. fragilis,* and *Vibrio* species can cause necrotizing infections.[25] Gas gangrene is myonecrosis caused by a *Clostridium* subspecies, most commonly *C. perfringens* (70%).[25] Gas in a wound is not necessarily indicative of gas gangrene caused by *C. perfringens.* Gram-negative organisms (e.g., *E. coli, Proteus* species, *Klebsiella* species) or anaerobic streptococci can produce gas in a wound. Air also could have been introduced at the time of the injury. Gas gangrene is characterized by acute onset of worsening pain that is usually out of proportion to the degree of injury. Clostridial myonecrosis (true gas gangrene), streptococcal gangrene (caused by group A β-hemolytic streptococci), and synergistic bacterial gangrene (caused by anaerobic and aerobic bacteria, usually gram-negative) are other terms used to describe necrotizing skin and soft tissue infections. Fournier's gangrene (a type of synergistic bacterial gangrene of the scrotum), nonclostridial crepitant gangrene (nonclostridial gas gangrene), and necrotizing fasciitis (all necrotizing soft tissue infections other than clostridial myonecrosis, or sometimes just streptococcal gangrene) are other commonly used terms.[25] The primary treatment for necrotizing soft tissue infections involves extensive débridement of the area to remove all necrotic tissue and drainage. Early fluid resuscitation and broad-spectrum antibiotics are also imperative.[26]

CASE 71-5

QUESTION 1: M.T., a 45-year-old alcoholic man who lives on the streets of the city, presents to the ED with a broken nose and facial lacerations, which he received after a fight outside one of the local taverns. On examination, in addition to the facial wounds, an area of severe inflammation, erythema, and necrosis is evident on his left calf. The area is very painful, crepitation is felt over the area, and a purulent discharge is present. M.T. states he believes the infection is because of a knife wound he experienced approximately 1 week ago. What antibacterial treatment should be provided?

In addition to setting the broken nose and suturing the facial lacerations, the clinician should evaluate the infection on M.T.'s calf. A Gram stain and culture of the purulent discharge should take place before initiating antimicrobial therapy. Because crepitus is present, the area should be incised, and a specimen of the infected tissue should be obtained for Gram stain and culture. Because the presence of crepitus may suggest a necrotizing infection, an immediate surgical consultation will be required for M.T. Redness, tenderness, and edema beyond the edges of the infection are frequently the only distinguishing features between necrotizing infections and simple cellulitis.[27] Pending the surgical evaluation, fluid resuscitation should be completed, and IV antibiotics initiated. Gas in the tissues could be caused by many organisms, and empiric broad-spectrum antibiotic therapy with coverage against gram-positive organisms, the Enterobacteriaceae, and *B. fragilis* should be started. Initial therapy with a carbapenem and anti-MRSA antibiotic (vancomycin or linezolid) should be used, with the addition of clindamycin if group A β-hemolytic streptococci are suspected. Clindamycin is often added for these streptococci, not for its antibacterial effects but for its ability to reduce production of bacterial toxins. Considering the risk for MRSA, either community- or hospital-acquired, empiric use of an antibiotic with activity against this organism is necessary.[27] If the patient was at low risk for MRSA, use of a carbapenem, extended-spectrum penicillin/beta lactamase inhibitor or tigecycline alone are effective.[29]

If a Gram stain of the infected tissue clearly shows the predominance of gram-positive cocci, consideration of narrowing the spectrum of antibiotic therapy is appropriate. Flesh-eating disease is usually a necrotizing fasciitis caused by virulent strains of group A streptococci. High-dose penicillin G (3 million units every 4 hours) plus clindamycin (900 mg IV every 8 hours) are the drugs of choice for this condition.[2,30] Although only experimental model data exist, the addition of clindamycin to penicillin is more effective in fulminant streptococcal infections than beta-lactam alone, potentially because it inhibits protein synthesis, which may reduce toxin expression by the bacteria, and cytokine response by the host.[2] Clindamycin may have adjunctive activities that contribute to reduced morbidity from gram-positive pathogens. In vitro evidence suggests that clindamycin suppresses toxin production by *S. aureus* isolates.[30]

Potential adjunctive therapy for streptococcal necrotizing skin infections include IV immunoglobulin G (IVIG) 2 g/kg as a single dose or 0.4 g/kg daily for 2 days. Alternative dosage regimens have included 1 g/kg on day 1 with 0.5 g/kg on days 2 and 3.[31] No clinical trials have proven the definitive benefit of IVIG, and the optimal dose, if used, is unknown. If it truly provides benefit, IVIG is thought to work by binding to the superantigens released by the streptococcal bacteria that are involved in the systemic effects of the infection.[31,32]

ERYSIPELAS

Erysipelas is a superficial skin infection caused by streptococci, predominantly group A, although groups C or G (and group B in children) also may cause the infection.[33,34] This skin infection affects approximately 1 in 1,000 persons per year, and is associated with diabetes mellitus, chronic venous insufficiency, and cardiovascular disease.[34] Erysipelas is diagnosed based on characteristics of the skin lesion and concurrent systemic symptoms.[33] The lesion is a continuous, indurated, edematous area, with a clearly defined raised edge.[34] Early in the course, the lesion is bright red, but it may turn to brown as the lesion ages or grows. The lesion spreads peripherally with no islands of unaffected tissue. The initial lesion results from a small break in the skin that becomes infected, although signs of the initial wound often are not evident. Aspiration of the lesion or a superficial swab is not recommended because this has not been shown useful in detecting the pathogen.[33] Patients with erysipelas have associated systemic symptoms of high fever, chills, frequent history of rigors, and general malaise. This constellation of systemic symptoms differentiates erysipelas from other local skin disorders.

CASE 71-6

QUESTION 1: D.D., a 70-year-old man, presents to the ED with a red, swollen face. He describes the area as "a swollen red spot" that has appeared during the past 2 days. He also describes feeling unwell for the previous 3 days and having a fever. On examination, D.D. has a bright red, shiny, edematous lesion on his right cheek that is 0.4 cm wide. It is a continuous lesion with a clearly demarcated border. What antibiotic therapy should be initiated for D.D.?

Erysipelas will respond promptly to antibiotics with activity against group A streptococci.[35] Oral penicillin V 250 to 300 mg (depending on available dosage form) every 6 hours or parenteral penicillin G (1 million units IV every 6 hours) generally reduce the systemic symptoms (e.g., fever, malaise) within 24 to 48 hours[35]; however, it will take several more days for the skin lesion to resolve. If D.D.'s condition does not improve within 72 hours after initiation of antibiotics, he should be instructed to return for reassessment. If D.D. has an allergy to penicillins, then clindamycin or an oral fluoroquinolone, such as moxifloxacin, is an alternative.[33,35] If the community has increased macrolide resistance to group A streptococci, these agents should not be part of empiric therapy. Antibiotic therapy should be continued for 10 days even if signs and symptoms resolve quickly to avoid a relapse, which could lead to chronic infection or scarring.

ACUTE TRAUMATIC WOUNDS

Although almost all traumatic wounds are contaminated with bacteria, routine oral antibiotic therapy is not indicated unless there is evidence of an infection. Contaminated wounds do become infected more often than uncontaminated wounds, but prophylactic antibiotic therapy does not appear to decrease the chance of infection.[36] For all traumatic wounds, aggressive wound care (e.g., irrigation, removal of foreign objects) is required. Randomized trials of prophylactic antibiotics in patients presenting to an ED for wounds other than bites found no evidence that oral antibiotics would protect against infection.[36]

CASE 71-7

QUESTION 1: J.K., a 25-year-old construction worker presents to the ED with a deep cut on his left forearm experienced when he accidentally put his hand through a plate glass window. Fourteen stitches are required to close the wound. Is oral antibiotic therapy required for J.K.?

A course of antibiotic therapy should be given to immunocompromised patients (e.g., those with diabetes mellitus, peripheral vascular disease, human immunodeficiency virus [HIV] or acquired immunodeficiency syndrome [AIDS], chronic corticosteroid use, leukopenia).[37] Other potential candidates for antibiotic therapy include wounds with pus, contamination by feces, and delays in cleansing (>3 hours) of the wound. Because J.K. has no risk factors, all that is required is removal of any glass fragments, irrigation, and suturing of the area.

CASE 71-8

QUESTION 1: K.M., a 7-year-old boy, presents 30 minutes after falling and scraping his elbow on the pavement. The father requests an antibiotic ointment for the wound. You look at his elbow and notice a mildly abraded, 1-inch square area. What treatment would you recommend?

All minor injuries, such as scratches, cuts, and abrasions, should be thoroughly cleaned with soap and water. The evidence on the use of a topical antibiotic as a preventive measure is contradictory, with some research demonstrating benefit but others lacking.[37] Some patients can experience skin sensitivities to topical antibiotics. K.M.'s wound should be thoroughly washed and inspected, but a topical antibiotic ointment would not be required.[36] Similarly, application of an antiseptic to the abrasion would not be recommended.[38]

ANIMAL BITE WOUNDS

Any wound caused by an animal that results in the skin being cut or punctured should be examined to ensure no underlying tissue damage has occurred. This is especially true in patients with bites of the hand or around other joints. The wound should be washed thoroughly with clean water as soon as possible after the bite.[37] Irrigation of the wound, including puncture sites, should be extensive to reduce the risk of infection. Obtaining specimens for cultures is not required, and wound irrigation should begin as soon as possible.

Animals have different oral flora, which alters the potential pathogens associated with bites. The most common pathogens in dog bites are β-hemolytic streptococci, staphylococci, *Pasteurella multocida*, anaerobic bacteria (particularly *Bacteroides* species), and *Fusobacterium* species.[39] For cat bites, the role of *P. multocida* appears more significant because this organism can be found in the oral flora of up to 75% of cats. Although antibiotic treatment is not required for some dog bites, reports of a greater than 75% incidence of infection after cat bites suggest that all patients with cat bites should receive antibiotics.[37] Because *P. multocida* often is resistant to penicillinase-resistant penicillins and first-generation cephalosporins, use of these agents in cat bites should be avoided.

CASE 71-9

QUESTION 1: P.J., a 14-year-old boy, presents to the ED 3 hours after being bitten on the leg by a neighbor's dog. He has a laceration, 14 cm long, on his medial calf. Four distinct puncture marks, suggestive of teeth marks, also are present on the calf. There is no suggestion of bone injury. P.J. was healthy before the attack and has no chronic illness. Should P.J. receive any treatment other than suturing of his laceration?

The standard of care for all bites involves copious irrigation of the wound.[39] P.J.'s wound should be evaluated for deep tissue injury, devascularization of any tissue, and bone injury. Loose suturing or closure with adhesive strips is appropriate for lacerations after irrigation.[37] Although the safety of closure of bite wounds has been debated, a good therapeutic response has been obtained after the closure of wounds.[37]

The need for antibiotics is controversial and guided by wound characteristics.[40] The patient should receive a course of antibiotics if the wound involves the hand or is near joints, if it involves deep punctures or is difficult to irrigate, if the patient is immunocompromised (e.g., diabetes, splenectomy), or if the wound is not well perfused. Antibiotics are not required for dog bites in which no deep tissue injury is present and the wound can be well irrigated, particularly if the wound is on the lower extremities in healthy adults or children.[37]

Prophylaxis for rabies is required only if the animal is from an area with endemic rabies or if the bite was the result of an unprovoked attack by a wild animal.[37] The local health board should be contacted to determine the recent rabies risk in the area. If P.J. has not received a tetanus toxoid booster within the past 5 years, a booster should be administered. If P.J. has never been immunized for tetanus, tetanus immune globulin should be administered in addition to the tetanus toxoid (see Tetanus Prophylaxis section below).

CASE 71-9, QUESTION 2: Because P.J. has several punctures that are difficult to irrigate, he is a candidate for antibiotic therapy. Which antibiotic(s) should he receive?

The selection of the appropriate antibiotic is based on the most likely pathogens from the specific animal bite. Although *P. multocida* often is considered the primary pathogen of dog bites, antibiotic coverage also must address the other common pathogens. Monotherapy with amoxicillin/clavulanate 500/875 mg orally every 12 hours is recommended.[37] If the patient is allergic to penicillin, tetracycline or doxycycline provides adequate coverage. Doxycycline is preferred over tetracycline because it is more convenient to administer (twice daily for doxycycline vs. four times a day for tetracycline); it can be used in patients with decreased renal function, may be taken with food, and is only slightly more expensive (in the generic form) than tetracycline. If the penicillin-allergic patient cannot take doxycycline, a fluoroquinolone, such as moxifloxacin 400 mg orally daily, could be used.[37] In all cases, patients should be instructed to watch for improvement; if the wound does not heal or it worsens within 48 hours, the patient needs to be re-evaluated. Antibiotic treatment should not extend beyond 5 days unless signs of an infection remain.

If the patient presents with an established infection, parenteral therapy is warranted if the infection is over a joint, has lymphatic spread, or involves the hand or head. If the patient has not responded to oral therapy, parenteral second-generation cephalosporins, such as cefoxitin 1 g IV every 6 hours, or a third-generation cephalosporin, such as ceftizoxime 1 g IV every

8 hours, have activity against *P. multocida*, streptococci, staphylococci, and anaerobes. The potential use of parenteral clindamycin or erythromycin is limited by poor activity against *P. multocida*. The poor activity of quinolones against anaerobes limits their use, despite good activity against *P. multocida*. Parenteral therapy should be continued until the infection has resolved, and therapy should then be continued with oral antibiotics. Alternative, but more expensive, therapies would include β-lactam/β-lactamase combinations or carbapenems. There is no evidence that these agents are superior to second- or third generation cephalosporins. If anaerobic infection is considered, the addition of metronidazole to the cephalosporin therapy may be warranted. Treatment should continue for at least 7 days or until all clinical signs of the infection have resolved.

HUMAN BITE WOUNDS

CASE 71-10

QUESTION 1: E.D., a 40-year-old man, presents with a sore arm 24 hours after receiving a bite to his left forearm by his neighbor in a "discussion over property boundaries." E.D. was previously healthy and has no chronic diseases. A 6 × 8-cm area of his left forearm is swollen and erythematous and includes several distinct puncture marks consistent with a human bite. No joint deformity or bone abnormality is detected on clinical examination. How should E.D. be treated?

Treating a human bite is similar to any other laceration, including cleansing, irrigating, exploring, débriding, draining, excising, and suturing, as required.[37] All human bites should be cleansed as soon as possible, and any lacerations or punctures irrigated copiously. Surgical exploration with débridement, drainage, or excision should be undertaken if deeper tissues may have been injured or if pus collection could have occurred. Exploration for damage to subcutaneous nerves, tendons, joints, or vascularity is particularly important in bites to the hand, especially the knuckles, because subsequent infections could seriously affect hand function. If E.D. had been seen within 12 hours of the injury, the wound could likely have been treated adequately with simple irrigation.[39,41] This is especially true if the human bite does not involve the hand. Because E.D. presented 24 hours after the injury, thorough exploration and irrigation of all lacerations or punctures are required. With evidence of pus accumulation in his wound, the area should be explored and drained. E.D. also should receive systemic antibiotic therapy to eradicate potential infecting organisms. If the wound is severe (i.e., involves subcutaneous tissues, a joint, or a large area) or if the patient is unlikely to be compliant with oral antibiotics, parenteral administration of antibiotics is required. The most common pathogens in human bites are β-hemolytic streptococci, *S. aureus*, *Eikenella corrodens*, and *Corynebacterium* subspecies.[39,42] Anaerobic bacteria also are commonly involved.[42] Treatment with a combination of penicillin G and a penicillinase-resistant penicillin is appropriate. Therapy with a penicillinase-resistant penicillin or a first-generation cephalosporin alone is not appropriate because *E. corrodens* commonly is resistant to these antibiotics.[42] Because the anaerobic flora of the mouth is often penicillinase-producing, alternative anaerobic coverage with amoxicillin–clavulanate may be required. If parenteral therapy is required, a second-generation cephalosporin with antianaerobic activity (e.g., cefoxitin) or a third-generation cephalosporin (e.g., ceftizoxime) is appropriate. Cefuroxime should not be used as single-agent therapy because it lacks activity against anaerobes and *E. corrodens*. Other third-generation cephalosporins and quinolones have good activity against *E. corrodens*, but not all of them can be recommended because of their inferior activity against anaerobic organisms. Moxifloxacin would be the preferred fluoroquinolone because it has good activity against the organisms associated with bite infections.[42] Azithromycin is the macrolide with the best activity against bite organisms. Alternative, but more expensive, parenteral therapy would include β-lactam/β-lactamase inhibitor combinations or carbapenems. Oral regimens for penicillin-allergic patients would include combinations of cotrimoxazole plus metronidazole, or a fluoroquinolone plus clindamycin or moxifloxacin monotherapy.[2]

Tetanus toxoid booster should be administered if E.D. has not received a booster in the past 10 years.

Tetanus Prophylaxis

Tetanus is a preventable disease through primary prophylaxis and appropriate wound management. Every child should receive primary prophylaxis of three separate doses of tetanus toxoid.[43] This provides adequate coverage for at least 10 years.[44] Tetanus can develop in patients who have not been immunized or who have not received a booster dose within the past 10 years. Patients at risk of developing tetanus are those with wounds contaminated with dirt, feces, soil, or saliva; those with puncture wounds; and those with wounds from missiles, crush injuries, burns, or frostbite.[37]

CASE 71-11

QUESTION 1: G.T., a 48-year-old woman, presents to the ED 1 hour after receiving a 2-cm laceration to her foot from stepping on a nail while walking around her neighborhood. Examination of the wound found it to be clean, with no subcutaneous extension. The wound was closed with superficial sutures, and no antibiotics, systemic or topical, were prescribed. Should G.T. receive tetanus prophylaxis?

If G.T. has received her primary tetanus immunization and had a booster dose within the previous 10 years, no additional tetanus prophylaxis is required for her wound (Table 71-3). If her primary immunization status is unknown or more than 10 years has elapsed since her last dose, a single 0.5-mL subcutaneous tetanus toxoid dose should be administered. If primary immunization is unknown or incomplete, G.T. should receive the initial 0.5-mL dose immediately and should be scheduled to complete the primary immunization during the next 2 months.

TABLE 71-3
Tetanus Prophylaxis in Routine Wound Management: Adults

History of Adsorbed Tetanus Toxoid	Clean, Minor Wounds		All Other Wounds[a]	
	Td[b]	TIG	Td[b]	TIG
Unknown or <3 doses	Yes	No	Yes	Yes
≥3 doses	No[c]	No	Yes[d]	No

[a] Including, but not limited to, wounds contaminated with dirt, feces, soil, and saliva; puncture wounds, avulsions, and wounds resulting from missiles; crushing, burns, frostbite.
[b] For children <7 years of age, diphtheria-tetanus-pertussis (DTP) is preferred to tetanus toxoid alone. For persons ≥7 years of age, Td is preferred to tetanus toxoid alone.
[c] Yes, if >10 years since last dose.
[d] Yes, if >5 years since last dose. (More frequent boosters are not needed and can accentuate the side effects.)
Td, tetanus and diphtheria toxoid; TIG, tetanus immune globulin.

For adults, the combination product of tetanus and diphtheria toxoid is the recommended treatment because this will enhance protection against diphtheria.

If G.T. had presented with a dirty wound (contaminated with dirt, feces, soil, or saliva) or if the wound had resulted from a burn, frostbite, missile (bullet), crush, or avulsion, she should receive passive tetanus immunization with tetanus immune globulin in addition to the tetanus toxoid described above. A single 250-unit intramuscular dose of tetanus immune globulin will provide passive immunization in addition to the active immunization produced from exposure to the tetanus toxoid (Table 71-3).

KEY REFERENCES AND WEBSITES

A full list of references for this chapter can be found at http://thepoint.lww.com/AT10e. Below are the key references for this chapter, with the corresponding reference number in this chapter found in parentheses after the reference.

Key References

Dryden MS. Complicated skin and soft tissue infections. *J Antimicrob Chemother*. 2010;65(Suppl 3):iii35. (1)

Jenkins TC et al. Skin and soft-tissue infections requiring hospitalization at an academic medical center: opportunities for antimicrobial stewardship. *Clin Inf Dis*. 2010;51:895. (13)

Lipsky BA et al. Diagnosis and treatment of diabetic foot infections. *Clin Infect Dis*. 2004;39:885. (21)

Liu C et al. Clinical practice guidelines by the Infectious Diseases Society of America for the treatment of methicillin-resistant *Staphylococcus aureus* infections in adults and children. *Clin Infect Dis*. 2011;52:e18. (7)

Looke D, Dendle C. Bites (mammalian). *Clin Evid*. 2010;7:914. (39)

Matthews PC et al. Clinical management of diabetic foot infection: diagnostics, therapeutics and the future. *Expert Rev Anti Infect Ther*. 2007;5:117. (19)

May AK et al. Treatment of complicated skin and soft tissue infections. *Surg Infect (Larchmt)*. 2009;10:467. (29)

Phan HH, Cocanour CS. Necrotizing soft tissue infections in the intensive care unit. *Crit Care Med*. 2010;38(Suppl):S460. (28)

Rhee P et al. Tetanus and trauma: a review and recommendations. *J Trauma*. 2005;58:1082. (43)

Sarani B et al. Necrotizing fasciitis: current concepts and review of the literature. *J Am Coll Surg*. 2009;208:279. (27)

Stevens DL et al. Practice guidelines for the diagnosis and management of skin and soft-tissue infections. *Clin Infect Dis*. 2005;41:1373. (2)

72 Prevention and Treatment of Infections in Neutropenic Cancer Patients

Richard H. Drew

CORE PRINCIPLES

	CHAPTER CASES
DEFINITIONS	
1 As a consequence of select cancer chemotherapies, patients experience neutropenia (defined as an absolute neutrophil count <500 cells/μL or anticipated to drop <500 cells/μL within 48 hours).	**Case 72-1 (Question 4)**
2 Fever (defined as a single oral temperature of ≥38.3°C [101°F] or a temperature of ≥38.0°C [100.4°F] for >1 hour) may be a sign of infection.	**Case 72-1 (Question 4)**
3 Bacteria are the primary pathogens associated with infection in febrile neutropenic patients (especially those occurring early).	**Case 72-1 (Questions 1, 6)**
CLINICAL PRESENTATION	
1 Fever is usually the earliest (and often the only) sign of infection.	**Case 72-1 (Question 4)**
2 In patients with documented infections, the most common sites are skin; mouth and throat; esophagus; sinuses; abdomen, rectum, and liver; vascular access; lungs; and urinary tract.	**Case 72-1 (Question 4)**
3 An accurate history (including the cancer type and treatment regimen, new signs of infection, antimicrobial prophylaxis, prior infections, and comorbidities) and complete physical examination should be completed.	**Case 72-1 (Question 5)**
4 Before antibiotics are initiated, two sets of blood cultures (with each set consisting of two culture bottles) should be obtained. Additional Gram stain and cultures (e.g., stool, urine, skin, intravenous site, and respiratory specimens) should also be obtained if such infections are suspected based on signs and symptoms.	**Case 72-1 (Question 5)**
5 Chest radiographs and oximetry should be completed if signs and symptoms point to the respiratory tract.	**Case 72-1 (Question 5)**
6 A complete blood count, serum electrolytes, coagulation, C-reactive protein, urinalysis, and assessment of organ function (e.g., liver and kidney function) should be assessed.	**Case 72-1 (Question 5)**
KEY TREATMENT INFORMATION	
1 Risk stratification should be undertaken to identify patients most likely to experience significant infection-related complications. Patients at highest risk include those with prolonged (>7 days) and profound (<100 cells/μL) neutropenia or select comorbidities (hypotension, severe mucositis interfering with swallowing or causing diarrhea, pneumonia, new-onset abdominal pain, hepatic or renal insufficiency, or neurologic changes).	**Case 72-1 (Questions 2, 3, 7)**

continued

KEY TREATMENT INFORMATION *CONTINUED*

2 Highest risk patients should be considered for antibacterial and antifungal prophylaxis.	**Case 72-1 (Questions 2, 3)**
3 In the absence of evidence of site- or pathogen-specific etiologies or clinical instability, initial empiric monotherapy is most commonly an antipseudomonal third-generation cephalosporin (e.g., ceftazidime), a fourth-generation cephalosporin (e.g., cefepime), or an antipseudomonal carbapenem (e.g., imipenem-cilastatin or meropenem). Additional agents may be added (such as vancomycin, an aminoglycoside, or fluoroquinolone) to initial therapy in patients who are hemodynamically unstable.	**Case 72-1 (Questions 7–10), Case 72-2 (Questions 1, 2)**

MONITORING PARAMETERS

1 The need for modification of the initial empiric therapy is dependent on the risk group (i.e., low- vs. high-risk), establishment of an infection site or causative pathogen, persistence or defervescence of fever, and clinical stability.	**Case 72-2 (Question 6)**
2 Defervescence of fever and clinical stability should guide early modifications of therapy (usually days 2–4).	**Case 72-3 (Questions 1, 2)**
3 Highest-risk patients unresponsive to initial empiric antibacterial therapy should be considered for the addition of antifungal therapy at days 4 through 7. In addition to coverage for *Candida* species, highest-risk patients with persistent or recurrent fever after 4 to 7 days of appropriate antibacterial therapy with prolonged (i.e., >10 days) neutropenia should be considered for antimold therapy. Low-risk patients who are clinically stable do not routinely need antifungal therapy.	**Case 72-3 (Questions 1, 2), Case 72-4 (Questions 1, 2)**
4 Antiviral therapy is generally restricted to patients with serologic or clinical evidence of viral infection.	**Case 72-4 (Question 4)**
5 All patients should be monitored for adverse events and drug interactions related to antibiotic therapy.	**Case 72-3 (Question 1)**

THERAPEUTIC CONTROVERSIES

1 The role of vancomycin as part of the initial empiric regimen remains controversial. In general, routine use of vancomycin as part of initial empiric therapy for fever in neutropenic patients without other evidence of infection should be discouraged (except in clinically unstable patients).	**Case 72-2 (Question 3)**
2 The ideal initial empiric antifungal agent is debatable. However, patients receiving fluconazole prophylaxis requiring addition of empiric antifungals should be considered for antifungals with activity against azole-resistant *Candida* species and mold infections.	**Case 72-4 (Questions 3, 4)**
3 Although hematopoietic colony-stimulating factors prevent neutropenia in high-risk cancer patients, use of these agents as treatment of febrile neutropenia unresponsive to antibiotics remains controversial.	**Case 72-1 (Question 3)**

Many patients with both solid tumor and hematologic malignancies have had their lives prolonged through therapeutic advances in chemotherapy, immunotherapy, and hematologic stem cell transplantation (HSCT). Despite such advances, infectious complications continue to be a major cause of morbidity and mortality in these patients. The prevention, detection, and management of infections in such immunocompromised hosts remain a major challenge.[1,2]

This chapter focuses on the prevention, diagnosis, and management of infectious complications in patients with neutropenia secondary to cancer chemotherapy. The following topics are addressed: risks and epidemiology of infection, principles of prophylactic antimicrobials, empiric initial antibacterial selection, modification and duration of therapy, empiric antifungal and antiviral use, and the use of hematopoietic growth factors.

RISK FACTORS FOR INFECTION

Patients are rendered immunocompromised when there is a significant disruption or deficiency of one or more of the host defenses as a result of the underlying disease or chemotherapy. These risk factors include neutropenia and impairment in both humoral (antibody and complement) and cell-mediated immune defenses. Disruption of barriers to infection resulting from chemotherapy-related damage to skin and mucosal barriers further increases the risk of infection. As a result, bacteria, fungi, viruses, and protozoa may infect various sites (depending on the specific immunodeficiency).

Neutropenia

Granulocytes, or granular leukocytes, represent an important defense against bacterial and fungal infections. *Neutropenia* (a reduction in the number of circulating granulocytes or neutrophils) predisposes the host to infections. The terms *granulocytopenia* and *neutropenia* are often used interchangeably. The degree of neutropenia is expressed in terms of the absolute neutrophil count (ANC) or the total number of granulocytes (polymorphonuclear leukocytes and band forms) present in the circulating pool of white blood cells (WBCs).

For purposes of guideline development and clinical trials, neutropenia is usually defined as an ANC less than 500 cells/μL or anticipated to drop to less than 500 cells/μL within 48 hours.[2–4] The risk of infection in the neutropenic patient is proportional to both the severity and duration of neutropenia.[5] In general, the risk of infection is low when the ANC exceeds 1,000 cells/μL, with the frequency and severity of infection inversely proportional to the ANC.[3,5] As the ANC drops to less than 500 cells/μL, the risk of infection rapidly increases. Conversely, recovery of the ANC is the most important factor determining the outcome of infectious complications in the neutropenic patient. Febrile patients with short durations of neutropenia ($\leq$7 days) or in whom neutropenia is not severe (<100 cells/μL) less frequently experience serious, life-threatening infections.[2,3] In contrast, patients with severe neutropenia lasting more than 7 days are at significant risk of infection.[2,3]

Damage to Physical Barriers

The intact skin and mucosal surfaces of the body constitute the host's primary physical defense against microbial invasion. The integrity of this physical barrier may be disrupted by tumor, treatment (e.g., surgery, radiation), or various medical procedures (e.g., insertion of intravenous [IV] or urinary catheters, venipuncture, measurement of rectal temperature). Device-related infections, including those associated with central venous catheters, are commonly caused by migration of skin flora (e.g., staphylococci) through the cutaneous insertion site. Infections secondary to damaged mucosal lining of the gastrointestinal (GI) tract such as mucositis (usually secondary to chemotherapy) are usually caused by enteric bacteria and fungi such as *Candida* species.

Alterations in the Immune System

Patients with immunoglobulin deficiencies (e.g., hypogammaglobulinemia, chronic lymphocytic leukemia, or splenectomy) are at increased risk for infections with encapsulated bacteria, which undergo antibody opsonization for efficient phagocytosis. Such bacteria include *Neisseria meningitidis, Haemophilus influenzae,* and *Streptococcus pneumoniae.* Hodgkin disease, organ transplantation, and human immunodeficiency virus (HIV) disease can disrupt the cellular immune system, increasing the risk for infections with obligate and facultative intracellular organisms such as mycobacteria, *Listeria, Toxoplasma,* viruses, and fungi. Certain hematologic malignancies and myelodysplastic syndromes may also be associated with immunodeficiencies secondary to replacement of leukocytes with malignant cells.

Some chemotherapeutic agents (such as fludarabine) have profound effects on both cellular and humoral defenses.[6,7] Corticosteroids exert their immunosuppressive effects on the cellular immune system, particularly at the T-lymphocyte and macrophage level. Therefore, patients receiving corticosteroids (such as HSCT recipients with graft-versus-host disease [GVHD]) have increased susceptibility to viral, bacterial, protozoal, and fungal infections.[8] Infectious complications secondary to glucocorticoids are dose-dependent. The risk of infection increases with daily doses greater than 10 mg or cumulative doses greater than 700 mg of prednisone or its equivalent.[8] Thus, patients receiving corticosteroids in either high doses or for prolonged periods are at increased risk for infections caused by opportunistic pathogens. Severe cell-mediated immunodeficiency may also be caused by GVHD and its treatment.[2,3,6] More recently, chemotherapeutic monoclonal options, such as alemtuzumab and bortezomib, significantly weaken the immune system, predisposing recipients to infection.[9,10]

Colonization or Prior Infection

Colonization is characterized as isolation of an organism from any particular site (e.g., stool, nasopharynx) without clinical signs of infection. Most infections in neutropenic patients are caused by either the host's endogenous microflora or hospital-acquired pathogens that have colonized the alimentary tract, upper respiratory tract, or skin. Therefore, microbial colonization can be a prerequisite to infection in neutropenic patients. This is perhaps best studied in patients colonized with methicillin-resistant *Staphylococcus aureus* (MRSA). Prior infection (especially in the pre-engraftment phase of HSCT recipients) is a risk factor for infection during immunosuppression, particularly for viral infections (such as cytomegalovirus [CMV], *herpes simplex* virus [HSV], and *varicella zoster* virus [VZV]). Infections with these pathogens during immunosuppression are generally considered to be a consequence of latent infection rather than new infection.[2,3,6,11,12]

Hematopoietic Stem Cell Transplantation

Transplantation of bone marrow predisposes patients to the development of opportunistic infections secondary to both intensive immunosuppressive therapy and transmission.[6] These infections may be acquired or may represent reactivation of latent host infection. The introduction of new therapeutic approaches for treatment of the underlying malignancy (including nucleoside analogs and monoclonal antibodies to CD20 and CD52), along with use of unrelated stem cell donors, has increased the potential for infections in these patients.[6] When compared with autologous or syngeneic HSCT recipients, allogeneic HSCT patients have an increased risk of infection, particularly in those patients undergoing therapy for GVHD.[6] The use of immunosuppressives after transplantation (such as corticosteroids, antithymocyte globulin, and alemtuzumab) also significantly increases the risk for infection.[6]

Radiation Therapy

Side effects associated with the use of radiation therapy for the treatment of malignancy (e.g., mucositis, skin breakdown, or reduction in blood counts) also predispose a patient with neutropenia to infection.

Functional Asplenia

The spleen is responsible for production of opsonizing antibodies, assisting in protection against encapsulated bacteria (such as *S. pneumoniae, H. influenzae,* and *N. meningitidis*). Functional asplenia may occur secondary to irradiation or as a complication of GVHD.[3]

MOST COMMON PATHOGENS

CASE 72-1

QUESTION 1: B.C., a 41-year-old woman, was admitted to the cancer center for placement of a central IV catheter for administration of chemotherapy to treat acute nonlymphocytic leukemia in relapse. She was diagnosed 2 years ago and was treated with cytarabine plus daunorubicin, which resulted in a complete remission for 33 months. This admission, she will be treated with high-dose cytarabine plus mitoxantrone for reinduction. What are the most likely pathogens to cause infection in patients like B.C. during periods of chemotherapy-induced neutropenia?

Bacteria are the primary pathogens associated with infection in febrile neutropenic patients, especially those occurring early.[13] Bacteremia (reported in approximately 25% of febrile neutropenic patients) is most often caused by aerobic gram-negative bacilli (including *Pseudomonas aeruginosa, Escherichia coli,* and *Klebsiella pneumoniae*) or aerobic gram-positive cocci (i.e., coagulase-negative staphylococci, *S. aureus,* enterococci, viridans streptococci).[14] Since the mid-1990s, the proportion of gram-negative infections has decreased with a proportional increase in gram-positive infections.[2,15] Gram-positive bacteria now account for approximately 60% to 70% of microbiologically documented infections in neutropenic cancer patients.[2,16] This is likely attributable (in part) to the frequent use of indwelling IV catheters, more-intensive chemotherapy, and widespread use of broad-spectrum antibiotics.

ONLINE CONTENT

For images of *Pseudomonas aeruginosa, Escherichia coli,* and *Klebsiella pneumonia,* go to http://thepoint.lww.com/AT10e.

S. aureus (including MRSA) and coagulase-negative staphylococci, streptococci (including *S. pneumoniae* and viridans streptococci), and *Corynebacterium* species are increasingly important pathogens.[16] Moreover, enterococcal infections (including vancomycin-resistant enterococci [VRE]) are increasing in frequency. Meningitis caused by the intracellular organism *Listeria monocytogenes* can be observed in patients with defective cellular immunity caused by disease or prolonged corticosteroid use. In general, anaerobic bacteria are an infrequent cause of infection in granulocytopenic patients with hematologic malignancies.[17] However, they should be suspected in patients with GI malignancies or with significant disruption of the GI tract.[17] *Clostridium difficile* is another anaerobic pathogen that may cause infection in this population.

Pneumocystis jiroveci (formerly known as *Pneumocystis carinii* or PCP) is a pathogen responsible for lung infections primarily in patients with HIV infection. However, PCP can also be responsible for lung infections in some cancer patients.[18,19] Seen predominantly in patients with solid tumors or hematologic malignancies receiving long-term corticosteroids, PCP may present as subacute, febrile, hypoxemic, and diffuse pulmonary involvement.[18,19]

Invasive fungal infections (IFIs) are a major cause of morbidity and mortality among neutropenic cancer patients and patients undergoing HSCT.[20,21] IFIs tend to occur later in the illness. Patients with prolonged neutropenia (>7 days) or with acute myelogenous leukemia (AML) undergoing intensive induction therapy, allogeneic HSCT recipients, and those undergoing therapy for GVHD are at increased risk of acquiring systemic fungal infections.[20,21] Up to 50% of patients who die during prolonged periods of neutropenia have evidence of deep-seated mycoses.[20] Before the use fluconazole prophylaxis in selected populations, *Candida* species were responsible for most invasive fungal infections. Today, invasive infections attributable to *Aspergillus* species and other molds are a major cause of IFI-related death (particularly in those with prolonged neutropenia and GVHD).[20,22] Recent reports of improved survival from IFIs are likely related to newer prophylactic and treatment options and advances in cancer chemotherapy.[23]

As previously stated, most viral infections in neutropenic cancer patients are caused by a reactivation of latent infection rather than new infection.[2,3,6,11,12] These may include HSV and VZV. Other viruses, such as CMV, can be either reactivation or newly acquired during HSCT. Respiratory viruses (e.g., respiratory syncytial virus [RSV], influenza, parainfluenza), GI viruses (such as rotavirus and norovirus), and other seasonal viruses may occasionally cause infection in this population.

RISK STRATIFICATION

Risk stratification to identify patients most likely to experience neutropenia has important implications for decisions about prevention, diagnostic strategies, empiric therapy (selection, route of administration, duration), and site of care.[2–4,6,11,12,24] In general, patients at highest risk of complications include those with prolonged (>7 days) and profound (<100 cells/μL) neutropenia or with select comorbidities (hypotension, severe mucositis interfering with swallowing or causing diarrhea, pneumonia, new-onset abdominal pain, hepatic or renal insufficiency, or neurologic changes).[3,4] In contrast, patients with shorter (≤7 days) anticipated durations of neutropenia without significant comorbidities are generally considered at low risk of complications of infection.[3,4] Patients without fever but exhibiting new signs of infection should also be treated as high risk. Presenting signs and symptoms, cancer type, chemotherapy regimen, medical comorbidities, and prior history of febrile neutropenia (especially if severe or prolonged) should also be considered. Patients with select solid tumors (breast, lung, colorectal, ovarian) and lymphoma most frequently experience neutropenic fever. Chemotherapeutic regimens associated with the highest (>20%) incidence are summarized in detail elsewhere[24] (see Section 17, Neoplastic Disorders).

Although several risk assessment tools have been proposed,[3,11,12] the Multinational Association for Supportive Care in Cancer (MASCC) index is often used.[25] Age of at least 60 years, presence of hematologic malignancies with a history of prior fungal infections, severe symptoms (particularly hypotension), inpatient site of care, and presence of chronic obstructive pulmonary disease are important variables that result in a low MASCC score, and (consequently) patients with any of these factors are considered at highest risk. Young patients (<20 years) with solid tumors and no or mild symptoms (including the absence of hypotension) or organ dysfunction are generally at low risk for complications.

PROPHYLAXIS AGAINST INFECTION

Infection Control

CASE 72-1, QUESTION 2: Should B.C. receive antimicrobial prophylaxis during the neutropenic period? If yes, which agents should be used?

Exogenous contamination can be prevented by strict protective isolation of patients in specially designed rooms that maintain a sterile environment. These laminar airflow rooms are ventilated with air that is passed through a high-efficiency particulate air filter, which removes greater than 99% of all particles larger than 3 μm. Total protective isolation is accomplished by strict isolation in conjunction with the administration of sterile food and water, local skin care, and intensive microbial surveillance. However, this regimen is burdensome, difficult to accomplish, and expensive, and is recommended only for high-risk patients (such as allogeneic HSCT recipients).[4] HSCT recipients and candidates undergoing conditioning therapy should avoid exposure to plants, flowers, and certain foods (such as uncooked fruits and vegetables), which increase the risk of exposure to fungi.[4,6] Close attention and adherence to adequate hand-washing procedures is essential. In addition, contact isolation is advocated in circumstances in which the patient may be colonized or infected with resistant organisms (such as MRSA, VRE, or multidrug-resistant gram-negative pathogens). Finally, isolating the patients from family or caregivers with potentially contagious respiratory viral illnesses is advocated.

Antimicrobial Prophylaxis

Early administration of oral antibiotics (both antibacterials and antifungals) during the afebrile, neutropenic period in select high-risk patients may result in a reduction in the number of febrile episodes and subsequent risk of infection. The goals of such prophylactic regimens are intended to reduce pathogenic endogenous microflora or prevent the acquisition of new microorganisms. The potential benefits of such prophylaxis must outweigh the risks of antibiotic-related adverse effects including drug interactions, the development of resistance, and the potential for superinfection.

In general, patients receiving standard chemotherapy, those with solid tumors, and neutropenia of fewer than 7 days are at lowest risk and should not routinely receive prophylaxis.[3,4] In contrast, allogeneic HSCT recipients and those with acute leukemia, receipt of alemtuzumab therapy, uncontrolled malignancy, pneumonia, GVHD requiring high-dose steroids, and either profound (ANC $\leq$100 cells/μL for >7 days) or prolonged (>10 days) neutropenia are at highest risk of infection and should receive antibacterial, antifungal, and (in select cases) antiviral prophylaxis.[3,4]

NONABSORBABLE ANTIBACTERIALS

Because the GI tract is an important reservoir of potential pathogens, gut decontamination has been investigated. Early studies focused on the use of nonabsorbable antimicrobials such as gentamicin, polymyxin B, and colistin to eradicate selected gram-negative bowel flora and lack of systemic toxicity. However, these nonabsorbable regimens are inconsistent in preventing infection and have an unpleasant taste. Of additional concern is the development of aminoglycoside resistance from the nonabsorbable aminoglycoside-containing regimens. Finally, colistin use has been identified as a risk factor for staphylococcal infections.[16] Therefore, use of nonabsorbable antibacterial agents has been replaced by oral, absorbable antibiotics.[3,4]

ABSORBABLE ANTIBACTERIALS

Although trimethoprim-sulfamethoxazole (TMP-SMX) decreases bacterial infections in neutropenic patients,[26,27] it may not reduce mortality in this patient population. In contrast, TMP-SMX prevents *P. jiroveci* pneumonia independent of the presence of neutropenia. The potential benefits of TMP-SMX prophylaxis must be carefully balanced against the potential for drug-induced bone marrow suppression, hypersensitivity reactions, hyperkalemia, nephrotoxicity, pancreatitis, the emergence of resistant organisms (e.g., *E. coli*), and the development of superinfections. In addition, leukemic patients receiving mucotoxic chemotherapy and TMP-SMX prophylaxis may be at increased risk for infections caused by viridans streptococci.[28,29] TMP-SMX prophylaxis should be used only in high-risk patients. Patients with malignancy at highest risk for experiencing *P. jiroveci* pneumonia (i.e., patients with acute lymphocytic leukemia receiving intensive chemotherapy, those with acquired immunodeficiency syndrome, allogeneic HSCT recipients, those receiving alemtuzumab, and patients with GVHD) should receive TMP-SMX prophylaxis.[3,6] Recipients of T-cell–depleting agents (e.g., fludarabine or cladribine), cancer patients receiving prolonged or high-dose corticosteroids (>20 mg of prednisone or its equivalent daily) should also be considered for prophylaxis with TMP-SMX.[6] In such settings, primary prevention should be continued for up to 6 months (in the case of HSCT recipients) or longer (in cases in which immunosuppression is continued). In the setting of alemtuzumab therapy, such prophylaxis would generally continue for at least 2 months and until the CD4 count exceeded 200 cells/μL.[3] In patients requiring PCP prophylaxis but unable to tolerate TMP-SMX, patients should be considered for either TMP-SMX desensitization, atovaquone, dapsone, or aerosolized pentamidine.[3,6]

The fluoroquinolones ciprofloxacin and levofloxacin are used by some centers as prophylaxis for adult patients at high risk of infection. Data regarding their use for preventing infection in neutropenic cancer patients have been summarized elsewhere.[30,31] Of concern, however, is the increasing frequency of gram-positive infections (including viridans streptococci) and resistant gram-negative bacilli (most notable in *P. aeruginosa* and *E. coli*)[34] in patients receiving fluoroquinolone prophylaxis.[28,29,32,33] Meta-analyses report reductions in mortality in high-risk patients receiving prophylaxis with these fluoroquinolones.[35] Because fluoroquinolone prophylaxis is offset by the emergence of resistant organisms, routine prophylactic use in neutropenic patients should generally be avoided.[4] However, those at highest risk of bacterial infections (i.e., those patients with an ANC $\leq$100 neutrophils/μL for >7 days) should be considered for fluoroquinolone prophylaxis until either the onset of fever (at which time empiric antibacterials would be started) or resolution of severe neutropenia.[4,6] Levofloxacin has been recommended over ciprofloxacin in patients at increased risk of oral mucositis-related infection with invasive viridans streptococci.[4] Regardless of the fluoroquinolone chosen, local resistance patterns should be closely monitored before such prophylaxis is chosen.

Because of the increased risk of invasive pneumococcal infections, select patient populations (notably asplenic patients, allogeneic HSCT recipients [owing to functional asplenia and impaired B-cell immunity], and those undergoing immunosuppression for GVHD) should be considered for prophylaxis with penicillin.[3] In patients with chronic GVHD, penicillin prophylaxis may be continued during the administration of immunosuppressives. In HSCT recipients, prophylaxis should begin 3 months after transplant and continue for 1 year after transplant.[3] Alternative prophylaxis should be considered in areas where penicillin resistance in pneumococci is significant.

ANTIFUNGALS

CASE 72-1, QUESTION 3: Should antifungal prophylaxis be used in B.C.? What is the role of hematopoietic growth factors?

Routine antifungal prophylaxis is not indicated in all patients with neutropenia. However, select patients are at increased risk of developing systemic fungal infections.[20] Because of the frequency with which such infections are encountered, difficulties in establishing a diagnosis, and poor response rates in patients with serious invasive infection who are immunocompromised, effective prophylactic strategies are necessary in these high-risk patients.

Nonabsorbable antifungal agents, such as oral nystatin,[36,37] clotrimazole,[38] and oral amphotericin B,[39] have been studied. Although oral amphotericin B and clotrimazole reduce the frequency of oropharyngeal candidiasis, none of these antifungals has a role as primary prophylaxis of invasive fungal infections.[6] In attempts to enhance activity while minimizing side effects associated with IV administration, aerosolized delivery of amphotericin B deoxycholate has been investigated for the prevention of invasive fungal infections in this patient population,[40] and aerosolized liposomal amphotericin B has been used in leukemic and HSCT patients.[41] Although promising, the optimal dose, delivery device, and duration for aerosol administration of amphotericin B preparations have not yet been determined.

The use of systemic antifungals for prophylaxis has been summarized elsewhere.[42] Many of the earlier studies evaluated the prophylactic role of IV amphotericin B.[43,44] In one such evaluation, amphotericin B 0.5 mg/kg given three times weekly was compared with fluconazole 400 mg/day in acute leukemia.[44] Although efficacy was similar in both groups, more side effects (i.e., infusion-related reactions, nephrotoxicity, and electrolyte disturbances) were observed with the amphotericin B regimen. There are limited published data on the efficacy of lipid-based formulations of amphotericin B (e.g., amphotericin B lipid complex, liposomal amphotericin B) for prophylaxis. One study compared liposomal amphotericin B versus a combination with fluconazole and itraconazole.[45] No significant differences were detected in terms of efficacy, but toxicity was noted more frequently in the patients receiving liposomal amphotericin B. Consequently, amphotericin B is generally discouraged for primary prophylaxis in high-risk patients, unless the patient is unable to receive other mold-active prophylactic agents.

Although early trials with miconazole and ketoconazole met with limited success, the availability of more-active, less-toxic antifungals has eliminated their use. In addition to in vitro activity against many *Candida* species (e.g., *Candida albicans*), itraconazole is active in vitro against *Aspergillus* species and reduces systemic *Candida* infections.[46,47,48] Although itraconazole oral solution demonstrates improved bioavailability over the capsule, it is associated with significant GI intolerance.[49,50]

Fluconazole prophylaxis decreases the frequency of both superficial (e.g., oropharyngeal candidiasis) and systemic fungal infections in HSCT patients[51,52] but not in patients with leukemia.[53–55] When fluconazole 400 mg/day was compared with placebo for fungal prophylaxis in bone marrow transplant recipients, it significantly reduced the incidence of invasive candidiasis and delayed the initiation of empiric amphotericin B from day 17 to day 21.[52] It is unknown, however, whether such patients who currently may experience a reduction in the degree and duration of neutropenia owing to the administration of colony-stimulating growth factors would also benefit. In contrast, in a study of patients with acute leukemia undergoing chemotherapy, fluconazole prophylaxis was not associated with a reduction in invasive fungal infections or need for empiric amphotericin B.[55] Although fluconazole is useful prophylactically, concern about its lack of reliable in vitro activity against molds limits its use in highest-risk patients. An increased frequency of isolation of non-albicans *Candida* (e.g., *Candida krusei, Candida glabrata, Candida parapsilosis*) has also been noted in some institutions.[56] Fluconazole may not have a significant role in these patients.[43]

Fluconazole is available as both oral and IV formulations, and its oral bioavailability is not significantly influenced by changes in gastric acidity. The IV formulation enables fluconazole to be administered to critically ill patients or patients who have difficulty swallowing. Despite such potential advantages, prophylactic fluconazole was inferior to itraconazole in allogeneic HSCT recipients.[49] In this trial, proven invasive fungal infections occurred in 6 of 71 (9%) itraconazole recipients and 17 of 61 (25%) fluconazole-treated patients. However, there were no differences in morality. In a similar trial in allogeneic HSCT patients, itraconazole was superior to fluconazole in the prevention of mold infections.[50] However, there was no difference in invasive fungal infections or mortality between treatments. Treatment-related hepatotoxicity and drug discontinuation because of side effects (predominantly GI intolerance) were more frequent in the group receiving itraconazole.

The extended-spectrum triazoles posaconazole and voriconazole have been evaluated as a prophylactic strategy. Posaconazole demonstrated improved survival, a reduction in proven or probable IFI, and a reduction in invasive aspergillosis when compared with standard prophylaxis (either itraconazole or fluconazole) for the prevention of fungal infection in patients undergoing chemotherapy for AML or myelodysplastic syndrome.[57] Posaconazole was also effective prophylaxis in allogeneic HSCT recipients undergoing therapy for GVHD.[58] Posaconazole is currently available only as an oral formulation, which limits its use in patients unable to take oral therapy. It requires divided daily doses, coadministration with high-fat meals, and avoidance of acid-suppressing proton-pump inhibitor therapy for optimal absorption.[59] Absorption of posaconazole may be reduced in patients with mucositis.[60] Although the efficacy of voriconazole in the treatment of invasive aspergillosis has been well documented (and represents the standard of care for treatment of this disease), published data to support its prophylactic use in adequately powered, controlled clinical trials are currently lacking.[61,62] A recent study compared prophylactic voriconazole and fluconazole in allogeneic HSCT patients.[63] No differences were observed in fungal-free survival rate rates at 180 days. Side effects (most notably hepatotoxicity, rash, phototoxicity) and the increased potential (relative to other azoles and the echinocandins) for drug interactions with voriconazole may limit its prophylactic use to patients at highest risk of mold infections. In addition, the use of IV voriconazole should be avoided in patients with significant renal impairment because of the potential toxicity of the vehicle. Although use of voriconazole has also been implicated in the emergence of pathogens such as zygomycosis in this patient population,[64] a definitive cause-and-effect relationship is lacking.

The echinocandins (e.g., caspofungin, micafungin, and anidulafungin) may be useful as a prophylactic strategy in high-risk patients. Micafungin has been compared with fluconazole in autologous and allogeneic HSCT recipients.[65] Based on a composite end point (which included absence of breakthrough fungal infection and absence of empiric modifications to the antifungal regimen owing to neutropenic fever), micafungin was found to be superior. Although breakthrough candidemia, survival, and adverse events were similar in both groups, a trend toward a reduction in invasive aspergillosis in the allogeneic HSCT population was noted in the micafungin group. Micafungin is currently US Food and Drug Administration (FDA)–approved for the prevention of *Candida* infections in HSCT patients.

The use of primary antifungal prophylaxis in cancer patients with neutropenia should be reserved for high-risk patients,[4] i.e., patients with hematologic malignancies (such as leukemia) and allogeneic HSCT. In patients receiving cytotoxic chemotherapy for solid tumors, antifungal prophylaxis may not be beneficial and may increase superinfection with resistant fungi. These latter patients should be managed with empiric antifungal therapy if they exhibit persistent fever and neutropenia. Patients with acute lymphocytic leukemia receiving remission- or salvage-induction chemotherapy are at intermediate risk, and should be considered for prophylaxis. Although autologous HSCT recipients may not routinely benefit from fungal prophylaxis, those with prolonged neutropenia, mucosal damage, or receipt of purine analogs should receive primary prophylaxis.[6] Acceptable options for prophylaxis against *Candida* species include fluconazole, itraconazole, voriconazole, posaconazole, micafungin, and caspofungin.[4] Of these options, fluconazole is the most commonly used agent. In the setting of colonization with fluconazole-resistant *Candida* species (such as *C. krusei*, *C. glabrata*), an echinocandin (such as micafungin) is preferred.[3,4,6,65] In contrast, patients with higher risk for mold infections (such as AML/MDS patients, or allogeneic HSCT recipients with GVHD) should be considered for prophylaxis with mold-active drugs (such as posaconazole, voriconazole, echinocandins, or amphotericin B) during periods of risk.[3,4,6] Mold-active agents are also recommended in the setting of anticipated periods of prolonged (at least 2 weeks) neutropenia, or prolonged neutropenia immediately before HSCT.[4] Prophylaxis is generally continued during the period of neutropenia. In HSCT recipients, prophylaxis should continue until day 75 after transplant or through induction therapy for patients with leukemia.[66] Patients with a history of documented *Aspergillus* infection undergoing intensive chemotherapy should be considered for voriconazole.[6] Although the addition of a second prophylaxis (e.g., caspofungin) may be considered, the benefits of combination therapy for secondary prophylaxis are unknown.

ANTIVIRALS

High-risk patients (e.g., seropositive for HSV undergoing allogeneic HSCT or induction or reinduction therapy for acute leukemia) should be given antiviral prophylaxis (e.g., acyclovir) for the first month after transplant or (for patients with acute leukemia) during periods of neutropenia.[3,4] Both oral or IV acyclovir and oral valacyclovir are appropriate and generally started at the beginning of chemotherapy. Although the optimal duration of therapy is unknown, prevention of latent infections may require up to 1 year after HSCT.[6] Published data for famciclovir for this indication are lacking. Patients experiencing HSV reactivation during treatment should also receive prophylaxis. Allogeneic HSCT patients who are seropositive for VZV should also be given prophylaxis until no longer immunocompromised,[4] particularly with receipt of either bortezomib or alemtuzumab.[3] Low-dose (i.e., 500 mg/day three times weekly) valacyclovir prophylaxis after a 35-day course of IV acyclovir is safe and effective in allogeneic HSCT recipients.[67] In addition, HSCT recipients at increased risk of CMV infection (e.g., CMV-seropositive patients and CMV-seronegative recipients with a CMV-seropositive donor, allogeneic HSCT recipients, and those receiving alemtuzumab) should be given either ganciclovir prophylaxis or pre-emptive therapy if early evidence of infection is observed. The role of valganciclovir as a prophylactic strategy in this population requires further evaluation.[68]

Respiratory tract infections caused by RSV, influenza, and parainfluenza are less commonly observed in patients with neutropenia. Although response to influenza virus vaccine may be attenuated, patients undergoing cancer treatment should receive annual vaccinations with inactivated influenza vaccine.[4] Whenever possible, the timing of such vaccinations may be best between cycles (>7 days after or >2 weeks before next treatment). In contrast, immunocompromised patients should not receive the intranasal live virus vaccine.[4]

Hematopoietic Growth Factors

Hematopoietic colony-stimulating factors (CSFs) such as granulocyte CSF (G-CSF; filgrastim), pegylated G-CSF (pegfilgrastim), or granulocyte-macrophage CSF (GM-CSF; sargramostim) are important adjuncts in cancer patients. Studies in cancer patients receiving myelosuppressive or myeloablative chemotherapy have demonstrated that concurrent use of the CSFs can reduce the duration of neutropenia. The selection of one CSF agent over another is often based on practitioner preference rather than clinical data.

Hematopoietic growth factors (more specifically G-CSF [filgrastim] or pegylated G-CSF [pegfilgrastim]) reduce the risk of chemotherapy-induced febrile neutropenia.[7,24,69–71] Risk factors for neutropenia include age (i.e., >65 years), medical history (including prior history of febrile neutropenic episodes, nutritional status, unstable comorbidities, and presence of active infections), disease characteristics (especially those involving bone marrow resulting in cytopenias), and myelotoxicity of the regimen (including both chemotherapy and radiation) used to treat the underlying malignancy.[24,69–71] Routine use should be discouraged in patients at low risk (<10%) of febrile neutropenia.[4,24,70] In contrast, guidelines advocate the use as primary prophylaxis in patients at high risk (>20%) of fever and neutropenia (based on either the chemotherapeutic regimen or other risk factors such as reduced marrow reserve [ANC <1.5] owing to radiotherapy of >20% marrow, concomitant HIV infection, or patients ≥65 years receiving cyclophosphamide, doxorubicin, vincristine, and prednisone or more aggressive chemotherapy regimens for non-Hodgkin lymphoma).[69,71] In such cases, use may not only affect ANC recovery, but may reduce fever, infection rate, and the need for IV antibiotics, shorten the time to hospital discharge, and prevent the need for dose reduction of chemotherapy in situations in which it would be detrimental. However, it has yet to be proven that hematopoietic growth factors improve tumor response or increase survival.[72] Data are also lacking to demonstrate a prophylactic benefit in the prevention of IFIs.[73] Administration is generally initiated after chemotherapy administration and continued until a sufficient and stable postnadir ANC recovery is established.[7] Pegylated G-CSF may be preferred in some settings owing to the convenience of single administration.[24,74] Secondary prophylaxis should be considered for patients who experienced life-threatening, neutropenic-related complications from prior cycles of chemotherapy (especially if primary prophylaxis was not administered), or for whom reductions in chemotherapy dose to avoid neutropenia may compromise treatment outcome and disease-free or overall survival.[7,69,71]

Other Agents

Although beyond the scope of this chapter, select vaccinations have also been recommended for both autologous and allogeneic HSCT recipients (primarily caused by a decline in antibody titers to many vaccine-preventable diseases).[6] These include (but are not limited to) administration of pneumococcal vaccine and *H. influenzae* vaccine. Live vaccinations should be avoided in this population. However, because immune response may be altered immediately after transplant, delays of up to 6 months are recommended for many vaccines. In addition, serologic testing of antibody response is recommended in selected settings.[6] In addition, although data to support use are sparse, IV immunoglobulins have been recommended for HSCT recipients with severe hypogammaglobulinemia (i.e., serum immunoglobulin G level

<400 mg/dL) and recurrent infections.[6] In contrast, granulocyte transfusions have not been proven to be effective in either prevention or treatment of infection in the neutropenic cancer patient.[75]

INFECTIONS IN NEUTROPENIC CANCER PATIENTS

Clinical Signs and Symptoms

CASE 72-1, QUESTION 4: Seven days after completing chemotherapy, B.C. experienced a fever of 102°F (orally). Vital signs are blood pressure, 109/70 mm Hg; pulse, 102 beats/minute; and respirations, 25 breaths/minute. Physical examination demonstrates a clear oropharynx without exudates or plaques. Chest and cardiac examination are normal. The exit site for the Hickman catheter is clean and nontender without signs of erythema or induration. The perineum and rectum are nontender, and no masses are noted. Laboratory data are as follows:

Hematocrit, 20%
Hemoglobin, 7 g/dL
WBC count, 1,400 cells/μL, with 3% polymorphonuclear leukocytes (PMNs), 1% band forms, 70% lymphocytes, and 22% monocytes
Platelet count, 17,000 cells/L
Blood glucose, 160 mg/dL
Serum creatinine (SCr), 1.1 mg/dL
Blood urea nitrogen (BUN), 24 mg/dL

What are the signs and symptoms of infection in B.C.? What are the most common sites and sources of infection in patients such as B.C.?

B.C. has an ANC of 48 cells/μL (1,400 WBCs/μL × [0.03 PMNs + 0.01 bands]) and is therefore at high risk for infection.

Fever in neutropenic patients is defined as a single oral temperature of at least 38.3°C (101°F) or a temperature of at least 38.0°C (100.4°F) for more than 1 hour in the absence of an obvious cause.[3,4] It is the earliest (and often the only) sign of infection in neutropenic patients, as typical signs can be modified or absent in this patient population.[4] However, only 48% to 60% of patients with febrile neutropenia have occult or documented infections.[3] Noninfectious sources of fever in the neutropenic cancer patient include inflammation, tumor progression, tumor lysis, adverse drug reactions, and transfusion reactions.[3,11,12] Signs and symptoms consistent with a diagnosis of infection without fever should be considered to be infection in the neutropenic host until proven otherwise.[3]

In patients with documented infections, the most common sites are skin, mouth, throat, esophagus, sinuses, abdomen, rectum, liver, vascular access, lungs, and urinary tract.[3,76] Although the lung is the most common site of serious infection in neutropenic cancer patients, fever and dry cough are often the only presenting signs of pneumonia.[76] The impaired inflammatory response results in scant sputum production, and sputum Gram stains often contain few PMNs. Radiologic evidence of a pulmonary infection can be minimal or absent, and the chest examination is frequently not diagnostic.[77] Pneumonia is associated with high mortality in neutropenic patients, particularly in the setting of bacteremia. In the presence of shock, a mortality rate of approximately 80% has been observed in these patients.[78]

Invasive procedures such as venipuncture, central IV catheter placement (e.g., Hickman catheter), and skin biopsies are associated with cellulitis and systemic infections. However, the typical signs and symptoms of infection (e.g., pain, heat, erythema, swelling) are often absent in part owing to inadequate granulocytes.[76] Colonization of these lesions may result in local infection and the potential for systemic dissemination of bacteria and fungi. Bacteremia occurs primarily from entry of bacteria through the skin or through unrecognized ulcerations in the GI and perirectal areas.

Confirmation of Infection

CASE 72-1, QUESTION 5: How can an infection be confirmed in patients such as B.C.?

Because of the frequent lack of physical signs and symptoms of infection, the clinician must obtain an accurate history (including the cancer type and treatment regimen, new signs of infection, antimicrobial prophylaxis, prior infections, and comorbidities) and conduct a careful physical examination at the first sign of fever. A detailed search for subtle signs and symptoms of inflammation at the most common sites, such as the oropharynx, bone marrow aspiration sites, lung, periodontium, skin, vascular catheter access sites, nail beds, and perineum (including the anus) is necessary. Before antibiotics are initiated, two sets of blood cultures (with each set consisting of two culture bottles) should be obtained.[3,4,11] Blood should also be obtained from central venous catheters to rule out catheter-related infection.[4] Additional Gram stain and cultures (e.g., stool, urine, skin, IV site, respiratory specimens) should be obtained depending on signs and symptoms.[4] The yield from such cultures, however, may be affected by the prior or concurrent administration of prophylaxis.[2] Chest radiographs and oximetry should be obtained in the presence of respiratory symptoms.[4] Respiratory virus testing should take place for patients with upper respiratory tract infection symptoms (i.e., coryza) or cough.[4] In settings in which pulmonary aspergillosis is suspected, further radiologic evaluations (such as computed tomography scans) should be considered.[22] A complete blood count, serum electrolytes, coagulation, C-reactive protein, urinalysis, and assessment of organ function (e.g., liver and kidney function) should be obtained to assist in drug dosing and monitoring for treatment-related toxicities.[4]

Recent advances have been made in nonculture-based diagnostic tests that help support (or in some cases eliminate) the diagnosis of infection in these patients.[79] Such studies include C-reactive protein[80–82] and procalcitonin.[82–84] However, these tests are not routinely ordered, and their role in the treatment of the neutropenic cancer patient has not yet been established.[4] Galactomannan (specific for aspergillosis)[85] and β-D-glucan testing may assist in the diagnosis of fungal infections.[86,87] Serial galactomannan testing has also been used pre-emptively to initiate antifungal therapy before overt signs and symptoms of invasive fungal infections occur.[88] In addition to other issues regarding sensitivity and specificity of these assays, both galactomannan and β-D-glucan are affected by prior or current receipt of antifungals.[22] At present, the use of these tests should be restricted to persistent fever despite other etiologic investigations.[4]

Significance of Colonization

CASE 72-1, QUESTION 6: Routine surveillance cultures of swabs taken from B.C.'s axillae, nasopharynx, and rectum grew *Corynebacterium jeikeium* (axillae), *S. aureus* (axillae and nasopharynx), and *Enterococcus faecium* (rectum). What is the significance of these culture results? Should

routine, serial surveillance cultures be performed in patients such as B.C.?

Several factors influence the colonization and subsequent infection by micro-organisms in cancer patients. Organisms isolated from infected patients can be found in endogenous flora or acquired during hospitalization.[89] Factors leading to colonization include staff-to-staff and patient-to-patient transmission (e.g., lack of frequent and adequate hand hygiene), direct transmission from the environment (e.g., inadequately disinfected bathtubs, sinks, toilet bowls), foods (e.g., raw fruits and vegetables), inhalation from contaminated fomites (e.g., respirators, ventilating systems), and IV access devices.

In addition to immunosuppression, the underlying malignancy and associated chemotherapy diminish the cancer patient's resistance to colonization and infection. For example, chemotherapy induces changes in the microbial binding receptors on epithelial cells in the oropharynx. This allows gram-negative bacilli to adhere to these surfaces, changing the composition of the oropharyngeal flora from a mixture of gram-positive aerobes and anaerobes to gram-negative aerobic bacteria.[90] Colonization with resistant organisms is enhanced by prior antibiotic administration, which may suppress the growth of normal anaerobic flora in the GI tract. This anaerobic suppression may promote the overgrowth of resistant micro-organisms.[90] For example, *P. aeruginosa* and *K. pneumoniae* are not commonly found in the stools of normal healthy adults, but they are recovered from the stools of hospitalized cancer patients.

Organisms that colonize cancer patients differ in their invasiveness and propensity to cause infection. For example, colonization with *P. aeruginosa* is more likely to result in infection than less virulent organisms (such as *E. coli* or *Staphylococcus epidermidis*).[91] However, if the host is profoundly impaired, organisms generally considered to be less virulent may become pathogenic.

The acquisition of and subsequent colonization by potentially pathogenic microbes may be detected by serial surveillance cultures of specimens obtained from various body sites such as the nasopharynx, axilla, urine, and rectum. Such surveillance cultures may be useful for infection control purposes. However, little clinically useful information is gained in the absence of infection. Therefore, surveillance cultures are generally restricted to select patients for infection control purposes. In such cases, culture of the anterior nares (for MRSA) or rectal samples (for VRE or multidrug-resistant gram-negative bacilli) may be performed.

In summary, B.C.'s surveillance culture results indicate that she is colonized with several potential pathogens associated with infection in the immunocompromised host, but these results are probably not useful in selecting empiric antibiotics for her fever.

EMPIRIC ANTIBIOTIC THERAPY

Rationale

CASE 72-1, QUESTION 7: Should B.C. be started on antibiotic therapy immediately? Is this rational in view of the fact that neither the source of her fever nor the pathogen has been established?

All febrile neutropenic patients or afebrile neutropenic patients with signs and symptoms of infection should undergo risk assessment for the possibility of a life-threatening infection. Once cultures are obtained, these patients should be emergently started on broad-spectrum antibacterials. Prompt institution should not be delayed if cultures cannot be obtained. Early studies confirmed high mortality in neutropenic patients with untreated gram-negative infections up to 24 to 48 hours after the onset of fever. Crude mortality rates secondary to *P. aeruginosa* bacteremia approached 91%.[91] Prompt use of empiric, broad-spectrum antibiotics has resulted in significant reductions in infectious mortality rates. These observations emphasize the need for rapid institution of empiric antibiotic therapy to prevent early morbidity and mortality.

Optimal Antibacterial Spectrum

CASE 72-1, QUESTION 8: What pathogen- and patient-specific factors should be considered when initiating empiric therapy for B.C.?

Despite continued development in antibacterial drugs, the empiric management of febrile neutropenic patients is complicated by the changing spectrum of bacterial pathogens and their antimicrobial susceptibilities. Empiric antibiotic regimens should provide broad-spectrum coverage against the potential gram-negative bacilli most commonly isolated from neutropenic cancer patients (e.g., *E. coli*, *K. pneumoniae*, *P. aeruginosa*), staphylococci, and viridans streptococci.[3,10] Because mortality from untreated bacteremia caused by *P. aeruginosa* is so high,[56] empiric regimens have traditionally included antimicrobials with antipseudomonal activity.

Selecting an initial empiric regimen for a given patient should take into account the patient's risk of infection, likely pathogens, infection site–specific antibiotic efficacy, and institutional susceptibility patterns. This point is especially true in areas experiencing a growing frequency of multidrug-resistant organisms, such as MRSA, VRE, and extended-spectrum β-lactamase (ESBL)-producing organisms (such as *K. pneumoniae* and *E. coli*).[15] Patient-related considerations should include medical stability, allergies, prior and concomitant antimicrobials, and organ dysfunction (e.g., renal or hepatic). Attempts should be made to identify low-risk patients for whom oral antimicrobial therapy may be an option. Finally, dosing schedules, acquisition costs, and the potential for significant toxicities should be considered. In addition to broad-spectrum activity, antibacterial regimens should be bactericidal against the infecting pathogen. However, no adequately controlled comparative trials of bacteriostatic versus bactericidal antibiotics have been conducted in humans.

In summary, many organisms, including those recovered from surveillance cultures, may be pathogens in B.C. Those associated with a high mortality rate during the first 48 hours should be empirically treated pending culture and sensitivity results. Therefore, an empiric regimen with optimal activity against commonly isolated gram-negative bacilli (including *P. aeruginosa*) should be promptly administered to B.C.

Initial Empiric Antibiotic Regimens

CASE 72-1, QUESTION 9: Given the lack of site-specific signs and symptoms of infection, what would be a reasonable initial empiric antibiotic regimen for B.C.?

Practice guidelines prepared by the National Comprehensive Cancer Network,[3] the Infectious Diseases Society of America,[4] and the European Society of Medical Oncology[11] identify antimicrobial options for the treatment of fever in the neutropenic cancer patient. The ideal antibiotic regimen for empiric management in this setting remains controversial. High-risk patients requiring IV therapy are often candidates for monotherapy regimens, including a third-generation cephalosporin (e.g., ceftazidime), a fourth-generation cephalosporin (e.g., cefepime), or an antipseudomonal carbapenem (e.g., imipenem-cilastatin or meropenem).[3,4,11,12] Additional antibiotics (such as fluoroquinolones, aminoglycosides, and vancomycin) may be added to address site-specific infections, resistant organisms, or clinically unstable patients.[4] Alternative parenteral regimens that have been investigated in this patient population include combinations (excluding those containing vancomycin) of an aminoglycoside (e.g., gentamicin, tobramycin, or amikacin) plus an antipseudomonal ureidopenicillin with or without a β-lactamase inhibitor (e.g., piperacillin-tazobactam), an aminoglycoside with an antipseudomonal cephalosporin (e.g., ceftazidime, cefepime), or an aminoglycoside in combination with an antipseudomonal carbapenem (e.g., imipenem-cilastatin or meropenem).[3,4,11,12] Combination β-lactam antibiotics offer no additional benefit, and some are potentially antagonistic. Comparisons of efficacy among studies are complicated by differences in the definitions of neutropenia, the incidence of documented infections, criteria used to assess clinical response, and statistical methodology.[92] No significant differences exist among any of these empiric approaches.

ORAL ANTIBIOTICS

Carefully selected (low-risk) adult febrile neutropenic patients may be candidates for oral antibiotic therapy, either as initial therapy or as follow-up to IV antibiotics (sequential therapy).[2,4,93,94] In general, patients considered for oral therapy must be without microbiological or clinical evidence of infection (other than fever), clinically stable, and closely observed. This would exclude patients with any of the following: serious comorbidities, inpatient acquisition of infection, uncontrolled malignancy, pneumonia, recent HSCT, dehydration, hypotension, chronic lung disease, abnormal liver (>3× upper limits of normal) or renal function (serum creatinine >2 mg/dL), ANC less than 100 cells/μL, or signs and symptoms lasting longer than 7 days.[4] An international collaborative study established and validated a risk scoring system in adults that incorporated these principles to identify low-risk patients for whom oral therapy may be an option.[25]

Oral ciprofloxacin in combination with amoxicillin-clavulanate is useful in low-risk adult patients with febrile neutropenia,[95,96] and is the most commonly used oral regimen.[4] Levofloxacin may be used in place of ciprofloxacin, and clindamycin may be used in place of amoxicillin-clavulanate if the patient is allergic to β-lactam antibiotics. Patients already receiving fluoroquinolones as prophylaxis should be excluded from receiving this regimen. Cefixime has been used effectively as an alternative regimen in low-risk pediatric patients initially receiving IV therapy,[97] but there is not adequate experience to recommend it at this time.

Low-risk patients with adequate home support (e.g., access to emergency facilities, phone access) and the desire for home treatment may be treated as an outpatient (with either IV or oral therapy). Therapy is usually initiated in a clinic or hospital setting.[4] Monitoring in the outpatient setting should include either home nursing or office visits daily for 3 days to review progress and to screen for problems. Patients who are stable and responding after the initial observation period may continue to receive monitoring by phone contact.

INTRAVENOUS MONOTHERAPY

CASE 72-1, QUESTION 10: Can any of the more potent, ESBLs be used as monotherapy in febrile neutropenic patients?

In general, monotherapy with an antipseudomonal β-lactam (such as an antipseudomonal cephalosporin, carbapenem, or β-lactam and β-lactamase combination) is advocated.[3,4] Additional agents are added to the initial regimen in the setting of complications (such as hypotension or pneumonia) or if antimicrobial resistance is either likely or confirmed.[4]

ANTIPSEUDOMONAL CEPHALOSPORINS

The antipseudomonal third-generation cephalosporin ceftazidime and the fourth-generation agent cefepime are well-established as monotherapy for febrile neutropenia. Ceftazidime has been found to be as effective as combination therapy. However, in some of these trials, the efficacy of ceftazidime in patients with documented staphylococcal and streptococcal infections was suboptimal. Select clinical trials have empirically added antistaphylococcal coverage with a glycopeptide (e.g., vancomycin) and have shown improved outcomes in these patients. In addition, pathogens (particularly gram-negative pathogens) that produce either type 1 β-lactamase or ESBL (e.g., *K. pneumoniae*) are not likely to respond to ceftazidime monotherapy. These organisms are more likely with prolonged hospitalization or receipt of antimicrobial therapy. Therefore, local in vitro susceptibilities of common gram-negative pathogens should be examined before the routine use of ceftazidime as monotherapy.

Cefepime is a fourth-generation cephalosporin with an FDA-approved indication for monotherapy for empiric management of infection in patients with febrile neutropenia. The potential advantage of this agent compared with third-generation cephalosporins is its low affinity for major chromosomally mediated β-lactamases. Compared with ceftazidime, cefepime has more potent activity in vitro against select gram-positive bacteria (methicillin-susceptible *Staphylococcus* species, viridans streptococci, and *S. pneumoniae*). Similar to ceftazidime, numerous randomized, comparative studies have evaluated the role of cefepime as monotherapy in both adults and children with febrile neutropenia. The improved gram-positive activity (relative to ceftazidime) may decrease the empiric need for vancomycin in some patients. However, this advantage is less likely in institutions with a high rate of MRSA because cefepime and other cephalosporins (with the exception of ceftaroline) are inactive against this pathogen. Although a meta-analysis published in 2007 suggested increased all-cause mortality in neutropenic patients treated empirically with cefepime,[98,99] subsequent analysis by the FDA concluded no such differences existed when compared with control patients.

CARBAPENEMS

The carbapenems are a unique class of antibiotics with broad-spectrum activity against numerous gram-positive and gram-negative bacteria, including anaerobes. In addition, carbapenems may be used in the setting in which the patient is at increased risk of ESBL-producing gram-negative pathogens (such as *K. pneumoniae* or *E. coli*). Imipenem (in combination with the dehydropeptidase inhibitor cilastatin) and meropenem are two currently available agents in this class that have been studied as monotherapy for febrile, neutropenic patients.

Clinical outcomes with imipenem-cilastatin monotherapy have been comparable with those of the β-lactam plus aminoglycoside combinations. Although effective, imipenem-cilastatin has generally been associated with a higher incidence of nausea and vomiting compared with ceftazidime or meropenem.[100,101] The GI side effects are generally dose related (3–4 g/day) and associated with the rate of IV administration. Therefore, dosages of 2 g/day (divided every 6 hours) are generally given to patients with normal renal function.

Meropenem has a broad spectrum of activity (comparable to that of imipenem-cilastatin) but is generally associated with fewer GI side effects. Meropenem monotherapy for febrile neutropenia has been evaluated in both adults and children, and the results have supported the value of meropenem as empiric monotherapy for use in febrile neutropenic patients. Meropenem may have advantages over imipenem-cilastatin in the treatment of central nervous system infections (owing to less associated seizure activity).

Although doripenem possesses comparable microbiologic activity, studies evaluating its administration in this population are lacking. Although ertapenem possesses microbiological activity comparable to that of the other carbapenems, it lacks in vitro activity against *Acinetobacter* species and *Pseudomonas,* including *P. aeruginosa*. Considering this lack of activity, ertapenem would not be appropriate as empiric therapy for febrile neutropenic patients. Agents with increased anaerobic activity (including carbapenems) might be used as empiric therapy in cases in which an intra-abdominal infection is suspected.

β-LACTAM/β-LACTAMASE INHIBITORS

Randomized trials have compared piperacillin-tazobactam monotherapy to various antibiotics. Published trials have documented that piperacillin-tazobactam is not inferior to cefepime in this patient population.[102,103] Although experience with this agent as monotherapy is limited relative to that for the antipseudomonal carbapenems and antipseudomonal cephalosporins, it is considered to be an adequate choice for monotherapy.[4] Higher doses of piperacillin-tazobactam (i.e., 3.375 g IV every 4 hours or 4.5 g IV every 6 hours in adult patients with normal renal function) should be used because of the risk of pseudomonal infections.[3] Piperacillin-tazobactam may interfere with the galactomannan assay used in the diagnosis of select IFIs, including aspergillosis.

In summary, several studies have demonstrated that monotherapy with an antipseudomonal β-lactam (cefepime, ceftazidime), select carbapenems (imipenem-cilastatin or meropenem), or the β-lactam/β-lactamase inhibitor combination drug piperacillin-tazobactam are appropriate as initial empiric monotherapy in febrile neutropenic patients.[4] There are no convincing data to support one choice over the others as empiric monotherapy. However, routine carbapenem use may be associated with increased drug acquisition cost (relative to cephalosporins) and increased potential for development of carbapenem resistance. Therefore, many institutions have elected to reserve the carbapenems for patients who have failed to respond to prior empiric therapy, have a history of infections with pathogens resistant to third- and fourth-generation cephalosporins, are clinically unstable, or have need for expanded anaerobic coverage.

ANTIMICROBIAL COMBINATIONS (EXCLUDING VANCOMYCIN)

CASE 72-2

QUESTION 1: B.L., a 13-year-old boy, presented with a 3-week history of "always being tired" and a persistent sore throat. Initial evaluation revealed anemia, thrombocytopenia, and a WBC count of 130,000 cells/L, with a predominance of immature lymphoblasts. Further evaluation demonstrated that B.L. had high-risk acute lymphocytic leukemia. Remission induction treatment was initiated with teniposide plus cytarabine followed by prednisone, vincristine, and L-asparaginase. Seven days after induction chemotherapy, B.L. experienced a fever (102°F) and chills. The ANC was 48 cells/μL. SCr and BUN were 1.0 mg/dL and 15 mg/dL, respectively. The physician wants to empirically start B.L. on ceftazidime plus gentamicin combination regimen. What is the role of this combination in the empiric management of febrile neutropenia? Are there any differences in efficacy between these combinations?

Before the introduction of third- and fourth-generation cephalosporins and carbapenems, the empiric use of antibacterial combinations in febrile neutropenic cancer patients was favored because these regimens offered a broader spectrum of activity against bacteria commonly infecting cancer patients.[3,104] In addition, these combinations offered the potential for an additive or synergistic effect.[104,105] However, infections in neutropenic patients have shifted largely from gram-negative to gram-positive pathogens, for which these traditional combination regimens have limited efficacy. Despite this concern, some clinicians continue to favor antibiotic combinations as initial empiric therapy, especially in patients who are clinically unstable.[3] It is unknown whether combination therapy prevents the emergence of resistance.

AMINOGLYCOSIDE PLUS β-LACTAM COMBINATIONS

Until the 1980s, most febrile neutropenic patients were treated with two-drug combination regimens that contained an aminoglycoside (gentamicin, tobramycin, or amikacin) plus a β-lactam antibiotic, such as antipseudomonal penicillin, or a third-generation cephalosporin. This combination is one of the most established empiric treatment regimens for the management of febrile neutropenia.

Numerous studies have been conducted to evaluate the efficacy of combination therapy of an aminoglycoside with an antipseudomonal cephalosporin (ceftazidime and cefepime).[3] Antipseudomonal penicillins plus β-lactamase inhibitors (in combination with an aminoglycoside) would also be considered a comparable regimen. A better outcome was demonstrated with full-course amikacin plus ceftazidime than with a short course (3 days) of amikacin plus a full course of ceftazidime.[106] However, the longer course of the aminoglycoside is likely to be associated with more toxicity.

Because carbapenem antibiotics are more frequently evaluated as monotherapy in this patient population, there are limited studies examining the combination of an aminoglycoside with either imipenem-cilastatin or meropenem. However, in one such evaluation, the combination of imipenem-cilastatin plus amikacin was found to be superior to imipenem-cilastatin monotherapy.[107] Carbapenems (in combination with aminoglycosides and vancomycin) have been recommended as empiric initial therapy for patients who are clinically unstable.

Aminoglycosides have generally been considered the backbone of combination regimens because of their potential for bactericidal action against various bacteria. However, the addition of an aminoglycoside is associated with increased costs for therapeutic monitoring. The benefit of an aminoglycoside for empiric therapy has not been consistently demonstrated.[107,108] In addition, there is an increased potential for the development of nephrotoxicity and ototoxicity.[108] This concern is especially relevant in patients receiving concomitant nephrotoxins (such as cisplatin and cyclosporine).

CASE 72-2, QUESTION 2: Seven days into therapy, despite rehydration, B.L.'s SCr and BUN rose to 2.0 g/dL and 45 mg/dL, respectively. Because B.L. has nephrotoxicity (believed to be secondary to the aminoglycoside), what other combination regimens (excluding those containing aminoglycosides) could be used? Are these regimens as effective as aminoglycoside-containing regimens?

DOUBLE β-LACTAM COMBINATIONS

Although numerous β-lactam combinations (usually consisting of either moxalactam or a cephalosporin plus an antipseudomonal penicillin) have been studied, overall response rates have not been significantly different from those of patients treated with aminoglycoside/β-lactam regimens. However, experience is limited with double β-lactam combinations in patients with neutropenia or patients with documented infections caused by *P. aeruginosa*.[109] Therefore, empiric therapy with double β-lactam regimens should not routinely be used.

OTHER COMBINATIONS

As previously stated, ciprofloxacin has been studied in combination with other antibacterials (either an aminoglycoside or a β-lactam, including an antipseudomonal penicillin) as initial empiric therapy for treatment of suspected infection in febrile neutropenic patients.[3,110–113] Ciprofloxacin in combination with clindamycin may also be useful in patients unable to receive β-lactam–containing combinations owing to the presence of immediate-type hypersensitivity reactions.[4] These studies, however, were associated with increased gram-positive infections in ciprofloxacin-treated patients. In addition, the in vitro activity of ciprofloxacin against *P. aeruginosa* has declined significantly (to <70% in many institutions). Therefore, if used as part of combination therapy, ciprofloxacin should be combined with an antimicrobial with favorable in vitro activity against this pathogen. Finally, the combination of aztreonam and vancomycin has been recognized as reasonable empiric combination therapy in patients with immediate-type hypersensitivity reactions to penicillin.[4]

EMPIRIC VANCOMYCIN

CASE 72-2, QUESTION 3: B.L. is begun on a two-drug regimen of ceftazidime and vancomycin. What is the rationale for adding vancomycin to the regimen?

As previously discussed, gram-positive bacteria are important pathogens in these patients. Because cephalosporins lack activity against methicillin-resistant staphylococci, vancomycin is often added to empiric regimens. A growing proportion of *S. aureus* infections are methicillin-resistant (as many as 60% in some institutions). However, widespread use of vancomycin has been associated with the rise in vancomycin resistance among gram-positive organisms, such as VRE. Furthermore, vancomycin intermediate–resistant *S. aureus* and rare case reports of *S. aureus* fully resistant to vancomycin have been reported. More recently, high trough concentrations of vancomycin (i.e., >15 mcg/mL) have recently been associated with a moderately increased risk of nephrotoxicity.

Primarily because of differences in the measured end points, the need for vancomycin as initial empiric therapy continues to be debated. For example, febrile neutropenic patients with cancer had more rapid resolution of fever, fewer days of bacteremia, and a lower frequency of treatment failure when vancomycin was added to an initial regimen of antipseudomonal penicillin plus an aminoglycoside.[114,115] Similarly, the addition of vancomycin to ceftazidime showed improved results compared with ceftazidime alone or with a three-drug combination.[116] However, other studies have concluded that mortality was not increased when vancomycin therapy was delayed.[117–120] The mortality from staphylococcal (generally coagulase-negative staphylococci) infections is generally considered to be low (<4%) during the first 48 hours after the onset of fever. In contrast, the mortality associated with viridans streptococcal infections is higher among patients who are not initially treated with vancomycin.[121] Some strains of viridans streptococci are either resistant or tolerant to penicillin.[121,122] In general, vancomycin would represent a reasonable alterative treatment of such infections, or in patients allergic to penicillins.

There continues to be considerable debate about whether vancomycin should be included in the initial empiric regimen for febrile neutropenic patients. In general, routine use of empiric vancomycin should be discouraged.[3,4] However, for institutions frequently isolating invasive gram-positive bacterial pathogens (e.g., those caused by viridans streptococci), vancomycin should probably be included in the initial empiric regimen.

Patients with clinically suspected catheter-related infections, skin or soft-tissue infections, or pneumonia, those receiving intensive chemotherapy (e.g., high-dose cytarabine) resulting in substantial mucosal damage, patients receiving prior fluoroquinolone or TMP-SMX prophylaxis, those with prior history of colonization with β-lactam–resistant pneumococci or MRSA or with gram-positive bacteria in blood cultures (before identification and susceptibility testing), and those with sepsis without an identified pathogen should also be considered for vancomycin therapy.[4] The addition of vancomycin to an aminoglycoside-containing regimen should be done with caution because data support an increased risk of aminoglycoside-induced nephrotoxicity in patients receiving these agents concomitantly with vancomycin.[123]

ALTERNATIVES TO VANCOMYCIN

Options exist for the treatment of invasive gram-positive infections. Linezolid is an oxazolidinone that can be administered IV or orally. A randomized, double-blind trial comparing the use of linezolid with vancomycin for empiric therapy demonstrated comparable safety and efficacy.[124] It is associated with thrombocytopenia and secondary neutropenia, especially when given for prolonged periods (i.e., >14 days). Considering the reduced bone marrow reserve in cancer chemotherapy patients, these adverse events are of particular concern. In addition, it is currently not recommended for patients with catheter-related infections (including bacteremia). The emergence of linezolid-resistant enterococci is of concern in this patient population. Therefore, its primary role in this patient population would be as a treatment for resistant or refractory gram-positive infections (such as MRSA or VRE). Quinupristin-dalfopristin is available for IV administration only, and concerns about potential drug interactions and patient tolerability (including myalgias and arthralgias) limit its use as empiric therapy in this setting. Daptomycin provides potent in vitro activity against many multidrug-resistant gram-positive pathogens (including VRE and MRSA), but requires IV therapy, should not be used for the treatment of pneumonia, and has not been studied in this patient population. Tigecycline possesses activity in vitro against both MRSA and VRE (in addition to many gram-negative and anaerobic pathogens). However, it lacks activity against *P. aeruginosa*, and therefore would not be considered a viable option for empiric monotherapy. Telavancin is a new lipoglycopeptide with potent activity in vitro against select gram-positive pathogens (including MRSA). However, experience to date in this population has not been published. Therefore, these alternative agents (most frequently daptomycin and linezolid) are generally reserved for situations in which vancomycin is inappropriate (because of resistance or intolerance).[3,4]

In the case of B.L., empiric use of vancomycin is not warranted based on the previous discussion, and it should be discontinued unless cultures indicate the need for this antibiotic.

ANTIBIOTIC DOSING, ADMINISTRATION, AND MONITORING CONSIDERATIONS

Intermittent versus Continuous versus Prolonged Infusion of Intravenous Antibiotics

CASE 72-2, QUESTION 4: Should B.L.'s antibiotics be given intermittently (i.e., divided doses) or as a continuous infusion?

β-Lactam antibiotics exhibit time-dependent (i.e., concentration-independent) pharmacodynamic activity, and in vitro models of infection suggest that prolonged exposure of bacteria to drug concentrations above the minimum inhibitory concentration is linked with improved bacterial killing and survival. On the basis of these observations and the poor prognosis of neutropenic cancer patients with bacteremia, noncomparative, open-label trials were conducted to evaluate the role of continuous infusions of β-lactams (i.e., ceftazidime) in the empiric treatment of suspected infection in cancer patients.[125–127] However, this method of administration would require an IV line dedicated for continuous drug administration and limit B.L.'s ability to receive intermittent tobramycin infusions unless additional IV ports or lines are available for use. In contrast to continuous infusions, prolonged infusions (i.e., 3–4 hours) of select β-lactams (notably carbapenems, third- or fourth-generation cephalosporins, or piperacillin-tazobactam) have shown promise in a variety of pharmacodynamic models of infection, specifically with elevated minimum inhibitory concentrations. Prolonged infusions of β-lactams also have the potential to reduce the total dose, and therefore result in cost savings. Although only limited clinical data exist to support such a strategy, such evaluations have not been tested specifically in the setting of infections in the neutropenic host.

Consolidated (Once-Daily) Aminoglycoside Dosing

CASE 72-2, QUESTION 5: What is the role of consolidated (once-daily) aminoglycoside dosing in febrile neutropenic patients such as B.L.?

Because of the concentration-dependent pharmacodynamic properties of aminoglycosides and the convenience of administration, studies have been conducted to describe both the pharmacokinetic properties and efficacy of consolidated dosing of aminoglycosides in animals and in neutropenic patients. Pharmacokinetic studies with amikacin[128,129] and gentamicin[130,131] have not revealed pharmacokinetic differences when compared with other populations. Several clinical studies have included consolidated aminoglycoside dosing for amikacin, gentamicin, and tobramycin.[132] However, most of the studies in this population were not designed to evaluate differences between consolidated aminoglycoside dosing compared with similar regimens using intermittent dosing. In general, the various studies suggest that consolidated dosing is as effective and possibly less nephrotoxic than traditional dosing. Therefore, consolidated dosing of aminoglycosides appears reasonable in empiric therapy of neutropenic patients.[132]

Outpatient Administration

Continued administration of antimicrobials in the outpatient setting has been suggested in a subset of low-risk patients. The criteria used to define eligibility for outpatient therapy are generally similar to those established and previously discussed for oral therapy. Therefore, outpatient administration of parenteral antibiotics can be considered in a subset of low-risk patients with close medical follow-up.[4]

HOST FACTORS INFLUENCING RESPONSE TO THERAPY

CASE 72-2, QUESTION 6: What factors may have influenced B.L.'s clinical response to antimicrobial therapy?

The most important prognostic determinants of a favorable outcome in patients with neutropenia and infection are the recovery of the granulocyte count and (for the patient with infection) proper selection of antimicrobial therapy. Patients with profound, persistent neutropenia (<100 cells/μL that does not rise during therapy or an initial ANC of 100–500 cells/μL that declines during therapy) respond to antibiotics less favorably than patients whose bone marrow recovers. The initial granulocyte count appears to be less important than the trend toward granulocyte recovery. Although other evidence of bone marrow recovery (such as the absolute phagocyte count, absolute monocyte count, or reticulocyte fraction) may precede the ANC target of 500 cells/μL by several days, they are not as widely used clinically. The site of infection also influences outcome. Septic shock and pneumonia are associated with high mortality in bacteremic neutropenic patients.

MODIFYING INITIAL EMPIRIC ANTIBIOTIC THERAPY

CASE 72-3

QUESTION 1: M.H., a 24-year-old woman with a recent diagnosis of ovarian cancer, exhibited neutropenia (ANC < 150 cells/μL) after chemotherapy. Five days after becoming neutropenic, she experienced a fever of 101°F and was begun on an empiric antibiotic regimen of ceftazidime 2 g IV every 8 hours. Although she remained febrile, her initial cultures remained negative at 48 hours. Should M.H. be continued on the same regimen, or should modifications be made? How do the culture results influence this decision? How long should empiric therapy be continued?

The need for modification of the initial empiric therapy is dependent on the risk group (i.e., low- vs. high-risk), establishment of an infection site or causative pathogen, persistence or defervescence of fever, and clinical stability. In the absence of worsening of clinical status or onset of new signs and symptoms of infection, 2 to 4 days of empiric treatment are generally required to determine initial efficacy after initiation of empiric antibiotics.[4] Defervescence in patients with hematologic malignancies, as well as HSCT recipients, may be delayed (up to 5 days). During this time, daily assessments should include history and physical examinations, review of laboratory results, assessment of response, and evaluation of any antibiotic-related toxicities. Adjustments to initial empiric antibiotic therapy should be made if a site-specific infection is identified, antimicrobial resistance is suspected or documented, or the patient's condition deteriorates.

Premature discontinuation of antibiotics may predispose these patients to recrudescence of bacterial infection and increase the risk of infection-related morbidity and mortality. Cancer patients with unexplained fever who became afebrile after empiric antibiotics were randomly assigned to continue or discontinue antibiotic therapy after 7 days.[133] The patients whose neutropenia resolved had no infectious sequelae regardless of whether antibiotics were continued or discontinued. However, for persistently neutropenic patients randomly assigned to continue or discontinue antibiotic therapy until their ANC was greater than 500 cells/μL, the percentages of patients remaining febrile without infections complications were 94% and 41%, respectively.

Documented Infections

CASE 72-3, QUESTION 2: On day 3, M.H.'s temperature is normal (97.6°C). However, two sets of blood cultures drawn 3 days ago have grown *S. aureus* resistant to methicillin and susceptible to vancomycin. Her ANC is 170 cells/μL. How should therapy be modified in M.H.? For how long should antibiotics be continued?

As previously stated, modification of initial empiric therapy should be made based on culture results as well as site-specific signs and symptoms of infection (Table 72-1). For example, anaerobic coverage (often with a carbapenem or piperacillin-tazobactam if not used for initial monotherapy) may be expanded in the setting of abdominal pain. Metronidazole or oral vancomycin should be initiated in the setting of diarrhea when *C. difficile* is suspected.[4] Vesicular lesions may be suggestive of viral infections (such as HSV or VZV) and may respond to the addition of acyclovir.[11] Suspected IV catheter infections should be managed with catheter removal (whenever possible), and this as well as skin and skin structure infections should be managed with treatment directed at MRSA.[4] For pneumonia, antibiotic coverage should be consistent with published guidelines for the treatment of health care–associated infections (see Chapter 64, Respiratory Tract Infections).[134] In the setting of severe or life-threatening pulmonary infections, antifungal therapy should also be included (see Table 72-1). Modifications of therapy may also be based on isolation of a resistant pathogen. For example, resistant gram-positive infections such as MRSA may be treated with vancomycin, linezolid, or daptomycin, whereas linezolid or daptomycin may be used for the treatment of VRE. For multidrug-resistant gram-negative pathogens, carbapenems are often used to treat ESBL-producing organisms, whereas carbapenemase-producing Enterobacteriaceae may require therapy with polymyxin, colistin, or tigecycline.

For patients with documented infections unresponsive to modification of therapy, new or worsening sites of infection should be suspected. Clinical, laboratory, and radiographic investigations should be undertaken or repeated. For hemodynamically unstable patients, antimicrobial therapy should be broadened and the patient should be considered for empiric antifungal therapy.[4] The duration of therapy is based on the infecting organism and site of infection (often up to 14 days), and should continue at least until the ANC are 500/μL or greater and rising.[4] If the patient has responded to an appropriate course of therapy but remains neutropenic, oral fluoroquinolone prophylaxis should be considered until the resolution of neutropenia.

No Etiology Identified

CASE 72-4

QUESTION 1: S.B. is a 55-year-old woman with chronic myelogenous leukemia. She was admitted to the hospital with a 4-day history of fevers and night sweats. On admission, her temperature was 102.3°F, and her WBC count was 100,000 cells/μL, with an ANC of 500 cells/μL. Blood and urine cultures were obtained, and ceftazidime was empirically started. For the next 3 days, S.B. remained persistently febrile and neutropenic. All cultures remained negative. How should she be treated?

Modification of therapy for unexplained fever is based on patient risk group, response to therapy, and clinical stability. In general, with defervescence and the patient stable or improving after initiation of therapy with no identifiable etiology, empiric therapy should be continued at least until the ANC is 500/μL or greater and rising.[4] For patients responding to initial therapy but with persisting neutropenia, one option is to continue therapy until the resolution of neutropenia.[3] Low-risk patients responding to empiric therapy receiving initial IV therapy can be considered for transition to combination oral antibiotics with ciprofloxacin plus amoxicillin-clavulanate if they are able to tolerate oral medications.[3,4]

Patients with persistent fever who are clinically stable do not routinely require a change in therapy unless guided by clinical changes or culture results.[3,4] However, outpatients with persistent fever should be hospitalized and receive IV therapy. Empiric addition of vancomycin in patients with persistent fever does not decrease the time to fever resolution in this population,[135] and should therefore be discouraged.[4] Empirical vancomycin should ultimately be discontinued in the absence of gram-positive infection.[4]

Hemodynamically unstable patients with a persistent fever without a clear source of infection should have their initial therapy modified to broaden coverage against resistant gram-positive and gram-negative organisms, as well as anaerobes.[3,4] Patients with initial monotherapy with ceftazidime or cefepime can be switched to vancomycin with an antipseudomonal carbapenem (such as imipenem-cilastatin or meropenem) in combination with either an aminoglycoside, aztreonam, or ciprofloxacin.[3,4] Antifungal therapy targeting *Candida* species should also be considered (see Case 72-4, Question 3).

CASE 72-4, QUESTION 2: S.B., on day 4, continues to feel "lousy" and has started to complain of abdominal pains. What is the significance of this complaint? Should her antibiotic regimen be modified again?

Because S.B. has new abdominal pains suggestive of enterocolitis, her antibiotic regimen should be modified. Although cefepime provides excellent coverage against the common gram-negative pathogens, it has limited activity against select gram-positive pathogens (e.g., MRSA or VRE) and anaerobes. A change from cefepime to imipenem-cilastatin or another broad-spectrum regimen with both aerobic and anaerobic activity should be considered.

ANTIFUNGAL THERAPY

CASE 72-4, QUESTION 3: S.B.'s antibiotic regimen was changed to imipenem-cilastatin. Despite the change, she

TABLE 72-1
Antibacterials in Patients With Neutropenia and Fever[a]

Condition	Therapy[b]
Initial Empiric Therapy	
Low Risk (Anticipated Neutropenia ≤7 Days, Clinically Stable, No Medical Comorbidities)	
Candidate for oral therapy	Adults: ciprofloxacin[a] + amoxicillin-clavulanate (alternate clindamycin if penicillin allergic)
	Children: cefixime
Requires IV therapy	(see *High-Risk* below)
High Risk (Anticipated Neutropenia >7 Days, Clinically Unstable, Or Medical Comorbidities)	
	Piperacillin-tazobactam, antipseudomonal carbapenem,[c] ceftazidime, or cefepime
	Clinically unstable: consider addition of aminoglycoside, fluoroquinolone, or vancomycin to regimen above
Modifications of Initial Therapy	
Unexplained Fever	
Defervescence with negative cultures	Continue antibiotics
	Low-risk patients: if IV therapy initially, consider switch to oral therapy
Persistent fever (2–4 days) without clinical or microbiological evidence of infection	Clinically stable: continue antibiotics
	Unstable: Hospitalize (if outpatient), IV therapy (if initially treated with oral), broaden antibacterial coverage to include anaerobes, resistant gram-negative rods, and resistant gram-positive organisms. Consider antifungal therapy for *Candida* species, or antimold therapy if previously receiving azole prophylaxis
	Consider empiric antifungal therapy on days 4–7, especially if neutropenia is expected to continue >7 days or the patient has other risk factors for fungal infections
	If initial regimen did not include vancomycin: re-evaluate risk factors for gram-positive infection, consider adding vancomycin
Documented Infection(s)	
Multidrug-resistant pathogen	MRSA: add vancomycin, linezolid or daptomycin
	VRE: add linezolid or daptomycin
	ESBLs: switch to a carbapenem carbapenemase-producing Enterobacteriacae: polymyxin-colistin or tigecycline
Head, Eyes, Ears, Nose, Throat	
Necrotizing ulceration, gingivitis	If initial regimen did not include anaerobic therapy (carbapenem or β-lactam/β-lactamase inhibitor; i.e., piperacillin-tazobactam), consider adding clindamycin or metronidazole or switch to antipseudomonal carbapenem (imipenem-cilastatin or meropenem)
	Consider adding antifungal or antiviral therapy
Oral vesicular lesions	Add antiviral therapy for Herpes simplex virus
Oral thrush	Add systemic (e.g., fluconazole) antifungal therapy
Sinus tenderness, periorbital cellulitis, nasal ulceration	If suspicion of mold infection: add lipid amphotericin B formulation. Vancomycin for periorbital cellulitis
	Reassess antistaphylococcal activity of empiric regimen; consider vancomycin
Gastrointestinal Tract	
Esophagitis	Add antifungal agent (see text); if no response, add acyclovir. Assess CMV risk and (if high) consider ganciclovir or foscarnet
Acute abdominal pain/perianal	If initial regimen did not include carbapenem or β-lactam/β-lactamase inhibitor (i.e., piperacillin-tazobactam), consider adding metronidazole, or switch to imipenem-cilastatin or meropenem. Assure pseudomonal coverage for perirectal infection
	For perirectal pain: consider enterococcal coverage for infection (not colonization)
	Consider antifungal
Diarrhea	Add metronidazole if *Clostridium difficile* documented or suspected. Oral vancomycin should be used for severe *C. difficile* infections
	Contact isolation of rotavirus documented
Liver abnormalities	Consider anaerobic and enterococcal coverage. Antifungal or antiviral therapy added based on results of diagnostic studies
Respiratory Tract	
Pneumonia	Add vancomycin or linezolid. Add an aminoglycoside and switch to antipseudomonal carbapenem
	PCP: institute TMP-SMX or (for sulfa-allergic patients) pentamidine
	Atypical pathogens *(Mycoplasma, Legionella)*. Add fluoroquinolone or macrolide
	CMV: add ganciclovir if high risk
	Consider influenza during outbreaks. Oseltamivir (preferred) or other directed therapies when indicated
Focal lesion on chest radiograph	If evidence of mold infection, add mold-active antifungal (such as voriconazole [preferred] or amphotericin B formulations)
	Consider growth factors (G-CSF, GM-CSF)
	Consider antibiotic coverage for pathogen causing atypical pneumonia
Vesicular lesions	HSV, VZV treatment: acyclovir, famciclovir, or valacyclovir
Cellulitis, wound infection	Consider adding vancomycin therapy
Vascular access device infection, tunnel tract infection	Remove catheter whenever possible. Add empiric vancomycin therapy. Adjust based on culture and susceptibility results

(continued)

Section 14 Infectious Disease

TABLE 72-1
Antibacterials in Patients With Neutropenia and Fever[a] (*Continued*)

Condition	Therapy[b]
Documented Infection(s) (continued)	
Central nervous system	Antipseudomonal β-lactam (cefepime, ceftazidime, meropenem [imipenem if meropenem not available]) + vancomycin. Add ampicillin if meropenem not used
Encephalitis	Consider high-dose acyclovir
Urinary tract	Change based on pathogen identification and susceptibility
Bloodstream infections	Gram-negative: add aminoglycoside and switch to antipseudomonal carbapenem Gram-positive: add vancomycin, linezolid or daptomycin

[a]Exclude option if patient received fluoroquinolone prophylaxis.
[b]All modifications should be based on clinical and microbiologic data.
[c]Antipseudomonal carbapenem is imipenem-cilastatin or meropenem. Doripenem provides comparable in vitro activity, but has not been investigated in this patient population.
CMV, cytomegalovirus; ESBL, extended-spectrum β-lactamase; G-CSF, granulocyte colony-stimulating factor; GM-CSF, granulocyte-macrophage colony-stimulating factor; HSV, herpes simplex virus; IV, intravenous; KPCs, *Klebsiella* producing carbapenemases, MRSA, methicillin-resistant *Staphylococcus aureus;* PCP, *Pneumocystis jiroveci;* TMP-SMX, trimethoprim-sulfamethoxazole; VRE, vancomycin-resistant enterococcus; VZV, varicella-zoster virus.
Source: National Comprehensive Cancer Network. Clinical Practice Guidelines in Oncology. Prevention and treatment of cancer-related infections (V2.2009). http://www.nccn.org/professionals/physician_gls/pdf/infections.pdf. Accessed June 21, 2010; Freifeld A et al. Clinical practice guideline for the use of antimicrobial agents in neutropenic patients with cancer: 2010 update by the Infectious Diseases Society of America. *Clin Infect Dis.* 2011;52:e56.

continues to have a low-grade fever and does not feel better. What is S.B.'s risk for having a systemic fungal infection? What is the significance of fungal infections in neutropenic cancer patients?

The incidence of invasive fungal infections in febrile neutropenic patients varies widely because of differences in definitions, methods of detection, patient populations, and prior use of antifungal prophylaxis. In general, patients with hematologic malignancies have a higher incidence of fungal infections than those with solid tumors.[136] Similar to the risk of bacterial infections, the risk of invasive fungal infections is also related to the degree and duration of neutropenia. Most fungal infections in neutropenic cancer patients are caused by *Candida* and *Aspergillus* species.[137–139] Other less common but important pathogenic fungi are those associated with zygomycosis (e.g., *Mucor* and *Rhizopus* species) and other emerging pathogens (non-albicans *Candida, Trichosporon beigelii, Malassezia* species, *Cryptococcus neoformans,* and *Fusarium* species).[137–139]

Early diagnosis and prompt treatment of such systemic fungal diseases are critical to patient survival. However, significant challenges exist in making an accurate and timely diagnosis of invasive fungal infections. Therefore, patients who are neutropenic with protracted (4–7 days) fever despite the administration of broad-spectrum antibiotics should be considered for empiric antifungal therapy, especially patients whose neutropenia is anticipated to exceed 7 days.[4,140] Considerations for earlier empiric antifungal therapy (i.e., days 2–4) should be made in patients with persistent fever and hemodynamic instability.[4]

Newer diagnostic tests (e.g., β-D-glucan tests or galactomannan assays), along with additional diagnostic support, may allow for early pre-emptive therapy.[141] Such approaches may also be used to support decisions to withhold empiric antifungal therapy. As an example, persistently febrile patients on appropriate antibacterials who are clinically stable without clinical or radiographic signs of fungal infection, have had negative serologic assays for invasive fungal infection, and have had no recovery of fungi from any body site may have empiric antifungal agents withheld.[4,88]

It is difficult to compare data among clinical trials evaluating empiric antifungal therapy in neutropenic cancer patients because of differences in trial design. Such differences may include inclusion of low-risk patients, lack of blinding, changes in concomitant antibacterials obscuring antifungal therapy end points, prior antifungal prophylaxis, use of composite end points of safety and efficacy, and different end point criteria.[136] Although select studies have also demonstrated that empiric antifungal therapy can decrease fungal-related deaths, overall mortality has not been affected.[20] This is the case particularly for patients with invasive disease and persistent neutropenia.

Considerations about the choice of empiric antifungals should include prior or current antifungal prophylaxis, risk of mold infections, risks of antifungal-related toxicities, drug interactions, route of administration, clinical stability, and costs.[20] Although prompting evaluation, fever alone does not necessarily indicate the need for intervention with an antifungal in hemodynamically stable patients receiving mold-active prophylaxis.[4] In patients requiring therapy, antifungal coverage should be directed at *Candida* species. Highest-risk patients with persistent or recurrent fever after 4 to 7 days of appropriate antibacterial therapy and anticipated to have prolonged (i.e., >10 days) neutropenia should be considered for antimold therapy.[4]

EMPIRIC AMPHOTERICIN B THERAPY

CASE 72-4, QUESTION 4: Should amphotericin B or acyclovir therapy be considered in S.B.?

Historically, amphotericin B deoxycholate (AmBD) was most commonly used in this setting because of its reliable activity in vitro against most *Candida* and *Aspergillus* species. Comparative trials have also evaluated the role of lipid-based formulations of amphotericin B in the treatment of suspected or documented infections in this population. Liposomal amphotericin B (LAmB),[142–145] amphotericin B lipid complex,[144] and amphotericin B colloidal dispersion[146] have demonstrated reductions in nephrotoxicity compared with AmBD. In addition, LAmB is least likely to be associated with infusion-related side effects.[143] Although there are limited data to suggest that the continuous infusion of AmBD may also reduce nephrotoxicity,[147] efficacy regarding this method of administration in patients with documented infections has not been established. Therefore, continuous infusion of AmBD cannot be routinely recommended at this time.

Considering the availability of other agents, empiric amphotericin B products is generally reserved for patients at highest risk of mold infections unable to receive alternative antifungals. When initiated as empiric therapy, amphotericin B administration is often preceded by attempts to minimize nephrotoxicity (e.g., saline loading) and premedications to minimize infusion-related reactions. Close monitoring of tolerability, renal function, and electrolytes is required during administration. When initiated, amphotericin B is generally continued (in the absence of a documented fungal infection) in a clinically stable patient until the resolution of neutropenia. Clinically stable patients without evidence of fungal infection but with persistent neutropenia often receive a 2-week course of therapy. Patients with documented (invasive) fungal infections are treated with variable durations of treatment, depending on the fungal diagnosis.

ALTERNATIVES TO AMPHOTERICIN B

In stable patients at low risk of mold infections or drug-resistant *Candida* species (e.g., *C. krusei* and some strains of *C. glabrata*), fluconazole may be preferable to amphotericin B.[4,148,149] Patients with suspected mold infections (e.g., aspergillosis), hemodynamic instability, or in whom an azole was used as prophylaxis should not receive fluconazole. Although itraconazole possesses enhanced activity in vitro against *Aspergillus* species and has reduced toxicity relative to amphotericin B, issues regarding tolerability with the oral solution, potential for cross-resistance with other azoles, lack of a parenteral treatment option, and considerations of alternative treatment options generally limit its usefulness. As previously discussed, posaconazole possesses a broad spectrum of activity in vitro against a variety of yeasts and molds. However, it is currently available only in an oral formulation. Voriconazole (an azole antifungal agent with increased activity against *Aspergillus* and non-albicans *Candida* relative to fluconazole) has been tested in this population. When compared with LAmB, voriconazole failed to meet the pre-established criteria for noninferiority.[145] However, some believe that voriconazole should be considered as an alternative to amphotericin B preparations for empiric therapy in patients requiring initial empiric antifungal therapy who are at increased risk of mold infections (owing to receipt of prior azole prophylaxis) or for those patients suspected of having invasive candidiasis.[140] Others continue to support the superiority of LAmB for empiric therapy in this population.[150] Because of the increased potential (relative to fluconazole) for drug interactions (including immunosuppressives and chemotherapy) and adverse events (e.g., phototoxicity, hepatotoxicity), voriconazole therapy should be monitored closely. IV use of voriconazole is contraindicated in patients with severe renal dysfunction. In addition, serum drug concentration monitoring for posaconazole and voriconazole may be considered in patients with suspected malabsorption.[4,6]

The echinocandins (e.g., caspofungin, micafungin, anidulafungin) possess in vitro activity against *Candida* species (including non-albicans *Candida*) and *Aspergillus* species. Caspofungin is at least as effective and better tolerated than LAmB as empiric therapy in this patient population.[151,152] Because of their safety profile and in vitro activity, echinocandins are often considered for patients requiring initial empiric antifungal therapy and who are at increased risk of mold infections (owing to receipt of prior azole prophylaxis). Caspofungin is currently FDA approved for such use. Published experience with other echinocandins (e.g., micafungin, anidulafungin) as empiric therapy in the febrile neutropenic patient is lacking at present.

In summary, empiric antifungal therapy is indicated for persistent (4–7 days) or recurrent fever on appropriate antibacterials if the duration of neutropenia exceeds 7 days.[4] Low-risk patients who are clinically stable do not routinely need antifungal therapy.[4] Persistently febrile patients who are clinically stable without computed tomography signs of infection and have no serologic or culture results suggestive of infection may have antifungal therapy withheld.[4] Patients receiving fluconazole prophylaxis requiring addition of empiric antifungals should be considered for antifungals with activity against azole-resistant *Candida* species and mold infections.[4] In the setting in which an antimold agent was used for prophylaxis, switching antifungal classes or conversion to IV therapy should be performed.[4]

ANTIVIRAL THERAPY

Empiric use of antiviral agents in the febrile neutropenic patient are not indicated without evidence of such disease.[4] In contrast, clinical evidence of HSV or VZV involving the skin or mucous membranes should be treated with antivirals (e.g., acyclovir, valacyclovir).[4] When oral therapy is used, valacyclovir is favored over acyclovir because of improved oral bioavailability and need for less-frequent dosing. With the exception of patients undergoing bone marrow transplantation,[153] CMV is an uncommon source of infection in the febrile neutropenic patient. However, ganciclovir, valganciclovir, foscarnet, or, less commonly, cidofovir treatment should be initiated in patients with documented CMV infections (antigenemia, polymerase chain reaction for CMV DNA, or detection of CMV mRNA). Because both ganciclovir and valganciclovir can cause or worsen existing neutropenia, caution and close monitoring is warranted when these agents are prescribed in this setting. Treatment with neuraminidase inhibitors (such as oseltamivir or zanamivir) may be initiated empirically for influenza in the setting of exposure or outbreaks if the patient is presenting with an influenzalike illness.[4] Likewise, if RSV is identified, appropriate antiviral therapy should be initiated.[4]

ANTIMICROBIAL ADJUVANTS

CASE 72-4, QUESTION 5: S.B. became afebrile 2 days after micafungin was initiated, yet she remained neutropenic with an ANC of 480 cells/μL. An induction chemotherapy regimen consisting of idarubicin plus cytarabine was initiated for her chronic myelogenous leukemia. Because the chemotherapy will further reduce her ANC 7 to 10 days after treatment, is there any way to facilitate marrow recovery and reduce the duration of neutropenia in S.B.?

As previously discussed, the duration of neutropenia is the most important factor affecting outcome in neutropenic cancer patients. Because of this, there has been considerable interest in enhancing the immune system in these patients.

Granulocyte Transfusions

One of the earliest approaches used to boost the patient's defense against infections was the transfusion of WBCs. In the 1970s, granulocyte transfusions were used adjunctively in patients with persistent neutropenia and documented infections who, despite appropriate antibiotics, failed to respond after 24 to 48 hours. This approach had limited value because of the difficulties in obtaining adequate cells for transfusion, as well as the problems with alloimmunization and risk of infection transmission. In addition, the questionable efficacy of WBC transfusions has decreased the use of this strategy.[154] Therefore, granulocyte transfusions are not routinely indicated in this population. However, patients with progressive bacterial or fungal infections unresponsive to appropriate antimicrobial therapy may be considered as candidates.[3]

Hematopoietic Growth Factors

Because these agents have not demonstrated a consistent and significant effect on other infection-related parameters (e.g., duration of fever, use of antibiotics, costs of treatment), routine use of CSFs as adjunctive therapy to antibiotics for febrile neutropenic patients should be avoided.[4,24,69] However, patients with high risks for infection-related complications may be considered for therapy.[3,69] Such risks include expected prolonged (>7 days) and profound (<100 cells/μL) neutropenia in clinically unstable patients unresponsive to initial empiric therapy, age older than 65 years, uncontrolled malignancy, pneumonia, sepsis and multiorgan dysfunction (characteristic of sepsis syndrome), and invasive fungal infection.[69]

Immunoglobulins

Data regarding the use of immunoglobulins as adjunctive therapy for the treatment of select infections in the neutropenic cancer patient are primarily limited to case reports. Patients with pneumonia secondary to CMV may benefit from adjunctive immunoglobulin therapy (in combination with ganciclovir). In addition, IV immunoglobulin G should be considered in those patients with hypogammaglobulinemia.

G-CSF administration, although likely to reduce the duration of her chemotherapy-induced neutropenia, is not indicated in S.B., who is otherwise stable.

KEY REFERENCES AND WEBSITES

A full list of references for this chapter can be found at http://thepoint.lww.com/AT10e. Below are the key references and websites for this chapter, with the corresponding reference number in this chapter found in parentheses after the reference.

Key References

Aapro MS et al. 2010 update of EORTC guidelines for the use of granulocyte-colony stimulating factor to reduce the incidence of chemotherapy-induced febrile neutropenia in adult patients with lymphoproliferative disorders and solid tumours. *Eur J Cancer.* 2011;47:8. (24)

Crawford J et al. Hematopoietic growth factors: ESMO Clinical Practice Guidelines for the applications. *Ann Oncol.* 2010; 21(Suppl 5):v248. (7)

de Naurois J et al. Management of febrile neutropenia: ESMO Clinical Practice Guidelines. *Ann Oncol.* 2010;21(Suppl 5):v252. (2)

Freifeld A et al. Clinical practice guideline for the use of antimicrobial agents in neutropenic patients with cancer: 2010 update by the Infectious Diseases Society of America. *Clin Infect Dis.* 2011;52:e56. (4)

Key Websites

National Comprehensive Cancer Network. Clinical Practice Guidelines in Oncology. Myeloid growth factors (v.1.2010). http://www.nccn.org/professionals/physician_gls/pdf/myeloid_growth.pdf. Accessed June 21, 2010. (70)

National Comprehensive Cancer Network. Clinical Practice Guidelines in Oncology. Prevention and treatment of cancer-related infections (V2.2009). http://www.nccn.org/professionals/physician_gls/pdf/infections.pdf. Accessed June 21, 2010. (3)

73

Pharmacotherapy of Human Immunodeficiency Virus Infection

Jessica L. Adams, Julie B. Dumond, and Angela D.M. Kashuba

CORE PRINCIPLES

		CHAPTER CASES
1	Acute retroviral syndrome is characterized by nonspecific symptoms such as fever, lymphadenopathy, rash, fatigue, and night sweats that coincide with an initial burst of viremia. These symptoms, as well as the presence of an opportunistic infection, and high-risk sexual or drug-using behaviors warrant human immunodeficiency virus (HIV) testing. After 6 to 12 weeks of infection, HIV can be diagnosed with use of the enzyme-linked immunosorbent assays (ELISA) and confirmed with Western blot tests. With testing earlier than 6 weeks, only an HIV RNA test will be positive.	**Case 73-1 (Question 1)**
2	HIV RNA viral load is measured to quantify the level of viral replication in the body and CD4 cell counts are followed to assess immune system function.	**Case 73-1 (Question 2)**
3	Initiation of antiretroviral therapy should be considered in all patients who are symptomatic, have CD4 counts less than 500, are pregnant, are coinfected with hepatitis B, or have HIV-associated nephropathy. Patients must also be willing to start therapy and to strongly adhere to their medication regimen. US Department of Health and Human Services (DHHS) guidelines provide recommendations for optimal antiretroviral therapy.	**Case 73-1 (Question 3)**
4	Goals of antiretroviral therapy include suppression of viral load, preservation and strengthening of the immune system, limitation of drug adverse events, promotion of adherence, and prevention of HIV-related morbidity and mortality.	**Case 73-1 (Question 4)**
5	General rules of therapy involve selection of highly active antiretroviral therapy–based regimen, optimization of the selected agents, and inclusion of quality of life in decisions.	**Case 73-1 (Questions 5, 6)**
6	After initiating a regimen, short-term goals include resolution of symptoms, at least a threefold (0.5 log) decrease in HIV RNA at 1 month, a tenfold decrease (1.0 log) in HIV RNA at 2 months, and an increase in CD4 count at 3 to 4 months. Long-term assessments include the monitoring of HIV RNA and CD4 count every 3 to 6 months to identify treatment failures, assessment of medication adherence, and determination of tolerability and quality of life.	**Case 73-1 (Questions 7, 8)**
7	General rules for changing failing regimens include switching to at least two new active drugs (although all new drugs are preferable), as quickly as possible after treatment failure to avoid accumulation of resistance mutations. To avoid the development of further resistance, a single drug should never be added to a failing regimen. If one drug must be discontinued, the whole regimen should be stopped simultaneously. Finally, previously failed regimens should never be restarted due to the potential of archived resistance mutations.	**Case 73-1 (Questions 9, 10)**
8	Considerations for treatment of antiretroviral-experienced patients include regimen tolerability, comorbid conditions, associated pharmacokinetic properties, antiretroviral histories, and resistance testing. Resistance testing should be performed when HIV RNA is greater than 1,000 copies/mL. Antiretroviral drug resistance is assessed through two methods; genotyping evaluates mutations in the virus genetic code, phenotyping involves growing virus in various concentrations of drug to determine viral susceptibilities. DHHS guidelines provide recommendations for treating antiretroviral-experienced patients.	**Case 73-2 (Question 1–3)**

continued

	CHAPTER CASES
9 Therapeutic drug monitoring is not routinely performed, but may be useful with failure associated with a previously fully suppressive regimen; for patients with uncharacterized drug interactions; those with questionable absorption, hepatic, or renal function; and for verification of suboptimal adherence.	**Case 73-3 (Question 1)**
10 Drug interactions between antiretrovirals and coadministered medications are common and should always screened with the addition of any new medication.	**Case 73-4 (Question 1)**
11 Antiretrovirals are used in pregnancy for the health of the mother and to prevent transmission of HIV to the child. There are specific DHHS guidelines for antiretroviral use in pregnancy.	**Case 73-5 (Question 1)**
12 The use of antiretrovirals for occupational (e.g., needle sticks) and nonoccupational (e.g., high-risk behaviors) postexposure prophylaxis may be warranted if initiated within 48 hours, but no longer than 72 hours after exposure. The Centers for Disease Control and Prevention guideline recommendations for the choice of antiretrovirals depends on the severity of the exposure and the specific patient.	**Case 73-6 (Question 1)**

INTRODUCTION

Potent combinations of antiretroviral drugs (also called highly active antiretroviral therapy [HAART]) have dramatically altered the natural progression of human immunodeficiency virus (HIV) infection, and significantly improved patients' quality of life. As a result, the number of new acquired immunodeficiency syndrome (AIDS)-related opportunistic infections and deaths has declined.[1,2] In most instances, the use of HAART has shifted HIV infection from a fatal disease to a manageable chronic disease. Most recent advances in HIV therapy include new and more potent antiretroviral agents in existing therapeutic drug classes, new antiretroviral agents in new therapeutic drug classes, and novel, potent combinations of antiretrovirals.

Although many patients will benefit from these new and more potent regimens, up to 25% of patients will fail therapy in the first year,[3] and approximately 25% will have to change regimens within the first year due to drug-related adverse events.[4] Other concerns include suboptimal patient compliance and the development of resistance, management of HAART failures, long-term adverse events, and the rampant spread of HIV throughout resource-poor countries.

This chapter focuses on the antiretroviral treatment of HIV infection. Although many therapeutic options exist, a thorough understanding of viral pathogenesis is essential for managing patients infected with HIV. By understanding the principles of therapy as they relate to viral pathogenesis, clinicians can rapidly assimilate new data as they become available. Consensus panel recommendations provide a framework for clinical decision making.[5–7] Given the complexity of therapy, this chapter focuses only on treatment of adult HIV infection; the reader is referred to the various consensus panel guidelines on treatment of perinatal transmission, pediatric HIV, and postexposure prophylaxis for both occupational and nonoccupational HIV exposures (**http://www.aidsinfo.nih.gov/**).

EPIDEMIOLOGY

Despite a dramatic decline in the number of AIDS-related opportunistic infections and deaths in industrialized countries,[2,8,9] infection with HIV remains a leading cause of death throughout the world. Access to newer, more potent antiretroviral regimens and monitoring are often limited by economics and politics. Infected patients residing in countries with a strong economic standing (North America, Western Europe, Australia, and New Zealand) have reasonable access to medications, whereas patients residing in countries with scarce resources (Africa, south and southeast Asia, the Pacific, and the Caribbean) do not. This is of significant concern given that most infected patients worldwide reside in these latter regions of the world.[8]

As of December 2009,[9] the worldwide estimate of persons living with HIV infection is 33.3 million: 30.8 million adults (52% of which are women) and 2.5 million children younger than 15 years of age. In 2009, it is estimated that 2.6 million people were newly infected with HIV and 1.8 million people died from AIDS. Two-thirds (68%) of all adults and children infected with HIV live in sub-Saharan Africa, and almost three-quarters (72%) of all adult and child deaths caused by AIDS occurred there in 2009. Encouragingly, the rate of new HIV infections has slowly declined: The number of new infections in 2009 was approximately 25% lower than in 2001 in 33 countries, 22 of which are in sub-Saharan Africa. A 20% decline in AIDS-related deaths in this region between 2004 and 2009 is partly attributed to increased access to HIV treatment.[9] Although these numbers show some improvement, there is great variability among countries and regions within Sub-Saharan Africa. Although treatment strategies are difficult to implement in developing countries because of social and political barriers and resource limitations, access to antiretroviral medications in low-income and middle-income countries increased 10-fold between 2003 and 2008 and an additional 30% between 2008 and 2009. Despite these advances, it was estimated that only about 37% of people eligible for treatment in sub-Saharan Africa in 2009 were able to access it.[9]

In the United States, the availability of antiretroviral therapy has resulted in a 67% decline in AIDS death rates between 1994 and 2007, but it is estimated that 18,000 people still die from AIDS each year and greater than about 20% to 25% are unaware that they are HIV-positive, and approximately 56,300 are infected each year. Racial and ethnic minorities continue to be disproportionately affected by HIV due to a complicated combination of poverty, disproportionate incarceration, and social and sexual network segregation.[10] Blacks, who only constitute 12% of the US population, account for 46% of cases in the United States and 45% of new infections yearly. Hispanics/Latinos, who constitute 15% of the US population account for 17% of people living with HIV in the United States and 17% of new infections yearly. Compared with white men and women, the lifetime risk of HIV seroconversion is 6 times higher in black men, 15 times higher in black women, 2 times higher in Hispanic/Latino men, and 4 times higher in Hispanic/Latino women.[11] Transmission through sexual intercourse remains a predominant route of infection, with unsafe sex between men accounting for approximately 53% of cases, and heterosexual intercourse accounting for approximately 31% of cases.[12–14] The proportion of women newly diagnosed worldwide increased dramatically from 15% in 1995 to 27% in 2004 and has remained steady at 27% through 2009. Additionally, patients older than 50 years of age represent a rapidly expanding group, both from new infections and as a result of effective antiretroviral therapy extending life expectancy.[11]

PATHOPHYSIOLOGY

Infection with HIV can be acquired through unprotected sexual intercourse (both anal and vaginal), injectable drug use, receipt of tainted blood products, and mother-to-infant transmission (both perinatal infection and postpartum through breast-feeding).[5] Infection can also be acquired from occupational exposures among health care workers after needle sticks or infected blood splashes from patients infected with HIV onto vulnerable mucosal membranes. Rarely has HIV infection been documented after oral sex.[12,13]

Unprotected sexual intercourse has accounted for approximately 80% of all documented HIV infections to date.[9] Transmission between sexual partners depends on a number of factors, including the HIV viral subtype, stage of infection in the index partner, genetic susceptibility to infection of the potential host, and the viral fitness (or pathogenicity) of the infecting strain. Infectivity via male-to-male receptive anal intercourse represents the greatest sexual risk factor followed by male-to-female vaginal transmission and then female-to-male penile transmission.[14]

During transmission, HIV binds to specific immune cells, including monocytes, macrophages, and T-cell lymphocytes (also known as CD4$^+$ T cells, helper T cells, or T cells).[14–18] These cells express specific receptor proteins known as CD4 receptors to which HIV binds. Once bound to the CD4 receptor, coreceptor proteins (CCR5, CXCR-4) are required for fusion of the viral membrane to the immune cell membrane.[19,20] CCR5 coreceptors are found on both monocytes and T lymphocytes, and are more abundant in patients newly infected with HIV.[20,21] CXCR-4 coreceptors are predominantly found on T lymphocytes and are more abundant in patients who have been on long-term antiretroviral therapy. The CD4–coreceptor complex causes conformational changes to key HIV proteins (gp41 and gp120) allowing for a more close association between the virus and host cell.[22,23] HIV fuses with the cell and releases its contents into the host cell's cytoplasm: this includes the virus's RNA and specific enzymes necessary for replication (Fig. 73-1; see online

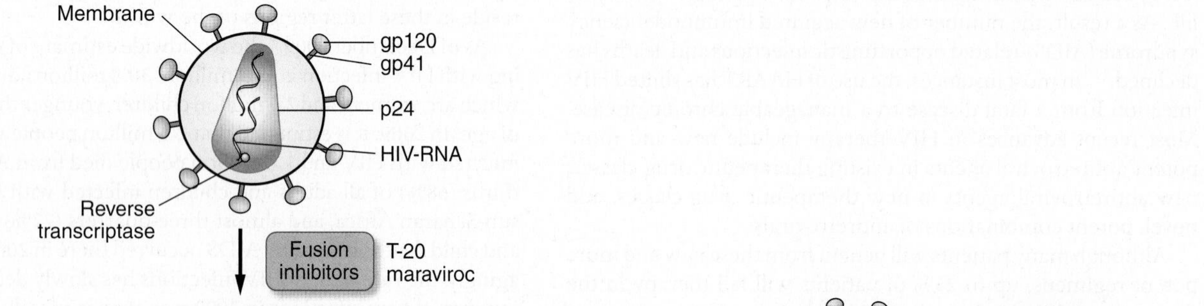

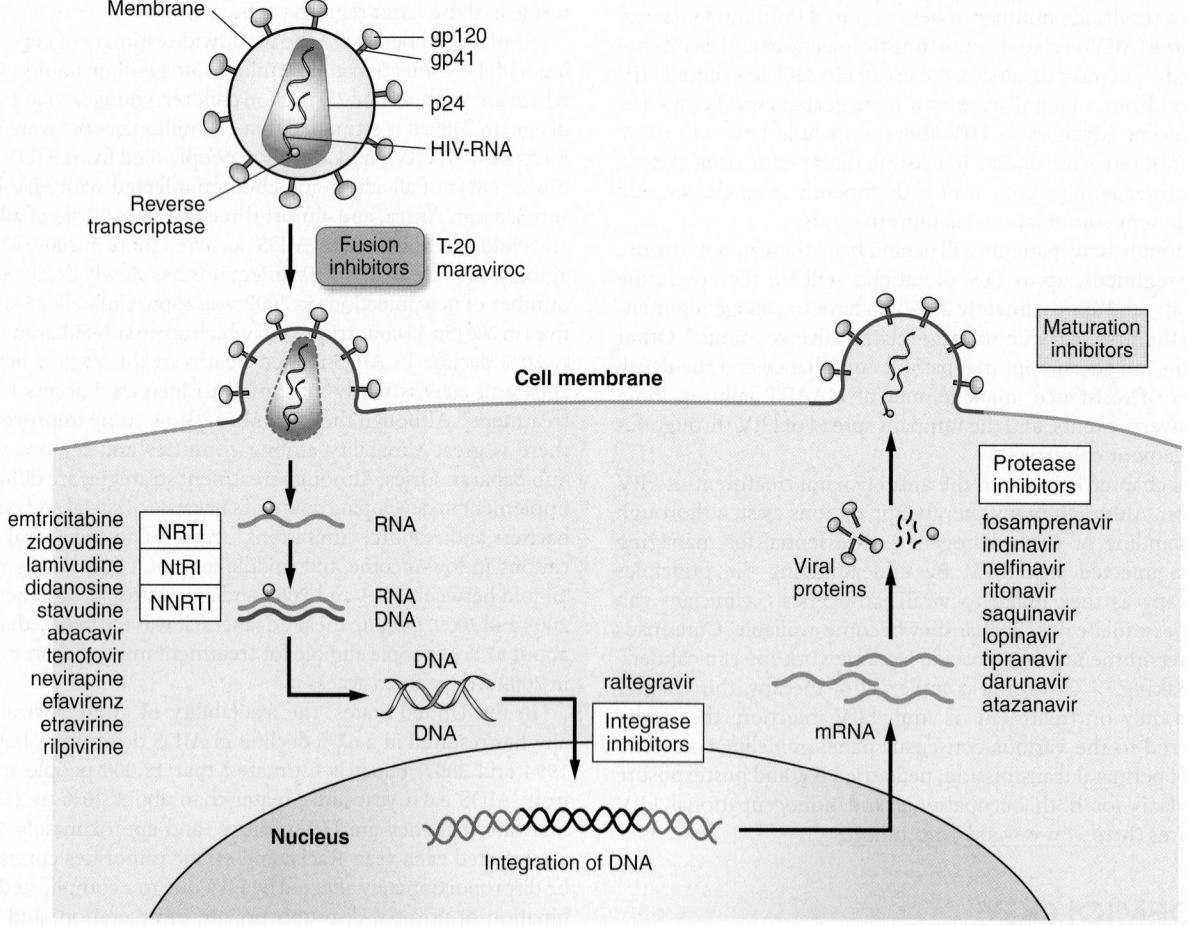

FIGURE 73-1 Schematic representation of the HIV-1 life cycle. Four classes of antiretroviral drugs are available at present. Fusion inhibitors inhibit the entry of virions into a new target cell. The step of reverse transcription can be targeted, using nucleoside nucleotide analogs or non-nucleoside reverse-transcriptase inhibitors (NRTIs, NtRTI, and NNRTIs, respectively). The class of integrase inhibitors prevent integration of viral DNA into host cell DNA. The class of protease inhibitors interferes with the last state of the life cycle, the proteolytic processing of the viral proteins, which results in the production of noninfectious particles. (Adapted with permission from Simon V, Ho DD. HIV-1 dynamics in vivo: implications for therapy. *Nat Rev Microb.* 2003;1:181.)

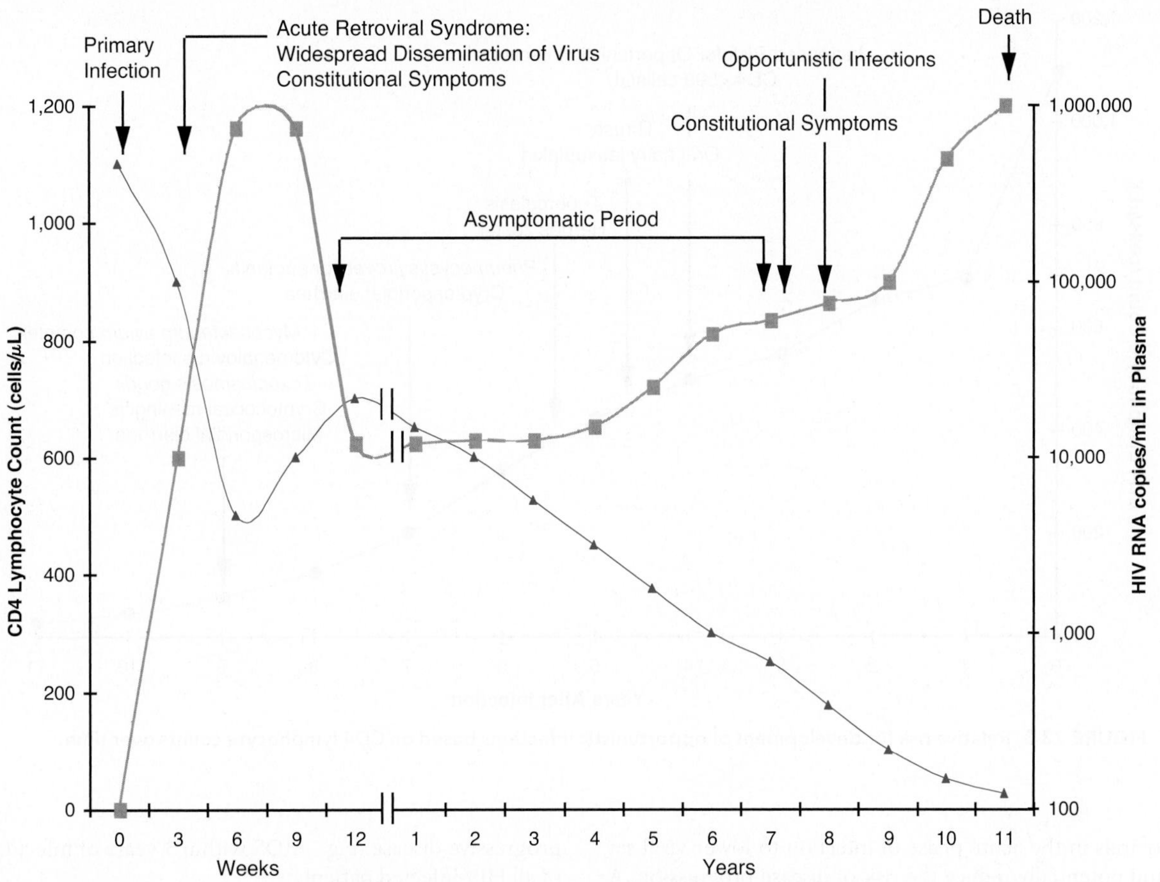

FIGURE 73-2 Sample disease course for an untreated HIV-infected individual showing the relationships among immunologic, virologic, and clinical outcomes over time. Constitutional symptoms include fever, night sweats, and weight loss. ■ Viral load values; ▲ CD4 T lymphocytes. (Source: Fauci AS et al. Immunopathogenic mechanisms of HIV infection. *Ann Intern Med.* 1996;124:654; Perelson AS et al. HIV-1 dynamics in vivo: virion clearance rate, infected cell life-span, and viral generation time. *Science.* 1996;271:1582.)

animated images of HIV lifecycle and where the drugs act, such as **http://www.sumanasinc.com/webcontent/animations/content/hiv.html** or **http://biosingularity.wordpress.com/2007/03/04/3d-animation-of-hiv-replication/**). The single-stranded viral RNA is transcribed via reverse transcriptase into a double-stranded proviral DNA that is subsequently incorporated into the host cell's genetic material via the integrase enzyme. HIV then uses the infected cell's machinery to translate, transcribe, and produce immature viral particles that bud and break from the infected cell. For these immature virions to become infectious, the HIV protease enzyme must cleave large precursor polypeptides into functional proteins.[24,25] Once complete, the mature virion is free to infect new host cells and subsequently produce more infectious virus.

Over time, HIV-infected host cells can be destroyed by a number of mechanisms: (a) a direct cytolytic effect of the virus (e.g., formation of syncytium induction, cellular dysfunction); (b) the identification and elimination of the infected cell by the host's immune response (e.g., via cytotoxic T-cell lymphocytes); or (c) the cell's natural life cycle coming to completion.[18] In addition, HIV infection can inhibit the production of new CD4$^+$ cells.[26]

Once a patient becomes infected, an initial burst of viremia occurs and causes latent infection in various tissues (e.g., lymph nodes) and cells (CD4, macrophages, and monocytes).[15,27] Most infectious HIV virions (~99%) reside inside lymph nodes and other immune-cell rich tissues found throughout the body.[15,16,28,29] The immune system reacts by producing antibodies against HIV; however, given the rapid production of new HIV particles and the development of many new viral strains (a result of the error-susceptible HIV reverse transcriptase), the antibody response is inadequate.[30] After this burst of viremia, a transient depletion of CD4$^+$ cells occurs (Fig. 73-2). Initially, patients may complain of nonspecific symptoms, such as fever, lymphadenopathy, rash, fatigue, and night sweats.[31,32]

This phase of infection is known as the acute retroviral syndrome.

ONLINE CONTENT

For a photo of a rash caused by acute HIV infection, go to http://thepoint.lww.com/AT10e.

In most cases, patients are unaware that they are infected. Within 6 months, the host's immune response is able to control the infection to a point where the number of virus particles produced per day equals the number of particles destroyed per day. This steady-state is often referred to as the patient's viral "set point."

The higher a patient's viral set point, the greater the risk for disease progression. This is because there is a greater chance for more widespread viral infection and immune cell destruction with a larger replicating viral population. Why some patients establish higher or lower viral set points is currently under investigation, but this may be a consequence of differences in immune responses, cellular receptor populations, viral subtypes, viral fitness, or a combination of these factors. This understanding of viral pathogenesis may lead to a new paradigm of therapy: using

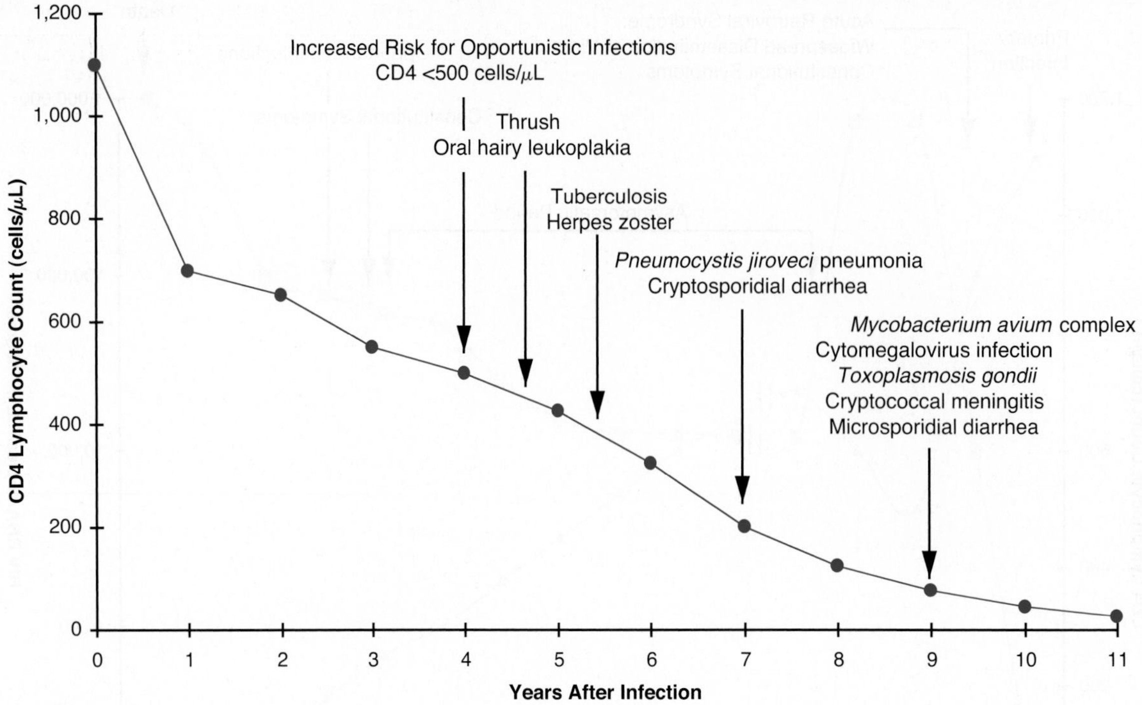

FIGURE 73-3 Relative risk for development of opportunistic infections based on CD4 lymphocyte counts over time.

antiretrovirals in the acute phase of infection to lower viral set points and potentially reduce the risk of disease progression. A significant challenge is to identify those patients with acute infection who have nonspecific symptoms.[33]

Once the initial burst of viremia has been controlled and the viral set point established, infection with HIV results in a constant battle between viral replication and suppression of that replication by the immune system. Mathematical models have calculated the production of HIV at 10 billion particles per day.[16,34–36] To keep the infection controlled, the body must produce an equal immune response. Over time, HIV depletes the body of T cells, which places the host at an increased risk for opportunistic infections (Fig. 73-3). Direct measurements of HIV RNA concentrations in plasma (also called "viral load") can predict disease progression (see subsequent discussion).[37–39] Higher viral load measurements represent an inability of the host to control viral replication, and a greater risk for immune cell destruction. Long-term "nonprogressors" (e.g., patients with asymptomatic HIV infection for >10 years; 5% of all HIV-infected patients) consistently have lower baseline viral loads than patients with rapidly progressive disease (e.g., AIDS within 5 years of infection; 20% of all HIV-infected patients).[40,41]

Without intervention, the natural progression of HIV infection results in depletion of 50 to 100 T cells/μL/year.[15,42] The severity of immune dysfunction, as evidenced by T-cell loss, is highly predictive of the potential for the development of specific types of opportunistic infections. For example, *Pneumocystis carinii* pneumonia rarely occurs when T-cell counts are greater than 200 cells/μL, whereas retinitis from cytomegalovirus infection infrequently occurs in patients with CD4 counts greater than 75 cells/μL (Figs. 73-2, 73-3). The diagnosis of AIDS is made when a significant amount of immune deterioration has occurred, either by depletion of $CD4^+$ cells to less than 200 cells/μL or because of the development of new opportunistic infections (Tables 73-1, 73-2). It is important to recognize that not every patient with HIV has a diagnosis of AIDS. On average, without appropriate drug therapy, death occurs within 10 to 15 years after infection.[15,43]

The interplay between viral load and CD4 T-cell counts is often compared with that of a train heading toward a particular

TABLE 73-1
1993 Revised Classification System for HIV Infection and the Expanded CDC Surveillance Case Definition for AIDS in Adults and Adolescents[a]

	Clinical Categories		
$CD4^+$ T-Cell Categories	(A) Asymptomatic, Acute (Primary) HIV	(B) Symptomatic, Not (A) or (C) Conditions	(C) AIDS-Indicator Conditions
500/μL	A1	B1	C1
200–499/μL	A2	B2	C2
<200/μL (AIDS indicator T-cell count)	A3	B3	C3

[a] The modifications to the prior 1986 Surveillance Case Definition, which have been included in the 1993 revision, include the use of CD4 cell count (<200 cells/μL) or CD4 cell percent (<14%) and the additional AIDS-indicating conditions of pulmonary tuberculosis, recurrent pneumonia, and invasive cervical cancer (see Table 73-2).
AIDS, acquired immunodeficiency syndrome; CDC, Centers for Disease Control and Prevention; HIV, human immunodeficiency virus.

TABLE 73-2
Conditions Included in the 1993 Surveillance Case Definition

Category A
Asymptomatic human immunodeficiency virus (HIV) infection
Persistent generalized lymphadenopathy
Acute HIV infection with accompanying illness or history of HIV infection
Category B
Bacillary angiomatosis
Candidiasis, oropharyngeal (thrush)
Candidiasis, vulvovaginal; persistent, frequent, or poorly responsive to treatment
Cervical dysplasia or carcinoma in situ
Constitutional symptoms, such as fever >38°C or diarrhea >1 month
Hairy leukoplakia
Herpes zoster (shingles), involving at least two distinct episodes or more than one dermatome
Idiopathic thrombocytopenic purpura
Listeriosis
Pelvic inflammatory disease, particularly if complicated by tubo-ovarian abscess
Peripheral neuropathy
Category C
Candidiasis of bronchi, trachea, or lungs
Candidiasis, esophageal
Cervical cancer, invasive
Coccidioidomycosis, disseminated or extrapulmonary
Cryptococcosis, extrapulmonary
Cryptosporidiosis, chronic intestinal (>1 month)
Cytomegalovirus disease (other than liver, spleen, or nodes)
Cytomegalovirus retinitis (with loss of vision)
Encephalopathy, HIV-related
Herpes simplex: chronic ulcer(s) (>1 month); or bronchitis, pneumonitis, or esophagitis
Histoplasmosis, disseminated or extrapulmonary
Isosporiasis, chronic intestinal (duration >1 month)
Kaposi sarcoma
Lymphoid interstitial pneumonia, pulmonary lymphoid hyperplasia, or both[a]
Lymphoma, Burkitt (or equivalent term)
Lymphoma, immunoblastic (or equivalent term)
Lymphoma, primary, of brain
Mycobacterium avium–intracellulare complex or *Mycobacterium kansasii*, disseminated or extrapulmonary
Mycobacterium tuberculosis, any site (pulmonary[b] or extrapulmonary)
Mycobacterium, other species or unidentified species, disseminated or extrapulmonary
Pneumocystis carinii pneumonia
Pneumonia, recurrent[b]
Progressive multifocal leukoencephalopathy
Salmonella septicemia, recurrent
Toxoplasmosis of brain
Wasting syndrome resulting from HIV

[a]Children <13 years of age.
[b]Added in the 1993 expansions of the acquired immunodeficiency syndrome surveillance case definition for adolescents and adults.

destination. If the destination is immune system destruction (and eventually death), then the T-cell count is the distance of the train from this destination, and the viral load (concentration of HIV RNA in plasma) is the speed of the train. As both higher speeds and shorter distances reach destinations faster, so does a high viral load and low T-cell count result in quicker onset of immune destruction (and death). Potent antiretroviral regimens decrease viral replication and dramatically alter the natural course of infec-

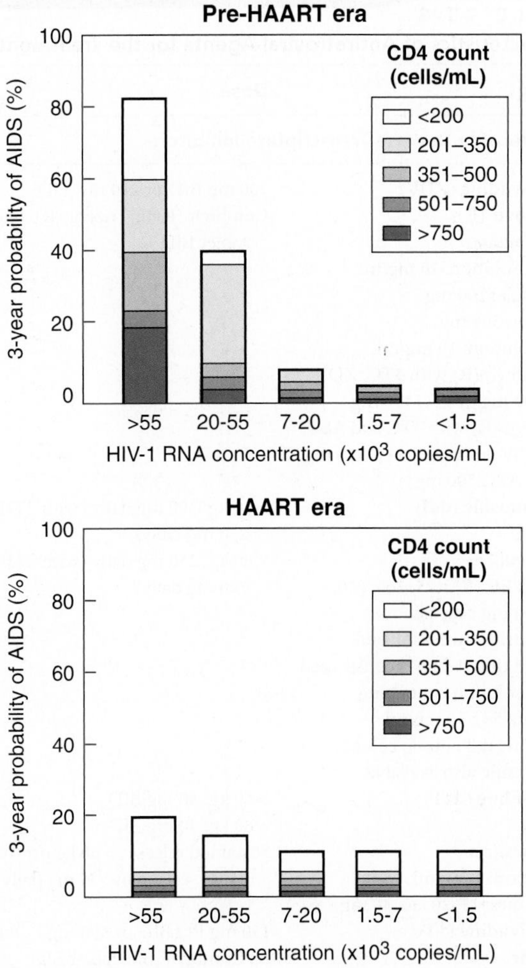

FIGURE 73-4 Prognosis according to CD4 cell count and viral load in the pre-HAART and HAART eras. (Adapted with permission from Egger M et al. Prognosis of HIV-1–infected patients starting highly active antiretroviral therapy: a collaborative analysis of prospective studies [published correction appears in *Lancet.* 2002;360:1178]. *Lancet.* 2002;360:119.)

tion by prolonging the time to opportunistic infection and death (Fig. 73-4).[44]

PHARMACOTHERAPY

Pharmacotherapy of HIV has been directed at inhibiting key areas of the HIV life cycle (Fig. 73-1 and animations found at http://www.sumanasinc.com/webcontent/animations/content/hiv.html or http://biosingularity.wordpress.com/2007/03/04/3d-animation-of-hiv-replication/; Table 73-3). Much research has been focused on agents that inhibit the reverse transcriptase enzyme. Nucleoside or nucleotide analog reverse transcriptase inhibitors (nucleoside RT inhibitors [NRTIs] include zidovudine, didanosine, lamivudine, abacavir, emtricitabine, and stavudine; nucleotide RT inhibitors (currently only include tenofovir), inhibit this enzyme by incorporating false nucleic acids into the newly forming proviral DNA.[45] This results in an HIV DNA strand that cannot continue to elongate. Non-nucleoside reverse transcriptase inhibitors (NNRTIs; nevirapine, delavirdine, efavirenz, rilpivirine, and etravirine), inhibit reverse transcriptase by directly binding to the enzyme itself, and prevent DNA transcription from RNA.[46] Protease inhibitors (PIs: saquinavir, fosamprenavir, nelfinavir, indinavir, lopinavir,

TABLE 73-3
Characteristics of Antiretroviral Agents for the Treatment of Adult Human Immunodeficiency Virus Infection[5,7]

Drug	Dose	Pharmacokinetic Parameters	Administration Considerations
Nucleoside Reverse Transcriptase Inhibitors			
Zidovudine (ZDV) **Retrovir (R)** *Preparations* Oral Solution: 10 mg/mL Capsule: 100 mg Tablet: 300 mg IV Solution: 10 mg/mL Combivir (R) with 3TC: ZDV 300 mg + 3TC 150 mg Trizivir (R) with 3TC and ABC: ZDV 300 mg + 3TC 150 mg + ABC 300 mg	300 mg BID or 200 mg TID Combivir (R) or Trizivir (R): one tablet BID	*Oral bioavailability:* 60% *Serum* $t_{1/2}$: 1.1 hours *Intracellular* $t_{1/2}$: 3 hours *Elimination:* hepatic glucuronidation; renal excretion of glucuronide metabolite	Can be administered without regard to meals (manufacturer recommends administration 30 minutes before or 1 hour after a meal)
Didanosine (ddI) **Videx** *Preparations* Videx EC (R): 125, 200, 250, 400 mg capsule Pediatric powder for oral solution (when reconstituted as solution containing antacid): 10 mg/mL Generic ddI enteric-coated capsule also available	>60 kg: 400 mg daily (with TDF, use 250 mg daily) <60 kg: 250 mg daily (with TDF, use 200 mg daily)	*Oral bioavailability:* 30%–40% *Serum* $t_{1/2}$: 1.6 hours *Intracellular* $t_{1/2}$: 25–40 hours *Elimination:* renal excretion ~50%	Food decreases absorption (↓ 55%); administer ddI on empty stomach (1 hour before or 2 hours after meal) Separate ATV and TPV/r administration by at least 2 hours
Stavudine (d4T) **Zerit** *Preparations* Solution: 1 mg/mL Capsules: 15, 20, 30, 40 mg	>60 kg: 40 mg BID <60 kg: 30 mg BID Sustained release: >60 kg use 100 mg daily; <60 kg use 75 mg daily	*Oral bioavailability:* 86% *Serum* $t_{1/2}$: 1.0 hour *Intracellular* $t_{1/2}$: 3.5 hours *Elimination:* renal excretion ~50%	Can be administered without regard to meals
Lamivudine (3TC) **Epivir** *Preparations* Solution: 10 mg/mL Tablets: 150 mg, 300 mg Combivir: 3TC 150 mg + ZDV 300 mg Epzicom: 3TC 300 mg + ABC 600 mg Trizivir: 3TC 150 mg + ZDV 300 mg + ABC 300 mg	150 mg PO BID or 300 mg PO daily As Combivir: one tablet BID As Epzicom: one tablet BID As Trizivir: one tablet BID	*Oral bioavailability:* 86% *Serum* $t_{1/2}$: 5–7 hours *Intracellular* $t_{1/2}$: 18–22 hours *Elimination:* 70% unchanged in urine	Can be administered without regard to meals
Emtricitabine (FTC) **Emtriva** *Preparations* Capsules: 200 mg Oral solution: 10 mg/mL Truvada: FTC 200 mg + TDF 300 mg Atripla: FTC 200 mg + TDF 300 mg + EFV 600 mg	200 mg daily for patients with calculated CrCl >50 mL/min Dose needs to be adjusted for renal dysfunction: CrCl 30–49 mL/min: 200 mg every 48 hours CrCl 15–29 mL/min: 200 mg every 72 hours CrCl <15 mL/min: 200 mg every 96 hours As Truvada: one tablet daily Truvada not for patients with CrCl <30 mL/min As Atripla: one tablet daily Atripla not for patients with CrCl <50 mL/min	*Oral bioavailability:* 93% *Serum* $t_{1/2}$: 10 hours *Intracellular* $t_{1/2}$: >20 hours *Elimination:* 86% recovered in urine	Can be administered without regard to meals
Tenofovir Disoproxil Fumarate (TDF) **Viread** *Preparations* Tablets: 300 mg Truvada: TDF 300 mg + FTC 200 mg Atripla: TDF 300 mg + FTC 200 mg + EFV 600 mg	300 mg daily for patients with CrCl >60 mL/min; Truvada: 1 tablet daily Atripla: 1 tablet daily	*Oral bioavailability:* 25% fasting; 39% with high-fat meal *Serum* $t_{1/2}$: 17 hours *Intracellular* $t_{1/2}$: >60 hours *Elimination:* primarily by glomerular filtration and active tubular secretion	Can be administered without regard to meals

(*continued*)

TABLE 73-3

Characteristics of Antiretroviral Agents for the Treatment of Adult Human Immunodeficiency Virus Infection[5,7] (*Continued*)

Drug	Dose	Pharmacokinetic Parameters	Administration Considerations
Nucleoside Reverse Transcriptase Inhibitors (*continued*)			
Abacavir (ABC) **Ziagen** *Preparations* Tablets: 300 mg Oral solution: 20 mg/mL Epzicom: ABC 600 mg + 3TC 300 mg Trizivir: ABC 300 mg + ZDV 300 mg + 3TC 150 mg	300 mg every 12 hours, or 600 mg daily Epzicom: one tablet daily Trizivir: one tablet BID	*Oral bioavailability:* 83% *Serum* $t_{1/2}$: 1.5 hours *Intracellular* $t_{1/2}$: 12–26 hours *Elimination:* alcohol dehydrogenase and glucuronyltransferase; 82% renal elimination of metabolites	Can be administered without regard to meals Alcohol raises abacavir exposure by 41% HLA testing required before administration
Non-Nucleoside Reverse Transcriptase Inhibitors[a]			
Nevirapine (NVP) **Viramune** *Preparations* Suspension: 50 mg/5 mL Tablets: 200 mg	200 mg PO daily × 14 days, then 200 mg PO BID	*Oral bioavailability:* >90% *Serum* $t_{1/2}$: 25–30 hours *Intracellular* $t_{1/2}$: unknown *Elimination:* metabolized by CYP2B6 and CYP3A4 (also a CYP3A4 inducer) with 80% excreted in urine as the glucuronide metabolite	Can be administered without regard to meals
Delavirdine (DLV) **Rescriptor** *Preparations* Tablets: 100, 200 mg	400 mg TID (four 100-mg tabs in at least 3 ounces of water to produce slurry); 200-mg tablets should be taken intact	*Oral bioavailability:* 85% *Serum* $t_{1/2}$: 5.8 hours *Intracellular* $t_{1/2}$: unknown *Elimination:* metabolized by CYP3A4 (also a CYP3A4 inhibitor) with 51% excreted in urine as metabolites	Can be administered without regard to meals
Efavirenz (EFV) **Sustiva** *Preparations* Capsules: 50, 100, 200 mg Tablets: 600 mg Atripla: EFV 600 mg + TDF 300 mg + FTC 200 mg	600 mg at bedtime Atripla one tablet at bedtime. Not for patients with CrCl <50 mL/min	*Oral bioavailability:* ~60%–70% *Serum* $t_{1/2}$: 40–55 hours *Intracellular* $t_{1/2}$: unknown *Elimination:* hepatically metabolized by CYP2B6 and CYP3A4 (also CYP3A4 mixed inhibitor/inducer)	Avoid taking with high-fat meals, concentrations ↑ 50% (increased risk for CNS toxicity) Take after a meal
Etravirine (ETV) **Intelence** *Preparations* Tablets: 100, 200 mg Complera: RPV 25 mg + TDF 300 mg + FTC 200 mg	200 mg BID	*Oral bioavailability:* unknown *Serum* $t_{1/2}$: 40 ± 20 hours *Intracellular* $t_{1/2}$: unknown *Elimination:* hepatically metabolized by CYP3A4, CYP2C9, CYP2C19 (also 3A4 inducer, 2C9 and 2C19 inhibitor)	
Rilpivirine (RPV) **Edurant** *Preperations* Tablets: 25 mg	25 mg daily	*Oral bioavailability:* not established *Serum* $t_{1/2}$: ~50 hours *Intracellular* $t_{1/2}$: unknown *Elimination:* hepatic metabolism primarily by CYP3A4 with 85% fecal excretion.	Take with moderate- to high-calorie meal (increases absorption 40%)
Protease Inhibitors			
Indinavir (IDV) **Crixivan** *Preparations* Capsule: 200, 333, 400 mg	800 mg every 8 hours (BID dosing ineffective when sole protease inhibitor) IDV/RTV: IDV 800 mg + 100 mg or 200 mg RTV BID	*Oral bioavailability:* 65% *Serum* $t_{1/2}$: 1.5–2 hours *Intracellular* $t_{1/2}$: unknown *Elimination:* hepatically metabolized via CYP3A4 (also inhibitor of CYP3A4)	Must be taken on empty stomach (1 hour before or 2 hours after a meal); may take with skim milk or low-fat meal Adequate hydration necessary (at least 1.5 L/24 hours of liquid) to minimize risk of nephrolithiasis
Ritonavir (RTV) **Norvir** *Preparations* Oral solution: 80 mg/mL Capsules: 100 mg	Current primary use is as a pharmacokinetic enhancer for other PIs, using 100–400 mg/d in one to two divided doses	*Oral bioavailability:* Not determined *Serum* $t_{1/2}$: 3–5 hours *Intracellular* $t_{1/2}$: unknown *Elimination:* extensive hepatic metabolism via CYP3A4 (also potent CYP3A4 inhibitor and mixed inhibitor/inducer of other isozymes)	Take with food if possible to improve tolerability Dose should be titrated upward to minimize gastrointestinal adverse events Refrigerate capsules but not liquid

(*continued*)

TABLE 73-3

Characteristics of Antiretroviral Agents for the Treatment of Adult Human Immunodeficiency Virus Infection[5,7] (*Continued*)

Drug	Dose	Pharmacokinetic Parameters	Administration Considerations
Protease Inhibitors (*continued*)			
Nelfinavir (NFV) **Viracept** *Preparations* Powder for oral suspension: 50 mg per one level scoop (200 mg per one level teaspoon) Tablets: 250 and 625 mg	750 mg TID or 1,250 mg BID	*Oral bioavailability:* 20%–80% *Serum* $t_{1/2}$: 3.5–5 hours *Intracellular* $t_{1/2}$: unknown *Elimination:* hepatic metabolism via CYP3A4	Administer with meal or light snack (exposure increased twofold to threefold)
Saquinavir (SQV) **Invirase** (hard gel capsules) *Preparations* Hard gel capsule: 200 mg Tablets: 500 mg	Unboosted saquinavir not recommended Saquinavir/ritonavir: 1,000/100 BID; 1,600/100 daily under investigation	*Oral bioavailability:* 4% (as the sole PI) *Serum* $t_{1/2}$: 1–2 hours *Intracellular* $t_{1/2}$: unknown *Elimination:* hepatic metabolism via CYP3A4 (inhibitor)	Take within 2 hours of a meal and take with RTV
Fosamprenavir (FPV) **Lexiva** Tablet: 700 mg	In ARV-naïve patients: FPV 1,400 mg BID or FPV 1,400 mg + RTV 200 mg daily or FPV 700 mg + RTV 100 mg BID In PI-experienced patients: FPV 700 mg + RTV 100 mg BID	*Oral bioavailability:* not determined *Serum* $t_{1/2}$: 7.1–10.6 hours (APV) *Intracellular* $t_{1/2}$: unknown *Elimination:* hepatic metabolism via CYP3A4 (inhibitor)	Can be taken without regard to meals but should not be taken with high-fat meals
Lopinavir (LPV)/ritonavir (RTV) **Kaletra** *Preparations* Tablet: LPV 200 mg + RTV 50 mg Solution: LPV 80 mg+ RTV 20 mg per mL	Two tablets or 5 mL BID or Four tablets or 10 mL daily (recommended for treatment-naïve patients only)	*Oral bioavailability:* not determined *Serum* $t_{1/2}$: 5–6 hours *Intracellular* $t_{1/2}$: unknown *Elimination:* hepatic metabolism via CYP3A4 (inhibitor)	Take with food (increases AUC by 48%). Tablet stable at room temperature
Atazanavir (ATV) **Reyataz** *Preparations* Capsules: 100, 150, 200, 300 mg	400 mg daily Atazanavir/RTV: 300/100 daily	*Oral bioavailability:* 60%–70% *Serum* $t_{1/2}$: 6–7 hours *Intracellular* $t_{1/2}$: unknown *Elimination:* hepatic metabolism via CYP3A4 (modest inhibitor)	Take with food, and avoid acid suppressing agents (which prevent ATV solubility and absorption)
Darunavir (DRV) **Prezista** *Preparations* Tablet: 300 mg, 600 mg	DRV 600 mg + RTV 100 mg BID	*Oral bioavailability:* 37% alone, 82% with RTV *Serum* $t_{1/2}$: 15 hours *Intracellular* $t_{1/2}$: unknown *Elimination:* hepatic metabolism via CYP3A4 (inhibitor)	Food ↑ C_{max} and AUC by 30%: administer with food
Tipranavir (TPV) **Aptivus** Capsules: 250 mg	TPV 500 mg + RTV 200 mg BID DO NOT USE WITHOUT RTV	*Oral bioavailability:* not determined *Serum* $t_{1/2}$: 6 hours *Intracellular* $t_{1/2}$: unknown *Elimination:* hepatic metabolism via CYP3A4 (inhibitor and inducer)	Administer with food to increase bioavailability
Entry Inhibitors			
Enfuvirtide (T-20) Fuzeon	90 mg SC BID in upper arm, thigh, or abdomen	*Oral bioavailability:* 84.3% compared with IV *Serum* $t_{1/2}$: 3.8 hours *Intracellular* $t_{1/2}$: not applicable *Elimination:* nonrenal, nonhepatic	Reconstitute with 1.1 mL sterile water for injection; gently tap vial for 10 seconds and then roll gently between hands to avoid foaming and ensure all drug is off vial walls After reconstitution, use immediately or refrigerate for 24 hours. Refrigerated T-20 should be brought to room temperature before injection.

(continued)

TABLE 73-3

Characteristics of Antiretroviral Agents for the Treatment of Adult Human Immunodeficiency Virus Infection[5,7] (*Continued*)

Drug	Dose	Pharmacokinetic Parameters	Administration Considerations
Chemokine Receptor Antagonists (CCR5)			
Maraviroc (MVC) **Selzentry** *Preparations* Tablet: 150, 300 mg	300 mg BID (with all NRTIs, NVP, TPV, ENF), 150 mg BID with CYP3A inhibitors (with or without a CYP3A inducer) including: protease inhibitors (except tipranavir/ritonavir), delavirdine, ketoconazole, itraconazole, clarithromycin, and other strong CYP3A inhibitors (e.g., nefazodone, telithromycin) 600 mg BID with CYP3A inducers (without a strong CYP3A inhibitor) including: Efavirenz, etravirine (TMC125), rifampin, carbamazepine, phenobarbital, and phenytoin	*Oral bioavailability:* ~33% *Serum* $t_{1/2}$: 14–18 hours *Elimination:* hepatic metabolism by CYP3A; 20% recovered in urine, 76% recovered in feces	Can be administered without regard to meals (high-fat meal decreases C_{max} and AUC by ~30%) Trofile assay must be performed before administration
Integrase Inhibitors			
Raltegravir (RAL) **Isentress** *Preparations* Tablet: 400 mg	400 mg BID	*Oral bioavailability:* not established *Serum* $t_{1/2}$: 9 hours *Elimination:* hepatic metabolism by UGT1A1 glucuronidation; 32% recovered in urine, 51% recovered in feces	Can be administered without regard to meals (high-fat meal decreases C_{max} by ~34% and increases AUC by ~19%)

[a] In clinical trials, the NNRTIs was discontinued because of rash in 7% of patients taking nevirapine, 4.3% of patients taking delavirdine, and 1.7% of patients taking efavirenz. Rare cases of Stevens-Johnson syndrome have been reported with all three NNRTIs.

ABC, abacavir; ARV, antiviral; ATV, atazanavir; AUC, area under the curve; BID, twice daily; CNS, central nervous system; CrCl, creatinine clearance; ddI, didanosine; d4T, stavudine; DLV, delavirdine; DRV, darunavir; EFV, efavirenz; ENF, enfuvirtide; ETV, etravirine; FPV, fosamprenavir; FTC, emtricitabine; HLA, human leukocyte antigen; IDV, indinavir; IV, intravenous; LPV, lopinavir; MVC, maraviroc; NFV, nelfinavir, NNRTI, non-nucleoside reverse transcriptase inhibitor; NRTIs, nucleoside reverse transcriptase inhibitors; NVP, nevirapine; PI, protein inhibitor; PO, orally; QID, four times daily; RAL, raltegravir; RPV, rilpivirine; RTV, ritonavir; SC, subcutaneously; SQV, saquinavir; 3TC, lamivudine; TDF, tenofovir disoproxil fumarate; TID, three times daily; TPV, tipranavir; TPV/r, tipranavir/ritonavir; T-20, enfuvirtide; ZDV, zidovudine.

atazanavir, ritonavir, tipranavir, and darunavir) directly bind to the catalytic site of HIV protease, inactivating the enzyme and preventing maturation of the HIV virion.[47,48] Unlike reverse transcription, which occurs early in the course of the HIV life cycle, protease enzyme activity occurs late in virion development. As a result, inactivation of the protease enzyme inhibits viral replication in any infected cell regardless of the current stage of HIV replication within that cell. In contrast, reverse transcriptase inhibitors can protect newly infected cells from becoming latently infected cells only before formation and insertion of proviral DNA into the host cell's genetic material. Subsequently, these agents provide no benefit for those infected cells that are actively producing new strains of virus.

Fusion inhibitors, such as enfuvirtide, prevent HIV and $CD4^+$ T cells from being pulled closer together after HIV binds to CD4 and CCR5 or CXCR-4 coreceptors. Enfuvirtide prevents fusion of the virus with the T-cell by binding to a double coil–coil complex at the gp41–gp120–CD4 receptor area.[49] The newest classes of antiretroviral agents are coreceptor blockers and integrase inhibitors. Maraviroc is a CCR5 coreceptor blocker which prevents HIV from fully binding to cells and causing infection.[50] Raltegravir is an integrase strand transfer inhibitor (INSTI) that prevents the integrase enzyme from integrating HIV DNA into the immune cell's genome.[51]

With the development of newer, more potent antiretroviral regimens, researchers have speculated about the possibility of complete eradication of HIV from an infected patient. This outcome may require complete inhibition of viral replication in all cells and body stores where HIV resides.[16] However, a barrier to eradication is the varying half-lives of cell populations (e.g., 1–2 days for peripheral T cells vs. 14 days for macrophages).[52,53] In addition, extremely long-lived infected T cells with half-lives lasting more than 6 to 44 months have been identified.[54,55] Thus, it may require complete suppression of HIV replication for 60 years or more to eradicate HIV infection completely from the body.[54–56] Another complicating factor is the potential for HIV to reside in sites that achieve low antiretroviral concentrations, thereby serving as sanctuaries for HIV replication (e.g., central nervous system [CNS], testes). Once therapy is discontinued, these sites could theoretically release unaffected virions and repopulate the host. As a result, research has shifted toward immune-based therapies that can identify and destroy HIV-infected cells, in addition to preventing HIV acquisition.

DIAGNOSIS

CASE 73-1

QUESTION 1: E.J. is a 27-year-old man who presents with new complaints of fevers, night sweats, weight loss, and white patches in his mouth. He states that these symptoms have been present for the past 4 to 6 weeks. E.J. admits to intravenous drug use in the past; however, he states that he has been "clean" for 3 years. E.J. is diagnosed with thrush caused by *Candida albicans*. HIV infection is suspected and consent for an HIV test is obtained. Why is HIV suspected and how is it confirmed?

In otherwise healthy, immunocompetent individuals, opportunistic infections, such as thrush, are rare because an intact cell-mediated immunity protects against infection. In immunosuppressed individuals, such as those infected with HIV, the immune system is significantly compromised and places patients at risk for opportunistic infections. Infections such as shingles (herpes zoster), tuberculosis, thrush, and recurrent candidal vaginal infections in an otherwise healthy person warrant further evaluation for the possibility of HIV infection. More advanced diseases, such as *Pneumocystis jiroveci* pneumonia, *Mycobacterium avium* bacteremia, and cytomegalovirus retinitis infections, among others, generally occur in patients with severely depressed immune systems and strongly suggest HIV infection. This suggestion is especially true for those patients with risk factors for HIV infection. Despite E.J.'s discontinuation of intravenous drugs, his prior use places him at risk for HIV infection. Given his social history and current clinical presentation, an HIV test is warranted.

Testing for HIV is based on detection of an antibody to the virus. The most commonly used methods include the enzyme-linked immunosorbent assays (ELISA) and confirmatory Western blot tests.[57,58]

ONLINE CONTENT

For an illustration showing the ELISA process, go to http://thepoint.lww.com/AT10e.

ELISA is highly sensitive and specific (>99%) and therefore represents a good screening test. Using this method, the patient's serum is placed in wells coated with HIV antigens. After incubation and washing, an enzyme-labeled antihuman antibody is added, followed by a substrate. If HIV antibodies are present, a color change takes place; this is confirmed with a spectrophotometer. Reactive ELISA is subsequently repeated and, if both tests are positive, a Western blot confirmatory test is performed. The Western blot involves the addition of the host's serum to known HIV antigens that have been separated by gel electrophoresis. After washing and incubation, antihuman immune globulins linked to an enzyme or radioactive probe are added. The spectrum of band patterns on the gel is then interpreted and compared with controls for HIV diagnosis.

Although these tests when used together are highly specific and sensitive, false-negative and false-positive findings occur.[59] The most troublesome is the situation in which a patient is truly infected with both ELISA and Western blot negative results, known clinically as acute HIV infection. The reason for this phenomenon is, once infected, it takes 1 to 2 months for a person to develop antibodies to HIV.[60] Because both of these tests rely on antibody detection, this "window" period of acute infection could result in a false-negative test finding for HIV. If this window period is suspected, an HIV polymerase chain reaction (PCR) test (a measure of HIV RNA or "viral load"; see subsequent discussion) can be ordered; measurements greater than 10,000 copies/mL are present only among patients who are HIV infected. Acute HIV infection is increasingly implicated in the sexual transmission of HIV (an increased HIV RNA increases the probability of transmission), and cost-efficient methods to detect acute infection using routine viral load measurements have been developed.[61] In all situations, a confirmatory Western blot test should be performed to rule out false-positive findings and mislabeled samples.

Results of the ELISA test take up to 1 to 2 weeks, and this delay means that patients must contact their providers for test results. According to the Centers for Disease Control and Prevention (CDC), in the year 2000 approximately one-third of individuals who tested positive for HIV did not return to the clinic to learn their results. Newer test methods have been developed that allow clinicians to supply definitive negative and preliminary positive results to patients within 20 minutes or less of screening, using whole blood, serum, plasma, or oral fluid.[62] The sensitivity and specificity of these new, rapid screening tests are comparable to those of ELISA. Similar to ELISA, a positive rapid test result should be confirmed by a supplemental test. The use of rapid HIV tests should be strongly considered when expected return rates for test results are low. The CDC has published guidelines on the use and quality assurance of these rapid HIV tests.[63]

SURROGATE MARKER DATA

CASE 73-1, QUESTION 2: E.J.'s ELISA and Western blot tests both return positive, and he is informed of his HIV status the next week at his follow-up examination. Before making any decisions regarding therapeutic options, what additional laboratory tests should be obtained? What cautions should be used when interpreting these values?

To determine whether therapeutic interventions are necessary, the severity of immune damage and potential for disease progression must be assessed. As stated previously, HIV predominantly infects and destroys T cells. The larger the viral load, the greater the risk for T-cell destruction and opportunistic infections. Therefore, quantitative measurements of E.J.'s HIV viral load and T-cell counts are necessary to "stage" the severity of infection, assess the risk for disease progression, and provide a reference point (i.e., baseline) for future therapeutic decisions.

Identification and measurement of T-lymphocyte subsets (e.g., CD4, CD8) are based on flow cytometry readings of fluorescent-labeled monoclonal antibodies.[5,43] These values can very widely on repeated laboratory evaluations, even in clinically stable patients. Patient samples can display up to 30% intralaboratory and interlaboratory variability.[5] In at least one study, sufficient interlaboratory variability existed to potentially result in conflicting treatment recommendations in 58% of patients (e.g., initiating therapy when T-cell counts fell <500 cells/μL).[64] Consequently, it is important to realize that assessment of T-cell measurements should always be interpreted as trends and not as individual values. Variability can also be minimized by using the same laboratory and by sampling patients at a consistent time of day.

The measurement of HIV viral load can be performed by one of three methods: reverse transcriptase–polymerase chain reaction (RT-PCR), branched-chain DNA assay, or nucleic acid sequence-based amplification.[65] Measurements using RT-PCR are obtained when viral RNA is amplified and counted. In contrast, branched-chain DNA amplifies and enumerates the signal from target probes attached to the viral RNA. Nucleic acid sequence-based amplification allows real-time, high throughput amplification of viral RNA. All methods report HIV RNA in plasma as the number of copies per milliliter, but have differing lower limits of quantitation.[5] It should be recognized that plasma viral RNA values measure the amount of free virus in the periphery and not the lymph nodes. Because viral concentrations are substantially greater in the lymph node, plasma measurements of HIV indirectly reflect spillover from replication in that compartment.[66,67]

Similar to CD4 counts, viral load measurements (copies/milliliter) can vary by as much as threefold (0.5 log) in either direction.[5] When obtaining a patient's baseline value, a number of issues must be considered. On initial infection with HIV, a burst of viremia occurs until the host's immune responses are able to control the infection. Consequently, viral load measurements obtained during the first 6 months of infection may not accurately reflect a true baseline value.[5] In addition, factors that activate the immune system, such as the development of a new opportunistic infection or immunizations,[68] can result in transient elevations of viral load measurements. In these situations, concentrations obtained within 4 weeks of the event may not accurately reflect the baseline viral load measurement.[5]

Some clinicians would recommend that at least two separate viral load measurements, which are obtained within 1 to 4 weeks of each other, be performed before making decisions regarding therapeutic options.[5] As with T-cell values, viral load measurements should be evaluated as trends.

In addition to quantifying the viral load, baseline resistance testing should be performed, using either genotypic or phenotypic testing,[5] to guide the selection of the initial regimen. Resistance testing is recommended in most clinical situations before beginning treatment, because the rate of transmission of virus resistant to at least one drug is estimated to be between 6% and 16% in European and American cohorts[69–71] (see Resistance, Viral Genotyping, Phenotyping, and Viral Fitness section for further discussion).

E.J. should have a baseline T-cell count, viral load measurement, and viral genotype obtained. A complete blood count, electrolyte panel, and renal and liver function tests should also be performed. If specific therapies are being considered, such as abacavir and maraviroc, specific testing is available to guide the appropriate use of these agents. HLA-B5701 screening is performed before starting a patient on abacavir due to an increased risk for exhibiting a hypersensitivity reaction in patients positive for this allele. Coreceptor tropism assay is performed before initiating maraviroc to determine whether the patient has a virus that predominantly uses CCR5 receptors (vs. ones that use primarily CXCR-4 receptors or ones that can use both).[5] These laboratory results help in selecting therapeutic options (see subsequent discussion) and establish baseline values in the event that problems are encountered in the future.

ANTIRETROVIRAL THERAPY

CASE 73-1, QUESTION 3: E.J.'s T-cell count and viral load measurement return at 225 cells/μL and 145,000 copies/mL (by RT-PCR assay), respectively. Should antiretroviral therapy be initiated?

In deciding to initiate antiretroviral therapy, it is important to consider both the potential benefits of therapy and the potential risk of therapy, including both short-term and long-term side effects and potential for the development of drug resistance (and cross-resistance; see subsequent discussion). Antiretroviral therapy should be offered to any patient who is symptomatic, regardless of T-cell count and viral load measurements. "Symptomatic" refers to any new opportunistic infection or increases in constitutional symptoms (e.g., fevers, night sweats, unexplained weight loss). These events suggest a faltering immune system that necessitates therapy. Additional clinical situations such as pregnancy, HIV-associated nephropathy, and hepatitis B necessitating treatment warrant the initiation of antiretroviral therapy regardless of surrogate marker data.[5] In patients who are asymptomatic, assessment of the patient's surrogate marker data (T-cell count, viral load measurements), concurrent medical conditions, medication adherence history (if any), and motivation to initiate therapy are necessary. The results of resistance testing should be considered before initiating therapy.

Knowledge of both the T-cell count and the baseline viral load values is necessary to "stage" the severity of infection. In otherwise healthy, immunocompetent persons, T-cell measurements are greater than 1,200 cells/μL. In patients who have been chronically infected with HIV, significant T-cell destruction occurs. When T-cell counts fall to less than 500 cells/μL, patients are at increased risk for opportunistic infections (Fig. 73-3). Data from both clinical trials and observational cohort studies have shown a clear benefit for antiretroviral therapy when CD4 cell counts are less than or equal to 350 cells/μL and many cohort analyses have shown benefit for starting therapy at CD4 counts less than or equal to 500 cells/μL.[3] Currently, the optimal time to initiate antiretroviral therapy in patients with CD4 cell counts greater than 500 cells/μL is unknown.

The risk of disease progression is closely tied to CD4 cell counts, with low CD4 counts (<200 cells/μL) predicting both short-term and long-term risk of disease progression.[72–74] High viral load (>100,000 copies/mL), increasing age, acquisition of infection through intravenous drug use, and a previous AIDS diagnosis also increase the risk of disease progression in observational cohorts. Based on these data, the US Department of Health and Human Services published guidelines on when to consider antiretroviral therapy in those infected with HIV (Table 73-4). These guidelines provide general principles for when to initiate therapy in an antiretroviral-naïve patient; however, they are not absolute. Most clinicians prefer to begin therapy before CD4 cell counts are less than 350 cells/μL, and many use less than 500 cells/μL as a point to begin discussions with the patient regarding initiating therapy. Increasing data from longitudinal cohort studies suggest that patients who begin HAART therapy at higher CD4 cell counts are more likely to achieve CD4 cell-count recovery than patients who begin at counts less than 200 cells/μL,[72–74] although the potential clinical implications of

TABLE 73-4
Indications for the Initiation of Antiretroviral Therapy in the Chronically HIV-1–Infected Patient[a]

Clinical Category	CD4+ T-Cell Count	Plasma HIV RNA	Recommendation
Symptomatic (AIDS, severe symptoms)	Any value	Any value	Treat
Asymptomatic	<350/μL	Any value	Treat
Asymptomatic	350–500/μL	Any value	Treatment should be offered
Asymptomatic	>500/μL	>100,000 copies/mL	Some clinicians may consider initiating treatment
Asymptomatic	>500/μL	<100,000 copies/mL	Many clinicians will decide to defer therapy

[a]The optimal time to initiate therapy in asymptomatic individuals with >500 CD4+ cells/μL is not known. This table provides general guidance rather than absolute recommendations for an individual patient. All decisions to initiate therapy should be based on prognosis as determined by the CD4+ T-cell count and plasma HIV RNA, the potential benefits and risks of therapy shown in Table 73-6, and the willingness of the patient to accept therapy.
AIDS, acquired immunodeficiency syndrome; HIV, human immunodeficiency virus.

this practice remain unknown. This finding, coupled with the ease of dosing and tolerability of new HAART regimens may tip the balance to early treatment. Thus, treatment is offered to patients with CD4 cell counts less than 500 cells/μL. In the case of CD4 cell counts greater than 500 cells/μL, many clinicians would defer treatment, unless viral load is very high (i.e., >100,000 copies/mL), which increases the potential for rapid CD4 cell-count decline, and the risk of disease progression. In this situation, clinicians may elect to offer therapy early to prevent further immune compromise.

The decision to initiate therapy should not be taken lightly nor should it be based solely on surrogate marker data. Antiretroviral regimens may improve the quality and duration of a patient's life, but they are not without significant risks. Once therapy is initiated, antiretroviral therapy is a lifetime commitment. For some patients, this may be a difficult realization, particularly if the patient is relatively healthy. In addition, the fear of adverse events and toxicities must also be overcome. These guidelines, therefore, should be used to initiate discussions with the patient regarding the risks and benefits of therapy. It is critical for practitioners to talk openly with patients about their fears and concerns and make an assessment about their motivation to initiate therapy and ability to adhere to a lifelong regimen. The patient should always make the final decision after careful discussions with the practitioner.

E.J. has a number of significant risk factors for disease progression. He is clinically symptomatic with oral thrush and nonspecific constitutional symptoms (e.g., fevers, night sweats, and weight loss). His surrogate maker data place him at risk for greater disease progression (T-cell count <500 cells/μL and viral load >100,000 copies/mL). Based on these values, E.J. should be counseled on his risk of disease progression, potential adverse events associated with both starting and deferring treatment, and his willingness to adhere to a regimen.

CASE 73-1, QUESTION 4: After careful discussions, E.J. agrees to initiate therapy. What should be the goals of therapy? What other factors or information needs to be considered in selecting an appropriate regimen?

Before developing a patient-specific regimen, it is important to recognize the benefits and limitations of therapy and identify obtainable and realistic goals.

Goals of Therapy

GOAL 1: MAXIMALLY AND DURABLY SUPPRESS VIRAL LOAD

Maximal viral suppression often results in significant increases in T-cell counts and improved clinical outcomes.[75] Based on our understanding of viral pathogenesis, this finding is not surprising. Lower amounts of replicating virus result in decreased risk for T-cell infection and destruction and, subsequently, a more intact immune response. Therefore, therapy should suppress viral replication to undetectable levels in the plasma (<50 copies/mL), for as long as possible.[5,7] The development of new antiretroviral agents with improved potency, low adverse event profiles, and more convenient dosing regimens (once or twice daily), makes viral suppression a reasonable goal in most patients, even those who previously have received multiple suboptimal regimens or failed therapy. In the treatment-experienced patient, however, special care must to given to designing a regimen that will suppress viral load, yet not contribute to the development of drug resistance that limits future treatment options. Consultation with an expert in antiretroviral resistance patterns is critical to designing a salvage regimen in such patients.

The development of drug resistance is also a consideration in the selection of regimens for patients who have not previously used antiretrovirals (antiretroviral naïve). In any given viral population, the potential exists for a spontaneous mutation to occur, which results in a resistant isolate. The larger the population, the greater the risk for mutations. HIV replication is a highly error-susceptible process, especially with the reverse transcriptase enzyme. Given the high rate of viral replication, the potential exists for the daily production of thousands of replication-competent viral mutations to each and every site on the HIV genome (~10,000 nucleotides in length).[6,36] Under selective pressures from inadequate antiretroviral therapies, spontaneously produced isolates with reduced susceptibility to the given regimen eventually flourish and repopulate the host. This fact is of particular concern given the potential for cross-resistance between antiretroviral agents (see the following discussion of resistance). Therefore, the use of a regimen that fully suppresses viral replication reduces the potential for mutations and the development of cross-resistance.

Although more than 20 US Food and Drug Administration (FDA)-approved antiretroviral agents are currently available to use in combination therapies, many of these agents display similar resistance profiles. Developing resistance to one or more agents in a given regimen may result in the loss of activity to other agents with similar resistance profiles (i.e., cross-resistance).[6] Whether or not drug resistance develops is determined by the genetic barrier associated with the individual antiretroviral drugs. Some drugs have low genetic barriers; that is, only one or two critical changes in the virus are necessary for resistance to occur. An example of a class of agents with a low genetic barrier is the NNRTIs. Only one critical point mutation in the viral genome is required for loss of activity for nevirapine, delavirdine, and efavirenz. This limitation is the reason for development of newer second-generation NNRTIs (etravirine) to improve the barrier to resistance. In contrast, the PIs have a wide genetic barrier which requires multiple changes to the viral genome to incur resistance.[6]

It should be recognized, however, that just because an agent has a low genetic barrier does not mean it is virologically inferior or less potent. Potent regimens containing NNRTIs are highly effective and provide durable treatment responses. The potency of the entire regimen[5] is critical to determining whether or not drug resistance develops. If viral replication is suppressed, the development of resistance will be minimal. When viral replication does occur, the greater the replication, the greater the risk for development of resistance. In those situations in which viral replication does occur, a inclusion of a drug with a low genetic barrier in the antiretroviral regimen may be risky and could result in the loss of activity of the drug, the development of cross-resistance to other drugs, or both. As a result, an antiretroviral regimen should be selected that has a high likelihood of suppressing viral replication and to which the patient will strictly adhere.

GOAL 2: PRESERVE AND STRENGTHEN THE IMMUNE SYSTEM

Decreasing viral replication usually leads to increased CD4 cell counts, which strengthens and preserves the immune system. With increased cell counts, patients are at lower risk for exhibiting opportunistic infections and death. With newer and improved regimens, strengthening and preserving the immune system may be possible even in treatment-experienced patients, although drug regimens must be designed carefully to prevent developing further resistance. Although full immune reconstitution may not be possible if the CD4 cell count is low for a long period of time, it is reasonable to try and restore immune function as fully

TABLE 73-5

Recommended Antiretroviral Agents for Initial Treatment of Established Human Immunodeficiency Virus Infection[a]

	Preferred	Alternatives
NNRTIs (one NNRTI + two NRTIs)	Efavirenz[b] + tenofovir/emtricitabine	Efavirenz + abacavir/lamivudine Rilpivirine/tenofovir/emtricitabine
PIs (one or two PIs + two NRTIs)	Atazanavir/ritonavir + tenofovir/emtricitabine Darunavir once daily/ritonavir + tenofovir/emtricitabine	Rilpivirine + abacavir/lamivudine Atazanavir/ritonavir + abacavir/lamivudine Darunavir/ritonavir + abacavir/lamivudine Fosamprenavir/ritonavir (once or twice daily) + abacavir/lamivudine or tenofovir/emtricitabine Lopinavir/ritonavir (coformulated once or twice daily) + abacavir/lamivudine or tenofovir/emtricitabine Raltegravir + abacavir/lamivudine
Integrase inhibitors	Raltegravir twice daily + tenofovir/emtricitabine	
Not recommended: Should not be offered	All monotherapies, dual-nucleoside regimens, triple-NRTI regimens	

[a] This table provides a guide to the use of available treatment regimens for individuals with no prior or limited experience on HIV therapy. In accordance with the established goals of HIV therapy, priority is given to regimens in which clinical trial data suggest the following: sustained suppression of HIV plasma RNA (particularly in patients with high baseline viral load), sustained increase in CD4+ T-cell count (in most cases >48 weeks), and favorable clinical outcome (i.e., delayed progression to AIDS and death). Additional consideration is given to the regimen's pill burden, dosing frequency, food requirements, convenience, toxicity, and drug interaction profile compared with other regimens. It is important to note that all antiretroviral agents have potentially serious toxic and adverse events associated with their use.

[b] Except during the first trimester of pregnancy or in women with high pregnancy potential (women who are trying to conceive or who are not using effective and consistent contraception).

[c] As an alternative in women with CD4+ T-cell counts <250 cells/μL and men with CD4+ T-cell counts ≤400 cells/μL.

[d] When used with tenofovir, atazanavir should be combined with ritonavir 100 mg/d.

AIDS, acquired immunodeficiency syndrome; HIV, human immunodeficiency virus; NRTI, nucleos(t)ide analog reverse transcriptase inhibitor; NNRTI, non-nucleos(t)ide analog reverse transcriptase inhibitor; PI, protease inhibitor.

as possible. Despite advances in drug therapy, it is important to remember that HIV remains an incurable condition.

GOAL 3: LIMIT DRUG ADVERSE EVENTS, PROMOTE ADHERENCE, AND IMPROVE QUALITY OF LIFE

Treatment with combination therapy has been shown to be highly effective in suppressing HIV replication and improving survival among patients who are HIV infected. Lifelong adherence to an antiretroviral regimen is required and can be a complex and difficult task,[4,75] although advances in coformulation of drug products and the advent of ritonavir-boosted protease inhibitors have simplified treatment considerably. Several once-daily regimens are recommended as first-line therapy (Tables 73-3 and 73-5). The patient's ability to adhere to therapy may, however, still be the difference between a regimen that fails and one that results in a clinical benefit. The first regimen generally provides the best chance for treatment success. Adverse events can make tolerating these regimens difficult, which can then affect drug adherence and response to therapy. Changes in body composition (known as lipodystrophy), increases in lipids and triglycerides, bone and joint fractures, increased risks for cardiac disease, and the development of lactic acidosis are serious concerns.[76] In addition, both acute and long-term adverse events can be fatal if not properly identified and managed.

LIMIT ADVERSE EVENTS

Metabolic complications from antiretroviral therapy include abnormal distribution of body fat, lipid abnormalities (e.g., hypercholesterolemia, hypertriglyceridemia, increases in low-density lipoprotein [LDL] and decreases in high-density lipoprotein [HDL]), and new-onset diabetes.[77–85] Coronary artery disease, myocardial infarctions, and vascular complications among relatively young patients (30–40 years old) taking HAART-containing regimens have been reported.[86–91] Large observational studies suggest an increased risk for cardiovascular disease among patients taking HAART, particularly among those receiving protease inhibitors.[78,92–94] Additionally, nucleoside analogs can inhibit mitochondrial DNA polymerase and, as a result, have been implicated in lipoatrophy.[95] Finally, metabolic abnormalities have also been reported in patients who are HIV infected before receiving HAART, and may also be a consequence of HIV infection or pre-existing metabolic disorders that are exacerbated by HAART.[79]

Up to 40% of patients on PI-based HAART are reported to experience impaired glucose tolerance due to significant insulin resistance.[96] Patients with type 2 diabetes mellitus are at increased risk, and PI-based regimens should be avoided in these patients.[79] Fasting glucose measures for all patients are recommended before and during therapy (e.g., every 3–6 months) with PI-based regimens.[79] Treatment of type 2 diabetes in HIV patients as a result of HAART therapy should be handled similarly to any other patient.

Elevations in serum levels of triglycerides, total cholesterol, and LDL, with mild decreases in HDL, are associated with HAART.[79,97,98] These abnormalities may be seen as early as 2 weeks after the initiation of therapy.[79] Although all PIs have been implicated, these laboratory abnormalities appear to occur more frequently in ritonavir-containing regimens, and less frequently in patients receiving atazanavir alone.[79] The NNRTIs can also cause lipid alterations, although their incidence is lower. Both efavirenz and nevirapine have been shown to increase HDL concentrations among patients receiving HAART. Nevirapine may have the least detrimental lipid profile (i.e., greater increases in HDL concentrations and less effect on LDL elevations).[99] Of the NRTIs, stavudine appears to affect lipid profiles to the greatest extent: two prospective clinical trials have shown greater increases in triglycerides and total cholesterol among patients receiving stavudine-based HAART compared with zidovudine- or tenofovir-based regimens.[100–101] The management of HAART-associated hyperlipidemias should be handled similarly to hyperlipidemia in other patients with close attention paid to preventing drug–drug interactions.

Up to 40% to 50% of patients have been reported to experience alterations in body composition (fat loss [arms, legs, face, buttocks] and fat accumulation [dorsocervical fatty deposits or "buffalo humps"], increased abdominal girth), although the exact rate is confounded by differences in definition and assessment.[79] Risk factors for this complication include higher baseline body mass index, increased duration of exposure to antiretroviral agents, lower CD4 nadir at time of initiation of HAART, increasing age, female sex, and prolonged duration of HIV infection. The nucleoside analogs are likely responsible for lipoatrophy, whereas the PIs are believed to be responsible for lipoaccumulation,[79] although it is difficult to precisely identify which class of agents is responsible for which adverse event because they are given in combination.

The causes of lipodystrophy are unknown. It appears that there is greater propensity for lipoatrophy by those nucleoside analogs which greatly inhibit mitochondrial DNA polymerase in vitro (e.g., stavudine). Although substituting stavudine with an alternate NRTI such as zidovudine, tenofovir, or abacavir is associated with significant increases in arm and leg fat, and decreases in trunk fat (using radiographic tests such as dual-energy x-ray absorptiometry, computed tomography scans), these improvements are so modest that they may not be clinically relevant.[80,102–106] The use of recombinant human growth hormone, an agent with lipolytic effects, decreases the size of buffalo humps and abdominal girth; however, the growth often returns once growth hormone therapy is stopped.[79] Tesamorelin, a growth hormone–releasing factor given as a 2-mg once daily subcutaneous injection, was approved in 2010. It is specifically indicated for the reduction of excess abdominal fat in HIV-infected patients with lipodystrophy.[107] Surgical excision or liposuction may be effective; however, recurrences, along with adverse events (intestinal perforation, intraperitoneal bleeding) have been reported.[108] For facial wasting, injection of fat or synthetic polymers into the recessed areas of the cheeks have shown good results but require frequent costly administration, and lack long-term safety data.[109,110]

Other important long-term complications include nucleoside-associated lactic acidosis, osteonecrosis, and osteopenia.[79] Lactic acidosis has been predominantly associated with the use of stavudine, but has been reported with other nucleoside analogs. This complication is managed by discontinuing therapy until lactate levels return to normal and then reinitiating therapy with a non-stavudine or non-nucleoside analog-containing HAART regimen.[5]

PROMOTE ADHERENCE

Data from studies evaluating nonadherence among those who are HIV infected shows that at least 10% of patients on PIs miss a dose each day and that at least 20% miss a dose every 2 days.[111] The exact degree of adherence required for clinical success is currently unknown, and patients should be counseled to always take their regimens as prescribed. The four most common reasons for skipping antiretroviral doses are: simple forgetfulness, a change in daily routine, being too busy with other things, and being away from home.[83,112] Factors associated with poor adherence include (a) the number of medications (the greater the number, the greater the likelihood of poor adherence); (b) the complexity of the regimen (special meal requirements, escalating or de-escalating doses, dose frequency); (c) special storage requirements; (d) interference of medication with lifestyle and daily activities; and (e) poor communication with primary care providers and other health care professionals. Comorbid psychiatric conditions, as well as substance abuse issues, are also significant barriers to adherence in the HIV infected population. Incorporating these factors into the selection of a patient-specific regimen may improve adherence and, subsequently, the chance for an improved clinical outcome and quality of life.

GOAL 4: PREVENT HUMAN IMMUNODEFICIENCY VIRUS–RELATED MORBIDITY AND MORTALITY

By successfully treating HIV (suppressing viral load and restoring immune function), patients are at decreased risk for acquiring HIV-associated opportunistic infections (Fig. 73-3). By achieving goals 1 through 3, goal 4 naturally follows, and truly this is the ultimate goal of the pharmacotherapy of HIV infection. With modern-day HAART therapy, patients infected with HIV are dying more frequently from non–HIV-related conditions common in the general population (i.e., cardiovascular disease, hepatic disease, non–HIV-associated malignancies).[113] Although this represents a significant achievement in care, it also provides increased complexity in caring for those who are both at risk for HIV-related illness and also receiving treatment for comorbid conditions. This increases the potential for drug–drug and drug–disease interactions.

CASE 73-1, QUESTION 5: On questioning, E.J. states that he has had two bouts of alcohol-induced pancreatitis in the past. The last episode was approximately 1 year ago. He admits to occasional binge drinking even though he knows it is not good for him. E.J. has no known drug allergies and is currently taking only temazepam periodically to help him sleep. His father has a history of coronary artery disease. He is employed as a construction worker and is extremely busy during the day, so he prefers to take medications only one time daily. His complete blood count, electrolyte, and liver and renal panel all return within normal limits. E.J. has no particular preference for a specific regimen and appears highly motivated to take control of his disease. What factors should be considered when selecting an appropriate antiretroviral regimen?

The selection of a patient-specific regimen can be a complex decision. Many potential combinations can be used, but a number of general principles should be followed.[5,7]

General Rules of Therapy

1. Initiate therapy when the potential clinical benefits outweigh the potential risks. Many of the current regimens reduce viral replication to less than detectable levels in most patients, and result in durable treatment responses. Reasons for the current improved response rates include the simplification of the regimens (e.g., fewer pills per day, less frequent dosing per day, use of fixed-dose combination products), improvement in overall potency of the regimens, and minimization of short-term side effects. Consequently, if the correct patient-specific HAART regimen is selected as initial therapy, the patient should be able to adhere to therapy and gain both a virologic and clinical benefit from the regimen.
2. Select the type of antiretroviral regimen. The use of combination HAART therapy should be the standard medical care for all patients. Monotherapy and the use of dual nucleoside-only–containing regimens should be avoided because initial viral suppression is not sustained. In general, three types of initial strategies (NNRTI-based, PI-based, or integrase inhibitor [INSTI]-based) are preferred (Table 73-6). All three types of regimens can produce sustained virologic response. Currently, no evidence definitively recommends one type over another, and the selection is dependent on patient-specific factors, such as concomitant disease states (i.e., hepatitis, diabetes, cardiovascular disease), and provider preference.
3. Avoid regimens with overlapping toxicities. In general, the concomitant use of the "D" NRTIs (didanosine [ddI] and stavudine [d4T]) should be avoided owing to an increased risk of

TABLE 73-6
Advantages and Disadvantages of Antiretroviral Components for Initial Antiretroviral Therapy[a]

ARV Class	Possible Advantages	Possible Disadvantages
Dual NRTI	• Established backbone of combination antiretroviral therapy • Less fat maldistribution and dyslipidemia than PI-based regimens	• Rare but serious cases of lactic acidosis with hepatic steatosis reported (d4T > ddI = ZDV > TDF = ABC = 3TC = FTC) • Low genetic barrier to resistance (single mutation confers resistance)
NNRTI	• Save PIs and RAL for future use • Long half-lives	• Low genetic barrier to resistance • Cross resistance among approved NNRTIs • Skin rash • Potential for cytochrome P-450 drug interactions • Transmitted resistance to NNRTIs more common than with PIs
PI	• Save NNRTIs for future use • Higher genetic barrier to resistance • PI resistance uncommon with failure (boosted PIs)	• Metabolic complications (fat maldistribution, dyslipidemia, insulin resistance) • Cytochrome P-450 substrates, inhibitors, and inducers (potential for drug interactions)
INSTI	Fewer drug-related adverse effects than efavirenz in studies with RAL Fewer drug–drug interactions than NNRTI-based or PI-based regimens	Less long-term experience in treatment-naïve patients than with boosted PI-based or NNRTI-based regimens Lower genetic barrier to resistance than boosted PI-based regimens

[a] Adapted from DHHS treatment guidelines January 2011.
ABC, abacavir; ARV, antiretroviral; ddI, didanosine; DHHS, Department of Health and Human Services; d4T, stavudine; FTC, emtricitabine; NNRTI, non-nucleoside reverse transcriptase inhibitors; NRTI, nucleoside reverse transcriptase inhibitor; PI, protease inhibitor; INSTI, integrase strand transfer inhibitor; RAL, raltegravir; TDF, tenofovir disoproxil fumarate; 3TC, lamivudine; ZDV, zidovudine.

pancreatitis and neuropathy. Atazanavir and indinavir can both cause severe hyperbilirubinemia, and concomitant use should be avoided.

4. Avoid regimens that are not virologically additive or synergistic. Zidovudine (ZDV) and d4T should not be used together because both in vitro and in vivo studies have shown these agents to be antagonistic. Lamivudine (3TC) and emtricitabine (FTC) should not be used together because they have similar resistance profiles, and concomitant use will not confer any additional virologic benefit. The use of tenofovir and ddI as initial therapy is not recommended due to the potential for virologic failure, suboptimal immunologic response, and the potential for development of drug resistance.
5. If PI-based HAART is desired, ritonavir-boosted regimens are preferred. Ritonavir, a potent inhibitor of cytochrome P-450 metabolism and P-glycoprotein activity, interacts significantly with a number of agents, including other PIs. This inhibition can be exploited to decrease the metabolism or increase the absorption of the other PIs. In some cases, such as in the use of lopinavir, tipranavir, and darunavir, the use of coadministered ritonavir is required for virologically relevant concentrations. The result is a regimen with more potent viral suppression than a regimen using either agent alone. In addition, this combination allows for more convenient once-daily or twice-daily dosing, often lowers the total daily pill burden, and removes the need for drug/food restrictions. Given that ritonavir can cause significant gastrointestinal side effects at increased doses and that only small amounts of ritonavir are needed to inhibit metabolism, low doses are sufficient (e.g., no more than 200 mg per dose). Because ritonavir interacts with a number of medications, concomitant medications may require dosage adjustments, depending on the severity of the interaction.[5,7]
6. Avoid regimens shown to be detrimental in specific patient populations. Examples include the use of efavirenz (pregnancy class D) in women of child-bearing potential not using reliable methods of birth control or in the first trimester of pregnancy. This is due to an association with teratogenic effects in animals. Nevirapine has the potential for hepatotoxicity in patients with higher baseline CD4 cell counts (>250 cells/μL for women, >400 cells/μL for men).

CASE 73-1, QUESTION 6: What initial antiretroviral regimen should E.J. receive?

When selecting a patient-specific regimen, the following steps should be followed.

STEP 1: DETERMINE WHICH HIGHLY ACTIVE ANTIRETROVIRAL THERAPY–BASED REGIMEN WILL BE USED

A careful review of the advantages and disadvantages of each interventional strategy should occur (Table 73-6). For example, efavirenz may be avoided for patients with a psychiatric history. Protease inhibitors may be less favored with a familial history or current medical condition consisting of coronary artery disease, hyperlipidemia, or diabetes mellitus.[76]

After discussions with E.J., it appears that he is highly motivated to take control of his disease and is willing to initiate therapy. Subsequently, the use of a combination regimen with either a PI-based, NNRTI-based or INSTI-based regimen is appropriate. Potential treatment options are listed in Table 73-5.

STEP 2: OPTIMIZE AGENTS IN THE REGIMEN

The next step requires the selection of agents for the regimen. In many situations, absolute contraindications and significant drug–drug interactions limit the agents available for use in the regimen. In this case, ddI is a relative contraindication given a history of alcohol abuse and pancreatitis. The remaining nucleoside or nucleotide reverse transcriptase inhibitors, including ZDV, 3TC, d4T, tenofovir (TDF), FTC, and abacavir (ABC), are all potential options. With respect to drug interaction issues, any NNRTI, PI, or INSTI can be administered safely with temazepam. Given his family history of coronary artery disease, a protease inhibitor may be a less favorable option.

STEP 3: QUALITY-OF-LIFE CONSIDERATIONS

When selecting a regimen, assessment of quality-of-life issues, potential adverse drug events, and patient preference should receive as much consideration as drug–drug interactions and absolute contraindications. In some situations, these issues could mean the difference between a regimen that is effective and one that is not. Considering E.J.'s lifestyle and work requirements, it is best to select a regimen that will minimally interfere with his daily activities. The selection of a regimen with once-daily or twice-daily dosing is appropriate (Table 73-3), although once-daily dosing might be preferred. The combination of nucleosides recommended as initial therapy can be given once daily, and is available as a coformulated product (Table 73-3). An example of a potential regimen is FTC plus TDF (dosed once daily) with efavirenz (the preferred first-line NNRTI). Using the same nucleoside agents, atazanavir/ritonavir or darunavir–ritonavir (both administered once daily) would be the preferred PI-based regimens. Raltegravir twice daily, in combination with nucleoside agents, is the preferred INSTI regimen.

CASE 73-1, QUESTION 7: E.J. is starting emtricitabine, tenofovir, and efavirenz (coformulated for once-daily dosing as Atripla). How should therapy be monitored? Are any additional laboratory tests necessary?

Short-Term Assessments

Three important criteria determine whether an antiretroviral regimen is effective: clinical assessment, surrogate marker responses, and regimen tolerability.[5,7] In patients who are clinically symptomatic (e.g., constitutional symptoms such as fatigue, night sweats, and weight loss; new opportunistic infections), the initiation of an appropriate antiretroviral regimen often results in resolution of symptoms, increased strength and energy, and improvement in overall well-being. In some patients, however, the effect may not be as prominent. A careful assessment of clinical symptoms should therefore be regularly performed at all follow-up appointments.

In all patients, repeat viral load and T-cell measurements are necessary. This early value allows clinicians to assess the magnitude of response and ensures declining viral load measurements. Therapy with an effective regimen will result in at least a threefold (0.5 log) and tenfold decrease (1.0 log) in viral load counts by weeks 4 and 8, respectively.[5,7] The viral load should continue to decline during the next 12 to 16 weeks and, in most patients, it will become undetectable.[5,7] Long-term response to therapy correlates with the magnitude of viral suppression on initiation of a regimen. The greater the suppression, the greater the durability of response to that regimen.[114–116] The speed and magnitude of suppression, however, can be affected by a number of factors, including clinical status of the patient (e.g., more advanced disease–low T-cell counts, high viral load value), adherence to therapy, and overall potency of the regimen.[5,7] When the virologic response is less than optimal, evaluation of compliance should be assessed, repeat viral load measurements performed, and drug concentrations of key antiretroviral agents evaluated for subtherapeutic values before considering a change in therapy.

In response to declining viral replication, T-cell destruction slows, and eventually cellular repopulation occurs. The magnitude of this T-cell increase can vary significantly, with some patients experiencing large increases (≥500 cells/μL) and others experiencing little or no change. Given that T-cell changes do not occur rapidly, once therapy is initiated, repeat T-cell counts should be obtained at 3-month to 4-month intervals.[5,7]

Drug failure (defined by either surrogate markers or clinical symptomatology) is associated with subtherapeutic serum antiretroviral concentrations. The most common reason for this finding is nonadherence to the prescribed regimen. Reasons for nonadherence must be quickly and adequately addressed (e.g., by education on the management of adverse events, optimizing dose-taking strategies, or switching to a better-tolerated regimen). Drug exposures can also be affected by the addition of new drugs or herbal products to a patient's regimen. Both garlic and St. John's wort have been shown to lower the exposure to non–ritonavir-boosted protease inhibitors.[5,7,117,118] In addition, certain medications require specific food requirements to ensure optimal exposure (Table 73-3). Therefore, careful evaluation of new prescription and over-the-counter drugs, nutraceuticals, and dosing habits should be performed at each follow-up visit. If after discussions with the patient, the clinician does not identify adverse events, adherence issues, and new drug interactions as potential causes of failure, then changing to another viable regimen should be considered. In some cases, therapeutic drug monitoring may assist in identifying physiologic factors such as malabsorption or rapid metabolism.

A seemingly worsening of symptoms may also occur after the initiation of potent antiretroviral therapies due to immune reconstitution.[119–121] In patients with advanced HIV disease (i.e., CD4 <100 cells/μL), significant immune dysfunction results in an inability to mount an appropriate response to subclinical infections. As a result, these infections replicate unimpeded and often undetected by the host (also known as quiescent disease). During the first 12 weeks of therapy, an increased immune response results from redistribution of memory cells[122–124] and inflammation at the site of infection occurs. The immune reconstitution syndrome can present in any organ system where quiescent disease exists (e.g., CNS, eyes, lymph nodes). Most cases occur within 1 to 4 weeks after the initiation of potent antiretroviral therapies. Although most reports of immune system reconstitution and inflammatory responses have been associated with concomitant opportunistic infections, the recurrence of drug-induced hypersensitivity reactions can also occur.[125]

CASE 73-1, QUESTION 8: After initiation of therapy, E.J.'s viral load values are 7,000 copies/mL at 4 weeks, and less than 50 copies/mL (undetectable) at 14 weeks. His T-cell counts have increased from 225 to 525 cells/μL. In addition, E.J. states that his night sweats and fevers have disappeared, he "feels great" and that he has had no drug-related problems. Is the therapy effective? How should therapy be monitored?

E.J.'s response to the emtricitabine, tenofovir, and efavirenz does indicate efficacy. Clinically, his symptoms have subsided and his overall health is much improved. His viral load measurements have responded appropriately and are now less than the level of assay detection. T-cell counts have increased by 300 cells/μL. Finally, E.J. has experienced no drug-related adverse events. Given the response to date, no changes are required and the current regimen should be continued.

Long-Term Assessments

Once the prescribed regimen has been stabilized, the long-term goals are to maintain maximal viral suppression, sustain clinical and immunologic improvements, and maintain drug tolerability. Periodic assessments should be made of viral load (every 3–4 months) and T-cell counts (every 3–6 months).[5,7] These surrogate marker data allow clinicians to monitor trends in viral activity and immunologic status and assist them in identifying early regimen failure. Clinical assessment of the patient and questioning of tolerability to the prescribed regimen should occur at the 3-month to 6-month follow-up visits.

Treatment Failure

CASE 73-1, QUESTION 9: E.J. has remained on FTC, TDF, and efavirenz for more than a year. To date, his T-cell counts have remained stable at 550 cells/μL, and his viral load measurements have remained less than the limit of assay detection. He presents with new complaints of fevers and malaise. E.J. reports that he has been compliant with therapy and has not started any new medications. Repeat laboratory tests now show E.J.'s viral load is 3,000 copies/mL and his T-cell count is 375 cells/μL (both repeated and validated). Should E.J.'s regimen be changed?

Up to 25% of patient on HAART fail therapy within the first year.[3] Reasons for failure are not fully known; however, risk factors include a history of low initial T-cell counts, high initial viral loads, and extensive use of antiretroviral agents.[3,4] Assessment of regimen failure should be based on: (a) clinical symptoms, (b) surrogate marker data, and (c) regimen tolerability and adherence.[5–7]

In many patients, the first sign of failure is a change in signs and symptoms. These changes can be subtle (e.g., increase in constitutional symptoms, new onset of oral thrush) or more severe (e.g., new opportunistic infections) and suggest a failing regimen and need to change therapy.

Assessment of efficacy should also involve evaluation of surrogate marker data (e.g., T cells and viral load). In many situations, changes to these markers occur before any noticeable clinical signs and symptoms. Therefore, careful evaluation of surrogate marker data may allow for intervention before any significant immune destruction occurs. Virologic failure, defined as new or continued viral replication despite appropriate antiretroviral therapy, suggests a failing regimen. For example, patients with repeated detection of virus in plasma after initial suppression to undetectable levels should be evaluated as potential treatment failures. In patients who do not achieve viral suppression to less than detectable levels, a significant increase in viral replication (defined as a threefold increase or greater) should also be viewed as a treatment failure.[5,6]

When assessing viral load, it is important to recognize that these values can increase from vaccinations or other concurrent infections (see Case 73-1, Question 2). Therefore, a thorough medical history should be taken to rule out other causes of increasing viral load. In addition, laboratory values should be interpreted as trends over time and not necessarily as individual measurements. A repeat viral load should be performed and evaluated within 4 weeks of the initial viral load increase. In some cases, transient viral "blips" occur (increases in viral load measurements just above the level of assay detection (e.g., 50–1,000 copies/mL), which become undetectable at the next visit.[126–128] The clinical significance of viral blips is unknown and, although they may not directly reflect treatment failure, they may represent near future viral breakthrough, either because of patient nonadherence or insufficient antiretroviral potency. Careful follow-up of these patients is required, as changes to the current HAART regimen may be necessary.

In response to increasing viral replication, T-cell destruction occurs. A significant decrease in CD4 cells is defined as a decrease of more than 30% in absolute numbers, or a decrease of 3% in percentage.[5,6] Persistently declining T-cell counts, with or without increasing viral load measurements, represent treatment failure and suggest a change in therapy is warranted.

Other potential causes for failure include nonadherence and drug–drug interactions. In the event of nonadherence, discussions regarding tolerability, number of doses missed, duration of nonadherence, and lifestyle changes should take place. The decision to reinitiate a prescribed regimen should take into account the future likelihood of adherence and the potential development of resistant strains. In those patients with a history of long-standing nonadherence, the success of reinitiating the prescribed regimen may be limited. Stopping all antiretrovirals for a patient imposed drug "holiday" poses less risk for the development of resistance than intermittent adherence to some or all of a regimen. The precise effect of the duration and extent of nonadherence on the development of resistance, however, has not been fully evaluated. For the virus to mutate, sufficient drug pressure must be placed on the virus. Some estimate this requires moderate patient adherence of 50%.

Significant drug interactions could also contribute to reduction in oral bioavailability or increased metabolism of the HIV medications leading to low serum concentrations, resulting in failure.[5,117,118] In addition, many medications require certain food requirements to allow maximal drug absorption. A careful review of all new medications and their potential for clinically significant drug interactions should be evaluated at all visits (Table 73-7).

Currently, E.J. has a number of signs and symptoms that suggest a failing regimen. E.J. is experiencing new symptoms of fevers and malaise not attributable to any other cause. E.J.'s viral load value has become detectable at 3,000 copies/mL without evidence of concurrent infections or vaccinations in the past 4 weeks. E.J.'s T-cell counts have declined from 550 cells/μL to 375 cells/μL. Finally, it appears that E.J. has been adhering to his therapy and has not started any new medications that could affect the efficacy of his current regimen. Therefore, a change in therapy is necessary.

CASE 73-1, QUESTION 10: What potential antiretroviral regimen(s) can be considered for E.J.?

In addition to the general rules of therapy described in Case 73-1, Question 5, other issues should be considered when selecting an alternative regimen for a patient failing therapy.[5,6]

GENERAL RULES FOR CHANGING THERAPIES

1. If possible, the new regimen should contain only antiretroviral agents to which the patient has not been exposed. If this is not possible, the new regimen should contain at least two new agents that are not currently contained in the failing regimen. The potential for cross-resistance between antiretroviral drugs should be considered when choosing new regimens, and therefore resistance testing should provide useful information (see Case 73-1, Question 12).
2. Given that antiretroviral drug resistance is more likely to occur with increased and prolonged viral replication in the presence of antiretroviral agents, changes to therapy should occur close to the time of treatment failure. Prolonged treatment with a failing regimen is likely to result in the accumulation of resistance mutations (particularly with protease inhibitors), which may limit future treatment options.
3. Resistance testing is recommended to guide the selection of future drug regimens. Optimally, testing via genotype, phenotype, or virtual phenotype should occur while the patient is taking the failing regimen, or within 4 weeks of discontinuation to increase the likelihood of detecting resistant isolates. These tests cannot reliably detect mutations at viral concentrations less than 1,000 copies/mL, and may have limited usefulness in patients with persistent low-level viremia.
4. To prevent the development of resistance, one new drug should never be added to a failing regimen. An exception to this rule is if the initial response to a first regimen has been

TABLE 73-7

Drugs That Should not be Coadministered With Antiretrovirals (at any dose unless otherwise indicated)[5]

	Cardiac Agents	Lipid-Lowering Agents	Anti-Infectants	Gastrointestinal Drugs	Psychotropic Agents	Anticonvulsants	Pulmonary Agents	Herbs	Others	ARV Agents
ATV ± RTV	Bosentan[a]	Lovastatin Pitavastatin Simvastatin	Rifampin Rifapentine Voriconazole[b]	Cisapride PPIs[c]	Midazolam Triazolam		Salmeterol Sildenafil (for PAH) Fluticasone[d]	St. John's wort	Alfuzosin Irinotecan Buprenorphine[e]	ETR NVP
DRV/r		Lovastatin Pitavastatin Simvastatin	Rifampin Rifapentine Voriconazole[b]	Cisapride	Midazolam Triazolam		Salmeterol Sildenafil (for PAH) Fluticasone[c]	St. John's wort	Alfuzosin	
FPV ± RTV	Flecainide Propafenone	Lovastatin Pitavastatin Simvastatin	Rifampin Rifapentine Voriconazole[b]	Cisapride	Midazolam Triazolam		Salmeterol Sildenafil (for PAH) Fluticasone[c]	St. John's wort	Alfuzosin	ETR
LPV/r		Lovastatin Pitavastatin Simvastatin	Rifampin Rifapentine Voriconazole[b]	Cisapride	Midazolam Triazolam	Carbamazepine[f] Phenobarbital[f] Phenytoin[f]	Salmeterol Sildenafil (for PAH) Fluticasone[c]	St. John's wort	Alfuzosin	
TPV/r	Amiodarone Flecainide Propafenone Quinidine	Lovastatin Pitavastatin Simvastatin	Rifampin Rifapentine Voriconazole[b]	Cisapride	Midazolam Triazolam		Salmeterol Sildenafil (for PAH) Fluticasone[c]	St. John's wort	Alfuzosin	ETR
EFV			Rifapentine Voriconazole[b]	Cisapride	Midazolam Triazolam			St. John's wort		Other NNRTIs
ETR			Rifampin Rifapentine			Carbamazepine Phenobarbital Phenytoin		St. John's wort	Clopidogrel	Unboosted PIs ATV/r, FPV/r, or TPV/r Other NNRTIs
NVP			Rifapentine Ketoconazole					St. John's wort		ATV ± RTV Other NNRTIs
MVC			Rifapentine					St. John's wort		

[a] Bosentan not recommended if ATV is unboosted.
[b] Do not coadminister with boosted PIs unless benefit outweighs risk and do not coadminister with EFV at standard doses (voriconazole 400 mg BID, EFV 300 mg daily).
[c] PPIs are not recommended if ATV is unboosted or in treatment experienced patients.
[d] Do not coadminister inhaled or intranasal fluticasone with boosted PIs unless benefit outweighs risk of systemic corticosteroid adverse effects.
[e] Do not coadminister with unboosted ATV.
[f] Not recommended if LPV/r is given once daily.
ATV, atazanavir; DRV/r, darunavir/ritonavir; EFV, efavirenz; ETR, etravirine; FPV, fosamprenavir; LPV/r, lopinavir/ritonavir; MVC, maraviroc; NVP, nevirapine; RTV, ritonavir; TPV/r, tipranavir/ritonavir.

inadequate (e.g., undetectable viral load at 16–20 weeks). In this situation, some clinicians may intensify therapy with an additional agent provided that the viral load measurements were trending downward since initiation of therapy.

5. If possible, a regimen that has failed in the past should not be reinitiated, as an isolate resistant to the failed regimen could continue to reside within various compartments of the body. If a regimen to which the patient had previously failed were restarted, unimpeded viral replication of the resistant strain would occur, repopulate the host, and eventually result in treatment failure. In some situations (e.g., patients with advanced disease, limited treatment options, and prior exposure to most antiretroviral agents), it may be necessary to reinitiate agents or regimens in combination with additional new agents with the goal of suppressing viral replication.
6. When treatment failure is a direct result of drug toxicity (rather than poor drug efficacy), the offending agent should be replaced with an alternative drug from a similar class, provided that the potential for cross-resistance is minimal.
7. If an agent in a given regimen must be stopped, it is recommended that all agents in the regimen be stopped and restarted simultaneously to prevent the development of resistance. An exception to this rule is when components of a regimen have differing half-lives, such as NNRTIs and NRTIs. In this situation, if all drugs are discontinued simultaneously, continued monotherapy exposure with the NNRTI is likely to result, due to the much longer NNRTI half-life. Consequently, many experts recommend continuing the NRTIs for 1 to 2 weeks past NNRTI discontinuation to provide combination therapy while the NNRTI is eliminated from the body (covering the "tail" of the pharmacokinetic profile).

It should be recognized that many alternative regimens are based on theoretical benefits or limited data. In addition, many potential options could be limited in some patients based on prior antiretroviral use, toxicity, or past intolerances. Therefore, the clinician should carefully discuss these issues with the patient before changing therapy.

Because E.J. is failing to respond to his current regimen, a new antiretroviral regimen must be chosen. In addition to selecting susceptible agents from resistance testing, the new regimen should take into consideration quality-of-life issues. In E.J.'s situation, it is reasonable to switch to a ritonavir-boosted PI regimen, with two or more nucleoside agents as dictated by the viral resistance profile.

Considerations in Antiretroviral-Experienced Patients

CASE 73-2

QUESTION 1: H.G. is a 46-year-old, HIV-positive man with an extensive history of treatment with a variety of antiretroviral agents. He took ZDV monotherapy in the late 1980s and early 1990s. When 3TC became available, he took the combination of ZDV and 3TC until he failed therapy about 15 years ago. At that time, he began experiencing ZDV-induced myopathies. Since that time, H.G. has been "on and off" various regimens without sustained clinical benefit. He is currently taking TDF, FTC, and lopinavir/ritonavir with a CD4 count and viral load measurement of 55 cells/μL and 48,000 copies/mL, respectively. These laboratory values have been stable for the last 9 months. How do patients with extensive antiretroviral histories differ from antiretroviral-naïve patients? Are there any special considerations when selecting therapeutic regimens for patients such as H.G.?

Patients who have been infected for 15 or more years may have been treated with many different regimens, both experimental and FDA-approved. As a result, many potential regimens have already been exhausted; thus, there are not many viable choices left. Many patients previously treated with multiple antiretroviral regimens will exhibit a decreased response and decreased durability to older protease inhibitors such as indinavir and nelfinavir.[5,6] Several newer agents, such as tipranavir, darunavir, etravirine, and enfuvirtide, have been developed specifically for highly treatment-experienced patients: These may achieve viral suppression in these patients. Maraviroc, the first CCR5 receptor antagonist approved by the FDA, is also an option for treatment-experienced patients infected with HIV-1 utilizing this coreceptor and failing current treatment. Maraviroc is not recommended for use in patients with dual-trophic viral populations (i.e., able to use CXCR-4 or CCR5 as coreceptors) or CXCR-4-trophic virus and, thus, patients with extensive treatment histories should undergo tropism testing before maraviroc is initiated. Additionally, raltegravir has a novel mechanism of action that allow for its use in patients with extensive reverse transcriptase or protease mutations. Some highly treatment-experienced individuals will have extensive resistance patterns that limit their therapeutic options. In such patients, full suppression of viral load and immune reconstitution may not be possible.[5,6]

Patients who have experienced several antiretroviral regimens present other unique challenges for clinicians and require consideration of the following factors.

1. *Regimen tolerability:* Patients with advanced HIV disease display decreased tolerability to many medications, including antiretroviral agents. Although this is not fully understood, it is probably a result of HIV-induced immune alterations and cytokine dysregulations. Subsequently, clinicians evaluating patients with advanced disease should be alert for possible drug-induced adverse events.
2. *Drug interactions:* Many patients with advanced disease take numerous medications for primary or secondary prophylaxis of various opportunistic infections, as well as other medications for comorbid disease states. Subsequently, the risk for a drug–drug interaction is increased. The addition of any new medication, either prescription or over-the-counter, should be carefully evaluated for potential interactions with the patient's current antiretroviral regimen (see Table 73-7). In addition, any change to the current antiretroviral regimen should also be checked against the patient's current medication list.
3. *Altered bioavailability:* Patients with advanced HIV infection may have unreliable absorption of many medications due to severe diarrhea, anorexia, weight loss, wasting, and gastric achlorhydria. As a result, the bioavailability of some agents, especially certain PIs that require specific dietary requirements, may be affected (Table 73-3). Any changes in dietary habits or bowel function should be carefully assessed in light of the potential impact on the antiretroviral regimen.
4. *Antiretroviral drug histories and resistance testing:* The most useful information to guide the choice of alternative regimens is a detailed drug history, in conjunction with appropriate resistance testing. Among patients with extensive prior antiretroviral use, it is critical to identify previously failed regimens and determine the precise cause of the failures. In an experienced patient who has taken many different regimens over a lifetime, the number of remaining viable agents and regimens may be limited. Therefore, it is important to determine whether prior regimens truly failed for virologic reasons or some other cause

(e.g., regimen intolerability or an inadequate trial period). In addition, detailed knowledge of regimen intolerabilities and which agent(s) caused the adverse event will help in the selection of a new appropriate regimen. In some situations, the offending agent may be reinitiated if the adverse event was minimal or can be appropriately managed.

RESISTANCE, VIRAL GENOTYPING, PHENOTYPING, AND VIRAL FITNESS

CASE 73-2, QUESTION 2: Will viral genotyping and phenotyping assist in selecting an appropriate therapeutic regimen for H.G.? What are these tests? What are their limitations and when should they be used? What is viral fitness, and does it have a role in clinical decision making?

Viral genotyping and phenotyping reveal resistance patterns to antiretroviral agents. Genotyping evaluates mutations in the virus's genetic material, whereas phenotyping assesses the ability of the virus to grow in the presence of increasing concentrations of antiretroviral agents. The three potential causes for the development of resistance are as follows.

1. Initial infection with a resistant isolate[69–71,129]
2. Natural selection of a resistant isolate as a consequence of inefficient, error-susceptible viral replication[36,130,131]
3. Generation of resistant isolates via selective pressures from antiretroviral therapies that do not fully suppress viral replication[6,132–141]

Mutations are generated when naturally occurring amino acids in the HIV genome are replaced with alternative amino acids. For example, resistance to 3TC occurs when the amino acid methionine (M) is replaced by valine (V) at the 184th amino acid in the protein chain.[142,143] This mutation is subsequently referred to as an M184V mutation. These amino acid substitutions change the proteins that are produced and may alter the shape, size, or charge of the viral enzyme's substrate or primer.[144–146] Subsequently, antiretroviral drug binding to the active site is decreased, affinity for natural substrates is increased, or there is an increased removal of the antiretroviral agent from the enzyme by the virus (known as pyrophosphorylation).[147] Whether a mutation results in a clinically resistant, less viable, or indifferent isolate depends on which amino acid(s) is replaced. In addition, certain mutations or combination of mutations have been shown to produce viral isolates that display increased sensitivity to various antiretroviral agents (known as hypersusceptibility). Alterations to certain key amino acids can also result in cross-resistance between various antiretrovirals.[6]

Two key enzymes have been extensively studied with regard to their potential for development of resistance: reverse transcriptase (RT) and protease. Replication by the RT enzyme is highly susceptible to errors. Given that the HIV genome is approximately 10,000 nucleotides in length and that mutations via the RT enzyme occur approximately once in every 10,000 nucleotides copied, it has been estimated that a mutation occurs with every viral replication cycle. With up to 10 billion particles of virus being produced per day, the potential exists for 1,000 to 10,000 mutations occurring at each site in the HIV genome every day.[35] Integrase resistance, including resistance mutations to raltegravir, exists, but has not yet been fully described, because use is not widespread.[51] Key mutations to the antiretroviral agents are identified in Figure 73-5 and are updated periodically by expert panels of clinicians.[6]

Over time, countless viral subpopulations known as "quasi-species" develop. In any given host, at any given time, many different quasi-species can exist. In addition, within any compartment of the body (e.g., CNS, testes, lymph nodes), many different quasi-species can also exist. Because these mutant strains represent only a small number of isolates in the total viral population, they must have some replicative disadvantage when compared with the "wild-type" virus.[138,139] Under selective pressures from antiretroviral therapies, however, these mutant isolates can replicate. For example, if wild-type viral replication is inhibited by an antiretroviral regimen, and if any one viral strain of the quasi-species is more fit for growth in the presence of that regimen, then the viral mutant will have a competitive advantage.[148] It should be recognized that for resistance to develop, viral replication must occur. When viral replication is completely inhibited, the development of resistant isolates is uncommon.

Genotypic analysis involves sequencing the viral genetic material via PCR amplification. Mutations are identified by analysis of key sequences of the RT or protease enzymes. These tests can be rapidly processed; however, they detect mutations present only in more than 25% of all HIV isolates in the body, and can only reliably detect resistance patterns in samples with HIV RNA greater than 1,000 copies/mL. Because pressures from antiretroviral therapies select resistant isolates, these tests may not provide information regarding rare, yet potentially clinically significant, isolates.[5,6]

Phenotypic analysis involves growing virus in the presence of various concentrations of drug and then determining viral susceptibilities (e.g., half-maximal inhibitory concentration [IC_{50}]). Phenotyping is limited because it evaluates only one viral isolate at a time and could fail to identify other clinically relevant isolates.[5] An additional methodology, known as the virtual phenotype, is also currently available, and compares the genotype information from a sample of interest to a large database of viral isolates where both genotype and phenotype have been performed.[5] This method is only as reliable as the databases from which the virtual phenotype is generated, and may be limited for newer agents with less available genotype-phenotype data.

Genotyping and phenotyping have the potential to provide useful information to clinicians who treat patients with HIV infection. Evidence to date suggests that these tests are effective at predicting which agents will not work, but they are less useful in predicting those that will work.[5,6,149] For example, if testing identifies resistance to an agent, it is highly unlikely this agent will be effective. If testing identifies an agent as susceptible, however, it does not necessarily predict that this agent will be effective. Clinical trials evaluating the use of genotyping and phenotyping for selection of alternative antiretroviral regimens have shown positive treatment responses.[5,6] As with all clinical decisions made for those who are HIV infected, careful assessment of the results in combination with the treatment history are essential for proper clinical decision making. Consultation with an expert in antiretroviral drug resistance patterns is highly recommended.

One other measure available to clinicians is "viral fitness" or "replication capacity." The genetic changes that occur in a virus to become resistant to antiretroviral therapy often impair the virus' ability to replicate.[41,150–152] This measure is called "fitness" and is quantified as replication capacity during phenotypic evaluation. During amplification of the virus before the phenotype is measured, the replication capacity of the virus is evaluated and compared to a reference wild-type, drug-sensitive virus. A virus with normal fitness has a replication capacity between 70% and 120% of the reference viral strain; isolates with values less than 70% are considered to be less fit than wild-type virus. In general, the more mutations that occur to the virus, the more compromised the virus becomes, and the lower the fitness (although, in

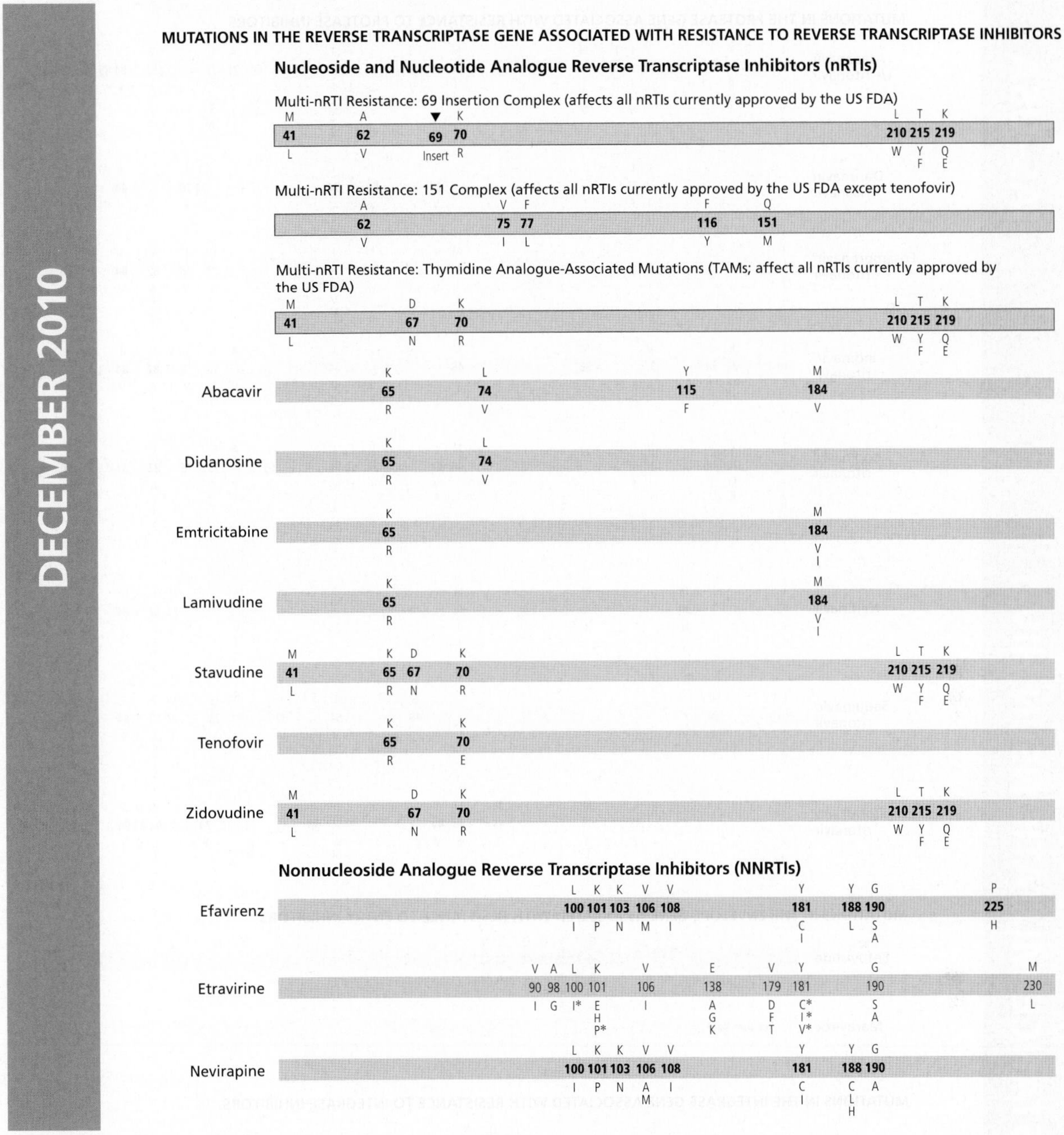
DECEMBER 2010
MUTATIONS IN THE REVERSE TRANSCRIPTASE GENE ASSOCIATED WITH RESISTANCE TO REVERSE TRANSCRIPTASE INHIBITORS
Nucleoside and Nucleotide Analogue Reverse Transcriptase Inhibitors (nRTIs)
Multi-nRTI Resistance: 69 Insertion Complex (affects all nRTIs currently approved by the US FDA)
M 41 L; A 62 V; 69 Insert; K 70 R; L 210 W; T 215 Y F; K 219 Q E
Multi-nRTI Resistance: 151 Complex (affects all nRTIs currently approved by the US FDA except tenofovir)
A 62 V; V 75 I; F 77 L; F 116 Y; Q 151 M
Multi-nRTI Resistance: Thymidine Analogue-Associated Mutations (TAMs; affect all nRTIs currently approved by the US FDA)
M 41 L; D 67 N; K 70 R; L 210 W; T 215 Y F; K 219 Q E
Abacavir
K 65 R; L 74 V; Y 115 F; M 184 V
Didanosine
K 65 R; L 74 V
Emtricitabine
K 65 R; M 184 V I
Lamivudine
K 65 R; M 184 V I
Stavudine
M 41 L; K 65 R; D 67 N; K 70 R; L 210 W; T 215 Y F; K 219 Q E
Tenofovir
K 65 R; K 70 E
Zidovudine
M 41 L; D 67 N; K 70 R; L 210 W; T 215 Y F; K 219 Q E
Nonnucleoside Analogue Reverse Transcriptase Inhibitors (NNRTIs)
Efavirenz
L 100 I; K 101 P; K 103 N; V 106 M; V 108 I; Y 181 C I; Y 188 L; G 190 S A; P 225 H
Etravirine
V 90 I; A 98 G; L 100 I*; K 101 E H P*; V 106 I; E 138 A G K; V 179 D F T; Y 181 C* I* V*; G 190 S A; M 230 L
Nevirapine
L 100 I; K 101 P; K 103 N; V 106 A M; V 108 I; Y 181 C I; Y 188 C L H; G 190 A

FIGURE 73-5 Mutations associated with resistance to the various classes of antiretroviral agents. Amino acid abbreviation: A, alanine; C, cysteine; D, aspartate; E, glutamate; F, phenylalanine; G, glycine; H, histidine; I, isoleucine; K, lysine; L, leucine; M, methionine; N, asparagine; P, proline; Q, glutamine; R, arginine; S, serine; T, threonine; V, valine; W, tryptophan; Y, tyrosine. (Reprinted with permission from the IAS–USA. Johnson VA, Brun-Vézinet F, Clotet B, Günthard HF, Kuritzkes DR, Pillay D, Schapiro JM, and Richman DD. Update of the Drug Resistance Mutations in HIV-1: December 2010. *Topics in HIV Medicine.* 2010;18(5):156–163. Updated information and User Notes are available at **www.iasusa.org.**) (*Continued*)

some situations, the interplay between mutations can result in a viral isolate that is relatively fit). Recent data have shown that, despite persistent viral replication, unfit viruses may not cause the same degree of immune destruction as fit viruses.[151] This finding is important for patients with limited treatment options because it may allow for continuation of a HAART regimen that is not completely suppressive, but that produces an unfit virus, with less T-cell depletion. In these situations, it may be best to keep patients on their current therapy despite measurable viral load measurements (provided their CD4 cell counts are stable) until newer treatment options become available.

Given H.G.'s extensive antiretroviral drug history and his current failure, a genotype, phenotype, or virtual phenotype will likely provide some insights into potential therapeutic options.

SPECIAL CIRCUMSTANCES

Discordant Surrogate Markers

CASE 73-2, QUESTION 3: H.G. was started on a regimen of tenofovir, 3TC, etravirine, and darunavir–ritonavir. During the following 6 months, H.G.'s T-cell counts increased to 325 cells/μL and his viral load value declined to 5,000 copies/mL. At the last two clinic visits, H.G.'s viral load (copies/mL) and CD4 counts (cells/μL) were 2,000/275 and less than 50/225, respectively. H.G. reports no new clinical complaints or adverse drug events. In addition, H.G. states

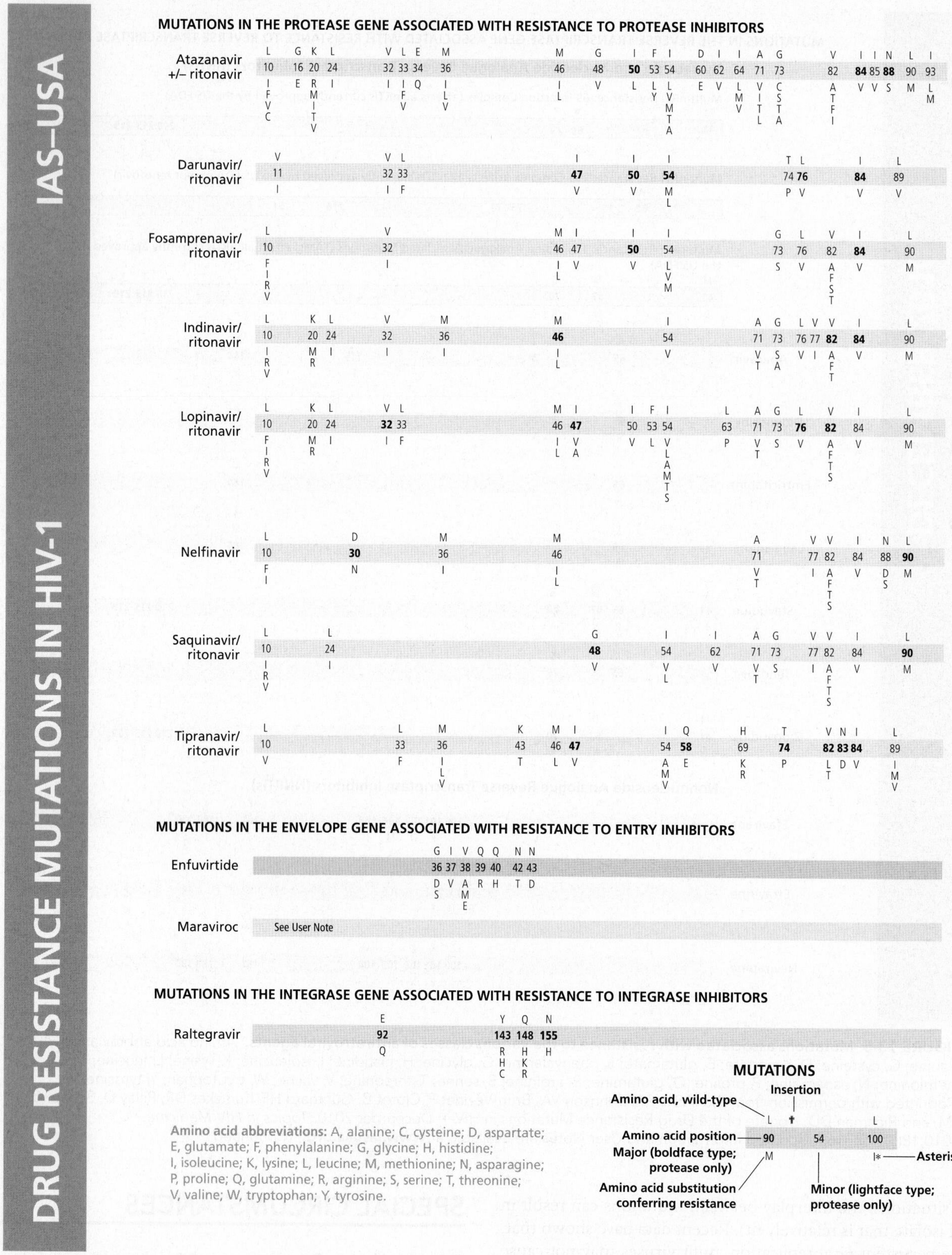

FIGURE 73-5 *(Continued)*

that he has been compliant with therapy. Are changes to therapy necessary?

In most cases, declines in viral load result in increases in CD4 cell counts, and increasing viral loads result in declining CD4 cell counts. In approximately 20% of cases, however, T cells decline along with viral load decline or T cells increase along with viral load increases.[5] These situations are referred to as discordant surrogate marker data.

In this situation, it may be wise to continue current treatment and monitor the patient closely, because changing or adding an additional drug may not increase CD4 cell counts.[5] When T-cell counts increase despite increasing viral load measurements, decisions regarding therapeutic options are unknown. Although these patients may derive clinical benefit from the current antiretroviral regimen for a short period of time, data suggest that long-term stability of the CD4 count is unlikely.[5] Because this may be an early warning sign of impending CD4 cell destruction, many clinicians would change antiretroviral therapies. Other clinicians, however, might follow patients carefully and change therapies at the first sign of T-cell declines or new clinical signs and symptoms. In these situations, other potential causes of viral load increases (e.g., recent infection, vaccination) should be carefully evaluated to prevent inappropriately changing a nonfailing regimen.

Therapeutic Drug Monitoring

CASE 73-3

QUESTION 1: P.P. is a 30-year-old HIV-positive man who has failed prior antiretroviral regimens. Based on phenotypic resistance testing, it appears that a regimen including lopinavir–ritonavir may be able to overcome the viral isolate's resistance pattern. Will plasma measurements of P.P.'s antiretroviral drug concentrations be useful? What measurement should be used, which agent(s) should be measured, and how should the samples be collected?

Pharmacokinetic evaluations of various antiretrovirals, including the NNRTIs, PIs, and raltegravir have shown wide interpatient variability in drug exposures among cohorts of patients taking the same dose of drug under the same conditions.[47,153–157] Many factors contribute to interpatient variability in drug exposure, such as pharmacogenetics, environment, different physiologic conditions, regimen adherence, and drug interactions. For most antiretrovirals, a drug exposure–response relationship exists (e.g., the higher the exposure, the faster and more prolonged the viral suppression). In addition, most antiretrovirals also have well defined exposure–toxicity relationships.

Therapeutic drug monitoring (TDM) is currently recommended for selected clinical situations.[156] In patients failing a first regimen, or a regimen that was initially fully suppressive, TDM may identify suboptimal drug concentrations. For patients with uncharacterized drug interactions and those with impairments in gastrointestinal, hepatic, or renal function, drug concentrations may help identify low or high exposure that can be corrected with a dosage adjustment. TDM may also be useful for assuring that a novel antiretroviral combination does not have any unpredictable adverse drug interactions. In treatment-experienced patients, knowledge of drug exposure with viral susceptibility may assist in designing an optimal dosage regimen. Conversely, patients experiencing toxicities thought to be concentration-dependent (e.g., neuropsychiatric effects of efavirenz) may benefit from TDM as well. Monitoring adherence and evaluating pharmacokinetics in special populations, such as pregnant women or pediatric patients, are additional indications for TDM.

Pharmacology experts currently recommend obtaining trough concentrations immediately before the next dose of a PI or an NNRTI. For efavirenz (which is usually taken in the evening), samples obtained 12 hours postdose will closely reflect the concentration at 24 hours postdose due to its long half-life. Many factors can affect the trough values of various antiretroviral agents. For proper interpretation of the concentrations, patients should provide a dosing history from the last several days, a list of concomitantly administered drugs to screen for interactions, and the exact time the last dose was taken. The exact time the TDM sample was collected should also be recorded. Another factor that can affect interpretation of drug concentrations over time is intrapatient variability. Although not fully evaluated, it appears that under stringent pharmacokinetic study conditions (e.g., study conditions in which dosing, concomitant food administration, drug interactions, and adherence all are controlled) the day-to-day variability of drug concentrations over time is minimal. Outside of a clinical study, however, where patients take their medications under conditions that vary from day to day, the concentrations could be highly variable at clinic visits over time, and several samples might be required to determine trends in the drug exposure before making a dose adjustment.[158] Finally, to minimize laboratory variability and error in measuring these concentrations, it is also recommended that a laboratory that routinely measures antiretrovirals and participates in both internal and external quality control programs be used. A list of such laboratories can be obtained from the Clinical Pharmacology Quality Assurance and Quality Control Program (https://www.fstrf.org/apps/cfmx/apps/cpqa/cpqaDocs/public/index.html).

In general, total drug concentration ranges for defining efficacy and toxicity have been developed for PIs and NNRTIs.[156] A limitation of obtaining total drug concentrations is that unbound, active drug fraction is not quantitated. These agents are generally highly protein-bound, and alterations in the bound or unbound fraction can contribute to both reduced efficacy and increased toxicity within accepted total drug concentration ranges. Despite this fact, total concentrations are generally used owing to technical challenges inherent in determining unbound drug concentrations, and because a reasonable relationship exists between these concentrations and clinical outcomes. The plasma or serum concentrations of NRTIs, however, may or may not be reflective of the active intracellular triphosphate moiety, but may be useful to measure in certain situations. Limitations to determining intracellular concentrations include the sophisticated processing of the cellular components before storage, the technical difficulty of the assay itself (generally only found in pharmaceutical companies and academic centers), and the limited availability of instrumentation to measure the low concentrations of these moieties (e.g., fmol/10^6 cells).

The interpretation of the drug concentration itself will vary according on the clinical situation. Among treatment-naïve patients with wild-type viral isolates, an assessment should be made whether the concentration lies within a range of the population concentrations—how that range is defined tends to be clinician-specific, but can be interquartile range, or a 90% confidence interval, among others. If the concentration is less than the desired cut-off, and the patient is not responding well to the therapy, the clinician should consider increasing the dose or using a pharmacokinetic-enhancing technique (e.g., adding ritonavir). If the concentration is higher than the cut-off, and the patient is experiencing drug toxicity, a dose reduction should be considered. Clinical trials evaluating TDM among antiretroviral-naïve patients initiating PI-based HAART have shown improved clinical responses compared with patients given standard of care without TDM. However, many of these improved responses were seen with older protease inhibitors such as indinavir and nelfinavir that had narrower therapeutic ranges than the newer antiretroviral drugs recommended as first line agents. A study performed assessing TDM of more recent PI-based HAART regimens in treatment experienced patients failed to show an overall benefit.[159]

Among patients with antiretroviral resistance, the interpretation of the concentration is much more complex and may require the additional assessment of phenotypic resistance data. Higher drug exposure may be needed for patients with drug-resistant viruses to achieve efficacy. Preliminary investigations have evaluated the ratio between drug exposure and viral susceptibility (in a similar fashion to the antimicrobial efficacy ratios of C_{min}/minimal inhibitory concentration [MIC] or area under the curve [AUC]/MIC), also called an inhibitory quotient. Interpretation of the current inhibitory quotient data is difficult, however, owing to the various methodologies used for its calculation.[156] Ongoing research is focused on standardizing calculation methods to improve the prediction of appropriate antiretroviral concentrations for maximal efficacy.

In the current case, assuring that P.P.'s lopinavir trough concentration is at least greater than the IC_{50} value from the phenotype may help improve his chances of optimal antiviral response. If P.P.'s response to treatment is inadequate (e.g., unsatisfactory decline in HIV RNA), then a concentration should be obtained from a trough sample, with a careful concomitant drug and dosing history, and sent to a reliable laboratory for analysis.

Drug Interactions

CASE 73-4

QUESTION 1: J.F. is a 37-year-old HIV positive man who has been taking emtricitabine, tenofovir, and atazanavir/ritonavir for the past 4 years. Lately, he has been experiencing heartburn and was diagnosed with gastroesophageal reflux disease (GERD). What needs to be considered when starting a new medication for J.F.'s acid reflux?

Drug interactions are very common with antiretrovirals and need to be considered when changing HIV-related or non-related drug regimens. In this case, stomach acid suppressants will significantly decrease the concentration of atazanavir as it requires an acid environment for complete dissolution.[51] If J.F.'s GERD needs treatment, H_2 receptor antagonists should be given either simultaneously with ritonavir-boosted atazanavir or at least 10 hours before administration of the antiretrovirals. A dose of famotidine or its equivalent should not exceed 40 mg twice a day (BID) for treatment-naïve patients, and famotidine 20 mg BID or its equivalent should not be exceeded in treatment-experienced patients. Additionally, atazanavir AUC exposures are decreased by 25% with concomitant tenofovir and C_{min} can be decreased 23% to 40%. Therefore, in treatment-experienced patients taking tenofovir, atazanavir should be given at an increased dose of 400 mg daily in combination with 100 mg of ritonavir. Proton pump inhibitors (PPIs) are not recommended for use in protease-inhibitor–experienced patients. In treatment-naïve patients who require a PPI, only atazanavir–ritonavir 300 mg/100 mg should be used, and separated from the PPI by 12 hours or more.[5]

Pregnancy and Breast-Feeding

CASE 73-5

QUESTION 1: T.D. is a 32-year-old woman infected with HIV whose antiretroviral therapy includes efavirenz, tenofovir, and emtricitabine. She has had a positive home pregnancy test result. Is her current antiretroviral regimen appropriate for use during pregnancy and for prevention of mother-to-child transmission?

The current perinatal HIV guidelines[75] recommend that women receiving and tolerating a currently suppressive regimen when they become pregnant continue on that regimen unless it contains efavirenz. Efavirenz is the only antiretroviral that is currently pregnancy category D and is not recommended in pregnancy or breast-feeding. It has been shown to be teratogenic in animal studies, particularly in the first trimester of pregnancy, and retrospective case reports of neural tube defects in humans have been documented.[160–163] Perinatal transmission prevention guidelines recommend lamivudine and zidovudine as first-line NRTIs and abacavir, didanosine, emtricitabine, and stavudine as alternative agents. Nevirapine is the recommended NNRTI if the CD4 count is less than 250/μL and lopinavir–ritonavir is the recommended protease inhibitor during pregnancy. Many of the pregnancy recommendations are based on those drugs which have the most safety and efficacy data available during pregnancy (both animal and human).[75]

In women who have a viral load persistently greater than 1,000 copies/mL, it is recommended that a planned 38-week cesarean section be performed to reduce the risk of mother-to-child transmission. In women with a viral load less than 1,000 copies/mL, there is little evidence to show that cesarean section decreases transmission rates compared to vaginal delivery. In this case, the decision is made at the discretion of the physician in consultation with the mother. Additionally, it is recommended that intravenous zidovudine be administered to the mother at 2 mg/kg intravenously (IV) for 1 hour at the onset of labor, then given as a continuous infusion of 1 mg/kg/hour during the intrapartum period (during labor and postpartum). Once delivered, it is recommended that oral zidovudine at 2 mg/kg every 6 hours be started in the infant immediately after birth and continued for 6 weeks. It is recommended that the infant undergo diagnostic virologic testing using either HIV DNA PCR or RNA virologic assays at a minimum at ages 14 to 21 days, 1 to 2 months, and 4 to 6 months. Antibody testing should not be performed on the infant because maternal HIV antibody crosses the placenta and will be detectable in all HIV-exposed infants up to 18 months of age.[75]

It is not recommended that HIV-positive women breast-feed their children in resource-rich settings where clean water and formula are reasonably available. The risk of transmission from breast-feeding is consistently higher than formula feeding even with the use of antiretroviral prophylaxis.[164]

Postexposure Prophylaxis

CASE 73-6

QUESTION 1: L.T. is a 47-year-old nurse at an HIV clinic. While drawing routine labs on a newly diagnosed HIV+ male patient, not yet started on HAART, she accidently stuck herself with a contaminated needle. Are interventions available to prevent L.T. from contracting HIV from the needlestick? What drugs should be utilized, and for how long?

Occupational postexposure prophylaxis (PEP) recommendations are dependent on the type of exposure and the risk factors associated with that exposure. For example, percutaneous exposure poses more of a concern than mucous membrane exposure. A needle stick with a large hollow-bore needle is higher risk that a solid needle, a deep penetrating wound is considered a high-risk exposure compared to a superficial injury, and a exposure to a large volume of infectious fluid is more concerning than exposure to a low volume. Patient-specific factors must also be considered, such as whether the HIV-positive patient is on HAART therapy and has a suppressed viral load or whether the HIV-positive patient currently has a high viral load.

Basic two-drug PEP is generally recommended for less severe percutaneous exposures (solid needle or superficial injury) from an HIV-positive patient who is suppressed on antiretrovirals, a patient with an unknown HIV status who has HIV risk factors, or for mucous membrane exposures. Basic two-drug PEP generally consists of two NRTIs such as zidovudine, stavudine, or tenofovir with lamivudine or emtricitabine.[165]

TABLE 73-8
Human Immunodeficiency Virus Internet Resources

Government Sites	AIDS Treatment/Advocacy Groups
American Foundation for AIDS Research: http://www.amfar.org	Project Inform: http://www.projinf.org
AIDSinfo from US DHHS: http://www.aidsinfo.nih.gov	San Francisco AIDS Foundation: http://www.sfaf.org/index.html
Centers for Disease Control and Prevention: http://www.cdc.gov	**Other Relevant Sites**
Consensus Panel Guidelines Online: http://www.aidsinfo.nih.gov	The AIDS Map: http://www.aidsmap.com
Government HIV Mutation Charts: http://hiv-web.lanl.gov	AIDS Education Global Information System: http://www.aegis.com
National Institute of Allergy and Infectious Diseases: http://www.niaid.nih.gov	Clinical Care Options: http://www.clinicalcareoptions.com
National Prevention Information Network: http://www.cdcnpin.org	HIV Drug Interactions: http://www.hiv-druginteractions.org
United Nations AIDS Website: http://www.unaids.org/	HIV and Hepatitis: http://hivandhepatitis.com
University Sites	HIV Pharmacology: http://www.hivpharmacology.com
Johns Hopkins AIDS Service: http://www.hopkins-aids.edu	HIV Resistance Web: http://www.hivresistanceweb.com
University of California, HIV/AIDS Program: http://hivinsite.ucsf.edu	HIV Treatment Information: http://www.i-base/info
University of Stanford HIV Drug Resistance Database: http://hivdb.stanford.edu/	Medscape: http://www.medscape.com
	Physician's Research Network: http://www.prn.org
	The Body for Clinicians: http://www.thebodypro.com
	Retrovirus Conference: http://www.retroconference.org

Expanded three-drug PEP is recommended for more severe percutaneous exposures (large-bore hollow needle or deep puncture wound) from suppressed HIV-positive patients and more-than-three–drug PEP is indicated for percutaneous exposures where the patient has a high viral load or acute infection or from similar patients if there is a large volume mucous membrane exposure. In these instances, the choice of agents to use for PEP is generally dependent on the patient's regimen and resistant profile.[165]

L.T. should start immediately on an expanded basic regimen of at least three drugs consisting of two of the NNRTIs recommended for basic two-drug PEP with the addition of a PI, preferably lopinavir–ritonavir. This entire regimen should be continued for a total of 4 weeks. It would also be a good idea to look at the specific patient from which the exposure occurred. If he had a great deal of known antiretroviral drug resistance, then L.T. may need to be put on different antiretrovirals according to the patient's resistance profile. HIV antibody testing using ELISA should be performed on L.T. at baseline exposure, 6 weeks, 12 weeks, and 6 months after exposure. She should also have baseline and follow-up labs performed to assess antiretroviral toxicity. At a minimum, these should include a complete blood count, renal and hepatic function tests, and fasting glucose while on the protease inhibitor. Additional laboratory tests should be performed based on the individual drugs chosen.[165]

Additional guidelines exist for non-occupational HIV exposures and follow similar risk and stratification treatment paradigms. In those instances where a person seeks care within 72 hours of exposure to blood, genital secretions or other potentially infected body fluids of persons known to be HIV-infected and the exposure represents a substantial risk for HIV transmission then the person is started on PEP in a similar fashion as with an occupation exposure and continued for 4 weeks with similar monitoring and HIV testing.[166]

KEEPING CURRENT

The management of HIV infection continues to evolve. Additional important emerging data are in HIV prevention and cure.

The overwhelming data presented at scientific meetings and in journals has made staying informed about current issues and new developments a daunting task. As a result, many clinicians, even those actively caring for patients who are HIV infected, remain cautious and often confused regarding therapeutic options.

New technologies for the dissemination of medical information are constantly evolving. The Internet has allowed clinicians worldwide to exchange ideas, teach new concepts, and obtain access to limited resources. In addition, many research centers, patient advocacy groups, and academic institutions have posted sites on the Internet that have resulted in access to large amounts of high-quality medical information. This new technology has also allowed, however, for the dissemination of incomplete, misleading, or inaccurate information. Therefore, clinicians must remain cautious and carefully evaluate the information obtained from various websites.

When evaluating the quality of a website, clinicians should look for a few basic standards.

- *Author qualifications.* Is the author qualified to write the article or perform the research? Is his or her affiliation or relevant credentials provided?
- *Attribution.* Are references provided to confirm statements? Is all relevant copyrighted information noted?
- *Currency.* When was the content posted? Is the website updated regularly?
- *Disclosure.* Who owns the website? Is there a conflict of interest between what is being posted and any commercial interest?

Any Internet site that fails to meet these basic competencies should be viewed with caution. In general, the most accurate and informative websites for HIV-specific information come from academic institutions, government organizations, medical societies, and patient advocacy groups. Table 73-8 lists high-quality websites that provide timely and accurate information. A periodic evaluation of these sites often provides sufficient information to stay up-to-date on current issues and controversies.

CONCLUSION

Despite significant advances made in the treatment of patients infected with HIV, a cure continues to be out of reach. Although the pharmacologic management of HIV is rapidly evolving, a basic understanding of viral pathogenesis and drug interactions provides a framework that can be used to evaluate new information as it becomes available.

United States during 1996.[1] This report represents the first calendar year in which the overall incidence of AIDS-associated OIs did not increase in the United States; the 1996 figure represented a decline of 6% compared with 1995. Patients with human immunodeficiency virus (HIV) infection are susceptible to an array of diseases, but most OIs are caused by a few common pathogens, including *Pneumocystis jiroveci (carinii)*, cytomegalovirus (CMV), fungi, and mycobacteria.[4]

For a visual of potential opportunistic infections, go to http://thepoint.lww.com/AT10e.

ONLINE CONTENT

The most recent data document esophageal candidiasis (360 patients) and *Pneumocystis jiroveci* pneumonia to be the most common OIs.[5]

The 1993 revised classification system for HIV infection and expanded surveillance case definition for AIDS included stratification for the CD4$^+$ lymphocyte count, as well as subgrouping by clinical categories (Table 74-1). These AIDS-defining OIs may also occur in asymptomatic HIV-infected patients (Table 74-1).[4]

The Natural History of Opportunistic Infections

THE DECLINE OF THE CD4 LYMPHOCYTE

Within the immune system, the CD4$^+$ lymphocyte functions as a "helper cell" that modulates the actions of the other key cellular components of the immune system. The eventual loss of CD4$^+$ lymphocytes is the underlying pathophysiology that leads to AIDS. (See Chapter 73, Pharmacotherapy of Human Immunodeficiency Virus Infection, and comprehensive immunology texts for a more detailed explanation of immune function and inflammation associated with HIV infection.) The infected CD4$^+$ lymphocyte can function normally for a time, but eventually becomes dysfunctional, as manifested by an abnormal response to soluble mitogens. It is this cellular functional deficit, compounded by the eventual decline in the absolute number of CD4$^+$ lymphocytes, that leads to OIs and neurologic dysfunctions. The CD4$^+$ count declines gradually during several years in the untreated HIV-infected person. The average rate of decline of CD4$^+$ lymphocyte cells (CD4 slope) is approximately 40 to 80 cells/μL/year in the absence of antiretroviral therapy. An accelerated decline in the CD4$^+$ count occurs at 1.5 to 2 years, just before an AIDS-defining diagnosis.[6] Without therapy, the course of infection averages approximately 10 years from the time of initial infection to an AIDS-defining diagnosis. However, some patients experience a rapid decline after the acute retroviral presentation, and 5% to 15% maintain a CD4$^+$ count of 500 for longer than 8 years; these patients are considered chronic nonprogressors.[7]

The CD4$^+$ count dictates the need for OI prophylaxis, influences the differential diagnosis of the OI, and is an independent indicator of prognosis. For these reasons, the CD4$^+$ count has become a primary surrogate marker of immune suppression and antiretroviral activity. HIV-1 RNA is the other clinical surrogate marker most predictive of survival and antiretroviral activity.

OIs range from relatively minor events (e.g., oral candidiasis or oral hairy leukoplakia) to sight-threatening episodes of CMV retinitis, or life-threatening *P. jiroveci (carinii)* pneumonia (PCP). The risk for specific OIs varies with the degree of

TABLE 74-1
Conditions Included in the 1993 Surveillance Case Definition

Category A
Asymptomatic HIV infection
Persistent generalized lymphadenopathy
Acute HIV infection with accompanying illness or history of HIV infection
Category B
Bacillary angiomatosis
Candidiasis, oropharyngeal (thrush)
Candidiasis, vulvovaginal; persistent, frequent, or poorly responsive to treatment
Cervical dysplasia/carcinoma in situ
Constitutional symptoms, such as fever >38°C or diarrhea >1 month
Hairy leukoplakia
Herpes zoster (shingles), involving at least two distinct episodes or more than one dermatome
Idiopathic thrombocytopenia purpura
Listeriosis
Pelvic inflammatory disease, particularly if complicated by tubo-ovarian abscess
Peripheral neuropathy
Category C
Candidiasis of bronchi, trachea, or lungs
Candidiasis, esophageal
Cervical cancer, invasive
Coccidioidomycosis, disseminated or extrapulmonary
Category C (*Continued*)
Cryptococcosis, extrapulmonary
Cryptosporidiosis, chronic intestinal (>1 month)
CMV disease (other than liver, spleen, or nodes)
CMV retinitis (with loss of vision)
Encephalopathy, HIV-related
Herpes simplex: chronic ulcer(s) (>1 month); or bronchitis, pneumonitis, or esophagitis
Histoplasmosis, disseminated or extrapulmonary
Isosporiasis, chronic intestinal (>1 month's duration)
Kaposi sarcoma
Lymphoid interstitial pneumonia and/or pulmonary lymphoid hyperplasia[a]
Lymphoma, Burkitt (or equivalent term)
Lymphoma, immunoblastic (or equivalent term)
Lymphoma, primary, of brain
Mycobacterium avium-intracellulare complex or *M. kansasii*, disseminated or extrapulmonary
Mycobacterium tuberculosis, any site (pulmonary[b] or extrapulmonary)
Mycobacterium, other species or unidentified species, disseminated or extrapulmonary
Pneumocystis carinii pneumonia
Pneumonia, recurrent[b]
PML
Salmonella septicemia, recurrent
Toxoplasmosis of brain
Wasting syndrome due to HIV

[a]Children <13 years old.
[b]Added in the 1993 expansions of the AIDS surveillance case definition for adolescents and adults.
CMV, cytomegalovirus; HIV, human immunodeficiency virus; PML, progressive multifocal leukoencephalopathy.

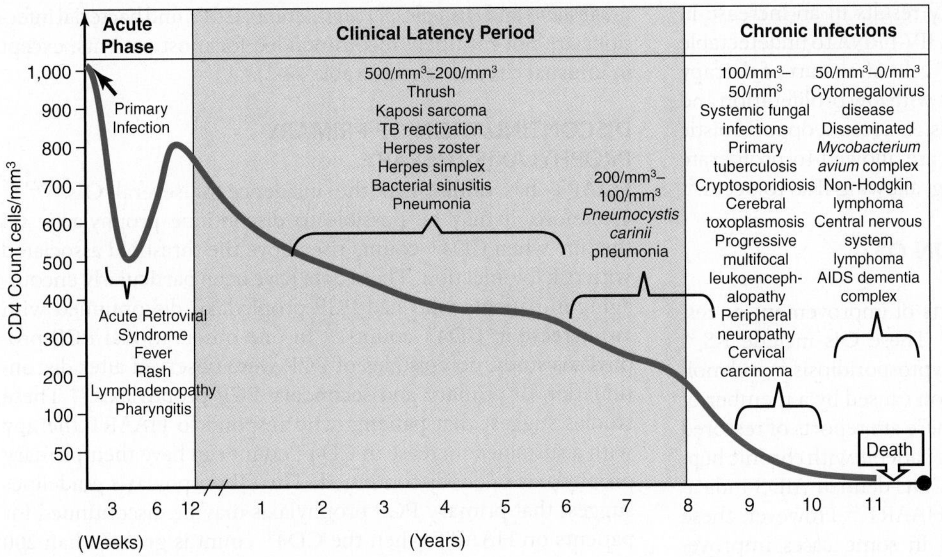

FIGURE 74-1 Natural history of CD4+ cell count in the average HIV patient without antiretroviral therapy, from the time of HIV transmissions to death. (Illustration by Mary Van, PharmD.)

immunosuppression.[8] Asymptomatic patients with moderate immunosuppression (CD4+ counts 200–500) may become infected with herpes viruses and *Candida* species or develop pneumonia, enteric infection, and meningitis with more common pathogens. Massive destruction of the immune system occurs when the CD4+ count drops below 200, which increases the risk for opportunistic pathogens (e.g., PCP), opportunistic tumors, wasting, and neurologic complications. With a CD4+ count of 50 to 100, invasive candidiasis, cerebral toxoplasmosis, cryptococcosis, and various protozoal infections are observed. When the CD4+ count falls below 50, the patient is in an advanced immunosuppressed state, which is associated with non-Hodgkin lymphoma, CMV, and disseminated *Mycobacterium avium* complex (MAC; Fig. 74-1). Without treatment, the median survival associated with a CD4+ count less than 200 is 3.1 years, and the time to an AIDS-defining infection ranges from 18 to 24 months.[6,8] With the implementation of HAART, the 3-year probability of AIDS has dramatically declined; however, much of this decline may be associated with the use of OI prophylaxis.[9]

THE EFFECT OF OPPORTUNISTIC INFECTIONS ON VIRAL LOAD AND SURVIVAL

Acute OIs upregulate HIV replication, resulting in higher HIV-1 RNA concentrations in the plasma and lymphoid tissues of HIV-infected patients. This enhanced replication is presumably caused by antigen-mediated activation of HIV-1 replication in latently infected cells. To assess the impact of OIs on survival, data from a cohort of 2,081 HIV-infected patients followed (in the pre–protease inhibitor era) for a mean of 30 months were analyzed.[10] CD4+ counts and incidence of opportunistic disease were used as independent variables. These investigators found that PCP, CMV, MAC, esophageal candidiasis, Kaposi sarcoma (KS), non-Hodgkin lymphoma, progressive multifocal leukoencephalopathy (PML), dementia, wasting syndrome, toxoplasmosis, and cryptosporidiosis were independently associated with death.[10] Additionally, data from a prospective longitudinal study of HIV infection in homosexual men initiated in 1984 (Multicenter AIDS Cohort Study) demonstrated that plasma HIV-1 RNA concentrations strongly predict the rate of decline of the absolute CD4+ count as well as clinical progression to AIDS and death.[11] More recent investigations in the era of HAART have demonstrated that CD4+ count is the strongest prognostic factor in patients starting therapy.[9]

IMPACT OF ANTIRETROVIRAL AGENTS ON THE NATURAL HISTORY OF OPPORTUNISTIC INFECTIONS

REDUCTION IN THE INCIDENCE OF OPPORTUNISTIC INFECTIONS AND DEATH

The introduction of protease inhibitors, combination therapy, prophylaxis therapy, and improved medical care has reduced the incidence of OIs and death resulting from AIDS in HIV-positive patients. HAART generally refers to an antiretroviral regimen that can be expected to reduce the viral load in antiretroviral-naïve patients to fewer than 50 copies/mL. A panel of experts convened by the US Department of Health and Human Services and the Henry J. Kaiser Family Foundation recommended HAART as the standard of care for all HIV-infected patients.[12] These potent antiretroviral agents and effective management of OIs have led to an improved quality of life and prolonged survival among HIV-infected US patients.[13] A significant decrease in the incidence of OIs and death was first reported in 1996, when preliminary data demonstrated that the addition of ritonavir to an existing reverse transcriptase regimen in severely immunocompromised patients decreased the incidence of OIs and death.[14] A recent analysis demonstrated both a decline in opportunistic infections (89 to 13.3 per 1,000 person-years) and opportunistic malignancies (23.4 to 3.0 per 1,000 person-years) from 1994 to 2007.[2]

CHANGES IN THE NATURAL HISTORY OF OPPORTUNISTIC INFECTIONS

OIs result from long-standing immunosuppression from HIV infection.[8] For example, before HAART, approximately 40% of all AIDS patients exhibited CMV retinitis, with the most cases occurring at CD4+ counts below 100. Since the implementation of HAART, a decrease in the incidence and progression of CMV retinitis have been noted.[15,16]

Ironically, HAART therapy also has been associated with a worsening or an unmasking of occult OIs in patients with advanced AIDS. When antiretroviral therapy strengthens the immune system, inflammatory symptoms in response to infection are more clinically pronounced.[13] This syndrome has been referred to as immune reconstitution inflammatory syndrome (IRIS). IRIS incidence is estimated to be 10% to 40% in patients starting antiretroviral therapy, based primarily on retrospective observational data.[17–20] During IRIS, there is typically a rapid increase in CD4+ lymphocytes; however, this does not represent fully function cells, but rather an increase in memory subtypes.

The initiation of HAART typically results in an increase in $CD4^+$ lymphocytes and a decrease in HIV-1 RNA to undetectable levels. This initial increase in $CD4^+$ T cells after start of therapy involves an increase in memory T cells with low proliferation and a decrease in functional or effector cells. As a result, opportunistic infections that are present in tissues are allowed to proliferate once the immune system is recovering, allowing IRIS to occur.[21]

IMPROVEMENT OR RESOLUTION OF OPPORTUNISTIC INFECTIONS

With the initiation of HAART, reports of improvement or resolution of some OIs can occur.[22–26] These OIs include KS,[26] PML,[24] CMV,[15,16] microsporidiosis, cryptosporidiosis,[23] and molluscum contagiosum,[25] a viral infection caused by a member of the *Poxviridae* family. Furthermore, there are reports of restored immunity and clinical improvement in patients with chronic hepatitis B infection (not classified as a CDC-defined AIDS indicator condition) with the initiation of HAART.[22] However, these infections were not eradicated, and in some cases improvement was only transient. Clinical resolution most likely results from immunologic improvement, and the protective immunity against OI is sustained only as long as HAART remains effective.

Pharmacotherapeutic Management of Opportunistic Infections

Successful pharmacotherapeutic management of OIs requires an understanding of the natural history of HIV-associated OIs, including the recognition that OIs occur with declining $CD4^+$ lymphocyte counts, the clinical presentation of each disease, diagnostic techniques, and effective treatment and preventive strategies.[27] Management issues, complicated by multiple-drug therapy for OIs and HIV suppression, include adherence, toxicities, resistance, drug interactions, and cost. HIV-infected patients are usually less tolerant to drugs such as flucytosine, trimethoprim-sulfamethoxazole (TMP-SMX), and pyrimethamine; however, alternative agents are available to overcome these barriers to treatment.

In 1995, the US Public Health Service (USPHS) and the Infectious Diseases Society of America (IDSA) issued guidelines for the prevention of OIs in HIV-infected patients; these were revised in 1997,[28] 1999,[29] and 2002.[30] Recommendations are included for preventing exposure to opportunistic pathogens, preventing first episodes of disease by chemoprophylaxis or vaccination (primary prophylaxis), and preventing disease recurrence (secondary prophylaxis). Additionally, in 2004, the CDC published the first edition guidelines for treatment of OIs.[31] In 2009, a combined set of guidelines for both prevention and treatment of more than 30 opportunistic infections was developed.[13] The most recent and any archieved guidelines can be found at www.aidsinfo.nih.gov.

PRIMARY PROPHYLAXIS

Primary prophylaxis is defined as therapy that is initiated before the appearance of an OI in high-risk asymptomatic persons to prevent the initial occurrence of an infection. Primary prevention of OIs is important, considering the inevitable immune depletion associated with chronic HIV infection.[27] PCP and MAC prophylaxis have significantly prolonged survival and delayed the onset of illness (see Prophylaxis sections for both PCP and MAC).[32,33]

The guidelines strongly recommend primary prophylaxis against PCP, toxoplasmosis, *Mycobacterium tuberculosis,* MAC, and varicella-zoster virus (VZV). Vaccinations to prevent *Streptococcus pneumoniae,* hepatitis B virus, hepatitis A virus, and influenza virus infection generally are recommended for all HIV-infected patients. Primary prophylaxis for fungal infections (*Cryptococcus neoformans* and *Histoplasma capsulatum*), CMV, and bacterial infections are not routinely recommended for most patients, except in unusual circumstances (Table 74-2).

DISCONTINUATION OF PRIMARY PROPHYLAXIS THERAPY

HAART has diminished the incidence of several OIs.[16,23,26] Therefore, it may be possible to discontinue prophylactic OI therapy when $CD4^+$ counts rise above the threshold associated with risk for infection. These data have been particularly encouraging in patients who had PCP prophylaxis discontinued with an increase in $CD4^+$ counts.[13] In one observational PCP prophylaxis study, no episodes of PCP were observed after discontinuation of primary and secondary PCP prophylaxis.[34] These studies suggest that patients who respond to HAART therapy with a sustained increase in $CD4^+$ count can have their primary prophylaxis safely discontinued. The OI prophylaxis guidelines suggest that primary PCP prophylaxis may be discontinued for patients on HAART when the $CD4^+$ count is greater than 200 for at least 3 months. Primary prophylaxis for MAC may also be discontinued when the $CD4^+$ count increases to greater than 100.[13] In addition, the guidelines suggest discontinuing primary prophylaxis for toxoplasmosis when the $CD4^+$ count increases to higher than 200 for at least 3 months.[13]

ACUTE THERAPY

Prompt diagnosis and immediate initiation of therapy are essential to the management of acute infections. Most common OIs can be classified into one of two groups. The first group consists of infections that can be treated by conventional or investigational agents. These include PCP, tuberculosis (TB), cryptococcosis, CMV, MAC, and histoplasmosis. Treatment may result in either effective or moderately effective resolution. These infections may recur if chronic suppressive or secondary prophylaxis is discontinued without an accompanying elevation in the $CD4^+$ count and viral load suppression. The second group includes pathogens for which no therapeutic regimen is currently effective. These include cryptosporidiosis, microsporidiosis, and PML.

SECONDARY PROPHYLAXIS OR CHRONIC SUPPRESSIVE THERAPY

Secondary prophylaxis is used to prevent recurrence of an OI once the patient has developed signs and symptoms of active infection. In some cases, secondary prophylaxis regimens can be discontinued after patients achieve a certain $CD4^+$ level. The USPHS and IDSA strongly recommend secondary prophylaxis for PCP, toxoplasmosis (reduced dosage), MAC, CMV, *Salmonella* species, and infections caused by endemic fungi and *C. neoformans.*[13]

DISCONTINUATION OF SECONDARY PROPHYLAXIS OR CHRONIC SUPPRESSIVE THERAPY

In 1999, the USPHS/IDSA guidelines first reported that stopping primary or secondary prophylaxis for certain pathogens was safe with HAART-related increases in $CD4^+$ count to specified threshold levels. The 2002 USPHS/IDSA guidelines expanded these recommendations to other pathogens. These recommendations are also included in the most recent 2009 USPHS/IDSA guidelines.[13] Criteria for discontinuing chemoprophylaxis are based on specific clinical studies and vary by duration of $CD4^+$ count increase and duration of treatment of the initial episode of disease (in the case of secondary prophylaxis).

Maintenance therapy for CMV can be discontinued safely in patients who have maintained a $CD4^+$ count of greater than 100 for greater than 6 months on HAART.[13,16] Whereas CMV retinitis typically reactivated less than 6 to 8 weeks after stopping CMV therapy in the pre-HAART era, these patients have remained

TABLE 74-2

Primary Prophylaxis of Opportunistic Infections in HIV-Infected Adults and Adolescents

		Preventive Regimens		
Pathogen	**Indication**	**First Choice**	**Alternatives**	**D/C Prophylaxis**
Strongly Recommended as Standard of Care				
Pneumocystis jiroveci (carinii)	$CD4^+$ count <200 or oropharyngeal candidiasis	TMP-SMX, 1 DS PO daily or TMP-SMX 1 SS PO daily	TMP-SMX 1 DS TIW Dapsone 50 mg BID or 100 mg/d; dapsone 50 mg daily + pyrimethamine 50 mg QW + leucovorin 25 mg PO QW; aerosolized pentamadine 300 mg QM via Respirgard II nebulizer, atovaquone 1,500 mg PO daily; atovaquone 1,500 mg PO + pyrimethamine 25 mg PO + leucovorin 25 mg PO daily	Patients on HAART with sustained CD4 >200 cells for ≥3 months may discontinue PCP prophylaxis. Reintroduce if $CD4^+$ <200.
Mycobacterium tuberculosis				
Isoniazid sensitive	+ diagnostic test for TB with no evidence of active TB, no prior treatment OR − diagnostic test for TB, close contact with person with active TB and no personal active TB OR History of untreated or inadequately treated TB and no evidence of active TB	Isoniazid 300 mg PO daily OR isoniazid 900 mg PO BIW × 9 months both with pyridoxine 50 mg PO daily	Rifampin 600 mg PO daily × 4 months or rifabutin dose adjusted for antiretroviral therapy × 4 months	
Drug-resistant TB	Same; high probability of exposure to isoniazid-resistant tuberculosis	Choice of drugs requires consultation with public health authorities	None	
Toxoplasma gondii	IgG antibody to *Toxoplasma* and $CD4^+$ count <100	TMP-SMX, 1 DS PO daily	TMP-SMX, 1 SS PO daily; TMP-SMX 1 DS PO TIW; dapsone 50 mg PO daily + pyrimethamine 50 mg PO QW + leucovorin 25 mg PO QW; dapsone 200 mg PO QW + pyrimethymine 75 mg PO QW + leucovorin 25 mg PO QW; atovaquone 1,500 mg PO daily with or without pyrimethamine 25 mg PO daily + leucovorin 10 mg PO daily	Patients on HAART with sustained $CD4^+$ >200 for ≥3 months may discontinue toxoplasmosis prophylaxis. Restart if $CD4^+$ <100–200.
MAC	$CD4^+$ count <50 after ruling out active infection	Azithromycin, 1,200 mg PO QW; clarithromycin 500 mg PO BID; azithromycin 600 mg PO BIW	Rifabutin, 300 mg PO daily	Patients on HAART with sustained $CD4^+$ >100 for ≥3 months may discontinue MAC prophylaxis. Restart if CD4 <50.
VZV	Significant exposure to chicken pox or shingles for patients who have no history of either condition or, if available, negative antibody to VZV	VZIG 125 international units per 10 kg (max of 635 international units) IM administered 96 hours after exposure		
Usually Recommended				
Streptococcus pneumoniae	$CD4^+$ >200	23-valent polysaccharide pneumococcal vaccine 0.5 mL IM	None	
HBV	All susceptible (anti-HBc-negative) patients	Hepatitis B vaccine 3 doses	None	

(continued)

TABLE 74-2
Primary Prophylaxis of Opportunistic Infections in HIV-Infected Adults and Adolescents (*Continued*)

Pathogen	Indication	Preventive Regimens: First Choice	Alternatives	D/C Prophylaxis
Usually Recommended (*continued*)				
Influenza virus	All patients (annually before influenza season)	Inactivated trivalent influenza virus vaccine 0.5 mL/y IM	Oseltamivir 75 mg daily (influenza A or B); rimantadine, 100 mg PO BID, or amantadine 100 mg PO BID (influenza A only)	
HAV	All susceptible (anti-HAV-negative) patient at increased risk for HAV or patients with chronic liver disease (including HBV or HCV)	Hepatitis A vaccine; 2 doses	None	
Not Recommended for Most Patients; Indicated for Use Only in Unusual Circumstances				
Bacteria	Neutropenia	G-CSF 510 mg/kg SC daily ×24 weeks or GM-CSF 250 mg/m^2 SC × 24 weeks	None	
Cryptococcus neoformans	CD4$^+$ count <50	Fluconazole 100–200 mg PO daily	Itraconazole 200 mg PO daily	
Histoplasma capsulatum	CD4$^+$ count <100, endemic geographic areas	Itraconazole 200 mg PO daily	None	
CMV	CD4$^+$ count <50 and CMV antibody positive	Valganciclovir 900 mg PO daily	None	

BID, twice a day; BIW, twice weekly; CMV, cytomegalovirus; DS, double strength; G-CSF, granulocyte colony-stimulating factor; GM-CSF, granulocyte-macrophage colony-stimulating factor; HAART, highly active antiretroviral therapy; HAV, hepatitis A virus; HBc, hepatitis B core; HBV, hepatitis B virus; IM, intramuscularly; INH, isoniazid; MAC, *Mycobacterium avium* complex; PO, orally; QM, monthly; QW, weekly; RIF, rifampin; SC, subcutaneously; SS, single strength; TIW, three times a week; TMP-SMX, trimethoprim-sulfamethoxazole; TST, tuberculin skin test; VZIG, varicella-zoster immune globulin; VZV, varicella-zoster virus.
Source: Kaplan JE et al. Guidelines for prevention and treatment of opportunistic infections in HIV-infected adults and adolescents: recommendations from the CDC, the National Institutes of Health, and the HIV Medicine Association of the Infectious Diseases Society of America. *MMWR Recomm Rep*. 2009;58(RR-4):1.

diseasefree for more than 30 to 95 weeks with concomitant HAART. Plasma HIV RNA levels varied among these patients, demonstrating that the CD4$^+$ count is the primary determinant of immune recovery to CMV. The decision to stop CMV prophylaxis should be made in consultation with an ophthalmologist and is influenced by factors such as the magnitude and duration of CD4$^+$ increases and viral load suppression, anatomical location of retinal lesions, and vision in the contralateral eye. Regular ophthalmic examination is critical.[13] Secondary PCP prophylaxis may be discontinued among patients whose CD4$^+$ counts have increased to greater than 200 for more than 3 months while on HAART. Secondary prophylaxis for disseminated MAC may be discontinued among patients who have completed 12 months of MAC therapy, have no signs or symptoms of MAC, and have had a CD4$^+$ count of greater than 100 for more than or equal to 3 months in response to HAART. Similarly, secondary prophylaxis for toxoplasmosis may be discontinued in patients who have completed initial therapy, have no signs or symptoms of infection, and have had CD4$^+$ counts of greater than 200 for more than 3 months. Using the same criteria, patients with cryptococcosis can discontinue secondary prophylaxis if they have had CD4$^+$ counts of greater than or equal to 200 for more than 6 months.

Although there are considerable data concerning the discontinuation of primary and secondary prophylaxis, there are no data regarding restarting prophylaxis if the CD4$^+$ count decreases again to levels at which the patient is likely to again be at risk for OIs. For primary prophylaxis, the same CD4$^+$ count threshold for stopping or restarting therapy is recommended. For PCP prophylaxis, the 2009 guidelines use a CD4$^+$ count of 200 as the threshold for restarting both primary and secondary prophylaxis. For toxoplasmosis the CD4$^+$ threshold is 100 to 200, and for MAC it is 50.[13]

PNEUMOCYSTIS JIROVECI PNEUMONIA

As an indication of the relative obscurity of this organism, no comprehensive text on PCP was available until 1983.[35] Since that time, this organism has been reclassified from a protozoan to a fungus on the basis of ribosomal RNA sequence comparisons. The morphologic resemblance of *P. carinii* to a protozoan has led to its life cycle being described as a cyst form, with up to eight sporozoites per cyst. The trophozoite or extracystic form has different staining characteristics (i.e., it does not stain with Toluidine Blue O or Grocott-Gomori stains) compared with the cyst or sporozoites. In addition, current literature refers to PCP as *Pneumocystis jiroveci* as opposed to the original terminology of *Pneumocystis carinii*. The former species is the one responsible for infectivity in humans. *Pneumocystis jiroveci* pneumonia is the second leading opportunitistic infection affecting HIV patients in the United States.[2] Hospitalizations and hospital mortality for AIDS-associated PCP has decreased signficiantly in the last 20 years; however, there has been a shift in the overall population at risk for PCP over time with a greater proportion of patients with PCP who are black, female, or from the Southern region of the United States.[36]

Clinical Presentation

CASE 74-1

QUESTION 1: J.R. is a 38-year-old, HIV-seropositive man who was diagnosed 5 years ago when he had an outbreak of herpes zoster. He refused antiretroviral therapy and was determined to treat himself using natural teas and herbs. J.R. developed a mild, nonproductive cough that has persisted for the last 4 weeks. He has also had a low-grade fever but denies any chills or pleuritic chest pain. His chest radiograph demonstrates a diffuse, symmetric, interstitial infiltrate. Arterial oxygen partial pressure (Pao_2) is 80 mm Hg. His last $CD4^+$ count approximately 3 months ago was 180 cells/μL and his viral load was 60,000 copies/mL. He refused primary PCP prophylaxis. After hypertonic saline nebulization for sputum induction and subsequent bronchoalveolar lavage, examination of the specimens with the modified Giemsa stain revealed both intracystic bodies and extracystic trophozoites. How is the clinical presentation of J.R. consistent with PCP?

The clinical features of PCP in AIDS patients differ from those of non-AIDS patients in that a more subtle onset, with mild fever, a cough, tachypnea, and dyspnea, is typically seen in HIV-infected patients.[13] J.R.'s low-grade fever and mild, nonproductive cough of 4 weeks' duration are consistent with this description of PCP. His history of HIV infection and the finding of trophozoites on Giemsa stain further support a diagnosis of PCP. The characteristic diffuse interstitial pulmonary infiltrates on J.R.'s chest radiograph are consistent with PCP. Limited data exist with regard to the latent state of *P. jiroveci* after host infection. Some investigators hypothesize that most persons are asymptomatic unless the host immune system becomes impaired. Others believe that the infection is caused by reinfection as opposed to reactivation.[37]

Antimicrobial Selection

CASE 74-1, QUESTION 2: A diagnosis of PCP is made and J.R. agrees to be treated. What patient factors are important to consider when selecting an antimicrobial? What would be a reasonable drug for J.R., and how might his course of PCP be monitored?

The treatment of acute PCP is determined by the degree of clinical severity on presentation. The arterial oxygen status on presentation is an important indicator of overall outcome. In one study, surviving patients had a mean Pao_2 of 70 mm Hg, whereas the mean Pao_2 of the nonsurvivors was 55 mm Hg.[37] Key factors to consider when initiating therapy for PCP include arterial blood gas findings, whether it is an initial or repeat episode of PCP, the need for parenteral therapy, and a prior history of adverse drug reactions or hypersensitivity. Concomitant therapy must also be considered.

Patients with PCP often can be classified as having mild, moderate, or severe disease, based on their oxygenation. Patients with mild PCP often have a room air alveolar-arterial (A-a) oxygen gradient of less than 35 or Pao_2 greater than 70 mm Hg, patients with moderate or severe disease have an A-a greater than 35 mm Hg or Pao_2 greater than 70 mm Hg. With the advent of corticosteroid use for moderate to severe cases of PCP (discussed later), it is useful to calculate the A-a gradient or Pao_2. The A-a gradient (normal range, 5–15 mm Hg) can be calculated as $P_{IO_2} - (1.25 \times Paco_2) - Pao_2$, where P_{IO_2} is the partial pressure of inspired oxygen (150 mm Hg in room air), and $Paco_2$ and Pao_2 are arterial levels of CO_2 and O_2, respectively, expressed in mm Hg.

Several other clinical tests have been used to identify and monitor PCP. The lactate dehydrogenase concentration in serum or bronchoalveolar lavage fluid has been used to diagnose and monitor therapy and to predict outcome of PCP. However, many patients have overlapping diseases, preventing lactate dehydrogenase from being used alone. Chest radiographs also vary with PCP. The most common picture is one of bilateral diffuse interstitial pneumonitis, but atypical patterns, such as pleural effusion, cavities, pneumatoceles, and nodules, may occur as well. A normal chest radiograph is associated with improved clinical outcome.

The natural course of PCP among untreated HIV-infected patients is progressive dyspnea and hypoxemia. Increasing patient age, subsequent episode of PCP, low hemoglobin, low partial pressure of oxygen breathing room air, the presence of medical comorbidity, and pulmonary KS are all early predictors of mortality from PCP at hospital admission.[38] Treatment of PCP in AIDS patients (compared with non–HIV-infected patients) indicates that a longer duration of therapy is needed.[35] Some patients may experience worsening hypoxemia during the first 3 to 5 days after treatment is initiated. This period of clinical worsening is least tolerated by those patients with moderate to severe PCP (Pao_2 <70 mm Hg). In sicker patients, this period may lead to respiratory failure and the need for intubation. Although many would associate the need for intensive care unit admission as a poor prognostic factor, many patients do well despite the need for mechanical ventilation and intravenous (IV) antibiotics. In light of the role of corticosteroids, patients with PCP and respiratory failure may be viewed as manageable if treated aggressively (Table 74-3).

TRIMETHOPRIM-SULFAMETHOXAZOLE

The decision to hospitalize a patient is based on the severity of his or her illness. Patients who present with mild PCP with reasonable oxygenation and without evidence of clinical deterioration can be managed as outpatients. Patients with reasonably good gas exchange (i.e., Pao_2 >70 mm Hg) but with signs of clinical deterioration most often are admitted to the hospital and given oxygen by nasal cannula and are usually started on IV TMP-SMX (15–20 mg/kg/day TMP, 75–100 mg/kg/day SMX) for 21 days.[13] The dosing of IV TMP-SMX must be modified in patients with renal dysfunction. TMP reversibly inhibits dihydrofolate reductase, and sulfamethoxazole competes with para-aminobenzoic acid in the production of dihydrofolate, synergistically blocking thymidine biosynthesis.

TMP-SMX is the drug of choice for PCP unless the patient has a history of life-threatening intolerance. In the treatment of PCP, TMP-SMX is either as effective as, or superior to, all alternative agents. A good response may be expected in more than 70% of patients receiving TMP-SMX. TMP-SMX is often prescribed orally because of its high bioavailability. The usual dose is 15 mg/kg (dosed by the TMP component) divided every 8 hours for 21 days. Because one double-strength tablet of TMP-SMX contains 160 mg TMP plus 800 mg SMX, a standard regimen is two double-strength tablets three times per day (or every 8 hours). Taking two double-strength tablets every 6 hours (eight double-strength tablets per day) does not improve efficacy and causes increased toxicity (gastrointestinal [GI] intolerance, nausea, vomiting, anorexia, and abdominal pain).

Although the TMP-SMX regimen is very efficacious, 25% to 50% of patients may be intolerant. Adverse effects include an erythematous, maculopapular, morbilliform rash, and, less commonly, severe urticaria, exfoliative dermatitis, and Stevens-Johnson syndrome. GI intolerance (nausea, vomiting, abdominal

TABLE 74-3
Treatment of *Pneumocystis jiroveci* Pneumonia

Regimen	Dose	Route	Adverse Effects/Comments
Approved			
TMP-SMX	15–20 mg/kg TMP (75–100 mg/kg SMX) daily administered IV or PO every 6–8 hours or 2 DS tabs TID	IV, PO	Hypersensitivity, hyperkalemia, rash, fever, neutropenia ↑LFTs, nephrotoxicity (15 mg/kg/d preferred to 20 mg/kg/d because of reduced toxicity)
Pentamidine isethionate	4 mg/kg IV daily for 60–90 minutes ×21 days	IV	Pancreatitis, hypotension, hypoglycemia, hyperglycemia, nephrotoxicity
Atovaquone[a]	750 mg BID with meals ×21 days (suspension)	PO	Headache, nausea, diarrhea, rash, fever, ↑LFTs
TMP[a] + dapsone	15 mg/kg/d	PO	Pruritus, GI intolerance, bone marrow suppression
	100 mg/d × 21 days	PO	Methemoglobinemia, hemolytic anemia (contraindicated in G6PD deficiency)
Clindamycin + primaquine	600 mg IV every 8 hours or 300–450 mg PO every 6 hours	PO or IV	Rash, diarrhea
	15–30 mg (base) daily × 21 days	PO	Methemoglobinemia, hemolytic anemia (contraindicated in G6PD deficiency)
Prednisone	Within 72 hours of anti-*Pneumocystis* therapy 40 mg every 12 hours × 5 days, then 40 mg daily × 5 days, then 20 mg/d × 11 days	PO	Initiation in patients with moderately severe or severe disease Pao_2 <70 mm Hg or A-a gradient >35 mm Hg

[a]Used only in mild to moderate PCP.
A-a, alveolar-arterial gradient; BID, twice a day; CNS, central nervous system; DS, double strength; GI, gastrointestinal; G6PD, glucose-6 phosphate dehydrogenase; IV, intravenous; PCP, *Pneumocystis jiroveci* pneumonia; PO, oral; Pao_2, arterial partial pressure of oxygen; LFTs, liver function tests; TMP-SMX, trimethoprim-sulfamethoxazole.

pain) is common. Hematologic side effects may include leukopenia, anemia, and thrombocytopenia. Neurologic toxicities, hyperkalemia, and hepatitis also may occur. Although increased doses, plasma concentration monitoring, and SMX metabolic capability (i.e., rapid or slow acetylation) have been considered, they have a limited role in the treatment of this disease.[39,40] Most patients who exhibit a mild hypersensitivity (skin rash) reaction can be managed with antipruritics or antihistamines without discontinuation of TMP-SMX. In some patients with mild hypersensitivity reactions, the agent can be restarted after the rash has resolved, using gradual dosage escalation or rapid oral desensitization to reduce adverse effects.[41] Patients with severe adverse reactions should be switched to another agent rather than being rechallenged with this drug.

Because J.R. seems to have a mild to moderate case of PCP (Pao_2, 80 mm Hg), has not previously experienced an episode of PCP, and has no history of adverse effects to TMP-SMX, an outpatient course of TMP-SMX would be reasonable.

ALTERNATIVES TO TRIMETHOPRIM-SULFAMETHOXAZOLE

CASE 74-1, QUESTION 3: J.R. experienced exfoliative dermatitis on day 7 of TMP-SMX treatment. What other drugs could be prescribed to treat his PCP?

Because J.R. presents with a serious adverse effect to TMP-SMX, it should be discontinued and he should not be rechallenged or desensitized. Instead, he should be treated with an alternative regimen (Table 74-3).

IV pentamidine isethionate can be used to treat acute PCP. The mechanism of action is unknown, but it may be related to interference with oxidative phosphorylation, inhibition of nucleic acid biosynthesis, or interference with dihydrofolate reductase. Pentamidine generally is more toxic than TMP-SMX.[42] In a 5-year review of 106 courses of IV pentamidine, 76 patients (72%) had adverse reactions (nephrotoxicity, dysglycemia, hepatotoxicity, hyperkalemia, and hyperamylasemia). Drug discontinuation occurred in 31 (18%) of the severe cases. Nephrotoxicity and hypoglycemia were the most common causes of drug discontinuation. Nephrotoxicity occurred in 25% to 50% of the patients with dehydration and concurrent nephrotoxic drugs among the risk factors. Hypoglycemia was noted in 5% to 10% of patients after 5 to 7 days of treatment, or several days after discontinuation of treatment. Hyperglycemia is a consequence of decreased β-cells and results in diabetes mellitus in 2% to 9% of patients. Other less common adverse effects and toxicities include thrombocytopenia, orthostatic hypotension, ventricular tachycardia, leukopenia, nausea, vomiting, abdominal pain, and anorexia.[42]

Patients receiving IV pentamidine should be monitored closely, and serum concentrations of glucose, potassium, blood urea nitrogen (BUN), and creatinine should be obtained daily or every other day during treatment. Other tests for periodic monitoring include a complete blood count (CBC), liver function tests (LFTs), amylase, lipase, and calcium.[42] Renal toxicity often responds to a reduction in the dosage of pentamidine to 3 mg/kg/day or 4 mg/kg every 48 hours (creatinine clearance <10 mL/minute); however, the drug should be discontinued in patients who exhibit signs and symptoms of pancreatitis. Risk factors for pentamidine-induced pancreatitis include prior episodes of pancreatitis and concurrent therapy with other drugs known to cause pancreatitis.

The exact mechanisms for elimination of pentamidine are not well understood. The drug is not excreted by renal mechanisms, and no metabolites have been identified. The half-life of pentamidine is prolonged with multiple dosing and may increase up to 12 days after the last dose. Nebulized pentamidine should not be considered as an alternative to IV pentamidine for treatment of PCP.[43]

Atovaquone suspension, 750 mg twice a day (BID), is available for treatment of mild to moderate PCP. Atovaquone interrupts protozoan pyrimidine synthesis and demonstrates activity against *P. carinii* and *Toxoplasma gondii* in animal models. Thus, this compound may benefit patients with more than one OI. Atovaquone is approved by the US Food and Drug Administration (FDA) for the treatment of mild to moderate PCP in patients intolerant of TMP-SMX. Atovaquone is also an alternative for primary and secondary prophylaxis for both PCP and toxoplasmosis.[13] Atovaquone is well tolerated compared with other PCP therapies. Adverse effects include rash, fever, elevated LFTs, and emesis. Atovaquone is safer, but less effective, than TMP-SMX in patients with mild to moderate PCP.[44] When compared with IV pentamidine in the treatment of mild to moderate PCP, atovaquone and pentamidine were equally efficacious; however, pentamidine was significantly more toxic.[45] Most atovaquone studies were performed using the moderately absorbed oral tablets; reformulation of this drug as a suspension has improved bioavailability by at least 30%. Concomitant administration of fatty foods with atovaquone doubles the absorption.

An oral regimen of dapsone plus TMP is another alternative to TMP-SMX. Dapsone- TMP can be used to treat mild to moderate PCP in patients intolerant of TMP-SMX. Dapsone is a sulfone antimicrobial that is used for leprosy. Although monotherapy (200 mg/day) with dapsone is ineffective for the treatment (not prophylaxis) of PCP, the addition of TMP (20 mg/kg/day) to dapsone (100 mg/day) is an effective alternative regimen.[46] In a small comparative trial of TMP-dapsone versus TMP-SMX, response rates of 93% and 90% were observed, respectively.[47] When dapsone is coadministered with TMP, the resulting plasma concentrations for both drugs are higher than when either drug is taken alone. In combination with TMP, a pyrimidine, synergistic inhibition of folic acid synthesis occurs.[48] Dapsone-TMP should not be used in sulfonamide-allergic patients with a history of type I hypersensitivity reaction, toxic epidermal necrolysis, or Stevens-Johnson syndrome. Dapsone is associated with hematologic toxicities, including hemolytic anemia, methemoglobinemia, neutropenia, and thrombocytopenia. Patients with glucose-6-phosphate dehydrogenase (G6PD) deficiency cannot detoxify hydrogen peroxide and are at an increased risk for hematologic toxicity from dapsone.

Success rates of 70% to 100% have been reported with clindamycin (600 mg IV every 6 hours or 600 mg orally three times a day [TID]) given in conjunction with 30 mg/day of primaquine base. Although skin rashes are common with this combination, these often subside with continued therapy. Some patients experience toxicities (fever, rash, granulocytopenia, and methemoglobinemia) requiring discontinuation.[49–51] As with dapsone, before starting primaquine patients should be screened for G6PD deficiency. Patients who test positive for G6PD deficiency are at risk for developing hemolytic anemia.

A double-blind efficacy and toxicity study of 181 patients with mild to moderate PCP compared three oral drug regimens: TMP-SMX versus dapsone-TMP versus clindamycin-primaquine. The doses of TMP-SMX and dapsone-TMP were weight-based, and the dosage of clindamycin-primaquine was 600 mg clindamycin TID and primaquine 30 mg/day. All patients with moderately severe PCP (A-a oxygen gradient >45) were treated with prednisone (40 mg BID for 5 days, then once daily for 3 weeks). Rash was the most frequent dose-limiting toxicity (TMP-SMX, 19%; dapsone-TMP, 10%; clindamycin-primaquine, 21%). Hematologic toxicities were observed more frequently in the clindamycin-primaquine arm. Elevated LFTs (five times above baseline) were more frequent in the TMP-SMX arm. The clindamycin-primaquine group demonstrated better quality of life scores at day 7, but by day 21 these differences became less significant.[46] TMP-SMX, dapsone-TMP, and clindamycin-primaquine demonstrated equal efficacy in patients with mild to moderate PCP.

J.R. should be hospitalized to better manage his severe adverse reaction and to complete his treatment of PCP. Because of his severe reaction to TMP-SMX, dapsone-TMP should not be administered because dapsone is a sulfone with risk of cross-reactivity in patients with severe sulfonamide allergies. IV pentamidine is an option for J.R., but its toxicity suggests that it should be reserved for patients with more severe PCP presentation. Atovaquone is a reasonable option for patients with mild PCP who are intolerant to TMP-SMX and have no evidence of GI dysfunction, but it is not as effective as TMP-SMX or IV pentamidine. Clindamycin-primaquine is as efficacious as TMP-SMX for the treatment of mild to moderate PCP and can be administered orally. Consequently, it is the drug of choice in this patient.

The decision was made to start J.R. on oral clindamycin-primaquine for his mild to moderate PCP. J.R. tested negative for G6PD deficiency and was treated with clindamycin-primaquine for 14 days, completing a 21-day course of PCP therapy (Table 74-3).

Initiation of Corticosteroids

CASE 74-1, QUESTION 4: Should J.R. receive corticosteroid therapy with PCP treatment? When should corticosteroids be initiated, and what would be a reasonable regimen for patients with PCP?

Corticosteroids have an important role in the management of patients with acute PCP who are clinically ill and have a low Po_2 (<70 mm Hg) or an A-a oxygen gradient greater than 35.[13] Many patients who are started on PCP therapy have an acute period of clinical deterioration, which may be associated with an acute inflammatory reaction to the rapid killing of *Pneumocystis.* Particularly among patients with moderate to severe PCP (A-a oxygen gradient >35 mm Hg or Pao_2 <70 mm Hg on room air), the use of prednisone during the first 72 hours of treatment may prevent fatal acute deterioration.[52] Corticosteroids may also have some benefit in patients exhibiting acute respiratory failure after 72 hours of conventional PCP therapy.[53] The recommended dosing of prednisone is 40 mg given orally BID for 5 days, then 40 mg/day for 5 days, and then 20 mg/day for 11 days, for a total of 21 days.[54] Patients requiring IV corticosteroids may receive methylprednisolone at 75% of the prednisone dose. The major concern using glucocorticoids is activation of latent infections (such as TB) or exacerbation of an active undiagnosed condition (especially fungal infections). However, the beneficial role of corticosteroids as adjunctive therapy outweighs the relative risk of short-term steroid use in this population.[55] More common side effects of short-term corticosteroids include ulcerative esophagitis, increased appetite, weight gain, sodium and fluid retention, headache, and elevated LFTs. While corticosteroids are being given, it may be prudent for patients with a history of candidiasis to receive suppressive fluconazole therapy; those with a positive TB skin test should receive suppressive TB therapy. Corticosteroids should be used with caution in the presence of uncontrolled diabetes, active GI bleeding, and uncontrolled hypertension.

Considering his mild hypoxemia (Pao_2 >70 mm Hg), J.R. is not a candidate for corticosteroid therapy.

Prophylaxis

CASE 74-1, QUESTION 5: J.R. was hospitalized and responded well to treatment. He now is a candidate for secondary prophylaxis. What secondary prophylaxis would be a good choice for J.R. when he is discharged from the hospital?

The early recognized efficacy of TMP-SMX prophylaxis[50] led to the eventual widespread application of prophylaxis and the development of guidelines for PCP prophylaxis (Table 74-2).[13]

HIV-infected patients not receiving HAART or *Pneumocystis* prophylaxis were associated with a PCP prevalence of 8.4%, 18.4%, and 33.3% at 6, 12, and 36 months, respectively, in patients with a $CD4^+$ count of less than 200.[56] These data have formed the basis on which patients receive PCP prophylaxis. In addition to patients with $CD4^+$ counts of less than 200, other patients at risk for PCP include those with a $CD4^+$ count of less than 14%, a history of an AIDS-defining illness, a history of oropharyngeal candidiasis, and possibly those with $CD4^+$ counts of 200 to 250.[13] J.R. refused primary prophylaxis and developed PCP. Because the expected relapse rate without prophylaxis among patients (before the use of protease inhibitors) is 66% at 12 months' follow-up, secondary prophylaxis is necessary for J.R. to prevent recurrence.

The same agents and dosing schedules are recommended for primary (before an acute event) and secondary (after an acute event) prophylaxis of PCP.[13] TMP-SMX, one double-strength tablet daily, is the most efficacious prophylactic regimen; a single-strength tablet daily is less toxic and nearly as efficacious. Patients with a history of non–life-threatening rash or fever due to TMP-SMX may benefit from rechallenge with the original (or half) dose, or a dose-escalation technique (desensitization regimen). Desensitization is preferred to switching to an alternative agent and is more successful than the direct rechallenge method.[57] Desensitization involves initiating very low doses of TMP-SMX and gradually increasing to the maximum dose over the course of days to weeks. In addition, patients who develop PCP while receiving prophylactic doses of TMP-SMX usually respond to full therapeutic doses for acute therapy. However, J.R. had a life-threatening reaction to TMP-SMX and should not be rechallenged or desensitized, and another agent should be chosen for prophylaxis.

The alternative agents used for prophylaxis include dapsone, dapsone plus pyrimethamine (with leucovorin), atovaquone suspension, and aerosolized pentamidine administered by the Respirgard II nebulizer (Table 74-2). TMP-SMX confers additional protection against toxoplasmosis and certain bacterial infections. Regimens containing dapsone plus pyrimethamine or atovaquone with or without pyrimethamine also protect against toxoplasmosis.[13] Although yet to be confirmed in clinical trials, other options include oral clindamycin-primaquine, intermittently administered IV pentamidine, oral pyrimethamine-sulfadiazine, and aerosolized pentamidine administered by other nebulizing devices.[13] TMP-SMX is more efficacious than dapsone or aerosolized pentamidine in the prevention of PCP.[58]

Extrapulmonary (e.g., lymph nodes, spleen, liver, bone marrow, adrenal gland, GI tract) *P. carinii* has been noted in patients receiving inhaled pentamidine prophylaxis,[59] a finding rarely observed with IV administration. In addition, aerosolized pentamidine alters the usual chest radiograph findings associated with PCP, potentially complicating the diagnosis of this disease. Upper lobe infiltrates, cystic lesions, pneumothoraces, cavitary lesions with nodular infiltrates, and pleural effusions have been associated with aerosolized pentamidine prophylaxis. Pentamidine prophylaxis is more expensive than TMP-SMX or dapsone but less expensive than atovaquone suspension.

The guidelines for primary prophylaxis suggest that prophylactic antimicrobial therapy can be discontinued when $CD4^+$ counts rise above the threshold associated with risk for infection (i.e., <200 for PCP).[13] Many studies support the practice of discontinuing secondary PCP prophylaxis in patients whose $CD4^+$ counts have increased to greater than 200 for at least 3 months.[13] A European cohort study found that primary PCP rates were very low in patients with CD4 counts of 101 to 200 cells/μL and a viral load less than 400 copies/mL regardless of prophylaxis, indicating that discontinuation of prophylaxis may be safe in patients with a CD4 count greater than 100 cells/μL who are on effective antiretrovirals.[60] The guidelines recommend that prophylaxis be reintroduced if the $CD4^+$ count decreases to less than 200, or if PCP recurs at a $CD4^+$ count of greater than 200.[13] J.R. responded well to his PCP treatment with clindamycin-primaquine in the hospital. However, because this regimen is unproven for secondary prophylaxis, it cannot be recommended. Considering his intolerance to TMP-SMX, the best selections would be dapsone (with or without pyrimethamine) or atovaquone suspension.

TOXOPLASMA GONDII ENCEPHALITIS

Clinical Presentation

CASE 74-2

QUESTION 1: W.O. is a 40-year-old man discovered to be HIV-positive during admission to a detoxification program for alcohol and heroin dependency. W.O. presented to the AIDS clinic with esophageal candidiasis, a $CD4^+$ count of 60 cells/μL (normal, approximately 1,000 cells/μL), a viral load of 150,000 copies/mL, and a *Toxoplasma* immunoglobulin G (IgG) titer of 1:256. W.O. was started on HAART therapy. He remained well until 2 years later, when he presented to the emergency department reporting two seizures in the past 24 hours. His medications at that time included daily zidovudine (AZT), lamivudine, lopinavir/ritonavir, and inhaled pentamidine 300 mg monthly. His temperature was 100.1°F, and he was observed to have difficulty walking. His $CD4^+$ count is 90 cells/μL (previously 230 cells/μL), viral load is 70,000 copies/mL (previously 4,000), and white blood cell (WBC) count is 4,200 cells/L (normal, 3,800–9,800). A magnetic resonance image (MRI) of the head reveals several ring-shaped lesions in the brain stem. *Toxoplasma* encephalitis is presumptively diagnosed. Should W.O. be isolated from other patients and health care workers to prevent the spread of this organism?

T. gondii is a parasitic protozoan that can infect people and is spread by environmental factors, such as the consumption of raw or undercooked meats and contact with cat feces. Immunocompetent persons infected with *T. gondii* may develop mild symptoms resembling infectious mononucleosis. However, these symptoms are generally transient and not associated with significant sequelae in immune competent patients (except in pregnant women). Recrudescent disease from *T. gondii* is problematic in patients with a suppressed cellular immune system, including those infected with HIV. Any HIV-positive patient infected with *T. gondii* is at risk for developing clinical disease, particularly at $CD4^+$ counts less than 100, as illustrated by W.O.[13] W.O. presents with encephalitis (an inflammation of the brain or brainstem), the most frequent manifestation of *T. gondii* in HIV-positive patients.

All HIV-infected patients should be tested for IgG antibody to *T. gondii* after HIV diagnosis to detect latent infection. In the United States, as many as 70% of healthy adults are seropositive to *Toxoplasma*. The prevalence of *Toxoplasma* encephalitis among HIV-positive patients varies depending on the geographic region. In the United States, only 3% to 10% of AIDS patients actually develop encephalitis. In countries such as France, El Salvador, and Tahiti, where uncooked meat commonly is ingested, seropositivity is greater than 90% by the fourth decade of life. *Toxoplasma* encephalitis may develop in as many as 25% to 50% of AIDS patients in these countries.[61]

The two major routes of transmission of *Toxoplasma* to humans are oral and congenital. W.O. need not be isolated from other patients and health care workers. HIV-infected patients should be advised not to eat raw and undercooked meat (internal temperature of meat should be at least 165°–170°F), especially patients who are IgG negative for *T. gondii*. Patients should wash their hands after touching uncooked meats and soil, and fruits and vegetables must be washed before eating. HIV-infected patients should avoid stray cats, keep their cats inside, and change the litter box daily. If no one else is available to change the litter box, patients should wash their hands thoroughly afterward.[13]

Diagnosis

CASE 74-2, QUESTION 2: Is there sufficient clinical evidence to establish a presumptive diagnosis of *Toxoplasma* encephalitis in W.O.?

The diagnosis of *Toxoplasma* encephalitis usually is presumptive because demonstration of cysts or trophozoites in brain tissue is required for a definitive diagnosis. The clinical signs and symptoms of *Toxoplasma* encephalitis can be either focal (indicating a specific region of the brain that is infected or inflamed) or generalized (indicating diffuse inflammation of the brain). *Toxoplasma* encephalitis usually occurs in patients with $CD4^+$ counts of less than 100. Serum titers of antibodies against *T. gondii* typically reflect past infection with the organism and unfortunately do not help delineate whether acute infection is present. In addition, cerebrospinal fluid (CSF) polymerase chain reaction for *Toxoplasma* is not always a reliable diagnostic tool. Without prophylaxis, 45% of seropositive HIV-infected patients experience encephalitis as a reactivation of a latent infection. Most patients with encephalitis have single or multiple ring-enhancing lesions demonstrated on computed tomography scan or MRI of the head. Brain biopsy is reserved for patients with symptoms of encephalitis who are seronegative and for those who do not respond to presumptive antitoxoplasmosis therapy.[62] Because of the nonspecific diagnosis of *Toxoplasma* encephalitis, a high index of suspicion for other causes of encephalitis (e.g., central nervous system [CNS] lymphoma or TB) should be maintained throughout the treatment period for presumed *Toxoplasma* encephalitis. W.O. has overwhelming clinical evidence suggestive of *Toxoplasma* encephalitis. He is HIV positive, has a $CD4^+$ count of less than 100, a positive *Toxoplasma* titer of 1:256 IgG, and a ring-shaped lesion in the brainstem on MRI. The development of this infection, in addition to the decline in $CD4^+$ T cells and the increase in plasma HIV RNA concentrations, may signal antiretroviral failure. W.O.'s current antiretroviral therapy should be reassessed, including his adherence to the regimen.

Prophylaxis

CASE 74-2, QUESTION 3: Should W.O. have been receiving prophylactic therapy for *T. gondii*?

Similar to many other OIs associated with HIV, therapy for toxoplasmosis can be categorized into primary prophylaxis, treatment of acute disease, and secondary prophylaxis. Primary prophylaxis is currently recommended in HIV-infected patients with $CD4^+$ counts of less than 100 who are also IgG positive for *T. gondii* (Table 74-2). Many of the agents used to prevent PCP have activity against *T. gondii:* TMP-SMX, dapsone-pyrimethamine-leucovorin, and atovaquone with or without pyrimethamine/leucovorin are effective as primary prophylaxis for *T. gondii*.[13] The increased use of prophylaxis with these agents has significantly decreased the incidence of *Toxoplasma* encephalitis.[2,13] The double-strength TMP-SMX tablet once daily is recommended as first-line prophylaxis. Data do not support the use of macrolides or aerosolized pentamidine for *Toxoplasma* prophylaxis. Similarly, data are conflicting regarding the efficacy of pyrimethamine as monotherapy for primary prophylaxis.[63,64]

Primary prophylaxis may be discontinued in patients who have responded to HAART with an increase in the $CD4^+$ counts to greater than 200 for more than 3 months. In addition, data supports reinstituting primary prophylaxis when $CD4^+$ counts drop below 200.

W.O. is currently receiving inhaled pentamidine for PCP prophylaxis. Because of the localized delivery of inhaled pentamidine, W.O. was at risk for the development of *Toxoplasma* encephalitis. Considering his $CD4^+$ count and IgG seropositivity, he should have received primary prophylaxis for *T. gondii*.

Treatment

ACUTE THERAPY

CASE 74-2, QUESTION 4: How should W.O.'s presumptive *Toxoplasma* encephalitis be treated?

Approximately 80% of patients with acute *Toxoplasma* encephalitis can be treated successfully with a combination of sulfadiazine 4 g/day in three or four daily divided doses and pyrimethamine as a single 200-mg loading dose, followed by 50 to 75 mg/day as a single daily dose plus leucovorin 10 to 25 mg orally every day.[13] Induction therapy should be continued for 6 weeks after resolution of symptoms (a treatment course of approximately 8 weeks) followed by maintenance therapy (secondary prophylaxis). Sulfadiazine toxicity may limit the completion of a full course of therapy in as many as 40% of patients.[65] However, successful desensitization has been documented.[66] W.O.'s clinical and radiologic response should be monitored closely and other diagnoses considered if there is no improvement.

Alternative therapy includes pyrimethamine plus leucovorin with clindamycin 600 to 900 mg IV every 6 hours or 600 mg orally every 6 hours for at least 6 weeks. One controlled trial compared the efficacy and tolerability of pyrimethamine plus sulfadiazine versus pyrimethamine plus clindamycin. Although both regimens were effective, pyrimethamine-sulfadiazine was superior to pyrimethamine-clindamycin. The rate of adverse events was similar with both regimens; however, pyrimethamine-clindamycin led to fewer discontinuations than pyrimethamine-sulfadiazine (11% vs. 30%, respectively).[67] Trimethoprim-sulfamethoxazole may be considered a treatment option, particularly in patients who cannot take an oral regimen because the only widely available parenteral sulfonamide is the sulfamethoxazole component of TMP-SMX. However, there is less in vitro activity and less clinical data to support the use of TMP-SMX as monotherapy for toxoplasmosis.[68] Additionally, anticonvulsants should be given to patients with *Toxoplasma* encephalitis and a history of seizures, and corticosteroids may be warranted for focal lesions or edema, but should be used cautiously.

CASE 74-2, QUESTION 5: W.O. is treated with sulfadiazine-pyrimethamine. What are the limitations to the use of the sulfadiazine component for the treatment of *Toxoplasma* encephalitis?

As with other sulfonamides in HIV patients, rashes commonly occur with sulfadiazine therapy.[65] Similar to TMP-SMX, various desensitization regimens have been recommended[41,66]; however, it may be simpler to use alternative regimens.

Renal function should be monitored throughout therapy. Elevated serum creatinine (SCr) levels, hematuria, or decreased urine output may occur secondary to sulfadiazine-induced crystalluria. The water solubility of sulfadiazine is less than that of other sulfonamides; therefore, hydration (2–3 L/day) is needed to prevent crystalline nephropathy, and aggressive hydration and alkalinization can be used in cases of crystal formation.

CASE 74-2, QUESTION 6: What toxicities are associated with the pyrimethamine component?

Pyrimethamine can suppress bone marrow function; thus, concomitant therapy with other medications that suppress marrow function (e.g., AZT or ganciclovir) may not be tolerated. Leucovorin (10–25 mg/day) is always given in conjunction with pyrimethamine to maintain bone marrow function, although it may not always be successful. Leucovorin doses can be increased to 50 to 100 mg/day in divided doses if needed to reverse bone marrow suppression.[13] Folic acid (not folinic acid) should be avoided because it can be used for growth by protozoal organisms, potentially antagonizing pyrimethamine-sulfadiazine activity.[69] Vitamin preparations containing large quantities of folic acid should be discontinued during therapy for *T. gondii*.

W.O. is not taking any medications that would make him particularly susceptible to the myelosuppressive effects of pyrimethamine and he is not neutropenic. Consequently, he should be given sulfadiazine and pyrimethamine.

SUPPRESSIVE THERAPY (SECONDARY PROPHYLAXIS)

CASE 74-2, QUESTION 7: Once W.O. has completed acute therapy for his *Toxoplasma* encephalitis, should he receive suppressive therapy?

Most antiprotozoal agents do not eradicate the cyst form of *T. gondii*. Therefore, patients should be administered lifelong suppressive therapy unless immune reconstitution occurs as a consequence of HAART.[13] A commonly used regimen for patients who cannot tolerate sulfonamides is pyrimethamine plus clindamycin. However, only the combination of pyrimethamine plus sulfadiazine provides protection against PCP as well. Additionally, two small studies of patients receiving maintenance therapy for *Toxoplasma* encephalitis have suggested that sulfadiazine-pyrimethamine is more effective than clindamycin-pyrimethamine or pyrimethamine alone.[67] The use of atovaquone with or without pyrimethamine is also effective as prophylaxis for both *Toxoplasma* and PCP, but is significantly more expensive and is only available as a less palatable liquid formulation.

Patients receiving secondary prophylaxis are at low risk for recurrence of *Toxoplasma* encephalitis, remain asymptomatic, and have a sustained increase in their CD4+ count to greater than 200 after more than 6 months of HAART therapy. Clinicians may obtain a brain MRI as part of the evaluation to determine the end point of therapy. Discontinuation of primary and secondary toxoplasmosis prophylaxis is safe if patients are receiving HAART and their CD4+ count has increased to greater than 200 for at least 3 months. Secondary prophylaxis should be reintroduced if the CD4+ count decreases to less than 200.[13]

W.O. will be continued on sulfadiazine-pyrimethamine for suppressive therapy for his *Toxoplasma* encephalitis because his CD4+ count has decreased to less than 100. W.O. is currently receiving aerosolized pentamidine for PCP prophylaxis, but because sulfadiazine-pyrimethamine is also protective against PCP, the aerosolized pentamidine can be discontinued. Clindamycin-pyrimethamine is an inferior option because it does not protect against PCP.[13]

ALTERNATIVE THERAPIES

CASE 74-2, QUESTION 8: What treatment options exist for patients who cannot tolerate sulfadiazine and do not wish to undergo desensitization?

Clindamycin can be substituted for sulfadiazine in the acute treatment of toxoplasmosis (900–1,200 mg IV every 6 hours or 600 mg orally [PO] every 6 hours) plus pyrimethamine and leucovorin at standard doses.[13] Monotherapy with atovaquone and the tetracyclines, doxycycline and minocycline, have been anecdotally effective. Combination therapy with pyrimethamine and leucovorin plus azithromycin (1.2–1.5 g/day), clarithromycin (1 g BID), or atovaquone (750 mg PO four times a day) similarly has shown promise in a limited numbers of patients.[13]

CYTOMEGALOVIRUS DISEASE

Diagnosis

CASE 74-3

QUESTION 1: P.Z., a 39-year-old man with AIDS, complains of floating spots, light flashes, and difficulty reading road signs when he drives. His most recent laboratory results were as follows:

BUN, 17 mg/dL
SCr, 0.8 mg/dL
CD4+ count, 40 cells/μL
Viral load, 80,000 copies/mL (3 months ago)
WBC count, 1,200 cells/L, with 63% polymorphonuclear neutrophil leukocytes

His current weight is 63 kg. P.Z.'s medications include tenofovir, emtricitabine, atazanavir, ritonavir, dapsone (PCP prophylaxis), and azithromycin (MAC prophylaxis). He has a history of hematologic intolerance to zidovudine and TMP-SMX. P.Z. is known to have a positive CMV IgG antibody titer. Funduscopic examination reveals alternating areas of hemorrhage and scar tissue (a "cottage cheese and ketchup" appearance) in the proximity of the retina in his left eye.

ONLINE CONTENT

For a visual of the presentation of CMV, go to http://thepoint.lww.com/AT10e.

What is the likely cause of P.Z.'s visual problems?

P.Z. has an inflammation of the retina (retinitis), most likely because of CMV. Many HIV patients have been previously infected with CMV, and reactivation typically occurs when CD4+ counts are less than 50. Before HAART, the prevalence of CMV disease in patients with AIDS was 30%.[13] Incidence of new cases of CMV end-organ disease has declined by 75% to 80% with the advent of HAART and is now estimated to be less than 6 cases per 100 person-years.[70] Although CMV can cause colitis, pneumonitis, esophagitis, hepatitis, and neurologic disease, retinitis is the most common manifestation of active infection in AIDS patients, accounting for 75% to 85% of CMV end-organ disease. One investigation describing patients with CMV retinitis in the post-HAART era found a diverse demographic group with infection; most of them had received HAART, and as expected they had very low $CD4^+$ counts.[71] In addition, characteristics of the disease in this group were similar to those in the pre-HAART era. Diagnosis is usually presumptive because biopsy is difficult given the inaccessibility of the retina. Serology is indicative of previous CMV infection but not active disease. Cultures (serum, urine, and saliva) may be useful for monitoring therapy, considering that patients frequently have disseminated CMV disease. Patients with positive cultures for CMV while receiving therapy may be at a higher risk for relapse.[72] Typically, the diagnosis of CMV retinitis is based on observations made during a dilated retinal examination and indirect ophthalmoscopy, as was done for P.Z. Lesions appear as fluffy, white retinal patches with retinal hemorrhage.

Once CMV retinitis is diagnosed, the patient should be thoroughly examined for extraocular CMV disease. P.Z. will require regular ophthalmologic examinations, along with retinal photographs, for life. As with HIV therapy, CMV DNA quantification in plasma or blood cells by polymerase chain reaction may have a role in evaluating treatment efficacy and predicting symptomatic development of CMV disease.[13]

Drug Therapy

CASE 74-3, QUESTION 2: What are the treatment options for CMV retinitis, and which one would be preferred for P.Z.?

Several treatment options exist for CMV retinitis: oral valganciclovir, IV ganciclovir, IV ganiclovir followed by oral valganciclovir, IV foscarnet, IV cidofovir, and ganciclovir intraocular implants with valganciclovir for induction and maintenance therapy. Alternatives include combined IV ganciclovir plus foscarnet, or intraocular injections of ganciclovir, foscarnet, or cidofovir.[13] The efficacy of combined parenteral ganciclovir and foscarnet is similar to monotherapy, but it is more toxic. This latter therapy should be reserved for patients with refractory disease (Table 74-4).[73]

Intraocular implants and intraocular injections of ganciclovir have similar efficacy in the treatment of CMV retinitis, but their benefit is localized to the infected eye and may lead to an increased risk of contralateral retinitis and extraocular CMV disease. Concomitant systemic anti-CMV therapy is, therefore, recommended (e.g., oral valganciclovir or IV ganciclovir). Use of ganciclovir intraocular implants with oral valganciclovir has shown to be more effective at preventing relapse of retinitis than IV ganciclovir and likely oral valganciclovir.[13] Therefore, many providers prefer this as first-line therapy in patients with immediate sight-threatening lesions, although others chose oral valganciclovir as first-line treatment. The choice of agents typically depends on drug efficacy, toxicity, stage of disease, and quality-of-life issues.

GANCICLOVIR

Ganciclovir is an acyclic nucleoside with CMV activity superior to acyclovir. Similar to other nucleosides, ganciclovir must be taken into cells and phosphorylated before it can compete with endogenous nucleotides for binding to viral DNA polymerase. Ganciclovir is poorly absorbed orally (bioavailability, approximately 5%–9%), and the oral form is no longer marketed. The disposition of ganciclovir is biexponential after IV administration (terminal half-life, approximately 2.5 hours). The total body clearance is highly dependent on glomerular filtration and tubular secretion.

The induction dose of ganciclovir is 5 mg/kg per dose every 12 hours IV for 14 to 21 days. The dose-limiting toxicity is bone marrow suppression, with neutropenia occurring in approximately 50% of patients. Thrombocytopenia is also observed. Absolute neutrophil counts (ANCs) and platelets should be monitored weekly during ganciclovir therapy. If the ANC falls to less than 1,000 cells/μL or the platelet count to less than 50,000/μL, the monitoring frequency should be increased to twice weekly.[27,74] Ganciclovir is also available as an intraocular implant (Table 74-4). Dosage adjustments must be made in patients with renal dysfunction (Table 74-5).

Patients who develop ganciclovir-induced bone marrow suppression can be given granulocyte colony-stimulating factor (G-CSF). Both G-CSF (filgrastim) and granulocyte-macrophage colony-stimulating factor (GM-CSF [sargramostim])[75,76] have been used successfully in stimulating production of WBC. Although neither of these agents is FDA-approved for this indication, use of the colony-stimulating factors may allow for continuation of sight-saving or life-prolonging therapy. Because GM-CSF may stimulate HIV replication in macrophage cell lines,[77] patients should receive concomitant antiretroviral therapy.

VALGANCICLOVIR

Valganciclovir is an oral monovalyl ester prodrug that is rapidly hydrolyzed to ganciclovir. The absolute bioavailability of ganciclovir from valganciclovir is 60%, and a dose of 900 mg results in ganciclovir blood concentrations similar to those obtained with a dose of 5 mg/kg of IV ganciclovir. Oral valganciclovir and IV ganciclovir are equally effective as induction therapy for newly diagnosed CMV retinitis in patients with AIDS.[78] The frequency and severity of adverse events were similar in the two groups. Based on these data, oral valganciclovir is as effective as and no more toxic than IV ganciclovir and the convenience of the oral route suggests it be the drug of choice for the long-term management of CMV retinitis in patients with AIDS.

CIDOFOVIR

Cidofovir is a nucleotide analog that is phosphorylated intracellularly to an active diphosphate metabolite. It is the most potent of all the available anti-CMV compounds and is active against herpes simplex virus (HSV) and VZV, including acyclovir-resistant isolates. Cidofovir does not require viral activation. Because nucleotide analogs do not require virally encoded kinases for their activity, they remain a treatment option for patients who have failed to respond to ganciclovir. Cidofovir is poorly absorbed orally (bioavailability, <5%) and has an intracellular half-life of 17 to 65 hours, resulting in once-weekly induction and every-other-week maintenance therapy. This feature substantially enhances the quality of life relative to foscarnet or ganciclovir, which must be administered much more frequently.

Eighty percent (80%) of this poorly soluble agent is excreted unchanged in the urine via filtration and tubular secretion. Cidofovir is nephrotoxic; however, administration of probenecid (2 g administered 3 hours before the start of infusion and two 1-g doses administered at 2 and 8 hours after infusion) blocks tubular secretion and reduces nephrotoxicity. Prehydration with 1 L of normal saline is required 1 hour before each dose and, if tolerated, repeated concomitantly with or after the cidofovir infusion. Because nephrotoxicity is the most significant dose-limiting toxicity, other nephrotoxic agents should be discontinued (e.g., nonsteroidal anti-inflammatory drugs, aminoglycosides), and renal function should be carefully monitored throughout therapy (BUN, SCr, proteinuria) (Table 74-4). Dosage adjustment must accompany any deterioration in renal function (Table 74-5).

TABLE 74-4
Treatment of Cytomegalovirus Retinitis[a]

	IV Ganciclovir	Valganciclovir	IV Foscarnet	Combination IV Ganciclovir and IV Foscarnet Sodium	Intraocular Ganciclovir Implant	IV Cidofovir
Dosing regimens	*Induction:* 5 mg/kg every 12 hours for 14–21 days	*Induction:* 900 mg every 12 hours for 14–21 days	*Induction:* 90 mg/kg every 12 hours for 14–21 days	*Prior ganciclovir induction:* both IV foscarnet 90 mg/kg every 12 hours and IV ganciclovir 5 mg/kg daily for 14–21 days	*Surgical:* intraocular implantation of ganciclovir (4.5 mg) implant releasing 1 mg/h (duration 68 months; then replacement required every 58 months)	*Induction:* 5 mg/kg every week for 2 weeks
	Maintenance: 5 mg/kg daily	*Maintenance:* 900 mg daily	*Maintenance:* 90–120 mg/kg daily; 750–1,000 mL of 0.9% saline or D_5W solution with each dose	*Maintenance:* both IV foscarnet 90–120 mg/kg and IV ganciclovir 5 mg/kg daily	*Maintenance:* 5 mg/kg every 2 weeks (*Note:* dose reduction to 3 mg/kg for SCr by 0.3–0.4 mg/dL above baseline; all doses given with probenecid and IV fluid)	
	Refractory disease induction: 7.5 mg/kg every 12 hours for 14–21 days	*Alternative regimen:* with ganciclovir intraocular implant 900 mg daily		*Prior foscarnet sodium induction:* both IV ganciclovir 5 mg/kg every 12 hours and IV foscarnet 90–120 mg/kg daily		
	Maintenance: 10 mg/kg daily (*Note:* dosage should be adjusted for creatinine clearance <70 mL/min; see Table 74-5)			*Reinduction:* IV ganciclovir 5 mg/kg and IV foscarnet 90 mg/kg every 12 hours for 14–21 days		
Select adverse effects	Neutropenia, thrombocytopenia, catheter sepsis	Same as ganciclovir	Nephrotoxicity, electrolyte abnormalities, anemia, catheter sepsis, nausea/irritability, genital ulceration	Same as IV ganciclovir and IV foscarnet	*Surgical complications:* transient blurred vision, infection, hemorrhage	Nephrotoxicity, neutropenia, probenecid adverse effects (rash, fever, nausea, fatigue), uveitis, alopecia, hypotonia
Important drug interactions	Neutropenia, with AZT, cancer chemotherapy didanosine levels	Same as ganciclovir	Nephrotoxicity with other nephrotoxic drugs (e.g., amphotericin B, aminoglycosides, IV pentamadine)	Same as IV ganciclovir and IV foscarnet		Nephrotoxicity with other nephrotoxic drugs (e.g., amphotericin B, aminoglycosides, IV pentamadine, NSAIDs) Probenecid: Level of most proximal tubular excreted drugs
Adjunctive therapy	G-CSF/GM-CSF effective for neutropenia	Same as ganciclovir	IV or oral hydration essential; potassium, calcium/magnesium supplements, antiemetics may be required	Same as both IV ganciclovir and IV foscarnet	Systemic anti-CMV therapy recommended (oral ganciclovir, 4,500 mg/d)	Probenecid and IV hydration essential; antiemetics, antihistamine, acetaminophen premedication commonly used for probenecid toxicity

Advantages	Systemic therapy; anti-HSV activity	Increased bioavailability and decreased pill count compared with PO ganciclovir	Systemic therapy; anti-HSV (acyclovir-resistant) activity; anti-HIV activity	Increased efficacy compared with either IV ganciclovir or IV foscarnet alone; improved response for relapsed disease	Longest time to retinitis progression in treated eye; no IV dosing or catheter required	Systemic therapy; no indwelling catheter required; infrequent dosing
Disadvantages	Hematologic toxicity; requires daily infusions; indwelling catheter	Must have adequate GI absorption; less clinical data than with ganciclovir	Nephrotoxicity; requires daily infusions/ indwelling catheter; supplemental hydration required; prolonged infusion time; requires infusion pump or controlled rate infusion device	Same as IV ganciclovir and IV foscarnet; prolonged daily infusion time and impact on quality of life	Fellow eye and extraocular disease; requires surgery; postintraocular surgical complications	Requires probenecid and IV hydration; probenecid toxicity; nephrotoxicity (may be prolonged)
Monitoring requirement	*Induction therapy:* (a) CBC with WBC differential, platelet count weekly; (b) SCr weekly *Maintenance therapy:* (a) CBC with WBC differential, platelet count weekly; (b) SCr every 24 weeks	Same as ganciclovir	*Induction therapy:* (a) SCr twice weekly; (b) serum Ca^{2+}, albumin Mg^{2+}, phosphates, and K^+ twice weekly; (c) Hgb and Hct weekly *Maintenance therapy:* (a) SCr weekly; (b) serum Ca^{2+}, albumin Mg^{2+}, phosphates, and K^+ weekly; (c) Hgb and Hct every 24 weeks	Same as both IV ganciclovir and IV foscarnet	No specific laboratory monitoring required for implant; if oral valganciclovir therapy is added, follow monitoring guidelines as outlined	Within 48 hours before each induction and maintenance: (a) SCr quantitation proteinuria; (b) WBC with differential cell count; monitor intraocular pressure and slit-lamp examination at least monthly
Precautions and contraindications	Moderate to severe thrombocytopenia (platelet counts $<25 \times 10^{10}$/L)	Same as ganciclovir	Concomitant use with other nephrotoxic drugs (e.g., amphotericin B, aminoglycosides, or IV pentamadine) or in patients with pre-existing moderate to severe renal insufficiency (SCr >168 mmol/L or creatinine clearance <50 mL/min)	Same as both IV ganciclovir and IV foscarnet	External ocular or nasolacrimal infection; patients with risk of postoperative intraocular infection	Same as IV foscarnet except parameters are baseline SCr level (>1.5 mg/dL) or creatinine clearance (<55 mL/min), or 2+ proteinuria (after IV fluid); discontinue therapy for 3+ proteinuria, if SCr level increases by 0.5 mg/dL above baseline, or intraocular pressure decreases by 50% of baseline value

[a] Fomivirsen intravitreal injection: *Induction therapy:* 330 mg (0.05 mL) every other week for 2 doses (days 1 and 15). *Maintenance dose:* 330 mg (0.05 mL) once every 4 weeks (monthly). *Primary adverse effects:* uveitis (ocular inflammation); increased intraocular pressure.

AZT, zidovudine; CBC, complete blood count; CMV, cytomegalovirus; G-CSF, granulocyte colony-stimulating factor; D_5W, 5% dextrose in water solution; GI, gastrointestinal; GM-CSF, granulocyte-macrophage colony-stimulating factor; Hct, hematocrit; Hgb, hemoglobin; HIV, human immunodeficiency virus; HSV, herpes simplex virus; IV, intravenously; NSAIDs, nonsteroidal anti-inflammatory drugs; PO, orally; SCr, serum creatinine; WBC, white blood cells.

Source: Whitley RJ et al. Guidelines for the treatment of cytomegalovirus diseases in patients with AIDS in the era of potent antiretroviral therapy: recommendations of an international panel. International AIDS Society-USA. *Arch Intern Med* 1998;158:957; Kaplan JE et al. Guidelines for prevention and treatment of opportunistic infections in HIV-infected adults and adolescents: recommendations from the CDC, the National Institutes of Health, and the HIV Medicine Association of the Infectious Diseases Society of America. *MMWR Recomm Rep*. 2009;58(RR-4):1; and product information.

TABLE 74-5
Dosage Adjustment for Cytomegalovirus Medications

Drug	Normal Dosage	CrCl (mL/min/1.73 m²)	Adjusted Dosage			
Cidofovir	*Induction dose:* 5 mg/kg IV QW × 2 doses	Increase in SCr of 0.3–0.4 above baseline	3 mg/kg per dose			
	Maintenance dose: 5 mg/kg IV QOW	Increase in SCr of 0.5 above baseline or 3+ proteinuria	Discontinue cidofovir			
		Cidofovir is contraindicated in patients with pre-existing renal failure: 1. SCr concentrations >1.5 mg/dL 2. Calculated CrCl of <55 mL/min 3. Urine protein 100 mg/dL (>2+ proteinuria)				
			Induction Dose		Maintenance Dose	
Foscarnet	*Induction dose:*	CrCl (mL/min/kg)	Low Dose	High Dose	Low Dose	High Dose
	IV every 8 hours to 90 mg/kg	>1.4	60 mg/kg every 8 hours	90 mg/kg every 12 hours	90 mg/kg every 24 hours	120 mg/kg every 24 hours
	IV every 12 hours	1.0–1.4	45 mg/kg every 8 hours	70 mg/kg every 12 hours	70 mg/kg every 24 hours	90 mg/kg every 24 hours
	Maintenance dose: 90–120 mg/kg	0.8–1.0	50 mg/kg every 12 hours	50 mg/kg every 12 hours	50 mg/kg every 24 hours	65 mg/kg every 24 hours
	IV daily	0.6–0.8	40 mg/kg every 12 hours	80 mg/kg every 24 hours	80 mg/kg every 48 hours	105 mg/kg every 48 hours
		0.5–0.6	60 mg/kg every 24 hours	60 mg/kg every 24 hours	60 mg/kg every 48 hours	80 mg/kg every 48 hhours
		0.4–0.5	50 mg/kg every 24 hours	50 mg/kg every 24 hours	50 mg/kg every 48 hours	65 mg/kg every 48 hours
		<0.4	Not recommended		Not recommended	
Ganciclovir			Maintenance dose			
	IV					
	Induction dose: 5 mg/kg every 12 hours	CrCl (mL/min)	Induction dose		Maintenance dose	
		>70	5 mg/kg every 12 hours		5 mg/kg every 24 hours	
	Maintenance dose: 5 mg/kg daily or 6 mg/kg daily × 5 d/wk	50–69	2.5 mg/kg every 12 hours		2.5 mg/kg every 24 hours	
		25–49	2.5 mg/kg every 24 hours		1.25 mg/kg every 24 hours	
		10–24	1.25 mg/kg every 24 hours		0.625 mg/kg every 24 hours	
		<10	1.25 mg/kg 3 × every week after hemodialysis		0.625 mg/kg 3 × every week after hemodialysis	
Valganciclovir	*Induction dose:* 900 mg PO BID	CrCl (mL/min)	Induction dose		Maintenance dose	
	Maintenance dose: 900 mg PO daily	40–59	450 mg BID		450 mg daily	
		25–39	450 mg daily		450 mg every other day	
		10–25	450 mg every other day		450 mg BIW	
		Hemodialysis	Not recommended		Not recommended	

BID, twice a day; BIW, twice a week; CrCl, creatinine clearnace; IV, intravenously; PO, orally; QOW, every other week; QW, weekly; SCr, serum creatinine; TID, three times a day; TIW, three times a week.

Source: Safrin S et al. Comparison of three regimens for treatment of mild to moderate *Pneumocystis carinii* pneumonia in patients with AIDS. A double-blind, randomized, trial of oral trimethoprim-sulfamethoxazole, dapsone-trimethoprim, and clindamycin-primaquine. ACTG 108 Study Group. *Ann Intern Med.* 1996;124:792; Lee BL et al. Dapsone, trimethoprim, and sulfamethoxazole plasma levels during treatment of *Pneumocystis* pneumonia in patients with the acquired immunodeficiency syndrome (AIDS). Evidence of drug interactions. *Ann Intern Med.* 1989;110:606; Kaplan JE et al. Guidelines for prevention and treatment of opportunisitic infections in HIV-infected adults and adolescents: recommendations from the CDC, the National Institutes of Health, and the HIV Medicine Association of the Infectious Diseases Society of America. *MMWR Morb Mortal Wkly Rep.* 2009;58(RR-4):1; and product information.

The CBC should be checked at baseline because neutropenia has been reported in approximately 20% of patients in clinical trials. Hypotony (reduction in intraocular pressure) and uveitis (inflammation of the uveal tract of the eye) have also been reported. Thus, monthly ophthalmologic examinations of the retina are necessary.[13]

The role of cidofovir is limited. Although it offers the advantage of weekly and biweekly dosing, its toxicity greatly limits its utility. Cidofovir appears to be as efficacious as foscarnet and ganciclovir in the treatment of CMV retinitis, but limited comparative studies have been performed. Finally, the efficacy of cidofovir in the treatment of extraocular CMV (e.g., GI disease, pneumonitis, encephalitis) remains to be established.

FOSCARNET

Foscarnet is a pyrophosphate analog that acts by selectively inhibiting viral DNA polymerases and reverse transcriptase. At doses currently recommended for induction therapy (60 mg/kg every 8 hours or 90 mg/kg IV every 12 hours), peak plasma foscarnet concentrations are higher than those which inhibit CMV in vitro (Table 74-4).[79] The dose-limiting toxicity of foscarnet is nephrotoxicity, probably because its poor solubility results in crystallization in nephrons.[74] In one trial, when compared to ganciclovir, patients treated with foscarnet survived approximately 4 months longer; however, foscarnet-treated patients with reduced creatinine clearance (<1.2 mL/minute/kg) had a poorer survival rate.[80]

Because P.Z. has a low ANC, the bone marrow–suppressive effects of ganciclovir and valganciclovir are of concern. Adjunctive therapy with G-CSF is an option. Because he has good renal function (SCr of 0.8 mg/dL), foscarnet or cidofovir probably would be preferred.

NEPHROTOXICITY

CASE 74-3, QUESTION 3: P.Z. will receive foscarnet, 90 mg/kg IV for 2 hours every 12 hours. How can the risk of nephrotoxicity be minimized?

During foscarnet therapy, adequate hydration is important to prevent nephrotoxicity. To establish diuresis, 750 to 1,000 mL of normal saline or 5% dextrose should be administered before the first infusion of foscarnet. With subsequent infusions, 500 to 1,000 mL should be administered, depending on the foscarnet dose. Careful dosage titration based on P.Z.'s estimated creatinine clearance may also minimize nephrotoxicity (Table 74-5). The SCr clearance should be measured at least twice weekly and the dosage recalculated if the creatinine clearance changes. CMV infection itself may also cause an acute increase in the SCr owing to acute interstitial nephritis. Drugs with nephrotoxic potential, such as amphotericin B or aminoglycosides, should be avoided.

ADVERSE EFFECTS

CASE 74-3, QUESTION 4: What toxicities other than nephrotoxicity have been associated with foscarnet therapy?

Hypocalcemia can occur because foscarnet, a pyrophosphate analog, can bind to unbound calcium. Electrolyte complications can be minimized by avoiding high foscarnet plasma concentrations. Therefore, foscarnet should be infused slowly for 1 to 2 hours.[81] Unbound serum calcium and phosphate levels should be monitored twice weekly during induction therapy and weekly during maintenance therapy, ideally when foscarnet is at its highest concentration. Fatal hypocalcemia has been reported in an AIDS patient receiving both foscarnet and parenteral pentamidine; thus, coadministration of these drugs should be avoided.[82]

Penile ulceration from foscarnet has been problematic, especially in uncircumcised men. Characterized as a fixed-drug eruption, careful attention to genital hygiene may minimize the potential for penile ulceration. Other adverse events associated with foscarnet include seizures, hypomagnesemia, anemia, nausea, fever, and rash. Twice-weekly albumin, magnesium, and potassium levels are required during induction therapy and then weekly during maintenance therapy. In general, patients tolerate foscarnet less well than ganciclovir.[81]

DOSAGE ADJUSTMENTS

CASE 74-3, QUESTION 5: After 12 days of foscarnet therapy, P.Z.'s SCr has increased from 0.8 mg/dL to 1.2 mg/dL despite the coadministration of 2 L of normal saline daily. What dosage adjustments should be made for the remainder of the foscarnet treatment?

Valganciclovir, ganciclovir, foscarnet, and cidofovir are highly dependent on renal elimination, and dosages (or dosing intervals) should be adjusted for even a modest reduction in renal function (Table 74-5). For example, the creatinine clearance threshold for dosage reduction of ganciclovir is 70 mL/1.73 m^2/minute; for dosage reduction of foscarnet, it is 1.6 mL/minute/kg. In contrast, the renal threshold for acyclovir and many other drugs is a creatinine clearance of less than 50 mL/minute. Therefore, careful monitoring of renal function is important throughout CMV therapy. P.Z.'s estimated creatinine clearance is 1.2 mL/minute/kg; therefore, his foscarnet induction dosage should be adjusted to 70 mg/kg IV every 12 hours (Table 74-5).[13]

GANCICLOVIR-FOSCARNET COMBINATION

In a prospective, randomized, controlled trial of patients with persistent or relapsed retinitis, ganciclovir and foscarnet monotherapy were compared with combination low-dose therapy.[73] Mortality and adverse effects were similar in all three groups. However, combination therapy was associated with significantly delayed time to retinitis progression when compared with foscarnet and ganciclovir monotherapy. However, the overall prolonged daily infusion time (up to 4 hours/day) and adverse effects were associated with decreased quality of life.[73] Consequently, combination therapy should be reserved for more refractory cases of CMV retinitis[83,84] (see Relapse or Refractory Cytomegalovirus Retinitis section).

Suppression Therapy

CASE 74-3, QUESTION 6: P.Z. completes 21 days of foscarnet induction therapy. How can his CMV retinitis be suppressed in the future?

The currently available antiviral agents used to treat CMV disease are not curative. After induction therapy, chronic maintenance therapy is indicated for the remainder of P.Z.'s life, unless immune reconstitution occurs as a result of HAART. Effective suppressive regimens include parenteral or oral ganciclovir, parenteral foscarnet, combined parenteral ganciclovir and foscarnet, parenteral cidofovir, and (for retinitis only) ganciclovir administration via intraocular implant or repetitive intravitreous injections of fomivirsen. Oral valganciclovir is approved for both acute induction and maintenance therapy, but the published clinical data are limited. In uncontrolled case series, repeated intravitreous injections of ganciclovir, foscarnet, and cidofovir have been shown to be effective for prophylaxis of CMV retinitis. However, because this therapy is effective only locally and does not protect the contralateral eye or other organ systems, it is usually combined with oral valganciclovir.

Foscarnet 90 mg/kg every 12 hours as IV induction for 14 to 21 days is usually followed by IV foscarnet 90 to 120 mg/kg/day as a single daily maintenance dose. The maintenance dose of 120 mg/kg/day is more efficacious, but likely more toxic than the lower maintenance dose.[85] Ganciclovir IV induction (5 mg/kg/dose every 12 hours) may be followed by IV ganciclovir maintenance (5 mg/kg/day 5–7 times per week). Cidofovir, with induction doses of 5 mg/kg IV each week for 2 weeks followed by a maintenance dose of 5 mg/kg IV every 2 weeks, offers a more convenient dosing schedule and negates the need for an indwelling IV catheter (Table 74-4).

Guidelines suggest that discontinuation of prophylaxis may be considered in patients with CMV retinitis who are taking HAART with a sustained (>6 months) increase in the CD4$^+$ count to greater than 100 to 150 and have remained disease free for more than 30 weeks. The decision to discontinue suppression should be based on the magnitude and duration of the CD4$^+$ increase and viral load suppression, the anatomical location of the retinal lesions, and the degree of vision loss.[13] All patients who have had anti-CMV maintenance therapy discontinued should continue to undergo regular ophthalmologic monitoring for early detection of CMV relapse as well as for immune reconstitution uveitis.

Relapse or Refractory Cytomegalovirus Retinitis

CASE 74-3, QUESTION 7: After 5 months of maintenance therapy with foscarnet, a routine funduscopic examination reveals retinal CMV disease progression. How should P.Z.'s retinitis be managed at this time?

Most patients with CMV not receiving HAART while undergoing maintenance treatment eventually relapse.[13] For the first relapse, repeat induction therapy followed by maintenance therapy with the same drug is beneficial in most patients. Because P.Z. has tolerated foscarnet therapy thus far, he should receive another course of induction therapy. After reinduction, P.Z. should receive a higher maintenance dosage (120 mg/kg/day).[30]

It is important to distinguish between relapse and refractory disease. Relapse, as in the case of P.Z., is defined as recurrence of clinically apparent viral activity and is usually caused by a decline in immune function, insufficient delivery of drug into the eye, or resistant CMV strains. Relapse can be effectively managed by repeat induction therapy of the same drug. If the relapse is caused by a resistant virus, the patient may benefit from a change in therapy. Ganciclovir-resistant CMV strains occur by two mechanisms. DNA polymerase mutation at the *UL54* gene is observed in approximately 20% of ganciclovir-resistant strains. This mutation usually confers resistance to cidofovir and, to a lesser extent, foscarnet.[13] Most ganciclovir-resistant CMV strains have *UL97* mutations. *UL97* mutations are incapable of monophosphorylating ganciclovir. Cidofovir and foscarnet are appropriate alternatives to treat strains with *UL97* mutations. Patients who receive extensive ganciclovir treatment (>6–9 months) may present with highly ganciclovir-resistant strains containing *UL54* and *UL97* mutations.[86] Cidofovir may be considered in most patients who relapse while receiving ganciclovir or foscarnet. Although ganciclovir-resistant and foscarnet-resistant strains of CMV have been reported, their precise role in the clinical failure of these regimens is not known. Because of the different mechanisms of action of ganciclovir and foscarnet, strains resistant to one drug may retain sensitivity to the other.[87] Resistant or relapsing CMV retinitis may be treated by administration of local ocular therapy via intravitreal injection of ganciclovir or foscarnet; ganciclovir intraocular implants are also a potential option (see Local Treatment section).

Refractory CMV retinitis is defined by disease progression because of ineffective therapy. This phenomenon is observed in two clinical situations: when the disease persists with minimal or no response during induction therapy, and when long-term control is inadequate with maintenance therapy. Refractory CMV disease has been defined in clinical trials as two relapses occurring within 10 weeks despite repeat induction and maintenance therapy. Treatment options for refractory CMV retinitis include reinduction with ganciclovir at higher dosages (7.5 mg/kg/dose every 12 hours, followed by maintenance doses of 10 mg/kg/day) or reinduction using combination therapy (IV ganciclovir plus foscarnet).[27] Refractory CMV retinitis can be treated with local ocular therapy via intravitreal injection of ganciclovir or foscarnet as well as intraocular implants.[88]

Local Treatment

INTRAVITREAL INJECTIONS

CASE 74-3, QUESTION 8: What is the role of intravitreal injections in CMV retinitis?

Intravitreal administration of ganciclovir or foscarnet through a small-gauge needle is a method of selectively delivering the drug to the site of infection. Ganciclovir and foscarnet doses of 0.2 to 2 mg and 1.2 to 2 mg, respectively, are administered two or three times per week for active disease, followed by weekly maintenance injections.[27] Potential complications of intravitreal injections include bacterial endophthalmitis, vitreous hemorrhage, and retinal detachment. Intravitreous therapy is relatively uncommon because intraocular implants are available. Importantly, in contrast with systemic therapy, local instillation of a drug is associated with a higher risk of CMV disease developing in the contralateral eye as well as extraocular sites (Table 74-4).

INTRAOCULAR GANCICLOVIR IMPLANTS

CASE 74-3, QUESTION 9: Is P.Z. a candidate for ganciclovir intraocular implants?

The intraocular implant is a surgically implantable delivery device capable of delivering ganciclovir into the vitreous humor at a constant rate of approximately 1 mcg/hr over a period of 5 to 8 months.[89] The implant delivers a much higher concentration into the vitreous cavity than can be achieved with systemic therapy. Implants may be an acceptable initial choice for newly diagnosed patients or patients with imminently sight-threatening disease. Surgical complications, such as retinal detachments, infections, and hemorrhage, can occur during or after the procedure. To reduce the risk of contralateral retinitis or extraocular CMV disease, patients receiving the intraocular implant should also be given oral valganciclovir (900 mg BID) (Table 74-4).[13]

P.Z. should be reinduced with foscarnet therapy and maintained on a higher foscarnet dose. Neither alternating regimens nor intravitreal administration of antiviral agents is appropriate at present.

Valganciclovir

CASE 74-3, QUESTION 10: What is the role of valganciclovir for initial CMV prevention?

Valganciclovir has replaced oral ganciclovir, which is no longer marketed. This agent yields an area under the curve approximately equivalent to that associated with the IV administration of ganciclovir. The maintenance dosage is two 450-mg tablets of valganciclovir once daily.

Data from clinical trials conducted with oral ganciclovir have been extrapolated to valganciclvor, and all references in the OI treatment guidelines to oral ganciclovir have been substituted with valganciclovir. The role of oral ganciclovir for primary prophylaxis of CMV retinitis has been evaluated in two studies.[90,91] Oral ganciclovir decreased the 1-year incidence of disease by approximately 50% in one study,[91] but was ineffective in another.[90] These two studies had important differences in study design that likely explain the disparate results. One cost-effectiveness study estimated that oral ganciclovir prophylaxis would cost more than $1.7 million per year of anticipated life expectancy.[92] Valganciclovir has not demonstrated a survival advantage in patients with $CD4^+$ count less than 50 using it for CMV primary prevention.[13] These issues, in addition to adverse effects such as neutropenia and anemia, the lack of proven survival benefit in HIV-infected patients, and the risk for inducing CMV resistance, are concerns that should be addressed when deciding whether to institute prophylaxis in individual patients. Prophylaxis with valganciclovir is not recommended as standard of care (Table 74-2).[13]

CRYPTOCOCCOSIS

Clinical Presentation and Prognosis

CASE 74-4

QUESTION 1: A.S., age 28, is infected with HIV. She weighs 48 kg. Her boyfriend was an IV drug user who died of AIDS 2 years ago. She presents with a fever (103°F) and a 2-week history of "splitting headaches." Laboratory test results include the following:

Hemoglobin, 11.2 g/dL
WBC count, 4,100 cells/μL
Platelets, 73,000/L
SCr, 0.9 mg/dL
Glucose, 94 mg/dL
$CD4^+$ count, 47 cells/μL

A.S. is highly nonadherent and has not been to the clinic in more than a year, at which time she was prescribed AZT, lamivudine, fosamprenavir, and ritonavir. Physical examination reveals no nuchal rigidity. With the exception of moderate lethargy, her neurologic examination is unremarkable. Her chest radiograph and three sets of blood cultures for bacteria and fungi are negative. A computed tomography scan is nondiagnostic. Lumbar puncture reveals the following CSF findings:

Glucose, 45 mg/dL
Protein, 90 mg/dL
WBC count, 10 cells/μL
Cryptococcal antigen titer, 1:2,048I
Intracranial pressure (ICP), 24 cm H_2O (normal, 8–22 cm H_2O)

How is A.S.'s clinical presentation typical of a patient with AIDS and cryptococcal meningitis? What is her likely prognosis?

In the pre-HAART era, cryptococcosis developed in approximately 6% to 10% of AIDS patients in the United States, with meningitis being the most common clinical presentation.[93] In the era of HAART and azole prophylaxis, a significant decline in the incidence of cryptococcosis has been observed.[93] Based on a 2010 cohort study, cryptococcosis is the second most common CNS infection associated with AIDS.[2] The initial portal of entry is the lungs, where the organism is normally contained by an intact immune system. Cryptococcal disease typically develops in patients with profound defects in cell-mediated immunity (i.e., $CD4^+$ counts <50). Unlike bacterial meningitis, cryptococcal CNS infection has a much more insidious onset; the most common symptoms are fever and headache. Less frequent signs and symptoms include nausea and vomiting, meningismus, photophobia, and altered mental status. Focal neurologic deficits and seizures are observed in less than 10% of patients. CSF glucose is decreased, whereas CSF proteins are usually elevated. CSF cryptococcal antigen titer and CSF culture are frequently positive. These findings, along with the clinical presentation, form the basis for the diagnosis. The overall outcome is poor, with a mean survival of 5 months in patients not receiving HAART. Relapse within 6 months occurs in 50% of patients who do not receive suppressive therapy. Altered mental status at baseline, CSF WBC count of less than 20 cells/μL, high CSF cryptococcal antigen titer (>1:1,000), and an elevated initial CSF opening pressure of greater than 20 cm H_2O have all been associated with a poor prognosis.[93]

A.S.'s $CD4^+$ count is 92. She has a temperature of 103°F and has experienced "splitting headaches" for about a week. Her clinical presentation is typical of an AIDS patient with cryptococcal meningitis. The CSF WBC count of 10 cells/μL, high cryptococcal antigen titer, and ICP greater than 20 cm H_2O suggest a poor prognosis.[94] If left untreated, cryptococcal meningitis is fatal.

Treatment

AMPHOTERICIN B

CASE 74-4, QUESTION 2: How should A.S.'s acute cryptococcal meningitis be managed?

The current treatment recommended for cryptococcal meningitis is amphotericin B, 0.7 mg/kg/day IV, plus flucytosine (100 mg/kg/day) given orally in four divided doses as induction therapy for 14 days. Once the patient is stable (e.g., afebrile, with resolution of symptoms), then consolidation therapy with oral fluconazole 400 mg/day for 8 weeks or until CSF cultures are sterile can be initiated. After consolidation therapy, daily suppressive therapy with fluconazole 200 mg should be continued indefinitely unless immune reconstitution occurs with HAART.[94] Lipid-based formulations of amphotericin B (specifically liposomal amphotericin, dosed as 4 to 6 mg/kg/day is also effective.[95,96]

Although the aforementioned regimen is highly effective, the ability to rapidly reduce A.S.'s ICP will also significantly improve her clinical course. Removal of 10 to 20 mL of spinal fluid by repeat lumbar puncture is recommended for patients with an ICP greater than 20 cm H_2O (A.S.'s ICP is 24 cm H_2O). An additional intervention to consider to reduce A.S.'s elevated ICP is the insertion of an intraventricular shunt.[13]

CASE 74-4, QUESTION 3: What is the evidence for adding flucytosine to amphotericin B in the acute treatment of A.S.? What are the disadvantages of this combination?

Amphotericin B binds to sterols in the fungal cell membrane, resulting in leakage of cytoplasmic contents. Flucytosine is an antimetabolite type of antifungal drug that is activated by deamination within the fungal cells to 5-fluorouracil. It inhibits fungal protein synthesis by replacing uracil with 5-flurouracil in fungal RNA, and it also inhibits thymidylate synthetase via 5-fluorodeoxy-uridine monophosphate, interfering with fungal DNA synthesis. Flucytosine, a purine analog, is approximately 10% converted to 5-fluorouracil, an antimetabolite, which is the mechanism for its potential bone marrow toxicity.

A classic prospective study conducted in HIV-negative patients favored the use of the combination.[97] The protocol randomly assigned patients to receive either amphotericin B monotherapy (0.4 mg/kg/day IV for 6 weeks followed by 0.8 mg/kg/day IV every other day for 4 weeks) or amphotericin B plus flucytosine (150 mg/kg/day orally divided every 6 hours) for 6 weeks. Fewer failures or relapses, more rapid CSF sterilization, and less nephrotoxicity occurred in the combination group, although overall mortality was no different. However, approximately one-fourth of the patients in the combination arm developed leukopenia, thrombocytopenia, or both.

If flucytosine is chosen as adjunctive therapy, renal function and CBCs should be monitored closely for these adverse effects. A.S. is at increased risk of granulocytopenia because of her HIV disease and her concomitant myelotoxic AZT therapy.

The comparative trial forming the basis for the current recommendations for treatment of acute cryptococcal meningitis in HIV-positive patients evaluated a higher dose of IV amphotericin B (0.7 mg/kg/day) with or without flucytosine given at a lower dose (25 mg/kg/dose PO every 6 hours) for 2 weeks.[94] The study evaluated 381 patients with an acute first episode of cryptococcal meningitis. The second part of this trial randomly reassigned stable or improved patients to either a fluconazole or itraconazole treatment arm for an additional 8 weeks as consolidation therapy. Sixty percent (60%) and 51% of patients receiving amphotericin B plus flucytosine, and amphotericin B alone, respectively, had sterile CSF cultures at 2 weeks of therapy. No significant differences were noted between groups in the percentage of patients who were culture-negative at 2 weeks. Importantly, the addition of flucytosine to amphotericin B was not associated with a significant increase in drug toxicities at 2 weeks. Fluconazole and itraconazole were similar in efficacy. However, multivariate analysis revealed two factors that were independently associated with a higher rate of CSF sterilization: the addition of flucytosine and the randomization to fluconazole. Consequently, amphotericin with flucytosine, followed by fluconazole, is the preferred initial regimen.

FLUCONAZOLE

CASE 74-4, QUESTION 4: Could A.S. be treated with fluconazole instead of amphotericin B for acute cryptococcal meningitis?

Fluconazole, one of the triazole antifungal agents, inhibits a fungal cytochrome P-450 enzyme necessary for the conversion of lanosterol to ergosterol. Without ergosterol, the fungal cell membrane becomes defective and loses its selective permeability properties. Unlike itraconazole, fluconazole is well absorbed orally even in the presence of an elevated gastric pH. Fluconazole has excellent CNS penetration and a good safety profile, but is likely a secondary choice in the initial treatment of cryptococcal meningitis. In a prospective, randomized, multicenter trial, the National Institute of Allergy and Infectious Diseases Mycoses Study Group and the AIDS Clinical Trial Group compared amphotericin B with 200 mg/day of oral fluconazole (after a 400-mg loading dose) for 10 weeks in 194 patients.[98] The dose of amphotericin B (mean dose, 0.4–0.5 mg/kg/day) and the possible addition of flucytosine were left to the discretion of the individual investigators. Although the overall mortality was similar (14% for amphotericin B vs. 18% for fluconazole), more fluconazole-treated patients died during the first 2 weeks of treatment (15% vs. 8%; $p = 0.25$). Furthermore, the median time to the first negative CSF culture in the successfully treated patients was shorter in the amphotericin B group compared with fluconazole (16 vs. 30 days). In a small, prospective, randomized trial of 20 male patients with AIDS, oral fluconazole (400 mg/day) for 10 weeks was compared with IV amphotericin B (0.7 mg/kg/day for 1 week, followed by the same dose three times weekly for 9 weeks) combined with flucytosine (150 mg/kg/day).[99] There were four deaths in the fluconazole group and none in the amphotericin B group ($p = 0.27$). Eight of the 14 patients in the fluconazole group failed to respond to treatment, whereas none of the amphotericin B patients failed to respond. The mean duration of positive CSF cultures was 41 days in the fluconazole group and 16 days in the amphotericin B group ($p = 0.02$). These results, taken together, have led most clinicians to choose amphotericin, with or without flucytosine, as initial treatment for severe cryptococcal meningitis. Although increased doses of fluconazole have been proposed, it is unknown whether these will result in improved outcomes. High doses of fluconazole are being investigated further for patients in the developing world where use of IV amphotericin may not always be feasible. Considering the severity of her meningitis, A.S. should be treated acutely with amphotericin and not fluconazole.

DURATION OF THERAPY

CASE 74-4, QUESTION 5: How long should treatment continue for A.S.'s cryptococcal meningitis?

Once A.S. completes 2 weeks of acute induction therapy with amphotericin B and flucytosine, she should be switched, if stable, to oral fluconazole 400 mg/day for consolidation therapy. Consolidation should be continued for an additional 8 to 10 weeks, followed by lifelong suppressive therapy with fluconazole 200 mg/day[94] (see Maintenance Therapy section).

MAINTENANCE THERAPY

CASE 74-4, QUESTION 6: Should A.S. receive maintenance therapy after successful treatment?

After induction and consolidation treatment of cryptococcal meningitis, A.S. and all AIDS patients should receive maintenance therapy indefinitely, unless immune reconstitution occurs as a result of HAART.[13,93,94] A higher relapse rate and a shorter life expectancy have been observed in patients who did not receive chronic secondary prophylaxis.[100] Fluconazole (200 mg once daily) has emerged as the suppressive treatment of choice. In a randomized, placebo-controlled trial of 61 AIDS patients, four recurrent cases of meningitis developed in the placebo group and none in the fluconazole group.[101] One multicenter, comparative trial randomized patients to receive either weekly amphotericin B 1 mg/kg/day IV or 200 mg/day of fluconazole orally.[102] Of 189 patients enrolled, 18% of the patients in the amphotericin B group relapsed, compared with 2% in the fluconazole group.

Serious toxicities were more frequent in the amphotericin B group.[94] The newer triazole antifungals, posaconazole and voriconazole, have limited experience as primary or maintenance therapy for patients with cryptococcosis, and are associated with many drug interactions with antiretroviral therapy.[13]

According to the OI guidelines,[13] adult and adolescent patients are at low risk for recurrence of cryptococcosis when they have completed a course of initial therapy, remain asymptomatic, and have a sustained increase (e.g., >6 months) in their $CD4^+$ counts to at least 200 after HAART. Thus, discontinuing chronic maintenance therapy among such patients is reasonable. Recurrences may occur, and some specialists recommend a repeat lumbar puncture to determine if the CSF is culture-negative before stopping therapy. Maintenance therapy should be reinitiated if the $CD4^+$ count decreases to less than 200.

Primary Prophylaxis

CASE 74-4, QUESTION 7: What is the role of primary prophylaxis in cryptococcal meningitis?*

Primary prophylaxis against cryptococcal disease in HIV-infected patients has been studied in a few clinical trials.[103,104] In one open-label study, fluconazole (100 mg/day) was administered to all patients (329 HIV-infected patients) with $CD4^+$ counts less than 68. These results were compared with 337 historical controls from the pre-HAART era.[104] Sixteen cases of cryptococcal meningitis occurred in the historical controls (4.8%) compared with only one case in the fluconazole group (0.3%). In a prospective, randomized AIDS Clinical Trial Group study, fluconazole 200 mg/day was compared with clotrimazole troches (10 mg five times a day) for the prevention of fungal infections in 428 patients with advanced HIV disease. After a median follow-up of 35 months, 32 cases of invasive fungal infection were confirmed. Of these, the majority (17 of 32) were cryptococcosis: 2 cases in the fluconazole group and 15 cases in the clotrimazole group. The greatest benefit derived from fluconazole was observed in patient with $CD4^+$ counts of less than 50.[104] However, no effect on survival was noted. A randomized, double-blind, placebo-controlled trial of fluconazole 200 mg 3 times weekly versus placebo in Ugandan adults with $CD4^+$ counts less than 200 found fluconazole prophylaxis to be effective prophylaxis against cryptococcal disease, with 18 patients in the placebo group developing cryptococcal disease versus 1 patient in the fluconazole group. There was no difference in all-cause mortality between the groups.[103]

Fluconazole resistance has been reported in HIV-infected patients receiving long-term therapy.[105] In addition to the potential for resistance, other concerns include the lack of survival benefits associated with prophylaxis, the possibility of drug interactions, and cost. In light of these concerns, the guidelines currently do not recommend primary prophylaxis for this disease (Table 74-2).[13] Fluconazole in a daily dose of 100 to 200 mg is reasonable for patients with a $CD4^+$ count of less than 50. An observational cohort study found no reduction in CNS OIs, such as cryptococcal meningitis, with the use of HAART that penetrated well into CSF.[106]

ADDITIONAL THERAPIES

CASE 74-4, QUESTION 8: What other acute therapies have been investigated for cryptococcal meningitis?

High-dose fluconazole alone (800–2,000 mg/day for up to 6 months) has been compared with high-dose fluconazole and flucytosine (100–150 mg/kg/day for 4 weeks) in multiple clinical trials.[107–109] These studies have shown that the combination fluconazole and flucytosine is superior to fluconazole alone in terms of both survival and CSF culture clearance. Combination fluconazole and flucytosine are useful because of their excellent oral bioavailability, cost effectiveness, and safety, which are particularly important in developing countries. Additionally, higher doses of fluconazole in these settings (1,800–2,000 mg/day) may be the best option for patients owing to the limitations of obtaining and administering flucytosine. Caution should be used when combining antiretroviral therapies such as nevirapine with fluconazole because of the risk of fluconazole failure or nevirapine toxicity.

MYCOBACTERIUM TUBERCULOSIS

Clinical Presentation

CASE 74-5

QUESTION 1: C.J., a 45-year-old male prison inmate with AIDS, presents with fever, cough, and occasional night sweats. A tuberculin purified protein derivative (PPD) skin test is negative, but C.J. is assumed to be anergic based on his response to other skin test antigens. Two acid-fast bacilli (AFB) sputum smears are also negative. Chest radiograph reveals hilar adenopathy with a questionable right middle lobe localized infiltrate. No cavitary lesions are seen. Why is infection with *M. tuberculosis* a strong possibility in C.J.? His antiretroviral medications include abacavir, lamivudine, and efavirenz. Three months ago his $CD4^+$ count was 320 cells/μL and his viral load was 5,200 copies/mL.

One-third of the global population is infected with *M. tuberculosis*, with 9 million new cases every year. Mortality is 2 million people annually, making TB the most common cause of death in HIV-infected patients worldwide.[110] The incidence of TB in the United States from 1985 to 1992 increased by 20%, approximately 40,000 more cases than expected.[111] Factors associated with this resurgence include the HIV epidemic, urban homelessness, drug abuse, and the dismantling of public-health TB-control resources. At that time, HIV disease was believed to be a major factor contributing to the emergence of multidrug-resistant *M. tuberculosis*. The recognized link between HIV and TB, along with an increase in clinical and public-health resources, has subsequently resulted in a decline in the incidence of TB in the United States.[111] Fortunately in 2008, incidence in the United States was 4.2 per 100,000 persons, the lowest reported rate since TB surveillance began.[111] Furthermore, *M. tuberculosis* strains resistant to isoniazid and rifampin, with or without resistance to other agents, have become a major public health concern.[110]

C.J. presents with fever, cough, night sweats, and a right middle lobe infiltrate with hilar adenopathy, consistent with TB. Furthermore, his HIV status in combination with his incarceration increases the probability of *M. tuberculosis* infection, including multidrug-resistant isolates. C.J. will be started with the standard four-drug regimen: isoniazid, rifampin (or rifabutin), pyrazinamide, and ethambutol.[13] (See Chapter 65, Tuberculosis, for a more comprehensive approach to TB treatment, and Table 74-6.)

CASE 74-5, QUESTION 2: Why are the negative tuberculin skin test, negative sputum smears for AFB, and lack of cavitary lesions in C.J. still consistent with *M. tuberculosis* infection?

TABLE 74-6

Tuberculosis Treatment Recommendations for Patients Coinfected with HIV and Tuberculosis

Induction	Maintenance	Comments
Rifampin-Based Therapy (no concurrent use of PIs or NNRTIs)		
INH/RIF (OR RFB)/PZA/EMB (or SM) daily or 2–3 × per week × 2 months	INH/RIF (or RFB) daily or 2–3 × per week (duration dependent on location of TB)	RIF-containing regimens used with caution with protease inhibitors and NNRTIs

EMB, ethambutol; INH, isoniazid; NNRTI, nonnucleoside reverse transcriptase inhibitor; PI, protease inhibitor; PZA, pyrazinamide; RFB, rifabutin; RIF, rifampin; SM, streptomycin.

Source: Kaplan JE et al. Guidelines for prevention and treatment of opportunisitic infections in HIV-infected adults and adolescents: recommendations from the CDC, the National Institutes of Health, and the HIV Medicine Association of the Infectious Diseases Society of America. *MMWR Morb Mortal Wkly Rep*. 2009;58(RR-4):1.

HIV-infected patients with CD4+ counts less than 200 commonly present with extrapulmonary tuberculosis, along with or in the absence of pulmonary disease. These extrapulmonary sites include lymph nodes, bone marrow, spleen, liver, CSF, and blood.[13] The chest radiograph in HIV-infected patients may reveal hilar or mediastinal adenopathy or localized infiltrates in the middle or lower lung fields.

In HIV-infected patients, it is unusual to see typical apical infiltrates or cavitations. Furthermore, concomitant PCP may confuse interpretation of chest radiographs. Finally, anergy (a state of immune unresponsiveness) is common in HIV disease. Thus, definitive diagnosis of TB rests on positive cultures from sputum or other tissue and body fluid specimens.[13] Unlike many other AIDS-related opportunitistic infections, CD4+ count is not a reliable predictor of increased risk for TB diseases, and patients can have relatively high CD4+ counts at the time TB develops.

HIV-INFECTED PERSONS: DRUG-SUSCEPTIBLE TUBERCULOSIS

CASE 74-6

QUESTION 1: K.D., a 26-year-old HIV-infected man, comes in for a routine clinic visit. It is discovered that he is a household contact of a person known to have active, untreated, drug-susceptible TB. His CD4+ count is 350 cells/μL. A tuberculin skin test (5 tuberculin units of PPD) and two other skin test antigens are administered, and he is instructed to return to the clinic in 48 hours. His PPD has been negative in the past, and he has demonstrated delayed hypersensitivity responsiveness. How should the results of K.D.'s skin tests be interpreted, and should he receive prophylaxis considering his known exposure to TB?

Current guidelines recommend 9 months of isoniazid prophylaxis (300 mg/day PO) plus pyridoxine (50 mg/day PO) for all HIV-infected persons who have at least a 5-mm induration reaction to PPD and no evidence of active TB (negative chest radiograph and no clinical symptoms), unless otherwise contraindicated and regardless of Bacillus Calmette-Guerin vaccination status.[13] The administration of Bacillus Calmette-Guerin vaccine to HIV-infected persons is contraindicated because of the potential to cause disseminated disease.[13] A greater than 5-mm reaction in HIV-infected persons is considered positive.[13] Few isoniazid prophylaxis failures have been reported, although this finding has not been systematically studied. Additional preferred regimens in instances of questionable compliance include isoniazid 900 mg twice weekly plus pyridoxine 50 mg twice weekly for 9 months, both administered under direct observed therapy. Persons who cannot take isoniazid or who have been exposed to a known isoniazid-resistant strain should use either rifampin or rifabutin alone for 4 months as alternatives, being mindful of potential drug interactions with antiretroviral therapy.[12,112] All HIV-infected persons, irrespective of age, PPD results, or prior course of chemoprophylaxis, should be given chemoprophylaxis if they are in close contact with persons who have active TB. Prophylaxis also should be given for anergic, HIV-infected persons who have been in contact with patients known to have active TB.[113] Before any prophylactic regimen is begun, active TB needs to be ruled out. K.D. should undergo chest radiography and clinical evaluation to rule out active disease. The CDC no longer recommends routine anergy testing in these patients.[13]

HIV-INFECTED PERSONS: PROTEASE INHIBITORS OR NONNUCLEOSIDE REVERSE TRANSCRIPTASE INHIBITORS

CASE 74-7

QUESTION 1: F.C., a 36-year-old HIV-infected woman, diagnosed 6 months ago, was found to have active TB (pulmonary infiltrates on chest radiographs, sputum AFB stain and culture positive, culture pansensitive). She is taking zidovudine, lamivudine, lopinavir/ritonavir, and fluconazole, and her CD4+ count is 300 cells/μL. What factors must be considered when selecting TB therapy for F.C.?

The use of protease inhibitors in the treatment of HIV patients coinfected with TB increases the potential for drug interactions with rifamycin derivatives (rifampin, rifabutin). Because the rifamycins are potent inducers of the hepatic cytochrome P-450 system (e.g., CYP3A4), they can induce metabolism of the protease inhibitors, resulting in subtherapeutic levels. Conversely, the protease inhibitors elevate rifamycin serum levels by inhibiting their metabolism and increasing toxicities, such as rifabutin-associated uveitis (inflammation of the uveal tract of the eye; see Chapter 65, Tuberculosis).

According to recent guidelines, rifampin should not be coadministered with any standard protease inhibitors (boosted or not with ritonavir), etravirine, nevirapine, and delavirdine.[12,112] Rifampin may be used with efavirenz at the standard 600-mg once-daily dose with close monitoring for virologic response to antiviral therapy. Some clinicians recommend an 800-mg dose of efavirenz for patients weighing greater than 60 kg.[12,112] When using rifampin with raltegravir the recommended dose of raltegravir is 800 mg BID, and patients should be monitored closely for virologic response. Coadministration of rifampin and maraviroc is not recommended, but if necessary, maraviroc should be dosed 600 mg BID (or, if coadministered with a strong CYP3A inhibitor, maraviroc 300 mg BID).[12] Rifabutin may be used in place of rifampin but should not be used with the saquinavir (without ritonavir) or delavirdine. Rifabutin should be given at 50% of the usual dose (i.e., reduce from 300 to 150 mg/day) with indinavir, nelfinavir, amprenavir, and fosamprenavir. Rifabutin should be used at 25% of the usual dose (i.e., 150 mg every other day or three times a week), with atazanavir, lopinavir/ritonavir, or any ritonavir-boosted protease inhibitor. When rifabutin is administered with indinavir as a single protease inhibitor, the dosage of indinavir should be increased from 800 mg every 8 hours to 1,000 mg every 8 hours or given as 800 mg twice daily with ritonavir 100 mg twice daily. It should be noted that rifabutin 150 mg 3 times weekly in combination with lopinavir/ritonavir has resulted in inadequate rifabutin levels and has led to acquired rifamycin resistance. Therefore, therapeutic drug monitoring of rifabutin is now recommended.[12,114] Rifabutin should be given with efavirenz at dosages of 450 to 600 mg/day. There are no data on using rifabutin with concomitant efavirenz plus a protease inhibitor. Rifabutin can be used in full doses with nevirapine and etravirine.[112] If etravirine is coadministered with a ritonavir-boosted protease ingibitor, rifabutin should not be coadministered.[12]

An open-label, randomized, controlled trial in South Africa assigned patients with both tuberculosis and active HIV infection to start antiretroviral therapy either during tuberculosis therapy or after the completion of tuberculosis therapy. The initiation of antiretroviral therapy during tuberculosis therapy significantly improved survival with similar rates of adverse effects.[115] When tuberculosis occurs in patients already on antiretroviral therapy, treatment for tuberculosis should be started immediately with modifications to antiretroviral therapy as necessary to minimize drug interactions while maintaining virologic suppression.

Discontinuing the protease inhibitor for F.C. is not an option considering the rapid viral replication and the risk of developing resistant isolates, especially considering that she recently was started on protease inhibitor therapy and is clinically responsive. A reduced dose of rifabutin (150 mg every other day or three times per week) is recommended when coadministered with lopinavir/ritonavir. Considering that F.C. is receiving lopinavir/ritonavir, she will be treated with a rifabutin-based regimen. She will receive isoniazid, rifabutin, pyrazinamide, and ethambutol daily for 8 weeks followed by isoniazid and rifabutin daily or twice weekly for 18 weeks. An alternative regimen could be isoniazid, rifabutin, pyrazinamide, and ethambutol daily for 2 weeks, then two times weekly for 6 weeks, followed by isoniazid and rifabutin twice weekly for 18 weeks. Considering the lopinavir/ritonavir-associated reduction in metabolism, rifabutin should be administered 150 mg every other day or three times weekly with concurrent therapeutic drug monitoring of rifabutin (Table 74-7).

TABLE 74-7
Recommendations for Coadministering Rifampin and Rifabutin with Nonnucleoside Reverse Transcriptase Inhibitors and Protease Inhibitors

Antiretroviral	Use in Combination With Rifabutin	Use in Combination With Rifampin	Comments
All ritonavir-boosted protease inhibitors	Dose as 150 mg every other day or 3 × per week. Therapeutic drug monitoring is recommended.	Do not coadminister	
Indinavir	Rifabutin 150 mg daily or 300 mg 3 × per week + indinavir 100 mg every 8 hours or consider ritonavir boosting.	Do not coadminister	
Nelfinavir	Rifabutin 150 mg daily or 300 mg 3 × per week	Do not coadminister	Coadministration of nelfinavir with rifampin is not recommended because rifampin markedly decreases concentrations of nelfinavir.
Fosamprenavir	Rifabutin 150 mg daily or 300 mg 3 × per week	Do not coadminister	
Atazanavir	Rifabutin 150 mg daily or 300 mg 3 × per week	Do not coadminister	
Nevirapine	Use caution at usual doses of rifabutin; however, there are no published clinical data	Do not coadminister	
Efavirenz	Rifabutin 450–600 mg 3 × per week unless coadministered with a protease inhibitor	Usual recommended dose of efavirenz is 600 mg daily. Some experts recommend increasing the efavirenz dose to 800 mg daily if efavirenz is used in combination with rifampin	
Etravirine	Rifabutin 300 mg daily unless coadministered with a boosted protease inhibitor, then do not coadminister	Do not coadminister	Etravirine
Maraviroc	Maraviroc 300 mg BID unless coadministered with a CYP3A4 inhibitor or inducer; rifabutin 300 mg daily	Coadministration not recommended; if used then dose maraviroc 600 mg BID unless coadministered with a CYP3A4 inhibitor then maraviroc 300 mg BID	Maraviroc
Raltegravir	No change in dosing	Raltegravir 800 mg BID and monitor closely for virologic response	

BID, twice a day; CYP3A4, cytochrome P-450 3A4.
Source: Panel on Antiretroviral Guidelines for Adults and Adolescents. Guidelines for the use of antiretroviral agents in HIV-1 infected adults and adolescents. Department of Health and Human Services. January 10, 2011; 1–166. http://www.aidsinfo.nih.gov/contentfiles/adultandadolescentgl.pdf.

MYCOBACTERIUM AVIUM COMPLEX DISEASE

Clinical Presentation

CASE 74-8

QUESTION 1: M.E., an HIV-infected 38-year-old woman with a history of IV drug use, presents with fevers, drenching night sweats, a poor appetite, and a 20-pound weight loss (> 15% of baseline) during the past 4 months. M.E. has refused all antiretroviral therapy for the past year because of drug intolerance. She has a past medical history of recurrent herpes zoster, PCP, and cryptococcal meningitis. Her current medications include one TMP-SMX double-strength tablet once daily and an occasional valacyclovir dose when she feels the herpes zoster "is beginning to start"; she refuses MAC prophylaxis therapy. Physical examination reveals a cachectic woman with mild hepatosplenomegaly. Pertinent laboratory test results include the following:

Hematocrit, 23%
WBC count, 3,500 cells/L, with 68% neutrophils, 2% bands, 22% lymphocytes, and 8% monocytes
Absolute CD4$^+$ count, 25 cells/μL
Viral load, 200,000 copies/mL
Aspartate transferase, 135 international units/L
Alanine aminotransferase, 95 international units/L
Alkaline phosphatase, 186 international units/L

Skin testing reveals anergy. The chest radiograph is unremarkable. Based on these findings, a presumptive diagnosis of MAC infection is made. Why is M.E.'s clinical presentation consistent with MAC infection?

Disseminated MAC infection is common in end-stage AIDS patients. On autopsy, MAC organisms are observed in the lungs and multiple other bodily tissues.[116] The predominant organism in HIV-positive patients is *M. avium* (>95% of typeable isolates).[13] The risk of developing disseminated MAC infection is strongly associated with a CD4$^+$ count of less than 100; the highest risk is in patients with a CD4$^+$ count less than 50.[13] Poor prognostic indicators include prior OI, high plasma HIV RNA levels, previous colonization of the respiratory or GI tract with MAC, and reduced in vitro lymphoproliferative immune responses to *M. avium* antigens.[13]

M. avium is a ubiquitous organism found in food, water, soil, and house dust. The most likely portal of entry is either the GI or respiratory tract. Sputum and stool samples frequently are colonized with MAC, although the significance of this finding remains controversial. Common presenting symptoms associated with MAC infection include fever, night sweats, anorexia, malaise, profound weight loss (>10% body weight), anemia, lymphadenopathy, and diarrhea.[13] M.E.'s fevers, drenching night sweats, poor appetite, 20-pound weight loss, and mild hepatosplenomegaly are consistent with MAC infection. In particular, her CD4$^+$ count of 25 puts her at risk for this OI.

Treatment

INITIATION

CASE 74-8, QUESTION 2: Why is it appropriate to initiate M.E.'s drug therapy before blood culture results have documented the presence of MAC?

Disseminated MAC is best diagnosed by peripheral blood cultures. However, initial testing often inclues AFB on a blood smear.[13] Conventional culture methods using solid media may have a turnaround time of as long as 8 weeks; however, radiometric broth systems signaling the release of carbon 15–labeled CO_2 from mycobacteria may detect bacterial growth in 7 to 10 days.[117] Identification of the organism (*M. tuberculosis* vs. atypical mycobacteria) by conventional biochemical methods may take weeks to months. Techniques using DNA probes make diagnosis possible within several hours.[117] Quantitative blood cultures have been useful to monitor the effects of drug therapy, but may not be practical on a routine clinical basis. Radiometric broth methods also may provide in vitro drug susceptibility in another 7 to 10 days. Even with the availability of all of these laboratory tests, results generally are not available for 2 to 3 weeks. In view of this lag time, empiric therapy should be initiated as quickly as possible. Although MAC is typically isolated from blood, the organism can also be demonstrated via acid-fast smears of lymph node, liver, or bone marrow biopsies. Because these organs are rich in monocytes (the target cells for MAC infection) the organism load may be high (up to 10^{11} colony-forming units/mL). Granuloma formation or inflammation may be absent because of profound suppression of cell-mediated immunity in end-stage AIDS patients.[117]

DRUG SUSCEPTIBILITY AS A BASIS FOR TREATMENT

CASE 74-8, QUESTION 3: Should M.E.'s therapy be based on in vitro drug susceptibility results?

Correlation between in vitro drug susceptibility results and clinical efficacy has not been clearly established for MAC. Numerous reasons may account for this finding. First, results are method-dependent; MAC isolates are more sensitive to antibiotics if broth is used rather than agar.[117,118] Second, current in vitro methods are cellfree, which does not take into account the intracellular nature of MAC infection. Thus, drugs with increased intracellular penetration may be useful clinically, even if in vitro minimum inhibitory concentration (MIC) data suggest otherwise. Conversely, drugs that have favorable MIC data may be ineffective clinically if they do not reach the intracellular environment.[118]

Drug susceptibility studies also may not correlate with clinical efficacy because in vitro results for individually tested drugs may show resistance, but combination therapy may be additive or synergistic. Finally, some antimycobacterial agents exhibit large differences between the MIC and maximum bactericidal concentration. This finding may reflect the difficulty in eradicating this organism, particularly in a severely immunocompromised host. Despite these limitations, in vitro drug susceptibility testing is only recommended for macrolide antibiotics because of the correlation with clinical outcomes.[119]

DRUG THERAPY

CASE 74-8, QUESTION 4: What drug regimens could be selected to treat M.E.?

The guidelines recommend a two-drug or three-drug MAC regimen, and at least one of these drugs must be a macrolide. Clarithromycin (500 mg PO BID) is the preferred agent; azithromycin is an alternative. Ethambutol (15 to 25 mg/kg/day PO) is recommended as the second agent. Several drugs can be used as the third agent, including rifabutin (300 mg/day), amikacin (10–15 mg/kg/day) and fluoroquinolones. The choice of the third agent depends on the severity of the illness including high mycobacterial loads, CD4$^+$ count less than 50, drug interactions, hepatic and renal function, patient tolerability, patient compliance, and cost. Amikacin (10–15 mg/kg/day) has been used in acute MAC therapy, but it is toxic and has a limited role in long-term therapy. Long-term therapy may be discontinued in patients who have completed a course of more than 12 months of treatment for MAC, remain asymptomatic, and have a sustained increase (e.g., >6 months) in their $CD4^+$ count to greater than 100 after HAART.[13]

The macrolides have potent activity versus MAC. Clarithromycin is the preferred agent as there is more clinical data in HIV-infected patients compared with azithromycin. In situations in which clarithromycin is not tolerable or significant drug interactions need to be avoided, azithromycin is an acceptable substitute.[13] Because monotherapy can lead to breakthrough bacteremia and resistance, MAC infections should be treated with a combination of at least two agents, including a macrolide plus ethambutol. Both macrolides demonstrate excellent intracellular penetration and have prolonged half-lives. GI toxicity (nausea, vomiting, diarrhea, abdominal pain, and anorexia) is the most frequent adverse effect with either agent. These effects may be dose-related. The dosage of clarithromycin is 500 mg orally twice daily, and the dosage of azithromycin is 500 mg/day. Doses of clarithromycin greater than 1 g/day in the treatment of MAC have been associated with increased mortality.[13]

Ethambutol (15–25 mg/kg/day orally) is preferred as the second agent. In a monotherapy study, 800 mg of ethambutol was more effective than either clofazimine or rifampin.[120] One or more of the following drugs can be added to the macrolide/ethambutol combination: rifabutin, amikacin, streptomycin, ciprofloxacin, levofloxacin, or moxifloxacin.[13]

Although four-drug regimens have been used, one study observed that a three-drug macrolide regimen (clarithromycin, ethambutol, rifabutin) was more effective than a four-drug regimen (ciprofloxacin, clofazimine, ethambutol, rifampin).[121] Benefits of the macrolide regimen included more rapid clearing of MAC bacteremia and a longer duration of survival. Rifabutin, at 600 mg/day, induced uveitis in approximately one-third of patients. Subsequently, the rifabutin dosage was lowered to 300 mg/day, and the incidence of uveitis decreased to 5.6%. Although clearance of bacteremia was superior at the higher rifabutin dose, no differences in survival were observed.

IRIS can also occur with MAC disease. IRIS-associated fever and lymphadenitis is difficult to differentiate from active MAC disease. IRIS most commonly occurs in patients with MAC and very low $CD4^+$ counts with the initiation of antiretroviral therapy. The disease is often self-limiting and requires no therapy; however, steroid therapy may be warranted in severe disease. For this reason, for patients not taking antiretroviral therapy, it may be warranted to administer MAC therapy for 2 weeks before initiation of antiretroviral therapy to minimize the risk of IRIS.[13]

M.E. is placed on a regimen of clarithromycin 500 mg twice daily and ethambutol 15 mg/kg/day. The choice to use two drugs, rather than three, is based on M.E.'s poor adherence profile. Other considerations for the addition of a third-line agent include the severity of the illness, potential drug interactions, tolerability, hepatic and renal function, and cost. M.E. must be counseled regarding the slow response to treatment. If she improves, therapy should be continued and HAART therapy should be reinstituted.

MONITORING THERAPY

CASE 74-8, QUESTION 5: How should M.E. be monitored?

The primary goals of MAC therapy are to eradicate or reduce the number of *M. avium* organisms, decrease symptoms, enhance quality of life, and prolong survival. M.E. should be monitored for symptomatic relief (temperature spikes and frequency of night sweats), as well as a microbiologic response (colony-forming units/mL). Clinical response, as well as a decline in quantity of mycobacteria, is expected in 2 to 4 weeks, but may be delayed in patients with extensive disease. If no clinical response is seen in 4 to 8 weeks, repeat blood cultures for MAC should be obtained along with repeat susceptibility testing for clarithromycin and azithromycin. If resistance is observed or suspected, two new drugs should be added based on susceptibility testing with or without the macrolide. If the organism is found to be susceptible to macrolides, therapy should be continued and adherence, absorption, tolerance, and drug interactions should be considered.[13] If the problem is determined to be drug absorption, IV agents can be considered. M.E. also should be followed for development of toxicities related to drug therapy. Furthermore, because many drugs used to treat MAC infections are associated with drug interactions, this issue must be considered each time a new drug is prescribed. In some cases, drug doses need to be modified or alternative drugs selected to prevent adverse events or therapeutic failures (Table 74-8).[13,119]

Prophylaxis

CASE 74-8, QUESTION 6: What drug(s) should be used to provide primary prophylaxis against MAC infection?

The most recent official guidelines recommend oral therapy with clarithromycin (500 mg BID) or azithromycin 1,200 mg every week or 600 mg twice weekly for persons with a $CD4^+$ count less than 50. Although the combination of azithromycin and rifabutin is more effective than azithromycin alone, the increased cost, adverse events, potential for drug interactions with rifabutin, and absence of a survival benefit preclude this regimen from being routinely recommended. If neither clarithromycin nor azithromycin is tolerated, rifabutin 300 mg/day may be used (Tables 74-2 and 74-9).[13]

Six hundred eighty-two patients with AIDS, $CD4^+$ counts less than 100, and negative MAC blood cultures were randomly assigned to receive clarithromycin (500 mg PO BID) or placebo.[33] The clarithromycin arm had a 69% reduction in MAC bacteremia and fewer (16% vs. 6%) cases of MAC infection. Significantly more patients in the clarithromycin arm survived during the 10-month follow-up (68% vs. 59%), with an accompanying longer median duration of survival. This trial was the first prospective MAC prophylaxis study demonstrating a survival benefit and a reduced risk of disseminated MAC infection.[33]

Azithromycin 1,200 mg every week, rifabutin 300 mg/day, and a combination of both drugs in the same doses were compared in patients with AIDS and $CD4^+$ counts less than 100. The incidence of MAC bacteremia was 13.9% in the azithromycin monotherapy arm, 23.3% in the rifabutin monotherapy arm, and 8.3% in the azithromycin plus rifabutin combination arm. Time to death was not significantly different among the treatments; however, the combination arm had an increased incidence of adverse drug effects. Although combination therapy was superior to azithromycin alone, its use is considered second-line because of the increased cost, toxicity, and lack of survival benefit.[122]

In a similar trial, patients with AIDS and $CD4^+$ counts less than 100 were randomly assigned to receive clarithromycin 500 mg twice daily, rifabutin 450 mg/day, or both.[123] In the midst of the trial, the rifabutin dosage was reduced to 300 mg/day because of a drug interaction with clarithromycin that resulted in rifabutin-induced uveitis. MAC bacteremia occurred in 9% of patients in the clarithromycin monotherapy arm, 15% of patients in the rifabutin monotherapy arm, and 7% of patients receiving the combination. Time to death was not significantly different among the arms, but the combination was more toxic.

TABLE 74-8
Drug Interactions with Tuberculosis and *Mycobacterium avium* Complex Medications

Affected Drug	Interacting Drug(s)	Mechanism	Recommendation
Atovaquone	Rifampin	Induction of metabolism drug concentrations	Concentrations might not be therapeutic; avoid combination or ↑ atovaquone dose
Clarithromycin	Ritonavir, indinavir	Inhibition of metabolism ↑ drug concentrations by 77% (with ritonavir) and 53% with indinavir	No adjustments needed in normal renal function; adjust if CrCl is <30 mL/min
Clarithromycin	Nevirapine	Induction of metabolism ↓ in clarithromycin AUC by 35%, ↑ in AUC of 14-OH clarithromycin by 27%	Effect on *M. avium* prophylaxis might be decreased; monitor closely
Clarithromycin	Rifabutin, rifampin	Induction of hepatic metabolism ↓ clarithromycin concentration 50% (with rifabutin) to 120% (with rifampin)	Clinical significance of ↓ clarithromycin levels unknown
Ketoconazole, rifampin	Isoniazid	↓ Serum concentration of ketoconazole	Possible antifungal treatment resistance
		↑ Hepatotoxicity	May consider discontinuing one or both agents if >5× baseline
Quinolones	Didanosine, antacids, iron products, calcium products, sucralfate	Chelation that results in marked ↓ in quinolone drug levels	Administer interacting drug ≥2 hours after quinolone
Rifabutin	Fluconazole	Inhibition of metabolism with significant ↑ in rifabutin drug levels	Monitor for rifabutin, toxicity such as uveitis, nausea, neutropenia
Antifungals, dapsone, methadone, theophylline, oral contraceptives, phenytoin, digoxin, warfarin (all drugs metabolized via CYP450)	Rifampin	Induction of metabolism-significant decrease in drug levels	Monitor drug levels (theophylline, phenytoin, digoxin) Monitor prothrombin time with warfarin Use alternative birth control method
Theophylline, warfarin, digoxin	Ciprofloxacin	Inhibition of metabolism theophylline levels, digoxin levels, anticoagulant effects	Monitor theophylline and digoxin levels and prothrombin time

AUC, area under the curve; CrCl, creatinine clearance; CYP450, cytochrome P-450 enzyme system.
Source: 1999 USPHS/IDSA guidelines for the prevention of opportunistic infections in persons infected with human immunodeficiency virus. U.S. Public Health Service (USPHS) and Infectious Diseases Society of America (IDSA). *MMWR Recomm Rep*. 1999;48(RR-10):1.

The decision to use clarithromycin or azithromycin (both first-line recommendations for primary prophylaxis) is based on patient compliance and the potential for drug interactions. Azithromycin (1,200 mg once weekly or 600 mg twice weekly) may be preferable for a patient who has difficulty with compliance. In contrast with clarithromycin, azithromycin does not affect the cytochrome P-450 enzyme system and is therefore less likely to interact with other drugs. M.E. would have benefited from MAC prophylaxis when her $CD4^+$ count decreased to less than 50.

TABLE 74-9
Drugs Commonly Used in the Treatment of *Mycobacterium avium* Complex Infection[a]

Agents	Dose	Toxicities
Initial Therapy Agents		
Clarithromycin	500 mg PO BID[b]	Nausea, vomiting, diarrhea, abdominal pain, serum transferase elevations, bitter taste
Azithromycin	500–600 mg/d PO	Nausea, vomiting, diarrhea, abdominal pain, serum transferase elevations
Ethambutol	15 mg/kg/d PO	Optic neuritis,[c] nausea and vomiting
Rifabutin[d]	300 mg/d PO	Nausea, vomiting, diarrhea, serum transferase elevations, hepatitis, neutropenia, thrombocytopenia, rash, orange discoloration of body fluids, uveitis Clearance of other drugs owing to hepatic microsomal enzyme induction[e]
Secondary Agents		
Ciprofloxacin	500–750 mg PO BID	Nausea, vomiting, diarrhea, abdominal pain, headache, rare insomnia, hallucinations, seizures
Amikacin	10–15 mg/kg/d IV	Nephrotoxicity, ototoxicity

[a]Macrolide plus ethambutol with or without rifabutin.
[b]Clarithromycin dose >500 mg BID is associated with increased mortality.
[c]Visual testing should be done monthly in patients receiving >15 mg/kg/d.
[d]Rifabutin dose 300–600 mg/d; but should not exceed 300 mg/d if given with clarithromycin or fluconazole.
[e]Common drug interactions include protease inhibitors (see Table 74-8).
BID, twice a day; IM, intramuscularly; IV, intravenously; PO, orally.

TABLE 74-10
Enteric Infections Associated with Infectious Diarrhea

Enteric Infections	Treatment
Fungal	
Candida albicans[a]	Fluconazole 100–400 mg PO daily; clotrimazole troches 10 mg PO 5×/d; nystatin suspension 4–6 mL QID; caspofungin 50 mg IV daily; micafungin 150 mg IV daily; anidulafungin 100 mg IV, then 50 mg IV daily; amphotericin B 0.3–0.5 mg/kg IV; liposomal or lipid amphotericin 3–5 mg/kg IV daily; voriconazole 200 mg BID; itraconazole solution 200 mg daily; posaconazole 400 mg PO BID
Histoplasmosis	Itraconazole 200 mg PO TID ×3 days, then 200 mg PO BID ×at least 12 months (liquid formulation has better absorption, limited data available on IV) *Alternative:* liposomal amphotericin 4 mg/kg daily or amphotericin B 0.7 mg/kg IV daily, then itraconazole 200 mg TID ×3 days, then BID ×12 months
Viral	
CMV	Ganciclovir 5 mg/kg IV BID ×21–28 days; foscarnet 40–60 mg/kg every 8 hours ×21–28 days (or oral valganciclovir)
HSV[a]	Valacyclovir 1 g PO BID; acyclovir 400 mg or acyclovir 5 mg/kg IV every 8 hours ×5–14 days
Bacterial	
Salmonella spp.	Ciprofloxacin 500–750 mg PO/IV BID 7 days to 6 weeks (depending on CD4$^+$ count) or TMP-SMX 5–10 mg/kg/d PO/IV BID ×2–4 weeks; levofloxacin 750 mg daily ×2–4 weeks;or third-generation cephalosporin treatment may be extended to 4–6 weeks
Shigella spp.	Ciprofloxacin 500 mg PO/IV BID ×3–14 days; TMP-SMX 1 DS PO BID ×3–7 days; azithromycin 500 mg ×1 day, then 250 mg daily ×4 days; antiperistaltic agents (atropine/diphenoxylate or loperamide) are contraindicated
C. jejuni	Ciprofloxacin 500 mg PO BID ×7 days or azithromycin 500 mg daily ×7 days
C. difficile	Metronidazole 250–500 mg PO QID ×10–14 days or vancomycin 125 mg PO QID 10–14 days; antiperistaltic agents (atropine/diphenoxylate or loperamide) are contraindicated
Protozoa	
Isospora	TMP-SMX 1 DS QID or 2 DS BID *Alternative:* pyrimethamine 50–75 mg with leucovorin 5–10 mg or fluroquinolone
Cyclospora	TMP-SMX 1 DS BID
Microsporidia	Albendazole 400 PO BID until CD4$^+$ >200 *Alternative:* itraconazole, nitazoxanide
Cryptosporidia	No effective treatment; paromomycin, nitazoxanide, octreotide, azithromycin (marginal benefits and no cure); best treatment approach is antiretroviral therapy to increase CD4$^+$ >100

[a] Primarily esophagitis.
BID, twice a day; DS, double strength; HSV, herpes simplex virus; IV, intravenously; PO, orally; QID, four times a day; TID, three times a day; TMP-SMX, trimethoprim-sulfamethoxazole.
Source: Jacobson MA et al. Retinal and gastrointestinal disease due to cytomegalovirus in patients with the acquired immune deficiency syndrome: prevalence, natural history, and response to ganciclovir therapy. *Q J Med.* 1988;67:473; Vakil NB et al. Biliary cryptosporidiosis in HIV-infected people after the waterborne outbreak of cryptosporidiosis in Milwaukee. *N Engl J Med.* 1996;334:19.

Patients whose CD4$^+$ count increases from 100 for more than 3 months may discontinue primary prophylaxis (Table 74-2). However, prophylaxis should be reintroduced if the CD4$^+$ count decreases to less than 100.[13]

ENTERIC INFECTIONS

CASE 74-9

QUESTION 1: A.B. is a 38-year-old woman with a 4-year history of HIV infection and a CD4$^+$ count of 160. She reports two or three watery, unformed bowel movements per day for approximately 6 weeks, with accompanying abdominal pain. She has refused antiretroviral therapy and is currently taking only one TMP-SMX double-strength tablet each day. What GI pathogens should be considered in the differential diagnosis in HIV-infected patients who develop diarrhea?

GI complications are common in HIV patients (e.g., enteric infections, gastric achlorhydria, pancreatitis, cholangitis, hepatitis, proctitis, KS, lymphoma, carcinoma, and HIV enteropathy). Enteric infections can be caused by fungal, viral, bacterial, or protozoan pathogens (Table 74-10). In general, clinical manifestations caused by GI infections appear with a decline in the CD4$^+$ count. Similar to A.B., most patients present with a change in bowel habits, predominantly diarrhea.[13] Acute diarrhea is defined as an episode of diarrhea less than 14 days in duration, and persistant diarrhea is diarrhea lasting more than 14 days.[124]

Viral Infections

Viruses that infect the GI tract of AIDS patients are unlike those associated with diarrhea in non–HIV-infected patients (e.g., rotaviruses, enteric adenoviruses, Norwalk agent, coronavirus, and coxsackieviruses). More common among HIV patients are CMV and HSV infections. Disseminated CMV infection is common in HIV-infected patients with advanced disease, and although retinitis is the most common CMV infection, as many as 5% to 10% of patients have GI involvement.[13] CMV usually involves the colon, and the common presentation is diarrhea. Tissue biopsy is preferred for a definitive diagnosis. CMV infection of the pancreas, liver, gallbladder, and biliary tree also has been described.[125] The IV agents used to treat CMV retinitis may also be used to treat CMV disease in the GI tract. In contrast with the treatment of CMV retinitis, therapy for colitis lasts 3 to 6 weeks. Data support the use of ganciclovir over foscarnet for CMV colitis, whereas the efficacy of cidofovir is unknown. Regular ophthalmologic screening for CMV retinitis is recommended for all patients with CMV GI tract disease.[27]

Bacterial Infections

Bacteria such as *Salmonella, Shigella,* and *Campylobacter* cause lower-GI disease in HIV patients, but these organisms are generally more virulent in HIV-negative patients. The frequency of acute infectious diarrhea caused by *Salmonella* for patients with AIDS is 5% to 15%. *Salmonella* bacteremia is considered an AIDS-defining diagnosis. The clinical features include fever and watery stools, with variable fecal WBCs. Diagnosis is made based on stool and blood cultures. In contrast with immunocompetent persons, antibiotics are recommended for treatment of *Salmonella* in HIV-infected patients; ciprofloxacin (500–750 mg BID for 2 weeks) is the preferred regimen. Alternative regimens include TMP-SMX (5–10 mg/kg/day TMP component IV or PO for 2–4 weeks), levofloxacin 750 mg daily or a third-generation cephalosporin. Bacteremia may be more frequent in HIV patients compared with non–HIV-infected patients and may recur despite antibiotic therapy. For patients with $CD4^+$ cell counts less than 200, a longer course of antibiotics may be needed. For recurrent disease, secondary prophylaxis should be continued for at least 6 months and possibly discontinued once patients respond to HAART.[13,124]

Another cause of acute infectious diarrhea in AIDS patients is *Shigella*. Person-to-person spread is the main route of transmission. *Shigella* causes dysentery, fever, and abdominal cramps that precede voluminous, watery stools. Bloody mucoid stools with fecal urgency may also develop. Fecal WBCs are common, and diagnosis is made by stool culture. Mild to severe cases of *Shigella* bacteremia have been reported, lasting an average of 7 days if untreated. Ciprofloxacin (500 mg PO BID) is the first line treatment with TMP-SMX (1 double-strength tablet PO BID for 3 days) or azithromycin as alternative options based on susceptibility patterns. Antiperistaltic agents are contraindicated. As with *Salmonella, Shigella* infections are associated with an increased frequency of bacteremia in HIV-infected patients who may require prolonged therapy (Table 74-10).[13]

C. jejuni is one of the three most common causes of acute infectious diahrrea in AIDS patients. *Campylobacter* enteritis is associated with a prodrome of fever, headaches, myalgia, and malaise 12 to 24 hours before diarrhea and abdominal pain. Diarrhea varies from loose bowel movements to voluminous, watery, and grossly bloody stools. Fecal leukocytes are variable, and the diagnosis is made by stool culture. *Campylobacter* enteritis is self-limiting, lasting only several days; however, some HIV-infected persons have symptoms lasting more than 1 week and may relapse if left untreated. Antibiotics are recommended for patients with high fevers, bloody stools, more than eight stools per day, and symptoms for more than 1 week without improvement. Ciprofloxacin (500 mg PO BID for 3–5 days) and aztithromycin 500 mg daily for 7 days are the preferred agents, pending susceptibility patterns. Quinolone resistance is increasing in prevalence, thus macrolides often must be used (Table 74-10). Patients with a bacteremia should be treated for at least 2 weeks, and a second agent should be considered.[13]

HIV-positive patients should take preventive measures against potential enteric pathogens. Close attention to hand hygiene is recommended, as is not handling or eating raw or uncooked poultry, fruits, vegetables, and nonpasteurized dairy products. Fortunately, the widespread use of TMP-SMX for PCP prophylaxis has reduced the frequency of these bacterial infections. Disseminated MAC disease, *M. tuberculosis, Helicobacter pylori,* and *C. difficile* also can cause diarrhea in HIV-infected patients.[13]

Protozoal Infections

Protozoal infections are a common cause of diarrhea among HIV-infected patients. Opportunistic protozoans such as *Cryptosporidium* and *Microsporidia* are well-known GI pathogens.

Cryptosporidium, a coccidioidin protozoan with a life cycle that occurs entirely within a single host, can be transmitted from animals to humans by fecal water contamination or person-to-person fecal–oral spread. HIV-infected patients should be advised to wash their hands after contact with fecal material (e.g., changing diapers), exposure to pets, gardening, or contact with soil, and they should avoid oral–anal sexual practices. HIV-infected patients also should avoid drinking water from lakes and swallowing water during recreational activities. In addition, outbreaks of cryptosporidiosis have been linked to municipal water supplies as infectious oocysts can persist in chlorinated water. HIV-infected patients should avoid eating raw oysters because the oocysts can survive in oysters for more than 2 months.[13] Intestinal cryptosporidiosis may be complicated by concurrent biliary involvement, leading to sclerosing cholangitis and pancreatitis, particularly in patients with low $CD4^+$ counts. Although the diagnosis of cryptosporidiosis formerly depended on intestinal tissue biopsy, newer techniques such as staining oocysts in stool (modified acid-fast methods) and fluorescent antibody assays have been developed. The best therapeutic prevention is initiation of HAART and prevention of severe immunosuppression. A MAC prophylaxis study suggested that clarithromycin and rifabutin also may prevent cryptosporidiosis. The treatment of cryptosporidiosis remains HAART and supportive case. Supportive care includes fluid and electrolytes, parenteral hyperalimentation, and antidiarrheal agents.

Nitazoxanide is an antimicrobial compound with activity against protozoans, helminths, and bacterial organisms. This drug has been approved for use by the FDA for treatment in children and adults. In HIV patients with $CD4^+$ counts greater than 150, 500 to 1,000 mg twice daily of nitazoxanide for 14 days had much higher rates of paracytological and clinical cure compared to placebo.[13]

Paromomycin is a poorly absorbed aminoglycoside antibiotic not specifically approved for treatment of cryptosporidiosis. Despite a moderate rate in several published trials, relapses were common with poor long-term success. Hence, paromomycin is not recommended for use in cryptosporidiosis.[13] Anti-diarrheal agents can be used for symptom management; however, these agents are not always completely effective. Octreotide is a long-acting somatostatin analog that has shown benefit in a limited number of patients. However, because of its expense, parenteral formulation, and similar efficacy to other anti-motility agents, its use is not recommended.[13]

Microsporidium (a ubiquitous, obligate intracellular protozoan parasite) can occur in HIV-infected patients, especially those with $CD4^+$ cell counts less than 100 and those without access to HAART. In addition infectious diarrhea, *Microsporidia* can cause other infections such as encephalitis, ocular infection, sinusitis, and myocitis. *Microsporidia* can be identified in intestinal biopsy specimens or stool samples using various lab techniques. The mainstay of treatment is HAART. Albendazole (400 mg PO BID for >3 weeks) has been found to be efficacious, but is not effective against all strains of *Microsporidia*. Itraconazole may be useful when combined with albendazole for some species.[13]

GI manifestations of HIV infection become increasingly common in the advanced stages of HIV infection. A.B. presents with chronic infectious diarrhea (two or three watery stools for >30 days). Review of her current medications (to rule out a medication source for diarrhea) revealed only low-dose TMP-SMX. CMV, MAC, *Microsporidia,* and *Cyclospora* are common in patients with a CD4$^+$ count less than 100. Stool analyses, including ova and parasites, AFB smears, bacterial culture, *C. difficile* toxin assay, and *Microsporidia* assay, were ordered. A fecal WBC examination was also ordered. The AFB smear of stool showed *Cryptosporidia* oocysts. It is recommended that A.B. be treated with antiretroviral therapy, therefore a discussion with the patient about her concerns with therapy should be intiated as HAART is by far the most effective treatment of *Cryptosporidia*. A.B. should be treated symptomatically with nutritional supplements and antidiarrheal agents.

ESOPHAGEAL DISEASE

CASE 74-10

QUESTION 1: P.J. is a 45-year-old, HIV-positive man who was started on AZT, lamivudine, and lopinavir/ritonavir when he was diagnosed 1 year ago. P.J. is a heroin user and has not been seen in the clinic since his initial presentation. He appears today complaining of difficult, painful swallowing and diffuse pain. On examination, localized white plaques are observed in the oral cavity. His CD4$^+$ count is 280 cells/μL. What is the most likely cause of this patient's dysphagia and odynophagia?

Esophagitis in HIV-positive patients is most commonly caused by *Candida*, but can also be caused by CMV, HSV, and aphthous ulcers. Symptoms include dysphagia, odynophagia, and thrush (with *Candida* infections). Oral ulcers are common with HSV, rare with *Candida*, and uncommon with CMV or aphthous ulcers. Pain is usually diffuse in *Candida* infections and more focused with HSV, CMV, and aphthous ulcers. Fever is primarily associated with CMV.[13]

Oral candidiasis is the most common opportunistic infection; however, overall rates have declined to 5% with the widespread use of HAART.[2] Patients with localized white plaques in the oral cavity likely have oral candidiasis (thrush) and should be started on antifungal therapy. Oral fluconazole (100 mg once daily) is considered the drug of choice for treatment of oropharyngeal candidiasis as it is more convenient and better tolerated than topical therapies. Patients may also be treated with local antifungal therapy (e.g., "swish and swallow" nystatin suspension, one teaspoon four or five times daily or clotrimazole troches four or five times daily). The preferred therapy for esophageal candidiasis is 14 to 21 days of fluconazole at higher doses (up to 400 mg PO or IV daily). Alternate therapies include amphotericin B, itraconazole, micafungin, and andulafungin.[13] Esophagitis in HIV-infected patients can be caused by CMV, with an incidence of less than 5% to 10% of patients with CMV end-organ disease. CMV esophagitis is confirmed via endoscopic biopsy demonstrating erythema and single or multiple discrete erosive lesions, usually located distally.[27] HAART is critical for immune reconstitution in patients with CMV esophagitis, and some providers may soley rely on immune recovery as treatment of mild CMV disease. Acute treatment of moderate to severe disease consists of ganciclovir 5 mg/kg IV per dose twice daily (or valganciclovir if patient has adequate gastrointestinal absorption) or foscarnet 40 to 60 mg/kg IV per dose every 8 hours for 3 to 4 weeks. Maintenance therapy may not always be necessary except in the case of recurrent disease.[13]

A presumptive diagnosis of *Candida* esophagitis can be made for P.J. because he presents with oral pharyngeal candidiasis, dysphagia, and odynophagia. P.J. should be empirically treated with fluconazole 200 mg/day for 14 to 21 days. If he is unresponsive to fluconazole, endoscopy with biopsy and culture should be performed to confirm the diagnosis as well *Candida* speciation. If candidiasis is confirmed, P.J. should be checked for medication adherence and potential drug interactions. If the patient is adherent and does not have malabsorption, parenteral amphotericin B or an echinocandin should be considered. In addition, higher doses of fluconazole could be considered before initiation of alternative IV therapy. Relapse is common in patients who do not receive secondary prophylaxis. Chronic suppressive therapy (fluconazole 100–200 mg/d) should be considered in patients responsive to fluconazole therapy who have frequent or severe recurrent esophagitis. However, there is increased probability of azole resistance with this practice.[13]

ACKNOWLEDGMENTS

The authors acknowledge Angela D.M. Kashuba, PharmD, Gene D. Morse, PharmD, Alice M. O'Donnell, PharmD, Marjorie Robinson, PharmD, and Mark J. Shelton, PharmD, for their contributions to this chapter in previous editions.

KEY REFERENCES AND WEBSITES

A full list of references for this chapter can be found at **http://thepoint.lww.com/AT10e.** Below are the key references and websites for this chapter, with the corresponding reference number in this chapter found in parentheses after the reference.

Key References

Buchacz K et al. AIDS-defining opportunistic illnesses in US patients, 1994–2007: a cohort study. *AIDS*. 2010;24:1549. (2)

Kaplan JE et al. Guidelines for prevention and treatment of opportunistic infections in HIV-infected adults and adolescents: recommendations from CDC, the National Institutes of Health, and the HIV Medicine Association of the Infectious Diseases Society of America. *MMWR Recomm Rep*. 2009;58(RR-4):1. (13)

[No authors listed]. 1993 revised classification system for HIV infection and expanded surveillance case definition for AIDS among adolescents and adults. *MMWR Recomm Rep*. 1992; 41(RR-17):1. (4)

Key Websites

Centers for Disease Control and Prevention. HIV/AIDS. **http://www.cdc.gov/hiv.** Accessed March 16, 2011.

Centers for Disease Control. Managing Drug Interactions in the Treatment of HIV-Related Tuberculosis. 2007. **http://www.cdc.gov/tb/publications/guidelines/TB_HIV_Drugs/default.htm.** Accessed March 16, 2011.

Panel on Antiretroviral Guidelines for Adults and Adolescents. Guidelines for the use of antiretroviral agents in HIV-1 infected adults and adolescents. Department of Health and Human Services. January 10, 2011; 1–166. **http://www.aidsinfo.nih.gov/contentfiles/adultandadolescentgl.pdf.** Accessed March 19, 2011. (12)

US Department of Health and Human Services. AIDS Info. **http://www.aidsinfo.nih.gov/.** Accessed March 16, 2011.

75 Fungal Infections

John D. Cleary, Stanley W. Chapman, and Margaret M. Pearson

CORE PRINCIPLES

	CORE PRINCIPLES	CHAPTER CASES
1	Due to increased numbers of immunocompromised patients, use of invasive devices, and an aging patient population, fungal infections are the fourth most common nosocomial infection.	
2	Yeast infections are generally easier to treat than mold infections. However, mortality is still significant for both types of infection even when treated appropriately.	
3	Most common risk factors for acquiring mycotic infections include immunocompromised host, use of broad-spectrum antibacterials, and breakdown of physical barriers including invasive catheterization.	
4	Diagnostic tools (i.e., serum galactomannan or β-glucan) can be useful as monitoring parameters for therapeutic outcomes assessment.	
5	The Infectious Disease Society of America (IDSA) and the Mycoses Study Group are important sources for guidelines and evidence-based approaches to therapy.	
6	Dermatophytic infection is most commonly associated with *Tinea* species and the most effective antifungal agents include itraconazole and terbinafine.	**Case 75-1 (Questions 1–3)**
7	Sporothrix is one of the most common fungal pathogens associated with subcutaneous infections and amphotericin and itraconazole are useful treatments.	**Case 75-2 (Questions 1–3)**
8	Candida represents the most common cause of systemic fungal infection in hospitalized patients. Candidemia must be treated promptly and appropriately. Delay in treatment or failure to ahere to IDSA guidelines results in a significant increase in mortality. Fluconazole and echinocandins are the most recommended therapies for disseminated candidiasis.	**Case 75-3 (Questions 1–4)**
9	Fluconazole, although reliable against *C. albicans*, is less reliable against certain non-albicans Candida species, including *C. glabrata* and *C kruzei*.	**Case 75-3 (Question 5)**
10	Conventional amphotericin is associated with significant infusion-related adverse events, nephrotoxicity, and electrolyte abnormalities. Consequently, other agents, including lipid-based amphotericin, triazoles, and echinocandins are drugs of choice for most deep-seated fungal infections.	**Case 75-3 (Questions 6–10)**
11	In patients with yeast identified in urine, selection of drug therapy for a simple candiduria versus organ infection as a result of disseminated candidiasis is complicated by difficulties with diagnostics.	**Case 75-4 (Question 1)**
12	Blastomycosis, histoplasmosis, and coccidiodes are associated with endemic infection from specific geographical areas. Long-term treatment with polyenes and/or azole antifungals is useful in the management of these diseases.	**Case 75-5 (Questions 1–3), Case 75-6 (Questions 1–3), Case 75-7 (Questions 1–3)**

continued

13	Aspergillus is the most significant fungal pathogen associated with severely immunocompromised patients. Aggressive, immediate treatment with voricononazole alone or in combination with other antifungals is the most effective therapy of disseminated disease.	Case 75-8 (Questions 1–3)
14	*Cryptococcus neoformans* is associated with opportunistic infection, particularly in acquired immunodeficiency syndrome (AIDS) and the central nervous system is a common site of infection. Initial treatment of meningitis in AIDS should include amphotericin plus flucytosine, followed by long-term fluconazole.	Case 75-9 (Questions 1–3)

Mycotic (fungal) infections are now the fourth most commonly encountered nosocomial infection. This increase can be attributed, in part, to the growing numbers of immunocompromised hosts as a result of organ transplants, cancer-chemotherapy–associated neutropenia, and acquired immunodeficiency syndrome (AIDS). This chapter reviews the mycology, diagnosis, and pharmacotherapeutics for common mycotic infections. For a more indepth presentation of the basic biology of fungi, as well as the epidemiology, pathogenesis, immunology, diagnosis, and monitoring of mycotic infections, see *Clinical Mycology*.[1] You are referred to other chapters including Chapter 62, Central Nervous System Infections; Chapter 63, Endocarditis; Chapter 67, Intra-Abdominal Infections; Chapter 70, Osteomyelitis and Septic Arthritis; and infections in immunocompromised patients with and without human immunodeficiency virus (HIV) infections; Chapter 73, Pharmacotherapy of Human Immunodeficiency Virus Infection.

MYCOLOGY

Morphology

The pathogenic fungi that infect humans are nonmotile eucaryotes that reproduce by sporulation and they exist in two forms: filamentous molds and unicellular yeasts. These forms are not mutually exclusive and, depending on the growth conditions, a fungus may exist in one or even both of these forms (Table 75-1).

TABLE 75-1
Organism Classification

Hyphae (Molds)
Hyalohyphomycoses
Aspergillus species, *Pseudallescheria boydii*
Dermatophytes: Epidermophyton floccosum, Trichophyton species, *Microsporum* species
Phaeohyphomycoses
Alternaria species, Anthopsis deltoidea, Bipolaris hawaiiensis, Cladosporium species, *Curvularia geniculata, Exophiala* species, *Fonsecaea pedrosoi, Phialophora* species, *Fusarium* species
Zygomycetes
Absidia corymbifera, Mucor indicus, Rhizomucor pusillus
Dimorphic Fungi
Blastomyces species, *Coccidioides species, Paracoccidioides* species, *Histoplasma* species, *Sporothrix* species
Yeasts
Candida species, *Cryptococcus neoformans*

For a visual of the microscopic appearance of various fungi, go to http://thepoint.lww.com/AT10e.

The dimorphic fungi (e.g., *Histoplasma capsulatum* and *Blastomyces dermatitidis*) grow as a mold in nature (27°C), but quickly convert to the parasitic yeast form after infecting the host (37°C). This mycelium-to-yeast conversion is an important factor in the pathogenesis of disease caused by these organisms. Other pathogenic fungi, such as *Aspergillus* species, grow only as a mold form, whereas *Cryptococcus neoformans* usually grows as a yeast form. *Candida* species grow with a modified form of budding whereby newly budded cells remain attached to the parent cells and form pseudohyphae. Fungi are aerobic and are easily grown on routine culture media similar to that used to grow bacteria. Most fungi grow best at 25°C to 35°C. Fungi that cause only cutaneous and subcutaneous disease grow poorly at temperatures greater than 37°C. This temperature-selective growth explains, at least in part, why these organisms rarely disseminate from a primary focus in the skin or subcutaneous tissues.

Classification

Fungal infections are best classified by the area of the body infected (Table 75-2). Superficial mycoses involve only the outermost keratinized layers of the skin (stratum corneum) and hair. The cutaneous mycoses extend deeper into the epidermis and may also infect the nails. The subcutaneous mycoses infect the dermis and subcutaneous tissues; entry into these sites is by inoculation or implantation of dirt or vegetative matter. The systemic mycoses cause disease of the internal organs of the body. Standard definitions that are useful in daily patient care for invasive fungal infections have been developed for epidemiologic and clinical trials. The guidelines are referenced under each infection. The respiratory tract is the most common primary portal of entry, and lung infection may be symptomatic or asymptomatic. Systemic infection with *Candida* usually results from a primary focus in the gastrointestinal (GI) tract or skin. In each case, the organism may spread hematogenously from the primary focus throughout the body, resulting in disseminated disease. The opportunistic mycoses occur primarily in the immunocompromised host and require immediate and aggressive treatment. The list of fungi that cause opportunistic infection has expanded, especially with the AIDS epidemic; however, the now commonplace use of highly active antiretroviral therapy has resulted in some decrease in this incidence.[2] The nonopportunistic fungi (primary pathogens) usually cause disease in the immunologically normal host. Some primary pathogens, however, result in unique clinical syndromes when infection occurs in the immunocompromised host, such as histoplasmosis in AIDS.[1]

biosynthesis inhibition is a faulty cell membrane with altered permeability. In general, the allylamines and older azoles are fungistatic. The newer triazoles (voriconazole, posaconazole) demonstrate fungicidal activity against some fungal species.[15] The clinical relevance of in vitro fungicidal versus fungistatic action is the subject of considerable debate. Nevertheless, it seems logical that fungicidal action, if it can also be achieved in vivo, is preferred in immunosuppressed hosts.

Lipopeptides, which are potent antifungal agents, include the structural class of echinocandins (anidulafungin, micafungin, and caspofungin). All share a common mechanism: They act by interfering with 1,3-β-D-glucan, preventing synthesis of essential cell wall polysaccharides that protect the cell from osmotic and structural stresses. The result is inhibition of fungal cell wall biosynthesis. Targeting the cell wall (as opposed to the cell membrane, which is the target of polyene, azole, and allylamine) results in selective inhibition of fungal versus mammalian cells; the fungal cell wall does not share target-associated toxicity with the mammalian cell wall.[16]

Antifungal Spectrum and Susceptibility Testing

The Clinical and Laboratory Standards Institute (CLSI) recommends standardized broth dilution (M27-A3) and disk diffusion (M44-A2, M44-S3, M51-A) methods for determining in vitro antifungal susceptibilities for yeasts.[17] These methods stipulate test medium, inoculum size and preparation, incubation time and temperature, end point reading, and quality control limits for AmB, flucytosine, fluconazole, ketoconazole, and itraconazole. Minimum inhibitory concentration (MIC) values for use in clinical interpretation are specified for fluconazole, itraconazole, and flucytosine against *Candida* species after 48 hours of incubation. For fluconazole and itraconazole, a susceptible-dose dependent (S-DD) breakpoint was developed based on data supporting a trend toward better response with higher drug levels for isolates with higher MIC.[18] The S-DD range is 16 mcg/mL and greater than 0.125 for fluconazole, and 32 mcg/mL and less than 0.5 mcg/mL for itraconazole. *Candida* isolates with MIC less than these ranges are considered susceptible, and isolates with MIC greater than these ranges are considered resistant. Owing to rapid development of resistance and limited data on correlation of MIC with outcome for flucytosine monotherapy, proposed interpretive breakpoints for this agent are based on a combination of historical data and results from animal studies. *Candida* isolates with a flucytosine MIC less than or equal to 4 mcg/mL are considered susceptible, isolates with MIC greater than 16 mcg/mL are considered resistant. Limitations of the M27-A methodology have precluded development of AmB interpretive breakpoints nor have interpretive criteria been proposed for ketoconazole MIC. Commercial kits are available for antifungal susceptibility testing which utilize broth microdilution, colorimetric, and agar-based techniques.[19—21]

An E-Test (AB Biodisk; Piscataway, NJ) is commercially available. Difficulties in end point determination using this method result from frequent, nonuniform growth of the fungus on the agar medium; yet, when properly performed, correlation between the E-Test and M27-A methods has been satisfactory for the azole antifungal agents against most *Candida*.[19] Other techniques under development for antifungal susceptibility testing for yeasts include flow cytometry and direct measurement of alterations in ergosterol synthesis.[20] Flow cytometry detects activity of the test antifungal drug through identification of subtle dosage-response effects on specific cell parameters as cells within the prepared innoculum pass through a beam of light. Test results may be available in as few as four hours. Interlaboratory reproducibility or correlation between test results and clinical outcomes have not been well studied.[21]

The CLSI-recommended standardized broth dilution method for determining in vitro antifungal susceptibilities for certain spore-producing molds, namely, *Aspergillus* species, *Fusarium* species, *Rhizopus* species, *Pseudallescheria boydii,* and *Sporothrix schenckii,* is the M38-A2 method.[15] An E-Test to evaluate mold susceptibilities is also commercially available (AB Biodisk) and correlates well with the CLSI M38-A method for AmB and itraconzole.[22] Colorimetric microdilution, flow cytometry, and agar-based testing methods are under development. Despite these recent advances, the determination of in vitro susceptibilities or resistance in clinical practice is of limited utility and not readily available for yeast or molds in most institutions.

Susceptibility testing for clinical isolates is not routinely recommended; however, published data on the susceptibility of the identified species of yeast or mold should guide the clinician's therapeutic choice. Clinical isolates from patients failing high-dose therapy (i.e., refractory oral pharyngeal candidiasis) or unusual pathogenic yeasts in patients with AIDS can be sent for testing.[20] Testing should be performed in a laboratory where the staff is trained in mycoses. Despite these limitations, certain generalities should be emphasized. First, AmB has broad in vitro activity and clinical efficacy against the yeasts and filamentous molds. The echinocandins have cidal activity in vitro versus *Candida* species and static activity for *Aspergillus* species; they are not active in vitro against *Cryptococcus* species and many endemic mycoses.[23] The azole antifungals are generally reliable against the yeasts and most dimorphic fungi. Additionally, itraconazole, voriconazole, and posaconazole have excellent in vitro activity against *Aspergillus* species, with associated clinical efficacy. Unlike other azoles, posaconazole is active in vitro and has some clinical efficacy against zygomycetes, for which previously only AmB formulations were therapeutic options.[24,25]

New Frontiers for Antifungal Therapy

Various investigative efforts have been directed toward both enhancing efficacy and reducing the toxicity of older antifungal drugs, including biochemical modifications of the agent, improved delivery systems, and combination therapy. Aerosol delivery of AmB products, itraconazole, voriconazole, and caspofungin in immunocompromised patients have been investigated for prevention of invasive pulmonary aspergillosis. Reduction in invasive pulmonary aspergillosis was demonstrated in a randomized, placebo-controlled trial of aerosolized liposomal AmB.[26] Additional well-designed clinical trials are still needed to establish the role of aerosolized delivery of antifungal agents. Optimal antifungal dose and nebulized system required for effective prophylaxis has yet to be established compared to traditional gastrointestinal regimens (Table 75-4).[27a,27b]

Identification of new antifungal compounds has been challenging. One significant barrier is that both mammalian cells and fungal cells are eukaryotes and share many similar biochemical processes, unlike bacterial cells, which are prokaryotes. Traditionally, the drug discovery process depended on the ability to detect compounds (either natural products or synthetic compounds) that selectively inhibit or destroy fungal cells. This process is accomplished by either or both of two approaches: (a) the evaluation of existing compounds (natural or synthetic) for potentially useful antifungal activity and (b) the design and synthesis of new compounds that selectively block fungal targets. Recent advances in genomic sequencing of *C. albicans, C. glabrata, A. fumigatus,* and *C. neoformans* have facilitated the search for

TABLE 75-4
Antimycotic Prophylaxis Regimens and Approximate Costs

Agent	Dose/Day	Formulation	Recommended Regimen	Cost ($)/day[a]
Selective GI Decontamination				
Amphotericin B	400 mg	Oral suspension	Swish and swallow QID	9.75
Nystatin	4–12 million units	Oral suspension	Swish and swallow QID	38.50–115.25
Systemic				
Clotrimazole	30–80 mg	Trouche	TID–QID	125–450
Ketoconazole	200–400 mg	Oral	Daily	0.75–1.50
Itraconazole	200–400 mg	Oral	Daily	18–36.25
Fluconazole	50–400 mg	Oral	Daily	4.50–35.25

[a] Average wholesale price, on average. Source: [No authors listed]. *Red Book*. Montvale, NJ: PDR Network, LLC; 2011.
GI, gastrointestinal; QID, four times daily; TID, three times daily.

new targets. Other less conventional drug discovery approaches include targeting known traditional virulence factors (e.g., adhesions, secreted enzymes). This approach is based on the principle that killing of the microbe need not occur for an anti-infective agent to be efficacious. Promising lead compounds include nikkomycins, sordarins, lytic peptides, hydroxypyridones, and cathelicidins. Nikkomycins inhibit chitin synthase. Chitin synthase catalyzes the polymerization of β-(1,4) linkages of *N*-acetyl glucosamine, which is critical to yeast cell membrane stabilization. Nikkomycin Z is undergoing phase I/II clinical trials as an orphan product for treatment of coccidioidomycosis.[28] Sordarins interfere with elongation factor-2, which is essential for protein synthesis, and lytic peptides and cathelicidins bind to cell membrane sterols, thereby reducing cell membrane stability. The mode of cathelicidin interaction with fungal cell walls is likely distinct as in vitro studies demonstrate activity in AmB-resistant and fluconazole-resistant strains. Along with direct actions against fungal cell walls, cathelicidins display indirect actions that modulate immune response.[29] The likely role of cathelicidin agents is in treatment of dermatophytosis and topical mycoses.[29,30] The inhibition of cellular uptake of essential compounds and loss of other compounds likely are secondary effects of an unknown primary mode of action for the hydroxypyridone antimycotics.[31] Sordarins, lytic peptides, hydroxypyridones, cathelicidins, and antibody-directed therapies (i.e., mycograb: antiheat shock protein 90), a novel approach usually reserved for extracellular pathogens,[32] are still in early development.

SUPERFICIAL AND CUTANEOUS MYCOSES

Tinea Pedis: Treatment

CASE 75-1

QUESTION 1: C.W., a 28-year-old male construction worker, is evaluated for a chronic case of "athlete's foot." He wears boots all day at work and notes intense itching of both feet throughout the day. He has been using tolnaftate powder for 1 week with no real therapeutic benefit. On examination, the web spaces between all the toes are white, macerated, and cracked. A few vesicles are also present over the dorsum of the foot at the base of the toes. Scrapings of the lesions examined as a potassium hydroxide preparation reveal branching, filamentous hyphae compatible with a dermatophyte infection. The diagnosis of athlete's foot is made. What therapeutic options are available for C.W.?

Selection of antifungal therapy should be based on the extent and type of infection.

For a visual of Tinea pedis, go to http://thepoint.lww.com/AT10e.

Superficial or cutaneous infections should initially be approached topically. Any follicular, nail, or widespread (>20% of body surface area) infection should be treated systemically under medical supervision owing to poor penetration of topical applications. Topical antifungals have been reviewed as a class by the FDA advisory review panel on over-the-counter (OTC) antimicrobial drug products and on an individual basis as newer products have been released. To receive a class I recommendation, each agent (or combination) must have been tested in well-designed clinical trials that show the drug microbiologically and clinically effective against dermatophytosis or candidiasis with insignificant toxicity (irritation). Class I agents are listed in Table 75-3. Class II agents (camphor, candicidin, coal tar, menthol, phenolates, resorcinol, tannic acid, thymol, tolindate) are considered to have higher risk–benefit ratios associated with their pharmacotherapy. Class III agents (benzoic acid, borates, caprylic acid, oxyquinolines, iodines, propionic acid, salicylates, triacetin, gentian violet) lack adequate scientific data to determine efficacy. Topical therapy with any class I agent applied twice daily to the affected area for 2 to 6 weeks should be adequate. Therapy should be titrated to response.

Because C.W. could continue tolnaftate powder for 2 to 6 weeks or switch to an antifungal cream or lotion (e.g., miconazole, terbinafine), these products should be applied to the web spaces between all the affected toes twice daily. C.W. should also be careful to use nonocclusive footwear (e.g., cotton rather than synthetic fiber socks, and leather rather than vinyl boots). Application of an absorbent or antifungal powder to his footwear would also be helpful (see Chapter 39, Dermatotherapy and Drug-Induced Skin Disorders).

Tinea Unguium (Onychomycosis): Treatment

CASE 75-1, QUESTION 2: If C.W. also suffered from an infection of the toenail (onychomycosis), what additional therapy could be offered to him?

Onychomycosis is typically caused by a dermatophyte, a hyphal fungi, or *Candida*.

For a visual of onychomycoses of the foot, go to http://thepoint.lww.com/AT10e.

Nail scrapings and culture should be performed to help plan initial therapy. Once culture results are known, therapy can be initiated with either terbinafine 250 mg/day or itraconazole 200 mg/day for 6 (fingernail) to 12 (toenail) weeks. In some cases, however, successful therapy of tinea unguium can require 3 to 6 months for fingernails and 6 to 12 months for toenails. Therapy should be considered successful when several millimeters of healthy nail have emerged from the nailfold to the margin of infected nail, or when a 25% reduction in size of the infected site has been achieved.

For dermatophyte nail or paronychial infections, griseofulvin therapy could be used if an azole or allylamine is contraindicated. Griseofulvin (microsized or ultramicrosized) administered orally at 10 mg/kg/day and titrated to response should be effective.[25] Owing to the large doses given for prolonged periods, C.W. should be monitored closely at each prescription refill for signs and symptoms of adverse reactions. The most common adverse events associated with terbinafine or itraconazole are headache, rash, and GI distress. Griseofulvin is more toxic, often causing hypersensitivity (urticaria, angioedema, type II hypersensitivity reactions), photosensitivity dermatitis, GI distress, and neurologic complications (headache, paresthesias, altered sensorium).[25]

Antimycotic pulse therapy is a novel approach to the treatment of onychomycosis. An FDA-approved alternative to daily therapy can now include a course of itraconazole 200 mg twice daily for 1 week in 2 consecutive months for fingernail infections. Double-blind, placebo-controlled trials revealed that this regimen was associated with a 77% clinical response and 73% mycologic response.[33] Overall responses and toxicity to therapy were more desirable with pulse regimens than with traditional regimens. Comparative studies demonstrate promising results for itraconazole pulse therapy for toenail infections[34] and fluconazole pulse therapy administered as a 150-mg to 450-mg dose once weekly for up to 12 months for mild disease.[35,36] Relapse rates after pulse (intermittent) terbinafine for 4 months have been frequent and longer courses of therapy are under study to enhance long-term efficacy.[37] Longer courses of therapy are being evaluated.

Removal of the nail as the sole therapy is not recommended because of the high relapse rate without concomitant systemic therapy. Likewise, IV antifungals are not indicated.

CASE 75-1, QUESTION 3: Describe the role of corticosteroids, antibacterials, or other additives to the antimycotic regimen in C.W.

Many patients with superficial, cutaneous, or nail fungal infections will have local inflammation and secondary bacterial infections. Inflammation is primarily a type IV hypersensitivity reaction. Topical corticosteroids in conjunction with antifungals can relieve itching and erythema secondary to inflammation. Bacterial (*Proteus* or *Pseudomonas* species) superinfection can also occur in these inflamed or macerated areas requiring concomitant topical antibacterial therapy. Pharmaceutical manufacturers of OTC preparations often combine a drying agent or astringent (e.g., alcohol, starch, talc, camphor) to their preparations to increase desquamation of the stratum corneum. Hyperhidrosis also can be relieved by these pharmaceutical additions. Such combination treatments should not be used routinely, however, because they increase the risk of toxicity and do not increase efficacy. If required for symptomatic relief, they should be used only for the initial days of treatment.

The affected web spaces between C.W.'s toes are macerated and cracked and vesicles are present at the base of his toes. A topical corticosteroid cream will probably facilitate the healing process and make him more comfortable during the first few days of antifungal therapy. The selection of topical corticosteroid formulations is presented in Chapter 39, Dermatotherapy and Drug-Induced Skin Disorders.

SUBCUTANEOUS MYCOSES

Sporotrichosis

TREATMENT OPTIONS

CASE 75-2

QUESTION 1: O.M., a 62-year-old man, has had a painless, slowly enlarging ulcer on his left hand for the past 4 months. He is an avid gardener, but can identify no antecedent local trauma. The primary lesion began as a red papule that slowly enlarged and then ulcerated. At the same time that the ulcer developed, O.M. also noted painless, red nodules that spread proximally up his arm. He denies any chills, fever, weight loss, or cough. The ulcer has slowly enlarged despite daily application of a povidone-iodine ointment and 2 weeks of cephalexin treatment. On physical examination, O.M. is afebrile. A 1.5-cm^2 ulcer is present on the dorsum of the left hand. Extending proximally from the ulcer is a palpable cord and multiple nontender, erythematous nodules distributed linearly up the forearm, elbow, arm, and axilla. A culture of this ulcer obtained 4 weeks ago is now growing *Sporothrix schenckii*. What is the recommended therapy for O.M.?

Sporothrix schenckii is the dimorphic fungi found in the soil and on many plants. Infection is usually secondary to inoculation into the skin from a thorn or sharp plant matter. *S. schenckii* infection most commonly causes lymphocutaneous disease (Fig. 75-1) as illustrated by this case. Rarely, extracutaneous disease may occur and usually involves the lungs, bones, or joints.

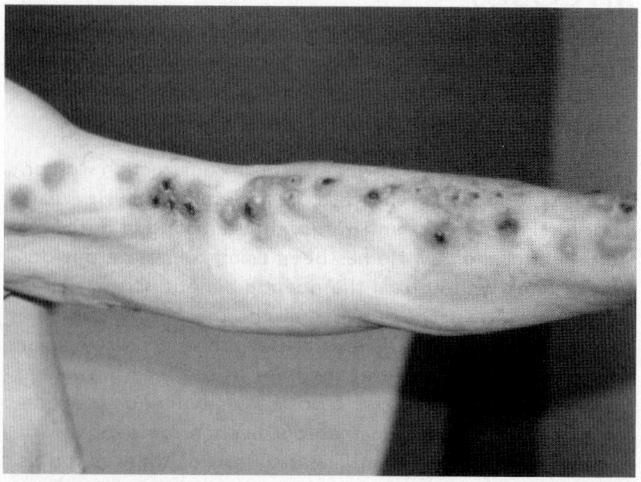

FIGURE 75-1 Lymphocutaneous sporotrichosis.

TABLE 75-5
Pharmacokinetic Properties of Systemically Active Antifungals

Characteristic	Imidazoles		Triazoles					Echinocandins			Other	
	MCZ[a]	*KCZ*[a]	*ITZ*[a]	*FCZ*[a]	*PCZ*[a]	*RCZ*[a]	*VCZ*[a]	*AFG*[a]	*CFG*[a]	*MFG*[a]	*5FC*[a]	*TBF*[a]
Absorption												
Relative bioavailability	<10	75[b]	99.8 (40)[b]	(85–92)[b]		ND	>90[d]	<10	<10	<10	75–90[b]	70
C_{max} (mcg/mL)	1.9	3.29	0.63	1.4	0.851	0.76	2.3–4.7[d]	7.5	12	7.1	70–80	1.34–1.7
T_{max} (hours)	1.0	2.6	4.0	1.0–4.0	3	ND	<2	1	1	1	<2	1.5
AUC[c] (mcg/hr/mL)	ND	12.9 (13.6)	1.9(0.7)	42	8.619	13.84–119.12	9–11 (13)[d]	104.5	97.63–100.5	59.9	ND	4.74–10.48
Distribution												
Protein binding (%)	91–93	99	99.8	11	ND	95	58	80	96.5	99.5	2–4	>99
CSF or serum concentration (%)	<10	<10	<10	60	ND	ND	~50	ND	ND	ND	60	<10
Excretion												
β $t_{1/2}$ (hours)	2.1	8.1[d]	17[d]	23–45	11.9	157	6	25.6	10	13	2.5–6.0	36
Active drug in urine (%)	1	2	<10	60–80	13	ND	<2	<1	2	1	0	80

[a] Given parameters are estimated from the administration of currently recommended doses. Miconazole (MCZ) 7.4–14.2 mg/kg/day (500–1,000 mg) parenterally; ketoconzole (KTZ) 2.8 mg/kg/day orally (200 mg); itraconazole (ITZ) 1.4–2.8 mg/kg/day orally (100–200 mg); fluconazole (FCZ) 0.7–1.4 mg/kg/day orally; voriconazole (VCZ) and posaconazole (PCZ) 400 mg twice daily orally, ravuconazole (RCZ) 400 mg/day orally; anidulofungin (AFG) 200 mg parenterally; caspofungin (CFG) 70(50) mg parenterally on day 1 (2–14); micafungin (MFG) 70 mg parenterally; flucytosine (5FC) 150 mg/day parenterally; and terbinafine (TBF) 250 mg/day orally.
[b] With meals (fasting), absorption altered by gastric acidity.
[c] Dose-dependent and/or influsion-dependent.
[d] Absorption decreased when administered with high-fat meal; C_{max} and AUC reduced by 34% and 24%, respectively.
AUC, area under the concentration-time curve; C_{max}, maximum concentration; CSF, cerebrospinal fluid; ND, no data; T_{max}, time of maximum concentration; $t_{1/2}$, half-life.

HEAT TREATMENT

In the 1930s and 1940s, local heat was applied to very mild plaque or lymphocutaneous disease. Germination rates of this dimorphic fungus actually can be decreased by increased temperature, and heat therapy 1 hour/day for 3 months is effective in 90% of patients with plaques (very mild disease).[38] Heat treatment could be particularly useful in pregnant patients when pharmacotherapy may be contraindicated.

ITRACONAZOLE

Itraconazole is more active in vitro against *S. schenckii* than other imidazoles or saturated solution of potassium iodide and efficacious in the therapy of sporotrichosis. Saturated solution of potassium iodide is seldom used for therapy secondary to treatment-limiting toxicity. Cure rates for sporotrichosis cutaneous and lymphocutaneous disease are greater than 90% with itraconazole 100 to 200 mg/day for 3 to 6 months. For extracutaneous disease, higher dosages of itraconazole (200 mg twice a day [BID]) for 1 to 2 years achieve response rates of 81%, but relapse frequently occurs (27%) after therapy is stopped.[38,39] Itraconazole is well tolerated in these patients. Patients with extracutaneous disease who are unable to tolerate the higher itraconazole dosages or whose disease continues to progress should be treated with AmB or a lipid-based amphotericin product. A total dose of 2.0 to 2.5 g is most often recommended if conventional AmB is used. Although voriconazole, posaconazole, and ravuconazole demonstrate in vitro activity against *S. schenckii* (albeit less than itraconazole), their role in the treatment of sporotrichosis has not been defined.[40] Neither ketoconazole nor fluconazole is effective in the treatment of sporotrichosis.

TERBINAFINE

Terbinafine has good in vitro activity against *S. schenckii* and has been used clinically with some success.[41] An unpublished clinical trial comparing 250 mg or 500 mg BID for 3 months for lymphocutaneous disease appeared clinically equivalent to itraconazole. Adverse reactions include GI distress (dysgeusia, dyspepsia, diarrhea), skin rash, and weight gain.

Therefore, in the case of lymphocutaneous disease; itraconazole 100 mg/day for a minimum of 3 months is the treatment of choice. If significant improvement is not observed in the first 6 weeks, the itraconazole dosage should be increased to 200 mg/day and continued for 6 months or until both the ulcer and lymphangitis have resolved. Most patients will respond to this dosage, but an occasional patient may require dosages of 300 or 400 mg/day.

Itraconazole Dosing

CASE 75-2, QUESTION 2: What instructions should O.M. receive for taking his itraconazole dose?

The peak serum concentrations of itraconazole capsules are ninefold higher when the drug is taken with food (0.18 mcg/mL with food vs. 0.02 mcg/mL in fasting subjects).[42] The influence of food on absorption appears to be independent of the food. High-carbohydrate meals decrease the absorption of itraconazole, and high-lipid content meals increase itraconazole absorption.[43] Patients who have difficulty eating (e.g., patients with AIDS, those with cancer receiving antineoplastic therapy) or with hypchlorhydria may not absorb a sufficient amount from the capsule to achieve therapeutic plasma concentrations after a typical oral dose.[44] Although itraconazole manifests nonlinear serum pharmacokinetics (i.e., administering the total dose in two divided doses is associated with higher peak serum concentrations than a single larger dose), there is no clinical benefit in splitting the dose. Therefore, O.M. could be instructed to take his itraconazole capsule with his highest-fat-content meal of the day or itraconazole solution could be substituted to improve absorption.

Itraconazole oral solution is a cyclodextrin formulation that has 55% bioavailability in a fed patient; this increases in a fasting patient (Table 75-5). Furthermore, bioavailability of this formulation is not affected by level of gastric acidity. Average serum concentration in a cohort of patients with advanced HIV infection was 2.7 mcg/mL after a 28-day twice daily dosing regimen.[45] O.M. should take his itraconazole solution on an empty stomach twice a day if this formulation is selected.

CASE 75-2, QUESTION 3: How would instructions for taking itraconazole capsules be modified if O.M. were achlorhydric as a result of medications or AIDS gastropathy? Should azole serum concentrations be monitored for an assessment of efficacy?

Itraconazole capsules, as with ketoconazole, require an acidic environment for dissolution and absorption. Thus, patients who are achlorhydric, either as a result of medications, surgery, or underlying disease (e.g., AIDS gastropathy) may not absorb itraconazole capsules adequately.[44,46] Use of ketoconazole in achlorhydric patients has historically required concomitant administration of 4 mL, 0.2 N hydrochloric acid aqueous solution.[47] Etching of tooth enamel by the acid can occur, thus other alternatives have been explored. The administration of ketoconazole and itraconazole with a low pH liquid (e.g., 8–16 fluid ounces of a carbonated cola beverage or orange juice) improves absorption in 65.2% of healthy patients who are achlorhydric or taking H_2-blockers (Table 75-6).[23,48–68]

Voriconazole does not require an acidic environment for adequate oral absorption, but voriconazole should be administered 1 hour before or after meals as high-fat meals may reduce voriconazole serum concentrations.[58] In contrast, posaconazole plasma levels are fourfold higher after administration with food or a high fat nutritional supplement.[69]

Because serum ketoconazole, itraconazole, and voriconazole concentrations less than 0.25 mcg/mL have been associated with treatment failures, therapeutic drug monitoring is justified in patients in whom therapy is failing. Similarly, posaconazole serum concentrations less than 0.7 mcg/mL have been associated with treatment failure. Serum antimycotic concentrations may be more easily monitored in the future as assays become available and correlations between concentration and efficacy and toxicity are more clearly established.[70]

SYSTEMIC MYCOSES

Candida Infection

CASE 75-3

QUESTION 1: L.K., a 21-year-old, 5-foot 8-inch, 170-pound, otherwise healthy man, was admitted to the hospital 16 days ago after a gunshot wound to the abdomen. He has undergone three exploratory laparotomies with repair and resection of damaged small intestine. He was placed on TPN to allow his bowel to rest and received stress doses of methylprednisilone on hospital day 6. Three days ago, he exhibited a fever of 39.1°C and chills; his blood pressure of 100/70 mm Hg had dropped more than 30 mm Hg

TABLE 75-6
Significant Drug Interactions

Antifungal	Interacting Agent(s)	Class[a]	Onset	Manifestation
AmB	Acetazolamide	2	R	Severe hyperchloremic acidosis secondary to additive or synergistic renal effects
	Chemotherapeutic agents			
	Doxorubicin, carmustine, cyclophosphamide, fluorouracil	2	D	Enhanced chemotherapeutic effect secondary to ↑ cellular uptake
	Cyclosporine	2	D	Enhanced nephrotoxitiy
	Digoxin	2	D	AmB-induced hypokalemia leading to ↑ digoxin toxicity
	Leukocyte transfusion	1	R	Severe pulmonary leukostasis with potential for respiratory failure
	NSAID	2	R	Additive or synergistic nephrotoxicity
	Pentamidine	2	D	Additive or synergistic nephrotoxicity
	Potassium-sparing diuretics	2	D	Spironolactone ↓ potassium requirements preventing hypokalemia in neutropenic patients receiving AmB
AFG, CFG	Cyclosporine	2	D	Cyclosporine ↑ AFG AUC by 22%; CFG AUC ↑ by 35%; elevations in transaminases (hepatic toxicity) seen with CFG
CFG	***CYP450 inducers***			
	Carbamazepine, phenytoin, mephenytoin, dexamethasone, efavirenz, nevirapine	3	D	↓ CFG concentrations through CYP450 induction; use of 70 mg of CFG should be considered
CFG	Rifampin	3	D	Hepatic uptake transporters of CFG might be induced by rifampin; administer CFG 70 mg/day when coadministered with rifampin
CFG	Tacrolimus	2	D	Tacrolimus peak blood concentrations ↓ by 20%; monitor tacrolimus whole blood trough concentrations and adjust dose as warranted
MFG	Nifedipine	3	D	Nifedipine serum concentrations ↑; monitor for adverse effects
MFG	Sirolimus	2	D	Sirolimus serum concentrations ↑; monitor for toxicity and reduce dose as warranted
Griseofulvin	**Sedative/hypnotics**			
	Benzodiazepines, ethanol, barbiturates	3	D	↑ Griseofulvin clearance with concomitant barbiturate or ethanol consumption
	Oral contraceptives	1	D	↓ Oral contraceptive efficacy
KI	ACE inhibitors	2	D	Hyperkalemia
	Lithium	2	D	Hypothyroidism
	Potassium-sparing diuretics	2	D	Hyperkalemia
Azole Antifungal Interactions				
Effect of other drugs on azole(s)				
Azole	**Interacting Agent(s)**	**Class**	**Onset**	**Manifestation**
KCZ	Isoniazid	2	D	↓ Serum antifungal concentration and potential treatment failure
KCZ	Anticholinergics	2	R	↓ Antifungal absorption; antifungal should not be administered concomitantly
KCZ	Sucralfate	2	R	20% ↓ in KCZ concentration
KCZ, ITZ	Didanosine	2	R	Acid neutralizing agents in didanosine prevent ITZ absorption; KCZ extrapolated
ITZ	Dexamethasone	2	D	Dexamethasone hepatically induces metabolism of ITZ
ITZ	Fluoxetine	3	D	Norfluoxetine inhibits CYP3A4, ↑ ITZ concentrations
ITZ	Micafungin	3	D	ITZ AUC and C_{max} ↑ by 22% and 11%; monitor for ITZ toxicity and reduce dose as warranted
FCZ	Hydrochlorthiazide	2	D	Significant ↑ in FCZ concentrations; changes attributed to ↓ FCZ renal clearance
KCZ, ITZ, FCZ	Antacids	2	R	Poor dissolution of dosage form, therefore ↓ azole availability; administer KCZ and ITZ 2 hours after antacid dose; note drug formulations containing antacid buffers
KCZ, ITZ, FCZ	H_2-blockers[b]	2	R	↓ Antifungal absorption; antifungal should not be administered with H_2-blockers
FCZ, PCZ, VCZ	Cimetidine	2	R	Alteration of gastric pH ↓ FCZ, and PCZ absorption; VCZ concentrations noted slightly ↑, possibly through nonspecific CYP450 inhibition by cimetidine

(continued)

TABLE 75-6
Significant Drug Interactions (*Continued*)

Azole	Interacting Agent(s)	Class	Onset	Manifestation
KCZ, ITZ, FCZ, VCZ	Carbamazepine	2	D	↓ ITZ serum concentrations and therapeutic failures have occurred; carbamazepine likely to significantly ↓ VCZ concentration via potent CYP450 induction; coadministration contraindicated
KCZ, ITZ, FCZ, VCZ	Rifampin	2	D	Rifampin-potent CYP450 inducer; significant ↓ in serum antifungal concentrations, potentially leading to treatment failure-doubling VCZ dose does not restore adequate antifungal exposure; coadministration contraindicated
PCZ	Esomeprazole	2	D	↓ PCZ concentrations; monitor for breakthrough fungal infections
PCZ	Metoclopramide	2	D	↓ PCZ concentrations; monitor for breakthrough fungal infections
VCZ	Barbiturates	3	D	Long-acting barbiturates likely to significantly ↓ VCZ concentrations; coadministration contraindicated
VCZ	St. John's wort	3	D	St. John's wort CYP450 and P-gp inducer; long-term use could lead to ↓ VCZ concentrations; concomitant use contraindicated
Azole effects on other drugs				
KCZ, ITZ	Corticosteroids	2	D	Twofold ↑ in serum methylprednisolone observed with concomitant KCZ; similar reaction with prednisone has been observed; ↑ systemic effects of inhaled budesonide after ITZ
ITZ	Fexofenadine	2	R	Significant ↑ fexofenadin AUC not related to dose of ITZ suggesting mechanism related to inhibition of gastrointestinal P-glycoprotein
KCZ, FCZ	Theobromines	2	R	Inhibition of theophylline absorption
FCZ	Oral contraceptives	1	D	↓ Oral contraceptive efficacy
KCZ, ITZ, FCZ, VCZ	Warfarin	1	D	↓ Warfarin protein binding and hydroxylation by liver (poor documentation) leading to ↑ in prothrombin time response; interaction with VCZ proposed via CYP2C9 inhibition
KTZ, FCZ, VCZ	Pimozide Quinidine	1	D	Azoles result in inhibition of metabolism of these drugs; ↑ plasma concentrations can lead to QT prolongation and rarely *torsade de pointes;* coadministration of VCZ contraindicated; coadministration of FCZ and terfenadine contraindicated
	Immunologic agents			
KCZ, ITZ, FCZ, PCZ, VCZ	Cyclosporine, sirolimus, tacrolimus	2	D	Azole inhibition of CYP3A4 produce significant ↑ in serum immunosuppressant concentration and ↑ toxicity; monitor cyclosporine and tacrolimus whole blood trough concentrations frequently during and at discontinuation of antifungal therapy. Coadministration of PCZ or VCZ and sirolimus contraindicated; data extrapolated for sirolimus and ITZ
KCZ, ITZ, FCZ,	Sulfonylureas	2	D	Significantly ↑ sulfonylurea concentrations; data extrapolated for VCZ
PCZ, VCZ, KCZ, ITZ, FCZ, PCZ, VCZ	Benzodiazepines	3	D	20% ↓ in chlordiazepoxide clearance demonstrated with KCZ. Inhibition of CYP3A4 by azole significantly ↑ serum concentrations of benzodiazepines metabolized by this enzyme; monitor adverse effects frequently and consider dose reduction
PCZ	Digoxin	1	D	↑ Plasma concentrations of digoxin; monitor digoxin plasma concentrations
FCZ, VCZ	NSAIDs	3	D	VCZ ↑ serum concentrations of ibuprofen and diclofenac; FCZ ↓ flubiprofen clearance by 55%; mechanism is CYP2C9 inhibition by FCZ and VCZ
PCZ, VCZ	Calcium channel blockers	3	D	↑ Plasma concentrations of calcium channel blockers metabolized by CYP3A4
PCZ, VCZ	Statins	2	D	VCZ inhibits lovastatin metabolism in vitro (CYP3A4 inhibition). PCZ ↑ simvastatin concentration ~10-fold; coadministration contraindicated; PCZ data extrapolated to other HMG-CoA reductase inhibitors; monitor for rhabdomyolysis
PCZ, VCZ	Vinca alkaloids	3	D	↑ Plasma concentrations of vinca alkoloids (CYP3A4 substrates) leading to neurotoxicity
PCZ, VCZ	Ergot alkaloids	1	D	Ergotism; coadministration of VCZ with ergot alkaloids contraindicated; data extrapolated to PCZ
VCZ	Methadone	2	D	R-methadone and S-methadone serum concentrations ↑ via VCZ inhibition of CYP2C9, CYP2C19, and CYP3A4; monitor for methadone toxicity (QT prolongation)
VCZ	Alfentanil, fentanyl, oxycodone	3	D	↑ Plasma concentration of opiates (CYP3A4 substrate); heterophoria and miosis noted with oxycodone; ↓ dose of opiates metabolized by CYP3A4 and monitor for repiratory and other opiate adverse effects

(continued)

TABLE 75-6
Significant Drug Interactions (*Continued*)

Azole	Interacting Agent(s)	Class	Onset	Manifestation
Two-way interactions				
KCZ, ITZ, FCZ, PCZ, VCZ	Phenytoin, mephenytoin	2	D	Phenytoin induction of UDP-G metabolism decreases PCZ concentrations; ↓ VCZ concentrations thought due to phenytoin as CYP2C9 substrate and CYP450 inducer; avoid concomitant phenytoin and PCZ use; ↑ VCZ maintenance dose Phenytoin serum concentrations ↑ after FCZ, PCZ, or VCZ administration; postulated mechanism via CYP3A4 inhibition; monitor plasma phenytoin concentrations
PCZ, VCZ	Rifabutin	2	D	↓ PCZ concentrations via UDP-6 induction; ↓ VCZ concentrations via potent CYP450 induction ↑ Rifabutin concentrations due to inhibition of CYP3A4 by PCZ and VCZ may ↑ rifabutin adverse effects; avoid concomitant PCZ and rifabutin; coadministration with VCZ contraindicated
PCZ, VCZ	Ritonavir	2	D	Ritonavir-potent CYP450 inducer and both substrate for and inhibitor of CYP3A4; ritonavir plasma concentractions ↑ by PCZ and ↓ by VCZ in dose-dependant manner; VCZ serum concentrations ↓ by ritonavir in dose-dependent manner; VCZ coadministration with high-dose ritonavir contraindicated and should be avoided with low-dose ritonavir
PCZ, VCZ	Efavirenz	1	D	Efavirenz is a CYP450 inducer, CYP3A4 substrate and inhibitor. Concomitant administration results in ↓ VCZ and ↑ efavirenz concentrations; if coadministered, ↑ VCZ dose and ↓ efavirenza dose; PCZ serum concentrations ↓ through UDP-6 induction of efavirenz; avoid concomitant PCZ and efavirenz; VCZ in vitro data for other non-nucleoside reverse transcriptase inhibitors; monitor for drug toxicity or antifungal failure
VCZ	Omeprazole	2	R	↑ Omeprazole and VCZ concentrations via CYP2C19 inhibition; reduce omeprazole doses of ≥40 mg by one-half. Metabolism of other proton pump inhibitors CYP2C19 substrates may also be inhibited by VCZ
VCZ	Oral contraceptives	2	D	↑ Oral contraceptive and VCZ concentrations via CYP2C19 inhibition; monitor for oral contraceptive and VCZ adverse events
VCZ	**HIV protease inhibitors** Saquinavir, amprenavir, nelfinavir	2	D	VCZ and protease inhibitors cause inhibition of CYP3A4 metabolism (in vitro); monitor patients for toxicity

[a] Classification: 1, major; 2, moderate; 3, minor.
[b] Clinically significant interaction that the authors recommend the reader should focus upon.
ACE, angiotensin-converting enzyme; AFG, anidulofungin; AmB, amphotericin B; AUC, area under the curve; CFG, casopfungin; CYP, cytochrome P; D, delayed; FCZ, fluconazole; HIV, human immunodeficiency virus; ITZ, itraconazole; KCZ, ketoconazole; KI, potassium iodide; MFG, micofungin; NSAID, nonsteroidal anti-inflammatory drugs; PCZ, posaconazole; R, rapid; UDP-G, uridine diphosphate 6-deoxygalactose; VCZ, voriconazole.

(systolic). Vancomycin and meropenem were promptly begun after obtaining blood cultures. Despite 3 days of antibiotics, he remains febrile. His physical examination reveals a Hickman catheter in the right subclavian vein that is functioning normally; no inflammatory changes are evident at the exit site. A single erythematous nodule about 0.5 cm wide is noted near the left wrist. The funduscopic examination of both eyes is normal. A chest radiograph is also normal. The white blood cell (WBC) count is currently 10,950 cells/μL and renal function is normal. What subjective and objective data in this case suggest a possible *Candida* infection?

EPIDEMIOLOGY

Although it is possible that L.K. might be infected with bacterial pathogens not susceptible to vancomycin and meropenem, the possibility of a candidal infection should be considered. *Candida* species are the most common nosocomial fungal pathogens. *Candida* species were responsible for 72.2% of mycoses in hospitalized cases, and *Candida albicans* accounted for 55% of these cases in the Centers for Disease Control, National Nosocomial Infections Surveillance System. Attributable mortality associated with disseminated candidiasis from all species is 38% and ~12% for extremely low birth weight neonates.[71] These statistics may underestimate the true occurrence because systemic candidiasis is difficult to diagnose. To reinforce this point, diagnosis of systemic candidal infection is made in 30% to 50% of neutropenic patients with hematologic malignancies at postmortem.[72] Therefore, the morbidity for systemic candidiasis may be even higher due to the limited ability to diagnose systemic disease.

CHARACTERISTICS

The diagnosis and monitoring of therapeutic outcomes for systemic candidal infection are difficult because the characteristics of systemic candidal infection are subtle. Salient clinical features include constitutional symptoms (e.g., fever, chills, hypotension) and evidence of end-organ dissemination, such as nodular erythematous skin lesions, endophthalmitis, liver abscess, and spleen abscess. In addition, 50% of patients or fewer will have a single positive *Candida* blood culture. The Mycoses Study Group utilizes a single positive culture from a sterile body site and hypotension (systolic blood pressure [SBP] <100 mm Hg or a SBP decrease >30 mm Hg) or abnormal temperature (<35.5°C or >38.6°C on one occasion or >37.8°C on two separate occasions more than

4 hours apart), or inflammation at a infected site as diagnostic criteria.

RISK FACTORS

Risk factors for candidemia include central venous catheters, broad-spectrum antibiotic use, extensive surgical procedures, *Candida* colonization, TPN, pancreatitis, neutropenia or neutrophil dysfunction, and immunosuppression (e.g., premature infants, burn patients, mannose-binding lectin deficiency, and patients with AIDS).[73]

L.K. has chills, a temperature of 39.1°C, and is hypotensive. He is probably immunosuppressed as a result of multiple surgical procedures and receipt of corticosteroids. His Hickman catheter is a possible portal of entry, and his broad-spectrum antibiotic therapy with vancomycin and meropenem should be adequate for most bacterial pathogens. Because L.K. still has manifestations of an infection despite 3 days of antibiotics, additional diagnostic studies are warranted.

DIAGNOSTIC TESTS

CASE 75-3, QUESTION 2: What diagnostic tests could be ordered for L.K. to evaluate a possible fungal infection?

The diagnosis of fungal infection may be made with varying levels of certainty. Sometimes, the diagnosis is absolutely certain, such as isolation of a pathogenic fungus from a clinical specimen in an immunocompromised patient. Such a finding is referred to as a definitive or microbiologically confirmed diagnosis. At other times, only a high probability of infection can be determined, that is, a presumptive diagnosis. To illustrate, a patient with a chest radiograph showing nodular lesions and a high complement fixation antibody against *H. capsulatum* would have a presumptive diagnosis of histoplasmosis. This finding may be as certain a diagnosis as is possible without performing a more invasive procedure to obtain lung tissue. In this event, a trial of drug therapy can be undertaken on the presumptive diagnosis alone. A diverse spectrum of tests is available for clinicians to diagnose and monitor therapeutic responses.

DIRECT EXAMINATION

Direct examination of the specimen is often useful in diagnosing fungal infection. Traditionally, the specimen is treated with 10% potassium hydroxide (KOH) to digest the cells and debris, resulting in clear visualization of the hyphae or yeast. Treatment of cerebrospinal fluid (CSF) specimens with KOH is not necessary because this fluid is naturally clear. India ink can be added to CSF to increase contrast and outline the organisms. Calcofluor white, a fluorescent fabric brightener that binds to fungi and fluoresces brilliantly when viewed under the ultraviolet microscope, also can be used to assist in recognition of fungal elements.

Histologic examination of biopsy specimens is an important tool for diagnosing and monitoring fungal infection, but identifying the exact fungus may be difficult. This is because only the tissue phase can be observed, and the fungal organisms in the specimen may be few. Because recognizing a fungus in hematoxylin-stained or eosin-stained sections may be difficult, a number of special stains have been developed.[73] Periodic acid–Schiff staining binds linked sugar groups in the fungal cell wall intensely magenta, thus making visualization of the fungal form easier. Likewise, several silver precipitation stains (e.g., Gomori methenamine silver) rely on the presence of a charged fungal surface to reduce oxidized silver to metallic silver. This process coats the fungus with a black layer, again outlining the form.[74] The mucicarmine stain imparts a deep red color to complex polysaccharides, such as mucin which can stain the thick capsule of *C. neoformans.* Because no other yeast has a positive mucicarmine stain, the definitive diagnosis of cryptococcosis can be made.[75] The size of the organism, manner of budding, and the presence or absence of septae all assist in the diagnosis.

Monoclonal antibodies against many fungi are now available. Immunohistochemical procedures using these sera on biopsy specimens allow for the identification of a number of fungal pathogens.[75] Reagents for in situ oligonucleotide probe hybridization to detect fungi in tissue are being developed and will also be extremely helpful.[76]

CULTURE

The most definitive method for diagnosing or monitoring a fungal infection is with culture. Specimens should be inoculated onto several different types of fungal media, some of which contain antibiotics to inhibit bacterial overgrowth. Swab specimens have a very low yield, especially for hyphal fungi and should be avoided in follow-up cultures. Yeast may grow rapidly and be isolated within 24 to 48 hours, but many fungi grow slowly and 4 to 6 weeks of incubation may be necessary to isolate and identify the organism. After growth, yeasts are usually recognized by their patterns of metabolic activity on a variety of substrates, whereas mycelial organisms may produce characteristic spores and fruiting bodies that are used for identification. Occasionally, a mycelial organism will be slow in producing recognizable spores, and immunologic testing for a characteristic isoantigen may be used for identification. A peptide nucleic acid fluorescense in situ hybridization test more rapidly identifies *C. albicans* from blood-culture bottles.[77] It is unclear how cost effective this test will be compared to traditional germ-tube testing.

ANTIGEN DETECTION

Fungi synthesize polysaccharides that cannot be broken down by human enzymatic systems. These polysaccharides can accumulate within the body and be excreted in the urine. These fungal antigens can be detected by using antibodies that specifically recognize a particular species of fungus, thereby providing a diagnosis. The most commonly used antigen detection test is a latex agglutination test for cryptococcal antigen. This assay can be performed on serum or CSF. Antigenemia is present in 80% to 100% of patients with culture-proved cryptococcal meningitis. This test can also be used to monitor patient response to therapy by determining the end point dilution for the positive reaction and following this end point over time as the patient is treated. If treatment is successful, the titer will decline.[78,79]

Tests (quantitative polymerase chain reaction, enzyme-linked immunosorbent assay [ELISA], latex agglutination) for other fungal antigens are not as well established. Latex particle agglutination tests to detect candidal antigens are available, but their utility has not been clearly demonstrated. Assays for detecting *H. capsulatum* antigen in serum and urine have been reported.[80] Antigen can be detected in the blood of 50% and in the urine of 80% to 90% of patients with systemic histoplasmosis. Patients with blastomycosis and paracoccidioidomycosis, however, may also have positive cross-reactions. The ELISA for detection of *Aspergillus* galactomannan antigen (Section 71-30) and *Candida* (1–3)-β-D-glucan are now marketed. The reported sensitivity (63%) and specificity (96%) of two consecutive (1–3)-β-D-glucan results greater than 7 pg/mL is clinically useful. Using these tests can result in a shorter time to diagnosis and leads to significantly shorter time of illness compared to other diagnostic tests. β-Glucan is most valuable for its negative predictive value.[81] Considering the presence of false-positives or false-negatives, it is unknown whether these assays will improve diagnostic capability for patients at risk for these infections. Increasing or decreasing values can be used to monitor clinical response to antifungal therapy.[77]

ANTIBODY DETECTION

Detection of antibody can be useful for some fungal diseases but not for others. Serologic diagnosis of systemic candidiasis is complicated because most people have anti-*Candida* antibodies. A rising titer is not specific for infection and may indicate only colonization. Furthermore, dissemination of *Candida* is most likely in people who are immunocompromised and, therefore, may not respond by producing antibody.[82] On the other hand, seropositivity can be demonstrated in more than 90% of patients with symptomatic histoplasmosis.[83] The most important serologic tests use the complement fixation, immunodiffusion, and enzyme immunoassay (EIA) techniques. Appropriate evolution of serologic results requires an understanding of the sensitivity, specificity, and predictive value of each methodology. In general, serologic tests allow only a presumptive diagnosis of mycotic infections.

Although any of the aforementioned tests could be ordered for L.K., a direct examination of his blood and urine specimens along with an assessment of signs and symptoms of disseminated candidiasis are reasonable first steps in his evaluation. A blood specimen from L.K. should also be cultured on different fungal media. Because a candidal infection is suspected, the culture could isolate *Candida* within 24 to 48 hours. Cultures and histopathologic examination of a biopsy specimen of skin lesions are often helpful not only in confirming a diagnosis of disseminated candidal infection but also in monitoring response to therapy. The other fungal tests previously described need not be ordered immediately and should await the results from direct examination and culture.

NECESSITY OF TREATMENT

CASE 75-3, QUESTION 3: The clinical laboratory reports that a single blood culture obtained from 2 days ago is growing *Candida* species. Why is therapy necessary in L.K. with only a single positive blood culture?

Case control studies of candidemia report an 85.6% mortality rate in untreated patients compared with a 41.8% mortality rate in patients who received early treatment. Isolation of *Candida* from a patient's bloodstream requires initiation of immediate antifungal therapy. Delays in therapy are associated with significant increase in mortality. In fact, delaying therapy 24 hours from the time a blood culture is positive or failure to follow Infectious Disease Society of America treatment guidelines increases mortality nearly 50%.[84–86] Elimination of risk factors may improve the clinical outcome of candidemia, and removal of central venous catheters reduces morbidity and mortality.[87,88] Although discontinuation of a centrally inserted catheter may complicate drug administration, it still should be removed. L.K.'s other risk factors (e.g., broad-spectrum antibacterials) are perhaps of even greater importance.

TREATMENT OPTIONS AND COMBINATION THERAPY

CASE 75-3, QUESTION 4: What therapeutic options are available to treat candidemia? Which option would be best for L.K.?

Therapeutic options are individualized and based on the competence of a patient's host defenses. In immunocompetent patients, AmB, an echinocandin, or a triazole decreases morbidity and mortality associated with this disease.[89–93] Echinocandins have been demonstrated as effective as AmB in neutropenic and nonneutropenic patients; however, AmB clears the bloodstream the most rapidly.[94,95] In the largest, well-controlled comparative trial, 206 nonneutropenic patients were randomly assigned to AmB 0.5 to 0.6 mg/kg/day or fluconazole 400 mg/day for 14 days. Mortality was less than 9% in both groups with no significant difference in successful outcomes (AmB, 80%; fluconazole, 72%). Less toxicity was noted in the fluconazole group, however.[90] Therefore, fluconazole 400 mg/day is as effective as AmB for nonneutropenic patients infected with susceptible *Candida*. Candidemic (or other mycotic infections discussed in this chapter) patients who are clinically stable and have no evidence of deep-seated infection should be initiated on a triazole or echinocandin for at least 14 days. Patients who cannot be treated with an echinocandin or azole can be treated with AmB 0.5 to 1.0 mg/kg/day or 3 to 5 mg/kg/day of a lipid formulation of AmB. A comparison of micafungin (100 mg or 150 mg) versus caspofungin revealed no difference with micafungin 100 mg and caspofungin after 10 days of therapy. However, micafungin 150 mg trended toward poorer responses.[96]

High-dose fluconazole (12 mg/kg/day) alone or in combination with AmB for a minimum of 3 days, followed by step-down therapy to fluconazole, were evaluated. Outcomes were not different between treatment groups and consistent with previously reported success rates. Notably, the fluconazole treatment group had higher Acute Physiology and Chronic Health Evaluation (APACHE II) scores, making evaluation of the comparison difficult.[94] In contrast, in another clinical trial, the combination of AmB and flucytosine was suggested to be more effective than single-agent therapy.[97,98] An AmB-containing regimen may be more effective in patients with APACHE II scores between 10 and 22.[94]

L.K. could be treated with an echinocandin, with the total duration based on clinical response and resolution of positive cultures (see Case 75-3, Question 6). Efficacy should be monitored using patient-specific signs and symptoms of candidemia. Combination therapy can be considered in those patients who are not responding clinically. More importantly, a complete examination for focal sites of infection (septic thrombi or intra-abdominal abscess) should take place. If eventually available as an adjunctive therapy, HSP90 antibody may be associated with improved outcomes in the future.[32]

CASE 75-3, QUESTION 5: This fungal species has now been identified as *C. non-albicans*. How does this affect the therapeutic options for L.K.?

Historically, isolation of a non-albicans *Candida* from blood has resulted in a therapeutic dilemma due to common in vitro resistance, which has been associated with poor clinical outcomes in animal models and uncontrolled case reports. Intrinsic resistance (*C. lusitaniae* to AmB, *C. parapsilosis* to echinocandins, and *C. kruseii* to fluconazole) or acquired resistance (*C. tropicalis* or *glabrata* against fluconazole) has been reported.[91,97,98] Acquired in vitro fluconazole drug resistance is probably associated with altered fungal cell membrane permeability, antifungal efflux pumps, and changes in CYP450 enzymes. In observational studies, fluconazole resistance in vitro has been 9%.[91,97,98] A large, multicenter study of 232 nonneutropenic patients was unable, however, to demonstrate a relationship between yeast MIC and patient outcome.[91] An inability to demonstrate a relationship is probably a result of a limited understanding or inadequate management of risk factors for infection. For example, the removal of a colonized IV catheter is probably a more important predictor of outcome than the MIC of the isolated yeast.

Therefore, the true rate of acquired clinical resistance to azoles and ultimate failure is unknown. Vigilant monitoring and aggressive therapy of infections caused by *Candida non-albicans* is recommended. In patients in whom susceptibilities are available, fluconazole should be avoided when the MIC is greater than 16 mcg/mL.

AMPHOTERICIN

DOSING

CASE 75-3, QUESTION 6: How should amphotericin B formulation be dosed and administered to L.K.?

The AmB dose and duration of therapy should be individualized based on the severity of infection and immunocompetence of the patient. Once the patient is stable, therapy should be changed to one of the applicable regimens discussed previously. The dose of AmB formulations should be based on lean body mass. Owing to the difficulty in measuring lean body mass, many clinicians, however, use ideal body weight. Tissues that contain large numbers of macrophages sequester significant amounts of AmB (liver, 17.5%–40.3%; spleen, 0.7%–15.6%; kidney, 0.6%–4.1%; lung, 0.4%–13%), but it does not distribute well into adipose tissue (<1.0%).[92,93] Because L.K. is 5-feet, 8-inches tall and not obese, his ideal body weight should be about 70 kg. Therefore, AmB 35 mg/day (0.5 mg/kg) should be initiated because L.K. is not clinically stable and may require increased doses. Half the full dose should be given on the first day of therapy and the full dose given on subsequent days. In more seriously ill patients, the full dose of AmB can be initiated immediately. Although the optimal dosing regimen to initiate AmB is not well established, most clinicians gradually titrate the dose upward to minimize infusion-related reactions. Peak AmB serum concentrations achieved after parenteral administration are a function of dose, frequency of dosing, and rate of infusion. When the AmB total dose is less than 50 mg, the serum concentration is directly proportional to the dose; doses greater than 50 mg are associated with a plateau in serum concentrations. After administration, AmB undergoes biphasic elimination: Peak serum concentrations drop rapidly (initial $t_{1/2}$, 24–48 hours), but low concentrations (0.5–1.0 mcg/mL) are detectable for up to 2 weeks (terminal $t_{1/2}$ 15 days).[99] The long terminal-elimination half-life has been used as a justification for the common practice of every-other-day AmB dosing, in which twice the daily dose is given every other day. Every-other-day regimens have not been carefully evaluated but are rationalized based on the potential for reduced nephrotoxicity. Administration of 0.5 mg/kg/day or 1.0 mg/kg every other day results in trough AmB concentrations with sufficient postdose antifungal effects that inhibit the common pathogenic fungi.[100] Once L.K.'s clinical status has improved, the potential for renal toxicity could outweigh the concerns of potential reduced efficacy, and implementation of AmB every-other-day therapy should be considered.

INFUSION REACTIONS

CASE 75-3, QUESTION 7: L.K. has no complaints except for fevers and shaking chills that occur during his 6-hour to 8-hour AmB infusion for the past 3 days. He has been receiving acetaminophen 650 mg 30 minutes before AmB infusion, but he has refused today's AmB dose. What measures can be taken to minimize these infusion-related reactions?

Adverse reactions, which are common with AmB administration, are best classified as infusion-related, dose-related, or idiosyncratic reactions. Infusion-related reactions include an acute symptom complex of fever, chills, nausea, vomiting, headache, hypotension, and thrombophlebitis. Dose-related reactions also can be acute (e.g., cardiac arrhythmias) or chronic (e.g., renal dysfunction with secondary electrolyte imbalances and anemia). Premedication to prevent AmB formulation infusion-related reactions and a test dose of AmB formulations are not needed for L.K. Most practices of premedicating are performed out of ritual rather than predicated on scientific study.[101] Test dosing with 1 mg before the first dose is not currently used because of the immeasurably low incidence of anaphylactoid reactions. Until clinical trials clarify the risk–benefit ratio of premedications, concomitant therapy should be restricted to acetaminophen for fever or headache and heparin to prevent thrombophlebitis when possible.

Many infusion-related reactions are mediated by AmB-induced cytokine (interleukin-1β, tumor necrosis factor, prostaglandin E_2) expression by mononuclear cells.[102,103] Hydrocortisone is extremely effective in suppressing cytokine expression[102] and it also blunts the fever and chills associated with AmB administration.[104] Hydrocortisone, however, does not reduce the frequency of chronic dose-related toxicity such as renal insufficiency, and corticosteroid-induced immunosuppression could decrease AmB fungicidal activity.[105] Nonsteroidal anti-inflammatory drugs (NSAIDs) also prevent fever, most likely by the suppression of prostaglandin E_2 expression.[106] NSAIDs, however, cannot be recommended for routine use because of their potential for additive nephrotoxicity when used with AmB.

The mild to moderate elevations in temperature and the other infusion-related symptoms usually subside when the infusion is completed, and tolerance to these effects develops over 3 to 5 days. L.K. initially should be counseled that these reactions will abate over the next few days without intervention. If assessment of the reactions suggests the need for more aggressive premedication, a short course of hydrocortisone 0.7 mg/kg prior to AmB or added to the infusion bag should be initiated.[104] Meperidine 25 to 50 mg by rapid IV infusion reduces AmB-induced rigors and can be repeated every 15 minutes as required while monitoring for signs and symptoms of opiate toxicity. Administration of an average meperidine dose of 45 mg has been found to resolve chills three times faster than placebo.[107]

Faster AmB infusion rates (<4–6 hours) are associated with the earlier onset of infusion-related reactions but not with more severe infusion reactions.[108,109] Many patients prefer rapid infusions (1–2 hours) because the infusion-related reactions abate quickly on completion of the AmB infusion. Electrocardiographic evaluations of 1-hour infusions indicate that this rate of amphotericin infusion is safe at currently recommended doses in patients without renal or heart disease. Rapid infusions are not safe in all patients, however, because cardiac arrhythmias appear to be dose and infusion rate related. If infused too rapidly, high serum concentrations of AmB can precipitate severe cardiac adverse events. Arrhythmias have been reported most often in patients who are anuric or who have previous cardiac disease.[110] Continuous infusion is not recommended based on the pharmacodynamics of this agent and the concentration dependence of activity.

NEPHROTOXICITY

CASE 75-3, QUESTION 8: On day 4 of therapy with AmB, L.K.'s serum creatinine (SCr) and blood urea nitrogen (BUN) are 2.3 mg/dL (SI units, 203.32 μmol/L) and 42 mg/dL (SI units, 14.99 mmol/L), respectively. How could AmB exacerbate L.K.'s renal dysfunction and how could it be prevented from worsening?

Renal dysfunction is the adverse event that most often limits treatment with AmB. The renal toxicity results from

AmB-mediated damage to renal tubules, which causes electrolyte wasting and disrupts the tubuloglomerular feedback mechanism. The clinical manifestations of AmB-induced renal damage include azotemia, renal tubular acidosis, hypokalemia, and hypomagnesemia.[101] Generally, AmB-related renal toxicity is reversible within 2 weeks after therapy has been discontinued. Administration of normal saline (250 mL) immediately before AmB administration reduces the risk for AmB-induced nephrotoxicity[111] and should be initiated before L.K.'s next dose. AmB should not be admixed with normal saline, however, because sodium causes AmB to precipitate into an inactive particulate in IV admixture formulations.[112] Other nephrotoxins should be avoided (especially diuretics) (Table 75-6) and patients with already compromised renal function should be closely monitored and alternate therapy should be considered.[112] Hypokalemia and hypomagnesemia also should be monitored closely. These measures to prevent further renal deterioration should be implemented and the AmB therapy continued cautiously in this patient with systemic candidiasis. Anemia, associated with decreased renal production of erythropoietin, should resolve after AmB is discontinued and need not be treated.[113]

CASE 75-3, QUESTION 9: L.K. has exhibited significant renal dysfunction resulting from acute tubular necrosis. How should his dose of systemic antifungal drugs be altered?

Renal elimination of the antimycotics varies tremendously. For systemically administered AmB, only 5% to 10% of unchanged drug is eliminated in urine and bile during the first 24 hours,[101] and no evidence indicates it is metabolized to a significant extent. Therefore, no substantial dosage adjustment is required for patients with chronic renal or hepatic failure. Although many clinicians will withhold AmB doses if acute renal dysfunction develops during therapy, concerns of drug-induced nephrotoxicity in L.K. must be balanced against the high likelihood of mortality in untreated patients with deep-seated infections.[70,72] Alternative systemic antifungal therapy (i.e., azoles or echinocandins) that is less nephrotoxic should also be considered. Dosing recommendations for echinocandins are unchanged in renal dysfunction or liver dysfunction except for caspofungin. For patients in moderate hepatic insufficiency (Child-Turcotte Pugh score 7–9), the maintenance caspofungin dose should be decreased to 35 mg/day. No data are available for caspofungin used in severe hepatic impairment and a further dosage reduction should be considered.

Ketoconazole and itraconazole undergo first-pass metabolism and have a biphasic dose-dependent elimination.[42,43] These agents are extensively metabolized and excreted in the bile; small amounts of unchanged drug are excreted in the urine, therefore no need exists to adjust dosages in patients with renal dysfunction or in patients undergoing dialysis.[114] Fluconazole and voriconazole, unlike ketoconazole and itraconazole, are not extensively metabolized. More than 90% of a fluconazole dose is excreted in urine, of which about 80% is measured as unchanged drug and about 20% as metabolites.[115] Because fluconazole is excreted primarily unchanged in the urine, dosages should be adjusted in patients with renal insufficiency (Table 75-5).[23,24,42–45,101,114–122] Fluconazole or voriconazole may be reasonable alternatives in L.K., but the dosage must be adjusted for renal function based on published nomograms.[116]

CASE 75-3, QUESTION 10: What is the role of an AmB formulated with a lipid?

Lipid formulations of AmB have been approved by the FDA for patients who are unable to tolerate generic AmB (Table 75-7). In addition, the admixture of AmB in 10% or 20% lipid emulsion has been used for treating systemic mycotic infections. The lipid carriers differ tremendously for each of the amphotericin formulations. The liposomal formulation is a spherical carrier that contains AmB both on the inside and outside of the vesicle. Imagine the lipid complex as a snowflake shape, and the colloidal dispersion shaped like a Frisbee with AmB bound to the structure. The differences in structure appear to have no effect on therapeutic outcome but confer different protection against amphotericin adverse effects.[123] AmB admixture with a lipid emulsion cannot be recommended until a stable formulation can be established.[124]

Limited data are available to assist in the management of this case. A single large controlled trial has evaluated AmB lipid complex for the treatment of disseminated candidiases. AmB 0.6 to 1.0 mg/kg/day for 14 days was slightly, but not significantly, superior to the lipid complex formulation at 5 mg/kg/day for mycologic efficacy (68% vs. 63%) or survival.[125] Renal dysfunction defined as a doubling in SCr, however, was 47% with AmB and 28% with this lipid formulation. Because of the significant cost, some health care facilities reserve lipid formulations for patients who have pre-existing renal dysfunction or those who have severe adverse reactions to generic AmB. However, most centers use lipid formulations as their formulary polyene due to patient acceptance and cost of AmB-associated renal dysfunction. Indications for the lipid formulations are further reviewed in the discussion of sections on aspergillosis and cryptococcosis.

ANTIMYCOTIC PROPHYLAXIS

CASE 75-3, QUESTION 11: What measures could have been undertaken to prevent invasive fungal infections in L.K.?

In 2005, the Mycoses Study Group Trial initially defined patients at high risk as patients who could benefit from prophylaxis. Trials are still underway assessing the efficacy of differing antifungals in those patients who have at least one of the primary risk factors: systemic antibiotics for previous 4 days or presence of a central venous catheter, and at least two secondary risk factors: dialysis or use of TPN during previous 4 days; inpatient surgery, pancreatitis, or more than one dose of systemic steroids or immunsuppressive within 7 days before ICU admission. Minimizing these risk factors is instrumental in preventing fungal infections. When such control is not possible, antifungal prophylaxis should be considered in high-risk populations (>10% candidemia incidence).[126]

Selective GI decontamination or systemic antimycotic pharmacotherapy can be used in high-risk, immunocompromised, or surgical patients to prevent the development of fungal infections and could have been used for L.K. In critically ill surgical patients, the risk of invasive infection, but not mortality, may be reduced by more than 50% with fluconazole prophylaxis.[127] Alternatively, a nonabsorbable antifungal such as AmB or nystatin are possible options. Oral AmB decreases systemic candidal infections threefold to fivefold in high-risk patients.[128] Yet the problems of unreliable antifungal stool concentrations,[129] decreasing azole cost associated with the availability of generics, and poor compliance have led to preferential azole use. Azoles are more effective in preventing oral pharyngeal candidiasis than placebo.[130,131] At the present time, no well-designed studies have compared azoles with polyene antifungals (e.g., AmB) for prevention of oropharyngeal or systemic candidiasis.

Prophylaxis could be initiated and continued until L.K. is no longer immunocompromised. If L.K. is discharged from the

TABLE 75-7
Amphotericin B Formulations

Category	Amphotericin B (Fungizone)	Amphotericin B Lipid Complex (Abelcet)	Amphotericin B Colloidal Dispersion (Amphotec)	Liposomal Amphotericin B (AmBisome)		Amphotericin B in Lipid Emulsion
FDA-approved indication	Life-threatening fungal infections Visceral leishmaniasis	Refractory or intolerant to AmB	Invasive Aspergillosis in patients refractory or intolerant to AmB	Empirical therapy in neutropenic FUO Refractory or intolerant to AmB Visceral leishmaniasis		NA
Formulation						
Sterol	None	None	Cholesterol sulfate	Cholesterol sulfate (5)[a]		Safflower and soybean oils
Phospholipid	None	DMPC and DMPG (7:3)[a]	None	EPC and DSPG (10:4)[a]		10–20 g/100 mL EPC >2.21 g/100 mL Glycerin >258 g/100 mL
Amphotericin B (Mole%)	34	33	50	10		Variable
Particle size (nm)	<10	1,600–11,000	122(± 48)	80–120		333–500
Manufacturer	Generic	Enzon	Intermune	Fujisawa Pharmaceuticals		Not applicable
Stability	1 week at 2–8°C or 24 hours at 27°C	15 hours at 2–8°C or 6 hours at 27°C	24 hours at 2–8°C	24 hours at 2–8°C		Unstable
Dosage and rate	0.3–0.7 mg/kg/d during 1–6 hours[b]	5 mg/kg/d at 2.5 mg/kg/hr	3–4 mg/kg/d during 2 hours	3–5[c] mg/kg/d during 2 hours		Investigational: 1 mg/kg/d during 1–8 hours
Lethal dose 50%	3.3 mg/kg	10–25 mg/kg	68 mg/kg	175 mg/kg		Unknown
Pharmacokinetic Parameters						
Dose	0.5 mg/kg	5 mg/kg × 7 days	5 mg/kg × 7 days	2.5 mg/kg × 7 days	5 mg/kg × 7 days	0.8 mg/kg/day × 13 d
Serum Concentrations						
Peak	1.2 mcg/mL	1.7 mcg/mL	3.1 mcg/mL	31.4 mcg/mL	83.0 mcg/mL	2.13 mcg/mL
Trough	0.5 mcg/mL	0.7 mcg/mL		4.0 mcg/mL		0.42 mcg/mL
Half-life	91.1 hours	173.4 hours	28.5 hours	6.3 hours	6.8 hours	7.75 hours
Volume of distribution	5.0 L/kg	131.0 L/kg	4.3 L/kg	0.16 L/kg	0.10 L/kg	0.45 L/kg
Clearance	38.0 mL/hr/kg	436.0 mL/hr/kg	0.117 mL/hr/kg	22.0 mL/hr/kg	11.0 mL/hr/kg	37.0 m/hr/kg
AUC	14 mcg/mL · hr	17 mcg/mL · hr	43.0 mcg/mL · hr	197 mcg/mL · hr	555 mcg/mL · hr	26.37 mcg/mL · hr

[a] Molar ratio of each component, respectively.
[b] No benefit for longer infusions.
[c] Doses greater than 10 mg/kg have no benefit.
AmB, amphotericin B; AUC, area under the curve; DMPC, dimyristoyl phosphatidycholine; DMPG, dimyristoyl phosphatidyglycerol; DSPG, distearolyphosphatidyglycerol; EPC, egg phosphatidylcholine; FDA, US Food and Drug Administration; FUO, fever of unknown origin; NA, not applicable.

hospital and treated as an outpatient, a systemic azole (imidazole or triazole) administered once daily is preferable to a polyene to improve adherence. To reemphasize, however, systemic therapy increases the risk of resistance, adverse effects, drug interactions, and potentially cost (Table 75-4).

Candiduria

TREATMENT

CASE 75-4

QUESTION 1: M.Y., a 24-year-old man, has been hospitalized in the surgical intensive care unit (ICU) with multiple traumatic injuries resulting from a motor vehicle accident. Shortly after admission, he underwent an exploratory laparotomy for a ruptured spleen and lacerated liver. He subsequently suffered respiratory and renal failure. M.Y. is currently intubated and on mechanical ventilation. Since admission, he has been nutritionally supported with central hyperalimentation and has been receiving broad-spectrum antibiotics (gentamicin, ampicillin, and metronidazole). A Foley catheter is in place. Two recent urinalyses (UAs) show budding yeast and cultures were positive for greater than 100,000 colony-forming units of *C. albicans*. M.Y. is currently afebrile, his funduscopic examination is normal, and no macronodular skin lesions are present. The WBC count is 8,900 cells/μL (SI units, WBC count, 8.9 × 10^9/L), and three sets of blood cultures drawn during the past 2 days are negative. How should M.Y.'s candiduria be treated?

It is difficult to differentiate among cystitis, urethritis, or systemic infection in the presence of funguria. Similarly, it is difficult to differentiate colonization from infection because candiduric patients are usually asymptomatic. Funguria cannot be used to determine the location or severity of invasion. Signs and symptoms of systemic disease should be monitored diligently until a diagnosis of colonization, cystitis, or urethritis is confirmed and the risk of dissemination is excluded.

Eradication of fungi in the urine (specifically *C. albicans*) should begin with removal of the indwelling urinary catheter and alleviation of risk factors for fungal disease. If catheter removal does not clear the urine within 48 hours, pharmacotherapy should be considered. If M.Y. is scheduled for a genitourinary procedure, he should receive systemic therapy because the rate of candidemia after surgery is high (10.8%) in candiduric patients. In addition, any patient at high risk for dissemination into the blood should be considered for treatment (e.g., patients with immunosuppression).[132]

Bladder irrigation with AmB has been used in the past at concentrations of 150 mcg/mL, however has limited clinical utility and is not recommended by the Infectious Diseases Society of America.[133] In two comparative studies, bladder irrigation for 5 days with AmB 50 mcg/mL was superior to fluconazole 100 mg/day as measured by microbiologic cure rates. Clinical cure rates at 2 to 4 weeks were equal—however, mortality rates were higher in the AmB-treated groups. It was suggested that AmB failures may have been associated with dissemination of yeast from the urinary tract.[134,135] Systemic antifungal therapy with flucytosine 100 to 150 mg/kg/day for 7 days[136] and azoles (fluconazole 0.6 to 1.4 mg/kg/day for 7 days)[137,138] also has been used in noncomparative or nonrandomized studies.

Blastomycosis

ETIOLOGY

CASE 75-5

QUESTION 1: C.P., a 17-year-old girl, is admitted to the hospital with a chronic pneumonia that has not responded to antibiotics. Three months ago, she began to exhibit a chronic cough that eventually became productive of purulent sputum, which was occasionally streaked with blood. Two months ago, she began to exhibit "boils" on her lower extremities and back, which drained spontaneously. She was hospitalized at another hospital but failed to respond to amoxicillin and clarithromycin. C.P. denies fever, chills, or night sweats, but has lost 11 pounds. Her temperature is 38.2°C. A 2-cm^2 subcutaneous, fluctuant, tender mass is seen over the right mandible and a second fluctuant mass about 4 cm wide on the lower back. Also, several 0.5-cm^2 to 1-cm^2 ulcers with heaped-up, hyperkeratotic margins are noted on the lower extremities (Fig. 75-2). Rales are heard at the right lung base. C.P.'s leukocyte count is slightly elevated at 13,500 cells/μL (SI units, WBC count, 13.5 × 10^9/L). A chest radiograph shows a masslike infiltrate in the right mid-lung field (Fig. 75-3). A wet preparation of ulcer scrapings and material aspirated from a subcutaneous abscess reveal numerous broad-based, budding yeast forms with refractile cell walls and multiple nuclei typical of *B. dermatitidis*.

Cultures of sputum, skin scrapings, and abscess material eventually confirmed the diagnosis. What was the likely portal of entry for C.P.'s disseminated blastomycosis? Why should it be treated?

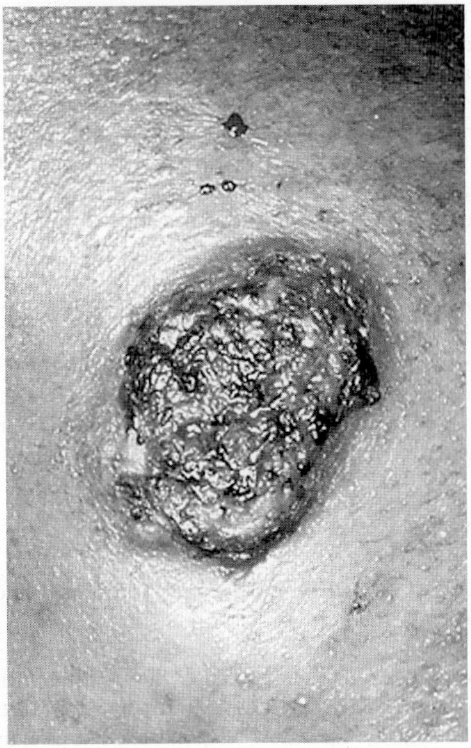

FIGURE 75-2 Disseminated *Blastomyces dermatitidis* skin ulcers.

Typical of the other endemic mycoses, the primary portal of entry for *B. dermatitidis* is the lungs. A pulmonary origin for C.P.'s infection is supported by her history of cough with purulent, blood-streaked sputum, followed a month later with cutaneous lesions on her legs and back. An acute pulmonary

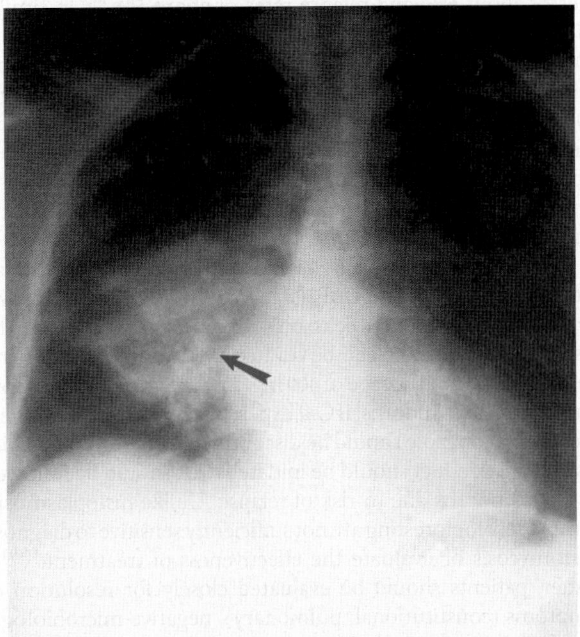

FIGURE 75-3 Chest radiograph of pulmonary *Blastomyces dermatitidis*.

infection is most often asymptomatic and, when symptomatic, usually requires only observation. Chronic pulmonary or extrapulmonary blastomycosis will develop in an unknown number of these patients. C.P.'s rales at the base of her right lung and persistent pneumonia unresponsive to antibacterials suggest a chronic pulmonary infection and need for treatment. Chronic pulmonary disease often presents with radiographic studies often mistaken for tuberculosis or cancer; the masslike infiltrate in her right lung on chest radiograph also is consistent with chronic pulmonary disease. Extrapulmonary infections can involve the skin (verrucous or ulcerative lesions), bone, genitourinary system (prostatitis, epididymo-orchitis), or central nervous system (CNS) (meningitis or brain abscess). If untreated, these chronic pulmonary or extrapulmonary infections are fatal in at least 21% of patients.[139] Because C.P. presents with pulmonary and cutaneous evidence of blastomycosis, she should be treated.

TREATMENT

CASE 75-5, QUESTION 2: What specific therapy should be initiated for C.P.?

Historically, AmB was considered the treatment of choice for blastomycosis and total doses of more than 2 g were associated with 97% cure rates, low relapse rates, but also, however, substantial associated toxicity.[139] Ketoconazole and itraconazole are safe, effective alternatives to AmB in patients with non–life-threatening, non-CNS infections. The NIAID-Mycoses Study Group[140] confirmed the effectiveness of azoles for the treatment of chronic pulmonary and extrapulmonary disease associated with blastomycosis and histoplasmosis. In uncontrolled evaluations of chronic pulmonary and extrapulmonary infections (excluding life-threatening or CNS), ketoconazole at dosages of 400 to 800 mg/day resulted in cure rates of about 89%, failure rates of about 6%, and relapse rates of about 5%.[140] In similar studies, itraconazole capsules 200 to 400 mg/day for a median of 6.2 months resulted in cure rates of 88% to 95%.[141] Fluconazole was ineffective at dosages less than 400 mg/day. Higher dosages (400–800 mg/day), however, are as effective as ketoconazole in non–life-threatening disease.[142] Although these trials are neither comparative nor controlled, itraconazole is less toxic than ketoconazole and with the best benefit (efficacy) to risk (toxicity) ratio.

C.P. has mild to moderate disease and can be treated with an initial itraconazole dosage of 200 mg/day. If no clinical improvement is seen within 2 weeks or if the disease progresses, the dosage of itraconazole can be titrated upward in 100-mg increments to a maximal dosage of 400 mg/day. Treatment should continue for at least 6 months. If C.P. experiences severe or meningeal disease, itraconazole should be discontinued and AmB or a lipid-based AmB product should be initiated. C.P. should be followed up for 12 months due to risk of relapse. Unlike histoplasmosis, skin and serologic testing are not sufficiently sensitive to diagnose blastomycosis or evaluate the effectiveness of treatment.[140,143] Rather, patients should be evaluated closely for resolution of symptoms (constitutional, pulmonary), negative microbiologic samples, and improvement in radiographic studies.

ANTIFUNGALS IN PREGNANCY

CASE 75-5, QUESTION 3: C.P. reports she has not menstruated in 3 months, and a urine pregnancy test is positive. How does this information change the therapeutic options for her?

The data on the safety of antimycotics for treating patients who are pregnant or lactating are limited, but comprehensively reviewed according to FDA categories of the teratogenic risks of drugs (see Chapter 49, Obstetric Drug Therapy).[144,145] The systemic azoles are categorized with risk factor C.[146] However, these agents should be avoided in pregnant or lactating women who are breast-feeding because of their potential teratogenicity and endocrine toxicity in the fetus or newborn. As with the azoles, griseofulvin and flucytosine have been classified with risk factor C. These agents should not be used in C.P. because the risk clearly outweighs the therapeutic benefit. Few or no data exist on the secretion of these agents in breast milk. Therefore, breast-feeding should be discouraged in women receiving these antifungal agents.

AmB and terbinafine are classified as risk factor B. Therapeutic agents in this category have no fetal risk based on animal studies or, when risk has been found in animals, controlled human studies have not confirmed the results. There are limited data regarding the use of terbinafine in pregnancy. Consequently, clinicians should avoid terbinafine use in pregnancy until published data support a B classification. Furthermore, considerable clinical experience with AmB in pregnant women has documented successful treatment of systemic mycoses with no excess toxicity to either the mother or fetus. Thus, AmB formulations have been the mainstay of antifungal therapy in pregnancy.

Histoplasmosis

TREATMENT

CASE 75-6

QUESTION 1: J.N., a 47-year-old man with severe rheumatoid arthritis, has been maintained on daily prednisone for the past 6 years; his current dosage is 20 mg/day. For the past 4 weeks, he has experienced daily fevers to 38.4°C, drenching night sweats, anorexia, and an 8.2-kg weight loss. His prednisone dosage was increased to 40 mg/day with little clinical effect. On admission to the hospital, J.N. appears chronically ill and has many of the stigmata of chronic steroid therapy. His temperature is 37.8°C with an associated rapid heart rate of 105 beats/minute. A shallow mouth ulcer is present on the hard palate. The liver is enlarged to a total span of 18 cm, and the spleen is palpable 3 cm below the left costal margin. Stool is positive for occult blood. A chest radiograph shows bilateral interstitial infiltrates (Fig. 75-4A). He is pancytopenic, with the following laboratory results:

Hematocrit, 29% (normal, 39%–45% SI units, 0.29)
WBC count, 3,500 cells/μL (normal, 4,000–11,000 cells/μL) (SI units, 3.5 × 10^9/L)
Platelet count, 78,000 cells/μL (normal, 130 to 400,000 cells/μL)
UA, 8 to 10 WBC/high-power field
SCr, 1.9 mg/dL (SI units, 167.96 μmol/L)
BUN, 42 mg/dL (SI units, 14.99 mmol/L urea)

The bilirubin is normal but the aminotransferases are elevated to about 1.5 times normal, and serum lactate dehydrogenase is 10 times greater than normal. A bone marrow aspirate and biopsy of the mouth ulcer reveals multiple, small intracellular yeast forms compatible with *H. capsulatum* in macrophages and polymorphonuclear leukocytes (Fig. 75-4B).

Section 14 Infectious Disease

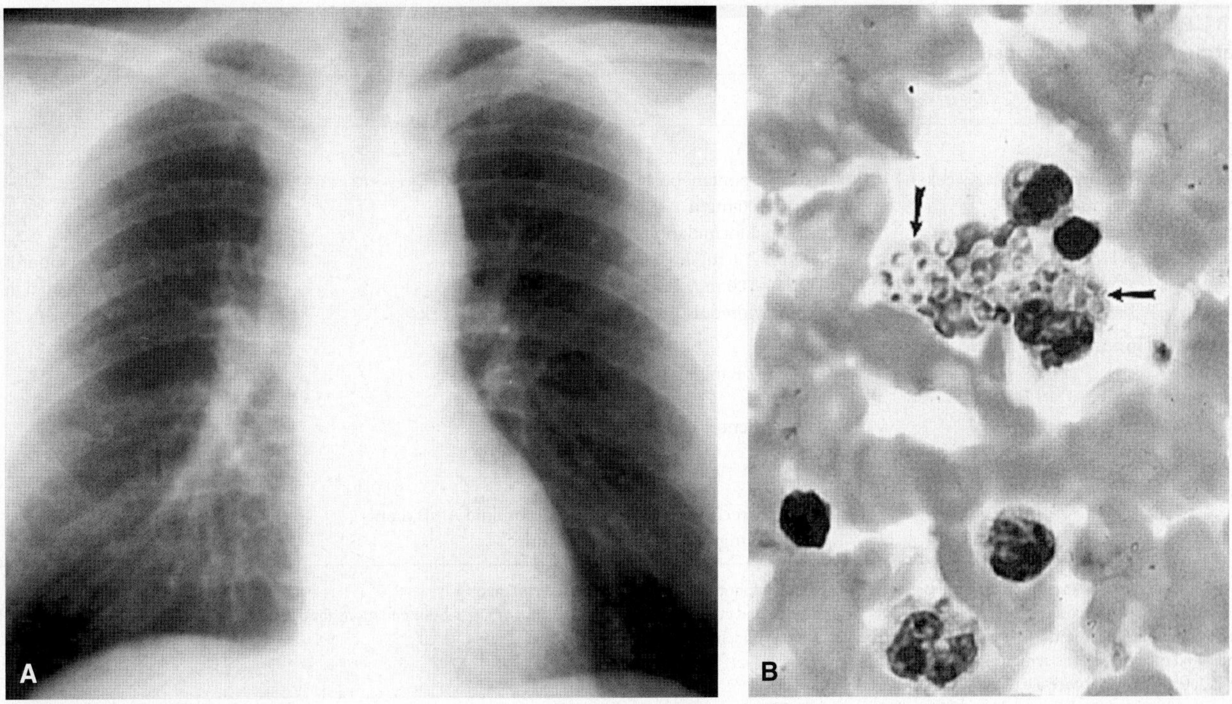

FIGURE 75-4 **Histoplasmosis infection.** **A:** Chest radiograph showing bilateral interstitial infiltrate. **B:** Gram stain of peripheral blood showing leukocytes with intracellular organisms.

ONLINE CONTENT

For a visual of the microscopic appearance of the mold phase of Histoplasma capsulatum, go to http://thepoint.lww.com/AT10e.

Cultures of blood and urine, bone marrow aspirate, and mouth ulcer biopsy grew *H. capsulatum*. What is the optimal antifungal therapy in this case of systemic *H. capsulatum*? What clinical parameters should be monitored to assess the efficacy and toxicity of J.N.'s therapy?

The treatment benefits of antifungal therapy in systemic histoplasmosis have not been well investigated. Treatment options for histoplasmosis are outlined in Table 75-8.[147] Accordingly, J.N. should be treated with an intravenous amphotericin product or itraconazole 2.8 mg/kg/day, and his course of therapy should be monitored for both efficacy and toxicity. The decision was made to use conventional amphotericin for J.N.

Blood and urine cultures, WBC and platelet counts (histoplasma is associated with pancytopenia), constitutional symptoms, serum lactate dehydrogenase, and hepatosplenomegaly are useful measures for evaluating outcome to antifungal therapy of J.N.'s histoplasmosis. Anemia and chest radiographs are poor measures of treatment response. Chest radiographs often reflect calcified granulomas in chronic disease with scarring, which rarely resolve even with extensive therapy. Therefore, evaluation of deterioration on radiograph but not of improvement is possible. In addition, AmB-induced renal disease with secondary anemia can confuse evaluation of disease resolution. Anemia must be excluded as a prognostic indicator in patients receiving AmB for durations of 3 weeks regardless of the dose.[113]

Diligent follow-up of patients is required because relapses occur in 5% to 15% of AmB-treated patients within 3 years. Relapses have occurred in patients who received less than 30 mg/kg total dose of AmB, or had concomitant untreated Addison disease, immunosuppression, vascular infections (endocarditis, grafts, aneurysms), or meningeal infections.[147] More than 90% of HIV-positive patients experience a relapse of histoplasmosis subsequent to adequate AmB therapy. A double blind trial in immunocompromised patients (HIV) revealed that liposomal AmB was superior to AmB deoxycholate. It is not known how itraconazole compares with liposomal AmB in those co-infected with HIV. If this patient was co-infected with HIV, a lipid based amphotericin may have been preferred.[148] Even the initiation of subsequent immunosuppressive therapy is of particular concern because of the potential for reactivation (relapse) and dissemination of histoplasmosis from dormant foci, especially in patients with residual granulomas. The residual disease has been hypothesized to lead to chronic inflammatory responses and secondary strokes.[149]

Potential adverse effects to AmB also should be monitored in J.N. (e.g., infusion-related reactions, nephrotoxicity, anemia, hypokalemia, neurotoxicity, thrombophlebitis). In addition, J.N.'s adrenal status should be monitored closely because of his long-term corticosteroid therapy and his histoplasmosis. Patients who are addisonian secondary to histoplasmosis infections appear to experience more episodes of AmB-induced acute hypotension.

AZOLE ADVERSE EFFECTS

CASE 75-6, QUESTION 2: After treatment with a total AmB dose of 750 mg, clinical improvement of J.N.'s histoplasmosis is subjectively and objectively documented. The clinician selected ketoconazole 400 mg/day as an oral substitute for his AmB regimen because of the patient's economic circumstances. Six weeks later, J.N. complains of impotence and wonders whether this could be caused by his medication. What is the likelihood that ketoconazole is the cause of J.N.'s impotence?

TABLE 75-8
Treatment of Histoplasmosis

Disease	Primary	Secondary
Acute Pulmonary		
Prolonged symptomatology (>2 weeks)	Resolves spontaneously	N/A
Immunocompromised[a]	ITZ 50–100 mg/d (3–6 months)[b]	AmB 0.3–0.5 mg/kg/d[b]
Respiratory distress	AmB lipid formulation 3–5 mg/kg/d[a]	AmB 0.3–0.5 mg/kg/d
(Pao_2 <70 mm Hg)	AmB 0.5–1.0 mg/kg/d (TD 250–500 mg) ± corticosteroids (methylprednisolone 0.5–1 mg/kg) × 1–2 weeks	ITZ 1.5–2.8 mg/kg/d (≥6 months)[b] ITZ (has not been investigated in life-threatening situations)
Chronic Pulmonary		
Active	ITZ (1.5–2.8 mg/kg/d 9 months)[b,c]	AmB 0.5 mg/kg/day[c]
Inactive		or KTZ 400 mg/day (≈6 mos)
Histoplasmoma	No treatment	N/A
Mediastinal fibrosis	Surgery[d]	N/A
Systemic Disease		
	AmB (TD recommended: 35 mg/kg) or lipid AmB then ITZ 2.8 mg/kg/d × up to 12 months[b]	Fluconazole 400–800 mg/d[e]

[a] Lipid formulations of amphotericin B are preferable to generic amphotericin B in HIV-infected patients.[148]
[b] Treatment should be continued until the patient is symptomfree and culture negative for 3 months. The recommendations for duration of therapy or total doses should be used only as guides for initial therapy based upon the IDSA 2007 Guideline.[147]
[c] Indicated only for serious symptoms (i.e., hemoptysis).
[d] ITZ 200 mg daily or twice a day for 6–18 months for most patients.
[e] Fluconazole should only be used in patients who cannot take ITZ.
AmB, amphotericin B deoxycholate; ITZ, itraconazole; KTZ, ketoconazole; TD, total dose.

Ketoconazole has been associated with more adverse reactions and greater potential for drug interactions compared with itraconazole and fluconazole. The most common side effects of ketoconazole, however, are nausea and vomiting. GI distress is dose-related, with fewer GI effects with 400 mg/day compared with 800 mg/day.[147] Endocrine and hepatic toxicities are the most significant adverse effects of ketoconazole. Dose-splitting from daily to twice daily may decrease nausea and vomiting. Dose-related endocrinologic toxicities (hypoadrenalism, oligospermia, and diminished libido) have been observed during ketoconazole therapy secondary to inhibition of mammalian sterol synthesis,[13,150] and usually resolve with drug discontinuation. Therefore, J.N.'s complaints of impotence might well be attributed to his ketoconazole. Liver enzymes should also be monitored because an approximate 10% risk exists of elevation in transaminases and an occasional case of serious hepatitis and hepatic failure.[13,150]

The triazoles—itraconazole, fluconazole, and voriconazole—are much better tolerated and require less monitoring than ketoconazole therapy. This result has been attributed to the greater affinity of the triazoles for fungal cytochrome enzymes and less interference with mammalian enzymes.[151] Itraconazole, fluconazole (6 mg/kg/day), and voriconazole do not exhibit antiandrogenic effects, and nausea and vomiting is less common when compared with imidazoles. Abnormal elevations in liver function have been reported in 2.7% of patients receiving voriconazole during clinical trials. Abnormalities in liver function tests may be associated with higher azole dosages or serum concentrations, but generally resolve either with continued therapy or dosage modification, including drug discontinuance. Liver function should be determined before and periodically throughout azole therapy because cases of serious hepatic reactions have been reported.[151] A unique adverse event associated with voriconazole is enhanced perception to light, which may be associated with higher plasma concentrations or doses. Generally, drug discontinuance is not required, although monitoring of visual acuity, visual field, and color perception is advised if therapy lasts longer than 28 days. Diarrhea, asthenia, flatulence, and eye pain have been reported with posaconazole therapy.[58] Based on these data, J.N. should be given a trial of itraconazole.

AZOLE DRUG INTERACTIONS

CASE 75-6, QUESTION 3: J.N. chose to continue his ketoconazole therapy. He now returns with Cushnoid signs and symptoms. What potential drug or disease state interaction could be implicated as a cause of this serious problem in J.N.?

Drug interactions with systemic azoles and polyenes varies from mild inconveniences to life-threatening events (Table 75-6). Historically, the interaction between azoles and nonsedating H_1-selective antihistamines has been serious leading to QT prolongation and ventricular arrhythmias.[152] Although it is possible that concomitant use of corticosteroids could reduce antifungal efficacy, no clinical trial has addressed this important question. Corticosteroid serum concentrations can double with concomitant use of ketoconazole, leading to recommendations to decrease the steroid dose by 50% when ketoconazole is used. The interaction has been suggested between glucocorticoids and other azoles.[153] In addition, dexamethasone has been demonstrated to increase the clearance of caspofungin.

Other significant drug interactions with the azole antifungals involve their ability to inhibit the CYP450 enzyme system. All five azoles inhibit CYP3A4, but with varying potency: Ketoconazole is the most potent inhibitor, followed by itraconazole and voriconazole, then posaconazole and fluconazole. In addition to the interactions documented in Table 75-6, numerous other agents are substrates to cytochrome CYP3A4, but have yet to be evaluated. Because azole antifungals could increase serum concentrations with associated potential toxicity, caution should be exercised during concomitant use. Adding complexity to voriconazole's interactions include its propensity to inhibit CYP2C9 and CYP2C19, two isoenzymes exhibiting polymorphism, thus increasing concentrations of CYP2C9 or CYP2C19 substrates. Conversely, agents that either induce or inhibit the CYP450 system may decrease or increase, respectively, antifungal drug concentrations. Posaconazole is a substrate for p-glycoprotein efflux and is metabolized via UDP glucuronidation; therefore, inhibitors or inducers of these clearance pathways may affect posaconazole concentrations.[61]

Coccidioidomycosis

SEROLOGIC TESTS

CASE 75-7

QUESTION 1: F.W., a 32-year-old Filipina woman and a lifelong resident of the Central Valley in California, is admitted to the hospital with a third recurrence of coccidioidal meningitis. Approximately 4 years ago, she was treated with a total AmB dose of 2.2 g, which resulted in a good clinical response. Nine months later, she relapsed and received a second course of AmB to a total of 1.6 g. She did well during the next 18 months and was able to return to work as a secretary. Over the past 4 months, however, F.W. has had chronic headaches, has been unable to concentrate at work, and is reported by family members to have a very labile personality. A computed tomography (CT) scan of the brain reveals mild hydrocephalus. An opening pressure of 19 mm Hg (normal, 10 mm Hg) was documented at lumbar puncture. Analysis of the CSF showed:

110 WBC/μL (normal, 0 WBC/μL)
Glucose, 18 mg/dL (normal, 60% of serum glucose)
Protein, 190 mg/dL (normal, <50 mg/dL)

Complement fixation antibodies were positive in the CSF at a titer of 1:32. How should serologic tests for coccidioidomycosis be interpreted?

The most important serologic tests for fungal infections use complement fixation (CF), immunodiffusion, and EIA techniques. Tests for complement fixing antibodies (i.e., CF) to the dimorphic fungi (Table 75-1) are well established and various antigens have been used. Coccidioidin is the mycelial phase antigen for *Coccidioides immitis*. Of patients with coccidioidomycosis, 61% will have coccidioidin CF titers of at least 1:32 and 41% will have titers of 1:64. Rising titers are a bad prognostic sign, and falling titers indicate clinical improvement. Therefore, F.W.'s CSF CF titer of 1:32 is consistent with active coccidioidomycosis. Immunodiffusion testing for coccidioidomycosis using coccidioidin reveals that seropositive results appear 1 to 3 weeks after onset of primary infection in 75% of patients and this positivity usually disappears within 4 months if the infection resolves.[154] IgG-specific and IgM-specific EIA using a combination of antigens for *C. immitis* have been developed. These tests offer sensitivities of more than 92% and specificities of 98% for serum and CSF. EIA reactivity appears earlier than CF reactivity.[155,156]

ANTIFUNGAL CENTRAL NERVOUS SYSTEM PENETRATION

CASE 75-7, QUESTION 2: What is a pharmacokinetic explanation for the treatment failure of F.W.? How might this problem be overcome?

F.W. has received prolonged parenteral AmB administration and the CSF still contains fungal organisms. Treatment failures in this case may partly be owing to the limited penetration of AmB into the CSF.[101] Because AmB is highly bound to lipid (90%–95%), CSF concentrations achieved are only 2% to 4% of the serum concentration[101,151]; peritoneal, synovial, and pleural fluid concentrations are less than 50% of the serum concentrations (Table 75-5). Flucytosine is not significantly bound to protein and penetrates the CSF, vitreous, and peritoneal fluids; its volume of distribution approximates that of total body water.[157] Flucytosine concentration in the CSF is 74% of the serum concentration, resulting in its extensive use in treatment of CNS mycoses, particularly cryptococcal meningitis. Flucytosine, however, has no activity in coccidioidomycosis and, therefore, cannot be used in F.W.

The volume of distribution of fluconazole approaches that of total body water,[158] and concentrations of fluconazole in CSF are approximately 60% of simultaneous serum concentrations. Ketoconazole penetrates CSF poorly, because it is highly bound to plasma proteins (>80%) and to erythrocytes (15%). Itraconazole is similar to ketoconazole in that it is greater than 99% protein bound. Itraconazole concentrates intracellularly in host alveolar macrophages, which may account for its efficacy against some fungal CNS infection despite its inability to penetrate into the CSF.[159] Echinocandins also poorly (<5%) penetrate into the CSF.[160] Reliable data on terbinafine and posaconazole penetration are currently unavailable. Therefore, fluconazole might be an alternative to CNS instillation of AmB based upon pharmacokinetic considerations.[161]

Fluconazole, investigated at dosages of 400 mg/day, is useful in patients with coccidioidomycosis meningitis. Similar to amphotericin, relapse rates are high once fluconazole therapy is stopped.[154] Oral itraconazole 200 mg twice daily was not found to be superior to fluconazole in a controlled trial of nonmeningitis disease; however, a trend toward greater efficacy was observed, particularly in skeletal disease.[162]

INTRATHECAL AMPHOTERICIN

CASE 75-7, QUESTION 3: What adverse events might be observed with the intrathecal administration of an antifungal in F.W.?

Augmentation of systemic antifungal administration with intraventricular or intrathecal administration may improve the outcome for antifungals with poor penetration into the CSF.[162–167] Intrathecal AmB doses in adults normally range from 0.25 to 0.5 mg diluted in 5 mL of 5% glucose.[154,159] A few studies suggest that doses larger than 0.7 mg improve the cure rate and decrease relapse.[161] Cisternal or intraventricular administration is recommended as the routes of choice because of flow characteristics of CSF from the ventricles to the spinal cord.[162–164] When lumbar administration has been necessary, agents are administered in a hypertonic solution of 10% glucose and the patient is placed in a Trendelenburg position in an attempt to improve distribution of the drug to the basilar meninges and ventricles and reduce local toxicity. Voriconazole, caspofungin, and the lipid amphotericin formulations have been used but not evaluated in controlled trials.

Cisternal antifungal administration has been associated with headaches, nausea, vomiting, cranial nerve paresis, and cisternal hemorrhage caused by needle trauma.[163,164–166] An Ommaya reservoir often is used to facilitate intraventricular administration of AmB. Common complications of these devices include shunt occlusion, bacterial colonization or bacterial meningitis, parkinsonian symptoms, and seizures.[163–167] In the past, lumbar administration was used because it is simpler, but it often must be discontinued because of chemical arachnoiditis, headache, transient radiculitis, paresthesia, nerve pulses, difficulty voiding, impaired vision, vertigo, and tinnitus.[167] Acute toxic delirium, demyelinating peripheral neuropathy, and spinal cord injury have also been reported.[168–170] Regardless of the substantial and serious adverse effects, intraventricular administration may be effective in treating patients with meningitis who have severe disease or who are pharmacologic nonresponders.

Aspergillosis

EMPIRIC THERAPY (NEUTROPENIC HOST)

CASE 75-8

QUESTION 1: M.Z., an otherwise healthy 29-year-old man, presented for allogeneic stem cell transplantation 12 days ago. He has had no serious complications associated with his chloroquine-induced aplastic anemia during his 7-month wait for transplant. On transplant days −5 to −2, induction therapy was initiated with cyclophosphamide (50 mg/kg) and total body irradiation, and then bone marrow from his HLA-antigen–compatible brother was infused on day 0. The onset of neutropenia was noted on day 3 and the WBC count was 50 cells/μL. M.Z. has complained only of stomatitis and diarrhea before day 5. On that morning, he was complaining of fever, chest pain, and headache. On physical examination, his temperature was 37°C. Empiric anti-infectives were added, but by day 8 he was not clinically improving. What therapeutic options should be considered for this patient?

Empiric antifungal therapy in a neutropenic host should be initiated when a patient is febrile for more than 96 hours on appropriate anti-infectives. Routine empiric therapy for a patient without evidence of deep-seated fungal infection historically has been AmB 0.3 to 0.6 mg/kg/day or fluconazole 200 to 400 mg/day until the absolute neutrophil count is greater than 500 cells/μL.[171] Therapy results in resolution of signs and symptoms in up to 64% of patients.

Because mold infections are of concern in this neutropenic patient population, drug therapy that is highly active against these organisms should be considered. Assessments of newer antifungals using a composite end-point for success have failed to show superiority over AmB formulations. A large, well-controlled, double-blind comparison of AmB 0.6 mg/kg/day was compared with liposomal AmB 3.0 mg/kg/day in febrile neutropenic patients. Patients who were febrile more than 96 hours and neutropenic (<500 cells/μL) experienced equal survival and clinical success of approximately 50% for both agents.[172] Success rates have been similar with other agents, including liposomal AmB (34%), caspofungin (34%),[173] voriconazole, or itraconazole.[174,175] It is important to remember that fever is a late and insensitive measure of infection. Prevention of breakthrough invasive fungal infection may be the most important indicator of an agent's efficacy. Using this measure comparing the various trials, voriconazole appears to be the most effective agent: voriconazole versus liposomal AmB (1.9% vs. 5%), AmB versus liposomal AmB (3.2% vs. 7.8%).[172,175] Selection of any of these expensive, however less toxic, agents should be weighed against the morbidity and mortality associated with invasive fungal disease.

CASE 75-8, QUESTION 2: What is the role of lipid formulations of AmB?

A motivation for developing these formulations was the observation that serum triglycerides and cholesterol decrease adverse drug reactions and may improve efficacy.[126,176] The advantage of the formulations (Table 75-7) is clear in the treatment of diseases such as aspergillosis, which require long-term therapy that can result in patient intolerance to generic AmB.[123] Multiple uncontrolled or retrospective trials have observed that all four past and current lipid formulations of AmB are less nephrotoxic and potentially more effective than AmB deoxycholate. A single large randomized, double-blind trial and a historical controlled trial support these observations.[161,177]

Few well-controlled prospective comparative trials exist to guide the decision-making process for fungal infections that require a shorter course of therapy. In addition to the data presented for candidemia (Case 75-3, Question 10), liposomal and lipid complex AmB have been evaluated for treatment of cryptococcal meningitis and histoplasmosis in patients infected with HIV.[148,178,179] Each lipid agent is safer and as or more effective than AmB deoxycholate. Considering the high acquisition cost and relatively low rates of toxicity with short course therapy, generic AmB could be selected over the lipid formulation unless a patient is clearly intolerant, requires extended therapy, or experiences a treatment failure. Longer courses, however, should use lipid-based products.

Of particular interest are the ongoing studies and case reports in which Intralipid 10% to 20% combined with AmB (1–2 mg/mL) is administered at a dosage of 1 mg/kg/day. This practice cannot be recommended until a prospective, randomized, controlled trial documents efficacy and reduced toxicity of these lipid emulsion–AmB formulations as compared with AmB alone. Current concerns are (a) the inability to formulate a pharmaceutically stable product,[180] (b) difficulty assessing whether inline filtering is required, and (c) the delivery of excessive calories.[181]

TREATMENT OF ASPERGILLOSIS

CASE 75-8, QUESTION 3: Chest auscultation on day 8 reveals right-sided rales with a friction rub. Chest radiograph shows a nodular infiltrate in the right middle lobe. Fiberoptic bronchoscopy identified eroded bronchioles with necrotic tissue, and methenamine silver nitrate stain of a biopsy sample revealed fragmented, closely septated hyphal bodies branched at 45-degree angles. The samples were sent to microbiology for cultures. All previous blood and sputum cultures have been negative, except that *Aspergillus niger* growing from sputum before admission was classified as a "contaminant." The diagnosis at this time is probable aspergillosis. What treatment steps should be taken?

Drug therapy should be approached by first determining whether the infection is likely to be invasive or noninvasive disease (Fig. 75-5). Most patients inhale *Aspergillus* species and never become symptomatic or exhibit only mild hypersensitivity pneumonitis. Invasive infections are more likely to occur in immunocompromised patients, especially those with prolonged neutropenia associated with stem cell transplantation. Allogeneic hematopoietic stem cell transplantation (HSCT) has a much greater infection rate and mortality compared with autologous HSCT.[182] A classic observation reported by radiology is a "halo" sign or a "crescent" sign identified on CT, highly suggestive of this infection. Additionally, an ELISA for a surface protein, galactomannan, has been reported to have high sensitivity in the diagnosis of invasive disease.[183] Positive serum results (optical density index >1.5) can be obtained as early as 17 days before clinical symptoms or radiologic signs. False-positive test findings have been associated with *Bifidobacterium* sp. colonization in pediatric gastrointestinal tracts other eukaryotic infections (i.e. *Trichosporon, Fusarium, Saccharomyces, Hisplasma,* or *Acremonium*), and administration of piperacillin-tazobactam or calcium gluconate, which is of concern for clinicians using this test for

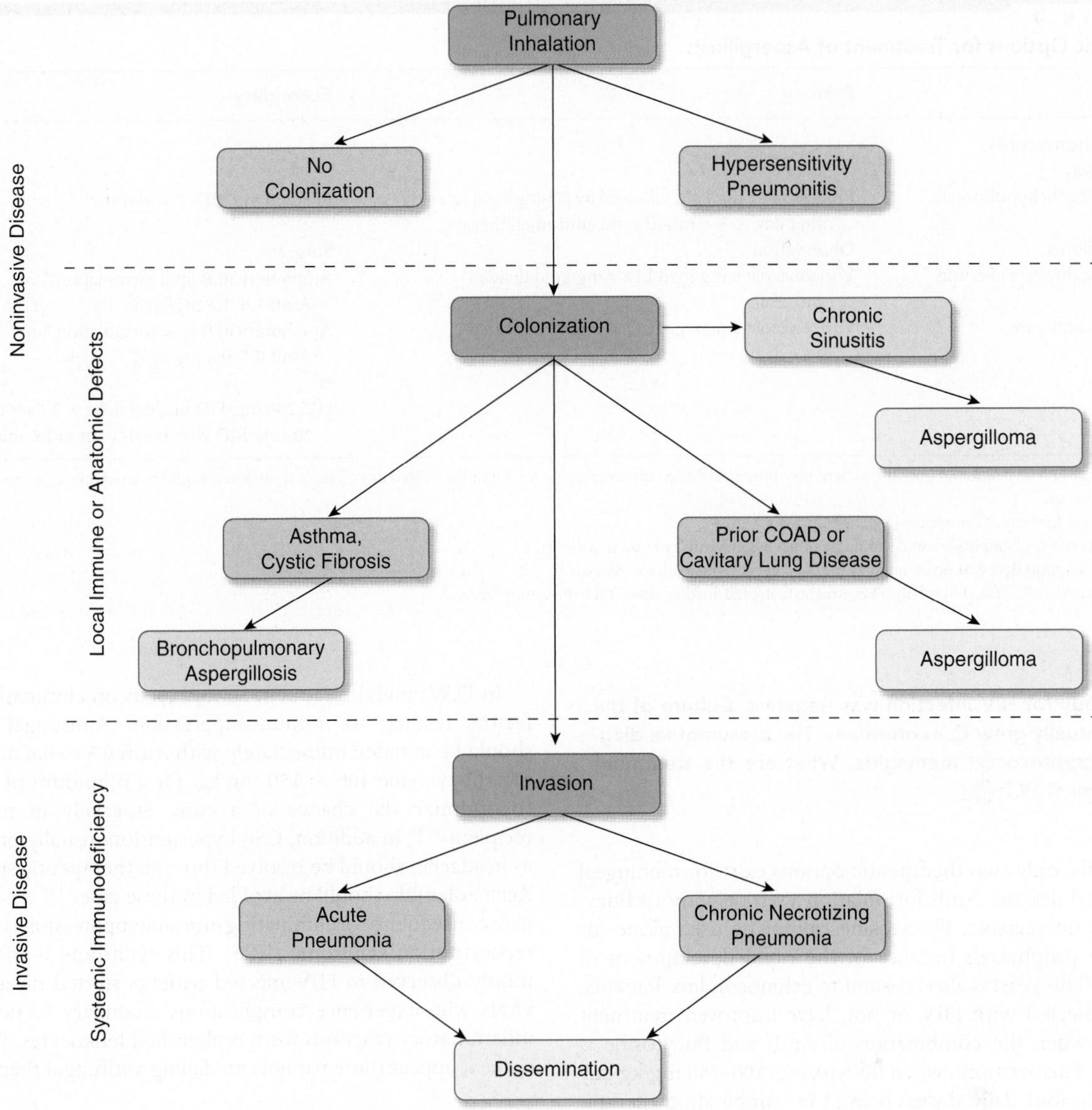

FIGURE 75-5 Classification of aspergillosis infections. COAD, chronic obstructive airway disease.

screening in areas with low case rates. This test is an excellent prognostic indicator for therapeutic outcome in confirmed cases or as a screen in areas with high case rates. The subjective and objective data in this case clearly represent invasive symptomatic disease necessitating aggressive treatment.

Aspergillosis is a model for invasive mold infections that have a propensity to invade blood vessels and tissue. Antimycotic pharmacotherapy should be initiated rapidly and aggressively (Table 75-9) in conjunction with removal or reversal of immunosuppression if possible. Definite or probable invasive aspergillosis should be treated with voriconazole or high-dose AmB formulation (liposomal AmB 3–5 mg/kd/day),[185] or combination therapy.[183] Combination of voriconazole and caspofungin for salvage therapy has been associated with reduced mortality when compared with voriconazole alone.[186] The optimal dose of liposomal AmB is still not known.[187] Despite early and intensive therapy, mortality from invasive aspergillosis can be greater than 50%.[188] In unresponsive patients, an AmB formulation in combination therapy with an echinocandin, flucytosine, rifampin, or itraconazole; or an echinocandin with voriconazole should be considered.[183,185,189,190] Flushing, rash, facial swelling, and pruritis can occur with caspofungin administration and is likely histamine-mediated. Less serious, but more frequent, adverse effects reported in patients receiving caspofungin include fever, elevations in serum transaminases, serum alkaline phosphatase, or both, and headache.[64]

Patients with mild to moderate *Aspergillus* should be treated with voriconazole.[174] Clinical and microbiologic cure rates of 50% to 71% have been reported for voriconazole or itraconazole-treated patients with invasive aspergillosis. Further studies are necessary to define the optimal dose, duration, and route of itraconazole in invasive forms of aspergillosis.

Cryptococcosis

CASE 75-9

QUESTION 1: D.W., a 48-year-old man, was hospitalized with fever and severe headache. His history was significant for Hodgkin lymphoma, which is in remission. Lumbar puncture revealed the following:

Opening pressure of 280 mm Hg (normal, 10 mm Hg)
WBC count, 50 leukocytes/μL (normal, 0 leukocytes/μL)
Positive India ink preparation
Cryptococcal antigen titer, 1:4,096

TABLE 75-9
Therapeutic Options for Treatment of Aspergillosis

Disease	Primary	Secondary
Hyalohyphomycetes		
Aspergillosis		
Allergic bronchopulmonary	Prednisone 1 mg/kg/d followed by 0.5 mg/kg/d or every other day × 3–6 months; no antifungal therapy	ITZ 200 mg BID × 4 months[a]
Aspergilloma	Observation	Surgery[b]
Systemic (invasive) Serious	Voriconazole 6 mg/kg/d LD, 4 mg/kg/d divided twice daily	Amphotericin B lipid formulation,[d] or AmB 1.0–1.5 mg/kg/d[c]
Mild or moderate	Voriconazole 6 mg/kg/d LD, 4 mg/kg/d divided twice daily	Amphotericin B lipid formulation,[d] or AmB 0.5–0.6 mg/kg/d[c] or ITZ 200 mg TID loading dose × 3 days then 200 mg BID with meals (6 months, minimum)

[a] Treatment should be continued until the patient is symptom-free and culture-negative for 3 months. Noted durations or total doses should be used only as a compass to help guide therapy.
[b] Indicated only for serious symptoms (e.g., hemoptysis).
[c] Lipid formulations of amphotericin B should be utilized preferentially in these patients.
[d] Liposomal amphotericin B at doses up to 15 mg/kg/d appear safe in phase I/II trials.[184]
AmB, amphotericin B; BID, twice daily; ITZ, itraconazole; LD, loading dose; TID, three times daily.

Serology for HIV infection was negative. Culture of the CSF eventually grew *C. neoformans*. The presumptive diagnosis is cryptococcal meningitis. What are the treatment options for D.W.?

Currently, only two therapeutic options exist for meningeal cryptococcal disease: AmB formulation with or without flucytosine and fluconazole. Flucytosine cannot be used alone for therapy or prophylaxis because of the rapid development of resistance. This yeast is also resistant to echinocondins. Patients, whether infected with HIV or not, have improved treatment outcomes when the combination of AmB and flucytosine is used.[191,192] Furthermore, when flucytosine (100–150 mg/kg/day divided into four daily doses) is used in combination therapy, the dose of AmB may be reduced to 0.3 to 0.6 mg/kg/day, which decreases the frequency of dose-related AmB toxicity. In patients who cannot be treated with flucytosine, the dosage of AmB must be increased to more than 0.6 mg/kg/day. AmB 1 mg/kg/day is more rapidly fungicidal than 0.7 mg/kg/day when used with 5FC. Liposomal AmB 3 mg/kg/day can and probably should be used instead of the non-lipid formulations in this disease.[193]

Fluconazole is an alternative to AmB in patients infected with HIV with cryptococcal meningitis. It is important to be mindful of the following caveats, however: Sterilization of the CSF occurs more rapidly and mortality is lower during the first 2 weeks of therapy in patients treated with AmB as compared with fluconazole.[176,194] Early mortality was especially high in fluconazole-treated patients who presented with altered mental status.[191,194,195] Thus, initial therapy of cryptococcal meningitis in patients with mental status changes should be initiated with AmB for at least 2 weeks or until the patient has stabilized clinically. At this point, fluconazole may be substituted at an initial dosage of 400 mg/day for up to 10 weeks. In HIV-infected patients, the dosage of fluconazole maybe reduced to a maintenance dosage of 200 mg/day that may need to be continued for life. Fluconazole 400 mg/day can be used in all other patients. Another alternative may include liposomal AmB 4 mg/kg/day for 21 days.[179] Until larger clinical studies have been completed, however, this regimen cannot be recommended over generic AmB (see Chapter 74, Opportunistic Infections in HIV-Infected Patients).[193]

In D.W., initial treatment should focus on elimination of all factors leading to immunosuppression. Antifungal therapy should be initiated immediately with AmB 0.3 to 0.6 mg/kg/day plus flucytosine 100 to 150 mg/kg/ for a minimum of 6 weeks to optimize the chance of a cure, especially in transplant recipients.[195] In addition, CSF hypertension, usually presenting as headache, should be resolved through therapeutic spinal tap. Acetazolamide should be avoided in these cases.[196] An unfortunate consequence of eliminating immune suppression is immune reconstitution syndrome (IRIS). This syndrome is most commonly observed in HIV-infected patients started on antiretrovirals who experience complications secondary to new onset inflammatory reactions from replenished leukocytes. IRIS may make it appear these patients are failing antifungal therapy.

CASE 75-9, QUESTION 2: What parameters should be monitored while D.W. is treated with flucytosine?

The most common side effect of flucytosine is GI distress (e.g., nausea, vomiting, diarrhea). Although flucytosine is not metabolized per se by mammalian cells, gut flora may be responsible for metabolism of flucytosine to fluorouracil. This toxic metabolite has been speculated to account, in part, for the GI distress and bone marrow toxicity associated with flucytosine therapy.[197] Other flucytosine adverse effects include leukopenia, thrombocytopenia, and hepatotoxicity. Dose-dependent bone marrow suppression, which can be fatal, generally is seen in patients whose serum concentration of flucytosine is greater than 100 mcg/mL. Thus, it is important to monitor blood concentrations and maintain concentrations below this level.[192,195] If assays for flucytosine serum concentrations are unavailable, signs and symptoms of bone marrow suppression or worsening renal function should result in a dosage reduction or discontinuation of the drug. Flucytosine is eliminated by glomerular filtration, with 80% to 95% of the dose excreted unchanged in the urine. Renal excretion of flucytosine is directly related to creatinine clearance, and dosages should be adjusted based on creatinine clearance to prevent accumulation to toxic concentrations in patients with renal impairment.[114] Patients with creatinine clearances of 10 to 40 mL/min should have the dosage of flucytosine reduced by 50% (usual dose, 37.5 mg/kg every 12 hours). For patients with creatinine clearance less than 10 mL/min, dosing should be initiated at 37.5 mg/kg/day, with frequent monitoring of flucytosine serum concentrations. Dosage adjustment and close monitoring also are required for patients receiving hemodialysis and it is recommended that the dose be given postdialysis.

CASE 75-9, QUESTION 3: When is combination antifungal therapy indicated?

In vitro results of antifungal combinations against many common mycotic pathogens have been variable. These incomplete and inconsistent findings have been attributed to variable incubation times, variable concentrations of antifungal agents, and the sequence of antifungal addition.[196] As a result, clinical decisions about combination therapy should be based on patient-specific in vivo evaluations. Because of the limited clinical data, combination antifungal therapy should be initiated cautiously. Except for the treatment of cryptococcal meningitis and disseminated aspergillosis, combination therapy should be reserved for cases of treatment failure (disseminated candidiasis) with no other established pharmacologic options for therapy or mold infections with high mortality rates.

KEY REFERENCES AND WEBSITES

A full list of references for this chapter can be found at **http://thepoint.lww.com/AT10e.** Below are the key references for this chapter, with the corresponding reference number in this chapter found in parentheses after the reference.

Key References

Herbrecht R et al. Voriconazole versus amphotericin B for primary therapy of invasive aspergillosis. *N Engl J Med*. 2002;347:408. (188)

Johnson PC et al. Safety and efficacy of liposomal amphotericin B compared with conventional amphotericin B for induction therapy of histoplasmosis in patients with AIDS. *Ann Intern Med*. 2002;137:105. (148)

Morrell M et al. Delaying the empiric treatment of candida bloodstream infection until positive blood culture results are obtained: A potential risk factor for hospital mortality. *Antimicrob Agents Chemother*. 2005;49:3640. (86)

Odom RB et al. A multicenter, placebo-controlled, double-blind study of intermittent therapy with itraconazole for the treatment of onychomycosis of the fingernail. *J Am Acad Dermatol*. 1997;36:231. (33)

Pappas PG, et al. Clinical practice guidelines for the management of candidiasis: 2009 update by the Infectious Diseases Society of America. *Clin Infect Dis*. 2009;48(5):503. (72)

Patel M et al. Initial management of candidemia at an academic medical center: evaluation of the IDSA guidelines. *Diagn Microbiol Infect Dis*. 2005;52:26. (85)

Pelz RK et al. Double-blind placebo-controlled trial of fluconazole to prevent candidal infections in critically ill surgical patients. *Ann Surg*. 2001;233:542. (127)

Perfect JR et al. Clinical practice guidelines for the management of cryptococcal disease: 2010 update by the Infectious Diseases Society of America. *Clin Infect Dis*. 2010;50(3):291. (193)

Rex JH et al. Antifungal susceptibility testing: practical aspects and current challenges. *Clin Microbiol Rev*. 2001;14:643. (20)

Shepard JR et al. Multicenter evaluation of the *Candida albicans/Candida glabrata* peptide nucleic acid fluorescent in situ hybridization method for simultaneous dual-color identification of *C. albicans* and *C. glabrata* directly from blood culture bottles. *J Clin Microbiol*. 2008;46:50. (77)

Stevens DA et al. Practice guidelines for diseases caused by *Aspergillus*. Infectious Diseases Society of America. *Clin Infect Dis*. 2000;30:696. (190)

76 Viral Infections

Milap C. Nahata, Neeta Bahal O'Mara, and Sandra Benavides

CORE PRINCIPLES

		CHAPTER CASES
1	Herpes simplex virus (HSV) encephalitis is associated with significant morbidity and mortality. Intravenous acyclovir for a 21-day period is the therapy of choice.	Case 76-1 (Questions 2, 4)
2	Neonatal herpes can present with mucocutaneous, ocular infection, as well as encephalitis and disseminated HSV infection. Transmission can be acquired during the first trimester of pregnancy or during vaginal delivery in an infected mother.	Case 76-2 (Questions 1, 2)
3	Herpes labialis is the most common oral-facial HSV infection and is usually self-limiting in an immunocompetent host. Patients who are immunocompromised must be treated with antiviral therapy, primarily oral or intravenous acyclovir or oral valacyclovir.	Case 76-3 (Question 1), Case 76-4 (Question 1)
4	Individuals with progressive varicella, those with extracutaneous complications, or those at high risk for developing complications to varicella infection benefit from antiviral therapy.	Case 76-7 (Question 1), Case 76-8 (Question 1)
5	The goal of pharmacotherapy treatment of herpes zoster is to reduce pain and duration of rash, and to prevent the development of postherpetic neuralgia (PHN). These outcomes can be accomplished with the use of oral acyclovir, famciclovir, or valacyclovir. For the treatment of PHN, topical capsaicin gels, creams and patches, topical lidocaine patches, and oral gabapentin and pregabalin are efficacious.	Case 76-9 (Questions 1, 3)
6	Neuraminidase inhibitors, such as zanamivir and oseltamivir, are indicated for the treatment of influenza if used within 48 hours after the onset of symptoms. Zanamivir is administered intranasally, with bronchospasm the most common adverse drug reaction. Oseltamivir is administered orally, with nausea, vomiting, and headache as common side effects.	Case 76-11 (Question 2)
7	Influenza vaccination is the most effective mechanism to prevent the flu. However, certain high-risk populations may require additional prophylaxis with oseltamivir or zanamivir.	Case 76-12 (Question 2)
8	Infants at high risk for severe disease caused by respiratory syncytial virus (RSV) should receive monthly intramuscular injections of palivizumab for a total of five doses during RSV season.	Case 76-14 (Questions 1, 2)
9	Hantavirus pulmonary syndrome, caused by the *Hantavirus*, is characterized by fever, myalgia, headache, and cough and can rapidly progress to acute respiratory distress syndrome (ARDS). Therapy is aimed at supportive care, although ribavirin has been used with some success.	Case 76-15 (Questions 1, 2)
10	West Nile virus can cause disease ranging from a febrile infection to encephalitis. Treatment is supportive; however, ribavirin and interferon-α-2b have been tried in this patient population. Clinical trials evaluating the use of immunoglobulin, monoclonal antibodies, and vaccines are ongoing.	Case 76-16 (Questions 1, 2)

continued

CHAPTER CASES

11 Severe acute respiratory distress syndrome (SARS) coronavirus (SARS-CoV) is associated with severe illness including fever, chills, rigor, myalgia, headache, diarrhea, sore throat, and rhinorrhea progressing to ARDS. SARS has a 10% case fatality rate with increased age associated with increased mortality. No cases have been reported in the world since 2004.	**Case 76-17 (Question 1)**
12 The common cold is the most prevalent viral infection. Numerous pathogens can cause this respiratory infection, including rhinovirus, coronavirus, parainfluenza, RSV, adenovirus, and enterovirus. There are currently no products that have been conclusively shown to prevent or treat the common cold.	**Case 76-18 (Question 1)**

Viral infections are common causes of human disease. An estimated 60% of illnesses in developed countries result from viruses, compared with only 15% from bacteria. These include the common cold, chickenpox, measles, mumps, influenza, bronchitis, gastroenteritis, hepatitis, poliomyelitis, rabies, and numerous diseases caused by the herpesvirus. Upper respiratory tract infections, such as the common cold or influenza, are among the most common reasons for visits to a health care professional.[1] Although most of these patients have a self-limiting illness, certain viral infections, such as influenza, can cause significant mortality, particularly in the elderly. During the worldwide Spanish influenza epidemic of 1918 to 1920, 20 to 100 million people died.[2] Although influenza vaccines reduce the morbidity and mortality associated with this disease, many other potentially severe viral infections, including herpes encephalitis and neonatal herpes, have no vaccine.

Substantial progress has been made in antiviral chemotherapy as a result of advances in molecular virology and genetic engineering. Antiviral agents can be designed to inhibit functions specific to viruses, which maximizes their therapeutic benefits and minimizes adverse effects.

Current technology also permits rapid diagnosis of viral diseases. It is now possible to make a specific diagnosis of several viral illnesses within hours to a few days; previously, a specific diagnosis often took days to months. These improved diagnostics have facilitated rapid selection of an appropriate antiviral drug.

This chapter describes the etiology, pathogenesis, and treatment of common viral infections. Specific case presentations illustrate the optimal use of antiviral drugs in patients with viral infections.

HERPES SIMPLEX VIRUS INFECTIONS

Herpes viruses are responsible for a wide spectrum of disease including acute life-threatening illness (herpes encephalitis and neonatal herpes), as well as more chronic, recurrent infection (genital herpes). Antivirals significantly decrease the morbidity and mortality in most of these infections.[3]

Herpes Encephalitis

Herpes simplex virus (HSV) encephalitis is the most common sporadic viral infection of the central nervous system (CNS). HSV encephalitis occurs in up to 500,000 people yearly, although this may be an underestimate owing to difficulties in diagnosis. It typically occurs in two populations, those 6 months to 20 years of age and those older than 50 years, and is characterized by the acute onset of fever, headache, decreased consciousness, and seizures. Any child with fever and altered behavior should be evaluated for HSV encephalitis. Without treatment, mortality approaches 70% and some morbidity takes place in 97% of survivors. Only 2.5% of patients recover sufficiently to lead normal lives.[3]

Herpes simplex virus type 1 (HSV-1) is the etiologic agent in most patients with herpes encephalitis, but herpes simplex virus type 2 (HSV-2) is more common in newborns. The infection may be localized to the brain or involve cutaneous and mucous membranes. Although any area of the brain can be involved, the orbital region of the frontal lobes and the temporal lobes are most often affected.

ONLINE CONTENT

For a photo of a herpes simplex lesion and an MR scan of a patient with encephalitis, go to http://thepoint.lww.com/AT10e.

Herpes encephalitis is often difficult to diagnose. A computed tomography (CT) scan is usually indicated to rule out other conditions, such as brain abscess or other space-occupying lesions. The CT or radionuclide scans may be unremarkable early in the course of the disease.

Cerebrospinal fluid (CSF) examination usually reveals pleocytosis (predominately lymphocytes) with 50 to 2,000 white blood cells (WBCs)/μL. Polymorphonuclear leukocytosis and red blood cells (RBCs) may also be seen. Many patients have an elevated protein level in the CSF (median, 80 mg/dL). The presence of antibody to HSV-1 is useful in making the diagnosis.

The electroencephalogram (EEG) is the most sensitive but least specific test. There are usually CT or brain scan abnormalities, but these may take a day or two longer to appear. The EEG, CT, and brain scan findings compatible with HSV encephalitis can be mimicked by other conditions, and a brain biopsy is required to clearly establish the diagnosis. Rapid diagnosis of herpes encephalitis by a polymerase chain reaction (PCR) assay of HSV DNA in the CSF is available at most medical centers. This is a highly sensitive, specific, and rapid method for diagnosing herpes encephalitis.[4]

CLINICAL PRESENTATION

CASE 76-1

QUESTION 1: R.F., a 7-year-old boy weighing 20 kg, was seen in the emergency department (ED) after a seizure. For the previous 3 days, R.F. had decreased appetite, headache, and fever (101°–102°F), and was lethargic and disoriented. His leukocyte count was 13,000/μL (SI units, 13×10^6/L) with a shift to the left. Ceftriaxone (50 mg/kg intravenously [IV] every 12 hours) and dexamethasone (0.15 mg/kg IV every 6 hours) were initiated for presumed bacterial meningitis. Phenobarbital (5 mg/kg IV every 24 hours) was given for seizure control. The CSF was normal, and no bacteria

could be cultured. Acyclovir 20 mg/kg IV every 8 hours was started immediately. A PCR analysis of HSV-1 was positive. What findings in R.F. are consistent with the diagnosis of herpes encephalitis?

Fever, headache, lethargy, and disorientation are common features of herpes encephalitis. As illustrated by R.F., the CSF examination can be normal in some patients. A negative CSF culture suggests the absence of a bacterial infection.[5] However, the positive HSV-1 DNA by PCR analysis confirms the diagnosis of herpes encephalitis.

TREATMENT: ACYCLOVIR

CASE 76-1, QUESTION 2: What is the treatment of choice for R.F.'s herpes encephalitis?

Two studies comparing acyclovir and vidarabine have demonstrated that IV acyclovir (10 mg/kg every 8 hours for 10 days) is the treatment of choice in patients with herpes encephalitis.[6,7] The 12-month all-cause mortality was 25% in the acyclovir-treated group and 59% in the vidarabine-treated group. Notably, nearly one-third of the acyclovir-treated patients returned to normal life, compared with only 12% of those treated with vidarabine.[8] Vidarabine is no longer marketed in the United States.

Acyclovir-resistant herpes is not an important consideration in the management of herpes encephalitis in most patients. However, resistant herpes is important in acquired immunodeficiency syndrome (AIDS) or other immunocompromised patients who receive multiple courses of acyclovir (see Chapter 72, Prevention and Treatment of Infections in Neutropenic Cancer Patients). Foscarnet and cidofovir have been successfully used in immunocompromised patients with acyclovir-resistant HSV.[9–12]

Acyclovir is the treatment of choice for R.F. because it has been shown to decrease morbidity in patients with herpes encephalitis. Acyclovir should be started as soon as HSV encephalitis is suspected because early initiation of therapy is associated with improved outcome. Therapy should be continued for at least 21 days.[13]

The role of corticosteroids in the treatment of herpes encephalitis is not well defined. One small, nonrandomized trial found that corticosteroid therapy, in combination with IV acyclovir, was associated with an improved outcome.[14] However, prospective, randomized trials are needed before routine use of corticosteroids can be recommended.[15]

ADVERSE EFFECTS

CASE 76-1, QUESTION 3: What adverse effects can occur with IV acyclovir therapy in R.F.? How should these be monitored, and how can they be minimized?

Acyclovir is a relatively safe drug, but renal toxicity associated with IV acyclovir is well described (Table 76-1). Blood urea nitrogen (BUN) and serum creatinine (SCr) levels can increase in 5% to 10% of patients; however, these changes are generally reversible. Acyclovir is relatively insoluble: maximal urine solubility at 37°C is 1.3 mg/mL. Consequently, the mechanism of acyclovir-associated renal disease is a transient crystal nephropathy, which may occur at high acyclovir concentrations.[8]

Other common adverse effects include gastrointestinal (GI) complaints such as nausea and vomiting and, less commonly, neurologic disturbances, including lethargy, tremors, confusion, hallucinations, and seizures.[8,16] Neurotoxicity appears to be more common in patients with impaired renal function and is reversible. Finally, IV acyclovir can cause phlebitis and pain at the injection site.[8] This complication can be minimized by

TABLE 76-1
Adverse Effects of US Food and Drug Administration-Indicated Drugs for Various Viral Infections

Drug	Adverse Effects
Acyclovir	Local irritation, phlebitis (9%); increased SCr, BUN (5%–10%); nausea, vomiting (7%); itching, rash (2%); increased liver transaminases (1%–2%); CNS toxicity (1%), hematologic abnormalities (<1%)
Amantadine	Nausea, dizziness (lightheadedness), insomnia (5%–10%); depression, anxiety, irritability, hallucination, confusion, dry mouth; constipation, ataxia, headache, peripheral edema, orthostatic hypotension (1%–5%); suicide ideation or attempt (<1%)
Cidofovir	Nephrotoxicity (53%); neutropenia (34%); rash (30%); headache (27%); alopecia (25%); anemia (20%); abdominal pain (17%); fever (15%); infection (12%); ocular hypotonia (12%); nausea, vomiting (8%); asthenia (7%); diarrhea (7%)
Famciclovir	Headache (6%–9%); nausea (4%–5%); diarrhea (1%–2%)
Foscarnet	Fever, nausea, vomiting (47%); renal dysfunction (33%); anemia (9%–33%); diarrhea (30%); headache (26%); electrolyte abnormalities (6%–15%); bone marrow suppression (10%); seizure (10%); anorexia (5%); abdominal pain (5%); mental status changes (5%); paresthesia, peripheral neuropathy (5%); cough, dyspnea (5%); rash (5%); first-degree AV block, ECG changes (1%–5%)
Ganciclovir	Increased SCr (35%–69%); anemia (15%–25%); neutropenia, pancytopenia, thrombocytopenia (5%–8%); abdominal pain, anorexia (15%); diarrhea (44%); nausea, vomiting (13%); retinal detachment, vitreous hemorrhage, cataracts, corneal opacification (6%–15%); neuropathy; rash
Oseltamivir	Nausea, vomiting (9%–15%); diarrhea (3%); abdominal pain (2%); dizziness, vertigo, insomnia (1%); self-injury and psychosis
Ribavirin	Worsening of respiratory status, bacterial pneumonia, pneumothorax, apnea, ventilator dependence; cardiac arrest, hypotension; rash; conjunctivitis
Rimantadine	CNS (insomnia, dizziness, headache, nervousness, fatigue); GI (nausea, vomiting, anorexia, dry mouth, abdominal pain) (1%–3%)
Trifluridine	Burning or stinging on instillation (4.6%); palpebral edema (2.8%); keratopathy; hypersensitivity reaction; stromal edema; hyperemia; increased intraocular pressure
Valacyclovir	Headache (14%); nausea (15%); vomiting (6%); dizziness (3%); abdominal pain (3%)
Valganciclovir	Neutropenia (27%); thrombocytopenia (6%); diarrhea (41%); nausea, vomiting (21%–30%); abdominal pain (15%); increased SCr (3%); insomnia (16%); peripheral neuropathy (9%); paresthesias (8%); ataxia, dizziness, seizures, psychosis, hallucinations, confusion, drowsiness (<5%); retinal detachment (15% during treatment of CMV retinitis); hypersensitivity
Zanamivir	Bronchospasm; decline in respiratory function, especially if underlying respiratory disease; nasal or throat irritation or congestion (2%); headache (2%); cough (2%); diarrhea (3%); nausea, vomiting (1%–3%)

AV, atrioventricular; BUN, blood urea nitrogen; CMV, cytomegalovirus; CNS, central nervous system; ECG, electrocardiogram; GI, gastrointestinal; SCr, serum creatinine.

administering acyclovir at a concentration of 5 mg/mL (maximum, 7 mg/mL).[16]

Renal function tests, including BUN, SCr, and urine output, should be monitored. To minimize the risk of acyclovir nephrotoxicity, R.F. should be well hydrated, and each acyclovir dose should be infused for 1 hour. In addition, the IV infusion site should be inspected for inflammation and pain, and R.F. should be asked about pain at the infusion site.

CONVERSION TO ORAL THERAPY

CASE 76-1, QUESTION 4: After 7 days of IV acyclovir, R.F. is alert, responsive, actively moving about, and eating a normal diet. The intern suggests switching him to oral acyclovir and discontinuing IV therapy. Why is this not appropriate?

Oral acyclovir therapy is inappropriate for R.F. On the basis of studies in adults, the absorption of acyclovir after oral administration is variable, slow, and incomplete. The relative bioavailability (F) of acyclovir is low ($F = 0.15–0.30$) and decreases with increasing doses.[17] The mean peak plasma concentration has ranged from only 0.83 to 1.61 mcg/mL after multiple acyclovir doses of 200 to 800 mg.[17] Thus, with only approximately 50% of acyclovir penetrating the blood–brain barrier, the concentrations of acyclovir in the CSF may be inadequate for R.F. There is only very limited information regarding the use of oral valacyclovir for therapy.[18] Therefore, therapy with IV acyclovir should be continued to complete a 21-day course (Table 76-2).

Neonatal Herpes

Most neonates acquire herpes from the infected genital secretions of the mother at delivery.[19] Most cases are caused by HSV-2 virus. The incidence ranges from 1 in 3,000 to 5,000 deliveries per year in the United States. The infection can present in one of three forms: localized to the skin, eye, and mouth (SEM) (45%); encephalitis (30%); or disseminated disease (25%). The effects of neonatal herpes can be devastating, and severe disabilities persist in many afflicted children.[19] With currently available antivirals, the mortality has ranged from 4% in those with CNS involvement to 29% in those with other disseminated disease.[19] Neonatal HSV-1 infections may also be acquired after birth through contact with family members with symptomatic or asymptomatic oral-labial HSV-1 infection or from nosocomial transmission. When the virus is transmitted from the mother, clinical evidence of infection in the neonate usually is present 5 to 17 days after birth. Although skin vesicles are the hallmark of infection, at least one-third to one-half of neonates never have skin lesions.[20] In 70% of patients, the disease may progress from isolated skin lesions to involve other organs, including the lungs, liver, spleen, CNS, and eyes.

Diagnosis can be made by direct fluorescent antibody examination of epithelial cells from the infant or the mother. Examination of the base of a vesicular lesion may show giant cells and intranuclear inclusions, which are characteristic of HSV infections. Serologic test results can make a diagnosis of neonatal herpes.

RISK FACTORS

CASE 76-2

QUESTION 1: S.P., an 18-year-old woman, was admitted to labor and delivery with premature rupture of the membranes. Four hours later, S.P. vaginally delivered a 2.5-kg baby boy, R.P., who had an estimated gestational age of 33 weeks. Twenty-four hours after delivery, S.P. reported the onset of vesicles in the genital area; she had a history of previous episodes of genital herpes. The last infection was during her first trimester of pregnancy. Is R.P. at risk of developing herpes infection?

R.P. is at risk of acquiring herpes infection because the mother had genital herpes during the first trimester and because he was delivered vaginally rather than by cesarean section.[21] The risk of a newborn acquiring the disease from an infected mother with primary disease is about 35%; that from a mother who has reactivation of disease is 3%.

TREATMENT: ACYCLOVIR

CASE 76-2, QUESTION 2: Ten days after birth, R.P. exhibited poor feeding patterns, irritability, and respiratory distress. Three days later, skin lesions appeared. How should R.P. be treated?

R.P. is manifesting signs of HSV infection and should be treated with antiviral therapy (Table 76-2). The drug of choice for neonatal herpes simplex virus infections is IV acyclovir.[19,20] Vidarabine was the first antiviral agent used in the treatment of neonatal HSV. Because of the drastic reduction in morbidity, it became the standard of therapy to which other antiviral agents were compared. In clinical trials comparing vidarabine with acyclovir, acyclovir was shown to be as effective as vidarabine in infants with SEM involvement, encephalitis, and disseminated HSV infection.[22] Although both agents were equally effective, acyclovir was safer and easier to administer, making it the standard of care for neonatal HSV.

ACYLOVIR ADMINISTRATION

CASE 76-2, QUESTION 3: What dosage of acyclovir should R.P. receive?

Although an IV dosage of 30 mg/kg given in three divided doses has been shown to be effective in the treatment of neonatal herpes, the use of 60 mg/kg is superior in decreasing morbidity and mortality. The higher dose of acyclovir is associated with a higher frequency of hematologic abnormalities, especially neutropenia.[19,23,24] The minimum duration of therapy should be 14 days for neonates with only SEM involvement, whereas longer courses (e.g., 21 days) are indicated in infants with CNS involvement or disseminated disease.[19]

The role of prolonged oral suppressive therapy in newborns with SEM involvement has been investigated. Acyclovir, given orally (PO) at 300 mg/m^2 per dose three times a day (TID), resulted in a reduction in the recurrences of lesions. Half of these patients developed neutropenia. One patient had lesions resistant to acyclovir.[25] Because the long-term benefits cannot be fully attributed to the use of suppressive acyclovir, suppressive therapy for patients with SEM involvement is not recommended.[26]

Oral-Facial Herpes (Herpes Labialis)

Both primary and recurrent oral-facial HSV-1 infections can be asymptomatic. Gingivostomatitis and pharyngitis are the most common clinical manifestations of a first episode of HSV-1 infection, and recurrent herpes labialis is most commonly caused by reactivated HSV infection. Clinical features include fever, malaise, myalgia, inability to eat, and irritability. Immunocompromised patients with oral-facial herpes have severe pain, extensive lesions, and prolonged viral shedding; thus, they are candidates for antiviral therapy.

TABLE 76-2
US Food and Drug Administration (FDA)–Indicated Drugs for Various Viral Infections

Disease	Drug	Dosage (Age Group)	Route	Duration
Herpes encephalitis	Acyclovir (Zovirax)[a]	>12 years: 10 mg/kg every 8 hours	IV	21 days
		3 months–12 years: 20 mg/kg every 8 hours	IV	21 days
Neonatal herpes	Acyclovir (Zovirax)	Birth–3 months: 10–20 mg/kg every 8 hours[a]	IV	14–21 days
Oral-facial herpes (for treatment of recurrent infection)	Acyclovir (Zovirax)	Adults: 400 mg 5×/d	PO	5 days
	Famciclovir (Famvir)	Adults: 1,500 mg	PO	1 dose
	Valacyclovir (Valtrex)	Adults: 2,000 mg BID	PO	1 day
Oral-facial herpes[b] (immunocompromised patients)	Acyclovir (Zovirax)	>12 years: 5 mg/kg every 8 hours	IV	7 days
		<12 years: 10 mg/kg every 8 hours	IV	7 days
	Famciclovir (Famvir)	Adults: 500 mg BID	PO	7 days
Herpes zoster[b] (immunocompetent patients)	Acyclovir (Zovirax)	Adults: 800 mg 5×/d	PO	7–10 days
	Famciclovir (Famvir)	Adult: 500 mg every 8 hours	PO	7 days
	Valacyclovir (Valtrex)	Adult: 1,000 mg every 8 hours	PO	7 days
Herpes zoster[b] (immunocompromised patients)	Acyclovir (Zovirax)	>12 years: 10 mg/kg every 8 hours	IV	7 days
		<12 years: 20 mg/kg every 8 hours	IV	7 days
Varicella (immunocompetent patient)	Acyclovir (Zovirax)	>40 kg: 800 mg QID	PO	5 days
		>2 years and <40 kg: 20 mg/kg (max 800 mg) QID	PO	5–10 days
Varicella (immunocompromised patients)	Acyclovir (Zovirax)	>12 years: 10 mg/kg every 8 hours	IV	7–10 days
		<12 years: 500 mg/m^2 every 8 hours	IV	7–10 days
Cytomegalovirus retinitis (immunocompromised patients)	Ganciclovir (Cytovene)	5 mg/kg every 12 hours; then 5 mg/kg/d or 6 mg/kg, 5 days a week	IV	14–21 days for induction; maintenance
	Cidofovir (Vistide)	5 mg/kg every week for 2 weeks, then every 2 weeks	IV	Maintenance
	Foscarnet (Foscavir)	90 mg/kg every 12 hours, then 90 mg/kg every day	IV	Induction for 2 weeks; maintenance
	Valganciclovir (Valcyte)	900 mg BID, 900 mg every day	PO	Induction for 21 days; maintenance
Influenza A	Amantadine[c] (Symmetrel)	>9 years: 100 mg BID	PO	10 days (treatment), 14–28 days (protection with vaccine), 90 days (protection without vaccine)
		1–9 years: 4.4–8.8 mg/kg/d but <150 mg/d	PO	
	Rimantadine[c] (Flumadine)	>14 years: 100 mg BID	PO	7 days (treatment, not approved for treatment in children) up to 6 weeks for prophylaxis
		1–13 years: 100 mg BID	PO	Up to 6 weeks for prophylaxis
		1–9 years: 5 mg/kg div. every day BID (max 150 mg/d)	PO	
Influenza A and B	Oseltamivir (Tamiflu)	>13 years (or >40 kg): 75 mg BID	PO	5 days (treatment)
		>13 years (or >40 kg): 75 mg every day	PO	10 days (prophylaxis) Up to 6 weeks (community outbreaks)
		24–40 kg: 60 mg BID 16–23 kg: 45 mg BID >1 year–15 kg: 30 mg BID	PO	5 days (treatment)
		24–40 kg: 60 mg every day 16–23 kg: 45 mg every day >1 year–15 kg: 30 mg every day	PO	10 days (prophylaxis)
	Zanamivir (Relenza)	>7 years: 10 mg (2 inhalations) BID	Inhalation	5 days (treatment)
		Adolescent and adult: 10 mg (2 inhalations) every day	Inhalation	10 days (prophylaxis) 28 days (community outbreak)
		>5 years: 10 mg (2 inhalations) every day	Inhalation	10 days (prophylaxis)
Respiratory syncytial virus	Ribavirin (Virazole)	6 g in 300 mL for 12–18 h/d	Inhalation	3–7 days

[a]FDA-approved dose is 10 mg/kg. Although doses of 15–20 mg/kg have been used, safety has not been established at these doses.
[b]Foscarnet 40 mg/kg IV every 8 hours is recommended for acyclovir-resistant herpes simplex virus or varicella-zoster virus.
[c]Amantadine and rimantadine are no longer recommended as drugs of choice for either prophylaxis or treatment of influenza A.
BID, twice a day; IV, intravenously; PO, orally; QID, four times a day.

Herpes labialis (cold sores) is the most common oral-facial HSV infection. Clinical features include pain or paresthesia and erythematous or papular lesions followed by vesiculation and swelling. These lesions usually crust and heal in the next few days. Viral cultures generally are positive within 2 to 3 days. Rapid diagnosis can be made by visualizing viral particles in vesicular fluid with electron microscopy or fluorescent antibody staining of cells from vesicles.

INDICATIONS FOR ANTIVIRAL TREATMENT

CASE 76-3

QUESTION 1: M.K., a 26-year-old man, experienced pain and erythematous skin lesions on his face and around his mouth during a 2-day period after contact with a person with active lesions. For the next 2 days, significant swelling was noted. He remembers similar episodes in the past. M.K. has no previous history of any other illness. Should he be treated with antiviral drugs?

Most patients with herpes labialis have a self-limiting benign course and heal within 10 days. Antiviral drugs (e.g., acyclovir, valacyclovir) are indicated only when the patient has a primary infection, an underlying illness, or a compromised immune system that may lead to prolonged illness or dissemination.

M.K. should not receive antiviral therapy. However, aspirin or acetaminophen can be considered for symptomatic relief. Although ice, ether, lysine, silver nitrate, and smallpox vaccine have been used to treat cold sores, no data support their efficacy.

CASE 76-4

QUESTION 1: P.L., a 16-year-old boy diagnosed with acute lymphocytic leukemia 8 months ago, is now admitted for a bone marrow transplant. Admission laboratory tests reveal that he has antibodies against HSV-1 and that 4 months ago, during a course of chemotherapy, he developed an oral-facial herpes infection. What is the significance of these findings for P.L., who is about to undergo a bone marrow transplant?

Immunosuppressed patients have more frequent and severe mucocutaneous HSV infections. Therefore, IV acyclovir should be considered to suppress the reactivation of oral-facial HSV infections.[27,28] Oral therapy with famciclovir is approved for use in HIV-infected patients,[29] but efficacy in other immunocompromised patients is not yet established.

ANTIVIRAL TREATMENT

CASE 76-4, QUESTION 2: P.L. did not receive antiviral therapy. Two weeks later, he developed malaise and painful oral-mucosal and skin lesions on his face. HSV was identified from the lesion by immunofluorescence. What is the treatment of choice for P.L.?

Acyclovir should be administered IV at 5 mg/kg every 8 hours for 7 days[8] or until the lesions are healed, followed by oral acyclovir 200 mg TID for about 6 months. In patients with marrow transplants and culture-proven recurrent mucocutaneous herpes simplex, oral acyclovir (400 mg five times daily for 10 days) is significantly more effective than placebo in reducing pain, virus shedding, new lesion formation, and lesion healing time.[30] Valacyclovir and famciclovir have also been used in the transplant population.[31]

CASE 76-5

QUESTION 1: N.B., a 43-year-old woman, experiences eight to ten cold sores a year. These are typically preceded by "colds" or sun exposure. She requests a prescription for acyclovir to prevent cold sores when she feels one coming on. What is the role of antiviral medications in the acute treatment and prevention in immunocompetent patients with recurrent herpes labialis?

Topical agents that are approved by the US Food and Drug Administration (FDA) for the treatment of recurrent herpes labialis in immunocompetent patients include acyclovir (Zovirax) 5% cream, docosanol (Abreva) 10% cream, and penciclovir (Denavir) 1% cream. Clinical trials demonstrate that each agent modestly decreases healing time of herpes lesions when started at the first sign or symptom of a cold sore.[32–38] Although penciclovir cream may be more effective than acyclovir cream, the benefit is small.[35,36] An advantage of docosanol compared with the other agents is that it is available without a prescription. The topical agents must be applied within 1 hour of the first sign or symptom of a cold sore and then every 2 hours for 4 days while awake.

Studies evaluating the use of oral antiviral agents have produced conflicting results. In some studies, oral antiviral medications can decrease the duration of pain and healing time in immunocompetent patients. One study demonstrated that oral acyclovir 200 mg five times daily for 5 days had no benefit. However, 400 mg five times daily for 5 days started within 1 hour of the development of a cold sore significantly decreased duration of pain and healing time in immunocompetent patients.[39] Valacyclovir 2 g at the first signs of a cold sore followed by 2 g 12 hours later, and famciclovir 1,500 mg as a single dose showed similar clinical efficacy.[40,41] No studies have directly compared the efficacy of the different oral antiviral medications.[42] Frequency of dosing and cost should be considered when choosing a particular agent.[17,43,44]

Daily suppressive therapy may be recommended in patients with six or more recurrences per year or in patients with severe episodes. In immunocompetent patients with six or more episodes of herpes labialis, oral acyclovir 400 mg twice a day (BID) for 4 months was more effective than placebo in decreasing the number of recurrences in patients with herpes labialis.[45] Valacyclovir, 500 mg once daily or 1,000 mg once daily, is efficacious in decreasing the number of recurrences.[46] Controlled trials of famciclovir for chronic suppressive therapy of herpes labialis have not been performed.

N.B. should be treated with either a topical antiviral medication or an oral antiviral for the acute episode of herpes labialis. She should be instructed to start treatment as soon as the first sign or symptom of the cold sore appears. If suppressive therapy is desired, N.B. should be treated with oral acyclovir or valacyclovir.

RESISTANCE

CASE 76-6

QUESTION 1: How should an acyclovir-resistant HSV infection be treated?

The incidence of acyclovir-resistant herpes is greater in immunocompromised patients compared with immunocompetent patients. Current estimates of HSV resistance in the immunocompromised population are about 5%; some populations, such as bone marrow transplant patients, have a resistance rate approaching 30%.[47,48] IV foscarnet 40 mg/kg every 8 hours is more effective and less toxic than IV vidarabine

15 mg/kg/day in patients with AIDS and mucocutaneous herpetic lesions unresponsive to IV acyclovir.[10] More concerning, however, are the reports of foscarnet-resistant HSV, particularly in the bone marrow transplant population.[49,50] Cidofovir has been used with moderate success in such cases. In patients with recurrent acyclovir-resistant genital herpes, limited evidence suggests that topical imiquimod 5% cream may be effective.[51]

VARICELLA-ZOSTER INFECTIONS

Chickenpox

Chickenpox used to be a common childhood infection, but the incidence has decreased by up to 84% in states with moderate rates of use of the varicella-zoster virus (VZV) vaccine since 1995.[52] This vaccine is now considered a routine childhood vaccine by the American Academy of Pediatrics. Unimmunized adolescents and adults who have not had chickenpox should also be vaccinated. Before the vaccine was available, approximately 3.5 million cases occurred per year in the United States: 60% of cases occurred in children 5 to 9 years of age, and 80% occurred in those younger than 10 years. Although it is a benign disease in most patients, complications and mortality (7 of 10,000 cases) can occur in patients younger than 5 years and older than 20 years, and in immunocompromised patients.

This is a contagious disease; the average incubation period is 14 to 16 days. Children are considered contagious from 1 to 2 days before the onset of rash until all vesicles have crusted (usually 4–6 days after the onset of rash).

ONLINE CONTENT

For a photo of a chickenpox rash, go to http://thepoint.lww.com/AT10e.

After household exposure, more than 90% of susceptible individuals become infected. Thus, a history of exposure is useful in making a diagnosis. A smear of cells scraped from the lesions will show multinucleated giant cells. Viruses also can be identified in vesicular lesions by electron microscopy, or antigen can be detected by countercurrent immunoelectrophoresis. Chickenpox is a primary varicella-zoster infection, whereas herpes zoster (shingles) is caused by reactivation of VZV.

CLINICAL PRESENTATION

CASE 76-7

QUESTION 1: A.V., a 10-year-old boy, was admitted to the hospital for evaluation and treatment of possible recurrent chickenpox with progressive lesions. According to his mother and his physician, he had a mild case of chickenpox at age 4 years and has not received the vaccine. At admission, A.V. had a 10-day history of progressive vesicular and pustular lesions that began on his neck and spread to his back, trunk, extremities, and face. Although he had been febrile (up to 40.5°C orally) for the past 3 days, his temperature on admission was 37°C. A.V. had episodes of vomiting during the 4 days before admission. On admission, he was alert, cooperative, and well oriented but had overt ataxia with abnormal cerebellar signs. Lesions consistent with VZV infection were extensive and confluent over the face, neck, chest, and back. Stages of lesions varied from tiny thin-walled vesicles with an erythematous base to umbilicated vesicles. Few crusted lesions were present. Blood analysis revealed the following results:

BUN, 9 mg/dL (SI units, 3.213 mmol/L)
SCr, 0.2 mg/dL (SI units, 15.25 μmol/L)
Serum aspartate aminotransferase, 65 international units/L (normal, 0–34; SI units, 1.084 mckat/L)
Serum alanine aminotransferase 122 international units/L (normal, 0–34; SI units, 2.034 mckat/L)

Because of the possibility of cerebellar involvement with VZV infection and possible underlying immunodeficiency, therapy with acyclovir 550 mg IV every 8 hours (1,500 mg/m^2/day) was instituted. Oral diphenhydramine was also prescribed for itching, but A.V. required only two doses on the first hospital day.

New lesions were noted on the second day of acyclovir therapy, but by the third day, no new lesions appeared and previous lesions were healing. The ataxia improved daily. He was discharged on day 7 with no further complaints of nausea and vomiting. Follow-up serologic evaluation demonstrated a fourfold rise in the optical density for the VZV enzyme-linked immunosorbent assay (ELISA) from day 20 to day 60 after the onset of infection. These results suggested primary VZV infection. Why is the use of acyclovir in A.V. appropriate?

ANTIVIRAL TREATMENT

Neonates, adults, immunocompromised hosts, patients with progressive varicella, and those with extracutaneous complications benefit from acyclovir therapy. Acyclovir is effective in preventing dissemination of VZV infection, accelerating cutaneous healing, decreasing fever and pain, and reducing mortality.[53,54] A.V. had a prolonged progressive course of varicella and demonstrated an extracutaneous manifestation of varicella infection (e.g., ataxia with abnormal cerebellar signs). Because of the concern of possible cerebellar involvement, the use of IV acyclovir was appropriate in A.V.

CASE 76-8

QUESTION 1: C.J., an 8-year-old boy, developed a case of chickenpox and was kept home from school. Four days later, his 15-year-old brother, K.J., began to exhibit similar symptoms. What is the role of acyclovir in immunocompetent patients with chickenpox? Should C.J. or K.J. be treated with acyclovir?

Three studies in children (2–18 years of age) have shown that oral acyclovir 20 mg/kg (when initiated within 24 hours of disease onset) four times a day (QID) for 5 to 10 days accelerates healing and decreases the formation of new lesions, fever, and itching. However, the benefit is modest (usually healing 1 day sooner than placebo) and does not reduce the complications of varicella.[55] Thus, the American Academy of Pediatrics does not consider routine use of acyclovir in healthy children justified, and it is not indicated for C.J.[56]

Adolescents and adults are more likely to develop complications (e.g., pneumonia, encephalitis) than children. Others at higher risk for developing complications include those with chronic cutaneous or pulmonary disease, patients receiving chronic salicylate therapy, and patients receiving short, intermittent, or aerosolized corticosteroid therapy.[56] In these patients, acyclovir therapy may be warranted. Acyclovir 800 mg PO QID for 5 days in adolescents and 800 mg PO five times daily for 5 days in adults (initiated within 24 hours of disease onset) decreases the number of lesions and reduces time for healing, fever, and itching.

The effect of acyclovir on prevention of severe complications is unknown.[57–59] Thus, acyclovir therapy should be considered in those at increased risk of severe chickenpox, for example, those like K.J. who are older than 14 years or those with chronic respiratory or skin disease.[60] There are no published clinical trials to support the use of famciclovir and valacyclovir in the treatment of chickenpox.

SUPPORTIVE TREATMENT

CASE 76-8, QUESTION 2: What is the role of supportive treatment in C.J. and K.J.?

Cool baths and application of calamine or other topical antipruritic agents may decrease itching. In severe cases, a systemic antipruritic and antihistamine preparation may be useful because some degree of sedation may be desired. In C.J. and K.J., aspirin should not be used because Reye syndrome has been associated with the use of salicylates in chickenpox or flulike illness (see Chapter 97, Pediatric Pharmacotherapy).

Shingles (Herpes Zoster)

Herpes zoster infections are caused by the reactivation of dormant VZV in the sensory neurons. Reactivation is believed to occur because of waning immunity. The incidence of herpes zoster is higher in immunocompromised patients (e.g., those with HIV or cancer or those receiving immunosuppressive medications), and the incidence of zoster increases with age. It tends to be more severe in the elderly.

Acute herpes zoster infection is characterized by pain, which is described as a deep aching or burning pain. It may be accompanied by excessive sensitivity to touch. Many patients exhibit a rash that presents initially as erythematous patches and progresses to vesicles that crust in 7 to 10 days. By 1 month, the rash is usually gone, but scarring can occur.

ONLINE CONTENT

For a photo of shingles, go to http://thepoint.lww.com/AT10e.

Postherpetic neuralgia (PHN) is associated pain that continues more than 1 month after the onset of the rash. It is estimated that 10% to 70% of patients experience PHN. PHN is the most common complication of acute herpes zoster, and its prevention is important because PHN pain is difficult to treat.

The goal of pharmacotherapy in acute herpes zoster is to inhibit viral replication to reduce pain and duration of rash. Ultimately, by inhibiting the virus, nerve damage can be prevented and the incidence and severity of PHN can be decreased. Unfortunately, no therapy can prevent all cases of PHN.

The herpes zoster vaccine (Zostavax) significantly reduces the incidence of herpes zoster and the associated resulting PHN (see Chapter 11, Vaccinations).

ANTIVIRAL THERAPY IN IMMUNOCOMPETENT PATIENTS

CASE 76-9

QUESTION 1: E.O. is a 72-year-old, previously healthy man who complains of a burning pain under his left arm for the last 2 days. The pain radiates across his chest. The pain is worse when the area is touched. This morning, he noticed a rash that starts under his arm and continues to his midline. Pertinent laboratory findings include BUN of 15 mg/dL (normal, 8–18; SI units, 5.4 mmol/L) and SCr of 2.0 mg/dL (normal, 0.6–1.2; SI units, 177 μmol/L). He has not received the herpes zoster vaccine. A diagnosis of herpes zoster is made. What therapy should be initiated?

Acyclovir is the standard antiviral agent against which new VZV therapies are compared. In immunocompetent patients, oral acyclovir 800 mg five times daily for 10 days is moderately beneficial in reducing acute pain during the first 28 days. Acyclovir therapy should be initiated within 72 hours of the onset of the rash. The benefit of acyclovir in reducing PHN and chronic pain is modest at best. Although a number of trials showed no benefit from acyclovir in reducing PHN, a meta-analysis of acyclovir treatment in herpes zoster concluded that acyclovir was effective, but that 6.3 patients would need to be treated to prevent 1 patient from having PHN 6 months after the outbreak of VZV.[61]

Famciclovir (Famvir) is approved for the treatment of acute herpes zoster infection. Famciclovir is rapidly absorbed and converted to the active drug penciclovir in the intestine. The bioavailability of famciclovir is greater than acyclovir, resulting in higher concentrations of active drug in the infected cells. In addition, the longer half-life of famciclovir allows for less frequent administration. Famciclovir 500 mg TID is as effective as acyclovir 800 mg five times a day in reducing the duration of acute pain and healing of the rash.[62] Although famciclovir does not decrease the incidence of PHN, it may reduce the duration of PHN.[63]

To overcome the poor oral bioavailability of acyclovir, valacyclovir (Valtrex), a prodrug of acyclovir, was developed. Valacyclovir is rapidly and extensively absorbed and converted to acyclovir after oral administration. Valacyclovir 1 g TID is as effective as acyclovir 800 mg five times a day in terms of reducing rash progression and time to rash healing, and valacyclovir is more effective than acyclovir in relieving zoster-associated pain.[64] Valacyclovir is comparable to famciclovir with respect to decreasing the duration of acute zoster-associated pain and PHN.[65]

E.O. should be started on acyclovir, famciclovir, or valacyclovir. Famciclovir or valacyclovir may be preferred because adherence with a three-times-daily regimen will likely be better than with acyclovir, which must be administered five times a day. Therapy should be initiated within 72 hours of the rash onset and continued for 10 days; the duration of therapy for famciclovir and valacyclovir is 7 days. Although therapy may not prevent PHN, it may decrease the duration of pain. Because these agents are renally eliminated, the dosage should be adjusted based on E.O.'s reduced creatinine clearance (Table 76-3).

For acute illness, E.O. may require pain control with medications such as nonsteroidal anti-inflammatory agents, opioids, or tramadol.[82,83] In addition, E.O. should be counseled to keep the area of the rash clean and dry, and to avoid topical antibiotics. If the rash worsens or fever develops, he should contact his health care professional.

CASE 76-9, QUESTION 2: Should E.O. receive a corticosteroid to treat or prevent the pain associated with herpes zoster?

The decision to use corticosteroids such as prednisone or prednisolone remains controversial.[84] A number of studies have examined the effect of steroids on pain during acute neuralgia and on the development of PHN. Early studies revealed that steroids are effective for both acute pain and PHN, but these studies were small and uncontrolled, and used various corticosteroid regimens. Most studies suggest relief of the acute pain but no decrease in PHN.[85–88] Adverse effects of the corticosteroids and the theoretical possibility of dissemination of herpes zoster

TABLE 76-3
Clinical Pharmacokinetics of Antiviral Drugs

Drug	Type of Patient	Peak Serum Concentration (mcg/mL)	VD	Elimination: % Recovered Unchanged in Urine	Elimination: Total Clearance	Elimination: Half-Life (hours)	Comments
Acyclovir[8,16,17,66–69]	Adults	3.4–22.9 (Based on a dose of 2.5–10 mg/kg IV) 0.83–1.61 (Based on a dose of 200–800 mg PO)	59 L/1.73 m^2	69–91	327 mL/min/1.73 m^2	2.5–3.3	Use 100% of recommended dose, but extend dosage interval to 12 and 24 hours if ClCr ranges from 25–50 and 10–25 mL/min/1.73 m^2, respectively; use 50% of recommended dose every 24 hours if ClCr ranges from 0–10 mL/min/1.73 m^2.
	Neonates	N/A	24–30 L/1.73 m^2	N/A	98–122 mL/min/1.73 m^2	3.2–4.1	
Amantadine[70]	Adults	0.2–0.5 (Based on a dose of 100–200 mg PO)	3–8 L/kg	52–88	2.5–10.5 L/h	20–41	Adjust doses in renal failure: 200 mg on day 1, then 100 mg/d if ClCr 30–50; 200 mg on day 1, then 100 mg every other day if ClCr 15–29; 200 mg every 7 days if ClCr <15 mL/min/1.73 m^2.
Famciclovir[44,71,72]	Adults	0.8–6.6 (Based on a dose of 125–1,000 mg PO)	1.1 L/kg	73–94[a]	0.37–0.48 L/h/kg	2.2–3.0	Use 100% of recommended dose, but extend dosage interval to 12 and 24 hours if ClCr ranges from 40–59 and 20–39 mL/min, respectively; use 250 mg every 24 hours if ClCr <20 mL/min.
Oseltamivir[73–76]	Adults	0.6–3.5[b] (Based on a dose of 75 mg PO)	23–26 L	99[b]	18.8 L/h	6.0–10	Use 75 mg/d in patients if ClCr 10–30 mL/min. The effect of hepatic impairment has not been determined.
	Pediatrics (1–12 years)	0.06–0.8[b] (Based on a dose of 2 mg/kg PO)	N/A	N/A	0.63 L/h/kg	3.2–7.8	Dosage recommendations are based on body weight and age. Use 30 mg BID if patient is 15 kg and 1–3 years, 45 mg if patient is 15–23 kg and 4–7 years, 60 mg if patient is 23–40 kg and 8–12 years, and normal adult dose if >40 kg and older than 13 years.
	Adolescents	N/A	N/A	N/A	0.32 L/h/kg	8.1	
Rimantadine[77]	Adults	0.2–0.7 (Based on a dose of 100–200 mg PO)	17–25 L/kg	20	20–48 L/h	25–32	Because it undergoes extensive metabolism, dose may have to be adjusted in patients with severe liver disease. Dose adjustments may also be necessary in elderly and in those with severe renal failure (ClCr <10 mL/min). Manufacturer recommends 50% reduction in such cases.
Valacyclovir[43,78] (See Acyclovir [prodrug of acyclovir])	Adults	5.7–6.7[c] (Based on a dose of 1,000 mg PO)	N/A	46–80[c]	N/A	2.5–3.3[c]	Use 100% of recommended dose, but extend dosage interval to 12 and 24 hours if ClCr ranges from 30–49 and 10–29 mL/min, respectively; use 500 mg every 24 hours if ClCr <10 mL/min.
Zanamivir[79–81]	Adults	0.02–0.1 (Based on a dose of 10 mg INH)	15.9 L	7–17	2.5–10.9 L/h	2.5–5.1	4%–17% of inhaled dose systemically absorbed. Although only limited studies with renal or hepatic impairment, dosing adjustment likely unnecessary.

[a]Pharmacokinetic properties of active metabolite penciclovir.
[b]Active metabolite oseltamivir carboxylate.
[c]Pharmacokinetic properties of active metabolite acyclovir.
BID, twice a day; ClCr, creatinine clearance; INH, inhalation; IV, intravenously; N/A, not available; PO, orally; VD, volume of distribution.

should be considered when deciding whether to initiate therapy. Because of recent studies demonstrating a lack of benefit in preventing PHN, the theoretical concerns of herpes zoster dissemination, and the beneficial effects of antiviral agents such as acyclovir, famciclovir, and valacyclovir for acute pain, corticosteroids should not be used in E.O.

CASE 76-9, QUESTION 3: Two months after the onset of the rash, E.O. continues to complain of pain. A diagnosis of PHN is made. What FDA-approved treatments for PHN should be prescribed for E.O.?

Although many different agents have been studied, the only FDA-approved treatments for PHN are topical capsaicin cream or gel, capsaicin patch 8% (Qutenza), topical lidocaine 5% patches (Lidoderm), and oral gabapentin (Neurontin) and pregabalin (Lyrica). Capsaicin depletes substance P, a mediator that transmits pain from the periphery to the CNS. The largest double-blind, placebo-controlled trial of capsaicin evaluated 143 patients with PHN for at least 6 months. After 6 weeks of treatment with capsaicin 0.075% cream, pain scores were reduced in 21% and 6% of the capsaicin and placebo groups, respectively. After the double-blind phase of the study ended, a subset of patients continued to use capsaicin cream for up to 2 years, and most patients experienced prolonged pain relief.[89] Capsaicin should be applied three or four times per day. Qutenza is a capsaicin patch, which is applied by a health care professional. The patch is applied for 1 hour and cannot be repeated more frequently than every 3 months. Lidocaine 5% patches have only been compared with placebo and have been shown to relieve pain for 4 to 12 hours after administration. Either capsaicin cream or gel or lidocaine patches can be considered as a first-line option for E.O. A common adverse effect is a burning sensation after application of capsaicin, which is intolerable in up to one-third of patients. The burning sensation usually lessens with continued use.

If lidocaine patches are prescribed, E.O. should be instructed to apply up to three patches to the painful area. Patients should be instructed to wear the patches for a maximum of 12 hours a day, and proper disposal of used patches should be emphasized. Even a used patch contains a large amount of lidocaine, and small children or pets could suffer serious consequences from chewing or swallowing a used patch.[90]

Pregabalin is approved for the treatment of PHN, but is associated with a greater risk of adverse effects. Pregabalin binds to a subunit of calcium channels, thereby decreasing calcium influx at nerve terminals and reducing the release of several neurotransmitters, including glutamate, norepinephrine, and substance P.[91] In clinical trials, dizziness was experienced by 29% of patients treated with pregabalin compared with 9% of placebo-treated patients; somnolence was noted in 22% of patients who received pregabalin compared with 8% of placebo-treated patients. Dizziness and somnolence usually occur soon after the pregabalin is started and is dose dependent.[91]

Other agents that have been used in the treatment of PHN include tricyclic antidepressants (e.g., amitriptyline, desipramine) and opioids.[92]

ANTIVIRAL THERAPY IN IMMUNOCOMPROMISED PATIENTS

CASE 76-10

QUESTION 1: R.F. is a 68-year-old woman with a chief complaint of vesicles on her face associated with severe pain. She has a history of polymyalgia rheumatica and possible temporal arteritis with headaches that are responsive to steroids. She had been having increasing headaches on the right side of her forehead 5 days before admission. Two days before admission, her family physician increased the dosage of prednisone from 30 mg/day to 60 mg/day. Vesicles developed on her face 1 day before admission. She was admitted for pain control and diagnosed with herpes zoster infection. Six hours after admission, R.F. began having visual hallucinations, hearing noises, and talking to herself. A lumbar puncture was performed with the following results:

WBCs, 3 (2 lymphocytes and 1 monocyte)
RBCs, 3
Protein, 84 mg/dL
Glucose, 86 mg/dL

VZV was isolated from the CSF. IV acyclovir was started at a dosage of 10 mg/kg every 8 hours. Why is antiviral therapy indicated in R.F.? Should her prednisone be continued or discontinued?

Antiviral therapy is indicated for R.F. Acyclovir may halt the progression of acute herpes zoster infection in immunocompromised hosts such as R.F., who has been taking large doses of corticosteroids.[93]

IV acyclovir 10 mg/kg every 8 hours is effective in severely immunocompromised patients. Alternatively, in less severely immunocompromised patients, oral therapy with acyclovir 800 mg five times a day, valacyclovir 1,000 mg TID, or famciclovir 500 mg TID, along with close monitoring, can be used.[94] Antiviral therapy is associated with more rapid clearance of the herpes zoster virus from vesicles. Acyclovir has little to no benefit in resolution of pain or prevention of PHN.[93] Initial data indicate that famciclovir or valacyclovir are effective in severe herpes zoster infection in an immunocompromised host.[95,96]

Systemic corticosteroids are of unproven usefulness and may slow the healing of lesions. Therefore, if possible, R.F.'s prednisone should be slowly tapered.

ACYCLOVIR TOXICITY

CASE 76-10, QUESTION 2: On the fourth day of acyclovir therapy, R.F. developed severe nausea and vomited three times. The laboratory data showed a BUN of 45 mg/dL (SI units, 16.07 mmol/L) and SCr of 3.2 mg/dL (SI units, 282.88 μmol/L) (baseline BUN, 10 mg/dL [SI units, 3.57 mmol/L] and SCr, 1.0 mg/dL [SI units, 88.40 μmol/L]). Why must R.F.'s acyclovir dosage be altered?

Nausea and vomiting have been reported with acyclovir therapy in patients with herpes zoster infections.[8] Similarly, elevations of SCr and BUN can occur in association with acyclovir therapy. This may be secondary to acyclovir crystallization in the renal tubules, particularly when fluid intake is inadequate (Table 76-1). Because R.F.'s creatinine clearance is between 10 and 25 mL/minute per 1.73 m^2, the acyclovir dosage interval should be extended to 24 hours. Every effort should be made to maintain adequate hydration for the duration of acyclovir therapy. (See Table 76-3 and Chapter 2, Interpretation of Clinical Laboratory Tests, for creatinine clearance calculation.)

INFLUENZA

Influenza is an acute infection caused by the virus of the Orthomyxoviridae family. Epidemics of influenza are usually

TABLE 76-4
Persons Who Should Receive the Influenza Vaccine[97]

- All persons 6 months of age or older
- Nursing home or chronic care facility residents
- Children and adults with chronic pulmonary or cardiovascular disease
- Children and adults who have required medical follow-up because of chronic metabolic diseases (e.g., diabetes mellitus), renal dysfunction, hemoglobinopathies, or immunosuppression (as a result of medications or diseases such as HIV)
- Children and adults who are at risk for aspiration (e.g., cognitive dysfunction, spinal cord injuries, seizures)
- Children (6 months–18 years) receiving long-term aspirin therapy
- Women who will be pregnant during influenza season
- Health care workers
- Household members of persons in high-risk groups (including contacts of infants and children 0–59 months)

TABLE 76-5
Influenza Vaccines[97]

Age	Dosage	Number of Doses
6–35 months	0.25 mL IM[a] inactivated vaccine or 0.2 mL IN[b] live vaccine	1 or 2[c]
36–59 months	0.5 mL IM[a] inactivated vaccine or 0.2 mL IN[b] live vaccine	1 or 2[c]
5–49 years	0.5 mL IM[a] inactivated vaccine or 0.2 mL IN[b] live vaccine	1 or 2[c]
50 years	0.5 mL IM[a] inactivated vaccine	1

[a] The recommended site is the deltoid muscle for adults and older children and the anterolateral aspect of the thigh in infants and young children.
[b] The live vaccine should not be used in patients with chronic pulmonary or cardiovascular disease and in those with underlying immunodeficiencies.
[c] Two doses given at least 1 month apart for children younger than 9 years who are receiving the vaccine for the first time.
IM, intramuscularly; IN, intranasally.

caused by the type A virus; type B virus is generally associated with more sporadic infection. Infection is transmitted by the inhalation of virus-containing droplets ejected from the respiratory tract of a person with influenza. It can be spread by direct contact, large droplets, or articles recently contaminated by nasopharyngeal secretions. The incubation period is typically 2 days (range, 1–4 days).

Influenza A viruses are classified into subtypes of hemagglutinin (H) and neuraminidase (N) surface antigens. Three subtypes of hemagglutinin (H1, H2, H3) and two subtypes of neuraminidase (N1, N2) have caused influenza in humans. Infection with a virus of one subtype may confer little or no protection against viruses of other subtypes. In addition, significant antigenic variation (antigenic drift) within a subtype may occur with time. Thus, infection or vaccination with one strain may not protect against a distantly related strain of the same subtype. This is why major epidemics of influenza continue to occur, and influenza vaccines must be reformulated each year with the most likely viral strains to maximize vaccine benefit.

The influenza vaccine is indicated for all individuals 6 months of age or older. However, there are a number of populations for which vaccination is vital. Persons at highest risk for influenza infection (Table 76–4) should receive the influenza vaccine each year. Each year's vaccine contains three virus strains (generally two type A and one type B) that are likely to circulate in the community for the upcoming season. The efficacy depends on the similarity of the components of the vaccine to the circulating viruses that year and the immunocompetence of the host. If there is a good match with the circulating viruses, the vaccine can prevent illness in approximately 70% to 90% of healthy adults and children. The vaccine is effective in preventing hospitalization and pneumonia in 70% of elderly persons living in the community and in 50% to 60% of elderly persons residing in nursing homes. However, the efficacy of the vaccine in preventing illness is less, i.e., 30% to 40% among the frail elderly. Despite the lower efficacy, vaccination is still associated with less severe illness and fewer complications in vaccinated individuals.

Individuals at high risk for transmission to patients include physicians, nurses, and other personnel in both hospital and ambulatory settings; employees of nursing homes and chronic care facilities; providers of home care services; and household members, including children. It is vital that all the above individuals should be vaccinated annually. However, considering the morbidity and mortality associated with influenza, all individuals should receive an annual influenza vaccination.

Table 76–5 describes the types of vaccines, dosage, number of doses, and route of administration. The optimal time for vaccine administration is between mid-October and mid-November because influenza activity peaks between late December and early March in the United States. Vaccinating an individual too early in the season could result in waning antibody concentrations before the influenza season is over. However, influenza vaccine should be offered throughout the influenza season, even if outbreaks of influenza have already been documented in the community.[97]

Because the parenteral influenza vaccine is an inactivated vaccine and contains no infectious viruses, it cannot cause influenza. The most common adverse effect is soreness at the administration site lasting for up to 2 days.[98] Fever, malaise, myalgia, and other systemic reactions occur infrequently; these may develop within 6 to 12 hours after the vaccine is given and persist for 1 to 3 days.[98,99] Immediate hypersensitivity to egg protein (hives, angioedema, allergic asthma, or systemic anaphylaxis) rarely occurs. Persons with anaphylactic hypersensitivity and those with acute febrile illness should not be given the vaccine. However, minor illnesses with or without fever are not contraindications for the influenza vaccine, particularly in children with a mild upper respiratory tract infection or allergic rhinitis. When the vaccine is contraindicated, a neuraminidase inhibitor (oseltamivir or zanamivir) should be used for prophylaxis.[97] Amantadine and rimantadine are no longer recommended for prophylaxis of influenza because of widespread resistance in the United States.

Clinically, it is impossible to differentiate between influenza A and B. Definitive diagnosis can be made by isolating the virus from throat washings or sputum and by a significant increase in antibody titers during the convalescent period.

Clinical Presentation

CASE 76-11

QUESTION 1: K.B., a 40-year-old woman, comes into the pharmacy claiming she has "the flu." She recently started a new job and is afraid she will lose her job if she misses too many days from work. What questions would you ask her to differentiate the common cold from an influenza infection?

Although it can be difficult to differentiate the common cold from influenza, there are some clues that may suggest one viral infection from the other. Influenza infections typically occur from December through March in the United States. Patients with influenza generally experience more systemic symptoms, such as fever higher than 102°F, headache, myalgia, and cough. Rhinorrhea, nasal congestion, and sneezing are more pronounced in patients with the common cold. Sore throat can occur with both a cold and the flu. Bacterial sore throat (e.g., strep throat) is somewhat differentiated from a viral sore throat in that a viral sore throat usually has a slower onset and the throat pain is less severe. Lymph nodes are only slightly enlarged and not tender in a viral sore throat, whereas with a bacterial sore throat, lymph nodes are large and tender.[100]

K.B. should be questioned about her symptoms and exposure to ill contacts, and investigation into whether influenza has been documented in the community should be performed to help differentiate an influenza infection from the common cold.

Treatment

CASE 76-11, QUESTION 2: K.B. describes symptoms consistent with an influenza infection for the past 24 hours. What treatment options exist for the treatment of influenza? Why is she a candidate for a neuraminidase inhibitor agent such as zanamivir or oseltamivir?

Persons with highly suspected influenza virus infection who are at high risk of developing complications (e.g., those with pre-existing cardiac or pulmonary disease, unvaccinated infants and children, elderly, immunocompromised) may benefit from antiviral therapy if started within 48 hours after the onset of symptoms. Treatment is recommended regardless of influenza vaccination status and severity of illness in all patients who develop symptoms of influenza and who require hospitalization within the initial 48 hours of symptoms. Treatment can be considered in patients who have had symptoms for longer than 48 hours, but the benefits are less well established. Treatment should be considered in outpatients at high risk of complications with illness that is not improving or in patients who request antiviral therapy within 48 hours of onset of symptoms. Therapy will shorten the duration of illness and decrease the risk for transmission to others in close contact with persons at high risk of complications secondary to influenza infection. The benefits are less clear in patients who have had symptoms longer than 48 hours.[101]

The neuraminidase inhibitors, zanamivir (Relenza) and oseltamivir (Tamiflu), are active against influenza A and B. These agents work by selectively inhibiting the enzyme neuraminidase, an enzyme necessary for viral replication and spread. Oseltamivir is currently indicated for the prevention and treatment of influenza in patients 1 year of age and older; zanamivir is indicated for the prevention of influenza in patients 7 years of age and older and for the treatment of influenza in patients 5 years of age and older.[73,79]

Zanamivir is available as an oral powder for inhalation. For the treatment of influenza infection in adults, 10 mg (two inhalations) BID for 5 days should be used. Patients should inhale two doses separated by at least 2 hours on the first day and then two doses separated by 12 hours on days 2 through 5.[79] Bronchospasm after use can occur, and if bronchodilators are also prescribed, the bronchodilator should be used before zanamivir.[79] Proper use of the delivery system (Rotadisk/Diskhaler) is important, and thus patients should be instructed on proper use, with a demonstration of delivery technique, by the pharmacist.

Oseltamivir is pharmacologically related to zanamivir but has significantly better oral bioavailability, allowing oral dosing. It is approved for children 1 year of age or older and for adults. The dosage of oseltamivir for the treatment of influenza in adults is 75 mg BID for 5 days.[73] Pediatric dosing recommendations are available, and oseltamivir is available as a suspension for use in the pediatric population. As with zanamivir, treatment with oseltamivir must be started within 48 hours of the onset of symptoms. Common side effects include nausea, vomiting, and headache.[73] Of concern, oseltamivir-resistant influenza has been reported.[102] In addition, there are reports, predominantly in children, of self-injury and delirium after the administration of oseltamivir.[103]

Resistance to amantadine and rimantadine has increased dramatically in recent years; consequently, these agents are no longer recommended for the routine prevention or treatment of influenza infections.[97]

When administered within 48 hours of onset of illness, zanamivir and oseltamivir reduce influenza symptoms by approximately 1 day.[104–106] Information regarding the effectiveness of the neuraminidase inhibitors in preventing serious complications of influenza, such as pneumonia or worsening of chronic diseases, is limited.[97] Considering the causative agent is unknown and symptoms have been present for only 24 hours, K.B. may benefit from a neuraminidase inhibitor. Oral oseltamivir is easier to administer than inhaled zanamivir. Although oseltamivir will not cure influenza, it may reduce the severity and duration of symptoms by about 1 day. She should be treated with a 5-day course of oseltamivir.

CASE 76-12

QUESTION 1: J.T., a 74-year-old man, is brought to the ED from a nursing home with chief complaints of fever (103°F), shaking chills, cough, headache, malaise, anorexia, and photophobia. He has been ill for the past 48 hours but is much worse this evening. On physical examination, he appeared flushed, his skin was hot and moist, and he was having difficulty breathing. Vital signs included blood pressure, 150/90 mm Hg; pulse, 108 beats/minute; respiratory rate, 22 breaths/minute; and temperature, 103°F. Rales were audible on auscultation of both lungs. A chest roentgenogram showed bilateral infiltrates but no consolidation. Blood gas studies showed significant hypoxia, with a PaO_2 of 50 mm Hg (SI units, 6.665 kPa) and a $PaCO_2$ of 50 mm Hg (SI units, 6.665 kPa). J.T.'s medical history was significant for chronic bronchitis and a stroke 16 months ago. Blood, sputum, and urine cultures were obtained, and J.T. was started on antibiotics (ceftriaxone 1 g IV every 24 hours and azithromycin 500 mg IV every 24 hours). Gram stain of the sputum sample showed many WBCs but no bacteria. He was started on oxygen therapy at 4 L/minute via nasal cannula. Twenty-four hours later, his respiratory symptoms worsened, and his arterial blood gases deteriorated slightly (PaO_2, 40 mm Hg [SI units, 5.332 kPa]; $PaCO_2$, 55 mm Hg [SI units, 7.332 kPa]). J.T. was intubated, and a sputum sample was obtained and sent to the virology laboratory. Three days later, influenza A virus was isolated from the sputum. Blood, urine, and sputum cultures were all negative for bacterial pathogens. Why is this presentation consistent with influenza infection? Is antiviral treatment indicated in J.T.?

Although symptoms of influenza may vary depending on age, most patients with influenza A have an abrupt onset of fever, chills, cough, and headache. In elderly patients such as J.T. and those with underlying diseases, the course of influenza can worsen quickly, and patients are more likely to require hospitalization.

Antiviral therapy in J.T. is inappropriate. None of the antiviral agents has been studied in patients presenting with symptoms after 48 hours of onset. In addition, the antiviral agents have shown efficacy only in uncomplicated influenza.[97]

Prevention

CASE 76-12, QUESTION 2: During the next 3 weeks, two other nursing home patients develop influenza A infections. What measures should be taken to prevent a further outbreak of influenza among other residents?

INFLUENZA VACCINES

The nursing home residents and staff should receive influenza vaccine plus chemoprophylaxis with oseltamivir or zanamivir. The Centers for Disease Control and Prevention (CDC) recommends immunization of all individuals 6 months of age or older, and especially those in high-risk groups (Table 76–4).[97] The top-priority groups include all individuals who are at high risk for influenza-related complications and their household contacts. Second in priority are otherwise healthy adults 50 years of age or older and children with chronic metabolic diseases severe enough to warrant regular follow-up during the preceding year. Any child younger than 9 years in which the vaccine is indicated requires two doses of the vaccine for optimal effectiveness. The first dose should be administered as soon as the vaccine becomes available, if possible by October, and the second dose is given before influenza infection is present in the community. Vaccination should continue throughout the season, and can continue as late as February or March, depending on the duration of influenza season. However, the efficacy of influenza vaccine is incomplete (70%).[107] Therefore, the oseltamivir or zanamivir should be used in high-risk individuals who may not develop an adequate antibody response (e.g., patients with advanced HIV infection, residents of nursing homes) to supplement the protection by vaccine.[97,101]

A live, attenuated influenza vaccine (FluMist) is an option for healthy, nonpregnant individuals between the ages of 2 and 49 years. In clinical studies with matched influenza strains, live, attenuated influenza vaccine was approximately 87% effective in preventing influenza in children and provided 85% efficacy in adults.[108] Advantages of the intranasal route of administration include ease of administration and patient acceptability of an intranasal preparation compared with an intramuscular (IM) injection. However, because the vaccine is live, viral shedding can occur for 2 or more days after vaccination. Consequently, patients who are immunosuppressed and close contacts of patients who are severely immunocompromised (including health care workers who care for them) should not receive the live vaccine. Others who should not receive the live vaccine include patients with asthma or other chronic disorders of the pulmonary or cardiovascular systems, those with chronic metabolic diseases such as diabetes, renal dysfunction, or hemoglobinopathies, and children or adolescents who are receiving aspirin or other salicylates.[97]

OSELTAMIVIR AND ZANAMIVIR

Analysis of clinical trials of oseltamivir in the prevention of influenza showed a decreased incidence of laboratory-confirmed influenza: 4.8% in the placebo group and 1.2% in the treatment group.[109] The incidence of influenza in a skilled nursing facility was 4.4% in the placebo group and 0.4% in the oseltamivir group. In addition, oseltamivir lowered the rate of infection in patients exposed to influenza at home from 12% to 1%. Zanamivir has also been found to be effective in preventing infection.[110,111]

Comparative studies between neuraminidase inhibitors have not been published. Considering that oseltamivir is available in an oral formulation, it is easier to administer in nursing home patients compared with zanamivir, which requires proper use of the delivery device and a coordinated inspiratory effort.

RESPIRATORY SYNCYTIAL VIRUS INFECTIONS

Respiratory syncytial virus (RSV) causes bronchiolitis and bronchopneumonia in infants younger than 2 years. More than one-half of affected infants are infected in the first 2 years of life. Of these infants, approximately 1% to 2% will require hospitalization.[112] Children who are severely premature, immunocompromised, or with underlying congenital heart disease or lung disease may be at increased risk of mortality because of RSV.[113] Patients with RSV infection before 3 years of age are at increased risk of wheezing and asthma during childhood.[114]

RSV infections usually occur in the winter. The chest radiograph and blood gases are often abnormal, and the virus can be isolated in the nasopharyngeal secretions.

Clinical Presentation and Ribavirin Therapy

CASE 76-13

QUESTION 1: J.R., a 6-month-old infant who is lethargic, tachypneic, and cyanotic, is brought to the ED. J.R.'s medical history is significant for congenital HIV. He has a fever (102°F), his breathing is labored, and wheezing is audible on expiration. The chest roentgenograms reveal a flattened diaphragm and hyperinflated lung parenchyma. Because of hypoxemia and hypercarbia, J.R. is placed on ambient oxygen to maintain the alveolar oxygen pressure at greater than 60 mm Hg. RSV is present in the respiratory secretions. What therapy is indicated for J.R.?

The goal of RSV therapy is to increase oxygen saturation and decrease airway resistance in patients such as J.R.[115] Treatment of RSV is highly individualized, depending on the presenting signs and symptoms and associated comorbidities. Oxygen is first-line therapy; however, decrease in airway resistance may be achieved with the use of bronchodilators or corticosteroids. However, bronchodilators have been associated with improvement in only 25% of patients with RSV and this improvement is minimal.[116] Two meta-analyses found no benefits associated with corticosteroids with respect to decreasing length of stay or disease severity.[117,118] The use of corticosteroids in the treatment of RSV is not recommended.[119]

Ribavirin (Virazole) is active against many DNA and RNA viruses, including RSV. However, its benefit remains controversial. Early studies with ribavirin showed significant clinical improvement compared with placebo in both healthy children and those with underlying disease.[120] These studies reported benefit in terms of clinical recovery and improvement in arterial oxygenation. Subsequent studies found ribavirin to be ineffective in patients with a variety of risk factors.[121,122] Consequently, the routine use in previously healthy infants and children has not been clearly established. Whether ribavirin decreases the long-term sequelae and severity of illness in high-risk groups (including premature infants, patients with bronchopulmonary dysplasia, congenital heart disease, cystic fibrosis, and immunodeficiency) has not been determined.[123] Current recommendations include consideration for use of ribavirin in infants with severe disease or those at risk for severe disease such as infants who may be immunocompromised or have hemodynamically significant cardiopulmonary disease.[119] Because J.R. has an underlying immunodeficiency, ribavirin may be considered if J.R.'s condition worsens.

ADMINISTRATION OF RIBAVIRIN

CASE 76-13, QUESTION 2: How is ribavirin administered, and what precautions should be taken during drug administration in J.R.?

Ribavirin is administered as an aerosol through a collision generator that generates particles small enough (1–2 μm wide) to reach the lower respiratory tract. The concentration of the ribavirin solution in the reservoir is 20 mg/mL (6 g in 300 mL of sterile water). The dose is administered over the course of 12 to 18 hours, although in nonventilated patients, 2 g during 2 hours TID (using a 60-mg/mL solution) has been successfully used.[121] Ribavirin therapy is continued for 3 to 7 days.[124]

Ribavirin is approved for use in patients requiring mechanical ventilation. However, ribavirin is hygroscopic, and aerosol particles can deposit in the tubing and around the expiratory valve of a ventilator. The precipitated drug can obstruct the expiratory valve and alter the peak end-expiratory pressure.[124] Ribavirin has been safely used in such patients,[125,126] but close monitoring of respiratory therapy is advised to prevent this problem. In addition to the inspection of tubing, modifications of standard ventilatory circuits have been suggested.[124]

ADVERSE EFFECTS

CASE 76-13, QUESTION 3: What are the important adverse effects of ribavirin?

The most common adverse effects of ribavirin are rash, initial mild bronchospasm, and reversible skin irritation.[127] Although long-term follow-up data are limited, a study evaluating the effects of ribavirin in patients 1 year after administration showed a reduction in the incidence and severity of reactive airway disease, as well as in hospitalizations related to respiratory illness.[128] Further long-term evaluation is still necessary.

Ribavirin is contraindicated in women who are or may become pregnant during exposure to the drug. Although there are no human data, ribavirin has been found to be teratogenic or lethal to embryos in nearly all animal species in which it has been tested. Teratogenesis was evident after a single oral dose of 2.5 mg/kg in hamsters and after daily oral doses of 10 mg/kg in rats. Malformation of the skull, palate, eye, jaw, skeleton, and GI tract have been documented in animals. Ribavirin has reduced the survival of fetuses and offspring of animals tested. It is lethal to rabbit embryos in daily oral doses as small as 1 mg/kg. There are no studies that address teratogenicity in humans, but hospital personnel who are pregnant or may become pregnant should avoid exposure to this drug.[124]

It is important to consider the environmental effects of ribavirin on the personnel involved with its administration. One study found no detectable plasma or urine concentrations of ribavirin in 19 nurses, whereas another reported its presence in the RBCs of a nurse caring for a patient who received ribavirin via oxygen tent.[129] The ribavirin concentration in the air was highest when it was administered via oxygen tent, followed by mist mask, and was lowest after administration via endotracheal tubes of mechanically ventilated patients. This has led to several recommendations: (a) ribavirin aerosol should be administered solely via endotracheal tube of mechanically ventilated patients in a closed filtered system[112]; (b) children receiving ribavirin should be placed in a containment chamber equipped with a high-efficiency particulate air filter exhaust in an isolation room with negative air pressure[124]; (c) disposable full-body coverings and either a powered air-purifying respirator or disposable particulate respirator should be made available to all health care personnel[124]; and (d) men and women planning to have children should not care for patients receiving ribavirin via oxygen tents.[129] Valeant Pharmaceuticals markets an aerosol delivery system for oxygen and ribavirin that decreases the liberation of ribavirin into the environment.[124]

Prevention

CASE 76-14

QUESTION 1: S.N. is a 7-month-old boy born prematurely at 31 weeks' gestation. He has chronic lung disease of prematurity (CLD) and uses oxygen at home. RSV season will begin next month. What treatments to prevent RSV infection are available? Why is S.N. a candidate for such treatment?

Palivizumab (Synagis), a humanized monoclonal antibody made from recombinant DNA, is active against RSV and is indicated for children at risk of severe RSV respiratory tract infections (e.g., infants with CLD or a history of premature birth before 35 weeks' gestation). The efficacy of palivizumab has been demonstrated in children with a history of prematurity or CLD.[130] Children receiving monthly IM injections of palivizumab for 5 months during RSV season had a reduction in RSV hospitalizations and intensive care admissions, and had shorter hospitalizations for RSV disease. Palivizumab has replaced the use of RSV-immunoglobulins in infants because it is easier to administer (IM vs. IV), does not interfere with the response of live vaccines such as measles-mumps-rubella or varicella vaccine, and is not likely to transmit blood-borne diseases because it is a synthetic product rather than one derived from human blood.[131] A second monoclonal antibody, motavizumab, is in phase 3 clinical trials and is 20 times more potent than palivizumab.[132,133] A noninferiority trial found palivizumab and motavizumab equally effective in preventing hospitalization.[134] However, motavizumab may have a higher incidence of allergic reactions than palivizumab.[134] Motavizumab is not currently approved in the United States.

Based on S.N.'s age and his CLD, he is a candidate for palivizumab therapy.[119]

PALIVIZUMAB DOSAGE AND ADMINISTRATION

CASE 76-14, QUESTION 2: How are the doses of palivizumab calculated, and how should it be administered?

The dose of palivizumab is 15 mg/kg given IM. The first dose is given before the start of the RSV season, and then monthly doses are given for a total of 5 months. In the Northern Hemisphere, the RSV season is typically November through April.

HANTAVIRUS INFECTIONS

Rodents are the primary reservoir hosts of *Hantavirus,* and in the United States, the deer mouse (*Peromyscus maniculatus*) is the main reservoir. These viruses apparently do not cause illness in the reservoir hosts, but infection in humans occurs when infected saliva, urine, and feces produced by the rodent are inhaled as aerosols. Most patients recall exposure to rodents or rodent feces within 6 weeks of the onset of illness.[135] Person-to-person transmission has not been documented.

The case definition includes clinical evidence of (a) febrile illness characterized by unexplained adult respiratory distress syndrome (ARDS) or acute bilateral pulmonary interstitial infiltrates, or (b) an autopsy finding of noncardiogenic pulmonary edema resulting from an unexplained respiratory illness. In addition, laboratory evidence consists of (a) a positive serology (i.e., presence of hantavirus-specific immunoglobulin [Ig] M or rising titers of IgG), (b) positive immunohistochemistry for hantavirus antigen in a tissue specimen, or (c) positive PCR for hantavirus RNA in a tissue specimen.[136] Hantavirus infection can cause three different clinical diseases: hemorrhagic fever with renal syndrome, nephropathia epidemica, and hantavirus pulmonary syndrome (HPS). Hemorrhagic fever with renal syndrome and nephropathia epidemica occur in Asian and European countries. HPS occurs only in the Western Hemisphere, including North America.[137] As of December 2009, there have been 537 cases of HPS in the United States, with 36% of the cases resulting in death.[138] Most have occurred in the southwestern United States during spring and summer.

Clinical Presentation

CASE 76-15

QUESTION 1: K.C., a previously healthy 55-year-old woman, presented with an abrupt onset of fever, cough, myalgia, and shortness of breath. K.C. lives in western Texas and has not traveled out of the state during the past 6 months. Diagnostic evaluation, including a complete blood count with differential and blood and sputum cultures, was negative. On day 3, K.C. remained febrile and had vomiting, hypotension, hypoxemia, and bilateral diffuse infiltrates on the chest radiograph.

Abnormal laboratory findings included a leukocyte count of 22,000/μL with a shift to the left, platelets 70,000/μL, and albumin concentration of 2 g/dL. K.C. suddenly developed ARDS. The hantavirus IgM ELISA titer performed at the CDC from K.C.'s serum specimen was elevated. What signs and symptoms are consistent with hantavirus infection?

The clinical features of patients with HPS include fever, myalgia, headache, and cough. Abdominal pain, nausea, or vomiting may also be present. The physical examination has been unreliable. Laboratory abnormalities may include leukocytosis, thrombocytopenia, and hypoalbuminemia. The chest radiograph may initially be normal but can progress rapidly to bilateral infiltrates and ARDS. Other viral pneumonias do not typically progress to ARDS as rapidly as hantavirus infections. Because of the nonspecific signs and symptoms, some patients may be misdiagnosed as having influenza.

Treatment

CASE 76-15, QUESTION 2: How should K.C. be treated?

Supportive treatment is important. Oxygen therapy and mechanical ventilation may be necessary. Hypotension can be treated with vasopressor agents and judicious use of IV crystalloids (i.e., 0.9% NaCl) to prevent worsening of pulmonary edema. Universal precautions and respiratory isolation should be instituted.[137]

There is no FDA-approved drug to treat hantavirus infections. Based on one study in 242 patients, IV ribavirin was more effective than placebo in reducing morbidity (oliguria and hemorrhage) and mortality. IV ribavirin was given as a loading dose of 33 mg/kg, followed by 16 mg/kg every 6 hours for 4 days and 8 mg/kg every 8 hours for the next 3 days.[139]

Two other clinical trials, however, did not show similar clinical efficacy in the treatment of HPS. One open-label trial conducted by the CDC showed a mortality rate of 47% in patients who received ribavirin compared with 50% to those who did not.[140] In addition, a small trial conducted at the National Institutes of Health could not demonstrate any benefit from ribavirin.[141] K.C. should receive supportive treatment, including vasopressors, fluids, oxygen, and mechanical ventilation, if necessary.

WEST NILE VIRUS

West Nile virus (WNV) was first identified in the United States in 1999 in New York City. Since then, the virus has had rapid geographic expansion and has infected individuals in all states in the continental United States.[142] Although WNV normally occurs in tropical climates, the increase in international travel and changes in weather patterns have led to its spread.

WNV is a member of the Flaviviridae family. Culicine mosquitoes (including *Culex pipiens, Culex restuans,* and *Culex quinquefasciatus*) are the vectors, and they infect both birds and humans.[143] Infection with the virus involves direct inoculation by the infecting mosquito. Birds are reservoir hosts. WNV can infect a number of vertebrates, including horses. Transmission usually occurs from a mosquito bite; however, reports indicate that transmission of the infection has occurred through transfusions, organ transplantation, placental transfer, and via breast milk.[144] Because of the seasonal variations in the life cycle of the mosquito, cases are most commonly seen during the summer and early fall.

Diagnosis is usually made by high clinical suspicion and laboratory tests. WNV can cause a wide range of illness, from an asymptomatic disease to West Nile fever to encephalitis or meningitis. Mortality is low except in the neuroinvasive forms of the infection. Mortality rates in the elderly, particularly those older than 70 years, can be nine times higher than in the general population.[145] The CDC laboratory criteria for diagnosis of WNV includes (a) isolation of the WNV antigen or genomic sequence from a tissue, blood, CSF, or other body fluids; or (b) WNV IgM antibody in a CSF sample; (c) a fourfold rise in the antibody titer to WNV; and (d) demonstration of an IgM or rising titers of IgG to WNV in a single serum sample.[146]

Clinical Presentation

CASE 76-16

QUESTION 1: A.G. is an 84-year-old woman. She is very active and runs the yearly flower festival in the community. She was brought to the ED by her granddaughter, who found her at home, confused and complaining of a headache, fatigue, and increasing muscle weakness. She is found to have a temperature of 103°F. Her Mini-Mental Status Examination score was 21 of 30. She has decreasing muscle strength and an erythematous, macular, papular rash on her arms and legs. The complete blood count and electrolytes were normal, with the exception of slightly decreased sodium. The CSF reveals increased WBCs, increased protein, normal glucose, and positive IgM antibody to WNV. A CT scan showed no abnormalities. What signs and symptoms are indicative of WNV encephalitis?

Acute signs and symptoms of WNV include sudden onset of fever, anorexia, weakness, nausea, vomiting, eye pain, headache, altered mental status, and stiff neck. A rash may be present on the arms, legs, neck, and trunk. The rash is typically erythematous, macular, and papular with or without morbilliform eruption. Laboratory parameters may show normal or elevated WBC counts. Low serum sodium concentrations may be seen in patients with encephalitis. CSF usually shows pleocytosis, mostly with an elevation of lymphocytes, elevated protein levels, and normal glucose levels. Magnetic resonance imaging (MRI) shows some enhancement of the leptomeninges or the periventricular areas in approximately one-third of patients, but no other abnormalities or evidence of acute disease are present on either CT or MRI examination.

With disease progression, further muscle weakness and hyporeflexia may be seen. Patients may progress to a diffuse, flaccid paralysis similar to Guillain-Barré syndrome. Ataxia, extrapyramidal symptoms, cranial nerve abnormalities, myelitis, optic neuritis, and seizures may be seen.

Treatment

CASE 76-16, QUESTION 2: What treatment options are available to A.G.?

Currently, treatment of WNV infection is supportive. Patients with febrile infection usually have a self-limiting course. In severe cases, patients with muscle weakness and signs of encephalitis will require admission to an intensive care unit, and many will need mechanical ventilation. The available antiviral medications do not have any activity against WNV in vivo, although ribavirin inhibits replication in vitro.[147] Combination therapy of high-dose ribavirin and interferon-α-2b has been used in patients with severe disease with limited success. Although optimal doses have not been established, the doses needed to inhibit the virus were 2 to 3 million units of interferon and 2,400 mg of ribavirin daily.[148–150] Clinical trials are ongoing to establish the safety and efficacy of intravenous immunoglobulin and humanized monoclonal antibodies. Additionally, several vaccines for the prevention of WNV infection are in various phases of clinical trials.

SEVERE ACUTE RESPIRATORY DISTRESS SYNDROME

Severe acute respiratory distress syndrome (SARS), a highly infectious disease, was first identified in China in early 2003. Since then, the viral syndrome has been reported in several countries in East Asia, North America (particularly Canada), South America, and Europe. As of April 2004, approximately 8,000 cases have been reported, with a case fatality rate of about 10%.[151,152] No cases of SARS have been reported worldwide since 2004. Many of the cases reported in Asia and Canada have been traced to a single index case, with outbreaks clustered in apartments, hotels, health care facilities, or biomedical facilities. There is some evidence to suggest that increased age (older than 60 years) may be associated with an increased mortality risk.[153]

The disease is easily spread by airborne microdroplets. Geography and a history of recent travel to affected areas are believed to be important to an individual's likelihood of contracting the disease. In a sample of 100 suspected patients in the United States, 94% traveled within the 10 days before illness onset to an area listed in SARS case definitions.[154] SARS is believed to be transmitted mostly by close contact with an infected person (e.g., sharing eating utensils, <3-foot conversations).

A novel coronavirus, SARS coronavirus (SARS-CoV), was isolated from patients and identified as the causative agent of SARS. Inoculations of a Vero E6 cell line with throat swab specimens from patients with the diagnosis of SARS showed cytopathologic features.[155] Although the natural reservoir of SARS-CoV has not been identified, the virus has been detected in the Himalayan masked palm civet, the Chinese ferret badger, and the raccoon dog.

Clinical Presentation

CASE 76-17

QUESTION 1: N.Z. is a 48-year-old Asian woman who returned 3 days ago from a business trip to Taiwan. Two days after her return, she complained of fatigue, myalgia, chills, and headache. On the third day, she awoke feeling feverish and diaphoretic. Her temperature was 101°F. She complained of a sore throat with cough and shortness of breath when she climbed stairs. She visited her local physician, who noted rales during chest auscultation. As there was concern for SARS, the patient was admitted and placed under quarantine in a local hospital. A chest radiograph revealed bilateral interstitial infiltrates. A routine pneumonia workup was performed with pulse oximetry, blood cultures, and sputum Gram stain and culture. Blood was also collected for antibody analysis. Complete blood count and clinical chemistries were obtained, and the tests were remarkable only for lymphopenia. What signs and symptoms in N.Z. suggest that this is a case of SARS?

The case definition established by the CDC includes clinical, epidemiologic, laboratory, and exclusion criteria.[156] Symptoms of early disease include fever, chills, rigor, myalgia, headache, diarrhea, sore throat, or rhinorrhea. Mild-to-moderate illness includes temperature higher than 100.4°F and clinical findings of lower respiratory illness such as cough or shortness of breath. Severe illness includes the previous criteria plus radiographic evidence of pneumonia or acute respiratory distress syndrome. N.Z. presents to her physician with severe respiratory illness.

Probable or likely exposure to SARS-CoV is a critical component of the SARS case definition. Travel to a location with documented or suspected recent transmission of SARS-CoV and close contact with a person with mild-to-moderate or severe respiratory illness in the 10 days before the onset of symptoms are defined as possible exposures to SARS-CoV. Likely exposure is defined as close contact with a person with confirmed disease or symptoms of disease. In N.Z.'s case, travel to Taiwan classifies her as having possible exposure.

For patients suspected of having SARS in the United States, laboratory diagnosis can be confirmed by an enzyme immunoassay detecting serum antibody to SARS-CoV, isolation of SARS-CoV from a clinical specimen, or detection of SARS-CoV RNA by a reverse transcriptase PCR. Both the enzyme immunoassay and the PCR are validated by the CDC. Information regarding the most recent criteria for laboratory diagnosis can be found at the CDC website.

Although the majority of cases of infection are self-limited, initial symptoms may be followed by hypoxemia, which may progress to the need for intubation and mechanical ventilation. Typically, patients do not manifest neurologic or GI symptoms.

Treatment

CASE 76-17, QUESTION 2: What treatment options are available to N.Z.?

Treatment for SARS during the 2002 through 2003 outbreak included broad-spectrum antibiotics, ribavirin, lopinavir/ritonavir, corticosteroids, interferon, and immunoglobulin.[157] Broad-spectrum antibiotics are recommended to cover other potential pathogens until infection attributable to SARS-CoV is confirmed. Ribavirin has been used in doses ranging from 400 mg IV every day to 2 g IV followed by 1 g IV every 6 hours with a duration of 4 to 14 days.[158] Interestingly, ribavirin does not inhibit SARS-CoV in vitro, and viral loads remained elevated after death despite therapy with ribavirin.[159,160] Furthermore, adverse drug reactions, including hemolytic anemia (61%), hypocalcemia (58%), and hypomagnesemia (46%), were common. Two of three in vitro studies of lopinavir and ritonavir showed activity against SARS-CoV. Lopinavir 400 mg PO BID with ritonavir 100 mg BID may be useful in the treatment of SARS, but data are limited.[157] Treatments with various corticosteroids, interferon, and immunoglobulin remain controversial. No treatment guidelines are available owing to the lack of prospective randomized controlled trials.

THE COMMON COLD

The most prevalent viral infection is the common cold. In the United States, approximately 62 million cases of the common cold occur annually.[161] An estimated 20 million and 22 million days of absence from work and school, respectively, occur. The frequency of the occurrence of a cold is greater in younger children and decreases with increasing age. Although the common cold is self-limiting, otitis media occurs in approximately 20% of children after infection.[162]

Many viruses have been isolated from patients with respiratory infections, but rhinovirus is the most common viral pathogen.[163] Rhinovirus accounts for approximately 34% of all respiratory illnesses. More than 100 different serotypes of rhinovirus exist, and the prevalence of each varies with time and geography. Other pathogens include coronavirus, parainfluenza, RSV, adenovirus, and enterovirus. Because of the number of pathogens known to cause the common cold, development of an effective vaccine remains difficult.

Treatment for the common cold is directed at pharmacologic treatment of symptoms. Nonsteroidal anti-inflammatory drugs, oral or intranasal decongestants, antihistamines, and antitussives may be used. However, these products provide minimal relief of symptoms and do not shorten the natural course of infection.[164–166] In pediatric patients younger than 4 years, the use of cough and cold medications is not recommended by the FDA because of the deaths associated with their use.[167–169] Currently, there are no specific antiviral treatments for the common cold.

Prevention

CASE 76-18

QUESTION 1: J.C. comes into the pharmacy asking for an herbal product that will help him prevent colds this upcoming cold season. He states that last year he had three colds and his neighbor had none. His neighbor had mentioned an herbal product he had been taking. J.C. cannot remember the name of the product but wonders whether there are any products that may be helpful.

Zinc

Zinc, a dietary supplement, has been studied in both the prevention and treatment of the common cold. The proposed mechanism of action is that the rhinovirus 3C protease is inhibited by zinc, and the inhibition of this enzyme prevents viral replication. In vitro, zinc has been shown to have antiviral activity. Several trials conducted in the past several decades have produced conflicting results on the benefits of zinc in decreasing symptom severity or duration. A meta-analysis found no clear evidence to support the use of zinc lozenges in the treatment or prevention of the common cold.[170,171] Patients who took zinc lozenges for the common cold complained of mouth irritation, unpleasant taste, feeling sick, and diarrhea. Zinc is not currently recommended for treatment or prophylaxis of the common cold.

Echinacea

Echinacea is an herbal product extracted from the *Echinacea* plant, which belongs to the Compositae family. Echinacea is believed to stimulate the immune system, specifically phagocytosis. Some clinical trials using echinacea have shown positive results in decreasing the incidence of infection when compared with placebo, but the results remain inconclusive. No benefits were shown in decreasing the severity and duration of the common cold when compared with placebo. In trials evaluating the effectiveness of echinacea in the treatment of the common cold, 9 of 16 trials found a decrease in the severity and duration of symptoms.[172] One study showed no benefit of echinacea versus placebo but did show an increased incidence of rash in the treatment group.[173] Because the current data are inconclusive and owing to the variability of echinacea concentrations in the available products, use of echinacea in the prevention and treatment of the common cold is not recommended.[174]

KEY REFERENCES AND WEBSITES

A full list of references for this chapter can be found at **http://thepoint.lww.com/AT10e.** Below are the key references and websites for this chapter, with the corresponding reference number in this chapter found in parentheses after the reference.

Key References

American Academy of Pediatrics Subcommittee on Diagnosis and Management of Bronchiolitis. Diagnosis and management of bronchiolitis. *Pediatrics*. 2006;118:1174. (119)

Chen N et al. Corticosteroids for preventing postherpetic neuralgia. *Cochrane Database Syst Rev*. 2010;(12):CD005582. (86)

Fiore AE et al. Prevention and control of influenza with vaccines: recommendations of the Advisory Committee on Immunization Practices (ACIP), 2010. *MMWR Recomm Rep*. 2010;59(RR-8):1. (97)

Harpaz R et al. Prevention of herpes zoster. Recommendations of the Advisory Committee on Immunization Practices (ACIP). *MMWR Recomm Rep*. 2008;57(RR-5):1. (85)

James SH et al. Antiviral therapy for herpesvirus central nervous system infections: neonatal herpes simplex virus infection, herpes simplex encephalitis, and congenital cytomegalovirus infection. *Antiviral Res*. 2009;83:207. (13)

[No authors listed]. American Academy of Pediatrics Committee on Infectious Diseases: the use of acyclovir in otherwise healthy children with varicella. *Pediatrics*. 1993;91:674. (60)

Vassilev ZP et al. Safety and efficacy of over-the-counter cough and cold medicines for use in children. *Expert Opin Drug Saf*. 2010;9:233. (168)

Key Websites

Centers for Disease Control and Prevention. All About Hantaviruses. Hantavirus Pulmonary Syndrome (HPS). http://www.cdc.gov/ncidod/diseases/hanta/hps/. Accessed January 21, 2011. (143)

Centers for Disease Control and Prevention. Severe Acute Respiratory Syndrome. http://www.cdc.gov/ncidod/sars/. Accessed January 21, 2011.

Centers for Disease Control and Prevention. West Nile Virus. http://www.cdc.gov/ncidod/dvbid/westnile/. Accessed January 21, 2011.

77 Viral Hepatitis

Curtis D. Holt

CORE PRINCIPLES

	CHAPTER CASES
1 Hepatitis A virus (HAV) is a worldwide, acute self-limited disease transmitted via the fecal-oral route. Hepatocyte injury is caused by a cytopathic and immunologic response, which can result in jaundice and increased liver function tests. Treatment measures are usually supportive and aimed toward prevention (pre-exposure and postexposure) through vaccination.	**Case 77-1 (Questions 1–3), Case 77-2 (Question 1), Case 77-3 (Question 1)**
2 Hepatitis B virus (HBV) is transmitted through percutaneous or perinatal exposure, blood, blood products, or sexual contact. HBV has an acute phase with resolution (or rarely, acute liver failure [ALF]) and a chronic phase. Over the course of decades, the chronic phase can lead to hepatic cirrhosis and death. Patients with chronic infection require treatment with pegylated interferons, interferons, nucleoside or nucleotide reverse transcriptase inhibitors. Several effective prophylactic strategies (immunoglobulin and nucleoside or nucleotide reverse transcriptase inhibitors) are used to prevent HBV reinfection.	**Case 77-4 (Questions 1–4), Case 77-5 (Questions 1, 2), Case 77-6 (Questions 1–3), Case 77-7 (Question 1), Case 77-8 (Question 1), Case 77-9 (Question 1), Case 77-10 (Questions 1, 2), Case 77-11 (Question 1), Case 77-12 (Questions 1–14)**
3 Hepatitis C virus (HCV) is transmitted through percutaneous or perinatal exposure, blood, blood products, or sexual contact. HCV has an acute phase and subsequent chronic phase (over the course of several decades) that can lead to cirrhosis, decompensated liver disease, and death. Acute clinical manifestations are similar to those for HAV and HBV. Treatment of acute HCV infection has been with interferon-based monotherapy, whereas chronic HCV infection is primarily managed with pegylated interferons plus ribavirin. Several agents (telaprevir, boceprevir) are under investigation.	**Case 77-13 (Questions 1–9), Case 77-14 (Question 1)**
4 Hepatitis D virus (HDV) is a small RNA virus that requires coinfection with HBV for replication. HDV infections are most likely in persons with percutaneous exposure. HDV leads to a much higher risk of ALF. Prevention strategies rely on successful immunization of HBV. In patients with chronic HDV infection, interferon and pegylated interferon (plus or minus ribavirin or oral antivirals) are implemented.	**(no cases)**
5 Hepatitis E virus is transmitted via the fecal-oral route, especially through contaminated water. Recovery from acute illness usually occurs; however, maternal mortality is significant. Treatment measures are limited, but ribavirin has been used in some patients.	**(no cases)**

Five distinctly separate hepatitis viruses cause liver disease. A sixth virus also has been identified, but has yet to be implicated in liver disease. Five of these viruses are RNA viruses, and one is a DNA virus. The individual viral types can be distinguished by serologic assays and, in some instances, by genotyping. Although progress in the area of disease prevention has occurred, advances in treatment have been limited because of the large amount of virus produced and its rapid mutation. People with chronic hepatitis C produce approximately 1 trillion virus particles daily, compared with 100 billion particles daily for those infected with chronic hepatitis B and 10 billion particles daily for those with human immunodeficiency virus (HIV) infection. This chapter reviews the virology, epidemiology, pathogenesis, clinical manifestations, diagnosis, natural history, prevention, and treatment strategies for viral hepatitis A through E.

TABLE 77-1
Hepatitis Nomenclature

Hepatitis Type	Antigen	Corresponding Antibody	Comments
A	Hepatitis A virus (HAV)	Hepatitis A antibody (anti-HAV)	RNA virus; present in stool and serum early in course of hepatitis A
B	Hepatitis B surface antigen (HBsAg)	Hepatitis B surface antibody (anti-HBs)	DNA virus; found in serum in >90% of patients with acute hepatitis B, anti-HBs appears after infection and confers immunity
	Hepatitis B core antigen (HBcAg)	Hepatitis B core antibody (anti-HBc)	Anti-HBc detected in serum during and after acute infection
	Hepatitis B envelope antigen (HBeAg)	HB envelope antibody (anti-HBe)	HBeAg correlates with infectivity; suggestive of active viral replication
C	Hepatitis C antigen (HCAg)	Hepatitis C antibody (anti-HCV)	RNA virus; previously known as posttransfusion NANB hepatitis
D	Hepatitis D antigen (HDAg)	Hepatitis D antibody (anti-HDV)	Defective RNA virus; requires presence of HBsAg
E	Hepatitis E antigen (HEAg)	Hepatitis E antibody (anti-HEV)	RNA virus present in stool; cause of enteric NANB hepatitis

NANB, non-A, non-B hepatitis.

CAUSATIVE AGENTS AND CHARACTERISTICS

Viral hepatitis is a major cause of morbidity and mortality in the United States.[1–3] At least six distinct agents are responsible for viral hepatitis. These hepatotrophic viruses are identified by the letters A through E as follows: (a) type A hepatitis caused by hepatitis A virus (HAV), (b) type B hepatitis caused by hepatitis B virus (HBV), (c) type C hepatitis caused by hepatitis C virus (HCV), (d) delta hepatitis caused by the HBV-associated hepatitis D virus (HDV), and (e) type E hepatitis caused by the hepatitis E virus (HEV) (Table 77-1). Hepatitis A through E viruses differ in their immunologic characteristics and epidemiologic patterns (Table 77-2) Fecal-oral transmission is the primary mode of infection for HAV and HEV, whereas percutaneous transmission is characteristic of HBV, HCV, and HDV.[1–3] Several other viruses primarily affect nonhepatic organ systems and may secondarily induce a hepatitislike syndrome. These include the Epstein-Barr virus (infectious mononucleosis); cytomegalovirus; herpes simplex viruses; varicella-zoster virus; and rubella, rubeola, and mumps viruses (Table 77-3).

Definitions of Acute and Chronic Hepatitis

Viral hepatitis can present as either an acute or chronic illness. Acute hepatitis is defined as an illness with a discrete date of onset with jaundice or increased serum aminotransferase concentrations greater than 2.5 times the upper limit of normal.[1–4] Acute infection lasts as long as, but not exceeding, 6 months.

Chronic hepatitis is an inflammatory condition of the liver that involves ongoing hepatocellular necrosis for 6 months or more beyond the onset of acute illness.[5–7] The causes of chronic hepatitis are shown in Table 77-3. The most common cause of chronic hepatitis is HBV or HCV.[1,3] Drug-induced and autoimmune chronic hepatitis occur less frequently, whereas metabolic disorders and HDV chronic hepatitis are relatively rare.[1–3,8–10] Neither HAV nor HEV infections cause chronic hepatitis.

Serologic Evaluation in Presumed Chronic Hepatitis

Serologies are useful in diagnosing viral hepatitis. Antibodies against hepatitis A virus (anti-HAV), hepatitis B surface antigen (HBsAg), and hepatitis C virus (anti-HCV) are useful diagnostic tests. A diagnosis of acute HAV infection includes the presence of immunoglobulin M (IgM) anti-HAV. If HBsAg is present, further testing for hepatitis B envelope antigen (HBeAg) and HBV-DNA confirms the presence of active viral replication and assesses the viral load. Testing for hepatitis D antibody (anti-HDV) also should be performed in patients with hepatitis B to evaluate the possibility of coexisting delta hepatitis. If serology is negative, rare but treatable causes of chronic active hepatitis should be excluded. These include alcoholic liver disease, Wilson disease, α_1-antitrypsin deficiency, and drug-induced chronic active hepatitis. Drugs associated with reversible chronic active hepatitis syndrome include methyldopa,[11] nitrofurantoin,[12] isoniazid,[13] and, rarely, sulfonamides[14] and propylthiouracil.[15]

HEPATITIS A VIRUS

Virology and Epidemiology

HAV is a 27-nm diameter, single-stranded RNA virus that is classified as a picornavirus in the *Hepatovirus* genus (Table 77-2).[2,16,17]

For an electron micrograph of HAV, go to http://thepoint.lww.com/AT10e.

HAV has a worldwide distribution.[1,2,17–20] The prevalence of infection is related to the quality of the water supply, level of sanitation, and age.[1,2,17–21] Incidence data are unreliable, however, because the disease is frequently mild and often unrecognized, resulting in underreporting.[1,2,17–21] The primary mode of transmission is person-to-person via the fecal-oral route.[1,2,17–26] The virus resists degradation by environmental conditions, gastric acid, and digestive enzymes in the upper gastrointestinal (GI) tract, thus, is readily spread within a population. Fecally contaminated water or also food is a significant mode of transmission.[1,2,17–25] Children are considered an important reservoir.[1,2,17–25]

In the United States, the reported incidence of HAV is 10.8 cases per 100,000, and it is usually associated with outbreaks in lower socioeconomic groups or common-source outbreaks (e.g., day-care centers).[1,2,17–22] Rates in males are greater than those in females by about 20%.[1,2,22] Children aged 5 to 14 years and Native

TABLE 77-2
Comparison of the Etiologic Forms of Hepatitis A, B, C, D, and E Viruses

Virus	HAV	HBV	HCV	HDV	HEV
Genome	RNA	DNA	RNA	RNA	RNA
Family	Picornavirus	Hepadnavirus	Flavivirus	Satellite	Hepeviridae
Size (nm)	27	42	30–60	40	32
Incubation (days) [mean]	15–50 [30]	45–180 [80]	15–160	21–140 [35]	15–65 [42]
Transmission					
Oral	Common	Rare	Rare	No	Yes, common
Percutaneous	Rare	Common	Common	Common	Unknown
Sexual	No	Common	Common	Common	No
Perinatal	No	Common	Rare	Common	Rare
Onset	Sudden	Insidious	Insidious	Insidious	Sudden
Clinical illness	70%–80% adults 5% children	10%–15%	5%–10%	10%	70%–80% adults
Icteric presentation					
Children	<10%	30%	25%	Unknown	Unknown
Adults	30%	5%–20%	5%–10%	25%	Common
Peak alanine aminotransferase (ALT) (units/L)	800–1,000	1,000–1,500	300–800	1,000–1,500	800–1,000
Incidence of acute liver failure (%)	<1	<1	<1	2–7.5	<1; higher in pregnant women
Serum diagnosis					
Acute infection	Anti-HAV IgM	HBsAg, anti-HBc IgM	HCV-RNA (anti-HCV)	Anti-HDV IgM	Anti-HEV IgG (seroconversion)
Chronic infection		HBsAg Anti-HBc IgG	Anti-HCV (ELISA) RIBA	Anti-HDV IgG	NA
Viral markers	HAV RNA	HBV DNA DNA polymerase	HCV RNA	HDV RNA	Viruslike particles
Immunity	Anti-HAV IgG	Anti-HBs	NA	NA	Anti-HEV IgG
Case-fatality rate	0.1%–2.7% 0.15%–1.7%	1%–3%	1%–2%	<1% coinfect	0.5%–4% 1.5%–21% pregnant women
Complete recovery	>97%	85%–97%	50%	90%	99%
Incidence of chronic infection	0%	2%–7% >90% neonates	50%	80% superinfect ≤5% coinfection	0%
Carrier state	No	Yes	Yes	Yes	No
Risk of hepatocellular carcinoma	No	Yes	Yes	Yes	No
Drug treatment	None	Pegylated interferon, interferon, tenofovir, entecavir, adefovir, telbivudine, lamivudine	Pegylated interferon + ribavirin, pegylated interferon, interferon, telaprevir, boceprevir	Pegylated interferon, interferon	None

ELISA, enzyme-linked immunosorbent assay; NA, not applicable; RIBA, recombinant immunoblot assay.

Americans have the highest incidence of HAV.[2,22] Vaccination in children (age 12–23 months and maintenance from 2 to 18 years) has resulted in a decline in the incidence of HAV infection to 1.9 cases per 100,000 population.[2,19,22] Similar rates of decline have been demonstrated in Native Americans and Hispanics. Additionally, cyclic outbreaks of HAV have been reported among users of injection and noninjection drugs and in men who have sex with men.[2,22] Considering the widespread presence of anti-HAV, the virus has a high attack rate, with 70% to 90% of those exposed ultimately becoming infected.[2,18,19,22]

The most common risk factors for acquiring HAV include close contact with a person positive for HAV (26%), employment or attendance at a day-care center (14%), injection drug use (11%), recent travel (4%), and association with a suspected food- or water-borne outbreak (3%).[1,2,18–26] Up to 42% of reported HAV infections have no known source for infection.[22] Exceedingly rare causes of HAV include transfusion of blood or blood products collected from donors during the viremic phase of their infection and from contact with experimentally infected nonhuman primates.[19,22] Percutaneous transmission is rare because no asymptomatic carrier state for HAV exists and the incubation period is brief.[1,2,18–26] Occupations at risk for HAV infection include sewage workers, hospital cleaning personnel, day-care staff, and pediatric nurses.[1,2,18–26] HAV is the most common preventable (e.g., vaccination) infection in travelers visiting locations with poor hygienic conditions.[1,26] Up to 22% of patients with acute HAV require hospitalization with an associated cost of more than $400 million annually.[17,22]

Pathogenesis

Although the exact mechanism of injury is unknown,[17,23,27] viral replication occurs within the liver.

TABLE 77-3
Etiologies of Chronic Hepatitis

Viral Infections
Hepatitis viruses (B, C, D)
Cytomegalovirus (CMV)
Epstein-Barr virus (EBV)
Rubella virus
Drug-Induced
Methyldopa
Nitrofurantoin
Isoniazid
Sulfonamides
Propylthiouracil
Metabolic Disorders
Wilson disease
α_1-Antitrypsin deficiency
Autoimmune hepatitis

ONLINE CONTENT

For a schematic of the replication cycle of HAV, go to http://thepoint.lww.com/AT10e.

Subsequent hepatocyte death results in viral elimination and eventual resolution of the clinical illness.

Natural History

HAV is typically a benign, self-limited infection, with recovery within 2 months of disease onset. Two atypical courses of acute HAV infection have also been described: prolonged cholestasis and relapsing hepatitis.[2,17] In patients with prolonged cholestasis, the duration of jaundice exceeds 12 weeks and is associated with pruritus, fatigue, loose stools, and weight loss. Aminotransferase concentrations during this period are less than 500 units/L. Relapsing or polyphasic HAV occurs in 6% to 12% of both adult and pediatric patients and is characterized by an initial phase of acute infection followed by remission (duration of 4–15 weeks), with subsequent relapse. Aminotransferase concentrations often normalize during the time of remission but increase to greater than 1,000 units/L with relapse. HAV RNA is detectable in the serum, and HAV is usually recovered from the stool during relapse. Fulminant hepatitis A is rare, occurring in 0.014% to 3.0% of the population infected with HAV, but often fatal.[2,17,28] Patients older than 40 years of age or younger than 11 years are more susceptible to HAV-induced fulminant hepatic failure (FHF) Additionally, low serum HAV RNA levels and high bilirubin levels are significantly associated with FHF, suggesting that HAV-related liver failure may be caused by a host immune response.[2,17,28] Chronic HAV does not exist. Typically, the course of HAV includes an incubation phase, an acute hepatitis phase, and a convalescent phase. Complete clinical recovery is usually seen within 2 months in 60% of patients and virtually all patients within 6 months after HAV infection.

Clinical Manifestations

CASE 77-1

QUESTION 1: E.T., a 34-year-old medical sales representative, presents to the emergency department (ED) with acute onset of jaundice and "dark urine." He was in good health until 2 weeks ago, when he noted feeling fatigued and weak, which he attributed to his demanding work schedule. He also recalled having a mild headache, loss of appetite, muscle pain, diarrhea, and low-grade fevers from 99°F to 101°F. He attributed these symptoms to the flu and took acetaminophen with plenty of fluids. His symptoms persisted until yesterday, when they seemed to resolve unexplainably. He then noted his urine was cola-colored. This morning, he noted jaundice of his eyes and skin and sought medical attention.

E.T.'s medical history includes a recent respiratory tract infection, treated successfully with levofloxacin. His social history is significant for frequenting the local oyster bar, where he regularly ingests raw oysters. He denies smoking and recent travel outside the United States, but admits to occasional alcohol consumption. E.T. has no history of sexual exposure, needle use, or transfusions. His current medications include oral (PO) diazepam 5 mg at bedtime (HS) as needed (PRN) for "muscle spasms," but he has not taken diazepam for "several months." He also has a seizure disorder sustained after a motorcycle accident 2 years before admission, for which he takes phenytoin 400 mg PO every HS.

Physical examination is significant for a well-developed, well-nourished man in no acute distress. He is alert and oriented, with a temperature of 99°F. His sclerae and skin are icteric, and his abdomen is positive for a tender, enlarged liver and right upper quadrant pain. Laboratory tests reveal the following values:

Hemoglobin (Hgb), 16 g/dL
Hematocrit (Hct), 44%
White blood cell (WBC) count, 5,500 cells/μL
Aspartate transaminase (AST), 120 units/L
Alanine aminotransferase (ALT), 240 units/L
Alkaline phosphatase, 86 units/L
Total bilirubin, 3.2 mg/dL
Direct bilirubin, 1.5 mg/dL
Phenytoin concentration, 12 mg/L (normal, 10–20 mg/L)

The albumin, prothrombin time (PT), blood glucose, and electrolytes all are within normal limits. E.T. is negative for anti-HCV, HBeAg, HBsAg, and hepatitis B core antibody (anti-HBc), but is positive for IgM anti-HAV. What clinical features and serologic markers are consistent with viral hepatitis in E.T.?

The incubation period for HAV is 15 to 50 days (average, 28) after inoculation (Table 77-2). The host is usually asymptomatic during this stage of the infection; thus, E.T. is beyond the inoculation phase of the disease. Because HAV titers are highest in the acute-phase fecal samples, the period of infectivity is 14 and 21 days before the onset of jaundice to 7 or 8 days after jaundice. Thus, E.T. should be considered infectious at this time. In HAV infections, acute-phase serum and saliva are less infectious than fecal samples, whereas urine and semen samples are not infectious. Family members and persons recently in immediate contact with E.T. should be notified.

The symptoms of acute viral hepatitis caused by HAV, HBV, HCV, HDV, and HEV are similar. The onset of symptoms in HAV infection, however, is less insidious than those seen with HBV and HCV infection.[2,17,23] Generally, symptoms of HAV infection present a week or more before the onset of jaundice. The likelihood of having symptoms is related to age. In children younger than 6 years of age, 70% of infections are asymptomatic, whereas older children and adults have symptomatic disease with jaundice occurring in more than 70% of cases.[2,17,23,29,30] E.T. has signs and symptoms of acute HAV infection, including the nonspecific prodromal symptoms of fatigue, weakness, anorexia, nausea, and

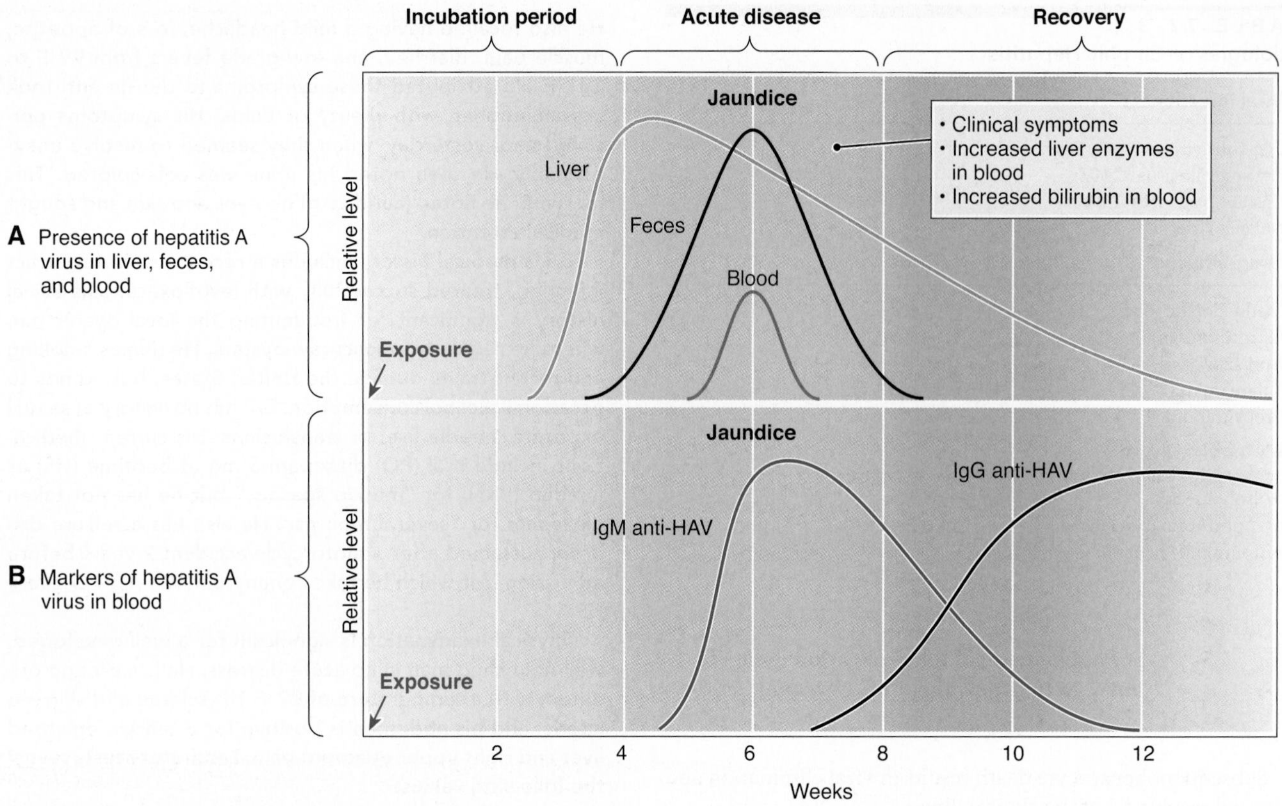

FIGURE 77-1 Typical course of hepatitis A. anti-HAV, antibody to HAV; HAV, hepatitis A virus. (Adapted with permission from Thomas H. McConnell, *The Nature of Disease Pathology for the Health Professions*, Philadelphia: Lippincott Williams & Wilkins, 2007.)

vomiting. Abdominal pain and hepatomegaly are common. Less common symptoms include fever, headache, arthralgias, myalgias, and diarrhea. Within 1 to 2 weeks of the onset of prodromal symptoms, patients may enter an icteric phase with symptoms, including clay-colored stools, dark urine, scleral icterus, and frank jaundice. The dark urine is caused by bilirubin, generally occurring shortly before the onset of jaundice. E.T. should be questioned about the presence of pale stools (light gray or yellow), which usually is observed during the icteric phase. His scleral icterus is strongly suggestive of viral hepatitis. Icteric infections usually occur in adults, and are 3.5 times more common than the nonicteric presentation that is seen in children.[2,17,23,29,30]

The results of E.T.'s liver function tests (LFTs) (e.g., elevations in AST, ALT, and bilirubin) also are consistent with viral hepatitis. Serum transaminase concentrations increase during the prodromal phase (usually ALT > AST) of HAV infection, peaking before the onset of jaundice. These concentrations are often greater than 500 units/L, and decline at an initial rate of 75% per week, followed by a slower rate of decline thereafter. Serum bilirubin peaks after aminotransferase activity and rarely exceeds 10 mg/dL. Bilirubin levels decline more slowly than aminotransferases and generally normalize within 3 months. Right upper quadrant tenderness, mild liver enlargement, and splenomegaly may also be present in patients with acute HAV infection.

Extrahepatic Manifestations

CASE 77-1, QUESTION 2: Are there any additional complications that E.T. could experience from his acute HAV infection?

With the appearance of jaundice, prodromal pruritus and extrahepatic manifestations can occur, usually in patients with a more protracted illness. Thus, E.T. should be monitored for additional manifestations of HAV infection, including immune complex–associated rash, leukocytoclastic vasculitis, glomerulonephritis, cryoglobulinemia (less likely than with HCV), and arthritis.

Diagnosis and Serology

Diagnostic methods for detecting HAV antigen and anti-HAV are listed in Figure 77-1. Detection of IgM to HAV in a patient who presents with clinical characteristics of hepatitis or in an asymptomatic patient with elevated transaminases is consistent with acute HAV infection. HAV IgG appears after IgM and is indicative of previous exposure and immunity to HAV, whereas a rising IgG is consistent with recent exposure.[2,17,23,30] Anti-HAV IgM is commonly present throughout the disease course (16–40 weeks), usually peaking early and declining to undetectable levels 3 to 4 months after the initial infection.[30,31] One-quarter of patients infected with HAV have IgM present for up to 6 months, and occasionally longer. HAV IgG appears early in the convalescent phase and is detectable for decades after the acute infection resolves, with a slowly declining titer.[17,23,30] Both enzyme-linked immunosorbent assay (ELISA) and radioimmunoassay methods of antibody detection are sensitive, specific, and reliable to diagnose acute HAV infection. E.T. has a positive IgM anti-HAV, consistent with acute HAV infection. E.T. has a negative IgM anti-HBc test, ruling out acute HBV infection.[17,23,30]

Treatment

GENERAL MEASURES

HAV infection is usually a self-limited disease. Drug treatment does not significantly alter the course of the disease. Acute viral hepatitis is generally treated on an outpatient basis as long as regular medical evaluation occurs. Patients should continue their normal activities as much as possible while avoiding physical exhaustion. Intravenous (IV) fluid and electrolyte replacement, nutritional support, and the use of antiemetics may be necessary in some patients. Antipyretics (acetaminophen) should not be used because the risk of FHF could increase. Considering that hemolysis or acute kidney injury are possible, a regular assessment of renal function with a complete blood count should also be performed. Patients should abstain from alcohol during the acute phase of the disease. After resolution of symptoms and serum biochemical abnormalities, moderate alcohol intake is no longer contraindicated.

Adjustment of Medication Doses

CASE 77-1, QUESTION 3: Should E.T.'s medications be adjusted during the acute phase of HAV infection?

Dosage adjustments for hepatically eliminated drugs in the setting of liver disease are difficult to predict. This is because hepatic metabolism is complex, involving numerous oxidative and conjugative pathways that are variably affected in hepatic disease. In renal disease, creatinine serves as an endogenous marker to predict the clearance of renally eliminated drugs. In hepatic disease, however, no reliable endogenous markers exist to predict drug hepatic clearance. Laboratory tests that approximate the synthetic function of the liver (albumin, PT) and biliary clearance (bilirubin) are used to estimate the degree of hepatic impairment, but these tests are not dependable in predicting alterations in pharmacokinetic parameters for hepatically metabolized drugs.

Unnecessary and potentially hepatotoxic medications should be avoided during the acute phase of the illness. When drug therapy is indicated with agents that undergo hepatic elimination, it is prudent to use the lowest doses possible to achieve the desired therapeutic effect. Data from small pharmacokinetic studies in patients with acute viral hepatitis are shown in Table 77-4.[31–49]

TABLE 77-4
Half-Life Data for Various Agents in Acute Viral Hepatitis Compared With Reference Normal Controls

	Half-life (hours)	
Drug[7]	**Normal Controls**	**Acute Viral Hepatitis**
Acetaminophen[31]	2.1	3.2
Aspirin[31]	0.4	No change[a]
Carbamazepine[32]	12	Increased
Chlordiazepoxide[33]	11.1	91
Chloramphenicol[34]	4.6	11.6
Clofibrate[35]	17.5	No change
Diazepam[36]	37.2	74.5
Lidocaine[37]	3.7	6.4
Lorazepam[38]	21.7	No change
Meperidine[39]	3.4	7
Nitrendipine[40]	2.2	No change
Norfloxacin[41]	4.3	No change
Oxazepam[42]	5.1	No change
Phenobarbital[43]	86	No change
Phenytoin[44]	13.2	No change
Quinine[45]	10	17
Rifampin[46]	2.5	6.5
Theophylline[47]	7.7	19.2
Tolbutamide[48]	5.9	4.0
Warfarin[49]	25	No change

[a] No change indicates that the difference between patients with acute viral hepatitis and normal control patients is not statistically significant.

E.T. should be advised to discontinue diazepam because this medication undergoes extensive hepatic biotransformation and limited data suggest this agent accumulates in the setting of acute viral hepatitis.[36] If E.T. should require drug therapy for muscle spasms, he should either decrease the diazepam dose or consider using an alternative agent (e.g., lorazepam) that does not accumulate in acute viral hepatitis.[38] Patients with acute viral hepatitis do not require phenytoin dosage adjustments.[44] Because E.T.'s plasma phenytoin concentration is within the desired therapeutic range, no dosage adjustment is needed.

Prevention of Hepatitis A

Prevention of hepatitis A infection can be achieved through immunoprophylactic measures. Immunoprophylaxis may be passive, active, or a combination of both. In passive immunization, temporary protective antibody in the form of immunoglobulin is administered. In active immunization, a vaccine is administered to induce the formation of protective antibody. Prophylaxis can be administered before (pre-exposure prophylaxis) or after exposure (postexposure prophylaxis).

Pre-Exposure Prophylaxis

CASE 77-2

QUESTION 1: M.D., a 22-year-old student, is preparing for a 2-week vacation to Thailand. He plans to travel 3 months from now and wonders whether he should receive prophylaxis for HAV.

IMMUNOGLOBULIN

Before hepatitis A vaccine was available, the sole therapy for pre-exposure prophylaxis of hepatitis A infection was immunoglobulin. Although passive immunization with immunoglobulin alone is highly effective in preventing HAV infection,[17,22] the duration of protection is short. When used for pre-exposure prophylaxis (e.g., in travelers who are allergic to a vaccine component or decide against vaccination), a dose of 0.02 mL/kg of immunoglobulin administered intramuscularly (IM) confers protection for less than 3 months, and an IM dose of 0.06 mL/kg confers protection for 5 months or longer.[22,23,30]

VACCINE

Active immunization with hepatitis A vaccine has largely supplanted the use of immunoglobulin for pre-exposure prophylaxis of infection caused by HAV. Formulations of inactivated hepatitis A vaccine available in the United States include Havrix and Vaqta. Both vaccines are formalin-inactivated preparations of attenuated HAV strains. The manufacturers use differing units to express antigen content of their respective vaccines. Havrix dosages are expressed in ELISA units, and Vaqta dosages are expressed as units of hepatitis A antigen.

Dosing Regimen

Havrix is available in two formulations that differ according to age: for persons 12 months to 18 years of age, 720 ELISA units (0.5 mL) per dose in a two-dose schedule; and for persons older than 19 years of age, 1,440 ELISA units (1.0 mL) per dose in a two-dose schedule (Table 77-5).[17,22,23,50–53] This vaccine is usually injected IM into the deltoid muscle with a booster dose administered 6 to 12 months later. The pediatric Havrix formulation (three-dose schedule) is no longer available. Vaqta is available in two formulations, and the formulations differ according to the person's age: for persons 12 months to 18 years of age,

TABLE 77-5
Recommended Doses of Hepatitis A Vaccines[22,50,52]

Age at Vaccination	Dose (Volume)[a]	Schedule (Months)[b]
Havrix		
Children 12 months–18 years	720 ELISA units (0.5 mL)	0, 6–12
Adults >19 years	1,440 ELISA units (1.0 mL)	0, 6–12
Vaqta		
Children 12 months–18 years	25 units (0.5 mL)	0, 6–18
Adults >19 years	50 units (1.0 mL)	0, 6

[a] Enzyme-linked immunosorbent assay (ELISA) units.
[b] Zero months represents timing of the initial dose; subsequent numbers represent months after the initial dose.

25 units (0.5 mL) in a two-dose schedule; for persons older than 19 years of age, 50 units (1.0 mL) per dose in a two-dose schedule (Table 77-5).[17,22,23,50–54] Likewise, this vaccine is usually injected IM into the deltoid muscle with a booster dose administered 6 to 18 months later.[22,50]

COMBINATION VACCINE

The US Food and Drug Administration (FDA) has also licensed a combined HAV and HBV vaccine (Twinrix) for use in persons aged 18 years or older.[17,22,54] Twinrix is composed of the same antigenic components used in Havrix and Engerix-B. Each dose of Twinrix contains at least 720 ELISA units of inactivated HAV and 20 mcg of recombinant HBsAg. Trace amounts of thimerosal (<1 mcg) are also present from the manufacturing process.

Primary immunization consists of three doses, given on a 0-, 1-, and 6- month schedule, the same that is used for single-antigen hepatitis B vaccine.[22,54] Any person 18 years of age or older having an indication for both hepatitis A and hepatitis B vaccine can be given Twinrix, including patients with chronic liver disease, users of illicit injectable drugs, men who have sex with men, and persons with clotting factor disorders who receive therapeutic blood products.[22,54] For international travel, hepatitis A vaccine is recommended; hepatitis B vaccine is recommended for travelers to areas of high or intermediate hepatitis B endemicity who plan to stay for longer than 6 months and have frequent close contact with the local population.[22,54]

At 1 month after completion of the three-dose series, seroconversion for anti-HAV (titer >20 milli-international units/mL) was elicited in 99.9% of vaccines, and protective antibodies against HBsAg (anti-HBs >10 milli-international units/mL) were elicited in 98.5% of vaccinees.[17,22,53,54] The persistence of anti-HAV and antibody to HBsAg (anti-HBs) after administration is similar to that after single-antigen hepatitis A and B vaccine administration at 4-year follow-up. Observed adverse effects were generally similar in type and frequency to those reported after vaccination with monovalent hepatitis A and B vaccines.[22,54]

Efficacy, Safety, and Duration of Response

The efficacy of the hepatitis A vaccine is well established, with protective efficacy of 94% to 100%.[17,22,53] The vaccine is well tolerated, with soreness at the injection site, headache, myalgia, and malaise as the most commonly reported adverse effects. A recent postmarketing surveillance study of more than 6 million doses of vaccine revealed less than 0.01% of patients reporting adverse events.[17,22]

The duration of protection has not been studied extensively; however, protective antibody titers persist for 5 to 6 years with Havrix and Vaqta.[17,22] However, protective antibody could be present for more than 20 years.[29,53,55] The US Advisory Committee on Immunization Practices (ACIP) has no recommendation regarding the need for booster doses at this time.

Indications

The ACIP recommends hepatitis A vaccination for several high-risk groups, including travelers to countries with high endemicity of infection (South and Central America, Africa, South and Southeast Asia, Caribbean, and the Middle East), travelers to countries with intermediate endemicity of infection (Eastern and Southern Europe and the former Soviet Union), children living in communities with high rates of hepatitis A infection and periodic hepatitis A outbreaks (Alaskan Native villages, American Indian reservations), men who have sex with men, IV drug users, researchers or persons who have occupational risk for hepatitis A (health care workers), persons with clotting factor disorders, and persons with chronic liver disease who are at increased risk for fulminant hepatitis A.[17,22,50] Thus, M.D. should receive either Havrix 1,440 ELISA units or Vaqta 50 units. This initial injection will provide adequate protection from HAV infection during his travel, and he can receive the booster injection on his return, at least 6 months after the first injection. If M.D. decides to travel within the next 2 weeks, he should receive both vaccination and immunoglobulin before departure.[17,22,55]

POSTEXPOSURE PROPHYLAXIS

CASE 77-3

QUESTION 1: L.W., a 26-year-old man, recently was diagnosed with HAV infection. He attends college and works part-time as a retail clerk. He lives with his healthy, 25-year-old wife and 10-month-old infant daughter. Which of L.W.'s contacts require postexposure prophylaxis for HAV?

Although immunoglobulin has been recommended in the past for unvaccinated people recently exposed to HAV, hepatitis A vaccine is effective in preventing secondary HAV infection in healthy people. A vaccine can be administered in healthy people age 12 months to 40 years within 14 days of exposure to HAV.[17,50,55] However, at this time, individuals outside of this age range or with significant comorbid conditions should receive immunoglobulin instead of the vaccine. Therefore, L.W.'s wife should receive prophylactic administration of HAV vaccine and his 10-month-old infect daughter should receive immunoglobulin at a dose of 0.02 mL/kg, administered IM as soon as possible but no later than 2 weeks after exposure. Contacts who have received a dose of hepatitis A vaccine at least 1 month before exposure do not need immunoglobulin, because protective antibody titers are achieved in greater than 95% of patients 1 month after vaccination.[17,22] Prophylaxis is not recommended for casual contacts at work or school.

Administration of immunoglobulin within 2 weeks of exposure to HAV is 80% to 90% effective in preventing acute HAV infection.[17,22,23] In most cases, when given early, immunoglobulin prevents both clinical and subclinical HAV illness. Protection after immunoglobulin administration is immediate and complete but short-lived. Other situations in which immunoglobulin administration may be indicated include hepatitis A infection in day-care centers and in settings with infected persons who prepare and serve food. Immunoglobulin is recommended for all staff and children in day-care settings when a case of hepatitis A virus infection is diagnosed among employees or attendees.[17,22,23] When a food handler is diagnosed with hepatitis A, immunoglobulin is recommended for other food handlers at the same location. Given the improbability of disease transmission to persons consuming food prepared or served by workers infected with hepatitis A, the routine administration of immunoglobulin in this setting is not recommended.[17,22,23]

When immunoglobulin is required for infants or pregnant women, preparations free of thimerosal should be used.[22] Although immunoglobulin does not impede the immune response to inactivated vaccines, oral poliovirus vaccine, or yellow fever vaccine, it may interfere with the response to live attenuated vaccines such as measles, mumps, rubella (MMR) vaccine and varicella vaccine. Therefore, MMR and varicella vaccine should be delayed for at least 3 months after administration of immunoglobulin for HAV prophylaxis. Immunoglobulin should not be given within 2 weeks after the administration of MMR or varicella vaccine. Finally, if immunoglobulin is administered within 2 weeks of MMR, the person requires revaccination, but not sooner than 3 months after the immunoglobulin administration for MMR. Serologic tests for varicella vaccination should be performed 3 months after immunoglobulin administration to determine whether revaccination is required.

HEPATITIS B VIRUS

Virology

HBV is a partially double-stranded DNA virus that is a member of the Hepadnaviridae family of viruses (Table 77-2).[2,3,56–59] Unlike HAV, HBV is antigenically complex, and results in an acute illness with or without a chronic disease state.

ONLINE CONTENT

For an illustration of HBV and a schematic of the HBV genome structure and mRNA transcripts, go to http://thepoint.lww.com/AT10e.

The life cycle of HBV is described in Figure 77-2. Elucidation of the HBV life cycle has resulted in opportunities for drug development. Of special importance, the HBV polymerase functions as both a reverse transcriptase (RT) for synthesis of the negative DNA strand from genomic RNA and as an endogenous DNA polymerase. Because the HBV polymerase is remotely related to the RT enzymes of retroviruses (e.g., HIV), some inhibitors of HIV polymerase or RT also have activity against the HBV polymerase. Thus, several RT inhibitors have been evaluated for treating and preventing HBV; however, rapid emergence of resistance occurs with many of these agents.

Epidemiology

Approximately 5% of the world's population is infected with HBV.[1–3,56,60–62] It is estimated that more than 1.25 million carriers (defined as persons positive for HBsAg for >6 months) occur in the United States, many of whom are immigrants from endemic areas and Alaskan natives (6.4%).[1–3,56,60–62] The incidence of acute HBV infection has declined in the United States.[1–3,56,60–62] This reduction has occurred in all age, racial, ethnic, and high-risk groups, but particularly in children and health care workers, groups with the highest rate of vaccination. Less high-risk behavior also has led to decreased transmission of infection. High-risk groups in the United States for acquiring HBV infection include certain ethnic groups (Alaskan natives, Pacific Islanders), first-generation immigrants from regions of high endemicity (Southeast Asia), injection drug users, gay men, black Americans (compared with white Americans), and males (more than females).[1–3,56,60–62] The most prominent risk factors associated with acute HBV infection include heterosexual contact (42%), men having sex with men (15%), and injection drug use (21%).[1–3,56,60–62] HBV vaccination opportunities include clinics for sexually transmitted disease (STD) (and contacts) and in prisons and holding centers for incarceration.

The epidemiology of chronic HBV infection is less well known; 0.2% of the US population is HBsAg positive.[1–3,56,60–62] Blacks are more likely to be HBsAg positive than whites, but the highest reported rates of HBsAg symptoms are among Asian Americans, especially those from China and Southeast Asia. In population-based surveys, HBV is responsible for 1% to 14%

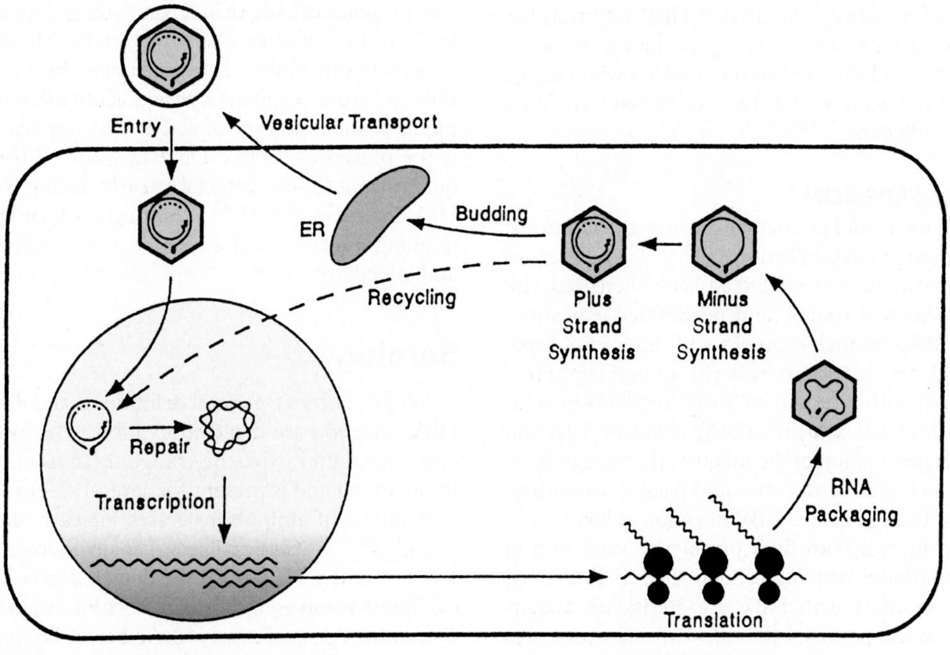

FIGURE 77-2 Life cycle of hepatitis B virus. ER, endoplasmic reticulum. (Reprinted with permission from Ganem D. Hepadnaviridae: the viruses and their replication. In: Fields BN, ed. *Fundamental Virology*. 3rd ed. Philadelphia, PA: Lippincott-Raven; 1996:1199.)

of chronic liver disease, with chronic infection more likely to develop in infants compared with adults.[5,6,56]

Transmission

HBV is transmitted by sexual contact, percutaneous or perinatal exposure, and close person-to-person contact allegedly through open cuts and sores, especially among children in hyperendemic areas. These modes of transmission of HBV are summarized in the following sections.

SEXUAL TRANSMISSION

Sexual activity is the most significant mode of HBV transmission worldwide, including North America, where the prevalence of infection is low.[1–3,56,60–62] Heterosexual intercourse accounts for the majority of US infections (26%). In heterosexuals, factors associated with an enhanced risk of HBV infection include duration of sexual activity, number of sexual partners, and history of STD. Sexual partners of injection drug users, sex workers, and clients of sex workers are at a very high risk for infection. Sexual partners of infected individuals are at high risk for infection, even in the absence of high-risk behavior. Between 0% and 3% of contact spouses or sexual partners and between 4% and 9% of household children are HBsAg positive. Because most patients with chronic HBV infection are unaware of their infection and are "silent carriers," sexual transmission is a significant mode of transmission. The use of condoms appears to reduce the risk of sexual transmission.[1–3,56,60–62]

From 1980 to 1985, a very high rate of HBV infection was observed in homosexual men, accounting for 20% of all reported cases of infection.[1–3,56,60–62] Multiple sexual partners, anal-receptive intercourse, and duration of sexual activity were the most common factors associated with HBV acquisition in this population. Current rates of HBV infection in this population have fallen and are estimated to be about 8%, possibly as a result of modifications of sexual behavior in response to HIV. Similar to heterosexuals, the use of condoms in this population may reduce the risk of sexual transmission.

BLOOD AND BLOOD PRODUCTS

Although the risk of transfusion-associated HBV infection has been greatly reduced with the screening of blood (tests for HBsAg and anti-HBc) and the exclusion of donors who engage in high-risk activities, it is estimated that 1 of 50,000 transfused units transmit HBV infection.[1–3,56,60–62]

PERINATAL TRANSMISSION

Early childhood exposure and perinatal exposure are additional modes of transmission of HBV infection.[1–3,56,60–62] High serum concentrations of virus have been linked with increased risk of transmission by vertical routes (and needlestick exposure). Infants born to HBeAg-positive mothers with high viral replication (>80 pg/mL) have a 70% to 90% risk of perinatal HBV acquisition compared with a 10% to 40% risk in infants born to mothers infected with HBV who are HBeAg negative. Infection generally occurs via inoculation of the infant at the time of birth or soon thereafter, and even with active and passive immunization, 10% to 15% of babies acquire HBV infection at birth.

In developing countries with high prevalence rates and in regions of the United States with high endemicity, children born to HBsAg-positive mothers with HBV are at risk for acquiring HBV infection in the perinatal period, with infection rates reported to be between 7% and 13%.[1–3,56,60–62] In addition, children of HBsAg-positive mothers who are not infected at birth remain at very high risk of early childhood infection, with 60% of those born to HBsAg-positive mothers becoming infected by the age of 5 years. The mechanism of the later infection, which is neither perinatal nor sexual, is not known however. Although HBsAg is detectable in breast milk, breast-feeding is not believed to be a primary mode of HBV transmission.

INJECTION DRUG USE

Recreational drug use in the United States and Europe is an important mode of HBV transmission, accounting for approximately 23% of all patients.[1–3,56,60–62] The risk increases with duration of recreational drug use; thus, serologic markers of ongoing or prior HBV infection are usually positive after 5 years of drug use.

OTHER MODES OF TRANSMISSION

Other risk factors for transmission of HBV include working in a health care setting, transfusion and dialysis, acupuncture, tattooing, travel, and living in institutions.[1–3,56,60–62] Sporadic cases of HBV transmission have been attributed to nonpercutaneous transmission by way of small breaks in the skin, biting, or mucous membranes. Although HBsAg is found in saliva, tears, sweat, semen, vaginal secretions, breast milk, cerebrospinal fluid, ascites, pleural fluid, synovial fluid, gastric juice, urine, and, rarely, feces of HBsAg-positive persons, only semen, saliva, and serum actually contain infectious HBV in experimental transmission studies. Kissing is not considered to be a significant means of HBV transmission, but biting could be.

Pathogenesis

Similar to HAV infection, clinical observations suggest that host immune responses are more important than virologic factors in the pathogenesis of liver injury.[56,63,64] Host cellular and humoral immune responses are linked to T lymphocytes, which enhance viral clearance from hepatocytes and cause liver injury.[56,63,64]

Diagnosis

The presence of HBsAg in serum is diagnostic for HBV infection. In 5% to 10% of acute cases in which the HBsAg levels fall below sensitivity thresholds of current assays, the presence of IgM anti-HBc in serum confirms a recent acute HBV infection. Another highly reliable marker of active HBV replication and diagnosis is the presence of HBV DNA in serum through qualitative or quantitative assays, detectable early during the course of acute HBV infection.[56–60,65–68] Persisting levels of HBV DNA indicate ongoing infection and a high degree of active viral replication and infectivity.

Serology

Serologic patterns, general definitions, and diagnostic criteria of HBV infection are depicted in Table 77-6. Within the first several weeks after exposure (range, 2–10 weeks), HBsAg appears in the blood and is present for several weeks before serum concentrations of aminotransferases increase and symptoms (Fig. 77-3).[56–60,65–68] Clinical illness usually follows HBV exposure by 1 to 3 months. HBsAg can be detected in serum until the clinical illness resolves and usually becomes undetectable after 4 to 6 months. Persistence of HBsAg beyond 6 months implies progression to chronic HBV infection. The antibody to HBsAg (anti-HBs) often appears after a short "window" period during which

TABLE 77-6
Common Serologic Patterns of Hepatitis B Virus Infection

HBsAg	HBeAg	Anti-HBs	Anti-HBe	Anti-HBc	Interpretation
+	+	−	−	−	Incubation period
+	+	−	−	+ (IgM)	Acute HBV infection (typical case); chronic HBV carrier with high infectivity
−	−	+	−	+ (IgG)	Recovery from HBV infection
+	−	−	−	+ (IgG)	Chronic HBV carrier; chronic hepatitis B
−	−	+	−	−	Successful immunization with HBV vaccine

Anti-HBc, hepatitis B core antibody; anti-HBe, hepatitis B envelope antibody; anti-HBs, hepatitis B surface antibody; HBeAg, hepatitis B envelope antigen; HBsAg, hepatitis B surface antigen; HBV, hepatitis B virus; IgG, immunoglobulin G; IgM, immunoglobulin M.

neither HBsAg nor anti-HBs are detectable. In most patients, anti-HBs persists for years after HBV infection, conferring immunity to reinfection (Fig. 77-3).

A soluble viral protein, HBeAg is detectable early during the acute phase of the disease and persists in chronic hepatitis B infection. HBeAg is a marker of active HBV replication, and its presence correlates with circulating HBV particles. The presence of both HBeAg and HBsAg indicates a high level of viral replication and infectivity and a need for antiviral therapy. Generally, seroconversion from HBeAg to hepatitis B envelope antibody (anti-HBe) results in a reduction in HBV DNA and suggests resolution of HBV infection. Some patients may, however, continue to have active liver disease and detectable serum HBV DNA levels as a result of the presence of wild-type virus or the presence of precore or promoter mutations that impair HBeAg secretion (HBeAg-negative patients).

Hepatitis B core antigen does not circulate freely in the bloodstream and is not measured. Anti-HBc, the antibody directed against hepatitis B core antigen, is usually detected 1 to 2 weeks after the appearance of HBsAg and just before the onset of clinical symptoms, and it persists for life. The detection of IgM anti-HBc is the most sensitive diagnostic test for acute HBV infection. During the recovery phase of infection, the predominant form of anti-HBc is in the IgG class. The presence of this antibody suggests prior or ongoing infection with HBV. Furthermore, in areas where HBV is not endemic, isolated detection of anti-HBc in a patient's serum may correlate with low levels of HBV DNA. The presence of HBV DNA may enhance the risk of transmission of HBV and progression to cirrhosis and hepatocellular carcinoma. Patients immunized against HBV do not develop anti-HBc; therefore, the presence of this antibody differentiates successful vaccination from actual HBV infection.

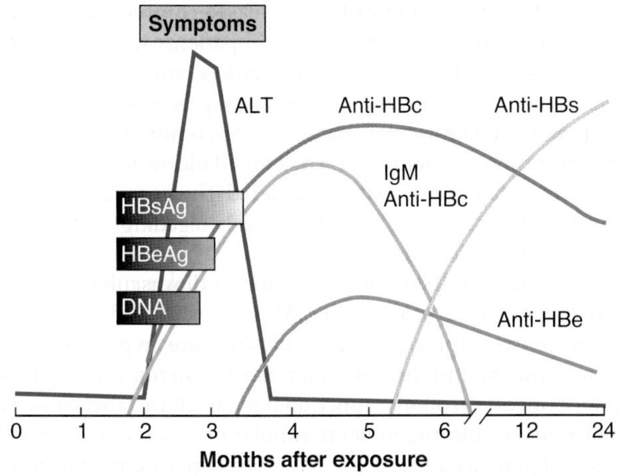

FIGURE 77-3 Sequence of events after acute hepatitis B virus infection with resolution. ALT, alanine aminotransferase; anti-HBc, hepatitis B core antibody; anti-HBe, hepatitis B envelope antibody; anti-HBs, hepatitis B surface antibody; HBeAg, hepatitis B envelope antigen; HBsAg, hepatitis B surface antigen; HBV DNA; hepatitis B virus DNA; IgM anti-HBc, immunoglobulin M antibody to hepatitis B core virus. Adapted with permission from Perrillo, R.P., & Regenstein, F.G. [1996]. Viral and immune hepatitis. In Kelley, W.N. [Ed.]. Textbook of internal medicine. [3rd ed.]. Philadelphia: J.B. Lippincott.

Natural History

Of those patients with acute HBV infection, only 1% develop FHF with associated coagulopathy, encephalopathy, and cerebral edema.[28,56,69,70] The cause of fulminant infection is a heightened immune response to the virus, in the absence of HDV or HCV coinfections. Patients with acute liver failure often have early clearance of HBsAg, which may complicate the diagnosis, but a positive IgM antibody to hepatitis B core antigen generally confirms the diagnosis.

Four phases of HBV infection are present: immune tolerance, immune clearance, low-level replication or nonreplication phase (inactive carrier), and reactivation phase. Up to 12% (average 5%) of immunocompetent patients acutely infected with HBV remain chronically infected (historically defined as detectable HBsAg in serum for 6 months or longer).[56–60,66–68] In these patients, HBsAg generally remains detectable indefinitely and anti-HBs fails to appear. The risk of chronicity after neonatally acquired infection is high (>90%), possibly because neonates have immature immune systems. Of infected neonates, 50% have evidence of active viral replication. Furthermore, patients who have a reduced ability to clear viral infections—including those receiving chronic hemodialysis, immunosuppression after transplantation, or chemotherapy, or patients with HIV infection—may have a greater risk for developing chronic HBV infection.[56,70] Ultimate outcomes are linked with the presence or absence of viral replication and by the severity of liver damage.[56,70] Approximately 50% of all chronic carriers have ongoing viral replication, especially with elevated aminotransferases, and 15% to 20% of these develop cirrhosis within 5 years.[56–60,70] Spontaneous loss of HBeAg (7%–20% per year) has been reported, possibly as a result of the use of antiviral therapy, whereas loss of HBsAg occurs less frequently (1%–2% per year). In general, chronic carriers remain infected throughout their life.[56–60,70] Five-year survival rates decline depending on the severity of disease (55% survival with cirrhosis).[71] Asymptomatic HBV carriers tend to have mild disease manifestations with few complications, even with a long period of follow-up. Finally, the risk of hepatocellular carcinoma (HCC) is increased up to 300 times in chronic carriers with active viral replication (HBeAg positive).[56,70,72–74]

TABLE 77-8
Recommended Doses of Currently Licensed Hepatitis B Vaccines[a61,84,85]

	Recombivax HB		Engerix-B	
Group	Dose (mcg)	(mL)	Dose (mcg)	(mL)
Birth to 10 years	—	—	10	(0.5)
Birth to 19 years	5	(0.5)	—	—
Children and adolescents 11–19 years	—	—	10	(0.5)
Adolescents 11–15 years[b]	10	(1.0)	—	—
Adults >20 years	10	(1.0)	20	(1.0)
Dialysis patients and other immunocompromised hosts	40	(1.0)	40[c]	(2.0)

[a] One dose administered three times: at time 0, 1 month, and 6 months.
[b] One dose administered two times: at 0 and 4–6 months.
[c] Two 1.0-mL doses administered at one site, in a four-dose schedule at 0, 1, 2, and 6 months.

Manufactured using recombinant DNA technology, Recombivax HB (10 mg HBsAg/mL) and Engerix-B (20 mg HBsAg/mL) are yeast-derived HBV vaccines that induce an immunologic response similar to the plasma-derived vaccine (no longer used). Because P.G. will come in contact with potentially infectious bodily secretions during her rotations, she should be immunized against hepatitis B with either Recombivax HB or Engerix-B.

DOSING REGIMEN

The recommended doses of available hepatitis B vaccines are shown in Table 77-8.[61,67,84,85] Relative potency comparisons are not clinically important because comparative trials using Recombivax HB and Engerix-B in the recommended dosages have demonstrated equivalent immunogenicity and tolerability. P.G. can be immunized with either product, provided she receives the manufacturer's recommended dosage with each injection.

Hepatitis B vaccine should be administered as an IM injection in the deltoid muscle of adults and children or in the anterolateral thigh muscle of neonates and infants. The immunogenicity of hepatitis B vaccine is significantly lower when injections are given in the buttocks, probably because the greater amount of fat tissue in the buttocks inhibits interfacing of vaccine and antigen-recognition leukocytes. The results of a small vaccination series suggest that healthy adults who do not respond to HBV injection to the buttocks have a significantly higher response when vaccinated in the arm. P.G. should be immunized with either Recombivax HB (10 mcg) or Engerix-B (20 mcg) administered as a 1-mL IM injection in the deltoid muscle.

EFFICACY

Recombinant yeast-derived vaccines (e.g., Recombivax HB, Engerix-B) produce similar results.[61,84,85] A protective antibody response has been defined as anti-HBs levels of at least 10 milli-international units/mL.[61,86] This threshold was derived from early HBV vaccine trials in homosexual men, in which vaccine recipients with serum antibody levels of at least 10 sample ratio units (SRU) were protected from HBV infection.[61,86,87] A serum antibody level of 10 SRU is roughly equivalent to 10 milli-international units/mL when the international standard is used. For this reason, an anti-HBs level of at least 10 milli-international units/mL is considered a protective antibody titer and is the standard used by the ACIP. Although HBV infections have occurred in vaccine recipients with a detectable immune response, almost all infections have been asymptomatic, identified only through the presence of anti-HBc. These infections have been limited largely to patients with no response or a poor response to vaccination.[61]

NONRESPONDERS

CASE 77-5, QUESTION 2: P.G. has completed her three-dose vaccination series with Engerix-B. Routine hepatitis serology testing, performed before volunteering for a drug study, reveals that P.G. is anti-HBs negative. Why did P.G. not respond to the hepatitis B vaccine, and how should she be managed?

Two important determinants of vaccine efficacy appear to be the age at vaccination and underlying immune function. In healthy recipients, the immune response to vaccination decreases with advancing age. In one study, 99% of patients age 0 to 19 years, 93% of those age 20 to 49 years, and 73% of those older than 50 years of age achieved protective anti-HBs levels (>10 SRU) after three doses of the hepatitis B vaccine.[61] Immunocompromised patients, including those receiving hemodialysis, those infected with HIV, or children receiving cytotoxic chemotherapy, respond poorly to the HBV vaccine.[61,84,85,87] Patients who smoke or are obese also have a reduced response.[61,84,85,87] P.G. has two risk factors for a poor response to the hepatitis B vaccine: she is older than 50 years of age and she is moderately obese (ideal body weight for her height is 50 kg).

Vaccine recipients who respond poorly to hepatitis B vaccine have been classified either as hyporesponders who can probably be protected by additional doses of vaccine or as true nonresponders. Patients with inadequate initial response to the HBV vaccine series should be revaccinated. Of hyporesponders (anti-HBs levels <10 milli-international units/mL), 50% to 90% achieve a protective level after a single booster injection or after repeating the entire three-dose series.[61,84,85,87,88] Of patients not responding to a primary vaccination series with Engerix B, 60% produced an immune response after a three-dose series with HBVax II (Recombivax), suggesting a repeat course with the alternative HBV vaccine may be a reasonable approach in some patients.[61,84,85,87] Revaccination of nonresponders (no detectable anti-HBs) is less successful, and protective levels, if achieved, are not sustained.[61] True nonresponders to HBV vaccination are rare in the immunocompetent population, and these persons may have a genetic predisposition toward nonresponsiveness.[61,84,85,87] P.G. should be revaccinated with a booster dose of hepatitis B vaccine. Her anti-HBs levels can be rechecked 1 month after the injection. If she still has not responded, it is reasonable to administer an additional two injections to complete a second vaccination series.

INTERCHANGEABILITY OF HEPATITIS B VIRUS VACCINES

CASE 77-6

QUESTION 1: T.M., a 32-year-old hospital laboratory technician, received the first two doses of hepatitis B vaccine with Recombivax HB. He has relocated recently and is due for the third injection. The employee health service at his new job uses only Engerix-B for hepatitis B vaccination. Can hepatitis B vaccines produced by different manufacturers be used interchangeably?

Although it is recommended that patients receive the complete vaccination series with the same product, it is not absolutely necessary. To determine whether a hepatitis B vaccination series initiated with Recombivax HB could be completed with Engerix-B, healthy adults received 10 mcg of Recombivax HB at baseline and 1 month. At 6 months, the subjects were randomly assigned to receive either Engerix-B 20 mcg or Recombivax HB 10 mcg. One month after the third dose, 100% of those who had received Engerix-B and 92% of those who had received Recombivax HB had protective anti-HBs levels.[61,84,85]

Chan et al.[89] studied the booster response to either recombinant hepatitis B vaccine or plasma-derived vaccine in children who had been vaccinated originally with the plasma-derived product (Heptavax-B). Children were randomly assigned to receive either 5 mcg of the plasma-derived vaccine or 20 mcg of Engerix-B. One month after the booster injection, all vaccine recipients had significant elevations in their anti-HBs titers, suggesting recombinant hepatitis B vaccines elicit an adequate booster response in persons who originally received the plasma-derived vaccine. According to the ACIP, the immune response from one or two doses of a vaccine produced by one manufacturer, when followed by subsequent doses from a different manufacturer, is comparable with that resulting from a full course of vaccination with a single vaccine.[61]

T.M. may complete the hepatitis B vaccine series with Engerix-B provided he receives the recommended dosage of 20 mcg administered as a 1-mL IM injection to the deltoid region.

DURATION OF RESPONSE

CASE 77-6, QUESTION 2: Does T.M. require a booster injection for sustained protection from HBV infection?

The duration of vaccine-induced immunity has been evaluated in many long-term studies.[61,84,85,87,90–94] The duration of detectable anti-HBs appears proportional to the peak antibody response achieved after vaccination, and protective anti-HBs levels were sustained in 68% to 85% of patients receiving the plasma-derived HBV vaccine from 6 to 12 years.[61,90–94] Importantly, the protective efficacy of the HBV vaccine in these trials was high, even in patients with anti-HBs levels less than 10 milli-international units/mL. HBsAg was only rarely detected, and most HBV events consisted of asymptomatic seroconversion to anti-HBc. These studies suggest that successful HBV vaccination is associated with long-lasting protection without the need for additional booster doses for up to 12 years.

The mechanism of sustained protection from HBV, despite low or undetectable anti-HBs levels, is thought to be related to the phenomenon of immunologic memory in previously sensitized B lymphocytes. This amnestic response, in combination with the long incubation period of HBV, may allow the synthesis of protective antibodies sufficiently quickly to block infection in patients rechallenged with HBV.[95]

In summary, no need exists for routine administration of HBV vaccine booster doses to immunocompetent persons after successful vaccination. Immunocompromised patients may require a persistent minimal level of protective antibody, and the ACIP does recommend annual antibody testing for patients receiving chronic hemodialysis with administration of a booster dose when antibody levels are less than 10 milli-international units/mL.[61] Based on available evidence, T.M. does not require a scheduled booster dose of hepatitis B vaccine.

INDICATIONS

CASE 77-6, QUESTION 3: Why is it appropriate for T.M. to be vaccinated with hepatitis B vaccine, and who else should be vaccinated with this vaccine?

The ACIP has recommended pre-exposure hepatitis B vaccination for the following high-risk groups: health care workers with exposure to blood, staff of institutions for the developmentally

TABLE 77-9

Recommended Schedules of Hepatitis B Vaccination for Infants Born to HBsAg (–) Mothers[61,84,85]

Hepatitis B Vaccine	Age of Infant
Option 1	
Dose 1	Birth (before hospital discharge)
Dose 2	1–2 months[a]
Dose 3	6–18 months[a]
Option 2	
Dose 1	1–2 months[a]
Dose 2	4 months[a]
Dose 3	6–18 months[a]

[a] Hepatitis B vaccine can be administered simultaneously with diphtheria-tetanus-pertussis, *Haemophilus influenzae* type b conjugate, measles-mumps-rubella, and oral polio vaccines.

disabled, hemodialysis patients, recipients of blood products, household and sexual contacts of HBV carriers, international travelers to HBV-endemic areas, injecting drug users, sexually active homosexual men, bisexual men, and inmates of long-term correctional facilities.[61,96,97] Because T.M. is a hospital laboratory technician, he is at high risk for exposure to HBV and should be vaccinated.

UNIVERSAL HEPATITIS B VACCINATION

In addition to the previously listed high-risk groups, all infants should receive hepatitis B vaccination. The practice of vaccinating only high-risk persons has resulted in little impact on the incidence of HBV disease. Populations at risk for HBV disease (injecting drug users, persons with multiple sexual partners) generally are not vaccinated before they begin engaging in high-risk behaviors. In addition, many persons who become infected have no identifiable risk factors for infection and thus would not be recognized as candidates for vaccination. A program designed to immunize children before they initiate high-risk behaviors is likely to have a greater impact in reducing the incidence of HBV infection. As a means to achieve this goal, the hepatitis B vaccine now is incorporated into the existing pediatric vaccination schedule. The first dose is administered during the newborn period (preferably before the infant is discharged from the hospital) but no later than 2 months of age.[61,97] The recommended vaccination schedule is shown in Table 77-9.

CASE 77-7

QUESTION 1: R.M. is a mother of two children aged 11 years and 2 months. Her infant daughter just received a second dose of hepatitis B vaccine as part of her routine well-baby care. R.M. wonders whether her son, who did not receive the hepatitis B vaccine during his normal childhood immunizations, should receive the vaccine now.

The Centers for Disease Control and Prevention (CDC) has addressed the issue of immunizing children and adolescents born before 1991 who are potentially at risk for hepatitis B infection. The current recommendations suggest that adolescents who have not received three doses of hepatitis B vaccine should initiate or complete the series at ages 11 to 15 years. A schedule of 0, 1 to 2, and 4 to 6 months is recommended.[61,96] It is anticipated that universal vaccination of all infants and previously unvaccinated adolescents aged 11 to 12 years, in addition to ongoing

TABLE 77-10
Guide to Postexposure Immunoprophylaxis for Exposure to Hepatitis B Virus[61,84,85]

Type of Exposure	Immunoprophylaxis
Perinatal	Vaccination + HBIG
Sexual	Vaccination + HBIG
Household contact	
Chronic carrier	Vaccination
Acute case	None unless known exposure
Acute case, known exposure	HBIG – vaccination
Infant (<12 months) acute case in primary caregiver	HBIG + vaccination
Inadvertent (percutaneous or permucosal)	Vaccination – HBIG

HBIG, hepatitis B immunoglobulin.

immunization of high-risk persons, will reduce the incidence of acute hepatitis B infection, hepatitis B-associated chronic liver disease, and HCC. R.M.'s son should receive either Recombivax HB 5 mcg or Engerix-B 10 mcg IM in the deltoid with repeat doses 1 to 2 months and 4 to 6 months from the initial injection.

ADVERSE EFFECTS

Hepatitis B virus vaccination generally has been well tolerated. The most common side effect is pain at the injection site, observed in 3% to 29% of patients. Transient febrile reactions (defined as temperature >99.9°F) occur in less than 6% of recipients, and other reactions, including nausea, rash, headache, myalgias, and arthralgias, are observed in less than 1% of recipients. Ongoing monitoring of vaccine safety by the FDA and CDC is assessed through the Vaccine Safety Datalink project and Vaccine Adverse Events Reporting System. On the basis of these reporting systems, additional "causal" adverse effects associated with vaccination include anaphylaxis (1 case per 1.1 million vaccine doses), Guillain-Barré syndrome, and multiple sclerosis. Additional rare adverse events that have been reported but remain to be validated are chronic fatigue syndrome, neurologic disorders (leukoencephalitis, optic neuritis, and transverse myelitis), rheumatoid arthritis, type 1 diabetes, and autoimmune disease.

POSTEXPOSURE PROPHYLAXIS

PERCUTANEOUS EXPOSURE

CASE 77-8

QUESTION 1: K.N., a 26-year-old medical student, presents to the ED after accidentally sticking herself with a contaminated needle while drawing blood from an HBsAg-positive patient. K.N. was not vaccinated previously and had no known prior episodes of hepatitis or liver disease. Her tetanus status is current. She weighs 56 kg. How should K.N. be treated for percutaneous exposure to hepatitis B?

After exposure to HBV, prophylactic treatment with hepatitis B vaccination and possibly passive immunization with hepatitis B immunoglobulin (HBIG) should be considered. The ACIP recommendations for postexposure immunoprophylaxis after hepatitis B exposure are shown in Table 77-10.

K.N.'s percutaneous exposure warrants active immunization with HBV and passive immunization with HBIG. The source of K.N.'s exposure is HBsAg positive, and K.N. had not been vaccinated previously with the hepatitis B vaccine. She should receive a single dose of HBIG 0.06 mL/kg (3.4 mL) as an IM injection in either the gluteal or deltoid region as soon as possible after exposure, preferably within 24 hours. HBIG is prepared from plasma of persons preselected for high-titer anti-HBs. The anti-HBs of HBIG in the United States is 1:100,000 as determined by radioimmunoassay. HBIG is superior to immunoglobulin in the prevention of hepatitis B infection after percutaneous exposure. K.N. also should receive active immunization with IM hepatitis B vaccine (at a separate site) simultaneously with HBIG. The second and third doses should be given 1 month and 6 months later. Passively acquired antibodies against hepatitis B virus from HBIG or immunoglobulin will not interfere with active immunization via hepatitis B vaccine.[97]

If the HBsAg status of the donor source of a percutaneous exposure is unknown, recommendations for prophylaxis of HBV infection depend on whether the donor source is at high risk or at low risk for being HBsAg positive. High-risk donor sources include homosexual men, IV drug abusers, patients undergoing hemodialysis, residents of mental institutions, immigrants from endemic areas, and household contacts of HBV carriers. Additional ACIP recommendations for hepatitis B prophylaxis after percutaneous exposure are shown in Table 77-11.

TABLE 77-11
Recommendations for Hepatitis B Prophylaxis After Percutaneous Exposure[61,84 85]

	Treatment When Source Is Found to Be		
Exposed Person	HBsAg-Positive	HBsAg-Negative	Unknown or Not Tested
Unvaccinated	Administer HBIG × 1[a] and initiate hepatitis vaccine	Initiate hepatitis B vaccine[b]	Initiate hepatitis B vaccine[b]
Previously vaccinated			
Known responder	Test exposed person for anti-HBs[c] 1. If inadequate, hepatitis B vaccine booster dose 2. If adequate, no treatment	No treatment	No treatment
Known responder	HBIG × 1[a] as soon as possible, repeat in 1 month *OR* HBIG × 1[a] plus one dose of hepatitis B vaccine	No treatment	If known high-risk source, may treat as if source were HBsAg positive
Response unknown	Test exposed person for anti-HBs[c] 1. If inadequate, HBIG × 1[a] plus hepatitis B vaccine booster dose 2. If adequate, no treatment	No treatment	Test exposed person for anti-HBs[c] 1. If inadequate, hepatitis B vaccine booster dose 2. If adequate, no treatment

[a] HBIG dose 0.06 mL/kg given intramuscularly.
[b] For dosing information, see Table 77-8.
[c] Adequate anti-HBs is ≥10 milli-international units.
HBIG, hepatitis B immunoglobulin; HBs, hepatitis B surface; HBsAg, hepatitis B surface antigen.

SEXUAL EXPOSURE

CASE 77-9

QUESTION 1: G.G. is a 20-year-old construction worker who had sexual contact with a partner who recently found out she was HBsAg-positive. What are the current recommendations for a person who has had sexual contact with an HBsAg-positive person?

Sexual transmission of HBV is an important cause of HBV infection, accounting for approximately 30% to 60% of all new cases annually.[56–60] Passive immunization with a single 5-mL dose of HBIG was found highly effective in preventing HBV infection after sexual exposure when compared with a control globulin (with no anti-HBs activity).[61,97] The CDC recommends that susceptible persons exposed to HBV through sexual contact with a person who has acute or chronic HBV infection should receive postexposure prophylaxis with 0.06 mL/kg of HBIG as a single IM dose within 14 days of the last exposure. Patients also should receive the standard three-dose immunization series with hepatitis B vaccine beginning at the time of HBIG administration.[97,98]

PERINATAL EXPOSURE

CASE 77-10

QUESTION 1: S.L., a 3.2-kg boy, was just born to an HBsAg-positive mother. Is S.L. at risk for acquiring HBV infection, and how should he be treated?

In many Asian and developing countries, perinatal (vertical) transmission accounts for most HBV infections. Infants born to HBV-infected mothers have a greater than 85% risk of acquiring HBV during the perinatal period. Of those who become infected, 80% to 90% become chronic HBsAg carriers.[56,74,99] Although fulminant cases have been reported, most hepatitis infections in neonates are asymptomatic. Despite the usually innocuous initial disease, significant adverse consequences are associated with chronic HBsAg carriage in neonates. Chronic hepatitis B infection is associated with chronic liver disease and has been clearly implicated as a major risk factor in the development of primary HCC.[56,72,73]

Mothers who are chronic carriers of HBV can transmit HBV to their infants. The risk is related to the presence of HBsAg and HBeAg (suggesting a high degree of viral replication and infectivity). The likelihood that S.L. will develop HBV infection is high. S.L. requires immediate therapy with HBIG (to provide immediate high titers of circulating anti-HBs) and simultaneous vaccination with hepatitis B vaccine (to induce long-lasting protective immunity). Screening pregnant women for the presence of HBeAg and administration of HBIG and hepatitis B vaccine is 85% to 98% effective in preventing HBV infection and the chronic carrier state.[56,60,62] This compares with a 71% efficacy rate for administration of HBIG alone. Simultaneous administration of HBIG and hepatitis B vaccine does not adversely affect the production of anti-HBs in neonates.[56,60,62]

Infants born to mothers who are HBsAg positive should receive simultaneous IM injections of the appropriate doses of hepatitis B vaccine (Table 77-9) and HBIG (0.5 mL) within 12 hours of birth. The injections should be administered at separate sites. S.L. should receive HBIG (0.5 mL) as soon as possible after birth, administered as an IM injection. He also should receive 0.5 mL of either Recombivax HB (5 mcg) or Engerix-B (10 mcg) as an IM injection at a separate site.

CASE 77-10, QUESTION 2: What would the management plan be if the HBsAg status of S.L.'s mother was unknown?

The ACIP has developed recommendations for the prevention of perinatal HBV infection. This includes the routine testing of all pregnant women for HBsAg during an early prenatal visit. HBsAg testing should be repeated late in the pregnancy for women who are HBsAg-negative but who are at high risk of HBV infection or who have had clinically apparent hepatitis. Women admitted for delivery who have not had prenatal HBsAg testing should have blood drawn for testing. While test results are pending, the infant should receive hepatitis B vaccine within 12 hours of birth (Table 77-8). If the mother is found later to be HBsAg positive, her infant should receive HBIG as soon as possible within 7 days of birth. The second and third doses of vaccine should be administered at 1 and 6 months, respectively. If the mother is found to be HBsAg negative, her infant should continue to receive hepatitis B vaccine as part of the routine vaccination series.[61]

Evaluation and Management of Patients With Chronic Hepatitis B Virus Infection

CASE 77-11

QUESTION 1: E.A. is a 55-year-old woman who presents to the hepatology clinic with a recent history of mild jaundice. Her previous medical history is unremarkable except for a blood transfusion she received during childbirth in 1988. What initial and follow-up tests should be performed to assess the extent of HBV infection in E.A.?

The evaluation of patients infected with chronic HBV is described in Table 77-12.[56–60] Initially, a thorough history and physical examination should be performed with greater emphasis placed on risk factors for coinfection, alcohol use, and family history of HBV and liver cancer. Laboratory tests should include assessment of liver disease, markers of HBV replication, and screening tests for HCV, HDV, or HIV. Vaccinations for hepatitis A should also be administered as described above. The decision to perform a liver biopsy should be made based on knowledge of a patient's age, the ALT level, HBeAg status, HBV DNA levels, and additional clinical features suggestive of chronic liver disease or portal hypertension. In patients who are not initially considered for treatment (inactive HBV carriers), a guideline for follow-up based on HBeAg status is described in Table 77-12. Periodic screening for HCC should also be performed in high-risk populations such as Asian men older than 40 and Asian women older than 50 years of age, persons with cirrhosis, persons with a family history of HCC, blacks older than 20 years of age, and any carrier older than 40 years of age with persistent or intermittent ALT or HBV DNA elevations.

CASE 77-12

QUESTION 1: C.R., a 48-year-old man, presents to the ED with jaundice, complaints of incapacitating fatigue, and vague intermittent abdominal pain for the past month. C.R. was diagnosed with hepatitis B 12 years before admission. His social history includes IV drug abuse (none for 2 years) and alcohol abuse (none for 2 years). Several weeks ago, C.R. noted darkening of his urine and yellowing of his eyes. Additionally, C.R. has a history of severe depression, managed with escitalopram.

Physical examination reveals a thin man in no apparent distress. He is afebrile, and his blood pressure, heart rate,

TABLE 77-12
Evaluation of Patients With Chronic Hepatitis B[58,60]

Initial evaluation
History and physical examination
Determine whether the patient will be committed to ongoing adherence with drug therapy and routine disease and treatment response monitoring (if needed)
Laboratory tests to assess liver disease (CBC, platelets, ALT, AST, bilirubin, prothrombin time/INR) and biopsy
Tests for HBV replication (HBeAg/anti-HBe, HBV DNA)
Tests to rule out coinfection (anti-HCV, anti-HDV, anti-HIV)
Tests to screen for HCC (AFP, and ultrasound for high-risk patients)
Suggested Follow-Up for Patients Not Considered For Treatment (HBeAg+,HBV DNA > 20,000 international units/mL, and normal ALT)
ALT every 3–6 months, increasing frequency if ALT becomes elevated
If ALT >2× ULN, recheck ALT every 1 to 3 months; consider liver biopsy if age >40 years, ALT borderline or mildly elevated on serial tests. Consider treatment if biopsy shows moderate or severe inflammation or significant fibrosis
If ALT >2× ULN for 3–6 months and HBeAg+, HBV DNA >20,000 international units/mL, consider liver biopsy and treatment
Consider screening for HCC in relevant population
Inactive HBsAg Carrier
ALT every 3 months for 1 year, if persistently normal, ALT every 6–12 months
If ALT >1–2× ULN, check serum HBV DNA level and exclude other causes of liver disease. Consider liver biopsy if ALT borderline or mildly elevated in serial tests or if HBV DNA persistently >20,000 international units/mL. Consider treatment if biopsy shows moderate or severe inflammation or significant fibrosis
Consider screening for HCC in relevant population

ALT, alanine aminotransferase; anti-HBe, hepatitis B envelope antibody; anti-HCV, hepatitis C antibody; anti-HDV, hepatitis D antibody; anti-HIV, human immunodeficiency virus antibody; APF, α-fetoprotein; AST, aspartate aminotransferase; CBC, complete blood count; HBeAg, hepatitis B envelope antigen; HBsAg, hepatitis B surface antigen; HBV, hepatitis B virus; HCC, hepatocellular carcinoma; INR, international normalized ratio; ULN, upper limit of normal.

and respiratory rate are within normal limits. Moderate scleral icterus is noted. The abdomen is soft and not distended. The liver is enlarged, nontender, and smooth with an edge palpable 5 cm below the costal margin and a span of 15 cm. The spleen is palpable. The cardiac, pulmonary, neurologic, and extremity examinations all are within normal limits.

C.R.'s laboratory evaluation is significant for the following:

Hct, 39%
Hgb, 11 g/dL
WBC count, 8.8 cells/μL
Platelets, 75,000/μL
PT, 15.4 seconds
INR, 2.1
AST, 326 units/L
ALT, 382 units/L
Alkaline phosphatase, 142 units/mL
Total bilirubin, 4.2 mg/dL
Albumin, 2.8 g/dL

Hepatitis serologic tests are positive for HBsAg, HBeAg, and anti-HBc and negative for IgM anti-HBc, IgM anti-HAV, and anti-HCV. HBV DNA is reported as greater than 200 pg/mL. A liver biopsy reveals periportal inflammation as well as piecemeal and bridging necrosis. What clinical findings does C.R. have that support the diagnosis of chronic HBV infection?

The chronic occurrence of jaundice and hepatosplenomegaly with significantly elevated AST and ALT in a young patient such as C.R. is suggestive of chronic hepatitis. Although alcoholic hepatitis secondary to long-term alcohol use is consistent with these clinical features, his serologic tests are positive for HBV. Hepatitis serology with positive HBsAg and HBeAg suggest ongoing viral replication and a high degree of infectivity.

Serum concentrations of aminotransferases can range from slightly abnormal to greatly elevated, with ALT concentrations generally greater than AST. Serum bilirubin concentrations greater than 3.0 mg/dL are common, serum concentration of alkaline phosphatase usually is increased, and the PT may be prolonged. Patients such as C.R. with a prolonged PT, thrombocytopenia, and low serum albumin concentration generally have a more severe form of chronic hepatitis and can be considered to have decompensated liver disease.

Liver biopsy is important for the diagnosis, treatment, and prognosis of patients with chronic hepatitis. C.R.'s liver biopsy reveals the classic triad of periportal inflammation as well as piecemeal and bridging necrosis. The liver biopsy and hepatitis serologic test results are consistent with a diagnosis of chronic HBV infection.

Treatment of chronic HBV infection requires knowledge of the natural history of the untreated disease and the potential benefits of intervention. Currently, seven agents are approved by the FDA for treating chronic HBV infection.

CASE 77-12, QUESTION 2: Does C.R. require treatment for chronic hepatitis secondary to hepatitis B?

The decision to treat C.R. depends on the severity of symptoms, the serum biochemistries, and the liver biopsy results. C.R. has evidence of severe chronic HBV infection. He is symptomatic with jaundice, severe fatigue, and abdominal pain, and the results of his LFTs and HBV DNA levels suggest his disease is advanced (decreased albumin, elevated PT, low platelets). Therefore, he should be treated to reduce the replication of HBV, resolve the hepatocellular damage, and prevent long-term adverse hepatic sequelae.[56–60,99]

GOALS OF THERAPY

CASE 77-12, QUESTION 3: What are the goals of therapy for chronic hepatitis secondary to HBV?

Progression of chronic hepatitis to cirrhosis is likely because of continued replication of the HBV. Loss of active viral replication usually is associated with a decrease in infectivity, a reduction in inflammatory cells within the liver, and a fall of serum aminotransferase activities into the normal range. The disappearance of detectable HBeAg and HBV DNA is considered an indicator of loss of active viral replication.

The goals of therapy in chronic HBV infection are to achieve sustained suppression of HBV replication and remission of liver disease.[56–60] Ultimately, achieving these goals should lead to resolving ongoing hepatocellular damage and reducing the development of cirrhosis and HCC.[56–60] Clinical trials for chronic HBV infection have used the following markers as end points for successful therapy: seroconversion from HBeAg positive to

TABLE 77-13
Definition of Response to Antiviral Therapy[56,58,60]

Category of Response	Characteristics
Biochemical response (BR)	Decrease in serum ALT to within the normal range
Virologic relapse (VR)	Decrease in serum HBV DNA to undetectable levels by PCR assays, and loss of HBeAg in HBeAg-positive patients
Primary nonresponse (not applicable to IFN therapy)	Decrease in serum HBV DNA by $<2\ \log_{10}$ international units/mL after at least 24 weeks of therapy
Virologic relapse (VR)	Increase in serum HBV DNA of 1 $\log_{10}$ international units/mL after discontinuation of treatment in at least two determinations more than 4 weeks apart
Histologic response (HR)	Decrease in histology activity index by at least 2 points and no worsening of fibrosis score compared with pretreatment liver biopsy
Complete response (CR)	Fulfill criteria of biochemical and virological response and loss of HBsAg

ALT, alanine aminotransferase; HBeAg, hepatitis B envelope antigen; HBsAg, hepatitis B surface antigen; HBV, hepatitis B virus; IFN, interferon; PCR, polymerase chain reaction.

HBeAg negative (with appearance of anti-HBe), reductions in serum aminotransferase activity, elimination of circulating HBV DNA, and improvement in liver histology. The elimination of HBsAg (termination of HBV carrier state) has been difficult to achieve in clinical trials. Additionally, the responses to antiviral therapy of chronic HBV can be categorized as biochemical, virologic, or histologic, and as on therapy or sustained off therapy (Table 77-13).

DRUG THERAPY

CASE 77-12, QUESTION 4: Would initiating therapy during the acute phase of the HBV infection have benefited C.R.?

Pharmacologic interventions in the management of acute hepatitis B have been disappointing. Early studies demonstrated a transient decrease in serum aminotransferase activity and bilirubin concentration associated with corticosteroids. More recent studies, however, have resulted in a higher incidence of relapse and mortality in patients receiving corticosteroids.[56–60,99] Other therapies, including HBIG and α-interferon, have been ineffective in managing acute viral hepatitis secondary to HBV.[56–60,99] Nucleoside and nucleotide RT inhibitors reduce HBV DNA levels in patients with chronic disease,[56–60,99–106] but their use in acute HBV infection requires further investigation. Thus, administration of antivirals during the acute phase of HBV infection is not recommended in C.R.

INTERFERONS

CASE 77-12, QUESTION 5: What drug therapy should C.R. receive to treat chronic HBV-associated infection?

Previously, the most effective agents for treating chronic hepatitis B have been interferons (IFNs),[56–60,107] which appear to activate their target cells by binding to specific cell surface receptors to induce synthesis of effector proteins.[107,108] These intracellular proteins induce the antiviral, antiproliferative, and immunomodulatory actions of the IFNs. Their antiviral activity possibly arises from their ability to abate viral entry into the host cells and modulate several steps of the viral replication cycle (e.g., viral uncoating, inhibition of messenger RNA, and protein synthesis). Several varieties of IFNs are commercially available. IFN-α2b (Intron-A) and pegylated IFN (PegIFN-α2a) remain the only FDA-approved IFNs for the treatment of chronic HBV infection. PegIFNs are also preferred for treatment of HCV infection (see Hepatitis C Virus section). These agents are known to have increased serum half-life, resulting in a prolonged antiviral effect.

Efficacy

Conventional Interferon. IFN-α is moderately effective in treating chronic hepatitis B in a small percentage of highly selected patients[56,107–110] (Tables 77-14, 77-15). HBeAg-positive patients with chronic HBV receiving IFN-α may experience a virologic response based on clearance of HBeAg (27%; range, 15%–41%) or HBV DNA (47%; range, 32%–79%) compared with 9% of untreated control patients. Normalization of ALT values is observed in 47% of IFN-α–treated patients versus 13% in untreated control patients. Clearance of HBsAg occurs in only 10% to 15% of patients after completion of therapy.[56,107–110]

Pegylated Interferon. PegIFNs have the advantage of more convenient dosing and additional viral suppression for patients with HBV. Clinical data suggest that these agents have slightly enhanced efficacy than standard IFN formulations (Tables 77-14, 77-15). PegIFN-α2a 180 mcg weekly was compared with PegIFN-α2a plus lamivudine 100 mg daily or lamivudine 100 mg daily.[111] At the end of the 24-week follow-up, significantly more patients who received PegIFN monotherapy or combination therapy than those who received lamivudine monotherapy had HBeAg conversion. PegIFN-α2a (alone or in combination) resulted in HBsAg conversion in 16 patients compared with none in the lamivudine monotherapy group ($p = 0.001$). Additionally, at the end of treatment, viral suppression was most pronounced in the group that received combination therapy. Similar results were reported in HBeAg-positive patients receiving PegIFN-α2b.[112] In the only published trial performed in HBeAg-negative patients, PegIFN-α2a 180 mcg weekly (n = 177) was compared with either PegIFN-α2a 180 mcg weekly plus 100 mg of lamivudine (n = 179) or 100 mg of lamivudine alone (n = 181). Viral suppression was greater in the combination group, but sustained response (HBV DNA and ALT levels at week 72) was comparable in the group that received PegIFN-α2a alone (or in combination), and superior to the lamivudine monotherapy group. Loss of HBsAg occurred in 12 patients in the PegIFN groups, as compared with none in the lamivudine group. Ultimately, the addition of lamivudine to PegIFN did not improve posttherapy response rates.[113]

Dosing Considerations

Standard IFN doses of 2.5 to 10 million units can be administered subcutaneously (SC) daily or three times weekly for 1 to 12 months. The manufacturer of IFN-α2b recommends 30 to 35 million units/week, administered SC or IM as 5 million units/day or 10 million units three times weekly. For children, the dose should be 6 million units/m^2 SC three times a week with a maximum of 10 million units. The recommended duration of therapy for patients who are HBeAg positive is for 16 to 24 weeks. HBeAg-negative HBV infection should be treated for at least 12 months and possibly for 24 months to enhance the rate of sustained response.[56–60,109] The recommended dose of PegIFN-α2a, the only pegylated IFN approved for the treatment of HBV infection in the United States, is 180 mcg SC weekly for 48 weeks.[56–60,109] It is possible that more severe flulike symptoms and headache occur with thrice-weekly dosing when compared with daily administration. In contrast, severe bone marrow suppression tends to occur less often with thrice-weekly administration.[109]

TABLE 77-14

Responses to Antiviral Therapies Among Treatment-Naïve Patients With Hepatitis B Envelope Antigen–Positive Chronic Hepatitis B[56,58,101,105–107]

	Standard IFN-α 5 million units every day or 10 million units three times a week (12–24 weeks)	Lamivudine 100 mg every day (48–52 weeks)	Adefovir 10 mg every day (48 weeks)	Entecavir 0.5 mg every day (48 weeks)	Telbivudine 600 mg every day (52 weeks)	Tenofovir 300 mg every day (48 weeks)	PegIFN-α 180 mcg every week (48/72 weeks)	PegIFN-α + lamivudine 180 mcg every week + 100 mg (48–72 weeks)
Loss HBV DNA	37%	40%–44%	21%	67%	60%	76%	25%	69%
Loss HBeAg	33%	17%–32%	24%	22%	26%	NA	30%/34%[a]	27%/28%[a]
HBeAg seroconversion	Difference of 18%	16%–21%	12%	21%	22%	21%	27%/32%[a]	24%/27%[a]
Loss HBsAg	7.8%	1%	0	2%	0%	3.2%	3%	3%
ALT normalization	Difference of 23%	41%–75%	48%	68%	77%	68%	39%	46%
Histologic improvement	NA	49%–56%	53%	72%	65%	74%	38%	41%
Durability of response	80%–90%	50%–80%[b]	90%[b]	69%[b]	80%[b]	NA	NA	NA

[a] Response at week 48/week 72 (24 weeks after stopping therapy).

[b] Lamivudine and entecavir—no or short duration of consolidation treatment; adefovir and telbivudine—most patients had consolidation treatment.

ALT, alanine aminotransferase; HBeAg, hepatitis B envelope antigen; HBsAg, hepatitis B surface antigen; HBV, hepatitis B virus; IFN-α, interferon-α; NA, not available; PegIFN-α, pegylated interferon-α.

TABLE 77-15

Responses to Antiviral Therapies Among Treatment-Naïve Patients With Hepatitis B Envelope Antigen–Negative Chronic Hepatitis B[56,58,101,105–107]

	Standard IFN-α 5 million units every day or 10 million units three times a week (6–12 months)	Lamivudine 100 mg every day (48–52 weeks)	Adefovir 10 mg every day (48 weeks)	Entecavir 0.5 mg every day (48 weeks)	Telbivudine 600 mg every day (52 weeks)	Tenofovir 300 mg every day (48 weeks)	PegIFN-α 180 mcg every week (48 weeks)	PegIFN-α + lamivudine 180 mcg every week + 100 mg (48 weeks)
Loss HBV DNA	60%–70%	60%–73%	51%	90%	88%	93%	63%	87%
ALT normalization	60%–70%	60%–79%	72%	78%	74%	76%	38%	49%
Histologic improvement	NA	60%–66%	64%	70%	67%	72%	48%[a]	38%[a]
Durability of response	10%–22%	<10%	5%	3%	NA	NA	20%	20%

[a] Posttreatment biopsies obtained at week 72.

ALT, alanine aminotransferase; HBV, hepatitis B virus; IFN-α, interferon-α; NA, not available; PegIFN-α, pegylated interferon-α.

Predictors of Response

CASE 77-12, QUESTION 6: Would C.R. be likely to respond to IFN-α therapy?

Certain patient variables can predict the response to therapy with standard and pegylated IFN-α. The most reliable predictor of a positive response to IFN-α in HBeAg-positive patients is pretreatment ALT and HBV DNA levels.[56–60,109] Patients with high pretreatment ALT levels (greater than twice the upper limit of normal) and HBV DNA levels less than 200 pg/mL (roughly equivalent to 56 million copies/mL on a polymerase chain reaction [PCR] assay) are more likely to respond to therapy.[56–60,109] HBeAg seroconversion with IFN treatment is associated with improved survival and reduced complications. Other predictors of a positive response include a short duration of disease, negative HIV status, and a high histologic activity index as demonstrated by liver biopsy.[56–60,109] HBV genotypes A and B may respond better than genotypes C and D.[56–60,109] No consistent predictor of sustained response in patients who are HBeAg negative exists. Thus, C.R. is not a reasonable candidate for IFN-α therapy. His liver biopsy is consistent with chronic disease, he has high pretreatment aminotransferase levels, his HBV DNA is greater than 200 pg/mL, and his duration of chronic hepatitis is long.

Adverse Effects

CASE 77-12, QUESTION 7: What are some additional reasons for avoiding IFN-α therapy in C.R.?

Adverse effects associated with standard and PegIFN-α therapy are similar and quite common. These have been categorized as early side effects that rarely limit the use of IFN, and late side effects that may necessitate dose reduction or discontinuation of therapy altogether.[56–60,107,109,114,115] The early side effects of IFN-α therapy generally appear hours after administration and resemble an influenzalike syndrome with fever, chills, anorexia, nausea, myalgias, fatigue, and headache. Virtually all patients receiving IFN-α experience these toxicities, and they tend to resolve after repeated exposure to the drug. Administration of IFN-α at bedtime may decrease the severity of early side effects. Acetaminophen can be used to treat early side effects of IFN-α therapy, but should be limited to 2 g/day to minimize the risk of hepatotoxicity. The late side effects usually are observed after 2 weeks of therapy and are more serious. These toxicities, which limit the use of IFN-α, include worsening of the influenzalike syndrome, alopecia, bone marrow suppression, bacterial infections, thyroid dysfunction (both hypothyroidism and hyperthyroidism), and psychiatric disturbances (emotional lability, irritability, depression, anxiety, delirium, and suicidal ideation). The use of IFN-α can also cause a flare (increase) in ALT levels in 30% to 40% of patients. These flares are considered to be a favorable prognostic indicator, but they have been reported to cause hepatic decompensation, especially in cirrhotic patients. C.R.'s history of severe depression should be considered a relative contraindication to treating him with IFNs. Furthermore, the use of IFNs in patients with decompensated liver disease may lead to FHF; thus, these agents, although approved for HBV, are not optimal for him.[28,69,109,114,115]

NUCLEOSIDE/NUCLEOTIDE ANALOGS

CASE 77-12, QUESTION 8: What other antiviral therapies are available to treat C.R.'s chronic HBV infection?

Although IFNs have been important in the treatment of chronic HBV infection, patients included in most clinical trials represented a highly select group of chronic HBV carriers. Specifically, patients with decompensated liver disease were excluded because they often have leukopenia and thrombocytopenia as a result of hypersplenism, which limits the dose of IFN that can be administered. In addition to the IFNs, the FDA has approved several antiviral agents for treatment of chronic hepatitis B infection (lamivudine, adefovir dipivoxil, entecavir, tenofovir disoproxil, and telbivudine) with at least two more (emtricitabine and clevudine) that may be approved in the near future.

Lamivudine

Lamivudine was the first nucleoside analog approved by the FDA for use in patients with compensated liver disease who had evidence of active viral replication and liver inflammation caused by chronic hepatitis B infection. Nucleoside analogs represent an alternative approach to treatment in patients with decompensated disease.[56–60,116–119] Lamivudine, the (–) enantiomer of 3-thiacytidine, is an oral 2-′,3 ′-dideoxynucleoside that inhibits DNA synthesis by terminating the nascent proviral DNA chain and interferes with the RT activity of HBV.[116,117] Lamivudine is well tolerated and reduces serum levels of HBV DNA.[56–60,103,104,118,119]

Lamivudine Resistance

CASE 77-12, QUESTION 9: What is the risk of development of lamivudine resistance in C.R.?

Considering the high rate of viral turnover and the error-susceptible nature of the polymerase (particularly the RT), acquisition of resistance mutations is common. The most common mutation leading to lamivudine resistance is a specific point mutation in the highly conserved methionine motif of the HBV polymerase.[56–60,120,121] In this mutation, the methionine residue is changed to a valine or isoleucine. These genotypic mutations in the YMDD locus associated with a reduced sensitivity to lamivudine occur after long-term therapy (e.g., 52 weeks). This motif is thought to be representative of the active site of the enzyme, similar to that associated with HIV RT, leading to lamivudine resistance.[56–60,103,104,118–121] Lamivudine-resistant HBV mutants generally are detectable after 6 months or more of continuous therapy. Integrated data from four studies show a 16% to 32% incidence at 1 year, increasing to 47% to 56% at 2 years of therapy and 69% to 75% at 3 years of therapy.[56–60,103,104,118–121] The presence of YMDD mutants results in a loss of the clinical response, a rise in ALT levels, and worsening of hepatic histology.[56–60] Reports of continued improvement despite lamivudine resistance exist, but the long-term consequences of viral resistance (including hepatic decompensation and exacerbation of liver disease) are substantial. Thus, lamivudine has limited clinical utility in patients with chronic HBV and is currently considered a second-line agent.

CASE 77-12, QUESTION 10: What other nucleoside or nucleotide therapies are available for managing C.R.'s chronic HBV infection?

Adefovir

Adefovir dipivoxil is approved for the treatment of chronic hepatitis B in adults with evidence either of active viral replication or of persistent elevations in serum aminotransferases (ALT or AST) or histologically active disease.[122] Adefovir dipivoxil is the oral prodrug of an acyclic nucleotide monophosphate analog, 9-(2-phosphonylmethoxyethyl)-adenine. The active drug is a selective inhibitor of numerous species of viral nucleic acid polymerases and RTs.

Previously, two trials reported the efficacy of adefovir for the treatment of patients who were HBeAg negative[123] and HBeAg positive[124] (Tables 77-14, 77-15). Adverse effects from adefovir included abdominal pain, diarrhea, dyspepsia, headaches, and nausea.

Resistance to adefovir occurs at a much slower rate compared with lamivudine. The cumulative probability of resistance in the HBeAg-negative patient trial was estimated to be 0%, 3%, 1%, 18%, and 29% at years 1, 2, 3, 4, and 5 years, respectively.[123] In the trial with HBeAg-positive patients, resistance was estimated to be 20% at 5 years.[124] Other reports have described adefovir resistance rates as high as 20% after 2 years of treatment.[58,122] Risk factors for adefovir resistance appear to be suboptimal viral suppression and sequential monotherapy. Thus adefovir should also be considered a second-line therapy for C.R.

Entecavir

Entecavir is an acyclic guanosine derivative with potent activity against HBV.[56–60,125–133] The drug inhibits HBV replication at three different steps: (a) the priming of HBV DNA polymerase; (b) the RT of the negative-strand HBV DNA from the pregenomic RNA; and (c) the synthesis of positive-strand HBV DNA. In vitro studies have shown that the drug is more potent than lamivudine and adefovir and is highly effective against lamivudine-resistant HBV mutants.

In two published phase III clinical trials, the efficacy of entecavir was reported in patients with HBeAg-positive[126] and HBeAg-negative[127] hepatitis B infection (Tables 77-14, 77-15). Patients with compensated liver disease who had not previously received a nucleoside analog were assigned to receive entecavir 0.5 mg or lamivudine 100 mg once daily for a minimum of 52 weeks. By week 48, HBeAg-positive patients receiving entecavir had higher rates of histologic (72% vs. 62%), virologic (HBV DNA undetectable by PCR; 67% vs. 36%), and biochemical (ALT normalization; 68% vs. 60%) responses when compared with lamivudine.[126] Of note, the seroconversion rates were similar among the two treatment groups (21% vs. 18%; entecavir vs. lamivudine, respectively). No viral resistance to entecavir was detected during the study period, but follow-up data suggest a low rate of resistance (3% by week 96 of therapy).[126] The authors concluded that entecavir was as safe and had significantly higher histologic, virologic, and biochemical response rates than HBeAg-positive patients treated with lamivudine. In patients who remained HBeAg positive with low levels of HBV DNA replication, a second year of entecavir and lamivudine therapy resulted in seroconversion in 11% and 13% of patients, respectively.[125]

In another trial of HBeAg-negative hepatitis B infection, patients received either entecavir 0.5 mg or 100 mg of lamivudine daily for a minimum of 52 weeks. At week 48, patients receiving entecavir had significantly higher rates of histologic (70% vs. 61%; $p < 0.01$), virologic (90% vs. 72%), and biochemical (78% vs. 71%) response rates.[127] No resistance was seen among patients receiving entecavir. Safety and adverse events were similar in the two groups. Thus, C.R. could receive entecavir 0.5 mg daily. As with all of the nucleoside agents, dosage adjustments should be implemented with changes in renal function (Table 77-16). Furthermore, entecavir may be used for lamivudine-refractory or -resistant patients. In these patients, lamivudine should be discontinued to reduce the risk of entecavir cross-resistance. The dose of entecavir used for lamivudine-resistant patients is 1.0 mg daily. In these patients, entecavir resistance has been reported to be 51% after 5 years of therapy. Thus, alternatives may be warranted for these patients.[56–60,120,121,132,133]

Telbivudine

Telbivudine is an orally available L-nucleoside analog with potent antiviral activity against HBV.[134,136] Patients with HBeAg-positive or HBeAg-negative chronic hepatitis B infection were randomly assigned to receive 600 mg of telbivudine or 100 mg of lamivudine once daily[136] (Tables 77-14, 77-15). The primary efficacy end point was noninferiority of telbivudine to lamivudine for therapeutic response (i.e., a reduction in serum HBV DNA levels to <5 log 10 copies/mL, along with a loss of HBeAg, or normalization of aminotransferase levels). Secondary end points included histologic response, change in HBV DNA, and HBeAg responses. At week 52, a higher proportion of HBeAg-positive patients receiving telbivudine than lamivudine had a therapeutic response (75.3% vs. 67.0%; $p = 0.005$) or a histologic response (64.7% vs. 56.3%; $p = 0.01$); telbivudine was also not inferior to lamivudine for these end points in HBeAg-negative patients. Elevated creatinine kinase levels were more commonly seen in the patients treated with telbivudine, whereas elevated ALT and AST levels were more common in those treated with lamivudine. Resistance rates were lower among the telbivudine group compared with the lamivudine group during the first year of therapy. The rates of HBeAg loss were similar between the telbivudine and lamivudine treatment groups (26% vs. 23%, respectively). With respect to resistance, telbivudine selects for mutations in the YMDD motif. Although resistance rates are lower than those reported with lamivudine, the resistance rate is substantial and increases at a high rate after the first year of therapy.[56–60,120,121] In the phase III trial, genotypic resistance after 1 and 2 years of therapy was observed in 4.4% and 21.6%, respectively, of HBeAg-positive and 2.7% and 8.6%, respectively, of HBeAg-negative patients who received telbivudine compared with 9.1% and 33%, respectively, of HBeAg-positive and 9.8% and 21.9%, respectively, of HBeAg-negative patients who received lamivudine.[56–60,120,121] Although telbivudine is more potent with lower rates of resistance than lamivudine, the rates of resistance are much greater than for entecavir. Thus, telbivudine is not an optimal choice for C.R.

Tenofovir

Tenofovir is approved for treatment of chronic HBV.[56–60,135,137,138] This agent is a potent nucleotide analog that is structurally similar, yet equipotent, but less nephrotoxic than adefovir. Clinical trials in HBeAg-positive and HBeAg-negative patients with chronic HBV infection have demonstrated the efficacy of tenofovir[137] (Tables 77-14, 77-15). In the first phase III trial of HBeAg-positive patients with compensated liver disease, a significantly higher proportion of tenofovir-treated patients had undetectable HBV DNA (76% vs. 13%), ALT normalization (68% vs. 54%), and HBsAg loss (3% vs. 0%) at the end of therapy. Histologic response rates and HBeAg conversion were similar between the two groups. Of note, at the end of therapy, patients in the adefovir group were switched to tenofovir, and any patient who had detectable HBV DNA by week 72 had emtricitabine added to their regimen with subsequent additional serologic benefit.

In the second trial, HBeAg-negative patients with compensated liver disease were given a similar regimen (300 mg of tenofovir or 10 mg of adefovir daily for 48 weeks).[137] By week 48, a higher percentage of tenofovir-treated patients had undetectable serum HBV DNA than those treated with adefovir (93% vs. 63%). The proportions of patients having ALT normalization (76% vs. 77%) or histologic response (72% vs. 69%) were similar. No patients in the study became HBsAg negative. Again, at week 48, patients receiving adefovir were switched to tenofovir. Patients in both groups who still had detectable HBV DNA by 72 weeks were given emtricitabine. Similar to the HBeAg-positive group, the change to tenofovir led to additional viral suppression in the patients initially treated with adefovir. In the previous

TABLE 77-16

Adjustment of Adult Dosage of Nucleoside/Nucleotide Analogs in Accordance With Creatinine Clearance[58,59,117,122,125,134,135]

Creatinine Clearance (mL/min)	Recommended Dose	
Lamivudine		
≥50	100 mg every day	
30–49	100 mg first dose then 50 mg every day	
15–29	35 mg first dose, then 25 mg every day	
5–14	35 mg first dose, then 15 mg every day	
<5	35 mg first dose, then 10 mg every day	
Adefovir		
≥50	10 mg daily	
20–49	10 mg every other day	
10–19	10 mg every third day	
Hemodialysis patients	10 mg every other week after dialysis	
Entecavir		
	Nucleoside naïve	Lamivudine refractory/resistant
≥50	0.5 mg every day	1.0 mg every day
30–49	0.25 mg every day or 0.5 mg every 48 hours	0.5 mg every day or 1 mg every 48 hours
10–29	0.15 mg every day or 0.5 mg every 72 hours	0.3 mg every day or 1 mg every 72 hours
<10 or hemodialysis or continuous ambulatory peritoneal dialysis	0.05 mg every day or 0.5 mg every 7 days	0.1 mg every day or 1 mg every 7 days
Telbivudine		
≥50	600 mg daily	
30–49	600 mg once every 48 hours	
<30 (not requiring dialysis)	600 mg once every 72 hours	
End-stage renal disease	600 mg once every 96 hours (give after dialysis)	
Tenofovir		
≥50	300 mg every 24 hours	
30–49	300 mg every 48 hours	
10–29	300 mg every 72–96 hours	
<10 (with hemodialysis)	300 mg once a week or after 12 hours of hemodialysis (give dose after dialysis)	
<10 without dialysis	No recommendation	

two trials, only 7 patients were observed to have virologic breakthrough during 96 weeks of therapy, but no tenofovir-resistant HBV mutations were detected. Current guidelines suggest and clinical data support tenofovir (300 mg PO every day) as a viable first-line agent for C.R.[56–60,138] Generally, tenofovir is well tolerated, but it has been reported to cause Fanconi syndrome, renal insufficiency, osteomalacia, and a decrease in bone density.[60,135] Similar to other agents in this class, the dose of tenofovir should be adjusted based on renal function[135,137,138] (Table 77-16). Recommendations for treatment of chronic HBV can be found in Table 77-17.

INVESTIGATIONAL AGENTS

The safety and efficacy of other antiviral agents for the treatment of chronic HBV infection, including emtricitabine 2*R*,5*S*-5-fluoro-1[2-(hydroxymethyl)-1,3-oxathiolan-5-yl]cytosine), and clevudine (1-(2-fluoro-5-methyl-L-arabinofuranosyl) uracil), are under investigation.[139,140] Emtricitabine has been associated with significantly higher rates of histologic, virologic, and biochemical responses at week 48 compared with placebo.[56,139] However, rates of HBeAg seroconversion were the same in both groups (12%), with emtricitabine resistance rates occurring in 13% of treated patients.[139] Clevudine is well tolerated with undetectable serum HBV DNA levels at the end of treatment in 59% of HBeAg-positive and in 92% of HBeAg-negative patients.[56,140] A unique characteristic of clevudine is the durability of viral suppression, which persists up to 24 weeks after therapy is discontinued.[140] However, it does not increase the rate of HBeAg seroconversion compared with placebo control patients, and it also may select for mutations in the YMDD motif.

Additional agents, such as glycosidase inhibitors, hammerhead ribozymes (short RNA molecules that possess endoribonuclease activity capable of degrading target RNA), and antisense phosphodiester oligodeoxynucleotides (short fragments of DNA that are complementary to HBV-RNA, which result in inhibition of RNA translation) are also under investigation.[2,56–60,141] Pending the results of these trials and the arrival of HBV protease inhibitors and cytokine therapies, combination antiviral therapy as demonstrated in patients with HIV may improve outcomes in patients with chronic HBV infection.

COMBINATION THERAPIES

CASE 77-12, QUESTION 11: If C.R. fails therapy with entecavir or tenofovir, is combination therapy appropriate?

Combination therapy for HIV and HCV is more effective than monotherapy. The potential for additive or synergistic antiviral effects and reduced or delayed rates of viral resistance may also be possible in patients with HBV infection. Several combination therapies have been evaluated (PegIFN and lamivudine, lamivudine and adefovir, lamivudine and telbivudine), but none are superior to monotherapy.[56–60] Combination therapy is superior to lamivudine monotherapy in reducing the rate of resistance in

TABLE 77-17

Recommendations for Treatment of Chronic Hepatitis B[56,58,60]

HBeAg	HBV DNA (PCR)	ALT	Treatment Strategy
+	>20,000 international units/mL	≤2× ULN	- Low efficacy with current treatment. - Observe, consider treatment when ALT becomes elevated. - Consider biopsy in persons >40 years, ALT persistently high normal to 2× ULN, or family history of HCC - Consider treatment if HBV DNA >20,000 international units/mL and biopsy shows moderate to severe inflammation or significant fibrosis
+	>20,000 international units/mL	≥2× ULN	- Observe for 3–6 months and treat if no spontaneous HBeAg loss - Consider liver biopsy before treatment if compensated - Immediate treatment if icteric or clinical decompensation (IFN-α/PegIFN-α, LAM, ADV, ETV, LdT, TNF may be used as initial therapy) - ADV not preferred owing to weak antiviral activity and high 1-year resistance rates - LAM, LdT not preferred owing to high rate of resistance - End point of treatment: seroconversion from HBeAg to anti-HBe - Duration of therapy: IFN-α: 16 weeks PegIFN-α: 48 weeks LAM, ADV, ETV, LdT/TNF: minimum 1 year, continue for at least 6 months after HBeAg seroconversion - IFN-α nonresponders/contraindications to IFN-α → TNF/EDV
–	>20,000 international units/mL	≥2× ULN	- IFN-α/PegIFN-α, LAM, ADV, ETV, TNF or LdT may be used as initial therapy, LAM and LdT not preferred owing to high rate of resistance - ADV not preferred owing to weak antiviral activity and high 1-year resistance rates - End point of therapy not defined - Duration of therapy: IFN-α/PegIFN-α: 1 year LAM, ADV, ETV, LdT, TNF: >1 year - IFN-α nonresponders/contraindications to IFN-α → TNF/EDV
–	>2,000 international units/mL	1–2× ULN	Consider liver biopsy and treat if liver biopsy shows moderate to severe necroinflammation or significant fibrosis
–	<2,000 international units/mL	≤ULN	Observe, treat if HBV DNA or ALT becomes higher
+/–	Detectable	Cirrhosis	Compensated: - HBV DNA >2,000 international units/mL—treat: LAM/ADV/ETV/LdT/TNF may be used as initial therapy; LAM and LdT not preferred owing to high rate of resistance - ADV not preferred owing to weak antiviral activity and high 1-year resistance rates - HBV DNA <2,000 international units/mL—consider treatment if ALT is elevated Decompensated: - Coordinate treatment with transplant center, LAM (or LdT) + ADV, TNF or ETV preferred. Refer for liver transplant
+/–	Undetectable	Cirrhosis	Compensated: observe Decompensated: refer for liver transplant

ADV, adefovir; ALT, alanine aminotransferase; ETV, entecavir; HBeAg, hepatitis B envelope antigen; HBV, hepatitis B virus; HCC, hepatocellular carcinoma; IFN-α, interferon-α; LAM, lamivudine; LdT, telbivudine; PCR, polymerase chain reaction; PegIFN-α, pegylated interferon-α; TNF, tenofovir; ULN, upper limit of normal.

patients. However, there is no such role for combination therapy for those agents (entecavir, tenofovir) associated with low resistance as monotherapy. Therefore, combination therapy is not appropriate for C.R. at this time.

LIVER TRANSPLANTATION

CASE 77-12, QUESTION 12: If C.R. fails therapy, continues to decompensate, and develops cirrhosis from his chronic HBV infection, what nonpharmacologic interventions are available?

One-year survival rates for patients with cholestatic or alcoholic liver disease who undergo liver transplantation are greater than 90% in most liver transplant centers.[142] Historical data for liver transplants in patients with chronic HBV infection indicated that the spontaneous risk for allograft reinfection was approximately 80%.[142–149] This reinfection rate was associated with the initial liver disease and the hepatitis B viral load at the time of transplantation, and with allograft failure, retransplantation, or death. However, with appropriate posttransplant HBV prophylactic management, overall survival rates of patients who receive a liver transplant for HBV-related cirrhosis now exceed 85% at 1 year and 75% at 5 years, making liver transplantation a viable alternative for C.R.

CASE 77-12, QUESTION 13: What are the current recommendations for prevention of recurrent HBV infection after liver transplantation?

The most efficacious approach to preventing HBV recurrence after transplantation historically was with high-dose IV HBIG given in the anhepatic and postoperative periods. Daily IV HBIG in the early postoperative period with maintenance of serum anti-HBs levels of 100 international units/L or more had an overall survival (84%) that approached that observed in other transplant recipients without HBV infection.[143] Furthermore, patients receiving long-term HBIG administration (>6 months) compared with patients receiving short-term HBIG (<6 months) had a lower risk for recurrent HBV infection (35% vs. 75%) and longer 3-year actuarial survival (78% vs. 48%).[143,144]

HEPATITIS B IMMUNOGLOBULIN DOSAGE, ADMINISTRATION, AND ADVERSE EFFECTS

Over the years, many liver transplant centers routinely administered immunoprophylaxis with IV HBIG 10,000 international units (10 vials, 50 mL in 250 mL of saline) given in the anhepatic (recipient liver excised) phase, then gave 10,000 international units (50 mL infused for 4–6 hours) for the next 6 days postoperatively.[142,144] HBIG (10,000 international units) was generally administered on a monthly basis for life, or discontinued if HBsAg becomes positive, indicating treatment failure.[144,146–148] This regimen was able to achieve trough anti-HBs titers of approximately 500 international units/L and up to 2,000 international units/L, which provided protection from HBV recurrence in the majority of transplanted patients. Patients who received HBIG oftentimes experienced a serum sicknesslike syndrome (fever, myalgias) managed by administering premedications (i.e., acetaminophen, benadryl), prolonging the HBIG infusion (up to 6 hours), or discontinuing HBIG therapy altogether.

Long-term concerns associated with HBIG administration included the potential for treatment failure (HBV reinfection from extrahepatic sites despite adequate anti-HBs titers), emergence of mutant viruses, and the prohibitive high cost of therapy (>$60,000/year).[144,146–148] Some data suggested that pharmacokinetic modeling and use of maintenance therapy with IM administration of HBIG (e.g., 2.5–10 mL every 2–3 weeks) after a reduced induction dose (e.g., 10,000 international units anhepatically, then 2,000 international units IV × six doses) could achieve similar outcomes and reduce the cost associated with IV administration of the drug.[148]

CASE 77-12, QUESTION 14: What is the role of oral antiviral agents in liver transplant recipients with HBV?

The nucleoside and nucleotide analogs, such as lamivudine, adefovir, entecavir, and more recently tenofovir, potentially prevent recurrence of HBV in patients who undergo transplants for chronic HBV infection.[144–149] Lamivudine monotherapy was proven successful in converting HBV DNA–positive patients to negative status before and after liver transplantation. Resistance in transplant and nontransplant recipients also has been observed.[120,121,144–149] Nucleoside analogs are not FDA-approved for this prophylaxis in the United States. Several transplant centers, however, have implemented clinical protocols that administer adefovir, entecavir, or tenofovir before transplantation to achieve undetectable viral loads (HBV DNA) at the time of transplant, then combine one of these agents with HBIG in the postoperative setting.[144–149] Ultimately, these management strategies have emerged as a clinical standard in the preoperative and early postoperative period because they are effective and have low rates of resistance. Future considerations for preventing recurrent HBV infection after transplantation include combining oral nucleoside (adefovir, entecavir) with nucleotide (tenofovir) analogs, thus avoiding HBIG altogether.[149]

HEPATITIS C VIRUS

Virology

HCV is recognized now as the most common cause of chronic NANB transfusion-associated hepatitis.[2,3,5,6,150–165] HCV is a single-stranded, 50-nm RNA virus related to the flaviviruses, a family that includes the yellow fever virus and two animal viruses (Table 77-2).[150,153,157]

In primates, HCV RNA is detectable within 3 days of infection, persisting in the serum during peak ALT elevation. Detection appears to be associated with the appearance of viral antigens in hepatocytes, the major site of HCV replication. The importance of extrahepatic sites for replication (e.g., mononuclear cells) has not been determined. Kinetic studies in HCV-infected patients have depicted a high viral turnover that may partially explain the rapid emergence of viral diversity in patients with chronic HCV infection and the persistence of the infection, through immune escape, after acute exposure. Mechanisms pertaining to viral packaging and release from the hepatocytes are poorly understood.

Epidemiology

The worldwide seroprevalence based on antibody to HCV (anti-HCV) is approximately 3%, with up to 180 million people infected chronically.[1,3,150,152,153,165] Geographic variations exist, from 0.4% to 1.1% in North America to 9.6% to 13.6% in North Africa.[1,3,150,152,153,165] The prevalence of anti-HCV in the United States has been estimated to be 1.8%, corresponding to an estimated 4.1 million persons infected nationwide. Of these, 2.7 million persons are chronically infected (based on positive HCV RNA), with approximately 230,000 new infections per year.[1,3,150,152,153,165] Of concern, HCV is the primary cause of death from liver disease and is the leading indication for liver transplantation in the United States.[1,3,150,152,153,165] Several studies indicate that mortality related to HCV (death as a result of liver failure or HCC) will continue to rise in the next two decades and will significantly impact health care costs.[1,3,150,152,153,165] HCV is the etiologic agent in more than 85% of cases associated with posttransfusional NANB hepatitis.[1,3,150,152,153,165] After HCV antibody screening of blood donors in the early 1990s, transfusion-related reports of HCV have been dramatically reduced, and non–transfusion-related cases have emerged (e.g., injection drug users).[150,153,165] Sporadic infection with HCV (infection without an identifiable risk factor) accounts for up to 40% of reported HCV infections.[150,153,165] HCV is transmitted through percutaneous (e.g., blood transfusion, needlestick inoculation, high-risk behavior)[150–153,165] and nonpercutaneous (e.g., sexual contact, perinatal exposure) routes.[150–153,164,165] The latter appears to occur to a lesser extent than with HBV.

HCV infection occurs among persons of all ages, but the highest incidence is among persons aged 20 to 39 years, with a male predominance. Blacks and whites have similar incidence rates of acute disease, whereas persons of Hispanic ethnicity have higher rates. In the general population, the highest prevalence rates of chronic HCV infection are found among persons aged 30 to 49 years and among males.[150–153,164,165] Unlike the racial or ethnic pattern of acute disease, blacks have a substantially higher prevalence of chronic HCV infection than do whites.

In the United States, the predominant HCV genotype is type 1, with subtypes 1a and 1b accounting for 70% of cases.[153–156,164,165] Knowledge of the genotype or serotype (genotype-specific antibodies) of HCV is helpful in making recommendations and counseling regarding therapy. Once the genotype is identified, it need not be tested again; genotypes do not change during the course of infection. Because HCV has a high mutation rate during replication, several so-called quasi-species, a heterogeneous population of HCV isolates that are closely related, may, however, exist in an infected individual.[150–153,165] The number of quasi-species increases during the course of infection, which allows HCV to escape the host's immune system, leading to persistent infection.

PERCUTANEOUS TRANSMISSION

Before the routine use of blood screening, the incidence of acute HCV infection among transfusion recipients in the 1970s was approximately 5% to 10%. Subsequently, blood donor screening using a first-generation anti-HCV test reduced the risk of transfusion-related hepatitis to 0.6% per patient and 0.03% per unit transfused.[153,156,165] After the use of more sensitive second- and third-generation assays for anti-HCV, the risk and incidence of transfusion-related hepatitis approaches that reported in hospitalized patients who have not received a transfusion.

The incidence of HCV infection is 48% to 90% among injection drug users, and the risk of acquiring the infection in these persons is as high as 90%.[153,156,165] Of injection drug users with acute NANB hepatitis, 75% are anti-HCV positive and, unlike transfusion-related hepatitis, the incidence of HCV infection associated with injection drug use has not declined.[153,156,165] Additional risk factors for HCV infection include the presence of HBV or HIV infection.[153,156,165] Other populations at risk for acquiring HCV include patients receiving chronic hemodialysis (up to 45%)[153,156,165] and health care workers (0% to 4% seroconversion after needlestick).[153,156,165]

NONPERCUTANEOUS AND SPORADIC TRANSMISSION

Nonpercutaneous transmission includes transmission between sexual partners and from mother to child. This route of transmission is less efficient compared with the percutaneous route, and is supported by data assessing sexual transmission of HCV. Sexual partners of index patients with anti-HCV have an incidence of HCV infection ranging from 0% to 27%, whereas low-risk (anti-HCV negative) index subjects without liver disease or high-risk behavior (injection drug use or promiscuity) have an incidence of anti-HCV of 0% to 7%.[153,156,165] In contrast, sexual partners of subjects with liver disease or high-risk behavior have an incidence of anti-HCV ranging between 11% and 27%.[153,156,165] Also, the sexual partners of homosexual men and promiscuous heterosexuals with HCV have shown an increase in anti-HCV positivity.

Compared with the high incidence of perinatal transmission of HBV from mothers to infants, perinatal transmission of HCV infection is relatively low; however, high titers of circulating HCV in the mother may enhance the risk of infection in the infant.[153,156,165] Additional concerns and areas for investigation related to mother-to-infant transmission of HCV include the timing of transmission (in utero, time of birth), the relative risk associated with breast-feeding, and the natural history of perinatally acquired infection.

In sporadic HCV infection, up to 40% of patients acquire HCV infection without a known or identifiable risk factor.[153,156,165] This type of HCV infection may be related to a prevalent nonpercutaneous or percutaneous route that has yet to be identified.

Pathogenesis

The pathogenesis of liver damage as a result of HCV infection most likely results from both direct and indirect immune-mediated responses instigated by the virus. Direct cellular injury may be caused by the accumulation of intact virus or viral proteins.[150,166,167] The direct mechanism of injury is supported by the observation that patients with high concentrations of HCV RNA (quantified through branched-chain DNA assay) have greater lobular inflammatory activity compared with those with minimal inflammation. Whether specific genotypes (i.e., 1, 1b, 2) are correlated with severe disease continues to be assessed. European data suggest that type 1 genotype is associated with higher viral replication, and infection with the type 1b genotype is associated with more progressive liver disease.[150,166–168] One reason why HCV genotype 1 may be more difficult to treat than genotypes 2 or 3 is that genotype 1 has a longer half-life (2.9 hours) than that of genotypes 2 or 3 (2.0 hours).[166,167,169,170] Viral half-life can be defined as the time for the original amount of virus to be decreased by half, or in this case, die. Other data do not support these findings and have shown that patients with type 2 genotypes have more severe liver disease.[166,167,169,170] Duration of infection is another factor that may be related to disease severity because the expression of genotypes may change with time, making the correlation between genotype and severity of disease problematic. Furthermore, immune-mediated mechanisms for hepatic injury have been based on the presence of $CD8^+$ and $CD4^+$ lymphocytes in portal, periportal, and lobular areas in patients with HCV infection.[170,171]

Diagnosis

Two classes of assays are used in the diagnosis and management of HCV. These include serologic assays that detect specific antibody to HCV (anti-HCV) and molecular assays that detect viral nucleic acid. These assays are not used to assess the severity of disease or predict prognosis in patients infected with HCV.

SEROLOGIC ASSAYS

A test for antibodies to HCV is the initial screening test for suspected HCV infection.[150,172–176] The two types of antibody tests are (a) the enzyme immunoassay (EIA) and the (b) recombinant immunoblot assay (RIBA). These serologic assays were developed using recombinant antigens derived from cloned HCV transcripts to substantiate a diagnosis of HCV. Predictive values of a positive third-generation EIA test are about 99% (in immunocompetent patients), which obviates the need for a confirmatory RIBA test in the diagnosis of patients with clinical liver disease.[150,172–176] A negative EIA test is adequate to exclude a diagnosis of chronic HCV infection in nonimmunocompromised individuals.[150,172–176] The clinical symptoms, changes in HCV RNA, and serologic changes in acute and chronic HCV infection are shown in Figure 77-4.

MOLECULAR ASSAYS

Several commercial assays are available for the detection (qualitative HCV RNA assays) or quantification (quantitative assays) of HCV RNA.[150] Over time, the qualitative assays have been found to be more sensitive than quantitative assays. However, with the recent availability of real-time PCR-based assays and transcription-mediated amplification, which has a detection limit of 10 to 50 international units/mL, there is no longer a role for qualitative assays.[150,172–176] A highly sensitive assay with this lower limit of detection can be used for monitoring throughout therapy.

BIOCHEMICAL MARKERS

Testing for serum ALT concentrations is not a sensitive marker for assessing disease activity and at best has a weak correlation with the histopathologic findings on a liver biopsy.[150–154,157] Nevertheless, serial determination of ALT as a function of time appears to be a better indicator of liver injury than is a single ALT test.

BIOPSY

Liver biopsy can determine the extent of liver injury caused by HCV.[150–154,157] Although some histologic findings are characteristic of HCV infection, such as portal lymphoid aggregates, steatosis, and bile duct injury, these alone are not sufficiently specific to establish a diagnosis of hepatitis C. Currently, no reliable, readily available tests exist to detect HCV antigens in the

and 3, respectively. In summary, PegIFN-α2a for 48 weeks, with or without adefovir, resulted in sustained HDV RNA clearance in about 25% of patients with HDV infection.

Other oral agents such as famciclovir, lamivudine, tenofovir/emtricitabine, or thymosin have not proven to be effective in clearing HDV.[300–303,308,315,316] Therefore, these agents cannot be recommended at this time.

In patients with decompensated cirrhosis caused by HDV, liver transplantation is the most appropriate intervention because IFN may precipitate hepatic decompensation.[143,300–303,307] The presence and amount of HBV DNA before transplantation is the most significant outcome marker, often predicting the posttransplant reinfection rate. Patients who receive a liver transplant for chronic HDV infection have a lower incidence of posttransplant HBV infection than do those with HBV infection alone (67% vs. 32%, respectively).[143] This is thought to be related to an inhibitory effect of HDV on HBV replication. Furthermore, 3-year survival is higher for patients with HDV cirrhosis than for patients undergoing transplantation for HBV cirrhosis alone (88% vs. 44%, respectively) and is similar to patients having liver transplantation for other indications.[143]

HEPATITIS E VIRUS

Virology, Epidemiology, Transmission, and Pathogenesis

HEV is an icosahedral, nonenveloped virus of the Hepeviridae family (Table 77-2).[2,317–329] The HEV genome is a single-stranded polyadenylated RNA and, unlike HAV, has an RNA genome that encodes for nonstructural proteins through overlapping open reading frames.[318] HEV sequences have been classified into four genotypes (1, 2, 3, and 4).[318,319,324,325] Genotype 1 consists of epidemic strains in developing countries; genotype 2 has been found in Mexico; genotype 3 has been associated with acute cases of hepatitis and with domestic pigs in the United States, European countries, and Japan; and genotype 4 has been found in Asian countries.

HEV occurs in endemic areas such as Africa, Southeast and Central Asia, Mexico, and Central and South America as both epidemic and sporadic infections.[317–326] Sporadic infections also occur in nonendemic areas and are usually associated with travel into areas of endemicity. The attack rate (the percentage of exposed patients who become infected) of HEV is low compared with HAV (1% vs. 10%, respectively). In endemic areas, outbreaks usually occur between 5 and 10 years apart and are often associated with times of heavy rainfall, after floods or monsoons, or after the recession of flood waters.[317–326] The overall case fatality rate for the general endemic population is 0.5% to 4%, whereas for reasons unknown, pregnant women have a much greater case fatality rate of 20%.[317–329] In particular, the fetal complication rate is increased, especially if the infection occurs in the third trimester of pregnancy.[317–329] The frequency of death in utero and immediately after birth is also greater than seen with acute hepatitis of other causes.[317–329]

Transmission of HEV is via the fecal-oral route, and the most common source of transmission is ingestion of fecally contaminated water.[317–326] Poor climactic conditions in conjunction with inadequate personal hygiene and sanitation have led to epidemics of HEV infection. Additional routes of transmission include consuming raw or undercooked meat of infected animals such as boar or deer and domestic animals such as pigs, vertical, and blood-borne transmission.[317–326]

Interference with the production of cellular macromolecules, alteration of cellular membranes, and alteration of lysosomal permeability are some of the proposed mechanisms of hepatic injury.[324] In addition, immune-mediated mechanisms are believed to be responsible for lysis of virally infected hepatocytes by direct lymphocyte cytotoxicity or antibody-mediated cytotoxicity.

ONLINE CONTENT

For an illustration of the proposed scheme of clinical, biochemical, virologic, and serologic events in acute hepatitis E infection, go to http://thepoint.lww.com/AT10e.

Diagnosis

Initial assays for detection of anti-HEV used electron microscopy to detect HEV antigen on the surface of HEV particles in stool and serum and immunohistochemistry to detect the antigen in liver tissue.[318,325,326] Fluorescent antibody-blocking assay is currently used to detect anti-HEV reacting to HEV antigen in serum, but although highly specific, this assay lacks sensitivity (50%) in acute HEV infection.[318,325,326] Additional cloning and sequencing of HEV has led to the development of Western blot assays and ELISA that detect anti-HEV by using recombinant expressed proteins from the structural region of the virus. RT-PCR has also been used to confirm the diagnosis of HEV by detecting HEV RNA from serum, liver, or stool.[318,325,326] Clinically, HEV is a diagnosis of exclusion.

Clinical Manifestations and Natural History

Typical HEV clinical symptoms include jaundice, dark urine, tender and enlarged liver, elevated liver enzymes, abdominal pain, nausea, vomiting, and fever. Protracted coagulopathy and cholestasis have also been reported in more severe cases, possibly related to genotype 4.[318,325,326] The incubation period after exposure is listed in Table 77-1. Two phases of illness exist, including a prodromal and preicteric phase.[318,325,326] Peak serum aminotransferase levels reflect the onset of the icteric phase and generally return to baseline by 6 weeks.[318,325,326] Stool is often positive for HEV RNA at the onset of the icteric phase and persists for an additional 10 days beyond this period. Viral shedding may occur for up to 52 days after the onset of icterus. Detection in the serum occurs during the preicteric phase, before detection of virus in the stool, and becomes undetectable after the peak in aminotransferase activity. Because HEV RNA is not detectable in the serum during symptoms, diagnostic tests using HEV RNA have limited utility, and a correlation between PCR detection and infectivity has not been observed. Serologically, HEV IgM becomes detectable before the peak rise in ALT, whereas antibody titers peak with peak ALT levels and subsequently decline. In most patients, HEV IgM is present for 5 to 6 months after the onset of illness. HEV IgG appears after HEV IgM and remains detectable for up to 14 years after acute infection; however, the duration of protective immunity has not been fully elucidated.[318,325,326]

In nonfatal cases, acute HEV hepatitis is followed by complete recovery without any chronic complications. There is protection from reinfection; however, the duration of protection is variable. Fulminant hepatitis has also been associated with HEV infection, mostly in pregnancy.[318,325,326] Maternal mortality was reported to be 1.5% for HEV infection occurring in the first trimester of pregnancy, 8.5% for those in the second trimester, and 21% for those infected in the third trimester.

A persistent form of HEV infection accompanied by chronic liver disease (occasionally progressing to cirrhosis) has been reported in solid-organ transplant recipients (liver, kidney, or pancreas).[330,331] Although infrequently encountered, these patients have HEV infection for more than 15 months after their acute infection. Chronic infection has led to portal hepatitis, fibrosis, and allograft loss in these patients.

Prevention and Treatment

No immunoprophylactic measures exist for HEV disease, and effective prevention strategies are dependent on improved sanitation in endemic areas. Travelers going to endemic areas should be educated regarding the risks of drinking water, eating ice, or eating uncooked shellfish or uncooked and peeled fruits and vegetables. Drinking water should be boiled to inactivate HEV. No vaccines or postexposure prophylaxis treatments are currently available to prevent HEV infection. However, results from a phase II randomized trial using 20 mcg of a recombinant 56-kDa truncated open reading frame-2 vaccine in young healthy men suggest that these agents could be effective in the prevention of HEV infection.[332] Others have reported limited success with oral ribavirin (12 mg/kg daily for 12 weeks) in a kidney and pancreas transplant recipient with chronic HEV infection.[333,334] Clearly, an appropriately designed clinical trial is required to define the role of ribavirin for chronic HEV infection.

SUMMARY

Viral hepatitis continues to be a significant worldwide infectious disease. To date, prevention strategies through universal vaccination are the most efficient methods for minimizing the incidence of HAV, HBV, and HDV. Patient education with respect to the common ways of spreading these infections may also result in behavioral modifications that reduce the overall incidence of infection. Once HBV and HCV progress to chronic infection, more efficacious and better-tolerated antiviral therapies are needed to treat these infections. Similarly, therapeutic modalities that reduce the progression of these diseases are necessary to prevent end-stage liver disease and the development of additional complications (encephalopathy, intractable ascites, coagulation disorders, and HCC). As a better understanding of viral replication is established, as well as appropriate models for study, new agents are becoming available. Furthermore, viral kinetics and genomic-based approaches may optimize responses to drug therapies, especially in HCV-infected patients. The economic impact and quality of life of these patients remains to be fully elucidated.

KEY REFERENCES AND WEBSITES

A full list of references for this chapter can be found at **http://thepoint.lww.com/AT10e.** Below are the key references and website for this chapter, with the corresponding reference number in this chapter found in parentheses after the reference.

Key References

Advisory Committee on Immunization Practices (ACIP) et al. Prevention of hepatitis A through active or passive immunization: recommendations of the Advisory Committee on Immunization Practices (ACIP). *MMWR Recomm Rep*. 2006;55(RR-7):1. (22)

Afdhal NH et al. Hepatitis C pharmacogenetics: state of the art in 2010. *Hepatology*. 2011;53:336. (240)

Aggarwal R. Hepatitis E: historical, contemporary and future perspectives. *J Gastroenterol Hepatol*. 2011;26(Suppl 1):72. (319)

Dienstag JL. Hepatitis B virus infection [published correction appears in *N Engl J Med*. 2010;363:298]. *N Engl J Med*. 2008;359:1486. (56)

Foster GR. Pegylated interferons for the treatment of chronic hepatitis C: pharmacological and clinical differences between peginterferon-alpha-2a and peginterferon-alpha-2b. *Drugs* 2010;70:147. (229)

Ghany MG et al. Diagnosis, management and treatment of hepatitis C: an update. *Hepatology*. 2009;49:1335. (150)

Lok A, McMahon BJ. Chronic hepatitis B: update 2009. *Hepatology*. 2009;50:661. (58)

Mast EE et al. A comprehensive immunization strategy to eliminate transmission of hepatitis B virus infection in the United States: recommendations of the Immunization Practices Advisory Committee (ACIP) Part II: immunization of adults [published correction appears in *MMWR Morb Mortal Wkly Rep*. 2007;56:1114]. *MMWR Recomm Rep*. 2006;55(RR-16):1. (61)

[No authors listed]. Recommendations for prevention and control of hepatitis C virus (HCV) infection and HCV-related chronic disease. Centers for Disease Control and Prevention. *MMWR Recomm Rep*. 1998;47(RR-19):1. (156)

Pawlotsky JM. The results of Phase III clinical trials with telaprevir and boceprevir presented at the Liver Meeting 2010; a new standard of care for hepatitis C virus genotype 1 infection, but with issues still pending. *Gastroenterology*. 2011;140:746. (275)

Rizzetto M. Hepatitis D: thirty years after. *J Hepatol*. 2009;50:1043 (301)

Seeff LB. The history of the "natural history" of hepatitis C (1968–2009). *Liver Int*. 2009;29(Suppl 1):89. (153)

Thompson AJV, McHutchison JG. Review article: investigational agents for chronic hepatitis C. *Aliment Pharmacol Ther*. 2009;29:689. (262)

Zoulim F, Locarnini S. Hepatitis B virus resistance to nucleos(t)ide analogues. *Gastroenterology*. 2009;137:1593. (121)

Key Website

American Association for the Study of Liver Diseases (AASLD). **http://www.aasld.org.**

78 Parasitic Infections

J.V. Anandan

CORE PRINCIPLES

	CHAPTER CASES
MALARIA	
1 Malaria is responsible for 300 to 500 million cases and annual deaths in excess of 1 million. Acute malaria usually presents as an abrupt onset of coldness and chills, followed by high fever, headache, nausea, and vomiting.	**Case 78-1 (Question 1)**
2 Falciparum malaria is the most severe form of malaria and has the highest mortality. The incidence of chloroquine resistance and serious complications associated with this plasmodium mandate immediate use of parenteral antimalarials and adjunctive supportive measures.	**Case 78-1 (Question 2)**
3 Pregnant women are at greater risk for malaria and its associated complications and should avoid travel to endemic areas. Malaria vaccines are under investigation, and their effectiveness and safety in children and pregnant women are being evaluated.	**Case 78-2 (Questions 1, 2)**
4 Multiresistant falciparum malaria, which may require combination therapy, has been reported in the Thai-Myanmar border, in New Guinea, and in West Africa.	**Case 78-3 (Question 1)**
5 Antimalarial drugs are associated with some significant adverse effects. Special attention needs to be directed to those who have glucose-6-phosphate deficiency when antimalarials are used.	**Case 78-4 (Questions 1, 2)**
AMEBIASIS	
1 Amebiasis is caused by *Entamoeba histolytic* and implicated in amebic dysentery and hepatic abscesses. Diagnosis of amebic dysentery may include the following information: history of travel, stool and biopsy specimens, and ultrasound to exclude liver abscesses. Treatment for amebiasis calls for a combination of agents with both luminal-acting and extraintestinal effects. Amebic cyst passers and pregnant women must be treated to avoid invasive disease and transmission of the infection.	**Case 78-5 (Questions 1, 2), Case 78-6 (Questions 1, 2), Case 78-7 (Question 1)**
GIARDIASIS	
1 The signs and symptoms of giardiasis could be insidious and vague, but patients usually present with diarrhea and bulky, foul-smelling stools along with confirmation of *Giardia lamblia*.	**Case 78-8 (Question 1)**
2 Negative stool samples for *G. lamblia* should result in further diagnostic testing. The major treatments for giardiasis are metronidazole and tinidazole.	**Case 78-8 (Questions 2, 3)**
ENTEROBIASIS	
1 The signs and symptoms of the infection may be subtle, but the specific diagnostic test for *Enterobius vermicularis* is the cellophane tape swab. Therapy for enterobiasis includes three different antihelminthic agents. Household measures to eradicate the infection need to be addressed.	**Case 78-9 (Questions 1–3)**

continued

CESTODIASIS	
1 Primarily this includes *Taenia saginata* and *Taenia Solium*, and symptoms of infections are nonspecific. It is critical to differentiate these two infections from other cestode infections. Praziquantel remains an effective agent for all species of Cestoidea. Cysticercosis, a complication caused by the larval cysts of *T. solium* that may be associated with central nervous system infection (neurocysticercosis), is serious and requires separate diagnostic testing and controversial therapy. Praziquantel, which is indicated for most cestodiasis, is well tolerated.	**Case 78-10 (Questions 1–4), Case 78-11 (Questions 1–3)**
PEDICULOSIS	
1 Head and body lice are associated wth dermatological reactions, which can be treated with a number of agents: pyrethrin, lindane, malathion, and ivermectin. Special attention needs to be focused on drug resistance, side effects of lindane, and lice decontamination measures.	**Case 78-12 (Questions 1–3)**
SCABIES	
1 Scabies produces pruritic rash and excoriations of the interdigital area of the upper and lower limbs. Treatment includes lindane, permethrin, and crotamiton. Clothes and personal items of the infected person and family members need to laundered (>50°C) to avoid reinfection.	**Case 78-13 (Question 1)**

MALARIA

Distribution and Mortality

Malaria is responsible for an estimated 300 to 500 million cases and annual deaths in excess of 1 million.[1–4] Millions of US travelers visit malaria-endemic areas each year.[2,3,5] The distribution of the four *Plasmodium* species of malaria varies worldwide, with *Plasmodium falciparum,* which has the highest mortality, primarily acquired in sub-Saharan Africa, Haiti, the Dominican Republic, the Amazon region in South America, and parts of Asia and Oceania.[3–5]

Life Cycle

Malarial infection is transmitted by the female mosquito of the genus *Anopheles,* which injects the asexual forms or sporozoites into the human host during a blood meal. After a lapse of 9 to 16 days and an asexual multiplication stage in the liver called *exoerythrocytic schizogony,* daughter cells, or merozoites, are released into the blood to infect red blood cells (RBCs). The merozoites develop into the characteristic ring or trophozoite forms in RBCs and then go through another asexual reproductive stage called *erythrocytic schizogony* to produce more merozoites. When the infected RBCs rupture, the merozoites invade new blood cells and repeat the erythrocyte cycle. In 1 to 2 weeks, a subpopulation of merozoites differentiates into the sexual forms, resulting in male and female gametocytes. If the gametocytes in the host blood are ingested by a female *Anopheles* mosquito during a blood meal, fertilization and an asexual division in the mosquito midgut will propagate the infective sporozoites to complete the cycle.

The characteristic malarial paroxysms of chills and fever usually coincide with the periodic release of merozoites and other pyrogens in the blood. In *P. falciparum* infections, this periodicity may not always be apparent. However, intervals of 48 hours between paroxysms are reported for *Plasmodium vivax, Plasmodium ovale,* and *P. falciparum* (tertian periodicity), and 72 hours for *Plasmodium malariae* (quartan periodicity). Unlike infections caused by *P. falciparum* and *P. malariae,* infections with *P. vivax* and *P. ovale* have a latent form of the exoerythrocytic phase that can persist in the host liver for months to years. This latent form can produce relapses of the erythrocytic infection (Fig. 78-1).

Epidemiology

Although malaria is endemic to the tropics, approximately 1,298 cases were diagnosed in the United States in 2008.[4] Of the 792 imported cases of malaria, 563 were acquired in Africa, 170 in Asia, 49 in the Americas, and 10 in Oceania.[3] Malaria transmission in the United States has occurred from the blood of immigrants and travelers, local transmission, military personnel, and rarely through blood transfusions.[2–5] Of *Plasmodium* identified in the United States, 41% of those represent *P. falciparum,* and 14.6% as *P. vivax. P. falciparum* was predominantly acquired in Africa.[3] One confirmed case of *P. knowlesi,* a species normally found in monkeys in Southeast Asia, was reported by the Centers for Disease Control and Prevention (CDC).[3] It is now thought that *P. knowlesi* can be transmitted to humans.[6] Transfusion malaria, particularly *P. malariae,* can persist in the blood without symptoms for extended periods.[7,8] Malaria can also be transmitted congenitally and through contaminated needles.[3,8,9]

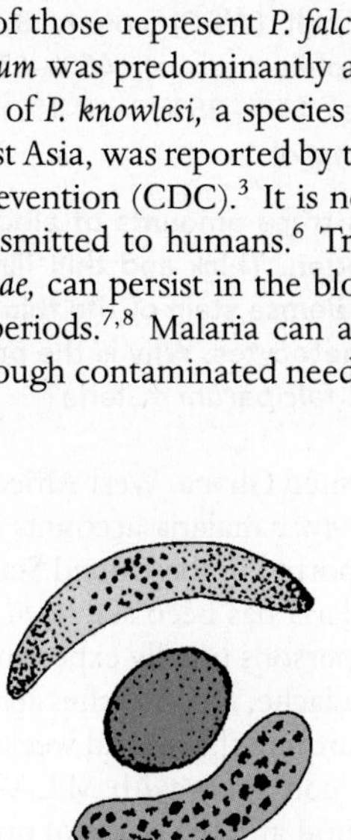

FIGURE 78-1 ***Plasmodium falciparum*** **gametocytes.**

Drug Resistance

Chloroquine-resistant *P. falciparum* (CRPF) is widespread and present in all malaria-endemic areas of the world except Mexico, the Caribbean, and Central America (north of the Panama Canal). Resistant strains have also ben reported in parts of the Middle East (Iran, Yemen, Oman, and Saudi Arabia).[10–14] *P. falciparum* malaria resistant to chloroquine and mefloquine has been isolated in Thailand, Cambodia, and Myanmar (Burma). Chloroquine-resistant *P. vivax* is an emerging problem in Papua New Guinea, Irian, Jaya (Indonesia), Myanmar, and Colombia.[9,11,14,15] Most fatal cases of imported malaria in the United States are the result of travelers' failure to comply with appropriate chemosuppressive regimens, delays in seeking treatment, misdiagnosis by physicians or laboratories, and inappropriate antimalarial regimens.[3,13] Prophylactic drug regimens for individuals traveling to endemic (drug-resistant *P. falciparum*) areas are problematic (see Case 78-3, Question 1).[10,11,15]

Acute Malaria

SIGNS AND SYMPTOMS

CASE 78-1

QUESTION 1: M.L., a 29-year-old male student, presents to the emergency department (ED) with complaints of malaise, myalgia, headache, and fever of 4 days' duration. A native of Ghana, West Africa, he recently visited his parents and returned to the United States 3 weeks ago. Two days before admission, he had an abrupt onset of coldness and chills, followed 1 hour later by a high fever, headache, nausea, and vomiting. The episode of chills and fever lasted about 24 hours, after which he became asymptomatic. On the afternoon of admission, he again had a bout of chills that preceded a fever of 40°C.

Physical examination reveals a slender black man who is acutely ill and complaining of severe abdominal pain. Abdominal examination reveals a soft, tender spleen that is slightly enlarged. Blood pressure (BP) is 110/70 mm Hg; pulse, 120 beats/minute; respiration rate, 32 breaths/minute; and temperature, 40°C. Laboratory findings include the following:

Hemoglobin (Hgb), 11 g/dL
Hematocrit (Hct), 34%
White blood cell (WBC) count, 3,300 cells/μL with 76% neutrophils (normal, 45%–65%), 23% lymphocytes (normal, 15%–35%), and 1% monocytes
Bilirubin, 1.0 mg/dL

Urinalysis reveals trace amounts of albumin and the presence of urobilinogen. Thick and thin films of M.L.'s blood are prepared. A Giemsa stain of the thin film demonstrates *P. falciparum* gametocytes. Why is the presentation of M.L. consistent with *P. falciparum* malaria?

M.L. recently visited Ghana, West Africa, where *P. falciparum* is endemic.[4,9,11] *P. vivax* malaria accounts for about 15% of all cases of malaria reported in the United States.[3] The prevalence of *P. falciparum* malaria has been stable, accounting for 41% of all cases.[3] Infected persons usually experience prodromal symptoms (primarily headache, muscle aches and pains, malaise, nausea, and vomiting) around the second week after exposure.[9,13,16] This time frame is consistent with M.L.'s onset of symptoms. The incubation period and the onset of primary symptoms for *P. falciparum* malaria can be delayed for months.[2,3,9,11,16] History of travel to an endemic area, the cyclical paroxysmal episodes of chills and fever, the presence of thrombocytopenia and jaundice, and the identification of *P. falciparum* gametocytes in M.L.'s blood confirm the diagnosis of malaria.

TREATMENT

CASE 78-1, QUESTION 2: How should the *P. falciparum* malaria in M.L. be treated? How would M.L.'s treatment differ from that used for other *Plasmodium* species?

P. falciparum malaria, the most severe form of malaria, has the highest mortality rate.[3,8,16–25] The fever spikes, unlike those associated with *P. vivax* and *P. ovale* malaria, normally are very high (40°–41°C), and complications (including confusion, vomiting, diarrhea, severe abdominal pain, hypoglycemia, renal failure, and encephalopathy) are common.[16–25]

QUINIDINE AND QUININE

M.L. is very ill and may be unable to tolerate oral medications because of nausea and vomiting. He should be admitted to an acute care unit and started on intravenous (IV) quinidine gluconate.[7,11,22,25–28] (For doses of IV quinidine, see Table 78-1.) If more than 48 hours of parenteral therapy is required, the dosage of quinidine should be reduced by one-third to one-half.[9,11,18,27]

Because IV quinidine is not routinely used in cardiology care, it may not be available in all hospitals. Because of the serious nature of *P. falciparum* malaria, small stocks of the drug should be kept on hand. Alternatively, the hospital should be prepared to acquire IV quinidine on short notice (contact Eli Lilly at 800-821-0538).[27] Oral quinine and clindamycin or the combination of atovaquone and proguanil (Malarone) can be used until IV quinidine is available.[4,7,27] Intravenous artesunate (a water-soluble hemisuccinate derivative of dihydroartemisinin) is an alternative agent for use in serious malaria for patients intolerant of quinidine or with unavailability of intravenous quinidine or with parasitemia greater than 10% at 48 hours.[9,26–28] Intravenous artesunate can be obtained from the CDC (Malaria Hotline: 770-488-7788 or after hours at 770-488-7100 for malaria clinician on call) as an investigational new drug (IND).[28] Intravenous artesunate is administered at 2.4 mg/kg per dose every 12 hours for 3 days (may be continued for longer periods if necessary) followed by oral atovaquone-proguanil, mefloquine, or clindamycin to complete a total of 7 days of therapy.[9,27,28]

If IV quinidine is used, M.L.'s electrocardiogram, BP, and serum glucose should be monitored closely.[7,9,18,22] Supportive care, including fluids, IV dextrose infusions (initially 50% concentration but subsequently 10%), electrolyte management, dialysis, blood transfusion, and mechanically assisted ventilation, is important adjunctive therapy in seriously ill patients.[7,9] Thick blood films should be examined at 24 and 48 hours to confirm or exclude the diagnosis. The serum concentration of quinidine should be determined once daily during the continuous infusion. Quinidine levels should remain between 4.6 and 9.2 μmol/L (2–6 mcg/mL). The quinidine infusion should be slowed or stopped if the QRS complex exceeds 25% of baseline, if hypotension is unresponsive to fluid challenge, or if the quinidine serum concentration is greater than 9.2 μmol/L.[9,18] When M.L. can be switched to oral therapy, he should receive oral quinine sulfate 650 mg every 8 hours to complete 3 to 7 days of total therapy.[9,27] The quinine is administered for 7 days if *P. falciparum* is acquired in Thailand.[27]

MANAGING CHLOROQUINE-RESISTANT MALARIA

If M.L. does not respond to the quinidine or quinine regimen within 48 to 72 hours (i.e., failure to reduce parasitemia by

TABLE 78-1
Drug Therapy of Parasitic Infection[2,7,9,10,11,14,18,22,26–29,32,35,36,39,57,61,64,79,82,100,107,110,111,116,119,120,124–126,130]

Drug of Choice	Dosage	Adverse Effects
Amebiasis (Including Cyst Passers)		
Asymptomatic		
Iodoquinol	*Adults:* 650 mg PO TID × 20 days	Rash, acne, thyroid enlargement
Or	*Children:* 30–40 mg/kg/d PO TID × 20 days	
Diloxanide furoate	*Adults:* 500 mg PO TID × 10 days	Flatulence, abdominal pain
Or	*Children:* 20 mg/kg/d PO TID × 10 days	
Paromomycin	*Adults:* 25–35 mg/kg/d PO TID × 7 days	Nausea, vomiting
	Children: Same as adults	
Mild to Moderate Gastrointestinal Disease		
Metronidazole	*Adults:* 750 mg PO TID × 10 days	Nausea, headache, metallic taste, disulfiram reaction
Or	*Children:* 35–50 mg/kg/d PO TID × 10 days	with alcohol, paresthesia
Tinidazole	*Adults:* 2 g once daily × 3 days	Metallic or bitter taste, anorexia, nausea, vomiting,
followed by	*Children:* 50 mg/kg (max. 2 g) × 3 days	epigastric discomfort, weakness, seizures, peripheral neuropathy
Iodoquinol	*Adults:* 650 mg PO TID × 20 days	Rash, acne, thyroid enlargement
	Children: 30–40 mg/kg/d PO TID × 20 days	
Severe Gastrointestinal Disease		
Metronidazole	*Adults:* 750 mg PO TID × 10 days	Nausea, headache, metallic taste, disulfiram reaction
Or	*Children:* 35–50 mg/kg/d PO TID × 10 days	with alcohol, paresthesia
Tinidazole	*Adults:* 2 g once daily × 5 days	Metallic taste or bitter taste, nausea, vomiting, epigastric
followed by	*Children:* 50 mg/kg/d (max. 2 g) × 5 days	discomfort, anorexia and weakness
Iodoquinol	*Adults:* 650 mg PO TID × 20 days	Rash, acne, thyroid enlargement
	Children: 30–40 mg/kg/d PO TID × 20 days	
Amebic Liver Abscess		
Metronidazole	*Adults:* 750 mg PO TID × 10 days	Nausea, headache, metallic taste, disulfiram reaction
Or	*Children:* 35–50 mg/kg/d PO TID × 10 days	with alcohol, paresthesia
Tinidazole	*Adults:* 2 g once daily × 5 days	
followed by	*Children:* 50 mg/kg (max. 2 g) × 5 days	
Iodoquinol	*Adults:* 650 mg PO TID × 20 days	Rash, acne, thyroid enlargement
Or	*Children:* 30–40 mg/kg/d PO TID × 20 days	
Diloxanide furoate[b]	*Adults:* 500 mg PO TID × 10 days	
Or	*Children:* 20 mg/kg/d PO TID × 10 days	
Paromomycin	*Adults:* 25–30 mg/kg/d PO TID × 7 days	Nausea, vomiting
	Children: Same as adults	
Ascariasis (Roundworm)		
Albendazole	*Adults and children:* 400 mg once	Nausea and headache
Or		
Mebendazole	*Adults and children:* 100 mg BID PO × 3 days	Diarrhea, abdominal pain
Enterobiasis (Pinworm)		
Mebendazole	*Adults and children:* 100 mg once; repeat in 2 weeks	Diarrhea, abdominal pain
Pyrantel pamoate	*Adults and children:* 11 mg/kg PO once (max. 1 g),	Nausea, headache, dizziness, rash, fever
Or	repeat in 2 weeks	
Albendazole	*Adults and children:* 400 mg once; repeat in 2 weeks	Abdominal pain, reversible alopecia, increased transaminases, rarely leukopenia
Filariasis		
Diethylcarbamazine	*Adults:* Day 1, 50 mg PO; day 2, 50 mg TID; day 3, 100 mg TID; days 4–14, 6 mg/kg/d in 3 doses	Severe allergic or febrile reactions, gastrointestinal disturbance, rarely encephalopathy
	Children: Day 1, 25–50 mg; day 2, 25–50 mg TID; day 3, 50–100 mg TID; days 4–14, 6 mg/kg/d in 3 doses	
Flukes (Trematodes)[a]		
Praziquantel	*Adults and children:* 75 mg/kg/d in 3 doses × 2 days (exceptions: *C. sinensis* and *P. westermani*, × 2 days)	Malaise, headache, dizziness, sedation, fever, eosinophilia
Giardiasis		
Metronidazole	*Adults:* 250 mg PO TID with meals × 5–7 days	Nausea, headache, metallic taste, disulfiram reaction
Or	*Children:* 15 mg/kg/d PO TID × 5–7 days	with alcohol, paresthesia
Quinacrine[b]	*Adults:* 100 mg PO TID × 5 days	Gastrointestinal yellow staining of skin and psychosis
	Children: 2 mg/kg TID × 5 days (max 300 mg/d)	
Nitazoxanide[c]	*Children:* 12–47 months	Abdominal pain, diarrhea, vomiting, and headache
	100 mg (5 mL) every 12 hours × 3 days	
	4–11 years	
	200 mg (10 mL) every 12 hours × 3 days	

(continued)

TABLE 78-1
Drug Therapy of Parasitic Infection[2,7,9,10,11,14,18,22,26–29,32,35,36,39,57,61,64,79,82,100,107,110,111,116,119,120,124–126,130] *(Continued)*

Drug of Choice	Dosage	Adverse Effects
Hookworm		
Mebendazole	*Adults and children:* 100 mg PO BID × 3 days	Diarrhea, abdominal pain
Lice		
1% Permethrin (NIX) *Or*	Topical administration	Occasional allergic reaction, mild stinging, erythema
Ivermectin	*Adults and children:* 200 mcg/kg × 3, day 1, day 2, and day 10	Fever, pruritus, sore lymph nodes, headache, joint pains, rarely hypotension
Leishmaniasis		
Sodium stibogluconate *Or*	*Adults:* 20 mg SB/kg IV or IM × 20–28 days *Children:* Same as adults	Gastrointestinal, malaise, headache arthralgias, myalgias, anemia, neutropenia, thrombocytopenia; ECG abnormalities (ST- and T-wave changes)
Liposomal Amphotericin B	*Adults:* 3 mg/kg/d (days 1–5) and 3 mg/kg/d (days 14 and 21) *Children:* Same as adult	Hypotension, chills, headache, anemia, thrombocytopenia, fever, and elevated serum creatinine
Malaria		
All Plasmodia except chloroquine-resistant		
Parenteral Therapy		
Quinidine gluconate *Or*	*Adults:* Loading dose 10 mg/kg of salt (6.2 mg base) diluted in 250 mL of normal saline and infused IV for 2 hours, followed by a continuous IV infusion of 0.02 mg/kg/min (0.012 mg base) for 72 hours; switch to oral quinine 650 mg every 8 hours as soon as possible	ECG: Q-T and QRS prolongation; hypotension, syncope, arrhythmias; cinchonism
Artesunate[d]	2.4 mg/kg per dose every 12 hours for 3 days. *Children:* Same as adults.	Pruritus, hypotension, dizziness, nausea, vomiting, diarrhea, and bitter metallic taste
Oral Therapy		
Chloroquine phosphate	*Adults:* 1 g (600 mg base), then 500 mg 6 hours later, then 500 mg at 24 and 48 hours later *Children:* 10 mg base (max. 600 mg base) then 5 mg base/kg 6 hours later, then 5 mg/base at 24 and 48 hours	Gastrointestinal, headache, pruritus, malaise, and cinchonism
Chemoprophylaxis		
Chloroquine phosphate	*Adults:* 500 mg (base) once weekly (beginning 1–2 weeks before departure and continuing through stay and up to 4 weeks after returning) *Children:* 5 mg/kg base once weekly up to adult dose (300 mg base)	Dose-related: vertigo, nausea, dizziness, light-headedness, headache, visual disturbances, toxic psychosis, and seizures
Chloroquine-Resistant Therapy (CRF)		
Mefloquine *Or*	*Adults:* 750 mg followed by 500 mg 12 hours later *Children:* 15 mg/kg followed 8–12 hours later by 10 mg/kg	Nausea, vomiting, abdominal pain, arthralgias, chills, dizziness, tinnitus, and A-V block
Atovaquone/proguanil *Or*	*Adults:* 2 tablets BID × 3 days *Children:* 11–20 kg: 1 adult tablet/d × 3 days; 21–30 kg: 2 adult tablets/d × 3 days; 31–40 kg: 3 adult tablets/d × 3 days; >40 kg: 2 adult tablets BID × 3 days	Rash, nausea, diarrhea, increased aminotransferases, cholestasis
Artemether 20 mg-lumefantrine 120 mg (Coartem)	3-day regimen of 6 doses based on body weight: initial dose, followed by 8 hours later and one dose twice daily × 2 days; 5–<15 kg: 1 tablet per dose; 15–<25 kg: 2 tablets per dose; 25–<35 kg: 3 tablets per dose; >35 kg: 4 tablets per dose	
Chemoprophylaxis-CRF		
Mefloquine *Or*	*Adults:* 250 mg once weekly beginning 1–2 weeks before departure, continuing through stay and for 1–4 weeks after return *Children:* <15 kg: 5 mg/kg once weekly; 15–19 kg: 1/4 tablet once weekly; 20–30 kg: 1/2 tablet once weekly; 31–45 kg: 3/4 tablet once weekly; >45 kg: 1 tablet once weekly	
Doxycycline	*Adults:* 100 mg daily beginning 1–2 days before departure continuing during stay and 1 week after return	Nausea, diarrhea, and monilial rash

(continued)

TABLE 78-1
Drug Therapy of Parasitic Infection[2,7,9,10,11,14,18,22,26–29,32,35,36,39,57,61,64,79,82,100,107,110,111,116,119,120,124–126,130] ***(Continued)***

Drug of Choice	Dosage	Adverse Effects
Quinine sulfate (Qualaquin)	*Adults:* 650 PO TID × 3 days	Cinchonism
Plus	*Children:* 25 mg/kg/d PO TID × 3 days	
Pyrimethamine-sulfadoxine (Fansidar)	*Adults:* 3 tablets at once (withhold until febrile episode) *Children:* 1/2–2 tablets (depends on age)[c]	Gastrointestinal, erythema multiforme, Stevens-Johnson syndrome, toxic epidermal necrolysis
Or		
Mefloquine	*Adults:* 1,250 mg once *Children:* 25 mg/kg once (>45 kg)	Dose-related: vertigo, nausea, dizziness, light-headedness, headache, visual disturbances, toxic psychosis seizures
Prevention of Relapses (*P. vivax* and *P. ovale*)		
Primaquine phosphate	*Adults:* 52.6 mg/d (30 mg base) × 14 days; this follows chloroquine or mefloquine regimen	Abdominal cramps, nausea, hemolytic anemia in G6PD
Scabies		
5% Permethrin (Elimite cream)	Topical administration	Rash, edema, erythema
Alternatives		
Ivermectin	*Adults:* 200 mcg/kg PO; repeat in 2 weeks	Nausea, diarrhea, dizziness, vertigo, and pruritus
Lindane (Kwell)	Apply topically once	Not recommended in pregnant women, infants, and patients with massively excoriated skin. Second-line therapy when other alternatives have failed.
Crotamiton 10% (Eurax)	Topically	Local skin irritation
Tapeworm[e]		
Praziquantel	*Adults and children:* 5–10 mg/kg PO × 1 dose	Malaise, headache, dizziness, sedation, eosinophilia, fever
Hydatid Cysts[f]		
Albendazole	*Adults:* 400 mg BID × 8–30 days, repeat if necessary *Children:* 15 mg/kg/d × 28 days, repeat if necessary (surgical resection may precede drug therapy)	Diarrhea, abdominal pain, rarely hepatotoxicity, leukopenia
Trichomoniasis		
Metronidazole	*Adults:* 2 g PO × 1 day or 250 mg PO TID × 7 days *Children:* 15 mg/kg/d PO TID × 7 days	Nausea, headache, metallic taste, disulfiram reaction with alcohol, paresthesia

[a]*Schistosoma haematobium, Schistosoma mansoni, Schistosoma japonicum, Clonorchis sinensis, Paragonimus westermani.*
[b]Quinacrine is available in the United States: Panorama Compounding Pharmacy, 6744 Balboa Blvd, Van Nuys, CA 91406 (1-800-247-9767). Diloxanide furoate is not available in the United States or Canada.
[c]Same dose is recommended in children with *Cryptosporidium parvum.*
[d]Obtained from CDC under an Investigational New Drug (IND) protocol for patients intolerant of intravenous quinidine or when intravenous quinidine is not readily available. Therapy should be followed by oral therapy with antimalarials (see above and text).
[e]*Diphyllobothrium latum* (fish), *Taenia solium* (pork), and *Dipylidium caninum* (dog), except for *Hymenolepis nana,* in which the dose is 25 mg/kg × 1 dose.
[f]*Echinococcus granulosus, Echinococcus multilocularis.* For neurocysticercosis: 400 mg BID 8–30 days.
BID, twice daily; ECG, electrocardiograph; G6PD, glucose-6-phosphate dehydrogenase; IM, intramuscularly; PO, orally; SB, Sodium stibogluconate; TID, three times daily.

25% of baseline and continued fever over this period), other adjunctive therapies must be considered.[9,27] One of the recommended drug treatments for CRPF infection, which is added to quinine therapy, is doxycycline 100 mg twice daily for 7 days (doxycycline should overlap the quinine for 2 to 3 days before the latter is discontinued) or clindamycin 900 mg three times a day for 5 days.[27] If the patient cannot tolerate oral doxycycline, IV doxycycline 100 mg every 12 hours can be substituted. An alternative in a patient who can tolerate oral therapy and has no contraindications (i.e., history of seizures, or endemic area where *P. falciparum* is resistant to the agent, e.g., Thailand, Myanmar, Vietnam, Laos, and Cambodia) is mefloquine 750 mg, which can be initiated followed by 500 mg 12 hours later.[9,27] M.L. may also be treated with the combination of atovaquone 250 mg and proguanil 100 mg (Malarone). The dose of atovaquone/proguanil is two tablets twice daily for 3 days.[9,27] Although exchange transfusion has been suggested as an adjunct therapy for serious *P. falciparum* malaria, the role of this intervention remains questionable.[11]

ONLINE CONTENT

For a narrated PowerPoint presentation titled "Red blood cell exchange (RBC) transfusion for severe falciparum malaria: Is it beneficial?", go to http://thepoint.lww.com/AT10e.

The CDC suggests parasitemia greater than 10%, altered mental status, nonvolume pulmonary edema, or renal complications for exchange transfusion to be considered (www.cdcgov/malaria/pdf/treatmenttable.pdf, accessed on August 12, 2010).

MANAGING OTHER *PLASMODIUM* SPECIES

A patient infected with one of the other species of *Plasmodium* (*P. vivax, P. ovale,* or *P. malariae*) should receive oral chloroquine phosphate (Aralen). The initial dose is 1 g (600 mg base) followed by 500 mg (300 mg base) 6 hours later; subsequently, 500 mg (300 mg base) is administered daily for 2 days.[27] For patients who cannot tolerate the oral doses of chloroquine, parenteral doses of quinidine can be administered (Case 78-1, Question 2 lists doses).[27] Patients with *P. ovale* and *P. vivax* also should be given primaquine to prevent relapses from the latent exoerythrocytic stages in the liver. The adult dosage of primaquine is 52.6 mg/day (30 mg base) for 14 days; this should follow the chloroquine regimen.[9,27]

CHEMOPROPHYLAXIS AND PREGNANCY

CASE 78-2

QUESTION 1: T.P., a male medical resident from Indonesia, is planning to visit his seriously ill mother. His wife, T.R., who

is 16 weeks pregnant, and their 4-year-old daughter will accompany him. What prophylactic medications for malaria should be administered to each member of the family?

All travelers to endemic areas should receive chemoprophylaxis for malaria. In Indonesia, including Papua New Guinea, all four types of malaria are present.[3,9,11] T.P. and his family may need prophylactic therapy for all malarial species, including a regimen that will protect them against CRPF infections. To verify whether a country is included in the CRPF list or to obtain other relevant information on malaria prophylaxis, T.P. should call the CDC Malaria Hotline, which provides a touch tone–activated, computer-assisted service (770-488-7788).[3,27] Pregnant women are at greater risk for malaria infection and its complications (including severe edema, hemolytic anemia, splenomegaly, premature labor, fetal distress, and stillbirth) and should be advised not to travel to areas endemic for malaria, if possible.[11,13,29–34] Current publications that provide updated information on parasitic diseases and immunization requirements include *Medical Letter, Morbidity and Mortality Weekly Reports, Health Information for International Travel,* and various Internet sites.[11,13,27]

CHLOROQUINE AND PRIMAQUINE PHOSPHATE

Chloroquine phosphate is an effective chemoprophylactic agent against all species of *Plasmodium* except drug-resistant *P. falciparum.* The adult dosage of chloroquine phosphate is 500 mg (300 mg base) once weekly beginning 1 week before departure and continuing for 4 weeks after last exposure. The pediatric dosage of chloroquine is 5 mg/kg base (8.3 mg chloroquine phosphate) once weekly beginning 1 week before departure and continuing for 4 weeks after exposure. A suspension of chloroquine in chocolate syrup can be prepared for children (5 mg/mL). Chloroquine prophylaxis is safe during pregnancy, and the benefits outweigh the risk of malaria and side effects.[9,13,27–33] Mefloquine and the combination of atovaquone/proguanil may be options for prophylaxis and treatment in pregnancy[29–34]; however, these are not recommended in the United States.[27]

By taking the chloroquine 1 week before travel, the patient can achieve adequate antimalarial chloroquine levels in the blood by the second week. A weekly dose of 0.5 g of chloroquine phosphate produces average plasma concentrations of chloroquine between 0.47 and 0.78 μmol/L. Most strains of *P. vivax* and *P. falciparum* are susceptible to plasma levels between 0.046 and 0.093 μmol/L, respectively.[7,18,35] Mefloquine (Lariam) 250 mg (salt) once weekly beginning 1 week before departure and continuing for 4 weeks after leaving the endemic area is an alternative regimen to chloroquine.[7,18,27,36] Mefloquine is not recommended during pregnancy or in children weighing 5 kg or less because the safety of this agent has not been fully established in these populations.[27] Recently, *P. vivax* was reported to be resistant to chloroquine in Indonesia and New Guinea, and despite the lack of data on mefloquine in pregnancy (T.R. is in the second trimester), T.R. may need this agent.[15,18,32,33,37,38] Chloroquine suppresses the asexual erythrocytic forms of the malaria parasite and has no action against the exoerythrocytic phase of *P. vivax* and *P. ovale.*[7,18] However, primaquine phosphate prevents relapses of *P. vivax* and *P. ovale* by inhibiting the exoerythrocytic stage; it also has a significant gametocidal effect against all species.[11,15,18] To prevent an attack after departure from an area where *P. vivax* and *P. ovale* are present, the clinician should also prescribe primaquine phosphate 52.6 mg/day (30 mg base) for 14 days to coincide with the last 2 weeks of the chloroquine regimen. Primaquine should not be administered to pregnant patients.[27] The major toxicity of concern, aside from the teratogenic risk, is hemolytic anemia in patients with RBC glucose-6-phosphate dehydrogenase (G6PD) deficiency.[7,18,36,39]

PROPHYLAXIS FOR CHLOROQUINE-RESISTANT *PLASMODIUM FALCIPARUM*

Prophylaxis for CRPF also can be achieved by taking mefloquine in the doses indicated above.[27] An alternative to mefloquine is doxycycline 100 mg/day beginning 1 day before travel and continuing for the duration of the stay and for 4 weeks after leaving the malarial area. Travelers such as T.P. should be advised to take measures to reduce contact with infected mosquitoes by wearing long-sleeved blouses or shirts and pants or trousers, applying insect repellent containing 31% to 35% N,N-diethyl-*meta*-toluamide (DEET) (e.g., HourGuard-12, Amway Corp.; DEET Plus, Sawyer Products), sleeping in a screened room, or using netting impregnated with permethrin.[30,34,37,40] An alternative to the mefloquine chemoprophylaxis regimen in CRPF areas is the combination of atovaquone 250 mg and proguanil 100 mg administered once daily 1 to 2 days before departure and continued for 1 week after return.[11,27] The pediatric formula (Malarone Pediatric) contains 62.5 mg of atovaquone and 25 mg of proguanil.[27] Instead of doxycycline, T.R. could take atovaquone/proguanil as chemoprophylaxis. The advantage of atovaquone/proguanil is that it can also be used as treatment. The recommended therapeutic dose of atovaquone/proguanil for CRPF is two tablets twice daily for 3 days.[27] Both prophylaxis and treatment of CRPF in nonimmune subjects and pregnant patients are complicated.[41–47] Pyrimethamine is teratogenic, and sulfonamides are contraindicated in early pregnancy; however, chloroquine, quinine, and quinidine have been suggested as safe during pregnancy.[2,8,27,29,32,33,39] Although not associated with abortions, low birth weight, neurologic retardation, or congenital malformations, mefloquine is associated with an increased risk of stillbirth.[27,34,39]

T.P. and T.R. should reconsider their decision to travel together because of the risks of malarial infection during pregnancy. In view of the recent report of *P. vivax* resistance to chloroquine in Indonesia, the family members should consider using mefloquine.[27] The risks and benefits of mefloquine in pregnancy (T.R. is in her second trimester) should be communicated to the family.[15,39] Physical barriers (e.g., clothes, mosquito nets), insect repellent, and minimizing the stay in the endemic area also decrease the likelihood of transmission.[29,34,48]

MALARIA VACCINE

CASE 78-2, QUESTION 2: Could T.R. be vaccinated as an alternative to chemoprophylaxis?

Currently, no vaccination is available. As a result of successful in vitro *P. falciparum* cultivation and advances in genetic engineering and monoclonal antibody research, some progress has been made, but this vaccine is years from approval.[49–54] The malaria plasmodium undergoes many transformations during its development, and each stage expresses a different plasmodial genome that generates a large number of antigens. The development of a malaria vaccine relies on the identification and characterization of these antigens and the subsequent production of monoclonal antibodies.[49,51]

At present, three types of vaccines against *P. falciparum* are under study: a merozoite vaccine that would induce immunity against the erythrocytic forms of plasmodia in the blood, a sporozoite vaccine that would protect against the exoerythrocytic or liver phase, and a gamete vaccine ("transmission blocking") that would prevent transmission of malaria in endemic areas.[49,50] When a vaccine for malaria is available, it is expected to provide an immune response for at least 1 year. The safety of these vaccines to the fetus and mother during pregnancy will require further evaluation.

MULTIDRUG-RESISTANT *PLASMODIUM FALCIPARUM* MALARIA

CASE 78-3

QUESTION 1: F.S., a permanent US resident of Cambodian origin, is planning to travel to the Thai-Kampuchean refugee camp. What antimalarial agents should he use for chemoprophylaxis?

F.S. is traveling to the Thai-Burma border, where *P. falciparum* malaria is epidemic. Chemoprophylaxis against malaria in this region of Southeast Asia has become progressively difficult to achieve because of the prevalence of *P. falciparum* strains resistant to chloroquine, pyrimethamine-sulfadoxine, quinine, and even mefloquine.[7,13,38,43,47]

F.S. will have to take chemoprophylaxis against both *P. vivax* and multidrug-resistant *P. falciparum*. Mefloquine 250 mg once weekly starting 1 week before travel and continuing weekly for the duration of the stay and for 4 weeks after leaving Thailand is recommended.[27] On return from his visit, primaquine phosphate should be added to F.S.'s regimen to prevent an attack of *P. vivax* because mefloquine has no effect on the exoerythrocytic phase of *P. vivax* (see Case 78-2, Question 1 for doses of primaquine).[27] Another alternative drug for prophylaxis against *P. falciparum* malaria for F.S. would be doxycycline 100 mg taken once daily 1 to 2 days before departure and continuing for 4 weeks after his return from Thailand.[9,11,27]

Ginghaosu, a plant extract (artemisinin compounds), has been used for many centuries in China for fever and malaria.[9,11,41–45,55–58] Artemisinin and its derivatives (artemether and artesunate) are rapidly effective even against CRPF strains.[7,18,55–58] The antimalarial agent halofantrine (Halfan) may be another alternative to mefloquine, but this agent has been associated with fatal arrhythmias.[27] Clinical trials of fosmidomycin, piperquine, lumefantrine, and other new antimalarial agents are ongoing.[14,15,47,55–60]

SIDE EFFECTS OF ANTIMALARIALS

CASE 78-4

QUESTION 1: A.K., a 36-year-old Malaysian man, presents with a 2-day history of fever, chills, and bouts of diarrhea after his return from west Malaysia, where he was visiting his parents for 3 weeks. A.K. did not take prophylaxis for malaria. A blood smear stained with Giemsa solution demonstrated *P. vivax*, and A.K. was given chloroquine 1 g (600 mg base) initially, to be followed by 500 mg (300 mg base) 6 hours later and 500 mg at 24 and 48 hours. On completion of the chloroquine regimen, A.K. was instructed to take primaquine 52.6 mg/day (30 mg base) for 14 days. However, A.K. presents to the ED a day later with complaints of abdominal pain, severe headache, vomiting, and a bitter taste in the mouth. What evidence does A.K. exhibit that is compatible with the toxicity of antimalarials?

The major side effects of chloroquine (e.g., nausea, abdominal pain, pruritus, vertigo, headache, and visual disturbances)[7,18,39] usually are associated with large doses such as those needed for A.K.'s therapy. The gastrointestinal (GI) complaints and severe headache experienced by A.K. are consistent with chloroquine therapy, and the bitter taste he described is experienced by all patients receiving chloroquine or other 8-aminoquinoline preparations. Because A.K. also will be taking primaquine after the course of chloroquine, he should be told that he probably will experience some GI upset with this drug as well. Abdominal cramps associated with primaquine may be relieved by antacids or by taking the drug after meals. The severe nausea and vomiting may have dehydrated A.K., and he should be encouraged to replenish his fluids. Table 78-1 lists the adverse effects of antimalarials.

GLUCOSE-6-PHOSPHATE DEHYDROGENASE DEFICIENCY

CASE 78-4, QUESTION 2: Why is A.K. at risk for primaquine sensitivity?

Primaquine sensitivity, or G6PD deficiency, is an inherited error of metabolism transmitted by a gene of partial dominance located on the X chromosome. Patients with this enzyme deficiency are susceptible to RBC hemolysis when receiving the 8-aminoquinolines, sulfonamides, *para*-aminosalicylates, nitrofurantoin, sulfone, aspirin, quinine, quinidine, nalidixic acid, and methylene blue.[27,36,39] G6PD in RBCs preserves glutathione in the reduced form by regenerating nicotinamide adenine dinucleotide phosphate (NADPH). Reduced glutathione protects RBC membranes from increased oxidant stress. Patients with low levels of glutathione and impaired regeneration of NADPH, as seen with G6PD deficiency, are susceptible to the oxidizing effect of drugs.[18,30,61–63] Hemolysis generally occurs on the third day of drug ingestion and is manifested by abdominal discomfort, anemia, and hemoglobinuria.[61]

The incidence of G6PD deficiency in the Southeast Asian refugee population is approximately 5.2%.[63] Because A.K. is a native of Malaysia and may have G6PD deficiency, he may be at risk of hemolysis if primaquine is ingested. Therefore, he should be screened for G6PD deficiency before treatment.

Although a number of simple and satisfactory screening tests for G6PD deficiency are available, the fluorescent spot test is the simplest, most reliable, and most sensitive. The spot test is based on the addition of a reagent containing NADPH to a hemolysate of the patient's RBCs. After an incubation period, the mixture is spotted on filter paper and examined under long-wave ultralight. Fluorescence of the mixture on the filter paper will indicate the presence of NADPH generated by G6PD. Patients with G6PD deficiency will have weak to no fluorescence detected. Large variants exist among those with the mutant gene, and if A.K. has a variant with relatively mild episodic clinical manifestations (variant A, with 10%–60% residual enzyme activity), he may be treated with primaquine at 45 mg/week for 8 weeks.[64]

AMEBIASIS

Prevalence and Mortality

Amebiasis, caused by the small protozoan parasite *Entamoeba histolytica* (Fig. 78-2), results in amebic dysentery and hepatic abscess.[65–69] Approximately 10% of the world's population (predominately in Latin America, Africa, and Asia) is infected, and about 100,000 die annually from this infection.[66,68] In the United States, amebiasis is considered endemic in 33% of immigrants from Mexico and Central and South America and in 17% of those from Asia and the Pacific Islands.[66,68] Most of these individuals are infected with *E. dispar* (80%) or *E. moshkovskii*, which are antigenically different strains from the pathogenic *E. histolytica* (10%)

PANIC DISORDER *CONTINUED*

2 Therapy for panic disorder includes CBT or medications such as SSRIs or benzodiazepines. Combination therapy with CBT and SSRIs or benzodiazepines or combinations of SSRIs and benzodiazepines can also effectively treat panic disorder. The duration of drug therapy and expected short- and long-term adverse effects such as jitteriness or sexual dysfunction should be discussed with the patient.	**Case 80-7 (Questions 2–4)**

SOCIAL ANXIETY AND SPECIFIC PHOBIAS

1 Both social anxiety and specific phobias involve fears that are excessive and lead to avoidance behaviors to minimize fear. Social anxiety involves a generalized and intense anxiety involving social interactions, whereas specific phobias involve intense fear associated with specific objects or situations (e.g., spiders or elevators). SSRIs are first-line treatments for social anxiety. Treatment goals and duration of treatment should be discussed with patients suffering from social anxiety or specific phobias.	**Case 80-8 (Questions 1–3)**

POSTTRAUMATIC STRESS DISORDER AND ACUTE STRESS DISORDER

1 Posttraumatic stress disorder (PTSD) and acute stress disorder occur in persons who have experienced a severely distressing traumatic event. Re-experiencing symptoms, avoidance, emotional numbing, and autonomic hyperarousal cause considerable psychological distress, as well as impairment in occupational functioning and personal relationships in PTSD.	**Case 80-9 (Question 1)**
2 Medications, primarily SSRIs, and CBT are used to treat PTSD. Adjunctive treatment for psychiatric comorbidities such as depression or sleep are often indicated. Treatment goals include reducing the core symptoms of PTSD and improving patient functioning.	**Case 80-9 (Questions 2, 3)**

OBSESSIVE–COMPULSIVE DISORDER

1 Obsessive–compulsive disorder (OCD) is characterized by chronic obsessions or compulsions. Obsessions and compulsions can be extremely disabling and usually consume at least an hour a day. OCD can be treated with medications, including SSRIs, clomipramine, or venlafaxine. Additionally, CBT combined with exposure therapy can effectively treat OCD. Psychotherapy can be combined with drug treatment for optimal therapy, although up to 40% of patients may continue to experience disabling symptoms even with optimized treatment.	**Case 80-10 (Questions 1–5)**
2 Owing to incomplete remission of symptoms with treatment in many patients suffering from OCD, augmentation strategies involving the combination of antidepressants or antidepressants with antipsychotics have been evaluated. Although augmentation with clomipramine or antipsychotics has achieved success in a sizable proportion of those not responding to monotherapy, care must be taken to monitor for increased adverse effects and drug–drug interactions.	**Case 80-11 (Questions 1–3)**

Anxiety can be described as an uncomfortable feeling of vague fear or apprehension accompanied by characteristic physical sensations. It is a normal reaction to a perceived threat to one's physical or psychological well-being. The anxiety reaction is normally provoked by stress of some sort and involves activation of neurobiological systems that, when activated, contribute to self-preservation. Anxiety serves the purpose of alerting us to take appropriate measures for dealing with stressful circumstances. Anxiety involves the perturbation of several different neural systems causing two basic components: mental features (e.g., worry, fear, difficulty concentrating) and physical symptoms (e.g., racing heart, shortness of breath, trembling, pacing). An activation of these same systems can also be caused by certain medical illnesses such as pheochromocytoma or hyperthyroidism or medications such as sympathomimetics, resulting in both the physical and psychological manifestations of anxiety. However, when the anxiety is attributable to an external cause such as a medical illness or a medication, the anxiety abates when the physiological cause is removed.[1]

If the anxiety is not the result of an external cause or is out of proportion to the actual threat or when the anxiety lasts far beyond the presence of the threat, anxiety may impair normal functioning and be classified as an anxiety disorder. The anxiety experienced by a person is excessive for the situation (in intensity or duration) or very distressing, to the point that it interferes with daily functioning. Pathological anxiety can be differentiated according to whether it occurs (a) as a primary anxiety disorder, (b) as a secondary anxiety disorder owing to medical causes or substances, (c) in response to acute stress (e.g., loss of a loved one, marital or financial problems), or (d) as a symptom associated with other psychiatric disorders. This differentiation can be difficult, but is important in guiding optimal treatment.

Classification and Diagnosis of Anxiety Disorders

The *Diagnostic and Statistical Manual of Mental Disorders,* Fourth Edition, Text Revision (DSM-IV-TR) classifies primary anxiety disorders into six types: generalized anxiety disorder (GAD), panic disorder, phobic disorders (including social anxiety disorder), obsessive–compulsive disorder (OCD), posttraumatic stress disorder (PTSD), and acute stress disorder.[1] Each disorder involves an unhealthy level of anxiety, but the characteristic type and severity of symptoms, as well as course of illness, vary from one disorder to another. Efficacy of drug and nondrug treatments also varies among disorders, indicating underlying biological differences. The DSM-IV-TR secondary anxiety disorders include "anxiety disorder due to a general medical condition" and "substance-induced anxiety disorder."[1] An anxiety disorder may occur in the absence of other psychiatric disorders, but it is often present in addition to other psychiatric disorders, such as mood disorders. Although anxiety disorders and mood disorders are classified separately in the DSM-IV-TR, a perusal of the criteria for both diagnostic categories reveals they have much in common, including fatigue, impaired concentration, restlessness, difficulties with sleep, and somatic symptoms. The main difference is that mood disorders have a prominent mood factor. Both anxiety and mood disorders appear to be associated with dysregulations in the limbic system of the brain, which is involved in emotion, learning, and memory.[2]

ONLINE CONTENT

For an illustration that shows the limbic system, go to http://thepoint.lww.com/AT10e.

Neurobiology of Anxiety

The limbic system is composed of a set of structures integral to behavior, including the two key structures, the hippocampus and the amygdala. Hippocampal brain circuits are essential for conversion of short-term to long-term memory and for spatial memory, whereas the amygdala circuits are involved with emotion and its expression. A neurocircuit arising from the output pathways of the central nucleus of the amygdala is believed to mediate fear and anxiety responses in humans.[3] Dysregulated or exaggerated output through various amygdala-related circuits may be a common element underlying the different anxiety disorders, but the specific type of dysfunction probably differs among the various disorders. If it is assumed a dysregulation of the stress response is the basis of anxiety disorders, then the genesis of anxiety is probably related primarily to interactions between neural pathways in and between the limbic system structures, the sympathetic nervous system, and the hypothalamic-pituitary-adrenocortical (HPA) axis.[2,4] It is becoming clear that neither anxiety nor depression is due solely to abnormalities of neurotransmitter systems because these systems regulate and are regulated by other neurocircuits. Many neurotransmitter systems interact to modulate the actions of the limbic pathways, including the monoamine neurotransmitters, epinephrine and norepinephrine (NE); corticotrophin-releasing hormone (CRH); the indoleamine, serotonin (5-HT); the inhibitory amino acid, γ-aminobutyric acid (GABA); the excitatory amino acid, glutamate; and the neuropeptides, cholecystokinin (CCK), neuropeptide Y, and substance P.[3,5]

Interaction of the Hypothalamic-Pituitary-Adrenocortical, Noradrenergic, and Serotonergic Systems

In the event of an acute threat, a fear stimulus is transmitted via the thalamus to the amygdala, which then projects to both the hypothalamus and the brainstem. This results in the peripheral reactions such as increased heart rate and heart stroke volume, and vasodilation of blood vessels carrying blood to the muscles. This is accompanied by a release of NE by the locus ceruleus (LC), the main nidus of NE cell bodies in the brain. Central release of NE results in vigilance and arousal, and the ability to focus attention on the threat and its stimulation in response to stress or fear produces arousal and symptoms of anxiety (tachycardia, tremor, sweating). NE innervation of the hippocampus results in an increased state of memory formation, whereas innervation of the amygdala potentiates the formation of aversive memories.[4] Normally, this is important in allowing us to encode emotionally laden memories, but when overactive, it may result in a constant state of arousal and hypervigilance.

During a perceived threat, CRH is released in the hypothalamus, and it activates the anterior pituitary to release adrenocorticotropic hormone (ACTH). This stimulates the release of glucocorticoid steroids from the adrenal cortex. Although short-term elevation of glucocorticoids allows the body to adapt to a stressful situation by supporting HPA activation and mobilizing energy stores, prolonged elevation of the same glucocorticoids impairs neural plasticity and may even result in neuronal death. Both the sympathetic system and the HPA axis responses are modulated by limbic brain circuits innervating the amygdala, hippocampus, and orbital/medial prefrontal cortex. CRH is expressed in the amygdala and LC as well as in the hypothalamus. CRH binds to at least two specific receptors in the brain, CR_1 and CR_2 receptors. These receptors modulate the actions of a variety of neurotransmitters, including NE, 5-HT, glutamate, and dopamine. When CRH is infused into the LC in rodents, it causes anxietylike behaviors.[2,4,6]

Although the inhibitory neurotransmitter 5-HT is involved in stress reactions, its role is not entirely clear. Serotonin has roles in sleep, appetite, memory, impulsivity, sexual behavior, and motor function, and seems to decrease aggressive behavior. The site of most 5-HT cell bodies in the brain is the raphe nuclei. There is considerable interconnectivity between the raphe nuclei and the LC, and they tend to mutually inhibit one another. Under normal circumstances, 5-HT connections from the hippocampus decrease activity in the amygdala, which would dampen fear and anxiety responses. However, under conditions of stress, the LC accelerates firing, inhibits the raphe nuclei firing, and increases CRH release—all of which sensitize the limbic system and cause arousal and sensitivity to memory of any stressful or aversive stimuli. This primes the system to a state of arousal to deal with the threat.[2]

A potential mechanism for anxiety states involves chronic NE overactivity combined with decreased activity in the 5-HT system.[2] For example, a minor fear response might be associated with a disproportionately large fear or aversion response. This would result in a chronic activation of the HPA axis. Chronically elevated corticosteroid levels have been shown to contribute to hippocampal and cerebral atrophy. Although the specific etiology of anxiety is only hypothesized, the current use of treatments activating the 5-HT system, or other inhibitory systems such as the GABA system, supports the hypothesis.

Epidemiology and Clinical Significance of Anxiety Disorders

As a group, anxiety disorders are the most common psychiatric illnesses. Epidemiologic surveys indicate 13% to 28% of Americans suffer from an anxiety disorder at some time in their lives, and similar prevalences have been noted in other parts of the world.[7,8] Anxiety disorders are more common in women than in men.[8]

Anxiety disorders are associated with a decrease in quality of life and psychosocial functioning, which affect marital, educational, and employment status. Although most anxiety disorders do not require inpatient hospitalization for treatment, their presence is associated with significant impairment in major areas of life functioning.[9]

Today, most anxiety disorders can be successfully treated with medications, cognitive or behavioral therapies, or combinations thereof. However, less than one-third of those affected seek help, and many who do are not properly diagnosed.[8] Most medical care for anxiety disorders is rendered in nonpsychiatric settings. Patients commonly present to primary-care providers complaining of physical symptoms that cannot be medically explained, leading to progression of the anxiety disorder. A significant portion of patients with anxiety do not believe in taking medication for emotional problems; others remain untreated because of an inappropriate diagnosis.[10]

Because anxiety is a feeling with which everyone is familiar, there is a tendency to trivialize the impact it can have on a sufferer's functioning and quality of life. An increased understanding about pathological anxiety is needed in society in general, and health care professionals in particular, so that people seek and receive the treatment they need. Practitioners must be knowledgeable about the clinical characteristics and treatment options for various disorders, and must be able to share this information with patients and other health care professionals. A list of consumer and professional resources for information about anxiety disorders and treatment can be found in Table 80-1.

TABLE 80-1
Resource Organizations for Anxiety Disorders

Anxiety Coach
5105 Tollview Drive Rolling Meadows, IL 60008 (847) 481-5251 Website: www.anxietycoach.com
Anxiety Disorders Association of America
8730 Georgia Avenue Silver Spring, MD 20910 (240) 485-1001 Website: www.adaa.org
Freedom From Fear
308 Seaview Avenue Staten Island, NY 10305 (718) 351-1717 Website: www.freedomfromfear.org
Mental Health America
2000 N. Beauregard Street, 6th Floor Alexandria, VA 22311 (800) 969-6642 Website: www.nmha.org/
Obsessive Compulsive Foundation
676 State Street New Haven, CT 06511 (203) 401-2070 Website: www.ocfoundation.org
PTSD Gateway
(877) 507-PTSD Website: www.ptsdinfo.org

Clinical Assessment and Differential Diagnosis of Anxiety

CASE 80-1

QUESTION 1: R.R., a 49-year-old woman, complains to her physician of having trouble sleeping, feeling tired and nervous, and worrying constantly. R.R. was divorced 2 years ago, and she retained custody of their 15-year-old daughter. Since her divorce, R.R. has returned to work as a nurse, but she worries constantly that she will not be able to earn enough money to support herself and her daughter. R.R. has hypertension, and she suffers from asthma and seasonal allergies. Her currently prescribed medications include hydrochlorothiazide, losartan, montelukast, albuterol, and pantoprazole. She also takes over-the-counter (OTC) loratadine and pseudoephedrine for allergies, naproxen for occasional back pain, and polyethylene glycol as needed (PRN) for constipation. R.R. drinks three or four cups of coffee each morning and one or two glasses of wine several nights each week to help her calm down when she has had a stressful day. She denies any history of psychiatric illness but states she has always been a "worrier." What factors should be considered in the clinical assessment and differential diagnosis of R.R.'s symptoms of anxiety?

A diagnostic decision tree such as that in Figure 80-1 can be used to assist the clinician in differentiating among various causes of anxiety and different anxiety disorders. According to DSM-IV-TR criteria for primary anxiety disorders, the symptoms should not be secondary to any medical (drug or disease) causes. As illustrated in Table 80-2, the potential non-anxiety disorder–related or secondary sources for anxiety symptoms are numerous.

SECONDARY CAUSES OF ANXIETY

A diagnosis of anxiety disorder attributable to a general medical condition is warranted when symptoms are believed to be the direct physiological consequence of a medical condition.[1] In patients such as R.R., medical illnesses must be considered as possible underlying precipitants of anxiety. A complete physical and laboratory workup, with a thorough medical and psychiatric history, is also needed to exclude other, possibly reversible causes before a primary anxiety disorder diagnosis is considered. Because the onset of anxiety disorders usually occurs in young adulthood (or earlier), new-onset anxiety in elderly persons often can be attributed to some medical or substance-related cause.

Hypoglycemia, hyperthyroidism, electrolyte abnormalities, and angina pectoris are notably associated with anxiety symptoms.[11] Individuals with chronic medical conditions such as chronic obstructive pulmonary disease (COPD), Parkinson disease, cardiomyopathy, post–myocardial infarction, Graves

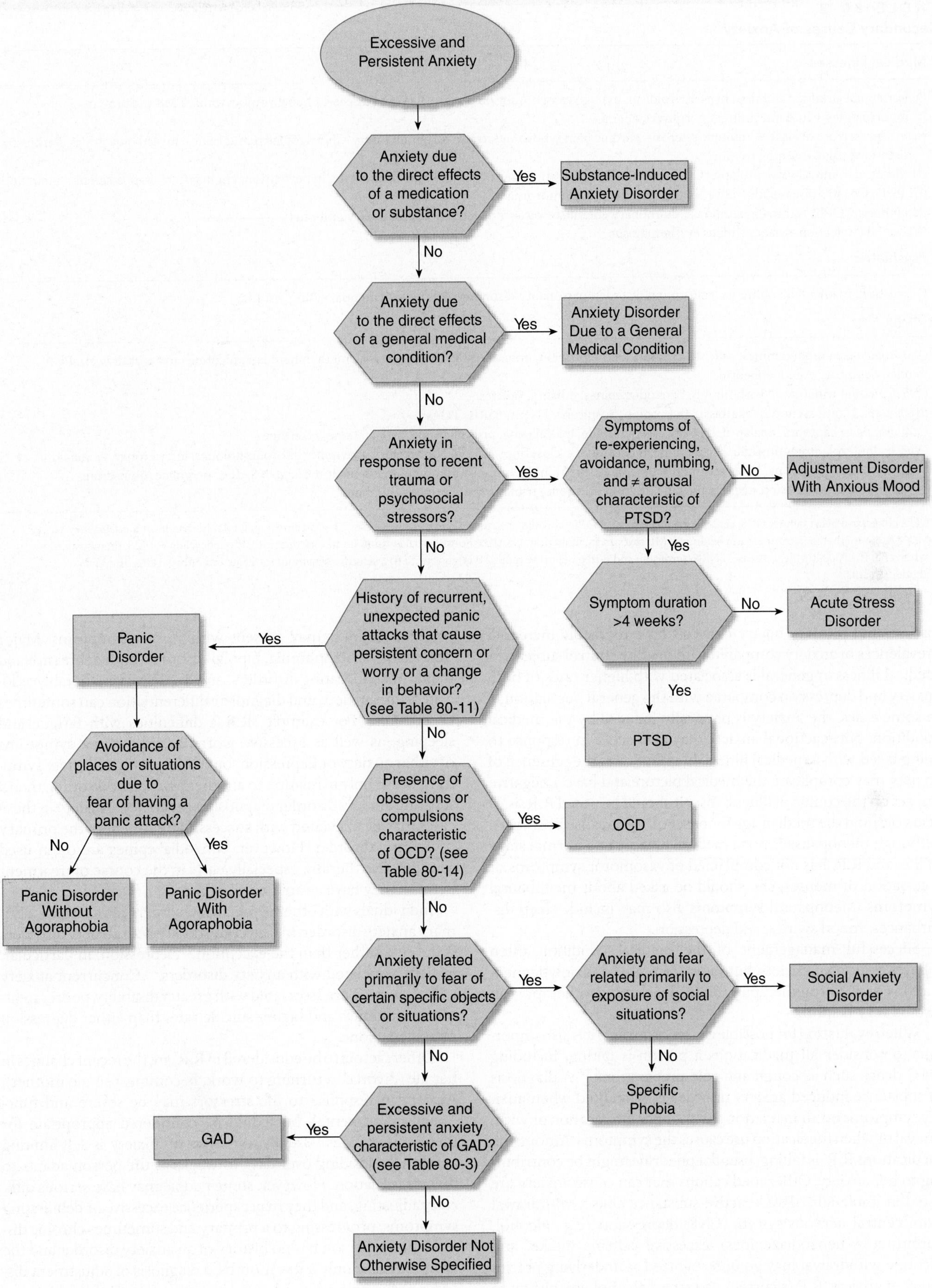

FIGURE 80-1 Diagnostic decision tree for anxiety disorders. GAD, generalized anxiety disorder; OCD, obsessive–compulsive disorder; PTSD, posttraumatic stress disorder.

TABLE 80-2
Secondary Causes of Anxiety

Medical Illnesses
Endocrine and metabolic disorders: hyperthyroidism, hypoglycemia, Addison disease, Cushing disease, pheochromocytoma, PMS, electrolyte abnormalities, acute intermittent porphyria, anemia
Neurologic: seizure disorders, multiple sclerosis, chronic pain syndromes, traumatic brain injury, CNS neoplasm, migraines, myasthenia gravis, Parkinson disease, vertigo, essential tremor
Cardiovascular: mitral valve prolapse, CHF, arrhythmias, post-MI, hyperdynamic β-adrenergic state, hypertension, angina pectoris, postcerebral infarction
GI: PUD, Crohn's disease, ulcerative colitis, irritable bowel syndrome
Respiratory: COPD, asthma, pneumonia, pulmonary edema, respirator dependence, pulmonary embolus
Others: HIV infection, systemic lupus erythematosus
Psychiatric
Depression, mania, schizophrenia, adjustment disorder, personality disorders, delirium, dementia, eating disorders
Drugs
CNS stimulants: amphetamines, caffeine, cocaine, diethylpropion, ephedrine, MDMA (Ecstasy), methylphenidate, nicotine (and withdrawal), PCP, phenylephrine, pseudoephedrine
CNS depressant withdrawal: barbiturates, benzodiazepines, ethanol, opiates
Psychotropics: antipsychotics (akathisia), bupropion, buspirone, SNRIs, SSRIs, TCAs
Cardiovascular: captopril, enalapril, digoxin, disopyramide, hydralazine, procainamide, propafenone, reserpine
Others: albuterol, aminophylline, baclofen, bromocriptine, cycloserine, dapsone, dronabinol, efavirenz, fluoroquinolones, interferon-α, isoniazid, isoproterenol, levodopa, lidocaine, mefloquine, metoclopramide, monosodium glutamate, nicotinic acid, NSAIDs, pergolide, quinacrine, sibutramine, statins, steroids, theophylline, thyroid hormone, triptans, vinblastine, yohimbine

CHF, congestive heart failure; CNS, central nervous system; COPD, chronic obstructive pulmonary disease; GI, gastrointestinal; HIV, human immunodeficiency virus; MDMA, 3,4-methylenedioxymethamphetamine; MI, myocardial infarction; NSAIDs, nonsteroidal anti-inflammatory drugs; PCP, phencyclidine; PMS, premenstrual syndrome; PUD, peptic ulcer disease; SNRIs, serotonin and norepinephrine reuptake inhibitors; SSRIs, selective serotonin reuptake inhibitors; TCAs, tricyclic antidepressants.

disease, and primary biliary cirrhosis have markedly increased prevalences of anxiety compared with healthy control subjects.[11] Medical illness in general is associated with higher rates of both anxiety and depression compared with the general population.[11] In some cases, the anxiety is physically induced by the medical condition, but reactional anxiety may also occur in response to being faced with a medical illness. In either case, the presence of anxiety may complicate the medical picture and have a negative impact on the course of illness. Also, it should be noted R.R. is 49 years old, and the median age for onset of menopause is 52 years. Although menopause is not a medical illness but a normal stage of life, and R.R. has not complained of vasomotor symptoms or a cessation of menses, she should be asked about menopausal symptoms. Menopausal symptoms also may include sleep disturbances, mood swings, and depression.

Successful management of the medical condition often relieves associated anxiety, but short-term use of anxiolytic medications or nondrug therapies (biofeedback, psychotherapy) can also be very helpful.

When evaluating for possible causes of anxiety, it is also important to consider all medications a person is taking, including OTC drugs such as cough and cold preparations.[12] A diagnosis of substance-induced anxiety disorder is warranted when anxiety symptoms occur in relation to substance intoxication or withdrawal or when medication use causes the symptoms. Among the medications R.R. is taking, pseudoephedrine might be contributing to her anxiety. Other medications that can cause anxiety are listed in Table 80-2. Psychoactive substance abuse, withdrawal from central nervous system (CNS) depressants (e.g., alcohol, barbiturates, benzodiazepines), excessive caffeine intake, and nicotine withdrawal may go unrecognized as underlying precipitants of anxiety. R.R.'s current pattern of alcohol use, although not excessive, may become problematic if she uses alcohol to self-medicate her anxiety symptoms.

Although anxiety is the hallmark characteristic of anxiety disorders, it is not unique to this diagnostic category. Virtually any psychiatric illness may present with anxiety symptoms. Major depression, schizophrenia, bipolar disorder (both depressive and manic phases), eating disorders, and dysthymia are notably associated with anxiety, and diagnostic differentiation can sometimes be difficult.[1] For example, R.R.'s difficulties with fatigue and sleeping, as well as excessive worry, may be target symptoms of either anxiety or depression, or possibly both. If anxiety symptoms occur only in relation to another psychiatric disorder, then a separate anxiety disorder diagnosis is precluded. Anxiety in these cases may be alleviated with successful treatment of the primary psychiatric disorder. However, benzodiazepines are often used as adjunctive therapy, especially early in the course of treatment because they have a rapid onset of action.

Individuals with other psychiatric disorders can also have a primary anxiety disorder. In fact, comorbidity with anxiety disorders is the rule rather than the exception.[7] Depression, in particular, is often associated with anxiety disorders.[13] Concurrent anxiety and depression are associated with greater disability, poorer treatment outcomes, and higher suicide rates than either depression or anxiety alone.

Other factors to be considered in R.R. are the recent changes in her life (divorce, returning to work, becoming a single mother). Anxiety in response to life stressors may be severe and functionally detrimental, but could be considered appropriate for the circumstances. Usually, this type of anxiety is self-limiting and brief, subsiding over days to weeks as the person adapts to the new situation. However, some people may have serious difficulty adjusting, and they may experience excessive or debilitating symptoms, progressing to a primary and sometimes chronic disorder. If the person has no history of an anxiety disorder and the symptoms last only a few months, a diagnosis of adjustment disorder with anxious mood may be appropriate. If the symptoms are severe and continue for a prolonged period, a primary anxiety disorder may be present. The initial onset of a chronic anxiety disorder often occurs during a stressful period. Short-term or intermittent therapy with anxiolytic medication or counseling can be extremely beneficial in helping persons cope during times of acute stress. In contrast, management of primary anxiety disorders usually requires more extended treatment.

In summary, the factors in R.R.'s case warranting further investigation before a primary anxiety disorder diagnosis can be made include her medical illness (asthma), possible onset of menopause, her use of pseudoephedrine and caffeine, possible depression, and her adjustment to the recent life changes. These factors need to be addressed, and treated if possible, before a diagnosis of an anxiety disorder can be made and an appropriate treatment plan defined.

GENERALIZED ANXIETY DISORDER

Epidemiology and Clinical Course

Generalized anxiety disorder is one of the most common anxiety disorders, with a lifetime prevalence of 3.9% to 6.6%.[1,8] Onset is usually gradual and may be associated with increased life stressors. GAD usually begins between the mid teens and mid-50s and the median age of onset is 31 years.[8] As such, GAD presents the latest of all anxiety disorders.[14] GAD is twice as common in women than in men, and affected women often experience premenstrual exacerbation of symptoms.[15] Whites are more likely to report anxiety symptoms than Asians, Hispanics, and African Americans.[16] The typical course of GAD is described as being chronic and recurrent, but much is unknown about the long-term course of illness. Without treatment, it appears that less than half of GAD cases undergo remission.

Most people with GAD have at least one other psychiatric disorder. Common comorbid disorders include panic or social anxiety disorder, simple phobia, OCD, and major depression.[7] GAD commonly precedes the development of these other disorders, and comorbidity is associated with marked disability, high utilization of health care resources, and relatively poor treatment outcomes.[8] Alcohol abuse and dependence are also common in GAD and frequently result from attempts at self-medication of anxiety symptoms.[17] The observation that GAD rarely occurs in isolation has prompted debate about whether it is a primary anxiety disorder or merely a prodromal or residual phase of another disorder. Lastly, recent evidence suggests that GAD itself may be a risk factor for suicidal ideation, particularly among women, even when comorbid substance abuse and depression are considered.[18]

Diagnostic Criteria

The DSM-IV-TR criteria for GAD are presented in Table 80-3. GAD is characterized by unrealistic or excessive anxiety and worry about life issues for 6 months or longer.[1] The patient usually has great difficulty controlling the worry, which is accompanied by at least three of the associated symptoms listed in Table 80-3. Although some physical symptoms are similar between GAD and other anxiety disorders, symptom course varies among disorders. If the anxiety is related solely to another anxiety disorder (e.g., obsession with germs, fear of social situations), a diagnosis of GAD is not warranted.

Etiology and Pathophysiology

Genetic factors play a significant role in the etiology of GAD. Genes involved in the hereditary development of GAD are believed to be the same as those for neuroticism and major depression, with environmental factors determining which disorder is expressed in an individual.[5,19,20] Biological studies in GAD have found abnormalities in noradrenergic, serotonergic, and CCK and GABA-A receptor function.[5] Several studies report decreased α_2-adrenergic receptors in GAD patients, and this is believed to represent downregulation of receptors in response to high catecholamine levels. Abnormally low levels of lymphocyte peripheral benzodiazepine receptors have been reported by several investigators.

TABLE 80-3
Diagnostic Criteria for Generalized Anxiety Disorder

1. Unrealistic or excessive anxiety and worry about life circumstances for at least 6 months, during which the person has been bothered more days than not by these concerns
2. Person has difficulty controlling anxiety and worry
3. Anxiety and worry are associated with at least three of the following symptoms:
   a. Restlessness or feeling keyed up or on edge
   b. Easy fatigue
   c. Difficulty concentrating or mind going blank
   d. Irritability
   e. Muscle tension
   f. Sleep disturbances
4. If another psychiatric disorder is present, the focus of the anxiety and worry is unrelated to it
5. Anxiety, worry, or physical symptoms cause significant distress or impairment in social, occupational, or some other important aspect of functioning
6. Disturbance is not attributable to the direct effects of a substance, medication, or general medical condition and does not occur only during the course of a mood disorder, psychotic disorder, or pervasive developmental disorder

Adapted with permission from American Psychiatric Association. *Diagnostic and Statistical Manual of Mental Disorders*. 4th ed. Text Revision. Washington, DC: American Psychiatric Association; 2000. Copyright © 2000 American Psychiatric Association.

Treatment of Generalized Anxiety Disorder

NONPHARMACOLOGIC TREATMENTS

Management of GAD can involve both nonpharmacologic and pharmacologic therapies. Nondrug treatments such as supportive psychotherapy, dynamic psychotherapy, cognitive therapy, relaxation training, and meditation are often helpful in relieving anxiety and improving coping skills.[21] Cognitive therapy is aimed at identifying negative thought patterns provoking or worsening anxiety and making them more positive. Cognitive behavioral therapy (CBT) has been associated with significant reductions in anxiety that are maintained for 6 to 12 months, as well as decreased psychiatric comorbidity in GAD.[21] Controlled comparisons of cognitive therapies and benzodiazepine treatment have reported comparable efficacies in GAD.[21] Although psychosocial treatments are commonly recommended as first-line therapy for GAD and other anxiety disorders, they are vastly underused because of cost (many insurance providers offer limited coverage for outpatient psychotherapy), time requirements, and a limited availability of trained therapists. The decline in use of psychosocial therapies for anxiety disorders also correlates with the explosion in medication options for treating anxiety disorders.

BENZODIAZEPINES

Benzodiazepines are widely prescribed anxiolytic agents, and their efficacy in treating GAD and other anxiety disorders, particularly in the short-term, is well established.[17] Benzodiazepines

TABLE 80-4
Clinical Comparison of Benzodiazepine Agents

Drug (Trade Name, Generic)	FDA-Approved Indications	Usual Dosage Range Through 65 Years of Age	Maximal Recommended Dosage Through 65 Years of Age	Approximate Dosage Equivalencies
Alprazolam (Xanax, Xanax XR, Niravam orally disintegrating tablets, Intensol oral solution, generic)	Anxiety, anxiety associated with depression, panic disorder	0.5–6 mg/d (up to 10 mg/d for panic disorder)	2 mg/d	1
Chlordiazepoxide (Librium, Limbitrol,[a] Librax,[b] generic)	Anxiety, preoperative anxiety, acute alcohol withdrawal	15–100 mg/d	40 mg/d	50
Clonazepam (Klonopin, Klonopin wafer, generic)	Anticonvulsant, panic disorder	0.5–12 mg/d	3 mg/d	0.5
Clorazepate (Tranxene, Tranxene-SD, generic)	Anxiety, alcohol withdrawal, anticonvulsant	15–60 mg/d	30 mg/d	15
Diazepam (Valium, Intensol oral solution, Injection solution, generic)	Anxiety, muscle relaxant, acute alcohol withdrawal, preoperative anxiety, anticonvulsant	4–40 mg/d	20 mg/d	10
Estazolam (ProSom, generic)	Sedative-hypnotic	1–2 mg HS	1 mg HS	2
Flurazepam (Dalmane, generic)	Sedative-hypnotic	15–30 mg HS	15 mg HS	30
Lorazepam (Ativan, oral solution, injection solution, generic)	Anxiety, anxiety associated with depression, anticonvulsant, premedication for anesthetic procedure	2–6 mg/d	3 mg/d	1.5–2
Oxazepam (Serax, generic)	Anxiety, alcohol withdrawal	30–120 mg/d	60 mg/d	30
Quazepam (Doral)	Sedative-hypnotic	7.5–15 mg HS	7.5 mg HS	15
Temazepam (Restoril, generic)	Sedative-hypnotic	15–30 mg HS	15 mg HS	30
Triazolam (Halcion, generic)	Sedative-hypnotic	0.125–0.25 mg HS	0.125 mg HS	0.25

[a] Combination product containing amitriptyline.
[b] Combination product containing clidinium bromide (classified as a gastrointestinal antispasmodic agent).
FDA, US Food and Drug Administration; HS, at bedtime.

offer rapid symptom relief with distinct clinical advantages compared with older agents such as barbiturates and alcohol. These advantages include more specific anxiolytic effects, lower fatality rates from acute toxicity and overdose (in monotherapy), improved tolerability, lower abuse potential, and fewer dangerous drug interactions. Use of older nonbenzodiazepine agents as anxiolytics is considered inappropriate because of the many advantages of benzodiazepines and other newer agents. Although preferred over these older agents, benzodiazepines are still associated with risks of dependence and withdrawal and are not recommended for the long-term management of GAD.

MECHANISM OF ACTION

Benzodiazepines have four distinct effects: anxiolytic, anticonvulsant, muscle relaxant, and sedative-hypnotic. These agents are used to treat a wide variety of medical and psychiatric conditions, including muscle spasms, seizures, anxiety disorders, acute agitation, and insomnia. Benzodiazepines with a rapid onset and short duration of action are commonly used to decrease anxiety and apprehension, as well as induce sedation before surgery and other medical procedures.

Benzodiazepines potentiate GABA by binding to sites on the central GABA-A receptor. There are four types of GABA-A receptors that are benzodiazepine sensitive; these receptors are distinguished by the type of α subunit they contain (α_1, α_2, α_3, or α_5).[22,23] Receptors with an α_1 subunit are the most abundant type and are widely distributed throughout the brain. Benzodiazepine action at the α_1-GABA-A receptors produces sedative and amnestic effects, whereas anxiolytic effects are associated with binding to the α_2-GABA-A receptor.[22,24] This latter type of GABA-A receptor is localized mainly in the limbic system, cerebral cortex, and striatum. GABA-A receptors with α_3 subunits are linked with noradrenergic, serotonergic, and cholinergic neurons.

Currently available benzodiazepine anxiolytics are not selective at any of the four GABA-A receptor subtypes. Research is aimed at developing benzodiazepine compounds with specific affinity for the α_2-GABA-A receptor, which would produce anxiolytic effects without tolerance or sedative and amnestic effects.[25,26]

CLINICAL COMPARISON OF BENZODIAZEPINES

Of the 13 benzodiazepines commercially available in the United States, 7 are marketed as antianxiety agents, and 6 as oral sedative-hypnotics. Indications reflect manufacturers' labeling decisions because anxiolytics can be effective sedatives and vice versa.

Table 80-4 compares the clinical profiles of marketed oral benzodiazepines. Midazolam is not included in Table 80-4. It is a short-acting, water-soluble benzodiazepine, indicated only for induction of sedation before surgery or for short diagnostic or endoscopic procedures. It is available as a parenteral or oral syrup formulation. Most benzodiazepines have unlabeled uses, including treatment of anxiety and agitation associated with medical or psychiatric illnesses; alcohol withdrawal; irritable bowel syndrome; premenstrual syndrome; chemotherapy-induced nausea and vomiting; catatonia; tetanus; involuntary movement disorders (restless legs syndrome, akathisia, tardive dyskinesia, essential tremor); and spasticity associated with various neurologic disorders (cerebral palsy, paraplegia).

ANTIDEPRESSANT AGENTS

Antidepressants are the recommended first-line treatment for most patients with anxiety disorder, even though benzodiazepines are still widely prescribed. One important distinction

TABLE 80-5
Summary of Comparative Medication Treatment Options for Anxiety Disorders

Disorder	First-Line Treatments[a]	Second-Line Treatments	Possible Alternatives
Generalized anxiety disorder	Venlafaxine XR Buspirone Benzodiazepines Paroxetine Escitalopram Duloxetine	Sertraline Citalopram	Tricyclic antidepressants[b] Pregabalin Fluoxetine Mirtazapine Atypical antipsychotics[c]
Panic disorder	Paroxetine Sertraline Fluoxetine Venlafaxine Alprazolam Clonazepam	Fluvoxamine Citalopram Escitalopram Clomipramine Lorazepam	Nefazodone[b] Mirtazapine Imipramine Valproic acid Diazepam
Social anxiety disorder	Paroxetine Sertraline Venlafaxine XR Fluvoxamine CR	Citalopram Escitalopram Fluoxetine Alprazolam Clonazepam	Phenelzine[b] Nefazodone Bupropion Duloxetine Gabapentin Pregabalin Atypical antipsychotics[c]
Posttraumatic stress disorder	Sertraline Paroxetine	Fluoxetine Fluvoxamine Venlafaxine XR Citalopram Escitalopram	Amitriptyline[b] Imipramine[b] Phenelzine[b] Mirtazapine Bupropion Nefazodone[b] Prazosin Atypical antipsychotics[c] Anticonvulsants
Obsessive–compulsive disorder	Paroxetine Fluoxetine Sertraline Fluvoxamine CR Fluvoxamine	Clomipramine[b] Venlafaxine Citalopram Escitalopram	Clonazepam[c] Antipsychotic agents[c]

[a] US Food and Drug Administration–approved indications.
[b] Documented efficacy, but not recommended for first-line treatment because of undesirable clinical properties (side effects, potential toxicity, drug interactions).
[c] Adjunctive therapy only.

between these two medication classes is that the anxiolytic effects of benzodiazepines occur almost immediately, whereas the effects of antidepressants occur gradually during several weeks. Therefore, it is common for short-term benzodiazepine therapy to be prescribed in combination with an antidepressant during initial treatment of many anxiety disorders.

Antidepressants were found to be effective in the treatment of anxiety disorders in the 1970s, when certain tricyclic antidepressants (TCAs) and monoamine oxidase inhibitors (MAOIs) were deemed useful in treating panic disorder. Clomipramine, a TCA, emerged as an effective treatment for OCD soon thereafter. As shown in Table 80-5, selective serotonin reuptake inhibitors (SSRIs) have since gained first-line status for treating all five primary anxiety disorders.[27] The distinction between anxiolytics and antidepressants is continually narrowing, particularly considering the common comorbid presentation of depression and anxiety.

Early controlled studies found trazodone, doxepin, imipramine, and amitriptyline comparably effective or superior to benzodiazepines in treating GAD.[17] Although benzodiazepines work quickly, and TCA treatment is often associated with initial increases in anxiety (especially with higher dosages), continued TCA therapy is usually effective if side effects are tolerated. However, TCAs are not widely used for treating anxiety disorders because attention has turned to other much safer and better tolerated antidepressants.

Paroxetine is the best-studied SSRI in GAD and is US Food and Drug Administration (FDA) approved for this indication. Paroxetine is superior to placebo and as effective as TCAs in treating GAD, with improved tolerability. Results from a large fixed-dose study suggest a paroxetine dosage of 20 mg/day is effective for most patients with GAD, although some patients may require doses up to 40 mg/day for optimal benefits.[28] Like TCAs, patients may experience an initial increase in anxiety during SSRI treatment, so lower-than-normal SSRI starting doses should be used in patients with GAD. A low paroxetine starting dose of 10 mg/day is recommended for the first week in patients with GAD to minimize initial side effects. Paroxetine maintenance therapy significantly decreases the risk of GAD relapse at 6 months.[29] The most common side effects of paroxetine in patients with GAD are sedation, nausea, dry mouth, constipation, asthenia, headache, and sexual dysfunction. With long-term therapy, weight gain may be problematic.

The combination serotonin and norepinephrine reuptake inhibitors (SNRIs), venlafaxine, and duloxetine are FDA-approved for the treatment of GAD. Newer SNRIs including milnacipran and venlafaxine's active metabolite, desvenlafaxine, have not been well studied in the management of anxiety. However, data suggest these agents may be useful for the treatment of anxiety symptoms associated with depression, although further randomized controlled trials are needed to confirm this finding.[30,31] Several large controlled studies have shown venlafaxine XR to be effective in reducing anxiety associated with depression, as well as in the treatment of GAD.[32–35] The recommended starting dose is 37.5 to 75 mg/day, and the effective dosage range for GAD is 75 to 225 mg/day.[34] Many patients respond to venlafaxine doses of 75 to 150 mg/day, although some may require up to 225 mg/day. The side effect profile of venlafaxine is similar to that of the SSRIs, with dose-related nausea being the most common, and this usually subsides after 1 to 2 weeks of continued therapy. Other common side effects of venlafaxine include dizziness, asthenia, dry mouth, sweating, and either sedation or insomnia. Significant increases in blood pressure are not usually seen within the dosage range used for GAD (75–225 mg/day), but can occur with higher doses. Long-term studies report sustained GAD response to venlafaxine during 6 months of continued treatment.[33] Duloxetine's effectiveness has been demonstrated in short- and long-term trials, with the latter citing a decrease in relapse of GAD in patients treated with 60 to 120 mg/day.[35–39] In the single trial with a venlafaxine XR comparison arm, both duloxetine and venlafaxine exhibited similar efficacy and tolerability.[36]

With regard to other SSRIs, escitalopram received FDA approval for GAD in late 2003, and preliminary reports suggest efficacy for citalopram.[27,40] Sertraline, fluvoxamine, and fluoxetine are reportedly effective in alleviating anxiety symptoms in patients with depression.[17,41,42] Fluoxetine may be more likely than other SSRIs to cause anxiety as an initial side effect.[27] Fluoxetine has been associated with poor response in depressed patients with prominent anxiety or psychomotor agitation in some studies, although others report it to be comparably effective and as well tolerated as other SSRIs in this population.[42,43]

Mirtazapine is a non-SSRI antidepressant that appears promising in the treatment of GAD, particularly in patients with comorbid major depression, but controlled studies are few.[44,45] It is unlikely to cause anxiety as a side effect, owing to its 5-HT receptor type-2 blocking activity. (See Chapter 83, Mood Disorders I: Major Depressive Disorders, for more information regarding the clinical use of various antidepressant agents.) As mentioned previously, lower initial doses of antidepressants are recommended to avoid acute worsening of anxiety symptoms. Slow titration and patient education regarding adverse reactions associated with antidepressants, including the black-box warning for suicidality, are also recommended.[46] Although decreases in anxiety symptoms during antidepressant treatment may appear within the first 2 weeks, response is gradual and generally continues for 8 to 12 weeks or longer. Therefore, optimal trials of antidepressants in GAD should allow at least 8 weeks of adequate doses before a lack of response is determined. Continued improvements may occur for 4 to 6 months in some GAD patients treated with antidepressants.[29,33]

Overall, advantages of antidepressants compared with benzodiazepines in treating GAD include their superior efficacy for cognitive symptoms such as excessive worry and their better efficacy for common comorbid disorders such as depression and other anxiety disorders. Antidepressants also lack potential for abuse and dependence, although most antidepressants can cause a withdrawal syndrome on abrupt discontinuation.

OTHER AGENTS USED TO TREAT GENERALIZED ANXIETY DISORDER

Buspirone was marketed in the United States as the first of a nonbenzodiazepine class of anxiolytics, the azapirones. This class differs pharmacologically and clinically from benzodiazepines.[17,47] Buspirone does not interact with GABA receptors and works as a partial agonist of the 5-HT type 1A receptor (i.e., it binds to the receptor but exerts a fraction of the effect of a full agonist).[48] This partial agonist activity results in reduced 5-HT neurotransmission. In addition, buspirone enhances dopaminergic neurotransmission by blocking presynaptic dopamine receptor-2 autoreceptors and also facilitates noradrenergic activity.[47] Buspirone is effective in treating cognitive anxiety symptoms and is not associated with abuse or dependence; however, it has a delayed onset of anxiolytic effects and is not appropriate for as-needed use.

Anticonvulsant medications, particularly pregabalin, a schedule V controlled substance, have recently received attention for the treatment of anxiety disorders. Pregabalin appears to be efficacious in managing somatic and psychic symptoms of GAD compared with active comparators, benzodiazepines and venlafaxine.[46,49] Pregabalin exhibits a dose–response effect that appears to plateau at 300 mg/day. Additionally, one long-term continuation study of up to 24 weeks suggests pregabalin 450 mg/day may be effective in preventing relapse compared with placebo.[50] Finally, atypical antipsychotics are being investigated as monotherapy and augmentation therapy in patients with GAD. Aripiprazole, olanzapine, quetiapine, risperidone, and ziprasidone have been studied for treatment-resistant GAD, in mostly small, open-label trials.[51] These agents may be useful in patients who fail to respond to first-line treatment options, or in patients with a comorbid psychotic illness.[52]

Clinical Presentation and Assessment of Generalized Anxiety Disorder

CASE 80-2

QUESTION 1: L.V., a 32-year-old man, has been employed as a teacher for the past 10 years. He has had an excellent work record until 8 months ago, when excessive absences and a tendency to become easily upset at students and coworkers became noticeable. On clinical assessment, L.V. complains of being "on edge," irritable, and tense, with frequent stomach upset and diarrhea. He has no history of mental illness; however, he admits to being stressed and worrying too much about "insignificant things." He cannot seem to control these symptoms regardless of how hard he tries. L.V. denies any symptoms indicative of panic disorder or OCD.

L.V.'s physical examination is unremarkable, and his family history is only notable for his sister who is described as a "nervous person." L.V. denies past or present use of any illicit substances and drinks three to four beers at social events, which he has not enjoyed recently. His mental status examination reveals the following:

- ***Appearance and behavior:* L.V. is neatly groomed and dressed and speaks coherently, but he constantly fidgets and taps his right foot.**
- ***Mood:* L.V. is anxious and worried about the clinician's evaluation and admits to occasionally feeling depressed and hopeless because of his anxiety. He often has difficulty falling asleep but generally remains asleep throughout the night.**
- ***Sensorium:* L.V. is oriented to person, place, and time.**
- ***Thoughts:* L.V. denies any auditory or visual hallucinations, or suicidal or homicidal ideation.**

L.V. states, at times, that he is unable to relax and startles easily, particularly in the classroom around his students. His work has been difficult for him lately, and the principal has told him that his job is in immediate jeopardy unless he improves his performance. L.V. states that he just wants to be able to perform his job like he used to and be able to "chill out" and get back to his old life. His insight and

judgment are good, and he is motivated to obtain treatment. The physician's provisional diagnosis is GAD. What clinical features of GAD are present in L.V., and how can his symptoms be assessed objectively?

L.V. exhibits the following target symptoms associated with GAD: excessive worry that is difficult to control, irritability, tension, and inability to relax. Other typical symptoms of anxiety present in L.V. include gastrointestinal (GI) problems (upset stomach and diarrhea), being startled easily, and fidgeting. These target symptoms are not necessarily diagnostic of any particular disorder, but other factors in association with these symptoms are consistent with GAD. The absence of physical or other psychiatric illnesses, as well as use of any illicit substances and lack of recent use of alcohol, excludes possible secondary causes of anxiety. The 8-month duration of symptoms is consistent with a diagnosis of GAD, and L.V.'s age is consistent with the usual onset of GAD. More importantly, the symptoms are causing significant occupational impairment for L.V. and interfering with his quality of life; therefore, a diagnosis of GAD is appropriate in L.V.

The Hamilton Anxiety Rating Scale (HAM-A) is a useful assessment tool to evaluate clinical anxiety, and it is the standard instrument used in GAD clinical trials. A HAM-A score of greater than 18 is generally correlated with significant anxiety, and a score of 7 to 10 is associated with remission.[53] The HAM-A can be used to assess baseline anxiety symptoms in patients such as L.V. and to monitor response throughout treatment. The Sheehan Disability Scale is a patient-rated instrument, which is commonly used to assess functional impairment caused by GAD and other anxiety disorders. A score of 1 reflects mild disability.[53]

Indications for and Selection of Treatment

CASE 80-2, QUESTION 2: Based on the information presented in L.V.'s case, how can it be determined whether treatment is indicated? What factors should be considered in choosing the most appropriate treatment for L.V.?

L.V. meets the diagnostic criteria for GAD and is suffering significant disability from his anxiety disorder. He also has insight into his illness and desires treatment that will enable him to improve his job performance and quality of life. Appropriate treatment of GAD can help achieve these goals and is therefore indicated for patients such as L.V.

Treatment options for GAD include both pharmacologic and nondrug therapies. Psychosocial treatments such as CBT can be effective in treating GAD, but use of these therapies alone is generally reserved for patients with mild-to-moderate symptoms. In L.V.'s case, prompt treatment is needed because his job is in immediate jeopardy owing to impairments associated with his anxiety. Therefore, pharmacotherapy in combination with psychological therapy, if available, is indicated in L.V.

Among potential drug therapies, the benzodiazepines, SSRIs (escitalopram and paroxetine), SNRIs (duloxetine and venlafaxine), and buspirone are all considered first-line treatments for GAD.[17,54] A primary consideration when choosing among these options is whether any comorbid psychiatric conditions are present. Antidepressants are good initial choices for patients with concurrent depression, which is common in GAD patients. They are also preferred over benzodiazepines in patients with past or present alcohol or substance abuse. Other medical or psychiatric disorders may also be present, which can guide selection toward a treatment that may be dually effective.

Another important consideration when selecting treatment for GAD is how quickly therapeutic effects are needed. Benzodiazepines reduce anxiety within a few hours, whereas antidepressants and buspirone have delayed onsets of anxiolytic effects. Medication cost is another potential factor, and generic benzodiazepines or SSRIs are inexpensive options.

In L.V.'s case, a benzodiazepine may be a good initial choice because of the need for quick symptom relief relating to his problems at work. L.V. is young and healthy with no past or present history of substance abuse or alcohol use that might make benzodiazepines unsuitable for him. Although L.V. drinks beer on occasion at social gatherings, he has not participated in these events recently, and he should continue to avoid alcohol if a benzodiazepine is initiated. GAD is often chronic, and antidepressants or buspirone are usually preferred to benzodiazepines for long-term treatment. Therefore, one of these agents would also be appropriate to use in this case. Combination benzodiazepine-SSRI therapy during initial treatment of anxiety disorders is well tolerated and may result in synergistic anxiolytic effects and quicker response.[55,56]

Benzodiazepine Treatment

FACTORS INFLUENCING BENZODIAZEPINE SELECTION

CASE 80-2, QUESTION 3: The physician decides to treat L.V.'s GAD with paroxetine and a benzodiazepine for quick control of his anxiety during the first several weeks until the onset of paroxetine's anxiolytic effects. What factors are important in the selection of a particular benzodiazepine agent for L.V.?

Of the available benzodiazepines, none have demonstrated clear superior efficacy in the treatment of GAD. However, certain agents have been used more extensively than others. Alprazolam is the most commonly used in the United States, followed by lorazepam, clonazepam, and diazepam. All four of these benzodiazepines have been successfully used in the treatment of GAD.

Because of similar overall anxiolytic efficacies of benzodiazepines, other factors must be considered when selecting one agent versus another. Benzodiazepines differ in their pharmacokinetic properties, and these are generally the main factors considered in drug selection (Table 80-6).

Benzodiazepines can be differentiated pharmacokinetically according to their elimination half-lives and their metabolism to active or inactive compounds (Fig. 80-2; Table 80-6). Diazepam (Valium) and chlordiazepoxide (Librium) have half-lives between 10 and 40 hours, and are metabolized by hepatic oxidative pathways to the active metabolite desmethyldiazepam (DMDZ). As shown in Figure 80-2, the prodrugs quazepam (Doral) and clorazepate (Tranxene) are also metabolized to DMDZ.[57] The metabolite DMDZ has a half-life of at least 100 hours, and chronic dosing of benzodiazepines that get converted to DMDZ can result in drug accumulation and prolonged clinical effects.[57] This can be especially detrimental in the elderly, those with liver disease, persons taking other drugs interfering with benzodiazepine metabolism, or those who are poor metabolizers. Although long durations of action make once-daily dosing possible, small, divided daily doses are often used clinically to minimize side effects.

Clonazepam undergoes various routes of hepatic metabolism, including oxidative hydroxylation, reduction, and acetylation.[57] Specific enzymes responsible for clonazepam metabolism have not been confirmed, but there is evidence it is a

TABLE 80-6
Pharmacokinetic Comparison of Benzodiazepine Agents

Drug	Elimination Half-Life (hours)[a]	Active Metabolites	Protein Binding	Pathway of Metabolism	Rate of Onset After Oral Administration
Chlordiazepoxide	>100	Desmethyldiazepam	96%	Oxidation	Intermediate
Diazepam	>100	Desmethyldiazepam	98%	Oxidation (CYP3A4, CYP2C19)	Very fast
Oxazepam	5–14	None	87%	Conjugation	Slow
Flurazepam	>100	Desalkylflurazepam, hydroxyethylflurazepam	97%	Oxidation	Fast
Clorazepate	>100	Desmethyldiazepam	98%	Oxidation	Fast
Lorazepam	10–20	None	85%–90%	Conjugation	Intermediate
Alprazolam	12–15	Insignificant	80%	Oxidation (CYP3A4)	Fast
Temazepam	10–20	Insignificant	98%	Conjugation	Intermediate
Triazolam	1.5–5	Insignificant	90%	Oxidation (CYP3A4)	Intermediate
Quazepam	47–100	2-Oxoquazepam, *N*-desalkyl-2-oxoquazepam	>95%	Oxidation	Fast
Estazolam	24	Insignificant	93%	Oxidation	Intermediate
Clonazepam	20–50	Insignificant	85%	Oxidation, reduction (CYP3A4)	Intermediate
Midazolam	1–4	None	97%	Oxidation (CYP3A4)	NA

[a]Parent drug + active metabolite.
CYP, cytochrome P-450; NA, not applicable.

substrate for cytochrome P-450 (CYP) 3A4.[58] The elimination half-life of clonazepam ranges from 20 to 50 hours, making once-daily dosing feasible. Orally disintegrating clonazepam tablets (Klonopin wafer) have been introduced and are indicated for the treatment of panic disorder. This product dissolves quickly on the tongue and can be taken without water when quick and easy administration is needed.

Alprazolam (Xanax, Niravam) and lorazepam (Ativan) have intermediate half-lives of 10 to 20 hours, and oxazepam (Serax) has a short to intermediate half-life of 5 to 14 hours. Alprazolam is a triazolobenzodiazepine metabolized by CYP3A4. Alprazolam, lorazepam, and oxazepam usually need to be taken on a three times a day (TID) to four times a day dosing schedule for sustained clinical effects, but an extended-release (XR) preparation of alprazolam allows daily or twice-daily dosing. Alprazolam XR may be associated with fewer CNS side effects than the immediate-release form because peak alprazolam blood levels are lower.[59] Also, a quickly dissolving tablet of alprazolam (Niravam) has been marketed. Lorazepam, temazepam, and oxazepam undergo phase 2 metabolism by glucuronidation and are believed to be substrates for the uridine diphosphate-glucuronosyltransferase 2B7 isozyme.[60] These agents are free of active metabolites and are unlikely to accumulate with chronic administration; they are preferred over long-acting agents in patients with liver disease and in the elderly. Unlike phase 1 oxidative metabolism, phase 2 glucuronidation processes do not appear to decline with age.[60]

Benzodiazepines are readily absorbed within 2 to 3 hours after oral administration.[57] They are widely distributed in the body and accumulate preferentially in lipid-rich areas such as the CNS and fat tissue. Lipid solubility varies among the agents, resulting in differences in rates of absorption and speed of onset, as well as duration of clinical effects (Table 80-6). Diazepam and clorazepate have the highest lipid solubilities and the quickest

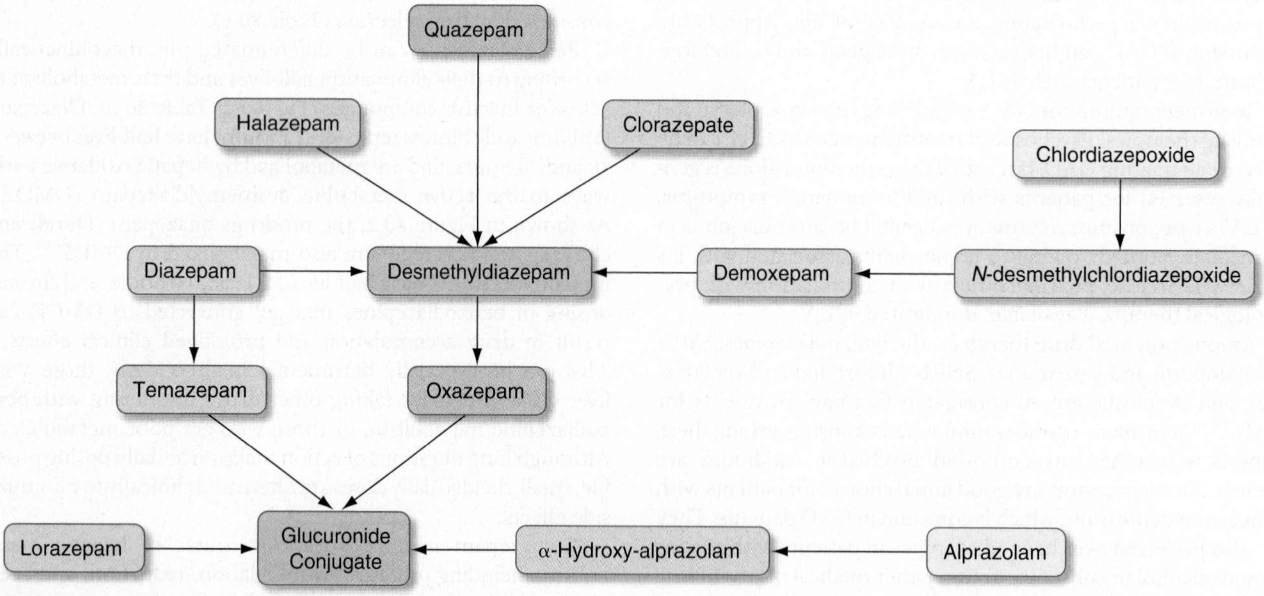

FIGURE 80-2 Metabolic pathways of benzodiazepines.

Section 15 Psychiatric Disorders

onset of action, which can be desirable when rapid anxiolysis is needed; however, both can produce a "drugged" or "high" feeling in some patients. Highly lipophilic benzodiazepines are also more quickly redistributed out of the brain, which decreases their duration of action acutely. For example, even though diazepam has a very long half-life, its clinical effects last for a shorter period than those of lorazepam, which has a relatively short half-life.

Diazepam, lorazepam, chlordiazepoxide, and midazolam are also available for parenteral (intravenous [IV] and intramuscular [IM]) administration[57] for treatment of severe agitation or seizures, or for induction of preoperative sedation and anxiolysis. IM injection of both chlordiazepoxide and diazepam can be very painful. Lorazepam is the preferred agent when IM dosing is needed for quick control of anxiety or agitation. The absorption of sublingual lorazepam, alprazolam, and triazolam (Halcion) is comparable to or slightly faster than oral absorption.[57]

Cost is another important factor in benzodiazepine selection. Brand-name benzodiazepines can be relatively expensive, but all are available in less costly generic versions, except the extended-release and quick-dissolving formulations. Potential drug interactions should also be considered in the selection of an agent because they can alter pharmacokinetics and clinical effects (see Case 80-4, Question 1).

Because L.V. is young and healthy and is not taking any other medications, the clinician could choose any benzodiazepine. Nevertheless, most clinicians still prefer to use shorter-acting high-potency agents such as lorazepam or alprazolam for patients such as L.V. Appropriate starting doses would be lorazepam 0.5 to 1 mg TID or alprazolam 0.25 to 0.5 mg TID. Dosages can be increased every 3 to 4 days, if needed, within the dosage ranges indicated in Table 80-4. L.V. should notice a decrease in his anxiety symptoms within the first few days of treatment. Prescription of a generic formulation is recommended to reduce treatment costs.

ADVERSE EFFECTS AND PATIENT COUNSELING

CASE 80-2, QUESTION 4: Alprazolam 0.25 mg TID is prescribed for L.V. in addition to paroxetine. What side effects may occur with benzodiazepine treatment, and how should L.V. be counseled regarding benzodiazepine therapy?

Overall, benzodiazepines are very safe and well-tolerated medications. Sedation and feelings of tiredness are the most common side effects of benzodiazepines, but sedation can also be beneficial in alleviating insomnia that often accompanies anxiety. Tolerance usually develops to the sedative effects of benzodiazepines within 1 to 2 weeks of continued treatment; consequently, benzodiazepine sedative-hypnotics are recommended for only short-term use.[61] Tolerance does not appear to develop to the anxiolytic or muscle relaxant effects of benzodiazepines.

Benzodiazepines can cause cognitive impairment and anterograde amnesia (decreased memory for new information after taking the drug), which is dose-related and reversible on medication discontinuation. Tolerance often develops to the cognitive adverse effects, but they can also persist throughout therapy in some patients.[62] Use of alcohol during benzodiazepine therapy greatly increases the risks for memory problems and sedation, as well as for other more dangerous effects, including respiratory depression. Elderly individuals are more sensitive to sedative, cognitive, and psychomotor effects of benzodiazepines, and tolerance to these effects may occur more slowly than in the nonelderly.[63]

Other psychomotor effects such as problems with balance, coordination, and delayed reaction time also can occur during benzodiazepine treatment.[57] These effects are also dose related, but usually subside within a few weeks of continued treatment. However, it is important to warn patients starting on benzodiazepine therapy about possible adverse psychomotor effects. Long-acting benzodiazepines taken the previous night may cause residual daytime effects and pose a hazard while driving the next day.

The link between benzodiazepine use and falls, especially in the elderly, is well documented and may result from a combination of balance impairment, sedation, and muscle relaxant effects.[64] Rapid dosage escalation and use of high doses have been identified as major risk factors, but even use of low doses of short-acting agents greatly increases the risk of falling in the elderly.[64,65] Although tolerance can develop to the psychomotor effects of benzodiazepines, elderly individuals may experience persistent impairment. Benzodiazepines should probably be considered second-line therapy in the ambulatory older population.

Respiratory depression is another potential adverse effect of benzodiazepines, but it is usually clinically relevant only in patients with severe respiratory disease, in overdose situations (see Case 80-5, Question 1), or when combined with alcohol or substances that depress breathing. It is recommended that benzodiazepines be avoided in patients with sleep apnea. Respiratory complications are encountered most often with IV administration. IV midazolam has been associated with a number of deaths owing to cardiorespiratory arrest during its use for conscious sedation, most often in patients premedicated with narcotics or in those with chronic obstructive airway disease. Severe respiratory depression has also occurred with the concurrent use of benzodiazepines and olanzapine (Zyprexa), loxapine (Loxitane), or clozapine (Clozaril).

Paradoxical disinhibition, with increased anxiety, irritability, and agitation, can occur infrequently with benzodiazepines.[57,66] Such effects have been mainly observed in elderly or developmentally disabled patients. Other unusual behaviors, such as increased anger, hostility, and violence, have been attributed to benzodiazepine use in a small number of cases.[43] Most of these reports were anecdotal and involved patients with pre-existing psychiatric disorders such as bipolar disorder, schizophrenia, or personality disorders. It is difficult to confirm benzodiazepines caused these paradoxical reactions because such disorders are commonly associated with behavioral problems, and benzodiazepines are often used in their treatment. Overall, there is no convincing evidence that benzodiazepines actually cause violent or suicidal behaviors, but there is some evidence to the contrary.[57,66]

In summary, L.V. should be told he may experience sedation and difficulties in thinking, concentration, or memory during the first week or so of therapy, but these side effects should resolve once he experiences some tolerance to the drug. He should be extremely careful while driving or performing other tasks requiring psychomotor skills, especially during the first week, and he should avoid the use of alcohol while he is taking benzodiazepines.

BENZODIAZEPINE ABUSE AND DEPENDENCE

CASE 80-2, QUESTION 5: Two weeks later, L.V. contacts his clinician to discuss a medication concern. He reports the medication has been extremely effective in relieving his anxiety, and he is currently taking paroxetine 20 mg every morning and alprazolam, 0.25 mg TID, as directed by his physician. However, his friend has told him he will become addicted to alprazolam, and he wonders whether he should stop taking it because of this concern. What potential for abuse and dependence is associated with benzodiazepines? How should L.V. be counseled regarding "becoming addicted" to alprazolam?

Concerns related to abuse and dependence are probably the major drawback to the clinical use of benzodiazepines. These agents are classified as schedule IV controlled substances, reflecting a relatively limited abuse and dependence liability. There may be differences within the class regarding abuse potential. Diazepam, alprazolam, and lorazepam are reported to be more likely to be abused than are oxazepam and chlordiazepoxide.[67] This difference is commonly attributed to the quicker onset of effect, which may be associated with a subjective euphoric sensation. The XR alprazolam formulation is reported to have a lower abuse potential than immediate-release alprazolam because of its slower onset of effect and lower maximal plasma concentrations.[59]

Abuse is characterized by drug use outside the therapeutic setting and implies recreational use combined with continued use despite negative consequences, dose escalation, and loss of control over use. Patients without a history of substance abuse who take benzodiazepines for therapeutic purposes are unlikely to escalate doses or use them in ways characteristic of abuse.[67]

The potential problems with benzodiazepine abuse and dependence can be avoided or minimized in several ways. First is the identification of patients who have a history of alcohol or substance abuse and using nonbenzodiazepine treatments in such cases.[67] Second, patients should be counseled about the anticipated duration of benzodiazepine use, the possibility of withdrawal symptoms, and the importance of gradual drug tapering when therapy is discontinued. The distinction between "addiction" and appropriate therapeutic use, which may be accompanied by some degree of physical dependence, should be explained.

L.V. should be advised that as long as the medication is helping his anxiety and he is taking it according to his physician's instructions, his use of alprazolam does not constitute addiction. However, his body may develop some physiological dependence to the drug, so if he stops taking alprazolam abruptly, he could experience increased anxiety and other withdrawal symptoms. When alprazolam is to be discontinued, the dose should be decreased gradually for a sufficient period to minimize withdrawal symptoms.

DURATION OF TREATMENT

CASE 80-2, QUESTION 6: Two weeks later at his clinic appointment, L.V. is still doing well and has shown further improvements in his GAD symptoms. He has been taking the prescribed alprazolam and paroxetine for 1 month, and his paroxetine has been increased to 20 mg/day during this time. How long should medication therapy continue?

GAD is a chronic disorder fluctuating in severity and often requires long-term treatment. Relapse after discontinuation of benzodiazepine monotherapy is reported to occur in 50% to 80% of GAD patients; however, some of these cases may actually involve benzodiazepine withdrawal.[68] These relapse rates also do not take into account the concurrent use of other medications that may prevent relapse, such as paroxetine. Although long-term use of benzodiazepines is generally safe and effective, it is desirable to limit treatment to the shortest duration necessary because of the physical dependence potential.[17] When benzodiazepines are used for acute anxiolytic effects during initiation of antidepressant treatment for GAD, they are commonly limited to short-term (2–6 weeks) therapy. L.V. has demonstrated good response after 1 month of combined alprazolam and paroxetine therapy. Because the anxiolytic effects of paroxetine usually occur between 2 and 4 weeks of therapy and he is taking a therapeutic paroxetine dose, it is appropriate to start discontinuing alprazolam at this time. L.V. is unlikely to experience significant withdrawal symptoms after only 1 month of treatment, but the dose should still be gradually decreased for several weeks, according to tolerability of the taper.[68] In patients who are treated with short-acting benzodiazepines for longer durations, switching to an equivalent dose of a longer-acting benzodiazepine, like diazepam, may simplify the withdrawal schedule.[69]

There is no consensus about the optimal duration of drug therapy for GAD. However, recent recommendations suggest effective medication treatment be continued for at least 6 to 12 months after response.[17] Continuation treatment with antidepressants significantly reduces the risk of GAD relapse in 6 months.[29,33] Therefore, paroxetine therapy should be continued for another 5 to 11 months in L.V.'s case. After that time, gradual paroxetine discontinuation may be considered, and reinstitution of treatment is warranted if relapse occurs.

SYMPTOMS AND MANAGEMENT OF BENZODIAZEPINE WITHDRAWAL

CASE 80-3

QUESTION 1: T.B., a 48-year-old woman, has been taking diazepam 40 mg/day for 7 months for its muscle relaxant effects after sustaining back and other injuries from a collision with her road bike and an automobile. Five days ago, T.B. was unable to refill her prescription for financial reasons. A brief mental status examination reveals mild confusion and irritability. Physically, T.B. is trembling and complains of nausea and insomnia. Her medical history indicates no current medical problems or psychiatric illnesses, and T.B. denies the use of tobacco, alcohol, or other drugs of abuse. How should T.B. be treated?

Because T.B. has not taken her prescribed diazepam for five days, it is likely she is experiencing a withdrawal syndrome from long-term benzodiazepine use. Her mental and physical symptoms are consistent with benzodiazepine withdrawal. The benzodiazepine withdrawal syndrome implies some degree of physical dependence, and its onset, duration, and severity can vary according to dose, duration of treatment, speed of withdrawal, and elimination half-life of the agent used.[67,68] Withdrawal symptoms that follow discontinuation of agents with short half-lives usually appear within 1 to 2 days and may be more intense and short-lived than after discontinuation of long-acting benzodiazepines. Withdrawal symptoms usually appear 4 to 7 days after discontinuation of long-acting agents and may last several weeks. Symptoms of benzodiazepine withdrawal, which are listed in Table 80-7, are generally mild when the drug is tapered gradually during discontinuation.[68] Rarely, serious symptoms such as seizures or psychosis may occur during benzodiazepine withdrawal. Risk factors for seizures include head injury, alcohol dependence,

TABLE 80-7
Symptoms of Benzodiazepine Withdrawal

Common	Less Common	Rare
Anxiety	Nausea	Confusion
Insomnia	Depression	Delirium
Irritability	Ataxia	Psychosis
Muscle aches or weakness	Hyperreflexia	Seizures
Tremor	Blurred vision	Catatonia
Loss of appetite	Fatigue	

electroencephalogram abnormalities, and use of other drugs that lower the seizure threshold.

Diazepam 10 to 20 mg orally should be administered and repeated within 1 to 2 hours if needed. Resumption of her previous diazepam dosage of 40 mg/day should effectively treat her withdrawal symptoms. However, because her acute injury occurred 7 months ago, it may be desirable to begin tapering diazepam.

Various dosage reduction regimens have been proposed for benzodiazepine discontinuation. Even when managing withdrawal from low-dose benzodiazepine use, doses should be reduced slowly for 4 to 16 weeks.[68] The rate of the drug taper should be individualized to the patient, but a general recommendation is a 10% to 25% decrease in the dosage every 1 to 2 weeks. The first half of the benzodiazepine taper (down to 50% of the original dose) is generally easier and can proceed more quickly than the last half of the taper.[68] In T.B.'s case, the discontinuation period may take several months.

In general, the same benzodiazepine the patient has been taking should be used to manage withdrawal. However, because withdrawal symptoms are more severe during discontinuation of short-acting compared with long-acting benzodiazepines, a long-acting agent can be substituted at an equivalent dosage and then tapered.[68,69] In difficult cases, adjunctive medications have been used to ease tolerability of the gradual withdrawal. Carbamazepine (Tegretol) has been effective in attenuating the symptoms of withdrawal from both benzodiazepines and alcohol. Propranolol decreases some physical withdrawal symptoms (tremor, tachycardia), but does not affect the associated anxiety or decrease the seizure risk.[68] CBT, combined with gradual drug taper, has also been effective in facilitating successful benzodiazepine discontinuation.

BENZODIAZEPINE DRUG INTERACTIONS

CASE 80-4

QUESTION 1: N.P., a 20-year-old female college student, has been taking alprazolam 1 mg TID for treatment of GAD for almost 1 year. She states alprazolam has been very helpful for her GAD, but complains to her physician she is feeling especially stressed. She is having trouble balancing the increased workload of higher-level courses with her social life, which includes a new relationship. She has no medical illnesses, but states she has suffered from several episodes of heartburn recently, which may be stress-related. She is also interested in starting an oral contraceptive. N.P. smokes two packs of cigarettes per day and drinks up to three 12-ounce caffeinated sodas per day. An oral contraceptive (Yaz) is prescribed, and ranitidine is recommended for treatment of heartburn. What potential drug interactions with alprazolam are present in this case?

Reported drug interactions with benzodiazepines are summarized in Table 80-8[70–76,78–79] and can be divided into two primary types: pharmacodynamic and pharmacokinetic. The most significant pharmacodynamic drug interactions involve other CNS depressants such as alcohol or barbiturates. These combinations can lead to additive CNS and respiratory depressant effects that can be deadly. Important pharmacokinetic drug interactions mainly involve agents that either inhibit or induce benzodiazepine metabolism.[77] Because benzodiazepines have a relatively wide margin of safety, elevated plasma levels or prolonged elimination half-lives are unlikely to cause serious toxicity. However, they can lead to increased sedative and psychomotor effects, which may be clinically significant in certain cases. Conversely, increased benzodiazepine metabolism by hepatic enzyme inducers may result in medication ineffectiveness. As indicated in Table 80-8, most pharmacokinetic drug interactions with benzodiazepines involve CYP3A4– or CYP2C19–mediated mechanisms.

In N.P.'s case, the most important drug interaction is between alprazolam and the newly prescribed oral contraceptive, Yaz. Estrogen-containing oral contraceptives can inhibit the CYP3A4 metabolism of benzodiazepines such as alprazolam, potentially resulting in increased side effects.[15,80] Thus, a reduction in the benzodiazepine dosage may be needed when oral contraceptives are added to ongoing benzodiazepine therapy, as in N.P.'s case. The clearance of benzodiazepines that undergo glucuronidation (lorazepam, oxazepam, and temazepam) can be accelerated by oral contraceptives, but this interaction is probably clinically insignificant.[15,60]

Cigarette smoking increases the clearance of some benzodiazepines (clorazepate, lorazepam, oxazepam), but has no effect on others (diazepam, midazolam, chlordiazepoxide).[81] Overall, the effect of smoking is unpredictable and is most likely to be important in patients who either stop or start smoking while taking a benzodiazepine. N.P. should be urged to quit smoking for the sake of her general health and to prevent substantial risks for serious cardiovascular events occurring in smokers taking oral contraceptives. If N.P. does quit, careful monitoring will be needed to determine whether any alprazolam dosage reduction is necessary.

N.P. should also be encouraged to decrease her soda consumption because caffeine can increase anxiety and possibly decrease the effectiveness of alprazolam. Caffeine has been shown to decrease diazepam concentrations by approximately 22%, but studies with other benzodiazepines are lacking.[77]

Another potentially clinically significant drug interaction occurs with the use of azole antifungals in combination with benzodiazepines. Azole antifungals are potent CYP3A4 inhibitors that can cause a 170% increase in the area under the curve of alprazolam.[82] Therefore, the dosage of alprazolam should be reduced by about one-third in patients receiving this combination.

BENZODIAZEPINE USE IN PREGNANCY AND LACTATION

CASE 80-4, QUESTION 2: At her clinic visit 2 years later, N.P. is doing very well. She has graduated from college, is happily married, and states she and her husband have decided to start a family. N.P. has discontinued her oral contraceptive in hopes of becoming pregnant soon, and has successfully quit smoking. N.P. continues to take alprazolam 0.5 mg twice daily (BID) to TID and wonders whether she should also stop taking this drug before she becomes pregnant. What is the teratogenic potential of alprazolam? What alternative treatments are available for the management of N.P.'s anxiety?

Early reports implicated diazepam in causing several birth deformities, including cleft lip or cleft palate and limb and digit malformations, but later studies failed to support this association.[83–85] Most benzodiazepine anxiolytics are classified as pregnancy category D, indicating there is some evidence of fetal risk but the benefits of the medication may outweigh these risks in certain patients.[83,85] Available evidence suggests benzodiazepine use during the first trimester increases the risk for oral clefts by approximately 2.4-fold, but the absolute risk is increased only 0.01%. Benzodiazepines have not exhibited strong teratogenic

TABLE 80-8
Drug Interactions With Benzodiazepines

Interacting Drug(s)	Effect on Object Drug	Clinical Significance or Comments
Hepatic enzyme inducers: carbamazepine, phenobarbital, phenytoin, and rifampin	Decreased Cps and clinical effects of benzodiazepines	Triazolam and midazolam may be ineffective in patients taking rifampin.[70] Carbamazepine greatly decreases the Cps and clinical effects of midazolam, alprazolam, and clonazepam, possibly rendering them ineffective.[71,72]
Hepatic CYP 3A4 inhibitors: ketoconazole, itraconazole, nefazodone, fluvoxamine, fluoxetine, erythromycin, clarithromycin, cimetidine, oral contraceptives, diltiazem, nelfinavir, indinavir, ritonavir, saquinavir, verapamil	Significantly increased Cps of benzodiazepines that undergo oxidative metabolism (alprazolam, triazolam, diazepam, chlordiazepoxide, clonazepam)	Benzodiazepine dosage reductions may be required because of increased clinical effects such as sedation and psychomotor impairment; effects are greatest on alprazolam, triazolam, and midazolam.[73] Ketoconazole and itraconazole should be avoided in patients taking alprazolam or triazolam.[74] Benzodiazepine dosage reductions are recommended when nefazodone, fluoxetine, or fluvoxamine are added to alprazolam, diazepam, or triazolam.[73]
Ritonavir	Initial inhibition of alprazolam and triazolam metabolism, followed by later induction of metabolism	Reduced benzodiazepine dosage is needed initially if ritonavir is added to therapy; a dosage increase may be required later.[75]
Grapefruit juice	Increased Cps of diazepam, alprazolam, and triazolam	Increased benzodiazepine clinical effects (sedation, psychomotor impairment) are possible.[73,76]
Omeprazole	Increased diazepam Cp and prolonged half-life	Increased benzodiazepine clinical effects (sedation, psychomotor impairment) are possible.[77]
Valproic acid, probenecid	Significantly decreased clearance of lorazepam	Lorazepam dosage reductions may be required.[78]
Estrogen-containing oral contraceptives	Decreased Cps of benzodiazepines that undergo glucuronidation (lorazepam, oxazepam, temazepam) and increased Cps of benzodiazepines that undergo oxidative CYP 3A4 metabolism (alprazolam)	Decreased or increased clinical effects of benzodiazepines are possible.[15,60,77]
Central nervous system depressants (alcohol, barbiturates, and opioids)	Increased central nervous system depressant effects of benzodiazepines (sedation, psychomotor impairment)	Avoid use of alcohol with benzodiazepines; exercise caution with use of other depressants.
Alprazolam	Increased digoxin Cp	Digoxin toxicity is possible; monitoring of digoxin level and possible digoxin dosage reduction are recommended.[79]
Benzodiazepines	Respiratory depression and adverse cardiovascular effects reported on addition of benzodiazepines in several patients taking clozapine	Caution with benzodiazepine use in patients taking clozapine.
	Possible decreased efficacy of levodopa in Parkinson disease	Drug interaction is not well established; monitor for possible effect.
	Increased or decreased efficacy of neuromuscular blocking agents	Drug interaction is not well established; monitor for possible effect.

Cp, plasma concentration; CYP, cytochrome P-450.

effects, but it is always advisable to avoid drug use during pregnancy when possible, especially in the first trimester.[83–85] In patients such as N.P., the benzodiazepine should be tapered and discontinued before she becomes pregnant. Nondrug treatments for her GAD such as relaxation therapy, meditation, biofeedback, or cognitive therapy may be helpful. If necessary, single or repeated small doses of benzodiazepines during the second and third trimesters are unlikely to have important adverse effects on the fetus. Alprazolam, lorazepam, and clonazepam in low doses are the preferred agents.[83,85] Chronic or large doses, especially of long-acting agents, should be avoided because they may accumulate in the fetus. Perinatal sequelae in newborns of mothers who took benzodiazepines during pregnancy include withdrawal symptoms, sedation, muscle weakness, hypotonia, apnea, poor feeding, impaired temperature regulation, low birth weight, and increased risk for preterm birth.[83,84]

Pregnancies are sometimes unplanned, and the clinical situation of unexpected pregnancy in a woman maintained on benzodiazepines can also arise. The general course of action in such cases is often to discontinue all medications immediately. However, it is unwise to abruptly stop benzodiazepine treatment in someone who has been receiving chronic therapy because the resultant withdrawal syndromes can be detrimental to both mother and child. Benzodiazepine dosages should be tapered as quickly as possible to the lowest dosage necessary and discontinued if possible. The postpartum period is a time of heightened risk for recurrence of anxiety disorders, and new mothers should be monitored carefully for signs of relapse.[86] Benzodiazepines are excreted readily in breast milk, and they should be avoided by nursing mothers.[87] If benzodiazepines are used, short-acting agents with no active metabolites are recommended to avoid sedation, poor feeding, withdrawal, and other effects in the infant.[85,88] (Also see Chapter 49, Obstetric Drug Therapy.)

BENZODIAZEPINE OVERDOSE AND USE OF FLUMAZENIL

CASE 80-5

QUESTION 1: S.P. is a 17-year-old boy who is brought to the hospital by his mother. S.P. is barely conscious, and his breathing is slow and shallow. His mother states he "took a whole bottle of diazepam" (5 mg, 30 pills) sometime during the previous night. S.P.'s medical history is significant for a severe head injury sustained from a car accident 8 months ago. He currently takes carbamazepine (Tegretol) 200 mg TID for seizure prophylaxis. S.P.'s mother believes diazepam is the only drug he ingested because no other medications are missing. What signs and symptoms are consistent with benzodiazepine overdose? Why is it inappropriate to administer the benzodiazepine antagonist, flumazenil, in this case?

Benzodiazepine overdose is characterized by respiratory and CNS depression, both of which are evident in this case (S.P. is almost unconscious, with slow and shallow breathing). Overdose with benzodiazepines as the sole ingested agent is rarely life threatening, and full recovery is the usual outcome.[89] Flumazenil is a benzodiazepine receptor antagonist effective in reversing sedation associated with benzodiazepine intoxication. Its effects on respiratory depression are inconsistent, but improved breathing may occur secondarily to increased consciousness.[89]

The primary use of flumazenil is in reversing benzodiazepine-induced conscious sedation (primarily with midazolam) in patients who have been sedated for minor surgical or diagnostic procedures. Use for this purpose is generally safe and effective, and facilitates patient recovery and discharge by decreasing the postprocedural monitoring period.[90] Flumazenil is also approved for treating benzodiazepine overdose, but this use is controversial because of potentially serious complications and questions about its cost-effectiveness.[90] Flumazenil administration does not appear to decrease mortality or length of hospital stay in cases of benzodiazepine overdose; therefore, its use for this purpose has become limited.[90]

There are several reports of seizures or cardiac arrhythmias (including fatalities) after the administration of flumazenil in comatose patients who had ingested multiple drugs.[89] These overdoses often included TCAs and carbamazepine. The anticonvulsant effects of benzodiazepines may protect against TCA-induced seizures, and the rapid reversal of their effects with flumazenil removes this protection. Flumazenil is contraindicated in overdoses of any agent that decreases the seizure threshold, such as TCAs. Toxicology screening and an electrocardiogram (ECG) should be performed before flumazenil is administered. Because of a risk of seizures, flumazenil should also be avoided in patients with increased intracranial pressure or a known history of seizures or head injury, in those who have been receiving chronic benzodiazepine therapy, and in patients with a history of recent illicit drug abuse (cocaine, heroin). Administration of flumazenil should occur only when acute seizure management measures are available.

Flumazenil reverses benzodiazepine-induced sedation or coma within 1 to 2 minutes after IV administration. The most common side effects include agitation, dizziness, nausea, general discomfort, tearfulness, anxiety, and a sensation of coldness.[89] Rapid or excessive infusion has been associated with tachycardia and hypertension. The elimination half-life of flumazenil is 41 to 79 minutes, and sedation may recur after 1 to 2 hours, especially when large doses of long-acting benzodiazepines are involved. Repeated flumazenil doses or an IV infusion may be indicated in these cases. Full recovery should be verified (3–4 hours of stable alertness) before patients are discharged after flumazenil administration, and they should be advised to avoid driving or performing other potentially hazardous activities for 24 hours. Flumazenil undergoes extensive hepatic metabolism, and dosage reductions are recommended in patients with liver dysfunction. Pharmacokinetics are not altered significantly by sex, age, or renal impairment.

Flumazenil is not appropriate in S.P.'s case because of his history of head injury and risk of posttraumatic seizures. Instead, management should involve general supportive measures and mechanical ventilation, if indicated. A psychiatric evaluation is also indicated in this case to identify and address the reasons for S.P.'s overdose.

PHYSIOLOGICAL VARIABLES INFLUENCING BENZODIAZEPINES

CASE 80-6

QUESTION 1: B.G., a 68-year-old man, is brought to the emergency department (ED) by his wife after being involved as the driver in a minor car accident. He has no physical injuries except for several small abrasions caused by the car airbag deployment. However, B.G. appears drowsy, is mildly confused, and has an unsteady gait. A toxicology screen reveals no alcohol or other substances, except for diazepam, which his physician prescribed several months ago. B.G.'s wife states he has been taking 1 tablet (5 mg) BID or TID, and it has been remarkably effective in improving his mood and anxiety. B.G., who is 5 feet 8 inches tall and weighs 250 pounds, is a recovering alcoholic with moderate liver disease caused by years of heavy drinking. He has successfully maintained his sobriety for nearly 2 years. In addition to diazepam, B.G. also occasionally takes OTC omeprazole and cimetidine for heartburn. It is determined B.G. is experiencing adverse effects of diazepam, probably caused by drug accumulation. What factors could be influencing disposition of diazepam in this patient?

Benzodiazepine pharmacokinetics can be affected by various physiological factors, listed in Table 80-9.[91–94] Several of these factors are present in this case and may have contributed to the accumulation of diazepam with resulting adverse consequences.

B.G.'s age may influence diazepam disposition. Reductions in both CYP3A4 and CYP2C19 activity have been reported to occur with aging. The glucuronidation metabolic pathways are minimally affected with age, so no such effect is seen with lorazepam or oxazepam.[60] Other factors contributing to longer benzodiazepine half-lives in the elderly include decreased hepatic blood flow and increased volumes of distribution of lipid-soluble compounds (owing to decreased muscle mass and increased fat); the latter can increase a drug's half-life in the absence of any clearance changes. As described in Case 80-3, Question 4, older patients

TABLE 80-9
Physiological Factors Influencing Benzodiazepine Pharmacokinetics

Factor	Physiological and Pharmacokinetic Effects	Clinical Significance or Comments
Aging	Increased elimination half-life as a result of increased Vd of all benzodiazepines[91]	Lower benzodiazepine dosages, and possibly less-frequent dosing intervals, recommended in the elderly
	Decreased clearance of benzodiazepines that undergo oxidative hepatic metabolism (Table 80-6)[92]	Benzodiazepines that undergo glucuronidation (lorazepam, oxazepam) preferred in the elderly
	Decreased plasma proteins may lead to increased free fraction of highly protein-bound benzodiazepines (Table 80-6)	Possible increased clinical effects
	Decreased gastric acidity may lead to increased rate of benzodiazepine absorption	Possible faster onset of clinical effects
Sex	Age-related decrease in hepatic oxidative metabolism of benzodiazepines more pronounced in men	Elderly men may require especially low benzodiazepine dosages
	Increased CYP 3A4 and CYP 2C19 activity in premenopausal women may result in higher clearance of drugs that undergo oxidative metabolism[15]	Possible decreased plasma benzodiazepine concentrations and shorter duration of clinical effects of oxidatively metabolized agents in premenopausal women
	Decreased glucuronidation in women may result in slower clearance of benzodiazepines metabolized by conjugation[15]	Women may have longer elimination half-lives of lorazepam and temazepam and may require less frequent dosing
	Increased Vd in women owing to lower lean body mass and increased adipose tissue[15]	Possible longer elimination half-lives in women, especially the elderly, and greater drug accumulation
	Lower plasma protein binding in women[15]	Clinical significance unknown
Obesity	Increased benzodiazepine elimination half-lives owing to increased Vd	Increased chance of drug accumulation in obese patients; dosage reductions may be indicated
Liver disease	Decreased clearance and increased elimination half-lives of long-acting benzodiazepines and alprazolam in cirrhosis and hepatitis; no changes with oxazepam or triazolam[60]	Avoid long-acting benzodiazepines, or use significantly lower doses to avoid drug accumulation
	Increased elimination half-life of lorazepam in cirrhosis but not acute hepatitis	Decreased lorazepam dose or increased dosing interval recommended in cirrhosis
Kidney disease	Decreased plasma protein binding may lead to increased free fraction of highly protein-bound benzodiazepines (Table 80-6)[93]	Dosage reductions may be necessary
Ethnicity	Decreased oxidative metabolism (via CYP 2C19) of diazepam and alprazolam in Asians[94]	Asians may require lower doses of diazepam, alprazolam, and possibly other benzodiazepines

CYP, cytochrome P-450; Vd, volume of distribution.

are more sensitive to the sedative and psychomotor effects of benzodiazepines. For these reasons, the recommended benzodiazepine dosages for patients older than 65 years are generally one-third to one-half of those used in healthy adults (Table 80-4).

Sex also may influence benzodiazepine clearance, but studies yield mixed results, likely because of wide interindividual differences.[15,95] In elderly patients, some investigators have found lower clearances of clorazepate, diazepam, and alprazolam in men compared with those in women.[95] Women have been reported to have higher CYP3A4 and CYP2C19 activities than men, which may partially explain these findings. Increased CYP3A4 activity in women disappears after menopause, which may necessitate the use of lower benzodiazepine dosages during the postmenopausal period. Women have slower glucuronidation metabolic processes than men, resulting in lower clearance of agents such as temazepam and oxazepam.[15,60]

Obesity and liver impairment are other physiological factors relevant to B.G.'s case. Obesity increases the volume of distribution of benzodiazepines and the extent of accumulation of long-acting agents. Significant changes in the elimination half-lives of lorazepam and oxazepam are not observed in obese patients. Liver dysfunction can reduce benzodiazepine elimination rates and prolong their half-lives, resulting in recommendations for decreased dosages. The pharmacokinetics of lorazepam, oxazepam, and temazepam are unaffected by liver disease.

Decreased protein binding of benzodiazepines can occur in patients with renal insufficiency, which may lead to increased free fractions of highly protein-bound agents. However, no significant changes in clearance or volume of distribution of free drug have been noted. Regarding ethnicity, up to 20% of Asians are CYP2C19 poor metabolizers. Decreased clearance of a variety of CYP2C19 substrates, including diazepam, has been reported in Asian subjects.[94]

In summary, the physiological factors that can alter benzodiazepine disposition in B.G. are his age, obesity, male sex, and liver disease. Accumulation of diazepam owing to these combined effects probably led to his mental status changes. In addition to these factors, cimetidine and omeprazole can both significantly impair the metabolism of diazepam, resulting in decreased clearance and increased side effects (Table 80-8).[77]

If continued benzodiazepine therapy is deemed necessary for B.G., lorazepam or oxazepam would be preferred agents because they are least affected by aging, obesity, liver disease, or drug interactions. Benzodiazepine dosage equivalencies, which are based on relative potencies, can be used to determine an equivalent dose for the selected agent (Table 80-4). However, these equivalencies are inexact, and dosing conversions should take patient variables and usual dosage ranges into consideration. For example, B.G. had been taking 10 to 15 mg/day of diazepam, so the calculated equivalent lorazepam dosage is 2 to 3 mg/day. Because of his age, a somewhat lower initial dose of 0.5 to 1 mg BID would be indicated, accompanied by careful monitoring for adverse effects or withdrawal symptoms. However, switching to a nonbenzodiazepine agent should be considered because this may be a better treatment option for B.G.

Buspirone Therapy

CASE 80-6, QUESTION 2: Several days after recovery from diazepam intoxication, B.G. expresses a desire to discontinue benzodiazepine use. He is being criticized by his fellow

Alcoholics Anonymous program members for taking a drug associated with dependency. The decision is made to switch B.G. from diazepam to buspirone. How does the clinical profile of buspirone compare with benzodiazepines?

Buspirone lacks CNS depressant effects, sedation, cognitive or psychomotor impairment, respiratory depression, and muscle relaxant or anticonvulsant effects.[48] This makes buspirone useful in older patients who may have a variety of chronic medical conditions. Buspirone is generally well tolerated, and possible side effects include mild nausea, dizziness, headache, and initial nervousness.[96] Some patients may experience mild drowsiness or fatigue on initiation. Unlike many antidepressants, buspirone does not adversely affect sexual functioning and has actually improved sexual functioning in some patients with GAD.[47] Buspirone has minimal potential for abuse and is not classified as a controlled substance. It does not produce physical dependence or withdrawal syndromes on discontinuation, even after long-term therapy.[48,97] It also does not interact with alcohol or other CNS depressants and is relatively safe in overdose.[48]

Buspirone is as effective as benzodiazepines such as alprazolam, oxazepam, lorazepam, diazepam, and clorazepate in the treatment of GAD.[96,97] Like antidepressants, buspirone is more effective than benzodiazepines in treating the cognitive symptoms of anxiety. However, the anxiolytic effects of buspirone have a more gradual onset than benzodiazepines. Initial effects are observed within the first 7 to 10 days, but 3 to 4 weeks may be needed for optimal results. Buspirone must be taken on an ongoing basis if it is effective, and the drug should not be taken "as needed."

SWITCHING FROM BENZODIAZEPINE TO BUSPIRONE THERAPY

CASE 80-6, QUESTION 3: How should B.G. be switched from benzodiazepine to buspirone therapy?

Because buspirone has no CNS depressant effects and is not cross-tolerant with the benzodiazepines, it is not effective in preventing or treating benzodiazepine withdrawal. Thus, when patients are converted from benzodiazepine to buspirone therapy, the benzodiazepine must be discontinued gradually. Because it takes several weeks for full therapeutic effects of buspirone to occur, it can be initiated before the benzodiazepine taper begins. This may indirectly ease benzodiazepine withdrawal by providing extra anxiolytic coverage during the benzodiazepine taper period.[98]

Buspirone is completely absorbed, but it undergoes extensive first-pass metabolism, which reduces its absolute bioavailability to approximately 5%.[48] Administration with food may significantly increase bioavailability by decreasing the first-pass effect. Buspirone has an active metabolite, 1-pyrimidinylpiperazine (1-PP), which is present in much higher concentrations than buspirone at therapeutic doses. 1-PP acts on the noradrenergic system rather than 5-HT and functions as an α_2-adrenergic antagonist. Some of the side effects of buspirone, such as nervousness, are attributed to this active metabolite.[48,99] The mean elimination half-life of buspirone is short, approximately 2 to 3 hours, but 1-PP is longer acting.

The clearance of buspirone is significantly reduced in patients with kidney or liver disease, but there is little change in side effects or tolerability.[48] Nevertheless, it is recommended that buspirone dosages be lowered in patients with compromised renal or hepatic function and that use of the drug be avoided in cases of severe impairment. Buspirone pharmacokinetics are

TABLE 80-10
Buspirone Drug Interactions

Interacting Drug(s)	Clinical Significance or Comments
CYP 3A4 inhibitors: nefazodone, fluoxetine, fluvoxamine, erythromycin, itraconazole, ketoconazole, diltiazem, verapamil, grapefruit juice, and ritonavir	Significant increases in buspirone Cp have been reported with these agents, but adverse clinical effects are not always apparent.
	Buspirone dosage reductions are recommended when coadministered with erythromycin, fluvoxamine, nefazodone, fluoxetine, or itraconazole.
Rifampin	Highly significant decreases in buspirone Cp; avoid concurrent use.
Haloperidol	Buspirone may increase haloperidol Cp, but one study found no interaction.
Monoamine oxidase inhibitors	Possible serotonin syndrome; avoid concurrent use.

Cp, plasma concentration; CYP, cytochrome P-450.

not significantly affected by age or sex; therefore, no dosage adjustments are needed in the elderly.[48]

Important drug interactions with buspirone are summarized in Table 80-10.[48] Buspirone is metabolized by CYP3A4, and coadministration of CYP3A4 inhibitors, including grapefruit juice, can result in significant increases in buspirone levels. In many cases, the half-life of buspirone remained unchanged, suggesting these interactions are mainly caused by inhibition of CYP3A4–mediated first-pass metabolism in the gut. Because of buspirone's extremely wide margin of safety and tolerability, even very large increases in its plasma levels may be clinically insignificant. Some hepatic enzyme inducers can render buspirone ineffective as a result of large increases in buspirone clearance. Buspirone should be avoided in patients taking MAOIs and used cautiously in combination with high-dose antidepressants because of the risk of serotonin syndrome.

Some studies suggest patients previously treated with benzodiazepines will not respond favorably to buspirone.[54,97] However, buspirone may provide benefit in this population as long as the benzodiazepine is tapered slowly enough to prevent withdrawal effects.[17] B.G. has been taking diazepam for several months and the drug needs to be withdrawn gradually during a period of at least several weeks. B.G. can be started on buspirone at this time. The usual recommended starting dosage of buspirone is 15 mg/day given in two to three divided doses, but a lower dosage (10 mg/day) is indicated in B.G. because of his liver disease. Twice-daily dosing is preferred to facilitate compliance and is comparable in efficacy and tolerability to three-times-daily dosing.[100] The daily dosage may be increased in 5-mg/day increments every 3 to 4 days. Optimal anxiolytic doses generally range from 20 to 30 mg/day, with 60 mg/day being the recommended maximum. There are no specific guidelines for adjusting dosages in patients with liver impairment; therefore, dosage titrations in B.G. should be made slowly, according to his response and side effects. Dividose 15-mg tablets are available; these tablets are scored and notched, so they may be broken into 5-, 7.5-, or 10-mg doses. A 30-mg Dividose tablet is also available, as well as generic buspirone products.

PANIC DISORDER

Diagnostic Criteria

The DSM-IV-TR criteria for panic disorder are presented in Table 80-11.[1] The hallmark characteristic of panic disorder is the occurrence of sudden and distinct panic attacks, which are marked by an overwhelming wave of symptoms and feelings listed in Table 80-11. At least four of these symptoms are required to fulfill criteria for a panic attack, and the term "limited symptom attack" refers to those events involving fewer than four symptoms. Three types of panic attacks have been defined with regard to the context in which they occur: unexpected or uncued panic attacks (the attack is not associated with a situational trigger); situationally bound panic attacks (the attacks invariably occur on exposure to a situational trigger); and situationally predisposed panic attacks (the attacks are more likely to, but do not invariably, occur on exposure to a situational trigger).[1]

The DSM-IV-TR criteria for panic disorder requires the occurrence of at least two unexpected or uncued panic attacks followed by persistent worry or concern about having another panic attack or a significant change in behavior related to the attacks. Although panic attacks are the hallmark symptom of panic disorder, their occurrence does not always indicate panic disorder.[1] Depressive disorders and other anxiety disorders can also be associated with occasional panic attacks. Situationally bound panic attacks are more characteristic of specific phobias or social anxiety disorder than panic disorder, and situationally predisposed panic attacks may occur in either panic or phobic disorders. Nocturnal panic attacks, which awaken a person from sleep, are almost always indicative of panic disorder. Because panic attacks occur unpredictably, they often lead to generalized anxiety or constant fear of sudden attacks. Two subtypes of panic disorder have been identified: without agoraphobia or with agoraphobia.[1] *Agoraphobia* refers to a fear of being in situations from which escape might be difficult or embarrassing in the event of a panic attack. Mild-to-moderate agoraphobia involves selective avoidance of certain places or situations such as shopping malls, theaters, grocery stores, elevators, and driving alone. Some agoraphobia sufferers may be unable to go anywhere unless accompanied by a companion. In severe cases of agoraphobia, the sufferer may become completely housebound.

TABLE 80-11
Diagnostic Criteria for Panic Disorder

1. Presence of at least two unexpected panic attacks, characterized by at least four of the following symptoms, which develop abruptly and reach a peak within 10 minutes:
   a. Palpitations, pounding heart, or accelerated heart rate
   b. Sweating
   c. Trembling or shaking
   d. Sensations of shortness of breath or smothering
   e. Feeling of choking
   f. Chest pain or discomfort
   g. Nausea or abdominal distress
   h. Feeling dizzy, unsteady, lightheaded, or faint
   i. Derealization or depersonalization
   j. Fear of losing control or going crazy
   k. Fear of dying
   l. Numbness or tingling sensations
   m. Chills or hot flushes
2. At least one of the attacks has been followed by at least one of the following symptoms for a duration of at least 1 month:
   a. Persistent concern about having another attack
   b. Worry about the implications or consequences of the attack
   c. Significant change in behavior because of the attack
3. Symptoms are not attributable to the direct effects of a medication, substance, or general medical condition
4. Panic attacks are not better accounted for by another psychiatric or anxiety disorder (e.g., phobias, obsessive–compulsive disorder)
5. May occur with or without agoraphobia (see text)

Adapted with permission from American Psychiatric Association. *Diagnostic and Statistical Manual of Mental Disorders*. 4th ed. Text Revision. Washington, DC: American Psychiatric Association; 2000. Copyright © 2000 American Psychiatric Association.

Epidemiology and Clinical Course

Approximately 28% of the general population experiences a single isolated panic attack at some time in their lives.[101] Approximately 10% to 12% of persons experience recurrent panic attacks that do not fulfill the diagnostic criteria for panic disorder; however, these persons can still be significantly affected. The estimated lifetime prevalence of panic disorder in America ranges from 4% to 5%.[101] Women are affected two to three times more often than men and are more likely to develop agoraphobia.[15] The onset of panic disorder usually occurs in the late teens to mid-30s, and new onset is rare in the elderly population.[8] Most persons report onset of the disorder at some particularly stressful time in their life; in women, this often includes the prenatal and postpartum periods.[15,86]

Panic disorder is accompanied by marked degrees of psychiatric comorbidity; 50% to 60% of patients suffer a major depressive episode at some point. Other common comorbid conditions include social anxiety disorder, GAD, OCD, PTSD, personality disorders, alcohol abuse, and bipolar disorder.[1,101,102] Patients with comorbid disorders have more severe symptoms, show slower and poorer response to treatments, are less likely to experience full remission, and have a greater suicide risk (particularly when depression or substance abuse are present) than those with panic disorder alone.[103,104] Panic disorder causes significant functional disability in areas of work, family relationships, and overall quality of life.[8,105]

Panic disorder is associated with very high rates of health care service utilization.[104] Because of the physical manifestations of panic attacks, repeated ED visits and costly diagnostic tests are common.[106] About 25% to 32% of patients making ED visits related to chest pain actually have panic disorder. The poor recognition of panic disorder in primary-care settings further increases use of medical services. Panic disorder is the underlying cause of symptoms in an estimated 10% to 30% of patients referred to specialty vestibular, respiratory, or neurology clinics, and up to 60% of those referred for cardiology consultation.[1] The vast majority of patients with panic disorder do not complain of feeling anxious and report only physical symptoms, such as chest pain, GI problems, headache, dizziness, and shortness of breath, which contributes to misdiagnosis.[106] It is not uncommon for patients to have been in the health care system for up to 10 years before they are correctly diagnosed.

The long-term course of panic disorder is highly variable.[1] Some patients experience episodic periods of remission and relapse, whereas others suffer almost continuously. One follow-up study found that 18% of patients still suffered from panic disorder after 15 years of initial treatment.[107]

Etiology and Pathophysiology

There is substantial evidence that panic disorder is biologically based. A neuroanatomical model for panic disorder has been proposed in which the anxiety and fear response to threatening stimuli are mediated through the amygdala.[5,108] Various projections from the amygdala, including the hypothalamus and the LC, trigger autonomic and neuroendocrine responses resulting in anxiety and panic attacks. Patients with panic disorder have a heightened anxiety sensitivity (fear of anxiety-related sensations), and a variety of substances and situations are capable of triggering the neural fear network, activating the anxiety and panic response.[108] Acute panic attacks are believed to be caused by dysregulated firing in the LC as described previously (see Neurobiology of Anxiety section), and hyperresponsiveness of the NE system may be an underlying cause for panic disorder.[109]

Experimental provocation of panic attacks is an important component of panic disorder research. Administration of certain substances induces panic attacks rather consistently in persons with panic disorder, but not in normal healthy subjects.[5,108] These substances include caffeine, NE, sodium lactate, hypertonic sodium chloride, high concentrations of carbon dioxide, yohimbine, flumazenil, and CCK-B agonists. Administration of effective medication treatments for panic disorder blocks the effects of these panic-inducing substances. Challenge studies such as these provide evidence for possible abnormalities in GABA-A receptor, NE, 5-HT, and CCK functioning that underlie panic disorders. Decreased GABA-A benzodiazepine binding sites, abnormal regulation of neuroactive steroids that modulate GABA-A receptors, hyperactivation of the HPA axis, and CCK-B receptor gene polymorphism are among the findings associated with panic disorder.[102,109]

Hypersensitivity to 35% CO_2 inhalation, as evidenced by precipitation of panic attacks, robustly identifies patients with panic disorder as well as those with other anxiety disorders such as OCD and GAD.[108] This association is specific enough that carbon dioxide hypersensitivity is considered a biological trait marker, at least for a subset of panic disorder patients. Effective treatment of panic disorder with medication significantly decreases the sensitivity to carbon dioxide inhalation.[110] Brain imaging studies also have demonstrated abnormal patterns of cerebral glucose metabolism in certain brain areas in patients with panic disorder.[108]

A familial occurrence of panic disorder has been noted; first-degree relatives of individuals with panic disorder have an 8- to 21-fold greater risk of panic disorder than relatives of unaffected persons.[1,19] Genetic and environmental influences both contribute to this familial pattern. The inherited component is believed to involve heightened anxiety sensitivity, which confers increased vulnerability for panic disorder. Heightened anxiety sensitivity in panic disorder has been associated with "catastrophic cognitions," in which harmless normal physical sensations are misinterpreted as being dangerous and cause fear.[111] These negative cognitive patterns are often unconscious and may be integral in potentiating recurrent panic attacks in a biologically predisposed individual.

Developmental experiences may also be important in the etiology of panic disorder. Several studies have shown distressing childhood events such as separation from parents and abuse are associated with markedly increased risks of developing panic disorder later in life.[108] Behavioral inhibition during childhood, characterized by excessive fear and avoidance of novel stimuli, is also extremely common in panic disorder patients. No one biological abnormality can explain panic disorder, and further research is needed to define the complex interplay of the various pathophysiological, genetic, and cognitive findings in this illness.

Treatment of Panic Disorder

Approximately 70% to 90% of patients with panic disorder can experience substantial relief with currently available treatments, which include both pharmacologic therapies and CBT.[1,102] Medications and CBT both are beneficial for reducing panic attacks initially, and their effects on phobic avoidance generally occur later. First-line medication treatments for panic disorder are SSRIs and venlafaxine.[111] Benzodiazepines also are effective but no longer recommended as first-line treatment because they do not treat concomitant depression and they possess abuse liability. Several TCA and MAOI antidepressants are also effective in treating panic disorder, but are reserved as second- or third-line options because of their clinical disadvantages compared with SSRIs. The heightened anxiety sensitivity common in panic disorder makes patients especially vulnerable to initial SSRI and TCA side effects, such as anxiety and agitation. For this reason, lower than usual starting doses of antidepressants are recommended in patients with panic disorder.

SELECTIVE SEROTONIN REUPTAKE INHIBITORS

Paroxetine, sertraline, fluoxetine, and venlafaxine are FDA approved for treating panic disorder. There is strong evidence other SSRIs (fluvoxamine, citalopram, escitalopram) are also effective.[27,40] Several large, controlled trials have demonstrated the superiority of paroxetine, sertraline, and fluoxetine versus placebo in reducing the frequency of panic attacks, anticipatory anxiety, and associated depression.[112,113] Although low starting dosages are recommended (10 mg/day for paroxetine and citalopram, 25 mg/day for sertraline, 5–10 mg/day for fluoxetine and escitalopram) to minimize side effects, higher doses are usually required for response. The recommended target dosage range of paroxetine, citalopram, and fluoxetine for panic disorder is 20 to 40 mg/day.[111,114] Recommended therapeutic ranges for sertraline and fluvoxamine are 100 to 200 mg/day. For escitalopram, a 10- to 20-mg/day dosage range is recommended. The initial dose of venlafaxine XR should be 37.5 mg/day, and the recommended therapeutic dose is 150 to 225 mg/day.[111]

Response to SSRIs and other antidepressants in panic disorder occurs gradually, over the course of several weeks. Reduced frequency of panic attacks usually begins within 3 to 4 weeks. A trial period of at least 6 weeks should be allowed to fully assess response, and continued improvements may be seen during a treatment period of 6 months or longer.[111]

BENZODIAZEPINES

The benzodiazepines alprazolam and clonazepam are FDA approved for treating panic disorder and are the most extensively studied agents of this class.[106,111,115] As previously described, specialized formulations of these agents (alprazolam XR, clonazepam wafer) have been introduced specifically for use in panic disorder. Other benzodiazepines such as diazepam and lorazepam appear to be as effective as alprazolam and clonazepam when they are used in equivalent doses.[111]

Optimal benzodiazepine dosing is an important issue in treating patients with panic disorder because these individuals may need higher doses for response than patients with other anxiety disorders.[116] This may be related to reduced sensitivity of benzodiazepine binding sites in panic disorder.[23] An alprazolam dosage range of 4 to 6 mg/day is effective for most panic disorder patients, but others may require up to 10 mg/day for optimal response. When clonazepam is used, the minimum effective dosage appears to be 1 mg/day, and most panic disorder patients do well in the range of 1 to 2 mg/day.

One problem with alprazolam use in panic disorder is breakthrough anxiety or panic attacks before the next scheduled dose because of its relatively short duration of action.[111] The total daily dose usually needs to be taken in three or four divided doses to minimize this effect. The extended-release alprazolam formulation (alprazolam XR) was developed to address this problem.[59]

It can be dosed once or twice daily and is associated with minimal interdose anxiety. It may have a lower abuse liability than immediate-release alprazolam, but this remains to be proven. Clonazepam is longer acting than standard-release alprazolam, and a twice-daily dosing schedule is usually sufficient. A switch to either clonazepam or extended-release alprazolam can be beneficial when breakthrough anxiety is a problem with immediate-release alprazolam. Patients with panic disorder are especially sensitive to benzodiazepine withdrawal effects. For this reason, clonazepam may be preferred over alprazolam in patients with panic disorder.[116]

TRICYCLIC ANTIDEPRESSANTS, MONOAMINE OXIDASE INHIBITORS, AND OTHER ANTIDEPRESSANTS

TCAs were the first medications widely used in the treatment of panic disorder. Imipramine and clomipramine are as effective as alprazolam, but are less well tolerated.[103,114] A small number of trials have evaluated desipramine and nortriptyline and have generally found them also to be effective for the treatment of panic disorder.[111] Well-conducted studies involving other TCAs are lacking. As stated previously, low starting dosages of TCAs (10 mg/day or less) are needed to minimize initial anxietylike side effects. Even so, many patients discontinue therapy because of poor tolerability. Imipramine should be slowly titrated up to an initial target dosage of 100 mg/day, and further increased up to 300 mg/day if needed.

Clomipramine appears to be more effective than other TCAs for panic disorder, perhaps because of its greater serotonergic effects.[117] The possibility of a therapeutic dosage window for clomipramine in panic disorder has been suggested, with dosages in excess of 80 mg/day being associated with a reduced likelihood of response.[117,118] Clomipramine seems to be most effective within the dosage range of 50 to 150 mg/day.[111]

Among the MAOIs, phenelzine (Nardil) is often heralded as being remarkably effective in the treatment of panic disorder, but this claim is based on studies conducted before the publication of the initial diagnostic criteria for panic disorder in 1980.[111] No recent MAOI studies are available to assess phenelzine's efficacy within the context of current diagnostic and treatment standards.

Although phenelzine is widely believed to be extremely effective, it is generally an option of last resort for treatment-refractory cases because of the many clinical disadvantages of MAOIs relative to other antidepressants (see Chapter 83, Mood Disorders I: Major Depressive Disorders). Preliminary reports suggest mirtazapine may also be beneficial in treating panic disorder.[111,116] This agent may be useful in patients who do not respond to SSRI therapy. Bupropion (Wellbutrin), buspirone, and trazodone are generally ineffective for panic disorder.[111]

MISCELLANEOUS AGENTS

Trials of propranolol, calcium-channel blockers, and clonidine have yielded mixed, but largely negative, results.[111] None of these agents are considered appropriate treatment options in panic disorder. Other medications that are reportedly effective in treating panic disorder include gabapentin, vigabatrin, tiagabine, valproic acid, olanzapine, and risperidone used in combination with an SSRI.[111] More information is needed before any of these can be recommended for the treatment of panic disorder.

NONPHARMACOLOGIC TREATMENTS

CBT, including exposure treatment and relaxation training, is also established as being effective in panic disorder.[102,111] The cognitive theory of panic disorder is based on the observed heightened anxiety sensitivity in these patients and asserts that physical anxiety sensations are misinterpreted as being serious or life threatening. These fears trigger a cycle of further worsening anxiety symptoms that finally progress to a panic attack. Reversing the cognitive component of this vicious cycle is an integral part of CBT and is important in producing lasting therapeutic effects of treatment.[111] Breathing retraining and exposure to fear cues are key components of behavioral therapy.

Some studies have found medications to be superior to CBT in the treatment of panic disorder, whereas others report opposite results.[111,118] Combining medication with CBT can be useful, especially in patients with severe agoraphobia or those who only partially respond to either treatment modality alone.[116,119]

Clinical Presentation and Differential Diagnosis of Panic Disorder

CASE 80-7

QUESTION 1: S.K., a 24-year-old female graphic artist, presents to the ED complaining of chest pain, difficulty breathing, dizziness, and nausea. She describes feeling "as if my head is going off in space and I am outside my body." She states she has been under extreme stress lately because of the poor economy, and conflicts with her landlord as a result of nonpayment of the rent on her art studio. S.K. fears she has had a heart attack or stroke brought on by her stressful life. S.K. recently visited her family physician for the same symptoms; however, a complete physical examination and laboratory workup yielded no abnormalities. She states her first "attack" occurred out of the blue about 5 months ago while she was shopping for oil paints at the art supply store, and she can never predict when they will occur. Since then, her symptoms have become more severe and frequent, and she has started isolating herself in her studio for fear they will return when she is in public. S.K. uses marijuana "to relax" and occasionally drinks alcohol (but only rarely). She has suffered from depression in the past and was hospitalized for one severe episode 2 years ago. An ECG is performed and found to be normal. The physician's diagnosis is panic disorder with agoraphobia. What clinical features of panic disorder does S.K. display, and what are the important factors in the differential diagnosis of panic disorder?

S.K. exhibits many typical characteristics of panic disorder. As illustrated in this case, the first panic attack typically occurs without warning while the person is involved in a normal everyday activity and lasts 10 to 30 minutes. Panic attacks are extremely terrifying and usually leave the sufferer feeling anxious and convinced something is medically wrong. As with S.K., it is not uncommon for persons to make ED visits after or during panic attacks, believing they have had a heart attack or other serious event. Unfortunately, panic disorder is often not recognized in primary-care settings, and no medical cause for the symptoms can be identified. Faced with findings that they are apparently healthy, persons may make repeated ED visits and consult different doctors and specialists in an attempt to uncover a physical explanation for their frightening symptoms.

S.K. exhibits the following target symptoms of panic disorder: chest pain, shortness of breath, dizziness, abdominal distress, and depersonalization ("my head is going off in space and I am outside my body"). Agoraphobia is present because she avoids leaving her studio because of her fear of having panic attacks. Other factors consistent with a diagnosis of panic disorder include her young age, female sex, and lack of abnormal physical findings. This case also illustrates the association between onset of panic disorder and stressful life events, its common association with depression, and the frequent lack of recognition of panic disorder in primary-care settings.

Because different substances or medical conditions can cause severe anxiety and panic, it is necessary to rule out these potential causes for panic disorder symptoms.[106] Notable triggers of panic attacks include caffeine, alcohol, nicotine, nonprescription cold preparations, cannabis, amphetamines, and cocaine (Table 80-2).[106] S.K. uses marijuana, which can be associated with panic symptoms. Although chronic moderate to severe use of marijuana may complicate the treatment of panic, it appears infrequent marijuana use does not adversely affect treatment.[120,121] S.K. does not endorse chronic, severe marijuana abuse, but if she does not adequately respond to treatment, this might be further explored. Medical illnesses that can cause panic attacks include thyroid dysfunction, asthma, COPD, mitral valve prolapse, and seizure disorders.[122] Panic attacks can also occur with other anxiety disorders. However, in these cases, the panic attacks usually occur on exposure to a feared object or situation (in phobic disorders), an object of obsession (in OCD), or a stimulus associated with a traumatic stressor (in PTSD). S.K. reports her panic attacks occur unexpectedly, and situationally bound or predisposed attacks are not evident; therefore, the features are consistent with panic disorder.

Treatment Selection for Panic Disorder, Selective Serotonin Reuptake Inhibitor Dosing Issues, and Combination Selective Serotonin Reuptake Inhibitor–Benzodiazepine Therapy

CASE 80-7, QUESTION 2: S.K. is referred to a psychiatrist who decides to initiate treatment with paroxetine 20 mg every morning. Three days later, S.K. calls the doctor complaining that her anxiety and panic attacks have greatly increased since she started taking paroxetine. The psychiatrist prescribes alprazolam 0.5 mg (tablets) and instructs S.K. to take one tablet as needed for the anxiety. What factors should be considered in the selection of an initial medication treatment for panic disorder? Why is the prescribed treatment for S.K. inappropriate?

An SSRI is an appropriate first-line treatment for most panic disorder patients.[115,116] In patients such as S.K. who have a history of depression, SSRIs may also help prevent relapse of depression. Patients with severe or distressing symptoms may initially require concurrent benzodiazepine therapy, which provides quick relief from anxiety and panic attacks until the therapeutic effects of SSRIs are evident. At that time, usually after several weeks, the benzodiazepine can be gradually discontinued. An SSRI-benzodiazepine combination is still the most commonly prescribed initial treatment, even though guidelines recommend monotherapy unless initial anxiety is extremely high.[123] Although benzodiazepines are generally avoided in patients with a history of substance abuse, use of low doses for a limited time may be appropriate for some patients with disabling symptoms, as long as there is no current substance (especially alcohol) abuse.[67,111,116] Because of the levels of distress and impairment caused by S.K.'s panic disorder, combined SSRI-benzodiazepine therapy would have been the preferred initial treatment. Scheduled benzodiazepine dosing is preferred over as-needed dosing schedule during initial therapy to prevent panic attacks.[116] Because panic attacks generally last less than 30 minutes, as-needed benzodiazepine is not helpful.

In choosing among SSRIs for the treatment of panic disorder, paroxetine or sertraline may be less anxiety-provoking in some patients than a more activating SSRI such as fluoxetine.[27] When paroxetine is used, a very low initial dose of 10 mg/day should be used. In S.K.'s case, the prescribed 20-mg/day starting dose was too high. Also, scheduled versus as-needed benzodiazepine dosing would have been preferred. After 2 to 4 weeks, the benzodiazepine can be gradually discontinued while the SSRI therapy is continued and gradually titrated to the target effective dose. The potential for drug interactions must also be kept in mind when SSRI-benzodiazepine combinations are used because certain SSRIs can inhibit benzodiazepine metabolism, leading to increased benzodiazepine side effects (see Benzodiazepine Drug Interactions section and Table 80-8).

Patient Counseling Information

Patients such as S.K. who are beginning SSRI therapy for the treatment of panic disorder should be counseled about possible increased anxiety during the first 1 or 2 weeks of treatment, as well as other common SSRI side effects, including nausea, headache, sexual dysfunction, and either insomnia or sedation. Because these are dose-related effects, patients should inform their clinician of any problems, and a dosage reduction may be indicated. These adverse effects (with the possible exception of sexual dysfunction) usually subside after 1 to 3 weeks of continued treatment. It is also important to inform patients it may take several weeks before beneficial effects of antidepressant treatment are seen, and 6 to 12 weeks or longer may be required for full response. Patients receiving benzodiazepines should be counseled about their use in providing anxiolytic coverage during the initial weeks of SSRI therapy, as well as their limited utility as long-term therapy. Other pertinent counseling information for benzodiazepine treatment should also be included (see Case 80-2, Question 4). The desired goals of therapy and likely duration of treatment should also be explained. Providing information about the nature of panic disorder, including reassurance that panic attacks are not life threatening, is also important. Many clinicians recommend patients keep a "panic diary" in which they record frequency of panic attacks, along with symptoms experienced during attacks.

Clinical Assessment and Goals of Therapy

CASE 80-7, QUESTION 3: S.K. refuses to continue paroxetine, so citalopram is prescribed instead. After 1 week of citalopram therapy at the initial dosage of 10 mg/day, S.K. is tolerating the medication well. The plan is to gradually increase citalopram to 20 mg, then to 40 mg/day during the next several weeks. S.K. is also taking alprazolam, 0.5 mg BID to TID. What are the desired goals of treatment in this case, and how can S.K.'s response to treatment be assessed?

Five domains in panic disorder have been identified in which treatment outcomes should be assessed: (a) frequency and severity of panic attacks, (b) anticipatory anxiety, (c) phobic avoidance behaviors, (d) overall well-being, and (e) illness-related disability in various areas (work, school, family).[111] The treatment goals in this case are first to stop S.K.'s panic attacks, then to reduce her anticipatory anxiety, followed by reversal of phobic avoidance.[53] These outcomes should allow her to more comfortably leave her studio when required and, secondarily, improve her overall functioning and quality of life.

Several different instruments have been used to assess outcomes of treatment in panic disorder.[53] In addition to the panic diary, others include the Fear Questionnaire, the Panic Appraisal Inventory, and the Panic Disorder Severity Scale. The latter is currently considered by many experts to be the most useful because it evaluates outcomes in all five identified target domains of panic disorder.[53,111]

Course and Duration of Therapy

CASE 80-7, QUESTION 4: After 3 months of citalopram therapy, S.K. reports she has had no panic attacks in the past month and her functioning has improved dramatically. She is currently taking 40 mg/day of citalopram and gradually stopped taking the alprazolam 3 to 4 weeks ago. S.K. reveals she is painting regularly, selling some of her paintings, and paying her rent, and she has begun dating again. S.K. is experiencing no significant side effects from citalopram except for some sexual dysfunction. She wonders how long she should continue taking it since she is doing so well. What is the recommended duration of treatment for panic disorder?

Long-term medication trials in panic disorder support the recommendation that treatment should continue for at least 6 to 12 months after acute response.[111,124] The benefits of maintenance pharmacotherapy in preventing relapse are well documented although the optimal duration of treatment is a subject of continued debate among panic researchers. Maintenance treatment gives patients time to resume normal lifestyles and to re-establish daily activities after acute cessation of panic attacks.

In this case, S.K.'s current citalopram dosage of 40 mg/day is appropriate because this is within the effective dosage range for panic disorder. Citalopram therapy should be continued at the current dosage for 3 to 6 more months. S.K.'s sexual dysfunction may decrease with continued treatment, otherwise, specific remedies for SSRI-induced sexual dysfunction may be tried (see Chapter 83, Mood Disorders I: Major Depressive Disorders). After a successful period of full remission, a trial of medication discontinuation may be attempted to determine whether continued treatment is necessary. Medication should not be stopped in patients who are experiencing stressful life events or substantial residual problems in any of the five domains. When a medication is discontinued, it should be withdrawn gradually for several months, regardless of the class. Because of the devastating impact panic disorder can have, reinstitution of drug treatment is indicated if relapse occurs. Long-term treatment with antidepressants, and benzodiazepines if necessary, is generally successful in maintaining treatment benefits without detrimental effects or dosage escalations. Panic disorder is accepted as an appropriate indication for long-term benzodiazepine therapy if necessary.[115]

SOCIAL ANXIETY DISORDER AND SPECIFIC PHOBIAS

Classification and Diagnosis of Phobic Disorders

The DSM-IV-TR category of phobic disorders includes two primary types: specific phobia and social phobia (also called social anxiety disorder).[1] The term *social anxiety disorder* is more commonly used and is the term used in this text. These disorders involve excessive or unreasonable fears and lead to avoidance behavior to minimize anxiety. The DSM-IV-TR criteria for phobic disorders are presented in Table 80-12.[1] The main difference between specific phobias and social anxiety disorder is that the former involves fear and avoidance of specific objects or situations, whereas the latter involves social situations.

TABLE 80-12
Diagnostic Criteria for Phobic Disorders

Social Anxiety Disorder (Social Phobia)

1. Marked and constant fear of one or more social situations in which the person is exposed to unfamiliar people or possible scrutiny by others and the person fears humiliation or embarrassment
2. Exposure to the situation provokes an immediate anxiety response
3. Person realizes the fear is excessive or unreasonable (not required in children)
4. Feared situation is avoided or endured with intense anxiety or distress
5. Fear or avoidance significantly interferes with the person's normal routine or activities or causes marked distress
6. In individuals younger than 18 years of age, the duration of the fear is at least 6 months
7. Anxiety or phobic avoidance are not better accounted for by another psychiatric disorder (e.g., fear of having a panic attack, obsessions that accompany OCD, trauma related to PTSD)

Specific Phobia

1. Marked and persistent fear of a specific object or situation that is excessive or unreasonable
2. Other criteria (2–7) listed previously for social anxiety disorder

OCD, obsessive–compulsive disorder; PTSD, posttraumatic stress disorder.
Adapted with permission from American Psychiatric Association. *Diagnostic and Statistical Manual of Mental Disorders*. 4th ed. Text Revision. Washington, DC: American Psychiatric Association; 2000. Copyright © 2000 American Psychiatric Association.

SOCIAL ANXIETY DISORDER

Social anxiety disorder manifests as an intense irrational fear of scrutiny or evaluation by others because of concerns about humiliation or being made to appear ridiculous.[1] The *generalized* type of social anxiety disorder refers to cases in which fears relate to most social situations (e.g., fear of general social interactions, speaking to people, attending social gatherings), whereas the *nongeneralized* type involves more specific phobias.[1] Public speaking is the most common nongeneralized type; others include speaking to strangers, eating in public, and using public restrooms. A defining feature of either type is that the fears and anxiety are confined to social situations, and patients are usually symptomfree when alone. Common symptoms seen in social anxiety disorder include blushing, muscle twitching, and stuttering, in addition to other typical symptoms of anxiety. Panic attacks may also occur in either specific phobia or social anxiety disorder on exposure to the feared object or situation. However, social anxiety disorder is differentiated from panic disorder and agoraphobia in that it involves the fear of humiliation and social scrutiny, rather than the fear of having a panic attack.

The DSM-IV-TR excludes a diagnosis of social anxiety disorder if the person fears public embarrassment as a result of some physical or medical condition. However, this criterion is controversial because it excludes social anxiety disorder that is caused by certain socially stigmatizing conditions, such as Parkinson disease, obesity, and physical disfigurement or deformity.[1] These cases are sometimes referred to as *secondary social anxiety disorder.*

SPECIFIC PHOBIAS

Specific phobias are classified into five subtypes: animal type (snakes, dogs, spiders), natural environment type (heights, water, storms), blood-injection type (blood, injury, medical procedures), situational type (flying, bridges, elevators), and others.[1] Exposure to the feared circumstance produces intense anxiety, sometimes to the degree of panic attacks, and avoidance of the stimuli is common. Significant impairment of functioning or marked distress must be present for a diagnosis of specific phobia to be warranted. For example, fear of flying might constitute a diagnosis of specific phobia in a person whose job requires airplane travel, but it would not impair functioning in someone who never has occasion to fly.

Management of specific phobias has traditionally involved avoidance of the stimuli. Medications generally are not considered beneficial, but CBT involving repeated exposure to the feared situation and systemic desensitization is effective. Computer-generated, virtual environment desensitization (virtual reality) therapy has been used successfully to reduce fears associated with flying and heights. Benzodiazepines not only effectively reduce anxiety associated with a phobic trigger, but they can also interfere with the efficacy of exposure therapies.

Social Anxiety Disorder

EPIDEMIOLOGY AND CLINICAL COURSE

In the United States, the lifetime and past-year prevalence of social anxiety disorder are approximately 12% and 7%, respectively.[125] The male to female prevalence ratio is approximately 2 : 3.[8] Social anxiety disorder usually begins early in life, with a mean onset between ages 14 and 16 years.[126] More than 50% of patients are affected before adolescence, and a history of shyness and behavioral inhibition throughout childhood is common.[126] Unless effectively treated, the clinical course is often chronic, unremitting, and lifelong, and only 20% to 40% of patients are reported to recover after 20 years of living with this condition.[125]

COMORBIDITY AND CLINICAL SIGNIFICANCE

Because social anxiety disorder usually begins during the teenage years, it can seriously interfere with development of normal social skills and abilities to form interpersonal relationships.[127] This leads to functional disabilities that may persist for a lifetime. Social anxiety disorder can interfere with achievement of full academic and career potentials and is associated with unemployment, lower levels of education, and dependence on public financial support systems.[8] Persons with social anxiety disorder are less likely to marry, and more than half report moderate-to-severe impairments in their abilities to carry out ordinary daily activities.[127]

Comorbidity in social anxiety disorder is high, with an estimated 70% to 90% of individuals having at least one other psychiatric disorder in their lifetime.[1,125,126] Common comorbid conditions include simple phobia, major depression, GAD, panic disorder, body dysmorphic disorder, and alcohol abuse. Because of its early onset, social anxiety disorder usually precedes the development of comorbid disorders. Alcohol is commonly used to decrease anxiety in social situations. The risk of suicide attempts is high, especially in those with both social anxiety disorder and another psychiatric illness, like depression.[8]

ETIOLOGY AND PATHOPHYSIOLOGY

Social anxiety disorder is a familial disease, but the relative contributions of genetic versus environmental influences have not been differentiated.[19] Early factors predisposing to its development include anxious behavior modeling in parents and parental overprotection.[1] Shyness in children, which is associated with later development of social anxiety disorder, has been linked to a specific genetic polymorphism of the serotonin transporter promoter region.[128]

Biological studies suggest the generalized and nongeneralized types of social anxiety disorder may have different underlying pathophysiologies. Nongeneralized social anxiety disorder may mainly involve disturbances in noradrenergic system functioning, whereas substantial evidence for dopaminergic and serotonergic dysfunction in the generalized form exists.[129,130] Abnormally low dopamine neurotransmission in generalized social anxiety disorder is supported by findings of significantly decreased dopamine-2 receptor binding; markedly reduced dopamine transporter densities; low levels of the dopamine metabolite, homovanillic acid; high rates of social anxiety disorder in persons who later develop Parkinson disease; and reports of emergence of social anxiety disorder during antipsychotic treatment.[129,130] Social anxiety disorder appears to be unique among the anxiety disorders in its association with dopamine system abnormalities. Pharmacologic challenge studies suggest 5-HT type-2 receptors are hypersensitive in patients with social anxiety disorder, and neuroimaging studies have found specific neural circuits to be activated in this illness.[129,131]

TREATMENT OF SOCIAL ANXIETY DISORDER

Early detection and treatment of social anxiety disorder are vital in reducing lifelong functional consequences and may prevent development of comorbid disorders. Because of the nature of the disorder, some sufferers are reluctant to seek treatment. Those who seek help, even in psychiatric settings, are rarely diagnosed and treated appropriately.[126] Pharmacotherapy has become first-line for social anxiety disorder. Nonpharmacologic treatments, particularly CBT,[132] can be beneficial. Data do not support the combined use of nonpharmacologic and pharmacologic treatments in the management of social anxiety disorder; clinicians should determine whether combined therapy would be useful on a case-by-case basis.[133]

SELECTIVE SEROTONIN REUPTAKE INHIBITORS

As with other anxiety disorders, SSRIs are considered the primary treatment option for most patients with social anxiety disorder.[126] Paroxetine, sertraline, fluvoxamine CR, and venlafaxine XR have received FDA approval for this indication.[134] Fluoxetine, citalopram, and escitalopram have also demonstrated efficacy in controlled clinical trials,[134–136] and preliminary evidence with duloxetine suggests this agent may be useful.[137]

Unlike patients with GAD and panic disorder, those with social anxiety disorder often tolerate standard antidepressant starting doses. Target effective SSRI doses for social anxiety disorder are within the normal antidepressant dosage ranges, and maximum doses may be required to ensure adequate response.[138] One fixed-dose study of paroxetine in social anxiety disorder found no overall difference in efficacy between 20, 40, and 60 mg/day.[139] Although some individuals may respond better to higher dosages, an adequate time should be allowed at 20 mg/day before the dosage is increased. Response to SSRI occurs gradually, and an adequate medication trial to assess response should last at least 8 to 10 weeks. Many who experience minimal response at week 8 may show a good response at week 12, and improvements have been found to continue throughout 16 weeks of treatment.[140]

OTHER ANTIDEPRESSANTS

The MAOIs phenelzine and tranylcypromine have also demonstrated marked efficacy for social anxiety disorder but are reserved for SSRI nonresponders.[126,134] Before SSRIs, phenelzine was considered the mainstay of pharmacotherapy for social anxiety disorder. The typically effective dosage ranges are 60 to 90 mg/day for phenelzine and 30 to 60 mg/day for tranylcypromine.

Case reports and open studies suggest other antidepressants, including nefazodone and bupropion, may be useful in treating social anxiety disorder, but controlled trials are needed to define their roles.[126] Imipramine is ineffective for social anxiety disorder, and TCAs are not among the recommended treatment options.[126,134] Likewise, one study found mirtazapine to be ineffective in this population.[141]

BENZODIAZEPINES

The high-potency benzodiazepines, clonazepam and alprazolam, may also be useful in some patients with social anxiety disorder. Clonazepam was markedly efficacious in one controlled study, whereas alprazolam showed only modest efficacy compared with placebo.[126,134] The usual effective dosage ranges are 1 to 3 mg/day for clonazepam and 1 to 6 mg/day for alprazolam. In contrast to the antidepressants, benzodiazepines have a quicker onset of therapeutic effects and can also be used on an as-needed basis before participation in stressful social situations. However, benzodiazepines can reduce the therapeutic effects of exposure therapy. Benzodiazepines are generally considered second-line therapy for social anxiety disorder, but in clinical practice, they are commonly used on an as-needed basis in combination with SSRI therapy.[134]

β-BLOCKERS AND OTHER MISCELLANEOUS AGENTS

β-Adrenergic receptor blockers reduce peripheral autonomic symptoms of anxiety, but they are not effective in treating generalized social anxiety disorder.[126] They are, however, useful for nongeneralized social phobia involving performance-related situations. Propranolol and atenolol are the two recommended agents and can be used on an as-needed basis to reduce performance anxiety. Small doses (10–80 mg of propranolol or 25–50 mg of atenolol) of either agent may be administered 1 to 2 hours before the performance to decrease symptoms such as tremors, palpitations, and blushing. A test dose should be tried before the actual occasion to assess tolerability. Various other medications, including pregabalin, gabapentin, tiagabine, levetiracetam, and atypical antipsychotics, like aripiprazole, olanzapine, and risperidone, have also been reported to be effective in the treatment of social anxiety disorder, but they are considered second- or third-line treatments.[46,134,138,142]

NONPHARMACOLOGIC TREATMENTS

Several studies have demonstrated CBT to be comparable to medications in the treatment of social anxiety disorder.[143] The cognitive therapy component is aimed at changing negative thought patterns, such as expectations of performing poorly and overconcern about negative evaluation by others.[143] These negative expectations lead to increased apprehension and anxiety, which further impair performance abilities. The behavioral therapy component, as in other anxiety disorders, involves repeated exposure to the feared social situations and practice performing in those situations. Cognitive-behavioral group therapies are especially beneficial in social anxiety disorder because group members can practice social interactions with one another. Although medications may work faster, CBT is believed to result in longer-lasting treatment gains.[143] Social skills training can also be beneficial in improving interpersonal communication skills.

CLINICAL PRESENTATION OF SOCIAL ANXIETY DISORDER

CASE 80-8

QUESTION 1: S.H., an 18-year-old man, is brought for psychiatric consultation by his mother who complains her son is extremely shy and she's concerned about his ability to "fit in" at college. S.H. was referred to the psychiatrist by his primary-care physician, who reports S.H. is physically healthy. S.H.'s mother states he is a very bright young man who made straight As in high school despite frequent absenteeism. He only has one close friend and has never been on a date. S.H.'s mother says during high school, S.H. rarely attended school social functions and spent much of his time in his room working on his computer. On graduation from high school, he received a full scholarship to a community college but is quite anxious about going and is debating whether he should turn down the scholarship. When questioned by the psychiatrist, S.H.'s face turns bright red, and his voice shakes when he speaks. S.H. admits his behavior is not normal but says he is afraid he might "do something stupid" when he is around people and becomes extremely embarrassed when he has to talk to anyone. He has wanted to ask a certain girl on a date for 3 years but experienced severe anxiety attacks on the few occasions he tried to approach her. S.H. is afraid of being turned down and believes no girl would ever want to date someone like him. The psychiatrist's diagnosis is social anxiety disorder. What clinical features of social anxiety disorder are present in S.H.?

S.H. exhibits many characteristic features of the generalized type of social anxiety disorder. S.H. admits he does not like being around people for fear of embarrassment, and he generally avoids social situations, which are classic traits of social anxiety disorder. Symptoms of blushing and shaking voice are also common in social anxiety disorder, as well as other typical anxiety symptoms such as palpitations, trembling, sweating, tense muscles, dry throat, hot/cold sensations, and a sinking feeling in the stomach. S.H. also displays hypersensitivity to rejection and low self-esteem, and he realizes his behavior and fears are unreasonable. These symptoms and S.H.'s young age are consistent with a diagnosis of social anxiety disorder.

S.H.'s case illustrates the substantial disability that can result from this illness. S.H.'s anxiety disorder has deprived him of normal social development, making friends, dating, participating in social functions regularly, and pursuit of higher education. Future impairments throughout S.H.'s life are likely to be significant unless his anxiety is treated successfully.

TREATMENT SELECTION FOR SOCIAL ANXIETY DISORDER

CASE 80-8, QUESTION 2: The physician decides to treat S.H. with sertraline 50 mg every morning. Is the prescribed pharmacotherapy appropriate in this case?

Because S.H.'s generalized social anxiety disorder is severely affecting his life, medication treatment is indicated. SSRIs are first-line therapy for treating social anxiety disorder, and sertraline is a good choice because it is FDA approved for this indication and available as a generic. Although not applicable in this case, sertraline is also effective for many other psychiatric disorders commonly seen in patients with social anxiety disorder. The sertraline starting dose of 50 mg/day is appropriate for S.H., and 50-mg increment dosage increases can be made every 4 weeks according to response, up to a maximum of 200 mg/day. Signs of response may be seen within 2 to 4 weeks, but 8 to 12 weeks is usually required for optimal results. If available, CBT may also be combined with pharmacotherapy for S.H.

GOALS AND DURATION OF TREATMENT

CASE 80-8, QUESTION 3: What are the goals of treatment in this case, and how can S.H.'s response to treatment be objectively assessed? How long should effective therapy be continued?

Three principle domains of treatment outcomes have been defined for social anxiety disorder: symptoms, functionality, and overall well-being.[53] It is recommended that all three of these areas are assessed because even if all anxiety symptoms disappear, treatment is not clinically significant unless functioning also improves. The clinician-rated Liebowitz Social Anxiety Scale and the patient-rated Sheehan Disability Scale can be used for measuring improvements in symptom and functional ability domains, respectively.[53] In S.H.'s case, the desired outcomes of treatment include reducing fear and avoidance of social situations, enabling him to comfortably interact socially and attend college, and improving his quality of life.

Several studies have examined relapse rates after double-blind discontinuation of effective treatment in social anxiety disorder.[134,140,143] Based on their results, relapse appears to be very common. Long-term studies have shown sertraline, paroxetine, escitalopram, and clonazepam prevent relapse of social anxiety disorder during continuation treatment. Therefore, pharmacotherapy should be continued for at least 1 year after response.[126,134] After that time, a trial of gradual medication discontinuation may be attempted, accompanied by close monitoring for signs of relapse.

POSTTRAUMATIC STRESS DISORDER AND ACUTE STRESS DISORDER

Diagnostic Criteria

PTSD and acute stress disorder occur in people who have experienced a severely distressing traumatic event. These disorders are characterized by symptoms of intrusive re-experiencing, avoidance features, emotional numbing, and symptoms of autonomic hyperarousal.[1] PTSD has been recognized most commonly in war veterans and was referred to as "shell shock" after World War I. However, PTSD also occurs in persons exposed to events such as natural disasters, serious accidents, criminal assault, rape, physical or sexual abuse, and political victimization (refugees, concentration camp survivors, hostages). The trauma does not have to involve physical injury to the PTSD victim. Witnessing someone else being injured or killed, being diagnosed with a life-threatening illness, and experiencing the unexpected death of a loved one are common types of trauma that may lead to PTSD.[1]

The DSM-IV-TR criteria for PTSD are presented in Table 80-13. PTSD is classified as having either an acute or delayed (after 6 months) onset in relation to the trauma; the latter is extremely rare.[1] Symptoms must persist for at least 1 month to meet the criteria for PTSD. *Acute stress disorder* is a separate diagnostic category in the DSM-IV-TR and refers to cases in which symptoms last less than 1 month (but at least 2 days).[1] It involves many of the same clinical features as PTSD, but there is an additional requirement of peritraumatic dissociative symptoms (numbing, derealization, depersonalization, amnesia, feeling dazed). In both PTSD and acute stress disorder, the symptoms must be severe enough to interfere with functioning.

TABLE 80-13
Diagnostic Criteria for Posttraumatic Stress Disorder

1. Person has experienced a traumatic event in which the individual witnessed, experienced, or was confronted with actual or threatened death, or serious injury to self or others, and to which the person responded with intense fear, helplessness, or horror
2. Traumatic event is re-experienced persistently in some way (e.g., dreams, nightmares, flashbacks, recurrent thoughts or images), or intense distress is experienced on exposure to stimuli associated with the traumatic event
3. Persistent avoidance of stimuli associated with the event and numbing of general responsiveness involving at least three of the following:
   a. Efforts to avoid thoughts, feelings, or conversations related to the trauma
   b. Efforts to avoid people, places, or activities that are reminders of the trauma
   c. Impaired recall of the traumatic event
   d. Decreased interest or participation in activities
   e. Feelings of detachment
   f. Restricted range of affect
   g. Sense of foreshortened future
4. Persistent symptoms of increased arousal (not present before the event) that include at last two of the following:
   a. Sleep disturbances
   b. Irritability or anger outbursts
   c. Difficulty concentrating
   d. Hypervigilance
   e. Exaggerated startle response
5. Duration of the disturbance (2–4) of at least 1 month
6. Disturbance causes significant impairment in some aspect of daily functioning

Adapted with permission from American Psychiatric Association. *Diagnostic and Statistical Manual of Mental Disorders*. 4th ed. Text Revision. Washington, DC: American Psychiatric Association; 2000. Copyright © 2000 American Psychiatric Association.

Epidemiology and Clinical Course

PTSD is associated with a lifetime prevalence in the general population of approximately 10% and up to 24% among deployed serviceman from Iraq and Afghanistan.[144] PTSD is twice as common in women, although overall, men are exposed to trauma more often.[145] Rates of PTSD are expected to rise as the frequency of traumatic events throughout the world continues to increase. An estimated 80% to 90% of individuals in the United States today will experience at least one event during their lifetime traumatic enough to lead to PTSD.[145]

Most people who are exposed to a traumatic event do not develop PTSD; approximately 90% of individuals experience a normal acute stress response to trauma and fully recover.[145] Risk factors for the development of PTSD include experiencing assaultive violence, more severe and chronic traumas, a history of depressive or anxiety disorders, lack of social support after the trauma, and experiencing dissociative or other intense symptoms during or soon after the trauma.[144–146] Previous exposure to trauma also increases the risk of developing PTSD after later traumas, and survivors of childhood sexual or physical abuse have been found to be especially vulnerable.[146,147] Among people exposed to various traumatic events, the overall conditional risks for PTSD are reported to be 6% for men and 13% for women.[144] In general, traumas involving personal assault (e.g., rape, combat) are associated with much higher conditional risks of developing PTSD than other types of trauma.

Overall, 79% to 88% of PTSD patients also suffer from other disorders in their lifetime, including major depression, alcohol or other substance abuse, GAD, panic disorder, and phobic disorders.[144,145,147–149] The suicide risk in PTSD is high and comparable to that seen in major depression.[124] PTSD causes significant functional disability and has been associated with school failure, teenage pregnancy, unemployment, marital instability, legal problems, and impaired performance in the workplace.[150]

The course of PTSD is highly variable. Most patients who meet criteria for PTSD 1 month after trauma show spontaneous recovery within 6 to 9 months.[148] PTSD continues for years in a significant minority, estimated at 10% to 25%, and some sufferers experience a lifelong course of illness. The overall median duration of PTSD is reported to be approximately 2 years, but has been found to be four times longer in women (4 years) than in men (1 year).[148]

Etiology and Pathophysiology

The effects of stress on the brain have been a topic of intensive research. Psychological trauma, especially that which occurs early in life or is chronic in duration, can cause persistent changes in various aspects of brain functioning and in neurobiological responses to stress.[151] Evidence of altered NE, 5-HT, glutamatergic, GABA system, HPA axis, neuroendocrine, substance P, and opioid system functioning has been found in PTSD.[152–155] Stress-induced hyperactivity of central noradrenergic systems is believed to lead to the generalized anxiety and autonomic hyperarousal associated with PTSD.[153] These symptoms may also be related to a supersensitivity of the HPA axis system in PTSD because affected patients have a blunted ACTH response to CRH and decreased basal cortisol levels, as well as increased numbers of glucocorticoid receptors.[152] A subset of PTSD patients appear to have an abnormally sensitized 5-HT system, and these patients may represent a neurobiologically distinct subgroup.[154]

Neuropsychological tests show reduced hippocampal volume is associated with cognitive and memory impairments in PTSD patients.[150] Functional neuroimaging studies in PTSD have found excessive activation of the amygdala and other brain areas in response to trauma-related stimuli.[151,156] Thus, the neurobiological consequences of stress and trauma result in both structural and functional changes in the brain. Genetic factors may also play a role in influencing vulnerability to the damaging effects of stress.[156]

Treatment of Posttraumatic Stress Disorder

Both medications and CBT are useful in treating PTSD. Nonpharmacologic therapies alone may be appropriate for initial treatment of mild PTSD, but pharmacotherapy, either alone or in combination with psychological therapies, is usually recommended for patients with moderate or severe illness.[146,147,150,157] When assessing various treatment options for PTSD, it is important to consider effects on all three core symptom clusters (re-experiencing or intrusive symptoms, avoidance or emotional numbing, hyperarousal symptoms). Not all PTSD treatments are effective for all three domains.

The preferred first-line medications in PTSD are SSRIs, but various other antidepressants may also be useful. Response to pharmacotherapy occurs very gradually, taking 8 to 12 weeks or longer. Partial response at 12 weeks of treatment may be followed by full remission after several more months of therapy; therefore, an adequate period should be allowed to fully determine response to a particular medication. Lack of improvement after 4 weeks of therapy indicates nonresponse, so alternative treatment strategies should be tried in these cases.[158] Early treatment during the first 3 months after a trauma may prevent the development of chronic PTSD; however, recent research focusing on discovering specific early pharmacologic interventions has been unsuccessful.[144,147]

SELECTIVE SEROTONIN REUPTAKE INHIBITORS

Sertraline and paroxetine are currently the only FDA-approved SSRIs for PTSD. Large controlled studies have demonstrated that both agents are effective and superior to placebo in reducing all three PTSD symptom clusters.[158] They also have beneficial effects on depression and general anxiety symptoms and have been associated with improvements in overall functioning and quality of life.[158] Fluoxetine also appears to be effective in treating PTSD in some patients, although study results have been mixed and the drug may lack significant efficacy for avoidance or numbing symptoms.[158] Male war veterans with long-standing combat-related PTSD have been noted to respond poorly to fluoxetine, compared with women and civilians, but this observation may apply to treatment of PTSD in general.[159,160] Citalopram, escitalopram, and fluvoxamine have shown efficacy in the treatment of PTSD in open trials, but randomized, double-blind, placebo-controlled studies have yielded negative results.[158,161] Venlafaxine XR has also demonstrated efficacy in one short-term and one long-term double-blind trial in PTSD, particularly for re-experiencing and avoidance or numbing symptoms, but not hyperarousal.[162,163] Finally, duloxetine has been implicated in worsening existing PTSD in one case.[164] However, one small, naturalistic study in treatment-resistant men suggests duloxetine may be effective in managing comorbid depression and PTSD.[165]

OTHER ANTIDEPRESSANTS

Several open studies and case reports suggest nefazodone, mirtazapine, and bupropion are effective in treating the core symptoms of PTSD.[155,166] Although supporting evidence for these antidepressants is not as strong as for sertraline and paroxetine, they may be considered appropriate alternatives to SSRIs in certain patients. The TCAs amitriptyline and imipramine and the MAOI phenelzine have also been found to be effective for PTSD in controlled trials, but these agents are generally not recommended because of their poor tolerability and safety profiles.[147] Because of the relatively high risk of suicide in PTSD, TCAs can be especially dangerous in this population.

MISCELLANEOUS AGENTS

Various other medications have been used successfully in limited numbers of PTSD cases. Anticonvulsants carbamazepine, valproate, topiramate, tiagabine, gabapentin, oxcarbazepine, vigabatrin, pregabalin, levetiracetam, and lamotrigine have been studied with inconsistent results, mostly in case series and open-label trials.[165] These agents may be effective in certain patients and can be useful for reducing irritability, impulsivity, and angry or violent outbursts.[166,167] Anticonvulsants may also be effective for intrusive, re-experiencing, and hyperarousal symptoms. Atypical antipsychotic agents (risperidone, clozapine, olanzapine) have been used effectively to treat PTSD-related psychotic symptoms and sleep disturbances. However, they do not appear to be useful for treating core PTSD symptoms, except as augmentation strategies, although results in this regard have been inconsistent.[46,166] The α_1-adrenergic antagonist, prazosin, is reported to decrease nightmares, increase sleep time, and reduce other core symptoms in patients with PTSD.[155,168] Conflicting evidence exists for the use of the β-adrenergic antagonist, propranolol, which has been studied in blocking memory consolidation and therefore may prevent PTSD if administered within hours of the traumatic event.[155] Larger studies are needed to determine whether this is a useful preventive option. Benzodiazepines are generally ineffective in treating PTSD, although they may be useful in managing sleep disturbances during the early weeks after trauma. Their use in PTSD should be limited to short-term therapy because chronic use may have detrimental effects.[169]

NONPHARMACOLOGIC TREATMENTS

Various types of psychosocial therapies have been used in the treatment of PTSD, including anxiety management training to help patients cope with stress.[169] Trauma-focused CBT and eye movement desensitization and reprocessing treatment have both demonstrated effectiveness in PTSD, and either of these treatments are recommended for all patients with PTSD.[144,157] Cognitive therapies seem to be most effective for symptoms of demoralization, guilt, and shame, whereas exposure therapies are better for reducing intrusive thoughts, flashbacks, and avoidance behaviors. Both cognitive and exposure therapies have been shown to be markedly and comparably effective in controlled PTSD trials, but exposure is probably more critical for optimal results.[147,150] Studies of combined psychosocial therapies and medication are inconclusive and require further investigation to determine superior effectiveness compared with either treatment strategy alone.[170]

Clinical Presentation of Posttraumatic Stress Disorder

CASE 80-9

QUESTION 1: D.D. is a 42-year-old woman who was attacked and raped in the driveway of her home as she was getting out of her car 1 month ago. She did not seek medical treatment at the time and waited several days before reporting the incident to anyone, including her family. She presents to her physician complaining that she cannot sleep and she is irritable, anxious, and depressed. When asked about any recent stressors in her life, she finally tells her doctor about the rape. D.D. has no history of psychiatric illness, admits her symptoms have appeared since the attack, and says she has never had any psychiatric problems until now. She states she has nightly nightmares and becomes extremely anxious every time she comes home and gets out of her car at night (which she avoids doing when possible). She is startled when the phone rings or when someone approaches her unexpectedly, and she literally freezes if she sees a man who bears any physical resemblance to her attacker. D.D. also states that memories of the rape often flash through her mind for no reason, although she tries hard not to think about it. The assailant has not been caught, and D.D. feels extremely guilty for not promptly reporting the crime. Her symptoms are interfering significantly with her ability to work and have put a strain on her marriage. What clinical features of PTSD does D.D. display?

Individuals with PTSD often present with nonspecific complaints indicative of a generalized anxiety, depression, or substance use disorder. They may not realize or want to reveal an association between their symptoms and the trauma experienced. Careful evaluation by the clinician is required to elicit a pattern suggestive of PTSD. D.D. displays many target symptoms of PTSD, including re-experiencing (nightmares, recurrent memories), avoidance of the activity reminding her of the trauma, and symptoms of increased arousal (sleep difficulties, irritability, exaggerated startle response). In addition, she is experiencing feelings of depression, distress, marital problems, and impairment in occupational functioning as a result of her symptoms. The lack of any previous psychiatric illness combined with the temporal relationship between the attack and her symptoms support the presence of PTSD as opposed to another anxiety or depressive disorder. Because her trauma occurred 1 month ago, her condition would be classified as acute-onset PTSD.

Treatment Selection and Selective Serotonin Reuptake Inhibitor Dosing

CASE 80-9, QUESTION 2: What factors are important in the selection of an initial treatment for D.D.?

Because D.D. is exhibiting moderate-to-severe PTSD symptoms, pharmacotherapy is indicated. Medication treatment can also be combined with CBT if it is available, but nonpharmacologic therapies alone are generally reserved for patients with mild symptoms. An SSRI is the preferred initial medication treatment for most patients.[158] Sertraline is an appropriate choice of treatment in this case and is FDA approved for PTSD. Low initial SSRI doses are recommended in PTSD, so sertraline can be started at 25 mg/day and gradually increased to the target dosage range of 100 to 150 mg/day, according to response and tolerability.[166] Regarding other SSRIs, studies suggest a paroxetine dose of 20 to 40 mg/day is effective for most PTSD patients; higher doses have not been associated with better response.[166] Persistent sleep complaints during the first month after a traumatic experience may predispose the patient to chronic PTSD, so management of sleep disturbances is an important component of initial PTSD treatment.[168] Low-dose adjunctive trazodone (25–50 mg at bedtime) would be a good choice in this case because it is safe, effective, and inexpensive.

Even in the absence of formal CBT, certain aspects of patient and family education are vital to the successful treatment of PTSD.[146,147] Providing information about the nature and prognosis of PTSD are important. The patient should be encouraged to talk with family and friends about the trauma because repeated retelling of the traumatic event is therapeutic and can help facilitate recovery. Significant others need to understand the importance of listening and of being tolerant of the patient's emotional reaction and persistent preoccupation with the experience. Peer support groups are widely available and can be beneficial in the recovery of trauma victims. Patients should be advised to try not to avoid things that remind them of the trauma, but rather to expose themselves to these situations as often as possible.

Clinical Assessment and Goals of Therapy

CASE 80-9, QUESTION 3: What are the goals of treatment in this case, and how can D.D.'s symptoms be objectively assessed?

The first goal of treatment of PTSD is to reduce the core symptoms of re-experiencing, avoidance, numbing, and hyperarousal. In D.D.'s case, these target symptoms include nightmares, intrusive memories, avoidance behaviors, irritability, hyperarousal, and sleep difficulties. Improvements should begin within the first 2 weeks and gradually continue over the course of 2 to 3 months. Secondary goals in this case include improving D.D.'s stress resilience, decreasing her work- and marriage-related disability, and improving her quality of life. Other general treatment goals in PTSD include decreasing detrimental behaviors (use of alcohol or substances, risky activities, violence) and treating comorbid psychiatric conditions.

Several different rating scales have been developed to assess response to treatments in PTSD.[53] The most commonly used clinician-rated scales are the Clinician Administered PTSD Scale and the Treatment Outcome PTSD Scale. The Clinician Administered PTSD Scale is most often used in clinical PTSD trials, whereas the Treatment Outcome PTSD Scale is shorter and easier to use in clinical practice. Patient-rated scales for evaluating PTSD symptoms include the Davidson Trauma Scale and the Impact of Events Scale. The Sheehan Disability Scale is often used to assess functional impairment attributable to PTSD.

Course and Duration of Treatment

Good treatment response in PTSD is more likely to occur when treatment is started within 3 months of the trauma.[147,150] There is no well-established definition of response in PTSD, but a decrease in symptoms by 30% to 50%, along with substantial functional improvement, is commonly used in clinical trials. Full recovery during treatment of PTSD is fairly uncommon, and partial responders to either medication or psychosocial therapies may benefit from adding another treatment modality. When an initial SSRI trial is ineffective, the patient may be switched to another SSRI or another antidepressant shown to be effective in PTSD.[166] Partial responders may benefit from the addition of a second medication, depending on which core symptoms predominate (see Treatment of Posttraumatic Stress Disorder section).

For patients who respond, treatment should be continued for an additional 6 to 12 months for acute cases (when symptoms were present <3 months before treatment) and 12 to 24 months for chronic cases (when symptoms lasted >3 months before treatment).[147] Long-term SSRI treatment can prevent relapse of PTSD, especially in those who show good response during the first 3 months of therapy.[169] When pharmacotherapy is discontinued, it should be withdrawn gradually over the course of 1 to 3 months.

OBSESSIVE–COMPULSIVE DISORDER

Diagnostic Criteria

The DSM-IV-TR criteria for OCD are presented in Table 80-14.[1] OCD is characterized by recurrent obsessions or compulsions, which are severe enough to be distressing, consume at least 1 hour a day, or significantly interfere with some aspect of functioning. An *obsession* is an intrusive or recurrent thought, image, or impulse that incites anxiety in the person and cannot be ignored or suppressed voluntarily. The most common obsessions include germs and contamination, pathological doubt, somatic concerns, need for order and symmetry, and religious, aggressive, or sexual thoughts.[171,172] A *compulsion* is a behavior or ritual that is performed in a repetitive or stereotypic way designed to reduce anxiety associated with obsessions or to prevent some future event or situation. However, the compulsions are not actually connected to the obsessions in any realistic way. Frequent compulsions include checking, cleaning, arranging symmetrically, ordering, hoarding, counting, and needing to ask questions or confess.[172] The obsessions and compulsions are unpleasant and disturbing to the sufferer and are not associated with pleasure or gratification. This feature distinguishes OCD from certain other detrimental behaviors (excessive gambling or shopping), which are often described as being "compulsive." Adults with OCD usually realize their rituals are senseless and excessive at some point, but children may not make this distinction.[1]

TABLE 80-14
Diagnostic Criteria for Obsessive–Compulsive Disorder

1. Presence of either obsessions or compulsions:
   Obsessions:
   (a) Recurrent and persistent ideas or thoughts are experienced, at some time during the disturbance, as intrusive and senseless
   (b) Thoughts, impulses, or images are not simply excessive worries about real life problems
   (c) Person attempts to ignore or neutralize the ideas or thoughts with some other thought or action
   (d) Person realizes the obsessions are the product of his or her own mind
   Compulsions:
   (a) Repetitive and intentional behaviors or mental acts are performed in response to the obsession or according to rigid rules
   (b) Behavior is designed to prevent or reduce distress or to prevent some dreaded event; however, the activity is clearly excessive and unrealistic to neutralize the situation
2. At some point during the disturbance, the person realizes that the obsessions and compulsions are excessive or unreasonable (not necessary in children)
3. Obsessions or compulsions cause marked distress, are time-consuming (>1 h/d), or significantly interfere with some aspect of daily functioning
4. Content of the symptoms is not related to another psychiatric disorder, and the disturbance is not attributable to the direct effects of a substance, medication, or general medical illness

Adapted with permission from American Psychiatric Association. *Diagnostic and Statistical Manual of Mental Disorders*. 4th ed. Text Revision. Washington, DC: American Psychiatric Association; 2000. Copyright © 2000 American Psychiatric Association.

OCD is a clinically heterogeneous disorder involving a wide range of symptoms. Five separate OCD symptom dimensions have been defined: symmetry obsessions and repeating, counting, and ordering compulsions; contamination obsessions and cleaning compulsions; hoarding obsessions and compulsions; aggressive obsessions and checking compulsions; and sexual or religious obsessions and related compulsions. Although specific symptoms in an individual may change with time, they usually remain within the same dimension.[173]

Epidemiology and Clinical Course

OCD once was believed to be a rare disorder, but epidemiologic studies reveal it affects between 2% and 3% of the worldwide population.[1,174] The overall lifetime prevalence is slightly higher in women, but men tend to have an earlier onset of illness (between ages 6 and 15 years) than women (between ages 20 and 29 years).[1,15,174] Many patients report having mild symptoms for years before full OCD emerges, and an estimated one-third to one-half of patients have onset during childhood or adolescence. Prepubertal OCD is three times more common in boys than in girls.[15] Women with OCD often have onset or worsening of OCD during pregnancy.[86] Regardless of sex, the severity of illness usually worsens during stressful life periods.

The course and severity of OCD are highly variable and unpredictable, with some persons only mildly or intermittently affected and others suffering severely and constantly throughout their lifetime. The natural course of untreated OCD was followed for a 40-year period in a group of 144 patients.[172] Although 83% of patients were improved at the end of the follow-up period, only 20% experienced full remission. Two-thirds of patients continued to have some OCD symptoms, and a progressive deterioration was observed in 10%. Observational studies suggest the long-term course of OCD may be improved substantially with appropriate treatment.[175,176] However, a portion of sufferers still experience a chronic and lifelong course.

OCD can have seriously detrimental effects on functional abilities and quality of life. In large-scale surveys, OCD patients report their symptoms significantly interfere with their abilities to socialize, study, work, make friends, and maintain good relationships with family and friends.[177] It is estimated that each person with OCD loses an average of 3 years' wages during his or her lifetime.[177] Quality-of-life ratings in OCD patients indicate marked impairments and are similar to those observed in patients with depression. Fortunately, treatment of OCD can be accompanied by significant improvements in quality of life and functional abilities.

Although several effective treatments are currently available for OCD, most patients do not seek treatment until the disorder is seriously affecting their lives. One study found OCD patients waited an average of 7.5 years after the onset of OCD before seeking medical evaluation for their disorder.[177] This may be because most OCD patients realize their symptoms are senseless, so they attempt to hide their disorder because of embarrassment. People with OCD often carry out their rituals privately and may be very successful at concealing their symptoms from others. Initial treatment for OCD is commonly sought outside psychiatric settings, and the obsessive–compulsive symptoms are often missed.

The general public and health care professionals need to recognize that OCD is a biological disorder for which effective treatments are available. Four simple questions are recommended for screening for potential OCD.[171] Do you have to wash your hands over and over? Do you have to check things repeatedly? Do you have recurrent distressing thoughts you cannot get rid of? Do you have to complete actions again and again or in a certain way? Clinicians in a variety of health care settings can incorporate these screening questions into their practice to use when possible signs of OCD are present. Health care providers should be prepared to provide education about the nature and treatability of OCD to suspected sufferers and to make appropriate treatment referrals in these cases.

Psychiatric Comorbidity and Obsessive–Compulsive Spectrum Disorders

As with other anxiety disorders, OCD is often accompanied by psychiatric comorbidity. Two-thirds of those with OCD experience major depression during their lifetime.[1,172] There is a higher-than-expected overlap of OCD with disorders such as specific and social phobias, GAD, panic disorder, schizophrenia, schizoaffective disorder, bipolar disorder, and eating disorders. Identification of comorbid conditions with OCD is important because it can influence choice of treatments. Obsessive–compulsive personality disorder, which is classified as an Axis II disorder, occurs in a small percentage of OCD patients. Despite their name similarities, obsessive–compulsive personality disorder does not involve true obsessions and compulsions (which are senseless and distressing to the sufferer). Rather, it is a personality pattern characterized by rigid and inflexible preoccupation with rules, lists, order, and perfectionism.[1] Although these personality traits cause problems, the person with the personality disorder does not view his or her behavior as abnormal or unreasonable.

The relation between tic disorders and OCD is particularly striking. Tics occur in 20% to 30% of OCD patients, and 5% to 7% have full Tourette syndrome, whereas 35% to 50% of Tourette syndrome patients exhibit OCD symptoms.[172] Individuals with OCD plus Tourette syndrome are believed to represent a genetically and pathophysiologically distinct subtype of illness.[172] These patients are more likely to be male and tend to have an earlier age at OCD onset (before age 10 years), more severe symptoms, and poorer response to SSRIs than those with OCD alone.[178]

Another childhood neurologic disorder commonly associated with OCD is Sydenham chorea. This is the neurologic variant of rheumatic fever, which is an autoimmune disease triggered by infection with group A β-hemolytic streptococcal pharyngitis. Reports describe children who developed sudden and severe tics and obsessive–compulsive symptoms after strep throat infections.[179] This condition, called PANDAS (pediatric autoimmune neuropsychiatric disorders associated with streptococcal infection), has been rapidly reversed by antibiotic or IV immunoglobulin treatment. Currently, the National Institutes of Health advises that immunotherapy be reserved for those participating in double-blind studies.[179] The possibility of a PANDAS correlation should be considered in any child who develops abrupt onset of obsessive–compulsive symptoms and has a history of pharyngitis within the past 6 months.

The term *obsessive–compulsive spectrum disorder* is used to describe recurrent or distressing thoughts or irresistible or repetitive behaviors.[180] These include somatoform disorders (body dysmorphic disorder [preoccupation with an imagined or slight defect in appearance], hypochondriasis), eating disorders (anorexia nervosa, bulimia nervosa, binge eating disorder), and impulse control disorders (trichotillomania [recurrent impulses to pull out one's hair], pathological gambling, compulsive nail biting, kleptomania, compulsive buying). Tourette syndrome and autism are also often included in this spectrum of disorders. Some of these disorders, such as body dysmorphic disorder, have much higher comorbidities with OCD than others. Like OCD, many patients with these conditions have shown good response to treatment with serotonergic antidepressants such as clomipramine and SSRIs.[180]

Etiology and Pathophysiology

A wealth of research has attempted to identify a specific biological explanation for OCD. Because OCD displays such clinical heterogeneity, there may be several distinct etiologies for different subtypes of illness. One leading hypothesis has focused on the role of 5-HT dysfunction, which is supported by the finding that primarily serotonergic medications are effective for OCD.[181] However, the multitude of studies involving 5-HT challenges and other methods for assessing central 5-HT function in OCD have resulted in inconclusive answers, and the exact role of 5-HT underlying OCD still has not been determined. Naturally occurring animal models of OCD have been observed in dogs (canine acral lick) and birds (feather picking disorder), and these conditions have been treated successfully with SSRIs.

More promising areas of OCD research involve structural and functional brain imaging studies.[181,182] These techniques are used to assess regional metabolic activity in different areas of the brain. Studies in OCD patients have identified abnormal hyperactivity (when compared with normal control subjects) in certain frontal lobe and basal ganglia regions, specifically the orbital frontal cortex, cingulate cortex, and head of the caudate nucleus.[182] Interestingly, these regional brain metabolic abnormalities normalize after successful treatment of OCD, and certain brain metabolism patterns may be associated with preferential response to SSRI versus CBT.[181,182] These findings have led to one current hypothesis that OCD is a neurologic disorder characterized by a hyperfunctioning circuit involving the aforementioned brain regions. In support of this hypothesis, neurosurgical techniques interrupting this circuit are often effective in the treatment of OCD. The mechanism of efficacy of the SSRIs may be related to desensitization of terminal 5-HT autoreceptors in the orbitofrontal cortex, which enhances 5-HT neurotransmission in this brain region.[181,182] Specific types of cognitive dysfunction have also been found, including problems with nonverbal memory, visuospatial skills, and visual attention.[181] Impairments in memory functioning have been correlated with the aforementioned structural abnormalities in OCD.

In addition to biological factors, twin and family studies support an effect of genetics on risk for OCD.[19] Heredity appears to be most important in early-onset OCD cases (before the age of 18 years) because familial aggregation has not been observed in OCD cases with a later age at onset.[183] Several studies suggest an association between OCD and specific polymorphisms in the serotonin transporter, 5-HT type 1Dβ and 5-HT type 2A receptor genes, but others have failed to replicate these findings.[184,185] Other candidate gene studies have linked OCD with functional polymorphisms in the catechol-*O*-methyltransferase, dopamine D_4-receptor genes, and a high-affinity neuronal/epithelial excitatory amino acid transporter gene.[185,186]

Treatment of Obsessive–Compulsive Disorder

Both medications and behavioral therapies are effective in the treatment of OCD. Behavioral therapy is vitally important for OCD, and the combination of drugs plus behavioral therapy provides optimal treatment. All medications consistently effective in the monotherapy treatment of OCD are potent inhibitors of serotonin reuptake. These include clomipramine and the SSRIs (fluvoxamine, fluoxetine, paroxetine, and sertraline). All five of these medications are FDA approved for the treatment of OCD in adults, and all except paroxetine are indicated for use in children with OCD. The SNRI venlafaxine is also effective for the treatment of OCD. Although duloxetine, desvenlafaxine, or milnacipran (other SNRIs) may ultimately show efficacy in the treatment of OCD, no well-controlled studies have been conducted evaluating these medications in the treatment of OCD.[187]

CLOMIPRAMINE

Clomipramine was the first drug with proven efficacy in treating OCD, and it was considered the standard first-line treatment for several years until the SSRIs gained popularity. Many large well-controlled studies have documented that clomipramine is far superior to placebo and significantly improves OCD symptoms in approximately 60% to 70% of patients.[172,188] Clomipramine is unique among TCAs in its effectiveness for OCD. This distinct property is attributed to its more potent effects on 5-HT reuptake inhibition compared with other TCAs. Clomipramine is often referred to as an SRI (serotonin reuptake inhibitor), not an SSRI, because its major active metabolite, desmethylclomipramine, is a potent inhibitor of NE reuptake. Clomipramine also blocks adrenergic, histaminergic, and cholinergic receptors similarly to other TCAs, resulting in an adverse effect profile similar to imipramine (see Chapter 83, Mood Disorders I: Major Depressive Disorders).

Although direct comparison studies have shown clomipramine to be similar in efficacy to various SSRIs in treating OCD, several meta-analyses have concluded clomipramine is superior to SSRIs overall.[188,189] However, clomipramine is less well tolerated than SSRIs, and patients may discontinue clomipramine treatment because of sedation, orthostatic hypotension, and anticholinergic side effects. Therefore, clomipramine is currently reserved as a second-line treatment option for patients who do not respond adequately to SSRI therapy.[188] Details about the clinical use of clomipramine are discussed in Case 80-11, Question 1.

SELECTIVE SEROTONIN REUPTAKE INHIBITORS AND VENLAFAXINE

SSRIs are the only first-line medication treatments for OCD. Double-blind, placebo-controlled studies have documented the efficacies of fluvoxamine, fluoxetine, paroxetine, and sertraline in the treatment of OCD.[190] Citalopram and escitalopram also are effective, but there is less evidence to support their use. There is no strong evidence to demonstrate that any one SSRI is more effective than the others in treating OCD, but some patients may respond to or tolerate one agent better than another.[190] Usual SSRI starting dosages can be used in OCD, but at least 4 weeks should be allowed before exceeding the targeted minimally effective dosages (fluvoxamine 200 mg/day, fluoxetine 40 mg/day, paroxetine 40 mg/day, and sertraline 100 mg/day).[190] Several controlled studies support the efficacy of venlafaxine in the treatment of OCD.[188] A recent trial comparing venlafaxine with clomipramine in OCD found these agents to be comparably effective, but venlafaxine was better tolerated.[191]

AUGMENTATION STRATEGIES

Other than venlafaxine, none of the other miscellaneous agents studied in OCD have demonstrated impressive efficacy as monotherapy. However, several agents appear to be useful as augmentation therapy to boost response to SSRIs or clomipramine in partial responders to these agents.[192] The combination of an SSRI plus clomipramine is one such option for patients who show partial response, although attention must be paid to potential drug interactions, which may lead to clomipramine toxicity (see Case 80-11, Questions 2 and 3).

Antipsychotic agents are useful for augmentation therapy. They may be particularly effective in patients with comorbid tic disorders, although recent reports suggest they are equally effective in patients without tics. Older first-generation antipsychotics, such as haloperidol and pimozide, are effective in augmenting response to fluvoxamine in controlled trials (conducted before the dangerous interaction between pimozide and CYP 3A4 inhibitors, such as fluvoxamine, was identified). Recent reports have focused on newer second-generation antipsychotics because these agents are generally preferred over first-generation antipsychotics and are better tolerated.[192,193] Risperidone (2–4 mg/day), olanzapine (10–20 mg/day), and quetiapine (up to 600 mg/day) have all been used successfully in treatment-resistant OCD to augment response to SSRIs.[192,194,195] The findings of studies, to date, suggest risperidone is more effective for this augmentation strategy than olanzapine or quetiapine. Of note, second-generation antipsychotics (risperidone, clozapine, olanzapine) have been reported to cause or worsen obsessive–compulsive symptoms in select patients with schizophrenia.[192] This effect is believed to be related to the 5-HT_2-receptor antagonistic activity of antipsychotics. Certain SSRI-antipsychotic combinations can increase antipsychotic plasma levels and side effects, particularly extrapyramidal symptoms. Pimozide should not be used in combination with clomipramine, fluoxetine, sertraline, or fluvoxamine because of the potential for cardiac QT interval prolongation.

MISCELLANEOUS AGENTS

A wide variety of other medications have been tried in the treatment of OCD, with varying degrees of success.

Benzodiazepines are generally not beneficial in treating OCD, although there are several reports of clonazepam being effective as adjunctive therapy or monotherapy.[172] Clonazepam appears to have serotonergic effects, which may explain its potential usefulness in OCD. This agent may be helpful in patients with prominent anxiety symptoms, but it may also interfere with the effectiveness of CBT and probably should not be used concurrently. As discussed, fluvoxamine and fluoxetine can significantly increase serum levels of clonazepam.

The MAOI phenelzine was one of the first medications studied for OCD. Early case reports of its use were favorable, but more recent findings suggest phenelzine is largely ineffective for OCD.[172]

NONPHARMACOLOGIC TREATMENTS

COGNITIVE BEHAVIORAL THERAPIES

CBT is an extremely important component of treatment for OCD and should be incorporated into the initial treatment plan whenever possible. CBT alone may be appropriate for mild OCD or in cases in which it is desirable to avoid medication (e.g., pregnancy, medical conditions). The combination of CBT and medication is generally superior to either treatment approach used alone.[171,172] Treatment gains achieved with CBT often are maintained long after its discontinuation, which is an advantage versus pharmacotherapy.[171]

The cognitive therapy component of CBT is aimed toward changing the detrimental thought patterns in OCD and is most helpful for obsessions such as scrupulosity, moral guilt, and pathological doubt. The behavioral therapy aspect, called exposure plus response prevention, involves exposure to feared objects or situations followed by prevention of the usual compulsive response. This type of therapy is most beneficial for patients with contamination fears, hoarding, and rituals involving symmetry, counting, or repeating. Because exposure plus response prevention is anxiety provoking and can be very distressing, many patients refuse to participate in it.

NEUROSURGERY

Neurosurgical treatment of OCD has been practiced since the 1950s and is considered an option of last resort in treatment-refractory patients. More recently, deep brain stimulation has also been used to treat OCD that is refractory to medications and psychotherapy. Anterior cingulotomy and anterior capsulotomy are the most commonly used surgical procedures. Indications for neurosurgery include severe disability from obsessive–compulsive symptoms and failed treatments (drugs and behavioral therapies) that have been tried systematically for at least 5 years.[196] Reported success rates of neurosurgery in OCD range from approximately 35% to 70%, and complications (including potential infections, personality changes, cognitive impairment, and epilepsy) appear to be rare. A recent, long-term, follow-up study of patients who underwent neurosurgery during the 1970s found therapeutic effects were maintained, but patients exhibited mild-to-moderate impairments in neuropsychological performance.[196,197] Deep brain stimulation requires the bilateral implantation of electrodes into the ventral caudate or ventral striatum targets. Although this procedure is still experimental, overall preliminary results are positive.[197]

Defining Response to Therapy

Response to medication treatment in OCD is gradual and often delayed. Initial improvements usually begin to appear within the first month, but maximal response may take as long as 5 to 6 months. Patients who show unsatisfactory response to lower SSRI dosages by weeks 4 to 9 should have their dosages gradually increased to the manufacturer's recommended maximum. A trial of 8 to 12 weeks at maximal tolerated medication dosages is recommended before determining response to a particular medication.

The primary goal of treatment in OCD is to decrease obsessions and compulsions to a level at which the person is able to function normally. Complete elimination of symptoms is rare with current treatments.[198] Most clinical trials in OCD define clinical response as a 25% to 35% reduction in Yale–Brown Obsessive–Compulsive Symptom Checklist (Y-BOCS) scores. Therefore, even those classified as responders may be left with 65% to 75% of their original symptoms, and this may or may not result in significant improvements in functioning or quality of life.

STRATEGIES FOR MANAGING PARTIAL RESPONSE AND NONRESPONSE

Current estimates are that approximately 40% to 60% of patients show clinically meaningful improvements in obsessive–compulsive symptoms during an initial (SSRI or clomipramine) medication trial, but only a small percentage exhibit marked response.[188] Unfortunately, a fairly large percentage of patients derive minimal or no benefit from an initial trial and require further tactics. Approximately 20% of those who fail a first SSRI trial subsequently respond to another agent in this class; therefore, switching to a second SSRI is usually recommended as the next step before initiating a trial of clomipramine.[171,188] However, clomipramine can be extremely effective in SSRI nonresponders, and it remains a useful treatment option despite its clinical disadvantages.

Partial responders to an initial SSRI trial may be better served by addition of one of the augmentation agents discussed in the previous section than by switching to a new medication. Also, inclusion of CBT is important for optimizing treatment with any medication. Neurosurgery is an option for severe treatment-refractory cases. Predictors of poor response to treatment in OCD include poor insight; hoarding or sexual or religious dimension symptoms; prepubertal onset of illness; and presence of comorbid personality, mood, or eating disorders.

Clinical Presentation and Assessment

CASE 80-10

QUESTION 1: R.G. is a 25-year-old woman whose husband complains she spends 1.5 hours a day cleaning the stove and takes four showers each day. The unusual behavior began about 1 year ago after the birth of their son but has continued to worsen, and R.G.'s husband states that he cannot deal with her "odd habits" any longer. R.G. recently lost her job as a secretary because of tardiness (it took her 3 hours to get ready for work) and spending too much time away from her desk in the ladies' room. R.G. admits that it is silly, but she has irresistible urges to make sure both she and her surroundings are completely free of germs so her child will not get sick. She also confines herself to one floor of their three-level house because she is afraid she will fall down the stairs while carrying her son. R.G. also states that she constantly has "what if" thoughts about horrible things happening to her family, which are very disturbing. The physician's diagnosis is OCD. What clinical features of OCD does R.G. display, and how can her symptoms be objectively evaluated?

R.G. displays many characteristic symptoms of OCD. The most commonly encountered clinical presentation of OCD involves excessive fear of contamination with dirt, germs, or toxins and repeated washing of hands or cleaning objects or surroundings. These persons also typically avoid touching possibly dirty objects (e.g., doorknobs, money) or shaking hands with people. Another common clinical presentation of OCD is the patient with pathological doubt who constantly worries something bad will happen because of his or her negligence. Individuals can be afraid they have failed to lock the door, turn off the stove, shut the refrigerator door, or secure the medicine cabinet from children. As a result, they continuously check and recheck their actions.

R.G. displays obsessions of contamination and pathological doubt, and compulsions of excessive cleaning and washing. These symptoms are time-consuming, cause significant distress, and have led to her unemployment and marital difficulties. As seen in this case, most persons present with a mixture of various obsessions and compulsions. R.G. also realizes her thoughts and behaviors are "silly," which most often is the case in OCD. This case also illustrates the onset of OCD during times of stressful or significant life events. Pregnancy, death of a relative, and marital discord have been identified as precipitating factors in the onset of OCD.[86,174,198]

The aforementioned Y-BOCS is a useful tool in the initial evaluation of those who present with symptoms of OCD and may be used in the objective assessment of R.G.'s symptoms. The Y-BOCS is a 10-item scale with a maximal possible score of 40; a score of more than 15 is generally considered to represent clinically significant obsessive–compulsive symptoms.[199] This scale is a standard tool for evaluating drug efficacy in OCD clinical trials and is often used in clinical practice to assess response to treatments. Other OCD assessment instruments include the National Institute of Mental Health Obsessive–Compulsive Scale, the Leyton Obsessional Inventory, and the self-rated Maudsley Obsessional–Compulsive Inventory. Special versions for use in children have been developed for the Y-BOCS and the Leyton Obsessional Inventory.

Selective Serotonin Reuptake Inhibitor Treatment of Obsessive–Compulsive Disorder

SELECTIVE SEROTONIN REUPTAKE INHIBITOR SELECTION AND DOSING

CASE 80-10, QUESTION 2: On assessment, R.G.'s Y-BOCS score is found to be 33. Her physician prescribes fluvoxamine and instructs R.G. to take 100 mg every morning for 1 week and then 200 mg every morning thereafter. He also refers R.G. to a psychologist to receive CBT. Is this initial choice of therapy appropriate?

SSRIs such as fluvoxamine are considered the best choice of initial pharmacotherapy for OCD. The primary differences between SSRIs involve pharmacokinetic properties and potential for drug interactions (see Chapter 83, Mood Disorders I: Major Depressive Disorders). Because there are no overall differences in efficacy among the four SSRIs approved for OCD, fluvoxamine is a suitable selection for R.G. However, the prescribed dosing instructions for R.G. are not appropriate. The initial recommended dosage for fluvoxamine in adults is 50 mg/day (25 mg in children), and it is best taken in the evening because it tends to be sedating. Using higher-than-necessary dosages can increase both adverse effects and medication costs, and these factors can lead to early termination of therapy. The dosage can be increased by 50-mg increments every 3 to 4 days according to patient tolerability, up to the initial targeted dose of 200 mg/day and a maximum of 300 mg/day.[190] Daily doses exceeding 100 mg should be given in two divided doses if once-daily dosing is not well tolerated.

ADJUNCTIVE COGNITIVE BEHAVIORAL THERAPY

The decision to include CBT in R.G.'s treatment plan is appropriate. The overall efficacy of these nonpharmacologic treatments is estimated to be 50% to 70% when used alone, and their use to complement pharmacotherapy is considered vital.[171] R.G.'s Y-BOCS score of 33 indicates a moderate-to-severe symptom severity, which provides further support for using a combined treatment approach. For R.G., exposure plus response prevention therapy might involve covering her hands with dirt and not allowing her to wash them for a certain time period. These behavioral techniques cause extreme anxiety and discomfort, which often lead to dropout from therapy or noncompliance with "homework assignments" (which involve continuation of the therapy principles outside the clinical setting), but are highly effective if the patient can adhere to treatment.

SELECTIVE SEROTONIN REUPTAKE INHIBITOR ADVERSE EFFECTS AND PATIENT COUNSELING

CASE 80-10, QUESTION 3: What patient counseling information should be provided to R.G. in conjunction with the prescribed treatments?

All OCD patients beginning treatment should be counseled that medication response occurs gradually and several weeks may elapse before beneficial effects become noticeable. It is important to emphasize that maximal response may take 3 months or longer and complete elimination of all symptoms is unlikely. It also is helpful to point out that a variety of other medications exist for those who do not respond adequately to an initial trial.

R.G. should be educated about possible fluvoxamine side effects, including nausea, sedation or insomnia, and headache. Medication should be taken with food to decrease these effects. Side effects are most common during the initial weeks of therapy, are usually dose related, and often subside with continued treatment. Other aspects of SSRI therapy, including additional adverse effects and their management and drug–drug interactions, are discussed in Chapter 83, Mood Disorders I: Major Depressive Disorders. Patients should be encouraged to report any problems to their treatment provider. The importance of adhering to prescribed therapies, both pharmacologic and behavioral, should also be stressed.

CASE 80-10, QUESTION 4: After 4 weeks, R.G. is taking fluvoxamine 200 mg daily and tolerating the medication well. She complains she has not noticed much improvement, and her Y-BOCS score is slightly decreased at 30. R.G. has been to the cognitive behavioral therapist twice but is reluctant to return because the therapy was so stressful. R.G. requests to be switched to a more effective medication, and she also asks to be given some alprazolam to help calm her anxiety during behavioral therapy sessions. What is the best course of action for R.G. at this point?

Switching to another medication is not recommended at this point because not enough time has elapsed to assess fluvoxamine's efficacy. R.G. is tolerating fluvoxamine well and has shown a mild improvement, so this medication should be continued for at least another 4 weeks. Additional counseling information should be provided to R.G. to emphasize the gradual response to treatment in OCD. An increase in fluvoxamine dosage, up to 250 or 300 mg/day, may be considered after several more weeks because some patients may respond better to higher dosages. If R.G.'s symptoms continue to cause significant functional impairment after 10 to 12 weeks of higher-dose fluvoxamine therapy, a change in treatment (e.g., switching to another SSRI or augmentation therapy) will be indicated.

R.G. should be encouraged to continue CBT to optimize the chance for successful treatment. An anxiety response is integral to the therapeutic benefits of behavioral therapies; because benzodiazepines can blunt this response, they may reduce their efficacy. Therefore, alprazolam should be avoided, and a temporary reduction in the intensity of behavioral therapy may be indicated instead. Fluvoxamine can also inhibit the CYP3A4-mediated metabolism of alprazolam, resulting in more pronounced effects from a given dose.

Course and Duration of Therapy

CASE 80-10, QUESTION 5: After 5 months of treatment, R.G. is happy to report her OCD is much improved (Y-BOCS score of 11). She still has intermittent obsessions related to contamination and doubting, but they are less intense than before. She is usually able to resist urges to clean and wash excessively and is using the stairs in their home with only mild discomfort. Her previous employer has agreed to let her return to her secretarial position when she is ready, and she plans to do so soon. R.G.'s husband is extremely pleased with her progress. Their primary question at this visit is whether treatment can be discontinued now because R.G. is doing so well. What recommendations should be provided regarding the long-term course of therapy for R.G.?

This case illustrates a common outcome of OCD treatment, in which some symptoms persist (as evidenced by a Y-BOCS score of 11), but significant improvements in functioning occur. It is currently recommended that effective treatment for OCD be continued for at least 1 year after response to reduce the risk of relapse. The effectiveness of maintenance pharmacotherapy in preventing relapse of OCD is well documented.[175,199] Therefore, continued drug treatment for at least 7 more months is indicated for R.G. Results from several studies suggest decreased medication doses (with SSRIs and clomipramine) during maintenance therapy are comparably as effective as full doses in preventing relapse.[199] If R.G. were experiencing any fluvoxamine-related problems, a decrease to the minimally effective dose (150 mg/day) during maintenance therapy might be recommended.

After a 1-year maintenance period, discontinuation of medication may be considered by carefully weighing the possible risks and benefits. When medication therapy for OCD is withdrawn, the dosage should be gradually decreased by approximately 25% every 1 to 2 months. Continuous monitoring for signs of relapse is required during this period. Gradual discontinuation also lessens the chance of the withdrawal syndrome often occurring after abrupt discontinuation of SSRI or TCA therapy (see Chapter 83, Mood Disorders I: Major Depressive Disorders). Long-term or even lifelong maintenance pharmacotherapy is usually recommended after two to four severe relapses or three to four less-severe relapses.

Clomipramine Treatment

DOSING GUIDELINES

CASE 80-11

QUESTION 1: K.T. is an 18-year-old Asian man who was diagnosed with OCD 2 years ago and also suffers from moderate depression. His physician plans to start him on clomipramine therapy because he has failed previous trials with paroxetine and fluvoxamine. Is clomipramine an appropriate choice of therapy for this patient? What recommendations can be made regarding initiation of clomipramine treatment?

Current guidelines recommend clomipramine be reserved for OCD patients who fail at least two SSRI trials; therefore, its choice for this patient is appropriate.[172] One precaution relevant to this case is that clomipramine, like other TCAs, is highly dangerous in overdose situations. Because K.T. is depressed, he should be evaluated carefully for any suicidal thoughts before starting clomipramine. If suicidal ideation is detected, it would be preferable to try another SSRI. This case also illustrates the common comorbidity of depression with OCD. Fortunately, most effective treatments for OCD fall into the antidepressant category, and drug treatment can be beneficial for both conditions. Nevertheless, the responses of depression and OCD to treatment are independent of one another, so depression may respond completely to a certain medication while OCD symptoms persist.[199]

Clomipramine should be initiated at a low dosage of 25 to 50 mg/day administered with meals. Divided daily doses are sometimes used initially to minimize side effects, but the total daily dose can be given at bedtime after dose titration. The pharmacokinetic parameters of clomipramine are comparable to those of other TCAs. Its average elimination half-life of approximately 24 hours makes once-daily dosing appropriate.[190,200]

The clomipramine dosage should be increased to an initial target range of 150 to 200 mg/day during 2 to 4 weeks, guided by patient tolerability. The maximal recommended daily dosage of clomipramine is 250 mg/day because of the sharply increased risk of seizures (2.1%–3.4%) with higher dosages as compared with the risk with dosages less than 250 mg/day (0.24%–0.48%).[201] Longer duration of clomipramine therapy may also increase the risk of seizures. Clomipramine should be used with caution in persons with a history of seizures, head injury, or any other factors that might lower the seizure threshold.

CLOMIPRAMINE SIDE EFFECTS AND MONITORING GUIDELINES

CASE 80-11, QUESTION 2: What guidelines should be recommended for monitoring the outcomes (both therapeutic and adverse) of clomipramine therapy?

Clomipramine is less well tolerated than the SSRIs and can cause a number of significant adverse effects, especially during the first few weeks of therapy. The most common side effects, reported in more than half of those taking clomipramine, include sedation, dry mouth, dizziness, and tremor.[201] Constipation, nausea, blurred vision, insomnia, and headache also occur frequently. K.T. should be advised these are not serious effects and that they usually subside with continued treatment.

Many patients receiving long-term clomipramine (and other TCA) therapy gain substantial amounts of weight. As with the SSRIs, sexual dysfunction can be a problem in both men and women. In men, clomipramine can cause ejaculation abnormalities, which can impair fertility. Patients taking clomipramine should also be counseled about the additive CNS depressant effects with alcohol and to be cautious about the possible sedative effects while driving or performing other potentially hazardous activities.

As with other TCAs, an ECG should be performed before starting clomipramine in individuals at risk for heart disease and in pediatric patients. Elevations in liver enzymes have been observed frequently during the first 3 months of clomipramine treatment, and baseline liver function tests should also be obtained before initiating treatment. The liver enzyme changes are reversible on discontinuation of clomipramine therapy.

No therapeutic range for plasma drug concentrations has been firmly established for clomipramine in OCD, but monitoring plasma levels may be clinically useful in certain patients to guide dosing and minimize drug toxicity. Clomipramine metabolism is highly variable from one person to the next, and it is difficult to accurately predict the resulting clomipramine level from any given dose. The initial hepatic metabolism of tertiary TCAs such as clomipramine involves demethylation through various isozymes, including CYP1A2, CYP2C19, and CYP3A4.[200,202] Both the parent drug (clomipramine) and the primary active metabolite (*N*-desmethylclomipramine) then undergo CYP2D6-mediated hydroxylation. Therefore, the metabolism of clomipramine will be affected by combination with any agent inhibiting CYP1A2, CYP2C19, CYP3A4, or CYP2D6. Clinically significant drug interactions are possible with several of the SSRIs, including fluoxetine, paroxetine, fluvoxamine, and sertraline (see Chapter 83, Mood Disorders I: Major Depressive Disorders).

Although various studies have failed to find a correlation between clomipramine plasma level and clinical response, the ratio of clomipramine to *N*-desmethylclomipramine may be important.[203] Clomipramine is primarily serotonergic, whereas *N*-desmethylclomipramine is more noradrenergic; higher levels of *N*-desmethylclomipramine relative to clomipramine have been associated with poorer clinical response. Factors impairing the CYP2D6-mediated elimination of *N*-desmethylclomipramine (concurrent medications that are potent CYP2D6 inhibitors, CYP2D6 poor metabolizers) may possibly decrease the efficacy of clomipramine by shifting the metabolic ratio in an undesired direction.

Asian patients such as K.T. have been found to have significantly decreased clearance of clomipramine and higher clomipramine to *N*-desmethylclomipramine ratios compared with whites, which may necessitate use of lower doses.[204] This is probably caused by a genetic polymorphism of either CYP2C19 or CYP2D6, which results in decreased metabolic capacity via these metabolic pathways in the Asian population. Careful monitoring for possible signs of toxicity should accompany dose increases, and the clomipramine plasma level should be checked in those patients (Asian or otherwise) who show unexpected effects with usual doses. An opposite effect has been described in ultra-rapid CYP2D6 metabolizers, in which unusually high clomipramine dosages may be required for therapeutic efficacy.

CLOMIPRAMINE AUGMENTATION

CASE 80-11, QUESTION 3: After 10 weeks of taking clomipramine 100 mg at bedtime, K.T. has shown partial response. He continues to experience mild-to-moderate anticholinergic side effects and frequent daytime fatigue. His plasma clomipramine level is relatively high for the given dose at 453 ng/mL (clomipramine plus desmethylclomipramine). The physician decides to add another drug to augment treatment. Considering K.T.'s current medication regimen and the evidence supporting the different augmentation strategies, which drug would be the best choice for K.T.?

Many different agents have been used to augment response to either an SSRI or clomipramine. An SSRI could be added to clomipramine. Of the SSRIs, fluvoxamine, fluoxetine, paroxetine, and sertraline are all approved as monotherapy for OCD, and any of these would be likely to augment therapy. However, when adding an SSRI to a TCA, the potential for drug interactions should always be considered. Clomipramine is metabolized by CYP1A2, CYP3A4, CYP2C19, and CYP2D6.[200,202,205,206] The CYP2D6 pathway is particularly important because it is the rate-limiting metabolic pathway for elimination of both clomipramine and desmethylclomipramine. Fluvoxamine, paroxetine, and fluoxetine are all important inhibitors of clomipramine metabolism. Sertraline also has the potential to cause a clinically significant interaction with clomipramine. Alternatively, escitalopram and citalopram would not be likely to cause a significant drug interaction, but evidence for their efficacy as augmenting agents in combination with clomipramine is lacking. A combination less likely to be associated with a drug interaction is the combination of clomipramine and a second-generation antipsychotic. Trials comparing the effectiveness of antipsychotic augmentation have been published, but most combined antipsychotics with SSRIs rather than clomipramine. Risperidone, olanzapine, and quetiapine have been studied in well-designed trials, whereas numerous publications have reported on the use of other antipsychotics as augmentation in SSRI treatment of OCD in case series or open trials. Unfortunately, most of the well-designed studies are small (<30 patients). However, a meta-analysis of the available data suggested risperidone was most effective (at a dose near 2 mg/day), and haloperidol was the next most effective agent.[193] Haloperidol would not be the optimal choice in K.T. because it inhibits clomipramine metabolism, and as a first-generation antipsychotic, it is associated with numerous side effects.

KEY REFERENCES AND WEBSITES

A full list of references for this chapter can be found at http://thepoint.lww.com/AT10e. Below are the key references and website for this chapter, with the corresponding reference number in this chapter found in parentheses after the reference.

Key References

ACOG Committee on Practice Bulletins—Obstetrics. ACOG Practice Bulletin: Clinical management guidelines for obstetrician-gynecologists number 92, April 2008 (replaces practice bulletin number 87, November 2007). Use of psychiatric medications during pregnancy and lactation. *Obstet Gynecol.* 2008;111:1001. (85)

American Psychiatric Association. *Diagnostic and Statistical Manual of Mental Disorders.* 4th ed. Text Revision. Washington, DC: American Psychiatric Association; 2000. (1)

American Psychiatric Association. *Practice Guideline for the Treatment of Patients With Obsessive-Compulsive Disorder.* Arlington, VA: American Psychiatric Association; 2007. (172)

Brawman-Mintzer O. Pharmacologic treatment of generalized anxiety disorder. *Psychiatr Clin North Am.* 2001;24:119. (17)

Davidson JR et al. A psychopharmacologic treatment algorithm for generalised anxiety disorder (GAD). *J Psychopharmacol.* 2010;24:3. (54)

Katzman MA. Current considerations in the treatment of generalized anxiety disorder. *CNS Drugs.* 2009;23:103. (52)

Mathew SJ et al. Recent advances in the neurobiology of anxiety; implications for novel therapeutics. *Am J Med Genet C Semin Med Genet.* 2008;148C:89. (6)

Muller JE et al. Anxiety and medical disorders. *Curr Psychiatry Rep.* 2005;7:245. (122)

Ravindran LN, Stein MB. The pharmacologic treatment of anxiety disorders: a review of progress. *J Clin Psychiatry.* 2010;71:839. (46)

Ravindran LN, Stein MB. Pharmacotherapy of PTSD: premises, principles, and priorities. *Brain Res.* 2009;1293:24. (155)

Shalev AY. Posttraumatic stress disorder and stress-related disorders. *Psychiatr Clin North Am.* 2009;32:687. (144)

Stein DJ et al. A 2010 evidence-based algorithm for the pharmacotherapy of social anxiety disorder. *Curr Psychiatry Rep.* 2010;12:471. (138)

Stein MB, Stein DJ. Social anxiety disorder. *Lancet.* 2008;371:1115. (133)

Key Website

Treatment of Patients With Panic Disorder. 2nd ed. **http://www.psychiatryonline.com/pracGuideTopic_9.aspx.** Accessed October 23, 2010. (111)

81 Sleep Disorders

Julie A. Dopheide and Glen L. Stimmel

CORE PRINCIPLES

	CHAPTER CASES
INSOMNIA AND RESULTING DAYTIME SLEEPINESS	
1 Asking the right questions to investigate the type of insomnia (i.e., trouble falling asleep, staying asleep, or early morning awakening), possible causes (lifestyle issues, drugs), resulting impairment, and concomitant conditions is essential to determine proper management.	**Case 81-1 (Questions 1, 2)**
2 Nonpharmacologic treatments such as sleep hygiene and cognitive-behavioral interventions are recommended first-line therapy for managing insomnia in a variety of patients owing to high efficacy and avoidance of medication side effects.	**Case 81-1 (Questions 3, 4)**
3 Pharmacologic treatments for insomnia are selected based on their efficacy, tolerability, onset and duration of effect, potential for next day hangover, and abuse potential.	**Case 81-1 (Questions 5–9)**
4 Insomnia concurrent with medical illness is frequently chronic (>1 month), and if left untreated, it may affect recovery from the medical condition. Treating both conditions at the same time is recommended.	**Case 81-2 (Questions 1–4)**
5 Insomnia concurrent with psychiatric illness requires optimization of psychiatric maintenance medications and the judicious use of hypnotic medications based on type of sleep complaint and substance abuse history.	**Case 81-3 (Questions 1–4)**
6 Managing insomnia in an elderly individual involves consideration of age-related pharmacodynamic and pharmacokinetic changes and counseling regarding realistic treatment expectations. Medication doses lower than those used in younger individuals should be prescribed.	**Case 81-4 (Questions 1–5)**
7 Neuropsychiatric disorders such as attention deficit hyperactivity disorder and autism spectrum disorders are associated with high rates of insomnia in children and adolescents. Melatonin has evidence for efficacy, whereas zolpidem studies show limited benefit and a notable risk of psychiatric side effects.	**Case 81-5 (Questions 1–3)**
8 If nonpharmacologic treatment is ineffective, diphenhydramine is considered safe for short-term use (<1 week) in pregnancy. Risks outweigh benefits for benzodiazepines and Z-hypnotics in pregnancy.	**Case 81-6 (Questions 1, 2)**
SLEEP APNEA	
1 Sleep apnea leads to excessive daytime sleepiness, fatigue, and increased risk of cardiovascular and cerebrovascular disease. Effective treatment with continuous positive airway pressure or surgical interventions can decrease cardiovascular disease and improve overall functioning and quality of life.	**Case 81-8 (Questions 1, 2)**
2 It is essential to avoid sedating medications in patients with sleep apnea because these agents interfere with mini-arousals that keep the patient alive.	**Case 81-8 (Question 3)**

continued

NARCOLEPSY

1	Narcolepsy is an incurable neurologic disease characterized by sleep attacks and cataplexy. Stimulants modafinil or armodafinil help decrease sleep attacks and promote daytime alertness but they do not help with cataplexy or nocturnal insomnia.	**Case 81-9 (Questions 1, 2)**
2	Sodium oxybate is effective for cataplexy and improves nocturnal sleep, but it has high abuse potential and has been associated with psychiatric side effects.	**Case 81-9 (Questions 3, 4)**

SOCIETAL IMPACT

The impact of sleep disorders on overall health, productivity, and quality of life has been increasingly appreciated. Untreated sleep disorders, including chronic insomnia, sleep apnea, periodic limb movements during sleep (PLMS), and narcolepsy, are all associated with diminished mental and physical functioning and poor quality of life.[1–3] Sleep research shows that chronic insomnia, for example, can predict untreated illness or may contribute to injury and illness.[1–5]

Chronic insomnia is associated with immune system dysregulation and the release of proinflammatory cytokines (interleukin [IL] 6 and tumor necrosis factor-α), a disruption of the hypothalamic-pituitary-adrenal axis, and a depletion of brain serotonin and other neurotransmitters.[5] Persons with insomnia are 10 times more likely to suffer from depression and 17 times more likely to have anxiety compared with people without insomnia.[4] Chronic insomnia is two to three times more common in individuals with high blood pressure, breathing difficulties, gastrointestinal (GI) disorders, cancer, and chronic pain, among other conditions.[6] Insomnia and excessive daytime sleepiness (EDS) in the elderly are leading predictors of institutionalization.[2]

In 2005, a National Institutes of Health (NIH) panel of sleep experts recommended a major shift regarding insomnia. The panel stated that insomnia is not just a symptom of a medical or psychiatric illness but a condition that contributes to the severity of that disease or disorder. Indeed, when insomnia is effectively treated, concomitant medical and psychiatric conditions, such as chronic pain or depression, are relieved along with improvement in functioning and quality of life. The relationship between insomnia and medical or psychiatric illness is bidirectional.[2,5] Instead of categorizing insomnia as either primary (with no other concomitant disorder) or secondary, it should be categorized as either primary or comorbid (insomnia that occurs concomitant with medical or psychiatric illness).[4]

Excessive sleepiness caused by a sleep disorder or sleep deprivation constitutes a serious public health hazard in health care workers, firefighters, police officers, truck drivers, and the general public.[7] An alert mind is crucial for maximal productivity in all occupations, particularly when driving is involved. A 2010 phone survey of 1,728 drivers conducted by the Automobile Association of America (AAA) found that 41% of respondents admitted to having fallen asleep at the wheel at some point in their lifetime.[8] Analysis of passenger car crashes from 1999 to 2008 found that 16.5% of all fatal crashes involved drowsy drivers.[8] Motor vehicle accidents also tend to peak during the early morning (1 AM to 6 AM) and mid afternoon (2 PM to 4 PM) hours—times when the circadian cycle for sleepiness is maximal.[7] College students with short sleep times (≤6 hours/night) had lower grade point averages than long sleepers (≥9 hours). Mid range sleepers (7–8 hours) were not significantly different from long sleepers.[9] Medical interns made 35.9% more errors in the medical intensive care and cardiac care units when working a 24-hour shift compared with those working 16 hours.[10] Medical resident shifts are now limited to 12 to 16 hours to improve patient safety.[10]

EPIDEMIOLOGY

Sleep Disorders

One in seven Americans has a longstanding sleep–wake disorder.[3,4,11–13] During the course of a year, approximately 30% of the population will experience insomnia, and approximately one-third of this group will consider the problem severe.[2,4] Insomnia is defined as requiring longer than 30 minutes to fall asleep, awakenings throughout the night without immediate return to sleep, early-morning awakening, or total sleep time decreased to less than 6 hours.[2,4,13] Insomnia is the most common sleep complaint, but the resulting daytime sleepiness and fatigue are troubling aftereffects. Insomnia is categorized into three general types: transient (lasting a few days), short-term (lasting <4 weeks), or chronic (persisting for ≥1 month). The resulting level of daytime impairment should be assessed to determine insomnia severity.[4,5,13,14]

Major sleep disorders in order of decreasing prevalence are listed in Table 81-1.[2,3] Nightmares, nocturnal leg cramps, and snoring are more benign sleep disorders. Nightmares occur in 5% to 30% of children 3 to 6 years of age, and approximately 2% to 6% of adults have weekly nightmares.[15] Sleepwalking occurs in 1% to 2% of the population. Complex sleep behavior disorders, such as driving or eating while still half-asleep, are uncommon to rare. These behaviors are more common in people taking hypnotic medications, and in these patients, counseling is needed.[15,16] In 2007, the US Food and Drug Administration (FDA) issued a black-box warning that applies to all medications marketed for insomnia. It warns of the risk of angioedema (facial

TABLE 81-1
Incidence of Major Sleep Disorders[3,4,11–13]

Sleep Disorder	Incidence (%)
Insomnia	30–35
Transient (few days)	
Short-term (up to 1 month)	
Chronic (>1 month)	
Sleep apnea	5–15
PLMS (nocturnal myoclonus)	5–15
RLS	5–15
Narcolepsy	0.06

PLMS, periodic limb movements during sleep; RLS, restless legs syndrome.

swelling), an allergic reaction, as well as complex sleep behaviors as described above.[16]

Hypnotic Use

Cognitive-behavioral therapy (CBT) is the preferred treatment for insomnia because of well-established efficacy, absence of drug side effects, and sustained benefit with time.[4,14,17–19] Hypnotic medications are recommended when nondrug interventions fail or cannot be implemented, or when rapid results are essential.[4,14,20]

Prescribing trends have shifted away from older benzodiazepine hypnotics toward newer benzodiazepine receptor–active "Z-hypnotics" (zaleplon, zolpidem, eszopiclone), sedating antidepressants (i.e., trazodone), and sedating antipsychotics such as quetiapine.[20] Age, sex, and socioeconomic status influence hypnotic prescribing. One study of 2,966 outpatient visits for insomnia or sleep complaint between 1996 and 2001 showed that 48% received a prescription for medication only—with no CBT. Z-hypnotics were prescribed at 25% of these visits. Factors that increased the likelihood of receiving a Z-hypnotic included female sex, concomitant psychiatric illness, and upper socioeconomic status.[21]

An analysis of 147,945 patient-visits for sleep difficulty between 1997 and 2002 in the United States showed that women were 1.5 times more likely to have insomnia-related visits. In all ages, the most frequently prescribed or recommended medications were either zaleplon or zolpidem (28.5%), and trazodone (32%). Temazepam was prescribed for 16% to 18% of patients, and triazolam and flurazepam were prescribed for 5% to 8% of patients.[22]

With aging, sleep typically changes in quality, partially because of sleep disruption related to chronic illnesses.[23,24] Elderly persons consume more sleep-promoting medications than younger adults. The 2003 National Sleep Foundation's "Sleep in America" poll found that 11% of older adults take prescription medications to promote sleep compared with 6% of younger adults.[23]

THE SLEEP STAGES

Normal Sleep

Each sleep stage serves a physiologic function and can be monitored in sleep laboratories by polysomnography. Polysomnography is the term used to describe three electrophysiologic measures: the electroencephalogram (EEG), the electromyogram, and the electro-oculogram. The pattern of brain waves, muscle tone, and eye movements can be used to categorize sleep as rapid eye movement (REM) sleep or nonrapid eye movement (NREM) sleep.[25,26]

Nonrapid Eye Movement Sleep

NREM sleep is divided further into four stages, with different quantities of time spent in each stage. Stage 1 is a transition between sleep and wakefulness known as *relaxed wakefulness,* which generally makes up approximately 2% to 5% of sleep. Approximately 50% of total sleep time is spent in stage 2, which is rapid-wave (alpha) or lighter sleep. Stages 3 and 4 are slow-wave (delta) or deep sleep. Stage 3 occupies an average of 5% of sleep time, whereas stage 4 constitutes 10% to 15% of sleep time in young, healthy adults. At sleep onset, the brain quickly passes through stage 1 and moves to stage 2. Muscle activity shuts down, and brain waves become less active. After a brief REM period, the brain moves into slow-wave sleep (NREM stages 3 and 4) approximately 1 to 3 hours after a person falls asleep. The body continually moves through all of the sleep stages over the course of the night (Fig. 81-1). REM periods become longer, and deep sleep lessens during the last half of the night.[25–27]

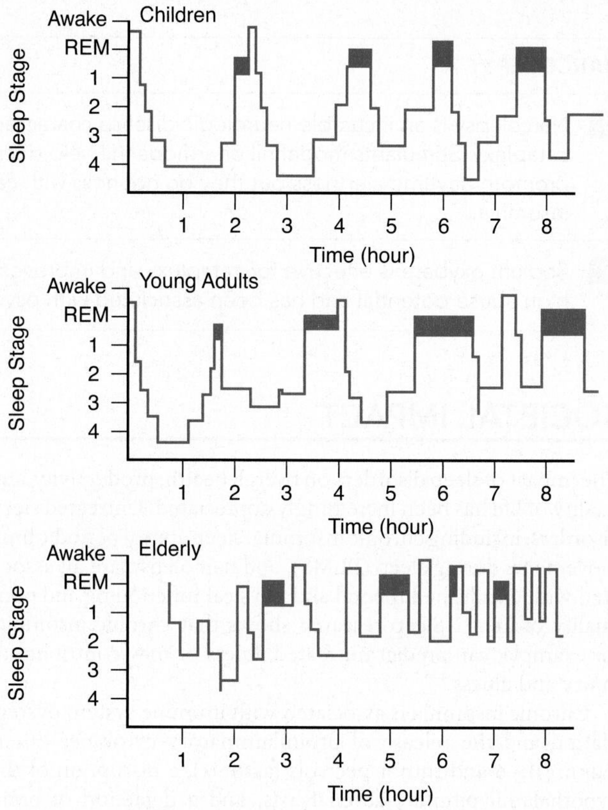

FIGURE 81-1 Normal sleep cycles.

NREM sleep stages differ qualitatively as well as quantitatively. The function of stage 1 is to initiate sleep. Stage 2 provides rest for the muscles and brain through muscle atonia and low-voltage brain wave activity. Arousability from sleep is highest during stages 1 and 2. In contrast, it is difficult to awaken someone during stages 3 and 4, or delta sleep. Delta sleep, also known as *restorative sleep,* is enhanced by serotonin, adenosine, cholecystokinin, and IL-1. The ability of IL-1 to promote slow-wave sleep supports a widely held theory linking deep sleep to the augmentation of immune function. Some hormones (e.g., somatostatin, growth hormone) are released mainly during slow-wave sleep. Deep sleep is most abundant in infants and children and tends to level off at approximately 4 hours a night during adolescence.[25,26] At age 65, deep sleep accounts for only 10% of sleep, and at age 75, it often is nonexistent.[25,27] Age-related increased awakenings, decreased deep sleep, and daytime sleepiness have been associated with increases in cortisol and the proinflammatory cytokine, IL-6.[5,24,26]

Rapid Eye Movement Sleep

Whereas NREM sleep is necessary for rest and rejuvenation, the purpose of REM sleep remains a mystery. REM sleep is also called *paradoxical sleep* because it has aspects of both deep sleep and light sleep. Body and brainstem functions appear to be in a deep sleep state as muscle and sympathetic tone drop dramatically. In contrast, neurochemical processes and higher cortical brain function appear active. Dreaming is associated closely with REM sleep, and when a person is awakened from REM, alertness returns relatively quickly.

Numerous physiologic functions are altered during REM sleep. Breathing is irregular, consisting of sudden changes in respiratory amplitude and frequency corresponding to bursts of REM. Temperature control is lost and the body temperature typically lowers. REM sleep brings on variability in heart rate, blood pressure (BP), cerebral blood flow, and metabolism. Cardiac output and urine volume decrease. Blood may become thicker as a result of autonomic instability and temperature changes.[26,28]

REM periods cycle approximately every 90 minutes throughout the night. Duration of REM increases in the last half of the night, becoming longer and more intense just after the time when body temperature is at its lowest, around 5 AM. Although the reason for the importance of REM sleep is unknown, it is clear that the human body needs REM sleep. When deprived of REM sleep, whether through poor sleep, drugs, or disease states, the brain and body try to catch up. REM rebound occurs, which may result in vivid dreams or an overall less restful sleep.[25–27]

Abnormal Sleep

Primary insomnia (difficulty sleeping not attributable to a drug, psychiatric disorder, or medical condition) can resemble a normal sleep pattern, but may be associated with an increased time to fall asleep, multiple awakenings, or decreased total sleep time. Polysomnographic readings evaluating insomnia secondary to psychiatric disorders can be markedly different. In depressive disorders, decreased REM latency (i.e., the time from sleep onset to the appearance of REM) is a classic finding. Acute psychotic disorders feature prolonged global sleeplessness, with sleep onset latency, fragmented sleep, and decreased slow-wave sleep. Medical disorders (e.g., arthritis, cancer, infections) can be associated with significantly altered sleep-stage patterns. Uncontrolled pain can result in frequent awakenings and decreased total sleep time. Oxygen saturation is at its lowest during REM sleep; therefore, less time in REM may be advantageous for patients with cystic fibrosis and other breathing disorders.[25,26,28]

Primary sleep disorders, including PLMS, can cause intermittent partial arousals out of stage 2 sleep and can impair the progress to slow-wave sleep. This may disrupt the quality of sleep and contribute to daytime impairment. Sleep apnea syndrome signals the brain to initiate multiple mini-arousals in response to breathing cessation during sleep and, therefore, decreases the quality of sleep. Patients with narcolepsy may have a unique pattern of sleep disruption because they fall almost immediately into REM sleep (instead of the usual 90-minute latency) and may experience an increased number of REM episodes.[3]

Although polysomnographic readings from sleep laboratories are interesting and can be useful diagnostic and assessment tools, they are not routinely available and the costs are not routinely reimbursable by insurers. A thorough history of sleep problems obtained through patient interviews, along with both physical and psychiatric evaluations, are the most widely used methods of patient assessment. Although acknowledging the usefulness of clinical assessment, certain patients with more serious sleep problems, such as sleep apnea, narcolepsy, or excessive daytime impairment, should have sleep laboratory evaluations.

NEUROCHEMISTRY OF SLEEP–WAKE CYCLE

Wakefulness- and Sleep-Promoting Neurochemicals

A basic understanding of brain neurochemistry is essential in understanding sleep disorders and the clinical use of hypnotics. Hypnotics exert their effects by modulating brain neurotransmitters and neuropeptides (e.g., serotonin, norepinephrine, acetylcholine, histamine, adenosine, and γ-aminobutyric acid [GABA]). The neuronal systems in which neurotransmitters and neuropeptides act to control the sleep–wake cycle lie in the brainstem, hypothalamus, and basal forebrain, with connections in the thalamus and cortex. Noradrenergic, histaminergic, and acetylcholine-containing neurons promote wakefulness as they modulate cortical and subcortical neurons. Excitatory amino acids, such as glutamate, and stimulating neuropeptides (e.g., substance P, thyrotropin-releasing factor, corticotropin-releasing factor) also promote wakefulness.[27] Hypocretin 1 and 2, also known as orexin A and B, are neuropeptides that modulate the sleep–wake cycle. Hypocretin 1 and 2 are deficient in people with narcolepsy and primary hypersomnia.[29,30]

Wakefulness and sleep are antagonistic states competing for control of brain activity. Sleep takes over as the wakefulness-maintaining neuronal systems weaken and sleep-promoting neurons become active. Serotonin-containing neurons of the brainstem raphe dampen sensory input and inhibit motor activity, promoting the emergence of slow-wave sleep.[5,25,27,31] Opiate peptides (e.g., enkephalin, endorphin) and GABA, an inhibitory neurotransmitter, also promote sleep.[27,31–33]

Drug-Induced Effects on Neurochemicals

The neurochemistry of sleep also can be understood by considering the effect of hypnotic drugs on specific neurotransmitters. GABA is facilitated when a benzodiazepine compound attaches to the GABA–chloride-ionophore complex and causes chloride channels to open and inhibit overexcited areas of the brain. GABA-facilitating hypnotics, such as benzodiazepines, induce sleep and decrease arousals between stages, providing more continuous stage 2 sleep. Benzodiazepines, however, also may decrease stage 4 slow-wave sleep and suppress REM, leading to REM rebound on abrupt discontinuation.[27,31,33–35] Some antihistamines promote sleep by blocking histamine-containing neurons involved in maintaining wakefulness. The excitatory effects of caffeine and other methylxanthines are attributed to their antagonism of adenosine receptors. Adenosine is a sleep-promoting neurotransmitter or neuromodulator.[27,30]

Neurotransmitter alteration may or may not affect REM sleep. Drug-induced noradrenergic and serotonergic modulation usually decreases REM sleep. An increase in dopaminergic neurotransmission can increase wakefulness but has no direct effect on REM sleep.[27,32] In contrast, increased cholinergic neurotransmission triggers REM sleep.[27,32] Cortisol decreases REM sleep in young and old with unpredictable effects on slow-wave sleep and increased wakefulness in the elderly.[5,25,34,36] It is useful to think of the brain centers, neurochemicals, and neuropeptides involved as an interactive network regulating our sleep–wake cycle. Certainly, drugs or disease states that alter neurotransmission can have significant impact on the sleep–wake cycle. Sensory input (visual and acoustic) works with the internal network and signals brain centers to either wake or sleep. Thus, darkness is a visual cue that prepares the brain for sleep. Similarly, bright light serves to prepare the brain for wakefulness.[25,37]

PATIENT ASSESSMENT

Questions to Ask Patients

The first step in patient assessment is to determine whether the sleep problem is difficulty falling asleep, difficulty maintaining

TABLE 81-2
Classification of Sleep Disorders[5,13,15]

Dyssomnias[a]
Intrinsic: idiopathic insomnia, narcolepsy, sleep apnea, periodic limb movements during sleep
Extrinsic: inadequate sleep hygiene, substance-induced sleep disorder
Circadian rhythm sleep disorders: jet lag, shift work, delayed sleep-phase syndrome
Parasomnias[b]
Arousal: confusional arousals, sleepwalking, sleep terrors
Sleep–wake transition disorders: sleep talking, nocturnal leg cramps
Associated with REM: nightmares, sleep paralysis, impaired sleep-related penile erections
Other: primary snoring, sudden infant death syndrome, sleep bruxism
Medical, Psychiatric, and Substance-Induced Sleep Disorders
Associated with mental disorders: mood disorders, anxiety disorders, psychotic disorders
Associated with neurologic disorders: Parkinson disease, Huntington disease, dementia
Associated with other medical disorders: heart disease, renal insufficiency, pulmonary disease
Associated with a substance: medication/substance abuse (e.g., phenylpropanolamine, cocaine)
Proposed Sleep Disorders
Menstrual-associated sleep disorder, pregnancy-associated sleep disorder, short or long sleeper

[a]Any sleep pattern that is abnormal (e.g., insomnia or excessive sleepiness).
[b]Any unusual behavior that emerges during sleep.

sleep, early-morning awakening, poor-quality sleep, or EDS. Answers to the questions, "How long does it take you to fall asleep, and how many hours do you sleep?" should be compared with the patient's normal sleep pattern to determine how it varies. Questions such as "How do you feel during the day: well rested, sleepy, or something else?" can help assess functional impairment. Not all patients need the same amount of sleep. Approximately 7 to 9 hours of sleep is optimal for most people: too much sleep can be as problematic as too little sleep.[13,25,38] The International Classification of Sleep Disorders and the Diagnostic and Statistical Manual of Mental Disorders, Fourth Edition, Text Revision (DSM-IV-TR) have categorized sleep disorders largely based on pathophysiology and presumed etiology rather than numbers of hours of sleep.[39,40] Four main categories of sleep disorders are useful for clinical assessment (Table 81-2). The next step in patient assessment involves investigating the possible causes of the sleep disorder and any concomitant conditions. All medical, psychiatric, drug, environmental, and social causes must be considered and treated along with the sleep disorder. The degree of functional impairment should be assessed to evaluate the severity of the disorder.

Setting Treatment Expectations

WHAT IS NORMAL SLEEP?

When patients seek treatment for insomnia, it is important that appropriate expectations are set. Both the patient and caregivers need to understand normal sleep and appropriate therapeutic end points.[38] Unlike what many patients expect, normal sleep is not immediate unconsciousness that lasts 8 hours without interruption every night. Rather, normal sleep is more appropriately viewed as some nights when sleep latency is a little longer, some nights with occasional interruptions in sleep, and some nights of 5, 6, or 7 hours rather than 8 hours of sleep. Attempts to treat sleep complaints will fail unless the patient understands that normal sleep means a return to a pattern of natural variations in sleep.[38]

Nonpharmacologic Treatment

Cognitive-behavioral therapies (CBTs) are the most effective interventions for insomnia according to the American Academy of Sleep Medicine and the NIH. These interventions can take 2 to 10 weeks to successfully implement based on the individual and the severity and chronicity of that person's insomnia; however, results are long-lasting. Table 81-3 lists established cognitive and behavioral interventions with brief descriptions in addition to some sleep-hygiene tips to include in patient counseling. Sleep-hygiene techniques have not been demonstrated as effective without adjunctive CBT.[4,14]

The sleep environment should be dark and comfortable, free from noise or distractions, and not too warm or too cold. Along with creating a sleep-friendly setting, establishing regular sleep hours, particularly a regular wake time, is necessary to condition the body to sleep. Even after a poor night's sleep, it is important for healthy sleepers to avoid daytime naps and stay awake until the regular sleep time. In some cases, brief (e.g., 20-minute) naps may be refreshing without disrupting nocturnal sleep. Phototherapy, bright light exposure for 30 minutes to 1 hour on awakening in the morning, is an additional tool that can help set the circadian rhythm for regular sleep–wake cycles.[14,20,37] Healthy sleep often can be facilitated by avoiding problem-solving activities (e.g., finances, crossword puzzles), strenuous physical exercise, or exciting movies while in bed. Exercise early in the day can improve sleep. Exercise should be completed before dinner time so that the body has a few hours to relax before it is time to sleep. Relaxation is the key to healthy sleep. If a patient finds himself or herself tossing, turning, or worrying, it is time to get out of bed and stretch, read, or listen to soft music to relax. Health care practitioners should remind patients to avoid large meals at bedtime because the digestion of heavy meals can impair sleep. Last,

TABLE 81-3
Nonpharmacologic Treatments for Insomnia[14,19]

1. Cognitive-behavioral therapy: most effective; can be from any trained provider.
   Cognitive: identify and stop thought patterns that interfere with sleep (e.g., "I'm never going to sleep" or allowing 15 minutes to review a worry list, then putting worries aside).
   Behavioral: stimulus control, sleep restriction, relaxation, paradoxical intention.
   (a) Stimulus control: train the brain to reassociate the bed and bedroom with sleep and re-establish a consistent sleep–wake schedule.
   (b) Sleep restriction: create "sleep-debt" by curtailing amount of time in bed, then increasing time in bed as sleep efficiency improves.
   (c) Relaxation therapy: progressive tensing and relaxing of muscles, yoga, stretching.
   (d) Paradoxical intention: encourage patient to engage in most-feared behavior, "staying awake," to reduce performance anxiety associated with trying to sleep.
2. Sleep hygiene: not considered effective on its own; useful adjunctive treatment.
   Avoid caffeine, stimulants, heavy meals, and alcohol at bedtime; exercise early in the day before dinner to relieve stress and prime brain for sleep. Turn the face of the clock away from view; establish a before-bedtime ritual, make sure bedroom is dark, quiet, comfortable

chemicals that can disrupt sleep (e.g., alcohol, caffeine, other stimulants) should be eliminated when possible.[14,20,22]

Pharmacologic Treatment

When rapid relief of transient or short-term insomnia is needed or when chronic insomnia persists despite nondrug therapeutic interventions, hypnotic medication is indicated. Benzodiazepine hypnotics or newer, benzodiazepine Ω-1 selective hypnotics, sometimes called "Z-hypnotics," are first-line therapies because they offer significantly greater efficacy than over-the-counter (OTC) products; they are safer than barbiturates and are more effective compared with sedating antidepressants.[4,20,41]

Some patients need pharmacologic treatment for insomnia but do not seek treatment from their health care providers.[4,21] Alcohol and OTC sleep aids containing antihistamines are widely used to self-medicate insomnia, although the results are less than ideal.[4,20]

The ideal hypnotic has a rapid onset of effect (within 20 minutes, the natural time to fall asleep), helps the patient sleep throughout the night, does not cause daytime impairment, and has no abuse potential. Currently, there are no ideal hypnotics. Hypnotics that act at benzodiazepine receptors come closest to the ideal.[42] Available agents vary in onset, duration, and potential for daytime impairment, mostly because of their individual pharmacokinetic profiles.[41,42] The selection of the appropriate hypnotic should consider the type of insomnia to be treated and the physiologic characteristics of the patient. For example, if someone cannot fall asleep but has no trouble staying asleep and wants no carryover effect into the next day, a rapid-acting hypnotic with a short half-life and no active metabolites is desirable.[20,42]

Less common sleep disorders are treated with a variety of medications as well as some nondrug therapies. PLMS and restless legs syndrome (RLS) can be relieved with dopamine agonists, opioids, gabapentin, or clonazepam.[3] Narcolepsy is best treated with planned naps, modafinil, stimulants, sodium oxybate, or select antidepressants.[3] Both sleep apnea and primary snoring can be worsened with central nervous system (CNS) depressants but usually improve with nondrug therapies such as continuous positive airway pressure (CPAP).[43] Sleep disturbances associated with medical and psychiatric diagnoses require special attention because a hypnotic can either improve or worsen the problem.[5,13]

INSOMNIA IN A NORMALLY HEALTHY PATIENT

CASE 81-1

QUESTION 1: E.P., a 31-year-old woman, is requesting a medication for treatment of her insomnia. She returned to California from Hong Kong 2 days ago and is now having difficulty getting to sleep. When she arrived in Hong Kong, she went to sleep immediately at 4 PM and awoke at 3 AM. Her sleep pattern adjusted during her 6-week visit in Hong Kong, but on returning to California, it now takes her 2 to 3 hours to fall asleep. She has difficulty awakening in the morning and, as a result, sleeps past noon. She needs to be alert during the day to fulfill her obligations as a school teacher. What information provided by E.P. is important in the assessment of her insomnia? What additional information should be obtained from E.P. to assist in the assessment of her sleep disturbance?

E.P. describes a time-zone shift or disruption in circadian rhythm, which is a common cause of transient insomnia. Her major complaint is difficulty falling asleep, because she reports no trouble staying asleep or awakening too early. It is important for E.P. not to be sedated during the day because she is a teacher. Additional information needed from E.P. includes the duration of insomnia, methods already tried to relieve insomnia and their efficacy, concomitant medications, coexisting medical or psychiatric problems, alcohol use, caffeine use, and current life stresses. E.P. should be advised that assessing all of the aforementioned information is necessary in treating her sleep problem.

CASE 81-1, QUESTION 2: In response to your additional questions, you learn that E.P. has no medical problems and takes no prescription medications. She has been taking pseudoephedrine at night for nasal stuffiness since returning from Hong Kong. She denies drinking alcoholic beverages and coffee but admits to recently increasing her tea intake to try to stay awake during the day. She denies a long history of insomnia, but adds, "I have not been able to sleep as well in my new apartment; I don't know why." What factors could be contributing to E.P.'s complaints?

Several factors are contributing to E.P.'s type of insomnia, which can be classified as circadian rhythm sleep disorder related to jet lag. Her circadian rhythm has been disrupted because of travel, but she also takes a stimulating decongestant (i.e., pseudoephedrine) and drinks a caffeine-containing beverage (i.e., tea). In addition, she sleeps in new surroundings that may require time for adjustment. All these factors can contribute to her difficulty in falling asleep. Circadian rhythm sleep disorder results from a mismatch between the sleep–wake schedule required by a person's environment and the circadian sleep–wake pattern.

NONPRESCRIPTION SLEEP AIDS

CASE 81-1, QUESTION 3: E.P. would like to purchase a nonprescription sleep medication. What would you recommend?

An individual risk-versus-benefit assessment is essential before recommending any medication, even OTC products. Most nonprescription sleep aids contain antihistamines such as diphenhydramine. Antihistamines can cause drowsiness and can help patients fall asleep. The ability to cause sedation does not necessarily lead to hypnotic efficacy. Some patients do not feel well rested the next day after taking an antihistamine, but instead feel slow, lethargic, and not mentally sharp. This "hangover effect" can be significant and may be related to the lipid solubility and central histaminic (H_1) and muscarinic blocking effects of the antihistamine.[20,41] Antihistamines with low lipid solubility (e.g., cetirizine, loratadine) do not cross the blood–brain barrier readily and do not cause sedation. Although diphenhydramine is the most common antihistamine found in nonprescription sleep medications, some preparations contain the antihistamines doxylamine or hydroxyzine. Tolerance can develop to the sedative effects of antihistamines after 3 to 7 days of continued use.[20,41,44] Because of a high incidence of daytime sedation and risk of cognitive impairment,[44] antihistamines are a poor choice for E.P., a teacher who must stay alert and functional throughout the day. Therefore, E.P.'s insomnia should be managed with nonpharmacologic interventions before initiating any drug therapy.

TIME-ZONE SHIFT: NONPHARMACOLOGIC TREATMENT VERSUS TRIAZOLAM OR Z-HYPNOTIC

CASE 81-1, QUESTION 4: Why is E.P. especially susceptible to the effects of time-zone shift (i.e., "jet lag"), and what counseling is needed?

Time-zone shift disrupts the natural circadian rhythm, which helps regulate sleep. E.P. traveled west, then east through multiple time zones. Symptoms and severity of jet lag are related to the direction traveled and the number of time zones crossed.[37] Individuals older than 50 years of age and those traveling eastward have more difficulty in adjusting their circadian rhythm to time-zone changes. Eastward travelers have difficulty falling asleep and westward travelers complain of difficulty staying asleep and early morning awakening.[37] Travelers should be made aware of the problem and should take steps to help their systems adjust. On arrival in the new time zone, travelers such as E.P. should reset their watches and participate in activities corresponding to the new time. Staying active until the new time-zone bedtime and avoiding naps and stimulants can be helpful.[37]

E.P. should be informed about the likely causes of her insomnia (i.e., jet lag, tea, pseudoephedrine, new surroundings). She also should understand that it may take 1 to 3 weeks for her system to readjust after traveling.[37] The importance of nonpharmacologic interventions to improve sleep (Table 81-3) should be emphasized. For E.P., it is necessary to pay particular attention to regulating her sleep cycle by awakening at the same time each day and resisting daytime naps even after a poor night of sleep. This process, called *chronotherapy,* regulates the internal time clock. In addition, an hour of bright light in the morning can serve as an environmental stimulus, normalizing the circadian rhythm.[37] If E.P.'s insomnia persists despite adhering to cognitive-behavioral interventions, a prescription hypnotic may be necessary.

CASE 81-1, QUESTION 5: E.P. asks whether she can try one of her husband's triazolam tablets. She notes, "He is immediately out like a light when he takes it, and I worry it may be too strong for me."

Short-acting hypnotics (Table 81-4)[45–47] like triazolam are effective to induce and regulate sleep if the stay will be relatively short (<5 days) and if critical activities must be accomplished during the first 48 hours after arrival at the destination.[37] Advantages of triazolam for E.P. include well-established efficacy, an onset of 15 to 30 minutes and no next-day impairment at recommended doses (0.25 mg, 0.125 mg for elderly). Women may be more affected from hypnotics than men, possibly because of greater oral bioavailability.[20,41] E.P. could ask her physician to prescribe triazolam 0.125 mg in case it is needed. Triazolam is less optimal than zaleplon or zolpidem for E.P. because it can cause impairment in new learning or anterograde amnesia. These effects can be sufficiently severe and result in the inability to remember new information learned on the trip.

REBOUND INSOMNIA RISK

Triazolam is also associated with rebound insomnia (i.e., daytime nervousness, jitteriness, and insomnia worse than before) if abruptly stopped after more than 7 to 10 days of continuous use. Of the benzodiazepine receptor–active hypnotics, triazolam is most commonly associated with rebound insomnia and withdrawal problems, likely related to its high binding affinity to the benzodiazepine–GABA–chloride-ionophore receptor complex.[41,48] Z-hypnotics such as zaleplon, zolpidem, and eszopiclone have fewer reports of rebound insomnia and anterograde amnesia at recommended doses because they are selective for the Ω-1 receptor and do not have significant anxiolytic effects compared with triazolam.[41] Also, triazolam's short half-life (2–5 hours) and rapid decrease in blood levels create the potential for withdrawal symptoms including anxiety and insomnia. Triazolam is highly effective in inducing sleep when used on an as-needed basis. Long-acting hypnotics, such as flurazepam, may prevent the traveler from awakening in the morning and should be avoided.

MELATONIN

CASE 81-1, QUESTION 6: E.P. states she would like to try melatonin for improved sleep but wonders whether it is safe and effective. What information is available on the safety and efficacy of melatonin for jet lag or other types of insomnia?

Melatonin is a naturally occurring hormone secreted by the pineal gland, located in the center of the brain. The pineal gland is connected to the retina via a nerve pathway that runs through the suprachiasmatic nucleus of the hypothalamus, the body's circadian clock. The pineal gland produces melatonin (a by-product of serotonin metabolism) only during the nocturnal phase of the circadian cycle and only in relative darkness.[37,41,49]

Several studies show melatonin has at least mild sleep-promoting properties when administered before the period of natural increase in endogenous melatonin (~10 PM to midnight). Studies in adults show melatonin causes significantly more sleepiness when taken at 8 PM compared with 11:30 PM, theoretically because the brain's receptors are already saturated with melatonin late at night.[37,41,49]

TABLE 81-4
Pharmacokinetic Properties of Hypnotics Acting at Benzodiazepine Receptors[33,34,41,45–47]

Active Substance	Lipid Solubility	T_{max} (hours)	Onset (minutes)	Half-Life (hours)	Duration (hours)[a]
Zaleplon	Moderate	1.1	30	1.1	1–2
Zolpidem	Low	1–2	30	2.5	2–4
Zolpidem ER	Low	2	45	2.8	3–5
Eszopiclone	Low	1–1.6	30–45	6	5–8
Triazolam	Moderate	1	15–30	2–5	2–4
Temazepam	Moderate	1.5–2.0	60–120	10–20	8–12
Flurazepam[b]					
Hydroxyethyl[b]	Low	1		2–3	
Aldehyde[b]	Low	1		1	
N-desalkyl[b]	Moderate	10	30–60	50–100	10–30

[a]Time the patient feels the effects after a single dose; usually approximates half-life with multiple doses; individual variability exists; and tolerance may develop with continued use, lessening the duration.
[b]Flurazepam metabolite.
T_{max}, time of maximum concentration.

Eight of ten clinical trials for jet lag found that melatonin, between 0.5 and 5 mg taken close to the target bedtime in the new time zone, decreased jet lag. A systematic review of ten clinical trials showed melatonin was more effective for travel eastward crossing multiple time zones.[49] Melatonin 0.5 to 10 mg has been found effective for entraining the circadian rhythms in blind people, alleviating insomnia in developmentally disabled, handicapped, or autistic spectrum children and adults, and treating short-term, initial insomnia in children with attention deficit hyperactivity disorder (ADHD).[41,49,50] It has no established effectiveness for chronic insomnia.[4] Consumers selecting melatonin should be advised that the safety and effectiveness of melatonin for long-term use have not been clearly established and the purity of melatonin is not regulated by the FDA. Melatonin side effects include sleepiness, headache, and nausea, although usual doses of melatonin 0.5 to 5 mg are well tolerated.[41,49,50] Melatonin use has been associated with reports of depression, liver disease, and vasoconstrictive, immunologic, and contraceptive effects.[41,49]

ONLINE CONTENT

For an illustration that explains the function of the suprachiasmatic nucleus, go to http://thepoint.lww.com/AT10e.

RAMELTEON

CASE 81-1, QUESTION 7: E.P. is concerned about using melatonin because it is not regulated by the FDA and the purity and product integrity cannot be guaranteed. Her doctor gave her a prescription for ramelteon 8 mg at bedtime. How does ramelteon compare with melatonin?

Ramelteon is a highly selective agonist for melatonin receptors 1 and 2 (MT 1, MT 2). Melatonin receptor 1 regulates sleepiness and MT 2 regulates phase shifts from day to night. The clinical significance of ramelteon's selectivity for MT 1 and MT 2 is not well described.[51] Ramelteon is approved by the FDA for insomnia characterized by difficulty falling asleep. Clinical studies in primary insomnia show it decreases the time to fall asleep by 10 to 19 minutes, and it increases total sleep time by 8 to 22 minutes.[51] One controlled trial showed it was superior to placebo in decreasing time to fall asleep during a 6-month period, although ramelteon's onset was 15 minutes faster than placebo after week one but only 9 minutes faster at 6 months.[52] Its half-life ranges from 1 to 2.6 hours. The half-life of its active metabolite, M II, is 2 to 5 hours. Ramelteon undergoes hepatic metabolism by cytochrome P-450 isoenzyme CYP1A2. Increases in serum concentration occur even with mild liver disease, so caution is recommended for patients who have at least moderate liver disease. Fluvoxamine inhibits CYP1A2, dramatically increasing the serum concentration of ramelteon, and coadministration with all potent CYP1A2 inhibitors should be avoided. The most common adverse events observed with ramelteon include headache (7%), dizziness (5%), somnolence (5%), fatigue (4%), and nausea (3%).[51]

No evidence of cognitive impairment, rebound insomnia, withdrawal effects, or abuse potential was noted in clinical trials. Adults with a history of sedative abuse took triazolam 0.25, 0.5, 0.75 mg, and ramelteon 16, 80, 160 mg, versus placebo for 18 days. Ramelteon demonstrated no potential for abuse or motor and cognitive impairment up to 20 times the recommended therapeutic dose, whereas triazolam demonstrated potential for abuse at all doses.[51,53]

Ramelteon is a reasonable option for patients with initial insomnia with no abuse potential and has little to no risk of next-day impairment. In the absence of published trials comparing ramelteon with other sedative-hypnotic agents, or in special populations such as those with insomnia and substance abuse, its place in therapy is unclear.

"Z-HYPNOTICS" (ZOLPIDEM, ZALEPLON, AND ESZOPICLONE)

CASE 81-1, QUESTION 8: It has been a month since her return, and E.P. continues to have difficulty falling asleep. What alternative medications (aside from triazolam and ramelteon) offer rapid onset, have low risk of daytime sedation, and can be administered safely for weeks to months if necessary?

Considering their rapid onset of action, Z-hypnotics (zaleplon, zolpidem, and eszopiclone) are all potential alternatives for E.P. They have varying degrees of selectivity for the Ω-1 receptor on the benzodiazepine receptor complex. This selectivity imparts hypnotic efficacy with no significant anxiolytic, muscle relaxant, or anticonvulsant effects. Consequently, Z-hypnotics have a lower risk of abuse, withdrawal, and tolerance compared with older nonselective benzodiazepines such as triazolam and temazepam. These attributes make Z-hypnotics more desirable for the treatment of chronic insomnia. Both zolpidem controlled-release and eszopiclone are FDA approved for chronic insomnia and are effective for up to 3 to 6 months of therapy.[45] Another potential advantage of Z-hypnotic's Ω-1 selectivity is little to no change in sleep architecture or sleep stages. Temazepam and flurazepam increase the percentage of stage 2 sleep but can suppress REM and stage 3 and 4 deep restorative sleep. In contrast, Z-hypnotics do not interfere with these sleep stages and have lower rates of uncomfortable REM rebound (vivid dreams, increased autonomic instability) on discontinuation.[45,46]

The Z-hypnotics differ with respect to pharmacokinetics and adverse events. Zolpidem, the first Z-hypnotic, was marketed in the United States in 1991. It is absorbed rapidly, reaches peak serum levels in 1.5 hours, and is eliminated rapidly with an average half-life of approximately 2.5 hours.[41] Zolpidem is metabolized by the oxidative cytochrome P-450 isoenzyme CYP3A4; therefore, drug interactions should be considered when zolpidem is coadministered with CYP3A4 inhibitors such as diltiazem or fluoxetine. Zolpidem has no active metabolites, and it has a low risk of residual daytime sedation in recommended doses.[45,46] It should be taken on an empty stomach for faster absorption. The usual adult dose of zolpidem is 10 mg at bedtime; elderly patients or patients such as E.P., who express concern that a medicine may be too strong, should begin with 5 mg at bedtime. Zolpidem controlled-release has no clear advantage over zolpidem, except that it may provide a slightly longer duration of sleep. Serum concentrations peak in 2 hours compared with 1.5 hours for immediate-release zolpidem, with an associated longer latency to effect.[42]

Zaleplon offers a shorter elimination half-life (1.1 hour) and duration of effect than zolpidem. It is least likely of all hypnotic agents to cause residual daytime sedation and has the least effect on memory and psychomotor performance. An assessment of psychomotor performance, arousal, memory, and cognitive functioning with zaleplon revealed no cognitive impairment.[45,46] The most common adverse effects with zaleplon include dizziness, headache, and somnolence.[54] In dose escalation studies using up to 60 mg, symptoms appear at approximately 30 minutes after dosing, peak at 1 to 2 hours, and are no longer evident after 4 hours. It can be taken in the middle of the night as long as the individual has 4 hours left in bed.[41] Zaleplon is metabolized primarily via aldehyde oxidase, CYP3A4 is a secondary route of metabolism, and there are no active metabolites; it has less potential for drug or food interactions compared with zolpidem or eszopiclone.[41]

Eszopiclone maintains efficacy with no evidence of tolerance after 6 months of continuous use, resulting in FDA approval for long-term use.[55] Hypnotic efficacy has been demonstrated for up to 6 months in younger patients taking 2 to 3 mg nightly, and in elderly patients taking 1 to 2 mg nightly, although only the higher range of doses significantly improved sleep maintenance. As with zolpidem and zaleplon, eszopiclone has a rapid onset of effect, but differs in that it has a longer duration of effect (Table 81-4). Time to maximal concentration (T_{max}) is delayed up to 1 hour when eszopiclone is administered after a high-fat meal, potentially delaying the onset of sleep.[55]

Eszopiclone has less receptor selectivity than either zaleplon or zolpidem, potentially resulting in some anxiolytic, amnestic, and anticonvulsant activity.[47] Among the three Z-hypnotic drugs, eszopiclone has a dose-related unpleasant bitter taste noted by 16% to 33% of patients.[55] Headache and dizziness were reported more commonly with eszopiclone than placebo, and at higher doses, next-day confusion and memory impairment were reported in up to 3% of patients.[45,55] Eszopiclone is primarily metabolized by CYP3A4, so drugs that induce or inhibit this isoenzyme can have an impact on metabolism and a clinical effect.[55]

E.P. needs a medication that will hasten sleep onset, but does not need continued drug effect later in the night. Both zolpidem and zaleplon are useful alternatives for E.P. because of their efficacy for her sleep onset difficulty. Among the Z-hypnotics, eszopiclone has the longest half-life and the greatest risk for next-day impairment.

CASE 81-1, QUESTION 9: Zolpidem immediate-release 5 mg is prescribed because of its rapid onset, low cost, and low risk for next-day impairment. E.P. expresses concern about possible adverse effects owing to its labeling as a Schedule IV controlled substance and the FDA warning of complex sleep behaviors such as night eating and night driving. How should E.P.'s concerns be addressed?

Patient counseling is most effective when it is interactive with both patient and practitioner actively listening to each other while exchanging information. It is best to begin by emphasizing the benefits of zolpidem to improve her sleep and daytime functioning. Next, E.P. should be reassured that zolpidem is generally well tolerated and she will be prescribed the lowest dose to minimize the likelihood of adverse effects. Counseling should include a discussion of common and potentially serious adverse effects along with management strategies. Common possible adverse effects include headache (28.4%), drowsiness (26.2%), fatigue (16.6%), and dizziness (14.0%).[45,54] GI side effects occurred in 1.7% of patients; this side effect is more common with Z-hypnotics compared with nonselective benzodiazepines. Confusion, disorientation, obsessive ideas, delirium, and psychosis occurred at a rate of 1% in postmarketing surveillance studies. Hallucinations, mostly visual, are more common in elderly patients, those taking high doses, or patients with impaired metabolism of zolpidem.[20] E.P. should be encouraged to report both effectiveness and all adverse effects to her clinician. Alcohol may be ingested 3 to 4 hours before taking zolpidem, but they should not be taken together because it may cause excessive side effects and interfere with E.P.'s sleep.

To address E.P.'s concern about the FDA's hypnotic warning, a reasonable response would be "rarely, individuals taking sleeping medication have been reported to be making phone calls, eating, having sex, or driving while half asleep. The risk for these potentially dangerous effects increase if consumers take a higher than recommended dose, or drink alcohol or mix hypnotics with other sedating medications."[16] Another rare allergic reaction is facial swelling (angioedema). All manufacturers of hypnotic medication are required to include this information in their package inserts.[16] E.P. should be encouraged to take zolpidem on an empty stomach 30 minutes before desired sleep time for the fastest onset of effect.

Although the abuse potential of Z-hypnotics is less than for nonselective benzodiazepines, they are problematic in active substance-abuse disorders. Z-hypnotics are Schedule IV controlled substances with more potential for abuse than ramelteon or sedating antidepressants, like trazodone. Tolerance and withdrawal effects have been reported with abrupt discontinuation of zolpidem, particularly with self-escalation of dose; thus monitoring and counseling are needed.

INSOMNIA IN A MEDICALLY ILL PATIENT

Insomnia and Effect on Sleep Stages

CASE 81-2

QUESTION 1: A.T., a 42-year-old woman with a 5-year history of hypothyroidism and a 2-year history of hypertension and chronic lower back pain, was just transferred from the intensive care unit (ICU) into a medical unit. Her cardiac status is considered "stable" 2 days after a myocardial infarction (MI). She is 5 feet 9 inches tall and weighs 72 kg. She is receiving aspirin (enteric-coated), levothyroxine, and felodipine. Her main complaint is insomnia, including difficulty falling asleep, difficulty maintaining sleep, and early-morning awakenings. A.T. reports insomnia for 6 weeks before admission, which worsened during the hospitalization. What type of insomnia does A.T. have, and how might the insomnia affect her health?

A.T.'s insomnia is considered chronic because she experienced it for 6 weeks before hospital admission. It is severe because it involves difficulty falling asleep, maintaining sleep, and early-morning awakening. Careful monitoring and effective treatment of A.T.'s sleep disturbance is crucial; studies show disrupted sleep can increase the risk of another adverse cardiac event owing to worsening autonomic instability and poor perfusion to the myocardium.[2]

Because normal sleep moves through all the stages of NREM and REM in a continuous cycle, a patient deprived of continuous sleep may not receive sufficient time in each sleep stage. When stage 2 is diminished, muscles have insufficient opportunity to rest and rejuvenate. If NREM stages 3 and 4 are eliminated, immune function and the healing process can be disrupted. If REM sleep is deprived or excessive, neurotransmitter function may be altered and physiologic homeostatic processes can be disrupted.[6,13,25]

Drug or Disease Etiologies

CASE 81-2, QUESTION 2: What individual drug or disease state factors should be assessed in A.T. before developing a treatment plan?

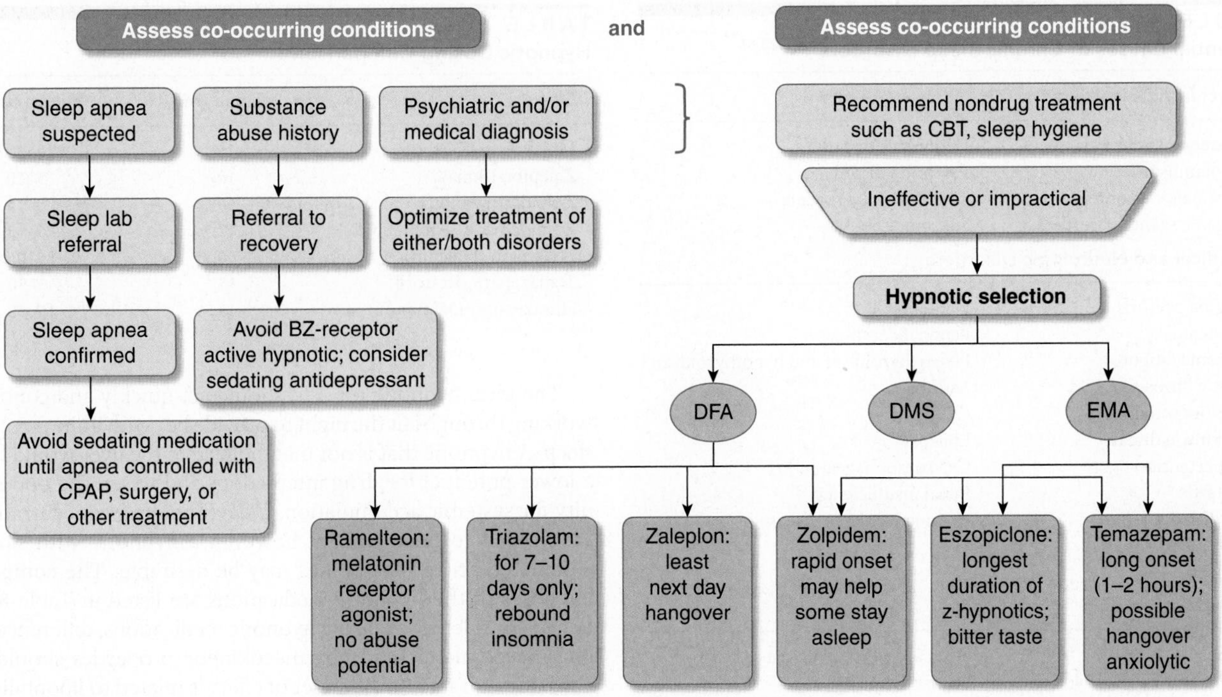

FIGURE 81-2 Algorithm for treatment of insomnia. DFA, difficulty falling asleep; DMS, difficulty maintaining sleep; EMA, early morning awakening.

The Insomnia Treatment Algorithm in Figure 81-2 is useful in systematically addressing A.T.'s sleep complaint. It calls for thoroughly evaluating all concomitant conditions and the type of insomnia in each patient. Numerous medical disorders and primary sleep disorders are associated with difficulty falling asleep and maintaining sleep (Tables 81-5, 81-6).[2,6,56] First, A.T. should be assessed for sleep apnea because hypnotics can be dangerous in untreated sleep apnea and untreated sleep apnea is a known etiology of cardiac disease (see Case 81-8, in the Sleep Apnea section). Second, A.T.'s pain management should be assessed for optimal efficacy. Acute post-MI pain adds to A.T.'s chronic lower back pain. Of patients with lower back pain, 50% experience chronic poor sleep patterns.[2,6] Third, A.T. was just transferred out of the ICU. Sleep deprivation in an ICU is common and is attributed to the continuous lighting, noise, and constant interventions. Sleep deprivation may prolong or worsen a disease process through diminished natural killer cell activity and decreased stages 3 and 4 of NREM sleep (when healing occurs).[5,13,41] Medications also may be contributing to A.T.'s insomnia (Table 81-5). Levothyroxine can overstimulate the CNS if given in excessive doses.[57] A.T.'s thyroid status should be re-evaluated to ensure appropriateness of the thyroid dose, especially considering her post-MI status. Calcium-channel blockers have been associated with occasional sleep disturbances; therefore, felodipine should be evaluated as a potential contributing factor.[57]

Another clue to a possible cause of A.T.'s sleep problem is her description of early-morning awakening, which could be related to hospital activity during these hours or to the presence of a major depressive disorder. A.T. requires psychiatric evaluation to rule out depression, which occurs in 33% to 88% of patients after an MI.[28] In general, patients with chronic illnesses are at increased risk of experiencing major depression, which typically presents with insomnia or hypersomnia. Interestingly, medical outcome studies of other chronic illnesses (cardiovascular, pulmonary, renal, neurologic disease) show a high prevalence of sleep disturbance even in those not suffering from depression.[2,6] Chronic insomnia related to multiple causes can be resistant to

TABLE 81-5
Potential Causes and Contributing Factors for Each Chronic Sleep Complaint[13]

Difficulty Falling Asleep (DFA)
Learned or conditioned activation (primary insomnia): restless legs syndrome (RLS)
Medications: methylphenidate, modafinil, fluoxetine, bupropion, steroid, β-blocker
Substances: caffeine, guarana, alcohol
Psychiatric disorders: schizophrenia, depression, anxiety disorder, bipolar disorder
Medical disorder: chronic pain, neuropathy, gastrointestinal disorder, cardiopulmonary disorders (particularly if in recumbent position)
Difficulty Maintaining Sleep (DMA)
Excessive time in bed
Psychiatric disorder: major depression, anxiety or bipolar disorder, substance abuse
Sleep-disordered breathing: sleep apnea, acute respiratory distress syndrome
Cardiac disease: atrial fibrillation, heart failure, angina
Neurologic disorder: dementia, Parkinson disease, multiple sclerosis
Early Morning Awakening (EMA)
Major depression
Advanced sleep-phase syndrome: learned or conditioned activation (primary insomnia)
Forced to get up because of family or work obligations
Excessive Daytime Sleepiness
Medications: clonidine, antihistamines, antipsychotic, antidepressant, benzodiazepine, chloral hydrate, opioid, anticonvulsant, α_1-adrenergic blockers
Obstructive sleep apnea, central sleep apnea, narcolepsy
Chronic sleep deprivation

TABLE 81-6
Potential Causes of Chronic Sleep Disorders[2,4,5,23,56]

Psychiatric Disorders	
Anxiety disorders	Depressive disorders
Bipolar disorder	Psychotic disorders
Personality disorders	Somatoform disorders
Organic mental disorders	Substance abuse
Medical and Neurologic Disorders	
Angina pectoris	Dementia
Bronchitis	Peptic ulcer disease
Chronic fatigue	Hyperthyroidism and hypothyroidism
Cystic fibrosis	Asthma
Huntington disease	COPD
Parkinson disease	Epilepsy
Hypertension	Gastroesophageal reflux
Arthritis	Renal insufficiency
Cardiac disease	Connective tissue disease
Chronic pain	
Cancer	
Sleep Disorders	
RLS	Sleep apnea (obstructive or central)
PLMS (nocturnal myoclonus)	Primary snoring
Circadian rhythm sleep disorder (jet lag, shift work, delayed sleep phase)	Narcolepsy
Drugs Associated With Sleep Disturbance	
Insomnia	Hypersomnia
Alcohol	Alcohol
Bupropion	Benzodiazepines
Fluoxetine	Antihypertensives
Sertraline	Clonidine
MAO inhibitors	α-Adrenergic blockers
TCA	ACE inhibitors
Thyroid supplements	β-Blockers
Calcium-channel blockers	Anticonvulsants
Decongestants	Analgesics
Appetite suppressants	Chloral hydrate
Theophylline	Antipsychotics
Corticosteroids	Antihistamines
Dopamine agonists	Opioids

ACE, angiotensin-converting enzyme; COPD, chronic obstructive pulmonary disease; MAO, monoamine oxidase; PLMS, periodic limb movements during sleep; RLS, restless legs syndrome; TCA, tricyclic antidepressants.

treatment; however, treatment of underlying causes increases the likelihood of insomnia resolution.

Comparing Available Hypnotics

CASE 81-2, QUESTION 3: A.T.'s pain is now under control, her levothyroxine dose is appropriate, and felodipine-induced sleep disturbance, sleep-disordered breathing, RLS, and PLMS have all been ruled out. A psychiatric evaluation finds that A.T. does not have major depression, but she is anxious about "life after a heart attack." She meets criteria for primary insomnia and adjustment disorder with anxiety. She continues to have trouble falling asleep and staying asleep. She will be discharged in 2 days. The pain management team suggests an adjunctive medication with anxiolytic properties that may also help with sleep. Which hypnotic is best for A.T., considering her individual clinical characteristics?

TABLE 81-7
Hypnotic Dosing Comparison

Drug	Dose (mg)	Range (mg)
Midazolam (Versed)	15	10–30
Zaleplon (Sonata)	10	5–10
Zolpidem (Ambien)	10	5–10
Zolpidem ER (Ambien CR)	12.5	6.25–12.5
Triazolam (Halcion)	0.25	0.125–0.25
Temazepam (Restoril)	15	7.5–30
Flurazepam (Dalmane)	15	15–30

The ideal hypnotic for A.T. should act quickly and continue working throughout the night to provide her with uninterrupted sleep. A hypnotic that is not metabolized in the liver would have a lower potential for drug interactions and lessen the opportunity for systemic accumulation. If daytime drug concentrations are needed to calm anxiety, however, a hypnotic with slowly eliminated active metabolites may be desirable. The comparable doses of the hypnotic medications are listed in Table 81-7. When considering available hypnotic medications, differences in pharmacodynamic and pharmacokinetic properties should be considered (Table 81-4). Onset of effect is related to lipophilicity, receptor binding affinity, and T_{max}.[41,42]

A nonselective benzodiazepine hypnotic is preferable in A.T. because of the need for anxiolytic properties in addition to hypnotic efficacy. Z-hypnotics are not effective anxiolytic agents. The pharmacodynamic and pharmacokinetic properties of triazolam have already been presented. Its rapid onset is an advantage for A.T.; however, the duration of action would not be sufficient to help A.T. stay asleep. In addition, it should not be used for longer than 7 to 10 days because of the greater potential for adverse effects with prolonged use and the possibility of significant rebound insomnia on withdrawal.[41] A.T. may require a hypnotic for more than 7 to 10 days, which is the maximal duration for triazolam use.

Flurazepam induces sleep within 15 to 45 minutes during chronic dosing. On the first night of use, however, flurazepam does not induce sleep as well as triazolam. It has intermediate fat solubility but depends on the plasma concentrations of its metabolite, *N*-desalkylflurazepam, for most of its activity.[41] *N*-desalkylflurazepam concentrations take approximately 24 hours to accumulate and induce sleep. Studies show flurazepam maintains efficacy in sleep induction for at least 30 days; *N*-desalkylflurazepam has weak receptor binding affinity and a long half-life, resulting in gradual elimination and little chance for rebound insomnia.[41] *N*-desalkylflurazepam can accumulate during chronic dosing and affect daytime cognition in some patients or compete for hepatic metabolism, resulting in altered levels of other hepatically metabolized medications.[41,57] Accumulation and daytime sedation can be therapeutic for some patients with daytime anxiety. A.T. has difficulty moving around during the day because of her chronic lower back pain, and oversedation from accumulation may impair her daytime functioning. Flurazepam is infrequently used because of the risk of next-day impairment; it is useful to explore other options.

Temazepam takes 1 to 2 hours to induce sleep. It has moderate fat solubility, similar to *N*-desalkylflurazepam, but it has a longer dissolution time. Temazepam takes 1.5 to 2 hours to reach peak plasma concentrations. Temazepam's longer dissolution time is caused by its large drug particle size in a gelatin capsule. The European product formulation, consisting of a solution in a wax matrix, induces sleep in 30 minutes.[41,58] A potential advantage for using temazepam in A.T.'s case is its lack of hepatic oxidative metabolism and intermediate duration of action of 8 to 12 hours.

It does not interfere with the metabolism of other hepatically metabolized drugs and it does not accumulate, minimizing the potential for daytime impairment relative to flurazepam.[34,41] The long onset of action may be of concern, although A.T. could take the drug an hour before bedtime to optimize timing for sleep.

For A.T., the most appropriate choice is temazepam. Temazepam's advantages are intermediate duration of activity that would keep her asleep throughout the night, anxiolytic benefit, and low risk of daytime impairment owing to no known active metabolites.[34,41]

Benzodiazepine Dependence and Tolerance

CASE 81-2, QUESTION 4: On further discussion with A.T., who prefers to try cognitive-behavioral interventions for anxiety reduction and sleep induction, temazepam 15 mg at bedtime is prescribed on an as-needed basis. A.T. will be monitored regularly as an outpatient for efficacy and tolerability. As A.T. is preparing to leave the hospital, her daughter, B.T., expresses concerns about the potential for physical dependence on temazepam and the risk of A.T. becoming an addict. How would you respond to her concerns?

Fear of dependence and addiction to medications is a concern among the general public. Television station "medical experts" and popular magazine "health sections," while providing information, may increase the potential for confusion, erroneous impressions, and misinformation. For health care practitioners, it becomes even more crucial to provide sound drug information in common, easy-to-understand terms.

An example of the practitioner's response may be, "I'm glad you have expressed a concern; it gives us a chance to discuss temazepam therapy before your mother leaves the hospital. Temazepam has been prescribed for a medical reason, to improve your mother's sleep and to aid in her healing process. One therapeutic benefit of temazepam is an 8-hour duration of effect. Your mother will be able to sleep throughout the night so that she is well rested during the day. It also may decrease her anxiety over not sleeping, and that puts less stress on her heart.

"The possible side effects of temazepam include sedation, unsteadiness, and dizziness. She should let her doctor know if she experiences any adverse effects. Right now, it is unclear how long your mother will be taking temazepam. Duration of therapy needs to be assessed on an ongoing basis. If your mother takes temazepam every night for more than 4 weeks, two things could happen: (a) she may develop a tolerance and it may not help her sleep anymore, or (b) her system may develop a dependence in which she may have worse insomnia if she does not take it. The primary concern is not addiction but the possible dependence. This means your mother should not change her dose or stop on her own. Any changes in dose or stopping must be done slowly and with her doctor's involvement. These two scenarios do not always occur and are not likely because your mother will be taking it on an as-needed basis. If one or the other does happen, some other intervention may be tried to help with her sleep, or the temazepam dose can be gradually decreased to prevent withdrawal problems. It is important to advise your mother to avoid alcohol, and report any decrease in effectiveness or any adverse effects to her health care practitioner."

Epidemiologic data indicate that benzodiazepines are widely used primarily for brief periods, but less commonly used on a long-term basis. Dependence can occur after continued use for 2 to 4 months.[35] Daily users for longer than 1 year tend to be older, medically ill, and chronically dysphoric and have panic disorder or chronic insomnia. Most chronic use appears to be medically appropriate and does not lead to dose escalation or abuse. Among chronic dysphoric patients, the indications are less clear, and dose escalation is noted sometimes without notable therapeutic benefit. Benzodiazepine hypnotics rarely are taken alone for pleasure, and generally are not likely to be abused. Among substance abusers, however, they frequently are taken as part of a polysubstance abuse pattern by alcoholics and narcotic, methadone, and cocaine users. In these groups, abuse is highly prevalent. Benzodiazepines are used to augment euphoria (narcotics and methadone users), to decrease anxiety and withdrawal symptoms (alcoholics), and to ease the "crash" from stimulant-induced euphoria (cocaine users).[36]

Physiologic dependence on benzodiazepines, resulting in a withdrawal and abstinence syndrome, develops usually after 2 to 4 months of daily use of the longer half-life benzodiazepines. Shorter half-life benzodiazepine use can result in physiologic dependence earlier (days to weeks) and may be associated with more withdrawal problems.[41,48] See Table 81-4 for a comparison of pharmacokinetic properties of hypnotics.

INSOMNIA AND PSYCHIATRIC DISORDERS

Stepwise Approach to Selecting a Hypnotic

CASE 81-3

QUESTION 1: P.H., a 35-year-old man, is hospitalized after a suicide attempt in which he cut his neck with a large kitchen knife. Before the suicide attempt, P.H. had been sober for 2 years. He is diagnosed with major depression, substance abuse, and alcohol dependence. His target symptoms include a 20-pound weight loss, low energy, social withdrawal, depressed mood, hopelessness, inability to experience pleasure, trouble falling asleep, and early-morning awakening. His medications include sertraline 50 mg daily, lansoprazole 30 mg daily, and a multivitamin daily, all started 5 days ago. After completing an interview with P.H., you learn that he was doing well until 2 months ago (3 months after stopping fluoxetine due to insomnia). He began to attend Alcoholics Anonymous groups more regularly, but his depression worsened. Two weeks before admission, he went on a drinking binge that ended with the suicide attempt. Currently, 5 days after his suicide attempt, P.H. reports feeling restless and sleeping only 3 to 4 hours a night. Use Tables 81-4 and 81-7 and Figure 81-2 to compare the clinically significant differences between available hypnotics and to demonstrate how such information can be used to develop a patient-specific treatment plan. What is the best approach to solving P.H.'s sleep problem?

The Insomnia Treatment Algorithm outlined in Figure 81-2 serves as a useful guide for the assessment and management of P.H.'s sleep complaint. Concomitant conditions and the type of insomnia (difficulty falling asleep, difficulty maintaining sleep, early-morning awakening) are assessed simultaneously. Possible causes or contributing factors are identified and treated. The type of insomnia can aid in treatment selection. Cognitive-behavioral interventions can be implemented if P.H. is willing and able to participate.

Factors to consider in the drug selection process include substance abuse history, and the need for rapid onset or long duration of effect. For example, agents with long-acting metabolites (e.g., flurazepam), may accumulate or cause daytime hangover. If the hypnotic has no hepatic metabolism, it will not be subject to drug interactions with other agents that are hepatically metabolized. If insomnia is chronic and resistant to hypnotic treatment, or if a low abuse potential agent is desired (e.g., for a person with an existing addictive disorder like P.H.), trazodone or another sedating antidepressant may be selected.

Sleep Disturbance of Depression

CASE 81-3, QUESTION 2: What type of insomnia does P.H. have, and how is it different from other types of insomnia?

P.H. has trouble falling asleep and early-morning awakening, and sleep time has decreased to 3 or 4 hours a night. He is diagnosed with major depression, and sleep difficulty is part of the disorder. Generally, initial insomnia and early-morning awakening are associated with depression, although difficulty maintaining sleep and next-day fatigue are common as well. P.H. is most bothered by trouble falling asleep, early-morning awakening, and next-day fatigue. Up to 65% of outpatients with major depression report one or more symptoms of sleep disturbance, whereas 90% of inpatients with depression like P.H. report insomnia.[59]

The insomnia of depression is likely related to a dysregulation of neurotransmitters, such as serotonin, norepinephrine, and dopamine, in addition to dysregulation of the hypothalamic-pituitary axis. All are involved in regulating mood and the sleep–wake cycle.[5,13] Neurotransmitter activity is modified by the effects of antidepressants on REM sleep. Most effective antidepressants (excluding trazodone and bupropion) suppress REM, causing increased REM latency and decreased total REM time.[32,59] Indeed, REM sleep deprivation can elevate mood.[59,60] Depressed patients deliberately deprived of REM sleep have had a reduction in depressive symptoms. In addition to effects on REM, antidepressants redistribute slow-wave sleep to more physiologically natural patterns, with increased intensity in the first half of the night.[60] Sedating antidepressants with serotonin 2 ($5\text{-}HT_2$) antagonist properties, such as trazodone and mirtazapine, alleviate insomnia and improve sleep architecture.[59]

Causes: Psychiatric and Alcohol and Substance Abuse

CASE 81-3, QUESTION 3: P.H. and the treatment team ask you what factors other than depression (i.e., medications, alcohol) may contribute to P.H.'s insomnia. How can his sleep problem be solved?

P.H. has been prescribed sertraline to treat his depression. Sertraline can cause insomnia in 15% to 30% of patients, and P.H. should be asked whether insomnia worsened after starting sertraline.[59] P.H. also was using alcohol before admission. Alcohol disrupts sleep, leading to more fragmented sleep.[56] All patients should be counseled to have their last alcoholic drink at least 3 hours before sleep. P.H. should avoid alcohol altogether given his history of abuse. Drug and alcohol withdrawal and the lingering "abstinence syndromes" often are associated with insomnia, although sometimes hypersomnia is the predominant symptom.[36,56]

Treatment

The treatment for P.H.'s insomnia should begin with patient education. P.H. should be informed that more than 90% of depressed patients have some sleep disturbance, either too little or too much, and his sleep should improve as depressive symptoms improve (in 2–8 weeks). Counseling on cognitive-behavioral interventions to improve sleep may be appropriate when P.H.'s depression begins to clear and he is more motivated to improve his sleep hygiene. In the meantime, the potential contribution of sertraline to his restlessness or insomnia should be assessed by confirming that the drug is being dosed in the early morning to minimize this effect. A sedating antidepressant such as mirtazapine may be preferred unless P.H.'s history includes a positive response with sertraline that would justify ongoing treatment. In some cases, dual antidepressant therapy is needed to achieve remission of depression (see Chapter 83, Mood Disorders I: Major Depressive Disorders).

HYPNOTICS

All antidepressants, including selective serotonin reuptake inhibitors (SSRIs), such as sertraline, can improve sleep as the depression lifts; however, SSRIs, bupropion, and monoamine oxidase inhibitors can all cause insomnia as well.[57,59,61] Analysis of residual symptoms in partially treated depressed patients taking SSRIs shows continuing insomnia is present in 44%, requiring additional interventions such as the addition of trazodone or mirtazapine. Prescribing a hypnotic short term or a sedating antidepressant is recommended for depressed patients with insomnia because a good night's sleep can improve treatment adherence and daytime functioning until antidepressant effects become apparent.[2,5]

In a study of 545 patients with major depression and insomnia taking fluoxetine in the morning, patients were randomly assigned to receive either eszopiclone 3 mg or placebo for 8 weeks. Concomitant eszopiclone resulted in improved sleep quality, faster antidepressant response, and significantly more responders and remitters at week 8 compared with placebo.[62] Unpleasant taste was the only adverse effect reported significantly more in the eszopiclone group versus the placebo group (22.7% vs. 0.7%). In separate studies, zolpidem and trazodone have demonstrated efficacy for residual insomnia in depressed patients with partial antidepressant response.[5]

Hypnotics that act at benzodiazepine receptors are not recommended for P.H. because of his drug use history and recent alcohol abuse. Nonselective benzodiazepines like temazepam can have a euphoric effect, are cross-tolerant with alcohol, and are likely to be abused by patients with alcohol and substance-abuse problems.[35,41] Abuse, dependence, and withdrawal reactions have been reported with Ω-1 selective Z-hypnotics (zolpidem, zaleplon, eszopiclone); therefore, neither class of drugs is appropriate for P.H.[45,54]

If the clinician determines that sertraline treatment is preferred over an alternate SSRI or mirtazapine, then trazodone may be added to alleviate insomnia.[63] The addition of trazodone to fluoxetine, bupropion, or monoamine oxidase inhibitors decreased time to sleep and increased duration of sleep but caused intolerable sedation in a few patients who received fluoxetine. Tolerance did not develop to the sedative effects of trazodone in short-term studies (<6 weeks) used adjunctively for depression; however, decreased benefit with time has been reported.[63] The $5\text{-}HT_2$ antagonist properties of trazodone at low dosages and its α-adrenergic blocking effects provide the rationale for its efficacy as a sedating agent.

ANTIDEPRESSANTS

CASE 81-3, QUESTION 4: What is the evidence for trazodone's use in managing insomnia? What other

antidepressants are used in the treatment of insomnia? Discuss the advantages and disadvantages of using sedating antidepressants for the treatment of insomnia in P.H.

Trazodone is not thought to be a highly effective antidepressant because most people cannot tolerate an effective dose (300–600 mg/day). Because of its sedating properties, trazodone has become a commonly prescribed adjunctive medication (50–200 mg/day at bedtime) to induce sleep while awaiting the onset of the primary antidepressant's effect. Trazodone's half-life is approximately 6.4 hours in younger adults and 11.6 hours in the elderly. It undergoes hepatic metabolism via CYP2D6 and CYP3A4, so inhibitors of these isoenzymes can increase blood levels and worsen side effects. The most common side effects of trazodone include drowsiness (29.1%), dizziness (21.9%), and dry mouth (17.7%). Cardiac arrhythmias are possible at doses greater than 200 mg/day, as is priapism, a painful prolonged erection that occurs in 1 of 1,000 to 10,000 men. Although priapism is considered rare, it can lead to impotence if untreated; therefore, P.H. should be counseled about priapism.[61,63]

In the only placebo-controlled trial of trazodone conducted in primary insomnia, investigators compared the hypnotic efficacy of trazodone and zolpidem with placebo in 306 adults (21–65 years of age). Subjects were randomly assigned to receive trazodone 50 mg, zolpidem 10 mg, or placebo nightly for 2 weeks. Sleep parameters were assessed using a subjective sleep questionnaire, which patients completed each morning and at weekly office visits.

Trazodone was found to be as effective as zolpidem for the first week of treatment, but during the second week, only zolpidem was more effective than placebo.[63] Tricyclic antidepressants (TCAs; e.g., amitriptyline, doxepin) were used to treat primary insomnia for years based on case reports describing efficacy in doses of 10 to 75 mg/night.[41,59] TCAs, however, increase the risk of cardiovascular problems and anticholinergic side effects in a dose-related manner (see Chapter 83, Mood Disorders I: Major Depressive Disorders).

Ultra-low-dose doxepin 3-mg and 6-mg tablets are now available for the treatment of insomnia characterized by difficulties with sleep maintenance. Doxepin is not a controlled substance, so it may be of value in patients with a history of substance abuse. Four clinical trials conducted in slightly more than 1,000 patients demonstrated doxepin's efficacy and safety in both younger adults and the elderly.[64] Doxepin demonstrated improved sleep efficiency during the final third of the night and in the seventh and eighth hours of sleep. Doxepin was well tolerated, with residual sedation and anticholinergic effects no different than placebo. There were no significant effects on next-day alertness, memory, or psychomotor function. Hypnotic efficacy with doxepin was demonstrated for up to 3 months. The primary disadvantage of this formulation of doxepin is its cost, with an acquisition cost of approximately $5.00 per tablet. It remains to be seen whether these low-dose studies will prompt increased use of generic doxepin 10 mg, and whether any advantages can be demonstrated in using the branded low-dose doxepin formulation.

For P.H., a TCA raises additional safety concerns. P.H. has a history of substance abuse and prior suicide attempts. Both are risk factors for future suicide attempts. TCAs are more toxic in overdose when compared with trazodone, and there are multiple reports of TCA plasma levels increasing to toxic levels when administered in combination with sertraline, particularly at sertraline doses greater than 100 mg/day (see Chapter 83, Mood Disorders I: Major Depressive Disorders).

Switching to mirtazapine as an antidepressant that offers more sedation is a reasonable consideration for P.H. If P.H. has a partial but significant response to sertraline at maximal tolerated doses and good tolerability except for insomnia at 4 weeks, mirtazapine can be added to facilitate remission. Mirtazapine has 5-HT_2 antagonist and antihistamine effects, which impart sedation, and it is safer than TCAs in overdose.[59] Mirtazapine is not associated with priapism, but it can cause weight gain.

INSOMNIA IN THE ELDERLY

CASE 81-4

QUESTION 1: S.D., a 77-year-old man, is seen for his initial geriatrics primary-care clinic visit. Vital signs include temperature, 98.8°F; heart rate, 58 beats/minute; respiratory rate, 18 breaths/minute; BP, 166/69 mm Hg; height, 5 feet 3 inches; and weight, 109 pounds. He was referred from an emergency department (ED) visit 4 days earlier with complaints of palpitations and anxiety. Before his ED visit, his medications included atenolol 50 mg daily, lorazepam 1 mg at bedtime, and saw palmetto 320 mg daily. At his ED visit, he stated he had taken lorazepam for sleep for more than 1 year, but did not take it the prior 2 nights and started feeling palpitations and anxiety. His electrocardiogram showed normal sinus rhythm at 67 beats/minute, and S.D.'s head computed tomography scan was negative for any hemorrhage. S.D. was told to not restart the lorazepam, but instead to take diphenhydramine 50 mg at bedtime. He took only one dose, felt "terrible" and fatigued for the next 2 days. On further questioning, he states that he falls asleep without difficulty, usually awakens two to three times each night to urinate, and often has difficulty falling back to sleep. In the past, lorazepam was helpful with his sleep difficulty. What considerations are important for the assessment and treatment of insomnia in an elderly patient such as S.D.?

Treatment of insomnia in the elderly represents a therapeutic dilemma. Recent evidence supports an increased need to treat insomnia in the elderly to reduce its potentially serious complications, yet many drug treatment options have potential for harm that may outweigh their benefit. Among the elderly, a review of community and epidemiology studies from a total of more than 43,000 subjects found insomnia in 17%, and it was 10% in studies with more stringent criteria.[65] In a large epidemiological study of sleep complaints in 9,282 individuals 65 years and older conducted by the National Institute on Aging, 57% of subjects indicated at least one sleep complaint occurring most of the time, 19% had difficulty falling asleep, 30% complained of awakening at night, and 19% complained of awakening too early.[66] Despite such high frequency of sleep complaints, these complaints are primarily thought to be more a marker of poor physical and mental health rather than caused by aging itself.[67,68]

The accepted wisdom is that age-related sleep changes begin to appear in early adulthood and progress steadily across the adult lifespan.[69] However, in a meta-analysis of 65 studies of quantitative sleep parameters across the lifespan of individuals from ages 5 to 102 without sleep complaint, most changes in sleep were found to occur by age 60.[70] Changes in sleep latency are small and subtle, with an overall increase between 20 and 80 years of less than 10 minutes. Increases in percentages of stage 1 and 2 sleep, as well as decreases in total sleep time, percentage of slow-wave and REM sleep, and REM latency, were significant with aging up to age 60, but only minimal changes were seen after age 60. Only sleep efficiency was found to continue to significantly decrease after age 60. Therefore, identifying factors underlying sleep complaints in the elderly is critical, and can lead to appropriate diagnosis and treatment. Elderly patients need not be resigned merely to getting the sleep that they do because they are "getting older."[69]

CASE 81-4, QUESTION 2: What are the more common underlying causes of sleep complaints in the elderly?

Common precipitants of acute insomnia in the elderly include acute medical illnesses, hospitalization, changes in the sleeping environment, medications, and acute or recurring psychological stressors. Chronic or long-term insomnia may be associated with a variety of underlying medical, behavioral, and environmental conditions, as well as a variety of medications.[71] Identification of treatable underlying causes should be the first step in management of insomnia, based on a medical and medication history, physical and mental status examination, and laboratory investigations including thyroid function, serum chemistry panel, and cardiopulmonary studies if indicated.[71,72] Special attention should be directed to chronic pain from any cause, advanced chronic obstructive pulmonary disease, chronic renal disease, neurologic disorders, and polyuria from urinary, prostate, or endocrine disorders. Medical conditions with a strong association with insomnia include Parkinson disease,[73] chronic pain conditions,[74,75] chronic obstructive pulmonary disease,[1,76] depression, and bipolar disorder, as well as primary sleep disorders such as RLS, sleep apnea, and circadian rhythm disorders.[2,23,67] The potential contribution of medications to the sleep complaint needs to be evaluated, and changes in medication or timing of administration should be considered. Many drugs with CNS effects can alter patterns of sleep and wakefulness, both during their use and their withdrawal.[23,68,77,78] Both prescribed and OTC medications must be evaluated. The more common drugs of concern include stimulants (caffeine, nicotine, and amphetamines), alcohol, activating antidepressants (fluoxetine, bupropion), pseudoephedrine, bronchodilators, β-blockers, calcium-channel blockers, corticosteroids, and dopamine agonists. Evening administration of drugs like diuretics may also contribute to nighttime awakenings and sleep complaints.

Psychological Versus Drug Treatments for Insomnia

CASE 81-4, QUESTION 3: Which nondrug therapy treatment options might be appropriate for S.D.?

CBT is an effective and safe alternative to drug therapy for insomnia, and has also been shown to be an effective augmenting treatment with drug therapy.[79] CBT limitations include that it is little known, not widely available, and more time-consuming than drug therapy. Both pharmacologic and nonpharmacologic approaches are effective for the short-term management of insomnia in late life, and current evidence suggests that sleep improvements are better sustained over time with behavioral treatment.[80] A comparative meta-analysis of 21 studies of pharmacotherapy and behavior therapy for persistent insomnia in adults found that both treatments similarly produced moderate to large improvements in number of awakenings, wake time after sleep onset, total sleep time, and sleep quality.[81] Behavior therapy, however, resulted in a greater reduction of sleep latency than pharmacotherapy. CBT was compared with pharmacotherapy (zolpidem) and its combination in 63 young and middle-aged adults with chronic sleep-onset insomnia.[82] There was a significant difference in percent change in improved sleep-onset latency (CBT 52%, combination therapies 52%, zolpidem 14%, placebo 17%). No significant differences were found among the groups in total sleep time. The authors concluded that CBT, alone or in combination with pharmacotherapy, was more effective than pharmacotherapy alone or placebo for the treatment of sleep-onset insomnia. Avoidance of medications with their associated costs, adverse effects, and drug interactions is the primary advantage of CBT. Disadvantages of CBT include possible longer time to effective treatment, higher initial cost, and relative paucity of trained providers in many areas.[83]

CASE 81-4, QUESTION 4: What are the concerns about the use of lorazepam in S.D.?

Two specific concerns need to be addressed about the risks most associated with benzodiazepines in the elderly—dependence and risk of falls. Concern about dependence and the nontherapeutic use of benzodiazepines has been an important factor in limiting the long-term treatment of insomnia with hypnotic drugs.[84] In insomnia patients specifically, the risks of dependence and recreational use of benzodiazepines are relatively low. Dose escalation appears to occur only when treatment is ineffective, or when the patient has a history of substance abuse or anxiety. Although still controversial, the risk of dependence and abuse associated with the newer nonbenzodiazepine drugs may be lower than that associated with benzodiazepine hypnotic drugs. An even greater concern with benzodiazepine use in the elderly is the risk of falls and subsequent hip fractures. Using 42 months of Medicaid health care claims data in New Jersey for more than 125,000 individuals older than 65 years, the association of hip fractures and benzodiazepine use was evaluated.[85] Compared with not being exposed to a benzodiazepine, exposure to any benzodiazepine was associated with a 54% higher rate of hip fracture, and after adjusting for potential confounding variables, benzodiazepine use was associated with a 24% higher rate of hip fracture. Use of short half-life benzodiazepines was found to be no safer than use of long half-life benzodiazepines, and the risk of hip fracture was highest during the first 2 weeks after starting a benzodiazepine. These findings support the usual recommendation that the elderly should be given lower doses than their younger adult counterparts, but they challenge the suggestion that only long half-life drugs should be avoided in the elderly owing to clearance concerns.

CASE 81-4, QUESTION 5: What are the concerns about the use of diphenhydramine in S.D.?

Sedating antihistamines are not recommended for treating insomnia in the elderly, as there is no evidence of sustained benefit and they pose significant risk of anticholinergic effects, notably cognitive impairment, dry mouth, urinary retention, and constipation.[77,83,86] A 2-week randomized, crossover trial compared diphenhydramine 50 mg with temazepam 15 mg in 20 elderly individuals with insomnia, 70 to 89 years of age.[87] Temazepam was significantly better than placebo on all sleep measures—sleep quality, total sleep time, number of awakenings, and sleep-onset latency. Diphenhydramine was significantly better than placebo only in reducing the number of awakenings. Both drugs were well tolerated, with similar numbers of adverse effects that were mostly mild and reversible. Although anticholinergic effects were not prominently seen in this study, individuals who may have been at risk for adverse events owing to anticholinergic effects were excluded. In addition to concerns about anticholinergic effects in the elderly, the duration of sedative effect efficacy from antihistamines has also been questioned. A randomized, double-blind, crossover study of diphenhydramine 50 mg and placebo for 4 days was conducted in 15 healthy men, aged 18 to 50 years.[88] Although diphenhydramine produced significant sedative effect on day 1 compared with placebo, by day 4, levels of sleepiness on diphenhydramine were indistinguishable from placebo. In addition, the impairment in performance with diphenhydramine seen on day 1 was completely reversed on day 4. The authors concluded that tolerance developed quickly with diphenhydramine and was complete by the end of day 3.

S.D.'s primary sleep complaint is related to his nocturia. He is self-treating his urinary symptoms with saw palmetto, which he did not mention at his ED visit (perhaps because no one asked whether he used any OTC or herbal medications). His primary treatment, therefore, must be directed at assessing and more successfully treating his nocturia. S.D. also likely experienced lorazepam withdrawal symptoms. The many potential risks associated with benzodiazepines in the elderly led to a valid decision to discontinue lorazepam. The choice of diphenhydramine was poor, however, not only because of its limited short-term efficacy but also because of its potential to worsen his urinary symptoms. Clinicians must ask patients about OTC and herbal medications they may be using to self-treat their symptoms. Like so many elderly patients, the best treatment of sleep complaints is to identify any underlying treatable cause, review and identify any sleep hygiene issues, and avoid the use of benzodiazepines and sedating antihistamines, whose risks often outweigh any benefit.

PEDIATRIC INSOMNIA

CASE 81-5

QUESTION 1: J.B. is an 11-year-old, 5 feet 1 inch, 62-kg boy with a diagnosis of ADHD and conduct disorder who presents to the clinic with trouble falling asleep and staying asleep. Current medications include methylphenidate (Concerta) 54 mg every morning for ADHD symptoms and risperidone 0.5 mg twice daily. Risperidone was prescribed for aggression associated with J.B.'s conduct disorder. A trial of a lower dose of methylphenidate resulted in re-emergence of ADHD symptoms, so his dose was increased back to 54 mg every morning 1 week ago. His mother had been giving him diphenhydramine 50 mg; the drug worked initially, but it is no longer effective. His mother requests a safe medication that will alleviate J.B.'s insomnia. What is the risk of sleep disturbances in children with psychiatric comorbidities?

Typical sleep need in children varies from 12 to 14 hours in children 1 to 3 years of age to between 8.5 and 9.5 hours in adolescents.[89] All major sleep disorders can occur in youth, and therefore evaluation for insomnia, RLS, PLMS, sleep apnea, and narcolepsy are needed whenever symptoms warrant. Trouble initiating and maintaining sleep are more common in children with ADHD (25%–50%) and autism spectrum disorders (44%–83%). Of infants and toddlers, 10% to 30% have bedtime sleep resistance that can be managed behaviorally with parental education. Inconsistent bedtime, falling asleep away from bed, fears, and psychiatric and medical conditions can all contribute to poor sleep in children.[89]

At least 5% to 10% of high school students have delayed sleep-phase syndrome, a physiologic condition in which they do not fall asleep until between 1 and 3 AM and they awaken between 9 AM and noon. School schedules dictate earlier awakening, resulting in chronic sleep deprivation. Poll data indicate that 28% of high school students fall asleep in school at least once a week, and 14% are late or miss school because of oversleeping.[89]

Behavioral interventions to promote good sleep habits (e.g., consistent bedtime and wake-time, before-bedtime ritual) should be initiated during childhood and continued throughout adolescence to promote a lifetime of healthy sleep. No hypnotics are FDA approved for insomnia in children and adolescents, and significant data are lacking to guide clinicians on medications to improve sleep in youth. Diphenhydramine, clonidine, melatonin, and chloral hydrate are commonly used in children and some adolescents; however, the use of Z-hypnotics is also increasing, although this class has not been well studied in this population.[90]

CASE 81-5, QUESTION 2: What is the evidence for the safety and efficacy of diphenhydramine, melatonin, clonidine, chloral hydrate, and benzodiazepine receptor–active hypnotics in children and adolescents?

Before recommending another medication, behavioral interventions such as establishing a before-bedtime ritual and waking at the same time daily should be encouraged. Diphenhydramine is the most commonly used sedative in children according to a survey of 800 pediatricians in four states.[90] It has been shown to decrease both time to fall asleep and awakenings in children and adults.[91] The lowest effective dose should be given to minimize anticholinergic side effects and impaired cognition. Increasing the dose of diphenhydramine could cause next-day hangover for J.B., impairing his ability to function optimally in school. Cyproheptadine is a sedating antihistamine that is sometimes given to children with ADHD who have poor appetite and insomnia.[92] J.B. is overweight and has no appetite problems; therefore, cyproheptadine would not be a good choice.[91,92]

Melatonin is a reasonable option to help J.B. fall asleep, but it may not help him stay asleep. Four trials involving approximately 250 children taking melatonin 2 to 6 mg/night administered 1 to 2 hours before bedtime was effective and well tolerated for weeks and months, but many of the children in the trials were stimulantfree. Headache and upset stomach were the most common side effects.[93] Children without ADHD who experience insomnia may benefit from melatonin as well according to small controlled trials.[94] Melatonin 0.3 to 5 mg given 1 to 2 hours before bedtime has been effective for delayed sleep-phase syndrome in adolescents.[95] There are two case reports describing efficacy for ramelteon as insomnia treatment in children with autism.[91]

After diphenhydramine, clonidine, an α_2-adrenergic agonist, is the most prescribed medication to improve sleep in youth despite the lack of data to support its safety and effectiveness for insomnia. Mostly, it is prescribed to treat difficulty initiating sleep. Dosing is 50 to 100 mcg at bedtime.[90] Common side effects include sedation, dry mouth, constipation, dizziness, and bradycardia.[96] Rebound hypertension is possible on abrupt discontinuation of regular use of clonidine. Clonidine could be tried, but it would cause additive hypotension with risperidone.

Z-hypnotics are increasingly prescribed for insomnia in youth despite a lack of clear therapeutic benefit. An NIH open-label dose-finding study in children with functionally impairing insomnia evaluated 0.125 mg/kg, 0.25 mg/kg, or 0.5 mg/kg zolpidem in 2- to 6-year-olds (n = 21), 7- to 12-year-olds (n = 22), and 13- to 18-year-olds (n = 22), respectively; sleep was measured via polysomnography, and zolpidem blood levels were obtained out to 12 hours after the dose. Time to fall asleep decreased by 5 minutes, total sleep time increased by 20 minutes, but sleep efficiency remained unchanged. As expected, younger patients metabolized zolpidem more efficiently. Compared with the 13- to 18-year-olds, the 2- to 6-year-olds had almost three times greater clearance, and the 7- to 12-year-olds had two times greater

O.R. reports diminished sleep quality, excessive snoring, gasping for air, and weight gain. Although a number of causes could be responsible for O.R.'s symptoms, one of the most serious is sleep apnea. Sleep apnea is a neurologic disorder characterized by mini-episodes of cessation of breathing, which can occur 10 to 200 times an hour. If there is a reduction in airflow but no cessation of breathing, it is called *hypopnea*. The brain responds to episodes of apnea and hypopnea with mini-arousals, waking the individual to stimulate breathing.[3,111,112] These frequent mini-arousals prevent the individual from obtaining quality sleep by not allowing sufficient time in deep, slow-wave sleep, or REM. Obstructive sleep apnea (OSA), the most common type, may be induced when extra body weight (note O.R.'s weight gain) places pressure on the throat and uvula, narrowing the space into which air must travel; this results in the difficulty in breathing and excessive snoring. Biochemically, proinflammatory cytokines such as C-reactive protein, tumor necrosis factor-α, and IL-6 have been associated with the pathogenesis of EDS and sleep apnea.[11,12,111]

Hypertension may be contributing to O.R.'s sleep difficulty. Several studies show an increased risk of sleep apnea in patients with hypertension, coronary artery disease, and cerebrovascular disease.[111,113] Although sleep apnea occurs in approximately 5% of women and 15% of men in the general population, it occurs in up to 40% of patients with hypertension.[113] Treatment of OSA can improve BP control and lead to more restful sleep. Of note, OSA occurs in nonobese individuals and in all ages, including infants.[11,43,111] Sleep-disordered breathing, including snoring, is a significant risk factor for hypertension even in young individuals of normal weight.[113]

Overnight evaluation by polysomnography (i.e., EEG, electro-oculogram, electromyogram) in a sleep laboratory would confirm or rule out sleep apnea and allow distinction between OSA and the less-common central sleep apnea.[43,111] Patients with central sleep apnea lack respiratory effort (i.e., the diaphragm does not move in attempts to take in air); they frequently gasp for air during the night.[111] Treatment of central sleep apnea requires continuous positive airway pressure (CPAP) as opposed to being alleviated through weight loss or anatomic manipulations. Central sleep apnea frequently occurs along with OSA.

For a video and an illustration about sleep apnea/CPAP, go to http://thepoint.lww.com/AT10e.

Drug Treatment Considerations

CASE 81-8, QUESTION 2: Results from the sleep laboratory study clearly document O.R.'s sleep problem as OSA. He experiences an average of 56 apneic episodes per hour. O.R.'s weight gain and inactivity probably contribute to the problem. Both are serious, potentially life-threatening conditions. Why should O.R.'s sleeping difficulties not be treated with a hypnotic medication?

Hypnotics, alcohol, or any CNS depressant can be lethal for patients with sleep apnea and should not be prescribed for O.R. CNS depressants interfere with the mini-arousals required to stimulate breathing once it has stopped. In this case, the sleep laboratory study may have saved O.R. from a potential life-threatening breathing disorder that could have been exacerbated by a hypnotic with CNS depressant activity.

OSA can be treated by tracheostomy, nasal surgery, tonsillectomy, uvulopalatoplasty, and either nasal or orally administered CPAP.[12,43,114] Weight loss and CPAP therapy are the most effective treatments and must be maintained for continued therapeutic efficacy.[11,111] In CPAP, the patient wears a lightweight mask to bed each night, and a constant flow of air is provided mechanically to prevent breathing cessation and to allow for more restful sleep. Although CPAP is effective for both OSA and central sleep apnea, the results are short lived, and apneic episodes typically reappear when CPAP therapy is stopped. Preliminary studies in individuals with nocturnal bradycardia and sleep apnea show that insertion of a permanent cardiac pacemaker significantly improved bradycardia and sleep apnea.[115] More studies are needed. At this time, the best treatment for O.R.'s hypertension and sleep apnea is weight loss and CPAP.

CASE 81-8, QUESTION 3: If weight loss, surgery, and CPAP are all ineffective or impractical, what drug treatments are potentially effective for O.R.'s sleep apnea?

Modafinil, an agent approved for narcolepsy, is also FDA approved to treat EDS caused by OSA or shift work sleep disorder. For O.R., it is best used as an adjunct to CPAP at doses of 200 to 400 mg in the morning.[116,117] Protriptyline, medroxyprogesterone, theophylline, and acetazolamide have been used successfully in small numbers of patients with sleep apnea.[117] A decrease in apneic episodes is statistically significant but not, however, clinically significant for most patients.[117] Fluoxetine and paroxetine show promise in treating sleep apnea by increasing upper-airway patency during sleep.[117,118] To date, no clinically significant improvement has been documented with either agent.

NARCOLEPSY

Narcolepsy is an incurable neurologic disorder characterized by irrepressible sleep attacks typically occurring three to five times a day.[119] These sleep attacks can intrude at any time during the individual's waking state. Narcolepsy may be present with or without cataplexy, although cataplexy is present in 60% to 90% of patients.[119] Cataplexy is the loss of muscle tone in the face or limb muscles and often is induced by emotions or laughter. Cataplexy can be subtle, with the patient limp and not moving, or dramatic, in which persons with narcolepsy collapse to the floor.[120] Hypnagogic hallucinations and sleep paralysis are other secondary symptoms not present in all persons with narcolepsy. Hypnagogic hallucinations are perceptual disturbances (i.e., auditory, visual, tactile) that occur while experiencing a sleep attack. The patient may see imaginary objects, hear sounds, or feel sensations. Sleep paralysis is a terrifying experience that can occur when falling asleep or when awakening. Patients are unable to move their limbs, to speak, or even to breathe deeply. Narcoleptics learn, however, that sleep paralysis episodes are benign and brief (lasting <10 minutes). Except for daytime sleepiness, these symptoms are thought to be expressions or partial expressions of REM sleep.[3,15,119]

Symptoms of narcolepsy often begin at puberty, but patients usually are not diagnosed until years later, in their late teens or early 20s. Early symptoms consist of excessive daytime sedation and poor sleep quality. The sleep cycle becomes progressively more erratic with frequent bursts of REM and decreased regularity of deep or slow-wave sleep. Polysomnography in a sleep laboratory is ideal to confirm narcolepsy. Sleep architecture is notably different. Instead of the 90-minute delay before

REM, individuals with narcolepsy progress directly into REM sleep.[3,119] A cerebrospinal fluid hypocretin 1 level of less than 110 pg/mL is also diagnostic for narcolepsy. Postmortem brain studies of patients with narcolepsy show 85% to 95% decrease in hypocretin-containing neurons.[119]

In the 1970s, genetic research in narcoleptic dogs (Doberman pinchers) and humans revealed that narcolepsy is associated with deficits in the hypocretin receptor-2 gene (*HCRTR2*).[3,29]

An autoimmune response of unknown origin is thought to damage hypocretin/orexin-secreting cells in the hypothalamus. Without functional hypocretin/orexin cells, the sleep–wake cycle is disrupted. Hypocretin/orexin are also involved in control of body weight, water balance, and temperature.[3,119] Hypocretin cell replacement therapy is under study.

Comparing Treatments

Optimal treatment of narcolepsy involves treating both sleep attacks and cataplexy. Schedule II controlled substances, methylphenidate and dextroamphetamine (Dexedrine), were the first drugs used to treat narcolepsy, with 65% to 85% of patients deriving significant improvements in wakefulness. Mixed amphetamine salts are also FDA approved for narcolepsy.[3] The mechanism of action of methylphenidate and amphetamines is related to increasing neurotransmission of dopamine and norepinephrine. Modafinil, a schedule C-IV controlled substance, is an effective treatment with less abuse potential. Its exact mode of action is not fully understood, but it is thought to increase wakefulness through noradrenergic, adrenergic, histaminergic, GABA-modulating, glutamatergic, and hypocretin/orexin-stimulating mechanisms.[3,116] Armodafinil is the dextroenantiomer of modafinil. Its therapeutic effect, side effect profile, half-life, and abuse potential are similar to those for modafinil.[119] In summary, these stimulating drugs decrease the number of sleep attacks, improve task performance, and increase the time to fall asleep, but they cannot eliminate sleep attacks altogether. Research is underway exploring the possible use of immunosuppression at the time of narcolepsy onset. One hypothesis suggests that immunosuppression therapy during a period of pathologic immune response could prevent or reduce damage to the hypocretin system that otherwise would lead to the development of narcolepsy.[3,119]

Cataplexy does not respond to psychostimulants or modafinil but may be lessened with low doses of antidepressants. TCAs (imipramine and clomipramine) were the first antidepressants used, but protriptyline, desipramine, and SSRIs (fluoxetine, sertraline, and paroxetine) are also used.[3] SSRIs and protriptyline offer the advantage of less daytime sedation, compared with tertiary TCAs. The effectiveness of antidepressants for the treatment of cataplexy is thought to be related to REM-suppressant effects. A Cochrane database review concluded that insufficient evidence exists to recommend antidepressants as effective treatments for cataplexy, given that most studies are small and uncontrolled. It should be recognized, however, that large-scale studies on such a rare disorder are difficult to conduct.[119] Antidepressants are not considered effective in decreasing sleep attacks.[3,119,121]

Sodium oxybate (Xyrem), a salt form of the CNS depressant γ-hydroxybutyrate, is the only FDA-approved treatment for cataplexy. Its therapeutic effects are related to decreased REM, improved sleep consolidation, and increased stage 3 and 4 slow-wave sleep.[3,120] In two randomized, double-blind, placebo-controlled trials, sodium oxybate 9 g/night (i.e., 450 mg at bedtime, then 450 mg 2 to 4 hours later), but not 3 or 6 g/night, significantly reduced the median frequency of cataplexy attacks by 69% in patients with narcolepsy, whereas 4.5 to 9 g for 8 weeks significantly reduced the median frequency of cataplexy attacks by 57% to 85% in a dose-related manner. Both trials showed 6% to 30% reduction in EDS as measured on the Epworth Sleepiness Scale and 20% to 43% reduction in daytime sleep attacks.[120] Because of a significant abuse potential, sodium oxybate is available only through restricted distribution, the Xyrem Success Program, by calling 1-866-997-3688 Orphan Medical. It is a Schedule III controlled substance.[119,120]

Mixed Amphetamine Salts and Fluoxetine

CASE 81-9

QUESTION 1: G.B., a 23-year-old man with narcolepsy, has been taking mixed amphetamine salts extended-release 60 mg in the morning for sleep attacks associated with narcolepsy, and fluoxetine 20 mg daily will be started to treat cataplexy. What are the potential risks of using both mixed amphetamine salts and fluoxetine to treat G.B.?

Anorexia, stomach pain, nervousness, irritability, insomnia, and headaches are common side effects of stimulant drugs.[3] Psychotic reactions can occur in narcoleptic patients taking stimulants at any dose; however, these symptoms resolve when the stimulant is discontinued. Hypertension and abnormal liver function are more serious complications of long-term stimulant use. Stimulants, even at high dosages (e.g., 80 mg methylphenidate), usually do not bring a patient to a normal level of alertness, and sometimes nocturnal sleep is disrupted. To prevent stimulant-induced insomnia, doses should be taken before 3 PM. Tolerance to the therapeutic effects of stimulants may, however, develop in some patients with narcolepsy.[3,119,122] Drug holidays may allow the patient to recapture therapeutic benefit; however, many patients opt for an increased stimulant dose instead. Exceeding maximal recommended doses of stimulant significantly increases the risk of psychosis, substance abuse, psychiatric hospitalization, tachyarrhythmia, and anorexia according to a case-control study in 116 patients with narcolepsy taking stimulants.[122]

Fluoxetine may improve cataplexy, but it can worsen nocturnal insomnia and contribute to restlessness, headache, nausea, and sexual side effects including anorgasmia.[59,121] In addition, fluoxetine is a potent CYP2D6 inhibitor resulting in higher levels of amphetamine.[123] G.B. should be monitored closely during the initiation of fluoxetine therapy, and the amphetamine dose should be lowered by 30% to 60% to minimize side effects and prevent toxicity. The optimal therapeutic dose of fluoxetine to manage cataplexy has not been established, but low doses may be effective and minimize the risk of side effects.

Modafinil and Sodium Oxybate

CASE 81-9, QUESTION 2: G.B. experiences intolerable nervousness, irritability, and nocturnal insomnia on mixed amphetamine salts and fluoxetine. There is no improvement in cataplexy with the addition of fluoxetine. He asks about switching to modafinil and sodium oxybate. Does the combination of modafinil and sodium oxybate offer any advantage for G.B.?

Modafinil's efficacy relative to other CNS stimulants has not been adequately assessed in controlled clinical trials; however, it has less potential for insomnia and adverse CNS reactions at recommended dosages between 200 and 400 mg/day administered in the morning.[4] It also has less abuse potential compared with stimulants and is a Schedule IV controlled substance. Headache was the only adverse experience rated significantly higher than placebo in 283 patients taking the recommended dose of either 200 or 400 mg/day of modafinil. Anorexia, nervousness, restlessness, and pulse and BP changes are dose-related side effects to discuss during counseling. The maximal tolerable single daily dose may be 600 mg/day, because 800 mg/day produced increased BP and pulse in one tolerability study.[124] Gradual dosage titration improves tolerability. Armodafinil, an active stereoisomer of modafinil, is effective at usual doses between 150 and 250 mg/day. It has a similar adverse effect profile as modafinil.[119]

Improved daytime wakefulness is an advantage of sodium oxybate compared with antidepressants. A controlled trial involving 278 patients showed an increase in slow-wave sleep (stages 3 and 4) and decreased nightly sleep disruption in patients taking sodium oxybate with modafinil compared with modafinil alone.[125] Sodium oxybate can be administered safely with stimulants and modafinil; however, coadministration with other CNS depressants, including hypnotic medication, is contraindicated because of the risk of respiratory depression.[120]

CASE 81-9, QUESTION 3: What counseling should G.B. receive as he switches to modafinil and sodium oxybate?

People taking modafinil should receive counseling regarding the potential for drug interactions. Modafinil induces CYP3A4 metabolism primarily in the gut; decreased levels of triazolam and ethinyl estradiol have been associated with modafinil coadministration.[126] Enzyme inhibition may also occur. Modafinil's inhibition of CYP2C19 is the proposed mechanism behind modafinil-associated clozapine toxicity.[127] Monitoring for drug interactions is crucial because modafinil and armodafinil are increasingly used for other indications, including daytime sleepiness associated with Parkinson disease, fibromyalgia, sleep apnea, fatigue associated with multiple sclerosis, and ADHD.[128–130]

Individuals taking sodium oxybate should take it on an empty stomach for maximal efficacy, and it should not be given to those with sleep-disordered breathing, sleep apnea, or an alcohol or substance abuse disorder.[120] Adverse effects include nausea, headache, dizziness, and enuresis. Safe coadministration of modafinil and sodium oxybate have been described in clinical trials[125]; however, cases of severe side effects including panic, psychosis, depression, and new-onset suicidal ideation have been described.[131] The risk of serious side effects versus benefits in managing cataplexy and nocturnal insomnia should be discussed with G.B. and his family. Close monitoring, particularly during the first weeks and months of treatment and when dosages are adjusted up or down, should be advised.[131] G.B. should be instructed how to properly administer sodium oxybate, drinking half immediately before bedtime and then setting his alarm for 4 hours to take the midnocturnal dose.

Naps and Other Behavioral Interventions

CASE 81-9, QUESTION 4: The benefits, possible risks, and importance of regular physician assessment have been explained to G.B., and he agrees to report efficacy and adverse effects to his primary-care provider regularly. G.B. is reminded to take the medicine at regular intervals along with daytime naps. Why are naps helpful in the treatment of G.B., and what other behavioral interventions are useful in treating narcolepsy?

Strategically timed 15- to 20-minute naps taken at lunch and then again at 5:30 PM can be refreshing for narcoleptics and increase their time between sleep attacks. Narcolepsy support groups are available and may help G.B. better cope with such a life-changing chronic illness. It also is important for G.B. to avoid alcohol and to regulate his bedtime and wake-up time in the attempt to normalize his sleep habits.[3,119]

KEY REFERENCES AND WEBSITES

A full list of references for this chapter can be found at http://thepoint.lww.com/AT10e. Below are the key references and websites for this chapter, with the corresponding reference number in this chapter found in parentheses after the reference.

Key References

Ahmed I, Thorpy M. Clinical features, diagnosis and treatment of narcolepsy. *Clin Chest Med.* 2010;31:371. (119)

Kushida CA et al. Practice parameters for the use of continuous and bilevel positive airway pressure devices to treat adult patients with sleep-related breathing disorders. *Sleep.* 2006;29:375. (43)

Morgenthaler T et al. Practice parameter for the psychological and behavioral treatment of insomnia: an update. An American Academy of Sleep Medicine report. *Sleep.* 2006;29:1415. (14)

[No authors listed]. NIH State-of-the-Science Conference Statement on manifestations and management of chronic insomnia in adults. *NIH Consens Sci Statements.* 2005;22:1. (4)

Wilson SJ et al. British Association for Psychopharmacology consensus statement on evidence-based treatment for insomnia, parasomnias and circadian-rhythm disorders. *J Psychopharmacol.* 2010;24:1577.

Key Websites

American Academy of Sleep Medicine. http://www.aasmnet.org/

American Sleep Apnea Association. http://www.sleepapnea.org/

National Sleep Foundation. http://www.sleepfoundation.org/

82

Schizophrenia

Jonathan P. Lacro, Sanaz Farhadian, and Rene A. Endow-Eyer

CORE PRINCIPLES

	CHAPTER CASES
1 The target symptoms of schizophrenia include positive and negative symptoms that determine change in clinical status and effectiveness of treatment. The course of schizophrenia begins with a prodrome, which then leads to episodic exacerbations; the disorder is generally associated with poor prognosis.	**Case 82-1 (Questions 1–3)**
2 The goals of treatment are to decrease immediate harm to patients and others around them and prolong the stable phase. Nonpharmacologic interventions should be incorporated into treatment plans.	**Case 82-1 (Questions 4–6)**
3 Selection of pharmacotherapy for patients with schizophrenia should depend on symptoms, nonadherence risk, and properties of medications such as efficacy, toxicity, personal and family history with medication, pharmacokinetic properties, drug–drug interactions, and economic factors.	**Case 82-1 (Questions 7–9, 15, 16, 22, 23)**
4 Extrapyramidal symptoms (acute dystonia, akathisia, parkinsonism) and tardive dyskinesia should be monitored and treated if necessary. The benefits and risks of long-term treatment for extrapyramidal symptoms should also be evaluated carefully and discussed with the patient.	**Case 82-1 (Questions 10–12, 17–21)**
5 Metabolic complications can be significant consequences of antipsychotic therapy. Body weight, waist circumference, fasting glucose, lipids, and blood pressure should be monitored as well as other cardiovascular risk factors.	**Case 82-1 (Questions 24–27)**
6 Clozapine is indicated for the treatment of patients with refractory schizophrenia. Weekly monitoring of blood counts are necessary because of the association between clozapine and life-threatening agranulocytosis.	**Case 82-1 (Questions 29–33)**
7 Female patients who are considering getting pregnant or are pregnant while on antipsychotic treatment should discuss the risks and benefits of pharmacologic treatment with their care providers. In some cases, treatment of schizophrenia symptoms with medications may be necessary to prevent harm to the patient and the fetus.	**Case 82-1 (Question 35)**
8 When treatment is necessary for children and adolescents, atypical antipsychotics and those with low potential for metabolic adverse effects should be used.	**Case 82-1 (Question 36)**

Schizophrenia is a debilitating and emotionally devastating illness with long-term impact on patients' lives. Many experts consider schizophrenia to be the most severe expression of psychopathology, encompassing significant disruptions of thinking, perception, emotion, and behavior. Schizophrenia is usually a lifelong psychiatric disability. Family relationships, social functioning, and employment are frequently affected, and periodic hospitalizations are common. The management of schizophrenia involves multiple strategies to optimize the patient's functional capacity, reduce the frequency and severity of symptom exacerbations, and reduce the overall morbidity and mortality from this disorder. Many patients require comprehensive and continuous care over the course of their lives.

EPIDEMIOLOGY

Schizophrenia has a low incidence of 2.4 to 6.7 per 1,000 persons.[1] Prevalence rates are similar throughout the world, but pockets of high prevalence have been reported in some areas. After adjusting for differences in diagnostic criteria for schizophrenia, similar prevalence rates across cultures have been observed. Although schizophrenia affects men and women with equal frequency, there are differences in the age of onset and course of illness.[2] Onset of schizophrenia usually occurs during late adolescence or early adulthood. Studies indicate that males are affected earlier than females by about 3 to 5 years. Males commonly exhibit schizophrenia between the ages of 15 and 25, whereas the illness affects females between the ages of 15 and 30, and a smaller group between ages 45 and 50.

ECONOMIC BURDEN

Mental health disorders constitute a large part of the global burden of disease, with schizophrenia being among the greatest causes of disability in the United States and the world. Unlike other chronic diseases such as diabetes and hypertension, which occur late in life, schizophrenia usually affects people when they are young, followed by a chronic course persisting throughout the patient's lifetime. Most people with schizophrenia experience multiple hospitalizations and generally require social assistance. Even during relatively stable phases of their illness, most people with schizophrenia require support ranging from a family member to daytime hospitalization. In 2002, total costs for schizophrenia patients in the United States averaged $62.7 billion annually, taking into account direct and indirect costs as well as unemployment costs.[3] Direct costs include hospitalization, rehabilitation, professional services, medication, and office visits. Indirect costs include loss of productivity caused by illness, disability, premature death, and economic burden to families.[3] The World Health Organization Global Burden of Disease study provides a comprehensive and comparable assessment of mortality and loss of health owing to diseases, injuries, and risk factors for all regions of the world. In their latest report, which provides estimates for 2004, neuropsychiatric conditions such as schizophrenia were among the top conditions accounting for disproportionately greater degrees of disability.[4] Persons afflicted by schizophrenia in the United States represent a disproportionately higher percentage of this country's permanently disabled population. In 2004, it was estimated that 70% of patients with schizophrenia receive medications through Medicaid. Because of the advent of newer atypical antipsychotics during the past 20 years, the cost of psychotropic medications now exceeds $10 billion annually.[5]

ETIOLOGY (NEUROBIOLOGY)

Schizophrenia is a complex disorder with multiple causes. Considering the lack of consistent neuropathology or biomarkers, current theories of the disorder have moved away from the view that it is a single entity, and toward a conceptualization of schizophrenia as a collection of etiologically disparate disorders with common clinical features. In this section, the genetic and environmental factors and the neuroanatomical and neurochemical features of schizophrenia are considered.

Genetic and Environmental Risk Factors

Studies have clearly established a familial predisposition for schizophrenia. Siblings of a proband with schizophrenia have a sevenfold to tenfold increased risk of the disorder; children born to a parent with schizophrenia have a 13-fold to 15-fold increased risk.[6] The risk is highest (40%–50%) in a monozygotic (identical) twin of a person with schizophrenia.[7] There is also higher concordance for schizophrenia in monozygotic twins compared with dizygotic twins, with respective rates being approximately 50% and 15%.[8] Because the concordance rate is not 100% in monozygotic twins or 50% in dizygotic twins, other nongenetic factors must contribute to the development of the disorder. Environmental factors such as prenatal difficulties (i.e., malnutrition in the first trimester of pregnancy or influenza in the second trimester), perinatal complications, and various nonspecific stressors may also influence the development of schizophrenia. Despite the evidence that schizophrenia is an inherited illness, a single "schizophrenia gene" has not been found. Risk for schizophrenia is, to some extent, genetically transmitted and is probably determined by multiple genes.[6]

Neuroanatomy

Computed tomography and magnetic resonance imaging brain studies of individuals with schizophrenia have shown enlarged ventricles, particularly the lateral and third ventricles. Other consistently reported findings include morphologic abnormalities involving the temporal, frontal, and parietal lobes, and the subcortical structures.[9,10] Findings include decreased neuronal volume and density, decreased synaptic connections, decreases in synaptophysin (a membrane protein of synaptic vesicles), and loss of microtubule-associated protein and synaptosomal protein in certain regions of the cortex.[11] The lack of gliosis in association with the neuroanatomical abnormalities in the brains of schizophrenia patients suggests that these changes occur neurodevelopmentally.[11] Functional imaging studies have demonstrated alterations in either cerebral perfusion or glucose metabolism in frontal, temporal, and basal ganglia areas of the brain.[10,12] In summary, neuroimaging studies have identified anatomical and functional abnormalities that affect different areas of the brain, particularly the prefrontal and temporal areas, corresponding with the impairments observed in schizophrenia. Medial temporal structures are important for the processing of sensory information, and abnormalities in this area may explain distortions in the interpretation of external reality that are characteristic of schizophrenia (i.e., delusions and hallucinations). The prefrontal cortex is responsible for some of the complex and highly evolved human functions, including the integration of information from other cortical areas. The prefrontal cortex is also largely responsible for the regulation of working memory, which involves maintaining information in temporary memory while that information is used for executive functions. Hence, these abnormalities in prefrontal areas could explain the deficits in working memory and attention that are often present in schizophrenia (i.e., cognitive impairment). Although research in this area has grown significantly in the last decade, many unanswered questions remain including whether or not such abnormalities are stable throughout the entire course of illness and may serve as predictors of pharmacologic response.

Neurochemistry

The discovery of the antipsychotic properties of chlorpromazine led to a fundamental understanding of the neurochemistry of schizophrenia. The finding that chlorpromazine and other antipsychotic drugs decrease dopamine activity by blocking specific postsynaptic receptors served as the foundation for the dopaminergic hypothesis of schizophrenia. Nearly all drugs that decrease dopamine activity decrease the positive symptoms of schizophrenia. Furthermore, the clinical efficacy of antipsychotic agents is roughly proportional to their affinity for a particular subtype of dopamine receptors, the D_2 receptor. Although other classes of dopamine receptors have been identified (e.g., D_1, D_3, D_4), this close relationship to clinical potency exists only for the D_2 receptor subtype.[13] Indirect evidence supporting the dopamine hypothesis is found in the observation that dopamine agonists such as amphetamine, levodopa, methylphenidate, and other aminergic agents can worsen schizophrenia symptoms in some patients.[14–16] Although these observations indicate that manipulating the dopaminergic system can regulate the positive symptoms of schizophrenia, they do not directly implicate a central excess of dopamine as the sole cause of schizophrenia symptoms. Excess dopaminergic activity in the mesolimbic system has been associated with the positive symptomatology of schizophrenia. This simplistic theory does not explain, for instance, cases of schizophrenia in which residual or negative symptoms predominate. The "hypofrontality theory" suggests that reduced or dysfunctional dopaminergic neurotransmission within the prefrontal cortex or mesocortical area of schizophrenic patients may be responsible for negative symptoms.[10,17] In addition to negative symptomatology, prefrontal dopaminergic dysfunction has been correlated with cognitive dysfunction, particularly in the area of working memory. It has also been proposed that a chronically low level of striatal dopamine release causes negative symptoms (caused by low levels of dopamine in the prefrontal cortex). The diminished dopamine release leads to an upregulation of dopamine receptors, resulting in supersensitivity to phasic dopamine release in the context of environmental stressors (exhibited behaviorally as positive symptoms).[18] This theory explains why dopamine-blocking drugs improve positive symptoms, but not negative symptoms.

Serotonin also seems to play a role in schizophrenia. Alteration in monoamine activity in the limbic circuit has been proposed as a possible link to the dopamine hypothesis of schizophrenia.[19] Serotonin receptors are abundant in mesocortical areas, and agonism at these receptor sites may have an inhibitory effect on dopaminergic receptors or dopamine release, possibly contributing to negative schizophrenia symptoms.

Another area of focus is the involvement of excitatory amino acids and the glutamate transmitter system in the pathogenesis of schizophrenia.[20] Decreased activation of *N*-methyl-D-aspartic acid (NMDA) or glutamate receptors may increase cortical dopamine release and produce a syndrome resembling schizophrenia. This hypofunctional NMDA receptor theory was supported by findings of low glutamate levels in the cerebrospinal fluid of persons with schizophrenia and by the observation that phencyclidine (PCP), an NMDA antagonist, could produce florid psychosis.[21] In utero exposure to excitotoxins or viruses has been proposed as a possible mechanism for destruction of NMDA receptors within the brain. The clinical effect of neuronal destruction may not be expressed until late adolescence or early adulthood (when symptoms of schizophrenia usually arise). γ-Aminobutyric acid (GABA), a major inhibitory neurotransmitter, may act as a third link between the neuromodulation of glutamate and dopamine receptors. It has been suggested that GABA receptor function may be impaired within the prefrontal region, resulting in abnormal NMDA receptor concentrations.[22] It has also been proposed that an imbalance between NMDA, GABA, and dopamine activity may cause the symptoms of schizophrenia. Studies examining the clinical effects of direct glycinergic agonists or inhibitors of glutamate uptake in persons with schizophrenia are needed to clarify the role of excitatory amino acid neurotransmission in this disorder.

Substantial progress has been made in neuropathological and neuroanatomical studies of schizophrenia. Insights from physiological imaging studies in living patients, studies of brain development and its genetic control, and pharmacologic studies using newer atypical antipsychotics are promising stepping stones that may lead to a better understanding of the pathogenesis of schizophrenia.

CLINICAL PRESENTATION

Historical Concept of Schizophrenia

Kraepelin[23] provided the first thorough description of symptoms that make up schizophrenia, which he called "dementia praecox" (a syndrome of cognitive and behavioral deficits that tend to appear early in life). Kraepelin emphasized that dementia praecox generally followed a chronic course with no return to the premorbid level of functioning. Kraepelin also noted that no single pathognomonic symptom or cluster of symptoms served to characterize dementia praecox, an illness he considered so mysterious that he referred to it as a disorder whose causes were shrouded in "impenetrable darkness." Bleuler[24] concurred with Kraepelin's initial description of schizophrenia, although he suggested that some patients did recover and subsequently could lead productive lives. For Bleuler, the most important and fundamental feature was a fragmentation in the formulation and expression of thought, referring to it as "loosening of associations." Bleuler described the "4 *A*'s" of schizophrenia, which include autism (preoccupation with internal stimuli), inappropriate affect (external manifestations of mood), loose associations (illogical or fragmented thought processes), and ambivalence (simultaneous, contradictory thinking). Thus, Bleuler focused on negative symptoms and thought disorganization rather than on the positive symptoms of schizophrenia, such as delusions and hallucinations. Another important contribution to the defining features of schizophrenia was Schneider's "first-rank" symptoms of schizophrenia.[25] First-rank symptoms include delusions, auditory hallucinations, thought withdrawal, thought insertion, thought broadcasting, and experiencing feelings or actions that are under someone else's control. Schneider's first-rank symptoms provided the framework for the systematic diagnostic criteria used today in psychiatry.

Diagnosis and Differential Diagnosis

The *Diagnostic and Statistical Manual of the American Psychiatric Association,* Fourth Edition, Text Revision (DSM-IV-TR), is the latest edition of the guide for diagnosis and classification of schizophrenia and other psychiatric disorders. Compared with previous DSM editions, the DSM-IV-TR places a greater emphasis on negative symptoms and the social and occupational dysfunction associated with schizophrenia.[7] Psychosis has many causes, and all must be excluded before the diagnosis of schizophrenia is made. In addition, a diagnosis can be made only if the DSM-IV-TR criteria are met (Table 82-1). Clinicians can misdiagnose psychotic patients when the diagnosis is based on presenting symptoms alone without regard to the longitudinal clinical course. An accurate diagnosis is important because treatments vary for psychoses with different origins. Schizophreniform disorder is similar to schizophrenia except that it lasts for more than 1 month but less than 6 months. Brief psychotic disorder is diagnosed when positive symptoms present suddenly and are present for greater than or equal to 1 day but less than 1 month. After the episode subsides, premorbid functioning usually returns. Various personality disorders, including schizotypal, schizoid, and paranoid types also can resemble schizophrenia; however, these disorders lack the chronic thought disturbances seen in schizophrenia. Bipolar disorder, manic or depressive phase, and major depression can have psychotic features that usually are mood congruent. Negative symptoms of schizophrenia such as akinesia, anergy, apathy, and

TABLE 82-1
DSM-IV-TR Criteria for Schizophrenia

A. Characteristic Symptoms

At least two (or more) of the following, each present for a significant portion of time during a 1-month period (or less if successfully treated). At least one of these should include 1–3:

1. Delusions
2. Hallucinations
3. Disorganized speech (e.g., frequent derailment or incoherence)
4. Grossly disorganized or catatonic behavior
5. Negative symptoms (i.e., restricted affect or avolition/asociality)

Note: Only one "A symptom" is required if delusions are bizarre or hallucinations consist of a voice keeping up a running commentary on the person's behavior or thought, two or more conversations with each other.

B. Social or Occupational Dysfunction

For a significant portion of the time since the onset of the disturbance, one or more major areas of functioning such as work, interpersonal relationships, or self-care is markedly below the level achieved before the onset (or when the onset is in childhood or adolescence, failure to achieve expected level of interpersonal, academic, or occupational achievement).

C. Duration

Continuous signs of the disturbance persist for at least 6 months. This 6-month period must include at least 1 month of symptoms (or less if successfully treated) that meet criterion A (i.e., active-phase symptoms) and may include prodromal or residual symptoms. During these prodromal or residual periods, signs of the disturbance may be manifested by negative symptoms or by two or more symptoms listed in criterion A present in an attenuated form (e.g., odd beliefs, unusual perceptual disturbances).

D. Schizoaffective Disorder and Mood Disorder Exclusion

Schizoaffective disorder and mood disorder with psychotic features have been ruled out because either (a) no major depressive, manic, or mixed episodes have occurred concurrently with the active phase symptoms or (b) if mood episodes have occurred during active phase symptoms, their total duration has been brief relative to the duration of the active and residual periods.

E. Substance or General Medical Condition Exclusion

The disturbance is not caused by direct physiological effects of a substance (e.g., drug of abuse or medication) or a general medical condition.

F. Relationship to a Pervasive Development Disorder

If there is a history of autistic disorder or another pervasive development disorder, the additional diagnosis of schizophrenia is made only if prominent delusions or hallucinations also are present for at least a month (or less if successfully treated).

Adapted with permission from American Psychiatric Association. *Diagnostic and Statistical Manual of Mental Disorders.* 4th ed. Text Revision (DSM-IV-TR). Washington, DC: American Psychiatric Press; 2000.

TABLE 82-2
Differential Diagnosis for Schizophrenia (DSM-IV-TR)

Drug-induced Psychoses

Amphetamine
Cocaine
Cannabis (marijuana)
Phencyclidine (PCP)
Lysergic acid diethylamide (LSD)
Anticholinergics

Primary Psychiatric Disorders

Brief psychotic disorder
Schizophreniform disorder
Bipolar affective disorder, manic type
Mood disorder with psychotic features

Personality Disorders

Schizotypal
Schizoid
Paranoid

Adapted with permission from American Psychiatric Association. *Diagnostic and Statistical Manual of Mental Disorders.* 4th ed. Text Revision (DSM-IV-TR). Washington, DC: American Psychiatric Press; 2000.

social withdrawal may resemble depression, but generally do not respond to antidepressant therapy. It is also important to differentiate extrapyramidal side effects of drugs, particularly akinesia seen with antipsychotic-induced parkinsonism, from the negative symptoms of schizophrenia. Common differential diagnoses are listed in Table 82-2.

Drug-induced psychosis is an important differential diagnosis when evaluating patients with symptoms resembling schizophrenia. Illicit drugs may cause psychotic symptoms in any individual, but do not cause schizophrenia in persons without a predisposition to mental illness or an underlying psychiatric disorder. Drugs causing acute psychotic symptoms include amphetamines, cocaine, cannabis, phencyclidine ("angel dust"), lysergic acid diethylamide, and ketamine. In addition, anticholinergic delirium can occur if excessive doses or combinations of therapeutic agents with anticholinergic properties are prescribed. A urine toxicology screen can help to evaluate the contribution of substance abuse to psychosis, but because of the risk of false-negative results, the quality and progression of the presenting symptoms and physical findings also must be considered to make an accurate diagnosis. A particularly difficult problem is evaluating the cause of psychosis in a patient with schizophrenia and concurrent drug abuse or alcohol abuse. Distinguishing between the two may not be possible until the patient becomes drug-free and residual symptoms are assessed. There are some differences in the presentation of drug-induced psychosis and schizophrenia. For example, chronic stimulant use usually does not present with a formal thought disorder. Cannabis psychosis may be differentiated from acute paranoid schizophrenia because patients with the former usually experience a subjective feeling of panic and retain insight into their problem.[26] Acute PCP ingestion can cause psychotic symptoms such as paranoia and acute catatonia, but other concomitant symptoms such as ataxia, hyperreflexia, nystagmus, and hypertension are not found in schizophrenia.

Target Symptoms

Schizophrenia is a complex disorder comprising different clusters of signs and symptoms. The characteristic symptoms of schizophrenia have often been conceptualized as falling into two broad categories: positive and negative (or deficit) symptoms. Positive symptoms can be further divided into two distinct groups, positive symptoms and disorganized symptoms. Positive symptoms include hallucinations (auditory, visual, olfactory, gustatory, tactile) and delusions (persecution, guilt, religion, mind control). Disorganized symptoms include disorganized speech, thought disorder (tangentiality, derailment, circumstantiality, incoherence) and disorganized behavior (clothing, appearance, aggression, repetitive actions). Positive symptoms are the most obvious and dramatic symptoms of schizophrenia and they

TABLE 82-3
Glossary of Commonly Used Terms in Schizophrenia

Affect: behavior (usually an expression of an emotion) observed by the interviewer. Common types of disturbances in affect include *restricted*—mild decrease in range and intensity of the expression of emotion; *blunted*—significant decrease in intensity of the expression of emotion; *flat*—absence of expression of emotion; *inappropriate*—incongruency between patient's affect and mood or behavior; and *labile*—abrupt shifts in expression of emotion.

Akathisia: syndrome consisting of subjective feelings of anxiety and restlessness, and objective signs of pacing, rocking, and an inability to sit or stand still for extended periods.

Akinesia: absence or decrease in voluntary movement; may be antipsychotic induced (extrapyramidal side effects) or a manifestation of negative symptoms of schizophrenia.

Alogia: impoverished thinking usually manifested through speech and language deficits. Speech is brief and lacks spontaneity; replies to questions are very concrete (*poverty of speech*). *Poverty of content* refers to speech that is adequate in amount, but is of little substance (overly abstract), repetitive, or stereotyped.

Anergy: lack of energy.

Anhedonia: loss of interest or pleasure.

Avolition: an inability to initiate and sustain goal-directed activities. The patient may sit for extended periods and show minimal interest in participating in social or work-related activities.

Circumstantiality: a form of disorganized speech characterized by "talking in circles" or taking an unusually long time in answering a question or expressing one's point of view.

Delusions: a false belief that is firmly held despite evidence to refute the belief. The belief does not qualify as a delusion if it is a cultural or religious belief accepted by a group of individuals. Types of delusions include grandiose, persecutory, and somatic type.

Executive function: the ability to design and carry out a solution to a plan when the solution is not obvious. Loss of executive function presents as failure to learn from past experience and failure to plan or organize life events.

Hallucination: a sensory perception (e.g., auditory, visual, somatic, tactile) experienced in the absence of external stimuli. Hallucinations may be recognized as false sensory perceptions in some, whereas others may believe that the experiences are reality based.

Loose associations: a form of disorganized, illogical speech characterized by unrelated words, phrases, and sentences used in a fashion that makes comprehension very difficult, if not impossible.

Mood: a pervasive and sustained emotion that is experienced by the patient. Examples include depressed, anxious, angry, or irritable mood.

Mood-congruent delusions or hallucinations: delusions or hallucinations that are consistent with a mood or behavior (e.g., delusions or hallucinations of death, guilt, or punishment in the presence of a depressed mood).

Mood-incongruent delusions or hallucinations: delusions or hallucinations that are not consistent with a mood or behavior (e.g., delusions or hallucinations of death, guilt, or punishment in the presence of mania).

Tangentiality: a form of disorganized speech in which answers are remotely or completely unrelated to questions, and patients' thoughts frequently shift in an unconnected fashion.

Thought broadcasting: a delusion that one's thoughts are being broadcast to others (e.g., a patient feels that others can read his or her mind).

Thought disorder: a general term often used to describe any type of abnormal thought process (e.g., delusion, loose association, conceptual disorganization).

Thought insertion: a delusion that one's thoughts are being inserted into one's mind by others.

are frequently what defines the illness for the general public. Negative symptoms, however, may be more important in the illness spectrum as its severity predicts long-term disability better than the severity of positive symptoms. Negative symptoms have been associated with functional impairment and include affective flattening, decreased thought and speech productivity (alogia), loss of ability to experience pleasure (anhedonia), decreased initiation of goal-directed behavior (avolition), and social withdrawal. Most patients with schizophrenia exhibit both positive and negative symptoms, although the dominance of one type over the other usually varies throughout the course of the illness. Younger patients tend to exhibit more positive symptoms, whereas in older patients negative symptoms predominate. Table 82-3 provides a glossary of commonly used terms in schizophrenia, and Table 82-4 lists positive and negative symptoms of schizophrenia.

Neurocognitive deficits, including problems with attention, memory, and concentration, are other frequently cited problems for people with schizophrenia. The most consistently identified deficits are observed on tasks measuring attention, information-processing speed, working memory, learning, and executive (frontal systems) functions.[27] These domains are not only commonly impaired in schizophrenia but they are also strongly associated with social and community functioning.[27] Although it is likely that the overall dysfunction observed in schizophrenia encompasses factors such as psychopathology, drug treatment, and social isolation, evidence suggests that cognitive impairments have a stronger relationship to long-term functional outcome than positive or negative symptoms.[27]

People with schizophrenia experience symptoms of depression and anxiety. These symptoms are often unnoticed by many clinicians and relatives of family members as they are too distracted by the patients' positive symptoms. Depression can also be obscured by negative symptoms, and both families and clinicians can consider the depression symptoms they see to be manifestations of negative symptoms; yet persons with schizophrenia are usually fully capable of acknowledging feelings of depression. Anxiety is a frequent complaint in schizophrenia and it has been suggested that its presence may lead to a poorer prognosis, precipitate violence and suicidal ideation, and that it can lead to

TABLE 82-4
Positive and Negative Symptoms of Schizophrenia

Positive	Negative
Psychosis	Psychomotor retardation
Hallucinations	Affective flattening
Delusions	Avolition
Disorganization	Lack of socialization
Disorganized speech (loose associations, tangential, blocking)	Alogia
Unusual behavior	Loss of emotional connectedness
Combativeness, agitation, and hostility	Loss of executive functions

increases in psychosis, disorganization, and depression—but this requires further study.

CASE 82-1

QUESTION 1: J.R. is a 26-year-old, single woman brought into the emergency department (ED) after police found her standing on a freeway overpass yelling "If I can't have my baby, no one can!" In the ED, she appears severely agitated, frequently screaming at the nurses and doctors, "You'll never take my baby!" On questioning, J.R. discloses that her Martian husband has been working with the government for the past 2 years to recruit her unborn baby into the space program. She just found out her father and roommate are also involved in this conspiracy, and no longer trusts them. She says her secret sources supply her with these messages via magazine and television ads. She reveals it was the voice of her dead mother that "told me to outsmart the baby stealers by killing myself."

J.R. has no history of a previous psychiatric illness and has never been hospitalized. She denies her current illness and says to the interviewer, "You are using this as an excuse to take my baby from me!" J.R. spent most of her childhood raised by her father because her mother was frequently hospitalized for episodes of psychosis. J.R.'s roommate of the past 3 years told the police her behavior has become increasingly odd during the last several months. J.R. works as a computer programmer, but more recently, she often skips work to stay home and watch television and has been spending her money on baby clothes and diapers. She no longer participates in her church group or sees her friends or family. She smokes 10 cigarettes/day and denies alcohol or illicit drug use.

J.R.'s physical and neurological examinations were unremarkable. Her body mass index is 27.2 kg/m^2. Her laboratory tests including a complete blood count (CBC) with differential, chem-10 panel, urinalysis, liver function tests (LFTs), and thyroid panel were within normal limits. Her lipid panel was abnormal:

Total cholesterol, 248 mg/dL
High-density lipoprotein (HDL), 34 mg/dL
Triglycerides (TG), 175 mg/dL
Low-density lipoprotein (LDL), 179 mg/dL

A urine drug screen and human chorionic gonadotropin (hCG) pregnancy test were both negative. An electrocardiogram (ECG) revealed a QTc of 460 milliseconds.

In an examination of J.R.'s mental status, under appearance and behavior J.R. is found to be a slightly overweight woman wearing raggedy clothes with multiple stains. She is easily agitated by the interviewer's multiple questions. She is suspicious of him and repeatedly asks, "Whom do you work for?" Under cognition and memory, J.R. is oriented to time, person, place, and situation. Her short-term memory is difficult to assess because of her uncooperativeness; her long-term memory appears to be intact. Under mood and affect, J.R. is anxious and frustrated. Her affect is blunted, with a minimal range of reactivity to her emotions. Under thought content, J.R. hears the voice of her dead mother and appears to be responding to this internal stimulus by having a conversation with herself. Under thought process, J.R.'s responses are tangential, answering the interviewer's initial question, and then straying off the topic with remarks such as "My roommate wants my baby. My baby loves music. My favorite music is punk rock. Do you play any instruments?" Under insight and judgment, both are poor as evidenced by J.R.'s denial of her illness and recent behavior that has led to her hospital admission. The provisional diagnosis is schizophrenia, paranoid type.

What target symptoms of schizophrenia are present in J.R.? How are target symptoms used to monitor treatment?

J.R. exhibits many of the classic symptoms of schizophrenia, including positive symptoms such as delusions (suspiciousness, being pregnant and in danger of losing her baby, thought insertion of receiving messages from magazine and television ads), auditory hallucinations of hearing her dead mother's voice, disorganization (disheveled appearance, tangential speech), and negative symptoms (self-isolating, avoiding church group and work). Other target symptoms include agitation, her recent changes in behavior, responding to internal stimuli, and impaired insight and judgment. These target symptoms are the basis of assessing a change in clinical status and monitoring J.R.'s response to medications.

Typical Course and Outcome

ONSET OF ILLNESS

CASE 82-1, QUESTION 2: What is the typical course and prognosis of patients with schizophrenia?

The onset of schizophrenia starts with the prodromal phase that begins with the first changes in behavior and lasts until the onset of psychosis.[28–30] It is characterized by a slow and gradual onset of signs and symptoms that can last weeks to years, but typically persists for at least a year.[28] Common prodromal signs and symptoms include anxiety, blunted affect, depression or dysphoric mood, irritability, loss of initiative, low energy, poor concentration, sleep disturbance, social isolation and withdrawal, and suspiciousness. Subthreshold or attenuated positive symptoms and mild disorganization (digressive, vague, overly abstract, or concrete thinking) may begin during the prodromal phase. Gradual deterioration in functioning commonly occurs. The prodrome is difficult to recognize; however, family members may interpret the earliest subtle changes as normal adolescence, a phase, relational problems, depression, or drug use. Some researchers have viewed the prodromal phase or "at-risk" mental state as an optimal point to begin pharmacologic intervention.[31] Research has shown that many patients are ill for months or even years before seeking treatment; this delay in treatment may influence long-term outcome and the occurrence of remission. Early recognition of the prodrome could lead to interventions that delay or prevent the emergence of psychosis. Eventually, a symptom characteristic of the active phase appears (Table 82-1, criterion A), marking the disturbance as schizophrenia.

COURSE OF ILLNESS

In contrast with the notion of an inevitable progressive deterioration in schizophrenia as proposed by Kraepelin, longitudinal studies of schizophrenia suggest that the course of illness is highly variable ranging from complete remission (i.e., a return to full premorbid functioning after a single psychotic episode) to continuous unremitting psychopathology and cognitive, social, and occupational dysfunction.[32–35] The majority suffers from episodic exacerbations and remissions with some degree of residual symptoms.[32–35] Of the patients with persistent symptoms, some seem to have a relatively stable course, whereas others show a progressive worsening associated with severe disability. Reported remission rates range from 10% to 60%, and a reasonable estimate is that 20% to 30% of all schizophrenia patients are able to lead somewhat normal lives. About 20% to 30% of patients continue to experience moderate symptoms, and 40% to 60% of patients remain significantly impaired by their disorder for their entire lives.[32] Early in the illness, negative symptoms may manifest as prodromal features. Subsequently, positive symptoms appear. Because these positive symptoms are particularly responsive to treatment, they typically diminish, but in many individuals negative symptoms persist between episodes of positive symptoms. As patients with schizophrenia age, the frequency and severity of acute episodes may decrease; however, negative symptoms may become more prominent, a state often referred to as "burn-out."[33]

PROGNOSIS

Predictors of an improved long-term outcome in patients with schizophrenia include female sex, a positive family history of an affective disorder, a negative family history of schizophrenia, good premorbid functioning, higher intelligence quotient, married marital status, acute onset of illness, fewer and shorter episodes, a phasic pattern of episodes and remissions (i.e., fewer residual symptoms), advancing age at onset, minimal comorbidity, paranoid subtype, symptoms that are predominantly positive (delusions, hallucinations) and not disorganized (thought disorder, disorganized behavior) nor negative, and an awareness and insight into the symptoms.[32,36–38] Despite modern treatment advancements, schizophrenia remains a severe disease with a relatively poor outcome. Many patients experience repeated hospitalizations and exacerbations of symptoms, and suicide attempts are relatively common. Individuals with schizophrenia have a 20% shorter life expectancy than the general population.[32] This is due in part to an increased incidence of general medical illness (such as diabetes and cardiovascular disease), poor attention to modifiable health risk factors (obesity, hypertension, dyslipidemia, hyperglycemia, metabolic syndrome, smoking, and substance abuse) and suicide.[32,39] Patients with schizophrenia have approximately a 50% lifetime risk for a suicide attempt and as many as 9% to 13% complete suicide.[40] Increased suicide risk has been observed early in the course of illness, with frequent relapse, and at around the time of admission or immediately after discharge from a psychiatric facility. Also, periods of increased psychosis, especially when paranoid delusions are prominent, a lack of insight, and a fear of mental deterioration seem to increase risk in this population. Nonspecific factors like depression, hopelessness, motor restlessness and agitation, impulsivity, and anxiety increase the risk for suicide in schizophrenia, as they do in other psychiatric illnesses.

CASE 82-1, QUESTION 3: What other factors in J.R.'s history are consistent with the diagnosis of schizophrenia, and what is her prognosis?

Other factors that are consistent with schizophrenia in J.R. include a young age of onset (typical age of onset is late adolescence to early 30s) and a positive family history (first-degree relative) with schizophrenia. Additionally, during the past several months, she has been exhibiting prodromal symptoms of loss of initiative, social isolation and withdrawal, and suspiciousness. J.R.'s prognosis is fair, as she has both positive and negative risk factors for a good recovery. Although she was young at the time of illness onset, had a positive family history for schizophrenia, and is slightly disorganized (tangential speech), her female sex, good premorbid functioning, and schizophrenia subtype (paranoid with primarily positive symptoms) predict a fair long-term prognosis. Of the multiple prognostic factors that influence outcome, the most important modifiable factor is proper treatment consisting of early identification, treatment with appropriate medications, family education, and psychosocial rehabilitation.[32]

TREATMENT

Schizophrenia is a chronic disease for which there is no cure. Pharmacotherapy can reduce symptoms to improve social and cognitive functions; however, patients often have multiple relapses and experience residual symptoms throughout their lives. Treatment can decrease acute symptoms, decrease the frequency and severity of psychotic episodes, and optimize psychosocial functioning between episodes. However, many patients require comprehensive care and lifelong treatment. Comprehensive care consists of pharmacologic, psychosocial, and rehabilitative treatment.

Goals of Treatment

The American Psychiatric Association Practice Guideline for the Treatment of Schizophrenia describes three phases of illness—acute, stabilization, and stable—for the purpose of integrating treatment.[32] Each phase uses different drug and nondrug strategies to achieve the desired therapeutic outcome. These phases are not always distinct or separate, but instead tend to overlap.

ACUTE PHASE

During the acute phase of illness, patients suffer from floridly psychotic symptoms such as delusions or hallucinations, are severely disorganized, and usually require hospitalization or are placed in a supervised outpatient setting. Negative symptoms become more severe during this phase as well. The initial treatment goal is to calm agitated patients who may be physical threats to themselves or others. Medication is usually required to achieve this outcome, although nondrug interventions such as emotional support from the staff and use of quiet areas can also be helpful. An antipsychotic should be initiated as soon as feasible because prolonged psychotic episodes are associated with a worsened course of illness.[32]

STABILIZATION PHASE

During the stabilization phase, acute symptoms gradually decrease in severity as the patient begins to stabilize. The goals of treatment during the stabilization phase of the illness are to reduce the likelihood of symptom exacerbation and to develop a plan for long-term treatment. The hope is that a patient will return to his or her premorbid level of functioning, although this is unlikely. Treatment should consist of a combination of pharmacologic and nonpharmacologic strategies. Treatment guidelines recommend that patients continue the same medication and dosage from which they received benefit from during the acute phase of illness. This treatment should be continued for at least 6 months.[32] During this phase, the individual is most vulnerable to relapse. Another concern during the stabilization phase is that clinicians, patients, and families may wrongly conclude that the antipsychotic stopped working if psychotic symptoms persist during this phase. For example, a patient may have suffered from hallucinations that were loud and derogatory before initiation of treatment; after 8 weeks of treatment, the voices might remain but become quieter and less demeaning. Because antipsychotics have been shown to provide gradual improvement during a period of months after the initial episode is treated, the current regimen should be continued.

either one alone.[83] However, rapid tranquilization is not necessarily more effective than traditional dosing methods, and is associated with a greater incidence of acute side effects such as dystonic reactions.[84,85] Rapid tranquilization can be achieved when repeated IM injections of high-potency antipsychotics or benzodiazepines are given until the patient is either adequately calmed, a maximum recommended daily dose is reached, or dose-limiting adverse effects such as acute dystonia (owing to antipsychotics), ataxia, or slurred speech (owing to benzodiazepines) occur. The most commonly used regimen is haloperidol 2 to 5 mg combined with lorazepam 2 mg injected IM every 30 to 60 minutes to a maximum of three doses.[86] Patients should be monitored for severe adverse events, particularly those patients with underlying medical or neurologic problems. Vital signs should be monitored and the dose should be held if clinically significant adverse effects occur.[31,85]

The concept of rapid tranquilization should not be confused with rapid neuroleptization, which implies the use of very high loading dosages of antipsychotics (i.e., administering a series of closely spaced IM doses during a period of hours) to produce a more rapid remission of psychotic symptoms.[86] The practice of rapid neuroleptization leads to a higher incidence of EPS without advantages in terms of efficacy when compared with the administration of lower doses of the same drugs, and hence is no longer recommended.[31] Because of the neurological risks associated with typical agents, use of atypical IM formulations have increased. Studies have shown that the US Food and Drug Administration (FDA)-approved IM formulations of the atypical agents (olanzapine, aripiprazole, and ziprasidone) seem to be better tolerated than typical agents and are equally effective as haloperidol and lorazepam in the acute treatment of agitation in patients with schizophrenia.[86–91]

CASE 82-1, QUESTION 8: How should pharmacotherapy be used to treat the acute phase of schizophrenia in J.R., and what should be done first to manage her acute symptoms?

J.R. is likely to refuse medications because of her paranoid symptoms; therefore, an IM formulation is a good choice for acute treatment. Aripiprazole 9.75 mg injection can be given to J.R. so that further assessment can be completed. Aripiprazole is a good choice because it is calming rather than sedating, and it has a lower propensity for EPS and TD compared with typical agents. Also, unlike ziprasidone IM, aripiprazole IM has not been associated with QTc prolongation nor has it been associated with hypotension, bradycardia with or without hypotension, tachycardia, and syncope, as with olanzapine IM.[92–94] Lorazepam 0.5 to 1 mg orally (PO) or IM every 4 to 6 hours as needed may be given to J.R. to control ongoing agitation; however, greater sedation and orthostatic hypotension have been observed with the combination of lorazepam and aripiprazole IM as compared with aripiprazole IM alone.[92] Subsequent doses of aripiprazole IM can be given every 2 hours if needed for agitation, up to a maximum of 30 mg/day.

CASE 82-1, QUESTION 9: J.R. was given a single dose of aripiprazole 9.75 mg IM. Her agitation responded to the first injection, but continues to be intermittent, and you are informed that this medication is not covered by J.R.'s health insurance plan. What is the next medication you would recommend for J.R.?

Because of J.R.'s continued agitation, she still requires an alternative antipsychotic that is available in an IM dosage form. Ziprasidone is not a good option for her because she already has QTc prolongation, and ziprasidone can further increase this interval and potentially cause life-threatening arrhythmias. Olanzapine also would not be appropriate for J.R. because of its high propensity to cause weight gain, dyslipidemia, and insulin resistance. Haloperidol 5 mg IM can be given every 1 hour as needed to J.R. to control her ongoing agitation. There is no maximum daily dose for haloperidol IM. Dosing of haloperidol is dependent on patient response and tolerability (i.e., oversedation, EPS, anticholinergic side effects).

LONG-ACTING INJECTABLES

Long-acting injectable antipsychotics are not recommended for acute psychotic episodes because these medications take months to reach a steady-state concentration and are eliminated very slowly.[32] Hence, it is difficult to correlate clinical effect with dosage, and it is extremely difficult to make dosage adjustments to manage side effects. However, long-acting injectable antipsychotics can be useful for maintenance therapy in patients with a history of nonadherence to their oral medication and in those who prefer the convenience of long-acting injections.[95] In addition, there is some evidence that patients administered long-acting antipsychotic injections will persist with therapy for longer periods than those prescribed oral medications.[95] In these situations, the oral form of available long-acting medication should be initiated first. If the oral form has been shown to be safe and effective, the patient can be converted to the long-acting form. Fluphenazine, haloperidol, risperidone, paliperidone, and olanzapine are available as long-acting injections. The benefits of long-acting injectable antipsychotics include consistent medication delivery and predictable bioavailability. However, a substantial proportion of patients feel that long-acting injections cause more shame and lead to more stigma than oral antipsychotics and they have feelings of loss of control when oral medications are substituted with injections.[96] Other patient concerns include injection site pain and needle phobia.

One notable adverse event unique to olanzapine long-acting injectable is postinjection delirium sedation syndrome (PDSS).[97] This syndrome is believed to be associated with accidental intravascular entry of a portion of the dose, likely after vessel injury during the injection process. This rapid release of a portion of the dose into the bloodstream results in higher-than-expected systemic olanzapine concentrations.[98] Afflicted patients experience symptoms consistent with an olanzapine overdose (i.e., sedation, confusion, slurred speech, altered gait, or unconsciousness). The onset of symptoms ranged from immediate to 3 to 5 hours postinjection, with a median onset time of 25 minutes after injection. Patients usually recovered within 1.5 to 72 hours and no clear risk factors have been identified. Olanzapine-induced PDSS is rare, having occurred in approximately 0.07% of injections or 1.4% of patients.[99] Because of the risk of PDSS after each injection, patients receiving long-acting olanzapine injection must be observed for at least 3 hours in a registered facility with ready access to emergency response services. In addition, the medication is available only through a restricted distribution program that requires enrollment of the prescriber, health care facility, patient, and pharmacy.[99]

PHARMACOKINETICS AND DRUG INTERACTIONS

Dosing considerations also have a major influence on safe and effective antipsychotic selections. Specific factors include the number of times a day a medication needs to be administered, the difference between a starting dose and a "target" therapeutic dose (i.e., titration required), and the risk for drug–drug interactions. The long half-life (12–24 hours) and active metabolites of most oral antipsychotic drugs allow for once-daily to twice-daily dosing.[100] Most antipsychotics achieve a steady-state concentration in 4 to 7 days, but it is important to understand that the onset of antipsychotic effect is not related to achieving steady state. Pharmacologic effects often persist for longer than

TABLE 82-9

Pharmacokinetic Comparisons of Antipsychotics

Antipsychotic Agent	Mean Half-Life (hours)	Major Cytochrome P-450 Pathway	Plasma Concentration Range
Chlorpromazine	24	2D6	Not well defined
Thioridazine	24	2D6	Not well defined
Perphenazine	9–12	2D6	Not well defined
Fluphenazine	18	2D6	0.2–2.8 ng/mL
Fluphenazine decanoate	8 days	2D6	0.2–2.8 ng/mL
Thiothixene	34	2D6	2–15 ng/mL
Haloperidol	18	2D6	4–12 ng/mL
Haloperidol decanoate	21 days	2D6	4–12 ng/mL
Loxapine	8	None	Not well defined
Trifluoperazine	18		Not well defined
Clozapine	16	1A2, 3A4	350–420 mcg/mL suggested
Risperidone	22	2D6	Not well defined
Olanzapine	30	1A2	>23.2 ng/mL at 12 hours after dose
Quetiapine	7	3A4	Not well defined
Ziprasidone	4–5	3A4	Not well defined
Aripiprazole	75–94	2D6, 3A4	Not well defined
Paliperidone	23	Limited 2D6, 3A4	Not well defined
Iloperidone	18–33	2D6, 3A4	Not well defined
Asenapine	24	UGT1A4, 1A2	Not well defined
Lurasidone	18	3A4	Not well defined

UGT1A4, uridine diphosphate glucuronosyltransferase 1 family, polypeptide A4.

Source: Facts & Comparisons eAnswers. http://online.factsandcomparisons.com/Viewer.aspx?book=DFC&monoID=fandc-hcp15080. Accessed January 19, 2011; Saphris [package insert]. Whitehouse Station, NJ: Schering Corporation, a subsidiary of Merck & Co, Inc; January 2011; Latuda [package insert]. Marlborough, MA: Sunovian Pharmaceuticals, Inc. a US subsidiary of Dainippon Sumitomo Pharma Co. Ltd; October 2010.

pharmacokinetics would imply. In some instances, treatment is initiated at a subtherapeutic dose and gradually titrated upward to an effective dose. This approach is taken to allow the patient to develop tolerance to adverse events such as sedation or orthostatic hypotension. In the case of acute agitation, antipsychotic doses are also often divided, despite the long half-lives of these drugs, so that the sedative effects are maintained over the day. Once a patient has been stabilized or has become tolerant to the adverse effects, the goal is to give medication once a day, usually at bedtime, to enhance medication adherence and increase tolerability.

Both pharmacokinetic and pharmacodynamic drug interactions can occur with antipsychotic agents. Cytochrome P-450 (CYP) enzymes, especially the 1A2, 2D6, and 3A4 isoenzymes, are responsible for the metabolism of many antipsychotics. Induction or inhibition of these enzymes by other drugs may result in clinically important drug interactions. Table 82-9 summarizes the metabolic pathways for commonly used antipsychotic drugs. In the case of clozapine, seizures can occur when drug interactions cause serum concentrations of clozapine to rise significantly. Examples of drugs that have the potential to cause serious interactions with antipsychotics include fluvoxamine (CYP1A2 inhibitor), erythromycin, ketoconazole, and ritonavir (CYP3A4 inhibitors), quinidine, fluoxetine, and paroxetine (CYP2D6 inhibitors), and cimetidine (multiple enzyme inhibition).[101] Conversely, inducers of drug metabolism such as carbamazepine or cigarette smoking (induces CYP1A2) can reduce the plasma concentrations of antipsychotic drugs.[102,103] Pharmacodynamic interactions may occur when medications with similar unwanted properties (e.g., orthostatic hypotension, anticholinergic effects, sedation) are concurrently prescribed. Pharmacokinetic and dosing information for the antipsychotics are provided in Tables 82-9 and 82-10.

PHARMACOECONOMIC CONSIDERATIONS

Drug-acquisition costs for atypical antipsychotics can be 100-fold higher than typical antipsychotics and concerns have been raised about the cost of atypical antipsychotics and whether their theoretical advantages over typical agents are worth their increased cost in the management of schizophrenia.[104] In 2005, annual expenditures on second-generation antipsychotics in the United States totaled $11.6 billion and represented approximately 10% of all US mental health expenditures.[104,105] Some, but not all, pharmacoeconomic studies with atypical antipsychotics show that these agents are at least cost neutral and may offer cost advantages compared with traditional agents when total mental health costs are considered.[5,106,107] Depending on the individual study, higher costs associated with atypical antipsychotics are offset by decreased numbers of hospital admissions, lengths of inpatient stay, and numbers of outpatient visits. Hence, drug costs should not be the sole factor considered when selecting an antipsychotic. The selection of a medication should be individualized and factors such as efficacy, side effects, patient acceptance, and total health care costs should be considered.[31,64,104]

ADVERSE EFFECTS

An important factor in the selection of an antipsychotic is the potential risk for adverse events such as EPS, anticholinergic side effects, cardiovascular effects, metabolic effects, and hyperprolactinemia. Table 82-7 compares antipsychotic agents with regard to the relative risk of these adverse effects.

Clinicians, when faced with any given side effect, should recognize the potential benefits of the current antipsychotic in managing symptoms, the severity of the side effect to the patient, and the potential risks and benefits of any intervention, particularly if a switch in antipsychotic medication is being considered. For mild side effects that cause little distress, the patient and clinician may opt to make no change and simply monitor the situation. With more severe or distressing side effects, options may include reducing the dose of the antipsychotic or prescribing a medication to treat the side effect (e.g., an anticholinergic drug to treat antipsychotic-induced parkinsonism), lifestyle changes (e.g., dietary change for constipation caused by an antipsychotic), or a switch to an alternative antipsychotic with a lower likelihood of causing the side effect in question. Switching to another

TABLE 82-10
Antipsychotic Relative Potency and Adult Dosing

Drug and Chemical Class	Dose Equivalence	Usual Starting Dose (mg/d)	Acute Phase Dosage (mg/d)	Maintenance or Stable Phase Dosage (mg/d)
Typical Agents—Phenothiazines				
Aliphatic type				
Chlorpromazine (Thorazine)	100	50–200	300–1,500[a]	150–800
Piperidine type				
Thioridazine (Mellaril)	100	50–200	300–800	150–600
Piperazine type				
Perphenazine (Trilafon)	10	4–16	32–64[a]	8–48
Trifluoperazine (Stelazine)	5	2–10	10–80	5–30
Fluphenazine (Prolixin)	2	2–10	5–80	2–20
Typical Agents—Nonphenothiazines				
Thioxanthene				
Thiothixene (Navane)	4	2–10	5–60[a]	5–30
Butyrophenone				
Haloperidol (Haldol)	2	2–10	5–100	2–20
Dibenzoxazepine				
Loxapine (Loxitane)	10	10–20	50–250	25–100
Dihydroindolone				
Diphenylbutylpiperidine				
Pimozide (Orap)	1	1–2	10–30	2–6
Atypical Agents				
Risperidone (Risperdal)	2	1–2	2–16	2–8
Clozapine (Clozaril)	50	12.5–25	150–900	150–600
Olanzapine (Zyprexa)	5	5–10	10–20	10–20
Quetiapine (Seroquel)	75	50–100	300–750	400–600
Ziprasidone (Geodon)	60	40–80	80–200	80–160
Aripiprazole (Abilify)	7.5	10–15	10–30	15–30
Paliperidone (Invega)	3	6	6–12	6–12
Iloperidone (Fanapt)	N/A	2	12–24	12–24
Asenapine (Saphris)	N/A	10	10–20	10–20
Lurasidone (Latuda)	N/A	40	40–80	40–80

[a] Dosages can be exceeded with caution, but high-dose therapy is rarely needed.
Source: Facts & Comparisons eAnswers. http://online.factsandcomparisons.com/Viewer.aspx?book=DFC&monoID=fandc-hcp15080. Accessed January 19, 2011; Saphris [package insert]. Whitehouse Station, NJ: Schering Corporation, a subsidiary of Merck & Co, Inc; January 2011; Latuda [package insert]. Marlborough, MA: Sunovian Pharmaceuticals, Inc. a US subsidiary of Dainippon Sumitomo Pharma Co. Ltd; October 2010.

antipsychotic should be done cautiously as potential benefits and risks of a treatment change are unpredictable.

If a change in antipsychotic medication is necessitated by side effects or insufficient efficacy, strategies may include an abrupt switch (abrupt cessation of the current drug, with abrupt introduction of the new one at the expected therapeutic dose), a gradual switch (slow downward adjustment of the dosage of the current medication, with slow upward adjustment of the dosage of the new drug) or an overlapping switch (abrupt introduction of the new medication overlapping with the current medication, followed by downward adjustment of the dosage of the previous medication).[108] None of these strategies has been demonstrated to be superior to another in terms of efficacy or safety, and the switch strategy depends on the clinical presentation.

EXTRAPYRAMIDAL SIDE EFFECTS AND TARDIVE SYNDROMES

EPS is a broad term that describes several types of acute and chronic drug-induced movement disorders. Acute dystonia, parkinsonism, and akathisia all occur early in treatment, whereas TD, tardive dystonia, and tardive akathisia have a late onset, usually after years of treatment. The acute forms of EPS usually develop soon after the initiation of antipsychotics, are dose-dependent, and are generally reversible soon after discontinuation of the offending agent.[34] It has been estimated that 60% of patients who receive typical antipsychotics experience some form of EPS acutely.[32] In general, typical agents are more likely to cause EPS than atypical agents when these medications are used at usual therapeutic doses. Among the currently available antipsychotic agents, clozapine and quetiapine have been associated with the lowest risk whereas high-potency typical antipsychotics have been associated with the highest risk for EPS.[64] The rising prescription rate of atypical antipsychotics (and decrease in use of the typical agents) has substantially reduced the incidence of EPS. Similarly, the risk of antipsychotic-induced TD is suggested to be lower with atypical agents compared with typical agents.[64,109,110] Most of the evidence documenting a decreased incidence of TD with atypical agents is derived from data and clinical experience with clozapine, risperidone, olanzapine, and quetiapine.

ACUTE DYSTONIA

CASE 82-1, QUESTION 10: J.R. received four doses of haloperidol 5 mg IM during 24 hours and was converted to

15 mg PO at bedtime. Her agitation resolved, but on day 2 of the admission she complained of a stiff neck and protruding tongue. Additionally, her nurse noted that she saw J.R.'s eyes roll back into her head. J.R. became very upset and wanted to leave the hospital and never take these medications again. No other medical conditions were noted. What evidence suggests that J.R. is experiencing an acute dystonic reaction?

Acute dystonia has the earliest onset of all the EPS symptoms. Most cases occur within the first few hours or days after initiation or dose increase of antipsychotic medication. Dystonia is characterized by sustained muscle contractions. Common presentations of antipsychotic-induced dystonia include a sudden onset of brief or sustained abnormal postures, including tongue protrusion, oculogyric crisis (eyes rolling back into head), trismus (spasm of the jaw), torticollis (torsion of the neck), opisthotonos (arching of back), and unusual positions in the trunk, limbs, and toes. Laryngeal dystonias are the most serious dystonias and are potentially fatal. Acute dystonia likely is caused by dysregulation of the dopamine system and imbalance between neurotransmitter systems after acute antipsychotic administration.[111] Risk factors include male sex and previous history of dystonia.[32] The sudden appearance of a stiff neck, protruding tongue, and eyes rolling back into the head in J.R. is consistent with acute dystonia. In addition, J.R.'s young age and use of a high-potency typical antipsychotic agent also place her at high risk for experiencing a dystonic reaction.

CASE 82-1, QUESTION 11: How should acute dystonia be treated in J.R.?

The initial goal of treatment is to relieve symptoms as soon as possible with either benztropine 1 to 2 mg or diphenhydramine 25 to 50 mg by IM injection. Although the intravenous (IV) route has a faster onset of action, it is not needed in J.R. because her reaction is not severe. If symptoms do not resolve within 15 to 30 minutes, then the dose should be repeated. If there are contraindications to the use of anticholinergic drugs, lorazepam 1 to 2 mg IM can be used. J.R. must be reassured that this is a temporary condition that can be prevented and treated. To prevent another reaction, J.R. should be given an oral anticholinergic drug for 2 weeks after this dystonic reaction.[112]

CASE 82-1, QUESTION 12: What is the next medication you would recommend for J.R., and what factors should be considered when selecting an antipsychotic for the acute and stabilization phases?

An antipsychotic prescribed at a therapeutic dose reflective of the needs during the stabilization phase should be started now. For pharmacologic treatment of schizophrenia in the acute phase, any of the atypical agents are appropriate choices. Although past experience with antipsychotics predicts therapeutic success in the selection of a regimen, J.R. does not have a past psychotropic medication history to guide drug selection. Because of the findings from her physical and laboratory examinations as well as her insurance restrictions, risperidone 2 mg at bedtime is an appropriate choice for the acute phase treatment for J.R. Some patients may require a lower starting dose of risperidone (e.g., 1 mg at bedtime) because of tolerability issues. The dose can then be titrated to clinical response, increasing the dose by 1 to 2 mg/day as tolerated.

CASE 82-1, QUESTION 13: J.R. has been acutely stabilized on risperidone 4 mg/day. When should her target symptoms start to respond to risperidone?

As a general rule, antipsychotic agents should be initiated and titrated during the first few days to an average effective target therapeutic dose unless the patient's physiological status or history indicates that this dose may result in unacceptable adverse events. During the first week, often known as the medicated cooperation stage, J.R. should respond to the calming properties of the antipsychotic and her symptoms of agitation. During the next 2 to 6 weeks, the improved socialization stage, J.R. should begin to observe hospital rules, attend ward meetings, and generally become more sociable. Severely ill schizophrenic patients with chronic disease may never reach this stage. The elimination of the thought disorder stage can occur within any time frame, but usually takes at least 2 to 3 weeks and up to several months to occur. During this stage, the core symptoms of schizophrenia such as delusions, hallucinations, and thought disturbance improve. If no improvement is observed after 3 weeks of risperidone 4 mg/day, then the dose should be increased slowly to 5 or 6 mg/day and J.R. should be observed for another 3 to 4 weeks. If necessary, the dose can be further increased up to 8 mg/day; however, doses greater than 6 mg/day are associated with greater incidence of EPS. The minimum duration of a trial before deeming it unsuccessful should be at least 4 weeks under ideal conditions (i.e., optimal therapeutic dose and medication adherent). This is based on an analysis of clinical trial data suggesting that the greatest amount of clinical improvement is observed in the first month of treatment and may be seen as early as the initial 2 weeks of treatment.[113–116] Dosing recommendations for the antipsychotics are provided in Table 82-10.

CASE 82-1, QUESTION 14: It is 6 months later and most of J.R.'s symptoms have improved. She is residing with her father and working part-time at her previous workplace. Although she is not troubled by any side effects, she sees no point in continuing her medication. Should risperidone be discontinued? What are the current practice guidelines regarding long-term treatment?

J.R. is clearly responding well to risperidone and has no side effects. To minimize her risk of relapse, she should continue her current regimen for at least another 6 months. If her symptoms remain stable and she maintains good psychosocial functioning (i.e., continues work, keeps close contact with social workers, attends medication groups), discontinuation of therapy can be considered.[32] When J.R. has been stabilized for approximately 1 year on risperidone 4 mg/day, the dose can be reduced by 20% every 3 to 6 months until it is discontinued or relapse occurs. If she exhibits recurrent target symptoms of schizophrenia or decompensation, then the dose should be increased to the previous effective dose or the medication should be restarted if it was discontinued. Most patients with schizophrenia will require life-long treatment with antipsychotics. For all patients receiving antipsychotics, it is important to determine the minimal effective dose to prevent recurrence while minimizing the risk of adverse effects.

CASE 82-1, QUESTION 15: Despite her psychiatrist's recommendations, J.R. discontinued her risperidone because she felt "cured" and was tired of taking pills every day. Three weeks later, she was readmitted to the hospital for a relapse

TABLE 82-11
Long-Acting Injectables (LAI)

	Dose	Frequency	Available	Comments
Haloperidol decanoate	10–20× oral Month 1: 20× Month 2: 15× Month 3: 10×	Every 4 weeks	50 mg/mL 100 mg/mL	1st injection NTE 100 mg Max: 3 mL/injection site *Sesame oil formulation
Fluphenazine decanoate	1.2× oral 12.5–25 mg	Every 3 weeks	25 mg/mL	Titrate by 12.5 mg increments Max: 100 mg/dose *Sesame oil formulation
Risperdal Consta	25 mg	Every 2 weeks	12.5 mg 25 mg 37.5 mg 50 mg	Overlap with PO ×3 weeks *Inject within 2 minutes of reconstituting Wait 4 weeks before ↑ dose Must refrigerate
Invega Sustenna	Day 1: 234 mg Day 8: 156 mg Then, 117 mg monthly	Every 4 weeks	39 mg/0.25 mL 78 mg/0.50 mL 117 mg/0.75 mL 156 mg/1 mL 234 mg/1.5 mL	3 mg oral = 39–78 mg IM 6 mg oral = 117 mg IM 12 mg oral = 234 mg IM
Zyprexa Relprevv	Weeks 1–8: 10 mg oral: 210 mg every 2 weeks or 405 mg every 4 weeks 15 mg oral: 300 mg every 2 weeks 20 mg oral: 300 mg every 2 weeks >8 weeks: 10 mg oral: 150 mg every 2 weeks or 300 mg every 4 weeks 15 mg oral: 210 mg every 2 weeks or 405 mg every 4 weeks 20 mg oral: 300 mg every 2 weeks	Every 2 weeks or Every 4 weeks	210 mg 300 mg 405 mg	Postinjection delirium or sedation may occur Must be given in health care facility with ready access to emergency response services. Patient must be observed for at least 3 hours by health care professional at the facility after each injection.

IM, intramuscular; NTE, not to exceed; PO, by mouth.

Source: Zyprexa Relprevv (olanzapine extended release injectable suspension) [package insert]. Indianapolis, IN: Eli Lilly and Company; 2010; Risperdal Consta (risperidone long acting injection) [package insert]. Titusville, NJ: Janssen, Division of Ortho-McNeil-Janssen Pharmaceuticals, Inc; 2011; Invega Sustenna [package insert]. Titusville, NJ: Janssen, division of Ortho-McNeil-Janssen Pharmaceuticals, Inc; March 2010.

and was restarted on risperidone by her treatment team. Is J.R. a candidate for a long-acting injection?

In patients who are nonadherent to medications, long-acting injections decrease the frequency of doses and decrease hospital readmissions. Because of her history of nonadherence, J.R. is a good candidate for receiving a depot product. Haloperidol, fluphenazine, risperidone, paliperidone, and olanzapine are all available in long-acting formulations. Because of her history of an acute dystonic reaction to oral haloperidol, haloperidol, fluphenazine and other high-potency antipsychotics should be avoided. J.R. had good response to risperidone in the past with good effectiveness and no side effects; therefore a long-acting formulation of risperidone is a good option. Paliperidone and olanzapine may be considered in the future if J.R. no longer receives benefit or begins to experience side effects with risperidone. Available long-acting options and selected clinical parameters are listed in Table 82-11.

CASE 82-1, QUESTION 16: J.R. has agreed to receive risperidone long-acting injection. How should this medication be started and how frequently should it be administered?

Before starting a patient on any long-acting injectable formulation, the patient should take the oral form of the medication first to ensure tolerability. Because J.R. is already taking oral risperidone with good effect and no side effects, she can immediately receive long-acting injectable risperidone. She should receive long-acting risperidone 25 mg IM in the gluteus or deltoid once every 2 weeks. Her oral risperidone should be continued at her current dose of 4 mg/day for 3 weeks after her initial long-acting injection and then discontinued. This overlap is required to provide coverage until release of the long-acting risperidone has begun. If J.R. does not respond to this dose, her dose may be increased to risperidone 37.5 mg IM after 4 weeks, up to a maximum dose of 50 mg IM every 2 weeks. Clinical effects from dose titrations may not be clear for 3 weeks because of the time release of the long-acting injection. Long-acting risperidone must be refrigerated until ready to administer.[117]

PARKINSONISM

CASE 82-1, QUESTION 17: Because of J.R.'s inability to regularly secure transportation to the outpatient clinic for her biweekly risperidone long-acting injections, she became noncompliant and suffered a return of her psychotic symptoms. Oral risperidone therapy was restarted at 4 mg at

bedtime. Because of her continued symptoms of thought insertion, thought broadcasting, and auditory hallucinations, her dose was subsequently increased to 6 mg at bedtime. Three weeks after this dose increase, J.R. returns stating that "the voices are softer and easy to ignore" but she complains about feeling "slow." On physical examination, you notice that she has a tremor in both hands at rest, as well as cogwheel rigidity in both arms. Can risperidone cause parkinsonism? What evidence suggests that J.R. has antipsychotic-induced parkinsonism?

The clinical presentation of antipsychotic-induced parkinsonism includes bradykinesia or akinesia, which may be associated with decreased arm swinging, a masklike face, drooling, decreased eye blinking, soft and monotonous speech, tremor (usually a rhythmic, resting tremor), and rigidity of the extremities, neck, or trunk (most identifiable in the limbs as a "cogwheel" rigidity during passive motion).[111,112] Symptoms of antipsychotic-induced parkinsonism can occur at any time, but usually develop within 4 weeks after antipsychotic initiation or a dose increase. Advanced age, antipsychotic dose and potency, and pre-existing EPS are the major risk factors for antipsychotic-induced parkinsonism.[111]

Reasons for the delay in onset between receptor blockade, which occurs within hours after initiating an antipsychotic, and development of symptoms are not well understood.[111,112] Atypical antipsychotics are the mainstay of the pharmacologic management of psychosis in patients vulnerable to developing antipsychotic-induced parkinsonism.

Although antipsychotic-induced parkinsonism is most commonly seen with the use of high-potency typical antipsychotics, it can still occur with atypical agents as well. Risperidone causes dose-related EPS, with higher frequencies observed at oral doses greater than 6 mg/day. The onset of symptoms within 3 weeks of her dose increase of risperidone suggests the EPS is caused by her medication change. The "slow" feeling may be indicative of akinesia or bradykinesia, and her symptoms of bilateral tremor and cogwheel rigidity are features of antipsychotic-induced parkinsonism.

CASE 82-1, QUESTION 18: How can J.R.'s antipsychotic-induced parkinsonism be treated?

In mild cases of antipsychotic-induced parkinsonism, immediate intervention may not be required if the movement disorder is not bothersome to the patient. For troublesome cases, as experienced by J.R., the simplest intervention is to reduce the antipsychotic dose to the lowest effective level or change to another agent with a lower propensity to cause EPS. In J.R.'s case, because of her partial response on risperidone, dose reduction is not an optimal choice. An alternative approach would be to add an antiparkinsonian agent to her drug regimen. Table 82-12 includes a list of medications used to treat antipsychotic-induced parkinsonism and akathisia.

Commonly used agents are anticholinergics. All anticholinergic antiparkinsonian agents are equally effective for antipsychotic-induced parkinsonism, although they differ in adverse events and duration of action. Trihexyphenidyl is the least sedating but more prone to abuse, whereas diphenhydramine is the most sedating. Benztropine has the longest duration and can be used once or twice a day if needed, whereas the others are commonly used three to four times daily. J.R. could be started on benztropine 1 mg twice a day orally. Alternatively, a switch to another antipsychotic with a lower risk of EPS may negate the need for an antiparkinsonian drug in J.R.

TABLE 82-12
Agents to Treat Antipsychotic-Induced Parkinsonism and Akathisia

Medication	Equivalent Dose (mg)	Dose/Day (mg/d)
Anticholinergic		
Benztropine (Cogentin)[a]	0.5	2–8
Biperiden (Akineton)[a]	0.5	2–8
Diphenhydramine (Benadryl)[a]	25	50–250
Procyclidine (Kemadrin)	1.5	10–20
Trihexyphenidyl (Artane)	1	2–15
Dopaminergic		
Amantadine	—	100–300
GABAminergic		
Diazepam (Valium)	10	5–40
Clonazepam (Klonopin)	2	1–3
Lorazepam (Ativan)[a]	2	1–3
Noradrenergic Blockers		
Propranolol (Inderal)	—	30–120

[a] Oral dose or intramuscular injection can be used.

CASE 82-1, QUESTION 19: J.R. is started on benztropine 1 mg twice a day, leading to resolution of her acute symptoms of parkinsonism. Does J.R. need to be continued on benztropine?

The long-term treatment of antipsychotic-induced parkinsonism with antiparkinsonian medication is controversial. The World Health Organization published a consensus statement recommending that the prophylactic use of anticholinergic medication in patients receiving antipsychotics should be avoided or used only in cases where alternative strategies have failed.[118] For J.R., an attempt to taper and discontinue the antiparkinsonian treatment should be initiated 6 weeks to 3 months after symptoms resolve. Unfortunately, many patients who exhibit antipsychotic-induced parkinsonism will continue to experience parkinsonian symptoms as long as they remain on the same antipsychotic. If that should occur with J.R., the potential benefits of a switch to an atypical agent that carries a lower EPS risk should be considered.

CASE 82-1, QUESTION 20: What risks are associated with long-term anticholinergic treatment?

The risks of anticholinergics include constipation, urinary retention, blurred vision, and dry mouth. They can also cause memory impairment, especially in older patients. Some patients experience tolerance to these adverse effects whereas others do not, even with chronic use. Patients sometimes abuse anticholinergic medications for their mood-elevating and hallucinogenic effects. Abuse may be confused with reluctance to discontinue antiparkinsonian medication because of the fear of recurrent EPS or ongoing symptoms.

CASE 82-1, QUESTION 21: What additional adverse effects should J.R. be monitored for during antipsychotic drug therapy?

Akathisia

Akathisia is a syndrome consisting of subjective feelings of restlessness or the urge to move and an objective motor component expressed as a semipurposeful movement most often involving the lower extremities (pacing, rocking, and an inability to sit or stand in one place for extended periods of time). Akathisia is observed in up to 50% of patients treated with typical antipsychotics and ranges from 5% to 15% of patients treated with atypical agents.[32] Akathisia is often extremely distressing to patients, is a common cause of medication nonadherence and may lead to dysphoria and possibly aggressive or suicidal behavior.[32] It is often difficult to distinguish from psychomotor agitation and worsening psychosis. Hence, the clinician must take care not to misdiagnose akathisia because an increase in antipsychotic dose could worsen this adverse event. It usually develops within days to weeks after initiating antipsychotic therapy.

The pathophysiology of akathisia is unclear, but much attention has focused on two theories.[111,112] One theory states that the mesocortical postsynaptic dopamine blockade leads to increased locomotor activity. An alternative theory claims that akathisia is caused by dopamine-antagonist–induced dysregulation of noradrenergic tracts that project from the locus ceruleus to the limbic system.

Akathisia is less responsive to treatment than are antipsychotic-induced parkinsonism and dystonia.[32] An initial pharmacologic approach in the management of antipsychotic-induced akathisia is a reduction in the original antipsychotic dose if that is feasible. If symptoms of psychosis return or if the akathisia persists, the addition of a β-blocking agent, an anticholinergic drug, or a benzodiazepine can be considered.[32,111,112,119]

Tardive Dyskinesia

TD is a syndrome characterized by involuntary choreoathetoid movements that occurs in individuals taking long-term antipsychotics.[120] The face (tics, blinking, grimacing), tongue (chewing, protrusion, tremor, writhing), lips (smacking, pursing, puckering), neck and trunk (torsion and torticollis), and limbs (toe tapping, pill rolling, and writhing) are commonly involved. The movements may be choreiform (rapid, jerky, nonrepetitive), athetoid (slow, sinuous, continual), or rhythmic (stereotypic) in nature.

Advanced age is the most consistently observed risk factor for the development of TD.[120] The annual incidence rates of developing TD are threefold to fivefold higher in older patients compared with younger adults.[121,122] Other risk factors include higher mean daily and cumulative antipsychotic doses, and presence of EPS early in treatment.[120–122] Although there is some indication that the risk of TD may be higher in women, nonwhites, patients with affective psychiatric disorders, and patients taking concomitant anticholinergic agents, these findings have not been consistently observed.[120]

For most patients, TD does not seem to be progressive or irreversible; it can be reversed with discontinuation of the antipsychotic agent. However, in some cases, TD is irreversible. The onset of symptoms tends to be subtle with a fluctuating course.[120] Most TD cases are relatively mild, however, a portion of patients (5%–10%) may experience a form of TD that is severe enough to impair functioning.[123] Severe oral dyskinesia may result in dental and denture problems that can progress to ulceration and infection of the mouth as well as muffled or unintelligible speech. Severe orofacial TD can impair eating and swallowing, which in turn could produce significant health problems. Gait disturbances owing to limb dyskinesia may leave patients vulnerable to falls and injuries.

Although the cause of TD is unknown, dopaminergic hypersensitivity, disturbed balance between dopamine and cholinergic systems, dysfunction of GABAergic and noradrenergic systems, and neurotoxicity via free radicals have been proposed.[120] Antipsychotic-induced TD needs to be differentiated from other causes that may present similarly. Tourette syndrome, dental problems, Huntington or Sydenham chorea, chorea of pregnancy, and systemic lupus erythematosus are among the disorders that have been associated with dyskinetic movements. In addition, medications such as metoclopramide, amoxapine, bromocriptine, levodopa/carbidopa, and pramipexole also can cause TD.[121] Spontaneous dyskinesia resembles TD but can occur in patients without previous exposure to antipsychotic medications.[120] This form of abnormal movement is noticeably more common in elderly patients. A movement disorder assessment is essential before treating patients with antipsychotic medications to avoid the potential diagnostic dilemma of differentiating spontaneous dyskinesia from antipsychotic-induced TD.

A temporal relationship between an antipsychotic dose change and movement severity should be evaluated when performing assessments. An increase in the antipsychotic dose can clinically suppress the symptoms, whereas a decrease in dose can transiently unmask the movements often called "withdrawal dyskinesia."[122,124] On the other hand, a dose increase may produce a temporary lessening of movement severity. Patients taking long-term antipsychotics should be evaluated for TD every 3 to 6 months and the findings documented in patient records to ensure continuity of care.

The primary management of TD is prevention. That is, antipsychotic drugs must be reserved to treat conditions known to respond (e.g., psychotic disorders such as schizophrenia, major depression with psychotic features, schizoaffective disorder), and the total dose and duration of treatment should be minimized. Numerous studies have evaluated various pharmacologic treatments of TD, but few therapies have produced more than slight to moderate benefit in clinical practice.[125] The two main strategies are discontinuation of the offending drug and switching to a drug with a lower EPS risk potential. Unfortunately, a majority of patients with schizophrenia require lifetime treatment with antipsychotics. Hence, switching to a medication with reduced TD liability such as clozapine or quetiapine is common if TD is severe enough to warrant a treatment change.[125–127] A number of other agents have been studied for their potential therapeutic effects on TD. Drugs that augment GABA neurotransmission (e.g., diazepam, clonazepam, valproic acid), adrenergic drugs (propranolol, clonidine), free-radical scavengers (vitamin E), and botulinum toxin A have all been used, with limited or inconsistent results.[120,125–128] These agents may be useful as adjunctive treatments when TD persists despite the use of atypical agents.

ANTICHOLINERGIC EFFECTS

Anticholinergic effects are more significant with low-potency typical antipsychotics, and with the atypical agents, clozapine and olanzapine. Clinically, patients complain of constipation, urinary retention, blurry vision, and dry eyes, mouth, and throat. Dry mouth and throat can cause several additional problems, including dental caries and weight gain if thirst is satisfied with high-sugar drinks. Oral fungal infections can also occur if gum or liquids with high sugar content are regularly consumed. The most serious complications from medications with anticholinergic properties are delirium and adynamic ileus. Interestingly, clozapine causes significant hypersalivation despite its anticholinergic effects. The mechanism is unknown, but it may be related to clozapine's augmentation of the adrenergic receptors that control salivation.[129] Although anticholinergic effects are a minor problem with high-potency typical agents, some patients may still have problems when anticholinergic antiparkinsonian agents are added to treat EPS.

CARDIOVASCULAR EFFECTS

Orthostatic Hypotension

Antipsychotic drugs can cause a variety of cardiovascular complications, but the most common problem is orthostasis from α_1-adrenergic blockade. Orthostasis is most likely to occur during the first few days of treatment or when increasing the dose of medication. Although tolerance usually occurs within 2 to 3 weeks, orthostasis necessitates slow dose titration early in treatment for patients who are particularly prone to this side effect.

Tachycardia

Tachycardia may occur as a result of the anticholinergic effects of antipsychotic medications on vagal inhibition, or secondary to orthostatic hypotension.[32] Clozapine produces the most pronounced tachycardia. If tachycardia is sustained or becomes symptomatic, low doses of a β-blocker such as atenolol or propranolol can be useful once an ECG has ruled out other medical causes.

Electrocardiographic Changes

ECG changes such as prolongation of the QT and PR intervals, ST-segment depression, and T-wave flattening have been observed with antipsychotics.[130] The most clinically important of these potential changes is prolongation of the QTc interval (which is the QT interval adjusted for heart rate) and has drawn the attention of the FDA. QTc prolongation may lead to the development of ventricular tachyarrhythmias such as torsades de pointes and ventricular fibrillation, which can cause syncope, cardiac arrest, or sudden cardiac death. All antipsychotics have the potential to prolong the QTc interval to varying degrees. In 2000, Pfizer, in consultation with the FDA, completed a study in which the QTc intervals of patients taking several antipsychotics at usual therapeutic dosages and in the presence of a metabolic inhibitor were compared (Fig. 82-2).[131] Thioridazine was shown to prolong the QTc interval at least 20 milliseconds longer than haloperidol, risperidone, olanzapine, or quetiapine. This led to a black-box warning on the FDA-approved product labeling stating that thioridazine has been shown to prolong the QTc interval in a dose-related manner and its use should be limited to patients who cannot be managed on other antipsychotics. In the same study, ziprasidone prolonged the QTc interval 5 to 15 milliseconds longer than did haloperidol, risperidone, olanzapine, or quetiapine. Unlike thioridazine, the ziprasidone effects were not dose-related. The exact point at which QTc prolongation becomes clinically dangerous is unclear. Because most reported cases of torsades de pointes have appeared in individuals with a QT interval greater than 500 milliseconds, discontinuation of the suspected offending agent has been recommended if the interval consistently exceeds 500 milliseconds. It is important to note that no patients in this study had QTc intervals exceeding 500 milliseconds or arrhythmias. Despite the fact that no increased risk of arrhythmia or sudden death has been demonstrated with ziprasidone, caution is warranted in patients with some types of cardiac disease and with an uncontrolled electrolyte disturbance. The coprescription of ziprasidone with other drugs that prolong the QT interval should be avoided. Under most clinical circumstances, however, ziprasidone may be safely used without ECG monitoring or other special precautions.

METABOLIC EFFECTS

Hyperprolactinemia

Before the introduction of atypical agents, prolactin elevation was unavoidable because all typical antipsychotics elevate serum prolactin by blocking the tonic inhibitory actions of dopamine in the tuberoinfundibular tract.[132] Differential risk for producing hyperprolactinemia has been observed with the atypical agents. According to the Schizophrenia Patient Outcomes Research Team treatment recommendations and summary statements, the relative risk for prolactin elevation in descending order is risperidone, paliperidone, typical antipsychotics, olanzapine, ziprasidone, quetiapine, clozapine followed lastly by

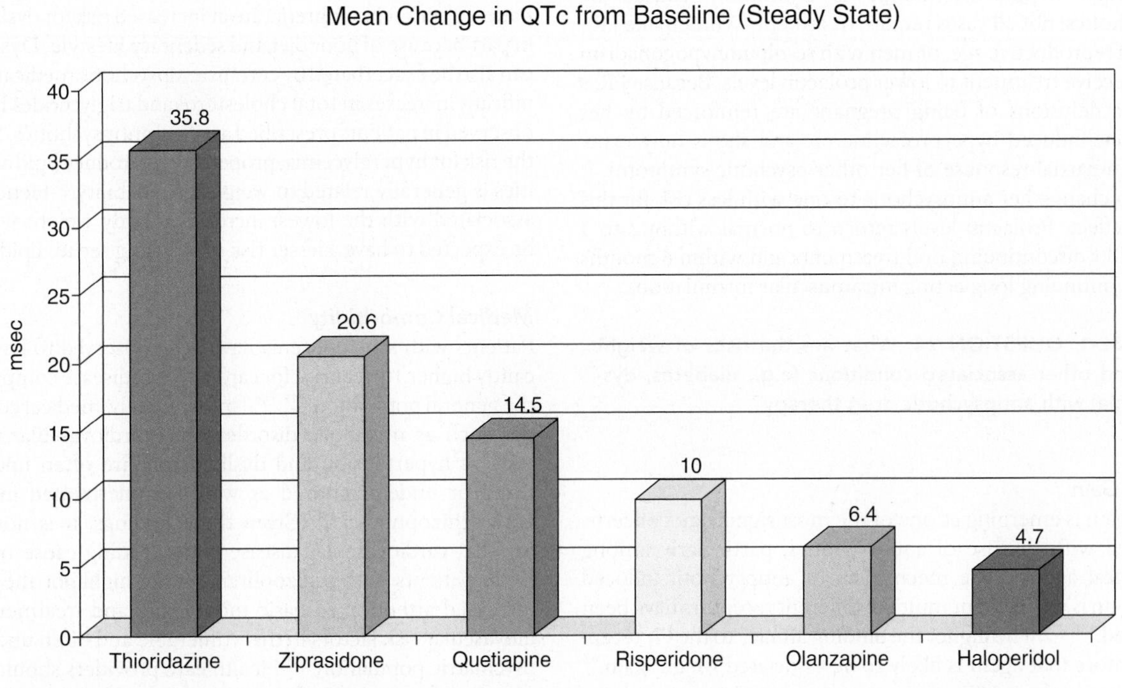

FIGURE 82-2 Comparison of QTc changes with antipsychotics. (Source: FDA Psychopharmacological Drugs Advisory Committee. 19 July 2000 Briefing Document for Zeldox Capsules [Ziprasidone HCl]. **http://www.fda.gov/ohrms/dockets/ac/00/backgrd/3619b1a.pdf.** Accessed June 29, 2011.)

aripiprazole.[64] Hyperprolactinemia is of clinical importance because it may lead to galactorrhea, gynecomastia, amenorrhea, anovulation, impaired spermatogenesis in males, decreased libido and sexual arousal, anorgasmia, and osteoporosis.[133] Hyperprolactinemia is not always associated with clinical symptoms. For example, Kleinberg et al.[134] failed to find an association between sexual dysfunction and risperidone-associated hyperprolactinemia. This may be a product of the multifactorial nature of sexual dysfunction or methodologic limitations in data collection. Patients often do not spontaneously report symptoms of sexual dysfunction and clinicians must remember to ask about these potential side effects.[135]

CASE 82-1, QUESTION 22: One week after starting benztropine, J.R.'s tremor and rigidity improved; however, she was still only experiencing a partial response to her risperidone. Her dose was further increased to risperidone 8 mg at bedtime. At her follow-up visit 3 weeks later, J.R. reports no longer hearing her mother's voice as much as she used to, and she misses it. "At least I won't be lonely once my baby is born. I'm so happy to be pregnant!" J.R. denies taking a pregnancy test, but is 1 week late for her menstrual period and she has been lactating. Laboratory tests reveal a negative hCG pregnancy test and an elevated prolactin level of 154 ng/mL. What could explain J.R.'s pregnancylike symptoms?

J.R. is experiencing antipsychotic-induced hyperprolactinemia, which is evident from her galactorrhea, amenorrhea, and elevated prolactin level. Prolactin elevation is attributable to dopamine receptor blockade in the tuberoinfundibular tract and is unavoidable with the typical antipsychotics. Risperidone and selected other atypical antipsychotics produce increases in prolactin levels that is equal to or greater than that seen with typical antipsychotics.

CASE 82-1, QUESTION 23: What should be done about J.R.'s hyperprolactinemia?

Although hyperprolactinemia is commonly caused by antipsychotics, not all cases require treatment. Women like J.R., who is of reproductive age, or men with resultant hypogonadism should receive treatment to lower prolactin levels. Because J.R.'s psychotic delusions of being pregnant are reinforced by her risperidone-induced hyperprolactinemia and she is only experiencing a partial response of her other psychotic symptoms, it is best to change her antipsychotic to one with less risk for this adverse effect. Prolactin levels return to normal within 2 to 3 weeks after discontinuing oral treatments and within 6 months after discontinuing long-acting intramuscular formulations.

CASE 82-1, QUESTION 24: What are the risks of weight gain and other associated conditions (e.g., diabetes, dyslipidemia) with antipsychotic drug therapy?

Weight Gain

Weight gain is emerging as one of the most significant concerns associated with the use of antipsychotics, particularly among the atypical agents. The mechanism of antipsychotic-induced weight gain is unclear, but multiple different receptors have been implicated.[136–138] The higher the binding affinity to the H_1 receptor, the more that agent is likely to be associated weight gain.[62] A mutation in the 5-HT_{2C} receptor gene may increase risk for weight gain from atypical antipsychotics. Unfortunately, a genetic test to predict which patients will gain weight from atypical antipsychotics is not available.[62,137] Another theory is the potential decreased signaling of 5-HT_{2A} and 5-HT_{2C}, increased calorie intake and appetite, or decreased metabolic rate.[62,138] Among the antipsychotics, weight gain is most common with clozapine and olanzapine compared with other atypical antipsychotics and medium-potency and high-potency typical antipsychotics.[62,139] In contrast, aripiprazole and ziprasidone have low risk for weight gain, and risk is intermediate with risperidone, paliperidone, and quetiapine.[64,139] The weight gain observed with clozapine and olanzapine is not dose-dependent and plateaus 6 to 12 months after treatment initiation.[140,141] Alternatively, other authors suggest that whereas antipsychotic-associated weight gain plateaus within the first several months of treatment with risperidone, quetiapine, and ziprasidone, it can continue for several years for clozapine and olanzapine.[135] The issue of weight gain has important clinical implications in light of its link with impaired glucose tolerance and type 2 diabetes, hyperlipidemia, and increased mortality.[142,143]

Hyperglycemia and Diabetes Mellitus

Hyperglycemia (with or without ketoacidosis, hyperosmolar coma, or death), as well as new-onset diabetes mellitus have been reported in patients treated with atypical antipsychotics. In general, the risk of hyperglycemia and new-onset diabetes mellitus for the various second-generation antipsychotics is proportional to their association with weight gain.[64,144] Therefore, olanzapine and clozapine are more likely to produce glucose elevation. It should be highlighted, however, that atypical antipsychotics may impair insulin sensitivity or glucose regulation independent of weight gain.[137,138] Developing precise risk estimates between atypical antipsychotic use and glucose abnormalities is complicated by the possibility of an increased background risk of diabetes mellitus in patients with schizophrenia. In light of this risk, any patient exposed to atypical antipsychotics should be monitored for subjective symptoms (i.e., polydipsia, polyuria, polyphagia, and weakness) and laboratory evidence (i.e., fasting blood glucose or hemoglobin A_{1c}) of hyperglycemia.

Dyslipidemia

Patients with schizophrenia are at increased risk for dyslipidemia, in part because of poor diet and sedentary lifestyle. Dyslipidemia can also be exacerbated by certain antipsychotic medications. Significant increases in total cholesterol and triglycerides have been observed in patients prescribed atypical antipsychotics. Similar to the risk for hyperglycemia, propensity to produce lipid abnormalities is generally related to weight gain liability.[62] Hence, agents associated with the lowest increase in body weight would also be expected to have a lesser risk of inducing serum lipid changes.

Medical Comorbidity

Patients with schizophrenia have been observed to have significantly higher 10-year risk for cardiac heart disease compared with the general population.[145,146] Unfortunately, medical comorbidities such as metabolic disorders and cardiovascular disorders such as hypertension and dyslipidemia are often underrecognized or underdiagnosed as well as undertreated in patients with schizophrenia.[147] Given these findings, it is not surprising that cardiovascular disease is the leading cause of mortality in patients with schizophrenia; they highlight the need for increased attention to basic monitoring and treatment of cardiovascular risk factors in this vulnerable and often underserved psychiatric population.[148] Health care providers should encourage all patients with schizophrenia to seek out a primary-care provider or receive annual health checks for routine physical monitoring.

CASE 82-1, QUESTION 25: After experiencing hyperprolactinemia, J.R.'s risperidone was discontinued. Benztropine was also discontinued at this time. She failed her next treatment trial of quetiapine 800 mg daily for 2 months, resulting in another hospital admission. During this hospitalization, she refused to initiate clozapine because of the weekly laboratory monitoring and was instead started on olanzapine and titrated up to 20 mg PO daily. What considerations should be taken on starting olanzapine for J.R.?

Multiple concerns should be taken into account before initiating olanzapine for J.R. She has previously experienced symptomatic hyperprolactinemia associated with risperidone treatment. Although olanzapine may cause a dose-related elevation of prolactin levels, this side effect occurs to a lesser extent than risperidone and typical antipsychotics. In comparison to other antipsychotics, olanzapine is associated with significant metabolic side effects such as weight gain and insulin resistance. J.R. has multiple risk factors for developing cardiovascular disease (i.e., overweight, smoker, high LDL and TG, low HDL), and olanzapine may not be an optimal antipsychotic owing to its metabolic adverse effects. Because J.R. has failed a number of different antipsychotics, olanzapine is an appropriate choice as long as she is monitored and treated for metabolic abnormalities.

CASE 82-1, QUESTION 26: How should the potential metabolic complications associated with olanzapine be monitored in J.R.?

J.R. should be informed about these potential metabolic complications, educated on prevention strategies such as healthy living (e.g., diet, exercise, weight loss) and routinely monitored. Guidelines recommend assessments at specific time points for weight, waist circumference, fasting glucose levels or hemoglobin A_{1c}, and lipid panels in patients treated with atypical agents (see Table 82-13).[100,144] J.R. should be encouraged to self-monitor her weight and report any significant weight fluctuations. Subjective evidence of a weight change may include a change in clothes or belt size. In addition, she should be routinely monitored for symptoms of hyperglycemia at every clinic visit. Appropriate therapeutic options should be initiated if abnormalities are observed.

CASE 82-1, QUESTION 27: J.R. has now been taking olanzapine 20 mg for 9 weeks. She reports her clothes have been tighter lately and she always wants to eat. At her last visit 2 months ago, J.R. weighed 148 pounds and now she weighs 158 pounds. J.R. is asking if her weight gain can be attributed to olanzapine, and if there is another medication she can take that does not have this side effect.

The cause of antipsychotic-induced weight gain is multifactorial and may include a change in food preferences, increased food or fluid intake, carbohydrate craving, or a lack of activity. It is plausible that her weight gain is related to olanzapine given its propensity to cause weight gain and the temporal relationship between recent weight gain and its introduction. J.R.'s weight gain should be taken seriously because it may contribute to medical conditions and psychosocial stigma. Significant weight gain may cause her to have a poor self-image leading to treatment nonadherence. Obese patients with schizophrenia are 2.5 times more likely to discontinue their medication than nonobese patients.[149] J.R. should be enrolled in a weight management program and she should be evaluated for switching to an antipsychotic medication with a lower weight-gain liability. Other considerations include adding a medication to prevent weight gain when an antipsychotic agent is initiated, and adding a medication during current antipsychotic therapy to promote weight loss.[43] Metformin has been found to attenuate and lower the weight-gain liability of olanzapine.[150,151] In one study, patients who received metformin 750 mg/day experienced greater weight loss, body mass index reduction, waist circumference reduction, and fasting insulin and insulin-resistance level reduction compared with those who received placebo with or without lifestyle changes.[150] In another study, weight, body mass index, waist circumference, and waist to hip ratios increased less in patients who received metformin and olanzapine compared with those who received olanzapine alone.[151] For J.R., switching to another antipsychotic with lower weight-gain liability and the addition of metformin may be considered; however, this decision must be balanced against her current response to olanzapine as well as the potential risks associated with any treatment changes.

CASE 82-1, QUESTION 28: What is neuroleptic malignant syndrome and how is this condition treated?

NEUROLEPTIC MALIGNANT SYNDROME

Neuroleptic malignant syndrome (NMS) is a rare but potentially lethal adverse effect of antipsychotic therapy. Cases of NMS have been linked to treatment with typical and atypical antipsychotics.[152,153] NMS can occur hours to months after the initial drug exposure, and the mortality rate is reported to be as high as 20%.[32] The incidence is estimated at between 0.02% and 3.23% of patients taking typical antipsychotic drugs.[153] The cardinal features include muscular rigidity, hyperthermia, autonomic dysfunction, and altered consciousness. Extrapyramidal dysfunction (e.g., rigidity) and akinesia usually develop initially

TABLE 82-13
Monitoring Protocol for Atypical Antipsychotics[a]

	Baseline	Week 4	Week 8	Week 12	Quarterly	Annually	Every 5 Years
Personal or family history	X					X	
Weight (BMI)	X	X	X	X	X		
Waist circumference	X					X	
Blood pressure	X			X		X	
Fasting plasma glucose	X			X		X	
Fasting lipids profile	X			X			X

[a] More frequent assessments may be warranted based on clinical status.

Reprinted with permission from American Diabetes Association et al. Consensus Development Conference on Antipsychotic Drugs and Obesity and Diabetes. *Diabetes Care.* 2004;27:596.

or concomitantly with a temperature elevation as high as 41°C. Autonomic dysfunction includes tachycardia, labile blood pressure, profuse diaphoresis, dyspnea, and urinary incontinence. The patient's level of consciousness may vary from alert to mutism, stupor, and coma. Other neurologic findings include sialorrhea, dyskinesia, and dysphagia. Symptoms usually develop rapidly during 24 to 72 hours. Creatine kinase, CBC, and LFTs are usually increased.

Treatment of NMS consists of discontinuation of the causative antipsychotic and supportive measures to treat hyperthermia and prevent dehydration (e.g., antipyretics, a cooling blanket, and IV fluids).[154] Secondary complications such as pneumonia and renal failure should be managed as they develop. If no improvement or worsening occurs after 1 to 3 days of observation and supportive therapy, a number of additional pharmacologic interventions should be considered.[154] NMS has been attributed to dopamine depletion caused by neuroleptic blockade of dopamine pathways in the basal ganglia and hypothalamus. For that reason, dopamine agonists such as amantadine or bromocriptine sometimes are beneficial. Dantrolene relaxes skeletal muscle and is specifically recommended for severe hyperthermia.

NMS is self-limiting and usually lasts 2 to 14 days after the oral antipsychotic is discontinued or longer after discontinuation of depot medications. After several weeks of recovery, treatment may be cautiously resumed with another atypical antipsychotic.[64]

CASE 82-1, QUESTION 29: Because of J.R.'s continued decompensation in mental status, her father placed her in a residential living facility for continuous care. For the past 5 years, her persistent psychotic symptoms have prevented her from maintaining employment or developing personal relationships with either her family or friends. Further, she has been admitted to the hospital three times during the previous 12 months for suicidal ideation brought on by command auditory hallucinations. During her current inpatient admission, she was given a diagnosis of antipsychotic-induced TD. Is J.R. a good candidate for clozapine?

Inadequate Response

J.R. meets criteria for treatment-resistant schizophrenia, and clozapine is the "gold standard" for the treatment of this type of patient. Clozapine is approved by the FDA for treatment of resistant schizophrenia, or when adverse effects such as TD and EPS preclude use of other antipsychotics. Because of J.R.'s progressive decline in social functioning, development of tardive dyskinesia, and inadequate response to multiple prior typical and atypical antipsychotics, clozapine should be considered.[155,156]

CASE 82-1, QUESTION 30: What side effect considerations would preclude using clozapine as a first-line therapy for any patient with schizophrenia? How should those side effects been managed?

Clozapine's side effect profile includes potentially life-threatening complications, which makes it one of the most difficult medications for providers to prescribe and for patients to accept in the management of schizophrenia. Although clozapine has been found to be a very effective antipsychotic, its side-effect burden and risk of agranulocytosis and associated requirement of white blood cell (WBC) monitoring often lead to multiple trials of other antipsychotics before initiating a clozapine trial.

Common side effects associated with clozapine include sedation, anticholinergic burden, sialorrhea, orthostasis, tachycardia, and metabolic abnormalities. Sedation is usually mild and transient in nature and can be minimized by using the lowest effective dose of clozapine or administering it before bedtime. Constipation is usually treated by increasing fluid and dietary fiber intake, exercise, and bulk-forming laxatives. Tachycardia that is sustained or becomes symptomatic may be treated with low doses of a β-blocker such as atenolol or propranolol provided that an ECG has ruled out other contributory medical causes. Despite its anticholinergic effects, clozapine causes significant hypersalivation. The mechanism is unknown but it may be caused by augmentation of the adrenergic receptors that control salivation.[157] Sialorrhea is most often worst at night, and may lead to social withdrawal, choking, or aspiration pneumonia.[158] Case reports have suggested that a scopolamine patch (1.5 mg/72 hours), ipratropium sublingual spray (0.03% or 0.06% given two sprays up to three times daily), atropine 1% ophthalmic solution (two drops swish and swallow twice daily[159]), botulinum toxin (150 international units injected into each parotid gland), and guanfacine (1 mg every morning) are effective in reducing or eliminating sialorrhea.[157,158,160–162] Other commonly used medications include clonidine, biperiden, benztropine, diphenhydramine, amitriptyline, terazosin, and propranolol; however, tolerance to these agents may develop.[157,162] Metabolic abnormalities should be addressed by diet and exercise, as well as pharmacotherapy if necessary.

Of greater concern is the fact that clozapine has been issued five black-box warnings from the FDA.[163] These include warnings for agranulocytosis, seizures, myocarditis, other adverse cardiovascular and respiratory effects, and increased mortality in elderly patients with dementia-related psychosis. The most serious side effect is potentially fatal agranulocytosis. Agranulocytosis occurs in about 1% and neutropenia in about 3% of patients taking clozapine.[164,165] The risk of both agranulocytosis and neutropenia is greatest early in treatment with most cases appearing during the first 3 months of treatment.[165] After 6 months, the risk for agranulocytosis decreases substantially, but has been observed in a single case 11 years into treatment.[164,166] Trends in the weekly tests showing a continual decline in WBC count, even if it remains greater than 3,000 cells/μL, require careful attention. Guidelines for responding to reduction in WBC are described in Table 82-14. Fortunately, most cases of agranulocytosis are reversible on discontinuation of clozapine with no persisting hematologic sequelae.

The risk of seizures with clozapine treatment is dose-related. Seizures occur in 1.0% of patients taking daily doses less than 300 mg, in 2.7% of patients taking between 300 and 600 mg, and 4.4% of those taking more than 600 mg.[167] The occurrence of seizures does not preclude continued use of clozapine, as reducing the dose and adding an anticonvulsant such as valproic acid can prevent recurrence in most patients. The patient may then be rechallenged with clozapine with the target dose decreased by 50%.

Clozapine-induced myocarditis is an uncommon but potentially fatal side effect. The risk of fatal myocarditis is most frequent in the first month of treatment with clozapine. It is often underrecognized because the initial presentation may resemble symptoms expected in a normal clozapine dose titration (i.e., tachycardia and fatigue). Because clozapine-induced myocarditis may rapidly progress to acute heart failure, it would be prudent to intervene if a patient exhibits new evidence of cardiovascular disease such as tachycardia, chest pain, or dyspnea, while taking clozapine.[168]

The warning related to "other adverse cardiovascular and respiratory effects" refers to orthostatic hypotension that may or may not be accompanied by syncope. Rarely, orthostasis may precipitate respiratory or cardiac arrest. To avoid this adverse effect, clozapine should be initiated at a low dose of 12.5 mg

TABLE 82-14
Clozapine Monitoring

Situation	Hematological Values for Monitoring	Frequency of WBC and ANC Monitoring
Initiation of therapy	WBC ≥3,500 cells/μL ANC ≥2,000 cells/μL NOTE: do not initiate in patients with (a) history of myeloproliferative disorder or (b) Clozaril (clozapine)-induced agranulocytosis or granulocytopenia	Weekly for 6 months
6 months–12 months of therapy	All results for: WBC ≥3,500 cells/μL ANC ≥2,000 cells/μL	Every 2 weeks for 6 months
12 months of therapy	All results for WBC ≥3,500 cells/μL ANC ≥2,000 cells/μL	Every 4 weeks for infinitum
Immature forms present	N/A	Repeat WBC and ANC
Discontinuation of therapy	N/A	Weekly for at least 4 weeks from day of discontinuation or until WBC ≥3,500 cells/μL and ANC >2,000 cells/μL
Substantial drop in WBC or ANC	Single drop or cumulative drop within 3 weeks of WBC ≥3,000 cells/μL or ANC ≥1,500 cells/μL	1. Repeat WBC and ANC 2. If repeat values are 3,000–3,500 cells/μL and ANC <2,000 cells/μL, then monitor twice weekly
Mild leukopenia or mild granulocytopenia	WBC 3,000–3,500 cells/μL or ANC 1,500–2,000 cells/μL	Twice weekly until WBC >3,500 cells/μL and ANC >2,000 cells/μL then return to previous monitoring frequency
Moderate leukopenia or moderate granulocytopenia	WBC 2,000–3,000 cells/μL or ANC 1,000–1,500 cells/μL	1. Interrupt therapy 2. Daily until WBC >3,000 cells/μL and ANC >1,500 cells/μL 3. Twice weekly until WBC >3,500 cells/μL and ANC >2,000 cells/μL 4. May rechallenge when WBC >3,500 cells/μL and ANC >2,000 cells/μL 5. If rechallenged, monitor weekly for 1 year before returning to the usual monitoring schedule
Severe leukopenia or severe granulocytopenia	WBC <2,000 cells/μL or ANC <1,000 cells/μL	1. Discontinue treatment and do not rechallenge patient 2. Monitor until normal and for at least 4 weeks from day of discontinuation as follows: • Daily until WBC >3,000 cells/μL and ANC >1,500 cells/μL • Twice weekly until WBC >3,500 cells/μL and ANC >2,000 cells/μL • Weekly after WBC >3,500 cells/μL and ANC >2,000 cells/μL
Agranulocytosis	ANC ≤500 cells/μL	Same as for severe leukopenia or severe granulocytopenia

Source: American Psychiatric Association. *Practice Guideline for the Treatment of Patients with Schizophrenia*. 2nd ed. 2004. http://www.guideline.gov/content.aspx?id=5217. Accessed June 28, 2011; Clozaril [package insert]. East Hanover, NJ: Novartis Pharmaceuticals; December 2010.

once or twice daily and titrated up slowly to a therapeutic dose. A slow titration schedule must be followed every time a patient is initiated on clozapine, whether it is initial treatment or reinitiation after the patient has been off clozapine for 2 or more days.

CASE 82-1, QUESTION 31: What procedures and laboratory tests needs to be done before starting J.R. on clozapine?

Before starting a patient on clozapine, it is necessary to obtain informed consent from the patient and register the patient, prescriber, and dispensing pharmacy with the clozapine registry. A baseline CBC with differential must also be drawn within 7 days before dispensing the medication. Although not required by the FDA, an ECG should be performed to assess for any pre-existing heart conditions. A physical examination should be performed at baseline, including measurements of height, weight, waist circumference, pulse, temperature, and blood pressure. Baseline laboratory tests should also include a hemoglobin A1c or fasting blood glucose, a fasting lipid panel, LFTs (e.g., aspartate aminotransferase and alanine aminotransferase), serum creatinine and blood urea nitrogen levels. Lastly, in women such as J.R., a pregnancy test should be performed.

CASE 82-1, QUESTION 32: How should clozapine be initiated in J.R.?

Whenever possible, clozapine should be initiated when a patient is medicationfree. However, if the patient is too ill to be taken off of all antipsychotic drugs before adding clozapine, the current medication can be discontinued after a therapeutic clozapine dose has been achieved. Alternatively, clozapine can be titrated upward while the first antipsychotic is slowly tapered downward. Benzodiazepines should not be used for early behavioral and anxiety control because their combined use with clozapine can lead to respiratory or cardiac arrest.

Clozapine can be started in an outpatient setting if patients are carefully monitored for tolerability, especially orthostasis. If baseline laboratory values are within normal limits and an informed consent is obtained, J.R. can start on clozapine 25 mg at bedtime. Her dose should be increased by 25 to 50 mg every day until the target dose of 300 mg/day is reached, the minimum dose at which most patients respond. Clozapine should be given in divided doses because of its risk of orthostasis; therefore, J.R. should receive 150 mg twice a day. J.R. may require higher doses because she is a smoker. Smoking induces clozapine's hepatic metabolism by increasing the activity of CYP1A2. If J.R. has

Key Websites

American Psychiatric Association. Treatment of Patients With Schizophrenia, Second Edition. http://www.psychiatryonline.com/pracGuide/pracGuideTopic_6.aspx.

National Institute for Health and Clinical Excellence. Schizophrenia (update). http://guidance.nice.org.uk/CG82.

US Food and Drug Administration. FDA Drug Safety Communication: Antipsychotic drug labels updated on use during pregnancy and risk of abnormal muscle movements and withdrawal symptoms in newborns. http://www.fda.gov/Drugs/DrugSafety/ucm243903.htm. Accessed March 17, 2011. (175)

Mood Disorders I: Major Depressive Disorders

83

Patrick R. Finley and Kelly C. Lee

CORE PRINCIPLES

MAJOR DEPRESSIVE DISORDER	CHAPTER CASES
1 Depression is a common and often chronic disorder that may manifest at anytime in one's life. Diagnostic criteria for major depression include a minimum of five symptoms persisting for at least two weeks. One of these symptoms must be either depressed mood or anhedonia. Suicidal ideation should be assessed in all patients.	**Case 83-1 (Questions 1, 2)**
2 A variety of treatment modalities are available for the management of depression. These include prescription medications, psychotherapy, and herbal preparations and dietary supplements. Prescription medications and/or psychotherapy are indicated for depressive symptoms that are moderate to severe in nature.	**Case 83-1 (Questions 3, 9)**
3 All of the prescription medications that are currently available are equally effective and possess the same delayed onset of therapeutic effects. Selection of an antidepressant is based on many factors, including previous response to medication, age, reproduction status, and both medical and psychiatric comorbidities.	**Case 83-1 (Questions 4–6, 12, 13)**
4 Antidepressants have also been associated with a wide variety of drug interactions and consideration should be made for the safety of combining medications as well.	**Case 83-1 (Questions 4–6, 14, 15)**
5 SSRIs are regarded as the initial treatment of choice for most depressed patients. They are inexpensive, effective for comorbid anxiety conditions, and possess a lower side-effect burden than other antidepressants overall. Side effects are generally mild and transient.	**Case 83-1 (Questions 5–10)**
6 The goal of antidepressant treatment is the complete amelioration of symptoms (i.e., remission). To achieve this, patients will need close and frequent follow-up, as well as individual titration and adjustment of their medication regimens. Once remission is achieved, the general recommendation is to continue the effective antidepressant regimen for a minimum of six months.	**Case 83-1 (Questions 9, 11)**
7 Because less than half of depressed patients will achieve remission with the first antidepressant selected, clinicians should have a comprehensive understanding of the role alternative antidepressants may have in optimizing outcomes. Clinicians should be familiar with augmentation strategies, as well as the merits of switching antidepressants in patients with an incomplete response.	**Case 83-2 (Questions 1–4)**
8 Depression in the elderly can be more difficult to recognize and treat than depression in younger patients. Medical etiologies of depressive symptoms must be ruled out and drug selection must take into consideration the potential interaction of medication-related adverse effects and medical comorbidities.	**Case 83-3 (Questions 1, 2)**

continued

MAJOR DEPRESSIVE DISORDER *CONTINUED*

9 The selection of antidepressants in patients with concomitant cardiac disease can be difficult given the wide spectrum of cardiac effects associated with antidepressants. Tricyclic antidepressants should be avoided in patients with cardiac conduction abnormalities. Plasma levels of tricyclic antidepressants may be helpful in monitoring adherence and toxicity.	**Case 83-4 (Questions 1–4)**
10 The relationship between diabetes and depression is bidirectional in that patients with depression are at increased risk for development of diabetes and patients with diabetes are also likely to suffer from depression. Management of both illnesses is critical for prevention of long-term complications from both diseases.	**Case 83-5 (Question 1)**
11 Patients with atypical features of depression are often treatment-resistant and tend to respond to monoamine oxidase inhibitors. Generally, monoamine oxidase inhibitors are reserved as last-line therapies and patients' ability to adhere to dietary restrictions must be considered prior to recommending these agents. Potentially fatal drug interactions can also occur with these drugs and must be carefully monitored.	**Case 83-9 (Questions 1–6)**
12 Psychotic depression is associated with increased morbidity and mortality more than other forms of depression and is often refractory to antidepressant monotherapy. Atypical antipsychotics may be effective in this population and somatic treatments such as electroconvulsive therapy have also been shown to be quite effective.	**Case 83-10 (Questions 1, 2)**

INTRODUCTION

Depression is a common, chronic, and potentially debilitating illness that has tempered the human condition since the beginning of recorded history. The ancient Egyptians, for instance, wrote about depression more than 3,000 years ago. In the First Book of Samuel (dated about 700 BC), Saul, the King of Israel, is overcome by an "evil spirit" that causes him to feel "incapacitated, guilt-ridden and hopeless," leading ultimately to his suicide.[1]

Cultures throughout history have speculated on the origin of depression. The ancient Greeks believed that depression was caused by an excess of bile. Hippocrates thoroughly described the condition as a somatic illness and is believed to have coined the term "melancholia," which literally translates to "black bile." During the Middle Ages, depression and other psychiatric illnesses were considered to be punishment or afflictions from a vengeful God rather than actual illness. At that time, the church and society believed depression to be the result of being weak minded or sinful. Even today, many people suffering from a depressive episode carry the stigma of "having a nervous breakdown," and medications may be viewed as a "crutch" to help cope with daily life. Throughout history, depression has affected the lives of many famous people, including Ludwig Van Beethoven, Meriwether Lewis, Abraham Lincoln, Charles Dickens, Winston Churchill, Ernest Hemingway, and Marilyn Monroe.[1]

Although many people experience "the blues" on occasion, the term "depression" is reserved in psychiatry to define a specific medical condition with distinctive biological and pharmacologic implications. Similarly, the term "clinical depression" is liberally applied in popular culture to a condition that approximates the psychiatric diagnosis of major depression. In general, depressive disorders are enormous health concerns that are often misdiagnosed or undertreated. The physical and social dysfunction associated with depression is profound and is believed to outweigh many other chronic medical conditions, including hypertension, diabetes, and arthritis.[2] The Medical Outcomes Study, for instance, determined that the degree of impairment in depressed individuals is comparable to that seen in patients with chronic heart disease.[3] The financial ramifications of depression are tremendous and place an overwhelming burden on our society. In 2000, the estimated cost of depression in the United States was $83.1 billion annually, with most of these costs ($51.5 billion) attributed to lost productivity and absenteeism in the workplace.[4]

Epidemiology

Since World War II, the lifetime incidence of depression has been rising steadily in studied populations. A recent investigation concluded that the annual incidence of mood disorders is approximately 10% in the adult population, and 1 in 15 adults (6.7%) will suffer from an episode of major depression during any 12-month period.[5] Various studies from Europe and the United States have estimated the lifetime prevalence to be 5% to 12% in men and 9% to 26% in women.[6] Although the incidence of depression is remarkably similar across various races and ethnic groups, the illness may be slightly more common in lower socioeconomic classes.[7]

The onset of depression occurs most commonly in the late 20s, but there is a wide range, and the first episode may actually present at any age. One prevailing misconception is that depression is more common among elderly individuals.[8] Epidemiologic evidence suggests that the incidence is slightly lower in older persons than in the general population, but certain subtypes may be more common (e.g., melancholia, depression with psychotic features), and new-onset depression that initially presents during geriatric years may carry a worse prognosis.

Genetic factors appear to play a major role in the cause of depression. The offspring of depressed individuals are 2.7 times more likely to have depression if one parent is afflicted, and 3.0 times more likely if both parents suffer from depression.[9] Concordance rates for monozygotic (identical) twins range from 54% to 65%, whereas the corresponding rates in dizygotic (fraternal) twins range from 14% to 24%.[10] Genetic factors may also predispose individuals to an earlier onset of depression (younger than 30 years of age).[11]

Alternatively, there is clear evidence that depression may occur as a result of stressful events (i.e., environmental factors) in one's life. These factors include a difficult childhood, physical or verbal abuse, pervasive low self-esteem, death of a loved one, loss of a job, and the end of a serious relationship. Acute depressive episodes are often attributed to a combination of environmental and genetic factors. For instance, individuals carrying a genetic predisposition to mood disorders may undergo a traumatic experience that ultimately triggers the manifestation of depressive symptomatology. Depression may also occur spontaneously among people who appear to lack any obvious genetic or environmental predisposition.

Diagnosis and Classification

Both the diagnosis and the classification of depression have undergone many transformations since Emil Kraepelin's biological model of the late 19th century. Kraepelin separated the functional psychoses into two groups: manic-depressive insanity and dementia praecox. Kraepelin's detailed descriptions of these two mental illnesses laid the foundation for modern psychiatry.[12] In 2000, the American Psychiatric Association (APA) published refined, standardized criteria for diagnosing depressive disorders in the *Diagnostic and Statistical Manual of Mental Disorders,* Fourth Edition, Text Revision (DSM-IV-TR).[13] Depressive disorders are classified under Mood Disorders in DSM-IV-TR and include major depressive disorder; single-episode or recurrent, dysthymic disorder; and depressive disorder, not otherwise specified. See Table 83-1 for the classification of mood disorders.

As previously stated, a major depressive disorder may manifest as a single episode, but it is more commonly a series of recurrent events. Thus, in most patients, depression is a chronic illness.[6] The frequency of recurrent episodes is highly variable, with some people experiencing discrete episodes separated by many years of relatively normal mood (i.e., euthymia), and others experiencing residual symptoms between episodes that may never completely remit. The risk of future episodes appears to increase disproportionately with the chronicity of the illness. For instance, after the first episode there is a 50% likelihood of a second episode. After the second, there is a 70% chance of a third, and with the third episode comes nearly a 90% incidence of a fourth.

Depressive disorders may be subclassified using cross-sectional symptom features, or specifiers, according to DSM-IV-TR.[13] For example, the phrase "with melancholic features" is used when patients possess primary neurovegetative symptoms, early morning awakening, marked psychomotor agitation or retardation, and significant anorexia or weight loss. Melancholia is often a more severe form of depression, and it often lacks apparent environmental triggers.[14] It may also be less likely than other forms of depression to remit spontaneously. The phrase "with atypical features" is used when depressive symptoms include weight gain, hypersomnia, leaden paralysis, or rejection sensitivity. When hallucinations or delusions occur in patients who are primarily depressed, the phrase "with psychotic features" is applicable to the mood disorder. Other diagnostic specifiers used in DSM-IV-TR include "chronic," "with catatonic features," and "with postpartum onset."

Dysthymic disorder is a type of depressive illness characterized by fewer symptoms than major depression, but the course is much more chronic with symptoms being present most of the time for at least 2 years. In practice, the distinction of major depression from dysthymia may be difficult to make and requires a detailed psychiatric history. The treatment for dysthymia has traditionally focused on psychotherapy, but recent evidence suggests that antidepressant medications may actually be more effective.[15]

TABLE 83-1
Classification of Mood Disorders

1. Mood Disorders
   - A. Depressive Disorders
     1. Major Depressive Disorder, Single Episode
     2. Major Depressive Disorder, Recurrent
     3. Dysthymic Disorder
     4. Depressive Disorder Not Otherwise Specified
   - B. Bipolar Disorders
     1. Bipolar Disorder, Single Episode
     2. Bipolar Disorder, Recurrent
     3. Cyclothymic Disorder
     4. Bipolar Disorder Not Otherwise Specified
   - C. Secondary Mood Disorder Due to Nonpsychiatric Medical Condition
   - D. Substance-Induced Mood Disorder
   - E. Mood Disorder Not Otherwise Specified

Adapted with permission from American Psychiatric Association. *Diagnostic and Statistical Manual of Mental Disorders.* 4th ed. Text Revision. Washington, DC: American Psychiatric Association; 2000.

TABLE 83-2
Selected Medical Conditions that May Mimic Depression

Central Nervous System	Women's Health
Alzheimer disease	Premenstrual dysphoric disorder
Cerebrovascular accident	Antepartum/postpartum
Epilepsy	Perimenopause
Multiple sclerosis	**Other**
Parkinson disease	Chronic fatigue syndrome
Cardiovascular	Chronic pain syndrome(s)
Cerebral arteriosclerosis	Fibromyalgia
Congestive heart failure	Irritable bowel syndrome
Myocardial infarction	Malignancies (various)
Endocrine	Migraine headaches
Addison disease	Rheumatoid arthritis
Diabetes mellitus (types 1 and 2)	Systemic lupus erythematosus
Hypothyroidism	

Differential Diagnosis

Symptoms of depression may be induced or exacerbated by numerous medical illnesses or medications (Tables 83-2 and 83-3). Consequently, DSM-IV-TR specifies that whenever an "organic cause" is temporally related to the onset of depressive symptoms, the patient does not fit the criteria for major depression, even if all other criteria are met.[13] The rationale for this stipulation is that if the medical illness is successfully treated or the offending agent is discontinued, the depressive illness would spontaneously resolve, eliminating the need for psychiatric intervention or somatic intervention. Although lists of medical illnesses or medications are helpful, the clinician should be aware that the actual evidence demonstrating an association between depression and specific organic causes is often very limited and anecdotal. If a medication or condition is suspected of

TABLE 83-3
Selected Medications that May Induce Depression

Cardiovascular Agents	Hormonal Agents
β-blockers[a] (?)	Anabolic steroids
Clonidine	Corticosteroids
Methyldopa	Gonadotropin-releasing hormone
Reserpine	Progestins
	Tamoxifen
Central Nervous System	**Others**
Barbiturates	Efavirenz
Chloral hydrate	Interferon
Ecstasy (MDMA)	Isotretinoin
Ethanol	Mefloquine
Varenicline	Levetiracetam

[a] Lipophilic beta-blockers (e.g., propranolol) may have higher risk but data are conflicting.

causing depression, the chronologic association should be investigated rigorously before other action is taken.

Clinical Presentation

For a diagnosis of major depressive disorder to be made, symptoms must be present for at least 2 weeks and must not be precipitated or influenced by a medical illness or medication (according to DSM-IV-TR criteria). Individuals must possess at least five symptoms, one of which is either depressed mood OR anhedonia (diminished interest or pleasure in activities). The other seven symptoms are as follows:

1. Change in appetite
2. Change in sleep
3. Low energy
4. Poor concentration (or difficulty making decisions)
5. Feelings of worthlessness or inappropriate guilt
6. Psychomotor agitation or retardation
7. Recurrent thoughts of suicide

The diagnostic criteria also stipulate that the mood disturbance must cause marked distress or result in clinically significant impairment of social or occupational functioning. Table 83-4 lists the specific criteria for a diagnosis of major depressive disorder.

Although low energy and changes in sleep or appetite are present in most depressed patients, the clinical presentation of depression can be highly variable. Many patients will readily express profound sadness or hopelessness, but others can project a more anxious or irritable appearance. Psychomotor agitation may be apparent, featuring wringing of the hands, grimacing, pacing, or cursing. Conversely, psychomotor retardation can be evident, with slowed speech or thinking, soft monotone voice, or minimal facial expression. Although the criteria for detecting major depression are identical in the elderly population as in the general population, the presentation may be slightly different than in younger individuals. Elderly patients may be less likely to acknowledge sadness or melancholy and choose to dwell instead on somatic complaints such as headache, insomnia, joint pain, dizziness, or constipation.[16] As a result, clinicians are advised to consider the possibility of depression whenever a person presents with vague, chronic symptoms of physical illness and unclear etiology.

TABLE 83-4
Diagnostic Criteria for Major Depressive Disorder

- At least five of the following symptoms have been present during the same 2-week period and represent a change from previous functioning. One of the symptoms must be either depressed mood or loss of interest/pleasure.
  - –Depressed mood most of the day, nearly every day
  - –Loss of interest in pleasurable activities most of the day, nearly every day
  - –Change in weight or appetite (increase or decrease) when not dieting
  - –Insomnia or hypersomnia nearly every day
  - –Fatigue or loss of energy nearly every day
  - –Diminished ability to think or concentrate, or indecisiveness
  - –Feelings of worthlessness or excessive or inappropriate guilt nearly every day
  - –Psychomotor agitation or retardation nearly every day
  - –Recurrent thoughts of death or suicidal ideation
- Symptoms cause clinically significant distress or impairment in social, occupational, or other important areas of functioning.
- Symptoms are not caused by an underlying medical condition or substance (e.g., medications or recreational drugs).

Adapted with permission from American Psychiatric Association. *Diagnostic and Statistical Manual of Mental Disorders.* 4th ed. Text Revision. Washington, DC: American Psychiatric Association; 2000.

Pathophysiology

Our understanding of the biological basis for depressive disorders has come a long way since Hippocrates first identified bile as a possible cause. Several modern theories addressing the origin of depression have evolved over the past three decades, focusing on neurotransmitter systems, including norepinephrine, serotonin, and dopamine (Fig. 83-1). As unique antidepressant medications are developed and our understanding of the mechanisms of pharmacologic action improves, other cogent theories of depression will undoubtedly evolve.

In the past, the monoamine hypothesis proposed that decreased synaptic concentrations of norepinephrine and/or serotonin caused depression. The norepinephrine depletion theory was originally based on the observation that reserpine, which depleted catecholamine stores in the central nervous system (CNS), was capable of causing depression.[17,18] This theory evolved into the permissive hypothesis, which emphasized a greater role for serotonin in promoting or "permitting" a decline in norepinephrine function. Specifically, this hypothesis suggests that low concentrations of serotonin or norepinephrine in the CNS precipitated depressive symptoms, whereas low levels of serotonin and increased activity of norepinephrine resulted in manic symptoms. Antidepressants were believed to relieve depression by inhibiting the reuptake of norepinephrine and/or serotonin from the synapse up into the neuron, and effectively increasing neurotransmitter concentrations in the synaptic cleft.[19]

Although these theories were initially helpful in enhancing our understanding of how antidepressants worked, there were multiple reasons to suspect that other mechanisms and systems were involved. First, antidepressants were capable of blocking the reuptake of neurotransmitters almost immediately after administration, yet several weeks lapsed before therapeutic effects were evident (i.e., delayed onset).[20] Second, synaptic concentrations of biogenic amines are not always decreased in depressed individuals and can actually be higher than those seen in normal controls.[21] Lastly, antidepressants in development can work via mechanisms that do not involve relative increases

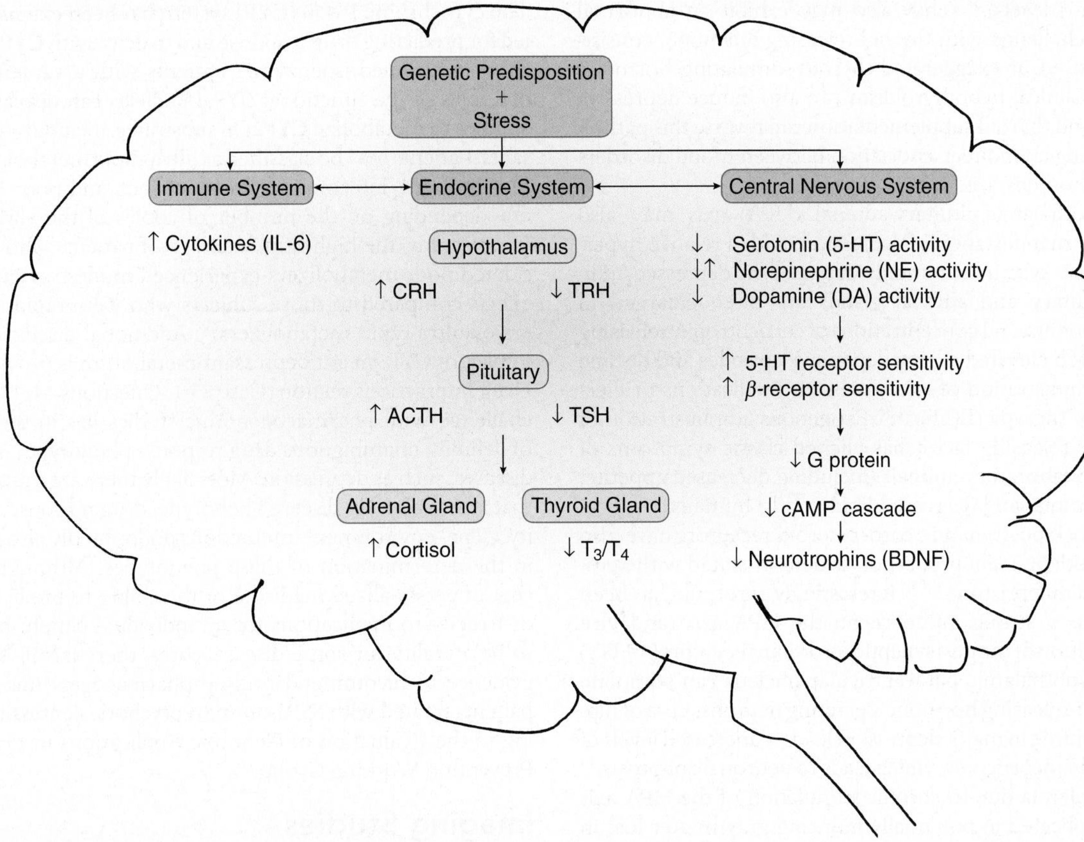

FIGURE 83-1 Influence of genetic and environmental factors on the immune system, endocrine system, and central nervous system. CRH, corticotropin-releasing hormone (also known as corticotropin-releasing factor [CRF]); TRH, thyrotrophin-releasing hormone; ACTH, adrenocorticotropic hormone; TSH, thyroid-stimulating hormone; T_3/T_4, triiodothyronine/thyroxine. (© JL Corbitt, PR Finley, 2003.)

in synaptic neurotransmitter concentrations. Such mechanisms include blockade of substance P, and antagonism of corticotropin-releasing factor or corticosteroid receptors.[22–24]

The dysregulation hypothesis has evolved more recently and suggests that depression, as well as other psychiatric disorders, is the result of a dysregulated neurotransmitter system. Such dysregulation may include (a) an impairment in the regulatory or homeostatic mechanisms, (b) an erratic basal output of neurotransmitters, (c) a disruption in normal periodicities (circadian rhythm), (d) a less selective response to environmental stimuli, (e) perturbation of the system resulting in a delayed return to baseline, and (f) restoration to efficient regulation through the use of pharmacologic agents.[25]

Depression has been associated with changes in presynaptic and postsynaptic receptor densities (or sensitivities) that have been described as being downregulated or desensitized.[26] Changes include a decrease in postsynaptic alpha-adrenergic receptor sensitivity, along with alterations in the sensitivities of the alpha-adrenergic, dopaminergic (D_2) and serotonin receptor subtypes (5-HT_{1A} and $5HT_{2A}$). For example, selective serotonin reuptake inhibitors (SSRIs) can increase the efficiency of serotonergic neurotransmission acutely (through reuptake blockade), but their therapeutic effects are linked temporally with increased release of serotonin through downregulation of presynaptic autoreceptors (5-HT_{1A}).[27]

Today, emphasis continues to be placed on serotonin, norepinephrine, and dopamine neurotransmitters, and additional attention is also being paid to their differential effects on specific depressive symptoms. For instance, appetite, sleep, libido, motor function, anxiety, and aggression all appear to be strongly influenced by serotonin transmission. Research evidence for serotonergic influence has demonstrated that the concentration of serotonin's primary metabolite (5-hydroxyindoleacetic acid [5-HIAA]) is decreased in the cerebrospinal fluid of depressed patients.[27] Low 5-HIAA concentrations have also been found in the cerebrospinal fluid of patients attempting suicide and may have a role in triggering other violent activities.[28] Dietary depletion of L-tryptophan, a serotonin precursor, has induced relapse in depressed patients previously responsive to SSRIs, and symptoms such as irritability and disrupted sleep/appetite appear to return preferentially.[29]

Alternatively, deficiencies in norepinephrine (and dopamine to some extent) are believed to mediate depressive symptoms such as anhedonia, decreased energy, memory impairments, and executive dysfunction.[30] Administration of α-methyl paratyrosine (which inhibits the synthesis of norepinephrine) has resulted in the return of these depressive symptoms among patients previously treated successfully with noradrenergic antidepressants.[31] The role of dopamine in mediating this constellation of symptoms has been implied through postmortem studies, neuroimaging results, and the demonstrated effectiveness of pure dopamine agonists (e.g., amantadine, pramipexole) in relieving depression.[32] Ultimately, it is still believed that a common circuitry is influenced by these various neurotransmitters, resulting in the clinical manifestation of depression.[31]

Neuroendocrine Findings

Along with dysregulated neurotransmitter systems, neuroendocrine abnormalities may contribute to the development of depression. Depressed patients often have abnormal thyroid function tests (including low triiodothyronine [T_3] and/or thyroxine [T_4] levels).[33] They also may exhibit an abnormal response to challenge with thyroid-releasing hormone, consisting of a blunted or exaggerated thyroid-stimulating hormone response.[34] Clinical hypothyroidism can also induce depressive symptoms, and thyroid supplementation can reverse this pathology, suggesting an indirect association between mood disorders and thyroid homeostasis.[35]

The hypothalamic-pituitary-adrenal (HPA) axis may also influence the manifestation of depression, with a relative hyperactivity of this system commonly reported in depressed individuals. Pituitary and adrenal glands are often enlarged in depressed patients, and concentrations of corticotropin-releasing factor are often elevated during depressive episodes and decline with the administration of antidepressant medications or electroconvulsive therapy (ECT).[24,36] Exogenous administration of corticotropin-releasing factor has elicited classic symptoms of depression in laboratory animals (including decreased appetite, anxiety, insomnia, and decreased libido).[37] In humans, medications that block postsynaptic corticosteroid receptors have also displayed antidepressant properties, as demonstrated with ketoconazole and mifepristone.[38,39] Interestingly, serotonin has been recognized as a strong influence on the HPA axis (and vice versa). Activation of the postsynaptic serotonin receptors (5-HT_2) along the hypothalamic paraventricular nucleus can stimulate corticotropin-releasing hormone–secreting neurons. Loss of hippocampal volume in major depression leads to increased levels of circulating glucocorticoids, which leads to neuronal apoptosis.[40] Hypercortisolemia due to chronic stimulation of the HPA axis has been implicated in potentially reducing gray matter loss in humans. It should be noted that the relationship between hippocampal volume and depression is not consistently observed and that various factors may affect these findings.[41] Corticosteroids can also modulate serotonin synthesis, metabolism, and reuptake.[24]

Not all of the evidence, however, supports a causative role of HPA overactivity in the manifestation of depression. The acute administration of high-dose corticosteroids, for instance, is more commonly associated with mood elevation (e.g., euphoria or hypomania), leading some to suggest that the exaggerated HPA response seen with depression is actually the body's attempt to overcome this mood disorder. Furthermore, HPA overactivity has not been observed in certain populations of depressed patients, such as adolescents and young adults. Given the strong association of depression with chronic inflammatory conditions, further exploration of the relationship of the HPA axis to depressive symptoms is imperative.

Genetic Studies

Over the last few years, significant scientific advances have been made in genetics and pharmacogenomics. Several genes have been implicated in predictive response or adverse effects to antidepressants. Pharmacodynamic targets have focused on serotonin transporters (5-HTTLPR), tryptophan hydroxylase enzymes 1 and 2 (TPH1 and TPH2), serotonin 1A (5-HT_{1A}) and 2A (5-HT_{2A}) receptors, brain-derived neurotrophic factor (BDNF), G-protein beta-3 subunit (GNB3), monoamine oxidase enzymes and p-glycoprotein; pharmacokinetic targets have been focused on polymorphic variations in CYP1A2, CYP2C19, CYP2D6, and CYP3A4 enzymes.[42–44] Variations in the serotonin transporter *SLC6A4* gene have been associated with remission and response rate in a meta-analysis of 1,435 patients.[43] Researchers found that patients with the *ss* genotype are less likely to reach remission during SSRI treatment and take longer to achieve 50% symptom improvement compared to those with the *ll* genotype. Asian patients had the most significant heterogeneity in response, although the association was also seen among white patients. The cytochrome P-450 (CYP) system has been extensively studied for predicting drug response and toxicity with CYP2D6 being the most studied isoenzyme. Patients with a variable number of copies of the functional *CYP2D6* alleles can display different abilities to metabolize CYP2D6 substrates, including antidepressants. Patients may be classified as ultra-rapid metabolizers, rapid metabolizers, intermediate metabolizers, and poor metabolizers, depending on the number of copies of the variant allele. In one study, the highest percentage of patients who were considered poor metabolizers experienced modest or marked side effects compared to those subjects who were rapid metabolizers or ultra-rapid metabolizers.[45] Additional discussion on the impact of CYP on antidepressant metabolism is provided in the Drug Interactions section (Case 83-1, Questions 14, 15). A major challenge with pharmacogenomic studies lies in the difficulty of defining unambiguous drug response phenotypes in complex diseases, such as depression. Most likely there are multiple genes that are involved in disease phenotype, drug response, and toxicity. Gene–environment interactions undoubtedly also play a role in the determination of these phenotypes. Although the concept of personalized medicine or the ability to predict response or toxicity to medications for an individual patient has proven to be a reality for some disease states, there is still insufficient evidence to recommend routine pharmacogenomic testing in patients treated with SSRIs for non-psychotic depression according to the Evaluation of Genomic Applications in Practice and Prevention Working Group.[46]

Imaging Studies

Imaging studies (including computed tomography, magnetic resonance imaging, positron emission tomography, and single-photon emission computed tomography) suggest that patients with depression have regional brain dysfunction, most often affecting the limbic structures and prefrontal cortex. Alterations in cerebral blood flow and/or metabolism in the frontal-temporal cortex and caudate nucleus are associated with common depressive symptoms such as dysphoria, anhedonia, hopelessness, and flat affect.[47] Increased firing of the amygdala in the left hemisphere has been linked in positron emission tomography studies with the future development of depression.[48] Because subtypes of depression have been linked to different regional dysfunctions, a network hypothesis has begun to emerge that may lead to improvements in depression diagnosis and targeted treatments.[49]

Patient Assessment Tools

Pharmaceutical care of the depressed patient requires specialized knowledge of the illness and treatments, as well as refined interviewing skills. To obtain specific information about the target symptoms of depression and to assess the therapeutic impact of psychotropic medications, effective and productive interpersonal communication is vital. The structured mental status examination is an established systematic way of assessing a patient's mental health (Table 83-5). Many functional domains are assessed in a mental status examination. Through this structured interview, the clinician has an observational basis for evaluating a patient's appearance, behavior, speech, mood, affect (i.e., outer manifestation of inner emotional states), sensorium, memory, and intellectual function.

For a more detailed discussion of the mental status examination and specific psychiatric interviewing techniques for depression, please refer to a narrated powerpoint presentation on depression assessment at http://thepoint.lww.com/AT10e or refer to other sources.[50,51]

TABLE 83-5
Mental Status Exam

General Appearance, Behavior, Speech
• Apparent age; appear ill or in distress? • Dress • General reaction to examination, negativism • Posture and gait • Unusual movements • Facial expression • Signs of anxiety • General level of activity • Repetitious activities (stereotypy, mannerisms, compulsions) • Disturbances of attention: distractibility • Speech: mute, word salad, echolalia, clang, neologisms
Mood and Affect
• Quality of prevailing mood; intensity and depth • Constancy of mood, patient-stated mood • Affect: range, appropriateness, lability, flatness
Sensorium
• Orientation for time, place, person, situation • Memory: recent and remote, immediate recall
Level of Intellectual Functioning
• An estimate of current intellectual functioning, not an estimate of original intellectual potential • General fund of information: presidents, oceans, governor, large cities, current events. Why does the moon appear larger than the stars? • Vocabulary • Serial 7 subtractions (also tests attention and sensorium)
Thought Processes
• Pattern of associations (tempo, rhythm, organization, distortions, excesses, deficiencies) • False perceptions (hallucinations, illusions, delusions, distortions of body image, depersonalization) • Thought content (what patient tells, main concerns, obsessive ideation) • Abstracting ability (tests by similarities, proverbs) • Judgment and insight

Adapted with permission from Carlat DJ. *The Psychiatric Interview. Practical Guides in Psychiatry*. Philadelphia, PA: Lippincott Williams & Wilkins; 2004.

Behavioral rating scales have been used for many years in drug efficacy studies and are widely advocated for routine use in the clinical arena today. Rating scales can be helpful in assessing the severity of mental illness, quantifying changes in target symptoms, and determining treatment efficacy, but they are not necessarily diagnostic. Rating scales can vary in length, content, and format, and can be completed by providers, patients, researchers, family members, or conservators. Numerous depression scales have been developed, including the Hamilton Rating Scale for Depression (HAM-D_{17} or HAM-D_{21}), the Beck Depression Inventory (BDI), the Hopkins Symptom Checklist, the Montgomery Asberg Depression Rating Scale (MADRS), the Center for Epidemiological Studies Depression (CES-D) Scale, the Patient Health Questionnaire (PHQ-9) (Fig. 83-2), and the Quick Inventory of Depressive Symptoms ($QIDS_{16}$ or $QIDS_{30}$; Fig. 83-3).[52–59] The HAM-D was initially designed to measure the efficacy of antidepressant medications given to severely depressed individuals in controlled clinical trials.[52] Over the years, this instrument emerged as the gold standard of depression rating scales, although many clinicians are unaware of its limitations. For instance, the HAM-D was never designed for routine use in the general ambulatory care patient population and fails to address a number of target symptoms required for a DSM-IV-TR diagnosis of major depression (e.g., low energy, poor concentration, hopelessness). The QIDS has emerged recently as a more valuable instrument in the hands of primary care providers. It contains a total of 16 items, can be completed within 10 to 15 minutes, and is available at no cost to clinicians. It has been validated and used extensively in clinical and research settings and is available in both clinician-rated and patient-rated formats. The CES-D is also available in an abbreviated format and has served as a useful screening instrument among elderly populations (Fig. 83-3, Table 83-6).[60]

Although depression symptoms are clearly associated with many biochemical and endocrine abnormalities, no laboratory tests are routinely assessed to aid the clinician in establishing a diagnosis of depression. For many years, the dexamethasone suppression test was used to confirm the diagnosis of depression, but now it is rarely used due to the high rate of false-positive findings. Attempts at correlating plasma concentrations of neurotransmitters with depression have not been successful, and urinary concentrations of monoamine metabolites are only weakly associated with depressive symptoms.

Nondrug Therapies for Depression

The successful treatment of depression provides a most formidable challenge to modern medicine. In addition to the emotional turmoil and social disability that a depressed individual endures, the illness can affect other disease states, slow the recovery process, or even promote complications.

Although pharmacologic intervention has become the primary treatment modality for relieving depressive symptoms, the efficacy and suitability of other therapeutic options should not be overlooked. Most experts now advocate a three-pronged approach to relieving and preventing depressive symptoms involving (a) psychotherapy, (b) medications, and (c) lifestyle adjustments. Because these interventions address different aspects of the illness at different stages in the recovery process, they work synergistically together, and a brief summary of these approaches can be found later in this chapter.

Psychotherapy

For the treatment of mild to moderate depression, psychotherapy has proved to be comparable to pharmacologic intervention and may be preferred by some patients. For the acute treatment of severe depression, antidepressants appear to be more effective than psychotherapy alone and have a more rapid onset of therapeutic action.[61] The beneficial effects of psychotherapy, however, may persist longer than medication-related benefits after the interventions have been formally discontinued. In addition, psychotherapy may be particularly beneficial for preventing relapse among patients who previously demonstrated a therapeutic response to antidepressants.[62] Overall, the combination of treatments is superior to either intervention alone, although the routine use of both modalities is often not feasible in today's health care environment.[61]

Several forms of psychotherapy are available, including cognitive-behavioral therapy, interpersonal therapy, and psychoanalytic and psychodynamic therapies. Cognitive-behavioral therapy, in particular, often focuses on identifying and reversing negative thought patterns that perpetuate depressed emotions. It has been studied extensively in the depression field and is now available in a manual-driven, evidence-based format. A more precise explanation and description of psychotherapeutic alternatives is beyond the scope of this textbook. However, clinicians in the field are strongly encouraged to develop familiarity

PATIENT HEALTH QUESTIONNAIRE-9 (PHQ-9)

Over the **last 2 weeks**, how often have you been bothered by any of the following problems? *(Use "☒" to indicate your answer)*	Not at all	Several days	More than half the days	Nearly every day
1. Little interest or pleasure in doing things	0	1	2	3
2. Feeling down, depressed, or hopeless	0	1	2	3
3. Trouble falling or staying asleep, or sleeping too much	0	1	2	3
4. Feeling tired or having little energy	0	1	2	3
5. Poor appetite or overeating	0	1	2	3
6. Feeling bad about yourself—or that you are a failure or have let yourself or your family down	0	1	2	3
7. Trouble concentrating on things, such as reading the newspaper or watching television	0	1	2	3
8. Moving or speaking so slowly that other people could have noticed? Or the opposite—being so fidgety or restless that you have been moving around a lot more than usual	0	1	2	3
9. Thoughts that you would be better off dead or of hurting yourself in some way	0	1	2	3

FOR OFFICE CODING ___0___ + ______ + ______ + ______

=Total Score: ______

If you checked off any problems, how difficult have these problems made it for you to do your work, take care of things at home, or get along with other people?

Not difficult at all	Somewhat difficult	Very difficult	Extremely difficult
☐	☐	☐	☐

FIGURE 83-2 Patient Health Questionnaire (PHQ-9). (Developed by Drs. Robert L. Spitzer, Janet B.W. Williams, Kurt Kroenke and colleagues, with an educational grant from Pfizer Inc. No permission required to reproduce, translate, display, or distribute.)

with these approaches, as well as general supportive counseling techniques, which can serve to promote the recovery process and decrease the likelihood of future episodes.[63]

Somatic Interventions

ECT is a safe, rapid-acting, and highly effective therapeutic intervention that continues to suffer, ostensibly, from a poor public image. ECT was enormously popular during the 1940s and 1950s and was used without discretion to treat a wide variety of psychiatric conditions. This practice waned with the advent of effective psychotropic medications, and with the accumulation of case reports describing fractures and severe cognitive impairment in treated patients. Since the 1950s, the ECT procedure has undergone considerable transformation and refinement.[64] Adjunctive medications are now routinely administered to prevent adverse effects and reduce morbidity (e.g., a short-acting barbiturate for general anesthesia, an anticholinergic agent to prevent bradycardia and to dry excessive airway secretions, succinylcholine to prevent fractures from tonic-clonic contractions). The electric stimulus itself is no longer applied in one steady current but now consists of a series of brief pulses that have been shown to decrease the severity of postictal headaches and memory impairment.

Fundamentally, ECT features the induction of generalized seizures through an electric current delivered by bilateral or unilateral electrode placement. Certain medications may raise seizure thresholds (benzodiazepines) or promote cognitive impairment (lithium) and should be discontinued before the procedure. Adverse effects are generally minimal and consist mainly

QUICK INVENTORY OF DEPRESSIVE SYMPTOMATOLOGY (SELF-REPORT)

THIS SECTION FOR USE BY STUDY PERSONNEL ONLY.

Questionnaire completed on visit date ☐ **or** specify date completed: ____________
DD-Mon-YYYY

Only the patient (subject) should enter information onto this questionnaire.

TICK THE ONE RESPONSE TO EACH ITEM THAT BEST DESCRIBES YOU FOR THE PAST SEVEN DAYS.

1. Falling Asleep:
- ☐0 I never take longer than 30 minutes to fall asleep.
- ☐1 I take at least 30 minutes to fall asleep, less than half the time (3 days or less out of the past 7 days).
- ☐2 I take at least 30 minutes to fall asleep, more than half the time (4 days or more out of the past 7 days).
- ☐3 I take more than 60 minutes to fall asleep, more than half the time (4 days or more out of the past 7 days).

2. Sleep During the Night:
- ☐0 I do not wake up at night.
- ☐1 I have a restless, light sleep waking up briefly a few times each night.
- ☐2 I wake up at least once a night, but I go back to sleep easily.
- ☐3 I wake up more than once a night and stay awake for 20 minutes or more, more than half the time (4 days or more out of the past 7 days).

3. Waking Up Too Early:
- ☐0 Most of the time, I wake up no more than 30 minutes before I need to get up.
- ☐1 More than half the time (4 days or more out of the past 7 days), I wake up more than 30 minutes before I need to get up.
- ☐2 I almost always wake up at least one hour or so before I need to get up, but I go back to sleep eventually.
- ☐3 I wake up at least one hour before I need to get up, and cannot go back to sleep.

4. Sleeping Too Much:
- ☐0 I sleep no more than 7-8 hours/night, without napping during the day.
- ☐1 I sleep no more than 10 hours in a 24-hour period including naps.
- ☐2 I sleep no more than 12 hours in a 24-hour period including naps.
- ☐3 I sleep more than 12 hours in a 24-hour period including naps.

5. Feeling Sad:
- ☐0 I do not feel sad.
- ☐1 I feel sad less than half the time (3 days or less out of the past 7 days).
- ☐2 I feel sad more than half the time (4 days or more out of the past 7 days).
- ☐3 I feel sad nearly all of the time.

Please complete <u>either</u> 6 <u>or</u> 7 (not both)

6. Decreased Appetite:
- ☐0 There is no change in my usual appetite.
- ☐1 I eat somewhat less often or lesser amounts of food than usual.
- ☐2 I eat much less than usual and only with personal effort.
- ☐3 I rarely eat within a 24-hour period, and only with extreme personal effort or when others persuade me to eat.

7. Increased Appetite:
- ☐0 There is no change from my usual appetite.
- ☐1 I feel a need to eat more frequently than usual.
- ☐2 I regularly eat more often and/or larger amounts of food than usual.
- ☐3 I feel driven to overeat both at mealtimes and between meals.

Please complete <u>either</u> 8 <u>or</u> 9 (not both)

8. Decreased Weight (Within the Last 14 Days)
- ☐0 I have not had a change in my weight.
- ☐1 I feel as if I have had a slight weight loss.
- ☐2 I have lost 1 kg or more.
- ☐3 I have lost 2 kg or more.

9. Increased Weight (Within the Last 14 Days)
- ☐0 I have not had a change in my weight.
- ☐1 I feel as if I have had a slight weight gain.
- ☐2 I have gained 1 kg or more.
- ☐3 I have gained 2 kg or more.

FIGURE 83-3 Quick Inventory for Depressive Symptomatology (self-report). (Reprinted with permission from Rush AJ et al. The 16-item Quick Inventory Of Depressive Symptomatology [QIDS], clinician rating [QIDS-C], and self-report [QIDS-SR]: a psychometric evaluation in patients with chronic major depression [published correction appears in *Biol Psychiatry.* 2003;54:585]. *Biol Psychiatry.* 2003;54:573.) (*continued*)

10. Concentration/Decision Making:

☐0 There is no change in my usual capacity to concentrate or make decisions.
☐1 I occasionally feel indecisive or find that my attention wanders.
☐2 Most of the time I struggle to focus my attention or to make decisions.
☐3 I cannot concentrate well enough to read or cannot make even minor decisions.

11. View of Myself:

☐0 I see myself as equally worthwhile and deserving as other people.
☐1 I am more self-blaming than usual.
☐2 I largely believe that I cause problems for others.
☐3 I think almost constantly about major and minor defects in myself.

12. Thoughts of Death or Suicide:

☐0 I do not think of suicide or death.
☐1 I feel that life is empty or wonder if it is worth living.
☐2 I think of suicide or death several times over the past 7 days for several minutes.
☐3 I think of suicide or death several times a day in some detail or I have made specific plans for suicide or have actually tried to take my life.

13. General Interest:

☐ 0 There is no change from usual in how interested I am in other people or activities.
☐ 1 I notice that I am less interested in people or activities.
☐ 2 I find I have interest in only one or two of my formerly pursued activities.
☐ 3 I have virtually no interest in formerly pursued activities.

14. Energy Level:

☐ 0 There is no change in my usual level of energy.
☐ 1 I get tired more easily than usual.
☐ 2 I have to make a big effort to start or finish my usual daily activities (for example, shopping, homework, cooking or going to work).
☐ 3 I really cannot carry out most of my usual daily activities because I just don't have the energy.

15. Feeling More Sluggish Than Usual:

☐ 0 I think, speak, and move at my usual rate of speed.
☐ 1 I find that my thinking is more sluggish than usual or that my voice sounds dull or flat.
☐ 2 It takes me several seconds to respond to most questions and I am sure my thinking is more sluggish than usual.
☐ 3 I am often unable to respond to questions without extreme effort.

16. Feeling Restless:

☐ 0 I do not feel restless.
☐ 1 I'm often fidgety, wringing my hands, or need to shift around when I am sitting.
☐ 2 I have impulses to move about and am quite restless.
☐ 3 At times, I am unable to stay seated and need to pace around.

I confirm that this information is accurate.	Patient's/Subject's initials:	Date:

QUICK INVENTORY OF DEPRESSIVE SYMPTOMATOLOGY (SCORE SHEET)

NOTE: THIS SECTION IS TO BE COMPLETED BY THE STUDY PERSONNEL ONLY.

______ Enter the highest score on any 1 of the 4 sleep items (1–4)
______ Item 5
______ Enter the highest score on any 1 of the appetite/weight items (6–9)
______ Item 10
______ Item 11
______ Item 12
______ Item 13
______ Item 14
______ Enter the highest score on either of the 2 psychomotor items (15 and 16)
______ **Total Score (Range: 0–27)**

FIGURE 83-3 *(Continued)*

Section 15 Psychiatric Disorders

TABLE 83-6
Comparison of Selected Depression Rating Scales

Instrument	Minimal	Mild	Moderate	Severe
Hamilton (HAM-D)—17-item (Clinician-rated)	<8	8–15	16–27	>27
Beck Depression Inventory (BDI)				
BDI (Clinician-rated)	<10	10–16	17–29	>29
BDI (Patient-rated)	<10	10–15	16–23	>23
Quick Inventory for Depressive Symptoms (QIDS)				
QIDS-C_{16} (Clinician-rated)	<6	6–10	11–15	>15
QIDS-SR_{16} (Patient-rated)	<6	6–10	11–15	>15
Patient Health Questionnaire (PHQ) (Patient-rated)	<10	11–14	15–19	>19
Montgomery-Asberg Depression Rating Scale (MADRS) (Clinician-rated)	<7	7–19	20–34	>34

of transient anterograde amnesia (i.e., difficulty remembering events around the time of the procedure), retrograde amnesia, confusion, headaches, and muscle aches. Cardiovascular effects (e.g., ventricular arrhythmias, myocardial infarction [MI]) are the most ominous sequelae, but these events are quite rare.

Many years of clinical experience have enabled clinicians to identify patient populations most likely to benefit from this intervention. Today, ECT is recommended for patients with treatment-resistant depression, severe vegetative depression, psychotic depression, and depression in pregnancy. Overall response rates are rather impressive, ranging from 70% to 90%, and ECT has the distinct advantage of inducing a therapeutic response within the first week or two of treatments.[65] The recommended frequency of ECT treatments is variable. Most institutions have used three sessions weekly to induce a therapeutic response acutely, although evidence suggests that twice-weekly sessions are better tolerated and more cost-effective.[66] The frequency of treatments thereafter (i.e., maintenance therapy) is unknown, although recent evidence suggests that ECT administered weekly for 1 month and less frequently thereafter may be as effective as aggressive pharmacotherapy in preventing relapse.[67]

Other somatic interventions have also been used successfully to treat depression. Transcranial magnetic stimulation (TMS) is a noninvasive procedure involving the application of an electrical stimulus across the scalp, which ultimately generates an electrical field in the cerebral cortex.[68] Unlike ECT, TMS does not generate an actual seizure, and it is very well tolerated, with common side effects consisting of transient scalp discomfort and headaches. Preliminary investigations successfully used repetitive high-frequency techniques in depressed subjects, and imaging studies have shown functional improvements consistent with antidepressant properties. However, two randomized sham-controlled studies of TMS, administered in the left dorsolateral prefrontal cortex, showed conflicting results.[69,70] In 2008, the US Food and Drug Administration (FDA) decided to allow the marketing of TMS for patients who failed a minimum of one prior antidepressant trial. However, some concerns remain regarding the scientific evidence supporting its use.[71] Vagus nerve stimulation involves the surgical implantation of an electrical device in the subcutaneous tissue below the clavicle, which sends an impulse along the left vagal nerve into the cerebral cortex.[72] This intervention has proven to be effective for intractable seizures. It is currently FDA-approved for the management of treatment-resistant depression, although the safety and cost effectiveness of this expensive approach have not been extensively studied.

Light therapy or phototherapy is particularly effective for relieving the irritability and malaise associated with seasonal affective disorder, a milder form of depression that has been attributed to decreases in natural sunlight found with seasonal variation.[73] Phototherapy is administered in the form of a light box delivering 1,500 to 10,000 lux for a period of 1 to 2 hours daily. It is generally well tolerated. Sleep deprivation may be an effective adjuvant to antidepressants and this therapy has been studied as a remedy for premenstrual dysphoric disorder. The goal of sleep deprivation is to gradually advance sleep cycles by altering wake schedules, ultimately minimizing the duration of rapid eye movement (REM) sleep.[74]

Lifestyle Adjustments

Any therapeutic approach to mood disorders should seek to reverse unhealthy or destructive lifestyle habits and promote other activities that may relieve stress and facilitate well-being. Alcohol, recreational drug use, and excessive caffeine consumption should be minimized (if not prohibited) in patients suffering from depression or anxiety disorders. Sleep habits should be evaluated and improved to ensure optimal rest. This also promotes the restoration of normal physiological and immunologic processes that can ward off chronic illness. Dietary factors should be modified to promote diverse, balanced, and nutritional eating habits.

Increased physical activity and sustained cardiovascular exertion can impart a variety of health benefits, including relief from mood disorders. Although investigations examining the effectiveness of exercise for depression have met with mixed results, exercise can regulate appetite, improve sleep patterns, increase energy, enhance self-esteem, and promote a return to euthymic status.[75] Exercise has been shown to increase circulating concentrations of serotonin in the periphery and enhance neurogenesis in the hippocampus.[76] Other activities may also serve to relieve stress and help patients acquire insights into their emotional well-being. These pursuits can range from daily journal writing ("journaling"), to prayer, meditation, yoga, and tai chi. Classes in mindfulness-based meditation, in particular, are offered at many medical centers, and the health benefits of this approach have been demonstrated in a wide range of medical conditions including cancer, chronic pain syndromes, and human immunodeficiency virus (HIV) illness.[77] Certain herbal remedies may also be effective and are discussed in Case 83-1, Question 3.

MAJOR DEPRESSIVE DISORDER

Diagnosis

CASE 83-1

QUESTION 1: A.R. is a 25-year-old woman who presents to the student health clinic for a routine physical examination. During her visit, A.R. states, "I've been feeling pretty down lately and just want to give up." Her physical examination is unremarkable, and all laboratory tests (complete

blood count with differential, chemistry panel, and thyroid function tests) are within normal limits. A human chorionic gonadotropin test is negative. Her medical history is noncontributory, the only prescription medication she has received is an oral contraceptive (which she has taken faithfully for the past 6 months), and she denies drinking alcohol or using other recreational substances.

When asked, A.R. states that she has had increasing periods of depressed mood during the past few months and often finds herself crying in the morning for no particular reason. She reports that she has no interest in her old hobbies (playing the piano, mountain biking, gardening). She is engaged to be married in 3 months but feels that she does not deserve to be a wife. During the past 2 months, her appetite has decreased, and she has lost 15 pounds. She feels overwhelmed about all of the plans that she needs to make for her wedding ("I don't even deserve a wedding this nice") and has difficulty sleeping, often waking in the middle of the night and being unable to fall back asleep. She has no energy during the day and finds it difficult to concentrate or make decisions. This is a major concern because she is a graduate student at the local university.

On examination, A.R. is an appropriately dressed woman who appears sad but who is alert, coherent, and logical. Her affect is constricted, apprehensive, and sad. Mood is depressed, and she admits having suicidal ideation but she has no specific plans. She is oriented to person, place, and time but shows some recent memory deficits. Her intelligence is estimated to be above average. Concentration and abstractions (e.g., "don't cry over spilled milk," "a rolling stone gathers no moss") are satisfactory. She denies hearing voices or other hallucinations. She has good insight and judgment into her illness. A.R. is asked to complete the QIDS-SR$_{16}$ and is given a total score of 15 (i.e., moderate to severe symptoms).

What signs and symptoms does A.R. have that support the diagnosis of major depressive disorder?

From A.R.'s history, she appears to be exhibiting a dysphoric or depressed mood as well as anhedonia (lack of interest in hobbies or pleasurable activities). In addition, she demonstrates frequent episodes of crying, decreased appetite (with an unintentional 15-pound weight loss), poor concentration, low energy, suicidal ideation, worthlessness, and inappropriate guilt. Her mental status examination is consistent with these target symptoms, revealing a constricted, sad affect (physical manifestation of inner emotional states) and frequent crying episodes during the interview.

Based on the DSM-IV-TR criteria (summarized in Table 83-7), A.R. has major depressive disorder. During the past 2 weeks, she has consistently exhibited at least five of the associated symptoms, one of which is depression or anhedonia. It does not appear that her symptoms are the result of any medical condition, medication, thought disorder, or uncomplicated bereavement. The anhedonia and vegetative symptoms (e.g., midnocturnal insomnia, decreased appetite, weight loss) are consistent with the depressive subtype of melancholia.

Suicide Assessment

CASE 83-1, QUESTION 2: What is the risk of A.R. hurting herself? How should suicidal ideation be assessed?

Patients with major depression should always be assessed for the presence of suicidal thoughts (e.g., "Do you ever feel like giving up?", "Are you thinking about hurting yourself?"). Suicide is viewed by the depressed patient as a remedy to insurmountable problems when all other options appear hopeless. Comments made by the patients alluding to suicide (e.g., "Life is not worth living anymore," "I am leaving and may never see you again") should be taken seriously. Misunderstandings about suicidal ideation abound in the general public. Common myths include the ideas that people are more likely to commit suicide if asked about it, that people who attempt suicide are just looking for attention, or that suicide is usually attempted after a sudden traumatic event.

Several factors may place a person at greater risk for a suicide attempt. A detailed plan, for instance, suggests a serious intent and a higher risk for completed suicide. The clinician should be concerned if a change takes place in A.R.'s personality (e.g., giving away possessions, making a will, purchasing a firearm, asking about the lethal dose of medications). Other risks for suicide include living alone, having a physical illness, being unemployed, being 15 to 24 years of age or older than 65 years of age, having a history of alcohol/drug abuse, or having a family history of suicide.[64] Gender plays a role as well, with women much more likely to attempt suicide, although men are more likely to complete the act.

The management of patients who are potentially suicidal depends on the attendant risk, incorporating many of the factors just cited. For patients who are actively suicidal, hospitalization is often necessary and may be facilitated against the patient's will in high-risk settings. Other life-saving interventions include establishing close contact with the patient's family and health care provider, convincing the patient to contract for his or her safety, ensuring that firearms and other lethal means are removed from the home, and avoiding antidepressants with a narrow therapeutic index (e.g., tricyclic antidepressants [TCAs]). Depressed patients surface in any health care environment, so all clinicians

TABLE 83-7
Depressive Disorder Target Symptom Mnemonic

D	SIG	E	CAPS
Depressed mood	Sleep (insomnia or hypersomnia) Interest (loss of, including libido) Guilt	Energy loss	Concentration (loss) Appetite (loss or gain) Psychomotor (agitation or retardation) Suicide (ideation)

Adapted with permission from Kellner CH et al. Continuation electroconvulsive therapy vs. pharmacotherapy for relapse prevention in major depression: a multisite study from the consortium for research in electroconvulsive therapy (CORE). *Arch Gen Psychiatry.* 2006;63:1337.

TABLE 83-8
Complementary and Alternative Medicine Treatments for Depression

Treatment Regimen	Efficacy	Toxicity	Dosing	Drug Interactions	Other Health Benefits
St. John's wort	Monotherapy: superior to placebo, comparable to antidepressants; best studied for mild–moderate depression Augmentation: no data available	Agitation, mania, sun sensitivity	900 mg PO daily (divided)	CYP3A4 inducer; weak evidence of 5-HT syndrome	—
S-Adenosyl-L-Methionine	Monotherapy: superior to placebo, comparable to antidepressants Augmentation: superior to placebo	Nausea, skin rashes, hypoglycemia, theoretical ↑ homocysteine levels	800–1600 mg PO daily	1 probable case of 5-HT syndrome (with clomipramine)	Osteoarthritis
Omega-3-Fatty Acids	Monotherapy: limited data available Augmentation: majority of trials positive	Fishy taste, regurgitation	1–2 g PO daily (EPA + DHA)	None	↓ CV risk; ↓ risk of obstetric complications
Folate	Monotherapy: no evidence available Augmentation: limited number of studies but positive results (esp in women); Methylfolate preferred due to superior CNS penetration (?)	Well tolerated; may mask pernicious anemia	Folic acid: 200–500 mg PO daily Methylfolate: 15–50 mg PO daily	None	Other health benefits: ↓ risk of pregnancy complications; reverse folate deficiency

Adapted with permission from Freeman MP et al. Complementary and alternative medicine in major depressive disorder: the American Psychiatric Association Task Report. *J Clin Psychiatry.* 2010;71:669.
5-HT, serotonin; CNS, central nervous system; CV, cardiovascular; CYP, cytochrome P-450; DHA, docosahexaenoic acid; EPA, eicosapentaenoic acid; PO, orally.

should have an emergency hotline or crisis telephone number readily available.

A.R. is at some risk for suicide, although she does not have a detailed plan at present. She should be monitored closely during the first few weeks of therapy by friends or family members. If her suicidal ideation becomes severe, A.R. should be admitted to a facility for her own safety. Unfortunately, it is not always possible to predict whether A.R. (or any depressed patient) will attempt suicide. Even with the most conservative precautions, a small percentage of patients complete their suicide attempts.

DRUG MANAGEMENT

Drug Selection: General Considerations

CASE 83-1, QUESTION 3: A.R. is diagnosed as follows: Axis I—major depressive disorder, single episode, with melancholic features; Axis II—none; and Axis III—none. A.R. is informed that a prescription medication would be recommended for her condition at this time, but she is hesitant to 'take anything strong just to control my mood swings.' She asks if there are any herbal medicines to treat her symptoms. How should she be advised?

Many people are reluctant to consider prescription medications for depression and will often explore other options on their own, perusing shelves at their local pharmacy or surfing the Internet for potential remedies. Historically, complementary and alternative medicine (CAM) approaches have not been subjected to the same rigorous standards of clinical evaluation as drugs in development, and the efficacy and toxicity of these compounds was largely unknown. Because the FDA does not routinely monitor the constituency of CAM products, the potency and purity of available preparations are highly variable as well. In the past decade, there have been substantial efforts to improve the methodology of CAM investigations and many large randomized controlled trials have been conducted. Recently, the APA published the report of a task force formed to scrutinize CAM remedies for depression (Table 83-8). Panel members focused on four oral preparations (as well as other somatic interventions) and reported that St. John's wort and SAMe had sufficient evidence to support their efficacy as monotherapy for depression, though the authors emphasized that treatment effects were more pronounced for mild symptoms than for severe psychopathology. Omega-3 fatty acids and folic acid could not be recommended as monotherapies but several positive augmentation (i.e., adjunctive therapy) trials have been published.

In discussing treatment options with A.R., she should be reminded that she has significant functional impairments and her symptoms are best described as moderate to severe. Given the seriousness of her depressive illness, she should be advised that prescription antidepressants are the treatment of choice for her condition. If she refuses to consider this option or psychotherapy, then A.R.'s clinician should review the safety and efficacy of CAM preparations and become familiar with brand name products that can be recommended. Consumer Lab and Natural Standard are two excellent Web-based resources in this regard.

CASE 83-1, QUESTION 4: A.R. recalls reading a popular national magazine which stated that "antidepressant medications don't work better than sugar pills." How effective are FDA-approved antidepressants?

In randomized controlled trials of antidepressants, a therapeutic response is usually apparent in 60% to 70% of subjects receiving active medication (therapeutic response typically defined as a $\geq$50% decline in depression rating scales). However, approximately 30% to 40% of subjects in these same trials will have a therapeutic response when assigned to placebo treatment, and the difference in respective treatment effects will often not reach a statistical level of significance. In the media, these negative trials have been cited as evidence that prescription antidepressants "don't work" but these results are largely a function of substantial limitations in study design, and the inherent difficulties in studying an illness with high spontaneous remission rates. For example, clinical trials with antidepressants are typically only 4 to 6 weeks in duration, preventing researchers from quantifying the high relapse rates generally seen with placebo responders after this brief time period. Similarly, all subjects have considerable contact with study researchers, which effectively serves as a psychosocial intervention, further increasing treatment response rates. Another important limitation relates to the patient populations typically included in antidepressant trials. Young men, with relatively severe symptoms and minimal medical comorbidity, are often overrepresented. This research cohort is obviously not representative of the vast majority of patients receiving antidepressants under "real world" conditions.

In an effort to explore the effectiveness of prescription antidepressants in actual clinical practice, a series of investigations known as the STAR*D (Sequenced Treatment Alternatives to Relieve Depression) trials have been conducted in recent years. The original multisite investigation enrolled nearly 3,000 patients from primary care clinics and mental health centers across the United States in an effort to determine the effectiveness of first-line treatments, as well as alternative agents and augmentation strategies.[78] All eligible patients received citalopram (average dose, 41.8 mg daily), and the results suggested that response rates are closer to 50%, and remission is achieved in 30% of patients treated under "real world" conditions.

CASE 83-1, QUESTION 5: A.R. ultimately agrees to a therapeutic trial of a prescription antidepressant. What are the drug options available for A.R.'s depressive symptoms? What considerations should be made when selecting antidepressant therapy?

At present, 26 medications have received FDA approval in the United States for the treatment of depression. They can be conveniently grouped into six categories:

1. SSRIs
2. Serotonin norepinephrine reuptake inhibitors (SNRIs)
3. Norepinephrine reuptake inhibitors (NRIs)
4. TCAs
5. Monoamine oxidase inhibitors (MAOIs)
6. Miscellaneous (e.g., trazodone, mirtazapine, atypical antipsychotics)

All available antidepressants are equally effective in the general depressed patient population, and all appear to have the same delayed onset of therapeutic effects. Because the response rates for all currently available antidepressants are comparable, other important considerations should influence decision-making (Tables 83-9 to 83-12). The first factor to consider is the patient's history of response to antidepressant drug therapy. If this history is unavailable (or the patient has never received an antidepressant before), the clinician should inquire about family history. If a first-degree relative had a successful course of antidepressant treatment with minimal adverse effects, that specific medication (or another from the same antidepressant class) would be a prudent choice for initial therapy.

The potential impact of an antidepressant on concurrent medical conditions or disease states is often considered next. For example, certain antidepressants (e.g., TCA, paroxetine, mirtazapine) are associated with significant weight gain and would not be desirable choices for obese patients. Similarly, bupropion should be avoided in patients with a history of seizures, and venlafaxine may not be ideal for patients with hypertension.

TABLE 83-9
Factors to Consider in Selecting an Antidepressant

- History of prior response (personal or family member)
- Safety in overdose
- Adverse effect profiles
- Patient age
- Concurrent medical/psychiatric conditions
- Concurrent medications (e.g., potential for drug interactions)
- Convenience (e.g., minimal titration, once-daily dosing)
- Cost
- Patient preference

Many clinicians select an antidepressant by matching the patient's presenting symptoms to the side-effect profile of antidepressant medications. For example, if a depressed patient is sleeping and eating excessively, and possesses little energy or motivation, the clinician may choose an agent that will address these baseline symptoms, perhaps through the enhancement of noradrenergic transmission (e.g., bupropion). Patients with substantial anxiety or irritability may benefit preferentially from antidepressants that facilitate serotonergic transmission (e.g., SSRI) because nearly 50% of patients with major depression are believed to be suffering from a concurrent anxiety disorder. Conversely, some clinicians hold the belief that an effective antidepressant will relieve all target symptoms eventually, regardless of the side effect profile. Nonetheless, tailoring antidepressant medications to a patient's presentation is a common practice that may minimize the initial side-effect burden and promote adherence.

Other important patient-specific factors to consider in the selection of an agent include safety in overdose, potential for drug interactions, ease of administration (once daily vs. divided doses), necessity for dose titration, cost, and patient preference.

Because A.R. is a student, the clinician may want to select an antidepressant that has minimal effects on alertness or cognitive function, such as an SSRI or bupropion. Of these two options, an SSRI may be preferred for A.R. because she is experiencing a significant decrease in appetite and insomnia, which may be exacerbated by bupropion.

Response Rates of Target Symptoms

CASE 83-1, QUESTION 6: A.R. is given a prescription for sertraline 50-mg tablets. She is instructed to take a half tablet (25 mg) for the first week and increase to a whole tablet daily thereafter. She is also asked to return to the clinic in 4 weeks for follow-up. How soon should A.R.'s target symptoms begin to resolve?

A similar delayed pattern of therapeutic response has been observed with all antidepressant medications. Traditionally, patients have been informed that approximately 4 to 6 weeks must elapse before they will experience any therapeutic benefit from medication. However, researchers in the field consider this a conservative estimate, gleaned from standard drug efficacy studies ill-suited to answer this question.[79] In such studies, patients often begin to show signs of clinical response during the first 1 or 2 weeks of active treatment, but because the difference from placebo is assessed every 7 days and will not ordinarily achieve statistical significance until the third or fourth week, these early response patterns are misinterpreted to suggest that it may take a month or more for patients to improve. Some experts have

TABLE 83-10
Pharmacology of Antidepressant Medications

Medication	Serotonin	Norepinephrine	Dopamine	Bioavailability (Oral)	Protein Binding	Half-Life (hours) (Active Metabolite)
Selective Serotonin Reuptake Inhibitors						
Fluoxetine	++++	0/+	0	80%	95%	24–72 (146)
Sertraline	++++	0/+	+	>44%	95%	26 (66)
Paroxetine	++++	+	0	64%	99%	24
Citalopram	++++	0	0	80%	<80%	33
Escitalopram	++++	0	0	80%	56%	27–32
Serotonin Norepinephrine Reuptake Inhibitors						
Venlafaxine	++++	+++	0	92%	25%–29%	4 (10)
Desvenlafaxine	+++	+++	0	80%	30%	11 (0)
Duloxetine	++++	++++	0	50%	>90%	12 (8–17)
Norepinephrine Reuptake Inhibitors						
Bupropion	0/+	+	+	>90%	85%	10–21
Tricyclic Antidepressants						
Desipramine	+	++++	0/+	51%	90%	12–28
Nortriptyline	++	+++	0	46%–56%	92%	18–56
Amitriptyline	++++	++++	0	37%–49%	95%	9–46 (18–56)
Imipramine	+++	++	0/+	19%–35%	95%	6–28 (12–28)
Doxepin	+++	+	0	17%–37%	68%–85%	11–23
Others						
Mirtazapine	+++	++++	0	50%	85%	20–40

0, negligible; +, very low; ++, low; +++, moderate; ++++, high.

TABLE 83-11
Adverse Effects of Antidepressant Medications

Medication	Sedation	Agitation/Insomnia	Anticholinergic Effects	Orthostasis	GI Effects (Nausea/Diarrhea)	Sexual Dysfunction	Weight Gain
Selective Serotonin Reuptake Inhibitors							
Fluoxetine	+	++++	0/+	0/+	++++	++++	+
Sertraline	+	+++	0/+	0	+++	+++	+
Paroxetine	+++	++	++	0	+++	++++	+++
Citalopram	++	++	0/+	0	+++	+++	+
Escitalopram	+	++	0/+	0	+++	+++	+
Serotonin Norepinephrine Reuptake Inhibitors							
Venlafaxine (Effexor)	++	++	+	0	+++	+++	+
Desvenlafaxine (Pristiq)	++	++	+	+	+++	++	0/+
Duloxetine (Cymbalta)	++	++	+	0	+++	++	0/+
Norepinephrine Reuptake Inhibitors							
Bupropion (Wellbutrin)	0	+++	+	0	+	0/+	0
Tricyclic Antidepressants							
Desipramine (Norpramin)	++	+	++	+++	0/+	+	++
Nortriptyline (Pamelor)	++	+	++	++	0/+	+	++
Amitriptyline (Elavil)	++++	0/+	++++	++++	0/+	++	+++
Imipramine (Tofranil)	+++	0/+	+++	++++	0/+	++	++
Doxepin (Sinequan)	++++	0/+	++++	++++	0/+	++	++
Others							
Mirtazapine (Remeron)	++++	0	++	0/+	+	0/+	+++

0, negligible; +, very low; ++, low; +++, moderate; ++++, high.

TABLE 83-12
Dosage Ranges and Costs of Commonly Prescribed Antidepressant Medications

Medication	Brand Name	Starting Dose (mg/day)	Maximum Dosage (mg/day)	Usual Dosage (mg/day)	Relative Cost[a]
Selective Serotonin Reuptake Inhibitors					
Fluoxetine	Prozac	10	80	10–20 mg daily	$[b]
Sertraline	Zoloft	25	200	50 mg daily	$[b]
Paroxetine	Paxil	10	50	10–20 mg daily	$[b]
Citalopram	Celexa	10	60	20 mg daily	$$[b]
Escitalopram	Lexapro	5	20	10 mg daily	$$$$
Serotonin Norepinephrine Reuptake Inhibitors					
Venlafaxine	Effexor XR	37.5	225	150 mg daily	$$$$
Desvenlafaxine	Pristiq	50	50	50 mg daily	$$$$
Duloxetine	Cymbalta	30	120	60 mg daily	$$$$
Norepinephrine Reuptake Inhibitors					
Bupropion	Wellbutrin SR	150	400	150 mg BID	$$$[b]
Bupropion	Wellbutrin XL	150	450	300 daily	$$$$[b]
Tricyclic Antidepressants					
Desipramine	Norpramin	25	300	200 mg half-strength	$
Nortriptyline	Pamelor	10–25	150	100 mg half-strength	$
Others					
Mirtazapine	Remeron	15	45	15–30 mg half-strength	$$[b]

[a] Based on average wholesale prices for usual therapeutic doses (April 2011).
[b] Price reflects cost of generic formulation.
$ = $0–25/month; $$ = $25–50/month; $$$ = $50–100/month; $$$$ = more than $100/month.
BID, twice a day; TID, three times a day.

contended, in fact, that trials uniquely designed to investigate the onset of therapeutic effect will conclusively show that patients exhibit substantial improvement during the first 2 weeks of treatment, and maximum improvement may not be evident for 4 weeks or more.[80] The pattern of patient response can also be generalized, with neurovegetative symptoms often the first to subside (e.g., altered sleep or appetite, decreased energy, excessive worrying and irritability). Cognitive symptoms are slower to respond, and 3 to 4 weeks or more may elapse before improvements are evident. These symptoms include excessive guilt or pessimism, poor concentration, hopelessness or sadness, and decreased libido.

A.R. should be counseled concerning this anticipated delay in therapeutic response and advised that optimal improvement may take at least 4 weeks. If she is not aware of this time frame, she may stop the medication prematurely, prolonging her distress and further delaying the recovery process.

Selective Serotonin Reuptake Inhibitors

ADVERSE EFFECTS

CASE 83-1, QUESTION 7: What are the most common side effects reported with SSRIs, and how should they be managed?

Although it is not accurate to say that SSRIs (or SNRIs) cause fewer side effects than TCAs, the adverse effects associated with these newer antidepressant classes are generally milder and less likely to lead to discontinuation.[81] Generally, SSRIs (and SNRIs) are less likely to exacerbate comorbid illnesses than TCAs. For this reason, SSRIs are often a better choice in medically complex patients.

As clinical experience accumulates with the SSRI (and SNRI) agents, a distinct side effect profile has emerged, consisting of gastrointestinal (GI) complaints, CNS disturbances, and sexual dysfunction. All of these medications may induce nausea, but this tends to be a transient effect that diminishes after the first week of treatment. Typically, SSRI-induced nausea occurs 1 to 2 hours after oral administration and is presumed to reflect a local irritant effect. For this reason, patients should always be advised to take the medication after a meal or snack, particularly during the first week of therapy. Nausea with SSRIs may also be mediated centrally through the stimulation of certain serotonin receptors (5-HT_{3C}) that activate the chemoreceptor trigger zone.[82] Nausea triggered by this mechanism has a more delayed onset, corresponding to the accumulation of medication until steady-state dynamics are reached, and often persists throughout the dosing interval. Patients who experience nausea mediated by CNS stimulation may benefit from dosage reduction or drug discontinuation.

SSRIs may also have transient and bothersome effects on bowel function. Unlike nausea, there does appear to be clinically relevant differences among SSRIs in this regard. Sertraline, fluoxetine, and citalopram have been associated with a 15% to 20% incidence of diarrhea.[83] Fortunately, the diarrhea often remits after 1 week of continued therapy and rarely requires an interruption of treatment. In contrast, paroxetine possesses a mild affinity for blocking muscarinic cholinergic receptors that can manifest as constipation, dry mouth, or urinary hesitancy. Thus, paroxetine use is often discouraged in patients with preexisting constipation or those receiving other medications with anticholinergic potential.

SSRIs can have myriad effects on the CNS, with disturbances in sleep being a primary concern. SSRIs can have significant but highly variable effects on sleep architecture. In sleep studies,

SSRIs have been shown to increase sleep latency and decrease sleep efficiency, often resulting in morning sleepiness or malaise. Many patients also notice that their dreams become more vivid and memorable, which may be an undesirable experience. REM stage sleep may be prolonged, resulting in less fitful sleep.[84] It should be emphasized, however, that sleep may eventually improve once the antidepressant properties of the medications are apparent and baseline depressive symptoms are relieved (e.g., midnocturnal insomnia).

Compared with older antidepressants, SSRIs are generally considered to be less sedating compounds, and there does appear to be a hierarchy among the individual agents. Fluoxetine, for example, is widely regarded as the most activating of the SSRIs, a property that may be desirable in anergic patients or undesirable in those who are agitated or have difficulty falling asleep.[85] For this reason, fluoxetine is usually administered in the morning after breakfast. However, it should be noted that fluoxetine is not necessarily activating for all patients. In fact, some find it to be slightly sedating or numbing. Daytime drowsiness can be experienced with fluoxetine, perhaps as a result of light, restless sleep. Sertraline, escitalopram, and citalopram have also been associated with comparatively more insomnia than sedation, but they are generally considered to be less activating than fluoxetine. The effects of paroxetine appear to be somewhat mixed, with approximately equal proportions of patients complaining of sedation and insomnia, respectively.

SSRIs have been associated with extrapyramidal side (EPS) effects, consisting of akathisia, dystonias, and parkinsonian symptoms that are qualitatively identical to those commonly seen with high-potency antipsychotics. Fortunately, the incidence of EPS effects is much lower than with antipsychotic agents.[86] Although EPS reactions have been documented with all SSRIs, most case reports have featured paroxetine. Because paroxetine has the highest affinity for serotonin receptors, this may lend support to the theory that these EPS effects are mediated through the indirect influence of serotonergic neurons on dopaminergic activity. In certain areas of the brain, serotonin and dopamine appear to have an inverse relationship, whereby central stimulation of serotonin receptors results in a net decline in dopaminergic transmission. Management of EPS effects induced by SSRI is identical with that of those precipitated by antipsychotics. Dystonias and parkinsonian side effects can be treated with anticholinergic agents and subsequent SSRI dosage reduction. Akathisia usually responds to a reduction in SSRI dosage and/or administration of low-dose β-blockers.

The deleterious effects of SSRI on sexual function were underappreciated in early clinical trials, but it is now widely recognized that these adverse effects are very common and potentially profound consequences of SSRI treatment that can often lead to medication nonadherence.[87] The reported incidence of sexual dysfunction ranges from 1.9% to 75%, reflecting the diversity of methods used for adverse event detection.[88,89] The actual incidence of SSRI-induced sexual dysfunction is approximately 30% to 50%, and it appears to be slightly more common in men, but the severity may be worse in women. Delayed orgasm is the most common sexual complaint attributed to SSRIs or SNRIs, and should be distinguished from decreases in desire or libido, which are considered to be an aspect of the psychopathology of depression itself. This iatrogenic effect on orgasms has actually been used to clinical advantage in men reporting premature ejaculation, but most patients find it undesirable.[90] All SSRIs are commonly implicated with sexual dysfunction, but there are several indirect lines of evidence suggesting that paroxetine and fluoxetine are the worst in this regard.[91,92] It also appears that this is a dose-dependent phenomenon, which may respond favorably to a decrease in daily dosage. Unlike the GI and CNS side effects reported with SSRIs, sexual dysfunction is not usually a transient adverse effect and must be addressed by clinicians if patients are to complete a full course of therapy.

CASE 83-1, QUESTION 8: Are there any other adverse effects of SSRIs about which A.R. should be aware?

In addition to GI, CNS, and sexual side effects, a variety of other, less-common adverse sequelae may jeopardize treatment. Dry mouth and headache occur with many antidepressants, and, although these somatic complaints are prevalent in the general population, placebo-adjusted rates suggest that SSRIs may induce this phenomenon.[83] Increased sweating has also been reported with SSRIs and can be particularly uncomfortable or embarrassing.[93] Dosage reduction may help relieve this adverse effect, and alpha-blockers (e.g., terazosin, prazosin) and anticholinergic antidotes have been used as well (e.g., benztropine or low-dose TCA at bedtime).[94,95] Bruxism, or teeth grinding, can also be an unfortunate consequence of SSRI treatment, leading to chipped or cracked teeth and generally poor dentition.[96] Often, patients may not be aware of this nocturnal effect and complain merely of a dull, persistent headache during the morning hours. This, too, may be a dose-dependent side effect of all SSRIs, and several antidotes have been prescribed (e.g., buspirone, benzodiazepines, gabapentin).[97,98] In small retrospective studies and several case reports, SSRIs have been linked to dilutional hyponatremia or syndrome of inappropriate antidiuretic hormone.[99,100] All SSRIs (and venlafaxine) have been associated with this phenomenon, and elderly patients appear to be uniquely at risk.

The long-term effects of SSRIs on body weight are variable and difficult to predict. It is worthwhile to recall that decreased appetite is one of the most common depressive symptoms and that a small weight gain after an antidepressant course may actually be viewed as a therapeutic effect of successful treatment. Conversely, early reports of weight loss with fluoxetine generated much optimism for the use of SSRIs in obesity, but longitudinal studies found this to be a brief, transient phenomenon.[101] All SSRIs have been reported to cause significant weight gain in long-term use, but it is a relatively rare phenomenon believed to be mediated by genetic markers that have not been conclusively identified. The exception is paroxetine, which has been implicated much more often than other SSRIs as a cause of weight gain. One long-term randomized controlled trial (RCT) compared the effects of fluoxetine, sertraline, and paroxetine on total body weight.[102] After 7 months of SSRI use, 25% of the patients receiving paroxetine gained a clinically significant amount of weight (defined as a >7% increase in total body weight) compared with 7% with fluoxetine and 4% with sertraline. Long-term studies with citalopram and escitalopram suggest that 3% to 5% of patients will experience a significant weight gain. Because weight gain may occur with any SSRI, it is best to monitor weight changes closely during long-term treatment and respond accordingly.

Epidemiological studies have also linked SSRIs and SNRIs with an increased risk for severe upper GI hemorrhage, though the absolute risk has been somewhat difficult to ascertain.[103] Recent trials suggest that the risk is modest but can be increased significantly by concurrent alcohol use or ingestion of NSAIDs.[104,105] The mechanism for SSRI-induced GI hemorrhage has been attributed to effects on decreasing platelet activation and aggregation. SSRIs and SNRIs should be avoided in patients with active GI bleeds, and the concurrent use of high-dose NSAID should be discouraged.

CASE 83-1, QUESTION 9: A.R. calls the clinic 2 weeks after her initial visit requesting a dosage increase. She reports that she has been taking 50 mg of sertraline every morning for the past week and has noticed considerable improvement in her sleep, appetite, and outlook ("Little things don't bother me so much anymore"), but believes she could be doing better. She still feels as though her mood and concentration could improve, and admits that she has yet to resume her exercise regimen ("I still don't have the energy"). She asks you if she could increase her dosage. What changes would you make to her antidepressant regimen at this time?

It is very important to establish realistic expectations for treatment with antidepressants from the beginning of therapy. Patients should be informed of the anticipated course of treatment and that the onset of side effects usually precedes that of therapeutic effects. Also, patients should be advised that, although antidepressants may relieve acute depressive symptoms and prevent relapse, they do not abolish environmental stressors, increase self-esteem, or reverse negative perceptions and emotions.

Dosing and prescribing patterns with SSRIs have changed since the first SSRI (fluoxetine) was introduced in the United States in 1988. In general, clinicians have come to realize that "one size fits all" prescribing philosophies and early aggressive dosing practices were largely unnecessary and often compromised medication adherence. Providers have found that lower dosages of SSRIs often suffice (e.g., 10 mg/day of fluoxetine, paroxetine, or citalopram) if patients are informed of the delayed onset of therapeutic effects and are closely monitored for tolerance and response. Because premarketing fixed-dose studies were rarely conducted with these lower dosages, it is difficult to endorse this practice empirically. However, there is evidence that daily doses as small as 5 mg of fluoxetine are more effective than placebo and comparable to 20 mg in a significant segment of the depressed populace.[106]

For A.R., many factors must be considered before increasing her dosage. She has been receiving the medication for only 2 weeks (25 mg daily for 1 week, 50 mg daily thereafter), and the improvement she is exhibiting in neurovegetative symptoms may indicate that resolution of cognitive symptoms is soon to follow. She should be reminded that the optimal effects of antidepressants may not be evident for 4 to 6 weeks. Furthermore, it is possible that the lack of improvement in her concentration and energy may be largely situational as the day of her wedding approaches. An increase in dosage at this time would not necessarily address these environmental factors and may serve only to increase the side-effect burden. Therefore, a reasonable recommendation would be to continue with the current daily dose of 50 mg and to re-evaluate the medication's effects when she returns to clinic in 2 weeks.

CASE 83-1, QUESTION 10: After 4 weeks of treatment with sertraline, A.R. is seen in the clinic and asked about side effects she has experienced. She recalls some mild nausea during the first week of treatment but continued to take the medication after breakfast (as directed) and noticed that this effect went away after approximately 3 or 4 days of therapy. She denies diarrhea, insomnia, or headache. Before leaving, she reluctantly admits that the only side effect she is currently experiencing is sexual ("I love my fiancé, but sex isn't as enjoyable anymore"). How should A.R.'s sexual side effect be managed?

TABLE 83-13
Management of SSRI-Induced Sexual Dysfunction

- Patience (may improve after 2–4 weeks)
- Reduced dosage (if possible)
- Drug holidays (sertraline, paroxetine, citalopram, escitalopram only)
- Antidotes
  - Bupropion SR 150 mg daily to BID
  - Sildenafil 50–100 mg daily PRN
  - Mirtazapine 7.5–15 mg at bedtime
  - Cyproheptadine 4–12 mg PRN (1 hour prior)
  - Methylphenidate 2.5–5.0 mg daily
  - Others: yohimbine, amantadine, buspirone, gingko
- Change of antidepressants (e.g., bupropion, mirtazapine)

BID, twice a day; PRN, as needed.

The detection and proper management of SSRI-induced sexual dysfunction can be one of the most important factors in ensuring medication adherence (Table 83-13). Clinicians may be uncomfortable asking patients about their sexual activities and satisfaction, but the high incidence of this side effect (and low likelihood of patients volunteering this information) necessitates a thoughtful and direct approach. Some patients acknowledge sexual dysfunction but decide that improvements in mood and overall health outweigh limitations in sexual performance; however, others simply stop the medication if the side effect is never addressed.

It may be wise to advise patients that sexual function may change over time, depending on the type and etiology of sexual dysfunction experienced. Depression itself is associated with a decreased libido in 70% to 90% of untreated patients.[107] This symptom will most likely subside with a successful course of antidepressant treatment. Delayed ejaculation or anorgasmia, however, may be caused by SSRIs and SNRIs, often persisting and jeopardizing treatment. Because A.R. has been taking the medication faithfully for the first 4 weeks and the time course is consistent with the SSRI effects, it is unlikely that the condition will spontaneously remit, and some action must be taken.

Ordinarily, one of the first options in managing sexual dysfunction is to reduce the dosage, but this may precipitate a recrudescence of the original depressive symptoms in some patients. In A.R.'s case, she is taking a relatively low therapeutic dosage of sertraline, and a further decrease may be risky. An alternative solution for A.R.'s problem may be to recommend drug holidays. Small open-label studies with short-acting SSRIs (e.g., sertraline, paroxetine) suggested that if patients skipped their doses on Friday and Saturday, sexual function would return to normal on the weekends.[108,109] Although this method was reported to be successful, it may also promote nonadherence with medication and lead to increased risk of relapse or withdrawal symptoms.

If the patient has had a therapeutic response to the antidepressant, the next option in this setting is to consider antidotes to SSRI-induced sexual dysfunction, and the most popular treatment at present is bupropion. Clinical reports and controlled investigations suggest that the addition of this antidepressant can be helpful for restoring sexual desire and may relieve delayed orgasm or anorgasmia in approximately 50% of patients.[110–112] This therapeutic effect has been demonstrated in depressed and nondepressed patients alike. A common dosing technique is to start with 150 mg of bupropion daily. If unsuccessful, the dose can be increased to 150 mg of bupropion sustained release (SR) twice daily after several days (or 300 mg of the extended release [XL] preparation). The mechanisms of SSRI-induced sexual dysfunction, and bupropion relief, are not well understood. Some researchers have theorized that delayed ejaculation or orgasm is mediated by a stimulation of postsynaptic 5-HT_2 or 5-HT_3 receptors, whereas others suggest that the indirect effects of SSRIs on dopamine may be involved.[113] Additional theories point to the inhibitory effects of SSRIs on prolactin or nitric oxide synthetase.[113]

Other remedies have been prescribed for SSRI-induced sexual dysfunction. A large randomized, controlled trial examined the impact of sildenafil on male patients suffering from this side effect.[114] Overall, 54% of patients randomly assigned to sildenafil found it be effective compared with a 4% response rate with placebo. Open-label trials of sildenafil in women experiencing SSRI-induced anorgasmia have also reported improvements, suggesting that controlled trials in this population are warranted.

Cyproheptadine, amantadine, buspirone, and yohimbine also have been used successfully to reverse delayed ejaculation or decreased libido, but the evidence for efficacy is limited.[115–117] One small double-blind study compared the effects of amantadine with buspirone or placebo among depressed patients experiencing sexual dysfunction on antidepressants.[118] All three study treatments improved sexual dysfunction to a comparable extent, and the only statistically significant finding was related to an increase in energy reported among patients receiving amantadine (vs. placebo). An open-label trial of Ginkgo biloba in men and women with sexual dysfunction reported very high success rates, but mixed results have been reported in clinical practice.[119] Mirtazapine is capable of blocking postsynaptic 5-HT_2 receptors and theoretically may relieve ejaculatory difficulties, but controlled trials have not been conducted. Finally, stimulants such as methylphenidate or dextroamphetamine may increase libido in SSRI-treated patients, but the potential for dependence and abuse discourages their routine administration.[120]

The onset of A.R.'s sexual dysfunction is consistent with the introduction of sertraline, and it appears, at this time, that her situation will not improve if she continues to take the SSRI. Because she is exhibiting some evidence of a therapeutic response, one would prefer to continue sertraline and discuss possible antidotes for sexual dysfunction with her (e.g., bupropion). A.R. states that she would prefer not to start another prescription medication to treat her problem, but she will "think about it."

DURATION OF TREATMENT

CASE 83-1, QUESTION 11: At 6 weeks, A.R. reports that her depressive symptoms are effectively in remission ("I feel like I have my old life back!"). Her energy has improved, and she is doing well in her studies and looks forward, once again, to her wedding day. How long should A.R. continue taking the antidepressant?

According to the guidelines issued by the Agency for Health Research and Quality, antidepressant treatment can be broken down into three stages (Table 83-14).[121] The first stage, acute treatment, lasts approximately 12 weeks; during this time, the clinician attempts to resolve the presenting symptoms and induce remission. The second stage is commonly called continuation treatment because the patient continues to receive the same antidepressant regimen that induced the initial treatment response, and the clinician attempts to keep the acute symptoms in remission. The duration of continuation treatment is variable (4–9 months after initial treatment or response), but it is recommended that all patients suffering from major depression complete these first two stages. Therefore, the minimum duration of treatment is 7 months. Alternatively, others have advocated that the minimum duration of treatment should be for 6 months after the complete resolution of symptoms.

TABLE 83-14
Duration of Antidepressant Treatment

Acute treatment phase:	3 months
Continuation treatment phase:	4–9 months
Maintenance treatment phase:	Variable

- Acute and continuation treatment recommended for all patients with major depressive disorder (i.e., minimal duration of treatment = 7 months)
- Decision to prescribe maintenance treatment is based on the following:
  - Number of previous episodes
  - Severity of previous episodes
  - Family history of depression
  - Patient age (worse prognosis if elderly)
  - Response to antidepressant
  - Persistence of environmental stressors
- Indefinite maintenance treatment is recommended if any one of the following criteria are met:
  1. Three or more previous episodes (regardless of age)
  2. Two or more previous episodes and age older than 50 years
  3. One or more and age older than 60 years

The third stage of treatment, maintenance treatment or prophylaxis, is not indicated for all patients, and the necessity of continuing medication beyond the first 6 to 7 months depends on many patient-specific factors. One must consider the number of previous episodes, family history of depression, patient's age, severity of presenting symptoms, response to therapy, and persistence or anticipation of environmental stressors. There are specific populations for whom indefinite pharmacologic treatment is advocated: (a) individuals with three or more previous episodes of major depression, (b) individuals older than 50 years with two or more previous episodes, and (c) individuals older than 60 years with one or more previous episodes.[121] Many experts believe that pharmacotherapy should also be continued indefinitely in all elderly people (older than 65 years) suffering from major depression, but research evidence to conclusively support this recommendation is currently lacking.[122]

Because A.R. is exhibiting a full therapeutic response to sertraline, the recommendation would be for her to continue with the effective dosage (50 mg/day) for at least 7 consecutive months. At the end of this time frame, the clinician should review with the patient those considerations that enter into the decision to continue treatment. Ultimately, the decision to continue antidepressant medications is left to the patient's judgment, and he or she should be well informed of the potential consequences of stopping treatment.

In the future, if A.R. decides to discontinue her antidepressant, she should be advised of potential withdrawal symptoms (Table 83-15). Abrupt discontinuation of chronic SSRI treatment (e.g., treatment >2 months) has been associated with dizziness, headache, anxiety, flulike symptoms, and paresthesias.[123] The onset of these symptoms is generally within 48 to 72 hours of stopping treatment, and effects may persist for at least 1 week. Withdrawal symptoms generally are mild and self-limiting but can be uncomfortable and alarming. Because of their relatively short half-life (and absence of long-acting metabolites), paroxetine, fluvoxamine, and venlafaxine have been associated with a more profound withdrawal presentation than other SSRIs and SNRIs. Due to its long-half life (and that of its active metabolite), fluoxetine has not been commonly associated with withdrawal symptoms. Nonetheless, it is advisable to taper slowly off all antidepressant medications after an extended treatment course to decrease the risk of withdrawal and subsequent relapse.[124]

TABLE 83-16
Drug Interactions of the Cytochrome P-450 System

Relative Rank	CYP1A2	CYP2C9/19	CYP2D6	CYP3A4
Offending Agent (inhibits enzyme)				
High	Fluvoxamine	*CYP2C9* Fluoxetine Fluvoxamine *CYP2C19* Fluvoxamine	Paroxetine Fluoxetine Duloxetine Bupropion	Fluoxetine (norfluoxetine) Fluvoxamine
Moderate	Fluoxetine Paroxetine	*CYP2C19* Fluoxetine Sertraline	Citalopram Escitalopram Sertraline	
Low	Citalopram Escitalopram Sertraline Venlafaxine Duloxetine Bupropion	*CYP2C9/19* Citalopram Escitalopram Paroxetine Sertraline Venlafaxine	Venlafaxine Mirtazapine	Citalopram Escitalopram Paroxetine Sertraline Venlafaxine Desvenlafaxine Duloxetine
Other Inhibitors				
	Quinolones (ciprofloxacin, enoxacin, etc.)	Modafinil (2C9, 2C19)	Fenfluramine	Macrolides (erythromycin, clarithromycin)
	Macrolides (erythromycin, clarithromycin)	Cimetidine (2C19)	Yohimbine	Cimetidine
	Grapefruit juice	Omeprazole (2C19) Imidazoles (2C9, 2C19) (ketoconazole, fluconazole)	Methadone Quinidine Celecoxib	CCB (verapamil, diltiazem) Imidazoles (ketoconazole, fluconazole) Protease inhibitors Grapefruit juice
Other Inducers				
	Cigarettes Caffeine St. John's wort	St. John's wort	Modafinil Phenytoin and phenobarbital Carbamazepine Rifampin Prednisone Testosterone	St. John's wort
Affected Agent (increased concentration)				
	TCA-tertiary amines (imipramine, amitriptyline)	*CYP2C9*	TCA-secondary amines (desipramine, nortriptyline)	Fluoxetine
	Phenothiazines (chlorpromazine)	Phenytoin	Fluoxetine	Sertraline
	Thiothixene Haloperidol Clozapine Olanzapine Caffeine	Tolbutamide Warfarin NSAIDs *CYP2C19* TCA-tertiary amines (imipramine, amitriptyline)	Paroxetine Venlafaxine Duloxetine Amphetamines Atomoxetine	Venlafaxine Modafinil Quetiapine Ziprasidone Aripiprazole
	Theophylline Propranolol	Citalopram Barbiturates	Risperidone Donepezil	Buspirone Benzodiazepines (triazolam, alprazolam)
	Tacrine	Propranolol Omeprazole	Codeine Hydrocodone Tramadol Dextromethorphan Chlorpheniramine β-blockers (propranolol, metoprolol)	Zolpidem Carbamazepine Donepezil CCB (verapamil, diltiazem, nifedipine) Sex hormones (estrogen) Corticosteroids Statins (lovastatin, simvastatin) Protease inhibitors Sildenafil

CCB, calcium-channel blockers; NSAIDs, nonsteroidal anti-inflammatory drugs; TCA, tricyclic antidepressant.

TABLE 83-17
Medications Associated with Serotonin Syndrome

Most Commonly Associated[a]
Monoamine oxidase inhibitors (selegiline, phenelzine, tranylcypromine)
Commonly Associated[a]
SSRI (all)
SNRI (all)
Clomipramine
Sibutramine
Occasionally Associated[a]
Tramadol
Meperidine
Linezolid
Dextromethorphan (high dose)

[a] The combination of any two medications from these categories should be strongly discouraged.

more drugs that enhance serotonin transmission[145] (Table 83-17). The syndrome includes a constellation of symptoms, including anxiety, shivering, diaphoresis, tremor, hyperreflexia, and autonomic instability (increased/decreased blood pressure and pulse rate).[146] Fatalities have been attributed to malignant hyperthermia.

With mild cases of serotonin syndrome, the symptoms ordinarily resolve 24 to 48 hours after the serotonergic agents have been discontinued. Supportive treatment is usually not necessary. For more severe reactions, various serotonergic antagonists, such as cyproheptadine, methysergide, and propranolol, have been used.[147–149] Dantrolene has been administered successfully to manage hyperthermia.[150]

Most case reports of serotonin syndrome (and most fatalities) have occurred with a combination of an MAOI and an SSRI, which is now considered an absolute contraindication. Other case reports involve the combination of an MAOI (or SSRI) with tryptophan, meperidine, SNRI, tricyclics, dextromethorphan, linezolid, and tramadol (Table 83-17).[145] One case of serotonin syndrome was reportedly induced by the combination of clomipramine with S-adenosylmethionine.[151] Serotonin syndrome has also been reported with concurrent administration of multiple SSRIs. Theoretically, the combination of an SSRI with St. John's wort may also precipitate this pharmacodynamic interaction, but more recent evidence has suggested that the MAOI properties of the herbal preparation are minimal with therapeutic doses. Nonetheless, a case series of five older patients who exhibited symptoms reminiscent of serotonin syndrome has appeared in the literature, and, given the degree of uncertainty that persists, this combination of antidepressant agents is best avoided.[152] The safety of combining an SSRI with certain migraine medications (e.g., sumatriptan) has not been elucidated, and clinicians are advised to avoid this combination if possible as well.

The combination of a phenylpiperazine (e.g., trazodone) with an SSRI may pose some concern because both classes of antidepressants augment serotonin activity in the CNS. Trazodone has been associated with serotonin syndrome in two incidences, one involving the coadministration of buspirone and the other associated with a concomitant MAOI.[146] However, in practice, trazodone has been commonly prescribed to patients receiving an SSRI for the treatment of insomnia, and no confirmed cases of serotonin syndrome have surfaced in the medical literature.[153]

Treatment-Resistant Depression

CASE 83-2

QUESTION 1: F.H. is a 55-year-old postmenopausal woman who presents to the women's health clinic after having suffered from multiple depressive episodes for the past 25 years. She reports that she has been hospitalized on three different occasions. Although F.H. is unable to recall details of any specific antidepressant trials, her prescription record reveals treatment with imipramine (100 mg/day), nortriptyline (75 mg/day), diazepam (10 mg/day), and fluoxetine (20 mg/day for the past 8 weeks). Eventually, she recalls that imipramine made her "dizzy and left a strange taste in my mouth" and that diazepam made her "even more depressed." She says that the fluoxetine may be "helping a little bit but I feel so jumpy and irritable that no one can stand me." F.H. has grown rather despondent over her situation ("I almost feel like giving up"). What would be the next reasonable step for managing F.H.'s depressive illness?

Pooled results of clinical trials suggest that the majority of patients with major depression receiving an adequate trial of any antidepressant will have a therapeutic response, traditionally defined as at least a 50% reduction in depressive symptoms. However, for a patient who is severely depressed, a 50% reduction in symptoms still leaves him or her with significant psychopathology and associated disability. Consequently, there has been a strong movement in recent years to consider full remission as the preferred therapeutic end point.[154] The recent STAR*D trials showed that after four stages of treatment (medication or psychotherapy), 33% of patients fail to reach remission.[155] In addition, with each course of antidepressants, people were less likely to achieve remission. One longitudinal investigation found that patients with residual symptoms were three times more likely to suffer relapse during the 12 months after treatment than those who had remitted.[156] Not surprisingly, patients with treatment-resistant depression have 40% higher direct medical costs than those without treatment-resistant depression, mainly due to medication and outpatient care costs.[157] Although remission can be generally defined as the virtual absence of residual depressive symptoms, it can also be quantified with a corresponding threshold value on a depression rating scale (e.g., QIDS <6; 17-item HAM-D <7).[154] The emphasis on achieving remission is to make patients feel well and not merely better, and providers must undertake a thorough, rational, and perhaps aggressive approach to optimize treatment and achieve this goal.

For F.H., the first step would be to confirm her diagnosis and rule out potential medical explanations for her distress. Iatrogenic causes should also be explored, such as recent changes in hormone replacement therapy. Persistent stressors or substance abuse patterns may be hindering her sustained recovery and should be addressed.

An assessment of F.H.'s attitude toward medication adherence is also vital, and her complete medical records should be obtained to verify the dose, duration, and results of previous antidepressant trials. It is critical to confirm that she received full therapeutic trials of the antidepressants that she was prescribed before considering other therapeutic options. A full therapeutic trial is considered to be a minimum of 4 weeks of treatment at a dosage shown to be clinically effective. Although some improvement may be noted during the first 1 or 2 weeks, maximal response is rarely evident until 4 weeks of treatment. In an open-label study with fluoxetine, patients who were not fully responsive after 3 weeks of treatment (20 mg/day) were randomly assigned to either continue with the original regimen or receive an increased dosage of fluoxetine (60 mg/day) for 5 additional weeks.[158] At the end of the study period, 49% of the patients receiving 20 mg converted to full responders, suggesting that 3 weeks is an inadequate period to confidently assess patient response. Because 50% of the patients receiving 60 mg/day converted to full responders, it may also be inferred that dosage increases are not necessary in many patients.

Drug Selection

SEROTONIN NOREPINEPHRINE REUPTAKE INHIBITORS

CASE 83-2, QUESTION 2: After a careful interview and workup, it was determined that F.H. is suffering from an acute episode of major depression with a probable history of dysthymia as well (i.e., double depression). She denies substance abuse, which is supported by a subsequent toxicology screen. From her medical chart and interview, it is confirmed that she received a therapeutic trial of nortriptyline and fluoxetine with inadequate clinical benefit. She is not interested in psychotherapy. Her provider decides to start venlafaxine (37.5 mg XR preparation daily). Is this a reasonable choice for F.H.?

Because 30% to 40% of patients will effectively achieve remission and about 20% to 25% of patients will stop an antidepressant because of side effects, it is safe to say that most patients started on a given antidepressant ultimately need a significant adjustment or change to their original regimen.[159] Clinicians, therefore, are obligated to have a thorough understanding of several antidepressant medications and classes if they are to facilitate successful outcomes.

In F.H.'s case, she has previously failed a therapeutic trial of nortriptyline and is currently expressing vague suicidality, so an alternate TCA would not be a reasonable choice (see full discussion of TCAs in the text that follows). Although she has also failed a fluoxetine trial, open-label studies and large controlled investigations suggest that 50% to 70% of patients who are unresponsive or intolerant of one SSRI will experience a therapeutic response to a different SSRI.[158,160,161] For example, in the STAR*D trial, patients failing an initial course of citalopram were just as likely to respond if they were randomly assigned to a subsequent trial of a different SSRI (sertraline) as they were to other antidepressant classes (venlafaxine and bupropion, specifically).[162] If a different SSRI is to be initiated, it may be wise to opt for one with fewer activating properties than fluoxetine (e.g., sertraline, paroxetine, citalopram, escitalopram) because F.H. is complaining of feeling jumpy and irritable. Alternatively, a medication from a different antidepressant class possesses the hypothetical benefit of a unique mechanism of action (e.g., venlafaxine, bupropion). Because of the severity of F.H.'s depressive symptoms, a sense of urgency should prevail and an alternate treatment is justified.

Venlafaxine was the first member of a relatively new class of antidepressants released in the United States known as SNRIs. Duloxetine, which possesses a very similar mechanism of action, was the second SNRI approved for the treatment of depression, and desvenlafaxine, the active metabolite of venlafaxine, recently became the third member of this class.[163] Studies in severe melancholic depression and treatment-resistant depression suggest that venlafaxine is at least as effective as other antidepressants in these populations, and it has emerged as a valuable alternative agent.[164–166] At dosages less than 150 mg/day, venlafaxine's therapeutic effects are mediated exclusively from the blockade of serotonin reuptake. Therefore, associated adverse effects at these dosages are qualitatively and quantitatively very similar to those found with SSRIs: GI distress, sleep disturbances, and sexual dysfunction. At higher dosages, effects on norepinephrine occur, and this can lead to the emergence of different adverse effects (e.g., tachycardia and hypertension). Duloxetine and desvenlafaxine enhance the activity of these two neurotransmitters as well, though their mechanism of action is not believed to be dose-dependent.[167]

Venlafaxine has a relatively brief plasma half-life (5–8 hours) and is demethylated to an active metabolite (*O*-desmethylvenlafaxine) that has a short half-life as well (11 hours). This metabolite, desvenlafaxine, was approved by the FDA in 2008 for the treatment of depression. Desvenlafaxine is commercially available as an extended-release tablet that has a similar mechanism of action as venlafaxine. It has no affinity for muscarinic, histaminic, cholinergic, or adrenergic receptors and has a terminal half-life of 11 hours.[168] Desvenlafaxine is not affected by CYP2D6 inhibitors; however, CYP3A4 inhibitors may reduce clearance of the drug.[168] Duloxetine also has a relatively short half-life (12 hours) and, as with the SSRIs, withdrawal reactions may occur when duloxetine is abruptly discontinued after chronic administration. Venlafaxine is not a potent inhibitor of cytochrome P-450 isoenzymes, so drug interactions are less of a concern than with certain SSRIs, but duloxetine is a moderate inhibitor of the CYP2D6 isoenzyme. All SNRIs have been associated with serotonin syndrome, so clinicians should be aware of the potentially dangerous drug combinations.[169]

For F.H., the choice of venlafaxine seems to be prudent. It is fairly safe in overdose, possesses a unique mechanism of action, and is generally less activating than fluoxetine (which had provoked some irritability in F.H.). In comparison to SSRIs, venlafaxine possesses a wide therapeutic range and ordinarily requires more dosage titration (which can increase resource utilization). A starting dose of 37.5 mg (XR) is reasonable, but baseline vitals should be recorded for F.H. with every dosage change in order to monitor the effect of this SNRI on her blood pressure and heart rate. Most patients respond to daily doses between 150 and 225 mg. Because F.H. is suffering from a relatively severe depression, it may be wise to increase her daily dose to 75 mg once she has exhibited good tolerance (i.e., after 4–7 days). In the event that F.H. has not exhibited a satisfactory response to 75 mg/day after 4 weeks, the dosage may be increased in increments of 37.5 to 75 mg every few weeks to a daily maximum of 225 mg. Although daily doses of the XL preparation above 225 mg are not recommended by the manufacturer, anecdotal success and relative safety have been reported for doses as high as 300 mg daily.[170]

OTHER AGENTS: BUPROPION AND MIRTAZAPINE

CASE 83-2, QUESTION 3: Are there any other antidepressants to consider if F.H. fails her venlafaxine trial?

Bupropion is an aminoketone with a mechanism of action that is clearly different from that of any other antidepressant that has received FDA approval. The direct effects of bupropion on serotonin transmission are negligible, but it may act by enhancing dopamine and/or norepinephrine activity.[171] At therapeutic dosages, bupropion has an attractive adverse effect profile, limited to occasional nausea and insomnia or jitteriness. Seizures, which were reported shortly after it was released in 1985, appear to be very unlikely with therapeutic dosing of bupropion, provided that patients are not predisposed (e.g., history of epilepsy, bulimia, or recent history of heavy drinking). Bupropion is one of the few antidepressants that may decrease appetite. A randomized, placebo-controlled investigation of bupropion in depressed obese patients observing caloric restriction found that bupropion was much more likely to induce significant weight loss than placebo.[172] After 26 weeks of treatment, 40% of the bupropion-treated patients lost more than 5% of their total body weight versus 16% with placebo. This weight loss was positively correlated with an improvement in depressive symptoms.

Bupropion is converted via the cytochrome CYP2B6 isoenzyme to an active metabolite (9 hydroxybupropion). Bupropion (and its metabolite) appears to have a moderate affinity for inhibiting the CYP2D6 isoenzyme, and significant elevations of venlafaxine and metoprolol have been demonstrated to occur with concurrent administration. Because of its short half-life (approximately 8 hours for the parent compound and 12 hours for the active metabolite), therapeutic doses of regular release bupropion must be administered in divided doses. The recommended starting dose is 100 mg twice a day (BID), increasing to 100 mg three times a day (TID) after at least 3 days. Individual doses must not exceed 150 mg and should be given at least 6 hours apart. An SR preparation is available though it is usually administered in multiple daily doses as well. For the SR formulation, initial daily doses are 150 mg every day, increased to 150 mg BID by the fourth day at the earliest. Individual doses of bupropion SR can be as large as 200 mg, and divided doses should be given at least 8 hours apart. More recently, a once-daily formulation has been developed (XL) and the package insert recommends initiating at 150 mg daily and increasing to 300 mg daily as early as the fourth day. Maximum daily doses are 450 mg for regular and XL products, and 400 mg for SR products.

Mirtazapine is a novel antidepressant capable of modulating serotonin and norepinephrine activity through a complex mechanism of action. In vitro studies reveal that mirtazapine is an antagonist at presynaptic α_2-autoreceptors and postsynaptic 5-HT_2 and 5-HT_3 receptors.[173] In addition, it appears to possess some mild inhibitory properties at serotonin reuptake transporters. Therefore, the net effect of mirtazapine is to enhance serotonin and norepinephrine albeit in a manner that is clearly distinct from any other antidepressants. In a comparative randomized trial with fluoxetine for moderate to severe depression, mirtazapine appeared to be much more effective than fluoxetine after 4 weeks of treatment (58% responders vs. 30% with fluoxetine; $p < 0.05$), but the differences were no longer significant at 6 weeks (63% vs. 54%; $p = 0.67$).[174]

The most common adverse effects experienced with mirtazapine are sedation and weight gain. Because mirtazapine has potent antihistaminergic effects, it can be quite sedating. Anecdotally, it has been reported that higher daily doses of mirtazapine (>30 mg) are less sedating than lower doses owing to an increase in noradrenergic effects. In addition to the substantial risk of increasing appetite and total body weight, mirtazapine has been associated with significant increases in total cholesterol and triglycerides.[175] The recommended starting dosage is 15 mg at bedtime, and the therapeutic dosage ranges from 15 to 45 mg/day.[175] Data from controlled trials have demonstrated safety and efficacy in doses up to 60 mg daily.[174,176]

Irreversible MAOIs (e.g., phenelzine, tranylepromine) may also be an alternative for patients who have failed multiple antidepressant trials. Like venlafaxine, TCAs, and mirtazapine, MAOIs are believed to relieve depressive symptoms by enhancing the activity of multiple neurotransmitters, which may be desirable for refractory cases. Because serious drug and dietary interactions are encountered with MAOIs, candidates for treatment should be chosen carefully; a full discussion of the clinical usefulness of MAOIs can be found in the Depression with Atypical Features section at the end of this chapter.

Antidepressant Augmentation

CASE 83-2, QUESTION 4: Three months later, F.H. reports that she feels less hopeless on venlafaxine XR (150 mg/day) and that her appetite has improved as well. However, she is still somewhat depressed and lethargic and attempts to increase her dosage have been limited by nausea and recurring insomnia. What pharmacologic options remain to help manage her refractory depression?

TABLE 83-18
Partial Response to Antidepressant Treatment Augmentation Strategies (with SSRIs)

Ensure completion of full therapeutic trial (4–6 weeks).
Ensure optimal dose of antidepressant.
Consider augmentation therapies:
- Bupropion
- Lithium
- Thyroid supplements
- Pindolol (?)
- Buspirone
- Atypical antipsychotics
- Modafinil
- Lamotrigine

SSRI, selective serotonin reuptake inhibitor.

Because F.H. has obtained considerable relief from her venlafaxine trial but is experiencing dose-limiting side effects, one would prefer to add a second medication (i.e., augmentation therapy) rather than changing antidepressants at this time (Table 83-18). A reasonable next step would be to augment her current venlafaxine regimen with another medication such as lithium, thyroid hormone, bupropion, or buspirone.

Lithium's antidepressant properties appear to apply to both unipolar and bipolar patients. Seven of nine antidepressant augmentation trials with lithium have reported positive therapeutic effects, usually within 1 week of achieving steady-state dynamics (i.e., 3–7 days of daily dosing).[177] Effective lithium blood levels are generally within the range used to treat bipolar disorder (0.5–1.2 mEq/L). As with the use of lithium therapy in bipolar disorder, all appropriate clinical monitoring parameters should be followed carefully (see Chapter 80, Anxiety Disorders).

Triiodothyronine (T_3) also has a long history of use in psychiatric circles for patients exhibiting partial or suboptimal responses to antidepressant monotherapy. Five of six RCTs support the use of T_3 supplementation for antidepressant augmentation, with an average effect size of 0.58 reported.[178] Triiodothyronine, at a dosage of 25 mg/day, can accelerate as well as augment antidepressant response, and superior effects have been reported in female patients, in particular. The response to the thyroid supplementation should be noticeable within 1 to 2 weeks, much like that found when lithium is used to augment therapy. Thyroxine (T_4) may also be effective with typical daily doses of 75 to 100 mcg daily often used. Whether T_3 is superior to T_4 has not been resolved, although one study seemed to indicate that more patients respond to T_3 than to T_4.[178] In the recently concluded STAR*D trials, T_3 was compared to lithium for antidepressant augmentation with citalopram in patients with two previous treatment failures.[179] Remission rates were modest for both agents in this challenging population (24.7% with T_3 vs. 15.9% with lithium) and there was no significant difference between these two therapies.

Bupropion has been used as augmentation therapy for many years and its use is supported by several open-label trials and one RCT.[180,181] Patients who continue to complain of fatigue, hypersomnia, or executive dysfunction on SSRI or SNRI therapy are excellent candidates for bupropion augmentation, and the combination treatment is usually well tolerated. In the STAR*D trial, augmentation with bupropion was compared to buspirone and both adjunctive treatment showed 30% remission rates. Buspirone may be of benefit to patients with residual symptoms of anxiety, in particular, and titration up to daily doses of 30 to 45 mg daily are often required. With F.H., one should be mindful that bupropion may increase her venlafaxine levels and hasten the return of GI and CNS effects.[112] Although the stimulating properties of bupropion may help relieve her lethargy, it may also exacerbate her insomnia.

Lamotrigine is FDA-approved for the treatment of bipolar depression. Like lithium, its clinical utility has also extended to the treatment of unipolar disorder although the evidence supporting its effectiveness is rather limited.[182] If indicated, lamotrigine should be initiated at a low dose of 25 mg at bedtime and slowly advanced to a target of 150 mg daily for a period of 6 to 8 weeks to minimize the potential for serious life-threatening rashes (e.g., 25 mg daily × 2 weeks, 50 mg daily × 2 weeks, 100 mg daily × 2 weeks, 150 mg daily thereafter). CNS side effects such as sedation, dizziness, and ataxia have also been commonly reported.

Among other options, pindolol is a unique β-blocker with intrinsic sympathomimetic properties that has received some attention as an augmenting agent.[183] Early open-label studies and one double-blind, controlled trial suggested that pindolol may enhance or accelerate the therapeutic effects of other antidepressants.[182–184] These benefits were attributed, in part, to the inhibitory effects that pindolol has on the 5-HT_{1A} autoreceptor.[185] A more recent double-blind placebo-controlled investigation enrolled 86 depressed patients, and, after 6 weeks of treatment, there was no statistical advantage to pindolol augmentation in terms of the onset or extent of antidepressant effect.[182] A 3-week, single-blind, crossover followed the initial study phase, and again no benefits from pindolol were evident. Given the obvious discrepancies in study results, further research appears warranted to adequately assess whether pindolol enhances response to SSRIs or other antidepressant medications.

Modafinil is FDA-approved for the treatment of narcolepsy, but it has been used extensively to increase energy and alertness, particularly among depressed patients. A large placebo-controlled RCT of modafinil was conducted among 311 subjects exhibiting a partial response to an SSRI.[186] Significant improvements were seen on sleepiness and fatigue scales, as well as overall depression scores, among patients randomly assigned to a fixed dose of modafinil 200 mg daily.

The use of atypical or second-generation antipsychotics for the management of treatment-resistant depression has become relatively common among mental health providers. Three atypical antipsychotics (aripiprazole, quetiapine, and olanzapine in combination with fluoxetine) have recently received FDA approval as adjunctive agents for treatment-resistant depression and others have been reported to be effective as well.[187] Generally, lower doses of second-generation antipsychotics have been successfully used in trials for depression (vs. schizophrenia) and relatively rapid improvement was evident. Given the high acquisition costs of these medications, and the significant risk of metabolic side effects that have been reported, clinicians must carefully weigh the risks and benefits of recommending this augmentation strategy.

The Elderly

CASE 83-3

QUESTION 1: R.M., a 71-year-old man, is brought in to see a primary care provider by his daughter with whom he has been living since the death of his wife 6 months ago. His daughter reports that R.M. had been in good health until his wife's death and that since then he has been keeping to himself, showing little interest in social activities. She reports that he used to be a happy, outgoing person but is now very irritable and becomes agitated over insignificant things. For the past 4 months, he has lost approximately 12 pounds and has trouble falling asleep. He used to be a voracious reader but seems uninterested in current events now. He appears to be confused or preoccupied at times and is incapable of understanding new concepts. His only documented medical problem is benign prostatic hypertrophy, and current medications consist of a stool softener and bulk laxative. Today's physical examination is normal, and the laboratory examination is significant only for a mildly elevated prostate-specific antigen of 10.0 ng/mL.

On examination, R.M. is perceived to be a thin, nervous, sad-appearing elderly man. He is oriented ×3. His response to questions is slow, and his volume of speech is reduced. Affect is sad. Mood is dysthymic. He shows mild impairments in his ability to think through problems and perform simple mathematical exercises. There is no evidence of delusions, hallucinations, or paranoia. He denies suicidal thoughts but feels hopeless at present and admits "there's no reason to live anymore." How does a depressive episode in late life, such as that in R.M., differ from an episode earlier in life?

Depression in late life is typically more difficult to recognize than depression in younger adults. Clinicians and patients may inappropriately attribute depressive symptoms to the "aging process" and minimize their significance. In addition, functional expectations are often lowered after retirement, making the degree of impairment difficult to evaluate. Because medical comorbidities are also more common in the elderly, depressive symptoms may be overlooked or misinterpreted in the workup as well.[188]

In general, the elderly present with the same depressive target symptoms as younger adults, which is reflected in the fact that DSM-IV-TR diagnosis for major depression in adults is not specific for age. However, qualitatively, the presentation of depression among the elderly may be quite different.[189] For instance, older patients are more likely to present with psychomotor retardation and are less likely to acknowledge "depression" per se, preferring instead to dwell on somatic concerns (e.g., poor sleep, low energy, changes in bowel function, bodily aches and pains). They are also much less likely to share or admit suicidal thoughts, and because elderly men have the highest suicide completion rate, an accurate assessment of depression and attendant risks is critical (see Drug Selection section).[190]

CASE 83-3, QUESTION 2: What is R.M.'s differential diagnosis? Should he receive antidepressant therapy?

In assessing nonspecific behavioral and cognitive symptoms in the elderly, a careful differential diagnosis between medical and other psychiatric disorders is essential because numerous medical illnesses can mimic depressive symptoms. Anemia, malignancies, congestive heart failure (CHF), and endocrine abnormalities may all present in a manner similar to that in depressive illness and can be ruled out only with a careful line of questioning and systematic physical workup.

One of the more difficult differential diagnoses in this setting involves the distinction of depression from dementia.[187,191] Like depression, patients with dementia may present with apathy, poor memory or concentration, reduced facial expression, and lack of spontaneous interaction. The illnesses are often comorbid, as 30% to 70% of patients with dementia also suffer from major depression.[191] Some experts have suggested, in fact, that new-onset depression in elderly patients may actually be part of a prodrome toward the manifestation of Alzheimer dementia.[191,192] A longitudinal cohort study found that among elderly patients suffering from an acute episode of major depression, 57% were ultimately diagnosed with Alzheimer dementia within the next 3 years.[187] Diagnostically, there are three notable differences between dementia and depression: (a) the symptoms (slow and subtle changes with dementia, rapid with depression), (b) orientation (markedly impaired with dementia, intact with depression), and (c) principal CNS impairment (short-term memory with dementia, concentration with depression).

DRUG SELECTION

A therapeutic trial of an antidepressant in a depressed individual with cognitive impairment may reverse the symptoms of the affective illness and restore functional capacity. Cognitive function may also improve to some degree. Moreover, because primary degenerative dementia is largely a diagnosis of exclusion, a successful trial of an antidepressant may help clarify the underlying pathological condition and is strongly recommended in patients with a positive personal or family history of mood disorders.[193] Although R.M.'s physical examination and laboratory workup were normal, a therapeutic trial of an antidepressant is warranted based on his current depressive target symptoms.

The overall efficacy of antidepressants in elderly patients is believed to be comparable to that observed in younger subjects, although the response to treatment is somewhat slower (i.e., 6-week therapeutic trial usually warranted). Similarly, the comparative therapeutic effects of individual antidepressants do not appear to differ qualitatively between elderly patients and the general population. The selection of antidepressants for geriatric depression, therefore, is quite similar to the process recommended for younger patients, although the presence of medical comorbidities and current medications will often have a greater influence on treatment plans due to the higher overall disease burden found in older patients. For example, the anticholinergic effects of certain antidepressants (TCA, paroxetine) may preclude their use in elderly patients suffering from narrow angle glaucoma, chronic constipation, or urinary hesitancy. The cognitive effects of antidepressants may also be more pronounced in elderly people due to differences in pharmacokinetic disposition (prolonged half-life) and pharmacodynamic properties (compromised integrity of blood–brain barrier). Although sedating antidepressants such as mirtazapine may serve to promote sleep in depressed patients suffering from insomnia, other geriatric clients may be candidates for more activating medications that can increase energy or enhance alertness (e.g., bupropion).

In the case of R.H., mirtazapine might be a judicious choice due to the fact that his appetite and sleep have diminished considerably during the past several months. A conservative starting dose of 7.5 mg at bedtime might be considered to enhance his ability to tolerate this new medication, although it is quite possible that eventual dosage increases might be required to achieve a therapeutic response.

Antidepressants and Cardiac Disease

CASE 83-4

QUESTION 1: B.H. is an obese 62-year-old man suffering from his first episode of major depressive disorder, melancholic subtype. He has an 8-year history of CHF (New York Heart Association functional class II) with an ejection fraction of 35% and atrial fibrillation. He is currently taking digoxin 0.25 mg orally daily and enalapril 10 mg orally BID. His CHF has been well controlled on this regimen, and he remains asymptomatic with regard to the CHF. His atrial fibrillation occurs about once every 6 months. All other laboratory parameters are within normal limits. His cardiologist believes that TCAs are the most effective antidepressants for melancholic depression. Are they any safety concerns in starting a TCA in this patient?

For many years, the TCAs were the most popular class of medications used to treat depression. The acquisition cost for TCAs was quite low, we had several decades of experience using them, and there continue to be providers who prefer antidepressant medications that enhance serotonin and norepinephrine for the treatment of severe or melancholic depression (i.e., dual-action antidepressants).[194] TCAs continue to be prescribed for other indications that are comorbid with depression as well (e.g., migraine prophylaxis, chronic pain). Unfortunately, TCAs cause a variety of adverse effects, ranging from bothersome (dry mouth, sedation, constipation) to serious (cardiovascular effects), which often prevent patients from receiving therapeutic doses of medication.[195] Patient adherence with prescribed medication may also be compromised with TCAs.[196]

The SSRIs have largely supplanted TCAs in their role as preferred agents for the treatment of mood disorders. The popularity of SSRIs can be attributed to numerous advantages over older compounds, including a lower side-effect burden, safety in overdose, less dosage titration, and patient preference. Results of a meta-analysis concluded that although the overall efficacy of the SSRI and TCA classes was comparable, primary care patients receiving an SSRI were much less likely to discontinue therapy prematurely due to side effects.[197] Although SSRIs were once more expensive than TCAs, most SSRIs are now available in generic formulations and are relatively inexpensive.

SIDE EFFECTS

CASE 83-4, QUESTION 2: B.H.'s cardiologist is concerned about the effect of a TCA on his cardiac status. What are the major adverse effects and toxicities of the TCAs, and how should these be managed?

The most common adverse effects of the TCAs are listed in Table 83-10. Anticholinergic effects are commonly encountered with the TCAs and may adversely affect adherence.[198] Although patients may develop tolerance to these effects, they may never disappear completely. Clinicians should be prepared to counsel patients about the appropriate way to manage these problems. Patients with dry mouth, for instance, may tend to drink excessive fluids to relieve discomfort. To minimize the inherent potential for weight gain with TCAs, patients should be advised to avoid caloric beverages and drink water or dietetic fluids instead. Sugarless gum or hard candy is often recommended as well.

TCAs also can be very sedating and are usually administered at bedtime to minimize functional impairments. Confusion or memory deficits may also occur with TCAs and can be particularly onerous in elderly patients. The secondary amines may be more tolerable in this regard, but all TCAs can impair concentration or alertness to some extent.

The impact of TCAs on cardiovascular function is a legitimate and serious concern. The most potentially dangerous adverse effect of the TCAs is their quinidinelike properties (type

IA) on prolonging cardiac conduction through the His-Purkinje system. This, in conjunction with positive chronotropic and adrenergic-blocking properties of the TCAs, can lead to reentry arrhythmias (e.g., torsades de pointes and other ventricular arrhythmias). In patients with pre-existing conduction defects and in overdose, there is a greater risk for cardiac arrhythmias.[199] Therefore, B.H. should receive a baseline electrocardiogram (ECG) before therapy.

Orthostatic hypotension is the most common and troublesome cardiovascular effect of the TCAs (as well as MAOIs) because it can result in significant morbidity and mortality.[200,201] Major clinical consequences of orthostatic hypotension include falls leading to bone fractures, lacerations, and even MI. Patients with CHF, such as B.H., are at greatest risk for experiencing orthostatic hypotension.

Imipramine and nortriptyline have been best studied with respect to their association with orthostatic hypotension. Amitriptyline, desipramine, doxepin, and clomipramine are also capable of producing it to varying degrees. Although systematic comparisons of the propensity of the TCAs to cause orthostatic hypotension are generally lacking, the tertiary amines (e.g., imipramine) may cause more severe orthostatic hypotension than the secondary amines (e.g., nortriptyline), and research evidence supports the contention that nortriptyline has the lowest risk for causing orthostatic hypotension among TCAs.[199,202]

CASE 83-4, QUESTION 3: Will the choice of antidepressant affect B.H.'s arrhythmia?

There are substantial differences among antidepressants (and antidepressant classes) in regard to overall cardiac safety and arrhythmogenic effects in particular. In general, the SSRIs appear to be relatively safe in patients with a history of arrhythmias or recent MI.[203] In a placebo-controlled investigation, hospitalized patients with unstable cardiac disease were randomly assigned to either sertraline or placebo.[204] Overall, both treatment arms were very well tolerated, and there was actually a lower risk of severe cardiac events reported in the sertraline group (vs. placebo). Retrospective data suggest that SSRIs may be somewhat cardioprotective in depressed patients with heart disease, a benefit that might be explained by their ability to decrease platelet activation.[205,206]

TCAs increase heart rate, probably via intrinsic anticholinergic properties that increase sinus node activity. Clinically, this effect is generally not significant, especially in medically healthy depressed patients.[207] However, it may be important in those with underlying conduction disease, coronary artery disease, or CHF. TCAs, when used at therapeutic dosages for the treatment of depression, decrease premature atrial and ventricular contractions in both depressed and nondepressed patients.[208,209] Antidepressants with class 1A antiarrhythmic activity (e.g., TCAs) may also have arrhythmogenic activity and thus increase the chances of ventricular arrhythmias and even sudden death. This effect on rhythm and conduction is believed to be related to the inhibitory effects of TCAs on the fast sodium channels and a decrease in Purkinje fiber action potential amplitude, membrane responsiveness, and slowed conduction.[209] Even nortriptyline, which is believed to be one of the safer TCAs in patients with heart disease, was associated with a greater risk for adverse cardiac events than paroxetine in an RCT.[210]

Bupropion and mirtazapine appear unlikely to affect cardiac rhythm or induce arrhythmias in susceptible patients.[203] Bupropion, however, should be used with caution in patients with pre-existing hypertension because of potential increases in BP.[211] Similarly, SNRIs do not appear to be arrhythmogenic, but increases in BP may be seen with higher dosages of venlafaxine in particular (>150 mg daily).[170] The nonselective MAOIs do not seem to affect rhythm significantly, although they can slow heart rate and can cause or worsen orthostatic hypotension.[212]

CASE 83-4, QUESTION 4: Are plasma concentrations clinically useful in monitoring antidepressant therapy? When should plasma antidepressant concentrations be obtained?

Attempts to demonstrate an association between plasma concentrations and therapeutic response for SSRIs, SNRIs, and NRIs have been largely unsuccessful. In contrast, the serum concentration of some TCAs correlates well with clinical response. Nortriptyline exhibits a curvilinear effect, whereas imipramine demonstrates a sigmoidal relationship between serum levels and clinical response.[213,214] Maximum benefit of imipramine is usually associated with serum levels of imipramine plus its demethylated metabolite, desipramine, in excess of 250 ng/mL. The relationship between plasma concentration of desipramine and clinical response is less clear, but a linear relationship is likely.[215] The most controversy surrounds amitriptyline; studies have shown a linear relationship, a curvilinear relationship, and no relationship between serum concentration and outcome.[216–218]

The APA Task Force on the Use of Laboratory Tests in Psychiatry recommends plasma concentration monitoring of TCAs when patients are elderly, not responding to therapy, nonadherent, experiencing adverse effects, or on multiple medications that may result in a possible drug interaction.[219] Plasma concentrations of imipramine, nortriptyline, and desipramine should be obtained after at least 1 week of a constant dosage when steady state has been achieved. Samples should be drawn 12 hours after the last dose has been administered. Routine therapeutic blood monitoring of other antidepressants is not recommended because information concerning their usefulness is limited; however, serum levels may be useful for evaluating adherence in some patients or ruling out serious toxicities.[220]

Antidepressants and Diabetes

CASE 83-5

QUESTION 1: B.L. is a 43-year-old woman who has become increasingly depressed during the past 4 months after the unexpected death of her father. She mentions that she was very upset immediately after his death, unable to sleep at night, and frequently crying at work. These symptoms have not abated during the past few months. She is slightly obese and has always been "borderline diabetic," but her blood sugar control has worsened since her father's death, and she has subsequently gained 30 pounds (HbA_{1c} = 8.2 last week, up from 6.1, 4 months ago). She is very upset that she has recently been diagnosed with type 2 diabetes and does not believe that she is capable of following the lifestyle modifications recommended. How strong is the association between depression and diabetes? Would an antidepressant be an appropriate treatment for her symptoms at this time, and, if so, which agent(s) would be recommended?

A potential association between depression and diabetes has been discussed in the medical literature for more than 300 years.[221] Results of a meta-analysis confirmed that diabetic patients are twice as likely to be suffering from depression than the general population, an association that appears to hold true for type 1 and type 2 diabetic illness.[222] Theories abound as to why diabetic patients become depressed, citing complex physiological, psychological, and social factors, and a precise explanation has not been elucidated. Depressed patients are also twice as likely to exhibit diabetes in comparison to nondepressed cohorts. One study of patients newly diagnosed with type 2 diabetes reported that more than 80% of this population had a documented episode of depression in their past.[223] It has also been established that depressed diabetic patients are much more likely to suffer long-term complications with this metabolic disorder, and successful treatment of depression has been demonstrated to improve glycemic indices.[224–226]

Successful treatment of mood disorders in patients with diabetes is important for several reasons. Patients with depression or diabetes are at risk for cardiovascular illness, and successful antidepressant treatment, therefore, may substantially decrease morbidity and mortality. Depressed patients are also much less likely to comply with treatment recommendations in general because of their hopelessness, cognitive impairment, and social isolation. As a result, they are three times more likely to stop taking their medications, leading to a worsening of diabetes and other medical conditions.[227] Most depressed patients also report a change in their appetite at baseline, which may lead to a compromise in blood sugar control. Moreover, decreases in energy and motivation may also sabotage diabetes treatment plans.

Although the number of clinical studies conducted with depressed diabetic patients is limited, antidepressants appear to have the same efficacy rates in both diabetic and nondiabetic populations.[226] Currently, there is no evidence to suggest that one class of antidepressant is more efficacious than another. Selection of an antidepressant in the diabetic population, therefore, rests largely on differences in adverse effect profiles, potential impact on diabetes complications, and potential for drug interactions.

One important consideration in selecting an antidepressant is the potential impact of the agent on appetite, blood sugar control, and total body weight. Although most research on the effects of antidepressants on glycemic control has been done in rats, important differences appear to exist among antidepressants in regard to weight gain potential.[228] As discussed previously, the risk of clinically significant weight gain appears to be highest with mirtazapine, TCAs, and MAOIs, and these medications should be avoided. Although SSRIs and SNRIs may occasionally induce weight gain in susceptible patients (estimated incidence of 3%–5%), this adverse effect appears to be of greatest concern with paroxetine (25% incidence). Bupropion may cause appetite suppression in some patients, which may be beneficial for the obese, but may also pose a theoretical concern about hypoglycemia in diabetic patients.

Because one of the long-term complications of diabetes is sexual dysfunction, this potential side effect of antidepressants should be considered. It should be emphasized, however, that erectile dysfunction and impotence are the sexual side effects most commonly encountered by male diabetics. Thus, although the SSRI may impair sexual performance by delaying or preventing orgasm, this impairment occurs at a different stage of the sexual process and would not necessarily preclude use of SSRIs. Diabetic neuropathies may also influence antidepressant selection. SNRIs have proven quite effective for the management of neuropathic pain, but the potential of these antidepressants to increase blood pressure or heart rate should be considered. Pharmacokinetic drug interactions between antidepressants and certain diabetes treatments should also be considered. For instance, many of the oral antidiabetic agents are substrates for metabolism by the cytochrome P-450 system. Inhibition of this metabolic step may precipitate a serious drug interaction by increasing plasma concentrations of the antidiabetic agents and enhancing hypoglycemic effects. Several of these agents are metabolized via the CYP2C9 isoenzyme (e.g., tolbutamide, glyburide, glipizide, rosiglitazone), and the administration of certain SSRIs (e.g., fluoxetine or fluvoxamine) may potentiate their effects. Repaglinide and some of the sulfonylureas are metabolized via the CYP3A4 isoenzyme, which may also be inhibited by fluoxetine or fluvoxamine.

For B.L., the depressive symptoms she experienced after her father's death may be considered a natural response to this serious loss. However, because her symptoms have persisted for longer than 2 months, her psychiatric illness would no longer be categorized as a grief reaction (or bereavement) and should be managed medically as an acute episode of major depression. If B.L. is amenable to an antidepressant, an SSRI that is unlikely to induce weight gain or potentiate drug interactions may be a prudent choice. Such agents would include sertraline, citalopram, or escitalopram.

Antidepressants and Epilepsy

CASE 83-6

QUESTION 1: C.B., a 20-year-old woman, was recently diagnosed with major depressive disorder, single episode. Since the age of 8 years, she has also experienced complex partial seizures. Her seizures have been difficult to control in the past (at least six seizures per month), but her condition has improved recently (none for 8 months) on a combination of carbamazepine and gabapentin. Are there any special considerations with regard to antidepressant selection in C.B.?

Although seizures are a relatively uncommon effect of antidepressant medications, they are frightening and serious when they occur. The overall risk of seizures with most antidepressants is quite low at therapeutic dosages, and, as a result, the precise risk is difficult to quantify with any statistical certainty.[229] Furthermore, the risk of new-onset seizures in the general population (i.e., not necessarily receiving antidepressants) is approximately 0.073% to 0.086% annually, suggesting the likelihood of occasional coincidental case reports.[230] Among the antidepressants marketed in the United States, imipramine may be the best studied, and the frequency of seizures was reported to be 0.1% among patients prescribed therapeutic dosages (≤200 mg/day).[231]

Generally, it is believed that drug-induced seizures are a dose-related phenomenon, so it is not surprising that most case reports of antidepressant seizures have involved overdose ingestions, most commonly with the TCAs. Seizures have been correlated to peak plasma concentrations of tricyclics (e.g., levels >1,000 ng/mL) and typically occur within 6 hours after the overdose.[232]

Although the specific antidepressant may also be of some importance in terms of seizure risk, there are significant methodologic difficulties that make it quite difficult to accurately compare seizure rates between specific agents. An older review cited amoxapine with the highest risk of seizures in overdose, followed by maprotiline and the TCAs (collectively).[233] Bupropion was withdrawn from the market in 1986 after the appearance of new-onset seizures in bulimic patients receiving the antidepressant as part of a placebo-controlled trial (4 of 69 subjects).[234] After a re-examination of the original dosing recommendations, bupropion was released again in 1989, and a new SR preparation appeared in 1998. Among the 3,100 patients to receive the new preparation for up to 1 year, the cumulative seizure risk was 0.15%.[235] Although SSRIs have been associated with seizures in acute overdose, the comparative risk encountered with dosages in the therapeutic range has not been determined.

Because of C.B.'s seizure history, choosing a medication with a low risk of seizures is prudent. Bupropion, for instance, is contraindicated in patients with a pre-existing seizure disorder. Because carbamazepine has a narrow therapeutic index and is metabolized primarily by the CYP3A4 isoenzyme, antidepressants that inhibit this enzyme, such as fluoxetine or fluvoxamine, should be avoided. Similarly, carbamazepine may induce the metabolism of certain TCAs, and it also possesses some of the cardiotoxic effects of these antidepressants (e.g., slowed conduction) further discouraging its use. Among the remaining alternatives, one may opt for an SSRI less likely to inhibit metabolic pathways (e.g., sertraline, citalopram) or venlafaxine.

Antidepressants and Acquired Immunodeficiency Syndrome

CASE 83-7

QUESTION 1: K.H., a 33-year-old HIV-positive woman, has been reasonably healthy during the past 2 years but she was recently diagnosed with acquired immune deficiency syndrome (AIDS) after an episode of oral candidiasis. During the past few months, she has noticed a loss of interest in life, accompanied by decreased energy, easy fatigability, and difficulty concentrating (she has to read a sentence several times before she can comprehend its meaning). She also reports a depressed mood but denies suicidal ideation. Her current medications are zidovudine, lamivudine, ritonavir, and oral clotrimazole troche. After a thorough medical workup, other opportunistic infections have been ruled out. What precipitating factors may be contributing to K.H.'s current symptoms of depression?

Patients with serious illnesses such as HIV/AIDS or certain cancers are faced with an extreme psychosocial stressor that can precipitate a depressive episode. Research evaluating the severity of emotional distress in persons with HIV has shown elevated anxiety, depression, social isolation, and suicidal ideation.[236] Chronic depression in AIDS patients has, in fact, been associated with an acceleration of the disease progression, as well as a significant reduction in the perceived quality of life (vs. nondepressed HIV-infected controls).[237,238] K.H. currently is, or will be, confronted with a number of psychological issues, including fear of developing an opportunistic infection, chronic somatic preoccupations, debilitation, anger, possible death at a young age, and reactive depression.[239,240]

Although K.H.'s target symptoms (fatigue, decreased concentration, and depressed mood) may represent a depressive episode secondary to psychosocial stressors, her differential diagnosis also includes HIV-1–associated cognitive/motor complex or dementia resulting from HIV disease (formally known as AIDS dementia complex).[241] HIV-associated dementia closely resembles the symptoms of a depressive disorder and is part of the Centers for Disease Control and Prevention classification system for HIV infection (category C).[242] Neoplasms and opportunistic infections of the CNS secondary to AIDS can also alter mental status. However, a thorough medical workup ruled out opportunistic infection in K.H.

CASE 83-7, QUESTION 2: Based on K.H.'s target symptoms, is she a candidate for antidepressant therapy? What considerations should be made when selecting antidepressant therapy for K.H.?

K.H. would benefit from antidepressant therapy to help ameliorate her target symptoms of decreased energy, lack of concentration, and depressed mood, regardless of whether it is a major depressive episode or direct HIV involvement within the CNS. Although antidepressant trials in the general HIV population are lacking (and particularly scarce among populations of women or underrepresented minorities), several factors should be taken into account when selecting antidepressant medication in an HIV/AIDS patient.[243,244] In general, comparative trials with conventional agents have been associated with high dropout rates because of adverse effects, suggesting that HIV/AIDS patients may be more vulnerable to toxic effects, or that lower doses of antidepressant medications should be considered.[245,246]

Drug interactions can be a primary concern because several of the protease inhibitors undergo metabolic transformation via the cytochrome P-450 system, primarily through the CYP3A4 and CYP2B6 isoenzymes. Therefore, fluoxetine and fluvoxamine are best avoided. Among the alternatives, SSRIs and TCAs have demonstrated comparable efficacy in the depressed HIV/AIDS population, but the side effect burden of SSRIs may be more tolerable to these patients. Bupropion has become increasingly popular in depressed HIV/AIDS patients, and the activating properties may be attractive in K.H. because of her fatigue and reduced energy.[247] Inhibition of bupropion metabolism has been demonstrated with concurrent administration of ritonavir, efavirenz, and nelfinavir, however, which may complicate its use under certain circumstances.[248] Some evidence suggests that low-dose psychostimulants (e.g., methylphenidate, dextroamphetamine) or modafinil may improve cognition and mood in patients with AIDS.[249] For appetite stimulation, mirtazapine would be a reasonable option in some AIDS patients, although the sedating potential should be carefully considered. An additional option may be ECT, which has been administered safely and effectively to the depressed AIDS population as well.[250]

ANTIDEPRESSANTS AND CHRONIC PAIN

CASE 83-8

QUESTION 1: D.C. is a 62-year-old woman with a history of fibromyalgia who has noted increased crying spells and a decreased interest in social activities during the course of the last 2 months. She attributes this downturn to the stress she is experiencing as she cares for her disabled mother who recently moved in with her. When asked, she also notes significant decreases in energy and concentration, and difficulties in falling and staying asleep.

In the past, D.C. recalls one previous episode of depression 8 years ago, shortly after her forced retirement from teaching, when she was treated initially with venlafaxine (discontinued due to agitation) and ultimately responded to a course of psychotherapy. Her past medical history is significant for fibromyalgia (diagnosed 7 years ago but continues to bother her on a daily basis; she rates pain at 3 of 10 currently), hypertension, hyperlipidemia, and new-onset alopecia (began last month). Her current medications include carisoprodol 350 mg BID, amlodipine 5 mg daily, atenolol 50 mg daily, and atorvastatin 10 mg daily. In addition, she started amitriptyline 50 mg at bedtime 2 months ago for her insomnia but noticed a 12-pound weight gain and recently discontinued. In the meantime, she has continued to see her therapist on a weekly basis during this time frame.

What considerations may influence treatment selection in this patient with chronic pain? What treatment would be recommended?

There is a strong and complex association between chronic pain syndromes and mood disorders. Epidemiological investigations reports that 30% to 54% of patients with chronic pain will satisfy the criteria for a depressive disorder, and anxiety disorders are commonly reported in this population as well. On the other hand, up to 80% of individuals with major depression will experience some symptoms of somatic pain, often presenting with pain as their chief complaint. Researchers have theorized that this comorbid phenomenon can be explained by deficiencies in the neurotransmitters serotonin and norepinephrine, which influence mood disorders in the prefrontal cortex and limbic system, as well as module pain sensitivity via descending projections down the spinal column. Other theories implicate elevations in cytokine activity, which commonly occur during the course of mood disorders, as well as mediating inflammatory activity occurring within the context of chronic pain.

Treatment plans for depressed patients with chronic pain should target both of these conditions in order to achieve optimal outcomes. In regards to the selection of antidepressants, preference is often given to medications that can address the unique cluster of symptoms associated with these comorbid conditions. For instance, antidepressant agents with pain-relieving properties and agents that promote sleep and relieve anxiety are often preferred. TCAs and SNRIs have proven to be quite effective for the management of neuropathic pain conditions, in addition to their benefits on anxiety and depression. Although is has been speculated that the analgesic effects of these agents are related to enhancements of both serotonin and norepinephrine activity, both of these classes of antidepressants are also potent sodium channel blockers, and it is this property that may contribute to their pain-relieving actions.

Given the heavy reliance upon medications to manage chronic pain drug interactions are often a major consideration in the selection of antidepressants. For example, the combination of serotonergic antidepressants (SSRIs or SNRIs) with the analgesic tramadol has been linked to many case reports of serotonin syndrome, and concomitant use of these agents should be discouraged. The potential of certain antidepressants to inhibit CYP2D6 isoenzymes (e.g., fluoxetine, paroxetine, duloxetine, bupropion) may also be a theoretical concern with certain opioid analgesics which are prodrugs and require metabolic transformation to generate the active species. These analgesics include codeine (metabolized to morphine), hydrocodone (active metabolite: hydromorphone), and oxycodone (oxymorphone), as well as tramadol (o-desmethyl tramadol). Patients who are receiving CYP2D6 inhibitors (or are poor metabolizers of CYP2D6 substrates) may require much higher doses of these analgesics to manage pain conditions.

D.C. appears to meet the criteria for an acute episode of major depression and medication is clearly indicated. Among the alternatives, SSRIs have not proven to be effective for neuropathic pain, and only limited evidence supports the use of an SNRI. TCAs are quite effective for certain pain conditions, as well as depression and anxiety. In the past, however, she has experienced significant weight gain with a low-dose TCA (50 mg amitriptyline) so other antidepressant classes may be preferred. An SNRI would be a good choice for the treatment of her depression, anxiety, and fibromyalgia. Given D.C.'s history of agitation from venlafaxine, an alternate SNRI, such as duloxetine, could be considered. However, duloxetine can inhibit CYP2D6 and this should be taken into consideration if other medication changes are considered in the future.

Depression With Atypical Features (Atypical Depression)

MONOAMINE OXIDASE INHIBITORS

CASE 83-9

QUESTION 1: G.R., a 38-year-old, 73-kg woman, presents at the university outpatient psychiatric clinic with a chief complaint of extreme lethargy and depressed mood more days than not for the past 6 weeks. During this period, she has also been sleeping too much and overeating (she says she has gained at least 10 pounds in this time frame). On interview, she also reports an intense fear of heights and consequently does not travel if it involves driving over a bridge or flying in an airplane. She reports that this episode seems to have started around the time of the break-up with her boyfriend, and she becomes extremely anxious and tearful in revealing this piece of her history. Her psychiatric history is consistent with at least two other similar depressive episodes, the first when she was 18 years old and the second occurring around age 25 years. Her physical examination and laboratory assessments are within normal limits. In the past, she has exhibited a poor response to trials of fluoxetine and nortriptyline. During her last episode, she responded to phenelzine 60 mg/day.

How does G.R.'s depressive condition manifest differently from melancholic depression?

G.R. suffers from hysteroid dysphoria, more commonly known as atypical depression (Table 83-19). DSM-IV-TR now refers to atypical depression as "depression with atypical features."[13] Traditionally, atypical depression has been regarded as a more persistent, debilitating, and treatment-resistant mood disorder. Patients with atypical depression tend to respond better to MAOIs than other antidepressant classes.[251]

The term atypical depression is generally applied to patients who fit the DSM-IV-TR criteria for major depressive disorder and suffer at least two of the following symptoms: (a) hypersomnia, (b) leaden paralysis (profound lethargy), (c) hyperphagia, or (d) pathological sensitivity to interpersonal rejection (rejection sensitivity). The features of atypical depression and melancholia are compared in Table 83-19.[252] G.R. appears to fit the diagnostic criteria for major depressive disorder in general, and the specific symptoms of hypersomnia, hyperphagia, and rejection sensitivity would support the descriptor "with atypical features."

TABLE 83-19

A Comparison of Atypical Depression and Melancholia

Feature	Atypical Depression	Melancholia
Onset	Teens (or younger)	Thirties (avg)
Sex	Females > males	Females > males
Course	Chronic	Episodic
Phenomenology		
Appetite/weight	Increased	Decreased
Sleep	Increased	Decreased
Energy	Low with leaden paralysis	Low
Reaction to rejection	Very sensitive	Indifferent
Treatment response	MAOI = SSRI = TCA	MAOI = TCA = SSRI

MAOI, monoamine oxidase inhibitor; SSRI, selective serotonin reuptake inhibitor; TCA, tricyclic antidepressant.

INITIATION

CASE 83-9, QUESTION 2: What role do MAOIs have in the current management of depression? Would this class of antidepressant be appropriate for G.R.? Outline a dosage titration and treatment plan.

TABLE 83-21
Seven Things Everyone Should Know About Depression

- **Depression is NOT a personality flaw or a weakness of character.**
  Depression has been associated with a chemical imbalance in the nervous system, which can be easily corrected with antidepressant medications and associated counseling.
- **All antidepressants are equally effective.**
  Approximately 65% of patients receiving a therapeutic trial of any antidepressant medication will have a beneficial response.
- **Most patients receiving antidepressants will experience some side effect(s) initially.**
  Identify an accessible health professional who can answer your questions.
- **Antidepressants should be taken at the same time daily.**
  This will make it easier for you to remember to take the medication and may also minimize side effects.
- **The response to antidepressants is delayed.**
  Several weeks may pass before you begin to feel better, and it may take 4 to 6 weeks before maximal benefits are evident.
- **Antidepressants must be taken for at least 6 to 9 months.**
  Even if you are feeling completely better, studies have shown that people who stop their medication during the first 6 months are much more likely to become depressed again.
- **Antidepressants are NOT addictive substances.**
  Antidepressants may elevate the moods of depressed individuals, but they do not act as stimulants and are not associated with craving or other abuse patterns. However, if certain antidepressants are discontinued abruptly, mild withdrawal reactions may occur.

KEY REFERENCES AND WEBSITES

A full list of references for this chapter can be found at http://thepoint.lww.com/AT10e. Below are the key references and websites for this chapter, with the corresponding reference number in this chapter found in parentheses after the reference.

Key References

Bostwick JM. A generalist's guide to treating patients with depression with an emphasis on using side effects to tailor antidepressant therapy. *Mayo Clin Proc.* 2010;85:538.

Carlat DJ. *The Psychiatric Interview.* Philadelphia, PA: Lippincott Williams & Wilkins; 2005. (51)

Chang T, Fava M. The future of psychopharmacology of depression. *J Clin Psychiatry.* 2010;71:971.

Cipriani A, et al. Comparative efficacy and acceptability of 12 new-generation antidepressants: a multiple-treatments meta-analysis. *Lancet.* 2009;373:746.

Mann JJ. The medical management of depression. *N Engl J Med.* 2005;353:1819.

Rush AJ et al. Acute and longer-term outcomes in depressed outpatients requiring one or several treatment steps: a STAR*D report. *Am J Psychiatry.* 2006;163:1905. (156)

Shelton RC, et al. Therapeutic options for treatment-resistant depression. *CNS Drugs.* 2010;24:131.

Taylor MJ, et al. Strategies for managing antidepressant-induced sexual dysfunction: systematic review of randomized controlled trials. *J Affect Disord.* 2005;88:241.

Trivedi MH et al. Evaluation of outcomes with citalopram for depression using measurement-based care in STAR*D: implications for clinical practice. *Am J Psychiatry.* 2006;163:28. (79)

Yonkers KA et al. The management of depression during pregnancy: a report from the American Psychiatric Association and the American College of Obstetricians and Gynecologists. *Gen Hosp Psychiatry.* 2009;31:403. (136)

Key Websites

The Macarthur Initiative on Depression and Primary Care. http://www.depression-primarycare.org.

National Alliance on Mental Illness. http://www.nami.org.

National Institute of Mental Health. http://www.nimh.nih.gov.

Natural Standard, the Authority on Integrative Medicine. http://www.naturalstandard.com.

Mood Disorders II: Bipolar Disorders

84

James J. Gasper

CORE PRINCIPLES

		CHAPTER CASES
1	Bipolar disorder is a relatively rare chronic progressive illness with an age of onset in the early 20s. It is characterized by recurrent mood episodes of mania and depression. Life stressors, substance use, and medications are common precipitants of these mood episodes.	**Case 84-1 (Questions 1–3)**
2	Manic episodes are characterized by elevated mood, irritability, inflated self-esteem, poor judgment, and excessive motor activity. Depressive episodes of bipolar disorder share the same diagnostic criteria as major depression.	**Case 84-1 (Questions 1, 4), Case 84-2 (Question 1), Case 84-7 (Question 1)**
3	Valproate, lithium, or atypical antipsychotics are appropriate first-line treatments for acute mania. Depending on the severity of symptoms these agents may be used alone or in combination.	**Case 84-1 (Question 5)**
4	Lithium, lamotrigine, or the combination of the two agents are appropriate first-line treatments for bipolar depression.	**Case 84-7 (Question 1)**
5	Maintenance treatment of bipolar disorder is imperative to prevent disease progression. The optimal approach is to continue the acute phase treatment with gradual simplification toward monotherapy with lithium, lamotrigine, or valproate. Atypical antipsychotics are appropriate alternative or adjunctive treatments.	**Case 84-8 (Questions 1, 2)**
6	Medications used to treat bipolar disorder have a wide range of side effects that may impact adherence. The history of response, patient preference, and long-term tolerability profile are important considerations when selecting an agent. Therapeutic blood level monitoring as well as laboratory monitoring for side effects is commonly required for certain medications.	**Case 84-1 (Questions 7, 8)**

INTRODUCTION

Bipolar disorder (BD), also known as manic-depression, is a severe life-threatening psychiatric condition that is commonly misdiagnosed and too often inappropriately treated.[1,2] BD is associated with high rates of health care utilization, suicidal behavior, and use of public assistance.[3] The global burden of BD is immense, exceeding many chronic diseases including human immunodeficiency virus, diabetes mellitus, and asthma.[4]

Diagnosis and Classification

Mood disorders like BD are diagnosed using the criteria established in the *Diagnostic and Statistical Manual of Mental Disorders*, fourth edition, Text Revision (DSM-IV-TR).[5] Discrete periods of mood disturbance associated with BD are defined as *manic episodes, hypomanic episodes, mixed episodes, or major depressive episodes.*

Manic or hypomanic episodes (Table 84-1) are periods of abnormally and persistently elevated, expansive, or irritable mood.[5] Hypomanic episodes are less intense than manic episodes, which are severe enough to impair functioning (self-care, occupational, social), complicate a medical condition, result in psychotic features, or require hospitalization.[5] Although manic and hypomanic episodes are characteristic symptoms of BD, it is depressive episodes that predominate and are ordinarily the initial presenting symptom.[6,7] BD and major depressive disorder share the same criteria for major depressive episodes (see Chapter 83, Mood Disorders I: Major Depressive Disorders).[5] A mixed episode is diagnosed when a patient meets criteria for both a major depressive episode and a manic episode concurrently for at least a 1-week period.[5]

A person who has experienced one or more manic or mixed episodes with or without a depressive episode is diagnosed as having *bipolar I disorder.* An individual who has experienced one or more episodes of both hypomania and depression (without a

TABLE 84-1
DSM-IV-TR Criteria for a Manic Episode[a]

1. A distinct period of abnormally and persistently elevated, expansive, or irritable mood, lasting $\geq$1 week (or of any duration if hospitalization is necessary).
2. During the period of mood disturbance, at least three of the following symptoms have persisted (four if the mood is only irritable) and have been present to a significant degree:
   - Inflated self-esteem or grandiosity
   - Decreased need for sleep (e.g., feels rested after only 3 hours of sleep)
   - More talkative than usual or pressure to keep talking
   - Flight of ideas or subjective experience that thoughts are racing
   - Distractibility (i.e., attention too easily drawn to unimportant or irrelevant external stimuli)
   - Increase in goal-directed activity (either social, at work, at school, or sexually) or psychomotor agitation
   - Excessive involvement in pleasurable activities that have a high potential for painful consequences (e.g., the person engages in unrestrained buying sprees, sexual indiscretions, or foolish business investing)
3. The symptoms do not meet the criteria for a mixed episode.
4. The mood disturbance is sufficiently severe to cause marked impairment in occupational functioning or in usual social activities or relationships with others, or to necessitate hospitalization to prevent harm to self or others, or there are psychotic features.
5. The symptoms are not caused by the direct physiologic effects of a substance (e.g., a drug of abuse, a medication, or other treatment) or a general medical condition (e.g., hyperthyroidism).

[a] Criteria for a hypomanic episode are identical to a manic episode; however, the symptoms need only be present for 4 days and are not severe enough to cause marked impairment in social or occupational functioning, necessitate hospitalization, or for psychotic features to be present.
Maniclike or hypomaniclike episodes that are clearly caused by somatic antidepressant treatment (e.g., medication, electroconvulsive therapy, light therapy) should not count toward a diagnosis of bipolar disorder.
Source: American Psychiatric Association. Mood disorders. In: *Diagnostic and Statistical Manual of Mental Disorders.* 4th ed. Text Revision. Washington, DC: American Psychiatric Association; 2000;362, 368.

history of manic or mixed episodes) is diagnosed as having *bipolar II disorder.*[5]

The diagnosis of a *cyclothymic disorder* is used for a person who has experienced at least 2 years of mood cycling characterized by numerous periods with hypomanic symptoms and separate periods with depressive symptoms that do not meet the criteria for a major depressive episode. *Bipolar disorder, not otherwise specified,* sometimes called *bipolar spectrum,* refers to disorders with features of mania or hypomania (and commonly depressive symptoms) that do not meet the criteria for a specific BD type.[5]

The DSM-IV-TR also uses a series of descriptors called *specifiers* to further characterize the course of illness and the most recent type of episode experienced by the individual. Recent episodes are first classified as hypomanic, manic, mixed, or depressed. They may be described further in terms of severity (mild, moderate, severe), the presence of psychotic features (in partial or full remission), with or without catatonic features, or with onset during the postpartum period. Other specifiers convey information regarding the pattern of illness. For example, some individuals experience major depressive episodes at a characteristic time of the year (usually the winter) or switch from depression to mania during a particular season. The related specifier is "with seasonal pattern," which applies only to the pattern of major depressive episodes. Other specifiers describe whether full recovery between episodes (i.e., with or without full interepisode recovery) occurs and whether individuals experience rapid cycling (four or more mood episodes per year).[5]

Epidemiology and Cost Burden

Using DSM-IV-TR criteria, the lifetime prevalence of bipolar I disorder is estimated to be 1%; bipolar II disorder is marginally more common at 1.1%.[8] The prevalence rate for the bipolar spectrum of illnesses, which include bipolar I, bipolar II, and subthreshold BD (i.e., not meeting full diagnostic criteria), is 4.4%.[8] Bipolar I and II are more common in women than in men, whereas subthreshold illness predominates in men.[8] The familial nature of BD has been well established with an 11-fold increased risk in first-degree relatives.[9] Twin studies add further support to the genetic linkage. Goodwin and Jamison report a 63% concordance rate (rate of illness in co-twin of affected proband) for monozygotic twins compared with 13% for dizygotic twins.[9]

The cost of BD in 2009 was reported to be $151 billion.[10] Direct costs, such as hospitalization, outpatient visits, and medications, accounted for 20% of the total. The remaining 80% was attributable to indirect costs such as lost productivity by patients and caregivers.

Clinical Signs and Symptoms

A manic episode usually begins with a change in sleep patterns along with mood elevation. Presenting symptoms include talkativeness, lack of sleep, and bursts of energy during which projects are begun but rarely completed. Mania often is characterized by thought disturbances exhibited by "flight of ideas" (rapid speech that switches among multiple ideas or topics) and delusions of grandeur (false beliefs of special powers, knowledge, abilities, importance, or identity). The behavior of manic patients is characterized as being intrusive, loud, intense, irritable, at times suspicious, and even challenging. Patients often exercise poor judgment, which may include spending large sums of money in business deals that ultimately fail, becoming sexually promiscuous, using substances, or failing to obey laws.

The symptoms of mania usually develop gradually over the course of several days to more than a week and are defined in three stages.[11] *Stage I* is characterized by euphoria, irritability, labile affect, grandiosity, overconfidence, racing thoughts, increased psychomotor activity, and an increase in the rate and amount of speech. This stage corresponds to an episode of hypomania. *Stage II* features increased dysphoria (a feeling of extreme discomfort and unrest), hostility, anger, delusions, and cognitive disorganization. This stage corresponds to acute mania. Many patients progress no further than this stage. Others may proceed to *stage III,* in which the manic episode progresses to an undifferentiated psychotic state. Individuals in stage III experience terror and panic, their behavior is bizarre, and psychomotor activity is frenzied. They may experience hallucinations. What were once simply disorganized thoughts become incoherent; disorientation to time and place occurs. Just as the manic episode gradually builds, it often declines in a gradual manner. Psychotic symptoms usually resolve first, whereas irritability, paranoia, and excessive behavior persist. Remaining symptoms such as talkativeness, seductiveness, and dysphoria slowly decrease with time.

Depressive episodes of BD share the diagnostic criteria with unipolar depression; however, the presentation of bipolar depression has some distinguishing features. In particular, bipolar depression (type I specifically) is more likely to be associated with mood lability, psychotic features, psychomotor retardation, and comorbid substance use.[12] This contrasts with unipolar depression, which is more likely to be associated with anxiety, agitation, insomnia, somatic complaints, and weight loss.[12]

Mixed episodes of BD, also known as *mixed mania,* are considered to be a variant of a manic episode during which patients experience both manic and depressive symptoms. Mixed episodes appear to be common, occurring in approximately 28% of patients presenting with mania.[11] A review by Salvatore et al. identified three important presentations of mixed episodes: *manic stupor, agitated depression,* and *unproductive mania.*[13] Manic stupor, "the most important of the mixed states," is characterized by mood elevation with a deficit in psychomotor activity (stupor) and slowed thoughts.[13] Agitated depression is depressed mood with psychomotor activation and flight-of-ideas. Unproductive mania consists of mood elevation, psychomotor activation, and thought retardation. Mixed states can occur abruptly or serve as a transitional phase to a depressed or manic episode. The duration may be short lived, lasting only days, or may take on a chronic course of weeks to months.

Course of Illness

The mean age of onset for the bipolar spectrum of illnesses is 21 years.[8] Bipolar I is the earliest in onset at age 18, compared with bipolar II at age 20 and subthreshold BD occurring at age 22.[8] Approximately 20% to 30% of new cases occur in children between 10 and 15 years old.[14,15] Late-life onset of BD is rare. After age 60, there is a sharp decrease in the new onset of BD; therefore, a presentation of mania at this age should alert the clinician to an underlying medical problem as the possible cause.[16]

Patients may present initially with mania, hypomania, depression, or a mixed episode. Nevertheless, it is important to note that 75% of patients report having had multiple episodes of depression before the development of a manic episode.[14] Not surprisingly, misdiagnosis (primarily as unipolar depression) is common, occurring in roughly 70% of patients.[14] Multiple physicians are often consulted for diagnostic evaluation. By some accounts one of four patients visit as many as five physicians before an accurate diagnosis is made. A significant contribution to misdiagnosis is the underreporting of manic symptoms, which are not considered to be particularly problematic by patients.[14]

BD is a recurrent illness; single episodes of mania occur in fewer than 10%.[5] Most suffer multiple episodes of mania, hypomania, or depression separated by periods of euthymia (normal mood) throughout the course of their lives. In the majority, mania occurs just before or immediately after a depressive episode.[5] There may be a 5- to 10-year period from the onset of illness until the first hospitalization or diagnosis of BD.[16]

The course of illness is characterized by the type of episode(s), duration of euthymic intervals, frequency of relapse, severity of episodes, and predominant syndrome (mania, hypomania, or depression). These factors do not remain fixed throughout an individual's illness. For instance, individuals may experience episodes of dysphoria and depression before ever experiencing hypomania or mania. Often, the euthymic interval and cycle length decrease with additional episodes. With time, a course of alternating recurrent depression interspersed with manic or hypomanic episodes and no intervening euthymic periods can develop.

A subtype of BD, termed *rapid cycling,* occurs in both bipolar I and II disorder and is defined as suffering four or more mood episodes per year. Rapid cycling is common, occurring in 20% of cases; women are more often affected than men.[17] The rapid cycling type of BD is often refractory to conventional treatment and carries significant morbidity and mortality because of rapid changes in mood states.

The prognosis, even for treated BD, is concerning, with 73% experiencing a recurrent mood episode within 5 years. Furthermore, nearly half continue to have significant mood symptoms between episodes, whereas less than 20% are euthymic or have minimal symptoms.[18]

Complications of Bipolar Illness

Patients with BD have higher rates of mortality from both natural and unnatural causes. Higher rates of natural deaths largely result from cardiovascular disease.[19] Suicide (primarily in depressive and mixed episodes) and excessive risk-taking behaviors (primarily during manic or hypomanic episodes) also contribute to the high mortality rate. The lifetime risk of suicide is 17% to 19%.[20] Previous suicide attempts and the presence of hopelessness are primary risk factors for completed suicide.[21] Nonlethal suicidal behavior also has risk factors that are multifactorial and include a family history of suicide, younger age at onset, greater severity of mood episodes, the presence of mixed states, rapid cycling, comorbid psychiatric conditions, and substance use.[21] Fortunately, overall mortality as well as deaths owing to suicide or cardiovascular disease are significantly reduced when BD is adequately treated.[18]

Substance use in BD is common, with approximately 42% having comorbid substance use disorders.[8] Rapid cyclers and those with dysphoric mania have the highest rates of substance use.[22] BD becomes difficult to treat in the face of active substance use. Constant intoxication and withdrawal not only impact the course of BD but masquerade as mood episodes. Symptoms are highly recurrent, and treatment resistance is common, as is violence and suicidal behavior.[23] The best outcome is achieved with aggressive simultaneous management of both BD and the concurrent substance use disorder.

Individuals with BD are likely to experience stress and upheaval in many areas of their lives, including relationships, employment, and finances. Of bipolar patients, 88% have been hospitalized once and 66% at least two times.[24] Patients with manic and depressive episodes have divorce rates that are twofold to threefold higher than those found in nonaffected populations. Patients often report having poor relationships with family members, and nearly 75% report that their family members have a limited understanding of BD.[14] Employment problems may result from bizarre, inappropriate, or unreliable behavior. In one study, 60% of patients reported being unemployed, 88% felt the disease affected how well they performed at work, and 63% felt that they were treated differently from their peers.[14] Financial and legal problems are tied to excessive spending, involvement in schemes, substance abuse, and risk-taking behavior.

Treatment Overview

Several North American guidelines and guideline updates exist for the treatment of BD. Only the Canadian Network for Mood and Anxiety Treatments (CANMAT) and the Texas Medication Algorithm Project have been recently updated.[20,25,26] The American Psychiatric Association Guidelines from 2002, although outdated, remain a useful reference for general information about the illness and time-tested treatments of BD.[16] The reader should be forewarned that the majority of published research and guidelines focus on bipolar type I disorder, particularly the management of acute manic or mixed episodes. There remains less published research and resultantly less consensus about the treatment of bipolar type II disorder, hypomanic episodes, bipolar depressive episodes, and relapse prevention (maintenance) strategies.

The goals of treatment across the phases of illness are manyfold, including the control of acute symptoms, symptomatic remission, return to a normal level of functioning, prevention of relapses, and prevention of suicide.[16] Both the acute treatment of manic and depressive episodes and the maintenance treatment for prevention of future episodes requires individualization of therapy. Treatment decisions should take into account presenting symptoms, history of response, patient preference, and comorbid medical or substance use conditions.

Initial treatment for hypomanic or manic episodes should be with one of the well-established antimanic agents such as lithium, valproate (VPA), or an atypical antipsychotic (AAP). In the case of mixed episodes, VPA or an AAP are preferred over lithium. During episodes of mania, short-term adjunctive use of benzodiazepines are often useful to reduce agitation and promote sleep.[16] In the case of severe manic symptoms or in those only partially responsive to an adequate trial of monotherapy (generally 1–2 weeks), a two-drug combination of lithium, valproate, or an AAP is recommended.[25] Carbamazepine (CBZ), oxcarbazepine, or a typical antipsychotic, alone or in combination with a preferred antimanic drug, are potential alternatives. For treatment-resistant cases, electroconvulsive therapy (ECT), clozapine, or a three-drug combination of lithium plus an anticonvulsant (CBZ, oxcarbazepine, VPA) plus an AAP are recommended. When drug combinations are used, the individual agents should possess different mechanisms of action.

Medications for the treatment of bipolar depression ideally produce an acute antidepressant response and prevent future depressive episodes, all while not inducing mania or mood cycling. Long-term tolerability is critical because of the chronic recurrent nature of depressive episodes in BD. First-line treatments include lithium or lamotrigine.[25,26] If monotherapy with either drug fails, then a second-line approach is to use the combination of lithium and lamotrigine. Third-line treatment includes quetiapine or the fixed olanzapine–fluoxetine combination (OFC), both of which have well-established efficacy but significant long-term risks for metabolic complications. Next, alternative two-drug combinations of lithium or lamotrigine plus quetiapine or OFC may be used.[25] Subsequent trials can include antidepressants such as selective serotonin reuptake inhibitors (SSRIs), bupropion, or serotonin and norepinephrine reuptake inhibitors (SNRIs) in combination with an antimanic agent.[25] Patients with severe depressive symptoms or who are treatment resistant can be considered for ECT.

Maintenance treatment of BD should include continuing the acute-phase treatment while periodically simplifying and moving toward monotherapy with lithium, VPA, or lamotrigine. Many AAPs are effective in maintenance treatment of BD; however, they must be used cautiously because of the long-term risk of metabolic complications.[27] Regardless of the regimen selected, medication adherence is critical to long-term recovery. Patients and caregivers must be actively engaged in discussing causes of nonadherence, including ambivalence, side effects, lack of insight, and a strong desire to maintain the euphoria and energy of manic episodes.[16] Patients should also be advised to maintain regular patterns of daily activities, a consistent sleep–wake cycle, meals, exercise routines, and other schedules to promote stability.

CLINICAL ASSESSMENT

Clinical Presentation and Diagnosis

CASE 84-1

QUESTION 1: H.M. is a 23-year-old man, accompanied to the clinic by his wife, A.M. She called the clinic before bringing him in and reported much of the following information. A.M. says that he was doing well until about 3 weeks ago, when his niece was killed in an automobile accident. At the funeral, he borrowed some "nerve pills" from his cousin. Since then, H.M. has been acting increasingly "wild." He has been staying up later at night and often bursts into the bedroom at 2 or 3 AM and loudly awakens A.M. Sometimes, he presents her with expensive gifts, which they cannot afford. He often jumps on the bed and starts singing her love songs in a loud voice. A.M. notes that H.M. then almost always demands sex, after which he sleeps for a few hours and then loudly gets up and leaves the house.

H.M. recently has experienced problems at work, where he is a snack delivery truck driver. During the last several weeks, he was noted to be loading his truck in a rapid and reckless manner. His boss received several reports that H.M. was driving unsafely and at high speeds. Store owners called to complain that he was giving away free cases of snacks to customers, and he often did not complete deliveries to the stores at the end of his route. Last week, when his boss called to express concern about his behavior, H.M. said he was quitting his job. He wrote an illegible resignation note, which was at least ten pages long, called an overnight air delivery service to send the note to his employer (who is located only 3 miles from his home), and then left the house before the driver arrived to pick it up. H.M. returned several hours later with a brand new car and wearing an expensive new suit, red cowboy boots, and a bright green hat with a large feather. He told A.M. that he had a new job, which was going to make him a millionaire. Last night, she found a large sum of money in his pants pocket when emptying the clothes hamper. He did not come home at all, but he called her at 4 AM to tell her to pack for Dallas, where he was going to become the new head coach of the professional football team.

On arriving at the clinic, H.M. insists, "I don't need no doc. I am supercalifragilistic!" He then bursts into song. He is dressed flamboyantly but needs a shave and shower. He gives the examiner (a stranger) a bear hug and has trouble sitting still, listening, or allowing others to talk. His speech is pressured and loud; he often fails to complete sentences or communicate entire ideas, and he is rhyming and punning. His mood obviously is elevated, but he becomes increasingly irritable throughout the examination. He insists he must get to Texas to sing the national anthem at a football game before the CIA can stop him; he then breaks down in tears. Within moments, he is again smiling and talking of money-making schemes. He is oriented to person and place, but thinks it is tomorrow. Intelligence seems average. When asked to interpret a proverb, H.M. becomes angry, throws a chair across the room, and yells, "Enough of this! Air Force One is waiting for me!" He then storms out of the office.

How is H.M.'s presentation consistent with the diagnosis of a manic episode?

The hallmark of a manic episode is changes in mood, behavior, cognition, and perception (Table 84-1).[11] H.M. demonstrates an elevated mood. He is exuberant and notes how great he feels. Nevertheless, manic patients often demonstrate lability in their mood, and they may become irritable and easily frustrated, especially when challenged. In this case, H.M. becomes irritable and resentful when questioned by the examiner. His quick displays of sadness and anger further demonstrate the volatility of his mood.

H.M. displays behavior and speech typical of acute mania. He has a reduced need for sleep, behaves recklessly, and is overactive. His speech is pressured, loud, and full of rhymes and puns, and he sings to express his emotions and skips from topic to topic in a flight of ideas. Behavior often is characterized as being excessive.

H.M. dresses flamboyantly, hugs his examiner, writes an unnecessarily lengthy letter of resignation, seeks an overnight courier service for local delivery, presents his wife with lavish gifts, and distributes merchandise to strangers.

Delusions are often present in acute mania and are grandiose in nature and deal with inflated abilities, self-importance, wealth, or special missions in life. H.M. makes unrealistic comments about his money-making schemes, his singing ability, his position as the coach of a professional football team, and his intended use of the presidential plane. Persecutory delusions may also be present, such as H.M.'s fear that the CIA is going to stop him.

Patients with acute mania are often disorganized and do not complete tasks. They tend to skip from idea to idea and scheme to scheme. In this case, H.M. neglects his hygiene, fails to complete his deliveries, and neglects sending out his resignation letter.

Precipitating Factors

CASE 84-1, QUESTION 2: What factors make H.M. vulnerable to the occurrence of a manic episode at this time?

The mean age of onset for BD is 21 years.[8] Thus, H.M. is at the age at which his disorder would likely first manifest itself. In addition, manic episodes are often precipitated by psychosocial stressors.[28] The death of H.M.'s niece may have served as a predisposing factor for the development of a manic episode.

A variety of medications and clinical states can induce or precipitate manic episodes (Table 84-2).[29–50] The drugs that most commonly precipitate mania affect monoamine neurotransmitters, such as antidepressants and stimulants.[29] Corticosteroids, anabolic steroids, isoniazid, levodopa, caffeine, and over-the-counter stimulants can induce or aggravate mania. Sleep loss also can be a significant cause of mania.[28] A reduction in sleep after the death of his niece could have contributed to the development of H.M.'s manic episode.

TABLE 84-2
Selected Drugs Reported to Induce Mania[29–50]

Anticonvulsants	Gabapentin, lamotrigine, topiramate
Antidepressants	Monoamine oxidase inhibitors, TCAs, SSRIs, SNRIs, bupropion, nefazodone, trazodone, mirtazapine
Antimicrobials	Clarithromycin, ofloxacin, cotrimoxazole, erythromycin, isoniazid, metronidazole, zidovudine, efavirenz
Antiparkinsonian drugs	Levodopa, amantadine, bromocriptine
Anxiolytics/hypnotics	Buspirone, alprazolam, triazolam
Atypical antipsychotics	Aripiprazole, olanzapine, quetiapine, risperidone, ziprasidone
CNS stimulants	Caffeine, cocaine, methylphenidate, amphetamine
Drugs of abuse	Marijuana, PCP, LSD
Endocrine	Corticosteroids, thyroid supplements, androgens
Herbals	St. John's wort, SAMe, ma-huang, omega-3 fatty acids, tryptophan
Sympathomimetics	Ephedrine, phenylpropanolamine, pseudoephedrine, phenylephrine
Miscellaneous	Cimetidine, tramadol, sibutramine

CNS, central nervous system; LSD, lysergic acid diethylamide; PCP, phencyclidine; SAMe, *S*-adenosyl-L-methionine; SNRI, serotonin and norepinephrine reuptake inhibitor; SSRI, selective serotonin reuptake inhibitor; TCA, tricyclic antidepressant.

CASE 84-1, QUESTION 3: If the "nerve pills" borrowed by H.M. were antidepressants, could they have contributed to the development of his manic episode?

All major classes of antidepressants including monoamine oxidase inhibitors, tricyclic antidepressants (TCAs), SSRIs, and SNRIs precipitate mania in an estimated 20% to 40% of patients with BD.[30] Despite this risk, up to 78% of patients with BD are treated with antidepressants (but only 56% receive mood stabilizers).[51] There are numerous case reports of mania or hypomania with antidepressant treatment, but few controlled studies, making it difficult to make comparisons across antidepressant classes. A comparison of the monoamine oxidase inhibitor, tranylcypromine, and the TCA, imipramine, found a similar rate of treatment emergent mania (21% and 25%, respectively).[52] A meta-analysis found a higher "switch" to mania rate for TCAs (11%) than for SSRIs (4%).[53] A controlled trial with bupropion, sertraline, and venlafaxine (all in combination with a mood stabilizer) found an overall switch rate of 19% during acute treatment and 37% during the continuation phase of the study with no difference among agents.[54] Antidepressants may also cause cycle acceleration, which effectively decreases the time between mood episodes. The risk for cycle acceleration may be heightened for patients who experience manic or hypomanic symptoms on antidepressants despite receiving antimanic treatment concurrently.[55] In the case of H.M., an antidepressant may have precipitated the manic episode or shortened his cycle, moving him into an episode of mania from a pre-existing state of depression or euthymic mood.[56] Any patient presenting with a manic or mixed episode should have all antidepressants discontinued.[20]

TREATMENT OF ACUTE MANIA

CASE 84-1, QUESTION 4: Why does H.M. require treatment?

Manic episodes have a number of severe complications. Left untreated, severe mania can result in confusion, fever, exhaustion, and even death. The impairment in judgment, the excesses, and the risk-taking that occur during manic episodes may be devastating. Detriments to relationships, careers, and finances and physical harm or loss of life may occur. Manic individuals may engage in illegal activities or behave in a manner that results in a violation of the law. H.M. drives recklessly; may have lost his job; spends excessive amounts of money on gifts, clothing, and automobiles; and plans to participate in a variety of money-making schemes. He has acquired a great deal of cash suddenly, perhaps from withdrawing all of his family's savings or from some type of illegal enterprise. Manic patients may engage in risky sexual encounters, leading to infection with sexually transmitted diseases including human immunodeficiency virus. Alcohol and drug abuse are common and may exacerbate or even precipitate mood episodes. Irritability, such as that demonstrated by H.M., can lead to episodes of violence, resulting in potential harm to the patient or to others. The goals of treatment are to reduce the severity and duration of the current mood episode as well as to prevent recurrence of future episodes.

Valproate (Divalproex, Valproic Acid)

CASE 84-1, QUESTION 5: What is the appropriate treatment for H.M.'s acute manic episode?

Depending on the type and severity of mania, first-line treatment includes lithium, VPA, AAPs (aripiprazole, quetiapine, risperidone, ziprasidone), or a combination of these agents.[25,26] Considering H.M.'s presentation, monotherapy with a first-line agent is appropriate. VPA is an ideal choice for H.M. considering the rapid onset, improved tolerability, and the established efficacy of this agent for preventing future mood episodes.[57]

DOSING AND MONITORING

CASE 84-1, QUESTION 6: VPA was chosen for the management of H.M.'s mania. How should VPA be initiated, and what baseline tests are necessary? How will H.M.'s response to therapy be monitored?

The initial dose of VPA for H.M. should be 250 mg three times per day.[16] The dosage should then be increased by 250 to 500 mg every 2 to 3 days to obtain steady-state serum VPA levels between 45 and 125 mcg/mL or a maximum dosage of 60 mg/kg/day.[58] An alternative strategy is to use an oral loading regimen of 20 to 30 mg/kg/day given on a three times a day schedule during an acute episode of mania. This approach has been used during inpatient management, and may result in a more rapid onset of effect.[59] The correlation between serum concentration and efficacy is not well established. VPA levels of 45 mcg/mL are the minimum threshold with higher concentrations offering greater benefit. In fact, those exceeding a serum concentration of 84 mcg/mL by the third day of treatment had greater early symptom improvement.[59] A pooled analysis demonstrated a linear relationship between serum concentration and efficacy with the greatest improvement found in patients with VPA levels in excess of 94 mcg/mL.[60] VPA levels greater than 125 mcg/mL are more often associated with side effects and should be avoided.[57]

Before VPA is initiated, baseline laboratory tests, including a complete blood count (CBC) with differential and platelets, and liver function tests should be obtained. H.M.'s baseline weight and neurologic status should be recorded. In premenopausal women who have not undergone surgical sterilization, a baseline pregnancy test is warranted. Attention should be given to any medications that might be administered concurrently. Interactions with aspirin, phenytoin, phenobarbital, lamotrigine, rifampin, warfarin, felbamate, and CBZ are cited frequently (also see Chapter 58, Seizure Disorders).

VPA should decrease the severity and duration of H.M.'s current manic episode, decrease the frequency of subsequent episodes, and increase his time spent in a euthymic state. Once treatment has started, H.M. should be monitored for response of his initial target symptoms, including grandiosity, decreased need for sleep, pressured speech, distractibility, and impulsivity. Symptom improvement with VPA can be expected in approximately 5 days.[61]

SIDE EFFECTS

CASE 84-1, QUESTION 7: What are the potential side effects of VPA therapy? How should H.M. be monitored for these possible effects?

H.M. should be monitored for potential dose-related adverse reactions of VPA including various gastrointestinal complaints (nausea, diarrhea, dyspepsia, anorexia), sedation, ataxia, tremor, benign hepatic transaminase elevations, and thrombocytopenia. Gastrointestinal complaints may be mitigated by reducing the dosage, changing to an extended-release preparation, or administering an antacid or histamine H_2-antagonist. Central nervous system effects such as ataxia and sedation may respond to dosage reduction, although sedation may resolve with continued treatment. If tremor is bothersome or interferes with the patient's functioning, dosage reduction or change to the extended-release preparation may provide relief.[62] Alopecia occurs in 0.5% to 12% of patients and may improve with dose reduction.[63] Small elevations in transaminases are considered benign; however, VPA should be discontinued if elevations are more than two to three times the upper limit of normal.

Weight gain occurs in up to 20% of patients receiving VPA.[57] The increase in body weight is particularly distressing to some patients and may contribute to medication nonadherence. Weight gain has been associated with VPA serum concentrations greater than 125 mcg/mL; therefore, dosage reduction may be helpful.[57] In women, VPA has been associated with the development of polycystic ovary syndrome.[64] Core features of polycystic ovary syndrome include oligomenorrhea and hyperandrogenism, which develop in about 10% of women with BD taking VPA.

There are several reports of VPA-induced hyperammonemic encephalopathy in psychiatric patients.[65,66] Patients presenting with coma or mental status changes should have serum ammonia and liver functions tests ordered. If VPA-induced hyperammonemic encephalopathy is suspected, then VPA should be discontinued. Other serious adverse events with VPA include fulminant hepatic failure, agranulocytosis, and pancreatitis. All of these adverse events require immediate discontinuation of therapy.

Once VPA therapy is initiated, liver function tests, VPA serum levels, and CBCs with differential and platelets should be monitored at least monthly for the first 3 months and every 3 to 6 months thereafter.[16] Body weight should also be determined at baseline and monitored monthly during therapy.

CASE 84-1, QUESTION 8: H.M. was titrated to a total daily VPA dosage of 2,500 mg/day and determined to have a steady-state plasma concentration of 95 mcg/mL after 1 month of treatment. A routine CBC with differential and platelet count was ordered at this time, and the following data were reported:

White blood cell count, 8.5 × 103/μL
Hemoglobin, 14.5 g/dL
Hematocrit, 43%
Red blood cells, 5.2 × 106/μL
Neutrophils, 59%
Lymphocytes, 27%
Monocytes, 6%
Eosinophils, 2%
Basophils, 0.5%
Platelets, 75 × 103/μL

How should H.M.'s VPA-induced thrombocytopenia be managed?

VPA-induced thrombocytopenia occurs in 18% of patients and is associated with female gender and higher VPA levels (>100 mcg/mL in women and >130 mcg/mL in men).[67] Clinicians should educate patients to look for signs such as easy bruising or bleeding. In most patients, thrombocytopenia is asymptomatic and responds to a lowering of the VPA dosage; complete discontinuation of the drug is usually unnecessary.[68] H.M.'s dosage should be reduced, and his platelet count should be monitored closely. In addition, he should be observed for reemerging symptoms of mania.

Lithium

PRELITHIUM WORKUP

CASE 84-2

QUESTION 1: C.N., a 21-year-old woman, was diagnosed with her first episode of mania 3 weeks ago. At that time, she was hospitalized and treated with lithium at a dose of 1,200 mg/day (serum level, 0.8 mEq/L). C.N.'s manic episode was stabilized, and after 10 days she was discharged from the hospital. She was scheduled to see her outpatient psychiatrist for follow-up 1 week later, but she failed to keep the appointment. Today, C.N. arrives at the emergency department at the request of her mother. C.N. is grabbing her mother's hair and kicking wildly as she is pulled from the car. She can be heard screaming "The FBI is after me, Mom! You want them to find me, don't you? I would have made it out of the country if you hadn't gotten in the way! I was going to marry Prince Charles and become the new queen of England." On evaluation, C.N.'s mood is irritable, and she is pacing around the interviewer. She is dressed in a short skirt and high heels and is wearing an excessive amount of makeup and costume jewelry. During the interview, she interrupts the examiner, smiles, and says in a loud, provocative voice, "Let's you and me get out of here!" Her mother states that after C.N. was discharged from the hospital, she lost her prescription and, within several days, stopped attending her classes at the local community college. She began staying out late, playing her radio loudly, and driving recklessly, finally hitting the side of the garage while parking early this morning. What laboratory tests are required before initiating lithium therapy for C.N.?

Because lithium can affect many organ systems, baseline laboratory values must be evaluated before therapy is initiated. These values will serve to determine whether future abnormal values are lithium related. Furthermore, various physiologic states may affect lithium's excretion or predispose one to lithium toxicity. In these cases, baseline laboratory tests are useful in determining contraindications to the use of lithium or conditions that require an adjustment in dosage. As a young, healthy female, C.N.'s prescreening laboratory battery should include electrolytes, blood urea nitrogen, creatinine, urine specific gravity, thyroid-stimulating hormone (TSH), thyroxine (T_4), and a CBC (Table 84-3). Also, a pregnancy test should be obtained before starting therapy.

TABLE 84-3
Routine Monitoring During Lithium Therapy

	Baseline	Every 1–3 Months	Yearly
CBC	X		
Electrolytes	X		X
Renal function[a]	X		X
ECG[b]	X		X
Urine	X		
Thyroid function	X		X
Lithium level[c]		X	
Weight or BMI	X		X
Pregnancy[d]	X		

[a] Monitor more often in patients with history of kidney disease.
[b] Patients ≥45 years or those with history of cardiac disease.
[c] Weekly monitoring during the first month of treatment is often recommended.
[d] Women of childbearing potential.
BMI, body mass index; CBC, complete blood count; ECG, electrocardiogram.

DOSING

CASE 84-2, QUESTION 2: C.N.'s baseline laboratory parameters were normal, and her pregnancy test was negative. How should lithium treatment for C.N. be initiated?

Because C.N. has previously responded to lithium and she does not have rapid cycling or mixed BD, she is likely to respond to lithium again. Although there are many strategies for calculating lithium dosage requirements, it is simplest to begin C.N. at a dosage of 300 mg twice daily. This is a common starting dose for a healthy adult patient.

Patients experiencing an acute manic episode require higher lithium levels compared with maintenance therapy. The goal for the acute management of C.N. is a serum level between 0.5 and 1.2 mEq/L.[16] Because lithium is not immediately effective, C.N.'s lithium dosage can be adjusted based on the results of lithium serum levels checked weekly until the manic episode resolves. As she recovers and enters the maintenance phase of treatment, both C.N.'s lithium dosage and her lithium levels will require re-evaluation (see Case 84-8, Question 1).

CASE 84-2, QUESTION 3: How long will it take for C.N. to get the full effect of lithium?

The half-life of lithium in a young patient with normal renal function is approximately 24 hours; therefore, steady-state concentrations are typically achieved in approximately 5 days. The onset of action is slow, taking as long as 1 to 2 weeks to fully exert its therapeutic effects.[16] Because of the delay in onset, it is appropriate to use an adjunctive medication to help reduce C.N.'s acute symptoms. Both benzodiazepines and antipsychotics have been used in this manner.[16] AAPs are preferred over typical antipsychotics (see also Chapter 82, Schizophrenia) and have been demonstrated to enhance efficacy and accelerate time to response when used in combination with lithium in acute mania.[27] Benzodiazepines work rapidly to reduce agitation, anxiety, and insomnia.[69]

SIDE EFFECTS

CASE 84-2, QUESTION 4: After 3 weeks of therapy, C.N. is demonstrating significant improvement in her sleep, impulsivity, delusions, and activity level. She has achieved her previous lithium carbonate dose of 1,200 mg/day, and her lithium level is 0.8 mEq/L. Today she is complaining to the nursing staff that she has developed a hand tremor. Soon after her physician arrives to evaluate her, C.N. asks to be excused so that she can go to the bathroom. How might C.N.'s presentation be related to her medication?

When considering side effect management early in lithium therapy, it becomes important to monitor lithium levels closely. When patients start to recover from acute mania, the rate of lithium clearance may decrease and patients may demonstrate an increase in lithium levels and worsening side effects (Table 84-4). This does not seem to be the case with C.N. because her lithium level is within the accepted range for the management of acute mania.

C.N. is complaining of a hand tremor. She should be interviewed and examined to determine its origin. In this case, the likely medication-related cause for the tremor would be lithium. Lithium-induced tremor occurs in 10% to 65% of treated patients and is characteristically rapid, regular, and fine in amplitude.[69,70] Often, this tremor occurs early in therapy and improves with

TABLE 84-4
Lithium Adverse Effects

Organ System	Clinical Presentation	Comments
Cardiovascular	ECG changes	T-wave suppression, delayed or irregular rhythm, increase in PVCs; SSNS; myocarditis
	Edema	Primarily ankles and feet; transient or intermittent; secondary to effects on sodium and carbohydrate metabolism; caution about diuretics and sodium restriction to avoid lithium toxicity
Dermatologic	Acne	Worsens
	Psoriasis	Treatment-refractory worsening
	Rashes	Maculopapular and follicular
Endocrine	Hypothyroidism	About 5% goiter; about 30% clinically significant hypothyroidism; may diminish sex drive
	Hyperparathyroidism	Clinically not significant
Fetus (teratogenic)	Tricuspid valve malformation, atrial septal defect	Ebstein anomaly
Gastrointestinal	Anorexia, nausea (10%–30%)	Usually early in treatment and usually transient; may be early sign of toxicity
	Diarrhea (5%–20%)	Slow-release preparations may help
Hematologic	Leukocytosis	May be useful in disorders such as Felty syndrome, iatrogenic neutropenia. May counter CBZ-induced leukopenia
Neurologic	Tremor (10%–65%)	Dose-related; men > women; worse with antidepressants and antipsychotics; reduce dose or use β-blocker
	Cognitive disruption (10%)	Worsens compliance; perceived as "mental dulling"
	Poor concentration or memory; fatigue or weakness	May be early toxicity; may mimic depression
Renal	Polyuria-polydipsia (nephrogenic diabetes insipidus)	May be an indication of morphological changes; requires adequate hydration

CBZ, carbamazepine; ECG, electrocardiogram; PVC, premature ventricular contraction; SSNS, sick sinus node syndrome.
Reprinted with permission from Janicak PG et al. Treatment with mood stabilizers. In: *Principles and Practice of Psychopharmacotherapy.* 4th ed. Philadelphia, PA: Lippincott Williams & Wilkins; 2006:426.

time. Caffeine, personal or family history of tremor, alcoholism, anxiety, antidepressants, antipsychotics, and possibly older age enhance the risk of lithium-induced tremor.[70] The tremor is more common in patients with higher serum concentrations and may be worse at times of peak lithium levels.[16] If C.N. is not bothered by the tremor and suffers no impairment, treatment is not necessary. If the tremor becomes problematic, her lithium dosage may be reduced or a β-adrenergic blocking agent can be added. Additionally, switching to a sustained-release lithium preparation may reduce peak serum levels and ameliorate tremors associated with peak concentrations.[16] Because it is early in treatment and C.N. has only a moderate lithium level, it is reasonable to add propranolol 10 mg three times a day rather than to reduce the lithium dosage (if an intervention is required). Propranolol usually is effective at dosages less than 160 mg/day.[70] C.N. should be educated about her tremor and instructed to minimize her caffeine consumption.

In addition, C.N. should be asked about her trip to the bathroom during this clinic visit because lithium may cause both diarrhea and polyuria. Polyuria and polydipsia are common, occurring in up to 60% of patients.[71] Nephrogenic diabetes insipidus is less common, affecting about 10% of patients on long-term treatment.[72] Nephrogenic diabetes insipidus is dose dependent, so C.N. can be told that a lower lithium dose may minimize the symptoms. Although the advantages of once-daily administration of lithium are not universally accepted, switching a stabilized patient to this schedule with its lower trough levels may help to reduce urine volume.[16] If C.N. were to fail to respond to either of these interventions, amiloride could be administered, which minimizes lithium's effect on free water clearance.[16,73]

If C.N.'s trip to the bathroom was because of diarrhea, lithium should be evaluated as a possible cause; up to 20% of patients started on lithium experience diarrhea, epigastric bloating, and sometimes stomach pain early in therapy.[74] Diarrhea from lithium is associated with high serum levels, once-daily dosing, and rapidly absorbed preparations; therefore, divided doses may help to alleviate the problem. Use of lower doses and switching to sustained-release preparations are alternative strategies that could be used if C.N. is experiencing diarrhea or polyuria. Her fluid status and lithium level also should be monitored closely. Dehydration leads to increased lithium reabsorption in the proximal tubule and could result in accumulation and lithium toxicity.

CASE 84-2, QUESTION 5: What should C.N. be told regarding potential renal damage from lithium?

C.N. should be informed that lithium can adversely affect her kidneys. Long term treatment has been associated with declines in kidney function and rarely end-stage renal disease.[75] Routine monitoring of renal function (Table 84-3) allows for the identification of patients with precipitous declines in glomerular filtration. In such patients, lithium should be discontinued to prevent progression to end-stage renal disease. Risk factors for renal insufficiency include episodes of lithium intoxication, medical conditions that impair glomerular filtration (e.g., hypertension, diabetes mellitus), and concurrent medications that are damaging to the kidney.[76] Communication with her physician about situations that increase the risk of lithium toxicity (see Case 84-2, Question 7) and cooperation with regular lithium and renal function monitoring can vastly reduce the risk of renal disease. Finally, C.N. must be informed that polyuria is not related to any of the more serious renal side effects.

PATIENT EDUCATION

CASE 84-2, QUESTION 6: What does C.N. need to know about lithium before she is discharged?

As with all drugs, C.N. should be instructed to disclose the medications she is taking to all of her health care providers. She should be informed that dehydration, fever, vomiting, or sodium-restricted diets could lead to increases in her lithium level. Therefore, she needs to drink plenty of fluids and eat a diet consistent in the amount of sodium.

C.N. should be instructed to contact her physician if she starts to experience any symptoms of lithium toxicity, including worsening tremor, slurred speech, muscle weakness or twitches, or difficulty walking. C.N. should be told to use caution in selecting over-the-counter medications. Specifically, she should be warned to avoid the use of preparations containing nonsteroidal anti-inflammatory drugs, which can increase lithium levels.[77] C.N. should know that caffeine can sometimes be troublesome in patients taking lithium, worsening tremor on a short-term basis and lowering lithium levels during the long term.[77] With regard to serum lithium level monitoring, C.N. needs to know that lithium levels usually are drawn approximately 12 hours after a dose of lithium. If she is taking lithium in the evening and the morning, she should take her evening dose and then report for a blood sample to be drawn in the morning before taking her morning dose.

TOXICITY

CASE 84-2, QUESTION 7: One day, C.N.'s mother calls, concerned that C.N. has been complaining of nausea, vomiting, and diarrhea for several days. During the past few hours, C.N. has become confused and has developed a coarse tremor and slurred speech. It has been 4 months since C.N.'s lithium level has been checked. The only change is that C.N. started taking ibuprofen recently for headaches. What action should be taken?

There is a strong possibility that C.N. is suffering from lithium toxicity, which can occur acutely from an overdose or insidiously from reduced lithium clearance. *Mild toxicity* at levels less than 1.5 mEq/L causes feelings of apathy, lethargy, and muscle weakness accompanied by nausea and irritability. *Moderate toxicity* occurs between 1.5 and 2.5 mEq/L with symptoms progressing to coarse tremor, slurred speech, unsteady gait, drowsiness, confusion, muscle twitches, and blurred vision. *Severe toxicity* at levels greater than 2.5 mEq/L can result in seizures, stupor, coma, renal failure, and cardiovascular collapse. C.N. seems to be experiencing moderate lithium toxicity. She should hold her lithium dose and be taken to the emergency department immediately, where stat laboratory tests, including a lithium level, electrolytes, and renal function tests, should be ordered. Intravenous solutions should be started to ensure that C.N. is hydrated adequately, and electrolyte abnormalities should be corrected promptly. Depending on the results of physical examination and laboratory tests, cardiac monitoring should be instituted. Her ibuprofen should be discontinued.

HYPOTHYROIDISM

CASE 84-2, QUESTION 8: After receiving lithium 1,200 mg/day for 1 year, C.N. returns complaining that the lithium is slowing her down. She is tired and has gained weight in recent weeks and thinks that she is becoming depressed. In the examining room, C.N. complains that the temperature is too cold. What is the most likely cause of C.N.'s complaints? What treatment should be instituted?

C.N.'s symptoms are consistent with those of hypothyroidism.

ONLINE CONTENT

For a graphic that shows the dominant clinical manifestations for hypothyroidism, see http://thepoint.lww.com/AT10e.

Lithium affects the incorporation of iodine into thyroid hormone, interferes with secretion of thyroid hormones, and may interfere with the peripheral conversion of T_4 to T_3 (triiodothyronine).[78] According to laboratory indices, the incidence of hypothyroidism in lithium-treated BD patients ranges from 28% to 32% compared with 6% to 11% in patients not taking lithium.[79] Risk factors for lithium-induced hypothyroidism include female sex, family history of hypothyroidism or thyroid illness in first-degree relatives, weight gain, elevated baseline TSH, pre-existing autoantibodies, an iodine-deficient diet, rapid cycling, and elevated lithium levels.[80] For women, the first 2 years of treatment is a period of heightened risk as well as for any patient starting lithium in middle age.[80]

Thyroid function tests should be ordered to evaluate C.N.'s current symptoms. If she is found to be hypothyroid, discontinuation of therapy is *not* necessary. She should receive levothyroxine in doses that normalize her thyroid function tests. Even if she has an elevated TSH with normal levels of T_3 and T_4, low-dose thyroid supplementation may help to resolve her symptoms, and prevent breakthrough depression.[78]

DRUG AND DIETARY INTERACTIONS

CASE 84-3

QUESTION 1: T.J., a 35-year-old man, is hospitalized and treated with lithium for a severe manic episode. He had a stable lithium level of around 0.84 mEq/L for several weeks, but his last two levels were 0.65 and 0.61 mEq/L without any change in his drug therapy. T.J. insists that he is taking the medication as prescribed. The nursing staff believes that he is compliant with his medication but notes that he is spending more time off the ward and in the cafeteria. What factors could contribute to a decrease in T.J.'s lithium levels?

Drug interactions are a common cause of changes in lithium levels, but there have been no changes in T.J.'s regimen (Table 84-5 provides a list of clinically significant drug interactions). Changes in formulation or brand may sometimes have an impact on lithium levels. Nevertheless, lithium is relatively well absorbed and has a long elimination half-life, so this usually does not result in large changes in the 12-hour postdose lithium level. Occasionally, patients switched from lithium citrate to solid dosage forms experience small changes in lithium levels.

T.J. should be questioned about his visits to the cafeteria because diet can have a major influence on lithium excretion. If T.J. is consuming large amounts of caffeinated beverages or salty snacks, a reduction in lithium levels could occur. Increases in dietary sodium intake and the ingestion of methylxanthines (e.g., caffeine, theophylline) can increase lithium clearance.[77]

Finally, acute mania can increase lithium clearance.[81] If T.J. was showing signs of a relapse, his decrease in lithium levels might be attributable to his return to a manic state.

TABLE 84-5
Lithium Drug Interactions of Clinical Significance

Drugs That Increase Lithium Levels	
NSAIDs	Many NSAIDs have been reported to increase lithium levels as much as 50%–60%. This probably is owing to an enhanced reabsorption of sodium and lithium secondary to inhibition of prostaglandin synthesis.
Diuretics	All diuretics can contribute to sodium depletion. Sodium depletion can result in an increased proximal tubular reabsorption of sodium and lithium. Thiazidelike diuretics cause the greatest increase in lithium levels, whereas loop diuretics and potassium-sparing diuretics seem to be somewhat safer.
ACE inhibitors	ACE inhibitors and lithium both result in volume depletion and a reduction in glomerular filtration rate. This results in reduced lithium excretion.
Drugs That Decrease Lithium Levels	
Theophylline, caffeine	Theophylline and caffeine may increase renal clearance of lithium and result in a decrease in levels in the range of 20%.
Acetazolamide	Acetazolamide may impair proximal tubular reabsorption of lithium ions.
Sodium	High dietary sodium intake promotes the renal clearance of lithium.
Drugs That Increase Lithium Toxicity	
Methyldopa	Cases of sedation, dysphoria, and confusion owing to the combined use of lithium and methyldopa have been reported.
Carbamazepine	Cases of neurotoxicity involving the combined use of lithium and carbamazepine have been reported in patients with normal lithium levels.
Calcium-channel antagonists	Cases of neurotoxicity involving the combined use of lithium and the calcium-channel blockers verapamil and diltiazem have been reported. Lithium interferes with calcium transport across cells.
Antipsychotics	Cases of neurotoxicity (encephalopathic syndrome, extrapyramidal effects, cerebellar effect, EEG abnormalities) have been reported owing to the combined use of lithium and various antipsychotics. The interaction may be related to increase in phenothiazine levels, changes in tissue uptake of lithium, or dopamine-blocking effects of lithium. Studies attempting to demonstrate this effect have yielded differing results.
Serotonin-selective reuptake inhibitors	Fluvoxamine and fluoxetine have been reported to result in toxicity when added to lithium. Sertraline has been reported to cause nausea and tremor in lithium recipients.

ACE, angiotensin-converting enzyme; EEG, electroencephalogram; NSAIDs, nonsteroidal anti-inflammatory drugs.

LITHIUM IN PREGNANCY

CASE 84-4

QUESTION 1: A.J., a 36-year-old woman, has been maintained successfully on lithium therapy for 5 years for BD. She asks whether she should stay on lithium because she plans to become pregnant in the near future.

Lithium has been associated with a variety of congenital malformations, including the rare cardiac malformation, Ebstein anomaly.[82] There is considerable disagreement about the importance of lithium as a teratogen. Lithium was originally thought to increase the risk of Ebstein anomaly 400 times; however, the risk is more likely 20 to 40 times higher than in the general population.[83] The current estimated overall risk for congenital malformations is approximately 4% to 12% (compared with 2% to 4% in controls).[84] Because malformations are most likely to occur in the first trimester of pregnancy, it is advisable for patients to avoid lithium, when possible, during this high-risk period.

In addition to cardiac malformations, infants exposed to lithium have been reported to have hypotonia, nephrogenic diabetes insipidus, and thyroid abnormalities.[82] Lithium administration during pregnancy increases the risk of premature delivery by a factor of two to three.[85] Unfortunately, the relative safety of other psychotropic agents commonly used in BD is either not ideal or unknown. VPA and CBZ are categorized as US Food and Drug Administration (FDA) category D during pregnancy; the general consensus is that these medications are genuine teratogens and should be avoided.[86] Lamotrigine has not been consistently associated with an increased risk of fetal anomalies thus far in available surveys, but the data are best regarded as preliminary at the present time. Typical antipsychotics are classified as pregnancy category C, suggesting that adverse morphologic outcomes are less common than with mood stabilizers. Data on AAPs are also preliminary, but it is worth noting that in a recent comparison of placental passage, olanzapine was associated with the highest exposure (72% ratio of umbilical cord-to-maternal plasma concentrations), followed by haloperidol (65%), risperidone (49%), and quetiapine (24%).[87] Olanzapine was also associated with the highest rates of low birth weight and neonatal intensive care unit admissions. For additional information on the safety of psychotropic medications see Chapter 58, Seizure Disorders, and all chapters in Section 15, Psychiatric Disorders, and Section 16, Substance Abuse.

A.J. and her physician should discuss her individual risks related to lithium treatment. In addition to the risks of teratogenicity, they must consider the harm that could result from the possible recurrence of episodes of mania or depression and the risks inherent in discontinuing lithium or switching to another antimanic agent. Also, A.J. should be actively involved in the decision-making process.

If A.J. and her physician decide that she is to remain on lithium, her levels must be monitored closely during pregnancy and her dosage adjusted periodically. Lithium clearance increases during the third trimester by 30% to 50%, resulting in a reduction in lithium levels and a need for dosage adjustment.[83] Approximately 16 to 18 weeks after conception, screening tests, high-resolution ultrasound, and fetal echocardiography can be used to determine whether cardiac defects have developed.[83] If possible, A.J.'s physician should consider decreasing the lithium dose before delivery to minimize lithium levels in the newborn and to offset the reduction in lithium excretion that occurs after delivery.[83]

If A.J. and her physician decide that she is to discontinue lithium, they must be prepared to deal with the risks of lithium discontinuation. Several cases of presumed rebound mania have occurred after abrupt cessation of lithium therapy. If lithium is to be discontinued in A.J., it should be gradually reduced over at least 4 weeks.

CASE 84-4, QUESTION 2: A.J. did not use lithium throughout her pregnancy. After delivery, A.J. and her physician decide to restart lithium. How soon can this take place?

Lithium can be restarted as soon as A.J.'s urine output is established and she is fully hydrated. However, this decision also may be affected by whether or not A.J. chooses to breast-feed her child because lithium passes into breast milk and is present in concentrations up to 72% of that found in the maternal blood.[82] Risks to the newborn include hypothyroidism, cyanosis, hypotonia, lethargy, and cardiac dysrhythmias. Hydration status must be closely monitored because lithium toxicity may develop during infantile illnesses. Thus, A.J. and her physician must discuss the advantages of breast-feeding versus the risks of exposing the newborn to lithium or withholding lithium during the postpartum period. A.J. should be informed that approximately 40% to 70% of women with BD experience affective episodes after delivery.[82]

If A.J. chooses to breast-feed while taking lithium, she should consider using infant formula when the child becomes ill because febrile illness, vomiting, and diarrhea can increase the risk of lithium toxicity. She also should be instructed to contact her pediatrician if the infant experiences diarrhea, vomiting, hypotonia, poor sucking, muscle twitches, restlessness, or other unexplained changes in behavior.

ATYPICAL ANTIPSYCHOTICS

CASE 84-5

QUESTION 1: D.W., a 34-year-old female singer and musician, recently experienced her fourth hospital admission for a manic episode. She also has psoriasis and asthma. A trial of lithium led to worsening of her psoriasis and unacceptable tremor, which interfered with her guitar playing. Use of β-blockers was not considered because of her asthma. She was subsequently switched to VPA monotherapy; however, tremor has again become problematic. Furthermore, she is concerned about her appearance because she has begun to experience weight gain and hair loss from the VPA. What other drugs are available for the treatment of acute mania?

AAPs are acceptable first-line choices for the treatment of acute mania. Three recent systematic reviews and meta-analyses support the efficacy of AAPs as a class.[88–90] Perlis et al. reviewed data from 12 randomized, placebo-controlled, monotherapy studies and 6 adjunctive studies and found a collective response rate of 53% for AAPs compared with 30% for placebo.[88] There was no difference in response between the individual AAPs. In adjunctive studies, the mean odds ratio was 2.4 for a 50% improvement with the addition of an AAP to a mood stabilizer (primarily lithium or VPA). Scherk et al. conducted a meta-analysis of 24 randomized controlled trials and found superiority of AAPs for acute mania in comparison to placebo and equal efficacy to lithium, VPA, and haloperidol.[89] In this analysis, the addition of an AAP to lithium, VPA, or CBZ was found to be more effective in reducing manic symptoms and yield less treatment discontinuation than lithium or the anticonvulsant alone. The results of a different meta-analysis specifically designed to evaluate combination treatment of AAPs with lithium or an anticonvulsant also found greater efficacy for the combined regimen.[90] In most combination therapy studies, AAPs were limited to patients having no response or only a partial response to lithium or an anticonvulsant. Thus, the utility of drug combinations as initial therapy cannot be directly assessed.

Although the AAPs seem to be equally effective for the treatment of acute mania, these agents differ in their adverse effect profiles (see also Chapter 82, Schizophrenia). A significant concern about the use of AAPs is the risk of metabolic complications, including weight gain, glucose dysregulation, and dyslipidemia. Clozapine and olanzapine have the highest risk for metabolic complications, quetiapine and risperidone are associated with an intermediate risk, and ziprasidone and aripiprazole seem to have the lowest risk.[27,91] Clozapine is also associated with significant safety concerns, including agranulocytosis, seizures, sialorrhea, anticholinergic side effects, and orthostasis. Efficacy data with clozapine are limited compared with the other AAPs, but clozapine seems to be effective in treatment-resistant mania and in long-term mood stabilization.[92–94] Several other AAPs (asenapine, iloperidone, paliperidone, and lurasidone) have recently been approved by the FDA, primarily for schizophrenia (with the exception of asenapine, which received an acute mania indication). The exact role of these agents for BD is yet to be determined.

Sedation is common with clozapine, olanzapine, and quetiapine, and this effect may be beneficial in the treatment of acute mania; however, sedation can also lead to nonadherence with long-term use.[95] Aripiprazole and ziprasidone are less sedating; thus, the adjunctive use of a benzodiazepine is often necessary in the acute management of mania. Adjunctive benzodiazepines may also benefit treatment of emergent akathisia, which occurs in 11% to 18% of patients treated with aripiprazole.[96,97] Ziprasidone may cause activation; however, this effect is attenuated at doses of 120 mg/day or more.[98] Results of the Clinical Antipsychotic Trials of Intervention Effectiveness study in schizophrenia suggest that risperidone may overall be the best tolerated of the AAPs, but this drug carries a higher risk for serum prolactin elevation and extrapyramidal symptoms.[99]

D.W.'s concern about her weight gain makes aripiprazole or ziprasidone rational choices for her manic episode. Aripiprazole should be started at 15 mg/day with the option to increase the dose to 30 mg/day. If ziprasidone is selected, it should be started at 40 mg twice daily with food and increased to 60 to 80 mg twice daily on the second day of therapy. In addition to symptom response, D.W. should be monitored for characteristic antipsychotic side effects, such as movement disorders, and metabolic complications. If D.W. fails to respond to the initially selected AAP, a switch to a different AAP may prove beneficial given the variability in individual response.[27] Table 84-6 provides dosing information for AAPs in acute mania.

CASE 84-5, QUESTION 2: What alternative agents are available for acute mania if lithium, VPA, or an AAP fail?

Anticonvulsants

CBZ represents an alternative treatment for the management of acute mania when lithium, VPA, and AAPs fail.[16,25,26] In 2005, the FDA approved the extended-release CBZ capsule for the treatment of acute manic and mixed episodes based on the results of two double-blind, randomized, placebo-controlled trials.[100] To enhance power, a pooled analysis of these two studies has been conducted.[101] The response rates at study end point were 52% for CBZ-treated patients and 26% for placebo-treated patients. Significant reductions in the Young Mania Rating Scale were achieved in both manic and mixed episodes. The mean final dose of extended-release CBZ was 707 mg/day. Despite demonstrated efficacy, CBZ remains a less than popular choice in BD. A study in an Oregon Medicaid population found that only 3% of patients with BD received CBZ (compared with 33% for VPA and 25% for lithium).[102] The risk of drug interactions and side effects are likely responsible for the low level of CBZ use.

CBZ should be started at 100 to 200 mg twice daily. The dose should be increased by 200 mg every 3 to 4 days until adequate serum levels have been reached.[16] Although no correlation between CBZ serum levels and response in BD has been established, serum levels greater than 12 mcg/mL are associated with sedation and ataxia. The recommended target serum level is from 4 to 12 mcg/mL.[16] Average daily doses for maintenance therapy range from 200 to 1,600 mg/day.

TABLE 84-6
Atypical Antipsychotic Dosing in Acute Mania

Atypical Antipsychotic	Initial Dose	Titration	Effective Dose Range
Aripiprazole	15 mg/d	Not required	15–30 mg/d
Asenapine	10 mg twice daily	5 mg twice daily	5–10 mg twice daily
Olanzapine	10–15 mg/d	5 mg/d	5–20 mg/d
Quetiapine	50 mg twice daily	50 mg twice daily	200–400 mg twice daily
Quetiapine XR	300 mg/d	300 mg/d	400–800 mg/d
Risperidone	2–3 mg/d	1 mg/d	1–6 mg/d
Ziprasidone	40 mg twice daily	20–40 mg twice daily	40–80 mg twice daily

Source: Abilify (aripiprazole) [package insert]. Tokyo, Japan: Otsuka Pharmaceutical; December 2010; Saphris (asenapine) [package insert]. Whitehouse Station, NJ: Merck & Company; November 2010; Zyprexa (olanzapine) [package insert]. Indianapolis, IN: Eli Lilly and Company; November 2010; Seroquel (quetiapine) [package insert]. Wilmington, DE: Astra Zeneca Pharmaceuticals; May 2010; Seroquel Extended Release (quetiapine fumarate) [package insert]. Wilmington, DE: Astra Zeneca Pharmaceuticals; May 2010; Risperdal (risperidone) [package insert]. Titusville, NJ: Janssen, LP; August 2010; Geodon (ziprasidone) [package insert]. New York, NY: Pfizer; November 2010.

Oxcarbazepine, a structural analog of CBZ, may be an option for the treatment of BD. Oxcarbazepine has some advantages over CBZ, including improved tolerability and fewer drug interactions; however, there is a paucity of well-designed clinical trials in BD.[103] Case reports, retrospective reviews, open-label trials, and small double-blind studies have found oxcarbazepine monotherapy or adjunctive treatment to be effective in acute mania.[103] The only well-designed study of oxcarbazepine in BD did not report a significant difference from placebo on the primary end point of mean reduction in Young Mania Rating Scale scores.[104]

Other anticonvulsants studied in mania include lamotrigine, gabapentin, topiramate, tiagabine, zonisamide, and levetiracetam. Initial open-label studies of lamotrigine in mania were promising, and there is one published double-blind trial to date that showed similar responses among lamotrigine, lithium, and olanzapine.[105,106] There are two unpublished trials of lamotrigine in mania, both of which were negative.[105] Currently, experts doubt that lamotrigine has any significant effect in acute mania.

The anticonvulsant gabapentin has been studied in BD. Open trials and case reports suggested adjunctive treatment with gabapentin was effective in manic, hypomanic, and depressive states of BD.[107–109] A more recent controlled trial found no benefit of gabapentin.[110] In this double-blind, placebo-controlled trial, gabapentin was administered as an adjunctive treatment in patients with bipolar I disorder whose current episode was manic, hypomanic, or mixed. At 12 weeks, gabapentin failed to show any significant benefit compared with placebo. In fact, the placebo group did significantly better than the gabapentin-treated patients.

Topiramate was also originally suspected to have antimanic effects based largely on open-label add-on studies.[111] However, in four double-blind, placebo-controlled trials, topiramate did not separate from placebo and was less effective than lithium in the treatment of acute mania.[112] Tiagabine, levetiracetam, and zonisamide have been studied in BD but lack adequate safety or efficacy data to receive any formal evaluation.

Combination Treatment

Despite the array of treatments available for the management of acute mania, large numbers of patients fail to respond to monotherapy, and combination therapy is becoming increasingly common.[113] Potentially useful combinations include lithium plus AAPs, VPA plus AAPs, and lithium plus VPA.[20,114] A combination to be avoided is CBZ and clozapine owing to the increased risk of hematologic adverse effects. Also combinations of CBZ with either olanzapine or with risperidone result in more side effects and decreased efficacy; therefore these combinations are not recommended.[26]

Benzodiazepines and Antipsychotics for Acute Agitation

CASE 84-6

QUESTION 1: M.B. is a 39-year-old man hospitalized for an acute manic episode, but is refusing all medications, reporting "I will be robbed of my superpowers." He is found pacing around the inpatient unit shouting orders for his release. When asked to return to his room by the nursing staff, he becomes agitated, picks up a chair, and begins swinging it wildly at anyone who approaches him. In the past M.B. experienced an acute dystonic reaction to haloperidol. M.B. has a medical history of diabetes mellitus and hypertension. What is an appropriate pharmacologic intervention for M.B.?

Benzodiazepines and antipsychotics are useful in treating agitation, irritability, and hyperactivity associated with acute manic episodes. Oral formulations are preferred and are favored by patients in psychiatric emergencies.[115] Oral dose delivery can be facilitated with liquid concentrates and orally disintegrating tablets. Uncooperative patients may require intramuscular (IM) injections of benzodiazepines or antipsychotics.[116] Traditionally, the combination of IM haloperidol and IM lorazepam has been used; however, the rapid-acting IM AAPs are becoming increasingly popular with improved tolerability versus typical antipsychotics. Currently, ziprasidone, aripiprazole, and olanzapine are available in rapid-acting IM dosage forms. IM ziprasidone at doses of 10 and 20 mg is effective in psychotic agitation.[117,118] IM aripiprazole at doses of 9.75 or 15 mg and IM olanzapine 10 mg are effective for manic or mixed-state agitation.[119,120] Repeat doses of IM ziprasidone, aripiprazole, and olanzapine can be administered 2 to 4 hours after the first dose, if needed. The concurrent use of a benzodiazepine with an antipsychotic is generally safe and potentially more effective than either agent alone. In the case of IM olanzapine, concurrent benzodiazepines should *not* be used because they may cause excessive sedation and cardiorespiratory depression.[121,122]

Lorazepam is the preferred benzodiazepine for acute manic agitation. Advantages of lorazepam include availability as both an IM and oral formulation (tablet and concentrate), lack of active metabolites, and safety in hepatic and renal impairment. The Expert Consensus Guideline recommends dosing lorazepam at 1 to 3 mg orally or 0.5 mg to 3 mg IM, with repeat doses at least 60 minutes apart. The maximal dose should not exceed 10 to 12 mg in the first 24 hours.[123] The primary concern regarding the use of benzodiazepines for agitated mania is sedation. The risk of abuse and addiction is minimized with short-term inpatient use.

M.B. is uncooperative and an immediate danger to others, thus warranting IM therapy. Because of M.B.'s history of acute dystonia to haloperidol, an IM AAP (such as olanzapine, ziprasidone, or aripiprazole) should be used. The combination of ziprasidone 10 mg IM and lorazepam 2 mg IM is an appropriate intervention. IM administration of aripiprazole and lorazepam may also be used. As M.B. becomes calmer and more receptive to treatment, he should be transitioned to oral therapy.

TREATMENT OF ACUTE BIPOLAR DEPRESSION

CASE 84-7

QUESTION 1: H.C., a 31-year-old woman, was hospitalized for treatment of an acute manic episode 3 months ago. She was discharged on VPA 1,750 mg/day with a favorable response. Recently, her parents have become concerned because H.C. has spent most of the day in bed starting about 2 weeks ago. When out of bed, H.C. sits on the couch without moving for hours. She only nibbles at the food her parents offer her. She has no other signs or symptoms of physical illness and has not taken any additional medications, alcohol, or drugs of abuse to her parents' knowledge. They report that H.C. was diagnosed with diabetes mellitus type 2 last year. So far her serum glucose has been controlled by diet. On further questioning, H.C.'s parents report that she has been intermittently tearful and expressed remorse for her behavior when she was manic. They also recall her as saying "I am as low as I can go, and I just want to die." Hence, they suspect she is suicidal. H.C.'s parents report that she is taking VPA as prescribed and that the last time she was this depressed the addition of lithium to VPA did not seem to help. Her VPA level on discharge was 84 mcg/mL. What change in H.C.'s treatment should be instituted at this time?

Bipolar depression is both recurrent and chronic, accounting for three-quarters of the time spent ill in BD.[124] The depression is often difficult to treat and puts patients at significant risk for suicide, which occurs at a rate 15 times greater than that of the general population.[125] Unfortunately, bipolar depression has received limited attention in research studies and suffers from a lack of consensus among guidelines.[126]

In bipolar depression, complete remission of symptoms is the primary goal of treatment. The ideal regimen should target acute depressive symptoms, decrease suicide risk, and prevent future mood episodes (both manic and depressive). These goals should be achieved without precipitating mania (switching) or mood cycling. Because simply addressing the acute depressive symptoms is often shortsighted in an illness with recurrent depressive episodes, the ability to prevent future depressive episodes and the long-term tolerability are important considerations.[127]

A logical first step in the management of bipolar depression is to verify adherence and optimize the dose of the current mood stabilizer.[20] For H.C., she is already on a therapeutic level of VPA; thus no change in dose is needed.

Lithium

Lithium remains a first-line treatment for bipolar depression.[25,26] The CANMAT guidelines recommend a level of 0.8 mEq/L or more for optimal response.[26] The benefit of lithium was demonstrated in seven of eight placebo-controlled crossover studies with a mean response rate of 76%.[128] Lithium may also be effective for preventing depressive episodes. A 6-year follow-up study of patients maintained on lithium found a reduction in the annual rate of depressive episodes by 46% and the time spent ill by 53%.[129] A meta-analysis of 1- or 2-year-long studies found a 22% relative risk reduction for a depressive relapse compared with placebo (risk ratio, 0.78; 95% confidence interval, 0.60–1.01).[130] The difference from placebo was not statistically significant.[130] Lithium was generally well tolerated, with fewer treated patients withdrawing from the study than those taking placebo. The only common side effects were somnolence, nausea, diarrhea, and hypothyroidism.[130] Beyond antidepressant effects in BD, lithium also has the vital benefit of reducing the risk of suicide, deliberate self-harm, and all-cause mortality.[131,132]

Lamotrigine

Lamotrigine is recommended as a first-line treatment for bipolar depression by both the Texas Medication Algorithm Project and CANMAT guidelines; however, more recent data from five double-blind, placebo-controlled trials has brought this recommendation into question.[25,26] These studies did not detect any benefit from lamotrigine on the primary end points (change in Hamilton Depression Rating Scale [HAM-D], or Montgomery Åsberg Depression Rating Scale [MADRS]) relative to placebo. An independent meta-analysis of the same five studies found significant (but only modest) benefits for lamotrigine with a relative risk of response of 1.27 for the HAM-D and 1.22 for the MADRS.[133] The ability of lamotrigine to reduce the risk of relapse to depression is less controversial. A pooled analysis of two long-term studies (up to 18 months) with lamotrigine found a 36% reduction in the risk of relapse to depression.[134] Lamotrigine was well tolerated with no difference from placebo in any side effect. Because lamotrigine has limited antimanic properties, patients with a history of severe, recent, or recurrent mania should only take lamotrigine in combination with an antimanic drug, such as lithium.[25]

The combination of lamotrigine and lithium may confer additional benefits on reducing depressive symptoms and should be considered as a second-line treatment for bipolar depression. Patients stabilized on lithium (predefined range of 0.6–1.2 mEq/L, mostly >3 months' duration) were randomly assigned to receive lamotrigine (200 mg/day) or placebo. The lithium–lamotrigine group had a response rate of 52% (based on MADRS scores) compared with 32% for the lithium–placebo group.[135] From the results of this study, clinical experience, and the need for long-term tolerability, the combination of lamotrigine and lithium is an appropriate treatment when monotherapy with these drugs has failed.

Atypical Antipsychotics

AAPs offer another option for the treatment of bipolar depression. Quetiapine has demonstrated efficacy in a total of four 8-week double-blind, placebo-controlled studies (300 mg/day or 600 mg/day).[136–139] Response rates ranged from 58% to 69% for the 300-mg dose, and 58% to 70% for the 600-mg dose. Both doses were commonly associated with sedation, somnolence, dry mouth, and dizziness. Clinically significant weight gain (≥7% of baseline weight) was detected in roughly 5% to 10% of subjects receiving quetiapine. No published trials exist for the use of quetiapine to prevent depressive relapses in BD.

The combination of olanzapine with fluoxetine is effective for patients with bipolar depression.[140] In a 7-week acute-phase treatment, OFC was superior to lamotrigine in symptom improvement but not significantly different in response rate (69% with OFC versus 60% with lamotrigine).[141] In an extension of this study (for a total of 6 months), OFC caused significant elevations in all metabolic parameters (weight, glucose, prolactin, cholesterol).[142] Most alarming was a 34% incidence of clinically significant weight gain in the OFC group (vs. 2% with lamotrigine). The rate of relapse to depression during the 6-month study was low and similar between OFC and lamotrigine (14% vs. 18%). The high risk of metabolic complications for quetiapine and OFC relegate these treatments to be used cautiously as third-line treatment options.

Aripiprazole does not appear to be effective for bipolar depression on the basis of two randomized, controlled trials.[143] Considering these findings, the CANMAT guidelines have listed aripiprazole as not recommended for acute bipolar depression.[26] Other AAPs have not been systematically studied in bipolar depression.

Antidepressants

The use of antidepressants in BD has been hotly debated. Some guidelines recommend restrictive use of antidepressants because of concerns of mood switching and cycle acceleration.[25] Other guidelines recommend early treatment with antidepressants, particularly SSRIs, to address the recurrent depressive episodes.[26] In either case, there is agreement that antidepressants should only be used in combination with antimanic agents such as VPA, lithium, or an AAP.[25,26] The largest controlled trial of antidepressant augmentation in bipolar depression was conducted as part of the Systematic Treatment Enhancement Program for Bipolar Disorder (STEP-BD) study. This study was a 26-week, double-blind, placebo-controlled trial comparing antidepressants (bupropion or paroxetine) with placebo as adjunctive treatment to an antimanic agent.[144] The primary end point of durable recovery (euthymia for 8 weeks) was achieved in 24% of antidepressant-treated subjects compared with 27% receiving placebo. There was no significant difference between groups in treatment emergent mood switch. A recent meta-analysis of 15 studies, primarily with bupropion or SSRIs, found that antidepressants were no more effective than placebo for acute (<16 weeks) bipolar depression.[145] This study also did not find an increased risk of mood switch.

Because H.C. did not respond to lithium in combination with VPA during her past depressive episode, an alternative first-line agent such as lamotrigine is a reasonable choice. OFC or quetiapine may compromise her type 2 diabetes control and thus are not appropriate options. Dosing of lamotrigine needs to account for H.C.'s concurrent use of VPA, which is known to inhibit the metabolism of lamotrigine. Therefore, the initial dose for H.C. is 25 mg every other day for weeks 1 and 2 followed by an increase to 25 mg/day for weeks 3 and 4. The dose can be increased to 50 mg/day for week 5, and then to a maximum of 100 mg/day beginning at week 6. In the absence of VPA the recommended target dose of lamotrigine is 200 mg/day. In patients taking enzyme inducers (e.g., CBZ), the target dose is 200 mg twice daily. The appropriate titration schedule must be followed for lamotrigine (see also Chapter 58, Seizure Disorders) because of the risk of skin rash, which may progress to the life-threatening Stevens-Johnson syndrome. The combination of lamotrigine and VPA is a risk factor for the development of a dangerous cutaneous reaction; therefore, H.C. should be instructed to contact her physician immediately if a skin rash develops.

MAINTENANCE THERAPY OF BIPOLAR DISORDER

CASE 84-8

QUESTION 1: R.L., a 33-year-old man, has been treated for an episode of acute mania with lithium 600 mg twice a day for 3 weeks. He is no longer overtly manic. Because of R.L.'s past episodes of depression and mania, his physician decides to institute prophylactic (maintenance) lithium therapy. What are the goals of maintenance lithium therapy for R.L.? How should he be monitored during this maintenance phase? How long should R.L. be maintained on lithium?

Recurrent mood episodes are associated with an increased risk for episode recurrence, decreased quality of life, poorer response to treatment, longer hospitalizations, and cognitive impairment.[20] Thus, early maintenance (prophylactic) treatment is indicated to prevent disease progression. Appropriate goals for maintenance therapy include an increase in the interval between episodes, a decrease in the frequency of episodes, and a reduction in the duration and severity of mood episodes. In most cases, patients will have been started on an acute treatment for a manic or depressive episode. These agents should generally be continued because abrupt switches in medications may predict poorer treatment outcomes.[20]

Lithium

The aforementioned meta-analysis (Case 84-7, Question 1) of long-term lithium therapy for relapse prevention in BD included five randomized, placebo-controlled studies.[130] Although lithium did not effectively reduce the risk of relapse to depression, it did reduce the risk of relapse to any mood episode (risk ratio, 0.66) and to manic episodes specifically (risk ratio, 0.62). The average risk of relapse to *any mood episode* on lithium was 40% versus 60% for placebo. The average risk of relapse to a *manic episode* was 14% for lithium versus 24% for placebo.

In the case of R.L., he should be continued on lithium. The target levels for maintenance therapy with lithium should be in the range of 0.5 to 0.8 mEq/L.[16] Higher levels ranging from 0.8 to 1.0 mEq/L are associated with a reduced number of relapses (compared with levels between 0.4 and 0.6 mEq/L) but also have an elevated risk of side effects.[146]

In addition to determining an appropriate maintenance lithium level for R.L., it is important to consider whether once-daily administration of lithium can improve adherence or side effects. During periods of dosage readjustment, R.L. will require monitoring of his lithium serum level more frequently. Once stabilized, the monitoring frequency can be reduced to quarterly. See Table 84-3 for recommended lithium monitoring guidelines.

CASE 84-8, QUESTION 2: What other maintenance treatments for BD are available should R.L. fail to respond to lithium?

Anticonvulsants

VPA and lamotrigine are reasonable alternatives to lithium that have shown efficacy in BD maintenance therapy. In the first controlled trial of VPA for the maintenance treatment of BD, patients were randomly assigned to receive VPA, lithium, or placebo and followed for 52 weeks.[147] The three groups did not differ with regard to the primary outcome of time to any

TABLE 84-7
FDA-Approved Medications for Bipolar Disorder

Drug	Mania	Mixed	Depression	Maintenance
Carbamazepine (extended-release capsule)	X	X		
Lamotrigine				X
Lithium	X			X
Valproate (divalproex sodium)	X	X		
Asenapine	X	X		
Aripiprazole	X	X		X
Olanzapine	X	X		X
Olanzapine–fluoxetine			X	
Quetiapine	X		X	X[a]
Quetiapine XR	X	X	X	X[a]
Risperidone long-acting injection				X
Risperidone	X	X		
Ziprasidone	X	X		X[a]

[a] Adjunct to lithium or valproate.
FDA, Food and Drug Administration.

mood episode. However, a lower percentage of patients discontinued treatment for any reason in the VPA group (62%) than lithium (76%) or placebo (75%); patients on VPA remained in the study longer (198 days) than patients on lithium (152 days) but not placebo (165 days). The mean VPA serum concentration was 85 mcg/mL. Lamotrigine has been studied rigorously in the maintenance treatment of BD. A pooled analysis of two placebo-controlled studies found that lamotrigine and lithium more than doubled the time to intervention (e.g., addition of pharmacotherapy or ECT) for any mood episode compared with placebo (see Case 84-7, Question 1).[148] The time to intervention was 197 days for lamotrigine, 187 days for lithium, and 86 days for placebo. Lithium preferentially prevented manic relapses, whereas lamotrigine preferentially prevented depressive episodes.

Atypical Antipsychotics

AAPs have become increasingly popular alternatives and adjunctive treatments for maintenance therapy of BD. To date, aripiprazole, olanzapine, quetiapine (adjunctive), risperidone long-acting injection, and ziprasidone (adjunctive) have received FDA approval for the maintenance treatment of BD (Table 84-7). Comparative studies of AAPs in BD maintenance are not available. The long-term risk of side effects, including metabolic complications, should be the primary consideration for selecting one AAP over another (see Case 84-5, Question 1).

CASE 84-8, QUESTION 3: What is the role of psychotherapy in BD?

Psychotherapy can have a profound effect on the prevention of acute illness, as well as a sustained effect on maintenance treatments. Excessive stress, for example, is often implicated in the onset of affective episodes, particularly early in the lifetime course of BD.[28] If individuals and their families can learn to avoid these triggers or to develop coping skills, the acute impact can be minimized and future episodes averted.

Therapy may also help the family to cope with the extreme emotions and disruption that are the hallmark of acute manic and depressive episodes. Violent outbursts, infidelity, financial debts, and loss of self-esteem may all be a byproduct of mood recurrence, and family members must come to terms with such calamities, as well as fears surrounding future episodes. Regular sleep–wake cycles seem vital to the maintenance of euthymic states; thus, improvements in sleep hygiene may be encouraged in these sessions. Last, sustained medication adherence must also be emphasized; individuals with BD will often stop their mood stabilizers in an effort to resume the "highs" of mania or because of the cumulative side effect burden of complex psychotropic regimens.

The specific psychotherapeutic approach to BD is generally quite similar to interventions offered to individuals with schizophrenia. Family-focused therapy seems to be quite effective, as are cognitive–behavioral, interpersonal, and social rhythm therapy. Collaborative care models have been extensively studied for unipolar depression in primary-care settings, but the effectiveness of collaborative care models for bipolar illness is less clear. In fact, in the STEP-BD trials collaborative care was the least effective.[149] Reported response rates were 77% with family-focused therapy, 64% with interpersonal and social rhythm therapy, 60% with cognitive–behavioral therapy, and 54% with collaborative care. Authorities contend that the collaborative care intervention was comparatively less intensive than the other three treatment modalities in this report.

CASE 84-8, QUESTION 4: Are there other treatment options for BD?

Although most experts advocate for regular physical activity to prevent bipolar mood swings, the body of literature supporting such an approach is very limited. Lifestyle surveys have demonstrated that people afflicted with BD are less likely to exercise and more likely to exhibit poor dietary habits than those without a serious mental illness.[150] Theoretically, exercise may improve dietary habits, regulate sleep, increase energy, and promote euthymic moods. As a result, increased physical activity would be expected to improve the prognosis of bipolar illness and should be encouraged at the very least for the physical health benefits.

Alternative Medicines

A wide variety of herbal preparations and dietary supplements has been studied for the treatment of BD. There has been considerable interest in the benefits of omega-3 fatty acid supplementation. A meta-analysis of double-blind, placebo-controlled

CHAPTER CASES

8 Most children with ADHD will continue to have symptoms of their illness well into their adult years, usually of the inattention subtype. There is a growing awareness that adults with ADHD have significant social and occupational impairments. Fortunately, medications used to treat ADHD in children appear to be equally effective in adults and should be widely advocated.

Case 85-3 (Question 2)

Although the diagnosis and treatment of attention deficit and hyperactivity disorder (ADHD) have been associated with considerable controversy, ADHD is a serious psychiatric condition that has been well described in the medical literature for more than two centuries.[1] There are highly effective pharmacological treatments that ameliorate the core symptoms of the illness. These agents are generally safe and have been shown to improve long-term prognosis.[2]

By definition, ADHD symptoms manifest early in childhood, and will persist into adulthood in the majority of cases. If left untreated, ADHD can produce significant impairments in academic performance and social functioning; adults with ADHD are often hindered in occupational settings as well.[3] Psychiatric comorbidities are commonly encountered among individuals suffering from ADHD, including developmental disorders, mood disorders, and substance abuse.

Although the effectiveness of pharmacological treatments for ADHD has been widely replicated, most children and adolescents with ADHD will receive suboptimal treatment for a variety of reasons, including parental reluctance to consider psychotropic medications, the perceived stigma of mental illness, and well-described deficiencies in the delivery of health care to persons with psychiatric conditions.[4] Ultimately, ADHD poses a huge economic burden to Western society with $1.6 billion attributed annually to direct treatment costs in the United States alone, and an estimated $2.6 billion loss associated with decrements in work productivity.[5]

Although hyperactivity has been recognized as a troublesome childhood behavior for perpetuity, ADHD was not formally described in the *Diagnostic and Statistical Manual of Mental Disorders* until the third edition was released in 1980.[6] Currently, there are three different types of ADHD specified in the *Diagnostic and Statistical Manual of Mental Disorders,* Fourth Edition, Text Revision (DSM-IV-TR): inattentive, hyperactive/impulsive, and both inattentive and hyperactive/impulsive.[7] Qualitatively the core symptoms of ADHD will differ according to sex, with boys more likely to exhibit the hyperactive/impulsive subtype (vs. girls).[8] These symptoms often change with time as hyperactive and impulsive behaviors recede during adolescence, and inattention predominates among adults with ADHD.[9]

Stimulants such as methylphenidate and amphetamines have been the mainstay of ADHD treatment in children for more than 30 years, and recent studies have demonstrated acute and long-term benefits in adolescents as well as adults.[10–12] Unfortunately, stimulants have not been consistently shown to decrease delinquency rates. They have also been implicated with rare but serious side effects, and they carry an elevated risk of diversion and abuse.[12–14] Pharmacological alternatives to stimulants have been identified in recent years and have proven to be useful, albeit primarily as second-line agents among individuals with medical or psychiatric comorbidities.[12] The benefits of behavioral modification have also been emphasized in recent years, and most experts now contend that the combination of pharmacotherapy with nonpharmacological interventions will generate the best long-term prognosis for individuals with this disorder.[2]

EPIDEMIOLOGY

ADHD is a chronic neurobehavioral disorder, with an overall estimated prevalence of 6% to 12% in school-aged children worldwide.[15] The Centers for Disease Control and Prevention analyzed data from the 2006 National Survey of Children's Health and reported that the incidence of ADHD diagnoses has risen annually by an average of 3% between 1997 and 2006.[8] In 2006, 7.4% of US children ages 4 to 17 years were diagnosed with ADHD. An ADHD diagnosis was reported approximately 2.8 times more frequently among boys than girls. It is hypothesized, however, that this sex predominance may be exaggerated because the conspicuous hyperactive subtype is more common in boys. As ADHD transitions into adulthood, the prevalence falls to 4.4% (standard error 0.6), with a higher risk found in previously married men who are unemployed and non-Hispanic white.[16]

PATHOPHYSIOLOGY

Etiology

ADHD is a heterogeneous behavioral disorder with current theories implicating a substantial genetic association, environmental causes, and psychosocial factors (e.g., socioeconomic status and family relationships).

Various abnormal genetic and neurochemical abnormalities are associated with ADHD. Family studies have demonstrated that the relative risk of ADHD is six to eight times higher among first-degree relatives of persons with ADHD compared with the general ADHD population.[17] Based on twin studies, ADHD is influenced strongly by genes with an estimated heritability of 0.75 to 0.91.[18] Several candidate genes associated with ADHD have been identified, such as the dopamine receptor, dopamine-transporter receptor, and serotonin transporter gene.[18,19] Despite a small causal effect, no single gene is responsible for the symptoms seen with ADHD, but rather these symptoms are likely the result of interactions among several genes, which influence multiple neurotransmitters, including serotonin, dopamine, and norepinephrine.[18]

Brain imaging studies have documented pathophysiologic differences in the premotor frontal cortex, caudate, and globus pallidus of children with ADHD compared with control children.[20] Functional magnetic resonance imaging studies have also shown hypoperfusion with memory tests in the anterior cingulate areas in ADHD patients.[21] This area of the brain is responsible for behavioral and functional abilities that may manifest in patients with ADHD as difficulties in organization, mood, motivation, self-regulation, and ability to retain specific information while performing a particular task, which are abilities referred to as executive functioning.

DIAGNOSIS

The diagnosis of ADHD is not dependent on a single test. To diagnose ADHD in a child, the DSM-IV-TR criteria (Table 85-1)

TABLE 85-1
***Diagnostic and Statistical Manual of Mental Disorders, Fourth Edition, Text Revision* Diagnostic Criteria for Attention Deficit Hyperactivity Disorder**

Inattention Factor
(Six or more of the following nine behaviors need to be present for ≥6 months in two or more settings, such as home, school, or physician's office.)
1. Careless mistakes or inattention to detail
2. Reduced attention span
3. Poor listener
4. Cannot follow instructions and does not complete tasks
5. Difficulty organizing tasks and activities
6. Avoids and/or dislikes chores or homework
7. Loses things needed for tasks and activities
8. Easily distracted by extraneous stimuli
9. Forgetful in daily activities
Hyperactivity/Impulsivity Factor
(Six or more of the following nine behaviors need to be present for ≥6 months in two or more settings, such as home, school, or physician's office.)
Hyperactivity
1. Fidgets with hands/feet or squirms in chair
2. Cannot remain seated in the classroom
3. Uncontrollable/inappropriate restlessness
4. Difficulty in engaging in play or leisure activities quietly
5. Often on the go and appearing driven by a motor
6. Excessive talking
Impulsivity
7. Blurts out answer prior to completion of question
8. Difficulty waiting turn
9. Interrupts or intrudes on others

Reprinted with permission from American Psychiatric Association. *Diagnostic and Statistical Manual of Mental Disorders, Fourth Edition, Text Revision* (DSM-IV-TR). Arlington, VA: American Psychiatric Association Press; 2000.

should be used along with a physical examination (including neurologic status), patient or parent interview, and primary-care provider interview. Other sources of valuable information include performance reports (e.g., report cards or job reviews) and ADHD rating scales scored in two different settings.[7]

To meet criteria for ADHD, the child must have six or more symptoms present in two different settings for a minimum of 6 months. Furthermore, there must be evidence that these symptoms were present before the age of 7 years. Based on these criteria, three types of ADHD are identified: predominantly inattentive, predominately hyperactive/impulsive, and combined, which account for 10% to 15%, 5%, and 80% of cases, respectively. For example, care providers will look for symptoms that have a negative impact on the child's education, career, relationships, or social life. The additional stipulation of symptoms present in multiple settings is believed to minimize the potential for overdiagnosis of ADHD and subsequent overmedication. On occasion, however, parents or teachers may pressure clinicians into writing stimulant prescriptions for a "let's see if it helps" trial. If the medication is helpful, they may assume incorrectly that the diagnosis of ADHD is validated.

Establishing a diagnosis of ADHD in an adult who has never been treated for the disorder during childhood is difficult. In adults, ADHD is a clinical diagnosis that relies on their recollection of ADHD symptoms as a child to which the DSM-IV-TR criteria validated for children are applied. Unlike teachers who are ordinarily familiar with the symptoms associated with ADHD in children, spouses, coworkers, and employers are often unfamiliar with ADHD as a disorder that can also affect adults. They may attribute the individual's difficulties to being lazy or to underachievement.

COMORBIDITY AND PROGNOSIS

Between the ages of 10 and 25 years, the signs and symptoms of ADHD decrease in frequency and severity by about 50% every 5 years but will generally persist into adulthood.[9] In the differential diagnosis of ADHD, it is critically important to distinguish ADHD from various behavioral, developmental, or medical conditions. Psychiatric comorbidity is more common with ADHD as up to 87% of children will be diagnosed with at least one additional psychiatric disorder and 67% have at least two or more disorders.[22] Other psychiatric conditions that frequently coexist or imitate symptoms of ADHD include conduct disorder, oppositional defiant disorder, Tourette syndrome, depression, and anxiety disorders, including obsessive–compulsive disorder. Of these conditions, anxiety disorders and mood disorders are most commonly misdiagnosed as ADHD. Family histories from first-degree relatives of probands with ADHD reveal increased rates of ADHD (25% concordance rate), polysubstance dependence, antisocial personality disorder, depression, and anxiety disorders.[23] Children with ADHD are at an increased risk of having antisocial behavior, depression, and polysubstance abuse problems as adults. ADHD symptoms persist into adulthood in the majority of patients.[12] Adults with ADHD are usually self-sufficient, but they have poorer academic performance, poorer job performance, and lower socioeconomic status than do their siblings. They also have more frequent divorces, job changes, and car accidents. Most adults with ADHD report a high level of subjective distress (79%) and interpersonal problems (75%).[24]

Medical conditions often complicate the diagnosis of ADHD and should be excluded before initiating treatment. These medical conditions include head injuries, seizure disorders, metabolic disorders, cerebral infection, toxic exposures (e.g., chronic lead exposure), sleep problems, substance abuse, and hyperthyroidism.

SIGNS AND SYMPTOMS

CASE 85-1

QUESTION 1: C.B., a 6-year-old boy, was brought into a child psychiatry clinic after his mother attended his first-grade school conference, where she was told that her son was having difficulty adjusting to first grade. C.B.'s mother reported that C.B. had always been a somewhat difficult child. As an infant, he was irritable and overactive. At 7 months, when he began crawling, he would disrupt the entire house. He was unable to follow through with parental instructions to keep his feet off the furniture, avoid standing on the tops of tables, and not walk through the living room carrying melting chocolate ice pop treats. He showed disruptive behavior and did not respond well to direction to put toys away, and he never seemed to be able to keep track of what was going on around him.

In preschool, C.B. was disruptive and impulsive, with noisy, attention-seeking behaviors that continued through first grade. He was oblivious to the pleas of teachers and teaching assistants to get him to sit still and pay attention. Often he would get up and run around the room. He could not stay on task on assignments for more than 5 minutes

and safety of modafinil for ADHD and determined the drug was effective but rejected its approval for ADHD based on concerns about safety. Twelve of 933 patients developed a skin rash, with one case thought to be Stevens-Johnson syndrome.[62]

Alternative Therapy

CASE 85-2

QUESTION 1: A.D., a 6-year-old first-grader with a diagnosis of ADHD, has responded well to methylphenidate (Concerta) treatment during the school year. His mother sends him off to his father and stepmother for his annual summer visit, with explicit directions regarding use of the medication. One month later, A.D. returns home with a full bottle of medication. As he bounces around the room, A.D. reports that his father and stepmother said he did not need these "poison pills." A.D.'s mother phones the stepmother to find that they put A.D. on the Feingold diet along with sugar restriction to control his behavior. What are the roles of diet and alternative therapies in the treatment of ADHD?

The Feingold diet is the most widely known dietary intervention used for the treatment of ADHD.[72] It is based on the theory that many children are sensitive to dietary salicylates and artificially added colors, flavors, and preservatives. The elimination of these substances from the diet has been proposed to improve learning and behavioral problems associated with ADHD. However, most randomized, controlled trials do not support the purported benefits of the Feingold diet.[73] Interestingly, a recent well-controlled prospective study in the United Kingdom did show a small but statistically significant increase in hyperactive behavior among children receiving juice fortified with six specific coloring agents commonly found in candy.[74]

In recent times there has been more interest in glutenfree diets, both for children with ADHD as well as those diagnosed with autism. Gluten is a proteinaceous compound that is found in wheat, barley, and rye. Researchers have theorized that the incomplete breakdown of gluten (and casein) in the gastrointestinal tract results in the formation of an opioidlike metabolite that ultimately accumulates in the central nervous system, precipitating opioid-type behaviors (e.g., inattention, dysphoria, and somnolence). Although there is much anecdotal support for glutenfree diets, there are no published controlled investigations of gluten-free diets for ADHD.[75] Another dietary intervention hypothesis is that the elimination of all dietary sugars will reverse the hyperactivity associated with ADHD. Claims of an association between sugar intake and hyperactivity have not been supported, however, even in those children who are reportedly sensitive to the effects of sugar.[76] However, a small study recently demonstrated the benefits of emphasizing low glycemic index foods at breakfast (vs. high glycemic index) on memory and attention.[77]

A plethora of dietary supplements have also been touted as effective remedies for treating and preventing ADHD, but convincing results derived from rigorous trials are currently lacking. For instance, the use of very high doses of vitamins or minerals has been promoted as a possible intervention, but all randomized, controlled trials conducted to evaluate the effectiveness of megavitamin therapy have been negative to date.[73] Omega-3 fatty acids have been considered as possible treatments for ADHD, based largely on population studies demonstrating an association between high dietary intake and a reduced risk of various neuropsychiatric disorders. Early pilot trials of omega-3 supplementation for ADHD were promising, but larger, well-controlled investigations have failed to find demonstrable benefit.[78] Similarly, there have been reports of zinc, iron, magnesium, *Hypericum* (St. John's wort), and gingko all relieving ADHD symptoms, but the evidence to support these interventions is very limited at the present time.[79]

There have been other somatic treatments aimed at relieving ADHD symptoms that may prove to be beneficial in the years ahead.[79] Several small randomized studies have reported benefits with neurofeedback, in which children are trained to modify certain brain activities demonstrated on electroencephalographic tracings (e.g., increased slow wave or alpha activity). Preliminary evidence also supports the exploration of meditation as an effective intervention for ADHD, particularly mindfulness-based methods that have proven to be particularly helpful for depression and chronic pain conditions. Proponents of acupuncture abound, although a recent systematic review failed to find any studies of sufficient rigor to include in their analysis.[80]

Tourette Syndrome

CASE 85-3

QUESTION 1: G.S. is a 6-year-old boy referred to the Tourette syndrome clinic by his pediatrician because of worsening motor (blinking, grimacing) and vocal (throat clearing, coprolalia, grunting) tics. He is treated successfully with clonidine 0.2 mg/day (in divided doses). However, his behavior and performance in school is still so poor that his teacher refers him to the school psychologist, who diagnoses ADHD, combined type. A trial of stimulant treatment is considered. His mother is concerned about treating his two disorders simultaneously with the clonidine and a stimulant. Can stimulants be used in children with both ADHD and Tourette syndrome?

α_2-Agonists (clonidine and guanfacine) and atomoxetine have been shown to reduce symptoms of both ADHD and tic disorders.[81] A large randomized, controlled trial supports the use of clonidine in the treatment of comorbid Tourette syndrome and ADHD.[40] The Tourette's Syndrome Study Group compared the effect of methylphenidate (mean, 26 mg/day), clonidine (mean, 0.25 mg/day), and the combination (methylphenidate ~26 mg/day plus clonidine mean, 0.28 mg/day) with placebo in the treatment of 136 children (7–14 years of age) diagnosed with ADHD and Tourette syndrome. Teacher ratings showed that both clonidine and methylphenidate used as individual treatments were more effective than placebo. However, the greatest improvement was seen with the combination therapy. Clonidine primarily benefited the symptoms of impulsivity and hyperactivity, whereas methylphenidate primarily benefited inattention. A meta-analysis of trials evaluating the efficacy of the clonidine for the treatment of children and adolescents with ADHD concluded that the effect size of the drug was modest (0.58) and less than that of the psychostimulants.[82] Despite its widespread use, there is only one randomized, controlled trial that documents the effectiveness of guanfacine in the treatment of patients diagnosed with ADHD and a tic disorder. Thirty-four medication-free elementary school–age children with ADHD and a tic disorder participated.[83] After 8 weeks of treatment with a dose of 1 mg of guanfacine three times a day, the children had a mean improvement of 37% in their total score on the teacher-rated ADHD Rating Scale, compared with 8% improvement for placebo. Continuous Performance Test commission errors decreased by 22% and omission errors by 17% in the treated group, compared with increases of 29% in commission errors and of 31% in omission errors in the placebo group. However, parent-rated hyperactivity on dextroamphetamine improved by 27% in the guanfacine group and 21% in the placebo group, an insignificant difference.

Adults with Attention Deficit Hyperactivity Disorder

CASE 85-3, QUESTION 2: G.S. returns to clinic 3 months later for a follow-up appointment. He is doing quite well with a combination of methylphenidate (Concerta 36 mg daily) and clonidine (0.2 mg/day in divided doses). His mother has been using the Iowa Connors Rating Scale for ADHD, which she was taught to use as a way to monitor her son's behavior. Her observational scores show him to have an approximate average score of 8 for the past week. This score is significantly decreased from a score of 24 at his initial workup. The teacher's scores on the rating scale are similar to the mother's scores.

G.S.'s mother asks the physician whether they could talk privately for a few minutes. She relates that she thinks she has been suffering from ADHD her "whole life." Although she has never been formally diagnosed (or treated) for ADHD, she recalls that she was very fidgety in school and had a hard time sitting at her desk for more than a few minutes. She says that she was a good student in spite of the fact that she had a difficult time paying attention and was often daydreaming during class. She also remembers being scolded by her parents often for forgetting to do her chores and was notorious for losing things (e.g., homework, bike locks, hats). As an adult, she continues to have a hard time maintaining her attention, although the hyperactivity aspect of her symptoms seems to have disappeared. A talented writer, she has switched jobs every year or so, either out of boredom or because of the fact that she tried to take on too many projects and inevitably failed. Socially, she continues to struggle with following conversations, and her friends often mention that she interrupts conversations to change subjects. Out of curiosity, she has filled out the Connors Rating Scale for herself and usually scores in the "moderately impaired" range. She even admits that she tried her son's Concerta once last month and hated it ("my heart was racing and I felt like I drank way too much coffee").

What is the natural course of ADHD through adulthood? What are the diagnostic criteria for ADHD, adult onset? Are the medications used to treat children with ADHD effective for adults as well?

It is estimated that two-thirds of children with ADHD will continue to have significant symptomatology as adults.[12] Often the hyperactivity/impulsivity aspect of the illness becomes less pronounced once the child hits adolescence, but the symptoms of inattention persist into adulthood.[9] Even though many of the children with ADHD may no longer satisfy strict diagnostic criteria for ADHD as adults, the severity and persistence of inattentive symptoms can continue to cause considerable social and functional disability. One investigation followed 128 children with ADHD for several years and reported that hyperactivity and impulsivity symptoms were seen to decline at a higher rate than inattention symptoms.[9] Among a cohort of 18- to 20-year-olds who had been followed for a minimum of 4 years, 40% continued to meet the *Diagnostic and Statistical Manual of Mental Disorders*, Third Edition, Revised criteria for ADHD and more than 90% continued to experience functional problems with inattention.[9] Other researchers have followed children with ADHD to adulthood by comparing the academic records of control subjects and ADHD adults. The latter had significantly higher rates of repeated grades, tutoring, placement in special classes, and reading disability.[84,85] Adults with ADHD have been found to achieve lower socioeconomic status and experience more work difficulties and more frequent job changes.[86] In a study comparing 172 ADHD adults with 30 non-ADHD adults, the adults with ADHD reported more psychological maladjustment, more speeding violations, and more frequent changes in employment.[87] More adults with ADHD had their driver's licenses suspended, had performed more poorly at work, and had quit or been fired from their job. Adults with ADHD also were more likely to have had multiple marriages.

At the present time, the diagnostic criteria for ADHD in adults are the same as for children and adolescents.[7] At least six symptoms of either hyperactivity/impulsivity or inattention must be present for a minimum of 6 months, impairing function in two or more settings. A diagnosis of ADHD in adults also requires evidence that symptoms were present before the age of 7, and it is this stipulation that has been a focus of much controversy as it is often difficult to retrospectively document the illness many years after the clinical presentation. One notable study compared the functional outcomes of adults with ADHD before age 7 with adults who had the requisite symptoms but lacked conclusive evidence of childhood onset. The investigators found no difference between the two groups in primary outcomes such as learning disabilities, arrests, motor vehicle accidents, and divorce.[88]

In 2013, the American Psychiatric Association is scheduled to publish the 5th version of the *Diagnostic and Statistical Manual of Mental Disorders*, and it has been reported to contain revised diagnostic criteria for ADHD, including a new stipulation that symptoms must be present before the age of 12 (as opposed to 7 in the current DSM-IV-TR).[89] Also, the diagnosis of ADHD in late adolescence or adulthood will likely require a minimum of four symptoms of hyperactivity/impulsivity or inattention (vs. six in the DSM-IV-TR).

Current treatment recommendations for ADHD in adults continue to support pharmacotherapy as the first-line option for moderate to severe symptoms.[12] Although benefits have been noted for psychotherapeutic approaches such as cognitive behavioral therapy and dialectic behavioral therapy, these interventions are recommended only for adults exhibiting suboptimal response to approved medications.[90,91]

A variety of medications have been reported to be beneficial for ADHD in adults including methylphenidate,[92] desmethylphenidate,[93] mixed amphetamine salts,[94] lisdexamphetamine,[95] desipramine,[96] bupropion,[54] atomoxetine,[97,98] and modafanil.[71] In general, the effect sizes for these ADHD medications in adults have been very similar to what has traditionally been reported in children. Faraone and Glatt recently conducted a meta-analysis of medications for ADHD in adults and found that long-acting stimulants were significantly more effective than nonstimulant drugs, but that the effectiveness of shorter-acting stimulants was comparable to the latter.[10] Major limitations in methodology were noted by the authors, however, including a relatively short study duration for all trials, considerable heterogeneity in study outcomes, and the absence of any investigations that compared active treatments. The authors also noted that lower doses appeared to be more effective for inattention than hyperactivity. For example, doses for immediate-release methylphenidate were more conservative (0.3 mg/kg per dose in adults) when inattention was the predominate feature. In contrast, doses of up to 0.6 mg/kg immediate-release methylphenidate were often necessary to optimally control the behavioral feature of the disorder in children.[99] These methylphenidate doses are consistent with 0.5 to 1.0 mg/kg/day doses found to be effective in children.[92]

	CHAPTER CASES
7 Marijuana is the most widely used illicit substance. The withdrawal syndrome is generally mild, characterized by anxiety, depression, irritability, and insomnia, and does not require treatment.	**Case 86-18 (Questions 1–3)**
8 Abused inhalants include volatile solvents, volatile nitrites, and nitrous oxide. Inhalant use is most common in younger individuals and produces a wide range of effects and toxicities, including CNS depressant effects, convulsions, asphyxiation, cardiotoxicity, and neurotoxicity.	**Case 86-19 (Questions 1–3)**

ADDICTION

CASE 86-1

QUESTION 1: R.L., age 26, was recently arrested for possession and driving under the influence (DUI) of methamphetamine. This is his second DUI offense in the last year. R.L. does not use methamphetamine daily, but admits to weekly use. Does R.L. meet the criteria for a diagnosis of methamphetamine abuse?

Physical addiction or dependence occurs when repeated administration of a drug causes an altered physiologic state (neuroadaptation). After neuroadaptation, a characteristic set of withdrawal symptoms occurs when the drug is abruptly discontinued. Psychological addiction or psychological dependence refers to a "maladaptive pattern of substance use leading to clinically significant impairment or distress."[1] Habituation is a state of either chronic or periodic drug use characterized by a desire (but not a compulsion) to continue using the drug, no tendency to increase the dose, and an absence of physical addiction despite some degree of psychological dependence. These conditions collectively are now thought of as addictive disease. A different clinical syndrome is associated with each drug, but all involve a chronic process with progressive deterioration of psychological and physiologic activity secondary to the habitual use of a drug. Although the neurochemistry of the addictive process is possibly the same for all drugs, the psychosocial and pharmacokinetic aspects vary from drug to drug. Evidence, consistent with models established for alcoholism, indicates that genetically inherited traits may result in expression of addictive disease when the person is exposed to certain drugs and other habituating psychic stimuli.[2]

ONLINE CONTENT

For a graphic that shows the role of opioids in the brain reward pathway, go to http://thepoint.lww.com/AT10e.

The *Diagnostic and Statistical Manual of Mental Disorders*, fourth edition (DSM-IV) cites criteria for substance-related disorders and divides them into two groups: the substance use disorders (including criteria for distinguishing between substance dependence and substance abuse, Table 86-1) and the substance-induced disorders (intoxication, withdrawal, and others).[1] In 2008, an estimated 22.2 million persons age 12 or older were classified with substance dependence or abuse in the past year according to DSM-IV criteria.[2]

The focus of this chapter is on the pharmacologic management of intoxication, overdose, and withdrawal states of various substances of abuse. It should be noted, however, that pharmacologic treatment is only one aspect of the management of addictive disorders. Detoxification is the first step in management and should be followed by individualized, culturally appropriate psychosocial treatment that is effective in the least restrictive and most cost-effective manner. A strong therapeutic alliance between care provider and patient based on a supportive, empathic, nonjudgmental, clinically appropriate relationship is predictive of successful therapy outcomes. Drug addiction is a complex disease that disrupts many if not all aspects of an individual's life. Therefore multimodal treatment is necessary. Psychosocial therapies that may or may not include pharmacologic agents consist of individual as well as group counseling, cognitive-behavioral therapies (learning triggers for use, new coping mechanisms, and relapse prevention), motivational enhancement therapies, family counseling, and voucher-based reinforcement therapy among others. These therapies are often augmented with involvement in support groups, such as 12-step programs.

R.L. has a pattern of methamphetamine use in situations in which it is physically hazardous, as well as two arrests in the last year for DUI. R.L. meets the DSM-IV criteria for substance abuse.

OPIOIDS

Abuse of opioids includes illicit drugs, such as heroin, and the nonmedical use of prescription pain relievers. According to the Drug Enforcement Administration (DEA), prescription pain relievers appear to be increasingly diverted from legitimate and illegitimate sources of supply via the Internet.[3] In the 2009 National Survey on Drug Use and Health, the rate of past month and past year use among persons age 12 years or older reporting nonmedical use of pain relievers was second only to marijuana and far surpassed those of cocaine and heroin. The survey reported 5.3 million Americans had used prescription pain relievers nonmedically in the past month.[4] The average per-milligram price nationwide for diverted oxycodone is $1.15.[5]

Heroin

CASE 86-2

QUESTION 1: D.J., age 28, has been "fixing" (injecting) two "quarter bags" ($25 worth) of "smack" (heroin sold on the street) daily for about a month. This "run" (daily use) began when he met a new "connection" (drug supplier) at a party. D.J. describes a steady supply of "Mexican tar." He explains he began smoking the heroin but has now progressed to injecting. What is "Mexican tar"?

Heroin is produced in four major source areas, South America, Mexico, Southeast Asia, and Southwest Asia. Mexico has been the predominant supplier to the west coast of the United States and is expanding distribution in eastern US markets as South American production has decreased.[3] Mexican heroin black tar is potent, 40% to 80% pure, but contains more plant impurities than the

TABLE 86-1

American Psychiatric Association, *Diagnostic and Statistical Manual of Mental Disorders*, Criteria for Substance Dependence and Substance Abuse[1]

Criteria for Substance[a] Dependence

A maladaptive pattern of substance use, leading to clinically significant impairment or distress, as manifested by three (or more) of the following, occurring at any time in the same 12-month period:

1. Tolerance, as defined by either of the following:
   a. A need for markedly increased amounts of the substance to achieve intoxication or desired effect
   b. Markedly diminished effect with continued use of the same amount of substance
2. Withdrawal, as manifested by either of the following:
   a. The characteristic withdrawal syndrome for the substance
   b. The same (or a closely related) substance is taken to relieve or avoid withdrawal symptoms
3. The substance is often taken in larger amounts or over a longer period than was intended
4. There is a persistent desire or unsuccessful efforts to cut down or control substance use
5. A great deal of time is spent in activities to obtain the substance, use of the substance, or recovery from its effects
6. Important social, occupational, or recreational activities are given up or reduced because of substance use
7. The substance use is continued despite knowledge of having a persistent or recurrent physical or psychological problem that is likely to have been caused or exacerbated by the substance (e.g., continued drinking despite recognition that an ulcer was made worse by alcohol consumption)

Criteria for Substance Abuse

A maladaptive pattern of substance use, leading to clinically significant impairment or distress, as manifested by one (or more) of the following, occurring at any time in the same 12-month period:

1. Recurrent substance use resulting in a failure to fulfill major role obligations at work, school, home
2. Recurrent substance use in situations in which it is physically hazardous
3. Recurrent substance-related legal problems
4. Continued substance use despite having persistent or recurrent social or interpersonal problems caused or exacerbated by the effects of the substance

[a] Substance is defined as any drug, including alcohol.

Source: American Psychiatric Association. *Diagnostic and Statistical Manual of Mental Disorders.* 4th ed., Text Revision (DSM-IV-TR). Washington, DC: American Psychiatric Publishing; 2000.

white powder refined heroin from Asia or South America.[6] The purity of available heroin enables a new, younger user population, who can smoke or snort this high-purity heroin and avoid the stigma and hazards associated with needle use. As the addiction progresses and the user's "habit" (amount used daily) increases, however, the user will often begin injecting the drug. The DEA estimates there are roughly 800,000 heroin addicts in the United States. The 2008 National Survey on Drug Use and Health, which does not survey institutionalized populations, and may therefore actually underestimate the true incidence, found the number of current heroin users in the United States was 213,000 in 2008.[2]

Heroin is often sold in glassine bags referred to as "dime" ($10) or "quarter" ($25) bags. A dime bag contains 40 to 50 mg of heroin.[6] Mexican tar, which looks and feels like sticky black roofing tar, is sold as a gummy, pasty chunk, the size of a matchhead, which is enough for two to five doses. The cost of a chunk of Mexican tar this size is $20 to $25. The cost of heroin dependence can range from $20 to $200/day, depending on the level of use. Some prescription opioid abusers will eventually switch to using heroin, as it is less expensive.

Heroin Addiction

CASE 86-2, QUESTION 2: D.J. developed a "big habit" (tolerance developed, and his daily requirement of drug to maintain euphoria had increased). He could not "hustle" (obtain by any means) any more cash on a daily basis. When he tried "kicking" (abrupt cessation of drug use) the drug "cold turkey" (without any therapy for withdrawal symptoms), he became "dope sick" (typical heroin withdrawal symptoms), which was extremely unpleasant. He has been "chipping" (using only occasionally) since his withdrawal. Is D.J. "hooked" (addicted)?

Abstinence precipitated a withdrawal syndrome in D.J.; therefore, he is by definition physically addicted to heroin. The powerful ability of the drug to rapidly alleviate withdrawal symptoms results in reinforcement to continue using the drug. D.J.'s ongoing desire to continue using heroin despite his inability to afford it and his all-day hustling constitutes a psychological dependence on heroin.

Noticeable opioid physical dependence is highly variable, but it is assumed that the potential for an abstinence syndrome exists after repeated administration for only a few days.[7]

OPIOID WITHDRAWAL

CASE 86-2, QUESTION 3: D.J. arrives at the detoxification clinic 10 hours after his last dose of heroin. He is sweating and shaking and keeps yawning. His pulse is 92 and his blood pressure is 130/86 mm Hg. Should he be treated for opioid withdrawal?

Six to 12 hours after the last dose of morphine or heroin (diacetylmorphine), patients addicted to heroin will typically experience symptoms of anxiety, hyperactivity, restlessness, and insomnia with yawning, sialorrhea, rhinorrhea, and lacrimation. There may also be profuse diaphoresis with concurrent shaking chills and pilomotor activity resulting in waves of gooseflesh of the skin (thus, the term *cold turkey*). Anorexia, nausea, vomiting, abdominal cramps, and diarrhea may occur. Severe back pain may accompany muscle spasms that cause kicking movements ("kicking the habit"). These symptoms are most severe 48 to 72 hours after the last opioid dose. D.J. is exhibiting typical heroin withdrawal symptoms, and supportive therapy would be appropriate.

During withdrawal, the heart rate and blood pressure may be elevated. Inadequate nutrition and hydration, combined with vomiting, sweating, and diarrhea, can result in marked weight loss, dehydration, ketosis, and acid–base imbalance. Rarely, cardiovascular collapse has occurred during the peak phase of opiate withdrawal.

The more dramatic symptoms of heroin withdrawal subside after 7 to 14 days of abstinence even without treatment; however, a return to complete physiologic equilibrium may require months or longer.[8]

The character, severity, and time course of withdrawal symptoms that appear when an opioid drug is discontinued depend on many factors, including the particular opioid, total daily dose, interval between doses, duration of use, intent of drug use, and the health and personality of the user. Unlike the withdrawal symptoms from sedative-hypnotic drugs, opioid withdrawal symptoms are seldom life-threatening.

ONLINE CONTENT **For a graph showing the pharmacokinetics and pharmacodynamics of a fast-acting opioid (heroin) compared to a slow-acting opioid (methadone), go to http://thepoint.lww.com/AT10e.**

WITHDRAWAL FROM DIFFERENT OPIOIDS

CASE 86-3

QUESTION 1: R.F., a 33-year-old man, says he is addicted to methadone, but hours after his last dose he does not exhibit any signs of opioid withdrawal. Why is this reasonable?

Physiologic withdrawal symptoms from all opioid drugs are qualitatively similar but quantitatively different in onset, duration, and severity. Opioids with shorter durations of action tend to produce brief, intense abstinence syndromes, whereas those eliminated from the body at much slower rates produce prolonged but milder withdrawal syndromes. The abstinence syndrome of methadone is consistent with that expected for a long-acting opioid. Methadone withdrawal symptoms generally do not become apparent until 36 to 48 hours after the last dose.[8] Although the symptoms are qualitatively similar to those of morphine and heroin, they are less severe overall but are most intense around the sixth day of abstinence, and persist for 14 days or more.[6] R.F. could be telling the truth because his methadone withdrawal symptoms would not be expected to occur until 2 to 3 days after his last dose.

Iatrogenic Dependence

CASE 86-4

QUESTION 1: J.B., a 21-year-old man who underwent surgery, required oxycodone 20 mg every 4 hours for 30 days. Is it possible that J.B. will become physically dependent on morphine?

As previously discussed, physical dependence occurs in any patient after a few days of continuous administration of an opioid. In the management of acute pain, opioid dependence is generally not clinically significant because the patient is tapered off narcotic analgesics naturally as the pain condition resolves. If the opioid is abruptly stopped, the patient may experience withdrawal symptoms; however, the intensity of those symptoms varies depending on the individual's physiology, as well as the dose and duration of use of the opioid. Although the exact dose and duration of opioid administration required to produce clinically significant physical dependence is not known, higher doses and longer times of administration are likely to produce more severe symptoms of withdrawal on cessation of opioid use.

Therapeutic physical dependence should not be confused with addiction. Physical dependence is defined as a neurobiological adaptation that occurs with chronic exposure, whereas addiction is a set of maladaptive behaviors involving adverse consequences owing to use of drugs, loss of control over drug use, and preoccupation with acquisition of the drug.[1] Physical dependence and tolerance (the need for increasing doses to achieve the initial effects of the drug) can occur in the setting of addiction, but are also expected, nonpathological sequelae of chronic opioid therapy.

ONLINE CONTENT **For a graph that shows induction of tolerance by increased metabolism of drug, go to http://thepoint.lww.com/AT10e.**

Most studies evaluating the occurrence of opioid addiction resulting from the therapeutic treatment of pain have concluded the risk is low.[9] Historically, a much greater problem has been the undertreatment of pain. It has been theorized that pain may actually reduce the risk of addiction by attenuating the euphoric effects of opioids.[9]

Certain pharmacologic properties, such as high potency, rapid onset and shorter duration of action, and water solubility, may increase the likelihood of abuse of that medication. Although all opioids have some abuse liability, some are intrinsically more abusable than others. For example, the controlled-release formulations have been promoted as less likely to cause addiction than immediate-release products, because when used as intended, the reinforcing properties of the opioid are reduced. When tablets, such as OxyContin, are crushed, however, the drug's controlled-release properties are compromised, and the result is much higher dosages than what is available in the immediate-release formulation tablets. Despite the manufacturer's attempts at altering the formulation of OxyContin to make it harder to tamper with, this product can still be abused. Mixed agonist–antagonist opioids (pentazocine, nalbuphine, butorphanol) and partial mu agonist opioids (buprenorphine, tramadol) have less potential for abuse and addiction than the pure mu agonists (e.g., morphine, hydromorphone, oxycodone); however, abuse and addiction to all has been observed.[9]

The term *pseudoaddiction* has been coined to describe the inaccurate interpretation of certain "drug-seeking behaviors" in patients who are inadequately treated for pain.[9] Their preoccupation actually reflects a need for pain relief, but is erroneously interpreted as addiction.

J.B. may experience a mild withdrawal syndrome on cessation of his morphine treatment, unless the doses are tapered. To avoid precipitating withdrawal in J.B., the oxycodone should be tapered by 20 mg/day.

Medical Complications

CASE 86-5

QUESTION 1: C.F., a 30-year-old woman, presented to the emergency department with violent shaking chills. She admitted that she was a heroin addict and was forced into "doing some cottons" because of an acute financial crisis. She now fears that she has "cotton fever." How should "cotton fever" be managed, and what other medical complications of heroin addiction might be suspected?

When heroin is prepared for self-administration, cotton is used as a filter to trap adulterants; thus, some of the drug remains trapped in the cotton. These crude filters are saved, and when money or drug availability is poor, water or other solvents are added to the "old cottons" to extract any remaining drug for intravenous (IV) use. "Cotton fever" is an acute febrile reaction. The onset is within 30 minutes of injection, with shaking chills, diaphoresis, postural hypotension, tachycardia, and low-grade fever. These symptoms are initially suggestive of sepsis, but most of the symptoms resolve without treatment in 2 to 4 hours, with complete recovery in 1 day. In the past, cotton fever was believed to be an allergic reaction to tiny cotton fibers injected with the drug, but a case report suggests that the causal agent is probably *Pantoea* (formerly *Enterobacter*) *agglomerans*, via a heat-stable endotoxin.[10] Cotton and cotton plants are heavily colonized with *P. agglomerans*.[11] IV drug users will often use the term *cotton fever* to describe any short-term illness characterized by fever, chills, aches, and pains. C.F. should have blood cultures performed and receive empiric therapy with a broad-spectrum antimicrobial, such as a third-generation cephalosporin.

According to the Drug Abuse Warning Network (DAWN), heroin is consistently among the top three drugs reported in emergency department visits and drug-related deaths.[12,13] Bacterial endocarditis, sepsis, embolism, septic and aseptic abscesses, thrombophlebitis, cellulitis, and necrotizing fasciitis have also resulted from both improper sterilization of injection apparatus and needles and poor injection techniques.

The common practice of sharing "works" (needle and syringe) between friends has resulted in transmission of various infectious diseases. Chief among those is viral hepatitis, specifically the hepatitis C virus (HCV). Approximately 3.2 million Americans are infected with HCV, and most of the cases resulted from injection drug use.[14] According to the Centers for Disease Control and Prevention (CDC), in the United States, human immunodeficiency virus (HIV) infection caused by injection drug use had an overall prevalence of 9% in men and 15% in women in 2008.[15] Other infectious diseases such as syphilis, tetanus, botulism, and malaria can be transmitted in a similar manner and should be considered when evaluating this patient.

Heroin Overdose

CASE 86-6

QUESTION 1: T.F., a 21-year-old man, was found unconscious after an alleged "OD" (overdose) on "smack" (heroin). He had a decreased respiratory rate of 4 breaths per minute, cyanosis, symmetrically "pinned" (maximally miotic or pinpoint) pupils, and a slightly decreased blood pressure, 117/72 mm Hg. He has one "fresh track" (needle puncture wound) and several "old tracks" (healed scars from needle puncture wounds) in the antecubital fossa area. What is the immediate treatment of choice for this patient?

Immediate treatment includes airway management, cardiorespiratory support, and opioid reversal with naloxone. Naloxone is a full opioid competitive antagonist that rapidly reverses the respiratory depression and hypotension associated with overdose. The preferred route of administration is IV; if access cannot be gained, it may be given intramuscularly (IM), subcutaneously (SC), or by endotracheal tube.[16]

Initial IV administration of 0.2 to 0.4 mg naloxone should be slow and should be discontinued if T.F. responds. It is not necessary to precipitate opioid withdrawal symptoms; the end point of naloxone therapy is a relative stabilization of the patient's vital signs. A naloxone-precipitated, sudden-onset withdrawal syndrome is more severe than the symptoms produced by abstinence alone. Repetitive doses should be given if the patient remains unresponsive, up to a maximal dose of 10 mg of naloxone.[16] If the patient still has not responded, the diagnosis of opioid overdose should be reconsidered.[16]

The duration of action of naloxone ranges from 20 to 60 minutes, depending on the dose and route of administration. Treatment of the methadone-overdosed patient will require serial dosing of naloxone every 20 to 60 minutes because the toxic effects of this long-acting opiate recur.[16] The patient must be carefully observed after the termination of naloxone therapy to detect any reappearance of opioid intoxication. An IV infusion of naloxone may be appropriate if high doses are needed or if the patient has recurrent respiratory depression.

Treatment of Opioid Dependence

CASE 86-7

QUESTION 1: A.X., a 27-year-old man, has been addicted to heroin for 3 years but is tired of the street scene and wants to "get clean" (complete abstinence). He can no longer afford his growing daily habit but is not sure he can stop using opioids. He seems willing and determined to receive treatment for his heroin dependence. What therapeutic options are available to him?

The ultimate goal of most detoxification programs is to transform the narcotic addict into a responsible, drug-free, emotionally stable, and productive member of society. Despite many claims, no program to date fulfils all of these goals. Furthermore, all programs either have a high recidivism rate or do not produce a drug-free state. Heroin addiction, or any other chronic, compulsive form of drug abuse, is a symptom of a wide range of problems in the addictive disease patient. Therefore, no single treatment modality can be universally applied to all patients.

Treatment options can be loosely divided into either *social model programs* or *medical model programs*. Either model may be inpatient or outpatient based. Social model programs use a nonmedical approach to detoxification and ongoing recovery. Detoxification usually involves the cold turkey method of abrupt cessation of the opioid without supportive therapy. Medical model programs are based on pharmacotherapeutic treatment managed by medical professionals and additionally offer recovery-oriented counseling. One therapeutic approach involves opioid substitution for detoxification or maintenance. Currently, methadone and buprenorphine are FDA-approved for these indications. Another approach involves symptomatic treatment of withdrawal. The mainstay of this approach is the α_2-agonist clonidine. A third approach uses rapid detoxification precipitated by an opioid antagonist under general anesthesia.

Methadone treatment for opioid dependence is federally regulated and is only available through specially licensed opioid treatment programs. The Drug Addiction Treatment Act of 2000 allows qualified physicians to prescribe Schedule III, IV, and V medications approved for the treatment of opioid dependence in an office-based setting.[17] Currently, only buprenorphine, a Schedule III medication, is approved for this indication.

With A.X.'s apparently strong psychological addiction to heroin (he does not know whether he can live without opioids) and his desire to be abstinent, it would seem appropriate to attempt gradual detoxification with intensive psychosocial counseling rather than maintenance therapy.

Substitution Pharmacotherapies for Opioid Dependence

METHADONE DETOXIFICATION

CASE 86-7, QUESTION 2: A.X. starts a methadone detoxification program at a local methadone clinic. He claims to have a $100/day habit. What is the recommended methadone dose for starting treatment?

Methadone is a synthetic, potentially addictive, orally acting opiate with a prolonged duration of action of 12 to 24 hours. Pharmacologically, it is qualitatively identical to morphine and other opioid analgesics. Pioneered by Dole and Nyswander,[18] methadone substitution was considered the treatment of choice for opioid addiction by many researchers. It continues to be widely used today, but methadone has emerged as a drug of abuse, and many deaths have resulted from its excessive use.[16] In 2005, there were 4,462 deaths from methadone overdose, compared with 1,456 in 2001.[19]

Purportedly, methadone (at a dose of 80–150 mg or more) blocks the euphoriant effects of other opioids without producing euphoria itself. This dose allegedly produces a high degree of cross-tolerance to other opioids so that it is extremely difficult to "get off" (obtain euphoria) with IV injection of other opioids. Addicts, however, have been able to obtain euphoria from doses of 60 to 100 mg of methadone. Furthermore, at lower maintenance doses of methadone that do not produce euphoria, addicts have been able to reach euphoric states through the concomitant IV administration of other opioids. The higher purity heroin available today has required even higher doses of methadone to achieve cross-tolerance.[20]

Methadone detoxification involves stabilizing the patient on a daily methadone dose that is determined by the patient's response based on objective symptoms of withdrawal. This may involve the use of standard rating scales for withdrawal, such as the Clinical Opiate Withdrawal Scale.[21] Initially, methadone may be given in 5-mg increments up to a total of 10 to 20 mg during the first 24 hours.[21] Larger methadone doses (i.e., a 20-mg starting dose) may be required for patients with larger habits. If initial withdrawal symptoms persist 2 to 4 hours after initial dose administration, the dose can be supplemented with an additional 5 to 10 mg. Federal regulations allow a maximum of 40 mg as an initial dose unless a program physician documents that 40 mg was insufficient to suppress opioid withdrawal symptoms.[22] Once a stabilizing dose has been reached (usually, 40–60 mg/day, but may be as high as 120 mg/day), methadone is tapered by 20% a day for inpatients or 5% a day for outpatients.[16,21,22] Studies have suggested that slow tapers are associated with better outcomes. The duration of the taper varies, but a period of 3 to 4 weeks is generally used. The gradual taper may last as long as 6 months. The most common side effects of methadone are constipation, sweating, and sexual dysfunction.[16,21] A Cochrane review of studies comparing methadone tapers with other detoxification methods (adrenergic agonists and other opioid agonists) found that programs vary widely in design, duration, and treatment objectives, but overall the effectiveness of the treatments was similar, with most patients relapsing to heroin use.[23] Persistent drug craving, often lasting months, probably accounts for the high relapse rate. Even temporary reductions in heroin use are seen as a benefit, however, because heroin use is associated with major health (HIV, hepatitis C) and social (crime) issues. Medical management of opioid dependence should be accompanied by psychosocial treatments, such as cognitive-behavioral therapies, behavioral therapies, and self-help groups, such as Narcotics Anonymous (NA).

A reasonable starting dose of methadone for A.X. would be 20 mg orally. An additional 5 to 10 mg could be administered after 2 to 4 hours for persistent withdrawal symptoms. The daily dose should be titrated upward every third day by 10 mg until he is stabilized on a methadone dose of 60 mg/day. The drug can then be tapered slowly (e.g., 3 mg/day) with A.X. as an outpatient during a period of 4 weeks, while attending counseling sessions and support group meetings.

BUPRENORPHINE DETOXIFICATION

CASE 86-7, QUESTION 3: A.X. heard about a medication called buprenorphine that can be used instead of methadone. How might this medication be used for A.X.?

Buprenorphine, a synthetic partial opioid agonist, was approved by the FDA in October 2002 for the treatment of opioid dependence. It is a partial agonist at mu receptors, and in opioid-dependent patients it prevents withdrawal symptoms. Because of its partial effects, it produces maximal "ceiling" analgesia with sublingual doses of 24 to 32 mg, a dosage equivalent to approximately 60 to 70 mg of oral methadone. This limits its use in the management of heroin addiction. Buprenorphine is associated with a milder withdrawal syndrome compared with full opioid agonists.

Buprenorphine has a long half-life owing to its prolonged occupancy of mu receptors, and it produces a relatively mild withdrawal when discontinued. It is believed to be a safer alternative to methadone because life-threatening respiratory depression is much less likely to occur than with a pure mu agonist, unless another central nervous system (CNS) depressant is taken concurrently. Most deaths involving buprenorphine have been caused by a combination of the drug with benzodiazepines.[24,25] Naloxone bolus doses often are ineffective in reversing respiratory depression caused by buprenorphine because of its prolonged occupancy on mu receptors. Evidence suggests that continuous infusion of naloxone is necessary to overcome buprenorphine-induced respiratory depression.[26]

Because buprenorphine is a schedule III medication, it can be prescribed in an office-based setting under the Drug Addiction Treatment Act of 2000. It is available as 2- and 8-mg tablets for sublingual use. The tablets contain buprenorphine hydrochloride alone (Subutex) or in combination with naloxone (Suboxone). The naloxone is poorly absorbed orally, and its presence in the combination tablets is to discourage the IV abuse of buprenorphine. Both tablet forms can be used in an inpatient setting, but Suboxone is preferred in the outpatient setting, to decrease the risk of diversion. When initiating buprenorphine, the first dose should not be given until more than 4 hours after the last dose of a short-acting opioid, such as heroin, or 24 hours after a long-acting opioid, such as methadone. As previously discussed, evaluation of objective opioid withdrawal signs may involve use of standard rating scales. Induction dosing should begin with 2 or 4 mg on the first day, which can be repeated every 2 to 4 hours if withdrawal symptoms subside and then reappear, up to a maximum of 8 mg. The dose can then be titrated the second day in 2- to 4-mg increments to a dose of 12 to 16 mg.[25] Higher doses during induction may precipitate withdrawal symptoms. In the inpatient setting, the patient may be stabilized on a relatively low daily dose (e.g., 8 mg/day) and then tapered in increments of 2 mg/day over the course of several days.[16] In the outpatient setting, the patient should be initially stabilized on a daily dose (probably 8–32 mg/day) of buprenorphine that suppresses withdrawal. The dose should then be gradually tapered during a period of 10 to 14 days. Buprenorphine is not associated with any significant adverse effects when used to manage opioid withdrawal. Buprenorphine detoxification should be accompanied by psychosocial treatments and support groups as mentioned.

A Cochrane review found that relative to clonidine, buprenorphine is more effective in alleviating opioid withdrawal symptoms; patients treated with buprenorphine stay in treatment longer, and are more likely to complete treatment.[8] The severity of withdrawal appears to be similar for withdrawal managed with buprenorphine or methadone, but withdrawal symptoms may resolve more quickly with buprenorphine. The authors of the meta-analysis concluded that although there is limited evidence comparing buprenorphine with methadone, both agents have similar effectiveness in the management of opioid withdrawal. Buprenorphine has a higher unit-dose cost compared with methadone. A subcutaneous implant preparation that delivers 6 months of buprenorphine (probuphine) is being investigated for the management of opioid withdrawal.

MAINTENANCE THERAPY

CASE 86-7, QUESTION 4: A.X.'s friend B.P. also attends the methadone clinic but is on methadone maintenance. How is methadone used in maintenance therapy? Which methadone maintenance alternatives are appropriate for A.X.?

Methadone maintenance is the most common form of pharmacologic treatment for opioid dependence. During methadone maintenance, heroin-dependent patients are stabilized on a dose of methadone that will be sufficient to suppress withdrawal symptoms for 12 to 24 hours without producing euphoria. Studies have shown that patients maintained on methadone doses of 60 mg or more had better outcomes than those maintained on lower doses.[20] Most patients do well on a dose range of 60 to 120 mg/day, although some patients require more and some require less.[22] Drugs that induce cytochrome-P450 (CYP) 3A4 enzymes (e.g., carbamazepine, phenobarbital, efavirenz, St. John's wort) can precipitate withdrawal in patients maintained on methadone. Drugs that inhibit CYP3A4 enzymes (e.g., erythromycin, diltiazem, ketoconazole, saquinavir) extend the duration of methadone's effects. The drug is administered in one daily oral dose to maintain daily contact with the patient. With the aid of daily counseling and rehabilitation, most clinicians attempt to detoxify the patient eventually from methadone as well. Patients who relapse repeatedly despite supportive treatment may require long-term maintenance therapy.

The ultimate goal of methadone maintenance is controversial. By enabling addicts to escape from the illicit drug scene, review their present lifestyles, and reorient their goals, rehabilitation becomes possible. Early enthusiasm for methadone maintenance has now been tarnished by its use in the same abuse patterns as other opioids. Methadone is now a desired substitute for heroin among the addict population, although the high it provides is generally considered inferior to that of heroin, codeine, and other opioids.

Whether rehabilitation occurs or is even possible is confused by the lack of clear and widely accepted goals of therapy. The addition of social objectives to the therapeutic medical goal of cessation of heroin self-administration further confuses the issue. Some people believe the patient must remain completely drug-free for life (including methadone) to consider the treatment program a success. Others see opioid addictive disease as a disorder in which some opioid (methadone for example) must always be administered to the addict to correct the underlying biochemical pathology before any social rehabilitation can occur.

Medical staffing problems and disruption of the patient's employment schedules brought about by the necessity for daily doses of methadone stimulated a search for alternative drugs to methadone. Take-home dosing, allowing patients to obtain more than a single day's dose of methadone for self-administration, has frequently led to drug diversion and heroin recidivism. Another alternative for maintenance therapy is buprenorphine (see Case 86-7, Question 3). Most patients can be stabilized on 8 to 32 mg/day of buprenorphine.[16]

Once stabilized, it may be possible to switch to alternate-day or three-times-a-week dosing schedules. As discussed, buprenorphine has the advantage of office-based availability, thus removing the stigma associated with attending a methadone clinic. There has been interest in developing office-based methadone treatment as well.

When levomethadyl acetate (removed from the US market in 2003 after reports of severe cardiac-related adverse events), buprenorphine, and high-dose methadone (60–100 mg) therapies were compared with low-dose methadone (20 mg), all three therapies were effective in treating opioid dependence and were superior to low-dose methadone.[27] Trials comparing 12 to 16 mg/day of buprenorphine with moderate doses of methadone (50–60 mg/day) have generally shown comparable outcomes, although higher doses of methadone (>80 mg) appear to be superior to buprenorphine. Buprenorphine may be best suited for patients with mild to moderate physical dependence. This is A.X.'s first attempt at detoxification from heroin; therefore, he would be a good candidate for a methadone or buprenorphine substitution and taper, rather than maintenance.

Pain Management

CASE 86-8

QUESTION 1: T.A., a 44-year-old man maintained on 120 mg daily of methadone, is in severe pain owing to a fractured femur. What type of analgesic, and how much, can be used safely in this patient?

Neuroplastic changes in pain perception occur with chronic opioid use and can result in increased pain sensitivity, or hyperalgesia. In addition, cross-tolerance to the analgesic effects extends to all opioids. Therefore, patients maintained on opioid agonist treatment for addiction may actually require higher doses of opioid agonist analgesics given at shorter intervals.[28] Furthermore, there is no evidence that the use of opioids for acute pain management increases the risk of relapse. Some experts believe that poor pain control itself is an important trigger for relapse.[28] Careful clinical assessment for objective signs of pain will decrease the clinician's concerns of being manipulated. For T.A., it would be appropriate to control his pain acutely using patient-controlled analgesia (PCA) with IV morphine. Given his narcotic tolerance, the initial PCA pump settings could include a 2-mg IV bolus dose of morphine with a 6-minute lock-out interval delivering a maximum of 20 mg/hour. T.A.'s pain should be evaluated, and the regimen adjusted as needed to achieve adequate control. T.A.'s usual maintenance dose of methadone should be continued while he is receiving morphine for his acute pain. Many clinicians would divide the daily dose (e.g., 30 mg every 6 hours) to avoid excessive peak levels of narcotic. Opioid withdrawal should be strictly avoided in this patient because it is associated with hypersensitivity to painful stimuli, followed by exaggerated catecholamine and anxiety responses. The partial antagonist–agonist narcotics pentazocine (Talwin), butorphanol (Stadol), and nalbuphine (Nubain) should be avoided because their narcotic antagonist properties may precipitate opioid withdrawal symptoms when used in a patient maintained on methadone.

There is less experience in treating acute pain in patients maintained on buprenorphine.[28] Buprenorphine's high affinity for the mu receptor risks competition with, or even displacement of, full opioid agonists. Naloxone should be readily available when opioid analgesics are used in a patient maintained on buprenorphine. Alternatively, the buprenorphine maintenance dose can be converted to methadone for the duration of opioid analgesia treatment.

T.A. should be reassured that his methadone will be continued and his pain aggressively treated. T.A.'s physician should consult with the methadone maintenance program to verify methadone dose and alert them to any controlled substances used in his treatment that may be detected with drug testing.

Methadone in Pregnancy

CASE 86-9

QUESTION 1: J.R., a 28-year-old woman, has been maintained on 100 mg of methadone daily for the past year. J.R.'s last menstrual period was 8 weeks ago, and she took a home pregnancy test yesterday, which was positive. She wants to keep the baby. What issues should the clinician address with J.R.?

Methadone has been accepted since the late 1970 s to treat opioid addiction during pregnancy.[22] Methadone maintenance was determined to be the standard of care for pregnant women with opiate addiction by a 1998 National Institutes of Health (NIH) consensus panel.[29] Currently, methadone is the only opioid medication approved by the FDA for medication-assisted treatment of opioid addiction in pregnant patients. Women maintained on methadone frequently have regular menstrual periods, ovulate, conceive, and have normal pregnancies. Heroin-addicted mothers, however, generally experience more complicated pregnancies because their lifestyles often predispose them to a poor general state of health and precludes adequate prenatal medical care.[25] Infants born to heroin-addicted mothers may also be exposed to other substances (e.g., alcohol, cocaine, tobacco). These infants tend to be smaller, to weigh less at birth, and to be born prematurely compared with the children of women not using opiates.[25] J.R. should be advised to continue her methadone and be referred to an obstetrician for prenatal care.

WITHDRAWAL DURING PREGNANCY

CASE 86-9, QUESTION 2: Are there alternatives to methadone in the treatment of opioid-dependence in pregnancy? Should methadone be continued in J.R.?

J.R. should continue methadone maintenance to avoid precipitating a withdrawal syndrome. Withdrawal from methadone is not recommended for pregnant women.[22] A structured methadone maintenance program that provides access to counseling and medical care is probably at least as beneficial to the pregnancy as the pharmacologic prevention of withdrawal. The dose of methadone should be titrated individually throughout the pregnancy. The neonate can be managed for either opioid-induced CNS depression or methadone withdrawal after delivery, as needed.

Methadone continues to be the standard of care for the management of opioid dependence in pregnancy; however, a growing body of evidence suggests buprenorphine may be a reasonably safe alternative.[16] Also some evidence suggests that infants born to buprenorphine-maintained women have a lower incidence of neonatal abstinence syndrome (NAS; see Case 86-9, Question 3) and shorter hospital stays.[30–32]

NEONATAL ADDICTION

CASE 86-9, QUESTION 3: Because methadone crosses the placental barrier, will J.R.'s infant exhibit opioid withdrawal symptoms after birth, and if so, how should they be managed?

Methadone crosses the placental barrier and can cause CNS and respiratory depression as well as opioid abstinence in the newborn. In general, the most common opioid NAS symptoms include restlessness, tremors, a high-pitched cry, hypertonicity, increased reflexes, regurgitation, tachypnea, diarrhea, and sneezing. Seizures are associated with, but not necessarily caused directly by, opioid withdrawal in the neonate. The withdrawal symptoms in the newborn may be delayed for up to 3 days.

Management of the neonate's opioid withdrawal syndrome entails careful attention to hydration with demand feeding and symptomatic care. Treatment of opioid NAS should begin when symptoms occur; prophylactic therapy is not recommended. Mild withdrawal symptoms generally do not need therapy, but moderate to severe symptoms may require 14 or more days of treatment.

Symptoms of physiologic addiction are usually apparent within 48 hours of birth. At this time, treatment can be initiated. Currently, NAS is treated with either morphine or phenobarbital. Studies have suggested that morphine is superior to phenobarbital in both decreasing time of treatment and need for higher intensity of care.[30,33,34] Morphine can be started at a dose of 50 mcg/kg given orally four times daily and titrated to control symptoms. Once the NAS symptoms have stabilized, the dose can be decreased daily by 20% until discontinuation of the drug. Phenobarbital is preferred for the treatment of NAS in cases of combined dependence or benzodiazepine dependence.[30] If used, phenobarbital is instituted in doses of 5 to 10 mg/kg/day in the first 24 hours, then tapered symptomatically, usually about 20% per day. If J.R.'s infant displays opioid withdrawal symptoms (e.g., feeds poorly, becomes tremulous or agitated), morphine at a dosage of 50 mcg/kg orally given four times daily would be an appropriate intervention. This dosage is given until symptoms stabilize and then gradually tapered (e.g., 20% each day) during the next week.

BREAST-FEEDING

CASE 86-9, QUESTION 4: Should J.R. breast-feed her infant?

Methadone is excreted into the breast milk of methadone-maintained mothers. The amount of methadone in the breast milk is unlikely, however, to have adverse effects on the infant.[35] Furthermore, studies have found minimal transfer of methadone into breast milk.[22] There are little data regarding the safety of buprenorphine in breast-feeding. One study found low levels of buprenorphine and its active metabolite, norbuphine, in infants' urine.[36] Breast milk offers advantages clearly beneficial to infants, and J.R. should be encouraged to breast-feed her infant.

Opiate Antagonist Treatments

CASE 86-10

QUESTION 1: A.J. is a 41-year-old anesthesiologist seeking rehabilitation and reinstatement of his medical license

after 5 years of fentanyl abuse. Are there any special considerations in chemical dependency treatment in health care providers? Would opiate antagonist treatment be appropriate for A.J.?

Research suggests that physicians consume more opioids, sedatives, and alcohol than the general public, but less tobacco.[37] The risk is largely based on access to drugs of abuse, and drug dependence is described as an occupational hazard for health care providers. Abuse of fentanyl by anesthesiologists and abuse of meperidine by nurses has long been recognized. Fentanyl (injectable as well as transdermal formulations) and meperidine are primarily, but not exclusively, drugs of abuse among health care providers. Hospice workers and veterinarians also have access to high-potency opioids. Studies have noted that substance use was highest in psychiatrists and emergency medicine physicians and lowest in surgeons and pediatricians.[37] Fentanyl is associated with rapid development of dependence, intense tolerance, and drug-seeking behavior in addicted physicians for a period of months rather than years.

A comprehensive assessment of addicted health care providers is necessary to determine whether professional impairment is present, and whether issues involving public health and safety or violations of ethical standards, such as professional boundary violations or improprieties, require that the heath care provider be reported to his or her respective medical board. A physician's registration with the federal DEA may need to be suspended. It generally is accepted that health care providers require longer durations of treatment because they are held to a higher standard of recovery owing to concerns of public safety, and they may be clever at concealing their illness.[37] Health care providers should have structured posttreatment monitoring for at least 5 years.

If opioid addiction results from a process of classic and instrumental conditioning and is positively reinforced by self-administration and drug-seeking behavior, then narcotic antagonists may break this addiction cycle. The narcotic antagonists naloxone and naltrexone can block the euphoriant effects of heroin and other opiates, prevent the development of physical dependence, and afford protection from opioid overdose deaths. Of these two antagonists, only naltrexone appears to have any practical utility. Naloxone (Narcan) is impractical because of its short duration of action and its variable potency when taken orally. Naltrexone (Trexan) is orally active and provides a dose-related duration of opioid blockade. An oral dose of 100 mg of naltrexone will block opiate effects for 2 days, and 150 mg for 3 days. Thus, dosing on Monday, Wednesday, and Friday is possible and convenient for the patient. Naltrexone is also available in an injectable extended-release formulation for once-monthly use.[38] Patients selected for naltrexone therapy must be opioid free to avoid precipitation of withdrawal. For heroin- or morphine-dependent patients, a 4- to 7-day wait is recommended, whereas methadone addiction requires a 10- to 14-day wait. Patients who are highly motivated to abstain have been most successfully treated with this drug. A.J. is a good candidate for naltrexone therapy because of his desire to become rehabilitated and his need to remain drug-free despite continued access to opioids at work.

Ultrarapid Opiate Detoxification

CASE 86-10, QUESTION 2: Before A.J. can start naltrexone therapy, he must undergo fentanyl detoxification. Would rapid detoxification during a few hours be preferable to the more traditional detoxification methods for A.J.?

Ultrarapid opiate detoxification (UROD) has been advocated to shorten the opioid detoxification period by precipitating withdrawal with an opioid antagonist. The opioid antagonist causes rapid stripping of agonist from opioid receptors. UROD is performed under heavy sedation or general anesthesia so the patient does not consciously experience the acute withdrawal symptoms. The protocols for UROD vary in terms of the setting of the procedure (inpatient or outpatient), opioid antagonist (naloxone, nalmefene, or naltrexone), anesthetic agent, adjunctive medications, and duration of anesthesia.[39]

The UROD procedure includes risks, such as vomiting with aspiration; cardiovascular complications, including cardiac arrest; pulmonary edema; and death.[39] Some patients have reported residual withdrawal symptoms for several days. Little information exists regarding referral to ongoing treatment or relapse rates after UROD.[40] One randomized, controlled trial found no benefit of UROD compared with safer, less-expensive treatments using buprenorphine and naltrexone or clonidine and naltrexone.[39] UROD has been criticized for being simply a "quick fix" that fails to address the underlying behavior changes necessary for recovery. Additionally, it subjects patients to possible morbidity and mortality when safer, established procedures are available. The high cost of UROD limits its accessibility. More studies are needed to evaluate the risks and benefits of this approach. UROD would probably not be recommended as a first-line detoxification method for A.J.

Symptomatic Therapy of Opioid Withdrawal

CASE 86-10, QUESTION 3: How can A.J.'s opioid withdrawal be managed symptomatically? He weighs 72 kg and his blood pressure is 130/80 mm Hg.

Methadone and buprenorphine treatments for addiction have limitations (prescribing restrictions, protracted withdrawal, drug of dependence), and many patients prefer an alternative. The discovery of the ability of the α_2-adrenergic agonist, clonidine, to ameliorate some of the opioid withdrawal symptoms, has led to its widespread use as a nonopioid alternative. Other α_2-adrenergic agonists (lofexidine, guanfacine, guanabenz acetate) have also been investigated.[41] Noradrenergic outflow from the locus ceruleus is increased during opioid withdrawal and is blocked by administration of mu agonist opioids. Symptoms of opioid withdrawal, therefore, are partly caused by excessive sympathetic activity in the locus ceruleus. Central α_2-adrenergic agonists act on presynaptic autoreceptors to inhibit locus ceruleus noradrenergic outflow during mu agonist opioid withdrawal, thereby significantly reducing some of the symptoms.

Clonidine is therefore best used in a multidrug regimen (Table 86-2). The four primary symptoms of opioid withdrawal are musculoskeletal aches and pains, anxiety, insomnia, and gastrointestinal disorders. Contraindications to clonidine use include diastolic blood pressure less than 70 mm Hg, concurrent dependence on sedative-hypnotics, and clonidine hypersensitivity or previous intolerance. The most common adverse effects are sedation and hypotension. A recent Cochrane review examined studies comparing clonidine with methadone taper and found no significant difference in efficacy between the two for the treatment of heroin or methadone withdrawal.[41] A separate Cochrane review did find buprenorphine to be more effective than clonidine in alleviating opioid withdrawal symptoms.[8]

A sublingual or oral test dose of 0.1 mg (0.2 mg for patients >91 kg) of clonidine is given: if diastolic blood pressure remains more than 70 mm Hg, additional doses may be instituted, usually

TABLE 86-2
Symptomatic Therapy of Opiate Withdrawal

Symptom	Medication	Dose
Bone or joint pain	Ibuprofen	800 mg every 8 hours with food as needed
Muscle pain or cramps	Methocarbamol	750 mg every 6 hours as needed
Insomnia	Trazodone	50–150 mg at bedtime
	Chloral hydrate	500–1,500 mg at bedtime
	Flurazepam[a]	30–90 mg at bedtime
	Doxepin	50–100 mg at bedtime
Gastrointestinal hyperactivity	Belladonna alkaloids with phenobarbital[b]	Two tablets every 8 hours as needed
	Dicyclomine[b]	20 mg every 6 hours as needed
Nausea	Prochlorperazine[b]	10 mg every 6 hours as needed
	Trimethobenzamide[b]	300 mg every 6 hours as needed

[a] Avoid in concurrent benzodiazepine dependence.
[b] Anticholinergic effects also alleviate rhinorrhea, sialorrhea, diaphoresis, and lacrimation.

as transdermal patches. Transdermal absorption of clonidine from patches (Catapres-TTS) avoids most of the problems encountered with oral therapy. The number of patches applied to a hairless area of the body (usually the upper back or scapular area) depends on the patient's lean body weight: <50 kg, clonidine 5 to 7.5 mg (two or three TTS-1 patches); 50 to 91 kg, 10 mg (two TTS-2 patches or one TTS-2 and two TTS-1 patches), and >91 kg, 10 to 15 mg (two or three TTS-2 patches). Patients weighing less than 73 kg should use two of the TTS-1 patches and one TTS-2 patch so that one TTS-1 patch can be removed in the event of hypotensive complications. Patches are left on for 7 days, replaced with half the dosage during the second week, and then discontinued. Alternatively, oral clonidine can be used at a dose of 0.1 to 0.2 mg/dose two to four times daily to a maximum of approximately 1 mg/day for 2 to 4 days after cessation of opioids, then tapered and discontinued by 7 to 10 days.[41]

Clonidine is also used in conjunction with naltrexone for rapidly withdrawing patients from opioid dependence. This technique has been shown to be safe and effective.[16] The withdrawal precipitated by naltrexone is avoided by pretreating the patient with clonidine. Limitations to this technique include the need to monitor the patient for the first 8 hours because of the potential severity of the precipitated withdrawal and the need for blood pressure monitoring. An advantage is the easy transition to opioid antagonist treatment.

A.J.'s blood pressure and drug history should be evaluated for clonidine therapy. Provided his diastolic blood pressure is greater than 70 mm Hg after the clonidine test dose, he can receive the clonidine patches (one TTS-2 and two TTS-1 patches) with additional medications to treat his withdrawal symptoms, along with daily intensive psychosocial counseling.

SEDATIVE-HYPNOTICS

The sedative-hypnotics are a diverse group of compounds with broad clinical uses, including anesthesia, treatment of anxiety, and treatment of insomnia. Ethanol, also a sedative-hypnotic agent, continues to be the most widely abused substance in the United States and is discussed in Chapter 87, Alcohol Use Disorders. Benzodiazepines, which have replaced barbiturates in clinical practice, have become the prototypical sedative-hypnotic drugs of abuse. Other abused sedative-hypnotic drugs include carisoprodol and γ-hydroxybutyric acid (GHB). Carisoprodol, a nonscheduled skeletal muscle relaxant, has an active metabolite meprobamate, a sedative-hypnotic agent with known abuse potential.[42] GHB is a putative neurotransmitter abused for its euphoric and sedative-hypnotic effects.

Abstinence Syndromes Associated With Sedative-Hypnotic Dependence

CASE 86-11

QUESTION 1: During a year of therapy for anxiety, B.J. increased his dose of alprazolam to two 1-mg tablets five times a day. He has admitted to "doctor shopping" and buying alprazolam on the street to maintain his daily habit. Will he experience withdrawal symptoms if he suddenly discontinues alprazolam?

Patients who have been on long-term courses of therapeutic doses of sedative-hypnotics often experience withdrawal symptoms on abrupt discontinuation of therapy. Withdrawal syndromes seen with sedative-hypnotics are similar to those seen with alcohol withdrawal and can include insomnia, anxiety, tremors, headaches, restlessness, nausea, vomiting, hypertension, tachycardia, hypersensitivity to light, sound, and touch, and perceptual distortions.[43] Generalized tonic-clonic seizures can occur as isolated seizures or as status epilepticus. The psychoses that develop resemble the delirium tremens produced by alcohol withdrawal and are usually characterized by disorientation, agitation, delusions, and hallucinations. During the delirium, hyperthermia and agitation can lead to exhaustion, rhabdomyolysis, cardiovascular collapse, and death. Abstinence from short-acting barbiturates and meprobamate produces symptoms that peak within 1 to 5 days. Discontinuation of short-acting benzodiazepines (e.g., lorazepam, oxazepam, alprazolam, temazepam) results in the abrupt onset of withdrawal symptoms, usually within 12 to 24 hours after the last dose. Long-acting agents, and those with active metabolites, have a gradual onset of milder withdrawal symptoms compared with the short-acting agents. Withdrawal symptoms after chronic use of long-acting benzodiazepines typically occur within 5 days of cessation and peak at 1 to 9 days after the last dose.[43]

B.J. has been abusing alprazolam, taking more than the recommended maximal dose. Likely, he will experience withdrawal, possibly including seizures, if he were to abruptly discontinue the alprazolam. His withdrawal from this medication should be medically managed. He should undergo an initial physical examination and plan to be absent from his place of employment for at least a week to begin detoxification.

TABLE 86-3
Hypnotic Dose Equivalent to 30 mg Phenobarbital[43]

Pure ethanol 30–60 mL	Clonazepam 1–2 mg	Pentobarbital 100 mg
Alprazolam 0.5–1 mg	Diazepam 10 mg	Secobarbital 100 mg
Butalbital 100 mg	Flunitrazepam 1–2 mg[a]	Temazepam 15 mg
Carisoprodol 700 mg	Lorazepam 2 mg	Triazolam 0.25–0.5 mg
Chlordiazepoxide 25 mg	Oxazepam 10–15 mg	Zolpidem 5 mg

[a] Not approved for use in the United States.
Source: Dickinson WE, Eickelberg SJ. Management of sedative-hypnotic intoxication and withdrawal. In: Ries RK et al. eds. *Principles of Addiction Medicine*, 4th ed. Philadelphia, PA: Lippincott Williams & Wilkins; 2009:573.

Treatment of Sedative Withdrawal

CASE 86-11, QUESTION 2: How should B.J.'s sedative-hypnotic dependence be treated?

In clinical practice, three general medication strategies are used for withdrawing patients from sedative-hypnotics: decreasing doses of the drug of dependence (tapering); substituting (and gradual taper) of phenobarbital for the drug of dependence; and the substituting (and gradual taper) of a long-acting benzodiazepine for the drug of dependence.[44] Gradual tapering of the drug of dependence is appropriate for patients with therapeutic dose dependence or those taking long-acting sedative-hypnotics, who are not currently abusing alcohol or other substances. A recent meta-analysis suggests that management of benzodiazepine monodependence by gradual taper is preferable to abrupt discontinuation.[45] The authors also noted that a potential value may exist with carbamazepine used as an adjunctive medication for benzodiazepine taper, but larger, controlled studies are needed. The patient who is abusing sedative-hypnotics already has a strong association between the drug of choice and certain desired effects. Therefore, to minimize exacerbating addictive disease, substitution and taper with a long-acting therapeutic agent is preferred. The pharmacologic rationale for phenobarbital substitution is that it is long acting, producing little changes in serum levels between doses, thereby preventing breakthrough withdrawal symptoms. Lethal doses are many times higher than toxic doses, and dysphoria occurs with elevated dose, rendering it undesirable for users. As a result, the abuse potential is low, and there is little to no street value.

The phenobarbital method is the one most generally applicable; it is widely used in drug treatment programs because it is the best choice for patients who have lost control of their benzodiazepine use or who are polydrug users. The technique described by Smith and Wesson in 1970 remains the gold standard for the management of sedative-hypnotic withdrawal. The method involves calculating a phenobarbital replacement dose for the total daily dose of the sedative-hypnotic being abused. The calculation is based on phenobarbital equivalents (Table 86-3). If multiple sedative-hypnotics are being used, the totals for each drug and alcohol (amount of pure ethanol) are summated. The total phenobarbital substitution dose should be given in divided doses, three or four times daily (to avoid dysphoria). Because the calculated dosage is an estimate based on patient history, which may be inaccurate, it is advisable to administer a test dose if the calculated replacement dose is more than 180 mg/day. The test dose, generally one-third the total dose, is given to the patient, who is then observed for 1 to 2 hours. The patient is observed for mitigation of withdrawal symptoms as well as signs of overmedication, such as somnolence or incoordination. Once an appropriate dose is determined, the patient is usually stabilized on that dose for 1 to 2 weeks. After stabilization, a gradual taper of phenobarbital is instituted, with dosages reduced by 15 mg weekly or every other week, or 10% of the current (starting) dose per week. For the last 25% to 35% of the taper, the rate is slowed to keep the patient stabilized. The taper should be held for a few days if withdrawal symptoms occur.[43]

B.J. has an addiction to alprazolam, and because it is a short-acting benzodiazepine, it is a poor choice for tapering his dosage. Phenobarbital should be substituted for alprazolam. His total dose of alprazolam is 10 mg/day, so he should receive 300 mg of phenobarbital divided three or four times a day. The total daily phenobarbital dose should be tapered by 10% of the dose per week as tolerated.

γ-Hydroxybutyric Acid

CASE 86-12

QUESTION 1: L.S., a 24-year-old woman, has been attending "raves" (all-night dance parties) every weekend for the past few months. She has been taking "liquid ecstasy" at these parties. What drug is she likely taking, and what are the risks with its use?

γ-Hydroxybutyric acid (GHB), commonly referred to as "liquid ecstasy," is a potent "club drug." Once available as an over-the-counter nutritional supplement, primarily used by bodybuilders, the FDA removed it from the retail market in 1990 because of widespread reports of poisoning. In 2000, it was classified as a schedule I drug; however, a GHB-containing product, sodium oxybate, is available as a schedule III prescription drug for the treatment of cataplexy associated with narcolepsy. GHB is simple to manufacture, and recipes abound on the Internet. GHB prodrugs, γ-butyrolactone (GBL) and 1,4-butanediol, have not been federally scheduled as of the date of this publication and are available for purchase on the Internet. GHB is found in mammalian brain tissue, where it is derived from conversion of its parent neurotransmitter, γ-aminobutyric acid (GABA).[46] It is believed to be a neurotransmitter. Experimental evidence suggests that the mechanism of action of exogenously administered GHB involves agonist activity at the $GABA_B$ receptor.[46]

γ-Hydroxybutyric acid has CNS depressant effects and is abused for its euphorigenic properties, disinhibition, and enhanced sensuality. Its psychic effects are similar to those of alcohol, and include increased libido, short-term anterograde amnesia, and a dreamy, altered sensorium. It has a steep dose-response curve, and common adverse effects include dizziness, nausea, weakness, agitation, hallucinations, seizures, respiratory depression, and coma. Its effects are synergistic with alcohol. GHB overdose may be fatal, and there is no antidote. Treatment for GHB overdose is primarily supportive.

Highly addictive, tolerance and physical dependence can occur with regular use of GHB, and a withdrawal syndrome has been seen in people who have taken high doses of it (~18 g/day or more, although doses are variable in solution form) with frequent dosing (every 1–3 hours).[46] Withdrawal symptoms can include muscle cramps, nausea, vomiting, tremor, anxiety, insomnia, tachycardia, restlessness, and delirium or frank psychosis. Death caused by pulmonary edema has been reported. Treatment of withdrawal involves supportive care, including use of benzodiazepines (e.g., lorazepam or diazepam) for sedation. Withdrawal can last up to 2 weeks.[46]

Misrepresented sometimes as a natural and safe hypnotic, the low therapeutic index and the unknown purity of illicit supplies, particularly when sold in solution, make GHB a potentially dangerous drug. Physical dependency is a possibility as well. L.S. should be educated about GHB's potential risks. If she chooses to use GHB, she should be encouraged not to drink alcohol or use other drugs, not to drive, and to be cautious about the amount she ingests.

CENTRAL NERVOUS SYSTEM STIMULANTS

Cocaine

Cocaine is a naturally occurring alkaloid derived from the *Erythroxylon coca* plant, found mainly in the Andes Mountains of South America. Cocaine was first isolated in the 1800s and was a common ingredient in tonics and elixirs of the 1900s. The Harrison Narcotic Act of 1914 prohibited nonmedical use, and in 1970 it became a schedule II controlled substance. It is the third most frequently used drug of abuse, after marijuana and the nonmedical use of prescription opioids. According to the 2008 National Survey on Drug Use and Health, nearly 37 million people in the continental United States have tried cocaine; 5 million people used cocaine within the previous year, and 1.9 million used cocaine at least once within a month before the survey.[2] Cocaine is a CNS stimulant and has vasoconstrictive and local anesthetic properties. Cocaine's stimulant effects are primarily caused by blockade of reuptake of dopamine, norepinephrine, and serotonin. It also facilitates the release of dopamine and norepinephrine. This results in an overall increase in availability of neurotransmitters. Cocaine also has other indirect effects on neurophysiology, including effects on the endogenous opioid systems.[47,48] Cocaine is associated with compulsive use. The powerful reinforcing effects of cocaine have been identified as occurring in brain regions rich in dopaminergic nerve terminals.

DOSAGE FORMS AND ROUTES OF ADMINISTRATION

CASE 86-13

QUESTION 1: C.H. and his friends bought an "eight ball" (one eighth of an ounce) of "blow" (powdered cocaine). C.H. has only snorted cocaine, but one of his friends suggests they cook up some "rocks" to smoke. What are the distinctions between the various dosage forms of cocaine and their respective routes of administration?

In the manufacture of cocaine, organic solvents are used to solubilize the alkaloidal bases from the leaves, which are then precipitated to form a sticky material, called "pasta" or "cocaine paste." The benzoylmethylecgonine (cocaine) in this "pasta" is separated from most of the other plant alkaloids, converted to the hydrochloride or other salts, precipitated, and dried. This product is the white cocaine hydrochloride powder usually seen in the illicit market. The final product is usually "stepped on" or "cut" (diluted) with various adulterants to increase profits for the dealers. According to the DEA, in 2009 the average purity of cocaine was down from 68.1% in 2006 to 46.2%.[3] Cocaine is usually purchased on the illicit market in quantities of gram or ounce increments. The cost varies geographically, but the average for 1 g of pure powdered cocaine is $174.03.[3]

Powdered cocaine is generally snorted. Usually 10 to 25 mg of powdered cocaine is placed on a mirror or flat surface, formed into a line, and then insufflated through a straw or rolled dollar bill. A typical low to moderate user may consume 1 to 3 g/week. Cocaine powder can also be used for IV injection. The highly water-soluble powder is usually mixed with water and injected. When cocaine is injected simultaneously with heroin, this is known as a "speedball."

Cocaine hydrochloride melts at a high temperature, destroying much of its psychoactivity in the process. Therefore, it is inefficient to smoke cocaine hydrochloride in this form. The use of "freebase" cocaine became popular during the late 1970s, as this form of cocaine has a lower melting point and can therefore be smoked, producing an intense rush. For freebase, the cocaine hydrochloride is dissolved into ethyl ether. When an alkali, such as bleach (sodium hypochlorite) or sodium bicarbonate, is added to this ethyl ether, the hydrochloride salt is cleaved from the free alkaloidal cocaine base. The sugars, salts, and some of the other water-soluble adulterants are precipitated out of solution, and the free alkaloidal base remains in the ethyl ether solution. When the ether is evaporated, the freebase of cocaine remains in a powder form. The synthesis of freebase is dangerous, and the resultant product may contain residual organic solvents, thus making it highly volatile and putting the user at risk of burns.

In the mid-1980s a safer, easier method for extracting the cocaine base supplanted the traditional freebase process. In the manufacture of "crack," cocaine hydrochloride is dissolved in water. When alkali (bleach or sodium bicarbonate) is added to this aqueous solution, the free alkaloidal base ("crack") precipitates out while the salts and some adulterants stay in aqueous solution. The precipitate is commonly referred to as a "rock." The size of the rock varies but generally ranges from one tenth of a gram to a half a gram. One gram of crack retails on average from $170 to $180, and the purity generally varies from 75% to 80%.[49]

ONLINE CONTENT

For a graph that shows plasma cocaine concentrations and levels of intoxication as a function of route of administration of the drug, go to http://thepoint.lww.com/AT10e.

PHARMACOKINETICS AND EFFECTS

CASE 86-13, QUESTION 2: C.H.'s friend gets some baking soda and water from the kitchen and proceeds to convert a few grams of their cocaine into "rock." After smoking a few "hits" (doses), C.H. feels euphoric, energized, and self-confident. Are these typical cocaine effects?

C.H. is describing the typical euphoria associated with cocaine use. Cocaine generally produces a euphoriant action with a rapid onset and short duration. Snorting cocaine generally produces euphoria and stimulation within 2 minutes; smoking produces these effects within 6 to 8 seconds. Cocaine has a short elimination half-life of approximately 30 minutes owing to its rapid metabolism by esterases in the plasma, liver, brain, and other tissues.[47] When alcohol and cocaine are consumed together, a metabolite, cocaethylene, is formed. Cocaethylene intensifies the euphoric as well as the toxic effects of cocaine. The risk of death from cocaethylene is 18 to 25 times greater than with cocaine alone.[50]

An initial relaxed, euphoric, gregarious, talkative, hyperactive state characterizes the "high" of cocaine. Additionally, the person may report increased interest in sexual matters, diminished short-term memory, periods of intense concentration on one limited subject, diminished hunger, hypervigilance, and a peculiar, slightly out-of-body sense of one's actions. Without additional doses of cocaine, these feelings usually resolve into a state of mild depression, fatigue, hunger, and sleepiness by 1 to 3 hours. Physiologic manifestations include mydriasis, sinus tachycardia, vasoconstriction with hypertension, bruxism, repetitive behavior, hyperthermia, and talkativeness. After a few hours, continuous self-administration of cocaine will begin to progress from euphoria to dysphoria and hallucinosis and then to psychosis. Some users engage in nonstop binges of self-administration until psychological toxicity develops.[51]

ADVERSE EFFECTS

CASE 86-13, QUESTION 3: C.H. and his friends continue to smoke crack for the next 10 hours. C.H. decides to go out for a pack of cigarettes and collapses on the sidewalk outside his apartment. A passerby calls 9-1-1, and C.H. is rushed to the nearest emergency department in a semiconscious state. What has likely happened to C.H.?

Cocaine is the most frequently mentioned illicit substance in emergency department visits. In 2007, 553,530 cocaine-related visits to an emergency department were reported in the United States.[12] The potential adverse effects associated with both acute and chronic use of cocaine are numerous and involve most organ systems in the body.

The cardiac complications associated with cocaine use include hypertension, arrhythmias, myocardial ischemia and infarction, dilated and hypertrophic cardiomyopathy, myocarditis, aortic dissection, and acceleration of atherosclerosis. These cardiac effects have occurred in individuals with and without underlying heart disease who have taken large or small doses by all routes of administration and may be associated with acute or chronic use. The cardiac events can occur before, during, or after other toxicities, such as seizures, and can be fatal. The mechanism of cocaine-induced myocardial infarction is most likely multifactorial, involving one or more of the following processes: coronary artery vasoconstriction, increased myocardial oxygen demand related to increased blood pressure and increased heart rate, increased platelet aggregation and thrombus formation, coronary vasospasm, and arrhythmia. The risk is greatest within the first hour after use.[52] Studies have shown 6% of patients presenting to emergency departments with chest pain after cocaine use have myocardial infarctions.[50–52]

The medical management of acute coronary syndromes differs when cocaine is the cause. Specifically, nonselective β-blocker therapy (i.e., propranolol) is contraindicated, thrombolysis should be used with caution, and nitroglycerine and benzodiazepines are part of first-line therapy.[50–52] In patients with cocaine-associated chest pain, a 12-hour observation period to rule out myocardial infarction or ischemia is probably sufficient before discharge from a medical facility.[51]

Cocaine has also been associated with cerebrovascular catastrophes. Stroke can occur as a result of increased blood pressure, vasoconstriction, or thrombosis. Seizures are another CNS complication. Seizures can occur with first use and are most often single, generalized tonic-clonic seizures. Most occur within 90 minutes of drug use, when drug plasma concentrations are highest.[47]

The route of cocaine administration also affects the nature of the adverse effects. For example, pulmonary complications, including pneumomediastinum, pneumothorax, pneumopericardium, acute exacerbation of asthma, diffuse alveolar hemorrhage, pulmonary edema, and "crack lung," are associated with smoking crack cocaine. Crack lung is a syndrome of acute pulmonary infiltrates associated with a spectrum of clinical and histologic findings.[50] Snorting cocaine can lead to perforation of the nasal septum because of the drug's local anesthetic and vasoconstrictive effects. IV use of cocaine has been associated with renal infarction, wound botulism, viral hepatitis, HIV infection, bacterial endocarditis, sepsis, and other infectious complications. C.H. could be suffering from cardiovascular, cerebrovascular, or pulmonary complications caused by his crack smoking. His emergency department workup should be thorough and directed by his symptoms.

COCAINE ADDICTION

CASE 86-13, QUESTION 4: C.H. is released from the emergency department and returns home to find his friend with more crack. They resume smoking and binge for the next 4 days. They run out of drugs and money, and C.H. begins to "crash." In desperation, he sells his skateboard to his neighbor for $20, buys another rock, smokes it, and feels good again. Is C.H.'s cocaine usage pattern consistent with cocaine dependence?

C.H. continues to use cocaine despite adverse consequences (emergency department visit), uses it compulsively, suffers withdrawal symptoms, and alleviates his symptoms with further use. Per the DSM-IV criteria for substance dependence, C.H. is addicted to cocaine.[1]

Prolonged or heavy use of cocaine has been associated with the development of tolerance to some of its central effects. Tolerance is caused by adaptive changes in the brain.[47] A withdrawal syndrome may follow long-term or binge use. The initial, acute symptoms, referred to as the "crash," consist of depression, fatigue, craving, hypersomnolence, and anxiety. Anhedonia and hyperphagia soon follow. Although most symptoms are mild and resolve within 1 to 2 weeks, the dysphoria and anhedonia can persist for weeks. These symptoms do not produce profound physiologic changes and are generally not life-threatening.[51]

TREATMENT OF ADDICTION

CASE 86-13, QUESTION 5: C.H. decides to get clean and seeks help from a detox clinic. What therapeutic options are available to him?

Most cases of simple cocaine withdrawal do not require medical treatment. However, multiple pharmacologic therapies to facilitate abstinence from cocaine have been, and continue to be, under investigation. Most studies have yielded variable results, and to date no drug exists that is proven effective in treating cocaine dependence.[16] Studies of dopamine agonists (amantadine, selegiline, levo-dopa/carbidopa, pergolide), antidepressants (desipramine, fluoxetine, bupropion), and carbamazepine have yielded inconsistent findings. Methylphenidate (Ritalin) has been investigated as "maintenance treatment" to satisfy the cocaine addict's desire for further enhancement of mood; however, methylphenidate also can stimulate a powerful craving for the more intense euphoria of cocaine and has significant abuse potential. Recent research shows promise for topiramate, baclofen, tiagabine, and modafinil, but these findings require replication.[16] A cocaine vaccine is currently under investigation. Psychosocial treatments focusing on abstinence have been effective in the treatment of cocaine dependence.[16] Cognitive-behavioral

psychotherapy in subjects with anxiety associated with advanced stages of cancer.

The effects of MDMA are mainly exerted by three neurochemical mechanisms: blockade of serotonin reuptake, stimulation of serotonin release, and stimulation of dopamine release.[60] The common psychological effects of MDMA intoxication include an overall heightened sense of empathy, interpersonal closeness, increased acceptance of others, and a powerful sense of well-being.[61] The experience is influenced by set and setting. The amphetaminelike side effects include mydriasis, tachycardia, sweating, increased energy and alertness, bruxism, nausea, and anorexia.[62] Users generally ingest MDMA in tablet form, and the onset of action is usually after 30 to 60 minutes. Some users take a "booster" dose after 2 hours. The usual duration of action of MDMA is 4 to 6 hours, and the half-life is approximately 8 hours. MDMA users in the rave scene often "stack" multiple doses, and polydrug use is common. The combined use of ecstasy and LSD is referred to as "candy flipping."[60]

R.X.'s feelings of love for everyone are consistent with the empathogenic effects of MDMA, whereas P.B. is enjoying the amphetaminelike effects of increased energy to dance all night.

ADVERSE EFFECTS

CASE 86-17, QUESTION 2: Several hours after taking MDMA, P.B. is still dancing. She begins to feel hot and realizes she is profusely sweating. On her way to the bar for a drink, she begins to feel confused and collapses to the floor. Her friends witness her having a seizure and call 9-1-1. What is happening to P.B.?

The rave scene, with its crowded conditions and often-high ambient temperatures, has contributed to many adverse effects associated with MDMA ingestion. Because of their increased physical activity, the ravers may become dehydrated. Additionally, supplies of MDMA have been notoriously unreliable. Many other drugs have been misrepresented as MDMA, including other phenethylamines such as 3,4-methylenedioxyamphetamine (MDA) and paramethoxyamphetamine (PMA); amphetamine; cocaine; opiates; ketamine; and dextromethorphan. The common polydrug use practiced at raves compounds the problem. Dextromethorphan taken at high doses for its dissociative properties competes with MDMA for hepatic metabolism, and its anticholinergic effects block perspiration, potentially leading to overheating.[58]

The most dangerous adverse physical effect of MDMA is hyperthermia. MDMA has a slight affinity for the 5-HT_2 receptor, and the increased body temperature may be the result of this activation.[60] The hyperthermia has led to rhabdomyolysis, and acute renal and hepatic failure, disseminated intravascular coagulation (DIC), and death.[63] DIC has been the most common cause of death. Treatment of hyperthermia involves cooling measures and IV fluids. Benzodiazepines (e.g., lorazepam 2 mg IM or IV) and dantrolene (1 mg/kg IV) may be helpful. Other adverse physical effects can include hypertension, cardiac arrhythmias, convulsions, cerebrovascular accident, hepatitis, and hyponatremia (from overingestion of water as a harm reduction measure to avoid hyperthermia).[62,63] In 2008, there were 17,865 emergency department visits associated with MDMA use. This represents less than 2% of all illicit drug reports.[64] Adverse psychological effects are also possible, including anxiety, depression, panic attacks, agitation, paranoia, and rarely psychosis. The treatment of these psychological adverse effects is the same as for those associated with the classic hallucinogens, including talk-down therapy and benzodiazepine administration. P.B. may be suffering from MDMA-induced hyperthermia and needs urgent medical evaluation.

LONG-TERM EFFECTS

CASE 86-17, QUESTION 3: R.X. has read in the newspaper that MDMA is associated with "brain damage" and is worried that she has caused permanent damage to her brain. What are the long-term effects of MDMA?

Animal studies have consistently demonstrated long-term MDMA-induced serotonin depletion. This has been evidenced by lower levels of serotonin, decreased metabolite levels, lowered levels of tryptophan hydroxylase, and loss of serotonin reuptake transporters.[58] MDMA damages serotonin axonal projections; axonal resprouting and regeneration do occur, but it is unclear whether these new projections are damaged. Despite this evidence of neurotoxicity, no associated functional changes have been demonstrated.[58,65]

Several retrospective studies in humans have claimed lowered cognitive performance in MDMA users compared with nonusers. These studies have serious methodologic flaws, including their retrospective design and failure to control for important confounding variables, such as other drug use and adulterant exposure and lifestyle factors.[58,65] Well-controlled, prospective clinical trials are required to establish definitively any risk associated with MDMA ingestion.

Use of MDMA does not appear to produce physical dependence, but some users may become psychologically dependent. Tolerance to the empathogenic effects develops rapidly and may last 24 to 36 hours. This may explain in part the more common practice of sporadic dosing of the drug.[51,61] No distinctive withdrawal syndrome has been described that would require pharmacologic treatment.

MARIJUANA

Marijuana is the most widely used illicit substance in the United States. In 2008, 102.4 million Americans reported using marijuana at some time in their lives, 25.7 million had used in the past year, and 15.2 million had used in the past month.[2] The main psychoactive ingredient in the *Cannabis sativa* plant is Δ-9-tetrahydrocannabinol (THC), although the plant is known to contain more than 70 cannabinoids.[66] In the United States, the dried, chopped leaves and flowers of the *Cannabis* plant (grass, pot, weed, green bud, chronic, mary jane) are rolled into a cigarette paper (marijuana cigarette, known as a joint or blunt; a "roach" is the butt of the marijuana cigarette) or smoked in a pipe or water pipe ("bong"). Each joint usually weighs 0.5 to 1 g, for a THC content of about 5 mg (very weak), 30 mg (average), or 150 mg (highest-quality sinsemilla). The sinsemilla (Spanish for "without seeds") growing technique involves separating the female plants from the males before pollination occurs. This results in female plants with higher amounts of THC, up to 14%.[67]

The raw resin of the *Cannabis* plant can be pressed into cakes, balls, or sticks, called hashish ("hash," "temple balls"), which is smoked or eaten. Hashish can contain up to 8% THC. The oils can be extracted from the plant with organic solvents to produce "hash oil," perhaps the most potent *Cannabis* derivative, with THC concentrations of up to 50%.[67] In 2007 the average price was calculated at $7.87 per gram or $233 per ounce.[68]

Researchers in cannabinoid neurobiology have discovered two cannabinoid receptors in the CNS: CB_1 and CB_2; however, additional receptors have been proposed. Research has demonstrated that the main pharmacologic and addictive effects are almost completely mediated by the CB_1 receptor.[67] In addition, five endogenous cannabinoids (endocannabinoids) that act at the cannabinoid receptors have been discovered.[69] The best known are arachidonic acid ethanolamide (anandamide) and 2-arachidonoylglycerol (2-AG).[69] Considerable evidence exists supporting the role of THC–opioid interactions with enhanced antinociception. Cannabinoids have been shown to release endogenous opioids, and cannabinoid receptors colocalize with substance P (the neurotransmitter responsible for transmitting pain information) receptors in the striatum. Subsequently, investigation of THC as an adjunct to opioid treatment of pain, prevention of opioid tolerance, and dependence is underway.[67]

Marijuana's therapeutic potential has been the center of much public controversy. Research on the effects of cannabinoids has led to several potential therapeutic uses, including relief of nausea and vomiting, appetite stimulation, and treatment of pain, epilepsy, glaucoma, and movement disorders (Parkinson disease, Huntington disease, Tourette syndrome, multiple sclerosis).[67,70] In 1999, the State of California passed the law SB847, which commissioned the University of California to establish the Center for Medicinal Cannabis Research (CMCR) to expand scientific knowledge on purported therapeutic usages of marijuana. The center's 2010 report to the California legislature and governor presented clinical trial findings demonstrating that cannabis has analgesic effects in pain conditions secondary to injury or disease and that cannabis reduces MS spasticity.[71] A synthetic form of THC, dronabinol, is available as prescription tablets, and a synthetic cannabinoid, nabilone (Cesamet), is available as capsules, but advocates of medicinal marijuana use argue that inhalation allows for faster onset and easier titration of the dose. In addition, nauseated patients want to avoid the oral route of administration. Future research may focus on developing a safer delivery system that will be reliable, rapid, and safe. An oromucosal spray, Sativex, derived from botanical material, is under investigation in the United States. The principal active components are THC and cannabidiol. This cannabis extract spray has been approved in Canada, and is also being used in the United Kingdom. A capsule formulation containing a mixed ratio of THC and cannabidiol produced by Cannador in Germany is also available.[67] Other alternative delivery methods may include vaporization, patches, and suppositories.

Effects

CASE 86-18

QUESTION 1: After school one day, P.H. is offered a joint by one of his friends. He smokes it and begins to feel lightheaded and euphoric. He begins laughing at everything around him. Thirty minutes later he and his friend become very hungry ("the munchies") and eat several candy bars. Which of P.H.'s symptoms are consistent with marijuana use?

The pharmacologic effects sought by most users of cannabis products are sedation, mental relaxation, euphoria, and mild hallucinogenic effects, and these effects depend on set and setting. Other common effects that are usually perceived as pleasurable include silliness, subjective slowing of time, gregariousness, hunger, and mild perceptual changes of all the senses that engender an absorbing fascination with music, eating, and other sensual and sensory activities. The state of mind generated is referred to as "stoned," "high," "loaded," "wasted," and many other colloquial terms. Smoking marijuana typically causes numbness and tingling of the extremities, light-headedness, loss of concentration, and a floating sensation in the first 3 or 4 minutes. Some of these effects are probably caused by the hyperventilation associated with deep inhalation of the smoke (referred to as a "hit" or "toke") and breath holding to allow maximal absorption from the lungs. During the first 10 to 30 minutes, the user may experience tachycardia (possibly palpitations), mild diaphoresis, conjunctival injection ("red eye"), drying of the mouth, weakness, postural hypotension, periods of tremulousness, incoordination, and ataxia along with euphoria and the mental effects described above. These effects usually resolve by 1 to 3 hours and are followed by a 30- to 60-minute period of sleepiness before complete clearing and return to normal consciousness. Oral ingestion of cannabis products may delay the onset of effects by 45 to 60 minutes and prolong the duration.[67] P.H. is experiencing euphoria, giddiness, and increased appetite, consistent with marijuana intoxication.

Adverse Effects

CASE 86-18, QUESTION 2: P.H. smokes more marijuana with his friend. He liked it so much the first time, he decides to take several "hits" this time. He begins to think his friend is laughing at him and notices his heart is beating rapidly. He starts to panic. Is P.H.'s reaction caused by the marijuana?

Consistent with its widespread use, marijuana was the second most frequently mentioned illicit substance in emergency department episodes in the United States in 2007. A total of 308,547 marijuana-related emergency department (ED) visits were reported in 2007.[12] These visits include marijuana in combination with other drugs. As the percentage of THC has increased in marijuana, so have the ED visits. The majority of ED visits are from unexpected reactions, such as anxiety, paranoia, and panic attacks. Despite these numbers, there are no documented cases of fatality in humans from marijuana overdose, and adverse effects tend to be self-limiting and often do not require medical treatment.

A syndrome consisting of anxiety, paranoia, depersonalization, disorientation, and confusion that can lead to panic states and incapacitating fear is perhaps the most frequently reported adverse effect of marijuana. Comforting reassurance (talk down) and reducing stressful stimuli can alleviate this condition. The dysphoria and anxiety usually resolve in a few hours or less with such an approach. More severe incidents that evolve into panic reactions that are not resolved by sympathetic counseling may be relieved with oral benzodiazepine therapy in a dose equivalent to 5 to 10 mg of diazepam.[51] These adverse psychological reactions to cannabis products commonly occur with inexperienced users, high doses, concomitant use of other psychoactive drugs, and overtly stressful situations. Severe reactions requiring pharmacologic therapy are rare.

Currently, there is much debate in the scientific community regarding the association of marijuana and psychosis. A review of the literature found that cannabis use increases the risk of developing psychotic disorders among vulnerable or predisposed individuals and negatively affects the course of pre-existing chronic psychosis.[66] Population statistics argue against a causal relationship.

Adverse physical effects can include slowed psychomotor responses and short-term memory loss. Slowed psychomotor responses have been shown in certain groups of acutely intoxicated subjects and chronic users. Short-term memory loss is a frequently documented acute, reversible effect of marijuana intoxication as well.

The paranoid ideation and panic reaction of P.H. could certainly be caused by the high dose and his inexperience with marijuana.

Long-Term Effects

CASE 86-18, QUESTION 3: P.H. continues to smoke marijuana daily. His parents discover his marijuana use and confront him, telling him it will make him stupid, unmotivated, and strung out, and may lead to the use of harder drugs. Are P.H.'s parents' concerns valid? What are possible long-term effects of marijuana use?

Chronic use of cannabis has been alleged to produce an "amotivational syndrome" characterized by apathy, lack of long-term goal achievement, inability to manage stress, and generalized laziness, but little scientific evidence supports such a syndrome.[67]

Cognitive impairment can occur after heavy marijuana use, but appears to be reversible with abstinence.[72] The impairment is more pronounced the longer the drug is used.[67] Other concurrent drug use may also contribute to cognitive impairment associated with marijuana use. Evidence of brain damage associated with marijuana use is equivocal.

The pulmonary complications of chronic heavy marijuana use are potentially significant. Chronic cough, sputum, wheezing, bronchitis, and cellular changes typical of chronic tobacco smokers are reported in chronic cannabis smokers.[67,73] THC has been shown to be a potent bronchodilator. Both oral and smoked THC were shown to produce significant bronchodilation when given to healthy subjects. The bronchodilatory response in asthmatics given THC has been shown to be less vigorous.[74] Tolerance to these effects can develop after some weeks, and chronic marijuana smoking results in increased airway resistance and decreased pulmonary function.[67] Many of the same carcinogens in nicotine cigarettes are also found in marijuana smoke. However, the International Agency for Research on Cancer found data regarding an increased risk of cancer from cannabis inconclusive.[67] *Aspergillus*-contaminated marijuana has been reported to cause pulmonary fungal infections in immunocompromised patients, who may be using the drug for its medicinal value.[75]

Tolerance to the psychoactive effects of marijuana does develop. Chronic users may not experience the full range of effects as new users unless they abstain for several days or weeks to regain initial sensitivity to the cannabis, and chronic users can tolerate large doses that generally are toxic to novices. Tolerance develops rapidly to both physiologic and psychological effects of cannabis. Dependence characterized by a physical withdrawal syndrome occurs after chronic high-dose use of cannabis. The withdrawal syndrome can involve anxiety, depression, irritability, restlessness, anorexia, insomnia and vivid or disturbing dreams, sweating, tremor, nausea, vomiting, and diarrhea.[51,67] Dysphoria and malaise similar to that experienced with influenza can also occur. The cumulative dose of cannabis and duration of use necessary to produce dependence is unknown. The withdrawal syndrome is generally mild and self-limiting, and pharmacologic treatments usually are not required.

Marijuana has been labeled as a "gateway drug," meaning that it will lead to the use of "harder" drugs, such as cocaine or heroin. Marijuana is the most widely used illicit drug, but use of drugs such as alcohol and tobacco often predates marijuana use. No studies have conclusively demonstrated a causal link between marijuana use and subsequent other drug use.[67]

P.H.'s parents' concerns are understandable, but not entirely accurate. They should attempt to educate P.H. about the true risks involved with marijuana use, such as interference with studies, risk of pulmonary complications, and possible risk of dependence.

INHALANTS

The introduction of anesthetics (nitrous oxide, chloroform, and ether) to medicine in the early 1800s also promoted the widespread and popular recreational use of these inhalants for mind-altering recreational purposes. Today, abused inhalants include a wide variety of chemicals that are found readily in homes or workplaces, or purchased at retail establishments. Inhalants are commonly subdivided into three main categories: the volatile solvents (mostly hydrocarbons); volatile nitrites (amyl, butyl, isobutyl, cyclohexyl); and nitrous oxide (laughing gas). The fumes or vapors of these liquids, or paste in the case of glue, are directly inhaled out of their containers ("sniffing"); poured onto a rag that is held to the nose ("huffing"); poured into a plastic bag ("bagging"); or merely cupped in the hands and inhaled. Aerosols and gaseous substances such as nitrous oxide are also used to inflate a balloon and then inhaled out of the balloon by the user. These products can also be ingested orally or sprayed directly into the mouth. Volatile solvents include gasoline, toluene, kerosene, alcohols, airplane glue, lacquer thinner, acetone (nail polish remover), benzene (nail polish remover, model cement), naphtha (lighter fluid), plastic cement, liquid paper (i.e., White Out, usually containing 1,1,1-trichloroethane, also trichloroethylene and perchloroethylene), and many others. The volatile nitrites, once widely available, are prohibited by the Consumer Product Safety Commission but can still be found, sold in small bottles, labeled as "video head cleaner" or "room odorizer." Amyl nitrite is used medically as a vasodilator for treatment of angina and requires a prescription. The volatile nitrites are commonly referred to as "poppers," because of the sound made when an ampule of amyl nitrite is broken open. The most commonly used inhalants are glue, shoe polish, toluene, and gasoline.[76] The use of multiple products is common. Silver and gold paints are popular because they contain more toluene than paints of other colors.[77]

In 2008, 22.2 million Americans reported using inhalants at some time in their lives, more than 2 million had used them in the past year, and 640,000 had used them in the past month.[2] Unlike other drugs of abuse, inhalant use is most common among younger individuals (consistently highest annual prevalence among 8th graders) and tends to decline as youth grow older. The decline likely reflects that other drugs become available and are substituted, and that the inhalants are seen as "kids" drugs. Abuse of inhalants is believed to be popular among children and adolescents because of their low cost, easy availability, rapid onset, and low threat of legal intervention. Additionally, they are easily concealed. The 2009 Monitoring the Future (MTF) study found that 12.5% of 8th, 10th, and 12th graders have abused inhalants.[78] The MTF and other national surveys of adolescents have found that after marijuana, inhalants are the second most widely used class of illicit drugs for 8th graders. Most inhalant users, however, have used alcohol or cigarettes previously.[79] These surveys, most of which are administered in schools, likely underestimate the true prevalence, as a small but high-risk group (incarcerated, homeless, and transient adolescents) are not included in the surveys.

Effects of Inhalants

CASE 86-19

QUESTION 1: H.K., a 14-year-old boy, has been pouring degreasing solvents, gasoline, and paint thinners onto a rag and "huffing" the fumes to produce intoxication. What clinical presentation might be expected in this young man?

Inhalant abuse includes a broad range of chemicals, and they likely have different pharmacologic effects. In fact, the mechanisms of action of the volatile inhalants are poorly understood. Nearly all have CNS depressant effects. Evidence from animal studies suggests the effects and mechanism of action of volatile solvents are similar to those of alcohol and sedative-hypnotics.[80]

Gases and vapors are rapidly absorbed when inhaled and, because of their high lipophilicity, tend to distribute preferentially to lipid-rich organs such as the brain and liver.[80] Expired air is the major route of elimination, and most are metabolized to some extent.

Inhalation of these products produces a temporary stimulation and reduced inhibitions before the depressive CNS effects occur. Acute intoxication is associated with euphoria, giddiness, dizziness, slurred speech, unsteady gait, and drowsiness.[77] As the CNS becomes more deeply affected, illusions, hallucinations, and delusions develop. The user experiences a euphoric, dreamy high that culminates in a short period of sleep. The intoxicated state lasts a few minutes, but users may continue to inhale repeatedly for several hours. Nitrous oxide is an antagonist of the NMDA subtype of the glutamate receptor.[53] Its pharmacologic effects are poorly understood. It produces euphoria and symptoms of intoxication similar to those described for the volatile solvents.

The major effect of the volatile nitrites is the relaxation of all smooth muscles in the body, including the blood vessels. This usually allows a greater volume of blood to flow to the brain. The onset of effects takes 7 or 8 seconds and the effects last about 30 seconds. A certain "rush" occurs, which may be followed by a severe headache, dizziness, and giddiness. The volatile nitrites are frequently used in the context of sexual activity, because of the effect of increased tumescence and relaxation of smooth muscle.[80]

Acute and Chronic Toxicities Associated With Inhalants

CASE 86-19, QUESTION 2: What acute and chronic complications may H.K. experience from inhalation of volatile solvents?

The wide variety of chemicals inhaled causes a tremendous range of toxicities. Toxicity depends on the chemical, and on the magnitude and duration of exposure. Complications can result from the effects of the solvents or other toxic ingredients, such as lead in gasoline. The lipophilicity of the volatiles enhances their toxicity. Injuries to the brain, liver, kidney, bone marrow, and particularly the lungs can occur, and they may result from the effect of heavy exposure or hypersensitivity. Inhalant abusers may develop irritation of the eyes, nose, and mouth, including rhinitis, conjunctivitis, and rash.[80] Methemoglobinemia has been associated with volatile nitrite use.

In 2007 the Drug Abuse Warning Network reported 7,920 emergency department visits were associated with inhalant use in the United States.[12] Deaths from inhalant use are well documented and may occur from overdose or trauma (falls, drowning, hanging). Death from overdose is often caused by respiratory problems or suffocation after CNS depression.[80] Deaths caused by asphyxiation, convulsions, coma, and aspiration of gastric contents have occurred.[77] Acute cardiotoxicity resulting in cardiac arrest may cause sudden death. Referred to as "sudden sniffing death," it is likely caused by sensitization of the myocardium to catecholamines, exacerbated by physical exercise, resulting in fatal ventricular arrhythmias.

Many of the inhalants produce neurotoxicity, which can range from mild impairment to severe dementia. Neurologic deficits include cognitive impairment, ataxia, optic neuropathy, deafness, and disorders of equilibrium. Loss of white matter, brain atrophy, and damage to specific neural pathways can result from chronic exposure to some inhalants. Some damage to the nervous system and other organs may be at least partially reversible when inhalant use is discontinued.[77] H.K. is at risk of acute injury including death. If he continues to abuse inhalants, he may suffer toxicities to major organs.

Inhalant Abuse and Dependence

CASE 86-19, QUESTION 3: Is H.K. likely to become addicted to volatile inhalants?

Compulsive use has been documented with inhalants, although inhalant abuse and dependence is a neglected area of research. Animal studies have shown some of the abused inhalants to have reinforcing properties.[80,81] The DSM-IV sets criteria for inhalant abuse and dependence, but does not provide for physiologic dependence, and it is unclear whether a true withdrawal syndrome occurs with chronic use of inhalants. Inhalant use is typically episodic in nature, and thus users may not be exposed to levels with sufficient frequency necessary to develop physical dependence or tolerance. H.K. is at risk for psychological dependence to inhalants.

ACKNOWLEDGMENT

The authors acknowledge James F. Buchanan, Howard E. McKinney, Gregory N. Hayner, Darryl S. Inaba, Jeffery N. Baldwin, and Blaine Benson for their authorship of previous editions of this chapter.

KEY REFERENCES AND WEBSITES

A full list of references for this chapter can be found at http://thepoint.lww.com/AT10e. Below are the key references and websites for this chapter, with the corresponding reference number in this chapter found in parentheses after the reference.

Key References

American Psychiatric Association. *Diagnostic and Statistical Manual of Mental Disorders.* 4th ed., Text Revision (DSM-IV-TR). Washington, DC: American Psychiatry Press; 2000. (1)

Inaba DS, Cohen WE. *Uppers, Downers, All Arounders: Physical and Mental Effects of Psychoactive Drugs.* 6th ed. Medford, OR: CNS Productions; 2007. (6)

Kleber HD et al; Work Group on Substance Use Disorders; American Psychiatric Association; Steering Committee on Practice

Guidelines. Treatment of patients with substance use disorders, second edition. American Psychiatric Association. *Am J Psychiatry.* 2007;164(4 Suppl):5. (16)

Lowinson JH, Ruiz P, Millman RB, Langrod JG, eds. *Substance Abuse: A Comprehensive Textbook.* 4th ed. Philadelphia, PA: Lippincott Williams & Wilkins; 2005. (7, 56, 58)

Ries RK, Fiellin DA, Miller SC, Saitz R, eds. *Principles of Addiction Medicine.* 4th ed. Philadelphia, PA: Lippincott Williams & Wilkins; 2009. (9, 20, 21, 37, 43, 47, 51, 53, 55, 67, 80)

Key Websites

Center for Substance Abuse Treatment. Treatment Improvement Protocol Series. Substance Abuse and Mental Health Services Administration. http://csat.samhsa.gov/publications.aspx.

Monitoring The Future: A Continuing Study of American Youth; The Regents of the University of Michigan. http://www.monitoringthefuture.org.

Substance Abuse and Mental Health Services Administration, Office of Applied Studies. Drug Abuse Warning Network: National Estimates of Drug-Related Emergency Department Visits, 2004–2008. http://dawninfo.samhsa.gov/data/report.asp?f = Nation/illicit/Nation_2008_Illicit_ED_visits_by_Drug. Accessed September 12, 2010. (64)

Substance Abuse and Mental Health Services Administration. Results from the National Survey on Drug Use and Health. Office of Applied Studies. http://oas.samhsa.gov/nhsda.htm.

US Department of Justice, National Drug Intelligence Center. National Drug Threat Assessment. http://www.justice.gov/ndic/topics/ndtas.htm.

Alcohol Use Disorders

George A. Kenna

87

CORE PRINCIPLES

	CHAPTER CASES
ALCOHOL USE DISORDER	
1 Alcohol use disorder is defined by acute and chronic alcohol use on a continuum from alcohol toxicity and alcohol abuse to alcohol dependence and alcohol withdrawal.	**Case 87-1 (Question 1), Case 87-2 (Question 1)**
ALCOHOL TOXICITY	
1 Alcohol toxicity is an acute, life-threatening condition that requires aggressive medical attention. Symptoms include a strong smell of alcohol, risk of aspiration, depressed and shallow respiration, and cardiac arrest. Management generally consists of respiratory support and a thorough diagnostic evaluation to rule out coingestion of other drugs or other underlying medical conditions that may also need attention.	**Case 87-1 (Questions 1–5)**
ALCOHOL WITHDRAWAL	
1 Alcohol withdrawal is the neurobiological syndrome associated with increased tolerance or physical dependence resulting from chronic alcohol consumption. This syndrome results in a continuum of signs or symptoms including paresthesias, headache, nausea, anxiety, shaking, increased heart rate and blood pressure, and seizures. Symptom-triggered assessment and treatment of alcohol withdrawal is extremely important to minimize seizures or even death in some at high risk.	**Case 87-2 (Questions 1–5)**
2 Treatment may be complicated not only by the physical or cognitive deterioration that can occur but also by the lack of attention to other serious medical or psychological conditions that could be contributing to, or resulting from, chronic alcohol use.	**Case 87-1 (Question 4), Case 87-2 (Questions 1, 3, 4), Case 87-5 (Question 2)**
3 Adjunctive treatments including fluid (e.g., normal saline solution), nutritional (e.g., thiamine, folic acid, multivitamins), and electrolyte (e.g., magnesium, potassium) replacement should also be initiated to address the physiological consequences of chronic alcohol use.	**Case 87-2 (Question 5)**
PHARMACOTHERAPY OF ALCOHOL DEPENDENCE	
1 Alcohol dependence is a chronic relapsing disorder that consists of signs of alcohol abuse (continued drinking despite alcohol-related physical, social, psychological, or occupational problems, or drinking in dangerous situations, such as while driving) to the extent that the person also experiences at least three of the following seven symptoms: neglect of other activities, excessive use of alcohol, impaired control of alcohol consumption, persistence of alcohol use, large amounts of time spent in alcohol-related activities, withdrawal symptoms, and tolerance of alcohol.	**Case 87-3 (Question 1)**

continued

PHARMACOTHERAPY OF ALCOHOL DEPENDENCE *CONTINUED*

2	Approved pharmacotherapies that include disulfiram, naltrexone (tablets and injection), and acamprosate should only be initiated after carefully evaluating the patient's commitment to abstinence, medical status, home care, psychosocial support, psychological status, and financial access to prescriptions.	**Case 87-3 (Question 2), Case 87-4 (Questions 1–4)**
3	Although research continues, other medications with off-label indications for alcohol dependence, including topiramate, ondansetron, baclofen, and sertraline, should be used only when the benefits clearly outweigh the risks given the patient's failure to respond to approved medications or their use is contraindicated.	**Case 87-5 (Questions 1–3)**
4	Follow-up includes assessing for continued alcohol abstinence, patient adherence, adverse effects, and drug interactions resulting from treatment.	**Case 87-6 (Question 1)**

ALCOHOL CONTENT AND DEFINITIONS

Beverages containing alcohol (ethanol) have a wide range of ethanol content. Alcoholic proof is a measure of how much ethanol is in an alcoholic beverage, and is twice the percentage of alcohol by volume (ABV), the unit that is commonly used as percent. This system dates to the 18th century, and perhaps earlier, when spirits were graded along with gunpowder. A solution of water and alcohol "proved" itself when it could be poured on a pinch of gunpowder and the wet powder could still be ignited. If the gunpowder did not ignite, the solution had too much water in it and the proof was considered insufficient. A "proven" solution was defined as 100 degrees proof (100).[1,2]

In the United States, the proof is twice the percentage of alcohol content measured by volume at a temperature of 60°F. Therefore "80 proof" is 40% alcohol by volume, and pure alcohol (100%) is "200 proof." One hundred percent ethanol does not stay 100% because it is hygroscopic and absorbs water from the atmosphere.

Alcohol is produced by yeast during the process of fermentation. The amount of alcohol in the finished liquid depends on the amount of sugar initially present for the yeast to convert into alcohol. Low-alcohol beer is beer with very low or no alcohol content. Legally, in the United States, beers containing up to 0.5% alcohol by volume can be called nonalcoholic. In some states (e.g., Minnesota, Colorado, and Utah), beer sold in supermarket chains and convenience stores must be less than 3.2% alcohol by weight (4% ABV). Alcohol content is generally listed by volume (e.g., a beer that is 4.0% ABV is about 3.2% by weight). Light beers range from 2% to about 4% ABV; beers range from 4% to 6% ABV; ales, stouts, and specialty brews can be as high as 10% ABV.

Depending on the strain of yeast, wines are produced at about 14% to 16% (28–32 proof), because that is the point in the fermentation process at which the alcohol concentration denatures the yeast. Since the 1990s, a few alcohol-tolerant "super yeast" strains have become commercially available, which can ferment up to 20%. Yeast organisms multiply as long as there is sugar to metabolize, gradually increasing the alcoholic content of the solution and killing off competing microorganisms, and eventually themselves. There are fortified wines with a higher alcohol concentration because stronger alcohol has been mixed with them. As this is usually done before fermentation is complete, these products contain a much higher quantity of sugar and therefore are typically sweet.

Stronger liquors are distilled after fermentation is complete to separate the alcoholic liquid from the remains of the source of sugar (e.g., grain, fruit). The idea of distillation is that a mixture of liquids is heated; the one with the lowest boiling point will evaporate first, followed by the one with the next lowest boiling point, and so on. Water and alcohol form a mixture called an *azeotrope* that has a lower boiling point than either one of them, so what distills off first is the mixture that is 95% alcohol and 5% water. Distilled liquor therefore cannot be stronger than 95% (190 proof). Other techniques can separate liquids that can produce 100% ethanol (called "absolute alcohol"), but they are used only for scientific or industrial purposes. A standard drink in the United States is considered to be 0.5 ounces or contain 15 g (0.5 fl oz of absolute alcohol) of alcohol. This is equal to 12 ounces (355 mL) of 5% beer, 5 ounces (148 mL) of 12% wine, or 1.5 ounces (44 mL) of 40% spirits.[1,2]

Epidemiology

Slightly more than half (51.1%) of Americans age 12 or older reported being current drinkers (at least one drink in the past 30 days) of alcohol in the 2008 National Survey on Drug Use and Health survey.[3] This translates to an estimated 127 million people, which is similar to the 2005 estimate of 126 million people (51.8%). More than 58 million people (23.3%) age 12 or older participated in binge drinking (five or more drinks on the same occasion; i.e., at the same time or within a couple of hours of each other, on at least 1 day in the past 30 days) in 2008. In 2008, heavy drinking (five or more drinks on the same occasion on each of 5 or more days in the past 30 days) was reported by 6.9% of the population age 12 or older.[3] In 2003, alcohol use disorder (AUD) in the United States accounted for 12,766 person-deaths in alcohol-related traffic crashes, constituting almost 30% of the total traffic crash fatalities,[4] although as of 2008, alcohol-related deaths had dropped.[3] In 2007, 19.3 million people age 12 or older needed treatment for their alcohol problems.[5]

Approximately 10% of Americans will be affected by alcohol dependence sometime during their lives.[6,7] In 2001 and 2002, the last year such statistics are available, prevalences of *Diagnostic and Statistical Manual of Mental Disorders,* Fourth Edition (DSM-IV)[8] alcohol abuse and dependence were estimated to be 4.7% and 3.8%, respectively.[9] Abuse and dependence were more common among males and among younger respondents. The prevalence of abuse was greater among whites than among African, Asian, and Hispanic Americans. The prevalence of dependence was higher in whites and Native and Hispanic Americans than in Asian Americans.[9]

Alcohol dependence is a chronic relapsing disorder with genetic, psychosocial, and environmental factors influencing its development and manifestations. Although treatment outcomes have improved, much remains to address unsuccessful treatment of alcohol abuse and dependence for many others.[10] As defined by the DSM-IV,[8] alcohol dependence is characterized by the preoccupation with alcohol use and by use despite adverse consequences, as well as evidence of signs of tolerance and withdrawal (see Chapter 86, Drug Abuse, Table 86-1).

Treatment of alcohol dependence consists mainly of psychological, social, and pharmacotherapy interventions aimed at reducing alcohol-related problems.[11] Treatment usually consists of two phases: detoxification and rehabilitation. Detoxification manages the signs and symptoms of withdrawal. Once detoxified, rehabilitation helps the individual avoid future problems with alcohol. Most rehabilitation treatments are psychosocial, consisting of individual and group therapies, residential treatment in alcohol-free settings, and self-help groups, such as Alcoholics Anonymous. Although psychosocial treatments show effectiveness in reducing alcohol consumption and in maintaining abstinence, reviews of treatment studies report 40% to 70% of patients return to drinking within the year after treatment.[12] The Agency for Health Care Research and Quality[13] concludes that there is a significant need both to improve current alcohol treatments and to develop new strategies.

Interest in using pharmacotherapies to improve treatments for alcohol dependence is growing.[14,15] The rationale for pharmacotherapy is based on several considerations. Advances in neurobiology have identified neurotransmitter systems that initiate and sustain alcohol drinking; pharmacologic modification of these neurotransmitters or their receptors may alter dependence.[16] Promising genetic research confirms that alcoholics are a heterogeneous population and that several gene variations can predispose some to increased alcohol use whereas other gene variations can confer protection.[16] Animal models have identified pharmacologic agents that reduce alcohol consumption in animals, suggesting similar agents could reduce alcohol consumption in humans. Finally, medications have improved the treatment of other addictive disorders, such as nicotine and opiate dependence, suggesting better pharmacotherapies may be developed for the treatment of alcoholism.

Risks and Benefits of Alcohol Consumption

The role of alcohol in the development of medical problems such as cardiovascular disease, hepatic cirrhosis, and fetal abnormalities is well documented. Alcohol use and abuse contribute to thousands of injuries, auto collisions, and violence.[17] Alcohol can dramatically affect worker productivity and absenteeism, family interactions, and school performance.[18] Some studies suggest, however, that individuals who abstain from using alcohol may also be at greater risk for a variety of conditions, particularly coronary heart disease (CHD), than people who consume small to moderate amounts of alcohol.[19]

A number of studies have documented an association between moderate alcohol consumption and lower risk for CHD[20] and myocardial infarction (MI).[21] Binge drinking after an MI, however, increases the risk of mortality.[22] US guidelines define moderate drinking as one drink or less daily for women or people age 65 and older, and two drinks or less per day for men.[23] An association between moderate drinking and lower risk of CHD does not mean that alcohol is the cause of the lower risk. A review of population studies indicates that the higher mortality risk among abstainers may be attributable to socioeconomic and employment status, mental health, and overall health, rather than abstinence from alcohol use.[24] Benefits of moderate drinking on CHD mortality are offset at higher drinking levels by increased risk of death because of other types of heart disease, cancer, cirrhosis, and trauma. The risk of a disease outcome from low to moderate drinking is less than the risk from either no drinking at all or heavier drinking. This produces a U-shaped curve when examining the association of alcohol consumption with rates of deaths from all causes.[19]

The exact mechanism by which alcohol use may be protective against morbidity in those with CHD is not clear. Some evidence indicates that different types of alcoholic beverages, such as red wines, which are high in tannins, may lower blood lipids and fats by increasing antioxidants.[22] Specifically, the mechanisms by which alcohol may reduce the risk of CHD include increasing levels of high-density lipoprotein cholesterol, decreasing levels of low-density lipoprotein cholesterol, prevention of clot formation, reduction in platelet aggregation, and lowering of plasma apolipoprotein(a) concentration, resulting in the attenuation of the formation of atheroma and decreasing the rate of blood coagulation.[25,26] It is also possible, however, that how a person drinks alcoholic beverages matters as well. For example, wines are ingested more slowly as they are typically consumed in moderate amounts with food. Binge drinking of any type of beverage, however, increases the risk of mortality from CHD in particular.[22]

NEUROSCIENCE AND NEUROBEHAVIOR

Pharmacokinetics and Pharmacology

When consumed in amounts typical of normal social drinking, the absorption of ethanol from the stomach, small intestine, and colon is complete; however, the rate is variable. Peak blood ethanol concentrations after oral doses in fasting subjects generally are reached in 30 to 75 minutes, but several factors can influence the rate and extent of absorption.[27] The most rapidly absorbed formulations are carbonated beverages containing 10% to 30% ethanol. In contrast, high concentrations of alcohol can produce vasoconstriction in the gastrointestinal (GI) mucosa, which results in slowed or even incomplete absorption of ethanol. Absorption of ethanol from the small intestine appears to be more rapid than any other part of the GI tract and does not depend on the presence or absence of food. Factors that control the rate of gastric emptying significantly control the rate of absorption by controlling the rate at which ethanol is delivered to the small intestine.[28,29] For example, food in the stomach slows the absorption of ethanol, probably by slowing gastric emptying. (For a presentation on the general pharmacology of alcohol's effects, to go **http://www.rsalectures.com/lovinger.html.**)

The level of intoxication achieved is not solely related to the plasma concentration. For any particular plasma concentration, greater cognitive impairment is seen during times when the plasma level is rising compared with when ethanol is primarily being eliminated. The degree of intoxication also appears to be directly related to the rate at which pharmacologically active plasma concentrations are attained. Alcohol negatively affects cognitive performance and has a differential effect on the descending versus ascending limb of the blood alcohol concentration curve. The latter finding may have important ramifications relating to the detrimental consequences of alcohol intoxication.[30]

The blood alcohol level (BAL) or blood alcohol concentration (BAC) is calculated using the weight of ethanol in milligrams and the volume of blood in deciliters. This yields a BAC expressed as

β-blocker or clonidine. The result of such adjuvant treatment may be a reduced sensitivity of the CIWA-Ar owing to a masking of the patient's autonomic manifestations of withdrawal. This could then lead to a higher likelihood of undermedicating the patient for withdrawal and may put the patient at higher risk for severe sequelae from withdrawal. Because of these exclusion criteria, the symptom-triggered approach has not been tested in such populations or those with histories of severe withdrawal including seizures or delirium. Therefore, traditional fixed-dose regimens are recommended in these populations.[80]

An effective approach is most likely to consider combining these two dosing strategies. For example, a low-risk patient (no history of AWS or AWD, the patient consumes low weekly amounts of alcohol and has no signs or symptoms of early AWS) receives a symptom-triggered regimen (e.g., lorazepam 1 mg every hour as needed). Alternatively, a high-risk patient (history of AWS, AWD, or withdrawal seizures, consumes large daily amounts of alcohol, has signs or symptoms of early AWS) receives fixed-dose lorazepam or diazepam with a tapering dose schedule and as needed benzodiazepine administration for uncontrolled alcohol withdrawal signs or symptoms.

CONTRAINDICATIONS, WARNINGS, AND INTERACTIONS

Elderly patients, those with hepatic or renal insufficiency, and those with medical (e.g., diabetes, cirrhosis) or other psychiatric illnesses (e.g., dementia) require close observation to prevent overmedication. In patients receiving calcium-channel blockers, β-blockers, and α_2-adrenergic agonists, some signs of withdrawal such as hypertension, tachycardia, and tremor may not be apparent.

SUMMARY

Patients with a history of severe withdrawal symptoms, withdrawal seizures, or delirium tremens; multiple previous detoxifications; concomitant psychiatric or medical illness; recent high levels of alcohol consumption; pregnancy; and lack of a reliable support network should be considered for inpatient treatment regardless of the severity of their symptoms.

Many clinicians have adopted lorazepam as the drug of choice to treat AWS because it has no active metabolites and has an intermediate elimination half-life. Therefore, alcoholic patients with liver disease are at less risk for developing toxicity from detoxification with lorazepam than other benzodiazepines. The choice of agent is primarily based on pharmacokinetics. Diazepam and chlordiazepoxide are long-acting agents that have been shown to be excellent in treating AWS. Because of the long half-life of these medications, withdrawal is smoother, and rebound withdrawal symptoms are less likely to occur. Lorazepam and oxazepam are intermediate-acting medications with excellent records of efficacy. Treatment with these agents may be preferable in patients who metabolize medications less effectively, particularly the elderly and those with liver failure. Lorazepam is the only benzodiazepine with predictable intramuscular absorption (if intramuscular administration is necessary). Rarely, it is necessary to use extremely high dosages of benzodiazepines to control the symptoms of alcohol withdrawal. Because clinicians often are reluctant to administer exceptionally high dosages, undertreatment of alcohol withdrawal is a common problem. Ultimately, controlled studies comparing the advantages and disadvantages of the various benzodiazepines in alcohol detoxification have not been performed, and no evidence exists to definitively support the use of lorazepam as the first-line agent in the treatment of AWS.

In most patients with mild to moderate withdrawal symptoms, outpatient detoxification is safe and effective, and costs less than inpatient treatment. If outpatient treatment is chosen, the patient and support person(s) should be instructed on how to take the prescribed medication, its side effects, the expected withdrawal symptoms, and what to do if symptoms worsen. Small quantities of the withdrawal medication, especially benzodiazepines, should be prescribed at each visit. Because close monitoring is not available in outpatient treatment, a fixed-schedule regimen should be used.

Given J.M.'s elevated liver enzymes, a reasonable approach would be to start with lorazepam. Shorter-acting agents, such as lorazepam, which do not undergo extensive hepatic metabolism, are more appropriate for patients with evidence of hepatic insufficiency. However, it should be noted that there is some evidence that baclofen may be a safe alternative for use in alcohol-dependent patients with liver cirrhosis[93] and may be comparable to diazepam for AWS[94]; yet more research is needed to validate these findings.

CASE 87-2, QUESTION 4: Is there an advantage to treating J.M. with an anticonvulsant given his history of seizures?

Anticonvulsants

EVIDENCE

Of anticonvulsant agents only carbamazepine demonstrates promise for a greater role in the treatment of alcohol withdrawal, although its place in treatment is not definitive.[91,95,96] Interest for its use includes the possibility that anticonvulsants in general may curb the *kindling* phenomenon suspected in withdrawal and may therefore be neuroprotective.[97] Kindling refers to long-term neuronal changes resulting from repeated detoxifications and may be associated with progressively worse AWS on subsequent detoxifications.[98] Additionally, anticonvulsants in general have a low abuse potential and a minimal effect on cognition,[99] whereas benzodiazepines may increase the level of alcohol craving and relapse to alcohol use after abstinence.[100] That said, with the exception of carbamazepine, the available evidence does not support the use of anticonvulsants in the management of AWS.[101] Benzodiazepines remain the drugs of choice for AWS.[91,102,103]

Carbamazepine is widely used in Europe for AWS, where it is considered comparable to benzodiazepines in terms of adverse events and is considered equally effective as lorazepam in decreasing the symptoms of alcohol withdrawal.[100] Although limited information is available on whether carbamazepine can reduce seizures or delirium associated with alcohol withdrawal in humans,[80] carbamazepine was found to be superior to lorazepam in preventing rebound withdrawal symptoms and reducing post-treatment drinking.[99] Also, patients treated with carbamazepine had a better success rate for subsequent rehabilitation than those treated with benzodiazepines. In that study, carbamazepine was dosed on a tapering schedule of 600 to 800 mg divided through day 1, down to 200 mg as a single dose on day 5. It was as equally efficacious as lorazepam in reducing most withdrawal symptoms during detoxification, and was better at reducing anxiety and promoting sleep.[95] It should be noted that this study involved patients with mild-to-moderate AWS who were treated on an outpatient basis. An earlier study among alcohol-dependent inpatients with severe withdrawal symptoms found that carbamazepine was equally safe and effective as oxazepam.[96] Overall, although there is insufficient evidence for the use of anticonvulsants for the treatment of AWS, some evidence does suggest that carbamazepine may be more effective in treating some aspects of alcohol withdrawal than benzodiazepines.[103]

The major concerns with the clinical use of carbamazepine are the risk of agranulocytosis or aplastic anemia, both potentially lethal conditions.[86] Additionally, in a study comparing carbamazepine with lorazepam, pruritus was the most frequent side effect in 18.9% of patients.[100] Strong evidence indicates human fetal risk with carbamazepine use (category D), which should only be considered if no other safer drugs can be used or are ineffective. Carbamazepine is not intended for outpatient use and can potentiate the sedative effects of alcohol.

SUMMARY

Currently, no specific indication exists for using anticonvulsants to treat alcohol withdrawal, yet because these agents are used internationally in the treatment of AWS, clinicians should be aware of this approach. Because gabapentin undergoes renal elimination, there is some advantage over lorazepam; however, support for gabapentin has been demonstrated in patients with mild to moderate AWS. At this time, no clear convincing evidence indicates an advantage to using an anticonvulsant over lorazepam. Anticonvulsants may offer advantages over benzodiazepines in some patients. Specifically, because they have low abuse potential and interact minimally with alcohol, anticonvulsants may be an option for outpatient treatment, particularly for those who are at sufficiently low risk not to require hospitalization. Although anticonvulsants may be useful for some patients, benzodiazepines are still the drugs of choice for most patients, including J.M.[104]

ADJUNCTIVE TREATMENTS

CASE 87-2, QUESTION 5: What adjunctive therapeutic support might be considered for J.M.?

The hydration, electrolyte (especially potassium and magnesium), and nutritional status of patients should be assessed at presentation. Support with IV fluids may be necessary in those patients with excessive losses through vomiting, sweating, and hyperthermia.[98] Thiamine and multivitamins should be routinely administered to patients in alcohol withdrawal. If IV fluids are given, to prevent precipitation of Wernicke's encephalopathy thiamine administration should precede that of glucose.[82] Alcohol-dependent patients are deficient of thiamine and have a higher risk for developing Wernicke's encephalopathy.[105] In 1881, Dr. Carl Wernicke, a Polish neurologist, described the condition as a triad of acute mental confusion, ataxia, and ophthalmoplegia. Korsakoff amnestic syndrome is a late neuropsychiatric manifestation of Wernicke's encephalopathy with memory loss and confabulation; hence, the condition is referred to as Wernicke-Korsakoff syndrome. It is most often seen in alcohol-dependent patients, but it can also be seen in disorders associated with malnutrition, e.g., long-term hemodialysis or patients with acquired immunodeficiency syndrome (AIDS). (For a presentation about the brain and cognitive effects of alcohol, go to http://www.rsalectures.com/sullivan.html.)

Thiamine deficiency results in a decrease in cerebral glucose utilization. The body usually stores about 3 weeks of thiamine with daily requirements of about 1.5 mg. Rapid correction of brain thiamine deficiency can occur with high plasma concentrations of thiamine, achieved by parenteral supplementation only because absorption of the oral thiamine by the GI tract is minimal (<5%), even with massive oral daily dosing.[105] According to the 2004 Evidence-Based Guidelines of the British Association of Psychopharmacology,[106] to prevent the neuropsychiatric effects of thiamine deficiency, patients should receive at least 100 mg IM on the first day, and patients should be taking 100 to 200 mg/day of thiamine for up to 30 days. Because parenteral thiamine supplementation has been associated with anaphylactic reactions, it is only recommended as a slow IV injection in the presence of resuscitation facilities, although some reviews cite lower grade evidence in favor of oral thiamine supplementation during outpatient detoxification.[107]

Several adjunctive medications, aside from the sedative-hypnotics, may serve ancillary roles in the therapy of AWS. Their selection should be based on treating specific symptoms associated with the syndrome. For instance, β-blockers (e.g., propranolol,[108] atenolol[109]) or α_2-adrenergic agonists (e.g., clonidine[110]) can be used for moderate to severe hypertension or other autonomic manifestations. These agents can, however, mask symptoms of severe withdrawal that may herald the onset of a seizure without providing any antiseizure activity. Antipsychotics (e.g., haloperidol) can be used for managing hallucinations and severe agitation, but care must be used because these drugs can reduce the seizure threshold.[85,104]

PHARMACOTHERAPY OF ALCOHOL DEPENDENCE

Screening for Alcohol Problems

CASE 87-3

QUESTION 1: R.M. is a 55-year-old man, weighing 140 pounds, who used to drink about 60 drinks a week before going through alcohol detoxification. R.M. is married and has a good job, and he is now committed to remain alcohol abstinent. R.M. heard about a drug called disulfiram from a friend and is interested in using this medication to help him abstain from drinking. Laboratory values obtained today include the following:

Sodium, 132 mEq/L	AST, 30 units/L
Potassium, 3.3 mEq/L	ALT, 35 units/L
CO_2, 22.6 mEq/mL	Uric acid, 9.1 mg/dL
Chloride, 109 mEq/L	Calcium, 8.7 mg/dL
BUN, 14 mg/dL	Magnesium, 1.7 mg/dL
Creatinine, 1.0 mg/dL	Albumin, 4.0 g/dL
Glucose, 123 mg/dL	Cholesterol, 255 mg/dL
Total bilirubin, 0.3 mg/dL	CK, 78 units/L
Direct bilirubin, 0.1 mg/dL	GGT, 30 units/L
ALP, 53 units/L	

What information should the clinician obtain to differentiate R.M.'s diagnosis to guide treatment?

Patients who are awake and cognitively responsive should be interviewed to assess their alcohol use history.[111] An accurate medical history, including laboratory test results, is the most important tool a clinician can use; however, patients commonly deny problems with alcohol use. The DSM-IV[8] defines the criteria necessary for a differential psychiatric diagnosis and provides insurance payors with diagnostic codes. In addition, several instruments are available to screen and delineate the extent of a patient's alcohol use. Ultimately, time and purpose for use are always major factors when deciding which instrument to use. The simplest screen to assess risk of alcohol abuse is to ask the patient, during the past year on how many occasions have you had five or more drinks (for a man) or four or more drinks (for a woman) at one time?[112] An affirmative answer would suggest that further follow-up of the patient's alcohol use history is needed. A second tool called the **C-A-G-E** consists of four questions: (1) Have you ever felt you should **c**ut down on your drinking?; (2) Have people **a**nnoyed you by criticizing your drinking?;

TABLE 87-5
Useful Screens for Assessing Alcohol Problems

The C-A-G-E Screening Questions (CAGE)
Have you ever felt you should *c*ut down on your drinking?
Have other people *a*nnoyed you by criticizing your drinking?
Have you ever felt *g*uilty about drinking?
Have you ever taken a drink in the morning to calm your nerves or get rid of a hangover (*e*ye opener)?

Methods for Determining Recent Alcohol Consumption
Acute consumption
- Blood alcohol concentration
- Urine (ethyl glucuronide)
- Saliva
- Breath alcohol concentration

Recent heavy consumption
- Gamma-glutamyl transferase (GGT)
- Carbohydrate-deficient tranferrin (CDT)
- Mean corpuscular volume (MCV)

(3) Have you ever felt bad or **g**uilty about your drinking?; (4) Have you ever felt you needed a drink first thing in the morning to steady your nerves or get rid of a hangover (**e**ye opener)? Positive responses to two questions suggest an alcohol problem (Table 87-5).[113] The Alcohol Use Disorders Identification Test (AUDIT), which was developed by the World Health Organization, has also been shown to be effective in screening individuals and distinguishing problem drinkers from others.[114]

For a related case study, go to **https://webmeeting.nih.gov/case4/.**

Treatment Aims

It is important to keep in mind that unknown numbers of people with alcohol dependence heal themselves. These people have had the ability to just stop drinking. For a good many other patients who need assistance and who meet diagnostic criteria for substance abuse or dependence, psychosocial approaches are the foundation of treatment for these patients (Table 87-6). By contrast, should the patient need pharmacologic support, then consideration of a medication plan is entirely appropriate.[115] (For a presentation on implementation of treatment strategies, go to **http://www.rsalectures.com/willenbring.html.**)

Pharmacotherapy

The pharmacologic treatments of alcohol dependence focus on relapse prevention once detoxification is complete and the patient has achieved a few days of abstinence. Treatment is intended to be an adjunct to psychosocial treatments (Table 87-6) and not used alone.[116] To date, disulfiram, acamprosate, and naltrexone tablet and injection have been US Food and Drug Admistration (FDA) approved for the treatment of alcohol dependence. In addition, several other drugs (Table 87-7)[117–127] have shown varying degrees of success.[116,128] (Table 87-8).[129–137] Much is still unknown about the long-term rates of abstinence, how long these drugs should be used once patients are in treatment, the optimal doses, and whether the drugs are more effective in men or women or for which specific subpopulations.[138]

CASE 87-3, QUESTION 2: Is disulfiram an appropriate agent to consider for R.M.?

TABLE 87-6
Psychosocial and Behavioral Interventions Used With AUD

Type of Therapy	Underlying Processes	Key Components
Cognitive behavioral therapy (CBT)	The foundation is the belief that by identifying and monitoring maladaptive thinking patterns, patients can reduce or eliminate negative feelings and substance use	Alter cognitive processes that lead to maladaptive behaviors of AUD Intervene in the behavioral chain that leads to substance use Help patients deal with acute or chronic substance craving Promote and reinforce the development of social skills and behaviors compatible with abstinence
Motivational enhancement therapy (MET)	Brief treatment is characterized by an empathetic approach in which the therapist helps to motivate the patient by asking about the pros and cons of the target behavior (e.g., substance use)	Develop discrepancy (e.g., comparing given behavior with peer norms) Elicit self-motivational statements Listen with empathy Avoid argumentation Support self-efficacy
Medical management (MM)	Brief 20-minute intervention by a health care professional (e.g., nurse, pharmacist, or physician)	Focus on medication adherence Monitor alcohol use Assess side effects Encourage 12-step meeting attendance Set goals Educate
Brief behavioral compliance enhancement therapy (BBCET)	Brief 10-minute intervention by a health care professional	Focus on medication adherence Monitor alcohol use Assess side effects Allow patient to set goal
12-Step facilitation	Any support group that is a self-help group. Commonly called Alcoholics Anonymous, for example	Find a support group one feels comfortable with Get a sponsor Work the 12 steps to recovery

AUD, alcohol use disorder.
Source: Miller WR et al. Mesa Grande: a methodological analysis of clinical trials of treatments for alcohol use disorders. *Addiction*. 2002;97:265.

TABLE 87-7
Selected Double-Blind, Placebo-Controlled Trials for Alcohol Dependence

Medication (dose)	Type of Agent	Weeks	Alcoholic Subtype	Drinking/ Nondrinking Days	Craving	Relapse
Disulfiram (1 mg, 250 mg)[117]	Aversive	52	AD	+	NR	NR
Naltrexone (50 mg)[118]	Opioid antagonist	12	AD	+	+/0	+
Naltrexone (50 mg)[119]	Opioid antagonist	12	AD	+	+	+
Acamprosate (1,998 mg)[120]	NMDA modulator	48	AD	+	0	+
Acamprosate (1,332 mg or 1,998 mg)[121]	NMDA modulator	24	AD	+	+	+
Fluoxetine (60 mg)[122]	SSRI	12	AD/Type A	0	NR	0
			AD/Type B	–	NR	0
Fluoxetine (60 mg)[123]	SSRI	12	AD/MD	+	NR	NR
Sertraline (200 mg)[124]	SSRI	14	AD/Type A	+	NR	0
			AD/Type B	0	NR	0
Ondansetron (4 mcg/kg)[125]	5-HT3 antagonist	12	Early onset	+	NR	NR
			Late onset	0	NR	NR
Topiramate (up to 300 mg)[126]	Mixed-action	12	AD	+	+	NR
Naltrexone (100 mg) or Acamprosate (3,000 mg) or both[127]	Opioid antagonist NMDA modulator	16	AD	–	NR	NR

+, medication significant compared with placebo ($p < 0.05$); –, significant difference favoring placebo; 0, no significant difference; AD, alcohol dependent; early onset, onset of alcohol problems <25 years; 5-HT3, serotonin type 3 receptor; late onset, onset of alcohol problems >25 years; MD, major depression; NMDA, *N*-methyl-D-aspartate; NR, data not reported; SSRI, selective serontonin reuptake inhibitor; Type A, later onset of alcohol-related problems, severe dependence, fewer childhood risk factors, alcohol-related problems, and psychopathological dysfunction; Type B, early onset of alcohol-related problems, increased number of childhood risk factors, family history of alcoholism, and greater severity of dependence.

DISULFIRAM

Disulfiram is an irreversible acetaldehyde dehydrogenase inhibitor that blocks alcohol metabolism, leading to an accumulation of acetaldehyde. Disulfiram reinforces an individual's desire to stop drinking by providing a disincentive associated with increased acetaldehyde levels, resulting in headache, palpitations, hypotension, flushing, nausea, and vomiting when patients consume alcohol. Although results from clinical trials are inconsistent, some consensus has developed that oral disulfiram reduces the number of drinking days.[116] Supervision of disulfiram administration leads to better outcomes, although not always of the order of a statistically significant effect.[128]

The primary predictor of success with disulfiram is the patient's commitment to total abstinence from alcohol. Although anecdotal reports of success are common, clinical evidence suggests disulfiram appears to be most effective for alcoholics who are involved in special high-risk situations (e.g., weddings, graduations) and is particularly effective when administration is supervised.[116]

Evidence

Controlled clinical trials of disulfiram have failed to demonstrate a consistent therapeutic benefit.[116] Double-blind, placebo-controlled studies using disulfiram are difficult because the psychological deterrent to use alcohol is experienced by both treatment groups and those who relapse will be unblinded when they experience the pharmacologic interaction.

In the most rigorous clinical trial conducted in a population of veterans, no significant difference in abstinence rates was demonstrated between patients taking placebo or 1 mg or 250 mg of disulfiram.[117] Patients randomly assigned to receive 250 mg of disulfiram daily drank less frequently (significantly fewer drinking days per year), however. Patients who were middle-aged and had social stability were more likely to benefit from disulfiram. In another trial in which administration was supervised, patients receiving disulfiram drank less alcohol and less frequently; however, on randomization, patients were unblinded to their drug.[139]

The efficacy of disulfiram compared with other drugs such as naltrexone is poorly studied.[140] Although no advantage was seen for combining disulfiram with naltrexone in dually diagnosed alcohol-dependent patients,[141] in one study disulfiram combined with acamprosate resulted in increased days of cumulative abstinence.[142]

Dosing

The recommended starting dose of disulfiram is 250 mg once daily, with a range of 125 to 500 mg/day.[141] If a patient drinks and does not experience a disulfiram-ethanol reaction, the dose can be increased to 500 mg, as a significant proportion of patients may not experience a disulfiram-alcohol reaction at the usual 250-mg daily dose.[143,144] Side effects are increased, however, at doses exceeding 250 mg. Dosing starts at least 12 to 24 hours after abstinence initiation (when the blood or breath alcohol concentration is zero). Treatment continues, depending on the particular needs of the individual, but is generally at least 90 days, and maintenance therapy may be required for years.

Contraindications, Warnings, and Interactions

Because of the intense cardiovascular and physical changes that occur in the disulfiram–ethanol interaction, disulfiram is contraindicated in patients with cardiac disease, coronary occlusion, cerebrovascular disease, and renal or hepatic failure. At somewhat higher doses, psychotic reactions have occurred. Many clinicians avoid disulfiram use in elderly patients or in those with any significant medical illness (e.g., diabetes). It is not definitive that disulfiram causes fetal abnormalities when administered during pregnancy,[145] but some data are found regarding limb reduction anomalies in infants born to disulfiram-treated mothers taking disulfiram during the first trimester of pregnancy.[146] As a result, disulfiram should only be used during pregnancy if the expected benefit to the mother and fetus is greater than the possible risk to the fetus; however, it should be avoided in the first trimester

TABLE 87-8
Recently Completed or Major Ongoing Drug Trials for Alcoholism

Drug	Pros	Cons	Comments
Sertraline 200 mg/d[129]	Selectively targeting LOA subtypes	Most likely little treatment benefit for EOA subtype	$N = 134$; EOA and LOA; significant interaction between LL alleles and sertraline but only in LOA group.
Topiramate 300 mg (maximal dose)[130,131]	Potentially mimics actions of alcohol without the reinforcement	Not tested in recently abstinent alcoholics; optimal dose unknown	$N = 368$; 14 weeks: 6-week titration, 8-week maintenance, and 7–16-day taper. Compared with placebo, topiramate significantly lowered % heavy drinking days ($p = 0.002$), drinks/drinking days ($p = 0.006$) and % of days abstinent ($p = 0.002$).
Ondansetron 4 mcg/kg twice a day[132]	Treatment matching in EOA based on SERT may result; nominal side effects	Most likely little treatment benefit for LOA subtype	$N = 304$ with LL 5-HTTLPR and the SS/SL SERT. Significant interaction between L′L′ genotype and ondansetron.
Ondansetron 4 mcg/kg twice a day and Topiramate 300 mg (maximal dose)	The combination of ondansetron and topiramate may be additive among EOA	Ondansetron dosing by weight does not easily translate to clinical practice	$N = 360$ 12 weeks; project still ongoing.
Aripiprazole 30 mg (maximal dose)[133]	Multiple mechanisms of action	No preclinical or clinical data; not tested in actively drinking alcoholics; optimal dose unknown	$N = 266$ 12 weeks; also received weekly psychotherapy. Discontinuations (40.3% vs. 26.7%) and treatment-related adverse events (82.8% vs. 63.6%) were higher with aripiprazole than placebo. No significant difference compared with placebo in % days abstinent ($p = 0.227$), % subjects without a heavy drinking day, or time to first drinking day. The aripiprazole group had fewer drinks per drinking day ($p < 0.001$).
Naltrexone injection 190 mg or 380 mg[134]	Increased adherence	Pain management	6 months; 380 mg of long-acting naltrexone ($n = 205$) or 190 mg of long-acting naltrexone ($n = 210$) or a matching volume of placebo ($n = 209$) each administered monthly and combined with 12 sessions of low-intensity psychosocial intervention. Compared with placebo, 380 mg of long-acting naltrexone resulted in a 25% decrease in the event rate of heavy drinking days ($p = 0.02$) and 190 mg of naltrexone resulted in a 17% decrease ($p = 0.07$). Sex and pretreatment abstinence each showed significant interaction with the medication group on treatment outcome, with men and those with lead-in abstinence both exhibiting greater treatment effects.
Naltrexone and Acamprosate 100 mg and 3 g (maximal doses)[127]	Targeting positive and negative reinforcement	Not tested in actively drinking alcoholics	$N = 1{,}383$; 16 weeks; patients receiving medical management with naltrexone, CBI, or both fared better on drinking outcomes, whereas acamprosate showed no evidence of efficacy, with or without CBI.
SR141716, Rimonabant[135]	Unique mechanism of action; potentially useful for nicotine cessation and weight loss	Little research on drugs that block the endocannabinoid system (i.e., potential side effects)	$N = 40$ laboratory study of non–treatment-seeking volunteers using cannabinoid-1 antagonist. 20 mg/day of rimonabant for 2 weeks has no effect on alcohol consumption in non–treatment-seeking heavy drinkers
Naltrexone and Sertraline[136]	Combination may yield better abstinence rates	Both drugs have gastrointestinal side effects	$N = 198$ Alaskan Native Americans; results suggest that combining sertraline with naltrexone is not better than naltrexone alone
Gabapentin as an adjunct to Naltrexone for alcoholism	Practical application to clinical practice		Examine whether alcoholics receiving naltrexone and adjunctive gabapentin will have fewer relapses than those treated with naltrexone alone. Project still ongoing.
Quetiapine XR 450 mg[137]	Some antipsychotics associated with reduced alcohol use	Side effects with quetiapine significantly greater than placebo	This study examined the efficacy of quetiapine XR 450 mg on the percentage of heavy drinking days in 224 heavy drinking patients. No significant results reported.
Aprepitant	NK1R antagonists may mediate stress response and decrease insula activation		Examine craving and fMRI changes in 120 comorbid PTSD and alcohol-dependent patients. Project still ongoing.

CBI, combined behavioral intervention; EOA, early-onset alcoholism; 5-HTTLPR, serotonin transporter polymorphism; fMRI, functional magnetic resonance imaging; L′L′, $long_A long_A$ 5-HTTLPR alleles; LOA, late-onset alcoholism; PTSD, posttraumatic stress disorderl SERT, sertraline; SS/SL, short-short 5-HTTLPR alleles/short-long 5-HTTLPR alleles.

(category C). No information is available about the safety of this medicine during breast-feeding.

Disulfiram can also be hepatotoxic and should be used cautiously in patients with liver disease. Liver function should be established at baseline and after 14 days of treatment, and a complete blood count (CBC) and liver function tests (LFTs) should be obtained every 6 months.[147]

R.M. has normal hepatic function; however, LFTs should be monitored at baseline and periodically during treatment. Although not all clinicians agree, most would recommend—at minimum—baseline LFTs: ALT, AST, and GGT and withholding disulfiram when LFTs are more than three times upper limits of normal.[147] If elevated, repeat LFTs every 1 to 2 weeks until normal, and then every 3 to 6 months if no elevations, with an awareness that increased LFT results may signal a return to drinking rather than disulfiram toxicity.[148,149] Persistently elevated LFTs may also indicate viral hepatitis (B or C), for which alcoholics have a higher risk, and thus the need to order a hepatitis profile. Currently no specific guidelines exist to determine whether a patient with elevated LFTs should or should not receive treatment for alcoholism. Many clinicians anecdotally feel that as long as a patient's hepatic function is closely monitored, a reduction in alcohol use will lead to more normalized LFTs. Wide ranges of psychiatric adverse effects include disorientation, agitation, depression, and behavioral changes such as paranoia, withdrawal and bizarre behaviors, and worsening of schizophrenia, especially at doses greater than 250 mg daily.[150,151] Disulfiram should be avoided or used very cautiously in persons with these conditions. Disulfiram can be used relatively safely at a dose of 250 mg daily in alcohol-dependent patients with concomittant psychiatric disorders, including schizophrenia.[141,152,153]

Disulfiram is a potent inhibitor of the CYP2E1 oxidase, and can interact with anticoagulants (warfarin), antiepileptics (phenytoin, carbamazepine), some benzodiazepines (e.g., diazepam but not lorazepam), and tricyclic antidepressants (amitriptyline, desipramine), potentially increasing the toxicity of these medications. Delirium can result in combination with monoamine oxidase inhibitors. Adverse effects with disulfiram that mimic the alcohol–disulfiram interaction can also occur with metronidazole and omeprazole.[154]

Patient Education

To receive optimal results with disulfiram, patients must receive regular counseling and be closely monitored for any changes in hepatic function. Patients should be advised that the involvement of significant others will facilitate their recovery. Having someone participate in helping to validate the administration process is known to lead to better outcomes. Discontinuation of disulfiram should occur only after consultation with the prescriber and counselor involved. Common side effects of disulfiram include drowsiness, particularly in the first few weeks of treatment, a metallic or garlic taste, and sexual dysfunction. The dose can be taken at bedtime if drowsiness or tiredness occurs.

Patients must stop the medication for at least 3 days (up to 14 days in some) before being exposed to products containing alcohol. What cannot be overlooked is that patients taking disulfiram must be informed about the dangers of consuming even small amounts of alcohol in foods, in over-the-counter medications, in mouthwashes, and in topical lotions. Also, it is important to verify that the patients understand the necessary precautions and the consequences of alcohol use. The patient should call the prescriber to report any respiratory difficulty, nausea, vomiting, decreased appetite, dark colored urine, or a change in pigmentation in the skin or eyes (primarily yellowing).

Summary

Generally, given the special circumstances needed for success, disulfiram is generally not the drug of choice for treating alcoholism. The social, medical, and psychiatric status of a candidate is an important consideration in the use of disulfiram. R.M. would appear to be a reasonable candidate for disulfiram given he has agreed to have his medication administration supervised (in this case by his wife), his steady employment, and his motivation to sustain abstinence. R.M. should also receive counseling and support services on a regular basis.

CASE 87-4

QUESTION 1: T.M. is a 60-year-old woman who weighs 105 pounds, is 63 inches tall, and is actively drinking about 40 to 50 drinks a week. Her CIWA-Ar score is 8. T.M. wants a medication that will gradually reduce her alcohol use over time so that she can drink socially with friends. T.M. has heard of acamprosate and asked for some samples but she was refused. Laboratory values obtained today include the following:

Sodium, 143 mEq/L	ALP, 80 units/L
Potassium, 4.2 mEq/L	AST, 30 units/L
CO_2, 25.2 mEq/L	ALT, 23 units/L
Chloride, 110 mEq/L	Uric acid, 3.3 mg/dL
BUN, 14 mg/dL	Calcium, 8.9 mg/dL
Glucose, 91 mg/dL	Albumin 4.5 g/dL
Creatinine, 1.2 mg/dL	Cholesterol, 195 mg/dL
Total bilirubin, 0.8 mg/dL	CK, 190 units/L
Direct bilirubin, 0.2 mg/dL	Magnesium, 1.9 mg/dL

Is acamprosate therapy appropriate for the treatment of T.M.'s alcohol use disorder?

ACAMPROSATE

Acamprosate (Campral) has multiple actions, but is principally a glutamate and GABA modulator. In vitro and in vivo studies in animals suggest that acamprosate interacts with GABA and glutamate to restore the imbalance of neuronal excitation[155] and inhibition[156] caused by chronic alcohol use. The key mechanism of action is considered to be as a weak functional antagonist of the glutamate NMDA receptor, possibly mediated through indirect modulation of the receptor site via antagonism at the mGluR5 receptor.[157] A series of meta-analyses and systematic reviews demonstrated that when used as an adjunct to psychosocial interventions, acamprosate improves drinking outcomes such as the length and rate of abstinence.[116,158–160] This effect is doubtful if acamprosate is not initiated quickly after a detoxification.[161,162] Evidence indicates that the effect of acamprosate on abstinence lasts after the treatment is stopped.[163] The success of acamprosate, however, seems limited to European trials as the two US trials both failed to demonstrate significant results on primary outcome measures.[127,164,165]

Acamprosate appears to be especially useful in a therapeutic regimen targeted at promoting abstinence and can be used in primary care settings as well as specialized addiction treatment programs.[166] Acamprosate has been studied in thousands of patients, primarily in Europe, and few contraindications to treatment exist. Little consistent information is found about patient characteristics that predict improvement while taking acamprosate. In a meta-analysis of all US and European studies, predictors of abstinence were motivation, readiness to change,

Patient Education

Naltrexone tablets have been demonstrated to be more effective when used in combination with CBT or some type of psychosocial therapy. Therefore, to obtain the optimal long-term benefit, patients must plan on meeting with a health care professional or counselor and enroll in a behavior modification or support group program such as Alcoholics Anonymous that supports their abstinence. Patients should be reminded not to use opioids or any medications not approved by the prescriber during treatment. Patients receiving naltrexone must be opioidfree from 7 to 10 days as substantiated with a urine drug test and should be asked to wear some kind of identifier for medical emergencies. Particularly with naltrexone injection, documentation to alert medical personnel of naltrexone treatment is needed in case of trauma necessitating pain management.

In a yearlong safety study, the most common side effects were nausea, dizziness, sedation, headache, anxiety, and blurred vision.[200] Should such side effects occur, reducing the dosage by one-half often reduces the side effects. Large doses (e.g., 200 mg) of naltrexone can cause liver failure. Patients should report excessive tiredness, unusual bleeding or bruising, loss of appetite, pain in the upper right part of the stomach, any discoloration of the skin or eyes, a change in stool color or urine, thoughts of suicide, or signs of pneumonia. Patients receiving extended-release naltrexone injection must also monitor the injection site for pain, swelling, tenderness, bruising, or redness that does not improve or even worsens within 2 weeks of the injection. These reactions may result in induration, cellulitis, abscess, sterile abscess, or necrosis. Some patients may need to be evaluated for surgical intervention.[200]

An important consumer consideration to note is cost. Naltrexone injection costs about $1,122 a month compared with less than $130 for a months' supply of 50-mg tablets. Because the injection is fairly new and expensive, some insurance plans might not pay for it, or it may be available on formulary but at a higher copay rate to the patient. This cost may represent a significant barrier to affordable treatment for many patients.

Summary

Naltrexone, CBT, or a support group would be appropriate for T.M. Current evidence suggests, however, that tablets rather than injection would be the most appropriate choice for T.M. Primary concerns would be poor hepatic function (which is normal in T.M.) or previous failure with the medication. The primary consideration in this case is that no significant difference has been seen in drinking outcomes in women who received naltrexone or placebo injections.[134] Although this perhaps anomalous result is still being investigated, sufficient support exists to prescribe naltrexone tablets to this patient. On the other hand, although everyone received a 1-hour low-intensity psychosocial intervention every other week, women compared with men in the control group reduced their alcohol use more than did men, suggesting that using a psychosocial approach such as CBT (Table 87-6) would also benefit T.M.[134]

COMBINATION PHARMACOTHERAPY

CASE 87-4, QUESTION 3: T.M. reduces her alcohol use substantially, but is still drinking. Is there any advantage to the combination therapy of acamprosate with naltrexone?

The rationale for combining medications, is that acamprosate reduces negative reinforcement and naltrexone attenuates positive reinforcement.[60] To test this hypothesis, a randomized, controlled study of 160 patients performed in Europe demonstrated that although combining naltrexone and acamprosate was more effective than either placebo or acamprosate alone, adding acamprosate was not significantly more effective than naltrexone alone.[183] In a much larger study, the COMBINE trial randomized more than 1,300 individuals in a double-blind fashion to receive placebo, naltrexone, or acamprosate alone or in combination with medical management or CBI.[127] Results from this study suggest that acamprosate has no significant effect on drinking versus placebo, either by itself or with any combination of the other treatments in the study. Furthermore, patients receiving placebo and medical management (MM) from a health care professional (Table 87-6) had better outcomes than patients receiving CBI (a CBT-like therapy that includes 12-step facilitation) alone. From the available evidence, it would not be reasonable to combine acamprosate with naltrexone.

ALTERNATIVE PHARMACOTHERAPY

CASE 87-5

QUESTION 1: W.W. is a 48-year-old male executive, who weighs 230 pounds and is 73 inches tall. He comes for help with his alcohol use, which he recognizes is out of control. He has previously tried disulfiram, naltrexone, and acamprosate, and does not want the naltrexone injection. Currently, W.W. is drinking 55 drinks a week. His CIWA-Ar score is 9 (although he does not appear to need inpatient detoxification). His laboratory work reveals the following:

Sodium, 134 mEq/L	ALP, 74 units/L
Potassium, 4.5 mEq/L	AST, 70 units/L
CO_2, 29.2 mEq/L	ALT, 89 units/L
Chloride, 97 mEq/L	Uric acid, 5.8 mg/dL
BUN, 14 mg/dL	Calcium, 10.0 mg/dL
Creatinine, 1.1 mg/dL	Albumin, 3.6 g/dL
Glucose, 151 mg/dL	Cholesterol, 189 mg/dL
Total bilirubin, 0.4 mg/dL	CK, 90 units/L
Direct bilirubin, 0.1 mg/dL	Magnesium, 2.3 mg/d

What other medications might be considered for use in W.W.?

Topiramate

Topiramate is an FDA-approved medication found to have multiple mechanisms of action, including enhanced $GABA_A$ inhibition that results in decreased dopamine facilitation in the midbrain, thought to be of potential benefit in the treatment of addiction.[201] Additionally, it causes antagonism of kainate to activate the kainate/AMPA glutamate receptor subtypes[202] and inhibition of type II and IV carbonic anhydrase isoenzymes.

EVIDENCE

Topiramate is not FDA-approved for the treatment of alcoholism. Because the drug has come off patent, it is unlikely the manufacturer will pursue an indication for topiramate in the treatment of alcohol dependence. A randomized, double-blind, placebo-controlled trial used an escalating dose from 25 to 300 mg/day of topiramate or matching placebo in 150 alcohol-dependent men and women during the first 8 weeks of a 12-week period.[126] Patients stayed at the same dose for the last 4 weeks of the study. All patients in the study received brief behavioral compliance enhancement therapy (BBCET) that was a 10- to 15-minute meeting with a health care professional that focused on resolving side effect issues and facilitated adherence (Table 87-6). Participants receiving topiramate reported significantly fewer drinks per day and drinks per drinking day, significantly fewer drinking days, significantly more days of abstinence, and significantly less craving than those on placebo. The evidence suggests that although abstinence was not a goal at the start of the topiramate study, the medication may be more beneficial during the abstinence initiation phase of treatment.[203] In a phase II clinical trial, the use of topiramate for alcohol dependence treatment was confirmed by outcomes demonstrating that topiramate recipients showed a significantly greater lowering of percentage of heavy drinking days and drinks per drinking day, and a higher percentage of days abstinent. Using a repeated-measures mixed model, topiramate showed even greater efficacy compared with placebo ($p < 0.001$) for all comparisons,[130] including quality of life.[131] In summary, topiramate shows great promise as a treatment for alcohol dependence, and it is unfortunate that there is no corporate interest to seek an indication for alcohol dependence.[204]

In the treatment of alcohol dependence, topiramate is titrated from 25 mg/day up to 300 mg/day over a 6-week period (100 mg in the morning; 200 mg in the afternoon) or to the patient's maximal tolerable dose. Abrupt discontinuation of topiramate has been associated with seizures in patients without a history of seizures, and for this reason, gradual withdrawal of the drug (e.g., a 25% decrease in the dosage every 4 days for 16 days) is recommended.

CASE 87-5, QUESTION 2: W.W. also reports a more than 2-week period of feeling worthless, suicidal ideation, a 29-pound weight loss during the last 6 weeks, hypersomnia, and lethargy. These symptoms have alternated with short periods (e.g., ~4 days) of feeling exhilarated, expansiveness, compulsive buying sprees, hyposomnia, and arguments with friends and coworkers. He does not report any psychotic episodes. How should patients with underlying psychiatric and alcohol use disorders be approached?

W.W. reports symptoms that appear consistent with bipolar II disorder (ruling out any other diagnosis) that would include a formal differential diagnosis of major depressive disorder and hypomania without psychosis. Clinicians must consider the potential for dual diagnosis disorders (e.g., depression, bipolar disorder, or schizophrenia) combined with substance dependence (e.g., as with alcohol). Tobacco and caffeine dependence are common. A significant number of individuals with mental health disorders also have an alcohol use disorder compared with the general population.[205] Increased comorbid conditions also lead to a poorer treatment prognosis.

Principles for the optimal treatment of patients with a dual diagnosis include the following: (a) flexibility (e.g., although the goal of treatment may be abstinence, for some patents movement in the right direction is just as important to keep the person engaged in treatment); (b) repetition (e.g., a constant refocusing of attention for avoiding alcohol and for confronting their psychiatric symptoms is a priority); and (c) counseling (e.g., matching patients to the appropriate intervention). These factors are all fundamental to long-lasting treatment success. Medications, when appropriate (e.g., early and vigorous drug intervention with nonaddictive medications), may also help the patient stay in treatment; however, every effort must be made to use medications that do not induce euphoria or cause dependence, and are effective and safe even during relapse.

Clinicians must distinguish between drug-induced and drug-related psychiatric disorders. Ideally, but often impractical, is to permit 3 to 4 weeks of abstinence to provide adequate information to determine the relationship of the alcohol use disorder with the psychiatric disorder. A complete drug use history, urinalysis, and blood or hair drug tests should be obtained. A comprehensive history, including age of onset of disorders, persistence of psychiatric illness during abstinence, and very importantly, family history, should provide adequate diagnostic information.

Patients with both drug use and psychiatric disorders constitute a substantial and challenging subpopulation. Treating the alcohol use disorder alone predicts a poorer outcome for other disorders including early relapse. Early and aggressive treatment for each condition should be implemented. Furthermore, care must be taken to ensure that the medications prescribed are safe if combined with alcohol.

A few studies have evaluated the effectiveness of mood stabilizers (e.g., lithium, carbamazepine, divalproex, atypical antipsychotics, and topiramate) in the treatment of comorbid bipolar disorder and alcohol dependence.[206,207] Some evidence suggests that topiramate may be helpful during the depressive phase of bipolar disorder,[207] perhaps as a result of reducing alcohol use.[208] Clinicians should monitor weight loss,[209] worsening depression, and suicidal ideation in patients using topiramate.[210] Although all antiepileptics have been associated with an increased risk of suicidality, topiramate has been found to have the lowest risk for suicidality.[211]

CASE 87-5, QUESTION 3: During an 8-week period, W.W. is taking 300 mg of topiramate a day and is only drinking 10 drinks a week. W.W. complains that he is experiencing pins and needles in his arms and hands. Is this related to symptoms of withdrawal or to topiramate?

It is likely that tingling in the extremities, called paresthesias, is a possible result of withdrawal from alcohol; however, the more probable reason for this occurrence (given the temporal relationship) is as a side effect of topiramate therapy. In addition to paresthesias, other prominent side effects include mental confusion, slowness in thinking, depression, and somnolence, which may be attenuated by titration when initiating therapy, and the development of renal calculi in about 1.5% of patients.[210] Adequate hydration is encouraged, particularly in patients who may be at risk for developing calculi.

CONTRAINDICATIONS, WARNINGS, AND INTERACTIONS

Topiramate is contraindicated in those hypersensitive to the drug. Topiramate should be used with caution in those who have a history of urolithiasis, paresthesias, secondary angle closure glaucoma, renal or hepatic impairment, and conditions or therapies that predispose to acidosis (e.g., renal disease, severe respiratory disorders, status epilepticus, diarrhea, surgery, ketogenic diet, or drugs). Monitoring for hyperchloremic non–ionic-gap metabolic acidosis is essential, and therefore baseline chemistry (e.g., HCO_3^- and pH) should be assessed and monitored regularly thereafter. Metabolic acidosis can cause symptoms such as tiredness and loss of appetite, or more serious conditions including arrhythmia or coma. Topiramate has been found to be teratogenic in animal studies and is a pregnancy category C medication.[210]

Concomitant use of oral contraceptives, phenytoin, carbamazepine, and valproic acid has been found to interact with topiramate.[154] Coadministration of another carbonic anhydrase inhibitor, such as acetazolamide, may increase the possibility of renal stone formation and should be avoided.

PATIENT EDUCATION

Patients should be advised not to adjust the dose or discontinue the medication without consulting a health care provider.

Unless otherwise instructed, to prevent kidney stones and dehydration, patients should maintain adequate hydration and be advised to drink 2 to 3 L/day of fluid. Patients may be at risk for decreased sweating and increased body temperature and should therefore monitor their exercise, particularly in hot weather. Topiramate can cause drowsiness, dizziness, changes in memory, a change in taste (particularly with carbonated beverages), vision changes (particularly associated with increased intraocular pressure), pressure to the touch, loss of appetite or unplanned weight loss, and sudden changes in mood.

SUMMARY

Evidence for the effectiveness of topiramate is promising, although more clinical research is needed on topiramate in efficacy and effectiveness trials, as well as determining the proper dose. Although W.W. has some liver impairment (AST and ALT twice the normal limit), some evidence supports the use of valproate as a good choice to treat the diagnosis of bipolar disorder and AUD in this particular patient[212]; drug levels must be monitored, however, because valproate is entirely metabolized by the liver. Topiramate, on the other hand, is renally metabolized and might be considered an adjunctive therapy if W.W. does not completely respond to the drug of first choice.

Baclofen

Baclofen is a possible alternative to topiramate for W.W., as like topiramate, it is not metabolized by the liver, but unlike topiramate, does not cause paresthesias. Baclofen promotes a balance between inhibition of release of GABA, mediated by presynaptic $GABA_B$ receptors, and inhibition of neuronal excitability, mediated by postsynaptic $GABA_B$ receptors.[213] Putatively, agonism of $GABA_B$ receptors also modulates mesolimbic dopamine neurons.[214] Baclofen is approved for use in the United States to reduce cramping, spasms, and muscle tightness.

EFFICACY

Baclofen has been promoted for investigation by the National Institute on Alcohol Abuse and Alcoholism (NIAAA) for alcohol dependence.[215] Studies show that baclofen is effective in reducing alcohol self-administration[216] and motivation to consume alcohol in rats.[217,218] In a double-blind, placebo-controlled trial using baclofen, alcohol-dependent patients reported less craving, drank on fewer days, and had higher rates of total abstinence than those receiving placebo.[219] Moreover, a double-blind, placebo-controlled trial in Italy evaluated the safety and effectiveness of baclofen in 84 alcohol-dependent patients with liver cirrhosis for 12 weeks and reported a significant difference in abstinence favoring the baclofen group.[93] On the other hand, a study performed in the United States reported no significant difference in alcohol-dependent patients.[220] Despite encouraging preclinical data and prior positive clinical trials with baclofen in Europe, the current trial did not find evidence that baclofen is superior to placebo in the treatment of alcohol dependence.

SUMMARY

Because baclofen is metabolized by the kidneys, it would be an alternative adjunct to topiramate to treat the AUD diagnosis in W.W. The evidence for baclofen is limited and should only be considered an alternative if other approved drugs failed or W.W. was known to be allergic to topiramate.

DRUG INTERACTIONS

CASE 87-6

QUESTION 1: T.C. is a 32-year-old man who has been diagnosed with alcohol dependence and depression. He reports recent weight loss (20 pounds in the last month), excessive "sluggishness," an increased need for sleep (10–12 hours a day), and feelings of guilt and worthlessness. His depression is likely substance induced, but the importance of his alcohol use is largely ignored. T.C.'s primary care provider plans to start sustained-release bupropion for depression. Laboratory tests were performed at the visit, but results are not yet available. What should be considered when prescribing bupropion or any other medication to T.C., and what simple information should T.C. be given?

Prescription drug use and interactions with alcohol are fairly common with individuals diagnosed with alcohol abuse or dependence disorders. Alcohol–prescription drug interactions in patients diagnosed with AUD have been found to be as high as 40%, with more than 20% taking medications with moderate to severe alcohol interactions.[221] The interaction of alcohol with the cytochrome-P450 enzyme system may be complex, and depends on duration of consumption. Notably, short-term consumption leads to a competitive inhibition of CYP2E1, whereas chronic use leads to induction of this enzyme. CYP2E1 induction leads to increased clearance of such drugs as alcohol itself, warfarin, diazepam, rifamycin, meprobamate, pentobarbital, and propranolol, with the effect on liver metabolism lasting for days to weeks after discontinuation of alcohol. More importantly, the CYP2E1 enzyme system converts several substances into highly toxic metabolites. These include cocaine, enflurane and methoxyflurane, isoniazid, phenylbutazone, and acetaminophen. Through induction of this alternate pathway of drug metabolism, otherwise safe doses of drugs may become hepatotoxic. Obviously, clinicians must consider the impact (e.g., on the liver) of prescribing drugs when patients are also abusing or dependent on alcohol.[154] (See Table 87-9 for more alcohol–drug interactions.)

Summary

An alternative to bupropion should be considered, particularly in light of the unavailability of T.C.'s laboratory test results. In this case, critical issues need to be considered, particularly hepatic function, which may be associated with an increased risk of seizures. Bupropion is extensively metabolized by the liver and should be used with extreme caution in patients with severe hepatic cirrhosis. In these patients, a reduced dose or frequency of administration is required, as peak plasma levels are substantially elevated, thereby increasing the risk of seizures. The dose should not exceed 150 mg every other day in patients with impaired hepatic function.[154] Additionally, patients should be told that the excessive use or abrupt discontinuation of alcohol may alter their seizure threshold, and bupropion is therefore contraindicated in patients undergoing abrupt discontinuation of alcohol. Patients have also reported lower alcohol tolerance during treatment with bupropion. Patients, in general, should be advised that the consumption of alcohol should be minimized or avoided.[222] Moreover, a recent study demonstrated that one-third of patients with AUD who were prescribed drugs were never advised not to take their prescribed medication with alcohol.[221] The study also reported that bupropion, serotonin reuptake inhibitors (SSRIs), and acetaminophen were the drugs most frequently involved in drug–alcohol interactions.

TABLE 87-9
Ethanol–Drug Interactions

Acetaminophen	Chronic excessive alcohol consumption increases susceptibility to acetaminophen-induced hepatotoxicity. Acute intoxication theoretically protects against acetaminophen toxicity because less hepatotoxic metabolite is generated.
Anticoagulants (oral)	Chronic ethanol consumption induces hepatic metabolism of warfarin, decreasing hypoprothrombinemic effect. Very large acute ethanol doses (>3 drinks/d) may impair the metabolism of warfarin and increase hypothrombinemic effect. Vitamin K-dependent clotting factors may be reduced in alcoholics with liver disease, also affecting coagulation.
Antidepressants	Enhanced sedative effects of alcohol and psychomotor impairment are possible. Acute ethanol impairs metabolism. Fluoxetine, paroxetine, fluvoxamine, and probably other serotonin reuptake inhibitors (SSRIs) do not interfere with psychomotor or subjective effects of ethanol.
Ascorbic acid	Ascorbic acid increases ethanol clearance and serum triglyceride levels and improves motor coordination and color discrimination after ethanol consumption.
Barbiturates	Phenobarbital decreases blood ethanol concentration; acute intoxication inhibits pentobarbital metabolism; chronic intoxication enhances hepatic pentobarbital metabolism.
Benzodiazepines	Psychomotor impairment increases with the combination.
Bromocriptine	Ethanol increases gastrointestinal side effects of bromocriptine.
Caffeine	Caffeine has no effect on ethanol-induced psychomotor impairment.
Calcium-channel blockers	Verapamil inhibits ethanol metabolism and increases intoxication.
Cephalosporin antibiotics	Ethanol produces flushing, nausea, headaches, tachycardia, and hypotension. Cephalosporin antibiotics that have an ethyltetrazolethiol side chain produce this disulfiramlike reaction (e.g., cefoperazone, cefamandole, cefotetan).
Chloral hydrate	Elevation of plasma trichloroethanol (a chloral hydrate metabolite) and blood ethanol may occur. Combined central nervous system (CNS) depression. Vasodilation, tachycardia, headache.
Chloroform	Ethanol increases chloroform hepatotoxicity.
Doxycycline	Chronic consumption of ethanol induces hepatic metabolism of doxycycline and may lower serum concentration of the antibiotic.
Erythromycin	Ethanol may interfere with absorption of the ethylsuccinate salt. Effects on other formulations are unknown.
Furazolidone	When ethanol is ingested, nausea, flushing, lightheadedness, and dyspnea may occur (i.e., a disulfiramlike reaction).
H_2 antagonists	Cimetidine potentiates ethanol effects. Increases peak plasma ethanol concentrations and area under the plasma ethanol concentration time curve. CNS toxicity from increased cimetidine serum concentration. Nizatidine and ranitidine may also increase blood alcohol levels slightly by inhibiting gastric alcohol dehydrogenase. Famotidine does not affect blood alcohol levels.
Isoniazid	Consumption of ethanol with isoniazid increases risk of hepatotoxicity. Tyramine-containing alcoholic beverages may cause hypertensive reaction.
Ketoconazole and metronidazole	When ethanol is ingested, nausea, flushing, lightheadedness, and dyspnea may occur (i.e., a disulfiramlike reaction may occur with metronidazole). A sunburnlike rash has been reported with ethanol consumption and ketoconazole. A similar reaction may occur with itraconazole, although no reports exist.
Meprobamate	Synergistic CNS depression may occur.
Metoclopramide	Enhances sedative effects of ethanol.
Monoamine oxidase inhibitors	Tyramine-containing alcoholic beverages (e.g., wines, beer) may cause a hypertensive crisis. Pargyline may inhibit aldehyde dehydrogenase and cause a disulfiramlike interaction with ethanol.
Narcotic analgesics	Volume of distribution of intravenous meperidine increases with increasing ethanol consumption. Clinical significance unknown. Potential for enhanced CNS depression.
Oral hypoglycemic agents	Chlorpropamide, tolbutamide, and tolazamide may cause flushing, lightheadedness, nausea, and dyspnea if alcohol is ingested (i.e., a disulfiramlike reaction).
Paraldehyde	Possible metabolic acidosis may occur.
Phenothiazines	Potentiates psychomotor effects of ethanol.
Quinacrine	Possibly inhibits acetaldehyde oxidation.
Salicylates	Increases gastric bleeding associated with aspirin; may increase chance of gastrointestinal hemorrhage.
Tetrachloroethylene	Combined CNS depression may occur.
Trichloroethylene	Flushing, lacrimation, blurred vision, and tachypnea may occur when patients exposed to trichloroethylene drink alcohol.

Adapted with permission from Ciraulo D, Shader RI, Greenblatt DJ, Creelman WL. *Drug Interactions in Psychiatry*. 3rd ed. Philadelphia, PA.: Lippincott Williams & Wilkins; 2006.

KEY REFERENCES AND WEBSITES

A full list of references for this chapter can be found at http://thepoint.lww.com/AT10e. Below are the key references and websites for this chapter, with the corresponding reference number in this chapter found in parentheses after the reference.

Key References

Amato L et al. Benzodiazepines for alcohol withdrawal. *Cochrane Database Syst Rev*. 2010;(3):CD005063. (91)

Anton RF et al. Combined pharmacotherapies and behavioral interventions for alcohol dependence: the COMBINE study: a randomized controlled trial. *JAMA*. 2006;295:2003. (127)

Johnson BA et al. Ondansetron for reduction of drinking among biologically predisposed patients: A randomized controlled trial. *JAMA*. 2000;284:963. (125)

Johnson BA et al. Topiramate for treating alcohol dependence: a randomized controlled trial. *JAMA*. 2007;298:1541. (130)

Kenna GA. Pharmacogenomics and the future of alcohol dependence treatment. In: Sher L, ed. *Research on the Neurobiology of Alcohol Use Disorders*. New York, N.Y.: Nova Publishers; 2008:79. (170)

Kenna GA et al. Review of topiramate: an antiepileptic for the treatment of alcohol dependence. *Curr Drug Abuse Rev.* 2009;2: 135. (204)

Kenna GA et al. Pharmacotherapy, pharmacogenomics and the future of alcohol dependence treatment. Part 2. *Am J Health Syst Pharm.* 2004;61:2380. (11)

Leggio L et al. Typologies of alcohol dependence. From Jellinek to genetics and beyond. *Neuropsychol Rev.* 2009;19:115. (138)

Ray LA et al. Naltrexone for the treatment of alcoholism: clinical findings, mechanisms of action, and pharmacogenetics. *CNS Neurol Disord Drug Targets.* 2010;9:13. (190)

Key Websites

Alcoholic Anonymous: http://www.aa.org.

The National Institute on Alcohol Abuse and Alcoholism: http://www.niaaa.nih.gov.

Research Society on Alcoholism: http://www.rsoa.org.

88

Tobacco Use and Dependence

Robin L. Corelli and Karen Suchanek Hudmon

CORE PRINCIPLES

		CHAPTER CASES
1	Cigarette smoking is the single most preventable cause of premature death in the United States, responsible for one in every five deaths. Smoking harms nearly every organ of the body, causing many diseases (including, but not limited to, cardiovascular disease, pulmonary disease, and cancers) and reducing the health of smokers in general. Quitting smoking has immediate as well as long-term benefits, reducing risks for diseases caused by smoking and improving health in general.	**Case 88-2 (Questions 1, 4), Case 88-3 (Question 1), Case 88-5 (Question 1), Case 88-6 (Question 1)**
2	Tobacco products are effective delivery systems for the drug nicotine. Nicotine is a highly addictive drug that activates the dopamine reward pathway in the brain that reinforces continued tobacco use. Nicotine withdrawal symptoms (e.g., irritability, anxiety, difficulty concentrating, restlessness, depressed mood, insomnia, impaired performance, increased appetite or weight gain, cravings) generally occur when nicotine is discontinued.	**Case 88-1 (Questions 2, 4), Case 88-3 (Question 1), Case 88-6 (Questions 1, 2)**
3	Constituents in tobacco smoke are associated with a number of clinically significant drug interactions.	**Case 88-4 (Questions 1, 3), Case 88-6 (Question 3)**
4	Tobacco dependence, a chronic disease that often requires repeated intervention and multiple attempts to quit, is characterized by physiological dependence (addiction to nicotine) and behavioral habit of using tobacco.	**Case 88-1 (Question 5), Case 88-2 (Question 3), Case 88-3 (Question 1)**
5	Numerous effective medications, as delineated in the Clinical Practice Guideline, are available for treating tobacco use and dependence. Most patients should be encouraged to use one or more first-line agents, which include the nicotine patch, nicotine gum, nicotine lozenge, nicotine nasal spray, nicotine oral inhaler, sustained-release bupropion, and varenicline. All first-line agents approximately double quit rates, and therefore the choice of therapy is based largely on contraindications, precautions, patient preference, and tolerability of the available dosage forms. In some cases, medications can be combined or used for extended durations. Although complementary therapies are available, these are not recommended because of insufficient evidence of efficacy.	**Case 88-1 (Questions 1–3), Case 88-2 (Questions 3, 4), Case 88-3 (Question 1), Case 88-4 (Question 2), Case 88-6 (Questions 1, 4)**
6	Comprehensive counseling, as defined by the Clinical Practice Guideline, includes asking about tobacco use, advising patients to quit, assessing readiness to quit, assisting patients with quitting, and arranging follow-up. This approach is referred to as "The 5 A's." Counseling and support can be provided a variety of ways, such as through individual counseling, group programs, telephone, or the Internet. Two components of counseling are especially effective and should be applied when assisting patients with quitting: practical counseling (problem solving or skills training) and social support delivered as part of treatment. Relapse is common, and clinicians should work with patients throughout the quit attempt to increase the chances for long-term abstinence.	**Case 88-1 (Questions 2, 5), Case 88-3 (Question 1), Case 88-5 (Question 1), Case 88-6 (Questions 1, 2, 4)**

continued

and by supplementing medication use with behavioral counseling as described later in this chapter.

Assisting Patients With Quitting

BEHAVIORAL COUNSELING STRATEGIES

According to the Clinical Practice Guideline,[8] five key components constitute comprehensive counseling for tobacco cessation: (a) asking patients whether they use tobacco, (b) advising tobacco users to quit, (c) assessing patients' readiness to quit, (d) assisting patients with quitting, and (e) arranging follow-up care. These steps are referred to as the "5 A's" and are described, in brief, as follows. Figure 88-2 can be used as a guide for structuring counseling interactions.

- ***Ask:*** Screening for tobacco use is essential and should be a routine component of clinical care. The following question can be used to identify tobacco users: *"Do you ever smoke or use any type of tobacco?"* At a minimum, tobacco use status (current, former, never user) and level of use (e.g., number of cigarettes smoked per day) should be assessed and documented in the medical record. Also, patients should be asked about exposure to secondhand smoke. Before imparting advice, consider asking the patient for permission to do so: *"Ms. Crosby, may I tell you why this concerns me?"*
- ***Advise:*** Tobacco users should be advised to consider quitting; the advice should be clear and compelling, yet delivered with sensitivity and a tone of voice that communicates concern and a willingness to assist with quitting. When possible, messages should be personalized by relating advice to factors such as a patient's health status, medication regimen, personal reasons for wanting to quit, or the impact of tobacco use on others. For example, *"I'm concerned because you are on two different inhalers for your emphysema. Quitting smoking is the single most important treatment to improve your breathing. I strongly encourage you to quit. Would you be interested in having me help you with this?"*
- ***Assess:*** Key to the provision of appropriate counseling interventions is the assessment of a patient's readiness to quit. Patients should be categorized as being (a) not ready to quit in the next month; (b) ready to quit in the next month; (c) a recent quitter, having quit in the past 6 months; or (d) a former user, having quit more than 6 months ago.[8,48] This classification defines the clinician's next step, which is to provide counseling that is tailored to the patient's level of readiness to quit. As an example for a current smoker: *"Mr. Malkin, what are your thoughts about quitting, and would you consider quitting sometime in the next month?"* The counseling interventions for patients who are ready to quit will be different from those for patients who are not considering quitting.
- ***Assist:*** When counseling tobacco users, it is important that clinicians view quitting as a process that might take months or even years to achieve, rather than a "now or never" event. The goal is to promote forward progress in the process of change, with the target end point being sustained abstinence from all nicotine-containing products.

When counseling patients who are not ready to quit, an important first step is to foster motivation. Some patients who are not ready to quit truly might not believe that they need to quit; however, most will recognize the need to quit but are simply not ready to make the commitment to do so. Often, patients have tried to quit multiple times and failed, and thus are too discouraged to try again. Strategies for working with patients who are not ready to quit involve enhancing motivation to quit,

STEP One: ASK about Tobacco Use

➲ Suggested Dialogue

- "Do you ever smoke or use any type of tobacco?"
- "I take time to talk with all of my patients about tobacco use—because it's important."
- "Medication X often is used for conditions linked with or caused by smoking. Do you, or does someone in your household smoke?"
- "Condition X often is caused or worsened by exposure to tobacco smoke. Do you, or does someone in your household smoke?"

STEP Two: Strongly ADVISE to Quit

➲ Suggested Dialogue

- Quitting is the most important thing you can do to protect your health now and in the future. I have training to help my patients quit, and when you are ready I would be more than happy to work with you to design a treatment plan.
- What are your thoughts about quitting? Might you consider quitting sometime in the next month?

Prior to imparting advice, consider asking the patient for permission to do so – e.g., "May I tell you why this concerns me?" {then elaborate on patient-specific concerns).

STEP Three: ASSESS Readiness to Quit

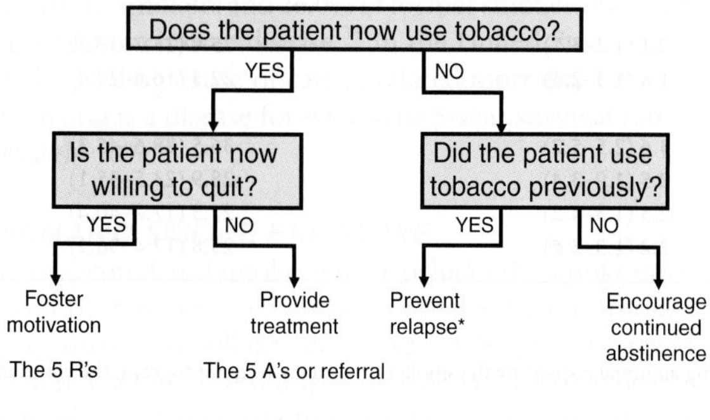
Does the patient now use tobacco?
YES
NO
Is the patient now willing to quit?
YES
NO
Did the patient use tobacco previously?
YES
NO
Foster motivation
Provide treatment
Prevent relapse*
Encourage continued abstinence
The 5 R's
The 5 A's or referral

* Relapse prevention interventions not necessary in the case of the adult who has not used tobacco for many years.

Fiore MC, Jaen CR, Baker TB, et al. Treating Tobacco Use and Dependence: 2008 Update. Clinical Practice Guideline. Rockville, MD: U.S. Department of Health and Human Services, Public Health Service. May 2008.

STEP Four: ASSIST with Quitting

✓ **Assess Tobacco Use History**
- Current use: type(s) of tobacco used, brand, amount
- Past use:
  - Duration of tobacco use
  - Changes in levels of use recently
- Past quit attempts:
  - Number of attempts, date of most recent attempt, duration
  - Methods used previously—What did or didn't work? Why or why not?
  - Prior medication administration, dose, compliance, duration of treatment
  - Reasons for relapse

✓ **Discuss Key Issues** (for the upcoming or current quit attempt)
- Reasons/motivation for wanting to quit (or avoid relapse)
- Confidence in ability to quit (or avoid relapse)
- Triggers for tobacco use
- Routines and situations associated with tobacco use
- Stress-related tobacco use
- Social support for quitting
- Concerns about weight gain
- Concerns about withdrawal symptoms

✓ **Facilitate Quitting Process**
- Discuss methods for quitting: pros and cons of the different methods
- Set a quit date: ideally, less than 2 weeks away
- Recommend completion of a Tobacco Use Log
- Discuss coping strategies (cognitive, behavioral) for key issues
- Discuss withdrawal symptoms
- Discuss concept of "slip" versus relapse
- Provide medication counseling: compliance, proper use, with demonstration
- Offer to assist throughout the quit attempt

✓ **Evaluate the Quit Attempt** (at follow-up)
- Status of attempt
- Inquire about "slips" and relapse
- Medication compliance and plans for discontinuation

STEP Five: ARRANGE Follow-up Counseling

✓ Monitor patients' progress throughout the quit attempt. Follow-up contact should occur during the first week after quitting. A second follow-up contact is recommended in the first month. Additional contacts should be scheduled as needed. Counseling contacts can occur face-to-face, by telephone, or by e-mail. Keep patient progress notes.

✓ Address temptations and triggers; discuss strategies to prevent relapse.

✓ Congratulate patients for continued success.

FIGURE 88-2 Tobacco-cessation counseling guide sheet. (Reprinted with permission from *Rx for Change: Clinician-Assisted Tobacco Cessation*. Copyright © 1999–2012. The Regents of the University of California. All rights reserved.)

TABLE 88-5
Enhancing Motivation to Quit: The "5 R's" for Tobacco Cessation Counseling

- **Relevance**—Encourage patients to think about the reasons why quitting is important. Counseling should be framed such that it relates to the patient's risk for disease or exacerbation of disease, family or social situations (e.g., having children with asthma), health concerns, age, or other patient factors, such as prior experience with quitting.
- **Risks**—Ask patients to identify potential negative health consequences of smoking, such as acute risks (shortness of breath, asthma exacerbations, harm to pregnancy, infertility), long-term risks (cancer, cardiac, and pulmonary disease), and environmental risks (promoting smoking among children by being a negative role model; effects of secondhand smoke on others, including children and pets).
- **Rewards**—Ask patients to identify potential benefits that they anticipate from quitting, such as improved health, enhanced physical performance, enhanced taste and smell, reduced expenditures for tobacco, less time wasted or work missed, reduced health risks to others (fetus, children, housemates), and reduced aging of the skin.
- **Roadblocks**—Help patients identify barriers to quitting and assist in developing coping strategies (Table 88-6) for addressing each barrier. Common barriers include nicotine withdrawal symptoms, fear of failure, a need for social support while quitting, depression, weight gain, and a sense of deprivation or loss.
- **Repetition**—Continue to work with patients who are successful in their quit attempt. Discuss circumstances in which smoking occurred to identify the trigger(s) for relapse; this is part of the learning process and will be useful information for the next quit attempt. Repeat interventions when possible.

Reprinted from Fiore MC et al. *Treating Tobacco Use and Dependence: 2008 Update. Clinical Practice Guideline.* Rockville, MD: Public Health Service, US Dept of Health and Human Services; 2008.

and this can be accomplished by applying the "5 R's"[8] (Table 88-5) and by offering to work closely with the patient in designing a treatment plan. Although it might be useful to educate patients about the pharmacotherapy options, it is inappropriate to prescribe a treatment regimen for patients who are not ready to quit. For patients who are not ready to quit in the next 30 days, encourage them to seriously consider quitting and ask the following questions:

1. *Do you ever plan to quit?*
   If the patient responds "no," the clinician should ask, *"What would have to change for you to decide to quit?"* If the patient responds "nothing," then offer to assist, if or when the patient changes his or her mind. If the patient responds "yes," the clinician should continue with question 2.
2. *What might be some benefits of quitting now, instead of later?*
   The longer a patient smokes, quitting generally becomes more difficult. Most patients will agree that there is never an ideal time to quit, and procrastinating a quit date has more negative effects than positive.
3. *What would have to change for you to decide to quit sooner?*
   This question probes patients' perceptions of quitting, which reveals some of the barriers to quitting that can then be discussed.

For patients who are ready to quit (i.e., in the next month), the goal is to work with the patient in designing an individualized treatment plan, addressing the key issues listed under the "Assist" component of Figure 88-2.[32] The first steps are to discuss the patient's tobacco use history, inquiring about levels of smoking, number of years smoked, methods used previously for quitting (what worked, what did not work and why), and reason(s) for previous failed quit attempts. Clinicians should elicit patients' opinions about the different medications for quitting and should work with patients in selecting the quitting methods (e.g., medications, behavioral counseling programs). Although it is important to recognize that pharmaceutical agents might not be appropriate, desirable, or affordable for all patients, clinicians should educate patients that medications, when taken correctly, can substantially increase the likelihood of success.

Patients should be advised to select a quit date. Ideally, this date will be within the next 2 weeks to allow sufficient time to prepare for the quit attempt, including mental preparation, as well as preparation of the environment, such as by removing all tobacco products and ashtrays from the home, car, and workspace and informing their family, friends, and coworkers about their upcoming quit attempt and requesting their support. Additional strategies for coping with quitting are shown in Table 88-6.[32] Patients should be counseled about withdrawal symptoms, medication use, and the importance of receiving behavioral counseling throughout the quit attempt. Finally, patients should be commended for taking important steps toward improving their health.

- ***Arrange:*** Because patients' ability to quit increases when multiple counseling interactions are provided, arranging follow-up counseling is an important, yet typically neglected, element of treatment for tobacco dependence. Follow-up contact should occur soon after the quit date, preferably during the first week. A second follow-up contact is recommended within the first month after quitting.[8] Periodically, additional follow-up contacts should occur to monitor patient progress, assess compliance with pharmacotherapy regimens, and provide additional support.

Relapse prevention counseling should be part of every follow-up contact with patients who have recently quit smoking. When counseling recent quitters, it is important to address challenges in countering withdrawal symptoms and cravings or temptations to use tobacco. A list of strategies for key triggers or temptations for tobacco use is provided in Table 88-6.[32] Importantly, because tobacco use is a habitual behavior, patients should be advised to alter their daily routines; this helps disassociate specific behaviors from the use of tobacco. Patients who slip and smoke a cigarette (or use any form of tobacco) or experience a full relapse back to habitual tobacco use should be encouraged to think through the scenario in which tobacco use first occurred and identify the trigger(s) for relapse. This process provides valuable information for future quit attempts.

PHARMACOTHERAPY OPTIONS

All smokers who are trying to quit should be encouraged to use one or more US Food and Drug Administration (FDA)-approved pharmacologic aids for cessation; potential exceptions that require special consideration include medical contraindications or use in specific populations for which there is insufficient evidence of effectiveness (i.e., pregnant women, smokeless tobacco users, light smokers, adolescents).[8] Currently, the FDA-approved first-line agents that have been shown to be effective in promoting smoking cessation include five NRT dosage forms, sustained-release bupropion, and varenicline.[8] Dosing information, precautions, and adverse effects for the first-line agents are shown in Table 88-7. Pharmacologic agents that have not

TABLE 88-6

Cognitive and Behavioral Strategies for Tobacco Cessation

Cognitive Strategies	
Focus on *retraining the way a patient thinks.* Often, patients deliberate on the fact that they are thinking about a cigarette, and this leads to relapse. Patients must recognize that thinking about a cigarette does not mean they need to have one.	
Review commitment to quit, focus on downside of tobacco	Reminding oneself that cravings and temptations are temporary and will pass. Announce, either silently or aloud, "I want to be a nonsmoker, and the temptation will pass."
Distractive thinking	Deliberate, immediate refocusing of thinking when cued by thoughts about tobacco use.
Positive self-talks, "pep talks"	Saying "I can do this" and reminding oneself of previous difficult situations in which tobacco use was avoided with success.
Relaxation through imagery	Centering of mind toward positive, relaxing thoughts.
Mental rehearsal, visualization	Preparing for situations that might arise by envisioning how best to handle them. For example, envision what would happen if offered a cigarette by a friend—mentally craft and rehearse a response, and perhaps even practice it by saying it aloud.
Behavioral Strategies	
Involve *specific actions to reduce risk for relapse.* For maximal effectiveness, these should be considered before quitting, after determining patient-specific triggers for tobacco use. Here, we list some behavioral strategies for several common cues or triggers for relapse.	
Stress	Anticipate upcoming challenges at work, at school, or in personal life. Develop a substitute plan for tobacco use during times of stress (e.g., breathe deeply several times, take a break or leave the situation, call a supportive friend or family member, perform self-massage, or use nicotine replacement therapy to manage situational cravings).
Alcohol	Drinking alcohol can lead to relapse. Consider limiting or abstaining from alcohol during the early stages of quitting.
Other tobacco users	Quitting is more difficult when around other tobacco users. This is especially difficult if there is another tobacco user in the household. When possible during the early stages of quitting, limit prolonged contact with individuals who are using tobacco. Ask coworkers, friends, and housemates not to smoke or use tobacco in your presence.
Oral gratification needs	Have nontobacco oral substitutes (e.g., gum, sugarless candy, straws, toothpicks, lip balm, toothbrush, nicotine replacement therapy, bottled water) readily available.
Automatic smoking routines	Anticipate routines that are associated with tobacco use and develop an alternative plan. Examples: *Morning coffee with cigarettes:* change morning routine, drink tea instead of coffee, take shower before drinking coffee, take a brisk walk shortly after awakening. *Smoking while driving:* remove all tobacco from car, have car interior detailed, listen to an audio book or talk radio, use oral substitute. *Smoking while on the phone:* stand while talking, limit call duration, change phone location, keep hands occupied by doodling or sketching. *Smoking after meals:* get up and immediately do dishes or take a brisk walk after eating, call supportive friend.
Postcessation weight gain	The majority of tobacco users gain weight after quitting. Most quitters will gain <10 pounds, but there is a broad range of weight gain reported, with up to 10% of quitters gaining as much as 30 pounds. Do not attempt to modify multiple behaviors at one time. If weight gain is a barrier to quitting, engage in regular physical activity and adhere to a healthful diet (as opposed to strict dieting). Carefully plan and prepare meals, increase fruit and water intake to create a feeling of fullness, and chew sugarless gum or eat sugarless candies. Consider use of pharmacotherapy shown to delay weight gain (e.g., nicotine gum, lozenge, or sustained-release bupropion).
Cravings for tobacco	Cravings for tobacco are temporary and usually pass within 5–10 minutes. Handle cravings through distractive thinking, take a break, change activities or tasks, take deep breaths, perform self-massage, or use nicotine replacement therapy.

received an approval from the FDA for smoking cessation but are recommended as second-line agents[8] include clonidine and nortriptyline.

FIRST-LINE AGENTS

NICOTINE REPLACEMENT THERAPY

NRT improves cessation rates by reducing the physical withdrawal symptoms associated with tobacco cessation while the patient focuses on modifying his or her behavior and coping with the psychological aspects of quitting. In addition, because the onset of action for NRT is not as rapid as that of nicotine obtained through smoking, patients become less accustomed to the nearly immediate, reinforcing effects of inhaled nicotine. A meta-analysis of 111 controlled trials, enrolling more than 43,000 participants, found that all NRT formulations (gum, inhaler, lozenge, patch, and nasal spray) result in statistically significant improvements in abstinence rates when compared with placebo. Patients using NRT are 1.6 times as likely to quit smoking than are those receiving placebo.[49] Figure 88-3[32] depicts the concentration–time curves for the various NRT formulations, compared with a cigarette and moist snuff (a smokeless form of tobacco).[50–52] It can be seen that of the five NRT dosage forms, the nicotine nasal spray reaches its peak concentration most rapidly. The nicotine gum, lozenge, and oral inhaler have similar concentration curves, and the nicotine transdermal patch

TABLE 88-7

Pharmacotherapy Options: Products; Precautions, Warnings, and Contraindications; Dosing; and Adverse Effects

NRT Formulations						
Gum	**Lozenge**	**Transdermal Patch**	**Nasal Spray**	**Oral Inhaler**	**Bupropion SR**	**Varenicline**
Product						
Nicorette,[a] Generic	**Nicorette (standard and mini),[a] Generic**	**NicoDerm CQ,[a] Generic[b]**	**Nicotrol NS[c]**	**Nicotrol Inhaler[c]**	**Zyban,[a] Generic**	**Chantix[c]**
OTC 2 mg, 4 mg	OTC 2 mg, 4 mg	OTC (NicoDerm CQ, generic) Rx (generic)	Rx Metered spray	Rx 10-mg cartridge	Rx 150-mg sustained-release tablet	Rx 0.5-mg, 1-mg tablet
Original, cinnamon, fruit, mint, orange	Cherry, mint	7 mg, 14 mg, 21 mg (24-hour release)	0.5 mg of nicotine in 50-μL aqueous nicotine solution	Delivers 4 mg of inhaled nicotine vapor		
Precautions, Warnings, and Contraindications						
• Recent (≤2 weeks) myocardial infarction • Serious underlying arrhythmias • Serious or worsening angina pectoris • Temporomandibular joint disease • Pregnancy[d] and breast-feeding • Adolescents (<18 years)	• Recent (≤2 weeks) myocardial infarction • Serious underlying arrhythmias • Serious or worsening angina pectoris • Pregnancy[d] and breast-feeding • Adolescents (<18 years)	• Recent (≤2 weeks) myocardial infarction • Serious underlying arrhythmias • Serious or worsening angina pectoris • Pregnancy[d] (Rx formulations, category D) and breast-feeding • Adolescents (<18 years)	• Recent (≤2 weeks) myocardial infarction • Serious underlying arrhythmias • Serious or worsening angina pectoris • Underlying chronic nasal disorders (rhinitis, nasal polyps, sinusitis) • Severe reactive airway disease • Pregnancy[d] (category D) and breast-feeding • Adolescents (<18 years)	• Recent (≤2 weeks) myocardial infarction • Serious underlying arrhythmias • Bronchospastic disease • Pregnancy[d] (category D) and breast-feeding • Adolescents (<18 years)	• Concomitant therapy with medications or medical conditions known to lower seizure threshold • Severe hepatic cirrhosis • Pregnancy[d] (category C) and breast-feeding • Adolescents (<18 years) **Warning:** • BLACK-BOXED WARNING for neuropsychiatric symptoms[e] **Contraindications:** • Seizure disorder • Concomitant bupropion (e.g., Wellbutrin) therapy • Current or prior diagnosis of bulimia or anorexia nervosa • Simultaneous abrupt discontinuation of alcohol or sedatives (including benzodiazepines) • Monoamine oxidase inhibitor therapy in previous 14 days	• Severe renal impairment (dosage adjustment is necessary) • Pregnancy[d] (category C) and breast-feeding • Adolescents (<18 years) **Warnings:** • BLACK-BOXED WARNING for neuropsychiatric symptoms[e] • Safety and efficacy have not been established in patients with serious psychiatric illness • Cardiovascular adverse events in patients with existing cardiovascular disease

(continued)

TABLE 88-7
Pharmacotherapy Options: Products; Precautions, Warnings, and Contraindications; Dosing; and Adverse Effects (*Continued*)

NRT Formulations						
Gum	**Lozenge**	**Transdermal Patch**	**Nasal Spray**	**Oral Inhaler**	**Bupropion SR**	**Varenicline**
Dosing[f]						
First cigarette ≤30 minutes after waking: 4 mg *First cigarette >30 minutes after waking:* 2 mg Weeks 1–6: 1 piece every 1–2 hours Weeks 7–9: 1 piece every 2–4 hours Weeks 10–12: 1 piece every 4–8 hours • Maximum, 24 pieces/day • Chew each piece slowly • Park between cheek and gum when peppery or tingling sensation appears (~15–30 chews) • Resume chewing when tingle fades • Repeat chew and park steps until most of nicotine is gone (tingle does not return; generally 30 minutes) • Park in different areas of mouth • No food or beverages 15 minutes before or during use • Duration: up to 12 weeks	*First cigarette ≤30 minutes after waking:* 4 mg *First cigarette >30 minutes after waking:* 2 mg Weeks 1–6: 1 lozenge every 1–2 hours Weeks 7–9: 1 lozenge every 2–4 hours Weeks 10–12: 1 lozenge every 4–8 hours • Maximum, 20 lozenges/day • Allow to dissolve slowly (20–30 minutes for standard; 10 minutes for mini) • Nicotine release may cause a warm, tingling sensation • Do not chew or swallow • Occasionally rotate to different areas of the mouth • No food or beverages 15 minutes before or during use • Duration: up to 12 weeks	*>10 cigarettes/day:* 21 mg/day × 4 weeks (generic) × 6 weeks (NicoDerm CQ) 14 mg/day × 2 weeks 7 mg/day × 2 weeks *≤10 cigarettes/day:* 14 mg/day × 6 weeks 7 mg/day × 2 weeks • May wear patch for 16 hours if patient experiences sleep disturbances (remove at bedtime) • Duration: 8–10 weeks	1–2 doses/hour (8–40 doses/day) One dose = 2 sprays (one in *each* nostril); each spray delivers 0.5 mg of nicotine to the nasal mucosa • Maximum –5 doses/hour or –40 doses/day • For best results, initially use at least 8 doses/day • Do not sniff, swallow, or inhale through the nose as the spray is being administered • Duration: 3–6 months	6–16 cartridges/day Individualize dosing; initially use 1 cartridge every 1–2 hours • Best effects with continuous puffing for 20 minutes • Initially use at least 6 cartridges/day • Nicotine in cartridge is depleted after 20 minutes of active puffing • Inhale into back of throat or puff in short breaths • Do NOT inhale into the lungs (like a cigarette) but "puff" as if lighting a pipe • Open cartridge retains potency for 24 hours • No food or beverages 15 minutes before or during use • Duration: 3–6 months	150 mg PO every morning × 3 days, then increase to 150 mg PO BID • Do not exceed 300 mg/day • Begin therapy 1–2 weeks *before* quit date • Allow at least 8 hours between doses • Avoid bedtime dosing to minimize insomnia • Dose tapering is not necessary • Can be used safely with NRT • Duration: 7–12 weeks, with maintenance up to 6 months in selected patients	Days 1–3: 0.5 mg PO every morning Days 4–7: 0.5 mg PO BID Weeks 2–12: 1 mg PO BID • Begin therapy 1 week *before* quit date. Alternatively, the patient can begin therapy and then quit smoking between days 8 and 35 of treatment. • Take dose after eating and with a full glass of water • Dose tapering is not necessary • Dosing adjustment is recommended for patients with severe renal impairment • Duration: 12 weeks; an additional 12-week course may be used in selected patients
Adverse Effects						
• Mouth or jaw soreness • Hiccups • Dyspepsia • Hypersalivation • Effects associated with incorrect chewing technique: –Lightheadedness –Nausea or vomiting –Throat and mouth irritation	• Nausea • Hiccups • Cough • Heartburn • Headache • Flatulence • Insomnia	• Local skin reactions (erythema, pruritus, burning) • Headache • Sleep disturbances (insomnia, abnormal or vivid dreams); associated with nocturnal nicotine absorption	• Nasal or throat irritation (hot, peppery, or burning sensation) • Rhinitis • Tearing • Sneezing • Cough • Headache	• Mouth or throat irritation • Cough • Headache • Rhinitis • Dyspepsia • Hiccups	• Insomnia • Dry mouth • Nervousness or difficulty concentrating • Rash • Constipation • Seizures (risk is ~0.1%) • Neuropsychiatric symptoms (rare; see PRECAUTIONS)	• Nausea • Sleep disturbances (insomnia, abnormal or vivid dreams) • Constipation • Flatulence • Vomiting • Neuropsychiatric symptoms (rare; see PRECAUTIONS)

[a]Marketed by GlaxoSmithKline.
[b]Transdermal patch formulation previously marketed as Habitrol.
[c]Marketed by Pfizer.
[d]The US Clinical Practice Guideline states that pregnant smokers should be encouraged to quit without medication based on insufficient evidence of effectiveness and theoretical concerns with safety. Pregnant smokers should be offered behavioral counseling interventions that exceed minimal advice to quit.
[e]In July 2009, the FDA mandated that the prescribing information for all bupropion- and varenicline-containing products include a black-boxed warning highlighting the risk of serious neuropsychiatric symptoms, including changes in behavior, hostility, agitation, depressed mood, suicidal thoughts and behavior, and attempted suicide. Clinicians should advise patients to stop taking varenicline or bupropion SR and contact a health care provider immediately if they experience agitation, depressed mood, and any changes in behavior that are not typical of nicotine withdrawal, or if they experience suicidal thoughts or behavior. If treatment is stopped because of neuropsychiatric symptoms, patients should be monitored until the symptoms resolve.
For complete prescribing information, refer to the manufacturers' package inserts.
NRT, nicotine replacement therapy; OTC, over-the-counter (nonprescription); Rx, prescription; SR, sustained-release.
Reprinted with permission from *Rx for Change: Clinician-Assisted Tobacco Cessation.*

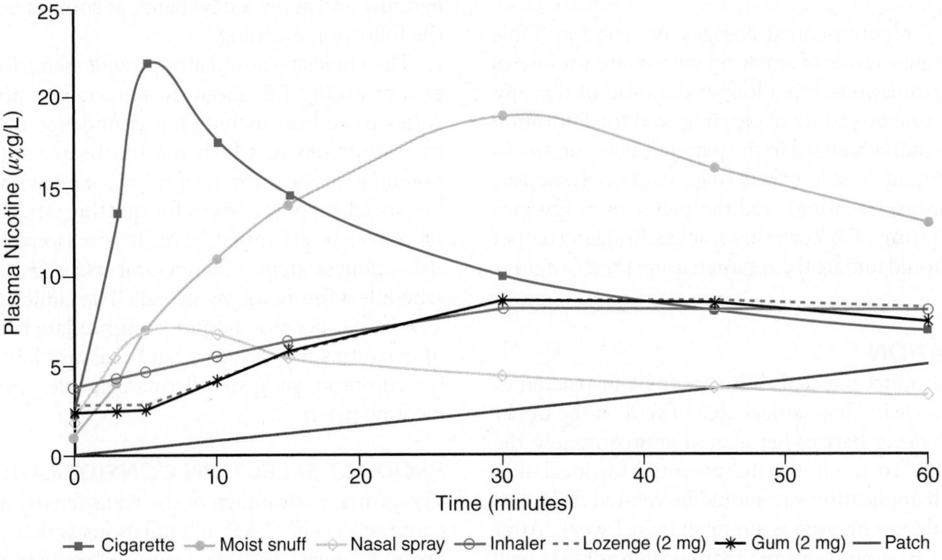

FIGURE 88-3 Plasma nicotine concentrations for various nicotine-containing products. (Reprinted with permission from *Rx for Change: Clinician-Assisted Tobacco Cessation.* Copyright © 1999–2012. The Regents of the University of California. All rights reserved. Plasma nicotine concentration curves derived from Choi JH et al. Pharmacokinetics of a nicotine polacrilex lozenge. *Nicotine Tob Res.* 2003;5(5):635; Schneider NG et al. The nicotine inhaler: clinical pharmacokinetics and comparison with other nicotine treatments. *Clin Pharmacokinet.* 2001;40(9):661; and Fant RV et al. Pharmacokinetics and pharmacodynamics of moist snuff in humans. *Tob Control.* 1999;8(4):387.)

has the slowest onset, but offers more consistent blood levels of nicotine for a sustained period.

SUSTAINED-RELEASE BUPROPION

Sustained-release bupropion is an atypical antidepressant medication hypothesized to promote smoking cessation by blocking the reuptake of dopamine and norepinephrine in the central nervous system[8] and possibly by acting as a nicotine receptor antagonist.[53] These neurochemical effects are believed to modulate the dopamine reward pathway and reduce cravings for nicotine and symptoms of withdrawal.[8] Use of sustained-release bupropion approximately doubles the long-term abstinence rate when compared with placebo.[8,54]

VARENICLINE

Varenicline, a cytisine analog, is a partial agonist that binds with high affinity and selectivity at $\alpha_4\beta_2$ neuronal nicotinic acetylcholine receptors.[55] The efficacy of varenicline in smoking cessation is believed to be the result of sustained, low-level agonist activity at the receptor site combined with competitive inhibition of nicotine binding. The partial agonist activity induces modest receptor stimulation, leading to increased dopamine levels, which attenuates the symptoms of nicotine withdrawal. In addition, by blocking the ability of nicotine to activate $\alpha_4\beta_2$ nicotinic acetylcholine receptors, varenicline inhibits the surges of dopamine release that are believed to be responsible for the reinforcement and reward associated with smoking.[55,56] Use of varenicline more than doubles the long-term abstinence rate when compared in clinical trials with placebo.[8,57]

SECOND-LINE AGENTS

Although not FDA-approved specifically for smoking cessation, the prescription medications clonidine and nortriptyline are recommended as second-line agents.[8] Lack of an FDA-approved indication for smoking cessation and less desirable side-effect profiles currently prohibit these agents from achieving first-line classification.[8]

PHARMACOTHERAPY FOR TREATING TOBACCO USE AND DEPENDENCE

Transdermal Nicotine Patch

CASE 88-1

QUESTION 1: T.B. is a 32-year-old woman who is enrolled in a worksite smoking-cessation program. During the previous group session, the cessation counselor discussed the various medications for cessation. T.B. has set her quit date for 1 week from today, and she is interested in starting the nicotine transdermal patch. She is currently smoking 1.5 packs per day (PPD), which is a reduction from the 2 PPD she had been smoking for the past 10 years. T.B. reports she smokes several cigarettes in succession immediately after waking in the morning. She takes no medications and has no medical problems. Which nicotine transdermal product should T.B. select, and how should it be used?

Transdermal nicotine delivery systems, available with or without a prescription, consist of an impermeable surface layer, a nicotine reservoir, an adhesive layer, and a removable protective liner. Although the transdermal delivery technology varies by manufacturer, nicotine is well absorbed, with 68% to 82% of the dose released from 24-hour patch formulations systemically bioavailable across the skin. Plasma nicotine concentrations from the patch rise slowly during 1 to 4 hours and peak within 3 to 12 hours after application.[22] Levels of nicotine achieved with the transdermal patch are lower and fluctuate less than do those achieved with tobacco products or other NRT formulations (Fig. 88-3).

The transdermal nicotine patch exhibits significantly improved abstinence rates relative to placebo (Table 88-4).[8,49] A meta-analysis of 25 randomized, controlled trials found treatment with the nicotine patch (6–14 weeks) approximately doubled the likelihood of long-term abstinence compared with placebo.[8]

DOSING

The manufacturers' recommended dosages are listed in Table 88-7. In general, higher levels of smoking necessitate the use of higher-strength formulations and a longer duration of therapy. Ultimately, the starting dose, rate of tapering, and total duration of therapy must be individualized to the patient's baseline smoking levels, development of side effects (e.g., nausea, dyspepsia, nervousness, dizziness, sweating), and the presence or absence of withdrawal symptoms. T.B. currently smokes 30 cigarettes per day, and thus she should initiate the regimen using the 21-mg/day patch.

PATIENT EDUCATION

Regardless of the product selected, T.B. should be instructed to apply the patch to a clean, dry, hairless area of skin on the upper body or the upper outer part of her arm at approximately the same time each day. To minimize the potential for local skin reactions, the patch application site should be rotated daily, and the same area should not be used again for at least 1 week. After patch application, T.B. should ensure that the patch adheres well to the skin, especially around the edges. The clinician should reassure T.B. that water will not reduce the effectiveness of the nicotine patch if it is applied correctly, and she may bathe, shower, swim, or exercise while wearing the patch. Finally, T.B. should be advised to discontinue use of the nicotine patch and contact a health care provider if skin redness caused by the patch does not resolve after 4 days; if the skin swells or a rash develops; if irregular heartbeat or palpitations occur; or if she experiences symptoms of nicotine overdose such as nausea, vomiting, dizziness, diarrhea, sweating, weakness, or rapid heartbeat.

ADVERSE REACTIONS

CASE 88-1, QUESTION 2: Ten days later, T.B. calls to complain of an itchy rash that she believes is caused by the nicotine patch. She noticed the rash yesterday when she removed the first patch from her left upper arm. This morning, after removing the second patch from her right upper arm, she noticed a similar rash. T.B. describes the skin on her right arm as slightly red but not swollen; the rash on her left arm has only a faint trace of pink discoloration. Her last cigarette was 2 days ago. How should T.B. be managed at this time?

The most common side effects associated with the nicotine patch are local reactions (erythema, burning, and pruritus) at the skin application site. These reactions are generally caused by skin occlusion or sensitivity to the patch adhesives. Rotating the patch application sites on a daily basis minimizes skin irritation; nonetheless, skin reactions to the patch adhesives occur in up to 50% of patch users. Fewer than 5% of patients discontinue therapy because of a skin reaction.[8]

T.B. appears to be experiencing a mild skin reaction and should be reassured that it is common for the skin to appear erythematous for up to 24 to 48 hours after the patch is removed. T.B. can apply topical hydrocortisone cream (0.5% or 1%) or triamcinolone cream (0.5%), or she can take an oral antihistamine for symptomatic treatment.[8] Because the rash on her left arm has nearly resolved, it is reasonable for T.B. to continue using the nicotine transdermal patch provided that the erythema is not too bothersome.

Other less common side effects associated with the transdermal nicotine patch include vivid or abnormal dreams, insomnia, and headache. Sleep disturbances likely result from nocturnal nicotine absorption. Patients experiencing troublesome sleep disturbances should be instructed to remove the patch before bedtime and apply a new patch as soon as possible after waking the following morning.[8]

The clinician should also provide behavioral counseling support by asking T.B. about the current quit attempt. Appropriate issues to address include her confidence in remaining tobacco free, situations in which she has been tempted to smoke and potential triggers for relapse, nicotine withdrawal symptoms, her social support system for quitting, and any other questions or concerns she might have. It is reasonable to review potential coping strategies (behavioral and cognitive; Table 88-6) and schedule a future follow-up call. The clinician should commend T.B. for her decision to quit, congratulate her for remaining free of cigarettes for 48 hours, and reassure her that skin irritation is a common, yet generally manageable, complication with the nicotine patch.

PRODUCT SELECTION CONSIDERATIONS

The primary advantage of the transdermal nicotine patch compared with other NRT formulations is that the patch is easy to use and conceal, releases a continuous dose of nicotine throughout the day, and requires administration only once daily. Disadvantages of the patch include a high incidence of skin irritation associated with the patch adhesives and the inability to acutely adjust the dose of nicotine to alleviate symptoms of withdrawal. Finally, patients with underlying dermatologic conditions (e.g., psoriasis, eczema, atopic dermatitis) should not use the patch because they are more likely to experience skin irritation.[8]

CASE 88-1, QUESTION 3: T.B. would like to discontinue the nicotine transdermal patch. She would like to purchase a nonprescription smoking-cessation medication and wants to know whether the gum or lozenge is an effective alternative.

Nicotine Gum

Nicotine polacrilex gum is a resin complex of nicotine and polacrilin in a chewing gum base that provides slow release and absorption of nicotine across the oral mucosa. The product is available in 2- and 4-mg strengths, and in multiple flavors (regular, cinnamon, fruit, mint, and orange). The gum has a distinct, tobaccolike, slightly peppery, minty, or fruity taste and contains buffering agents (sodium carbonate and sodium bicarbonate) to increase the salivary pH, which enhances the buccal absorption of nicotine. The amount of nicotine absorbed from each piece is variable, but when used properly, approximately 1.6 mg and 2.2 mg of nicotine is absorbed from each 2-mg and 4-mg piece of gum, respectively.[22] Peak plasma concentrations of nicotine are achieved approximately 30 minutes after chewing a single piece of gum and then slowly decline thereafter (Fig. 88-3). Patients using short-term (6–14 weeks) or long-term (>14 weeks) treatment with nicotine gum are significantly more likely to remain abstinent compared with those receiving placebo (Table 88-4).[8]

DOSING

Table 88-7 outlines the manufacturers' recommended dosing schedule for the nicotine gum. The recommended dosage of the nicotine gum is based on the "time to first cigarette" (TTFC) of the day. Having a strong desire or need to smoke soon after waking is viewed as a key indicator of nicotine dependence.[58] Therefore, patients who smoke their first cigarette of the day within 30 minutes of waking are likely to be more highly dependent on nicotine and require higher dosages than those who delay smoking for more than 30 minutes after waking (Table 88-7).

Specifically, if the TTFC is 30 minutes or less, therapy should be initiated with the 4 mg gum. If the TTFC is more than 30 minutes, therapy should be initiated with the 2 mg gum. During the initial 6 weeks of therapy, patients should use 1 piece of gum every 1 to 2 hours while awake. In general, this amounts to at least 9 pieces of gum daily. The "chew and park" method described here allows for the slow, consistent release of nicotine from the polacrilin resin. Patients can use additional pieces of gum (to the daily maximum of 24 pieces per day) if cravings occur between scheduled doses. In general, patients who smoke a greater number of cigarettes per day will require more nicotine gum to alleviate their cravings than will patients who smoke fewer cigarettes per day. It is preferable to use the gum on a fixed schedule of administration, tapering during 1 to 3 months rather than using it as needed to control cravings.[8]

PATIENT EDUCATION

Proper chewing technique is crucial when using the nicotine gum. Patients should be instructed to chew the gum slowly until a peppery, minty, or fruity taste or a slight tingling sensation in the mouth is detected; this varies but generally occurs after about 15 chews. When the taste or tingling sensation is noted, the patient should "park" the gum between the cheek and gum to allow absorption of nicotine across the buccal mucosa. When the taste or tingling dissipates (generally after 1–2 minutes), the patient should resume chewing slowly. When the taste or tingle returns, the patient should stop chewing and park the gum in a different area in the mouth. Rotating the gum placement site within the mouth helps decrease the incidence of oral irritation. The chew and park steps should be repeated until most of the nicotine is extracted; this generally occurs after 30 minutes and becomes obvious when chewing no longer elicits the characteristic taste or tingling sensation.

Patients should be warned that the absorption and therefore the effectiveness of nicotine gum might be reduced by acidic beverages (e.g., coffee, juices, wine, soft drinks),[59] which transiently reduce the salivary pH. To prevent this interaction, patients should be advised not to eat or drink (except water) for 15 minutes before or while using the nicotine gum.

ADVERSE REACTIONS

The most common side effects associated with use of the nicotine gum include unpleasant taste, mouth irritation, jaw muscle soreness or fatigue, hypersalivation, hiccups, and dyspepsia. Many of these side effects can be minimized or prevented by using proper chewing technique.[8] Patients should be warned that chewing the gum too rapidly may result in excessive release of nicotine, leading to lightheadedness, nausea, vomiting, irritation of the throat and mouth, hiccups, and indigestion.

PRODUCT SELECTION CONSIDERATIONS

Advantages of nicotine gum include the fact that this formulation may be used to satisfy oral cravings and the 4-mg strength might delay weight gain.[8] For these reasons, the gum may be particularly beneficial for patients who have weight-gain concerns or for patients who report boredom as a trigger for smoking. The gum might also be advantageous for patients who desire flexibility in dosing and prefer the ability to self-regulate nicotine levels to manage withdrawal symptoms. Some patients may find that the viscous consistency of the gum makes it difficult to use because it sticks to dental work. Others may find it difficult or socially unacceptable to chew the gum so frequently. Nicotine gum should not be used by patients with temporomandibular joint (TMJ) conditions.

Nicotine Lozenge

The nicotine polacrilex lozenge is a resin complex of nicotine and polacrilin in a sugarfree, light mint, or cherry-flavored lozenge. The product is available in 2- and 4-mg strengths, which are meant to be consumed like hard candy or other medicinal lozenges (e.g., sucked and moved from side to side in the mouth until fully dissolved). Because the nicotine lozenge dissolves completely, it delivers approximately 25% more nicotine than does an equivalent dose of nicotine gum.[50] Like the nicotine gum, the lozenge also contains buffering agents (sodium carbonate and potassium bicarbonate) to increase salivary pH, thereby enhancing buccal absorption of the nicotine. Peak nicotine concentrations of nicotine with the lozenge are achieved after 30 to 60 minutes of use and then slowly decline thereafter (Fig. 88-3). In a trial evaluating the formulation currently available in the United States, the nicotine lozenge approximately doubled the 6-month abstinence rates compared with placebo (23.9% vs. 12.3%).[60] A meta-analysis of five studies using either the nicotine lozenge (nicotine polacrilin) or sublingual tablet (not available in the United States) concluded that the odds of abstinence at 6 or more months was 2.0 with the tablet or lozenge relative to placebo (95% CI, 1.6–2.5).[49]

DOSING

Table 88-7 outlines the manufacturers' recommended dosing schedule for the nicotine lozenge. Like the nicotine gum, the lozenge is dosed based on the TTFC. Patients who smoke their first cigarette of the day within 30 minutes of waking should use the 4-mg strength lozenge, and patients who smoke their first cigarette of the day more than 30 minutes after waking should use the 2-mg strength lozenge. Patients are more likely to succeed if they use the lozenge on a fixed schedule rather than as needed. During the initial 6 weeks of therapy, patients should use 1 lozenge every 1 to 2 hours while awake. In general, this amounts to at least 9 lozenges daily. Patients can use additional lozenges (up to 5 lozenges in 6 hours or a maximum of 20 lozenges per day) if cravings occur between scheduled doses.

PATIENT EDUCATION

Similar to the gum, the nicotine lozenge is a specially formulated nicotine delivery system that must be used properly for optimal results. The lozenge should be allowed to dissolve slowly in the mouth; when nicotine is released from the polacrilin resin, a warm, tingling sensation may be experienced. The patient should occasionally rotate the lozenge to different areas of the mouth to reduce the potential for mucosal irritation. When used correctly, the lozenge should completely dissolve within 30 minutes. Patients should be counseled not to chew or swallow the lozenge because this increases the incidence of gastrointestinal-related side effects.

Because the nicotine in the lozenge is dissolved in saliva and absorbed through the buccal mucosa, patients should be cautioned that the effectiveness of the nicotine lozenge may be reduced by acidic beverages such as coffee, juices, wine, or soft drinks. As recommended for the nicotine gum, patients should be advised not to eat or drink (except water) for 15 minutes before or while using the nicotine lozenge.

ADVERSE REACTIONS

In general, the nicotine lozenge is well tolerated. The most common side effects include nausea, hiccups, cough, dyspepsia, headache, and flatulence. Patients who use more than one lozenge at a time, continuously use one lozenge after another, or chew or swallow the lozenge are more likely to experience dyspepsia or hiccups.

PRODUCT SELECTION CONSIDERATIONS

The nicotine lozenge is similar to the nicotine gum formulation in that it may be used to satisfy oral cravings, the 4-mg strength might delay weight gain,[8,59] and patients can self-titrate therapy to acutely manage withdrawal symptoms. Because the lozenge does not require chewing, many patients find this to be a more discrete nicotine delivery system. The disadvantages of the lozenge are the fact that it requires frequent dosing, and the gastrointestinal side effects (nausea, hiccups, and heartburn) may be bothersome.

T.B. has expressed interest in either the nicotine gum or lozenge formulation for her quit attempt. Both agents are effective, and the choice of therapy is dependent on the patient's perceptions and expectations regarding treatment, including the ability to comply with the regimen, previous experience with cessation medications, and other concerns (e.g., adverse effects, weight gain, cost of medications). T.B. would be a candidate for either agent provided she is able to comply with the frequent dosing schedule (one lozenge or piece of gum every 1–2 hours while she is awake). T.B. smokes her first cigarette of the day immediately after waking in the morning and she smokes approximately 30 cigarettes/day; this smoking pattern suggests a higher degree of nicotine dependence, and therefore T.B. would benefit from a higher dose of NRT. T.B. should initiate treatment with the 4-mg strength of either the nicotine lozenge or nicotine gum dosed every 1 to 2 hours while she is awake and tapered according to the schedule outlined in Table 88-7.

Postcessation Weight Gain

CASE 88-1, QUESTION 4: T.B. is very concerned about gaining weight after she quits smoking. Is weight gain common after quitting, and if so, how can this be prevented?

Most tobacco users gain weight after quitting, and clinicians should neither deny the likelihood of weight gain nor minimize its significance.[8] For nearly all patients, the health risks associated with postcessation weight gain are negligible compared with the risks of continued smoking.

Studies suggest that most quitters gain fewer than 10 pounds, but there is a broad range of weight gain reported, with up to 10% of quitters gaining as much as 30 pounds.[8] In general, women tend to gain more weight than men. In a study of nearly 6,000 smokers who were followed for 5 years after quitting, the average weight gain during the follow-up period was 19.2 and 16.7 pounds among women and men, respectively.[61] For men and women, subgroups that are more likely to gain weight after quitting are African Americans, younger tobacco users (younger than 55 years), and heavier tobacco users (those smoking more than 25 cigarettes per day).

The weight-suppressing effects of tobacco are well known. However, the mechanisms to explain why most successful quitters gain weight are not completely understood. Smokers have been found to have an approximately 10% higher metabolic rate compared with nonsmokers.[62] Increased postcessation caloric intake might result from an increase in appetite, improved sense of taste, or a change in the hand-to-mouth ritual through the substitution of tobacco with food.

In general, a patient is less likely to be successful if he or she attempts to change multiple behaviors at once. For most patients, strict dieting to prevent weight gain, especially during the early stages of quitting, is generally not recommended.[8] T.B. should be counseled that the average weight gain of fewer than 10 pounds is less detrimental to her overall health than is continued smoking. Although exercise interventions have not been shown to reduce weight gain among quitters,[63] it should not be ruled out as a recommendation for T.B. because she expresses significant concern about weight gain, and this might be a barrier to her quitting. As such, it is reasonable for the clinician to recommend that T.B. engage in some form of physical activity, such as walking 30 minutes daily. Even small changes, such as taking the stairs instead of the elevator, or parking toward the end of a parking lot instead of in the closest spot, can make a difference. Furthermore, T.B. should be advised to plan her meals in advance to avoid binge eating, increase her water intake to create a feeling of fullness, chew sugarless gum, and limit alcohol consumption. T.B. may consider pharmacotherapy options that have been shown to delay weight gain—according to the Clinical Practice Guideline, this would include the 4-mg nicotine gum or lozenge or sustained-release bupropion.[8] It is important to note, however, that once the medication is terminated, most quitters gain, on average, an amount of weight that is comparable to that which would have been gained in the absence of medication.[8]

Relapse Back to Smoking

CASE 88-1, QUESTION 5: During a follow-up contact, the clinician learns that T.B. smoked half a pack of cigarettes at a party over the weekend and has relapsed to her previous smoking levels after not having smoked for more than a month. How should the clinician respond?

The clinician should thank T.B. for being honest about her smoking and ask whether she is comfortable discussing the circumstances during which the smoking occurred. At the time of her smoking, where was she, who was she with, how did she get access to cigarettes, and how was she feeling at the time? What, specifically, were the triggers for her relapse (e.g., alcohol, depression, friends who were smoking around her)? It is important that the clinician help the patient to use this information as part of the learning process, but it also is important to focus on the "positive," such as T.B.'s ability to have remained tobacco free for more than 1 month. Four weeks after quitting, most physical effects of nicotine withdrawal have completely resolved, and thus, the relapse trigger for T.B. likely was psychological or situational and could be abated through application of effective coping techniques. After an informative discussion about the situation in which the smoking occurred, it is important that the clinician work with the patient in identifying strategies for avoiding relapse in the future (Table 88-6).

Smoking and Cardiovascular Disease

CASE 88-2

QUESTION 1: P.J. is a 62-year-old man admitted for an elective coronary artery bypass graft (CABG) procedure. His medical history is significant for angina, hypertension, dyslipidemia, peripheral vascular disease (PVD), and allergic rhinitis. He underwent a bilateral carotid endarterectomy procedure 2 years ago and had iliac artery angioplasty with stent placement 5 years ago for PVD. P.J.'s social history is significant for tobacco use (2 PPD) and alcohol (3–4 drinks/day). He is approximately 10 pounds overweight. His preoperative laboratory results are significant for a total cholesterol of 270 mg/dL (desirable, < 200), low-density lipoprotein cholesterol (LDL-C) of 163 mg/dL

(optimal, <70), high-density lipoprotein cholesterol (HDL-C) of 35 mg/dL (low, <40), and triglycerides of 350 mg/dL (normal, <150). His medications before admission include atenolol 50 mg daily, aspirin 81 mg daily, isosorbide dinitrate 20 mg TID, atorvastatin 20 mg daily, fluticasone nasal spray (50 mcg/spray) 1 spray/nostril daily, and nitroglycerin 0.4 mg sublingually as needed. Which of P.J.'s chronic medical conditions may be caused or exacerbated by his tobacco use?

A wealth of evidence suggests that cigarette smoking is a major cause of cardiovascular disease and is responsible for approximately 128,000 premature cardiovascular-related deaths each year.[5] Smoking is known to accelerate the process of atherosclerosis, leading to chronic cardiovascular disorders, including coronary heart disease, cerebrovascular disease, PVD, aortic aneurysm, and congestive heart failure.[3] In addition, smoking substantially elevates the risk for acute cardiovascular events, including sudden death, myocardial infarction (MI), stroke, and reocclusion of coronary or peripheral vessels after graft surgery or angioplasty.[3,64]

There are numerous plausible pathophysiological mechanisms by which tobacco smoking contributes to the development of cardiovascular disease.[7] Oxidant gases and other compounds in tobacco smoke are believed to induce a hypercoagulable state characterized by increased platelet aggregation and thrombosis, which substantially increases the risk of MI and sudden death.[64,65] The carbon monoxide in smoke reduces the amount of oxygen available to tissues and organs, including myocardial tissue, and may reduce the ventricular fibrillation threshold.[64] Smoking may accelerate atherosclerosis through effects on serum lipids; smokers tend to have higher levels of total cholesterol, LDL-C, and triglycerides and lower HDL-C than nonsmokers.[3] Smoking increases the levels of inflammatory mediators (C-reactive protein, leukocytes, and fibrinogen), which might contribute to the development and progression of atherosclerosis.[66] Finally, smoking stimulates the release of neurotransmitters (e.g., epinephrine, norepinephrine) that increase myocardial workload and induce coronary vasoconstriction, leading to ischemia, arrhythmias, and sudden death.[3,64]

P.J.'s hospital admission for a CABG procedure for coronary heart disease and angina, as well as previous procedures for peripheral vascular disease (angioplasty with stent placement) and cerebrovascular disease (bilateral carotid endarterectomy), are all conditions associated with chronic tobacco use. His elevated total cholesterol, LDL-C, and triglycerides, and reduced HDL-C levels are consistent with smoking-induced dyslipidemia. Cigarette smoking in combination with P.J.'s other established cardiovascular risk factors (hypertension, dyslipidemia) have synergistically increased his risk for serious cardiovascular disease.[3,64] Fortunately, the effects of smoking on lipids, coagulation, myocardial workload, and coronary blood flow appear to be reversible, and P.J.'s risk of developing further cardiovascular-related complications will markedly decrease if he is able to quit smoking.[37,67] A meta-analysis of 20 studies determined that smoking cessation is associated with a 36% reduction in the risk of death among patients with established coronary heart disease. The reduced mortality risk associated with quitting smoking is comparable to that observed with other established secondary preventative approaches such as therapies for hyperlipidemia and hypertension.[68] The clinician should approach this hospitalization as an opportunity to assist P.J. with quitting smoking.[8] Furthermore, published data suggest that initiation of intensive cessation counseling interventions for hospitalized patients is effective in achieving long-term abstinence.[69]

Noncigarette Forms of Tobacco

CASE 88-2, QUESTION 2: The cardiothoracic surgeon has strongly advised P.J. to quit smoking. P.J. would like to know whether cutting down to one to two cigars a day is an acceptable alternative to his current one to two packs of cigarettes per day.

The adverse health effects of cigar smoking have been well described and include an increased risk of cancer of the lung, oral cavity, larynx, esophagus, and pancreas. In addition, cigar smokers who inhale deeply are at increased risk for developing cardiovascular disease and chronic obstructive pulmonary disease (COPD).[70,71] Cigarette smokers who switch to smoking only cigars decrease their risk of developing lung cancer, but their risk is markedly higher than if they were to quit smoking altogether.[71]

Cigar weight and nicotine content vary widely from brand to brand and from cigar to cigar. Most cigars range in weight from about 1 to 22 g, and a typical cigarette weighs less than 1 g. The nicotine content of ten commercially available cigars studied in 1996 ranged from 10 to 444 mg. In comparison, US cigarettes have a relatively narrow total nicotine content range (mean, 13.5 ± 0.1 mg) per cigarette.[72] Relating these data, Henningfield and colleagues concluded that it is possible for one large cigar to contain as much tobacco as an entire pack of cigarettes and deliver enough nicotine to establish and maintain dependence.[73]

P.J. should be counseled that switching from cigarette smoking to low-level daily cigar smoking is not acceptable given his significant underlying cardiovascular disease. The amount of nicotine delivered by one to two cigars per day is capable of sustaining his dependence on nicotine. Furthermore, former cigarette smokers are more likely to inhale deeply, which further increases the risk of cancer and cardiovascular and pulmonary disease. The clinician should strongly advise P.J. to quit smoking cigarettes and that switching to cigars is not a safe alternative.

CASE 88-2, QUESTION 3: P.J. is willing to quit completely, but he is worried because he has tried to quit smoking "hundreds of times" and has never been able to quit for longer than 1 week. He expresses a desire for a medication to assist him during this quit attempt. He has tried the nicotine gum and transdermal patch during three previous quit attempts. He did not like the gum because it made his jaw sore. He had temporary success with the nicotine patch but found it to be less flexible than the gum. For example, when he needed extra nicotine during stressful situations, he could not apply a second patch. What treatment alternatives are reasonable for P.J.?

P.J. has inadequately responded to treatment with the transdermal patch and experienced intolerable jaw soreness with the nicotine gum. Newer formulations of the nicotine gum are less viscous, and therefore easier to chew, than earlier formulations of the gum; however, other options are available. First-line treatment options that he has not tried include the nicotine lozenge (see Case 88-1, Question 3), nicotine nasal spray, nicotine inhaler, sustained-release bupropion, varenicline, or an effective combination of first-line agents (see Case 88-3, Question 1).

Nicotine Nasal Spray

The nicotine nasal spray is an aqueous solution of nicotine available in a metered-spray pump for administration to the nasal mucosa. Each actuation delivers a metered 50-μL spray

Miscellaneous		Arsenic trioxide (Trisenox)	Causes morphological changes and DNA fragmentation characteristic of apoptosis	IV	Metabolism primarily hepatic; elimination primarily renal	Myelosuppression; cardiac effects; agitation, anxiety, depression, dizziness; dermatitis, pruritus; nausea, vomiting, diarrhea; electrolyte abnormalities
	Substituted urea	Hydroxyurea (Hydrea, Droxia)	Holds cells of the cell cycle in the G_1 or pre-DNA synthesis stage	PO	Well absorbed; hepatic metabolism; elimination primarily renal	Myelosuppression; hyperpigmentation of skin; nausea, vomiting, diarrhea
	Retinoids	Tretinoin (Vesanoid)	Produces an initial maturation of the primitive promyelocytes	PO	Well absorbed; highly protein bound; hepatic metabolism; primary renal elimination; moderate fecal elimination	RA-APL syndrome (fever, dyspnea, respiratory distress, edema, multiorgan failure); dizziness, paresthesia, anxiety, depression, insomnia, confusion, agitation, intracranial hypertension; hemorrhage; malaise; nausea, vomiting
	Rexinoid	Bexarotene (Targretin)	Activates transcription factors that regulate the expression of genes that control cellular differentiation and proliferation	PO	Highly protein bound; hepatic metabolism; primary hepatobiliary elimination	Lipid abnormalities; hypothyroidism; nausea; rash; leucopenia; headache; edema

CNS, central nervous system; CSF, cerebrospinal fluid; CYP, cytochrome; dCK, deoxycytidine kinase; DHFR, dihydrofolate reductase; DNA, deoxyribonucleic acid; GARFT, glycinamide ribonucleotide formyltransferase; IV, intravenous; MESNA, 2-mercaptoethane sulfonates sodium; PO, oral; RA-APL, retinoic acid–acute promyelocytic leukemia; RNA, ribonucleic acid; SC, subcutaneous; SIADH, syndrome of inappropriate antidiuretic hormone; TS, thymidylate synthase.

resistant to chemotherapy. In patients with large tumors showing a plateaulike growth curve, the fraction of cells killed with each treatment is usually low. The ability of this model to predict cell kill adequately is also limited by the need to administer chemotherapy in cycles (e.g., every 2, 3, or 4 weeks) in humans to allow normal cells to recover from the toxic effects of chemotherapy. During the recovery period, tumor cells can start to replicate again.

Therefore, successful treatment requires administration of the next cycle of therapy before the tumor has grown to its previous size. The objective of successive chemotherapy cycles is a further decrease in size of tumor mass. Other factors that influence cell kill include dose intensity, schedule, drug resistance, tumor site, and a patient's performance status.

Dose Intensity

Dose intensity is defined as the chemotherapy dose per unit time during which treatment is given (e.g., mg/m^2/week). Drug resistance might be overcome by escalating the dose intensity of drugs. This can be increased by (a) increasing the dose of chemotherapy per cycle, (b) shortening the interval between cycles, or (c) both. Unnecessary lengthening of the interval between successive cycles of chemotherapy or decreasing the dose can negatively affect treatment outcomes. Evidence suggests that reducing a dose can cause treatment failure in patients with chemotherapy-sensitive tumors who are having their first chemotherapy treatment.[41] A direct relationship between dose intensity and response rate also has been reported in several human tumors, including breast cancer, lymphomas, advanced ovarian cancer, and small-cell lung cancer.[42,43] Dose-dense treatment schedules have been designed to decrease the time between chemotherapy cycles, based on the theory that this would be more effective in reducing the residual tumor burden between treatments than escalating doses.[44] However, dose-intensive therapy has not consistently improved the overall cure rate of most solid tumors.

The dose intensity for most chemotherapy regimens is limited by the major dose-related toxicity, bone marrow suppression. To minimize this toxicity and administer higher doses, patients may receive hematopoietic growth factors, autologous stem cell transplantations, and altered schedules of drug delivery.[45,46]

Schedule Dependency

Chemotherapy is administered in cycles, with recovery periods between the cycles. A cycle of chemotherapy can last one or more days. A typical course of chemotherapy usually consists of several cycles of chemotherapy. How often the cycles are repeated depends on the type of cancer being treated and the drugs being used. This, in part, determines the schedule of administration.

The schedule of chemotherapy administration is additionally an important determinant of response. It influences dose intensity largely by affecting toxicity.[41] In some circumstances, changing the administration schedule can reduce the toxicity sufficiently to allow patients to receive higher total doses or more frequent courses of therapy, thereby increasing the dose intensity. The optimal schedule is also influenced by the pharmacokinetics of the agent. For example, phase-specific agents exert their cytotoxic effects only when the cell is in a particular phase of the cell cycle. If a phase-specific agent with a short half-life is administered by intravenous bolus, a significant number of tumor cells will probably not cycle through the vulnerable phase of the cell cycle during exposure to the agent. Comparatively, the same agent administered by frequent intravenous bolus or continuous infusion could expose more cells to the agent during the vulnerable phase.[47]

Drug Resistance

CASE 89-7

QUESTION 1: B.C. is a 39-year-old man with an aggressive non-Hodgkin lymphoma (NHL). At the time of diagnosis, B.C. had enlarged cervical lymph nodes, dyspnea, and a large mediastinal mass noted on chest x-ray examination. Chemotherapy was initiated with cyclophosphamide, doxorubicin, vincristine, prednisone, and rituximab. After the first cycle of chemotherapy, B.C.'s lymphadenopathy was greatly reduced. Chest x-ray examination repeated after the second cycle of therapy showed marked improvement. When he returned for his fifth cycle of chemotherapy, recurrent lymphadenopathy was noted, and the chest radiograph confirmed enlargement of the mediastinal mass. Why is B.C.'s cancer growing despite continued chemotherapy, and how should his treatment be altered?

Most likely B.C.'s cancer is now growing because the tumor has become resistant to the chemotherapy; therefore, it would be wise to discontinue the current regimen. Biochemical resistance to chemotherapy is the major impediment to successful treatment with most cancers.[41] Resistance can occur de novo in cancer cells or develop during cell division as a result of mutation.[41] In 1979, a proposed mathematical model predicted that tumor cells mutate to drug resistance at a rate related to the genetic instability of the tumor.[48] Thus, the probability that a tumor mass will contain resistant clones is related to both the rate of mutation and the size of the tumor. Many specific mechanisms now have been identified by which cancer cells resist the activity of cytotoxic agents.

Some cell lines that become resistant to a single chemotherapy agent may also be resistant to structurally unrelated cytotoxic compounds. This phenomenon is called *pleiotropic drug resistance* or *multidrug resistance* (MDR).[49] Cell lines that display this type of resistance generally are resistant to natural product cytotoxic agents such as the vinca alkaloids, antitumor antibiotics, epipodophyllotoxins, camptothecins, and taxanes. The primary mechanism believed to be responsible for MDR is an increase in efflux transporters such as P-glycoprotein in the cell membrane. These proteins mediate efflux of the chemotherapy agent, causing a decreased accumulation of drug within the cell (the site of drug activity).[49] Other transport proteins (e.g., breast cancer resistance protein) have been implicated in resistance to chemotherapy, as well.[50]

Drugs known to inhibit P-glycoprotein (e.g., verapamil, cyclosporine, quinidine) have been investigated as potential adjunctive therapies to reduce resistance. Dosages of the agents required to inhibit P-glycoprotein have been associated with significant morbidity. Substantial improved efficacy is, as of yet, unproved with P-glycoprotein inhibitors. A second type of MDR is resistance caused by changes or mutations of drug targets, for example the altered binding of topoisomerase II, an enzyme that promotes DNA strand breaks in the presence of anthracyclines and epipodophyllotoxins.[51] Because of the likelihood of MDR, B.C. should receive a chemotherapy regimen that does not include agents transported from tumor cells by the MDR mechanism. An alternative regimen, such as gemcitabine or oxaliplatin, with or without rituximab, may be a reasonable option as this regimen is active against NHL and these drugs are not known substrates for various efflux transporters.

Tumor Site

The cytotoxic effects of chemotherapy agents are related to the time the tumor is exposed to an effective concentration of the agent (i.e., concentration × time [C × T]). The drug dose,

TABLE 89-13
Monoclonal Antibodies[a]

Agent (Trade Name)	Mechanism of Action	Major Toxicities
Alemtuzumab (Campath)	Targets CD52 cell surface antigen; binding leads to lysis of CD52-positive leukemic cells	Hypersensitivity reactions; myelosuppression, pancytopenia, opportunistic infection, nausea, vomiting, dyspnea, hypotension
Bevacizumab (Avastin)	Inhibits development of new blood vessels (angiogenesis) by binding to and inhibiting vascular endothelial growth factor (VEGF) from interacting with receptors	Hypertension, diarrhea, constipation; bleeding, thrombosis; gastrointestinal perforation; impaired wound healing; proteinuria; infusion reactions
Cetuximab (Erbitux)	Inhibits cell proliferation by preventing activation of the epidermal growth factor receptor (EGFR)	Anaphylactic or hypersensitivity reactions; papulopustular skin rash; asthenia; nausea, vomiting, hypomagnesemia
Denileukin diftitox (Ontak)	Fusion protein containing diphtheria toxin and IL-segments; directs cytocidal action of diphtheria toxin to IL-2 receptor–expressing cells leading to inhibition of protein synthesis and cell death	Nausea, vomiting, diarrhea, fatigue, peripheral edema, pruritus, hypersensitivity reactions, rigors, capillary leak syndrome, loss of visual acuity
Ibritumomab tiuxetan (Zevalin)	Yttrium-90 (Y-90)-linked to rituximab; binds to the CD20 antigen on malignant B lymphocytes; releases radiation (β particles), which induces cell damage and death	Infusion reactions (hypotension, angioedema, hypoxia, bronchospasm); asthenia, chills, nausea; myelosuppression; see major toxicities for rituximab
Ofatumumab (Arzerra)	Mediates immune effector functions by binding the CD20 molecule to result in B-cell lysis	Cough, diarrhea, dyspnea, fatigue, nausea, neutropenia, anemia, hypersensitivity reactions, pyrexia, rash, infections
Panitumumab (Vectibix)	Same as cetuximab	Papular-pustular rash, pruritus, hypersensitivity reactions, abdominal pain, diarrhea, hypomagnesemia, nausea, paronychia
Rituximab (Rituxan)	Lyses B cells by recruiting immune effectors against the CD20 antigen	Tumor lysis; hypersensitivity reactions; mucocutaneous reactions; lymphopenia
Tositumomab (Bexxar)	Iodine-131 (I-131)-linked to rituximab; binds to the CD20 antigen on malignant B lymphocytes; releases radiation and induces apoptosis, complement or antibody-dependent cell cytotoxicity; inducing cell damage and death	Hypersensitivity reactions; myelosuppression; hypothyroidism; nausea, vomiting, abdominal pain, diarrhea; myelodysplastic syndrome, acute leukemia; see major toxicities for rituximab
Trastuzumab (Herceptin)	Inhibits proliferation of human tumor cells that express HER2 proto-oncogene	Cardiomyopathy; diarrhea; nausea, vomiting; hypersensitivity reaction

[a]All monoclonal antibodies are administered intravenously.

and are also used in other solid tumors. Figure 89-4 depicts key signaling molecules involved in angiogenesis and lists representative agents designed to inhibit these signals. Table 89-14 provides the tyrosine kinase inhibitors currently approved by the US Food and Drug Administration to treat malignancies.[38]

COMBINATION THERAPY WITH TARGETED AGENTS

The optimal activity of adding targeted agents to cytotoxic chemotherapy is difficult to predict. Knowledge about how to combine targeted agents with chemotherapy is limited, although clinical investigations are ongoing. See subsequent chapters for specific discussion of the use of targeted therapy with chemotherapy in solid tumor and hematologic malignancies.

OTHER TARGETED AGENTS

As more information is learned regarding signal transduction pathways and cellular growth and proliferation, more drugs are being developed that target these key molecules. Histone deacetylase inhibitors, mTOR inhibitors, and proteasome inhibitors are examples of new drugs that have novel mechanism(s) of action. Table 89-15 lists these and other targeted agents currently approved by the US Food and Drug Administration to treat malignancies.[38]

Endocrine Therapy

Endocrine therapy can be used to treat several common cancers, including breast, prostate, and endometrial cancers, which arise from hormone-sensitive tissues (Table 89-16). These tumors grow in response to endogenous hormones that trigger growth signals by binding to specific receptors located on a cell membrane or within the cytoplasm of a cell. Current endocrine therapies inhibit tumor growth by blocking the receptors or by eliminating the endogenous hormone feeding the tumor. (Note: Interruption of hormonal secretion also can be achieved through surgical removal of hormone-producing organs.) Not all tumors arising from hormone-sensitive tissues respond to endocrine manipulation. Lack of response may be associated with hormone-resistant tumor cells or inadequate suppression of the endogenous feeding hormones.[54]

Biologic Response Modifiers

Biologic response modifiers are substances that either boost or restore the ability of the immune system to fight cancer, infections, or other diseases.[35] Biologic response modifiers may include monoclonal antibodies (discussed in more detail above), vaccines, and growth factors (e.g., interferon-α and interleukin 2).

VACCINES

Vaccines are biologic response modifiers that may be used to treat cancers. They are immunotherapies meant to stimulate the body's immune response to cancer cells (usually after the patient is diagnosed). Sipuleucel-T (Provenge) has recently been

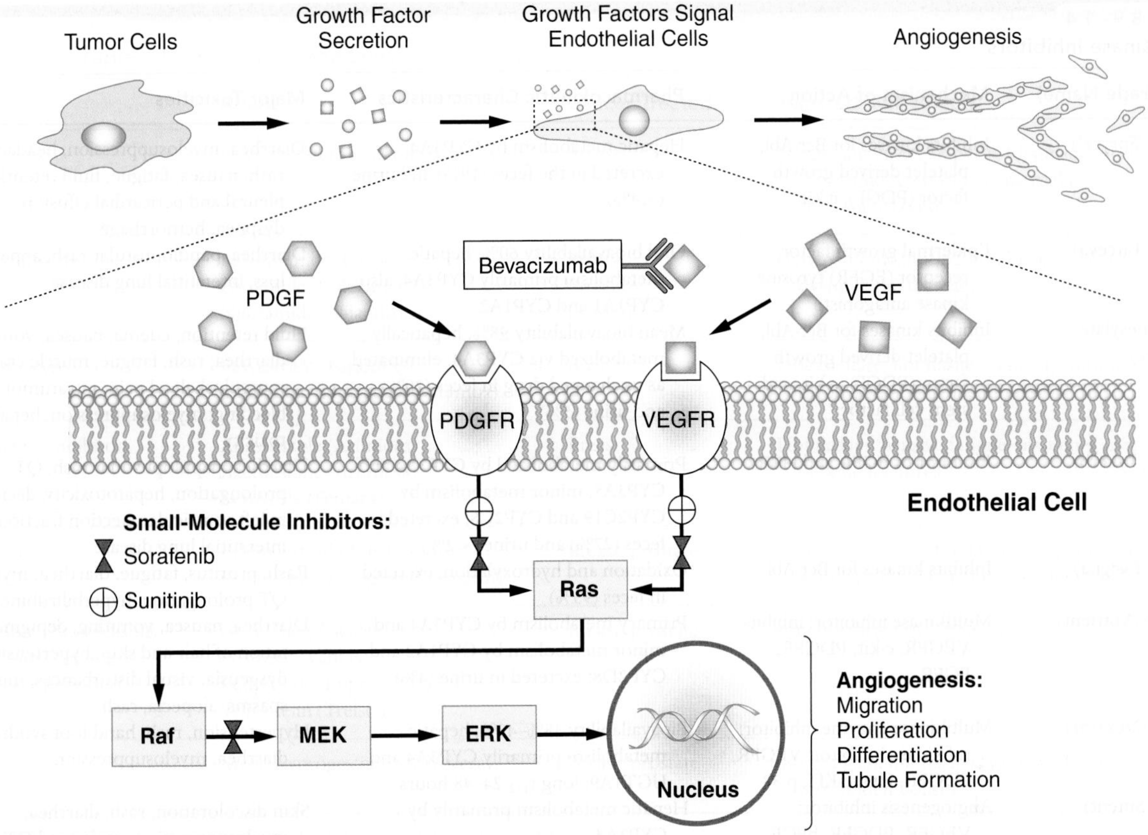

FIGURE 89-4 Angiogenesis and representative antiangiogenic agents. Tumor cells signal new blood vessel formation through secretion of growth factors such as vascular endothelial growth factor (VEGF) and platelet-derived growth factor (PDGF), which interact with and activate receptors (PDGFR, VEGFR) for tyrosine kinase signaling within the endothelial cells. Subsequent cascade signaling downstream activates the cell nucleus and initiates angiogenesis through endothelial cell proliferation, migration, differentiation, and tubule formation. Representative agents that block this signaling process are shown as bevacizumab (monoclonal antibody that blocks VEGF), and sorafenib and sunitinib (small-molecule inhibitors) that block several different targets associated with the angiogenic process. Raf, Ras, MEK, and ERK are kinase enzymes. Also see Figure 89-1 for additional details.

approved for patients with metastatic prostate cancer that is resistant to prior hormone therapy, and others are under evaluation in phase III clinical trials.[55] An individual's immune system plays a crucial role in developing or eradicating cancer. Normally, an intact immune system can protect the host against malignant cells and infectious pathogens, but current evidence shows that individuals with "weakened" immune systems are at an increased risk of developing cancer.

INTERFERON-α

The first recombinant cytokine to become available for the treatment of cancer was interferon-α. This interferon affects tumor cells through several different mechanisms, including (a) a direct antiproliferative effect; (b) an immunomodulatory effect on natural killer cells, T cells, B cells, and macrophages; (c) an induction of tumor cell antigens; and (d) a differentiating effect on tumor cells. Interferons also possess antiangiogenic effects.[15] Current studies show that interferon-α has antitumor effects against several human malignancies, including melanoma and renal cell carcinoma.[56] Interferon-α is sometimes given in combination with radiation therapy, other biologic response modifiers, or chemotherapy agents.

INTERLEUKIN 2

Interleukin 2 is a recombinantly produced lymphokine that has numerous immunoregulatory functions. In normal cells, interleukin 2 stimulates both T- and B-cell proliferation and differentiation.[57] The idea for interleukin 2 use to treat cancer arose from the observation that lymphoid cells incubated with interleukin 2 developed the capacity to lyse tumor cells.[58,59] This observation led to the development of some adoptive immunotherapies. Initial studies showed that patients with advanced tumors, such as renal cell carcinoma and melanoma, experienced tumor regression after receiving interleukin 2. Subsequent studies using high dosages of interleukin 2 also reported responses in similar patient populations with advanced disease.[59–61] High-dose interleukin 2 therapy is accompanied by significant, dose-related toxicity and is only administered in supervised settings. The most serious toxicities (hypotension, pulmonary edema, oliguria, increased bilirubin) occur secondary to a diffuse capillary leak that develops during interleukin 2 therapy. These toxicities usually resolve promptly after discontinuing therapy.

If H.P. is in fact diagnosed with stage IV adenocarcinoma of the lung, he may receive other agents besides just cytotoxic chemotherapy during the course of treatment for his disease. For specific discussion of which noncytotoxic agents H.P may receive, refer to Chapter 94, Lung Cancer.

Administration

SYSTEMIC

Systemic cytotoxic chemotherapy is most commonly administered by the intravenous route, either as a bolus injection

	CHAPTER CASES
8 Several anticancer agents carry severe risks of nephrotoxicity and bladder toxicity for which preventative measures are necessary. Cisplatin is one of the most nephrotoxic. Preventative strategies for cisplatin nephrotoxicity include normal saline hydration, mannitol, and amifostine, and methotrexate-induced nephrotoxicity may be prevented with alkalinization of the urine and leucovorin rescue. Ifosfamide-induced hemorrhagic cystitis may be prevented with concomitant use of mesna.	**Case 90-8 (Questions 1, 2), Case 90-9 (Questions 1–3)**
9 Many anticancer medications demonstrate organ-specific toxicities, such as pulmonary fibrosis caused by bleomycin and transaminitis caused by cytarabine. Specific treatments for resolution of these toxicities do not exist, rather, supportive care for symptoms is necessary. If adverse effects do not resolve, discontinuation of therapy or dose modifications may be warranted.	**Case 90-10 (Questions 1–4), Case 90-11 (Question 1)**
10 Many anticancer agents cause long-term complications after therapy, including treatment-related acute myeloid leukemia, lymphomas, bladder cancer, and bone sarcoma. The risks of secondary malignancies should be considered in assessing the adverse-effect profile and risks and benefits of specific types of therapy.	**Case 90-12 (Questions 1, 2)**
11 Cytotoxic chemotherapy is potentially gonadotoxic with use of specific agents. Sex, age, agent, and cumulative dose are factors in determining the risk of infertility. Methods of preserving fertility should be discussed with patients before initiating therapy.	**Case 90-13 (Question 1), Case 90-14 (Questions 1–3)**

Cytotoxic and targeted anticancer agents are toxic to cancer cells and also to various host tissues and organs. The adverse effects of anticancer therapies can be classified as common and acute toxicities, specific organ toxicities, and long-term complications. Common and acute toxicities generally occur as a result of inhibition of host-cell division. Host tissues most susceptible to cytotoxic agents include tissues with renewal cell populations, such as lymphoid tissues, bone marrow, and epithelium of the gastrointestinal (GI) tract and skin. Some other common and acute toxicities (e.g., nausea and vomiting, hypersensitivity reactions) frequently occur in patients shortly after therapy. Specific organ toxicities often are attributed to a unique uptake or a selective toxicity of the anticancer agent to the organ. Long-term complications are toxicities that occur months to years after anticancer therapy. These long-term toxicities occur secondary to continued immunodeficiencies or from permanent damage to the organ cells from the specific therapy. Regardless of the type of toxicities observed, most are classified for severity by the National Cancer Institute (NCI) Common Terminology Criteria for Adverse Events. This classification creates a common method for classification of events in clinical trials and for management of toxicities that occur for patients receiving standard of care regimens.[1] These criteria may be accessed at the National Cancer Institute website (http://ctep.cancer.gov/protocolDevelopment/electronic_applications/ctc.htm#ctc_40).

The toxicities associated with anticancer therapies are the most important factors limiting the use of potentially curative doses. Therefore, all discussions regarding the benefits of anticancer agents must include a discussion of toxicities associated with their use. Concerns regarding the toxicities of therapy include the incidence, predictability, severity, and reversibility of the adverse effects. In addition, the specific agent, dose intensity, and treatment duration can influence the incidence of several adverse effects. Although the incidence and predictability may be well defined in specific patient populations, the incidence often varies depending on individual susceptibility. The specific adverse effects that an individual patient will experience may be difficult to predict. Because several toxicities have well-defined characteristics, clinicians should be aware of the most common adverse effects.

Clinicians should also be aware of patient-specific factors, such as the stage of disease, concomitant illnesses, and concurrent medications, which could cause signs or symptoms that mimic the adverse effects associated with anticancer therapy. Many patients have disease involvement which may impair organ function. In addition, most patients with cancer receive many other medications, including antibiotics and analgesics, that may cause additional adverse effects or interact with anticancer agents. When a patient reports a new symptom, it may be difficult to determine whether it is secondary to anticancer therapy, concurrent medications, or disease progression.

COMMON AND ACUTE TOXICITIES

Hematologic Toxicities

EFFECTS ON BONE MARROW

The bone marrow contains a population of pluripotent stem cells capable of self-renewal and differentiation into any mature blood cell. Their progeny commit to either the myeloid or the lymphoid cell line. The myeloid stem cell further commits to developing into an erythrocyte (red blood cell), megakaryocyte (platelet), or granulocyte (white blood cell).

After committing to a particular cell line, bone marrow precursor cells undergo a series of divisions (mitosis) to increase the number of cells. The cells then undergo several developmental stages to mature and differentiate into their final forms (postmitotic) and leave the bone marrow. The total time required for a cell to pass through the mitotic and postmitotic pool under normal resting conditions is approximately 10 to 14 days. This process is regulated by several cytokines; although many cytokines have been identified, only a few growth factors are now produced through recombinant DNA technology. These growth factors can expand the mitotic pool and accelerate maturation and differentiation. Ultimately, these growth factors decrease the total time spent in these stages to approximately 5 to 7 days.

The development and circulating life span of hematopoietic cell lines determine the severity of the depression of that cell line (nadir, lowest point) and the time course of peripheral cytopenias. Because red blood cells (RBCs) survive approximately 120 days in the peripheral blood, clinically significant anemia is unlikely if production is impaired for a short period of time. Instead, anemia usually develops slowly after several courses of cytotoxic therapy. In contrast, platelets survive approximately 10 days, and granulocytes survive only 6 to 8 hours. Hence, granulocytopenia generally occurs before thrombocytopenia, but both may be observed after the first or subsequent courses of cytotoxic chemotherapy. The clinician may have to adjust the subsequent chemotherapy dosage based on nadir depth and slow recovery. Life-threatening granulocytopenia or thrombocytopenia often necessitates some action to minimize the risk of adverse effects with additional courses of cytotoxic chemotherapy. To diminish these effects, one can reduce the dose, delay therapy until recovery, or administer colony-stimulating factors (CSFs). The availability of CSFs provides an alternative approach to preventing severe granulocytopenia.

MYELOSUPPRESSION

CASE 90-1

QUESTION 1: J.T., a 68-year-old, 59-kg man with no significant past medical history, presents to the university hospital with complaints of cough and shortness of breath (SOB). Chest radiograph reveals a lesion in the right upper lobe; surgical resection and cytologic examination are positive for non–small-cell lung cancer (NSCLC). A workup for metastases is negative. J.T. is diagnosed with early-stage (stage II) NSCLC. His physicians plan to initiate adjuvant chemotherapy of carboplatin targeted to an area under the concentration-time curve (AUC) of 6 mg/mL × minute on day 1 and paclitaxel 200 mg/m^2 on day 1. Discuss the toxicities that might be expected to occur with this regimen. What effects on the bone marrow can be anticipated and how might they clinically appear in J.T.? What factors can influence the incidence and severity of these adverse effects? When can J.T. expect these effects to occur?

Although several toxicities are commonly associated with carboplatin and paclitaxel, the most predictable and severe toxicity associated with this regimen is myelosuppression. This chemotherapy regimen can significantly affect any cell line, including RBCs, neutrophils, and platelets, and the cytopenias can cause significant morbidity or mortality. Decreased RBCs can cause anemia, and patients usually present with fatigue and decreased exercise tolerance. Having low neutrophil counts significantly increases a patient's risk for bacterial infections. Moreover, reduced platelets can cause thrombocytopenia, which can cause bleeding from the GI and genitourinary tracts.

Both patient-related and agent-related factors can significantly influence the degree of cytopenia a patient faces after cytotoxic therapy. Agent-related factors include the specific agent, dose intensity, and dose density. Because most anticancer treatments are not given as a single agent, the effects of concurrent cytotoxic therapies may intensify the myelosuppressive effect of an individual agent. Host factors that specifically may affect the cellularity of the bone marrow compartment also influence the degree of cytopenia. They include the following:

1. Patient age. Younger patients are generally better able to tolerate cytotoxic chemotherapy than elderly patients because they have a more cellular marrow with a decreased percentage of marrow fat.
2. Bone marrow reserve. Certain diseases might present with tumor cells in the bone marrow, such as leukemias and some lymphomas, in which case the bone marrow does not have a healthy reserve of normal hematopoietic cells to help in the recovery process.
3. The degree of myelosuppression from previous cytotoxic chemotherapy, radiation therapy, or both. Prior cytotoxic chemotherapy and radiation therapy to fields involving marrow-producing bone (pelvic bone and sternum) reduce bone marrow reserves.
4. The ability of the liver or kidney to metabolize and excrete the compounds administered. If agents are administered to patients with specific organ insufficiencies (i.e., renal or hepatic), slower clearance, resulting in increased systemic exposure, can occur. This can cause greater toxicities, including longer cytopenias.

These factors, along with the kinetics of the stem cells, can help clinicians predict the severity and duration of cytopenia observed after therapy.

With most myelosuppressive agents, the patient's white blood cell (WBC) and platelet counts begin to fall within 5 to 7 days of cytotoxic therapy administration, reach a nadir within 7 to 10 days, and recover within 14 to 26 days. Phase-specific cytotoxic chemotherapy agents, such as the vinca alkaloids and antimetabolites, cause a fairly rapid onset of cytopenia that recovers faster than those occurring after treatment with phase-nonspecific agents, such as alkylating agents and anthracyclines. For poorly understood reasons, nitrosoureas typically produce severe, delayed neutropenia and thrombocytopenia 4 to 6 weeks after therapy. Other agents that exhibit this pattern include mitomycin and mechlorethamine. All of these anticancer agents exert their cytotoxic effects during the resting phase of the cell cycle. The nitrosoureas as well as mitomycin and mechlorethamine can cause two neutropenic nadirs; the first nadir occurs at the conventional time expected for phase-nonspecific agents and the second nadir occurs approximately 4 to 6 weeks after therapy. Many combination regimens with these agents are therefore given for 6-week cycles to avoid treatment before the second nadir. However, most other myelosuppressive regimens can be safely given every 3 to 4 weeks. The majority of the targeted therapies do not suppress bone marrow production, because they are designed to inhibit a specific molecular pathway rather than proliferating cells in general. Because of their minimal myelosuppressive effects, they may be desirable agents to add to regimens that are known to cause cytopenias.

Each of the agents included in J.T.'s regimen have marked myelosuppressive activity. His elderly age may place him at higher risk for exhibiting myelosuppression. J.T. should be carefully counseled to contact his physician or report to the emergency department if he experiences signs or symptoms of an infection (including fever) or bleeding. Typically, these symptoms occur 10 to 14 days after the first day of chemotherapy.

PREVENTION OF NEUTROPENIA

CASE 90-1, QUESTION 2: About 9 days after the first course of cytotoxic chemotherapy, J.T. experienced a severe sore throat and fever. He was admitted to the hospital and treated with intravenous (IV) antibiotics. At the time, his WBC count was 300 cells/μL; absolute neutrophil count (ANC), 50 cells/μL; platelets, 102,000 cells/μL; and

hemoglobin (Hgb), 11 g/dL. His fever resolved after 3 days, and all cultures were negative for bacterial growth. It is now 3 weeks after chemotherapy, and he is scheduled to receive a second course. Should he receive the same doses he was given initially?

One option would be to reduce (usually by 25%) the dose of each agent for all subsequent cycles. Although a dose reduction can clearly cause less neutropenia, it can also compromise the response and survival of patients with chemotherapy-sensitive tumors. Because J.T.'s cancer (i.e., early-stage NSCLC), is both chemosensitive and potentially curable, a dosage reduction is undesirable. To minimize the risk of neutropenia with future therapy, CSFs can be administered to J.T. to prevent potential complications associated with neutropenia.

Prophylactic administration of CSFs can be used to reduce the myelosuppressive effects of cytotoxic chemotherapy. Three CSFs—granulocyte colony-stimulating factor (G-CSF [filgrastim]), granulocyte-macrophage colony-stimulating factor (GM-CSF [sargramostim]), and a pegylated long-acting form of filgrastim, pegfilgrastim—are available in the United States. These products were approved by the US Food and Drug Administration (FDA) to enhance neutrophil recovery after chemotherapy. Pegfilgrastim was developed with the aim of providing the same pharmacologic benefit as filgrastim while offering the advantage and convenience of fewer injections. Evidence-based clinical practice guidelines for the use of CSFs have been developed by the American Society of Clinical Oncology (ASCO).[2] These guidelines recommend primary prophylaxis for all patients receiving chemotherapy regimens that have been previously reported to cause an incidence of approximately 20% febrile neutropenia. A CSF used in these patients can reduce both the incidence of febrile neutropenia and need for hospitalizations and broad-spectrum antibiotics. However, CSF usage has not been shown to lead to better tumor response or higher overall survival. Two randomized phase III clinical trials have shown that the risk of neutropenic fever is reduced when primary prophylaxis is used in regimens with a known incidence of approximately 20% neutropenia. In one trial, 928 patients with breast cancer receiving docetaxel 100 mg/m^2 every 21 days were randomly assigned to receive placebo or pegfilgrastim 6 mg subcutaneously (SC) 24 hours after chemotherapy. Patients who received pegfilgrastim had a lower incidence of febrile neutropenia (1% vs. 17%, respectively) and hospitalizations (1% vs. 14%, respectively).[3] A trial in patients ($n = 171$) with SCLC receiving a dose-intense regimen containing cyclophosphamide 1,000 mg/m^2 on day 1, doxorubicin 45 mg/m^2 on day 1, and etoposide 100 mg/m^2 on days 1 to 3 every 21 days was conducted. Patients were randomly assigned to receive prophylactic antibiotics with or without filgrastim. The rate of febrile neutropenia over all five cycles was 32% with prophylactic antibiotics without filgrastim versus 18% with antibiotics and filgrastim.[4] A meta-analysis of 17 randomized trials including 3,493 adult patients with solid tumors and lymphomas showed that the use of filgrastim as primary prophylaxis reduced the risk of febrile neutropenia and improved the rate of full-dose cytotoxic chemotherapy given on schedule. Additionally, the investigators in the meta-analysis observed a significant reduction in the risk of infection-related mortality.[5] Because the regimen J.T. received does not typically produce a 20% incidence of febrile neutropenia, a CSF was not recommended for him after his first course of cytotoxic chemotherapy. Now that J.T. has experienced febrile neutropenia and he has a potentially curable malignancy, a CSF is indicated with subsequent courses of chemotherapy to prevent additional febrile episodes.

DOSING OF COLONY-STIMULATING FACTORS

CASE 90-1, QUESTION 3: How should a CSF be dosed in J.T. to reduce the severity of chemotherapy-induced neutropenia?

The recommended initial dose of filgrastim is 5 mcg/kg/day as a single daily SC injection, and of sargramostim, 250 mcg/m^2/day SC. Pegfilgrastim is given once per cycle as 6 mg SC in adult patients regardless of patient weight. The ASCO guidelines state that rounding the dose of either weight-based filgrastim or sargramostim to the nearest vial size may enhance patient convenience and reduce cost without clinical detriment. Because commercially available vials contain either 300 or 480 mcg of filgrastim, adult patients weighing less than 75 kg should receive 300 mcg daily and adult patients weighing more than 75 kg should receive 480 mcg daily.[2] Because of differences in commercially available vial sizes, the weight breakpoint for sargramostim is slightly different; patients who weigh more than 60 kg should receive 500 mcg daily and patients who weigh less than 60 kg should receive 250 mcg daily.

The ASCO guidelines also recommend a shorter duration of treatment than the manufacturers. The manufacturers recommend that therapy with filgrastim or sargramostim continue until the patient's neutrophil count is greater than 10,000 cells/μL after the expected chemotherapy nadir. This is based on the observation that the neutrophil count falls roughly 50% after discontinuing a CSF. The risk of bacterial infection is highest, however, in patients with neutrophil counts of less than 500 to 1,000 cells/μL; patients with neutrophil counts greater than 500 to 1,000 cells/μL are not thought to be at high risk for experiencing bacterial infections. Thus, many clinicians elect to discontinue the CSF when the neutrophil count reaches 2,000 to 4,000 cells/μL after the chemotherapy nadir. This reduces the number of treatment days and the cost associated with therapy while concurrently reducing the excessive risk for bacterial infections. The ASCO guidelines support this recommendation to discontinue CSF earlier.

Many patients prefer a convenient single injection of pegfilgrastim over the daily injections of the other two, but one could question if it is as efficacious. Two pivotal, randomized, blinded multicenter phase III trials compared the efficacy of single-dose pegfilgrastim to filgrastim daily in the prevention of chemotherapy-induced neutropenia in patients with high-risk stage II through IV breast cancers.[6,7] The patients ($n = 310$[6]; $n = 157$[7]) received four cycles of doxorubicin 60 mg/m^2 and docetaxel 75 mg/m^2 chemotherapy on day 1 of each cycle and were randomly assigned to either single-dose pegfilgrastim on day 2 or filgrastim 5 mcg/kg/day from day 2 until the ANC was greater than 10,000 cells/μL up to 14 doses. In one study, the pegfilgrastim dose was fixed to 6 mg[7] and in the other, it was based on weight (100 mcg/kg).[6] The primary end point was duration of severe grade 4 neutropenia (ANC $<$500 cells/μL in cycle 1). Secondary end points included the severity of ANC nadir, time to recovery, incidence of grade 4 neutropenia and incidence of febrile neutropenia. For either trial, no significant difference in duration of grade 4 neutropenia was seen between the pegfilgrastim and filgrastim groups (1.7 vs. 1.8 days, respectively,[6] and 1.8 vs. 1.6 days, respectively[7]). The incidence of severe neutropenia after chemotherapy was similar in both arms. Patients who received pegfilgrastim had lower incidence of febrile neutropenia during four cycles of chemotherapy[6,7] than patients receiving filgrastim. In the larger of the trials, this difference was clinically significant ($p = 0.029$). The time to ANC recovery was defined as the time from chemotherapy administration until the ANC increased to greater than 2,000 cells/μL. In the larger phase III trial,[6] the mean time to recovery was 9.3 days in the

venous thromboembolic events when used in the treatment of multiple myeloma and other diseases.[43–45] Prophylaxis may be warranted during chemotherapy, although various strategies have only been explored in small, uncontrolled trials. A review of strategies including low-molecular-weight heparin or warfarin provides further explanation.[43] Bevacizumab is associated with both arterial thrombosis and bleeding events. A retrospective analysis of five trials of patients receiving chemotherapy for colorectal, breast, or NSCLC showed a 3.8% incidence of arterial thrombosis in patients receiving chemotherapy and bevacizumab versus 1.7% in chemotherapy alone.[46] Most bleeding events associated with bevacizumab are minor. However, severe major bleeding events have been reported in patients with metastatic colorectal cancer. Moreover, life-threatening pulmonary hemorrhage and hemoptysis have been described in those with squamous NSCLC; therefore, its use is restricted to those patients with nonsquamous NSCLC.[47] Different types of thrombotic events have been identified in patients receiving bevacizumab for other types of cancers.[48]

Other factors can cause patients to experience thrombosis. Many patients receiving cancer chemotherapy often have other illnesses that may predispose them to exhibiting thrombosis. In addition, surgical procedures and bed rest can increase the risk of thrombosis. Clinicians should maintain a high index of suspicion when a patient with cancer presents with signs or symptoms of thrombosis. Several reviews summarize risk factors and recommendations and provide further insight for specific clinical scenarios.[43,49,50]

Gastrointestinal Tract Toxicities

The GI tract may be second only to bone marrow in its susceptibility to toxic effects produced by cytotoxic chemotherapy. GI toxicities include nausea and vomiting, oral complications, esophagitis, and lower bowel disturbances.

NAUSEA AND VOMITING

Nausea and vomiting are common and serious toxicities associated with many cytotoxic and targeted anticancer agents. Anticancer agents or their metabolites may stimulate dopamine or serotonin receptors in the GI tract, the chemoreceptor trigger zone, or the central nervous system (CNS), which ultimately act on the vomiting center. Emesis most commonly occurs on the first day of chemotherapy and often persists for several days thereafter.[51] Most patients who receive traditional cytotoxic chemotherapy agents require antiemetics before and after chemotherapy for several days to control these symptoms. The most appropriate antiemetic regimen is based on patient-specific and agent-specific factors. Some of the targeted therapy agents carry some risk of emetogenicity, although it is generally milder. Guidelines are beginning to incorporate these targeted agents into their emetogenic classification schema based on incidence of nausea and vomiting in clinical trials (see Chapter 6, Nausea and Vomiting, for antiemetic algorithms and emetogenic potential of the cancer agents).

COMPLICATIONS OF THE ORAL CAVITY

Complications of the oral cavity include mucositis (or stomatitis), xerostomia (dry mouth), infection, and bleeding. The incidence of severe oral mucositis varies with the anticancer therapies given. Doxorubicin and continuous-infusion fluorouracil are among the agents at highest risk for causing severe mucositis. Virtually all patients who receive myeloablative hematopoietic cell transplantation (HCT) or have radiation therapy to the head and neck experience oral complications.[52] These toxicities occur because of the nonspecific effects of chemotherapy on cells undergoing rapid division, including the cells of the mouth that undergo rapid renewal with a turnover time equal to 7 to 14 days. Cytotoxic therapy reduces the renewal rate of the basal epithelium and can cause mucosal atrophy, as well as glandular and collagen degeneration.[52,53] Radiation therapy to the head and neck also causes mucosal atrophy by decreasing cell renewal. Radiation can also cause fibrosis of the salivary glands, muscles, ligaments, and blood vessels, and damage to the taste buds.[53] The combined effects of chemotherapy and radiation therapy on the oral mucosa can also cause infection and bleeding in the oral cavity. Infection and bleeding occurs when treatment causes bone marrow suppression, including thrombocytopenia and neutropenia. Because the oral mucosa is highly vascular and frequently traumatized, bleeding occurs commonly with thrombocytopenia. In addition, cytotoxic chemotherapy and neutropenia can alter the extensive microbial flora harbored in the oral cavity, thus leading to oral infections. Oral complications often compound one another. For example, xerostomia can accelerate the development of mucositis as well as the formation of dental caries and local infection. Mucositis can clearly predispose the oral cavity to local bleeding and infection, as well as systemic infections leading to sepsis. These oral complications can also cause varying degrees of discomfort and adversely affect the patient's ability to eat, which potentially may lead to a compromised nutritional status. Topical treatments of oral complications are reviewed extensively in guidelines.[54]

For a table that summarizes topical treatments of oral complications, see Online Table 90-1 at http://thepoint.lww.com/AT10e.

XEROSTOMIA

CASE 90-2

QUESTION 1: J.B. is a 55-year-old man with newly diagnosed, locally advanced head and neck cancer. His planned therapy includes cisplatin and fluorouracil given with concurrent radiation for a total of 6 weeks after surgical resection. A review of systems suggests that J.B. has poor oral hygiene, and a decision is made to consult the dental department of the university hospital before initiating radiation and chemotherapy. Is J.B. at risk for experiencing oral complications of chemotherapy? Is there anything that should be completed at this point to decrease his risk?

J.B. is at high risk for several of the oral complications previously described. Xerostomia, one of the most frequent side effects of radiation therapy to the head and neck, occurs secondary to radiation-induced changes to the salivary glands. Evidence supports a direct relationship between the dose of radiation to the salivary glands and the extent of glandular changes.[55] In most patients treated with less than 6,000 rad, radiation-induced changes to the salivary glands are reversible within 6 to 12 months after the end of therapy. J.B. will also be receiving chemotherapy agents (i.e., cisplatin) that can cause xerostomia and enhance the toxicity to the salivary glands. Clinically, xerostomia has been caused by as little as two to three radiation doses of 200 rad.[55]

Damage to the salivary glands causes various effects, including a loss of salivary buffering capacity, lower salivary pH, no mechanical flushing, decreased salivary immunoglobulin A, and reduction of saliva production. In addition, xerostomia can alter the sense of taste, causing some patients to lose their ability to differentiate between sweet and salty foods and others to report a bitter taste. Xerostomia also commonly causes caries. Caries and decalcification may become sufficiently severe to compromise tooth integrity and cause fracture. Because saliva is no longer available to help clear bacteria from the mouth, xerostomia also predisposes patients to infection secondary to the increases in oral bacteria.

Amifostine

Amifostine, an organic thiophosphate chemoprotectant agent, is approved to reduce the incidence of moderate to severe xerostomia in patients having postoperative radiation treatment for head and neck cancer when the radiation region includes a substantial portion of the parotid glands. A randomized, clinical trial demonstrated that the incidence of xerostomia was reduced by about 30% in patients receiving 200 mg/m^2 as a 3-minute IV infusion 15 to 30 minutes before each fraction of radiation.[56] Guidelines published by ASCO support the use of amifostine to reduce the incidence of acute and late xerostomia in patients receiving fractionated radiation therapy without concurrent chemotherapy for head and neck cancer.[57] Amifostine cannot, however, prevent xerostomia from occurring in all patients. Amifostine is not used widely for the prevention of radiation-induced xerostomia secondary to its cost and adverse effect profile. Intravenous amifostine can cause nausea and vomiting as well as hypotension. Subcutaneous administration of the agent causes fewer GI effects and less hypotension, but increases the risk of injection site reactions. Because of these toxicities, more than 20% of patients discontinue amifostine before completing their radiation.[56] J.B. will not receive amifostine as part of his prevention of xerostomia. The high cost of amifostine in combination with its toxicities have decreased its use in current practice.

Other Treatments and Prevention

If xerostomia occurs, treatment strategies can include stimulation of existing salivary flow and replacement of lost secretions. Relatively low doses of systemically administered pilocarpine (5–10 mg orally three times daily) may stimulate salivary flow and produce clinically significant benefits in patients with postradiation xerostomia.[58] Results demonstrating pilocarpine's benefit are inconsistent. Dose-related adverse effects include cholinergic effects, such as sweating, rhinitis, headache, nausea, and abdominal cramps. Sucrose-free hard candy and sugar-free chewing gum can also stimulate salivation, but these treatments are typically considered oral comfort agents. Saliva substitutes can also provide oral comfort to patients with xerostomia. Commercially available saliva substitutes generally are recommended for use before meals and at bedtime. They are available in several formulations, including sprays, rinses, and chewing gums. Patients who find one product or formulation unacceptable or unsuccessful may benefit from experimenting with other formulations or product lines. Studies have shown that salivary substitutes containing carboxymethyl cellulose or hydroxyethyl cellulose are more effective in relieving dryness than water-based or glycerin-based solutions.[59,60]

Prevention of radiation-induced caries is best accomplished by aggressively using fluorides.[61] Generally, acidulated fluorides are the most effective, although neutral fluorides may be more acceptable to patients with mucositis. Patients are instructed to rinse daily for 1 minute with 5 to 10 mL of a fluoride rinse. Stannous fluoride gels 0.4% or sodium fluoride gel 1.1% tooth brushing agents may be also be used by patients to minimize their risk of caries. Meticulous attention to oral hygiene with regular dental checkups and avoidance of sucrose is essential to minimize the development of caries.

In general, a dentist should see patients who will be receiving radiation therapy to the head and neck or chemotherapy agents with a high risk of oral complications before starting therapy. This includes patients with hematologic malignancies who will most likely experience severe myelosuppression for prolonged periods. Oral evaluation before therapy, intervention to eliminate potential sources of infection or irritation before therapy, and preventive measures taken during therapy can dramatically decrease the frequency of oral complications.[52,61] Given J.B.'s risk factors including the dose of radiation he will receive and concomitant therapy with cisplatin, a dental examination is indicated before initiating therapy.

MUCOSITIS AND STOMATITIS

CASE 90-2, QUESTION 2: J.B. successfully completed his first 2 weeks of combined chemotherapy and radiation therapy; however, 3 days into his third week, he complains of generalized burning, discomfort, and pain on the ventral surface of his tongue. On clinical observation, both the ventral surface of his tongue and the floor of his mouth appear erythematous, and several discrete lesions are present in both areas. What is the most likely explanation for J.B.'s new onset of symptoms? What treatment is indicated at this time?

J.B.'s symptoms are consistent with therapy-related stomatitis or oral mucositis.

ONLINE CONTENT

For photos of mucositis, see http://thepoint.lww.com/AT10e.

Mucositis occurs as a nonspecific effect of chemotherapy and radiation therapy on the basal epithelium of the mouth. Nonkeratinized mucosa is affected most often. Thus, the buccal, labial, and soft palate mucosa; the ventral surface of the tongue; and the floor of the mouth are the most common sites of involvement. Although lesions are usually discrete initially, they often progress to produce large areas of ulceration. The lesions typically do not progress outside the mouth, but they may extend to the esophagus and involve the entire GI tract. The terms of stomatitis and oral mucositis may be used interchangeably. Mucositis may occur anywhere along the full GI tract. Signs and symptoms generally occur about 5 to 7 days after chemotherapy or at almost any point during radiation therapy. The antimetabolites (e.g., methotrexate, fluorouracil, and cytarabine) and the antitumor antibiotics are the chemotherapy agents that most commonly produce direct effects on the epithelial cells of the GI tract. Lesions generally regress and resolve completely in approximately 1 to 3 weeks, depending on their severity.

In severe cases, mucositis may require parenteral opioid analgesics for relief. Other signs or symptoms include decreased ability to eat and speak. Mucositis may be confused with an oral infection, or mucositis and oral infections may occur concurrently. Local and systemic bacterial, fungal, or viral infections can occur and can cause a characteristic lesion; however, the lesion's appearance usually does not always correlate with the infectious agent. This particularly occurs in patients with neutropenia who cannot mount a full inflammatory response. In these individuals, the clinical appearance of an infected lesion may be muted relative to the presence or number of pathogens. Under normal conditions, the mucosa provides a natural barrier to the entry of normal oral flora, but the ulcerated mucosa allows pathogens access to the bloodstream. The patient could experience life-threatening infection or sepsis in addition to a local infection.

Treatment

Treatment of mucositis is palliative. Topical anesthetics, including viscous lidocaine or dyclonine hydrochloride 0.5% or 1%, are often recommended. Equal portions of lidocaine, diphenhydramine, and magnesium-containing or aluminum-containing antacids can be used for their anesthetic and astringent properties. Many institutions compound mouthwash products containing these ingredients as well as antibiotics, nystatin, or corticosteroids. Corticosteroids provide anti-inflammatory properties, and the antibiotics and antifungals provide antibacterial or antifungal properties. Another topical agent, sucralfate, may provide some benefit by coating the lesion and reducing discomfort. All of these topical products provide symptom control only, and data supporting superior efficacy of one product over another in relieving pain are lacking. Furthermore, these topical products are only effective in oral and throat lesions because lesions lower in the GI tract are not reached with these local products.

All the topical anesthetic-containing preparations are recommended for use as "swish-and-spit" preparations. Generally, 5 to 10 mL is used three to six times a day. The longer the patient can hold the solution in the mouth, the longer the contact, and, theoretically, the better the symptom relief. Therefore, patients should be advised to hold and swish the solution around the mouth for as long as possible before spitting it out. The risk of systemic effects from topical anesthetic preparations are slim if patients were to swallow them, however, large quantities swallowed could induce sedation and possible arrhythmias. Other palliative treatment options include topical benzocaine and ice chips. For small localized lesions, ointments such as benzocaine may be applied after the affected area has been dried with a sponge. Patients may also find ice chips soothing by allowing them to melt in their mouth. Most patients, however, require systemic analgesics to alleviate the pain. Online Table 90-1 lists topical products used to treat oral complications, and text Table 90-1 provides guidelines to manage mucositis.

Gelclair is a bioadherent oral gel containing polyvinylpyrrolidone, hyaluronic acid, and glycyrrhetinic acid (but no alcohol or anesthetic agent). It provides an adherent barrier over the mucosal surfaces, thereby shielding oral lesions from the effect of food, liquids, and saliva.[62] Controlled clinical data are lacking. In a study of 20 patients with head and neck cancer undergoing radiation therapy presenting with mucositis, Gelclair was compared with standard of care, including sucralfate and lidocaine. No significant difference was found between the Gelclair and standard of care in relieving general pain.[63]

J.B. appears to have a mild case of stomatitis or mucositis at this time. J.B. should be encouraged to maintain good mouth care by keeping his mouth clean. Additionally, topical anesthetics are indicated for J.B. Topical lidocaine or a mixture of topical lidocaine with diphenhydramine and an antacid, 5 to 10 mL swish and spit three to six times per day should be recommended. If the lesions progress during the next several days, systemic opioids may be necessary. J.B. should also be carefully assessed for local infections within his mouth.

TABLE 90-1
Guidelines for the Management of Mucositis

1. Remove dentures to prevent further irritation and tissue damage.
2. Maintain gentle brushing of teeth with a soft toothbrush.
3. Avoid mouthwashes or rinses that contain alcohol because they may be painful and cause drying of the mucosa. Consider normal saline or sodium bicarbonate oral swishes.
4. Lubricants, such as artificial saliva, may loosen mucus and prevent membranes from sticking together. Avoid mineral oil and petroleum jelly because they can be aspirated.
5. Apply local anesthetics for localized pain control, especially before meals (may add an antacid or an antihistamine). Systemic opioid analgesics may be required to control pain associated with severe mucositis. Acetaminophen is often avoided because it may mask fevers in neutropenic patients, and ibuprofen is often avoided because it may cause more bleeding in patients with thrombocytopenia.
6. Ensure that adequate hydration and nutrition are maintained:
   - Eat a bland diet, avoiding spiced, acidic, and salted foods.
   - Avoid rough food; process in a blender if necessary.
   - Use sugar-free gum or sugar-free hard candy to stimulate salivation and facilitate mastication.
   - If necessary, provide intravenous nutritional support.
   - Avoid extremely hot or cold foods.
   - Use shakes with nutritional supplements or ice cream.

Prevention

CASE 90-2, QUESTION 3: Could J.B.'s mucositis have been prevented?

Historically, treatment of chemotherapy-induced and radiation-induced mucositis has been aimed at reducing symptoms once they occur and avoiding further trauma to the oral mucosa. Cryotherapy has been marginally effective in reducing the severity of chemotherapy-induced mucositis.[64] Ice chips are placed in the mouth 5 minutes before chemotherapy begins and retained for 30 minutes. Theoretically, this will reduce blood flow to the mouth, thereby protecting the dividing cell population from toxins. Chlorhexidine gluconate 0.12% also may reduce the frequency and severity of mucositis infection,[65,66] although not all studies have shown a benefit. This solution should be used twice daily as a rinse. Side effects include occasional burning (thought to be caused by the product's alcohol content, which can be reduced by diluting it with water) and superficial brown tooth staining, which polishes off easily. Chlorhexidine may reduce the frequency and severity of mucositis by eliminating microorganisms in the oral cavity.

Despite these prophylactic measures, none of these aforementioned methods have a definitive benefit. To date, the only medication with proven efficacy is palifermin, a keratinocyte growth factor, approved for patients with hematologic malignancies undergoing HCT to reduce the incidence and duration of severe oral mucositis. Efficacy was established in a phase III multicenter, randomized, placebo-controlled double-blind trial ($n = 212$) comparing palifermin 60 mcg/kg/day IV starting 3 days before the conditioning regimen and continuing days 0, 1, and 2 of transplant with placebo. Palifermin demonstrated a difference in the incidence of severe mucositis of 63% versus 98%, respectively, and duration of mucositis of 6 days versus 9 days, respectively.[67] Palifermin has been studied in other clinical scenarios including a phase II trial in patients with squamous cell head and neck cancer receiving daily radiation with cisplatin and continuous infusion fluorouracil. Patients ($n = 99$) were randomly assigned palifermin 60 mcg/kg or placebo once weekly for 10 doses. Palifermin was well tolerated, but did not reduce the morbidity including mucositis, dysphagia, or xerostomia compared to placebo.[56] A randomized, placebo-controlled, evaluation of palifermin in allogeneic transplant patients ($n = 60$) receiving cyclophosphamide or total body irradiation conditioning regimens observed a trend toward reduced mucositis in the palifermin group (73%) compared to the placebo group (90%), however this did not demonstrate statistical significance. Palifermin was well tolerated.[68] Palifermin's use is limited thus far secondary to a complex administration schedule and high cost. It has not shown proven efficacy in other patient populations at risk for mucositis. Guidelines provide further recommendations.[57] Other methods for decreasing the incidence and severity of mucositis symptoms include reducing the dose of radiation or cytotoxic therapy, but doing so comes at the risk of compromising treatment outcomes. Mucositis remains the dose-limiting toxicity for several anticancer regimens. Unfortunately, there are no prevention strategies that would reduce the chance of J.B. experiencing mucositis from his chemotherapy and radiation, and thus treatment for J.B. is targeted towards relief of symptoms.

ESOPHAGITIS

Cytotoxic chemotherapy and radiation therapy can also damage the mucosal lining of the esophagus. Although dysphagia is a common symptom reported by patients with esophagitis, other causes of dysphagia should be excluded. Because patients receiving myelosuppressive cytotoxic therapy may exhibit infectious esophagitis, bacterial, viral, and fungal cultures should be completed to search for infectious causes before starting treatment for esophagitis. Symptomatic management of esophagitis is similar to the management of mucositis. Other treatment modalities, including behavioral modifications (e.g., elimination of acidic and irritating foods) and other medications (e.g., histamine-2 [H_2] receptor antagonist, antacids, and proton pump inhibitors) may help reduce esophageal irritation and improve comfort. Patients with severe esophagitis should be carefully monitored to ensure adequate oral hydration and nutritional intake, and instructed to avoid acidic or irritating foods. Symptoms should resolve in 1 to 2 weeks as myelosuppression resolves.

LOWER GASTROINTESTINAL TRACT COMPLICATIONS

Lower GI tract complications associated with anticancer therapy include malabsorption, diarrhea, and constipation. These complications may be related to structural changes that occur to the GI tract after cytotoxic or radiation therapy. Several investigators noted villus atrophy and cessation of mitosis within GI crypts in patients and animals treated with combination cytotoxic therapy.[69–71] Other investigators noted swelling and dilation of mitochondria and endoplasmic reticulum and shortening of the microvilli. These or other changes to the small and large bowel can cause decreased absorption of medications that are primarily absorbed in the upper portion of the small intestine.

Cytotoxic-induced intestinal changes also may be responsible for diarrhea, which frequently occurs with regimens containing irinotecan, high-dose cytarabine, or fluorouracil. Unlike diarrhea, constipation is rare. The vinca alkaloids, which produce colicky abdominal pain, constipation, and adynamic ileus caused by autonomic nerve dysfunction (see Neurotoxicity section), can cause chemotherapy-induced constipation. Additionally, constipation is a problematic side effect of therapy with thalidomide. Constipation should be treated prophylactically with stool softeners and mild stimulants. The true incidence of diarrhea and constipation associated with chemotherapy is difficult to discern, because many medications (e.g., opioid analgesics, antiemetics, antacids) and clinical conditions (e.g., immobility, spinal cord compression) commonly associated with cancer and anticancer therapies can cause these symptoms as well.

DIARRHEA

CASE 90-3

QUESTION 1: B.G., a 60-year-old woman with recurrent colorectal cancer refractory to FOLFOX (fluorouracil, leucovorin, and oxaliplatin), is beginning her first course of cetuximab and irinotecan. What instructions should she receive regarding the management of diarrhea if she experiences this complication?

Irinotecan can cause severe diarrhea, both early and late, in the course of therapy. The early-onset and late-onset diarrhea appear to be mediated by different mechanisms. Early-onset diarrhea (within 24 hours after treatment) may be mediated by parasympathetic stimulation. Patients often report other cholinergic symptoms, such as rhinitis, increased salivation, miosis, lacrimation, diaphoresis, flushing, and abdominal cramping as well. These symptoms can be prevented or managed with atropine IV or SC 0.25 to 1 mg. Late-onset diarrhea (generally occurring >24 hours after treatment) can be prolonged leading to dehydration, electrolyte imbalances, and significant morbidity. The mechanism of late diarrhea is not completely understood, but is likely multifactorial resulting from direct effects on the GI mucosa, secretory factors, and dysmotility.

Patients should promptly receive loperamide 4 mg with the first episode of diarrhea and repeat doses of 2 mg every 2 hours until 12 hours have passed without a bowel movement.[72] For patients who do not respond to initial therapy, some clinicians recommend higher doses equal to 4 mg every 2 hours. The maximum dose of loperamide (16 mg in 24 hours) does not apply for irinotecan-induced diarrhea. Fluid and electrolyte replacement should also be administered, if necessary. With the potential severe complications associated with irinotecan-associated diarrhea, prompt treatment cannot be overemphasized.

If a patient fails to respond to adequate doses of loperamide, the somatostatin analog, octreotide, can be used to manage the diarrhea. Randomized trials comparing loperamide with octreotide in patients with acute leukemia or those undergoing HCT found loperamide to be more effective.[73,74] Nevertheless, some evidence shows that octreotide may be used to successfully manage diarrhea associated with fluorouracil and other high-dose chemotherapy regimens.[75,76] These findings have been inconsistent. A trial in patients with colorectal cancer receiving chemoradiation failed to show benefit of decreasing diarrhea with long-acting octreotide.[76] Octreotide produces antisecretory activity in the gut and promotes the absorption of sodium, chloride, and water from luminal content. Patients should receive doses ranging from 100 to 2,000 mcg SC three times daily or 20 to 40 mg of long-acting octreotide.[75,76] Although responses seem to correlate with octreotide dose, more studies are needed to determine the optimal dose. Based on current evidence, octreotide should be limited to second-line therapy for cytotoxic therapy-associated diarrhea.

B.G. should be counseled on the diarrhea that is often seen with irinotecan. She should be instructed to call her clinic number if she starts experiencing any diarrhea within 24 hours after administration of irinotecan so she can receive prompt atropine therapy. Additionally, she should be given a prescription and instructions for loperamide administration for diarrhea occurring beyond the initial 24 hours after chemotherapy.

Dermatologic Toxicities

Dermatologic toxicities associated with anticancer therapies chemotherapy include alopecia, hyperpigmentation, radiation recall, photosensitivity, nail changes, hand-foot syndrome, acneiform rashes, hypersensitivity reactions, and extravasations. Several reviews serve as excellent references.[77–80]

ALOPECIA

CASE 90-4

QUESTION 1: C.W. is a 45-year-old woman with recently diagnosed breast cancer, who underwent lymph node dissection and lumpectomy. She will receive 20 fractions or courses of radiation therapy to the affected breast. She will also receive chemotherapy to minimize her risk of recurrence. She is in the clinic today to receive the first of four cycles of doxorubicin and cyclophosphamide (AC). Although C.W. had minimal problems with surgery, she particularly fears receiving combination chemotherapy. You counsel C.W. about the most common toxicities by reviewing the likelihood and management of myelosuppression, nausea, and vomiting. C.W. is appropriately attentive as you discuss these issues with her; however, her overriding concern is whether or not she will lose her hair. Is C.W.'s concern typical of most cancer patients? How would you respond?

C.W.'s concern regarding hair loss is typical of cancer patients starting chemotherapy. In fact, several investigators have reported that hair loss ranks second only to nausea and vomiting as a patient's greatest fear. Because hair bulb cells replicate every 12 to 24 hours, the cells are susceptible to various cytotoxic chemotherapy agents. Normally, hair follicles independently move cyclically through phases of growth (anagen), involution or transition (catagen), and rest (telogen). Although most persons normally lose about 100 scalp hairs a day, patients with cancer can lose substantially more. Because approximately 85% to 90% of hair follicles are in the anagen phase, chemotherapy agents may partially or completely inhibit mitosis or impair metabolic processes in the hair matrix. These effects can cause a thinned or weakened hair shaft or failure to form hair. Even mild trauma, such as normal hair grooming or rubbing the head on a pillow, can fracture the thinned hair shaft and cause hair loss. Hair loss usually begins 7 to 10 days after one treatment, with prominent hair loss noted within 1 or 2 months.

ONLINE CONTENT

For a photo showing alopecia, go to http://thepoint.lww.com/AT10e.

Other terminal hairs, such as beards, eyebrows, eyelashes, and axillary and pubic hair can be affected; however, these effects are somewhat variable, depending on the rate of mitosis and the percentage of hairs in the anagen phase.[81,82]

C.W. should be informed about the expected onset of hair loss, and she should be reassured that alopecia caused by cytotoxic chemotherapy is reversible. She can expect her hair to begin regenerating 1 to 2 months after therapy is completed. The color and texture of her hair may be altered; the new hair may be lighter, darker, or curlier as it regrows.

ONLINE CONTENT

For a table that lists the agents most commonly associated with severe alopecia, see Online Table 90-2 at http://thepoint.lww.com/AT10e.

PREVENTION OF ALOPECIA

Several interventions have been proposed to prevent scalp hair loss during chemotherapy. These procedures attempt to prevent chemotherapy agents from circulating to the hair follicles with either an occlusive scalp tourniquet or an ice cap that produces a localized hypothermia and vasoconstriction. Recognizing that such devices create a refuge for tumor cells, these procedures are contraindicated in patients with hematologic malignancies and in others at risk for scalp metastases. Concerns regarding the efficacy and safety of these devices have prevented them from availability in the US market.[81,83]

C.W.'s concern is a legitimate one expressed by many patients with cancer, not just patients with breast cancer. C.W. is likely to experience near or complete hair loss, depending on the thickness of her hair and its growth rate. She should be told how to minimize the effect of alopecia on her appearance through the use of hair pieces or stylish head scarves, turbans, or hats. She also should be referred to volunteer groups and organizations that can help her through this difficult time. Hair pieces are tax deductible as a medical expense and are covered by some health insurance policies. If C.W. thinks she will use a hair piece, she should be advised to select a wig before hair loss begins.

NAIL AND SKIN CHANGES

CASE 90-4, QUESTION 2: Besides alopecia, what other skin or nail changes should C.W. anticipate?

Several skin and nail changes have been associated with cytotoxic and targeted anticancer agents, which C.W. may find disturbing.

ONLINE CONTENT

For a photo that shows nail changes after chemotherapy, go to http://thepoint.lww.com/AT10e.

The major consequences of these toxicities are cosmetic, however, and they usually resolve within 6 to 12 months after discontinuing or completing therapy. Online Table 90-2 provides agents associated with nail changes.

NAIL CHANGES

The growth of fingernails and toenails is arrested in a manner similar to hair growth. A reduction or a cessation of mitotic activity in the nail matrix causes a horizontal depression of the nail plate. Within weeks, these pale horizontal lines ("Beau's lines") begin to appear in the nail beds. They are most commonly seen in patients receiving chemotherapy for more than 6 months. These growth arrest lines move distally as the nail grows and normally disappear from the fingernails in approximately 6 months. Nail changes including hemorrhagic onycholysis, discoloration, and acute exudative paronychia are seen in approximately 40% of patients receiving paclitaxel and docetaxel.[77] Some other nail pigmentation changes that can occur after therapy with cyclophosphamide, fluorouracil, daunorubicin, doxorubicin, and bleomycin are less well understood.[84,85] Brown or blue lines deposit as horizontal or vertical bands in the nails. These lines are seen more commonly in dark-skinned patients. As with Beau's lines, these pigmentation lines generally grow out with the nail.

DERMATOLOGIC PIGMENT CHANGES

Dermatologic pigment changes are among the most common and least well understood side effects of chemotherapy. Hypopigmentation has been reported occasionally in patients receiving cytotoxic therapy, but hyperpigmentation is more frequently reported. Usually, hyperpigmentation is not associated with an identifiable cause or systemic toxicity. It usually occurs after treatment with a wide variety of cytotoxic agents, including anthracyclines, alkylating agents, and antimetabolites. Most agents cause a diffuse, generalized hyperpigmentation, but the pigmentation changes can also be localized, involving only the mucous membrane, hair, or nails. Busulfan, cyclophosphamide, fluorouracil, dactinomycin, and hydroxyurea are examples of specific agents that can cause widespread cutaneous hyperpigmentation.[77]

Various chemotherapy agents can cause diverse patterns of hyperpigmentation. A peculiar serpiginous hyperpigmentation can occur over veins used to administer fluorouracil and bleomycin.[86,87] Some investigators have attributed this phenomenon to a subclinical phlebitis. Hyperpigmentation has also been noted over pressure points after the use of bleomycin. Thiotepa has been reported to cause hyperpigmentation in areas of skin occluded by bandages, which may be caused by secretion of thiotepa in sweat.[88] Interestingly, skin contact with thiotepa has been reported to cause hypopigmentation.[89] Topical contact with mechlorethamine and carmustine also has caused hyperpigmentation.[90,91] Although hyperpigmentation reactions commonly affect the skin, some rare reactions are noted in hair. Methotrexate can cause hyperpigmented banding of light-colored hair. This phenomenon has been described in a patient receiving intermittent high-dose methotrexate and has been referred to by some investigators as the "flag sign" of chemotherapy.[92] To minimize a patient's concern regarding these pigment changes, they should receive counseling before treatment.

As previously stated, pigment changes that occur in patients receiving cytotoxic chemotherapy are basically a cosmetic concern. It is important to anticipate these distressing side effects and educate patients in appropriate cases. At this time, C.W. should receive counseling, explaining that these side effects may occur because she will be receiving several agents that have been implicated in producing diffuse, as well as localized, cutaneous nail hyperpigmentation. She should be reassured that pigment changes usually resolve with time.

HAND-FOOT SYNDROME

Some patients receiving chemotherapy may exhibit tender, erythematous skin on the palms of their hands and sometimes on the soles of their feet. Patients may also complain of tingling, burning, or shooting sensations in their hands or feet usually not described as painful. These signs and symptoms may resolve after several days, or they may progress to bullous lesions that can desquamate. This reaction is referred to as chemotherapy-associated acral erythema or the palmar-plantar erythrodysesthesia syndrome. Agents most commonly reported to cause this reaction include cytarabine, fluorouracil, doxorubicin, liposomal doxorubicin, methotrexate, capecitabine, and hydroxyurea. Additionally, both sunitinib and sorafenib, vascular endothelial growth factor (VEGF) tyrosine kinase inhibitors, have been associated with hand-foot syndrome.[93–95] No specific therapy exists for hand-foot syndrome. Discontinuation of the medication will help to resolve the reaction. After resolution, the medication may be initiated at a lower dose.

ACNEIFORM–ERYTHEMATOUS RASH

The most common toxicities reported with the epidermal growth factor receptor (EGFR) inhibitors and EGFR monoclonal antibodies are skin related and are probably due to inhibition of the tyrosine kinase pathways in EGFR-dependent tissues, including keratinocytes in the skin. Erlotinib and lapatinib are small molecule tyrosine kinase inhibitors that target the intracellular domain of the EGFR, and cetuximab and panitumumab are monoclonal antibodies that target the extracellular domain of EGFR. These agents are associated with skin toxicities. Skin effects occur in greater than 50% of patients who receive these treatments and are dose-dependent. A pustular or maculopapular eruption typically appears on the upper body, face, and scalp in the first 1 to 2 weeks of treatment.

ONLINE CONTENT

For photos of acneiform rash, go to http://thepoint.lww.com/AT10e.

The rashes are predominantly grade 1 or 2 in severity, may be associated with dry skin and itching, and completely resolve without sequelae when the drug is discontinued.[79,96] Evidence suggests that the severity of the skin rash is associated with increased efficacy of this class of agents. In a retrospective analysis of a phase III trial in patients with NSCLC receiving erlotinib, those who experienced a rash had a significantly longer survival time than those who did not. Survival was reported to be 1.5 months in patients with no development of skin rash versus 8.5 months in those with grade 1 rash, and 19.6 months in patients exhibiting a grade 2 or 3 rash.[97] Evidence of a correlation between skin rashes and higher response rates has also been observed in patients receiving cetuximab for colorectal cancer.[98] No supportive therapy has, however, been proven to reduce or prevent this bothersome side effect. Several small trials have evaluated therapeutic options for relief or treatment of the acneiform rash, and have not demonstrated positive findings. Moisturizing creams, steroid creams, sunscreen, antibiotics (e.g., topical clindamycin or systemic tetracyclines), and topical calcineurin inhibitors (e.g., pimecrolimus cream) have been used to manage the effects with varying results. Patients are also advised to minimize sun exposure. All of these agents have demonstrated activity in some patients, but none have worked consistently in all. Therefore, if one agent is not successful, alternative agents should be tried.[96,99,100]

DRY SKIN

Many cytotoxic anticancer agents (especially bleomycin, hydroxyurea, and fluorouracil) can cause dry skin with fine scaling on the surface. Normally, sebaceous and sweat glands provide lipids, lactates, and other products that contribute to the pliability and moisture retention of the stratum corneum. In patients receiving cytotoxic therapy, the dry skin may be caused by the cytostatic effect of agents on sebaceous and sweat glands. Topical application of emollient creams may provide some symptomatic relief of this dryness.

INTERACTIONS WITH RADIATION THERAPY

CASE 90-4, QUESTION 3: C.W. recently completed her course of total breast radiation therapy. She plans to leave for a 1-week vacation in Florida 3 days after this clinic visit. Are there any interactions between radiation therapy and sunlight exposure with cytotoxic anticancer agents? Are there any specific precautions C.W. should take, or signs and symptoms of toxicity that she should know about?

The interactions between cytotoxic therapy and radiation therapy or ultraviolet (UV) light (from both external beam and natural sources) can be divided into radiation sensitization, radiation recall, photosensitivity reactions, and sunburn reactivation (Table 90-2).

Several excellent reviews are available that describe each of these interactions in detail. A discussion of the important

TABLE 90-2
Chemotherapy-Associated and Radiation-Associated Reactions

Radiation Sensitivity Reactions		
Bleomycin	Doxorubicin	Hydroxyurea
Dactinomycin	Fluorouracil	Methotrexate
Etoposide	Gemcitabine	
Radiation Recall Reactions		
All of the above plus		
Vinblastine	Epirubicin	Capecitabine
Etoposide	Paclitaxel	Oxaliplatin
	Docetaxel	
Reactions with Ultraviolet Light		
Phototoxic Sensitivity		
Dacarbazine	Thioguanine	Methotrexate
Fluorouracil	Vinblastine	Mitomycin
Sunburn Reactivation		
Methotrexate		

Source: Payne AS et al. Dermatologic toxicity of chemo-therapeutic agents. *Semin Oncol.* 2006;33:86; Yeo W, Johnson PJ. Radiation-recall skin disorders associated with the use of antineoplastic drugs: pathogenesis, prevalence, and management. *Am J Clin Dermatol.* 2000;1:113; Alley E et al. Cutaneous toxicities of cancer therapy. *Curr Opin Oncol.* 2002;14:212.

principles of the interaction between radiation therapy and cytotoxic therapy follows.[101–103] A synergistic interaction between a small number of cytotoxic agents and radiation therapy results in an enhanced radiation effect. This may be caused by an agent's ability to interfere with radiation repair. Radiation therapy can alter the molecular structure of DNA, but excision repair allows cells to remove small, damaged portions of one strand of DNA and insert new bases using the other strand as a template. This repair mechanism requires several enzymes, including DNA polymerase. Cytotoxic therapy agents can interfere with some of the enzymes and synthetic mechanisms needed to repair damaged cells. Although the synergistic effects of radiation therapy and cytotoxic therapy are often exploited therapeutically for the treatment of solid tumors, these reactions can inadvertently cause undesirable reactions in non-tumor tissues, such as the skin, esophagus, lung, and GI tract. The skin is the most common target of radiation reactions.

These reactions can produce severe tissue necrosis, which can compromise organ function and delay or mandate discontinuation of future treatment courses. These reactions may be further classified as either radiation sensitivity or radiation recall reactions. The primary distinction between radiation sensitivity reactions and radiation recall reactions lies in the temporal relationship between radiation therapy and chemotherapy. Generally, sensitivity reactions occur when chemotherapy is given concurrently or within 1 week of radiation therapy. In comparison, recall reactions occur several weeks to years after radiation therapy, when the administration of chemotherapy induces an inflammatory reaction in tissues previously treated with radiation. Radiation recall is independent of previous, clinically apparent radiation damage.

For a photo of Radiation Recall/Dermatitis, go to http://thepoint.lww.com/AT10e.

Not surprisingly, the chemotherapy agents that have been associated with radiation recall reactions are the same as those that cause radiation sensitivity reactions. Management of reactions is supportive and consists primarily of topical agents including corticosteroids.[101,103–106]

Because UV light has sufficient energy to cause photochemical changes in biologic molecules, cytotoxic agents can interact with it. The subsequent reactions are usually less severe than reactions that occur with radiation therapy, and they may be caused by a different mechanism. Photosensitivity reactions, defined as enhanced erythema responses to UV light, have been reported with specific agents (text Table 90-2). Methotrexate can also reactivate sunburns, causing a similar, but less-severe reaction compared with the radiation recall reactions described previously. The reaction can be more severe than the initial sunburn, resulting in severe blisters, and it usually occurs only in patients who receive large doses of methotrexate. Although the precise incidences of photosensitivity reactions caused by chemotherapy agents are unknown, they may be more common than generally believed. For example, photosensitivity may account for many of the erythematous periodic rashes attributed to allergy.[77,107]

C.W. received doxorubicin which can interact with radiation therapy. Although not commonly reported, doxorubicin also can cause some increased erythema in the specific area of skin treated with radiation. Because C.W. may have an increased risk for a photosensitivity reaction, she should be advised to avoid direct exposure to the sunlight for several days to a week after chemotherapy. Although no data exist regarding the efficacy of sunscreens in this patient population, C.W. should be advised to use a protective sunscreen with a high sun protective factor when she cannot avoid sun exposure. Protective clothing and a hat can provide additional protection for C.W. Furthermore, she should periodically assess her skin's reaction to the sun with intermittent periods of rest and observation throughout the day.

CASE 90-4, QUESTION 4: How will C.W. know if she has a radiation reaction? How should she be treated if such a reaction occurs?

If C.W. has a radiation reaction, she will experience "easy burning" and erythema or redness, followed by dry desquamation. With a more severe reaction, small blisters (vesicles) and oozing can develop. Necrosis with persistent painful ulceration can also occur in severe cases. Postinflammatory hyperpigmentation or depigmentation may follow. Treatment options vary, depending on reaction severity. Milder cases can be treated with topical steroids in an emollient cream base and cool wet compresses. Necrosis and ulcers are notoriously difficult to treat, however, because radiated skin does not heal well. Ulcers are often treated with surgical debridement to keep the ulcer clean. Even when the ulcers are clean, exudation and bacterial contamination can be persistent. Radiation reactions that occur in tissues other than the skin (e.g., the lungs, esophagus, GI tract) often are treated with oral corticosteroids, although data regarding the efficacy of these agents in ameliorating the symptoms or reducing the extent of damage are lacking. If C.W. experiences any of these signs or symptoms, she should immediately seek medical attention.

IRRITANT AND VESICANT REACTIONS

CASE 90-4, QUESTION 5: C.W. complained of pain and burning at the injection site immediately after the administration of her third course of IV chemotherapy with doxorubicin and cyclophosphamide. She described the sensation as being distinctly different from the mild discomfort she had experienced with previous courses. Physical examination of the injection site revealed mild erythema and slight

TABLE 90-3
Chemotherapeutic Drugs Reported to Produce Local Toxicities

Potential Vesicants	
Dactinomycin	Epirubicin
Daunorubicin	Streptozocin
Doxorubicin	Vinblastine
Idarubicin	Vincristine
Mechlorethamine	Paclitaxel
Mitomycin	Oxaliplatin
Potential Irritants	
Carmustine	Etoposide
Cisplatin	Mitoxantrone
Dacarbazine	Melphalan
Vinorelbine	Vindesine
Cyclophosphamide	Teniposide

Source: Goolsby TV, Lombardo FA. Extravasation of chemotherapeutic agents: prevention and treatment. *Semin Oncol.* 2006;33:139; Doellman D et al. Infiltration and extravasation: update on prevention and management. *J Infus Nurs.* 2009;32:203.

induration. What types of local reactions can occur after the administration of chemotherapy?

Several distinct types of local reactions (ranging from transient local irritation to severe tissue necrosis of the skin, surrounding vasculature, and supporting structures) have been reported after cytotoxic chemotherapy[78,108] (text Table 90-3). Some reactions are characterized by immediate local burning, itching, and erythema. Some patients may also experience a "flare" reaction along the length of the vein used for treatment. More severe reactions, including irritation of the vein (or phlebitis) caused by the irritant properties of an agent or a diluent, and possibly extravasation, can occur after cytotoxic chemotherapy.[78,108] Extravasation, a potentially serious local reaction, is seen in approximately 1% of chemotherapy administration and occurs when IV medications are accidentally administered into the surrounding tissue, either by leakage or by a needle puncturing the vein, causing direct exposure and damage to surrounding tissues.

ONLINE CONTENT

For a photo that shows the infiltration of chemotherapy into a hand, go to http://thepoint.lww.com/AT10e.

Reactions resulting from the extravasation of agents with vesicant or irritant properties are more severe. All agents with vesicant properties potentially can produce devastating reactions. Agents known to bind to DNA (i.e., the anthracyclines) have the propensity to produce the most severe damage. Treatment with a cytotoxic agent with these properties can produce phlebitis and pain; however, extravasations can cause severe local irritation or soft tissue ulcers, depending on the agent and the amount and concentration of the extravasated drug. In addition, no clear agreement exists regarding the vesicant potential of many cytotoxic chemotherapy agents, and various references may categorize agents differently based on their vesicant or irritant properties. Initially, it may be impossible to distinguish a local irritant reaction from a vesicant extravasation; therefore, if an agent with vesicant or irritant properties has been administered, the reaction should be treated as a potential extravasation.

Patients who experience an extravasation can show a range of different signs or symptoms. Infiltration of a vesicant into tissue often produces a severe burning sensation that may persist for hours. In some cases, no immediate symptoms or signs are evident. However, in the days to weeks that follow, the skin overlying the extravasation site may become reddened and firm. The redness may gradually diminish or progress to ulceration and necrosis.[108]

CASE 90-4, QUESTION 6: What factors in C.W. increase her risk of extravasation, and what administration techniques and precautions can minimize these risks?

Several factors have been associated with an increased risk of extravasation and subsequent tissue damage after administration of cytotoxic chemotherapy. Risk factors include generalized vascular disease commonly found in elderly and debilitated patients or in patients who have undergone frequent venipuncture and treatment with irritating chemotherapy (the latter causes venous fragility and instability or decreased local blood flow); elevated venous pressure, which typically occurs in patients with an obstructed superior vena cava or venous drainage after axillary dissection; prior radiation therapy to the injection site; recent venipuncture in the same vein; use of injection sites over joints, which increases the risk of needle dislodgement; and others.[78,108]

Tissue damage may be more severe if extravasation occurs in areas with only a small amount of subcutaneous tissue (e.g., the back of the hand or wrist) because wound healing is more difficult and exposure of deeper structures, such as the tendons, is increased.[108] These risks have led to the increased use of central catheters in patients receiving vesicant chemotherapy.

C.W. has several risks for extravasation. She had an axillary lymph node dissection for her breast cancer, which places her at higher risk for obstructed venous drainage. Additionally, she has had multiple venous punctures, and she is a thin woman with relatively small amounts of subcutaneous tissue.

Extravasations of agents with vesicant properties can produce devastating tissue damage that can potentially cause loss of an extremity or death. To prevent significant morbidity or mortality, major emphasis must be placed on prevention. All caretakers who administer agents with vesicant or irritant properties should be skilled in IV drug administration and receive special instruction before administering these agents. The patient also must be told how agent administration should feel and to report immediately any change in sensation, including pain, burning, or itching.

ONLINE CONTENT

For a table that includes recommendations to reduce the risk of local complications during cytotoxic agent administration, see Online Table 90-3 at http://thepoint.lww.com/AT10e.

CASE 90-4, QUESTION 7: C.W.'s oncology nurse believes that the doxorubicin may have extravasated during administration. How should this be managed? Do management strategies differ for other vesicant agents?

Immediate management of a potential vesicant extravasation should include stopping the injection if the entire agent has

TABLE 90-4
Suggested Procedures for Management of Suspected Extravasation of Vesicant Drugs

1. Stop the infusion immediately, but do not remove the needle. Any drug remaining in the tubing or needle, as well as the infiltrated area, should be aspirated.
2. Contact a physician as soon as possible.
3. If deemed appropriate, instill an antidote in the infiltrated areas (via the extravasated intravenous needle if possible).
4. Remove the needle.
5. Apply ice to the site and elevate the extremity for the first 24 to 48 hours (if vinca or podophyllotoxin, use warm compresses).
6. Document the drug, suspected volume extravasated, and the treatment in the patient's medical record.
7. Check the site frequently for 5 to 7 days.
8. Consult a surgeon familiar with extravasations early so that the surgeon can periodically review the site, and, if ulceration begins, the surgeon can rapidly assess if surgical debridement or excision is necessary.

Source: Goolsby TV, Lombardo FA. Extravasation of chemotherapeutic agents: prevention and treatment. *Semin Oncol.* 2006;33:139; Doellman D et al. Infiltration and extravasation: update on prevention and management. *J Infus Nurs.* 2009;32:203.

not been administered. Various other recommended measures may minimize vesicant exposure and subsequent tissue damage (Table 90-4). These include application of cold compresses to the extravasation site and elevation of the extremity. Cold compresses have been shown to cause vasoconstriction, which can help to localize the extravasation and allow time for local vessels to displace the extravasated agent, whereas warm compresses are thought to induce vasodilation, increase drug distribution and absorption, therefore decreasing the concentration of the offending agent around the immediate site. Warm compresses are recommended for vinca alkaloids and epipodophyllotoxins.[78,108] With the exception of these two classes of agents, cooling has been shown more effective than warm compresses. Specific antidotes thought to inactivate the extravasated chemotherapy have been suggested; however, many of these antidotes are based on observations in few patients or animal models, and their effectiveness, in many cases, is unsubstantiated. Antidotes recommended in some guidelines may actually worsen tissue damage (e.g., sodium bicarbonate for doxorubicin). Recommended treatments for suspected extravasation of vesicant agents are outlined in Table 90-5.[78,108]

Dexrazoxane has been established as a reliable antidote for anthracycline extravasations. Dexrazoxane, an iron chelator, was studied based on evidence that it protects cardiac tissue from anthracycline-induced toxicities. Two prospective, multicenter, single-arm trials were conducted in a total of 54 evaluable patients with anthracycline extravasations. In 98.2% of patients, surgical intervention was avoided and 71% of patients were able to continue treatment regimen without any delays. Hospitalization of 41% of patients was necessary secondary to their extravasation. Toxicities included myelosuppression, increased liver function tests, nausea, and pain at the dexrazoxane infusion site.[109] Based on these results, dexrazoxane is approved for the treatment of anthracycline extravasations. Dexrazoxane is given once daily for 3 days at a dose of 1,000 mg/m^2 IV on days 1 and 2, and 500 mg/m^2 IV on day 3. Because it is an agent that should be used as soon as possible and within 6 hours of extravasation, it is recommended to keep a dexrazoxane kit readily available. Dexrazoxane kits for extravasation come with significant cost because they might not be used before the expiration date for the product. Because of this, the manufacturer has developed replacement strategies if the kit expires before use.[110]

TABLE 90-5
Recommended Extravasation Antidotes

Class/Specific Agents	Local/Systemic Antidote Recommended	Specific Procedure
Alkylating Agents	1/6-M solution sodium thiosulfate	Mix 4 mL 10% sodium thiosulfate USP with 6 mL of sterile water for injection, USP for a 1/6-M solution. Into site, inject 2 mL for each mg of mechlorethamine or 100 mg of cisplatin extravasated.
Cisplatin[a]		
Oxaliplatin		
Mechlorethamine		
Mitomycin-C	Dimethyl sulfoxide 99% (w/v)	Apply 1–2 mL to the site every 6 hours for 14 days. Allow to air dry; do not cover.
Anthracyclines	Cold compresses	Apply immediately for 30–60 minutes on first day.
Doxorubicin	Dexrazoxane	Once daily for 3 days. First dose should be given within the first 6 hours.
Daunorubicin		Day 1: 1,000 mg/m^2 IV
		Day 2: 1,000 mg/m^2 IV
		Day 3: 500 mg/m^2 IV
Vinca alkaloids	Warm compresses	Apply immediately for 30–60 minutes, then alternate off/on every 15 minutes for 1 day.
Vinblastine	Hyaluronidase	
Vincristine		Inject 150 units into site.
Epipodophyllotoxins[a]	Warm compresses	Apply immediately for 30–60 minutes, then alternate off/on every 15 minutes for 1 day.
Etoposide	Hyaluronidase	Inject 150 units into site.
Taxanes	Cold compresses	Apply immediately for 30–60 minutes every 6 hours for 1 day.
Docetaxel	Hyaluronidase	Inject 150 units into site.
Paclitaxel		

[a] Treatment indicated only for large extravasations (e.g., doses one-half or more of the planned total dose for the course of therapy).
IV, intravenous; w/v, weight per volume.
Source: Goolsby TV, Lombardo FA. Extravasation of chemotherapeutic agents: prevention and treatment. *Semin Oncol.* 2006;33:139; Doellman D et al. Infiltration and extravasation: update on prevention and management. *J Infus Nurs.* 2009;32:203; Totect (dexrazoxane injection) [package insert]. Rockaway, NJ: Topo Target USA, Inc.; 2009.

TABLE 90-7
Prophylaxis and Treatment of Hypersensitivity Reactions From Anticancer Drugs

Prophylaxis
IV access must be established.
BP monitoring must be available.
Premedication
Dexamethasone 20 mg PO and diphenhydramine 50 mg PO 12 and 6 hours before treatment, then the same dose IV immediately before treatment.
Consider addition of H_2 antagonist with schedule similar to dexamethasome.
Have epinephrine and diphenhydramine readily available for use in case of a reaction.
Observe the patient up to 2 hours after discontinuing treatment.
Treatment
Discontinue the drug (immediately if being administered IV).
Administer epinephrine 0.3 mg IM or SC minutes until reaction subsides.
Administer diphenhydramine 50 mg IV.
If hypotension is present that does not respond to epinephrine, administer IV fluids.
If wheezing is present that does not respond to epinephrine, administer nebulized albuterol solution.
Although corticosteroids have no effect on the initial reaction, they can block late allergic symptoms. Thus, administer methylprednisolone 125 mg (or its equivalent) IV to prevent recurrent allergic manifestations.

BP, blood pressure; IV, intravenous; PO, orally.

is preceded by methods to prevent or minimize hypersensitivity reactions. General recommendations for preventing hypersensitivity reactions are found in Table 90-7. Pretreatment with corticosteroids and diphenhydramine significantly decreases the frequency and severity of hypersensitivity reactions; however, the effect of H_2 receptor antagonists and epinephrine remains controversial. Because the success of these preventive measures depends on the cause of the reaction (immunologic or anaphylactoid), the aforementioned characteristics of type I reactions should be used to assess the underlying pathogenesis. In addition, other chemicals present in the formulation or other agents administered concomitantly with the chemotherapy can cause the hypersensitivity reaction. Potential allergens included in the diluent or formulation of chemotherapy agents include Cremophor EL (present in paclitaxel), polysorbate 80 (present in docetaxel), benzyl alcohol (present in the parenteral form of methotrexate, cytarabine, and etoposide), and methoxypolyethylene glycol (present in liposomal doxorubicin). Recognizing potential allergens can significantly affect treatment of the current reaction and minimize the risk of future reactions.

PACLITAXEL PROTEIN-BOUND PARTICLES

To reduce the hypersensitivity reactions observed with paclitaxel, paclitaxel protein-bound particles (Abraxane), an albumin-bound formulation of paclitaxel, has been created. Because paclitaxel protein-bound particles formulation is Cremophor EL–free and less likely to cause hypersensitivity than traditional paclitaxel, it is not necessary to premedicate patients with steroids and antihistamines. The albumin-bound formulation is approved for patients with metastatic breast cancer after failure of a previous regimen containing an anthracycline. Doses between the two agents are not comparable; the recommended dose of paclitaxel protein-bound particles is 260 mg/m^2 IV every 21 days for six cycles. Although fewer hypersensitivity reactions are associated with this formulation, myelosuppression remains a dose-limiting toxicity.[113,114]

SPECIFIC ORGAN TOXICITIES

Neurotoxicity

SPECIFIC AGENTS

CASE 90-6

QUESTION 1: A.L., a 39-year-old woman with acute lymphocytic leukemia, has been admitted to the hospital for induction chemotherapy. Methotrexate 3 g/m^2 IV once on day 1, cytarabine 2 g/m^2 IV every 12 hours on days 2 and 3 for four doses, vincristine 2 mg IV on days 1 and 8 for two doses, and dexamethasone 20 mg orally daily for 5 days are ordered. Laboratory data obtained on admission include a WBC count of 120,000 cells/μL, with 9% neutrophils, 11% lymphocytes, and 80% blasts. On day 3, A.L. is confused and she has difficulty performing a finger-to-nose neurologic examination. On day 10, she complains of numbness in her hands and feet. In addition, the clinician notes an eyelid lag and ataxia. A.L. also complains of severe constipation. What signs and symptoms of neurotoxicity is A.L. experiencing? Should the leukemia regimen be modified for future courses?

METHOTREXATE, CYTARABINE, AND VINCRISTINE

Methotrexate causes little or no neurotoxicity when administered orally or intravenously in doses less than 1 g/m^2; however, high-dose IV methotrexate (usually >1 g/m^2) can occasionally cause acute encephalopathy. The encephalopathy that occurs after therapy with methotrexate is usually transient and reversible. Some patients may experience a progressive leukoencephalopathy after high-dose IV methotrexate. The risk of leukoencephalopathy increases with higher cumulative doses of methotrexate and concomitant cranial radiation therapy.[144,145] Posterior reversible encephalopathy syndrome has also been associated with high dose methotrexate and intrathecal methotrexate. Chemical meningitis can occur with intrathecal administration of methotrexate and, less frequently, myelopathy or paraplegia may be observed[146] (see Chapter 91, Pediatric Malignancies). Patients receiving intrathecal therapy or high-dose methotrexate should be carefully monitored for signs and symptoms associated with neurotoxicity.

High doses of cytarabine (>1 g/m^2 in multiple doses) are associated with CNS toxicity in 8% to 37% of patients.[147,148] These neurotoxicities are dose-related and schedule-related. Doses greater than 18 g/m^2 per course increase the frequency of neurotoxicity. Older patients are more susceptible than younger patients, and the prevalence seems higher in subsequent versus initial courses of therapy. As illustrated by A.L., neurotoxicity may become evident within a few days after treatment with cytarabine and, most commonly, the neurotoxicity is manifested by a generalized encephalopathy with symptoms such as confusion, obtundation, seizures, and coma. Cerebellar dysfunction, presenting as ataxia, gait and coordination difficulties, and dysmetria (inability to arrest muscular movement when desired and lack of harmonious action between muscles when executing voluntary movement), is also commonly observed in patients receiving high-dose cytarabine therapy. These neurologic symptoms may partially resolve over days to weeks after discontinuation of therapy. Other neurologic toxicities reported

Dexrazoxane is a chemoprotectant that reduces the incidence and severity of cardiomyopathy. It is indicated in women with metastatic breast cancer who have received a cumulative doxorubicin dose of 300 mg/m^2. The recommended dosing ratio of dexrazoxane to doxorubicin is 10:1 slow IV push 30 minutes before starting doxorubicin. Currently, the ASCO guidelines do not support the routine use of dexrazoxane in patients unless a plan exists to continue doxorubicin beyond a total cumulative dose greater than 300 mg/m^2.[57] Clinical trials are evaluating the benefits of dexrazoxane in children and patients receiving other anthracyclines. Some evidence supports the use of dexrazoxane in patients receiving epirubicin.[226]

To reduce cardiotoxicity, doxorubicin that is encapsulated in liposomes can be given instead. A phase III trial of women ($n = 509$) with metastatic breast cancer showed that efficacy with liposomal pegylated doxorubicin may be similar to conventional doxorubicin with decreased cardiotoxicity.[227] A review and meta-analysis of 55 randomized control trials in patients receiving anthracyclines showed that the risk of cardiotoxicity was significantly decreased with liposomal doxorubicin versus conventional doxorubicin (odds ratio, 0.18; 95% confidence interval, 0.08–0.38).[228] The majority of patients were women with advanced breast cancer. Despite reduced cardiotoxicity, liposomal doxorubicin has not replaced standard doxorubicin in current treatment regimens secondary to high cost and lack of evidence showing equivalency. An established equivalent dose of liposomal preparations to conventional doxorubicin is not confirmed and is variable depending on the disease state and regimen.

D.A.'s CHF may have been prevented with continuous infusion doxorubicin or the use of dexrazoxane; however, because he had not approached a cumulative dose that warranted alternative strategies, this would not have been part of the standard management plan for a patient receiving their first several cycles of ABVD.

MANAGEMENT

CASE 90-7, QUESTION 4: How should D.A.'s doxorubicin-induced CHF be managed clinically?

Anthracycline-induced CHF presents similarly to other forms of biventricular CHF and occurs between 0 and 231 days after the last dose of doxorubicin (mean, 33 days). Anthracycline-induced CHF should be treated with a similar approach to cardiomyopathy induced by other means. Often these measures are ineffective. The clinical course varies, with some patients showing stable disease and others showing improvement. Before cardiotoxicity was a widely recognized toxicity, the course of anthracycline-induced CHF was characterized by a rapid progression that generally led to death in a few weeks. The clinical outcome is better now, perhaps because anthracycline therapy is promptly discontinued after initial presentation and there are better treatments for CHF. These include the use of spironolactone, β-blockers, angiotensin-converting enzyme (ACE) inhibitors, angiotensin II receptor blockers, and diuretics, which have decreased morbidity and mortality in non–anthracycline-induced CHF. Enalapril was evaluated to determine whether it would prevent cardiac function decline in a randomized, double-blind, placebo-controlled study of pediatric cancer patients who were at least 2 years out from treatment with anthracyclines and had evidence of CHF. Patients received enalapril at 0.05 mg/kg/day and this dose was progressively escalated to 0.10 mg/kg/day, and finally 0.15 mg/kg/day if there were no side effects. Although enalapril did not increase exercise intolerance, it did increase left ventricular end-systolic wall stress in the first year of treatment. Side effects included dizziness, hypoten-

with cytarabine include progressive leukoencephalopathy and chemical meningitis. Intrathecal administration of cytarabine can also cause a chemical meningitis.[146,149] Leukoencephalopathy typically presents with progressive personality and intellectual decline, dementia, hemiparesis, and, sometimes, seizures. These neurotoxicities also can occur after treatment with other chemotherapy agents.

Asparaginase and PEG-aspargase, the pegylated formulation of asparaginase, can cause encephalopathy, which presents most commonly as lethargy and confusion.[150] This agent is also used in acute lymphocytic leukemia regimens. Severe cerebral dysfunction occurs occasionally, and patients may present with stupor, coma, excessive somnolence, disorientation, hallucination, or severe depression. Symptoms can occur early (within days of administration of asparaginase) or late, depending on the treatment schedule.[151,152] The suspected mechanism is the direct neurocytotoxic effect of aspartic acid, glutamic acid, and ammonia. The neurotoxicity is usually reversible with the acute syndrome clearing rapidly, and a delayed syndrome lasting several weeks.

A.L.'s symptoms most likely are the result of CNS toxicity caused by both high-dose methotrexate and cytarabine. A decision regarding further treatment with these agents is complicated because omitting a dose or decreasing the dose of either of these agents could compromise the likelihood of a complete remission. High-dose cytarabine cerebellar toxicity may be irreversible. Therefore, the clinician may decide to discontinue cytarabine in A.L.'s future regimens. Additionally, modifications of methotrexate including dose reductions may be necessary in future therapy for A.L.

Other agents that produce an encephalopathic toxicity include fluorouracil, fludarabine, nelarabine, procarbazine, and ifosfamide (Table 90-8). Recognition of neurotoxicity resulting from cytotoxic chemotherapy is often difficult because of comorbid conditions such as metastatic disease and other paraneoplastic syndromes, but it is important in assessing the need for potential dose modifications or even discontinuation of the agent. Several reviews provide detailed explanations of signs and symptoms, mechanisms, and potential treatments for chemotherapy-induced neurotoxicities.[153,154]

FLUOROURACIL

Fluorouracil can cause acute cerebellar dysfunction characterized by the rapid onset of gait ataxia, limb incoordination, dysarthria, and nystagmus.[155,156] Cerebellar dysfunction occurs in approximately 5% to 10% of patients receiving fluorouracil at all treatment schedules in common use and can present weeks to months after beginning therapy. A more diffuse encephalopathy presenting as headache, confusion, disorientation, lethargy, and seizures can also occur. These symptoms can be reversed if fluorouracil is discontinued or the dose is reduced. Reports of cerebellar ataxia has also been reported with capecitabine, an oral prodrug of fluorouracil.[157,158] Other neurotoxicities observed with fluorouracil include rare reports of optic neuropathy and decreased vision.

INTERFERON-α

Interferon-α can cause a neurologic complex characterized by headache and encephalopathy (weakness, confusion, lethargy). The symptoms occur in one-third of patients receiving interferon and can cause severe reactions in 10%. Severe reactions include coma, obtundation, major depression, and suicidal behavior. Elderly patients receiving high dosages may be more susceptible to these effects. Symptoms typically begin after several weeks of therapy and usually resolve within 3 weeks after dose attenuation or discontinuation of therapy. If further treatment is warranted, lower doses should be used.[159]

FLUDARABINE AND NELARABINE

Fludarabine can cause severe neurotoxicity when used at doses greater than 90 mg/m^2 for 5 to 7 days.[160–162] Symptoms include altered mental status, photophobia, amaurosis (blindness that usually is temporary without change in the eye itself), generalized seizures, spastic or flaccid paralysis, quadriparesis, and coma. Patients may progress to death even when therapy is discontinued. This neurotoxicity, however, is not common with the current recommended dosage of 25 mg/m^2/day for 5 days. Mild neurologic symptoms are typically reported, but severe neurotoxicity,[162,163] and optic demyelination occurs only occasionally.[164] Patients with signs or symptoms suggestive of significant neurotoxicity should receive a neurologic examination and, if warranted, therapy should be discontinued without rechallenging with a dose reduction. Nelarabine, a newer purine analog has dose-limiting neurotoxicity, and 18% to 37% of patients in phase II trials showed severe grade 3 or 4 neurotoxicities.[165,166] The clinical presentation includes severe somnolence, convulsions, and peripheral neuropathy ranging

TABLE 90-8
Neurotoxicity of Selected Chemotherapeutic Agents

Acute Encephalopathy	Chronic Encephalopathic Syndrome	Cerebellar Neuropathy	Peripheral Neuropathy	Cranial Neuropathy	Arachnoiditis (Intrathecal Therapy)	Autonomic Neuropathy	SIADH
Asparaginase	Cytarabine	Cytarabine	Bortezomib	Fluorouracil	Cytarabine	Vinblastine	Cyclophosphamide
Cisplatin	Methotrexate	Cisplatin	Cisplatin	Ifosfamide	Methotrexate	Vincristine	Vinblastine
Cytarabine	Nelarabine	Fludarabine	Docetaxel		Thiotepa	Vinorelbine	Vincristine
Fludarabine	Thiotepa	Fluorouracil	Fluorouracil				Vinorelbine
Ifosfamide		Ifosfamide	Ifosfamide				
Methotrexate			Lenalidomide				
Nelarabine			Nelarabine				
Procarbazine			Paclitaxel				
			Thalidomide				
			Vinblastine				
			Vincristine				
			Vinorelbine				

SIADH, syndrome of inappropriate secretion of antidiuretic hormone.
Source: Sul JK, Deangelis LM. Neurologic complications of cancer chemotherapy. *Semin Oncol.* 2006;33:324; Meyer M. Neurotoxicity of chemotherapy agents. In: Perry MC, ed. *The Chemotherapy Source Book.* 3rd ed. Philadelphia, PA: Lippincott Williams & Wilkins; 2001:504; Arranon (nelarabine injection) [package insert]. Research Triangle Park, NC: GlaxoSmithKline; 2009; Hildebrand J. Neurological complications of cancer chemotherapy. *Curr Opin Oncol.* 2006;18:321.

a patient's left ventricular ejection fraction (LVEF), which is a measure of the heart's systolic function by ECHO, radionuclide cardiac angiography (multiple gated acquisition [MUGA]) or endomyocardial biopsy. The use of MUGA for early detection of doxorubicin-induced cardiac dysfunction has been investigated extensively.[202] MUGA can accurately detect functional cardiac status, but it is not particularly sensitive in detecting patients who have early myocyte damage. Augmenting the MUGA with exercise appears to give a more accurate picture of functional cardiac reserve. Because myocyte damage usually occurs days to weeks after treatment with doxorubicin, the MUGA should be obtained just before, rather than just after, a course of the agent. Although guidelines vary, most suggest regular cardiac function assessment by evaluation of LVEF by either ECHO or MUGA.

D.A. should have received a baseline assessment of his LVEF either by ECHO or MUGA before his first cycle of ABVD. During courses of therapy, LVEF monitoring for D.A. would not have been routinely recommended unless he was approaching his lifetime cumulative dose or there were clinical signs or symptoms of CHF. Because D.A. presented before his fifth cycle of ABVD with symptoms of CHF, another ECHO should be performed, and his doxorubicin should be discontinued.

Additional assessments should be obtained when a patient shows signs or symptoms of CHF or when low-risk patients receive cumulative doxorubicin doses greater than 450 mg/m^2 or high-risk patients receive greater than 350 mg/m^2, if additional doses are planned. Most guidelines recommend stopping doxorubicin or obtaining an endomyocardial biopsy when there is an absolute decrease in the LVEF of greater than 10% to 20%, the LVEF is less than 40%, or the LVEF fails to increase greater than 5% with exercise. Endomyocardial biopsies, along with a quantitative assessment of morphologic changes, provide the most specific evaluation of myocardial damage induced by anthracyclines. Progressive myocardial pathology is graded on a scale (the Billingham score) of 0 (no change from normal) to 3 (diffuse cell damage in >35% of total number of cells with marked change in cardiac ultrastructure).[203] Abnormal MUGA findings and the appearance of signs and symptoms of CHF correlate with biopsy scores. Usually, a significant change in cardiac function is not seen with scores less than 2 to 2.5. Several investigators have evaluated the predictive value of this technique. With a score of 2, a patient has less than a 10% chance of experiencing heart failure if 100 mg more of doxorubicin is given.[204–206] There are occasional false-negative biopsy findings, and fatal CHF has been encountered in at least one patient with a relatively normal (1.0) biopsy score.[207] The most significant risk associated with endomyocardial biopsy is perforation of the right ventricle with associated tamponade; this occurs rarely and depends largely on the experience of the individual performing the biopsy.

DAUNORUBICIN

Daunorubicin differs structurally from doxorubicin only by hydroxylation of the fourteenth carbon. Unlike doxorubicin, daunorubicin is primarily used to treat hematologic malignancies, such as acute myeloid leukemia. Doxorubicin became favored to treat solid tumors because daunorubicin caused excessive mucositis and myelosuppression when patients received antileukemic dosages to treat these tumors.[208] Cardiac toxicities are similar for both drugs, however, although somewhat higher cumulative doses of daunorubicin are typically tolerated.[209] Risk factors for CHF appear to be the same, and similar assessments should be undertaken to monitor for cardiotoxicity.

IDARUBICIN

Idarubicin is an anthracycline that is approved for the treatment of acute leukemias. Although idarubicin appears less cardiotoxic

TABLE 90-9
Anticancer Agents Requiring Dosage Modifications or Dosage Omissions in Renal Insufficiency

Bleomycin	Lenalidomide
Capecitabine	Lomustine
Carboplatin	Melphalan
Carmustine	Methotrexate
Cisplatin	Mitomycin
Cytarabine	Pemetrexed
Dacarbazine	Pentostatin
Fludarabine	Topotecan
Ifosfamide	

Source: Kintzel PE, Dorr RT. Anticancer drug renal toxicity and elimination: dosing guidelines for altered renal function. *Cancer Treat Rev.* Jan 1995;21:33; Launay-Vacher V et al. Prevalence of renal insufficiency in cancer patients and implications for anticancer drug management: the renal insufficiency and anticancer medications (IRMA) study. *Cancer.* 2007;110:1376; Li YF et al. Systemic anticancer therapy in gynecological cancer patients with renal dysfunction. *Int J Gynecol Cancer.* 2007;17:739.

potassium, urinary pH, protein, and glucose should be monitored closely in patients receiving these agents. Because the reversibility of the lesions is reported to be highly variable and a significant number of patients who exhibit severe renal toxicity with these agents require dialysis,[250] patients should discontinue treatment with these agents if they show any changes in serum creatinine or electrolytes.

Proteinuria

Bevacizumab, an anti-VEGF monoclonal antibody, is associated with proteinuria and the reported incidence ranges from 21% to 46% of patients. Mechanisms for this toxicity include microcirculatory angiogenesis and inhibition of nitric oxide synthesis. This may lead to an increase in peripheral resistance and endothelial dysfunction. Glomerular injury from VEGF inhibition may also lead to renal thrombotic microangiopathy and glomerulonephritis. Severe nephrotic syndrome has been observed in 1% to 2% of patients.[255,256] Patients receiving bevacizumab should be monitored routinely for proteinuria by dipstick urinalysis. The manufacturer recommends that patients with a 2+ or greater urine dipstick reading undergo further assessment with a 24-hour urine collection. Additionally, it is recommended to delay further administration of bevacizumab when greater than 2 g of proteinuria in 24 hours is observed. Therapy may be reinitiated when the proteinuria observed is less than 2 g in 24 hours. Proteinuria is most often mild in patients and is usually reversible upon discontinuation of the agent. The highest incidence of severe proteinuria requiring permanent discontinuation has been seen in patients with metastatic renal cell carcinoma.[257]

Acute Tubular Obstruction

METHOTREXATE

CASE 90-9

QUESTION 1: J.R., a 15-year-old boy with osteogenic sarcoma of the right knee, was treated with amputation of his right leg. His leg is now healed and chemotherapy consisting of high-dose methotrexate with leucovorin rescue, doxorubicin, dactinomycin, bleomycin, cisplatin, and ifosfamide is planned. The dose of methotrexate is 15 g/m^2 IV administered during 4 hours. What precautions are necessary to prevent the renal and other toxicities associated with high-dose methotrexate therapy in J.R.?

Methotrexate normally is not nephrotoxic, although 90% of the agent is excreted unchanged in the urine; however, acute tubular obstruction can occur with high-dose methotrexate if appropriate precautions are not taken. Acute tubular obstruction is caused by tubular precipitation of methotrexate, which is poorly soluble at a pH less than 7.0. To prevent this, J.R. should receive hydration and brisk diuresis to produce urine output of 100 to 200 mL/hour for at least 24 hours after administration. A urine pH greater than 7.0 usually can be ensured by administration of 25 to 50 mEq/L sodium bicarbonate within the hydration fluid. Acetazolamide, a carbonic anhydrase inhibitor, promotes urinary bicarbonate excretion and is used by some clinicians at doses of 500 mg two to four times daily to assist in maintaining a urinary pH greater than 7.0. J.R.'s urine output and pH must be monitored closely to prevent acute tubular obstruction during this period.[258] In addition, intrapatient and interpatient variability in methotrexate clearance is considerable, particularly with high doses of methotrexate therapy. Renal excretion of methotrexate is a complex process involving glomerular filtration, tubular reabsorption, and secretion. Acute tubular obstruction associated with high-dose methotrexate therapy can be prevented only by appropriate attention to optimal urinary output before, and for at least 24 hours after, high-dose methotrexate administration and urinary alkalization.[258]

If J.R. has existing renal insufficiency, methotrexate excretion will be decreased, leading to higher systemic exposure. As a result, myelosuppression and mucositis can become more problematic. Leucovorin (folinic acid) is a reduced form of folic acid given after methotrexate administration to selectively rescue normal cells from adverse effects such as myelosuppression and mucositis. Because leucovorin is already in reduced form, it can bypass the action of dihydrofolate reductase and not interfere with methotrexate's inhibition of this enzyme. Therefore, it is important that leucovorin rescue is initiated within 24 to 48 hours after the high-dose methotrexate infusion. Blood concentrations of methotrexate obtained within 24 hours after the infusion often are not predictive of concentrations at 48 hours. Therefore, methotrexate concentrations between 24 and 48 hours after infusion must be monitored in J.R. and in all patients receiving high-dose therapy. Methotrexate levels are necessary to guide leucovorin dosing. Leucovorin rescue does not affect the renal clearance of methotrexate.

Hemorrhagic Cystitis

IFOSFAMIDE

CASE 90-9, QUESTION 2: J.R. also is receiving ifosfamide. What unique bladder toxicity occurs with ifosfamide that requires attention before its administration?

PATHOGENESIS

Ifosfamide is a structural analog of cyclophosphamide belonging to the oxazaphosphorine class of antitumor alkylating agents, which must be hydroxylated and activated by the cytochrome P-450 3A4/3A5 and 2B6 enzymes in the liver. The 4-hydroxy metabolite spontaneously liberates acrolein, which is excreted in high concentrations in the urine. Acrolein is responsible for urotoxicity causing a direct irritation of the bladder mucosa. Both ifosfamide and cyclophosphamide can produce cystitis, which ranges from mild to severe bladder damage and hemorrhage. Cystitis is characterized by tissue edema and ulceration followed by sloughing of mucosal epithelial cells, necrosis of smooth muscle fibers and arteries, and culminating in focal hemorrhage.

CLINICAL PRESENTATION

Patients with oxazaphosphorine-induced hemorrhagic cystitis initially go through an asymptomatic stage characterized by

TABLE 90-13
Select Anticancer Agents[a] Requiring Dose Modification in Hepatic Dysfunction

Fluorouracil	Methotrexate
Daunorubicin	Paclitaxel
Docetaxel	Vinblastine
Epirubicin	Vincristine
Etoposide	

[a] The agents listed in this table are examples and are not meant to be an exhaustive list of agents that may need dose adjustments. Additionally, specific dose reductions may depend on multiple factors including treatment goals (curative versus palliative), performance status, and specific protocols.
Source: Field KM et al. Part I: Liver function in oncology: biochemistry and beyond. *Lancet Oncol.* 2008;9:1092; Field KM, Michael M. Part II: Liver function in oncology: towards safer chemotherapy use. *Lancet Oncol.* 2008;9:1181.

disease and do not necessarily correlate with hepatic function. Serum levels of proteins produced by the liver (e.g., ferritin, albumin, prealbumin, or retinol-binding protein) also may be helpful in assessing liver function. The decision to continue or discontinue chemotherapy in patients with apparent hepatic dysfunction can be difficult. If the chemotherapy is the suspected cause, therapy should be withheld until LFTs are within normal ranges. The clinician should also consider alternative (nonhepatotoxic) chemotherapy for future treatment. In addition, agents that are cleared predominantly via the liver may require dosage adjustments and should be administered cautiously (Table 90-13). J.A.'s cytarabine is likely responsible for his elevated liver enzymes. Therefore, costly workup should be deferred to allow recovery of liver function. Recovery should occur within 2 weeks of chemotherapy. If full recovery does not occur, further therapy (agents, doses, or both) may require modifications.

Long-Term Complications of Anticancer Therapy

SECOND MALIGNANCIES AFTER ANTICANCER THERAPY

ACUTE MYELOID LEUKEMIA

CASE 90-12

QUESTION 1: T.D., a 55-year-old woman, was diagnosed with an early-stage breast cancer and successfully treated with radical mastectomy followed by four cycles of adjuvant AC (doxorubicin 60 mg/m^2 IV on day 1, cyclophosphamide 600 mg/m^2 IV on day 1). Eighteen months after her breast cancer therapy was completed, T.D. presents to her primary care physician with complaints of fatigue, SOB, easy bruising, and sinusitis. A peripheral blood smear shows a WBC count of 120,000 cells/μL with a differential of greater than 90% leukemic blasts and a bone marrow biopsy confirms acute myeloid leukemia (AML). Subsequent cytogenetic analysis revealed abnormalities involving chromosome 11q23. What factors support the diagnosis of anticancer-therapy–associated acute leukemia in T.D.?

Acute leukemia has been associated with cytotoxic therapies used to treat hematologic malignancies, solid tumors, and nonmalignant diseases.[303] AML has been reported after combination chemotherapy that involves topoisomerase inhibitors, including etoposide and anthracyclines. These leukemias usually occur 1 to 3 years after the completion of chemotherapy, and myelodysplasia does not usually occur before the leukemia. Other characteristics include chromosomal abnormalities involving chromo-

some 11c
widespre
as Hodgk
Acute
who hav
ally occu
Myelodys
occurs in
all alkylat
to be the
classes of
nificant a
treatmen
ation ther
Several ac
ing acute
Evider
phoid ma
strong. In
rather tha
Hodgkin
after antic
ciated wi
daily oral
after treat
tumors in
sidered co
T.D.'s
doxorubic
for her acu
induced r
ciated wit
cytogenet
patients w
and have
plastic sy
11q23 are
malities fi
abnormal
of chemot
leukemia.

CASE 90
of T.D. v
patients

Therap
less effecti
plete remi
imens are
associated
70% to 80
92, Hemat
High-d
with AML
series, how
of short du
lated case r
and those
The be
tion. In pa
for a curab
treatment-
the benefit
as more is

complaints of brief episodes of painful urination, frequency, and hematuria. The symptoms may subside over a period of several days or weeks after discontinuing the agent. The course of oxazaphosphorine-induced hemorrhagic cystitis usually is relatively benign, although death from massive refractory hemorrhage has occurred.[259] Factors that may predispose J.R. to hemorrhagic cystitis include IV administration and the doses he is receiving.

PREVENTION

Historically, forced hydration was the primary method used to prevent hemorrhagic cystitis in patients treated with cyclophosphamide therapy. Theoretically, hydration flushes the toxic acrolein metabolite out of the bladder so that insufficient contact time is available to set up the tissue reaction. The more urotoxic agent, ifosfamide, was introduced to the market with a uroprotective agent, mesna. This agent contains a free thiol group, which can neutralize the oxazaphosphorine metabolite, acrolein, in the bladder. When administered in an appropriate dosing schedule, mesna can prevent the bladder toxicity completely, and thus use of mesna is the current standard of care.[250,259]

ASCO recommends a parenteral mesna dose of 20% of the ifosfamide dose given at zero, 4, and 8 hours after ifosfamide (for a total mesna dose of 60% of the ifosfamide dose).[57] The goal is to maintain prolonged mesna concentrations within the urinary tract that are uroprotective. Repeated administration is required because mesna has a much shorter elimination half-life (<1 hour) than ifosfamide. If patients receive a continuous infusion of ifosfamide, a different dosing strategy for mesna is required. To prolong mesna's protective effects, ASCO guidelines recommend an IV bolus mesna dose that is 20% of the ifosfamide dose, followed by continuous infusion that is an additional equivalent of 40% given for 12 to 24 hours after the end of the ifosfamide infusion.[250] This regimen ensures that mesna remains in the bladder for an extensive amount of time after the end of the ifosfamide infusion.

Various other mesna dosing schedules are clinically used, but no trials have compared the different regimens. Many clinicians use a 1:1 mg dose of mesna to ifosfamide when administered by continuous infusion. The dosing guidelines become less well-defined, however, when patients receive higher dosages of ifosfamide (>2.5 g/m^2). The lack of data and the unique pharmacokinetic properties of ifosfamide have caused some concerns about the current dosing guidelines. The pharmacokinetics of ifosfamide are nonlinear. For example, the elimination half-life associated with doses of 2.5 g/m^2 is 6 to 8 hours, whereas with doses of 3.5 to 5 g/m^2 it is 14 to 16 hours. The current recommendations for mesna administration enable protection for approximately 12 hours after an IV bolus; thus, with higher dosages of ifosfamide, mesna should be infused beyond the recommended 8 hours after ifosfamide to maintain bladder protection.[250,259] Also, concern exists that the 4-hour dosing interval used with lower doses may be inadequate to maintain sufficient mesna concentrations within the bladder. To ensure maximal protection against urotoxicity, ASCO currently recommends more frequent or prolonged mesna dosage regimens to account for its short half-life.[250] Ifosfamide and mesna are compatible in solution; therefore they can be infused together, offering greater patient convenience.

Because mesna works in the bladder, frequent urination may diminish its efficacy. Several authors have suggested that the frequency of mesna doses be adjusted based on frequency and amount of urination.[260–262] Although forced hydration has been the mainstay for prevention of cyclophosphamide-induced hemorrhagic cystitis, it is unnecessary and potentially disadvantageous when mesna is used. This is because forced hydration can increase urination and thus the evacuation of mesna from the bladder.

Mesna is usually given IV, but an oral formulation is available. The oral bioavailability of mesna is approximately 50%; therefore, patients should receive twice the standard IV dose (e.g., oral mesna 40% of the ifosfamide dose) 2 hours before and 4 and 8 hours after ifosfamide.[262] Others have recommended that an oral dose also be given with the ifosfamide dose. Many centers administer the first dose of mesna IV followed by oral doses at 4 and 8 hours, particularly in the outpatient clinic setting.[57] All patients receiving cyclophosphamide should receive saline diuresis or forced saline diuresis to protect urothelial tissue. When patients receive cyclophosphamide for an HCT, it is at high dose; therefore, they receive mesna and hydration. Other practices to prevent this complication include hyperhydration and the use of continuous bladder irrigation. Data comparing these methods are controversial and report varying rates of hematuria and severe hemorrhagic cystitis. These recommendations are currently supported by the ASCO consensus guideline[57] (see Chapter 96, Hematopoietic Cell Transplantation). J.R. will receive mesna at a dose of 20% of the ifosfamide dose given immediately before ifosfamide, and at 4 and 8 hours after ifosfamide (for a total mesna dose of 60% of the ifosfamide dose).

CASE 90-9, QUESTION 3: If J.R. exhibits hemorrhagic cystitis, how should it be treated?

TREATMENT

Once hemorrhagic cystitis develops, the agent causing the disorder must be discontinued and vigorous hydration started. If gross hematuria occurs, a large-bore urinary catheter should be inserted to avoid obstruction of the urethra by clots. Some clinicians also use continuous silver nitrate irrigation, local instillation of formalin or alum, or electrocauterization of bladder blood vessels to control bleeding. There is no consensus as to which of these methods is superior. If these measures fail, surgical intervention may be necessary to divert urine flow away from the bladder.[259]

Pulmonary Toxicities

BLEOMYCIN AND OTHER AGENTS

CASE 90-10

QUESTION 1: J.A., a 54-year-old man with stage III Hodgkin disease has received ABVD (doxorubicin 25 mg/m^2 IV days 1 and 15, bleomycin 10 units/m^2 IV on days 1 and 15, vinblastine 6 mg/m^2 IV on days 1 and 15, and dacarbazine 375 mg/m^2 IV on days 1 and 15) for six cycles. He presents to the clinic 6 months after his last cycle with dyspnea, a nonproductive cough, and fever. Chest radiograph showed diffuse bilateral infiltrates; his respiratory rate was 36 breaths/minute; and his arterial blood gases (ABG) were as follows:

pH, 7.50
P_{O_2}, 62 mm Hg
P_{CO_2}, 28 mm Hg
O_2 saturation, 92%

What are the possible causes of his new pulmonary findings?

J.A. is at risk for several processes that could produce diffuse pulmonary infiltrates and dyspnea. He is immunosuppressed secondary to his lymphoma and the therapy; therefore, J.A. has

TABLE 90-10
Chemotherapy-Induced Pulmonary Toxicity (*Continued*)

Drug	Histopathology	Clinical Features
Methotrexate[280–283] Delayed	Nonspecific changes, occasional fibrosis	No evidence that it is d weekly schedules m toxicity than month *Clinical presentation:* he prodrome, dyspnea, hypoxemia, tachypn eosinophilia, cyanos of patients, interstiti ↓ diffusing capacity, ventilatory defect
Noncardiac pulmonary edema	Acute pulmonary edema	Occurs very rarely 6–1 IT methotrexate
Pleuritic chest pain		Not related to other m toxicities or serum le occur with each cour *Clinical presentation:* rig occasional pleural eff of lung, thickened pl
Mitomycin[276]	Similar to bleomycin	*Clinical presentation:* dys basilar rales, hypoxer interstitial or finely n ↓ diffusing capacity
Procarbazine[123,124]	Hypersensitivity pneumonitis with eosinophilia and interstitial fibrosis	*Clinical presentation:* nau cough, dyspnea with ingestion, bilateral in and pleural effusion
Vinblastine[270]	Hyperplasia, dysplasia, interstitial edema, and fibrosis	Associated with concom with mitomycin *Clinical presentation:* acu distress, bilateral infil

BP, blood pressure; FVC, forced vital capacity; IT, intrathecal; PO, oral; SOB, shortness of breath.

extensive workup to determine whether they require immediate attention for tumor involvement of the liver or possible infection. In addition, patients should discontinue any nonessential medications that can potentially cause hepatotoxicity. The clinician may also discontinue chemotherapy if this is the suspected cause.

Several anticancer agents, including cytarabine, have been associated with hepatocellular damage and are reviewed in detail (Table 90-12).[288–302] Some agents commonly associated with hepatotoxicity include asparaginase, carmustine, cytarabine, mercaptopurine, methotrexate, irinotecan, oxaliplatin, clofarabine and imatinib. All of these drugs come in contact with the liver by entering the liver's blood supply; the liver uniquely receives a dual blood supply from the portal and superior mesenteric veins. The liver detoxifies or inactivates noxious substances and metabolizes many anticancer agents. The exact mechanisms by

which unkno with tl ing he tions, (tral he cles se hepato

Sev ture ar and bil receivi indices

Section 17 Neoplastic Disorders

TABLE 90-11
Common Causes of Elevated Liver Function Tests in Patients With Cancer

Primary or metastatic tumor involvement of the liver
Hepatotoxic drugs (e.g., cytotoxics, hormones [estrogens, androgens], antimicrobials [trimethoprim-sulfamethoxazole, voriconazole])
Infections (e.g., hepatic candidiasis, viral hepatitis)
Parenteral nutrition
Portal vein thrombosis
Paraneoplastic syndrome
History of liver disease (including hepatitis B and hepatitis C)

TABL
Hepato

Drug
Aspara
Busulf
Carmu
Clofara
Cytara
Etopos
Imatini
Mercap
Methot
Strepto

Levine J et al. Fertility preservation in adolescents and young adults with cancer. *J Clin Oncol.* 2010;28:4831. (312)

Rizzo JD et al. American Society of Clinical Oncology/American Society of Hematology clinical practice guideline update on the use of epoetin and darbepoetin in adult patients with cancer. *J Clin Oncol.* 2010;28:4996. (23)

Sahni V et al. Chemotherapy-associated renal dysfunction. *Nat Rev Nephrol.* 2009;5:450. (250)

Sioka C, Kyritsis AP. Central and peripheral nervous system toxicity of common chemotherapeutic agents. *Cancer Chemother Pharmacol.* 2009;63:761. (153)

Smith TJ et al. 2006 update of recommendations for the use of white blood cell growth factors: an evidence-based clinical practice guideline. *J Clin Oncol.* 2006;24:3187. (2)

Tan EH, Chan A. Evidence-based treatment options for the management of skin toxicities associated with epidermal growth factor receptor inhibitors. *Ann Pharmacother.* 2009;43:1658. (99)

Vahid B, Marik PE. Pulmonary complications of novel antineoplastic agents for solid tumors. *Chest.* 2008;133:528. (264)

Wolf S et al. Chemotherapy-induced peripheral neuropathy: prevention and treatment strategies. *Eur J Cancer.* 2008;44:1507. (182)

Key Websites

American Society of Clinical Oncology (ASCO). http://www.asco.org.

American Society of Hematology (ASH). http://www.hematology.org.

Cancer Therapy Evaluation Program, National Cancer Institute. Common Terminology Criteria for Adverse Events (CTCAE). http://ctep.cancer.gov/protocolDevelopment/electronic_applications/ctc.htm.

Oncology Nursing Society (ONS). http://www.ons.org.

Section 17 Neoplastic Disorders

91

Pediatric Malignancies

David W. Henry, Mark T. Holdsworth, and Nicole A. Kaiser

CORE PRINCIPLES

		CHAPTER CASES
1	Micrometastases are present in most solid tumors at the time of diagnosis. Neoadjuvant therapy was designed to treat micrometastatic disease before surgery, in hopes of increasing survival. Although it is not clear whether neoadjuvant therapy increases survival, residual viable tumor serves as a marker of response to chemotherapy and neoadjuvant therapy may reduce tumor size to allow more surgical options in the patient.	Case 91-3 (Question 1)
2	When monitoring therapy in children, one has to remember the age-related differences in measured parameters and large differences in size. Blood pressures are lower, and heart rates and respirations are higher in younger children. Intake and output need to be considered in relationship to the patient's size.	Case 91-1 (Question 3)
3	It is important to adjust creatinine clearance measurements or estimates to adult size (i.e., per 1.73 m^2) to correctly adjust drug doses for renal function in children.	Case 91-1 (Question 4)
4	Infants have larger body surface area–weight ratios than older children. Further, organ function changes rapidly during the first year of life. Therefore, chemotherapy dosing guidelines in protocols generally specify how to calculate doses for smaller children and infants (i.e., converting to mg/kg dosing from mg/m^2, or halving doses).	Case 91-2 (Question 2)
5	Leucovorin, when used with methotrexate, reduces methotrexate-related toxicities. In treating children with high-dose methotrexate and leucovorin rescue, serum methotrexate concentrations are measured so that leucovorin will be discontinued at the correct time. Fluid accumulation in the patient or drug interactions can slow methotrexate excretion and require prolonged leucovorin rescue.	Case 91-3 (Questions 3, 4)
6	Rhabdomyosarcoma is a soft tissue tumor of skeletal muscle origin, and it is the most common soft tissue sarcoma of childhood, occurring in 3.5% of all children with cancer. The two most common histologic types in children are embryonal and alveolar. Using the combination of vincristine, dactinomycin, and cyclophosphamide with local control of surgery or radiation is associated with an approximate 75% failure-free survival for patients with nonmetastatic disease.	Case 91-4 (Question 1)
7	Acute lymphoblastic leukemia (ALL) involves replacement of normal bone marrow elements due to abnormalities in cellular proliferation. Signs and symptoms relate to the deficiency in normal bone marrow elements.	Case 91-5 (Question 1)
8	Important prognostic variables in ALL are based on clinical and laboratory findings, including age and white blood cells (WBC) at diagnosis, sex, race, immunologic classification, cytogenetics, and early treatment response/minimal residual disease.	Case 91-5 (Question 1)
9	The treatment of ALL is divided into phases, including remission induction therapy, central nervous system (CNS) preventative therapy, consolidation/intensification phases, and maintenance therapy. All phases are different, each using multiple agents, schedules, and toxicity.	Case 91-5 (Questions 3, 5, 6, 11–13)

continued

may not reflect the total leukemia burden in the body. It is estimated that these measures of early response may detect up to 25% of children at risk for early relapse.[155] Rapid early response has been defined as clearance of bone marrow blasts by day 15 of induction, whereas slow early response refers to the converse. Whether patients are rapid or slow early responders is now being used to determine the type and intensity of further chemotherapy because slow early responders benefit from more intensive postinduction chemotherapy.[156] Other groups have examined response to initial treatment with a 7-day course of prednisone (initiated before the start of systemic induction chemotherapy) in children with high-risk ALL. Prednisone-poor response, defined as patients with greater than 1,000 blast cells/μL in peripheral blood after 7 days, was a predictor of poor outcome and was used to intensify induction therapy, with a consequent improvement in eventfree survival.[157]

MINIMAL RESIDUAL DISEASE

Several investigators have examined the prognostic value of detecting minimal residual disease (MRD) in bone marrow samples through the use of sophisticated PCR and flow-cytometric–based assays. A variety of lymphoblast characteristics, including gene fusion transcripts, immunophenotype, and antigen receptor gene rearrangements, may be relied on for MRD detection in children with ALL. Although specific fusion transcripts can be relied on as PCR targets in only one-third of childhood ALL cases, clonal antigen receptor gene rearrangements occur in virtually all cases.[154] Using various techniques, approximately 50% of children with ALL are MRD positive at the completion of induction therapy, and roughly 45% of these patients will experience a relapse. The association for a negative test for MRD at the completion of induction therapy appears stronger because it has a negative predictive value of 92.5% and a positive predictive value of 44.5%. In patients positive for MRD, there is a continuous decrease in MRD during the months of chemotherapy treatment. Persistence of MRD beyond 4 to 6 months or re-emergence of MRD is almost always predictive of future relapse.[158] It is now established that the presence of MRD is an important prognostic factor, regardless of the patient's initial WBC count or age at presentation.[154] Recently, a large study of the prognostic value of MRD for day 7 blood samples and for bone marrow samples at both the end of the induction and consolidation phases demonstrated that MRD at the end of the induction phase was the most important predictor of prognosis when compared to other laboratory and clinical factors. Day 7 MRD findings had additional prognostic value.[159] Data from this study for end of induction MRD demonstrated major differences in eventfree survival as follows: 88% for MRD negative, 59% for MRD of 0.01% to 0.1%, 49% for MRD of 0.1% to 1% and 30% for MRD greater than 1%. MRD predicted relapse that occured early in treatment and late relapses as well. Monitoring of MRD is now established in the management of childhood ALL and is being used to risk-stratify treatment in current front-line leukemia studies.

ADDITIONAL VARIABLES

Several additional variables may determine the prognosis of children with ALL. A complete discussion of these factors is beyond the scope of this text, but a few of these deserve brief mention. In addition to having an increased risk for developing ALL, children with Down syndrome are at a slightly greater risk for treatment failure. Their adverse outcome has been ascribed to an excess of therapy-related toxicities, especially associated with high-dose methotrexate.[160] One variable that has not been traditionally considered a prognostic factor is nutritional status. Although this is usually not an important variable in the United States and in developed nations, it may be a significant factor in underdeveloped countries, which are home to the majority of the world's children. In several trials, the outcome in childhood ALL was significantly worse for malnourished patients, and in at least one trial, the most important predictor of relapse was malnutrition.[161] This may be related to a decrease in patient tolerance to chemotherapy. A malnutrition prevalence rate of up to 50% for children with ALL in underdeveloped countries has been reported. When compared with socioeconomic status, malnutrition was more closely related to prognosis than was poverty. It appears that height for age is a more reliable predictor of prognosis than weight for age, suggesting that chronic stunting is more important than acute wasting in malnourished patients.[161]

These prognostic variables can be used to assign patients to various categories based on their risk of relapse. These categories are important in determining the therapy that patients should receive. Although there is considerable agreement regarding the importance of certain variables in assigning patients to a defined risk group (e.g., age, initial WBC, MRD findings, translocations), institutions that treat ALL may differ in their definitions of what constitutes high-risk, intermediate-risk, and low-risk patients. This makes it difficult to compare treatment results from different institutions or treatment groups. Last, newer prognostic variables, especially rapidly evolving cytogenetic and MRD prognosticators, complicate the comparisons of treatment regimens over time.

OVERVIEW OF TREATMENT

The treatment for pediatric ALL is organized into different phases of chemotherapy. Treatment begins with induction therapy, which typically includes three or four systemic agents in addition to CNS preventative therapy. The intensity of induction therapy is based on the biology of the ALL, and today the main variables used for determining this phase of therapy are the child's age and WBC count at diagnosis. Induction therapy is designed to induce a complete remission, and typically lasts 28 days. After induction therapy, the next phase of therapy can be defined as postinduction therapy, and consists of a number of different cycles of chemotherapy referred to by such terms as consolidation, delayed intensification, and interim maintenance therapy. This phase of intensive chemotherapy usually uses combination approaches that are somewhat different than induction therapy, and that are designed to kill leukemia cells in the cell cycle that were not destroyed by induction therapy. This phase of therapy is continuing to undergo substantial revision as studies determine which therapy components are optimal for various patients. The duration and intensity of the postinduction phase of therapy is tailored based on certain prognostic features of the leukemia as outlined above. The third phase of therapy is termed the maintenance phase, and represents the longest phase of chemotherapy for these patients, often taking approximately 2 years to complete. Maintenance therapy is typically less intensive than the previous phases, and consists mostly of continuous oral chemotherapy with infrequent intravenous and CNS therapy. In general, treatment intensity diminishes from the induction/consolidation phase to the maintenance phase.

REMISSION INDUCTION THERAPY

ALLOPURINOL AND MERCAPTOPURINE INTERACTION

CASE 91-5

QUESTION 1: J.B. is a 4-year-old Hispanic boy presenting with a 2-week history of an upper respiratory tract infection and a 1-week history of otitis media. His symptoms have worsened, and he now presents with a nosebleed and fatigue. Physical examination reveals appreciable pallor and

hepatosplenomegaly. A CBC with differential reveals a normochromic, normocytic anemia with the following:

Hematocrit (Hct), 15.7%
Hgb, 5.7 g/dL
WBC count, 4,300 cells/μL
Platelet count, 13,000 cells/μL

A differential on the WBC count reveals 82% lymphocytes (normal, 30%–40%), 7% neutrophils (normal, 50%–60%), and 11% lymphoblasts (normal, 0%). Based on these findings, a bone marrow biopsy is performed, which reveals 95% lymphoblasts. A diagnosis of ALL is made. The immunologic class is early pre–B cell based on CD10 and CD19 positivity. Radiography of the chest does not reveal a mediastinal mass, and a lumbar puncture shows that there are no leukemic lymphoblasts in the cerebrospinal fluid. J.B. is hydrated, alkalinized, and treated with oral allopurinol 200 mg/m²/day, with a plan to institute induction therapy the next day. (For a discussion of the use of allopurinol in induction chemotherapy for the prevention of tumor lysis syndrome [TLS], also see Tailoring of Postinduction Therapy section). Within a few days, J.B. will be treated with several drugs for his leukemia. Do any of the agents that are likely to be used in J.B. exhibit significant drug interactions with allopurinol?

Xanthine oxidase, the enzyme inhibited by allopurinol, also converts mercaptopurine to 6-thiouric acid.[162] Thus, allopurinol may markedly increase the plasma concentrations of oral mercaptopurine by inhibiting first-pass metabolism, and this may lead to toxicity.[163] This potentially serious drug interaction is usually irrelevant for most patients with ALL because these agents are rarely used together. Allopurinol is usually used early in the first week of induction therapy, and patients do not receive mercaptopurine until they finish induction therapy in most contemporary childhood ALL protocols.

GOAL OF INDUCTION

CASE 91-5, QUESTION 2: What is the goal of the induction therapy that J.B. will receive?

The goal of induction therapy is complete remission (i.e., the inability to detect leukemic cells in the peripheral blood or the bone marrow by morphologic microscopic evaluation). J.B.'s peripheral blood values must be within the normal range, and the bone marrow must reveal less than 5% lymphoblasts. This definition also assumes the absence of lymphoblasts in the cerebrospinal fluid (CSF). In addition, based on what is now known regarding MRD, achievement of an MRD measurement of less than 0.01% by the end of induction therapy (i.e., day 29) would now be an additional goal of this first phase of therapy. Although these findings indicate an adequate response to chemotherapy, they do not indicate a cure. Most patients have a total of 10^{12} cells at diagnosis, and successful induction regimens reduce this cell load by 99% to 10^{9}.[164,165] Therefore, continuation of therapy will be required for J.B. to further reduce the leukemic cell population and to increase his chances of long-term survival. Without continuation of therapy, the majority of patients with ALL will relapse within a few months.[166]

INDUCTION COMBINATION CHEMOTHERAPY

CASE 91-5, QUESTION 3: Which agents should be used to achieve complete remission?

TABLE 91-7
Systemic Induction Regimens for Childhood Acute Lymphocytic Leukemia

Agent	Route	Dose/Schedule
Three-Drug Induction Regimen		
Prednisone	PO	40 mg/m²/d × 28 days
or		
Dexamethasone[a]	PO	6 mg/m²/d × 28 days
with		
Vincristine	IV	1.5 mg/m²/wk (max 2 mg) × 4 doses
and		
Asparaginase	IM	10,000 units/m² 3 times weekly × 9 doses
or		
Pegaspargase	IM	2,500 units/m² × 1 dose
And (if Four-Drug Induction)		
Daunorubicin	IV	25 mg/m² on days 2, 8, 15

[a] Denotes that this agent is only used in three-drug induction regimens (see text).
IM, intramuscularly; IV, intravenously; PO, orally.
Source: Bostrom BC et al. Dexamethasone versus prednisone and daily oral versus weekly intravenous mercaptopurine for patients with standard-risk acute lymphoblastic leukemia: a report from the Children's Cancer Group. *Blood.* 2003;101:3809; Clavell LA et al. Four-agent induction and intensive asparaginase therapy for treatment of childhood acute lymphoblastic leukemia. *N Engl J Med.* 1986;315:657; Balis FM et al. Differences in cerebrospinal fluid penetration of corticosteroids: possible relationship to the prevention of meningeal leukemia. *J Clin Oncol.* 1987;5:202; Hurwitz CA et al. Substituting dexamethasone for prednisone complicates remission induction in children with acute lymphoblastic leukemia. *Cancer.* 2000;88:1964; Ortega JA et al. L-asparaginase, vincristine, and prednisone for induction of first remission in acute lymphocytic leukemia. *Cancer Res.* 1977;37:535; Reiter A et al. Chemotherapy in 998 unselected childhood acute lymphoblastic leukemia patients: results and conclusions of the multicenter trial ALL-BFM 86. *Blood.* 1994;84:3122; Kaplan RS, Wiernik PH. Neurotoxicity of antineoplastic drugs. *Semin Oncol.* 1982;9:103.

The agents most commonly used in remission induction therapy are vincristine, prednisone, dexamethasone, asparaginase, pegaspargase, and daunorubicin (Table 91-7). The prednisone or dexamethasone dose is not routinely tapered at the end of induction treatment.[167–170] More recently, dexamethasone has begun to supplant prednisone as the corticosteroid used during induction therapy or throughout therapy. This is based on earlier work showing that dexamethasone has greater CSF penetration.[171] In patients with standard-risk ALL, a randomized comparison of dexamethasone to prednisone for induction therapy showed a lower CNS relapse rate in the dexamethasone group.[169] However, the use of a 28-day course of dexamethasone during induction for patients with high-risk ALL was also associated with an increased risk of infectious complications, in particular, sepsis and toxic deaths.[172] This has led to removal or alteration of dexamethasone use during induction therapy in high-risk patients. It is plausible that the addition of dexamethasone to a more intensive chemotherapy backbone that is used for induction therapy of high-risk ALL may significantly increase the risk of infection in this more myelosuppressive regimen. In addition to the choice of corticosteroids, the efficacy of the long-acting polyethylene glycol (PEG) asparaginase has been compared with the short-acting native *Escherichia coli* asparaginase. One study demonstrated a comparable degree and duration of systemic asparagine depletion with PEG as compared to native asparaginase. However, unlike native asparaginase, PEG did not result in asparagine depletion within the CNS. It is unclear whether this could have an impact on CNS relapse in children receiving contemporary chemotherapy regimens.[168] With regard to immunogenicity, PEG asparaginase is less likely to induce high antiasparaginase antibody titers, which are in turn associated with lower asparaginase activity. This resulted in an almost complete avoidance of the silent inactivation noted to occur in approximately 30% of patients receiving native asparaginase.[173]

No chemotherapy drug meets the criteria of an ideal agent (i.e., toxic to leukemic cells only and active in all phases of the cell cycle). Corticosteroids, vincristine, and various asparaginase products come closest to this ideal in terms of activity, primarily against lymphocytic leukemia, because these agents are selectively toxic to the leukemia cells while sparing normal bone marrow elements. To improve the success in attaining complete remission, additional agents have been added to vincristine, prednisone, and asparaginase (Table 91-7). The most frequently used additional agent is an anthracycline, such as daunorubicin or doxorubicin. Use of at least a three-drug induction regimen is the current standard of care for children at low or intermediate risk of relapse and results in improvements in both remission rate and duration versus less intensive therapy.[174–176] Currently, a four-drug regimen, or an even more intensive induction regimen consisting of more than four drugs, and often for a duration of more than 4 weeks, is used for children at high risk of relapse and adult ALL patients.[167,177–179]

If complete remission is not achieved with three agents by the end of induction, patients are treated with additional agents (e.g., an additional 2–4 weeks of daunorubicin and prednisone; initiation of cytarabine with additional asparaginase; vincristine and prednisone for 1–2 weeks). Because this occurs rarely, there is no consensus about the most effective agents or schedules to use in this situation. Most of these patients have a decreased survival and a higher relapse rate.

Intensive induction treatment has benefits for the majority of children with ALL. This treatment strategy supports the hypothesis of Goldie and Coldman[180] that intensification of early treatment may decrease the chance that drug resistance will develop. This may therefore increase the proportion of long-term relapse-free survivors. Induction therapy is determined based on clinical findings such as age at diagnosis and initial WBC count. Based on these prognostic variables, J.B. is a patient with a low risk of relapse. A three-drug induction regimen consisting of vincristine, dexamethasone, and pegaspargase is recommended to optimize his chances for long-term diseasefree survival.[168,169,173] Additional laboratory testing (e.g., bone marrow analysis for remission and MRD) will be relied on to design his postinduction therapy.

VINCRISTINE TOXICITY

CASE 91-5, QUESTION 4: J.B. is discharged from the hospital during the second week of induction chemotherapy. Results of his CBC and differential indicate that he is responding well to his chemotherapy (i.e., WBC count 2,600 cells/μL, neutrophils 69%, lymphocytes 22%, platelets 229,000 cells/μL, Hct 28.6%, blastocytes 0). However, during the third week of induction chemotherapy, J.B. exhibits severe abdominal pain. It is discovered that he has not had a bowel movement in 6 days. J.B. has also been exhibiting "acting out" behaviors in recent days. How might these symptoms be explained?

The use of vincristine is associated with an autonomic neuropathy, which may substantially reduce GI motility[181]; in severe cases, paralytic ileus may result. Constipation is often accompanied by colicky abdominal pain, which may be quite distressing.[182] These symptoms usually become apparent 3 to 10 days after drug administration and resolve over several days. Prophylactic use of a stool softener (docusate) or laxative (polyethylene glycol) may lessen the severity of J.B.'s constipation and facilitate regular defecation. This regimen should have been instituted soon after the first dose of vincristine.

J.B.'s emotional changes are likely the result of the dexamethasone he is receiving. Emotional lability, sleep disturbances, depressed mood, and listlessness have occurred during corticosteroid therapy in children with ALL.[183] These behavioral changes can be quite disruptive, and parents should be prepared for them in advance. Oral promethazine can be used to help mitigate severe behavioral changes associated with dexamethasone. Behavioral disturbances typically resolve within 2 weeks after corticosteroid discontinuation.[183]

INTRATHECAL CHEMOTHERAPY PROPHYLAXIS

CASE 91-5, QUESTION 5: In addition to the aforementioned drugs, J.B. also receives intrathecal (IT) chemotherapy for CNS prophylaxis with methotrexate at the beginning (week 1) and end (week 4) of induction therapy. What is the purpose of IT chemotherapy?

IT or CNS preventive therapy decreases the chance of relapse within the CNS and increases J.B.'s chance of long-term survival. Before CNS preventive therapy was routine, the CNS was the most common site of leukemic relapse and thus predicted bone marrow relapse.[184,185] Patients at greatest risk for CNS relapse include those with very high initial WBC counts, T-cell ALL, and infants.[186,187] However, because all patients with ALL are at risk for CNS relapse, one of the largest incremental improvements in diseasefree survival has been the routine use of CNS preventive therapy.[84] Because many antileukemic agents do not distribute well into the CSF, this area becomes a sanctuary site for leukemic lymphoblasts. The aim is to eradicate any CNS leukemic lymphoblasts present at diagnosis and to prevent the emergence of a relapse within the CNS.

CENTRAL NERVOUS SYSTEM PREVENTIVE THERAPY OPTIONS

CASE 91-5, QUESTION 6: What are the various treatments available for CNS preventive therapy? What determines which one is chosen for J.B.?

All treatment protocols for childhood ALL use some form of CNS preventive therapy, although different regimens are used. The first successful CNS prophylaxis treatments were 2,400 cGy of craniospinal radiation with or without IT methotrexate, which markedly reduced the CNS relapse rate.[188] To avoid the myelosuppression and reductions in spinal growth due to craniospinal irradiation, the standard CNS preventive therapy was modified to 2,400 cGy of cranial irradiation, along with IT methotrexate. However, the adverse effects of cranial irradiation remained problematic. These included decreased intellectual function, dysfunctions of the neuroendocrine system, and poorer psychosocial functioning.[189–191] As a result, clinicians sought alternative, potentially safer forms of CNS preventive therapy. For example, lower doses (1,800 cGy) of cranial irradiation were combined with IT methotrexate to reduce the CNS effects, which proved to be equivalent to 2,400 cGy in preventing CNS relapse.[187,192] Nevertheless, because concerns regarding the long-term toxicity of cranial radiation remain, especially for younger children, it is currently reserved for patients with detectable CNS disease on presentation, some patients with T-cell ALL, and patients with CNS relapse. Currently, CNS preventative therapy includes IT methotrexate alone, triple IT chemotherapy (methotrexate, cytarabine, and hydrocortisone), or IT methotrexate combined with systemic-dose–intensified methotrexate.[193–195]

Because patients differ in their risk for developing CNS leukemia, CNS preventive therapy should be tailored accordingly. Children with low-risk and intermediate-risk ALL have equivalent CNS protection rates with either cranial radiation or IT chemotherapy, as long as adequate intensive systemic therapy is provided.[196,197] Patients at low or intermediate risk of relapse may be treated with either triple IT chemotherapy or IT methotrexate, depending on the institutional protocol.[196] A randomized study comparing treatment outcomes in a large sample of children with ALL found some differences between triple IT chemotherapy and IT methotrexate when compared in the postinduction phase. Interestingly, the triple IT regimen was associated with a lower rate of CNS relapse but a higher rate of bone marrow and testicular relapses, suggesting that this regimen may alter detection of recurrent disease.[198]

Some high-risk children who are early responders to chemotherapy and who do not have CNS disease on presentation may also obtain adequate CNS protection with IT methotrexate alone.[199] Currently, most patients with T-cell disease still receive cranial radiation therapy as a component of their CNS preventive therapy, although with current intensive systemic therapy a radiation dose of 1,200 cGy appears to provide adequate CNS protection.[84]

INTRATHECAL CHEMOTHERAPY: CHRONIC ADVERSE EFFECTS

CASE 91-5, QUESTION 7: What are the chronic adverse effects of intrathecal chemotherapy?

The chronic toxicities of IT chemotherapy are now being determined. When examined for effects on growth, triple IT chemotherapy demonstrated no effect on the final height achieved by children in contrast to a reduced final height in patients receiving cranial irradiation.[200] Limited evidence suggests that IT chemotherapy may be associated with some neuropsychological deficits. At least one study of patients receiving IT chemotherapy without cranial irradiation has demonstrated deficits in higher-order cognitive function tasks and learning disabilities in mathematics.[201] Another study has demonstrated that children who were treated with IT chemotherapy before age 5 years had deficits in the cerebellar-frontal brain subsystem and in neuropsychological performance.[202] It is unclear whether these deficits translate into significant long-term consequences.

INTRATHECAL METHOTREXATE DOSE

CASE 91-5, QUESTION 8: J.B. is at a low risk for CNS relapse, and the decision is made to treat him with IT methotrexate. What dose of IT methotrexate should J.B. receive?

High chemotherapy concentrations can be attained within the CSF with relatively low doses because the CSF volume of distribution is small in contrast to the peripheral plasma volume (140 mL vs. 3,500 mL).[203,204] Drug exposure is also maximized by the longer half-life of most drugs in the CSF.[205] The approach used for IT dosing differs from systemic administration, the latter of which is based on body weight or body surface area. CSF methotrexate concentrations appear to correlate better with patient age than size.[206] The CSF volume in children approaches that of an adult by the age of 3 years. Because CSF volume does not correlate with body surface area, IT doses based on body size result in subtherapeutic concentrations in young children and potentially toxic concentrations in older children and adults. The age-based dosing regimens shown in Table 91-8 are less neurotoxic and are associated with a lower rate of CNS relapse than doses based on size.[207] Using this dosing regimen, J.B.'s dose of IT methotrexate should be 12 mg. If triple intrathecal therapy were used, the doses of IT cytarabine and hydrocortisone would be 24 and 12 mg, respectively. These latter doses are also based on age, but no literature exists to support how they were derived. Nevertheless, empiric evidence supports their efficacy.[198]

TABLE 91-8

Dosage Regimen for Intrathecal Chemotherapy Based on Patient Age

Patient Age (years)	Methotrexate (mg)	Hydrocortisone (mg)	Cytarabine (mg)
<1	6	6	12
1	8	8	16
2	10	10	20
3	12	12	24
≥9	15	15	30

Source : Lobel JS et al. Methotrexate and asparaginase combination chemotherapy in refractory acute lymphoblastic leukemia of childhood. *Cancer.* 1979;43:1089.

DANGERS OF INTRATHECAL VINCRISTINE

CASE 91-5, QUESTION 9: J.B.'s triple IT methotrexate is to be administered on the same day as his vincristine dose. Are there any special precautions that should be taken when these medications are administered in close proximity?

Inadvertent administration of vincristine into the intrathecal space is almost uniformly fatal,[208–210] although there is at least one report of a patient in whom death but not serious sequelae was prevented.[211] Despite widespread educational efforts in hospitals and clinics, and numerous precautionary measures, deaths from the inadvertent IT administration of vincristine still occur.[212] The clinical course in patients mistakenly given IT vincristine has typically progressed from backache and headache on day 1, muscle weakness (generalized) on day 2, apnea on day 5, loss of evidence of electroencephalographic activity by days 7 to 9, and death on day 12.[208] To avoid the tragedy of IT vincristine administration, vincristine should be admixed separately from IT medications, specially labeled and mixed as a small volume parenteral (i.e., minibag) rather than in a syringe, and preferably delivered to the patient area for IV infusion after the administration of IT medications.

ONLINE CONTENT

For a video that shows the dangers of inadvertent IT administration of vincristine, go to http://thepoint.lww.com/AT10e.

ACUTE ADVERSE EFFECTS OF INTRATHECAL METHOTREXATE

CASE 91-5, QUESTION 10: J.B. experiences severe nausea and vomiting after his IT methotrexate treatment. Is this common after IT chemotherapy? What can be done to decrease this toxicity for future IT chemotherapy treatments?

Several acute toxicities have been reported after IT chemotherapy. Acute arachnoiditis may occur 12 to 24 hours after injection, resulting in headaches, nausea, vomiting, and various other signs of increased intracranial pressure.[213] Severe symptoms occurred in 4 of 91 children receiving combination IT chemotherapy.[214] IT methotrexate alone produces these side effects in 38% of cases.[215] Fortunately, these reactions are usually self-limiting and can be reduced by use of doses based on patient age.[207]

Nausea and vomiting due to IT chemotherapy is usually mild to moderate in severity.[216] The emetogenic effect of IT chemotherapy is likely the result of direct contact between the chemotherapy and the chemoreceptor trigger zone. IV ondansetron (a 5-HT_3 antagonist) at a dose of 0.15 mg/kg before and 3 to 4 hours after IT chemotherapy or 0.3 mg IV × 1 dose before IT chemotherapy can significantly reduce the incidence and severity of nausea and vomiting secondary to triple IT chemotherapy.[216] Without antiemetic protection, only 22% of children receiving IT chemotherapy had no vomiting. With the addition of ondansetron, complete protection from vomiting rose to 69%.[216] The efficacy of ondansetron IV when chemotherapy is administered IT is consistent with animal data demonstrating that 5-HT_3 antagonists administered directly into the brainstem can block the emetic response of systemically administered chemotherapy.[217]

Rarely, a form of methotrexate neurotoxicity resulting in either paraplegia or necrotizing leukoencephalopathy may occur.[218–220] Leukoencephalopathy is associated with cranial irradiation given before or during IT therapy.[220] The preservatives in the chemotherapy diluents (methylhydroxylbenzoate and benzyl alcohol) rather than the chemotherapy agents are believed to be responsible for the paraplegia. This emphasizes the importance of diluting IT chemotherapy with a preservative-free diluent.[218] In addition, acute seizures associated with IT methotrexate have been reported. It also has been shown that methotrexate can increase the CSF concentration of homocysteine, as a consequence of decreased CSF folate. It is known that homocysteine can be metabolized to excitatory neurotransmitters that are agonists of the *N*-methyl-D-aspartate (NMDA) receptor, leading to seizures.[221,222] It is possible that known NMDA receptor antagonists (e.g., dextromethorphan) may decrease the risk of seizures in patients who experience this toxicity.[222]

TAILORING OF POSTINDUCTION THERAPY

CASE 91-5, QUESTION 11: An analysis of the chromosomes from J.B.'s bone marrow reveals the TEL-AML1 translocation and a DNA index of 1.0. His MRD findings reveal the following: Blood on day 8 is less than 1% and bone marrow on day 29 shows 0.15%. Based on his day 29 (end of induction) bone marrow positive MRD finding, J.B. is scheduled to receive a more aggressive postinduction chemotherapy regimen despite the presence of the TEL-AML1 translocation. This treatment is chosen because MRD findings are more predictive of the chance for relapse than are his cytogenetics. Although J.B. had bone marrow aspirations performed at day 8 and at the completion of induction treatment on day 29 that both indicated a complete morphologic remission, his MRD findings at the end of induction take precedence in defining his further therapy. After completion of the induction phase, J.B. was scheduled to receive an intensified phase of postinduction chemotherapy known as augmented interim maintenance. What is the purpose of postinduction treatment, and what are some examples of effective regimens for this phase of treatment?

Postinduction chemotherapy consists of a variety of combinations of different agents typically given on a 2 to 6 week treatment cycle. These different phases of postinduction therapy are known as consolidation, interim maintenance, and delayed intensification.

Postinduction treatment has proved to be an important strategy for the prevention of relapse in children with ALL and has helped produce eventfree survival of greater than 80% in low-risk childhood ALL.[84,223] To date, the optimum postinduction regimens have yet to be determined. However, a few interesting findings from investigations of consolidation therapy are briefly mentioned. A comparison between methotrexate 1 g/m^2 IV (intermediate-dose methotrexate) and low-dose (180 mg/m^2 divided into six doses) oral methotrexate revealed an approximate 4.4% increase in continuous complete remission with the higher-dose regimen.[223] This study is considered to be one of the pivotal trials demonstrating the superiority of higher-dose methotrexate in childhood ALL.[84] Although this difference was statistically significant, it may not have been clinically significant because leukoencephalopathy also occurred in 4.5% of children treated with the higher-dose regimen, compared with 0.6% of those treated with low-dose methotrexate. Although this study was not designed to examine differences in sex, female patients failed to benefit from the higher-dose regimen. This study has also been criticized for using the same leucovorin dosage with both methotrexate regimens because it is known that a lower-dose oral regimen without leucovorin may result in RBC concentrations similar to that achieved with higher-dose methotrexate with leucovorin.[224] A more recent trial comparing either longer duration or more intensive postinduction regimens for children with high-risk ALL found that a higher intensity treatment regimen improved outcome, whereas the longer duration regimen did not. In this study, the higher intensity postinduction treatment was made up of greater use of PEG-asparaginase, vincristine, and escalating-dose methotrexate (Table 91-9). Intermediate-dose

TABLE 91-9
Acute Lymphoblastic Leukemia Postinduction Regimen Components

Schedule	Reference
Vincristine 1.5 mg/m^2 IV on days 0, 10, 20, 30, and 40	
Methotrexate 100 mg/m^2 IV on days 0, 10, 20, 30, and 40 (escalate by 50 mg/m^2 per dose if tolerated) PEG-asparaginase 2,500 units/m^2 IM on days 1 and 21 Methotrexate IT on days 0 and 30	226
Cyclophosphamide 1 g/m^2 IV on days 0 and 28 Cytarabine 75 mg/m^2 SC or IV on days 1–4, 8–11, 29–32, and 36–39 Mercaptopurine 60 mg/m^2 PO daily on days 0–13, and 28–41 Methotrexate IT on days 1, 8, 15, and 22 PEG-asparaginase 2,500 units/m^2 IM on days 14 and 42 Vincristine 1.5 mg/m^2 IV on days 14, 21, 42, and 49	226
Methotrexate 1 g/m^2 IV for 24 hours, every 3 weeks × 6 doses Vincristine 1.5 mg/m^2 IV on weeks 8, 9, 17, and 18 Prednisone 40 mg/m^2 PO daily × 7 days on weeks 8 and 17	224
Dexamethasone 10 mg/m^2 PO daily on days 0–7, 14–20 Vincristine 1.5 mg/m^2 IV on days 0, 7, and 14 PEG-asparaginase 2,500 units/m^2 IM on day 3 Doxorubicin 25 mg/m^2 IV on days 0, 7, and 14	226

IV, intravenously; IM, intramuscularly; PO, orally; SC, subcutaneously; IT, intrathecally.

methotrexate was not used in the study likely due to the substantial rate of leukoencephalopathy previously observed. For most patients, intermediate-dose methotrexate treatment has been supplanted by other types of dose-intensive postinduction treatment strategies in contemporary pediatric ALL treatments.[225]

It is not uncommon for newer postinduction regimens to lead to complications, given the baseline treatment intensity of many contemporary ALL treatments. For example, a trial evaluating the addition of either intensified asparaginase or cytarabine to intermediate-dose methotrexate in standard-risk ALL patients failed to show any incremental benefit in eventfree survival over that achievable with methotrexate alone, although the cytarabine regimen resulted in an increase in both infectious morbidity and hospitalizations.[226] Some examples of postinduction regimens are provided in Table 91-9.[169,177,223,225–227]

ESCALATING METHOTREXATE DOSES

CASE 91-5, QUESTION 12: J.B. is now receiving postinduction therapy, and one of the components is interim maintenance with escalating-dose methotrexate. This treatment consists of vincristine and methotrexate dosed every 10 days, and PEG-asparaginase dosed twice during the 40-day treatment course as outlined in Table 91-9. Methotrexate serum concentrations are not monitored after the administration of each dose of methotrexate during this phase of therapy. Rather, determinations as to whether to give the next methotrexate dose and whether it should be increased by 50 mg/m^2 are determined by his clinical exam and laboratory values. The rationale behind this phase of therapy is to deliver maximal tolerated doses of methotrexate that are tailored to an individual patient's tolerance. What would be appropriate laboratory and clinical exam parameters for increasing methotrexate dosing in this regimen, and what should be done for patients whose laboratory values are not in the range required for a dosing increase? What potential complications could occur in a patient receiving this methotrexate regimen without appropriate lab monitoring?

Sample guidelines for escalating methotrexate dosing in the interim maintenance phase are as follows:

- If the ANC is greater than 750 cells/μL and platelets are greater than 75,000 cells/μL, escalate the methotrexate dose by 50 mg/m^2 more than the dose administered previously.
- If the ANC is greater than 500 cells/μL but less than 750 cells/μL or platelets are greater than 50,000 cells/μL but less than 75,000 cells/μL, then the dose of methotrexate should be the same as was previously administered.
- If the ANC is less than 500 cells/μL, platelets less than 50,000 cells/μL, or the patient exhibits grade III mucositis, then further methotrexate dosing is held; when resumed, methotrexate dosing is re-initiated at 80% of the previous dose.
- Methotrexate dosing would also be held for increases in serum creatinine (e.g., 1.5 times baseline creatinine), increases in hepatic transaminase levels (e.g., greater than 10 times the upper limit of normal), or hyperbilirubinemia (i.e., >2 mg/dL).

Because escalating methotrexate treatment does not include leucovorin rescue or methotrexate concentration monitoring, the only means by which to determine whether a patient is tolerating methotrexate is by careful monitoring of clinical and laboratory parameters. Without following such guidelines, severe methotrexate toxicity could occur. Such toxicity typically consists of myelosuppression and mucositis. In more severe cases, both renal and hepatic toxicity could occur. This type of escalating dosing is only possible because most children have excellent renal function and thus have fairly predictable methotrexate clearance. However, with higher doses of methotrexate (e.g., 1 g/m^2), all patients would require both leucovorin rescue and methotrexate concentration monitoring until the drug is adequately cleared.

MAINTENANCE CHEMOTHERAPY REGIMENS

CASE 91-5, QUESTION 13: After completion of his induction and postinduction treatments, J.B. is scheduled to receive maintenance (continuation) treatment for a total therapy duration of 2.5 years from the start of his induction therapy. His parents question why treatment will be of such a long duration and ask whether this is necessary because J.B. is already in remission. What is the purpose of J.B.'s maintenance or continuation treatment for ALL? Which agents should be used in J.B. for this phase of therapy?

Maintenance or continuation treatment sustains the complete remission achieved from induction chemotherapy. Early trials have shown that without maintenance treatment, the majority of ALL patients will relapse.[166] Patients who have successfully responded to induction and postinduction therapy may still have a high leukemic cell burden (although undetectable), which must be eradicated by additional treatment. This is supported by the results of bone marrow biopsies from patients who have experienced relapse after several months to years of treatment. The cytogenetic characteristics of the leukemic cells in relapsed patients are identical to those at the time of diagnosis.[228,229] Maintenance therapy is also supported by the results of MRD studies, which demonstrate that some amount of measurable leukemic cells are still present months after the completion of induction therapy.[154,159]

Drugs that are effective during induction therapy cannot, by themselves, sustain remission during maintenance therapy.[102] However, other agents are effective in sustaining a complete remission. Two of the most effective drugs are mercaptopurine and methotrexate.[174,230] Methotrexate is most effective and least toxic when administered intermittently, usually on a weekly basis in oral doses of 20 mg/m^2/week. Mercaptopurine is effective and well tolerated orally when dosed daily, usually at a dose of 50 to 75 mg/m^2/day.

Other agents have been added to standard maintenance therapy with mercaptopurine and methotrexate to improve remission duration and to increase a patient's chances for long-term survival. There is evidence that monthly pulses of vincristine and prednisone offer advantages (lower bone marrow and testicular relapse rates) in standard-risk patients as well.[231] At present, most contemporary treatment regimens for childhood ALL have intensified induction and postinduction phases during approximately the first 6 months.[177,178,223,226,227] These early intensive treatments typically are followed by a less intensive maintenance therapy consisting of methotrexate and mercaptopurine in combination with periodic IT chemotherapy treatments, either with or without intermittent vincristine/prednisone pulses.[177,178,223,226,227]

The available evidence suggests that a patient like J.B. with standard-risk ALL will benefit from use of daily mercaptopurine 50 to 75 mg/m^2 orally (PO) and weekly methotrexate 20 mg/m^2 PO or IV, along with periodic pulse therapy with vincristine 1.5 mg/m^2 for 1 day and either prednisone 40 mg/m^2 or dexamethasone 6 mg/m^2 PO for 7 days every 4 weeks. In addition, IT methotrexate should be repeated every 8 to 12 weeks.

DOSING OF METHOTREXATE AND MERCAPTOPURINE MAINTENANCE

CASE 91-5, QUESTION 14: After 8 weeks of maintenance therapy with the aforementioned regimen, J.B. has had an ANC that has ranged between 2,000 and 3,500 cells/μL for more than 6 weeks. Other hematologic and chemistry findings are also within normal limits. Should any changes in his maintenance therapy be considered at this time? Are there any potential problems with mercaptopurine and methotrexate that could explain his ANC values? Could normal ANCs increase his risk of treatment failure?

Diurnal variation of methotrexate concentration and marked interpatient variability in absorption and metabolism of mercaptopurine have been described, which may explain the varied response among patients to standard doses.[232–234] Most patients are able to tolerate full doses of mercaptopurine, which is inactivated by the enzyme thiopurine-*S*-methyltransferase (TPMT). It is known that approximately 89% to 94% of patients have high TPMT activity, 6% to 11% have intermediate activity, and 0.3% have deficient activity. Patients with deficient TPMT activity experience severe and even fatal toxicity with standard mercaptopurine doses and require very low doses (approximately 10 mg/m^2 three times per week) for avoidance of profound myelosuppression.[235,236]

Patients receiving half doses of these agents have shorter remission durations[237]; however, even those who tolerate maximal protocol dosages may also be at greater risk of relapse.[114] Patients who are able to tolerate maximal doses without significant myelosuppression may require doses that are higher than protocol initiation doses. Investigations, including studies of intracellular concentrations of active metabolites, have not found the pharmacokinetics of mercaptopurine or methotrexate to be predictive of outcome in children with ALL.[238–240] However, one of these trials demonstrated that dose intensity of mercaptopurine was a significant predictor of eventfree survival.[238] In addition, studies have shown that higher WBC or ANC values during maintenance therapy are associated with an increased risk of relapse.[230,241] Because bioavailability is a concern for both agents and because some patients, particularly males, may be able to tolerate higher dosages without toxicity, doses are often adjusted upward based on ANC. Some protocols allow for dosage increases of methotrexate or mercaptopurine every 4 to 6 weeks to maintain a target ANC in the range of 300 to 2,000 cells/μL.[238,239] This is usually accomplished by alternately increasing the doses of mercaptopurine and methotrexate by 25%. In this situation, dose increases of one of these agents are performed every 4 to 6 weeks.

J.B. has a normal ANC and is tolerating therapy; therefore, it is reasonable to attempt to intensify his chemotherapy dosing. For J.B., this means an increase in mercaptopurine from 50 mg/day to a daily schedule alternating 50 mg with 75 mg, or an increased methotrexate dose from 20 to 25 mg/week. Although parenteral administration of methotrexate provides more predictable levels and improved compliance, it does not consistently improve the results of therapy.[240,242] To assess whether J.B. is receiving an adequate dose, weekly WBC counts are essential. This allows his treatment team to accurately appraise the adequacy of his dose and to follow his disease status to ensure that remission is continuing. If an inadequate degree of myelosuppression is demonstrated, J.B.'s compliance should be investigated because decreased compliance is a frequent problem in the therapy of childhood ALL.[243–245] At least one investigation has found improved compliance with evening administration of mercaptopurine.[243]

DURATION OF THERAPY

CASE 91-5, QUESTION 15: How long should J.B.'s maintenance therapy be continued?

Most centers treat children with ALL until a total therapy duration of approximately 2.5 years is reached.[246,247] Extending maintenance treatment to 5 or 6 years adds no benefit.[246,247] Other data suggest that a shorter duration of 18 months may be adequate for girls, but not for boys.[248] Most patients who experience relapse do so during therapy or within the first year of completing therapy. After the second year of therapy and for every year thereafter, relapses become much less common, but are occasionally observed. Some centers are exploring whether more intensive treatment protocols could decrease the duration of maintenance treatment because the current duration is based on data from less aggressive protocols. Until there is more conclusive evidence regarding the duration of ALL maintenance therapy, patients with J.B.'s characteristics should receive chemotherapy for approximately 2.5 years.

HIGH-RISK ACUTE LYMPHOBLASTIC LEUKEMIA TREATMENT

PREVENTION OF TUMOR LYSIS SYNDROME

CASE 91-6

QUESTION 1: N.B. is a 12-year-old Hispanic boy with a 4-week to 5-week history of an enlarging right-sided neck mass. On physical examination, he is found to have a 6 × 3 cm right neck mass with extension to the nape of the neck. Radiography of the chest indicates an anterior mediastinal mass. The CBC reveals a WBC count of 62,000 cells/μL (43% lymphoblasts, 27% neutrophils, and 27% lymphocytes), Hct of 41.5%, and platelet count of 83,000 cells/μL. Other pertinent laboratory results are uric acid of 15.1 mg/dL and LDH of 1,636 units/L. A bone marrow biopsy confirms the diagnosis of ALL and shows that 85% of the bone marrow is replaced by leukemic lymphoblasts. The leukemic cells are T lymphoblasts, and their DNA index is 1.0. A lumbar puncture reveals a few cells within the CSF that are terminal deoxynucleotidal transferase negative, but are rather suspicious.

N.B. is started on rasburicase 0.2 mg/kg/day for 1 to 3 days (instead of allopurinol, hydration, and alkalinization). Because N.B. is diagnosed with T-cell ALL, he is begun on an intensive protocol. The induction regimen consists of six drugs, including prednisone 40 mg/m^2/day PO on days 1 to 29; vincristine 1.5 mg/m^2 IV weekly for 5 weeks; cyclophosphamide 1 g/m^2 on day 1 and 600 mg/m^2 on day 22; doxorubicin 50 mg/m^2 on day 1; cytarabine 100 mg/m^2/day via continuous infusion for 5 days starting on day 22; and asparaginase 10,000 units/m^2 intramuscularly (IM) on days 27, 29, and 31. Triple IT therapy of methotrexate 15 mg, cytarabine 30 mg, and hydrocortisone 15 mg will be administered weekly for 6 weeks. Why was rasburicase used instead of standard TLS preventive strategies?

Allopurinol is the standard prophylactic regimen for TLS; however, despite its use some high-risk patients with large tumor burdens may still exhibit urate nephropathy. Patients with a significant elevation in uric acid or renal dysfunction may not derive significant early benefit from the allopurinol, which is designed to prevent the formation of additional uric acid and to aid in its excretion. Significant elevations in uric acid or renal dysfunction may even delay the initiation of chemotherapy. Rasburicase is a recombinant form of urate oxidase, the enzyme that catalyzes the conversion of uric acid to the more water-soluble allantoin, and is an alternative to allopurinol. Rasburicase produces a dramatic reduction in uric acid within 4 hours of administration. Uric acid is often reduced below the normal range, and additional daily doses are not necessary if uric acid normalizes and remains within normal limits. Given N.B.'s significantly elevated uric acid and large tumor mass, he is at high risk for TLS and is a good candidate for initial management with rasburicase. Rasburicase obviates the need for allopurinol, hydration, and alkalinization.[249]

LONG-TERM COMPLICATIONS

CASE 91-6, QUESTION 2: N.B. achieves a complete remission based on the results of a bone marrow specimen on day 29. His parents are concerned about the doxorubicin because they have heard about heart problems with this drug. His protocol includes significant doses of this agent throughout his treatment plan. They ask about the likelihood for cardiac toxicity, what might be done to screen for it, and whether any preventive strategies exist that might be of value. What are the recommended screening tools and preventive strategies for anthracycline cardiotoxicity in children?

The relationship between cumulative anthracycline dose and cardiotoxicity is well established; a dramatic increase in congestive heart failure (CHF) is observed at cumulative doses larger than 450 mg/m^2.[84,250] However, because this is a median dose for cardiotoxicity, limiting the total dose to this threshold will not protect all patients. At least one study has demonstrated that both biochemical and echocardiographic abnormalities can be seen in childhood cancer survivors after lower cumulative anthracycline doses.[251] Although some early reports suggested reversibility in children, subsequent follow-up data confirm a worsening of CHF over time.[252–255] Late-occurring cardiotoxicity (i.e., years after completion of chemotherapy) has been reported in children.[255,256] The investigators for one of these studies used a very sensitive echocardiography technique and reported that the majority of patients had either abnormal contractility or afterload.[256] Another group of investigators used a less sensitive echocardiography technique and reported a lower incidence of cardiotoxicity, although the rate of abnormalities was shown to increase substantially with longer patient follow-up.[255] Recent prospective studies of long-term cardiac function after anthracycline therapy in children show a continual decrement in left ventricular function years after chemotherapy.[257] It is currently unclear what the long-term risk of CHF is in children. Close patient follow-up is important for early detection, although currently used screening tools such as echocardiography detect only functional damage and have not demonstrated value in preventing CHF. Newer nuclear medicine probes are promising for early detection of anthracycline-induced cardiotoxicity and may be used in the future for identifying children before the development of functional deficits.[258] Dexrazoxane, an intracellular iron chelator, has been studied for its effectiveness in preventing anthracycline-induced CHF in adults.[259,260] However, because there was a decreased antitumor response in dexrazoxane-treated patients in one of these trials, it was subsequently studied at a reduced dose. It has been approved for use only in women with breast cancer who have received a cumulative anthracycline dose of 300 mg/m^2. In one small trial in children with sarcoma, dexrazoxane decreased the risk of cardiotoxicity and improved tolerance of higher cumulative anthracycline doses.[261] However, the left ventricular ejection fraction declined in both groups receiving higher cumulative anthracycline doses. A more recent study using serum troponin T elevations as a surrogate marker for cardiac damage demonstrated that children with ALL randomly assigned to receive dexrazoxane with each dose of doxorubicin were less likely to have elevations of troponin T levels, but eventfree survival was not different between the group receiving dexrazoxane versus those receiving doxorubicin alone. Also, it is unclear whether these differences in serum troponin T will translate into differences in cardiotoxicity because the study did not report the results of echocardiography.[262] In summary, whether dexrazoxane circumvents the long-term risk of anthracycline-induced CHF in children is unclear. Some degree of long-term cardiotoxicity or CHF risk in children may be unavoidable when an anthracycline is used, even if it is combined with dexrazoxane. Because anthracyclines are an important component of many ALL treatment protocols and have figured significantly into the improved survival rates achieved in high-risk patients in recent years, the benefits seem to outweigh the risks in these patients at present. Although N.B. will be monitored closely for cardiac deterioration, there is currently no proven way to completely eliminate the risk of cardiotoxicity, although restricting children to a cumulative dose of less than 300 mg/m^2 has resulted in a low frequency of late occurring cardiotoxicity.[263]

CASE 91-6, QUESTION 3: His parents also ask about other potential long-term sequelae from his treatment. What are other long-term sequelae that N.B. is at risk of experiencing?

Many survivors of childhood ALL therapy lose bone mineral density.[264–268] This has been attributed to both corticosteroids and cranial radiation therapy. Studies of osteonecrosis in childhood ALL demonstrate an overall incidence of 1.1% to 1.8%.[265,266] However, patient age at the time of treatment is an important risk factor with an incidence of 0.2% in children younger than 10 years, but 8.9% in patients 10 years and 16.7% in those 15 years. Most patients experienced osteonecrosis in two or more joints. There is a fairly clear relationship between the cumulative dose of corticosteroid received and the incidence of osteonecrosis. An increased risk of fractures during chemotherapy has also been reported in children with ALL.[268] The risks of bone pathology in survivors of childhood ALL argue in favor of close monitoring as well as optimization of mineral supplementation.

ASPARAGINASE-RELATED COMPLICATIONS

CASE 91-6, QUESTION 4: After completing induction therapy, N.B. is scheduled to receive a 25-week consolidation therapy consisting of vincristine/prednisone pulses, along with doxorubicin 30 mg/m^2 every 3 weeks, in addition to oral mercaptopurine and three IV doses of methotrexate 5 g/m^2 on weeks 7, 10, and 13. Weekly asparaginase at a dose of 25,000 units/m^2 IM will also be given weekly for the first 20 weeks. Is this the usual dose of asparaginase? What is the therapeutic value of asparaginase treatment in patients with T-cell leukemia?

This dosage of asparaginase is higher than that usually used in the treatment of lower risk ALL (6,000–10,000 units/m^2). This is based on a study of T-cell ALL, in which patients were randomly assigned to receive asparaginase 25,000 units/m^2 IM every week or not for 20 doses. There was a significant improvement in continuous complete remission at 4 years for those who had received the additional high-dose asparaginase therapy (68% vs. 55%). This provided evidence that patients with

T-cell ALL may achieve long-term remission rates similar to those of other ALL immunologic subtypes.[139] At present, studies are being conducted to replace native *E. coli* asparaginase with PEG asparaginase to decrease the potential for immunogenicity. Furthermore, the addition of high-dose methotrexate has increased relapsefree survival rates to approximately 80% in patients with T-cell ALL.

CASE 91-6, QUESTION 5: Two weeks after his vincristine, doxorubicin, prednisone, mercaptopurine regimen and 5 days after his fifth dose of asparaginase, N.B. exhibits severe epigastric abdominal pain and hyperglycemia. N.B. has been having normal bowel movements and does not have abdominal distension. The serum amylase is markedly elevated to 450 international units/L. Which agent is likely responsible for N.B.'s abdominal pain? What other complications are associated with asparaginase?

ASPARAGINASE-RELATED PANCREATITIS

Pancreatitis has been noted in children after the administration of asparaginase.[269] As illustrated by N.B., this often presents as abdominal pain accompanied by an elevated serum amylase and hyperglycemia. Insulin may be required to control the hyperosmotic, nonketotic hyperglycemia that may result.[270,271] The pancreatitis is occasionally severe, and fatalities have been reported.[272] Unfortunately, the serum amylase may not predict whether patients will experience acute fatal pancreatitis.[272] N.B.'s pancreatitis secondary to asparaginase makes further treatment with this agent inadvisable.[273] Because this reaction is not a hypersensitivity reaction, further therapy with the Erwinia form of asparaginase is also not recommended. N.B. may be treated with supportive care and insulin therapy. He should recover fully and be able to receive further chemotherapy but without the asparaginase.

ASPARAGINASE-RELATED HYPERSENSITIVITY REACTIONS

Hypersensitivity reactions to asparaginase are common, occurring in 20% to 35% of patients, but they are usually mild, generally presenting as urticarial eruptions.[270] Premedication does not appear to prevent subsequent reactions in most patients.[274] Severe anaphylactoid reactions may occur and can be fatal.[275] Clinical reactions correlate better with asparaginase-specific IgG rather than IgE antibodies, and severe hypersensitivity reactions can be explained in most instances by complement activation.[276,277] Anaphylactoid reactions appear to be less common when asparaginase is administered intramuscularly.[278,279] This is because the slow absorption of asparaginase after IM administration results in delayed, less severe acute reactions. Because these reactions can be delayed, prolonged monitoring is recommended after IM asparaginase.[280] Most serious hypersensitivity reactions tend to occur after the patient has received several doses.

A significant number of patients receiving asparaginase as a component of ALL treatment test positive for antiasparaginase IgG antibodies, and antibody concentrations are significantly higher in patients who experience a hypersensitivity reaction.[274] Patients who are receiving asparaginase may also experience "silent" immune clearance (a type of hypersensitivity), which results in a rapid clearance of asparaginase from the plasma but without an allergic reaction.[281–283] Patients with silent immune clearance may not obtain benefit from asparaginase and may be at greater risk for treatment failure.[284] More recently, the prevalence of antibodies to asparaginase has been investigated. It was demonstrated that asparaginase antibody titers were present in 61% of patients receiving native *E. coli* asparaginase during induction therapy (including 29% with silent hypersensitivity). It was also shown that the majority (73%) of patients with detectible antibodies to asparaginase did not have measurable asparaginase activity in their serum. Preliminary analysis from this study also demonstrated a relationship between antibody titers and outcomes, with patients with silent hypersensitivity more likely to have an adverse outcome.[285] Because premedication usually does not prevent future reactions and because of the possibility that patients who exhibit hypersensitivity may derive no benefit from asparaginase, it appears that the best course of action is to switch patients from the *E. coli* preparation to an alternate asparaginase preparation.

ASPARAGINASE PREPARATIONS

Asparaginase is available from two natural sources, *E. coli* and *Erwinia*. These two preparations are not 100% cross-reactive, so the *Erwinia* product may be substituted for the *E. coli* product when hypersensitivity reactions occur.[286] However, one should be aware that cross-reactions occur in 17% to 26% of patients.[170,287] Because of the shorter half-life of the *Erwinia* product, a dosage increase of *Erwinia* asparaginase is necessary to equal the activity of the *E. coli* product.[288] Of note, patients receiving equivalent doses of *Erwinia* asparaginase have a poorer remission rate and survival than those patients receiving the *E. coli* asparaginase.[289] In contemporary protocols, the dose of *Erwinia* asparaginase is typically about 2.5 times greater than the *E. coli* asparaginase dose. The incidences of rash and silent immune clearance appear to be equivalent for these two preparations.[286]

Asparaginase is also available in a modified form known as pegaspargase. This agent is formed by covalently linking monomethoxy PEG to *E. coli* asparaginase. Pegaspargase has a prolonged half-life of 5.8 days compared with 1.2 days for *E. coli* asparaginase and appears to be safe and effective, even in patients with prior reactions to *E. coli* and *Erwinia* asparaginase.[290] The prolonged half-life allows for less frequent (i.e., every 2 weeks) dosing of PEG asparaginase than for the natural source asparaginase products (i.e., three times a week).[282] Asparaginase compounds derived from different *E. coli* strains may differ in both enzyme activity and half-life. At least one study has reported an unexpected mortality rate in childhood ALL associated with an assumption of equivalence among different *E. coli* asparaginase preparations.[291]

ASPARAGINASE-INDUCED COAGULATION DISORDERS

Asparaginase is known to cause decreases in albumin, fibrinogen, and α and β globulins, owing to its effects on general protein synthesis, which can result in inhibition of the synthesis of various clotting factors.[292,293] Asparaginase may also produce abnormalities in coagulation-inhibition and fibrinolytic system, along with deficiencies in antithrombin III and plasminogen.[292,293] This complex series of events can result in coagulopathies, occasionally leading to cerebral hemorrhage or infarction.[170,292–294] Some have suggested monitoring markers of the coagulation-inhibiting and fibrinolytic system to identify patients at risk for severe coagulation disturbances,[292] but no prospective studies support this practice. A higher risk of thrombotic events has been observed among children with central venous catheters or a genetic predisposition.[295,296] There is also a greater risk of thromboembolism in children receiving native asparaginase in combination with prednisone versus dexamethasone, perhaps due to greater inhibition of prostaglandin and thromboxane synthesis by the latter agent.[297]

Relapsed Acute Lymphoblastic Leukemia

PROGNOSIS

CASE 91-7

QUESTION 1: About 17 months after his initial diagnosis, N.B. undergoes a routine lumbar puncture as part of his planned maintenance therapy. Analysis of the CSF indicates the presence of numerous lymphoblasts. A CBC reveals the following:

Hct, 29.5%
Platelet count, 120,000 cells/μL
WBC, 5,300 cells/μL, with 45% lymphocytes, 50% neutrophils, and 5% bands

A bone marrow biopsy confirms relapsed ALL, with 53% lymphoblasts. What are N.B.'s chances of achieving a second remission and long-term survival? Are there specific features about N.B.'s relapse which confer a worse prognosis?

N.B. is asymptomatic at the time of relapse, as are most patients experiencing a relapse of ALL. Most of these patients are diagnosed by routine CBCs or lumbar punctures. Although ALL patients typically have excellent responses to treatment after relapse, 20% to 25% of patients will relapse again, and most will not be long-time survivors. Routine bone marrow biopsies may identify bone marrow relapses before they become evident on a CBC, but it has not been demonstrated that earlier identification of bone marrow relapse by morphologic criteria impacts long-term survival.[298–301]

At least 80% of relapsed ALL patients will achieve a second remission with salvage chemotherapy.[298,299,302] Unfortunately, bone marrow relapse in childhood ALL is associated with poor long-term survival and most patients will not be cured of their disease.[298–302] Rates of 5-year diseasefree survival vary from 6% to 60% for patients with bone marrow relapse, and are dependent on multiple variables.[298–300, 303–305] N.B.'s situation has several features which confer a worse prognosis on relapse including male sex, both marrow and CNS relapse, T-cell disease, and relapse less than 18 months from initial diagnosis.[300,301]

TREATMENT OF RELAPSED ACUTE LYMPHOBLASTIC LEUKEMIA

CASE 91-7, QUESTION 2: Which treatments could be used in an attempt to attain a complete remission and improve N.B.'s chances of long-term survival?

Agents used in salvage regimens are similar to those used in high-risk ALL regimens. In general, treatment usually consists of an intensive four-agent induction regimen of vincristine, prednisone, daunorubicin, and asparaginase. This is accompanied by radiation therapy to sites of local relapse (e.g., testis, CNS) and IT chemotherapy.[304–306] After this regimen has been completed, the patient may continue with courses of intensification therapy, continuation therapy, and IT therapy.[304,305] Relapsed regimens will include more intensive chemotherapy including high-dose methotrexate and high-dose cytarabine as well as etoposide and cyclophosphamide. High-dose methotrexate has excellent penetration into the central nervous system and can be used to treat and prevent CNS leukemia relapses. High-dose cytarabine (HiDAC, 3 g/m^2 every 12 hours for four doses) in conjunction with standard-dose asparaginase may be used to induce a remission in patients who fail reinduction therapy. This approach has been successful in approximately 40% of patients, although the median duration of second remission was only 3 months.[307] The selection of a salvage regimen will depend on how intensive the patient's initial therapy was, whether or not the relapse occurred while on therapy, and sites of relapse. In N.B.'s case, his regimen should include intensive therapy, preferably with chemotherapy drugs and regimens to which he has not been previously exposed, because his relapse occurred while he was on therapy. Additionally, he will have CNS radiation and intrathecal chemotherapy aimed at treating his specific sites of relapse.

CASE 91-7, QUESTION 3: N.B.'s family is quite concerned about the poor prognosis associated with his relapse and inquire about the role of hematopoietic cell transplantation (HCT) in his relapse treatment. Should he be considered for HCT at this point? Knowing the potential morbidity and mortality associated with allogeneic transplantation, would autologous transplant be a more appropriate option for N.B?

Allogeneic HCT is emerging as a superior treatment option for children with relapsed ALL who have high-risk and intermediate-risk features. In patients who receive a matched sibling HCT during their second complete remission for relapsed ALL, eventfree survival rates of 48% at 7 years and 52% at 5 years have been reported versus chemotherapy alone producing 9% eventfree survival at 7 years and 22% at 5 years.[308,309] Autologous HCT does not appear to be superior to standard chemotherapy for children with ALL in second remission, and should not be offered.[310,311] N.B.'s family should be offered the option of allogeneic HCT and his family should be tested for an appropriate sibling match, as this offers lower morbidity than an unrelated donor. Because his outcome in transplant improves if performed during a second complete remission, he should begin reinduction chemotherapy while HCT is being arranged. If HCT does not prove to be a feasible option for N.B., novel therapies may be considered. Nelarabine is a purine analogue approved for the treatment of relapsed T-cell leukemias and lymphomas and has shown response rates (complete and partial remission) as high as 55% in pediatric populations.[312,313]

PEDIATRIC NON-HODGKIN LYMPHOMA

Lymphomas are a collection of diseases originating in cells and organs of the immune system. Lymphomas account for approximately 10% to 15% of all childhood malignancies, but they are less common in children than in adults. Children younger than 16 years account for only 3% of all lymphoma cases. The malignancy can occur in any lymphoid cell at any level of differentiation and appears to be a consequence of a genetic alteration. Non-Hodgkin lymphoma (NHL) is the most common form of lymphoma in children younger than 10 years of age, whereas Hodgkin lymphoma is most common in children 15 to 19 years of age. This section will focus on NHL. Considerable progress has been made in the treatment of children with NHL, and currently approximately 80% are cured.[314]

Classification

Numerous classification systems for NHL exist, and there is considerable variation in terminology among these systems.[315–318] Pediatric NHLs are best classified using histopathology, which divides them into three different categories: B-cell lymphomas, lymphoblastic lymphomas, and anaplastic large cell lymphomas.[314] This is a narrower range of histologic types than in adults.

Lymphoblastic lymphomas account for approximately 30% of childhood NHLs, B-cell lymphomas for about 50%, and large cell lymphomas for the remainder.[314] The lymphoblastic lymphomas are usually immature T cells that are histologically identical to the cells of ALL. The distinction between lymphoblastic lymphoma and ALL is made on the basis of bone marrow involvement, with ALL being diagnosed if there is greater than 25% bone marrow infiltration. This distinction is made by the amount of bone marrow infiltration that is present at the time of diagnosis. B-cell lymphomas may be further divided into Burkitt, Burkittlike, and large B-cell lymphomas. Anaplastic large cell lymphomas may be T cell or null cell in origin.

Clinical Presentation

Pediatric patients with NHL may present with a number of different symptoms, many of which are related to the type of NHL. In general, these symptoms differ from those in adults because of the propensity of pediatric NHLs to be extranodal in origin in contrast to the common nodal presentation of adult NHL.[314] Patients with lymphoblastic lymphoma commonly present with a mediastinal mass or pleural effusions.[314] They also may have pain, dyspnea, or swelling of the face and upper arms if superior vena cava obstruction is present. Lymphoblastic lymphoma also has a predilection for the bone marrow and the CNS.[319,320] Lymphadenopathy in patients with lymphoblastic lymphoma tends to be supradiaphragmatic. Patients with B-cell NHL typically present with an abdominal tumor, abdominal pain, an alteration in bowel function, and possibly nausea and vomiting.[321] In addition, many patients with B-cell NHL present with bone marrow involvement.[314] Lymphadenopathy in these patients typically occurs below the diaphragm in the inguinal or iliac area. Anaplastic large cell lymphomas may involve the gut or unusual sites such as the lung, skin, face, or CNS.[314]

Staging

Several staging systems for pediatric NHLs are used.[321] A commonly used staging system for pediatric NHL is the St. Jude staging system.[314] This staging system includes four stages, with stage I being a single tumor or a single nodal area, and higher stages including cases with regional involvement or more than one anatomical site involved. The highest stage (stage IV) refers to patients with bone marrow or CNS involvement. The main predictor of outcome in pediatric patients with NHL has historically been determined by tumor burden at presentation.[322] However, with modern chemotherapy regimens that are tailored to the extent of disease, patients with higher-stage disease may achieve a similar eventfree survival to that achieved in patients with lower-stage disease.[314,323] A higher LDH is correlated with greater tumor burden. It has also been demonstrated that serum LDH greater than or equal to 500 to 1,000 units/L was a significant predictor of poorer outcome.[314]

Overview of Treatment

LYMPHOBLASTIC (T CELL)

The primary treatment for all stages and histologic types of pediatric NHL is combination chemotherapy because it is a generalized disease at the time of diagnosis.[314] A wide variety of chemotherapy agents have activity in childhood NHL. At present, the best results to date are reported by the BFM group, with an estimated 5-year eventfree survival of approximately 92% (Table 91-10).[323] This regimen uses an intensive scheme of multiagent chemotherapy administered during 24 months. Patients with lymphoblastic lymphoma require longer treatment duration than patients with B-cell or anaplastic large cell lymphoma. This chemotherapy plan is similar to that used in the treatment of ALL and is designed to deliver continuous or weekly therapy. All patients with lymphoblastic lymphoma are given CNS preventive therapy, regardless of stage. Few patients with lymphoblastic lymphoma present with limited disease (stages I and II), thus making it difficult to conduct adequate studies in this patient population. Attempts to shorten the duration of therapy for patients with limited-stage disease have been unsuccessful, although less-intensive therapy is administered to patients with early-stage disease on some protocols.[314]

B CELL

The main differences between the treatment of lymphoblastic and B-cell lymphoma are the use of more agents and longer treatment duration in the former. The trend in the treatment of B-cell lymphomas has been toward short-duration, intensive therapy with alkylating agents in conjunction with high-dose antimetabolite therapy (e.g., methotrexate, cytarabine). Chemotherapy is administered in rapid succession with limited recovery from neutropenia (i.e., ANC 500 cells/μL) between cycles. Patients with localized B-cell lymphomas respond as adequately to a four-drug regimen (consisting of cyclophosphamide, vincristine, methotrexate, and prednisone) as they do to more aggressive regimens.[314]

Evidence suggests that a 6-month course is as efficacious as an 18-month course for patients with localized B-cell lymphomas.[314] Studies indicate that even 6 months of chemotherapy may be unnecessary for patients with limited-stage disease because it has been demonstrated that maintenance treatment offered no additional benefit after 9 weeks of combination chemotherapy.[314] Contemporary chemotherapy regimens include varying degrees of treatment intensity from three to seven cycles, depending on whether the tumor is completely resected, on bone marrow and CNS involvement, and the serum LDH.[324]

With the addition of high-dose methotrexate, ifosfamide, etoposide, and HiDAC to the standard regimen, patients with stage III disease are now achieving survival rates comparable to those of patients with limited-stage disease.[324] Patients with bone marrow disease also benefit from these intensive therapeutic strategies and have achieved impressive survival rates of approximately 80%.[314] Currently, patients with advanced-stage disease are treated with a total of six to eight cycles of chemotherapy, and these treatment protocols achieve superior results to those of a much longer duration (e.g., 1–2 years) used previously.[314,324,325] Although rituximab is now a standard therapy component for B-cell lymphomas in adults, it has yet to be routinely used in frontline treatment in the pediatric arena. Case reports demonstrate the utility of this agent when added to a standard chemotherapy backbone for children with relapsed disease.[326,327]

LARGE CELL

Large cell lymphomas have responded well to both types of regimens.[314,328,329] Thus, the use of shorter, less complicated, B-cell protocols is appropriate. Patients who fail to respond may be treated with additional courses of their prescribed protocol in hopes of eventually inducing a response. Patients who relapse may be reinduced with intensive chemotherapy, but their prognosis for long-term survival is unfavorable.

TABLE 91-10
BFM Group Treatment Protocols for T-Cell Lymphoblastic Lymphoma

Drug	Dose	Days of Administration
Induction Protocol I (All Stages)		
Prednisone (PO)	60 mg/m^2	1–28, then taper
Vincristine (IV)	1.5 mg/m^2 (max 2 mg)	8, 15, 22, 29
Daunorubicin (IV for 1 hour)	30 mg/m^2	8, 15, 22, 29
L-asparaginase (IV[a] for 1 hour)	10,000 international units/m^2	12, 15, 18, 21, 24, 27, 30, 33
Cyclophosphamide[b] (IV for 1 hour)	1,000 mg/m^2	36, 64
Cytarabine (IV)	75 mg/m^2	38–41, 45–48, 52–55, 59–62
6-Mercaptopurine (PO)	60 mg/m^2	36–63
Methotrexate (IT)	12 mg	1, 15, 29, 45, 59
Protocol M (Typically Stages I and II)		
Mercaptopurine (PO)	25 mg/m^2	1–56
Methotrexate (IV)	5 g/m^2	8, 22, 36, 50
Methotrexate (IT)	12 mg	8, 22, 36, 50
Reinduction Protocol II (Stages III and IV Only)		
Dexamethasone (PO)	10 mg/m^2	1–21, then taper
Vincristine (IV)	1.5 mg/m^2 (max 2 mg)	8, 15, 22, 29
Doxorubicin (IV for 1 hour)	30 mg/m^2	8, 15, 22, 29
L-asparaginase (IV[a] for 1 hour)	10,000 international units/m^2	8, 11, 15, 18
Cyclophosphamide[b] (IV for 1 hour)	1,000 mg/m^2	36
Cytarabine (IV)	75 mg/m^2	38–41, 45–48
Thioguanine (PO)	60 mg/m^2	36–49
Methotrexate (IT)	12 mg	38, 45
Maintenance (All Stages)		
Mercaptopurine (PO)	50 mg/m^2	Daily until month 24 of therapy
Methotrexate (PO)	20 mg/m^2	Weekly until month 24 of therapy

[a]This agent is typically administered intramuscularly in most treatment protocols in the United States.
[b]With mesna.
Note. IT methotrexate doses were adjusted for children younger than 3 years. Ten percent (10%) of the 5 g/m^2 methotrexate dose in Protocol M was given for 30 minutes, and 90% was given as a 23.5-hour continuous IV infusion. Leucovorin rescue: 30 mg/m^2 IV at hour 42; 15 mg/m^2 IV at hours 48 and 54.
Additional doses are given on days 8 and 22 for CNS-positive patients.
CNS, central nervous system; IT, intrathecally; IV, intravenously; PO, orally.
Source: Watanabe A et al. Undifferentiated lymphoma, non-Burkitt's type: meningeal and bone marrow involvement in children. *Am J Dis Child* 1973;125:57.

Lymphoblastic Lymphoma

ACUTE TREATMENT

CASE 91-8

QUESTION 1: D.B., a 16-year-old girl, presents with a history of shortness of breath and chest pain for 3 weeks before admission. A mediastinal mass is found, and a biopsy confirms a lymphoblastic (T-cell) lymphoma. Radiography of the chest reveals a right pleural effusion. Laboratory values show the following results:

Erythrocyte sedimentation rate, 35
WBC count, 22,000 cells/μL
Uric acid, 7 mg/dL
LDH, 1,259 units/L

The bone marrow, CNS, and abdomen are negative for lymphoma. How should D.B. be managed acutely? Besides chemotherapy, what types of adjunctive therapies should be initiated to minimize the acute effects of treatment?

Given D.B.'s shortness of breath and chest pain, it is likely that her mediastinal mass may be obstructing the superior vena cava. To alleviate this obstruction, the most appropriate course of action is to decrease the tumor mass by initiating chemotherapy as soon as possible. Radiation therapy offers no additional benefit in patients such as D.B. with a tumor such as NHL, which is highly responsive to chemotherapy.[314,330] Because of the high cell kill that will result from the initial chemotherapy treatment, TLS and uric acid nephropathy is possible. However, the risk of this complication is probably greater in patients with B-cell NHL in whom the fraction of cells in S phase is higher.[331,332]

Alkaline diuresis and allopurinol should be instituted before chemotherapy to prevent TLS. Because D.B. has a pleural effusion, fluids may collect in this third space, resulting in weight gain and decreased urine output. Thus, in addition to placement of a chest tube with suction, D.B. should be given diuretics to maintain an adequate urine output. To minimize intravascular volume depletion and maintain electrolyte balances, fluid input and output, body weight, and electrolyte panels should be monitored daily. These values should be used to make appropriate adjustments in D.B.'s electrolyte and fluid balance.

ADVERSE EFFECTS

CASE 91-8, QUESTION 2: D.B. is treated with the BFM combination chemotherapy regimen. Due to her intrathoracic mass, her disease is characterized as stage III. She is to receive induction therapy (Induction Protocol I) for 8 weeks,

as outlined in Table 91-10. Which acute adverse effects are D.B. likely to experience with these agents? How can they be monitored, minimized, and treated?

Several toxicities are expected with these chemotherapy agents. For vincristine, both constipation and neuropathy are likely to appear during or after the 4 weeks of therapy.[181] Constipation can be prevented or minimized by use of stool softeners with or without a laxative.[333] Neuropathy may be painful (especially when jaw pain occurs) but can be managed with mild analgesic regimens consisting of NSAIDs or acetaminophen with codeine. Both toxicities are self-limiting and are not reasons to discontinue or decrease the dosage of vincristine unless neuromuscular toxicity, as evidenced by motor weakness, develops. As outlined previously, asparaginase can cause several types of toxicities, most of which are not thought to be preventable.

Prednisone is likely to increase D.B.'s appetite and may cause gastritis, although divided doses will help decrease stomach upset. In addition, prednisone-induced behavioral disturbances are common.[183] Unlike prednisone and vincristine, daunorubicin, cyclophosphamide, cytarabine, and mercaptopurine produce significant myelosuppression. Leukopenia is common, with the nadir occurring in approximately 8 to 14 days and recovery occurring by approximately day 21 after administration. Because the goal of induction therapy is achievement of remission, doses of daunorubicin will not be held for uncomplicated myelosuppression during the first 4 weeks of induction therapy, although during the latter 4 weeks, the combination of cyclophosphamide, cytarabine, and mercaptopurine are typically held until hematologic recovery occurs.

Hemorrhagic cystitis may occur with cyclophosphamide, but it is usually associated with high-dose therapy or with prolonged administration, which D.B. is not receiving. Vigorous IV hydration to maintain urine output of approximately 50 to 100 mL/m^2/hour should reduce the risk of this toxicity at this dose. In addition, this chemotherapy protocol also includes mesna, which will bind to urotoxic metabolites of cyclophosphamide and also reduce the risk of hemorrhagic cystitis. Because most of the induction regimen will be administered on an outpatient basis, patients or parents should be instructed to report signs or symptoms of infection (e.g., febrile episodes) immediately so that proper treatment may be instituted as soon as possible. To decrease the risk of hemorrhagic cystitis, parents should be instructed to report whether patients are urinating regularly after cyclophosphamide.

Nausea and vomiting are likely to be induced by both daunorubicin and cyclophosphamide/cytarabine.[334] D.B.'s chemotherapy regimen includes a corticosteroid (prednisone), which may provide some antiemetic activity during the initial 4 weeks.[335] However, to maximize tolerance to her chemotherapy, D.B. should receive a 5-HT_3 serotonin antagonist. Ondansetron may be used in this setting and is more effective than metoclopramide when either is combined with a corticosteroid. D.B. is unlikely to require additional corticosteroids during the first 4 weeks of induction therapy. However, during the second portion of induction, D.B. will benefit from a few doses of dexamethasone at 10 mg/m^2 PO or IV at the time of cyclophosphamide administration.[334]

CENTRAL NERVOUS SYSTEM PROPHYLAXIS

CASE 91-8, QUESTION 3: What is the importance of CNS prophylaxis for D.B., and what type of treatment regimen is typically used?

All pediatric patients with lymphoblastic lymphoma should receive some form of CNS prophylaxis. Although lymphoblastic lymphoma rarely presents with CNS involvement, as illustrated by D.B., it was a common site of relapse before CNS prophylaxis was included as a routine part of the chemotherapy regimen.[319,320] Recurrence of NHL within the CNS is rare when intrathecal methotrexate or cytarabine are given.[314] D.B. will be treated with intrathecal methotrexate periodically, as outlined in Table 91-10.

MYELOSUPPRESSION AND HEMATOPOIETIC RECOVERY

CASE 91-8, QUESTION 4: After completion of induction therapy, the chemotherapy plan for D.B. consists of protocol M and reinduction protocol II, as outlined in Table 91-10. How should D.B.'s hematopoietic recovery be managed, and what guidelines may be used to determine when it is appropriate for her to receive the next sequence of the treatment cycle? Would D.B. benefit from a colony-stimulating factor to aid with hematopoietic recovery?

Protocol M will likely not produce significant myelosuppression because leucovorin rescue will reduce the myelosuppression from the high-dose methotrexate. The most challenging problems with this phase of treatment will be to confirm that the methotrexate has been properly eliminated and to continue aggressive hydration, alkalinization, and leucovorin dosing until the methotrexate level is nontoxic. Due to D.B.'s pleural effusion at the time of diagnosis, it should be confirmed that this has resolved before administration of high-dose methotrexate to avoid significantly delayed clearance because the pleural effusion could allow for third spacing of high doses of methotrexate. Pleural effusions are a relative contraindication to high-dose methotrexate. Methotrexate elimination has high interpatient and intrapatient variability, and necessitates close monitoring of methotrexate concentrations and renal function after each dose.

Protocol II will result in significant myelosuppression. However, as with protocol I, dosing of doxorubicin will not be held for uncomplicated myelosuppression. Similarly, during the second phase of this protocol, dosing of cytarabine and thioguanine will also not be held for uncomplicated myelosuppression. However, before initiating the second phase on day 36, clinicians will assure adequate hematologic recovery, typically defined as an ANC greater than 750 cells/μL and platelets greater than 100,000 cells/μL. It is unlikely that D.B. will benefit from a colony-stimulating factor during these phases of therapy. When myelosuppressive chemotherapy is given fairly continuously, as is the case with protocol II, there is little room for inserting doses of colony-stimulating factors on days where myelosuppressive chemotherapy is not being administered.

KEY REFERENCES AND WEBSITES

A full list of references for this chapter can be found at http://thepoint.lww.com/AT10e. Below are the key references and websites for this chapter, with the corresponding reference number in this chapter found in parentheses after the reference.

Key References

Bassen R, Hoelzer D. Modern therapy of acute lymphoblastic leukemia. *J Clin Oncol.* 2011;29:532.

Boissel N et al. Should adolescents with acute lymphoblastic leukemia be treated as old children or young adults? Comparison of the French FRALLE-93 and LALA-94 trials. *J Clin Oncol.* 2003;21:774. (107)

Borowitz MJ et al. Clinical significance of minimal residual disease in childhood acute lymphoblastic leukemia and its relationship to other prognostic factors: a Children's Oncology Group study. *Blood.* 2008;111:5477. (159)

Burger B et al. Osteonecrosis: a treatment related toxicity in childhood acute lymphoblastic leukemia (ALL) experiences from trial ALL-BFM 95. *Pediatr Blood Cancer.* 2005;44:220. (266)

Fernandez CV et al. Intrathecal vincristine: an analysis of reasons for recurrent fatal chemotherapeutic error with recommendations for prevention. *J Pediatr Hematol Oncol.* 1998;20:587. (212)

Holdsworth MT et al. Acute and delayed nausea and emesis control in pediatric oncology patients. *Cancer.* 2006;106:931. (334)

Hurwitz CA et al. Substituting dexamethasone for prednisone complicates remission induction in children with acute lymphoblastic leukemia. *Cancer.* 2000;88:1964. (172)

Kearney SL et al. Clinical course and outcome in children with acute lymphoblastic leukemia and asparaginase-associated pancreatitis. *Pediatr Blood Cancer.* 2009;53:162. (273)

Lipshultz SE et al. Chronic progressive cardiac dysfunction years after doxorubicin therapy for childhood acute lymphoblastic leukemia. *J Clin Oncol.* 2005;23:2629. (49)

Link MP, Weinstein H. Malignant non-Hodgkin's lymphomas in children. In: Pizzo PA, Poplack DG, eds. *Principles and Practice of Pediatric Oncology.* 6th ed. Philadelphia, PA: Lippincott Williams & Wilkins; 2010. (314)

Mahoney DH et al. Intermediate-dose intravenous methotrexate with intravenous mercaptopurine is superior to repetitive low-dose oral methotrexate with intravenous mercaptopurine for children with lower-risk B-lineage acute lymphoblastic leukemia: a Pediatric Oncology Group phase III trial. *J Clin Oncol.* 1998;16:246. (223)

Maris JM. Recent advances in neuroblastoma. *N Engl J Med.* 2010;362:2202.

McNeil DE et al. SEER update of incidence and trends in pediatric malignancies: acute lymphoblastic leukemia. *Med Pediatr Oncol.* 2002;39:554. (121)

Nguyen K et al. Factors influencing survival after relapse from acute lyphoblastic leukemia: a Children's Oncology Group Study. *Leukemia.* 2008;22:2142. (301)

Oeffinger KC et al. Chronic health conditions in adult survivors of childhood cancer. *N Engl J Med.* 2006;355:1572. (12)

Pizzo PA, Poplack DG, eds. *Principles and Practice of Pediatric Oncology.* 6th ed. Philadelphia, PA: Lippincott Williams & Wilkins; 2010.

Pollock BH. Where adolescents and young adults with cancer receive their care: does it matter? *J Clin Oncol.* 2007;25:4522. (11)

Pui C et al. Biology, risk stratification, and therapy of pediatric acute leukemias: an update. *J Clin Oncol.* 2011;29:551.

Rosoff PM. The two-edged sword of curing childhood cancer. *N Engl J Med.* 2006;355:1522. (13)

Schmiegelow K et al. The degree of myelosuppression during maintenance therapy of adolescents with B-lineage intermediate risk acute lymphoblastic leukemia predicts risk of relapse. *Leukemia.* 2010;24:715. (230)

Seibel NL et al. Early postinduction intensification therapy improves survival for children and adolescents with high-risk acute lymphoblastic leukemia: a report from the Children's Oncology Group. *Blood.* 2008;111:2548. (225)

Key Websites

Childhood Cancer Survivor Study. www.stjude.org/ccss

Children's Oncology Group Cure Search. Screening and management guidelines for survivors. www.survivorshipguidelines.org

92 Adult Hematologic Malignancies

Lynn Weber, Steve Stricker, Casey B. Williams, and Katie A. Won

CORE PRINCIPLES

	CHAPTER CASES
ACUTE MYELOID LEUKEMIA	
1 Acute myeloid leukemia (AML) generally appears suddenly and progresses rapidly. Death as a result of infection or bleeding occurs within weeks to months if the patient is not effectively treated.	**Case 92-1 (Questions 1, 2)**
2 Although more than 60% of patients treated for AML achieve complete remission after induction therapy, the median duration of the remission is only about 12 to 18 months, and only 20% to 40% of patients have a diseasefree survival (DFS) exceeding 5 years. Short remissions have been attributed to proliferation of clinically undetectable leukemic cells. Thus, the rationale for administering chemotherapy after remission is to eradicate these residual cells.	**Case 92-1 (Questions 6, 7)**
3 The incidence of AML increases with advancing age. At age 40 years, there is only 1 case of AML per 100,000, but the annual incidence increases to 15% at age greater than 75 years. The prognosis of patients with AML is directly related to age.	**Case 92-1 (Question 8)**
4 Elderly patients do not tolerate intensive induction and postremission chemotherapy as well as younger patients. Older patients often have comorbid medical conditions and a poor performance status, which are associated with worse outcomes with conventional therapy.	**Case 92-1 (Question 8)**
5 In younger patients, failure to achieve remission or disease relapse remains the major cause of treatment failure. This reflects both the failure of current salvage regimens and the absence of effective strategies to secure long-term DFS in those patients who achieve a second hematologic remission. A wide range of salvage options have been studied, but with less than 50% of patients achieving a second remission and median survival ranging from 3 to 12 months, there remains considerable room for improvement.	**Case 92-2 (Question 1)**
CHRONIC MYELOGENOUS LEUKEMIA	
1 Many patients are asymptomatic at presentation but are evaluated because of an abnormally high leukocyte count. The cytogenetic hallmark of chronic myelogenous leukemia (CML) is the Philadelphia chromosome, which is present in more than 95% of cases. The chromosomal translocation generates a fusion gene called BCR-ABL that becomes inappropriately expressed, leading to CML. Identifying the Philadelphia chromosome is important in confirming the diagnosis of CML.	**Case 92-3 (Question 1)**
2 Hematopoietic stem cell transplantation is the only curative therapy for CML, but it is seldom recommended as first-line therapy for patients in chronic-phase CML. Imatinib, nilotinib, and dasatinib are all small-molecule tyrosine kinase inhibitors of BCR-ABL protein, and are all approved as initial first-line treatment.	**Case 92-3 (Question 3)**

continued

CHRONIC LYMPHOCYTIC LEUKEMIA	
1 Common treatment regimens for chronic lymphocytic leukemia (CLL) in patients without significant comorbidities include combinations of rituximab with fludarabine, cyclophosphamide, or bendamustine. Patients unable to tolerate a purine analog are treated with single-agent rituximab, chlorambucil-prednisone, or pulse steroids.	**Case 92-4 (Question 3)**
2 Infectious complications are common in patients with CLL. For recurrent infections, immune globulin treatment may be indicated. Vaccinations to prevent influenza and pneumococcus are indicated. Live vaccines including varicella zoster virus must be avoided.	**Case 92-4 (Question 5)**
MULTIPLE MYELOMA	
1 Multiple myeloma (MM) generally begins as a benign condition known as monoclonal gammopathy of undetermined significance. This condition may precede MM by years before transforming into a malignant disorder with clinical manifestations.	**Case 92-5 (Question 1)**
2 Induction therapy followed by hematopoietic cell transplantation in eligible patients is the standard of care and has increased overall survival in MM patients.	**Case 92-5 (Question 2)**
3 Supportive care of MM patients includes the prevention and treatment of skeletal disease, and should be considered in conjunction with induction therapy.	**Case 92-5 (Question 3)**
4 MM is not generally curable, even with maintenance therapy. Therefore, relapse usually occurs, and salvage therapies are commonly used.	**Case 92-5 (Questions 4, 5)**
LYMPHOMA	
1 Non–Hodgkin lymphomas (NHLs) arise from either B, T, or natural killer cells; approximately 80% are B-cell neoplasms. Aggressive NHLs are potentially curable and are typically treated with rituximab, cyclophosphamide, doxorubicin, vincristine, and prednisone.	**Case 92-6 (Questions 1, 2)**
2 Indolent NHLs respond well to therapy but the disease eventually recurs and is generally incurable.	**Case 92-7 (Question 2)**
3 Hodgkin lymphoma (HL) is a highly curable, chemotherapy-sensitive disease, and administration of full doses given on schedule is critical. The most commonly used regimen includes doxorubicin, bleomycin, vinblastine, and dacarbazine.	**Case 92-8 (Question 2)**

ACUTE MYELOID LEUKEMIA

Epidemiology

Acute myeloid leukemia (AML, also known as acute myelogenous leukemia and, less commonly, as acute non–lymphocytic leukemia) consists of a group of relatively well-defined hematopoietic neoplasms involving precursor cells committed to the myeloid line of cellular development.

In the United States and Europe, the incidence has been stable at 3 to 5 cases per 100,000. AML is the most common acute leukemia in adults and accounts for approximately 80% of cases in this group of neoplasms. In contrast, AML accounts for less than 10% of acute leukemias in children younger than 10 years of age. In adults, the median age at diagnosis is approximately 67 years. The incidence increases with age with approximately 1.3 and 12.2 cases per 100,000 for those younger than or older than 65 years, respectively. The male to female ratio is approximately 5:3.[1,2] See the surveillance, epidemiology, and end results (SEER) data for AML at http://seer.cancer.gov/statfacts/html/amyl.html#prevalence.

Pathophysiology

AML is characterized by a clonal proliferation of myeloid precursors with a reduced capacity to differentiate into more mature cellular elements. As a result, there is an accumulation of leukemic blasts in the bone marrow, peripheral blood, and occasionally in other tissues, with a variable reduction in the production of normal red blood cells, platelets, and mature granulocytes. The proliferation of malignant cells, along with a reduction in normal hematopoietic cells, results in a variety of systemic consequences including anemia, bleeding, and an increased risk of infection. Please refer to the following patient education video for

TABLE 92-1
Pretreatment Molecular Entities Shown to Predict Disease Outcome in Adults With Acute Myeloid Leukemia and a Normal Karyotype

Gene	Mutation Frequency (%)	Prognosis
NPM1	45–63	Favorable
FLT3	23–33	Poor
C/EBPa	8–19	Favorable
MLL	5–30	Poor

Source: Baldus CD et al. Clinical outcome of de novo acute myeloid leukaemia patients with normal cytogenetics is affected by molecular genetic alterations: a concise review. *Br J Haematol.* 2007;137:387.

additional information: http://www.careflash.com/video/acute-myeloid-leukemia.

Based on karyotype status (characterization of the chromosome such as shape, type, or number), two major groups of AML can be identified: (a) those with an abnormal karyotype, which accounts for approximately 50% to 60% of patients, and (b) those that demonstrate a normal karyotype by conventional cytogenetic testing, which accounts for the remainder of AML patients.[3,4]

Among patients with an abnormal karyotype, 25% have balanced (no gain or loss of chromosomal material) translocations, e.g., t(8;21), t(15;17), or inv(16), and 27% showed unbalanced (gain or loss of genetic material) abnormalities, e.g., −5/del(5q), −7/del(7q), or complex karyotype. Within the normal cytogenetic category, 45% to 63% have *NPM* (nucleophosmin) mutations (localized on chromosome 5, band q35), 23% to 33% show *FLT3* (FMS-like tyrosine kinase 3) mutation (localized on chromosome 13, band q12), 5% to 30% have *MLL* tandem duplications (localized on chromosome 11, band q23), and 8% to 19% have *C/EBP* (CCAAT enhancer binding protein) α mutations (localized on chromosome 19, band q13.1).[5]

The outcomes of patients with an abnormal karyotype are generally poor regardless of the molecular findings. However, the prognosis of patients with normal karyotype in the presence of each of these mutations is different as shown in Table 92-1. Patients with a normal karyotype and an *NPM* mutation alone have a favorable prognosis, with 60% surviving longer than 11 years.[6] In contrast, the presence of a normal karyotype with either *FLT3* or *MLL* mutations is generally associated with a poor prognosis. In addition, the coexistence of *FLT3* and *NPM* mutations does not improve the prognosis.[5]

Clinical Presentation and Diagnosis

Patients with AML generally present with symptoms related to complications of pancytopenia (e.g., anemia, neutropenia, and thrombocytopenia), including weakness and easy fatigability, infections of variable severity, and hemorrhagic findings such as gingival bleeding, ecchymoses, epistaxis, or menorrhagia. Combinations of these symptoms are common. It is often difficult to date the onset of AML precisely, at least in part because individuals have different symptomatic thresholds for seeking medical attention. It is likely that most patients have had more subtle evidence of bone marrow involvement for weeks, or perhaps months, before diagnosis. This can sometimes make the distinction between de novo leukemia and leukemia associated with a prior hematologic disorder such as a myelodysplastic syndrome somewhat arbitrary.

Although a presumptive diagnosis of AML can be made by examination of the peripheral blood smear when there are circulating leukemic blasts, a definitive diagnosis usually requires a bone marrow aspiration and biopsy. Morphologic, immunophenotypic, cytogenetic, and molecular studies must be performed in every case. The information derived from these studies is critical for making the correct diagnosis as well as determining prognosis.

Overview of Treatment

Once the diagnosis of AML is established, induction chemotherapy is given with the goal of rapidly restoring normal bone marrow function. Treatment regimens and outcomes differ between younger and older adults. Although there is no clear dividing line between younger and older adults when dealing with AML, in most studies "older adults" is defined as older than 60 years of age.

The objective of induction therapy is to reduce the total body leukemia cell population from approximately 10^{12} to less than the cytologically detectable level of about 10^9 cells. It is generally assumed, however, that a substantial burden of leukemia cells persists undetected (i.e., presence of "minimal residual disease"), leading to relapse within a few weeks or months if no further therapy were administered. The traditional goal of treatment of AML is to produce and maintain a complete remission. Criteria for this are platelet count higher than 100,000 cells/μL, neutrophil count higher than 1,000 cells/μL, and bone marrow specimen with less than 5% blasts.[7]

The most commonly used induction regimens for AML are the "7+3" regimens, which combine a 7-day continuous intravenous (IV) infusion of cytarabine (100 or 200 mg/m^2/day) with a short infusion or bolus of an anthracycline given on days 1 through 3. The most commonly used anthracycline in this regimen is daunorubicin, but idarubicin may be used instead.

Sixty to 80% of adult patients with newly diagnosed AML will attain a complete remission with intensive induction chemotherapy. However, without additional cytotoxic therapy, virtually all of these patients will relapse within a median of 4 to 8 months. In contrast, patients who receive postremission therapy may expect 4-year survival rates as high as 40% in young and middle-aged adults with good-risk disease.[8] High-dose cytarabine (HiDAC) has been the consolidation chemotherapy of choice for more than a decade for younger patients with good- or intermediate-risk disease. Attempts to improve on survival rates attained with HiDAC by substituting other agents with different mechanisms of action have not been successful.[9] For patients with an abnormal karyotype or with adverse molecular mutations, consolidation with HiDAC followed by an allogeneic hematopoietic cell transplant (HCT) with a suitably matched donor is the treatment of choice whenever possible. For patients older than 75 years of age, there is no specific standard of care except to enroll in a clinical trial when available. For the large number of patients who are 60 to 75 years of age, most clinicians will base induction and consolidation therapy recommendations on a patient's performance status, patient's wishes, and prognostic factors such as cytogenetics and mutation analysis.[10]

Twenty to 30% of young adult patients and 50% of older adult patients with newly diagnosed AML will fail to attain a complete response (CR) with intensive induction chemotherapy as a result of drug resistance or death. In addition, a large percentage of patients who initially attain a CR will relapse. The therapy that provides the best chance to cure a patient with relapsed or refractory AML is an allogeneic HCT. The best outcomes appear to be with a myeloablative preparative regimen administered after attaining a CR. However, some patients may be cured with myeloablative HCT even without attaining a CR although their chance of long-term survival is reduced. Nonmyeloablative preparative regimens are considered for patients who are not candidates for myeloablative HCT but have attained a CR.[11] See Chapter 96, Hematopoietic Cell Transplantation, for a complete discussion of HCT for leukemia. Please refer to the following online reference for more details about the treatment and prognosis of AML: http://www.cancer.gov/cancertopics/pdq/treatment/adultAML/healthprofessional/page4.

Signs and Symptoms

CASE 92-1

QUESTION 1: J.V., a 35-year-old man, presented to the emergency department with increasing fatigue and fever and an inability to eat. This past week, a peripheral blood smear (complete blood count [CBC]) revealed a white blood cell (WBC) count of 180,000 cells/μL with a differential of more than 90% leukemic blasts (normal, 0%), a hemoglobin (Hgb) of 7.8 g/dL, and a platelet count of 46,000 cells/μL. A bone marrow aspirate and biopsy confirmed the diagnosis of AML (FAB-M2, myeloid with maturation; 60% blasts, myeloperoxidase positive; CD13 and CD33 positive). All serum chemistry values were within normal limits, with the exception of potassium (K), 3.2 mEq/L; phosphorus, 5.5 mg/dL; and lactate dehydrogenase (LDH), 3,500 units/mL. Physical examination was remarkable for oral leukoplakia from oral candidiasis and poor dentition. Which signs and symptoms exhibited by J.V. are consistent with AML?

J.V.'s symptoms of increasing fatigue and fever of 1 week's duration are consistent with a rapid reduction in red blood cells leading to anemia (Hgb, 7.8 g/dL) and a low neutrophil count leading to infection (oral candidiasis). Although his WBC count is high, the differential reveals that more than 90% are blasts, which are immature, nonfunctional cells of myeloid or lymphoid origin. Circulating blast cells are typically not present in early chronic leukemias or mild-to-moderate infections. However, blasts may be observed on the peripheral blood smear in patients with anemia associated with primary bone marrow dysfunction (myelodysplastic syndromes). Blasts are also present in patients with severe infection, stress, or trauma, and in those with chronic myelogenous leukemia (CML) in transformation to acute leukemia. J.V.'s platelet count is also low, which may lead to bleeding or bruising. Collectively, these are presenting signs and symptoms of acute leukemia.

J.V.'s symptoms are consistent with either AML or acute lymphocytic leukemia (ALL). However, patients with ALL also commonly present with lymphadenopathy and hepatosplenomegaly, which J.V. does not have. It is important to distinguish between these two disorders because treatment regimens differ greatly. AML is more common in adults than in children. Because J.V. is 35 years old it is more likely that he has AML. For additional information on ALL, see Acute Lymphoblastic Leukemia of Childhood section in Chapter 91, Pediatric Malignancies.

Classification and Diagnosis

For a definitive diagnosis of AML, the bone marrow aspirate must contain more than 20% leukemic blast cells. A normal bone marrow aspirate would typically contain less than 5% blasts. Eight major variants of AML are defined by the French-American-British (FAB) classification system based on morphologic characteristics. More recently, the World Health Organization (WHO) has developed a classification system that expands the number of AML subtypes and better incorporates genotypic information, which is important in determining prognosis.[12]

ONLINE CONTENT

For a PowerPoint presentation that includes additional information about AML, go to http://thepoint.lww.com/AT10e.

Cells of myeloid origin commonly contain myeloperoxidase enzymes and express surface markers CD13, CD33, CD14, and CD15. Specific clonal chromosomal abnormalities are associated with several AML subtypes. These aberrations include gains or losses of whole chromosomes on the long (q) or short (p) arms, as well as a variety of structural rearrangements (e.g., translocations, inversions, insertions). A number of cytogenetic abnormalities in AML are associated with molecular-clinical syndromes, which are now under investigation at the genetic level. The translocation t(15;17) is the cytogenetic hallmark of acute promyelocytic leukemia (APL or AML-M3). This translocation splits the retinoic acid receptor gene on chromosome 17 and blocks expression of retinoic acid–controlled genes required for cell differentiation. Treating patients who have APL with all-*trans* retinoic acid (ATRA, tretinoin) has resulted in complete morphologic responses. This example shows how defining cytogenetic or chromosomal abnormalities in acute leukemia can be critical to understanding its pathophysiology and identifying optimal treatments. Currently, three chromosomal abnormalities are recognized as being associated with a better prognosis[13,14]: t(8;21), t(15;17), and inversion (inv) 16. In contrast, several chromosomal abnormalities have been associated with a relatively poor prognosis, including inv 3, deletion (del) 5, del(5q), del(7), and del(7q); trisomy 8; and complex (three or more unrelated cytogenetic abnormalities) cytogenetics. Additionally, molecular abnormalities such as *FLT3*, which is generally unfavorable, and *NPM1* and *C/EBPa*, which are generally favorable, are central in the evaluation of AML patients.[15] These findings are increasingly being used to guide treatment decisions. For example, patients with cytogenetic and molecular findings associated with a poor prognosis may be considered for more aggressive postremission therapy such as high-dose chemotherapy with HCT. Other poor prognostic signs in AML include age older than 60 years at the time of diagnosis, a pre-existing hematologic disorder (e.g., myelodysplastic syndrome), prior exposure to a chemotherapy agent (e.g., a secondary leukemia), and poor baseline performance status.[16]

J.V. has FAB-M2 (myelomonocytic) AML. Approximately 10% to 20% of patients with FAB-M2 acute leukemia have a translocation of t(8;21)(q22;q22).[13] This translocation is usually seen in young patients such as J.V. and is associated with a better response to therapy. J.V.'s bone marrow has been sent for cytogenetic and molecular analysis; however, results will not be available for approximately a week. Although neither the cytogenetic nor the molecular analysis will alter the planned induction therapy for J.V., these findings in combination with other prognostic features, as discussed previously, will influence postremission therapy recommendations.

Treatment

GOAL OF THERAPY

CASE 92-1, QUESTION 2: What is the goal of treatment, and what type of therapy is indicated for J.V. at this time?

The leukemic cells populating J.V.'s blood are abnormal and incapable of fighting infection. Their rapid proliferation is suppressing red blood cell and megakaryocyte production in the bone marrow. J.V. is at substantial risk for life-threatening infections and bleeding complications. The goal of the initial chemotherapy is to clear the bone marrow and peripheral blood of all blast cells in the hope that normal blood cell components can regenerate.

INDUCTION THERAPY

Standard induction chemotherapy for AML includes an anthracycline (either daunorubicin or idarubicin) and cytarabine, an antimetabolite. One commonly used regimen includes daunorubicin 90 mg/m^2/day on days 1 to 3 as an IV bolus injection, plus cytarabine 100 mg/m^2/day as a continuous IV infusion on days 1 to 7.[17] This combination (7 + 3) is one of the most effective chemotherapy regimens used to treat adult AML, with CR rates of 60% to 80%.[13] Continuous infusions of cytarabine are preferred because these regimens produce higher response rates than bolus injections during induction therapy.[18,19] Using higher doses of cytarabine by increasing the number of days of therapy to 10, doubling the daily dose to 200 mg/m^2, and using (HiDAC) (0.5–6.0 g/m^2/day) has not shown consistent improvement in CR rates or survival.[20] Adding etoposide for 7 days may increase the CR rate, response duration, and survival in patients younger than 55 years.[21] However, other investigators have not shown a benefit with the addition of etoposide to the standard 7 + 3 induction regimen.[22]

If a patient presents with a very high WBC count, he or she may experience complications associated with hyperviscosity of the blood (e.g., ringing ears, stroke, blindness, or headache as a result of impaired oxygen delivery to the central nervous system [CNS], pulmonary infarction). Because it may take several days for cytarabine and daunorubicin to substantially decrease the WBC count, the patient may receive hydroxyurea 2 to 4 g orally (PO) or undergo leukapheresis to rapidly reduce the WBC count. Leukapheresis is not routinely done unless the patient is experiencing symptoms of hyperviscosity or has a WBC 100,000 cells/μL or greater on diagnosis.

Because J.V.'s initial WBC was 180,000 cells/μL, leukapheresis was initiated together with concomitant hydroxyurea 2 g twice daily. Approximately 12 hours after initiating leukapheresis, J.V.'s WBC had decreased to 85,000 cells/μL, and he was stable enough to proceed to induction therapy with daunorubicin and cytarabine. The leukapheresis and hydroxyurea were subsequently discontinued.

TRETINOIN AND ARSENIC TRIOXIDE FOR ACUTE PROMYELOCYTIC LEUKEMIA

CASE 92-1, QUESTION 3: Would induction therapy for other subtypes of AML differ from that described previously?

Induction therapy with 7 + 3 is standard for all types of AML, with one exception: APL or AML-M3. APL is uniquely characterized by the t(15;17) translocation that fuses the *PML* gene on chromosome 15 to the retinoic acid receptor-alpha (*RAR-α*) gene on chromosome 17. In clinical trials, ATRA has induced complete remission in approximately 90% of patients with APL.[23] Serial bone marrow aspirations after initiation of ATRA therapy demonstrate progressive differentiation without hypoplasia.[23,24] Unfortunately, ATRA typically induces brief remissions. A number of trials have investigated combination treatment with chemotherapy and ATRA.[25,26] Current evidence supports the use of concurrent ATRA plus conventional chemotherapy for induction, with ATRA starting 2 days before chemotherapy. In addition, postremission therapy should include at least two cycles of an anthracycline-based regimen.[26,27] Maintenance therapy with intermittent ATRA has been shown to decrease the relapse rate.[25,28]

ATRA therapy, although avoiding life-threatening myelosuppression, can produce significant toxicities, including the retinoic acid syndrome (RAS), which manifests as fever, weight gain, respiratory distress, lung infiltrates, pleural or pericardial effusion, hypotension, and acute renal failure.[29] If RAS develops, corticosteroid therapy (dexamethasone 10 mg twice a day for at least 3 days) should be initiated.[30] In patients receiving concurrent ATRA and chemotherapy, ATRA may be stopped if the patient has received ATRA for at least 20 days or if symptoms of RAS are life-threatening or not improving with dexamethasone. Patients with leukocytosis seem to be more likely to experience RAS. Concurrent use of chemotherapy and ATRA has been reported to reduce the likelihood of RAS.[30] ATRA also causes dryness of the lining of the mouth, rectum, and skin; hair loss; skin rash; blepharon conjunctivitis; corneal erosions; muscle weakness; nail changes; depression; elevated liver enzymes; and high cholesterol. Despite the risk of serious complications and death during induction therapy, the long-term diseasefree survival (DFS) rate of patients with APL is superior compared with other AML subtypes. Approximately 75% of patients who receive ATRA-based induction and maintenance therapy are alive 3 to 5 years after diagnosis.[28]

COMPLICATIONS OF INDUCTION THERAPY

Tumor Lysis Syndrome

CASE 92-1, QUESTION 4: Twenty-four hours after J.V.'s induction chemotherapy was initiated, the following laboratory values were obtained:

WBC count, 78,000 cells/μL
K, 5.3 mEq/L
Phosphorus, 6.0 mg/dL
Uric acid, 9.8 mg/dL
Calcium, 6.0 mg/dL
Creatinine, 1.6 mg/dL

Why have these laboratory values changed so suddenly? Could this have been minimized or prevented? How should these metabolic disturbances be managed?

J.V. presented with a very high number of peripheral blood blasts. On administration of chemotherapy, patients with a hypercellular bone marrow and high number of blast cells can have a rapid lysis of the blast cells and the release of cellular contents. This can result in tumor lysis syndrome (TLS), which is associated with metabolic abnormalities such as hyperuricemia, hyperphosphatemia, hypocalcemia, and uremia. These disturbances may lead to arrhythmias and acute renal failure. In most cases, TLS occurs 12 to 24 hours after chemotherapy is initiated. TLS may occur after therapy for other malignancies, particularly in those with a high tumor burden, such as high-grade lymphomas and ALL. TLS rarely occurs after therapy for solid tumors.

Patients should receive IV hydration (3–4 L/day) beginning 24 to 48 hours before chemotherapy to maintain renal perfusion, optimize the solubility of tumor lysis products, and compensate for fluid losses caused by fever or vomiting. Alkalinization of the urine with the addition of sodium bicarbonate to the IV fluids may also reduce or prevent uric acid from precipitating in the renal tubules and collection ducts by maintaining the urate in its ionized state, but is not currently recommended for all patients. This is because the increased pH may increase the risk of precipitating calcium phosphate in both soft tissue and kidney tubules, and it may aggravate hypocalcemia.[31,32]

Allopurinol, a xanthine oxidase inhibitor that blocks the metabolism of uric acid, should be started before chemotherapy to prevent or minimize the complications of TLS. The recommended adult dosage is 300 to 600 mg/day. J.V.'s serum uric acid and electrolytes should be monitored at least two to three times a day for 24 to 48 hours after initiating chemotherapy. If severe abnormalities occur, more aggressive measures should be initiated. Allopurinol may be discontinued if the serum uric acid is within normal limits, the LDH has normalized, and the WBC count is low. Rasburicase, a recombinant urate oxidase product, can also be used as prophylaxis in patients who are at high risk of developing TLS or for the treatment of patients who present with or develop TLS. Rasburicase acts as a catalyst in the enzymatic oxidation of uric acid to allantoin, which is five to ten times more soluble than uric acid and undergoes rapid renal excretion. The recommended dose of rasburicase for both prevention and treatment of TLS is 0.2 mg/kg/dose IV. Rasburicase results in a rapid reduction in serum uric acid (within 4 hours of administration) and is generally well tolerated.[33] Most of the clinical data for rasburicase is in the pediatric population; however, data suggest that rasburicase is equally effective in adults.[33,34] In many adult centers, doses of 3 or 6 mg are commonly used.[35–39] Although rasburicase has demonstrated excellent efficacy and tolerability, its optimal role in the prevention and management of hyperuricemia in adults remains to be defined because of its high cost and lack of a randomized trial comparing its effect with other interventions.

Although J.V.'s serum potassium was low on admission, it has increased significantly as a result of TLS. For this reason, replacement potassium therapy by any method is not recommended before chemotherapy in patients in whom TLS is highly likely. In extreme circumstances, dialysis may be required to correct severe metabolic and electrolyte disturbances associated with TLS. J.V.'s kidneys continued to function throughout. Even though J.V.'s creatinine was above the normal range, his urine output did not decline substantially and he was able to proceed without further intervention.

Myelosuppression

CASE 92-1, QUESTION 5: J.V. received allopurinol therapy and aggressive hydration throughout his induction chemotherapy. The metabolic abnormalities gradually resolved as his WBC count declined and tumor lysis diminished. What other complications may occur during induction therapy and can they be treated?

Patients receiving cytarabine and daunorubicin induction therapy develop profound anemia, granulocytopenia (e.g., WBC count <100 cells/μL), and thrombocytopenia (<20,000 platelets/μL) shortly after therapy is initiated, which usually persist for approximately 21 to 28 days. Additionally, all infectious complications must be considered life-threatening in severely immunocompromised patients such as J.V.

Filgrastim (granulocyte colony-stimulating factor [G-CSF]) and sargramostim (granulocyte-macrophage colony-stimulating factor [GM-CSF]) stimulate leukemic cells as well as normal granulocyte precursors in vitro; however, several studies have demonstrated that these agents, when used as an adjunct to AML chemotherapy, are safe and do not adversely affect disease outcome.[40,41] Most studies have demonstrated that colony-stimulating factors (CSFs) can modestly decrease the length of profound neutropenia, and sometimes reduce the incidence of infection-related morbidity, the duration of systemic antibiotic and antifungal therapy, and the number of hospitalization days. Despite the reduction in short-term neutropenia-related complications, administration of CSFs after induction chemotherapy does not appear to have an impact on the rate of CR or the long-term outcomes of the disease. Refer to Chapter 90, Adverse Effects of Chemotherapy and Targeted Agents, for additional information about CSFs.

Severe thrombocytopenia may result in bleeding episodes that range in severity from oozing gums to massive hemorrhage. Serious bleeding complications can usually be avoided if patients receive platelet transfusions when their platelet counts decrease to less than 10,000 cells/μL or when patients experience bleeding. Currently, there are no data to support the use of interleukin (IL)-11 (oprelvekin) or investigational thrombopoietic agents in this setting.

Other common drug-induced complications that may occur during induction therapy include nausea and vomiting, mucositis, fever, and skin rash (see Chapter 6, Nausea and Vomiting, Chapter 7, Pain and Its Management, and Chapter 90, Neoplastic Disorders and Their Treatment: General Principles, for additional information and their management).

Postremission Therapy

RATIONALE

CASE 92-1, QUESTION 6: After completion of his induction chemotherapy, J.V.'s WBC count fell to less than 100 cells/μL and his platelet count fell to 5,000 cells/μL. He received platelet transfusions approximately every 2 to 3 days to prevent bleeding complications. On day 9, he developed a fever of 38.8°C. He was started immediately on empiric, broad-spectrum antibiotic therapy for fever and neutropenia, and it subsequently resolved. On day 29, his WBC count was 5,600 cells/μL with a normal differential, and his platelet count was 168,000 cells/μL. He received packed red blood cell transfusions on two separate occasions when his Hgb fell to less than 8 mg/dL. A repeat bone marrow aspirate showed no evidence of persistent leukemia, and J.V. was told that his leukemia was in remission. Nevertheless, his hematologist recommended additional chemotherapy, and J.V. questions why this is necessary. Is postremission therapy necessary, and if so, what therapeutic options are available to J.V.?

Although greater than 60% of patients treated for AML achieve CR after induction therapy, the median duration of the remission is only about 12 to 18 months, and only 20% to 40% of patients have a DFS exceeding 5 years.[20] Short remissions have been attributed to proliferation of clinically undetectable leukemic cells. Thus, the rationale for administering chemotherapy after remission is to eradicate these residual cells.

In adult AML, postremission therapy (also referred to as consolidation therapy) includes three to four cycles of chemotherapy. Clinical trials have shown that high-dose postremission therapy results in a higher percentage (30%–40%) of long-term (>2–5 years) diseasefree survivors than either no or low-dose postremission chemotherapy in patients generally younger than 60 years of age.[42,43] Postremission therapy regimens usually include HiDAC alone or in combination with one or more agents such as an anthracycline or etoposide. Patients 60 years of age and older or those with comorbid disease may not be able to tolerate this intensive postremission therapy. In these circumstances, the risk of life-threatening toxicity may outweigh the potential benefits of postremission chemotherapy. Allogeneic HCT has also been studied in the postremission treatment of AML and is addressed in Chapter 96, Hematopoietic Cell Transplantation.

In an effort to prolong survival, chemotherapy (thioguanine, methotrexate) and biologics (IL-2) for a prolonged period have been investigated. This is often referred to as maintenance therapy. With the exception of APL, maintenance chemotherapy has not been shown to improve survival in adult AML. In conclusion, J.V. should receive consolidation therapy after HiDAC induction because this has been shown to give him the best chance of long-term survival. Additionally, because J.V. was fortunate enough to be diagnosed with good-risk disease, he will not require an allogeneic HCT. He will be followed closely with at least bimonthly CBCs and a bone marrow biopsy at least every year for 5 years after consolidation. This close follow-up is vital for catching relapse as early as possible with the intent of going immediately to an allogeneic HCT and minimizing additional reinduction therapy if relapse occurs.

HIGH-DOSE CYTARABINE

CASE 92-1, QUESTION 7: Because J.V. does not require an allogeneic HCT at this time, his hematologist recommends three courses of HiDAC as postremission therapy. One week after he was declared to be in remission, J.V. is readmitted to the hospital to receive HiDAC 3 g/m^2 every 12 hours, over 3 hours, on days 1, 3, and 5. What are the potential acute and delayed toxicities associated with HiDAC, and how can these effects be prevented?

At conventional dosages of 100 to 200 mg/m^2/day, adverse effects associated with cytarabine include myelosuppression, fever, and skin rashes. Occasionally, liver enzymes rise transiently. The side effect profile for HiDAC (>1 g/m^2/day) by contrast is very different and can produce major cerebellar, ocular, and skin toxicities.[44,45]

CEREBELLAR AND OCULAR TOXICITY

Cerebellar toxicity is a significant problem in patients receiving HiDAC therapy. See Chapter 90, Adverse Effects of Chemotherapy and Targeted Agents, for details regarding cerebellar toxicity. Ocular toxicity results from damage to the corneal epithelium, occurring when cytarabine penetrates the epithelium through the anterior chamber of the eye or tears. Symptoms include conjunctivitis, excessive lacrimation, "burning" ocular pain, photophobia, and blurred vision. Artificial tears (two drops every 4–6 hours) administered concurrently with HiDAC generally prevents these symptoms. Corticosteroid eye drops can be used as an alternative to artificial tears or if symptoms of conjunctivitis occur.[46]

DERMATOLOGIC TOXICITY

Dermatologic toxicity may manifest as a rash covering most of the body or plantar-palmar erythrodysesthesia (PPE).

ONLINE CONTENT

For a photo of cytarabine-induced PPE, go to http://thepoint.lww.com/AT10e.

This is commonly seen several days after the start of the cytarabine, but may occur days to weeks after therapy. Desquamation of the palms and soles can occur with PPE, causing significant pain and allowing for pathogenic organisms to enter the body.[47] Treatment varies, but most suggest stopping the cytarabine if the rash or PPE is severe. Other strategies include minimizing tight-fitting shoes and socks if the feet are involved, as well as protecting the affected areas from further damage.

ACUTE MYELOID LEUKEMIA IN THE ELDERLY

CASE 92-1, QUESTION 8: Would recommendations for induction and postremission therapy differ if J.V. were elderly (60 years of age or older)?

As mentioned earlier, the incidence of AML increases with advancing age. At age 40 years, there is only 1 case of AML per 100,000, but the annual incidence increases to 15% at ages older than 75 years. The prognosis of patients with AML is also directly related to age. Older patients are generally less able to tolerate intensive induction and postremission chemotherapy. Older patients often have comorbid medical conditions and a poor performance status, which are directly associated with worse outcomes with conventional AML therapy.[48,49]

Many single-institution and cooperative group studies exclude elderly patients with AML or treat them on a separate less-intensive protocol. Elderly patients are often judged to be poor-risk candidates for intensive chemotherapy without objective review of available criteria. Because the median age of patients with AML and myelodysplastic syndrome is 67 years, the results of regimens studied in younger patients may not be applicable to the elderly. Some hematologists believe that it is most appropriate to offer older patients supportive care only, low-intensity therapy, or investigational treatment. Others believe that moderately intensive chemotherapy is beneficial in some candidates. However, most physicians feel uncomfortable offering intensive chemotherapy to elderly patients because of the high risk of induction mortality. Several studies have addressed the outcome of elderly patients.[50–56]

An analysis of 2,657 Medicare beneficiaries older than 65 years of age with AML may accurately reflect past experience with this population better.[57] The mortality rate was 86% and 94% at 1 and 2 years after diagnosis, respectively. Only 30% of these patients received any form of IV chemotherapy in the 2 years after diagnosis. The study did not distinguish between intensive induction chemotherapy and palliative therapy. Nevertheless, 89% of all patients required hospitalization, and they spent 31% of their remaining days in either a hospital or skilled nursing facility. The high rate of hospitalization is likely owing to the consequences of bone marrow failure caused by the AML, even in the absence of cytotoxic chemotherapy. Nevertheless, many believe aggressive therapy is warranted in most elderly patients given the rapid progression of the disease, and certain death within weeks if the disease is not treated.

The selection of postremission therapy is difficult in elderly patients because they have a higher risk of morbidity and mortality, and more important, no clinical trials have demonstrated the benefit of postremission therapy specifically in the elderly. The intensity of the regimens must often be attenuated because there is risk of serious toxicities. This is particularly true with HiDAC therapy because of the increased risk of cerebellar toxicity in the elderly. Studies have shown that postremission therapy with low-dose cytarabine (100 mg/m^2 by continuous infusion for 5 days) is as effective as HiDAC and better tolerated in elderly patients.[42]

Refractory or Resistant Acute Myeloid Leukemia

CASE 92-2

QUESTION 1: A.W., a 55-year-old man, is approximately 40 days after induction therapy with 7 + 3. Initially, his counts recovered on day 25, and a bone marrow biopsy

on day 28 revealed less than 5% blasts; therefore, he was in remission. Thereafter, a recent CBC showed a significant drop in his platelet count from 150,000 cells/μL on day 30 to 90,000 cells/μL 10 days later. A subsequent bone marrow biopsy reveals 60% blasts, confirming the diagnosis of relapsed AML. What are treatment options for A.W. at this time?

In younger patients, failure to achieve remission or disease relapse remains the major cause of treatment failure. This reflects both the failure of current salvage regimens and the absence of effective strategies to secure long-term DFS in those patients who achieve a second hematologic remission. A wide range of salvage options have been studied, but with less than 50% of patients achieving a second remission and median survival figures ranging from 3 to 12 months, there remains considerable room for improvement.[58]

The treatment of relapse in a patient younger than 75 years of age with a good performance status generally comprises one of several salvage options, including clofarabine, intermediate-dose cytarabine to HiDAC, or combination regimens such as fludarabine, cytarabine, and G-CSF (FLAG), or cladribine, cytarabine, and G-CSF (CLAG), followed by allogeneic HCT.

A recently completed phase III trial from the Southwest Oncology Group showed a significantly higher fatal toxicity rate in patients who received gemtuzumab ozogamicin in combination with standard induction therapy or as consolidation therapy alone.[59] These disappointing results prompted the US Food and Drug Administration (FDA) to remove commercially available gemtuzumab ozogamicin from the US market, thereby eliminating a therapeutic option for initial and relapsed or refractory AML.

Future Chemotherapy in Acute Myeloid Leukemia: Targeted Therapies?

CASE 92-2, QUESTION 2: The results of A.W.'s cytogenetic and molecular analysis show that his leukemia is *FLT3* positive. What would be the next step for A.W.?

Whereas some clinical factors have an impact on response to treatment, it is the cytogenetic and molecular heterogeneity of AML that is the major determinant of treatment success or failure. For A.W., the finding that his AML has a mutation in the *FLT3* gene portends a poor likelihood of long-term survival without new therapies. The estimated 5-year survival is approximately 10% to 15% among patients with an *FLT3* internal tandem duplication mutation.[60]

FLT3 is a receptor tyrosine kinase (TK) that is mutated in 25% to 30% of AML cases, and is associated with a poor disease outcome. Therefore, it is an attractive molecular target for the development of new therapeutics. Although more than 20 molecules have been reported to have inhibitory activity against FLT3,[61] only a few of them are currently in phase II or III clinical trials to assess their efficacy in AML patients: midostaurin,[62,63] lestaurtinib,[64,65] and sorafenib.[66]

To date, FLT3 inhibitors have shown only modest efficacy as monotherapy in patients with relapsed or refractory disease. However, in vitro studies suggest synergism between FLT3 inhibitors and conventional chemotherapy. As a result, several clinical trials are ongoing to investigate the combination of FLT3 inhibitors in combination with conventional chemotherapy like daunorubicin and cytarabine along with hypomethylating agents such as decitabine and azacitidine with the hope of improving the outcomes of patients with *FLT3* mutations in both the initial and relapse setting.[67]

For A.W., the best option would be to enroll in an investigational trial that incorporates one of the available FLT3 inhibitors with chemotherapy. If a trial is not available, then HiDAC or a combination regimen containing clofarabine or fludarabine followed by an allogeneic HCT would be his best option.

ONLINE CONTENT

For a PowerPoint presentation about the treatment of FLT3 positive AML, go to http://thepoint.lww.com/AT10e.

CHRONIC MYELOGENOUS LEUKEMIA

Epidemiology and Pathophysiology

CML is a myeloproliferative disorder characterized by unregulated stem cell proliferation in the bone marrow and an increase in mature granulocytes in the peripheral blood. The median age of diagnosis is 50 to 60 years, and there is an annual incidence of 1.0 to 1.5 per 100,000 patients.[68] Although seldom seen in pediatric leukemia, CML accounts for 15% of adult leukemia cases.[69] The estimated 7- to 10-year survival rate is 80% to 85%, since the introduction of TK inhibitors.

Clinical Presentation and Diagnosis

Presenting symptoms include fatigue, abdominal pain, fever, anorexia, and weight loss. On physical examination, the most common finding is splenomegaly. Approximately 25% to 50% of patients are asymptomatic at presentation, and the initial suspicion for CML is based solely on an abnormal CBC.[70] Bone marrow biopsy reveals the cytogenetic hallmark of CML, the Philadelphia chromosome, which is present in more than 95% of cases.[71] Cytogenetic analysis reveals a translocation of chromosomes 9 and 22 t(9;22)(q34;q11).[72] This translocation creates a new protein (BCR-ABL) that has unregulated TK activity, thereby promoting leukemia development. The three major mechanisms that have been implicated in the malignant transformation by unregulated TK include abnormal cell cycling, inhibition of apoptosis, and increased proliferation of cells.[72] Identification of the Philadelphia chromosome helps confirm the diagnosis of CML and helps with monitoring the efficacy of treatment. The natural history of CML can be divided into three distinct phases: chronic phase, accelerated phase, and blast phase. Greater than 90% of patients are diagnosed in chronic phase, which is the earliest phase of the disease.

Treatment

The ultimate goal of therapy is to cure patients of their disease, and allogeneic HCT remains the only curative therapy for CML to date. However, HCT is associated with a substantial risk of morbidity and mortality. Therefore, TK inhibitors are first line therapy in most patients even though they are not curative. The primary goals of the TK inhibitors are to prolong survival, prevent progression of disease, and attain a complete hematologic or cytogenetic remission. Imatinib, nilotinib, and dasatinib are TK inhibitors that achieve complete hematologic and cytogenetic response rates and are first-line treatment options in chronic-phase CML patients. Nilotinib and dasatinib are approved for the treatment of patients with resistant

TABLE 92-2
Definition of Complete and Partial Hematologic Response in Chronic Myelogenous Leukemia

	Partial Response	Complete Response
Peripheral leukocyte count	$<10 \times 10^9$/L	$<10 \times 10^9$/L
Platelet count	<50% pretreatment count (but $>450 \times 10^9$/L	$<450 \times 10^9$/L
Immature cells	Present	Absent
Splenomegaly	Present (but <50% pretreatment extent)	Absent

Source: NCCN National Comprehensive Cancer Network. Clinical Practice Guidelines in Oncology: Chronic Myelogenous Leukemia. 2012; V1.2012. http://www.nccn.org/professionals/physician_gls/f_guidelines.asp. Accessed May 2, 2011.

Philadelphia chromosome–positive chronic- or accelerated-phase CML. Treatment for patients who progress from chronic to accelerated or blast phase is determined based on mutational changes in the BCR-ABL protein and bone marrow cytogenetics. Owing to the sustained response rates achieved by the TK inhibitors, the exact timing of HCT is controversial, although patients in the accelerated or blast phase at presentation or those progressing during TK inhibitor therapy are generally referred for HCT.[73] Historically, patients undergoing transplantation in the accelerated and blast phases achieved a 40% and 10% 5-year, leukemiafree survival, respectively.[69,73]

Quantitative polymerase chain reaction assay is used to monitor BCR-ABL transcript levels for early detection of recurrence of the CML disease. Increased transcript levels at 6 and 12 months after transplant are associated with a 43% increased risk of relapse compared with a 3% risk of relapse in patients without level elevations.[69] For those who relapse after HCT, initiation of a TK inhibitor has improved long-term outcomes. Additional information regarding HCT and the preparative regimens used for patients undergoing allogeneic HCT for CML can be found in Chapter 96, Hematopoietic Cell Transplantation.

Assessment of response to CML therapies are based on both hematologic (Table 92-2) and cytogenetic (Table 92-3) responses. Response definitions were created when interferon was the primary treatment for CML, leading some clinicians to use major molecular response as another marker of response.[70] Major molecular response is defined as undetectable BCR-ABL mRNA by polymerase chain reaction assay and a greater than 3-log decrease in BCR-ABL mRNA.[69]

TABLE 92-3
Definition of Cytogenetic Response in Chronic Myelogenous Leukemia

Cytogenetic Response	Philadelphia (Ph) Chromosome–Positive Metaphase Cells (%)
Complete	0
Partial	1–35
Major (includes complete and partial responses)	0–35
Minor	>35

Source: NCCN National Comprehensive Cancer Network. Clinical Practice Guidelines in Oncology: Chronic Myelogenous Leukemia. 2012; V1.2012. http://www.nccn.org/professionals/physician_gls/f_guidelines.asp. Accessed May 2, 2011.

Signs and Symptoms

CASE 92-3

QUESTION 1: S.E., a 66-year-old white woman, recently had a routine CBC drawn during her annual checkup. Her CBC showed a WBC count of 60,000 cells/μL with 90% neutrophils, a hematocrit of 32%, and a platelet count of 300,000 cells/μL. The only pertinent physical finding was splenomegaly. On further workup, a bone marrow aspirate revealed a hypercellular marrow with less than 10% blasts. Cytogenetic analysis confirmed a diagnosis of Philadelphia chromosome–positive CML. Explain S.E.'s high WBC count. What are the possible clinical consequences of these abnormal values?

Approximately 40% to 50% of patients are asymptomatic at presentation, and the initial suspicion for CML is based solely on an abnormal CBC.[70] However, if symptomatic, patients may complain of fatigue, abdominal pain, fever, anorexia, and weight loss. The most common physical finding is splenomegaly, which results from increased activity of the reticuloendothelial system to remove the increased numbers of WBCs. Approximately 50% to 70% of patients present with a leukocyte count greater than 100,000 cells/μL. Consequences of hyperleukocytosis and hyperviscosity may include priapism, headaches, tinnitus, and cerebrovascular accidents. The presence of the Philadelphia chromosome is critical in the diagnosis of CML since the majority of cases will have this cytogenetic abnormality.

Clinical Course and Prognosis

CASE 92-3, QUESTION 2: What is the prognosis for S.E. and others with newly diagnosed CML?

Early in the disease (chronic phase), patients exhibit leukocytosis and associated symptoms as described previously. Chronic phase is defined as less than 10% blasts and promyelocytes in the bone marrow and peripheral blood.[71] The duration of the chronic phase may range from a few months to many years. Because symptoms may be nonspecific and relatively minor, CML may remain undiagnosed until patients progress into more advanced stages. The annual transition rate from chronic phase to accelerated phase is 5% to 10% in the first 2 years and 20% in subsequent years.[71] Common signs and symptoms suggestive of this transition include increased leukocytosis, anemia, increased splenomegaly, fever, and bone pain. Because less than 10% blast cells are present in S.E.'s bone marrow, she is in the chronic phase of the disease. Therefore, S.E.'s prognosis is good and her projected 8-year overall survival (OS) is 85% if treated with the TK inhibitor imatinib.[74]

During the second phase of the disease, the accelerated phase, leukocytosis progresses (despite therapy), and an increased number of immature leukocytes (blasts) appear in the peripheral blood. Patients may report significant symptoms. The estimated 4-year OS is 53% for accelerated-phase CML patients started on the TK inhibitor imatinib.[71] The accelerated phase will generally progress to the blast phase in less than 6 weeks if not treated. The final phase of the disease (blast phase or blast crisis) is characterized by a predominance of immature cells. Blast crisis is defined as more than 20% blasts in the peripheral blood or bone marrow by the WHO or more than 30% blasts in the blood or bone marrow with or without extramedullary disease by the International Bone Marrow Transplant Registry.[69–71] During this phase, CML is indistinguishable from AML with the exception of cytogenetics. In blast crisis, patients often experience bone pain, fatigue, fever, infections, and bleeding complications. The blast phase is often refractory to conventional induction chemotherapy regimens for AML, and the median survival is approximately 6 months.[68]

Treatment

CASE 92-3, QUESTION 3: What therapy is appropriate for S.E.'s chronic-phase disease?

HYDROXYUREA

As mentioned above, the ultimate goal of therapy for CML is cure, and allogeneic HCT remains the only curative therapy. However, in newly diagnosed patients who present with very high leukocyte counts (>100,000 cells/μL), the initial goal of therapy is to immediately reduce leukocytosis and its related symptoms.[71] In patients presenting with a leukocyte count greater than 20,000 cells/μL, hydroxyurea is still the most common agent used for initial leukocyte reduction. Treatment is initiated with 2 g/day PO, and the dosage is titrated to a WBC count of less than 20,000 cells/μL with a goal of 5,000 to 10,000 cells/μL.[71] A small dosage decrease often permits a considerable rise in leukocyte count in 1 or 2 days. Hydroxyurea is well tolerated and is relatively free of nonhematologic side effects. Although effective for initial control of high leukocyte counts, hydroxyurea is inferior to other treatments for long-term control of CML. Because S.E. presented with a WBC of 60,000 cells/μL, she will receive hydroxyurea for 3 to 5 days before transitioning to a TK inhibitor.

TYROSINE KINASE INHIBITORS

In 2001, the FDA approved imatinib mesylate (400 mg PO daily), a first-generation TK inhibitor, for the treatment of patients with CML. Since that time, two second-generation TK inhibitors, dasatinib (100 mg PO daily) and nilotinib (400 mg PO twice daily), have been approved. In the current National Comprehensive Cancer Network (NCCN) Guidelines, imatinib, nilotinib, and dasatinib are first-line treatment options for patients presenting with chronic-phase CML.[69] The following online video discusses the current treatment strategies for CML: http://www.youtube.com/watch?v=MGqyY57uTvU.

Imatinib occupies the adenosine triphosphate binding site of several TK molecules and prevents phosphorylation of substrates that are involved in regulating the cell cycle. Approval was based on the pivotal International Randomized Study of Interferon and STI571 (IRIS) trial, which compared imatinib with the combination of interferon (IFN)-α plus low-dose cytarabine in patients with newly diagnosed CML in the chronic phase. A total of 1,106 patients were randomly assigned to either imatinib (400 mg PO daily) or IFN plus cytarabine.[75] All primary and secondary end points of the trial, including rates of complete hematologic remission, major and complete cytogenetic response, and freedom from progression to the accelerated phase or blast crisis, demonstrated superiority of imatinib versus IFN plus cytarabine. In addition to superior efficacy, imatinib was very well tolerated. The most common toxicities reported with imatinib are superficial edema, nausea, muscle cramps, and rashes. More mature data from this trial, with a median follow-up of 60 months, demonstrated an 89% OS of patients who received imatinib as initial therapy.[76] This landmark trial clearly showed the superiority of imatinib compared with IFN plus cytarabine in the treatment of patients with newly diagnosed CML in chronic phase. Based on these results, TK inhibitors are now first-line standard of care for patients with newly diagnosed CML in chronic phase.

Dasatinib binds the BCR-ABL protein in the active confirmation, making it 325 times more potent than imatinib.[74] Approval was based on the international DASISION (Dasatinib versus Imatinib study in treatment-naïve CML patients) trial, which compared dasatinib 100 mg PO once daily with imatinib 400 mg PO once daily with food in a randomized 1 : 1 fashion in 519 patients with chronic-phase CML.[77] The primary objective of complete cytogenetic response at 12 months and the secondary objective of a major molecular response by 12 months were statistically superior for dasatinib versus imatinib. Dasatinib demonstrates a similar safety profile compared with imatinib, with a higher incidence of pleural effusion and thrombocytopenia and a lower incidence of rash and diarrhea.[74]

Nilotinib is structurally similar to imatinib but 30 times more potent as a result of an improved structural fit in the receptor pocket.[74] Approval was based on the international ENESTnd (Evaluating nilotinib efficacy and safety in clinical trials—newly diagnosed patients) trial, which randomly assigned 846 patients with chronic-phase CML in a 1:1:1 fashion to either imatinib (400 mg PO once a day with food) or nilotinib (300 mg or 400 mg PO twice a day). The primary objective of major molecular response at 12 months and the key secondary objective of a complete cytogenetic response by 12 months were statistically superior for both doses of nilotinib compared with imatinib.[78] Nilotinib demonstrates a similar safety profile compared with the other TK inhibitors, with a higher incidence of rash, headache, pruritus, and alopecia and a lower incidence of nausea, diarrhea, vomiting, edema, and muscle spasm.[78]

Clinicians and patients must carefully evaluate the potential risks and benefits of each treatment modality to make the best therapeutic decision for each individual situation. Because S.E. presented in chronic-phase CML, initiation of imatinib, nilotinib, or dasatinib are appropriate choice. Imatinib 400 mg once daily will be initiated.

Relapsed and Refractory Disease

CASE 92-3, QUESTION 4: On routine follow-up at 6 months, cytogenetics analysis of S.E.'s bone marrow demonstrates 10% Philadelphia chromosome–positive cells (partial cytogenetic response). Therefore, her imatinib dose is increased to 400 mg twice a day. Six months later, a repeat bone marrow biopsy continues to show 10% Philadelphia chromosome–positive cells, demonstrating continued partial cytogenetic response. Her WBC count is normal. Because the disease appears to be refractory to the higher imatinib dose, what treatment options are available for S.E.?

Although primary hematologic resistance is rare, primary cytogenetic resistance at 6 months is seen in 15% to 25% of patients started on imatinib therapy. Primary cytogenetic resistance is defined as failure of the patient to achieve any level of cytogenetic response at 6 months, major cytogenetic response at 12 months, and complete cytogenetic response at 18 months.[69] Resistance that occurs outside of these parameters is classified as secondary resistance. In secondary resistance, disease progression is multifactorial and thought to be largely related to mutational changes in the BCR-ABL protein. Based on the 6-year follow-up data from the IRIS trial, progressionfree survival was 91% for patients who achieved a complete cytogenetic response compared with 58% in patients achieving a minor cytogenetic response.[79] As in S.E.'s case, dose escalation of imatinib from

TABLE 92-4
Binet Classification

Stage	Lymphocytosis[a]	Anemia[b]	Thrombocytopenia[c]	Number of Involved Nodes (Max 5)[d]	Median Survival (Years)
A	+	–	–	<3	12
B	+	–	–	≥3	7
C	+	±	±	Any	2–4

[a]Lymphocytes $>5 \times 10^9$/L in peripheral blood and >30% of total cells in the bone marrow.
[b]Hemoglobin <11 g/dL in men and <10 g/dL in women excluding immune-mediated etiology.
[c]Platelets <100,000/μL.
[d]Maximum of five—cervical, axillary, inguinal, spleen, and liver—are counted as one area.
Source: Binet JL et al. A new prognostic classification of chronic lymphocytic leukemia derived from a multivariate survival analysis. *Cancer.* 1981;48:198.

400 mg daily to 400 mg twice daily is the preferred option for patients presenting with cytogenetic resistance at 6 months as demonstrated by a suboptimal cytogenetic response.[69] Low levels of residual disease demonstrate the need for chronic TK inhibitor therapy generally for the lifetime of the patient owing to the high risk of relapse on discontinuation.[80] Dasatinib or nilotinib are more active than imatinib for patients who have mutational changes in BRC-ABL. Because S.E. has not responded to the higher dose of imatinib, dasatinib 100 mg daily or nilotinib 400 mg twice daily would be appropriate treatment options for S.E.'s cytogenetic relapse. She should be continued on therapy indefinitely, assuming she responds, along with continued routine cytogenetic evaluations.

CHRONIC LYMPHOCYTIC LEUKEMIA

Epidemiology and Pathophysiology

Leukemias are hematologic malignancies that are derived from cytogenetic alterations in hematopoietic cells and are classified based on the cell of origin (myeloid or lymphocytic) and clinical course. Chronic lymphocytic leukemia (CLL) is a disorder of mature but functionally incompetent lymphocytes. Lymphomas are also disorders of lymphocytes; therefore, some molecular abnormalities are shared between the diseases.

CLL is the most common type of leukemia in adults, with approximately 15,000 new cases annually and 4,400 deaths.[81] CLL is a disease of the older population, and the median age at diagnosis is 65 years, with 90% of patients older than age 50 at diagnosis.[82,83] CLL is characterized by overproduction of functionally incompetent B-cell lymphocytes derived from a single stem cell clone in the bone marrow. These lymphocytes accumulate in the blood, bone marrow, lymph nodes, and spleen.

Presentation, Diagnosis, and Overview of Treatment

Chronic leukemias follow a relatively insidious onset and course compared with acute leukemias. Approximately 40% of patients are asymptomatic at presentation and are diagnosed by routine CBC (lymphocytosis, anemia, or thrombocytopenia).[64] Symptomatic patients commonly experience night sweats, fatigue, weight loss, fever, and painful lymphadenopathy. Patients often seek medical attention for infection caused by immune suppression or bleeding caused by thrombocytopenia.

Predicting the clinical course of CLL remains a challenge as some patients experience an indolent course and maintain a good quality of life, whereas others experience more aggressive disease and debilitation. Therefore, survival is variable and depends on the stage of disease at diagnosis. CLL is staged based on peripheral lymphocyte counts; enlargement of lymph nodes, liver, and spleen; and the presence of anemia or thrombocytopenia. The two most commonly used staging systems in clinical practice are shown in Tables 92-4 and 92-5. The Rai classification is the most clinically useful because it contains prognostic information (Table 92-5). Low-risk patients (Rai stage 0) have survival similar to that of age-matched control subjects. Intermediate-risk patients (stages I and II) have shorter survival, and high-risk patients (stages III and IV) have poor prognosis. The Binet system (Table 92-4) is based on the number of involved sites, platelets, and hemoglobin and provides prognostic information.

Selection of therapy is in part determined by the presence or absence of cytogenetic abnormalities such as del(11q) or del(17p), comorbidities, and age. Common first-line therapies are

TABLE 92-5
Modified Rai Classification

Risk	Stage	Lymphocytosis[a]	Anemia[b]	Thrombocytopenia[c]	Lymphadenopathy	Hepatomegaly or Splenomegaly	Median Survival (Years)
Low	0	+	–	–	–	–	10
Intermediate	I	+	–	–	+	–	7
	II	+	–	–	±	+	
High	III	+	+	–	±	±	1.5–4
	IV	+	±	+	±	±	

[a]Lymphocytes >5,000/μL in peripheral blood and >30% of total cells in the bone marrow.
[b]Hemoglobin <11 g/dL excluding immune-mediated etiology.
[c]Platelets <100,000/μL
Source: Rai KR et al. Clinical staging of chronic lymphocytic leukemia. *Blood.* 1975;46:219.

chlorambucil with or without prednisone; bendamustine and rituximab; and cyclophosphamide and prednisone with or without rituximab in patients older than or equal to 70 years. Fludarabine, cyclophosphamide, and rituximab (FCR) and fludarabine and rituximab are commonly used in patients younger than 70 years. Relapsed disease is often treated with combinations of the same drugs used for initial treatment. Although patients with CLLs may survive for years with suppressive therapies, these disorders are curable in only a fraction of patients who are candidates for immune-based approaches using chemotherapy and HCT.

Signs and Symptoms

CASE 92-4

QUESTION 1: G.R., a 66-year-old man, presents to his physician with a persistent semiproductive cough and increased fatigue. A routine CBC revealed an Hgb of 13.0 g/dL, a WBC count of 34,000 cells/μL (80% lymphocytes), and a platelet count of 175,000 cells/μL. Blood pressure was 120/70 mm Hg, heart rate 64 beats/minute, and respiratory rate 23 breaths/minute. He was afebrile. Physical examination was unremarkable. He was prescribed azithromycin for possible community-acquired pneumonia and scheduled for a return visit in 3 weeks. At that time, his CBC results were Hgb 13.2 g/dL, WBC count 32,000 cells/μL (82% lymphocytes), and platelets 168,000 cells/μL. Physical examination was unchanged, the chest radiograph was clear, and his cough had resolved. G.R. was referred to a hematologist for evaluation of his persistent lymphocytosis. What is the most likely cause of persistent lymphocytosis in G.R.?

CLL is usually included in the differential diagnosis of any adult with persistent lymphocytosis (>5,000 lymphocytes/μL in peripheral blood). Additional causes of lymphocytosis include transient reactions to acute infections and viruses such as influenza or mononucleosis, as well as other hematologic malignancies, including lymphoma and ALL.

To differentiate between benign and malignant lymphocytosis, examination of the peripheral blood or bone marrow morphology by a hematologist or pathologist may be required. Patients with CLL commonly have lymphocytosis in both the peripheral blood and bone marrow, whereas patients with other disorders have a high percentage of atypical lymphocytes in the peripheral blood alone. The absence of fever or additional signs of infection without significant diagnostic or physical examination findings, together with the presence of mature peripheral blood lymphocytes, make CLL the most likely diagnosis for G.R. Immunophenotyping and cytogenetics of involved cells are required to establish the diagnosis and to provide prognostic information and determine therapy. Bone marrow biopsy with aspirate may be useful to determine the definitive diagnosis.[84]

Staging and Prognosis

CASE 92-4, QUESTION 2: G.R.'s bone marrow examination reveals normal cellularity with greater than 40% of nucleated cells lymphocytes. The immunophenotype indicates that peripheral blood lymphocytes are predominately B cells and are positive for CD5, CD19, and CD20. A diagnosis of CLL is confirmed. Is G.R.'s presentation consistent with CLL? What is the prognosis for G.R.'s disease? What treatment is indicated at this time? G.R.'s cells were sent for routine cytogenetic analysis, which revealed a chromosome abnormality (deletion 11q). How does this affect his management?

G.R. has fatigue, infection, and lymphocytosis without lymphadenopathy, and these are consistent with low-risk CLL based on his Modified Rai stage. Given his stage, G.R. has an expected survival of at least 10 years.[82,85]

An accepted treatment modality for early-stage disease includes a conservative, watchful waiting approach. No clear advantage has been demonstrated in treating asymptomatic patients in early-stage disease with alkylator-based chemotherapy as compared with deferred treatment.[86] The survival of patients with smoldering CLL is similar to an age- and sex-matched normal population.[87,88]

There is significant heterogeneity in the clinical course of CLL that is in part attributable to the biological differences between tumors. Scientific advances have led to the discovery of chromosomal abnormalities (deletions 11q or 17p), gene mutations (unmutated immunoglobulin variable region and p53), and serum or cell surface markers (increased β_2 microglobulin, zeta-associated protein-70, and CD38 expression) that may confer poor prognosis.[89–92] The deletion 13q is the most common cytogenetic abnormality, occurring in 55% of patients, and it has a favorable prognosis (survival >10 years). The deletion 11q and deletion 17p occur in 18% and 7%, respectively, with shorter survival times of approximately 7 and 3 years, respectively. Current national guidelines take into account some of these factors in their treatment recommendations.

Despite his early stage by the Modified Rai classification, G.R. had an 11q deletion, conferring a worse prognosis; he would be encouraged to start treatment. However, as a result of having minimal symptoms, G.R. chooses to delay treatment until he becomes symptomatic.

Treatment

CASE 92-4, QUESTION 3: G.R. returns to the hematologist every 3 months and has no new symptoms or infectious complications for about 2 years. At that time, physical examination reveals enlargement of cervical, inguinal, and axillary lymph nodes; hepatomegaly; and splenomegaly. His WBC has increased from 34,000 cells/μL 6 months ago to 68,000 cells/μL today (85% lymphocytes). His Hgb is 11.7 g/dL, and his platelet count is 140,000 cells/μL. What treatment is now indicated?

Indications for treatment initiation in CLL include significant anemia or thrombocytopenia, progressive disease demonstrated by lymphadenopathy, hepatomegaly, splenomegaly, a lymphocyte doubling time of less than 6 months, persistent B symptoms (fever, night sweats, and weight loss), threatened end-organ function, and recurrent infection. Patient performance status, comorbid conditions, pharmacoeconomic variables, and social support should all be taken into consideration when selecting treatment. Cytogenetic results will also be considered. Because G.R. has experienced significant lymphadenopathy and hepatosplenomegaly, he should initiate treatment at this time to prevent further deterioration of his hematologic and immune function.

INITIAL THERAPY

CHLORAMBUCIL

Therapy for CLL has historically included use of an alkylating agent, most often oral chlorambucil or cyclophosphamide, with or without prednisone. A variety of daily and intermittent dosing schedules have been reported. The overall response (OR) rate to chlorambucil was approximately 40% to 60%, but only 3% to 5% achieved a CR.[82] Chlorambucil use has diminished, and the use of purine analogs, such as fludarabine and cladribine, is more common in clinical practice; however, chlorambucil with or without prednisone is recommended for patients older than or equal to 70 years, or in younger patients if they have significant comorbidities.[93]

FLUDARABINE

Fludarabine is now considered the single most active agent in the treatment of CLL. Fludarabine monotherapy at a dose range of 25 to 30 mg/m²/dose IV × 5 days has shown a 70% to 80% OR rate, and CR rates of 20% to 30% with increased progression-free survival (PFS).[94–96] Fludarabine may have improved OS compared with chlorambucil, but results are inconsistent across studies.[97–99] Toxicities associated with fludarabine are typically mild and include fever and immunosuppression. Increased incidence of infection and autoimmune hemolytic anemia are also associated with fludarabine therapy. Infection prophylaxis should be considered in elderly patients and patients with advanced disease or renal dysfunction.

Fludarabine has been combined with other chemotherapy and monoclonal antibodies, including cyclophosphamide and rituximab, in an effort to prevent multidrug resistance and increase response. Although combination regimens including fludarabine have demonstrated higher response rates and PFS, no difference in OS has been consistently demonstrated.[100–102] Additional toxicities of the combination regimens include higher rates of leukopenia, thrombocytopenia, nausea, vomiting, and alopecia.

CLADRIBINE

The response to cladribine, a synthetic purine nucleoside, is superior to chlorambucil, with OR and CR rates comparable to single-agent fludarabine.[103] A typical dose and schedule is 0.14 mg//kg/day IV over 2 hours for 5 days every 28 days for 3 to 6 cycles. The toxicity profile is similar to fludarabine. Although cladribine in combination with cyclophosphamide with or without mitoxantrone achieved higher CR rates and less multidrug-resistant clones, no significant improvement in OS has been demonstrated.[104] A higher percentage of grade 3 to grade 4 neutropenia was seen with the combination regimens compared with cladribine alone.

BENDAMUSTINE

Bendamustine, a nitrogen mustard/alkylating agent, was approved in 2008 for the treatment of CLL. In clinical studies it has been shown to be superior to chlorambucil with OR and CR rates of 68% and 31%, respectively.[105] A typical dose and schedule is 100 mg/m² IV on days 1 and 2. Toxicities include infusion reactions and myelosuppression. It is often used in combination with rituximab and primarily in patients older than or equal to 70 years or those with comorbidities.

RITUXIMAB

Rituximab is a chimeric human–murine anti-CD20 monoclonal antibody. The CD20 surface antigen is expressed on a high percentage of CLL cells. Rituximab monotherapy as initial therapy for untreated patients at a dose of 375 mg/m² weekly for four doses yielded OR rates of 58% and CR rates of 9%; these are lower than those seen with cytotoxic therapy, with a disappointing duration of response.[106] Therefore, rituximab monotherapy is reserved for patients with significant comorbidity. Generally it is used in combination therapy with cytotoxic agents.

COMBINATION REGIMENS

A regimen for initial treatment is the combination of FCR. In a study of first-line treatment of CLL, patients were treated with fludarabine 25 mg/m² IV on days 1 to 3, cyclophosphamide 250 mg/m² IV on days 1 to 3, and rituximab 375 mg/m² IV on day 1 of cycle 1, escalated to 500 mg/m² in subsequent cycles. CR was attained by 44% of patients, OR in 90%.[101] Toxicity of this regimen included infusion-related reactions, nausea, vomiting, and myelosuppression. Grade 3 or 4 neutropenia was noted in 34% of treatment courses, with an infection rate of 25%. FCR is recommended in patients younger than 70 years without significant comorbidities or older patients without comorbidities, and in any patient with the unfavorable del(17p) cytogenetic abnormality.[93]

Results for a bendamustine plus rituximab (BR) combination regimen have recently been reported. In a study of 117 patients with previously untreated CLL, patients were given bendamustine 90 mg/m² IV on days 1 and 2, and rituximab 375 mg/m² IV on day 1 of cycle 1, escalated to 500 mg/m² in subsequent cycles for up to 6 cycles. OR was 90% and CR 33%.[107] Trials are ongoing to compare this combination with FCR as first-line therapy for CLL patients who are able to tolerate combination chemotherapy. The BR regimen, like chlorambucil with or without prednisone, is commonly used in patients older than or equal to 70 years or in younger patients with comorbidities.

ALEMTUZUMAB

Alemtuzumab is a humanized conjugated anti-CD52 monoclonal antibody and a first-line treatment option for CLL.[93] Initial doses of 3 mg, titrated to 10 mg, and, ultimately, 30 mg, were administered either subcutaneously or IV three times weekly for up to 12 weeks. In comparison with chlorambucil, alemtuzumab had a CR rate of 24% versus 2% with chlorambucil. However, there was no difference in OS.[108] Toxicities associated with alemtuzumab include infusion-related reactions (rigors, fever, dyspnea), neutropenia, and infectious complications.[109,110] Alemtuzumab is usually given to older patients or those with comorbidities. The role of alemtuzumab maintenance after cytotoxic therapy is also under investigation.[111]

In summary, first-line therapy for patients older than or equal to 70 years old or with significant comorbidities generally includes BR, or chlorambucil plus prednisone. For younger patients without comorbidities, three-drug combinations such as FCR may be offered. G.R. is now 68 years old with no significant comorbidities and is likely to tolerate treatment with FCR.

CASE 92-4, QUESTION 4: G.R. receives FCR as initial CLL therapy. After the third cycle, he has complete regression of his lymphadenopathy and hepatosplenomegaly, and his WBC count decreases to 9,000 cells/μL. He finishes six cycles in total. G.R. comes to clinic 1.5 years after completion of therapy. A CBC is obtained that reveals a WBC count of 55,000 cells/μL (70% lymphocytes), Hgb of 10 g/dL, and platelet count of 90,000 cells/μL. On physical examination, G.R. is found to have cervical, inguinal, and axillary lymphadenopathy with no palpable splenomegaly. He complains of excessive fatigue and fever. Therefore, G.R. has recurrent disease. What therapies may be helpful to him at this point?

RELAPSED OR REFRACTORY THERAPY

Second-line therapy should be selected based on criteria similar to those used for initial management. Relapsed patients are classified as treatment-sensitive if the disease relapses more than 3 years after treatment, or refractory if the disease relapses within

2 years of treatment.[93] G.R.'s relapse occurred less than 2 years from completion of therapy. He is classified as refractory to his first-line regimen. He is still younger than 70 years old with minimal comorbidities and is a candidate for aggressive second-line treatment.

TREATMENT-SENSITIVE

Treatment-sensitive patients are retreated with the same regimen given for first-line therapy as long as they are expected to tolerate treatment. For patients who are older than 70 years old or those who have comorbidities, the regimen may be changed to one with less toxicity. These less toxic regimens include dose-reduced FCR, chlorambucil-prednisone, BR, single-agent alemtuzumab, single-agent rituximab, or cyclophosphamide-prednisone-rituximab.[93]

TREATMENT-REFRACTORY

Treatment-refractory patients will be offered a regimen containing at least one anticancer agent not previously given. For patients older than 70 years old with comorbidities, options include chemoimmunotherapy combinations: dose-reduced FCR, dose-reduced pentostatin-cyclophosphamide-rituximab, chlorambucil-prednisone, BR, and high-dose methylprednisolone-rituximab. Other options are alemtuzumab, ofatumumab, and dose-dense rituximab. Patients younger than 70 years old without significant comorbidities have several options, including combination chemotherapy, chemoimmunotherapy, and monoclonal antibodies and consideration of allogeneic HCT.[93,112]

Alemtuzumab as a single agent is FDA-approved for the treatment of refractory CLL and may be used regardless of age and presence of comorbidities.[113] The OR rate is approximately 30%, with a 0% to 2% CR rate and an OS of 16 to 27.5 months.[114,115] Activity has been demonstrated in patients who relapsed after or were refractory to alkylator or purine analog therapy, including those with the del(17p) cytogenetic mutation, which is associated with resistance to most cytotoxic agents.[113] Alemtuzumab is least effective in patients with bulky (>5 cm) disease.[116]

Major toxicities of alemtuzumab include infusion-related events, infections, and cytopenias. The occurrence of opportunistic infections, including *Pneumocystis carinii* [now *P. jiroveci*] pneumonia and cytomegalovirus (CMV) in as many as 15% to 25% of patients treated with alemtuzumab, warrants the use of prophylactic therapy. An increased risk of infection occurs 3 to 8 weeks after treatment, which corresponds to the T-cell nadir. Viral prophylaxis for herpes infections (e.g., acyclovir or equivalent) should be continued for at least 2 months after completion of therapy, and *P. jiroveci* pneumonia prophylaxis (e.g., sulfamethoxazole-trimethoprim) should be continued until the CD4 count is at least 200 cells/μL.[117,118]

Younger patients with relapsed disease or high-risk features may benefit from allogeneic HCT. Both clinical and molecular remissions have been reported after autologous HCT, with a 4-year survival of 42%.[119] Allogeneic HCT is the only curative treatment for CLL to date. However, the high risk of treatment-related morbidity and mortality must be considered. Patients with relapsed CLL after fludarabine therapy or with high-risk features should be referred to a transplant center to determine candidacy.[112]

In conclusion, G.R.'s disease relapsed within 18 months of completing initial therapy and is treatment refractory; therefore, he should receive a second-line regimen, which includes an agent he has not been previously exposed to. G.R. received FCR as his initial treatment; therefore, the BR regimen is a good choice for him now. In addition, he is younger and in relatively good health and should tolerate combination therapy.

Infectious Complications

CASE 92-4, QUESTION 5: Six weeks after the initiation of alemtuzumab, G.R. complains of progressive shortness of breath and fever. On questioning, he reveals that he quit taking his trimethoprim-sulfamethoxazole and valacyclovir because "I felt fine." Radiography of the chest reveals bilateral infiltrates. G.R. is admitted to the hospital for further evaluation and treatment. A CBC reveals a WBC count of 22,000 cells/μL (80% lymphocytes) and an absolute neutrophil count of 800 cells/μL, Hgb of 11 g/dL, and platelet count of 70,000 cells/μL. Quantification of serum immunoglobulins reveals profound hypogammaglobulinemia. What are the possible causes of G.R.'s pneumonia, and what treatment is indicated?

Infections contribute significantly to morbidity and mortality in patients with CLL. The immune compromise of CLL is attributable to immunoglobulin deficiency, abnormal T-cell function, neutropenia and chemotherapy, which contribute to the increased rate of both common and opportunistic infections.[120] Up to 80% of patients will develop an infectious complication; therefore, the use of IV immune globulin, antibacterials (trimethoprim-sulfamethoxazole), and antivirals (acyclovir for herpes simplex virus) and vaccinations (influenza, pneumococcal, live vaccines) are common. Opportunistic infections are particularly common in patients receiving a purine analog or alemtuzumab therapy, and ganciclovir prophylaxis may be given. The most commonly reported opportunistic infection associated with alemtuzumab is CMV reactivation. The use of supplemental IV immune globulin for prophylaxis of future infection is often used in patients with low immunoglobulin levels (IgG <500 mg/dL) and recurrent infections requiring hospitalization.[113]

ONLINE CONTENT

For a table titled "Types of infections in patients with chronic lymphocytic leukemia undergoing immunosuppressive therapy," go to http://thepoint.lww.com/AT10e.

Hospitalization is warranted for G.R. so he can receive broad-spectrum antimicrobials for neutropenic fever and a thorough workup for opportunistic etiologies. Because G.R. has a significant pulmonary infection requiring hospitalization with a documented hypogammaglobulinemia, prophylactic IV immune globulin therapy should be considered to prevent future infections.

MULTIPLE MYELOMA

Incidence and Epidemiology

Multiple myeloma (MM) is defined as a malignancy of "plasma cells," terminally differentiated B lymphocytes responsible for the production of antibodies and for the rapid response of the immune system to antigen exposure.[121,122] The abnormal proliferation and accumulation of plasma cells leads to excessive antibody (immunoglobulin) production, typically IgG or IgA. A variety of laboratory and clinical manifestations can be seen in MM and are related to the extent of excessive monoclonal immunoglobulin (M-protein) production, plasma cell infiltration, and immune deficiency. In the United States in 2010, there were an estimated 20,180 new diagnoses of MM. The average age at diagnosis is 70 years (98% of patients are 40 years or older) and 55% of patients are male.[121,123] The disease occurs twice as often in African Americans compared with whites and has increased in incidence each decade since the 1970s.[121]

Pathophysiology

Although MM may present as a de novo diagnosis, most cases are believed to arise from a benign precursor condition known as monoclonal gammopathy of undetermined significance (MGUS). MGUS is characterized by the accumulation of abnormal clonal plasma cells and may be differentiated from MM by the serum concentration of M-protein (<3 g/dL) and the lack of clinical manifestations typically associated with MM (osteolytic bone lesions, hypercalcemia, renal dysfunction, etc.).[124] By way of a complex multistep process involving a variety of genetic events and changes in the plasma cell's microenvironment, a transformation from MGUS to smoldering MM or symptomatic MM occurs at a rate of approximately 1% of patients per year.[125,126] Cellular events promoting the growth of malignant plasma cells, i.e., induction of angiogenesis, suppression of immunity, and the production of osteoclast-activating factors (e.g., IL-6, tumor necrosis factor, parathyroid hormone-related peptide), occur during the conversion of benign plasma cells to their malignant counterparts.[127,128]

Smoldering myeloma represents an indolent form of the disease in which patients produce M-protein (>3 g/dL) at a level consistent with the diagnosis of MM or have greater than 10% plasma cells in the bone marrow but remain asymptomatic.[127] Smoldering myeloma progresses to MM at a rate of 10% per year for the first 5 years after diagnosis, 3% per year for the next 5 years, and 1% per year for the next 10 years.[127]

Clinical Presentation, Diagnosis, and Treatment

Patients presenting initially with symptomatic MM frequently complain of bone pain, fatigue, and recurrent infections resulting from immune suppression. These patients may also have end-organ damage, including hyper<u>c</u>alcemia, <u>r</u>enal dysfunction, <u>a</u>nemia, and <u>b</u>one lesions (which may be remembered using the pneumonic *CRAB*). The final diagnosis requires confirmation of abnormal M-protein production and serum β_2 microglobulin concentration. Because MM is not generally considered to be a curable malignancy, the goal of treatment is to achieve and maintain a clinical response through the combination of induction therapy, HCT, and maintenance therapy. See the following video for more general information on MM: **<u>http//www.youtube.com/watch?v=uxdgFn1ZMRk.</u>**

Clinical Presentation

CASE 92-5

QUESTION 1: B.B. is a 62-year-old, otherwise healthy, man who presents with acute musculoskeletal chest and back pain after performing light maintenance work. He was initially prescribed muscle relaxers and over-the-counter nonsteroidal anti-inflammatory drugs (NSAIDs), but has achieved little relief. Computed tomography (CT) scan of the spine reveals osteolytic bone lesions from T6 to T11. Further workup reveals an Hgb of 7 g/dL, serum calcium of 11.8 mg/dL, and serum creatinine of 2.0 mg/dL. Serum and urine protein electrophoresis show M-protein typed as IgG-kappa of 5.3 g/dL. A serum β_2 microglobulin was 4.4 mg/L. Bone marrow biopsy reveals 90% plasma cells with normal cytogenetics. Skeletal survey shows additional lesions in the ribs. A diagnosis of MM stage II is made. Is this presentation consistent with the diagnosis of MM?

B.B. presents with a number of the classic features of MM. Bone pain and skeletal disease are common and occur when plasma cells infiltrate the bone marrow and secrete osteoclast-activating factors. Plain radiographic films will reveal osteopenia or multiple osteolytic bone lesions (punched out areas on radiographs). Hypercalcemia and pathological fractures often accompany the osteolytic lesions associated with this disease. When plasma cells infiltrate the bone marrow, they can also lead to a normocytic normochromic anemia in up to 70% of patients. Comparatively, neutropenia and thrombocytopenia are rarely present at the time of diagnosis. Renal dysfunction is generally attributable to deposition of kappa or lambda light chains of immunoglobulin in the distal tubule, and up to 40% of patients have or will develop renal insufficiency with the disease.[129] In most patients with MM, only light chains are found in the urine. Myelomas that overproduce light chains are most commonly associated with renal dysfunction. Renal dysfunction can be further complicated by dehydration secondary to hypercalcemia, the use of NSAIDs for pain relief, and the use of contrast dyes in radiographic evaluation. B.B. should receive hydration with a sodium chloride–containing solution to restore euvolemia and reduce his calcium; he should avoid NSAIDs and other nephrotoxic therapies. Another feature that may accompany MM is hyperviscosity syndrome, more commonly seen with IgA subtype. Hyperviscosity causes CNS, renal, cardiac, and pulmonary symptoms and complications. Plasmapheresis may be used emergently to alleviate life-threatening cases. Patients may experience recurrent infections as a result of depressed production of other immunoglobulin classes, leading to an inability to opsonize bacteria.

TABLE 92-6
Diagnostic Criteria for Plasma Cell Disorders[a]

Multiple Myeloma

1. Presence of a serum or urinary monoclonal immunoglobulin protein
2. Presence of clonal plasma cells in the bone marrow or a plasmacytoma
3. Presence of end-organ damage related to plasma cell proliferation, including:
   Elevated calcium (1 mg/dL above the upper limit of the normal range, or >11 mg/dL)
   Renal insufficiency (creatinine >1.9 mg/dL)
   Anemia (2 g/dL below the lower limit of the normal range, or <10 g/dL)
   Bone lesions (lytic lesions or osteoporosis with compression fractures)

Asymptomatic (Smoldering) Multiple Myeloma

1. Serum monoclonal immunoglobulin >3 g/dL or bone marrow plasma cells >10%
2. No end-organ damage related to plasma cell proliferation

Monoclonal Gammopathy of Undetermined Significance (MGUS)

1. Serum monoclonal immunoglobulin <3 g/dL
2. Bone marrow plasma cells <10%
3. No end-organ damage related to plasma cell proliferation

[a]All criteria must be met.
Source: International Myeloma Working Group. Criteria for the classification of monoclonal gammopathies, multiple myeloma and related disorders: a report of the International Working Group. *Br J Haematol*. 2003;121:749.

Diagnosis and Staging

Diagnostic criteria for all plasma cell disorders is shown in Table 92-6. B.B. clearly meets the criteria for MM. Two staging systems have been used for patients with MM. The older Durie-Salmon system, developed in 1975, relies on the extent of M-protein production, serum creatinine, hemoglobin, serum calcium, and presence and number of bone lesions.[130,131] More recently, a large international study demonstrated that staging and prognosis can be predicted reliably from serum β_2 microglobulin (a light chain protein expressed on all nucleated cells) and albumin (Table 92-7). Based on the International Staging System, B.B.'s serum β_2 microglobulin, is consistent with stage II MM.

TABLE 92-7
International Staging System for Multiple Myeloma

Stage I—β_2 microglobulin <3.5 mg/L and serum albumin ≥3.5 g/dL
Stage II—neither stage I nor stage III
Stage III—β_2 microglobulin ≥5.5 mg/L

Source: Greipp PR et al. International staging system for multiple myeloma. *J Clin Oncol.* 2005;23:3412.

Treatment

INITIAL THERAPY

CASE 92-5, QUESTION 2: The decision is made to begin B.B. on treatment with a regimen including bortezomib, lenalidomide, and dexamethasone. What advantages and disadvantages does this regimen have compared with others?

Patients who meet the diagnostic criteria for MM and who are symptomatic are candidates for systemic chemotherapy (Table 92-8). Choice of induction therapy is based on the patients' eligibility for HCT. When possible, the most effective treatment is induction chemotherapy to achieve a complete clinical response (defined by elimination of M-protein in plasma and elimination of plasma cells in the bone marrow) followed by autologous

TABLE 92-8
Multiple Myeloma Treatment Regimens

Regimen	Agents	Comments
Induction Therapy		
Eligible for High-Dose Chemotherapy With Autologous HCT		
RVD	Lenalidomide 25 mg PO daily, days 1–14 Bortezomib 1.3 mg/m^2 IV days 1, 4, 8 and 11 Dexamethasone 40 mg PO daily, days 1–2, 4–5, 8–9, 11–12 Repeat cycle every 21 days	Antithrombotic prophylaxis is recommended with lenalidomide. Antiviral prophylaxis with acyclovir is recommended with bortezomib.
VTD	Bortezomib 1.3 mg/m^2 IV days 1, 4, 8, and 11 Thalidomide 200 mg PO daily Dexamethasone 40 mg PO daily, days 1–4 and 9–12 Repeat cycle every 21 days	Thalidomide should be given in the evening to minimize sedation. Antithrombotic prophylaxis is recommended.
Bortezomib + Dexamethasone	Bortezomib 1.3 mg/m^2 IV days 1, 4, 8, and 11 Dexamethasone 20 mg PO daily, days 1–2, 4–5, 8–9, 11–12 Repeat cycle every 21 days	
Ineligible for High-Dose Chemotherapy With Autologous Stem Cell Support		
MPB	Melphalan 9–12 mg/m^2 PO daily, days 1–4 Prednisone 60 mg/m^2 PO daily, days 1–4 Bortezomib 1.3 mg/m^2 IV days 1, 4, 8, 11, 22, 25, 29, 32 for the first 4 cycles, then days 1, 8, 22, 29 in subsequent cycles	
MPT	Melphalan 4 mg/m^2 PO daily, days 1–7 Prednisone 40 mg/m^2 PO daily, days 1–7 Thalidomide 100 mg PO daily Repeat cycle every 28 days	Melphalan should be given on an empty stomach owing to variable absorption when administered with food.
MP	Melphalan 8–10 mg/m^2 PO daily, days 1–4 Prednisone 60 mg/m^2 PO daily, days 1–4 Repeat cycle every 28–42 days	
Salvage Therapy		
Bortezomib	Bortezomib 1.3 mg/m^2 IV days 1, 4, 8, and 11 Repeat cycle every 21 days	Dose reduction to 1 mg/m^2 may be necessary in patients with neuropathy or thrombocytopenia. Addition of dexamethasone may be required in patients who do not respond.
Bortezomib + liposomal doxorubicin	Bortezomib 1.3 mg/m^2 IV once Liposomal doxorubicin 30 mg/m^2, day 4 Repeat cycle every 21 days	
Lenalidomide + dexamethasone	Lenalidomide 25 mg PO daily, days 1–21 Dexamethasone 40 mg PO daily, days 1–4, 9–12, 17–20 for the first four cycles, then days 1–4 only in subsequent cycles	Consider prophylactic antithrombotics.

CIV, continuous intravenous infusion; HCT, hematopoietic cell transplantation; IV, intravenously; MP, melphalan and prednisone; MPB, melphalan, prednisone, and bortezomib; MPT, melphalan, prednisone, and thalidomide; PO, orally; RVD, lenalidomide, bortezomib, and dexamethasone; VTD, bortezomib, thalidomide, and dexamethasone.

HCT.[132] Many patients are not eligible to receive HCT, however. Determination of HCT eligibility includes consideration of patient age (typically 65 years of age or younger) and comorbidities. In the case of B.B., his age (62 years) and relative good health make him a candidate for further consideration of HCT as a component of his MM management. Those who are eligible for HCT should not be treated with agents such as melphalan, which may compromise the ability to collect a sufficient number of hematopoietic cells necessary to perform the autologous HCT. Although a number of drugs have shown efficacy in treating patients with MM, the most current NCCN Clinical Practice Guidelines recommend bortezomib, lenalidomide, and dexamethasone as initial induction therapy.[133]

The proteosome inhibitor bortezomib represents a novel class of agents for the treatment of MM. Bortezomib acts by inhibiting the 26S proteosome, a multienzyme complex responsible for regulation of proteins that promote cell survival, stimulate growth, and reduce susceptibility to programmed cell death.[134] Bortezomib is generally dosed as 1.3 mg/m^2 on days 1, 4, 8, and 11 of a 3-week cycle in combination with thalidomide, lenalidomide, and/or dexamethasone. Patients should be monitored for common adverse events, including fatigue, diarrhea, mild nausea, thrombocytopenia, and peripheral neuropathy (the most common cause of discontinuation of bortezomib in clinical trials).[135] Reactivation of herpes zoster has been observed in greater than 10% of patients treated with bortezomib; therefore, consideration should be given to prophylactic use of acyclovir in these immunocompromised patients.[136,137] An additional benefit of bortezomib is the ability to induce responses in MM patients with poor prognosis, such as the high-risk cytogenetic abnormalities del(13) and t(4;14).[138]

Lenalidomide, an oral immunomodulatory agent with antiangiogenic properties, is also effective in patients with MM. The dose of lenalidomide is most commonly 25 mg daily for 14 days of a 3-week cycle. Common adverse events include hematologic toxicities, muscle weakness, fatigue, and rash.[139] Less commonly, lenalidomide has been associated with thromboembolic events, and venous thrombotic embolism prophylaxis is recommended. Several recent cooperative group studies have revealed a small but concerning risk of secondary malignancies, including AML. Although this concern should not prohibit the use of lenalidomide, patients should be closely monitored, and practitioners should be aware of this risk. As an analog of thalidomide, concerns about teratogenicity prohibit the use of lenalidomide during pregnancy and make it available only through a restricted distribution program. In comparison with lenalidomide, thalidomide is less potent and has a less favorable toxicity profile, with sedation and peripheral neuropathy being common in addition to constipation and thrombotic events. Like lenalidomide, thalidomide is only available via a restricted access prescription program.

Dexamethasone is moderately effective as MM induction therapy alone and in combination, and has significant adverse effects, including hyperglycemia, insomnia, and increased infection risk. However, the combination of lenalidomide (Revlimid), bortezomib (Velcade), and dexamethasone (RVD) has demonstrated efficacy in early-phase clinical trials with an overall response rate of 100% in patients with newly diagnosed MM.[140] In addition to the exceptional response rate, RVD is well tolerated with sensory neuropathy, fatigue, and hematologic toxicities being the most commonly reported adverse events. Additional combination induction regimens in HCT-eligible patients include bortezomib, thalidomide, and dexamethasone; bortezomib and dexamethasone; bortezomib, doxorubicin, and dexamethasone; and lenalidomide and dexamethasone. Independent of the choice of induction regimen, patients commonly receive 3 to 6 cycles of treatment before HCT.[141]

In patients ineligible for autologous HCT, melphalan-based regimens are appropriate for induction therapy. Melphalan and prednisone (MP) was the first regimen to show significant activity in myeloma, but it rarely produces a complete remission. The addition of thalidomide to MP (MPT) was compared with MP in patients 60 to 85 years of age.[142] OR and CR rates were significantly improved with MPT (76% and 16%, respectively) compared with MP (48% and 2%, respectively). In addition, 2-year eventfree survival was superior in patients receiving MPT compared with MP (54% vs. 27%). Thromboembolic events seen in the early part of the trial in patients receiving MPT led to the use of enoxaparin 40 mg subcutaneously daily, which reduced thromboembolism from 20% to 3%. Other toxicities seen more commonly with MPT included peripheral neuropathy, constipation, and infection, necessitating discontinuation of thalidomide in 33% of patients before the completion of 2 months of therapy. Subsequently, the VISTA trial demonstrated the superiority of MP combined with bortezomib (MPB) as compared with MP. Time to disease progression and 3-year OS rates in previously untreated MM patients significantly favored MPB.[143,144] MPB has also been associated with better outcomes in patients with high-risk cytogenetics and poor renal function.[143,144] Peripheral neuropathy, gastrointestinal symptoms, and herpes zoster reactivation were more common in patients receiving MPB. Both MPT and MPB are proven to be superior to the historical standard MP and should be considered as standard of care treatment options in transplant-ineligible patients. Superior outcomes have been associated with RVD; therefore, this combination is appropriate induction therapy.

HEMATOPOIETIC CELL TRANSPLANTATION

Efforts to improve the outcome of MM treatment have led to the investigation of high-dose chemotherapy (e.g., melphalan 200 mg/m^2) with autologous HCT and nonmyeloablative preparative regimens with allogeneic HCT. Randomized comparisons of autologous HCT and conventional chemotherapy in previously untreated patients younger than 65 years have been conducted.[145–147,148] All patients received two to six cycles of conventional chemotherapy before randomization to autologous HCT or standard chemotherapy. Most trials reported higher response rates and improved survival in patients randomly assigned to receive autologous HCT. Younger age, chemosensitive disease, and fewer pretransplant therapies have emerged as important predictive factors for response to autologous HCT. Autologous HCT is regarded as the current treatment of choice for eligible patients with MM who achieve CR after induction therapy.[132,149] The use of allogeneic HCT in MM is a potentially curative option, but has been associated with excessive mortality. Nonmyeloablative allogeneic regimens (which use lower doses of chemotherapy) are generally associated with fewer regimen-related toxicities than full allogeneic transplants, but allow for a graft-versus-tumor effect that eradicates residual disease (see Chapter 96, Hematopoietic Cell Transplantation). Initial trials have been encouraging, particularly in patients who are not heavily pretreated and those with chemotherapy-sensitive disease.[150–152] B.B. will receive three cycles of RVD and will be evaluated for HCT.

BISPHOSPHONATES

CASE 92-5, QUESTION 3: Zoledronic acid 4 mg IV over 15 minutes every 28 days is ordered for B.B. What is the rationale for bisphosphonate therapy in the presence of normal serum calcium? What benefits and toxicities are associated with bisphosphonate therapy?

Osteolytic bone lesions or osteopenia occur in nearly 80% of all patients with MM and represent one of the most significant challenges to quality of life in this patient population.[125] Although these bone manifestations of MM may occur throughout the body, they are most commonly identified in the vertebral column, where they may lead to clinically significant issues, including fracture.[121]

The efficacy of pamidronate and zoledronic acid for the prevention of skeletal fractures in MM patients with osteolytic bone lesions or osteopenia has been established, and guidelines for their use have been developed.[153] Equivalent efficacy with monthly infusion has been shown with pamidronate 90 mg and zoledronic acid 4 mg. Zoledronic acid can be given in 15 minutes, whereas pamidronate is given for 2 hours. Because bisphosphonates can negatively affect kidney function, serum creatinine should be monitored monthly and urine albumin measured every 3 months. Higher doses and shorter infusion times have been associated with renal damage; patients with creatinine clearances between 30 and 60 mL/minute should receive reduced doses of zoledronic acid. In patients with baseline creatinine values of more than 3 mg/dL, pamidronate 90 mg over the course of 4 to 6 hours is recommended. Bisphosphonate therapy should be held in patients who have creatinine elevations above the normal baseline by 0.5 mg/dL or more until renal function returns to baseline. Osteonecrosis of the jaw is a rare but serious complication of bisphosphonate therapy that appears to increase in likelihood with prolonged treatment. Baseline dental examinations and avoidance of invasive dental procedures during therapy are recommended. The use of zoledronic acid has been associated with a 9.5-fold increased risk of osteonecrosis of the jaw compared with pamidronate. All patients with responsive or stable disease should be strongly considered for bisphosphonate discontinuation after 2 years of treatment.

Denosumab is a monoclonal antibody to the RANK-ligand receptor resulting in reduced bone resorption and localized bone destruction. With fewer side effects than the bisphosphonates and lack of renal toxicity, denosumab has demonstrated efficacy in patients with osteolytic bone lesions from MM.[153] Denosumab cannot be recommended at this time to replace bisphosphonates in the management of MM patients because of an increased risk of mortality observed in a planned subgroup analysis.[154]

B.B. is a candidate for bisphosphonate therapy with zoledronic acid 4 mg IV every 28 days because he has osteolytic disease in the spine and ribs.

MAINTENANCE THERAPY

CASE 92-5, QUESTION 4: B.B. receives three cycles of RVD, followed by autologous HCT. He returns to clinic today 8 weeks after HCT. Should he receive any additional treatment at this time?

Given the near certainty that MM will progress after autologous HCT, there exists a growing need for effective maintenance therapy. Two phase III studies have evaluated the benefit of lenalidomide in this setting. The CALGB 100104 study used a starting dose of 10 mg daily (allowing for escalation to 15 mg/day) for 21 of 28 days per month compared with placebo. The time to progression was 42.3 months for patients receiving lenalidomide versus 21.8 months for the placebo arm.[155] When compared with placebo in the IFM 2005-02 trial, lenalidomide 10 to 15 mg/day increased PFS by 18 months (42 months vs. 24 months).[156] Although thalidomide also has demonstrated efficacy as maintenance therapy, lenalidomide may be preferred as a result of its improved toxicity profile. Consideration should also be given to which drugs patients are exposed to during the entire course of treatment for MM beginning with induction therapy. One study evaluating the use of thalidomide during induction therapy as well as in maintenance therapy after HCT reported an increased response rate and improved 5-year eventfree survival but no improvement in OS and increased toxicity.[157] These results have suggested that sequencing of therapies may be important in the management of MM. Further study is warranted to determine whether patients treated with one drug during induction should be treated with a different drug for maintenance therapy.

The decision was made that B.B. would receive maintenance therapy with lenalidomide 10 mg daily until disease progression was documented.

Relapsed and Refractory Disease

CASE 92-5, QUESTION 5: Four years after autologous HCT, B.B. is found to have relapsed disease. What other therapies may offer benefit for his myeloma?

In those patients presenting with relapsed or refractory MM more than 6 months after the completion of initial induction therapy, it is reasonable to re-treat using the same drug regimen. For those patients with early relapse or refractory MM, consideration should be given to treatment with bortezomib or lenalidomide-containing regimens. In a comparison with dexamethasone alone, patients receiving bortezomib had a longer time to disease progression (6.2 months vs. 3.5 months) and longer OS, leading to a recommendation to halt the dexamethasone arm and allow those patients to receive single-agent bortezomib.[135] Bortezomib may be combined with pegylated liposomal doxorubicin, resulting in prolonged time to disease progression as compared with bortezomib alone (9.3 months vs. 6.5 months).[158] Common toxicities of the combination regimen include neutropenia, thrombocytopenia, diarrhea, and fatigue. Although bortezomib alone may be better tolerated than the combination with pegylated liposomal doxorubicin, the combination is more efficacious.

In addition to demonstrating efficacy as initial therapy of patients with MM, the combination of lenalidomide and dexamethasone has also been evaluated in patients with relapsed or refractory disease. Two pivotal phase III trials evaluating the combination versus dexamethasone alone demonstrated significant benefit of the combination with regard to OR (60% vs. 21.9%), CR rate (15% vs. 2%), time to disease progression (13.4 months vs. 4.6 months), duration of response (15.8 months vs. 7 months), and OS.[159]

The NCCN considers bortezomib alone or in combination with pegylated liposomal doxorubicin and the combination of lenalidomide and dexamethasone as the preferred regimens for the management of patients with relapsed or refractory MM.[133]

LYMPHOMA

Epidemiology, Pathophysiology, and Etiology

The lymphomas are a heterogeneous group of hematologic malignancies that originate in lymphoid tissues and arise from malignant transformation of lymphocytes (B cells, T cells, or natural killer cells). A lymphoma may arise within single or multiple lymph nodes or in extranodal sites involving the lymphoid tissue of the gastrointestinal tract, CNS, or other sites. The two major types of lymphomas are non–Hodgkin lymphoma (NHL) and Hodgkin lymphoma (HL) and it is estimated that these hematologic malignancies account for greater than 70,000 new cases annually, with eight times as many patients affected by NHL compared with HL.[160] In women, the incidence rate of HL has been rising compared with men, who have maintained a stable rate of disease for the past several decades.[160] NHL occurs at all ages, but risk increases with age, and individuals are commonly diagnosed in their 60s. HL can occur at any age, although 43.8% of cases occur in patients younger than 34 years of age, and 27.7% occur in patients older than 55 years.

NHL represents a spectrum of diseases marked by different pathological features, natural history, response to treatment, and prognosis. NHL is divided into categories based on cell of origin (B [80%–85%], T [15%–20%], or natural killer [rare]), histology (low, intermediate, or high grade), immunophenotypic characteristics, cytogenetic abnormalities, and natural history. Table 92-9 gives the World Health Organization classification of Non–Hodgkin lymphomas. NHL is further categorized as indolent or aggressive. Indolent NHLs generally carry a good prognosis, with a median survival of 10 years; however, it is not curable in advanced stages. Aggressive NHL has a much shorter natural history than indolent NHL, but it is cured in 30% to 60% of patients.

HL is classified into two distinct diseases, classical HL and lymphocyte-predominant HL. Classical HL accounts for 95% of all HL and is further divided into four subtypes, with the most common subtype being nodular sclerosis, representing about two-thirds of cases. HL is highly curable, with 75% to 80% of patients achieving long-term remission.

The etiology of NHL is unknown, although genetics, environmental and occupational exposures, viral disease (human immunodeficiency virus [HIV], CMV, hepatitis C virus), and immune suppression have been proposed to be associated in some studies. Other studies have shown a higher risk of NHL in individuals with close family members with NHL. There is also a possible genetic predisposition to HL. Jews and individuals

TABLE 92-9
World Health Organization Classification of Non–Hodgkin's Lymphoma

Precursor B- and T-Cell Neoplasms	**Mature T-Cell and NK Cell Neoplasms**
Precursor B-lymphoblastic leukemia/lymphoma	T-cell prolymphocytic leukemia
Precursor T-lymphoblastic leukemia/lymphoma	T-cell large granular lymphocytic leukemia
Mature B-Cell Neoplasms[a]	Chronic lymphoproliferative disorder of NK cells
Chronic lymphocytic leukemia/small lymphocytic lymphoma	Aggressive NK cell leukemia
B-cell prolymphocytic leukemia	Systemic EBV-positive T-cell lymphoproliferative diseases of childhood
Lymphoplasmacytic lymphoma/Waldenström macroglobulinemia	Hydroa vacciniformelike lymphoma
Splenic marginal zone B-cell lymphoma	Adult T-cell leukemia/lymphoma
Hairy cell leukemia	Extranodal NK/T-cell lymphoma, nasal type
Splenic B-cell lymphoma/leukemia, unclassifiable	Enteropathy-type T-cell lymphoma
Splenic diffuse red pulp small B-cell lymphoma	Hepatosplenic T-cell lymphoma
Hairy cell leukemia-variant	Subcutaneous panniculitislike T-cell lymphoma
Plasma cell neoplasms	Mycosis fungoides
Monoclonal gammopathy of undetermined significance (MGUS)	Sézary syndrome
Plasma cell myeloma	Primary cutaneous CD30-positive T-cell lymphoproliferative disorders:
Solitary plasmacytoma of bone	Primary cutaneous anaplastic large cell lymphoma
Extraosseous plasmacytoma	Lymphomatoid papulosis
Monoclonal immunoglobulin deposition diseases	Primary cutaneous peripheral T-cell lymphomas, rare subtypes
Extranodal marginal zone B-cell lymphoma (MALT lymphoma)	Primary cutaneous gamma-delta T-cell lymphoma
Nodal marginal zone B-cell lymphoma	Primary cutaneous CD8-positive aggressive epidermotropic cytotoxic T-cell lymphoma
Follicular lymphoma	Primary cutaneous CD4-positive small/medium T-cell lymphoma
Primary cutaneous follicle center lymphoma	Peripheral T-cell lymphoma, not otherwise specified
Mantle cell lymphoma	Angioimmunoblastic T-cell lymphoma
Diffuse large B-cell lymphoma (DLBCL)	Anaplastic large cell lymphoma, ALK-positive
T-cell/histiocyte-rich large B-cell lymphoma	Anaplastic large cell lymphoma, ALK-negative
Primary DLBCL of the central nervous system	**Immunodeficiency-Associated Lymphoproliferative Disorders**
Primary cutaneous DLBCL, leg type	Lymphoproliferative diseases associated with primary immune disorders
EBV-positive DLBCL of the elderly	Lymphomas associated with HIV infection
DLBCL associated with chronic inflammation	Posttransplant lymphoproliferative disorders (PTLD)
Lymphomatoid granulomatosis	Plasmacytic hyperplasia and infectious mononucleosis—like PTLD
Primary mediastinal (thymic) large B-cell lymphoma	Polymorphic PTLD
Intravascular large B-cell lymphoma	Monomorphic PTLD
ALK-positive large B-cell lymphoma	Classic Hodgkin lymphoma type PTLD
Plasmablastic lymphoma	Other iatrogenic immunodeficiency-associated lymphoproliferative disorders
Large B-cell lymphoma arising in HHV8-associated multicentric Castleman disease	
Burkitt lymphoma/leukemia	
B-cell lymphoma, unclassifiable, with features intermediate between DLBCL and Burkitt lymphoma	
B-cell lymphoma, unclassifiable, with features intermediate between DLBCL and classic Hodgkin lymphoma	

MALT, mucosa-associated lymphoid tissue; ALK, anaplastic lymphoma kinase; HHV8, human herpesvirus-8; NK, natural killer; EBV, Epstein-Barr virus; HIV, human immunodeficiency virus.
[a]B- and T/NK-cell neoplasms are grouped according to major clinical presentations (predominantly disseminated/leukemic, primary extranodal, predominantly nodal).
Reprinted with permission from DeVita VT et al, eds. *DeVita, Hellman, and Rosenberg's Cancer: Principles and Practice of Oncology.* 9th ed. Philadelphia, PA: Lippincott Williams & Wilkins; 2011.

with first-degree relatives with HL have a higher risk of disease. Other evidence suggests an association with prior Epstein-Barr virus infections and *BCL2* translocations.

Clinical Presentation and Diagnosis

Presentation of fast-growing, aggressive NHL, such as diffuse large B-cell (DLBC) lymphoma is variable; most patients present with lymphadenopathy and extranodal involvement. Presentation can involve one or more lymph nodes and, sometimes, extralymphatic organs. The most common extranodal sites include the gastrointestinal tract, skin, bone marrow, sinuses, or CNS. Fever (>38°C), night sweats, and weight loss (>10% of body weight in 6 months) are defined as B symptoms and are generally associated with more advanced or aggressive disease. Approximately one-third of patients with aggressive lymphomas will report B-symptoms.[161] Excisional or incisional lymph node biopsy, bone marrow biopsy, morphology, and immunophenotyping are used to confirm and classify an NHL diagnosis. Patients with indolent NHLs such as follicular or marginal zone lymphoma typically present with slow-growing, painless, generalized lymphadenopathy that can be either transient or persistent.

Individuals with HL will also present with lymphadenopathy typically in a contiguous pattern, whereas lymph nodes are more likely to present in a noncontiguous pattern in NHL. Extranodal lymphoid involvement in HL is less common than in NHL. In more than 90% of individuals the disease is located above the diaphragm at the time of initial diagnosis. They may also complain of B symptoms, fatigue, pruritus, cough, loss of appetite, and abdominal discomfort. The diagnosis of classic HL is made by the presence of Reed-Sternberg cells in a lymph node biopsy.

Treatment

Aggressive and highly aggressive B-cell NHLs are potentially curable. Patients with localized, nonbulky (<10 cm) stage I or II DLBC lymphoma without B symptoms are typically treated with rituximab, cyclophosphamide, doxorubicin, vincristine, and prednisone (R-CHOP) for three to six cycles with or without radiotherapy. For patients with advanced disease (bulky stage II or stage III or IV disease), R-CHOP for six cycles is the standard of care. Patients with stage III or IV aggressive NHL should also be encouraged to participate in clinical trials.

Indolent NHLs such as follicular lymphoma typically progress slowly; the disease may wax and wane, and median survival is 8 to 12 years after diagnosis.[161] Depending on the extent of disease, patient symptoms, and age, treatment may take a wait and watch approach, radiation alone, rituximab, or combination systemic chemotherapy. If treated, localized disease (defined as nonbulky stage I or II) generally includes radiation with or without systemic therapy. Approximately half of patients with localized disease will remain lymphomafree at 10 years with radiation therapy alone, and the addition of chemotherapy has not been shown to improve OS.[93,161] If treated, advanced disease (bulky stage II, stage III, or stage IV) is individualized based on age, performance status, comorbid disease states, disease progression, and future transplant possibility. Treatment is controversial because observation alone is associated with a 5-year survival of more than 75%.[162] Treatment of advanced disease usually consists of chemotherapy (cyclophosphamide, doxorubicin, vincristine, and prednisone [CHOP], cyclophosphamide, vincristine, and prednisone [CVP], or bendamustine) plus rituximab.

HL is highly responsive to treatment, with up to 95% of patients achieving complete remission with initial treatment. Initial treatment may include radiation, combination chemotherapy, or combined chemotherapy and radiation. The standard of care for patients with HL is doxorubicin, bleomycin, vinblastine, and dacarbazine (ABVD) owing to its demonstrated superiority over other combination chemotherapy regimens,[93] although other regimens such as Stanford V are used. HL has an excellent prognosis, with 75% to 80% of newly diagnosed adult patients achieving long-term remission. Prognosis depends on a number of factors, including the presence of systemic symptoms, disease stage, and the presence of bulky masses. In patients who relapse, the disease remains highly responsive to therapy. Patients with relapsed disease have two main treatment options: salvage chemotherapy with or without radiation therapy, or high-dose chemotherapy with stem cell support. HL treatment can be associated with serious long-term effects; therefore, minimization of late toxicities is an extremely important consideration in selection of a treatment regimen.

Non–Hodgkin Lymphoma

CLINICAL PRESENTATION

CASE 92-6

QUESTION 1: R.G., a 49-year-old woman, presents with complaints of swollen lymph nodes and occasional fevers and night sweats during the past month. Physical examination reveals marked cervical, supraclavicular, and inguinal lymphadenopathy. Laboratory values are normal with the exception of a mild anemia (Hgb, 11 g/dL) and an elevated LDH. HIV and hepatitis B surface antibody and antigen are negative. Excisional biopsy of a supraclavicular lymph node and immunophenotyping confirms a diagnosis of DLBC non–Hodgkin lymphoma (NHL). Flow cytometry is positive for CD10, CD19, and CD20 surface markers. Her bone marrow biopsy is negative for lymphoma. How common is NHL, and what are R.G.'s signs and symptoms, and what is her stage?

Approximately 65,000 new cases of NHL are diagnosed annually, making it the sixth most common new cancer in both men and women in the United States.[160] More than 80% of NHLs are B-cell neoplasms, with follicular and DLBC lymphoma as the most common subtypes, accounting for 31% and 22%, respectively[163] (Table 92-10).

Hundreds of lymph nodes can be found throughout the body, and they are designed to process antigens present in the lymphatic system. Each one consists of a capsule, cortex, medulla, and sinuses, with anatomical and functional compartments, such as follicular (germinal) centers, follicular mantle, and interfollicular and medullary areas (Fig. 92-1). The growth pattern of lymphoma is described as follicular when malignant B cells take over normal germinal centers of lymph follicles. When the normal architecture of the lymph node is replaced by a uniform population of neoplastic lymphocytes, the growth pattern is described as diffuse. Morphologic features of the lymph node, such as cell type, size, and appearance, are important because they establish the specific subtype of lymphoma and are helpful in determining the best treatment.[164]

CELLULAR CLASSIFICATION OF NON–HODGKIN LYMPHOMA

Historically, the main classification systems used for NHLs were the Working Formulation classification and the Revised European–American Lymphoma (REAL) classification. The Working Formulation classification classified NHLs into three broad groups (low, intermediate, and high grade) based on the morphology and clinical behavior of the disease; the REAL classification included morphology, immunophenotype, cytogenetics,

TABLE 92-10
Presenting Clinical Features of the Common Non–Hodgkin Lymphomas

	Frequency %	Age (yrs)	Stage % 1	2	3	4	Extranodal Involvement %	Bone Marrow Involvement %	B-Symptoms %	GI Involvement %	Elevated LDH %	International Prognostic Index % 0/1	2/3	4/5
Diffuse Large B-Cell	31	64	25	29	13	33	71	16	33	18	53	35	46	9
Follicular	22	59	18	15	16	51	64	42	28	3	30	45	48	7

Source: *J Clin Oncology*, 1998, Aug 16 (8):2780. Uses Revised European & American Lymphoma Classification.

and clinical groupings—indolent, aggressive, and highly aggressive lymphomas. The WHO updated the REAL classification, recognizing three categories of lymphoid malignancies based on morphology and cell lineage.[93,165] Currently, the WHO classification is the primary system for categorizing lymphoid neoplasms.

Lymphomas are common hematologic cancers in adults, and R.G. has one of the more common types. R.G. has swollen lymph nodes and occasional fevers and night sweats, which are highly consistent with NHL. Immunophenotyping of her lymph nodes confirms DLBC lymphoma. She is classified as having an aggressive, mature B-cell neoplasm.

STAGING AND PROGNOSIS

Staging is important for the selection of therapy. The Ann Arbor Staging System (Table 92-11) is used to stage lymphoma based on the results of the bone marrow biopsy, distribution, and number of involved sites; presence or absence of extranodal involvement; and presenting constitutional symptoms. In general, stage I or II is referred to as limited disease, whereas stage III or IV is considered advanced disease. Because of the wide range of outcomes in patients with lymphoma, even within histologic subtypes, factors that predict both response to treatment and outcomes are used to determine overall prognosis and need for aggressive therapy. The International Prognostic Index was designed to determine predictors of response and survival for aggressive lymphomas. Performance status greater than 2, age greater than 60 years, serum LDH above the upper limit of normal, advanced stage disease, and greater than two extranodal involved sites are associated with poorer survival.

Flow cytometry for R.G. is positive for surface markers CD10, CD19, and CD20, which is consistent with DLBC lymphoma, a type of aggressive lymphoma. Based on the Ann Arbor Staging System, R.G. has advanced stage IIIB disease because of the presence of lymph nodes on both sides of her diaphragm and B symptoms (fever and night sweats). R.G. has an elevated LDH and advanced stage disease, which are associated with lower survival rate. Patients with stage IIIB disease are generally treated with systemic chemotherapy.

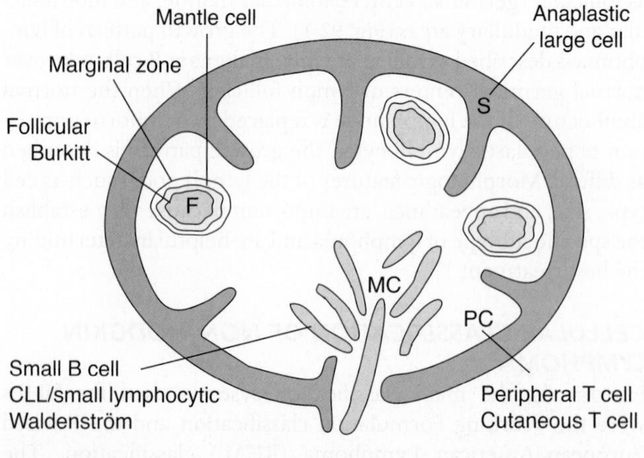

FIGURE 92-1 Sites of origin of malignant lymphomas in a lymph node according to anatomical and functional compartments of the immune system. CLL, chronic lymphocytic leukemia; F, follicles, or germinal centers; MC, medullary cords; PC, paracortex, or interfollicular areas; S, sinuses.

TREATMENT

AGGRESSIVE NON–HODGKIN LYMPHOMA

CASE 92-6, QUESTION 2: R.G. consults with a hematologist and elects to receive combination chemotherapy consisting of cyclophosphamide, doxorubicin, vincristine, and prednisone with rituximab (R-CHOP) every 21 days for six cycles. She will then be referred to a radiation oncologist to determine whether she will receive additional benefit from radiation therapy. Is R-CHOP considered standard initial therapy? What are the adverse effects that might occur in R.G.?

TABLE 92-11
Ann Arbor Staging System

Stage	Description[a]
I	Involvement of a single lymph node region or a single extralymphatic organ or site (IE)
II	Involvement of two or more lymph node regions on the same side of the diaphragm (II) or localized involvement of an extralymphatic organ or site (IIE)
III	Involvement of lymph node regions on both sides of the diaphragm (III) or localized involvement of an extralymphatic organ or site (IIIE) or spleen (IIIS) or both (IIISE)
IV	Diffuse or disseminated involvement of one or more extralymphatic organs with or without associated lymph node involvement. Bone marrow and liver involvement are always stage IV

[a]Identification of the presence or absence of symptoms should be noted with each stage designation: A, asymptomatic; B, fever, sweats, weight loss greater than 10% of body weight.

Reprinted with permission from DeVita VT et al, eds. *DeVita, Hellman, and Rosenberg's Cancer: Principles and Practice of Oncology*. 9th ed. Philadelphia, PA: Lippincott Williams & Wilkins; 2011.

Aggressive lymphomas are potentially curable. Patients with nonbulky, localized stage I or II DLBC lymphoma are typically treated with R-CHOP for three to six cycles with or without radiation. For individuals with advanced disease, defined as bulky stage II or stage III or IV disease, six cycles of R-CHOP are commonly used.[93] However, patients with advanced disease should also be considered for a clinical trial.

The Groups d'Étude des Lymphomas de l'Adult compared the 5-year follow-up of CHOP with R-CHOP in newly diagnosed DLBC lymphoma patients 60 to 80 years of age. Rituximab is a chimeric human monoclonal antibody to the B-cell surface antigen CD20. Although the exact mechanism is unknown, rituximab is believed to induce lysis through complement-mediated destruction, antibody-dependent cytotoxicity, and induction of apoptosis working in synergy with chemotherapy.[166] Eventfree survival, PFS, DFS, and OS were all higher in the R-CHOP arm. No additional significant long-term toxicity was apparent.[167] Because these results have been confirmed in both young and elderly patients, R-CHOP has become the standard of care in the United States.[168,169,170]

The effect of dose intensity (reduction of treatment interval from 3 weeks to 2 weeks) on response was investigated in a study comparing R-CHOP every 14 days (RCHOP-14) with traditional R-CHOP every 21 days (RCHOP-21). Growth factor support with G-CSF was required in the every 14-day arm to prevent myelosuppression and treatment delay. A total of 1,048 patients were randomly assigned to one of the two treatment arms, and 82% of patients receiving RCHOP-21 completed the study compared with 89% of patients receiving RCHOP-14. Grades III and IV toxicities were similar in both arms, with a slightly higher neutropenia (57%) and infection rate (22%) in the patients receiving RCHOP-21 compared with those receiving RCHOP-14 at 31% and 17%, respectively.[171] Although final analysis was not performed regarding OS, radiological response rates were the same in both arms at 47%, and the authors concluded that RCHOP-14 can be given as safely and effectively as RCHOP-21.[171] However, RCHOP-21 remains the most commonly used regimen.

The standard dose of rituximab is 375 mg/m^2 given IV in a variety of dosing schedules. An infusion-related complex consisting of fever, chills, and rigors may occur during rituximab infusion, necessitating premedication with acetaminophen and diphenhydramine. Other less common infusion-related symptoms include nausea, urticaria, pruritus, bronchospasm, angioedema, and hypotension. These reactions generally occur within 30 minutes to 2 hours from the start of the infusion (typically, the first dose) and resolve if the infusion is slowed or interrupted. Another less common side effect associated with rituximab is tumor lysis syndrome, which occurs mostly in patients with a high number of circulating CD20-positive cells. Before rituximab therapy, hepatitis B surface antigen and hepatitis B core antibody testing should be performed, and patients testing positive should receive empiric antiviral therapy during chemotherapy treatment to prevent hepatitis reactivation.[172]

Safety precautions associated with the chemotherapy medications included in the CHOP regimen include documentation of a normal cardiac ejection fraction (EF) before administration of doxorubicin and peripheral neuropathy assessments at baseline and throughout treatment owing to the administration of vincristine. Because of the increased risk of fetal abnormalities associated with cyclophosphamide in particular, a pregnancy test should be done before chemotherapy initiation. Antiemetics should be given before chemotherapy administration to prevent nausea or vomiting, and a bowel regimen should be initiated to prevent constipation. Prophylaxis with a CSF after chemotherapy should be considered in patients at high risk for febrile neutropenia.

R-CHOP would be considered standard treatment for R.G. because she has advanced stage IIIB disease. She should have baseline evaluation of EF and routine assessments for peripheral neuropathy attributable to vincristine. Supportive-care treatments of antiemetics, stool softener, and possibly filgrastim to prevent fever and neutropenia will be needed for R.G.

CASE 92-6, QUESTION 3: R.G. has a CR to R-CHOP therapy demonstrated by restaging studies performed after her third and sixth cycles of treatment, and did not receive radiation therapy after R-CHOP. Every 3 months, she has a follow-up examination for disease recurrence. At her 15-month follow-up visit, she has radiographic evidence of disease recurrence in her abdomen. What treatment options are available to R.G. at this time?

High-dose chemotherapy immediately followed by autologous HCT should be considered for patients who relapse after conventional chemotherapy. Salvage chemotherapy regimens are administered before HCT to ensure the disease is sensitive to additional cytotoxic therapy. Regimens use non–cross-resistant agents such as ifosfamide, carboplatin, and etoposide (ICE) with or without rituximab; dexamethasone, cytarabine, and cisplatin (DHAP) with or without rituximab; and etoposide, methylprednisolone, cytarabine, and cisplatin (ESHAP) with or without rituximab. Patients who previously responded to conventional therapy and demonstrated chemosensitive disease at relapse have the best outcome from autologous HCT. Allogeneic HCT may be considered in those not considered good candidates for autologous HCT.[93] R.G. received three cycles of R-ICE chemotherapy, to which her disease was highly responsive, and then a sufficient number of her stem cells were collected for autologous HCT.

CASE 92-6, QUESTION 4: How does treatment differ for highly aggressive NHL?

Highly aggressive NHL, such as lymphoblastic or Burkitt lymphoma, progresses very rapidly and commonly metastasizes to the CNS.[164] The majority of adult patients can be cured with an aggressive combination therapy. Regimens such as R-CHOP may not be intensive enough to prevent progression between cycles of therapy. Therefore, regimens similar to those for ALL are used because they provide more continuous exposure to more intensive chemotherapy. The hyperfractionated cyclophosphamide, vincristine, doxorubicin, and dexamethasone regimen, alternating with high-dose methotrexate and cytarabine, has a CR rate of 91%.[173] These regimens must include CNS prophylaxis with intrathecal methotrexate or cytarabine.[164] These patients are at increased risk for TLS and should be treated with allopurinol, vigorous IV hydration, and electrolytes.

INDOLENT LYMPHOMA

Clinical Presentation

CASE 92-7

QUESTION 1: D.J. is a 64-year-old healthy man who presents to his physician complaining of low-grade fevers and a constant "bloated feeling," despite taking over-the-counter aluminum hydroxide and famotidine. He was otherwise asymptomatic, denying recent weight loss or night sweats. On physical examination, axillary adenopathy was found. An excisional biopsy and pathological examination revealed follicular B-cell lymphoma, a type of indolent lymphoma. Laboratory values are normal. CT scans of the

chest, abdomen, and pelvis showed axillary and mediastinal lymphadenopathy. D.J. has stage II disease, with a low follicular lymphoma International Prognostic Index score of 2, for which he receives radiation therapy alone. D.J. remains asymptomatic for 3 years. However, now he develops abdominal and splenic lymphadenopathy, night sweats, and weight loss during a 2-month period. What treatment options are available for D.J.?

Recurrent, chemotherapy-sensitive disease is common for the indolent NHLs. Chemotherapy options include single-agent rituximab with a CR rate of 15% and OR rate of 64%, which may be extended by maintenance rituximab.[174] No improvement in OS has been reported. Rituximab, in combination with chemotherapy regimens such as CHOP or CVP, achieves higher CR rates and extends the duration of response.[175,176] Other options include purine analogs alone or in combination, such as fludarabine, mitoxantrone, and dexamethasone with or without rituximab, or oral alkylating agents such as chlorambucil or cyclophosphamide.[93,177] A recently available option is bendamustine, which is commonly combined with rituximab (BR). The OR rate and OS were similar to R-CHOP, but the BR patients had significantly longer PFS.[178] The NCCN Practice Guideline recommends treatment with a rituximab-containing regimen unless contraindicated, although definitive evidence supporting a survival advantage is lacking.[93] An echocardiogram reports D.J.'s EF as 40%. Therefore, a non–anthracycline-containing regimen (R-CVP) was selected to minimize cardiotoxicity because D.J. will be at higher risk.

CASE 92-7, QUESTION 2: D.J. is now 6 years out from his initial diagnosis. His disease was stable for 2 years after response to treatment with R-CVP. However, his most recent CT scan shows progression of his disease. The decision is made to administer more therapy, this time using rituximab alone. His daughter read on a lymphoma website that radioimmunotherapy and transplantation are potential treatments. She asks whether these options would be appropriate for D.J.

D.J.'s disease is typical of indolent NHLs in that they respond to therapy, but the disease eventually recurs and is generally incurable. Because these lymphomas are generally chemotherapy-sensitive, relapsed disease can be treated with the same modalities as first-line treatment. Retreatment with rituximab has been found to be efficacious without additional toxicities.[179] Radioimmunoconjugates are monoclonal antibodies that target CD20-positive lymphoma cells. These antibodies are linked to radioisotopes, enabling delivery of local radiation therapy. Although radioimmunotherapy may be used as a first-line therapy, it is most often used in the setting of relapsed disease.[180,181] Both iodine-131 [^{131}I]-tositumomab and yttrium-90 [^{90}Y]-ibritumomab tiuxetan have been developed to treat follicular lymphomas. Both contain anti-CD20 antibodies with β-emitting radioisotopes. [^{131}I]-Tositumomab also emits gamma irradiation.

Patients are candidates for radioimmunoconjugates if they have less than 25% bone marrow involvement and platelet counts greater than 100 × $10^3/\mu$L because of the significant hematologic toxicity associated with radioimmunotherapy. Response rates are higher than those seen with rituximab therapy alone. However, because of complicated administration procedures that are required for these agents and high cost, this treatment has not been widely used clinically. To protect the thyroid from the adverse effects of radioactive iodine, patients receiving [^{131}I]-tositumomab should also receive a saturated solution of potassium iodide (two drops PO three times a day) at least 24 hours before the first dose is administered and then continued for 14 days after therapy. Because low-level radiation exposure is a concern, patients receiving either agent should be counseled to properly dispose of body fluids, carefully attend to personal hygiene, and limit their social contact for up to 7 days after administration. Hematologic toxicity can occur 7 to 9 weeks after administration, with a median duration of neutropenia and thrombocytopenia of approximately 3 weeks.[180]

High-dose chemotherapy followed by autologous HCT has a higher PFS and OS than standard therapy (R-CHOP or other).[182] Patients in second remission should be referred for transplant evaluation, but HCT requires careful patient selection because of the high risk of morbidity and mortality.[183] D.J. is not a transplant candidate because of his advanced age and EF and will continue to receive conventional therapies.

Hodgkin Lymphoma

CLINICAL PRESENTATION AND PROGNOSIS

CASE 92-8

QUESTION 1: J.R. is a 55-year-old man with complaints of painless swelling around his collarbone, fever, night sweats, cough, and an unintentional 20-pound weight loss in the past 6 months. Radiography of the chest revealed a small mediastinal mass, and a CT scan of the neck, chest, abdomen, and pelvis confirmed cervical and mediastinal lymph node enlargement, as well as multiple enlarged lymph nodes in the perisplenic and inguinal areas. A bone marrow biopsy was positive for lymphoma cells. Excisional biopsy of the cervical lymph node revealed nodular sclerosing HL with Reed-Sternberg cells. Laboratory values are normal. HIV and hepatitis B surface antibody and antigen are negative. Is this a typical presentation for HL? What is J.R.'s stage and prognosis?

Presentation of HL can be limited to a single lymph node or to an extralymphatic organ or site, or it can involve multiple lymph nodes and extralymphatic organs. In general, the more extensive the involvement, the higher the stage of disease. In newly diagnosed patients, the tumor is staged to assist in treatment selection. The international staging classification is the Cotswolds classification which is a modification of the Ann Arbor Staging System. The Cotswolds staging classification is shown in Table 92-12.[172] Several factors unfavorably impact prognosis, including older age, certain histology (mixed cellularity or lymphocyte depleted), high erythrocyte sedimentation rate, presence of B symptoms and bulky mediastinal disease increasing number of nodal sites and extranodal lesions. Therefore, HL is usually further classified into three groups based on stage and symptoms; *early stage favorable* (stage I or II with no unfavorable factors), *early stage unfavorable* (stage I or II with any unfavorable factors such as large mediastinal adenopathy, B symptoms, numerous sites of disease, or significantly elevated erythrocyte sedimentation rate), and *advanced stage* disease (stage III or IV).

J.R.'s symptoms are those typical of HL, mainly lymphadenopathy, fever, night sweats, and weight loss. He also has bone marrow involvement and mediastinal mass. J.R. has diffuse or disseminated involvement of one or more extranodal organs with lymph node involvement and B symptoms; therefore, he has stage IVB (advanced stage) disease.

HL is one of the few malignancies that is typically curable, even in the advanced stages. An analysis of 5,000 patients with advanced-stage HL identified seven prognostic factors, each of

TABLE 92-12

Cotswolds Staging Classification For Hodgkin Lymphoma

Stage	Description
I	Involvement of a single lymph node region or lymphoid structure (e.g., spleen, thymus, Waldeyer's ring) or involvement of a single extralymphatic site (IE).
II	Involvement of two or more lymph node regions on the same side of the diaphragm (hilar nodes, when involved on both sides, constitute stage II disease); localized contiguous involvement of only one extranodal organ or site and lymph node region(s) on the same side of the diaphragm (IIE). The number of anatomic regions involved should be indicated by a subscript (e.g., II3).
III	Involvement of lymph node regions on both sides of the diaphragm (III), which may also be accompanied by involvement of the spleen (IIIS) or by localized contiguous involvement of only one extranodal organ site (IIIE) or both (IIISE).
III_1	With or without involvement of splenic, hilar, celiac, or portal nodes.
III_2	With involvement of para-aortic, iliac, and mesenteric nodes.
IV	Diffuse or disseminated involvement of one or more extranodal organs or tissues, with or without associated lymph node involvement.
	Designations Applicable to Any Disease Stage
A	No symptoms.
B	Fever (temperature, >38°C), drenching night sweats, unexplained loss of >10% body weight within the preceding 6 months.
X	Bulky disease (a widening of the mediastinum by more than one-third or the presence of a nodal mass with a maximal dimension >10 cm).
E	Involvement of a single extranodal site that is contiguous or proximal to the known nodal site.
CS	Clinical stage.
PS	Pathologic stage (as determined by laparotomy).

Reprinted with permission from DeVita VT et al, eds. *DeVita, Hellman, and Rosenberg's Cancer: Principles and Practice of Oncology*. 9th ed. Philadelphia, PA: Lippincott Williams & Wilkins; 2011.

which show an annual reduction in survival by 7% to 8% yearly. These adverse prognostic factors include age older than 45 years, serum albumin level less than 4 g/dL, Hgb less than 10.5 g/dL, male sex, stage IV disease, WBC greater than 15,000 cells/μL, and lymphocyte count less than 8% of total WBC count or lymphocyte count less than 600 cells/μL.[172,184] J.R. has three of these prognostic factors (age >45 years, male, stage IV disease), totaling an annual reduction in survival of 23%.

TREATMENT

CASE 92-8, QUESTION 2: J.R. is scheduled to begin chemotherapy with the ABVD regimen. His EF is 60%. Is this the optimal initial treatment? What information should be included in his medication counseling?

Chemotherapy regimens (with or without radiation therapy) are commonly used to treat early and advanced-stage disease owing to the increased risk of heart disease, pulmonary toxicity, and secondary malignancies associated with radiation. Multiple combination chemotherapy regimens have been developed for HL, including ABVD; mechlorethamine, vincristine, procarbazine, and prednisone (MOPP); bleomycin, etoposide, doxorubicin, cyclophosphamide, vincristine, procarbazine, and prednisone (BEACOPP); and the Stanford V regimen (mechlorethamine, doxorubicin, etoposide, vincristine, vinblastine, bleomycin, and prednisone). In direct comparison with MOPP, ABVD has been shown to have an improved OS and a lower risk of both short- and long-term toxicities, including myelosuppression, infertility, and secondary leukemias; therefore, ABVD is the preferred treatment compared with MOPP.[185–187] Although promising results have been obtained with BEACOPP and Stanford V, they have not been compared with ABVD in well-designed, long-term studies evaluating survival and toxicity.

NCCN guidelines recommend that patients with stage IA through IIA (favorable disease) receive ABVD with radiation or the Stanford V regimen with radiation.[172] Individuals with stage I to II (unfavorable disease) receive ABVD chemotherapy or Stanford V followed by radiation. For patients like J.R. with stage IVB (advanced) disease, chemotherapy is always used and ABVD or Stanford V is recommended, and radiation may be administered in certain individuals. J.R. will receive treatment with up to six cycles of ABVD. If he has a complete remission after six cycles, no further therapy will be given. J.R will likely not receive radiation because he does not have a bulky mediastinal mass on initial presentation.

Traditionally, patients with any of the histologic subtypes of HL have been treated in a similar fashion. One exception is nodular lymphocyte-predominant HL, which consistently expresses CD20 antigen. A small phase 2 study of 22 treated and untreated patients showed an OR rate of 100% with a complete remission rate of 41% to rituximab 375 mg/m^2 weekly for four doses.[188] Based on this and several other studies demonstrating rituximab's benefit in patients with CD20-positive lymphocyte-predominant HL, rituximab combination chemotherapy (such as ABVD, CHOP), with or without radiation, is now considered standard of care.[172]

HL is a chemotherapy-sensitive disease, and administration of full doses given on schedule is critical. Cycles of ABVD are given every 28 days, and all patients should continue treatment for two cycles beyond documentation of complete remission. Late effects of HL therapy are a major concern, particularly secondary malignancies, cardiovascular disease, hypothyroidism, and fertility issues.[189] Safety precautions associated with the chemotherapy medications included in the ABVD regimen include documentation of a normal cardiac EF before administration of doxorubicin and pulmonary function testing at baseline owing to risk of bleomycin-induced lung injury. Treatment-related cardiotoxicity is usually observed 5 to 10 years after completion of treatment, and therefore long-term follow-up is important. Patients should be monitored for pulmonary symptoms or abnormal pulmonary function tests or chest radiographs. If pulmonary changes occur, bleomycin should be discontinued from further treatment; deletion does not appear to reduce long-term survival.[190] Patients receiving ABVD are at high risk for neutropenia because of the administration of dacarbazine and vinblastine, and patients will be at increased risk of infections. Prophylaxis or treatment of neutropenia using a CSF has not been shown to improve OS or event-free survival in HL patients.[191] The NCCN recommends against dose reductions or delays based on neutropenia and does not recommend the use of growth factors routinely.[172]

In conclusion, J.R. has classical HL, and ABVD is considered a first-choice regimen, especially because he has normal EF before treatment. Pulmonary function should be monitored during the course of therapy. Because he is 55 years of age, it is unlikely that fertility is a major concern; however, he still should be warned. He will be at risk for acute toxicities such as nausea and vomiting, neutropenia, and infections, as well as long-term toxicities including secondary malignancies, hypothyroidism, and increased risk of cardiovascular disease.

RELAPSED DISEASE

CASE 92-8, QUESTION 3: J.R. achieved a complete remission and received a total of six cycles of full-dose ABVD. Two years after completion of chemotherapy, a routine follow-up radiograph of the chest revealed enlarged lymph nodes, which were subsequently biopsied and found to be recurrent disease. What treatment should J.R. receive?

Patients with relapsed HL have two main treatment options: high-dose chemotherapy with autologous stem cell support or salvage chemotherapy with or without radiation therapy. Prognostic and patient-specific factors may assist in determining which avenue is optimal. Patients whose recurrence occurs less than 1 year after initial therapy and who have stage III or IV disease at relapse need more aggressive therapy if age and performance status permit.[192] Most patients will be treated with high-dose chemotherapy and autologous HCT. Before undergoing transplantation, most patients will receive cytoreductive therapy depending on what initial therapy was given. Regimens such as ESHAP, DHAP, or ICE are often considered, along with others, although the optimal regimen is not known. DFS for patients who relapse 1 year or later after initial therapy and are treated with salvage chemotherapy is 45% at 20 years.[193] Patients who undergo high-dose chemotherapy and autologous HCT have an improved eventfree survival and PFS, but no difference in OS from those who receive conventional chemotherapy alone.[194,195] Freedom from treatment failure at 3 years was significantly better for patients given high-dose chemotherapy and autologous stem cell transplantation (55%) than for those given conventional chemotherapy (34%; $p = 0.019$).[195] J.R. will be referred for autologous HCT; however, he will receive a salvage regimen before transplantation. Harvesting of autologous stem cells will need to be coordinated around his pretransplant salvage chemotherapy.

KEY REFERENCES AND WEBSITES

A full list of references for this chapter can be found at http://thepoint.lww.com/AT10e. Below are the key references and websites for this chapter, with the corresponding reference number in this chapter found in parentheses after the reference.

Key References

Burnett A et al. Therapeutic advances in acute myeloid leukemia [published correction appears in *J Clin Oncol.* 2011;29:2293]. *J Clin Oncol.* 2011;29:487. (17)

Cervantes F et al. Practical management of patients with chronic myeloid leukemia. *Cancer.* 2011 Mar 16.

Dimopoulos MA et al. Long-term follow-up on overall survival from the MM-009 and MM-010 phase III trials of lenalidomide plus dexamethasone in patients with relapsed or refractory multiple myeloma. *Leukemia.* 2009;23:2147. (158)

Hallek M. Chronic lymphocytic leukemia for the clinician. *Ann Oncol.* 2011; 22(Suppl 4):iv54. (112)

Kindler T et al. FLT3 as a therapeutic target in AML: still challenging after all these years. *Blood.* 2010;116:5089. (67)

Kyle R et al. American Society of Clinical Oncology 2007 clinical practice guidelines update on the role of bisphosphonates in multiple myeloma. *J Clin Oncol.* 2007;25:2464. (152)

Marcucci G et al Molecular genetics of adult acute myeloid leukemia: prognostic and therapeutic implications [published correction appears in *J Clin Oncol.* 2011;29:1798]. *J Clin Oncol.* 2011;29:475. (16)

Munshi NC, Anderson KC. Plasma cell neoplasms. In: DeVita VT et al, eds. *Cancer: Principles and Practice of Oncology.* 8th ed. Philadelphia, PA: Lippincott Williams & Wilkins; 2008:2305. (121)

Ng AK et al. Long-term complications of lymphoma and its treatment. *J Clin Oncol.* 2011;29:1885. (188)

Palumbo A, Anderson K. Multiple myeloma. *N Engl J Med.* 2011;364:1046. (125)

Palumbo A et al. Oral melphalan, prednisone, and thalidomide compared with melphalan and prednisone alone in elderly patients with multiple myeloma: randomised controlled trial. *Lancet.* 2006;367:825. (142)

Pollyea DA, et al. Acute myeloid leukaemia in the elderly: a review. *Br J Haematol.* 2011;152:524. (49)

Rathore B, Kadin ME. Hodgkin's lymphoma therapy: past, present, and future. *Expert Opin Pharmacother.* 2010;11:2891.

Richardson P et al. Bortezomib or high-dose dexamethasone for relapsed multiple myeloma. *N Engl J Med.* 2005;352:2487. (135)

Richardson P et al. Lenalidomide, bortezomib, and dexamethasone combination therapy in patients with newly diagnosed multiple myeloma. *Blood.* 2010;116:679. (140)

Rosti G, et al. Second-generation BCR-ABL inhibitors for front-line treatment of chronic myeloid leukemia in chronic phase. *Crit Rev Oncol Hematol.* [Epub ahead of print]

Riches JC et al. Chronic lymphocytic leukemia: an update on biology and treatment. *Curr Oncol Rep.* 2011 Jul 20. [Epub ahead of print].

Sawas A et al. New therapeutic targets and drugs in non-Hodgkin's lymphoma. *Curr Opin Hematol.* 2011;18:280.

Key Websites

American Society of Hematology. *Hematology. Education Program Book.* 2010. http://www.asheducationbook.org.

The National Comprehensive Cancer Network. NCCN Guidelines for Treatment of Cancer. Non–Hodgkin's Lymphomas. Version 3.2011. http://www.nccn.org.

93

Breast Cancer

Kellie L. Jones

CORE PRINCIPLES

	CHAPTER CASES
1 Mammography and clinical breast examinations are important screening modalities for breast cancer.	**Case 93-1 (Question 1)**
2 Prevention can include both surgery (prophylactic mastectomy) and chemoprevention. Tamoxifen and raloxifene are two agents approved for breast cancer prevention.	**Case 93-1 (Question 2)**
3 Breast cancer is the most common cancer diagnosed in American women. Many risk factors have been associated with the development of breast cancer; however, the two most common risk factors are sex and age.	**Case 93-2 (Question 1), Case 93-3 (Question 1)**
4 A painless mass is a common presenting symptom for patients. To diagnose the disease and determine the histology, a mammogram and biopsy are performed. Staging is also performed to determine the extent of disease.	**Case 93-3 (Questions 2–4)**
5 Tumor-specific prognostic factors are evaluated such as hormonal status (estrogen and progesterone receptor status) and human epidermal growth factor receptor 2 (HER2) status. The results help guide treatment selection.	**Case 93-3 (Question 5)**
6 Local and systemic treatment can include surgery, radiation, hormonal therapy, chemotherapy, or biologic therapy.	**Case 93-3 (Questions 6–9)**
7 Early-stage disease is highly curable. In the adjuvant setting (after surgery), patients will receive hormonal therapy (if estrogen receptor/progesterone receptor-positive) or possibly chemotherapy, depending on the size of the disease and the presence of positive axillary lymph nodes.	**Case 93-3 (Questions 7–9)**
8 Adjuvant chemotherapy can include anthracyclines, cyclophosphamide, and taxanes. Biologic therapy such as trastuzumab can be incorporated if the patient has HER2-positive disease.	**Case 93-3 (Questions 6–8)**
9 Metastatic disease is considered incurable. Decisions regarding therapy will depend on the hormonal status of the tumor, toxicities from previous treatment, or other pre-existing comorbidities. Therapies could include systemic therapy (hormonal therapy, chemotherapy, or biologic therapy) or local treatment (radiation therapy or surgery).	**Case 93-4 (Questions 1–5)**

BREAST CANCER

Incidence, Prevalence, and Epidemiology

Breast cancer is the most common malignancy in American women and is second to lung cancer in mortality rates. It arises from the tissues of the breast, usually the ducts (tubes that carry milk to the nipple) and lobules (glands that make milk). In 2010, it was estimated that 209,060 women would be diagnosed with breast cancer and approximately 40,230 were expected to die from their disease.[1] Approximately 1,970 cases were estimated to be diagnosed in men, indicating it is not a disease solely of women.[1] The incidence rates of breast cancer have continued to decline from 1999 through 2004 due to the decreased use of hormone-replacement therapy. This decline follows the results of the Women's Health Initiative study, which demonstrated increased risk of breast cancer in those receiving hormone-replacement therapy.[2] One in eight women are expected to develop the disease over the course of their lifetime. However, this frequently quoted statistic may overestimate the risk of breast cancer because it is derived from women who live to be 110 years of age.

If breast cancer is diagnosed early, it is curable. The likelihood of diagnosing breast cancer is increased by the use of standardized screening methods. Currently, many different guidelines are available for breast cancer screening including recommendations from the American Cancer Society, National Comprehensive Cancer Network, and the US Preventative Services Task Force. All recommend combination modalities of screening because no one test is considered conclusive.

Breast cancer can be prevented in patients who are considered at high risk of developing breast cancer. Both surgical and pharmacologic options are available. Prophylactic mastectomies can be successfully completed; however, they do not provide a 100% guarantee of the prevention of breast cancer.[3] Pharmacologic therapies have been approved for the prevention of breast cancer including tamoxifen and raloxifene.[4,5] Two large studies in high-risk women demonstrated decreased incidences in breast cancer in those women who received tamoxifen or raloxifene for 5 years.

Pathophysiology

The breast itself is composed of many different structures including fat, muscle, ducts, and lobules (Figure 93-1). Lobules arise from glandular tissue that forms into a spoke-like formation

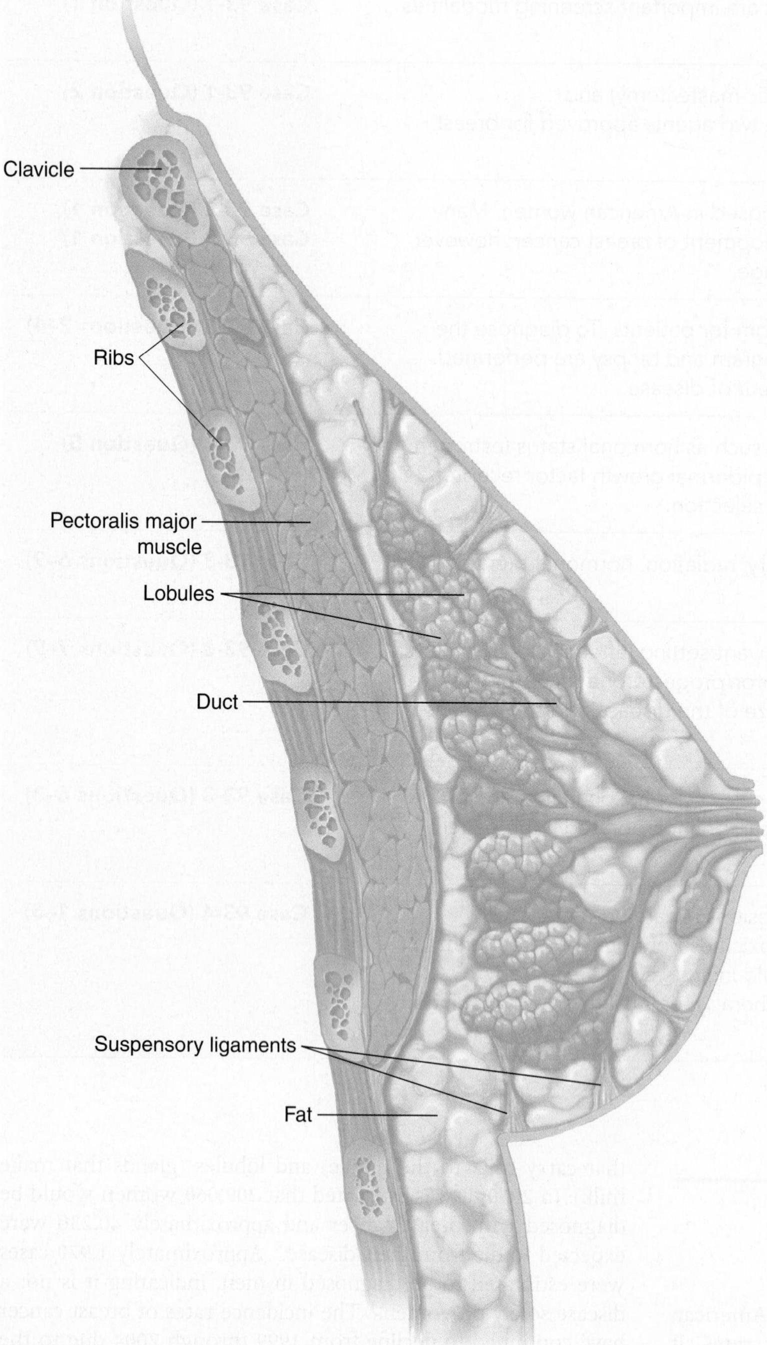

FIGURE 93-1 Anatomy of the breast. (Asset provided by Anatomical Chart Co.)

to constitute a lobule of two layers of epithelial cells. The ducts connect the milk-secreting lobules to the nipple.[6] A breast cancer is defined by where the tumor cells originate. The two most common histologic types of breast cancer are ductal and lobular carcinoma. Ductal tumors may either be classified as invasive ductal carcinoma if it has invaded through the basement membrane of the duct, or ductal carcinoma in situ (DCIS), if it has not. Likewise, lobular tumors may be classified similarly (i.e., invasive lobular carcinoma or lobular carcinoma in situ [LCIS]). Other types of breast cancers include inflammatory (which will be discussed later in the chapter) and rare histologies such as tubular or medullary carcinomas or sarcomas.

Overview of Treatment and Diagnosis

The treatment of breast cancer includes multiple modalities. Surgery, radiation therapy, hormonal therapy, chemotherapy, and biologic therapy can all be used in many different combinations based on a patient's specific disease. If therapy is given before surgery it is called neoadjuvant therapy and if treatment is administered after surgery it is termed adjuvant therapy. Therapy is determined based on the stage of disease. Staging is completed by evaluating the size of the tumor (either on clinical examination or from the surgical specimen), the extent of positive lymph nodes (evaluated on physical examination and with surgical removal through an axillary lymph node dissection), and the extent of disease (which is evaluated with radiologic examinations including computed tomography [CT] scan of the chest, abdomen, and pelvis and a bone scan to identify any metastatic disease).

Early-stage disease is highly curable whereas metastatic disease is not. The 5-year survival for localized, early-stage disease is approximately 98%. Most patients will present with early-stage disease. Many present with a painless lump found upon breast examination (either by themselves or by a clinician) or with a lump found on routine mammogram. In patients with stage II or III disease, the 5-year survival is approximately 83%, and for those with stage IV disease, the 5-year survival is approximately 26%. Patients who present with metastatic disease typically present with symptoms of their disease based on the metastatic site (such as bone pain with bone metastases or shortness of breath with lung metastases). In patients with metastatic disease, the goal is palliation of symptoms and improvement in quality of life.

SCREENING

CASE 93-1

QUESTION 1: M.P. is a 42-year-old woman with no personal history of breast cancer. She has a cousin who was diagnosed with breast cancer at the age of 65 years. M.P. is in her doctor's office today to discuss routine breast cancer screening. Based on M.P.'s personal and family history, would M.P. be considered an average risk or high-risk patient and what modalities of screening are recommended for average and high-risk patients?

For the average-risk patient, screening involves a clinical breast examination, mammography, and a breast self-examination (if the woman chooses to do so). Although the risk of breast cancer is low in one's 20s, these breast examinations allow a woman to become more familiar with her body and better able to discern changes at older ages. In the current American Cancer Society (ACS) guidelines, it states that women may choose to do breast self-examinations regularly, occasionally, or not at all.[7] Clinical breast examinations are recommended to begin between the ages of 20 to 39 years at least every 3 years and then annually starting at the age of 40 during the woman's regular health examination.

Screening mammography has been the gold standard for breast cancer for many decades. Based on the ACS guidelines, screening should be initiated at the age of 40 years and annually thereafter. Recently, there has been controversy regarding the utility of mammography and when screening should begin (40 or 50 years of age). This controversy stemmed from recommendations by the US Preventative Services Task Force (USPSTF).[8] Their recommendation was based on a cumulative review of all mammography trials for breast cancer screening. When evaluating breast cancer mortality, the relative risk reduction increases in women ages 40 to 49 years who were screened with mammography, but the greatest relative risk reduction was in women ages 60 to 69 years. Based on these data, the USPSTF concluded that for women in the younger age group, the benefits did not outweigh the harms of increased anxiety, radiation exposure, and inconvenience due to false positives. The task force further recommended that women aged 50 to 74 years only needed biennial screening rather than annual screenings. Although the relative risk reduction is lower in younger women, the ACS as well as all of the other organizations who publish breast cancer screening guidelines did not change their recommendation of annual mammography starting at the age of 40 years. One positive outcome from these controversial recommendations was the heightened awareness to the general public of the breast cancer screening guidelines.

M.P. has no first-degree relatives with breast cancer, or other family members affected by early breast cancer. M.P. is an average-risk patient and she should start standard screening modalities and intervals of testing with annual mammograms and clinical breast examinations. She may also decide to do breast self-examinations.

Individuals considered high risk (a) have a known *BRCA* gene mutation, (b) are untested for the *BRCA* gene mutation but have a first-degree relative with a *BRCA* mutation, (c) have a lifetime risk of experiencing breast cancer of approximately 20% to 25% or more based on risk estimation models, or (d) have a strong family history of breast cancer.[7] Screening with breast magnetic resonance imaging (MRI) is recommended in high-risk individuals. Annual mammography and breast MRIs should be initiated starting at the age of 30 years. An MRI allows a radiologist to see a contrasted view of the breast and is more sensitive to detecting breast cancer. In addition, breast tissue in younger patients can be denser due to higher levels of estrogen, making mammography less sensitive.[9] M.P. does not have an immediate family history of breast cancer, so no additional screening should be done in her case.

PREVENTION

CASE 93-1, QUESTION 2: M.P. works at her local hospital as a nurse and is volunteering this year at their breast cancer awareness seminar that is offered by her hospital. She was asked to prepare a talk for the event about breast cancer awareness. She wants to discuss breast cancer prevention. What are the common modalities of breast cancer prevention that M.P. should address and what chemopreventative agents should she include?

Prevention is key with any cancer. Women who are considered high risk for breast cancer may decide to undergo prophylactic mastectomy with reconstruction as an alternative to living with the prospect that they may develop breast cancer in their life. This modality of prevention is very successful, but does not completely eliminate the risk for developing breast cancer.[3]

Chemoprevention is also another option. Two agents approved for prevention are tamoxifen and raloxifene. The Breast Cancer Prevention Trial (or P1 trial) was conducted in more than 13,000 high-risk women (women were randomly assigned into three groups: those older than 60 years, women between 35 and 59 years of age with an increased risk of breast cancer based on a score of at least 1.66 as determined by the Gail risk model, or women older than 35 years with a history of LCIS, a risk factor for developing invasive breast cancer).[4] Women received tamoxifen 20 mg daily or placebo for 5 years of therapy. Tamoxifen significantly decreased the risk of developing breast cancer ($p < 0.00001$). In addition, this study illustrated toxicities associated with tamoxifen therapy especially in women older than 50 years of age. In those patients, a higher risk of deep vein thrombosis, stroke, pulmonary embolism, and endometrial cancers were identified.[4]

Raloxifene, a selective estrogen receptor modulator (SERM), is approved for chemoprevention in breast cancer. This originated from observations made in osteoporosis studies with raloxifene where patients who had received raloxifene therapy had a decreased risk of breast cancer. With this information, a large randomized chemoprevention trial of more than 19,000 postmenopausal women was conducted evaluating the use of raloxifene 60 mg daily compared to tamoxifen 20 mg daily for 5 years.[5] There was no difference in the number of invasive breast cancers diagnosed in the two treatment arms (relative risk, 1.02; 95% confidence interval, 0.82–1.28). Interestingly, more noninvasive breast cancers were identified in the raloxifene group (80 cases) compared with tamoxifen (57 cases); however, the clinical significance of this difference is unknown. The tamoxifen arm reported more hot flashes and uterine cancer and the raloxifene arm demonstrated fewer thromboembolic events, cataracts, but more musculoskeletal problems and weight gain. Raloxifene was considered as effective as tamoxifen with less toxicity such as thromboembolic events and uterine cancer. Based on the results of this trial, raloxifene received an indication for chemoprevention in high-risk women. M.P. should include information on both tamoxifen and raloxifene in her talk.

RISK FACTORS

CASE 93-2

QUESTION 1: B.W., a 59-year-old woman, is found to have a 2.2-cm mass in the upper, outer quadrant of her left breast during a routine screening mammogram. The rest of her physical examination is unremarkable, and she has no complaints. All laboratory values, including the complete blood count and liver function tests are within normal limits. A chest x-ray is negative. B.W. reports that she had her first menstrual cycle at the age of 10 years and has had regular periods since that time. She is married but has never been pregnant. What are B.W.'s risk factors for developing breast cancer?

Many different risk factors have been identified and are associated with the development of breast cancer. However, in greater than 50% of patients, there are no identifiable risk factors except increased age and female sex[10] (Table 93-1). One's risk increases with each decade of life and the median age of diagnosis is between 60 and 65 years of age. If the patient has had a previous history of breast cancer or atypical hyperplasia from previous breast biopsies, this increases her risk of developing breast cancer.

Breast cancer is a hormonally mediated disease and many risk factors are associated with hormonal influences. Early menarche (generally defined as younger than 12 years of age) and late menopause (generally defined as older than 55 years of age) exposes a woman to more estrogen throughout her lifetime, increasing her risk. Based on the results of the Women's Health Initiative, the use of hormone-replacement therapy was shown to increase one's risk of breast cancer.[11] Nulliparity, or having children after the age of 30 years, has been associated with an increased risk. Oral contraceptives have long been thought to increase the risk of breast cancer; however, investigators have refuted this claim based on more recent data.[12] Earlier forms of oral contraceptives contained much higher doses of estrogen compared with products today. The dose of estrogens in those products was thought to increase a woman's risk of developing breast cancer. However, a meta-analysis demonstrated no difference in risk no matter the dose of estrogen in the oral contraceptives.[12] Hereditary breast cancers (one or more first-degree relatives with the disease) only account for approximately 10% of breast cancer cases; however, these individuals have the highest risk of developing breast cancer.[13]

B.W. has risk factors that increased her risk of developing breast cancer. B.W. started menses early at the age of 10 years and therefore has been exposed longer to estrogen and she does not have any children. She is also 59 years of age and the risk of breast cancer increases with each decade of life. Therefore, all of these are considered risk factors for B.W.

TABLE 93-1
Risk Factors for Developing Breast Cancer

Known Risk Factors
Gender: Female > male
Personal history of breast cancer
Family history of breast cancer (first-degree relatives)
Benign breast "cancer" (i.e., atypical hyperplasia)
Early menarche (<12 years of age), late menopause (>55 years of age)
Late first pregnancy ($\geq$ 30 years) or no pregnancy
Advancing age
Long-term use of hormone-replacement therapy (estrogen)
Previous chest wall irradiation
Possible Risk Factors
Alcohol
Obesity
High-fat diet

Source: Carlson RW et al. Invasive breast cancer. *J Natl Compr Canc Netw.* 2011;9:136; Chlebowski RT et al. Influence of estrogen plus progestin on breast cancer and mammography in healthy postmenopausal women: the women's health initiative randomized trial. *JAMA.* 2003;289:3243.

INHERITED BREAST CANCER MUTATIONS

CASE 93-3

QUESTION 1: C.D., a 37-year-old woman, is found to have a 2.2-cm mass in the outer quadrant of her right breast during a mammogram. All of her laboratory values were normal and her chest x-ray was negative. Her family history is significant in that her mother died of breast cancer at the age of 42 years and her 44-year-old sister had a breast tumor removed 5 years ago. With C.D.'s family history, what genetic testing could be performed for her or for anyone else in her family? If C.D. did not have a family history of breast cancer, what other tests could be conducted to estimate her risk of developing breast cancer?

C.D. has two first-degree relatives with early-age breast cancer. This would indicate an inherited genetic mutation. Genetic testing for the presence of *BRCA1* and *BRCA2* mutations should be discussed with C.D. A person with a *BRCA1* mutation has a

40% to 85% lifetime risk of developing breast cancer and a 25% to 65% risk of ovarian cancer. *BRCA2* mutation carriers have the same risk of breast cancer but lower risk for ovarian cancer (15%–20%).[14] One population with a high incidence of *BRCA* mutations are those of Ashkenazi Jewish descent, where 1 in 50 individuals are *BRCA* carriers.[15] C.D. should meet with a genetic counselor to discuss risks and benefits of genetic testing for her and her family members.

An average risk patient (high-risk patients were previously described in the Screening section) can assess their risk of developing breast cancer by using validated risk tools. One such instrument is the Gail model, which takes into account numerous factors such as age at menarche, age of first live birth, presence of atypical hyperplasia, and number or previous breast biopsies. This model is available on-line (www.cancer.gov/bcrisktool/). Other models that have been validated include BRCAPRO and the Breast Cancer Risk Assessment Tool.[16,17] BRCAPRO is a statistical program that uses information from both affected and unaffected relatives to predict the likelihood if a person would have an inherited mutation in *BRCA1* or *BRCA2*.[14] This tool would be used in an individual with a high risk of developing breast cancer. There are numerous resources for patients and family members to help understand their risk of developing breast cancer. Concerned individuals should have a conversation with their physician regarding their risk of breast cancer and the utility of these risk assessment tools based on their personal and family history.

Clinical Presentation

CASE 93-3, QUESTION 2: What are the typical signs and symptoms of breast cancer and does C.D. have any?

Typical presentation involves the identification of a painless lump on clinical examination by a health care professional, by the patient, or visualization of a painless lump on mammography. Other symptoms are nipple discharge or retraction, or skin changes of the breast.[18] Less than 10% of patients will present with metastatic disease. Symptoms on presentation can reflect their metastatic disease (i.e., back pain: bone metastases; headaches/nausea/vomiting: brain metastases; dyspnea: lung metastases; or abdominal pain: liver metastases).[18] C.D. had a painless lump identified on mammogram as her presenting sign.

Diagnosis

CASE 93-3, QUESTION 3: After the identification of C.D.'s breast mass on mammogram, what diagnostic procedures should be done to determine C.D.'s type and stage of breast cancer?

Workup for breast cancer includes radiographic examinations, patient history, and a physical examination. If a mass is palpated, a mammogram is completed to identify the abnormality. A breast ultrasound can also be added after the mammogram to differentiate fluid-filled cysts (which are usually benign) versus discreet masses. Once identified, a biopsy would then be performed to diagnose the disease. This is achieved with a core biopsy—the standard method used to obtain a tissue sample. This procedure uses a large bore needle for tissue collection and can distinguish invasive versus noninvasive disease. Other methods are available for tissue diagnosis such as fine-needle aspiration and excisional biopsy, but the core biopsy is considered the standard approach.[18]

ONLINE CONTENT

For a short video on the differences in biopsy methods, courtesy of CancerQuest (http://www.cancerquest.org), go to http://thepoint.lww.com/AT10e.

Full radiologic testing should also be completed including a CT scan of the chest, abdomen, and pelvis, and bone scan to assess for metastatic disease. The most common places for breast cancer to metastasize are the bone, lung, liver, lymph nodes, and brain.[19] Evaluation for brain metastases will usually be performed if the patient is experiencing signs and symptoms such as blurry or double vision, uncontrolled nausea/vomiting, headaches, and unsteady gait. These tests are used to determine the extent and stage of the disease and ultimately help determine the prognosis and treatment of the patient. C.D. will need to undergo a biopsy and full staging with a CT scan of the chest, abdomen, and pelvis and a bone scan.

Types of Breast Cancer and Staging

CASE 93-3, QUESTION 4: C.D. had a core biopsy performed which revealed invasive ductal carcinoma. Other staging tests included a CT scan of the chest, abdomen, and pelvis and a bone scan. All tests were negative. Physical examination revealed ipsilateral lymph node involvement. Mammogram revealed a 2.2-cm mass in the left breast. What are the common types of breast cancer and what stage is C.D.'s breast cancer?

The histology of breast cancer is typically divided into two categories: invasive and noninvasive (in situ) disease. Invasive ductal carcinoma is the most common type found (~75% of cases) and invasive lobular carcinoma is second (~5%–10%). The noninvasive tumors are less common (DCIS and LCIS).[18] Other less common histologies include medullary, mucinous, tubular, and papillary. One of the most aggressive forms of breast cancer is inflammatory breast cancer, which is distinctly different from the other types of breast cancer mentioned. Breast cancer can take years to develop into a mass that is identifiable on physical examination or mammogram. In contrast, the onset of inflammatory breast cancer is sudden and can develop in weeks. Presentation includes a breast that looks "inflamed," red, and has the look of an orange peel (peau d'orange). The diagnosis may be delayed because the skin has the appearance of cellulitis. Antibiotics are typically prescribed first; however, the symptoms do not improve with treatment.[20]

Staging is conducted to evaluate the extent of disease. This is completed to understand a patient's prognosis and to help to determine the best treatment course. Staging of breast cancer is determined using the TNM (T, tumor size; N, nodal status; M, any site of metastatic disease) classification. This information is determined by both clinical and pathologic examination. In 2002, the breast cancer staging system was updated by the American Joint Commission on Cancer.[21] Stage I disease involves small tumors (<2 cm) with no lymph node involvement and is highly curable (~98% 5-year survival). Stage II includes small tumors with lymph node involvement or larger tumors (>2 cm and ≤5 cm) with no lymph node involvement. Stage III tumors are larger (>5 cm) with lymph node involvement with a 5-year survival of approximately 80%. Stage IV disease has metastasized to other distant organs and has the poorest prognosis with a 5-year survival of approximately 26% (Table 93-2).[18,21] Most patients will present with stage I or II disease due to routine screening. Based on C.D.'s clinical staging, she is considered to have stage II disease

TABLE 93-2
American Joint Committee on Cancer Staging for Breast Cancer

Stage	T	N	M
0	Tis	N0	M0
I	T1	N0	M0
II	T0–T3	N0–N1	M0
IIIA	T0–T3	N1–N2	M0
IIIB	T4	N0–N2	M0
IIIC	Any T	N3	M0
IV	Any T	Any N	M1

M, metastatic disease; N, presence of lymph nodes; N0, no lymph node involvement; N1, movable ipsilateral lymph nodes; N2, ipsilateral axillary lymph nodes (fixed or matted); or clinical ipsilateral internal mammary nodes with no axillary lymph node involvement; N3, ipsilateral infraclavicular lymph nodes, clinical ipsilateral internal mammary lymph nodes, clinical axillary lymph nodes, or ipsilateral supraclavicular lymph nodes with or without axillary or internal mammary lymph node involvement; T, tumor size; Tis, carcinoma in situ; T1, ≤2 cm; T2, >2 to 5 cm; T3, >5 cm; T4, any size with skin invasion or direct invasion to the chest wall.
Source: Singletary SE et al. Revision of the American Joint Committee on Cancer Staging System for Breast Cancer. *J Clin Oncol.* 2002;20:3628.

based on the size of her disease and the involvement of ipsilateral lymph nodes.

Prognostic Factors

CASE 93-3, QUESTION 5: Further pathologic analysis of C.D.'s breast tumor reveals estrogen receptor (ER)-positive and progesterone receptor (PR)-positive disease. Human epidermal growth factor receptor (HER2) testing of the tumor was negative. What prognostic factors are evaluated in all breast cancer patients?

In addition to staging, other prognostic factors should be evaluated to help determine a patient's treatment course. Prognostic factors such as size of the tumor and lymph node status are important. Large tumor size leads to worse prognosis than smaller tumor size, and presence of disease in the lymph nodes leads to worse prognosis than disease-negative nodes. Further, presence of a high number of positive lymph nodes is directly related to a poorer prognosis. Pathologic testing of the breast tumor gives important prognostic factors such as ER and PR and HER2 status.[22] Tumors that are ER or PR positive tend to denote a slower-growing, indolent disease and have a more favorable prognosis than ER/PR-negative disease. Approximately two-thirds of breast cancer patients diagnosed have ER/PR-positive disease. If a patient has ER/PR-positive disease, hormonal therapy is a treatment option. Tumors that are HER2-positive generally denote more aggressive disease. Approximately 25% of breast cancers test positive for HER2 gene amplification. Although this is indicative of a more aggressive disease, it is a positive predictor for response to trastuzumab therapy (which targets the HER2 protein).[23]

HER2 positivity is determined by two different methods, immunohistochemistry or fluorescence in situ hybridization (FISH). Either method could be used to determine HER2 status. Immunohistochemistry determines the overexpression of the HER2 protein and results are reported as 1+, 2+, and 3+. Patients with 3+ overexpression are considered positive for HER2 and will respond to trastuzumab therapy. If a patient is determined to have 2+ overexpression (an equivocal test), then further testing would be conducted with FISH. FISH testing evaluates the HER2 gene amplification by denoting a ratio of the number of gene copies of HER2 compared to the control and only those patients with positive FISH testing will respond to trastuzumab therapy.[22,23]

Other pathologic tests are completed such as nuclear grade (which determines the degree of differentiation of the tumor cells) as well as tests to evaluate the growth fraction of the disease (such as S-phase fraction, Ki-67, and mitotic index). Clinicians use all of these factors (positive and negative) to determine a patient's prognosis and treatment course.

Other tools allow clinicians to make a more individualized approach (i.e., hormonal therapy alone, chemotherapy alone, or a combination of chemotherapy and hormonal therapy) to treatment. One such tool is Adjuvant!online (www.Adjuvantonline.com), which can be used in early-stage breast cancer patients after surgery to evaluate their individual risk factors and determine treatment benefit versus risk of recurrence. The tool uses clinical factors to estimate an individual's percent risk reduction in recurrence after adjuvant treatment (the benefit with hormonal therapy alone versus the benefit of hormonal therapy and chemotherapy). In addition, genetic profiling has led to the creation of gene arrays to evaluate a patient's risk of recurrence based on their treatment course. Many patients today present with early-stage disease, which is highly curable. Clinicians can use these tests to determine which patients should receive more or less therapy based on their recurrence score. One such test is the Oncotype DX assay for patients with ER/PR-positive and lymph node negative disease and assigns a patient a recurrence score. Based on the score, clinicians and patients can decide the best treatment course such as hormonal therapy alone versus the combination of hormonal therapy and chemotherapy.[24]

Treatment

CASE 93-3, QUESTION 6: C.D. was diagnosed with a stage II, ER-positive and PR-positive, HER 2-negative, invasive ductal carcinoma of the left breast. Her staging workup was negative as indicated previously with a negative CT scan of the chest, abdomen, and pelvis and a negative bone scan. Based on this information what would be C.D.'s treatment course?

LOCAL TREATMENT (SURGERY AND RADIATION THERAPY)

Surgery is the definitive treatment in early-stage breast cancer. Many years ago, a more radical approach to the surgical removal of breast cancer was used. This approach, called a radical mastectomy, involved the removal of the entire breast, both the major and minor pectoralis muscle, and a full axillary lymph node dissection on the side of the breast cancer. Increased morbidity was associated with this approach such as shoulder dysfunction and a poor cosmetic appearance. Today, a modified radical mastectomy is used that removes the entire breast along with an axillary lymph node dissection while leaving the pectoralis muscles intact. This approach leads to equivalent survival compared with the radical surgery.[25] Radiation may be offered in addition to a modified radical mastectomy if the tumor is greater than 5 cm in size, if the patient has greater than four positive lymph nodes, or if positive tissue margins were present after surgery.[26,27] This further improves the local control of the disease.

Conservative approaches to surgery, such as lumpectomy, segmental mastectomy, or quadrantectomy, are also available. If a patient has a small tumor and wishes to preserve the breast, this surgical approach could be used; however, not all patients are candidates for this procedure. Those who are not candidates can include those with multicentric disease (numerous tumors throughout the breast), large tumors in relation to the size of the breast, and inflammatory breast cancer.[18] If the decision is to proceed with breast-conserving surgery, the patient must also undergo adjuvant radiation therapy. Because the surgery only removes the primary tumor, the rest of the breast should be treated with radiation therapy to prevent recurrence of disease. Similar survival rates are observed with modified radical mastectomy versus breast conserving surgery plus radiation therapy.[25,28] C.D. could either undergo breast-conserving surgery plus radiation therapy or a modified radical mastectomy, but with C.D.'s family history she may also choose to undergo bilateral mastectomies to prevent the development of contralateral breast cancer.

Larger tumors do not preclude a patient from undergoing breast-conservative surgery. However, to be eligible for this surgery, patients would receive neoadjuvant chemotherapy to help shrink the tumor to a size conducive to breast-conserving techniques. Neoadjuvant chemotherapy also allows the oncologist to assess response to treatment while the tumor is still in place and allows the opportunity to discontinue a particular chemotherapy regimen if the patient is not responding. Most patients will respond to chemotherapy; however, for those who do not, further chemotherapy (with a different regimen) or radiation therapy may be offered.[29]

The presence and extent of nodal disease is assessed through an axillary lymph node dissection. This involves the removal of at least ten lymph nodes on the same side of the primary tumor to assess for the presence of breast cancer. Lymph node dissection may result in lymphedema, thromboembolism, and infection.[30,31] Sentinel lymph node biopsy is one way to avoid the comorbidities associated with the axillary lymph node dissection. In this procedure, a blue dye (labeled with a radiocolloid) is injected around the breast tumor. Time is given for the dye to drain from the tumor to the lymph nodes. The surgeon is able to identify the sentinel nodes because of the presence of radiocolloid and the blue color. The breast (and presumably the cancer) drains first into the sentinel lymph nodes. Only one or two of the sentinel lymph nodes will be removed, reducing the risk of lymphedema, thromboembolism, and infection.

ONLINE CONTENT

For a video discussing sentinel lymph node biopsy, courtesy of CancerQuest http://www.cancerquest.org), go to http://thepoint.lww.com/AT10e.

Many consider this procedure the standard of care for assessment of the axillary lymph nodes.[29,32–34]

SYSTEMIC THERAPY (CHEMOTHERAPY, HORMONAL THERAPY, AND BIOLOGIC THERAPY)

Surgery and radiation therapy eradicates most tumor cells; however, microscopic disease is difficult to detect and treat locally. Microscopic cancer deposits can migrate through the body and serve as sites for disease recurrence. To diminish the chance of recurrence, systemic adjuvant chemotherapy, hormonal therapy, or biologic therapy is given. The determination of which single modality or combination of therapies is based on the patient's prognostic factors: ER/PR status and HER2 positivity. As mentioned earlier, tools such as the Oncotype DX genetic assay can estimate risk recurrence based on these tumor specific characteristics and assist in determination of therapy.

The size of the tumor and other prognostic factors are also evaluated to determine the course of therapy; see Table 93-3. The National Comprehensive Cancer Network provides treatment guidelines to help guide treatment planning.[29] Patients with small tumors (0.6–1 cm) and negative lymph nodes can be further divided into two groups based on favorable and unfavorable prognostic features. Favorable prognostic features would include hormone-positive disease. These patients can be offered hormonal therapy without chemotherapy. Those individuals with poor prognostic features (tumors with lymphatic invasion, high nuclear grade, hormone-receptor–negative, or HER2-positive disease) would be offered chemotherapy with or without trastuzumab therapy.[18]

Tumors greater than 1 cm in size are generally treated with systemic chemotherapy. Patients with ER/PR-positive disease are usually also treated with hormonal therapy. Biologic therapy with trastuzumab is added to chemotherapy if the patient has HER2-positive disease and assuming there are no contraindications such as cardiac disease. Patients should be fully informed of the absolute benefit of chemotherapy, because in those with early-stage disease the benefit from chemotherapy could be as low as 2% to 3%. The Early Breast Cancer Trialists Collaborative Group conducts an overview analysis every 5 years on the effects of chemotherapy and hormonal therapy in breast cancer randomized trials. In 2005, the 15-year survival updates were published. Although no standard regimen has been identified, combination regimens are superior to single-agent therapy (recurrence rates and mortality for combination chemotherapy, respectively: hazard ratio [HR], 0.77; $p < 0.00001$ and HR, 0.83; $p < 0.0001$, respectively; single-agent therapy recurrence rates and mortality: HR, 0.86; $p = 0.001$ and HR, 0.96; $p = 0.4$, respectively).[35]

Looking back at C.D.'s tumor characteristics, she has stage II (2.2 cm with lymph node involvement), ER-positive, PR-positive, and HER2-negative breast cancer. Based on this information, C.D. would be a candidate for surgery and chemotherapy (based

TABLE 93-3
Overview of the Selection of Adjuvant Treatment

	Adjuvant Hormonal Therapy		Adjuvant Chemotherapy†
Lymph node negative disease	ER/PR (+)	ER/PR (–)	
<0.5 cm	Yes	No	No
0.6 – 1 cm*	Yes	No	Consider
>1 cm	Yes	No	Yes
Lymph node positive disease	ER/PR (+)	ER/PR (–)	
	Yes	No	Yes

*Consider Oncotype DX testing: Low recurrence score (<18) = adjuvant hormonal therapy; intermediate recurrence score (18–30) = adjuvant hormonal therapy +/– chemotherapy; high recurrence score (≥ 31) = adjuvant hormonal therapy + chemotherapy
†Give trastuzumab therapy if the patient is HER2 (+) and no contraindications
Source: National Comprehensive Cancer Network. Clinical practice guidelines in oncology. Breast Cancer. v2. http://www.nccn.org. Accessed June 20, 2011.

on the tumor size and lymph node–positive disease), followed by hormonal therapy due to her ER/PR-positive disease.

ADJUVANT CHEMOTHERAPY

CASE 93-3, QUESTION 7: C.D. underwent a left modified radical mastectomy and axillary lymph node dissection. She had 2 of 15 lymph nodes positive for disease. Her adjuvant treatment will consist of chemotherapy (due to the larger size of the tumor and positive lymph nodes). What are typical adjuvant chemotherapy regimens for the treatment of early-stage breast cancer, and what should C.D. receive?

Many different combination chemotherapy regimens are used in the adjuvant setting (Table 93-4). Anthracycline-containing regimens are commonly used. Doxorubicin or epirubicin in combination with an alkylating agent, cyclophosphamide plus or minus fluorouracil are typical regimens. In the most recent Early Breast Cancer Trialist Cancer Group analysis, anthracycline regimens had significantly lower recurrence rates and death compared to traditional cyclophosphamide, methotrexate, fluorouracil (recurrence rate ratio, 0.89; $p = 0.001$ and cancer death rate ratio, 0.84; $p < 0.00001$, respectively).[35] Taxane-containing regimens are also used although the most recent analysis did not include taxanes as this class of agents is relatively new in the adjuvant setting. Future updated analyses will include results with the use of adjuvant taxanes. A large pooled analysis demonstrated improved diseasefree ($p < 0.00001$) and overall survival ($p < 0.0001$) with the addition of a taxane.[36] The optimal taxane regimen has yet to be identified and the full benefit of the utility of taxane therapy in lymph node–negative disease is yet to be determined; however, the benefit is apparent in lymph

TABLE 93-4
Common Adjuvant Chemotherapy Regimens

Regimen	Schedule (No. of Weeks Between Cycles)	Number of Cycles
Cyclophosphamide (C) Methotrexate (M) 5-Fluorouracil (F), classic (oral)	4	6
CMF (intravenous)	3	9–12
Cyclophosphamide (C) Doxorubicin (A) 5-Fluorouracil (F) (oral)	4	6
Cyclophosphamide (C) Doxorubicin (A) 5-Fluorouracil (F)	3–4	6
Cyclophosphamide (C) Epirubicin (E) 5-Fluorouracil (F)	3	6
Docetaxel (T) Doxorubicin (A) Cyclophosphamide (C)	4	6
Doxorubicin (A) → Cyclophosphamide (C) Methotrexate (M) 5-Fluorouracil (F)	3 → 3	4 → 8
Doxorubicin (A) Cyclophosphamide (C)	3	4–6
Doxorubicin (A) Cyclophosphamide (C) → Paclitaxel (P)	3 → 3	4 → 4
Doxorubicin (A) → Paclitaxel (P) → Cyclophosphamide (C)	3 → 3 → 3	4 → 4 → 4
Dose dense* Doxorubicin (A) Cyclophosphamide (C) → Paclitaxel (P)	2 → 2	4 → 4
Dose dense* Doxorubicin (A) → Paclitaxel (P) → Cyclophosphamide (C)	2 → 2 → 2	4 → 4 → 4

A, adriamycin; C, cyclophosphamide; E, epirubicin; F, fluorouracil; M, methotrexate; P, paclitaxel; T, docetaxel; →, followed by;
*Dose dense, given every two weeks instead of every 3 weeks. See source document for specific dosing.
Source: National Comprehensive Cancer Network. Clinical practice guidelines in oncology. Breast Cancer. v2. http://www.nccn.org. Accessed April 22, 2011.

node–positive disease. Taxanes should be incorporated in the treatment regimen of those with lymph node–positive disease.

Congestive heart failure is a well-known toxicity associated with anthracycline chemotherapy. If a patient has heart failure or other pre-existing cardiac disease, anthracyclines must be used cautiously. To avoid potential toxicity, taxane regimens such as docetaxel and cyclophosphamide have been compared to standard anthracycline-containing regimens, doxorubicin and cyclophosphamide. After 7 years of follow-up, both diseasefree and overall survival were significantly better in the taxane arm compared with the anthracycline arm (81% vs. 75%; $p = 0.033$ and 87% vs. 82%; $p = 0.032$, respectively).[37] Although the results are encouraging, these data do not have the track record of the anthracycline-containing regimens that are still considered the mainstay of therapy for adjuvant chemotherapy in early-stage breast cancer. Studies are currently underway to identify specific populations that may not respond to anthracycline therapy, thereby avoiding the risk of cardiac toxicity in these individuals.[38] If these specific cases are identified, more nonanthracycline-based chemotherapy regimens will be incorporated into clinical practice. Based on C.D.'s lymph node–positive breast cancer, a typical adjuvant chemotherapy regimen would consist of doxorubicin and cyclophosphamide (AC) or fluorouracil and doxorubicin and cyclophosphamide (FAC) given every 3 weeks for four cycles followed by a taxane such as paclitaxel weekly for 12 weeks (see Table 93-4 for commonly used adjuvant chemotherapy regimens).

Trastuzumab therapy can be incorporated into a patient's adjuvant chemotherapy regimen if the tumor is HER2-positive. Trastuzumab was first studied in the metastatic setting and demonstrated improved overall survival when added concurrently with chemotherapy.[39] Because of its robust activity in the metastatic setting, it was then studied in early breast cancer to see if the same benefit could be achieved. Two large trials were conducted concurrently addressing different questions regarding the use of concurrent, sequential, and maintenance trastuzumab.[40] Patients received the classic AC regimen for four cycles followed by paclitaxel weekly either given sequentially or concurrently. Trastuzumab therapy was started after the completion of the AC regimen to reduce potential cardiac toxicities associated with doxorubicin and trastuzumab.[40] The results of these trials were combined and published in full. Diseasefree and overall survival were significantly improved with the addition of trastuzumab (52% decrease in recurrence rates, $p < 0.0001$; and 33% reduction in mortality, $p = 0.015$, respectively).[40] Four-year follow-up data continued to demonstrate significant improvements with trastuzumab compared to chemotherapy alone. Based on these data, trastuzumab was approved for use in early-stage, HER2-positive disease after the completion of AC therapy followed by sequential paclitaxel therapy for 1 year.[40] The use of maintenance trastuzumab is being further studied in the HERA Trial (Herceptin Adjuvant Trial).[41] In that trial, patients are randomly assigned to complete 1 or 2 years of maintenance trastuzumab therapy. Results have not been published to date. One year of trastuzumab therapy is the current standard of practice for maintenance therapy in the adjuvant setting. Because C.D. does not have HER2-positive disease, trastuzumab therapy should not be used.

CHEMOTHERAPY TOXICITY

CASE 93-3, QUESTION 8: C.D. is to undergo four cycles of AC chemotherapy followed by weekly paclitaxel for 12 weeks. What are the common toxicities associated with this treatment course? If the tumor was HER2-positive and C.D. received trastuzumab, what toxicities would be associated with its use?

Doxorubicin is an anthracycline chemotherapy. It works through multiple mechanisms, but inhibition of topoisomerase II may be most important.[42] By inhibiting this enzyme, double-strand DNA breaks occur. Common toxicities include myelosuppression, nausea/vomiting, and alopecia. A well-known toxicity of anthracyclines is the risk of cardiomyopathy due to the formation of oxygen free radicals and doxorubicin metal complexes. These toxicities can be acute (with symptoms similar to an arrhythmia or myocardial infarction) or chronic (with a patient demonstrating symptoms of congestive heart failure).[43] The risk of cardiotoxicity increases with larger anthracycline cumulative doses.[44] With the typical doses of anthracyclines used in the adjuvant setting, a patient will not reach the cumulative doses known to increase the risk of cardiotoxicity. If a patient has underlying cardiac dysfunction, baseline evaluation of ejection fraction either through an echocardiogram or multigated acquisition scan should be completed.[45,46] Other known risk factors for the development of anthracycline-induced cardiotoxicity include age older than 70 years, hypertension, pre-existing coronary artery disease, and previous cardiac irradiation, or previous anthracycline exposure, and may warrant cardiac evaluation.[47]

Cyclophosphamide is an alkylating agent that works by forming cross-links in DNA, thus inhibiting DNA synthesis.[42] Common toxicities are nausea/vomiting, myelosuppression, and alopecia. The alkylating agents, although rare, are also associated with a risk of secondary leukemias.

Paclitaxel, a taxane chemotherapy, derived from the Pacific yew tree, works by binding to the β-tubulin subunit of microtubules preventing disassembly and ultimately causing inhibition of mitosis. Common toxicities associated with paclitaxel include nausea/vomiting, myelosuppression, neuropathy, and hypersensitivity reactions due to the cremaphor solvent in paclitaxel. All patients should be premedicated with dexamethasone and H_1 and H_2 blockers to prevent hypersensitivity.[48]

Trastuzumab is a monoclonal antibody targeted against the extracellular HER2 protein. The classic toxicity associated with trastuzumab is cardiac toxicity, but is different than that with anthracyclines. Trastuzumab cardiotoxicity is considered reversible and believed to be a result of HER2 blockade (HER2 signaling is responsible for cardiomyocyte growth, repair, and survival).[49–51] In those patients who will receive long-term trastuzumab therapy, baseline cardiac function should be evaluated similar to doxorubicin and then periodically with echocardiogram or multigated acquisition scan during therapy. C.D. does not have a history of cardiac disease, so a baseline cardiac evaluation before AC therapy may not occur. C.D. should be counseled on the common toxicities associated with her chemotherapy, such as myelosuppression, nausea/vomiting, alopecia, neuropathy, cardiomyopathy, and hypersensitivity reactions.

HORMONAL THERAPY

CASE 93-3, QUESTION 9: After the completion of adjuvant chemotherapy, C.D. will receive hormonal therapy because her disease is ER/PR-positive. What are the common adjuvant hormonal regimens used? What regimen would be appropriate for C.D.?

Breast cancer is a hormonally mediated disease and therapies that alter hormonal levels are an integral component to the treatment plan. This therapy is offered to patients with ER/PR-positive disease. Therapeutic options include SERMs, luteinizing hormone–releasing hormone (LH-RH) agonists, and aromatase

TABLE 93-5
Aromatase Inhibitors

Type	Dose	Toxicities
Nonsteroidal		
Anastrozole	1 mg daily PO	Common toxicities: myalgias/arthralgias, hot flashes, osteoporosis
Letrozole	2.5 mg daily PO	
Steroidal		
Exemestane	25 mg daily PO	

PO, orally.
Source: Jones KL, Buzdar AU. A review of adjuvant hormonal therapy in breast cancer. *Endocr Relat Cancer.* 2004;11:391; Buzdar AU, Howell A. Advances in aromatase inhibitors: clinical efficacy and tolerability in the treatment of breast cancer. *Clin Cancer Res.* 2001;7:2620.

inhibitors (AIs). Given this number of choices, menopausal status of the patient is used to guide selection of therapy.

Traditionally, tamoxifen has been the gold standard for adjuvant hormonal therapy. Tamoxifen is a SERM, which works by blocking estrogen from binding to the estrogen receptor. It does not alter estrogen production. Tamoxifen has antiestrogenic activity in the breast, although it has estrogenic effects in other areas such as bone.[52,53] Tamoxifen can be used in both premenopausal and postmenopausal women and is given 20 mg orally daily for 5 years based on the data from the National Surgical Adjuvant Breast and Bowel Project B-14 trial.[54,55] Tamoxifen should be initiated after chemotherapy because it can antagonize the antitumor activity of chemotherapy if given concurrently.[56] Common toxicities associated with therapy are hot flashes and vaginal discharge. More thrombosis, pulmonary embolisms, and strokes can occur in patients (older than 50 years of age) receiving tamoxifen compared to placebo (risk ratio, 1.60, 3.19, 1.59, respectively).[4]

Ovarian suppression is an alternative therapy for premenopausal patients as the ovaries are the largest source of estrogen. This is typically achieved through the use of LH-RH agonists. Surgery or radiation can also induce ovarian ablation; however, surgery is irreversible but offers an immediate effect where as radiation may offer an incomplete response and slower onset.[57] If a woman would like to maintain fertility throughout chemotherapy, a thorough discussion with her physician should occur. Studies with the use of LH-RH agents have been tested as a means to preserve fertility but have shown mixed results.[58]

Postmenopausal patients also have the option of AI therapy. Aromatase inhibitors inhibit the production of estrogen by preventing the conversion of androstenedione and testosterone to estrone and estradiol. There are two classes of agents: nonsteroidal AIs (anastrozole and letrozole) and the steroidal AI, exemestane. These agents are highly selective for the aromatase enzyme and have less toxicity than tamoxifen and other hormonal agents. Aromatase inhibitors should only be used in postmenopausal women. If used in the premenopausal setting, initial surges of estrogen occur due to the body's compensation mechanisms (i.e., hypothalamic-pituitary axis) and negative feedback loop. Table 93-5 provides a list of AIs.[59–61] If used as single therapy, AIs are given for 5 years.

The optimal hormonal therapy regimen for the adjuvant setting has not been identified. In premenopausal women, the options are 5 years of tamoxifen therapy plus or minus ovarian suppression with an LH-RH agonist. If, after 2 to 3 years, the patient is postmenopausal, then 2 to 3 years of an AI may be given to complete a total of 5 years of therapy. If the patient is postmenopausal at the beginning of adjuvant hormonal therapy, an option would be to take an AI for 5 years. There have been no prospective comparisons of the AIs with each other; therefore, any can be used as first-line treatment.[60,61] Another clinical option is 5 years of tamoxifen and then if the patient is postmenopausal after the end of 5 years, an additional 5 years of an AI can be given. This was found beneficial in an extended study of hormonal therapy (the BIG 1–98 trial). At the 2.4-year follow-up, additional letrozole therapy was associated with a superior 4-year diseasefree survival (93% with extended letrozole vs. 87% in the tamoxifen arm; $p < 0.001$).[62] Table 93-6 lists adjuvant hormonal therapy options.[29]

C.D. is premenopausal, so she would start with tamoxifen therapy. If after 2 to 3 years of therapy, C.D. becomes postmenopausal, then she could continue the tamoxifen for a total of 5 years or convert to an AI to complete a total of 5 years of therapy. Because of her age, she will likely continue to be premenopausal after chemotherapy and be maintained on 5 years of tamoxifen. If she completes 5 years of tamoxifen therapy and is postmenopausal at that time, then extended use of an AI for an additional 5 years would be recommended. Ovarian suppression with an LH-RH agonist can also be added because she is premenopausal to chemically suppress her ovarian function.

TABLE 93-6
Overview of Adjuvant Hormonal Therapy

	Option 1	Option 2	Option 3
Premenopausal at time of therapy initiation (Patients can complete one of 3 different options)	Tamoxifen × 5 years ± LH-RH agonist or ovarian ablation	If still premenopausal after 2–3 years of tamoxifen therapy, complete a total of 5 years of tamoxifen. If postmenopausal after 2–3 years: A. Complete 5 years of tamoxifen followed by 5 additional years of an AI OR B. Convert to an AI × 2–3 years for a total of 5 years of hormonal therapy	If still premenopausal after 5 years of tamoxifen: Stop therapy If postmenopausal after 5 years of therapy give AI × 5 additional years
Postmenopausal at time of therapy initiation	1. Any AI × 5 years OR 2. Tamoxifen × 5 years OR 3. Tamoxifen × 2–3 years then AI to complete a total of 5 years OR 4. Tamoxifen × 4–6 years then an AI for 5 additional years		

AI, aromatase inhibitor; LH-RH, luteinizing hormone–releasing hormone.
Source: National Comprehensive Cancer Network. Clinical practice guidelines in oncology. Breast Cancer. v2. http://www.nccn.org. Accessed April 22, 2011.

Treatment

CASE 93-4

QUESTION 1: T.R. is a 65-year-old, postmenopausal woman diagnosed with breast cancer at the age of 48 years. At the time of diagnosis she was premenopausal. She underwent surgery with a modified radical mastectomy and was found to have a 1.5-cm invasive ductal carcinoma of the right breast. She had two of ten lymph nodes positive. Her breast cancer was ER-positive, PR-positive, and HER2-negative. T.R. went on to complete adjuvant chemotherapy with AC therapy for four cycles followed by weekly paclitaxel for 12 weeks. After completion of her chemotherapy, she received 5 years of tamoxifen therapy. Ten years after completing her therapy, she experiences pain in her right arm and rib cage. A bone scan revealed metastatic breast cancer. What would be an appropriate treatment regimen for T.R. at this time?

Early-stage breast cancer is curable. However, if a patient develops metastatic disease, the goal of treatment shifts from cure to palliation and stabilization of disease. Treatment is offered to improve quality of life and alleviate symptoms from treatment or disease. The mean survival time after diagnosis of metastatic disease is approximately 2 to 4 years; however, this can range from months to many years depending on the site of the metastases.[63] The choice of therapy is based on the site of disease and other factors that help guide therapy such as ER/PR status. Endocrine therapy is more likely to be effective in patients with bone-only disease whereas chemotherapy may be used when there is visceral disease (i.e., liver or lung). Patients with organ involvement tend to have more rapidly growing disease that generally requires therapy with a quicker onset of action such as chemotherapy.[18] Common sites of metastases include liver, lung, brain, bone, and lymph nodes.

In addition to systemic therapy (chemotherapy and/or hormonal therapy), the clinician needs to determine whether or not local therapy (such as radiation or surgery) would be appropriate for a patient. Radiation therapy can be used to target painful bone metastases, to prevent further tumor growth, and to relieve pain. Surgery may be performed on bones with impending fractures, spinal cord compression, or brain metastases for palliation. These modalities of treatment only affect the local site of disease, so a combination of local and systemic therapy would need to be administered to fully treat the patient. Chemotherapy generally offers a much quicker onset of action compared to hormonal therapy. If a patient is experiencing worsening symptoms such as shortness of breath due to lung metastases or increased abdominal pain due to liver metastases, the use of chemotherapy may be preferred over hormonal therapy.[64] Disease recurrence greater than 5 years after diagnosis illustrates a more indolent-growing disease and is a favorable prognostic factor. Tumors with ER/PR-positive characteristics would also be considered a good prognostic factor. Once therapy is initiated, response to therapy should be monitored periodically. Tumor markers such as CA.27.29 and CA.15.3 are commonly monitored in metastatic breast cancer. In addition, radiologic evaluation of disease progression (such as a CT scan of the chest, abdomen, and pelvis or bone scan depending on the sites of disease) would be conducted. A clinical examination in combination with radiologic tests and tumor markers are assessed to determine response to therapy. Based on T.R.'s metastatic bone disease and ER/PR-positive tumor characteristics, the use of hormonal therapy would be the most appropriate agent to initiate. T.R. received tamoxifen therapy in the adjuvant setting. Because she progressed after taking tamoxifen therapy, this would not be reinitiated. An AI would be started because she is postmenopausal and should be continued until there is evidence of progression of disease via radiologic findings or increases in tumor markers.

CASE 93-4, QUESTION 2: T.R. is started on anastrozole 1 mg orally daily. What are the other hormonal agents that can be used in the treatment of metastatic breast cancer?

Hormonal therapy in the metastatic setting can provide long progressionfree survival in patients. If the patient responds for a long period of time, the likelihood of response to another hormonal agent is high.[64] A patient may take multiple hormonal therapies before ever having to receive chemotherapy. As before, the decision regarding which hormonal agent to use is based on one's menopausal status. If the patient is premenopausal the options include tamoxifen and LH-RH agonists; however, if the patient has received these agents in the adjuvant setting, they would not be used again in the metastatic setting. Aromatase inhibitors are indicated for use in first-line therapy in the metastatic setting. If an AI is chosen as the first-line agent in the metastatic setting, use of another AI after progression would include one from another category (i.e., nonsteroidal vs. steroidal AI). For example, if anastrozole was used as first-line therapy for metastatic disease, then when the patient progresses, exemestane can be used.

Many other hormonal agents are available for use. The pure antiestrogen, fulvestrant, is the only drug in a unique category of agents. It exerts its mechanism via binding and blocking of the estrogen receptor and downregulates the number of estrogen receptors. Fulvestrant is administered as an intramuscular injection and is dosed 250 mg once a month. It is approved for use after failure of tamoxifen therapy in the metastatic setting.[65] This is an alternative for patients with compliance issues due to its once-monthly dosing. Other hormonal agents used in metastatic disease are megestrol acetate, progestins, and high-dose estrogens (higher doses have been found to inhibit cancer cell growth). These agents were used routinely before the approval of AIs. Now they are reserved for use after multiple hormonal therapy failures due to the toxicities associated with these therapies such as weight gain, vaginal bleeding, and thromboembolic events.[60]

T.R. was started on anastrozole therapy. She could have been initiated on any of the AIs. If her disease progresses, options include sequential exemestane, then fulvestrant, and then other agents such as megestrol acetate, high-dose estrogens, or androgens. The goal is to continue T.R. on multiple lines of hormonal therapy (as long as she is responding) before administering chemotherapy.

Prevention of Skeletal Events

CASE 93-4, QUESTION 3: In addition to anastrozole therapy, what other supportive care medicines should be added to T.R.'s regimen?

Patients with bone metastases are commonly treated with bisphosphonate therapy to decrease the risk of skeletal-related events (i.e., pathologic fractures, spinal cord compression, need for surgery, or radiation to the bone). Bisphosphonates act by inhibiting bone resorption. This ultimately will halt osteoclastic activity leading to stabilization of bony involvement, prevention of fractures, and reduction in calcium levels.[66,67] Bisphosphonates used are pamidronate 90 mg intravenously (IV) for 2 hours and zolendronic acid 4 mg IV for 15 minutes. Both of these can be administered once a month. Bisphosphonates are typically well tolerated although they may cause nausea, increased bone pain,

the nodes would be sampled for presence of the disease and to confirm staging. J.W. appears to have limited disease, and so lobectomy would be recommended for him. For patients whose primary tumor or lymph node involvement extends to the proximal bronchus or proximal pulmonary artery, or crosses the major fissure, then a more extensive pneumonectomy is performed. Therefore, surgery is the treatment of choice, and final staging during surgery will guide further adjunct treatments. The tumors can often spread to mediastinal lymph nodes, and for those who have spread of the disease to this location (stage IIIA), then neoadjuvant chemotherapy can be recommended to reduce the tumor burden prior to surgery. If neoadjuvant therapy is chosen, the regimen is usually similar to those used in the adjuvant setting (Table 94-5).[18–21] Therefore, surgery is the primary treatment modality for patients with stages I, II, and early stage III disease. J.W.'s disease appears to be localized; therefore, surgical removal of the tumor would be indicated, and neoadjuvant chemotherapy would not be indicated since there does not appear to be disease in the mediastinum.[22]

CASE 94-1, QUESTION 3: J.W. was referred to a thoracic surgeon for resection. A right upper lobe lobectomy was performed with lymph node dissection. The pathology report revealed a 3.2 × 4 cm adenocarcinoma with three associated peribronchial lymph nodes containing cancer cells. Lymph nodes sampled from the mediastinum demonstrated no cancer. The patient's tumor was staged as a T2N1M0 (stage 2A) NSCLC. Now that the tumor is removed and staging of the disease is finalized, what additional therapy, if any, is recommended now?

Although NSCLC tumors are minimally responsive to chemotherapy, evidence from several studies (Table 94-5) shows that adjuvant treatment enhances patient survival, and therefore should be considered as part of the treatment plan for the patient.

TABLE 94-5
Adjuvant Chemotherapy Regimens for Non–Small Cell Lung Cancer

Regimen	Schedule
Cisplatin, days 1 and 8 Vinorelbine, days 1, 8, 15, 22	Every 28 days for four cycles[18]
Cisplatin, day 1 Vinorelbine, days 1, 8, 15, 22	Every 28 days for four cycles[19,20]
Cisplatin, day 1 Vinorelbine, days 1, 8	Every 21 days for four cycles[18]
Cisplatin, day 1 Etoposide, days 1–3	Every 28 days for four cycles[20]
Cisplatin, days 1, 22, 43, 64 Vinblastine, days 1, 8, 15, 22, then every 2 weeks after day 43	Every 21 days for four cycles[20]
Paclitaxel on, day 1 Carboplatin, day 1	Every 21 days[21]
Other Acceptable Regimens	
Cisplatin, day 1 Gemcitabine, days 1, 8	Every 21 days[22]
Cisplatin, day 1 Docetaxel, day 1	Every 21 days[23]
Pemetrexed, day 1 Cisplatin, day 1 for nonsquamous NSCLC	Every 21 days for four cycles[22]

NSCLC, non–small cell lung cancer.

Though adjuvant treatment is often recommended, results from two other studies indicate that adjuvant treatment is not always effective.[24] This suggests that there is a need to identify subsets of patients who would likely benefit from treatment, and one group that does not seem to gain benefit are those with stage I disease. In the CALGB 9633 study, patients were randomly assigned to receive carboplatin and paclitaxel or placebo, and a survival benefit was observed for those receiving chemotherapy. However, this survival was not uniform across the entire cohort. Subgroup analysis showed that adjuvant chemotherapy should not be considered standard of care for patients with stage IB disease, unless the tumor size is greater than 4 cm. Collectively, these studies show that patients with stages II and IIIA disease gain the most benefit from adjuvant chemotherapy.[21] As summarized in Table 94-5, this chemotherapy usually includes cisplatin, or if the patient is unable to tolerate it, then carboplatin. A second agent, usually selected from one of those listed in Table 94-5, is added as doublet therapy, and the goal is for patients to receive four cycles. Toxicity often becomes worse beyond four cycles and benefits are diminished thereafter. Therefore, chemotherapy is beneficial, but has its limitations.

Radiation therapy is frequently used in the treatment of malignancies including later stages of NSCLC and also SCLC (described subsequently); however, it has no proven benefit for the treatment of early stage disease. The PORT Group conducted a meta-analysis from nine randomized trials to evaluate the possible role of postoperative radiotherapy in patients with completely resected NSCLC. There were 707 deaths among 1,056 patients assigned postoperative radiotherapy and 661 among 1,072 assigned surgery alone (hazard ratio, 1.21 [95% confidence interval, 1.08–1.34]). This 21% relative increase in the risk of death with radiotherapy is equivalent to a reduction in overall survival from 55% to 48%. Subgroup analysis showed that the increased risk of death was greatest for patients with stage I/II, N0 or N1, but no clear evidence for those with stage III, N2 disease.[25] Separately, another postoperative radiotherapy study was conducted, using data from 7,465 patients in the Surveillance, Epidemiology, and End Results database. The investigators for this study also found no benefit for radiotherapy, especially for patients with N1 and N0 nodal disease. However, an increase in survival was associated with radiotherapy for patients who had N2 nodal disease.[26] Hence, based on these two studies, radiation therapy is harmful for patients with early stage disease, but patients with higher stage NSCLC may benefit from the treatment.

In summary, adjuvant chemotherapy is recommended for all patients found to have stage II or III NSCLC at surgery, as well as for larger (>4 cm) tumors. Multiple prospective phase 3 studies have shown that platinum-based chemotherapy after surgery will increase the survival rate of patients after surgery by about 10%. Because J.W. has Stage IIA disease, four cycles of a platinum-based doublet regimen would be indicated after surgery; however, he should not receive radiotherapy at this time.

CASE 94-1, QUESTION 4: After surgery, J.W. saw both a medical oncologist and a radiation oncologist to discuss additional therapies. The radiation oncologist advised the patient that no radiation was needed, and that studies have demonstrated that for patients with stage 1 or 2 NSCLC, radiation leads to a surprising decrease in survival after surgery. Participation in a clinical trial was also discussed with J.W. The patient agreed to participate in the study and was randomly assigned to receive a platinum-based chemotherapy regimen along with bevacizumab. What place in therapy do targeted agents have?

As will be discussed later in this chapter, targeted therapies such as anti-angiogenesis and anti-EGFR therapies are useful for the treatment of advanced stage NSCLC. However, their role has not been established for patients like J.W. who have early stage disease. Currently, a large international phase 3 study (ECOG 1505) is investigating the role of adding anti-angiogenic therapy with bevacizumab to standard platinum-based adjuvant chemotherapy.[27]

Late-Stage Non–Small Cell Lung Cancer

CASE 94-2

QUESTION 1: L.L., an 85-year-old woman, presented with mild cough productive with non-bloody sputum. There was associated fever and shortness of breath. She was initially seen by primary care physicians who treated her with antibiotics for possible pneumonia; however, the radiogram of the chest obtained showed persisting infiltrate in the left upper lung. This was later confirmed on a CT scan that showed the presence of a 6 × 3 × 3.6 cm mass in the left upper lobe. Tumor extended to left superior hilum. There were also mediastinal adenopathy and multiple pulmonary nodules seen in the right upper lobe with associated scarring, the largest of them measuring 14 × 9 mm in the right upper lobe anteriorly. Transbronchial biopsy led to a diagnosis of adenocarcinoma with pathologic grade 3 out of 4. The PET scan confirmed the presence of metabolic activity in the left primary tumor mass and right apical lesion as well. Because of the spread of disease to contralateral lung, disease was staged as IV. Pertinent patient history included hypertension and hyperlipidemia. The patient also had a hemangioma of the brain resected in 1950, and a history of cervical cancer treated with abdominal hysterectomy in 1952. She has never been a smoker. Upon evaluation, she was found to have hemoglobin slightly low at 11.3 g/dL with white blood cell count of 5,200 cells/μL and a platelet count of 245,000/μL. The electrolytes showed normal sodium 143 mEq/L, normal potassium of 4.4 mEq/L, and creatinine 1.08 mg/dL, with estimated creatinine clearance of 48 mL/minute. Performance status 0–1. What are the treatment options for patients such as L.L. with advanced (stage IIIB and IV) disease?

SURGERY

In general, tumors in patients with stage IIIB and IV disease are inoperable. These tumors often invade the carina, great vessels, vertebral bodies, more distant lymph nodes, metastases, and are frequently associated with malignant pleural effusions. Hence, combined modality treatments such as chemotherapy and radiation are the preferred treatments for patients with advanced stage disease.[28,29] Surgery to remove solitary metastatic sites may also be considered.

RADIATION

Radiotherapy is the primary local treatment (i.e., definitive radiotherapy) for inoperable NSCLC, and is also used as a palliative modality for patients with incurable disease. For tumors classified as stage III, radiotherapy is often given concurrently with chemotherapy, as this has been shown to be superior to both radiation alone and also sequential radiation followed by chemotherapy.[22] The radiation dose, in combination with chemotherapy, usually ranges between 60 Gy and 65 Gy, given in 2-Gy fractions. Metastases may also be treated locally with radiotherapy. For example, brain metastases, spinal cord compression, and impending fractures of weight-bearing bones can be treated with radiation or surgery before systemic therapy commences. In contrast to patients with stage III disease, those with stage IV disease usually receive local treatment with radiotherapy first, followed by chemotherapy, because therapy given concurrently is often not well tolerated by patients with this stage of disease.

CHEMOTHERAPY

Patients with advanced disease and good performance status usually benefit from chemotherapy. Similar to early stage disease, these tumors often respond to treatment with platinum-based doublet cytotoxic combination therapy, which refers to treatment with either cisplatin or carboplatin plus a second cytotoxic agent. These doublets may also include targeted treatments such as bevacizumab or cetuximab (Table 94-6).[30–35] Many of these platinum doublet regimens are associated with similar response rates and survival to one another. They differ in their toxicity profiles and cost, and until recently, these considerations were the only means available to guide treatment decisions.

NSCLC was treated as a single disease despite recognition of its histologic and molecular heterogeneity, but recent clinical trials demonstrate that histology is an important factor for individualizing treatment based either on safety or efficacy outcomes. Hence, once the biopsy is obtained, it is crucial to differentiate the histiologic subtype (i.e., squamous vs. nonsquamous). The role of histology in the management of advanced NSCLC is reviewed more extensively elsewhere.[36] In developed countries, an increasing incidence of adenocarcinoma and a decline in squamous cell carcinomas has been observed in recent years. This appears to be correlated to declines in smoking rates. Many agents are effective against all histiologic types, such as cisplatin, carboplatin, gemcitabine, and paclitaxel. However, other agents such as bevacizumab and pemetrexed are only indicated for use in patients who have the nonsquamous histology. Squamous cell histology is associated with increased risk for severe pulmonary hemorrhage

TABLE 94-6
Representative Regimens for Advanced or Metastatic Non–Small Cell Lung Cancer

Regimen	Schedule
Cisplatin, day 1 Paclitaxel, day 1	Every 21 days[30]
Cisplatin, day 1 Gemcitabine, days 1, 8, 15	Every 28 days[30,31]
Cisplatin, day 1 Docetaxel, day 1	Every 21 days[30]
Paclitaxel, day 1 Carboplatin, day 1	Every 21 days[30]
Cisplatin, day 1 Vinorelbine, days 1, 8 Cetuximab weekly Nonsquamous histology	Every 21 days[32]
Cisplatin, day 1 Gemcitabine, days 1, 8 Bevacizumab, day 1	Every 21 days[33]
Paclitaxel, day 1 Carboplatin, day 1 Bevacizumab, day 1	Every 21 days[34]
Pemetrexed, day 1 Cisplatin, day 1	Every 21 days[31]
Erlotinib daily for known EGFR mutation status	Until disease progression or unacceptable toxicity[35]

EGFR, epidermal growth factor receptor.

compared with adenocarcinoma.[37] For pemetrexed, significant association between improved efficacy and the nonsquamous subtype has been reported.[38,39]

Characterization of advanced NSCLC tumors at the molecular level has also recently become part of clinical practice. It is recommended that tumor tissues from patients with nonsquamous histology tumors should be analyzed for the presence of EGFR mutation status.[22] Tumors that are positive for EGFR somatic mutations are often more responsive to erlotinib therapy, and evidence also suggests that this would be a preferred treatment, rather than cytotoxic chemotherapy, for the first-line setting. This analysis is limited to patients with stages IIIB or IV disease, because there is yet no proven benefit for erlotinib in patients with earlier-stage disease and EGFR mutations.[40] For the advanced disease setting, therefore, treatment decisions are becoming more individualized on the basis of tumor histology and somatic mutations. As more targeted therapies, designed to inhibit other targets, are approved it is likely that their use will be based upon at least some of these same principles.

Patients who respond to treatment or achieve stable disease after four to six cycles may be given maintenance therapy. The intention of such additional treatment would be to prolong the response and survival made possible by first-line treatment, while minimizing the chances for toxicity associated with platinum-based doublet regimens. Maintenance therapy differs from second-line therapy in that second-line treatment is only used when the patient has progressed during or after first-line treatment or is unable to tolerate it. Maintenance may be given as continuation maintenance, which refers to the use of one of the agents given in first line. Often, biologic agents that were given as part of the first line regimen (e.g., bevacizumab or cetuximab) are continued due to their better tolerability relative to the cytotoxic agents.[34,41] Pemetrexed may also be given as continuation maintenance treatment, though there is not a uniform consensus to support its use in this setting, according to the National Comprehensive Cancer Network guidelines.[22] Overall, continuation maintenance is associated with an improvement in progression-free survival, but not overall survival. Alternatively, the agent may be different from those used in first-line treatment, and is referred to as switch maintenance. Pemetrexed, erlotinib, and docetaxel are three agents for which there is supportive clinical trial data in the switch-maintenance setting.[22,38,42] The first two agents are associated with an improvement in overall survival, and have an indication for use in this setting. Maintenance therapy is reviewed more extensively elsewhere.[43]

PALLIATION

Patients with metastatic NSCLC receive benefit from palliative care early after diagnosis, rather than waiting until end-of-life care. This palliative care includes helping the patient deal with the psychosocial aspects of their disease through methods such as counseling (e.g., expectation of treatment outcomes and affordability of treatment). In a study of patients with metastatic disease, subjects were randomly assigned to receive either early palliative care integrated with standard oncologic care vs. standard oncologic care alone. Patients assigned to early palliative care experienced a better quality of life and survival (11.6 months vs. 8.9 months) than patients assigned to standard care alone. They also experienced fewer depressive symptoms (16% vs. 38%). The results show that palliative care is appropriate and potentially beneficial when it is introduced at the time of diagnosis at the same time as other benefical therapies.[44]

In conclusion, L.L. would not likely receive benefit from surgical removal of the primary tumor or metastatic site. Instead, radiation and chemotherapy are the definitive treatments of choice because these modalities are more effective for controlling disease that has already spread. If this option is chosen, the radiation should be given prior to the chemotherapy (Table 94-6) to minimize toxicity for this patient with stage IV disease. Consideration for palliative care would also be beneficial.

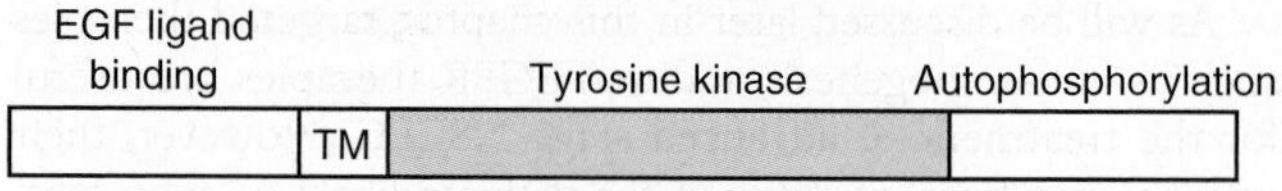

FIGURE 94-1 Tumor epidermal growth factor receptor. Mutations in the tyrosine kinase domain (Exons 18-21) render tumors more sensitive to the antitumor effects of small-molecule kinase inhibitors such as erlotinib. Once treatment with erlotinib has begun, other mutations can arise that are associated with reduced sensitivity. TM = transmembrane domain.

CASE 94-2, QUESTION 2: The tumor tissue was sent out for analysis of presence of EGFR mutation. What characteristics for L.L. would prompt a decision to send a tumor specimen for analysis of EGFR mutation?

The mutations that have been described reside in exons 18–24 (amino acids 718–964) of the tyrosine kinase domain of the EGFR gene (which behaves as an oncogene). Of those, 90% reside in exon 19 or 21 (Figure 94-1).[45] The role of these mutations are thought to constitutively activate the receptor. Such an activated receptor is likely to be important for the pathogenesis of the disease by tumors. Exon 19 deletions are associated with longer median time to disease progression than L858R mutations, suggesting that all mutations are not equivalent with respect to tyrosine kinase responsiveness.[35,46]

The importance of this analysis is underscored by the fact that patients with EGFR-mutation–positive advanced stage tumors respond better to treatment with erlotinib than they do with conventional chemotherapy.[35] Further, erlotinib is better tolerated than doublet platinum-based therapies; therefore, patients with EGFR-mutation–positive tumors would be expected to experience better outcomes related to both tumor response and tolerability. Soon after erlotinib was approved by the US Food and Drug Administration (FDA), investigators noticed that patients who were women, Asian, and nonsmokers tended to respond to erlotinib therapy more frequently than other populations. However, it was subsequently realized that presence of mutations in EGFR was a better predictor of response to erlotinib therapy than demographic factors and smoking status. The prevalence of EGFR mutations is between 10% and 15% for the overall population, but is 35% in white nonsmokers, and 65% for Asian nonsmokers.[47] Hence, the probability that L.L., a nonsmoking white woman, has a tumor with this somatic mutation is higher than for other categories of patients such as smokers or men. Further, the observed incidence of these mutations is less than 3% for patients with squamous cell histology; therefore, it is not recommended to test patients with this histology.[22] L.L. was diagnosed with adenocarcinoma, which is a nonsquamous subtype, and mutation testing is thus warranted on that basis alone.

The question arises that patients who fall into the category with multiple clinical predictors of response could be started empirically on erlotinib therapy without the need to test for EGFR mutations. In L.L.'s case, she would be classified as having three of these clinical predictors: female, nonsmoker, and adenocarcinoma. However, studies with populations of patients from developed countries with NSCLC showed that those who had three or more of these characteristics experienced a 49% response rate, whereas those with sensitizing EGFR mutations experienced much higher 67% response rate.[35] This indicates that EGFR mutation is a better predictor of response to erlotinib therapy than presence of multiple clinical predictors.

Application of this EGFR testing is useful for small molecule tyrosine kinase inhibitors (e.g., erlotinib), but not for antibody molecules (e.g., cetuximab) that also block EGFR. The antibody molecules function to block the receptor externally to the cell surface, and they also stimulate immune responses (e.g., antibody-dependent cell-mediated cytotoxicity, complement) against the tumor. It is likely that even without presence of the mutation(s), the antibody molecule still binds, and can function through several mechanisms to promote an anti-tumor effect. Small molecule inhibitors, however, also bind receptor internally to the cell surface and can inhibit the active ATP binding region, which is constitutively activated in tumors with EGFR mutations. For L.L., it is standard of care to send the tumor specimen for EGFR mutation analysis.

CASE 94-2, QUESTION 3: Analysis of tumor tissue detected L858R mutation in exon 21, which is commonly associated with high sensitivity to the EGFR tyrosine kinase inhibitor (TKI) erlotinib.[35] L.L. was then started on erlotinib therapy and within 8 weeks of therapy she had obtained a partial response. What benefit from erlotinib therapy can L.L. expect in terms of prolonged survival?

Although there is short-term benefit for patients with EGFR-mutation–positive tumors to receive erlotinib, it is not yet clear if there is a longer-term benefit. The response rate for erlotinib treatment is approximately 67%, time to disease progression is 11.8 months, and overall survival is approximately 24 months. As of yet, there are no data to support that treatment with small molecule inhibitors prolongs overall survival, relative to doublet platinum-based therapy. It is much easier to demonstrate an effect on tumor response and time to progression (such as with erlotinib) than it is for overall survival in most cancer studies. Showing improvement in overall survival is difficult because study subjects who are randomly assigned to one arm of a study can exhibit progressive disease, and could hypothetically cross over to receive the competing treatment once they are classified as off study. The competing treatment could prolong overall survival and confound interpretation of the overall survival benefit for the test treatment (e.g., erlotinib). Further study is required to establish the benefit of erlotinib treatment on overall survival. There is also no evidence to show that addition of erlotinib to chemotherapy is superior to either treatment alone. Hence, at this time, treatment for L.L. (single-agent erlotinib) would be expected to prolong her progression-free survival, but it is not yet known if erlotinib prolongs overall survival.

CASE 94-2, QUESTION 4: As mentioned earlier, patients with stage IV NSCLC should receive radiotherapy prior to chemotherapy, provided they can tolerate aggressive treatment. However, L.L. did not receive radiotherapy. What characteristic about this patient might preclude her from receiving radiation prior to erlotinib?

The rationale for omitting radiotherapy has more to do with the likely toxicity of the combination of radiation and chemotherapy, rather than any characteristics of L.L. She clearly has good performance status, and there is no indication of comorbidities other than moderate renal dysfunction therefore she would likely tolerate aggressive chemotherapy. Two recent clinical trials suggest that radiotherapy and small molecule EGFR inhibitor therapy may not be safe to give either sequentially or together. Both studies were conducted with the EGFR small molecule inhibitor, gefitinib, a quinazoline with similar properties to erlotinib. In the first study, gefitinib versus placebo was given after a platinum-based concurrent radiotherapy regimen. Enrollment for this phase III study was stopped early due to the results of an interim analysis showing median survival time for those getting placebo (35 months) was greater than for those getting gefitinib (23 months). The gefitinib arm was associated with an increased number of pulmonary deaths.[48] The second study was a phase I study evaluating the safety of concurrent gefitinib, docetaxel, and three-dimensional conformal radiotherapy. Dose-limiting pulmonary toxicity was observed in this second study.[49] For both studies, the EGFR inhibitor was given concurrently and/or after cytotoxic chemotherapy and radiotherapy. Therefore, the toxicity may be the result of all three (cytotoxic chemotherapy, radiotherapy, and EGFR inhibitor). Radiotherapy delivered to the lungs is associated with pulmonary fibrosis and small molecule EGFR inhibitor therapy is associated with the development of pneumonitis. Though definitive proof does not exist for this interaction, it would not be advisable to give L.L. radiotherapy prior to her erlotinib treatment.

CASE 94-2, QUESTION 5: If L.L.'s tumor was classified as having wildtype EGFR instead, what treatment should L.L. receive?

If the biopsy results had shown that the tumor EGFR was wildtype (i.e., no mutation), then L.L. would be considered for a platinum-based doublet such as one shown in Table 94-6. Because her disease is nonsquamous, the adjunct agent selected would most likely be pemetrexed. Scagliotti et al. randomly assigned patients with advanced-stage NSCLC to receive either cisplatin plus gemcitabine versus cisplatin plus pemetrexed. Although the median survival time was similar between the two arms, there were differences depending on tumor histology. Patients who received pemetrexed and had adenocarcinoma experienced a median overall survival of 12.6 months, whereas those who received gemcitabine had shorter survival. In contrast, those with squamous carcinoma who received pemetrexed experienced a 9.4-month median overall survival, whereas those who received gemcitabine had longer survival.[31] Therefore, if L.L.'s tumor had been wildtype for EGFR, she could receive cisplatin and pemetrexed as first-line treatment because her disease is adenocarcinoma. Consideration could also be given for using cisplatin and paclitaxel together with bevacizumab. As mentioned previously, the latter agent is approved for use only in patients with nonsquamous cell NSCLC.[34] Those who respond to treatment with four to six cycles of cytotoxic therapy can receive maintenance therapy afterward.

CASE 94-2, QUESTION 6: As discussed in Chapter 90, Adverse Effects of Chemotherapy and Targeted Agents, the adverse effect profiles for cisplatin and carboplatin differ from each other. If a platinum-based regimen had been selected instead of erlotinib for L.L., what characteristics about L.L. could be used to guide the selection of carboplatin versus cisplatin?

Cisplatin is predominantly associated with ototoxicity, nephrotoxicity, and neurotoxicity, whereas carboplatin is predominantly associated with myelosuppression. This would be her first cycle of chemotherapy; therefore, she is not expected to have depleted reserves of myeloid progenitor cells. Her estimated creatinine clearance is 48 mL/minute and based upon this, would be considered to have moderate renal impairment. In this case, carboplatin may be preferred over cisplatin because it is associated with less renal toxicity and it is dosed according to the Calvert formula, which accounts for renal function:

$$\text{Total Carboplatin dose (mg)} = \text{AUC (GFR} + 25) \qquad \textit{(Eq. 94-1)}$$

AUC is the area under the concentration-time curve and GFR is glomerular filtration rate.[50] A typical dose of carboplatin in this setting would be determined based on an AUC to account for renal function instead of the typical weight (or m^2)-based dosing. AUC targets are commonly 4 to 6 mg/mL · minute for most doublet regimens. If a patient with moderate renal function were to receive a fixed dose that is similar to that given to a patient with normal renal function, then systemic exposure would be higher. This higher exposure could result in greater toxicity, notably greater myelosuppression. By dosing the drug according to the patient's renal function, the risk for overdosing a patient with decreased renal function is minimized. Personnel, usually in the pharmacy, must calculate the actual dose that should be prepared. For example, if L.L.'s carboplatin dose is ordered as 5 mg/mL · min, then her dose would be calculated as dose = 5 mg/mL · minute (48 mL/min + 25), which is 365 mg. In contrast, if her renal function were within normal range for estimated creatinine clearance (e.g., 100 mL/minute), her carboplatin dose would be 625 mg (~70% higher). Several different methods may used to estimate renal function, such as the Cockroft and Gault equation, and the dose calculations will differ according to the method chosen. Usually, the choice of method is institution-specific, because there is no evidence to show that one estimation method is superior to the other. By consistently using the same formula, providers reduce variability in systemic exposure and thus increase the predictability of tolerance to the drug. If the patient's GFR is estimated based upon serum creatinine measurements by the isotope dilution mass spectrometry method, then the GFR should be capped to a maximum of 125 mL/minute, because serum creatinine values can be underestimated when they fall below 0.7 mg/mL, as can happen in some patients. The FDA issued this safety alert to avoid administration of high doses to patients with normal renal function and thus likely avoiding drug-related toxicity.[51]

In conclusion, L.L. should receive erlotinib as first-line therapy. If her tumor had contained wildtype EGFR (instead of mutant), or if her disease becomes refractory to erlotinib, then a platinum-based doublet (i.e., cisplatin or carboplatin) could be considered. She has moderate renal impairment; therefore, an agent such as cisplatin would not be favored because it is associated with a high incidence of renal toxicity. Carboplatin would be a safer choice because the dose would be selected based upon her renal function, and is associated with a lower incidence of renal toxicity than cisplatin.

CASE 94-2, QUESTION 7: L.L. experienced minor grade diarrhea and skin rash and otherwise tolerated erlotinib treatment very well without any impact on her daily activities and quality of life. L.L. continued erlotinib therapy, and at 9 months there is no evidence of disease progression. The plan is to continue this therapy until the disease relapses.

In general, therapy with erlotinib is well tolerated, especially relative to cytotoxic chemotherapy. Diarrhea and rash are the two most common adverse effects of EGFR TKI therapy.[52] The diarrhea can be treated with loperamide in most cases. Rash requires intervention in approximately one-third of cases, and it is desirable to treat it with agents such as 2% topical clindamycin, minocycline, or doxycycline, and topical 1% hydrocortisone (discussed in Chapter 90, Adverse Effects of Chemotherapy and Targeted Agents). Erlotinib dose reduction (in 50-mg decrements) could also be considered, although this would likely shorten the anticancer benefit experienced with this agent.[53]

As mentioned earlier, NSCLC is primarily a disease in those older than 60 years. L.L. is 85 years old, and there is concern that patients, particularly more than 80 years old, may not tolerate cytotoxic chemotherapy as well as younger patients. Hence, elderly patients are often undertreated. However, recent studies suggest that survival benefits are greater in elderly patients who receive doublet therapy versus single agent.[54] More studies of various regimens are needed that would focus on treatment of elderly patients, particularly effects on survival, quality of life, and tolerability. Such studies would investigate the best clinical parameters that enable prediction of response and tolerability to therapies, and also the doses associated with the best outcomes. Because the majority of patients have wildtype EGFR, cytotoxic chemotherapy is first-line. Therefore, considerations must be given to patient preferences, co-morbidities, and performance status. It is not uncommon for those with advanced age to live alone. Caretakers who could help the patient monitor for and treat adverse effects of chemotherapy (dehydration from diarrhea or vomiting, febrile neutropenia, etc.) would be an essential consideration, particularly in this population. Even though L.L. is able to continue treatment beyond 9 months, most patients eventually exhibit progressive disease within 1 to 2 years. These patients can often be re-biopsied. Approximately 40% of these cases develop secondary mutations in EGFR (T790M) that render the tumor resistant to erlotinib treatment.[55] At such time, consideration can be given for second-line treatment, and if there is concern regarding tolerability of combination cytotoxic chemotherapy, then single agent therapy would be another second option.

Small Cell Lung Cancer

EPIDEMIOLOGY

Small cell lung cancer (SCLC) accounts for approximately 15% of all lung cancer histology, and affects both sexes in equal distribution. The disease is much more highly attributable to smoking than NSCLC. As the numbers of people who smoke have decreased in the United States since its peak in the 1960s, the incidence of SCLC has also declined. Relative to NSCLC, these tumors generally have a more rapid doubling time, a higher growth fraction, and early development of widespread metastases. As a consequence, SCLC is highly sensitive to chemotherapy and radiotherapy; however, most patients eventually die from recurrent disease.[56,57]

PATHOPHYSIOLOGY

SCLC is a malignancy thought to be derived from neuroendocrine cells in the bronchus. SCLC is readily diagnosed on small specimens such as bronchoscopic biopsies, fine needle aspirates, core biopsies, and cytology. As the name suggests, these tumors consist of small cells with limited volume of cytoplasm, poorly defined cell borders, and finely granular chromatin.[58] The cells may be round, oval, or spindle-shaped, and, as previously mentioned, the mitotic count is high. Other characteristics, which may enable characterization as SCLC include immunoreactivity for cytokeratin (AE1/AE3), epithelial membrane antigen, thyroid transcription factor 1, and selected markers of neuroendocrine differentiation (CD56, chromogranin, and synaptophysin). The diagnosis is not based solely upon the presence of the latter, because approximately 10% of NSCLC also stain positively for these markers. Hence, the diagnosis of SCLC requires microscopic evaluation of tissue histology, and tests for presence of molecular markers may also aid in the diagnosis.[1]

CLINICAL PRESENTATION

SCLCs usually arise centrally (i.e., in the chest region) and present as a large hilar mass with bulky mediastinal lymphadenopathy that can cause cough and dyspnea. Very rarely do patients diagnosed with SCLC present with the primary tumor located in the lung periphery, as can be the case with NSCLC. Due to smoking, patients with lung cancer may have had previously existing symptoms such as cough and even dyspnea that are related to presence of other smoking-related diseases such as COPD. Therefore, these previously existing symptoms may not prompt patients to seek medical attention except in the further management of the underlying condition.

DIAGNOSIS AND OVERVIEW OF TREATMENT

In general, diagnostic procedures are similar to those used to diagnose NSCLC. Staging of SCLC is used to determine prognosis and treatment. The median overall survival for patients with limited stage disease ranges from 17 to 26 months and, for extensive stage, 3 to 12 months.[59] (These data were collected from an analysis of 14 studies of SCLC, thus wide ranges for survival are reported.) Surgery (e.g., thoracotomy) is appropriate for less than 5% of patients with early-stage disease, mainly due to the tendency for these tumors to be bulky and to metastasize quickly. The limited role for surgery, therefore, enables the use of a simple two-stage system instead of the TNM system used for other solid tumors. In the Veterans Administration Lung Study Group staging system, limited stage disease is defined as disease confined to the ipsilateral hemithorax and encompassed in a tolerable radiation field, and extensive disease is defined as disease beyond the ipsilateral hemithorax including malignant pleural, pericardial effusion or hematogenous metastases.[60] As discussed subsequently, patients with limited stage disease are treated with a combined modality approach (i.e., chemotherapy and radiation), and extensive stage, chemotherapy. Only approximately 30% of patients present with limited stage, and the rest with extensive stage disease.[61]

CLINICAL PRESENTATION AND PATHOPHYSIOLOGY OF SMALL CELL LUNG CANCER

CASE 94-3

QUESTION 1: M.W. is a 63-year-old woman who presented to her primary doctor with complaint of heartburn and pain in the right side of her upper abdomen; she also had a feeling of gas in the stomach. In addition, she noticed a 20-pound weight loss within three months, although she attributed this to changes in her diet. She was not complaining of any coughing. There was no shortness of breath. The evaluation with chest radiogram demonstrated the presence of a large mass in the right parahilar region with extension to the mediastinum and significant mediastinal adenopathy with narrowing of the trachea and its displacement to the left by the mass. The follow-up PET-CT scan confirmed presence of that large mass and no other areas of abnormality within the abdomen or pelvis. Patient also had a brain MRI which showed no evidence of metastatic disease. After that, the patient had a bronchoscopic evaluation and a biopsy of the mediastinal mass. Pathology came back positive for small cell lung carcinoma histology. Having disease only limited to the chest and mediastinum, the patient was diagnosed with limited stage SCLC. Peripheral blood chemistry, LDH, and counts were normal. What features of M.W.'s disease are suggestive for SCLC?

M.W.'s chief complaints were heartburn and pain in the upper right side of her abdomen, not necessarily common symptoms of SCLC. Location of the tumor is a determining factor in specific symptoms that a patient can experience, and can serve as an indicator of the invasiveness of the disease. Although M.W. did not complain of cough, her presentation is representative of patients diagnosed with this disease in that the tumor was centrally located with spread to the mediastinum. She also experienced weight loss, and although she attributed this to her diet, it is a symptom experienced by patients with rapidly growing disease, and associated with appetite suppression.

CASE 94-3, QUESTION 2: What potential complications might patients such as M.W. experience during the course of their disease?

M.W. did not experience all of the symptoms that are frequently found in patients. Fatigue, especially together with decreased physical activity, is a common complaint as well as hemoptysis.[62] Owing to the central location of most of these tumors, approximately 10% of patients can experience superior vena cava syndrome (SVCS). This is a very serious complication and requires immediate medical attention as a result of the growing tumor impinging upon the superior vena cava. This can restrict blood return to the heart, resulting in head and facial swelling.[63,64]

ONLINE CONTENT

For a visual of the superior vena cava syndrome, go to http://thepoint.lww.com/AT10e.

One-third of patients have some degree of atelectasis present.[65] A peripheral location or chest wall involvement by the tumor is uncommon. Rarely, SCLC presents as a solitary pulmonary nodule.

Patients with SCLC frequently experience paraneoplastic syndromes as a result of their disease, and these often differ from patients who have NSCLC. For example, patients with NSCLC have a higher tendency to develop hypertrophic pulmonary osteoarthropathy and hypercalcemia. On the other hand, patients with SCLC have higher incidence rates for syndrome of inappropriate antidiuretic hormone (SIADH), Cushing syndrome, and neurologic paraneoplastic syndrome. The serum concentrations of antidiuretic hormone are often elevated in SCLC, but few of these cases fulfill the criteria for SIADH and are mostly asymptomatic. In some cases, ectopic production of atrial natriuretic factor contributes to the disorder in sodium homeostasis. Because SCLC is usually responsive to cytotoxic agents, the treatment of choice for hyponatremia is chemotherapy. If further management is needed (i.e., if the cancer is nonresponsive to chemotherapy or symptomatic), fluid restriction, intravenous hypertonic saline, and treatment with demeclocycline are options, depending on severity.[1] The serum concentrations of adrenocorticotropic hormone are elevated in approximately half of patients with lung cancer, but Cushing syndrome develops in only 5% of those with SCLC. Low serum sodium and Cushing syndrome are both poor prognostic indicators for the disease.[1]

Unlike M.W., most patients already have metastatic disease at diagnosis, and the most common sites include bone, liver, adrenal glands, and brain. Bone pain may or may not occur, depending on the nature of the metastases to the afflicted area. Patients with hepatic and adrenal lesions do not usually experience symptoms, even if they have elevations of bilirubin, alkaline phosphatase, or hepatic transaminases. In contrast, brain metastases are symptomatic in more than 90% of cases, and patients can often present with central nervous system complications (e.g., seizures) as the first sign of the disease.[1]

TREATMENT MODALITIES FOR SMALL CELL LUNG CANCER

CASE 94-3, QUESTION 3: M.W. reads about various treatments for her disease online. What is the utility for each of the three treatment modalities (i.e., surgery, radiation, and chemotherapy) for the treatment of her disease?

SURGERY

As mentioned earlier, surgery has a very limited role as part of the treatment for patients with SCLC. In general, patients with tumors larger than 3 to 7 cm and presence of any disease in the lymph nodes or distant metastases do not benefit from surgery.[66] The percentage of patients who fit this category is less than 5%. If surgery is chosen, the procedure usually includes lobectomy with mediastinal nodal dissection and sampling. Thereafter, patients would receive adjuvant radiation and chemotherapy and then prophylactic cranial irradiation as described in the subsequent sections.

RADIATION

SCLC is responsive to radiation therapy; therefore, it is useful in treating patients with limited stage disease. These treatments are usually given as fractionated doses over the course of 2 to 4 weeks, and total dosage targets range between 45 and 70 Gy. Three-dimensional conformal radiation (intensity modulated radiation therapy) is the preferred method, and the radiation is delivered from an external source concurrently with multidimensional imaging to assure tumor movement of less than 1 cm is achievable (movement as a result of breathing during the procedure). See **http://www.slideshare.net/fovak/igrt-srt-for-lung-cancer** for more information.[67–69] In addition to their cytotoxic effects, many chemotherapeutic agents also sensitize tumors to radiation. Hence radiotherapy should start concurrently with chemotherapy, usually at the first or second cycle. Due to the high incidence of metastases to the brain (i.e., greater than 50% of patients with SCLC), prophylactic cranial irradiation is the standard of treatment for patients with limited stage and extensive stage diseases. The total dosage for this ranges between 25 and 30 Gy given for 10 to 15 fractions.[70,71]

CHEMOTHERAPY

The proliferative indices for SCLC cells are high, and early metastatic spread is common. Therefore, systemic chemotherapy is the treatment of choice because it is effective for tumor cells progressing through the cell cycle and its utility for treating metastases. Shown in Table 94-7[69,72–75] are the commonly used representative first-line treatment regimens for limited stage and extensive stage diseases. In general, most of the regimens are platinum-based combinations with etoposide or, less commonly, irinotecan (the latter proven to be efficacious in Japanese patients). If a tumor response is observed, the benefit is usually seen early during the treatment course. Prolongation of treatment beyond six cycles is usually not recommended for this disease because the maximum effect of the treatment is achieved in this time frame. Further, toxicity after treatment with these agents accumulates and diminishes the overall benefit to the patient beyond six courses[76,77] Hence, treatment is usually stopped after four to six cycles and the patient is closely monitored for recurrence of the disease afterward.

TABLE 94-7
Representative Chemotherapy Regimens for Small Cell Lung Cancer

Limited Stage SCLC (maximum 4–6 cycles)
Cisplatin, day 1 Etoposide, days 1, 2, 3, and then every 21 days[69]
Carboplatin, day 1 Etoposide, days 1–4, then every 21 days[72]
Extensive Stage SCLC (maximum 4–6 cycles)
Cisplatin, day 1 Etoposide days 1–4, then every 21 days[72]
Carboplatin, day 1 Etoposide, days 1, 2, 3, then every 21 days[73]
Cisplatin, day 1 Irinotecan days 1, 8, 15, then every 28 days[74]
Cisplatin, day 1 Irinotecan days 1, 8, then every 21 days[75]
Chemotherapy for Relapsed Disease[58]
Clinical trial preferred
If relapse occurs <2–3 months after first-line and PS 0–2: ifosfamide, paclitaxel, docetaxel, gemcitabine, irinotecan, or topotecan
If relapse occurs >2–3 months up to 6 months: topotecan (oral or IV), irinotecan, paclitaxel, docetaxel, oral etoposide, vinorelbine, gemcitabine, or cyclophosphamide/doxorubicin/vincristine
If relapse occurs >6 months: original regimen

PS, performance status; SCLC, small cell lung cancer.

As mentioned previously, SCLC has a very high rate of recurrence; therefore, second-line therapy is usually implemented. Several choices of agents are available as shown in Table 94-7, and the selection is dependent on the overall condition of the patient (e.g., performance status, toxicity from previous regimen) and the length of time after the first line regimen was completed. Many of these agents are given as single agent therapy except for the CAV regimen. In general, a recurrence that occurs within 6 months of treatment with first-line therapy is considered resistant and other agents are selected. If recurrence occurs after 6 months, then the same agents used for the first-line regimen may be used again. To date, no targeted agents are approved for use in treating SCLC.

In conclusion, M.W.'s disease would not be a good candidate for surgical removal because there is lack of proven benefit. Small cell lung tumor cells proliferate rapidly; therefore, they are usually responsive to chemotherapy and radiation treatment. This systemic therapy would also be favored because the tumor tends to metastasize quickly and it provides a way to eradicate disease that may have spread.

TREATMENT WITH CHEMOTHERAPY AND RADIATION

CASE 94-3, QUESTION 4: M.W. begins therapy with intravenous cisplatin on day 1 combined with etoposide on days 1 to 3 given in a 21-day cycle. Four to six cycles are planned,

and she will also receive concurrent radiation.[78,79] For M.W., what is the goal of therapy? What objective baseline data should be acquired prior to starting treatment? What monitoring parameters should be utilized?

The goal of therapy for a patient with limited stage disease such as M.W. would be to increase overall survival and achieve a potential cure. In patients with limited stage disease, response rates of 70% to 90% are expected after a regimen such as the one M.W. is receiving, whereas response rates of 60% to 70% are expected for patients with extensive stage disease.[57] If M.W. had been diagnosed with extensive stage disease, then the goals would have been to increase overall survival and for palliation. Given the complications that can arise as a result of SCLC, treatment could be used to minimize these adverse events. For example, radiotherapy is often used in treating patients with SVCS, because it would reduce tumor size and enable resumption of more normal blood flow. Therefore, if a patient has acceptable performance status (e.g., 0–2) and minimal to no comorbidites, then treatment such as the one that M.W. is receiving is the best course of action.

A treatment regimen such as cisplatin and etoposide plus radiation is tolerated by most patients, especially because the number of cycles is usually limited to six. However, administration of these cytotoxic agents is associated with several adverse effects, some of which can be life-threatening. Hence, the clinician is expected to anticipate these events, and plan treatment accordingly to minimize complications. The patient is receiving cisplatin, which causes several different adverse effects such as renal insufficiency, sensory neuropathy, ototoxicity, and is considered highly emetogenic (refer to Chapter 90, Adverse Effects of Chemotherapy and Targeted Agents). Hydration and diuresis are required with cisplatin doses greater than 40 mg/m^2 to maintain a urine output of 100 to 150 mL/hour before administration of the drug. Mannitol is frequently added to cisplatin in order to force dieuresis. The intravenous fluids are supplemented with KCl and $MgSO_4$. Monitoring of serum creatinine, electrolytes including magnesium and calcium is performed usually before each infusion of chemotherapeutics. An appropriate antiemetic regimen must be implemented to prevent both acute and delayed nausea and vomiting. For etoposide, neutropenia is usually the dose-limiting toxicity. Therefore, monitoring of absolute neutrophil count is important and if the counts do not recover in a timely manner (i.e., before the next dose) then delays in treatment or dosage reductions occur. In phase III clinical trials for this regimen, grade 4 leukopenia occurred in approximately 35% to 40% of patients, and any grade fever and infection in greater than 20%.[68,69] Therefore, consideration must be given toward the use of colony stimulating factors to manage this latter event, usually after radiation is completed (refer to Chapter 90, Adverse Effects of Chemotherapy and Targeted Agents).

In conclusion, the goal of M.W.'s therapy is a potential cure. Hydration with fluids supplemented with KCl and $MgSO_4$ must be initiated prior to cisplatin therapy to prevent cisplatin-induced renal toxicity. During therapy, clinicians must observe for decreased ANC due to etoposide, and may need to implement delays in therapy or use of a colony stimulating factor (e.g., granulocyte colony-stimulating factor). Supportive care such as antiemetics during therapy to prevent or manage cisplatin-associated acute and delayed phase nausea and vomiting will also be essential.

CASE 94-3, QUESTION 5: M.W. tolerated therapy very well, with mild esophagitis and cough during treatment. She did not experience any vomiting due to good aggressive antiemetic use, nor did she exhibit any neuropathy or hearing loss. What adverse conditions that M.W. experienced are associated with her treatment?

Both esophagitis and cough are likely attributable to radiation effects. If esophagitis worsens to grade 3 or more, patients can lose the ability to swallow and may require a feeding tube. During therapy, cough can develop and patients can become concerned that it is a sign of worsening of the disease. Radiation-induced pneumonitis, acute (in first 3 months) and chronic (4–12 months), can be a frequent cause of the new onset of cough, which can be ameliorated with corticosteroid treatment.

CASE 94-3, QUESTION 6: After two cycles of chemotherapy with concurrent radiotherapy, CT scan indicates a partial response. Therefore, an additional four cycles of cisplatin and etoposide were planned. How is the course of M.W.'s disease likely to proceed?

The chances for long-term survival greater than 5 years is very low, even for the patient with no other comorbidities and limited stage disease such as M.W. At the completion of chemotherapy, M.W. should be offered therapy with prophylactic cranial irradiation because brain metastases occur in greater than 50% of patients with SCLC. Prophylactic cranial irradiation not only reduces the incidence of metastatic disease but also increases overall survival. Within a year of completing therapy, most patients experience progressive or relapsed disease. The duration of the remission is the single largest predictor of outcome, and patients are classified as having either sensitive or refractory disease, depending on length of this duration. Approximately half of those tumors that are deemed sensitive in this setting respond to second-line therapy. Therefore, most SCLC tumors become resistant to therapy either during first-line or salvage therapy. Patients can also exhibit second primary tumors, especially NSCLC, during the course of the disease.

KEY REFERENCES AND WEBSITES

A full list of references for this chapter can be found at http://thepoint.lww.com/AT10e. Below are the key references and websites for this chapter, with the corresponding reference number in this chapter found in parentheses after the reference.

Key References

DeVita VT et al, eds. *DeVita, Hellman, and Rosenberg's Cancer: Principles and Practice of Oncology*. 8th ed. Philadelphia, PA: Lippincott Williams & Wilkins; 2008. (1)

Doll R et al. Mortality in relation to smoking: 50 years' observations on male British doctors. *BMJ*. 2004;328:1519. (12)

Jemal A et al. Cancer statistics, 2010. *CA Cancer J Clin*. 2010;60:277. (3)

Langer CJ et al. The evolving role of histology in the management of advanced non-small-cell lung cancer. *J Clin Oncol*. 2010; 28:5311. (36)

Peto R et al. Smoking, smoking cessation, and lung cancer in the UK since 1950: combination of national statistics with two case-control studies. *BMJ*. 2000;321:323. (11)

Socinski MA, Bogart JA. Limited-stage small-cell lung cancer: the current status of combined-modality therapy. *J Clin Oncol*. 2007;25:4137. (79)

Subramanian J, Govindan R. Lung cancer in never smokers: a review. *J Clin Oncol.* 2007;25:561. (13)

Key Websites

National Cancer Comprehensive Network. Small cell lung cancer. NCCN guidelines for the treatment of SCLC. http://www.nccn.org/professionals/physician_gls/f_guidelines.asp. Accessed January 4, 2011. (58)

National Cancer Comprehensive Network. Non–small cell lung cancer. NCCN guidelines for the treatment of SCLC. http://www.nccn.org/professionals/physician_gls/f_guidelines.asp. Accessed January 4, 2011. (22)

National Cancer Institute. New Surgeon General's report outlines how tobacco smoke causes disease. http://www.cancer.gov/ncicancerbulletin/121410/page2. Accessed November 4, 2010.

95

Colorectal Cancer

Sachin R. Shah and Julian Hoyt Slade, III

CORE PRINCIPLES

		CHAPTER CASES
1	Family history, patient-specific factors, and environmental factors are identified as risk factors for colorectal cancer. Environmental factors could be modified to reduce the risk of colorectal cancer.	**Case 95-1 (Question 1)**
2	Early detection of colorectal cancer through screening reduces cancer-related mortality. Most patients at low risk of colorectal cancer are recommended to begin screening at the age of 50 years.	**Case 95-1 (Question 2)**
3	Patients may be asymptomatic at diagnosis or have nonspecific symptoms. Carcinoembryonic antigen (CEA) may be elevated in patients with colorectal cancer, but it cannot be used alone for diagnosis.	**Case 95-2 (Questions 1, 2)**
4	Adjuvant combination chemotherapy with 5′-fluorouracil (5′-FU) and oxaliplatin is currently considered the standard of care for patients with stage III colorectal cancer after surgery with curative intent.	**Case 95-2 (Question 3)**
5	All patients diagnosed with localized colorectal cancer should undergo routine surveillance visits with their oncologist for a period of 5 years after completion of their definitive therapy.	**Case 95-2 (Question 6)**
6	During the last decade newer chemotherapy agents (oxaliplatin, irinotecan) and targeted therapies (bevacizumab, cetuximab, panitumumab) have doubled the overall survival of patients with metastatic colorectal cancer. Fluoropyrimidine (5′-FU or capecitabine) remains the key agent in the first-line treatment of advanced cancer. The right combination and sequencing of these agents is vital to improving the care of patients with colorectal cancer.	**Case 95-3 (Question 1)**
7	Utilization of specific predictive markers helps maximize the desired outcome in colorectal cancer. Patients with tumor expressing wild-type-*KRAS* gene receive significant survival benefit from anti–epidermal growth factor receptor (EGFR) monoclonal antibody therapy.	**Case 95-3 (Question 4)**
8	Myelosuppression, diarrhea, and peripheral neuropathy are potential dose-limiting toxicities associated with chemotherapy agents used in the treatment of colon and rectal cancers. Prevention strategies, diligent monitoring, and adequate supportive-care measures are vital to effective toxicity management and should be used to maintain patient safety and enhance quality of life.	**Case 95-2 (Questions 4, 5), Case 95-3 (Question 3)**
9	Severe, life-threatening adverse effects are uncommon, but potential hazards are associated with targeted colorectal cancer therapies and avoiding their use is warranted in patients at increased risk of experiencing these complications. Prevention and treatment strategies are available for common adverse effects such as hypertension associated with bevacizumab use or EGFR inhibitor–induced dermatologic toxicity.	**Case 95-3 (Questions 3, 5, 6)**
10	Certain genetic variants of key enzymes involved in the catabolism of 5′-FU and irinotecan are associated with increased toxicity from these agents. The clinical utility of identifying these variants in an effort to avoid or manage these toxicities continues to be elucidated.	**Case 95-3 (Question 2)**

COLORECTAL CANCER

Epidemiology, Etiology, and Pathophysiology

Colorectal cancer is the malignant growth of tumor that begins from the inner wall of the colon or rectum. According to the American Cancer Society, colorectal cancer is the third most common cancer in the United States for both men and women.[1] In 2010, approximately 142,570 individuals are expected be diagnosed with colorectal cancer, and it is the second leading cause of cancer-related deaths after lung cancer.[1] The overall incidence of colorectal cancer has been in decline for the past two decades primarily as a result of early detection through screening and removal of colorectal polyps, which are often considered precursors to the disease. There has been significant improvement in the survival of patients with colorectal cancer as well. Patients diagnosed with colon cancer in 1975 had a 5-year relative survival rate of 52% and in 2005, 66%.[1] During the last decade, new agents and better predictive markers have enabled improvement in the detection, safety, and survival of patients with colorectal cancer.

The formation of colorectal cancer is a multistep process. It begins with an abnormal growth of tissue known as a polyp originating from the innermost wall of the colon. The process of transformation from a benign polyp to malignant disease can take several years. Once this transformation occurs, the cancer begins to spread through the wall of the colon or rectum, where it can eventually invade the blood, lymph nodes, or other organs directly. The vast majority of colon and rectal cancers are classified as adenocarcinomas, meaning that they arise from the glandular tissue responsible for producing the secretions of the gastrointestinal tract. Approximately two-thirds of these cancers will arise from the colon, and the remainder will form in the rectum. Colorectal cancer is among the few cancers that can be prevented by removal of precancerous tissue; therefore, early detection is crucial.

The etiology of colorectal cancer is complex, involving patient-specific, environmental, and genetic factors. Of these, age is considered the most important risk because greater than 90% of patients diagnosed are older than 50 years of age.[1] Other patient-specific risk factors are male sex, history of previous colonic polyps, and inflammatory bowel disease (ulcerative colitis or Crohn's disease). Environmental factors like a diet consisting primarily of red meat, high fat, and low fiber can also increase the risk of colorectal cancer, as can a sedentary lifestyle, obesity, excessive alcohol consumption, and long-term smoking.[2,3] Smoking, particularly early in life, has been shown to increase the risk of developing colorectal cancer. In addition, patients who smoked more than 12 pack-years of cigarettes before the age of 30 are at increased risk of recurrence after a diagnosis of stage III colon cancer.[4] Therefore, smoking is also associated with overall worse long-term outcomes for those already diagnosed with the disease. Inherited genetic mutations can increase the risk of colorectal cancer. Specific inherited syndromes include hereditary nonpolyposis colon cancer (HNPCC), also known as Lynch syndrome, and familial adenomatous polyposis (FAP).[5] HNPCC accounts for 5% to 10% of colorectal cancers. It is an autosomal dominant disorder that has an early age of onset. Unlike FAP, there are no distinctive clinical features present in the asymptomatic patients, who are carriers of the HNPCC gene. Therefore, patients with HNPCC are diagnosed later in life compared with FAP. Patients with FAP are diagnosed by their late teens or early 20s. FAP is an autosomal dominant disorder accounting for 0.5% of all colorectal cancer cases.[6] Mutation of the adenomatous polyposis coli (*APC*) gene is responsible for FAP. Screening for these patients is recommended at an early age (i.e., 12 years old), and total colectomy is recommended when colon polyps are detected.

Regular consumption of milk or calcium may decrease the risk of colorectal cancer.[1] In addition, use of aspirin or nonsteroidal anti-inflammatory drugs (NSAIDs) may reduce the risk of colorectal cancer for some patients.[7,8] Celecoxib, a cyclooxygenase-2 inhibitor, is US Food and Drug Administration (FDA) approved for the treatment of patients with known FAP.[9] However, the routine use of NSAIDs for the prevention of colorectal cancer is not recommended because of concerns of toxicity.

Clinical Presentation and Diagnosis

Symptoms associated with the development of colon and rectal cancers are often subtle and can mimic "generalized" symptoms associated with numerous other benign conditions. Although they can certainly accompany a diagnosis of colorectal cancer, abdominal pain, constipation, diarrhea, bloating, and other sudden changes in bowel habits are often nonspecific making it difficult to attribute to an underlying malignant process. Furthermore, patients whose cancers are detected during a screening procedure may report being completely asymptomatic. Although symptoms can be nonspecific, they may include a change in bowel habits such as prolonged constipation or diarrhea, "pencil-thin" stools, rectal bleeding, abdominal pain or bloating, or tenesmus. Unintentional weight loss, anemia, and weakness may also be present, particularly in advanced stages of the disease. A diagnosis is made once a colonoscopy or sigmoidoscopy is performed and a biopsy is obtained to confirm the presence of cancer. Additional diagnostic procedures would be performed before initiating treatment including a computed tomography (CT) scan of the chest, abdomen, and pelvis as well as laboratory collection of blood to obtain a baseline carcinoembryonic antigen (CEA) level. These will be useful in determining the extent of disease and providing a means to monitor for its recurrence or progression after treatment. For cancers of the rectum, an endoscopic ultrasound may be performed to aid in the preoperative or clinical staging of the tumor. Definitive or pathological staging for all tumors of the colon and rectum takes place during surgical resection.

Treatment Overview

The therapeutic modalities available to the patient with colorectal cancer are similar to those used in other solid tumors. Surgery, radiation, and chemotherapy have roles in both localized and advanced disease, but just how each of these strategies is used depends on the location and extent of disease as well as the goal of therapy. In general, surgery is preferred for patients with stages I, II, and III disease, and selected patients with metastatic stage IV disease. Radiation is usually reserved for patients with rectal cancer. This chapter will primarily focus on the use of systemic therapy (i.e., chemotherapy and targeted therapy) for patients diagnosed with colon or rectal cancer. Colorectal cancer is unique in that the depth of invasion of the primary tumor and not its size is a primary factor for determining its stage. This depth of penetration into the wall of the colon represents the "T" of the TNM system that is used in the staging and classification of solid tumors. Like other solid tumors, the remaining components of this classification system are lymph node involvement and metastatic spread (Fig. 95-1).[10] Staging of the tumor affects the strategy clinicians use when formulating a therapeutic plan with the patient. Colon and rectal cancers are staged in the exact same manner; however, rectal tumors lie in closer

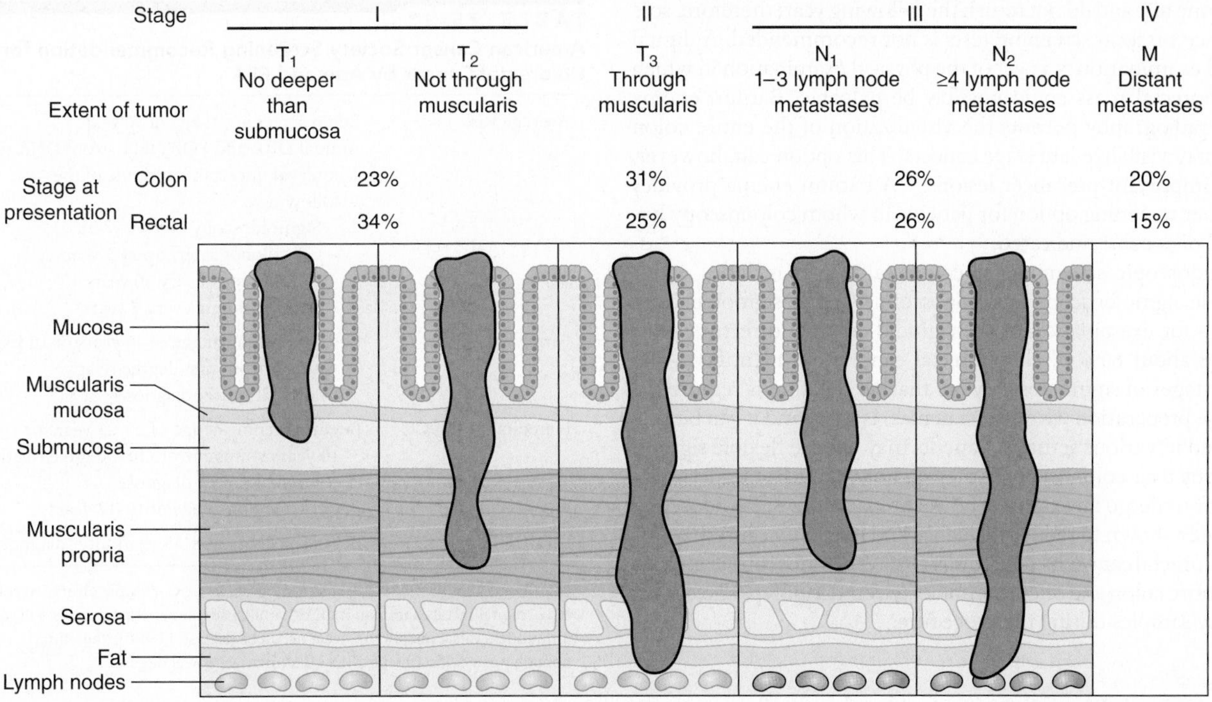

FIGURE 95-1 Colorectal cancer staging with % initial presentation for each stage. Going from left to right, colorectal tumors usually develop in the lumen of the gastrointestinal tract, and invade through the tissue (e.g., muscularis), eventually reaching lymphatic tissue. Once tumor has reached this later stage, the likelihood for metastases increases. (Adapted with permission from Fauci AS et al, eds. *Harrison's Principles of Internal Medicine.* 17th ed. New York, NY: McGraw-Hill; 2008. STAT!Ref Online Electronic Medical Library. http://online.statref.com/document.aspx?fxid=55&docid=913. Accessed October 25, 2010.)

proximity to the anal sphincter, therefore the risk of localized treatment failure and of recurrence at the initial site of disease is increased. An area of controversy in the management of colon cancer is whether or not all patients with stage II disease should receive adjuvant therapy. Although the routine use of adjuvant chemotherapy in this setting is not recommended, it should be considered for stage II patients with the following high-risk features: T4 lesions, bowel obstruction or local perforation at presentation, poorly differentiated histology, lymphovascular invasion, inadequate lymph node sampling, and positive margins after surgery.[11]

ETIOLOGY

CASE 95-1

QUESTION 1: O.B., a 35-year-old woman, recently learned that her 68-year-old father was diagnosed with colon cancer. O.B. is obese and smokes a half-pack of cigarettes per day. She loves eating out and spends most of her evening watching TV at home. O.B. would like to know the risk factors for colorectal cancer. She also would like to know whether there is anything she can do to reduce her risk of developing colorectal cancer in the future.

O.B. is at an increased risk of developing colorectal cancer given her family history of colon cancer. In addition, she is obese, lives a sedentary lifestyle, and smokes. She eats out, but no information is given about her diet. There are modifiable risk factors, which she could address to lower her risk of developing colorectal cancer. O.B. can lose weight through exercise and adopt a high-fiber, low-fat diet. Daily intake of milk, vegetables, and fruits can provide an adequate supply of calcium and antioxidants. In addition, she can stop smoking, which can help reduce the risk of colorectal as well as other cancers.

SCREENING

CASE 95-1, QUESTION 2: O.B. would like to know whether there is a way to screen for colorectal cancer. If there is, does this method detect cancer early? Her father had a colon cancer diagnosis; therefore, O.B. wonders when she should get screened for colorectal cancer.

Colon and rectal cancers are among the few cancers that can be prevented by removal of precancerous tissue; therefore, early detection is crucial. As described above, formation of colorectal cancers is a multistep process, and the early precancerous tissue is identifiable and can be removed. Colorectal cancer is not always asymptomatic, but early detection of colorectal cancer through screening has been proven to reduce mortality. A variety of screening methods exist, including fecal screening tests, digital rectal examination, barium enemas, endoscopy, and CT colonography. Fecal screening tests are designed to detect occult blood in the stool, and they are inexpensive and noninvasive and can be performed at home. Fecal screening tests have been shown to reduce colorectal cancer–related mortality by 33%.[12] There are two main types of tests, the fecal occult blood test (FOBT) and fecal immunochemical test (FIT). One-time testing with FOBT (standard or sensitive test) has a 33% to 75% sensitivity for detecting cancer.[13] The FIT uses antibodies to detect human hemoglobin or other blood components. Compared with FOBT, the FIT has no drug or food interactions and a 60% to 85% sensitivity for detecting colorectal cancer.[13] Specificity of FIT tends to be higher (97%) than that of FOBT. Even though FIT has the advantage of fewer requirements of testing and no dietary interactions compared with FOBT, both out-of-pocket and total cost is a concern. The wide range of sensitivity is a major limitation for both. Therefore, adherence to regular screening is important to improve sensitivity of the test. Many patients have only one test and do not return the following year; therefore, sole reliance on fecal screening tests is not recommended. A digital rectal examination is a part of the physical examination in which an anorectal mass could possibly be palpable. Barium enema with radiography permits the visualization of the entire colon and may visualize late-stage cancers. This option can, however, miss important precancer lesions.[14] A barium enema provides another screening option for patients in whom colonoscopy has failed or is contraindicated.

Endoscopic screening for colorectal cancer includes either flexible sigmoidoscopy or colonoscopy. Flexible sigmoidoscopy allows for examination of the sigmoid colon and rectum only, where about 60% of all colorectal cancers are identified. The advantages of sigmoidoscopy are that no sedation is required, a simple preparation (two Fleet enemas) is used, and it can be performed in various settings. Patients may choose flexible sigmoidoscopy over colonoscopy if they do not want to go under sedation or undergo an extensive bowel preparation. Sigmoidoscopy has been shown to reduce incidence and mortality caused by distal colorectal cancer by 60% to 80%.[15,16] A colonoscopy examines the entire colon and offers the ability to remove polyps and obtain biopsy samples during the procedure.

ONLINE CONTENT

For a photo of a pedunculated polyp, go to http://thepoint.lww.com/AT10e.

Because cancerous lesions detected by any of the other tests will ultimately necessitate an examination by colonoscopy, it is considered the gold standard. A relatively new method known as CT colonography provides two- and three-dimensional images of the colon. As with endoscopic procedures, it requires complete bowel preparation to remove feces from the intestine.

ONLINE CONTENT

For a patient handout for colonscopy preparation, go to http://thepoint.lww.com/AT10e.

This screening test has the ability to detect 90% of polyps that are 10 mm or larger in diameter.[17] If suspicious lesions are visible, biopsies would be obtained in a separate procedure (e.g., colonoscopy), and this represents a limitation to CT colonography. CEA is a tumor marker that has been evaluated as a screening tool, but its primary utility is in monitoring response to treatment, and not screening.

The American Cancer Society, the US Multi-Society Task Force on Colorectal Cancer, and the American College of Radiology have jointly published screening recommendations for the early detection of colorectal cancer.[13] According to their recommendations any man or woman at average risk of developing colorectal cancer should begin screening at age of 50 years (Table 95-1). Patients at average risk of developing colorectal cancer will not have genetic predisposition or history of a family member with colorectal cancer. In addition, patients in this category will have no history of polyps, previous history of colorectal cancer, inflammatory bowel disease, chronic ulcerative colitis, or Crohn's colitis.

O.B. is a 35-year-old woman with a first-degree relative with a diagnosis of colon cancer at the age of 68. It is less likely she would develop colorectal cancer through a hereditary syndrome because her father was diagnosed after the age of 50. She does, however, have nearly double the life time risk of developing colorectal cancer because a first-degree relative had colorectal cancer.[18] Because O.B.'s father had colorectal cancer diagnosed at or above the age of 60, she is at increased risk for developing the disease and should consider initiating a colorectal screening program at the age of 40.[13]

TABLE 95-1

American Cancer Society Screening Recommendation for Colorectal Cancer by Age and Risk

Average Risk	Begin screening at age of 50 years Annual DRE **and** FOBT/FIT (stool DNA test, interval uncertain) **and** one of the following: – Sigmoidoscopy every 5 years – CT colonography every 5 years – Colonoscopy every 10 years – Barium enema every 5 years
Family History	Begin screening at age of 40 years or 10 years younger from first-degree relative colorectal cancer diagnosis
Hereditary HNPCC	Begin screening at age of 20–25 years **or** 10 years younger from first-degree relative colorectal cancer diagnosis
FAP	Begin screening at age of 10–12 years
IBD, CUC, or CC	Begin screening at 8–15 years after diagnosis

CC, Crohn's colitis; CT, computed tomography; CUC, chronic ulcerative colitis; DRE, digital rectal examination; FAP, familial adenomatous polyposis; FIT, fecal immunochemical test; FOBT, fecal occult blood test; HNPCC, hereditary nonpolyposis colon cancer; IBD, inflammatory bowel disease.

Clinical Presentation

CASE 95-2

QUESTION 1: B.R. is a 66-year-old white man who was in his usual state of health until recently, when he decided to visit his general practitioner owing to progressively worsening gastrointestinal symptoms including abdominal cramping and changing bowel habits. He admits to also having some blood in his stool at times, which he attributes to his hemorrhoids. His family history is notable for a paternal uncle with gastric cancer. He occasionally drinks alcohol and has never smoked nor used illicit or recreational drugs. On physical examination he is a well-nourished, well-developed man who is afebrile, alert and oriented, and in no apparent distress. He has no palpable masses and no hepatomegaly, and his abdomen is soft and nontender with normal active bowel sounds. The rest of his review of systems is unremarkable. His performance status is excellent. He does have a history of type II diabetes mellitus and hypercholesterolemia, which are both controlled on his current medication regimen. Vital signs and laboratory values obtained are as follows:

Blood pressure, 108/71 mm Hg
Heart rate, 95 beats/minute
Respiratory rate, 18 breaths/minute
White blood cell (WBC) count, 4.8×10^3 cells/μL
Hemoglobin, 11.6 g/dL
Hematocrit, 35.1%
Platelet count, 208×10^3 cells/μL
Total bilirubin, 0.3 mg/dL
Serum creatinine, 0.8 mg/dL
Blood urea nitrogen, 15 mg/dL
Alkaline phosphatase, 61 international units/L
Lactate dehydrogenase, 366 international units/L
Albumin, 4.2 g/dL
Hemoglobin A1C, 6.2%

Are any of the symptoms that B.R. is exhibiting associated with colorectal cancer?

Although the symptoms B.R. is describing are nonspecific in nature, the changes in bowel habits in addition to the blood in his stools are symptoms associated with the development of colorectal cancer. Given his age, symptoms, and lack of prior cancer screening, additional workup is warranted with one of the screening modalities mentioned earlier in this chapter, preferably colonoscopy.

CASE 95-2, QUESTION 2: If B.R. did have colon or rectal cancer, could it be diagnosed with CEA alone?

CEA was first described in 1965. It was detected in fetal colon and colon adenocarcinoma; therefore CEA was named carcinoembryonic antigen.[19] It is a tumor marker that is detected in the blood. It has been suggested that CEA may act as an adhesion molecule that facilitates malignant colon cancer cell interaction with healthy tissue and promotes tumor dissemination.[19] It has a high specificity (87%) for detecting occult colorectal cancer, but very low sensitivity (36%). Therefore, it is not a good diagnostic tool for B.R. It has been suggested that CEA values increase as the disease stage increases. Therefore, stage IV colorectal cancer patients are more likely to present with higher concentrations of CEA compared with stage II patients. In addition, a higher proportion of patients with advanced stages presents with elevated CEA compared with earlier stages. One study used a CEA threshold of 5 mg/mL, and it showed that 3%, 25%, 45%, and 65% of patients had Dukes stage A, B, C, and D colorectal cancer at this threshold, respectively.[20] Also, a CEA level greater than 5 mg/mL before surgery is a poor prognostic indicator.[21] Therefore, CEA levels are routinely recommended during diagnostic and presurgery workup. The CEA is primarily used to monitor for the recurrence of disease after treatment. About 80% of recurrences are identified by CEA monitoring.[22] Healthy smokers are likely to have twice the CEA level compared with nonsmokers. Administration of 5′-fluorouracil (5′-FU)–containing therapy can cause false elevation of CEA without disease progression.

Chemotherapy for Localized Colorectal Cancer

ADJUVANT THERAPY

CASE 95-2, QUESTION 3: After a colonoscopy, B.R. is found to have a moderately differentiated adenocarcinoma of the colon lying 18 cm from the anal verge invading through the muscularis propria with lymphovascular invasion and involvement of 8 of 25 regional lymph nodes. A CT scan of his chest, abdomen, and pelvis shows no evidence of metastatic disease. A baseline CEA level of 8.0 ng/mL (normal range, 0–3.0 ng/mL for nonsmokers and 0–6.0 ng/mL for smokers) is reported. After surgical resection, would B.R. benefit from adjuvant chemotherapy? Which chemotherapy agents or regimen gives B.R. the best chance to avoid a future recurrence?

B.R. has extensive lymph node involvement, and this means he has stage IIIC disease (Table 95-2), which places him at a high risk of recurrence; therefore, he should receive adjuvant chemotherapy after surgery. The goal of adjuvant therapy is to eradicate any residual, undetectable disease left behind after surgery and to reduce his risk of recurrence.

Historically, 5′-FU combined with leucovorin was considered the standard chemotherapy for adjuvant treatment of stage III colon cancer. Leucovorin stabilizes the binding of an active metabolite of 5′-FU known as fluorodeoxyuridine monophosphate to its intracellular target thymidylate synthase, ultimately enhancing the cytotoxicity of 5′-FU. Single-agent capecitabine, an oral prodrug of 5′-FU, offers convenient administration and is as effective as intravenous (IV) bolus 5′-FU modulated with leucovorin.[23] Because the enzyme involved in the final conversion of capecitabine to 5′-FU is expressed more prominently in cancerous cells compared with healthy cells, further biomodulation of capecitabine to enhance activity with leucovorin is not required. At present, single-agent therapy is typically considered for patients with a poor performance status or those who are unable to tolerate or possess a contraindication to combination therapy. Combinations of irinotecan with 5′-FU have been studied but are not currently recommended for use in the adjuvant setting owing to the lack of survival benefit and an increase in treatment-related morbidity.[24–26]

A combination of 5′-FU and oxaliplatin is considered the current standard of care in the adjuvant setting for patients with stage III disease, as several landmark trials have shown this strategy can improve diseasefree survival and reduce the relative risk of disease recurrence by 20% to 23%.[27,28] There are several 5′-FU and oxaliplatin regimens used in clinical practice. The choice is based on differences in toxicity and convenience because these regimens use different administration strategies for 5′-FU. For example, some regimens with 5′-FU administer the drug for a short 10- to 30-minute bolus infusion, whereas others specify a much longer continuous infusion, spanning several days. 5′-FU has a very short half-life and must be metabolically activated; therefore, infusing the drug for a prolonged period results in greater formation of the active metabolite and, theoretically, greater antitumor effect. The shorter infusion, however, is more convenient for the patient and caregiver.

The toxicity profiles vary according to the length of infusion. Efforts to reduce adverse effects observed with continuous infusions have resulted in the evolution of multiple dosing strategies collectively referred to as FOLFOX regimens.

ONLINE CONTENT

For an audio file explaining the FOLFOX acronym and evolution of the FOLFOX regimen, go to http://thepoint.lww.com/AT10e.

Each is considered equally effective, differing only in toxicity patterns. Adjuvant capecitabine combined with oxaliplatin (Xeloda) (XELOX) has recently been evaluated in patients with stage III disease, and has also proven to be safe and effective in this setting.[29] A list of commonly used adjuvant regimens is presented in Table 95-3. Combination therapy in the form of FLOX, XELOX, or FOLFOX should be considered for B.R., noting that a FOLFOX regimen is often clinically recommended based on a superior tolerability profile.

The initial cycle of B.R.'s adjuvant chemotherapy should begin approximately 4 to 6 weeks after his surgery and continue for a total of 6 months.

ADVERSE EFFECTS OF 5-FU AND OXALIPLATIN

CASE 95-2, QUESTION 4: B.R. is scheduled to receive a modified FOLFOX6 (mFOLFOX6) regimen in the adjuvant setting. What potential adverse effects should B.R. be made aware of before receiving this regimen? Are any dose-limiting side effects associated with this therapy? Are there

TABLE 95-2
Colorectal Cancer Staging

T, N, M Definitions

Primary Tumor (T)

TX Primary tumor cannot be assessed
T0 No evidence of primary tumor
Tis Carcinoma in situ: intraepithelial or invasion of lamina propria[a]
T1 Tumor invades submucosa
T2 Tumor invades muscularis propria
T3 Tumor invades through the muscularis propria into pericolorectal tissues
T4a Tumor penetrates to the surface of the visceral peritoneum[b]
T4b Tumor directly invades or is adherent to other organs or structures[b,c]

Regional Lymph Nodes (N)[d]

NX Regional lymph nodes cannot be assessed
N0 No regional lymph node metastasis
N1 Metastasis in 1–3 regional lymph nodes
N1a Metastasis in one regional lymph node
N1b Metastasis in 2–3 regional lymph nodes
N1c Tumor deposit(s) in the subserosa, mesentery, or nonperitonealized pericolic or perirectal tissues without regional nodal metastasis
N2 Metastasis in 4 or more regional lymph nodes
N2a Metastasis in 4–6 regional lymph nodes
N2b Metastasis in 7 or more regional lymph nodes

Distant Metastasis (M)

M0 No distant metastasis
M1 Distant metastasis
M1a Metastasis confined to one organ or site (for example, liver, lung, ovary, nonregional node)
M1b Metastases in more than one organ or site or the peritoneum

Anatomic Stage/Prognostic Groups

Stage	T	N	M	Dukes[e]	MAC[e]
0	Tis	N0	M0	—	—
I	T1	N0	M0	A	A
	T2	N0	M0	A	B1
IIA	T3	N0	M0	B	B2
IIB	T4a	N0	M0	B	B2
IIC	T4b	N0	M0	B	B3
IIIA	T1–T2	N1/N1c	M0	C	C1
	T1	N2a	M0	C	C1
IIIB	T3–T4a	N1/N1c	M0	C	C2
	T2–T3	N2a	M0	C	C1/C2
	T1–T2	N2b	M0	C	C1
IIIC	T4a	N2a	M0	C	C2
	T3–T4a	N2b	M0	C	C2
	T4b	N1–N2	M0	C	C3
IVA	Any T	Any N	M1a	—	—
IVB	Any T	Any N	M1b	—	—

NOTE: cTNM is the clinical classification, pTNM is the pathologic classification. The y prefix is used for those cancers that are classified after neoadjuvant pretreatment (for example, ypTNM). Patients who have a complete pathologic response are ypT0N0cM0, which may be similar to Stage Group 0 or I. The r prefix is to be used for those cancers that have recurred after a diseasefree interval (rTNM).

[a] Tis includes cancer cells confined within the glandular basement membrane (intraepithelial) or mucosal lamina propria (intramucosal) with no extension through the muscularis mucosae into the submucosa.

[b] Direct invasion in T4 includes invasion of other organs or other segments of the colorectum as a result of direct extension through the serosa, as confirmed on microscopic examination (for example, invasion of the sigmoid colon by a carcinoma of the cecum) or, for cancers in a retroperitoneal or subperitoneal location, direct invasion of other organs or structures by virtue of extension beyond the muscularis propria (that is, a tumor on the posterior wall of the descending colon invading the left kidney or lateral abdominal wall; or a mid or distal rectal cancer with invasion of prostate, seminal vesicles, cervix, or vagina).

[c] Tumor that is adherent to other organs or structures, grossly, is classified cT4b. However, if no tumor is present in the adhesion, microscopically, the classification should be pT1-4a depending on the anatomical depth of wall invasion. The V and L classifications should be used to identify the presence or absence of vascular or lymphatic invasion, whereas the PN site-specific factor should be used for perineural invasion.

[d] A satellite peritumoral nodule in the pericolorectal adipose tissue of a primary carcinoma without histologic evidence of residual lymph node in the nodule may represent discontinuous spread, venous invasion with extravascular spread (V1/2), or a totally replaced lymph node (N1/2). Replaced nodes should be counted separately as positive nodes in the N category, whereas discontinuous spread or venous invasion should be classified and counted in the Site-Specific Factor category Tumor Deposits (TD).

[e] Dukes B is a composite of better (T3 N0 M0) and worse (T4 N0 M0) prognostic groups, as is Dukes C (any T N1 M0 and any T N2 M0). MAC is the modified Astler-Coller classification.

Used with the permission of the American Joint Committee on Cancer (AJCC). Chicago, IL. The original source for this material is the *AJCC Cancer Staging Manual*, Seventh Edition (2010) published by Springer-Verlag, New York, www.springer.com

TABLE 95-3

Select Regimens Used in the Treatment of Localized Colon and Rectal Cancers[a]

Regimen Name	Dosing of Chemotherapy Agents	Cycle Description
Colon and Rectal Adjuvant Regimens		
Roswell Park	Leucovorin 500 mg/m² IV for 2 hours; One hour after starting the leucovorin administer: 5′-Fluorouracil 500 mg/m² IV bolus Administered on days 1, 8, 15, 22, 29, and 36, followed by 2 weeks off	Cycle length = 56 days Repeat × 3 cycles
Mayo Clinic	Leucovorin 20 mg/m² IV bolus daily on days 1–5; 5′-Fluorouracil 425 mg/m² IV bolus daily on days 1–5	Cycle length = 28 days Repeat × 6 cycles
Simplified Infusional Biweekly 5′-FU/LV[b]	Leucovorin 400 mg/m²/d IV for 2 hours on day 1 5′-Fluorouracil 400 mg/m² IV bolus on day 1, then 5′-Fluorouracil 1,200 mg/m²/d IVCI × 2 days (total 2,400 mg/m² IVCI for 46–48 hours)	Cycle length = 14 days Repeat × 12 cycles
Capecitabine	Capecitabine 1,000–1,250 mg/m²/d PO BID days 1–14	Cycle length = 21 days Repeat × 8 cycles
FLOX	Leucovorin 500 mg/m² IV for 2 hours; One hour after starting the leucovorin administer: 5′-Fluorouracil 500 mg/m² IV bolus Administered on days 1, 8, 15, 22, 29, and 36 Oxaliplatin 85 mg/m² IV for 2 hours Administered on days 1, 15, and 29	Cycle length = 56 days Repeat × 3 cycles
$FOLFOX_4$	Oxaliplatin 85 mg/m² IV for 2 hours day 1 Leucovorin 200 mg/m²/d IV for 2 hours on days 1 and 2 5′-Fluorouracil 400 mg/m²/d IV bolus on days 1 and 2 5′-Fluorouracil 600 mg/m²/d IVCI for 22 hours on days 1 and 2	Cycle length = 14 days Repeat × 12 cycles
$mFOLFOX_6$	Oxaliplatin 85 mg/m² IV for 2 hours day 1 Leucovorin 350–400 mg/m²/d IV for 2 hours on day 1 5′-Fluorouracil 400 mg/m² IV bolus on day 1, then 5′-Fluorouracil 1,200 mg/m²/d IVCI × 2 days (total 2,400 mg/m² IVCI for 46–48 hours)	Cycle length = 14 days Repeat × 12 cycles
XELOX[c]	Capecitabine 1,000 mg/m² PO BID days 1–14 Oxaliplatin 130 mg/m² IV every 21 days	Cycle length = 21 days Repeat × 8 cycles
Rectal Regimens Combined With Radiation		
Infusional 5′-FU	5′-Fluorouracil 225–300 mg/m² IVCI	Daily throughout radiation or Monday–Friday throughout radiation
Capecitabine	Capecitabine 825 mg/m² PO BID	Daily throughout radiation or Monday–Friday throughout radiation

[a] Disclaimer: Please consult specific regimen protocol for exact dosing recommendation.
[b] Recommended as an option in NCCN guidelines.
[c] Not in current NCCN recommendations, but data are available supporting its use in stage III disease.
BID, twice daily; 5′-FU, 5′-fluorouracil; IV, intravenous; IVCI, intravenous continuous infusion; LV, leucovorin; NCCN, National Comprehensive Cancer Network; PO, orally.

any preventive measures that can be taken to limit the severity of these adverse effects?

The goal of therapy in this setting is a cure; therefore, clinicians typically try to remain aggressive and limit chemotherapy dose reductions or delays while trying to maintain an acceptable toxicity profile. Although generally considered mild, there are a number of chemotherapy-related toxicities that may occur during adjuvant therapy or after its completion. Because B.R. will receive a combination of 5′-FU and oxaliplatin in the adjuvant setting, the toxicities of these agents should be discussed before initiation of therapy.

The toxicity of 5′-FU will vary depending on its dose, route, and schedule of administration. At doses used in the treatment of colorectal cancer, bolus administration is associated with more severe neutropenia and mucositis whereas continuous infusion administration is associated with more severe palmar-plantar erythrodysesthesia or hand-foot syndrome (HFS)

ONLINE CONTENT

For a narrated PowerPoint presentation with photos of HFS and information about its incidence, prevention, and treatment, go to http://thepoint.lww.com/AT10e.

HFS is managed primarily with supportive-care measures such as the application of topical moisturizers in addition to temporary withdrawal of fluorouracil-based therapy to allow time to heal. Once the wound has healed or decreased in its severity, fluorouracil-based therapy is often resumed at a reduced dose. Severe neutropenia is typically managed with chemotherapy dose reductions or delays, and in some cases clinicians may use daily administration of granulocyte colony-stimulating factors such as filgrastim or sargramostim until recovery of a patient's absolute neutrophil count. Severe mucositis is uncommon, but mild symptoms can be managed with supportive-care measures such as mild narcotic pain medications or mouthwashes that contain a local anesthetic such as lidocaine. Strategies for preventing this complication are also important and include stressing the importance of good oral hygiene and avoidance of harsh substances, which may irritate the oral mucosa or inhibit saliva production, such as alcohol, alcohol-based mouthwashes or rinses, spicy foods, and anticholinergic medications. As is the case with many fluorinated pharmaceutical agents, 5′-FU causes photosensitivity, which may result in mild to severe sunburns after sun exposure. Therefore, during his adjuvant therapy, B.R. should avoid prolonged exposure to direct sunlight and use a sun block of SPF-15 or higher during outdoor activities.

If oral capecitabine were chosen to substitute for the IV formulation of 5′-FU, the differences with regard to toxicity should be explained. Capecitabine undergoes enzymatic conversion to 5′-FU in the tumor and is usually given daily for 14 days; therefore, it has a similar toxicity profile to continuous infusion 5′-FU. However, it is usually associated with a greater incidence and severity of HFS and diarrhea compared with continuous infusions. Often the decision of which fluorouracil-based therapy to choose is multifactorial owing to the nuances of clinical practice. Potential factors that play a role in the agent chosen can include, but are not limited to, toxicity differences, institutional resources (pump availability, etc.), insurance coverage, and patient preference. Additional factors that could influence the selection of a capecitabine-based regimen include the presence of renal impairment and relevant drug–drug interactions, particularly concomitant warfarin use.

Oxaliplatin is the newest member of the platinum family of antineoplastics, and it offers a different antitumor profile and resistance pattern than cisplatin or carboplatin. Of the three agents, oxaliplatin is highly active against colorectal tumors. Myelosuppression, primarily neutropenia and thrombocytopenia, and neurotoxicity are dose-limiting toxicities associated with its use.[30] Oxaliplatin causes an acute, reversible neuropathy consisting of either paresthesias or dysesthesias and in some instances muscle spasms. One particular phenomenon that is distressing for patients is an involuntary laryngopharyngeal dysesthesia that can create the sensation of an inability to swallow or breathe. The acute phenomenon is reported to occur in greater than 90% of patients receiving oxaliplatin.[28,31] Although our understanding of the event is limited, it is known to be triggered by direct contact with anything cold. This sensitivity to cold as well as the aforementioned reactions generally occur within minutes of receiving the infusion and can persist up to 7 days. Avoidance of cold objects, including the eating or drinking of cold foods and beverages, should be emphasized to B.R. after each dose of oxaliplatin. The use of gloves, socks, and scarves can also be recommended, especially in cold weather. B.R. should be reassured that the intensity of this reaction diminishes daily after treatment and usually resolves within a week. Delayed neurotoxicity may also occur and is potentially irreversible. This chronic neuropathy is a cumulative, dose-dependent effect. It initially develops in the distal extremities and slowly progresses in a glove and stocking distribution pattern. It is typically characterized by a persistent sensation of numbness, tingling, or burning in the extremities.

Hypersensitivity reactions have also been observed with oxaliplatin use, but the appearance of the reaction is arbitrary in that it can manifest with any dose, and although it usually occurs during the infusion, delayed reactions are possible. The severity of these allergic reactions can range from mild itching or flushing to anaphylaxis. After a reaction, mild cases are often managed through premedication with antihistamines or corticosteroids (e.g., diphenhydramine 50 mg IV or orally with or without hydrocortisone 50 mg 15 minutes before oxaliplatin IV) in addition to prolonging the infusion of oxaliplatin. More-severe reactions generally warrant discontinuation of the drug; however, there are reports in which desensitization protocols have been used successfully, allowing for continued administration.[32,33] Regardless of what is chosen, this strategy accompanies all subsequent doses of oxaliplatin.

The primary role of chemotherapy in this setting is to reduce the risk of relapse and prolong diseasefree survival by eradicating residual, undetectable disease. A total of 6 months of adjuvant therapy is considered the current standard of care after surgery with curative intent (12 cycles of an every 2-week regimen like FOLFOX, or 8 cycles of an every 3-week strategy like single-agent capecitabine) owing in large part to data from select adjuvant trials as well as the results obtained after multivariate analyses of these trials. In short, the truly optimal duration for any given patient in this setting is unknown because the patients are technically diseasefree after their resection.

PERIPHERAL NEUROPATHY

CASE 95-2, QUESTION 5: After eight cycles of adjuvant therapy, B.R. begins complaining of a constant numbness and tingling in the toes on his left foot that is not interfering with his daily activities but is described as more of a nuisance. Which drug is most likely responsible for this, and what course of action should be taken?

The timing of the symptoms that B.R. is experiencing is indicative of the cumulative toxicity oxaliplatin exerts on peripheral sensory nerves. As explained earlier, the severity of this condition can worsen with continued doses of oxaliplatin and is not readily reversible; therefore, it is imperative that clinicians and patients work together to minimize its negative impact on various activities of daily living such as buttoning a shirt, walking up or down stairs, or realizing whether one's foot is actually touching the brake pedal as the car approaches a red light. The incidence of delayed neurotoxicity causing functional impairment has been reported to exceed 15% after cumulative doses of 780 mg/m^2.[31] Early evidence suggested that use of IV infusions of calcium and magnesium with oxaliplatin attenuates the acute symptoms and perhaps delays the onset and intensity of the chronic manifestations of this neurotoxicity.[34] Controversy as to whether this strategy is practical in the adjuvant setting exists because of concerns of decreased tumor response rates and other measures of effectiveness. Another strategy uses a "stop-and-go" approach to limit exposure to oxaliplatin while retaining its antitumor effects and has been shown to be beneficial in delaying the development of peripheral neuropathy.[35] In this approach, oxaliplatin is withdrawn from therapy in patients with metastatic disease and is reinitiated when disease progression is noted. However, this strategy was used in patients with metastatic disease, and although effective, it is impractical in the adjuvant setting.

Because B.R. has completed 8 of a planned 12 cycles of his adjuvant therapy and because his symptoms just started, are confined to one extremity, and are not interfering with his daily activities, the reaction would be graded as relatively mild in its severity at this point. He will likely benefit most from continued administration of oxaliplatin at a reduced dosage with diligent monitoring of his neuropathy. Several small trials have been conducted to evaluate the effectiveness of certain pharmaceutical agents in the management of chemotherapy-induced peripheral neuropathy. These trials have focused on either the prevention or treatment of chemotherapy-induced peripheral neuropathy and as a whole have yielded disappointing results; however, some of these agents have been shown to alleviate neuropathic pain in other chronic pain syndromes like diabetic neuropathy, and they could be considered as adjunctive options for the management of B.R.'s symptoms. Given his age and lack of contraindications, a tricyclic antidepressant such as nortriptyline or amitriptyline, or an anticonvulsant such as gabapentin could be considered as these agents have proven beneficial and are recommended as initial therapy in other neuropathic pain settings.[36] It is important to note that when using adjunctive agents such as these to manage neuropathic pain, doses typically require upward titration after initiation. This strategy enables the clinician to find the dose that provides the greatest benefit. It is important to explain to the patient that these agents may take several weeks before a response is seen. Symptom relief generally requires continued daily use of these agents on a scheduled basis; however, it is important to consider weaning them with time if neuropathic symptoms continue to improve.

Clinical Surveillance for Recurrence

CASE 95-2, QUESTION 6: After completing his treatment, how often and for how long should B.R. be monitored for recurrence of his disease?

Because the majority of recurrences occur within the first 2 to 3 years after completion of adjuvant therapy, both the American Society of Clinical Oncology and the National Comprehensive Cancer Network have published guidelines that address the importance of patient follow-up and surveillance after definitive therapy for localized disease.[37,38] Both organizations agree that patients treated definitively for localized disease should be monitored regularly for at least 5 years. Should B.R. remain disease-free throughout this 5-year surveillance period, he will be considered cured of his cancer. Because most recurrences occur relatively soon, his surveillance visits will be more frequent for the first 2 years. Given his treatment, B.R. should have a history and physical examination performed every 3 to 6 months for the first 2 years, then semiannually thereafter. He should also have a CEA level obtained every 3 to 6 months for the first 2 years, then semiannually thereafter. He should also have a CT scan of his chest, abdomen, and pelvis performed at least annually for 3 years. Another colonoscopy should be performed within a year of his surgical resection or approximately 1 year from his original colonoscopy, and then repeated again in 3 years. During the surveillance period, development of a concerning symptom on physical examination, an abnormality on a CT scan, or a rise in CEA level above the upper limit of normal (3 ng/mL for nonsmokers or 6 ng/mL for smokers) would necessitate B.R. to undergo evaluation for disease recurrence. After the 5-year surveillance period, B.R. will remain at increased risk for recurrent disease; therefore, he should resume screening for colorectal cancer every 5 years, which is more frequent than the every 10 years recommended for an average-risk patient.

Chemotherapy for Metastatic Colorectal Cancer

CASE 95-3

QUESTION 1: K.T. is a 64-year-old man treated approximately 2 years ago with adjuvant chemotherapy for colon cancer. On a routine surveillance visit, his CT scan shows a colon mass, two discrete liver nodules, and a nodule in the left lung that are consistent with metastatic disease. The biopsy of the liver was positive for adenocarcinoma of the colon. K.T. is feeling well and has been asymptomatic. No cytogenetics on the tumor was performed at this time. K.T.'s CBC and chemistry values were as follows:

WBC count, 7.8 $\times$ 10^3 cells/μL
Hemoglobin, 13.2 g/dL
Platelet count, 252 $\times$ 10^3 cells/μL
Serum creatinine, 1.1 mg/dL
Blood urea nitrogen, 15 mg/dL
Aspartate aminotransferase, 28 units/L
Alanine aminotransferase, 35 units/L
Alkaline phosphatase, 135 units/L
Total bilirubin, 0.8 mg/dL

K.T.'s CEA concentration was 22 ng/mL. What is the role of chemotherapy now that K.T. has a metastatic recurrence?

Of those who present initially with localized, resectable disease, 30% will subsequently have metastatic disease. Among patients with newly diagnosed colorectal cancer, 25% will present with metastatic disease. Therefore, metastatic disease affects a substantial number of patients.

Significant treatment advances have been made in the last 10 years for cases of advanced colorectal cancer such that the median overall survival is currently close to 2 years in treated patients.[39–41] Treatments include single-agent therapy (irinotecan, 5′-FU, capecitabine), combination chemotherapy, and the use of monoclonal antibodies (bevacizumab, cetuximab, and panitumumab). Irinotecan, 5′-FU, and leucovorin regimens (IFL, FOLFIRI), and oxaliplatin, 5′-FU, and leucovorin (FOLFOX) combinations for the initial treatment of metastatic colorectal cancer have been studied. Patients treated with FOLFOX had response rates, times to disease progression, and overall survival rates that were superior to those observed for patients treated with IFL or IROX (irinotecan, oxaliplatin). Although overall survival is the gold standard therapeutic end point, it is difficult to control for patients who progress on one arm of the study, and then switch to receive the other treatment(s). Therefore, even though overall survival results were superior, the investigators were unable to account for second-line therapies, which could affect survival.[42] Nevertheless, this trial established the evidence for the replacement of the IFL regimen with FOLFOX as the first-line chemotherapy for patients with metastatic disease. Other first-line regimens for metastatic disease include FOLFIRI (5′-FU, irinotecan, leucovorin), XELOX (capecitabine, oxaliplatin), and XELIRI (capecitabine, irinotecan); however, the optimal sequencing of these agents within a regimen are unclear, which has led to differences in clinical practice. Therefore, the decision regarding the choice of combination therapy for first- or second-line therapy is based on prior therapy, quality of life, pre-existing toxicities, and comorbid conditions. Surgery is typically not an option in extensive metastatic disease.

In the past 7 years, biologic therapies targeting vascular endothelial growth factor (bevacizumab) and epidermal growth factor receptor (EGFR; cetuximab and panitumumab), have been incorporated into the treatment of many cases of metastatic colorectal cancer. The addition of bevacizumab to IFL or FOLFOX significantly improved response rate and overall survival.[40,43] Cetuximab, a chimeric monoclonal antibody against the extracellular domain of EGFR, is active as a single agent or in combination with irinotecan even in patients with irinotecan-refractory malignancies.[44,45] In first-line setting, addition of cetuximab or panitumumab to FOLFIRI or FOLFOX has only provided modest improvement, except in patients with *KRAS* wild-type tumor.[46,47] Panitumumab, a fully human monoclonal antibody also targeting the extracellular domain of EGFR, is active as monotherapy for refractory metastatic disease when compared with best supportive care. Panitumumab has been studied in combination with either irinotecan- or oxaliplatin-based regimen and shows modest response.[48,49] The trials of combining cetuximab or panitumumab with bevacizumab and chemotherapy have resulted in poor progressionfree survival and increased toxicity to the patients.[50,51] Therefore, FOLFOX, FOLFIRI, XELOX, or XELIRI in combination with bevacizumab is considered first-line treatment options for patients with metastatic colorectal cancer.

K.T. has stage IV colon cancer with metastasis to the liver and lung. The goal of therapy for K.T. is prolongation of survival. At this point, K.T.'s cancer is not curable. Because tumor cytogenetics was not performed, K.T.'s *KRAS* status is unknown. Therefore, EGFR monoclonal antibody at this point is not considered a first-line treatment option. K.T. should receive combination chemotherapy. This chemotherapy could be 5′-FU or capecitabine in combination with oxaliplatin or irinotecan. Addition of bevacizumab to this regimen will further improve response rate and survival of K.T. In this case, K.T. is scheduled to receive FOLFIRI plus bevacizumab regimen, which is given every 2 weeks. He will receive this chemotherapy regimen until disease progression. The FOLFIRI plus bevacizumab is given as bevacizumab 5 mg/kg IV for 10 to 30 minutes, leucovorin 200 mg/m^2 IV for 2 hours, irinotecan 180 mg/m^2 IV for 90 minutes, and 5′-FU 400 mg/m^2 bolus on day 1. 5′-FU 2400 mg/m^2 is infused for 46 hours starting after completion of the bolus 5′-FU.

HEPATIC METASTASES

Colorectal-related metastases most commonly arise in the liver. In one-third of cases, the metastases are synchronous and in two-thirds, metachronous. Synchronous means metastasis occurring simultaneously, and metachronous means metastases occur as separate occurrences, which could have two separate primary colorectal cancers. Surgical resection, if possible, is the most effective treatment modality for potential long-term survival in colorectal patients with isolated liver metastases.[52] Many patients, however, could potentially benefit from regional therapy. Because liver metastases derive most of their blood supply from the hepatic artery, direct administration of anticancer drugs into the artery provides high drug concentrations to the area of tumor involvement. Hepatic intra-arterial administration of 5′-FU, floxuridine, or other chemotherapeutic agents has been extensively studied in patients with metastases confined to the liver.[53] This localized therapy is usually restricted to treatment centers that have expertise for this modality. The major limitation for such treatment is that undetected metastases located elsewhere would not be exposed to the agents as they would after IV administration. Because K.T. clearly has disease that involves the liver and lung, he should receive systemic chemotherapy for his disease. Hepatic intra-arterial treatment would not be effective for K.T.'s lung metastases.

Pharmacogenomics of Irinotecan and 5′-FU

CASE 95-3, QUESTION 2: Fourteen days after receiving FOLFIRI plus bevacizumab, K.T. presented to the emergency room complaining of fever (101.2°F). On further evaluation, K.T. was identified as having febrile neutropenia with a WBC count of 1.2×10^3 cells/μL and an absolute neutrophil count of 650 cells/μL. He was admitted to the hospital for treatment. Is there an accurate method for predicting this outcome in K.T.? Can K.T. continue to receive this therapy?

Recent discoveries in the field of pharmacogenomics have identified several important genetic variations (polymorphisms) that partly account for between-patient differences regarding tolerability and efficacy of drug therapies. This pharmacogenomic profiling may, therefore, prove beneficial in guiding therapeutic decisions.[30] Genotyping tests that assess for the presence of polymorphisms are available, and these may help in predicting the resultant activity of key enzymes that metabolize 5′-FU and irinotecan before administration. Presence of one or more of these polymorphisms may result in an enzyme(s) with decreased ability to metabolize the drug, resulting in potentially severe toxicities.

Dihydropyrimidine dehydrogenase (DPD) is the rate-limiting enzyme that metabolizes 5′-FU.[54] Approximately 5% of patients will poorly metabolize 5′-FU, which in some cases is attributable to genetic polymorphisms. However, the presence of a genetic polymorphism of this enzyme does not always translate into a functional decrease in enzyme activity and poor metabolism.[55] Multiple tests are currently available to assess for DPD polymorphisms. Currently, screening for DPD polymorphisms is not recommended as a standard of care before receiving 5′-FU–based chemotherapy for colorectal cancer.[21] Some advocates of genetic testing before 5′-FU therapy suggest that individuals heterozygous for the DPD intron 14 splice site polymorphism receive lower doses and those homozygous for the polymorphism receive alternative therapy to reduce toxicity.

Polymorphisms in the thymidylate synthase *TYMS* gene have also been investigated. Uridine diphosphate glucuronosyltransferase (UGT) enzymes are responsible for the glucuronidation of bilirubin and other endogenous substrates as well as drugs and other toxins.[56] The enzyme UGT1A1 is responsible for the glucuronidation of SN-38, the active metabolite of irinotecan. Reductions in glucuronidation and accumulation of SN-38 are associated with greater toxicity. Of the known genetic polymorphisms of UGT1A1, one polymorphism in particular (UGT1A1*28) has been associated with decreased glucuronidation of SN-38, and several studies have demonstrated an association between this polymorphism and the subsequent development of toxicity, primarily severe neutropenia.[57,58] A dose reduction is recommended before initiating therapy with irinotecan if the polymorphism is present. Although not consistently observed among trials, severe diarrhea has also been observed with genetic polymorphisms of UGT1A1.[59] Limited laboratories with the ability to perform these tests and the lack of consensus guidelines that outline how to use the results represent some of the challenges that currently restrict their widespread use in clinical practice; however, practitioners should still exercise caution when treating patients with either a known or suspected deficiency in DPD or UGT1A1.

K.T. should receive empiric antibiotic therapy, and his chemotherapy should be held until both his fever and neutropenia resolve. Because he did not experience febrile neutropenia with his previous adjuvant therapy it is unlikely he would harbor a DPD deficiency. A dose reduction of 5′-FU could be considered. More importantly, a reduction of his irinotecan dose is warranted before resuming his chemotherapy to reduce the risk of fever and neutropenia with consecutive cycles. The FDA-approved Invader UGT1A1 molecular assay is commercially available to detect the UGT1A1*28 polymorphism. If it is known that a patient has this polymorphism, an empiric reduction in the dose of irinotecan is recommended; however, its use is not generally recommended for determining reductions of subsequent doses of irinotecan after a toxic event.

Adverse Effects of 5′-FU, Irinotecan, and Bevacizumab

CASE 95-3, QUESTION 3: K.T. was discharged from the hospital after 4 days without identification of any infection. K.T. presents to clinic to receive a second cycle of FOLFIRI plus bevacizumab. He is now more cognizant of chemotherapy's adverse effects. He states that after his first cycle of chemotherapy, he also experienced abdominal cramping followed by profuse watery bowel movements for 3 days. He reported periods of nose bleeds lasting up to 2 weeks as well, which he never had in the past. The following laboratory values were also noted:

WBC count, 4.5 × 10^3 cells/μL
Hemoglobin, 12.5 g/dL
Platelet count, 210,000 cells/μL
Serum creatinine, 1.3 mg/dL

What can be done to alleviate or avoid these symptoms? K.T. would like to know more information about side effects of chemotherapy agents he is receiving.

The incidence of irinotecan-induced diarrhea varies depending on the dosing schedule used and its combination with other chemotherapeutic agents. Trials in metastatic colorectal cancer have reported rates of grade 3 or 4 diarrhea of 20% to 30% depending on which irinotecan-based regimen is used.[60,61] The active metabolite of irinotecan, SN-38, is capable of producing acute abdominal cramping and diarrhea, which is a cholinergic-mediated process. Administration of subcutaneous or IV atropine at doses typically lower than those used in the cardiac setting is recommended for the treatment of acute diarrhea caused by irinotecan. The occurrence of diarrhea can also be delayed; thus, the use of an oral antidiarrheal is recommended if this occurs. A regimen of oral loperamide 4 mg with the first loose bowel movement, followed by 2 mg every 2 hours during the day or 4 mg every 4 hours in the evening, is recommended until the patient is diarrheafree for a period of 12 hours.[62] If severe diarrhea symptoms persist for more than 48 hours, in spite of these measures, patients should be instructed to seek emergency medical attention. Insufficient hydration resulting from diarrhea may lead to electrolyte losses and life-threatening consequences.

The key adverse effects of 5′-FU, oxaliplatin, and irinotecan are discussed under Case 95-2, Questions 3 and 4, and Case 95-3, Question 2. Although bevacizumab may share some overlapping toxicities with traditional chemotherapy, the majority of its effects are unique. Therefore, this agent may be safely administered concurrently with chemotherapy. Although cytotoxic agents are associated with myelosuppression, antiangiogenesis agents such as bevacizumab do not target proliferating cells. Hence, they do not cause this type of severe toxicity. Bevacizumab has been associated with less than 3% of grade 3 or 4 bleeding events in clinical trials.[44,63] The epistaxis K.T. is experiencing with this cycle of chemotherapy may be attributed directly or indirectly to his current regimen. Although 5′-FU and irinotecan may also cause bleeding, this is usually related to their myelosuppressive effects on platelet progenitors. Because K.T. has a platelet count of 210,000 cells/μL on his recent laboratory work, this bleeding is more likely associated with bevacizumab use. Although not well understood, the mechanism for bevacizumab-induced epistaxis is likely related to its effect on blood vessel homeostasis. The severity of bleeding can vary from mild, reversible symptoms (such as epistaxis that is sporadic and controlled with supportive measures) to severe, life-threatening bleeding requiring more extensive interventions.[64]

In addition to bleeding, bevacizumab may cause serious and potentially life-threatening toxicities, including wound-healing complications, gastrointestinal perforation, congestive heart failure, arterial and venous thromboembolism, leukoencephalopathy syndrome, proteinuria, and hypertension.[64] Therapy should be interrupted for severe bleeding events or for patients who are either recovering from or planning to undertake a major surgical procedure as the incidence of wound dehiscence is increased significantly in the perioperative period because of its antiangiogenic effects. Although surgery is not planned for K.T., it would be necessary to stop the drug at least 4 to 6 weeks before invasive surgical procedures because bevacizumab has a long half-life and could affect wound healing. Likewise, it is recommended to delay the start of bevacizumab after surgery to give the surgical wound sufficient time to heal first.[65]

Predictive Molecular Tumor Markers

CASE 95-3, QUESTION 4: About 10 months into his treatment, K.T. had a CT scan that suggested progression of the liver and lung masses. Cytogenetic analysis of tissue from his old tumor biopsy was requested. The cytogenetic results suggested wild-type *KRAS* and no mutation of *BRAF*. What should be the best second-line treatment option for K.T.'s metastatic disease?

The ultimate goal of treatment is to individualize therapy based on patient and tumor characteristics. This is now possible as a result of better understanding of the pathophysiology of colorectal cancer and availability of newer targeted therapies. Prognostic markers provide information on disease outcome regardless of treatment provided. Predictive markers provide information on disease outcome based on treatment provided. These predictive markers facilitate specific treatment decision making to improve the desired outcome. For patients with metastatic colorectal cancer, the presence of the *KRAS* mutation is one of the most important predictive molecular markers identified. The *KRAS* mutation occurs in approximately 35% of colon cancer cases.[66] Whereas *KRAS* gene status has no prognostic value, it does provide important predictive value when anti-EGFR monoclonal antibodies like cetuximab and panitumumab are considered.[67] Patients whose tumors express mutated *KRAS* do not receive treatment benefit with either of these agents. On the contrary, patients with tumor expressing wild-type *KRAS* gene will often receive benefit from the anti-EGFR monoclonal antibody therapy. Studies show significant improvement in the response rate and the diseasefree survival in patients with wild-type KRAS compared with those with mutated *KRAS* tumor receiving cetuximab or panitumumab.[48,49,68] *BRAF* is another molecular marker, which is a downstream effector of *KRAS*. Early data suggest that patients with wild-type *KRAS*, but mutated *BRAF*, may not benefit from anti-EGFR monoclonal antibody therapy.[69,70] Therefore, *BRAF* gene status analysis is considered in patients with wild-type *KRAS* tumor.

Typically adjuvant chemotherapy in colon cancer is only supported for stage III cancer and not stage II. At the same time, experts believe that there are some high-risk patients with stage II colon cancer who may benefit from adjuvant chemotherapy. The question is how best to identify these, few, high-risk patients. Microsatellite instability is one of the predictive markers that may be used for adjuvant chemotherapy decision making for patients with stage II colon cancer. Clinicians may use nonmolecular markers. For example, development of hypertension while receiving bevacizumab suggests that the drug is displaying a systemic effect, most likely on blood vasculature. As a second example, development of papular-pustular (acneiform) skin rash while receiving anti-EGFR monoclonal antibody therapies is also indicative of systemic effects. For both cases, studies have shown that patients who experienced these specific adverse events while on treatment were more likely to respond to treatment.[44,46,71] This would imply that those who experience these adverse effects should remain on therapy. Unfortunately, effective treatments to manage these effects have yet to be thoroughly tested in clinical trials.

K.T. has not received anti-EGFR monoclonal antibody–based chemotherapy. A tumor tissue analysis now reveals that it contains wild-type *KRAS* and negative *BRAF* cytogenetics. Therefore, K.T. may receive benefit from anti-EGFR monoclonal antibodies. In addition, irinotecan in combination with cetuximab has synergistic activity; therefore, a regimen of irinotecan and anti-EGFR (cetuximab or panitumumab) combination would be a good choice.

Epidermal Growth Factor Receptor–Inhibitors

INFUSION-RELATED REACTIONS

CASE 95-3, QUESTION 5: K.T. will receive the following combination chemotherapy regimen: irinotecan 125 mg/m^2 IV on day 1 and day 8 plus cetuximab 400 mg/m^2 IV as an initial loading dose on day 1 of the first cycle followed by 250 mg/m^2 IV weekly. Each cycle is to be repeated every 3 weeks. Within minutes of receiving the initial cetuximab infusion, K.T. becomes hypotensive and begins having difficulty breathing. What measures should be taken as quickly as possible?

The incidence of grade 3 or 4 infusion-related reactions reported in clinical trials is less than 3.5% with cetuximab and even less for panitumumab.[45,71,72] Because cetuximab is a chimeric monoclonal antibody, the higher incidence of reactions is not surprising. Therefore, cetuximab administration requires premedication with diphenhydramine, whereas panitumumab does not.[44] Although the incidence estimate for hypersensitivity is less than 5%, these reactions may be underestimated, especially in the middle southern region of the United States where a higher incidence has been observed.[73] It is not currently known why there is a greater propensity for severe hypersensitivity reactions in patients in this region of the country. Unlike cetuximab, panitumumab is not currently approved for use in combination with chemotherapy. However, studies are under way to assess this more thoroughly, and there are data to support its use when combined with chemotherapy in the metastatic setting.[48] Because of the severe nature of the reaction experienced by K.T., rechallenging with cetuximab at this point would be contraindicated. Because panitumumab is a fully humanized monoclonal antibody with a much lower incidence of severe hypersensitivity reactions and no documentation of cross-reactivity with cetuximab, it could be considered as a substitute for cetuximab, but currently data to support this are limited to case reports.

DERMATOLOGIC REACTIONS

CASE 95-3, QUESTION 6: Assuming K.T. continued EGFR therapy, what is the most common adverse effect he is likely to experience? How can this toxicity be minimized?

In addition to diarrhea, dermatologic toxicity related to EGFR therapy occurs in more than 90% of metastatic colorectal cancer patients treated with these agents. As mentioned earlier, rash is often a predictor of response to treatment; however, published response rates for this agent are less than 90%. EGFR skin reactions typically occur within 7 to 10 days of therapy, and most often present as a maculopapular rash on the face or upper torso of patients.[44] The rash may cause discomfort and reduce quality of life. Both cetuximab and panitumumab have recommendations for dose reductions or the withholding of therapy based on rash severity. Collaborative efforts have been made across clinical disciplines to develop treatment strategies for EGFR-induced dermatologic toxicities based on their severity. One such multidisciplinary guideline has suggested a stepwise approach to treatment based on severity of symptoms.[74] Strategies for preventing or limiting the severity of EGFR dermatologic toxicities have also been explored, including the use of a daily regimen of skin moisturizer, sunscreen, topical 1% hydrocortisone cream, and doxycycline.[75] In addition to their antimicrobial properties, the tetracycline class of antibiotics possesses anti-inflammatory properties and antiproliferative effects on lymphocytes, which makes it a reasonable class of agents to consider given the proposed mechanisms involved in EGFR rash development. A strategy focused on skin moisturization and protection combined with a daily application of hydrocortisone cream and the administration of doxycycline 100 mg twice daily or another tetracycline derivative could be considered for K.T.

CHEMOTHERAPY AND RADIATION FOR EARLY-STAGE RECTAL CANCER

Approximately one-third of newly diagnosed colorectal cancers originate from the rectum.[1] The differentiation between cancers of the colon and rectum lies in their location and their propensity for recurrence at or near the site of origin after treatment. If the location of B.R.'s tumor had been within 12 to 15 cm from the anal verge, he would have been diagnosed with rectal cancer (Case 95-2). The main difference between rectal cancer and colon cancer treatment lies primarily in patients with stage II or stage III disease. Unless contraindicated, radiation therapy is incorporated into the treatment plan of patients with stage II or stage III disease of the rectum. In addition, slightly different surgical techniques are used, and a short course of 5′-FU or capecitabine chemotherapy is administered in combination with the radiation until it is complete. When combined with chemotherapy, radiation can significantly reduce local recurrence rates.[75–77] An area of debate is the timing of chemoradiotherapy and whether it should be started before (neoadjuvant) or after surgery (adjuvant). Both strategies appear to be equally effective, so other issues are considered when choosing one modality over the other. Adjuvant chemoradiotherapy may avoid overtreatment of disease, whereas a neoadjuvant approach of chemoradiotherapy before surgery has the advantage of potentially shrinking the tumor and giving the surgeon a greater chance of obtaining negative margins, perhaps allowing for a less radical procedure and preservation of the anal sphincter. Another difference between tumors of the rectum and colon is the vascular drainage by the venous system. The colon is drained by the mesenteric veins of the hepatic portal system, whereas more distal portions of the rectum are drained by veins that empty into the inferior vena cava. This plays a role in the initial site of metastatic development for each disease. Although the liver is the most common overall site of colorectal cancer metastasis, when compared with the colon, cancers of the distal rectum are more likely to metastasize to the lungs because of the differences in their respective vasculature.

KEY REFERENCES AND WEBSITES

A full list of references for this chapter can be found at http://thepoint.lww.com/AT10e. Below are the key references for this chapter, with the corresponding reference number in this chapter found in parentheses after the reference.

Key References

Andre T et al. Oxaliplatin, fluorouracil, and leucovorin as adjuvant treatment for colon cancer. *N Engl J Med.* 2004;350:2343. (28)

Desch CE et al. Colorectal cancer surveillance: 2005 update of an American Society of Clinical Oncology practice guideline [published correction appears in *J Clin Oncol.* 2006;24:1224]. *J Clin Oncol.* 2005;23:8512. (37)

Giantonio BJ et al. Bevacizumab in combination with oxaliplatin, fluorouracil, and leucovorin (FOLFOX4) for previously treated metastatic colorectal cancer: results from the Eastern Cooperative Oncology Group Study E3200. *J Clin Oncol.* 2007;25:1539. (40)

Gressett SM, Shah SR. Intricacies of bevacizumab-induced toxicities and their management. *Ann Pharmacother.* 2009;43:490. (64)

Innocenti F et al. Genetic variants in the UDP-glucuronosyltransferase 1A1 gene predict the risk of severe neutropenia of irinotecan. *J Clin Oncol.* 2004;22:1382. (58)

Kuebler JP et al. Oxaliplatin combined with weekly bolus fluorouracil and leucovorin as surgical adjuvant chemotherapy for stage II and III colon cancer: results from NSABP C-07. *J Clin Oncol.* 2007;25:2198. (27)

Lacouture ME et al. The SERIES clinic: an interdisciplinary approach to the management of toxicities of EGFR inhibitors. *J Support Oncol.* 2006;4:236. (74)

Levin B et al. Screening and surveillance for the early detection of colorectal cancer and adenomatous polyps, 2008: a joint guideline from the American Cancer Society, the US Multi-Society Task Force on Colorectal Cancer, and the American College of Radiology. *CA Cancer J Clin.* 2008;58:130. (13)

Loupakis F et al. *KRAS* codon 61, 146 and *BRAF* mutations predict resistance to cetuximab plus irinotecan in *KRAS* codon 12 and 13 wild-type metastatic colorectal cancer. *Br J Cancer.* 2009;101:715. (70)

Sauer R et al. Preoperative versus postoperative chemoradiotherapy for rectal cancer. *N Engl J Med.* 2004;351:1731. (76)

Sobrero AF et al. EPIC: phase III trial of cetuximab plus irinotecan after fluoropyrimidine and oxaliplatin failure in patients with metastatic colorectal cancer. *J Clin Oncol.* 2008;26:2311. (72)

Tan BR, McLeod HL. Pharmacogenetic influences on treatment response and toxicity in colorectal cancer. *Semin Oncol.* 2005;32:113. (30)

Tournigand C et al. OPTIMOX1: a randomized study of FOLFOX4 or FOLFOX7 with oxaliplatin in a stop-and-Go fashion in advanced colorectal cancer—a GERCOR study. *J Clin Oncol.* 2006;24:394. (35)

Twelves C et al. Capecitabine as adjuvant treatment for stage III colon cancer. *N Engl J Med.* 2005;352:2696. (23)

96 Hematopoietic Cell Transplantation

Kathleen G.E. Green and John R. Rogosheske

CORE PRINCIPLES

		CHAPTER CASES
1	Hematopoietic cell transplantation (HCT) is a life-saving medical procedure involving the infusion of hematopoietic stem cells into a patient, the HCT recipient, to treat malignant and nonmalignant diseases and/or restore normal hematopoiesis and lymphopoiesis.	**Case 96-1 (Question 1), Case 96-2 (Question 1)**
2	In autologous HCT, the donor and recipient are the same individual, eliminating the need for pretransplantation and posttransplantation immunosuppression. Autologous hematopoietic cells must be obtained (i.e., harvested) before the myeloablative preparative regimen is administered and subsequently stored for administration after the preparative regimen.	**Case 96-1 (Questions 2, 3)**
3	Posttransplantation pharmacotherapy for autologous HCT includes hematopoietic growth factors to stimulate the proliferation of committed progenitor cells and to accelerate hematopoietic recovery.	**Case 96-1 (Question 6), Case 96-2 (Question 8)**
4	Common complications after autologous HCT are infections and organ failure, which occur in less than 5% of patients. The most common cause of death after autologous HCT is recurrence of the primary disease.	**Case 96-1 (Question 5)**
5	Allogeneic HCT involves the transplantation of hematopoietic stem cells obtained from a donor's bone marrow, peripheral blood progenitor cells, or umbilical cord blood to a patient. The donor for an allogeneic HCT may be an unrelated or related individual. Histocompatibility determination between donors and recipients must be performed through human leukocyte antigen (HLA) typing. The preparative regimen is, in part, determined by the degree of mismatch between the donor and the recipient.	**Case 96-2 (Questions 2, 3)**
6	The function of the preparative regimens for autologous HCT is to eradicate residual malignancy. The function of the preparative regimen in allogeneic HCT is to eradicate the residual malignancy but also to provide immunosuppression, allowing the transplanted stem cells to grow and create a graft-versus-tumor effect.	**Case 96-1 (Question 4)**
7	Choice of preparative regimens for HCT depends on factors such as underlying disease, degree of HLA matching, stem cell source, patient age and comorbid conditions. Preparative regimen differ in intensity and are distinguished as myeloablative or nonmyeloablative.	**Case 96-2 (Questions 5, 6)**
8	Posttransplantation immunosuppressive therapy is necessary for allogeneic HCT to prevent both graft rejection and acute and/or chronic graft versus host disease (AGVHD/CGVHD). Some immunosuppressants require therapeutic drug monitoring to ensure effectiveness while minimizing toxicity.	**Case 96-2 (Question 7), Case 96-4 (Question 1), Case 96-5 (Questions 1–9)**
9	Posttransplantation complications of myeloablative preparation regimens such as hemorrhagic cystitis, mucositis, and venoocclusive disease require pharmaceutical management.	**Case 96-2 (Questions 8, 9), Case 96-3 (Questions 1–9)**

continued

		CHAPTER CASES
10	Opportunistic infections are a major cause of morbidity and mortality after myeloablative and nonmyeloablative HCT. The primary pathogens vary based on the time posttransplant, and include bacterial, fungal, and viral species.	**Case 96-6 (Questions 1–3), Case 96-7 (Questions 1–5)**
11	Long-term complications of HCT include CGVHD, endocrine dysfunction, and secondary cancers.	**Case 96-5 (Questions 7–9), Case 96-8 (Question 1)**

OVERVIEW

Worldwide, more than 32,000 autologous and 25,000 allogeneic hematopoietic stem cell transplantations (HCTs) are performed annually.[1] HCT is a medical procedure involving the administration of chemotherapy followed by infusion of hematopoietic stem cells into a patient (the HCT recipient) to treat disease and/or restore normal hematopoiesis and lymphopoiesis. The first HCTs were allogeneic bone marrow transplants (BMT) with myeloablative (high dose) chemotherapy.[2]

Bone marrow contains multipotent stem cells and postthymic lymphocytes, which are responsible for long-term hematopoietic reconstitution, immune recovery, and graft-versus-host disease (GVHD).[2]

ONLINE CONTENT

For an illustration that shows hematopoietic stem cell differentiation, go to http://thepoint.lww.com/AT10e.

Subsequently, the "dose intensity" concept for cancer treatment was expanded to autologous HCT. Autologous HCT, or infusion of a patient's own hematopoietic stem cells, allows for the administration of higher doses of chemotherapy, radiation, or both to treat cancer.[2,3] In autologous HCT, the hematopoietic stem cells "rescue" the patient from otherwise dose-limiting hematopoietic toxicity, although undetectable malignant cells may be reinfused into the patient. During the 1990s, there was an improved understanding of the graft-versus-tumor (GVT) effect, where the donor's cytotoxic T lymphocytes suppress the recipient's malignancy. The use of the GVT effect in treatment led to reduced-intensity or nonmyeloablative preparative regimens. These less-toxic preparative regimens expand the availability of allogeneic HCT to patients whose pre-existing medical condition(s) or greater age excludes them as candidates for myeloablative regimens.[4–6]

HCT is the only treatment available to many patients; however, it is associated with considerable morbidity and mortality, with approximately 40% of advanced cancer patients who undergo HCT dying of complications.[2] The basic schema for HCT is illustrated in Figure 96-1. The combination of chemotherapy and/or radiation administered before infusion of hematopoietic stem cells is referred to as the preparative or conditioning regimen.[2] Although the preparative regimen uses the same agents that are used in conventional chemotherapy regimens, the doses are higher. The purpose of the preparative regimen is to eradicate the residual malignancy and, in the setting of an allogeneic HCT, to suppress the recipient's immunity, therefore agents are selected for these properties.[2] Only myeloablative preparative regimens are used for autologous HCT, whereas myeloablative, reduced-intensity, or nonmyeloablative preparative regimens may be used with allogeneic HCT. Myeloablative preparative regimens involve administration of near-lethal doses of chemotherapy and/or radiation which myeloablate the bone marrow; this is generally followed by a 1-day to 2-day rest and then infusion of hematopoietic stem cells. Myeloablative preparative regimens have significant regimen-related toxicity and morbidity, and thus are usually limited to healthy, younger (i.e., usually younger than 55 years) patients.[7] Alternatively, reduced-intensity or nonmyeloablative transplantations are performed with the hope of curing more cancer patients with less preparative regimen–related toxicity and of using the GVT effect that allows an early mixed chimerism, or combination of host and donor hematopoietic cells, to take advantage of the donor lymphocyte induced tumor eradication (see Graft-versus-Tumor section). For most chemotherapy-based preparative regimens, the rest period is necessary to allow for elimination of toxic metabolites from the chemotherapy that could damage infused cells. After chemotherapy and radiation, a period of pancytopenia lasts until the infused hematopoietic stem cells re-establish functional hematopoiesis. This process is called engraftment and is commonly defined as the point at which a patient can maintain a sustained absolute neutrophil count (ANC) of more than 500 cells/μL and a sustained platelet count of at least 20,000/μL lasting 3 consecutive days without transfusions.[8] Graft rejection occurs when the patient cannot maintain functional hematopoiesis and may occur after autologous or allogeneic HCT.

There are various sources of hematopoietic stem cells that can be used for HCT. The key properties of the hematopoietic stem cells are their ability to engraft, the speed of engraftment, and the durability of the engraftment.[9] Peripheral blood progenitor cell transplant (PBPCT) has essentially replaced BMT as the preferred stem cell source for autologous HCT and is being increasingly

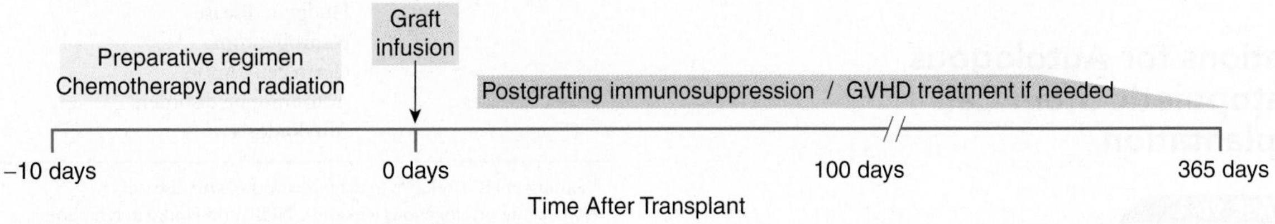

FIGURE 96-1 Basic schema for hematopoietic stem cell transplantation. Day 0 = bone marrow, peripheral blood progenitor cell, or umbilical cord blood infusion. Postgraft immunosuppression or graft-versus-host disease (GVHD) prophylaxis for allogeneic grafts only.

TABLE 96-1
Comparison of Types of Hematopoietic Cell Transplants

	Myeloablative		Nonmyeloablative
Risk[a]	Autologous	Allogeneic	Allogeneic
Relapse after HCT	+++	+	+
Rejection	–	+	++
Delayed engraftment	++	+	+
GVHD	–	+	++
Infection	+	++ to +++[b]	++ to +++[b]
Transplant-related morbidity	+	+++	++
Transplant-related mortality	+	++	+
Cost of procedure	++	+++	++ to +++

[a] Risk varies depending on underlying disease, patient characteristics, and previous medical history.
[b] Risk of infection increases with intensity and duration of immunosuppression and/or chronic GVHD.
GVHD, graft-versus-host disease; HCT, hematopoietic cell transplants.

used in the allogeneic setting.[9] Umbilical cord transplant (UCT) has increased the availability of allogeneic HCT to those in need of an urgent HCT or to those for whom suitable donors are not found.[2] Umbilical cord blood is rich in hematopoietic stem cells but has a limited number of hematopoietic stem cells; thus, both hematologic and immunologic reconstitution is delayed in UCT.[2]

The type of HCT performed depends on a number of factors, including type and status of disease, availability of a compatible donor, patient age, performance status, and organ function. Characteristics of autologous and allogeneic transplantation, with either myeloablative or nonmyeloablative preparative regimens, are compared in Table 96-1.[2] Many diseases are treated with autologous or allogeneic HCT and are listed in Table 96-2.[2] Modifications to the basic schema for HCT are necessary based on the immunologic source (i.e., allogeneic or autologous) and the anatomical source (i.e., bone marrow, PBPCs, or umbilical cord blood) of the hematopoietic stem cells infused.

AUTOLOGOUS HEMATOPOIETIC STEM CELL TRANSPLANTATION

The defining characteristic of autologous HCT is that the donor and the recipient are the same individual. Consequently, pretransplantation and posttransplantation immunosuppression is unnecessary. Autologous hematopoietic stem cells must be obtained (i.e., harvested) before the myeloablative preparative regimen is administered and subsequently stored for administration after the preparative regimen. Essentially, these hematopoietic stem cells are administered as a rescue intervention to re-establish bone marrow function and avoid long-lasting, life-threatening marrow aplasia that results from the myeloablative preparative regimen.[10] Although one might expect the autologous graft to be contaminated, incomplete tumor eradication by the high-intensity treatment prior to transplant remains the main cause of relapse after transplant.[11]

Indications for Autologous Hematopoietic Stem Cell Transplantation

CASE 96-1

QUESTION 1: P.J., a 46-year-old man, has diffuse large B-cell non-Hodgkin lymphoma (NHL) in first relapse after a complete remission of 1 year. An 80% reduction in measurable disease is noted after two cycles of dexamethasone, high-dose cytarabine, and cisplatin (DHAP) salvage chemotherapy. P.J.'s bone marrow biopsy and lumbar puncture are negative for malignant cells. Is a myeloablative preparative regimen with autologous HCT indicated for P.J.?

Autologous HCT is used to treat a variety of malignancies (Table 96-2). NHL and multiple myeloma are the most common indications for this procedure and represent more than two-thirds of all autologous HCT.[2] Patients with NHL are more frequently treated with an autologous HCT than with an allogeneic

TABLE 96-2
Diseases Commonly Treated with Hematopoietic Stem Cell Transplantation[a]

Allogeneic	
Nonmalignant	Aplastic anemia
	Thalassemia major
	Severe combined immunodeficiency disease
	Wiskott-Aldrich syndrome
	Fanconi anemia
	Inborn errors of metabolism
Malignant	AML
	Acute lymphoblastic leukemia
	Chronic myeloid leukemia
	Myelodysplastic syndrome
	Myeloproliferative disorders
	NHL
	Hodgkin disease
	Chronic lymphocytic leukemia
	Multiple myeloma
	Juvenile myelomonocytic leukemia
Autologous	
Malignant	NHL
	Multiple myeloma
	AML
	Hodgkin disease
	Neuroblastoma
	Germ-cell tumors
Other diseases	Autoimmune disorders
	Amyloidosis

[a] Timing of HCT relative to diagnosis varies with disease.
AML, acute myelogenous leukemia; NHL, non-Hodgkin lymphoma.
Source: Copelan EA. Hematopoietic stem-cell transplantation. *N Engl J Med.* 2006;354:1813; Vaughan W et al. The principles and overview of autologous hematopoietic stem cell transplantation. *Cancer Treat Res.* 2009;144:23.

HCT because autologous HCT has equivalent or superior survival to allogeneic HCT.[12,13] However, the usefulness of reduced-intensity preparative regimens with allogeneic HCT is currently being evaluated for the treatment of NHL because of the potential advantages of a graft-versus-lymphoma effect and of using donor hematopoietic stem cells that have not been previously exposed to cytotoxic chemotherapy.[4–6] Nearly all patients who undergo autologous HCT have failed standard chemotherapy regimens; therefore, their hematopoietic stem cells have been exposed to prior chemotherapy leading to less abundant and viable stem cells.

The most appropriate patient population and timing for autologous HCT in the treatment of NHL are being defined. A significant percentage of patients with aggressive NHL are cured with conventional chemotherapy alone. Adding autologous HCT to initial combination chemotherapy does not improve outcomes in patients with aggressive NHL.[14–16] The primary use of autologous HCT is aggressive, relapsed NHL that is still chemotherapy-sensitive.[17] In a randomized, controlled trial,[18] autologous BMT, compared with conventional chemotherapy with DHAP, resulted in a 5-year eventfree survival of 46% versus 12%, respectively ($p = 0.001$). Overall 5-year survival was 53% in the BMT group and 32% in the conventional chemotherapy patients ($p = 0.038$).[18]

Whereas HCT is delayed until relapse after primary treatment in NHL, in some malignancies, autologous HCT is indicated as primary therapy to improve overall survival and progressionfree survival.[17,19–20]

Prospective studies comparing preparative regimens, stem cell mobilization techniques, and stem cell source (i.e., BMT vs. PBPCT) are not available; however, autologous PBPCT has become the preferred source of stem cells, most likely owing to the improved outcomes with PBPCT in other disease settings.[21] Because PBPCT cells are continuously circulating in the blood, their number is too low to easily collect the amount needed in transplant. Mobilization refers to the techniques used to move the stem cells out of the bone marrow compartment, increasing their numbers in circulation. This can be accomplished using growth factors or chemotherapy (see Mobilization and Collection of Autologous Peripheral Blood Progenitor Cells section).

P.J. has minimal residual disease that has demonstrated chemotherapy sensitivity (i.e., he had an 80% response to chemotherapy). His long-term prognosis will be improved with autologous PBPCT rather than further conventional chemotherapy, as described previously. Thus, autologous PBPCT is indicated, owing to the greater likelihood that higer dose chemotherapy may eradicate his tumor. As discussed subsequently, additional chemotherapy and mobilization procedures will be required to ensure P.J. a successful transplantation.

Harvesting Autologous Hematopoietic Stem Cells

CASE 96-1, QUESTION 2: What is the best way to harvest and preserve harvested hematopoietic stem cells for P.J.?

PBPCs have essentially replaced bone marrow at many HCT centers, accounting for 98% of autologous transplants in adults from 2004 to 2008,[1] because PBPCs result in more rapid engraftment than bone marrow and therefore fewer days of neutropenia.[9] Because the harvest occurs before administering the preparative regimen, autologous hematopoietic stem cells must be cryopreserved.[2] Hematopoietic stem cells are usually frozen below −120°C and used within a few weeks; although, when frozen, they are viable for years.[2] Dimethylsulfoxide (DMSO) is the cryopreservative commonly used to protect hematopoietic stem cells from damage during freezing and thawing. Infusion of hematopoietic stem cells stored in DMSO can be associated with toxicities due to the DMSO itself. During infusion, DMSO is associated with skin flushing, nausea, diarrhea, dyspnea, hypotension, arrhythmias, and, rarely, anaphylactic reactions.[22] The presence of undetectable tumor cells in the transplanted cells contributes to relapse of hematologic cancers; unfortunately, purging the grafts of tumor cells does not improve survival.[2]

Relative to a bone marrow graft, a PBPC graft requires less invasive collection methods and contains up to five times more hematopoietic stem cells than a bone marrow harvest. This results in a PBPC graft having more rapid neutrophil and platelet recovery (i.e., a shorter duration of neutropenia or thrombocytopenia), fewer platelet transfusions, fewer days of intravenous (IV) antibiotics, and a shorter duration of hospitalization compared to a bone marrow graft. Thus, the shift to the use of PBPCs instead of bone marrow for autologous HCT is primarily because of the more rapid engraftment and less invasive collection methods.[21] Therefore, it would be best for P.J. to undergo pheresis for PBPC collection. These cells would be bathed in DMSO and frozen to −156°C.

Mobilization and Collection of Autologous Peripheral Blood Progenitor Cells

CASE 96-1, QUESTION 3: For PBPC mobilization, P.J. received one dose of cyclophosphamide 4 g/m² IV on day 1, followed by filgrastim 10 mcg/kg/day subcutaneously (SC) beginning on day 2 and continuing through completion of pheresis. Twelve days after receiving cyclophosphamide, P.J.'s white blood cell (WBC) count recovered to 3,000 cells/μL and pheresis was begun. An adequate number of PBPCs is collected after two pheresis sessions. P.J.'s cells are processed and stored. What was the rationale for administering filgrastim and cyclophosphamide? What determines the duration of pheresis?

There is a low number of PBPCs in the peripheral circulation. Thus, mobilizing PBPC from the marrow compartment and increasing their numbers in the peripheral circulation is necessary to collect sufficient numbers of PBPCs for clinical use. Mobilization leads to collection of sufficient numbers of autologous PBPCs in most patients, although a minority of patients may still have poor mobilization.[21]

PBPCs are obtained by administering a mobilizing agent(s) followed by pheresis, which is an outpatient procedure similar to dialysis.[9] Hematopoietic growth factors (HGFs) alone or in combination with myelosuppressive chemotherapy are used to mobilize of PBPCs.[21] The HGF granulocyte-macrophage colony-stimulating factor (sargramostim) and granulocyte colony-stimulating (G-CSF) factor (filgrastim) are used as mobilizing agents for PBPC collection.[21,23] Both HGFs reliably mobilize PBPCs, with filgrastim providing a higher PBPC yield.[21] The most frequently used filgrastim doses for autologous PBPC mobilization are in the range of 10 to 24 mcg/kg/day SC.[21,23] This is a higher dose than used for prevention of neutropenia after standard chemotherapy. PBPC yield is higher when pheresis is started at day 5 (vs. day 6), with the optimal yield being around 10 hours after filgrastim administration.[21]

Myelosuppressive chemotherapy stimulates stem cell and progenitor cell proliferation. The combination of chemotherapy with filgrastim enhances PBPC mobilization relative to filgrastim alone.[21] The chemotherapy also treats the underlying malignancy, but increases the risk of neutropenia.[21] Examples of PBPC mobilization chemotherapy regimens include single-agent cyclophosphamide or melphalan. No mobilization chemotherapy regimen is clearly superior, which has led to incorporating PBPC mobilization into a cycle of disease-specific chemotherapy, such as using a single cycle of R-ICE (rituximab, ifosfamide, carboplatin, etoposide) therapy as the mobilization regimen for a NHL patient whose disease is responsive to R-ICE treatment.[21] By administering chemotherapy to the patient, the body's repair mechanism accelerates the cell division of stem cells and releases them into the circulation. This is a delicate balance, because the more chemotherapy that is given to mobilize the stem cells, the greater the potential for damage to the stem cells and a decreased yield at collection. Stem cell toxic agents, such as melphalan and carmustine, should be avoided because they lower the quantity and quality of PBPCs.[21] The HGF is initiated 24–72 hours after completion of chemotherapy. Pheresis begins when the peripheral WBC count recovers to greater than 1 to 3 $\times 10^3$ cells/μL.[21]

Plerixafor, a new inhibitor of the CXCR4 chemokine receptor, was approved by the US Food and Drug Administrations (FDAs) in 2008 for use in stem cell mobilization in conjunction with G-CSF. Inhibition of the CXCR4 blocks the ligand, chemokine SDF-1, from binding to the CXCR receptor. Because it can't bind to the CXCR4 receptor, the SDF-1 remains in blood circulation. SDF-1 is a chemoattractant agent for HSC; its presence in circulation causes rapid HSC migration to the peripheral blood.[21] In two randomized studies, 59% of NHL patients and 72% of multiple myeloma patients had sufficient $CD34^+$ cell collection for autologous transplant using plerixafor and G-CSF in four or fewer pheresis sessions, compared to 24% and 34%, respectively, in those using G-CSF alone.[24] $CD34^+$ cells are hematopoietic multipotent cells that express the CD34 antigen on their surface and are capable of self renewal. The function of the CD34 antigen is not fully understood. What is known is that it is an adhesion molecule involved in promoting the adherence of HSC to the bone marrow microenvironment as well as in the process of allowing T cells to enter lymph nodes. Plerixafor is administered to the patient approximately 11 hours prior to each pheresis beginning four days after initiation of daily G-CSF 10 mcg/kg. There is no consensus as to this agent's role in autologous transplant, though it will likely be used in patients whose cancer is resistant to chemotherapy mobilization and where G-CSF mobilization alone is insufficient.

Pheresis is continued daily until the target number of PBPCs per kilogram of the recipients' weight is obtained.[21] For adult recipients, the number of cells infused that express the CD34 antigen (i.e., $CD34^+$ cells) is the most reliable indicator of an adequate PBPC collection and predictor of durable engraftment.[21] The CD34 antigen is expressed on 1% to 4% of human marrow cells. It is expressed on virtually all unipotent and multipotent colony-forming cells and on precursors of colony-forming cells, but not on mature peripheral blood cells.[25] A variety of different thresholds have been identified as the minimal number of $CD34^+$ cells needed for an autologous PBPCT to produce rapid and complete (i.e., WBC, red blood cell [RBC], platelet) engraftment in adults. The minimum threshold range has varied from 1 to 3 $\times 10^6$ $CD34^+$ cells/kg of recipient weight, with more rapid platelet and neutrophil engraftment occurring with greater than or equal to 5 to 8 $\times 10^6$ $CD34^+$ cells/kg of recipient weight.[21]

There are a number of factors that can affect the yield of $CD34^+$ cells. The timing and amount of myelosuppressive treatments received prior to mobilization, both chemotherapy and radiation, negatively impact mobilization. The type of chemotherapy, number of different regimens, and overall duration of chemotherapy treatment affect the ability to collect stem cells. Additionally, hypocellular marrow and refractory disease can lead to a poor PBPC harvest.[21] There is a paucity of information regarding the parameters associated with engraftment in children undergoing an autologous PBPCT.[26] After pheresis, the cells are cryopreserved, stored, thawed, and infused into the patient as described in the Harvesting Autologous Hematopoietic Stem Cells section. Because P.J. has been in remission for a year after initial treatment for his disease, received no radiation treatment, and his salvage therapy did not contain alkylating agents, his cell collection can be expected to be good and of short duration.

Myeloablative Preparative Regimens

CASE 96-1, QUESTION 4: What are the goals and characteristics of agents used for myeloablative preparative regimens in patients like P.J.?

The primary goal of P.J.'s high-dose, myeloablative preparative regimen followed by autologous transplant is to eradicate residual malignancy that is not treatable with standard chemotherapy. With autologous HCT, there is no need for immunosuppression because the donor and recipient are genetically identical.[2] Combination chemotherapy with multiple alkylating agents constitutes the most common high-dose regimens before autologous HCT. Alkylating agents are used because they exhibit a steep dose–response curve for various malignancies to overcome resistance to treatment, and are characterized by dose-limiting bone marrow suppression.[3] Ideally, combinations of antineoplastics should have nonhematologic toxicities that do not overlap which are not life threatening. Examples of common myeloablative regimens are illustrated in Table 96-3.[27–31] The early and late toxicities to myeloablative regimens are listed in Table 96-4.

Complications of Autologous Hematopoietic Cell Transplantation

CASE 96-1, QUESTION 5: What complications must be anticipated as a consequence of autologous HCT? How can these be minimized? How can treatment be provided in an outpatient setting?

The most common cause of death after autologous HCT is the primary disease.

To view a pie chart that shows the autologous causes of death, go to http://thepoint.lww.com/AT10e.

Concerning toxicities are infection and organ failure, each occurring in less than 5% of patients. Because autologous HCT is not complicated by profound immunosuppression or GVHD, supportive care strategies differ from allogeneic HCT in the early and late recovery periods. Isolation and use of laminar air flow rooms are unnecessary, although many centers continue to provide care for patients undergoing autologous HCT in high-efficiency particulate air (HEPA) filtered rooms. The use of autologous PBSCT is associated with shorter periods of neutropenia and less need for clinical resources. Thus, some HCT centers have developed programs that incorporate outpatient care into the initial recovery; these programs also offer cost savings to the payer for health services.[32,33] Successful outpatient

TABLE 96-3
Representative Myeloablative Preparative Regimens Used in Hematopoietic Stem Cell Transplantation

Type of HCT	Disease State	Regimen	Dose/Schedule
Allogeneic[27]	Hematologic malignancies[a]	CY/TBI	CY 60 mg/kg/d IV on 2 consecutive days before TBI 1,000–1,575 rads fractionated for 1–7 days
Autologous[28,29,30]	Acute and chronic leukemias	BU/CY	BU adult 1 mg/kg/dose PO or 0.8 mg/kg/dose IV every 6 hours for 16 doses BU children <12 kg 1.1 mg/kg/dose IV every 6 hours for 16 doses CY 50 mg/kg/d IV daily for 4 days or 60 mg/kg/d IV daily for 2 days after BU
Autologous[31]	Non-Hodgkin lymphoma, Hodgkin disease	BEAM (carmustine/etoposide/cytarabine/melphalan)	Carmustine 300 mg/m^2/d IV, 1 dose Etoposide 200 mg/m^2/d BID IV for 3 days Cytarabine 100 mg/m^2/d IV BID for 4 days Melphalan 140 mg/m^2 1 dose

[a] Includes acute myelogenous leukemia, acute lymphocytic leukemia, chronic myelogenous leukemia, non-Hodgkin lymphoma, and Hodgkin disease.
BID, twice a day; BU, busulfan; CY, cyclophosphamide; IV, intravenously; PO, orally; TBI, total body irradiation.

care during administration of a myeloablative preparative regimen and the neutropenic period requires careful development and implementation of the necessary supportive care strategies to prevent or minimize infection, chemotherapy-induced nausea and vomiting (CINV), pain, and bleeding, along with admission criteria for more severe complications. This gives an example of an antiemetic order set for HCT recipients.

For an example of an antiemetic order set for HCT recipients, go to http://thepoint.lww.com/AT10e.

Use of prophylactic oral antibiotics and once-daily IV antibiotics to prevent or treat febrile neutropenia have facilitated outpatient care and prevented many patients from being hospitalized.[34]

For a table showing factors that favor a low risk for severe infection in neutropenic patients and a table regarding antibiotic use in neutropenic patients, go to http://thepoint.lww.com/AT10e.

TABLE 96-4
Common Toxicities Associated with Myeloablative Allogeneic Hematopoietic Stem Cell Transplantation

Early Posttransplant (<100 days)	Late Posttransplant (>100 days)
Febrile neutropenia	Increased susceptibility to infections
Nausea, vomiting, diarrhea	Endocrine disorders (hypothyroidism, hemorrhagic cystitis, infertility, growth retardation)
Mucositis	
Veno-occlusive disease	
Renal dysfunction	
Cardiotoxicity	Neurocognitive changes
Pneumonitis	Secondary malignant neoplasms
Graft rejection	Chronic GVHD
Acute GVHD	Cataracts

GVHD, graft-versus-host disease.

In addition, outpatient care during autologous HCT demands that HCT centers have appropriate resources, facilities, and staff to provide 24-hour patient care coverage. Patients undergoing outpatient care must meet eligibility criteria, including the availability of caregivers 24 hours a day and housing within close proximity to the HCT center.

Hematopoietic Growth Factors After Autologous Peripheral Blood Progenitor Cell Infusion

CASE 96-1, QUESTION 6: Ten days after the collection of PBPC, P.J. is admitted for his autologous BMT. He receives a myeloablative preparative regimen with cyclophosphamide, carmustine, and etoposide with an autologous PBPC graft. An order is written to begin filgrastim 5 mcg/kg/day SC, beginning on day 0 and continuing until the ANC has recovered to 500 cells/μL for 2 consecutive days. What is the rationale for filgrastim in P.J. after the transplant procedure?

Autologous HCTs, regardless of the stem cell source, are associated with profound aplasia due to the myeloablative preparative regimen (Table 96-3). Aplasia typically lasts 20 to 30 days after an autologous BMT and 7 to 14 days after an autologous PBPCT.[21] During this period of aplasia, patients are at high risk for complications such as bleeding and infection. Filgrastim and sargramostim exert their effects by stimulating the proliferation of committed progenitor cells, and, once engraftment occurs, hematopoietic recovery may be accelerated.

Several factors need to be considered when discussing the role of HGF in accelerating engraftment after HCT. First, the anatomical source of hematopoietic stem cells predicts the degree of benefit. The greatest benefit is enhanced neutrophil recovery and decreased use of associated resources in the setting of autologous BMT. The benefits of the HGF have been shown in several large multicenter, randomized, double-blind, placebo-controlled trials.[35–37] The majority of the trials suggest HGF administration is associated with a shorter time to neutrophil engraftment (by 4–7 days), less infectious complications, and shorter hospitalization after autologous BMT.[35,36,38] Survival is equivalent in those who received an HGF or a placebo.[35,37]

Although studies in the autologous PBPCT setting note more rapid neutrophil recovery after HGF use, others report no difference in infection rates and minimal decreases in associated resource use such as the duration of hospitalization.[36,38–40] In addition, sargramostim administration had no benefit (i.e., neutrophil and platelet engraftment) over placebo after autologous PBPCT in one trial.[41] Several large randomized trials have demonstrated that sargramostim in both autologous BMT and PBSCT had significant recovery of neutropil counts compared to placebo.[36,42,43] Although clinical practice guidelines for HGF support their use after autologous transplant, pharmacoeconomic analyses are needed to further evaluate the true benefit of HGFs after autologous PBPCT.

Filgrastim is preferred for accelerating neutrophil engraftment in clinical practice. The reason most commonly cited is the desire to avoid febrile reactions associated with sargramostim, which complicate interpretation of febrile neutropenia. Although sargramostim or filgrastim theoretically may stimulate proliferation of leukemia myeloblasts, no evidence to date suggests that the incidence of leukemia relapse is higher in patients who receive these HGFs after autologous or allogeneic HCT.[41,44] This may be due to the fact that patients with leukemia are usually in remission at the time of HCT. Thus, the population of residual leukemia cells is probably minimal.

Although both filgrastim and sargramostim successfully hasten neutrophil recovery, neither agent stimulates platelet production or augments platelet recovery.[35,36] This is an important consideration because thrombocytopenia is often a cause of prolonged hospitalization in the HCT patient. Successful engraftment of all hematopoietic stem cell lines will likely require combinations of growth factors that work in concert to augment hematopoiesis. However, epoetin alpha and interleukin (IL)-11 have only been used experimentally in the HCT patient. At this time, there is no established role for either agent in the care of these patients. In summary, P.J. is undergoing autologous PBPCT for the treatment of a lymphoid malignancy. Thus, either sargramostim or filgrastim is an acceptable option for accelerating engraftment. Whether the addition of either agent will reduce infection and improve other clinically relevant outcomes is debatable.[23] A complete blood cell (CBC) count with differential should be obtained daily. Filgrastim should be continued until neutrophil recovery is achieved.

ALLOGENEIC HEMATOPOIETIC STEM CELL TRANSPLANTATION

Allogeneic HCT involves the transplantation of hematopoietic stem cells obtained from a donor's bone marrow, PBPCs, or umbilical cord blood to a patient. Fifty-one percent (51%) of all transplants performed in North America in 2008 used unrelated donors.[1] Thus, to understand the application of and complications after allogeneic HCT, a working knowledge of immunology and the major histocompatibility complex (MHC) and human leukocyte antigen (HLA) in humans is necessary.

Indications for Allogeneic Hematopoietic Stem Cell Transplantation

CASE 96-2

QUESTION 1: B.S., a 22-year-old man, has AML in first remission after induction chemotherapy with standard doses of cytarabine and daunorubicin and consolidation with high-dose cytarabine. B.S. has poor risk cytogenetics, with abnormalities of 11q23 and inversion 3. Thus he will receive an allogeneic HCT as part of postremission therapy. HLA typing performed on family members has identified a fully HLA-matched sibling donor. B.S. returns to the clinic today for a pretransplantation workup. At this time, his physical examination is noncontributory. All laboratory values are within normal limits. A bone marrow biopsy reveals less than 5% blasts. B.S. has a normal electrocardiogram and cardiac wall motion study. His renal, hepatic, and pulmonary function tests are normal. Is an allogeneic HCT indicated for B.S.?

B.S. has a diagnosis of AML, which is one of the most common indications for allogeneic HCT.[2] The primary indications for allogeneic HCT include treatment of otherwise fatal diseases of the bone marrow or immune system (Table 96-2). The optimal role and timing of allogeneic HCT, in contrast to other therapies, remains controversial,[45] especially because treatment options for AML have increased. The National Comprehensive Cancer Network treatment guidelines for AML include the use of allogeneic HCT. A matched sibling or alternative donor (e.g., matched unrelated donor) HCT is recommended as part of postremission therapy in patients with preceding hematologic disease (e.g., myelodysplasia, secondary AML) or poor risk cytogenetics, as in the case of B.S.[46] Current research efforts focus on the use of reduced-intensity preparative regimens and the utility of HCT relative to novel targeted agents in the hope of improving the outcome of allogeneic HCT.[46] B.S. is eligible for allogeneic HCT by virtue of his cytogenetics and the availability of a histocompatible donor. In addition, he meets age and organ function eligibility requirements and is in complete remission with minimal residual disease.

Histocompatibility

CASE 96-2, QUESTION 2: Why is histocompatibility important in selection of the donor in patients like B.S. who undergo an allogeneic HCT?

Because the tissue transplanted in allogeneic HCT is immunologically active, there is potential for bidirectional graft rejection.[2] In the first scenario, cytotoxic T cells and NK cells belonging to the host (recipient) recognize MHC antigens of the graft (donor hematopoietic stem cells) and elicit a graft rejection response. This results in ineffective hematopoiesis (i.e., inadequate ANC and/or platelet counts) posttransplant. In the second scenario, immunologically active cells in the graft recognize host MHC antigens and elicit an immune response, referred to as GVHD. Therefore, an essential first step for patients eligible for HCT is finding an HLA-compatible graft with an acceptable risk of rejection and GVHD.

Graft rejection is least likely to occur with a syngeneic donor, meaning that the recipient and host are identical (monozygotic) twins. Identical twins occur spontaneously in nature in approximately 1 in 100 births; thus, it is unlikely that a patient would have a syngeneic donor. In those patients without a syngeneic donor, initial HLA typing is conducted on family members because the likelihood of a complete histocompatibility match between unrelated individuals is remote. Siblings are the most likely to be histocompatible within a family. However, only 25% of potential HCT recipients have an HLA-identical sibling.[47]

Determination of histocompatibility between potential donors and the patient is completed before allogeneic HCT.[48] Initially, HLA typing performed using blood samples and compatibility for class I MHC antigens (HLA-A, HLA-B, and HLA-C) is determined through serologic and DNA-based testing methods.[47] In vitro reactivity between donor and recipient can also be assessed in mixed lymphocyte culture, a test used to measure compatibility of the MHC class II antigens (HLA-DR, HLA-DP, HLA-DQ).[47] Currently, most clinical and research laboratories are also performing molecular DNA typing using polymerase chain reaction (PCR) methodology to determine the HLA allele sequence.[47] A donor–recipient pair with different HLA antigens (i.e., "antigen mismatched") always has different alleles, whereas pairs with the same allele always have the same antigen and are termed "matched." However, some pairs have the same HLA antigen but different alleles and are thus "allele mismatched."[49] (See Chapter 34, Kidney and Liver Transplantation, for additional discussion of histocompatibility.)

Lack of an HLA-matched sibling donor can be a barrier to allogeneic HCT. The use of alternative sources of allogeneic hematopoietic stem cells, such as related donors mismatched at one or more HLA loci, or phenotypically (i.e., serologically) matched unrelated donors are used.[50] Establishment of the National Marrow Donor Program has helped increase the pool of potential donors for allogeneic HCT.[50] Through this program, an HLA-matched unrelated volunteer donor might be identified. Recipients of an unrelated graft are more likely to experience graft failure and acute GVHD relative to recipients of a matched-sibling donor.[51] Thus, work is ongoing to identify factors that predict graft failure or GVHD to improve the availability and safety of unrelated donor transplants[52] (see Graft Rejection section).

The preparative regimen or GVHD prophylaxis with immune suppressant may be altered based on the mismatch between the donor and the recipient. The risk of graft failure decreases with better matches, and although mismatching in a single HLA allele does not appear to impact overall survival, mismatching in more than one allele significantly impairs overall survival, with the most important alleles to match being HLA-A, HLA-B, HLA-C, and HLA-DRB1.[53–55]

Eligibility criteria for allogeneic HCT vary between institutions. Having a matched sibling donor is no longer a requirement for allogeneic HCT, because improved immunosuppressive regimens and the National Marrow Donor Program have allowed an increase in the use of unrelated or related matched or mismatched HCT.[50] Potential donors also include haploidentical donors, who are a parent, sibling, or child of a parent with only one identical HLA haplotype. HCT with a haploidentical donor was initially associated with high rates of graft failure and GVHD, but recent technological advances have improved outcomes. Haploidentical HCT involves another alloreactive mechanism involving NK cells, which may be associated with reduced relapse rates in acute myelogenous leukemia (AML) patients.[2]

Normal renal, hepatic, pulmonary, and cardiac functions are necessary for eligibility at most centers. Historically, patients older than 55 years were excluded from allogeneic HCT because they were more likely to succumb to transplantation-related complications. However, many centers are now considering patients up to 65 years old and basing their selection criteria on physiological rather than biological age.

Harvesting, Preparing, and Transplanting Allogeneic Hematopoietic Stem Cells

CASE 96-2, QUESTION 3: What methods can be used to harvest hematopoietic stem cells from B.S.'s histocompatible sibling and prepare them for transplant? Are there any advantages to the use of bone marrow, PBPCs, or umbilical cord blood as a source for hematopoietic stem cells?

The method of harvesting allogeneic hematopoietic stem cells varies according to the site of harvest (i.e., bone marrow, peripheral blood, or umbilical cord blood). ABO incompatibility increases the complexity of HCT, but is not an obstacle to HCT. The hematopoietic stem cells may need additional processing to reduce the RBC infused with the HCT product if the donor and recipient are ABO incompatible, which occurs in 30% to 40% of sibling donor HCTs and is higher in unrelated donor HCT.[56] Various strategies posttransplant used to manage blood support for ABO-incompatible HCT recipients include the infusion of donor type fresh frozen plasma to provide a non-cellular source of A or B antigens, as well as transfusing type volume reduced RBCs and platelets or O RBCs to minimize the risk of immune-mediated hemolytic anemia and thrombotic microangiopathic syndromes.[56]

BONE MARROW

Harvesting bone marrow entails a surgical procedure in which marrow is obtained from the iliac crests. Allogeneic bone marrow is obtained from the donor under local or general anesthesia on day 0 of BMT.[2] The number of nucleated marrow cells harvested varies depending on disease being treated, conditioning regimen, and pre-infusion manipulation, and is usually 1 to 3×10^8 infused cells/kg of recipient weight.[26] These cells are obtained through multiple aspirations of marrow from the posterior iliac crests, processed to remove fat or marrow emboli and are usually immediately infused intravenously into the patient like a blood transfusion. If immediate transplant is not possible, the bone marrow is frozen until it can be infused. Once infused into circulation, through the mechanism of the chemokine SDF-1/CXCR4 receptor, the stem cells migrate to the bone marrow compartment where they will eventually reside. Bone marrow is the primary graft source for allogenic transplant in children, accounting for 60% of HCT in this population with PBPCs and cord blood accounting for the remainder. In adults, bone marrow accounts for less than 20% of stem cells in HCT.[1]

PERIPHERAL BLOOD PROGENITOR CELLS

Peripheral blood has replaced marrow for allogeneic HCT in adults.[2,57] Marrow stem cells continuously detach, enter the circulation, and return to the marrow; thus, the peripheral blood is a convenient source of hematopoietic stem cells. The number of PBPCs is estimated by using the cell surface molecule CD34 as a surrogate marker. The number of circulating $CD34^+$ cells in blood is increased by mobilizing them from the marrow. The most commonly used regimen to mobilize allogeneic (healthy) donors is a 4-day to 5-day course of filgrastim, 10 to 16 mcg/kg/day SC, followed by pheresis on the fourth or fifth day when peripheral blood levels of $CD34^+$ cells peak.[19] An adequate number of hematopoietic stem cells is usually obtained with one to two pheresis collections. The optimal number of $CD34^+$ required is 4 to 10×10^6 cells/kg of recipient body weight for a HLA identical sibling donor transplant with haploidentical transplants requiring greater numbers.[20,58,59] Higher cell doses have been associated with not only more rapid engraftment but also fewer fungal infections and improved overall survival.[60] Hematopoietic stem cells obtained from the peripheral blood are processed like bone marrow–derived stem cells and may be infused immediately into the recipient or frozen for future use. Allogeneic donation of PBPC has a similar level of physical discomfort to bone marrow donation; however, PBPC donation leads to quicker recovery.[58] The donor may experience musculoskeletal pain, headache, mild increases in hepatic enzyme or lactate dehydrogenase levels due to filgrastim administration, and hypocalcemia due to citrate accumulation, which decreases ionized calcium concentrations during pheresis.[61]

Compared to bone marrow, PBPC infusions are associated with quicker neutrophil and platelet engraftment.[2] In patients with a hematologic malignancy and a matched sibling donor, PBPCT is also associated with lower relapse rates and increased diseasefree survival rates.[62] However, PBPC grafts contain more T cells than do bone marrow grafts.[2] Therefore, PBPCT has a similar incidence of acute GVHD, but an approximately 20% higher incidence of extensive stage and overall chronic GVHD.[62]

UMBILICAL CORD BLOOD

Blood from the umbilical cord and the placenta is rich in hematopoietic stem cells but limited in volume.[63] Thus, UCT offers an alternative stem cell source to those patients who do not have a suitable related donor. After consent is obtained, the cord blood cells are obtained in the delivery room after birth and, typically after the delivery of the placenta.[64]

For a video that shows the harvesting and transplanting of cord cells, go to http://thepoint.lww.com/AT10e.

The cord blood is then processed, and if it matches certain pre-established criteria (e.g., minimum nucleated cell content, sterility) a sample is sent for HLA typing and cryopreserved for future use. An estimated 20,000 HCTs with cord blood donors have been performed, with more than 300,000 cord blood units banked worldwide. It is unclear how long cryopreserved cord blood is viable.[65]

HCT with an unrelated cord blood donor has several potential advantages over unrelated marrow or PBPC donors.[63] Specifically, (a) cord blood is readily available, which leads to a more rapid time to HCT; (b) lack of stem cell exposure to the thymus allows for greater degrees of HLA disparity as compared to bone marrow or PBPC, making it easier to find a graft in particular for patients with rare haplotypes[64]; and (c) despite the less stringent HLA matching, mismatched cord blood cells are less likely to cause GVHD while still maintaining GVT activity. The less stringent HLA requirements also increase the likelihood of identifying a suitable allogeneic donor, which is particularly beneficial for minority populations who are underrepresented in adult registries and often lack matched stem cell sources. Outcomes in umbilical cord blood recipients are improved with fewer HLA mismatches and greater numbers of $CD34^+$ cells.[66] However, the limited number of hematopoietic stem cells in cord blood is a disadvantage in particular when considering adult patients.[67] In order to overcome the cell dose limitation and improve engraftment, researchers have been studying combining two cord blood units in graft,[68] co-infuse a cord blood unit with highly purified $CD34^+$ cells from haploidentical donors,[69] and ex vivo expansion of cord blood progenitors,[70] delivery of the cord blood unit directly into the bone marrow space,[71,72] and priming of cord blood with agents that may facilitate homing to the bone marrow.[73]

Retrospective and prospective data have shown that UCT from a related or unrelated donor is effective in children with cancer and nonmalignant conditions.[74–78] Neutrophil and platelet engraftment is slower in UCT, with a lower risk of acute and chronic GVHD and similar survival rates relative to a BMT. In children with acute leukemia cord blood yields similar outcomes as unrelated bone marrow and has become part of the standard of care in many centers.[74]

As an adequate cell dose is critical for engraftment after cord blood transplantation and the cell dose of a single cord blood unit is limited, progress in the field of cord blood transplantation for the treatment of adults has been slower.[67] However, recent data showed that when a single cord blood unit with an adequate cell dose is available, the outcomes of adults with leukemia are similar to those with receiving unrelated bone marrow or peripheral blood grafts.[79] Moreover, for those adults with leukemia who do not have a single cord blood unit with a suitable cell dose, the use of two partially matched cord blood units to compose the graft also provides outcomes similar to that of related and unrelated donors.[80] These data associated with the promising outcomes when using UCB in the context of reduced-intensity conditioning has significantly increased the utilization of cord blood as a source of hematopoietic progenitors for the treatment of adult patients.[81,82]

In summary, the utilization of cord blood as a source of hematopoietic stem cells for transplantation has substantially expanded in the last decade. Novel methodologies to improve engraftment, promote immune reconstitution, and improve outcomes after cord blood transplantation are under investigation and are likely to further extend its availability to patients who require a potentially curative allogeneic transplant but lack a suitable related donor.

Therefore, it is most reasonable to harvest PBPCs from B.S.'s sibling to use for his myeloablative HCT because his sibling is fully HLA-matched. A PBPC transplant is preferred to BMT due to the expectations of increased speed of neutrophil and platelet engraftment and disease-free survival rate and lower relapse rate.

Graft-versus-Tumor Effect

CASE 96-2, QUESTION 4: What is the GVT effect? Which tumors are most responsive to this effect?

GVT refers to the phenomonon where the donor's cytotoxic T lymphocytes suppress or eliminate the recipient's malignancy. Initial clinical evidence of a GVT effect came from the observation that patients with GVHD had lower relapse rates compared with those who did not.[83,84] This suggested a GVT effect due to the donor lymphocytes. Lymphocyte involvement in GVT was further supported by the effectiveness of donor lymphocyte infusions in treating patients who experienced relapse of their malignancies after allogeneic HCT.[85,86] Eradication of the recurrent malignancy is due to either specific targeting of the tumor antigens or to GVHD, which may affect cancer cells preferentially. Different illnesses vary in their responsiveness to donor lymphocyte infusions, with chronic myelogenous leukemia (CML) and acute leukemias being the most and least responsive, respectively.[87] Patients with certain solid tumors (e.g., renal cell carcinoma) also appear to benefit from a GVT effect.[88] These data gave rise to the use of reduced-intensity and nonmyeloablative preparative regimens, which rely on the GVT effect.

Preparative Regimens for Allogeneic Hematopoietic Stem Cell Transplantation

MYELOABLATIVE PREPARATIVE REGIMENS

CASE 96-2, QUESTION 5: What is the rationale for using myeloablative preparative regimens for patients like B.S. who are to receive an allogeneic HCT? What types of regimens are used, and what is recommended for B.S.?

The combination of chemotherapy and/or radiation used in allogeneic HCT is referred to as the preparative or conditioning regimen. The rationale for high-dose myeloablative preparative regimens is similar to that discussed in the Autologous Hematopoietic Stem Cell Transplantation section. Specifically, infusion of hematopoietic stem cells restores hematopoiesis induced by dose-limiting myelosuppression of chemotherapy, maximizing the potential value of the steep dose–response curve to alkylating agents and radiation,[3] and suppressing the host immune system. The preparative regimen is designed to eradicate immunologically active host tissues (lymphoid tissue and macrophages) and to prevent or minimize the development of host-versus-graft reactions. In contrast, a myeloablative preparative regimen may not be necessary if a histocompatible allogeneic HCT is performed on a patient with a poorly functioning immune system (e.g., severe combined immunodeficiency disease).[89] In the absence of a functioning immune system, the likelihood of a host-versus-graft reaction to histocompatible donor hematopoietic stem cells is small. Similarly, patients undergoing syngeneic transplantation do not require immunosuppressive preparative regimens before HCT because the donor and the patient are genetically identical. Thus, the preparative regimen is tailored to the primary disease and to HLA compatibility between the recipient–donor pair.

Examples of common preparative regimens for allogeneic HCT are shown in Table 96-3.[18,28,90] Table 96-4 lists the common toxicities associated with myeloablative allogeneic HCT. Most allogeneic preparative regimens for the treatment of hematologic malignancies contain cyclophosphamide, radiation, or both. The combination of cyclophosphamide and total body irradiation (TBI) was one of the first preparative regimens used, and it is still used widely today. This regimen is immunosuppressive and has inherent activity against hematologic malignancies (e.g., leukemias, lymphomas). TBI is myeloablative and immunosuppressive, does not have cross-resistance to chemotherapy, and also reaches sites not affected by chemotherapy (e.g., the central nervous system).[2] Toxicity to TBI is considerable and although fractionating its dose reduces toxicity, research is ongoing to identify newer methods of selective radiation with increased specificity.[2] The toxicity of TBI and the scarcity of facilities for its delivery have led to the development of radiationfree preparative regimens. Modifications of the cyclophosphamide-TBI preparative regimen include replacing TBI with other agents (e.g., busulfan) and adding other chemotherapeutic or monoclonal agents such as alemtuzumab to the existing regimen. These measures are designed to minimize the long-term toxicities associated with TBI (e.g., growth retardation in children, cataracts) or to provide additional antitumor activity. In the case of a mismatched allogeneic HCT with an increased chance of graft rejection, antithymocyte globulin (ATG) may also be added to the preparative regimen to further immunosuppress the recipient.

The optimal myeloablative preparative regimen for allogeneic HCT is challenging to study because several indications for HCT (e.g., thalassemia, Fanconi anemia) are so infrequent that it is infeasible or cost-prohibitive to conduct clinical trials adequately powered to detect clinically relevant differences. However, the long-term outcomes of busulfan/cyclophosphamide (BU/CY) and CY/TBI in patients with AML and CML have been compared in a meta-analysis of four clinical trials.[91] Equivalent rates of long-term complications were present between the two preparative regimens, except for a greater risk of cataracts with CY/TBI and alopecia with BU/CY. Overall and diseasefree survival rates were similar in patients with CML, although there was a trend for improved diseasefree survival with CY/TBI in AML patients.

Based on these data, the CY/TBI preparative regimen is preferred for B.S. because he has AML with poor cytogenetics and has a matched sibling available. Because of the high relapse rates seen in AML, myeloablative allogeneic transplant is indicated in first remission for patients less than 60 years old with good performance status due to the decrease in likelihood of achieving a complete response to reinduction chemotherapy and the expected reduced duration of a second remisison.

REDUCED-INTENSITY OR NONMYELOABLATIVE PREPARATIVE REGIMENS

CASE 96-2, QUESTION 6: Describe the rationale for nonmyeloablative preparative regimens. Is B.S. a candidate for such a regimen?

The regimen-related toxicity of a myeloablative preparative regimen (Table 96-4) limits the use of allogeneic HCT to younger patients who have minimal comorbidities. Because many patients with hematologic malignancies are older, myeloablative HCT cannot be offered to a substantial portion of patients.[92] An improved understanding of the GVT effect led to the development of strongly immunosuppressive but not myeloablative (i.e., a reduced-intensity or nonmyeloablative) preparative regimens.[2] Now, reduced-intensity preparative regimens account for 30% of allogeneic transplants.[57] More than 60% of patients receiving reduced-intensity preparative regimens are older than 50 years.[1,57]

There is a wide spectrum of reduced-intensity preparative regimens, with the nonmyeloablative regimens causing the least amount of myelosuppression. In general, more intensive preparative regimens are required for engraftment in the setting of unrelated donor or HLA-mismatched related HCT.[93] Reduced-intensity regimens do not completely eliminate the host's normal hematologic and malignant cells and therefore depend on the GVT effect to eradicate remaining cancer. Thus, these preparative regimens may be preferable in those malignancies in which immunologic elimination of the malignant stem cells is possible.[2] The newly transplanted donor cells slowly replace host hematopoiesis, and elicit GVT effects.[88] After engraftment, mixed chimerism is generally present as evidenced by the ability to detect both donor-derived and recipient-derived hematopoietic cells. If the graft is rejected, typically only recipient cells are present. After a reduced-intensity preparative regimen, mixed chimerism (defined as 5%–95% donor T cells present in the peripheral blood) between the host and recipient develops, allowing for a GVT effect as the primary form of therapy. Chimerism is evaluated to monitor disease response and engraftment posttransplant. Chimerism is assessed within T cells and granulocytes in the peripheral blood and bone marrow using conventional (e.g., using sex chromosomes for opposite sex donors) and molecular (e.g., variable number of tandem repeats for same sex donors) methods. The methods used to characterize chimerism after HCT are reviewed elsewhere.[94–96] A few months after HCT, donor lymphocytes can be infused (called a "donor lymphocyte infusion") to augment the GVT activity.[2] The use of donor lymphocyte infusions is dependant on the availability of the donor and is highly center specific. The challenge is to maximize the GVT effect while minimizing the risk of GVHD. Therefore, GVHD prophylaxis, although different from that used with myeloablative regimens, is still necessary to minimize GVHD.

Reduced-intensity preparative regimens lead to lower treatment-related mortality rates, but they may be offset by higher relapse rates.[97] Slow-growing cancers (e.g., chronic lymphocytic leukemia) appear to be most susceptible to the GVT effect.[2] The safety and efficacy of these regimens have led to their wider application to nonmalignant conditions.[2] Because most of the data for reduced-intensity preparative regimens are derived from older patients or those with comorbid conditions, they cannot be compared with data for myeloablative preparative regimens.[97] It is unclear if reduced-intensity preparative regimens improve long-term survival of patients with malignant or nonmalignant diseases who are younger or without comorbid conditions. Prospective controlled trials are needed with stratification based on comorbidities, disease characteristics, pretransplant therapy, and hematopoietic stem cell source.[97]

There is a paucity of data regarding the optimal source of hematopoietic stem cells after reduced-intensity preparative regimens. Most case series have combined data from PBPC and marrow grafts. But some data suggest that, compared to bone marrow grafts, PBPC is associated with quicker engraftment, earlier T-cell chimerism, longer progression-free survival, and a lower risk of graft rejection.[98,99]

B.S. is young and healthy enough to receive a myeloablative allogeneic HCT. Presently, reduced-intensity HCT is only indicated as first-line therapy for patients ineligible for myeloablative regimens due to age, extensive prior treatments, or other contraindications. It is not an option for B.S.

Posttransplantation Immunosuppressive Therapy

CASE 96-2, QUESTION 7: What is the rationale for immunosuppressive therapy after an allogeneic HCT? What is recommended for B.S.?

After infusion of hematopoietic stem cells, immunosuppressive therapy is administered to prevent or minimize GVHD. Patients receiving syngeneic transplants or a T-cell–depleted histocompatible allogeneic transplant generally do not receive posttransplantation immunosuppressive therapy. In syngeneic transplantation, the donor and the patient are genetically identical, and GVHD should not be elicited. In T-cell depleted transplantation, the volume of donor T cells infused into the patient is usually insufficient to elicit a significant graft-versus-host reaction.[85,100] Numerous immunosuppressive agents given alone or in combination have been evaluated for the prevention of GVHD. Commonly used regimens after myeloablative HCT include cyclosporine or tacrolimus administered with a short course of low-dose methotrexate.[101] GVHD prophylaxis varies in reduced-intensity protocols and doses can be found at (Table 96-5).[102] Corticosteroids may also be used to prevent GVHD, but they are more commonly used to treat GVHD. In allogeneic HCT recipients without GVHD, immunosuppressive therapy is slowly tapered and discontinued over the course of 6 months to 1 year because of immunologic tolerance. Over time, the immunologically active tissue between host and recipient become tolerant of one another and cease recognizing the other as foreign. In contrast, solid organ transplant recipients usually continue immunosuppressive therapy for the duration of the recipient's life.

B.S. is receiving a myeloablative preparative regimen with allogeneic transplant and will receive cyclosporine administered for 6 months, followed by a taper, with a short course of methotrexate 15 mg/m^2 on day +1 and 10 mg/m^2 on day +3, +6, and +11 for posttransplantation immunosuppression. This combination regimen will lower the risk of GVHD. Assuming B.S. does not experience any serious complications, he will likely be immune suppressant free by 9 months posttransplant. The cyclosporine will require therapeutic drug monitoring.

TABLE 96-5

Common Reduced Intensity Preparative or Nonmyeloablative Regimens and Post Grafting Immunosuppresion[102]

Preparative Regimens	Postgrafting Immunosuppression
Fludarabine 30 mg/m^2/d IV on 3 consecutive days (−4, −3, −2), TBI 2 Gy as single fraction on day 0	Cyclosporine 6.25 mg/kg PO BID, days −3 to day +100 with taper from day +100 to +180
Fludarabine 25 mg/m^2/d IV for 5 days and melphalan 90 mg/m^2/d IV for 2 days	Mycophenolate mofetil 15 mg/kg PO BID or TID, day +0 to +40 with taper from day +40 to +90
Fludarabine 25–30 mg/m^2/d IV for 3–5 days, busulfan ≤9 mg/kg/total dose	Tacrolimus to maintain trough blood concentration of 5–10 ng/mL with methotrexate 5 mg/m^2/d IV days +1, +3, +6, +11

BID, twice a day; IV, intravenous; PO, orally; TBI, total body irradiation; TID, three times a day.

COMPARISON OF SUPPORTIVE CARE STRATEGIES BETWEEN AUTOLOGOUS AND ALLOGENEIC MYELOABLATIVE HEMATOPOIETIC STEM CELL TRANSPLANTATION

CASE 96-2, QUESTION 8: How do supportive care strategies used for myeloablative preparative regimens with an autologous graft differ from an allogeneic graft? What supportive care will B.S. likely require?

Supportive care strategies common to patients receiving a myeloablative preparative regimen, regardless of whether they have received an autologous or allogeneic HCT, include use of indwelling central venous catheters; blood product support; and pharmacologic management of CINV, mucositis, and pain. These similarities are a function of the side effects of a myeloablative preparative regimen.

Because of the different needs for immunosuppression with an autologous and allogeneic HCT, the supportive care differs. Allogeneic HCT patients experience an initial period of pancytopenia followed by a more prolonged period of immunosuppression, which substantially increases the risk of bacterial infections, but more importantly, fungal, viral, and other opportunistic infections.[8] The risk of infection increases as additional immunosuppressive therapy is incorporated to prevent or treat GVHD. Supportive strategies designed to minimize infection during immunosuppression are essential after allogeneic HCT (see Infectious Complications section).

B.S. received a myeloablative allogeneic transplant; therefore, he will have a central venous catheter inserted at admission. He will most likely require multiple RBC and platelet transfusions until hematopoiesis of donor erythrocytes and thrombocytes occurs. He is at increased risk of infection because he will be myelosuppressed for months after the transplant. Also, if he were to aquire GVHD, additional supportive care would be required. GVHD prophylaxis with cyclosporine and methotrexate will place him at risk for additional drug-related toxicities that will require monitoring. Had he received an autologous transplant the duration of neutropenia would be less, no immunosuppressive medications would be required, and the risk of developing complications from GVHD would have been avoided.

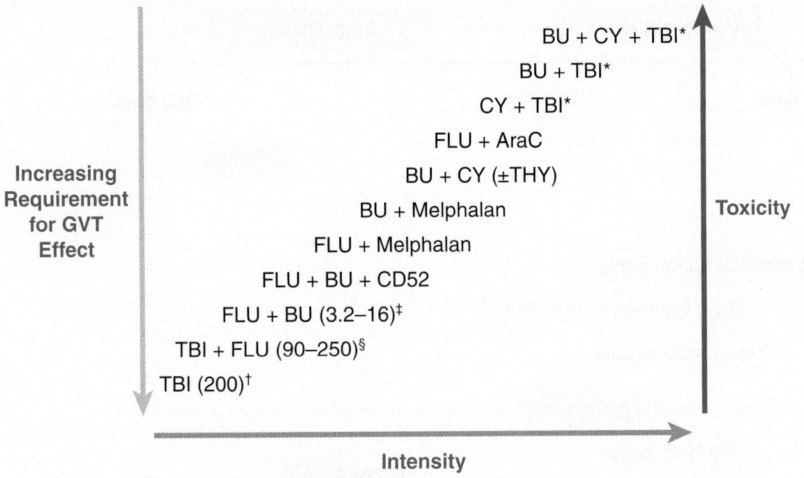

FIGURE 96-2 Partial spectrum of preparative regimens of various intensities, their impact on toxicity, and their dependance on graft-versus-tumor (GVT) effects for success of hematopoietic stem cell transplantation. AraC, cytarabine; BU, busulfan; CD52, anti-CD52 antibody (alemtuzumab); CY, cyclophosphamide; FLU, fludarabine; TBI, total body irradiation; THY, thymoglobulin. *TBI >1,200 cGy; †200 cGy; ‡3.2–16 mg/kg; §90–250 mg/m^2. (Adapted with permission from Deeg HJ et al. Optimization of allogeneic transplant conditioning: not the time for dogma. *Leukemia*. 2006;20:1701.)

COMPARISON OF SUPPORTIVE CARE STRATEGIES BETWEEN ALLOGENEIC MYELOABLATIVE AND NONMYELOABLATIVE HEMATOPOIETIC STEM CELL TRANSPLANTATION

CASE 96-2, QUESTION 9: How do supportive care strategies used for myeloablative and nonmyeloablative preparative regimens with an allogeneic graft differ?

Nonmyeloablative HCT is the least myelosuppressive reduced-intensity regimen (Fig. 96-2). A direct comparison of the toxicities with a myeloablative and nonmyeloablative preparative regimen is difficult because the latter is offered only to patients who are not candidates for myeloablative allogeneic HCT. These preparative regimens differ substantially in terms of the chemotherapy agents used (Tables 96-3 and 96-5) and the degree of myelosuppression. Nonmyeloablative HCT may have a different time pattern for infectious complications but there is a similar incidence and severity of acute GVHD. Nevertheless, comparisons between the preparative regimens are challenging because of the differences in the pre-HCT health of the recipients.[93] Clinical research is focusing on designing optimal preparative regimens with acceptable efficacy and toxicity (i.e., mixed chimerism, disease response). Thus, relative to myeloablative HCT, the preparative regimens and immunosuppression used after graft infusion are more variable for reduced-intensity or nonmyeloablative HCT (Table 96-5).

COMPLICATIONS ASSOCIATED WITH HEMATOPOIETIC STEM CELL TRANSPLANTATION

CASE 96-3

QUESTION 1: K.M. is a 36-year-old woman with CML in accelerated phase. After her initial diagnosis, a successful search for an unrelated 6/6 HLA-matched allogeneic donor was conducted. K.M. is being admitted for myeloablative allogeneic PBPCT. Orders for K.M.'s preparative regimen are written as follows: busulfan, 16 mg/kg total dose to be administered for 4 days (1 mg/kg per dose orally [PO] every 6 hours for 16 doses, days −7, −6, −5, and −4). Cyclophosphamide 60 mg/kg/day IV to be administered on days −3 and −2. Day −1 is a "rest" day, followed by infusion of PBPC on day 0. What toxicities associated with myeloablative preparative regimen should be anticipated in K.M.? Are they similar to those anticipated after standard-dose chemotherapy?

Myelosuppression is a frequent dose-limiting toxicity for antineoplastics when administered in conventional doses used to treat cancer. However, because myelosuppression is circumvented with hematopoietic rescue in the case of patients receiving HCT, the dose-limiting toxicities of these myeloablative preparative regimens are nonhematologic (i.e., extramedullary) in nature. The toxicities vary with the preparative regimen used. Most patients undergoing HCT experience toxicities commonly associated with chemotherapy, such as alopecia, mucositis, CINV, infertility, and pulmonary toxicity (see Chapter 90, Adverse Effects of Chemotherapy and Targeted Agents). However, these drug-related toxicities are magnified in the HCT population.

Table 96-4 depicts a range of toxicities that can occur after myeloablative preparative regimen for HCT, and Figure 96-3 depicts the time course for complications after HCT. Selected toxicities are discussed in the following sections.

Busulfan Seizures

CASE 96-3, QUESTION 2: In addition to her preparative regimen, the following supportive care agents and monitoring parameters are prescribed for K.M.: On the day of admission (day −8), administer levetiracetam 500 mg PO twice daily from days −8 to −3. Busulfan pharmacokinetic blood sampling is to occur after dose 1 to a target busulfan concentration at steady state (C_{SS}) greater than 900 ng/mL. Begin normal saline hydration 3,000 mL/m^2/day 4 hours before cyclophosphamide and continue for 24 hours after the last cyclophosphamide dose. Mesna is to be given concurrently with cyclophosphamide as 10% of the cyclophosphamide dose administered intravenously 30 minutes before starting the cyclophosphamide dose, then as 100% of cyclophosphamide dose administered as a continuous IV infusion for 24 hours after each dose of cyclophosphamide. Beginning on day −5, weigh patient twice daily, check fluid input and urinary output every 4 hours, and monitor urine for RBCs daily until 24 hours after the last cyclophosphamide dose. If urine output drops below

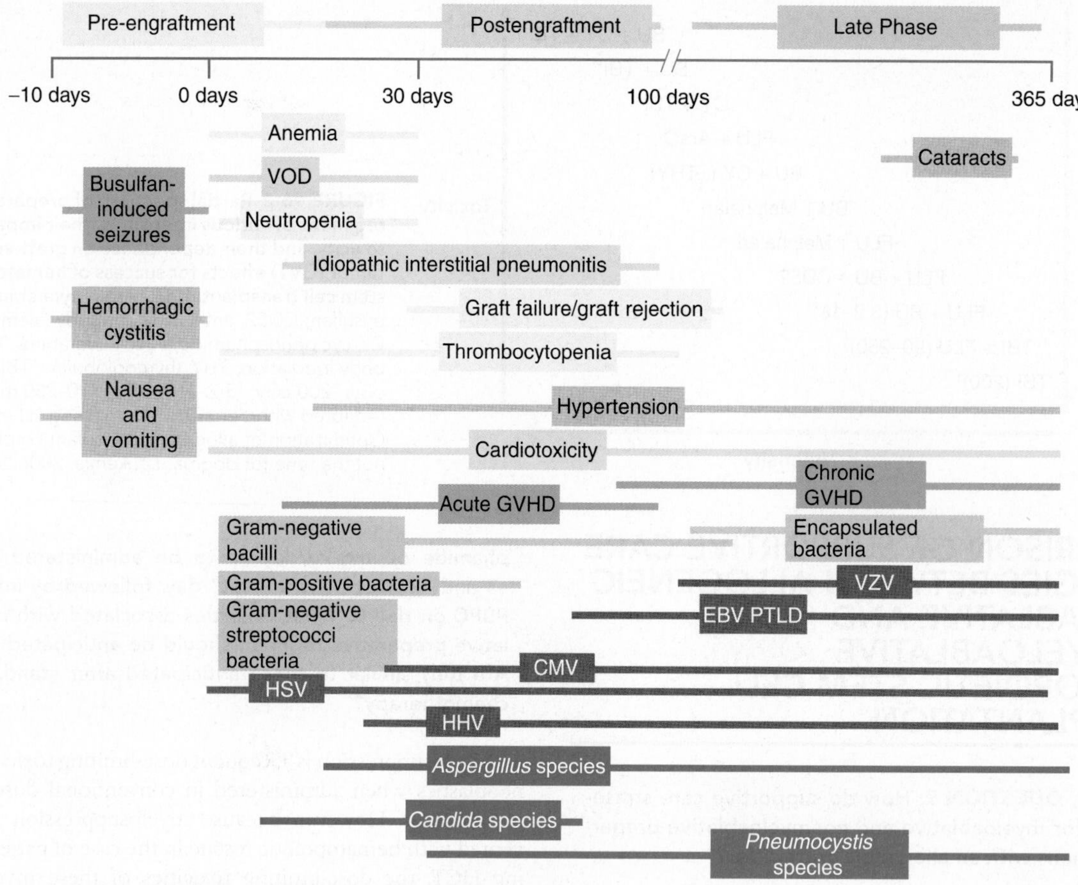

FIGURE 96-3 Complications after hematopoietic stem cell transplantation (HCT) by time for patients undergoing myeloablative allogeneic HCT only. CMV, cytomegalovirus; EBV, Epstein-Barr virus; GVHD, graft-versus-host disease; HHV, human herpes virus; HSV, herpes simplex virus; PTLD, posttransplantation lymphoproliferative disease; VOD, veno-occlusive disease; VZV, varicella-zoster virus.

300 mL for 2 hours, administer an IV bolus of 250 mL normal saline and give furosemide 10 mg/m², not to exceed 20 mg IV. What is the rationale for these supportive care therapies and monitoring parameters prescribed for K.M. as they relate to busulfan therapy?

Seizures occur in approximately 10% of patients receiving high-dose busulfan for HCT preparative regimens. Busulfan is highly lipophilic and readily crosses the blood–brain barrier with an average cerebrospinal fluid : plasma ratio of 1 or higher. Seizures are probably a direct neurotoxic effect,[103] therefore seizure prophylaxis is used. Many HCT centers have moved from phenytoin to levetiracetam for seizure prophylaxis, although benzodiazepines (e.g., lorazepam or clonazepam) also have been used.[104] Seizure prophylaxis is started at least 12 hours before the first busulfan dose and is usually discontinued 24 to 48 hours after administering the last busulfan dose. Seizures can occur despite the use of seizure prophylaxis, but they usually do not result in permanent neurologic deficits.

Adaptive Dosing of Busulfan

CASE 96-3, QUESTION 3: What dosing strategies can be used to minimize busulfan toxicities?

Wide interpatient variability in the clearance of both oral and IV busulfan, along with the identified concentration–effect relationships, has led to adaptive dosing of busulfan. The clearance of IV busulfan adjusted for weight exhibited interpatient variability with a coefficient of variation (standard deviation/mean) of 25% in 59 patients.[29] Oral busulfan exhibited a similar coefficient of variation of 21% in 279 adult patients.[105] Weight, disease, and age are factors that may influence the clearance of oral busulfan.[105]

In patients receiving BU/CY, adaptive dosing of busulfan to achieve a target plasma level minimizes veno-occlusive disease (VOD), while improving engraftment and relapse rates.[30,106–107] The pharmacodynamic relationships are briefly reviewed here; however, more complete reviews of these relationships after oral busulfan administration are available elsewhere.[108,109] When reviewing pharmacodynamic data for busulfan, close attention should be paid to their interpretation because of the potential changes in the concentration–effect relationships between busulfan C_{SS} and outcome in each patient population and for each preparative regimen. Most studies have shown a pharmacodynamic relationship in patients receiving the BU/CY preparative regimens. One must also pay close attention to the units used in these studies. Data are represented as area under the plasma concentration time curve (AUC) or C_{SS}. AUC data are easily converted to C_{SS} (C_{SS} = AUC/dosing interval). Results are expressed as μM-minute or ng/mL; an AUC of 1,500 μM-minute is roughly equivalent to a C_{SS} of 1,025 ng/mL based on busulfan's molecular weight of 246.

Hepatic VOD was observed more frequently in patients receiving BU/CY with a busulfan C_{SS} greater than 925 to 1,025 ng/mL. In BU/CY regimens, busulfan C_{SS} greater than 600 ng/mL favors engraftment, although contradictory data exist. Higher busulfan concentrations (C_{SS} >900 ng/mL) were associated with lower relapse rates in adult CML patients receiving BU/CY before HLA-matched grafts, with acceptable rates of VOD. Thus, a busulfan C_{SS} greater than 900 ng/mL is targeted for K.M. because she has CML.

IV busulfan is commonly used in combination with cyclophosphamide as a preparative regimen before allogeneic HCT for CML. The FDA-approved dose is 0.8 mg/kg IV every 6 hours for 16 doses, which is similar to the oral busulfan dose of 1 mg/kg with assuming a fraction absorbed of 90%.[110] IV busulfan, at 0.8 mg/kg of actual body weight or 29 mg/m^2 of body surface area produces an average AUC of 1,200 μM-minute, within a wide range of 900 to 1,500 μM-minute in 80% of patients.[111] The product labeling states "high busulfan AUC values (>1,500 μM-minute) may be associated with an increased risk of developing hepatic VOD," which has resulted in many HCT centers instituting adaptive dosing of IV busulfan to achieve an AUC commonly between 900 to 1,350 μM-minute after the first dose to minimize VOD and graft failure and maximize disease recurrence.[112] (See Case 96-3, Questions 7–9 for information on VOD.)

To minimize adverse events from IV busulfan, an AUC is obtained with the first dose of busulfan to analyze K.M.'s exposure. Samples are drawn at the end of the 2-hour infusion, then 1, 2, and 4 hours after the first sample. Many centers are not capable of analyzing IV busulfan levels; therefore, prior arrangements must be made for timely analysis of these samples in order to adjust the dose after the second or third dose if needed. K.M.'s AUC comes back 12 hours later at 1,225 μM-minute and, therefore, her dose is not changed. Had the AUC been greater than 1,350 μM-minute; her dose could have been adjusted using the following formula: Adjusted dose (mg) = Actual Dose (mg) × Target AUC (μM · min)/Actual AUC (μM · min)

Hemorrhagic Cystitis

CASE 96-3, QUESTION 4: What is the rationale for these supportive care therapies and monitoring parameters prescribed for K.M. as they relate to cyclophosphamide therapy?

In HCT patients receiving cyclophosphamide, moderate to severe hemorrhagic cystitis occurs in 4% to 20% of patients receiving hydration alone.[113] The putative bladder toxin is acrolein, a metabolite of cyclophosphamide.[114] Mesna donates free thiol groups to bind acrolein. American Society of Clinical Oncology (ASCO) Guidelines for the Use of Chemotherapy and Radiotherapy Protectants recommends the use of mesna plus saline diuresis or forced saline diuresis to lower the incidence of urothelial toxicity with high-dose cyclophosphamide in the setting of HCT.[115] It is important to note that hematuria or hemorrhagic cystitis can occur despite the use of any of these methods.

The optimal mesna dose with high-dose cyclophosphamide in preparation for myeloablative HCT is unknown. A variety of different regimens have been used, including intermittent bolus dosing (mesna dose 20%–40% of cyclophosphamide dose, administered for up to five doses) or continuous infusion regimens (mesna dose 80%–160% of cyclophosphamide dose).[113,116,117] Mesna should be continued for 24 to 48 hours after the last cyclophosphamide dose, such that mesna is present within the bladder to donate free thiol groups at the same time as the urotoxic metabolite acrolein. After IV administration of mesna, most of it (i.e., 60%–100%) is excreted within the urine over the course of 4 hours.[118] Cyclophosphamide has an average half-life of 7 hours after administration of 60 mg/kg,[119] and acrolein may be present within the urine for 24 to 48 hours after cyclophosphamide administration.[120]

Thus, K.M. is receiving hydration with normal saline and mesna, administered as a continuous infusion, to minimize her risk of hemorrhagic cystitis due to cyclophosphamide. K.M. should be monitored for any RBCs present in the urine, along with her urinary output, to allow for rapid intervention if hemorrhagic cystitis occurs.

Chemotherapy-Induced Gastrointestinal Effects

CASE 96-3, QUESTION 5: What other end-organ toxicities must be watched for? Should any medications be ordered for K.M. to prevent and treat the gastrointestinal (GI) effects associated with myeloablative therapy?

Preparative regimens for myeloablative HCT result in other end-organ toxicities, such as renal failure[121] and idiopathic pneumonia syndrome.[122] Lung injury post HCT has a mortality rate greater than 60%. Risk factors include TBI, allogeneic HCT, and acute GVHD, which suggest that donor lymphocytes target the lung.[123] Tumor necrosis factor, induced by GVHD and damage to the intestinal mucosa, contributes to lung injury by promoting the release of inflammatory cytokines which can travel through circulation to the lungs. Lung injury may be decreased by prompt treatment with etanercept (which inhibits tumor necrosis factor) and corticosteroids.[2]

The preparative regimen causes most patients to be nauseated and anorexic until day +10 to +15. CINV in HCT recipients can be due to highly emetogenic chemotherapy agents (see Chapter 6, Nausea and Vomiting), TBI administration, and poor control of CINV prior to HCT. Thus, patients such as K.M. who are undergoing a myeloablative HCT should be given prophylaxis with a serotonin antagonist plus a corticosteroid.[124]

ONLINE CONTENT

For a table of serotonin antagonists daily prior to preparative regimen chemotherapy, go to http://thepoint.lww.com/AT10e.

ASCO guidelines state that the use of the neurokinin receptor 1 antagonist, aprepitant, should be considered, although evidence to support its use in HCT patients is lacking.[124] Because aprepitant is a moderate inhibitor of cytochrome P-450 3A4, it may theoretically interact with the preparative regimen especially cyclophosphamide. Well-controlled studies evaluating its efficacy, along with its potential for causing drug interactions, are needed.[124] The serotonin antagonist ondansetron may increase cyclophosphamide clearance in breast cancer patients undergoing a myeloablative HCT[125,126]; however, further work is needed to identify the clinical implications of this finding because, to date, cyclophosphamide concentrations have not been consistently associated with clinical outcomes in patients undergoing a myeloablative HCT.[110,27]

Most patients receiving a myeloablative preparative regimen experience mucositis due to its effects on rapidly dividing cells of the oral epithelium. The use of methotrexate, as GVHD prophylaxis, also contributes to mucositis.[127] Oral mucositis causes nausea and anorexia. (For a picture of mucositis and other dental and oral complications of cancer treatment, go to **http://www.oralcancerfoundation.org/dental/dental-complications.htm.**)

In severe cases, parenteral opioid analgesics for pain relief[128] and total parenteral nutrition to prevent the development of nutritional deficits may be needed. Because mucositis can be worsened by superinfection, good oral hygiene should be practiced. Soft toothbrushes should be used and replaced often.[129] Oral mucositis can be decreased with the use of recombinant human keratinocyte growth factor palifermin. The Multinational Association of Supportive Care in Cancer and International Society for Oral Oncology Guidelines recommend palifermin to prevent mucositis for patients with hematologic malignancies receiving myeloablative chemotherapy and TBI with autologous HCT. Palifermin 60 mcg/kg/day is given for 3 days immediately prior to administering the preparative regimen and for 3 days after infusion of the hematopoietic stem cell graft (i.e., days 0, +1, +2).[129] In these patients, palifermin lowered the incidence and average duration of clinically meaningful oral mucositis. The incidence of blood-borne infections and the use of parenteral opioids were also diminished in patients using palifermin.[130]

Myelosuppression and Growth Factor Use

CASE 96-3, QUESTION 6: An order is written to begin filgrastim on day 0 and to continue administration until the ANC has recovered to 500/μL for 2 consecutive days. Is this therapy appropriate for K.M.?

The use of hematopoietic growth factors (HGFs) after infusion of allogeneic PBPC is controversial and is not recommended by ASCO Guidelines.[23] Administration of HGFs after allogeneic graft infusion decreases the duration of neutropenia, but has not been demonstrated to decrease cost, length of hospitalization, or antibiotic use. HGF administration may increase the incidence of severe GVHD and lower survival.[131] K.M. is receiving an allogeneic PBPC graft and thus should not receive filgrastim.

Veno-Occlusive Disease of the Liver

CASE 96-3, QUESTION 7: K.M.'s pretransplantation admission laboratory values are within normal limits. Her weight on admission is 80 kg. During the first 5 days after marrow infusion, K.M.'s weight begins to increase by approximately 0.5 kg/day, her inputs exceed her outputs by about 500 to 1,000 mL/day, and she is mildly febrile with an axillary temperature of 38°C. Blood and urine cultures are all negative. On day +6, her weight is 85 kg. Laboratory values on day +7 are significant for the following:

Total bilirubin, 1.5 mg/dL
Aspartate aminotransferase (AST), 40 units/L
Alkaline phosphatase, 120 units/L

By day +10, K.M. is complaining of midepigastric, right upper quadrant pain, and a liver that is tender to palpation. During the next few days, K.M. begins to look icteric. Her liver function tests continue to rise slowly, until day +18 when they reach the following peak values:

Total bilirubin, 5.0 mg/dL,
AST, 150 units/L
Alkaline phosphatase, 180 units/L

On day +18, K.M.'s weight is 90 kg. "Rule out VOD of the liver" is included on her problem list in the medical record. What is VOD?

Hepatic VOD is a life-threatening complication of HCT.[127] The incidence of VOD varies considerably, ranging from 5.3% to 54%, mainly due to differences in the preparative regimens.[127] Preparative regimens including busulfan, cyclophosphamide, and/or TBI greater than 13.2 Gy have been associated with higher VOD rates.[27,132] Although the pathogenesis is not understood completely, the key event is toxic injury to the sinusoidal endothelial cells. Involvement of the hepatic venules is not essential to developing the clinical signs and symptoms; thus, the term "sinusoidal obstruction syndrome" has been proposed in place of VOD.[133] The endothelial damage initiates the coagulation cascade, induces thrombosis of the hepatic venules, and eventually leads to fibrous obliteration of the affected venules.[127] The cardinal histologic features are marked sinusoidal fibrosis, necrosis of pericentral hepatocytes, and narrowing and eventual fibrosis of central veins.[133] In patients with VOD, early microscopic changes include subendothelial swelling, leading to several physiological changes, including narrowing of hepatic venules and necrosis of centrizonal hepatocytes.[127]

CLINICAL PRESENTATION

CASE 96-3, QUESTION 8: What signs and symptoms in K.M. are consistent with a diagnosis of VOD?

The signs and symptoms associated with VOD are hyperbilirubinemia (≥2 mg/dL), weight gain (>5% above baseline), hepatomegaly, azotemia, elevated alkaline phosphatase, ascites, elevated AST, and encephalopathy.[134] Insidious weight gain exceeding 5% of baseline is usually the first manifestation of impending VOD, occurring in more than 90% of patients within 3 to 6 days after marrow infusion.[135] Weight gain is caused by sodium and water retention, as evidenced by decreased renal sodium excretion. This is usually distinguished from cyclophosphamide-induced syndrome of inappropriate secretion of antidiuretic hormone by the time course relative to administration of the preparative regimen. Hyperbilirubinemia, which also occurs in virtually all patients, follows the onset of weight gain and usually appears within 10 days after hematopoietic stem cell infusion. In more than half of the patients, the peak bilirubin concentration is greater than 6 mg/dL. Other liver function test abnormalities usually occur after hyperbilirubinemia and include elevations in AST and alkaline phosphatase. Ascites, right upper quadrant pain, and encephalopathy lag behind changes in liver function tests and develop within 10 to 15 days after infusion of hematopoietic stem cells.[135]

A clinical diagnosis of VOD is made when two of the following features occur within the first 20 days of HCT: (a) hyperbilirubinemia (total serum bilirubin >2 mg/dL); (b) hepatomegaly or right upper quadrant pain; and (c) sudden weight gain.[135] To make a clinical diagnosis of VOD, the features listed previously must occur without other causes of post-HCT liver damage, including GVHD, viral hepatitis, fungal abscesses, and drug reactions. A clinical diagnosis can be confirmed histologically via liver biopsy; however, these are often not performed due to the increased risk of bleeding due to thrombocytopenia.

In summary, the signs and symptoms consistent with VOD in K.M. include insidious weight gain, hyperbilirubinemia, and right upper quadrant pain. The onset and timing of these signs and symptoms are consistent with VOD and occurred without other causes of hepatic toxicity. K.M. received a myeloablative preparative regimen containing cyclophosphamide and busulfan which is known to be associated with VOD.

PREVENTION AND TREATMENT

CASE 96-3, QUESTION 9: What is the likelihood that K.M. will recover from her VOD? How should she be treated?

The overall mortality for patients who experience VOD varies considerably (i.e., 0%–67%) due to the variable definitions of VOD.[127] Patients with greater weight gain and elevations in total bilirubin are more likely to die of VOD when compared to patients with less severe weight gain and elevations in total bilirubin.[127] Severe VOD is usually accompanied by multi-organ system failure, and these patients rarely die from liver failure itself but from renal and cardiopulmonary complications.[127]

Risk factors for severe and/or fatal VOD have been identified in the hope of preventing this condition or its progression through early treatment. Although various risk factors have been identified, their association is variable, and conflicting reports of their association can be found. The most important risk factors are the preparative regimen, TBI dose, high systemic exposure to busulfan and/or cyclophosphamide, and liver inflammation and fibrosis pre-HCT.[127]

Various pharmacologic methods to prevent VOD have been evaluated. One such method is altering the preparative regimen. The substitution of fludarabine (FLU) for cyclophosphamide in combination with busulfan (i.e., BU/FLU) and the use of reduced-intensity regimens with agents with low hepatic toxicity appear to lower VOD risk.[2,127,136,137] VOD rates are lower with IV busulfan compared to oral busulfan due to the eliminaton of the first-pass effect on the liver.[138,139] Individualizing chemotherapy doses for busulfan or cyclophosphamide may also lower VOD rates. There is high interpatient variability in their metabolism and clearance, associations between systemic exposure, and toxicity and response (a pharmacodynamic relationship); however, these relationships vary with preparative regimens.[108,140] The association of VOD with busulfan concentrations is discussed in the Adaptive Dosing of Busulfan section. Single-agent ursodiol (600 mg/day PO) used for prophylaxis has been associated with a lower incidence of VOD[141,142] or with a lower frequency of total bilirubin greater than 3 mg/dL.[143] Ursodiol, which is a bile acid, most likely minimizes cholestasis but cannot prevent toxic liver injury.[127] Prostaglandin E1 and anticytokine strategies, specifically pentoxifylline, have been ineffective in preventing VOD in clinical trials.[127]

Most patients with VOD (70%–85%) spontaneously recover; thus, the mainstay of treatment is managing sodium and water balance, and paracentesis, in severe cases, for ascites that is associated with pain and pulmonary compromise.[127] Volume expanders such as albumin and colloids may be used to maintain intravascular volume, spironolactone may be used to minimize extravascular fluid accumulation, and protein restriction and lactulose may be used if encephalopathy develops. Unfortunately, improved outcomes with these measures have not been confirmed. In patients with severe VOD and multiorgan failure, available treatment options are limited. Thrombolytic therapy with recombinant human tissue plasminogen activator and heparin have had mixed results in terms of efficacy, and can cause fatal intracerebral or pulmonary bleeding.[127] Defibrotide (DF), an investigational drug, has shown promising results in the treatment of VOD.[144–146] Defibrotide, a ribonucleotide, has antithrombotic, anti-ischemic, and thrombolytic activity without producing significant systemic anticoagulation. In a compassionate use trial of 88 patients with severe VOD and associated organ dysfunction, 36% of patients had complete resolution of VOD and 35% survived past day 100 after HCT.[146]

Although the use of DF in treating VOD appears to be effective, little is known about whether prophylactic DF could be beneficial in high risk patients. Corbacioglu et al. explored this question in children with malignant infantile osteopetrosis undergoing stem cell transplantation. Previously 7/11 or 63.6% ($n = 20$) of the children in their center between 1996 and 2001 experienced VOD. DF prophylaxis was initiated in 9 consecutive patients between 2001 and 2005 and in this group 1/9 (11.1%) was diagnosed with moderate VOD suggesting a significant benefit from prophylactic DF. To further explore this question a US National Institutes of Health–sponsored prospective randomized trial has been undertaken to answer the question as to whether prophylactic DF is superior to therapeutic DF in children at high risk for experiencing VOD during stem cell transplantation.[147]

Because K.M. does not meet the criteria for severe VOD, she should be managed conservatively with fluid restriction and spironolactone for fluid diuresis. Her signs and symptoms should resolve during the next 2 weeks. Because she has mild VOD, she is likely to recover completely without sequelae.

Graft Rejection

CASE 96-4

QUESTION 1: E.R. is a 65-year-old woman diagnosed with myelodysplastic syndrome. Past medical history is significant for type I diabetes and renal dysfunction. After her initial diagnosis, a search for a completely HLA-matched unrelated donor was conducted. A donor was found in the National Marrow Donor Registry and E.R. will receive a non-myeloablative allogeneic HCT using bone marrow from an unrelated male donor. E.R.'s preparative regimen is as follows: fludarabine, 30 mg/m²/day on days −4, −3 and −2, and 2 Gy TBI on the day of marrow infusion with postgrafting cyclosporine and mycophenolate mofetil. It is now day +28 and E.R.'s CBC shows the following:

WBC count, 500 cells/μL
Differential, no granulocytes or monocytes detected
Platelets, 100,000/μL
Hematocrit (Hct), 30%

Donor T-cell chimerism is <5%. What is E.R. experiencing, and how should she be treated?

Reduced-intensity regimens typically consist of fludarabine in combination with an alkylating agent or low-dose TBI (Fig. 96-2). With the nonmyeloablative fludarabine/TBI regimen, there is minimal neutropenia, thrombocytopenia, and other nonhematologic toxicity, thus it may be given as a outpatient procedure.[2] Engraftment is usually evident within the first 30 days in patients receiving a nonmyeloablative preparative regimen; however, rejection can occur after initial engraftment.[5] A mixed chimerism generally develops after nonmyeloablative HCT but E.R. has low donor T-cell chimerism on day +28, placing her at high risk of graft rejection.

Graft rejection is less common after allogeneic versus autologous HCT because the donor PBPC or marrow is unmanipulated and free from the damaging effects of prior chemotherapy. However, graft rejection still occurs particularly after nonmyeloablative allogeneic HCT. A delicate balance between host and donor effector cells must be established with myelosuppressive chemotherapy and immune suppressants since excessive host-versus-graft effects may lead to graft rejection. The incidence of graft rejection is higher in patients with aplastic anemia and in patients undergoing HCT with histoincompatible marrow or T-cell–depleted marrow. Graft rejection is uncommon in leukemia patients receiving myeloablative preparative regimen with a histocompatible allogeneic donor. There are limited therapeutic options for the treatment of graft rejection. A second HCT is the most definitive therapy, assuming donor cells are available, although the toxicities are formidable.[148] In patients receiving myeloablative allogeneic HCT, graft rejection is best managed with immunosuppressants such as antithymocyte globulin. In patients receiving a reduced-intensity regimen, graft rejection may require a second HCT.

E.R. received nonmyeloablative conditioning, and thus she should have mixed chimerism posttransplant. However, because she has fewer than 5% donor T cells she will not benefit from the GVT effect due to the lack of the donor's cytotoxic T lymphocytes that suppress the recipient's malignancy. Current research is focusing on quantitative chimerism monitoring, specifically evaluating the percent donor chimerism, which may be a tool on which to base clinical interventions.[95] Donor chimerism is evaluated in different cell types (e.g., T cells, NK cells, granulocytes) although cell type most predictive of outcome is not known. The changes in the percent donor chimerism over time posttransplant, termed "engraftment kinetics," are influenced by several factors such as type of HCT conditioning, stem cell source, and intensity of postgrafting immunosuppression.[95,149] A balance between the recipient's and donor's cells is needed to maximize the GVT effect, which lowers the risk of relapse while minimizing the risk of GVHD.[95,149]

E.R. is at high risk of graft rejection and therefore may not benefit from the transplant. A trial of discontinuing cyclosporine and mycophenolate mofetil, in an attempt to shift the balance toward donor graft growth and away from recipient T-cell growth, is an option. E.R.'s T-cell chimerism should be monitored periodically, and hematopoietic function should be monitored with daily CBCs and a bone marrow biopsy every 2 weeks.

GRAFT-VERSUS-HOST DISEASE

GVHD is caused by activation of donor lymphocytes leading to immune-mediated damage to the recipient. Histocompatibility differences between donor and recipient necessitate posttransplantation immunosuppression after allogeneic HCT because considerable morbidity and mortality are associated with graft rejection and GVHD. Therefore, postgrafting immunosuppression or GVHD prophylaxis is used after allogeneic HCT. However, because allogeneic transplantation offers the potential for a GVT effect in which immune effector cells from the donor recognize and eliminate residual tumor in the recipient, research is focusing on immune suppression manipulations that allow sufficient GVT effects while not increasing the risk of graft rejection and GVHD.[4]

GVHD is the most important complication of allogeneic HCT, and limits the use of this lifesaving treatment.[2,150] GVHD can occur after allogeneic HCT, regardless of the preparative regimen used. The pathophysiology of GVHD is not completely understood, but the current view of its development is described by a three-step process, including (a) the preparative regimen results in tissue damage and release of inflammatory cytokines into the circulation; (b) both recipient and donor antigen presenting cells and inflammatory cytokines trigger activation of donor-derived T cells; and (c) the activated donor T cells mediate cytotoxicity through a variety of mechanisms, which leads to tissue damage characteristic of acute GVHD.[151]

GVHD has traditionally been divided into two forms (i.e., acute or chronic) based on clinical manifestations. Acute GVHD damages the skin, GI tract, and liver and usually occurs in the first 100 days after allogeneic HCT.[2] In contrast, chronic GVHD may affect almost any organ system, closely resembles several autoimmune diseases, and usually occurs after day 100. A late-onset acute GVHD occuring after day 100 is possible; however, in these individuals acute and chronic GVHD symptoms may both be present. This additional syndrome is included in the National Institutes of Health classification system for GVHD because these symptoms are common after allogeneic transplants.[152]

The majority of the data regarding the prevention and treatment of GVHD have been obtained after myeloablative preparative regimens. Therefore, the subsequent section refers only to trials conducted in recipients of a myeloablative allogeneic HCT.

Acute Graft-versus-Host Disease

RISK FACTORS

CASE 96-5

QUESTION 1: M.P., a 22-year-old, 70-kg man, undergoes a one-antigen mismatched allogeneic HCT from his sister for the diagnosis of Philadelphia chromosome—positive (Ph^+) AML. After a myeloablative preparative regimen of CY/TBI, the following immunosuppressive regimen is ordered: cyclosporine 2.5 mg/kg every 12 hours from day −3 until tolerating oral medications, then switch to cyclosporine 4 mg/kg PO every 12 hours until day +50. Methotrexate 15 mg/m^2 IV on day +1, then 10 mg/m^2 on days +3, +6, and +11. What factors are associated with an increased risk of acute GVHD?

The single most important factor associated with the development of GVHD is the degree of histocompatibility between donor and recipient.[2] Clinically relevant grade II–IV acute GVHD occurs in 20% to 50% of HLA-matched sibling grafts and 50% to 80% of HLA-mismatched sibling or HLA-identical unrelated donors.[153] The onset of acute GVHD is earlier and severity is increased in mismatched grafts relative to matched grafts, and also in matched unrelated donors relative to matched sibling donors.[51,154] Other factors that increase the risk of experiencing acute GVHD include increasing recipient (and possibly donor) age, greater intensity of the preparative regimen, use of PBPC rather than bone marrow, and donor/recipient sex mismatch.[151] UCT have a lower risk of acute GVHD.[155–157]

M.P. is receiving allogeneic bone marrow from a (a) female sibling donor that is (b) mismatched at one HLA antigen. These two factors increase his risk of exhibiting acute GVHD. Therefore good immune suppressive therapy is critical in preventing its development.

CLINICAL PRESENTATION

CASE 96-5, QUESTION 2: On day +14, the time at which engraftment occurred, M.P. is noted to have a diffuse macular papular rash on his arms, hands, and front trunk. He does not have diarrhea, and his liver function tests are within normal limits. At the onset of his rash, M.P.'s empiric antibiotics are changed from cefepime to imipenem. Despite the change in antibiotics, M.P.'s rash persists. How is M.P.'s presentation consistent with acute GVHD?

The primary targets of immune-mediated destruction of host tissue by donor lymphocytes in acute GVHD are the skin (the most frequently affected organ, with 81% of patients experiencing symptoms), followed by the GI tract and the liver in 54% and 50% of patients receiving myeloablative transplants, respectively.[158,153] Acute GVHD of the skin usually manifests as a diffuse maculopapular pruritic rash that starts on the palms of the hands, soles of the feet, or the face. In more severe cases, skin

TABLE 96-6
Modified Glucksberg Grading of Acute Graft-versus-Host Disease

Organ Stage	Skin[a]	Liver	Intestinal Tract[b]
1	Maculopapular rash <25% of body surface	Bilirubin 2–2.9 mg/dL	500–1,000 mL/d diarrhea or biopsy-proven upper GI involvement
2	Maculopapular rash 25%–50% body surface	Bilirubin 3–6 mg/dL	1,000–1,500 mL/d diarrhea
3	Maculopapular rash >50% body surface	Bilirubin 6.1–15 mg/dL	1,500–2,000 mL/d diarrhea
4	Generalized erythroderma with bullae	Bilirubin >15 mg/dL	>2,000 mL/d diarrhea or severe abdominal pain with or without ileus

[a] Extent of rash determined by "rule of nines."
[b] Diarrhea volume applies to adults.
Source: Cutler C, Antin JH. Manifestations and treatment of acute graft-versus-host disease. In: Blume KG et al, eds. *Thomas' Hematopoietic Cell Transplantation*. 4th ed. Malden, MA: Blackwell; 2009:1291.

GVHD can progress to a generalized total body erythroderma, bullous formation, and skin desquamation.

For photos of GVHD, go to http://thepoint.lww.com/AT10e.

The earliest symptoms of acute GVHD of the GI tract are usually loss of appetite followed by nausea and vomiting.[127] Abdominal pain and watery or bloody diarrhea also occur, which can result in electrolyte abnormalities, dehydration, or ileus in severe cases. (To view a video of a small intestine endoscopy for GVHD, go to http://daveproject.org/viewfilms.cfm?film_id=102.) Liver GVHD usually follows skin and/or GI GVHD. Clinical symptoms of liver GVHD include a gradual rise in total bilirubin, alkaline phosphatase, and hepatic transaminases.[127] Acute GVHD is usually not evident until the time of engraftment, when donor lymphoid elements begin to proliferate. The skin is usually the first organ to be involved. The onset of liver or GI GVHD usually lags behind the onset of skin GVHD by approximately 1 week and infrequently occurs without skin GVHD.

Acute GVHD must be distinguished accurately from other causes of skin, liver, or GI toxicity in the HCT patient. For example, a maculopapular rash, which may occur as a manifestation of an allergic reaction to antibiotics, usually begins on the trunk or upper extremities and rarely presents on the palms of the hands or soles of the feet. Diarrhea can be caused by chemotherapy, radiation, infection, or antibiotic therapy.[127] However, diarrhea caused by the preparative regimen is rarely bloody and usually resolves within 3 to 7 days after discontinuation of drugs and radiation. Diarrhea caused by infectious agents such as *Clostridium difficile* or cytomegalovirus (CMV) should be distinguished from GVHD. Liver GVHD must be distinguished primarily from VOD and, to a lesser extent, hepatitis induced by drugs, blood products, or parenteral nutrition.[127] Although liver function test abnormalities between these syndromes are similar, liver GVHD is rarely associated with insidious weight gain or right upper quadrant pain.[127] A tissue biopsy of the affected organ in conjunction with clinical evidence is the only way to definitively diagnose acute GVHD, though biopsy of the gut and liver is rarely done due to the increased risks associated with thrombocytopenia early in the posttransplant phase. Acute GVHD is associated with characteristic histologic changes to affected organs. A staging system based on clinical criteria is used to grade acute GVHD. The severity of organ involvement is determined first (Table 96-6), and then an overall grade is established based on number and extent of involved organs (Table 96-7).

M.P. developed a rash at the time of engraftment that could have been consistent with either an antibiotic-induced rash or acute GVHD. Although it was appropriate to change antibiotics, the fact that M.P.'s rash did not improve is suggestive of acute GVHD. M.P.'s rash is present on 36% of his body, but because there are no signs of GI or liver involvement at this time, M.P. is likely to have grade I GVHD (Tables 96-6 and Table 96-7).

IMMUNOSUPPRESSIVE PROPHYLAXIS

CASE 96-5, QUESTION 3: Why did M.P. receive prophylactic immunosuppressive therapy with cyclosporine and methotrexate?

GVHD is a leading cause of morbidity and mortality after allogeneic HCT. Without post-HCT immunosuppression, serious acute GVHD would occur in almost every allogeneic HCT recipient.[2] The most common method used to minimize GHVD risk is to administer postgrafting immunosuppressive therapies. However, these immunosuppressive regimens are associated with significant toxicity and a higher risk of relapse in patients with acute leukemia who are at high risk of relapse.[159] The latter is most likely due to diminished GVT effect due to the immune suppression. This inverse relationship between acute GVHD and leukemic relapse has been observed in multiple studies.[4] Patients with acute leukemias at high risk for relapse may receive

TABLE 96-7
Modified Glucksberg versus International Bone Marrow Transplant Registry Overall Grading of Acute Graft-versus-Host Disease Severity

Organ Stage	Skin	Liver	Gut
Glucksberg Grading			
I—Mild	Stage 1–2	None	None
II—Moderate	Stage 3 or	Stage 1 or	Stage 1
III—Severe		Stage 2–3 or	Stage 2–4
IV—Life threatening	Stage 4 or	Stage 4	—
IBMTR Grading			
A—Mild	Stage 1	None	None
B—Moderate	Stage 2	Stage 1 or 2	Stage 1 or 2
C—Severe	Stage 3	Stage 3	Stage 3
D—Life threatening	Stage 4	Stage 4	Stage 4

Source: Cutler C, Antin JH. Manifestations and treatment of acute graft-versus-host disease. In: Blume KG et al, eds. *Thomas' Hematopoietic Cell Transplantation*. 4th ed. Malden, MA: Blackwell; 2009:1291.
IBMTR, International Bone Marrow Transplant Registry.

TABLE 96-8
Combination Immunosuppression Regimens for Prophylaxis of Acute Graft-versus-Host Disease in Myeloablative Transplant

Drug	Dosing Examples
Cyclosporine/short-term methotrexate	1.5 mg/kg IV or 4 mg/kg (Neoral) PO every 12 hours, days –1 to +50, then taper 5% per week and discontinue by day +180 Methotrexate 10 mg/m^2 IV, days +3, +6, +11
Tacrolimus/short-term methotrexate[101]	Tacrolimus 0.03 mg/kg/d continuous IV infusion or 0.12 mg/kg/d PO BID Methotrexate 15 mg/m^2 IV day +1; 10 mg/m^2 IV, days +3, +6, +11
Cyclosporine/methotrexate/prednisone	Cyclosporine 5 mg/kg/d IV continuous infusion, days –2 to +3, then 3–3.75 mg/kg IV until day +35; then 7 mg/kg/d (Neoral) PO, dose adjusted to cyclosporine concentrations (via radioimmunoassay) of 200–400 ng/mL. Taper by 20% every 2 weeks; then discontinue by day +180 Methotrexate 15 mg/m^2 IV day +1; 10 mg/m^2 IV days +3, +6 Methylprednisolone 0.5 mg/kg/d IV day +7 until day +14; then 1 mg/kg/d IV until day +28; then prednisone 0.8 mg/kg/d PO until day +42; then taper slowly and discontinue by day +180

BID, twice a day; IV, intravenous; PO, orally.

single-agent prophylaxis for acute GVHD because the development of mild acute GVHD may produce a robust GVT effect. However, most patients today receive multi-drug GVHD prophylaxis.

Historically, acute GVHD was prevented with single-drug therapy using ATG, cyclophosphamide, methotrexate, or cyclosporine.[160–162] ATG binds nonspecifically to mononuclear cells and depletes hematopoietic progenitor cells in addition to lymphocytes. Consequently, ATG is generally avoided as a prophylactic agent due to the risk of graft failure.[160] The risk of GVHD is greatly reduced by two-drug combination immunosuppression (Table 96-8). Although the most widely published regimen is short-course methotrexate plus cyclosporine,[162] there is no national consensus with regard to the most effective regimen. Several randomized clinical trials have compared tacrolimus and short-course methotrexate with cyclosporine plus short-course methotrexate in patients undergoing allogeneic HCT using HLA-matched siblings[163,164] and unrelated donors.[101] Recipients of matched-sibling grafts treated with tacrolimus had a lower incidence of grade II to IV acute GVHD, but a similar incidence of chronic GVHD.[163] Overall survival was lower in the tacrolimus group as a result of more toxic deaths in patients with advanced stage disease; however, a higher number of advanced stage disease patients in the tacrolimus/methotrexate group make the results of this trial somewhat difficult to interpret.[163]

Subsequently, the International Bone and Marrow Transplant Registry conducted a matched control study, which suggested that the survival difference between the two arms of tacrolimus plus short-course methotrexate and cyclosporine plus short-course methotrexate was in fact due to the imbalance in the underlying risk factors.[164] In patients receiving HLA-matched or slightly mismatched unrelated grafts, those given tacrolimus had a lower incidence of grade II to IV acute GVHD, a similar incidence of chronic GVHD and similar diseasefree and overall survival rates.[101] Patients with advanced hematologic malignancies were excluded from this study. Both regimens are currently used in allogeneic HCT after myeloablative preparative regimens.

More recently, the use of mycophenolate mofetil (MMF) has been studied in allogeneic transplants with myeloablative conditioning, and when used in combination with cyclosporine appears to have similar incidence of acute GVHD and 100-day survival as methotrexate/cyclosporine, yet significantly less severe mucositis and more rapid neutrophil engraftment than the methotrexate/cyclosporine arm.[165,166] MMF is now commonly used in clinical practice in combination with cyclosporine or tacrolimus.

Several studies have compared triple-drug with two-drug immunosuppression. The incidence of acute GVHD has been similar or lower with triple-drug regimens, but infectious complications are higher, and overall survival is similar to two-drug regimens.[167–169]

M.P. received acute GVHD prophylaxis with a two-drug regimen of short-course methotrexate and cyclosporine, the most common regimen for myeloablative allogeneic conditioning regimens. Using two drugs with different mechanisms of immunosuppression, one blocking the activation of T cells (cyclosporine), and the other (methotrexate) blocking the division and clonal expansion of activated T cells, is more effective in decreasing the likelihood of GVHD than one of these agents alone.

CASE 96-5, QUESTION 4: What principles are used in dosing medications used for acute GVHD prophylaxis?

Although the various combination immunosuppressive regimens vary slightly by drug, dose, and combination, several guidelines are consistent throughout all regimens. First, cytotoxic agents used for prophylaxis of acute GVHD (methotrexate) are withheld or given in reduced doses if mucositis is severe or the patient experiences excessive fluid retention or excessive delay in neutrophil recovery.[162,167] Fluid retention sites act as a depot for methotrexate accumulation, increasing duration of exposure. In this case, methotrexate levels are drawn and, if excessive, the drug is held and leucovorin is administered until the level is immeasurable. Methotrexate for GVHD prophylaxis can delay engraftment, increase the incidence and severity of mucositis, and cause liver function test elevations. The methotrexate dose is reduced in the setting of renal or liver impairment.[162,170] Because of these concerns some centers use MMF in place of methotrexate.

The calcineurin inhibitors (i.e., cyclosporine, tacrolimus) should be initiated before or immediately after donor cell infusion (day –3 to 0) when used for GVHD prophylaxis. This schedule is recommended because of the known mechanism of action of these agents, which entails blocking the proliferation of cytotoxic T cells by inhibiting production of helper T-cell–derived IL-2. Administering cyclosporine before the donor cell infusion allows inhibition of IL-2 secretion to occur before a rejection response has been initiated.

Cyclosporine is usually administered intravenously until the GI toxicity from a myeloablative preparative regimen has resolved (e.g., for 7–21 days).[162] This is because GI effects of the preparative regimen (e.g., CINV, diarrhea) and GVHD affect the oral absorption of microemulsion cyclosporine and may result in inconsistent blood concentrations.[171] Most centers use the microemulsion oral formulation (Neoral) or other new generic microemulsion formulations that have improved bioavailability. With the microemulsion oral formulation, an IV to PO dosing ratio of 1:2 or 1:3 is appropriate. The most common ratio used when converting tacrolimus from IV to oral is 1:4. Emperic dose adjustments may be required when patients are receiving concomitant medications that affect cytochrome P-450 3A or P-glycoprotein, which are involved in the metabolism and transport of the calcineurin inhibitors (e.g., voriconazole). Thus, careful monitoring for drug interactions with the calcineurin inhibitors is warranted.[172]

The dose of cyclosporine or tacrolimus is adjusted based on serum drug levels and the serum creatinine (SCr) concentration. Doses are usually reduced by 50% if the SCr concentration doubles above baseline and is withheld for SCr concentrations greater than 2 mg/dL.[162,173] Although the calcineurin inhibitors do not contribute to myelosuppression, common adverse effects to these agents include electrolyte abnormalities, neurotoxicity, hypertension, and/or nephrotoxicity (which may lead to an impaired clearance of methotrexate).[103]

Corticosteroids are seldom used in combination immunosuppressive regimens. Administering corticosteroids early in the posttransplantation period (e.g., around day 0) paradoxically increases the incidence of GVHD when used in combination with methotrexate and cyclosporine.[174] Additionally, corticosteroids in combination prophylaxis regimens are associated with several adverse effects, including infectious complications, hyperglycemia, and an increased incidence of hypertension. Reserving corticosteroids for treatment of GVHD is supported by a randomized study which found no difference between a regimen of cyclosporine and methotrexate and one with methylprednisone added in a triple drug combination.[169]

Tapering schedules for GVHD prophylaxis vary widely among institutions. The general goal is to keep calcineurin inhibitor doses stable to day +50, and then slowly taper with the intent of discontinuing all immunosuppressive agents by 6 months after HCT. By this time, immunologic tolerance has developed, and patients no longer require immunosuppressive therapy.

ADAPTIVE DOSING OF CALCINEURIN INHIBITORS

CASE 96-5, QUESTION 5: On day +18, a cyclosporine concentration is measured right before the morning dose (trough) and is reported as 392 ng/mL. Why are cyclosporine concentrations being obtained for M.P.?

The role of pharmacokinetic monitoring of the calcineurin inhibitors in HCT patients is not well defined but is commonly performed because of the established pharmacodynamic associations within solid organ transplant recipients. It is standard practice for HCT centers to adjust cyclosporine or tacrolimus doses based on trough blood concentrations.[175] An association between cyclosporine concentrations and acute GVHD was not found in early studies; however, other studies have suggested that cyclosporine trough concentrations for 12-hour dosing of 200 to 400 ng/mL in adult patients minimize the risk of acute GVHD and the risk of cyclosporine-induced nephrotoxicity.[176–178] For continuously infused cyclosporine, higher target blood concentrations of 300 to 500 ng/mL have been required to prevent GVHD in order to provide an equivalent AUC of exposure to intermittent dosing.[179,180] It is important to note that cyclosporine-induced nephrotoxicity may occur despite low or normal concentrations of cyclosporine and may be a consequence of other drug- or disease-related factors known to influence the development of nephrotoxicity (e.g., concurrent use of other nephrotoxic agents, sepsis). Additionally, recent studies suggest that trough concentrations do not correlate well with exposure to cyclosporine, and that a peak level is better correlated to the $AUC_{(0-12)}$. A peak concentration of greater than 800 ng/mL may be required to prevent GVHD. Despite this, the data are limited and the routine use of peaks for therapeutic drug monitoring is not recommended.[181] Desired tacrolimus trough concentrations are 5 to 15 ng/mL. Tacrolimus concentrations greater than 20 ng/mL have been associated with increased risk of toxicity, primarily nephrotoxicity.[175,183] Adjustments in tacrolimus dosing for increased SCr should be made in a manner similar to that described for cyclosporine.

It is reasonable to adjust M.P.'s doses to maintain cyclosporine trough concentrations between 200 and 400 ng/mL, as in all patients undergoing allogeneic HCT with a myeloablative preparative regimen. Recommendations for dose adjustments should be based on cyclosporine concentrations and SCr level. Dosage adjustments should be made for changes in the SCr, regardless of cyclosporine concentration, as recommended previously. No standard dosage adjustment schedule exists, but most centers adopt their own standardized approach. M.P. has a normal SCr, and his cyclosporine trough is 392 ng/mL. Therefore, his cyclosporine dose should be maintained and the trough repeated in a few days. It may be repeated sooner if an interacting drug is added or discontinued, or if there are toxicity concerns.

TREATMENT OF ESTABLISHED ACUTE GRAFT-VERSUS-HOST DISEASE

CASE 96-5, QUESTION 6: In the third week posttransplant, M.P. experiences a pruritic rash on his shoulders and neck which spreads to the palms of his hands and looks like a sunburn. On day +19, the suspicion of acute skin GVHD is confirmed by biopsy. On the same day, M.P. experiences 1,000 mL of diarrhea during the next 24 hours and is noted to have a bilirubin of 2.8 mg/dL. He is started on methylprednisolone 35 mg IV every 6 hours. What is the rationale for methylprednisolone therapy in M.P.?

Preventing the development of GVHD is the most effective way to treat this HCT complication. In patients who develop GVHD, first-line treatment is a corticosteroid added to their current immune suppression regimen.[151] For this reason GVHD and its treatment cause profound immunodeficiency.[2,182] The combination of GVHD and infectious complications are leading causes of mortality for allogeneic HCT patients.

The route of corticosteroid administration is determined by the severity of the GVHD. Those patients with only skin involvement of less than 50% of their body surface area may be treated with topical steroid creams, while involvement of other organs, or stage 3 or 4 skin disease, require systemic steroids. A complete response occurs in up to 25% to 40% of patients, with a lower likelihood of response in more severe cases of acute GVHD.[151,184] Patients with mild to moderate (grades I–III) acute GVHD who respond to initial therapy have a significantly better survival advantage than patients with severe acute GVHD who do not respond to initial therapy. Patients who do not respond to therapy or have ongoing severe GVHD usually die from a combination of GVHD and infectious complications.[185]

Corticosteroids used in the treatment of acute GVHD are generally tapered based on response. There is no consensus on the optimal method for tapering the corticosteroids[182] and the tapering rate depends on the patient. Patients who experience acute GVHD or who experience flares of existing GVHD during a tapering trial will have their dosages increased or tapered more slowly as tolerated.

Because M.P. had objective evidence of established acute GVHD he was given systemic IV corticosteroids. This was appropriate because single-agent corticosteroids are considered the therapy of choice for established acute GVHD.[186] Corticosteroids indirectly halt the progression of immune-mediated destruction of host tissues by blocking macrophage-derived IL-1 secretion. IL-1 is a primary stimulus for helper T-cell–induced secretion of IL-2, which in turn is responsible for stimulating proliferation of cytotoxic T lymphocytes. The recommended dosage of methylprednisolone for the treatment of established acute GVHD is 1 to 2 mg/kg/day, given intravenously or orally in divided doses for a minimum of 14 days, followed by a tapering schedule that is determined by response.[185] This is an example of an acute GVHD treatment order set. The dosage of methylprednisolone in M.P., approximately 2 mg/kg/day, is consistent with these recommendations. Trials that compared higher doses of corticosteroids (i.e., 10 mg/kg/day) to 2 mg/kg/day as initial treatment of acute GVHD showed no advantage.[187] Monitoring for rash, diarrhea, and bilirubin levels to asses acute GHVD response should occur every 3 to 5 days.[151] M.P. was receiving cyclosporine for GVHD prophylaxis at the time the acute GVHD developed. Although the cyclosporine was not effective in preventing the GVHD it is typical for patients to remain on their prophylactic immune suppressants.

ONLINE CONTENT

For an example of an acute GVHD treatment order set, go to http://thepoint.lww.com/AT10e.

A significant portion of patients do not respond to corticosteroids, and they are said to have steroid-refractory GVHD.[151] The timing of treatment response varies among the organs affected by GVHD and patients. If GVHD symptoms worsen during 3 days of treatment and if the skin does not improve by 5 days, it is unlikely that a response will be achieved in a timely manner, and secondary therapy should be considered.[151] Patients with steroid-refractory acute GVHD have a poor prognosis. A variety of medications are being studied for "salvage" or secondary therapy. The salvage therapy depends on the organs affected. For example, phototherapy is used as salvage therapy for skin GVHD and nonabsorbable corticosteroids are used for GI GHVD. Other options for salvage therapy include ATG, denileukin diftitox, MMF and TNF-α blockers (e.g., infliximab, etanercept).[151,188] The most effective dose, timing, or combination of these salvage therapies is still unknown.

M.P. should be evaluated for response to methylprednisolone after 4 to 7 days. If his acute GVHD has improved or stabilized, he should be continued on therapy at this dose for a total of 14 days. If M.P. responds to therapy, his methylprednisolone dose should be tapered slowly over a minimum of 1 month, and he should be monitored for any evidence of recurrent GVHD. If the GVHD flares during his steroid taper as evidenced by worsening skin reactions, increased bilirubin, or increased diarrhea volume, the dose should be increased again until his disease is stable; the subsequent taper should be initiated at a slower rate. If M.P. fails to respond to first-line therapy with methylprednisolone, he should receive salvage therapy.

Chronic Graft-versus-Host Disease

CLINICAL PRESENTATION

CASE 96-5, QUESTION 7: **M.P. was successfully treated for his acute GVHD, is no longer taking corticosteroids, and is currently tapering off his cyclosporine. On day +200, M.P. comes to clinic for follow-up after a 2-week vacation in Florida. On examination, M.P. is found to have a mild skin rash on his arms and legs, hyperpigmentation of the tissue surrounding the eyes, and white plaquelike lesions in his mouth. He is also complaining of dry eyes. Laboratory tests reveal an increased alkaline phosphatase and total bilirubin concentration. What is the most likely cause of M.P.'s findings?**

Chronic GVHD, the most common late complication of allogeneic HCT, occurs in 20% to 70% of patients surviving more than 100 days.[189] Chronic GVHD is a major cause of nonrelapse morbidity and mortality.[2] Risk factors for chronic GVHD include recipient, donor, and transplant factors. Nonmodifiable recipient risk factors include older age, certain diagnoses (e.g., CML), and lack of an HLA-matched donor. Modifiable factors that may lower the risk of chronic GVHD include selecting a younger donor, avoiding a multiparous female donor, using umbilical cord blood or a bone marrow graft rather than PBPC, and limiting the $CD34^+$ and T-cell dose infused.[189] Development of acute GVHD is a major predictor of chronic GVHD; 70% to 80% of those with grade II to IV acute GVHD develop chronic GVHD.[189]

Chronic GVHD is not a continuation of acute GVHD.[189] Traditionally, the boundary between the two was based on time, but now they are classified based on different clinical symptoms.[189] Signs and symptoms of chronic GVHD in various organ systems are listed in Table 96-9.

ONLINE CONTENT

For CGVHD photos, go to http://thepoint.lww.com/AT10e.

A consensus guideline for the diagnosis and scoring of chronic GVHD has been published.[152] The diagnosis of chronic GVHD requires (a) being distinct from acute GVHD, (b) having at least one diagnostic clinical sign of chronic GVHD or at least one distinctive manifestation confirmed by pertinent biopsy or other relevant tests, and (c) exclusion of other possible diagnoses. The clinical scoring system uses a numerical value of 0 to 3, with more severe symptoms having a higher number. A global score is calculated by including the number of organs involved and the severity within each affected organ. The global score reflects the expected effect of chronic GVHD on the patient's performance status and can be used to evaluate whether treatment with systemic immunosuppression is required. The grading and prognosis of chronic GVHD can define and predict high-risk patient groups.[190] These patients could then benefit from the development of new treatment options as well as improve comparability between publications.

The signs and symptoms of chronic GVHD in M.P. include a rash in sun-exposed areas of the skin, hyperpigmentation of tissues surrounding his eyes, white plaquelike lesions in the mouth, dry mucous membranes, and increased alkaline phosphatase and total bilirubin levels. These symptoms appeared after a period of complete resolution of acute GVHD and during a taper of the cyclosporine. Thus, M.P. has moderate involvement,[152] quiescent chronic GVHD.

PHARMACOLOGIC MANAGEMENT

CASE 96-5, QUESTION 8: **M.P. is started on prednisone 1 mg/kg PO daily for the treatment of his chronic GVHD. His cyclosporine taper is stopped, and the dosage is raised to therapeutic concentrations. Is this therapy rational? What other agents are available to treat chronic GVHD?**

TABLE 96-9

Selected Signs and Symptoms of Chronic Graft-versus-Host Disease[a]

Affected Organ	Diagnostic	Distinctive	Other Features[b]	Seen With Both Acute and Chronic GVHD
Eyes		New-onset dry, gritty, or painful eyes[c]	Photophobia	
		Cicatricial conjunctivitis	Periorbital hyperpigmentation	
		Keratoconjunctivitis sicca[c]		
		Confluent areas of punctuate keratopathy, tear formation, dry eyes, burning, photophobia	Erythema of the eyelids with edema	
Gastrointestinal tract	Esophageal web		Pancreatic insufficiency	Anorexia
	Stricture or stenosis in the upper to mid third of the esophagus[d]			Nausea
				Vomiting
				Diarrhea
				Weight loss
				Failure to thrive (infants and children)
Liver				Total bilirubin, alkaline phosphatase >2 × upper limit of normal[d]
Lung	Bronchiolitis obliterans diagnosis with lung biopsy	Bronchiolitis obliterans diagnosed with pulmonary function tests and radiology[c]		Bronchiolitis obliterans organizing pneumonia
Skin	Poikiloderma	Depigmentation	Seat impairment ichthyosis	Erythema
	Lichen planuslike features		Keratosis pilaris	Maculopapular rash
				Pruritus
	Sclerotic features		Hypopigmentation	
	Morphealike features		Hyperpigmentation	
	Lichen sclerosuslike features			

[a] Signs and symptoms for hematopoietic and immune differences, as well as for nails; scalp and body hair; mouth; genitalia; muscles, fascia, and joints; and other organs, are also described by Filipovich et al.[152]
[b] Part of chronic GVHD symptomatology if the diagnosis is confirmed.
[c] Diagnosis of chronic GVHD requires biopsy or radiology confirmation (or Schirmer's test for eyes).
[d] Infection, drug effects, malignancy, or other causes must be excluded.
GVHD, graft-versus-host disease.

There is no specific prophylactic therapy for chronic GVHD and the optimal treatment remains controversial. The mainstay of therapy for chronic GVHD is long-term immunosuppressive therapy. Survival for patients with chronic GVHD is improved by extended corticosteroid therapy, although there are multiple long-term adverse effects associated with the corticosteroids.[189,191] A typical regimen is prednisone 1 mg/kg/day, administered orally in divided doses for 14 days and then converted slowly to alternate-day therapy by increasing the "on-day" and decreasing the "off-day" dose until a total of 1 mg/kg/day on alternate days is administered.[191] Alternate-day therapy is preferred to minimize adrenocortical suppression. Once therapy is initiated, 1 to 2 months may pass before an improvement in clinical symptoms is noted. Therapy is usually continued for 9 to 12 months and then slowly tapered after signs and symptoms of chronic GVHD have resolved. The median duration of treatment has been reported to be 23 months.[192] If chronic GVHD worsens during the tapering or after discontinuation of prednisone, immunosuppressive therapy is restarted. Other potential approaches for patients with refractory chronic GVHD include MMF, daclizumab, sirolimus, pentostatin, and extracorporeal photochemotherapy.[191]

When immunosuppressive therapy is administered for long periods, the patient must be monitored closely for chronic toxicity. Cushingoid effects, aseptic necrosis of the joints, and diabetes can develop with long-term corticosteroid use. Other severe complications include a high incidence of infection with encapsulated organisms and atypical pathogens such as *Pneumocystis jiroveci (P. Jiroveci)* pneumonia, CMV, and herpes zoster.

Thus, it is reasonable to start M.P. on single-agent prednisone for chronic GVHD treatment at 1 mg/kg daily for 2 weeks and then convert to every other day as described herein.

ADJUVANT THERAPIES

CASE 96-5, QUESTION 9: Suggest some adjuvant therapies that should be instituted in a patient like M.P. with chronic GVHD.

Patients who are being treated for chronic GVHD should receive trimethoprim-sulfamethoxazole for prophylaxis of *P. jiroveci* and encapsulated organisms, such as *Streptococcus pneumoniae* and *Haemophilus influenzae*. Ensuring optimal prophylactic antibiotics in chronic GVHD patients is critical because infection is the primary cause of death during treatment.[192] Artificial tears and saliva may improve lubrication and decrease the occurrence of cracking and fissures in mucous membranes. If nutritional intake is poor, consultation with a clinical nutritionist and use of oral nutritional supplementation may be advisable. Patients should be instructed to apply sunscreens to exposed areas whenever prolonged sun exposure is anticipated. Liver function abnormalities have been improved by up to 30% with the use of ursodiol as bile acid displacement therapy.[141–143] Calcium supplements, estrogen replacement, or other antiosteoporosis agents should be considered in women or other patients at risk for fracture or bone loss while receiving prolonged regimens with immunosuppressant therapy.[194] Patient education regarding the gradual resolution of symptoms such as skin sclerosis, fatigue and muscle weakness, anticipated duration of therapy, and importance of compliance with oral immunosuppressive therapy is essential.

INFECTIOUS COMPLICATIONS

Opportunistic infections are a major cause of morbidity and mortality after myeloablative and nonmyeloablative HCT. There are three general periods of infectious risk (Fig. 96-3). During the early period pre-engraftment, particularly for patients undergoing myeloablative HCT, the primary pathogens are aerobic bacteria, *Candida* spp., and herpes simplex virus (HSV). Chemotherapy-induced mucosal damage creates a portal of entry into the bloodstream for many organisms, such as viridans group *Streptococcus*, *Candida*, and aerobic gram-negative bacteria. Catheter-associated infections have become the leading cause of bacteremia, most notably in the early posttransplant period.[190,192] The routine use of antiviral prophylaxis has decreased the incidence of HSV. Respiratory viruses such as respiratory syncytial virus, influenza, adenovirus, and parainfluenza are increasingly recognized as pathogens causing pneumonia, particularly during community outbreaks of infection.[195] To reduce potential exposure of HCT recipients to these pathogens, visitors and staff members with signs and symptoms of a viral respiratory illness may not be allowed direct contact with patients.

A potential advantage of reduced-intensity or nonmyeloablative preparative regimens is reduced toxicity of the preparative regimen compared to myeloablative HCT. Reduced intensity or nonmyeloablative preparative regimens frequently do not result in true neutropenia,[5] and the incidence of mucositis during the early period is reduced.[196] In a matched controlled study the incidence of bacteremia during the first 30 days post HCT in the nonmyeloablative recipients was significantly reduced compared to myeloablative recipients.[196] Moreover, nonmyeloablative HCT recipients experienced significantly fewer infections attributable to mucositis during the early period.

The second or middle (Fig. 96-3) period of infectious risk includes the time from engraftment to posttransplantation day +100. Pathogens such as CMV, adenovirus, and *Aspergillus* are common. CMV, adenovirus, *Aspergillus*, and *P. jiroveci* frequently cause interstitial pneumonitis. Patients undergoing reduced intensity or nonmyeloablative preparative regimens that experience acute GVHD and are treated with corticosteroids have a similar risk of infection during this time period as those undergoing myeloablative HCT.[196]

During the late period (after day +100), the predominant pathogens are the encapsulated bacteria (e.g., *S. pneumoniae*, *H. influenzae*, *Neisseria meningitidis*), fungi, and varicella-zoster virus (VZV). The encapsulated bacteria commonly cause sinopulmonary infections. The risk of infection during this late period is increased in patients with chronic GVHD as a result of prolonged immunosuppression.

Because of the morbidity associated with opportunistic infection in HCT recipients, optimal pharmacotherapy for prevention and treatment is critical. In 2000, the US Centers for Disease Control and Prevention (CDC) published guidelines for prevention of opportunistic infection in HCT recipients.[8] These guidelines were constructed from available data by an expert panel from the CDC, the Infectious Disease Society of America, and the American Society for Blood and Marrow Transplantation. In 2009 an update to the guidelines were published.[197] The following discussion incorporates recommendations from the CDC guidelines and also provides information on the pharmacotherapy of opportunistic infections in all types of HCT.

Prevention and Treatment of Bacterial and Fungal Infections

CASE 96-6

QUESTION 1: S.D. is a 26-year-old woman with Ph$^+$ acute lymphocytic leukemia in first complete remission who is admitted for allogeneic myeloablative HCT. The following orders are written: Admit to a room with a positive-pressure HEPA filter. Flush double-lumen Hickman catheter per protocol. Immunosuppressed patient diet as tolerated. Begin fluconazole 400 mg PO every 24 hours and levofloxacin 500 mg PO every 24 hours on admission. Begin ceftazidime 2 g IV every 8 hours with first fever when ANC is less than 500 cells/μL. Transfuse 2 units of packed RBCs for hematocrit less than 25% and 1 unit of single-donor platelets for platelet count less than 20,000/μL. What is the rationale for these supportive measures?

As a result of disease-related immunosuppression, intensive preparative regimens, and posttransplantation immunosuppressive therapy, patients undergoing allogeneic HCT require careful vigilance for regimen-related toxicities and intensive supportive care directed at maintaining adequate blood counts, preventing or treating infection, and providing optimum nutrition.

Placement of a double-lumen or triple-lumen central venous catheter (e.g., Hickman, Groshong, Broviac, Neostar) is mandatory in all patients.

ONLINE CONTENT

For an illustration of a triple-lumen catheter, go to http://thepoint.lww.com/AT10e.

The need for prolonged administration of chemotherapy, blood products, antibiotics, parenteral nutrition, and adjunctive medications precludes the use of peripheral access sites. The use of a central venous catheter allows delivery of maximum concentrations of all medications into a high-flow blood vessel. Administration time is reduced and daily fluid infusion is minimized.

After administration of the preparative regimen and before successful engraftment, allogeneic myeloablative HCT patients undergo a period of pancytopenia lasting from 2 to 6 weeks. During this time, patients may require multiple RBC and platelet transfusions. Packed RBCs and platelets are usually given for a hematocrit less than 25% and a platelet count less than 10,000/μL or 20,000/μL. Transfusions with multiple blood products put patients at risk for blood product–derived infection (e.g., CMV, hepatitis). In addition, sensitization to foreign leukocyte HLA antigens (alloimmunization) may cause immune-mediated thrombocytopenia. Thus, blood-product support in the myeloablative allogeneic HCT patient must incorporate strategies that reduce the risk of viral infection and alloimmunization. Effective methods include minimizing the number of pretransplant infusions, using single-donor rather than pooled-donor blood products, irradiating blood products, and filtering blood products with leukocyte reduction filters.

Patients receiving reduced intensity or nonmyeloablative preparative regimens may or may not experience neutropenia and generally have reduced requirements for blood products. In

TABLE 96-10
Foods Posing Infection Risk in Neutropenic Patients

High-Risk Foods to Avoid When Neutropenic	Infection Risk
Salad	Gram-negative bacillus including *Pseudomonas aeruginosa* and *Campylobacter*
Tomatoes, radishes, celery, and carrots	*Pseudomonas aeruginosa*
Raw eggs	*Campylobacter jejuni, Salmonella*
Unpasteurized cheeses	*Listeria monocytogenes*
	Enterococci
Cold, loose meats	*Listeria, Clostridium perfringens, Campylobacter jejuni*
Undercooked meat	*Salmonella, Listeria, Escherichia coli*
Uncooked nuts	*Aspergillus niger, Aspergillus flavus*
Black pepper/uncooked herbs and spices	*Aspergillus* sp
Raw shellfish/sushi	*Vibro vulnificus*, Norwalk virus
Bottled water	*Pseudomonas, Cytophaga, Campylobacter*
Prepared foods that are cooked and then eaten chilled	*Listeria*
Ice machines	*P. aeruginosa, Stenophomonas maltophilia*

fact, many centers perform reduced intensity or nonmyeloablative HCT in the outpatient setting and admit patients to the hospital only for complications requiring more aggressive management.

Several measures are recommended to minimize the risk of infection in autologous and allogeneic myeloablative HCT patients. Private reverse isolation rooms equipped with positive-pressure HEPA filters and adherence to strict handwashing techniques reduce the incidence of bacterial and fungal infections.[8] To reduce exposure to exogenous sources of bacteria in immunosuppressed patients, low microbial diets (Table 96-10) may be instituted on hospital admission, and visitors are prohibited from bringing plants or flowers into the patient's room. Patients are encouraged to maintain good oral hygiene because the mouth can be a source of bacterial or fungal infection. Frequent (4–6 times daily) mouth rinses with sterile water, normal saline, or sodium bicarbonate are effective.[8] Brushing or flossing teeth is avoided during periods of thrombocytopenia and neutropenia.

Aggressive use of antibacterial, antifungal, and antiviral therapy, both prophylactically and for documented infection, is an important aspect of patient management. Antibiotics with a broad gram-negative spectrum may be instituted prophylactically once the patient becomes neutropenic (ANC $<1{,}000$ cells/μL), or empirically after the patient is neutropenic and experiences fever (oral temperature $>38°$C). Some transplant centers administer a prophylactic fluoroquinolone such as levofloxacin on admission especially if the neutropenic period is expected to extend beyond 7 days.[198–202]

For a table regarding antibiotic use in neutropenic patients, go to http://thepoint.lww.com/AT10e.

Fluoroquinolone prophylaxis significantly reduces the incidence of gram-negative bacteremia but generally does not affect mortality.[8] Concerns regarding prophylactic fluoroquinolone use include the emergence of resistant organisms and an increased risk of streptococcal infection.[8,203] In fact, the incidence of viridians group of streptococci has been increasing.[8,204] To decrease the possibilities of selecting out resistance, when the neutropenia has resolved the fluroquinolone should be discontinued. Prophylactic antibiotics (e.g., penicillin, vancomycin) are not recommended due to their lack of proven efficacy in preventing streptococcal infections and the concern about antibiotic-resistant bacteria.[8] Regardless of prophylactic strategies, patients who become febrile during neutropenia should immediately receive broad-spectrum IV antibiotic(s) (e.g., ceftazidime, cefepime, or imipenem) and prophylaxis should be discontinued.[8,205]

Antifungal prophylactic agents are commonly used in HCT recipients. S.D. is prescribed fluconazole 400 mg/day on admission because prophylactic use until day +75 posttransplantation decreases the incidence of systemic fungal infection and fungal death in patients undergoing transplantation.[206,207] The use of prophylactic fluconazole has been linked to reports of breakthrough infections with resistant fungi such as *C. glabrata* and *Aspergillus*.[208,209] Itraconazole has improved activity in vitro against fluconazole-resistant fungi. In a randomized trial, allogeneic HCT patients treated with prophylactic itraconazole (200 mg IV every 24 hours or oral solution 200 mg twice a day [BID]) experienced significantly fewer invasive fungal infections than those treated with fluconazole (400 mg every 24 hours). Although there was a trend toward fewer fungal deaths in the itraconazole-treated patients, overall mortality was similar. Itraconazole was associated with more frequent GI side effects (e.g., nausea, vomiting).[210] Clinically, most centers use fluconazole instead of itraconazole prophylaxis.[210,211]

When mold prophylaxis is required either posiconazole or voriconazole may be used. If S.D. were to require mold prophylaxis, voriconazole 200 mg twice daily would be a good choice. Published data supporting the use of newer mold-active agents for antifungal prophylaxis are limited. Micafungin (50 mg IV every 24 hours) and fluconazole (400 mg IV every 24 hours) were compared in a randomized, double-blind study of patients undergoing HCT. Overall success was defined as the absence of suspected, proven, or probable systemic fungal infection through the end of therapy and as the absence of proven or probable systemic fungal infection through the end of the 4-week posttreatment period. The overall efficacy was greater in the patients who received micafungin (80.0% vs. 73.5% in patients treated with fluconazole, $p = 0.03$). Fewer episodes of aspergillosis occurred in patients treated with micafungin. Patient tolerability of the regimens was similar.[212] Voriconazole 200 mg twice daily was compared to fluconazole 400 mg once daily in a randomized double-blind trial for prevention of invasive fungal infections in standard risk HCT. No significant differences were seen in fungus-free survival, relapsefree status, and overall survival at 6 months. Toxicities were similar and there was a trend toward reduced aspergillus infections and less empiric antifungal therapy in the voriconazole arm.[213] Supportive measures such as prophylaxtic antibiotics, positive pressure HEPA filter rooms, and immunosuppressed diet decrease infection risk and bridge the gap while the patient's new immune system takes hold.

Prevention of Herpes Simplex Virus and Varicella-Zoster Virus

CASE 96-6, QUESTION 2: On routine screening before transplantation, S.D. is found to be HSV-seropositive (≥1.11 index value) and VZV-seropositive (≥1 index value). How will this affect her management?

Up to 70% of HSV-seropositive patients undergoing myeloablative allogeneic HCT will experience reactivation of HSV.[214] Prophylactic acyclovir is commonly used in HSV-seropositive patients undergoing allogeneic or autologous HCT to prevent viral reactivation.[8,215] Dosing regimens for prophylactic acyclovir vary widely; the dose of IV acyclovir is typically 250 mg/m^2 IV every 12 hours, whereas oral doses of acyclovir range from 600 mg/day to 1,600 mg/day.[8] The recommended duration of acyclovir prophylaxis for HSV varies from day +30 to day +365 posttransplantation or longer, depending on the specific type of HCT and other risk factors. Valacyclovir, a prodrug of acyclovir with improved bioavailability, provides sufficient blood concentrations to prevent HSV in patients with mucositis or gastrointestinal acute GVHD.[216] Prophylactic valacyclovir is commonly used at a dose of 500 mg PO every 12 hours.[217,218]

Varizella zoster virus-seropositive patients are at risk for developing herpes zoster, particularly after day +100 posttransplanation.[216] Prophylactic acyclovir reduces the risk of VZV reactivation.[219] As with prophylaxis for HSV reactivation, the optimum duration of VZV prophylaxis is controversial, often extending to day +365 posttransplantation or longer.

Patients who are HSV-seronegative or VZV-seronegative rarely exhibit primary HSV or VZV infection and are therefore not administered prophylactic acyclovir. If HSV does occur, lesions usually appear on the oral mucosa, nasolabial mucous membranes, or genital mucocutaneous area and can be managed with acyclovir at standand treatment doses.

Because S.D. is HSV and VZV seropositive, she is at risk for viral reactivation and should receive prophylactic acyclovir 400 mg PO twice daily, beginning four days prior to transplant and continuing until her ANC is greater than 2,500 cells/μL for at least two days.

Prevention of Cytomegalovirus Disease

CASE 96-6, QUESTION 3: S.D. is also CMV-seropositive. What is the significance of this finding, and what measures can be taken to prevent reactivation of CMV?

CMV has the ability to establish lifelong latent infection after primary exposure. In immunocompromised patients, the virus may reactivate, resulting in asymptomatic shedding or the development of CMV disease. The incidence of CMV infection (defined as isolation of the virus or detection of viral proteins or nucleic acid in any body fluid without clinical symptoms) and CMV disease (signs and symptoms consistent with CMV invasion into a tissue) in HCT recipients is 15% to 60% and 20% to 35%, respectively. The most common manifestations of CMV disease after allogeneic HCT are pneumonitis, fever, and GI infection.[220]

In the CMV-seronegative HCT recipient, primary CMV infection or disease can be prevented by selecting a CMV-seronegative donor and using only blood products from CMV-seronegative donors. No anti-CMV prophylaxis is required in these recipients. In patients who are CMV-seropositive or who have received a CMV-seropositive graft, antiviral drugs are essential to minimize morbidity associated with CMV reactivation or secondary infection. Two general strategies are possible. Universal prophylaxis involves the administration of ganciclovir from the time of engraftment until approximately day +100 posttransplantation. This strategy significantly decreases the incidence of CMV infection and disease compared with placebo.[221] However, prophylactic ganciclovir therapy is associated with neutropenia in 30% of patients, which contributes to an increased risk of invasive bacterial and fungal infections.[221,222] Neutropenia secondary to ganciclovir may lead to interruptions in antiviral therapy or necessitate administration of filgrastim daily or several times per week to maintain adequate neutrophil counts.

Pre-emptive therapy, or risk-adjusted therapy, is the most commonly used strategy for preventing CMV disease after allogeneic HCT.[216,223] Using this strategy, patients begin therapy only if they have early reactivation of CMV detected through shell vial cultures, assay of blood for CMV antigens (e.g., pp65), or viral nucleic acid using the PCR. Using preemptive therapy selectively administers ganciclovir to only those HCT patients at greatest risk for development of CMV disease.[224–226] Antigenemia-based pre-emptive therapy is as effective as universal ganciclovir prophylaxis for prevention of CMV disease and is associated with reduced CMV mortality.[222,227–230] The induction dose of ganciclovir is typically 5 mg/kg IV every 12 hours for 7 to 14 days, followed by a maintenance dose of 5 mg/kg IV daily until 2 to 3 weeks after the last occurrence of antigenemia or until day +100 posttransplantation.[8] Pre-emptive therapy limits patient exposure to the potential toxicity of ganciclovir and thus reduces overall cost.[219] Recent data suggest that oral valganciclovir is a safe and effective alternative to ganciclovir for pre-emptive therapy.[231,232] Foscarnet may also be administered in lieu of ganciclovir, but its use is complicated by nephrotoxicity and electrolyte wasting.[230,233] Monitoring and correction of electrolyte and fluid imbalances are essential when foscarnet is initiated.

ONLINE CONTENT

To see a preprinted order set for ganciclovir, valganciclovir, and foscarnet treatment at time of reactivation/positive tests, go to http://thepoint.lww.com/AT10e.

Cidofovir is used to treat CMV in HCT patients but is reserved for use when ganciclovir or foscarnet have failed.[234] Dose-related renal dysfunction limits the number of patients able to receive cidofovir. Renal imparment can be seen after only 1 to 2 doses.[235,236] An advantages of cidofovir is its infrequent dosing making it conducive to clinic administration. Monitoring renal function, electrolytes, WBC, and intraocular pressure are essential monitoring parameters.

ONLINE CONTENT

To see a preprinted order set for cidofovir treatment at time of reactivation/positive tests, go to http://thepoint.lww.com/AT10e.

Autologous HCT recipients who are CMV-seropositive pretransplant should receive antiviral treatment pre-emptively as described previously.[8,237] Nonmyeloablative or reduced intensity HCT recipients should also receive pre-emptive antiviral treatment. Because host T cells may persist in the peripheral blood for up to 6 months after reduced intensity or nonmyeloablative preparative regimens, their presence may provide some protection against early CMV disease. A matched controlled study comparing the incidence and outcome of CMV infection in myeloablative and nonmyeloablative HCT demonstrated that although the time to onset of CMV antigenemia was similar in the two groups, fewer nonmyeloablative HCT recipients experienced CMV disease in the early period.[238] The overall 1-year incidence of CMV disease was also similar, suggesting that nonmyeloablative HCT recipients are at increased risk for exhibiting late CMV disease (>100 days after transplantation) compared to their myeloablative counterparts.[238] It is therefore recommended that nonmyeloablative HCT patients receive pre-emptive antiviral therapy and be monitored for development of CMV antigenemia for 1 year after HCT.[238,239]

S.D.'s absolute neutrophil count recovers to greater than 1,000 cells/μL on day +20, and on day +32, her weekly surveillance blood sample is positive for CMV by PCR. Pre-emptive ganciclovir induction is initiated at 5 mg/kg IV every 12 hours for two weeks followed by maintenance dosing of 5 mg/kg daily. After 3 weeks of therapy, S.D.'s surveillance samples are negative and ganciclovir is discontinued. Weekly surveillance sampling continues until day +100. If surveillance samples again become positive for CMV, ganciclovir therapy should be reinstituted.

Diagnosis and Treatment of *Aspergillus* Infection

RISK FACTORS

CASE 96-7

QUESTION 1: A.W., a 60-kg, 165-cm, 15-year-old boy, is day +79 after a matched, unrelated, nonmyeloablative PBPC transplant for acute lymphocytic leukemia in third complete remission. He presents to the clinic for evaluation of a temperature of 102.3°F and a 3-day history of nonproductive cough. Significant medical history includes skin and GI GVHD (stable on his current regimen of cyclosporine, mycophenolate mofetil, and prednisone) and congestive heart failure believed to be secondary to anthracycline exposure. A.W. has chronic low-grade nausea and hypomagnesemia necessitating daily IV hydration with magnesium supplementation. Relevant laboratory values are as follows:

Na, 138 mEq/L
K, 4.2 mEq/L
Cl, 100 mEq/L
CO_2, 23 mEq/L
Blood urea nitrogen, 18 mg/dL
SCr, 0.8 mg/dL
Total bilirubin, 0.6 mg/dL
Mg, 1.5 mg/dL
WBC count, 3,500 cells/μL
Platelets, 78,000/μL
ANC, 1,810 cells/μL
Hemoglobin, 10.8 g/dL

He was CMV-seropositive and HSV-seropositive before HCT. Oral medications include cyclosporine 275 mg every 12 hours, MMF 900 mg every 12 hours, prednisone 60 mg every morning and 12.5 mg every evening (tapering), trimethoprim-sulfamethoxazole (TMP/SMX) 160 mg/800 mg BID on Monday and Tuesday, fluconazole 400 mg every morning, valacyclovir 500 mg BID, digoxin 0.125 mg every 12 hours, enalapril 10 mg every 12 hours, and One-a-Day Plus vitamin every morning.

On physical examination, A.W. is a chronically ill–appearing child with "moon" face, dry skin with thickened areas, a pleural friction rub, and thinning hair. Blood cultures, urinalysis, and chest x-ray are obtained. Chest x-ray reveals several small cavitary lesions worrisome for fungal disease. A.W. is admitted for further workup and management of presumed *Aspergillus* infection. What risk factors does A.W. have for developing an infection with *Aspergillus*?

Invasive molds (most commonly *Aspergillus* spp., but also *Fusarium* spp., *Scedosporium*, and *Zygomycetes*) are an increasing cause of morbidity and mortality after allogeneic and autologous HCT.[208]

ONLINE CONTENT

For a picture showing invasion of tissue by *Aspergillus* species, go to http://thepoint.lww.com/AT10e.

Factors contributing to this trend include (a) more effective prevention of bacterial and viral infection which promote mold overgrowth, as described previously; and (b) the use of fluconazole prophylaxis, which has reduced the incidence of candidemia and Candida-related mortality.[206–208,240,241] *Aspergillus* infection is reported in up to 26% of HCT recipients, and the mortality rate of invasive aspergillosis (IA) is 74% to 92%.[242]

Several risk factors for development of invasive fungal infection have been identified.[240,241] Given that neutrophils are critical for host defense, prolonged neutropenia is considered the single most important predictor of infection at all time points after HCT.[209,240] GVHD (acute and chronic) and treatment with corticosteroids are also important risk factors, particularly for aspergillosis occurring between day +40 and day +100 posttransplantation, presumably as a result of neutrophil dysfunction.[240,241,243] In addition, the widespread use of fluconazole prophylaxis (400 mg/day) for prevention of invasive candidiasis in transplant patients since the early 1990s has led to a substantial increase in the incidence of IA and also fluconazole-resistant *Candida* species such as *Candida* krusei and *Candida glabrata*.[240,243,244]

A.W. is receiving corticosteroid treatment for GVHD and fluconazole prophylaxis. These therapies increase his risk for exhibiting IA.

TREATMENT

CASE 96-7, QUESTION 2: A.W. undergoes bronchoalveolar lavage to identify the organism responsible for his pulmonary infection. Pathological examination of the fluid obtained reveals septate, branching hyphae, and culture results confirm the diagnosis of *Aspergillus fumigatus* infection. CT scans are negative for extrapulmonary involvement. A.W. is started on amphotericin B lipid complex (ABLC) at a dose of 300 mg IV daily. How is aspergillosis usually diagnosed, and what are the acceptable alternatives for treating this infection?

ONLINE CONTENT

For a video of a narrated BAL procedure, go to http://thepoint.lww.com/AT10e.

Early diagnosis and treatment of IA, which rely on tissue or fluid obtained from the infected site followed by aggressive antifungal therapy, may improve patient survival.[245] Although the lower respiratory tract is frequently the primary focus of infection, *Aspergillus* may invade blood vessels and spread hematogenously to other organs, including the brain, liver, kidneys, spleen, and skin.[246] Head, chest, abdomen, and pelvic computed tomography scans assist in assessing the extent of disease, treatment options, and overall prognosis. Cultures of respiratory tract secretions lack sensitivity for detecting *Aspergillus*, and the medical condition of the patient may preclude invasive diagnostic procedures altogether. Many clinicians have adopted the European

Organization for Research and Treatment of Cancer criteria for diagnosis of proven, probable, and possible IA.[247]

Newer diagnostic tests based on the detection of fungal antigens or metabolites, such as galactomannan, 1,3-β-D-glucan, and fungal DNA detection by PCR, are being developed. Galactomannan is a polysaccharide component of the *Aspergillus* cell wall that is released during fungal cell growth. Galactomannan detection by enzyme-linked immunoassay (GM-EIA) has proved to be a sensitive and specific tool for early detection of *Aspergillus* infection. The test is useful not only for serum samples but also for bronchoalveolar lavage and cerebrospinal fluid. Concomitant antifungal therapy may cause false-negative GM-EIA results, whereas antibiotics of fungal origin (e.g., piperacillin/tazobactam) have been associated with false positives.[242,248]

ANTIFUNGALS

Outcomes for patients with IA after HCT are often poor, with approximately 20% of patients alive after 1 year.[240] Treatment success depends not only on the use of intensive antifungal agents but also on recovery of the host immune system and/or reduction of immunosuppression.[245,249] Conventional amphotericin B (c-AmB) at a dose of at least 1 mg/kg/day has traditionally been the gold standard antifungal therapy for IA. Response rates with c-AmB monotherapy range from 28% to 51%, depending on the severity of the underlying immunosuppression; however, 65% of responders eventually die of their infection.[245] Moreover, toxicity, particularly renal, associated with c-AmB frequently limits the dose and duration of therapy. Fortunately, the lipid derivatives of amphotericin B, broad-spectrum triazoles, and echinocandins are available as alternatives to c-AmB.

Three lipid formulations of amphotericin B have been marketed: ABLC (Abelcet), liposomal amphotericin B (L-AmB; AmBisome) and amphotericin B colloidal dispersion (ABCD; Amphotec currently unavailable at the time of this writing). Practice guidelines for use of these agents in HCT patients have been published.[250] Studies of lipid amphotericin B formulations as monotherapy for patients with IA who have failed or are intolerant to c-AmB therapy demonstrate response rates of 23% to 71%, regardless of which formulation is used. No randomized trials show superiority of lipid amphotericin B products over c-Amb for IA.[249] Doses most commonly used in the studies are 5 mg/kg/day for ABLC and L-AmB and 4 to 6 mg/kg/day for ABCD. The lipid formulations of amphotericin B are clearly less toxic than c-AmB, with L-AmB being the least toxic.[251]

Three broad-spectrum triazole agents (itraconaole, voriconazole, posaconazole) are available for patients who are refractory to or intolerant of amphotericin B therapy. Oral itraconazole capsules were approved in 1992, followed later by the oral solution and an IV formulation. In an early compassionate use trial of IA unresponsive to amphotericin B, 27% of patients had a complete response to itraconazole, and another 35% experienced improvement in their infection.[252] Patients who had undergone HCT had response rates similar to patients who were less immunocompromised. Unfortunately, oral itraconazole capsules exhibit erratic absorption, and the IV form is complicated by the risk of drug precipitation in the IV line.[249] In addition, itraconazole is a potent inhibitor of common CYP isoforms and also has negative inotropic properties.[253,254]

Voriconazole was approved in 2002. An advantage of voriconazole is excellent (96%) oral bioavailability; however, like itraconazole, the drug is a potent inhibitor of cytochrome P-450 enzymes. Voriconazole has been compared to c-AmB in a randomized, unblinded trial as primary therapy for established IA in an immunocompromised host.[255] The primary objective was to demonstrate the noninferiority of voriconazole compared with c-AmB after 12 weeks of therapy in patients with definite or probable IA. Patients received voriconazole 6 mg/kg IV every 12 hours × two doses followed by 4 mg/kg IV every 12 hours for at least 7 days, followed by oral voriconazole 200 mg every 12 hours or c-AmB at a dose of 1 to 1.5 mg/kg/day. Patients refractory to or intolerant of initial therapy could receive other antifungal drugs. Of 144 evaluable patients who received voriconazole, 76 (52.8%) had a partial or complete response compared to 42 of 133 (31.6%) patients treated with c-Amb. The median duration of therapy for patients treated with voriconazole was 77 days, and 52 of 144 patients switched to an alternative agent. In contrast, the median duration of therapy for patients receiving c-AmB was 10 days, and 107 of 133 patients switched to another agent (most commonly, a lipid formulation of amphotericin B). The survival rate at 12 weeks in the voriconazole group was 70.8% compared to 57.9% in the c-Amb group ($p = 0.02$). These results of initial therapy with voriconazole indicate superior response and improved survival compared to c-AmB in immunocompromised patients, such as allogeneic HCT recipients, with IA. Voriconazole-treated patients also experienced fewer drug-related adverse effects.

Posaconazole was approved in 2006. This broad-spectrum triazole is available only as a variably absorbed oral suspension, and like itraconazole and voriconazole, is a cytochrome P-450 3A4 inhibitor. Posaconazole has the lowest minimum inhibitory concentration of any available triazole against *Aspergillus* spp., including *Aspergillus* terreus, and it is the only triazole with useful activity against the *Zygomycetes*. Published clinical experience with posaconazole is limited; however, in an open-label externally controlled trial in patients with IA refractory to or intolerant of other therapies, the overall success rate was 42% in posaconazole-treated patients compared to 26% for controls ($p = 0.006$).[256]

Echinocandin antifungal agents (caspofungin, micafungin, and anidulafungin) inhibit the synthesis of β-(1,3)-glucan, an important component of the fungal cell wall. No prospective randomized trials document the efficacy of any echinocandin for primary therapy of IA, and only caspofungin is approved for salvage therapy. An open-label, noncomparative trial evaluated the efficacy of caspofungin in 69 patients with IA who had failed or were intolerant of at least 7 days of standard antifungal therapy.[257] Patients received 70 mg IV of caspofungin on day 1 followed by 50 mg IV daily. Of the 63 evaluable patients, 26 (43%) responded favorably to treatment. Twenty-six of 52 patients (50%) who had received at least 7 days of therapy had a favorable response. In another open-label, noncomparative trial, Denning et al. evaluated the safety and efficacy of micafungin (alone or in combination) in patients with proven or probable IA. Eighty of 225 patients (35.6%) had a favorable response. Most patients received combination therapy; the 34 patients treated with monotherapy had a similar response rate.[258]

In summary, the number of agents available to manage IA has expanded greatly in the past few years. Although some experts believe that voriconazole is the drug of first choice, considerable controversy still exists regarding acquiring resistance, selecting out other species of molds, and side effect tolerance due to the lack of definitive studies. Therapy should be tailored to the individual patient based on response, tolerability, and cost.

ANTIFUNGAL TOXICITIES

CASE 96-7, QUESTION 3: Despite premedication with acetaminophen and diphenhydramine, A.W. experiences significant chills and rigors with his ABLC infusions. In addition, he is having daily temperatures exceeding 39°C. On

day 5 of therapy, morning laboratory tests reveal the following:

SCr, 1.4 mg/dL
K, 2.7 mEq/L
Mg, 1.4 mg/dL

What expected adverse reactions of ABLC-based therapy does A.W. demonstrate?

The most troublesome side effect of amphotericin B therapy is nephrotoxicity. Up to 80% of patients treated with conventional amphotericin B will experience an episode of altered renal function.[259] The mechanism of amphotericin B nephrotoxicity is complex and poorly understood. It most likely results from afferent vasoconstriction leading to cortical ischemia and a subsequent decrease in glomerular filtration rate, as well as defective acid secretion by the renal tubule. Risk factors for nephrotoxicity include concomitant administration of other nephrotoxic drugs such as aminoglycosides, cyclosporine, cisplatin, and radiocontrast dye; prolonged duration of therapy; history of chronic renal disease; male sex; and a mean daily dose greater than or equal to 35 mg.[260]

The lipid derivatives of amphotericin B were developed with the goal of reducing nephrotoxicity, and each is significantly less nephrotoxic compared to conventional c-AmB.[250,261–264] Furthermore, patients treated with c-AmB who experience nephrotoxicity and are then switched to a lipid formulation frequently show improvement in renal function. It is difficult to determine the true incidence of nephrotoxicity associated with the lipid products because most trials evaluate their use in patients who have received prior c-AmB therapy. In addition, many trials do not control for other factors known to reduce the risk of nephrotoxicity, including sodium loading and IV fluid boluses administered before c-AmB infusion. Nonetheless, clinical experience confirms the reduced incidence of nephrotoxicity with these products, and they are recommended as first-line therapy for patients at high risk for nephrotoxicity or in whom baseline renal function is impaired.

Other toxicities of amphotericin B include infusion-related reactions (fever, chills, rigors, hypotension, hypoxia), hypokalemia, hypomagnesemia, nausea, and anemia. Premedications such as acetaminophen, diphenhydramine, and/or hydrocortisone are typically administered before each dose to lessen or prevent the infusion-related reactions, with mixed results. Patients may also develop tolerance. Fortunately, there appears to be a reduced incidence of infusion-related reactions when the lipid products are used. Significant hypokalemia and hypomagnesemia may persist well beyond discontinuation of amphotericin B. Most patients require daily potassium and magnesium supplementation, particularly if they require prolonged antifungal treatment. A.W. is experiencing nephrotoxicity from ABLC as reflected in the elevated SCr and changing electrolye pattern representing wasting of potassium and magnesium into the urine.

LENGTH OF ANTIFUNGAL THERAPY AND COMBINATION ANTIFUNGAL THERAPY

CASE 96-7, QUESTION 4: In response to A.W.'s rise in SCr, his physician elects to discontinue ABLC and begin voriconazole 6 mg/kg IV every 12 hours × two doses, followed by 4 mg/kg IV every 12 hours, plus caspofungin 70 mg IV on day 1 and 50 mg IV daily thereafter. What is the rationale for combination therapy, and how should the patient be monitored? How long should A.W. receive antifungal therapy for his IA?

Common toxicities reported with voriconazole include reversible visual disturbances (blurred vision, altered color perception, photophobia, visual hallucinations), skin reactions (rash, pruritus, photosensitivity), elevations in hepatic transaminase enzymes and alkaline phosphatase, nausea, and headache.[255,265,266] Caspofungin has fewer adverse effects. Vein irritation and headache are most common; dermatologic reactions related to histamine release (flushing, erythema, wheals) have also been reported. Increased hepatic transaminase enzymes occur in approximately 6% of patients treated with caspofungin.[257] A.W. should be monitored for changes in liver function and counseled regarding the potential visual side effects of voriconazole.

Data supporting improved outcomes with two-drug combinations of triazoles, echinocandins, and polyenes in patients with IA are sparse. However, in vitro and animal data suggest that an echinocandin plus voriconazole or a polyene may be synergistic.[267–270] Given the overall poor prognosis of IA in severely immunocompromised patients, many practitioners are choosing to treat patients with two-drug combination therapy. Voriconazole in combination with caspofungin is thus a reasonable alternative for A.W., particularly in view of the ABLC toxicity he is experiencing. With the discontinuation of ABLC, A.W.'s renal function is expected to resolve.

The optimum duration of antifungal therapy for treatment of IA is unestablished.[249] Important considerations include the status of the patient's immune system and the extent of response to treatment. Many clinicians continue aggressive antifungal therapy until the infection has stabilized radiographically and then proceed with less aggressive "maintenance" therapy (e.g., single-agent oral voriconazole) until restoration of the immune system has taken place. It is not uncommon for a patient to require several months of antifungal therapy for effective management of IA.

Prevention of *Pneumocystis jiroveci* Pneumonia

CASE 96-7, QUESTION 5: A.W. is receiving TMP/SMX, one double-strength tablet PO BID on Monday and Tuesday. What is the rationale for its use?

P. jiroveci is a common pathogen that causes *Pneumocystis* pneumonia (PCP) in patients who have undergone allogeneic HCT. PCP is a potentially lethal infection, and therefore prophylaxis is routinely administered. The optimum prophylactic regimen has not been established, but most centers administer TMP/SMX for PCP prophylaxis.[8] Dapsone or aerosolized pentamidine are alternatives for patients who are allergic to sulfonamides or do not tolerate TMP/SMX for other reasons such as hematologic toxicities. PCP prophylaxis is usually begun after neutrophil recovery because (a) PCP most commonly occurs after engraftment, and (b) TMP/SMX is potentially myelosuppressing. Patients should be closely monitored for unexplained neutropenia or thrombocytopenia.

ISSUES OF SURVIVORSHIP AFTER HEMATOPOIETIC STEM CELL TRANSPLANTATION

CASE 96-8

QUESTION 1: H.O. is a 32-year-old woman who received a BU/CY preparative regimen and an HLA-matched sibling

BMT for treatment of chronic phase CML at age 21 years. H.O. received her BMT more than 10 years ago, is disease-free, and has not had chronic GVHD for 9 years. Her only medication is one multivitamin tablet PO daily. What issues of cancer survivorship are of concern to H.O.?

A greater proportion of HCT recipients are surviving their cancer diagnosis without evidence of their primary malignancy, but they are at risk for long-term physical and emotional sequelae of their cancer treatments.[2] Because most long-term HCT survivors are no longer under the care of an HCT center, their health care providers may be unfamiliar with the complications of HCT. To facilitate the clinical care of long-term HCT recipients, recommendations for screening and preventative practices have been created for adult and pediatric HCT survivors.[271,272] These guidelines should facilitate the provision of health care to HCT recipients. The following paragraphs describe various concerns associated with the morbidity of long-term HCT survivors.[271–273] Long-term HCT survivors should be regularly screened, or take preventative steps regarding immunity, secondary malignant neoplasm, oral complications from GVHD or radiation, and liver, respiratory, endocrine, ocular, skeletal, nervous system, kidney, vascular, and psychosocial function.

Immune function can take more than 2 years to recover, even after discontinuation immunosuppressants.[274] Treatment of GVHD exacerbates immune system defects, necessitating prophylaxis and vigilant monitoring for infectious complications. Fevers should be rapidly assessed and treated to prevent a fatal infection. Recipients of HCT also lose protective antibodies to vaccine-preventable diseases. Therefore, HCT survivors need to be revaccinated for selected infectious diseases with due consideration for the risk of vaccination.

For a vaccination table, see http://thepoint.lww.com/AT10e.

HCT survivors have a greater risk of secondary malignant neoplasms.[2] An increased incidence of cancer of the skin, oral mucosa, brain, thyroid, and bone is observed after allogeneic HCT, and an increased incidence of myelodysplasia and acute leukemia can occur after autologous HCT for NHL.[2] HCT survivors should avoid carcinogens (e.g., tobacco) and be screened for secondary malignant neoplasms indefinitely.[2] Long-term impairment of end-organ function may be due to the preparative regimen, infectious complications (either autologous or allogeneic grafts), and posttransplantation immunosuppression (allogeneic grafts only).[271,273] Endocrine dysfunction, specifically of the thyroid, gonads, and growth velocity, is common.[271,272] Adrenal insufficiency can result from long-term corticosteroids therapy used to treat GVHD. Infertility is commonly observed after myeloablative HCT secondary to the high doses of alkylating agents and radiation administered. Frequently, men become azoospermic, and chemically induced menopause develops in women.[2] However, pregnancies have occurred after HCT.[2] Up to 60% of HCT recipients have osteopenia, most likely resulting from gonadal dysfunction and corticosteroid administration; avascular necrosis due to corticosteroids can also occur.[275] A significant portion (15%–40%) of HCT survivors exhibit pulmonary dysfunction with variable symptoms (e.g., restrictive, chronic obstructive lung disease) from multiple causes.[275] Hepatitic infections can occur in HCT recipients through blood transfusions or, more commonly, because recipients or donors have a latent hepatitis viral infection. The prevalence of chronic hepatitis C ranges from 5% to 70% in long-term HCT survivors.[276] Because of this, cirrhosis and its complications may become an important late complication of HCT.[276] Hepatic dysfunction can also result from iron overload, which may occur secondary to multiple PRBC transfusions administered during aplasia after myeloablative preparative regimens and before HCT. Alopecia is a common late effect with BU/CY, as are cataracts with CY/TBI.[91]

H.O. should be routinely monitored for signs of relapse and chronic GVHD. To lower the risk of infectious complications, she should be counseled to obtain prompt medical care for fevers or signs of an infection, and she should be revaccinated if she has not done so since receiving her myeloablative HCT. Thorough evaluation of end-organ function, including renal, hepatic, thyroid, and ovarian function, should be assessed at regular intervals. In addition, her bone mineral density should be determined, and H.O. should be counseled on preventive measures for osteopenia (e.g., calcium supplementation). In addition to standard cancer screening tests, H.O. should be closely monitored for secondary malignant neoplasms.[2]

KEY REFERENCES AND WEBSITES

A full list of references for this chapter can be found at http://thepoint.lww.com/AT10e. Below are the key references and websites for this chapter, with the corresponding reference number in this chapter found in parentheses after the reference.

Key References

Appelbaum FR et al. Haematopoietic cell transplantation as immunotherapy. *Nature.* 2001;411:385. (4)

Copelan EA et al. Hematopoietic stem-cell transplantation. *N Engl J Med.* 2006;354:1813. (2)

Pasquini MC, Wang Z. Current use and outcome of hematopoietic stem cell transplantation: CIBMTR Summary Slides. Center for International Blood and Marrow Transplant Research. http://www.cibmtr.org/ReferenceCenter/SlidesReports/SummarySlides/pages/index.aspx. Accessed December 9, 2010. (1)

Blume KG et al, eds. *Thomas' Hematopoietic Cell Transplantation.* 4th ed. Malden, MA: Blackwell; 2009. (21, 22, 47, 56, 59, 64, 94, 103, 127)

Key Websites

Health Resources and Services Administration (HRSA). http://www.hrsa.gov/. Accessed March 18, 2011.

International Bone Marrow Transplant Registry (IBMTR) and Autologous Blood and Marrow Transplant Registry (ABMTR). http://www.ibmtr.org/. Accessed March 18, 2011.

National Marrow Donor Program. http://www.marrow.org/. Accessed March 18, 2011.

American Society for Blood and Marrow Transplantation (ASBMT). http://www.asbmt.org/. Accessed March 18, 2011.

97

Pediatric Pharmacotherapy

Marcia L. Buck

CORE PRINCIPLES

	CHAPTER CASES
GROWTH AND DEVELOPMENT	
1 Children undergo considerable physiologic changes between birth and adulthood. Although most follow the same general pattern of growth, the timing of maturation varies from child to child.	**Case 97-1 (Question 1), Table 97-1**
PHARMACOKINETIC DIFFERENCES	
1 All aspects of pharmacokinetics are affected by growth and development. Drug absorption is altered by a variety of mechanisms, with the most significant differences noted during the first months of life.	**Case 97-2 (Question 1), Case 97-3 (Questions 1–4)**
2 Drug distribution is affected by changes in relative organ size, body water content, fat stores, plasma protein concentrations, acid–base balance, cardiac output, and tissue perfusion. The greatest degree of change occurs during the first year of life.	**Case 97-3 (Questions 5, 6), Table 97-2**
3 Metabolic function is highly dependent on patient age. This has been demonstrated in a number of recent studies, which have identified significant differences in half-life during infancy, childhood, and adolescence.	**Case 97-4 (Questions 1–4)**
4 Elimination is reduced during infancy, resulting in slower rates of clearance for many commonly used drugs. Glomerular filtration rate increases throughout childhood. Use of creatinine clearance as an estimate of glomerular filtration rate requires different equations than those used in adults.	**Case 97-5 (Questions 1, 2), Case 97-6 (Question 1)**
5 Adolescence is not simply a link between childhood and adulthood; it is a distinct period of significant physiologic change. The effects of puberty can alter the efficacy or toxicity of many drugs administered during this period.	**Case 97-7 (Question 1)**
PHARMACODYNAMIC DIFFERENCES	
1 Although less well understood than pharmacokinetic differences between children and adults, there are significant age-related effects on pharmacodynamics as well. Children may exhibit differences in both therapeutic response and adverse effect profiles.	**Case 97-8 (Question 1), Case 97-9 (Questions 1, 2)**
MEDICATION DOSING IN CHILDREN	
1 The differences in pharmacokinetics and pharmacodynamics observed in children influence the choice of drug dose and dosing interval. For most dose calculations, weight is used to account for growth and development.	**Case 97-10 (Question 1)**

continued

MEDICATION DOSING IN CHILDREN *CONTINUED*

2	All pediatric prescriptions and medication orders must be checked for the appropriateness of the dose, route, and frequency with a pediatric dosing reference.	**Figure 97-1**

PREVENTING MEDICATION ERRORS IN CHILDREN

1	Children are at a greater risk for medication errors than adults, as a result of the need to calculate drug doses and alter dosage formulations.	**Case 97-10 (Question 2)**
2	Electronic prescribing, standardization of drug doses and concentrations, and the introduction of smart-pump technology have been shown to reduce errors in many children's hospitals. One of the most effective methods to avoid errors is the inclusion of pediatric pharmacists in the medication ordering and review process.	**Case 97-10 (Question 3), Table 97-3**

INCREASING PEDIATRIC MEDICATION INFORMATION

1	A number of governmental programs are increasing the availability of pediatric medication information and improving the ability of pediatric health care professionals to provide safe and effective drug therapy for children.	**Case 97-10 (Question 4)**

Providing care for children can be one of the most challenging, but rewarding, aspects of pharmacy practice. Although a relatively small number of health care providers pursue specialty training in pediatrics and work exclusively with children, most clinicians will provide care for children every day in the community or hospital setting. According to recent population estimates, approximately one-quarter of the US population is younger than 20 years of age, with 7% younger than 5 years of age.[1] Although most children are healthy, this segment of the population still uses a significant amount of health care resources. In a recent telephone survey, one in five parents reported giving their child one or more prescription medications within the previous week.[2] A survey conducted in pediatricians' offices found that 53% of children left their visit with a prescription.[3]

Pediatrics, as a specialty, encompasses a very diverse patient population. Patients range in age from premature neonates to adolescents and can vary in weight by 100-fold, from a 0.5-kg premature neonate to a 50-kg 16-year-old. Further complicating the care of children is the relative lack of information on drug dosing and monitoring. Because of the small numbers of children requiring medical treatment and the difficulty in conducting research in these patients, fewer than half of the drugs currently available in the United States are approved by the Food and Drug Administration (FDA) for pediatric use.[4,5] As a result, as many as 60% of all prescriptions written by pediatricians are for "off-label" uses.[6] Dosing and monitoring information for off-label uses is often based on case series and clinical trials published in the medical literature and may not be readily available in general drug references.

Health care providers caring for children must be capable of assessing the appropriateness of drug doses for this diverse population and providing recommendations for dosage adjustments and patient monitoring with limited resources. This requires knowledge of the pharmacokinetic and pharmacodynamic differences between children and adults and how these differences impact both therapeutic and adverse drug effects.

GROWTH AND DEVELOPMENT DURING CHILDHOOD

CASE 97-1

QUESTION 1: C.J. is a 4-month-old, 6.5 kg baby boy who has recently started teething. His parents ask for advice on a medication to alleviate C.J.'s pain. What factors will influence the decision, and what medication and dosing regimen would be appropriate for C.J.?

Children undergo considerable physiologic changes between birth and adulthood. Although many changes are easily observed, such as the ability to walk or the development of language, others are less evident. C.J.'s analgesic dose will be based on his age and weight, as estimates of the numerous pharmacokinetic and pharmacodynamic differences between children and adults. To discuss the changes that occur with growth and development, pediatric patients are typically grouped by age (Table 97-1). These definitions are helpful to provide a consistent framework for dosing recommendations, but it should be kept in mind that they are arbitrary and can oversimplify the differences among individual patients. Although children tend to grow and develop

TABLE 97-1
Commonly Used Age Definitions

Premature neonate	Born at <36 weeks' gestational age
Term neonate	Born at ≥36 weeks' gestational age
Neonate	Birth–1 month of age
Infant	>1 month–1 year of age
Child	>1 year–11 years of age
Adolescent	12–16 years of age

in a relatively similar manner, the timing of maturation varies from child to child. Children do not grow in a predictable, linear fashion, but rather in periodic bursts, with additional variation caused by differences in genetic predisposition, nutritional intake, and environment.[7] Research on the impact of growth and development on pharmacokinetics and pharmacodynamics, often referred to as developmental pharmacology, has grown considerably during the past several decades, improving our ability to optimize the efficacy of drug therapy in children while minimizing adverse effects.

The most appropriate analgesic for C.J. would be acetaminophen. Aspirin is no longer used as an analgesic in children because of its association with Reye syndrome, a rare condition causing mitochondrial damage and resulting in hepatic failure. Nonsteroidal anti-inflammatory drugs, such as ibuprofen, are not recommended for use in infants younger than 6 months of age because of an increased risk for renal impairment. C.J. should receive an acetaminophen dose of 10 to 15 mg/kg given every 4 to 6 hours as needed, with no more than five doses given in a 24-hour period. Based on his age and weight, an appropriate recommendation for C.J. would be to give 65 mg of the concentrated infant acetaminophen drops by mouth every 6 hours as needed. If C.J. continues to need medication for more than 24 hours, his parents should contact C.J.'s primary health care provider.

PEDIATRIC PHARMACOKINETIC DIFFERENCES

All aspects of pharmacokinetics are affected by growth and physical maturation, beginning during gestation (pregnancy) and ending in adulthood. These changes are complex, and their timing can vary widely from patient to patient.

Drug Absorption

ORAL DRUG ABSORPTION

CASE 97-2

QUESTION 1: A.H., a 1.5-kg, 4-week-old infant girl born at 29 weeks' gestational age, is being treated with phenobarbital for seizures associated with a period of asphyxia at birth. She is currently receiving a maintenance dose of 7.5 mg (5 mg/kg) given intravenously (IV) once daily. The team wishes to transition her to oral therapy now that she is receiving full enteral feeds. A trough serum phenobarbital concentration obtained during IV therapy was 17.5 mcg/mL, within the desired range of 15 to 40 mcg/mL. Switching the patient to phenobarbital elixir 7.5 mg given orally once daily results in a serum concentration of only 8.9 mcg/mL after 1 week of therapy. What factors might explain the lower concentration, and how should A.H. be managed?

Enteral absorption of drugs is altered at birth and does not approximate adult patterns for several months.[7,8] Gastric fluid volume is greatly reduced at birth. Gastric acid production is decreased, giving the neonate a higher, nearly neutral pH in the stomach. This results in a greater absorption of acid-labile drugs such as penicillin G and erythromycin, but reduced absorption of weakly acidic drugs such as phenobarbital and phenytoin. Gastric acid output increases during the first 1 to 2 weeks of life, but only reaches adult values at 2 to 3 years of age. Transport of bile acids into the gastrointestinal lumen and pancreatic enzyme production are also reduced, further altering the absorption of pH-sensitive drugs and reducing enterohepatic recirculation. Amylase activity is minimal at birth and remains low until the third month of life.[9] Pancreatic lipase activity is detectable by 32 weeks' gestational age, but remains low at birth and throughout the next 2 to 3 months. In contrast, gastric lipase is present at birth and accounts for a greater percentage of fat absorption during early life. In addition to these differences, neonates are also born with relatively sterile gastrointestinal tracts. Normal bacterial colonization typically occurs within days for term infants, but may be delayed in premature infants who reside in the more sterile environment of an intensive care unit. The effectiveness of drugs that rely on gastrointestinal flora for activation or degradation may be significantly altered during this period.

Gastric emptying time is delayed and intestinal transit time is prolonged at birth, but both quickly increase within the first few days of life as contractions in the stomach become more coordinated and intestinal contractions become more frequent, stronger, and sustained. Premature infants have delayed development of normal gastric emptying and intestinal transit, as shown in a study of acetaminophen dosing in which premature infants at 28 weeks' gestational age had a 2-hour delay in absorption compared with older infants.[10] Adult values for gastric emptying and intestinal transit time are generally reached by 4 to 8 months of age.

For drugs absorbed through passive diffusion, reduced splanchnic blood flow during the first weeks of life can reduce the rate and extent of absorption by altering concentration gradients across the intestinal villi.[7] Reduction in blood flow may also place neonates at risk for damage to the gut lining from hyperosmolar drug formulations. As a result, many institutions delay use of the enteral route for drug administration until the patient is receiving at least one-quarter to half of their nutritional needs through enteral feedings. This allows dilution of drug doses and may reduce the risk for mucosal damage. Lower levels of metabolic enzyme activity in the intestine may reduce first-pass metabolism of drugs given enterally.[11,12] Boucher and colleagues found that the bioavailability of zidovudine decreased from 89% in neonates during the first 2 weeks of life to 61% in older infants, reflecting increased first-pass metabolism in the older patients.[12] Intestinal enzymatic activity does not approach adult values until 2 to 3 years of age.

The lower phenobarbital serum concentration after A.H. was placed on enteral therapy is most likely the result of reduced drug absorption in the gastrointestinal tract, resulting from the higher gastric pH and reduced splanchnic blood flow. The maintenance phenobarbital dose for A.H. should be increased to achieve a trough serum concentration within the desired range. An increase of the oral dose to 10 mg would be appropriate, with a plan to obtain a trough concentration within 3 to 5 days. Although this value will not yet reflect the steady-state concentration, due to the long half-life of the drug, it will be useful to guide additional dosing changes.

INTRAMUSCULAR DRUG ABSORPTION

CASE 97-3

QUESTION 1: C.B. is a 3.6-kg newborn boy, born at 39 weeks' gestational age, who was transferred to the newborn nursery after delivery. Routine care for neonates during the first hours of life generally includes administration of erythromycin eye ointment for prevention of neonatal ophthalmia and 1 mg of phytonadione (vitamin K_1) given intramuscularly (IM) to prevent vitamin K–deficiency bleeding of the newborn. C.B.'s parents question the need to give

their baby a shot so soon after birth. How would you explain the rationale for giving phytonadione IM rather than orally?

In the United States, phytonadione is typically given by IM injection after birth. Drug administration by IM injection typically results in a delay in time to reach peak serum concentrations in neonates. This delay is related to reduced muscle size, weaker muscle contractions, and an immature vasculature resulting in more erratic blood flow to and from the muscle.[7,8] Although considered a disadvantage when rapid absorption is needed, such as with antibiotic administration, the delay in systemic absorption after IM injection is used as an advantage for the administration of phytonadione after birth. The delayed absorption from muscle results in a depotlike effect, providing a slow release of the drug into the systemic circulation until the infant's dietary intake is adequate to maintain necessary vitamin K serum concentrations.[13] A similar delay in drug absorption may occur with subcutaneous injection because of the lower percentage of body fat in neonates. The delay in absorption seen with IM and subcutaneous administration becomes negligible after the first months of life. When counseling C.B.'s parents, it will be important to stress the benefit of the slower absorption of vitamin K with IM administration compared with the rapid absorption and clearance of a single oral dose. A single IM injection of vitamin K will protect their son from bleeding until he is approximately a month old, when he should be taking in enough breast milk or infant formula to maintain adequate vitamin K concentrations.

TRANSDERMAL DRUG ABSORPTION

CASE 97-3, QUESTION 2: C.B. is scheduled for a circumcision before discharge. The surgical site will be prepped with a 10% povidone–iodine solution. What factors influence the absorption of medications via this route in the neonatal patient? Based on these factors, how should the povidone–iodine be applied to minimize toxicity?

In contrast to enteral, IM, and subcutaneous administration, transdermal or percutaneous administration results in greater drug absorption in neonates than it does in older children and adults. Enhanced absorption results from a greater skin to body surface area ratio, approximately three times that of adults, as well as a thinner stratum corneum, better epidermis hydration, and greater perfusion.[7,8] The greater degree of percutaneous absorption in infants has resulted in significant toxicity. Hexachlorophene, when used routinely to bathe infants, has resulted in seizures and is now considered contraindicated in this age range. Application of povidone–iodine as a topical disinfectant before surgery has been linked to neonatal thyroid dysfunction and, as a result, is now used only in limited quantities for brief periods to limit percutaneous iodine absorption. In spite of the knowledge of this adverse effect, cases continue to be reported in the medical literature.[14] Even relatively common topical products can produce systemic toxicity. Frequent use of diaper rash products containing hydrocortisone can produce suppression of the hypothalamus-pituitary-adrenal axis in as little as 2 weeks.

Cleaning and disinfecting the skin before surgery in a neonate requires special attention to the selection of agent, surface area affected, and the length of skin contact. For C.B., a 10% povidone–iodine solution should be gently applied to the penis and surrounding skin immediately before surgery and removed as soon as the 5- to 10-minute circumcision has been completed to minimize the risk for systemic toxicity resulting from enhanced percutaneous iodine absorption.

CASE 97-3, QUESTION 3: Are transdermal anesthetics an appropriate option for use before C.B.'s procedure?

Both 4% lidocaine and EMLA (eutectic mixture of local anesthetics) cream, which contains lidocaine and prilocaine, are widely used as topical anesthetics for infants and children before venipuncture, IV catheter placement, or circumcision. Both have been shown in clinical trials to be safe and effective.[15] The low concentration of the active ingredients and the limited duration of contact, 30 to 60 minutes, prevent excessive systemic absorption when applied to intact skin. Either analgesic cream would be appropriate for C.B. EMLA should be applied an hour before the start of the circumcision, while 4% lidocaine cream should be applied 30 minutes before the procedure. A thin layer of cream should be applied, without an occlusive dressing, and the baby diapered until the start of the procedure. The cream should be completely removed before the application of the 10% povidone–iodine solution.

Other transdermal medications should be avoided or used with caution for only limited periods in infants. After the first year of life, transdermal application becomes a more useful route of administration for several medications. Methylphenidate and clonidine patches are used in the treatment of attention deficit hyperactivity disorder (ADHD), and both lidocaine and fentanyl patches are used for the treatment of children with severe pain.

RECTAL DRUG ABSORPTION

CASE 97-3, QUESTION 4: A week after C.B.'s discharge from the hospital, he is brought into the emergency department after becoming lethargic and febrile at home. His parents have tried giving him oral acetaminophen, but he is vomiting and unable to take liquids. Is rectal administration of acetaminophen an acceptable option for C.B. in the hospital after he has been stabilized?

Rectal administration is a useful route of drug delivery for many pediatric patients. Most drugs are well absorbed by this route, but the strong rectal contractions in infants can result in an inability to retain suppositories for the length of time needed to achieve optimal absorption.[7,8] Gels and liquid dosage preparations that do not require an extended time for dissolution are better options. Rectal diazepam gel is often used by parents of children with seizure disorders to provide rapid control of worsening seizures while awaiting emergency medical personnel. In a recent observational trial of 358 children, the median time from administration of rectal diazepam by a parent to cessation of seizures was 4.3 minutes.[16]

Rectal acetaminophen would be a viable option for C.B. It is rapidly absorbed through this route. Many drug dosing references recommend a slightly higher rectal acetaminophen dose (10–20 mg/kg) to account for a potentially lower bioavailability.

Drug Distribution

Growth and development also affect drug distribution. Organ size, body water content, fat stores, plasma protein concentrations, acid–base balance, cardiac output, and tissue perfusion all change throughout childhood, altering the pattern of distribution and extent of drug penetration.[7] The greatest degree of change occurs during the first year of life.

CASE 97-3, QUESTION 5: In the emergency department, C.B. is refusing to breast-feed and is having difficulty

breathing. Neonatal sepsis with possible meningitis is suspected. Laboratory values and vital signs include the following:

Temperature, 39.4°C
Heart rate, 202 beats/minute (normal 107–182 beats/minute)
Blood pressure, 85/62 mm Hg (normal systolic 70–75 mm Hg, diastolic 50–55 mm Hg)

He currently weighs 3.4 kg and appears slightly dehydrated. His parents report that C.B. has had fewer wet diapers than usual during the last 24 hours. What physiologic differences in the neonatal period would affect your choice of empiric antibiotics for the treatment of neonatal central nervous system infections?

Empiric antibiotic therapy for sepsis and meningitis for C.B. typically consists of ampicillin and an aminoglycoside. Although not commonly used in adults because of the relatively low degree of penetration across the blood–brain barrier, this combination is very effective in the neonatal period when drug distribution into the central nervous system is much higher. Constituting only 2% of total body weight in an adult, the brain makes up 10% to 12% of the weight of an infant. As a result, the brain serves as a much larger potential compartment for drug distribution. In addition, the percentage of systemic blood flow that reaches the cerebral vasculature is greater. These factors, along with a potential for greater passive diffusion of drugs across the functionally immature blood–brain barrier, can result in higher drug concentrations within the central nervous system of infants compared with older children and adults.[7,8] This can produce both benefit and risk to the infant. Drugs given to treat meningitis or seizures are more likely to achieve therapeutic concentrations within the central nervous system, but there is also a greater potential risk for drug-induced neurotoxicity.

BODY WATER

One of the most significant differences in drug distribution during childhood is the decrease in total body water content with increasing age. Approximately 85% of a premature newborn's weight and 70% to 80% of a term newborn's weight is body water, compared with only 60% to 65% in a 1-year-old.[7,8] After a year of age, the percentage declines to 50% to 60% and remains relatively constant. Extracellular water decreases in a similar manner, from 40% to 45% in the newborn to 20% to 25% by the end of the first year of life. Intracellular water content, however, remains relatively stable. These changes result in a much greater distribution of highly water-soluble drugs, such as the aminoglycosides or linezolid, and a reduced accumulation of highly lipid-soluble drugs, such as amphotericin, amiodarone, benzodiazepines, or digoxin.

The pharmacokinetic profile of gentamicin has been well described in infants and children as a result of its role in empiric antibiotic therapy for neonatal sepsis and meningitis. The volume of distribution of gentamicin in premature neonates ranges from 0.5 to 0.7 L/kg, reflecting the higher extracellular water content at this age. This value falls to 0.4 L/kg by the end of the first year of life and further declines to 0.2 to 0.3 L/kg by adulthood.[17] As a result of their higher volume of distribution, the weight-based dose for an infant is often much higher than a comparable dose in an adult. Based on C.B.'s age and weight, the *Pediatric Dosage Handbook*,[17] one of the most widely used pediatric drug references, recommends an ampicillin dose of 170 mg (50 mg/kg) given IV every 6 hours and a gentamicin dose of 8.5 mg (2.5 mg/kg) given IV every 8 hours. Using these same weight-based doses in a 70-kg adult would result in doses much higher than the typical recommended adult dose.

BODY FAT

Whereas the effects of growth and development on changes in body water content are well defined and typically require adjustments in drug dosing only during infancy, the effects of changes in body fat are not yet well understood. Body fat increases throughout gestation and infancy. A premature neonate may have as little as 1% to 2% body fat, whereas a term infant will have closer to 10% to 15% body fat. A 1-year-old will have a body fat of 20% to 25%, similar to that of an adult. Children following normal growth patterns have relatively little change in their body fat percentage between the second year of life and the onset of puberty. However, the increasing rate of childhood obesity has generated concern about the efficacy and safety of current weight-based dosing strategies.[18] In a 2010 retrospective study of 699 children between 5 and 12 years of age admitted to a children's hospital during a 6-month period, overweight children (defined as having a body mass index greater than the 85th percentile for age) accounted for 33% of the admissions.[19] Evaluation of their medication orders revealed that 8.5% of the doses ordered were for less than the recommended dose, whereas 2.8% were for an excessive dose. The need to make dosage adjustments in these children remains controversial; little research has been done to document the effects of childhood obesity on the pharmacokinetics and pharmacodynamics of commonly used pediatric medications.

PROTEIN BINDING

CASE 97-3, QUESTION 6: On the third day of admission, the microbiology laboratory reports the culture and sensitivity results for C.B. Although the cerebrospinal fluid and urine cultures were negative, the peripheral blood culture grew *Escherichia coli*. The organism appears to be sensitive to a wide range of antibiotics, including penicillins, cephalosporins, gentamicin, and sulfamethoxazole-trimethoprim. What would your recommendation be for C.B.'s continuing treatment?

Many of the drugs that would treat C.B.'s infection are highly protein bound. Plasma protein binding is reduced in neonates as a result of decreased circulating levels of both albumin and α_1-acid glycoprotein, as well as decreased binding affinity.[7,8,11] With the known susceptibilities and their long history of efficacy and safety, continuing C.B.'s current ampicillin and gentamicin regimen for 7 to 10 days would be an appropriate choice. Although ampicillin is known to be present in higher unbound concentrations in infants compared with adults (Table 97-2), use of standard dosing recommendations for C.B. based on age should be

TABLE 97-2
Examples of Drugs Present in Greater Unbound Concentrations in Neonates Than in Adults

Alfentanil	Penicillin G
Ampicillin	Phenobarbital
Ceftriaxone	Phenytoin
Cefuroxime	Propranolol
Diazepam	Salicylates
Digoxin	Sulfonamides
Lidocaine	Teicoplanin
Ketamine	Theophylline
Morphine	Thiopental
Nafcillin	Valproic acid

adequate to prevent toxicity. Sulfamethoxazole-trimethoprim would not be appropriate. Administration of drugs with a high binding affinity for albumin, such as the sulfonamides, during the neonatal period can result in competition with bilirubin for binding sites. The resulting increase in unbound bilirubin can lead to kernicterus, neurologic damage caused by deposition of bilirubin in the brain, primarily in the basal ganglia.[20] For this reason, sulfonamides are not recommended for neonates and are not approved by the FDA for use in infants younger than 2 months of age. Ceftriaxone, another possible option for C.B., also is known to be highly protein bound. Although approved for use in neonates, it is contraindicated in those with hyperbilirubinemia. As a precaution, many hospitals restrict its use in the neonatal population to only those patients who have infections resistant to other antibiotics.

The clinical impact of changes in protein binding can be difficult to predict. Separation and measurement of the unbound (free) fraction can be used to guide therapy for drugs such as valproic acid or phenytoin, but this process is more labor-intensive and expensive and, as a result, may not be available at all hospitals. Larger blood sample volumes may also be required, which can lead to excessive blood loss in premature infants. An estimation of the unbound concentration can be made from total serum drug concentrations, but may not be accurate in infants. Methods to estimate unbound serum valproic acid concentrations from total concentrations that were developed for adults have been found to be ineffective in predicting free levels in neonates and infants.[21]

Metabolism

Much of the research currently being conducted in developmental pharmacology is focused on changes in metabolic function.[7,8,11,22–49] Our understanding of the ontogeny of metabolic enzymes is improving rapidly, as in vitro data gathered from studies quantifying hepatic microsomal proteins and determining levels of enzymatic activity are combined with information obtained through pharmacokinetic and pharmacogenomic research. It is clear that the onset of function varies among enzymes; whereas some exhibit metabolic activity in utero, others demonstrate activity only after several months of life. The development of metabolic enzyme function continues during the first years of life and does not appear to be complete until after puberty. There appears to be considerable interpatient variability. Enzyme development can be affected by the underlying health of the child, nutritional status, and exposure to substrate. Metabolic activity also reflects genetic polymorphisms, just as in adults.

PHASE I DRUG METABOLISM

CASE 97-4

QUESTION 1: N.M. is a 1.38-kg, 3-week-old girl who was born at 28 weeks' gestational age. She has recently been started on nasogastric feedings, but has had repeated episodes of emesis and is not producing regular stools. Erythromycin is recommended to increase her gastric motility. What can you tell your team about the ability of N.M. to metabolize this drug? What dose of erythromycin should be chosen for N.M.?

Phase I reactions, which include oxidation, reduction, hydroxylation, and hydrolysis, develop at varying rates during childhood, resulting in the wide range of half-lives reported for many drugs. The cytochrome P-450 (CYP) 3A enzymes, which play a major role in drug metabolism, including that of erythromycin, develop early in life.[7,8,11,22–27] The earliest isozyme in this group to show activity is CYP3A7, the primary metabolic enzyme present in utero. It has been found on the endoplasmic reticulum of fetal hepatocytes by the end of the first trimester and serves a role in the transformation of fetal dehydroepiandrosterone and the detoxification of retinoic acid derivatives transferred from maternal serum across the placenta.[22,23,25–27] Enzymatic activity of CYP3A7 declines rapidly after birth, with a 50% reduction during the first month of life. Levels continue to decline at a slower rate through the next 6 months and are typically undetectable after 1 year of age. As levels of CYP3A7 decline, CYP3A4 and CYP3A5 levels rise. Although present during fetal development, the level of CYP3A4 activity is nearly 100-fold less than that of CYP3A7 until after birth.[22,27] Increases in CYP3A4 occur slowly, with a very gradual increase between the first month and the end of the first year of life. Levels continue to increase during childhood, but may not reach adult values for several years. Development of CYP3A5 function is highly variable among infants and children and does not appear to be related to patient age.

It can be anticipated that N.M. will have a slower rate of erythromycin metabolism as a result of lower levels of CYP3A4 activity, so a more conservative approach to dosing is often used. An oral erythromycin dose of 7 mg (5 mg/kg) given every 8 hours would be an appropriate starting dose for N.M. In addition to increasing the risk for adverse effects, higher serum erythromycin concentrations can lead to greater inhibition of CYP3A4. This may place N.M. at risk for toxicity from accumulation of other drugs metabolized via CYP3A4, such as fentanyl and midazolam.

Upregulation of CYP2D6 appears to begin in the last stage of gestation as a part of the complex transition of the baby to extrauterine life.[22–24,28] In fetal liver tissue samples obtained early in gestation, CYP2D6 activity has been reported to be only 1% to 5% of adult values.[22] Earlier studies suggested that levels of enzymatic activity remained low during infancy, but more recent research has demonstrated that CYP2D6 activity increases rapidly during the third trimester, and by the second week of life, values are similar to values in adults.[23] CYP2D6 levels remain relatively constant throughout childhood. The impact of genetic polymorphisms of CYP2D6 on elimination half-life in children is comparable to that demonstrated in adults, and appears to play a greater role in determining metabolic function than ontogeny.[23,24,28] A recent study of atomoxetine response in children and adolescents with ADHD found that CYP2D6 poor metabolizers had greater increases in heart rate and blood pressure and impaired weight gain compared with extensive metabolizers taking comparable doses, reflecting higher serum concentrations with the poor metabolizer phenotype.[29]

The enzymatic activity of CYP2C9 and CYP2C19 develops throughout childhood.[22,23,30] Studies of fetal hepatocytes demonstrated CYP2C9 activity at only 1% of adult values from 8 to 24 weeks' gestation, with an increase to 10% to 20% between 25 and 40 weeks. Enzyme activity continues to increase after birth, reaching 25% of adult values by approximately 5 months of age. Unlike other enzymes, CYP2C9 activity remains at only 50% of adult values until after puberty. The development of CYP2C9 activity is illustrated by the change in the rate of metabolism of phenytoin with advancing age. The apparent (calculated Michaelis–Menten) half-life of phenytoin in premature infants is approximately 75 hours, compared with 20 hours in a term neonate and 8 hours in a 2-week-old.[31]

Development of CYP2C19 function also occurs in utero, with enzyme activity 10% to 20% that of adults at birth.[23] Enzymatic activity increases gradually during the first 3 months of life to near full adult values. As with CYP2D6, genetic polymorphisms for CYP2C9 and CYP2C19 play an important role in determining individual patient response. Population modeling of pantoprazole pharmacokinetics in term neonates and premature infants revealed a longer elimination half-life than that reported in adults, supporting the lower levels of CYP2C19 activity in this age group.[32] The study also demonstrated significantly greater drug concentrations in the patients who had the poor metabolizer genotype.

The ontogeny of CYP2E1 has been studied in conjunction with the ability of infants to metabolize acetaminophen. Fetal hepatic CYP2E1 concentrations are typically undetectable during the first trimester, but begin to increase during the second trimester.[33] Levels are approximately 10% to 20% of adult values at birth. Enzyme concentrations continue to increase at a more gradual pace, until by 3 months of age, CYP2E1 expression becomes similar to that in adults. The increase in CYP2E1 metabolic capacity, along with maturation of glucuronidation, is responsible for the changing patterns of acetaminophen metabolite formation during infancy.

CASE 97-4, QUESTION 2: N.M. is now tolerating her enteral feedings and was recently extubated. However, she has had increasing episodes of apnea, a pause in breathing of 20 seconds or greater frequently present in premature newborns, during the past 2 days. Based on current dosing guidelines, you have recommended a caffeine citrate loading dose of 20 mg/kg given IV to be followed by a maintenance dose of 5 mg/kg given once daily to treat her apnea.[34] While reviewing the dosing information, you note that the elimination half-life for caffeine in neonates is approximately 70 to 100 hours, whereas the half-life for older infants, children, and adults is only 5 hours. What would explain that dramatic difference in half-life?

The changing elimination half-life of caffeine reflects the onset and maturation of CYP1A2 activity. The metabolism of caffeine during infancy has been extensively studied because many neonates are exposed in utero as a result of maternal intake and premature infants often receive caffeine for the treatment for apnea.[22–23,34,35] Studies have shown that CYP1A2 activity is negligible in fetal liver tissue and in newborns who were not exposed to it in utero.[35] The lower levels of enzymatic activity result in a longer caffeine half-life and allow once-daily dosing.[36] In contrast, newborns exposed to caffeine during gestation have higher levels of CYP1A2 activity at birth. Enzymatic activity rises progressively during the first months of life. By 6 months of age, it may exceed adult values, giving the infant a caffeine half-life of only 4 to 5 hours and necessitating more frequent dosing.

CASE 97-4, QUESTION 3: While N.M. was receiving mechanical ventilation during her first weeks of life, she was sedated with an infusion of midazolam. Many IV products, including some brands of midazolam, contain benzyl alcohol as a preservative and are labeled "Not for Use in Infants." What is the rationale for restricting the use of benzyl alcohol in the neonatal population?

Alcohol dehydrogenase, another Phase I enzyme, is present in utero, but in concentrations less than 5% of adult values.[23] Enzymatic activity does not approach functional maturity until approximately 5 years of age. The lack of alcohol dehydrogenase activity has a profound impact on the ability of newborns to metabolize benzyl alcohol, a common preservative in injectable drug products. In 1982, five neonates died after developing gasping respirations that progressed to respiratory failure, severe metabolic acidosis, renal and hepatic failure, thrombocytopenia, and cardiovascular collapse.[37] All of the infants had been repeatedly exposed to benzyl alcohol as a preservative in IV flush solutions. This toxicity, termed *gasping syndrome,* resulted from accumulation of the parent compound, as well as the benzoic acid metabolite. Another series of ten patient deaths was reported from a second institution.[38] From these case series, the threshold for toxicity was estimated to be a total daily exposure of 99 mg/kg/day. Within months of these reports, the FDA issued a safety alert calling attention to this reaction and recommending use of preservativefree products or preparations with alternative preservatives in newborns.[39] This change in practice led to the virtual elimination of gasping syndrome and brought to light the significance of differences in neonatal metabolism on drug toxicity. Pediatric clinicians continue to be vigilant for benzyl alcohol exposure, as several drugs routinely used in premature and critically ill neonates are not available in preservative-free preparations.[40]

PHASE II DRUG METABOLISM

Phase II reactions, including glucuronidation, sulfation, and acetylation, also undergo change throughout childhood. Present in low levels in fetal hepatic and renal tissues, the uridine 5′-diphosphate glucuronosyltransferase (UGT) enzymes responsible for the glucuronidation of both drugs and endogenous substances have minimal metabolic activity. A gradual increase in UGT expression occurs in the first 6 months of life, but still remains lower than that of adults for the first 2 to 3 years of life. Genetic polymorphisms produce additional variation in UGT expression.[11,22,23,41–44] The reduced ability of infants to perform glucuronidation has been known for many years as a result of the chloramphenicol "gray baby syndrome." Chloramphenicol was a widely used antibiotic during the 1950s. Within several years of its introduction, case reports began to appear in the medical literature describing emesis, abdominal distension, and cyanosis followed by cardiovascular collapse in infants given the drug.[46] The mechanism for this toxic effect was later found to be reduced activity of UGT2B7, the primary enzyme responsible for chloramphenicol metabolism, that allowed accumulation of the parent compound.[23,41]

CASE 97-4, QUESTION 4: N.M. also received morphine as an infusion during mechanical ventilation. Careful attention is needed when administering opioids to neonates to avoid drug accumulation. What differences in metabolism might affect the dosing requirements of morphine in the premature neonate such as N.M.?

Glucuronidation of morphine to morphine-6-glucuronide and morphine-3-glucuronide via UGT2B7 can be demonstrated in premature neonates born as early as 24 weeks' gestational age, but at a much slower rate than that of term neonates.[23,43,47,48] Studies of fetal liver microsomes have confirmed the presence of UGT2B7, with a rate of enzymatic activity only 10% to 20% of adult values.[22] Morphine metabolism increases rapidly during the last trimester of intrauterine life and the first weeks after birth. Clearance has been estimated to increase fourfold between 24 and 40 weeks' postconceptional age, but remains substantially slower than that of adults until approximately 3 years of age.[47,48]

Sulfation is a more important pathway in the metabolism of morphine during early infancy than later in life. Unlike UGT enzymes, sulfotransferases (SULT) develop extensively in utero, reaching levels of enzyme activity similar to that of adults at birth.[22,23,49] Intrauterine expression of SULT1A1, which is responsible for fetal metabolism of thyroid hormones, SULT2A1, the enzyme that metabolizes steroid hormones, and SULT1A3, which metabolizes catecholamines, occurs early in gestation and remains relatively constant thereafter. Not all SULT enzyme development takes place in the liver. Expression of SULT2A1 occurs primarily in the fetal adrenal gland.

The reliance on sulfation during infancy is found with several drugs besides morphine, including catecholamines, thyroid hormones, theophylline, and acetaminophen. Glucuronidation of acetaminophen via UGT1A6 and UGT1A9 is decreased in infants, and as a result, the primary route of acetaminophen metabolism is formation of sulfate conjugates for the first year of life.[23,45] Glucuronide pathways begin to predominate later in infancy and eventually surpass sulfation as the predominate route for acetaminophen metabolism.

Because of the slower rate of morphine clearance in neonates, particularly those born prematurely, morphine should be initiated at lower doses than those recommended for older infants and children. An appropriate starting dose for N.M.'s morphine infusion would be 0.005 to 0.01 mg/kg/hour. N.M. should be closely monitored for adverse effects, including hypotension, respiratory depression after extubation, and constipation.

Elimination

CASE 97-5

QUESTION 1: E.C. is a 1.85-kg infant girl born at 30 weeks' gestation. As with the other neonates described earlier, she is started on empiric antibiotic therapy with ampicillin and gentamicin shortly after birth. E.C. is given ampicillin 50 mg/kg IV every 12 hours and gentamicin 2.5 mg/kg IV every 24 hours. In the next bed, N.M., now 2 months old and 2.6 kg, is on the same regimen for a fever and elevated white blood cell count during the past 24 hours. N.M. is given ampicillin 50 mg/kg IV every 6 hours and gentamicin 2.5 mg/kg IV every 8 hours. What is the rationale for the differences in these patients' dosing intervals?

GLOMERULAR FILTRATION

Like the liver, the kidneys are not fully developed at birth. The ability to filter, excrete, and reabsorb substances is not maximized until 1 year of age.[7,8,50,51] At birth, full-term neonates have an average glomerular filtration rate (GFR) of only 2 to 4 mL/minute/1.73 m^2; in premature infants, the value may be even lower (0.6–0.8 mL/minute/1.73 m^2). There is a rapid rise in GFR during the first 2 weeks of life, with values increasing to 20 to 40 mL/minute/1.73 m^2 as a result of increased renal blood flow, increased function of the existing nephrons, and the appearance of additional nephrons, all of which may be timed to coincide with birth.[51] GFR increases to 80 to 110 mL/minute/1.73 m^2 by 6 months of age and continues to increase in a linear manner until it approaches adult values of 100 to 120 mL/minute/1.73 m^2 by 1 year of age. The impact of this increase in GFR can be seen in the neonatal dosing recommendations for many renally eliminated drugs, including the aminoglycosides and vancomycin. To account for reduced renal function, most pediatric references use a combination of patient weight and age (postnatal, postconceptional, or postmenstrual) to determine gentamicin dosing in neonates.[17] As a premature newborn, E.C. is likely to have significantly reduced glomerular filtration. E.C.'s gentamicin regimen will consist of the standard neonatal dose (2.5 mg/kg) given at a less frequent interval than that of 2-month-old N.M. to compensate for her renal insufficiency.

TUBULAR SECRETION

The elimination of ampicillin is also affected by changes in the rate of tubular secretion.[7,8,50] Like GFR, tubular secretion is reduced immediately after birth, but gradually increases during the first year of life. In addition to the penicillins, a reduction in tubular secretion also results in a prolonged elimination half-life for cephalosporins, furosemide, and digoxin. Digoxin has been used for many years in the management of supraventricular tachycardia in neonates. The half-life of digoxin decreases from approximately 30 to 40 hours in a term neonate to 20 to 25 hours in a 1-year-old as renal function matures. Selection of a digoxin dose must take into account the difference in elimination. The recommended oral digoxin maintenance dose for a neonate is 5 mcg/kg/day, whereas a 2-year-old would need to receive twice that amount to achieve target serum digoxin concentrations.[52] Ampicillin doses are typically adjusted by lengthening the dosing interval to compensate for reduced tubular secretion. E.C. (a newborn delivered at 30 weeks' gestation) would be dosed every 12 hours, whereas an older child such as N.M. would be expected to clear ampicillin more rapidly and would be dosed every 6 hours.

CASE 97-5, QUESTION 2: How should renal function be assessed in E.C. and N.M.?

As with adults, renal function should be closely monitored in children and drug doses adjusted accordingly. Unlike adults, blood urea nitrogen and serum creatinine values are not always useful as indicators of renal function. In the first days after birth, serum creatinine values reflect maternal creatinine transferred through the placenta and may appear falsely elevated. After the first week, serum creatinine values are typically low as a result of less muscle mass, especially in premature neonates, and may not accurately represent renal function.[8] Urine output is often used as an additional measure of renal function in this population. Diaper weights can be used to estimate output in E.C. and N.M., with values greater than 1 mL/kg/hour considered adequate renal function. At the time of initiation of therapy, if both babies are maintaining urine output values greater than 1 mL/kg/hour, the dosing regimens recommended in the *Pediatric Dosage Handbook*[17] can be used without further alteration. If urine output falls, the dosing intervals of both antibiotics may require adjustment. A trough serum gentamicin concentration should be obtained to further guide dosing.

CASE 97-6

QUESTION 1: H.G. is a 10-year-old boy admitted with osteomyelitis in his left ankle. The team plans to treat H.G. with vancomycin for 6 weeks. He is 140 cm (55 inches) tall and weighs 32 kg (70 pounds). His serum creatine is 0.5 mg/dL (normal for age 0.5–1.5 mg/dL). Determine H.G.'s creatinine clearance.

After infancy, serum creatinine may be used to estimate clearance. The equations used in adults, such as Cockroft-Gault, Jellife, or the Modification of Diet in Renal Disease (MDRD), are not appropriate for patients younger than 18 years of age.[8,53,54] There are several equations designed for pediatric use; one of the most common is the method described by Traub and Johnson[53,54]:

$$CL_{Cr} = (0.48 \times Ht)/S_{Cr} \qquad \textit{(Eq. 97-1)}$$

where CL_{Cr} is creatinine clearance (mL/minute/1.73 m^2), Ht is height (cm), and S_{Cr} is serum creatinine (mg/dL).

Using this method, H.G. has a calculated creatinine clearance of 134 mL/minute/1.73 m^2, indicating normal renal function. As with patients of any age, this equation should be used only as an estimate of renal function. It should be interpreted with caution in patients with little muscle mass or those who are dehydrated.

Pharmacokinetic Changes During Puberty

CASE 97-7

QUESTION 1: A.M. is a 16-year-old, 67-kg boy with osteosarcoma. He has received morphine for pain throughout his numerous hospitalizations for surgery and chemotherapy during the past 2 years, requiring an infusion rate as high as 0.5 mg/kg/hour. During this period, he has also progressed through puberty and is now a mature adult male. During his last admission, it was noted that his pain was well controlled on an adult morphine infusion rate of 10 mg/hour, equivalent to 0.15 mg/kg/hour. It was noted by the medical team that A.M.'s morphine infusion requirements were actually lower than in earlier admissions, although his pain scores have been unchanged. What might explain the change in A.M.'s response to morphine?

Although developmental pharmacology has traditionally focused on the differences in neonatal pharmacokinetics, there is growing interest in the influence of puberty on drug disposition.[55–57] Adolescence is not simply a link between childhood and adulthood, but is a distinct period of significant physiologic change. Hormonal fluctuations and sexual maturation can alter the efficacy or toxicity of many drugs administered during this period. Drug distribution can be altered as a result of an increase in body fat. Rapid increases in serum protein concentrations that occur during puberty alter drug binding characteristics.[56] Renal function, as measured by GFR, may exceed average adult values, resulting in rapid clearance of renally eliminated drugs such as aminoglycosides and vancomycin. Metabolic activity changes as well.[57] A study conducted in adolescents receiving morphine during a sickle cell crisis revealed a reduction in drug clearance with advancing sexual maturation.[58] Postpubertal adolescents, such as A.M., had weight-normalized clearance values 30% lower than younger patients during early puberty, suggesting a possible reduction in UGT2B7 activity. The titration of A.M.'s morphine must encompass not only the changes in drug clearance resulting from growth and development but also the progression of his disease and his need for pain control. Assessment of pain, using frequent self-report or a standardized pain scale, as well as heart rate, blood pressure, and respiratory rate, is essential for appropriate adjustment of A.M.'s morphine infusion.

A second example comes from a recent study of lopinavir pharmacokinetics in children who exhibited identified age- and sex-related differences in drug clearance.[59] When normalized for weight, there was no significant difference in clearance between prepubertal boys and girls. After the age of 12, boys had a mean rate of lopinavir clearance 39% greater than girls. The area under the concentration–time curve in boys was only half that of the girls. The authors suggest that this difference may reflect a reduction in CYP3A4 in girls that becomes apparent only with sexual maturation. Similar sex-related results have been reported in lopinavir studies conducted in adults. Caffeine metabolism via CYP1A2 has also been found to differ by sex in adolescents.[60] The rate of *N*-demethylation slows in both sexes after puberty, but appears to decrease earlier in puberty for girls than for boys. Other investigators have identified pharmacokinetic changes during adolescence with acetaminophen, alprazolam, carbamazepine, digoxin, isoniazid, lamotrigine, lorazepam, and theophylline.[56]

PEDIATRIC PHARMACODYNAMIC DIFFERENCES

Although not as well studied as pharmacokinetics, developmental changes in pharmacodynamics during growth may have equally significant effects on response to drug therapy in children.

CASE 97-8

QUESTION 1: S.L. is a 0.725-kg infant boy with an estimated gestational age of 24 weeks. He was brought to the neonatal intensive care unit immediately after birth with severe hypotension. A dopamine infusion was started at a rate of 10 mcg/kg/minute and quickly titrated to 20 mcg/kg/minute without significant benefit. What might explain S.L.'s lack of response, and how should his hypotension be managed?

Maturational changes in receptor conformation, density, and affinity, as well as signal transduction, can result in clinically significant differences in response to common therapies.[61] Although a dopamine infusion of 20 mcg/kg/minute will produce an adequate increase in myocardial contractility and elevate systemic vascular resistance in most children and adults, infants may not have a significant change in cardiovascular response. Infants have long been suspected to be relatively resistant to the effects of β-adrenergic agonists, including dopamine, dobutamine, and epinephrine. Recent research suggests the lack of response is related to a relative reduction in adrenergic receptor density or a downregulation of receptors within the myocardium of premature and critically ill neonates.[62] A higher dopamine infusion rate, up to 40 mcg/kg/minute, may be necessary to achieve an adequate blood pressure for S.L. If the dopamine is increased, S.L.'s extremities must be closely monitored for any signs of excessive peripheral vasoconstriction. Supplemental therapy with hydrocortisone, at a dose of 0.7 mg (1 mg/kg) IV every 8 hours, may also be used to manage his hypotension.

CASE 97-9

QUESTION 1: You will be counseling the parents of E.S., a 7-year-old girl with refractory seizures as a result of Lennox-Gastaut syndrome, on the use of lamotrigine. While preparing for your discussion, you note in the manufacturer's prescribing information a black-box warning regarding the risk for serious skin rashes. The incidence is listed as 0.8% in children 2 to 16 years of age, but only 0.3% in adults.[63] What might explain the difference in the incidence of an adverse effect by age?

Differences in pharmacodynamics resulting from growth and development can alter more than just therapeutic response. A drug's adverse effect profile may be distinctly different during childhood. A classic example of this phenomenon is the higher incidence of serious dermatologic reactions, including toxic epidermal necrolysis, in children taking lamotrigine compared with that of adults.[64–66] This was first suspected during initial pediatric clinical trials and appeared to be associated with rapid dose titration during the first several months of treatment, which had been based on previous studies in adults.[65] The slower dose escalation, now recommended for pediatric patients, is starting E.S.'s lamotrigine dose at 0.15 mg/kg/day and increasing by 0.15- to

0.3-mg/kg/day increments every 2 weeks, should reduce the likelihood for these reactions.

CASE 97-9, QUESTION 2: What is the possible mechanism(s) for the increased risk for toxicity with lamotrigine in children such as E.S.?

Research has led to several theories for the greater incidence of serious dermatologic reactions in children. Some investigators have suggested that this is a dose-related toxicity more evident in children who have a limited capacity to metabolize lamotrigine through glucuronidation to its inactive metabolites.[65] This theory, however, does not explain why other patient groups known to have higher serum lamotrigine concentrations during treatment, such as the elderly, are not at increased risk. Others have speculated that this represents an immune-mediated hypersensitivity response, as many of the affected patients reported have had previous reactions with other antiepileptic drugs.[66] Children with refractory seizures, such as those with Lennox-Gastaut syndrome, who are often treated with multiple agents beginning in the first years of life may be more likely to develop hypersensitivity. Although the mechanism underlying the age-related difference in the incidence of lamotrigine-associated rashes is not yet well understood, the importance of patient counseling is clear. The caregivers of all children receiving lamotrigine should be made aware of the risk and the need to seek medical care as soon as any signs of rash or erythema are noted.

MEDICATION DOSING IN CHILDREN

CASE 97-10

QUESTION 1: A.K. is a 7-year-old, 20-kg boy recently diagnosed with ADHD. After developing insomnia when treated with methylphenidate, he was switched to clonidine by his pediatrician. The recommended starting dose for clonidine in children is 5 mcg/kg/day divided and given in two to four doses.[67] His prescription is for clonidine 0.05 mg by mouth twice daily. Because A.K. does not yet swallow tablets easily, he will need a solution made from the tablets. It will be prepared from a published extemporaneous formulation with a final concentration of 0.1 mg/mL. What steps are necessary to ensure the accuracy of this prescription?

The differences in pharmacokinetics and pharmacodynamics observed in children influence the choice of dose and dosing interval.[68] Because incorporating all of these variables would result in dosing calculations too difficult for practical use, weight has traditionally been chosen as the single best estimate of growth. Pediatric drug references provide most doses in units per weight, such as mg/kg/day or mcg/kg/dose. Among the exceptions to this are chemotherapeutic agents, which are dosed by body surface area, incorporating height as an additional variable. Because of the difficulty in accurately determining height (or length) in young children, it is not commonly used for other drugs.

Age can be an important variable, especially for premature infants, in whom it can be used to account for differences in volume of distribution and elimination half-life. For example, neonatal gentamicin dosing is often based on a rubric of gestational or postconceptional age, postnatal age, and weight.[17] A recent study of clonidine clearance in the early postnatal period suggests that both age and weight should be used to optimize clonidine doses in newborns being treated for neonatal abstinence syndrome.[69] In the future, pediatric dosing recommendations for many drugs may be based on more than just weight to incorporate new pharmacokinetic data.[70]

Medication orders or prescriptions with doses outside of the dosing range listed in a pediatric drug reference should always be questioned for appropriateness. Older children and adolescents should transition to adult dosing whenever the calculated weight-based dose exceeds the usual adult dose. When evaluating a pediatric prescription or medication order, determining whether the dose is appropriate for the patient's weight is not the only step undertaken by the pharmacist (Fig. 97-1). As with all patients, allergies, underlying diseases, and concomitant therapy must be taken into account as well.

A.K.'s clonidine dose of 0.05 mg twice daily is equivalent to 5 mcg/kg/day, the appropriate starting dose for a child. Using a 0.1-mg/mL extemporaneous solution, his dose will be 0.5 mL twice daily. The label on A.K.'s clonidine bottle should include the concentration of the formulation, as well as the dose in both mg and mL. Before the start of treatment, A.K.'s parents should be counseled about the drug, the dose, and potential adverse effects. They should be given or have access to an oral dosing syringe or spoon to accurately measure the dose.

PREVENTING MEDICATION ERRORS IN CHILDREN

CASE 97-10, QUESTION 2: After 2 days of therapy, A.K. returns to his pediatrician's office with his parents. He is lethargic and feels dizzy when getting out of bed. His blood pressure is 90/54 mm Hg (normal for age and weight is 99/59 mm Hg), suggesting a possible clonidine overdose. As you begin to investigate the potential cause of A.K.'s symptoms, what factors may have led to an error in A.K.'s case?

Medication errors pose a significant risk for infants and children.[71–75] Whereas the rate of medication errors reported in studies of adults is approximately 5%, rates in many pediatric studies have ranged from 10% to 15%.[71–73] The need to calculate weight-based doses can lead to mathematical errors. In A.K.'s case, the dose must be multiplied by the patient's weight, divided into individual doses, and converted from micrograms to milligrams. Unit conversions and decimal point errors are particularly dangerous in pediatrics, because a 10-fold overdose of a drug with a narrow dosing range such as clonidine, digoxin, morphine, or fentanyl can be fatal.[76] In addition to prescribing errors, dosage formulation manipulation, such as the preparation of an extemporaneous liquid in this case, increases the risk for drug preparation errors. Oral liquid medications also present a risk for administration errors. Health care providers and caregivers in the home must be aware of the potential for errors and the need for precise dose measurement. A.K.'s medical history must include information on how the clonidine had been prepared by the pharmacy as well as how his parents were preparing and administering his doses.

CASE 97-10, QUESTION 3: What steps could have been taken to prevent the medication error that occurred with A.K.?

There are a number of methods to reduce the potential for medication errors, including recommendations from the Joint Commission and the Institute for Safe Medication Practices (Table 97-3).[71,74,75,77–84] Use of standard concentrations

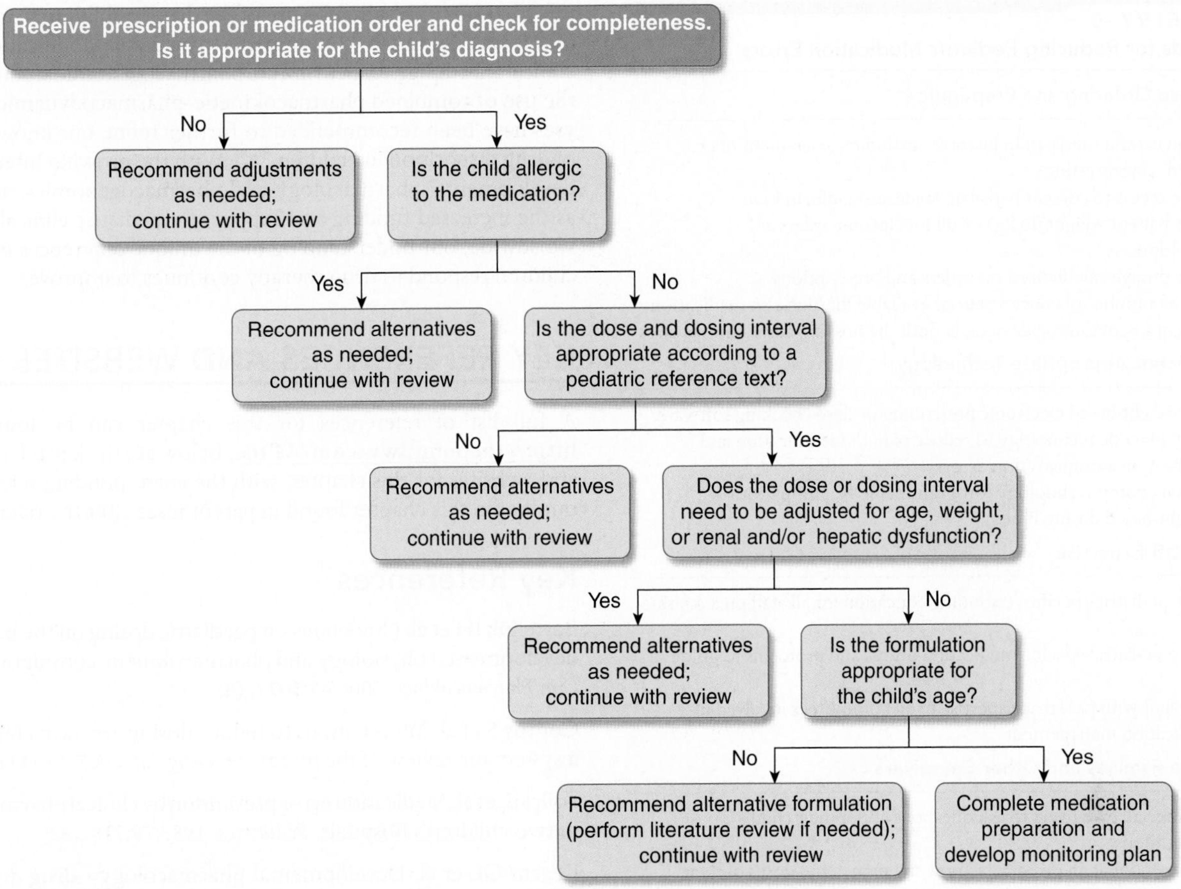
Receive prescription or medication order and check for completeness.
Is it appropriate for the child's diagnosis?
No
Yes
Recommend adjustments as needed; continue with review
Is the child allergic to the medication?
Yes
No
Recommend alternatives as needed; continue with review
Is the dose and dosing interval appropriate according to a pediatric reference text?
No
Yes
Recommend alternatives as needed; continue with review
Does the dose or dosing interval need to be adjusted for age, weight, or renal and/or hepatic dysfunction?
Yes
No
Recommend alternatives as needed; continue with review
Is the formulation appropriate for the child's age?
No
Yes
Recommend alternative formulation (perform literature review if needed); continue with review
Complete medication preparation and develop monitoring plan

FIGURE 97-1 Evaluation of pediatric prescriptions and medication orders. (Modified with permission from the American College of Clinical Pharmacy. Buck ML. Pediatric pharmacotherapy. In: Carter BL et al, eds. *Pharmacotherapy Self-Assessment Program*. 3rd ed. Module 9: Pediatrics. Lenexa, KS: American College of Clinical Pharmacy; 2000:189.)

for IV products and oral liquids, smart pump technology, bar-coding, and electronic prescribing with clinical decision support tools have been found to significantly reduce errors in pediatric hospitals.[77–81] In the outpatient setting, medication errors can be reduced by the inclusion of patient-specific information on prescriptions, including diagnosis and patient weight.[83] The product label, whether it is a prescription or over-the-counter medication, should include all the information needed to correctly prepare and administer the dose. Caregivers should have access to the appropriate tools for measuring liquid medications, such as oral dosing spoons or syringes, and the opportunity to practice preparing a dose under the supervision of a health care provider to ensure that they are able to prepare the dose correctly.[84]

ONLINE CONTENT

For an illustration of measuring devices for medication, go to http://thepoint.lww.com/AT10e.

One of the most effective methods to prevent medication errors has been to include pharmacists in the medication ordering and review process. The value of pharmacists in reducing pediatric medication errors was demonstrated by Folli et al. in 1987.[82] In this landmark study, clinical pharmacists performed prospective evaluations of medication orders at two children's hospitals for a 6-month period. The overall rate of medication errors detected by the pharmacists averaged 4.7 per 1,000 medication orders. Of these, 5.6% were considered potentially lethal. The majority of the errors (64.3%) occurred in children younger than 2 years of age. The most common type of error identified by the pharmacists was incorrect dosage. The authors concluded that pharmacy intervention had a significant effect on medication error prevention, a finding that resulted in the expansion of pediatric clinical pharmacy services in many institutions. Pharmacists in the community provide the same benefit when reviewing pediatric prescriptions and play a significant role in caregiver medication education.

INCREASING AVAILABILITY OF PEDIATRIC MEDICATION INFORMATION

CASE 97-10, QUESTION 4: Although the dose of clonidine for the treatment of ADHD is available in most pediatric dosing references, it is not found in the manufacturer's prescribing information (package insert) for the drug because the treatment of ADHD it is not currently an FDA-approved indication. What is being done to increase the availability of pediatric drug information?

Although the availability of pediatric drug information has been limited in the past, several recent initiatives from the FDA are increasing the number of clinical trials being conducted in infants and children. The Pediatric Exclusivity Program, part of the FDA Modernization Act of 1997, was developed to address the lack of pediatric study data, including medication prescribing information.[85–87] The Exclusivity Program provides pharmaceutical manufacturers with incentives to study their products in

TABLE 97-3
Methods for Reducing Pediatric Medication Errors

Improve Ordering and Preparation
Perform careful medication histories, including assessment of oral liquid concentrations
Provide access to current pediatric medication information
Include patient weight (in kg) on all medication orders and prescriptions
Include dosage calculations on orders and prescriptions
Limit the number of concentrations available for high-risk medications
Use accurate measuring devices, in both the hospital and home settings
Implement Appropriate Technology
Adopt weight-based electronic prescribing or dose-checking software
Employ barcode technology to reduce patient identification and medication administration errors
Use smart pump technology (programmable IV pumps with weight-based dosing limits)
Use Staff Expertise
Provide pediatric-specific continuing education for all staff on a routine basis
Develop pediatric-specific medication orders and protocols to guide care
Assign staff with pediatric expertise to all committees involved in medication management
Involve Families and Other Caregivers
Encourage all caregivers to ask questions about their child's medications
Recommend that all caregivers know the names and doses of their children's medications or carry information about their medications
Remind caregivers to include nutritional supplements, herbal or complementary therapies, and over-the-counter medications when giving a medication history
Ensure that caregivers can accurately prepare the medication dose

IV, intravenous.

children, including a 6-month extension at the end of a drug's patent life if a pediatric study is conducted.[85,86] The 1998 Pediatric Rule gave the FDA the ability to require manufacturers to conduct clinical trials of drugs that would be used in a significant number of patients. The Best Pharmaceuticals for Children Act of 2002 extended the previous incentives and created a mechanism for funding studies of older, off-patent medications that are often used in children. The emphasis on the needs of pediatric patients has not been limited to just the United States. In 2007, the World Health Organization passed a resolution calling for better medications for children and initiated their "Make Medicines Child-Sized" program with the goal of increasing medication availability for all children.[87]

These programs have been successful in adding pediatric dosing and adverse effect information to the prescribing information of many drugs routinely used in children. As of August 2011, the FDA had issued 407 written requests for pediatric studies, and 185 drugs had been granted a patent extension under the Exclusivity Program.[85] An assessment of the first 7 years of the program found that 50% of the studies conducted resulted in the new information supporting the use of the drug in children.[86] In spite of this success, much work remains to be done. Modifications in clinical trial design to incorporate pharmacogenomic studies and the use of combined pharmacokinetic–pharmacodynamic analyses have been recommended to further refine our knowledge of drug disposition in children.[86,87] With the growing interest in developmental pharmacology and pharmacogenomics, as well as the increased funding and support for pediatric clinical trials worldwide, our understanding of the unique differences in how children respond to drug therapy continues to improve.

KEY REFERENCES AND WEBSITES

A full list of references for this chapter can be found at http://thepoint.lww.com/AT10e. Below are the key references and websites for this chapter, with the corresponding reference number in this chapter found in parentheses after the reference.

Key References

Bartelink IH et al. Guidelines on paediatric dosing on the basis of developmental physiology and pharmacokinetic considerations. *Clin Pharmacokinet*. 2006;45:1077. (8)

Conroy S et al. Interventions to reduce dosing errors in children: a systematic review of the literature. *Drug Saf*. 2007;30:1111. (71)

Folli HL et al. Medication error prevention by clinical pharmacists in two children's hospitals. *Pediatrics*. 1987;79:718. (82)

Kearns GL et al. Developmental pharmacology—drug disposition, action, and therapy in infants and children. *N Engl J Med*. 2003;349:1157. (7)

Leeder JS et al. Understanding the relative roles of pharmacogenetics and ontogeny in pediatric drug development and regulatory science. *J Clin Pharmacol*. 2010;50:1377. (24)

MacLeod S. Therapeutic drug monitoring in pediatrics: how do children differ? *Ther Drug Monit*. 2010;32:253. (87)

Taketomo CK et al. *Pediatric Dosage Handbook*. 18th ed. Hudson, OH: Lexi-Comp, Inc; 2011. (17)

Traub SL, Johnson CE. Comparison of methods of estimating creatinine clearance in children. *Am J Hosp Pharm*. 1980;37:195. (53)

Key Websites

American Academy of Pediatrics. Ages and Stages. http://www.healthychildren.org

The Joint Commission. Sentinel event alert: preventing pediatric medication errors. http://www.jointcommission.org/sentinel_event_alert_issue_39_preventing_pediatric_medication_errors./ (74)

U.S. Department of Health and Human Services, Food and Drug Administration. Pediatric Drug Development. http://www.fda.gov/Drugs/DevelopmentApprovalProcess/DevelopmentResources/ucm049867.htm. (85)

98

Pediatric Fluid, Electrolytes, and Nutrition

Michael F. Chicella and Jennifer W. Chow

CORE PRINCIPLES

	CHAPTER CASES
1 Fluid requirements and calories normalized to body weight are much greater in very small children than in older children and adults. It is important to understand how to calculate the normal fluid and caloric needs of children, and how fluid and caloric needs change with changes in clinical status.	**Case 98-1 (Questions 1, 2), Case 98-2 (Questions 1–3), Case 98-3 (Questions 1–3), Tables 98-1–98-6**
2 Human milk is the ideal food for a human infant. In addition to meeting the infant's nutritional requirements, human milk provides the infant with protection against a wide variety of infectious diseases and noninfectious disorders. Solid foods are generally introduced at 4 to 6 months of age, and pure cow's milk is generally introduced after 1 year.	**Case 98-4 (Questions 1, 2, 4, 5)**
3 Infant formula is available in three different formulations: cow's milk-based, soy-based, and protein hydrolysate (elemental). Cow's milk-based formulas are the standard for most infants. Soy-based and protein hydrolysate formulas are primarily intended for infants who are intolerant of cow's milk-based formulas. Other therapeutic formulas are available or can be made for infants with disease states that preclude the use of one of these three main types of formula.	**Case 98-4 (Question 3), Case 98-5 (Question 1), Case 98-6 (Questions 2, 3), Table 98-7**
4 Growth assessment is an important focus of pediatric health care, especially during the first year of life. With the exception of the intrauterine period, the most rapid growth occurs during the first year.	**Case 98-6 (Question 1)**
5 Parenteral nutrition in infants and children is usually initiated below estimated caloric needs and advanced as tolerated over the course of 3 or more days until goal caloric needs are met.	**Case 98-6 (Question 4)**
6 Parenteral nutrition can be used to supply sufficient nutrients to promote healing and a normal rate of growth in sick infants and children. However, parenteral nutrition is associated with clinically significant risks and complications.	**Case 98-7 (Questions 1–5, 7–9), Table 98-8**
7 Specialized pediatric amino acid solutions are available for infants younger than 1 year of age. These products were designed to produce plasma amino acid patterns closely matching those of human milk–fed infants.	**Case 98-7 (Question 6)**
8 Irreversible liver damage can occur with long-term parenteral nutrition. Liver disease associated with parenteral nutrition usually presents as an elevated direct (conjugated) hyperbilirubinemia and can occur as early as 2 weeks after beginning parenteral nutrition.	**Case 98-7 (Questions 10, 11)**
9 A number of modifications can be made to the patient's parenteral nutrition regimen to alleviate or slow the progression of cholestasis. The initiation of enteral feeding, even if limited to low-volume trophic feeding, appears to be the most effective method for preventing cholestasis.	**Case 98-7 (Question 11)**

Adequate nutrition is an essential component of the health maintenance of children, and, in part, has been responsible for the dramatic reduction of infant mortality seen in the United States during the 20th century. Clinical experience has confirmed the value of optimal nutrition in resisting the effects of disease and trauma and in improving the response to medical and surgical therapy. The metabolic demands of rapid growth and maturation, in addition to the low nutritional reserves present during infancy, make the potential benefit of good nutrition to critically ill pediatric patients even greater.

Breast-feeding is the ideal method of feeding an infant and should be continued for at least the first year of life whenever possible. When this is not feasible, various infant formulas are available that provide appropriate nutrients for infants using the oral route. A pediatric patient who has a functioning intestinal tract, but is unable to achieve adequate oral intake, can be fed enterally using a tube inserted into the stomach or small intestine. Indications for providing specialized enteral nutrition include malnutrition, malabsorption, hypermetabolism, failure to thrive, prematurity, and disorders of absorption, digestion, excretion, or utilization of nutrients.

Despite the many formulas and feeding techniques available, several medical and gastrointestinal (GI) dilemmas that limit the use of the GI tract for nutritional support can occur in infants and children. Premature infants with severe respiratory disease, congenital abnormalities of the GI tract, or necrotizing enterocolitis are typical candidates for support with parenteral nutrition (PN). Older children with short bowel syndrome, severe malnutrition, intractable diarrhea, or inflammatory bowel disease have been treated successfully with PN therapy. Pediatric patients receiving chemotherapy for the treatment of malignancies or bone marrow transplant and children with severe cardiac failure also have been successfully rehabilitated with PN.

Many disorders that adversely affect nutrient intake or absorption also have an adverse impact on fluid and electrolyte status. Consequently, fluid, electrolyte, and nutrient management should be approached in an integrated manner. This chapter reviews selected aspects of fluid and electrolyte management and nutrition therapy for the pediatric population.

FLUID AND ELECTROLYTE MAINTENANCE

Management of fluid and electrolyte disturbances involves providing normal daily maintenance requirements and replacing deficits and ongoing losses. To design rational fluid therapy, it is necessary to know the normal composition of body water, and to understand the routes through which water and solutes are lost from the body and the effects of disease and medications on water and electrolytes. Sodium-containing fluids are often referred to as fractions of normal saline (NS) (0.9% NaCl). Normal saline contains 154 mEq/L of sodium chloride.

Calculation of Maintenance Fluid and Electrolyte Requirements

CASE 98-1

QUESTION 1: P.J., a 2-day-old, 3.5-kg term female infant has developed abdominal distension, and her oral feedings have been stopped. Calculate a maintenance fluid and electrolyte prescription for her. Her serum electrolytes include the following:

Sodium, 137 mEq/L
Potassium, 4.2 mEq/L
Chloride, 105 mEq/L
CO_2, 23 mEq/L

While P.J. receives nothing by mouth (NPO), her fluid and electrolyte needs must be met intravenously. Estimate her requirements.

General recommendations for calculating maintenance fluid have not changed significantly since first outlined by Holliday and Segar in 1957.[1] Similarly, electrolyte and nutrient replacement is still based on guidelines published in 1988 by Greene et al.[2] Fluid, electrolyte, and nutrient requirements on the basis of weight are provided in Table 98-1. Although a commercially available intravenous (IV) solution will be used, each component of the solution can be calculated separately. Using the guidelines in Table 98-1, P.J.'s maintenance requirements can be estimated as follows:

Fluid: $100 \text{ mL/kg/day} \times 3.5 \text{ kg} = 350 \text{ mL/day}$ or 15 mL/hour *(Eq. 98-1)*

Sodium: $2\text{–}4 \text{ mEq/kg/day} \times 3.5 \text{ kg} = 7\text{–}14 \text{ mEq/day}$ *(Eq. 98-2)*

Potassium: $2\text{–}3 \text{ mEq/kg/day} \times 3.5 \text{ kg} = 7\text{–}10.5 \text{ mEq/day}$ *(Eq. 98-3)*

Fluid and electrolyte requirements can be met by infusing a solution of 5% dextrose with one-quarter NS (38 mEq/L) and 20 mEq/L of KCl at 15 mL/hour. This provides 12 mEq (3.4 mEq/kg/day) of NaCl and 7 mEq (2 mEq/kg/day) of KCl in 360 mL (103 mL/kg/day) of fluid per day.

ONLINE CONTENT

For narrated PowerPoint slides on calculation of fluid and electrolyte requirements for P.J., go to http://thepoint.lww.com/AT10e.

Alteration of Maintenance Fluid and Electrolyte Requirements

CASE 98-1, QUESTION 2: On the third day of life, P.J.'s indirect bilirubin is 15.2 mg/dL (normal, 0.6–1.05 mg/dL). It is decided to use phototherapy lights to treat her hyperbilirubinemia. How should P.J.'s maintenance fluids be modified?

Table 98-2 details situations that alter maintenance fluid needs. Phototherapy lights will increase P.J.'s insensible losses and will increase her maintenance fluid needs by 10% to 20%. This can be met by increasing her IV fluid rate to 17 mL/hour (116 mL/kg/day).

Fluid and electrolyte requirements can also be altered when fluid and electrolyte losses are increased or when excretion is impaired. When abnormal fluid losses are present from any of the sources listed in Table 98-2, they must be given back to the patient daily. Replacement fluid is generally 1 mL for every 1 mL lost, but can be more or less based on the patient's clinical status. In general, a solution of one-half NS with 20 mEq of KCl per liter is used to replace upper GI tract losses; however, the electrolyte content of GI secretions varies widely. The composition of a replacement fluid can be estimated based on knowledge of the usual electrolyte distribution of the fluid type being lost. Estimates are listed in Table 98-3. If serum electrolyte concentrations are abnormal, indicating that the replacement fluid is

TABLE 98-1
Daily Parenteral Nutrient Requirements in Children

Nutrient	Weight/Age	Requirement
Fluid	<1.5 kg	150 mL/kg
	1.5–2.5 kg	120 mL/kg
	2.5–10 kg	100 mL/kg
	10–20 kg	1,000 mL + 50 mL/kg for each kg >10 kg
	>20 kg	1,500 mL + 20 mL/kg for each kg >20 kg
Calories	Up to 10 kg	100 kcal/kg
	20 kg	1,000 kcal + 50 kcal/kg for each kg >10 kg
	>20 kg	1,500 kcal + 20 kcal/kg for each kg >20 kg
Protein[a]	Infants	2–3 g/kg
	Older children	1.5–2.0 g/kg
	Adolescents and older	1.0–1.5 g/kg
Fat[b]	Infants and children	Initially 0.5–1 g/kg then increase by 0.5–1 g/kg (maximum of 3 g/kg in preterm neonates, 4 g/kg older infants and children) (≥4% of calories as linoleic acid)
	>50 kg	One 500-mL bottle (100 g fat)
Electrolytes and Minerals[c]		
Sodium	Infants and children	2–4 mEq/kg
Potassium	Infants and children	2–3 mEq/kg
Chloride	Infants and children	2–4 mEq/kg
Magnesium	Preterm and term infants	0.25–0.5 mEq/kg
	Children >1 year (or >12 kg)	4–12 mEq
Calcium	Preterm and term infants	2–3 mEq/kg
	Children >1 year (or >12 kg)	10–20 mEq
Phosphorus	Preterm and term infants	1.0–1.5 mmol/kg
	Children >1 year (or >12 kg)	10–20 mmol
Trace Elements		
Zinc	Preterm infants	400 mcg/kg
	Term infants	
	<3 mos	250 mcg/kg
	>3 mos	100 mcg/kg
	Children	50 mcg/kg (up to 5 mg)
Copper	Infants and children	20 mcg/kg (up to 300 mcg)
Manganese	Infants and children	1 mcg/kg (up to 50 mcg)
Chromium	Infants and children	0.2 mcg/kg (up to 5 mcg)
Selenium	Infants and children	2 mcg/kg (up to 80 mcg)

Vitamins	Preterm Infants <2.5 kg (2 mL/kg MVI Pediatric)	Term Infants and Children <11 years (5 mL MVI Pediatric)	Children >11 years (10 mL MVI-12)
Vitamin A	280 mcg/kg	700 mcg	1 mg
Vitamin D	160 international units/kg	400 international units	200 international units
Vitamin E	2.8 mg/kg	7 mg	10 mg
Vitamin K[d]	80 mcg/kg	200 mcg	None
Thiamine	0.48 mg/kg	1.2 mg	3 mg
Niacin	6.8 mg/kg	17 mg	40 mg
Riboflavin	0.56 mg/kg	1.4 mg	3.6 mg
Pyridoxine	0.4 mg/kg	1 mg	4 mg
Vitamin B_{12}	0.4 mcg/kg	1 mcg	5 mcg
Biotin	8 mcg/kg	20 mcg	60 mcg
Vitamin C	32 mg/kg	80 mg	100 mg
Folic acid	56 mcg/kg	140 mcg	400 mcg

[a] "Infant" amino acids contain histidine, taurine, tyrosine, and cysteine, which are essential in infants but not older patients.

[b] Because linoleic acid represents 54% of the fatty acid in soy bean oil and 77% in safflower oil, 7% to 10% of calories must be provided as fat emulsion. This can be given daily over the course of 24 hours (preferred in patients predisposed to sepsis and preterm infants) or two to three times weekly.

[c] These doses are guidelines and all patients should be evaluated individually for appropriateness of dosing. For example, patients with short bowel syndrome may require large doses of magnesium, and patients with renal insufficiency may require none to low amounts of potassium, calcium, phosphorous, and magnesium.

[d] For patients receiving MVI-12, it may be desirable to add vitamin K.

MVI, multivitamin.

Source: Holliday MA, Segar WE. The maintenance need for water in parenteral fluid therapy. *Pediatrics.* 1957;19(5):823–832[1]; Greene HL, Hambidge KM, Schanler R, Tsang RC. Guidelines for the use of vitamins, trace elements, calcium, magnesium, and phosphorus in infants and children receiving total parenteral nutrition: report of the Subcommittee on Pediatric Parenteral Nutrient Requirements from the Committee on Clinical Practice Issues of the American Society for Clinical Nutrition [published corrections appear in *Am J Clin Nutr.* 1989;49(6):1332; *Am J Clin Nutr.* 1989;50(3):560]. *Am J Clin Nutr.* 1988;48(5):1324–1342.[2]

TABLE 98-2
Situations That Alter Maintenance Fluid Requirements

Situation	Mechanism	Extent of Change (%)
Extreme prematurity	↑ Skin losses	Varies
Radiant warmer use	↑ Insensible water loss	20–40
Diarrhea or vomiting	↑ GI loss	Varies
Fever	↑ Insensible water loss	10–15/°C
Renal dysfunction	↑ or ↓ renal loss	Varies
Hyperventilation	↑ Pulmonary evaporative loss	Varies
Phototherapy for hyperbilirubinemia	↑ Insensible water loss	10–20
GI tract suction or ostomy	↑ GI loss	Varies
Mechanical ventilation	↓ Insensible water loss	20–30

GI, gastrointestinal.

not appropriate, a sample of the fluid lost from the patient can be analyzed for electrolyte content, and electrolyte replacement fluid can be individualized.

The requirements for fluid and calories normalized to body weight are much greater in very small children than in older children and adults as can be seen in Table 98-1. This is because infants have a much larger body surface area relative to weight, lose more fluid through evaporation, and dissipate more heat per kilogram than their older counterparts. Furthermore, very low-birth-weight (VLBW) infants cannot concentrate urine and are at increased risk for dehydration if inadequate fluids are provided.

Dehydration

CASE 98-2

QUESTION 1: H.S. is a 2-year-old lethargic girl with a 2-day history of vomiting and minimal oral intake. Yesterday, she required only three diaper changes instead of her usual eight and has needed only one change today. Her vital signs are as follows:

Temperature, 39°C
Pulse, 140 beats/minute (normal, 80–130 beats/minute)
Respiratory rate, 30 breaths/minute (normal, 30–35 breaths/minute)
Blood pressure (BP), 80/45 mm Hg (normal, 80–115 mm Hg systolic and 50–80 mm Hg diastolic)

On physical examination, her eyes appear sunken, her mucous membranes are dry, and her skin is dry and cool to touch. Although she is crying, there are no tears, and the skin over her sternum tents when pinched. Her weight today is 11.4 kg; 3 weeks ago, it was 12.9 kg. What do these findings represent? What immediate treatment should be provided?

H.S.'s lethargy, decreased urine output, tearless crying, dry mucous membranes, dry skin with fever, sunken eyes, mild tachycardia with low normal blood pressure, and poor skin turgor are all signs of dehydration. This is consistent with her 2-day history of vomiting and poor intake. Her weight loss of 1.5 kg gives a further clue to the extent of dehydration. Dehydration or fluid loss is determined most accurately by weight loss. Because 1 g of body weight is approximately equal to 1 mL, her fluid deficit is estimated to be 1,500 mL. The percentage dehydration is estimated using the following formula:

$$\%\ \text{Dehydration} = \text{Normal body weight} - \frac{\text{Actual body weight}}{\text{Normal body weight}} \times 100 \quad \text{(Eq. 98-4)}$$

If recent weights are unavailable, the extent of dehydration can be approximated from physical findings as described in Table 98-4. Tachycardia and marginal blood pressure dictate the need for immediate IV rehydration. Normal serum sodium concentration ranges from 135 to 145 mEq/L of sodium; thus, normal saline approximates the sodium concentration of plasma and is often used as a volume expander. In this patient, 10 to 20 mL/kg of normal saline (12.9 kg × 10 to 20 mL/kg = 129 to 258 mL) should be infused as rapidly as possible to establish normal blood pressure. For symptomatic patients, including those with seizures, the serum sodium concentration should be increased acutely only to the degree necessary to abate symptoms.

CASE 98-2, QUESTION 2: Calculate H.S.'s fluid and electrolyte needs. Her serum electrolyte results were as follows:

Sodium, 128 mEq/L (normal, 135–145 mEq/L)
Potassium, 3.1 mEq/L (normal, 3.5–5 mEq/L)
Chloride, 88 mEq/L (normal, 102–109 mEq/L)
HCO_3^-, 30 mEq/L (normal, 22–29 mEq/L)

In addition to normal maintenance fluids, H.S. must be provided with fluids and electrolytes to replace her deficit secondary to dehydration and compensate for increased insensible water loss because of fever. Each component of the fluid can be calculated separately, using Equations 98-5 to 98-7.

$$\text{Fluid deficit} = \text{Weight loss (kg)} \times 1{,}000\ \text{mL/kg} \quad \text{(Eq. 98-5)}$$

$$\text{Fever adjustment} = 10\% \times \text{Maintenance for each } ^\circ\text{C} \geq 30^\circ\text{C} \quad \text{(Eq. 98-6)}$$

$$(\text{CD} - \text{CO}) \times F_d \times \text{Weight} = \text{mEq required} \quad \text{(Eq. 98-7)}$$

where *CD* is the concentration of sodium desired (mEq/L), *CO* is the concentration observed (mEq/L), F_d is the apparent

TABLE 98-3
Body Fluid Volumes and Electrolyte Content

Source	Volume (L/d)	Na^+ (mEq/L)	K^+ (mEq/L)	Cl^- (mEq/L)	HCO_3^- (mEq/L)
Salivary glands	1.5 (0.5–2)	10 (2–10)	26 (20–30)	10 (8–18)	30
Stomach	1.5 (0.1–4)	60 (9–116)	10 (0–32)	130 (8–154)	—
Duodenum	(0.1–2)	140	5	80	—
Ileum	3 (0.1–9)	140 (80–150)	5 (2–8)	104 (43–137)	30
Colon	—	60	30	40	—
Pancreas	(0.1–0.8)	140 (113–185)	5 (3–7)	75 (54–95)	115
Bile	(0.05–0.8)	145 (131–164)	5 (3–12)	100 (89–180)	35

TABLE 98-4
Clinical Signs of Dehydration

Severity	Dehydration (%)	Psyche	Thirst	Mucous Membranes	Tears	Anterior Fontanel	Skin	Urine Specific Gravity
Mild	<5	Normal	Slight	Normal to dry	Present	Flat	Normal	Slight change
Moderate	6–10	Irritable	Moderate	Dry	±	±	±	Increased
Severe	10–15	Hyperirritable to lethargic	Intense	Parched	Absent	Sunken	Tenting	Greatly increased

distribution factor as a fraction of body weight (Table 98-5), and weight is the baseline weight before illness (kg). In consideration of both maintenance needs and current deficits, fluid and electrolyte requirements for H.S. would be estimated as follows.

FLUID

$$\begin{aligned} \text{Maintenance} \quad & 1{,}000\text{ mL} + (50 \times 2.9) = 1{,}145\text{ mL} \\ \text{Fever} \quad & 2^\circ\text{C} \times 0.1\,(1{,}145) = 229\text{ mL} \\ \text{Deficit} \quad & 1.5\text{ kg} \times 1{,}000\text{ mL/kg} = 1{,}500\text{ mL} \\ & \text{Total fluid} = 2{,}874\text{ mL} \end{aligned} \quad \text{(Eq. 98-8)}$$

SODIUM

$$\begin{aligned} \text{Maintenance} \quad & 3\text{ mEq/kg} \times 12.9\text{ kg} = 38.7 \\ \text{Deficit} \quad & (135 - 128\text{ mEq/L}) \times 0.6\text{ L/kg} \times 12.9\text{ kg} = 54.2 \\ & \text{Total sodium} \sim 93\text{ mEq} \end{aligned} \quad \text{(Eq. 98-9)}$$

CHLORIDE

H.S. has a mild metabolic alkalosis as evidenced by her serum chloride of 88 mEq/L and her serum bicarbonate of 30 mEq/L. This is most likely because of the loss of hydrogen and chloride in her vomitus. Thus, both the sodium and potassium replacements should be administered as chloride salts.

POTASSIUM

Potassium is primarily an intracellular ion. It moves in and out of cells in exchange for hydrogen ions to maintain a normal blood pH. Therefore, in metabolic alkalosis, the intracellular shift of potassium will decrease the serum potassium concentration. When the pH normalizes, as will occur with rehydration, the hydrogen ions will move intracellularly and the potassium will move extracellularly, thus causing the serum potassium concentration to increase. Additionally, potassium is also excreted by the kidney in exchange for hydrogen ion conservation. These factors make the serum potassium concentration difficult to interpret. Intravascular volume depletion causes hypoperfusion of the kidney and can result in acute renal failure; therefore, the prudent approach is to give no potassium until urine output is clearly established. Then, only maintenance doses of potassium should be administered until a normal acid–base and fluid status are established and the serum potassium can be assessed more accurately. Hence, H.S. should receive approximately 26 to 39 mEq of potassium (2–3 mEq/kg × 12.9 kg) once urine flow is established.

TABLE 98-5
Electrolytes and Apparent Distribution

Electrolyte	F_d (L/kg)
Sodium	0.6–0.7
Bicarbonate	0.4–0.5
Chloride	0.2–0.3

F_d, apparent distribution factor as a fraction of body weight.

Administration of Fluid Requirements

CASE 98-2, QUESTION 3: How should these calculated needs be given?

Requirements for the first 24 hours of parenteral fluid therapy should provide approximately 2,875 mL of fluid to account for maintenance fluid needs, fever replacement, and deficit replacement. In addition to fluid, at least 93 mEq of sodium (maintenance needs plus deficit replacement) should be provided in the first 24 hours. It is important to provide sufficient amounts of sodium and water.

Rehydration fluids are usually dispensed in volumes less than the 24-hour requirement. This is to prevent wasting IV fluids caused by changes in electrolyte needs during replacement therapy. Because this patient requires approximately 3 L of fluid, only 1 L would be prepared initially, and this would likely consist of dextrose 5% and 0.2% NS (or greater). Approximately 15 mEq/L of potassium would be added to the next liter of IV solution if the patient had a reasonable urine output.

The infusion rate should be calculated to provide one-third of the daily maintenance fluid plus one-half of the deficit replacement during the first 8 hours. The remainder of the maintenance fluid (adjusted for fever) and deficit replacement should be administered during the next 16 hours. Usually, serum electrolytes are monitored every 6 to 8 hours during rehydration therapy to ensure that appropriate electrolytes are being provided. Usually, the concentration of serum electrolytes is monitored frequently during fluid replacement therapy of deficits. In general, the serum sodium concentration should not be increased by more than 10 to 12 mEq/L/day. After the initial fluid deficits are replaced, the infusion rate of the IV fluid would be decreased to 48 mL/hour (1,152 mL or approximately maintenance fluid rate).

Dehydration Associated with Diarrhea

CASE 98-3

QUESTION 1: S.B. is a 4-month-old, 5.9-kg boy presenting with a 4-day history of diarrhea (five to eight large, liquid stools each day). On a well-child visit 4 weeks ago, his weight was 6 kg. Since the onset of diarrhea, he has only been receiving oral rehydration fluids. Physical examination reveals the following:

Temperature, 39.8°C
Pulse, 110 beats/minute (normal, 80–160 beats/minute)
Respirations, 45 breaths/minute (normal, 20–40 breaths/minute)

BP, 100/58 mm Hg (normal, 75–105 mm Hg systolic and 40–65 mm Hg diastolic)

His skin is pale, warm, and dry. He is very irritable, and his mucous membranes are dry. S.B.'s laboratory values are as follows:

Sodium, 159 mEq/L
Potassium, 3.3 mEq/L
Chloride, 114 mEq/L
CO_2, 12 mEq/L
Blood urea nitrogen (BUN), 22 mg/dL
Creatinine, 0.9 mg/dL

Correlate S.B.'s history and physical findings with the reported laboratory values.

Diarrheal fluid losses commonly contain high concentrations of bicarbonate, accounting for S.B.'s metabolic acidosis. This, in turn, has resulted in a rapid respiratory rate as the body attempts to compensate for the acidosis by eliminating carbon dioxide. The increased insensible water losses of fever and tachypnea have resulted in the loss of water in excess of sodium, producing hypernatremia.

CASE 98-3, QUESTION 2: How should S.B.'s dehydration be managed?

S.B. has relatively normal vital signs and will not require rapid fluid replacement to correct hypotension. Hypernatremia in S.B. indicates fluid losses in excess of sodium and this should be corrected. With hypernatremia, the central nervous system (CNS) increases intracellular osmolarity load to prevent intracellular dehydration of cells in the CNS. Rapid correction of hypernatremia can cause excessive movement of water into the cells of the CNS and has been associated with seizures. Therefore, S.B.'s fluid and electrolyte deficits should be corrected over the course of 2 to 3 days at a consistent rate, rather than rapidly. In general, serum sodium should not be decreased more than 2 mEq/hour (maximum, 15 mEq/L/day).

S.B.'s requirements are estimated using the same methods described previously. First, the approximate extent of dehydration must be estimated. S.B.'s weight of 6 kg at the time of his well-child visit at 3 months of age was at the 50th percentile. If his growth has continued at this rate, his current pre-illness weight should be approximately 6.5 kg.[3] This weight should be used to calculate his maintenance requirements. Thus, his water deficit is approximately 0.6 L, or 9%. Using this approximation, his fluid and electrolyte requirements can be estimated as follows.

FLUID

Maintenance	6.5×100 mL/kg = 650 mL/24 hours
Fever	$1.8°C \times 0.1$ (650 mL) = 117 mL/24 hours
	600 mL/3 days = 200 mL/24 hours
Deficit	Total daily needs = 967 mL or 40 mL/hour

(Eq. 98-10)

SODIUM

Maintenance	3 mEq/kg $\times$ 6.5 kg = 19.5 mEq/24 hours
Deficit	This is calculated as total body deficit (normal – actual)
Normal	145 mEq/L $\times$ 0.6 L/kg $\times$ 6.5 kg = 566 mEq
Actual	159 mEq/L $\times$ 0.6 L/kg $\times$ 5.9 kg = 563 mEq
Deficit	= 3 mEqor 1 mEq/day

(Eq. 98-11)

POTASSIUM

As discussed in Case 98-2, Question 2, the serum potassium value of 3.3 mEq/L may not be indicative of S.B.'s total body potassium status. A metabolic acidosis in S.B. should have facilitated the movement of hydrogen ions into the cells and the movement of potassium from the intracellular to the extracellular space. Thus, the serum potassium of 3.3 mEq/L probably indicates a total body deficit. Therefore, a maintenance potassium dosage of 13 to 20 mEq/day (approximately 2 to 3 mEq/kg) of potassium should be added to the intravenous fluid. Serum electrolytes should be measured every 8 to 12 hours, and the intake of all electrolytes should be readjusted based on the results.

BICARBONATE

With metabolic acidosis, bicarbonate should be administered as well. No maintenance amount is customarily given, but deficit replacement is calculated in a manner similar to that used for sodium (Table 98-5). The volume of distribution of bicarbonate is 0.5 L/kg. For S.B. the bicarbonate deficit is as follows:

$$\begin{aligned}\text{Calculated Deficit Requirement} &= (\text{Normal} - \text{Actual}) \times \text{Vd} \times \text{Wt}\\ &= (23 - 12)\ \text{mEq/L} \times 0.5\ \text{L/kg} \times 6.5\ \text{kg}\\ &= 36\ \text{mEq}\end{aligned} \quad \text{(Eq. 98-12)}$$

Initially, about half this amount should be added to the intravenous fluid and replaced during the first 8 to 12 hours. His serum electrolytes then should be reassessed, and the dosages adjusted accordingly. The entire bicarbonate deficit need not be replaced at once because other compensatory mechanisms will contribute to endogenous bicarbonate sparing.

CASE 98-3, QUESTION 3: Recommend an appropriate replacement fluid for S.B.'s therapy.

S.B.'s fluid and electrolyte maintenance requirements and deficits should be corrected with dextrose 5% and approximately 0.2% NS with half as the chloride salt and half as $NaHCO_3$. An infusion of this solution at 43 mL/hour should correct approximately one-half the calculated fluid and bicarbonate deficits within 24 hours in addition to his normal daily doses. After he urinates, 15 mEq/L KCl can be added to the next liter of solution to provide approximately 2.6 mEq/kg/day to this patient. The concentration of serum electrolytes should be measured often, and the concentration of electrolytes in the replacement fluid should be adjusted every 8 to 12 hours based on laboratory results. The amount of fluid replacement should be modified based on whether this patient's diarrhea has resolved and fever has subsided.

Rehydration of the dehydrated patient may be achieved by either the oral or intravenous route. In some patients, vomiting may preclude effective oral rehydration. If the losses are diarrheal and no problem with vomiting exists, the oral route may be a cost-effective alternative to the parenteral route. Various solutions have been used to rehydrate children orally. In an asymptomatic dehydrated child, the sodium concentration of an oral rehydration fluid should contain at least 70 mEq/L of sodium.[4]

The composition of several products is shown in Table 98-6. A glucose concentration of 2% optimizes water and electrolyte absorption from the GI tract[4]; more concentrated glucose solutions can worsen rather than ameliorate diarrhea. Use of the oral route and the more concentrated sodium solutions may allow safe rehydration of hypernatremic dehydration in a shorter time frame than the 2 to 3 days previously noted.[4]

S.B.'s output must be measured to account for ongoing fluid loss. This often is accomplished by weighing the baby's diapers when they are dry and again when they are full. Composition of additional replacement fluids can be determined by using the average composition of the patient's losses (Table 98-3). As an alternative, the composition of the losses can be determined by actual laboratory measurement. If prolonged therapy is

TABLE 98-6
Composition of Oral Rehydration Products[4]

Product	Na^+ (mEq/L)	K^+ (mEq/L)	Cl^- (mEq/L)	Bicarbonate Source (mEq/L)	Carbohydrate (%)
Enfalyte	50	25	45	34 citrate	3
Rehydralyte	75	20	65	30 citrate	2.5
Pedialyte	45	20	35	30 citrate	2.5
Gatorade	23.5	<1	17	—	4.6
WHO salts	90	20	80	30 bicarbonate	2

WHO, World Health Organization.

necessary, specific analyses are recommended because of the wide range of normal values for diarrheal stool and other GI tract fluids. Because frequent adjustments may be necessary, replacement fluid should be administered separately if PN is being used as a maintenance solution.

INFANT ENTERAL NUTRITION

Caloric requirements of infants can be estimated using the formula provided in Table 98-1. The American Heart Association has suggested that infant feeding be divided into three stages.[5] In the nursing period, only liquids are provided. During the transitional period, solid foods are introduced, but human milk, or commercially prepared infant formula, still provides the major source of the infant's caloric and nutrient supply. In the modified adult period, most nutrition is derived from the solid foods consumed by other household members.

At birth, the human GI tract is adapted for the consumption of a human milk–based diet. Intestinal lactase is present from 36 weeks' gestation and exhibits its maximal activity during infancy. Pancreatic amylase secretion is low, and the bile salt pool is decreased relative to that of older persons, resulting in decreased fat absorption.[6] Human milk provides nutrients in their most usable form for the developing GI tract.

Human Milk Feeding

CASE 98-4

QUESTION 1: M.E. is a 1-day-old full-term infant. M.E.'s mother will breast-feed her infant. What are the nutritional implications of this decision for M.E.?

Human milk is the ideal food for a human infant and should be encouraged to be continued for the first year of life as long as mutually desired by both mother and child.[7] There are three phases to human milk production. During the first 5 days of lactation, a viscous, yellow liquid known as *colostrum* is produced. Colostrum is rich in protein, minerals, and other substances (e.g., immunoglobulins). During the next 5 days, transitional milk is produced; in the last phase, mature human milk is produced. The exact nutritional content of human milk varies from mother to mother; however, mature human milk provides sufficient protein, minerals, and calories regardless of the mother's nutritional status. Mature human milk generally provides 70 kcal/100 mL, and fat accounts for more than 50% of the caloric content.[8] The fat in human milk is highly digestible and absorbable.[8] An additional 40% of calories is provided as carbohydrates, primarily in the form of lactose, and the remaining 10% is provided as protein. Whey and casein are the two primary proteins in mature human milk, with whey being the major protein component (whey-to-casein ratio of 60:40).[9] Human milk is of such biologic quality and bioavailability that adequate growth can be attained with a lower overall intake of protein than is provided by commercially prepared infant formulas, which contain lower whey-to-casein ratios.[9]

The iron content of human milk is inadequate for term infants; however, supplementation generally is unnecessary in the breast-fed infant.[10] Regardless of maternal status, the vitamin D content of human milk is inadequate. Thus, M.E. will require 400 international units of vitamin D while she is exclusively breast-fed.[11]

Additionally, human milk provides the infant with protection against a wide variety of infectious diseases, including otitis media, diarrhea, pneumonia, and bronchiolitis. Evidence further suggests that human milk provides protection against noninfectious disorders, such as allergies, inflammatory bowel disease, insulin-dependent diabetes mellitus, and sudden infant death syndrome.[7,8] Human milk contains immunologically active cellular components and antibodies. These include secretory IgA, both T and B lymphocytes, macrophages, and neutrophils.[7,8] The lipases and amylase present in human milk may facilitate digestion of fat and carbohydrates in the still developing GI tract. Proteins present in human milk serve as carriers for trace minerals and facilitate their absorption.[9] Oligosaccharides and glycopeptides may promote the colonization of the GI tract by *Lactobacilli* and decrease colonization by *Bacteroides, Clostridia,* enterococci, and gram-negative rods, all of which may be pathogenic.[8]

CASE 98-4, QUESTION 2: What potential complications are associated with breast-feeding? What instructions should be given to M.E.'s mother?

Complications associated with breast-feeding are few; however, there are some potential problems. "Breast milk jaundice" associated with an indirect (unconjugated) hyperbilirubinemia can occur in the breast-fed infant during the first week of life, and generally resolves by the fourth week of life. Although the infant's skin, sclera, and palate become yellow, this is generally not a dangerous condition. Nevertheless, if the bilirubin level becomes too high, the infant could develop an encephalopathy known as kernicterus. However, it is generally not necessary for the mother to stop breast-feeding while the infant has jaundice. The American Academy of Pediatrics (AAP) recommends that infants nurse at least 8 to 12 times daily while jaundiced.[12] Some maternal infections have the potential to be transmitted to the infant during breast-feeding. Human immunodeficiency virus (HIV) and human T-lymphotropic virus 1 (HTLV-1) can be transmitted via breast milk, and, therefore, maternal infections with these viruses are contraindications to breast-feeding.[7,8] Other viruses, such as herpes simplex virus, can be transmitted if contact with active lesions occurs during breast-feeding. Similarly, some medications taken by the mother are detectable in her breast milk. Only a few agents (e.g., antineoplastics, radiopharmaceuticals, ergot alkaloids, iodides, atropine, lithium, cyclosporine, chloramphenicol, bromocriptine), however, are absolute contraindications to breast-feeding.[7,8] (See Chapter 49, Obstetric Drug Therapy, for additional information concerning the transfer of medications and chemicals into breast milk.)

CASE 98-4, QUESTION 3: M.E.'s mother suffers from migraine headaches, which have increased in frequency since M.E.'s birth. M.E.'s mother takes an ergot alkaloid for the acute management of her headaches and therefore has

TABLE 98-7
Infant Formulas

Cow's Milk-Based Formulas	Soy-Based, Lactosefree Formulas	Protein Hydrolysate, Elemental, Premature Infant Formulas
Enfamil with iron	Isomil	Alimentum
Similac with iron	Nursoy	Nutramigen
Gerber Good Start	ProSoBee	Pregestimil
	Alsoy	NeoCate
	Gerber Soy Plus	Neosure Advance
	Similac Sensitive	Enfamil Premature with Lipil
		Similac Special Care

decided not to breast-feed M.E. She will be using infant formula instead. How are these products prepared and how do they differ from human milk?

Because of the excretion of ergot alkaloids into breast milk and the risk for toxicity to the infant, it is advisable to either select an alternative medication or discontinue breast-feeding and use an infant formula. Examples of infant formulas are provided in Table 98-7. According to AAP guidelines for commercially prepared infant formula composition, formula should provide 20 kcal/ounce, osmolality should be between 300 and 400 mOsm/L, protein quantity should be a minimum of 1.8 g/100 kcal and should not exceed 4.5 g/100 kcal, and fat quantity should be between 3.3 and 6 g/100 kcal, supplying between 30% and 54% of calories. Infant formulas generally begin with a cow's milk base; however, intolerance to pure cow's milk has resulted in several modifications. The predominant protein in cow's milk is casein, which is more difficult for infants to digest than the human milk protein, whey. Consequently, infant formulas generally have less casein than cow's milk, although not to the level of human milk. The casein present in cow's milk formulas also may be heat denatured to improve its digestibility. In addition, the fat source in cow's milk is replaced by one of several vegetable oils, allowing for easier digestion. Last, the carbohydrate source in cow's milk-based formula is supplemented with lactose or sucrose because the lactose content of cow's milk is only 50% to 70% of that in human milk. Soy-based and protein hydrolysate formulas are available for infants who are intolerant of cow's milk-based formulas.

Soy-based formulas use soybean as the protein source.[13] The soy is heat-treated to enhance protein digestibility and improve the bioavailability of some nutrients. Although nutrients, such as methionine, zinc, and carnitine, are still present, their concentrations are relatively low. Therefore, the manufacturer routinely adds methionine to all soy-based formulas. Zinc and carnitine may not be added, and exogenous supplementation may be necessary. Soy-based formulas substitute sucrose, corn syrup, or a combination of the two for lactose as the carbohydrate source. Additionally, soy protein formulas are more expensive than cow's milk-based formulas. The AAP recommends that the use of soy-based formula be limited to patients with primary lactase deficiency (galactosemia), patients with secondary lactose intolerance from enteric infections or other causes, vegetarian families in which animal protein formulas are not desired, and infants who are potentially cow's milk protein allergic, but who have not demonstrated clinical manifestations of allergy. Long-term use of soy-based formulas in premature and low-birth-weight infants should not be recommended. Soy-based formulas have aluminum contamination, and have been associated with the development of rickets. Soy-based formulas are also not recommended for infants with documented allergic reactions to cow's milk protein because of the potential for cross-antigenicity between the two proteins. Additionally, soy protein formulas are not recommended for the routine management of colic.

Elemental formulas, made with hydrolysate formulas, are another option for infants who are intolerant of cow's milk-based formulas. The milk proteins (i.e., casein and whey) are heat-treated and enzymatically hydrolyzed to enhance digestibility of protein hydrolysate formulas, which are fortified with additional amino acids that are lost during processing. As with soy protein formulas, protein hydrolysates substitute sucrose, tapioca, or corn syrup for lactose as the carbohydrate source. Protein hydrolysate formulas often include significant amounts of medium-chain triglycerides because they are easily absorbed. Because the proteins are extensively hydrolyzed, these formulas probably are the least allergenic of the infant formulas and, therefore, may be appropriate for infants with true allergy to cow's milk protein. Nevertheless, prospective studies on the safety of such a substitution in human infants have not been undertaken because it would be unethical to intentionally expose infants with documented allergies to a potential allergen. Protein hydrolysate formulas are the least palatable of the available pediatric formulas, and are more costly than other formulas.[14]

Infant formula is available from the manufacturers in three forms: ready-to-feed formula, powder for reconstitution, and concentrated liquid. The ready-to-feed form is the most convenient but also the most expensive. The powder and the concentrated liquid are less expensive; however, both require that predetermined amounts of boiled water be added before use. To save money, some parents will dilute infant formula to a greater extent than is recommended to make the formula last longer. This practice should be discouraged because excessive free water intake by infants younger than 1 year of age may result in hyponatremia and, ultimately, seizures. Similarly, supplementing an infant's diet with free water, for whatever reason, may also result in hyponatremia and seizures and should be discouraged. Periodically, manufacturing problems can occur, resulting in the recall of a product from the market.[15] Therefore, it is important for the patient's health care providers to stay abreast of manufacturers' recalls.

Introduction of Pure Cow's Milk

CASE 98-4, QUESTION 4: At 2 months of age, M.E. is found to have a hematocrit (Hct) of 33% (normal, 35%–45%). After questioning her mother, you learn that M.E. was taken off infant formula 1 month ago and changed to whole cow's milk to decrease food costs. How are these two findings related, and how should M.E. be managed?

Pure cow's milk, straight from the dairy counter in the grocery store, is not recommended for infants younger than 1 year of age. Unlike human milk, the iron in cow's milk is present in inadequate concentrations and absorbed poorly from the human GI tract. For this reason, most infant formulas are fortified with iron. Cow's milk has been associated with GI blood loss in infants younger than 140 days of age.[16] When the milk is heated to a higher temperature than the usual pasteurization temperature, as it is in formula preparation, the association of cow's milk with GI bleeding is no longer present; therefore, the component responsible for the blood loss appears to be a heat-labile protein. Furthermore, cow's milk contains excessive amounts of solute that cannot be eliminated by the immature kidney. Also, cow's milk does not contain taurine, an amino acid that is important in retinal development.

To treat M.E.'s anemia, iron should be added to her diet. This can be done by changing back to an iron-fortified infant formula, feeding her an iron-fortified cereal, or giving a therapeutic ferrous sulfate liquid medication. The appropriate iron replacement dose for severe anemia is 4 to 6 mg/kg/day of elemental iron in divided doses with follow-up of the infant's hemoglobin and hematocrit.

Introduction of Solid Foods

CASE 98-4, QUESTION 5: At 4 months of age, M.E.'s mother asks about the introduction of "baby foods" into M.E.'s diet. How should the clinician respond?

Human milk or commercially prepared infant formula provides adequate nutrition for an infant for the first 12 months of life. Introduction of solid foods before the age of 4 months, although common in the past, is discouraged because the younger infant is unprepared to swallow foods other than liquids. Solids (first cereals, then fruits and vegetables) should be introduced when the child has good control of the head and neck movements (i.e., usually at the age of 4–6 months).[5] Preferably, one new food should be introduced at a time, at 1-week intervals, to allow assessment of food allergy.

Therapeutic Formulas

CASE 98-5

QUESTION 1: L.B. is a 2-week-old infant whose newborn screen is positive for phenylketonuria (PKU). Discuss the concepts behind the production of therapeutic formulas and the dietary management of patients with inborn errors of metabolism. How should L.B.'s diet be modified?

Inborn errors of metabolism are disorders in which an enzyme or its cofactor is absent or insufficient to meet metabolic demands.[17] As a result, one or more precursor compounds in a metabolic pathway can accumulate before the defective step. Correspondingly, one or more metabolic products that normally would have been generated after the defective step in the metabolic pathway are not sufficiently available.

The dietary management of metabolic errors is based on the following strategies:

- Reduce the intake of a precursor compound that cannot be metabolized.
- Supplement the deficient compounds that would have been produced if the normal metabolic pathway had not been blocked.
- Add a substrate that provides an alternative pathway for elimination of an accumulated toxin.

Therapeutic formulas are designed to reduce the intake of precursor compounds or to provide the deficient metabolic end product.

When hydroxylation of phenylalanine to tyrosine does not take place, phenylalanine accumulates in the blood and results in mental retardation. Because PKU has been diagnosed in L.B., his diet should be modified using a formula containing little or no phenylalanine (e.g., Periflex Infant). The tyrosine deficiency of PKU also can be managed by the addition of tyrosine to the phenylalaninefree therapeutic formulas that are available for patients with PKU. When L.B. progresses to solid foods, it will be important to limit or avoid foods that contain high levels of protein such as eggs and soybeans.

Other metabolic errors present in infancy include galactosemia (galactose cannot be metabolized to glucose), homocystinuria (methionine is not converted to cysteine), urea cycle disorders (ammonia detoxification is impaired), and maple syrup urine disease (metabolism of the branched-chain amino acids leucine, isoleucine, and valine is blocked).

These metabolic errors are managed by manipulating the diet.[17] In galactosemia, the carbohydrate source should not contain galactose or lactose. In homocystinuria, methionine should be present only in quantities sufficient to meet basic requirements, and cysteine should be supplemented. In the urea cycle disorders, protein often is provided only as essential amino acids, and a high-energy diet is provided to maximize the formation of nonessential amino acids from nitrogen and to minimize ammonia production. In maple syrup urine disease, natural protein is fed in small quantities to provide the minimal requirement of branched-chain amino acids, and a branched-chain amino acid–free supplement is added to provide adequate protein intake.

Route of Administration

Nutritional support using the GI tract is the preferred approach when possible. Enteral nutrition provides several advantages. First, interposition of the GI mucosa between the nutrient supply and the circulation allows absorptive function to provide a homeostatic control. Second, the flow of nutrients from the GI tract to the liver via the portal circulation before reaching the systemic circulation also assists homeostatic control. Third, the lack of enteral nutrition allows normal GI tract flora to overgrow and translocate into the blood, ultimately resulting in bacteremia. Finally, the intestinal mucosa depends on intraluminal absorption for much of its energy supply. Hence, provision of at least a small amount of enteral feeding, referred to as trophic feeds, helps to ensure a healthy GI tract and may facilitate advancement to full enteral feedings at the appropriate time.[18]

Normal oral feeding is the most basic method for patients who are willing and able to eat or drink. Patients whose GI motility, structure, and function are normal but whose oral feeding is prevented by an altered state of consciousness, uncoordinated sucking and swallowing, or other conditions that prevent adequate oral ingestion can be fed by a GI tube in intermittent boluses or by continuous infusion.

Bolus tube feedings more closely mimic the normal state. They periodically distend the stomach, which aids in gastric secretion and emptying. When bolus tube feeding is undertaken, the volume of formula or expressed breast milk required to provide sufficient calories for a 24-hour period is administered through the tube in equal aliquots every 2, 3, 4, or 6 hours. The frequency of administration depends on the patient's age, gastric capacity, and the infant's ability to maintain a normal serum glucose concentration between feedings. In general, younger and more premature infants require more frequent feedings. Intolerance to bolus tube feedings can be manifested as diarrhea, gastroesophageal reflux with emesis, or poor motility. Poor motility usually is apparent when large volumes of feeding, referred to as residuals, remain in the stomach when the next feeding is due.

Continuous tube feedings can be given at a constant rate of infusion by pump into the stomach or duodenum when bolus feedings have failed. This approach may be better tolerated by premature infants and children with diarrhea.

Patients with intrinsic GI disease (Table 98-8) or malabsorption may require total or supplemental PN. Concurrent administration of low-volume, trophic enteral feedings may provide important nutrients to the gut mucosa even when the parenteral route supplies all of the necessary systemic nutrients.[18] Administration of PN into a peripheral vein is limited to those patients

TABLE 98-8
Indications for Parenteral Nutrition Support

Extreme prematurity
Respiratory distress
Congenital GI anomalies
Duodenal atresia
Jejunal atresia
Esophageal atresia
Tracheoesophageal fistula
Pyloric stenosis
Congenital webs
Hirschsprung disease
Malrotation
Volvulus
Abdominal wall defects
Omphalocele (herniation of viscera into the umbilical cord base)
Gastroschisis (defect of abdominal wall, any location except umbilical cord)
Congenital diaphragmatic hernia
Necrotizing enterocolitis
Chronic diarrhea
Inflammatory bowel disease
Chylothorax
Pseudoobstruction
Megacystic microcolon
Abdominal trauma involving viscera
Adverse effects of treating neoplastic disease
Radiation enteritis
Nausea and vomiting
Stomatitis, glossitis, and esophagitis
Anorexia nervosa
Cystic fibrosis
Chronic renal failure
Hepatic failure
Metabolic errors

GI, gastrointestinal.

expected to require parenteral feeding only for a short time (i.e., 2 weeks) because the amount of nutrients that can be safely infused peripherally is limited. In patients who require long-term PN, the IV solution is more concentrated and must be administered into a central vein.

Nutritional Assessment

CASE 98-6

QUESTION 1: T.C. is a 4-month-old, lethargic boy. On examination, he has a moderately distended abdomen and dry mucous membranes. No other remarkable abnormalities are noted. His weight is 6.5 kg (50th–75th percentile for age). Previously, when he was 2 months old, T.C. weighed 5.6 kg (75th percentile for age), and his length was 57 cm (50th percentile for age). His mother reports that for the past 5 to 7 days, he has had five to eight large, liquid stools per day. His infant formula has not changed. He is to be hospitalized for evaluation of his diarrhea and weight loss and for fluid and nutritional management.

After correction of his initial fluid and electrolyte deficits, an assessment of his nutritional status shows the following:

Weight, 6.5 kg (50th–75th percentile)
Length, 62 cm (50th percentile)
Albumin, 3.8 g/dL (normal, 4–5.3 g/dL)
Prealbumin, 7 mg/dL (normal, 20–50 mg/dL)

How would you assess T.C.'s nutritional status?

Growth assessment is an important focus of pediatric health care, especially during the first year of life. With the exception of the intrauterine period, the most rapid growth occurs during the first year. On average, a normally growing infant gains approximately 30 g/day. Typically, healthy infants weigh approximately three times their birth weight by their first birthday.

The patient's nutritional status should be assessed before beginning a nutritional support regimen and reassessed at regular intervals during the course of treatment. If the patient previously was well nourished, the goal is to maintain that status until a normal diet can be resumed. In a child who was previously malnourished, an effort should be made to promote "catch-up" growth and to normalize the biochemical nutritional measures. One in five children admitted to the hospital experience acute or chronic malnutrition.[19] Malnutrition in children is a risk factor for decreased social skills and impaired intellectual development.[20]

Factors used to determine nutritional status in children include dietary history, weight, height, and visceral protein measurements (e.g., albumin, prealbumin). Other measurements used in adults, such as 24-hour creatinine excretion, 24-hour nitrogen excretion, and nitrogen balance, are reserved for older children because complete collections of urine are difficult to obtain and because the percentage of non–urea nitrogen present in urine is variable in infants.

Anthropometric measurements can also be used to assess T.C.'s nutritional status. Height, weight, and head circumference are used to determine nutritional status in infants and children. Standards for these measurements have been derived from pediatric patients in the United States and compiled into graphs referred to as growth curves (http://www.cdc.gov/growthcharts).[3] An individual patient's measurements are compared with the graph of normal values for that specific age group. As prematurely born infants age, a standard growth curve adjusted for prematurity can be used. Using these measurements, comparisons with standards are possible: weight for age, height for age, and weight for height.[3] A weight that is below the fifth percentile for the patient's height is considered an indication of acute malnutrition. Similarly, a height and weight that are below the fifth percentile for the patient's age indicate chronic malnutrition. It is important to consider the height and weight of the child's parents because genetics are important determinants of the height and weight that a child may ultimately achieve. Additionally, the revised growth charts include the body mass index (BMI) for age for children older than 2 years. The BMI helps identify children at risk for obesity and type 2 diabetes, two problems that have recently become concerns in children.[3]

Numerous biochemical indices are also used in the assessment of nutritional status. Of these, the most readily available and widely used is the serum albumin concentration. Although a low serum albumin can be a specific indicator of protein-calorie malnutrition, its long half-life (20 days)[19] makes it an insensitive indicator for developing and resolving malnutrition.

Prealbumin can also function as a biochemical marker of nutritional status.[19] Because of its shorter half-life, prealbumin has the advantage of being more sensitive than albumin to acute nutritional changes, and it is still useful when exogenous albumin infusions are given.[19]

CASE 98-6, QUESTION 2: After initial IV rehydration and receiving nothing by mouth (NPO) for 48 hours, T.C.'s stool output has decreased dramatically. Is this characteristic of infants with chronic diarrhea? How should T.C.'s enteral diet be initiated?

A prompt decrease in stool output when enteral intake is stopped is typical of infants with chronic diarrhea. Nonetheless, evaluation of bowel function and adaptation has shown that enteral nutrition is superior to PN with regard to histologic recovery, improvement of D-xylose absorption, protein absorption, and disaccharidase activity.[21] In fact, improvement in histology or absorptive function might not occur until enteral nutrients are given.[18] Thus, for T.C., every effort should be made to provide some nutrition enterally.

The enteral regimen should be initiated with a lactosefree formula, such as an elemental formula or a soy-based formula. Although any soy-based formula would be appropriate, Isomil DF is a soy-based formula with added fiber that is indicated for infants with diarrhea. Infants with chronic diarrhea can have small bowel mucosal damage and decreased disaccharidase activity.[4] Carbohydrate absorption depends on digestion of disaccharides and polysaccharides to monosaccharides through disaccharidase activity in the intestinal lumen. Substitution of free glucose orally may overcome the problem of carbohydrate digestion and absorption. Administration of large amounts of oral glucose should be limited, however, because of its osmotic effect and potential to worsen diarrhea. Furthermore, incompletely absorbed carbohydrate is available to colonic bacteria for fermentation, the end products of which can produce diarrhea through colonic irritation.

Unlike carbohydrate, protein rarely causes diarrhea, but the mucosal damage present in patients with chronic diarrhea, such as T.C., can reduce the absorptive surface area so that protein malabsorption may occur. This can be minimized through the administration of a formula containing protein in the form of dipeptides and tripeptides, which are absorbed more efficiently than free amino acids.

Dilution of hypertonic formulas to half strength may improve formula tolerance. The concentration is increased in a stepwise fashion to full strength if there is no carbohydrate malabsorption and if stool output is not excessive. Tolerance may be improved by continuous infusion of the enteral product. If enteral refeeding results in the return of diarrhea, fluid and electrolytes must be replaced with an equal volume of an IV solution of similar electrolyte composition to the stool loss.

CASE 98-6, QUESTION 3: How can T.C.'s tolerance to the formula and his recovery of intestinal function be assessed?

Malabsorption or formula intolerance can be assessed by stool studies, which would include assessing for the presence of reducing substances and stool pH. Lactose is a reducing sugar and its presence in stool is an assessment of carbohydrate absorption. The bacterial fermentation products of malabsorbed carbohydrates can result in a decreased stool pH, which suggests malabsorption. To further evaluate carbohydrate absorption, D-xylose may be given orally; a blood sample is drawn 4 to 5 hours later to determine the amount absorbed. This test may be of initial prognostic value in predicting which patients will require prolonged courses of treatment.[21] More than 5% of ingested fat in a stool collection (typically obtained for 3 days) is indicative of fat malabsorption. All these tests can be evaluated during outpatient visits to guide the refeeding process.

Once the diarrhea has resolved, standard infant formula feedings should be established using an enteral elemental or soy-based formula. Regardless of the time chosen, a gradual stepwise conversion is suggested. A small volume of standard formula is substituted for an equal volume of elemental or soy-based formula, and the substitution volume is increased daily until the elemental or soy-based formula is eliminated completely from the regimen. If a specific nutrient intolerance has been identified, a standard formula that does not contain that nutrient must be selected. For example, a patient with cow's milk protein intolerance may require a soy protein formula or an elemental formula.

Pediatric Parenteral Nutrition

The basic requirements for a parenteral nutrient regimen are listed in Table 98-1. These guidelines for the initiation of a nutrient regimen should be individualized to specific patient needs. The correct regimen for any specific patient is that which supplies sufficient nutrients to promote a normal rate of growth without toxicity. In particular, patients with ongoing, abnormal nutrient losses may require much larger doses of certain nutrients. Individualization of the nutrient prescription cannot be overemphasized. Many of the requirements listed in Table 98-1 apply to nutrients administered by the enteral route as well. In some instances, the absorption of a particular nutrient from the GI mucosa is incomplete, and enteral requirements are substantially higher. This is particularly true of the major minerals (calcium, magnesium, and iron) and trace elements.

Indications

Parenteral nutrition is indicated for any infant or child unable to take in sufficient nourishment to maintain normal growth. Some specific indications are listed in Table 98-8.

VERY LOW-BIRTH-WEIGHT INFANTS

Extremely premature or VLBW infants require specialized nutritional support for two distinct reasons. First, the third trimester in utero is a time of rapid growth and accumulation of protein, glycogen, fat, and minerals.[22] The infant born in the very early stages of the third trimester does not accumulate these stores and, therefore, must receive nutrients earlier than a more mature infant. Second, extreme prematurity is associated with poor coordination of the suck and swallow reflex, poor GI motility, and incomplete absorption. Therefore, enteral nutrients may need to be administered via an orogastric or nasogastric tube, and PN supplementation probably will be needed. PN, especially of amino acids, should be initiated soon after birth to duplicate intrauterine growth and prevent a catabolic state in the first few days of life. The fetus has a continuous supply of amino acids that is immediately stopped after preterm birth.[23] A standardized solution containing amino acids and dextrose can be used for infants weighing less than 1 kg in the first 24 hours of life. There has been some reluctance to administer amino acids this soon after birth because of increased risk of hyperammonemia, uremia, and metabolic acidosis. Several studies, however, have shown early introduction of amino acids is safe, provides a positive nitrogen balance, and promotes better health outcomes.[24,25]

RESPIRATORY DISTRESS

Respiratory distress may preclude the ability to consume sufficient nutrients enterally because high respiratory rates prevent coordinated breathing and swallowing. In infants who are hypoxic, or at high risk for hypoxia, aggressive enteral feedings during the acute phase of their illness can increase the likelihood of bowel ischemia. Often, these situations are resolved in 3 to 5 days, but this can rarely be predicted at the outset. Trophic feedings (1–5 mL/hour) are often implemented to maintain GI tract integrity. Nutritional support in such cases is initiated by giving parenteral fluids, which provide dextrose as a caloric source. This allows the infant to conserve endogenous energy substrates, an important consideration for the VLBW infant whose entire body composition may contain as little as a 3- to 4-day energy supply.[22] PN should be initiated as soon as it becomes clear the enteral feeding will not be possible for at least 3 to 5 days, or when several days have elapsed and no clear time frame can be determined for the establishment of enteral feeding. Although a short course (5 days or less) of PN may be used, the quantity of nutrients supplied during the process of initiation and gradual increase to full requirements is so low that extremely short courses may be difficult to justify. Peripheral PN using fat emulsion as a significant source of calories, however, can provide up to 70 kcal/kg and, with appropriate types and amounts of protein, result in modest weight gain and nitrogen equilibrium.

GASTROINTESTINAL ANOMALIES

Infants with GI anomalies often require PN because the implementation of enteral feedings may be delayed. For example, GI tract atresias or stenosis can obstruct, or partially obstruct, the lumen of the GI tract. This prevents or slows the passage of fluids and nutrients and can result in vomiting, depending on the location of the obstruction. Similarly, infants with necrotizing enterocolitis have zones of ischemic bowel and are at risk for bowel perforation if fed enterally.[26] Infants with these disorders need PN until the viability of the entire GI tract can be assured.

CHRONIC RENAL FAILURE AND HEPATIC DISEASE

Chronic renal or hepatic disease requires modification of a normal diet to account for the impaired elimination of nitrogenous waste or impaired protein metabolism. Careful caloric supplementation with a reduced amount of protein may permit normal growth while minimizing excess urea production in an infant with renal failure.

CASE 98-6, QUESTION 4: Approximately 48 hours after discharge from the hospital, T.C. returns to the emergency department with abdominal distension and bloody diarrhea. He is diagnosed with post gastroenteritis syndrome. T.C. cannot receive nutrients enterally, and PN is to be initiated because he is nutritionally depleted. Describe how a regimen of PN should be instituted in T.C. What aspects of his disease may alter specific nutrient needs?

When initiating PN, the protein (amino acids), glucose (dextrose), fat (lipids or fat emulsion), fluid, and electrolyte, mineral, and vitamin components of the regimen are managed as separate entities. In addition, the route of PN delivery is important to consider because the amount of glucose, potassium, and calcium must be limited if the infusion is given peripherally. In general, 12.5% dextrose, 40 mEq/L potassium, and 10 mEq/L calcium are the maximal amounts that should be provided by infusion into a peripheral vein. These nutrients can be increased if a central venous catheter is placed. The fluids, electrolytes, minerals, and vitamins are initiated at full daily maintenance doses after correction of any pre-existing abnormalities. Protein should be initiated at full daily doses in term infants and children with normal renal and hepatic function. Glucose and fat are started at lower doses and increased daily until requirements are reached.

Protein should be started in T.C. at full daily requirements of 2 to 3 g/kg/day. Azotemia and acidosis have occurred in infants receiving more than 4 g/kg/day of protein; however, these complications are rare at the recommended dosage. Parenteral glucose administration is initiated at 5 to 8 mg/kg/minute (7.2–11.5 g/kg/day). At normal maintenance fluid rates, 10% dextrose represents a generally well-tolerated starting solution for patients of virtually any age or size, except the VLBW infant. In T.C.'s case, the dextrose concentration will begin and continue at 10% because of the peripheral catheter limitations. This concentration will provide 7.3 mg/kg/minute. If a central catheter later becomes necessary, the concentration can be increased by 5% each day until the caloric requirement is met. This increase should be accompanied by blood and urine glucose monitoring. If the blood glucose is 150 mg/dL or greater, or if the urine glucose exceeds "trace" amounts, the PN infusion rate should be decreased by at least 25% and a second IV solution should be added to provide needed fluids and electrolytes. Alternatively, the dextrose concentration can be decreased or insulin can be infused concomitantly and titrated to a desired serum glucose concentration of 120 to 140 mg/dL.

Fat emulsion should be initiated at 1 g/kg/day and increased daily by 0.5 to 1 g/kg/day until the maximal dosage of 3 g/kg/day is reached. The daily fat dose should be infused at a constant rate because fats are better tolerated when infused over the course of 24 hours.[27] Serum triglycerides should be monitored every other day while the dose of fat is being increased. Patients with a fasting triglyceride concentration of 150 mg/dL or less may have their fat dose increased. In patients who are receiving inadequate calories, triglycerides may be elevated because endogenous fats are being mobilized. If the triglyceride concentration is greater than 150 mg/dL, the serum sample must be examined visually. A clear sample with a mildly elevated triglyceride concentration probably indicates the use of endogenous fat stores for energy. Conversely, a turbid or lipemic sample indicates the patient's inability to use the amount of intravenous fat administered. In this case, further increases in the fat dose should be delayed until triglyceride concentrations decrease.

Special Considerations and Complications

CASE 98-7

QUESTION 1: J.H., a 4-day-old boy, was born at 31 weeks' gestation. His birth weight was 1,950 g, and he now weighs 2,000 g. On the first day of life, he was given a commercial preterm infant formula by orogastric tube in gradually increasing quantity with supplemental IV fluids. Now, on the fourth day of life, he has a distended abdomen and his stools contain bright red blood. An abdominal radiograph shows pneumatosis intestinalis (gas within the intestinal wall seen on x-ray). All enteral feedings are stopped (NPO). What do these findings represent? What are the implications for J.H.'s nutritional management?

Abdominal distension, bloody stools, and pneumatosis intestinalis are characteristic of necrotizing enterocolitis historically.[28] The causes of this disorder are unclear, but it occurs more often in premature than in term infants; it can occur in clusters of cases, rarely is seen before enteral feeding is instituted, and can be associated with rapid increases in enteral intake.[29] Because J.H. will receive antibiotics for 10 to 14 days and remain NPO, he requires PN. The planned duration of the regimen makes central venous access a necessity.

GOALS OF LONG-TERM SUPPORT

CASE 98-7, QUESTION 2: The following day, intestinal perforation requires the resection of two-thirds of J.H.'s distal jejunum and one-third of his ileum, with creation of a jejunostomy. The ileocecal valve and the entire colon are left intact. During the operation, a central venous catheter is placed. What is the goal of PN for J.H.?

J.H. will be NPO for a prolonged time. Therefore, the goals of his PN must be to promote normal growth as well as healing of his diseased gut and surgical wounds. Because J.H. is a premature infant, it will be difficult to predict how well he will tolerate PN. VLBW infants tolerate normal doses of pediatric amino acids without difficulty; however, some clinicians initiate protein at a lower daily dose (e.g., 1.0 g/kg/day) and advance by 0.5 g/kg/day each day until a goal of 2 to 3 g/kg/day is achieved. Fat should be started at 0.5 to 1 g/kg/day and increased by 0.5 g/kg/day up to 3 g/kg/day. Glucose should be initiated at 5 to 10 g/kg/day and increased by 2 to 3 g/kg until the desired caloric intake is achieved. Appropriate doses of electrolytes and minerals may be started immediately using the guidelines listed in Table 98-1.

FAT EMULSIONS: COMPLICATIONS

CASE 98-7, QUESTION 3: What must be considered in making decisions regarding fat administration in J.H.?

Although J.H. can receive adequate calories using only glucose and crystalline amino acids, he will require fat to provide a more physiologic diet and to prevent essential fatty acid deficiency (EFAD), which develops quickly in low-birth-weight infants who have little fat reserve. J.H. should receive a minimum of 5% of his total caloric requirement as fat emulsion to minimize the risk of EFAD. Ideally, his nutrition regimen will provide approximately 40% of calories from fat, which is similar to what is provided by human milk.

Infusions of fat emulsion have been associated with impaired oxygen transport and pulmonary ventilation-perfusion mismatch. This adverse effect occurs more often when the dose of fat is 4 g/kg or greater and is infused for a relatively short (4 hours) period. Current practice is to increase gradually the doses of fat from 0.5 to 1 g/kg/day up to a maximum of 4 g/kg/day and to infuse the fat emulsion over the course of 24 hours to minimize the likelihood of pulmonary problems and to promote clearance.

It is unclear whether IV fat administration is detrimental to patients with sepsis. Infusion of fat emulsion has resulted in lymphocyte and neutrophil death.[30] On the other hand, the linoleic acid in IV fat is the precursor to arachidonic acid, prostaglandins, thromboxane, interleukins, and immune-mediating cells. Theoretically, this may minimize bacteremia. Necrotizing enterocolitis, intestinal perforation, and surgery predispose J.H. to sepsis. Therefore, he should have his IV fat infused at an appropriate dose over the course of 24 hours. Because fat clearance can be impaired during infection, it is also prudent to monitor his triglyceride concentrations.

Free fatty acids can displace bilirubin from its albumin binding sites, thereby placing the infant at risk for kernicterus.[31] Therefore, before advancing the fat dose, the total bilirubin and direct bilirubin should be measured. Patients with an indirect bilirubin (total bilirubin minus direct bilirubin) of 10 mg/dL or less whose albumin levels are normal are at low risk for kernicterus. Indirect bilirubin usually peaks before 1 week of age. After the risk for indirect hyperbilirubinemia has passed, the fat dose can be increased as recommended in Table 98-1. The infusion of 1 g/kg over the course of 24 hours is associated with minimal risk for decreased bilirubin binding[31]; however, rapid infusion of this same dose can displace bilirubin from albumin binding sites. Given the low level of indirect bilirubin found on routine monitoring and the planned fat infusion rate, J.H. should not be at risk for kernicterus.

Egg phospholipids are used to emulsify fats; therefore, patients with a known allergy to eggs (e.g., fever, chills, urticaria, dyspnea, bronchospasm, chest pain) should not receive fat emulsion.

GLUCOSE INTOLERANCE

CASE 98-7, QUESTION 4: Because J.H. is a premature infant, PN is initiated using 5% glucose, 2.5 g/kg/day of amino acids, and 0.5 g/kg/day of fat emulsion. The volume of PN should be 240 mL based on a maintenance fluid requirement of 120 mL/kg (Table 98-1). On the second day, he receives 10% glucose, 2.5 g/kg/day of amino acids, and 1 g/kg/day of fat. On the third day, glucose is increased to 15%, amino acids remain at 2.5 g/kg/day, and fat emulsion is increased to 1.5 g/kg/day. On the fourth day, glucose is increased to 20%, amino acids remain at 2.5 g/kg/day, and fats are increased to 2 g/kg/day. After this solution has been infused for 8 hours, his urine test yields 1% for glucose (normal, no glucose) and his blood glucose level is 210 mg/dL (normal, 120 mg/dL). Explain this new finding and the problems it may cause. How should hyperglycemia be managed?

Maximal glucose oxidation rates in milligrams per kilograms per minute are inversely related to age, and decrease from 15 to 18 mg/kg/minute in neonates and young infants to 4 to 5 mg/kg/minute in adults. In full-term neonates and infants receiving maintenance fluids (100 mL/kg/day), glucose concentrations can be started at 10 g/kg/day (equivalent to dextrose 10%) and advanced by 5 g/kg (equivalent to dextrose 5%) every 24 hours up to approximately 25 g/kg/day (equivalent to dextrose 25%). In preterm neonates, such as J.H., dextrose is started at a lower dose and advanced at smaller increments, usually 2 to 3 g/kg/day. Glucose tolerance varies significantly, so each patient should be considered individually.

At J.H.'s prescribed fluid rate of 10 mL/hour, 20% glucose represents 16.7 mg/kg/minute of glucose. The hyperglycemia and glycosuria probably have occurred because the increases in the infusion rate have exceeded J.H.'s ability to adapt to the glucose dose. Patients who have been euglycemic on their glucose dose and then become glucose intolerant should be evaluated, however, for other causes, such as infection and addition of exogenous corticosteroids. Hyperglycemia and glycosuria can result in serum hyperosmolarity, osmotic diuresis, and dehydration. Regardless of the cause, the hyperglycemia should be treated by reducing the glucose administration rate. The rate of the PN infusion can be decreased further if hyperglycemia continues or increased if the hyperglycemia resolves.

When the PN order is written for the subsequent days, the glucose increases should be made in smaller amounts up to the full daily maintenance calorie requirements. Frequent blood and urine glucose monitoring must be continued. Severe glucose intolerance in patients who require PN can be managed with insulin to normalize serum glucose. Although insulin is compatible with PN solutions, it does adsorb to glass, polyvinyl chloride, and filters, resulting in decreased delivery of insulin.[32] Frequently, pediatric patients have changing insulin requirements that prevent the addition of insulin to PN solutions. A separate continuous infusion of regular insulin (initial dose, 0.05 to 0.1 units/kg/hour) titrated to control serum glucose concentrations offers a practical solution to minimize waste of the PN solution.[33] It is essential to discontinue the insulin infusion if the PN solution is discontinued to avoid hypoglycemia.

EFFECTS OF BRONCHOPULMONARY DYSPLASIA AND MECHANICAL VENTILATION

CASE 98-7, QUESTION 5: J.H. remains dependent on a ventilator because of his immature lungs. How could J.H.'s respiratory disease influence his nutritional regimen?

After 28 days of age, J.H.'s ventilator dependence defines him as having bronchopulmonary dysplasia (BPD), a chronic lung disease of infancy. Historically, BPD is characterized by an increase in resting energy expenditure, increased work of breathing, and period and then restarted and gradually increased to the desired rate, will decrease the length of time the liver is exposed to PN. VLBW infants, however, may become hypoglycemic even with very gradual decreases in infusion rate, so this option should be used with care. In any event, a short time off PN (e.g., 2 hours) should be attempted.

The trace elements provided by the formulation should be examined. Both copper and manganese are enterohepatically recycled and may accumulate in liver disease. Manganese can also contribute to hepatotoxicity and should be removed from J.H.'s PN solutions. Studies have not established when removal of copper and manganese is warranted. The inappropriate removal of copper could lead to anemia, osteopenia, and neutropenia. Therefore, decreasing the copper dose and monitoring serum concentrations of both copper and manganese should guide therapy.

Recently, case reports have demonstrated that using intravenous fat emulsion derived from fish oil rather than soy oil may reverse liver damage in infants with PN-associated cholestasis. Fish oil is high in eicosapentaenoic and docosahexaenoic acids, which do not impair bile flow and may actually diminish fat accumulation in the liver.[47]

Pharmacologic interventions have had limited success in the management of PN-associated cholestasis. Phenobarbital has not been shown to be effective in reducing or reversing PN-associated cholestasis.[48] Ursodiol 10 to 20 mg/kg/day has been used successfully in the treatment of other cholestatic liver diseases, and preliminary reports indicate that it may also improve PN-associated cholestasis in children.[49] Ursodiol, a naturally occurring nontoxic bile acid, presumably works by displacing and replacing the endogenously produced, potentially toxic bile salts that accumulate with cholestasis.

Sincalide is part of the endogenous hormone cholecystokinin (CCK), and may improve signs of PN-associated cholestasis. CCK is secreted in the small intestine in response to meals and stimulates gallbladder contraction and increases intestinal motility. In PN-dependent patients, such as J.H., endogenous CCK secretion is diminished. For J.H., the dose of sincalide would be 0.12 mcg/kg/day.[50]

The antibiotic metronidazole also appears promising in the prevention of PN-associated cholestasis in adults. Metronidazole inhibits the bacterial overgrowth in the GI tract that occurs with intestinal stasis. The bacteria are responsible for increased formation of hepatotoxic bile acids such as lithocholate; 25 mg/kg/day of metronidazole has been shown to be effective.[51]

CASE 98-7, QUESTION 11: Project the course of J.H.'s liver disease if PN is discontinued and enteral feedings are instituted within 2 weeks. What may occur if enteral feedings cannot be instituted?

It is difficult to predict a successful wean from PN. Historically, success has been associated with longer length of intact small intestine. Additionally, studies in children with short bowel syndrome have shown that serum citrulline levels may predict the ability to successfully wean a patient from PN. Citrulline is a free amino acid that is produced by the small bowel enterocytes. Therefore, it may be warranted to measure J.H.'s serum citrulline level before weaning from PN.[52]

If PN can be discontinued soon after the onset of cholestasis, the prospects for J.H. to recover normal hepatic function are good. Jaundice usually resolves within 2 weeks after PN is discontinued, and the biochemical abnormalities normalize soon thereafter.[43] The pathologic changes observed on biopsy resolve even more slowly. Biopsy evidence of cholestasis has been observed for up to 40 weeks after resolution of clinical and serologic evidence of hepatic disease.[43]

If enteral feedings cannot be instituted successfully, the prognosis for J.H.'s liver function is not as good. Studies have demonstrated that infants receiving PN for 90 days or more had biopsy evidence of irreversible liver damage.[43] Thus, it clearly is advantageous to convert J.H.'s nutrition to the enteral route as soon as he tolerates such a change.

KEY REFERENCES AND WEBSITES

A full list of references for this chapter can be found at http://thepoint.lww.com/AT10e. Below are the key references for this chapter, with the corresponding reference number in this chapter found in parentheses after the reference.

Key References

Greene HL et al. Guidelines for the use of vitamins, trace elements, calcium, magnesium, and phosphorus in infants and children receiving total parenteral nutrition: report of the Subcommittee on Pediatric Parenteral Nutrient Requirements from the Committee on Clinical Practice Issues of the American Society for Clinical Nutrition [published corrections appear in *Am J Clin Nutr.* 1989;49(6):1332; *Am J Clin Nutr.* 1989;50(3):560]. *Am J Clin Nutr.* 1988;48(5):1324. (2)

Gura KM et al. Reversal of parenteral nutrition-associated liver disease in two infants with short-bowel syndrome using parenteral fish oil: implications for future management. *Pediatrics.* 2006;118(1):e197. (47)

Hay WW Jr et al. Workshop summary: nutrition of the extremely low birth weight infant. *Pediatrics.* 1999;104(6):1360. (24)

Heird WC et al. Intravenous alimentation in pediatric patients. *J Pediatr.* 1972;80(3):351. (22)

Heird WC et al. Pediatric parenteral amino acid mixture in low birth weight infants. *Pediatrics.* 1988;81(1):41. (37)

Helms RA et al. Comparison of a pediatric versus standard amino acid formulation in preterm neonates requiring parenteral nutrition. *J Pediatr.* 1987;110(3):466. (38)

Holliday MA, Segar WE. The maintenance need for water in parenteral fluid therapy. *Pediatrics.* 1957;19(5):823. (1)

Kelly DA. Intestinal failure-associated liver disease: what do we know today? *Gastroenterology.* 2006;130(2 Suppl 1):S70. (43)

King C et al; Centers for Disease Control and Prevention. Managing acute gastroenteritis among children oral rehydration, maintenance, and nutritional therapy. *MMWR Recomm Rep.* 2003;52(RR-16):1. (4)

Section 18 Pediatrics

Common Pediatric Illnesses

99

Michelle Condren and Mark Haase

CORE PRINCIPLES

		CHAPTER CASES
1	Medication administration to children can be challenging. For oral administration, dosing syringes or droppers should be used rather than household spoons or cups. The administration of medications by any route may require special techniques in an uncooperative child.	**Case 99-1 (Question 1)**
2	Teething often results in drooling, salivation, and pain leading to irritability. Therapy is supportive, using teething aids and systemic acetaminophen or ibuprofen. Topical benzocaine products are not recommended due to the risk for methemoglobinemia.	**Case 99-2 (Questions 1, 2)**
3	Diaper dermatitis presents as a mild red rash that often progresses to increased redness and lesions outside the diaper area. Barrier creams are recommended for initial treatment with the addition of a topical antifungal for dermatitis lasting longer than 3 days and spreading outside the diaper area.	**Case 99-3 (Questions 1, 2)**
4	Fever in children may be the result of a common viral infection, but could also be an indicator of a more serious bacterial infection or lead to complications such as febrile seizures. Proper management depends in large part on accurate assessment.	**Case 99-4 (Questions 1, 2)**
5	The treatment of cough and cold symptoms in children younger than 6 years of age is generally supportive with nasal saline, hydration, and humidification. Over-the-counter agents have little proven effectiveness and have been associated with severe adverse effects owing to inadvertent overdoses during parental administration.	**Case 99-5 (Question 1)**
6	Constipation can be defined by a delay or difficulty in stooling for at least 2 weeks duration. Constipation is most commonly functional, and may be managed with behavioral modification or drug therapy.	**Case 99-6 (Question 1)**
7	Gastroenteritis, although usually self-limiting, may result in clinically significant dehydration in infants and children. Assessment of the degree of dehydration is important in determining whether oral rehydration is appropriate or hospital admission with intravenous rehydration is required.	**Case 99-7 (Questions 1–4)**
8	Gastroesophageal reflux is a common disorder in young infants. Most will require no intervention. Some, however, will require feeding modifications and possibly drug therapy, including acid-suppressing or prokinetic agents.	**Case 99-8 (Questions 1, 2)**
9	Otitis media is a middle ear infection associated with effusion, rapid symptom development, and evidence of middle ear inflammation. Options for therapy include antibiotic management and watchful waiting, the choice of which depends on the age of the child and severity of disease. Amoxicillin (or amoxicillin/clavulanate) remains the antibiotic of choice despite the high incidence of penicillin nonsusceptible *Streptococcus pneumoniae*.	**Case 99-9 (Questions 1–3)**
10	Acute pharyngitis may be caused by respiratory viruses or bacteria, most commonly *Streptococcus pyogenes*. Treatment goals for bacterial pharyngitis include resolution of symptoms and prevention of rheumatic heart disease. Amoxicillin is the antibiotic of choice for bacterial pharyngitis.	**Case 99-10 (Questions 1, 2)**

Children represent more than 25% of the population and receive an average of three prescription medications before 5 years of age. According to the Slone Survey, between 1998 and 2007, 56% of children younger than 12 years of age had taken at least one medication in the previous week.[1] Prescription medications accounted for only 20% of cases; thus, the use of over-the-counter (e.g., nonprescription) medications was most prevalent. The most predominant over-the-counter medications used were acetaminophen, pseudoephedrine, ibuprofen, dextromethorphan, antihistamines, and iron. The most prevalent prescription medications were amoxicillin and albuterol. The prevalence of chronic medication use for dyslipidemia, hypertension, type 2 diabetes, and attention deficit hyperactivity disorder have increased in recent years, illustrating that chronic disease management is becoming more important in pediatric medicine.[2,3] Given the prevalence of medication use in children, it is essential that health care providers be prepared to educate families and children on the appropriate use of over-the-counter and prescription medications.

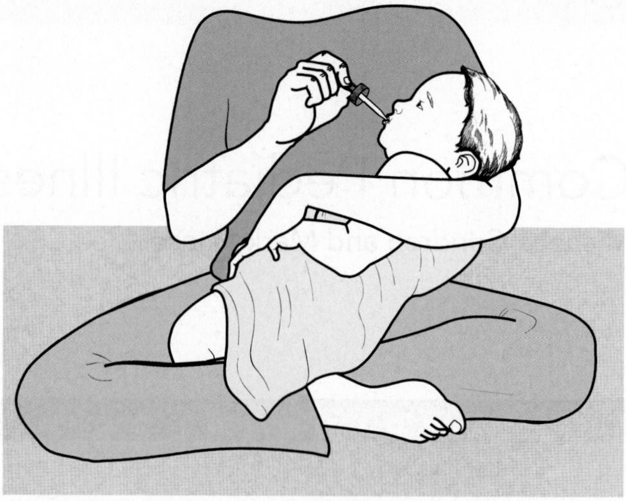

FIGURE 99-1 Administration of oral liquid medication to a young child. (1) Premeasure the medication and have it within reach. (2) Hold the child in your lap, placing one of the child's arms behind your back and both of the child's legs between your legs. Restrain the child's other arm securely with your nondominant arm. (3) Tilt the child's head back slightly, pressing gently on the child's cheeks to open the mouth. Using your dominant hand, aim the dropper or syringe between the rear gum and cheek. Administer small amounts of medication (1–2 mL) at a time, making sure the baby swallows.

ADMINISTERING MEDICATION TO CHILDREN

CASE 99-1

QUESTION 1: M.B., a 16-month-old girl weighing 9 kg, has been diagnosed with an ear infection. She will be receiving antipyrine/benzocaine ear drops every 4 hours as needed for pain and amoxicillin (400 mg/5 mL) 5 mL by mouth every 12 hours. What tips for successfully administering these medications should be recommended?

Oral Medications

The administration of oral medications to a young child or infant often requires two adults: one to gently restrain the child while the other rapidly and accurately administers the medication. If only one adult is available, one can restrain the arms and legs of the child in a swaddling blanket or large towel as depicted in Figure 99-1. For a video of how to swaddle, see http://www.eugenepeds.com/swaddling.html.

The administration device (syringe or dropper) that generally accompanies a liquid medication product provides the most accurate measurement of the desired dose. For infants, liquid medications are most easily administered to the back cheek in 1- to 2-mL amounts with an oral syringe. Household teaspoons should not be used to measure medications because teaspoons are of variable sizes and hold 3 to 8 mL of a liquid. Studies have shown that parents have more difficulty accurately delivering doses using dosing cups than other devices.[4] In some situations, crushed tablets or capsule contents mixed in small amounts (1–2 teaspoons) of food (e.g., chocolate pudding, applesauce, ice cream, jelly, chocolate syrup) offer an alternative to liquid formulations. The taste of liquid dosage formulations generally is improved by refrigeration and flavoring agents, and "chasers" (i.e., popsicle, chocolate syrup, or a flavored drink after a dose) also are helpful. Although medications can be delivered in small amounts (10–15 mL) of liquid in a bottle (juice, milk, formula), doses should not be diluted into an entire scheduled feeding or prepared ahead of time in batches in anticipation of future administration. Limiting the volume more likely facilitates delivery of the entire dose, and adding the medication to a feeding bottle immediately before delivery minimizes the potential of drug instability. Drug interactions with foods and dairy products also should be considered before drugs are added to feeding formulas. Most children are able to swallow tablets at 5 to 8 years of age. Duplicate supplies of medication should be provided to the caregiver when midday doses are required for children who attend school or childcare in the event a dose is dropped. Children of all ages should be encouraged and praised for their cooperation in taking their medicine. Rewards and positive reinforcements can be useful to gain cooperation in an older child.

For M.B.'s amoxicillin, the parents should be given a dosing syringe and shown how to measure 5 mL. If M.B. is uncooperative with medication administration, she may need to be restrained and the medication delivered in 1- to 2-mL increments. The parents should be ready to provide M.B. with something that tastes good immediately after administering the medication.

Ear, Nose, and Eye Drops

Otic, ophthalmic, and nasal medications usually need to be administered to infants and young children in a different manner than adults. Otic medications should be instilled by pulling the auricle down and out in infants and young children, whereas older children should have the auricle of the ear held up and back to straighten the ear canal. During the instillation of nose and eye drops, position infants and toddlers with their head lower than the rest of the body because gravity assists in dispersing the medication. This can be achieved by laying the infant across a bed with the shoulders projecting over the edge of the bed. Restraining the infant often is required during the administration of ophthalmic formulations. When administering the eye medication (Fig. 99-2; see also http://www.eugenepeds.com/giving-eye-drops.html for a video of how to give eye drops), the caregiver must be cautious to avoid injury to the eye caused by sudden movements of the infant. The technique of placing the hand which holds the eye medication on the forehead of the infant during administration can help to minimize eye injury because the hand holding the eye dropper will move when the infant's head moves.

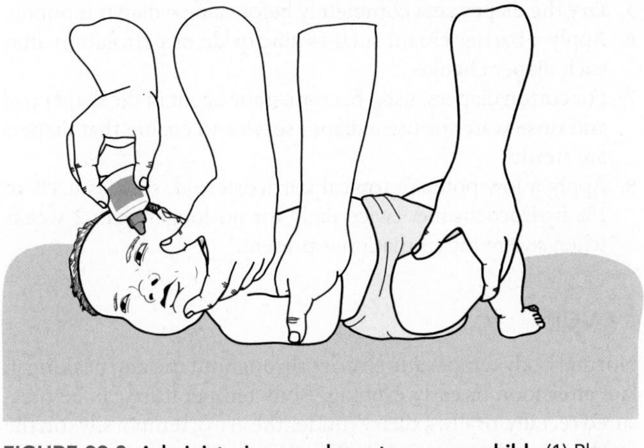

FIGURE 99-2 **Administering eye drops to a young child.** (1) Place the child on a flat surface. Enlist the help of a second adult to restrain the child or swaddle the child as described in the video clip referenced in the text. (2) Holding the child's head steady, gently pull the eyelids apart. The hand that is holding the medication dropper can rest on the child's head while administering the medication to minimize the potential for injury to the eye if the child's head moves abruptly. Administer the medication as directed.

To minimize fear and improve cooperation during instillation of eye, nose, or ear drops, the procedure should be explained to the child as simply as possible. It is best to warm the medication in your hand for a few minutes before administration because medications can feel cold inside the ears or nose even when stored at room temperature.

For the administration of ear drops to M.B., she should be lying down with the affected ear up. The auricle should be pulled down and out and the ear drops placed in the ear canal. She should remain in that position for at least 1 minute. See **http://www.gosh.nhs.uk/gosh_families/information_sheets/medicines_ear_drops_spray/medicines_ear_drops_spray_video_wmv.html** for a video of how to give ear drops.

INFANT CARE

Teething

The growth and development of teeth begin as early as the sixth week of embryonic life. Calcification of the enamel and dentin begins at 4 months of gestation. Normal eruption of primary or deciduous teeth rarely begins before 4 to 5 months of age and usually is completed by 30 months of age.[5] Although premature infants usually experience delayed eruption of their deciduous teeth, their first tooth appears (based on postconceptual age) at about the same time as term infants.[5] In many full-term infants, however, teeth do not erupt until the end of the first year. Delayed eruption of all teeth can reflect systemic or nutritional disturbances (e.g., hypothyroidism, hypopituitarism, rickets).[5] Early eruption is less common and also can be associated with medical conditions (e.g., hyperthyroidism, precocious puberty, long-term corticosteroid therapy).

SIGNS AND SYMPTOMS

CASE 99-2

QUESTION 1: C.J., a 6-month-old girl weighing 7 kg, has become increasingly irritable and has been waking up four to five times a night. She is drooling excessively and biting on hard objects constantly. A brief examination of C.J.'s mouth shows red and tender gums. No teeth are present, and C.J. is afebrile. Her mother is concerned that C.J.'s teething has caused a secondary illness. What would be a likely explanation for these symptoms?

C.J.'s regular sleeping pattern has been disturbed by symptomatic teething. As the teeth penetrate the gums, the site can become tender. This process generally is associated with increased salivation. Bacterial invasion through a break in the tissue or under a gingival flap covering the teeth can cause inflammation and edema, but teething itself does not cause systemic disturbances.[5] Restlessness, increased salivation, thumb-sucking, gum-rubbing, and decreased appetite commonly accompany teething.

MANAGEMENT OF TEETHING

CASE 99-2, QUESTION 2: What course of treatment can be suggested for C.J.?

Gentle irrigation with water often relieves the inflammation around a gum flap. A topical anesthetic can be rubbed gently on the mucous membranes overlying C.J.'s erupting tooth with a cotton-tipped applicator. Local anesthetics, however, should not be used long-term, and topical products containing lidocaine should not be used for symptomatic relief of teething because absorption of lidocaine can lead to systemic toxicity. Alcohol-free products containing 7.5% or 10% benzocaine (e.g., Baby Orajel gel, Orabase Baby Teething Gel) have been reported to cause methemoglobinemia and should not be used.[5,6] Giving the child a blunt, firm object to chew is helpful, and wrapping cracked ice in a soft cloth also can hasten tooth eruption and relieve pain. Rubber teething rings of various shapes can be beneficial, but trauma from the teething ring might lead to angular cheilitis, cracking, or soreness at the corners of the mouth. Water-containing rings can become contaminated with bacteria and should be avoided.

Ibuprofen and acetaminophen are commonly prescribed for younger children to relieve pain associated with the eruption of primary dentition. Ibuprofen's anti-inflammatory effects last for about 6 to 8 hours and might be especially helpful for C.J. at bedtime. Pediatric dosing is 5 to 10 mg/kg/dose beginning at 6 months of age. If ibuprofen is selected, C.J. should receive ibuprofen 40 mg/mL infant drops, 1 mL every 6 to 8 hours as needed. The recommended acetaminophen dose is 10 to 15 mg/kg every 4 to 6 hours as needed. If acetaminophen is chosen for C.J., she should receive 160 mg/5 mL suspension, 2.5 mL every 4 to 6 hours as needed. Topical aspirin should never be used because it can cause oral chemical burns. Oral aspirin is not used because of its association with Reye syndrome, a condition consisting of encephalopathy and fatty degeneration of the liver. Systemic analgesics are explained in greater detail in the fever section of this chapter.

Diaper Rash

ETIOLOGY

Diaper dermatitis is commonly encountered in pediatric practice, occurring in up to 35% of infants at any given time. Although the pathogenesis of diaper dermatitis is not well defined, a number of factors (e.g., chemical irritants, friction, bacteria) have been associated with skin inflammation in the diaper area. In particular, skin wetness and pH have been implicated in diaper dermatitis, and wetness appears to have greater influence than that of pH. Overhydration of the skin increases the permeability of low molecular weight compounds and exacerbates the effects of friction.[7] Cloth diapers covered with plastic pants or disposable diapers with plastic outer linings decrease air circulation and increase moisture in the diaper area and should be avoided.[8] Residual chemicals or laundry detergents in the diaper (cloth or disposable), as well as soaps, medications, or lotions that have been applied directly to the infant's skin, also have roles in the development of diaper rash.

CLINICAL PRESENTATION

Four clinical presentations of dermatitis are associated with diaper wear:

1. A mild, scaling rash in the perianal area
2. A sharply demarcated confluent erythema
3. Ulceration distributed through the diaper area
4. A beefy red confluent erythema with satellite lesions, vesiculopustular lesions, and diffuse involvement of the genitalia

TREATMENT

CASE 99-3

QUESTION 1: K.G., a 3-month-old infant, has had a severe diaper rash for the past 4 days. The very inflamed and tender area is confined to the diaper area, and vesicular satellite lesions are present on the periphery of the erythematous area. K.G.'s mother uses only cloth diapers and has not changed soap or her normal pattern of diaper care since K.G. was born. What is the likely cause of K.G.'s diaper rash and what treatments are appropriate?

K.G.'s rash is consistent with a candidal infection, which typically is beefy red and associated with vesicular satellite lesions. Presence of a rash for longer than 3 days and diffuse involvement of the genitalia and inguinal folds also are characteristic of this form of diaper rash. K.G.'s rash can be treated with 1% clotrimazole or 2% miconazole cream applied to the inflamed area four times daily until it has resolved. Nystatin (100,000 units/g) ointment can be applied, but often is not as effective as the imidazole antifungals because of increasing resistance of *Candida* species to nystatin.

CASE 99-3, QUESTION 2: What steps would you recommend for K.G.'s mother to treat her diaper rash and prevent recurrence?

Removal of stool and urine from the diaper area by gentle rinsing with plain water and more frequent diaper changes often help to alleviate diaper rashes. Wiping the baby with diaper wipes that contain alcohol can sting, further irritating the involved area, and should be avoided until the rash has resolved. A good protective agent containing zinc oxide or petrolatum (e.g., Desitin) can be applied with each diaper change to create a barrier to irritants and seal out moisture. Powdered protective agents (e.g., cornstarch, talc) can minimize friction caused by diapers, but should be used cautiously because the infant can aspirate powder particles and develop a chemical pneumonia.[9] When used, powders should be shaken into the diaper or applied close to the body, away from the baby's face. Other prevention and treatment measures appropriate for K.G. include the following:

1. Change the diaper as soon as it is wet or at least every 2 to 4 hours during the day.
2. Keep the diaper area clean (e.g., nightly baths until resolved).
3. Use superabsorbent disposable diapers at night.
4. Expose the diaper area to air as often as possible.
5. Dry the diaper area completely before a new diaper is put on.
6. Apply a barrier cream such as zinc oxide or petrolatum after each diaper change.
7. For cotton diapers, use a bacteriostatic agent in the diaper pail and rinse water or use a diaper service to ensure that diapers are sterile.
8. Apply a low-potency topical corticosteroid, such as 0.5% to 1% hydrocortisone, twice daily for no longer than 2 weeks when severe inflammation is present.[5]

Fever

Normal body temperature varies throughout the day, peaking in late afternoon or early evening. Body temperature can be measured rectally, orally, axillary (under the arm), temporally (on the forehead) and tympanically. Rectal temperatures are most reliable in infants younger than 3 months of age. Oral measurements of temperature are not appropriate in children younger than 3 years of age because it is difficult for young children to maintain a tight seal around the thermometer.

Although references differ, fever can be defined as an axillary temperature greater than 37.5°C (99.5°F), or a core temperature greater than 38°C (100.4°F).[10] Rectal and tympanic measurements are typically 0.3° to 0.6°C (0.5°–1°F) higher than an oral reading, whereas axillary measurements are lower by the same amount. (Fahrenheit temperatures can be converted to or from centigrade temperatures by the formula $°F = 1.8°C + 32$.)

Children with fevers might not have other signs or symptoms of an illness. Any child younger than 2 months of age who develops a fever requires a complete evaluation (e.g., blood culture, urinalysis) because clinical manifestations of a serious infection often are subtle, nonspecific, and not predictive of the extent or severity of illness.[11] In this situation, antibiotic therapy usually is initiated while awaiting laboratory results. Children 3 to 36 months of age with a temperature greater than or equal to 39°C (102.2°F) and white blood cell (WBC) counts less than 5,000/μL or greater than 15,000/μL are at increased risk for bacteremia.[11] Children of any age with a temperature greater than 41°C should be evaluated not only for bacteremia, but also for possible meningitis. Blood cultures, lumbar puncture, urinalysis, and chest radiograph should be considered on an individual basis to help determine the etiology of infection. Febrile immunocompromised children and febrile children with functional or anatomic asplenia are at increased risk for sepsis or fulminant infections (e.g., *Streptococcus pneumoniae, Salmonella* species, *Escherichia coli*) and should receive prompt antibiotic therapy.[12]

Febrile Seizures

CASE 99-4

QUESTION 1: R.B., a 12-month-old, 10-kg baby boy, was well yesterday until his mother noticed that he felt warm to her touch later in the afternoon. For the past 24 hours, he has remained warm and is fussy and less active. A rectal temperature 15 minutes ago was 39°C. Because her other two children experienced febrile seizures, his mother is concerned R.B.'s temperature will continue to rise and put R.B at risk for febrile seizures. Is this a valid concern?

Febrile seizures occur in approximately 2% to 4% of children 6 months to 5 years of age who have temperature elevations greater than 38°C.[12] The etiology and pathogenesis are unknown, and there is no evidence that the rate of temperature increase is important.[13] Genetic predisposition also appears to be a factor because febrile seizures occur with greater frequency among family members.[14] Febrile seizures are of two types:

simple and complex. Simple febrile seizures last less than 15 minutes and do not have significant focal features. Complex febrile seizures have a longer duration, occur in series, and are associated with focal changes. Typically, febrile seizures occur within the first 24 hours of a febrile episode.[13,14] Although R.B. is in the age group at greatest risk for having a febrile seizure, he has been febrile for more than 24 hours, and a seizure is unlikely during this illness.

TREATMENT

CASE 99-4, QUESTION 2: How should R.B.'s fever be treated?

Acetaminophen is the most common antipyretic agent used in children. The usual dose, oral or rectal, is 10 to 15 mg/kg/dose (100 to 150 mg) administered every 4 to 6 hours as needed to a maximum of 90 mg/kg/day.[12,15] Ibuprofen is administered as 5 to 10 mg/kg/dose (50 to 100 mg) orally every 6 to 8 hours as needed to a maximum of 40 mg/kg/day. Ibuprofen is as effective as acetaminophen as an antipyretic and is associated with a low incidence of adverse effects.[16,17] Although renal failure has been reported after ibuprofen use in children,[18,19] the risk of renal impairment is small with short-term use and not greater than that with acetaminophen.[17,19]

Acetaminophen or ibuprofen should be effective in lowering R.B.'s fever. Acetaminophen typically has been considered to be a first-line drug in children. Dosing errors have occurred when teaspoonful quantities of acetaminophen infant drops (80 mg/0.8 mL) were given instead of the liquid formulation (160 mg/5 mL) or when regular-strength tablets (325 mg) have been substituted for chewable children's tablets (160 mg). To reduce the risk for dosing errors, in 2011, the Consumer Healthcare Products Association (a group of leading manufacturers and distributors of nonprescription medications) voluntarily converted to a single 160 mg/5 mL acetaminophen concentration. However, providers should continue to question caregivers about the dosage form of acetaminophen they have at home, concurrent use of any other products containing acetaminophen, and whether cumulative doses are within the recommended range. Recent data have suggested ibuprofen may be a more effective alternative to acetaminophen for R.B. and should be used first.[20] It is available in two liquid formulations (infant drops, 40 mg/mL; children's suspension, 100 mg/5 mL) and a chewable tablet (100 mg). Adverse effects are limited when ibuprofen is used in recommended doses for short-term antipyresis. Some data suggest that combination therapy with acetaminophen every 4 to 6 hours and ibuprofen every 6 to 8 hours may be more effective in reducing time with fever in the first 24 hours.[20] Aspirin therapy is not recommended for treatment of fever in children or adolescents with chickenpox, gastroenteritis, or respiratory viral infections because of its link with Reye syndrome.[21,22]

Cough and Cold

Another common diagnosis in children is viral upper respiratory infection or the common cold. Preschool children generally experience between six and eight colds each year.[23] Children with a cold often present with sore throat, nasal congestion, rhinorrhea, sneezing, cough, and irritability.

CLINICAL PRESENTATION AND TREATMENT

CASE 99-5

QUESTION 1: J.K. is a 3-month-old, 5.3-kg infant who began having nasal congestion, rhinorrhea, and cough yesterday. She has had no fever and is eating well, but did not sleep well last evening. J.K.'s mother called her pediatrician and was told that J.K. most likely has a cold caused by a virus. J.K.'s mother would like to know which cold medications would be appropriate to manage J.K.'s symptoms.

A cool-mist humidifier can increase the amount of moisture in room air and decrease irritation in the upper airway when humidity is low. Saline nose drops followed by bulb suctioning can help to clear the nasal passages in J.K. who is younger than 6 months of age. It is especially important to do this before feedings. A decongestant, however, should not be prescribed for J.K. because of her age and the potential for adverse effects. If J.K. were older and a topical nasal decongestant was needed, phenylephrine would be preferred over oxymetazoline and xylometazoline because of its lesser association with toxicity (e.g., sedation, convulsions, insomnia, coma) in children younger than 6 years of age.[24,25] Neither antihistamines, antitussives, nor guaifenesin should be recommended for J.K. as there is no evidence of their efficacy and unintentional overdoses are common in this age group. Antihistamines are not effective for rhinorrhea caused by the common cold and should not be recommended. Antitussives are likely not effective and should not be used if the child's cough is productive. Expectorants, such as guaifenesin, also are not effective, and evidence is insufficient to support the use of vitamin C, zinc, or echinacea in children for treatment or prevention of the common cold.

Several hundred over-the-counter medications for upper respiratory symptoms are available, and about 95 million units of these products are sold each year in the United States. Nevertheless, the safety and effectiveness of these cough and cold medications in children have yet to be proved.[26] The Centers for Disease Control and Prevention (CDC) reported that 1,519 children younger than 2 years of age were admitted to emergency departments in 2004 to 2005 because of overdoses and other problems associated with cough and cold medicines. Furthermore, according to the US Food and Drug Administration (FDA), 54 deaths in children were linked to the use of decongestants (e.g., pseudoephedrine, phenylephrine, ephedrine) and 69 deaths to antihistamines (e.g., diphenhydramine, brompheniramine, chlorpheniramine) from 1969 to September 13, 2006. Most of these deaths occurred in children younger than 2 years of age, and some of the fatalities occurred in children who received overdoses that might have been the result of inadvertent administration of multiple medications containing the same ingredient.

An FDA advisory committee in 2007 voted to recommend that over-the-counter cold and cough medications not be used in children younger than 6 years of age. In 2008, the Consumer Healthcare Products Association announced that many manufacturers would voluntarily modify their labels to exclude recommendations for children younger than 4 years of age.[26] Owing to reports of toxicity and death related to over-the-counter cough and cold products, the CDC has recommended that caregivers avoid giving these products to children younger than 2 years of age unless advised by a clinician.[27] If deemed necessary by a physician for older children, nonprescription cough and cold medications containing single ingredients should be selected to minimize the potential for adverse effects and administration of multiple products with similar ingredients. Of note, parents often misunderstand labeling of over-the-counter products, placing the child at risk for dosing errors.[28] It is critical that health care providers educate caregivers on the proper use and administration of these medications to children. Treatment of J.K.'s symptoms should include the use of a cool-mist humidifier in the room and saline nasal drops followed by suctioning before feedings.

Constipation

Chronic constipation is defined as delay or difficulty in stooling for at least 2 weeks' duration.[29] It accounts for 3% of annual visits to pediatrician offices, and up to a quarter of referrals to gastroenterologists.[30] Beyond the neonatal period, constipation is most commonly idiopathic or functional and may be related to a diet low in fiber, lack of time or routine for toileting, or passage of a painful stool resulting in a fear of defecating. Stool retention over time may result in encopresis (involuntary fecal soiling). Other causes of constipation include anatomic (fissures), neurogenic (Hirschsprung disease), hypotonic (cerebral palsy), and endocrine (cystic fibrosis, hypothyroidism) disorders.[30] Medications such as opioids, antacids, and anticonvulsants, among others, can also contribute to constipation. It is important that constipation be managed appropriately as it can have negative effects on growth and development, has been linked to gastrointestinal distress, and adversely impacts quality of life.[30] In addition, constipation in childhood can remain a problem into adulthood.[31]

CLINICAL PRESENTATION AND TREATMENT

CASE 99-6

QUESTION 1: R.J., a 2-year-old, 15-kg boy, has had abdominal pain for several weeks. On average he has one stool weekly, and he cries each time because of pain. R.J. eats regular table food and has 2 glasses of whole milk each day. After obtaining a thorough history and performing a physical examination, the physician determines that R.J. has functional constipation. What treatment measures are appropriate to relieve and prevent R.J.'s constipation?

Before maintenance therapy can be initiated, disimpaction of the patient is necessary. Although no controlled studies compare efficacy of the oral and rectal routes, oral therapy (mineral oil, polyethylene glycol, bisacodyl) is preferred because it is less invasive and might achieve better adherence than rectal therapy (phosphate soda enemas, mineral oil enemas, glycerin suppositories in infants, bisacodyl suppositories in older children).[30] After disimpaction, a combination of behavioral, dietary, and medication therapies should be initiated to promote regular stool production and prevent reimpaction. Dietary interventions include adequate fluid and fiber intake. The impact of cow's milk on constipation is not known with certainty. Some data suggest no link,[30] but more recent literature hints at causation.[31,32] This needs to be confirmed with a prospective trial. Medications (e.g., polyethylene glycol 3350, mineral oil, lactulose, sorbitol) should be titrated to produce one to two soft stools daily, and stimulant laxatives might be needed intermittently. Although no clear recommendation for one maintenance medication has been given over others, recent data suggest that polyethylene glycol may be the most effective and best tolerated in children.[33–37] The recommended dosing of medications for treatment of constipation is listed in Table 99-1. Appropriate initial therapy for R.J. could include eliminating or limiting milk intake, and polyethylene glycol 0.5 to 1.5 g/kg/day (7.5–15 g). Practically, this would be half to one 17-g packet administered daily in 4 to 8 ounces of water or other beverage.

Vomiting and Diarrhea

Vomiting and diarrhea, two commonly encountered complaints in pediatric practice, usually are self-limiting, but severe cases can result in serious complications (e.g., dehydration, metabolic disturbances, and even death). Infants and young children are particularly susceptible to more severe complications.

PATHOGENESIS AND PRESENTATION OF VOMITING

Vomiting or emesis is defined as forceful expulsion of gastrointestinal (GI) contents through the mouth or nose; nonforceful expulsion of GI contents is considered regurgitation. In newborns, regurgitation of small amounts of breast milk or formula after feeding, especially when burping, is common. In most cases, regurgitation usually resolves by 1 to 2 years of age and rarely causes a problem.[38] Extensive evaluation of regurgitation is not needed in a child who is growing well. Other causes of vomiting during the newborn period include pyloric stenosis, gastroesophageal reflux, overfeeding, food intolerance, and GI obstruction. Beyond the neonatal period, the most common cause of vomiting is infection. Vomiting in infants and children also can be caused by central nervous system (CNS) disease (e.g., intracranial tumors), metabolic disease (e.g., urea cycle disorder), inflammatory bowel disease, and ulcers. Conditions causing emesis in older infants and children range from viral gastroenteritis to

TABLE 99-1
Medications for the Treatment of Constipation[29]

Medication	Initial Dosage	Comments
Osmotic Agents		
Polyethylene glycol	0.5–1.5 g/kg/day	0.5 g/kg initial dose; titrate to effect; do not exceed 17 g/day
Lactulose	1–3 mL/kg/day once or twice daily	
Sorbitol	1–3 mL/kg/day once or twice daily	Less expensive than lactulose
Barley malt extract	2–10 mL/240 mL of milk or juice daily	Useful for infants drinking from a bottle
Magnesium hydroxide	1–3 mL/kg/day using 400 mg/5 mL	Infants are at risk for hypermagnesemia
Phosphate enema	≥2 years of age: 6 mL/kg up to 135 mL	Electrolyte abnormalities more common in children with renal failure or Hirschprung disease. Avoid in children <2 years.
Lubricant		
Mineral oil	>1 year of age: Disimpaction: 15–30 mL/y of age up to 240 mL daily Maintenance: 1–3 mL/kg/day	Better tolerated if chilled. Avoid in children <1 year. Lipoid pneumonia may occur if aspirated.
Stimulants		
Senna	2–6 years of age: 2.5–7.5 mL/day 6–12 years of age: 5–15 mL/day	Not recommended for chronic use
Bisacodyl	≥2 years old: 0.5–1 suppository or 1–3 tablets per dose	Not recommended for chronic use
Glycerin suppositories	1 suppository per dose	Preferred stimulant for children <2 years of age

TABLE 99-2
Causes of Vomiting in Infants and Children[39]

Causes	Other Signs and Symptoms
Drug Induced	
Cancer chemotherapy	Nausea
Narcotics	
Theophylline or aminophylline	
Antibiotics	
Alcohol	
Anesthetics	
Toxic ingestion	
Metabolic or Endocrine Disorders	Alteration in behavior
Infectious Diseases	Fever
Otitis media	Symptoms of otitis media
Meningitis	Stiff neck, toxic appearance
Appendicitis	Abdominal pain
Urinary tract infection or pyelonephritis	Dysuria, frequency, and urgency in older children
Viral or bacterial gastroenteritis	Diarrhea
Mechanical Obstruction	
Bowel obstruction	Abdominal distension, green emesis
Pyloric stenosis	Projectile nonbilious vomiting Abdominal pain
Inflammatory	
Pancreatitis	
Inflammatory bowel	Diarrhea
Peptic ulcer disease	Black or red vomitus
Psychologic	
Chemotherapy	
Bulimia	
Miscellaneous	
Gastroesophageal reflux	Usually self-limited; indications for evaluation include recurrent pneumonia, poor growth, gastrointestinal blood loss, dysphagia, or heartburn
Increased intracranial pressure	Mental status alteration
Head injury or trauma	History of trauma, mental status changes
Food or milk intolerance	Irritability, loose stool, blood in stool, or allergy

more severe illnesses, such as bowel obstruction or head injury, which require immediate medical attention (Table 99-2).[39] Acute vomiting also can result from medication or toxic ingestions. In teenagers, migraine, pregnancy, and psychological disorders (e.g., bulimia) have been associated with vomiting.

PATHOGENESIS AND PRESENTATION OF DIARRHEA

Diarrhea refers to an increase in frequency, volume, or liquidity of stool when compared with normal bowel movements. In developing countries, diarrhea is a common cause of death in children younger than 5 years of age. In the United States, gastroenteritis accounts for approximately 1 to 2 million physician visits, more than 200,000 hospitalizations, and about 300 deaths each year.[40]

Acute diarrhea in infants and children generally is abrupt in onset, lasts a few days, and usually is caused by viruses. (See Chapter 66, Infectious Diarrhea for infectious diarrhea of other origins.) Diarrhea is considered chronic if it is longer than 2 weeks in duration, and it can be caused by malabsorption, inflammatory disease, infection, alteration of intestinal flora, milk or protein intolerance, and drugs, among other causes.[41]

Infants and children are at high risk for morbidity and mortality secondary to diarrhea for several reasons. Dehydration can occur easily as acute net intestinal fluid losses are relatively much greater in young children than in adults. This may result from inefficient transport systems in the developing intestine. In addition, the percent of total body water in children is higher than in adults; thus, they are more susceptible to body fluid shifts. Total body water changes from 80% of total body weight in premature infants to 70% in term infants and 60% in adults. Finally, the renal capacity to compensate for fluid and electrolyte imbalances in the infant is limited compared with that of adults.[42]

VIRAL GASTROENTERITIS

CASE 99-7

QUESTION 1: J.R., a 15-month-old male 10-kg infant, had one loose stool and began vomiting this morning but has not had a fever. On questioning, you discover that many children attending day care with J.R. are experiencing vomiting, diarrhea, and low-grade temperatures. How should J.R.'s vomiting be treated?

Routine use of antiemetics for acute vomiting in children is not recommended because masking of symptoms may delay diagnosis of a treatable illness. In addition, the safety and efficacy of the antiemetics, including metoclopramide, promethazine, trimethobenzamide, and dimenhydrinate, have not been demonstrated.[43] In particular, promethazine is contraindicated in children younger than 2 years of age because of the risk of fatal respiratory depression. Ondansetron does decrease vomiting, and it increases oral intake and decreases the need for intravenous (IV) rehydration; however, the utility of ondansetron in gastroenteritis needs consideration because this effect may not be sustained and the drug has not been shown to consistently decrease hospital admission.[44–46]

Parents should be taught the signs and symptoms of gastroenteritis and vomiting that are sufficiently serious to warrant medical attention. The child's primary-care provider should be contacted if the child is toxic appearing, exhibits unusual behavior or signs of an ear infection, experiences abdominal pain or distension, or has red or black vomitus or stool, or if there is a history or suspicion of toxic ingestion or head trauma. Medical evaluation also is necessary for infants younger than 6 months of age, when persistent vomiting or high-volume diarrhea is present, or when chronic medical conditions or prematurity are involved. Because fever can accompany vomiting in viral gastroenteritis, any fever occurring in a neonate warrants medical attention, as well as in older infants and children when fever becomes prolonged or changes in pattern.

When communicating with a health care provider about a vomiting child, it is helpful if the parents have knowledge of the child's fluid intake, and the frequency and volume of vomiting and urination. The amount of vomitus can be estimated by the following rule of thumb: one tablespoon makes a spot 4 inches wide and a quarter-cup makes a spot approximately 8 inches wide.

Vomiting associated with gastroenteritis usually resolves in 24 to 48 hours. Infants are particularly susceptible to the development of fluid and electrolyte abnormalities; therefore, fluid and electrolyte replacements are critically important.

J.R., who is early in the course of gastroenteritis, must receive sufficient fluids to prevent dehydration. Oral hydration therapy can be successful when given in small volumes, even if J.R. is still vomiting. For example, 5 to 10 mL can be administered every 5 to 10 minutes, and the volume can be gradually increased as tolerated. Volumes equal to estimated fluid deficit (usually 50–100 mL/kg) should be given over the course of 2 to 4 hours. For each diarrheal stool, an additional 10 mL/kg (150 mL) of oral electrolyte solution should be given. If diarrhea or vomiting recurs, 10 mL/kg and 2 mL/kg (30 mL) of an oral rehydration solution (ORS) can be administered for each stool or emesis, respectively.[46] J.R.'s clinical condition should continue to be monitored by his caregiver. If stool output exceeds 10 mL/kg/hour, ORS might not be sufficient, and the health care provider should again be contacted. ORS should only be abandoned in children with intractable vomiting, loss of consciousness, or bowel obstruction, or if the child is in shock. Most infants will tolerate oral hydration when small amounts are given frequently. Using a spoon or oral syringe to administer the fluid may be more effective than using a nipple or cup. As dehydration is corrected, the frequency of vomiting typically decreases. Once rehydration has been achieved, fluids other than ORS and a diet appropriate for age may be started.[46] Breast milk or formula should be given as tolerated.

Assessment of Dehydration

CASE 99-7, QUESTION 2: On the second day of illness, J.R. develops a mild fever and diarrhea that has increased in frequency and water content. How can the severity of J.R.'s diarrhea be assessed?

To determine the severity of dehydration and whether hospitalization may be needed, consider the following questions:

1. Does the child have any of the following signs and symptoms of severe dehydration: deeply sunken eyes, parched mucous membranes, significantly prolonged capillary refill (this can be assessed by applying enough pressure on the nail bed to cause blanching; refill time of approximately 1 second is normal); cool, mottled extremities; crying without tears; oliguria or anuria; weak or thready pulses; lethargy; poor oral intake; deep respirations; history of seizures or convulsions; a fever without perspiration; or thirst?
2. Are a large number of copious stools still being produced (>10 mL/kg/hour)? Is bowel obstruction a possibility?
3. Is there a risk of dehydration from inadequate monitoring, or is the parent unable to care for the child? Specific inquiries should be made about the number and consistency of stools in children with diarrhea.

Estimating the degree of dehydration is particularly valuable in assessing the patient with diarrhea: weight loss is a good criterion. A 3% to 9% weight loss is considered mild to moderate dehydration, whereas more than 9% is considered severe dehydration.[43] (See Chapter 98, Pediatric Fluid, Electrolytes, and Nutrition, for information about IV replacement therapy in children with 10% or more dehydration.)

Oral Replacement Therapy

CASE 99-7, QUESTION 3: J.R. was evaluated by his pediatrician and was not considered to be sufficiently dehydrated to warrant hospitalization. How might J.R.'s fluids and electrolytes be managed on an outpatient basis?

The goal of J.R.'s treatment should be focused on the prevention of dehydration and the restoration and maintenance of adequate fluid and electrolyte balance. Mild to moderate diarrhea without dehydration generally is managed at home by continued age-appropriate feeding. Fluid losses in stools can be replaced with a glucose-containing ORS. Glucose provides calories and enhances salt and water absorption in the small intestine through mechanisms that usually are unimpaired in many toxin-induced diarrheas. Parents formerly were instructed to prepare salt and sugar solutions at home; however, frequent errors in the preparation of these solutions resulted in exacerbation of problems with fluid and electrolyte balance. Oral glucose–electrolyte formulations (e.g., Pedialyte) designed to enhance glucose and sodium absorption are commercially available and should be used in infants and young children. Gatorade is an alternative for older children, but carbonated beverages and fruit juices do not contain sufficient sodium to replace diarrheal losses. Rehydration and maintenance solutions can be made more palatable with sugar-free flavorings (e.g., Kool-Aid, Crystal Lite).

The World Health Organization (WHO) formerly promoted use of an oral replacement solution (WHO formula) containing sodium (90 mEq/L), potassium (20 mEq/L), bicarbonate (30 mEq/L), chloride (80 mEq/L), and 2% glucose for the widespread management of acute diarrhea in third-world countries. The WHO formula, which had a 90% successful rehydration rate for the management of diarrhea, contained a high concentration of sodium because secretory diarrhea (e.g., cholera) is associated with substantial loss of sodium. Malabsorptive diarrheas, such as those associated with rotavirus infections, are associated with much lower loss of sodium (<40 mEq/L). Although commercially available ORS contain less sodium than the WHO formulation, these preparations were equally effective as the WHO formula, even when used to treat the high-sodium losses associated with cholera. Furthermore, these lower sodium-containing formulations were associated with less vomiting, lower stool output, and reduced need for IV infusions in non–cholera-associated gastroenteritis. As a result, the WHO, in 2002, promoted a new formulation that consists of 75 mEq/L sodium and a total osmolarity of 245 mOsm/L.[43,45] Glucose is added to oral electrolyte solutions to enhance glucose-coupled sodium transport; however, concentrations greater than 3% can impair sodium absorption because the glucose-coupled sodium transport system becomes saturated at this concentration and any additional glucose acts as an osmotically active solute in the bowel lumen. The electrolyte content of commonly used ORS is provided in Table 99-3. Assuming J.R.'s fluid deficit is 50 to 100 mL/kg, he should receive 750 to 1,500 mL of ORS in the course of approximately 4 hours. In addition, he should receive an extra 150 mL for each diarrheal stool and 30 mL for each emesis that occurs. If stool output continues at a pace that cannot be matched with oral replacement, or signs and symptoms of severe dehydration occur, J.R. should be referred to his pediatrician again.

REINSTITUTION OF ORAL FEEDINGS

Previously, feeding during an episode of viral gastroenteritis has been delayed because of the malabsorption that typically occurs during and after these bouts. The malabsorption, however, is self-limiting, and substantial amounts of carbohydrate, protein, and fat can still be absorbed. The reinstitution of a regular diet, therefore, should not adversely affect mild diarrhea and can be beneficial.[46] Parents are encouraged to continue feeding their children using age-appropriate diet while avoiding simple sugars, which can increase osmotic load and worsen diarrhea. Continuation of oral feeding, despite diarrheal episodes, minimizes the development of protein and energy deficits; facilitates the maintenance and repair of intestinal mucosa; promotes recovery of brush border membrane disaccharidases; decreases the duration of illness; and improves nutritional status.[45,46] Although lactose

TABLE 99-3
Oral Electrolyte Solutions[43]

	Compositions			
Solution	Sodium (mmol/L)	Potassium (mmol/L)	Carbohydrate (mmol/L)	Osmolarity
Rehydration				
Rehydralyte	75	20	140	305
WHO formula (1975)	90	20	111	311
WHO formula (2002)	75	20	75	245
Maintenance				
Enfalyte	50	25	167	200
Pedialyte	45	20	139	250
Home Remedies				
Apple juice	0.4	44	667	730
Gatorade	20	3	255	330
Ginger ale	3	1	500	540
Chicken broth	250	8		500
Cola	1.6		622	730

WHO, World Health Organization.

intolerance can occur with viral gastroenteritis, most children with mild diarrhea can tolerate full-strength animal milk, animal milk–based formula, and breast milk. If the child becomes lactose intolerant during this illness, a lactosefree formula may be substituted for 2 to 6 weeks until GI lactase production returns to normal. Specific diets are often recommended during diarrhea (e.g., BRAT [bananas, rice, applesauce, toast]). Although these diets occasionally can be useful, the nutritional value of these foods is relatively low, and they do not provide optimal nutrition compared with complete diets with fats and proteins.[45,46] Once J.R. has been adequately rehydrated, he may resume his normal diet. However, the caregivers must take care to avoid juices and other foods with simple sugars, which may worsen diarrhea.

Drug Therapy

Medications play a minor role in the treatment of acute infantile diarrhea because most episodes are self-limiting. Antibiotics are recommended when systemic bacteremia is suspected, when immune defenses are compromised, when a persistent enteric infection is sensitive to antibiotics, or when *Shigella, Campylobacter, Vibrio cholerae, Clostridium difficile,* and certain *Escherichia coli* strains are isolated.[46,47] In general, antidiarrheal preparations are not recommended for infants or children because they have little effect on acute diarrhea, are associated with side effects, and direct attention away from the use of oral hydration therapy.[45,46] Drugs such as loperamide that alter GI motility should be avoided, especially in children with high fever, toxemia, or bloody mucoid stools, because they may worsen the clinical course of the bacterial infection. Bismuth subsalicylate preparations, which possess antisecretory and antimicrobial effects, have not been shown to provide clinical benefit and are not recommended.[45] Adsorbents, such as kaolin-pectin or attapulgite, adsorb bacterial toxins and water and lessen the symptoms of diarrhea by producing more formed stools, but there is no evidence of effectiveness and they are not recommended.[45] Zinc supplementation (10–20 mg for 10–14 days) has been recommended by the WHO for the treatment and prevention of diarrheal disease in children in developing countries; however, its mechanism of action, best method of administration, and efficacy in different populations are not yet well understood.[43,48]

Probiotics, live microbial products containing species of *Lactobacillus, Bifidobacterium, Saccharomyces,* and *Streptococcus,* can improve the balance of intestinal flora and diminish the effect of enteric pathogens. These microbes are thought to exert their beneficial effects through various mechanisms including producing antibacterial chemicals, competing with enteric pathogens, inhibiting the adhesive capabilities of pathogens, altering toxins or toxin receptors, and upregulating interleukin-mediated T-cell response.[48,49] Probiotics are most useful in infectious gastroenteritis when used early in the course of disease. Lactobacilli are the most well studied species and have been the most consistently effective in clinical trials. It appears that efficacy of the different species may depend on the specific strain, the dose, and the timing of administration, although it is generally accepted that dosage forms with at least 10^6 to 10^9 colony-forming units and above are required.[45,48] The manufacture of probiotics is not regulated by the FDA; therefore, the organism count per dose might be based on the number present at the time of production and not at time of expiration, and the labeling might incorrectly identify the species of organism. Probiotics are not recommended for use in immunocompromised individuals because systemic infections after use of these products have been reported.[43] For J.R., a *Lactobacillus* preparation administered for 5 days may provide some modest clinical benefit, although the benefit is most pronounced in rotavirus diarrhea, which has not been documented in his case.

GASTROESOPHAGEAL REFLUX

Gastroesophageal reflux (GER) is a common disorder, with 50% to 67% of infants experiencing recurrent vomiting and regurgitation during the first 4 months of life.[50] Most reflux in infants is believed to be caused by transient relaxations of the lower esophageal sphincter (LES). Infants also might be predisposed to reflux because of their body positioning (e.g., slumped over in a car seat or lying supine); their consumption of a liquid feeding that exceeds the volume capacity of the stomach; and in premature infants, a decrease in peristaltic activity.[51] Infants and young children also might have undiagnosed underlying conditions that predispose them to reflux (e.g., neurologic disorders, hiatal hernia, hypertrophic pyloric stenosis, cow's milk protein allergy).[52] Of cases of reflux in infants, 80% are benign and resolve by 18 months of age,[53] and reflux in older children resolves in a timeframe similar to that of adults. If untreated, GER can result in esophageal strictures, GI hemorrhage, or chronic respiratory disease from the aspiration of GI contents. Studies evaluating the relationship between GER disease (GERD) and asthma or *Helicobacter pylori* have shown mixed results.[54–57]

Clinical Presentation

In infants, the vomiting and regurgitation of GER occur frequently, and other symptoms often are nonspecific (e.g., failure to thrive [FTT], recurrent pneumonia, apnea, dysphagia, reactive airway disease, apparent life-threatening events [ALTE], hematemesis, anemia).[58] A thorough diagnostic workup generally is not necessary in a healthy infant with functional GER presenting as recurrent vomiting; empiric drug therapy can be initiated after the diagnosis is made based on clinical findings and after other causes of vomiting have been eliminated.[58] Further diagnostic evaluations, however, are indicated for infants and children presenting with additional symptoms of GERD (e.g., FTT, irritability, ALTE, respiratory difficulties).[53] Esophageal pH monitoring, endoscopy, and biopsy can be considered, although results of pH monitoring will not consistently correlate with the severity of symptoms in infants.[58] Multichannel intraluminal impedance measurements, which detect the extent of movements of stomach contents to the esophagus, can be used to detect nonacid reflux as well as acid reflux.[58] It is not clear whether the combination of pH and impedance measurements will provide more useful data for diagnosis and monitoring response to therapy, although recent data suggest efficacy.[59] New diagnostic tools such as a pH capsule inserted during endoscopy could provide another option for safe monitoring of reflux in children.[60] Further evaluations (e.g., barium contrast radiography) might be necessary if anatomic abnormalities (e.g., strictures, pyloric stenosis) are suspected.[58]

Treatment

Because uncomplicated GER usually resolves spontaneously in infants, therapy should focus on providing symptom relief and maintaining normal growth.[53] The goals of therapy are to lessen symptoms, heal esophagitis, and prevent complications in infants and children with pathologic GER so that surgery can be avoided.[53] Infants and young children with underlying neurologic problems (e.g., cerebral palsy) are unlikely to have spontaneous resolutions of GER and frequently require aggressive antireflux therapies and surgical intervention.

POSITIONAL AND DIETARY MEASURES

CASE 99-8

QUESTION 1: S.B., a 3-month-old, 6-kg, 60-cm breastfed male infant, has a 2-week history of regurgitation after each feeding. The pediatrician noted that S.B. had not gained weight since his last visit 1 month earlier. The presumptive diagnosis is FTT secondary to GER, and S.B. was referred to a pediatric gastroenterologist. The gastroenterologist admitted S.B. to the hospital and confirmed the diagnosis using 24-hour pH monitoring. How should S.B. be treated initially?

S.B. can be treated conservatively because he does not present with life-threatening complications.[58] First, caregiver feedings should be observed to rule out regurgitation caused either by overfeeding or by inappropriate feeding techniques. Sometimes infants with milk protein allergies can have a similar clinical presentation; therefore, a change to a soy protein formula or hypoallergenic formula should be tried.[58] Interventions to modify an infant's body positioning or to modify infant feedings with milk thickeners are not proven to be effective, but are reasonable to undertake.[61,62] Maintaining S.B. at a 60-degree angle during the day while sitting and at a 30-degree position at night should be implemented in an effort to promote clearance of acid from the esophagus and to minimize reflux after meals. Milk thickeners (most commonly rice cereal in the United States) and more frequent, smaller feedings also are worthwhile interventions, although thickened formula could lead to increased coughing during feeding. Mild cases of GER often can be treated successfully by dietary measures alone, as well as by propping infants in an upright position during, and 1 hour after, feedings. Although the placement of infants in a face-down prone position during sleep can reduce reflux, the greater risk of sudden infant death syndrome (SIDS) in infants younger than 12 months of age outweighs the benefits of such positioning.[58] Older children and adolescents should follow the recommended dietary guidelines (i.e., avoidance of caffeine, chocolate, spicy foods) for adults.

DRUG THERAPY

The efficacy of pharmacologic therapy in altering the course of uncomplicated GER in infants has not been proven.[58] In infants or children who present with nonspecific symptoms or complications, such as S.B., acid-suppression therapy or prokinetic therapy is warranted even in the absence of documented esophagitis.[58] When esophagitis is present, acid suppression is always recommended to aid in the healing process; however, these agents alone do not rectify the causes of the GER.[58] The various agents to treat infant GER are listed in Table 99-4.[63–74]

ACID-SUPPRESSANT AGENTS

Antacids

Chronic antacid therapy is generally not recommended for the treatment of GER in infants and young children because infants treated with aluminum-containing antacids can accumulate sufficient aluminum to cause osteopenia and neurotoxicity.[58,63,73] In addition, information on other antacids in infants is limited; nevertheless, antacids can provide short-term relief of symptoms in older children and adults.

Proton-Pump Inhibitors

Proton-pump inhibitors (PPI) are superior to histamine-2 receptor antagonists (H_2RA) in relieving symptoms and in promoting healing of significant esophagitis from GER in infants, young children, and adults.[58,74,75] PPI control both basal and meal-stimulated acid secretion, which may in part explain their superior efficacy. The incidence of adverse effects in children from PPI is similar to that reported in adults.[65,76] Despite concerns about the long-term use of PPI, untoward effects have not been observed from their use for up to 11 years.[77] In children, increased metabolism and decreased bioavailability necessitate larger milligram per kilogram doses to maintain acid suppression than adults; thus, titration of dose to response is necessary, particularly for treatment of esophageal erosions.[61,78] Although most clinicians dose PPI once a day, multiple, divided daily doses can prevent acid breakthrough and better promote healing.[74] Omeprazole, lansoprazole, and esomeprazole are available in extended-release capsules, which can be separated, opened, and sprinkled on soft foods. Omeprazole and esomeprazole are also available as granules for an oral suspension. Suspension formulations for both omeprazole and lansoprazole have been extemporaneously compounded and evaluated for stability. Esomeprazole has also been recently approved for use in children with GERD aged 1 to 11 years and has been studied and reviewed extensively.[75,79,80]

Histamine$_2$-Receptor Antagonists

Histamine$_2$-receptor antagonists (H_2RA) reduce histamine-stimulated acid secretion, but have limited effects on acid secretion by other chemical mediators and other stimuli. In randomized, controlled trials, H_2RA in infants and children relieved symptoms and facilitated the healing of esophageal tissue.[66,67] Tolerance to the acid-suppressant activity of H_2RA for a relatively short time ($<$30 days), however,[68,69] can limit their use for long-term treatment of esophagitis. Oral liquid formulations are available for most H_2RA. Ranitidine also is available in an effervescent tablet.

PROKINETIC AGENTS

Metoclopramide, a dopamine antagonist with cholinergic and serotonergic effects, accelerates gastric emptying, increases LES pressure, enhances esophageal clearance, and accelerates transit time in the small bowel; however, its effects on vomiting and esophageal pH in children with GER has been equivocal.[70,71] Additionally, metoclopramide has been associated with

TABLE 99-4
Oral Drugs Used to Treat Gastroesophageal Reflux in Infants[58,63–72]

Agent	Mode of Action	Oral Dosage
Acid-Suppressing Agents		
Antacids (aluminum or magnesium hydroxide)	Neutralizes acid	0.5–1.0 mL/kg/dose before and after feeding (maximum, 15 mL/dose)
Proton-Pump Inhibitors	Decrease acid secretion via inhibition of gastric hydrogen-potassium adenosine triphosphatase	
Omeprazole		5 mg daily (5 kg–<10 kg) 10 mg daily (10 kg–≤20 kg) 20 mg daily (>20 kg) 1 mg/kg daily or twice daily (alternate dosing)
Esomeprazole		10–20 mg daily (1–11 years) >1 mg/kg/day has not been evaluated
Lansoprazole		15 mg daily (weight ≤30 kg) 30 mg daily (weight >30 kg)
Pantoprazole		20 mg daily (0.5–1 mg/kg/day)
H_2 Receptor Antagonists	Blocks H_2-receptors; ↓ acid secretion	
Cimetidine		40 mg/kg/day divided QID
Famotidine		0.5–1 mg/kg/day divided daily or BID
Nizatidine		5–10 mg/kg/day divided BID
Ranitidine		4–10 mg/kg/day divided TID or QID
Prokinetic Agents		
Bethanechol	Cholinergic agent; stimulates peristalsis ↑ ↑ LES pressure; ↑ gastric emptying; ↑ colonic motility ↑ Gastric emptying; ↑ LES pressure; augments esophageal clearance	0.1–0.2 mg/kg/dose QID given 30–60 minutes before feeding and HS
Metoclopramide	Dopamine antagonist	0.1–0.2 mg/kg/dose QID given 30 minutes before feeding and HS
Erythromycin	Motilin agonist stimulates smooth muscle contraction	1–3 mg/kg/dose QID
Surface-Active Agents		
Sucralfate	Forms paste and adheres to damaged esophageal mucosa	40–80 mg/kg/day divided QID

BID, twice daily; HS, at bedtime; LES, lower esophageal sphincter; QID, four times daily; TID, three times daily.

significant CNS (i.e., restlessness, drowsiness, extrapyramidal) effects and rare reports of gynecomastia and galactorrhea. Erythromycin increases GI motility by increasing smooth muscle contractions through its motilin agonistic activity, and it has been used as a prokinetic agent for GER in children when acid suppression therapy alone was ineffective.[81] Erythromycin-induced development of infantile hypertrophic pyloric stenosis, arrhythmias, and potential changes in bacterial resistance patterns, however, limit its use for GER. The cholinergic agonist, bethanechol, reportedly reduces vomiting episodes in infants with GER[40,58,82]; however, its role in treating GER in infants is limited because of its potential to induce bronchospasm and to stimulate gastric acid secretion. The lack of a suitable commercially available formulation of bethanechol for young infants necessitates its extemporaneous compounding. Baclofen, which decreases transient LES relaxations through its γ-aminobutyric acid (GABA) agonist actions, could be a future therapeutic option for GER, pending further study.[83] Generally, prokinetic agents only are marginally effective in the management of GER.

SURFACE-ACTIVE AGENTS

Sucralfate was equally effective as cimetidine for use in esophagitis[84]; however, its use for GER is more limited because of concern about the adverse effects of aluminum-containing products in infants.

CASE 99-8, QUESTION 2: Four weeks after instituting positional and dietary measures, S.B. continues to vomit and still has not been gaining weight. On physical examination, the gastroenterologist notes bilateral wheezes; endoscopy rules out esophagitis. What would be the next step of therapy?

The treatment of S.B. can include acid-suppression therapy and a prokinetic agent. Acid-suppression therapy in children who have complications from GER can be implemented by a step-up approach in which treatment is initiated with an H_2RA followed by a PPI if no improvement is noted, or through a step-down approach involving a PPI followed by an H_2RA for maintenance therapy. However, initial therapy with PPI is preferred,[58] and S.B. may be treated with omeprazole 5 mg daily. Granules for suspension may be mixed in 10 mL of water and administered orally.

The effectiveness of acid suppression for managing symptoms of GER in children is not as well documented as it is for healing esophagitis; however, acid suppression is believed to play a useful role for symptom control, particularly for managing the respiratory symptoms.[58] If additional symptom control is desired, metoclopramide 0.6 mg (0.1 mg/kg/dose) four times daily, 30 minutes before meals and at bedtime can be initiated for S.B. This dose can be adjusted based on his response, with close observation for adverse effects. Treatment should be continued for at least 3 to 4 months, although the optimal duration of therapy is unknown. If S.B. requires additional drug therapy to control symptoms of GER beyond 18 months to 2 years of age, surgery should be considered because GER is unlikely to resolve spontaneously after this age.[85] Surgery might be considered earlier if S.B. fails medical therapy or if he develops an esophageal stricture, apnea, or recurrent respiratory disease.[58]

Acute Otitis Media

Acute otitis media (AOM) is the most common reason for antimicrobial use in children, and is associated with expenditures of $350 per episode and, cumulatively, almost $3 billion annually.[86] Acute otitis media is most common from the ages of 3 months to 3 years, although the highest incidence occurs between 6 and 9 months of age. Most children will have had at least one episode by the time they reach 1 year of age.[87] Incidence is higher in the winter months, concurrent with viral upper respiratory illnesses. Several risk factors for AOM have been identified and include age younger than 2 years, early colonization of pathogens and onset of AOM, day-care attendance, bottle propping, cleft palate, immune compromise, and Down syndrome. Other factors such as smoke exposure, bottle feeding, pacifier use, and ethnicity have not been consistently found to increase risk of AOM.[88,89]

Eustachian tube dysfunction, either from intermittent causes such as upper respiratory infections or permanent causes such as cleft palate, is the primary condition required for the development of AOM. This results in a defect in the eustachian tube's ability to equilibrate middle ear pressure. Thus nasopharyngeal contents, including bacteria, may be aspirated into the middle ear. This process is more likely in infants and young children who have shorter, flatter eustachian tubes.[88] Changes in pressure can also cause increased vascular permeability, resulting in an effusion. Viral infections contribute by enhancing bacterial transfer from the nasopharynx and adherence to the middle ear.[88]

Streptococcus pneumoniae, nontypeable *Haemophilus influenzae,* and *Moraxella catarrhalis* colonize the nasopharynx early in childhood, and thus are the most common pathogens causing AOM.[87] Historically, these pathogens have been implicated in 25% to 50%, 15% to 30%, and 3% to 20% of cases of AOM, respectively.[90] The pneumococcal conjugate vaccine (PCV7) has been shown to decrease the overall incidence of AOM, the recurrence of AOM, and the need for tympanostomy tube insertion.[86,87,89] However, administration of the PCV7 vaccine has resulted in important changes. Epidemiologic studies have found a decrease in the incidence of AOM caused by pneumococcus while at the same time noting an increase in episodes caused by *Haemophilus influenzae* and *Moraxella catarralis.*[86,87] Other studies have demonstrated an increase in the incidence of pneumococcal serotypes not found in the PCV7 vaccine,[86,91,92] as well as increased microbial resistance of these nonvaccine serotypes.[91] These studies were used to guide the development of a 13-valent pneumococcal conjugate vaccine, which was approved in 2010. The new PCV13 vaccine includes six of the serotypes that had been shown to produce more than 60% of non-PCV7 vaccine strain invasive infections. The 13-valent preparation has replaced PCV7,[93] although monitoring for further changes in the epidemiology of pneumococcal infections will be important.

CASE 99-9

QUESTION 1: C.D. is a 7-month-old, 8-kg infant who during the last 2 days has developed cough and rhinorrhea, became irritable and at times inconsolable, and now has a temperature of 102.4°F (39.1°C). Physical examination shows bulging, dark, yellow opaque tympanic membranes bilaterally. This is the first time he has had these symptoms. What signs and symptoms does C.D. exhibit that are consistent with acute otitis media, and how should AOM be diagnosed?

TABLE 99-5
Evidence of Middle Ear Effusion and Inflammation on Otoscopic Examination[90]

Middle Ear Effusion
Bulging tympanic membrane
Lack of tympanic membrane mobility
Presence of air-fluid level in middle ear
Otorrhea
Middle Ear Inflammation
Obvious erythema of tympanic membrane
Pain specific to the ear preventing normal activity and sleep

Very often, as in this patient case, otitis media is preceded by an upper respiratory tract infection. These viral infections often will produce otitis media with effusion (OME), which typically will cause no more than temporary mild hearing loss. If AOM develops, more signs and symptoms will usually arise. These symptoms can include otalgia (infants may pull on or rub the ears), fever, irritability, and otorrhea.[86,90] Unfortunately, aside from otorrhea, these symptoms are nonspecific and may be present in many children who do not have AOM. As a result, a definitive diagnosis may not be easily obtained with symptoms alone. Diagnosis should be confirmed on visualization of the middle ear.

In 2004, the American Academy of Pediatrics (AAP) and the American Academy of Family Physicians (AAFP) published guidelines on the diagnosis and management of acute otitis media that stated that a diagnosis of AOM requires acute symptom onset, middle ear effusion, and signs and symptoms of inflammation.[90] Pneumatic otoscopy should be used to confirm the presence of effusion. Middle ear effusion can be differentiated from AOM in that, whereas both present with bulging tympanic membranes, in AOM, the middle ear fluid is more often dark yellow or red.[88,90] Other diagnostic tools may be used. Tympanometry uses sound waves to measure the compliance of the tympanic membrane. In acoustic reflectometry, the absorption of sound waves by the tympanic membrane provides information about the middle ear in that an effusion will cause more sound to be reflected back than a normal ear.[88] Table 99-5 lists ways in which middle ear effusion and inflammation can present. C.D.'s fever and irritability along with fluid in the middle ear and bulging, dark yellow tympanic membranes are consistent with the diagnosis of acute otitis media.

CASE 99-9, QUESTION 2: How should C.D.'s otitis media be treated?

The 2004 AAP/AAFP recommendations provide for the option to observe without treatment or to treat with antibiotics, depending on the age of the patient, the certainty of the diagnosis, and severity of disease.[90] Severe illness consists of otalgia, irritability, fussiness, lethargy, less interest in eating, and a temperature of at least 39°C, whereas nonsevere illness is described by milder symptoms and fever less than 39°C. A certain diagnosis is made when all three criteria for AOM are present. Generally, infants 6 months of age and younger should receive antibiotic therapy in all cases. Infants and children 6 months to 2 years of age can be managed with observation for 48 to 72 hours in the case of an uncertain diagnosis and if illness is not severe. Children 2 years of age and older can be managed with observation even in the case of a certain diagnosis, although illness should be nonsevere.[90]

C.D. appears to have a certain diagnosis and severe disease based on his symptoms and a fever greater than 39°C, so antibiotic therapy is indicated. Despite pneumococcal penicillin resistance rates ranging from 30% to 70%, initial therapy in most children with nonsevere disease should still be amoxicillin at a dose of 80 to 90 mg/kg/day.[87,88] Amoxicillin is still effective against susceptible and intermediately resistant pneumococcus, it is affordable and palatable, and it has a narrow spectrum of activity.[87] However, because C.D. has severe disease, he should receive amoxicillin/clavulanate at a dose of 360 mg by mouth twice daily (90 mg/kg/day), using the ES or XR formulation. Oral cephalosporins, including cefdinir, cefuroxime, or cefpodoxime, are options in patients with a non–type I allergy to penicillin, and macrolides such as azithromycin or clarithromycin may be used in those with type I allergies to penicillin.

ONLINE CONTENT

For a narrated PowerPoint presentation on antimicrobial management of AOM, see http://thepoint.lww.com/AT10e.

It is important to recognize that although the oral cephalosporins generally provide good activity against *H. influenzae, M. catarrhalis,* and penicillin-susceptible *S. pneumoniae,* they are not effective against penicillin-nonsusceptible pneumococcal isolates.[94–98] Additionally, penicillin resistance does not necessarily confer resistance to amoxicillin.[99] Macrolides have also been shown to be less effective than amoxicillin/clavulanate.[100]

Whichever treatment course is taken in a patient (observation or antibiotic therapy with amoxicillin or amoxicillin/clavulanate), effectiveness is assessed for 48 to 72 hours. If the treatment is effective, the patient should defervesce, irritability should decrease, and normal activity should resume (e.g., eating, sleeping). If observation is ineffective, treatment with amoxicillin or amoxicillin/clavulanate is recommended. If amoxicillin or amoxicillin/clavulanate is ineffective for C.D., ceftriaxone 400 mg (50 mg/kg) intramuscularly for 1 or 3 days is recommended. Tympanocentesis may be useful if ceftriaxone fails, and clindamycin can be used if pneumococcus is strongly suspected or proven to be the pathogen.[96]

Two recent studies have been published that may provide strong support for the recommendation to treat all children with a certain diagnosis, regardless of age or severity.[101,102] Both trials compared amoxicillin/clavulanate with placebo in children with certain diagnoses, and in both trials patients receiving active drug saw a decrease in the duration of illness. The results of these trials may impact the new guidelines for the diagnosis and management of acute otitis media, which are currently under revision.

CASE 99-9, QUESTION 3: How should C.D.'s otalgia be managed?

Ear pain is a common feature of AOM, and it should be addressed regardless of the decision to use antibiotics or not. Acetaminophen 120 mg (15 mg/kg) or ibuprofen 80 mg (10 mg/kg) can provide adequate relief, and are first-line agents in the management of otalgia.[90] Topical agents such as benzocaine can provide benefit as well, particularly in older children. Home remedies such as the application of heat or cold may also be helpful.[90] For example, a washcloth can be soaked with very warm water, wrung out, and placed over the ear for comfort for 15 minutes several times per day.

Acute Pharyngitis

Acute pharyngitis is most common in children 5 to 15 years of age and is rare before 3 years of age. The etiology is typically viral, but bacteria such as group A streptococci (GAS, *Streptococcus pyogenes*), groups C and G streptococci, *Neisseria gonorrhoeae, Mycoplasma pneumoniae,* and *Chlamydia pneumoniae* may also cause pharyngitis in children.[103] The majority of attention is directed toward the detection and management of GAS infections as, untreated, they may lead to rheumatic fever, a complication progressing to permanent heart disease.

CASE 99-10

QUESTION 1: P.J., a 6-year-old boy weighing 23.4 kg, presents to the pediatrician's office complaining of fever, sore throat, and headache. His mother reports that he initially complained of sore throat about 12 hours ago. His temperature this morning was 102°F. He has had no other symptoms. He takes no medications and has no known drug allergies. Physical examination reveals erythematous tonsils and throat, as well as an enlarged anterior cervical lymph node. Are P.J.'s symptoms more consistent with GAS or viral pharyngitis?

Findings suggestive of GAS tonsillopharyngitis include sudden onset of throat pain, fever, headache, abdominal pain, nausea, vomiting, tonsillopharyngeal edema, enlarged anterior cervical lymph nodes, soft palate petechiae, and a scarlatiniform rash.[103] Symptoms that increase the likelihood of a viral cause include rhinorrhea, cough, conjunctivitis, and viral rash. P.J. is lacking associated symptoms that would suggest a viral cause and has more symptoms of GAS pharyngitis, but confirmatory testing is needed.

DIAGNOSIS

As clinical and physical findings are not definitive for GAS pharyngitis, confirmatory testing is important to determine the need for antibiotic therapy. A rapid antigen test is recommended and, if positive, treatment is initiated. If negative, a throat culture should also be obtained and treatment initiated if the culture grows GAS. Rheumatic fever can be effectively prevented if treatment is started within 9 days from the start of the illness.

TREATMENT

CASE 99-10, QUESTION 2: A rapid antigen test for GAS is performed for P.J. and is positive. What treatment should be initiated at this time?

Penicillins remain the agents of choice for GAS pharyngitis. Either oral penicillin, oral amoxicillin, or intramuscular benzathine penicillin may be used. Amoxicillin suspension is more palatable than penicillin and has the advantage of a once-daily dosing regimen. Intramuscular penicillin is a one-time dose that is helpful in those at risk for nonadherence. In patients with a type I hypersensitivity to penicillins, azithromycin, clarithromycin, or clindamycin may be used. In those with a non–type I allergy to penicillin, a first-generation cephalosporin may be considered. The regimens and doses recommended by the American Heart Association are summarized in Table 99-6.[104] Although there is little reported GAS resistance to penicillin, some patients have a decreased clinical response and may respond better to cephalosporins. This is often seen in patients who are GAS carriers and those who may have other bacteria-causing infection. Patients are no longer contagious 24 hours after the first antibiotic dose.[103]

P.J. should receive amoxicillin (400 mg/5 mL), 12.5 mL (1,000 mg) every 24 hours for 10 days. For pain relief, he may also receive as-needed doses of acetaminophen (160 mg/5 mL),

TABLE 99-6
Medication Regimens for the Treatment of Streptococcal Pharyngitis and Prevention of Rheumatic Fever[103,104]

Medication	Dose	Duration
Amoxicillin	50 mg/kg once a day (maximum 1 g)	10 days
Penicillin VK	≤27 kg: 250 mg 2 or 3 times a day >27 kg: 500 mg 2 or 3 times a day	10 days
Benzathine penicillin G	≤27 kg: 600,000 units IM >27 kg: 1,200,000 units IM	Once
For Patients with Penicillin Allergy		
Cephalexin	12.5–25 mg/kg (up to 500 mg) twice a day	10 days
Cefadroxil	15 mg/kg (up to 1 g) twice a day	10 days
Clindamycin	10 mg/kg three times a day (maximum 1.8 g per day)	10 days
Azithromycin	12 mg/kg once a day (maximum 500 mg)	5 days
Clarithromycin	7.5 mg/kg twice a day (maximum 250 mg per dose)	10 days

IM, intramuscular.

10 mL every 6 hours, or ibuprofen (100 mg/5 mL), 10 mL every 6 hours.

Those with a history of rheumatic fever, characterized by acute generalized inflammation of the heart, joints, brain, or skin, should receive long-term antibiotic prophylaxis to prevent further complications from streptococcal infections. Recommended medications and dosing regimens are summarized in Table 99-7.[105,106] Patients with acute carditis and residual heart disease should receive treatment for 10 years or until 40 years of age, whichever is longer.[103] Patients with an episode of carditis but without residual heart disease should receive treatment for 10 years or at least until 21 years of age.[103] Patients who had rheumatic fever without carditis should receive treatment for 5 years or at least until 21 years of age.[103]

TABLE 99-7
Medication Regimens for the Prevention of Recurrent Rheumatic Fever[103]

Medication	Dose	Frequency
Benzathine penicillin G	≤27 kg: 600,000 units IM >27 kg: 1,200,000 units IM	Every 4 weeks
Penicillin V	250 mg oral	Twice a day
Sulfadiazine	≤27 kg: 0.5 g oral >27 kg: 1 g oral	Once a day
If allergic to above agents		
Erythromycin[105]	250 mg oral	Twice a day
Clindamycin[106]	75 mg oral	Twice a day

IM, intramuscular.

KEY REFERENCES AND WEBSITES

A full list of references for this chapter can be found at http://thepoint.lww.com/AT10e. Below are the key references and website for this chapter, with the corresponding reference number in this chapter found in parentheses after the reference.

Key References

American Academy of Pediatrics Subcommittee on Management of Acute Otitis Media. Diagnosis and management of acute otitis media. *Pediatrics.* 2004;113:1451. (90)

Coker TR et al. Diagnosis, microbial epidemiology, and antibiotic treatment of acute otitis media in children. *JAMA.* 2010;304:2161. (86)

Gerber MA et al. Prevention of rheumatic fever and diagnosis and treatment of acute streptococcal pharyngitis: a scientific statement from the American Heart Association Rheumatic Fever, Endocarditis, and Kawasaki Disease Committee of the Council on Cardiovascular Disease in the Young, the Interdisciplinary Council on Functional Genomics and Translational Biology, and the Interdisciplinary Council on Quality of Care and Outcomes Research: endorsed by the American Academy of Pediatrics. *Circulation.* 2009;119:1541. (103)

Ishimine P. The evolving approach to the young child who has fever and no obvious source. *Emerg Med Clin North Am.* 2007; 25:1087. (11).

Markman L. Teething: facts and fiction. *Pediatr Rev.* 2009;30:359. (5)

Nield LS, Kamat D. Prevention, diagnosis, and management of diaper dermatitis. *Clin Pediatr (Phila).* 2007;46:480. (8)

Vandenplas Y et al. Pediatric gastroesophageal reflux clinical practice guidelines: joint recommendations of the North American Society for Pediatric Gastroenterology, Hepatology, and Nutrition (NASPGHAN) and the European Society for Pediatric Gastroenterology, Hepatology, and Nutrition (ESPGHAN). *J Pediatr Gastroenterol Nutr.* 2009;49:498. (58)

Key Websites

Consumer Healthcare Products Association. *Voluntary codes and guidelines of the Consumer Healthcare Products Industry.* Program on OTC oral pediatric cough and cold medicines. http://www.chpa-info.org/scienceregulatory/voluntary_codes.aspx. Accessed December 16, 2010. (27)

Neonatal Therapy

100

Donna M. Kraus and Jennifer Tran Pham

CORE PRINCIPLES

	CHAPTER CASES
RESPIRATORY DISTRESS SYNDROME	
1 Respiratory distress syndrome (RDS) is a major cause of morbidity and mortality in preterm neonates, resulting from pulmonary surfactant deficiency; it is characterized by atelectasis, hypoxemia, decreased lung compliance, small airway epithelial damage, and pulmonary edema.	**Case 100-1 (Question 1)**
2 Beractant, calfactant, and poractant alfa are exogenous surfactants used in the prevention and treatment of RDS in preterm infants. These agents have been shown to improve oxygenation and lung compliance and decrease the need for supplemental oxygen and mechanical ventilation.	**Case 100-1 (Questions 2–6)**
BRONCHOPULMONARY DYSPLASIA	
1 Bronchopulmonary dysplasia (BPD) is the most common form of chronic pulmonary disease in infants; it is caused by lung immaturity, surfactant deficiency, oxygen toxicity, barotrauma, and inflammation and is characterized by tachypnea, retractions, and wheezing.	**Case 100-2 (Question 1)**
2 The management of BPD includes supplemental oxygen therapy, mechanical ventilation, and pharmacologic interventions including diuretics, bronchodilators, and corticosteroids.	**Case 100-2 (Questions 2, 3)**
3 Infants with BPD are at higher risk for experiencing cardiorespiratory problems including pneumonia, pulmonary hypertension, left ventricular hypertrophy, and neurologic and developmental abnormalities.	**Case 100-2 (Questions 4, 5)**
PATENT DUCTUS ARTERIOSUS	
1 Preterm neonates are at high risk for patent ductus arteriosus (PDA), a serious cardiovascular disorder, which may present with tachycardia, wide pulse pressure, bounding pulses, and systolic murmur. Complications of PDA include pulmonary edema and heart failure. PDA places the neonate at high risk for BPD, intraventricular hemorrhage, and necrotizing enterocolitis.	**Case 100-3 (Questions 1–3)**
2 Medical management of PDA includes fluid management, correction of anemia, treatment of hypoxia and acidosis, and pharmacologic therapy with prostaglandin inhibitors (indomethacin or ibuprofen) to close the ductus.	**Case 100-3 (Questions 4–9)**
NECROTIZING ENTEROCOLITIS	
1 Necrotizing enterocolitis (NEC) is the most common life-threatening nonrespiratory condition in newborns and is characterized by abdominal distension, bloody stools, metabolic acidosis, and bowel perforation.	**Case 100-4 (Question 1)**
2 The management of NEC includes parenteral nutrition, intravenous antibiotics, and bowel resection. Interventions including trophic feedings, breast milk, and probiotics may be used to decrease the incidence of NEC.	**Case 100-4 (Questions 2–6)**

continued

NEONATAL SEPSIS AND MENINGITIS	
1 Bacterial sepsis can be classified as early-onset (caused by pathogens colonized from the maternal genital tract) or late-onset sepsis (caused by nosocomial pathogens). Clinical signs can be subtle and nonspecific especially in preterm infants.	**Case 100-5 (Question 1)**
2 Selection of empiric intravenous antibiotics is the same for sepsis and meningitis and will depend on nosocomial pathogens commonly isolated in the neonatal intensive care unit, antibiotic resistance patterns, and underlying neonatal risk factors.	**Case 100-5 (Question 2)**
CONGENITAL INFECTIONS	
1 Congenital infections including herpes simplex virus, syphilis, and cytomegalovirus may result in fetal death, congenital anomalies, serious central nervous system sequelae, intrauterine growth retardation, or preterm birth; if suspected, appropriate diagnostic tests and treatment should be started immediately.	**Case 100-6 (Question 1)**
APNEA OF PREMATURITY	
1 Pharmacologic treatment of apnea of prematurity includes the use of methylxanthines, specifically caffeine and theophylline, which decrease apneic episodes via both central and peripheral effects.	**Case 100-7 (Question 1)**
2 Caffeine offers several advantages over theophylline for the treatment of apnea including a wider therapeutic index, fewer adverse effects, prolonged half-life, once-daily dosing, and lack of the need for routine serum drug concentration monitoring.	**Case 100-7 (Questions 2, 3)**
NEONATAL SEIZURES	
1 Neonatal seizure activity is a common manifestation of a life-threatening underlying neurologic process. Initial therapy is focused on the treatment of the underlying cause (e.g., hypoglycemia, hypocalcemia, infection) and may not include antiepileptic drug therapy.	**Case 100-8 (Questions 1–3)**
2 Common antiepileptic medications used to treat neonatal seizure activity are phenobarbital, phenytoin, and lorazepam.	**Case 100-8 (Questions 4, 5)**

NEONATAL THERAPY

The rational use of medications in neonates depends on an appreciation of both the physiological immaturity and the developmental maturation that influence neonatal drug disposition and pharmacologic effects. Much progress has been made to decrease neonatal mortality and improve survival of more premature and lower-birth-weight newborns. Neonates, particularly those of extremely low-birth-weights (ELBW), pose a pharmacotherapeutic challenge to the clinician. The alterations of body composition, weight, and size, as well as physiological and pharmacokinetic parameters, that occur with normal growth and maturation during the first few months of life are greater than at any other time. Although the amount of neonatal drug information is increasing, the overall lack of well-designed pharmacokinetic and pharmacodynamic studies still hinders the clinical use of many drugs in this population. This is especially true for newborns of the lowest birth weights (<750 g). An understanding of common neonatal terminology (Table 100-1) is important because every newborn is evaluated and classified at birth according to birth weight, gestational age, and intrauterine growth status.[1] Pharmacokinetic parameters, pharmacodynamics, and dosing recommendations often are specified according to these terms.[2] Important neonatal pharmacokinetic differences are reviewed in Chapter 97, Pediatric Pharmacotherapy. This chapter focuses on the safe and effective use of medications for common neonatal medical conditions.

RESPIRATORY DISTRESS SYNDROME

Respiratory distress syndrome (RDS) is a major cause of morbidity and mortality in preterm neonates, affecting approximately 50,000 infants in the United States each year.[3] This clinical syndrome is characterized by respiratory failure with atelectasis, hypoxemia, decreased lung compliance, small airway epithelial damage, and pulmonary edema. The principal cause of RDS is pulmonary surfactant deficiency. Pulmonary surfactant decreases the surface tension at the air–fluid interface in the alveoli and prevents alveolar collapse. Surfactant also facilitates the clearance of pulmonary fluid, prevents pulmonary edema, and stabilizes alveoli during aeration. At birth, the clearance of residual fetal lung fluid is accompanied by an increase in pulmonary

TABLE 100-1
Common Neonatal Terminology[1,2]

Term	Definition
Gestational age (GA)	*By dates:* The number of weeks from the onset of the mother's last menstrual period until birth *By examination:* Assessment of gestational maturity by physical and neuromuscular examination; gestational age estimates the time from conception until birth
Postnatal age (PNA)	Chronologic age after birth
Postconceptional age (PCA)	Gestational age plus postnatal age
Corrected age	Postconceptional age in weeks minus 40; represents postnatal age if neonate had been born at term (40 weeks' gestational age)
Preterm	<38 weeks' gestational age at birth
Term	38–42 weeks' gestational age at birth
Postterm	≥43 weeks' gestational age at birth
Extremely low-birth-weight (ELBW)	Birth weight <1 kg
Very low-birth-weight (VLBW)	Birth weight <1.5 kg
Low-birth-weight (LBW)	Birth weight <2.5 kg
Small for gestational age (SGA)	Birth weight <10th percentile for gestational age
Appropriate for gestational age (AGA)	Birth weight between 10th and 90th percentiles for gestational age
Large for gestational age (LGA)	Birth weight >90th percentile for gestational age

blood flow, which facilitates the transition from fetal to adult circulation.[3]

In the fetus, endogenous cortisol stimulates the synthesis and secretion of pulmonary surfactant at 30 to 32 weeks' gestational age.[4] However, sufficient amounts of pulmonary surfactant for normal lung function are not present before 34 to 36 weeks' gestation.[5] Therefore, the incidence and severity of RDS increase as gestational age decreases. RDS occurs in less than 20% to 30% of neonates born at 30 to 31 weeks' gestational age, but in 50% of neonates born at 26 to 28 weeks' gestational age.[3]

Without adequate amounts of surfactant, the surface tension within the alveoli is so great that the alveoli collapse (atelectasis), resulting in poor gas exchange (e.g., hypoxemia, hypercapnia). Low lung compliance also results, and large inspiratory pressures are needed to aerate the lungs. Unfortunately, the extremely compliant neonatal chest wall makes it difficult to create the large negative inspiratory pressures necessary to open the alveoli. This results in an increased work of breathing and alterations of ventilation and perfusion (V/Q mismatch).[3]

Aeration of the surfactant-deficient lung also results in the cyclic collapse and distension of bronchioles, with resultant bronchiolar epithelial injury and necrosis. This epithelial damage causes pulmonary edema by allowing fluid and proteins to leak from the intravascular space into the airspaces and interstitium of the lung. The necrotic epithelial debris and proteins then form fibrous hyaline membranes.[3] Hyaline membranes and pulmonary edema further impair gas exchange.

The inadequate oxygenation and ventilation and increased work of breathing caused by RDS may result in the need for assisted positive-pressure ventilation. Complications of RDS may be related to mechanical ventilation and include pulmonary barotrauma (e.g., pneumothorax, pulmonary interstitial emphysema [PIE]), intraventricular hemorrhage (IVH), patent ductus arteriosus (PDA), retinopathy of prematurity (ROP), and chronic lung disease or bronchopulmonary dysplasia (BPD).[3]

Clinical Presentation

CASE 100-1

QUESTION 1: L.D., an 700-g male, was born at 25 weeks' gestational age via cesarean section as a result of placenta abruption to a 38-year-old gravida 6 para 5 woman with gestational diabetes. Apgar scores were 3 at 1 minute, 5 at 5 minutes, and 8 at 10 minutes. Thirty minutes after birth, L.D. appears cyanotic and has retracting respirations with grunting and nasal flaring. His heart rate (HR) is 160 beats/minute and respiratory rate (RR) is 65 breaths/minute. An arterial blood gas (ABG) on 100% oxygen by nasal cannula is as follows:

pH, 7.26
P_{CO_2}, 50 mm Hg
P_{O_2}, 45 mm Hg
Base deficit, 7

L.D. is intubated immediately and placed on positive-pressure–assisted ventilation. A catheter is inserted in his umbilical artery for frequent ABG monitoring, and an umbilical vein catheter is inserted for central venous access. L.D.'s chest radiographic shows RDS (see http://www.adhb.govt.nz/newborn/teachingresources/radiology/CXR/RDS/RDS.jpg for a radiograph of an infant with RDS). Ampicillin 50 mg/kg every 12 hours and gentamicin 5 mg/kg every 48 hours are ordered intravenously (IV) to rule out sepsis. What is an Apgar score? What risk factors does L.D. have for RDS? What signs and laboratory data are consistent with RDS?

An Apgar score is a method of evaluating the physical condition of a newborn infant immediately after birth. It consists of five clinical signs including HR, respiratory effort, muscle tone, skin color, and reflex irritability. Each sign can receive a score of 0 to 2 points with a total possible score of 10 points. A score of 7 to 10 is considered normal, whereas scores of 0 to 3 require immediate resuscitation. The Apgar score is routinely done at 1 and 5 minutes of life and is repeated every 5 minutes until a total score of at least 7 is achieved. (For a video of how to assign an Apgar score to newborns, go to http://online.wsj.com/video/assigning-an-apgar-score-to-newborns/9B7B09A9-1B12-4C65-92BA-D4C6DFA35BBA.html?mod=googlewsj.) L.D.'s Apgar scores of 3 and 5 at 1 and 5 minutes indicate that he may have experienced some perinatal asphyxia, most likely secondary to maternal placenta abruption. L.D.'s risk factors for RDS are prematurity, male sex, perinatal asphyxia, cesarean section, and maternal gestational diabetes. Other risk factors include second-born twins and maternal-fetal hemorrhage.[3,6] Clinical signs and laboratory data consistent with RDS in L.D. include tachypnea, cyanosis, retracting respirations, grunting, nasal flaring, hypoxemia, hypercapnia, and a mixed respiratory and metabolic acidosis.[3,6] Clinical manifestations classically present within the first 6 hours of life.[6]

Tachypnea, the first sign of respiratory distress, is an attempt to compensate for the inadequate ventilation, hypercapnia, and acidosis. L.D.'s retracting respirations (the use of intercostal, subcostal, suprasternal, or sternal accessory muscles) reflect the increased work of breathing necessary to maintain ventilation. His nasal flaring decreases resistance during inspiration and increases oxygenation. Grunting is the result of forceful exhalation against a partially closed glottis in an effort to prolong expiration and maximize oxygenation. Grunting also increases intrathoracic pressure during expiration in an attempt to stabilize the alveoli and prevent atelectasis. L.D.'s cyanosis, hypoxemia, hypercapnia, and mixed respiratory and metabolic acidosis are consequences of inadequate oxygenation and poor ventilation and are consistent with RDS.[3]

Treatment

CASE 100-1, QUESTION 2: What treatments should be initiated for L.D.'s respiratory insufficiency?

Before L.D. is treated for RDS, other causes of respiratory distress must be ruled out. For example, infections (particularly group B streptococcal sepsis or pneumonia) often present with respiratory distress. Because it is difficult to distinguish between RDS and infection, all infants with severe RDS should receive antibiotics. L.D. was started empirically on antibiotics, and a complete evaluation of possible sepsis should be performed.

L.D. should be intubated and exogenous surfactant should be administered intratracheally as soon as possible. Human surfactant is synthesized and secreted by type II alveolar epithelial cells of the lung. It contains 80% phospholipids, 8% neutral lipids, and 12% proteins.[7] The major surface-active component is dipalmitoylphosphatidylcholine (DPPC), also known as colfosceril or lecithin. However, this phospholipid slowly adsorbs to the air–fluid interface in the alveoli. Other phospholipids (e.g., phosphatidylcholine, phosphatidylglycerol), and four surfactant apoproteins (SP-A, SP-B, SP-C, and SP-D) enhance spreadability and surface adsorption.[5,8] Adsorption and surface spreading of the surfactant in the alveoli are important determinants of surface-tension activity. SP-A and SP-D both play a role in immune regulation and providing host defense. SP-A may also help to regulate alveolar surfactant reuptake and metabolism.[5] SP-B and SP-C are the two most important apoproteins responsible for promoting adsorption and surface spreading of the surfactant in the alveoli to form a phospholipid monolayer.[7] Surfactant apoprotein B (SP-B) is thought to be the most critical protein for surfactant activity.

Natural surfactants are derived from bovine or porcine lung lipid or lavage extracts, or from human amniotic fluid. Modified natural surfactants are lung lipid extracts supplemented with phospholipids or other components.[8] Currently, three surfactant products are commercially available for clinical use in the United States: beractant (Survanta) is a modified natural surfactant, and both calfactant (Infasurf) and poractant alfa (Curosurf) are natural surfactants. Beractant and calfactant are US Food and Drug Administration (FDA) -approved for the prevention (i.e., prophylaxis) of RDS, and all three products are approved for the treatment (i.e., rescue therapy) of RDS.[9–11]

Beractant is prepared by mincing bovine lung, which contains lung surfactant and phospholipids from lung cells. During the extraction process, cholesterol is removed and synthetic DPPC is added to improve surface activity. Surfactant apoprotein B (SP-B) is removed with cholesterol. As a result, beractant contains only trace amounts of SP-B (<0.5% of total protein). Ninety-nine percent of the protein in beractant is SP-C.[12,13] Although the amounts of SP-B are low, beractant is still effective because of the presence of DPPC, the major surface-active component of surfactant.

In contrast, calfactant is extracted from washings of newborn calves' lungs; therefore it contains fewer contaminating lung cell components. Forty percent of the protein in calfactant is SP-B and 60% is SP-C. Poractant alfa is extracted from washings of pigs' lungs and is purified by liquid gel chromatography to remove neutralized lipids such as cholesterol. As with calfactant, no synthetic DPPC is added to poractant alfa.[11] It is composed of 99% lipids and 1% apoproteins (SP-B [45%] and SP-C [55%]). Neither beractant, calfactant, nor poractant alfa contain SP-A (refer to Table 100-2 for comparisons).[9–11]

CASE 100-1, QUESTION 3: What are the effects of exogenously administered surfactant that can be expected in L.D.?

Oxygenation and lung compliance rapidly and markedly improve after the administration of surfactant to L.D. It should be expected that supplemental oxygen and mechanical ventilation may need to be significantly reduced. The increased lung compliance and decreased need for high inspiratory pressures result in a dramatic decrease in the incidence of pneumothorax and PIE. Survival in treated infants increases by approximately 40% regardless of birth weight or gestational age, and neonatal mortality from RDS is decreased to approximately 20%.[14] Other complications of RDS such as severe BPD, IVH, and PDA have not been decreased consistently with surfactant therapy. Although the severity of ROP was decreased with the use of exogenous surfactants, overall incidence is unchanged.[14]

CASE 100-1, QUESTION 4: Which surfactant is appropriate and when should it be administered to L.D.?

PRODUCT SELECTION

To date, there are eight trials comparing the three natural surfactants; four trials compared beractant with calfactant and the other four compared beractant with poractant alfa.[12,15] In the trials comparing beractant with calfactant, infants treated with calfactant required significantly less supplemental oxygen and mean airway pressures (MAP), but only during the acute phase of respiratory distress.[12,15] The overall duration of mechanical ventilation and supplemental oxygen use and the incidence of death, BPD, and secondary outcomes, including pneumothorax, were not significantly different between the two groups. However, when administered as prophylaxis, infants less than 600 g treated with calfactant had a significantly higher mortality compared with the beractant group.[12,15] The percentage of infants requiring two or more doses were not significantly different between surfactants.[15]

Four randomized trials compared poractant alfa with beractant.[12,15] Treatment with poractant alfa was associated with a significantly faster weaning of supplemental oxygen, peak inspiratory pressure (PIP), and MAP; fewer days on oxygen, mechanical ventilation, and hospital stay; and a decreased number of required additional doses.[12,15] The higher initial dose of poractant alfa 200 mg/kg may have accounted for the decrease in repeat dosing in the poractant alfa group. In addition, mortality at 36 weeks' postconceptional age (PCA) was significantly lower in the poractant alfa 200 mg/kg group compared with the beractant group.[12,15] The incidence of BPD and other secondary outcomes was not significantly different between the two groups. Two studies have evaluated the cost-effectiveness of different surfactant products for the treatment of RDS.[12,15] Both of these studies reported significant cost savings associated with poractant alfa compared with beractant. Infants treated with poractant alfa required fewer additional doses than those treated with beractant.

Based on these comparative trials, the natural surfactants (calfactant and poractant alfa) seem to have a longer duration of effect and require less supplemental oxygen and MAP than the modified natural surfactant, beractant. All-cause mortality and mortality

TABLE 100-2
Comparison of Currently Marketed Surfactant Products[9–11]

Variable	Calfactant (Infasurf)	Poractant Alpha (Curosurf)	Beractant (Survanta)
Type and source	Natural surfactant, calf lung wash	Natural surfactant, porcine lung mince extract	Modified natural surfactant, bovine lung mince extract
Phospholipids	Natural DPPC with mixed phospholipids	Natural DPPC with mixed phospholipids	Natural and supplemented DPPC with mixed phospholipids
Proteins	Calf proteins SP-B and SP-C	Porcine proteins SP-B and SP-C	Bovine proteins SP-B and SP-C
Dispersing and adsorption agents	Proteins SP-B and SP-C	Proteins SP-B and SP-C	Proteins SP-B and SP-C
Indications	Prophylaxis and rescue therapy	Rescue therapy	Prophylaxis and rescue therapy
Criteria for prophylaxis	Premature infants <29 weeks' gestational age at high risk for RDS	Not approved	Birth weight <1,250 g or evidence of surfactant deficiency
Recommended dose	3 mL/kg (phospholipids 105 mg/kg)	*Initial dose:* 2.5 mL/kg (phospholipids 200 mg/kg); *Repeat dose:* 1.25 mL/kg (phospholipids 100 mg/kg)	4 mL/kg (phospholipids 100 mg/kg)
Recommended regimen for prophylaxis	Give first dose ASAP after birth, preferably within 30 minutes; repeat every 12 hours up to a total of three doses if infant remains intubated or repeat as early as 6 hours up to a total of four doses if infant remains intubated and requires $FIO_2 \geq 0.3$ with $PaO_2 \leq 80$ mm Hg	Not approved	Give first dose ASAP after birth, preferably within 15 minutes; repeat as early as 6 hours up to a total of four doses if infant remains intubated and requires $FIO_2 \geq 0.3$ with $PaO_2 \leq 80$ mm Hg
Criterion for rescue therapy	Infants ≤72 hours of age with confirmed RDS who require endotracheal intubation	Infants with confirmed RDS who require endotracheal intubation	Infants with confirmed RDS who require endotracheal intubation
Recommended regimen for rescue therapy	Give first dose ASAP after RDS diagnosed, repeat every 12 hours up to a total of three doses if infant still remains intubated or repeat as early as 6 hours up to a total of four doses if infant still remains intubated and requires $FIO_2 \geq 0.3$ with $PaO_2 \leq 80$ mm Hg	Give first dose ASAP after RDS diagnosed, repeat every 12 hours up to a total of three doses if infant remains intubated and requires mechanical ventilation with supplemental oxygen	Give first dose ASAP after RDS diagnosed, preferably by 8 hours postnatal age; repeat as early as 6 hours up to a total of four doses if infant remains intubated and requires $FIO_2 \geq 0.3$ with $PaO_2 \leq 80$ mm Hg
Recommended administration technique	Administer through side-port of ETT adapter via ventilator, divide dose into two aliquots with position change *or* through disconnected ETT via 5F catheter, divide dose into four aliquots with position change	Administer through disconnected ETT via 5F catheter, divide dose into two aliquots with position change	Administer through disconnected ETT via 5F catheter, divide dose into four aliquots with position change
Special instructions	Gentle swirling of the vial may be necessary for redispersion; warming to room temperature is not necessary; do not shake	Warm to room temperature before use, do not shake	Warm to room temperature before use; do not shake
Stability	If warmed to room temperature for <24 hours, unopened, unused vials may be returned once to refrigerator; single-use vial contains no preservative, discard unused portion	If warmed to room temperature for <24 hours, unopened, unused vials may be returned only once to refrigerator; single-use vial contains no preservative, discard unused portion	If warmed to room temperature for <24 hours, unopened, unused vials may be returned only once to refrigerator; single-use vial contains no preservative, discard unused portion
Cost per vial	\$413.64 (3 mL), \$732.12 (6 mL)[a]	\$418.71 (1.5 mL), \$819.70 (3 mL)[a]	\$459.60 (4 mL), \$813.46 (8 mL)[a]

[a] Average wholesale price according to *2010 Red Book*.
ASAP, as soon as possible; DPPC, dipalmitoylphosphatidylcholine; ETT, endotracheal tube; F, French; FIO_2, fractional inspired oxygen; PaO_2, partial pressure of oxygen; RDS, respiratory distress syndrome.

(at 36 weeks' PCA) were also significantly lower in the poractant alfa group when compared with beractant or calfactant.[12,15] In addition, cost-analysis studies also reported significant cost savings associated with poractant alfa. The incidence of BPD and other secondary outcomes are not different between natural and modified natural surfactants. Based on these findings, it appears that treatment with natural surfactants for infants with or at risk for RDS results in better clinical outcomes and that poractant alfa seems to be the favorable surfactant therapy and should be initiated in L.D.

Surfactant should be administered by qualified physicians with the presence of nursing and respiratory therapy personnel.[14] (For a video on surfactant administration, go to **http://www.youtube.com/watch?v=hkUdH01sLmA&feature=related.**) Neonates receiving beractant or poractant alfa need to be disconnected from the ventilator before surfactant administration.[9,11] As a result, clinicians transiently increase both the fraction of inspired oxygen (FIO_2) and PIPs before disconnecting the ventilator. Calfactant, on the other hand, has the advantage of flexible administration techniques. It can be administered intratracheally via a catheter passed through the endotracheal tube (ETT) with brief interruptions in ventilation (as with beractant and poractant alfa) or via a side-port adapter into the ETT without disconnecting the ventilator.[10]

TIME OF ADMINISTRATION

Surfactant therapy can be administered as prophylactic (i.e., within 10–30 minutes after birth) or rescue treatment (given to those with established RDS within 12 hours of life). Early rescue is defined as the administration of surfactant within the first 2 hours of life; late rescue is defined as treatment after more than 2 hours of life. Theoretically, the first dose of surfactant should be given before the newborn's first breath or before positive-pressure ventilation.[13,14] This would avoid the early lung injury in RDS that can interfere with surfactant distribution, bioavailability, and effectiveness.[8] This strategy, however, increases the cost of care because newborns who might never experience RDS would be intubated and treated unnecessarily.[6,8] In addition, delivery room treatment may interfere with resuscitation and stabilization of the neonate.[13]

Prophylactic surfactant therapy has been shown to decrease the incidence and severity of RDS, mortality, pneumothorax, PIE, and the combined variable of BPD or death, compared with rescue treatment.[14] When early versus late rescue therapy was compared, similar findings were reported (except for RDS), favoring those treated with early rescue therapy.[16] No differences were found in the incidence of BPD, IVH, PDA, or ROP between prophylactic and rescue therapy. Despite the favorable effects of prophylactic therapy, most clinicians would administer surfactant only after RDS is established, as rescue therapy. In addition, most of the studies were conducted when antenatal steroids were not commonly used. Therefore, the current potential benefits of prophylactic or early rescue may be less than what were reported in these studies.

Mechanical ventilation can be avoided by using the "INSURE" (INtubate–SURfactant–Extubate) technique in infants who require surfactant therapy. Randomized trials have shown this technique to reduce the need for mechanical ventilation and subsequent BPD.[17] Because surfactant works better if given earlier in the course of RDS, it is important to determine who is at highest risk for RDS. Unfortunately, the exact criteria to clinically determine high-risk newborns are still unclear. In summary, surfactant treatment should be administered as soon as clinical signs of RDS appear. Early therapy avoids progression of the disease and the potential for decreased surfactant effectiveness. Prophylactic administration in the delivery room should be reserved for extremely premature neonates who are at the highest risk for RDS.[13] Because L.D. has clinical, laboratory, and radiographic findings consistent with RDS, a dose of 2.5 mL/kg (200 mg/kg phospholipid) of poractant alfa should be administered to L.D. intratracheally immediately within 1 hour of age.

CASE 100-1, QUESTION 5: Within 1 hour of poractant alfa administration, L.D.'s oxygenation improved and the FiO_2 was weaned from 100% to 60%. Ten hours later, the ABGs revealed the following:

pH, 7.36
PCO_2, 45 mm Hg
PO_2, 80 mm Hg
Base deficit, 2
O_2 saturation, 94% on the following ventilator settings: FiO_2, 0.60; intermittent mechanical ventilation (IMV), 30; PIP, 14; and positive end-expiratory pressure (PEEP), +4

Should another dose of poractant alfa be administered?

The response to a single dose of surfactant usually is transient; thus, more than one dose is needed. Response to surfactant therapy can be variable, especially in preterm newborns weighing less than 750 g.[8] Reasons for lack of response include surfactant inhibition by proteins that have leaked into the alveolar spaces, inactivation of surfactant by inflammatory mediators (free oxygen radicals, proteases), presence of conditions that can decrease surfactant effectiveness (e.g., pulmonary edema), or poor delivery of surfactant to the alveoli (owing to atelectasis). The degree of responsiveness to surfactant also decreases with increasing postnatal age.[8,13,14]

Although the indications for subsequent doses of surfactant have varied in investigational studies, persistence of respiratory failure is the major clinical indicator for retreatment. A second dose of poractant alfa should be given to L.D. because he still requires mechanical ventilation with relatively high inspiratory pressures and supplemental oxygen ($FiO_2 \geq 0.3$) to maintain an arterial PO_2 of at least 50 mm Hg and oxygen saturation of 90%. In a recent Cochrane review, multiple surfactant doses were associated with a decreased incidence of neonatal death and pneumothorax compared with a single dose.[18] In practice, despite these potential benefits associated with multiple doses, most infants require only one dose of surfactant. This may be related to advances in neonatal and perinatal management and an increased use of antenatal steroids.

CASE 100-1, QUESTION 6: What complications of surfactant treatment is L.D. at risk of experiencing?

The most common adverse effects of surfactant therapy are related to the method of administration.[13] Surfactant is administered directly into the lungs via the ETT by using a catheter or a side-port adapter connected to the ETT. During administration, L.D. may experience bradycardia and oxygen desaturation secondary to vagal stimulation and airway obstruction.[9–11] These adverse events might require temporary discontinuation of surfactant administration and increased ventilator support.

Surfactant therapy may increase the risk of pulmonary hemorrhage in L.D. Although the exact mechanism is unknown, surfactant may increase pulmonary blood flow through the ductus arteriosus, increase pulmonary microvascular pressures, and cause hemorrhagic pulmonary edema. The benefits of surfactant therapy, however, far outweigh the increased risk of pulmonary hemorrhage.

Neonates who are given surfactant can be at greater risk for apnea that requires methylxanthine treatment. Surfactant-treated neonates can be weaned from ventilator support sooner and, therefore, might display apnea more easily. Individual trials with natural surfactants have suggested an increased incidence of sepsis and necrotizing enterocolitis (NEC), but most studies have not validated these findings. No difference in the incidence of NEC or apnea treated with methylxanthines was noted between calfactant and beractant.[12]

BRONCHOPULMONARY DYSPLASIA

CASE 100-2

QUESTION 1: J.T. is a 7-week-old, 1.4-kg female who was born at 25 weeks' gestation. Her medical history includes RDS, episodes of sepsis and pneumonia, and 5 weeks of parenteral nutrition. J.T. has also failed extubation numerous times and is currently requiring mechanical ventilation with an FiO_2 of 0.5. Current vital signs are as follows:

RR, 60 breaths/minute
HR, 150 beats/minute
BP, 80/55 mm Hg
O_2 saturation, 90%

On physical examination, J.T. has intercostal and subcostal retractions, shallow breathing, and an expiratory wheeze. Bilateral diffuse haziness with lung hyperinflation, focal emphysema (with bleb formation), atelectasis, and irregular fibrous streaks are seen on chest radiograph. J.T. is currently receiving enteral feedings with a preterm 24-cal/ounce formula at 28 mL every 3 hours. Based on these findings, the diagnosis of BPD is made. What is the pathogenesis of BPD? What risk factors for BPD does J.T. have? What clinical signs and laboratory evidence of BPD are apparent in J.T.?

BPD (also known as chronic lung disease) is the most common form of chronic pulmonary disease in infants. The disease develops in newborns who require supplemental oxygen and positive-pressure ventilation for RDS or other primary lung disorders. A severity-based definition of BPD has been developed by the National Institute of Child Health and Human Development.[19] For infants born at less than 32 weeks' gestational age, assessment of BPD is performed at 36 weeks' PCA or at the time of discharge. Mild BPD is defined as a need for supplemental O_2 in excess of 21% for at least 28 days but not at 36 weeks' PCA or discharge; moderate BPD as a need for supplemental O_2 for at least 28 days plus treatment with less than 30% O_2 at 36 weeks' PCA or discharge; and severe BPD as a need for supplemental O_2 for at least 28 days plus treatment with at least 30% O_2 or positive-pressure ventilation at 36 weeks' PCA or discharge. For infants born at 32 weeks' gestational age or older, the above definitions are different only in that assessments are conducted at 56 days of life rather than 36 weeks' PCA.[19] BPD is a significant cause of infant morbidity and mortality. Approximately 14,000 new cases of BPD occur in the United States each year.[20] The overall incidence of BPD is 23% and is inversely related to gestational age and birth weight. Infants with birth weights between 501 and 750 g have a 57% incidence of BPD compared with a 6% incidence in infants with birth weights between 1,251 and 1,500 g.[20] An annual decrease of 3.3% in the incidence of BPD has been reported between 1993 and 2006. However, a significant annual increase in hospital length of stay (3.9%) and charges (4.9%) for neonates with BPD has also occurred. The decrease in BPD was coincident with an increase in noninvasive respiratory support (i.e., continuous positive airway pressure [CPAP]), but may also have been influenced by changes in the definition of BPD during the late 1990s to early 2000s.[21]

Pathogenesis and Clinical Manifestations

The cause of BPD seems to be multifactorial. Lung immaturity, surfactant deficiency, oxygen toxicity, barotrauma or volutrauma, and inflammation all play important roles. Premature infants, especially those at less than 26 weeks' gestation, are at a higher risk for BPD owing to lung immaturity.[22] Surfactant deficiency (which causes severe RDS) and the immature parenchymal structure of the lung and chest wall contribute to the development of BPD. Oxygen therapy, which causes a release of free oxygen radicals, is directly associated with the pathogenesis of BPD. Prolonged exposure to high oxygen concentrations and free oxygen radicals causes tissue damage, alveolar-capillary leaks, and atelectasis with resultant impaired gas exchange and pulmonary edema.[22] This may lead to the chronic pulmonary fibrotic changes seen in infants with BPD. In term infants, the lungs contain antioxidant enzymes that help to protect the lung from damage produced by free oxygen radicals. However, in preterm infants, the concentration of antioxidant enzymes may be low or absent. Therefore, premature infants are more susceptible to develop BPD than term infants.

Barotrauma secondary to positive-pressure ventilation is also a major factor in the pathogenesis of BPD, independent of oxygen toxicity.[22] Barotrauma is caused by repetitive distension of the terminal airways during mechanical ventilation. This results in disruption of the epithelium and an increase in capillary permeability to proteinaceous fluid. The severity of lung injury is related to the amount of positive peak pressure used. Volutrauma is also involved in the pathogenesis of BPD and is caused by high tidal volume ventilation and overdistension. Volutrauma may be related to unusually high peak inflation pressures compared with lung compliance. The combined iatrogenic insults of oxygen toxicity and barotrauma or volutrauma, both inflicted on an immature lung for an extended time, can worsen lung damage.

The inflammatory process in the lung is activated by oxygen toxicity, barotrauma or volutrauma, or other injury. This results in the attraction and activation of leukocytes (e.g., neutrophils, macrophages), which may cause further release of inflammatory mediators, elastase, and collagenase.[23] Elevated levels of elastase and collagenase can destroy the elastin and collagen framework of the lung. α_1-Proteinase inhibitor, a major defense against elastase activity, may be inactivated by free oxygen radicals. Therefore, the combined elevated levels of elastase and the decreased activity of α_1-proteinase inhibitor may enhance lung injury and lead to the development of BPD.

Infants who exhibit BPD also have elevated levels of cytokines such as platelet-activating factor, leukotrienes, tumor necrosis factor, and fibronectin.[22] These agents, combined with the activated leukocytes, cause significant lung damage with breakdown of capillary endothelial integrity and capillary leakage. Furthermore, the increased fibronectin levels found in tracheal aspirate samples of infants with early BPD may predispose them to exhibit pulmonary fibrosis.[22]

Infection and nutrient deficiency may also play a role in the pathogenesis of BPD. Pathogens such as *Ureaplasma, Chlamydia,* or cytomegalovirus may cause chronic infection and contribute to the development of BPD. Studies have shown direct correlations between *Ureaplasma* colonization and the presence of BPD.[20,22] Deficiencies in nutrients such as vitamin A (retinol) or trace elements such as zinc, copper, and selenium (which are integral components of the antioxidant enzyme structure) may also play a role in the pathogenesis of BPD.

J.T. has two of the most important risk factors for BPD, low birth weight and decreased gestational age. She is also at risk for BPD owing to mechanical ventilation, oxygen toxicity, and fluid excess (160 mL/kg/day). Other risk factors include male sex, white ethnicity, and persistent PDA.[20,24]

BPD is characterized by tachypnea with shallow breathing, intercostal and subcostal retractions, and expiratory wheezing as demonstrated in J.T. Other signs and symptoms include rales, rhonchi, cough, airflow obstruction, airway hyperreactivity, increased mucus production, hypoxemia, and hypercarbia.[23] J.T.'s chest radiograph shows evidence of BPD, including focal emphysema (with bleb formation), atelectasis, bilateral diffuse haziness (interstitial thickening) with increased expansion of the lungs (hyperinflation), and irregular fibrous streaks. Mucous plugging, sepsis, and pneumonia can also develop in BPD infants on chronic mechanical ventilation. Infants with severe BPD eventually experience cardiovascular complications such as pulmonary hypertension, cor pulmonale, systemic hypertension, and left ventricular hypertrophy. In addition to chronic

TABLE 100-3
Pharmacologic Management of Bronchopulmonary Dysplasia[2,23,24,26–30]

Drug Therapy	Dosage Regimen
Diuretics	
Chlorothiazide	*Neonates and infants <6 months:* PO: 20–40 mg/kg/d in two divided doses; maximum dose: 375 mg/d
Furosemide	PO: 1–4 mg/kg/dose every 12–24 hours IV: 1–2 mg/kg/dose every 12–24 hours *Nebulized:* 1 mg/kg/dose diluted to a final volume of 2 mL with NS (use IV form)
Hydrochlorothiazide	*Neonates and infants <6 months:* PO: 2–3 mg/kg/d in two divided doses; maximum dose: 37.5 mg/d
Spironolactone	PO: 1–3 mg/kg/d every 12–24 hours
Inhaled Bronchodilators	
Albuterol	0.03–0.06 mL/kg/dose of 0.5% solution (0.15–0.3 mg/kg/dose) diluted to 1–2 mL of NS; give via nebulization every 2–6 hours or PRN; minimum dose: 0.25 mL (1.25 mg); maximum dose: 1 mL (5 mg)
Ipratropium bromide	*Neonates:* 0.125 mL/kg/dose of 0.02% solution (25 mcg/kg/dose) diluted to 2–2.5 mL of NS; give via nebulization every 8 hours *Infants:* 0.625–1.25 mL of 0.02% solution (125–250 mcg/dose) diluted to 2–2.5 mL of NS; give via nebulization every 8 hours
Inhaled Corticosteroids	
Beclomethasone dipropionate	2 puffs (40 mcg/puff) via face mask and spacer every 12 hours OR 2 puffs (80 mcg/puff) via face mask and spacer every 12 hours
Budesonide	0.25–0.5 mg; give via nebulization every 12 hours
Fluticasone	2–4 puffs (44 mcg/puff) via face mask and spacer every 12 hours

IV, intravenous; NS, normal saline; PO, oral; PRN, as needed.

respiratory and cardiovascular complications, infants with BPD have significant growth, nutritional, and neurodevelopmental problems.

Management

CASE 100-2, QUESTION 2: What nonpharmacologic and therapeutic agents should be used to manage BPD in J.T.?

The medical management of infants with BPD includes supplemental oxygen therapy, mechanical ventilation, fluid restriction, nutritional management, and various pharmacologic interventions. Supplemental oxygen administered via mechanical ventilation, CPAP, or nasal cannula should be provided to maintain an oxygen saturation of 88% to 94% and prevent hypoxemia.[24,25] Fluids should be restricted to 120 to 130 mL/kg/day to prevent congestive heart disease and pulmonary edema. Because infants with BPD have a 25% increase in caloric expenditure (owing to the increased work of breathing), hypercaloric formulas (e.g., 24 or 27 cal/ounce) may be used to optimize calories while restricting fluid intake.[23] If this increased energy is not provided, infants are at risk for undergoing a catabolic state that places them at higher risk of experiencing more severe BPD (inadequate nutrition may potentiate the toxic effects of oxygen toxicity and barotrauma). The goal of nutritional therapy is to produce weight gains of 10 to 30 g/day, which can usually be accomplished by providing 140 to 160 kcal/kg/day.[22,23] If infants do not tolerate enteral feedings, parenteral alimentation should be substituted until the gastrointestinal (GI) tract becomes more functional. Because J.T. is on a 20-cal/ounce formula, switching her to a hypercaloric formula (i.e., 24 or 27 cal/ounce) would help to optimize her weight gain. Her fluids should be restricted to 168 to 182 mL/day (120–130 mL/kg/day).

PHARMACOLOGIC THERAPY

The treatment of BPD consists of multiple-drug therapy, which includes diuretics, bronchodilators, and corticosteroids. Despite the advancement of drug therapy, none of these drugs have been shown to reverse pulmonary damage in infants with BPD. Instead, they are used primarily to reduce clinical symptoms and to improve lung function. Pharmacologic therapy and dosage regimens for the management of BPD are shown in Table 100-3.[2,23,24,26–30]

DIURETICS

Infants with BPD are particularly prone to pulmonary edema from cardiogenic and noncardiogenic factors. Left ventricular failure may worsen the already existing right ventricular failure. Pulmonary vascular permeability is increased because of the disruption of the alveolar-capillary unit and causes an increased amount of fluid in the interstitium. Although the precise mechanism in the treatment of BPD is unknown, diuretics help to reduce interstitial lung water.[24,27] In addition, diuretics lower pulmonary vascular resistance and improve gas exchange, thereby reducing oxygen requirements. The most commonly used diuretics are furosemide, thiazides, and spironolactone. Furosemide is the drug of choice because of its potent diuretic effect. In addition, it increases lymphatic flow and plasma oncotic pressure and decreases pulmonary interstitial edema. In several studies, the use of furosemide in infants with BPD was associated with short-term improvement in lung compliance and oxygenation, decreased total pulmonary resistance, and facilitation in ventilator weaning.[23,27] However, a meta-analysis did not support all of these findings. The chronic use of furosemide in infants older than 3 weeks of age with BPD was associated with significant improvements in oxygenation and lung compliance only.[27] The effects of furosemide on the duration of oxygen requirement and mechanical ventilation, length of hospital stay, mortality, and the incidence of BPD could not be assessed owing to limited data. Infants may exhibit tolerance to furosemide after a few days of therapy. This may be a result of the contraction in extracellular volume, which can lead to a compensatory increase in water and sodium reabsorption in the renal tubules. In addition to questionable clinical outcome, furosemide can have significant adverse effects including hypochloremia, hypokalemia, and hyponatremia. Furthermore, volume depletion, hypercalciuria, nephrocalcinosis, osteopenia, and ototoxicity may also occur.[23,27] Excessive fluid loss or hypochloremia may result in metabolic alkalosis and worsen respiratory acidosis. Some of these adverse effects may be reduced by using alternate-day furosemide therapy or nebulized furosemide.[27] Neither of these regimens were associated with electrolyte imbalances, and both were shown to significantly increase lung compliance and decrease pulmonary resistance.[27]

Thiazide diuretics (e.g., hydrochlorothiazide) in combination with a potassium-sparing diuretic (e.g., spironolactone) can improve lung function and decrease oxygen requirements with increased diuresis.[23,27] Although less potent than furosemide, the combination of these two diuretics can reduce the incidence of hypokalemia commonly associated with loop or thiazide diuretics. Adverse effects commonly seen with a combination of a thiazide and spironolactone include hyponatremia, hyperkalemia or hypokalemia, hypercalciuria, hyperuricemia, hyperglycemia, azotemia, and hypomagnesia.[23] Thiazides alone can also be added to furosemide to help overcome the rapid tolerance associated with furosemide. In summary, despite insufficient evidence of long-term efficacy and the potential for adverse effects, diuretics are often used in the management of BPD to provide short-term improvement in pulmonary edema and reduce the need for ventilatory support.

Generally, infants with BPD who are treated with diuretics are started on furosemide, but are changed to a combination diuretic (spironolactone/hydrochlorothiazide) if long-term treatment is needed to avoid adverse effects. Suggested indications for initiating furosemide therapy include (a) 1-week-old infants with early BPD and ventilator dependency, (b) infants with stable BPD who significantly worsen owing to fluid overload, (c) infants with chronic BPD who do not improve, and (d) infants requiring an increased fluid intake to provide adequate calories.[22] Because J.T. has chronic BPD and is not improving (i.e., she has not been able to be weaned off the ventilator), furosemide 2 mg/kg given every 12 hours enterally may be considered. J.T. should be monitored and treated for electrolyte disturbances while on furosemide.

CASE 100-2, QUESTION 3: One week after starting furosemide, J.T. still requires high ventilatory settings and is unable to be weaned from the ventilator. What other therapeutic agents may be considered to treat J.T.'s BPD?

INHALED BRONCHODILATORS

Infants in the early stages of BPD generally have airway hyperactivity and smooth muscle hypertrophy. They are also at higher risk for bronchoconstriction owing to increased airway resistance secondary to hypoxia. Therefore, the use of bronchodilators may be helpful in these infants. β_2-Agonists such as albuterol have been shown to provide short-term improvements (4 hours) in lung compliance and pulmonary resistance owing to bronchial smooth muscle relaxation.[23,31] However, inhaled bronchodilators are not effective in all infants with BPD. Infants in the late stages of BPD may have severe pulmonary damage and fibrotic changes. Only half of these infants demonstrate a decrease in pulmonary resistance after albuterol therapy.[32] In addition, tolerance may develop with prolonged administration.[23] Therefore, inhaled bronchodilators should be reserved for infants who clearly demonstrate improvements during therapy. Currently, there are no well-designed studies evaluating the chronic use or long-term outcome of using inhaled bronchodilators in BPD infants. Despite the lack of meaningful long-term clinical outcomes associated with β_2-agonists and the variable results, their use continues to be very common in preterm infants with BPD. Further studies evaluating the efficacy and safety of long-term inhaled bronchodilator therapy are needed.

Inhaled anticholinergics such as ipratropium bromide have produced short-term benefits (approximately 4 hours) in infants with BPD by improving pulmonary function.[24,27] Inhaled anticholinergics, which relax bronchial smooth muscle and decrease mucus secretion, are generally reserved for infants who fail or are intolerant to albuterol, or as an adjunct to albuterol if clinical improvement is not seen.[23] The combined therapy of albuterol and ipratropium may be more effective than either drug alone.[23,24] The adverse effect profile of ipratropium is minimal because the drug is poorly absorbed.

A major problem with inhaled bronchodilators is their method of administration and drug delivery. Inhaled bronchodilators can be given by jet or ultrasonic nebulization or via a metered-dose inhaler (MDI).[27] For ventilator-dependent infants receiving MDIs, the MDI is connected to an adapter that is attached to the ventilator circuit and ETT. MDIs can also be given through bag ventilation via the ETT. For nonventilated infants, the MDI can be given using a valved holding chamber device and a face mask.

Compared with MDIs, nebulization of inhaled bronchodilators has several disadvantages. Loss or inefficient delivery of drug and cooling of the inspired oxygen mixture may occur with nebulization. In several studies in neonates, MDIs with a spacer provided more efficient delivery of inhaled bronchodilators and greater improvements in oxygenation and ventilation; smaller doses and a shorter treatment time were also used.[33,34] Furthermore, when comparing the three different devices, the MDI with spacer and the ultrasonic nebulizer are more efficient in delivering aerosols to neonates than the jet nebulizer.[27] In addition, MDIs are less expensive than nebulization. Therefore, the use of MDIs with an appropriate spacing device is preferred for most infants.

CORTICOSTEROIDS

Corticosteroids, particularly dexamethasone, have been used extensively for the prevention and treatment of BPD. Mechanisms of action of corticosteroids include (a) reduction of polymorphonuclear leukocyte migration to the lung, (b) reduction of lung inflammation, (c) inhibition of prostaglandin, leukotriene, tumor necrosis factor, and interleukin synthesis, (d) reduction of elastase production, (e) stimulation of surfactant synthesis, (f) reduction of vascular permeability and pulmonary edema, (g) enhancement of β-adrenergic receptor activity, (h) reduction of pulmonary fibronectin (which can reduce the risk of interstitial fibrosis), and (i) stimulation of serum retinol concentrations.[2,23] Treatment with dexamethasone (initiated at ~7 days of life) in infants with documented BPD or with clinical signs and chest radiograph findings consistent with BPD reduces the release of inflammatory mediators, improves pulmonary mechanics and clinical status, facilitates weaning from mechanical ventilation, and decreases the duration of oxygen therapy.[22,23,35] However, in most studies, dexamethasone therapy did not significantly reduce the duration of hospitalization or improve survival in infants with BPD.[23,27,35,36]

Systemic dexamethasone is associated with many serious short-term adverse effects, including hyperglycemia, increased

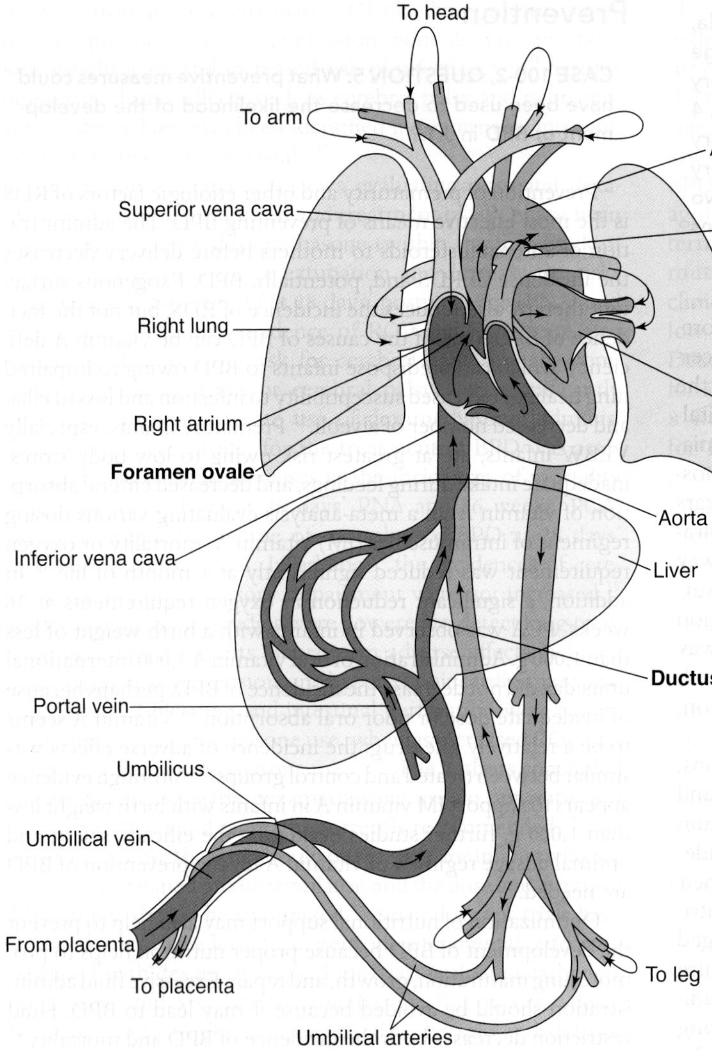

FIGURE 100-1 Fetal circulation. (Adapted with permission From Nettina, Sandra M., MSN, RN, CS, ANP, *The Lippincott Manual of Nursing Practice*, 7th ed. Lippincott Williams & Wilkins, 2001.)

Pulmonary vasoconstriction, along with compression of pulmonary blood vessels by unexpanded fetal lung mass, results in a high pulmonary vascular resistance and decreased pulmonary blood flow. This decreased pulmonary blood flow is acceptable in utero because the lungs essentially are nonfunctional. Large amounts of blood, however, must be pumped through the placenta where gas exchange occurs.

Maximally oxygenated blood (Po_2, 30–35 mm Hg) flows from the placenta to the fetus through the umbilical vein (Fig. 100-1). Approximately 50% of the umbilical venous blood is shunted away from the liver through the ductus venosus and directed into the inferior vena cava. Blood from the inferior vena cava and superior vena cava then enters the right atrium. Most of the blood from the inferior vena cava, which is well oxygenated, is directed in a straight pathway across the right atrium through the foramen ovale directly into the left atrium. It then enters the left ventricle through the mitral valve and is pumped through the ascending aorta and into the vessels of the head and forelimbs. Thus, the fetal brain is preferentially perfused with blood containing a higher amount of oxygen. Deoxygenated blood returning from the head region via the superior vena cava enters the right atrium and is directed through the tricuspid valve into the right ventricle, where it then is pumped into the pulmonary artery. Most of this blood is diverted through the ductus arteriosus into the descending aorta and then through the two umbilical arteries to the placenta. A small percentage of the blood flows to the lower extremities and then is returned to the heart via the inferior vena cava.[46]

Changes at Birth

At birth, major circulatory changes result from umbilical cord clamping, aeration and expansion of the lungs, and an increase in arterial Po_2. These changes are important in the transition from a fetal to an adult circulation. When the umbilical cord is clamped, blood flow decreases through the ductus venosus. Clamping of the umbilical cord also results in a twofold increase in systemic vascular resistance. This increase in systemic vascular resistance increases aortic, left ventricular, and left atrial pressures and cardiac output. Pulmonary pressures and blood flow also change. After the neonate's first breath, the lungs expand, oxygenation improves, and pulmonary vascular resistance immediately drops. This increases pulmonary blood flow, causing a decrease in pulmonary arterial, right ventricular, and right atrial pressures.[46]

If hypoxia occurs after delivery, pulmonary vasoconstriction results and the neonate may experience pulmonary hypertension with a persistence of the fetal circulation. This is termed persistent pulmonary hypertension of the newborn or persistent fetal circulation. Oxygenation of these neonates is extremely difficult because of the pulmonary vasoconstriction and resultant decreased pulmonary blood flow. Administration of oxygen and correction of acidosis, hypotension, and hypercapnia are important initial treatment measures. Patients with persistent hypoxia require intubation and mechanical ventilation. Nitric oxide gas, inotropic agents (to support blood pressure and perfusion), oral sildenafil, and inhaled or IV prostacyclin (epoprostenol) may also be used. Severe cases may require extracorporeal membrane oxygenation.[47]

Closure of the Foramen Ovale

Because of the decreased right atrial pressure and increased left atrial pressure that occur after birth, blood attempts to flow down the pressure gradient from the left atrium through the foramen ovale into the right atrium. This is in the opposite direction from what occurs in fetal life. The small, valvelike flap that lies over the foramen ovale on the left side of the atrial septum closes over the foramen ovale opening when the pressure in the left atrium exceeds the pressure in the right atrium. Closure of this flap prevents further flow through the foramen ovale. As long as the pressure in the left atrium is higher than that in the right atrium, the foramen ovale remains functionally closed, until it closes anatomically.

Closure of the Ductus Arteriosus

Closure of the ductus arteriosus is more complex and depends on many factors. In utero, patency of the ductus arteriosus is maintained through the combined vasodilatory effects of a low Po_2 and high concentrations of prostanoids, particularly prostaglandin E_2 (PGE_2) and prostacyclin.[48] After birth, the smooth muscles of the ductus arteriosus constrict as arterial oxygenation increases and concentrations of placentally derived prostaglandins, particularly PGE_2, decrease.[48] In utero, the Po_2 of the ductal blood is 18 to 22 mm Hg, whereas after birth in a term neonate, it is approximately 100 mm Hg.[46] Normally, the ductus arteriosus of a term neonate functionally closes within the first few days of life (i.e., in 82% of infants within 48 hours of life and in 100% of infants within 96 hours of life). Anatomical closure of the ductus occurs within 2 to 3 weeks of life. When the ductus arteriosus fails to close, it is called patent ductus arteriosus (PDA). In a term neonate, a PDA beyond the first few days of life generally is permanent. It usually is secondary to an anatomical defect in the wall of the ductus arteriosus and requires surgical ligation. In contrast, a PDA in a preterm neonate may persist for weeks and still close spontaneously.

When a PDA is present, the direction and amount of shunting through this opening are determined by the pressure gradient between the systemic and pulmonary circulations. Usually, blood flows from the aorta into the pulmonary circulation. Because systemic vascular resistance and aortic pressure are increased, and pulmonary vascular resistance and pulmonary arterial pressure are decreased after birth, blood pumped from the left ventricle into the aorta flows from the aorta (a high-pressure area) through the PDA and into the pulmonary artery (a lower-pressure area). This flow is called left-to-right shunting and is in contrast to the right-to-left shunting that occurs through the PDA during fetal life.

Although the persistence of a PDA is pathological, it is necessary for the survival of patients with cyanotic congenital heart disease while awaiting corrective or palliative cardiac surgery. These patients have congenital cardiac defects that depend on the ductus arteriosus to maintain cardiac output and systemic perfusion (e.g., coarctation of the aorta, aortic stenosis, and hypoplastic left heart syndrome) or to provide pulmonary blood flow and maintain systemic oxygenation (e.g., pulmonary artery atresia or severe stenosis and tricuspid atresia). Patency of the ductus arteriosus can be maintained pharmacologically with a continuous infusion of alprostadil (PGE_1). The initial starting dose of PGE_1 is 0.05 to 0.1 mcg/kg/minute and may be increased gradually, if needed, every 15 to 30 minutes up to 0.2 mcg/kg/minute until achievement of clinical response. Continuous infusion doses up to 0.4 mcg/kg/minute have also been used by several centers. PGE_1 infusion should be reduced to the lowest effective dose once patency of the ductus arteriosus is achieved.[2] Doses as low as 0.01 mcg/kg/minute may be effective.

Clinical Presentation

CASE 100-3

QUESTION 1: T.S. is a 750-g female who was born at 25 weeks' gestational age to a 22-year-old gravida 2 para 1 woman. One hour after birth, T.S. exhibited symptoms of RDS, and two doses of beractant were given within the first 24 hours of life. After the second dose of beractant, T.S.'s respiratory function greatly improved, and no further doses of beractant were required. On the third day of life, the nurse noticed that T.S. had tachycardia, a systolic murmur, a hyperactive precordium, and a widened pulse pressure. Her lungs sounded "wet." In addition, the nurse noted that T.S.'s combined IV fluid rates total 160 mL/kg/day instead of the desired fluid intake of 120 mL/kg/day. Current vital signs and ABGs are as follows:

HR, 190 beats/minute
RR, 65 breaths/minute
BP, 55/23 mm Hg
O_2 saturation, 89%
pH, 7.22
Pco_2, 55 mm Hg
Po_2, 77 mm Hg
Base deficit, 10

Ventilator support is increased to compensate for T.S.'s deteriorating respiratory status. Echocardiography is performed and shows a moderate-size PDA with significant left-to-right shunting. The chest radiograph shows pulmonary edema and an enlarged heart. What risk factors for PDA does T.S. have?

T.S. has two major risk factors for developing a symptomatic PDA: prematurity and RDS. The occurrence of a PDA is inversely proportional to gestational age and birth weight. The incidence of PDA is approximately 45% in premature infants with a birth weight of less than 1,750 g, but can be as high as 80% in premature infants with a birth weight of less than 1,200 g.[49] In contrast, the incidence of PDA in term infants is only 0.06%.[48] Preterm neonates are at a higher risk for PDA than term newborns because the smooth muscle of the immature ductus is more sensitive to the dilatory effects of prostaglandins and less sensitive to the constrictive effects of increased oxygen tension. In addition, circulating concentrations of PGE_2 are often elevated in premature infants owing to the decreased pulmonary metabolism of prostaglandins. These factors contribute to the delayed closure of the ductus arteriosus in premature infants. With advanced gestation, the ductus is less responsive to the relaxant effects of prostaglandins and is more sensitive to the constricting effects of oxygen.[50]

RDS also increases the risk for PDA. Exogenous surfactant, especially prophylactic use, also may increase the risk of symptomatic PDA.[50,51] PDA can further complicate the course of RDS.[50,52] T.S.'s course is typical of a preterm neonate with resolving RDS. T.S.'s pulmonary function improved after surfactant administration. Consequently, pulmonary vascular resistance decreased and the degree of left-to-right shunting across the ductus arteriosus increased, causing a deterioration in respiratory status. In addition, the excess fluid that T.S. received is an iatrogenic factor that may have increased the shunting across the PDA, aggravating the degree of pulmonary congestion.[50]

CASE 100-3, QUESTION 2: How is T.S.'s presentation consistent with that of PDA?

T.S.'s clinical presentation is related to the increased pulmonary blood flow, decreased systemic perfusion, and left ventricular volume overload that resulted from the shunting of left ventricular cardiac output through the PDA into the lungs. To compensate for the inadequate peripheral perfusion, HR increases. This results in an increase in cardiac output and a greater left-to-right shunt through the PDA, creating a vicious cycle. The widened pulse pressure (the difference between systolic and diastolic pressures, 32 mm Hg) is a result of diversion of aortic blood flow through the PDA, which is causing the bounding pulses. The systolic murmur, which is not always present, is the result of turbulent blood flow through the ductus arteriosus occurring as the pulmonary vascular resistance decreases. Tachycardia, hyperactive precordium, and a continuous murmur are results of the left-to-right shunting through the ductus arteriosus during systole.[53]

CASE 100-3, QUESTION 3: What are the potential complications of this hemodynamically significant PDA in T.S.?

The increased pulmonary blood flow and resultant pulmonary edema will worsen T.S.'s respiratory disease and increase the need for ventilatory support. The higher ventilatory settings (increase in MAP and FIO_2) place T.S. at risk for having BPD. If the PDA is left untreated, T.S. may experience congestive heart failure secondary to an increased left ventricular end-diastolic volume. A hemodynamically significant PDA also places T.S. at risk for IVH and NEC.[50]

Treatment

CASE 100-3, QUESTION 4: How should T.S.'s PDA be managed?

The initial medical management for T.S.'s symptomatic PDA is supportive care, which includes fluid management (e.g., fluid restriction and diuretic therapy), correction of anemia, and treatment of hypoxia and acidosis. Although excessive fluid administration may increase the risk of PDA, fluid restriction alone is unlikely to result in ductal closure. T.S.'s fluid intake should be restricted to 100 to 120 mL/kg/day (approximately 80% of total fluid maintenance requirements) to avoid worsening of her pulmonary edema and to prevent congestive heart failure.[50] Furosemide 1 mg/kg IV push should also be given to T.S. immediately to treat her pulmonary edema. In addition to fluid management, correction of anemia is important. Low concentrations of hemoglobin result in an increased cardiac output, which may worsen the infant's cardiac function. Anemia not only increases the demand of left ventricular output to ensure adequate oxygen delivery to the tissues, but may also increase the magnitude of the left-to-right shunt by decreasing the resistance of blood flow through the pulmonary vascular bed.[50] Maintaining a hematocrit level of more than 40% to 45% is often recommended. Because of T.S.'s gestational age, birth weight, and size of PDA, it is unlikely that she will respond to these general measures alone. Therefore, T.S. requires pharmacologic treatment with indomethacin or ibuprofen.

NONSTEROIDAL ANTI-INFLAMMATORY DRUGS

Both indomethacin and ibuprofen are available in injectable form for the treatment of PDA. These drugs nonspecifically inhibit prostaglandin synthesis, thereby eliminating the vasodilator effects of the PGE series on the ductus arteriosus, allowing the ductus to close. Indomethacin has been used clinically for more than 25 years for the treatment of PDA. However, because of its adverse effects, other prostaglandin inhibitors, such as ibuprofen, have been studied for PDA closure. Results indicate that ibuprofen is as effective as indomethacin in closing the ductus and causes significantly less of a decrease in renal, mesenteric, and cerebral blood flow. In a recent meta-analysis comparing ibuprofen with indomethacin, ibuprofen reduced the risks of NEC and transient adverse effects on renal function (e.g., oliguria, elevations of serum creatinine [SCr]).[54] However, the incidence of mortality, BPD, and IVH were similar for both drugs. Unfortunately, no long-term follow-up studies of ibuprofen exist. These studies are needed to determine whether ibuprofen or indomethacin is the drug of choice for PDA closure.[54] Based on the studies currently available, ibuprofen may be preferred in patients who have or are at risk for decreased renal function. The initial dose of ibuprofen lysine is 10 mg/kg followed by two doses of 5 mg/kg given at 24-hour intervals. If urinary output decreases to less than 0.6 mL/kg/hour, the second or third doses should be held.[2]

Unfortunately, not every infant who is treated with a nonsteroidal anti-inflammatory drug (NSAID) responds with constriction of the ductus arteriosus; therefore, surgical ligation of the PDA may be required. Ligation generally is reserved for neonates who do not respond to pharmacologic therapy or those in whom drug therapy is contraindicated.[50]

CASE 100-3, QUESTION 5: Because of a manufacturer's product recall and temporary shortage of ibuprofen, a decision is made to treat T.S. with indomethacin for closure of her PDA. What is the dose of indomethacin for T.S., and what route should be used for its administration?

The route of choice for indomethacin is IV; enteral indomethacin is less effective. This reduced effectiveness may be related to the formulation of the suspension and decreased, erratic enteral absorption. In addition, the use of enteral indomethacin has been associated with NEC.[55]

A large interpatient variability of indomethacin pharmacokinetics occurs in preterm neonates. Serum concentrations do not correlate consistently with therapeutic or adverse effects. Furthermore, the optimal therapeutic serum concentration is not yet defined.[56] Although many dosage regimens have been reported, dosing guidelines from the National Collaborative Study are commonly used.[52] Three indomethacin doses are given in 12- to 24-hour intervals, with the first dose equal to 0.2 mg/kg IV in all neonates. Because indomethacin clearance is directly proportional to postnatal age, the second and third doses are determined by postnatal age at initiation of indomethacin therapy. If onset of treatment was at less than 2 days' PNA, neonates receive 0.1 mg/kg/dose; if initiation of therapy occurred at 2 to 7 days' PNA, neonates receive 0.2 mg/kg/dose; and if therapy began at more than 7 days' PNA, neonates receive 0.25 mg/kg/dose. Second and third doses are administered at 12- to 24-hour intervals. No specific guidelines exist regarding which patients receive every-12-hour versus every-24-hour dosing; however, the individual dosing interval generally is determined by the neonate's urine output. If urine output remains greater than 1 mL/kg/hour after an indomethacin dose, then the next dose may be given in

12 hours. If urine output is less than 1 mL/kg/hour but greater than 0.6 mL/kg/hour, then the dosing interval may be extended to 24 hours. Doses should be held if urine output is less than 0.6 mL/kg/hour. T.S. should receive three doses of indomethacin 0.15 mg (0.2 mg/kg/dose) given every 12 hours, as long as her urine output remains greater than 1 mL/kg/hour. If T.S.'s urine output decreases, then the dosing interval should be adjusted as outlined above.

Other indomethacin dosing regimens have been evaluated more recently for the treatment of PDA in preterm infants. An initial dose of 0.2 mg/kg followed by either 0.1 or 0.2 mg/kg for two doses at 12- to 24-hour intervals has been used. In a study measuring serum concentrations, higher doses of indomethacin were required in older neonates (>10 days' PNA).[57] This may be owing to an increased indomethacin clearance in these infants. Because rapid IV administration of indomethacin can decrease cerebral, mesenteric, and renal blood flow, longer infusion rates of 20 to 30 minutes are recommended. Continuous infusion of indomethacin (for 36 hours) seems to reduce these adverse effects. However, data regarding effectiveness are inconclusive, and additional studies are needed.[58]

Response to NSAID therapy can be determined by assessing the clinical signs of PDA such as tachycardia, widened pulse pressure, bounding pulses, heart murmur, and the ability to wean from ventilator support. In certain cases, echocardiography may be performed to confirm closure of a PDA.

CASE 100-3, QUESTION 6: What clinical and laboratory data should be monitored during T.S.'s indomethacin therapy?

Before initiating indomethacin therapy, T.S. should receive an echocardiogram to rule out ductal-dependent congenital heart disease and to confirm the presence of a PDA. In addition, an SCr and blood urea nitrogen (BUN) should be obtained from T.S. before indomethacin therapy because nephrotoxicity is the most common adverse effect. Infants receiving indomethacin can experience transient oliguria with increased SCr. This occurs as a result of indomethacin-induced decreases in renal blood flow and glomerular filtration rate.[55] Dilutional hyponatremia may occur secondary to either decreased urine output or decreased free water diuresis owing to increased antidiuretic hormone activity. Treatment of hyponatremia should be aimed at decreasing free water intake through fluid restriction rather than by sodium supplementation. Typically, renal function normalizes within 72 hours after the last dose of indomethacin. In general, indomethacin therapy is contraindicated in neonates with renal failure, urine output less than 0.6 mL/kg/hour, or an SCr of 1.8 mg/dL or greater.[55]

Furosemide, which increases renal prostaglandin synthesis, has been suggested to help prevent indomethacin-associated renal toxicity. However, by increasing prostaglandins, furosemide may theoretically decrease ductal closure. Currently, studies do not support the routine use of furosemide in preterm neonates who receive indomethacin for the treatment of PDA. Furosemide is also contraindicated in patients who are dehydrated.[59] In addition to monitoring renal function and serum electrolytes, serum concentrations of aminoglycosides, digoxin, and other renally eliminated drugs should be monitored carefully. Indomethacin therapy may decrease renal drug clearance and cause accumulation of these agents, which may require a dosage reduction.[60]

A platelet count should also be obtained from T.S. before therapy because indomethacin may decrease platelet aggregation. Thrombocytopenia (platelet count, <50,000/μL) is a contraindication to indomethacin therapy.[52] In cases of thrombocytopenia, indomethacin may be withheld temporarily until platelets can be transfused. Other potential contraindications to indomethacin therapy include active bleeding and clinical evidence of NEC because GI bleeding, perforation, and NEC have been reported with indomethacin use.[50] These GI effects may be related to decreases in intestinal blood flow usually seen with rapid IV infusions. Grades II to IV IVH also are frequently quoted as contraindications to indomethacin therapy; however, indomethacin treatment probably is not associated with progression of IVH. In fact, prophylactic treatment with indomethacin may be associated with a decrease in the incidence of severe IVH (grades III and IV).[50,51]

CASE 100-3, QUESTION 7: When is the best time to initiate an NSAID for symptomatic treatment of T.S.'s PDA?

Conflicting data exist on when to initiate indomethacin or ibuprofen therapy for the treatment of symptomatic PDA. Some centers may opt to treat within the first 2 to 3 days of life (early symptomatic PDA) when infants initially present with clinical signs of PDA (i.e., murmur, widened pulse pressures, tachycardia). Others may not treat until clinical signs of congestive heart failure are present (late symptomatic PDA; 7–10 days of life).[51] Both treatment strategies (early and late) significantly decrease the incidence of PDA, but both cause significant transient reduction of urine output and SCr elevation. In some studies, infants receiving early treatment of indomethacin had significant reductions in the incidence of BPD and NEC and the need for surgical ligation.[51] In contrast, one study found that final PDA closure rates and the need for surgical ligation were comparable in early versus late indomethacin-treated neonates. In fact, spontaneous closure was observed in 43% of the late treatment group, which may indicate unnecessary treatment in the early group. In addition, renal adverse effects and ventilatory requirements were higher in the infants treated early.[61] Thus, early administration of indomethacin should not be used routinely; however, it is usually given to preterm neonates at high risk for having a large PDA. Clinically these recommendations can also be applied to ibuprofen. Because T.S. is an ELBW neonate with RDS, she is at high risk for exhibiting a large PDA. She also has clinical signs of a PDA and, thus, should be treated as soon as possible.

CASE 100-3, QUESTION 8: The physicians were able to decrease T.S.'s ventilator support within the first 12 to 24 hours after starting indomethacin treatment. After 3 to 4 days of gradual and consistent ventilator weaning, the ventilator settings could not be decreased further. During the next 2 to 3 days, T.S.'s respiratory status deteriorates, and she requires increased ventilator support. T.S. now has tachycardia, a widened pulse pressure, bounding pulses, and a hyperactive precordium. Repeat echocardiogram shows a small-to-moderate PDA. Current data include the following:

BUN, 10 mg/dL
SCr, 1.1 mg/dL
Sodium, 134 mEq/L
Potassium, 4.9 mEq/L
Chloride, 97 mEq/L
Urine output, 2.3 mL/kg/hour
Fluid intake, 130 mL/kg/day
Platelets, 180,000/μL

Why did PDA recur in T.S., and how should it be managed?

Successful closure of the PDA with indomethacin occurs in 70% to 90% of infants; however, ductal reopening or recurrence can occur in 20% to 35% of infants who initially respond to indomethacin.[62] Recurrence of PDA occurs especially in lower birth-weight infants. Several reasons might explain T.S.'s transient response to indomethacin. Recurrence of PDA is inversely proportional to gestational age; the incidence of ductal reopening is significantly higher in infants younger than 26 weeks' gestational age compared with infants born at 27 weeks' gestation or more (37% versus 11%, respectively).[63] The higher recurrence in younger gestational age neonates may be related to resumption of PGE_2 production after indomethacin serum concentrations decline and heightened sensitivity of the immature ductus arteriosus to the dilating effects of PGE_2.[50,62] This is particularly important in ventilator-dependent patients such as T.S. because mechanical ventilation increases circulating vasodilating prostaglandins. Furthermore, the rate of ductal reopening is independent of indomethacin serum concentrations, but seems to be related to the timing of indomethacin therapy, PNA, and the amount of fluid intake 24 hours before indomethacin treatment.[63] The rate of recurrence is lower in infants who were treated with indomethacin within the first 48 hours of life compared with those receiving treatment after 7 days of life.[50] Because anatomical closure of a PDA may be delayed for a couple of weeks, it is not surprising that the ductus arteriosus reopened in T.S. after her initial response to indomethacin.

Although controversial, prolonged indomethacin therapy may prevent recurrences and allow for permanent closure of the ductus arteriosus. Several prolonged treatment regimens have been successful in preventing ductal reopening.[50,62] One such regimen (indomethacin 0.2 mg/kg/dose IV every 12 hours for three doses, followed by 0.2 mg/kg/dose every 24 hours for five doses) was able to significantly decrease the recurrence of PDA from 47% to 10% in neonates less than 1,500 g without increasing toxicity. The need for surgical ligation also was decreased significantly.[62] However, some studies report an increased mortality in infants receiving prolonged therapy (seven doses) compared with those receiving the short course (three doses).[50] Furthermore, a recent meta-analysis demonstrated that prolonged therapy (six to eight doses) did not improve PDA closure, retreatment, reopening, or surgical ligation rates. Although prolonged courses were shown to decrease transient renal dysfunction, a significantly higher incidence of NEC was observed. Thus, the routine use of prolonged courses of indomethacin is not currently recommended.[64] Select use of prolonged therapy may be used. Individual patient response needs to be considered, especially in ELBW neonates. The optimal duration of indomethacin therapy and dosing regimen need to be identified.

T.S. remains ventilator-dependent and is at increased risk for exhibiting BPD. Because she has no contraindications to indomethacin therapy, a second course of indomethacin (0.1–0.2 mg/kg/dose every 12–24 hours for three to five doses) should be considered.[62] If the PDA fails to respond to this prolonged regimen or if it recurs again after an initial response, and T.S. remains ventilator-dependent, surgical ligation most likely will be required to permanently close the PDA.

Prophylactic Administration

CASE 100-3, QUESTION 9: Could prophylactic NSAID administration have prevented the development of a symptomatic PDA in T.S.?

Prophylactic indomethacin therapy is defined as the administration of indomethacin within 24 hours of life to newborns who are at risk of experiencing a symptomatic PDA.[65] However, routine prophylaxis would unnecessarily expose a large number of newborns to indomethacin (and its adverse effects), as PDA closure may occur spontaneously without treatment. Prophylactic use of indomethacin has short-term benefits; it significantly decreases the incidence of PDA and IVH (grades III and IV) and the need for PDA surgical ligation.[65] Unfortunately, most studies have not shown that prophylactic ductal closure with indomethacin decreases the incidence of death, BPD, NEC, or neurodevelopmental disabilities. Additionally, infants receiving prophylactic therapy have a higher incidence of severe oliguria or anuria, albeit transient.[65] Therefore, routine prophylactic administration is usually not warranted. It may be considered, however, in some neonatal units that do not have easy access to cardiac diagnostic and therapeutic services or that have a high incidence of IVH. Typically, preterm neonates, particularly those at high risk for experiencing a large PDA (e.g., ELBW neonates), are treated as soon as clinical signs appear.

Prophylactic ibuprofen therapy (administered at <24 hours of life) significantly decreases the incidence of PDA and the need for rescue pharmacologic treatment and surgical ligation.[66] However, it does not appear to decrease BPD, IVH, NEC, or mortality, and may increase the risk of renal dysfunction and sepsis. Because of the lack of long-term follow-up studies with the current ibuprofen lysine product, prophylactic ibuprofen therapy for the prevention of PDA is not recommended at this time.[66]

NECROTIZING ENTEROCOLITIS

CASE 100-4

QUESTION 1: C.D., a 15-day-old female neonate, was born at 28 weeks' gestational age with a birth weight of 908 g. Her postnatal course has been complicated by RDS, sepsis, and a large PDA for which she required intubation and mechanical ventilation, one dose of beractant, a 7-day course of ampicillin and gentamicin, and indomethacin. Enteral feedings with a standard preterm 24-cal/ounce formula were started on day 4 of life at 5 mL every 3 hours (44 mL/kg/day). Feedings were increased by 5 mL/feed on days 5 through 7 to 20 mL/feed every 3 hours on day 7 of life (176 mL/kg/day). This morning, C.D. exhibited a distended abdomen, bloody stools, multiple episodes of apnea that required reintubation and assisted ventilation, and metabolic acidosis. ABG results revealed the following:

pH, 7.15
PCO_2, 67 mm Hg
PO_2, 55 mm Hg
Base deficit, 10

An abdominal radiograph revealed pneumatosis intestinalis (the presence of gas in the intestinal submucosa). C.D. is to take nothing by mouth (NPO), and gentamicin 4 mg/kg IV infusion every 36 hours and ampicillin 50 mg/kg IV push every 12 hours are restarted. What clinical signs of NEC does C.D. have? What is the pathogenesis of NEC, and what risk factors for NEC does C.D. have?

NEC, a type of acute intestinal necrosis, is the most common life-threatening nonrespiratory condition, affecting 1,200 to 9,600 newborns in the United States each year.[67] The rate of hospitalization associated with NEC is 1.1 per 1,000 live births.[68] Approximately 62% to 94% of NEC occurs in premature infants; however, NEC can infrequently occur in full-term neonates.[69] NEC occurs in 3% to 15% of neonatal intensive care unit (ICU) admissions and has a mortality rate of 25% to 33%; approximately 25% of survivors experience long-term complications.[70,71] In addition, about 34% to 50% of infants with NEC require surgical intervention.[67] The total cost for caring for infants with NEC is about $500 million to $1 billion per year in the United States.[69] In addition, infants with NEC required longer hospitalizations (60 days longer if surgery is needed and 20 days longer if surgery is not needed) compared with infants without NEC. The age of onset of NEC is inversely related to gestational age and birth weight; the greater the gestational age of the infant at birth, the sooner the onset of NEC. Although NEC is less common in term infants, it usually develops within 3 to 4 days of birth. In contrast, infants born at approximately 30 weeks' gestation acquire NEC at a mean PNA of 20 days. Thus, preterm infants are at a risk for NEC for a longer time.[69,70] Although C.D. is extremely premature, she experienced NEC early (at 11 days of age), most likely because of the aggressive advancement of feedings.

C.D. has several clinical signs of NEC, including abdominal distension, bloody stools, apnea, metabolic acidosis, and pneumatosis intestinalis on abdominal radiograph. Gastric retention of feedings, respiratory distress, occult blood in stools, lethargy, temperature instability, thrombocytopenia, and neutropenia also may occur. NEC may progress to bowel perforation, peritonitis, sepsis, disseminated intravascular coagulopathy (DIC), and shock. On an abdominal radiograph, the presence of gas in the intestinal mucosa or in the portal venous system is diagnostic of NEC, and free air in the abdomen is observed with bowel perforation. (Go to **http://rad.usuhs.edu/medpix/new_topic.html?mode=single&recnum=9539&table=card&srchstr=&search=#images** for images of NEC.) Although these radiographic findings confirm the diagnosis of NEC, a lag time may occur between the initial clinical signs of NEC and radiologic confirmation.

NEC can evolve slowly during a period of 24 to 48 hours, from a clinically benign course to an advanced stage of shock, peritonitis, and widespread intestinal necrosis. Although NEC can affect any part of the GI tract, most of the disease is confined to the ileum and colon. A staging system, which categorizes severity according to systemic, intestinal, and radiologic signs, has been developed to permit a more consistent evaluation and treatment of patients.[72] Stages IA and IB NEC include neonates and infants with suspected disease or rule out NEC. These patients may have mild GI problems such as delayed gastric emptying and emesis, temperature instability, apnea, bright red blood from the rectum, or a mild ileus. Infants with stages IIA and IIB have definite NEC and usually present with abdominal distension, bloody stools, and the presence of pneumatosis intestinalis on radiograph. Infants in stage IIB NEC may also exhibit metabolic acidosis and thrombocytopenia. C.D.'s presentation is most consistent with stage IIB NEC. Infants with stages IIIA and IIIB (advanced disease) are severely ill with clinical signs, including peritonitis, ascites, shock, severe metabolic and respiratory acidosis, and DIC. Those with stage IIIB have intestinal perforation. Pneumatosis intestinalis, caused by hydrogen production from bacterial translocation into the bowel wall, is a classic and diagnostic radiographic finding of NEC. Because pneumatosis intestinalis may be hard to detect on radiographs, some infants can experience severe NEC needing surgery without having radiographic findings. Therefore, new criteria including biomarkers of NEC may be needed to help diagnosis NEC sooner and prevent its progression.

The pathogenesis of NEC is unknown, but seems to be multifactorial. Most likely, NEC results from the effects of intestinal bacteria and other factors on injured intestinal mucosa (Fig. 100-2). Inflammatory mediators such as platelet-activating factor, tumor necrosis factor-α, interleukin 1β, and interleukin 8 may also contribute to mucosal damage.[69,71] The neonatal intestinal mucosa is prone to injury for the following reasons: (a) increased permeability to potentially harmful substances, such as bacteria and proteins; (b) decreased immunologic host defenses, including low concentrations of immunoglobulin A in intestinal mucosa; and (c) decreased nonimmunologic defenses, such as decreased concentrations of proteases and gastric acid. Furthermore, inappropriate initial microbial colonization may also contribute to the pathogenesis of NEC in preterm neonates, especially because NEC does not occur until after 1 week of life, at a time when the gut has been colonized with anaerobic bacteria. In addition, numerous factors (both prenatal and postnatal) can cause injury to the neonatal intestinal mucosa and increase the risk for NEC.[69,71] Prenatal maternal factors include eclampsia, prolonged rupture of membranes, fetal distress, maternal cocaine use, and cesarean section. Postnatal factors include prematurity, low birth weight, ischemia or hypoxemia, asphyxia, hypotension, respiratory distress, apnea, malnutrition, infection, hemodynamically significant PDA, congenital GI anomalies, cyanotic heart disease, toxins, hyperosmolar substances (e.g., feedings, medications), rapid advancement of enteral feedings, exchange transfusions, and the presence of umbilical catheters.[69–71] Medications such as corticosteroids, indomethacin, and H_2-blockers and prolonged empiric IV antibiotic use have also been associated with an increase risk of NEC.[69,73] However, the most significant clinical risk factor for NEC is prematurity.[72]

C.D. has several risks for developing NEC, which include prematurity (gestational age of 28 weeks), ELBW (908 g), history of infection, and RDS requiring mechanical ventilation. Furthermore, C.D. not only was given a hyperosmolar formula (24 cal/ounce instead of 20 cal/ounce) but her feedings were advanced aggressively. These two factors may also contribute to the development of NEC. More than 90% of infants with NEC have received enteral feedings, although NEC also occurs in infants who have never been fed.[71] Enteral feedings (breast milk or formulas) serve as substrates for bacterial proliferation in the gut. As a result, reducing substances, organic acids, and hydrogen gas are produced by bacterial fermentation of these nutrients. Although studies have shown that rapid advancements in the volume of feeds (30 mL/kg/day versus 15–20 mL/kg/day) were associated with an increased risk of NEC, a systematic review reported that infants advanced at a rate of 30 to 35 mL/kg/day reach full enteral intake and regain birth weight significantly earlier than infants advanced at 10 to 20 mL/kg/day without increasing the risk of NEC or NEC with perforation.[74] Similarly, older studies reported that early initiation of feeds might increase the risk of NEC; however, a recent review failed to confirm these findings. In fact, infants who were fed earlier (within 4 days of birth) had a significant reduction in the number of days on parenteral nutrition. C.D. was started at a much higher initial feeding volume (44 mL/kg/day) and aggressively increased by 44 mL/kg/day, which may have increased the risk of NEC. If C.D. were appropriately fed, she would have reached full feedings in 7 to 14 days instead of 4 days. Last, the presence of PDA and the use of indomethacin for the treatment of PDA may also have contributed to NEC in C.D. through decreased mesenteric blood flow with resultant ischemia and intestinal mucosal injury.[70]

Treatment

CASE 100-4, QUESTION 2: How should C.D. be managed?

Significant abdominal distension may compromise respiratory function and blood flow to the intestines. Therefore, as soon as NEC is suspected, feedings should be stopped immediately

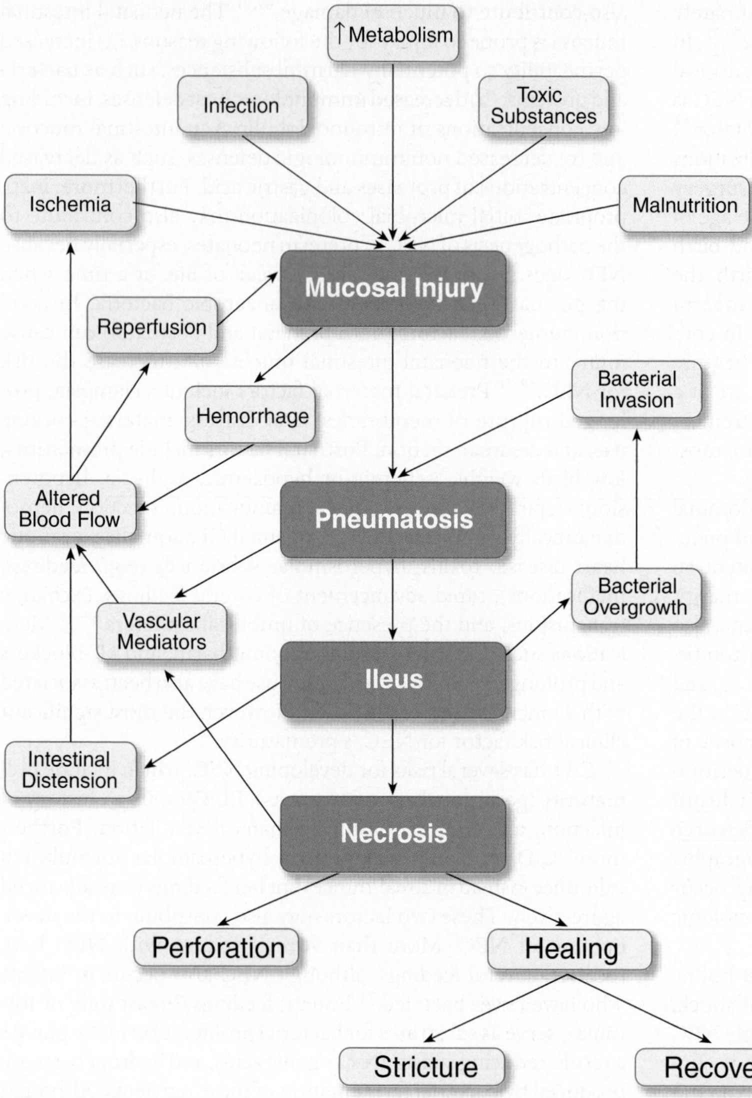

FIGURE 100-2 Necrotizing enterocolitis (NEC). This schematic is a composite of the theories about factors believed to be involved in the pathogenesis of NEC. The progression of this disease is denoted in large type. The factors believed to initiate or propagate the disease process are in smaller type. (Adapted with permission from Crouse DT. Necrotizing enterocolitis. In: Pomerance JJ, Richardson CJ, eds. *Neonatology for the Clinician*. Norwalk, CT: Appleton & Lange; 1993:364.)

and an orogastric tube with low intermittent suction placed to decompress the abdomen. C.D.'s vital signs and abdominal circumference should be closely monitored for disease progression. A complete blood count and platelet count should be obtained frequently to monitor for neutropenia and thrombocytopenia. Blood, urine, and stool cultures should be obtained, and parenteral antibiotics should be started as soon as possible; 20% to 30% of infants with NEC have associated bacteremia. Radiographic examinations should be routinely performed at least every 4 to 8 hours or as needed to evaluate the progression of the disease. In infants with stage I NEC, antibiotic therapy is usually given for 3 days pending culture results and clinical signs. Once the diagnosis of NEC is ruled out, antibiotics may be discontinued.[72] Enteral feedings can then be initiated slowly. However, if the diagnosis of NEC is made, antibiotics are continued and parenteral nutrition is initiated at that time. Infants require 7 to 14 days of bowel rest (NPO). The length of antibiotic therapy and bowel rest in infants with documented NEC (stages II or III) is determined by the severity of systemic illness (e.g., metabolic acidosis, thrombocytopenia). C.D. has stage IIB disease and needs to be NPO for at least 10 to 14 days; she requires total parenteral nutrition during that time, and the surgery team should be notified at this point. Infants with stage III disease may also require fluid resuscitation, administration of inotropic agents such as dopamine and dobutamine, and surgical intervention, especially for those with perforated NEC.[70] Two large multicenter trials reported no significant differences in survival rate, duration of hospitalization, and dependence on parenteral nutrition (assessed 90 days postoperatively) between primary peritoneal drainage versus laparotomy with bowel resection in preterm infants with perforated NEC.[75,76] However, a systematic review reported an increase of more than 50% in mortality in infants who had undergone peritoneal drainage versus laparotomy.[69] In addition, infants who had undergone laparotomy had a significantly reduced risk of death or neurodevelopmental impairment at 18 to 22 months' follow-up compared with those in the peritoneal drainage group. Despite the type of surgical interventions, up to 50% of ELBW infants who require surgery will die.[69]

CASE 100-4, QUESTION 3: C.D. just completed a 7-day course of ampicillin and gentamicin. Is it appropriate to restart these antibiotics?

The selection of antibiotics for NEC depends on the common micro-organisms observed in an individual neonatal unit and their sensitivities. Many organisms have been implicated in NEC, including Enterobacteriaceae (e.g., *Escherichia coli*, *Klebsiella* species), *Pseudomonas*, *Staphylococcus aureus* (in rare cases, methicillin resistant), *Staphylococcus epidermidis*, *Clostridium*, enteroviruses, and rotaviruses.[72,77] For most cases of NEC, treatment with a broad-spectrum penicillin, such as ampicillin, and an aminoglycoside (e.g., gentamicin) is appropriate.

However, in some nurseries, *S. epidermidis* is the most common cause of neonatal nosocomial infections. Increases in *S. epidermidis*–associated NEC also have been reported. Therefore, vancomycin and an aminoglycoside may be used as routine treatment in some nurseries or in specific patients at risk for *Staphylococcus* infections (e.g., neonates with central catheters or prolonged ICU stays). Vancomycin may be more appropriate than ampicillin because vancomycin has coverage against methicillin-resistant *S. epidermidis,* as well as enterococcal and streptococcal species. Because C.D. has been hospitalized for longer than 1 week and weighs less than 1,000 g, vancomycin and gentamicin may be more appropriate, especially if her neonatal ICU has a high incidence of staphylococcal nosocomial infections. C.D. should be treated with parenteral antibiotics for 10 to 14 days.

Other antibiotic combinations used to treat NEC include cefotaxime and vancomycin, and cefotaxime and ampicillin. The combination of cefotaxime and vancomycin has been shown to prevent severe peritonitis and death and reduce the need for surgery in less than 2,200-g birth-weight neonates with NEC, whereas gentamicin and ampicillin have not. Suppression of aerobic fecal flora by the combination of cefotaxime and vancomycin, but not by ampicillin and gentamicin, may explain these findings.[77] Therefore, if C.D. is not responding to vancomycin and gentamicin, consideration should be made to replace gentamicin with cefotaxime.

CASE 100-4, QUESTION 4: Two days later, C.D. exhibits peritonitis with ascites, hypotension, worsening metabolic acidosis, neutropenia, and DIC. IV fluids and dopamine are administered for the hypotension, fresh-frozen plasma and whole blood are given to treat the coagulopathy, and morphine 0.05 mg/kg IV push every 4 hours as needed is started for pain control. Free air in the abdomen is observed on abdominal radiograph. Blood and urine cultures have had no growth for 48 hours. What additional antimicrobial coverage should be provided?

Peritonitis secondary to intestinal perforation may be polymicrobial, involving both aerobes and anaerobes. Therefore, an antimicrobial agent with anaerobic activity should be added to C.D.'s current regimen.[70] Empiric anaerobic coverage is recommended in infants with definite NEC, stage II or III.[77] The two most commonly used agents are clindamycin and metronidazole.[71,77] Routine use of clindamycin in the treatment of NEC has not decreased the incidence of intestinal gangrene, perforation, or death. In addition, it has been associated with an increased incidence of abdominal strictures.[77] There are no studies to demonstrate the efficacy of metronidazole in this patient population, but the lack of reports documenting adverse effects in preterm infants has made it the agent of choice in some hospitals.

Complications and Prognosis

CASE 100-4, QUESTION 5: C.D. is taken urgently to the operating room, and 40 cm of necrotic ileum is removed along with the ileocecal valve. What long-term nutritional problems is C.D. likely to have?

The most common postoperative complications of NEC are intestinal strictures (up to 20%) and short-bowel syndrome (25%).[67,71] C.D. is at risk of experiencing short-bowel syndrome, a condition of malabsorption and malnutrition that results from surgical removal of a significant portion of the small intestine. The most important factors that determine short-bowel syndrome are the length of the remaining small intestine and the presence of the ileocecal valve. Because C.D. has had a majority of her ileum and her ileocecal valve removed, she most likely will suffer from short-bowel syndrome.

Because the terminal ileum is an important site for absorption of vitamins, trace minerals, and nutrients, C.D. will be at risk for decreased absorption of these substances. C.D. also will have a faster GI transit time and diarrhea because her ileocecal valve was removed. (The ileocecal valve plays a major role in controlling intestinal transit time.) Absorption of enterally administered medications also may be decreased in patients with short-bowel syndrome. As C.D. starts to receive most of her nutrition enterally, she should be monitored for fat malabsorption and other nutritional deficiencies (e.g., deficiencies in vitamins A, B_{12}, D, E, and K), and supplemented accordingly.

Owing to advances in earlier diagnosis and aggressive treatment, approximately 65% to 75% of all infants with NEC survive.[71] However, infants with NEC are significantly more likely to have neurodevelopmental impairment (e.g., cerebral palsy); those requiring surgical management are at higher risk.

Prevention

CASE 100-4, QUESTION 6: What could have been done to prevent NEC in C.D.?

Several interventions may decrease the incidence of NEC. Enteral feedings in preterm infants can be withheld for several weeks and parenteral nutrition initiated. Intestinal priming or trophic feeding (i.e., using a small amount of full-strength formula or breast milk for several days to stimulate GI mucosal development) has been shown to decrease the incidence of NEC compared with infants with advancement of feedings.[71,74] Because breast milk provides antibodies, growth factors, and cellular immune factors, it may reduce the incidence of NEC. In fact, NEC was six to ten times less common among infants fed human milk exclusively than in those fed formula alone, and three times less common in those fed a combination of human milk and formula than in those fed formula alone.[71] In a recent study, a significant decrease in the incidence of NEC and NEC requiring surgical intervention was observed in infants who were exclusively fed with a human milk-based diet compared with a combination of human milk- and formula-based diets.[78] In contrast, the use of hyperosmolar formulas or medications can cause osmotic injury to the bowel and may result in NEC. Maternal steroids (commonly used to accelerate fetal lung maturation) can decrease the incidence of NEC owing to a maturational effect on the microvillous membranes.

Although prophylactic enteral administration of antibiotics (i.e., gentamicin or vancomycin) has been shown to decrease the incidence of NEC, its routine use is not recommended.[71] Infants with NEC may be infected with different types of organisms, and treatment with one enteral antibiotic may not provide adequate antibacterial coverage in these infants. In addition, prophylactic use of these antibiotics has been associated with the emergence of resistant organisms, especially with long and repeated courses.[69,71]

Probiotics are live, nonpathogenic microbial preparations that colonize the intestine and have a beneficial effect on the health of the host. Probiotic micro-organisms commonly used are strains of *Lactobacillus* and *Bifidobacterium*. In a recent Cochrane review, enteral administration of probiotics has been shown to significantly decrease the risk of severe NEC and death and to shorten the time to full feedings in VLBW infants.[79] One major concern is that exposing immunologically immature VLBW infants to probiotics may potentially increase the risk for infections. Although the Cochrane review did not find an increased risk for infections in neonates receiving probiotics, one individual study did identify a significant risk of sepsis in infants weighing less than 750 g.[79] Other controversies exist. Most studies did not evaluate the effects of probiotics in ELBW infants, the population at greatest risk for NEC. The optimal type of probiotic (species, strains, single or combined, live or killed) and the timing, dosage, and duration of therapy are still unknown. Little is known regarding the benefits of probiotics in infants who are exclusively or partially fed breast milk. Furthermore, there is currently no product in the United States that has the appropriate regulatory mechanisms in place to ensure the quality of the product. Lastly, the long-term effects of probiotics for the prevention of NEC in VLBW infants are unknown. Therefore, clinical studies are needed to address these issues, and if probiotics are administered to VLBW infants for the prevention of NEC, careful surveillance of mortality, NEC, and emergence of resistant strains will be necessary. When C.D. is ready to be fed, breast milk (if available) should be used in place of formula to help prevent future risk of NEC. Although probiotics have been shown to significantly decrease the incidence of NEC, their use cannot be recommended for C.D. at this time.

NEONATAL SEPSIS AND MENINGITIS

CASE 100-5

QUESTION 1: J.E., a 28-week gestation, 850-g male, was born to a mother with prolonged rupture of membranes (> 72 hours). The newborn's mother is febrile with a white blood cell (WBC) count of 20 × $10^3/\mu L$ and differential of 70% segmented neutrophils, 20% bands, 7% lymphocytes, and 3% monocytes. J.E. had Apgar scores of 3 at 1 minute, 4 at 5 minutes, and 7 at 10 minutes after birth. Mechanical ventilation was instituted, and J.E. was admitted to the neonatal ICU. Vital signs on admission were as follows:

HR, 190 beats/minute
Temperature, 35.8°C
BP, 56/33 mm Hg

Blood and urine cultures are pending. Significant laboratory data include the following:

WBC 2,400 cells/μL with a differential of 25% segmented neutrophils, 15% bands, 45% lymphocytes, 10% monocytes, 4% eosinophils, and 1% basophils
Platelets, 45,000/μL
C-reactive protein (CRP), 5 mg/dL

What is the etiology and pathogenesis of neonatal sepsis? What risk factors for sepsis does J.E. have? What clinical signs and laboratory evidence of sepsis are apparent in J.E.?

Bacterial sepsis significantly contributes to neonatal morbidity and mortality. Neonates, especially preterm newborns, are at increased risk for infections and should be considered immunocompromised. The neonate's decreased immune function (e.g., immature function of neutrophils, lower amounts of immunoglobulin) also results in a reduced ability to localize infections. Once a tissue site becomes infected, bacteria can spread easily, resulting in disseminated disease. In addition, the lack of opsonic antibodies in preterm infants such as J.E. increases the susceptibility to infections caused by bacteria with polysaccharide capsules (e.g., group B streptococcus, *E. coli*, *Haemophilus influenzae* type B).[80]

The incidence of neonatal sepsis is inversely proportional to birth weight and gestational age and ranges from 6 to 9 cases per 1,000 live births. However, the incidence is much higher in VLBW neonates (~25%).[81] Risk factors (as demonstrated in J.E.) include prematurity, low birth weight, male sex, and predisposing maternal conditions (e.g., prolonged rupture of membranes, maternal fever, elevated maternal WBC or left shift, chorioamnionitis, and urinary tract infection).[82,83] Despite treatment, mortality rates for neonatal sepsis can be as high as 30% to 50%, with the highest mortality observed in newborns less than 1,500 g.[84] Meningitis occurs as a complication of bacterial sepsis in 10% to 30% of septic neonates[84] and has a mortality rate of 20% to 50%, depending on the pathogen.[82] Long-term sequelae of meningitis have been reported in about 20% to 60% of survivors and include hearing loss, abnormal behavior, developmental delay, cerebral palsy, focal motor disability, seizure disorders, and hydrocephalus.[80,85]

Common Pathogens

The fetal environment within the amniotic membranes is normally sterile until the onset of labor and delivery. Once the membranes are ruptured, the infant may be at risk for colonization of micro-organisms from the maternal genital tract. Many of these organisms do not cause infection in the mother, but may be detrimental to the infant. Early-onset neonatal sepsis (sepsis that presents during the first 5–7 days of life) usually is caused by organisms acquired from the maternal genital tract. The most common pathogens found in early-onset neonatal sepsis are group B streptococcus (50%) and *E. coli* (20%). Other primary pathogens include *Listeria monocytogenes, Enterococcus,* and other gram-negative bacilli (e.g., *H. influenzae, Klebsiella pneumoniae*). Late-onset sepsis (sepsis presenting after 5–7 days' PNA) usually is caused by these primary organisms or by nosocomial pathogens, such as coagulase-negative staphylococci (CONS), particularly *S. epidermidis, S. aureus, Pseudomonas* species, anaerobes, and *Candida* species.[86] The presence of IV catheters (umbilical or central) and duration of parenteral hyperalimentation are major risk factors for nosocomial septicemia.[86,87] Other risk factors include prematurity, low birth weight, prolonged hospital stay, prior antibiotic use, lipid emulsion, use of H_2-blockers, invasive procedures, GI disease (including NEC), the presence of other indwelling devices (e.g., ETTs, ventriculoperitoneal shunts), and nasal CPAP.[81,87]

Seventy percent of late-onset sepsis in VLBW infants is caused by gram-positive organisms, with CONS being the most common pathogen (68%); *S. aureus, Enterococcus* species, and group B streptococcus account for the remainder.[88] The emergence of CONS (such as *S. epidermidis*) as the most common pathogen is most likely related to the increased survival of extremely premature neonates with a resultant prolonged hospital stay and an increase in the associated risks of infection (i.e., placement of umbilical, central venous, and arterial catheters, use of hyperalimentation). Clinically, before continuation of antibiotic therapy, it is important to distinguish whether patient isolates of CONS are the result of colonization of the catheters or IV tubing or represent true bacteremia.

Neonatal sepsis may present with nonspecific or subtle signs, especially in VLBW infants.[82] The most common signs are poor feeding, temperature instability, lethargy, or apnea.[82,84] Other signs of neonatal sepsis include glucose instability (hypoglycemia or hyperglycemia), tachycardia, dyspnea or cyanosis, tachypnea, diarrhea, vomiting, feeding intolerance, abdominal distension, metabolic acidosis, and abnormal WBC.[82] Clinical signs and laboratory evidence of neonatal sepsis observed in J.E. include tachycardia (HR, 190 beats/minute), hypothermia (temperature 35.8°C), leukopenia (WBC, 2.4 × $10^3/\mu L$), neutropenia (absolute neutrophil count of 960/μL), a left shift in the differential (i.e., an immature-to-total neutrophil ratio [I/T] of 0.38), thrombocytopenia (platelets, 45,000/μL), and an elevated CRP (5 mg/dL). Hypothermia is more common than fever in neonatal sepsis, especially in preterm newborns. However, if fever is present, it is strongly associated with bacterial infection. Neutropenia, especially with a left shift (as seen in J.E.) can be a sign of WBC depletion from bone marrow owing to overwhelming sepsis. An elevated WBC also can indicate a neonatal infection, but may be less specific. The I/T ratio, defined as band forms plus any earlier cells divided by the total neutrophil count (including early cells), has been shown to be useful in diagnosing neonatal sepsis. An I/T ratio of less than 0.3 is normal.[83] CRP, an acute-phase reactant protein associated with tissue injury in response to an inflammatory process, may also be included as part of a sepsis workup. A CRP level of more than 1 mg/dL indicates inflammation and possible infection.[83] In infants with bacterial infection, serum CRP levels begin to increase 6 to 8 hours after the onset of the illness and peak after 2 to 3 days.[89] Therefore, because of the delayed response, the use of CRP for evaluation of early-onset sepsis is not of great value. Serial CRP levels obtained during 2 to 3 days of illness may aid in the determination of duration of empiric antibiotic therapy. Empiric antibiotic therapy may be discontinued in infants with normal serial CRP levels in the absence of any clinical signs suggestive of sepsis. However, elevated CRP levels can be found in other clinical conditions such as viral infection, ischemic tissue injuries, hemolysis, or chorioamnionitis. Therefore, CRP levels should be used with caution as the sole diagnostic criteria for sepsis or bacteremia. Late signs of neonatal infection include jaundice, hepatosplenomegaly, and petechiae.[82] A bulging fontanel, posturing, or seizures indicate meningitis, although these CNS signs are not always present when meningitis exists.

Bacterial meningitis should always be considered in infants with neonatal sepsis; up to 25% of neonates with bacteremia can have bacterial meningitis.[80] The major pathogens causing neonatal sepsis are also the primary pathogens that cause neonatal meningitis. Seventy-five percent of neonatal meningitis is caused by group B streptococcus and *E. coli*, with *L. monocytogenes* being the third most common organism.[84] The definitive diagnostic method for bacterial meningitis is lumbar puncture. Lumbar puncture should be performed in infants with a positive blood culture, abnormal neurologic signs, an elevated WBC or left shift, or the presence of bacterial antigen in the urine.[90] A lumbar puncture is not needed in neonates receiving empiric antibiotics solely because of maternal risk factors.[89] However, it is important to note that a negative blood culture does not dictate the absence of bacterial meningitis. Approximately 1 of every 4,000 live births has culture-proven bacterial meningitis, and 15% to 50% of infants with bacterial meningitis may have a negative blood culture.[89] The cerebrospinal fluid (CSF) should be tested with a Gram stain, cell counts with differential, glucose and protein levels, and bacterial culture. Normal CSF cell counts and protein concentrations are different for neonates compared with older children and adults. For example, the CSF protein concentration in a healthy neonate is about two to three times that of an adult and decreases with age; preterm infants may have higher levels.[80] Neonatal CSF cell counts are also difficult to interpret because values observed with meningitis may overlap with normal neonatal values. The diagnosis of neonatal sepsis is confirmed by isolation of the pathogen from blood, urine, CSF, or other body sites. Latex agglutination tests that detect antigens (e.g., bacterial cell wall fragments) of group B streptococcus, *E. coli, S. pneumonia, N. meningitidis,* and *H. influenzae* type B in body fluids can facilitate a prompt diagnosis, especially in patients who previously were treated with antibiotics.

Treatment of Sepsis and Meningitis

CASE 100-5, QUESTION 2: What antibiotic regimen should be prescribed for J.E.?

Empiric treatment with appropriate IV antibiotics must be initiated immediately in J.E. Significant morbidity or fatality would occur if antibiotics were withheld until a diagnosis was confirmed by culture results (in 24–72 hours). This is especially true in patients in whom meningitis is suspected. The initial empiric antibiotic treatment of choice for early-onset neonatal sepsis and meningitis is ampicillin plus an aminoglycoside (Tables 100-4, 100-5).[2,91–93] These antibiotics are used because they (a) are bactericidal against the common neonatal pathogens; (b) penetrate into the CNS; (c) are relatively safe; and (d) have proven clinical efficacy. If the culture is positive for group B streptococcus, ampicillin should be replaced with high-dose penicillin G because of its higher activity against group B streptococcus. If meningitis is highly suspected, gentamicin may be replaced by a third-generation cephalosporin (i.e., cefotaxime) owing to greater CSF penetration compared with aminoglycosides.

Therefore, ampicillin 45 mg every 12 hours IV plus an aminoglycoside (e.g., gentamicin 4.2 mg every 48 hours IV) should be started in J.E. for suspected neonatal sepsis and possible meningitis. Meningitic doses of ampicillin should be used in J.E. until meningitis can be ruled out. Ampicillin is active against group B streptococci, group D streptococci, *Listeria,* and most strains of *E. coli.* Aminoglycoside antibiotics (e.g., gentamicin or tobramycin) usually are active against gram-negative bacilli. In addition, aminoglycosides may provide synergy with ampicillin against *Listeria* and group B streptococci.[83] Selection of the specific aminoglycoside should be determined by antibiotic

TABLE 100-4
Gentamicin Dosing Guidelines for Neonates and Infants[2,92]

Traditional Dosing		
Age	**Weight**	**Dosing Regimen**
GA <38 weeks	<1,000 g	3.5 mg/kg/dose every 24 hours
PNA 0–4 weeks	<1,200 g	2.5 mg/kg/dose every 18–24 hours
PNA ≤7 days	≥1,200 g	2.5 mg/kg/dose every 12 hours
PNA >7 days	1,200–2,000 g	2.5 mg/kg/dose every 8–12 hours
PNA >7 days	>2,000 g	2.5 mg/kg/dose every 8 hours
Extended-Interval Dosing		
Age	**≤29 Weeks GA**	**30–34 Weeks GA**
PNA 0–7 days	5 mg/kg/dose every 48 hours	4.5 mg/kg/dose every 36 hours
PNA 8–28 days	4 mg/kg/dose every 36 hours	4 mg/kg/dose every 24 hours
PNA ≥29 days	4 mg/kg/dose every 24 hours	4 mg/kg/dose every 24 hours

GA, gestational age; PNA, postnatal age.

TABLE 100-5

Antimicrobial Dosage Regimens for Neonates: Dosages and Intervals of Administration[2,91–93]

	Weight <1,200 g	Weight 1,200–2,000 g		Weight >2,000 g	
Drug	**0–4 Weeks (mg/kg)[a]**	**0–7 Days (mg/kg)[a]**	**8–28 Days (mg/kg)[a]**	**0–7 Days (mg/kg)[a]**	**8–28 Days[a] (mg/kg)[a]**
Amphotericin B					
Deoxycholate	1 every 24 hours	1 every 24 hours	1 every 24 hours	1 every 24 hours	1 every 24 hours
Lipid complex/ Liposomal	5 every 24 hours	5 every 24 hours	5 every 24 hours	5 every 24 hours	5 every 24 hours
Ampicillin					
Meningitis	100 every 12 hours	100 every 8 hours	75 every 6 hours	50 every 8 hours	75 every 6 hours
Other diseases	25 every 12 hours	25 every 12 hours	25 every 8 hours	25 every 8 hours	25 every 6 hours
Cefazolin	25 every 12 hours	25 every 12 hours	25 every 12 hours	25 every 12 hours	25 every 8 hours
Cefepime	30 every 12 hours	50 every 12 hours	30 every 12 hours[b]	50 every 12 hours	30 every 12 hours[b]
Cefotaxime[c]	50 every 12 hours	50 every 12 hours	50 every 8 hours	50 every 12 hours	50 every 8 hours
Ceftazidime[c]	50 every 12 hours	50 every 12 hours	50 every 8 hours	50 every 12 hours	50 every 8 hours
Ceftriaxone[c]	25 every 24 hours	50 every 24 hours	50 every 24 hours	50 every 24 hours	75 every 24 hours
Clindamycin	5 every 12 hours	5 every 12 hours	5 every 8 hours	5 every 8 hours	5 every 6 hours
Erythromycin	10 every 12 hours	10 every 12 hours	10 every 8 hours	10 every 12 hours	13.3 every 8 hours
Fluconazole	6 every 72 hours	12 every 48 hours	12 every 24 hours	12 every 48 hours	12 every 24 hours
Linezolid	10 every 12 hours	10 every 12 hours	10 every 8 hours	10 every 8 hours	10 every 8 hours
Meropenem[c]	20 every 12 hours	20 every 12 hours	20 every 8 hours	20 every 8 hours	30 every 8 hours
Metronidazole	7.5 every 48 hours	7.5 every 24 hours	7.5 every 12 hours	7.5 every 12 hours	15 every 12 hours
Oxacillin	25 every 12 hours	25 every 12 hours	25 every 8 hours	25 every 8 hours	37.5 every 6 hours
Nafcillin	25 every 12 hours	25 every 12 hours	25 every 8 hours	25 every 8 hours	37.5 every 6 hours
Penicillin G					
Meningitis	50,000 U every 12 hours	50,000 U every 12 hours	50,000 U every 8 hours	50,000 U every 12 hours	50,000 U every 8 hours
Other diseases	25,000 U every 12 hours	25,000 U every 12 hours	25,000 U every 8 hours	25,000 U every 12 hours	25,000 U every 8 hours
Piperacillin/tazobactam	50 every 12 hours	75 every 12 hours	75 every 8 hours	75 every 12 hours	75 every 8 hours
Ticarcillin or Ticarcillin/ clavulanate	75 every 12 hours	75 every 12 hours	75 every 8 hours	75 every 12 hours	75 every 8 hours
Vancomycin	15 every 24 hours[d]	15[e]	15[e]	15[e]	15[e]

[a] Postnatal age.
[b] Cefepime should be given at 30 mg/kg/dose every 12 hours for the first 2 weeks of life then increase to 50 mg/kg/dose every 12 hours (or 50 mg/kg/dose every 8 hours for *Pseudomonas* infections or meningitis).
[c] Higher dosage may be needed for meningitis.
[d] If weight <750 g and postnatal age <14 days, use 10–12.5 mg/kg every 24 hours.
[e] If ≤26 weeks' PCA, use every 18 hours; if 27–34 weeks' PCA, use every 12 hours; if >35 weeks' PCA, use every 8 hours.

resistance patterns within the neonatal ICU. Amikacin should be reserved for gram-negative organisms resistant to gentamicin and tobramycin. Aminoglycoside regimens need to be designed to achieve safe and therapeutic serum concentrations (traditional dosing regimens: gentamicin and tobramycin, peak 6–8 mcg/mL, trough <2 mcg/mL; amikacin peak 20–30 mcg/mL, trough <10 mcg/mL) and to aim for a peak concentration that is more than eight times greater than the minimum inhibitory concentration (MIC) of the organism being treated.[94] If extended-interval aminoglycoside dosing is used, peak gentamicin and tobramycin serum concentrations of 10 to 12 mcg/mL and trough concentrations of less than 1 mcg/mL may be reasonable, depending on the MIC.

Extended-interval aminoglycoside dosing (also known as once-daily dosing or single-daily dosing) has been widely used in the adult population. Aminoglycoside antibiotics display concentration-dependent killing of bacteria. Rationale for the use of extended-interval aminoglycoside dosing include (a) enhancement of bacterial killing by providing a higher peak serum concentration to MIC ratio, (b) provision of a prolonged postantibiotic effect, and (c) minimization of adaptive postexposure microbial resistance.[95]

Because of these beneficial effects, the use of extended-interval aminoglycoside dosing has been studied in the neonatal population. However, most of the studies, which included term and preterm infants, evaluated serum gentamicin concentrations and potential adverse effects but not clinical efficacy or cure rates.[95,96] Furthermore, most studies used extended-interval aminoglycoside dosing for short periods, for example, during the workup to rule out neonatal sepsis (i.e., 72-hour duration). Studies included only a limited number of neonates who received extended-interval aminoglycoside dosing to actually treat documented neonatal infections.

As expected, the use of extended-interval aminoglycoside dosing resulted in higher peak and lower trough serum concentrations in these neonates compared with traditional multiple-daily dosing. Two meta-analyses reported clinical efficacy of extended-interval aminoglycoside dosing compared with conventional dosing in neonates.[95] In one review, only one of nine trials reported treatment failure in two neonates; no differences in ototoxicity or nephrotoxicity were found between the two dosing methods. In the second meta-analysis, which included six studies in neonates, there was no difference in efficacy or toxicity between the two dosing methods of aminoglycoside in neonates. However, currently there are no neonatal studies evaluating optimal regimens to achieve the best peak serum concentration to MIC ratio. In addition, other neonatal-specific factors, such as the neonate's immature immune function and a potential decreased postantibiotic effect, have not been adequately addressed. Therefore, large, well-designed studies evaluating the clinical efficacy and safety of extended-interval aminoglycoside dosing for the treatment of gram-negative infections in neonates are required before routine use of extended-interval aminoglycoside dosing can be recommended.

In some nurseries, a third-generation cephalosporin (e.g., cefotaxime or ceftriaxone), instead of an aminoglycoside, is added to ampicillin for initial empiric treatment of early-onset neonatal sepsis and meningitis.[81,87,94] The spectrum of activity of these third-generation cephalosporins includes many gram-negative organisms and group B streptococci. However, third-generation cephalosporins do not have sufficient activity against *Listeria* or group D streptococci. Therefore, these agents must be used in combination with ampicillin for empiric neonatal therapy. Ceftriaxone should be avoided in neonates with hyperbilirubinemia owing to bilirubin displacement from albumin-binding sites. Ceftriaxone has also been associated with sludging in the gallbladder and cholestasis.[2,94] In addition, calcium-ceftriaxone precipitates have been found in the lungs and kidneys of neonates when ceftriaxone was administered with calcium-containing solutions. Several fatalities have been reported; ceftriaxone should not be administered within 48 hours of calcium-containing solutions or products.[94] Hence, cefotaxime is the preferred cephalosporin for neonatal use.

The third-generation cephalosporins have advantages over the aminoglycosides, including better CNS penetration, the elimination of serum concentration measurements, and less nephrotoxicity. However, these cephalosporins do not significantly improve clinical or microbiological end points compared with the standard ampicillin and gentamicin regimen. In fact, overuse of cefotaxime during the first few days of life has been associated with an increased risk of death compared with the use of gentamicin.[94] Furthermore, extensive use of the third-generation cephalosporins in neonatal ICUs may lead to rapid emergence of resistant gram-negative bacilli (e.g., *Enterobacter cloacae, Pseudomonas aeruginosa,* and *Serratia* species) and vancomycin resistance in enterococci. Also, prolonged treatment has been associated with an increased risk of neonatal candidiasis.[94] In contrast, only rare cases of gentamicin resistance have been reported.[81] Thus, combinations such as ampicillin and cefotaxime should be reserved for the following situations: (a) neonatal ICUs in which aminoglycoside resistance to gram-negative enteric bacilli is of concern, (b) neonatal ICUs in which serum concentrations of aminoglycosides cannot be measured, and (c) specific neonates in whom aminoglycoside therapy could be of concern (e.g., neonates with known renal failure).

Therapy for late-onset sepsis or meningitis is directed toward nosocomial pathogens plus the primary pathogens of early-onset infection. Selection of initial antibiotic therapy should consider the specific neonatal ICU's nosocomial pathogen and antibiotic resistance patterns, as well as the neonate's risk factors, clinical condition, and previous antibiotic therapy. CONS is now the most common pathogen of late-onset neonatal nosocomial septicemia.[97] Because of the high incidence of methicillin-resistant CONS, vancomycin has been used as the drug of choice for empiric therapy for suspected late-onset neonatal sepsis. However, widespread use of vancomycin has led to the emergence of vancomycin-resistant *Enterococcus* and *S. aureus.* Therefore, the routine use of vancomycin as empiric therapy for nosocomial neonatal sepsis should be discouraged. The highly selective use of vancomycin for neonatal CONS septicemia results in low morbidity and mortality, while significantly reducing vancomycin use. Guidelines for the selective use of vancomycin should be tailored according to individual neonatal ICU's nosocomial pathogens, susceptibility patterns, and patient risk factors, clinical condition, and antibiotic history. Therefore, if J.E. had a central venous catheter and presented with a late-onset sepsis, initial antibiotic therapy should include an aminoglycoside (for gram-negative coverage) plus either an antistaphylococcal penicillin (e.g., nafcillin, methicillin) or vancomycin (for activity against *S. aureus* and *S. epidermidis*). Vancomycin is used in place of the antistaphylococcal penicillin in neonatal units with methicillin-resistant *S. aureus* and for selective use to cover *S. epidermidis* (a CONS) as outlined.[97]

For systemic fungal infections, amphotericin B is considered the initial treatment of choice.[84] Because of the high incidence of *Candida* species colonization (up to 60%), with up to 20% progressing to invasive fungal infections in VLBW infants, prophylactic antifungal agents may be used to prevent *Candida* colonization and infection in these infants.[98] In a recent meta-analysis, prophylactic fluconazole in preterm neonates significantly decreased the incidence of fungal colonization and invasive fungal disease in the fluconazole-treated infants compared with placebo.[98] Infants of 27 weeks' gestational age or less and weighing less than 1,000 g benefited most from prophylactic fluconazole. In addition, overall mortality and *Candida*-related mortality were significantly lower in the fluconazole-treated group. Significant adverse events and emergence of resistant *Candida* species were similar in both groups. Despite these findings, routine use of prophylactic antifungal therapy is not recommended and should be reserved for those units with a high incidence of fungal infections. Because uncommon organisms are not suspected in J.E., the regimen of ampicillin 45 mg IV every 12 hours plus gentamicin 4.2 mg IV every 48 hours is appropriate.

Once a pathogen is isolated, the antimicrobial susceptibilities should be evaluated and the drug therapy modified appropriately. Blood, CSF, or urine cultures should be repeated to document bacterial sterilization after 24 to 48 hours of appropriate therapy. J.E. should be evaluated carefully for the development of serious bacterial complications such as meningitis, osteomyelitis, abscess formation, or endocarditis.

DURATION OF THERAPY

As long as there is no evidence of meningitis or other focal infection (e.g., abscess formation), the duration of therapy for most systemic bacterial infections is 7 to 10 days (or approximately 5–7 days after significant clinical improvement). Antibiotic therapy may need to be continued for 14 to 21 days if the neonate's clinical response is slow or if multiple organ systems are involved.[84] If cultures are negative at 72 hours and the infant does not have any clinical or laboratory signs of sepsis, antibiotics can be discontinued. In neonates presenting with signs of severe infection followed by improvement after initiation of antibiotics, therapy may be continued despite negative cultures.

If CSF cultures are positive, repeat CSF cultures should be obtained daily or every other day in J.E. to document when the CSF becomes sterilized. The duration of therapy for neonatal meningitis depends on the clinical response and duration of positive CSF cultures after therapy is initiated. Appropriate antibiotics should be continued for a minimum of 14 days after the CSF is sterilized. This is equivalent to a duration of antibiotic therapy for a minimum of 21 days for gram-negative organisms and at least 14 days for gram-positive pathogens.[82,84] As a general rule, it takes longer to sterilize the CSF of neonates infected by gram-negative enteric bacilli (72 hours) than those infected by gram-positive bacteria (36–48 hours).[82] Although surgical placement of a ventricular reservoir for intraventricular administration of an antibiotic (usually an aminoglycoside) has been used to treat meningitis not responding to IV antimicrobial therapy, the Neonatal Meningitis Cooperative Study group reported no beneficial effect of this method of administration in infants with gram-negative meningitis. In fact, infants treated with intraventricular gentamicin had a threefold increase in mortality rate compared with infants treated solely with IV antibiotics.[84]

TORCH Titers

CASE 100-6

QUESTION 1: S.Y., a 2,000-g female, was born at 34 weeks' gestational age by vaginal delivery. S.Y.'s birth was complicated by prolonged rupture of membranes (>72 hours), a difficult labor and delivery, and fetal distress requiring a fetal scalp monitor. On physical examination, S.Y. is an extremely irritable newborn with a RR of 60 breaths/minute. Several vesicular skin lesions located on the scalp and around the eyes are noted. Conjunctivitis also is present. S.Y. is placed on supplemental oxygen, and ABGs are obtained. Blood, CSF, and urine were cultured for bacteria and fungus, and S.Y. was started on ampicillin 100 mg IV every 12 hours and gentamicin 9 mg IV every 36 hours to rule out sepsis. Antimicrobial therapy will not be altered until culture results are available. What other tests and information are needed for S.Y. at this time?

Certain bacteria, viruses, and protozoa can cause fetal infections that may result in fetal death, congenital anomalies, serious CNS sequelae, intrauterine growth retardation, or preterm birth.[99] The primary organisms that cause these infections can be remembered by the acronym, TORCH: toxoplasmosis; other (i.e., syphilis, gonorrhea, hepatitis B, listeria); rubella; cytomegalovirus; herpes simplex. Because of the potential severity of these diseases, newborns who display any signs of infection (e.g., irritability, fever, thrombocytopenia, hepatosplenomegaly) need to be evaluated for these intrauterine and perinatally acquired infections. The diagnosis of each of these infections should be considered separately. A complete infectious disease workup should include specific antibody titer measurements to

TABLE 100-6
Selected Congenital and Perinatal Infections in the Neonate[2,85,99–103]

Organism	Primary Clinical Manifestations	Treatment of Proven or Highly Probable Disease
Herpes simplex	Cutaneous vesicles, keratoconjunctivitis, microcephaly, CNS infection, hepatitis, pneumonitis, prematurity, respiratory distress, sepsis, convulsion, chorioretinitis	*Acyclovir:* 20 mg/kg every 8 hours IV × 14–21 days *Ocular involvement:* Acyclovir IV plus topical therapy: 1%–2% trifluridine, 1% iododeoxyuridine, or 3% vidarabine
Toxoplasmosis	Chorioretinitis, ventriculomegaly, microcephaly, hydrocephaly, intracranial calcifications, ascites, hepatosplenomegaly, lymphadenopathy, jaundice, anemia, mental retardation	Sulfadiazine 100 mg/kg/d in two divided doses PO for 1 year *and* pyrimethamine 2 mg/kg/d × 2 days then 1 mg/kg/d for 2–6 months then 1 mg/kg QOD to complete 1 year of therapy *and* leucovorin (folinic acid) 5–10 mg 3 times/wk × 1 year
Treponema pallidum	*Early:* Osteochondritis, periostitis, hepatosplenomegaly, skin rash (maculopapular or vesiculobullous), rhinitis, meningitis, IUGR, jaundice, hepatitis, anemia, thrombocytopenia, chorioretinitis *Late:* Hutchinson triad (interstitial keratitis, VIIIth-nerve deafness, Hutchinson teeth), mental retardation, hydrocephalus, saddle nose, mulberry molars	Aqueous crystalline penicillin G × 10 days IV (preferred) or IM: ≤7 days postnatal age: 50,000 units/kg every 12 hours >7 days postnatal age: 50,000 units/kg every 8 hours *OR* Procaine penicillin G 50,000 units/kg/d IM every 24 hours × 10 days
Hepatitis B	Prematurity; usually asymptomatic; long-term effects include chronic hepatitis, cirrhosis, liver failure, hepatocellular carcinoma	*Perinatal exposure (maternal HbsAg-positive):* HBIG 0.5 mL IM and hepatitis B vaccine IM (different IM sites) within 12 hours after birth; repeat hepatitis B vaccine at 1 and 6 months
Rubella	*Early:* IUGR, retinopathy, hypotonia, hepatosplenomegaly, thrombocytopenic purpura, bone lesions, cardiac effects *Late:* Hearing loss, mental retardation, diabetes *Rare:* Myocarditis, glaucoma, microcephaly, hepatitis, anemia	Supportive care
Cytomegalovirus	Petechiae, hepatosplenomegaly, jaundice, prematurity, IUGR, increased liver enzymes, hyperbilirubinemia, anemia, thrombocytopenia, interstitial pneumonitis, microcephaly, chorioretinitis, intracranial calcifications *Late:* Hearing loss, mental retardation, learning and motor abnormalities, visual disturbances	IV ganciclovir (optimal dose and duration not established; preliminary data suggests doses of 12 mg/kg/d divided every 12 hours for 6 weeks)
Neisseria gonorrhoeae	Ophthalmia neonatorum, scalp abscess, sepsis, arthritis, meningitis, endocarditis	*Nondisseminated (including ophthalmia neonatorum):* Ceftriaxone 25–50 mg/kg IV or IM × 1 (maximum dose: 125 mg); alternative for ophthalmic neonatorum: cefotaxime 100 mg/kg IM or IV × 1; use saline eye irrigations for ophthalmia neonatorum *Disseminated:* Ceftriaxone 25–50 mg/kg IV or IM every 24 hours; cefotaxime 25–50 mg/kg IV or IM every 12 hours Duration of therapy: • Arthritis or septicemia: 7 days • Meningitis: 10–14 days Use cefotaxime if hyperbilirubinemic

CNS, central nervous system; HBIG, hepatitis B immune globulin; HbsAg, hepatitis B surface antigen; IM, intramuscular; IUGR, intrauterine growth retardation; IV, intravenous; PO, oral; QOD, every other day.

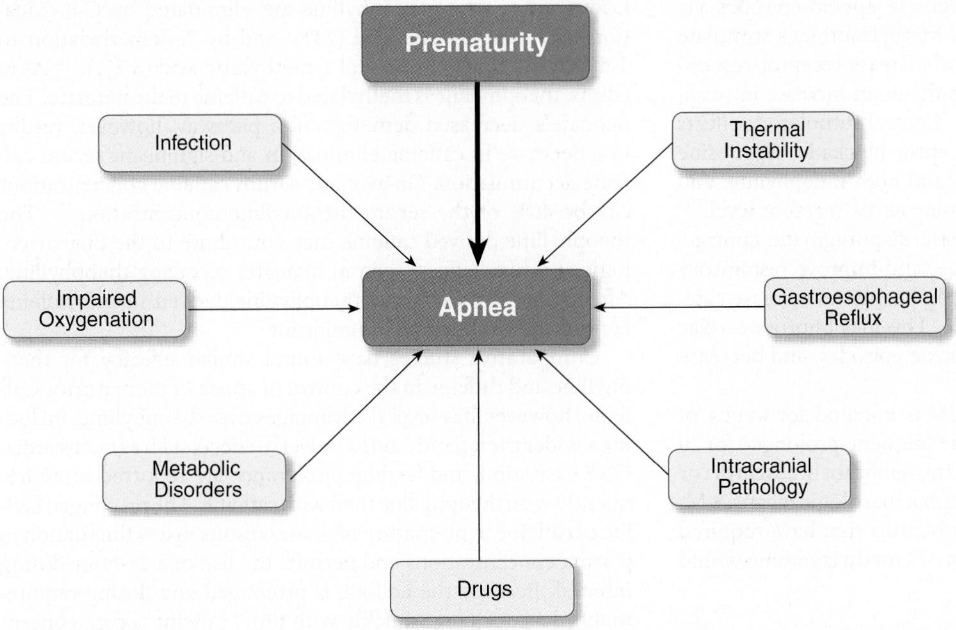

FIGURE 100-3 Causes of apnea in the neonate. (Adapted with permission from Martin RJ et al. Pathogenesis of apnea in preterm infants. *J Pediatr.* 1986;109:738.)

the suspected organisms rather than sending a single serum sample for TORCH titer measurement.[99]

Primary clinical manifestations and treatment for selected congenital infections are listed in Table 100-6.[2,85,99–103] The clinical signs of these infections may overlap, and concurrent infection with two or more micro-organisms is possible. The detection of congenital infections often is difficult because many neonates are asymptomatic at birth. Therefore, prenatal maternal screening and accurate evaluation of maternal history for risk factors are very important. Other organisms that can cause congenitally acquired infections include human immunodeficiency virus, human parvovirus, varicella-zoster virus, and measles virus.[99]

When congenital infections are suspected, appropriate diagnostic tests for each suspected organism should be performed. Viral cultures of the urine, oropharynx, nasopharynx, stool, and conjunctiva and a complete maternal history along with the results of recent maternal vaginal cultures also should be obtained.[99] Measurements of immunoglobulin M levels specific for each possible organism under consideration are also recommended. S.Y. has signs of a congenital infection (respiratory distress, skin rash, and conjunctivitis). Because of the nature of S.Y.'s skin rash (i.e., vesicular), infection with the herpes simplex virus (HSV) should be highly suspected. Skin vesicles, conjunctiva, oropharynx, nasopharynx, rectum, urine, and CSF should be cultured for HSV and other organisms known to cause congenital infections. Rapid diagnostic testing using tissue scrapings from vesicles and fluorescein-conjugated monoclonal HSV antibody can also be performed. Other appropriate tests for the diagnosis and workup of suspected congenital infections also should be performed (e.g., liver enzymes, prothrombin time, partial thromboplastin time, electroencephalogram [EEG], computed tomography scan, or magnetic resonance imaging).[99]

APNEA OF PREMATURITY

Apnea in neonates is a life-threatening condition that occurs more frequently in premature newborns and newborns of lower birth weights. Only 7% of infants 34 to 35 weeks' gestational age have apnea.[104] In contrast, the incidence of apnea has been reported to be 78% in infants 26 to 27 weeks' gestational age and 84% in infants with birth weights less than 1,000 g.[105] Although several definitions exist, clinically significant apnea may be defined as cessation of breathing for at least 15 seconds, or less, if accompanied by bradycardia (HR <100 beats/minute), significant hypoxemia, or cyanosis.[104,106,107] Pallor or hypotonia also may occur.

In neonates, apnea may be caused by a severe underlying illness, drugs, or prematurity itself (Fig. 100-3). Appropriate patient history, physical examination, and laboratory tests must be evaluated to rule out other causes of apnea before the diagnosis of apnea of prematurity can be made.[106] It is especially important to rule out sepsis before apnea of prematurity is presumed. If an etiology other than prematurity is identified, therapy would be directed toward that specific cause. For example, antibiotics are used to treat neonatal sepsis with secondary apnea.

Apnea of prematurity is classified into three types: central, obstructive, and mixed. Approximately 40% of apneic episodes are of central origin (i.e., no respiratory effort), 10% are caused by obstruction, and 50% are attributable to both (i.e., mixed events).[106] Although these terms imply separate mechanisms, obstruction and airway closure may be important in all three types (even "central"). Treatment of apnea of prematurity includes the use of supplemental oxygen, gentle tactile stimulation, environmental temperature control, methylxanthines, nasal CPAP, and positive-pressure ventilation.

CASE 100-7

QUESTION 1: S.M., a premature male newborn of 29 weeks' gestational age, had a birth weight of 995 g. On day 2 of life, he experienced seven episodes of apnea followed by bradycardia with HR as low as 85 beats/minute. These episodes lasted 20 to 30 seconds and required administration of oxygen and tactile stimulation. Three prolonged episodes required bag-and-mask ventilation. Between apneic spells, the newborn seemed well; physical examination and laboratory tests were normal for gestational age. Appropriate cultures were drawn for a septic workup, and ampicillin and gentamicin were initiated. How should S.M.'s apnea be managed?

Methylxanthines, specifically caffeine and theophylline (or aminophylline), are widely accepted as the initial pharmacologic approach for the treatment of idiopathic apnea of prematurity.[104,106] These agents decrease apneic episodes via both central and peripheral effects. Methylxanthines stimulate the medullary respiratory center and increase receptor responsiveness to carbon dioxide. This results in an increase in respiratory drive and minute ventilation. Central stimulatory effects may be mediated by adenosine receptor blockade. Adenosine is a known inhibitor of respiration, and both theophylline and caffeine competitively inhibit adenosine at the receptor level.[104] Peripherally, methylxanthines increase diaphragmatic contractility, decrease diaphragmatic fatigue, and improve respiratory muscle contraction. In addition, methylxanthines increase catecholamine release and metabolic rate. This may improve cardiac output and oxygenation, lessen hypoxic episodes, and decrease apneic spells.

Methylxanthine therapy generally is initiated for apnea of prematurity when apneic episodes are frequent, prolonged for 20 seconds or greater, are accompanied by significant bradycardia or cyanosis, or are not controlled by nonpharmacologic means. S.M. has had prolonged apneas with bradycardia that have required supplemental oxygenation. Initiation of a methylxanthine would be appropriate at this point.

CASE 100-7, QUESTION 2: How does caffeine compare with theophylline with regard to its pharmacokinetics, efficacy, and toxicity? What treatment and dose should be selected for S.M.?

The plasma clearance of caffeine is considerably lower, and the half-life is extremely prolonged in the premature newborn (72–96 hours).[2] The low clearance is a reflection of the decreased neonatal hepatic metabolism and a resultant dependence of elimination on the slow urinary excretion. As a result, caffeine can be dosed once daily (every 24 hours) in the neonate. In the preterm neonate, the amount of caffeine excreted unchanged in the urine is 85%, compared with less than 2% in adults. Adult urinary metabolite patterns are seen by 7 to 9 months of age.[108] The half-life of caffeine decreases with increasing PCA,[109] and plasma clearance reaches adult levels after 3 to 4.5 months of life.[110] As a result of the maturational changes, doses usually need to be adjusted after 38 weeks' PCA.

Protein binding of theophylline is decreased in term newborns (36%) compared with adults (65%).[111] The decreased protein binding along with an increased tissue distribution results in a larger volume of distribution of theophylline in neonates. This larger volume of distribution results in larger loading-dose requirements to attain similar serum concentrations. Like caffeine, theophylline clearance in preterm newborns (17.6 mL/hour/kg) is much slower than that observed in young children 1 to 4 years of age (100 mL/hour/kg).[111] As a result, smaller theophylline maintenance doses are required in neonates. Theophylline clearance increases dramatically during the first year of life, approaching adult values at 55 weeks' PCA.[112] Theophylline clearance and therefore maintenance doses increase with increasing PCA. Adjustment of maintenance doses is especially important in infants at 40 to 50 weeks' PCA when the greatest maturational changes in theophylline clearance occur.[112]

In adults, theophylline is eliminated primarily via hepatic metabolism by C-8 oxidation to 1,3-methyluric acid (39% of a dose) and by *N*-demethylation to 3-methylxanthine (16%) and 1-methyluric acid (20%).[113] Small amounts of theophylline are eliminated unchanged in the urine (13%), and 6% of the dose is *N*-methylated to caffeine.[113,114] In contrast, the primary route of theophylline elimination in neonates is renal excretion of unchanged drug (55%).[112] Hepatic metabolism of theophylline (especially *N*-demethylation) is decreased in the neonate. Lower amounts of theophylline are eliminated by C-8 oxidation to 1,3-methyluric acid (24%) and by *N*-demethylation to 3-methylxanthine (1.4%) and 1-methyluric acid (8.2%).[112] As in adults, theophylline is methylated to caffeine in the neonate. The neonate's decreased demethylation pathway, however, results in a decrease in caffeine elimination and significant serum caffeine accumulation. On average, serum caffeine concentrations can be 40% of the serum theophylline concentration.[112] The theophylline-derived caffeine may contribute to the pharmacologic and toxic effects seen in neonates receiving theophylline. After 50 weeks' PCA, the theophylline-derived serum caffeine concentrations become insignificant.

Comparative studies have found similar efficacy for theophylline and caffeine in the control of apnea of prematurity. Caffeine, however, has several advantages over theophylline, including a wider therapeutic index. Adverse effects such as tachycardia, CNS excitation, and feeding intolerance are reported more frequently with theophylline than with caffeine. The prolonged half-life of caffeine in premature neonates results in less fluctuation in plasma concentrations and permits the use of a 24-hour dosing interval. Because the half-life is prolonged and dosing requirements do not change quickly with time, caffeine serum concentrations do not need to be routinely monitored. The great majority of preterm neonates achieve caffeine plasma concentrations within the therapeutic range (5–20 mcg/mL) if they receive standard doses.[110] Caffeine serum concentrations may be obtained in select neonates (e.g., patients with clinical signs of toxicity or with intractable apnea). IV loading doses of 20 mg/kg caffeine citrate (10 mg/kg caffeine base), followed 24 hours later by maintenance doses of 5 to 8 mg/kg caffeine citrate (2.5–4 mg/kg caffeine base) given daily are recommended. Loading doses of caffeine citrate should be given IV for 30 minutes using a syringe infusion pump. Maintenance doses can be administered IV for 10 minutes or given orally.[2] Because of the longer half-life, infants receiving caffeine must be monitored for a longer time (e.g., for 7–10 days) for adverse effects if toxicities occur and for efficacy once the medication is discontinued. Now that a preservativefree caffeine citrate product is available in the United States, its use has greatly increased. It is important to remember that another IV caffeine product is marketed in the United States as the sodium benzoate salt. Benzoic acid has been associated with the gasping syndrome and also may displace bilirubin from albumin-binding sites.[2] Because of these toxicities, the caffeine sodium benzoate product should not be used in neonates.

The short- and long-term safety and efficacy of caffeine to treat apnea of prematurity in VLBW infants were studied in a large, randomized, placebo-controlled trial.[45,115] Caffeine significantly decreased the frequency of BPD.[45] Infants who received caffeine were able to have positive airway pressure discontinued 1 week sooner than those receiving placebo. Although caffeine reduced weight gain, the effect was only temporary (during the first 3 weeks of therapy). No significant short-term effects of caffeine on death rates, ultrasonographic signs of brain injury, or NEC were identified. In a follow-up study at 18 to 21 months' corrected age, caffeine significantly improved the rates of survival without neurodevelopmental disability; no difference in death rates was observed between caffeine and placebo, but the incidences of cerebral palsy and cognitive delay were both decreased in infants receiving caffeine.[115]

Although oral theophylline (aminophylline) and caffeine are considered to be well absorbed in the neonate, many neonates initially have feeding problems when apnea and bradycardia are present. Therefore, therapy is usually initiated with the IV route, and an oral nonalcoholic solution can be used when the neonate is stable and tolerating oral feedings. The injectable caffeine citrate product may be administered orally. It should also be remembered that, depending on the specific product used, aminophylline is 80% to 85% theophylline.

The generally accepted therapeutic range of theophylline for apnea of prematurity is 6 to 12 mcg/mL. This range is lower than that which is normally accepted for the treatment of asthma (5–15 mcg/mL) for several reasons: (a) the higher free fraction of theophylline found in neonates results in a higher free concentration at any given total concentration; (b) there is a significant accumulation of the unmeasured active metabolite, caffeine; and (c) a different mechanism of action for theophylline is being exploited for apnea (i.e., central stimulation versus bronchodilation for asthma). An aminophylline IV loading dose of 6 to 7 mg/kg (4.8–5.6 mg/kg of theophylline) produces theophylline levels of approximately 6.4 to 7.5 mcg/mL. Most centers use initial maintenance doses of aminophylline in the range of 1 to 2 mg/kg/dose given every 8 to 12 hours, with the lower doses in this range used in younger, more premature infants. For IV administration in neonates, aminophylline should be diluted to 1 mg/mL and infused for 20 to 30 minutes.[2] Lower doses as recommended by the FDA guidelines (theophylline 1 mg/kg every 12 hours for preterm neonates <24 days' PNA) result in serum concentrations less than 5 mcg/mL in most infants younger than 40 weeks' PCA.[116] Concomitant drug therapy and disease states (e.g., hepatic or renal dysfunction) also should be taken into consideration when selecting initial theophylline doses.

Serum theophylline concentrations should be monitored 72 hours after initiation of therapy or after a change in dosage. Serum concentrations of theophylline also should be measured if the infant experiences an increase in the number of apneic episodes, signs or symptoms of toxicity, or a significant increase in weight. In asymptomatic neonates, once steady-state levels are obtained, theophylline concentrations may be monitored every 2 weeks.

Because of the many advantages of caffeine over theophylline, S.M. should be given 20 mg of caffeine citrate (10 mg caffeine base) as an IV loading dose for 30 minutes. Maintenance doses of 5 mg of caffeine citrate (2.5 mg caffeine base) every 24 hours should be started 24 hours after the loading dose.

CASE 100-7, QUESTION 3: Outline a pharmacotherapeutic monitoring plan for S.M. that includes monitoring parameters for efficacy and toxicity and duration of therapy.

The goal of methylxanthine therapy for S.M. is to decrease the number of episodes of apnea and bradycardia. Continuous monitoring of HR and RR is required for proper evaluation. The time, duration, and severity of episodes, activity of the infant, and any necessary intervention performed should be documented. Relationships between the apneic episodes and the feeding schedule and volume of feeds, as well as the dosing schedule, should be examined. Apnea of prematurity usually resolves by 34 to 36 weeks' PCA; however, it may persist in some infants up to or beyond 40 weeks' PCA.[104,106] In general, the younger the gestational age of the infant at birth, the older the PCA at cessation of apnea. Apnea of prematurity frequently persists beyond 36 weeks' PCA in infants born at 28 weeks' gestational age or less, and persists beyond 40 weeks' PCA in 22% of infants born at 24 weeks' gestational age. Therefore, methylxanthine therapy usually is discontinued at 34 to 36 weeks' PCA provided that the infant has not been having apneic spells. Infants requiring therapy for longer periods may be discharged home on methylxanthines with apnea monitors.

Methylxanthine toxicities noted in neonates include tachycardia, agitation, irritability, hyperglycemia, feeding intolerance, gastroesophageal reflux, and emesis or occasional spitting up of food. Tachycardia is the most common toxicity and usually responds to a downward adjustment of the theophylline dose. Tachycardia may persist for 1 to 3 days after dosage reductions owing to the decreased elimination of caffeine. Seizures also have been reported with accidental overdoses. Methylxanthine toxicity can be minimized with careful dosing and appropriate monitoring of serum concentrations.

NEONATAL SEIZURES

CASE 100-8

QUESTION 1: F.H., a term female newborn (weight 3.5 kg), has a history of perinatal asphyxia. Apgar scores were 0, 1, 4, and 7 at 1, 5, 10, and 15 minutes, respectively. Maternal history is negative for drug abuse. Twenty-four hours after birth, F.H. begins to have rhythmic clonic twitching of the right hand, repetitive chewing movements, fluttering of the eyelids, and occasional pendulum-like movements of the extremities that resemble swimming motions. How should F.H.'s seizure activity be evaluated?

Seizure activity may be difficult to recognize in the term or premature neonate. Because of the immaturity of the cortex, neonatal seizures rarely are generalized tonic-clonic events, but can be clonic (focal or multifocal), tonic (focal or generalized), myoclonic (focal, multifocal, or generalized), or subtle in nature.[117,118]

ONLINE CONTENT

For videos of neonatal seizures, go to http://thepoint.lww.com/AT10e.

Subtle seizures include activities such as abnormal oral-buccal-lingual movements; ocular movements; swimming, pedaling, or stepping movements; and occasionally apnea. In addition, autonomic nervous system signs such as changes in HR, BP, respirations, skin color, oxygenation, salivation, or pupil size may occur.[119] Clinical neonatal seizures may or may not be associated with EEG changes.

Neonatal seizure activity is a common manifestation of a life-threatening underlying neurologic process (Table 100-7)[118–122]; therefore, initial efforts may not include antiepileptic drug therapy.[120] Definitive treatment is directed toward specific identified etiologies. The acute evaluation of neonatal seizures includes assessment of the infant's airway, breathing, and circulation and a review of the infant's history, physical examination, and laboratory studies. Every neonate with seizure activity should have a bedside determination of glucose; laboratory determinations of serum electrolytes, including sodium, BUN, glucose, calcium, and magnesium; blood gases; bilirubin; and an infectious disease workup, including complete blood cell count with platelets, blood culture, urine culture, lumbar puncture with CSF analysis (cell count, protein, glucose), and CSF culture.[117,118] Treatment with antiepileptic drugs is indicated after correction of known electrolyte abnormalities. Antiepileptic drug therapy can be initiated while laboratory test results are pending, as long as hypoglycemia has been corrected.

If these tests do not reveal any abnormalities, an EEG, metabolic disease workup (e.g., serum ammonia, lactate, and pyruvate; serum and urine amino and organic acids), and screening of blood and urine for drugs can be performed.[117,119]

TABLE 100-7
Causes of Neonatal Seizures[118–122]

Metabolic or electrolyte imbalance
Alterations in calcium, glucose, magnesium, or sodium concentrations
Inborn errors of metabolism (e.g., pyridoxine-responsive seizures)
Cerebrovascular injury
Hypoxic or ischemic encephalopathy
Arterial and venous ischemic stroke
Hemorrhage (intracerebral, intraventricular, subarachnoid, or subdural)
CNS infection
Bacterial meningitis
Viral meningoencephalitis
Congenital infections
Drug-related causes
Adverse effects from drugs administered before, during, or after delivery
Withdrawal after maternal drug use
Other
Cerebral dysgenesis
Genetic or syndromic disorders
Familial seizure disorders
Early myoclonic encephalopathy

Intrauterine infections associated with congenital neurologic abnormalities and seizures can be identified by obtainment of TORCH titers. Cranial ultrasounds, computed tomography scans, and magnetic resonance images may be obtained to identify infarcts, hemorrhages, calcifications, or cerebral malformations that may cause seizure activity.[118]

CASE 100-8, QUESTION 2: F.H. is found to have adequate ventilation and circulation. An IV line is established; blood cultures and serum chemistries, including calcium and magnesium, are obtained. A Chemstrip reveals a blood glucose of 20 mg/dL. What is your assessment and recommendation at this time?

Hypoglycemia seems to be the cause of F.H.'s seizure activity. Hypoxic ischemic encephalopathy secondary to asphyxia, however, is the most common cause of neonatal seizures.[118] Hypoxic ischemic encephalopathy can be associated with metabolic abnormalities such as hypoglycemia, hypocalcemia, and hyponatremia (owing to inappropriate secretion of antidiuretic hormone). The definition of clinically significant hypoglycemia in neonates remains controversial, as normal blood glucose depends on a variety of factors, including gestational age, birth weight, feeding status, body stores, and other disease states.[121] Historically, hypoglycemia was defined as a whole blood glucose less than 20 mg/dL for premature infants and less than 30 mg/dL for term infants during the first 72 hours of life and less than 40 mg/dL for any neonate after 72 hours of age. However, in clinical practice, a blood glucose less than 40 mg/dL in a neonate of any age would be treated.[121] F.H. should receive an IV bolus dose of 7 mL (2 mL/kg) of dextrose 10% (200 mg/kg) given in 2 to 3 minutes, followed by a continuous infusion of dextrose 10% at an initial dose of 12.6 to 16.8 mL/hour (6–8 mg/kg/minute or 3.6–4.8 mL/kg/hour).[118] Serum glucose levels should be monitored, and the dextrose infusion should be titrated as needed. If hypoglycemia persists, possible causes such as islet tumor of the pancreas, adrenal insufficiency, and inborn errors of metabolism should be investigated. Corticosteroids, glucagon, and diazoxide have been used to treat persistent hypoglycemia.[121]

Treatment of Hypocalcemia and Hypomagnesemia

CASE 100-8, QUESTION 3: F.H. receives 7 mL (700 mg) of 10% dextrose solution IV, and an IV infusion of glucose at 8 mg/kg/minute is initiated. A repeat Chemstrip reveals a blood glucose of 80 mg/dL, but F.H. continues to have seizure activity. F.H.'s laboratory results come back with the following results:

Sodium, 137 mEq/L
Potassium, 4.3 mEq/L
CO_2, 22 mEq/L
Chloride, 104 mEq/L
BUN, 7 mg/dL
SCr, 0.7 mg/dL
Glucose, 25 mg/dL
Magnesium, 1.0 mEq/L
Calcium, 6.5 mg/dL

What should be done next to control F.H.'s seizures?

F.H. also has hypocalcemia and hypomagnesemia, both of which may cause seizure activity. Neonatal hypocalcemia is defined as a serum calcium less than 7.5 mg/dL in preterm and less than 8 mg/dL in term infants[119] or an ionized serum calcium less than 3 mg/dL. Hypomagnesemia (defined as a serum magnesium <1.5 mEq/L) is rare but may coexist with hypocalcemia. Hypomagnesemia should be suspected when hypocalcemia cannot be corrected despite large doses of calcium.

F.H. should receive calcium gluconate 700 mg (200 mg/kg) given slowly IV as a 10% solution[119] and magnesium sulfate 25 to 50 mg/kg/dose (0.2–0.4 mEq/kg/dose) IM as a 50% solution or IV as a dilute solution (maximal concentration, 100 mg/mL) administered for 2 to 4 hours.[2] Doses of calcium gluconate and magnesium sulfate may be repeated based on serum determinations. If IV calcium is administered too quickly, vasodilation, hypotension, bradycardia, and cardiac arrhythmias may occur. Calcium gluconate may be administered IV at a maximal rate of 50 mg/minute while monitoring HR, BP, and electrocardiogram.[2] The IV site should be closely monitored for signs of infiltration because extravasation may result in severe dermal necrosis.

Treatment With Antiepileptic Drugs

CASE 100-8, QUESTION 4: Despite normalization of her laboratory tests, F.H. continues to have seizure activity. Phenobarbital 35 mg IV push for 1 minute is administered. Ten minutes later, F.H. continues to have intermittent seizure activity. Describe a pharmacotherapeutic plan to control F.H.'s seizure activity.

Phenobarbital is the initial antiepileptic drug of choice for neonatal seizures; phenytoin and lorazepam usually are considered the second and third drugs of choice.[118,122] Because of the large volume of distribution of phenobarbital in neonates (approximately 1 L/kg), large initial loading doses of 20 mg/kg are required to produce therapeutic serum concentrations (Table 100-8).[123] Because F.H. received only a 10-mg/kg dose (35 mg) of phenobarbital, an additional 10 mg/kg should be given now. Phenobarbital should be administered IV at a rate of 1 mg/kg/minute or less,[2,118] so a 35-mg dose should be given for at least 10 minutes, not in 1 minute. Rapid administration of phenobarbital may cause respiratory depression, apnea, or hypotension. If F.H. continues to have seizure activity after a total phenobarbital loading dose of 20 mg/kg, additional 5- to 10-mg/kg loading doses may

TABLE 100-8
Pharmacotherapy of Neonatal Seizures[a,2,123]

Drug	Loading Dose	Maintenance Dose	Therapeutic Concentration
Phenobarbital	*IV: Initial:* 20 mg/kg then 5–10 mg/kg every 15–20 minutes if needed until total load of 40 mg/kg	*IV PO: Initial:* Premature: 3 mg/kg/d Term: 4 mg/kg/d May need to ↑ to 4–5 mg/kg/d by 2–4 weeks of therapy	20–40 mcg/mL
Phenytoin	*IV:* 15–20 mg/kg	*IV: Initial:* 5 mg/kg/d May need to ↑ to ≥10 mg/kg/d by 2–4 weeks of therapy	8–15 mcg/mL
Lorazepam	*IV:* 0.05–0.1 mg/kg	May repeat doses if needed every 10–15 minutes	
Midazolam	*IV:* Initial bolus dose of 0.15 mg/kg has been used in some studies; however, for safety reasons, this bolus dose should not be given if the neonate has received an IV dose of a benzodiazepine	*IV continuous infusion: Initial:* 0.05 mg/kg/h; ↑ by 0.025 mg/kg/h increments; usual maximum 0.4 mg/kg/h; some studies reported neonates who required doses up to 1 mg/kg/h	
Levetiracetam	Dose not established; studies have used the following: *IV:* Initial: 10 mg/kg given twice daily	*IV:* ↑ dose by 10 mg/kg/d over 3 days to 30 mg/kg/d given in two divided doses; additional increases up to 45–60 mg/kg/d have been used	
Pyridoxine	*IV:* 50–100 mg	*IV PO:* 20–50 mg/d; ↑ dose PRN with age	
Valproic acid	*PO:* 20 mg/kg	*PO:* 10 mg/kg/dose every 12 hours	40–50 mcg/mL

[a] See text for comments on appropriate IV administration and monitoring.
IV, intravenous; PO, oral; PRN, as needed.

be given every 15 to 20 minutes as needed up to a total loading dose of 40 mg/kg. Ventilatory support may be required when using these higher doses, and serum phenobarbital concentrations should be monitored. Phenobarbital's therapeutic effect of controlling neonatal seizures plateaus at serum concentrations of 40 mcg/mL; adverse effects increase at higher serum concentrations.[124]

If seizure activity is not controlled in F.H. (despite optimal phenobarbital loading doses), a phenytoin loading dose of 70 mg (20 mg/kg) should be administered IV at a rate of 0.5 to 1 mg/kg/minute or less.[2,118] Rapid IV administration of phenytoin may cause cardiac arrhythmias, bradycardia, or hypotension. Phenytoin may cause severe damage to tissues if extravasation occurs. Therefore, BP, HR, electrocardiogram, and the IV site of infusion should be monitored. Fosphenytoin, the diphosphate ester salt of phenytoin, is available in the United States for IV and IM use in adults.[2] Fosphenytoin is a water-soluble prodrug of phenytoin that undergoes conversion by plasma and tissue esterases to phenytoin, phosphate, and formaldehyde. Because of its greater water solubility, the IV preparation does not contain propylene glycol, and thus fosphenytoin may have fewer cardiovascular adverse effects associated with IV administration. Unfortunately, appropriate clinical studies of fosphenytoin in neonates have not yet been conducted. Unanswered concerns about the neonatal handling of formaldehyde also exist. Currently, routine use of fosphenytoin in neonates cannot be recommended. Studies assessing the safety, efficacy, and optimal dosing are needed.

Lorazepam IV should be used to treat F.H.'s seizures if they are unresponsive to phenobarbital and phenytoin.[117,118,122] Lorazepam is preferred over diazepam owing to its longer duration of effect and fewer pharmaceutical adjuvants. Lorazepam (especially in combination with phenobarbital) may cause respiratory and CNS depression. RR, BP, and HR should be monitored. Doses should be diluted with an equal volume of 5% dextrose in water, normal saline, or sterile water for injection before IV use and administered slowly for 2 to 5 minutes.[2]

If seizure activity continues in F.H., continuous IV infusion of midazolam or IV or oral levetiracetam should be considered.[119,123,125] Although the IV formulation of levetiracetam is not approved for use in neonates, some neonatal centers use the pediatric oral dosing recommendations for the IV route because the two forms are bioequivalent.[2] However, the optimal neonatal dose of levetiracetam has not been established. Neonatal reports have used doses based on studies in pediatric patients.[123] Given that levetiracetam is primarily excreted via the kidney (66% of a dose is excreted as unchanged drug in the urine) and that the renal function of neonates is decreased compared with that of older infants, prudence dictates using conservative dose titration and close monitoring of adverse effects. Oral carbamazepine, primidone, lamotrigine, topiramate, and valproic acid (IV, oral) have also been used to treat neonatal seizures in limited numbers of patients.[117,118,122] Because the risk of valproic acid–associated hepatotoxicity is higher for patients younger than 2 years of age, this drug is not a preferred agent for use in neonates.[2] IV pyridoxine should be considered when seizure activity persists. Pyridoxine is a cofactor required for the synthesis of the inhibitory neurotransmitter γ-aminobutyric acid (GABA). Patients with pyridoxine dependency require higher amounts of pyridoxine for proper GABA synthesis. Pyridoxine dependency is a rare disorder, but should be considered in neonates with seizure activity unresponsive to antiepileptic drug therapy. Lifelong supplementation of pyridoxine is required in these patients.[119]

CASE 100-8, QUESTION 5: F.H.'s seizure activity stopped after receiving a total loading dose of 105 mg of phenobarbital and 70 mg of phenytoin. A serum phenobarbital concentration of 35 mcg/mL and a phenytoin concentration of 17 mcg/mL were measured 1 hour after the phenytoin loading dose (2 hours after the last phenobarbital loading dose). How should maintenance doses of antiepileptic drugs be instituted in F.H.?

It is not surprising that F.H. required both phenobarbital and phenytoin to control her seizures. Although phenobarbital and phenytoin are equally effective, neonatal seizures are controlled in fewer than 50% of neonates with either agent alone. When both agents are used together, neonatal seizures are controlled in approximately 60% of neonates.[126]

F.H. should be placed on maintenance doses of both phenobarbital and phenytoin because both drugs were needed to control her seizure activity. Because the half-life of phenobarbital is prolonged in neonates (about 100–150 hours), maintenance doses can be instituted 24 hours after the loading dose at 3 to 4 mg/kg/day[119,127] as a single daily dose (Table 100-8). Although this newborn is term, she should receive a lower dose of phenobarbital (2.5–3 mg/kg/day) because of her history of asphyxia. Asphyxiated neonates have impaired phenobarbital clearance and therefore require lower maintenance doses than nonasphyxiated neonates to achieve similar phenobarbital serum concentrations.[128] Maintenance doses of phenytoin (3–4 mg/kg/day given in divided doses every 12 hours) may be initiated 12 to 24 hours after the loading dose. Serum concentrations of these agents should be monitored periodically because maintenance dose requirements increase with time, usually by weeks 2 to 4 of therapy.[127] This may be related to a normal maturation of hepatic enzyme systems with age or induction of cytochrome P-450 enzymes. In neonates, oral phenytoin is poorly absorbed and should be avoided in the acute setting. A routine 25% increase in the dose is needed when converting IV phenytoin to oral to attain similar serum concentrations. In addition, after 2 to 4 weeks of age, dosing intervals of every 8 hours may be needed.

It should be remembered that phenytoin is a highly protein-bound drug. In neonates, protein binding of phenytoin is decreased. This results in an increased free fraction and suggests that total phenytoin therapeutic serum concentrations in newborns should be 8 to 15 mcg/mL rather than the 10 to 20 mcg/mL as accepted in children and adults.[2] In addition, bilirubin can displace phenytoin from albumin binding sites. A positive correlation between total bilirubin concentrations and free fraction of phenytoin has been described. Unbound phenytoin was reported to be approximately 20% in neonates when bilirubin concentrations were 20 mg/dL (compared with 10% normally).[129] Thus, total phenytoin serum concentrations must be interpreted carefully in neonates, and measurement of unbound phenytoin may be required in neonates with hyperbilirubinemia.

The optimal duration of anticonvulsant treatment of neonatal seizures has not been clearly established. Because of the potential long-term toxicities of these medications and the low risk of seizure recurrence, anticonvulsants are generally discontinued before discharge if the neonate's neurologic examination and EEG are normal. Neonates who continue receiving anticonvulsants are reassessed periodically after discharge (e.g., at 1 and 3 months of age and then every 3 months).[118] Thus, the duration of anticonvulsant medications is individualized based on the infant's neurologic examination and EEG.

KEY REFERENCES AND WEBSITES

A full list of references for this chapter can be found at http://thepoint.lww.com/AT10e. Below are the key references and websites for this chapter, with the corresponding reference number in this chapter found in parentheses after the reference.

Key References

Engle WA et al. Surfactant-replacement therapy for respiratory distress in the preterm and term neonate. *Pediatrics*. 2008;121:419. (14)

Pickering LK et al, eds. *2009 Red Book: Report of the Committee on Infectious Diseases*, 28th ed. Elk Grove Village, IL: American Academy of Pediatrics; 2009. (85)

Taketomo CK et al. *Pediatric and Neonatal Dosage Handbook*, 18th ed. Hudson, OH: Lexi-Comp; 2011. (2)

Thompson AM, Bizzarro MJ. Necrotizing enterocolitis in newborns: pathogenesis, prevention and management. *Drugs*. 2008;68:1227. (71)

Watterberg K et al. Policy statement—postnatal corticosteroids to prevent or treat bronchopulmonary dysplasia. *Pediatrics*. 2010;126:800. (38)

Key Websites

American Heart Association, Congenital Heart Defects. http://www.heart.org/HEARTORG/Conditions/CongenitalHeartDefects/Congenital-Heart-Defects_UCM_001090_SubHomePage.jsp.

Cochrane Neonatal Group. http://neonatal.cochrane.org/.

The Congenital Heart Information Network. http://www.tchin.org/.

Neonatology on the Web. http://www.neonatology.org/.

NICHD- The Eunice Kennedy Shriver National Institute of Child Health & Human Development. http://www.nichd.nih.gov/cochrane/.

Care of the Critically Ill Child

101

Elizabeth Anne Farrington and Marcia L. Buck

CORE PRINCIPLES

		CHAPTER CASES
1	The most frequent cause of cardiac arrest in pediatric patients is a terminal result of respiratory failure or shock, not a primary cardiac event.	**Case 101-1 (Question 1)**
2	Developmental changes and immaturity of the respiratory system make respiratory distress the most common reason for hospital admission in the first year of life. Nasal flaring and grunting are unique features of the respiratory examination in infants that indicate respiratory distress. The normal respiratory rate in children changes over time, therefore the respiratory rate that would be of concern varies based on the age of the patient.	**Case 101-2 (Questions 1, 2)**
3	Oxygen should be administered immediately in a child where respiratory difficulty is suspected. Once the decision is made to intubate the patient, the choices for pharmacotherapy of intubation vary based on the cardiovascular stability of the patient, whether the stomach is empty or full, and the underlying cause of the respiratory distress.	**Case 101-2 (Questions 3, 4)**
4	Hypovolemic shock is the most common type of shock seen in pediatric patients. Septic, obstructive, and cardiogenic shock occur in children but are less common. The initial treatment of all forms of shock is the same. A pediatric patient can present with compensated or decompensated shock. There are physiologic differences in the pediatric patient's response to hypovolemia, with hypotension being the last physiologic change during decompensation.	**Case 101-3 (Questions 1, 2)**
5	Infants have low glycogen stores, so are at high risk for the development of hypoglycemia when they have poor oral intake or during conditions of stress. Because hypoglycemia may cause seizures and is linked to poor neurologic outcome, all critically ill infants should have a point-of-care glucose testing on presentation. If identified, hypoglycemia must be treated promptly.	**Case 101-3 (Question 3)**
6	Due to the immature immune system in the infant, the incidence of septic shock is the highest in the first year of life. Patients with underlying medical conditions have a higher mortality rate than previously healthy children who experience sepsis.	**Case 101-4 (Question 1)**
7	Due to physiologic changes during childhood, the definitions of sepsis and systemic inflammatory response syndrome (SIRS) are different in children and adults. Tachycardia and tachypnea, pivotal to the adult definition of SIRS, are common presenting symptoms of many pediatric disease processes and are not solely indicative of sepsis. Unlike adult guidelines, temperature variation and leukocyte abnormalities are included in the pediatric definitions. There are also specific definitions based on patient age: newborn, neonate, infant, toddler and preschool-aged child, school-aged child, and adolescent.	**Case 101-4 (Question 2)**
8	Septic shock can be further defined by the patient's response to fluid resuscitation and catecholamine administration. These factors, as well as physiologic differences in neonatal and pediatric cardiovascular physiology compared with adults, affect not only the choice of therapy but also drug dosing and monitoring.	**Case 101-4 (Questions 3–6)**

continued

		CHAPTER CASES
9	Neonates with ductal-dependent congenital heart disease (CHD) may not be diagnosed immediately after birth. These patients may present with symptoms of being either in respiratory distress, in cardiogenic or obstructive shock, or in a combination of both. It is essential to consider CHD in any neonate who presents with these symptoms.	**Case 101-5 (Question 1)**
10	Traumatic brain injury (TBI) is the leading cause of mortality in children and leads to significant morbidity among survivors. The anatomical differences of the child's brain render it more susceptible to certain types of injuries after head trauma. Causes vary by age, with non-accidental trauma seen most commonly in the first year of life. Quick assessment of the patient on presentation to emergency services is needed for appropriate diagnosis, stabilization, and treatment.	**Case 101-6 (Questions 1–3)**
11	Placement of a ventriculostomy will allow for measurement of intracranial pressure (ICP) and drainage of cerebral spinal fluid. The ability to measure ICP will assist in the evaluation of the efficacy of treatments. Cerebral perfusion pressure (CPP) also must be monitored closely in patients with TBI. Goal CPP values vary by age. Standard therapies to reduce ICP include CSF drainage, medically induced hypertension, and hyperosmolar therapy with mannitol or hypertonic saline. When standard therapies fail, barbiturate coma, therapeutic hypothermia, or decompressive craniectomy may be considered.	**Case 101-6 (Questions 4–6)**
12	Treatment and/or prevention of early posttraumatic seizures has been shown to improve outcomes, but long-term use of anticonvulsant medications (greater than 7 days) has not been shown to improve outcomes and is associated with adverse effects.	**Case 101-7 (Question 1)**

Much of pediatric practice is dedicated to assisting the child in making the transition from the intrauterine environment through infancy, childhood, and adolescence to adulthood. One of the greatest challenges in managing pediatric patients is recognizing the numerous physiologic changes that take place during this time and understanding how they affect assessment and management of the patient. The definition and presentation of many disease states encountered in the critical care setting, including respiratory depression, supraventricular tachycardia, hypotension, and shock, vary based on the age of the patient as a result of these physiologic variations. There are also newborn emergencies that are unique to the physiologic transitions that occur in the first month of life.

Pediatric health care providers practicing in critical care settings such as the emergency department or pediatric intensive care unit (PICU) must be adept at incorporating these physiologic differences into medication selection, dosing, and monitoring to optimize patient care.

The epidemiology of patients admitted to either the pediatric emergency department or PICU differs from that typically seen in adult critical care settings.[1,2] In an evaluation of 361 children presenting to an emergency department, the most common medial reasons for admission were cardiocirculatory causes (32%), neurological conditions (26%), and respiratory causes (23%).[1] Cardiocirculatory causes included hypovolemic, septic, cardiac, and anaphylactic shock. Neurological conditions consisted primarily of seizures, status epilepticus, and meningitis or encephalitis. The most common respiratory cause for admission was respiratory syncytial virus (RSV) bronchiolitis, followed by pneumonia, pleural effusions, and croup. Eighteen percent (18%) of the patients were admitted after trauma. Diabetic ketoacidosis accounted for 6% of admissions. Other diagnoses included intoxications, near drowning, snake bites, and burns. Assessment of the most common causes for PICU admission has provided similar results. In a review of 1,149 children admitted during a 2-year period to the PICU of a university-affiliated children's hospital, the majority (38%) were diagnosed with cardiovascular diseases, followed by respiratory illnesses (28%), other medical causes (10%), neurologic illness (8%), and trauma (8%). Another 7% were admitted for postoperative care.[2]

PEDIATRIC CARDIOPULMONARY RESUSCITATION

In marked contrast to pediatric cardiac arrest, adult cardiac arrest studies have focused on the diagnosis and treatment of ventricular fibrillation (VF) in both inpatient and out-of-hospital cardiac arrest. Studies showed that VF was the most common initial dysrhythmia in adults with sudden death; in some reports, the prevalence of VF was 60% to 85%. Cardiac arrest due to VF or pulseless ventricular tachycardia as the initial cardiac rhythm occurs in only 5% to 15% of pediatric inhospital and out-of hospital cardiac arrest.[3] In contrast to adults, cardiac arrest in infants and children does not usually result from a primary cardiac cause; more often it is the terminal result of progressive respiratory failure or shock. Therefore, it is essential to recognize and treat pediatric patients admitted with respiratory distress, pneumonia, and shock aggressively to prevent the development of systemic hypoxemia, hypercapnia, and acidosis that may then progress to bradycardia, hypotension, and eventually cardiorespiratory arrest.

ONLINE CONTENT

For illustrations of cardiopulmonary resuscitation on an infant and an older child, go to http://thepoint.lww.com/AT10e.

CASE 101-1

QUESTION 1: Paramedics are transporting C.W., a 5-month-old, 5-kg infant with respiratory distress who stops breathing en route to the hospital. The patient is bag-mask–ventilated with cardiopulmonary resuscitation in progress. On arrival in the emergency department, the patient is apneic, asystolic, and pulseless. The infant has no intravenous (IV) access. After brief bag-mask ventilation, the patient is intubated with an endotracheal tube (ETT). A colorimetric carbon dioxide capnometer detector device confirms proper ETT placement. Findings now include breath sounds that are equal bilaterally and good chest movement with ventilation, although there is still no pulse palpable without chest compressions and no heart sounds are heard. An electrocardiogram shows asystole. Oxygen saturation is not obtainable. What medication is needed for C.W. at this point in his resuscitation?

Epinephrine is the drug of choice for the management of pediatric asystole.[3] Ventilation and chest compressions should be continued for C.W. and while one responder is attempting IV access, another may administer the first dose of epinephrine down the ETT using a higher dose of 0.5 mg (0.1 mg/kg prepared from the 1:1,000 or 1 mg/mL concentration) to account for reduced absorption. If two attempts at IV line placement are unsuccessful, an intraosseous (IO) catheter should be inserted into the proximal tibia. Blood may be obtained through the IO needle to perform a rapid glucose check and sent for further studies. After reassessment of the airway, ventilation and chest compressions should be continued. Subsequent doses of epinephrine can be administered every 3 to 5 minutes though the IO line, using the appropriate IV/IO dose of 0.05 mg (0.01 mg/kg using the 1:10,000 or 0.1 mg/mL concentration).

RESPIRATORY DISTRESS

Respiratory distress, related to problems at all levels of the respiratory tract from the nose to the lungs, is a frequent occurrence in children.[4] (For a video that shows some of the signs of respiratory distress in an infant, go to http://www.youtube.com/watch?v=42jJ18fkZ0Y.) The nose provides nearly half the total airway resistance in children. Infants under 2 months are obligate nasal breathers and their nose is short, soft, and small with nearly circular nares. The nares will double in size from birth to 6 months but they can easily be occluded from edema, secretions, or external pressure. Simply clearing the nasal passageways with saline and bulb suctioning can significantly improve an infant's respiratory condition. Other physiologic reasons for a high incidence of respiratory failure in infants and children are small and collapsible airways, an unstable chest wall, inadequate collateral ventilation for alveoli, poor control (tone) of the upper airway (particularly during sleep), tendency for the respiratory muscles to fatigue, reactivity of the pulmonary vascular bed (increased sensitivity of the vasculature, particularly in young infants), an inefficient immune system, genetic disorders or syndromes, and residual problems related to premature birth such as bronchopulmonary dysplasia.

CASE 101-2

QUESTION 1: T.F. is a 7-month-old, previously healthy 12-kg infant who presents to the emergency room with a 3-day history of upper respiratory tract symptoms. His mother states that he is having increasing difficulty breathing and has not wanted to drink or eat. On examination, he has a respiratory rate of 70 breaths/minute, an O_2 saturation of 90% on 100% FIO_2 via nasal cannula, nasal flaring and grunting, and both intercostal and suprasternal retractions. Initial viral screening reveals positive results for RSV and his chest x-ray is consistent with RSV bronchiolitis. He was agitated and fussy at first presentation, but during the last 30 minutes his respiratory rate has decreased to 40 breaths/minute with a reduction in retractions and he has become somnolent. What developmental changes in the lung explain why a routine viral infection could result in the need for an emergency room visit in a 7-month-old previously healthy child?

The most common reason for admission to the hospital in the first year of life is respiratory distress. This can be explained by the numerous physiologic differences seen in an infant. Although all the conducting airways are present at birth and the airway branching pattern is complete, the airways are small.[5] The airways will increase in size and length throughout childhood. Not only are the airways smaller in an infant but supporting airway cartilage and elastic tissue are not developed until school age. For these reasons, the child's airways are susceptible to collapse and may easily become obstructed as a result of laryngospasm, bronchospasm, and edema or mucus accumulation. Normal airway resistance is the highest in infants as it is inversely proportional to $1/\text{radius}^4$. Therefore, any airway narrowing from bronchospasm, edema, or mucus accumulation will significantly increase the airway resistance and increase the infant's work of breathing. The cartilaginous ribs of the infant and young child are twice as compliant as the bony ribs of the older child or adult. During episodes of respiratory distress the infant's chest wall will retract further than a patient with a bony ribcage. This will reduce the patient's ability to maintain functional residual capacity (FRC) or increase tidal volume, thus further increasing the patient's work of breathing.

The respiratory muscles consist of muscles of the upper airway, the lower airway, and the diaphragm. They contribute to expansion of the lung and maintenance of airway patency. Lack of development of the small airway muscles may render young infants less responsive than older children to bronchodilator therapy. Lastly, the intercostal muscles are not fully developed until school age, so they act primarily to stabilize the chest wall during the first years of life. Because the intercostal muscles have neither the leverage nor the strength to lift the rib cage in the young child, the diaphragm is responsible for the generation of tidal volume. Therefore, anything that impedes diaphragm movement, such as a large stomach bubble, abdominal distension, or peritonitis, can result in respiratory failure in the young child.

CASE 101-2, QUESTION 2: What respiratory signs and symptoms are present in T.F. and how to they define the patient's respiratory status? What are potential causes of T.F.'s respiratory distress?

To assess a patient for respiratory distress one should evaluate four areas: respiratory rate and effort, work of breathing, quality and magnitude of breath sounds, and the patient's mental status. Normal respiratory rates vary with age (Table 101-1). A respiratory rate greater than 60 breaths/minute is abnormal in a child of any age, but most concerning in an older child. An abnormally slow or decreasing respiratory rate may herald respiratory failure. Intercostal, subcostal, and supracostal retractions increase with increasing respiratory distress. Although increased

TABLE 101-1
Normal Respiratory Rates and Definition of Tachypnea for Children, by Age

Age	Respiratory Rate (breaths/min)	Tachypnea (breaths/min)
Newborn–2 months	30–60	>60
2 months–12 months	25–40	>50
1–3 years	20–30	>40
3–6 years	16–22	>40
7–12 years	14–20	>40
>12 years	12–20	>40

retractions are seen in infants, they have decreased efficiency of respiratory muscle function during the first years of life; therefore the benefit in infants is reduced. Decreasing respiratory rate and diminished retractions in a child with a history of distress may signal severe fatigue. Nasal flaring is an effort to increase airway diameter and is often seen with hypoxemia. T.F. demonstrates all of these physiologic signs of respiratory distress. In addition to these findings, some infants will exhibit an expiratory grunting noise. This noise is produced by the child's involuntary effort to counter the loss of FRC by closing their glottis on active exhalation. Grunting produces positive end-expiratory pressure (PEEP) in an effort to prevent airway collapse. An expiratory grunt is mechanistically similar to "pursed lip breathing" in adults with chronic dyspnea. An expiratory grunt is classically seen in the presence of extensive alveolar pathology and is considered a sign of serious disease.

There are numerous causes of respiratory distress in infants and children. Table 101-2 summarizes common respiratory noises in children and their site of origin which may provide clues to the clinical cause. The most common causes of respiratory failure in infants and children are infectious diseases, asthma, malignancies, trauma (both accidental and nonaccidental), poisonings, foreign body aspiration, anatomical upper airway obstruction, cardiogenic shock, and untreated left to right intracardiac shunts. Respiratory syncytial virus is among the most common causes of respiratory distress in infants and young children, leading to an estimated 90,000 hospitalizations each year.[6] Although RSV can occur at any age, it is most severe in children under 2 years of age such as T.F. Prematurity, as well as chronic respiratory

TABLE 101-2
Common Airway Noises, Site of Origin, and Clinical Causes in Children

Respiratory Noise	Definition	Site of Origin	Common Clinical Causes: Acute	Common Clinical Causes: Persistent
Wheeze	A high-pitched, continuous musical noise, often associated with prolonged expiration (can occur with inspiration or expiration)	Intrathoracic airways	Intermittent asthma/viral-induced wheeze	Persistent asthma
Rattle	This sound is the result of excessive secretions in the large airways, which are presumably moving with normal respirations	Either or both intrathoracic and extrathoracic airways	Acute viral bronchitis	Chronic sputum retention (neuromuscular disorders)
Stridor	This is predominately an inspiratory noise and indicates obstruction to airflow in the extrathoracic airways (upper airways obstruction) (can occur with inspiration or expiration)	Extrathoracic airways	Acute laryngotracheobronchitis (or viral croup)	Laryngomalacia
Snore	The noise arises from an increase to airflow through the upper airways, predominately in the region of the nasopharynx and oropharynx; it is more obvious during inspiration, but may be audible throughout the respiratory cycle	Oronasopharyngeal airway	Acute tonsillitis/pharyngitis	Chronically enlarged tonsils and adenoids, obstructive sleep apnea
Snuffle/Snort	These terms describe respiratory noises emanating from the nasal passages; these noises are audible in both inspiration and expiration and are often associated with visible secretions from the nares	Nasal passage/nasopharynx	Acute viral head cold	Allergic rhinitis
Grunt	This sound occurs with closure of the glottis during active exhalation	Alveoli/lung parenchyma	Any alveolar pathology in infants and small children	None

For examples of some of these airway noises, go to the following web links:

- Wheeze: http://www.youtube.com/watch?v=YG0-ukhU1xE&feature=related
- Rattle/rhonchi: http://www.youtube.com/watch?v=QPBZOohj2a0&feature=related
- Stridor:
  - Toddler: http://www.youtube.com/watch?v=Zkau4yHsLLM&feature=related
  - Infant: http://www.youtube.com/watch?v=73zUjcCzgqA&NR=1
- Grunt: http://www.youtube.com/watch?v=aptwttJ6y_4

disease and congenital heart disease, increase the risk for severe RSV bronchiolitis requiring hospitalization.

CASE 101-2, QUESTION 3: T.F. is no longer consistently maintaining oxygen saturation values above 90% on nasal cannula O_2. How should T.F. be managed?

Oxygen should be administered immediately in any patient where respiratory difficulty is suspected. Infants and children consume 2 to 3 times more oxygen per kilogram of body weight than adults under normal conditions and even more when they are ill or distressed. T.F. responded well to oxygen administered via nasal cannula in the emergency department, but is now increasingly somnolent and has a decreased respiratory rate along with decreased oxygen saturation values—all signs of impending respiratory failure. The specific indications for intubation in infants and children are as follows:

1. Apnea
2. Acute respiratory failure (Pa_{O_2} <50 mm Hg in patient with F_{IO_2} >0.5 and Pa_{CO_2} >55 mm Hg acutely)
3. Need to control oxygen delivery, with institution of PEEP or to provide accurate delivery of F_{IO_2} greater than 0.5
4. Need to control ventilation to decrease work of breathing, control Pa_{CO_2}, or to administer neuromuscular blocking agents
5. Inadequate chest wall function, as in patients with neuromuscular disorders such as Guillain-Barré syndrome, spinal muscular atrophy, or muscular dystrophy
6. Upper airway obstruction
7. Protection of the airway of a patient whose protective reflexes are absent, such as those with head trauma

Based on the diagnosis of acute respiratory failure and the need to control oxygen delivery, T.F. should be intubated and placed on mechanical ventilation.

MEDICATIONS FOR INTUBATION AND MECHANICAL VENTILATION

ONLINE CONTENT

For illustrations depicting intubation of an infant, see http://thepoint.lww.com/AT10e.

CASE 101-2, QUESTION 4: What pharmacologic agents are recommended when intubating a pediatric patient? Develop a plan for the medications to be used during intubation of T.F.

After the decision is made to proceed with intubation, the next decision needs to be whether pharmacologic agents are appropriate. Most pediatric patients require sedation before laryngoscopy and intubation. The goal is to depress the infant or child's level of consciousness sufficiently to produce appropriate conditions for intubation. Pharmacologic therapy is used to produce adequate sedation, analgesia, and amnesia plus a blunting of the physiologic response to airway manipulation. Intubation in the awake state can elicit protective reflexes that trigger tachycardia, bradycardia, and elevation of blood pressure, increased intracranial pressure, intraocular pressure, cough, and bronchospasm. Pharmacologic control promotes a smoother intubation with less physiologic stress for the patient who often is already in a compromised state. Ideally, this should be accomplished while producing minimal hemodynamic compromise.[7]

There are many factors to be considered when choosing agents for intubation: the onset of action of the agent, the patient's hemodynamic status, the need to prevent increased intraocular or intracranial pressure that may be caused with intubation, and whether the stomach is full or empty. A wide variety of medications may be used for pediatric sedation, each with its own risk and benefits (Table 101-3).[7] In general, agents that act rapidly and are eliminated quickly are ideal. Often drug choices are made based on the clinician's experience with a particular drug and the immediate availability of the drug. Most importantly, the drug regimen chosen must be based on the patient's physiologic state. Agents with adverse effects that would exacerbate any underlying medical conditions must be avoided. Narcotics used in combination with anxiolytics are used commonly. To produce optimal conditions for intubation, T.F. could be given 12 mcg of fentanyl (1 mcg/kg) and 1.2 mg of midazolam (0.1 mg/kg) IV before the procedure to provide sedation and analgesia. Both agents are relatively short-acting and reversible if difficulties arise with ETT placement.

Patients with inadequate relaxation despite adequate sedation may require neuromuscular blockade, although these agents are not without risk. In a patient with a partial airway obstruction, neuromuscular blockade may worsen pharyngeal collapse, potentially resulting in complete airway obstruction. Therefore, neuromuscular blocking agents should only be used if the clinician is absolutely certain that adequate ventilation can be provided or that the patient can be intubated. If adequate chest rise and oxygen saturation cannot be readily maintained with bag-mask ventilation, neuromuscular blockers should not be used. Infants and children younger than 5 years have a high vagal tone, therefore are more likely to exhibit bradycardia when intubated. Instrumentation of the airway can directly stimulate vagal receptors and induce bradycardia. In these patients it is prudent to administer atropine 0.02 mg/kg (minimum 0.1 mg) before intubation to blunt the autonomic response. Lidocaine (1–1.5 mg/kg/dose with a maximum dose of 100 mg) may be administered intravenously to blunt the airway protective reflexes elicited by instrumentation. This may be particularly useful in a patient with elevated intracranial pressure (ICP).

In the asthmatic patient, drugs that release histamine (e.g., morphine, atracurium, or thiopental) and have the potential to produce laryngospasm or bronchospasm should be avoided. The beneficial bronchodilatory side effects of ketamine, however, make it a useful choice in these patients. In a child with increased ICP, the choice of pharmacologic agent depends on the hemodynamic status of the patient. Thiopental or pentobarbital is an excellent choice in the hemodynamically stable patient whereas etomidate is preferred if the patient is unstable or hypovolemia is suspected. Etomidate should not be used routinely in pediatric patients as a single dose administered for intubation has the potential to produce adrenal inhibition.[8] In children and adults with septic shock, etomidate administration is associated with a higher mortality rate.[8–10]

In all cases of intubation, preoxygenation is carried out to increase the available oxygen in the lungs during the procedure, thus giving the practitioner some buffer time to intubate the patient. However, in patients with an elevated ICP or pulmonary vascular hypertension, hyperventilation is recommended to also produce hypocarbia. A summary of specific patient conditions and recommended agents for intubation can be found in Table 101-4. In an infant or child with a full stomach, the risk of aspiration of gastric contents is high. Rapid sequence intubation (RSI) is used when there is an aspiration risk, such as the child with a full stomach, and there is no concern of a difficult intubation.[11] The goal of RSI is to gain airway control with an ETT as quickly as possible to prevent aspiration. The patient is preoxygenated

TABLE 101-3
Pharmacologic Agents Used for Pediatric Intubation and Continuous Sedation

Drug	Route	Dose	Onset	Duration	Benefits	Adverse Effects
Narcotics						
Morphine	IV	0.1 mg/kg/dose (max: initial dose 2 mg) may repeat to a maximum total dose of 15 mg Neonates: 0.05 mg/kg/dose **Continuous infusion** Children: 20–50 mcg/kg/h Neonates: 15 mcg/kg/h Premature neonates: 10 mcg/kg/h	Peak: 20 minutes	2–4 hours in neonates	Reversible (naloxone)	Histamine release. Respiratory depression hypotension, peripheral vasodilatation, euphoria, dysphoria, itching, central nausea and vomiting, decreased response to hypercarbia
Fentanyl	IV	1–3 mcg/kg/dose (max: initial dose 100 mcg, may repeat to a total dose of 5 mcg/kg or 250 mcg) **Continuous infusion** 1–3 mcg/kg/h (max: initial dose 50–100 mcg/h) CHD patient with an open chest: 5 mcg/kg/h	1–3 minutes	30–90 minutes	Rapid onset, short acting, reversible (naloxone), relatively stable hemodynamic profile	Bradycardia, respiratory depression, decreased response to hypercarbia, acute chest wall rigidity, itching
Benzodiazepines						
Diazepam	IV	0.05 mg/kg/dose (max: 5 mg) may repeat in 0.05-mg/kg increments (max: 1 mg) to a total maximum dose of 10 mg	0.5–2 minutes	3 hours	Reversible (flumazenil)	Respiratory depression, lacks analgesic properties, hypotension and bradycardia, Local irritation, pain
Lorazepam	IV	0.05–0.15 mg/kg/dose (max: 4 mg)	15–30 minutes	0.5–3 hours	Reversible (flumazenil)	Respiratory depression, lacks analgesic properties, hypotension and bradycardia
Midazolam	IV/IM	0.05–0.15 mg/kg/dose (max: initial dose 2 mg, may repeat in 1-mg increments to a total dose of 5 mg) **Continuous infusion** 0.05–0.1 mg/kg/h (max: initial dose 2 mg/h)	1–5 minutes	20–30 minutes	Rapid onset, short acting, provides amnesia, reversible (flumazenil)	Respiratory depression, lacks analgesic properties, hypotension and bradycardia
	IN	0.1–0.3 mg/kg/dose (max: 10 mg) Use the 5-mg/mL concentration	2–5 minutes	30–60 minutes		
	PO	0.5–0.75 mg/kg/dose (max:10–20 mg)	30 minutes	2–6 hours		
Barbiturates						
Pentobarbital	IV	2 mg/kg/dose (max: 100 mg). May repeat in 1-mg/kg/dose increments to a total dose of 7 mg/kg. Do not exceed 200 mg total dose **Continuous infusion** 0.5–1 mg/kg/h	1 minute	15 minutes	Decreases intracranial pressure	Cardiovascular and respiratory depression
	IM/PO/PR	2–6 mg/kg/dose	IM: 10–15 minutes PR/PO: 15–60 minutes	1–4 hours		
Thiopental	IV	2–3 mg/kg/dose, repeat as needed	30–60 seconds	5–20 minutes	Ultrashort acting barbiturate Decreases intracranial pressure	Cardiovascular and respiratory depression

(continued)

TABLE 101-3

Pharmacologic Agents Used for Pediatric Intubation and Continuous Sedation (*Continued*)

Drug	Route	Dose	Onset	Duration	Benefits	Adverse Effects
Miscellaneous						
Ketamine	IV	1 mg/kg/dose every 5 minutes titrated to effect **Continuous infusion** 0.5–1 mg/kg/h	1–2 minutes	10–30 minutes	Rapid onset, airway protective reflexes stay intact, no hypotension or bradycardia Bronchodilation is useful to intubate asthmatics	Increases airway secretions and laryngospasm (blunted with atropine). Elevated intracranial and intraocular pressure. Emergence reactions are possible.
	IM	4–5 mg/kg/dose	3–5 minutes	12–25 minutes		
	PO	6–10 mg/kg (mixed in cola or other beverage)	30 minutes	30–60 minutes		
Etomidate	IV	0.3 mg/kg/dose initially, then 0.1 mg/kg/dose every 5 minutes to titrate to effect	10–20 seconds	4–10 minutes	Rapid onset Short acting Stable hemodynamic profile, decreased ICP	Potential for adrenal inhibition, nausea, and vomiting on emergence
Propofol	IV	1–2 mg/kg/dose initially, then 0.5–2 mg/kg/dose every 3–5 minutes to titrate to effect **Continuous infusion** Infants and children: 50–150 mcg/kg/min Adolescents: 10–50 mcg/kg/min	30–60 seconds	5–10 minutes	Intravenous general anesthetic, rapid onset and recovery	Cardiovascular and respiratory depression, contraindicated in patients with egg allergy, pain on injection
Dexmedetomidine	IV	0.5–1 mg/kg/dose **Continuous infusion** 0.4–0.7 mcg/kg/h Doses as high as 2.5 mcg/kg/h have been used	30 minutes	4 hours	Minimal to no respiratory depression	Hypotension and bradycardia Use with caution in patients with advanced heart block
Neuromuscular Blockers						
Succinylcholine	IV	1 mg/kg/dose	30–60 seconds	4–7 minutes	Rapid onset Short duration	Potentiates hyperkalemia. Contraindicated in head trauma (↑ ICP), crush injury, burns, hyperkalemia. May induce neuroleptic malignant syndrome
Vecuronium	IV	0.1 mg/kg/dose **Continuous infusion:** 0.1 mg/kg/h	1–3 minutes	30–40 minutes	Cardiovascular stable	Slower onset Longer duration of action
Rocuronium	IV/IM	0.6–1 mg/kg/dose	60–75 seconds	20–30 minutes	Cardiovascular stable	
Reversal Agents						
Naloxone	IV	For opioid overdose: 0.1 mg/kg/dose (max: 2 mg) For reversal of mild respiratory depression: 0.01–0.02 mg/kg/dose (max: 0.4 mg) may repeat every 2–3 minutes	2 minutes	20–60 minutes	Rapid onset	Shorter duration than most opioids, therefore repeated doses may be needed
Flumazenil	IV	0.01 mg/kg/dose (max: 0.2 mg), may repeat 0.005 mg/kg/dose at 1-minute intervals to a max total dose of 1 mg	1–3 minutes	6–10 minutes	Rapid onset	Shorter duration than most benzodiazepines, therefore repeated doses may be needed

CHD, congenital heart disease; ICP, intracranial pressure; IM, intramuscular; IN, intranasal; IV, intravenous; PO, oral.

TABLE 101-4
Management Examples of Specific Patient Cases

Condition	Treatment Goal During Intubation	Medications
Full stomach	Prevent passive regurgitation and aspiration after airway protective reflexes lost	Rocuronium, succinylcholine
Bronchospasm	Eliminate or treat stimuli that would induce or increase bronchospasm	Ketamine, vecuronium, lidocaine, atropine
Increased intracranial pressure	No increase in heart rate or blood pressure	Thiopental/pentobarbital, etomidate, vecurinium, rocuronium, lidocaine
Pulmonary vascular hypertension	Avoid decreased pulmonary blood flow	Midazolam, fentanyl, vecuronium
Hypocalemia or depressed cardiac output	Maintain blood pressure without heart rate changes	Etomidate or midazolam with fentanyl

via face mask as bag-mask ventilation cannot be used as it causes gastric distension. Once all necessary intubation equipment is ready, rapidly acting sedative, analgesic, and paralytic medications are administered simultaneously. Cricoid pressure must be maintained until the ETT is in place and confirmed to provide adequate protection from aspiration. An end-tidal CO_2 detector should be attached to the ETT after intubation to confirm proper placement in the trachea. Colorimetric end-tidal CO_2 devices change color from purple to yellow to confirm the presence of exhaled CO_2 and tracheal placement.

Endotracheal intubation and mechanical ventilation can be painful, frightening, and anxiety provoking, especially in a young child. To improve patient comfort, relieve anxiety, and lessen the work of breathing, anxiolytics, sedatives, analgesics are frequently administered once the patient is intubated and mechanically ventilated. Maintenance of adequate sedation is essential. Selection of appropriate agents is based on the physiology of the patient. Guidelines for the use of continuous infusions are outlined in Table 101-3. In the paralyzed patient, neuromuscular blockade neither alters consciousness nor provides analgesia; therefore adequate sedation and analgesia are essential. Providing effective analgesia and sedation to the pediatric patient depends on accurate ongoing efforts to assess the intensity of the patient's pain or anxiety. The assessment of pain and anxiety in infants and critically ill children who are unable to communicate relies heavily on physiologic and behavioral responses. A number of pain and sedation tools have been developed and validated specifically for use in children.[12] No single standard measure gives a complete qualitative or quantitative measure. Selection of an appropriate tool is based on the child's age, underlying medical condition, and cognition level. It is essential that these tools are utilized to evaluate the adequacy of the ICU sedation. Policies and procedures need to be in place for the appropriate selection and use of each tool, in addition to training of all health care professionals to appropriately use each tool. The goal is to use the minimum amount of sedation needed to adequately sedate the intubated child, while minimizing adverse effects.

PEDIATRIC SHOCK

CASE 101-3

QUESTION 1: M.M., a 3-month-old, 6-kg male infant presents with a history of decreased oral intake and progressive lethargy. Physical examination revealed an irritable infant with a respiratory rate of 50 breaths/minute, heart rate of 150 beats/minute, blood pressure of 80/50 mm Hg, and temperature of 39°C. He has cool extremities with a capillary refill of 3 seconds. The mother reports that her baby has had no wet diapers for the last 4 hours. A small purpuric rash has appeared on his trunk in the last half hour since the parents left home to bring him to the emergency room. Initial electrolytes obtained in the emergency room on placement of IV access were as follows:

Sodium, 136 mEq/L
Potassium, 4.9 mEq/L
Chloride, 111 mEq/L
CO_2 content, 13 mEq/L
Blood urea nitrogen, 31 mg/dL
Serum creatinine, 0.8 mg/dL
Serum glucose 50 mg/dL

What type of shock might M.M. be experiencing?

Shock may be classified as hypovolemic, distributive, cardiogenic, or obstructive. Based on his presentation, M.M. is most likely presenting with hypovolemic shock, the most frequent type of shock seen in pediatric patients. Hypovolemic shock occurs when circulating intravascular volume decreases to a point at which adequate tissue perfusion can no longer be maintained. Hypovolemia causes a decrease in preload and adversely affects cardiac output. Initially, hypovolemia activates peripheral and central baroreceptors that cause catecholamine-mediated vasoconstriction and tachycardia. This initial response can maintain adequate circulation and blood pressure even after acute loss of as much as 15% of the circulating blood volume. Shock results from inadequate blood flow and oxygen delivery to meet the metabolic demands of the tissues.[3] Shock will progress from an initial compensated state to decompensated. Typical signs of compensated shock include tachycardia, cool and pale distal extremities, prolonged (>2 seconds) capillary refill, weak peripheral pulses compared with central pulses, and normal systolic blood pressure. As shock progresses, the patient will exhaust his ability to compensate. The patient will exhibit signs of inadequate end organ perfusion, including depressed mental status, decreased urine output, metabolic acidosis, tachypnea, weak central pulses, and mottling of extremities. M.M. shows evidence of having progressed to this later stage, with lethargy and decreased urine output.

CASE 101-3, QUESTION 2: How should M.M. be initially managed and monitored?

All patients presenting with shock should be placed on high-flow oxygen while their initial evaluation is being performed. Initial volume resuscitation in all forms of shock is the same. It is recommended to push isotonic crystalloid fluid (normal saline or lactated Ringer's solution) in 20 mL/kg boluses administered over

5 minutes. Immediately reassess the patient for signs of improved perfusion, using clinical criteria such as reduction in heart rate, improvement of blood pressure, capillary refill, quality of pulses, and mental status. If the clinical signs of shock persist, another 20 mL/kg of isotonic fluid should be administered, reaching, if necessary, at least 60 mL/kg within the first 15 to 30 minutes of treatment.[3,13] Therapeutic end points of fluid resuscitation in patients with shock are capillary refill less than 2 seconds, normal pulses with no difference between central and peripheral pulses, warm limbs, urine output greater than 1 mL/kg/hour, normal mental status, decreased lactate as measured on arterial blood gases (ABG), and increased base deficit. Children normally have a lower blood pressure than adults and are better able to preserve adequate blood pressure by vasoconstriction and increasing heart rate; therefore, blood pressure by itself is not a reliable end point for evaluating the adequacy of resuscitation. Hypotension is the last thing to occur in pediatric shock states. The definition of hypotension, defined as the 5% for systolic blood pressure for age in the 2010 Pediatric Advanced Life Support guidelines[3] is as follows:

- less than 60 mm Hg in term neonates (0 to 28 days)
- less than 70 mm Hg in infants (1 month to 12 months)
- less than 70 mm Hg + (2 × age in years) in children 1 to 10 years of age
- less than 90 mm Hg in children older than or equal to 10 years of age

Fluid resuscitation should be continued until clinical improvement is clear or there is clinical evidence of hypervolemic state as evidenced by rales, a gallop rhythm, or hepatomegaly. Further discussion of the management of hypovolemia and dehydration in children can be found in Chapter 98, Pediatric Fluid, Electrolytes, and Nutrition. M.M. should receive a bolus 120 mL normal saline IV infused over 5 minutes, followed by assessment of perfusion status to ascertain improvement. If he has not demonstrated significant improvement, the fluid bolus should be repeated until adequate perfusion is seen and blood pressure is stable at greater than 70 mm Hg.

CASE 101-3, QUESTION 3: As noted earlier in the case, M.M. is hypoglycemic with a blood glucose of only 50 mg/dL. What are the concerns associated with hypoglycemia during pediatric shock and how should M.M be managed?

Hypoglycemia often develops in infants during episodes of stress, including shock, seizures, and sepsis. Infants have high glucose needs and low glycogen stores, which make hypoglycemia a risk in a critically ill infant, especially one with poor enteral intake. Point-of-care glucose testing should be performed in any critically ill infant with a history of poor oral intake. One should not wait to obtain serum chemistries. Aggressive fluid resuscitation recommended for hypovolemia and shock will only exacerbate hypoglycemia. Most importantly, hypoglycemia needs to be prevented during cardiopulmonary and trauma resuscitation because it may cause seizures and has been linked with poor neurologic outcome.[3,13] Hypoglycemia in pediatric patients must always be promptly identified and treated. After diagnosis, the patient should be managed with a bolus of 0.5 to 1 g/kg of glucose or 5 to 10 mL/kg of a 10% dextrose solution as required to achieve a serum glucose greater than 100 mg/dL. Neonates, especially premature neonates, are more prone to intraventricular hemorrhage with rapid changes in serum osmolarity than older infants and children, therefore 0.2 g/kg or 2 mL/kg of 10% dextrose is recommended in this population until the target serum glucose is achieved. M.M. should be given 30 mL (5 mL/kg) of 10% dextrose IV for 1 to 2 minutes, followed by reassessment of his serum glucose. Treatment may be continued until his serum glucose is within the normal range for his age (60–105 mg/dL). After stabilization, maintenance therapy should be initiated with fluids containing 10% dextrose.

SEPSIS AND SEPTIC SHOCK IN INFANTS AND CHILDREN

Septic shock can be a mixture of hypovolemic, cardiogenic, and distributive shock. In a recent population-based study of children in the United States with severe sepsis (defined as bacterial or fungal infection with at least one acute organ dysfunction), Watson et al. reported an incidence of severe sepsis of 5.3 cases per 1,000 in children younger than 1 year and 0.2 cases per 1,000 children between 5 and 15 years of age.[14] The mortality rate in this study was 10.6%, significantly lower than that reported for adult patients with severe sepsis and septic shock (approximately 30% and 50%, respectively). This dramatic improvement in outcome has been attained through a better understanding of the physiology of shock. The use of aggressive fluid resuscitation and the implementation of time-sensitive goal-directed therapies, as well as the application of technologic advances in respiratory, cardiovascular, renal, and nutritional support, and improved antibacterial, antiviral, and antifungal therapy, has resulted in improved survival in infants and children with septic shock and the resultant multisystem organ failure.[3,15–20]

Infants and young children are at a higher risk of severe systemic illness after infection than adults. Despite new developments in vaccine technology, rates of sepsis have not declined. This phenomenon is most likely as a result of cases occurring in infants before complete immunization. Infants are particularly vulnerable to infections for several reasons.[20] Passive immunity is normally conveyed from the mother to the fetus through transmission of immunoglobulins during the last trimester. As a result, premature neonates are immunoglobulin-deficient. Even the full-term neonate has decreased polymorphonuclear leucocyte function and small polymorphonuclear storage pools compared with older children and adults, as well as decreased ability to synthesize new antibodies. Lastly, neonates cannot make and deliver adequate amounts of phagocytes to sites of infection. This leaves them particularly vulnerable to polysaccharide-carrying bacteria and explains why, historically, *Haemophilus influenzae, Streptococcus pneumoniae,* and *Nisseria meningiditis* caused the majority of significant infections in the first years of life. Low immunoglobulin levels also make the infant susceptible to viral infections. Stores of maternal immunoglobulin are depleted at approximately 2 to 5 months of age. Adult levels of immunoglobulin are not typically achieved until 4 to 7 years of age. As the result of these physiologic differences, as well as differences in bacterial resistance patterns, the list of most likely pathogens in children with sepsis differ from those of adults. Table 101-5 lists common pediatric pathogens and appropriate empiric antibiotic coverage. Antibiotics should be administered within 1 hour of diagnosis, after the collection of appropriate cultures.[13]

As in adults, baseline health status also affects the likelihood of a child exhibiting severe sepsis. Watson et al. found that 49% of cases of sepsis occurred in children who had underlying illnesses which may place them at risk of higher morbidity and mortality.[14] At the Children's Hospital of Pittsburgh, the mortality rate for children who were previously healthy was 2% compared with 12% in children with chronic illnesses.[21]

TABLE 101-5

Causative Pathogens and Recommended Treatments for Pediatric Sepsis

Age or Risk Factor	Microorganism	Empiric Antibiotic Coverage
Age <30 days	*Listeria monocytogenes* *Escherichia coli* Group B *Streptococcus* Gram-negative enteric organisms	ampicillin + aminoglycoside or ampicillin + cefotaxime acyclovir (if patient presents with seizures, until HSV ruled out)
Age 1 to 3 months	*L. monocytogenes* *E. coli* Group B *Streptococcus* *Haemophilus influenzae* *Streptococcus pneumoniae* *Neisseria meningiditis*	ampicillin + TGC ± vancomycin[a]
Age >3 months	*H. influenzae* *S. pneumoniae* *N. meningiditis*	TGC ± vancomycin[a]
Immunocompromised child	*Pseudomonas aeruginosa* *Staphylococcus aureus* *Staphylococcus epidermidis*	ceftazidime or cefepime or piperacillin/tazobactam + vancomycin[a]
Child with a ventriculoperitoneal shunt	*S. aureus* *S. epidermidis* Gram-negative enteric organisms	TGC ± vancomycin[a]

[a] Dosed to maintain trough vancomycin serum concentrations of 15–20 mcg/mL.

HSV, herpes simplex virus; TGC, third-generation cephalosporin (i.e., cefotaxime, ceftriaxone, or ceftizoxime).

CASE 101-4

QUESTION 1: J.B., a 6-year-old, 20-kg girl, presented to the pediatric emergency department in acute distress. She was stabilized with oxygen via nasal cannula and fluid resuscitation before being transferred to the PICU for further management. On presentation to the PICU, she is lethargic and unable to follow commands, with warm, dry, slightly mottled skin and sluggish capillary return. She is febrile to 39.5°C and has a respiratory rate of 21 breaths/minute, a heart rate of 154 beats/minute, and a blood pressure of 76/55 mm Hg. Initial laboratory values are notable for a white blood cell count of 21 × $10^3/\mu L$. Her parents report that she has not urinated since the previous evening. Does J.B. meet the criteria for septic shock?

In an effort to develop a consensus definition of the pediatric sepsis continuum including systemic inflammatory response syndrome (SIRS), infection, sepsis, severe sepsis, septic shock, and multisystem organ dysfunction syndrome, a group of international experts in the fields of adult and pediatric sepsis and clinical research gathered in 2002. A panel was chosen consisting of published pediatric critical-care physicians and scientists with clinical research experience in pediatric sepsis.[16] Because the clinical variables used to define SIRS and organ dysfunction are greatly affected by the normal physiologic changes that occur as children age, the group first defined six clinically and physiologic age categories for defining SIRS criteria (Table 101-6). Premature infants were not included as their care occurs primarily in neonatal intensive care units and not PICUs. Before discussing treatment, it is important that the practitioner understand the terms used to define sepsis. In 1992, SIRS was proposed by the American College of Chest Physicians and the Society of Critical Care Medicine (SCCM) to describe the nonspecific inflammatory process occurring in adults after trauma, infection, burns, pancreatitis, and other diseases.[22,23] Sepsis was defined as SIRS associated with infection. The SIRS criteria were developed for use in adults; it was not until 2005 that a consensus definition was published for SIRS in children (Table 101-7).[24] A separate pediatric definition for SIRS was essential. Tachycardia and tachypnea, pivotal to the adult definition of SIRS, are common presenting symptoms of many pediatric disease processes. To better distinguish SIRS from other diseases, the pediatric definition also includes temperature and leukocyte abnormalities as criteria. Numeric values for each criterion were also established to account for the different physiology in children. Table 101-8 gives the age-specific cutoffs for each criterion.

Temperature is one of the main criteria of the pediatric SIRS definition. A core temperature greater than 38.5°C or less than 36°C may indicate serious infection. Hypothermia is more likely to occur in infants. A core temperature is one measured by either rectal, bladder, oral, or central catheter probe. Temperatures taken via the tympanic, toe, or another auxiliary route are not sufficiently accurate. Temperature may also be documented by a reliable source at home within 4 hours of presentation to the hospital or physician's office. If environmental overheating, such as that produced by overbundling, is suspected, the child should be returned to a neutral temperature environment, unbundled, and the temperature retaken in 15 to 30 minutes.

Meeting the SIRS criteria in children requires the presence of an abnormal temperature, either hypothermia or hyperthermia, or an abnormal leukocyte count in the presence of tachypnea and tachycardia. Sepsis is defined as the proven or suspected infection in the setting of SIRS. Severe sepsis is defined as sepsis in the

TABLE 101-6

Pediatric Age Groups Definitions for Severe Sepsis

Age Category	Definition
Newborn	0 days to 1 week
Neonate	1 week to 1 month
Infant	1 month to 1 year
Toddler and preschool	2 to 5 years
School-age child	6 to 12 years
Adolescent and young adult	13 to <18 years

Reprinted with permission from Goldstein B et al. International pediatric sepsis consensus conference: definitions for sepsis and organ dysfunction in pediatrics. *Pediatr Crit Care Med.* 2005;6(1):3

TABLE 101-7

Definitions of Systemic Inflammatory Response Syndrome, Infection, Sepsis, Severe Sepsis, and Septic Shock in Children

SIRS	The presence of at least two of the following four criteria, one of which must be abnormal temperature or leukocyte count: • Core temperature of >38°C or <36°C (must be measured by rectal, bladder, oral, or central catheter probe) • Tachycardia defined as at least 2 standard deviations above normal for age in the absence of external stimulus, chronic drugs or painful stimuli; or otherwise persistent elevation for a 0.5- to 4-hour time period OR for children <1 year old: bradycardia, defined as a mean heart rate <10% percentile for age in the absence external vagal stimulus, β-blocker drugs, or congenital heart disease; or otherwise unexplained depression in a half-hour period • Mean respiratory rate >2 standard deviations above normal for age or mechanical ventilation for an acute process not related to underlying neuromuscular disease or receipt of general anesthesia • Leukocyte count elevated or depressed for age (not secondary to chemotherapy-induced neutropenia) or >10% immature neutrophils
Infection	A suspected or proven (by positive culture, tissue stain, or polymerase chain reaction test) infection caused by any pathogen OR a clinical syndrome associated with a high probability of infection. Evidence of infection includes positive findings on clinical examination, imaging, or laboratory tests (e.g., white blood cells in a normally sterile body fluid, perforated viscus, chest radiograph consistent with pneumonia, petechial or purpuric rash, or purpura fulminans)
Sepsis	SIRS in the presence of or as a result of suspected or proven infection
Severe sepsis	Sepsis plus one of the following: cardiovascular organ dysfunction OR acute respiratory distress syndrome OR dysfunction of two or more other organs, as defined in Table 101-9
Septic shock	Severe sepsis with cardiovascular dysfunction, as defined in Table 101-9

SIRS, systemic inflammatory response syndrome.
Adapted with permission from Goldstein B et al. International pediatric sepsis consensus conference: definitions for sepsis and organ dysfunction in pediatrics. *Pediatr Crit Care Med.* 2005;6(1):4.

setting of acute respiratory distress syndrome, cardiovascular organ dysfunction, or two or more acute organ dysfunctions (respiratory, renal, hematologic, neurologic or hepatic). The definitions of organ dysfunction have also been modified for children (Table 101-9). Carcillo et al. defined pediatric septic shock (SS) as the presence of tachycardia and poor perfusion, including decreased peripheral pulses compared with central pulses; altered alertness; capillary refill greater than 2 seconds; mottled or cool extremities; or decreased urine output.[16] This definition of pediatric SS does not include hypotension as required in adults because children will often maintain their blood pressure until they are severely ill. Shock may occur long before hypotension occurs. J.B. exhibits the majority of the criteria for pediatric SS, including lethargy, fever, tachycardia, decreased perfusion, and decreased urination.

CASE 101-4, QUESTION 2: What physiologic differences may need to be taken into account when developing a management strategy for J.B.?

There are developmental differences in the hemodynamic response to sepsis in newborns, children, and adults. Practitioners in the PICU may encounter all age ranges thus must be familiar with the clinical differences seen between age groups as it may affect therapy. Adults and children have different adaptive responses that must be considered when selecting therapeutic management. Adolescent patients pose a unique challenge as they may present with either types of symptoms. Among adult patients, the most common hemodynamic alterations include diminished systemic vascular resistance (SVR) and elevated cardiac output (CO). SVR is diminished due to decreased vascular responsiveness to catecholamines, alterations in α-adrenergic receptor signal transduction, and the elaboration of inducible nitric oxide synthase. In general, adults with SS have myocardial dysfunction with a decreased ejection fraction; however, CO is preserved or increased through two compensatory mechanisms: tachycardia and reduced SVR.

Unlike SS in adults, pediatric SS is associated with severe hypovolemia, and children frequently respond well to aggressive fluid resuscitation. Pediatric patients demonstrate diverse hemodynamic profiles during fluid-refractory SS: 58% have low cardiac indexes responsive to inotropic medications with or without vasodilators, 20% exhibit high cardiac index and low SVR responsive to vasopressor therapy, and 22% present both vascular and cardiac dysfunctions necessitating the use of vasopressors and inotropic support.[25] Pediatric patients such as J.B. are different from adults with SS in that low CO, not low SVR, is associated with increased mortality. In fact, studies suggest that the majority of children showed some degree of cardiac dysfunction on presentation after fluid resuscitation.[13,18] Many

TABLE 101-8

Age-Specific Vital Signs and Laboratory Variables

Age Group	Heart Rate[a] (beats/min)		Respiratory Rate (breaths/min)	Leukocyte Count[a] (per $10^3/\mu L$)	Systolic Blood Pressure[a] (mm Hg)
	Tachycardia	Bradycardia			
0 days to 1 week	>180	<100	>50	>34	<65
1 week to 1 month	>180	<100	>40	>19.5 or <5	<75
1 month to 1 year	>180	<90	>34	>17.5 or <5	<100
2 to 5 years	>140	n/a	>22	>15.5 or <6	<94
6 to 12 years	>130	n/a	>18	>13.5 or <4.5	<105
13 to <18 years	>110	n/a	>14	>11 or <4.5	<117

[a] Lower limits of the normal range for heart rate, leukocyte count, and systolic blood pressure for the 5th percentile and upper limits for the for the 95th percentile.
Reprinted with permission from Goldstein B et al. International pediatric sepsis consensus conference: definitions for sepsis and organ dysfunction in pediatrics. *Pediatr Crit Care Med.* 2005;6(1):4

TABLE 101-9

Organ Dysfunction Criteria

Cardiovascular Dysfunction

Despite administration of isotonic intravenous fluid bolus 40 mL/kg in 1 hour

- Decrease in BP (hypotension) <5th percentile for age or systolic BP <2 standard deviations below normal for age[a] OR
- Need for vasoactive drug to maintain BP in normal range (dopamine >5 mcg/kg/min or dobutamine, epinephrine, or norepinephrine at any dose) OR
- Two of the following:

  Unexplained metabolic acidosis: base deficit >5 mEq/L

  Increased arterial lactate >2 times upper limit of normal

  Oliguria: urine output <0.5 mL/kg/h

  Prolonged capillary refill: >5 seconds

  Core to peripheral temperature gap >3°C

Respiratory[b]

- Pao_2/Fio_2 <300 in absence of cyanotic heart disease or preexisting lung disease OR
- $Paco_2$ >65 torr or 20 mm Hg over baseline $Paco_2$ OR
- Proven need[c] or >50% Fio_2 to maintain saturations >92% OR
- Need for nonelective invasive or noninvasive mechanical ventilation[d]

Neurologic

- Glasgow coma scale (see Table 101-12) <11 OR
- Acute change in mental status with a decrease in Glasgow Coma Scale ≥3 points from abnormal baseline

Hematologic

- Platelet count <80,000/μL or a decline of 50% in platelet count from highest value recorded in the past 3 days (for chronic hematology/oncology patients) OR
- International normalized ratio of >2

Renal

- Serum creatinine >2 times upper limit of normal for age or twofold increase in baseline creatinine

Hepatic

- Total bilirubin ≥4 mg/dL (not applicable for newborn) OR
- ALT 2 times upper limit of normal for age

ALT alanine transaminase; BP, blood pressure.

[a] See Table 101-8.

[b] Acute respiratory distress syndrome must include a Pao_2/Fio_2 ratio <200 mm Hg, bilateral infiltrates, acute onset, and no evidence of left heart failure. Acute lung injury is defined identically except the Pao_2/Fio_2 ratio must be <300 mm Hg.

[c] Proven need assumes oxygen requirement was tested by decreasing flow if required.

[d] In postoperative patients, this requirement can be met if the patient has exhibited an acute inflammatory or infectious process in the lungs that prevents him or her from being extubated.

Adapted with permission from Goldstein B et al. International pediatric sepsis consensus conference: definitions for sepsis and organ dysfunction in pediatrics. *Pediatr Crit Care Med.* 2005;6(1):5.

require a change in their inotropic and vasopressor management, or the addition of another agent during the first hours of treatment, emphasizing that the hemodynamic status in children can change rapidly.[13,16–18]

SS in the neonatal patient differs from that seen in older children. The relative ability of infants and children to augment CO through increased heart rate (HR), as seen in adults, is limited by their pre-existing elevated HR, which precludes proportionate increases in HR without compromising diastolic filling time. In adults, ventricular dilation is a compensatory response used to maintain CO. However, the increased connective tissue content of the infant's heart and diminished content of actin and myosin limits the potential for acute ventricular dilation. Neonatal SS can be further complicated by the physiologic transition from fetal to neonatal circulation. Sepsis-induced acidosis and hypoxia can increase pulmonary vascular resistance and thus arterial pressure, thereby maintaining the patency of the ductus arteriosus. This results in persistent pulmonary hypertension (PPHN) of the newborn and persistent fetal circulation. Neonatal SS with PPHN will increase the workload on the right ventricle, leading to right ventricular failure, tricuspid regurgitation, and hepatomegaly. Therefore, therapies directed at reversing right ventricular failure by reducing pulmonary artery pressures are commonly needed in neonates with fluid refractory SS and PPHN.

Based on her mottled dry skin, sluggish capillary refill, and decreased urination, it is evident that J.B. has inadequate perfusion. She should receive aggressive fluid resuscitation, beginning with a fluid bolus of 400 mL (20 mL/kg) normal saline or lactated Ringer's solution IV administered over 5 minutes. She should be reassessed immediately after the bolus to evaluate perfusion status as described previously. The 400 mL fluid bolus should be repeated until adequate perfusion has been established.

INITIAL MANAGEMENT OF PEDIATRIC SEPTIC SHOCK

Since the landmark study by Rivers in 2001 demonstrated a 33% reduction in mortality in adult patients with sepsis when they were aggressively treated with fluid resuscitation, blood transfusion, and inotropic therapy within 6 hours of admission, goal-directed therapy has been advocated for all patients who present in SS.[15] The components of early goal-directed therapy include respiratory support along with prompt resuscitation of poor perfusion through administration of IV fluids and appropriately targeted inotropic and vasopressor therapy, early empiric antimicrobial therapy, drainage of the infection whenever possible, and continuous monitoring of the patient's hemodynamic status.[13,15–19]

CASE 101-4, QUESTION 3: J.B. has received one bolus of normal saline in the pediatric emergency department,

but is still showing evidence of being hypoperfused. Her hemoglobin on admission to the PICU is 10 g/dL. Should she continue to receive traditional IV fluid replacement with normal saline or should other agents be considered to maximize perfusion and oxygenation?

There are no data to suggest a significant difference in survival rates in pediatric patients after resuscitation with colloids, including blood products, compared with crystalloid fluids.[26] The choice of fluid is less important than the volume administered. Adequate volume is necessary to sustain cardiac preload, increase stroke volume, and improve oxygen delivery. Both crystalloids and colloids, specifically packed red blood cells (PRBC), have equal effects on improving stroke volume. In addition, both restore tissue perfusion to the same degree if they are titrated to the same level of filling pressure.

Administration of blood products also differs among institutions. The optimal hemoglobin for infants and children in SS has not been established. In the early management of sepsis in adults, maintaining hemoglobin of 7 to 9 g/dL to improve oxygen carrying capacity has been documented to improve sepsis survival by improving tissue perfusion. Anemia in sepsis has been associated with increased mortality, but so has the administration of blood products.[27] Based on the limited data available, SCCM has recommended that hemoglobin concentrations in adults be maintained at 7 to 9 g/dL.[13] As pediatric data are even more limited, it is necessary to extrapolate from the adult literature suggesting maximizing tissue oxygen delivery if there is evidence of poor tissue perfusion. Once tissue hypoperfusion, acute hemorrhage, or lactic acidosis has resolved, PRBC transfusion should be considered only when the hemoglobin is less than 7 g/dL.[13,28] At this time, there is no indication for administration of blood products to J.B. Fresh frozen plasma may be infused to correct abnormal prothrombin time (PT) and partial thromboplastin time (PTT) values, but should not be rapidly infused because of the risk for acute hypotensive effects caused by vasoactive kinins and high citrate concentration. There is no literature to suggest that 5% albumin administration improves outcome in regards to sepsis mortality. Albumin administration may be considered in patients who are hypoalbuminemic, but routine use of albumin is not recommended.[29]

As described previously for the management of hypovolemic shock, patients with SS should be reassessed for signs of improved perfusion using clinical criteria such as reduction in heart rate, improvement of blood pressure, capillary refill, quality of pulses, and mental status with each fluid bolus. If the clinical signs of shock persist, another 20 mL/kg of isotonic fluid should be administered reaching, if necessary, 60 mL/kg within the first 15 to 30 minutes of treatment.[3,13,17] Some children with SS require as much as 200 mL/kg in the first hour.[17] Patients remaining in shock despite fluid resuscitation are given inotropic support to attain normal blood pressure for age and capillary refill time of less than 2 seconds. Every hour that goes by without implementing these therapies in associated with a 1.5-fold increased risk of mortality. Patients who do not respond rapidly to initial fluid boluses or those with insufficient physiologic reserve should be considered for invasive hemodynamic monitoring. Invasive monitoring of central venous pressure (CVP) is instituted to ensure that the satisfactory right ventricular preload is present, typically using a goal of 10 to 12 mm Hg, and that oxygen carrying capacity is optimized by PRBC transfusion to correct anemia to a goal hemoglobin concentration greater than 7 g/dL.[13,17]

Up to 40% of a child's CO may be required to support the work of breathing during SS; therefore, in the presence of respiratory distress, elective intubation and mechanical ventilation can be used to allow redistribution of blood flow from respiratory muscles toward other vital organs. Intubation is not without adverse effects; it is imperative that patients receive adequate fluid resuscitation before intubation as the change from spontaneous breathing to positive-pressure ventilation will decrease the effective preload to the heart, further decreasing cardiac output. Ventilation may reduce left ventricular afterload that may be beneficial in patients with low cardiac index and high SVR. In addition it may provide an alternative method to alter acid base balance. If sedatives and analgesics are used for intubation, choice of agents that do not cause further vasodilation is critical.

Although laboratory studies rarely affect the management of SS in the first hour of therapy, patients should have laboratory studies sent routinely assessing for hematologic abnormalities, metabolic derangements, or electrolyte abnormalities that may contribute to morbidity. A peripheral white blood count may aid in the choice of broad-spectrum antibiotics and hemoglobin and platelet count will help in assessing the need for early blood transfusion. A type and screen should be sent to the blood bank to prepare for any necessary transfusions. Electrolyte abnormalities are common in sepsis; recognition and treatment of metabolic abnormalities such as hypoglycemia and hypocalcemia will improve outcome. A disseminated intravascular coagulation panel, including PT, PTT, and fibrinogen, will aid in assessing the severity of illness. If abnormalities exist, they may need to be corrected before performing invasive procedures. Lastly, an arterial or venous blood gas will determine the adequacy of ventilation, oxygenation, and severity of acidemia.[17]

Unfortunately, clinical response to fluid resuscitation is a relatively insensitive indicator for the completeness of restoration of microvascular blood flow. Success of adequate fluid resuscitation can be guided by additional parameters: invasive blood pressure monitoring, CVP, measurement of mixed venous oxygen saturation (Svo_2), measurement of blood lactate, and urine output. An elevated serum lactate level suggests tissue is inadequately perfused and undergoing anaerobic metabolism, even in patients who are not hypotensive. Because low CO is associated with increased O_2 extraction, Svo_2 can be used as an indirect indicator of whether CO is adequate to meet tissue metabolic demand. If tissue oxygen delivery is adequate, then Svo_2 should be greater than 70%.[17] In the goal-directed study by Rivers, maintenance of Svo_2 was greater than 70% by use of blood transfusion to a hemoglobin of 10 g/dL and inotropic support to increase CO resulted in a 40% reduction in mortality compared with patients where only mean arterial pressure and CVP were monitored.[15] de Oliveria et al. reproduced this finding in children with SS, reducing mortality from 39% to 12% when directing therapy to a goal Svo_2 saturation greater than 70%.[18]

CARDIOVASCULAR DRUG THERAPY

Pharmacologic support in children with SS must be individualized as different hemodynamic abnormalities exist in pediatric patients, and the primary hemodynamic abnormalities may change with time and progression of the patient's disease (Table 101-10). Twenty percent (20%) of children present with predominant vasodilatory shock, referred to as "warm" shock. This form of shock is associated with vasodilation and capillary leak, but normal or elevated CO. The patients have strong pulses, warm extremities, good capillary refill, and tachycardia. In warm shock, using a vasopressor such as dopamine, norepinephrine, phenylephrine, or vasopressin to promote vasoconstriction would provide the most benefit. Fifty-eight percent (58%) of children present with "cold shock" or a poor CO state. These patients

TABLE 101-10
Summary of Selected Vasoactive Agents

Agent	Dose Range	Peripheral Vascular Effects			Cardiac Effects	
Vasopressors						
		α	β_1	β_2		
Dobutamine	2–10 mcg/kg/min	1+	3–4+	1–2+	Less chronotrophy and arrhythmias at lower doses; chronotropic advantage compared with dopamine may not be apparent in neonates	
Dopamine	2–4 mcg/kg/min	0	0	0	Splanchnic and renal vasodilator, increasing doses create increasing α-effect	
	4–8 mcg/kg/min	0	1–2+	1+		
	>10 mcg/kg/min	2–4+	1–2+	2+		
Epinephrine	0.03–0.1 mcg/kg/min	2+	2–3+	2+	β_2 effects with lower doses	
	0.2–0.5 mcg/kg/min	4+	2+	3+		
Norepinephrine	0.05–0.5 mcg/kg/min	4+	2+	0	Increases systemic resistance, moderate inotrophy	
Phenylephrine	0.05–0.5 mcg/kg/min	4+	0	0	Increases systemic resistance, moderate inotrophy	
Vasodilators						
Nitroprusside	0.5–8 mcg/kg/min	Donates nitric oxide to relax smooth muscles and dilate pulmonary and systemic vessels			Indirectly increases cardiac output by decreasing afterload	Reflex tachycardia
Nitroglycerine	0.5–10 mcg/kg/min	As a nitric oxide donor may cause pulmonary vasodilation and enhance coronary vasoreactivity after aortic cross-clamping			Decreases preload; may decrease afterload, reduces myocardial work in relation to change in wall stress	Minimal
Miscellaneous Agents						
Milrinone	50 mcg/kg load; then 0.25–1 mcg/kg/min	Systemic and pulmonary vasodilator			Diastolic relaxation (lusitrophy)	Minimal tachycardia
Vasopressin	0.003–0.002 units/kg/min OR 18–120 milliunits/kg/h	Potent vasoconstrictor			No direct effect	None known

have vasoconstriction, increased cardiac afterload, and a high SVR. This is clinically manifested as weak pulses, cool extremities, slow capillary refill, and hepatic and pulmonary congestion. Using an inotrope with or without a vasodilator would be most beneficial in cold shock (e.g., dobutamine, epinephrine, or milrinone). Careful assessment of clinical response is critical as a combination of warm and cold shock, with a low SVR and poor CO, occur in approximately 22% of children.

CASE 101-4, QUESTION 4: Despite adequate fluid resuscitation, intubation, and mechanical ventilation, J.B.'s condition has continued to decline. During the past 30 minutes, her systolic blood pressure has ranged between 72 and 79 mm Hg (normal for age, > 84 mm Hg). What would be an appropriate next step for the management of J.B.'s shock?

Vasopressors are required in shock unresponsive to initial fluid resuscitation.[3,13,17] In pediatric SS, the initial agent of choice has typically been dopamine.[13,17] Dopamine has direct and indirect effects on dopamine receptors, α-adrenergic receptors, and β-adrenergic receptors on both the heart and peripheral vasculature. One of the mechanisms of dopamine action is enhancement of endogenous catecholamine release. In severe septic states, presynaptic vacuoles may be depleted of norepinephrine, which may explain why dopamine may have diminished activity. In addition, infants younger than 6 months of age may not have developed their component of sympathetic innervations; therefore they have reduced releasable stores of epinephrine.

Some studies have raised the concern of increased mortality with the use of dopamine. One possible explanation is the ability of dopamine to reduce the release of hormones from the anterior pituitary gland, such as prolactin, through stimulation of the dopamine D_2 receptor, thus reducing cell-mediated immunity and inhibition of thyrotropin-releasing hormone release, worsening impaired thyroid function known to occur in critical illness. Although most clinicians continue to use dopamine as their drug of choice for initiating inotropic therapy in pediatric SS, some prefer low-dose norepinephrine as a first-line agent for those children with fluid-refractory hypotensive hyperdynamic shock.[17]

J.B. should be started on dopamine at a rate of 5 mcg/kg/minute, with further titration of the dose in increments of 2.5 mcg/kg/minute every 3 to 5 minutes until the goal of improved perfusion and/or a normal blood pressure for age is achieved.[3] The maximum recommended dose of dopamine is 20 mcg/kg/minute; higher doses may contribute to increased myocardial oxygen demand without much improvement in vasopressor activity.

CASE 101-4, QUESTION 5: J.B. dopamine has been steadily increased throughout the day. Her dose is currently at 20 mcg/kg/minute, but she continues to have refractory hypotension with a systolic blood pressure of 70 mm Hg. On physical examination, she is pale with cool, dry skin.

Her hemoglobin remains at 10 g/dL. Central venous pressures are now being measured and range from 6 to 9 mm Hg. What alternative to dopamine should be considered for J.B.?

Dopamine-resistant shock is diagnosed after titration of dopamine to 20 mcg/kg/minute with the persistence of signs and symptoms of shock. Patients with dopamine-resistant shock should be reassessed to evaluate fluid status and hemoglobin, with additional fluids or PRBC given as needed to improve tissue oxygen. Measurement of CVP can be performed to assess intravascular volume status with the goal of achieving a CVP of 8 to 12 mm Hg, and SvO_2 can be used as a marker of cardiac output (provided that the hemoglobin is within the normal range), along with the clinical examination. Dopamine-resistant shock commonly responds to epinephrine or norepinephrine.

Epinephrine

Epinephrine is a direct agent that is naturally produced in the adrenal gland and is the principal stress hormone with widespread metabolic and hemodynamic effects. It possesses both inotropic and chronotropic effects. Epinephrine is a reasonable choice for the treatment of patients with low CO and poor peripheral perfusion as it increases HR and myocardial contractility. Depending on the dose administered, epinephrine may exert variable effects on SVR. At doses less than 0.3 mcg/kg/minute, epinephrine exerts greater β_2-adrenergic receptor activation, resulting in vasodilation in skeletal muscle and cutaneous vascular beds, shunting blood flow away from the splanchnic circulation.[17] At higher doses, α_1-adrenergic receptor activation becomes more prominent and may increase SVR and heart rate. For patients with markedly elevated SVR, epinephrine (0.05–0.3 mcg/kg/minute) may be administered simultaneously with a vasodilator. Epinephrine increases glucogenesis and glycogenolysis, resulting in elevated serum blood glucose concentrations. Children receiving epinephrine infusions should have serum glucose monitored closely.

Norepinephrine

Norepinephrine is a direct agent and is naturally produced in the adrenal gland. It is a potent vasopressor that redirects blood flow away from skeletal muscle to the splanchnic circulation even in the presence of decreased cardiac output. Norepinephrine has been used extensively to elevate SVR in septic adults and children. If the patient's clinical state is characterized by low SVR (a wide pulse pressure with diastolic blood pressure less than one-half of the systolic blood pressure), norepinephrine (0.05–0.3 mcg/kg/minute) is recommended. Approximately 20% of children with volume-refractory SS have a low SVR. In children who are intubated and receiving sedatives or analgesics, the incidence of low SVR may be higher. The additional afterload imposed by norepinephrine may substantially compromise CO in patients with impaired contractility. In patients with both impaired or marginal CO and decreased SVR, it may be necessary to support myocardial contractility through the addition of an agent such as dobutamine.[13,17]

Vasopressin

Although not a recommendation in the 2010 Pediatric Advanced Life Support guidelines, vasopressin has been suggested as an alternative therapy for refractory cardiac arrest or hypotension due to a low SVR in children whose epinephrine infusion exceeds 1 mcg/kg/minute.[3] Vasopressin exerts its hemodynamic effects via the $V_{1\alpha}$ receptor, promoting an increase in intracellular calcium in the peripheral vasculature, thus enhancing vasoconstriction and restoring systemic vascular tone. In a preliminary case series, vasopressin at a dose of 0.3 to 2 milliunits/kg/minute (18-120 milliunits/kg/hour) improved blood pressure and urine output in patients with catecholamine-refractory vasodilatory shock and allowed weaning of catecholamines once treatment was initiated.[30] In a more recent analysis conducted by the American Heart Association, however, vasopressin use was associated with a lower rate of return to spontaneous circulation.[31] At this time, the use of vasopressin in critically ill children remains controversial.[3,13,17]

Dobutamine

Dobutamine is a nonselective β_2-adrenergic agonist, which produces improved contractility, chronotrophy, and some degree of lusitrophy, or improved myocardial relaxation. The β_2 activity can lead to peripheral vasodilation and this must be considered before its use in a patient who may already be hypotensive. If hypotension does exist, it should be used in combination with other vasopressor therapy. Dobutamine should be considered in the patient who has signs and symptoms or laboratory values consistent with poor tissue perfusion, but has an adequate blood pressure to tolerate some degree of vasodilation. It should be initiated at a rate of 2.5 mcg/kg/minute and titrated in increments of 2.5 mcg/kg/minute every 3 to 5 minutes to a maximum infusion rate of 20 mcg/kg/minute.[3,17] Careful attention to the patient's blood pressure is critical. Improved perfusion, decreased lactate, and an increased SvO_2 will help determine appropriate dosing.

Vasodilators

Vasodilator medications are occasionally required in the treatment of septic pediatric patients with markedly elevated SVR and normal or decreased CO. Vasodilators decrease SVR and improve cardiac output by decreasing ventricular afterload. Nitroglycerin or nitroprusside may be used for this indication. They each have a short half-life; therefore if hypotension occurs, it can be rapidly reversed by stopping the infusion. Both drugs can be infused at an initial rate of 0.5 mcg/kg/minute and titrated in increments of 0.5 mcg/kg/minute to a maximum infusion rate of 5 to 10 mcg/kg/minute.[3] If nitroprusside is used, it is necessary to observe for sodium thiocyanate accumulation in the setting of renal failure, and cyanide toxicity with hepatic failure or with prolonged infusions (more than 72 hours) of greater than 3 mcg/kg/minute. If a patient has tolerated short-term infusions of either of these agents, milrinone may be considered as an alternative for long-term therapy. Milrinone is a phosphodiesterase type III (PDE III) inhibitor that produces its hemodynamic effects by inhibiting the degradation of cyclic AMP in smooth muscle cells and cardiac myocytes. PDE III inhibitors work synergistically with catecholamines, which produce their hemodynamic effects by increasing the production of cyclic AMP. Milrinone, at a dose of 0.25 to 0.75 mcg/kg/minute, is useful in the treatment of infants and children with diminished CO, impaired myocardial contractility, and decreased SVR.[13,32] The primary concern with milrinone is its relatively long half-life of 2 to 6 hours, which requires several hours for the patient to reach steady-state. To achieve target serum concentrations more rapidly, a loading dose of 50 mcg/kg may be administered for 10 to 30 minutes before the start of the infusion. Administration of a loading dose must be done with caution in children with sepsis and shock as it may precipitate hypotension, requiring volume infusion and/or vasopressor infusion. Administering the loading dose over several hours may avoid this adverse effect.

J.B. remains hypotensive despite adequate fluid administration and a dopamine infusion at the maximum rate. After reassessing her laboratory parameters to determine if additional fluid or blood products are needed, J.B. should be started on epinephrine at 0.05 mcg/kg/minute. The dose may then be titrated upward in 0.05- to 0.1-mcg/kg/minute increments every 3 to 5 minutes as needed to achieve the desired clinical response or to the usual maximum of 2 mcg/kg/minute. Higher doses have been used in some pediatric cases, but may not always provide additional benefit.[3]

CORTICOSTEROID ADMINISTRATION IN PEDIATRIC SEPTIC SHOCK

CASE 101-4, QUESTION 6: J.B. is currently receiving epinephrine at an infusion rate of 0.35 mcg/kg/minute, but she continues to have refractory hypotension with a systolic blood pressure of 70 mm Hg. Is there a role for hydrocortisone replacement in J.B.? What would be the appropriate method for assessing adrenal insufficiency and the appropriate dose for replacement?

Although adjunctive corticosteroid therapy in patients in septic shock has not made a significant difference in outcome in all studies published to date, replacement may be of benefit in some patients.[33–35] In a recent study, 77% of children with septic shock admitted to two PICUs for a 6-month period exhibited adrenal insufficiency.[35] Due to the limited evidence of their efficacy and safety in children, corticosteroids should be reserved for those with catecholamine-resistant shock, severe septic shock and purpura, children who have previously received steroid therapies for chronic illness, children with pituitary or adrenal abnormalities, and those who previously received etomidate.[5–7,13,33–35] Assessment of serum cortisol should be used to guide treatment. There are no strict definitions, but adrenal insufficiency in adults with catecholamine-resistant shock has been defined as a random cortisol level of less than 18 mcg/dL or an increase in cortisol of less than or equal to 9 mcg/dL at 30 or 60 minutes after an adrenocorticotropic hormone stimulation test.[33] Similar values have been recommended for assessment of serum cortisol in children with SS.[13]

If J.B. has a random cortisol of 10 mcg/dL in the face of catecholamine-resistant hypotension, a trial of hydrocortisone is warranted. Published guidelines for hemodynamic support of pediatric and neonatal patients in septic shock recommend 0.5 to 1 mg/kg IV every 6 hours (with a maximum dose of 50 mg).[16] Using this regimen, J.B. should be treated with 10 to 20 mg IV every 6 hours. As an alternative, some clinicians use a regimen of a single 50-mg/m^2 loading dose, followed by the same dose (50 mg/m^2) divided into four doses and given every 6 hours.[13]

ADJUNCTIVE THERAPIES

Stress-Related Mucosal Bleeding

The use of prophylaxis to prevent stress-related mucosal bleeding, although common in adult ICU patients, is not as widely used in PICUs. Studies conducted to date have provided a wide range of gastrointestinal tract bleeding rates in children, ranging from 10% to 50%, with rates of clinically significant bleeding of approximately 1% to 4%.[36,37] Several investigators have identified thrombocytopenia, coagulopathy, organ failure, and mechanical ventilation as important risk factors for gastrointestinal bleeding, similar to studies conducted in adults. A recent systematic review suggested that critically ill pediatric patients may benefit from prophylaxis; however, the results were limited by the small number of controlled studies available.[37]

Thrombosis Prophylaxis

Patients admitted to the PICU can range from newborns to young adults. Unlike adults, there are no data on the use of subcutaneous heparin or low-molecular weight heparins as prophylaxis to prevent deep venous thrombosis (DVT) in children. However, when children reach puberty, the hormone changes that take place appear to increase their risk of thrombosis to that of adults. Although no published guidelines or consensus papers exist to guide therapy at this time, all pubescent adolescents should be considered for DVT prophylaxis. Most cases of thrombosis in infants and young children are associated with long-term use of central venous catheters. Unfortunately, a study evaluating low-dose heparin infused at 10 units/kg/hour did not prevent catheter-related thrombosis in infants after cardiac surgery.[38] It is important to note that the dose of heparin used in this study was less than the anticoagulant dose recommended for infants and children (15 to 25 units/kg/hour). At this time, the routine use of DVT prophylaxis in children remains controversial.

CONGENITAL HEART DISEASE

CASE 101-5

QUESTION 1: J.F. is a 3-week-old, 3.5-kg male infant who was seen by his physician with a history of poor feeding and increased work of breathing. On admission, he was mottled, and grunting, and had severe retractions. The physician referred him to the emergency department of the local children's hospital where his temperature was 40.8°C, heart rate was 200 beats/minute, respiratory rate was 80 breaths/minute, and oximetry saturation was between 60% and 70%; he had very poor peripheral perfusion. Blood-gas analysis results were as follows:

pH, 6.96,
P_{CO_2}, 35 mm Hg
Base deficit, 29 mmol/L

Chest radiography showed cardiomegaly and pulmonary edema. J.F. has presented with symptoms of both respiratory failure and shock. Based on his age, the severity of his hypoxemia, and evidence of cardiomegaly, congenital heart disease (CHD) is suspected. Echocardiography reveals coarctation of the aorta. What initial therapies are needed to stabilize J.F.?

With the neonate's first breath, changes in oxygen tension and a reduction in endogenous prostaglandin E_2 production stimulate closure of the ductus arteriosus (DA), the connection between the pulmonary artery and aorta that allows shunting of blood to the aorta during fetal circulation. Functional closure of the DA typically occurs within the first 10 to 14 hours of life, but complete anatomic closure may not occur until 2 to 3 weeks of age. Prematurity, acidosis, and hypoxia prolong the time to closure. In infants with ductal-dependent CHD, closure of the DA results in inadequate delivery of oxygenated blood to the systemic circulation (Table 101-11). These infants will present just as any other patient in shock. The immediate goal in evaluating a cyanotic neonate is to differentiate between cardiac and noncardiac causes. The classic hyperoxia test is carried out by

TABLE 101-11
Ductal-Dependent Congenital Heart Lesions

Lesions that depend on flow via the ductus arteriosus to maintain systemic circulation
Hypoplastic left heart syndrome (HLHS)
Coarctation of the aorta
Critical aortic stenosis
Interrupted aortic arch
Total anomalous pulmonary venous return (TAPVR) with obstruction
Lesions that depend on flow via the ductus arteriosus to maintain pulmonary circulation
Pulmonary atresia with intact ventricular septum
Critical pulmonic stenosis
Tricuspid atresia
Tetrology of Fallot (TOF)
Epstein anomaly
Lesions that depend on flow via the ductus arteriosus to maintain adequate mixing of the pulmonary and systemic circulations
Truncus arteriosus
Transposition of the great vessels (TGV)
Total anomalous pulmonary venous return (TAPVR) without obstruction

obtaining an ABG, then placing the patient on 100% oxygen for 10 minutes and then repeating the ABG. If the cause of cyanosis is pulmonary, the $Pa{O_2}$ should increase by 30 mm Hg, but if the cause is cardiac, there should be minimal improvement in the $Pa{O_2}$. If the patient is too unstable, one could place a pulse oximeter and place the patient on 100% $F{IO_2}$. With administration of oxygenation, there will typically be at least a 10% increase in oxygen saturation in neonates with pulmonary disease, but those with ductal-dependent CHD will have minimal or no improvement.

If the neonate's oxygen saturation or $Pa{O_2}$ fail to improve and CHD is suspected, an infusion of alprostadil, prostaglandin E_1 (PGE_1), should be initiated at a rate of 0.05 to 0.1 mcg/kg/minute.[39] Infusion of PGE_1 maintains patency of the DA and allows blood to reach the descending aorta, bypassing the cardiac defect. Apnea is a common adverse effect of PGE_1, occurring in 10% to 20% of patients, so age-appropriate equipment for intubation and mechanical ventilation should be immediately available before starting treatment and throughout therapy.[40] Within 10 to 15 minutes after starting an alprostadil infusion, there should be an improvement in the patient's oxygen saturation. The dose may then be titrated to optimize ductal flow and minimize dose-related adverse effects. The infusion is typically continued until corrective cardiac surgery can be performed. J.F. should receive fluid boluses as needed to correct his dehydration and will require intubation. In addition, he should be started on PGE_1 at a rate of 0.05 mcg/kg/minute, with subsequent titration of the dose to open and maintain the DA until the time of surgery.

PEDIATRIC TRAUMATIC BRAIN INJURY

Among children, traumatic brain injury (TBI) is the leading cause of mortality and leads to significant morbidity among survivors. Each year more than 400,000 children in the United States suffer a TBI requiring an emergency department visit, resulting in 30,000 hospitalizations and 3,000 deaths.[41] The most common mechanisms of injury differ by patient age. Children less than 4 years old most often suffer injuries due to child abuse, falls, and motor vehicle collisions (MVC). Child abuse, or nonaccidental trauma (NAT), sadly represents up to two-thirds of severe TBI in some series. Although it is difficult to obtain accurate data, in a population-based study from North Carolina the incidence of TBI due to NAT in the first 2 years of life was 17 per 100,000 person-years.[42] According to the National Center on Shaken Baby Syndrome, this translates to approximately 1,300 children per year in the United States who experience severe head trauma from child abuse. In school-aged children, those 5 to 12 years of age, pedestrian–motor vehicle collision and bicycle-related injuries are among the more common causes of severe injuries. For adolescents, MVC replace falls as the leading cause of all injuries, followed by assault and sports-related injuries.

CASE 101-6

QUESTION 1: K.B. is an 8-week-old, 4-kg male infant who was brought to an urgent care clinic by his 17-year-old mother. She stated that he would not wake up for his usual 7:00 PM feeding that evening. He had been in his usual state of health that morning. She fed him his usual bottle, changed his diaper, and laid him down for a nap. She left him in the care of her 19-year-old boyfriend and went to work. At the clinic, the infant was floppy and unarousable. There were no bruises or other signs of injury, but the anterior fontanel was bulging. His pupils were 3 mm and responded sluggishly to light. When prompted, the boyfriend stated that K.B. fell off the couch early in the morning but only cried for a few minutes. After some comforting, he went back to playing. He fed well the remainder of the day and was taking his evening nap when the mother returned from work. The urgent care clinic suspected NAT and transferred K.B. to the closest hospital with pediatric critical care services. What physiologic differences place K.B. at greater risk for severe TBI than an older child? What risk factors or associations for NAT can you identify in this case?

The anatomical differences of the infant's brain render it more susceptible to certain types of injuries after head trauma.[43] Infants such as K.B. and young children have large, heavy heads. The head is unstable because of its relative size to the rest of the body. If an infant or young child falls a significant distance, is ejected during an MVC, or is thrown from a bicycle after colliding with an automobile, the head will tend to lead (i.e., the infant or child will fly head first) and severe head injuries will occur when the head ultimately strikes the ground or another object. The infant's weak neck muscles also allow for greater movement when the head is acted on by acceleration/deceleration forces. The skull is thinner during infancy and early childhood, providing less protection for the brain and allowing forces to transfer more effectively across the shallow subarachnoid space. The base of the infant's skull is relatively flat, which also contributes to greater brain movement in response to acceleration/deceleration forces. In addition, the infant's brain has a higher water content (approximately 88% vs. 77% in an adult), which makes the brain softer and more prone to acceleration/deceleration injury. The water content is also inversely related to the myelination process, and the higher percentage of unmyelinated brain makes it more susceptible to sheer injuries. The infant brain is typically fully myelinated by 1 year of age. As the result of these physiologic differences, there are differences in the pathology after pediatric TBI by age group. In infants and young children, diffuse injury, such as diffuse cerebral swelling, and subdural hematomas are more common than focal injury, such as contusions, that are typically seen in older

TABLE 101-12
Modified Glasgow Coma Scale

Eye Opening

Score	≥1 year	0–1 year
4	Opens eyes spontaneously	Opens eyes spontaneously
3	Opens eyes to verbal command	Opens eyes to shout
2	Opens eyes in response to pain	Opens eyes in response to pain
1	No response	No response

Best Motor Response

Score	≥1 year	0–1 year
6	Obeys command	N/A
5	Localizes pain	Localizes pain
4	Flexion withdrawal	Flexion withdrawal
3	Flexion abnormal (decorticate)	Flexion abnormal (decorticate)
2	Extension (decerebrate)	Extension (decerebrate)
1	No response	No response

Best Verbal Response

Score	> 5 years	2–5 years	0–2 years
5	Oriented and able to converse	Uses appropriate words	Cries appropriately
4	Disoriented and able to converse	Uses inappropriate words	Cries
3	Uses inappropriate words	Cries and/or screams	Cries and/or screams inappropriately
2	Makes incomprehensible sounds	Grunts	Grunts
1	No response	No response	No response

Source: Chung CY et al. Critical score of Glasgow Coma Scale for pediatric traumatic brain injury. *Pediatr Neurol.* 2006;34:379.

children and adults. The typical pattern of hypoxic-ischemic injury in infants and young children after NAT is rarely seen in older children and adults who are victims of abuse.

Goldstein et al. have published risk factors for NAT based on data gathered from several earlier reports.[44] They found that victims of inflicted head injury tended to be younger, more often from families of poorer socioeconomic backgrounds, and were more likely to have parents who were younger than 18 years of age and who had never been married. In addition, a history inconsistent with physical findings was strongly associated with the presence of inflicted head injury. Additional risk factors reported as associated with NAT are alcohol or drug abuse, previous social service intervention, or a past history of child abuse, in combination with either retinal hemorrhages or an inconsistent history or physical examination. These investigators found this combination was 100% predictive of child abuse in children admitted to a PICU. K.B. met many of these risk factors: he is young, has an unmarried parent who is younger than 18, and is from a low socioeconomic background. In addition, his injuries appear inconsistent with the history of falling from a couch. A fall of approximately 3 feet is required to cause significant head injury to an infant or child; a standard couch is 18 inches from the floor.[45]

CASE 101-6, QUESTION 2: K.B. was transferred immediately to the emergency department at a local hospital. The O_2 saturation on room air was 100%, blood pressure 90/63 mm Hg, and HR 120 beats/minute. The initial Glasgow Coma Scale (GCS) score on presentation was 7, with 2 for eye opening in response to pain, 4 for withdrawing to pain, and 1 for no verbal response. What test or assessment tools are useful for evaluating the extent of K.B.'s injuries? Which are best for predicting his outcome?

The ability to evaluate the severity of TBI is essential to appropriately direct care, predict outcomes, and compare results to evaluate and improve patient care. Initial symptoms on presentation have been found to have little or no correlation with injury severity after TBI. The GCS is a widely accepted method in initially evaluating and characterizing trauma patients with head injuries (Table 101-12). The scale is composed of visual, motor, and verbal components, with lower scores representing more serious injuries. The severity of TBI may be characterized as mild (GCS 13–15), moderate (GCS 9–12), or severe (GCS 3–8) on presentation; however, continued evaluation of GCS scores is the best way to track the patient's clinical progress. K.B.'s GCS of 7 on admission puts him in the category of severe TBI.

The radiologic examination of choice for immediate assessment of a child with severe TBI is a noncontrast cerebral computed tomography (CT) scan. Most children with severe TBI undergo immediate CT imaging to delineate their injuries as soon as they have been fully assessed and sufficiently stabilized to permit safe transport to the radiology suite. If the brain injury does not need immediate surgical intervention, the patient's care is continued in the PICU with the implementation of therapies designed to minimize secondary brain injury. In a retrospective review of 309 children presenting with TBI, Chung et al. found that GCS was more useful in predicting survival among pediatric victims of TBI than CT findings and the presence of injuries to other organ systems.[46] In addition, they identified that a GCS score of less than 5, rather than a score of less than 8 as used in adults, was the threshold at which the patient was more likely to have a poor outcome. The authors also found that head CT findings of swelling or edema and subdural and intracerebral hemorrhage were associated with worse outcomes than subarachnoid or epidural hemorrhage.

Retinal hemorrhages are frequently, although not always, observed in inflicted head injury in infants and young children.

These hemorrhages are the result of sheer forces disrupting vulnerable tissue interfaces. The vitreous body is adherent to the retina in early childhood; shaking can cause retinal hemorrhaging throughout multiple tissue layers, extending to the periphery of the retina. This pattern is unique to "shaken baby syndrome." Although useful for diagnosis, the ocular examination is often deferred initially when evaluating an infant or child for TBI, as the medications used to facilitate funduscopy will preclude the use of pupillary reactivity as a tool to monitor evolving intracranial events.

According to the American Academy of Pediatrics guidelines on imaging for NAT, a skeletal survey is strongly recommended in all cases of suspected physical abuse in children under the age of 24 months.[47] A skeletal survey consist of films of the extremities, skull, and axial skeletal images. Follow-up radiographs of the ribs to assess for healing fractures not seen in the acute phase may be helpful 2 to 3 weeks after the skeletal survey. As with the eye examination, the skeletal survey is often delayed until the child is more stable.

CASE 101-6, QUESTION 3: After assessment by the emergency room physician, K.B. was intubated using rocuronium and pentobarbital, placed on an F_{IO_2} of 100% and sent for a CT scan. The CT reveals a subdural hematoma and cerebral swelling. On arrival to the PICU, K.B.'s vital signs are as follows:

Blood pressure, 85/58 mm Hg
HR, 125 beats/minute
Respiratory rate on the ventilator, 20 breaths/minute

Temperature was 36.9°C. What are the next goals for stabilization of K.B.?

The initial management of a child with a head injury should focus on the basics of resuscitation: assessing and securing the airway, ensuring adequate ventilation, and supporting circulation.[48] In addition, the goals of treatment of TBI are directed toward protecting against secondary brain insults (SBI) which can exacerbate neuronal damage and brain injury. SBI are often the result of systemic hypotension, hypoxia, hypercarbia, anemia, and hyperglycemia. Aggressive treatment strategies are needed to prevent and/or treat these conditions to decrease morbidity and improve neurologic outcome after TBI in children. The criteria for tracheal intubation include hypoxemia not resolved with supplemental oxygen, apnea, hypercarbia (Pa_{CO_2} >45 mm Hg), a GCS score less than or equal to 8, a decrease in GCS greater than 3 compared with the initial score, cervical spine injury, loss of pharyngeal reflex, or any clinical evidence of herniation. K.B. was intubated in the emergency room based on his presenting GCS of 7. All patients should be assumed to have a full stomach and cervical spine injury, so the intubation should be carried out using a rapid sequence intubation using appropriate short-acting sedatives and muscle relaxants (Tables 101-3 and 101-4).

After intubation, K.B.'s ventilatory goals include 100% oxygen saturation, normocarbia (35–39 mm Hg), and no hyperventilation, as confirmed by ABGs, end-tidal CO_2 monitoring, and chest radiographs showing tracheal tube in good position. Unless he has signs or symptoms of herniation, prophylactic hyperventilation (Pa_{CO_2} <35 mm Hg) should be avoided.[48] Hyperventilation causes cerebral vasoconstriction, which decreases cerebral blood flow and subsequent blood volume. Although it will lower ICP, hyperventilation may result in ischemia. Furthermore, respiratory alkalosis caused by hyperventilation makes it more difficult to release oxygen to the brain, shifting the oxygen–hemoglobin curve to the left. Short-term use of hyperventilation, however, may be useful in preventing herniation while other medical therapies are implemented. In addition to mechanical ventilation, the head of the bed should be kept in the neutral position and jugular venous obstruction should be avoided to prevent ICP elevation. Elevation of the head of the bed to thirty degrees usually decreases ICP.

Assessment and reassessment of the patient's circulatory status, including central and peripheral pulse quality, capillary refill, heart rate, and blood pressure, is critical. Hypotension after pediatric TBI is associated with increased morbidity and mortality.[48] Initial treatment of hypotension in the head-injured child is similar to that described earlier for pediatric shock; however, the goal systolic blood pressure in the TBI patient is typically higher: equal to or greater than the 50th-75th percentile for age, sex, and height. Systolic blood pressure less than the 75th percentile has been associated with a fourfold increase in the risk for poor outcome after severe TBI, even when values were 90 mm Hg or greater.[49] This suggests a possible benefit of a higher blood pressure target until ICP or cerebral perfusion pressure (CPP) monitoring is in place to guide therapy. As a result of the need for higher SBP, norepinephrine and phenylephrine, agents with greater vasopressor effects, are more frequently used in this patient population.[50]

The solution of choice for IV maintenance fluids in children with TBI is normal saline for children older than 1 year of age and 5% dextrose with normal saline for infants. Because hyperglycemia is known to worsen SBI, initial IV fluids for children should not contain dextrose. Infants are an exception, as their low glycogen stores make them prone to hypoglycemia, especially with poor oral intake. Hypoglycemia can also worsen neurologic outcome and should be avoided. Frequent assessment of blood glucose either by point-of-care testing or on an ABG is recommended.

Fever increases metabolic demands and is associated with worse outcomes after TBI. Treatment for K.B. should include 60 mg of acetaminophen (15 mg/kg) orally or rectally every 6 hours as needed and a cooling blanket when necessary. Ibuprofen should be avoided as it may increase the risk of bleeding. Patients who are hypothermic on arrival should only be actively rewarmed if there is hemodynamic instability or bleeding thought to be exacerbated by hypothermia. Serum electrolytes and osmolarity should be monitored regularly in K.B., along with accurate assessment of urine output. This is important to identify the development of either syndrome of inappropriate antidiuretic hormone or diabetes insipidus. Both have been reported to occur after pediatric TBI.[48]

CASE 101-6, QUESTION 4: K.B. has been intubated and placed on mechanical ventilation with an ABG showing that he is maintaining goal parameters. He is receiving fentanyl at 1 mcg/kg/hour and a midazolam infusion at 0.05 mg/kg/hour. The head of the bed is raised 30 degrees and his head is midline, supported by a head roll. K.B. has both a pulse oximeter and an end-tidal CO_2 monitor for continuous evaluation of his oxygenation and CO_2. Blood pressure is being maintained at the 75th percentile for age, height, and sex. What is the next step in monitoring head injury in K.B.?

One of the most significant consequences of SBI is the development of intracranial hypertension. The presence of an open fontanel or sutures in an infant with severe TBI does not preclude the development if intracranial hypertension or negate the utility of ICP monitoring. ICP monitoring is recommended for any child presenting with a GCS of 8 or less.[51] When possible, placement of a ventriculostomy catheter provides accurate pressure monitoring and allows for acute drainage of cerebrospinal fluid (CSF) for treatment of elevated ICP and assessment of CPP. The CPP value is calculated by subtracting the ICP from the mean arterial pressure (MAP),

$$(CPP = MAP - ICP) \qquad (Eq.\ 101\text{-}1)$$

This value is important as an indication of blood flow and oxygen that reach the brain. Maintaining CPP requires optimization of MAP with fluid therapy, and if necessary, vasoactive drugs. In the case of ICP elevation, inotropic or vasopressor agents may be used to optimize CPP by increasing MAP, even to the point of relative systemic hypertension. In adults, a CPP of 60 to 70 mm Hg is usually targeted.

There are no data that correlate CPP in infants to outcome. There are, however, pediatric TBI studies showing that CPP values ranging from 40 to 70 mm Hg are associated with a favorable outcome and that a CPP less than 40 mm Hg is associated with poor outcomes.[51] Because infants and children normally have a lower MAP and ICP, the SCCM Pediatric Fundamental Critical Care Support course recommends the following CPP ranges: 40 to 50 mm Hg in infants, 50 to 60 mm Hg in children, and 60 to 70 mm Hg in adolescents.[52] This is more specific than the 2003 pediatric recommendations that recommend a CPP greater than 40 mm Hg and an "age-related continuum" of CPP from 40 to 65 mm Hg in infants and adolescents be maintained.[48]

CASE 101-6, QUESTION 5: The neurosurgeon has placed a ventriculostomy in K.B., and his initial ICP is 25 mm Hg. His other vitals are as follows:

Blood pressure, 83/50 mm Hg
HR, 140 beats/minute
Temperature, 38.5° C

His pulse oximeter still reads 100% and the $ETCO_2$ monitor reads 35 mm Hg. Sedative infusions are unchanged: fentanyl 1 mcg/kg/hour and midazolam 0.05 mg/kg/hour. The pediatric intensivist has placed a central line, and the CVP is 10 mm Hg. What is K.B.'s calculated CPP? What interventions are recommended to treat this ICP elevation?

Uncontrolled increased ICP is very deleterious and must be aggressively treated as soon as possible to reduce cerebral ischemia. In this setting, the goal of any therapy is to lower ICP enough to increase CPP and improve cerebral oxygenation. All initial treatments should be reassessed for efficacy, including treatment of fever, avoidance of jugular venous outflow tract obstruction, maintenance of normovolemia and normocarbia, and provision of sedation and analgesia. The latter is of considerable importance, as anxiety and pain have been shown to increase ICP. K.B. appears to be euvolemic by CVP measurement, is normocapnic, and his O_2 saturation is 100%. He is febrile, however, so measures should be taken to treat the elevated temperature. Although he is receiving continuous sedation, additional bolus doses of sedatives should be given whenever needed. Because K.B. has an elevated CPP in spite of these initial therapies, the best option would be to drain CSF. This will provide an immediate, but transient, decrease in ICP. K.B. may have CSF drained until an ICP value of 15 mm Hg is reached; it should never be drained to 0 mm Hg because edema and diffuse brain swelling could cause an obstruction in the lateral ventricles. When a ventriculostomy is in place and CSF is frequently drained it is important to replace the CSF drained with an equal amount of normal saline. Draining of large amounts of CSF without IV normal saline replacement is associated with the development of hypochloremic metabolic alkalosis. Drainage of CSF in K.B. will provide a CPP in the 40- to 50-mm Hg range. If the ICP increases again, two interventions are recommended, either the addition of a vasopressor to increase SBP or institution of hyperosmolar therapy.

Hyperosmolar therapy may be useful in preventing the ICP from exceeding 20 mm Hg and in maintaining normal CPP. Mannitol has long been the standard of care for management of elevated ICP.[48] Although extensively used since 1961 to control elevated ICP, mannitol has never been compared with placebo. Mannitol reduces ICP by reducing blood viscosity, which promotes reflex vasoconstriction of the arterioles by autoregulation, thus decreasing cerebral blood volume and ICP. This mechanism is rapid, but transient, lasting about 75 minutes and requiring an intact autoregulation. It also produces an osmotic effect by increasing serum osmolarity, causing the shift of water from the brain cell to the intravascular space. Although this effect is slower in onset (15–30 minutes), the osmotic effect last up to 6 hours. Mannitol is a potent osmotic diuretic; osmotic diuresis should be anticipated and fluid resuscitation available to avoid hemodynamic compromise. A Foley catheter is recommended in these patients for accurate measurement of urine output. Mannitol is excreted unchanged in the urine; serum osmolarity should be maintained lower than 320 mOsm/L to avoid the development of mannitol-induced acute tubular necrosis.

Although mannitol has traditionally been the drug of choice for reducing elevated ICP, hypertonic saline (3% sodium chloride) is gaining favor. The main mechanism of action of hypertonic saline is an osmotic effect similar to mannitol. Hypertonic saline exhibits several other theoretical benefits such as restoration of normal cellular resting membrane potential and cell volume, inhibition of inflammation, stimulation of atrial natriuretic peptide release, and enhancement of cardiac output.[48] The theoretical advantage over mannitol is that hypertonic saline can be administered in a hemodynamically unstable patient without the risk of a subsequent osmotic diuresis. Continuous infusions of 0.1 to 1 mL/kg/hour of hypertonic saline titrated to maintain an ICP less than 20 mm Hg have been used successfully in children.[53] Serum osmolarity and serum sodium increase when this regimen is used, but sustained hypernatremia and hyperosmolarity appear to be generally well tolerated. Another potential concern with the use of hypertonic saline is central pontine myelinolysis that has been reported with rapid changes in serum sodium. Currently clinical trials have shown no evidence of demyelinating disorders.

To bring his ICP values down to the normal range (<20 mm Hg), K.B. may be given mannitol at an IV dose of 2 to 4 g (0.5–1 g/kg) administered over 20 to 30 minutes. The effects of mannitol on ICP should be evident within 15 minutes. This dose may be repeated every 4 to 6 hours as needed. If intermittent mannitol fails to bring his ICP down adequately, K.B. may be given hypertonic saline, beginning at 0.1 mL/kg/hour. Dosing of either agent should be guided by regular assessment of serum electrolytes and osmolarity.

CASE 101-6, QUESTION 6: K.B. has been in the PICU for 24 hours. Initial treatment allowed K.B. to maintain a CPP of 50 mm Hg and an ICP less than 20 mm Hg the majority of the day. He is receiving 3% sodium chloride combined with maintenance IV fluids, giving him a serum sodium of 166 mEq/L. Intermittent ICP spikes have responded to intermittent 4-g doses of mannitol; however, the most recent serum osmolarity is 330 mOs/L. What options remain to treat increased ICP in K.B.?

Two nonsurgical options are included in the TBI guideline: barbiturate coma and therapeutic hypothermia.[48] Barbiturates exert neuroprotective effects by reducing cerebral metabolism, lowering oxygen extraction and demand, and alternating vascular tone. Barbiturate serum levels poorly correlate with clinical efficacy, therefore monitoring of electroencephalographic (EEG) patterns for burst suppression is recommended. Burst suppression also represents near-maximum reduction in cerebral metabolism and cerebral blood flow. A pentobarbital loading dose of 10 mg/kg/dose may be administered over 30 minutes, followed by a continuous infusion of 1 mg/kg/hour. Additional loading doses, in 5-mg/kg/dose increments, may be necessary to achieve burst suppression. The primary disadvantage of barbiturate coma is the risk for myocardial depression and hypotension. In addition, the long-term effect on neurologic outcome is unknown. The TBI guideline states that high-dose barbiturate therapy may be considered in hemodynamically stable patients with salvageable severe head injury and refractory intracranial hypertension.[48]

Posttraumatic hyperthermia is defined as a core body temperature greater than 38.5°C, and hypothermia is defined as a temperature of less than 35°C. Although most clinicians agree that hyperthermia should be avoided in children with TBI, the role of hypothermia is unclear. Potential complications associated with hypothermia are increased bleeding risk, arrhythmias, and increased susceptibility to infection. A multicenter, international study of children with severe TBI randomly assigned to hypothermia therapy initiated within 8 hours after injury (32.5°C for 24 hours) or to normothermia (37°C) was recently published.[52] The study reported a worsening trend with hypothermia therapy: 31% of the patients in the hypothermia group had an unfavorable outcome, compared with 22% of the normothermia group. There were several methodological problems with this study. Although the investigators screened patients within 8 hours, the mean time to initiation of cooling was 6.3 hours, with a range of 1.6 to 19.7 hours. In addition, the protocol included a rapid rewarming of 0.5°C every 2 hours so that the patients were normothermic by a mean of 19 hours or 48 hours postinjury. They found that the ICP was significantly lower in the hypothermia group during the cooling period, but that it was significantly higher than the normothermic group during rewarming. Another larger trial conducted by the US pediatric traumatic brain injury consortium is underway which may clarify the utility of cooling in children. Patients will be cooled within 6 hours of TBI and remain cooled for 48 hours. The pediatric TBI guideline states that despite the lack of clinical data, hypothermia may be considered in the setting of refractory hypertension.[48]

Decompressive craniectomy, removal of a section of skull to allow room for brain swelling without herniation, is another option for managing pediatric TBI patients who fail to respond to standard therapies. A randomized trial of early decompressive craniectomy in children with TBI and sustained intracranial hypertension revealed that 54% of the surgically treated patients had a favorable outcome compared with only 14% of the medically treated group.[54] Additional case series have confirmed that patients who receive a decompressive craniectomy have improved survival and neurologic outcomes compared with those undergoing medical management alone.[55] As with barbiturate coma and therapeutic hypothermia, decompressive craniectomy is not without risk. A recent study reported an increased risk of posttraumatic hydrocephalus, wound complications and epilepsy in children with severe TBI.[56] Further studies are needed to establish the timing, efficacy and safety of this management strategy. The pediatric TBI guideline states that decompressive craniectomy should be considered in pediatric patients with severe TBI, diffuse cerebral swelling, and intracranial hypertension refractory to intensive medical management.

CASE 101-7

QUESTION 1: L.B. is an 18 kg, 6-year-old child hit by a car while riding her bicycle. When emergency medical services arrived they witnessed a 2-minute tonic-clonic seizure. GCS at the scene was 11. Should L.B. receive anticonvulsant medication after her TBI?

Posttraumatic seizures (PTS) are classified as early (occurring within 7 days after injury) or late (occurring after 7 days). In the immediate period after severe TBI, seizures increase the brain metabolic demands, increase ICP and are associated with SBI. Therefore, it would be prudent to prevent PTS in the period when the patient is at highest risk of SBI. Infants and children are reported to have a greater risk of early PTS compared with adults. Children younger than 2 years of age have almost a threefold greater risk of early PTS after TBI than children between 2 and 12 years of age. In addition to age, a low GCS (8–11) has been linked to an increased risk of early PTS. The pediatric TBI guideline states that prophylactic antiseizure therapy may be considered as a treatment to prevent early PTS. No prophylactic anticonvulsant therapy is recommended to prevent late PTS.[48]

The majority of the published studies in children have used phenytoin for PTS prophylaxis. Both phenytoin and carbamazepine have been reported to reduce the incidence of PTS in adults. Two recent studies, one retrospective and one prospective, have also evaluated the effectiveness of levetiracetam for seizure prophylaxis in severe TBI in adults.[57,58] Although both studies indicate that levetiracetam was equally effective to phenytoin in preventing PTS after TBI, one study was small and retrospective and the second, although prospective, reported an incidence of PTS that was significantly lower than that reported in the literature. There are currently no studies of levetiracetam for PTS prophylaxis in children. Due to the seizure witnessed at the scene, her young age, and her initial GSC score of 11, L.B. meets the criteria for prophylaxis. An appropriate regimen for L.B. would be phenytoin 45 mg given orally three times daily (7.5 mg/kg/day) for 7 days.

KEY REFERENCES AND WEBSITES

A full list of references for this chapter can be found at http://thepoint.lww.com/AT10e. Below are the key references and websites for this chapter, with the corresponding reference number in this chapter found in parentheses after the reference.

Key References

Adelson PD et al. Guidelines for the acute medical management of severe traumatic brain injury in infants, children, and adolescents. Pediatr Crit Care Med. 2003;4(3 Suppl):S1. (48)

Brierley J et al. Clinical practice parameters for hemodynamic support of pediatric and neonatal septic shock: 2007 update from the American College of Critical Care Medicine [published correction appears in *Crit Care Med.* 2009;37:1536]. *Crit Care Med.* 2009;37:666. (17)

de Oliveria CR et al. ACCM/PALS haemodynamic support guidelines for paediatric septic shock: an outcome comparison with and without monitoring central venous oxygen saturation. *Intensive Care Med.* 2008;34:1065. (18)

Dellinger RP et al. Surviving sepsis campaign guidelines for management of severe sepsis and septic shock [published correction appears in *Intensive Care Med.* 2008;34:783]. *Intensive Care Med.* 2007;32:858. (13)

Kleinman ME et al. Part 14: Pediatric advanced life support. 2010 American Heart Association Guidelines for Cardiopulmonary Resuscitation and Emergency Cardiovascular Care. *Circulation.* 2010;122 (Suppl 3):S876. (3)

Namachivayam P et al. Three decades of pediatric intensive care: who was admitted, what happened in intensive care, and what happened afterward. *Pediatr Crit Care Med.* 2010;11:549. (2)

Key Websites

International Liaison Committee on Resuscitation (ILCOR). Consensus 2010 Documents. www.ilcor.org. Accessed May 15, 2011.

The Surviving Sepsis Campaign. Guidelines for Management of Severe Sepsis and Septic Shock. www.survivingsepsis.com/implement/resources/guidelines. Accessed May 15, 2011.

Geriatric Drug Use

102

Jiwon Kim and May Mak

CORE PRINCIPLES

	CHAPTER CASES
AGE-RELATED PHYSIOLOGICAL, PHARMACOKINETIC, AND PHARMACODYNAMIC CHANGES	
1 Age-associated physiologic changes are associated with pharmacokinetic and pharmacodynamic alterations of drugs in older adults. Decline in drug metabolism and excretion and exaggerated response to drugs are important considerations in drug therapy of the elderly.	**Case 102-1 (Questions 1–4)**
2 Adverse drug events are one of the most important problems associated with drug use in older adults.	**Case 102-2 (Question 1)**
DISEASE-SPECIFIC GERIATRIC DRUG THERAPY	
1 Elderly patients have multiple chronic conditions and take numerous medications. They need to be educated on their disease states and be aware of potential adverse effects and drug interactions. Consulting with their physicians and pharmacists and behavioral modification are good places to start.	**Case 102-3 (Questions 1, 2)**
2 Pharmacologic treatments of heart failure in the elderly include a diuretic, β-blocker, an angiotensin-converting enzyme (ACE)-inhibitor or angiotensin receptor blocker (ARB), with or without digoxin and spironolactone. Benefits should be weighed against risks based on the patient's concurrent conditions.	**Case 102-3 (Questions 3–6)**
3 Elderly patients should be aggressively treated for elevated cholesterol to prevent coronary heart disease (CHD). The drug of choice for treating hyperlipidemia in the elderly is the class of statins. Combination with other classes of agents is considered only if necessary and based on concurrent disease states and potential adverse effects and drug interactions.	**Case 102-3 (Questions 7, 8)**
4 First-line therapy for prevention of coronary artery disease (CAD) includes acetylsalicylic acid (ASA) and β-blockers. Other agents are considered based on concomitant diseases and relative indications.	**Case 102-3 (Question 9)**
5 Hypertension should be treated in the elderly according to the guidelines set forth for the general adult population. Monitoring is essential to prevent excessively low blood pressure, bradycardia, and orthostatic hypotension.	**Case 102-3 (Question 10)**
6 The glycosylated hemoglobin (Hgb A_{1c}) goal may be higher for elderly patients who have hypoglycemia. Pharmacologic therapies for diabetes are recommended based on level of hyperglycemia and relative contraindications.	**Case 102-3 (Question 11)**

continued

DISEASE-SPECIFIC GERIATRIC DRUG THERAPY *CONTINUED*

7	Depression is the most common psychiatric disorder in the elderly, who often present with atypical symptoms of significant depression. Selective serotonin reuptake inhibitors are generally better tolerated than other agents and are considered first-line therapy for older adults.	**Case 102-4 (Questions 1, 2)**
8	Asthma in the elderly can be induced by several precipitating factors, and the management of asthma in older adults does not differ significantly from that for younger individuals. However, coexisting chronic medical conditions, exaggerated systemic adverse drug reactions, and decrease in hand strength or arthritis must be considered when managing drug therapy for asthma in the elderly.	**Case 102-5 (Questions 1–3)**
9	Pneumonia is the leading infectious cause of mortality in the elderly, who typically present with atypical symptoms of lower respiratory infection. Influenza and pneumococcal vaccinations are beneficial in the prevention of pneumonia in the older population.	**Case 102-6 (Questions 1–3)**
10	Urinary tract infection is the most common bacterial infection in the elderly. Oral antibiotics are appropriate for most older patients with symptomatic infection.	**Case 102-7 (Question 1)**
11	Arthritis is the most common cause of disability in the elderly and there are several analgesic agents available for the management of osteoarthritis. Safe and appropriate use of these analgesic medications is important as older adults are at increased risk of adverse drug reactions, including gastrointestinal complications associated with nonsteroidal anti-inflammatory drugs.	**Case 102-8 (Questions 1, 2)**

LONG-TERM CARE FACILITIES

1	Federally mandated responsibilities of pharmacists in long-term care facilities include monthly medication regimen review for appropriateness of drug therapy. Provision of pharmaceutical care in long-term care facilities helps to minimize medication errors, adverse drug reactions, and inappropriate prescribing.	**Case 102-9 (Questions 1, 2)**

DEMOGRAPHIC AND ECONOMIC CONSIDERATIONS

Demographic changes and US medical progress in the last half of the 20th century have created imperatives to improve our knowledge about the health care and drug therapy of older adults. The Federal Interagency Forum on Aging-Related Statistics published an updated chart book, which provides the most current information on the health and well-being of older Americans in the United States (Table 102-1).[1]

The oldest-old category (i.e., those older than 85 years of age) is going to have the greatest impact on the health care system because the number of people in this group has increased faster than any other age category. This group will triple its size by 2040, which is more than double the growth rate of the next fastest-growing category.[2] By 2050, at least half of Americans will live to age 85; they will number almost 19 million and make up 5% of the total US population.[3] Because the frail elderly are often dependent and in ill health, they require the highest level of health services. They have the highest health care expenditures, hospitalization rates, and home health visits.[1]

Approximately 1.3 million US residents 65 years of age or older in 2004 resided in long-term care facilities (LTCFs).[4] Elderly LTCF residents are predominantly women, 75 years and older, white non-Hispanic, and widowed. Although the prevalence of functional disability in the elderly is expected to be reduced,[5] the national expenditure for long-term care services for the elderly is expected to grow through the year 2040.[4] Of older adults who live at home, about 10% in the 65- to 74-year-old age group and up to 50% in the over-85 age group require assistance with everyday activities.[2] Informal care from children and other relatives provides the majority of assistance that allows disabled older adults to live in the community.[1] Thus, it is important to include the caregiver in the counseling and monitoring of daily activities when feasible.

Health care for the elderly is increasingly based on a prospective reimbursement system in institutional settings. Managed-care practices aim to minimize high-cost hospitalizations by shifting care to lower-cost alternatives, such as home health care, assisted living, and hospice care. The escalating costs and affordability of medications is a national concern, especially in the Medicare population. The Medicare Prescription Drug Improvement and Modernization Act of 2003 provided voluntary prescription drug insurance benefits, known as Medicare Part D, to improve older adults' access to prescription drugs. Medicare Part D implementation is associated with up to a 13% increase in drug use in older adults and up to an 18% decrease in patient out-of-pocket costs.[6]

AGE-RELATED PHYSIOLOGICAL, PHARMACOKINETIC, AND PHARMACODYNAMIC CHANGES

An important determinant of drug-related problems in the elderly is an increased physiological vulnerability to adverse drug

TABLE 102-1
Profile of Older Americans

Current Status of the Older Population

- The older population, persons age 65 years and older, numbered 39 million in 2008, representing 13% of the US population. This means that since 1900, the percentage of Americans age 65 years and older tripled (4.1% in 1900 to 13% in 2008), and their numbers have increased more than 10-fold (from 3.1 million to 39 million in 2008).
- There are more women than men in the older population. Among persons 65 years old in 2008, 58% were women. In the oldest old group, 67% of persons age 85 years and older were women.
- The older population is getting older. The 85 and older age group grew from just over 100,000 in 1900 to 5.7 million in 2008.
- The expected number of years of life increased by approximately 60% since 1900. In 2007, life expectancy was 80.4 years for women and 75.4 years for men.
- In 2008, the most common and costly health conditions among all persons age 65 and older were heart disease, diabetes, stroke, and cancer.
- Among all persons age 65 and older, the five leading causes of death are heart disease, cancer, stroke, chronic lower respiratory diseases, and diabetes.

Future Growth of the Older Population

- Although the rate of growth slowed during the 1990s because of the relatively small number of births during the Great Depression of the 1930s, the most rapid increase is expected between the years 2010 and 2030, when the baby boomer generation reaches age 65.
- By 2030, there will be about 72 million older persons, representing 20% of the total US population. The population age 85 years and older will grow from 5.7 million in 2008 to 19 million by 2050.

Source: Federal Interagency Forum on Aging-Related Statistics. Older Americans 2010: key indicators of well-being. Federal Interagency Forum on Aging-Related Statistics. Washington, DC: US Government Printing Office; July 2010.

reactions and an impaired ability to recover from drug-induced insults. The progressive decrease in the ability of each organ system to maintain homeostasis in the face of challenge is a definition of physiological aging.[7] Homeostatic mechanisms in the cardiovascular and nervous systems are less efficient, drug metabolism and excretion decrease, body tissue composition and drug volume of distribution change, and drug receptor sensitivity may be altered. Age-associated changes are progressive, occurring gradually over the course of a lifetime, rather than abruptly at any given age (e.g., 65 years of age).

Absorption

Changes in the gastrointestinal (GI) tract with age may influence drug absorption. Gastric pH increases, intestinal blood flow diminishes, and some impairment of both active and passive transport mechanisms occurs.[8] However, the significance of these changes is not clear. One study found nearly 90% of healthy, independently living elders (ages, 65–96 years) were able to acidify gastric contents (pH 3.5), even in the basal unstimulated state.[9]

Transdermal administration is becoming increasingly common and is used for several medications prescribed to older adults. Alterations in the stratum corneum and lipid composition of the skin, changes in sebaceous gland activity, and changes in the dermis and epidermis may affect drug absorption.[10] Lipophilic drugs (e.g., estradiol) appear to be less affected by aging than do hydrophilic compounds (e.g., acetylsalicylic acid [ASA]).[11]

The following generalizations can be concluded: the extent of absorption via the oral route is similar in older patients and in young adults, the rate of absorption is reduced or unaltered in older patients, and drugs that undergo first-pass metabolism are absorbed more completely in the older patient. Changes in transdermal absorption of drugs have not been sufficiently studied; thus, close monitoring is warranted.

CASE 102-1

QUESTION 1: I.W., a 75-year-old woman, 5′4″, 120 pounds, with a serum creatinine concentration of 1.9 mg/dL, has an acute exacerbation of heart failure (HF). She is given furosemide 40 mg orally, but this produces little increase in urine output or resolution of her symptoms.

What might be an explanation for I.W.'s lack of response to furosemide and how might the desired response to furosemide be achieved?

The extent of furosemide absorption is not changed in older patients, but the rate of absorption is slowed. This results in a diminished efficacy of the drug because active secretion into the urine (rate of entry) must reach the steep portion of the sigmoid dose–response curve for maximal effect of the drug.[12] I.W. should be given a 40-mg dose of furosemide intravenously to bypass the problem of decreased rate of absorption. High sodium intake or concurrent use of nonsteroidal anti-inflammatory drugs (NSAIDs) can also decrease the effectiveness of furosemide. Further increases in the dose of furosemide may be necessary, with consideration of a continuous infusion in patients with severe chronic renal insufficiency (see Chapter 31, Chronic Kidney Diseases).[12]

Distribution

There are a number of age-related changes that can affect the distribution of drugs in the body, including a decrease in cardiac output. This decline in cardiac output is accompanied by an increase in peripheral vascular resistance and a proportional decrease in hepatic and renal blood flow. However, noninstitutionalized older adults who are free of coronary artery disease or other debilitating health problems exhibit little age-related declines in cardiac output.[13] Body composition undergoes changes during normal aging. Total body water and lean body mass both decline with age, and total fat content increases between 18 and 85 years from 18% to 36% in men and from 33% to 48% in women.[14,15] Thus, the volume of distribution (Vd) of drugs that are distributed primarily in body water or lean body mass (e.g., lithium, digoxin) is decreased in older adults; unadjusted dosing can result in higher blood levels. Conversely, the Vd of highly lipid-soluble drugs, such as long-acting benzodiazepines (e.g., diazepam), may be increased, thereby delaying maximal effects or leading to accumulation with continued use.[16] Factors with special applicability in older patients that may affect binding include protein concentration, disease states, coadministration of other drugs, and nutritional status. Serum albumin concentrations fall progressively for each decade beyond 40 years of age, reaching a mean of 3.58 g/dL in those older than 80 years of age.[17] Decreased albumin concentrations are important because albumin is a major site of drug binding. Increases in α_1 glycoprotein in older patients[18] affect the binding of weak bases such as lidocaine and propranolol.

Altered Protein Binding

CASE 102-1, QUESTION 2: I.W. is brought to the emergency department (ED) for evaluation of a "shaking spell." In the ED, another "spell" is observed, starting with shaking of the left arm and progressing into a generalized tonic-clonic

seizure. A loading dose of phenytoin 1,000 mg is given intravenously (IV) for 30 minutes. I.W. is admitted to the neurology unit for further evaluation and given phenytoin 300 mg by mouth (PO) at bedtime. Is the phenytoin regimen appropriate for I.W.? What laboratory tests should be ordered, and how often should these be monitored?

I.W. received a recommended phenytoin loading dose of 17 mg/kg (normal, 15–20 mg/kg) and is receiving the usual daily maintenance dose. A serum sodium concentration should be obtained to rule out a hyponatremia-induced seizure, and a serum albumin concentration should be obtained because of phenytoin's high (90%) protein binding. A serum phenytoin concentration should be measured before I.W. is discharged from the hospital to document that the desired therapeutic serum concentration has been achieved. A follow-up, steady-state serum phenytoin concentration should be obtained in 10 to 14 days to determine whether the current dose is appropriate. The serum phenytoin concentration should be monitored periodically thereafter and whenever an adverse drug reaction or seizure occurs.

CASE 102-1, QUESTION 3: The serum albumin concentration is 2.2 g/dL, sodium is 140 mEq/L, and the serum phenytoin concentration is 15 mcg/mL. I.W. complains of drowsiness and has a wide-based, unsteady gait. What is the likely cause of her symptoms?

I.W. could have a phenytoin free-fraction percentage of up to 18%, compared with the normal value of 10%, because of her low serum albumin concentration.[19] This would produce an equivalent phenytoin concentration of 27 mcg/mL, explaining I.W.'s symptoms (assuming her serum phenytoin concentration is at steady state). In I.W.'s case, free phenytoin (unbound phenytoin) concentration monitoring would be appropriate, if available, and her dosage should be adjusted accordingly.

Metabolism

I.W.'s phenytoin metabolism may be affected by factors known to influence hepatic drug metabolism, which include disease states, concurrent drug use, nutritional status, environmental compounds, genetic differences, sex, liver mass, and blood flow. Liver mass declines and hepatic blood flow decreases 45% between the ages of 25 and 65.[20] Compounds undergoing phase I metabolism (reduction, oxidation, hydroxylation, demethylation) have a decreased or unchanged clearance, whereas compounds metabolized by phase II processes (conjugation, acetylation, sulfonation, glucuronidation) have no change in clearance with age.[20] Drugs with high hepatic-extraction ratios, such as the nitrates, barbiturates, lidocaine, and propranolol, may have reduced hepatic metabolism in older adults.[21]

Excretion

Age-related changes in renal function result in more adverse drug events than any other age-related physiological alteration. Compounding these changes in the kidney are the arteriosclerotic changes and a declining cardiac output that decrease renal perfusion by 40% to 50% between the ages of 25 and 65. This is accompanied by a corresponding decrease in glomerular filtration and urea clearance.[22] Urine concentrating ability declines with age, as does renal sodium conservation.[23,24] Tubular secretory capacity and creatinine clearance may also be reduced.[25,26] The kidney loses functioning cells with age, and histologic studies reveal a decline in the absolute number of nephrons.[27] Significant variability can occur in the rate of decline in renal function in a minority of elderly patients.[28]

TABLE 102-2

Drugs Highly Dependent on Renal Function for Elimination[a]

Acetazolamide	Clonidine	Methotrexate
Acyclovir	Colistimethate	Metoclopramide
Allopurinol	Digoxin	Nadolol
Amantadine	Enalapril	Phenazopyridine
Amiloride	Fluconazole	Penicillins (most)
Aminoglycosides	Fluoroquinolones (most)	Procainamide
Amphotericin B	Furosemide	Pyridostigmine
Atenolol	H_2 blockers (most)	Spironolactone
Aztreonam	Imipenem	Sulfamethoxazole
Captopril	Lisinopril	Thiazides
Cephalosporins (most)	Lithium	Trimethoprim
		Vancomycin

[a] This list is not comprehensive; for additional details, see Arnoff GR, et al., eds. *Drug Prescribing in Renal Failure: Dosing Guidelines for Adults.* 5th ed. Philadelphia, PA: American College of Physicians; 2007.

The plasma half-life is prolonged for a number of renally excreted drugs in "healthy" older adults. The highest-risk drugs are those that depend entirely on the kidney for elimination. Examples of these are listed in Table 102-2.

Age-related changes in renal function can be evaluated using creatinine clearance, an estimate of glomerular filtration rate. The Cockcroft-Gault equation is used most commonly in the majority of clinical settings to estimate creatinine clearance.[29] Many controversies exist with regard to the use of this equation. One relates to whether the actual or lean body weight should be used.[30,31] The use of lean body weight may reflect serum creatinine (SCr) production more accurately because creatinine is produced in muscle mass, which is decreased in older patients. In addition, the Cockcroft-Gault equation depends on SCr concentration and tubular secretion of creatinine, which results in overestimation of renal function in older individuals with chronic kidney disease.

CASE 102-1, QUESTION 4: For renally cleared drugs that require dosage adjustment for I.W., is the Cockcroft-Gault equation an appropriate tool to estimate I.W.'s renal function?

I.W.'s serum creatinine is 1.9 mg/dL and the calculated creatinine clearance using the Cockcroft-Gault equation is 22 mL/minutes. The equation was derived from a predominantly male veteran population who had a single measured 24-hour creatinine clearance.[29] This method overestimates I.W.'s renal capacity to clear renally eliminated drugs, although it remains the most commonly used method to determine drug dosage based on estimated glomerular filtration rate. Other assessments of the renal function, including urine output, should be considered when assessing drug dosage adjustments in older individuals such as I.W., and close monitoring of adverse drug reactions should be followed.

Table 102-3 provides a composite picture of the age-related physiological changes, disease states, and pharmacologic factors that affect pharmacokinetic processes in older adults.

PHARMACODYNAMIC CHANGES

Homeostasis and Postural Hypotension

Pharmacodynamic changes can be defined as alterations in concentration–response relationships or receptor sensitivity.

TABLE 102-3
Changes Affecting Pharmacokinetic Parameters

Parameter	Physiological Changes	Disease States	Pharmacologic Factors
Absorption (bioavailability, first-pass metabolism)	Gastric pH Absorptive surface Splanchnic blood flow GI motility Gastric emptying rate	Achlorhydria, diarrhea, gastrectomy, malabsorptive syndromes, pancreatitis	Drug interactions, antacids, anticholinergics, cholestyramine, food
Distribution	Cardiac output TBW Lean body mass Serum albumin α_1-Acid glycoprotein Body fat Altered relative tissue perfusion	HF, dehydration, edema, ascites, hepatic failure, malnutrition, renal failure	Drug interactions, protein-binding displacement
Metabolism	Hepatic mass Enzyme activity Hepatic blood flow	HF, fever, hepatic failure, malignancy, malnutrition, thyroid disease, viral infection or immunization	Dietary makeup, drug interactions, insecticides, alcohol, smoking, induction of metabolism, inhibition of metabolism
Excretion	Renal blood flow GFR Tubular secretion Renal mass	Hypovolemia, renal insufficiency	Drug interactions

GFR, glomerular filtration rate; GI, gastrointestinal; HF, heart failure; TBW, total body water.

Adverse drug reactions that are mild or nonexistent in younger patients may be significant in older adults because of inefficient homeostatic adjustments. For example, the higher rate of orthostatic hypotension observed in older patients is often the result of impaired baroreceptor function and a failure of cerebral blood flow autoregulation. Orthostatic hypotension occurs in 20% of ambulatory patients older than 65 years of age and in 30% of those older than 75,[32] and it is often aggravated by drugs with sympatholytic activity (e.g., α-adrenergic blocking agents, phenothiazines, tricyclic antidepressants [TCAs]), volume-depleting drugs (e.g., diuretics), and vasodilating agents (e.g., nitrates, alcohol).[33] In one study of 100 geriatric psychiatric outpatients, almost 40% complained of dizziness and falling, which were attributed to psychotropic medications.[34] Patients with impaired cardiac output and taking concurrent diuretic therapy are especially vulnerable. Also, aging impairs balance and posture maintenance, and drug effects on posture control may contribute to drug-induced falls in older adults.[35] Table 102-4 reviews the therapeutic agents commonly associated with adverse drug reactions that may affect the mobility of older patients.

TABLE 102-4
Adverse Drug Reactions That May Affect Mobility of the Older Patient

Medication Class	Adverse Drug Reaction
TCAs	Orthostatic hypotension, tremor, cardiac arrhythmias, sedation
Benzodiazepines and sedative hypnotics	Sedation, weakness, coordination, confusion
Narcotic analgesics	Sedation, coordination, confusion
Antipsychotics	Orthostatic hypotension, sedation, extrapyramidal effects
Antihypertensives	Orthostatic hypotension
β-Adrenergic blockers	Ability to respond to work load

TCAs, tricyclic antidepressants.

Receptor Sensitivity

An exaggerated response to some drugs (e.g., warfarin) may reflect an intrinsic, age-related change in receptor sensitivity.[36,37] The aging central nervous system (CNS) is particularly vulnerable to qualitative and quantitative alterations in drug response. The aging brain loses a significant number of active cells during later life, and some brain atrophy is a common finding in older adults. Normal aging also involves a reduction in cerebral blood flow and oxygen consumption, and increased cerebrovascular resistance.[38] Cholinergic neurons in the neocortex and hippocampal areas of the brain decrease with age. Drugs with anticholinergic properties are associated with memory loss, confusion, and other cognitive impairments in older patients. Several examples of therapeutic classes with anticholinergic properties are listed in Table 102-5.

TABLE 102-5
Categories of Anticholinergic Drugs That Can Induce Confusion in Older Patients

Therapeutic Class	Examples (Brand Name)
Antispasmodic	Belladonna (generic) Oxybutynin (Ditropan XL) Dicyclomine (Bentyl)
Antiparkinson	Benztropine (Cogentin)
Antihistamine	Diphenhydramine (Benadryl) Chlorpheniramine (Chlor-Trimeton)
Antidepressant	Paroxetine (Paxil) Amitriptyline (Elavil) Imipramine (Tofranil)
Antiarrhythmic	Quinidine
Antipsychotic	Olanzapine (Zypexa) Clozapine (Clozaril) Asenapine (Saphris)
Hypnotic	Hydroxyzine (Vistaril)
OTC agents	Antidiarrheals Doxylamine Cold remedies

OTC, over the counter.

Both central and peripheral responsiveness of adrenergic receptors decline with aging.[39] Monoamine-oxidase activity increases with normal aging, and this is reflected by a decline in norepinephrine and dopamine levels in aging brains.[40] The decline in CNS dopamine synthesis is associated with increased sensitivity to dopamine blocking agents (e.g., antipsychotics). However, β-receptor sensitivity to both β-agonists and β-antagonists decreases, even if the number of β-receptors does not decrease in older patients.[41,42] Because these neurologic and biochemical reserves are reduced as a normal consequence of aging, iatrogenic behavioral disorders are relatively common in older adults, and drugs are one of the most common causes of sudden, unexplained mental impairment in the older adult.

PROBLEMS ASSOCIATED WITH DRUG USE IN OLDER ADULTS

ONLINE CONTENT

For a narrated PowerPoint presentation that discusses strategies to evaluate medication therapy in an older adult, go to http://thepoint.lww.com/AT10e.

Polypharmacy

Multiple medication use is the primary cause of drug-related adverse events in the older population according to the Centers for Disease Control and Prevention.[43] Polydrug therapy thrives under conditions in which multiple chronic diseases exist in patients with communication problems, especially when the prescriber is under pressure to be time efficient. These factors can lead to misdiagnoses and unclear drug indications. For these reasons, monitoring drug therapy in these patients is not only challenging but imperative. Busy health care providers often assign a low priority to nursing home patients in terms of individual attention, and much of the prescribing of medications and follow-up is done by telephone. Duplicative prescribing within the same drug class often occurs, and unrecognized drug side effects are treated with more drugs. With minimal actual patient contact, prescribers may continue drugs in patients long after the original problem has resolved to avoid the inconvenience of meticulous dosage adjustments and follow-up monitoring. Careful medication regimen review is essential to identify potentially unnecessary or inappropriate medications and to systematically taper and discontinue these agents, with attentive monitoring of the older person.[44,45]

Adverse Drug Events

An adverse drug event includes preventable and nonpreventable events and accounts for errors related to prescribing and administration. The combining of several medications can also increase the risk of clinically significant drug–drug interactions and subsequent adverse drug events in the elderly. Nearly 1 in 25 community-dwelling older adults is potentially at risk for a major drug–drug interaction.[46] Age per se is not an independent risk factor for adverse drug events, but rather, increased risk is derived from age-related factors (e.g., physiological changes), chronic disease states, use of different health care providers, and inappropriate prescribing.

Twenty-eight percent of hospitalizations of older persons are a result of adverse drug events and poor medication adherence.[47] Adverse drug reactions in older patients cared for in the community may be as high as 35%.[48] An estimated 32,000 hip fractures, 163,000 cases of drug-induced cognitive impairment, and 61,000 cases of neuroleptic-induced parkinsonism occur annually in all elderly.[47]

TABLE 102-6
Predictors of Adverse Drug Events

- More than four prescription medications
- Length of stay in hospital longer than 14 days
- More than four active medical problems
- Admission to a general medical unit vs. a specialized geriatric ward
- History of alcohol use
- Lower mean Mini-Mental State Examination score (confusion, dementia)
- Twenty-four new medications added to medication regimen during hospitalization

Source: Budnitz DS, et al. National surveillance of emergency department visits for outpatient adverse drug events. *JAMA*. 2006;296:1858; Gray SL, et al. Adverse drug events in hospitalized elderly. *J Gerontol A Biol Sci Med Sci*. 1998;53:M59; and Gurwitz JH, et al. Incidence and preventability of adverse drug events among older persons in the ambulatory setting. *JAMA*. 2003;289:1107.

Adverse drug events can be difficult to detect in older patients because they often present atypically and with nonspecific symptoms, such as lethargy, confusion, lightheadedness, or falls. Nevertheless, most adverse reactions represent extensions of a drug's pharmacologic effect, have identifiable predictors, and are preventable (Table 102-6).[49–51] Adverse drug reactions remain a significant problem, with some experts placing the direct health care costs for adverse drug reactions at more than $3 billion annually.[52]

ADVERSE DRUG REACTIONS IN OLDER PATIENTS

CASE 102-2

QUESTION 1: S.E., an 85-year-old woman, 5′2″ and 102 pounds, with a serum creatinine of 1.6 mg/dL, is admitted for chest pain and shortness of breath, and to rule out myocardial infarction (MI). Her physician is concerned about oversedation with narcotics and prescribes ketorolac 30 mg every 6 hours IV. She has a history of severe HF and angina for which she takes lisinopril 10 mg daily, furosemide 40 mg daily, aspirin 81 mg daily, and isosorbide mononitrate 30 mg daily. The lisinopril dosage is increased to 20 mg daily, and the furosemide dosage is also increased to 40 mg twice daily. Her blood pressure (BP) is 110/66 mm Hg, and her urine output has been 20 to 30 mL/hour for 4 hours since ketorolac was initiated. What risk factors are present in S.E. for drug-induced renal problems?

S.E. has a number of risk factors for the development of drug-induced acute renal failure. Angiotensin-converting enzyme (ACE) inhibitors are indicated for HF management and improve renal function by increasing cardiac output. However, they can diminish efferent arteriole glomerular capillary filtration pressure and precipitate acute renal failure in predisposed patients. A 13% incidence of azotemia has been reported in LTCF residents started on a short course of NSAID treatment.[53] A low serum sodium concentration, high-dose diuretics, diabetes, severe HF (i.e., New York Heart Association [NYHA] class IV), use of a long-acting ACE inhibitor, and concurrent NSAID use are all risk factors for drug-induced acute renal failure (see Chapter 30, Acute Kidney Injury). Patients with these risk factors should be monitored closely when an ACE inhibitor is initiated and when the dosage of an ACE inhibitor is increased (see Chapter 19, Heart Failure). Renal prostaglandins (PGE_2, PGI_2) increase or help maintain renal blood flow when renal function is compromised by intrinsic renal disease, HF, liver disease with ascites, or hypertension; therefore, the use of a prostaglandin inhibitor such as ketorolac places S.E. at an increased risk for acute renal failure.

Furthermore, the ketorolac dose is excessive for S.E. based on the recommended maximal dose of 15 mg every 6 hours for elderly patients.[54]

DISEASE-SPECIFIC GERIATRIC DRUG THERAPY

Cardiovascular Disease in the Ambulatory Older Patient

CASE 102-3

QUESTION 1: T.M. is a 78-year-old woman who comes to a "brown bag" session at the local senior center. She reports recently feeling "sluggish" and dizzy. She lives at home alone on a modest, fixed retirement income. T.M.'s chronic medical problems include coronary artery disease (CAD), HF, hypertension, diabetes, and hyperlipidemia. She states that different specialists prescribe her "a lot of medications," but she does not know their names. She admits to skipping her medications periodically when she does not feel well. T.M. usually maintains an active social life, visiting her friends and attending the local seniors' luncheons. She is interested in natural medicines, and self-medicates with nonprescription medications and herbal remedies that her friends also take. Because of the recent weakness, however, she has not gone out as much. Review of her brown bag reveals the following items: glyburide 2.5 mg twice daily, hydrochlorothiazide 25 mg daily, atenolol 50 mg daily, niacin 500 mg three times a day, ASA 325 mg as needed, digoxin 0.25 mg daily, isosorbide dinitrate (ISDN) 20 mg four times a day, nitroglycerin (NTG) 0.4 mg sublingual (SL) as needed, captopril 25 mg three times a day, furosemide 40 mg twice daily, acetaminophen 500 mg as needed, verapamil 60 mg four times a day, multivitamins with minerals, calcium carbonate 500 mg three times a day, hawthorn tincture 20 drops twice daily, ibuprofen 200 mg as needed, pioglitazone 30 mg daily, and dandelion 10 mL twice daily. She also drinks a glass of red wine with dinner and several cups of licorice tea with breakfast and lunch. What initial steps are necessary for safe and effective management of T.M.'s drug therapy?

Like many ambulatory older patients who are being treated for multiple chronic medical conditions, T.M. is at high risk for drug-induced problems secondary to nonadherence, medication errors, prescribing from multiple providers, self-medicating, and polypharmacy. She is representative of more than nine million older adults who live at home alone. The isolated community-dwelling older patient is typically female and 75 years of age or older, has multiple medical issues, and takes multiple medications.[55] With rising life expectancy, the increased complexity of managing multiple morbidities has put nonhospitalized elderly individuals at higher risk of experiencing adverse drug reactions. Many of these individuals lack close support and a daily routine, and limited time awareness makes adherence to complicated medication regimens more difficult in this population. Another group of older individuals at higher risk of having adverse drug reactions is those who are recently discharged from the hospital. The postdischarge period is often a time of confusion, and the elderly may have difficulty coping and sorting out new versus replacement or duplicate drugs. A summary of the various factors contributing to nonadherence in the older patient is presented in Table 102-7.[56]

T.M. needs a primary-care provider to coordinate her medical care and to evaluate the new-onset sluggishness and dizziness.

TABLE 102-7
Factors Influencing the Inability to Adhere With a Medication Regimen

Three chronic conditions
More than five prescription medications
Twelve medication dosages per day
Medication regimen changed four times during the past 12 months
Three prescribers involved
Significant cognitive or physical impairments (e.g., memory, hearing, vision, color discrimination, child-resistant containers)
Living alone in the community
Recently discharged from the hospital
Reliance on a caregiver
Low literacy
Medication cost
Demonstrated poor adherence history

Source: Lamy PP. The elderly, communications, and compliance. *Pharm Times*. 1992;58:33; Bero LA, et al. Characterization of geriatric drug-related hospital readmissions. *Med Care*. 1991;29:989.

She should also be advised to establish a client–patient relationship at a specific pharmacy for all her medications to be on one profile for continuous assessment. Furthermore, T.M. should be counseled to discontinue alcohol, which can interact with several of her current medications and worsen her conditions. Finally, assessment of the risk for medication-related problems (MRPs) is highly recommended by doing a medication review such as the brown bag event, medication therapy management,[57] or using validated tools such as a self-administered questionnaire to identify potential for MRPs.[58]

CASE 102-3, QUESTION 2: T.M. presents to the multidisciplinary geriatric care team on the advice of pharmacists at the brown bag session. During the intake interview, she admits to selective adherence with many medications based on how they make her feel and their costs. Her wine intake with dinner is 8 to 12 ounces most days of the week. She also has not taken her furosemide and potassium supplement because she feels that they are contributing to her sluggishness and dizziness. She is using hawthorn and dandelion instead because they have improved her neighbor's breathing and swelling problems. T.M.'s medical history and physical examination are as follows: 78-year-old white woman, 5′6″, 189 pounds. Vital signs are as follows: BP, 168/82 mm Hg; heart rate (HR), 54 beats/minute; temperature, 98.7°F; and respiratory rate, 18 breaths/minute. Pertinent laboratory values are as follows:

Serum creatinine, 1.5 mg/dL
Blood urea nitrogen, 35 mg/dL
Sodium, 153 mEq/L
Potassium, 3.1 mEq/L
Magnesium, 1.5 mEq/L
Glucose, 250 mg/dL
Glycosylated hemoglobin (Hgb A_{1c}), 9.5%
Total cholesterol, 259 mg/dL
Low-density lipoprotein, 140 mg/dL
High-density lipoprotein, 40 mg/dL
Triglycerides, 200 mg/dL
Proteinuria
Digoxin level, 1.5 ng/mL

Electrocardiogram showed sinus bradycardia with an old anterior MI. Echocardiogram showed an ejection fraction (EF) of 25%. Her problem list includes new-onset sluggishness and fainting, chest pain and shortness of breath (SOB)

on exertion, 3(+) pitting edema bilaterally, NYHA class II–III HF, hypertension, type 2 diabetes, obesity, excessive alcohol intake, CAD, and hyperlipidemia. What factors may be contributing to T.M.'s feeling of sluggishness and dizziness?

T.M.'s sluggishness and dizziness are most likely caused by her low heart rate, somewhat dehydrated state, and multiple medications that have the potential for producing weakness. Specifically, digoxin 0.25 mg daily is considered a high dose for an elderly patient who has moderate kidney compromise. A level of 1.5 ng/mL is excessive because the therapeutic range is 0.5 to 1.2 ng/mL for HF; therefore, the digoxin dose should be lowered to 0.125 mg daily.[59] If the HF is controlled, one can try discontinuing digoxin to evaluate the actual benefit of this agent. T.M.'s supplements usage need to be carefully assessed, as they can contribute to her dizziness. Although hawthorn has been approved for use by the German Commission E in NYHA class II HF, it may have additive hypotensive and bradycardic effects when used with other cardiac medications. It may also increase digoxin's toxicity and should be discontinued.[60,61] In addition, dandelion can produce mild diuretic, hypokalemic, and hypoglycemic effects. Its use needs to be monitored closely in T.M., who has a history of hypokalemia, hypertension, heart failure, and diabetes.[62] Furthermore, the licorice tea has mineralocorticoid properties and may cause blood pressure elevation, salt and water retention, and low potassium levels (increasing the risk of digoxin toxicity), all of which are already present in T.M.[63] In general, elderly patients should be advised not to self-medicate with supplements without clear indications. Finally, atenolol and verapamil can both lower the heart rate and contribute further to the sluggishness. Switching atenolol to an extended-release β-blocker indicated for heart failure should help, and verapamil can be discontinued at this point because it may not have benefits for T.M. other than for hypertension.

HEART FAILURE

CASE 102-3, QUESTION 3: What is appropriate management for T.M.'s stage of HF?

On the basis of the history of an old MI and low EF, T.M. is in stage B of the American College of Cardiology/American Heart Association classification scheme (see Chapter 19, Heart Failure). Heart failure is a common cause of morbidity and mortality in older patients. The standard therapy for HF typically consists of three or more medications (diuretics, β-blockers, and ACE inhibitors, or angiotensin receptor blockers [ARBs], with or without digoxin and spironolactone). Although such a patient is symptomatically relieved with diuretics, the recommended therapy for stage B includes an ACE inhibitor, or ARB, or a β-blocker (if post-MI). Routine use of multiple medications in the treatment of HF with coexisting medical conditions makes close monitoring of drug therapy essential. Concurrent behavior modification with weight loss and salt restriction will also allow better control of the HF.[64]

DIURETICS

CASE 102-3, QUESTION 4: Is the combination of furosemide and hydrochlorothiazide the most appropriate diuretic regimen for T.M.?

Loop diuretics are generally more effective than thiazides; furosemide is also preferred in T.M. because hydrochlorothiazide is less effective in moderate to severe renal compromise (creatinine clearance <30 mL/minute).[65] Furthermore, the combination of furosemide and hydrochlorothiazide (HCTZ) is duplicative in diuretic action and may be excessive. Discontinuing the HCTZ will likely help with T.M.'s hypokalemia and slightly dehydrated state. Regular monitoring of serum creatinine, urea nitrogen, sodium, and potassium is essential while on diuretics. The need for potassium supplementation will depend on the resultant level after T.M. adheres to furosemide while being maintained on an ACE inhibitor. Elderly patients often dislike taking diuretics because of the frequent need to urinate. T.M. may be advised to take the furosemide later during the day after she returns from her social engagements.

ACE INHIBITORS AND ANGIOTENSIN RECEPTOR BLOCKERS

CASE 102-3, QUESTION 5: T.M. has been taking captopril 25 mg three times a day. Is this an appropriate choice of ACE inhibitor for T.M.?

Blockade of the renin-angiotensin-aldosterone system is essential in the management of HF. However, three times daily dosing of captopril is inconvenient and may contribute to poor adherence. A more suitable ACE inhibitor may be ramipril, initiated at 1.25 to 2.5 mg daily.[66] Alternatively, fosinopril 5 to 10 mg daily may also be desirable based on its 50% hepatic and 50% renal elimination profile.[67] However, if an intolerable cough develops, then an ARB such as losartan can be substituted and initiated at 25 mg daily and titrated up to 100 mg as needed.[68] Although previous studies have supported the addition of an ARB to ACE inhibitor therapy based on a lower mortality and hospitalization rate compared with an ACE inhibitor alone,[69] more recent data present concerns about the use of combination therapy in the elderly owing to higher risk of hyperkalemia and worsening renal function.[70]

β-BLOCKERS

CASE 102-3, QUESTION 6: T.M. is being treated with atenolol 50 mg daily. Is this an appropriate choice of β-blocker for T.M.?

The β-blockers carvedilol, metoprolol, and bisoprolol have been proven to reduce morbidity and mortality in patients with HF.[71–73] One of these agents should be considered in patients with HF, unless the patient is in stage IV HF, in which β-blockers are not beneficial.[74] In T.M.'s case, atenolol should be discontinued for two reasons. It is renally cleared and may contribute to excessive sluggishness in an elderly patient with compromised kidney function. Atenolol is also not indicated for HF. Carvedilol or carvedilol extended-release and extended-release metoprolol succinate have similar reductions in mortality, and either agent is appropriate and similarly effective in the management of HF in T.M.

CORONARY HEART DISEASE AND HYPERLIPIDEMIA

CASE 102-3, QUESTION 7: T.M. does not take her niacin because she experienced unbearable facial flushing. Despite her history of MI, she does not believe that cholesterol and "heart disease" are major health concerns for a woman. Are women older than age 65 at different risk of death owing to coronary heart disease (CHD) compared with their male counterparts, and is it important to manage cholesterol in an elderly woman with CHD?

Elevated total cholesterol (TC) levels have been shown to increase the risk for CHD in older adults. Among the elderly of ages 65 to 74 years, 10.9% of men and 24.2% of women have TC greater than 240 mg/dL. For those 75 years of age or older, 9.6% of men and 18.6% of women have TC greater than 240 mg/dL. Overall, 81% of elderly people who die of CHD are age 65 or older. Although male sex is an independent risk factor for CHD, more women than men die from heart attacks within a few weeks because these events occur in women at an older age.[75] The significantly higher rate of hypercholesterolemia in women seems also to predict a higher CHD risk than for men later in life. Therefore, it is important to treat dyslipidemia aggressively in all elderly patients, and not necessarily relax the treatment goals for women. With the 60 to 79-year-old age group, women begin to have an equivalent cardiovascular risk level as their male counterparts. For the 80+ year-old age group, the percentage of women with cardiovascular disease (86.7%) actually surpasses that of men (80.1%).[75]

T.M. is a 78-year-old with history of MI (positive CHD event), diabetes (CHD risk equivalent), and hypertension (HTN), dyslipidemia, and albuminuria (additional risk factors). All together these risk factors confer a 10-year CHD risk greater than 20%.[76]

CASE 102-3, QUESTION 8: What is an optimal therapeutic plan for management of T.M.'s hyperlipidemia?

T.M.'s treatment plan should begin with lifestyle and dietary modifications. Based on a high CHD risk level, she should be started with aggressive lipid-lowering therapy with an LDL goal of less than 100 mg/dL (optimal <70 mg/dL)[76] and a TG goal of less than 150 mg/dL for diabetic patients.[77] Statins are the drugs of choice. An adequate dose is able to lower LDL up to 60% and the TG up to 35%.[77] However, the relative benefits of statin therapy should be weighed against the potential risk of adverse reactions. Liver transaminases should be monitored on a regular basis. Although rare, myopathy with increased levels of muscle enzymes (creatine kinase >10× upper limit of normal) or rhabdomyolysis (myopathy and serum creatinine elevation) warrant discontinuation of these agents.[78] The hydrophilic statins pravastatin, rosuvastatin, and pitavastatin are not metabolized significantly by the cytochrome P-450 system and may present fewer side effects and lower potential of drug interactions.[78] If combination therapy is indicated, ezetimibe can be added to further reduce the levels of LDL and TG without escalating the dose and potential side effects of a statin.[79] Combination of a statin with niacin is less preferred owing to intolerable side effects of flushing and a slightly higher chance of myopathy and hyperglycemia when effective dosages are used.[80] The addition of fibrates to statins has become controversial in patients with diabetes, as shown recently in the ACCORD lipid trial. The addition of fenofibrate to simvastatin in patients with diabetes did not reduce the rate of fatal CHD events, nonfatal MI, or nonfatal stroke compared with those who received only simvastatin.[81] A statin titrated properly should bring the LDL and TG levels to target levels in T.M. In case combination therapy is necessary, then ezetimibe is preferred over niacin and fibrates in this patient. Finally, because alcohol can increase triglycerides as much as 50%, abstinence is strongly recommended.[82]

CASE 102-3, QUESTION 9: What other interventions should be implemented to optimize management of T.M.'s CAD?

Any strategy to optimize her CAD management should take into consideration the patient's functional status, comorbidities, and risks versus benefits. T.M. is still experiencing anginal pain on her current regimen, possibly caused by more advanced disease or inability to adhere to the four-times-daily regimen of ISDN. She should be evaluated for coronary vessel disease and appropriate antiplatelet therapy initiated if necessary. A once-daily long-acting nitrate preparation (isosorbide mononitrate [ISMN]) may be better suited for her, with sublingual NTG available as needed. T.M. should be maintained on first-line CAD therapy of aspirin and β-blockers because aspirin is indicated for MI prevention and β-blockers may also be beneficial for HF. To prevent further endothelial injury from the atherosclerosis that leads to plaque rupture, statins are indicated as described previously. ACE inhibitors (ramipril) have been shown to reduce mortality and to provide secondary prevention in CAD, particularly among those 65 years or older, and thus should be part of the regimen because ACE inhibitors also have benefits for T.M.'s HF and HTN, as well as diabetic nephropathy.[83] Although calcium-channel blockers are indicated in CAD, they have not been proven beneficial for HF; therefore, verapamil may be held at this time while the other agents are being optimized.

HYPERTENSION

CASE 102-3, QUESTION 10: T.M. has uncontrolled hypertension. How should this be managed in light of her advanced age?

T.M.'s blood pressure is well above the goal of less than 130/80 mm Hg for diabetic patients as set forth by the American Diabetes Association (ADA) and the Seventh Report of the Joint National Committee on Prevention, Detection, Evaluation, and Treatment of High Blood Pressure (JNC VII).[77,84] (See Chapter 14, Essential Hypertension.) Hypertension is present in more than two-thirds of individuals older than 65 years of age.[75] Despite having the highest prevalence of hypertension, only a small percentage of this population is controlled or adequately treated for their blood pressure.[84] Treatment of elderly patients should be based on the guidelines for the general adult population. T.M. is also a patient with compelling indications as defined by JNC VII, such as diabetes mellitus (DM), HF, and CAD. In such a patient, the use of a diuretic, ACE inhibitor or ARB, or β-blocker in appropriate combination may improve morbidity and mortality outcomes.[85] The HYVET study has shown that a mean reduction of blood pressure from a baseline of 173/91 mm Hg by 15/6 mm Hg in patients 80 years or older resulted in a 30% reduction in stroke, a 39% reduction in rate of death from stroke, a 23% reduction in the rate of death from cardiovascular causes, and a 64% reduction in the rate of heart failure.[86] Although adequate dosing and combination therapy may be essential in achieving blood pressure control in the elderly population, close monitoring is also necessary to avoid systolic blood pressure (SBP) less than 120 mm Hg based on the recent findings from the ACCORD BP trial. Intensive target of SBP less than 120 mm Hg did not reduce fatal and nonfatal major cardiovascular events but increased the incidence of adverse effects.[87] Serious side effects of aggressive BP lowering include hypotension, bradycardia, hypokalemia, and elevated SCr, and these effects must be diligently monitored. For T.M. it is recommended that adequate doses of furosemide, and ramipril or losartan with close monitoring, be the main therapeutic approach for her HTN. Extended- or controlled-release formulations of metoprolol or carvedilol should be considered as it has been deemed beneficial for HF. Verapamil in sustained-release formulation is only beneficial for CAD and HTN, and should not be used based on T.M.'s unstable HF.[84]

Diabetes in the Elderly

CASE 102-3, QUESTION 11: T.M. reports that she frequently feels lightheaded and shaky after she takes the

glyburide. She admits to not taking glyburide regularly because it also causes rapid heartbeats. What is an optimal therapeutic plan for the management of T.M.'s diabetes?

Comprehensive diabetes education needs to be initiated, stressing the importance of weight loss, self-monitoring of blood glucose, alcohol abstinence, and medication adherence. A 5% to 10% weight loss will improve her glucose control and cardiovascular status.[77] T.M.'s alcohol consumption and self-reported erratic meal schedule may be contributing to the hypoglycemia (in addition to the glyburide), as well as to the worsening of her hypertension and HF. The daily recommended allowance of alcohol is no more than two drinks (24 ounces of beer, 10 ounces of wine, or 3 ounces of 80-proof liquor) for men and no more than one drink for women. In T.M.'s case, this would be 5 ounces of wine (or 12 ounces of beer or 1.5 ounces of 80-proof alcohol).[88] Glyburide is also a long-acting sulfonylurea and is associated with severe hypoglycemia more commonly than other sulfonylureas because of its active metabolites. In general, the elderly are more susceptible, even at low doses, to hypoglycemia. In addition, they may not be able to recognize symptoms of hypoglycemia. Among the second-generation sulfonylureas, glipizide or glimepiride are better choices. However, meglitinides, such as repaglinide or nateglinide are preferred over the sulfonylureas in the elderly population because they do not require dose adjustment in renal compromise and also allow for a more flexible meal pattern because they are taken with each meal and can be skipped if a meal is skipped. Any new diabetes medication should be initiated in low doses and gradually titrated upward to avoid hypoglycemic episodes and to achieve glycemic goals in accordance with ADA guidelines.[77] The current treatment algorithm for diabetes states that metformin with lifestyle modification is the initial management approach.[89] However, metformin is contraindicated in T.M. because of a serum creatinine greater than 1.4 mg/dL. When metformin is contraindicated or inadequate, sulfonylureas or basal insulin can be added to achieve a hemoglobin A_{1c} goal of less than 7%. Less validated therapies include pioglitazone and exenatide or liraglutide.[90] However, pioglitazone should be avoided in T.M. owing to her history of HF. Incretin mimetics may work to prevent progressive beta cell exhaustion and insulin deficiency. Sitagliptin or saxagliptin (dipeptidyl peptidase inhibitors) do not promote hypoglycemia and should be considered early on during the disease state. Their dosages, however, need to be adjusted if the creatinine clearance is less than 50 mL/minutes.[91] In general, the priority of diabetes management in the elderly population should be on reduction of cardiovascular risks with strict control of blood pressure and lipids in addition to avoidance of hypoglycemic events. Therefore, an Hgb A_{1c} goal of less than 8% may be acceptable in some elderly patients who are prone to have hypoglycemia.[92] Injections such as exenatide, liraglutide, or pramlintide should be reserved unless a patient's Hgb A_{1c} remains above 8% while adhering to an appropriately titrated oral combination regimen. It is recommended that glyburide and pioglitazone be discontinued, and repaglinide and sitagliptin or basal insulin such as glargine should be initiated for T.M.'s diabetes. Finally, comprehensive screening of diabetic complications should be done routinely to decrease morbidity and mortality.[77]

Depression and the Older Patient

Significant depression is the most common mental illness among older adults older than 65 years of age, occurring in about 15%; it is a source of significant morbidity and mortality in this population.[93] Unfortunately, depression remains underrecognized and undertreated, even though it is a major risk factor for suicide in the elderly, who have a suicide death rate that is higher than the national average.[94,95] Older patients may be at increased risk for depression because of the high prevalence of comorbid medical conditions (i.e., stroke, cancer, MI, rheumatoid arthritis, dementia, Parkinson disease, DM).[96] Refer to Chapter 83, Mood Disorders I: Major Depressive Disorders, for further discussion of risk factors for depression and potential drug-induced causes. Most patients are treated in the primary-care setting.[95]

CASE 102-4

QUESTION 1: J.W. is a married, 5′8″, 110-pound, 79-year-old woman who presents for a psychiatric evaluation. Her husband says she just has not been herself lately. The changes in J.W. began on a family vacation 6 months earlier when she got lost on the cruise ship. Since that incident, she has become increasingly anxious and has developed insomnia. Although she does not feel sad or "depressed," she generally does not feel well. J.W.'s normally positive attitude toward life has become pessimistic. Her husband confirms that she has become more forgetful and no longer enjoys eating. In fact, she has lost 18 pounds during the past 2 months. J.W. no longer does her volunteer work at the local children's center. She says she wants to die because she is no longer the person she used to be, but she denies having any specific suicidal thoughts. Her medical history is significant for diabetes and hypertension, which are both well controlled on glipizide 5 mg every morning and hydrochlorothiazide 25 mg daily. Her medical evaluation and physical examination are unremarkable. Laboratory results and head computed tomography scan are within normal limits. J.W. is diagnosed as having a major depressive episode. What symptoms of depression are present in J.W.?

J.W.'s presenting symptoms are typical of major depression in an older patient, which is commonly quite different from that of younger depressed patients. Criteria set forth in the *Diagnostic and Statistical Manual of Mental Disorders, Fourth Edition*, for diagnosing depression were developed using younger subjects and may not be applicable to the older depressed patient.[97,98] Older patients are less likely to report suicidal thoughts, but are more likely to experience weight loss as a symptom of depression. Anxiety, irritability, somatic complaints, or a withdrawal from normal activities, as exhibited by J.W., may be more significant features in late-life depression than depressed mood. Memory problems, such as J.W.'s forgetfulness, may be attributable to a lack of concentration or effort stemming from her depression. This is distinct from dementia, which manifests itself predominantly with impairment in short- and long-term memory (see Chapter 103, Geriatric Dementias). Therefore, depressed mood cannot be relied on for determining whether an older patient has a depressive disorder.[94] Table 102-8 lists atypical depressive symptoms that may be found in older adults. The presence of any one of these symptoms should be considered a red flag and should prompt further evaluation for major depression.

CASE 102-4, QUESTION 2: J.W.'s physician decides to prescribe an antidepressant. Which antidepressants are preferred for use in older adults?

Selection of an antidepressant drug for elderly patients must take into consideration age-related changes in pharmacokinetic, pharmacodynamic, and physiological parameters that make this population more vulnerable to adverse effects. Although the

TABLE 102-8
Atypical Depressive Symptoms in the Older Adult

Agitation, anxiety, or worrying
Reduced initiative and problem-solving capacities
Alcohol or substance abuse
Paranoia
Obsessions and compulsions
Irritability
Somatic complaints
Excessive guilt
Marital discord
Social withdrawal
Cognitive impairment
Deterioration in self-care

Source: Sable JA, et al. Late-life depression: how to identify its symptoms and provide effective treatment. *Geriatrics*. 2002;57:18.

available antidepressants are equally effective, selective serotonin reuptake inhibitors (SSRIs) are better tolerated than older agents, such as the tricyclic antidepressants. Therefore, low-dose SSRIs should be considered first-line therapy for older patients. Of course, this does not preclude the use of sound clinical judgment that incorporates the patient's history of response, comorbidities, and the drug's side effect profile. J.W. should start taking a low-dose SSRI, such as citalopram 10 mg daily, with gradual dose titration to achieve control of her depressive symptoms. Table 102-9 lists recommended starting doses for antidepressants in older patients. Full antidepressant response may take twice as long in older patients compared with younger patients; it may take 8 to 12 weeks before assessment of J.W.'s full response can be made.[99]

Asthma and Chronic Obstructive Pulmonary Disease in the Elderly

Epidemiologic studies estimate the prevalence of asthma in the elderly to be between 6.5% and 17% and even higher for chronic obstructive pulmonary disease (COPD).[100,101] Although many patients have a history of childhood asthma that persists into adulthood, a significant proportion (up to 48%) are diagnosed with asthma after age 65.[102] Rates of hospitalization for asthma are highest in the older population, and asthma-related mortality for adults age 65 to 74 years is higher compared with younger adults, possibly because of underdiagnosis and undertreatment of the disease.[103] Symptoms of asthma, including wheezing, cough, chest tightness, and dyspnea are similar in both older and younger patients (see Chapter 23, Asthma). However, because the elderly are more likely to have coexisting medical conditions (e.g., HF, angina, COPD, gastroesophageal reflux disease [GERD]) with symptoms that mimic asthma, accurate diagnosis and assessment of severity is often more difficult.[104]

Chronic obstructive pulmonary disease is a lung disease caused by chronic bronchitis or emphysema seen largely in those older than 65 years. This chronic condition is a major cause of morbidity and mortality in the older population,[105] but it is often undiagnosed because patients tend to accept worsening pulmonary function as part of the "normal" aging process or may be less aware of the symptoms of airflow obstruction.[106,107] Drug therapy for COPD in the elderly does not differ significantly from standard management regimens (see Chapter 24, Chronic Obstructive Pulmonary Disease). However, older patients with pulmonary disease and coexisting medical problems may be more sensitive to the adverse effects of pharmacologic agents.

TABLE 102-9
Antidepressant Dosing in Older Adults

	Initial Dosage	Maximum Dosage
Citalopram	10 mg every day	40 mg every day
Escitalopram	5 mg every day	20 mg every day
Fluoxetine	5 mg every day	40 mg every day
Fluvoxamine	25 mg at bedtime	200 mg at bedtime
Paroxetine	10 mg every day	40 mg every day
Sertraline	25 mg every day	150 mg every day
Mirtazapine	7.5 mg every day	45 mg every day
Bupropion	37.5 mg twice a day	75 mg twice a day
Duloxetine	20 mg every day	40 mg every day
Venlafaxine	25 mg twice a day	225 mg every day
Desvenlafaxine	50 mg every day	400 mg every day

CASE 102-5

QUESTION 1: J.C., a 67-year-old woman, 5′6″, 145 pounds, presents to the ED with complaints of shortness of breath for the past 2 days. She was in her usual state of health until 4 days ago when she exhibited flulike symptoms consisting of fever, cough, and mild wheezing. J.C. has a history of asthma, diabetes, hypertension, headache, and GERD. Her current medications include glipizide 5 mg daily, lisinopril 10 mg daily, metoprolol 50 mg twice daily, lansoprazole 30 mg daily, ibuprofen 200 mg every 6 hours as needed for headache, albuterol metered-dose inhaler (MDI) 2 puffs four times a day as needed for SOB, and fluticasone HFA (44 mcg) MDI 2 puffs twice daily. Her drug regimen has been unchanged for the past 2 years, and she reports taking all medications as prescribed. The only recent change has been the need for albuterol every 3 to 4 hours for coughing and wheezing during the past few days. What factors (including medications) may have contributed to her acute asthma exacerbation?

Management of acute asthma exacerbations in previously stable elderly asthmatics should begin with a review of the medication history for asthma-inducing agents. Aspirin and other NSAIDs are known to induce acute bronchoconstriction in approximately 3% to 5% of adult asthmatics.[108] J.C. should be queried about her previous (especially recent) use of ibuprofen in relation to her asthma symptoms. If she reports worsening of her asthma after ingestion of ibuprofen, further use of aspirin and NSAIDs should be avoided. Alternative agents for pain control include acetaminophen or selective cyclo-oxygenase (COX) -2 inhibitors (e.g., celecoxib).[109] Nonselective β-blockers, including topical ophthalmic formulations, can precipitate acute bronchoconstriction and should be avoided in patients with reactive airway disease. Although cardioselective β-blockers are generally considered safe for use in patients with asthma, it is important to recognize that cardioselectivity may be lost with higher dosages. Because J.C. has been taking low-dose metoprolol (a cardioselective agent) for years without problem, this medication is unlikely to be contributing to her current asthma exacerbation. One of the most important triggers for asthma exacerbations is respiratory infection (particularly viral). J.C. reports the recent onset of symptoms consistent with influenza, and this is likely precipitating her current pulmonary symptoms. As a future prophylactic measure, J.C. should be counseled to receive the influenza vaccine annually. In addition, because she is older than 65 years, she should receive a one-time pneumococcal vaccine to reduce the risk of developing pneumococcal pneumonia.

CASE 102-5, QUESTION 2: Are the medication regimens used to treat asthma in elderly patients different from those used in children and younger adults? Should J.C.'s asthma regimen be changed?

Medications used in the management of persistent asthma in the elderly are similar to those used in younger patients and consist of bronchodilators in combination with anti-inflammatory agents (see Chapter 23, Asthma). The primary difference relates to drug selection and monitoring, which may be more complicated in the elderly because of the greater likelihood of coexisting medical conditions and increased potential for drug–disease and drug–drug interactions.

Inhaled β_2-agonists are an important class of drugs used to treat asthma in all age groups. The low incidence of drug interactions and reduced side effect profile make inhaled β_2-agonists ideal for use in the older asthmatics. However, both inhaled and oral β_2-agonists can cause dose-dependent systemic side effects, such as tremor, tachycardia, hypokalemia, and arrhythmias, which are of particular concern in patients with cardiac conditions.[110] Inhaled corticosteroids are the preferred treatment for all forms of persistent asthma and, in general, are well tolerated by older patients. However, elderly patients receiving high-dose therapy are at an increased risk for osteoporosis, cataracts, skin thinning, and bruising.[111] In addition to the well-known complications associated with systemic corticosteroid use (see Chapter 44, Rheumatoid Arthritis), these agents can acutely cause confusion, agitation, and hyperglycemia.

J.C. is currently maintained on low doses of an inhaled corticosteroid (fluticasone) in combination with a short-acting β_2-agonist (albuterol), and this is an appropriate regimen for a patient with mild-persistent asthma. J.C.'s asthma control should be re-evaluated within the next 3 months. If her asthma symptoms are not well controlled, she may benefit from an increase in her fluticasone dose or the addition of a long-acting inhaled β_2-agonist (salmeterol or formoterol). Because J.C. is postmenopausal, she is at risk for osteoporosis; calcium and vitamin D supplementation should be initiated.

CASE 102-5, QUESTION 3: J.C. was admitted to the hospital and given intravenous methylprednisolone for 4 days. She is discharged home with glipizide 5 mg daily, lisinopril 20 mg daily, fluticasone HFA (44 mcg) 2 puffs twice daily, albuterol 2 to 4 puffs every 4 hours as needed, and prednisone 40 mg daily for 7 days. What are some of the important counseling points for J.C. regarding her discharge medications?

Appropriate use of MDIs is difficult for most patients, but may be particularly problematic in the elderly population because of decreased hand strength or arthritis, difficulty timing actuation to inhalation, or impaired mental function. The use of spacer or holding chamber devices can alleviate this problem by minimizing the coordination necessary for proper use of an MDI, resulting in improved pulmonary drug delivery. In addition, spacers may reduce the incidence of systemic and local (cough, hoarseness, thrush) side effects associated with inhaled corticosteroids. J.C. should be discharged with a spacer device to use with her albuterol and fluticasone MDIs. Even though J.C. previously used an MDI, she should be asked to demonstrate her MDI technique and reinstructed, if necessary, to ensure she is using the inhaler and spacer correctly. If J.C. is unable to correctly use her MDIs with a spacer, use of nebulized solutions, breath-activated inhalers, or dry-powdered delivery devices should be considered. Although J.C. is prescribed prednisone for a short course, counseling for J.C. should also include more frequent monitoring of blood glucose while she is taking systemic corticosteroid therapy because of her diabetes.

Infectious Diseases in the Elderly

Infections are among the most common problems in the elderly and are a significant cause of morbidity and mortality. Infections are also one of the most frequent reasons for hospitalization of older ambulatory persons.[112] Antibiotic therapy for an infection in the elderly is often delayed because they present with atypical signs and symptoms. The older population is also more likely to have polymicrobial infections than younger people, and treatment duration is usually longer because of other comorbidities present in this population.[113]

PNEUMONIA

CASE 102-5, QUESTION 4: Three days after J.C. is discharged from the hospital, she presents again to the ED. This time, she is accompanied by a neighbor who noted that J.C. suddenly became forgetful and confused and continues to have difficulty breathing. Her neighbor reports that J.C. has been staying in bed the past 2 days and has not eaten much. J.C. has a low-grade fever, and chest examination reveals faint breath sounds with light crackling rales over her right lung base. A chest radiograph confirms the diagnosis of pneumonia. How is J.C.'s clinical presentation consistent with community-acquired pneumonia in the elderly?

Pneumonia is the leading infectious cause of mortality in the elderly, who have a 5- to 10-fold increased risk of developing pneumonia compared with younger adults.[114] Most patients admitted to hospital for the treatment of community-acquired pneumonia (CAP) are elderly.[115] Risk factors for CAP in the elderly include alcoholism and asthma, but other medical conditions common in older populations, such as dementia, HF, cerebrovascular disease, and chronic obstructive lung disease, can also increase the risk of pneumonia in this population.[116] *Streptococcus pneumoniae,* the most common cause of CAP in the elderly, is responsible for up to 50% of cases.[117–119] Viral pneumonia is the second most common cause of lower respiratory infection in older ambulatory patients. Respiratory symptoms and fever are often subtle or absent in older patients with pneumonia; instead, like J.C. they may present only with altered mental status (delirium, acute confusion, memory problems) or a decline in functional status. Delirium or acute confusion is a common presentation in elderly patients who may have new-onset lower respiratory infection.

CASE 102-5, QUESTION 5: How should J.C. be treated for her respiratory infection?

In many cases, management of pneumonia in the elderly requires hospitalization because they are at greater risk for mortality and complications. Early empiric antibacterial therapy is particularly important for older patients with pneumonia (see Chapter 64, Respiratory Tract Infections). J.C. should be hospitalized again and treated aggressively for pneumonia with broad-spectrum IV antibiotics. The recommended first-line agents for the treatment of hospitalized patients are β-lactams and macrolides (e.g., ceftriaxone and azithromycin), with fluoroquinolone monotherapy (e.g., levofloxacin or moxifloxacin) as an alternative agent.

PREVENTION

CASE 102-5, QUESTION 6: After 7 days of hospitalization, J.C. is discharged home with an oral antibiotic to finish the 14-day course of therapy. What preventive measures are available to J.C. after she is discharged?

Both influenza and pneumococcal vaccinations are beneficial in the prevention of pneumonia in the older population.[120,121] Among the elderly residents of nursing homes, influenza vaccine was found to be up to 60% effective in preventing pneumonia and hospitalization, and it was up to 70% effective in preventing hospitalization of ambulatory older adults. Among the respiratory viruses, influenza virus causes the greatest morbidity and mortality.[122] Influenza virus damages respiratory epithelial cells, decreases cell-mediated immunity, and exacerbates or worsens many chronic underlying medical conditions common to the older population. Oseltamivir is effective for the early treatment of influenza and for prophylaxis against influenza. Although oseltamivir is effective in the prevention of influenza, vaccination should be the primary prophylactic intervention. The pneumococcal vaccine has been shown to be effective in preventing pneumococcal bacteremia in those older than 65 years of age, although the reduction in the risk of pneumonia with pneumococcal vaccine is questionable.[123,124] Pneumococcal vaccine is nonetheless recommended in all adults age 65 and older to prevent bacteremia. Pneumococcal vaccination is generally given one time; if the vaccination was administered before the age of 65, however, another pneumococcal vaccine should be given. J.C. should be offered both influenza and pneumococcal vaccines after she is discharged from the hospital.

URINARY TRACT INFECTION

CASE 102-6

QUESTION 1: A.H. is a 72-year-old Hispanic woman who is currently wheelchair-bound because of pain in her right hip. Her granddaughter brings A.H. to the geriatric clinic because she has recently developed urinary incontinence. Her granddaughter reports that A.H. has been feeling weak the past 2 days and fell while getting out of the wheelchair. A urinalysis indicates the presence of a urinary tract infection (UTI), and A.H. is prescribed a 7-day course of ciprofloxacin 250 mg PO twice daily. Is this drug therapy appropriate?

Urinary tract infection is the most common bacterial infection in the elderly.[125] The frequency of bacteriuria in ambulatory older adults is 10% to 30% in women and 5% to 10% in men. These figures are even higher in elderly people residing in LTCFs. Impaired voiding with residual urine in older women and obstructive uropathy from prostatic disease in older men predispose them to bacteriuria. The severity of UTI in the older population ranges from mild cystitis to life-threatening urosepsis; both are more difficult to treat because of resistant organisms and age-related decreases in host defenses. The majority of UTIs in the older population do not present typically, but there are often nonspecific manifestations such as decline in functional status, cognitive impairment, weakness, falls, and urinary incontinence.[126] A.H.'s presentation (weakness, urinary incontinence, and a recent fall) is consistent with this pattern. As with most UTIs, those in the elderly are caused primarily by *Escherichia coli*. However, other species of bacteria such as *Klebsiella* species, *Proteus* species, and *Enterococcus* species are also frequently involved (see Chapter 68, Urinary Tract Infections).[127]

Oral antibiotics, such as sulfamethoxazole-trimethoprim or fluoroquinolones, are appropriate for most elderly patients with symptomatic UTI.[128] One study suggests that fluoroquinolones are significantly better tolerated than sulfamethoxazole-trimethoprim for the treatment of UTI in elderly women.[129] There was better clinical resolution at the end of the therapy, and the incidence of drug-related adverse events was significantly lower in women treated with a fluoroquinolone. This study suggests that a fluoroquinolone, including ofloxacin, ciprofloxacin, and levofloxacin, may be the preferred agent for a broad range of UTIs in the elderly and should be considered as initial therapy in the majority of the older population. Ciprofloxacin is a reasonable choice for A.H. because *E. coli* is the most likely causative agent and fluoroquinolones are well tolerated in the elderly.

The most important effect of age on antibiotic therapy for UTI is impaired renal function. Many older patients have limited renal function reserve because of prostatic disease or chronic UTIs. Nitrofurantoin should not be used in those patients with significantly impaired renal function owing to increased risk of peripheral neuropathy and acute pneumonitis, which may occur more frequently in geriatric patients. For those patients requiring IV therapy for UTI, such as the elderly people residing in LTCFs whose therapy is often guided by the culture and sensitivity of the causative organism, aminoglycosides pose a distinct disadvantage in older patients because of their drug-related nephrotoxicity and the need for serum drug-level monitoring.[130]

Osteoarthritis Pain

Arthritis is the most common cause of disability in people older than 75 years of age, with prevalence rates up to 30%.[131] It is also the most common cause of immobility in the older population, resulting in confinement in bed or to the house. Osteoarthritis, also called degenerative joint disease, is the most common type of joint disease in the older population. Its prevalence increases with age. Nonpharmacologic management of osteoarthritis, such as physical therapy and occupational therapy, have been shown to decrease pain and improve function in patients with osteoarthritis, both alone or in combination with appropriate analgesics.[130]

CASE 102-7

QUESTION 1: C.W., a 71-year-old retired school teacher, has been suffering from osteoarthritis of his hands for 5 years. He is an active older adult who enjoys volunteer work at the local hospital. He presents to the geriatric clinic with increased arthritis pain, which is uncontrolled by his current pain medication. He also complains of increased heartburn and gastric reflux symptoms. He also takes several other medications for his diabetes, hypertension, hypercholesterolemia, and GERD. C.W.'s current medications include glipizide 10 mg daily, verapamil sustained-released 240 mg daily, atorvastatin 10 mg daily, famotidine 20 mg twice daily, docusate sodium 100 mg twice daily, and ibuprofen 200 mg four times a day as needed. What modifications can be made to his drug regimen to better control his arthritis pain and minimize side effects from his pain medication?

Acetaminophen is the drug of choice for mild to moderate arthritis pain (see Chapter 43, Osteoarthritis). For elderly patients with reduced hepatic function or for those with a history of alcohol abuse, the maximal dose should be reduced 50% to 75%.[132] Acetaminophen is preferred over NSAIDs in the elderly because of its low renal and gastrointestinal toxicity. C.W.'s past medication history should be reviewed. If he has not tried acetaminophen in the past for his arthritis pain, acetaminophen 1 g three times a day should be initiated. Older patients with osteoarthritis pain often find relief from NSAIDs, which should be used with caution because of their potential GI complications and renal toxicity. In a group of United Kingdom older adults age 65 or older, for example, the risk of GI complications was found to be 4.03 per 1,000 patient-years, compared with 1.36 for all individuals 25 or older.[133] Up to 2% of older persons maintained on NSAID therapy are hospitalized because of serious GI complications, and up to 30% of all peptic ulcer–related hospital admissions and mortality in those older than 65 years are associated with chronic NSAID use. NSAID-associated renal toxicity is not as common as GI toxicity, but advanced age is one of the major risk factors.[134] Renal toxicities of NSAIDs in the elderly include sodium and water retention and increased risk for hypertension.[135] Thus, ibuprofen may be contributing to C.W.'s increased GERD symptoms and to his hypertension. Nonacetylated salicylates, such as salsalate, can be used if acetaminophen does not provide adequate pain relief. Compared with NSAIDs, nonacetylated salicylates have less renal and GI toxicity. Currently available selective COX-2 inhibitor celecoxib is preferred in older patients because it is less likely to cause GI complications than nonselective agents; however, the risk of adverse renal events is equivalent.[135] A COX-2 inhibitor or the addition of a more potent gastroprotective agent such as a proton-pump inhibitor to ibuprofen are options for C.W., who may experience reduced GI symptoms with equally effective pain relief.

CASE 102-7, QUESTION 2: C.W. reveals that he has tried acetaminophen without much relief of his pain. He is prescribed celecoxib and tries it for several months, but his pain continues and he is still experiencing GI distress. What other pain medication options does C.W. have?

For moderate to severe chronic pain caused by osteoarthritis, the topical analgesic, capsaicin, has been shown to provide temporary pain relief. However, capsaicin requires multiple daily applications for effective management of pain, and optimal efficacy takes 4 to 6 weeks of continued use. Diclofenac topical gel also provides faster onset of relief but requires multiple daily applications for persistent pain. Glucosamine and chondroitin have also been shown to decrease osteoarthritis pain and delay progression of the disease.[136] Glucosamine 1,500 mg combined with 1,200 mg chondroitin daily is recommended and is well tolerated by most elderly patients. However, glucosamine may increase the insulin resistance in diabetic patients, and C.W. should be counseled to monitor his blood glucose more closely when initiating this agent. Another option for C.W. is a long-acting opioid medication combined with acetaminophen, which can provide relief from pain with minimal adverse drug effects (see Chapter 7, Pain and Its Management). Codeine and tramadol are "weak" opioids that have ceiling effects and generally do not provide adequate analgesia. The use of propoxyphene should be avoided in the elderly because of its limited efficacy and the risk for neural and cardiac toxicity.[137] In November 2010, propoxyphene and all combination products containing propoxyphene were voluntarily withdrawn from the US market owing to the risk of serious and potentially fatal cardiac rhythm abnormalities. Meperidine should also be avoided in older adults because of its high potential for CNS side effects, especially in those with reduced renal function. C.W. is a candidate for opioid therapy. He should be started on the lowest dose of a short-acting formulation on a scheduled regimen and counseled on the adverse drug reactions. Constipation may be a particular problem because he is also taking verapamil, which can also cause significant constipation. The elderly are also at increased risk for constipation as a result of age-related reduced bowel motility. To prevent opioid-associated constipation in C.W., prophylactic laxatives and stool softeners should be started at the initiation of opioid therapy. Bulk laxatives are ineffective and should be avoided. He should be counseled to drink adequate fluids as well.[137]

LONG-TERM CARE FACILITIES

The LTCF environment is governed in part by the Omnibus Budget Reconciliation Act (OBRA), as well as by numerous other laws and regulations, which are contained in the federal Centers for Medicare and Medicaid Services (CMS) publication, States Operations Manual (SOM). The federal mandates include monthly review of each resident's medication profile to determine the following:

1. Is each drug clearly indicated?
2. If indicated, is it being dosed and administered appropriately?
3. Are the laboratory results and vital signs being done appropriately, and are they available for adequate evaluation of therapy?
4. Are any real or potential problems with drug side effects or interactions present?
5. What specific recommendations can be made to optimize this resident's drug therapy?
6. If neuroleptic agents are being prescribed, has their use been justified and is the therapy being monitored?
7. Have therapeutic goals been established for chronic drug therapies?
8. Are any unnecessary drugs present?

The findings of the medication regimen review, including medication discrepancies, errors, and adverse drug reactions, must be reported to the patient's physician who must respond to any recommendations in a timely manner. The American Society of Consultant Pharmacists publishes detailed information concerning standards of practice in the LTCF environment.[138]

CASE 102-8

QUESTION 1: As a new consulting pharmacist to a 60-bed, skilled nursing facility, several multiple-drug use problems become apparent during initial chart reviews. A typical case is D.M., an 82-year-old man who has resided there for the past month. D.M.'s past medical history is significant for hypertension, depression, constipation, long-standing mild cognitive impairment that is now worsening, and dizziness. In the nurses' notes, it is documented that D.M. had a fall when getting out of bed last week.

At admission, D.M.'s weight was 165 pounds; BP, 100/60 mm Hg; pulse, 85 beats/minute; and temperature, 98.6°F. Subsequent vital signs are not recorded systematically into his medical record. Sporadic documentation in the nurses' notes indicates little change from admission values. No laboratory information is available at this time. D.M. has no known allergies.

Current medications include amlodipine 10 mg daily, diltiazem CD 240 mg daily, hydrochlorothiazide 25 mg daily, quetiapine 300 mg daily, lorazepam 0.5 mg every 8 hours as needed for anxiety, docusate sodium 100 mg twice daily, milk of magnesia 30 mL daily, temazepam 15 mg at bedtime, and acetaminophen one to two 325-mg tablets every 4 to 6 hours as needed for pain. D.M. follows a 2-g sodium diet.

D.M. is ambulatory and takes his meals in the facility's cafeteria. He is not in any acute distress, but the nurses'

notes indicate that D.M. is often confused and complains of dizziness when ambulating. His weight has decreased 4 pounds since being admitted. What should be expected of this LTCF with respect to medication monitoring?

Under the CMS-mandated regulations, the establishment of goals of antihypertensive therapy and monitoring for these goals are required. D.M.'s blood pressure should be measured and documented in his medical record with a signature and date on a regular basis. D.M.'s dizziness, a symptom of orthostatic hypotension, may be caused by overtreatment of his hypertension as evidenced by his low admission blood pressure. Orthostatic hypotension occurs in more than half of frail, elderly LTCF residents and is most common when patients first arise, indicating that this may have been the cause of D.M.'s recent fall. D.M. is currently being inappropriately treated with two calcium-channel blockers. Discontinuation of one of them should reduce this patient's dizziness and help prevent future falls. Because D.M. is being treated with a diuretic, he should have a chemistry panel drawn to check for electrolyte abnormalities.

CASE 102-8, QUESTION 2: What deficiencies can be found in the review of D.M.'s case?

In the admission workup, D.M. was described as having a longstanding history of mild cognitive impairment, but subsequent nursing notes suggest that his symptoms of disorientation and confusion worsened quickly after admission. Chronic dementia is not normally characterized by rapid deterioration of mental acuity (see Chapter 103, Geriatric Dementias). This should raise the suspicion that a reversible factor could be responsible for D.M.'s mental decline. Overprescribing of psychotropic drugs in institutionalized elderly patients is well documented.[134,139] The cognitive impairment of chronic degenerative dementia can be greatly exaggerated by D.M.'s treatment with lorazepam, temazepam, and quetiapine, especially with the higher than recommended dosages. Benzodiazepines may also increase the risk of falls and bone fractures in the geriatric population. Antipsychotics are some of the most commonly prescribed drugs in nursing home residents. It is only appropriate to use these agents if the patient's behavior is (a) a danger to themselves or others (including staff), (b) impairing the patient's daily functioning, (c) interfering with the staff's ability to care for them, or (d) causing distress to the patient (i.e., frightening hallucinations). Unfortunately, antipsychotics are often unnecessarily prescribed for anxiety, insomnia, confusion, and failure to conform to the institution's standards for behavior. Antipsychotic use in older adults has been shown to be associated with a 1.7-fold increased risk of all-cause mortality compared with nonusers. Primary reasons for death were heart failure, sudden cardiac death, or pneumonia.[140] Federal regulations require that these drugs be used for a specified condition, at the lowest possible dosage, and for the shortest possible time. The regulations also mandate tapering of the dose and careful documentation of all clinical assessments that justify the ongoing need for antipsychotics.

In light of the atypical deterioration of D.M.'s cognitive function, the doses of all psychotropic medications should be gradually tapered down to the lowest effective dose. A baseline assessment of D.M.'s cognitive function and psychiatric status should be performed by a geriatrician, psychiatrist, or clinical psychologist to establish the presence or absence of psychotic behavioral disturbances or depression. If any of these disorders are present, then each should be managed with a single drug, titrated to the appropriate therapeutic dose. In accordance with established immunization practices, D.M., other LTCF residents, and staff members should receive an annual influenza vaccine. A pneumococcal vaccination should also be administered to D.M. if he has not previously received one.

KEY REFERENCES AND WEBSITES

A full list of references for this chapter can be found at **http://thepoint.lww.com/AT10e.** Below are the key references and websites for this chapter, with the corresponding reference number in this chapter found in parentheses after the reference.

Key References

American Diabetes Association. Standards of medical care in diabetes—2010 [published correction appears in *Diabetes Care.* 2010;33:692]. *Diabetes Care.* 2010;33(Suppl 1):S11. (77)

American Geriatrics Society Panel on Pharmacological Management of Persistent Pain in Older Persons. Pharmacological management of persistent pain in older persons. *J Am Geriatr Soc.* 2009;57:1331. (132)

Anderson JL et al. ACC/AHA 2007 guidelines for the management of patients with unstable angina/non ST-elevation myocardial infarction. Executive Summary. A report of the American College of Cardiology/American Heart Association Task Force on Practice Guidelines [published correction appears in *J Am Coll Cardiol.* 2008;51:974]. *J Am Coll Cardiol.* 2007;50:e1. (83)

Bowie MW, Slattum PW. Pharmacodynamics in older adults: a review. *Am J Geriatr Pharmacother.* 2007;5:263. (36)

Brown AF et al. Guidelines for improving the care of the older person with diabetes mellitus. *J Am Geriatr Soc.* 2003;51(5 Suppl Guidelines):S265. (92)

Chobanian AV et al. The Seventh Report of the Joint National Committee on Prevention, Detection, Evaluation, and Treatment of High Blood Pressure: the JNC 7 report [published correction appears in *JAMA.* 2003;290:197]. *JAMA.* 2003;289:2560. (84)

Cusack BJ. Pharmacokinetics in older persons. *Am J Geriatr Pharmacother.* 2004;2:274. (10)

Expert Panel on Detection, Evaluation, and Treatment of High Blood Cholesterol in Adults. Executive Summary of the Third Report of The National Cholesterol Education Program (NCEP) Expert Panel on Detection, Evaluation, and Treatment of High Blood Cholesterol in Adults (Adult Treatment Panel III). *JAMA* 2001;285:2486. (76)

Federal Interagency Forum on Aging-Related Statistics. Older Americans 2010: key indicators of well-being. Federal Interagency Forum on Aging-Related Statistics. Washington, DC: US Government Printing Office; July 2010. (1)

Gill SS et al. Antipsychotic drug use and mortality in older adults with dementia. *Ann Intern Med.* 2007;146:775. (140)

Jessup M et al. 2009 Focused Update: ACCF/AHA Guidelines for the Diagnosis and Management of Heart Failure in Adults. A report of the American College of Cardiology Foundation/American Heart Association Task Force on Practice Guidelines: developed in collaboration with the International Society for Heart and Lung Transplantation. *Circulation.* 2009;119:1977. (64)

Kane RL et al. *Essentials of Clinical Geriatrics.* 6th ed. New York, NY: McGraw-Hill; 2009. (7)

Krum H et al. Effects of initiating carvedilol in patients with severe chronic heart failure: results from the COPERNICUS Study. *JAMA.* 2003;289:712. (73)

Moberley SA et al. Vaccines for preventing pneumococcal infection in adults. *Cochrane Database Syst Rev.* 2008;(1):CD000422. (121)

Nichol KL et al. Effectiveness of influenza vaccine in the community-dwelling elderly. *N Engl J Med.* 2007;357:1373. (122)

Gerstein HC. Effects of ramipril on cardiovascular and microvascular outcomes in people with diabetes mellitus: results of the HOPE study and MICRO-HOPE substudy. Heart Outcomes Prevention Evaluation Study Investigators [published correction appears in *Lancet.* 2000;356:860]. *Lancet.* 2000; 355;253. (66)

Key Websites

American Geriatrics Society. **http://www.americangeriatrics.org.**

American Heart Association. **http://www.americanheart.org.** (75)

American Society of Consultant Pharmacists. **http://www.ascp.com.**

US Department of Health and Human Services. Dietary Guidelines for Americans, 2005. **http://www.health.gov/dietaryguidelines/dga2005/document/default.htm.** (82)

Geriatric Dementias

103

Nicole J. Brandt and Bradley R. Williams

CORE PRINCIPLES

	CHAPTER CASES
DEMENTIA	
1 Dementia is a syndrome that exhibits multiple cognitive deficits that compromise normal social or occupational function. There are numerous etiologies such as Alzheimer disease (AD), dementia with Lewy bodies (DLB), and vascular disease, which require a comprehensive evaluation to define a potential diagnosis.	**Case 103-1 (Question 1)**
ALZHEIMER DISEASE	
1 AD is a chronic, progressive, neurodegenerative disorder that results from neuropathological findings, such as neurofibrillary tangles or β-amyloid plaques that interfere with cholinergic transmission, as well as other neurochemical changes in the brain.	**Case 103-1 (Questions 1–3)**
2 AD has multiple risk factors such as age, family history, Down syndrome, head trauma, hypertension, and mild cognitive impairment, yet the exact etiology is still unknown.	**Case 103-1 (Question 2)**
3 Treatment for AD currently is symptomatic management, not disease altering, and focuses on neurotransmission (e.g., cholinergic system).	**Case 103-1 (Question 4)**
4 Cholinesterase inhibitors may be used as monotherapy or in combination with an *N*-methyl-D-aspartate antagonist for patients in the moderate to severe stage of AD.	**Case 103-1 (Questions 4–6)**
5 Monitoring for treatment efficacy should focus on cognition, function, and possibly behaviors, whereas treatment toxicity should look for common adverse effects such as gastrointestinal complaints with cholinesterase inhibitors.	**Case 103-1 (Question 5)**
LEWY BODY DEMENTIAS	
1 Lewy body dementias have similar neuropathology noted with α-synuclein aggregates found in Lewy bodies and neuritis (α-synucleinopathies), which typically present with parkinsonian findings as well as associated symptoms such as falls and visual hallucinations.	**Case 103-2 (Question 1)**
2 Cholinesterase inhibitors have demonstrated symptomatic benefit in patients with Lewy body dementias, yet monitoring for worsening of motor symptoms such as tremor is needed.	**Case 103-2 (Question 2)**
VASCULAR DEMENTIAS	
1 Vascular dementia is a broad classification of cognitive disorders caused by vascular disease, and notable multiple risk factors include advancing age, diabetes mellitus, small vessel cerebrovascular disease, hypertension, heart disease, hyperlipidemia, cigarette smoking, and alcohol use.	**Case 103-3 (Questions 1, 2)**
2 Treatment for vascular dementia strives to control the underlying modifiable risk factors owing to limited efficacy and controversial evidence with cholinesterase inhibitors.	**Case 103-3 (Question 3)**

continued

BEHAVIORAL DISTURBANCES IN DEMENTIA

1	When evaluating a dementia patient with behavior disturbances, the first step is to ensure that the problem is not caused by an unrecognized medical problem or adverse effect of a medication.	**Case 103-4 (Question 1), Case 103-5 (Question 1)**
2	Nonpharmacologic strategies are effective for managing many behavior disturbances and should be attempted before using medications to manage behavior.	**Case 103-4 (Questions 1–4)**
3	Delusions and hallucinations are common behaviors in dementia patients, yet the use of antipsychotics for these symptoms are not approved by the US Food and Drug Administration and have been associated with the increased risk of stroke and mortality in this patient population.	**Case 103-4 (Question 2)**
4	Wandering is a safety concern that often does not respond to pharmacologic intervention; instead, other strategies such as environmental modifications are used.	**Case 103-4 (Question 3)**
5	Antidepressants such as selective serotonin reuptake inhibitors have shown promise in addressing depressive symptoms, as well as screaming and irritability.	**Case 103-4 (Question 4)**
6	Caregiver support is essential to maintaining a dementia patient safely in his or her home as long as possible.	**Case 103-1 (Questions 3, 5), Case 103-4 (Question 5)**

GERIATRIC DEMENTIAS

With the continuing growth in the elderly population, the incidence and prevalence of cognitive disorders continues to rise.[1,2] Alzheimer disease (AD) is the most common cause of dementia, and accounts for more than half of all diagnosed cases.[3–5] Vascular dementias (VaDs), dementia with Lewy bodies (DLB), and Parkinson disease with dementia (PDD) are the next most common dementias, with frontotemporal dementia, pseudodementia, and other forms occurring less often.[4,6] AD is currently the fifth leading cause of death for people age 65 years and older and the sixth leading cause of death for all people in the United States.[2,7]

Incidence and Prevalence

It is estimated that 5.4 million Americans have AD, including approximately 13% of people age 65 years and older and 43% of people age 85 years and older. Of these, more than 3.4 million are women. Prevalence is greater among both African Americans and Hispanics compared with whites.[2] The annual incidence of AD in the United States rises from 53 per 1,000 among people age 65 to 74 years to 170 per 1,000 for those age 75 to 84 years, and to 231 per 1,000 for those at least 85 years of age.[8] Worldwide prevalence has been estimated to be as high as 24.3 million, with 8.4 million new cases annually.[1,9] Projections into the mid-century include a worldwide prevalence of more than 81 million, with cases in undeveloped countries occurring at about three times the rate as in developed countries.[9] In the United States, AD accounts for nearly 70% of cases; VaDs account for 17.4%, with the remaining 12.6% attributable to DLB, frontotemporal dementia, and other forms.[5] Life expectancy after a diagnosis of AD is reduced by as much as 69% for those diagnosed before age 70 years and by 39% for those diagnosed after age 90 years.[10]

The cost of dementia is staggering. Annual costs for Medicare recipients with dementia average $19,304, compared with $6,720 for those without dementia. For Medicaid recipients with dementia, the annual costs are $8,419, compared with $915 for those without dementia. The annual direct costs, in 2010 dollars, of treating a dementia patient are $42,072 annually, compared with $13,515 for an older adult without dementia. This translates to an estimated annual direct cost for dementia care of $183 billion for the year 2011.[2]

Clinical Diagnosis

Dementia is a syndrome that exhibits impaired short- and long-term memory as its most prominent feature. Multiple cognitive deficits that compromise normal social or occupational function must be present before dementia can be diagnosed (Table 103-1).[11] Commonly, forgetfulness is the primary complaint of patients or the first symptom noted by the family.[12] Family members or others may note several symptoms that should prompt a medical evaluation (Table 103-2).[12,13] Memory loss often accompanies several diseases or disorders in elderly individuals. Therefore, a medical history, physical examination, and medication history are essential in excluding systemic illness or medication toxicity as causes of the dementia (Table 103-3).[13–16] Laboratory and other tests to assist in differentiating dementia from other disorders are listed in Table 103-4. In patients with primary degenerative dementia, or AD, test results will generally be normal; evidence of cerebrovascular disease is present in patients with VaDs.

Brain imaging, such as a computed tomography (CT) scan or magnetic resonance imaging (MRI), can be useful in establishing the presence of a dementia, but neither is diagnostic. A CT scan is useful when a space-occupying lesion, such as a tumor, is suspected as a possible cause. An MRI scan is capable of identifying small infarcts, such as those found in some VaDs, and atrophy of subcortical structures such as the brainstem.[15]

Several simple tests, including the Folstein Mini-Mental State Exam (MMSE), Memory Impairment Screen (MIS), Mini-Cognitive Assessment Instrument (Mini-Cog), and Brief

TABLE 103-1
Diagnostic Criteria for Alzheimer Dementia

1. The presence of multiple cognitive deficits manifested by both:
   - Impaired memory (ability to learn new information or to retrieve information previously learned), and
   - At least one of the following:
     Aphasia (language difficulties)
     Apraxia (diminished ability to perform motor activities in the presence of intact motor function)
     Agnosia (inability to recognize or name objects despite intact sensory function)
     Disruption of executive function (diminished ability to plan, organize)
2. The previous deficits significantly interfere with normal work or social activities and represent a decline from previous ability to function
3. The previous deficits cannot be attributed to any of the following:
   - Central nervous system conditions that cause progressive cognitive or memory impairment (e.g., cerebrovascular disease)
   - Systemic conditions known to cause dementia (e.g., hypothyroidism, neurosyphilis, HIV infection)
   - Substance-induced conditions (e.g., drug toxicity)
4. The deficits do not occur exclusively during the course of a delirium. The disturbance is not better accounted for by another axis I disorder (schizophrenia, major depressive disorder)

HIV, human immunodeficiency virus.
Adapted with permission from American Psychiatric Association. *Diagnostic and Statistical Manual of Mental Disorders-IV-TR*. Washington, DC: American Psychiatric Association; 2000.

Interview of Mental Status (BIMS), are appropriate for initial screening of people with suspected cognitive impairment.[17–20] These tests rapidly assess multiple domains, typically including orientation, registration, attention and calculation, recall, and language. Patients with dementia exhibit deficits in multiple areas. Those who score below the normal range on the MMSE or other screens, or who exhibit symptoms characteristic of dementia receive further testing (Tables 103-1 and 103-2). A somewhat more detailed screen, the Blessed Dementia Scale, evaluates daily functional capacity (e.g., shopping, performing household tasks), activities of daily living (e.g., eating, dressing, toileting), and personality. The Blessed Information-Memory-Concentration Test evaluates orientation, memory, and concentration.[21] All screening tests are subject to limitations. Therefore, additional psychometric testing is often ordered to further establish the presence and type of dementia.[2,13,15]

Dementias may be classified as cortical or subcortical, according to the areas of the brain preferentially affected by the disorder. AD, a typical cortical dementia, disrupts the cerebral cortex. Patients with cortical dementias display impaired language rather than impaired speech, a learning deficit (amnesia), reduced higher cortical functions (e.g., inability to perform calculations, poor judgment), and an unconcerned or disinhibited affect.

TABLE 103-2
Symptoms Suggesting Dementia

Symptom	Evidence
Difficulty learning or retaining new information	Repeats questions; difficulty remembering recent conversations, events, etc.; loses items
Unable to handle complex tasks	Cannot complete tasks that require multiple steps (e.g., difficulty following a shopping list)
Impaired reasoning	Difficulty solving everyday problems; inappropriate social behavior
Impaired spatial orientation and abilities	Gets lost in familiar places; difficulty with driving
Language deficits	Problems finding appropriate words (e.g., difficulty with naming common objects)
Behavior changes	Changes in personality; suspiciousness

Adapted from Costa P et al. Recognition and initial assessment of Alzheimer's disease and related dementias. Clinical Practice Guideline No. 19. Rockville, MD: U.S. Department of Health and Human Services, Public Health Service, Agency for Health Care Policy and Research. AHCPR Publication No. 97-0702. November 1996.

TABLE 103-3
Causes of Dementia Symptoms

Central Nervous System Disorders	Systemic Illness	Medications
Adjustment disorder	Cardiovascular	Anticholinergic agents
(e.g., inability to	disease	Anticonvulsants
adjust to	Arrhythmia	Antidepressants
retirement)	Heart failure	Antihistamines
Amnestic syndrome	Vascular occlusion	Anti-infectives
(e.g., isolated	Deficiency states	Antineoplastic agents
memory	Vitamin B_{12}	Antipsychotic agents
impairment)	Folate	Cardiovascular agents
Delirium	Iron	Antiarrhythmics
Depression	Infections	Antihypertensives
Intracranial causes	Metabolic disorders	Corticosteroids
Brain abscess	Adrenal	H_2-receptor antagonists
Normal pressure	Glucose	Immunosuppressants
Hydrocephalus	Renal failure	Narcotic analgesics
Stroke	Thyroid	Nonsteroidal anti-
Subdural hematoma		inflammatory agents
Tumor		Sedative hypnotics and
		anxiolytics
		Skeletal muscle relaxants

TABLE 103-4
Dementia Screening Tests

Test	Rationale for Testing
Complete blood count with sedimentation rate	Anemic anoxia, infection, neoplasms
Metabolic screen	
Serum electrolytes	Hypernatremia, hyponatremia; renal function
Blood urea nitrogen, creatinine	Renal function
Bilirubin	Hepatic dysfunction (e.g., portal systemic encephalopathy, hepatocerebral degeneration)
Thyroid function	Hypothyroidism, hyperthyroidism
Iron, vitamin B_{12}, folate, vitamin D	Deficiency states (vitamin B_{12}, folate neuropathies, vitamin D deficiency), anemias
Stool occult blood	Blood loss, anemia
HIV and RPR	Infection
Urinalysis	Infection, proteinuria
Chest roentgenogram	Neoplasms, infection, airway disease (anoxia)
Electrocardiogram	Cardiac disease (stagnant anoxia)
Brain scan	Cerebral tumors, cerebrovascular disease
Mental status testing	General cognitive screen
Depression testing	Depression, pseudodementia

Subcortical dementias such as PDD primarily affect the basal ganglia, thalamus, and brainstem. Deficits include abnormal motor function, disrupted speech patterns rather than language difficulties, forgetfulness (impaired recall), slowed cognitive function, and an apathetic or depressed affect.[16]

ALZHEIMER DISEASE

Etiology

A definitive cause for AD has yet to be determined. Several risk factors, however, have been identified. Advancing age is the primary risk factor for AD; other risks include head trauma, metabolic syndrome, diabetes, hypertension, and family history.[13,22,23]

Genetics plays a significant role in the development of Alzheimer-type dementia. The high familial occurrence of Alzheimer dementia has been linked to autosomal-dominant traits on chromosomes 21, 14, and 1.[24,25] A gene that encodes for amyloid precursor protein (APP), a normal protein, is located on chromosome 21. An abnormal fragment of APP, discussed below, appears to be responsible for much of the neuronal damage in AD. A defect on chromosome 14 has been identified as the locus for the presenilin-1 gene, which codes for an inherited form of AD. The presenilin-2 gene, located on chromosome 1, also codes for an inherited form. Despite a strong genetic link in some pedigrees, the great majority of AD cases are sporadic.[25,26] The more common sporadic form appears to be linked to a susceptibility gene, apolipoprotein E, which occurs in three isoforms.[25] APP, a normal protein found throughout the body (e.g., platelets and peripheral lymphocytes), maps on chromosome 21 and plays a pivotal role in AD neuropathology. Because of overproduction or transcription errors, an abnormal subunit (i.e., β-amyloid) is produced.[25] Mutations on chromosomes 14 (presenilin-1 gene) and 1 (presenilin-2 gene) and the presence of apolipoprotein $\epsilon4$ allele code for alterations in the processing of APP. The abnormal cleavage of APP produces a 42–amino acid form of β-amyloid (Aβ) that demonstrates a higher toxicity than other amyloid forms.[25]

Apolipoprotein E (ApoE), a protein that is involved in cholesterol and phospholipid metabolism, plays a role in the development of sporadic, late-onset AD. The ApoE gene possesses three alleles: $\varepsilon2$, $\varepsilon3$, and $\varepsilon4$. The $\varepsilon3$ allele is most common, the $\varepsilon2$ allele appears to be protective against AD, and the $\varepsilon4$ allele increases the risk for AD.[25] The presence of ApoE-4, the protein coded for by the $\varepsilon4$ allele, appears to increase the deposition of Aβ and promote its change to a more pathological configuration.[25] The presence of one or two copies of ApoE4 increases the risk of developing AD twofold or fivefold, respectively.[26] Aβ, which differs from amyloid protein found in other regions of the body, appears to contribute to neuronal death through a combination of apoptosis, a direct toxic effect, and an increased risk for damage owing to oxidative and metabolic stresses.[25,27]

Neuropathology

ONLINE CONTENT

For an illustration of tissue changes in AD, go to http://thepoint.lww.com/AT10e.

Although brain atrophy is the most obvious finding among patients with Alzheimer-type dementia, it is not diagnostic for AD or other dementias because some degree of atrophy accompanies normal aging. Atrophic changes induced by AD are found primarily in the temporal, parietal, and frontal areas of the brain; the occipital region, primary motor cortex, and somatosensory areas are generally unaffected (Fig. 103-1).[4,27]

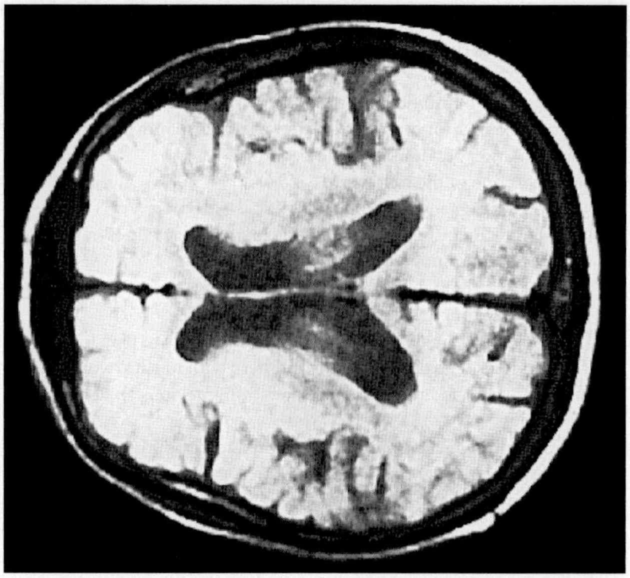

FIGURE 103-1 Alzheimer disease: magnetic resonance imaging scan. Ventricles are enlarged, and there is generalized atrophy, with greater atrophy present near the temporal areas.

Neuronal changes in the cerebral cortex associated with AD include neurofibrillary tangles, neuritic plaques, amyloid angiopathy, and granulovacuolar degeneration. These changes lead to loss of neurons and synapses (Fig. 103-2).[24] Neurofibrillary tangles (NFTs) are found primarily in the pyramidal regions of the neocortex, hippocampus, and amygdala, but they are also noted in areas of the brainstem and locus ceruleus.[4,27] Tangles are a prominent feature of Alzheimer-type dementia, but can be found in several other brain disorders (e.g., Down syndrome, postencephalitic Parkinson disease) and even in normally aging brains, although they are generally less numerous and histologically different.[24] NFTs are composed of paired helical filaments, combinations of fibrils with a characteristic width and contour, containing a tau protein with an abnormal pattern of phosphate deposition. They are highly immunoreactive and are most likely to form in large pyramidal neurons. NFTs typically begin in

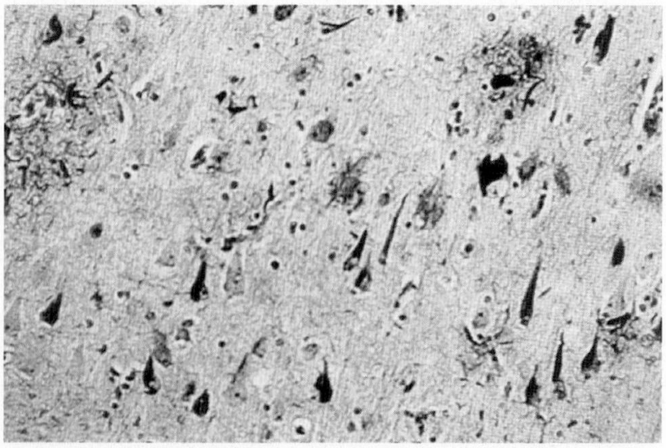

FIGURE 103-2 Numerous plaques (large, round bodies) and tangles (tear-shaped bodies) are found throughout the cortex in Alzheimer-type dementia.

the transentorhinal cortex and spread to the limbic cortex and the neocortex.[4,24] Neuritic plaques are spherical bodies of tissue composed of granular deposits and remnants of neuronal processes.[4] The typical neuritic plaques of AD are spherical structures between 50 and 200 μm wide and exhibit a three-tiered structure: a central amyloid core, a middle region of swollen axons and dendrites, and an outer zone containing degenerating neuritic processes.[24] Plaques contain APP, which can be cleaved by a defective metabolic process to form Aβ.[25] In addition to Aβ, plaques also contain protein, ApoE, and acute-phase inflammatory proteins such as α_1-chymotrypsin and α_2-macroglobulin.[24] Although Aβ is found in both normal and AD subjects, NFTs occurring in the plaques of nondemented subjects do not contain the abnormal protein seen in individuals with dementia.[4] The deposition of amyloid in neuritic plaques correlates with the severity of AD, and the density of cortical plaques is associated with decreased choline acetyltransferase and the severity of cognitive impairment.[4] Aβ has been identified in plaques associated with Down syndrome and in both familial and sporadic forms of dementia of the Alzheimer type.[25] The pathological process of AD development may begin as early as 20 to 30 years before any disease symptoms appear.[4,25,28]

Granulovacuolar degeneration is the other major histologic finding in AD. It consists of clusters of intracytoplasmic vacuoles that contain tiny granules. The vacuoles appear to be specifically located in the pyramidal neurons of the hippocampus. Granulovacuolar degeneration can also occur, albeit rarely, in individuals without dementia.[4,16,24] The loss of cortical neurons that originate in the nucleus basalis and project into the cerebral cortex is the most significant histopathological consequence of AD.[27] Cell loss, granulovacuolar degeneration, and neurons with NFTs are concentrated in this area.[16,24]

Accompanying these changes are decreased concentrations of several neurotransmitters and enzymes. Choline acetyltransferase levels are reduced 60% to 90% in the cortical and hippocampal regions.[24] Acetylcholine and acetylcholinesterase (AChE) are also decreased, whereas muscarinic receptors in the cortex and hippocampus remain at normal levels or are moderately decreased. Nicotinic receptor proteins are also reduced in patients with Alzheimer-type dementia when compared with age-matched controls. Decreased choline acetyltransferase activity has been correlated with plaque density and disease severity. Cortical synapse loss, especially in the midfrontal region, is associated with disease severity.[4,25–27]

Changes affecting AChE have significant implications for the management of AD symptoms. Many isoforms of AChE have been identified; they possess identical amino acid sequences, but display different posttranslational modifications, predominate at diverse anatomical and microanatomical locations, and function in different ways. The predominant form of AChE in the cortical and hippocampal regions of humans is G4, a tetrameric form that is membrane bound. The monomeric form, G1, is found in a much lower concentration. There is a selective loss of the G4 form in patients with AD, allowing the G1 form to assume greater importance.[29] Although cholinergic activity is most significantly affected by Alzheimer-type dementia, other neurochemical systems are also altered. Norepinephrine, serotonin, and γ-aminobutyric acid receptors are affected.[24,25]

Clinical Presentation and Diagnosis

CASE 103-1

QUESTION 1: C.L., a 63-year-old woman, complains of increasing memory problems during the past 2 years. She states that she began writing reminder notes to herself, but she often forgot to look at them. Eventually, she began to lose items around her house, forget appointments, and fail to pay some important bills. During the past 2 to 3 months, she has had difficulty following a shopping list and has become disoriented in the store. One week ago, she became agitated when she heard the low-battery alarm in her smoke detector. C.L. admits to becoming increasingly depressed about her memory problems but denies appetite or sleep changes or suicidal ideation. She also denies hallucinations, delusional thoughts, or symptoms of anxiety.

C.L.'s medical history is significant for type 2 diabetes mellitus, which is controlled by diet, and bilateral open-angle glaucoma, treated with latanoprost 0.005%, one drop in each eye at bedtime. Her family history is negative for stroke and positive for diabetes mellitus and hypertension. She reports that two or three of her maternal relatives had "memory problems" and that one aunt was diagnosed with AD 5 years ago.

Physical examination reveals a moderately obese woman who is well dressed and groomed. Her blood pressure (BP) is 140/86 mm Hg supine and 132/82 mm Hg standing, with pulse rates of 74 beats/minute and 78 beats/minute, respectively. She is alert and oriented to place and person. During the interview, she is reserved but becomes easily irritated with the physician.

The Folstein MMSE score was 23/30, with errors in orientation, attention, and calculation (inability to spell "world" backward), recall, and language (difficulty with word finding). The rest of the physical examination was within normal limits.

What additional evaluation steps should be considered for C.L.?

Before any conclusions can be reached, potentially reversible causes for C.L.'s impaired cognition must be evaluated. Although she displays several trigger symptoms associated with dementia (Table 103-2), including problems learning new information, difficulty with complex tasks (shopping), impaired reasoning (recognizing the smoke alarm battery warning), and increased irritability, it cannot be assumed that C.L. has a dementia. Several systemic diseases and other disorders can cause cognitive impairment, as shown in Table 103-3.

C.L. should undergo a battery of laboratory tests to rule out anemia, cardiac and renal disease, thyroid abnormalities, and tumors. In addition, she should receive thorough neuropsychological testing, including depression screening and more in-depth assessment of her cognitive function. The testing should be conducted by clinicians who are skilled in cognitive assessment, as educational and cultural factors can influence an individual's performance on these tests.[30]

CASE 103-1, QUESTION 2: C.L. is referred by her physician for additional testing. Laboratory tests performed include renal and liver chemistries, thyroid function tests, hemoglobin A_{1c}, vitamin B_{12} and folate levels, syphilis and HIV tests, complete blood cell count with sedimentation rate, and urinalysis. All results were normal with the exception of a fasting glucose level of 150 mg/dL and a hemoglobin A_{1c} of 8.4%. Chest radiograph and electrocardiogram were normal. Neurologic examination revealed no deficits. Depression testing revealed a sad, mildly anxious individual who was not depressed. Her score on the Blessed Dementia Scale was 25/33, with deficits in personality,

memory, concentration, and habits. What is the most probable diagnosis for C.L.?

C.L.'s score of 23/30 on the Folstein MMSE is consistent with mild cognitive impairment or early dementia as evidenced by errors in orientation, calculation, recall, and language.[17] Personality and habit changes and deficits in memory and concentration are revealed in C.L.'s score on the Blessed Dementia Scale.[21] Secondary medical causes of cognitive impairment can be eliminated by C.L.'s generally normal physical examination and laboratory test results. C.L.'s fasting glucose and glycosylated hemoglobin levels are mildly elevated, but cannot account for her significant cognitive decline. Diabetes is a risk factor for AD; it increases the likelihood that she has AD.[30] MRI or CT scanning may be useful in many cases to help eliminate brain pathology, such as stroke.[30] A positron emission tomography (PET) scan or a single photon emission computed tomography (SPECT) scan may be useful to help locate specific areas of pathology and assist with a differential diagnosis, but are not required.[31] Secondary psychiatric causes for C.L.'s decline can also be discounted. Although she is sad and anxious, the absence of alterations in appetite or sleep patterns, absence of suicidal thoughts, and the results of psychologic testing indicate C.L. is not depressed. She is fully conscious, alert, and oriented to place and person. She exhibits no psychotic behavior and no evidence of delirium.

C.L.'s slowly progressive decline and its impact on her social and occupational function (forgetting appointments, failing to pay bills), normal physical examination and laboratory findings, and family history meet the *Diagnostic and Statistical Manual of Mental Disorders,* Fourth Edition (DSM-IV) criteria for dementia (Table 103-1). Her history and course to date satisfy the criteria for AD and do not indicate a likely alternative explanation for her condition. Thus, C.L. can be classified as probable AD according to the criteria established by the National Institute of Neurological and Communicative Disorders–Alzheimer's Disease and Related Disorders Association Task Force (Table 103-5).[32] She also meets the criteria for probable AD according to proposed revised diagnostic criteria.[33]

TABLE 103-5

Revised Criteria for Dementia of the Alzheimer Type

Definite DAT
- Clinical criteria for probable DAT
- Histopathological evidence for DAT (autopsy or biopsy confirmed)

Probable DAT
- Dementia established by clinical examination and documented by mental status testing
- Confirmation of dementia by neuropsychologic tests (e.g., Blessed Dementia Scale and other tests)
- Insidious and gradual onset during a period of months to years
- History of worsening cognition established by observation or report
- Initial and most prominent cognitive deficits are evidenced by problems in either of the following categories:
  - Amnestic presentation, which includes impaired learning or inability to retain recently learned information, plus evidence of impairment in at least one other cognitive domain
  - Nonamnestic presentations, including (a) language, with deficits in word-finding; (b) visuospatial, with deficits in ability to recognize objects, impaired face recognition, or other similar impairments; (c) executive dysfunction, evidenced by impaired reasoning, judgment, and problem solving. All are accompanied by deficits in other cognitive domains
- Absence of evidence of significant cerebrovascular disease, core features of dementia with Lewy bodies, or other dementia syndromes or conditions that could have a substantial negative effect on cognition

Possible DAT
- Atypical onset, presentation, or progression of dementia with an unknown etiology
- Presence of a systemic or other brain disease capable of producing dementia, but not believed to be the cause of the dementia
- Gradually progressive decline in one intellectual function in the absence of another identifiable cause

Unlikely DAT
- Sudden onset
- Focal neurologic findings (e.g., deep tendon reflexes, hemiparesis)

DAT, dementia of the Alzheimer type.
Source: McKhann G et al. Clinical diagnosis of Alzheimer's disease: report of the NINCDS-ADRDA Work Group under the auspices of Department of Health and Human Services Task Force on Alzheimer's Disease. *Neurology.* 1984;34:939; McKhann G et al. The diagnosis of dementia due to Alzheimer's disease: recommendations from the National Institute on Aging–Alzheimer's Association workgroups on diagnostic guidelines for Alzheimer's disease. *Alzheimers Dement.* 2011;7:263.

CASE 103-1, QUESTION 3: C.L.'s children are very concerned about the family history for dementia. They ask whether there are any tests they should receive at this time to determine their risk. What should they be told?

Although there is a strong genetic association with AD, such instances account for a small minority of cases.[25] There is no apparent family history of Down syndrome. Mutations in the presenilin-1 and presenilin-2 genes are associated with only a small fraction of AD cases.[25] Although several potential biomarkers have been identified, they have not been sufficiently validated to be considered reliable predictors for the development of AD.[2,33,34]

Prognosis

CASE 103-1, QUESTION 4: What is the likely prognosis for C.L.?

AD follows a predictable course that may progress over the course of 10 years or more.[2,10] Two common rating scales for dementia are the Global Deterioration Scale and the Clinical Dementia Rating Scale. According to the Global Deterioration Scale (Table 103-6), C.L.'s impaired social functioning, anxiety, and objective cognitive decline as well as her continued ability to concentrate and perform some complex skills, combined with her preserved affect and social interaction, are consistent with the features of stage three dementia of the Alzheimer type. This stage of AD is generally associated with a period of mild cognitive decline.[35] The more general Clinical Dementia Rating Scale also places C.L. in the category of mild dementia.[36] Clinical diagnoses of AD using clinical criteria for probable AD have a sensitivity of up to 90% when compared with autopsy-confirmed cases, when diagnosed using appropriate criteria and assessment methods.[4,30,34]

Because of technologic advances, it is possible to diagnose dementia earlier and to keep patients alive into the final stages of the disease.[37] The early diagnosis of AD in C.L. will allow her condition to be followed closely. To ensure the most favorable outcome, C.L. should receive a thorough assessment beyond her dementia. This should include evaluation of her daily function (i.e., ability for self-care), comorbid medical conditions, medications, living arrangements, safety, and potential for abuse and neglect. Attention also should be given to C.L.'s caregivers and support system.[38,39] She should be reassessed every 6 months to both document disease progression and ensure that she is

TABLE 103-6
Stages of Dementia of the Alzheimer Type

Stage of Cognitive Decline	Features
No cognitive decline	Normal cognitive state
Very mild cognitive decline	Forgetfulness, subjective complaints only; no objective decline
Mild cognitive decline	Objective decline through psychiatric testing; work and social impairment; mild anxiety and denial
Moderate cognitive decline	Concentration, complex skills decline; flat affect and withdrawal
Moderately severe cognitive decline	Early dementia; difficulty in interactions; unable to recall or recognize people or places
Severe cognitive decline	Requires assistance with bathing, toileting; behavioral symptoms present (agitation, delusions, aggressive behavior)
Very severe cognitive decline	Loss of psychomotor skills and verbal abilities; incontinence; total dependence

Adapted from Reisberg B et al. The global deterioration scale for assessment of primary degenerative dementia. *Am J Psychiatry.* 1982;139:1136.

receiving the most appropriate care. At some point, care at home may become unrealistic. At that time, C.L. should be moved into a sheltered environment (e.g., residential-care facility or nursing home) before suffering an injury caused by her poor judgment (e.g., failing to dress properly for the weather, falling). In the later stages, interventions ranging from tube feedings to life support may prolong life, yet prove to be controversial.[40] Death in the late stage of AD is commonly associated with the development of infections such as pneumonia, urinary tract infections, or decubitus ulcers.

Treatment

For a narrated PowerPoint presentation discussing over-the-counter medications and nutritional supplements used for dementia, go to http://thepoint.lww.com/AT10e.

CASE 103-1, QUESTION 5: What is an appropriate initial treatment strategy for C.L.?

Maintaining independence as long as possible is an important goal in treating a patient with dementia. Keeping patients in familiar surroundings allows them to function without the added burden of having to attempt to adapt to a strange environment. C.L. appears to be functioning reasonably well at home, although her forgetfulness is causing some problems for her. She is still eating well (her laboratory testing indicated no deficiencies in total protein or albumin, vitamin B_{12}, or folic acid) and performing normal daily activities such as dressing, grooming, bathing, and toileting. Some regular supervision from family members, neighbors, or household help will ensure that C.L. remains safe in her own home.

C.L.'s diabetes mellitus and general medical condition should also be monitored closely. Because both hyperglycemia and hypoglycemia can impair cognitive processes, either complication can exacerbate her memory problems. Concurrent diseases and many medications can reduce function and increase cognitive impairment in demented patients, so any new findings in C.L. must be evaluated carefully to distinguish new problems from a worsening of her dementia.

C.L.'s family needs to be educated about what to expect as her dementia progresses. They should be referred to the Alzheimer's Association (www.alz.org) and to the Family Caregiver Alliance (www.caregiver.org). Both organizations provide a wealth of information and community resources, including caregiver support groups. They also should be encouraged to enroll in the MedicAlert + Alzheimer's Association Safe Return program, which provides 24-hour nationwide emergency response for people with dementia who wander or suffer a medical emergency. C.L.'s family should include her in any advance planning, seek legal advice regarding advance directives and durable power of attorney for health care and finance, and conduct estate planning to avoid having to perform these tasks when C.L. is no longer competent to participate.[38]

Currently, there are three agents available for the symptomatic treatment of AD. All agents inhibit AChE, the enzyme that is primarily responsible for the metabolism of acetylcholine. Some agents also inhibit butyrylcholinesterase (BChE), which metabolizes acetylcholine to a minor degree but becomes more prominent in AD.[29] Cholinesterase inhibitors (ChEI) have been shown to improve cognition and function, and delay symptom progression in people with dementia. Cholinergic-related effects, particularly in the gastrointestinal (GI) tract, are the most common adverse effects cause by all of the agents.[41] The first agent available, tacrine, is no longer marketed because of significant cholinergic adverse effects, risk of hepatotoxicity, and an inconvenient dosing schedule.

DONEPEZIL

Donepezil is a piperidine derivative that is somewhat selective for central AChE. It reversibly inhibits cholinesterase activity. Donepezil is highly bioavailable and exhibits a long half-life, allowing it to be given as a single daily dose. It is highly protein bound, primarily to albumin (Table 103-7).[42]

Donepezil may improve cognition, global function, and behavioral symptoms across all stages (mild, moderate, and severe) of AD. In a multicenter, double-blind, placebo-controlled trial, subjects with mild to moderately severe AD improved during a 12-week treatment period.[43] Subjects taking 10 mg of donepezil at bedtime improved their cognitive function as measured by the Alzheimer's Disease Assessment Scale-Cognitive Subscale (ADAS-Cog), and their overall function as measured by the Clinician's Interview-Based Impression of Change with caregiver input (CIBIC-Plus).[44,45] A 24-week multicenter, placebo-controlled trial using dosages of 5 mg/day and 10 mg/day demonstrated similar results. Both 5- and 10-mg doses were superior to placebo; adverse effects were less common with the 5-mg dose.[46] A long-term, open-label follow-up study to these trials demonstrated that donepezil effects may persist for almost 3 years.[47] Interruption or discontinuation of donepezil treatment was followed by a return of cognition and function to baseline or below.

Donepezil is the only ChEI currently indicated for the severe stage of AD. A 6-month, double-blind, parallel group, placebo-controlled study in patients with severe AD (MMSE 1–10) demonstrated an improvement in the Severe Impairment Battery[48] and Modified Alzheimer's Disease Cooperative Study activities of daily living inventory for severe AD. The domains that showed a significant improvement versus placebo were language, praxis, visuospatial, bowel/bladder function, and ability to get dressed. There were no differences noted in the neuropsychiatric inventory for behavioral issues associated with dementia.[49] A 23-mg dose of donepezil was recently approved for patients in the moderate to severe stages of AD. Small improvements were seen in

TABLE 103-7

U.S. Food and Drug Administration–Approved Drugs for Alzheimer Disease (AD)

Generic Drug (Brand Name) and Mechanism	Dosage Form and Dosage	Indication and Effect	Adverse Effects	Other
Donepezil HCl (Aricept) Reversibly inhibits AChE, primarily in CNS	Aricept – Tablets 5 mg – Tablets 10 mg – Tablets 23 mg Aricept RDT – Tablets, orally disintegrating 5 mg – Tablets, orally disintegrating 10 mg Mild to moderate Alzheimer disease: Adults: PO: 5 mg once daily; may increase to 10 mg once daily after 4 to 6 weeks. Severe Alzheimer Disease: Adults: PO: Start with 5 mg once daily. Increase to 10 mg once daily after 4 to 6 weeks. A dosage of 23 mg once daily may be given after the patient has been on 10 mg once daily for at least 3 months. General Dosing Information: • Orally disintegrating tablets are bioequivalent to tablets. • Administer in the evening, just before bedtime. • May be taken without respect to food. • Allow the oral disintegrating tablet to dissolve on the tongue and follow with water.	Treatment of mild to severe dementia of the Alzheimer type. Small improvements in cognition and function occur within 12–24 weeks; benefits may last for at least 2 years.	Cholinergic effects, particularly affecting the GI tract (nausea, anorexia, diarrhea); headache; bradycardia may occur.	Completely bioavailable and may be given as a single daily dose owing to long half-life (70 hours). Metabolized by CYP3A4 isoenzymes.
Galantamine HBr (Razadyne and Razadyne ER) Reversibly inhibits AChE, primarily in CNS; also stimulates nicotinic receptors at a site distinct from that of acetylcholine	Razadyne – Tablets 4 mg (as base) – Tablets 8 mg (as base) – Tablets 12 mg (as base) – Oral Solution 4 mg/mL Razadyne ER – Capsules, extended-release 8 mg (as base) – Capsules, extended-release 16 mg (as base) – Capsules, extended-release 24 mg (as base) Immediate-Release Tablets and Oral Solution: Adults: PO: 4 mg twice daily. May increase to 8 mg twice daily after 4 weeks. A further increase to 12 mg twice daily may be attempted after minimum of 4 weeks at previous dose. Extended-Release Capsules: Adults: PO: 8 mg/d. Increase to 16 mg/d after min 4 weeks. A further increase to 24 mg/d may be attempted after minimum of 4 weeks at previous dose. General Dosing Information: • Administer immediate-release tablets and oral solution twice daily, preferably with morning and evening meal. • Administer extended-release tablets once daily in the morning, preferably with food. Renal/Hepatic Function Impairment: In patients with moderately impaired hepatic function (Child-Turcotte-Pugh score 7–9) and those with moderate renal function impairment, the dose should not exceed 16 mg/d. Not recommended for patients with severe renal (CrCl less than 9 mL/min) or severe hepatic function impairment (Child-Turcotte-Pugh score 10–15).	Treatment of mild to moderate dementia of the Alzheimer type. Small improvements in cognition and function occur within 12–24 weeks. Benefits may last for more than 1 year.	Cholinergic effects, particularly affecting the GI tract (nausea, anorexia, diarrhea); headache; bradycardia may occur.	Highly bioavailable. Initial dose is not therapeutic; slow titration increases tolerability. Metabolized by CYP2D6 and CYP3A4 isoenzymes.

Rivastigmine tartrate (Exelon) Pseudo-irreversible inhibitor of AChE and butyrylcholinesterase, primarily in the CNS	Exelon • Capsules 1.5 mg (as tartrate) • Capsules 3 mg (as tartrate) • Capsules 4.5 mg (as tartrate) • Capsules 6 mg (as tartrate) • Solution, oral 2 mg/mL (as tartrate) Exelon • Patch, transdermal 4.6 mg/24 h • Patch, transdermal 9.5 mg/24 h Alzheimer Disease, Parkinson Disease Dementia: Adults: Transdermal: Start with 4.6 mg/24 h patch. After a minimum of 4 weeks at the initial dose, increase the dose to 9.5 mg/24 h patch (recommended max, 9.5 mg/24 h). If adverse reactions (e.g., diarrhea, nausea, vomiting) cause intolerance to treatment, stop treatment for several days, then restart at the same or next lower dose. If treatment is stopped for more than several days, restart treatment with 4.6 mg/24 h patch and titrate to 9.5 mg/24 h after a minimum of 4 weeks. Dementia of the Alzheimer Type: Adults: PO: 1.5 mg twice daily initially, then dose may be increased by increments of 1.5 mg twice daily at intervals of 2 weeks or more (max, 6 mg twice daily). Dementia Associated With Parkinson Disease: Adults: PO: 1.5 mg twice daily initially, then dose may be increased by increments of 1.5 mg twice daily at intervals of 4 weeks or more (max, 6 mg twice daily). Switching from Capsules or Oral Solution to Transdermal Patch: Adults: Transdermal: Patients receiving an oral dose of less than 6 mg of rivastigmine daily can be switched to 4.6 mg/24 h patch. Patients receiving an oral dose of rivastigmine 6 to 12 mg daily may be switched directly to 9.5 mg/24 h patch. When switching from oral administration to patch, it is recommended that the first patch be applied on the day after the last oral dose. General Dosing Information: Capsules and oral solution: • Administer with meals in divided doses in the morning and evening. • Use the provided syringe to withdraw the prescribed amount of oral solution. • Oral solution may be swallowed directly from the syringe or mixed with a small glass of water, cold fruit juice, or soda. Stir the mixture before drinking. • Oral solution and capsules may be interchanged at equal doses. Transdermal patch: • Apply patch once daily to clean, dry, hairless, intact, healthy skin. • Apply patch to an area that will not be rubbed against tight clothing. • The recommended sites for application of patch are the upper or lower back. If these sites are not accessible, patch can be applied to chest or upper arm. • Do not apply patch to an area that is red, irritated, or cut. • To avoid irritation, change the site of patch application daily. Avoid application to the same spot for at least 14 days. • Apply patch by pressing firmly until the edges stick. • The patch can be used in situations that include bathing and hot weather. • Do not apply patch to areas where cream, lotion, or powder has recently been applied. • The patch should be replaced every 24 hours. • Used transdermal system should be folded, with the adhesive surface pressed together, and discarded safely.	Treatment of mild to moderate dementia of the Alzheimer type; treatment of mild to moderate dementia associated with Parkinson disease. Small improvements in cognition and function occur within 12–24 weeks. Benefits may last for more than 1 year.	Cholinergic effects, particularly affecting the GI tract (nausea, anorexia, vomiting, diarrhea); headache; bradycardia may occur.	Highly bioavailable. Therapeutic effect greatly exceeds biological half-life (1 hour), allowing for twice-daily dosing. Metabolized by hydrolysis. Initial dose is not therapeutic; administration with food and slow titration are necessary to increase tolerability.

(continues)

TABLE 103-7

U.S. Food and Drug Administration–Approved Drugs for Alzheimer Disease (AD) (*Continued*)

Generic Drug (Brand Name) and Mechanism	Dosage Form and Dosage	Indication and Effect	Adverse Effects	Other
Memantine Immediate- and Extended-Release (Namenda and Namenda XR) Uncompetitive antagonist of the *N*-methyl-D-aspartate type of glutamate receptors	Namenda – Tablets 5 mg – Tablets 10 mg – Solution, oral 2 mg/mL Namenda XR – Capsules, ER 7 mg – Capsules, ER 14 mg – Capsules, ER 21 mg – Capsules, ER 28 mg Adults: Immediate Release: PO: Start with 5 mg daily. Increase the dose in 5-mg increments to 5 mg twice daily, 15 mg/d (5 and 10 mg as separate doses), and 10 mg twice daily. The minimum recommended interval between dose increases is 1 week. ER: PO: Start with 7 mg daily. Increase the dose in 7-mg increments to a maximum of 28 mg daily. The minimum recommended interval between dose increases is 1 week. Conversion from immediate-release to ER: PO: Patients taking immediate-release 10 mg twice daily may switch to ER 28 mg once daily the day after the last dose of an immediate-release 10-mg tablet. Renal Function Impairment: Adults: Immediate Release: Severe renal impairment (CrCl 5 to 29 mL/min): PO: A target dosage of 5 mg twice daily is recommended. Patients taking 5 mg twice daily may switch to ER 14 mg once daily the day after the last dose of an immediate-release 5-mg tablet. Mild to moderate renal impairment (CrCl 30 to 79 mL/min): PO: No dosage adjustment is recommended. ER: Severe renal impairment (CrCl 5 to 29 mL/min): PO: A target dosage of 14 mg/d is recommended. Mild to moderate renal impairment (CrCl 30 to 79 mL/min): PO: No dosage adjustment is recommended. General Dosing Information: • Administer without regard to meals. • ER capsules can be taken intact or may be opened, sprinkled on applesauce, and then swallowed. The entire contents of each capsule should be consumed; the dose should not be divided. Swallow capsules whole. The capsules should not be divided, chewed, or crushed. • Refer to the patient information for instructions on how to use the oral solution dosing device.	Treatment of moderate to severe dementia of the Alzheimer type. Small improvements in cognition and function as well as less burden on caregivers.	Well tolerated, yet can cause headaches, dizziness, insomnia, and agitation.	Can be used as monotherapy or in conjunction with cholinesterase inhibitors.

AChE, acetylcholinesterase; BID, twice daily; CNS, central nervous system; CrCl, creatinine clearance; CYP, cytochrome P-450; ER, extended release; GI, gastrointestinal; ODT, orally disintegrating tablets; PO, orally; QID, four times daily.

Source: Wilkinson DG et al. Cholinesterase inhibitors used in the treatment of Alzheimer's disease: the relationship between pharmacological effects and clinical efficacy. *Drugs Aging.* 2004;21:453; Masterman D. Cholinesterase inhibitors in the treatment of Alzheimer's disease and related dementias. *Clin Geriatr Med.* 2004;20:59; Winblad B et al. Donepezil in patients with severe Alzheimer's disease: double-blind, parallel-group, placebo-controlled study [published corrections appear in *Lancet.* 2006;367:1980; *Lancet.* 2006;368:1650]. *Lancet.* 2006;367:1057; Farlow MR et al. Effectiveness and tolerability of high-dose (23 mg/d) versus standard-dose (10 mg/d) donepezil in moderate to severe Alzheimer's disease: a 24-week, randomized, double-blind study. *Clin Ther.* 2010;32:1234; Williams BR et al. A review of rivastigmine: a reversible cholinesterase inhibitor. *Clin Ther.* 2003;25:1634; Farlow M et al. A 52-week study of the efficacy of rivastigmine in patients with mild to moderately severe Alzheimer's disease. *Eur Neurol.* 2000;44:236; Grossberg G et al. Safety and tolerability of the rivastigmine patch: results of a 28-week open-label extension. *Alzheimer Dis Assoc Disord.* 2009;23:158; Scott LJ, Goa KL. Galantamine: a review of its use in Alzheimer's disease. *Drugs.* 2000;60:1095; Becker M et al. The effect of cholinesterase inhibitors on risk of nursing home placement among Medicaid beneficiaries with dementia. *Alzheimer Dis Assoc Disord.* 2006;20:147; Wallin AK et al. Donepezil in Alzheimer's disease: what to expect after 3 years of treatment in a routine clinical setting. *Dement Geriatr Cogn Disord.* 2007;23:150; Jarvis B, Figgitt DP. Memantine. *Drugs Aging.* 2003;20:465; Tariot PN et al. Memantine treatment in patients with moderate to severe Alzheimer disease already receiving donepezil: a randomized controlled trial. *JAMA.* 2004;291:317; Monograph Summary for Donepezil HCl Oral and Rivastigmine Tartrate Oral. http://online.factsandcomparisons.com/ComparativeMonographSummary.aspx?drillDownType=SBS&selectedDrugs=47180|65654&unSelectedDrugs=|47180|65654|129123|91778|93939&searchSections=1|3|4|5|7|8|. Accessed June 29, 2011; Monograph Summary for Galantamine Hydrobromide Oral and Memantine HCl Oral. http://online.factsandcomparisons.com/ComparativeMonographSummary.aspx?drillDownType=SBS&selectedDrugs=91778|93939&unSelectedDrugs=|47180|65654|129123|91778|93939&searchSections=1|3|4|5|7|8|. Accessed June 29, 2011.

the Severe Impairment Battery, and there was no improvement in the CIBIC-Plus when compared with the 10-mg dose. More than 30% of the high-dose group and nearly 18% of the low-dose group failed to complete the 24-week trial.[50]

The most common adverse effects of donepezil are associated with cholinergic activity. They tend to be mild to moderate in nature and resolve with stabilization of the dose.[43,46] In a 144-week extension trial of donepezil, the most frequently encountered adverse effects were nausea, diarrhea, and headache.[47] In clinical trials, however, adverse effects were the primary reason for withdrawal from studies, with an overall dropout rate of 29% in the treatment groups.[41]

RIVASTIGMINE

Rivastigmine is a carbamate derivative that inhibits both AChE and BChE activity. BChE provides an alternative pathway for acetylcholine metabolism. Rivastigmine inhibits the activity of both cholinesterases, primarily in the central nervous system.[51] Its AChE inhibition is greater for the G1 as compared with the G4 form.[29] The drug binds to the esteratic sites of the AChE and BChE molecules and slowly dissociates. Because of this, it is often referred to as a "pseudoirreversible" inhibitor.[52] Rivastigmine's biological half-life is approximately 1 hour, but because its slow dissociation extends its activity for at least 10 hours, it can be dosed twice daily. Rivastigmine is bound approximately 40% to serum proteins and is metabolized via hydrolysis to renally excreted inactive compounds.[51] Rivastigmine absorption is nearly complete, but because it undergoes a significant first-pass effect, the resultant bioavailability is approximately 36% (Table 103-7).

In two large clinical trials conducted in patients with mild to moderately severe AD, rivastigmine improved cognition, the ability to perform daily activities, and global function over the course of 24 weeks.[52,53] In each multicenter, double-blind, placebo-controlled trial, subjects were randomly assigned to receive placebo or low-dose (1–4 mg/day) or high-dose (6–12 mg/day) rivastigmine in two divided doses during a 26-week period. In one study, subjects in both dosage groups demonstrated statistically significant improvement after 26 weeks on the ADAS-Cog and CIBIC-Plus scales.[52] In the other trial, only those subjects taking 6 to 12 mg/day improved on the same scales.[53] An open-label extension study that included subjects from both previous studies found that subjects taking 6 to 12 mg/day of rivastigmine had significantly better cognitive function after 1 year than did subjects who had originally received placebo.[54]

Adverse effects typically include nausea, vomiting, diarrhea, and other cholinergically mediated GI effects.[51] They are most common when rivastigmine is taken on an empty stomach or when the dose escalation is too rapid. Headache, dizziness, and fatigue are also common adverse effects. Increasing the dose by 1.5 mg twice daily at 4-week intervals increases drug tolerability and reduces the frequency and severity of GI side effects. Adverse effect severity appears to be less problematic with a transdermal formulation that delivers 4.6 or 9.5 mg/24 hours, which correspond to 6- and 12-mg daily doses of the oral formulation.[55]

GALANTAMINE

Like other agents used to treat AD, galantamine enhances cholinergic activity by inhibiting AChE. However, it also stimulates nicotinic receptors at a site distinct from that stimulated by acetylcholine, an action that does not rely on the presence of acetylcholine. This action is referred to as allosteric modulation.[29] Galantamine is rapidly and completely absorbed, reaches peak serum levels in less than 2 hours, and has a half-life of approximately 5 hours. It exhibits low protein binding and has a large volume of distribution. Galantamine is metabolized primarily by cytochrome P-450 (CYP) isoenzymes CYP2D6 and CYP3A4, and is eliminated in the urine (Table 103-7).[56]

Clinical trials have shown galantamine to be effective for the symptomatic treatment of mild to moderate AD. Doses of 16 and 24 mg/day produced clinically meaningful improvement in ADAS-Cog and CIBIC-Plus scores during a 5-month, randomized, placebo-controlled trial.[57] A similar trial conducted in Europe and Canada that evaluated patients for 6 months used doses of 24 and 32 mg/day. Both doses were more effective than placebo, but patients in the 32-mg/day group exhibited more adverse effects.[58] A 6-month, open-label extension trial showed that patients treated with galantamine 24 mg/day maintained ADAS-Cog scores throughout the entire 12 months of the study.[58]

As with the other ChEI, cholinergic effects in the GI tract are the most commonly encountered adverse effects. Nausea, diarrhea, vomiting, and anorexia were the most frequent events encountered during clinical trials.[29,41] They were typically present during the dose escalation phases of the studies. A dose titration interval of 4 weeks reduces the severity of adverse effects and increases tolerability.

C.L. is in the mild stage of the disease, so a ChEI is an appropriate choice.[38] It is unlikely that a ChEI will produce a dramatic or long-lasting improvement in C.L.'s cognitive abilities. Systematic reviews of ChEI therapy have consistently concluded that these agents provide modest benefits, at best, in the majority of patients.[41,59] Treatment, however, may slow her cognitive decline, help maintain her ability to care for herself for 1 year or more, and reduce the risk for nursing facility placement for as much as 2 years.[60] Beneficial effects may occur for as long as 3 years, and patients who start therapy earlier may experience greater benefit than those who delay treatment.[61,62] The choice of drug is based on the agent most likely to produce a positive response with the fewest adverse effects. Ease of adherence must also be considered. All agents exhibit similar adverse effect profiles. Rivastigmine may be less prone to drug interactions because of its metabolic pathway.[51] It is also available as a transdermal patch that is applied daily. Whereas the oral formulation of rivastigmine requires an initial, nontherapeutic titration dose to reduce the severity of adverse effects, the initial transdermal dosage is therapeutic.[55] Donepezil and galantamine extended-release can be given as a single daily dose and are available as generic equivalents. They can be given at bedtime, which may make cholinergic side effects less troublesome. Donepezil is an appropriate agent for C.L.

CASE 103-1, QUESTION 6: How should treatment with donepezil be instituted in C.L., and how should therapy be monitored?

C.L. should receive donepezil 5 mg at bedtime. She should be monitored for cholinergic side effects (particularly nausea and diarrhea), insomnia, headache, and dizziness, the adverse effects most commonly reported in clinical trials.[43,46] Her family and physician should look for improvements in her memory, orientation, and ability to concentrate on complex tasks, such as shopping. She may also become less irritable. After 1 month, her physician should assess her for adverse effects.[38] If she has not improved noticeably after 4 to 6 weeks, the dose of donepezil may be increased to 10 mg at bedtime.

If her condition does not respond to donepezil after a 6-month trial, or she is unable to tolerate the donepezil, it is reasonable to switch C.L. to another ChEI. Both rivastigmine and galantamine have additional mechanisms of action that might prove beneficial. Rivastigmine is started at a dose of 1.5 mg twice daily with meals to slow absorption and improve tolerability. The dose may be increased at 2-week intervals by 1.5 mg twice daily, up to the maximal dose of 6 mg twice daily; however, the transdermal formulation is better tolerated and may be preferable by avoiding a titration phase. Galantamine can be started at 4 mg twice daily or 8 mg daily (extended-release) and increased every 4 weeks by 8 mg, up to a maximal dose of 24 mg daily. As with oral rivastigmine, the initial dose is not therapeutic.[56] Taking galantamine with meals may improve tolerability of GI effects. If a trial of a second agent does not improve or stabilize a patient's condition, there is no value in attempting a third agent.

C.L. should have routine reassessment of her daily function, cognition, and behavior at 6-month intervals.[38] Close attention also must be paid to her other medical conditions, and her family should be provided ongoing support, such as through an AD caregiver support group.

MEMANTINE

CASE 103-1, QUESTION 7: C.L. tolerated donepezil 10 mg well, with the exception of some mild nausea and occasional loose stools. She was once again able to engage in normal activities with the help of reminder notes and became much less irritable according to her family.

One year later, C.L. is exhibiting some decline in her cognition and is becoming more disoriented, particularly in the afternoon and evening. Her physician considers her to now be in the moderate stage of AD. What other drug therapy strategies may be appropriate for C.L.'s worsening AD?

There are two treatment options that can be tried at this time. One option is to further titrate up the donepezil dose to 23 mg a day as mentioned above with some limited clinical efficacy.[47] Another option is to use an *N*-methyl-D-aspartate (NMDA) antagonist, which has been shown to reduce the release of glutamate in the central nervous system that can lead to excitotoxic reactions and cell death in AD and other neurodegenerative disorders.[63] Memantine is an noncompetitive NMDA receptor antagonist with moderate affinity and voltage-dependent binding. It is completely absorbed after oral administration, reaches peak serum concentrations in 3 to 8 hours, and is moderately protein bound (Table 103-7).

Two large clinical trials have evaluated memantine in subjects with moderate to severe AD. A dose of 10 mg/day for 12 weeks increased functional ability (e.g., dressing, toileting, participating in group activities) and reduced care dependence compared with placebo.[63] A 28-week trial using a dose of 20 mg/day improved CIBIC-Plus scores, activities of daily living, and global function compared with placebo.[64] Overall, the benefits of memantine are modest.[65] The combined use of memantine and a ChEI has been shown to be superior to a ChEI alone by improving daily function in individuals with moderate to severe dementia.[66–69] Common adverse effects include diarrhea, insomnia, dizziness, headache, and hallucinations.[63] C.L. should be started on memantine 5 mg daily, with the dosage increased in weekly intervals by 5 mg/day, up to a dose of 10 mg twice daily.[63] As an alternative, she can be started on the extended-release formulation given in weekly escalating doses of 7, 14, 21, and 28 mg daily (Table 103-7).

LEWY BODY DEMENTIAS

Etiology

Lewy bodies are hyaline-containing inclusion bodies typically found in people with Parkinson disease. Recently, attention has been given to distinguish DLB and PDD to help further research.[70] It is known that up to 25% of patients with dementia have Lewy bodies in the brainstem and cortex (particularly in the limbic and paralimbic cortices and frontal and temporal lobes).[4,71] Concentrations are found in the substantia nigra, locus ceruleus, hypothalamus, basal nucleus of Meynert, and neocortex. There is decreased dopamine in the basal ganglia and a loss of choline acetyltransferase (and thus, acetylcholine) in the basal nucleus of Meynert.[4] Many of these patients display extrapyramidal signs without the classic presentation of Parkinson disease.[6] The role of α-synuclein is a common biological theme in both DLB and PDD, with α-synuclein aggregates found in Lewy bodies and neurites.

Clinical Presentation

CASE 103-2

QUESTION 1: J.F. is a 72-year-old woman who was diagnosed with mild cognitive impairment 6 months ago. She had been increasingly forgetful and confused for about 1 year before the diagnosis. Approximately 3 months ago, J.F. and her family decided that J.F. should move in with them so she would not be left alone. Since moving in with the family, her son has noted that she seems "spaced out" at times. Some days, she appears to be very clear and not confused; other days she is very forgetful and requires assistance with daily tasks. Her daughter-in-law reported that J.F. has been unsteady on her feet at times and has fallen twice. She notes at times she moves very slowly and has difficulty initiating movement. Recently, J.F. reported seeing people coming out of the painting on the wall (a European street scene), stating that "they were walking all through the house trying to steal anything that can be hidden in a coat pocket."

At the physician visit, J.F. was found to be medically stable. Vital signs, serum chemistries, and complete blood cell count were within normal limits. Her MMSE score was 21/30. During the review of systems, J.F.'s daughter-in-law had to answer some questions because J.F. appeared either not to hear them or to ignore them. On physical examination, she demonstrated mild cog-wheeling rigidity bilaterally, bradykinesia, and masked facies; she did not display a resting tremor. What is the most likely explanation for J.F.'s presentation?

Given her physical health, inability to live alone because of impaired cognition, and MMSE score, J.F. meets the criteria for dementia. Her rigidity, bradykinesia, and masked facies are consistent with early Parkinson disease (see Chapter 57, Parkinson Disease and Other Movement Disorders). There have been revised criteria for the clinical diagnosis of DLB (Table 103-8).[72] J.F. exhibits all the central features, two core features, and the supportive feature of repeated falls. Her presentation is consistent with probable DLB versus PDD because of her temporal sequence and lack of well-established diagnosis of Parkinson disease.

Treatment

CASE 103-2, QUESTION 2: What is an appropriate treatment for J.F.?

To date, ChEIs are the only treatment strategy for the cognitive symptoms of both PDD and DLB. All ChEIs have demonstrated symptomatic benefit in patients with DLB.[73,74] The largest randomized, placebo-controlled trials have used rivastigmine (up to 12 mg/day) in subjects with mild to moderate disease,

TABLE 103-8
Revised Diagnostic Criteria for Dementia with Lewy Bodies

1. *Central features (essential for a diagnosis of possible or probable DLB):* Dementia is defined as a progressive cognitive decline that interferes with normal social or occupational function. There is prominent or persistent memory impairment usually evident with progression but not necessarily present in the early stages. Deficits on tests of attention, executive function, and visuospatial ability may be especially prominent.
2. *Core features (two core features are sufficient for diagnosis of probable DLB, one for possible DLB):* (a) Fluctuating cognition with pronounced variations in attention and alertness, (b) recurrent visual hallucinations that are typically well formed and detailed, and (c) spontaneous features of parkinsonism.
3. *Suggestive features (if one or more is present in the presence of one or more core features, a diagnosis of probable DLB can be made. In the absence of core features, one or more suggestive features are sufficient for possible DLB. Probable DLB should NOT be diagnosed on the basis of suggestive features alone):* (a) Rapid eye movement sleep behavior disorder, (b) severe neuroleptic sensitivity, and (c) low dopamine transporter uptake in basal ganglia demonstrated by SPECT or PET imaging.
4. *Supportive features (commonly present but not proven to have diagnostic specific):* (a) Repeated falls and syncope; (b) transient, unexplained loss of consciousness; (c) severe autonomic dysfunction; (d) hallucinations in other modalities; (e) systematized delusions; (f) depression; (g) relative preservation of medial temporal lobe structures with reduced occipital activity; (h) generalized low uptake on SPECT/PET perfusion scan with reduced occipital activity; and (i) abnormal (low uptake) MIBG myocardial scintigraphy.
5. A diagnosis of DLB is less likely in the presence of cerebrovascular disease, presence of any other physical illness or brain disorder, or if parkinsonism only appears for the first time at stage of severe dementia.
6. Need to evaluate the temporal sequence of symptoms to differentiate between DLB and PDD. DLB should be diagnosed when dementia occurs before or concurrently with parkinsonism. PDD should be used to describe dementia that occurs in the context of well-established Parkinson disease (generally the 1-year rule between the onset of dementia and parkinsonism should be followed in the diagnosis).

DLB, dementia with Lewy bodies; PDD, Parkinson disease dementia; PET, positron emission tomography; SPECT, single photon emission computed tomography.
Adapted from references McKeith IG et al. Consensus guidelines for the clinical and pathologic diagnosis of dementia with Lewy bodies (DLB): report of the consortium on DLB international workshop. *Neurology.* 1996;47:1113; McKeith IG et al. Diagnosis and management of dementia with Lewy bodies: third report of the DLB Consortium [published correction appears in *Neurology.* 2005;65:1992]. *Neurology.* 2005;65:1863.

and this medication has received US Food and Drug Administration (FDA) indication for PDD. Rivastigmine was reported to worsen tremor in 10% of the patients with PDD, yet overall there was not a statistically significant difference between groups.[70] Rivastigmine treatment has demonstrated improvements in apathy, anxiety, delusions, and hallucinations when titrated appropriately to doses of 6 to 12 mg daily.[75] Dose initiation, titration, and monitoring are conducted in the same manner as when ChEIs are used for the treatment of AD.

J.F.'s symptoms of Parkinson disease should be fully evaluated, and appropriate treatment, such as levodopa/carbidopa, should be started (see Chapter 57, Parkinson Disease and Other Movement Disorders). Because several medications for parkinsonism can have psychiatric effects, it is important to monitor for adverse effects such as worsening psychosis and cognition. Typical antipsychotics, such as haloperidol, may worsen her extrapyramidal symptoms (EPS) and should be avoided. Novel atypicals, namely, quetiapine and clozapine, may be less likely to exacerbate the parkinsonism but should be instituted after a trial of a ChEI or if more acute symptom control of behaviors is required.[70,72]

VASCULAR DEMENTIAS

Etiology

VaD is a broad classification of cognitive disorders caused by vascular disease. The most common cause of VaD is occlusion of cerebral blood vessels by a thrombus or embolus, leading to ischemic brain injury.[76] In the majority of cases, the dementia syndrome is the result of multiple individual cerebral infarcts, a single infarct in an area related to cognitive function, or diffuse white matter lesions in the subcortex.[16] A number of diseases, including atherosclerosis, arteriosclerosis, and vasculitis, lead to the production of emboli and thrombi that potentially occlude brain vessels. Hemorrhagic phenomena and disorders such as hypertension or cardiac disease can produce episodes of cerebral ischemia or hypoxia and are responsible for some cases of VaD.[14,76,77] Specific risk factors for VaDs include advancing age, diabetes mellitus, small vessel cerebrovascular disease, hypertension, heart disease, hyperlipidemia, cigarette smoking, and alcohol use.[23,77–79]

Neuropathology

VaDs are typically subcortical. Most patients with multi-infarct dementia (MID) have blockage of multiple blood vessels and infarction of the cerebral tissue supplied by those vessels.[77] When the distribution of a large artery or medium-size arteriole is blocked, focal neurologic deficits can result (see Chapter 59, Cerebrovascular Disorders). Depending on the area affected, there may be significant cognitive impairment. More often, however, a patient may have experienced transient ischemic attacks (TIAs) or multiple microinfarcts that have remained unrecognized.[77] Patients with subcortical VaDs often exhibit small, deep ischemic infarcts in arterioles of the basal ganglia, thalamus, and internal capsule.[6,77] A history of atherosclerosis, diabetes mellitus, or hypertension is often present without a history of stroke.[4,77,79] MRI scans can be very useful in diagnosing VaDs because areas of cerebral infarction are easier to visualize than they are with CT scanning (Fig. 103-3).[16,30] Lesions in white matter may occur in as many as 85% of patients with VaD. Deep white matter lesions known as leukoaraiosis often include demyelination and may represent early changes in dementia.[77] Although patients with Alzheimer-type dementia may also exhibit leukoaraiosis, it is much more prevalent in those with MIDs.[6] Because of the etiologic factors involved, VaD typically has an earlier onset than AD, and affects more men than women.

Clinical Presentation

CASE 103-3

QUESTION 1: D.V., a 73-year-old man, is accompanied by his daughter for evaluation of "fuzzy thinking." Although his chief complaint is impaired memory, he denies significant impact on his daily routine. D.V. states his memory problem began 2 years ago after a dizzy spell and subsequent fall. However, his daughter states that the impairment began approximately 1 year before that episode. The memory loss has been slowly progressive. D.V. states that he feels useless because of his memory problems and his "boring" daily

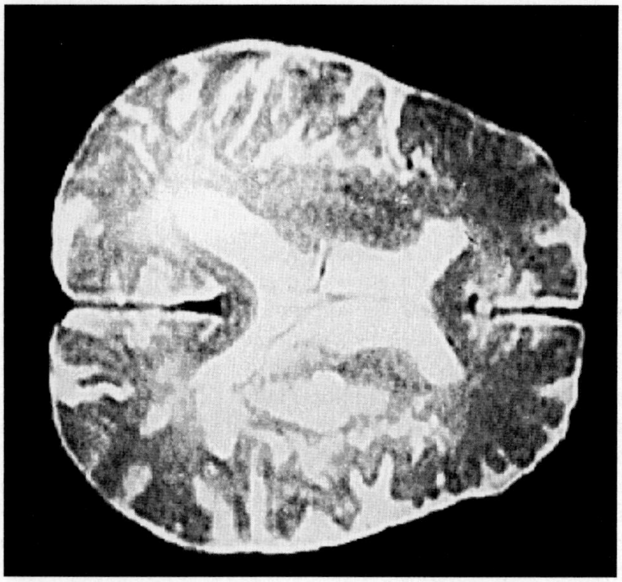

FIGURE 103-3 A large stroke is visible to the right of the ventricles. There is evidence of atrophy in the right temporal area.

routine. Although D.V. is generally independent, he relies on his daughter for assistance with most financial matters. He has voluntarily quit driving because of a lack of confidence in his abilities. D.V.'s daughter reports that according to her mother, D.V. is sometimes disoriented at night when he awakens to urinate. He has no history of urinary incontinence. D.V. has a questionable history of TIAs, but no focal neurologic deficits. He has a long history of mild hypertension, which is treated with a diuretic. He drinks alcohol occasionally and smokes about half a pack of cigarettes per day. His medical history is unremarkable except for the possible TIAs, hypertension, and a mildly enlarged prostate. His family history is positive for diabetes and heart disease.

On physical examination, D.V. is found to be a mildly obese man who is well dressed and groomed, alert, and oriented to person. His BP is 160/92 mm Hg sitting and 168/95 mm Hg standing. Cardiac examination is normal. Neurologic findings include somewhat diminished extraocular movements laterally and slightly asymmetric reflexes, with right greater than left. Muscle tone is normal in the lower extremities. He has a mild shuffling gait. Vibratory sensation is diminished but within normal limits for his age. His score on the Folstein MMSE was 22/30, including errors in orientation and recall. His score on the Blessed Dementia Scale was 16/33, with errors in memory and orientation. Psychologic evaluation found him to be mildly depressed.

A full laboratory analysis was generally within normal limits. D.V.'s serum potassium (3.8 mEq/dL) and sodium (138 mEq/dL) were in the low normal range, and his blood urea nitrogen (18 mg/dL) was in the upper normal range. Serum total cholesterol was 246 mg/dL, and fasting triglycerides were 230 mg/dL. A chest radiograph revealed a mildly enlarged heart; his electrocardiogram was normal. An MRI scan indicated generalized atrophy with enlarged ventricles, periventricular white matter ischemic changes, bilateral basal ganglion lacunar infarcts, and small cortical infarcts in the right parietal lobe. What subjective and objective evidence exists for a diagnosis of dementia in D.V.?

D.V.'s major complaint is "fuzzy thinking" and impaired memory that he attributes to his dizzy spell and fall. However, his family began to note problems a full year before that episode, with progression over time. Although D.V. denies that his impairment significantly affects his daily routine, he has voluntarily stopped driving and relies on his daughter for assistance with financial matters. His memory difficulties appear to have affected his mood and made him feel useless. D.V. is disoriented at night when he awakens to urinate. These factors satisfy the DSM-IV criteria for interference with normal activities.[11]

Multiple deficits are present on both the Folstein MMSE[17] (orientation, recall) and on the Blessed Dementia Scale[21] (memory, orientation), indicating impaired short- and long-term memory. D.V.'s inability to drive reflects poor judgment behind the wheel of a car; a disturbance of higher cortical function is indicated by his need for assistance with financial matters. There is no evidence of a delirium being present. Evidence of an organic cause is provided by the MRI scan.

Diagnosis

CASE 103-3, QUESTION 2: What type of dementia does D.V. have?

There is sufficient evidence to indicate that D.V. suffers from a VaD. Although DSM-IV provides diagnostic criteria for VaD (Table 103-9), it is not clear that D.V. satisfies the requirements.[11] VaDs commonly present suddenly after a cerebrovascular insult. This is followed by a period of stability and further declines after additional episodes, in a stepwise pattern. Cognitive impairments are variable and depend on the area of the brain affected by the insult.[11,16]

With the exception of the dizzy spell and fall, D.V.'s deterioration has had a pattern that resembles a downhill slide rather than stepwise decline. Although his cognitive deficits are "patchy" (e.g., he appears to have no language difficulty), they are not particularly prominent. D.V. displays some neurologic signs and symptoms, including diminished extraocular movements, asymmetric reflexes, and a mild shuffling gait, but they are subtle and might be easily missed by an untrained observer as being

TABLE 103-9
Diagnostic and Statistical Manual of Mental Disorders, 4th Edition, Criteria for Vascular Dementia

1. The presence of multiple cognitive deficits manifested by both
   - Impaired memory (ability to learn new information or to retrieve information previously learned)
   - At least one of the following:
     Aphasia (language difficulties)
     Apraxia (diminished ability to perform motor activities in the presence of intact motor function)
     Agnosia (inability to recognize or name objects despite intact sensory function)
     Disruption of executive function (diminished ability to plan, organize)
2. The previous deficits significantly interfere with normal work or social activities and represent a decline from previous ability to function
3. Focal neurologic deficits (e.g., hyperactive deep tendon reflexes, gait disturbances, weak extremities) or laboratory evidence indicating cerebrovascular disease (e.g., multiple infarctions of the cortex or white matter) judged to be etiologically linked to the disorder
4. The deficits do not occur exclusively during the course of a delirium

Adapted with permission from American Psychiatric Association. *Diagnostic and Statistical Manual of Mental Disorders-IV-TR*. Washington, DC: American Psychiatric Association; 2000.

related to a dementia. Reliance solely on the clear presence of diagnostic criteria may often lead to a missed diagnosis.[30] The Hachinski Ischemic Scale ranks signs and symptoms associated with cognitive impairment of cerebrovascular origin and is used to help differentiate between AD and VaD.[77] According to this scale, D.V.'s nocturnal confusion, depression, hypertension history, and focal neurologic signs and symptoms are sufficient to indicate VaD.

D.V.'s history and clinical presentation do not suggest dementia caused by a single large stroke or several small strokes. Large strokes produce significant motor damage, typically on one side of the body (the side contralateral to the stroke). Multiple smaller strokes cause prominent motor deficits in discrete areas controlled by the affected areas. Neither of these patterns describes D.V.'s condition. However, he is clearly exhibiting signs of dementia and has significant cerebrovascular disease. He possesses several risk factors for a VaD, including hypertension, smoking, and hyperlipidemia. His MRI indicates a lacunar state, with multiple small infarcts in the deep penetrating arterioles at the base of the brain, particularly in the basal ganglia, internal capsule, thalamus, and pons (see Chapter 59, Cerebrovascular Disorders). These MRI findings are consistent with D.V.'s long-standing hypertension and neurologic presentation.

Because diagnostic criteria for VaDs are vague, arriving at a specific diagnosis is difficult. Therefore, diagnostic criteria (Table 103-10) have been proposed for ischemic VaD, providing a structure for the most common type of these disorders.[76] According to this diagnostic scheme, D.V. suffers from probable ischemic VaD.

Treatment

CASE 103-3, QUESTION 3: How should D.V. be managed?

Several treatment options that modify risk factors for VaDs are available.

TABLE 103-10
Proposed Diagnostic Criteria for Ischemic Vascular Dementia

Definite IVD (requires histopathological examination of the brain)
- Clinical evidence of dementia
- Pathological confirmation of multiple infarcts, some extracerebellar

Probable IVD
- Dementia
- Evidence of at least two ischemic strokes by history, neurologic signs, or neuroimaging, or a single stroke with clearly documented temporal relationship to the dementia onset
- Supporting evidence of multiple infarcts in regions affecting cognition, history of transient ischemic attacks or vascular risk factors, elevated Hachinski score

Possible IVD
- Dementia, plus one or more of the following:
  - History or evidence of a single stroke (but not multiple strokes) without clearly documented temporal relationship to dementia onset
  - Binswanger disease (without multiple strokes), including all of the following:
    - Early-onset urinary incontinence unexplained by urologic disease, or gait disturbance not explained by peripheral cause
    - Vascular risk factors
    - Extensive white matter change on neuroimaging

IVD, ischemic vascular dementia.
Adapted from Chui HC et al. Criteria for the diagnosis of ischemic vascular dementia proposed by the State of California Alzheimer's Disease Diagnostic and Treatment Centers. *Neurology.* 1992;42(3 Pt 1):473.

SMOKING CESSATION

D.V. should be counseled to stop smoking because cigarette smoking reduces cerebral blood flow and increases the risk for stroke. Among smokers with MID, cessation of cigarette use improves cognitive performance.[80]

ANTIHYPERTENSIVE THERAPY

Hypertension and hyperlipidemia, both present in D.V., are additional risk factors for stroke and VaD. Control of systolic hypertension reduces the risk of stroke by 36% in elderly patients,[81] and maintaining the systolic BP between 135 and 150 mm Hg is associated with improved cognition among MID patients. A systolic BP that exceeds 150 mm Hg indicates inadequate control, whereas a systolic BP less than 135 mm Hg may lead to inadequate cerebral perfusion.[82] As in nondemented individuals, nonpharmacologic treatment (e.g., diet, weight loss, exercise) is an essential component. The antihypertensive agent must be chosen carefully in this population to maximize compliance and minimize adverse reactions.[83] Both thiazide diuretics and β-adrenergic blockers may increase lipid levels, a potential complication in D.V. α-Adrenergic blockers and sympatholytic agents may cause depression or impair cognitive activity. Calcium-channel blockers or angiotensin-converting enzyme inhibitors are acceptable because they are well tolerated by elderly patients and may help preserve renal function in patients with diabetes mellitus (see Chapter 14, Essential Hypertension). Dihydropyridine calcium-channel blockers have been shown to improve cognition in patients with dementia and reduce the risk of dementia in elderly patients with isolated systolic hypertension.[84] Because D.V. has benign prostatic hyperplasia, he may benefit from the use of an α-adrenergic blocking agent, such as doxazosin 1 mg at bedtime or terazosin 1 mg at bedtime (see Chapter 104, Geriatric Urologic Disorders). Evidence indicating an increased risk for negative cardiac outcomes, however, makes the α-adrenergic blocking agents less attractive choices.[85] The use of a vasodilating calcium-channel blocker, such as amlodipine 5 mg/day, is an appropriate first choice. An angiotensin-converting enzyme inhibitor such as benazepril 10 mg/day is an appropriate alternative. Both agents exhibit the advantage of once-daily dosing over some other agents within their respective classes. This feature is important for maximizing adherence in patients with declining memory.

ANTIPLATELET THERAPY

Prophylaxis against future cerebrovascular events is indicated in VaD, but few studies that have looked specifically at individuals with dementia are available. Cerebral perfusion and cognitive performance were improved in MID patients receiving aspirin 325 mg/day for 1 year when compared with a control population.[86] Guidelines from the American Heart Association and the American Stroke Association recommend the use of antiplatelet therapy in patients with a history of TIA or atherothrombotic stroke that is not of cardiogenic origin. Aspirin in doses of 50 to 325 mg/day, clopidogrel 75 mg daily, or aspirin 50 mg/dipyridamole 200 mg twice daily are all effective treatments for stroke prophylaxis.[87] Warfarin is recommended after cardioembolic cerebral ischemic events. However, only aspirin has been studied specifically in VaD patients. Aspirin 325 mg daily is an appropriate first choice for D.V.

CHOLINESTERASE INHIBITORS

Deficits in cholinergic transmission and nicotinic receptor binding abnormalities have been noted in VaD.[4,88] Early clinical trials with donepezil,[89] galantamine,[90] and rivastigmine[91] have demonstrated improvement in cognition and daily function among patients with VaD. As of yet, however, the use of these agents remains investigational and controversial. Because the use of these agents is not FDA-approved for VaD, D.V. and his family should have a thorough discussion with his physician regarding the potential risks and benefits when considering ChEI treatment for him.

MANAGING FUNCTION

D.V. should be referred for physical and occupational therapy for an assessment of his strength, gait, and daily function. Physical therapy can help him maintain his strength. Occupational therapy can provide him with equipment and strategies to adapt to his dizziness and avoid falls. In addition, the use of reminder notes and labels around the house will assist him in maintaining his independence.

BEHAVIORAL DISTURBANCES IN DEMENTIA

Several types of behavioral disturbances may develop during the course of a dementia and occur in almost all patients, particularly during the later stages (Table 103-11).[35,38] Behavior symptoms include a wide range of disturbances, including agitation, apathy, wandering, verbal and physical aggression, and psychotic symptoms.[38] Agitation in dementia has been described as excessive motor activity with a feeling of inner tension that may lead to related symptoms such as anxiety, irritability, motor restlessness, and abnormal vocalization.[92] Sleep disorders and mood disorders, such as anxiety and depression, also are common.[93] Agitation and anxiety are often managed best with nonpharmacologic treatment. Pharmacologic interventions are appropriate when nondrug therapies are unsuccessful or the behavior is severe. Nonpsychologic behaviors such as wandering and inappropriate motor activity respond better to environmental modification than to drug therapy.[38,93] The first step in evaluating altered behavior in patients with dementia is to ensure that the problem is not the result of an unrecognized medical problem or caused by an adverse effect of a medication (see Chapter 102, Geriatric Drug Use).

Agitated Behaviors

For a narrated PowerPoint presentation discussing nonpharmacologic management of behavior disturbances, go to http://thepoint.lww.com/AT10e.

TABLE 103-11
Behavior Disturbances in Dementia

Behavior	Typical Presentation	Nonpharmacologic Treatment	Pharmacologic Treatment
General strategies		Safety-proof living areas Issue one-step commands for directions Maintain a daily routine of activities Avoid arguing incorrect statements Avoid startling the patient Limit unusual or overly stimulating environments	
Anxiety	Excessive worrying, sleep disturbances, rumination	Listen to, and acknowledge frustrations Redirection Exercise Engage in enjoyable activities Sleep hygiene practices Limit noise and distractions	Trazodone Buspirone (if no insomnia) Short-acting benzodiazepine SSRI antidepressant
Depression	Withdrawal, loss of appetite, irritability, restlessness, sleep disturbances	Exercise Engage in meaningful activities	Trazodone SSRI antidepressant
General agitation and restlessness	Repeated questions, wandering, pacing	Distraction and redirection Break down tasks into simple steps Provide enclosed area for exercise	Often unresponsive to medications
Paranoid behaviors	Delusions (often of theft), hallucinations, misperceptions	Reassurance Distraction, rather than confrontation Remove potential sources of confusion (e.g., mirrors and other reflective surfaces)	Atypical antipsychotic, if not responsive to other strategies and person is fearful to self or others SSRI antidepressant, if associated with withdrawal, tearfulness, themes of loss
Aggressive behaviors	Physical or verbal aggressiveness toward others, excessive yelling and screaming, manic features	Identify the precipitating cause or situation Focus on the patient's feelings and concerns Avoid getting angry or upset Maintain a simple, pleasant, and familiar environment Use music, exercise, etc., as a calming activity Shift the focus to another activity	Anticonvulsant, such as divalproex or carbamazepine, possibly in combination with an atypical antipsychotic

Adapted from California Workgroup on Guidelines for Alzheimer's Disease Management. *Guideline for Alzheimer's Disease Management: Final Report:* State of California, Department of Public Health; April 2008; Teri L et al. Nonpharmacologic treatment of behavioral disturbance in dementia. *Med Clin North Am.* 2002;86:641; Tariot PN et al. Pharmacologic therapy for behavioral symptoms of Alzheimer's disease. *Clin Geriatr Med.* 2001;17:359; Herrmann N, Lanctôt KL. Pharmacologic management of neuropsychiatric symptoms of Alzheimer disease. *Can J Psychiatry.* 2007;52:630; Gray KF. Managing agitation and difficult behavior in dementia. *Clin Geriatr Med.* 2004;20:69; Binetti G et al. Delusions in Alzheimer's disease and multi-infarct dementia. *Acta Neurol Scand.* 1993;88:5; Teri L et al. Exercise plus behavioral management in patients with Alzheimer disease: a randomized controlled trial. *JAMA.* 2003;290:2015.

CASE 103-4

QUESTION 1: T.G., a 62-year-old man, has recently been diagnosed with AD, for which he takes donepezil 10 mg at bedtime. He also has hypertension that is treated with hydrochlorothiazide 12.5 mg daily and amlodipine 5 mg daily. He no longer takes his daily walks around the neighborhood because he is afraid he will get lost; instead, he follows his wife around the house as she does her daily chores. Other times, he paces throughout the house. He also expresses worry about the burden he will place on his family as his condition worsens. Recently, he has had episodes of incontinence and awakens four to five times during the night to urinate. His concerns contribute to his nighttime awakenings, making him quite tired during the day. How should T.G.'s agitation and anxiety be managed?

Anxiety and unfocused activity are common problems in the early stages of dementia. Agitation is a general term that, while commonly used, is subject to wide interpretation. It typically is used to describe specific behaviors such as restlessness, irritability, or unfocused motor activities. Patients are aware of their progressive cognitive decline and have sufficient insight to understand the consequences. T.G.'s shadowing of his wife indicate insecurity and anxiety; pacing through the house is an example of restlessness and unfocused behavior. T.G. is exhibiting anxiety, as evidenced by his worry about placing a burden on his family. His poor sleep is attributable to both nocturia and anxiety.

If T.G.'s behavior represents a sudden or rapid change, his physician should first evaluate him for a medical condition such as infection, pain, or a medication-related problem. Although T.G. has been taking hydrochlorothiazide without difficulty, he may no longer be recognizing the cues to urinate. The drug should be discontinued; if his blood pressure rises, the amlodipine dose can be increased. This may help with his incontinence, nocturia, and disturbed sleep.

Once medical problems have been ruled out or corrected, he should be evaluated using a systematic approach, as behavior problems are part of a chain of events. T.G. may be described as "agitated," but his behavior is shadowing his wife and pacing through the house. The behavior has an antecedent; because he has a dementia, he may be unable to initiate a meaningful or enjoyable activity on his own, and consequently he becomes bored. The consequence of his boredom is that he annoys his wife and paces the house. This represents what often is termed an "A-B-C" approach, for *antecedent, behavior, consequence.*[93] Pacing is a demonstration of unfocused energy. T.G.'s wife can give him simple tasks to perform, such as drying dishes, folding laundry, or simple gardening, to help channel his energy. It also may relieve his anxiety and insecurity. She also could accompany him on walks to alleviate his fear of getting lost. She may want to consider enrolling him in an adult day-care program. This would give him meaningful activity that might help him use up his excess energy and sleep better at night. It also will provide her with some respite and avoid or delay caregiver burnout. Appropriate strategies to manage agitated behaviors without medication are listed in Table 103-11.

When nonpharmacologic interventions are not successful in reducing anxiety, irritability, and similar behaviors, medications can be considered. Benzodiazepines are the most commonly used anxiolytics and will address T.G.'s insomnia and anxiety. However, they are associated with several negative outcomes in the elderly, including confusion, amnestic syndromes, ataxia, and falls.[94,95] Long-acting benzodiazepines are generally considered inappropriate for geriatric patients because age-associated accumulation increases the risk of acute toxicity.[96] Benzodiazepines with short half-lives, such as lorazepam or oxazepam, may be used, if necessary, but only for a short term and with caution.[95]

Trazodone is a sedative antidepressant that is effective for insomnia and agitated behaviors in patients with AD.[94,97] Treatment is started at 25 mg at bedtime and may be increased to a dose of 250 mg/day in divided doses. Another alternative treatment is buspirone, which does not cause the cognitive impairments associated with the benzodiazepines. Dosage begins at 5 mg three times daily and may be increased up to 15 mg three times daily. However, buspirone will not concurrently manage T.G.'s insomnia because it has no sedative effect, and there is no reliable evidence that it is efficacious in anxiety associated with dementia.[95] Citalopram has been shown to reduce agitated behaviors in people with dementia and could be used.[98]

If the nondrug strategies are ineffective in reducing T.G.'s insomnia and agitation, trazodone should be initiated at a dose of 25 mg at bedtime. It may be increased by 25 mg/day at 5- to 7-day intervals, up to 100 mg. Doses above 100 mg/day should be split into two daily doses.

Psychosis

CASE 103-4, QUESTION 2: T.G.'s mental status continues to decline to the point that he requires help with bathing and dressing. During a physician visit, he accuses his wife and children of stealing from him. He also cannot locate his coin collection, which he placed in a "safe" location when his memory began to decline; during the night, he rummages through the house looking for it. He believes his family has been plotting to steal his assets and then turn him out onto the street. T.G.'s son reports that T.G. has been verbally abusive and has threatened several members of the family recently. How should T.G.'s paranoid behavior be managed?

Delusions and hallucinations are common among individuals with dementia. Paranoid symptoms, often accompanied by aggression, have been reported in more than half of dementia patients.[97] Delusions typically involve suspicion of theft by family members, which may be secondary to the patient's inability to remember where valuable items were placed and incorrectly concluding that they were stolen.[99] Another common delusion is the misidentification of people or objects.[100] Capgras syndrome, the belief that a person has been "replaced" by an identical-looking impostor or the belief that photographs or television pictures are real individuals, may occur in almost half of demented individuals.[99]

There are a few behavioral interventions that could be tried first before resorting to medications, which produce limited benefits and are accompanied by significant risk.[101,102] The first step is to conduct a person-centered examination of the symptoms. Several questions need to be answered. What is the significance or meaning of these behaviors to T.G? (For example, he cannot locate items that are valuable to him, and does not recall where they are.) What triggers his thoughts and outbursts? (He may assume the items were stolen, and believes that his family, knowing their location, has taken them for their own gain.) How is the family's response further angering him? (If the family searches for and finds the items, it may reinforce his delusion that they stole them.) The family should be educated that paranoid behavior is common in dementia, and that it is likely to pass as the disease progresses. Depending on how fixed the paranoia is, distraction or redirection, such as changing the subject to something more pleasant, or initiating a pleasant activity, could resolve the problem. Regardless of the strategy, they need to be taught not to argue or debate with T.G. but to share his concern. When these strategies fail, then, depending on severity, it may be necessary to resort to medication.

Paranoid symptoms respond best to antipsychotic agents, although these are not highly effective, and no single antipsychotic is more effective than any other. Delusions, hallucinations, aggression, and uncooperativeness symptoms respond best, but overall improvement occurs in only a minority of patients.[95,102] The CATIE-AD trial compared olanzapine, quetiapine, risperidone, and placebo for the treatment of psychosis, aggression, and agitation for up to 36 weeks in patient with AD. Improvement was noted in 32%, 26%, 29%, and 21%, respectively. The authors concluded that efficacy of the agents was offset by adverse effects.[102] There are no antipsychotic medications that are approved by the FDA for use in the management of behavior symptoms in people with dementia. Black-box warnings are present for all agents because of the increased risk for stroke and mortality when used in this population.[101,103,104] Consequently, any use of these drugs in a person with dementia is for an unapproved use and requires a full discussion between the physician, patient, and caregivers.

The risks and potential benefits of therapy must be carefully weighed for T.G. before determining the appropriate treatment. The choice of an antipsychotic agent is determined by the symptoms displayed by the patient as well as the potential for adverse effects. T.G. is experiencing a delusion of theft, suspiciousness, and aggressive behavior. It is possible that the verbal abuse and threats are consequences of fear brought on by the false belief that his family is stealing from him and plans to abandon him.

T.G. has no major contraindications to the use of any antipsychotic agent, and his target symptoms will probably respond to any of the available agents. Therefore, a therapeutic trial is appropriate. The choice can be made according to which antipsychotic agent is least likely to cause intolerable adverse effects. Risperidone has been evaluated in a case series and in a large double-blind, placebo-controlled trial.[105,106] In the case study series, symptoms improved in half of the patients taking dosages ranging from 0.5 mg every other day to 3 mg twice daily. However, 50% also experienced EPS, even at the lowest dosage used.[105] Subjects in the double-blind trial received either placebo or risperidone at dosages of 0.5 mg/day, 1 mg/day, or 2 mg/day for 12 weeks. Daily doses of 1 or 2 mg reduced psychosis and improved behavior, but EPS and somnolence were common adverse effects.[106] Low doses of olanzapine, 5 to 15 mg/day, were superior to placebo for reducing agitation, aggression, and psychosis during a 6-week study among nursing facility residents.[107] Somnolence and gait disturbances were the most common adverse effects. Quetiapine has been shown to reduce agitated and psychotic behaviors at doses of 100 to 200 mg/day.[108] Clozapine poses significant risk for hematologic toxicity and requires careful monitoring. Because T.G. does not have cardiovascular or cerebrovascular risk factors and does not have gait or balance problems, either risperidone 0.25 mg at bedtime or quetiapine 25 mg at bedtime can be initiated. Doses of risperidone may be increased by 0.25 mg/day in weekly intervals, up to 2 mg/day; quetiapine doses can be increased by 25 mg/day, up to 200 mg/day in divided doses. Once his behavior has stabilized, the medication should be continued for about 3 months. At that time, the dose should be decreased in weekly intervals to determine whether the medication is still required. T.G. should be monitored closely for adverse effects, including EPS, which can occur with the atypical antipsychotics.[95,109]

Aggressive Behaviors

CASE 103-4, QUESTION 3: After 3 months, T.G.'s delusions have subsided, but he continues to be verbally abusive and often displays angry, emotional outbursts, especially when he requires help with bathing or toileting. At other times, he is withdrawn and apathetic. He has also been found wandering in the neighborhood on three occasions. These behaviors persist despite treatment with quetiapine 100 mg twice daily. What alternative treatments can be attempted?

Although psychotic symptoms respond to antipsychotic agents, many other behaviors do not. Up to 90% of patients with dementia exhibit at least one disruptive behavior such as angry outbursts, screaming, and abusive language, and many display multiple aggressive behaviors.[95] As many as 32% exhibit moderate to severe behaviors.[95] Such behaviors are typically directed at caregivers, precipitated by receipt of assistance with activities of daily living such as bathing and toileting, and increase in frequency with dementia severity.[93,110] Several of these behaviors may be merely defensive responses to perceived threats in cognitively impaired individuals.[110] Behavioral disturbances must be addressed because they can have a negative effect on the patient's ability to perform activities of daily living.[93]

Some behaviors exhibited by T.G. are not likely to respond to medications. Wandering is typically unaltered by the use of medications unless the patient is oversedated. Nonpharmacologic treatments, such as periods of physical exercise and rest, or environmental modification is much more effective.[93,97,111] T.G.'s reactions to assistance with bathing and toileting may be caused by confusion and fear. Breaking the tasks down to step-by-step procedures, accomplished individually, often helps modify aggressive behaviors.[38]

Verbal abuse and aggressiveness place both the patient and the caregiver at risk for injury, and may lead to abuse. In these situations, the patient and the caregiver may each be a precipitator or a target of abuse.[112] In some small studies, anticonvulsant agents have been shown to reduce rage and aggressive behaviors in patients resistant to treatment with antipsychotics. Carbamazepine and valproic acid (including divalproex) are the most well-studied agents.[95,109] Although initial trials were promising, later studies did not establish efficacy. The lack of benefit plus concerns about toxicities with each agent have led to recommendations that these agents not be used.[95,109] The addition of an antidepressant medication may be helpful, as described below. Wandering typically does not respond to pharmacologic intervention. Appropriate strategies include environmental modification, such as placing child-safety locks on exit doors; providing activities and other distractions; and having a safety plan, such as the Safe Return program. As described for his paranoid behavior, a person-centered evaluation using the A-B-C approach should be conducted to determine the cause and effects of his aggressiveness. If T.G.'s aggressive behaviors continue, his family may need to consider obtaining in-home assistance or placement in an assisted-living facility designed for the care of patients with dementia.

Depression

CASE 103-4, QUESTION 4: How should T.G.'s social withdrawal and apathy be treated?

Depression often accompanies dementia and may significantly impair a patient's functional capacity, cognitive abilities, and communication.[95,109] T.G. is withdrawn and apathetic, symptoms suggestive of depression. Screaming and irritability may be considered symptoms of depression in individuals with dementia, perhaps reflecting feelings of loneliness, boredom, or the need for attention.[113] Because a definite diagnosis of depression relies heavily on a patient interview and response to questions, a formal diagnosis in patients with dementia is difficult.

Therefore, patient observation is an important component for making a clinical evaluation. It is possible that he is reacting to a sense of loss of not only his memory and function, but also a loss of self. He also may feel isolated by the inability to communicate with others or participate in the outside world. Helping him to engage in meaningful activities and social engagement, perhaps as simple as going on a walk or attending adult day care, may help alleviate his apathy and reverse his withdrawal. Such a strategy is appropriate to try before considering an antidepressant.

The selective serotonin reuptake inhibitors have not been well studied in patients with dementia, but are effective antidepressants with adverse effects that are better tolerated than those of the tricyclic antidepressants. Sertraline, in doses of 50 to 150 mg/day, was superior to placebo in reducing depression in AD patients during a 12-week trial.[114] Citalopram has also demonstrated effectiveness in small trials; in contrast, fluoxetine and fluvoxamine have not demonstrated benefit.[95,109] Either sertraline 50 mg daily or citalopram 10 mg daily are reasonable choices to treat T.G.'s symptoms of depression if he does not respond to nonpharmacologic strategies. He should be reassessed in 1 month; if he has not responded, the dose may be increased. Dosages may be increased weekly up to a maximum of 150 mg/day or 20 mg/day, respectively. A full therapeutic trial requires a minimum of 3 months.

Social Support

CASE 103-4, QUESTION 5: T.G.'s family indicates that caring for him at home has become so burdensome that they are considering placing him in an institution. What social support services are available to families facing this decision?

Institutionalization is a typical outcome for patients in the late stages of dementia. The total care required to manage a dementia patient usually becomes unmanageable for most families as the disease progresses. Caregiver stress is often exacerbated by the patient's declining memory, inability to communicate, physical decline, and incontinence, as well as the caregiver's loss of freedom and depression. Caregivers commonly experience anger, helplessness, guilt, and worry, and suffer from physical stressors such as fatigue and illness.[38]

Outside assistance is essential to families caring for a patient with dementia. Families should be referred to the Alzheimer's Association as soon as a diagnosis of dementia is received. The association has local affiliates in most major cities. The book *The 36-Hour Day* is a valuable resource for families as well.[115] It describes the symptoms, behaviors, and problems that can be encountered when caring for a patient with dementia.

Support groups, individual and family counseling, and other sources of support are useful and may help families cope for a longer period. However, the key intervention to reduce caregiver stress is respite care, which allows a family time away from the responsibilities of taking care of a frail individual. Respite care brings a person into the home or allows the patient to go to a day-care center or similar environment on a regular schedule. Such programs may delay the need to institutionalize a patient.[38,39,115]

PSEUDODEMENTIA

Clinical Presentation and Diagnosis

CASE 103-5

QUESTION 1: G.Y., an 86-year-old woman, lives alone in a low-income housing unit. For the past 6 weeks, she has become disoriented and confused. A neighbor brought her to the hospital after finding her wandering through the neighborhood in her nightclothes. She eats only one meal a day—a frozen potpie—because she generally forgets to eat her other meals. Several bills remain unpaid. She has difficulty sleeping and expresses little desire to live because "all my friends are gone." Her score on the Folstein MMSE is 18/30 with multiple deficits. Most errors are attributable to answers of "I don't know" or "I can't." She currently takes clonidine 0.1 mg three times daily for hypertension, oxybutynin 10 mg twice daily for overactive bladder, hydrocodone/acetaminophen 7.5 mg/750 mg one tablet every 8 hours as needed for pain, and zolpidem 10 mg at bedtime as needed for insomnia. What subjective and objective data support a diagnosis of pseudodementia in G.Y.?

DEPRESSION

G.Y. clearly exhibits cognitive impairment as evidenced by her symptoms of confusion and disorientation, forgetting to eat, wandering, and a low score on the Folstein MMSE.[17] However, the rapid course of her decline, her lack of effort on mental status testing, and the medications she is taking, all of which may affect cognition in older adults, suggest that her impairment might be secondary to causes other than true dementia.

Depression is the most common cause of pseudodementia, accounting for at least 50% of cases. Depressive symptoms in G.Y. include self-neglect, insomnia, loss of desire to live, and lack of effort on mental status testing. When given a mental status screening test, depressed patients tend to give "I don't know" as their answers, which reflects a lack of effort or an inability to cooperate, consistent with a depressed mood.

MEDICATIONS

Medications are often responsible for cognitive impairment in older adults, accounting for dementia symptoms in approximately 12% of patients with cognitive impairment. Psychotropic medications, analgesics, antihypertensives, corticosteroids, and anticholinergic agents are often implicated (see Chapters 83, Mood Disorders I: Major Depressive Disorders, and Chapter 102, Geriatric Drug Use).

Treatment

CASE 103-5, QUESTION 2: What is the proper treatment for G.Y.'s pseudodementia?

Initial therapy should consist of the discontinuation of her medications, all of which may be contributing to her cognitive decline. Her clonidine, oxybutynin, and possibly zolpidem and hydrocodone (pending patterns of use) would need to be tapered to prevent medication withdrawal adverse events. Overall, the medications are relatively short-acting, and her mental status should improve significantly within 48 hours. At that time, her hypertension, overactive bladder, insomnia, and pain can be re-evaluated and more-appropriate therapy instituted, if warranted.

G.Y. should be evaluated for depression, and psychotherapy should be initiated if she is in fact depressed. She should also be referred to a social services agency or senior center to provide her with assistance and to offer her opportunities for social interaction.

ACKNOWLEDGEMENT

The authors gratefully acknowledge Debra Cherry, PhD, for her contribution to the section titled Behavioral Disturbances in Dementia.

KEY REFERENCES AND WEBSITES

A full list of references for this chapter can be found at http://thepoint.lww.com/AT10e. Below are the key references and websites for this chapter, with the corresponding reference number in this chapter found in parentheses after the reference.

Key References

Alzheimer's Disease Facts and Figures 2011. Chicago, IL: Alzheimer's Association; 2011. (2)

California Workgroup on Guidelines for Alzheimer's Disease Management. *Guideline for Alzheimer's Disease Management: Final Report*: State of California, Department of Public Health; April 2008. (38)

Gray KF. Managing agitation and difficult behavior in dementia. *Clin Geriatr Med*. 2004;20:69. (97)

Mace NL, Rabins PW. *The 36-Hour Day: A Family Guide to Caring for People with Alzheimer Disease, Other Dementias, and Memory Loss in Later Life*. 4th ed. Baltimore, MD: Johns Hopkins University Press; 2006. (115)

Mattson MP. Pathways towards and away from Alzheimer's disease. *Nature*. 2004;430:631. (25)

McKhann G et al. The diagnosis of dementia due to Alzheimer's disease: recommendations from the National Institute on Aging–Alzheimer's Association workgroups on diagnostic guidelines for Alzheimer's disease. *Alzheimers Dement*. 2011;7:263. (33)

Schneider LS et al. Effectiveness of atypical antipsychotic drugs in patients with Alzheimer's disease. *N Engl J Med*. 2006;355:1525. (102)

Teri L et al. Nonpharmacologic treatment of behavioral disturbance in dementia. *Med Clin North Am*. 2002;86:641. (93)

Key Websites

Alzheimer's Association. http://www.alz.org.

California Association of Area Agencies on Aging. http://www.c4aging.org.

Family Caregiver Alliance. http://www.caregiver.org.

MedicAlert + Alzheimer's Association Safe Return. http://www.alz.org/safetycenter/we_can_help_safety_medicalert_safereturn.asp.

National Institute on Aging. Alzheimer's Disease Education and Referral Center (ADEAR). http://www.niapublications.org/adear.

104

Geriatric Urologic Disorders

Michael R. Brodeur

CORE PRINCIPLES

CORE PRINCIPLES	CHAPTER CASES
URINARY INCONTINENCE	
1 Urinary incontinence is a common condition in older adults and can be classified as acute or persistent. Persistent incontinence can further be classified as urge, stress, overflow, or functional.	**Case 104-1 (Questions 1, 2)**
2 Urge incontinence is managed with nonpharmacologic interventions, such as a toileting schedule, and the use of anticholinergic medications.	**Case 104-1 (Questions 3, 4)**
3 Stress incontinence is managed with local estrogens, tricyclic antidepressants, and duloxetine.	**Case 104-2 (Questions 1, 2)**
BENIGN PROSTATIC HYPERPLASIA	
1 Benign prostatic hyperplasia (BPH) is the most common urologic condition in aging men. A wide range of signs and symptoms occurs in BPH that causes patients to seek care.	**Case 104-3 (Questions 1–3)**
2 Management of BPH includes the use of α_{1A}-adrenergic receptor antagonists and 5α-reductase inhibitors, either alone or in combination. Nonpharmacologic treatment and surgery may also be considered for some patients. In general, the use of over-the-counter medications should not be used to treat symptomatic BPH.	**Case 104-3 (Questions 4–7)**
ERECTILE DYSFUNCTION	
1 Erectile dysfunction (ED) is a condition that can be a result of neurogenic, hormonal, or vascular disorders. It is therefore essential that a complete urologic workup is conducted to assess the underlying pathophysiology. Underlying conditions should be addressed and treated before symptomatic therapy is initiated.	**Case 104-4 (Questions 1–6)**
2 Treatment for ED consists of a variety of pharmacologic agents, which include phosphodiesterase inhibitors, intracavernous injections, and alprostadil.	**Case 104-4 (Questions 7–14)**

URINARY INCONTINENCE

Neurophysiologic Considerations

The bladder can be thought of as a "balloon" with a narrow outlet, wrapped with a muscular layer, the detrusor muscle. The detrusor and the bladder outlet functions are coordinated neurologically to allow for storage and expulsion of urine.[1] The detrusor muscle is innervated by the parasympathetic nervous system, and the bladder neck is innervated by the sympathetic nervous system (α-adrenergic) (Fig. 104-1). The proximal smooth muscle (internal) sphincter in the bladder neck also is innervated through the sympathetic nervous system (α-adrenergic). The distal striated muscle (external) sphincter of the urethra is supplied by the somatic nervous system.

Urine storage is the result of detrusor muscle relaxation and closure of both the internal and external sphincters. Detrusor relaxation is accomplished by central nervous system (CNS) inhibition of the parasympathetic tone; sphincter closure is mediated by a reflex increase in α-adrenergic and somatic activity. Voiding occurs when detrusor contraction is coordinated with sphincter relaxation. Detrusor contraction is mediated by the parasympathetic nervous system, and relaxation requires inhibition of somatic and sympathetic nerve impulses to the outlet. The

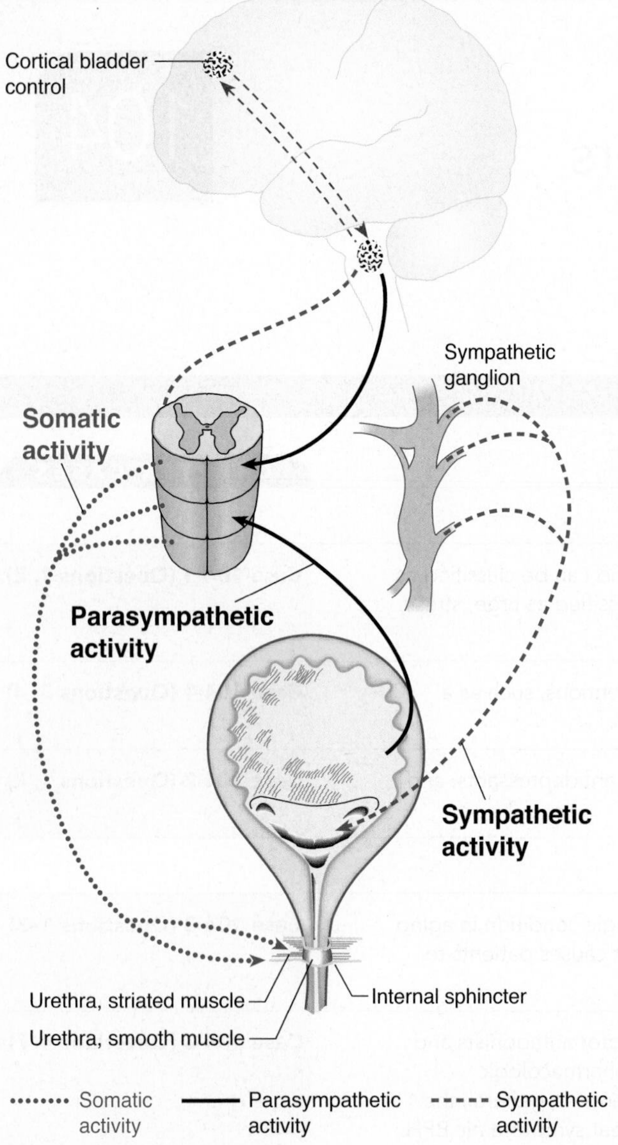

FIGURE 104-1 Neurologic bladder control. Three major components are involved in urine storage and release. (1) Central nervous system: Inhibition from the frontal lobe (cortical) micturition center permits bladder relaxation and filling, and sphincter closure to prevent leakage of urine. When cortical inhibition ceases (i.e., the patient wants to urinate), the brainstem (pontine) micturition center sends impulses down the spinal cord to the detrusor muscle, resulting in muscle contraction. (2) Bladder: Increase in bladder volume stimulates proprioception receptors in the bladder wall, and sensory impulses are transmitted through the sacral nerves (S2–S4 roots) to trigger bladder contraction. This stimulus for bladder contraction is under inhibitory control by the central nervous system frontal lobe as described previously. Cholinergic stimulation results in bladder contraction. (3) Bladder outlet: The two major factors in maintaining urethral pressure are the internal and external sphincters. Internal sphincter: α-Adrenergic stimulation causes muscle contraction, preventing flow of urine. External sphincter: It consists of striated muscle under voluntary control. Contraction prevents flow of urine. Estrogen deficiency in women can result in decreased competence of the internal and external sphincters. (Source: Ferri FF, Fretwell MD. *Practical Guide to the Care of the Geriatric Patient.* 2nd ed. St. Louis, MO: CV Mosby; 1992; Andersson KE, Wein AJ. Pharmacology of the lower urinary tract: basis for current and future treatments of urinary incontinence. *Pharmacol Rev.* 2004;56:581.)

bladder capacity is ~300 mL in the elderly and ~400 mL in young adults. The relationship between the detrusor and the outlet is coordinated by a micturition center located in the CNS, perhaps in the pons.[2] The cortex and diencephalon also permit inhibition of what would otherwise be a reflex contraction of the detrusor muscle in response to bladder distension.

Age-Related Changes

Aging affects the lower urinary tract in several ways (Table 104-1), including both structural and functional changes. Bladder capacity, the ability to postpone voiding, urethral and bladder compliance, maximal urethral closure pressure (the maximal difference between the urethral and the intravesical pressure), and urinary flow rate all are reduced with normal aging.[2,3] For women, these changes are correlated with the postmenopausal decline of estrogen production. Estrogen has trophic effects on the epithelium and on tissues lining and surrounding the urethra, bladder outlet, and vagina. Atrophy of these tissues can result in friability, inflammation, susceptibility to infection, diminished periurethral blood flow, and prolapse of pelvic structures. All of these effects can precipitate symptoms of urinary incontinence. For men, the age-related changes in the prostate gland are responsible for many of the changes in urination. The most common age-related change, in both women and men, is involuntary bladder contractions (detrusor motor instability). These involuntary bladder contractions occur in up to 20% of asymptomatic, neurologically normal, continent elderly patients.[4–7]

In many elderly persons, nocturia is a common complaint and may stem from age-related increases in nocturnal urine production.[8] Each of these changes predisposes people to incontinence, but none alone precipitates it. This predisposition to incontinence, together with the increased likelihood that an older person will be subjected to additional pathologic, physiologic, or pharmacologic insults, underlies the higher incidence of incontinence in the elderly. The onset or exacerbation of incontinence in an older person is likely to be caused by a precipitating factor outside the lower urinary tract.[9] Correspondingly, reversal of the precipitating factor may be sufficient to restore continence without correction of the underlying urologic abnormality.

Urinary incontinence, both acute and chronic, is a common disorder among elderly individuals, affecting approximately 50% of the institutionalized elderly and 30% to 61% of older women and 3% to 23% of older men living in the community.[10] Neurologic impairment, immobility, female sex, and history of hysterectomy are independent risk factors for incontinence. Incontinence has economic costs, and medical (e.g., cystitis, urosepsis, pressure sores, perineal rashes, falls) and psychosocial (e.g., embarrassment, isolation, depression, predisposition to institutionalization) consequences. Nevertheless, incontinence often is a neglected condition. Patients may not report incontinence to their primary-care providers because of embarrassment or misconception regarding treatment. Incontinence is not an inevitable consequence of aging. It is a pathologic condition that, when

TABLE 104-1
Age-Related Changes in Urologic Function

↓ Bladder capacity
↑ Residual urine
↑ Uninhibited bladder contractions
↑ Nocturnal sodium and fluid excretion
↓ Urethral resistance in women
↑ Urethral resistance in men
Weakness of pelvic floor muscles in women

TABLE 104-2
Causes of Incontinence

Resnick's Mnemonic: DIAPPERS	
D	Delirium and dementia
I	Infections
A	Atrophic vaginitis, atrophic urethritis, atonic bladder
P	Psychological causes, depression
P	Pharmacologic agents
E	Endocrine (diabetes, hypercalcemia, hypothyroidism)
R	Restricted mobility
S	Stool impaction

Source: Ouslander JG, Bruskewitz R. Disorders of micturition in the aging patient. *Adv Intern Med.* 1989;34:165; Ouslander JG. Management of overactive bladder. *N Engl J Med.* 2004;350:786; Ouslander JG. Urinary incontinence. In: Osterweil D et al, eds. *Comprehensive Geriatric Assessment*. New York, NY: McGraw-Hill; 2000:555.

rationally approached, usually can be ameliorated or cured, often without invasive tests or surgery and almost invariably without an indwelling catheter (Table 104-2).[11,12]

Classification

Urinary incontinence can be classified several different ways. The two most basic types of urinary incontinence are (a) *acute* (or *transient*) and *reversible* and (b) *chronic* and *persistent*. Persistent urinary incontinence (PUI), which refers to incontinence that is not acute and occurs for a long time, can be classified further into four subgroups: (a) urge, (b) stress, (c) overflow, and (d) functional.

ACUTE INCONTINENCE

Urinary incontinence that is of relatively recent onset or associated with an acute medical problem should prompt a review for reversible factors. These include the following: (a) cystitis, atrophic vaginitis, and urethritis; (b) heart failure; (c) polyuria from diabetes; (d) delirium and acute confusional states; (e) immobility; and (f) medication side effects (discussed subsequently). The management of acute forms of urinary incontinence depends on the identification and elimination of the reversible factor.

For women with urethritis and atrophic vaginitis with irritative voiding symptoms, estrogen replacement can be very helpful. An intravaginal estrogen cream is administered nightly for 7 days, followed by at least once-a-week application.[13] In keeping with the Women's Health Initiative trial, serious risks, including breast cancer and cardiovascular disease, appear to outweigh long-term benefits of systemic combination of hormone therapy. Therefore, topical therapy is preferred.[14]

DRUG-INDUCED URINARY INCONTINENCE

Several medications are associated with acute-onset urinary incontinence, including diuretics, α-adrenergic agonists (e.g., pseudoephedrine), α-adrenergic antagonists (e.g., terazosin), anticholinergics, and neuroleptics.

Reports of female stress incontinence from α_1-adrenergic receptor antagonists, which have a relaxant effect on urethral smooth muscle, have appeared in the medical literature.[15–17] In one study, the incidence of genuine stress incontinence was significantly higher in women taking prazosin (86.2%) than in the group without prazosin (65.7%; $p < 0.01$). In 55% of the women contacted in the prazosin group, urinary incontinence was reduced or cured by prazosin withdrawal.[18] There was a significant increase in functional urethral length, maximal urethral closure pressure, and abdominal pressure transmission to the urethra after prazosin withdrawal. In one case report, switching from doxazosin to enalapril briefly reduced the female patient's stress incontinence; however, she experienced a persistent dry cough (from the enalapril) that continued to cause episodic stress incontinence. Her cough and stress incontinence resolved when she was switched to amlodipine.[19]

PERSISTENT URINARY INCONTINENCE

URGE INCONTINENCE

Urge incontinence, the most common form of incontinence affecting the elderly, occurs when involuntary voiding is preceded by a warning of a few seconds to a few minutes. Urge PUI is characterized by precipitous urine leakage, most often after the urge to void is perceived. Urge PUI can be caused by a variety of genitourinary and neurologic disorders. It most often, but not always, is associated with detrusor motor instability (involuntary contraction of the bladder) or detrusor hyperreflexia (detrusor motor instability caused by a neurologic disorder). The most common causes are local genitourinary conditions, such as cystitis, urethritis, tumors, stones, bladder diverticula, and outflow obstruction. Neurologic disorders, such as stroke, dementia, parkinsonism, and spinal cord injury, can be associated with urge PUI.[9] Overactive bladder is a medical syndrome defined by symptoms of urgency, with or without urge urinary incontinence, usually with frequency and nocturia. By definition, overactive bladder is a syndrome and not a diagnosis.

STRESS INCONTINENCE

Stress incontinence, the involuntary leakage that occurs when an abrupt increase in intra-abdominal pressure ("stress," e.g., coughing, sneezing, laughing, lifting) overcomes urethral resistance. Stress incontinence is common in elderly women but uncommon in men (unless the sphincter has been damaged during a transurethral resection of the prostate (TURP) or a prostatectomy). Typical stress PUI is characterized by daytime loss of small to moderate amounts of urine, infrequent nocturnal incontinence, and a low postvoid residual volume in the absence of a large cystocele. Stress incontinence can be diagnosed by the "tissue test" in which a tissue is placed just below the urethra and the patient is asked to cough, resulting in the loss of a small amount of urine. The usual cause of stress PUI is urethral hypermobility owing to weakness and laxity of pelvic floor musculature, but other conditions, such as sphincter incompetence, urethral instability, or stress-induced detrusor instability, occasionally are responsible.[2] Obesity or TURP in men also can predispose individuals to stress incontinence. Many factors have been suggested to contribute to the development of urinary stress incontinence in women, including estrogen deficiency and a genetic defect in the connective tissue in such patients. The prevalence of urinary stress incontinence among first-degree relatives of patients with urinary incontinence is three times ($p < 0.005$) that of matched control groups of women without micturition disorders.[20]

OVERFLOW INCONTINENCE

Overflow incontinence occurs when the weight of urine in a distended bladder overcomes outlet resistance. Leakage of small amounts of urine is common throughout the day and night. The patient may complain of hesitancy, diminished and interrupted flow, a need to strain to void, and a sense of incomplete emptying. The bladder usually is palpable, and the residual urine volume is large. If the cause is neurologically mediated, control of the perianal sphincter may be impaired.[21]

Overflow incontinence results from an anatomic outlet obstruction or an acontractile (or atonic) bladder.[9] Common causes are benign prostatic hyperplasia (BPH), urethral stricture, bladder-sphincter dyssynergia, diabetic neuropathy, fecal impaction, and anticholinergic medication use.

FUNCTIONAL INCONTINENCE

Functional incontinence occurs when a continent individual is unable or unwilling to reach the toilet to urinate. Common causes are musculoskeletal disorders, muscle weakness, impaired mental status, use of physical restraints, psychological impairment, environmental barriers, and medications (e.g., sedatives, neuroleptics).

Clinical Presentation and Evaluation

CASE 104-1

QUESTION 1: H.K., an 83-year-old female resident of a nursing facility with moderate dementia, had urinary incontinence 3 years before admission. She has been managed with adult diapers (briefs) and bladder training. What objective and subjective data are needed to determine the pathophysiology (and hence the classification) of H.K.'s urinary incontinence?

The rationale for the clinical evaluation of H.K. is to classify the imbalance between bladder pressure and bladder sphincter resistance and, as a result, institute appropriate medical or surgical management of her urinary incontinence.

Documentation of H.K.'s urinary incontinence is accomplished most easily by keeping an incontinence record. Observations should be recorded every 2 hours regarding whether she is wet or dry, as well as associated symptoms or circumstances. A record maintained for 3 to 4 days will facilitate assessment of the voiding pattern. Knowledge of the voiding pattern can be used to design bladder training programs and to detect iatrogenic causes (e.g., diuretic ingestion, use of restraints). Successful bladder training relies on estimating when the bladder is full.

Physical examination, including a neurologic assessment, of H.K. is needed to determine the cause and classification of her urinary incontinence. Clinical findings may identify specific pathophysiologic abnormalities. H.K. should have a thorough pelvic examination to determine the contribution of atrophic vaginitis, uterine prolapse, and bladder anatomy. Funneling of the bladder neck suggests stress incontinence, and palpation of the bladder suggests overflow incontinence. The presence of physical restraints or musculoskeletal disability would suggest functional incontinence.

H.K.'s bladder should be catheterized immediately after urination to determine residual urine volume. Alternatively, if a bladder ultrasound is available, the volume can be measured noninvasively. Volumes in excess of 50 mL are abnormal and may indicate obstruction or an adynamic detrusor muscle. Although urodynamic studies are widely recommended and used, little evidence suggests that these produce clinically useful data for institutionalized geriatric patients. A urinalysis, blood chemistries, renal function, and postprandial glucose tests should be performed. An abnormal urinalysis may suggest pathology (e.g., infection) that can be managed medically. Urinary tract infection is common in the incontinent patient.

Treatment options exist for each type of urinary incontinence (Table 104-3). Proper evaluation should guide the clinician in choosing the optimal course of drug therapy. Drug therapy should be based on sound principles of neurophysiology, urology, and pharmacology. Drug therapy is directed at decreasing bladder contractility (detrusor instability) or increasing bladder outlet resistance (bladder neck and proximal urethra).

TABLE 104-3
Drug Therapy of Persistent Urinary Incontinence

Type	Treatment With Initial Doses
Urge	Oxybutynin 2.5 mg every day to TID; 5–30 mg XL
	Oxybutynin transdermal patch 1 patch 2×/wk
	Oxybutynin 10% topical gel 1 g every day
	Tolterodine 1–2 mg every day; 2–4 LA every day
	Trospium 20 mg BID; 60 mg ER every day
	Darifenacin 7.5 mg every day
	Solifenacin 5 mg every day
	Fesoterodine 4 mg every day
Stress	Pseudoephedrine 15–30 mg BID–TID
	Imipramine 25 mg every day
	Vaginal estrogen cream 0.5–1.0 g two to three times/wk
	Duloxetine 40–80 mg every day or BID
Overflow	Terazosin 1–5 mg every day (usually at bedtime)
	Doxazosin 1–8 mg every day
	Tamsulosin 0.4–0.8 mg every day
	Alfuzosin 10 mg every day
	Silodosin 4–8 mg every day
	Bethanechol 10 mg TID
Functional	None

BID, twice daily; LA, long acting; TID, three times daily; XL, extended release.

CASE 104-1, QUESTION 2: The incontinence record maintained by the nursing staff indicates that H.K. has urinary urges quite frequently, resulting in urine leakage. Throughout the day and night, H.K. urinates four to five times. Physical examination reveals atrophic vaginitis, no funneling of the bladder neck, and no bladder distension. H.K. does have a history of stroke. The urinalysis is normal, as are the blood chemistries. Postvoiding bladder scan revealed a residual urine volume of 30 mL. What is the pathophysiology and classification of H.K.'s incontinence?

Most neuropathic disease processes can change bladder function. As illustrated by H.K., a cerebrovascular accident is commonly associated with bladder dysfunction and incontinence in the elderly. Neurologic injury above the level of the micturition center in the spinal cord, in most cases, results in bladder spasticity. Sacral reflexes are intact, but loss of inhibition from higher CNS centers results in spastic bladder and inappropriate sphincter behavior. The degree of spasticity varies between the bladder and sphincter, as well as from patient to patient with the same CNS lesions. H.K. has a spastic detrusor muscle resulting from an unchecked sacral reflex. H.K.'s bladder dysfunction is classified as urge urinary incontinence of the persistent type.

Nonpharmacologic Therapy

A number of nonpharmacologic options are available that may help improve the symptoms of PUI. The first step is to educate patients about bladder function, appropriate fluid intake, and avoidance of caffeine and other bladder irritants. The patient can then keep a bladder diary in which they record their fluid intake, voiding pattern, and incontinence episodes. Bladder training refers to scheduled voiding, urge-suppression techniques, and pelvic muscle exercises. Scheduled voiding can be used in both cognitively intact and impaired individuals. The patient is instructed to void on a schedule (e.g., every 2 hours), thereby minimizing the volume of urine in the bladder and making incontinence episodes less likely. The same principle can be used in cognitively impaired patients by prompting them to toilet.

Urge-suppression techniques can be used to retrain the bladder; the scheduled toiletings are adjusted for longer or shorter times, depending on the patient's voiding pattern. The goal is to achieve an interval during which the patient is continent and does not need to void. In most patients, this is approximately 2 hours. Pelvic floor muscle exercises, also known as Kegel exercises, work by increasing the strength and tone of the pelvic floor muscles. In randomized trials, incontinence episodes were reduced by 54% to 75% compared with 6% to 16% with no treatment.[22] The patient should receive adequate instruction on how to identify the pelvic floor muscles and then practice these exercises three times a day.

CASE 104-1, QUESTION 3: What nonpharmacologic therapy should be recommended for H.K.?

H.K. should have a comprehensive review of her medications completed to determine any temporal relationship between medications and incontinence episodes. She should then be placed on a toileting schedule in which she is prompted to void every 2 hours. The nursing staff should continue to keep a bladder diary in which they record fluid intake and when she is wet and dry. This information can be used to tailor her toileting schedule to make sure H.K. has the best outcome while at the same time being practical, based on staffing at the institution. Because of H.K.'s moderate dementia, the teaching of pelvic floor muscle exercises may not be feasible.

Drug Therapy

ANTICHOLINERGIC AGENTS

CASE 104-1, QUESTION 4: What drug therapy should be prescribed for H.K.?

H.K. has detrusor instability that may respond to anticholinergic drug therapy if nonpharmacologic measures do not produce desired results. The major neurohormonal stimulus for physiologic bladder muscle contraction is acetylcholine-induced stimulation of postganglionic parasympathetic cholinergic receptor sites on bladder smooth muscle. Atropine and atropinelike substances depress true involuntary bladder contractions of any etiology by the interaction at the muscarinic receptor.[23] Of the five known muscarinic subtypes (M_1 through M_5), M_3 appears to be the most clinically relevant in the human bladder. M_2 muscarinic receptors are the predominant subtype (comprising about 80% of all muscarinic receptors); however, contraction of smooth muscle, including muscles in the urinary bladder, is mediated mainly by M_3 receptors. M_3 receptors are also involved in contraction of the gastrointestinal smooth muscle, saliva production, and iris sphincter function.[24] Inhibition of the muscarinic receptors in the urinary bladder results in decreased urinary bladder contraction, increased residual urine volume, and decreased detrusor muscle pressure.

OXYBUTYNIN CHLORIDE

Oxybutynin is available as an oral immediate-release tablet, an extended-release tablet, a transdermal system, and a topical gel. Oxybutynin is commonly used to produce an anticholinergic effect in the lower urinary tract. Oxybutynin has been described as a strong independent smooth muscle relaxant with local anesthetic activity and anticholinergic effects.[23,25] This agent has been used successfully to depress uninhibited detrusor contractions in patients with and without neurogenic bladder dysfunction. Oxybutynin improves total bladder capacity, neuropathic voiding dysfunction, and bladder filling pressure.[26,27] The oral dosage of oxybutynin chloride suggested for the elderly is 2.5 mg up to three times a day; in some cases, the dosage may need to be increased to 5 mg three times a day. Because oxybutynin is a tertiary-amine anticholinergic compound and also blocks central M_1 receptors, the potential for CNS toxicity increases as the dose is increased. Compared with oral propantheline bromide 15 mg three times a day, a full dose of oral oxybutynin (5 mg three times a day) in one study produced a good response more frequently.[28] Once-daily, controlled-release oxybutynin at doses of 5 to 30 mg reduced the number of incontinence episodes.[29,30] Maximal benefit was demonstrated by maintenance week 4 and was sustained as long as the patient continued therapy.[31]

The transdermal system contains 36 mg of active drug and delivers 3.9 mg of oxybutynin per day when dosed twice a week.[32] The transdermal system should be protected from moisture and humidity. Common side effects from the transdermal system at the application site are pruritus (14%) and redness (8.3%). A comparison study of immediate-release oxybutynin and the transdermal system indicated that patients using the transdermal system experienced fewer side effects. Dry mouth was reported in 38% of the oxybutynin transdermal system users in contrast to 94% of those who used immediate-release tablets.[33] Oxybutynin is also available as a 10% topical gel in 1-g unit dose sachets. One sachet is applied per day to the abdomen, thigh, upper arm, or shoulder. Application site reactions were reported in 5.4% of patients, and dry mouth was reported in 6.9% of patients.[34]

TOLTERODINE TARTRATE

Tolterodine is a competitive muscarinic receptor antagonist (anticholinergic) that is relatively selective for M_2 and M_3 receptors. It is indicated for the treatment of overactive bladder symptoms of urinary frequency or urge incontinence. At doses of 1 to 2 mg twice a day, compared with a placebo, the number of urinary voids per 24 hours decreased ($p = 0.0045$), the volume of urine per void increased ($p < 0.001$), and the mean number of incontinence episodes decreased by 50% ($p < 0.19$).[35] No clinical or electrocardiographic evidence was seen of significant cardiac adverse events in the group studied. Tolterodine has greater selectivity for the bladder than the salivary glands in vivo, which is not attributable to muscarinic receptor subtype selectivity.[36] Thus, tolterodine is much less potent in inhibiting salivation, suggesting that it may have less propensity to cause dry mouth in clinical use. The onset of pharmacologic action of tolterodine is less than 1 hour, and therapeutic efficacy is maintained during long-term treatment. In comparative trials, tolterodine and oxybutynin are equivalent in terms of efficacy, but tolterodine is better tolerated.

Despite short terminal half-lives of 2 to 3 hours and 3 to 4 hours for tolterodine and its active 5-hydroxy metabolite, respectively, twice-daily dosing is effective because of the drug's long pharmacodynamic effects.[37] Dosage adjustment is recommended in the presence of hepatic impairment and during concurrent therapy with drugs that inhibit cytochrome P-450 (CYP) 2D6 and CYP3A4 isozymes. The usual dose for the elderly is 1 to 2 mg twice daily of the immediate-release or 2 to 4 mg daily of the extended-release formulation.

FESOTERODINE

Fesoterodine is an antimuscarinic prodrug that is converted into the active metabolite 5-hydroxymethyl tolterodine, which is the same active metabolite as that of tolterodine. The efficacy and safety of fesoterodine appear comparable to that of tolterodine.[38] The recommended starting dosage of fesoterodine is 4 mg once daily. The dose may be increased to 8 mg in patients with an insufficient response. Patients with severe renal impairment (creatinine clearance <30 mL/minute) or those taking a strong CYP3A4 inhibitor should not take more than 4 mg per day.

Stromal hyperplasia in the prostate periurethral glands is one of the earliest microscopic findings in men with BPH.[64] As men increase in age, testosterone serum concentrations decrease and the peripheral conversion of testosterone to estrogen increases. At one time, estrogens were thought to initiate stromal hyperplasia, which in turn induces epithelial hyperplasia. It is now known, however, that estrogens do not have a direct effect on the development of BPH and prostatic carcinoma, but progesterone does play a role in their pathogenesis. Progesterone receptors have been shown to exist in prostate stromal cells, whereas estrogen receptors were essentially nonexistent.[70]

Pathophysiology and Clinical Presentation

CASE 104-3

QUESTION 1: G.M., a 72-year-old man, presents to the emergency department with severe lower abdominal discomfort of 4 days' duration. His history consists of having increasing difficulty initiating urination, a significant decrease in the force of his urinary stream, occasional midstream stoppage, and postvoid dribbling. Physical examination is unremarkable except for the abdominal and rectal examination. Abdominal examination reveals distension, tenderness, and increased dullness in the hypogastrium with a large mass, believed to be the bladder. On rectal examination, the prostate is found to be severely enlarged, firm, and rubbery without nodules or undue hardness. G.M. gives a history of nocturia (approximately four to five times a night) and daytime urinary frequency (eight to ten times a day). G.M. indicates that when he is able to urinate he has a weak stream and difficulty maintaining flow, and does not feel relieved. Laboratory findings are as follows:

Blood urea nitrogen (BUN), 45 mg/dL
Serum creatinine (SCr), 3.2 mg/dL
Serum prostatic acid phosphatase, 3 units/L
Serum prostate-specific antigen (PSA), 7.1 ng/mL

A urethral catheter was inserted, and 900 mL of urine was obtained. G.M. subsequently was scheduled for a urologic workup. What is the pathophysiologic basis for G.M.'s symptoms?

Symptoms of BPH can be both obstructive and irritative, and descriptions of the symptoms need a frame of reference for standardization. The Boyarsky index, a questionnaire consisting of nine questions to quantify the severity of BPH, has been developed.[71] Five questions are designed to assess obstructive symptoms and four to assess irritative symptoms. Although some limitations to the use of this questionnaire (Table 104-4) may exist, it is one of the most common measures used to quantify symptoms in BPH studies, and it correlates well with the pathophysiology of BPH.[64] The format of the Boyarsky index is designed to help the clinician educate the patient about the obstructive and irritative symptoms of BPH. The Boyarsky index was the first of three patient questionnaires developed to quantitatively assess BPH and the effectiveness of individual treatment.[68] As such, this questionnaire has been used in numerous clinical trials to measure the outcome of interventions. The Boyarsky index is not useful in comparing different treatment therapies among BPH patients because it has not been sufficiently validated for this purpose; rather, it is useful in evaluating an individual's response to therapy.

The Multidisciplinary Measurements Committee of the American Urologic Association (AUA) also has published a urinary symptom index for prostatism (Table 104-5).[72] The index is useful to assess the baseline severity of prostatism, disease progression, and effectiveness of different therapies. The AUA symptom index allows comparison among therapies and is the preferred questionnaire for BPH research. It has been validated through internal consistency reliability, constructive reliability,

TABLE 104-4
Benign Prostatic Hyperplasia Symptom Scoring System (Boyarsky Index)[a]

Nocturia	
0	Absence of symptoms
1	Urinates 1 time/night
2	Urinates 2–3 times/night
3	Urinates ≥4 times/night
Daytime Frequency	
0	Urinates 1–4 times/d
1	Urinates 5–7 times/d
2	Urinates 8–12 times/d
3	Urinates ≥13 times/d
Hesitance (lasts ≥1 minute)	
0	Occasional (≤20% of the time)
1	Moderate (20%–50% of the time)
2	Frequent (≥50% of the time)
3	Always present
Intermittency (lasts ≥1 minute)	
0	Occasional (≤20% of the time)
1	Moderate (20%–50% of the time)
2	Frequent (≥50% of the time)
3	Always present
Terminal Dribbling (at end of voiding)	
0	Occasional (≤20% of the time)
1	Moderate (20%–50% of the time)
2	Frequent (≥50% of the time)
3	Always present (may wet clothes)
Urgency	
0	Absence
1	Occasionally difficult to postpone urination
2	Frequently difficult to postpone urination
3	Always difficult to postpone urination
Impairment of Size and Force of Urinary Stream	
0	Absence
1	Impaired trajectory
2	Most of the time size and force are restricted
3	Urinates with great effort and stream is interrupted
Dysuria	
0	Absence
1	Occasional burning sensation during urination
2	Frequent (>50% of the time) burning sensation
3	Frequent and painful burning sensation during urination
Sensation of Incomplete Voiding	
0	Absence
1	Occasional sensation
2	Frequent (>50% of the time) sensation
3	Constant and urgent sensation, no relief on voiding

[a] Symptom scoring provides the clinician with a tool to measure the relative need for, and efficacy of, different interventions. No specific score is associated with the need for a specific intervention. A low symptom score in the absence of significant urine retention generally indicates that medical management can be attempted before considering surgical intervention.

TABLE 104-5
American Urological Association Urinary Symptom Index for Prostatism

Symptom	Score: Not at All	< 1 in 5 Times	< 1/2 the Time	=1/2 Time	> 1/2 the Time	Almost Always
1. Over the past month or so, how often have you had a sensation of not emptying your bladder completely after you finished urinating?	0	1	2	3	4	5
2. Over the past month or so, how often have you had to urinate again less than 2 hours after you finished urinating?	0	1	2	3	4	5
3. Over the past month or so, how often have you found you stopped and started several times when you urinated?	0	1	2	3	4	5
4. Over the past month or so, how often have you found it difficult to postpone urination?	0	1	2	3	4	5
5. Over the past month or so, how often have you had a weak urinary stream?	0	1	2	3	4	5
6. Over the past month or so, how often have you had to push or strain to begin urination?	0	1	2	3	4	5
7. Over the past month or so, how many times did you most times typically get up to urinate from the time you went to bed at night until the time you got up in the morning?	0 times	1 time	2 times	3 times	4 times	5 times
Interpretation of AUA Symptom Index						
AUA Symptom Score = Sum of questions 1–7 = ___________________						
Mild prostatism ≤7 Moderate prostatism 8–18 Severe prostatism >18 Highest possible score 35						

AUA, American Urological Association.
Reprinted with permission from Longe RL, Calvert JC. *Physical Assessment: A Guide for Evaluating Drug Therapy*. Vancouver, WA: Applied Therapeutics 1994.

test-retest reliability, and criterion reliability.[68] The AUA index, however, may not be BPH specific.[73] When 101 men and 96 women between the ages of 55 and 79 used the AUA index, urinary symptoms and severity of urinary symptoms were similar in both groups. Therefore, symptoms associated with prostatism can be associated with aging as well as BPH. The National Institutes of Health convened a chronic prostatitis workshop to come to consensus on a new classification system for the diagnosis and management of prostatitis.[74] This group developed a symptom index that provides a valid outcome measure for men with prostatitis. This index attempts to quantify the pain and discomfort associated with prostatism, and should help differentiate prostatism from prostatic hyperplasia. The symptom index is self-administered.

G.M. presents with obstructive symptoms consistent with BPH as follows: (a) a history of difficulty in initiating urination (hesitancy), (b) a decrease in urinary force, (c) occasional midstream stoppage, (d) postvoiding dribbling, and (e) a feeling of incomplete bladder emptying. The common obstructive symptom of decreased force and size of urine stream is caused by urethral compression from prostate gland hyperplasia. Hesitancy, another obstructive symptom, is the result of the bladder detrusor muscle taking a longer time to generate the initial increased pressure to overcome urethral resistance. Urinary stream intermittency is caused by the inability of the bladder detrusor muscle to sustain the increased pressure until the end of voiding. Terminal dribbling and incomplete emptying occur for the same reason, but also may be caused by obstructive prostatic tissue at the bladder neck, causing a "ball-valve" effect.

G.M. also has a history of classic irritative symptoms that are consistent with BPH as follows: (a) nocturia approximately four to five times a night and (b) daytime urinary frequency of eight to ten times a day. Incomplete emptying of the bladder results in shorter intervals between voiding, explaining the complaint of frequency. Also, a large prostate gland provokes the bladder to trigger a voiding response more frequently. This response is more pronounced if the prostate is growing intravesically and compromising the bladder volume. The bladder detrusor muscle becomes hypertrophied as a result of the greater bladder residual urine volume, which can result in increased detrusor muscle excitability. Clinically, this excitability may result in bladder instability. The symptoms of urinary frequency are more pronounced at night because cortical inhibitions are lessened and bladder sphincter tone is more relaxed during sleep. Obstructive symptoms are associated more with an enlarged prostate, and the predominance of irritative symptoms could suggest voiding dysfunctions in addition to those of BPH.

Urinary incontinence is not a common symptom of BPH. With advanced BPH, a large residual volume of urine in the bladder weakens the bladder sphincter and allows the escape of small amounts of urine when the bladder is full. As the residual bladder volume increases, the ureters will dilate, resulting in stasis of urine in the ureters. The end result may be ascending hydronephrosis caused by the transmission of high pressure to nephrons, which produces renal damage (Fig. 104-2). This can account for abdominal discomfort and flank pain during voiding and ascending urinary tract infections.

Acute urinary retention in BPH can occur as a result of increasing size of the prostate gland. Independent of gland size, drugs may precipitate acute urinary retention. Drugs, such as alcohol, anticholinergic agents, α-adrenergic agents, and neuroleptics, all have been associated with acute urinary retention in men with BPH. Commonly, when advanced BPH is present, acute urinary retention is exacerbated if the patient does not void at the first sign of urgency. G.M. is not taking any drugs commonly associated with urinary retention.

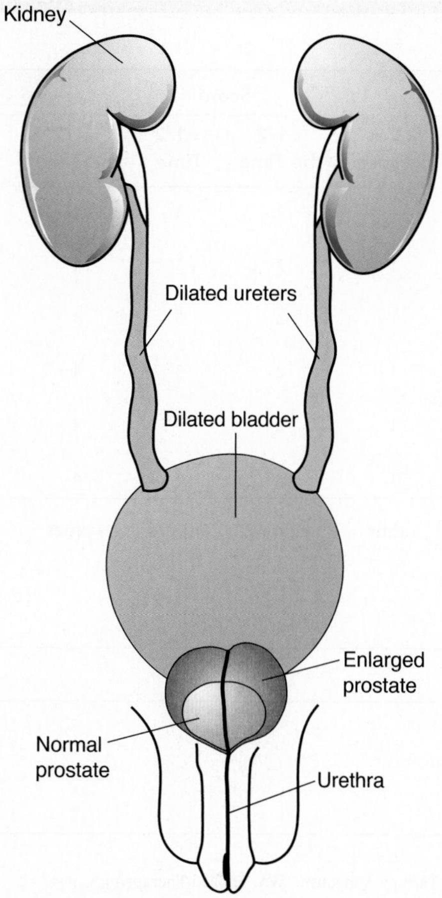

FIGURE 104-2 Flow of urine is interrupted by compression from a prostate that has enlarged from normal size. In this diagram, the ureters and bladder are dilated by backed-up urine.

Clinical Findings

CASE 104-3, QUESTION 2: What objective findings in G.M. are associated with BPH?

G.M. presents with classic symptoms of BPH. The increasingly severe symptoms culminated in an episode of acute urinary retention as evidenced by inability to void and lower abdominal discomfort. Objective symptoms associated with G.M.'s BPH include (a) abdominal tenderness with increased dullness in the hypogastrium; (b) the finding of an enlarged bladder; (c) an enlarged, firm, and rubbery prostate gland; and (d) a return of 900 mL of urine via urinary catheter. The normal serum acid phosphatase, slightly elevated PSA, and digital rectal examination of the prostate suggest that G.M. does not have prostatic carcinoma at this time (see the Prostate-Specific Antigen section later in this chapter). The elevated BUN and SCr may suggest hydronephrosis as a result of his BPH.

CASE 104-3, QUESTION 3: What additional tests should be completed to evaluate G.M.?

URINALYSIS

Because patients with BPH also may have a urinary tract infection, a urinalysis with microscopic examination is essential. It is mandatory that G.M. give a urine specimen for urinalysis before the digital rectal examination of the prostate gland because examination of the prostate causes prostatic secretions to be expelled into the urethra, which may contaminate the urine specimen and make it difficult to determine the source of an infection. The presence of white blood cells and bacteria in the urine necessitates a workup for infection. Similarly, hematuria requires a workup for urinary tract pathology other than BPH. Because BPH also can cause hydronephrosis, renal function, and serum electrolytes should be evaluated.

DIGITAL RECTAL EXAMINATION

A serum PSA followed by a digital rectal examination of the prostate remains a fundamental part of evaluating a man with prostatism. The prostate examination should determine the size, shape, consistency, and nodularity of this gland. Prostatic hyperplasia results in a large, palpable prostate with a smooth mucosal surface rectally. The discernment of the right and left prostate lobes is lost in BPH. The digital rectal examination of a patient with BPH commonly finds asymmetry of the prostate, with one side being larger than the other. Prostatic enlargement can be in both an anteroposterior and a superoinferior direction. As a result, on digital rectal examination, the upper extent of prostate hyperplasia is not palpable. Occasionally, the degree of enlargement felt by digital rectal examination may be misleading because a substantial portion of enlargement may be intravesicular. The consistency of the gland may be soft or firm, depending on the predominance of glandular or fibromuscular elements.[75] The presence of firm-to-hard nodules, irregularities, induration, or a stony, hard prostate suggests possible prostate cancer. In those cases in which the prostate gland size or shape may be questioned, the patient should have a transrectal ultrasound (TRUS) to determine the gland volume.

PROSTATE-SPECIFIC ANTIGEN

PSA is a glycoprotein enzyme (molecular weight, 33,000) that is secreted in the cytoplasm of the prostatic cells; it aids in the liquefaction of semen. Some claim that this enzyme is specific for prostate origin, although a few isolated instances of elevation in nonprostate tumors have been reported. PSA correlates reasonably well, on average, with prostate weight owing to benign prostate glandular hyperplasia.[76] Prostate cancer, however, produces approximately 10 times the amount of PSA on a tissue volume basis than does BPH.[77] Men 50 years of age or older have been encouraged to have an annual measurement of serum PSA and a digital rectal examination as a basic screen for prostate cancer and to monitor the growth of the prostate gland. Several investigators have proposed age-adjusted PSA reference ranges, which reflect the size of the prostate gland (Table 104-6).[78–80] Studies have resulted in several formulas that try to adjust the PSA for the effect of BPH. The best-known formula for predicting the PSA level (PSA serum density) is as follows[81]:

$$\text{PSA (in ng/mL or mcg/mL)} = 0.12 \times \text{gland volume (in mL by TRUS)} \qquad \textit{(Eq. 104-1)}$$

$$\text{TRUS gland volume} = \text{prostate height} \times \text{width} \times \text{length} \times 0.523 \qquad \textit{(Eq. 104-2)}$$

TABLE 104-6
Age-Adjusted Prostate-Specific Antigen Values

Age Range (years)	PSA Upper Limit (ng/mL)	PSA Density
40–49	2.5	0.08
50–59	3.5	0.10
60–69	4.5	0.11
70–79	6.5	0.13

PSA, prostate-specific antigen.

The PSA result for G.M. is slightly above the upper limit for his age. As such, he should have a TRUS to determine the prostate gland volume and, hence, the PSA density. Once the prostate gland volume is determined, the significance of his PSA level of 7.1 ng/mL can be determined.

Drug Therapy

α_1-ADRENERGIC RECEPTOR ANTAGONISTS

CASE 104-3, QUESTION 4: What drug therapy should be prescribed to treat G.M.'s prostatic hyperplasia?

G.M. most likely will be scheduled for a TURP, because he presents with acute urinary retention and hydronephrosis owing to a moderately enlarged prostate gland (i.e., >40 g and <80 g). He should be started and maintained on an α_1-adrenergic receptor antagonist to reduce the tension of the bladder neck, the prostate adenoma, and the prostatic capsule. Similarly, he should receive a 5α-reductase inhibitor to induce atrophy of the prostate gland and halt progression of the disease.

The prostatic capsule and hyperplastic prostate have plentiful α_{1A}-adrenergic receptors. The three known subtypes of the α_1-adrenergic receptor are α_{1A}, α_{1B}, and α_{1D}. Inhibiting the α_{1A}-adrenergic receptors can reduce the smooth muscle tone of the prostatic urethra, thereby reducing the functional component of urethral constriction and obstruction.

TERAZOSIN

Terazosin, a long-acting α_1-adrenergic receptor antagonist, has significantly reduced obstructive symptoms and improved urinary flow rates at doses of 1 to 5 mg/day.[68,82] The α_1-blockade alone does not account for the long-term clinical responses exerted by this drug in the treatment of BPH. Terazosin has been shown to induce prostate smooth muscle cell apoptosis, resulting in reduced urinary symptoms. Terazosin (and doxazosin) has a quinazoline nucleus, which may account for this effect. Tamsulosin, which is not a quinazoline, does not induce prostate smooth muscle cell apoptosis.[83]

In most patients, the dose of terazosin will need to be increased to 5 to 10 mg/day to obtain desired results. Orthostatic hypotension, however, may occur in the beginning days of therapy or during dosage adjustment periods. In patients who, for whatever reason, stop their terazosin therapy for 2 or more days, therapy should be reinstituted cautiously to avoid the "first-dose" adverse effect of syncope.

Terazosin has demonstrated sustained improvement in BPH symptom scores for a 30-month period. Only 10% of the patients experienced treatment failure.[68] In this long-term study, the systolic blood pressure in normotensive and hypertensive patients was decreased by 4 and 18 mm Hg, respectively. Apparently, terazosin typically only lowered the blood pressure significantly in the hypertensive patients.

DOXAZOSIN

Doxazosin, another quinazoline derivative, is a long-acting α_1-adrenergic receptor antagonist structurally related to prazosin and terazosin (Table 104-3). Doxazosin originally was prescribed primarily for hypertension and currently is not considered a first-line antihypertensive agent. (For a discussion of the current use of α-blockers in hypertension, see Chapter 14, Essential Hypertension.) Hypertension and BPH are linked by the sympathetic nervous system. As with terazosin, doxazosin improves urinary flow rates and symptoms in patients with BPH. These effects have been demonstrated in controlled clinical studies, within weeks, and for the long-term. Doxazosin should be started at 1 mg/day. After 1 to 2 weeks, the dose can be increased over several weeks to 8 mg/day. As with other long-acting α_1-adrenergic receptor antagonists, the first dose should be taken at bedtime to minimize lightheadedness and syncope (the first-dose effect), and the blood pressure of the patient should be monitored periodically during therapy. Most patients require between 4 and 8 mg/day for effective control of the urinary symptoms of BPH. Dosages greater than 4 mg/day are associated with a greater frequency of dizziness, orthostatic hypotension, and syncope.[82,84]

TAMSULOSIN

Tamsulosin, a nonquinazoline, is a long-acting selective α_{1A}-adrenergic receptor antagonist similar to doxazosin, terazosin, and prazosin. Tamsulosin and its metabolites are more specific for the prostatic α_{1A}-adrenergic receptors than any of the other α_1-adrenergic receptor antagonists.[85] Apparently, tamsulosin and its metabolites are less specific for the vascular α_{1A}-adrenergic receptors, and therefore cause less orthostatic hypotension than the other agents in the class. Consequently, no need exists to titrate tamsulosin to the recommended daily dose range of 0.4 to 0.8 mg. Coadministration of tamsulosin with antihypertensives does not require dosage adjustment of the antihypertensives. Tamsulosin is very effective in treating bladder outlet obstruction associated with BPH.[86,87]

More than 90% of tamsulosin is absorbed after oral administration of a 0.4-mg dose under fasting conditions. Administration with food decreases the bioavailability by 30% and increases time to peak plasma concentration. Tamsulosin is hepatically metabolized by CYP isozymes, CYP3A4 and CYP2D6.[88] Impaired renal function increases the total tamsulosin plasma concentration by approximately 100% during steady-state administration. Because active, unbound drug levels are not affected, no dose modification is required in renally impaired patients with symptomatic BPH.[89] As with all α_1-adrenergic receptor antagonists, tamsulosin does not affect the PSA and must be taken indefinitely to maintain its therapeutic effect.[90]

ALFUZOSIN

Alfuzosin is another quinazoline α_1-adrenergeric receptor antagonist. It displays a lower rate of hypotensive effects than doxazosin and terazosin. A lack of penetration of alfuzosin into the brain has been hypothesized to contribute to the decreased CNS effects such as somnolence. Unlike tamsulosin, alfuzosin will not cause ejaculatory dysfunction; the incidence is comparable to placebo.[90] Alfuzosin is available as an extended-release tablet that has a recommended daily dose of 10 mg given after the same meal each day.

SILODOSIN

Silodosin is another α_1-adrenergeric receptor antagonist that is selective the for the α_{1A}-receptor in the lower urinary tract. Silodosin has a strong affinity for prostatic tissue and is 20 times more "uroselective" than tamsulosin.[91] Whether this effect has any influence on its therapeutic efficacy remains to be seen until a long-term clinical trial with another selective α-blocker is conducted. The most common side effect with silodosin is retrograde ejaculation, reported in 21% of patients in an open-label extension study.[92] Silodosin is available as 4- and 8-mg capsules, and the recommended dose is 8 mg once daily. In patients with a creatinine clearance of less than 50 mL/minute, the dose should be decreased to 4 mg once daily.

Older α-blockers such as phenoxybenzamine and prazosin are rarely used because of their side effect profile.

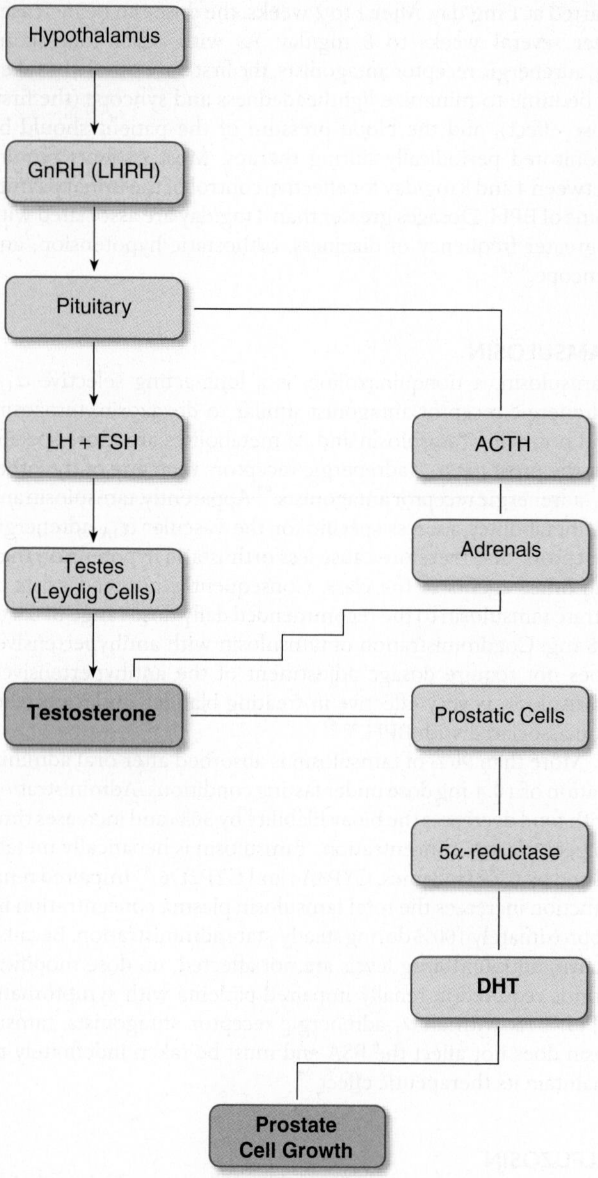

FIGURE 104-3 Pituitary-gonadal axis: endocrine basis for control of benign prostatic hyperplasia. The pituitary-gonadal axis plays an important role in prostatic growth. Neurons in the preoptic area of the hypothalamus secrete gonadotropin-releasing hormone (GnRH), also known as luteinizing hormone-releasing hormone (LHRH). LHRH is a small peptide that interacts with surface receptor sites on the plasma membrane of the pituitary cells. LHRH stimulates the pituitary to release both luteinizing hormone (LH) and follicle-stimulating hormone (FSH). LH secretion causes the Leydig cells of the testicle to produce testosterone. Testosterone appears to inhibit LHRH at the hypothalamic level and LH at the pituitary level. The adrenals only contribute approximately 1% of circulating testosterone. Testosterone diffuses into the prostatic cells, where it is converted to dihydrotestosterone (DHT) by 5α-reductase. DHT binds to steroid receptor complexes in the nucleus of the prostate, which causes cell growth. ACTH, corticotropin. (Reprinted with permission from Berry SJ et al. The development of human benign prostatic hyperplasia with age. *J Urol.* 1984;132:474.)

ANDROGEN SUPPRESSION

Considerable information has accrued concerning the endocrine basis for control of BPH (Fig. 104-3), the effect of age on hormone dynamics in men, and the hormonal changes in the hyperplastic human prostate. Maintenance of morphology and functional activity of the adult human prostate is controlled by, and dependent on, androgens. Prostatic regression after androgen deprivation is an active process that requires the synthesis of macromolecules.[93] As a result of androgen deprivation, the loss of stromal and epithelial prostate cells is disproportionate, with four times greater loss of epithelial cells. Testosterone serves as the prohormone for the two active metabolites, DHT and 17-β-estradiol. Testosterone is metabolized to DHT by the enzyme 5α-reductase (types 1 and 2). Thus, conversion of testosterone to DHT precludes its conversion to estrogen by the aromatase enzyme, and the relative activity of these two enzymes is of paramount importance in prostate homeostasis.[94]

Although the mean plasma testosterone level in men falls after the age of 60, the level of testosterone in subjects with BPH and age-matched control subjects is not different.[95] Moreover, the onset of BPH starts some 10 to 20 years before the plasma testosterone levels decrease. The serum concentration of DHT is increased, however, in men with BPH.[93,96,97] The mechanism responsible for accumulation of DHT has not been established, but a significant increase in 5α-reductase activity occurs, which is known to produce DHT.[98,99]

One other major hormonal change associated with aging is the increased formation of estrogen from circulating androgens in both the testes and the peripheral adipose tissue. Androgen conversion to estrogen via aromatase begins in men at approximately the third decade of life and increases with age,[100] but the plasma estrogen concentration is the same in men with BPH and age-matched control subjects without BPH.[96] Estrogen receptors are abundant in stroma cells,[101,102] more so in patients with prostatic carcinoma than in patients with BPH.[103] Estrogen stimulation of stromal tissue was once believed to explain the prostatic growth that continued with age despite the decline in testosterone secretion by the testes. Progesterone receptors, however, appear to be more abundant than estrogen receptors in the stromal and epithelial cells of prostate tissue of patients with BPH. Thus, progesterone may play a more important role in the pathogenesis of BPH than estrogen. The known effect of DHT in initiating the BPH process is believed to be augmented by estrogen.[104] The number of prostate androgen receptors can be increased by estrogens and can be reversed by the administration of antiestrogens.[95] The increase in androgen receptors induced by estrogens may allow for continued androgen-mediated growth despite the declining amount of testosterone produced with advancing age.

5α-REDUCTASE INHIBITORS

FINASTERIDE

Finasteride, a competitive inhibitor of 5α-reductase (type 2), decreases the conversion of testosterone to DHT, the principal androgen responsible for stimulation of prostatic growth. After 7 days of treatment with all doses of finasteride, prostatic tissue DHT declined to 15% or less of control levels, and the testosterone concentration increased in a reciprocal manner.[105] When finasteride was administered in 1- and 5-mg doses to men with BPH for a total of 12 months, the symptom score and urinary flow improved significantly. Finasteride 5 mg daily decreased the median prostate volume by 24% and improved the maximal urinary flow rate by 2.9 mL/second.[106] Adverse effects in the finasteride groups occurred in less than 5%, and side effects, such as decreased libido and ejaculatory dysfunction, were dose related.[107] The efficacy of daily finasteride 5 mg was evaluated in 298 men for 24 months.[108] A slight improvement compared with the results reported at the end of the 12-month period was noted. The median DHT levels had declined by 74.5% compared with 69.3% at 12 months, and prostate volume declined by 25.2% compared with 21.2% at 12 months. Patient symptom scores indicated slightly more improvement at 24 months compared with 12 months. Obstructive symptom scores were responsible for most of the improved symptoms reported. The prevalence of sexual adverse experiences at 24 months was similar to that at 12 months. In those men who experienced finasteride-induced sexual dysfunction, 50% will experience resolution after discontinuing the medication.[109] Inhibition of DHT by 5α-reductase inhibitors does not affect testosterone-mediated functions on muscle mass, libido, or spermatogenesis. Thus, finasteride has an acceptable safety profile, halts disease progression, and improves the quality of life in patients with moderate BPH disease (i.e., enlarged prostate with symptoms of urinary obstruction, but not acute urinary retention). Finasteride improves objective pressure flow parameters after 1 year of therapy, and efficacy appears to be greatest in patients with large prostates (>40 g).[110] For those who do respond, the drug must be continued indefinitely because DHT serum concentrations return to pretreatment levels within 14 days of discontinuing finasteride, and prostate size returns to pretreatment levels within 4 months.[111,112]

Unlike leuprolide, finasteride does not affect the histologic features of BPH and prostate cancer.[113] Morphologic evaluation of patients treated with finasteride with symptomatic BPH having adenectomy showed a reduction in the size of the prostate and an increase in the stroma to epithelial and stroma to lumen ratios.[114]

DUTASTERIDE

Dutasteride is a competitive inhibitor of both types 1 and 2 5α-reductase isoenzymes. An advantage of dutasteride compared with finasteride is the additional inhibition of 5α-reductase (type 1) in the peripheral tissues, which produces a further decline in serum DHT. In a prospective study of 2,951 men with moderate to severe BPH, dutasteride 0.5 mg/day decreased DHT serum levels by 90% at 1 month in 58% of patients. At 24 months, 85% of those treated with dutasteride were noted to have a 90% reduction of serum DHT.[115] Correspondingly, the patients noted reduction in urinary symptoms as early as 3 months after treatment and a significant ($p < 0.001$) reduction in symptoms by the sixth month when compared with those treated with placebo. Common side effects of dutasteride are similar to those of finasteride: impotence (4.7%), decreased libido (3.0%), ejaculation disorder (1.4%), and gynecomastia (1.0%).

COMBINATION THERAPY

Owing to different mechanisms of action, it is a reasonable strategy to combine an α_1-adrenergic receptor antagonist that will work quickly to provide symptomatic relief with a 5α-reductase inhibitor that will take longer to reduce prostate size.

This strategy has been supported by the Medical Therapy of Prostate Symptoms (MTOPS) and Combination of Avodart and Tamsulosin (CombAT) trials. The MTOPS trial studied 3,047 men with moderate to severe BPH and demonstrated that combination therapy was superior to monotherapy with either an α-blocker or a 5α-reductase inhibitor in improving symptoms and urinary flow rate. The risk of clinical progression of BPH was reduced by 39% in patients treated with doxazosin alone, by 34% in patients treated with finasteride alone, and by 66% in patients treated with combination therapy.[116] The CombAT trial studied 4,844 men with risk factors for BPH progression such as larger prostates (>30 g) and higher serum PSA concentrations (1.5–10 mcg/L). Combination therapy reduced the relative risk of acute urinary retention or BPH-related surgery by 65.8% compared with tamsulosin and by 19.6% compared with dutasteride. In addition, for those patients who completed the study, the mean change in the International Prostate Symptom Score from baseline to year 4 was significantly higher for the combination therapy compared with tamsulosin or dutasteride alone.[117] Adverse drug events are more common with combination therapy, but study withdrawal rates are less than 5% and similar among treatment groups. A commercially available combination of dutasteride 0.5 mg and tamsulosin hydrochloride 0.4 mg was introduced in 2010.

Effect of Androgen Suppression on Prostate-Specific Antigen

CASE 104-3, QUESTION 5: G.M. has an annual PSA test. Will androgen suppression alter his results?

The possibility that antiandrogen treatment of BPH could adversely affect the interpretation of the PSA screening test for prostate cancer is of concern. For example, androgen suppression with leuprolide acetate reduces prostate volume primarily by inducing involution of the epithelial elements of the prostate.[118] Because PSA primarily is produced by the epithelial cells of the prostate, these drugs can alter serum and prostate concentrations of PSA.[119] Finasteride 5 mg/day also can reduce the serum PSA level by 50%.[120] Dutasteride reduces total serum PSA by approximately 40% after 3 months of treatment and by approximately 50% after 24 months.[115] The serum PSA level reduction is predictable, however, and serum PSA levels can be recalculated during hormonal treatment for BPH. Nevertheless, patients receiving a 5α-reductase inhibitor should have (a) a digital rectal examination of their prostate periodically, (b) a PSA level measured, and (c) any suspicious findings investigated immediately.[108] Androgen suppression therapy is not contraindicated in BPH solely on the basis of its effect on serum PSA levels.[68]

CASE 104-3, QUESTION 6: G.M asks whether there are nonprescription treatments available that are effective for BPH. What over-the-counter medications are available for prostate disorders?

Two agents, saw palmetto and pygeum, have been promoted for the treatment of BPH. Saw palmetto is an herbal product obtained from the fruit of the *Serenoa repens* tree. The active ingredients are phytosterols; β-sitosterol and β-sitosterol-3-*O*-glucosides are the most abundant. Saw palmetto has antiandrogen activity. Several trials have shown that it significantly improves BPH symptoms[121–124] to a degree similar to finasteride.[125] The dose most often studied is 320 mg a day in one or two divided doses. Pygeum (*Pygeum africanum* bark extract) has been observed to moderately reduce urinary symptoms associated with enlargement of the prostate gland at a dose of 75 to 200 mg/day.[126] Pygeum has been well tolerated in most studies; however, the safety has not been extensively or systematically studied. Herbal products may be tried by men with mild symptoms that would usually be managed by watchful waiting; however, the use of complementary and alternative medicines for BPH is not currently recommended by the AUA guidelines.[127]

Nonpharmacologic Treatment

TRANSURETHRAL RESECTION OF THE PROSTATE

CASE 104-3, QUESTION 7: What are the options if drug therapy does not work for G.M.? When should prostate surgery be undertaken in general?

G.M.'s subjective and objective findings, particularly the acute urinary retention and hydronephrosis, collectively indicate the

TABLE 104-7

Common Procedures for the Management of Benign Prostatic Hyperplasia

Therapy	Brief Description	Comments
Transurethral resection of the prostate (TURP)	A resectoscope is inserted into the urethra and obstructing tissue is removed a piece at a time.	Post-TURP syndrome: potentially life-threatening, caused by the absorption of irrigating fluid. Cerebral edema and seizures may result from hypervolemia and hyponatremia. Late complications: erectile dysfunction (up to 30%), urinary incontinence, and bladder neck contractures, retrograde ejaculation.
Transurethral incision of the prostate (TUIP)	Shallow incisions in the prostatic urethra area relieve bladder outflow obstruction.	Advantageous in high-risk patients such as the elderly because it can be performed under local anesthesia.
Transurethral dilation of the prostate (TUDP)	Balloon catheter is positioned in the prostatic urethra and inflated.	Appropriate for men with smaller prostates who wish to avoid potential side effects of other procedures.
Visual laser ablation of the prostate gland (VLAP)	Laser is used to partially remove obstructing prostate.	Used in men with smaller prostates.
Transurethral microwave hyperthermia	Local microwave hyperthermia, delivered transurethrally or transrectally.	Not as effective as surgical therapy but can be completed as an outpatient procedure in 1 hour.

need for a TURP. G.M. has been advised by his urologist that a TURP is the treatment of choice given the severity of his presentation (e.g., large prostate gland with acute urinary retention) and that the procedure will relieve his symptoms, allow him to lead a relatively normal life, and avoid sequelae of prolonged obstruction.

TURP provides significant relief of BPH symptoms in 86%, 83%, 75%, and 75% of patients at 3 months, 1 year, 3 years, and 7 years, respectively.[128] Of patients with severe BPH, 93% report reduced symptoms 1 year after a TURP.[129] The TURP is considered the gold standard for the treatment of BPH and is used in 90% of patients with symptoms of residual urine or acute urinary retention.[64] As a result, surgical alternatives are always compared with the outcome studies of TURP.

The need for a TURP in G.M.'s situation is fairly clear. In most cases, however, the need for a TURP is less clear because the symptoms do not inevitably worsen and men often are willing to live with their symptoms. Therefore, clinicians need to be able to talk with patients and help them answer the question of whether the discomfort, risk, and problems during the postsurgical recovery period are outweighed by the high probability that surgery will relieve symptoms. After conditions that clearly require surgery have been ruled out, the severity of a patient's symptoms and the degree to which they interfere with living a normal life are the dominant factors in any decision to proceed with prostate surgery. Because surgery for prostate enlargement most often is performed to improve the patient's quality of life, clinicians must counsel patients and help them make the decision. For a comparison of common surgical treatments, refer to Table 104-7.

SEXUAL DYSFUNCTION

As individuals are living longer there is a growing interest in maintaining one's sexual health throughout later life. A nationally representative study concluded that the majority of older adults are engaged in sexual activity and regard sex as an important part of life.[130] Most studies show that sexual activity among the elderly depends on the life pattern and past experiences of good or poor sexual function in each patient. Elderly patients may experience physiologic changes and encounter additional interference with sexual activity because of disability, disease, and medications.

Poor health often is cited by elderly women as a reason for not participating in sexual activity, and among men, erectile dysfunction (ED) is the leading cause of decline in activity.[131,132] The major factors that correlate with reduced sexual activity include an older spouse, poor mental or physical health, marital difficulties, previous negative sexual experiences, and negative attitudes toward sexuality in the aged.[133] During the postmenopausal years, women undergo substantial physiologic changes (see Chapter 51, The Transition Through Menopause).

The major physiologic event of natural menopause is a decrease in estrogen production. Little doubt exists that a decline in estrogen production is associated with many of the physiologic changes causing elderly women to report a low interest in sexual activity. The medical literature is replete with research and data on elderly male sexual dysfunction, but little, if any, data exist on female sexual dysfunction.

Male Sexual Dysfunction

Aging men may experience andropause, a syndrome consisting of weakness, fatigue, reduced muscle and bone mass, impaired hematopoiesis, oligospermia, sexual dysfunction, and psychiatric symptoms.[134] The relationship between declining testosterone and andropause is not firmly established. Free testosterone levels begin to decline at the rate of 1% per year after age 40 years. By the age of 60 years, 20% of men have levels below the lower limit of normal.[135] The physiologic and psychological effects of declining hormone levels in men are less dramatic than those experienced by women.

Sexual function is considered an interaction among motivation, drive, desires, thoughts, fantasies, pleasures, experiences (referred to as the *libido*), penile vasocongestion, erection, orgasmic contractions, and ejaculations (referred to as *potency*).[136,137] Testosterone plays an important role in male libido and sexual behavior, and may play some role in penile erection. Elderly men show a strong correlation between advancing age and diminishing bioavailable serum testosterone levels.[138] Testosterone progressively declines after the seventh decade, partly because of testicular and hypothalamic-pituitary dysfunction.[139]

Male sexual dysfunction, denoting the inability to achieve a satisfactory sexual relationship, may involve inadequacy of erection or problems with emission, ejaculation, or orgasm. *Erectile dysfunction* is the inability to achieve and maintain a firm erection sufficient for satisfactory sexual performance.[140] *Premature ejaculation* refers to uncontrolled ejaculation before or shortly after entering the vagina. *Retarded ejaculation* usually is synonymous with delayed ejaculation. *Retrograde ejaculation* denotes backflow of semen into the bladder during ejaculation caused by an incompetent bladder neck mechanism.

For an illustration that shows the lateral view of the urinary bladder, prostate, seminal gland, and male genital organs, go to http://thepoint.lww.com/AT10e.

ED, once regarded as a psychosocial disorder, today is regarded as caused by a variety of medical, psychological, and lifestyle factors. It is an age-related condition, with about 50% of men older than 40 years of age experiencing some degree of ED.[141] As the population ages, it is estimated that the worldwide prevalence of ED will be approximately 322 million in 2025.[142]

Approximately 80% of all cases of ED now are thought to be related to organic disease and subject to numerous influences.[136,143–145] In one study, neurologic and vascular disorders were the primary causes of ED among elderly men, and psychogenic factors were the cause in less than 10%.[138] The single most common etiology for erectile failure in the elderly is severe atherosclerosis (e.g., vascular disease and diabetes mellitus).[138] Cardiovascular disease, hypertension, diabetes mellitus, elevated low-density lipoprotein cholesterol, and cigarette smoking are associated with a greater probability of complete ED in men.[146] Therefore, prevention of cardiovascular disorders by interventions such as low-fat and low-cholesterol diets and abstinence from tobacco should minimize the development of ED.

Because ED is more likely in male patients with coronary artery disease, the understanding of the cardiovascular stresses involved with sexual intercourse can aid in patient management. Cardiac and metabolic expenditures during sexual intercourse vary depending on the type of sexual activity. Healthy males with their usual female partners generally achieve a peak heart rate of 110 beats/minute with woman-on-top coitus and an average peak heart rate of 127 beats/minute with man-on-top coitus.[147] There is significant individual variation in cardiovascular response, when measured as oxygen uptake and metabolic expenditures, for man-on-top coitus.

In a study of medication-free patients with coronary artery disease who were in New York Heart Association functional class I or II, sexual activity was compared with near-maximal exercise treadmill test.[148] Electrocardiographic changes representing ischemia during intercourse were found in one-third of the patients; however, two-thirds of these patients remained asymptomatic. All patients with ischemia during coitus also demonstrated ischemia during exercise treadmill testing. The average heart rate during coitus was 118 beats/minute, with some patients attaining a heart rate of 185 beats/minute at orgasm. Intercourse in patients with coronary artery disease may provoke increased ventricular ectopic activity that is not necessarily elicited by other stimuli.[149] These electrocardiographic changes and associated symptoms can be abolished with the use of β-blockers.[150] Sexual activity is a likely contributor to the onset of myocardial infarction only 0.9% of the time.[151] Coital death is rare, accounting for 0.6% of sudden death cases.[152] The hemodynamic changes associated with sexual activity may be far greater with an unfamiliar partner, in unfamiliar settings, and after excessive eating and alcohol consumption.

Erectile Dysfunction

PATHOGENESIS

Erection involves the neurologic, psychological, hormonal, arterial, and venous systems. Evidence indicates that more than 80% of the cases of ED are because of organic causes, of which vascular disease is the most common (Table 104-8).[153] In most elderly male sexual dysfunction studies, 50% involve vascular problems, and 30% relate to diabetes mellitus.[154]

TABLE 104-8
Causes of Erectile Dysfunction

Atherosclerosis	Penile Raynaud's phenomenon
Neurologic	Cerebrovascular accident Spinal cord damage Autonomic neuropathy Peripheral neuropathy
Endocrine	Diabetes mellitus Hypogonadism Prolactinomas Hyperthyroidism Hypothyroidism
Iatrogenic	Pelvic radiation Lumbar sympathectomy Prostatectomy Renal transplantation Spinal cord resection
Psychogenic	Performance anxiety Depression Widower syndrome
Neurogenic	Diabetes Spinal cord injury Cauda equina lesions Polyneuropathy Myelopathy Multiple sclerosis Dorsal nerve dysfunction from alcohol abuse or parkinsonism Radical pelvic surgery

Source: Morley JE, Kaiser FE. Sexual function with advancing age. *Med Clin North Am.* 1989;73:1483; Whitehead ED et al. Diagnostic evaluation of impotence. *Postgrad Med.* 1990;88:123.

NEUROGENIC DISORDERS

ED can be caused by damage to the brain, spinal cord, cavernous or pudendal nerves, terminal nerve endings, and the receptors (Table 104-8). Approximately 95% of patients with upper motor neuron lesions resulting from spinal injury are capable of erection through the reflexogenic mechanism,[155] whereas only 25% of patients with complete lower motor neuron lesions can have erections through the psychogenic mechanism.[155] With incomplete lesions, up to 90% of patients in both groups retain erectile ability. Patients who have a cerebrovascular accident, dementia, epilepsy, Parkinson disease, or a brain tumor most likely experience erectile failure through loss of sexual interest or overinhibition of the spinal erection centers.[156]

HORMONAL DISORDERS

The incidence of ED with a hormonal cause has been estimated to be 5% to 35%, depending on which medical specialty is reporting the finding.[157] The most common hormonal disorder associated with ED in the elderly is diabetes mellitus. Depending on the severity and duration of diabetes, the prevalence of ED ranges from 20% to 85%.[158]

Other hormonal disorders, such as hypothyroidism, hyperthyroidism, Addison disease, and Cushing syndrome, are associated with ED. Patients with hypogonadism caused by pituitary or hypothalamic tumors, antiandrogen therapy, or orchiectomy experience ED. These patients can have a normal erection from visual stimulation, however, indicating that the erectile mechanism is intact.[159]

VASCULAR DISORDERS

Atherosclerosis is the leading vascular disease associated with male ED. The age of onset of coronary artery disease parallels the onset of ED, indicating a generalized atherosclerotic etiology for the ED.[160] The degree of arteriolar narrowing and clinical presentation, however, differ from patient to patient. Some patients can have severe coronary artery disease but retain the capability of a full erection. As long as the arterial flow into the penis exceeds the venous outflow, the patient can be potent. Narrowing of the arterial lumen lowers pressure in the cavernous arteries, and poor arterial flow can only partially fill the sinusoidal system. Overall, the partial filling of the sinusoidal system causes inadequate expansion of the sinusoidal wall, resulting in partial compression of the venules. The net effect is a partial erection, difficulty in maintaining an erection, or the most common complaint, early detumescence.

SIGNS AND SYMPTOMS

CASE 104-4

QUESTION 1: F.M., a 66-year-old man, was referred to a urologist because he was experiencing a loss of interest in sexual activity. He describes the inability to maintain a firm erection for the past 6 months in more than 75% of sexual attempts with his sexual partner. Physical examination was unremarkable except for an enlarged prostate gland and evidence of pubic and axillary hair loss. Vital signs were as follows:

Blood pressure, 160/95 mm Hg
Pulse, 88 beats/minute
Respirations, 14 breaths/minute
Temperature, 98.7°F

Current medications include ramipril 5 mg/day and glyburide 5 mg/day. F.M.'s medical history is positive for cigarette smoking, hypertension, and diabetes mellitus. Significant laboratory results include the following:

Random blood sugar, 200 mg/dL
SCr, 1.5 mg/dL
BUN, 22 mg/dL
Free testosterone level, 30 pg/mL (normal, 52–280 pg/mL)
Luteinizing hormone (LH), 4 milliunits/mL (normal, 1–8 milliunits/mL)
Follicle-stimulating hormone (FSH) level, 40 milli-international units/mL (normal, 4–25 milli-international units/mL)
Serum prolactin level, 28 ng/mL (normal, < 20 ng/mL)

What signs and symptoms does F.M. have that would suggest the need for a complete medical workup for ED?

F.M. presents with the complaint of loss of interest in sexual activity and the inability to maintain a full erection during greater than 75% of sexual encounters with his partner. On physical examination, F.M. is found to have a noticeable loss of pubic and axillary body hair. With longstanding androgen deficiency, there may be loss of hair in the androgen-dependent areas of the body, fine wrinkling of the skin around the mouth and eyes, noticeable loss of muscle mass and strength, altered body-fat distribution, and osteoporosis. In contrast, overt hypogonadism results in a change in the pattern of pubic hair from the male diamond shape to the female inverted triangle appearance. At this point, it appears that F.M.'s loss of pubic and axillary hair is the result of androgen deficiency, with the cause yet to be determined. The laboratory results for gonadal function coincide with what is expected in an elderly man with ED (see Case 104-4, Question 4).

UROLOGIC WORKUP

CASE 104-4, QUESTION 2: What clinical evaluations and laboratory tests should be included in the medical workup of F.M. to determine the cause of his ED?

A detailed medical and sexual history and thorough physical examination are essential in the evaluation of sexual dysfunction. General medical history and physical examination should consider drug-induced ED (Table 104-9)[161–179] along with other causes (Table 104-8). Hormonal and metabolic screening should be included with the history and physical examination.

Although laboratory-based diagnostic procedures are available, sexual function may be best assessed in a naturalistic setting with patient self-report techniques. One such self-reporting tool, the International Index of Erectile Function, has been demonstrated to address the relevant domains of male sexual function (erectile function, orgasmic function, sexual desire, intercourse satisfaction, and overall satisfaction), is psychometrically sound, and has been linguistically validated in ten languages.[180]

F.M.'s endocrine status should include assessment of his diabetes, thyroid function tests, and a serum lipid profile. Neuropathy and atherosclerosis are common findings among male patients with diabetes mellitus, and both are potential causes of ED. Patients experiencing hypothyroidism may have decreased libido, and hypothyroidism is associated with hyperprolactinemia, which can result in an inhibition in the release of testosterone. Elevated serum lipids (e.g., total cholesterol, triglycerides) may be associated with significant vascular damage that could contribute to erectile dysfunction. Diabetes mellitus is best evaluated with hemoglobin-A_{1c} and fasting blood glucose tests.[181]

The serum concentrations of free testosterone, prolactin, and LH should be evaluated. Testosterone, as with all other hormones secreted into the plasma, is available to tissues only in the free form (i.e., unbound to serum proteins, particularly the sex hormone–binding globulin). Only 1% to 2% of testosterone is free and physiologically active; therefore, measurement of the unbound serum testosterone provides the best estimate of biologically available testosterone. Low testosterone serum concentrations are associated with primary and secondary hypogonadism. Primary hypogonadism is associated with testicular disease (e.g., Leydig cell tumors), whereas secondary hypogonadism is the result of pituitary or hypothalamic disease.

The serum prolactin concentration should be determined because a high serum concentration of prolactin inhibits release of testosterone from the testes. Therefore, a low serum testosterone concentration may be caused by hyperprolactinemia. Hyperprolactinemia may be caused by prolactin adenomas, diabetes mellitus, or drug therapy (e.g., neuroleptics, metoclopramide).

LH stimulates testicular steroidogenesis and secretion of testosterone. LH increases the conversion of cholesterol to pregnenolone, a precursor of testosterone. FSH is required for spermatogenesis in early puberty, but is not a required gonadotropin for the maintenance of spermatogenesis in adult men. Normal testicular function depends on stimulation by the gonadotropin LH, which is secreted by the anterior pituitary gland. Consequently, a low normal serum concentration of LH is associated with secondary hypogonadism.

In patients with symptoms of prostatic disease, expressed prostatic secretions (EPS) should be examined because prostate inflammation has been associated with ejaculatory dysfunction. During prostatic inflammation, the EPS contains leukocytes and macrophages, and microscopic examination of the EPS can determine the degree of prostate inflammation. The presence of

TABLE 104-9
Common Drug-Induced Alterations in Sexual Response

Drug Categories	Clinical Considerations
Antihypertensives	
Diuretic thiazides	Temporal association with sexual dysfunction. Reported incidence varies between 0% and 32%[161–164]; however, impotence generally is not considered common. Mechanism believed to be a "steal syndrome" whereby blood is routed from erectile tissues to skeletal muscle.[165]
Spironolactone	Associated with ↓ libido, impotence, and gynecomastia. Mechanism may be hormone related. Incidence is dose related and reported to be 5%–67%[165] and much more commonly encountered than with the thiazides. May be owing to antiandrogen effects of drug.
Sympatholytics	
Methyldopa	Central action mediated causing vasodilation resulting in erectile dysfunction. Reported incidence: 10%.[165,166] Also ↓ libido.
Clonidine	Induces erectile dysfunction. Mechanism similar to methyldopa and other central α_2-agonists. Incidence reported to be 4%–70% and dose related.[167–169] Also ↓ libido.
Guanabenz, guanfacine	Incidence and mechanism believed to be similar to other central α_2-agonists.
Nonselective β-Blockers	
Propranolol	Associated with erectile dysfunction and ↓ libido. Mechanism believed to be caused by ↓ vascular resistance and central effects. Erectile dysfunction reported to begin at doses of 120 mg/d. Incidence may be as high as 100% at higher dosages.[166,170,171]
Selective β-Blockers	
Atenolol, metoprolol, pindolol, timolol	Incidence of erectile dysfunction is significantly less than nonselective β-blockers.[172]
α-Blockers	
Doxazosin, prazosin, terazosin	Associated with erectile dysfunction and priapism.[166,168] Reported incidence: 0.6%–4%.[166] Mechanism is local α_1-blockade resulting in vasodilation. Erectile dysfunction and priapism appears to be unique to the nonspecific α_1-antagonists.
Phenoxybenzamine	Associated with priapism, retrograde ejaculation, and inhibited emissions during erection. Effects are dose related.[173,174]
Direct Vasodilators	
Hydralazine	Associated with erectile dysfunction. Mechanism is vascular smooth muscle relaxation. Incidence not reported.[173]
Calcium-Channel Blockers	
Nifedipine	Associated with erectile dysfunction. Mechanism believed to be vasodilation and possibly muscle relaxation. Reported incidence: <2%.[175]
Diltiazem, verapamil	Similar to nifedipine. Reported incidence: <1%.
Antiarrhythmics	
Class 1A Disopyramide	Associated with erectile dysfunction in patients treated for ventricular arrhythmias. Incidence not reported. Mechanism believed to be caused by strong anticholinergic effect.[165,173]
Anticonvulsants	
Carbamazepine, phenytoin	May be associated with sexual dysfunction through decreasing DHEA, which is a precursor to testosterone, estrogen, and pheromones.[19]
Antidepressants	
Selective serotonin reuptake inhibitors	Drugs with prominent serotonin agonist effects commonly cause delayed ejaculation and anorgasmia. The reported incidence for delayed ejaculation among men is 2% to 12%; for anorgasmia among women users, the incidence appears to be <3%. This adverse effect is directly dose related.[19]
Tricyclic antidepressants, monoamine oxidase inhibitors	Associated with impairment of sexual performance in both male and female: ↓ libido, anorgasmia, retrograde ejaculation, erectile dysfunction. Mechanism believed to be caused by anticholinergic and serotonergic effects. Incidence not reported; several case studies in the literature.[165]
Trazodone	Associated with priapism in men and ↑ libido in women. Mechanism similar to TCA. Incidence not reported but believed to be dose related.[165] (Note: The literature reports that overall there is less sexual dysfunction with desipramine than with other antidepressants.)
Antipsychotics	
Phenothiazines	Frequently associated with sexual dysfunction. Commonly, ↓ libido is reported. Mechanism is owing to hyperprolactinemia secondary to central dopamine antagonism. Thioridazine is the most often reported offender. Erectile and ejaculatory pain are very common with this drug class; the α-antagonism and anticholinergic effects are responsible. Priapism is common with this drug group, owing to the peripheral α-blockade property. Incidence for all sexual dysfunction with this drug class: approximately 50% of users.[165]

(continued)

between the use of antihypertensives and hypoglycemic drugs with ED, clinicians must look at the individual drugs themselves and the conditions for which they are prescribed. Sexual dysfunction is not likely to occur with ramipril, or any of the other angiotensin-converting enzyme inhibitors, or with the hypoglycemic agent glyburide. Although ramipril is an antihypertensive, its pharmacologic effects do not contribute to a decline in libido or cause ED (an advantage that angiotensin-converting enzyme inhibitors have compared with other antihypertensive medications). Similarly, the pharmacologic action of glyburide does not contribute to F.M.'s decreased libido or ED. In most sexual dysfunction cases, it is less likely that the medication is the direct cause of the problem; rather, it is the medical condition for which the drugs were prescribed. The ability of a drug to induce sexual dysfunction simply is an extension of its pharmacologic actions. As a general rule, drugs that manipulate the sympathetic or the parasympathetic system, both centrally and peripherally, are associated with sexual dysfunction.

CASE 104-4, QUESTION 6: What factors most likely are contributing to F.M.'s ED?

F.M. is a patient with hypertension and diabetes who smokes cigarettes. Those three factors are more likely to be the cause of F.M.'s sexual dysfunction than are his medications. Again, in the MMAS,[136] cigarette smoking combined with hypertension was determined to be the most significant cause of ED. Diabetes mellitus is the most common hormonal disorder associated with ED in the elderly population.[195] The continued loss of interest in sexual activity experienced by F.M. most likely is the result of having experienced ED during past and present sexual events.

F.M.'s subjective and objective findings are common among elderly men. His sexual dysfunction is caused by atherosclerosis and possible neuropathy secondary to diabetes mellitus. Because cigarette smoking is no doubt contributing to F.M.'s ED, cessation should be encouraged; some improvement can be expected.[165] There is no need to alter F.M.'s drug regimen.

MANAGEMENT

CASE 104-4, QUESTION 7: What are the primary therapeutic considerations for F.M.?

Essentially, there are three levels to the management of ED. Level 1 includes lifestyle and drug therapy modifications. Specifically, the patient should be instructed to modify smoking and alcohol use. The patient's drug regimen should be checked periodically to ensure that drugs associated with ED are not being prescribed. If necessary, psychosocial counseling should be provided. After careful consideration, oral medications for management of ED should be instituted. If level 1 therapies have failed or are not acceptable to the patient, then level 2 therapy is instituted. These interventions include a vacuum constriction device to elicit an erection, intracavernosal injections, or transurethral inserts. Level 3 management involves placement of a penile prosthesis.

PHARMACOTHERAPY

Any therapy directed at male sexual dysfunction must include the elimination of drugs causing adverse sexual effects. Drug therapy is directed primarily toward treatment of ED and includes hormonal therapy, bromocriptine, prostaglandin E_1, sildenafil, tadalafil, vardenafil, and apomorphine.

PHOSOPHODIESTERASE-5 INHIBITORS

CASE 104-4, QUESTION 8: Would phosophodiesterase-5 inhibitor therapy be appropriate for F.M.? What are its side effects and contraindications? Does it interact with other drugs?

F.M. has diabetes mellitus and atherosclerosis and therefore is a candidate for treatment with a phosphodiesterase-5 (PDE-5) inhibitor.[211] These agents are orally active and selective inhibitors of cyclic guanosine monophosphate–specific PDE-5, the predominant phosphodiesterase isoenzyme metabolizing cyclic guanosine monophosphate in the corpus cavernosum. They facilitate an erection in response to sexual stimulation by enhancing the nitric oxide–induced relaxation of corpus cavernosal smooth muscle. The results of double-blind, placebo-controlled clinical trials in men with ED of various causes have demonstrated that PDE-5 inhibitors significantly improve erectile function and the rate of successful sexual intercourse, with therapeutic outcomes approaching those of normal men of the same age.[212–214]

F.M. should be counseled on the adverse effects of PDE-5 inhibitors. The vasodilating action of PDE-5 inhibitors affects both the arteries and the veins, so the most common side effects are headache and facial flushing.[215] PDE-5 inhibitors cause a small decrease in both systolic and diastolic blood pressures, but clinically significant hypotension is rare. Studies of PDE-5 inhibitors and nitrates taken together show much greater drops in blood pressure. For that reason, PDE-5 inhibitors are contraindicated in patients taking long-acting nitrates or short-acting nitrate-containing medications.[143] In phase II/III studies before US Food and Drug Administration (FDA) approval, more than 3,700 patients received sildenafil and almost 2,000 received placebo in double-blind and open-label studies. Approximately 25% of patients had hypertension and were taking antihypertensive medications, and 17% were diabetic. In these studies, the incidence of serious cardiovascular adverse effects was similar in the double-blind sildenafil group, the double-blind placebo group, and the open-label group. Twenty-eight patients had experienced a myocardial infarction. When adjusted for patient-years of exposure, no significant differences were seen in the myocardial infarction rates between the sildenafil and the placebo group, and no deaths were attributed to sildenafil.[216,217] In an analysis of 67 double-blind, placebo-controlled trials of sildenafil, the overall frequency of death was comparable between the sildenafil-treated patients (13 of 8,691; 0.15%) and placebo group (7 of 6,602; 0.11%).[218] Nevertheless, several deaths caused by myocardial infarction or arrhythmia have been associated with the use of sildenafil.[219] Deaths associated with sildenafil (and presumably other PDE-5 inhibitors) are most likely caused by increased cardiac workload in patients with unstable angina.[220]

Transient visual anomalies (mostly blue-green color-tinged objects, increased sensitivity to light, and blurred vision) have been reported in patients taking PDE-5 inhibitors, especially at higher dosages. These visual effects appear to be related to the weaker inhibiting action of PDE-5 inhibitors on the enzyme phosphodiesterase-6, which regulates signal transduction pathways in the retinal photoreceptors. In patients with inherited disorders of retinal phosphodiesterase-6, such as retinitis pigmentosa, PDE-5 inhibitors should be administered with extreme caution. In 2005, the FDA recommended that all PDE-5 inhibitors include a precaution in their labeling regarding the risk of nonarteritic anterior ischemic optic neuropathy as a cause of decreased vision including permanent vision loss. There have been only a handful of reports of nonarteritic anterior ischemic optic neuropathy in postmarketing surveillance, and most patients had underlying risk factors.[221] Clinicians should advise patients to discontinue the use of all PDE-5 inhibitors and seek medical attention in the event of sudden vision loss in one or both eyes.

The vasodilator actions of nitrates are profoundly amplified with concomitant use of PDE-5 inhibitors. This interaction likely applies to all nitrates and nitric oxide donors, regardless of their predominant hemodynamic site of action. They also may potentiate the inhaled form of nitrate, such as amyl nitrite, and therefore are contraindicated in patients using this product. Dietary sources of nitrates, nitrites, and L-arginine (the substrate from which nitric oxide is synthesized) do not contribute to the circulating levels of nitric oxide in humans and, therefore, are unlikely to interact with PDE-5 inhibitors. The anesthetic agent, nitrous oxide, is eliminated unchanged from the body, mostly via the lungs, within minutes of inhalation. It does not form nitric oxide in the human body and does not itself activate guanylate cyclase. As such, no contraindication exists to its use after administration of PDE-5 inhibitors. The concomitant use of nitrates and the PDE-5 inhibitors is contraindicated although some differences in the nitrate-free period do exist based on the pharmacokinetic profile of the PDE-5 inhibitor. After 24 hours, the administration of nitrates can once again be considered in patients using vardenafil and sildenafil; however, this should be extended to 48 hours in patients using tadalafil.

CASE 104-4, QUESTION 9: Which PDE-5 inhibitor should be recommended for F.M.?

SILDENAFIL

The typical dose of sildenafil is 50 mg orally, taken 1 hour before sexual activity. However, it may be taken anywhere from 4 hours to 30 minutes before sexual activity. The maximal recommended dosing frequency is once per day. The following factors are associated with increased plasma levels of sildenafil: age older than 65 years (40% increase in area under the curve), hepatic impairment (e.g., cirrhosis, 80% increase), severe renal impairment (creatinine clearance <30 mL/minute, 100% increase), and concomitant use of potent CYP3A4 inhibitors (e.g., erythromycin, ketoconazole, itraconazole, 200% increase). Because higher plasma levels may increase both the efficacy and the incidence of adverse events, a starting dose of 25 mg should be considered in these patients. The dose may be increased to 100 mg or reduced to 25 mg. Because F.M. is older than 65 years of age, he should be started on 25-mg tablets of sildenafil. The dose may be increased under strict supervision.

Sildenafil is metabolized by both the CYP2C9 pathway and the CYP3A4 pathway. Thus, inhibitors of the CYP3A4 isoenzyme, such as erythromycin or cimetidine, may lead to competitive inhibition of its metabolism; however, CYP3A4 is a high-capacity pathway. The effects of erythromycin or cimetidine on the half-life and physiologic effects of sildenafil are not known, but clinicians should be warned about the potential interaction.

Inadequate physical sexual stimulation while using any of the PDE-5 inhibitors can lead to treatment failure. Adequate sexual stimulation is needed to trigger the events leading to erection.[222] PDE-5-inhibitors cannot initiate an erection; they can only assist in the process. Some patients may need several attempts at sexual stimulation before they are successful with intercourse.

TADALAFIL

Similar to sildenafil, tadalafil is a selective inhibitor of PDE-5. Tadalafil has several times more affinity for PDE-5 than sildenafil.[223] Tadalafil and vardenafil, however, have minimal or no effect on visual disturbance (impairment of blue-green color discrimination), which is a well recognized side effect of sildenafil.[224] Tadalafil's extended half-life of 17.5 hours relative to sildenafil most likely precludes its use in patients with angina or hypertension. Tadalafil is metabolized by the hepatic CYP3A4 isozyme. Food has no effect on the oral absorption of tadalafil in contrast to sildenafil (bioavailability decreased by 29%). Tadalafil may be advantageous in a subset of patients, based on its shorter onset of action (16 minutes) and 24-hour duration of action.[225] Specifically, patients with psychogenic or neurogenic ED and those with stable cardiovascular systems may prefer tadalafil because it offers the potential for multiple sessions of intercourse with a single daily dose.

VARDENAFIL

Vardenafil is the third FDA-approved oral PDE-5 inhibitor for treatment of ED. The warnings regarding the use of nitrates while taking vardenafil are similar to the warnings for sildenafil. Patients using vardenafil may experience headache, flushing, or rhinitis; the incidence of these side effects are dose related.[226] Vardenafil is metabolized by the hepatic CYP3A4 isozyme and has a reported half-life of 5 hours.[227] Thus, drugs known to inhibit the CYP3A4 isozyme have the potential to prolong its half-life. Vardenafil 10 mg does not impair the ability of patients with stable coronary artery disease to exercise at levels equivalent to or greater than that attained during sexual intercourse.[228]

F.M. has hypertension that most likely would be affected by tadalafil; therefore, extreme caution is advised. Perhaps the shorter-acting sildenafil or vardenafil would be the PDE-5-inhibitor drug of choice for F.M.

TESTOSTERONE

CASE 104-4, QUESTION 10: Should F.M. be treated with testosterone?

Primary hypogonadism with severely deficient serum levels of bioavailable testosterone is the only appropriate indication for the use of androgen hormone therapy.[170] The goal of androgen-replacement therapy is to restore potency and libido by maintaining normal serum levels of testosterone.[229] Testosterone has no benefit in the treatment of eugonadal or mildly hypogonadal elderly men and actually may enhance the growth of undiagnosed adenocarcinoma of the prostate or cause further ED.[143] In eugonadal men, testosterone enhances the rigidity of the erection, but does not change the penile circumference.[230] F.M. would not be a candidate for testosterone therapy.

CASE 104-4, QUESTION 11: Which type of patient would benefit from testosterone therapy?

Unless testosterone deficiency is severe, for example, if free testosterone serum levels are less than 7 to 8 pg/mL, testosterone replacement therapy will not improve the success rate of intercourse.[231] Testosterone replacement in patients with primary hypogonadism generally restores libido and potency. In some patients with secondary hypogonadism caused by disorders of the hypothalamus or pituitary, GnRH analogs can be administered to differentiate between hypothalamic and pituitary abnormalities and to correct testosterone deficiency.[229] Libido and potency then are restored.

CASE 104-4, QUESTION 12: How should testosterone be used as a treatment for ED?

Testosterone-replacement therapy is available in several formulations, including gels, transdermal patches, and intramuscular injection. Because of poor drug bioavailability, oral testosterone-replacement therapy is less effective than parenteral testosterone in achieving normal serum testosterone levels. Oral administration also is associated with a higher incidence of hepatotoxicity and adverse serum lipid effects.[143,175] A long-acting testosterone intramuscular formulation, such as the enanthate or cypionate ester, is still considered the regimen of choice for the treatment of primary hypogonadism. A dose of 50 to 400 mg should be administered intramuscularly every 2 to 4 weeks. Side effects of testosterone therapy include early gynecomastia, increases in hematocrit (sometimes to the point of polycythemia), and fluid retention that may worsen hypertension or heart failure.

Results of several studies have demonstrated that serum testosterone levels are normalized while using transdermal testosterone applications.[176,232–234] The system normalizes DHT to testosterone ratios and reduces LH levels toward the normal range. The transdermal testosterone is well tolerated, with application site reactions such as pruritus, burnlike blisters, and erythema being the most commonly reported event. The adhesive side of the patch should be applied to a clean, dry area of the skin on the back, abdomen, upper arms, or thighs. The patient should be instructed to avoid application over bony prominences or on a part of the body that may be subject to prolonged pressure during sleep or sitting (e.g., the deltoid region of the upper arm, the greater trochanter of the femur, and the ischial tuberosity); do not apply to the scrotum. The sites of application should be rotated, with an interval of 7 days between applications to the same site. The area selected should not be oily, damaged, or irritated.

Topical testosterone gel should be applied once daily in the morning to clean, dry skin on the upper arms, shoulders, or abdomen. Topical testosterone gel is available as a 1% gel. The dose can be as high as 100 mg/24 hours. After the gel has dried on the site of application, it should be protected with clothing to prevent transfer to a nonuser. The patient's hands should be washed.

Commonly reported adverse effects in chronic users include acne, edema, gynecomastia, and dermatologic reactions to injections or transdermal applications of testosterone. The most serious risk of prolonged testosterone use is prostate carcinoma, although the association between high concentrations of testosterone and the risk of prostate carcinoma is controversial.[235–237] Three studies suggest that testosterone-replacement therapy is relatively safe in hypogonadism.[238–240] Baseline assessment of the prostate should be done before starting testosterone-replacement therapy. This should consist of a TRUS, digital palpation of the prostate gland, and analysis of the PSA, hemoglobin, and hematocrit levels.

BROMOCRIPTINE

CASE 104-4, QUESTION 13: Because F.M.'s prolactin serum concentration is 28 ng/mL, should bromocriptine be prescribed to decrease his hyperprolactinemia and treat his ED?

Hyperprolactinemia may be treated with the ergot alkaloid bromocriptine. Normalization of the serum prolactin level is mandatory if potency is to be restored. Even with normalization of prolactin levels, approximately 50% of elderly male patients are unable to achieve erectile function and desire.[175,229] Bromocriptine therapy may be initiated with twice-daily 1.25-mg doses taken with meals to minimize gastrointestinal upset. Thereafter, doses may be increased weekly, at a rate of no more than 2.5 mg/day. Because bromocriptine is associated with dizziness, drowsiness, hypotension, and cerebrovascular accidents, the patient should be forewarned.[143,229]

F.M. is not a candidate for treatment with bromocriptine because he does not have secondary hypogonadism, and his ED probably is secondary to atherosclerosis associated with his hypertension, diabetes, and cigarette smoking. Normalizing the prolactin serum level in F.M. would not correct his problem. Furthermore, the elevation of F.M.'s serum prolactin concentration is not significant enough to warrant drug therapy. With only a 50% (or less) response rate to bromocriptine in elderly men, the risk of adverse reactions (e.g., dyskinesia, dizziness, hallucinations, dystonia, confusion, cerebrovascular accidents) outweighs the benefit of this drug therapy.

CASE 104-4, QUESTION 14: What other drug therapy is available for F.M.?

Before the advent of the PDE-5-inhibitors, intracavernosal and intraurethral administration was the only nonsurgical option for ED. Prostaglandin E_1 (alprostadil) is available for intracavernosal injection, as a urethral insert (referred to as medicated urethral system for erection), and as a topical cream. All of these pharmaceutical preparations have been shown to be efficacious for men with ED,[140,241,242] with users reporting successful intercourse 65% of the time. Phentolamine, papaverine, and vasoactive intestinal peptide are also available for intracavernosal injection. Adverse events from these therapies include priapism, pain at the injection site, and penile fibrosis after long-term use.

KEY REFERENCES AND WEBSITES

A full list of references for this chapter can be found at http://thepoint.lww.com/AT10e. Below are the key websites for this chapter, with the corresponding reference number in this chapter found in parentheses after the website.

Key Websites

Agency for Healthcare Research and Quality. Urinary Incontinence in Adults: Clinical Practice Guideline Update. http://www.ahrq.gov/clinic/uiovervw.htm. Accessed November 30, 2010.

American Urologic Association. http://www.auanet.org.

American Urological Association. Clinical Guideline on the Management of BPH (2010 update). http://www.auanet.org/content/guidelines-and-quality-care/clinical-guidelines.cfm?sub=bph. Accessed November 30, 2010. (127)

American Urological Association. Clinical Guideline on the Management of Erectile Dysfunction (2006 update). http://www.auanet.org/content/guidelines-and-quality-care/clinical-guidelines.cfm?sub=ed. Accessed November 30, 2010.

National Association for Continence. http://www.nafc.org.

Simon Foundation for Continence. http://www.simonfoundation.org.

105

Osteoporosis

Rebecca A. Rottman-Sagebiel

CORE PRINCIPLES

		CHAPTER CASES
1	Osteoporosis is a condition of low bone mass and deterioration of bone tissue leading to bone fragility and potentially fracture with many preventable and inherent risk factors.	**Case 105-1 (Question 1)**
2	Prevention and treatment of osteoporosis focus on modifying preventable risk, providing adequate dietary supplementation of calcium and vitamin D, increasing bone mineral density, and reducing fracture rates.	**Case 105-1 (Questions 1–3), Case 105-2 (Question 2)**
3	Pharmacologic therapy is reserved for those patients with a hip or vertebral fracture, individuals with a T-score less than or equal to −2.5 at the femoral neck or spine once secondary causes have been excluded, and individuals with low bone mass with a 10-year probability of greater than or equal to 3% risk of hip fracture or greater than or equal to 20% risk of major osteoporotic fracture.	**Case 105-2 (Questions 3–7)**
4	Initial therapy with oral bisphosphonates is recommended unless patients are unable to take or have relative contraindications to oral bisphosphonate therapy.	**Case 105-2 (Question 7)**
5	Estrogen/progesterone therapy, selective estrogen receptor modulators, parathyroid hormone, denosumab, and calcitonin are alternative therapies for prevention and/or treatment of postmenopausal osteoporosis.	**Case 105-2 (Questions 3–7), Case 105-3 (Questions 1, 2)**
6	Duration of treatment with antiresorptive and/or anabolic therapy has remained controversial, secondary to concerns for oversuppression of bone turnover markers and the potential for the development of osteosarcomas, respectively.	**Case 105-2 (Question 7)**
7	Prevention and treatment of osteoporosis secondary to prolonged glucocorticoid therapy should be incorporated into a patient's treatment plan with considerations for dosage and duration of glucocorticoid therapy, the patient's individual risk factors, sex, and age.	**Case 105-4 (Questions 1–3)**
8	Pharmacological therapies to be considered for osteoporosis treatment in men include oral and intravenous bisphosphonates and parathyroid hormone.	**Case 105-5 (Questions 1–5)**

INCIDENCE, PREVALENCE, AND EPIDEMIOLOGY

The term osteoporosis is derived from the Greek words osteon (bone) and poros (pore).[1] The World Health Organization (WHO) defines it as a disease "characterized by low bone mass and microarchitectural deterioration of bone tissue, leading to enhanced bone fragility and a consequent increase in fracture risk."[2] A WHO working group defined osteoporosis as "the presence of bone mineral density (BMD) or a T-score that is 2.5 standard deviations (SD) or more below the mean peak value in young, healthy adults."[3,4] Osteopenia, a lesser degree of bone loss, is defined as a T-score that is between 1 and 2.5 SD lower than the mean peak value in young, healthy adults.

Osteoporosis can be classified as primary or secondary. Primary osteoporosis can be further defined as type 1 or 2. Type 1, postmenopausal osteoporosis, is associated with increased cortical and cancellous bone loss resulting from increased bone resorption, typically occurring during the first 3 to 6 years after menopause. Postmenopausal osteoporosis is manifested by vertebral fractures, distal radius fractures, hip fractures, and even an increased tooth loss secondary to osteoporosis of the mandible. Type 2, senile osteoporosis, occurs in both women and men 75 years of age and older with a female to male ratio of 2:1.[5,6]

TABLE 105-1
Risk Factors Associated With the Development of Osteoporosis

↑Age Female sex Caucasian or Asian Family history Small stature Low weight	Predisposing medical problems (e.g., chronic liver disease, chronic renal failure, hyperthyroidism, primary hyperparathyroidism, Cushing syndrome, insulin dependent diabetes, gastrointestinal resection, malabsorption, irritable bowel disease, chronic obstructive pulmonary disease, and acquired immune deficiency syndrome or human immunodeficiency virus)
Early menopause or oophorectomy Sedentary lifestyle ↓Mobility Low calcium intake Excessive alcohol intake Cigarette smoking	Drugs (e.g., corticosteroids, long-term anticonvulsant therapy [phenytoin or phenobarbital], excessive use of aluminum-containing antacids, long-term high-dose heparin, furosemide, excessive levothyroxine therapy)

Cortical and cancellous bone losses are proportional. These persons are at greatest risk for hip, pelvic, and vertebral fractures.

Secondary osteoporosis results from use of various medications or the presence of particular disease states (Table 105-1). This type of osteoporosis can occur at any age and is equally common in men and women.

Osteoporosis is a major health problem that affects approximately 10 million people in the United States, with 80% of the affected population being women 50 years of age and older. Another estimated 34 million Americans, 50 years and older, are at increased risk for osteoporosis, according to the National Osteoporosis Foundation (NOF).[6] The incidence for osteoporosis increases with age; 30% of women 80 years of age or older develop osteoporosis without medical intervention.[7]

Annually, more than 1.5 million osteoporosis-related fractures occur in elderly Americans.[6,8] Osteoporosis-related fracture sites predominantly include the vertebrae (often referred to as compression fracture), distal radius, and hips (examples include intertrochanteric and intracapsular hip fractures).

ONLINE CONTENT

For visuals of compression fractures and intertrochanteric hip fractures, go to http://thepoint.lww.com/AT10e.

Approximately 50% of women and 20% of men aged 50 years and older will sustain an osteoporosis-related fracture in their lifetime.[6] Patients who suffer hip fractures have a 10% to 20% higher mortality rate and 2.5-fold increased risk of future fractures relative to persons of the same sex and similar age without fractures.[6] In addition, hip fractures result in a multitude of complications for the elderly, including prolonged hospitalization, decreased independent living, depression, fear of future falls, and lifelong disability.

ONLINE CONTENT

To view a radiograph that shows a hip replacement in one hip and pins in the other, go to http://thepoint.lww.com/AT10e.

An estimated 20% require long-term nursing home placement and approximately 60% are unable to regain their prefracture level of independence.[6] Vertebral fractures may be painless or result in pain that usually lasts less than 3 months. The initiating injury may be as minor as a cough or turning over in bed. Vertebral collapse or deformity can result in loss of height, kyphosis, abdominal protuberance, decreased pulmonary function, and chronic back pain.

ONLINE CONTENT

For a visual of the causes of kyphosis, go to http://thepoint.lww.com/AT10e.

The annual direct cost for treating osteoporosis and osteoporosis-related fractures in the United States is estimated at $14 billion to $20 billion per year for fracture related costs alone. This figure will continue to rise (potentially even triple) in the next 30 years if prevention and early intervention measures do not reduce the incidence of osteoporosis.[6,8,9] Thus, the impact of osteoporosis on the health care system as the "baby-boomer" generation ages and life spans increase is potentially staggering.

Etiology

Structurally, bone is either cortical or cancellous (trabecular), with the adult skeleton containing 80% cortical and 20% cancellous bone. Dense cortical bone forms the outer shell of the skeleton, and porous cancellous bone forms the interior structures in a honeycombed fashion. The proportions of cortical and cancellous bone vary at different sites in the skeleton, with cortical bone predominating in long bones (~90%) except at their ends, which are predominantly cancellous. This type of bone is also found in the vertebrae and distal forearms. A balance between osteoblast and osteoclast activity results in a continuous remodeling process; osteoclasts resorb bone, whereas osteoblasts help reform bony surfaces and fill bony cavities.[6]

Bone mass peaks during the third decade of life. Around 35 years of age, cortical bone gradually begins to decrease 0.3% to 0.5% per year in both women and men.[10] In menopause, the decline in 17β-estradiol concentrations further accelerates cortical bone loss by 2% to 3% per year that is superimposed on age-related bone loss. This loss gradually decreases during the next 8 to 10 years.[10] Hormone-related, accelerated bone loss can also occur after surgical oophorectomy. Longitudinal data suggest that estrogen may play an important role in the development of osteoporosis in men as well.[11] Serum testosterone concentration has been evaluated in many studies; its effects on bone metabolism have been controversial, with more recent data suggesting that it does have direct beneficial effect on bone, but to a lesser extent than estrogen. Other hormones regulated by the hypothalamic-pituitary-gonadal axis (e.g., progesterone, follicle-stimulating hormone, inhibins, oxytocin, and prolactin) are also being studied for their effects on the skeletal system.[9,12,13]

Cancellous bone loss begins between the ages of 30 and 35 years with yearly decreases in women of 0.6% to 0.8% (linear decrease) or approximately 2% (curvilinear decrease) for a period of a few years, likely associated with a decrease in estrogen levels during perimenopause and early menopause.[5,10] Age-related cancellous losses in women appear approximately a decade earlier than cortical bone loss. The effect of menopause on cancellous bone loss is controversial; many studies indicate an increased rate of loss, whereas others do not.[5] Thus, early cancellous bone loss in conjunction with postmenopausal decreases in cortical and cancellous bone may lead to increased vertebral and distal forearm fractures, which predominate early after menopause.[10] Men begin to lose bone mass after 30 years of age. Cortical bone in the proximal radius, as well as cortical and cancellous bone in the distal radius, lose content at a rate of approximately 1% annually.[14] Spine and hip density also decline with increasing age.[15,16]

ONLINE CONTENT

To view a radiograph of osteoporotic hips, go to http://thepoint.lww.com/AT10e.

Women may lose as much as 50% of cancellous and 30% of cortical bone over their lifetimes, whereas men may lose only 30% and 20%, respectively.[17,18] In addition, women may have an increased risk for osteoporosis because throughout life they have 30% less bone mass than men of a similar age.[19]

Pathophysiology

Bone remodeling in humans occurs constantly, replacing the entire human skeleton every decade. The process is regulated by both systemic and local regulators of bone cell activity.[20] Bone remodeling normally is a continuous process that occurs in discrete skeletal foci called bone-remodeling units. Local regulators that determine osteoclast differentiation and activity include the receptor activator of nuclear factor-κB ligand (RANKL) and osteoprogenerin. Osteoblast-derived RANKL binds to the osteoclast RANK receptor to facilitate osteoclast differentiation and resorptive activity. The B cells produce a decoy receptor osteoprogenerin (OPG) that competitively antagonizes RANKL by binding to it and preventing osteoclast stimulation. This process begins with bone resorption that is initiated by osteoclasts excavating lacuna found on the surface of cancellous bone, or it occurs when cavities are formed in cortical bone (Fig. 105-1). Enzymes, specifically transforming growth factor-β (TGF-β), produced in this process dissolve bone mineral and proteins serving as a chemoattractant for osteoblast precursors to the sites where resorption has occurred.[20,21] Osteocytes, cells in the bones, have growth factors that display direct and indirect effects on bone turnover.[20] This occurs as collagen fills in bone cavities, which then are calcified.[17]

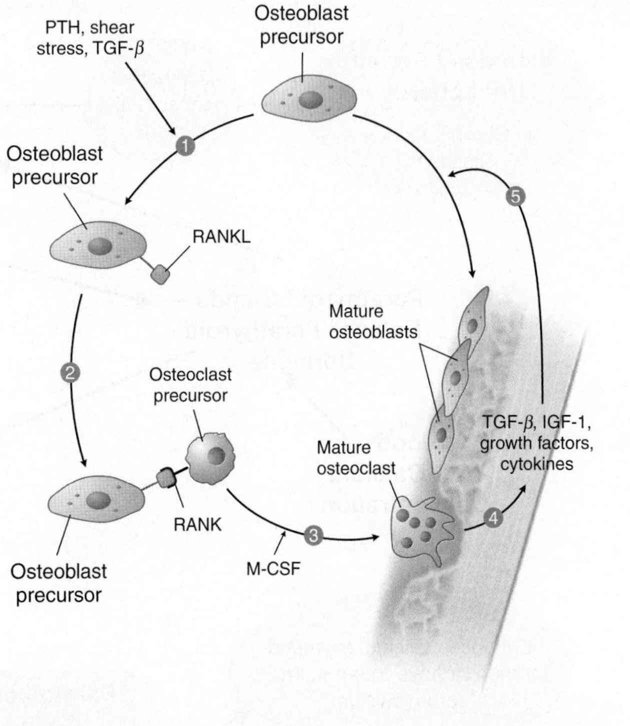

FIGURE 105-1 The bone remodeling cycle at the cellular level. In normal young adults, the bone removed by the osteoclasts is replaced completely by the osteoblasts. 1.) Local regulators simulate osteoblast precursors to interact with RANKL. 2.) Differentiation of osteoclast activity occurs when RANKL binds to the RANK receptor. 3.) Osteoclasts are matured through the binding and with the assistance of other factors to begin resorption. 4.) During the resorption phase, enzymes are released. 5.) These enzymes stimulate osteoblast precursor binding and osteoblast maturation leading to bone formation at the sites osteoclasts have excavated. (Reprinted with permission from Golan DE, Tashjian AH, Armstrong EJ. *Principles of Pharmacology: The Pathophysiologic Basis of Drug Therapy*, 2nd Edition. Baltimore: Wolters Kluwer Health, 2008.)

Calcium and vitamin D are important nutrients required for bone growth. Parathyroid hormone, glucocorticoid hormones, calcitonin, estrogen, and testosterone are all factors involved in bone remodeling.[20–22] Parathyroid hormone (PTH) and glucocorticoid hormones have been associated with bone resorption, whereas calcitonin, estrogen, and testosterone have been associated with bone formation.[23] The small intestine is the site for the absorption of dietary calcium, the kidneys reabsorb calcium in the tubular system, and the skeletal system serves as a reservoir for calcium. Calcium is primarily regulated by the actions of PTH, vitamin D, and calcitonin. The parathyroid gland releases PTH in response to low serum calcium levels, which in turn facilitates the mobilization of calcium and phosphate from bone and stimulates reabsorption of calcium through the tubular system in the kidneys.[24] Vitamin D aids in intestinal absorption of calcium as well as phosphorus and magnesium. Increases in vitamin D levels decrease PTH levels. Vitamin D also increases bone resorption to prevent symptomatic hypocalcemia.[25] Calcitonin is released in response to high serum calcium levels. Calcitonin decreases intestinal absorption of calcium and phosphorus, enhances calcium excretion in the kidneys, and prevents bone resorption (Fig. 105-2).[26]

Overview of Drug Therapy

Osteoporosis is a condition of low bone mass and deterioration of bone tissue, thus preventative measures with adequate intake in calcium and vitamin D should be incorporated into all treatment plans. For postmenopausal women with low bone mass and significant risks for the development of a fracture, preventative pharmacological therapies can be incorporated into the treatment plan with estrogen and progesterone therapy, selective estrogen receptor modulators (SERMs; e.g., raloxifene), and bisphosphonates (e.g., alendronate). For women suffering with postmenopausal osteoporosis, pharmacological treatment with either antiresorptive agents (SERMs, bisphosphonates, calcitonin, or RANKL inhibitors [e.g., denosumab]) or anabolic agents (e.g., parathyroid hormone) are recommended depending on the patient's risk factors and the severity of osteoporosis. Glucocorticoid-induced osteoporosis management varies depending on the duration and dosage of glucocorticoid therapy and risk factors. For patients requiring prevention or treatment, bisphosphonates and parathyroid hormone are the mainstays of therapy. Osteoporosis is a condition affecting both women and men, with mortality rates after hip fracture higher in men than women, thus pharmacological therapy is also warranted for men. Treatment options for osteoporosis in men include bisphosphonates and parathyroid hormone.

Risk Factors

CASE 105-1

QUESTION 1: T.J., a 28-year-old, thin white woman, is worried about developing osteoporosis. Her 75-year-old

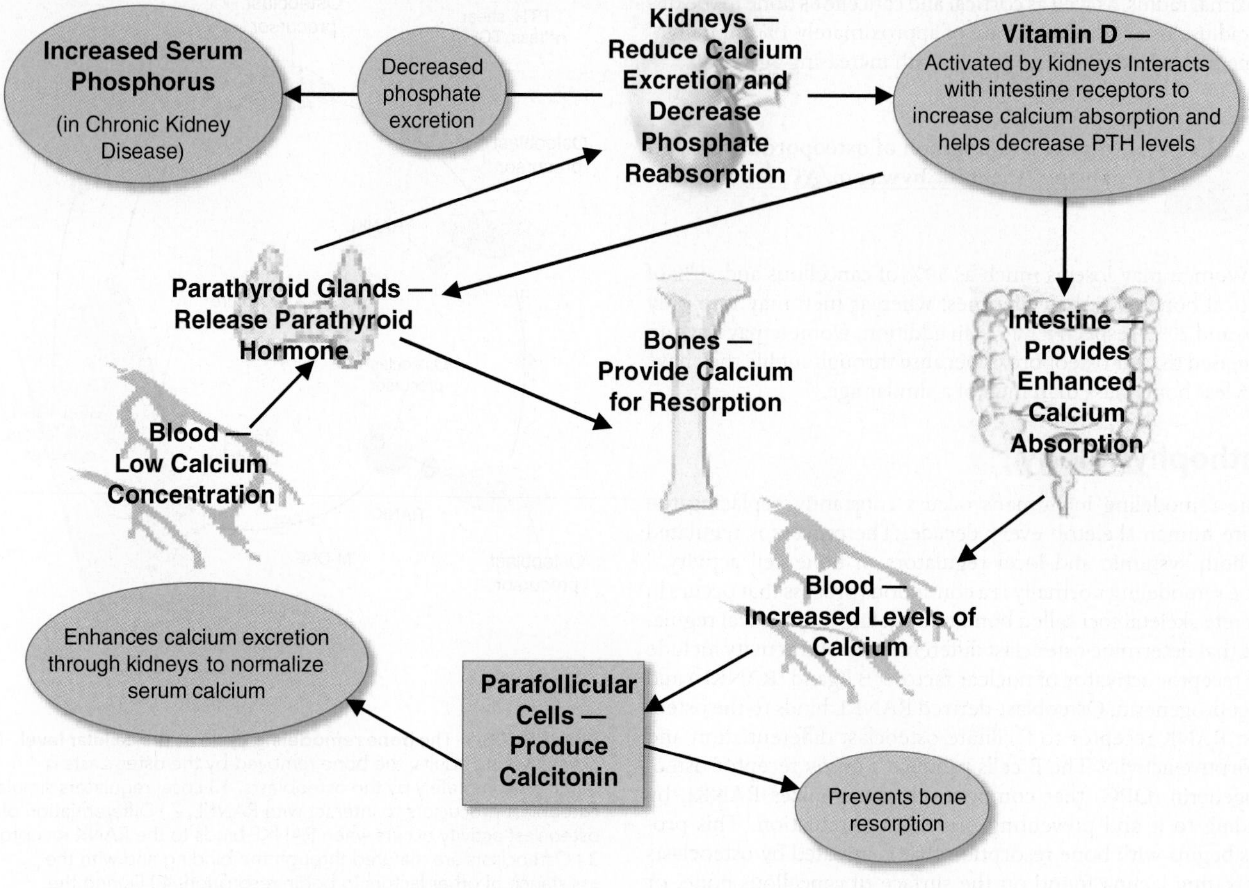

FIGURE 105-2 Pathway for calcium homeostasis with involvement from parathyroid hormone, vitamin D, and calcitonin.

maternal grandmother has osteoporosis and recently her postmenopausal mother (age 53) was told that she was at increased risk for osteoporosis. T.J. is 5 feet 2 inches tall, weighs 108 pounds, and is in good health. She jogs and occasionally does aerobic exercise. Her diet typically consists of cereal for breakfast, a sandwich for lunch, and meat with vegetables for dinner. Her only milk consumption consists of 1 cup of skim milk on her cereal. She occasionally has a dairy product for lunch or dinner. T.J. takes no medications, vitamins, or calcium supplement routinely. She occasionally takes a medication for headache or menstrual cramps. She does not smoke and occasionally drinks alcohol. Does T.J. have an increased risk for developing osteoporosis?

Table 105-1 lists risk factors associated with the development of osteoporosis. T.J. has several risk factors that could increase her risk for osteoporosis. She is a white woman of small stature and low weight, has a positive family history, and has a low calcium intake.

Prevalence of osteoporosis in the United States varies with ethnicity. White and Hispanic Americans are at greater risk for osteoporosis than other ethnic groups (e.g., black women of African ancestry), especially those who are of small stature, such as T.J., and those who are proportionally underweight for their height.[26] The significance of heredity as a risk factor for osteoporosis has been studied. Genetic association studies have identified polymorphisms in the vitamin D receptor, estrogen receptor (ER)α, Col1a1, bone morphogenetic proteins, signaling pathways, and various other bone-related proteins and receptors.[27] Data from a meta-analysis of 16 studies revealed conflicting results on the association of polymorphisms and fracture risk.[28] Women with a first-degree relative with osteoporosis typically have low bone mass.[29]

MOBILITY AND PHYSICAL ACTIVITY

Immobility owing to prolonged bedrest has been associated with decreased bone mass. Conversely, weight-bearing exercise helps prevent bone loss. Exercise throughout life helps maintain skeletal mass and may help reduce bone loss in postmenopausal women. Exercise appears to stimulate osteoblastic activity to help maintain bone mass.[30] Thirty minutes of weight-bearing exercise three times weekly has shown improvements in bone density and a reduced hip fracture risk in older women.[31]

CIGARETTE SMOKING AND ALCOHOL INGESTION

Although T.J. does not smoke and only occasionally ingests alcohol, it is important to include questions concerning cigarette and alcohol use when obtaining a medical history from a person at risk for osteoporosis. Women who smoke have an increased risk for fractures compared with nonsmokers.[32] Cigarette smokers may have impaired calcium absorption and lower 17β-estradiol levels; however, the mechanisms are unknown for effects on bone mass.[33]

Excessive alcohol use by both women and men may predispose them to low BMD. Moderate alcohol consumption has been associated with increased BMD in postmenopausal women.[33] Consuming more than two alcoholic drinks daily significantly increases the fracture risk according to other available literature.[34] The proposed mechanism may be a direct effect of alcohol on osteoblasts, or it may be secondary to nutritional

TABLE 105-2
Calcium Content of Selected Foods

Food	Serving Size	Calcium (mg)
Dairy Products		
Milk, dry nonfat	1 cup	350–450
Yogurt, low-fat	1 cup	345
Milk, skim	1 cup	300
Milk, whole	1 cup	250–350
Cheese, cheddar	1 oz	211
Cheese, cottage	1 cup	211
Cheese, American	1 oz	195
Cheese, Swiss	1 oz	270
Ice cream or ice milk	1/2 cup	50–150
Fish		
Sardines, in oil	8 med	354
Salmon, canned (pink)	3 oz	167
Fruits and Vegetables		
Calcium-fortified juices	1 cup	100–350
Spinach, fresh cooked	1/2 cup	245
Broccoli, cooked	1 cup	100
Collards, turnip greens	1/2 cup	175
Soybeans, cooked	1 cup	131
Tofu	1 oz	75
Kale	1/2 cup	50–150

compromise that could result in impaired calcium and vitamin D intake with subsequent decrease in bone formation.[35] Alcoholics may also be at risk for increased falls.

DIETARY INTAKE

Calcium, in conjunction with vitamin D, is needed to strengthen bones, increase bone mass, and decrease fracture rates. Girls and women such as T.J. need adequate calcium intake to achieve and help maintain optimal bone mass, but the typical American diet is low in calcium. The National Academy of Sciences published recommendations for calcium intake based on age. They recommend 1,000 mg/day of elemental calcium for women younger than 51 years of age.[36] The National Institutes of Health (NIH) recommend the same amount of calcium for women in this age group.[37] Calcium is best ingested from the diet (Table 105-2), but if the diet is low in calcium, supplements can be used (Table 105-3; see Case 105-1, Questions 2, 3). A diet high in caffeine, protein, phosphorus, and sodium has been associated with an increased risk of fractures by adversely effecting calcium balance.[38] However, many studies have found conflicting results.[37–43]

TABLE 105-3
Percentage of Calcium in Various Salts

Salt	Percent Calcium
Calcium carbonate	40
Tricalcium phosphate (calcium phosphate, tribasic)	39
Calcium chloride	27
Dibasic calcium phosphate dehydrate	23
Calcium citrate	21
Calcium lactate	13
Calcium gluconate	9

OTHER POTENTIAL RISKS

Various medications and medical conditions that have been associated with the development of secondary osteoporosis are listed in Table 105-1.

Prevention

PREMENOPAUSAL WOMEN

CASE 105-1, QUESTION 2: Although T.J. is premenopausal, what recommendations could be made to decrease her future risk of developing osteoporosis?

T.J.'s course of action should be to maximize her peak bone mass and prevent or decrease bone loss. This may be accomplished by ingesting a nutritious diet with adequate calcium and vitamin D and developing a lifelong exercise program.

EXERCISE

T.J. should be encouraged to participate regularly in weight-bearing exercises such as jogging, walking, running, biking, tennis, or weight-lifting and to continue appropriate exercise for her age throughout life. Aerobic training is important in controlling weight, increasing cardiorespiratory endurance, and decreasing the risk for cardiovascular disease.

Young women such as T.J. should be informed that excessive exercise can cause amenorrhea. Women with exercise-induced amenorrhea have been reported to have decreased bone mineralization and an increased risk for fractures.[44]

DIETARY INTAKE

Vitamin D helps regulate calcium by a complex interaction that involves PTH (see also Chapter 31, Chronic Kidney Diseases) as well as direct effects on bone. Studies have shown improvement in muscle strength and balance as well as reduced risk of falls with vitamin D supplementation.[33] Adult requirements for vitamin D range from 600 international units daily for individuals under 70 years of age to 800 international units for those older than 70 years of age. The NOF recommends vitamin D doses of 800 to 1000 international units daily in all postmenopausal women.[33] T.J. should be able to obtain adequate vitamin D intake from her diet and exposure to sunlight. Other sources of vitamin D include liver and fatty fish. She could also take a multivitamin daily that contains at least 400 international units of vitamin D. Studies found that when vitamin D is taken in conjunction with calcium supplementation, bone loss can be reduced; however, the effectiveness of vitamin D alone for fracture prevention is unclear.[33,45] Higher-than-recommended doses could lead to increased risks, including hypercalciuria and hypercalcemia.[33]

T.J.'s diet should be calcium-enriched to ensure that she receives 1,000 mg/day of elemental calcium, optimally from dietary sources.[6,33] Because dairy products are the major source of dietary calcium in the United States, T.J. should select low-fat or nonfat dairy products to decrease her caloric intake and minimize her fat intake when possible. If T.J. were lactose intolerant, she could select dairy products containing lactase. Although nondairy sources may contain lower amounts of calcium, they may be included in a diet plan to increase calcium content, especially when a woman cannot or will not use dairy products (Table 105-2). The ingestion of foods rich in phytates (e.g., cereal grains, legumes, and nuts) may decrease calcium absorption.

If T.J. cannot meet her daily calcium requirement from dietary sources, she can use a calcium supplement. Table 105-3 lists the percentage of elemental calcium available from selected calcium salts. See Case 105-1, Question 3, for further information on calcium supplements.

Currently, no evidence exists that magnesium supplementation prevents osteoporosis. People who might need extra magnesium beyond that found in their diets most likely are elderly women or individuals with gastrointestinal (GI) disease.[33] A few studies have been conducted to evaluate the effects of vitamin K on bone mineral density with mixed results. There is no strong evidence to suggest more than recommended supplementation to prevent osteoporosis.[33] Isoflavones are a class of phytoestrogens found in soybeans and red clover. The current data, mostly from small studies of short duration, are insufficient to support the use of isoflavones for osteoporosis prevention.[33]

SMOKING CESSATION

A woman who smokes should be encouraged to stop because cigarette smoking is associated with lowered BMD and increased fracture risk as well as other health problems.[33]

CASE 105-1, QUESTION 3: If T.J. needs a calcium supplement, which calcium salt should be recommended?

Calcium carbonate is usually the calcium salt recommended for women such as T.J. because it is reasonably priced and contains the highest percentage of elemental calcium (40%); allowing fewer tablets per day to meet daily calcium requirements. If T.J. needs a calcium supplement, she should be advised to take it in divided doses (e.g., 500–600 mg/dose) to maximize absorption. Calcium should be taken with fluids during or after meals that are low in fiber to increase absorption. The absorption of medications such as tetracyclines, iron, and quinolones may be decreased when taken with calcium. T.J. should be informed that the most common adverse effects of calcium are constipation, GI irritation, and flatulence. Doses exceeding 2,500 mg/day of elemental calcium can result in hypercalcemia, hypercalciuria, and possibly, urinary stones. If T.J. or any family member has a history of urinary stones, she should remain under medical supervision.

POSTMENOPAUSAL WOMEN

CASE 105-2

QUESTION 1: T.J.'s mother, M.J., age 53, is also a woman of small stature and low weight. She occasionally walks in the evenings. She currently is taking a calcium supplement to maintain her total calcium intake (dietary plus supplementation) of about 1 g/day. She takes omeprazole (over-the-counter) for her gastroesophageal reflux disease (GERD) and occasional acetaminophen for headaches. M.J. was a cigarette smoker but stopped in her late twenties and rarely drinks alcohol. She is in good health with no gynecologic surgery or major diseases. M.J. does admit to having a strong family history of breast cancer. Her last menstrual period was 6 months ago, but she began experiencing menstrual irregularity 2 years ago. M.J. has been experiencing some menopausal symptoms (hot flushes), but states that they are mild and occur only at night. M.J., worried about developing osteoporosis, decided to make an appointment with her gynecologist to discuss preventive measures. A dual-energy x-ray absorptiometry (DXA) measurement of her spine was administered, which noted her T-score to be –2.0 and a Z-score of –1.0. In addition to the DXA, what other information should be obtained to determine whether she is at risk for developing osteoporosis or already has osteoporosis?

A full medical history, including medications, and physical examination, including height, are needed in addition to a risk factor analysis. Other diagnostic tests should be obtained if needed.

From her history and risk factor analysis, it is determined that M.J. shares similar risk factors for osteoporosis with her daughter. In addition, she is early in the postmenopausal phase, has GERD, and was a previous smoker. M.J. has no loss of height, does not complain of back pain, and does not have signs of kyphosis, all of which may be signs of osteoporosis. Women can lose 1 to 1.5 inches in height as part of the normal aging process, secondary to shrinking of intervertebral disks.[33] Biochemical markers of bone turnover are not needed for M.J. at this time (e.g., alkaline phosphatase, calcium levels, phosphorus levels, bone-specific alkaline phosphatase, osteocalcin, cross-linked C-terminal telopeptide, and N-telopeptide) as they may be more helpful when treatment is to be started and during treatment to determine response as well as for drug development.[6,46]

The North American Menopause Society (NAMS) recommends a BMD measurement in women such as M.J. who are older than 50 years of age if one or more risk factors for fracture are present (e.g., weight <127 pounds, fracture [other than skull, facial bone, ankle, finger or toe] after menopause, first-degree relative with a history of a vertebral or hip fracture), smoking, rheumatoid arthritis, and women with excessive alcohol consumption.[33] The NOF recommends BMD testing for women 50 to 69 years of age when risk factors for osteoporosis are present and both NAMS and NOF recommend screening for women older than 65 years of age, in the absence of risk factors for osteoporosis, and postmenopausal women who present with fractures to confirm diagnosis and severity of disease.[6] Medicare has specific guidelines for covering BMD testing and physicians should refer to the most recent guidelines.

Differential absorption of x-rays from two different energies determines the amount of mineral in a given region with a DXA. One x-ray energy source is blocked by the patient while the other x-ray energy source passes completely through, with higher density bone blocking both x-rays. Lower density bone or soft tissue allows x-rays to be transmitted. X-ray energies completely transmitted are sent to a computer which then translates compiled data into an image with density measurements in grams per centimeter squared (g/cm^2), with pencil beam and fan beam DXA machines being the most commonly used.[47] Central DXA of hip, spine, and femoral neck remain the preferred measurement for definitive diagnosis.[6,33]

Although DXA is the gold standard for determining BMD, other methods can be used for screening but should not be used for diagnosis or to follow a patient's response to therapy[33] (Table 105-4). For postmenopausal women who are not receiving medications for osteoporosis prevention, a DXA may be useful no more frequently than every 2 to 5 years because the rate of bone loss is approximately 1% to 1.5% per year.[33] T-score values are supported by both the NAMS and NOF for diagnosis. The Z-score can be useful when looking for secondary causes contributing to low BMD, with a Z-score of less than –2 suggesting low BMD for chronological age.[6,47] In addition, it has been estimated that for every one point decrease in SD from the mean T-score, a 10% to 15% change can occur in BMD. The magnitude of this change can be translated into a 1.5-fold to 3-fold change in risk for fractures.[33]

Another tool health care providers can use when determining fracture probability is the WHO Fracture Risk Assessment Tool (FRAX). FRAX is a computer-based algorithm that provides models for the assessment of fracture probability in women and men using easily obtained clinical risk factors for fracture and death to estimate a 10-year fracture probability. FRAX can be used alone or in conjunction with BMD. FRAX incorporates different ethnicities as well as many clinical risk factors (e.g., age,

TABLE 105-4
Techniques for Measuring Bone Mineral Density

Technique	Abbreviation	Measurement Sites
Dual-energy x-ray absorptiometry	DXA	Hip, spine, total body bone mineral density
Peripheral dual-energy x-ray absorptiometry	PDXA	Forearm, fingers, heel
Peripheral quantitative computed tomography	PQTC	Forearm
Quantitative ultrasound	QUS	Heel, shin
Quantitative computed tomography	QCT	Spine
Single-energy x-ray absorptiometry	SXA	Heel

smoking, physical inactivity, height, weight, prior fracture, parental history of hip fracture, long-term use of glucocorticoids, and comorbid conditions that have been associated with decreases in BMD).[48–52] FRAX has been validated in 11 different cohorts and is a major achievement in terms of understanding and measuring fracture risk; however, it should not replace clinical judgment for treatment. There are several limitations to FRAX, including that it excludes certain variables (vitamin D deficiency, bone turnover markers, falls, etc.), it does not take into account single versus multiple fractures, it considers fracture risk constant over time (not variable as many studies have shown), it should only be used in treatment-naïve patients, the BMD input is limited to femoral neck, if BMD is entered then secondary osteoporosis does not apply (does not take into account multiple risk factors), it requires Internet access for use, and it assumes that the relationship between BMI and mortality is the same among all ethnic groups. Despite these limitations, the incorporation of FRAX into clinical practice increases the likelihood of patients in need of treatment receiving therapy.[51] FRAX can be found at http://www.shef.ac.uk/FRAX.[48]

CASE 105-2, QUESTION 2: What preventive measures would help decrease M.J.'s likelihood of developing osteoporosis?

EXERCISE

Although M.J. goes for walks occasionally, she should begin an aerobic and weight-bearing exercise program appropriate for her age and physical condition because exercise (particularly weight-bearing exercise) is important for maintaining healthy bones. (Also see Case 105-1, Question 2).

DIETARY INTAKE

As with T.J., it is important for M.J. to have adequate vitamin D intake from her diet and exposure to sunlight. The recommended daily allowance of vitamin D for women between 51 and 70 years of age is 600 international units/day, and those older than 70 years of age an intake of 800 international units/day may be needed.[33] Many experts feel this is not sufficient and the NOF recommends 800 to 1,000 international units/day.[33] This may be achieved from ingesting foods that contain vitamin D (e.g., fortified milk, fatty fish) or from ingesting a daily multiple vitamin containing vitamin D. For individuals with limited exposure to sunlight, vitamin D supplementation may be needed. Patients with renal or hepatic disease may need supplementation with active vitamin D metabolites, which are available by prescription only. The expert consensus opinion has made recommendations for serum 25(OH) vitamin D levels for bone health. Levels less than 20 ng/mL (50 nmol/L) suggest insufficiency, whereas levels of 29 to 32 ng/mL (70 to 80 nmol/L) suggest adequate stores. There is currently no justification to attempt to achieve serum 25(OH) vitamin D levels above 60 ng/mL (150 nmol/L).[33] (For further information, see Case 105-1, Question 2.)

Because of her postmenopausal status and other risk factors, M.J. should increase her current intake of elemental calcium to at least 1,200 mg/day.[36] Although calcium has antiresorptive activity, its use alone by postmenopausal women is not an alternative to estrogen/progestin therapy (EPT), estrogen therapy (ET), bisphosphonates, or a SERM for osteoporosis prevention. Calcium supplementation does help delay BMD loss in postmenopausal women and its use reduces the risk of hip fractures by 25% to 70%.[53] (Also see Case 105-1, Questions 2, 3.)

ESTROGEN/PROGESTIN THERAPY

Previously, EPT would have been considered first-line prevention for osteoporosis in a postmenopausal woman such as M.J., who has an intact uterus and is at risk for osteoporosis based on risk factors and T-score. Approved indications for use of these products include prevention, but not treatment, of postmenopausal osteoporosis, with the recommendation that agents be used for the shortest duration possible (e.g., duration of menopausal symptoms).[54] Studies have not been conducted to evaluate fracture rate reduction in less than standard doses of EPT or ET[27] (also see Chapter 51, The Transition Through Menopause). Since the publication of the Heart and Estrogen/Progestin Replacement Study (HERS) I[55] and HERS II[56] and the NIH Women's Health Initiative (WHI),[57] health care providers are less likely to prescribe EPT or ET for the sole purpose of osteoporosis prevention or to continue its use after a woman no longer needs EPT or ET for postmenopausal symptoms such as hot flushes.

ESTROGEN EFFICACY ON BONE MINERAL DENSITY AND FRACTURE RATE

CASE 105-2, QUESTION 3: M.J. is considering hormone therapy. What effect does estrogen have on BMD in a postmenopausal woman such as M.J. and can EPT or ET decrease fracture rates?

The primary effect of estrogen on BMD is related to its antiresorptive activity, which decreases bone loss and lowers fracture rates. Estrogen receptors (ER) are proteins that bind estrogens with high affinity and specificity.[58] Researchers have identified different ER, including α, β, and γ.[59] ER act on the reproductive organs, however, α and β also affect cardiovascular organs and bone.[60] Although not fully understood, the interplay between estrogens and their receptors may stimulate osteoblast activity and the secretion of insulinlike growth factor 1 and transforming growth factor-β. In addition, estrogens possibly inhibit interleukin-1 (IL-1), IL-6, and the release of tumor necrosis factor. Both ER-α and ER-β have been isolated from primary osteoblastic cells of neonatal rats, which, if translatable to humans, shows that both ER may have beneficial effects on BMD.[61] Estrogen may also affect calcium absorption and vitamin D receptors in osteoblasts.

An estimated 10% to 15% of a woman's bone mass is estrogen-dependent[62]; therefore, estrogen appears to effectively delay or prevent osteoporosis in postmenopausal women.[33] The addition of a progestin to ET for women with a uterus does not appear to decrease estrogen efficacy for osteoporosis prevention. More than 50 randomized, placebo-controlled clinical trials have shown that EPT or ET can increase BMD by 4% to 6% in the spine and 2% to 3% in hips.[33] These levels of BMD also have been noted to be maintained after 3 years of therapy.[33,63]

In observational studies, EPT or ET appears to reduce fracture rates in postmenopausal women. In one meta-analysis, hip-fracture risk was reduced by 25% for postmenopausal women who had used EPT or ET.[64] A second meta-analysis found that the use of EPT or ET for at least 1 year significantly reduced nonvertebral fracture risk (relative risk [RR], 0.73; 95% confidence interval [CI], 0.56–0.94). This effect on fracture rate was somewhat reduced in women who began EPT or ET after age 60 years.[65]

The Study of Osteoporotic Fractures, a large prospective cohort study, showed decreased risks for wrist and nonspinal fractures in estrogen users who were older than 65 years of age and decreased risks in the incidence of hip fractures in those older than 75.[66] The relative risk for nonspinal fractures in postmenopausal women who were current estrogen users versus those not receiving EPT or ET was 0.66 and 95% CI was 0.24 to 0.64.[67]

In a randomized, placebo-controlled trial that enrolled 2,763 postmenopausal women (HERS), a different outcome was noted. No reduction in fracture risk was observed, even after 4 years of EPT (conjugated estrogen [CEE] 0.625 mg/day and medroxyprogesterone acetate 2.5 mg/day). Women enrolled in HERS had histories of cardiac disease, but many were at low risk for fractures because they did not have osteoporosis. Women were enrolled in HERS to determine whether EPT use would decrease the incidence of cardiovascular disease—fracture risk was a secondary observation.[55]

The National Osteoporosis Risk Assessment Study and the Million Women Study, both large observational studies by design, found that EPT or ET provided significant relative-risk reductions in fracture.[68,69] These results were confirmed by the WHI with both the EPT and ET arms, showing significant risk reductions in hip, vertebral, and total fractures compared with placebo.[57,70]

CONTRAINDICATIONS TO ESTROGEN USE

CASE 105-2, QUESTION 4: Does M.J have any contraindications to the use of EPT or ET?

Contraindications to EPT or ET include pregnancy; active or history of deep vein thrombosis or pulmonary embolism; active or recent (e.g., within the past year) arterial thromboembolic disease (e.g., stroke, myocardial infarction); undiagnosed abnormal genital bleeding; known, suspected, history of breast cancer; known or suspected estrogen-dependent neoplasia; liver dysfunction or disease; or known hypersensitivity to the product or any of its ingredients.[71] In addition, women with a history of asthma, diabetes mellitus, migraine, epilepsy, systemic lupus erythematous, porphyria, and hepatic hemangiomas may have their disease exacerbated by the use of EPT or ET. Thus, women with any of the previously mentioned diseases should be monitored closely by their physicians for potential problems with therapy.[71] Patients on EPT or ET are at increased risk for cancer, including endometrial (if not on EPT), breast (for EPT), and ovarian cancer as well as increased cardiovascular events, thromboembolic disease, stroke, gallbladder disease, and dementia (also see Chapter 51, The Transition Through Menopause). M.J. has a strong family history of breast cancer and starting her on EPT therapy is not the treatment of choice to prevent osteoporosis.

ADVERSE EFFECTS

CASE 105-2, QUESTION 5: What are potential adverse effects of estrogens and progestins administered to a postmenopausal woman such as M.J.?

Estrogen-related adverse effects include nausea, vomiting, dizziness, weight gain, breast tenderness, and breast enlargement. She must also be educated about the possible return of uterine bleeding if she begins using EPT. Used alone, ET produces dose-dependent uterine bleeding; women who received 0.625 mg/day of CEE had a 1% to 4% incidence.[71] Addition of a progestin cyclically increases the incidence of uterine bleeding, normalizes the bleeding pattern, and reduces breakthrough bleeding. The continuous administration of both hormones decreases the incidence of bleeding, but breakthrough bleeding may continue for 6 months to 1 year until the endometrium becomes atrophic.

Adverse effects associated with progestin use may depend on the type of progestin prescribed, but typically include edema, increased breast size, mastalgia, rash, acne, hirsutism, alopecia, headaches, and psychological effects (e.g., irritability, fatigue, mood swings, depression).[71]

Other Prevention Modalities

SELECTIVE ESTROGEN RECEPTOR MODULATORS

RALOXIFENE

CASE 105-2, QUESTION 6: Should a SERM, such as raloxifene, be considered for the prevention of osteoporosis in M.J.?

Raloxifene, a SERM, may be an alternate therapeutic choice for M.J. SERMs are pharmaceutical agents that are "hormone-related" or "designer estrogens" that have estrogen agonist, antagonist, or both activities in various tissues where estrogen receptors are present. These compounds are also structurally diverse. For example, benzothiophene analogs, such as raloxifene, have agonistic (estrogenic) effects on bone and serum lipid profiles and antagonistic (antiestrogenic) effects on endometrial and breast tissues. Triphenylethylene analogs, such as tamoxifen, have agonistic effects on bone, serum lipid profiles, and endometrial tissue, and antagonistic effects on breast tissue.

Raloxifene at a dose of 60 mg/day is the only SERM currently approved by the US Food and Drug Administration (FDA) for the prevention and treatment of postmenopausal osteoporosis.[72] Raloxifene's agonist activity on bone tissue is believed to occur through a reduction in bone resorption and a decreased rate of bone turnover, which then results in increased BMD. The effects appear to be mediated through action as an estrogen agonist at ER in bone. Raloxifene activity may be mediated through transforming growth factor-$\beta 3$ (TGF-$\beta 3$) and suppression of cytokine IL-6.[73]

Data supporting raloxifene's effect on BMD were collected in three clinical osteoporosis prevention trials that were conducted in North America (544 women), Europe (601 women), and internationally (619 women, all of whom had undergone hysterectomy).[72,73] The trials were all randomized, double-blind, placebo-controlled studies that lasted 2 years. Participants were postmenopausal women 45 to 60 years of age. All received calcium supplementation, and women in the treatment groups received raloxifene 60 mg/day; the international study also included a CEE arm (0.625 mg/daily). The results of these studies showed loss of approximately 1% BMD among women in the placebo groups. In contrast, those in the raloxifene groups had an increase in BMD of 1.3% to 2.4% in the hips, 1.6% to 2.5% in femoral neck, 1.3% to 2.7% in the trochanter, 1.3% to 2.4% in the intertrochanter, and 1.8% to 2.4% in the lumbar spine. The increase in BMD in the hips of women in the CEE arm of the international study was twice that noted for raloxifene.

The Multiple Outcomes of Raloxifene Evaluation (MORE) trial enrolled 7,705 postmenopausal women 31 to 80 years of age. Of these, 5,129 were randomly assigned to either a 60 mg/day or 120 mg/day raloxifene group and the remainder were in the placebo group.[74] MORE trial outcomes after 3 years were as follows for BMD: femoral neck BMD increased 2.1% (60 mg/day group) and 2.4% (120 mg/day group) versus placebo, with spinal BMD increases of 2.6% and 2.7% in the raloxifene groups, respectively, compared with placebo. The RR for vertebral fractures was 0.7 (95% CI, 0.5–0.8) for those in the 60 mg/day group, whereas those in the 120 mg/day group had an RR of 0.5 (95% CI, 0.4–0.7), translating into a 38% and 41% reduction in vertebral fracture rate for the 60 mg/day and 120 mg/day groups, respectively.[75] No significant difference in nonvertebral fractures was noted among groups.

Sambrook et al.[76] conducted EFFECT (Efficacy of Fosamax versus Evista Comparison Trial), a randomized, double-blind, double dummy multicenter international study including 487 postmenopausal women with low bone density of the spine or hip (T-score ≤2.0) to determine efficacy and tolerability of alendronate and raloxifene. Patients were randomly assigned to either alendronate or raloxifene. After 1 year, BMD increased in both the alendronate and raloxifene groups in the lumbar spine (4.8% vs. 2.2%, respectively) and total hip (2.3% vs. 0.8%, respectively). Tolerability and GI effects were similar in both groups; however, significantly higher reports of vasomotor symptoms came from the raloxifene group.[76]

The CORE Study assessed the effects of raloxifene on breast cancer for an additional 4 years beyond the 4-year MORE trial. A substudy assessed lumbar spine and femoral neck BMD at 7 years, including 386 women (127 placebo, 259 raloxifene) who did not take other bone-active agents from the fourth year of MORE and who were at least 80% compliant with the study medication in CORE. When comparing MORE baseline BMD, after 7 years, raloxifene significantly increased lumbar spine (4.3% from baseline, 2.2% greater than placebo) and femoral neck (1.9% from baseline, 3% greater than placebo) BMD, with BMD significantly above MORE baseline at all time-frames observed at both sites.[77]

A paradox still exists regarding how raloxifene can decrease vertebral fractures by up to 41% while increasing BMD by only 2% to 3%, rates that are lower than those noted for ET, EPT, or alendronate. In addition, raloxifene has not been observed to have a positive effect on hip fractures. It has been postulated that the antifracture effect of raloxifene on vertebral fractures occurs secondary to its normalization of the high turnover rate of cancellous bone, which then prevents further disruption of bone microarchitecture.[78,79] This probably occurs through raloxifene binding at estrogen β-receptor sites that are predominant in cancellous bone whereas the α-receptor is predominantly in cortical bone.[78,79] Thus, bone type and estrogen receptors are different in the hips compared with vertebrae. In addition, a less potent antiresorptive agent, such as raloxifene, may help prevent vertebral fractures but not hip fractures because the threshold for preventing osteoclastic activity in cancellous bone (which is predominant in vertebrae) may be lower than in cortical bone (which predominates in hips). For these reasons, it may require a more potent antiresorptive agent to increase BMD in the hips.

Raloxifene might be considered for osteoporosis prevention in a woman such as M.J., even with her strong family history of breast cancer. This latter recommendation is based on results from the MORE trial. A 76% decrease was noted in risk for invasive breast cancer in postmenopausal women with osteoporosis (mean age, 66.5 years) who received raloxifene for 3 years.[80] A total of 7,705 women were assigned to raloxifene groups (60 mg twice daily or 60 mg daily) or a placebo group. Of those enrolled in either raloxifene group ($n = 5{,}129$), only 13 cases of breast cancer were reported versus 27 that occurred in the 2,576 women in the placebo group. M.J. could be a candidate for raloxifene for prevention of osteoporosis if her FRAX score is at least 3% risk of hip fracture or at least 20% risk of major osteoporotic fracture.[6,14] If M.J. is to start raloxifene she should speak with her physician before stopping raloxifene if her vasomotor symptoms worsen. Studies have shown that discontinuing raloxifene therapy resumes bone loss.[77,81]

Dosing and Pharmacokinetics

If M.J. were to use raloxifene, she should take 60 mg once daily without regard for food.[72] Raloxifene is approximately 60% absorbed and undergoes extensive glucuronide conjugation, resulting in a 2% absolute bioavailability. Some circulating raloxifene glucuronide conjugates are converted back to the parent compound.[72] Raloxifene and its monoglucuronide conjugates are highly protein-bound. Raloxifene is primarily excreted in feces, with less than 0.2% excreted unchanged and less than 6% eliminated in urine as glucuronide conjugates.[72] There appear to be no differences in pharmacokinetics based on age or sex. Raloxifene has a mean half-life of 27.7 hours after a single dose and 32.5 hours after multiple doses.[72]

Contraindications and Potential Drug Interactions

Raloxifene is contraindicated in women who are pregnant or may become pregnant. It is also contraindicated for women with an active or previous history of venous thromboembolic events.[72] Patients with hepatic dysfunction may need dosage adjustments, although more information is needed to clarify doses needed.[72] Cholestyramine, when coadministered with raloxifene, may decrease raloxifene absorption by 60% because of its effects on enterohepatic cycling.[72] Women who may be receiving warfarin as well as raloxifene should be monitored closely.[72] This may also be true for some other highly protein-bound medications.

Adverse Effects

Adverse effects include an increased risk for venous thromboembolic disease and an increase in hot flushes (25% in postmenopausal raloxifene users vs. 18% in those receiving placebo).[72] The greatest risk for thromboembolic events is during the first 4 months of therapy.[72] To decrease the risk of thrombosis associated with immobilization, raloxifene should be discontinued for at least 72 hours before immobilization such as that associated with surgery. M.J. is still experiencing hot flushes which could be exacerbated by raloxifene, so she should be counseled extensively on this potential side effect.

BISPHOSPHONATES

CASE 105-2, QUESTION 7: Should a bisphosphonate be considered for the prevention of osteoporosis in a woman such as M.J.?

Another alternative treatment option for M.J. would be a bisphosphonate, such as alendronate sodium, risedronate sodium, ibandronate, or zoledronic acid. These agents are approved for both the prevention and treatment of osteoporosis in postmenopausal women, with oral bisphosphonates being considered first line therapy by both NAMS and NOF.[6,33] Alendronate, risedronate, and zoledronic acid are also approved for osteoporosis in men, glucocorticoid-induced osteoporosis prevention, and treatment.[82–85] Aminobisphosphonates decrease bone resorption, resulting in decreased fracture rates in postmenopausal women who are at risk for osteoporosis. Amino groups in these newer generation bisphosphonates appear to increase selectivity for the antiresorptive surfaces of bone. Bisphosphonates have high affinities for bone hydroxyapatite and can be incorporated into bone; in doing this, they can interfere with osteoclast-mediated bone resorption. Because of their incorporation into bone, bisphosphonates have long half-lives, estimated to be 1 to 10 years. Unlike etidronate (a non-aminobisphosphonate), aminobisphosphonates do not inhibit bone mineralization, which could lead to osteomalacia.[82–85]

BONE MINERAL DENSITY EFFICACY

A study of the efficacy and safety of oral alendronate (5 mg/day) for osteoporosis prevention in early postmenopausal women[86] showed BMD increases in the spine of 2.9% at 5 years for women receiving alendronate, although total body bone density was increased only 0.3%. In a 2-year prevention study in postmenopausal women younger than 60 years,[87] placebo, 2.5 mg/day alendronate, 5 mg/day alendronate, and EPT were compared. An increased BMD in the spine, total hip, and total body were observed in the alendronate groups versus the placebo group. Results from the 5 mg group were as follows: lumbar spine, 3.5%; hip, 1.9%; and total body, 0.7%. These results were better than for those in the 2.5 mg group but lower than those who received estrogen; BMD for the hormone replacement therapy group was 1% to 2% greater than for the alendronate 5 mg group.

Another study found that women (ages 55–81 years) diagnosed with postmenopausal osteoporosis who were in an alendronate study group (alendronate 5 mg/day for 2 years followed by 10 mg/day for 1 year) had reduced risk for fractures at various anatomic sites compared with those in the placebo group.[88] For new vertebral fractures, the RR was 0.53 (95% CI, 0.41–0.68); hip, 0.49 (95% CI, 0.23–0.99); and wrist, 0.52 (95% CI, 0.31–0.87). The Fracture Intervention Trial (FIT) was a multicenter, placebo-controlled trial that enrolled 2,027 women between the ages of 55 and 81 years who had vertebral fractures and reduced BMD.[89] These women received placebo or alendronate 5 mg/day for 2 years and 10 mg/day during the third year. When compared to placebo, BMD increased by 6.2% in the spine and 4.7% in the total hip region after 3 years. During 3 years, 18.2% of the placebo group and 13.6% of the alendronate group had fractures.

Black et al. combined the data from the previous two studies to give overall information from the FIT. These investigators believed this was appropriate because fracture reduction rates in both studies with the use of alendronate were similar. The pooled information from 3 to 4 years of alendronate versus placebo resulted in the following fracture risk data: hip RR 0.47 (95% CI, 0.26–0.79); radiographic vertebral RR 0.52 (95% CI, 0.42–0.66); clinical vertebral RR 0.55 (95% CI, 0.36–0.82); and all clinical fractures RR 0.70 (95% CI, 0.59–0.82). The investigators concluded from these data that women with osteoporosis (T-score <–2.5), with or without previous vertebral fractures who took alendronate, had reduced risk for fractures.[90]

A meta-analysis was used to determine the nonvertebral fracture rate in postmenopausal women with osteoporosis who had been treated for at least 3 years with placebo or alendronate (doses used in the five trials ranged from 1–20 mg/day).[91] The overall results showed a 12.6% incidence of nonvertebral fracture in the placebo groups and a 9.0% incidence in the alendronate groups. This resulted in a RR of 0.71 (95% CI, 0.502–0.997) for those receiving alendronate.[91]

Several studies have addressed the effects of risedronate on BMD. In a study of women 40 to 60 years of age (early postmenopausal) who had normal BMD for age, those receiving risedronate 5 mg/day for 2 years had BMD increases of 5.7% in lumbar spine and 5.4% in the hip compared with women taking placebo.[92] In another study, postmenopausal women (mean age 69 years) who were older than those mentioned in the previous study had increases in BMD of 4.3% in the spine and 2.8% in the femoral neck when risedronate use was compared with placebo over 3 years.[93]

Ibandronate has been shown to have beneficial effects on BMD. McClung et al. evaluated the effects of ibandronate in early postmenopausal women resulting in a significantly increased BMD in the lumbar spine (1.9%) versus placebo (–1.9%) and total hip (1.2%) versus placebo (–0.6%) after 2 years.[94] Follow-up from the Once Monthly Ibandronate as Effective as Daily Ibandronate for Osteoporosis (MOBILE) study revealed that the monthly ibandronate dose of 150 mg significantly improved BMD over the 2.5 mg daily dose in the lumbar spine (6.6% vs. 5%) after 2 years of treatment.[95] Ibandronate was also studied as an intravenous (IV) formulation of 3 mg administered every 3 months. One-year results from the Dosing Intravenous Administration (DIVA) study improved BMD in the lumbar spine (4.5% vs. 3.5%) and the total hip (2.1% vs. 1.5%) to a similar if not greater degree than daily oral tablets.[96]

Zoledronic acid was initially approved for the treatment of osteoporosis but did receive FDA approval for prevention of osteoporosis with the exception that the infusion be administered every 2 years instead of annually after results from unpublished studies in postmenopausal women with osteopenia. One study that included 224 women with osteopenia up to 5 years after menopause found that after 2 years the group that received a one time dose of zoledronic acid 5 mg IV infusion or placebo had a total hip BMD increase of 2.6% versus a 2.1% reduction in the placebo group.[97] Another study of 357 osteopenic women more than 5 years after menopause found that one dose of zoledronic acid 5 mg IV infusion increased BMD after 2 years by 2.1% versus a 1% reduction in the placebo group.[97]

Many studies show the benefits of bisphosphonates not only in the prevention of osteoporosis-related fractures by increasing BMD but also for the treatment of osteoporosis. Many of these studies have been conducted for 3 years with at least one for 7 years,[98] with a 3-year extension.[99] This latter study extension noted that during years 8 through 10, a total of 247 women receiving either alendronate 5 mg/day or 10 mg/day had similar safety and tolerance profiles as women in placebo groups. Spinal BMD increased by 2.3% in the 10 mg/day group and 1.2% in the 5 mg/day group; hip and total body BMD was maintained, if not slightly improved, at levels that were noted at 7 years; and forearm BMD was maintained in the 10 mg/day group but decreased slightly in the 5 mg/day group. Women who took alendronate for 5 years, but thereafter were in a placebo group, maintained their spinal and total body BMD for 5 years. Ten-year cumulative spinal BMD was 13.7% for the 10 mg/day group and 9.8% for the 5 mg/day group. Rates of nonvertebral fractures between years 8 and 10 were 8.1% for the 10 mg/day group, 11.5% for the 5 mg/day group, and 12.0% for the group who had been on alendronate for 5 years and off alendronate for 5 years.

LENGTH OF TREATMENT

No consensus is currently available on how long to continue bisphosphonate therapy. Long-term treatment with bisphosphonates might lead to accumulation within the bone and over-suppression, which may lead to an increase fracture risk. In the Fracture Intervention Trial Long-term Extension (FLEX), a randomized trial, 1,099 of the original FIT trial participants did not have T-scores less than –3.5 or BMD lower than their FIT baseline levels. Statistically significant bone loss occurred (2% to 3% more than those who took alendronate for 10 years) when women were switched to placebo after 5 years of alendronate therapy; however, BMD remained well above FIT baseline. A gradual rise was seen in biochemical markers of bone turnover as well as a slightly higher risk of clinically detected vertebral fractures, suggesting that women at high risk for vertebral fracture or with T-scores less than −3.5 may benefit from continued bisphosphonate therapy.[100–102] The VERT-NA study evaluated fracture reduction in women with a prior vertebral fracture who had received risedronate for 3 years compared to placebo. One year after discontinuing therapy, BMD was still above baseline BMD in the risedronate group and vertebral fracture rate was reduced (46%) when compared to the placebo arm, however, there was no difference in nonvertebral fractures between the groups.[100–102] The FLEX and VERT-NA studies suggest that women with good response to bisphosphonate therapy who are not at high risk for fracture may be able to take a "drug holiday" (e.g., 1 year off therapy) after 3 to 5 years of treatment. Women who are able to reach a T-score of greater than −2.5 may be able to discontinue therapy for several years.[100–102]

CONTRAINDICATIONS AND PRECAUTIONS

Although no dosage change is recommended for a patient with mild to moderate renal failure, aminobisphosphonate use is not recommended for patients with significant renal insufficiency (e.g., creatinine clearance <35 mL/minute for alendronate and zoledronic acid, <30 mL/minute for risedronate and ibandronate). Hypocalcemia should be corrected before beginning therapy. Caution is warranted in patients who have any upper GI problem (e.g., esophageal disease, dysphasia, duodenitis, or ulcers).[85]

CASE 105-2, QUESTION 8: If M.J. begins bisphosphonate therapy, how should she be counseled?

Adverse Effects

Common adverse effects associated with the use of bisphosphonates include GI symptoms, such as acid regurgitation, dysphagia, abdominal distension, gastritis, nausea, dyspepsia, flatulence, diarrhea, and constipation. Although rare, esophageal adverse effects, such as esophagitis, esophageal ulcers, and erosions, have occurred and have been followed by esophageal stricture.[82–85] In addition, musculoskeletal pain, headaches, and rash have been noted. Osteonecrosis of the jaw (ONJ) or "death of tissue" or "dead jaw" can occur if blood loss in bone tissue is temporarily or permanently impaired, resulting in the eventual collapse of the bone. Patients taking oral bisphosphonates are at risk for the development of ONJ; however, most patients with ONJ are cancer patients receiving chemotherapy and concurrent high-dose IV bisphosphonate therapy. Cases have been reported in patients on oral bisphosphonate therapy with active dental disease and recent dental procedures.

Adverse events reported in zoledronic acid have been similar to that of oral bisphosphonates, with decreased incidence of GI adverse events. Acute phase reactions including fevers, flulike symptoms, headache, and arthralgias primarily occur within the first 3 days after the infusion and the incidence decreases with subsequent doses. Increased incidence of atrial fibrillation was noted to be greater than placebo in clinical trials.[85]

More recently, concern has emerged regarding atypical fractures occurring (subtrochanteric and femoral shaft fractures) while receiving long-term bisphosphonate therapy. Several case series and multiple individual case reports have been published. Patients may describe prodromal pain in the thigh or leg weeks to even months before the fracture occurring or be asymptomatic. The radiographic findings have all been similar in these occurrences. Bone biopsies of some of these patients show very low bone turnover markers, but this can even occur with short-term bisphosphonate use.[103] Black et al. conducted a secondary analysis from the results of three large trials, the FIT (alendronate for 3 to 4.5 years), FLEX (alendronate treatment for 10 years), and HORIZON (zoledronic acid for 3 years) trials, to look specifically at the occurrence of atypical fractures. There were a total of 12 fractures in 10 patients in the subtrochanteric or femur, for a combined rate of 2.3 per 10,000 patient-years. The hazard ratio was 1.03 (95% CI, 0.06–16.46) in the FIT trial, 1.5 (95% CI, 0.25–9) in the FLEX trial, and 1.33 (95% CI, 0.12–14.67) in the HORIZON trial when compared with placebo.[104] Currently, there is not enough evidence to hold bisphosphonate therapy for patients that have osteoporosis; however, if a patient has suffered an atypical fracture it would be reasonable to not continue therapy with bisphosphonates.[103,104]

Dosing

For prevention of osteoporosis, alendronate can be prescribed 5 mg daily or 35 mg weekly, risedronate 5 mg daily, 35 mg once weekly, 75 mg twice monthly on consecutive days, or 150 mg once monthly, and ibandronate 2.5 mg daily or 150 mg once monthly. It might be more convenient to take the medication once weekly or once monthly, and this might also increase adherence to therapy. Patients should be instructed to take most bisphosphonates with 6 to 8 ounces of water early in the morning on arising and at least 30 minutes (60 minutes for ibandronate) before ingesting food, beverage, or other medications. Risedronate is also available as a 35-mg extended-release formulation that should be taken once weekly after breakfast. Patients should not lie down, but should stay fully upright for at least 30 minutes (60 minutes for ibandronate) after ingesting an oral bisphosphonate to prevent esophageal irritation or ulceration and to ensure appropriate bioavailability. Patients should ingest adequate calcium and vitamin D, but should not take the calcium or vitamin D at the same time as the oral bisphosphonates.[82–84] Zoledronic acid is approved as a single 5-mg infusion given once every 2 years for no less than 15 minutes through a separate vented infusion line.[85]

M.J.'s diagnosis of GERD may preclude her use of oral bisphosphonate therapy for prevention of osteoporosis, but she would be a candidate for zoledronic acid for prevention of osteoporosis if indicated. M.J. did not have a previous vertebral or hip fracture and her T-score of −2.0 resulted in a calculated FRAX score 10-year probability of 0.9% for hip fracture and 6.3% for a major osteoporosis–related fracture. The current guidelines from the NOF and NAMS recommend pharmacologic therapy be reserved for those patients with a hip or vertebral fracture, individuals with a T-score of −2.5 or less at the femoral neck or spine once secondary causes have been excluded, and individuals with low bone mass with a 10-year probability of at least 3% risk of hip fracture or at least 20% risk of major osteoporotic fracture. At this time, M.J. should not be considered for pharmacological therapy for prevention of osteoporosis, but she should maintain adequate intake of calcium and vitamin D, as well as implement an exercise program and continue to avoid risk factors for osteoporosis.[6,33]

Treatment

CASE 105-3

QUESTION 1: T.J.'s 75-year-old grandmother, M.B., was diagnosed with osteoporosis 5 years ago when she broke her distal forearm. In addition, she has lost 2 inches in height (current height 5 feet and weight 100 pounds) and has mild kyphosis. M.B. denies severe back pain but occasionally uses acetaminophen or ibuprofen for mild back pain.

When used intranasally, calcitonin is dosed at 200 international units daily in alternating nares; given subcutaneously or intramuscularly, the dose is 100 international units/day.[120] A patient using calcitonin should have adequate intake of calcium and vitamin D.

Adverse effects associated with intranasal calcitonin include nasal symptoms, such as rhinitis and epistaxis. Other adverse effects include arthralgia, headache, and back pain. When calcitonin therapy is administered by injection, adverse effects such as flushing, nausea, and vomiting, as well as local irritation at the injection site (10%), can occur.[120,125] Flushing typically occurs on the hands and face and is noted in approximately 2% to 5% of patients. Nausea and vomiting occur in about 10% of patients. These latter reactions most commonly occur when therapy is initiated and usually subside with time. Injectable calcitonin should be refrigerated when not in use. The intranasal preparation should be refrigerated until it is opened for use; thereafter, it is stable for 30 days at room temperature.[125]

OTHER THERAPIES

CASE 105-3, QUESTION 2: What other possible alternatives or additive therapies for the treatment of postmenopausal osteoporosis are available for M.B.?

PARATHYROID HORMONE

Parathyroid hormone works differently from other medications discussed thus far because it stimulates new bone formation and activates remodeling, which then results in increased BMD and connectivity in cancellous more than cortical bone. This can be accomplished by administration of recombinant human PTH in women with postmenopausal osteoporosis.[33,126,127] Despite an incomplete understanding of the mechanisms for PTH, it is known that PTH stimulates the conversion of preosteoblasts to osteoblasts within the first month of treatment, peaking 6 to 9 months after daily administration.[128] In one study of 1,637 postmenopausal women who had previously sustained vertebral fractures, therapy (19 months of PTH 20 or 40 mcg daily subcutaneously) resulted in a reduction of new vertebral fractures by 65% and 69%, respectively, and reduced new nonvertebral fractures by 53% and 54%, respectively.[129]

The FDA has approved the PTH derivative teriparatide for use by women and men with osteoporosis who do not adequately respond to other therapies. In addition, those diagnosed as having severe osteoporosis and who are at an increased risk for fracture may be considered for therapy. Teriparatide 20 mcg should be given once daily subcutaneously in the thigh or abdomen. Initial administration should be given when the patient can sit or lie down. Teriparatide pens are stable for up to 28 days, including the first injection. The remaining medication should be discarded after 28 days. Teriparatide should be stored under refrigeration at 2°C to 8°C (36°F–46°F) and injected immediately on removal from refrigeration. After use, the pen should be recapped and protected from light. Safety and efficacy with teriparatide is limited beyond 2 years and therapy is not recommended after 2 years at this time.[130]

Because osteosarcomas were noted in study animals that received teriparatide, the FDA has required a black box warning for this medication.[130] This information may also be found in a medication guide that should be given to all patients receiving teriparatide. Studies have confirmed that BMD gains noted in the hip and spine decline after discontinuation with an approximate 2% loss in spinal BMD and 17% loss in trabecular BMD.[128,131] Black et al. conducted a trial in women who were randomly assigned to alendronate or placebo after 1 year of parathyroid hormone treatment. Patients receiving alendronate exhibited a further increase in BMD of approximately 6% after the first year of therapy, whereas BMD declined in the placebo group.[131] Similar effects were noted when estrogen therapy was started after discontinuing PTH,[132] suggesting that antiresorptive therapy should be started after discontinuation of PTH to preserve BMD.

Adverse effects reported include hypercalcemia, leg cramps, nausea, and dizziness. Orthostatic hypotension may occur within 4 hours of administration and spontaneously resolves after a few minutes to hours for the first several doses. Patients should immediately sit or lie down if symptoms occur.[130]

DENOSUMAB

Denosumab is a human monoclonal antibody that targets RANKL, which has been shown to be a necessary part of bone-resorbing osteoclasts. Denosumab has been hypothesized to increase the risk of cancer or infections as RANK and RANKL are members of the tumor necrosis superfamily expressed by many lymphoid cells. Clinical trials conducted to date have not shown significant increases in either cancer or infections.[133,134]

Cummings et al. conducted the FREEDOM (Denosumab for Prevention of Fractures in Postmenopausal Women with Osteoporosis) trial, a randomized, placebo-controlled, multicenter trial, with 7,868 postmenopausal women with osteoporosis (BMD <–2.5 to –4.0) at the lumbar spine or total hip using denosumab 60 mg subcutaneously every 6 months or placebo. Denosumab reduced vertebral fractures by 2.3% versus 7.2% in the placebo group (RR 0.32; 95% CI, 0.26–0.41) as well as reducing the risk of hip fractures with a cumulative incidence of 0.7% in the denosumab group versus 1.2% in the placebo group (hazard ratio, 0.6; 95% CI, 0.37–0.97) for a relative decrease of 40% and 20%, respectively.[134]

Brown et al. conducted a multicenter, double-blind randomized study in 1,189 postmenopausal women with T-score less than or equal to –2.0 at the lumbar spine or total hip receiving denosumab 60 mg subcutaneously every 6 months or alendronate 70 mg weekly in a 1:1 ratio to determine safety and efficacy of denosumab. BMD was assessed at various sites at month 1, 3, 6, 9, and 12. BMD increased by 3.5% versus 2.6% at the total hip after 12 months of therapy in the denosumab and alendronate groups, respectively. Markers of bone turnover were also further suppressed in the denosumab group. All skeletal sites showed improvement over alendronate at the end of 12 months of therapy with no increase in adverse events.[135]

Kendler et al. performed a multicenter, international, double-blind, double-dummy randomized trial in 504 postmenopausal women 55 years of age or older with T-score of –2.0 to –4.0 who had been receiving alendronate for at least 6 months. Alendronate 70 mg weekly was taken for 1 month and patients were then randomly assigned to continue alendronate or receive denosumab 60 mg subcutaneously every 6 months for 12 months. BMD at the total hip increased by 1.9% versus 1.05% in the denosumab and alendronate groups, respectively. Statistically significant gains over alendronate were noted at all sites (lumbar spine, femoral neck, total hip, and distal one-third of the radius). Markers of bone turnover were significantly decreased at all points in time in the denosumab group when compared to the alendronate group.[136]

Denosumab is FDA-approved for the treatment of postmenopausal women with osteoporosis who are at high risk for fracture with a dosage of 60 mg subcutaneously every 6 months. Prefilled syringes should be stored under refrigeration and administered at room temperature by a health care provider in the upper arm, upper thigh, or abdomen.[137] Patients should be taking calcium and vitamin D daily and those patients with hypocalcemia must be corrected before starting denosumab. Most common adverse reactions include back pain, pain in extremity, hypercholesterolemia, musculoskeletal pain, and cystitis.[137] Pancreatitis, ONJ, cellulitis, and rashes have all been been reported in clinical trials and patients should seek medical treatment if these conditions present. Patients should also be monitored for bone oversuppression.[137]

Glucocorticoid-Induced Osteoporosis

CASE 105-4

QUESTION 1: T.J.'s father, D.J, age 56 years, was diagnosed with rheumatoid arthritis 10 years ago. D.J. has been experiencing increased swelling and tenderness in his hands and feet for the past 2 years. D.J. made an appointment with his physician who noted that D.J.'s laboratory findings and imaging were suggestive of further progression of his rheumatoid arthritis. D.J. has been taking methotrexate, sulfasalazine, and hydroxychloroquine for the past 5 years and is not interested in starting injectable therapy at this time but would like to try an alternative treatment that will help alleviate his pain quickly. D.J.'s physician would like to have BMD testing performed before initiating prednisone 10 mg daily. D.J. is curious about why he will need a DXA test. What should D.J.'s physician tell him?

Prednisone is classified as a glucocorticoid steroid. Glucocorticoids have several possible mechanisms that contribute to bone loss resulting in osteoporosis. Glucocorticoids have been linked to decreases in serum estrogen and testosterone and increases in bone urine calcium excretion and decreased calcium absorption. Glucocorticoids have direct action on bone cells, decreased serum testosterone, and decrease muscle, which result in decreased bone formation. Both the increase in bone resorption and decrease in bone formation lead to decreased bone volume, resulting in a more rapid bone loss than other medications that have been associated with bone loss.[138–140] Glucocorticoids are not thought to affect bone-resorbing activity of mature osteoclasts, because they do not have functioning glucocorticoid receptors.[141] Decreases in BMD can be seen as soon as 3 to 6 months after glucocorticoid initiation; however, fracture risk appears to be contributed to by glucocorticoid duration and dose, but is independent of BMD.[142–144] After discontinuation of glucocorticoid therapy, BMD begins to increase.[145]

CASE 105-4, QUESTION 2: Are any medications available to prevent osteoporosis in D.J.?

BISPHOSPHONATES

Alendronate, risedronate, and zoledronic acid are FDA-approved for the prevention and treatment of glucocorticoid-induced osteoporosis (GIOP). They are thought to prevent glucocorticoid-induced osteoclast apoptosis; however, this theory has been challenged, suggesting that glucocorticoids may overcome the proapoptotic effects of bisphosphonates. Another thought is that bisphosphonates may prolong the life of osteoblasts.[140,146,147]

Saag et al. looked at alendronate 5-mg and 10-mg doses versus placebo and found that BMD in the lumbar spine increased in both alendronate groups and BMD declined in the placebo group 2.1%, 2.9%, and –0.4%, respectively, over 48 weeks. Total body, trochanter, and femoral neck bone mass also increased in the alendronate groups. Vertebral fractures were lower in the alendronate groups versus placebo (2.3% vs. 3.7%),[148] with benefits of alendronate seen after 2 years.[149] Risedronate is also effective in the prevention and treatment of GIOP. Reid et al. conducted a 1-year study with risedronate versus placebo in patients taking greater than 7.5 mg of prednisone daily for 6 or more months. They found increases in both lumbar spine and femoral neck (2.7% and 1.8%, respectively), with no change in BMD in patients taking placebo.[150] Black et al. conducted a noninferiority study of zoledronic acid 5 mg IV versus risedronate 5 mg oral daily. In the study, 833 women and men were randomly assigned to either group and were treated for 1 year. Zoledronic acid increased BMD by 2.06% in the spine compared to 0.64% in the risedronate group. In the group who had been on glucocorticoids for a longer period of time, BMD in the spine increased by 4.06% in the zoledronic acid group and 2.71% in the risedronate group. Bone turnover markers were suppressed further in the zoledronic acid group; however, no difference in fracture occurred between groups.[140]

PARATHYROID HORMONE

Teriparatide is also approved for GIOP. The approval came before completion of a 36-month trial conducted by Saag et al. comparing teriparatide 20 mcg subcutaneously daily versus alendronate 10 mg oral daily. The study included 400 men and women, primarily with rheumatological conditions. Teriparatide increased spinal BMD 7.2% versus 3.4% in the alendronate group after 18 months of therapy. Hip BMD increased 3.8% in the teriparatide group versus 2.4% in the alendronate group. Differences between groups were noted as early as 6 months. At 36 months, teriparatide continued to increase BMD in both the spine, hip, and femoral neck to a greater extent than alendronate; however, it is approved for 24 months of therapy.[140,151]

CASE 105-4, QUESTION 3: What recommendations should D.J.'s physician share with him for preventing osteoporosis?

The American College of Rheumatology (ACR) recommends preventative therapy in patients taking glucocorticoids based upon risk factors, sex, and age. Categories are broken down by low, medium, and high risk. The ACR recommends the following for all patients taking glucocorticoid therapy for at least 3 months:[144]

- Calcium, 1,200 to 1,500 mg daily
- Vitamin D, 800 to 1000 international units daily; also check 25(OH) vitamin D levels
- Bisphosphonate therapy (bisphosphonate, depending on the level of risk and dose of glucocorticoid)
- Assessment of fragility fractures
- Exercise program (appropriate for individual patient, including fall-risk assessment)
- BMD screen if greater than 3 months of glucocorticoid therapy will be needed
- Smoking cessation
- Limit alcohol to less than or equal to 2 drinks per day

D.J. is currently without contraindications to bisphosphonate therapy. D.J. should be counseled on the proper administration and adverse effects of bisphosphonates (see Case 105-2, Question 8). D.J. should be encouraged to incorporate 30 minutes of weight-bearing exercise into his daily routine. More information on specific recommendations from the ACR 2010 guidelines for GIOP for individual patients can be found at http://www.rheumatology.org/practice/clinical/guidelines/GIOP_Guidelines_Nov_2010.pdf.[144]

CASE 105-5

QUESTION 1: D.J. presents to his physician 1 year later and is found to be in good health. D.J. is concerned about the development of osteoporosis in his wife's father. J.B., age 77, has become frailer and is falling occasionally. His wife, M.J., is osteopenic and his wife's mother, M.B., has osteoporosis. D.J. knows osteoporosis occurs often in women, but was not aware that osteoporosis (excluding drug-induced) can occur in men. Should D.J. be concerned about osteoporosis in J.B.?

Osteoporosis is less common in men than in women; however, about 1.5 million men in the United States have osteoporosis, with another 3.5 million at risk.[152] Projections suggest that 17% of men who reach 90 years of age will exhibit osteoporosis.[153] Although reasons are still unknown, mortality rates after hip fracture are higher in men than in women, with patients having a previous distal radius fracture correlating with a high absolute risk for hip fractures in men.[154]

CASE 105-5, QUESTION 2: D.J. knows that BMD loss in both his wife and her mother has been attributed to a decrease in hormones. Is hormone loss the same cause of osteoporosis in men?

Bone loss for men may begin in their thirties with an estimated 1% loss of BMD occurring at the distal radius, with spinal content decreasing more quickly.[14,15] Many risk factors contribute to osteoporosis in men (Table 105-1), however, a decrease in androgen and estrogen production are the primary hormonal contributors to the development of osteoporosis in this population.[14,15]

Androgens and Estrogens

Androgen production, specifically, serum testosterone concentrations, decreases with age. These decreased concentrations are thought to decrease bone formation and increase resorption. Testosterone has been linked to decreases in BMD, whereas dihydrotestosterone has not been linked.[155] Despite testosterone's importance for skeletal health in men, research is now suggesting that estrogen may play a more important role in skeletal biology.[156] Khosla et al. found two genes required for estrogen effects; estrogen receptor α and aromatase.[157] ER-α are found on osteoblasts, osteoclasts, and stem cells in bone. Aromatase is present in osteoblasts and stem cells in bone.[158] The absence of these genes results in an inability to convert androgen into estrogen.[159,160] Replacement of estrogen in aromatase deficiency showed significant increases in bone mass and markers of bone turnover normalized.[160]

CASE 105-5, QUESTION 3: Should J.B. be given supplementation for hypogonadism if his testosterone levels are low?

Hypogonadism may be a major contributor of bone loss in men with low serum estradiol being the main contributor.[11] It would be appropriate for J.B.'s physician to order serum testosterone levels. Snyder et al. found that replacing testosterone (then converted to estrogen), increased bone density by 5.9% when pretreatment serum testosterone levels were less than 200 ng/dL (normal, 300–1,000 ng/dL).[161]

CASE 105-5, QUESTION 4: How is osteoporosis diagnosed in men?

The WHO criteria were established for diagnosing postmenopausal women with osteoporosis.[2] To date, no specific diagnostic criteria have been established specifically for men. Currently, diagnosis of osteoporosis in men can be made when a T-score is less than −2.5 until further definitions of osteoporosis are established by the NOF and the International Osteoporosis Foundation. The NOF recommends that all men the age of 70 or older receive BMD testing.[6]

CASE 105-5, QUESTION 5: What therapies are available to treat osteoporosis in men?

FDA-approved therapies include oral (e.g., alendronate and risedronate) and intravenous bisphosphonates (e.g., zoledronic acid) and parathyroid hormone.[82,83,85] Orwoll et al. conducted a double-blind randomized trial with alendronate 10 mg daily or placebo for 2 years in 241 men with osteoporosis. One-third of the population had low serum free-testosterone levels. BMD increased by 7.1% versus 1.8% in the lumbar spine, 2.5% versus −0.1% in the femoral neck, and 2% versus 0.4% in the total body for in the alendronate and placebo groups respectively. Incidence of new vertebral fractures was less in the alendronate group (0.8%) when compared with placebo (7.1%).[162]

A study with risedronate was conducted by Boonen et al. in a multinational, randomized, double-blind, placebo-controlled trial for 2 years. It included 284 men randomly assigned in a 2:1 fashion to risedronate 35 mg weekly or placebo, respectively. All patients received calcium and vitamin D supplementation. Lumbar spine BMD increased 4.5% over placebo in the risedronate group. There was no difference between groups in vertebral and nonvertebral fractures, but bone turnover markers were significantly lower in the risedronate group.[163]

Zoledronic acid received FDA approval in 2008 after results from a study were submitted to the FDA, but the study was not published until 2010. Orwoll et al. conducted a multicenter, double-blind, active-controlled, parallel-group study including 302 men randomly assigned to once-yearly zoledronic acid 5 mg IV infusion or oral alendronate 70 mg weekly and followed them for 2 years. All patients received calcium and vitamin D supplementation. The results of the study confirmed noninferiority of zoledronic acid to alendronate with similar BMD response and suppression of bone turnover markers. BMD at the lumbar spine increased by 6.1% in the zoledronic acid group versus 6.2% in the alendronate group with other sites showing similar BMD increases between groups.[164]

Orwoll et al. also conducted a multicenter, randomized, double-blind, placebo-controlled trial in 437 men with BMD less than 2 SD lower than the young adult male mean BMD. Patients received teriparatide 20 mcg subcutaneously daily, 40 mcg subcutaneously daily, or placebo with calcium and vitamin D supplementation for a median duration of 11 months. Lumbar spine BMD increases were noted after 3 months with increases of 5.9% in the 20 mcg group and 9.0% in the 40 mcg group by study end. Increases were also seen in bone turnover markers in the 20 mcg and 40 mcg groups. The study was halted early after findings of osteosarcomas in rats during routine testing.[165]

Investigational Agents

In the next few years, new agents should be approved for the prevention and treatment of osteoporosis; examples of these new agents are the SERMs bazedoxifene, lasofoxifene, ospemifene, and arzoxifene for postmenopausal osteoporosis.

STRONTIUM RANELATE

Strontium ranelate has antiresorptive and mild anabolic effects. The exact mechanism of action remains unknown. Strontium has been shown to decrease the risk of spine and nonspine fractures (35%–49%), as well as increase BMD in the spine and femoral neck (14% and 8%, respectively). Studies have been conducted for up to 3 years. Nausea and vomiting have been associated with oral dissolved strontium, which abated after 3 months of therapy.[166,167]

KEY REFERENCES AND WEBSITES

A full list of references for this chapter can be found at **http://thepoint.lww.com/AT10e.** Below are the key references and websites for this chapter, with the corresponding reference number in this chapter found in parentheses after the reference.

Key References

Black DM et al. Bisphosphonates and fractures of the subtrochanteric or diaphyseal femur. *N Engl J Med.* 2010;362:1761. (104)

Black DM et al. Effects of continuing or stopping alendronate after 5 years of treatment: the Fracture Intervention Trial Long-Term Extension (FLEX): a randomized trial. *JAMA.* 2006;296:2927. (100)

Brown JP et al. Comparison of the effect of denosumab and alendronate on BMD and biochemical markers of bone turnover in postmenopausal women with low bone mass: a randomized, blinded, phase 3 trial. *J Bone Miner Res.* 2009;24:153. (135)

Cummings SR et al. Effect of alendronate on risk of fracture in women with low bone density but without vertebral fractures: results from the Fracture Intervention Trial. *JAMA.* 1998;280:2077. (89)

Grossman JM et al. American College of Rheumatology 2010 recommendations for the prevention and treatment of glucocorticoid-induced osteoporosis. *Arthritis Care Res (Hoboken).* 2010;621515. (144)

Syed FA, Ng AC. The pathophysiology of the aging skeleton. *Curr Osteoporos Rep.* 2010;8:235. (27)

[No authors listed]. Management of postmenopausal osteoporosis: 2010 position statement of the North American Menopause Society. *Menopause.* 2010;17:25. (33)

Weiss AJ et al. The skeletal subsystem as an integrative physiology paradigm. *Curr Osteoporos Rep.* 2010;8:168. (21)

Key Websites

National Osteoporosis Foundation. Clinician's Guide to Prevention and Treatment of Osteoporosis. **http://www.nof.org/sites/default/files/pdfs/NOF_ClinicianGuide2009_v7.pdf.** Accessed May 15, 2011. (6)

World Health Organization. WHO Fracture Risk Assessment Tool. **http://www.shef.ac.uk/FRAX/.** Accessed May 15, 2011. (52)

Drug Index

Note: Page number followed by *f* and *t* indicates figure and table respectively.

Subject Index

Note: Page number followed by *f* and *t* indicates figure and table respectively.

Subject Index